PROFESSIONAL

2019

ICD-10-CM
Professional
for Hospitals

The complete official code set

Codes valid from October 1, 2018
through September 30, 2019

Power up your coding
optum360coding.com

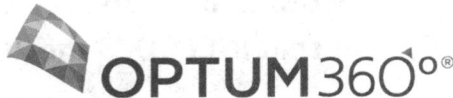

Publisher's Notice

The *ICD-10-CM Professional for Hospitals: The Complete Official Code Set* is designed to be an accurate and authoritative source regarding coding and every reasonable effort has been made to ensure accuracy and completeness of the content. However, Optum360 makes no guarantee, warranty, or representation that this publication is accurate, complete or without errors. It is understood that Optum360 is not rendering any legal or other professional services or advice in this publication and that Optum360 bears no liability for any results or consequences that may arise from the use of this book.

Acknowledgments

Marianne Randall, CPC, *Product Manager*
Karen Schmidt, BSN, *Technical Director*
Anita Schmidt, BS, RHIT, AHIMA-approved ICD-10-CM/PCS Trainer, *Clinical Technical Editor*
Anne Kenney, BA, MBA, CCS, *Clinical Technical Editor*
Karen Krawzik, RHIT, CCS, AHIMA-approved ICD-10-CM/PCS Trainer, *Clinical Technical Editor*
Peggy Willard, CCS, AHIMA-approved ICD-10-CM/PCS Trainer, *Clinical Technical Editor*
Leanne Patterson, CPC, *Clinical Technical Editor*
Stacy Perry, *Manager, Desktop Publishing*
Lisa Singley, *Project Manager*
Tracy Betzler, *Senior Desktop Publishing Specialist*
Hope M. Dunn, *Senior Desktop Publishing Specialist*
Katie Russell, *Desktop Publishing Specialist*
Kate Holden, *Editor*

Our Commitment to Accuracy

Optum360 is committed to producing accurate and reliable materials.

To report corrections, please visit www.optum360coding.com/accuracy or email accuracy@optum.com. You can also reach customer service by calling 1.800.464.3649, option 1.

Anita Schmidt, BS, RHIT, AHIMA-approved ICD-10-CM/PCS Trainer

Ms. Schmidt has expertise in Level I Adult and Pediatric Trauma hospital coding, specializing in ICD-9-CM, ICD-10-CM/PCS, DRG, and CPT coding. Her experience includes analysis of medical record documentation, assignment of ICD-10-CM and PCS codes, DRG validation, as well as CPT code assignments for same-day surgery cases. She has conducted coding training and auditing, including DRG validation, conducted electronic health record training, and worked with clinical documentation specialists to identify documentation needs and potential areas for physician education. Most recently she has been developing content for resource and educational products related to ICD-10-CM and ICD-10-PCS. Ms. Schmidt is an AHIMA-approved ICD-10-CM/PCS trainer, and is an active member of the American Health Information Management Association (AHIMA) and the Minnesota Health Information Management Association (MHIMA).

Anne Kenney, BA, MBA, CCS

Ms. Kenney has expertise in ICD-10-CM/PCS, ICD-9-CM, DRG, and CPT coding. Most recently she has been developing content for ICD-10-CM and ICD-10-PCS applications. Her prior experience in a major teaching hospital includes assignment of ICD-9-CM codes and DRGs, CPT code assignments, and determining physician evaluation and management levels for inpatient, emergency department, and observation cases. Ms. Kenney is an active member of the American Health Information Management Association (AHIMA) and the Minnesota Health Information Management Association (MHIMA).

2019 ICD-10-CM Official Guidelines for Coding and Reporting

Optum360 is pleased to provide you with this 2019 ICD-10-CM codebook that INCLUDES the 2019 Official Guidelines for Coding and Reporting.

Contents

Preface

ICD-10-CM Official Preface

This FY 2019 update of the International Statistical Classification of Diseases and Related Health Problems, 10th revision, Clinical Modification (ICD-10-CM) is being published by the United States government in recognition of its responsibility to promulgate this classification throughout the United States for morbidity coding. The International Statistical Classification of Diseases and Related Health Problems, 10th Revision (ICD-10), published by the World Health Organization (WHO), is the foundation of ICD-10-CM. ICD-10 continues to be the classification used in cause-of-death coding in the United States. The ICD-10-CM is comparable with the ICD-10. The WHO Collaborating Center for the Family of International Classifications in North America, housed at the Centers of Disease Control and Prevention's National Center for Health Statistics (NCHS), has responsibility for the implementation of ICD and other WHO-FIC classifications and serves as a liaison with the WHO, fulfilling international obligations for comparable classifications and the national health data needs of the United States. The historical background of ICD and ICD-10 can be found in the Introduction to the International Classification of Diseases and Related Health Problems (ICD-10), 2010, World Health Organization, Geneva, Switzerland.

ICD-10-CM is the United States' clinical modification of the World Health Organization's ICD-10. The term "clinical" is used to emphasize the modification's intent: to serve as a useful tool in the area of classification of morbidity data for indexing of health records, medical care review, and ambulatory and other health care programs, as well as for basic health statistics. To describe the clinical picture of the patient the codes must be more precise than those needed only for statistical groupings and trend analysis.

Characteristics of ICD-10-CM

ICD-10-CM far exceeds its predecessors in the number of concepts and codes provided. The disease classification has been expanded to include health-related conditions and to provide greater specificity at the 6th and 7th character level. The 6th and 7th characters are not optional and are intended for use in recording the information documented in the clinical record.

ICD-10-CM extensions, interpretations, modifications, addenda, or errata other than those approved by the Centers for Disease Control and Prevention are not to be considered official and should not be utilized. Continuous maintenance of the ICD-10- CM is the responsibility of the aforementioned agencies. However, because the ICD-10-CM represents the best in contemporary thinking of clinicians, nosologists, epidemiologists, and statisticians from both public and private sectors, when future modifications are considered, advice will be sought from all stakeholders.

All official authorized addenda since the last complete update (October 1, 2018) have been included in this revision. For more detailed information please see the complete official authorized addenda to ICD-10-CM, including the "ICD-10-CM Official Guidelines for Coding and Reporting," and a description of the ICD-10-CM updating and maintenance process.

What's New for 2019

Official Updates

The National Center for Health Statistics (NCHS), a section of the Centers for Disease Control and Prevention (CDC), is the agency charged with maintaining and updating ICD-10-CM. The 2019 official addendum was posted to the Centers for Medicare and Medicaid Services (CMS) website on June 11, 2018, identifying the changes to the ICD-10-CM code set for fiscal 2019. A summary of changes is provided below:

48 Codes Changed from Valid to Invalid

Note: Validity changes are the result of new codes being added to the classification, changing a previously valid code to an invalid code, creating a new subcategory.

C43.11	C43.12	C4A.11	C4A.12	C44.102
C44.109	C44.112	C44.119	C44.122	C44.129
C44.192	C44.199	D03.11	D03.12	D04.11
D04.12	D22.11	D22.12	D23.11	D23.12
E72.8	E78.4	F53	G51.3	G71.0
H57.8	I63.8	K35.2	K35.3	K35.89
K61.3	K83.0	M79.1	N35.8	N35.9
O86.0	P02.7	P04.1	P04.8	P74.2
P74.3	P74.4	Q51.2	Q93.5	R82.99
R93.8	Z04.8	Z13.4		

3 Codes Deleted from the Classification

T81.4XXA	Infection following a procedure, initial encounter
T81.4XXD	Infection following a procedure, subsequent encounter
T81.4XXS	Infection following a procedure, sequela

279 New Codes Added

C43.111	Malignant melanoma of right upper eyelid, including canthus
C43.112	Malignant melanoma of right lower eyelid, including canthus
C43.121	Malignant melanoma of left upper eyelid, including canthus
C43.122	Malignant melanoma of left lower eyelid, including canthus
C4A.111	Merkel cell carcinoma of right upper eyelid, including canthus
C4A.112	Merkel cell carcinoma of right lower eyelid, including canthus
C4A.121	Merkel cell carcinoma of left upper eyelid, including canthus
C4A.122	Merkel cell carcinoma of left lower eyelid, including canthus
C44.1021	Unspecified malignant neoplasm of skin of right upper eyelid, including canthus
C44.1022	Unspecified malignant neoplasm of skin of right lower eyelid, including canthus
C44.1091	Unspecified malignant neoplasm of skin of left upper eyelid, including canthus
C44.1092	Unspecified malignant neoplasm of skin of left lower eyelid, including canthus
C44.1121	Basal cell carcinoma of skin of right upper eyelid, including canthus
C44.1122	Basal cell carcinoma of skin of right lower eyelid, including canthus
C44.1191	Basal cell carcinoma of skin of left upper eyelid, including canthus
C44.1192	Basal cell carcinoma of skin of left lower eyelid, including canthus
C44.1221	Squamous cell carcinoma of skin of right upper eyelid, including canthus
C44.1222	Squamous cell carcinoma of skin of right lower eyelid, including canthus
C44.1291	Squamous cell carcinoma of skin of left upper eyelid, including canthus
C44.1292	Squamous cell carcinoma of skin of left lower eyelid, including canthus
C44.131	Sebaceous cell carcinoma of skin of unspecified eyelid, including canthus
C44.1321	Sebaceous cell carcinoma of skin of right upper eyelid, including canthus
C44.1322	Sebaceous cell carcinoma of skin of right lower eyelid, including canthus
C44.1391	Sebaceous cell carcinoma of skin of left upper eyelid, including canthus
C44.1392	Sebaceous cell carcinoma of skin of left lower eyelid, including canthus
C44.1921	Other specified malignant neoplasm of skin of right upper eyelid, including canthus
C44.1922	Other specified malignant neoplasm of skin of right lower eyelid, including canthus
C44.1991	Other specified malignant neoplasm of skin of left upper eyelid, including canthus
C44.1992	Other specified malignant neoplasm of skin of left lower eyelid, including canthus
D03.111	Melanoma in situ of right upper eyelid, including canthus
D03.112	Melanoma in situ of right lower eyelid, including canthus
D03.121	Melanoma in situ of left upper eyelid, including canthus
D03.122	Melanoma in situ of left lower eyelid, including canthus
D04.111	Carcinoma in situ of skin of right upper eyelid, including canthus
D04.112	Carcinoma in situ of skin of right lower eyelid, including canthus
D04.121	Carcinoma in situ of skin of left upper eyelid, including canthus
D04.122	Carcinoma in situ of skin of left lower eyelid, including canthus
D22.111	Melanocytic nevi of right upper eyelid, including canthus
D22.112	Melanocytic nevi of right lower eyelid, including canthus
D22.121	Melanocytic nevi of left upper eyelid, including canthus
D22.122	Melanocytic nevi of left lower eyelid, including canthus
D23.111	Other benign neoplasm of skin of right upper eyelid, including canthus
D23.112	Other benign neoplasm of skin of right lower eyelid, including canthus
D23.121	Other benign neoplasm of skin of left upper eyelid, including canthus
D23.122	Other benign neoplasm of skin of left lower eyelid, including canthus
E72.81	Disorders of gamma aminobutyric acid metabolism
E72.89	Other specified disorders of amino-acid metabolism
E75.26	Sulfatase deficiency
E78.41	Elevated Lipoprotein(a)
E78.49	Other hyperlipidemia
E88.02	Plasminogen deficiency
F12.23	Cannabis dependence with withdrawal
F12.93	Cannabis use, unspecified with withdrawal
F53.0	Postpartum depression
F53.1	Puerperal psychosis
F68.A	Factitious disorder imposed on another
G51.31	Clonic hemifacial spasm, right

279 New Codes Added (continued)

Code	Description
G51.32	Clonic hemifacial spasm, left
G51.33	Clonic hemifacial spasm, bilateral
G51.39	Clonic hemifacial spasm, unspecified
G71.00	Muscular dystrophy, unspecified
G71.01	Duchenne or Becker muscular dystrophy
G71.02	Facioscapulohumeral muscular dystrophy
G71.09	Other specified muscular dystrophies
H01.00A	Unspecified blepharitis right eye, upper and lower eyelids
H01.00B	Unspecified blepharitis left eye, upper and lower eyelids
H01.01A	Ulcerative blepharitis right eye, upper and lower eyelids
H01.01B	Ulcerative blepharitis left eye, upper and lower eyelids
H01.02A	Squamous blepharitis right eye, upper and lower eyelids
H01.02B	Squamous blepharitis left eye, upper and lower eyelids
H02.151	Paralytic ectropion of right upper eyelid
H02.152	Paralytic ectropion of right lower eyelid
H02.153	Paralytic ectropion of right eye, unspecified eyelid
H02.154	Paralytic ectropion of left upper eyelid
H02.155	Paralytic ectropion of left lower eyelid
H02.156	Paralytic ectropion of left eye, unspecified eyelid
H02.159	Paralytic ectropion of unspecified eye, unspecified eyelid
H02.20A	Unspecified lagophthalmos right eye, upper and lower eyelids
H02.20B	Unspecified lagophthalmos left eye, upper and lower eyelids
H02.20C	Unspecified lagophthalmos, bilateral, upper and lower eyelids
H02.21A	Cicatricial lagophthalmos right eye, upper and lower eyelids
H02.21B	Cicatricial lagophthalmos left eye, upper and lower eyelids
H02.21C	Cicatricial lagophthalmos, bilateral, upper and lower eyelids
H02.22A	Mechanical lagophthalmos right eye, upper and lower eyelids
H02.22B	Mechanical lagophthalmos left eye, upper and lower eyelids
H02.22C	Mechanical lagophthalmos, bilateral, upper and lower eyelids
H02.23A	Paralytic lagophthalmos right eye, upper and lower eyelids
H02.23B	Paralytic lagophthalmos left eye, upper and lower eyelids
H02.23C	Paralytic lagophthalmos, bilateral, upper and lower eyelids
H02.881	Meibomian gland dysfunction right upper eyelid
H02.882	Meibomian gland dysfunction right lower eyelid
H02.883	Meibomian gland dysfunction of right eye, unspecified eyelid
H02.884	Meibomian gland dysfunction left upper eyelid
H02.885	Meibomian gland dysfunction left lower eyelid
H02.886	Meibomian gland dysfunction of left eye, unspecified eyelid
H02.889	Meibomian gland dysfunction of unspecified eye, unspecified eyelid
H02.88A	Meibomian gland dysfunction right eye, upper and lower eyelids
H02.88B	Meibomian gland dysfunction left eye, upper and lower eyelids
H10.821	Rosacea conjunctivitis, right eye
H10.822	Rosacea conjunctivitis, left eye
H10.823	Rosacea conjunctivitis, bilateral
H10.829	Rosacea conjunctivitis, unspecified eye
H57.811	Brow ptosis, right
H57.812	Brow ptosis, left
H57.813	Brow ptosis, bilateral
H57.819	Brow ptosis, unspecified
H57.89	Other specified disorders of eye and adnexa
I63.81	Other cerebral infarction due to occlusion or stenosis of small artery
I63.89	Other cerebral infarction
I67.850	Cerebral autosomal dominant arteriopathy with subcortical infarcts and leukoencephalopathy
I67.858	Other hereditary cerebrovascular disease
K35.20	Acute appendicitis with generalized peritonitis, without abscess
K35.21	Acute appendicitis with generalized peritonitis, with abscess
K35.30	Acute appendicitis with localized peritonitis, without perforation or gangrene
K35.31	Acute appendicitis with localized peritonitis and gangrene, without perforation
K35.32	Acute appendicitis with perforation and localized peritonitis, without abscess
K35.33	Acute appendicitis with perforation and localized peritonitis, with abscess
K35.890	Other acute appendicitis without perforation or gangrene
K35.891	Other acute appendicitis without perforation, with gangrene
K61.31	Horseshoe abscess
K61.39	Other ischiorectal abscess
K61.5	Supralevator abscess
K82.A1	Gangrene of gallbladder in cholecystitis
K82.A2	Perforation of gallbladder in cholecystitis
K83.01	Primary sclerosing cholangitis
K83.09	Other cholangitis
M79.10	Myalgia, unspecified site
M79.11	Myalgia of mastication muscle
M79.12	Myalgia of auxiliary muscles, head and neck
M79.18	Myalgia, other site
N35.016	Post-traumatic urethral stricture, male, overlapping sites
N35.116	Postinfective urethral stricture, not elsewhere classified, male, overlapping sites
N35.811	Other urethral stricture, male, meatal
N35.812	Other urethral bulbous stricture, male
N35.813	Other membranous urethral stricture, male
N35.814	Other anterior urethral stricture, male, anterior
N35.816	Other urethral stricture, male, overlapping sites
N35.819	Other urethral stricture, male, unspecified site
N35.82	Other urethral stricture, female
N35.911	Unspecified urethral stricture, male, meatal
N35.912	Unspecified bulbous urethral stricture, male
N35.913	Unspecified membranous urethral stricture, male
N35.914	Unspecified anterior urethral stricture, male
N35.916	Unspecified urethral stricture, male, overlapping sites
N35.919	Unspecified urethral stricture, male, unspecified site
N35.92	Unspecified urethral stricture, female
N99.116	Postprocedural urethral stricture, male, overlapping sites
O30.131	Triplet pregnancy, trichorionic/triamniotic, first trimester
O30.132	Triplet pregnancy, trichorionic/triamniotic, second trimester
O30.133	Triplet pregnancy, trichorionic/triamniotic, third trimester
O30.139	Triplet pregnancy, trichorionic/triamniotic, unspecified trimester
O30.231	Quadruplet pregnancy, quadrachorionic/quadra-amniotic, first trimester
O30.232	Quadruplet pregnancy, quadrachorionic/quadra-amniotic, second trimester

279 New Codes Added (continued)

O30.233	Quadruplet pregnancy, quadrachorionic/quadra-amniotic, third trimester
O30.239	Quadruplet pregnancy, quadrachorionic/quadra-amniotic, unspecified trimester
O30.831	Other specified multiple gestation, number of chorions and amnions are both equal to the number of fetuses, first trimester
O30.832	Other specified multiple gestation, number of chorions and amnions are both equal to the number of fetuses, second trimester
O30.833	Other specified multiple gestation, number of chorions and amnions are both equal to the number of fetuses, third trimester
O30.839	Other specified multiple gestation, number of chorions and amnions are both equal to the number of fetuses, unspecified trimester
O86.00	Infection of obstetric surgical wound, unspecified
O86.01	Infection of obstetric surgical wound, superficial incisional site
O86.02	Infection of obstetric surgical wound, deep incisional site
O86.03	Infection of obstetric surgical wound, organ and space site
O86.04	Sepsis following an obstetrical procedure
O86.09	Infection of obstetric surgical wound, other surgical site
P02.70	Newborn affected by fetal inflammatory response syndrome
P02.78	Newborn affected by other conditions from chorioamnionitis
P04.11	Newborn affected by maternal antineoplastic chemotherapy
P04.12	Newborn affected by maternal cytotoxic drugs
P04.13	Newborn affected by maternal use of anticonvulsants
P04.14	Newborn affected by maternal use of opiates
P04.15	Newborn affected by maternal use of antidepressants
P04.16	Newborn affected by maternal use of amphetamines
P04.17	Newborn affected by maternal use of sedative-hypnotics
P04.1A	Newborn affected by maternal use of anxiolytics
P04.18	Newborn affected by other maternal medication
P04.19	Newborn affected by maternal use of unspecified medication
P04.40	Newborn affected by maternal use of unspecified drugs of addiction
P04.42	Newborn affected by maternal use of hallucinogens
P04.81	Newborn affected by maternal use of cannabis
P04.89	Newborn affected by other maternal noxious substances
P35.4	Congenital Zika virus disease
P74.21	Hypernatremia of newborn
P74.22	Hyponatremia of newborn
P74.31	Hyperkalemia of newborn
P74.32	Hypokalemia of newborn
P74.41	Alkalosis of newborn
P74.421	Hyperchloremia of newborn
P74.422	Hypochloremia of newborn
P74.49	Other transitory electrolyte disturbance of newborn
Q51.20	Other doubling of uterus, unspecified
Q51.21	Other complete doubling of uterus
Q51.22	Other partial doubling of uterus
Q51.28	Other doubling of uterus, other specified
Q93.51	Angelman syndrome
Q93.59	Other deletions of part of a chromosome

Q93.82	Williams syndrome
R82.991	Hypocitraturia
R82.992	Hyperoxaluria
R82.993	Hyperuricosuria
R82.994	Hypercalciuria
R82.998	Other abnormal findings in urine
R93.811	Abnormal radiologic findings on diagnostic imaging of right testicle
R93.812	Abnormal radiologic findings on diagnostic imaging of left testicle
R93.813	Abnormal radiologic findings on diagnostic imaging of testicles, bilateral
R93.819	Abnormal radiologic findings on diagnostic imaging of unspecified testicle
R93.89	Abnormal findings on diagnostic imaging of other specified body structures
T43.641A	Poisoning by ecstasy, accidental (unintentional), initial encounter
T43.641D	Poisoning by ecstasy, accidental (unintentional), subsequent encounter
T43.641S	Poisoning by ecstasy, accidental (unintentional), sequela
T43.642A	Poisoning by ecstasy, intentional self-harm, initial encounter
T43.642D	Poisoning by ecstasy, intentional self-harm, subsequent encounter
T43.642S	Poisoning by ecstasy, intentional self-harm, sequela
T43.643A	Poisoning by ecstasy, assault, initial encounter
T43.643D	Poisoning by ecstasy, assault, subsequent encounter
T43.643S	Poisoning by ecstasy, assault, sequela
T43.644A	Poisoning by ecstasy, undetermined, initial encounter
T43.644D	Poisoning by ecstasy, undetermined, subsequent encounter
T43.644S	Poisoning by ecstasy, undetermined, sequela
T74.51XA	Adult forced sexual exploitation, confirmed, initial encounter
T74.51XD	Adult forced sexual exploitation, confirmed, subsequent encounter
T74.51XS	Adult forced sexual exploitation, confirmed, sequela
T74.52XA	Child sexual exploitation, confirmed, initial encounter
T74.52XD	Child sexual exploitation, confirmed, subsequent encounter
T74.52XS	Child sexual exploitation, confirmed, sequela
T74.61XA	Adult forced labor exploitation, confirmed, initial encounter
T74.61XD	Adult forced labor exploitation, confirmed, subsequent encounter
T74.61XS	Adult forced labor exploitation, confirmed, sequela
T74.62XA	Child forced labor exploitation, confirmed, initial encounter
T74.62XD	Child forced labor exploitation, confirmed, subsequent encounter
T74.62XS	Child forced labor exploitation, confirmed, sequela
T76.51XA	Adult forced sexual exploitation, suspected, initial encounter
T76.51XD	Adult forced sexual exploitation, suspected, subsequent encounter
T76.51XS	Adult forced sexual exploitation, suspected, sequela
T76.52XA	Child sexual exploitation, suspected, initial encounter
T76.52XD	Child sexual exploitation, suspected, subsequent encounter
T76.52XS	Child sexual exploitation, suspected, sequela
T76.61XA	Adult forced labor exploitation, suspected, initial encounter
T76.61XD	Adult forced labor exploitation, suspected, subsequent encounter
T76.61XS	Adult forced labor exploitation, suspected, sequela

279 New Codes Added (continued)

T76.62XA	Child forced labor exploitation, suspected, initial encounter
T76.62XD	Child forced labor exploitation, suspected, subsequent encounter
T76.62XS	Child forced labor exploitation, suspected, sequela
T81.40XA	Infection following a procedure, unspecified, initial encounter
T81.40XD	Infection following a procedure, unspecified, subsequent encounter
T81.40XS	Infection following a procedure, unspecified, sequela
T81.41XA	Infection following a procedure, superficial incisional surgical site, initial encounter
T81.41XD	Infection following a procedure, superficial incisional surgical site, subsequent encounter
T81.41XS	Infection following a procedure, superficial incisional surgical site, sequela
T81.42XA	Infection following a procedure, deep incisional surgical site, initial encounter
T81.42XD	Infection following a procedure, deep incisional surgical site, subsequent encounter
T81.42XS	Infection following a procedure, deep incisional surgical site, sequela
T81.43XA	Infection following a procedure, organ and space surgical site, initial encounter
T81.43XD	Infection following a procedure, organ and space surgical site, subsequent encounter
T81.43XS	Infection following a procedure, organ and space surgical site, sequela
T81.44XA	Sepsis following a procedure, initial encounter
T81.44XD	Sepsis following a procedure, subsequent encounter
T81.44XS	Sepsis following a procedure, sequela
T81.49XA	Infection following a procedure, other surgical site, initial encounter
T81.49XD	Infection following a procedure, other surgical site, subsequent encounter
T81.49XS	Infection following a procedure, other surgical site, sequela
Y07.6	Multiple perpetrators of maltreatment and neglect
Z04.81	Encounter for examination and observation of victim following forced sexual exploitation
Z04.82	Encounter for examination and observation of victim following forced labor exploitation
Z04.89	Encounter for examination and observation for other specified reasons
Z13.30	Encounter for screening examination for mental health and behavioral disorders, unspecified
Z13.31	Encounter for screening for depression
Z13.32	Encounter for screening for maternal depression
Z13.39	Encounter for screening examination for other mental health and behavioral disorders
Z13.40	Encounter for screening for unspecified developmental delays
Z13.41	Encounter for autism screening
Z13.42	Encounter for screening for global developmental delays (milestones)
Z13.49	Encounter for screening for other developmental delays
Z20.821	Contact with and (suspected) exposure to Zika virus
Z28.83	Immunization not carried out due to unavailability of vaccine
Z62.813	Personal history of forced labor or sexual exploitation in childhood
Z83.430	Family history of elevated lipoprotein(a)
Z83.438	Family history of other disorder of lipoprotein metabolism and other lipidemia
Z91.42	Personal history of forced labor or sexual exploitation

143 Code Descriptions Revised

Note: Each code is listed with its revised description only. Please refer to the full FY 2019 official addenda code files at https://www.cdc.gov/nchs/icd/icd10cm.htm for the specific changes made to the codes listed.

E67.1	Hypercarotenemia
E72.53	Primary hyperoxaluria
F68.10	Factitious disorder imposed on self, unspecified
F68.11	Factitious disorder imposed on self, with predominantly psychological signs and symptoms
F68.12	Factitious disorder imposed on self, with predominantly physical signs and symptoms
F68.13	Factitious disorder imposed on self, with combined psychological and physical signs and symptoms
H04.201	Unspecified epiphora, right side
H04.202	Unspecified epiphora, left side
H04.203	Unspecified epiphora, bilateral
H04.209	Unspecified epiphora, unspecified side
H04.221	Epiphora due to insufficient drainage, right side
H04.222	Epiphora due to insufficient drainage, left side
H04.223	Epiphora due to insufficient drainage, bilateral
H04.229	Epiphora due to insufficient drainage, unspecified side
I63.219	Cerebral infarction due to unspecified occlusion or stenosis of unspecified vertebral artery
I63.239	Cerebral infarction due to unspecified occlusion or stenosis of unspecified carotid artery
I63.333	Cerebral infarction due to thrombosis of bilateral posterior cerebral arteries
I63.343	Cerebral infarction due to thrombosis of bilateral cerebellar arteries
J84.848	Other interstitial lung diseases of childhood
K43.5	Parastomal hernia without obstruction or gangrene
L98.495	Non-pressure chronic ulcer of skin of other sites with muscle involvement without evidence of necrosis
L98.496	Non-pressure chronic ulcer of skin of other sites with bone involvement without evidence of necrosis
L98.498	Non-pressure chronic ulcer of skin of other sites with other specified severity
M26.621	Arthralgia of right temporomandibular joint
M50.01	Cervical disc disorder with myelopathy, high cervical region
M50.11	Cervical disc disorder with radiculopathy, high cervical region
M50.21	Other cervical disc displacement, high cervical region
M50.31	Other cervical disc degeneration, high cervical region
M50.81	Other cervical disc disorders, high cervical region
M50.91	Cervical disc disorder, unspecified, high cervical region
M86.621	Other chronic osteomyelitis, right humerus
M86.622	Other chronic osteomyelitis, left humerus
M86.629	Other chronic osteomyelitis, unspecified humerus
N63.0	Unspecified lump in unspecified breast
O00.212	Left ovarian pregnancy with intrauterine pregnancy
Q66.89	Other specified congenital deformities of feet
R40.2330	Coma scale, best motor response, abnormal flexion, unspecified time
R40.2331	Coma scale, best motor response, abnormal flexion, in the field [EMT or ambulance]

143 Code Descriptions Revised (continued)

R4Ø.2332 Coma scale, best motor response, abnormal flexion, at arrival to emergency department

R4Ø.2333 Coma scale, best motor response, abnormal flexion, at hospital admission

R4Ø.2334 Coma scale, best motor response, abnormal flexion, 24 hours or more after hospital admission

S62.626A Displaced fracture of middle phalanx of right little finger, initial encounter for closed fracture

S62.626B Displaced fracture of middle phalanx of right little finger, initial encounter for open fracture

S62.626D Displaced fracture of middle phalanx of right little finger, subsequent encounter for fracture with routine healing

S62.626G Displaced fracture of middle phalanx of right little finger, subsequent encounter for fracture with delayed healing

S62.626K Displaced fracture of middle phalanx of right little finger, subsequent encounter for fracture with nonunion

S62.626P Displaced fracture of middle phalanx of right little finger, subsequent encounter for fracture with malunion

S62.626S Displaced fracture of middle phalanx of right little finger, sequela

S62.627A Displaced fracture of middle phalanx of left little finger, initial encounter for closed fracture

S62.627B Displaced fracture of middle phalanx of left little finger, initial encounter for open fracture

S62.627D Displaced fracture of middle phalanx of left little finger, subsequent encounter for fracture with routine healing

S62.627G Displaced fracture of middle phalanx of left little finger, subsequent encounter for fracture with delayed healing

S62.627K Displaced fracture of middle phalanx of left little finger, subsequent encounter for fracture with nonunion

S62.627P Displaced fracture of middle phalanx of left little finger, subsequent encounter for fracture with malunion

S62.627S Displaced fracture of middle phalanx of left little finger, sequela

S62.628A Displaced fracture of middle phalanx of other finger, initial encounter for closed fracture

S62.628B Displaced fracture of middle phalanx of other finger, initial encounter for open fracture

S62.628D Displaced fracture of middle phalanx of other finger, subsequent encounter for fracture with routine healing

S62.628G Displaced fracture of middle phalanx of other finger, subsequent encounter for fracture with delayed healing

S62.628K Displaced fracture of middle phalanx of other finger, subsequent encounter for fracture with nonunion

S62.628P Displaced fracture of middle phalanx of other finger, subsequent encounter for fracture with malunion

S62.628S Displaced fracture of middle phalanx of other finger, sequela

S62.629A Displaced fracture of middle phalanx of unspecified finger, initial encounter for closed fracture

S62.629B Displaced fracture of middle phalanx of unspecified finger, initial encounter for open fracture

S62.629D Displaced fracture of middle phalanx of unspecified finger, subsequent encounter for fracture with routine healing

S62.629G Displaced fracture of middle phalanx of unspecified finger, subsequent encounter for fracture with delayed healing

S62.629K Displaced fracture of middle phalanx of unspecified finger, subsequent encounter for fracture with nonunion

S62.629P Displaced fracture of middle phalanx of unspecified finger, subsequent encounter for fracture with malunion

S62.629S Displaced fracture of middle phalanx of unspecified finger, sequela

S62.654A Nondisplaced fracture of middle phalanx of right ring finger, initial encounter for closed fracture

S62.654B Nondisplaced fracture of middle phalanx of right ring finger, initial encounter for open fracture

S62.654D Nondisplaced fracture of middle phalanx of right ring finger, subsequent encounter for fracture with routine healing

S62.654G Nondisplaced fracture of middle phalanx of right ring finger, subsequent encounter for fracture with delayed healing

S62.654K Nondisplaced fracture of middle phalanx of right ring finger, subsequent encounter for fracture with nonunion

S62.654P Nondisplaced fracture of middle phalanx of right ring finger, subsequent encounter for fracture with malunion

S62.654S Nondisplaced fracture of middle phalanx of right ring finger, sequela

S62.655A Nondisplaced fracture of middle phalanx of left ring finger, initial encounter for closed fracture

S62.655B Nondisplaced fracture of middle phalanx of left ring finger, initial encounter for open fracture

S62.655D Nondisplaced fracture of middle phalanx of left ring finger, subsequent encounter for fracture with routine healing

S62.655G Nondisplaced fracture of middle phalanx of left ring finger, subsequent encounter for fracture with delayed healing

S62.655K Nondisplaced fracture of middle phalanx of left ring finger, subsequent encounter for fracture with nonunion

S62.655P Nondisplaced fracture of middle phalanx of left ring finger, subsequent encounter for fracture with malunion

S62.655S Nondisplaced fracture of middle phalanx of left ring finger, sequela

S62.656A Nondisplaced fracture of middle phalanx of right little finger, initial encounter for closed fracture

S62.656B Nondisplaced fracture of middle phalanx of right little finger, initial encounter for open fracture

S62.656D Nondisplaced fracture of middle phalanx of right little finger, subsequent encounter for fracture with routine healing

S62.656G Nondisplaced fracture of middle phalanx of right little finger, subsequent encounter for fracture with delayed healing

S62.656K Nondisplaced fracture of middle phalanx of right little finger, subsequent encounter for fracture with nonunion

S62.656P Nondisplaced fracture of middle phalanx of right little finger, subsequent encounter for fracture with malunion

S62.656S Nondisplaced fracture of middle phalanx of right little finger, sequela

S62.657A Nondisplaced fracture of middle phalanx of left little finger, initial encounter for closed fracture

S62.657B Nondisplaced fracture of middle phalanx of left little finger, initial encounter for open fracture

S62.657D Nondisplaced fracture of middle phalanx of left little finger, subsequent encounter for fracture with routine healing

S62.657G Nondisplaced fracture of middle phalanx of left little finger, subsequent encounter for fracture with delayed healing

S62.657K Nondisplaced fracture of middle phalanx of left little finger, subsequent encounter for fracture with nonunion

S62.657P Nondisplaced fracture of middle phalanx of left little finger, subsequent encounter for fracture with malunion

S62.657S Nondisplaced fracture of middle phalanx of left little finger, sequela

S62.658A Nondisplaced fracture of middle phalanx of other finger, initial encounter for closed fracture

S62.658B Nondisplaced fracture of middle phalanx of other finger, initial encounter for open fracture

143 Code Descriptions Revised (continued)

S62.658D Nondisplaced fracture of middle phalanx of other finger, subsequent encounter for fracture with routine healing

S62.658G Nondisplaced fracture of middle phalanx of other finger, subsequent encounter for fracture with delayed healing

S62.658K Nondisplaced fracture of middle phalanx of other finger, subsequent encounter for fracture with nonunion

S62.658P Nondisplaced fracture of middle phalanx of other finger, subsequent encounter for fracture with malunion

S62.658S Nondisplaced fracture of middle phalanx of other finger, sequela

S62.659A Nondisplaced fracture of middle phalanx of unspecified finger, initial encounter for closed fracture

S62.659B Nondisplaced fracture of middle phalanx of unspecified finger, initial encounter for open fracture

S62.659D Nondisplaced fracture of middle phalanx of unspecified finger, subsequent encounter for fracture with routine healing

S62.659G Nondisplaced fracture of middle phalanx of unspecified finger, subsequent encounter for fracture with delayed healing

S62.659K Nondisplaced fracture of middle phalanx of unspecified finger, subsequent encounter for fracture with nonunion

S62.659P Nondisplaced fracture of middle phalanx of unspecified finger, subsequent encounter for fracture with malunion

S62.659S Nondisplaced fracture of middle phalanx of unspecified finger, sequela

S99.101A Unspecified physeal fracture of right metatarsal, initial encounter for closed fracture

S99.101B Unspecified physeal fracture of right metatarsal, initial encounter for open fracture

S99.101D Unspecified physeal fracture of right metatarsal, subsequent encounter for fracture with routine healing

S99.101G Unspecified physeal fracture of right metatarsal, subsequent encounter for fracture with delayed healing

S99.101K Unspecified physeal fracture of right metatarsal, subsequent encounter for fracture with nonunion

S99.101P Unspecified physeal fracture of right metatarsal, subsequent encounter for fracture with malunion

S99.101S Unspecified physeal fracture of right metatarsal, sequela

S99.132A Salter-Harris Type III physeal fracture of left metatarsal, initial encounter for closed fracture

S99.132B Salter-Harris Type III physeal fracture of left metatarsal, initial encounter for open fracture

S99.132D Salter-Harris Type III physeal fracture of left metatarsal, subsequent encounter for fracture with routine healing

S99.132G Salter-Harris Type III physeal fracture of left metatarsal, subsequent encounter for fracture with delayed healing

S99.132K Salter-Harris Type III physeal fracture of left metatarsal, subsequent encounter for fracture with nonunion

S99.132P Salter-Harris Type III physeal fracture of left metatarsal, subsequent encounter for fracture with malunion

S99.132S Salter-Harris Type III physeal fracture of left metatarsal, sequela

T81.11XA Postprocedural cardiogenic shock, initial encounter

T81.11XD Postprocedural cardiogenic shock, subsequent encounter

T81.11XS Postprocedural cardiogenic shock, sequela

V00.821A Fall from baby stroller, initial encounter

V00.821D Fall from baby stroller, subsequent encounter

V00.821S Fall from baby stroller, sequela

V00.822A Baby stroller colliding with stationary object, initial encounter

V00.822D Baby stroller colliding with stationary object, subsequent encounter

V00.822S Baby stroller colliding with stationary object, sequela

V00.828A Other accident with baby stroller, initial encounter

V00.828D Other accident with baby stroller, subsequent encounter

V00.828S Other accident with baby stroller, sequela

Y92.000 Kitchen of unspecified non-institutional (private) residence as the place of occurrence of the external cause

Y93.23 Activity, snow (alpine) (downhill) skiing, snowboarding, sledding, tobogganing and snow tubing

Z40.03 Encounter for prophylactic removal of fallopian tube(s)

Z68.43 Body mass index (BMI) 50-59.9, adult

Z77.123 Contact with and (suspected) exposure to radon and other naturally occurring radiation

Z77.29 Contact with and (suspected) exposure to other hazardous substances

Discontinued Notations

Optum360 removed the *PDxCC or PDxMCC Condition* icons from the 2019 *ICD-10-CM Professional for Hospitals: The Complete Official Code Set*. The decision to remove the icons was based on the proposed rule published in the *Federal Register*, volume 83, number 88, May 7, 2018 ("Hospital Inpatient Prospective Payment Systems for Acute Care Hospitals and Long Term Care Hospital Prospective System and Proposed Policy Changes and Fiscal Year 2019 Rates") found at https://www.gpo.gov/fdsys/pkg/FR-2018-05-07/pdf/2018-09581.pdf.

The purpose of the principal diagnosis as its own CC or MCC was to ensure consistent MS-DRG assignment between the ICD-9 and ICD-10-MS-DRGs. The Centers for Medicare and Medicaid Services (CMS) stated it is no longer necessary to replicate MS-DRG assignment across the ICD-9 and ICD-10 versions of the MS-DRGs. CMS believes there may be more effective indicators of resource utilization than the special logic used to assign clinical severity to a principal diagnosis based on data analysis. Therefore, CMS proposed removing the special logic in the Grouper and deleting the tables containing the lists of principal diagnosis as its own MCC and principal diagnosis as its own CC codes from the ICD-10 MS-DRG Definitions Manual for FY 2019.

Proprietary Updates

The following proprietary features have also been added:

- New LTCH icon identifying ICD-10-CM codes that are considered severe wound diagnoses

- 300+ new definitions that describe, in lay terms, a specific condition or disease process

- 75+ new acute care hospital coding tips

- Updated *AHA Coding Clinic* references through second quarter 2018

- Conversion table of ICD-10-CM codes

- Coding examples in the chapter-specific guideline sections, specific to the acute care hospital setting

Conversion Table of ICD-10-CM Codes

Code Assignment Beginning 10/1/2018	Previous Code(s) Assignment	Code Assignment Beginning 10/1/2018	Previous Code(s) Assignment
C43.111	C43.11	E75.26	E75.29
C43.112	C43.11	E78.41	E78.4
C43.121	C43.12	E78.49	E78.4
C43.122	C43.12	E88.02	E88.09
C4A.111	C4A.11	F12.23	F12.288
C4A.112	C4A.11	F12.93	F12.988
C4A.121	C4A.12	F53.0	F53
C4A.122	C4A.12	F53.1	F53
C44.1021	C44.102	F68.A	F68.10
C44.1022	C44.102	G51.31	G51.3
C44.1091	C44.109	G51.32	G51.3
C44.1092	C44.109	G51.33	G51.3
C44.1121	C44.112	G51.39	G51.3
C44.1122	C44.112	G71.00	G71.0
C44.1191	C44.119	G71.01	G71.0
C44.1192	C44.119	G71.02	G71.0
C44.1221	C44.122	G71.09	G71.0
C44.1222	C44.122	H01.00A	H01.001 and H01.002
C44.1291	C44.129	H01.00B	H01.004 and H01.005
C44.1292	C44.129	H01.01A	H01.011 and H01.012
C44.131	C44.19	H01.01B	H01.014 and H01.015
C44.1321	C44.19	H01.02A	H01.021 and H01.022
C44.1322	C44.19	H01.02B	H01.024 and H01.025
C44.1391	C44.19	H02.151	H02.101-H02.106; H02.109
C44.1392	C44.19	H02.152	H02.101-H02.106; H02.109
C44.1921	C44.192	H02.153	H02.101-H02.106; H02.109
C44.1922	C44.192	H02.154	H02.101-H02.106; H02.109
C44.1991	C44.199	H02.155	H02.101-H02.106; H02.109
C44.1992	C44.199	H02.156	H02.101-H02.106; H02.109
D03.111	D03.11	H02.159	H02.101-H02.106; H02.109
D03.112	D03.11	H02.20A	H02.201 and H02.202
D03.121	D03.12	H02.20B	H02.204 and H02.205
D03.122	D03.12	H02.20C	H02.201, H02.202, H02.204 and H02.205
D04.111	D04.11	H02.21A	H02.211 and H02.212
D04.112	D04.11	H02.21B	H02.214 and H02.215
D04.121	D04.12	H02.21C	H02.211, H02.212, H02.214 and H02.215
D04.122	D04.12	H02.22A	H02.221 and H02.222
D22.111	D22.11	H02.22B	H02.224 and H02.225
D22.112	D22.11	H02.22C	H02.221, H02.222, H02.224 and H02.225
D22.121	D22.12	H02.23A	H02.231 and H02.232
D22.122	D22.12	H02.23B	H02.234 and H02.235
D23.111	D23.11	H02.23C	H02.231, H02.232, H02.234 and H02.235
D23.112	D23.11	H02.881	H02.89
D23.121	D23.12	H02.882	H02.89
D23.122	D23.12	H02.883	H02.89
E72.81	E72.8		
E72.89	E72.8		

Code Assignment Beginning 10/1/2018	Previous Code(s) Assignment	Code Assignment Beginning 10/1/2018	Previous Code(s) Assignment
H02.884	H02.89	N35.912	N35.9
H02.885	H02.89	N35.913	N35.9
H02.886	H02.89	N35.914	N35.9
H02.889	H02.89	N35.916	N35.9
H02.88A	H02.89	N35.919	N35.9
H02.88B	H02.89	N35.92	N35.9
H10.821	H10.89	N99.116	N99.114
H10.822	H10.89	O30.131	O30.101
H10.823	H10.89	O30.132	O30.101
H10.829	H10.89	O30.133	O30.101
H57.811	H57.8	O30.139	O30.101
H57.812	H57.8	O30.231	O30.201
H57.813	H57.8	O30.232	O30.201
H57.819	H57.8	O30.233	O30.201
H57.89	H57.8	O30.239	O30.201
I63.81	I63.8	O30.831	O30.801
I63.89	I63.8	O30.832	O30.801
I67.850	I67.89	O30.833	O30.801
I67.858	I67.89	O30.839	O30.801
K35.20	K35.2	O86.00	O86.0
K35.21	K35.2	O86.01	O86.0
K35.30	K35.3	O86.02	O86.0
K35.31	K35.3	O86.03	O86.0
K35.32	K35.3	O86.04	O86.0
K35.33	K35.3	O86.09	O86.0
K35.890	K35.89	P02.70	P02.7
K35.891	K35.89	P02.78	P02.7
K61.31	K61.3	P04.11	P04.1
K61.39	K61.3	P04.12	P04.1
K61.5	K61.3	P04.13	P04.1
K82.A1	K81.0	P04.14	P04.1
K82.A2	K82.2 and K81.9	P04.15	P04.1
K83.01	K83.0	P04.16	P04.1
K83.09	K83.0	P04.17	P04.1
M79.10	M79.1	P04.1A	P04.1
M79.11	M79.1	P04.18	P04.1
M79.12	M79.1	P04.19	P04.1
M79.18	M79.1	P04.40	P04.49
N35.016	N35.014	P04.42	P04.49
N35.116	N35.114	P04.81	P04.8
N35.811	N35.8	P04.89	P04.8
N35.812	N35.8	P35.4	P35.8 and A92.5
N35.813	N35.8	P74.21	P74.2
N35.814	N35.8	P74.22	P74.2
N35.816	N35.8	P74.31	P74.3
N35.819	N35.8	P74.32	P74.3
N35.82	N35.8	P74.41	P74.4
N35.911	N35.9	P74.421	P74.4

Code Assignment Beginning 10/1/2018	Previous Code(s) Assignment	Code Assignment Beginning 10/1/2018	Previous Code(s) Assignment
P74.422	P74.4	T76.52XS	T76.22XS
P74.49	P74.4	T76.61XA	T76.11XA
Q51.20	Q51.2	T76.61XD	T76.11XD
Q51.21	Q51.2	T76.61XS	T76.11XS
Q51.22	Q51.2	T76.62XA	T76.12XA
Q51.28	Q51.2	T76.62XD	T76.12XD
Q93.51	Q93.5	T76.62XS	T76.12XS
Q93.59	Q93.5	T81.40XA	T81.4XXA
Q93.82	Q93.89	T81.40XD	T81.4XXD
R82.991	R82.99	T81.40XS	T81.4XXS
R82.992	R82.99	T81.41XA	T81.4XXA
R82.993	R82.99	T81.41XD	T81.4XXD
R82.994	R82.99	T81.41XS	T81.4XXS
R82.998	R82.99	T81.42XA	T81.4XXA
R93.811	R93.8	T81.42XD	T81.4XXD
R93.812	R93.8	T81.42XS	T81.4XXS
R93.813	R93.8	T81.43XA	T81.4XXA
R93.819	R93.8	T81.43XD	T81.4XXD
R93.89	R93.8	T81.43XS	T81.4XXS
T43.641A	T43.621A	T81.44XA	T81.4XXA
T43.641D	T43.621D	T81.44XD	T81.4XXD
T43.641S	T43.621S	T81.44XS	T81.4XXS
T43.642A	T43.622A	T81.49XA	T81.4XXA
T43.642D	T43.622D	T81.49XD	T81.4XXD
T43.642S	T43.622S	T81.49XS	T81.4XXS
T43.643A	T43.623A	Y07.6	Y07.59
T43.643D	T43.623D	Z04.81	Z04.8
T43.643S	T43.623S	Z04.82	Z04.8
T43.644A	T43.624A	Z04.89	Z04.8
T43.644D	T43.624D	Z13.30	Z13.8
T43.644S	T43.624S	Z13.31	Z13.8
T74.51XA	T74.21XA	Z13.32	Z13.8
T74.51XD	T74.21XD	Z13.39	Z13.8
T74.51XS	T74.21XS	Z13.40	Z13.4
T74.52XA	T74.22XA	Z13.41	Z13.4
T74.52XD	T74.22XD	Z13.42	Z13.4
T74.52XS	T74.22XS	Z13.49	Z13.4
T74.61XA	T74.11XA	Z20.821	Z20.828
T74.61XD	T74.11XD	Z28.83	Z28.89
T74.61XS	T74.11XS	Z62.813	Z62.810
T74.62XA	T74.12XA	Z83.430	Z83.49
T74.62XD	T74.12XD	Z83.438	Z83.49
T74.62XS	T74.12XS	Z91.42	Z91.410
T76.51XA	T76.21XA		
T76.51XD	T76.21XD		
T76.51XS	T76.21XS		
T76.52XA	T76.22XA		
T76.52XD	T76.22XD		

Introduction

History of ICD-10-CM

The ICD-10-CM classification system was developed by the National Center for Health Statistics (NCHS) as a clinical modification to the ICD-10 system developed by the World Health Organization (WHO), primarily as a unique system for use in the United States for morbidity and mortality reporting. Although ICD-10 replaced ICD-9 for use in coding and classifying of mortality data from death certificates beginning January 1, 1999, ICD-10-CM implementation was postponed many years until legislation to replace ICD-9-CM, volumes 1 and 2, with ICD-10-CM was approved.

ICD-10 is the copyrighted product of the World Health Organization (WHO), which has authorized the development of a clinical modification (CM) of ICD-10 for use in the United States. However, all modifications to the ICD-10 must conform to WHO conventions for ICD. The development of ICD-10-CM included comprehensive evaluation by a Technical Advisory Panel and extensive consultation with physician groups, clinical coders, and other industry experts.

The ICD-10-CM draft and crosswalk between ICD-9-CM and ICD-10-CM were made available on the Centers for Medicare and Medicaid Services (CMS) website for public comment. The initial public comment period extended from December 1997 through February 1998. A field test for ICD-10-CM was conducted in the summer of 2003 jointly by the American Hospital Association (AMA) and the American Health Information Management Association (AHIMA). Public comments and suggestions were reviewed and additional modifications to ICD-10-CM were made. Revisions were made to ICD-10-CM based on the established update process for ICD-10-CM (the ICD-10-CM Coordination and Maintenance Committee) and the World Health Organization's ICD-10 (the Update and Revision Committee).

These revisions to ICD-10-CM have included:

- Information relevant to ambulatory and managed care encounters
- Expanded injury codes
- Creation of combination diagnosis/symptom codes to reduce the number of codes needed to fully describe a condition
- The addition of 6th and 7th character classifications
- Incorporation of common 4th and 5th character classifications
- Classifications specific to laterality
- Classification refinement for increased data granularity

This new structure allows for further expansion than was possible with the ICD-9-CM classification system.

The Department of Health and Human Services (HHS) published the final rule regarding the adoption of both ICD-10-CM and ICD-10-PCS in the January 16, 2009, *Federal Register* (45 CFR part 162 [CMS—0013—F]). The initial compliance date for implementation of ICD-10-CM and ICD-10-PCS as a replacement for ICD-9-CM was set at October 1, 2013. On April 17, 2012, the Department of Health and Human Services (HHS) released a notice to postpone the date by which certain health care entities have to comply with International Classification of Diseases, 10th Revision diagnosis and procedure codes (ICD-10). The compliance date for implementation of ICD-10-CM and ICD-10-PCS as a replacement for ICD-9-CM was changed to October 1, 2014. On April 1, 2014, Congress enacted the Protecting Access to Medicare Act of 2014, which contained a provision to delay the implementation of ICD-10-CM/PCS by at least one year, prohibiting the Department of Health and Human Services (HHS) from adopting the ICD-10-CM/PCS code sets as the mandatory standard until October 1, 2015. Eventually, the ICD-10-CM/PCS code sets were implemented in their entirety on October 1, 2015, and ICD-9-CM, volumes 1 and 2, were retired.

ICD-10-CM for Hospitals: The Complete Official Code Set

ICD-10-CM for Hospitals: The Complete Official Code Set 2019 includes information relevant to both acute care and long term care hospitals and many of the features described below were added in direct response to requests from our subscribers.

As you review the content, you will find the following:

- Optum360 Exclusive feature — Check Placeholder Alert symbol, indicating the need for one or more "filler" X character assignments in the 5th and/or 6th character position to appropriately assign a required character in the 7th character position
- Optum360 Exclusive feature — Key word differentiation by the use of a green font that highlights the differentiating terms in similar code descriptions in a given category
- Optum360 Exclusive feature — Exclusive *following* references and Check Additional Character symbol in the indexes. The *following* references (designed and used exclusively by Optum360) help coders locate those alphanumeric codes that are out of sequence in the tabular section.
- Optum360 Exclusive feature — Exclusive shaded guides in the index that help users easily follow the indent levels for the subterms under a main term
- Illustrations throughout the tabular list and at the back of the book that feature anatomy and terminology included in the ICD-10-CM classification system
- Optum360 Exclusive feature — Detailed muscle/tendon tables that correspond with codes in chapters 13 and 19
- The complete ICD-10-CM Official Guidelines for Coding and Reporting, published by the U.S. Department of Health and Human Services and approved by the cooperating parties (American Health Information Management Association, National Center for Health Statistics, Centers for Medicare and Medicaid Services, American Hospital Association)
- Optum360 Exclusive feature — Official chapter-specific guidelines with coding examples specific to the hospital setting at the beginning of each chapter
- Exclusive color coding, symbols, and footnotes that alert coders to coding and reimbursement issues, including the majority of the Medicare code edits and identification of conditions that significantly affect MS-DRG or MS-LTC-DRG assignment
- A searchable data file for complication and comorbidity (CC) exclusions with a reference beneath applicable codes to make it easier to determine complications and comorbidities excluded from a particular principal diagnosis
- All official ICD-10-CM codes, indexes, notes, footnotes, and symbols
- Check 4th, 5th, 6th, and 7th character symbols that identify codes that require the addition of a 4th, 5th, 6th, or 7th character for code specificity and validity
- Color coding and symbol legend at the bottom of each page

Please review "How to Use *ICD-10-CM Professional for Hospitals*" in this manual to learn about the features that will help you assign and report correct codes, ensuring appropriate reimbursement.

This International Classification of Diseases, 10th Revision, Clinical Modification (ICD-10-CM) is being published by the United States Government in recognition of its responsibility to promulgate this classification throughout the United States for morbidity coding. This code book represents an adaptation of ICD-10 that was created specifically for use in the United States. Revisions to ICD-10-CM will be made based on the established update process for ICD-10-CM (the ICD-10-CM Coordination and Maintenance Committee) and the World Health Organization's ICD-10 (the Update and Revision Committee).

Use of Official Sources

The *ICD-10-CM Professional for Hospitals* contains the official U.S. Department of Health and Human Services, Tenth Revision, Clinical Modification (ICD-10-CM) codes, effective for the current year.

Much of the color coding and many of the symbols and footnotes that identify coding and reimbursement issues are derived from official federal government sources, including Medicare Code Editor (MCE), version 35, ICD-10 MS-DRG Definitions Manual Files, version 35, and the *Federal Register*, volume 83, number 88, May 7, 2018 ("Hospital Inpatient Prospective Payment Systems for Acute Care Hospitals and the Long-Term Care Hospital Prospective Payment System and Proposed Policy Changes and Fiscal Year 2019 Rates; Proposed Rule").

For the most current files related to IPPS please refer to the following:

https://www.cms.gov/Medicare/Medicare-Fee-for-Service-Payment/ AcuteInpatientPPS/IPPS-Regulations-and-Notices.html.

Steps to Correct Coding

1. Before beginning to use this code book, review section I.A., "Conventions for the ICD-10-CM," and section I.B., "General Coding Guidelines," of the ICD-10-CM Official Guidelines for Coding and Reporting.

2. Look up the main term in the alphabetic index and scan the subterm entries as appropriate. Review continued lines and additional subterms that may appear in the next column or on the next page.

3. Note all parenthetical terms (nonessential modifiers) that help in code selection but do not affect code assignment. Shaded vertical guidelines in the index are provided to help determine the indentation level for each subterm in relation to the main terms.

4. Pay close attention to the following instructions in the index:
   - "See," "see also," and "see category" cross-references
   - "With"/"without" notes
   - "Omit code" notes
   - "Due to" subterms
   - Other instructions found in note boxes, such as "code by site"
   - *Following* references and Check Additional Character symbol in the indexes. The *following* references (designed and used exclusively by Optum360) help coders locate those alphanumeric codes that are out of sequence in the tabular section.

5. Do not code from the alphabetic index without verifying the accuracy of the code in the Tabular List. Locate the code in the alphanumerically arranged Tabular List.

6. To determine the appropriateness of the code selection and proper coding, read all instructional material:
   - "Includes" and both types of "Excludes" notes
   - "Use additional code" and "code first underlying disease" instructions
   - "Code also"
   - 4th, 5th, and 6th character requirements and 7th character extension requirements
   - CC Exclusions
   - Age and sex symbols

7. Consult the official ICD-10-CM guidelines, which govern the use of specific codes. These guidelines provide both general and chapter-specific coding guidance.

8. Confirm and assign the correct code.

Organization

This book is organized in the following manner:

Introduction

The introductory material in this book includes the ICD-10-CM Official Preface, the history of ICD-10-CM as well as an overview of the classification system.

Official ICD-10-CM Conventions and Guidelines

Included in this section are the *2019 Official Guidelines for Coding and Reporting.* This section also provides an explanation of the conventions and guidelines regulating the appropriate assignment and reporting of ICD-10-CM codes. This coding guidance is presented by the National Center for Health Statistics (NCHS), a governmental agency of the Centers for Disease Control and Prevention (CDC), within the United States Department of Health and Human Services (DHHS).

Alphabetic Index to Diseases

The Alphabetic Index to Diseases is arranged in alphabetic order by disease — by specific illness, injury, eponym, abbreviation, or other descriptive diagnostic term. The index also lists diagnostic terms for other reasons for encounters with health care professionals.

Neoplasm Table

The Neoplasm Table provides the proper code based upon histology of the neoplasm and site.

Table of Drugs and Chemicals

The Table of Drugs and Chemicals lists the drug and the specific codes that identify the drug and the intent. No additional external cause of injury and poisoning code is assigned in ICD-10-CM.

Index to External Causes

The Alphabetic Index to External Causes of injuries is arranged in alphabetic order by main term indicating the event.

Tabular List of Diseases

ICD-10-CM codes and descriptors are arranged numerically within the Tabular List of diseases within 21 separate chapters according to body system or nature of injury and disease. Classifications which were previously considered supplemental to ICD-9-CM (e.g., V codes and E codes) are incorporated into the Tabular Listing of ICD-10-CM as individual chapters. Chapters 20, "External Causes of Morbidity," and 21, "Factors Influencing Health Status and Contact with Health Services," include chapter-specific guidelines.

Illustrations

This section includes illustrations of normal anatomy with ICD-10-CM specific terminology.

ICD-10-CM Acute Care and Long-Term Care Hospital Data Files

To save space in this coding manual and provide more comprehensive references for the user, Optum360 has provided searchable data files for certain features in this manual. These data files can be accessed at the following:

http://www.optum360coding.com/ProductUpdates/

Two data files are available for FY 2019; the titles and passwords to each of these are provided below:

- CC Exclusions Data File

    Title: "2019 ICD-10-CM for Hospitals CC Excludes Data File"

    Password: OptumCCExcl19

- POA Exempt Data File

    Title: "2019 ICD-10-CM for Hospitals POA Exemption Data File"

    Password: OptumPOAExempt19

Overview of ICD-10-CM Official Conventions

This is an overview of the ICD-10-CM official conventions, which are general rules for the use of the classification system, independent of the guidelines. The official conventions and instructions of the classification, which take precedence over the guidelines, are incorporated within the alphabetic index and tabular list as instructional notes and are applicable regardless of the health care setting. For the full version of the official conventions, see the ICD-10-CM Official Guidelines for Coding and Reporting, section I.A., which is included in this book.

Format

ICD-10-CM is divided into two main parts: the index, an alphabetical list of terms and their corresponding code, and the Tabular List, a sequential, alphanumeric list of codes divided into chapters based on body system or condition. The index contains the Index to Diseases and Injuries (main index) and the Index to External Causes of Injury. Also included in the main Index is the Neoplasm Table and a Table of Drugs and Chemicals.

The Tabular List contains categories, subcategories, and valid codes. ICD-10-CM is an alphanumeric classification system. The 1st character of a three-character category is a letter. The 2nd and 3rd characters may be numbers or alpha characters. A three-character category without further subclassification is equivalent to a valid three-character code. Subcategories are either four or five characters. Subcategory characters include either letters or numbers. Codes may be three, four, five, six, or seven characters in length, in which each level of subdivision after a category is a subcategory. The final level of subdivision is a valid code. The final character in a code may be either a letter or a number.

The ICD-10-CM uses the letter "X" as a placeholder. A placeholder "X" is used as a 5th character placeholder at certain six character codes to allow for future expansion, without disturbing the 6th character structure. For instance, an initial encounter for accidental poisoning by penicillin is coded to T36.ØX1A. The "X" in the 5th character position is a placeholder, or filler character.

Similarly, certain categories have applicable 7th character extensions. In these cases, the 7th character extension is required for all codes within the category, or as otherwise instructed in the tabular list notations. 7th character extensions must always be the last character in the data field. If a code is not a full six characters in length, a dummy placeholder "X" must be used to fill in the empty characters when a 7th character extension is required.

Punctuation

[ ]   In the Tabular List, brackets are used to enclose synonyms, alternative wording, or explanatory phrases. In the index, brackets are used to identify manifestation codes.

( )   Parentheses are used in both the index and tabular list to enclose nonessential modifiers; supplementary words that may be present or absent in the statement of a disease or procedure without affecting the code number to which it is assigned.

:   Colons are used in the tabular list after an incomplete term that needs one or more of the modifiers following the colon to make it assignable to a given category.

Abbreviations

NEC

The abbreviation NEC, "Not elsewhere classifiable" represents "other specified" in the ICD-10-CM. An Index entry that states NEC directs the coder to an "other specified" code in the Tabular List. Codes titled "Other" or "Other specified" in the Tabular List (usually a code with a 4th or 6th character 8 and 5th character 9) are for use when the information in the medical record provides detail for which a specific code does not exist.

NOS

The abbreviation NOS, "Not otherwise specified," in the Tabular List may be interpreted as "unspecified." Codes in the Tabular List with "Unspecified" in the title (usually a code with a 4th or 6th character 9 and 5th character Ø) are for use when the information in the medical record is insufficient to assign a more specific code.

Typeface

Boldface

Boldface type is used for main term entries in the alphabetic index, and all codes and descriptions in the Tabular List.

General Notes

The following conventions and notes appear only in the Tabular List of Diseases:

Includes Notes

The word INCLUDES appears immediately under certain categories to further define, clarify, or give examples of the content of a code category.

Inclusion Terms

Lists of inclusion terms are included under certain codes. These terms indicate some of the conditions for which that code number may be used. Inclusion terms may be synonyms with the code title, or, in the case of "other specified" codes, the terms may also provide a list of various conditions included within a classification code. The inclusion terms are not exhaustive. The index may provide additional terms that may also be assigned to a given code.

Excludes Notes

ICD-10-CM has two types of excludes notes. Each note has a different definition for use. However, they are similar in that they both indicate that codes excluded from each other are independent of each other.

Excludes 1

An EXCLUDES 1 note is a "pure" excludes. It means "NOT CODED HERE!" An Excludes 1 note indicates mutually exclusive codes: two conditions that cannot be reported together. For example, a congenital form of a disease may not be reported with the acquired form of the same condition. The code excluded should never be reported with the applicable codes listed above the excludes notation.

An exception to the Excludes1 definition is the circumstance when the two conditions are unrelated to each other. If it is not clear whether the two conditions involving an Excludes1 note are related or not, query the provider. For example, code F45.8, Other somatoform disorders, has an Excludes1 note for "sleep related teeth grinding (G47.63)," because "teeth grinding" is an inclusion term under F45.8. Only one of these two codes should be assigned for teeth grinding. However psychogenic dysmenorrhea is also an inclusion term under F45.8, and a patient could have both this condition and sleep related teeth grinding. In this case, the two conditions are clearly unrelated to each other, and so it would be appropriate to report F45.8 and G47.63 together.

Excludes 2

An EXCLUDES 2 note means "NOT INCLUDED HERE." An Excludes 2 note indicates that although the excluded condition is not part of the condition it is excluded from, a patient may have both conditions at the same time. Therefore, when an Excludes 2 note appears under a code, it may be acceptable to use both the code and the excluded code together if supported by the medical documentation.

Note

NOTE The term "NOTE" appears as an icon and precedes the instructional information. These notes function as alerts to highlight coding instructions within the text.

Default Codes

In the Index, the default code is the code listed next to the main term. The default code represents the condition most commonly associated with the main term. This code may be assigned when documentation does not facilitate reporting a more specific code. Alternatively, it may provide an unspecified code for the condition.

Syndromes

Follow the Alphabetic Index guidance when coding syndromes. In the absence of index guidance, assign codes for the documented manifestations of the syndrome.

And

When the term "and" is used in a narrative statement or code title, it may be interpreted as "and/or."

With

The word "with" or "in" should be interpreted to mean "associated with" or "due to" when it appears in a code title, the Alphabetic Index (either under a main term or subterm), or an instructional note in the Tabular List. The classification presumes a causal relationship between the two conditions linked by these terms in the Alphabetic Index or Tabular List. These conditions should be coded as related even in the absence of provider documentation explicitly linking them, unless the documentation clearly states the conditions are unrelated or when another guideline exists that specifically requires a documented linkage between two conditions (e.g., sepsis guideline for "acute organ dysfunction that is not clearly associated with the sepsis"). For conditions not specifically linked by these relational terms in the classification or when a guideline requires that a linkage between two conditions be explicitly documented, provider documentation must link the conditions in order to code them as related.

The word "with" in the Alphabetic Index is sequenced immediately following the main term, not in alphabetical order.

See and See Also

The instruction "See" following a main term in the alphabetic index indicates that another term must be referenced in order to locate the correct code. The instructional note "See also" simply provides alternative terms that may be useful in determining the correct code but are not necessary to look up if the main term supplies the appropriate code.

Instructional Notes Used in the Tabular List

In the tabular section, the following instructional notes appear in red type for emphasis:

Code First/Use additional/In diseases classified elsewhere code:

These instructional notes provide sequencing instruction. They may appear independently of each other or to designate certain etiology/manifestation paired codes. These instructions signal the coder that an additional code should be reported to provide a more complete picture of that diagnosis.

In etiology/manifestation coding, ICD-10-CM requires the underlying condition to be sequenced first, followed by the manifestation. In these situations, codes with "In diseases classified elsewhere" in the code description are never permitted as a first-listed or principal diagnosis code and must be sequenced following the underlying condition code.

Code Also:

A "code also" note alerts the coder that more than one code may be required to fully describe the condition. The sequencing depends on the circumstances of the encounter. Factors that may determine sequencing include severity and reason for the encounter.

Code Assignment and Clinical Criteria

Diagnosis code assignment must be based on the provider's diagnostic statement that the condition exists and is not based on clinical criteria used by the provider to establish the diagnosis. Conflicting documentation must be queried.

Additional Annotations

Code-Level Notations

The tabular section of ICD-10-CM has various colors, symbol, and other tabular annotations that may help in code selection, provide clinical or coding information, or alert the coder to reimbursement issues affected by the diagnosis code assignment. Some codes may have more than one annotation. For quick reference to the meanings of the colors and symbols, look at the color/symbol legend at the bottom of each page in the tabular list.

Italics

Italicized type is used for all exclusion notes and to identify manifestation codes, those codes that should not be reported as first-listed (principal) diagnoses.

Color Coding/Symbols

New Code

This ● icon identifies the codes that are new to the classification system for the current year. The new code icon is to the left of the code.

Revised Code Title

This ▲ icon to the left of a code alerts the user to a change in that code's title. This change may be as simple as adding or removing punctuation, which may or may not change the intent of the code, to adding or removing specific terms from a code description that completely alter the circumstances in which the code would be used.

Revised Text

The revised text ►◄ "bow ties" alert the user to changes in parenthetical notes for the current year. Revised text may include the following:

* A change in a current parenthetical description
* A change in the code(s) associated with a current parenthetical note
* A change in how a current parenthetical note is classified (e.g., an Excludes 1 note that changed to an Excludes 2 note)
* Addition of a new parenthetical note(s) to a code

Deleted Text

~~Strikethrough~~ on code description(s) and/or code note(s) indicates a deletion from the classification for the current year.

Additional Characters Required

☑4ᵗʰ This symbol indicates that the code requires a 4th character.

☑5ᵗʰ This symbol indicates that the code requires a 5th character.

☑6ᵗʰ This symbol indicates that the code requires a 6th character.

☑7ᵗʰ This symbol indicates that the code requires a 7th character.

> ☑5ᵗʰ **H60.3 Other infective otitis externa**
>   ☑6ᵗʰ **H60.31 Diffuse otitis externa**
>   **H60.311 Diffuse otitis externa, right ear**
>   **H60.312 Diffuse otitis externa, left ear**
>   **H60.313 Diffuse otitis externa, bilateral**
>   **H60.319 Diffuse otitis externa, unspecified ear**

☑x7ᵗʰ This symbol indicates that the code requires a 7th character following the placeholder "X". Codes with fewer than six characters that require a 7th character must contain placeholder "X" to fill in the empty character(s).

> ☑x7ᵗʰ **T16.1 Foreign body in right ear**

Key Word

Green font is used throughout the Tabular List of Diseases to differentiate the key words that appear in similar code descriptions in a given category or subcategory.

For example, refer to the list of codes below from category H55:

> ☑4ᵗʰ **H55 Nystagmus and other irregular eye movements**
>   ☑5ᵗʰ **H55.0 Nystagmus**
>   **H55.00 Unspecified nystagmus**
>   **H55.01 Congenital nystagmus**
>   **H55.02 Latent nystagmus**
>   **H55.03 Visual deprivation nystagmus**
>   **H55.04 Dissociated nystagmus**
>   **H55.09 Other forms of nystagmus**

The portion of the code description that appears in green font in the tabular list helps the coder quickly identify the key terms and the correct code. This convention is especially useful when the codes describe laterality, such as the following codes from subcategory H40.22:

> ☑6ᵗʰ **H40.22 Chronic angle-closure glaucoma**
>   Chronic primary angle-closure glaucoma
>   ☑7ᵗʰ **H40.221 Chronic angle-closure glaucoma, right eye**
>   ☑7ᵗʰ **H40.222 Chronic angle-closure glaucoma, left eye**
>   ☑7ᵗʰ **H40.223 Chronic angle-closure glaucoma, bilateral**
>   ☑7ᵗʰ **H40.229 Chronic angle-closure glaucoma, unspecified eye**

The key word convention is used only in those categories in which there are multiple codes with very similar descriptions with only a few words that differentiate them.

Medicare Code Edits

Medicare Administrative Contractors (MACs) and many payers use Medicare code edits to check the coding accuracy on claims. The coding edit information in this manual is used for acute care and long-term care hospital admissions and has been updated to reflect v35 changes to the Medicare Code Editor (MCE) and ICD-10 MS-DRG Definitions Manual as well as changes identified in *Federal Register*, volume 83, number 88, May 7, 2018 ("Hospital Inpatient Prospective Payment Systems for Acute Care Hospitals and the Long-Term Care Hospital Prospective Payment System and Proposed Policy Changes and Fiscal Year 2019 Rates; Proposed Rule").

The Medicare code edits for diagnoses are listed below:

* Invalid diagnosis or procedure code
* External causes of morbidity codes as principal diagnosis
* Duplicate of PDx
* *Age conflict
* *Sex conflict
* *Manifestation code as principal diagnosis
* *Questionable principal diagnosis
* *Unacceptable principal diagnosis
* Invalid age
* Invalid sex
* Invalid discharge status
* *Wrong procedure performed

Starred edits above are identified in this manual by color bars, symbols, or footnotes as described on the following pages.

Age and Sex Edit

The age and sex edits below are used to detect inconsistencies between the patient's age and/or sex and the patient's diagnosis. The following edit symbols appear in the tabular list to the right of the code description.

N Newborn Age: 0

These diagnoses are intended for newborns and neonates and the patient's age must be 0 years.

N47.Ø Adherent prepuce, newborn	N♂

P Pediatric Age: 0-17

These diagnoses are intended for children and the patient's age must be between 0 and 17 years.

L21.1 Seborrheic infantile dermatitis	P

M Maternity Age: 12-55

These diagnoses are intended for childbearing patients between the age of 12 and 55 years.

OØ2.9 Abnormal product of conception, unspecified	M♀

A Adult Age: 15-124

These diagnoses are intended for patients between the age of 15 and 124 years.

R54 Age-related physical debility	A

Frailty   Senile asthenia
Old age   Senile debility
Senescence
  EXCLUDES 1 age-related cognitive decline (R41.81)
         sarcopenia (M62.84)
         senile psychosis (FØ3)
         senility NOS (R41.81)

♂ Male diagnosis only

Q98.Ø Klinefelter syndrome karyotype 47, XXY	♂

♀ Female diagnosis only

N35.12 Postinfective urethral stricture, not elsewhere classified, female	♀

Manifestation Code

These codes appear in italic type, with a ***blue color bar*** over the title. A manifestation code cannot be reported as a first-listed or principal diagnosis. By definition, a manifestation code represents a demonstration of some aspect of an underlying disease, which is separately classifiable. In the alphabetic index, these codes are listed as the secondary code in brackets. The underlying disease code is listed first.

G32.89 *Other specified degenerative disorders of nervous system in diseases classified elsewhere*

    Degenerative encephalopathy in diseases classified elsewhere

Unacceptable Principal Diagnoses

Unacceptable principal diagnoses will appear with a **gray color bar** over the code title. These codes do not describe a current illness or injury, but a circumstance which influences a patient's health status. They are considered an unacceptable principal diagnosis for *inpatient* admission.

✓7ᵗʰ T48.5X5 Adverse effect of other anti-common-cold drugs

Questionable Admission Diagnoses

Questionable admission diagnoses will appear with a **yellow color bar** over the code title. These codes, although not unacceptable as a PDx, may be considered a "questionable admission" when used as PDx in an acute care hospital.

E66.Ø9 Other obesity due to excess calories

Wrong Procedure Performed Edit

A **red color bar** over the code title indicates the Wrong Procedure Performed edit. This edit was created to identify cases in which wrong surgeries occurred. Any claim with a code from the Y65.51-Y65.53 will be denied and returned to the provider. A surgical or other invasive procedure is considered to be a wrong procedure if:

- The procedure was performed on the wrong site
- The procedure was performed on the wrong patient, or
- The incorrect procedure was performed on a patient.

Y65.51 Performance of wrong procedure (operation) on correct patient

    Wrong device implanted into correct surgical site
    EXCLUDES 1 *performance of correct procedure (operation) on wrong side or body part (Y65.53)*

ICD-10 MS-DRG Definitions Manual Edits

An MS-DRG or MS-LTC-DRG is assigned based on specific patient attributes, such as principal diagnosis, secondary diagnoses, procedures, and discharge status. The attributes (edits) provided in this manual are only those directly related to ICD-10-CM diagnoses and are used for acute care and long-term care hospital admissions.

H1-H14 Hospital Acquired Condition (HAC)

These codes identify conditions that are high cost or high volume or both, are either a complication or comorbidity (CC) or major complication or comorbidity (MCC) that as a secondary diagnosis results in assignment of a case to a higher-paying MS-DRG. These conditions are reasonably preventable through the application of evidence-based guidelines. If the condition is not present on admission (meaning it developed during the hospital admission), the case will not group to the higher-paying MS-DRG based solely upon the reporting of the HAC code. Many of these HACs are conditional, and are based on reporting the specific diagnosis code(s) in combination with certain procedure codes, notated in footnotes.

Note: Hospital-acquired conditions do not impact MS-LTC-DRG assignment.

The HAC icon with the specific HAC table number in which this code is classified appears to the right of the code description. The comprehensive list of HAC tables that coincide with these icon numbers appears in appendix I of this book.

N15.1 Renal and perinephric abscess	MCC H6

    CC Excl: PDX collection 919

CC CC Condition

This symbol designates a complication or comorbidity diagnosis that may affect DRG assignment. A complication or comorbidity diagnosis, CC condition, is defined as a significant acute disease, a significant acute manifestation of a chronic disease, an advanced or end-stage chronic disease, or a chronic disease associated with systemic physiological decompensation and debility that have consistently greater impact on hospital resources.

A CC icon appears to the right of the code description.

G9Ø.59 Complex regional pain syndrome I of other specified site	CC

MCC **MCC Condition**

This symbol designates a major complication or comorbidity diagnosis that may affect DRG assignment. An MCC condition meets the same criteria as a CC condition but is associated with a higher acuity level and hospital resource consumption is expected to be higher than that for a CC condition. There are fewer conditions that meet the criteria as an MCC than those for a CC condition.

An MCC icon appears to the right of the code description.

> ✓7ᵗʰ **S35.238** Other **injury of inferior mesenteric artery**   **MCC**

CC Excludes Notations

The assignment of an MS-DRG or MS-LTC-DRG often depends on the presence or absence of a secondary diagnosis code that is designated as an MCC or CC. However, in some instances the MCC or CC designation for that secondary diagnosis code is negated due to its relationship with the principal diagnosis.

To save space in this coding manual and provide a more comprehensive reference for the user, the CC Exclusion notations have been restructured. Instead of the individual codes being listed in the reference, which can in many cases be extensive, only the principal diagnosis collection (PDX collection) number is provided. A PDX collection contains a specific list of ICD-10-CM codes and their official descriptions that when used as principal diagnosis would render the MCC/CC designation ineffective. Each PDX collection is provided in an easily searchable data file which can be accessed at the following:

https://www.optum360coding.com/ProductUpdates/
Title: "2019 ICD-10-CM for Hospitals CC Excludes Data File"
Password: OptumCCExcl19

Similar to the parenthetical notes, the CC Exclusion notations are provided at the category, subcategory, and/or code level. If a CC Exclusion notation is found at the category or subcategory level, all the CC and/or MCC codes in that category or subcategory share the same PDX collection listed in that notation. For example:

> ✓5ᵗʰ **G43.6** Persistent **migraine** aura with cerebral infarction
> Code also the type of cerebral infarction (I63.-)
> **CC Excl: For CC codes in subcategory G43.6,**
> **unless otherwise noted:** PDX collection 584

There are four codes with a CC designation in subcategory G43.6; the CC Excludes notation applies to all four codes.

Often a CC exclusion reference is specific to laterality for CC/MCC codes in a category or subcategory. Where possible, a CC exclusion reference is placed at the category or subcategory level with the PDX collection identified for the right, left, or unspecified side. For example:

> ✓4ᵗʰ **S58** Traumatic amputation **of elbow and forearm**
> An amputation not identified as partial or complete should be coded to complete.
> EXCLUDES1 *traumatic amputation of wrist and hand (S68.-)*
> The appropriate 7th character is to be added to each code from category S58.
> A   initial encounter
> D   subsequent encounter
> S   sequela
>
> **CC Excl: For CC codes in category S58:**
> **Right side:** PDX collection 1266
> **Left side:** PDX collection 1267
> **Unspecifiedside:** PDXcollection1268

All CC codes that are specific to the right side in category S58 are excluded from being a CC for any principal diagnosis found in PDX collection 1266.

Where possible a "see" reference may also be used, referring the user to a previously designated CC excludes notation. For example:

> ✓5ᵗʰ **S72.0** Fracture of **head and neck** of femur
> EXCLUDES2 *physeal fracture of upper end of femur (S79.0-)*
> AHA: 2016, 3Q, 16
>
> **CC Excl: For CC/MCC codes in subcategory S72.0:**
> **Right side:** See code S72.001
> **Left side:** See code S72.002
> **Unspecified side:** See code S72.009

If users want to know the principal diagnoses to which code S72.022 Displaced fracture of epiphysis (separation) (upper) of left femur, may not function as a CC or MCC, they would be referred to the CC excludes notation under code S72.002.

Note: CC Excludes notations in chapters 13 and 19 apply to 7th character A, unless otherwise noted.

Certain codes may also have no principal diagnosis codes to which they would be excluded from functioning as a CC or MCC. These are identified as follows:

> **I16.1** Hypertensive emergency   **CC**
> **CC Excl:** No Excl

HIV **HIV-related Condition**

This symbol indicates that the condition is considered a major HIV-related diagnosis. When the condition is coded in combination with a diagnosis of human immunodeficiency virus (HIV), code B20, the case will move from MS-DRG/MS-LTC-DRG 977 to MS-DRGs/MS-LTC-DRGs 974-976.

The HIV icon appears to the right of the code description.

> **G96.9** Disorder of central nervous system, unspecified   **HIV**

Medicare Advantage Risk Adjustment Edits

Medicare Advantage plans provided as part of the Medicare Part C program uses a risk-adjustment model to plan for future healthcare costs to Medicare Part C participants. The risk-adjustment model measures disease burden by designating certain ICD-10-CM diagnosis codes as falling into hierarchical condition categories (HCC). The HCC information in this manual has been updated to reflect the CMS-HCC model category for v22 of the CMS-HCC risk-adjustment software.

HCC **CMS-HCC Condition**

This symbol indicates that the condition is considered a CMS-HCC diagnosis. All HCC conditions that are appropriately documented are used in the risk-adjustment model for Medicare Advantage to provide a means of comparing quality of care across Medicare Part C participants as well as predict future healthcare costs.

The HCC icon appears to the right of the code description.

> **Y62.2** Failure of sterile precautions during **kidney dialysis**   **HCC**
> **and other perfusion**

Long-Term Care Prospective Payment Program Edits

The Consolidated Appropriations Act, 2016, and the 21st Century Cures Act allow temporary exception from the site-neutral payment rates for patients discharged from certain long-term care hospitals with a severe wound. The edit information in this manual has been updated to reflect FY2018 changes.

SW **Severe Wound Diagnosis**

This symbol indicates that the condition is considered a severe wound diagnosis. Depending on the facility from which the patient is discharged, these conditions may not require that the payment rate for that admission be adjusted.

The SW icon appears to the right of the code description.

L89.000	Pressure ulcer of unspecified elbow, unstageable	HCC SW

Other Code-Level Notations

AHA This symbol precedes official citations from AHA's *Coding Clinic for ICD-10-CM/PCS*. Similar to the parenthetical notes, AHA references are placed in a hierarchical pattern at the chapter, code block, category, subcategory, or valid code level. This means that the information found in the reference applies to one or more codes depending on where the citation is placed.

The citations appear in purple type and are listed with the most current citation first. *Coding Clinic* citations included in this edition have been updated through second quarter 2018.

I15.1	Hypertension secondary to other renal disorders
	AHA: 2016, 3Q, 22

DEF This symbol precedes a definition of a condition or disease.

The definition appears in purple type directly under the code.

✓5ᵗʰ M51.4	Schmorl's nodes
	DEF: Irregular bone defect in the margin of the vertebral body that causes herniation into the end plate of the vertebral body.

TIP This symbol precedes coding advice that is not readily available within the ICD-10-CM classification. It may relate official coding guidelines, indexing nuances, or advice from *AHA's Coding Clinic for ICD-10-CM/PCS*.

The tip appears in brown type under the code.

P15.8	Other specified birth injuries
	TIP: Use for any injury of newborn from scalpel.

Footnotes

Certain codes in the tabular section have a numerical superscript located to the upper left of the code. This numerical superscript corresponds to a specific footnote description. For example:

[1] I49.01	Ventricular fibrillation	MCC HCC

The footnote 1 indicates "MCC = Only if patient is discharged alive." This means that ventricular fibrillation is considered a major complication or comorbidity that may affect DRG assignment only if the patient is discharged alive. Otherwise ventricular fibrillation is assigned as a non-MCC condition. In previous editions, the footnote description was provided at the bottom of the same page on which the numerical superscript was found. For convenience, beginning with the 2019 edition, the footnote descriptions are no longer provided on the tabular page but have been placed on the front cover. The following list identifies the meaning of each footnote number in the Tabular List of diseases:

1 These codes are considered major complication/comorbidity (MCC) conditions only if the patient is discharged alive.

2 This condition is considered an MCC only when reported as an initial encounter for an open fracture (7th character B or C specific to category).

3 This condition is considered a CC only when reported as an initial encounter for a fracture (7th character A, B, or C specific to category) or a subsequent encounter for nonunion or malunion fracture (7th character K, M, N, P, Q, or R specific to category).

4 This condition is considered a CC only when reported as a subsequent encounter for a nonunion or malunion fracture (7th character K, M, N, P, Q, or R specific to category).

5 This condition is considered a CC only when reported as an initial encounter or subsequent encounter (7th character A or D).

6 This condition is considered an HCC when reported as initial encounter (7th character A, B, or C specific to category).

7 This condition is considered an HCC when reported as initial encounter (7th character A or B specific to category) or as a sequela.

8 This condition is considered an HCC when reported as a sequela.

Chapter-Level Notations

Chapter-Specific Guidelines with Coding Examples

Each chapter begins with the Official Guidelines for Coding and Reporting specific to that chapter, where provided. Coding examples specific to inpatient care settings have been provided to illustrate the coding and/or sequencing guidance in these guidelines.

Muscle and Tendon Table

ICD-10-CM categorizes certain muscles and tendons in the upper and lower extremities by their action (e.g., extension or flexion) as well as their anatomical location. The Muscle/Tendon table is provided at the beginning of chapter 13 and chapter 19 to help users when code selection depends on the action of the muscle and/or tendon.

Note: This table is not all-inclusive, and proper code assignment should be based on the provider's documentation.

Index Notations

 Subterms under main terms may continue to next column or page. This warning statement is a reminder to always check for additional subterms and information that may continue onto the next page or column before making a final selection.

Following References

The Index includes following references to assist in locating "out-of-sequence" codes in the tabular list. "Out-of-sequence" codes contain an alphabetic character (letter) in the 3rd or 4th character position. These codes are placed according to the classification rules — the placement of the codes according to condition — not according to alphabetic or numeric sequencing rules.

Examples:

Carcinoma (malignant) (*see also* Neoplasm, by site, malignant)
  neuroendocrine (*see also* Tumor, neuroendocrine)
    high grade, any site C7A.1 (*following* C75)
    poorly differentiated, any site C7A.1 (*following* C75)

In the tabular rubric, C7A is included after rubric C75 and before C76.

Gout, chronic (*see also* Gout, gouty) M1A.9 ☑ (*following* M08)
  drug-induced M1A.20 ☑ (*following* M08)
    ankle M1A.27- ☑ (*following* M08)
    elbow M1A.22- ☑ (following M08)

In the tabular rubric, M1A is included after rubric M08 and before M10.

Discontinued Notations

PDxCC **PDxCC Condition**

PDxMCC **PDxMCC Condition**

Optum360 removed the *PDxCC or PDxMCC Condition* icons from the 2019 *ICD-10-CM Professional for Hospitals: The Complete Official Code Set*. The decision to remove the icons was based on the proposed rule published in the *Federal Register*, volume 83, number 88, May 7, 2018 ("Hospital Inpatient Prospective Payment Systems for Acute Care Hospitals and Long Term Care Hospital Prospective System and Proposed Policy Changes and Fiscal Year 2019 Rates") found at https://www.gpo.gov/fdsys/pkg/FR-2018-05-07/pdf/2018-09581.pdf.

The purpose of the principal diagnosis as its own CC or MCC was to ensure consistent MS-DRG assignment between the ICD-9 and ICD-10-MS-DRGs. The Centers for Medicare and Medicaid Services (CMS) stated it is no longer necessary to replicate MS-DRG assignment across the ICD-9 and ICD-10 versions of the MS-DRGs. CMS believes there may be more effective indicators of resource utilization than the special logic used to assign clinical severity to a principal diagnosis based on data analysis. Therefore, CMS proposed removing the special logic in the Grouper and deleting the tables containing the lists of principal diagnosis as its own MCC and principal diagnosis as its own CC codes from the ICD-10 MS-DRG Definitions Manual for FY 2019.

2019 ICD-10-CM Official Guidelines for Coding and Reporting

Narrative changes appear in **bold** text

Items <u>underlined</u> have been moved within the guidelines since the FY 2018 version

Italics are used to indicate revisions to heading changes

The Centers for Medicare and Medicaid Services (CMS) and the National Center for Health Statistics (NCHS), two departments within the U.S. Federal Government's Department of Health and Human Services (DHHS) provide the following guidelines for coding and reporting using the International Classification of Diseases, 10th Revision, Clinical Modification (ICD-10-CM). These guidelines should be used as a companion document to the official version of the ICD-10-CM as published on the NCHS website. The ICD-10-CM is a morbidity classification published by the United States for classifying diagnoses and reason for visits in all health care settings. The ICD-10-CM is based on the ICD-10, the statistical classification of disease published by the World Health Organization (WHO).

These guidelines have been approved by the four organizations that make up the Cooperating Parties for the ICD-10-CM: the American Hospital Association (AHA), the American Health Information Management Association (AHIMA), CMS, and NCHS.

These guidelines are a set of rules that have been developed to accompany and complement the official conventions and instructions provided within the ICD-10-CM itself. The instructions and conventions of the classification take precedence over guidelines. These guidelines are based on the coding and sequencing instructions in the Tabular List and Alphabetic Index of ICD-10-CM, but provide additional instruction. Adherence to these guidelines when assigning ICD-10-CM diagnosis codes is required under the Health Insurance Portability and Accountability Act (HIPAA). The diagnosis codes (Tabular List and Alphabetic Index) have been adopted under HIPAA for all healthcare settings. A joint effort between the healthcare provider and the coder is essential to achieve complete and accurate documentation, code assignment, and reporting of diagnoses and procedures. These guidelines have been developed to assist both the healthcare provider and the coder in identifying those diagnoses that are to be reported. The importance of consistent, complete documentation in the medical record cannot be overemphasized. Without such documentation accurate coding cannot be achieved. The entire record should be reviewed to determine the specific reason for the encounter and the conditions treated.

The term encounter is used for all settings, including hospital admissions. In the context of these guidelines, the term provider is used throughout the guidelines to mean physician or any qualified health care practitioner who is legally accountable for establishing the patient's diagnosis. Only this set of guidelines, approved by the Cooperating Parties, is official.

The guidelines are organized into sections. Section I includes the structure and conventions of the classification and general guidelines that apply to the entire classification, and chapter-specific guidelines that correspond to the chapters as they are arranged in the classification. Section II includes guidelines for selection of principal diagnosis for non-outpatient settings. Section III includes guidelines for reporting additional diagnoses in non-outpatient settings. Section IV is for outpatient coding and reporting. It is necessary to review all sections of the guidelines to fully understand all of the rules and instructions needed to code properly.

Section I. Conventions, general coding guidelines and chapter specific guidelines

The conventions, general guidelines and chapter-specific guidelines are applicable to all health care settings unless otherwise indicated. The conventions and instructions of the classification take precedence over guidelines.

A. Conventions for the ICD-10-CM

The conventions for the ICD-10-CM are the general rules for use of the classification independent of the guidelines. These conventions are incorporated within the Alphabetic Index and Tabular List of the ICD-10-CM as instructional notes.

1. **The Alphabetic Index and Tabular List**
   The ICD-10-CM is divided into the Alphabetic Index, an alphabetical list of terms and their corresponding code, and the Tabular List, a structured list of codes divided into chapters based on body system or condition. The Alphabetic Index consists of the following parts: the Index of Diseases and Injury, the Index of External Causes of Injury, the Table of Neoplasms and the Table of Drugs and Chemicals.
   See Section I.C2. General guidelines
   See Section I.C.19. Adverse effects, poisoning, underdosing and toxic effects

2. **Format and Structure:**
   The ICD-10-CM Tabular List contains categories, subcategories and codes. Characters for categories, subcategories and codes may be either a letter or a number. All categories are 3 characters. A three-character category that has no further subdivision is equivalent to a code. Subcategories are either 4 or 5 characters. Codes may be 3, 4, 5, 6 or 7 characters. That is, each level of subdivision after a category is a subcategory. The final level of subdivision is a code. Codes that have applicable 7th characters are still referred to as codes, not subcategories. A code that has an applicable 7th character is considered invalid without the 7th character.
   The ICD-10-CM uses an indented format for ease in reference.

3. **Use of codes for reporting purposes**
   For reporting purposes only codes are permissible, not categories or subcategories, and any applicable 7th character is required.

4. **Placeholder character**
   The ICD-10-CM utilizes a placeholder character "X". The "X" is used as a placeholder at certain codes to allow for future expansion. An example of this is at the poisoning, adverse effect and underdosing codes, categories T36–T50.
   Where a placeholder exists, the X must be used in order for the code to be considered a valid code.

5. **7th Characters**
   Certain ICD-10-CM categories have applicable 7th characters. The applicable 7th character is required for all codes within the category, or as the notes in the Tabular List instruct. The 7th character must always be the 7th character in the data field. If a code that requires a 7th character is not 6 characters, a placeholder X must be used to fill in the empty characters.

6. **Abbreviations**
   a. **Alphabetic Index abbreviations**
      NEC "Not elsewhere classifiable"
      This abbreviation in the Alphabetic Index represents "other specified." When a specific code is not available for a condition, the Alphabetic Index directs the coder to the "other specified" code in the Tabular List.
      NOS "Not otherwise specified"

This abbreviation is the equivalent of unspecified.

   b. **Tabular List abbreviations**
      NEC "Not elsewhere classifiable"
      This abbreviation in the Tabular List represents "other specified". When a specific code is not available for a condition, the Tabular List includes an NEC entry under a code to identify the code as the "other specified" code.
      NOS "Not otherwise specified"
      This abbreviation is the equivalent of unspecified.

7. **Punctuation**
   [ ] Brackets are used in the Tabular List to enclose synonyms, alternative wording or explanatory phrases. Brackets are used in the Alphabetic Index to identify manifestation codes.
   ( ) Parentheses are used in both the Alphabetic Index and Tabular List to enclose supplementary words that may be present or absent in the statement of a disease or procedure without affecting the code number to which it is assigned. The terms within the parentheses are referred to as nonessential modifiers. The nonessential modifiers in the Alphabetic Index to Diseases apply to subterms following a main term except when a nonessential modifier and a subentry are mutually exclusive, the subentry takes precedence. For example, in the ICD-10-CM Alphabetic Index under the main term Enteritis, "acute" is a nonessential modifier and "chronic" is a subentry. In this case, the nonessential modifier "acute" does not apply to the subentry "chronic".
   : Colons are used in the Tabular List after an incomplete term which needs one or more of the modifiers following the colon to make it assignable to a given category.

8. **Use of "and"**
   See Section I.A.14. Use of the term "And"

9. **Other and Unspecified codes**
   a. **"Other" codes**
      Codes titled "other" or "other specified" are for use when the information in the medical record provides detail for which a specific code does not exist. Alphabetic Index entries with NEC in the line designate "other" codes in the Tabular List. These Alphabetic Index entries represent specific disease entities for which no specific code exists so the term is included within an "other" code.

   b. **"Unspecified" codes**
      Codes titled "unspecified" are for use when the information in the medical record is insufficient to assign a more specific code. For those categories for which an unspecified code is not provided, the "other specified" code may represent both other and unspecified.
      See Section I.B.18 Use of Signs/Symptom/Unspecified Codes

10. **Includes Notes**
    This note appears immediately under a three character code title to further define, or give examples of, the content of the category.

11. **Inclusion terms**
    List of terms is included under some codes. These terms are the conditions for which that code is to be used. The terms may be synonyms of the code title, or, in the case of "other specified" codes, the terms are a list of the various conditions assigned to that code. The inclusion terms are not necessarily exhaustive. Additional terms found only in the Alphabetic Index may also be assigned to a code.

12. **Excludes Notes**
    The ICD-10-CM has two types of excludes notes. Each type of note has a different definition for use but they are all similar in that they indicate that codes excluded from each other are independent of each other.

    a. **Excludes1**
       A type 1 Excludes note is a pure excludes note. It means "NOT CODED HERE!" An Excludes1 note indicates that the code excluded should never be used at the same time as the code above the Excludes1 note. An Excludes1 is used when two conditions cannot occur together, such as a congenital form versus an acquired form of the same condition.

       An exception to the Excludes1 definition is the circumstance when the two conditions are unrelated to each other. If it is not clear whether the two conditions involving an Excludes1 note are related or not, query the provider. For example, code F45.8, Other somatoform disorders, has an Excludes1 note for "sleep related teeth grinding (G47.63)," because "teeth grinding" is an inclusion term under F45.8. Only one of these two codes should be assigned for teeth grinding. However psychogenic dysmenorrhea is also an inclusion term under F45.8, and a patient could have both this condition and sleep related

teeth grinding. In this case, the two conditions are clearly unrelated to each other, and so it would be appropriate to report F45.8 and G47.63 together.

b. Excludes2

A type 2 Excludes note represents "Not included here." An excludes2 note indicates that the condition excluded is not part of the condition represented by the code, but a patient may have both conditions at the same time. When an Excludes2 note appears under a code, it is acceptable to use both the code and the excluded code together, when appropriate.

13. Etiology/manifestation convention ("code first", "use additional code" and "in diseases classified elsewhere" notes)

Certain conditions have both an underlying etiology and multiple body system manifestations due to the underlying etiology. For such conditions, the ICD-10-CM has a coding convention that requires the underlying condition be sequenced first, if applicable, followed by the manifestation. Wherever such a combination exists, there is a "use additional code" note at the etiology code, and a "code first" note at the manifestation code. These instructional notes indicate the proper sequencing order of the codes, etiology followed by manifestation.

In most cases the manifestation codes will have in the code title, "in diseases classified elsewhere." Codes with this title are a component of the etiology/ manifestation convention. The code title indicates that it is a manifestation code. "In diseases classified elsewhere" codes are never permitted to be used as first-listed or principal diagnosis codes. They must be used in conjunction with an underlying condition code and they must be listed following the underlying condition. See category F02, Dementia in other diseases classified elsewhere, for an example of this convention.

There are manifestation codes that do not have "in diseases classified elsewhere" in the title. For such codes, there is a "use additional code" note at the etiology code and a "code first" note at the manifestation code, and the rules for sequencing apply.

In addition to the notes in the Tabular List, these conditions also have a specific Alphabetic Index entry structure. In the Alphabetic Index both conditions are listed together with the etiology code first followed by the manifestation codes in brackets. The code in brackets is always to be sequenced second.

An example of the etiology/manifestation convention is dementia in Parkinson's disease. In the Alphabetic Index, code G20 is listed first, followed by code F02.80 or F02.81 in brackets. Code G20 represents the underlying etiology, Parkinson's disease, and must be sequenced first, whereas code F02.80 and F02.81 represent the manifestation of dementia in diseases classified elsewhere, with or without behavioral disturbance.

"Code first" and "Use additional code" notes are also used as sequencing rules in the classification for certain codes that are not part of an etiology/ manifestation combination.

See Section I.B.7. Multiple coding for a single condition.

14. "And"

The word "and" should be interpreted to mean either "and" or "or" when it appears in a title.

For example, cases of "tuberculosis of bones", "tuberculosis of joints" and "tuberculosis of bones and joints" are classified to subcategory A18.0, Tuberculosis of bones and joints.

15. "With"

The word "with" or "in" should be interpreted to mean "associated with" or "due to" when it appears in a code title, the Alphabetic Index **(either under a main term or subterm),** or an instructional note in the Tabular List. The classification presumes a causal relationship between the two conditions linked by these terms in the Alphabetic Index or Tabular List. These conditions should be coded as related even in the absence of provider documentation explicitly linking them, unless the documentation clearly states the conditions are unrelated or when another guideline exists that specifically requires a documented linkage between two conditions (e.g., sepsis guideline for "acute organ dysfunction that is not clearly associated with the sepsis").

For conditions not specifically linked by these relational terms in the classification or when a guideline requires that a linkage between two conditions be explicitly documented, provider documentation must link the conditions in order to code them as related.

The word "with" in the Alphabetic Index is sequenced immediately following the main term, not in alphabetical order.

16. "See" and "See Also"

The "see" instruction following a main term in the Alphabetic Index indicates that another term should be referenced. It is necessary to go to the main term referenced with the "see" note to locate the correct code.

A "see also" instruction following a main term in the Alphabetic Index instructs that there is another main term that may also be referenced that may provide additional Alphabetic Index entries that may be useful. It is not necessary to follow the "see also" note when the original main term provides the necessary code.

17. "Code also" note

A "code also" note instructs that two codes may be required to fully describe a condition, but this note does not provide sequencing direction. The sequencing depends on the circumstances of the encounter.

18. Default codes

A code listed next to a main term in the ICD-10-CM Alphabetic Index is referred to as a default code. The default code represents that condition that is most commonly associated with the main term, or is the unspecified code for the condition. If a condition is documented in a medical record (for example, appendicitis) without any additional information, such as acute or chronic, the default code should be assigned.

19. Code assignment and Clinical Criteria

The assignment of a diagnosis code is based on the provider's diagnostic statement that the condition exists. The provider's statement that the patient has a particular condition is sufficient. Code assignment is not based on clinical criteria used by the provider to establish the diagnosis.

B. General Coding Guidelines

1. Locating a code in the ICD-10-CM

To select a code in the classification that corresponds to a diagnosis or reason for visit documented in a medical record, first locate the term in the Alphabetic Index, and then verify the code in the Tabular List. Read and be guided by instructional notations that appear in both the Alphabetic Index and the Tabular List.

It is essential to use both the Alphabetic Index and Tabular List when locating and assigning a code. The Alphabetic Index does not always provide the full code. Selection of the full code, including laterality and any applicable 7th character can only be done in the Tabular List. A dash (-) at the end of an Alphabetic Index entry indicates that additional characters are required. Even if a dash is not included at the Alphabetic Index entry, it is necessary to refer to the Tabular List to verify that no 7th character is required.

2. Level of Detail in Coding

Diagnosis codes are to be used and reported at their highest number of characters available.

ICD-10-CM diagnosis codes are composed of codes with 3, 4, 5, 6 or 7 characters. Codes with three characters are included in ICD-10-CM as the heading of a category of codes that may be further subdivided by the use of fourth and/or fifth characters and/or sixth characters, which provide greater detail.

A three-character code is to be used only if it is not further subdivided. A code is invalid if it has not been coded to the full number of characters required for that code, including the 7th character, if applicable.

3. Code or codes from A00.0 through T88.9, Z00-Z99.8

The appropriate code or codes from A00.0 through T88.9, Z00-Z99.8 must be used to identify diagnoses, symptoms, conditions, problems, complaints or other reason(s) for the encounter/visit.

4. Signs and symptoms

Codes that describe symptoms and signs, as opposed to diagnoses, are acceptable for reporting purposes when a related definitive diagnosis has not been established (confirmed) by the provider. Chapter 18 of ICD-10-CM, Symptoms, Signs, and Abnormal Clinical and Laboratory Findings, Not Elsewhere Classified (codes R00.0 - R99) contains many, but not all, codes for symptoms.

See Section I.B.18 Use of Signs/Symptom/Unspecified Codes

5. Conditions that are an integral part of a disease process

Signs and symptoms that are associated routinely with a disease process should not be assigned as additional codes, unless otherwise instructed by the classification.

6. Conditions that are not an integral part of a disease process

Additional signs and symptoms that may not be associated routinely with a disease process should be coded when present.

7. **Multiple coding for a single condition**

In addition to the etiology/manifestation convention that requires two codes to fully describe a single condition that affects multiple body systems, there are other single conditions that also require more than one code. "Use additional code" notes are found in the Tabular List at codes that are not part of an etiology/manifestation pair where a secondary code is useful to fully describe a condition. The sequencing rule is the same as the etiology/manifestation pair, "use additional code" indicates that a secondary code should be added**,** if known.

For example, for bacterial infections that are not included in chapter 1, a secondary code from category B95, Streptococcus, Staphylococcus, and Enterococcus, as the cause of diseases classified elsewhere, or B96, Other bacterial agents as the cause of diseases classified elsewhere, may be required to identify the bacterial organism causing the infection. A "use additional code" note will normally be found at the infectious disease code, indicating a need for the organism code to be added as a secondary code.

"Code first" notes are also under certain codes that are not specifically manifestation codes but may be due to an underlying cause. When there is a "code first" note and an underlying condition is present, the underlying condition should be sequenced first, if known.

"Code, if applicable, any causal condition first" notes indicate that this code may be assigned as a principal diagnosis when the causal condition is unknown or not applicable. If a causal condition is known, then the code for that condition should be sequenced as the principal or first-listed diagnosis.

Multiple codes may be needed for sequela, complication codes and obstetric codes to more fully describe a condition. See the specific guidelines for these conditions for further instruction.

8. **Acute and Chronic Conditions**

If the same condition is described as both acute (subacute) and chronic, and separate subentries exist in the Alphabetic Index at the same indentation level, code both and sequence the acute (subacute) code first.

9. **Combination Code**

A combination code is a single code used to classify:

> Two diagnoses, or
>
> A diagnosis with an associated secondary process (manifestation)
>
> A diagnosis with an associated complication

Combination codes are identified by referring to subterm entries in the Alphabetic Index and by reading the inclusion and exclusion notes in the Tabular List.

Assign only the combination code when that code fully identifies the diagnostic conditions involved or when the Alphabetic Index so directs. Multiple coding should not be used when the classification provides a combination code that clearly identifies all of the elements documented in the diagnosis. When the combination code lacks necessary specificity in describing the manifestation or complication, an additional code should be used as a secondary code.

10. **Sequela (Late Effects)**

A sequela is the residual effect (condition produced) after the acute phase of an illness or injury has terminated. There is no time limit on when a sequela code can be used. The residual may be apparent early, such as in cerebral infarction, or it may occur months or years later, such as that due to a previous injury. Examples of sequela include: scar formation resulting from a burn, deviated septum due to a nasal fracture, and infertility due to tubal occlusion from old tuberculosis. Coding of sequela generally requires two codes sequenced in the following order: the condition or nature of the sequela is sequenced first. The sequela code is sequenced second.

An exception to the above guidelines are those instances where the code for the sequela is followed by a manifestation code identified in the Tabular List and title, or the sequela code has been expanded (at the fourth, fifth or sixth character levels) to include the manifestation(s). The code for the acute phase of an illness or injury that led to the sequela is never used with a code for the late effect.

See Section I.C.9. Sequelae of cerebrovascular disease

See Section I.C.15. Sequelae of complication of pregnancy, childbirth and the puerperium

See Section I.C.19. Application of 7th characters for Chapter 19

11. **Impending or Threatened Condition**

Code any condition described at the time of discharge as "impending" or "threatened" as follows:

> If it did occur, code as confirmed diagnosis.

If it did not occur, reference the Alphabetic Index to determine if the condition has a subentry term for "impending" or "threatened" and also reference main term entries for "Impending" and for "Threatened."

If the subterms are listed, assign the given code.

If the subterms are not listed, code the existing underlying condition(s) and not the condition described as impending or threatened.

12. **Reporting Same Diagnosis Code more than Once**

Each unique ICD-10-CM diagnosis code may be reported only once for an encounter. This applies to bilateral conditions when there are no distinct codes identifying laterality or two different conditions classified to the same ICD-10-CM diagnosis code.

13. **Laterality**

Some ICD-10-CM codes indicate laterality, specifying whether the condition occurs on the left, right or is bilateral. If no bilateral code is provided and the condition is bilateral, assign separate codes for both the left and right side. If the side is not identified in the medical record, assign the code for the unspecified side.

When a patient has a bilateral condition and each side is treated during separate encounters, assign the "bilateral" code (as the condition still exists on both sides), including for the encounter to treat the first side. For the second encounter for treatment after one side has previously been treated and the condition no longer exists on that side, assign the appropriate unilateral code for the side where the condition still exists (e.g., cataract surgery performed on each eye in separate encounters). The bilateral code would not be assigned for the subsequent encounter, as the patient no longer has the condition in the previously-treated site. If the treatment on the first side did not completely resolve the condition, then the bilateral code would still be appropriate.

14. **Documentation** *by Clinicians Other than the Patient's Provider*

Code assignment is based on the documentation by patient's provider (i.e., physician or other qualified healthcare practitioner legally accountable for establishing the patient's diagnosis). There are a few exceptions, such as codes for the Body Mass Index (BMI), depth of non-pressure chronic ulcers, pressure ulcer stage, coma scale, and NIH stroke scale (NIHSS) codes, code assignment may be based on medical record documentation from clinicians who are not the patient's provider (i.e., physician or other qualified healthcare practitioner legally accountable for establishing the patient's diagnosis), since this information is typically documented by other clinicians involved in the care of the patient (e.g., a dietitian often documents the BMI, a nurse often documents the pressure ulcer stages, and an emergency medical technician often documents the coma scale). However, the associated diagnosis (such as overweight, obesity, acute stroke, or pressure ulcer) must be documented by the patient's provider. If there is conflicting medical record documentation, either from the same clinician or different clinicians, the patient's attending provider should be queried for clarification.

For social determinants of health, such as information found in categories Z55-Z65, Persons with potential health hazards related to socioeconomic and psychosocial circumstances, code assignment may be based on medical record documentation from clinicians involved in the care of the patient who are not the patient's provider since this information represents social information, rather than medical diagnoses.

The BMI, coma scale, NIHSS codes **and categories Z55-Z65** should only be reported as secondary diagnoses.

15. **Syndromes**

Follow the Alphabetic Index guidance when coding syndromes. In the absence of Alphabetic Index guidance, assign codes for the documented manifestations of the syndrome. Additional codes for manifestations that are not an integral part of the disease process may also be assigned when the condition does not have a unique code.

16. **Documentation of Complications of Care**

Code assignment is based on the provider's documentation of the relationship between the condition and the care or procedure**,** unless otherwise instructed by the classification. The guideline extends to any complications of care, regardless of the chapter the code is located in. It is important to note that not all conditions that occur during or following medical care or surgery are classified as complications. There must be a cause-and-effect relationship between the care provided and the condition, and an indication in the documentation that it is a complication. Query the provider for clarification, if the complication is not clearly documented.

17. Borderline Diagnosis

If the provider documents a "borderline" diagnosis at the time of discharge, the diagnosis is coded as confirmed, unless the classification provides a specific entry (e.g., borderline diabetes). If a borderline condition has a specific index entry in ICD-10-CM, it should be coded as such. Since borderline conditions are not uncertain diagnoses, no distinction is made between the care setting (inpatient versus outpatient). Whenever the documentation is unclear regarding a borderline condition, coders are encouraged to query for clarification.

18. Use of Sign/Symptom/Unspecified Codes

Sign/symptom and "unspecified" codes have acceptable, even necessary, uses. While specific diagnosis codes should be reported when they are supported by the available medical record documentation and clinical knowledge of the patient's health condition, there are instances when signs/symptoms or unspecified codes are the best choices for accurately reflecting the healthcare encounter. Each healthcare encounter should be coded to the level of certainty known for that encounter.

If a definitive diagnosis has not been established by the end of the encounter, it is appropriate to report codes for sign(s) and/or symptom(s) in lieu of a definitive diagnosis. When sufficient clinical information isn't known or available about a particular health condition to assign a more specific code, it is acceptable to report the appropriate "unspecified" code (e.g., a diagnosis of pneumonia has been determined, but not the specific type). Unspecified codes should be reported when they are the codes that most accurately reflect what is known about the patient's condition at the time of that particular encounter. It would be inappropriate to select a specific code that is not supported by the medical record documentation or conduct medically unnecessary diagnostic testing in order to determine a more specific code.

19. Coding for Healthcare Encounters in Hurricane Aftermath

a. Use of External Cause of Morbidity Codes

An external cause of morbidity code should be assigned to identify the cause of the injury(ies) incurred as a result of the hurricane. The use of external cause of morbidity codes is supplemental to the application of ICD-10-CM codes. External cause of morbidity codes are never to be recorded as a principal diagnosis (first-listed in non-inpatient settings). The appropriate injury code should be sequenced before any external cause codes. The external cause of morbidity codes capture how the injury or health condition happened (cause), the intent (unintentional or accidental; or intentional, such as suicide or assault), the place where the event occurred, the activity of the patient at the time of the event, and the person's status (e.g., civilian, military). They should not be assigned for encounters to treat hurricane victims' medical conditions when no injury, adverse effect or poisoning is involved. External cause of morbidity codes should be assigned for each encounter for care and treatment of the injury. External cause of morbidity codes may be assigned in all health care settings. For the purpose of capturing complete and accurate ICD-10-CM data in the aftermath of the hurricane, a healthcare setting should be considered as any location where medical care is provided by licensed healthcare professionals.

b. Sequencing of External Causes of Morbidity Codes

Codes for cataclysmic events, such as a hurricane, take priority over all other external cause codes except child and adult abuse and terrorism and should be sequenced before other external cause of injury codes. Assign as many external cause of morbidity codes as necessary to fully explain each cause. For example, if an injury occurs as a result of a building collapse during the hurricane, external cause codes for both the hurricane and the building collapse should be assigned, with the external causes code for hurricane being sequenced as the first external cause code. For injuries incurred as a direct result of the hurricane, assign the appropriate code(s) for the injuries, followed by the code X37.0-, Hurricane (with the appropriate 7th character), and any other applicable external cause of injury codes. Code X37.0- also should be assigned when an injury is incurred as a result of flooding caused by a levee breaking related to the hurricane. Code X38.-, Flood (with the appropriate 7th character), should be assigned when an injury is from flooding resulting directly from the storm. Code X36.0.-, Collapse of dam or man-made structure, should not be assigned when the cause of the collapse is due to the hurricane. Use of code X36.0- is limited to collapses of man-made structures due to earth surface movements, not due to storm surges directly from a hurricane.

c. Other External Causes of Morbidity Code Issues

For injuries that are not a direct result of the hurricane, such as an evacuee that has incurred an injury as a result of a motor vehicle accident, assign the appropriate external cause of morbidity code(s) to describe the cause of the injury, but do not assign code X37.0-, Hurricane. If it is not clear whether the injury was a direct result of the hurricane, assume the injury is due to the hurricane and assign code X37.0-, Hurricane, as well as any other applicable external cause of morbidity codes. In addition to code X37.0-, Hurricane, other possible applicable external cause of morbidity codes include:

> W54.0-, Bitten by dog
>
> X30-, Exposure to excessive natural heat
>
> X31-, Exposure to excessive natural cold
>
> X38-, Flood

d. Use of Z codes

Z codes (other reasons for healthcare encounters) may be assigned as appropriate to further explain the reasons for presenting for healthcare services, including transfers between healthcare facilities. The ICD-10-CM Official Guidelines for Coding and Reporting identify which codes maybe assigned as principal or first-listed diagnosis only, secondary diagnosis only, or principal/first-listed or secondary (depending on the circumstances). Possible applicable Z codes include:

> Z59.0, Homelessness
>
> Z59.1, Inadequate housing
>
> Z59.5, Extreme poverty
>
> Z75.1, Person awaiting admission to adequate facility elsewhere
>
> Z75.3, Unavailability and inaccessibility of health-care facilities
>
> Z75.4, Unavailability and inaccessibility of other helping agencies
>
> Z76.2, Encounter for health supervision and care of other healthy infant and child
>
> Z99.12, Encounter for respirator [ventilator] dependence during power failure

The external cause of morbidity codes and the Z codes listed above are not an all-inclusive list. Other codes may be applicable to the encounter based upon the documentation. Assign as many codes as necessary to fully explain each healthcare encounter. Since patient history information may be very limited, use any available documentation to assign the appropriate external cause of morbidity and Z codes.

C. Chapter-Specific Coding Guidelines

In addition to general coding guidelines, there are guidelines for specific diagnoses and/or conditions in the classification. Unless otherwise indicated, these guidelines apply to all health care settings. Please refer to Section II for guidelines on the selection of principal diagnosis.

1. Chapter 1: Certain Infectious and Parasitic Diseases (A00-B99)

a. Human Immunodeficiency Virus (HIV) Infections

1) Code only confirmed cases

Code only confirmed cases of HIV infection/illness. This is an exception to the hospital inpatient guideline Section II, H.

In this context, "confirmation" does not require documentation of positive serology or culture for HIV; the provider's diagnostic statement that the patient is HIV positive, or has an HIV-related illness is sufficient.

2) Selection and sequencing of HIV codes

(a) Patient admitted for HIV-related condition

If a patient is admitted for an HIV-related condition, the principal diagnosis should be B20, Human immunodeficiency virus [HIV] disease followed by additional diagnosis codes for all reported HIV-related conditions.

(b) Patient with HIV disease admitted for unrelated condition

If a patient with HIV disease is admitted for an unrelated condition (such as a traumatic injury), the code for the unrelated condition (e.g., the nature of injury code) should be the principal diagnosis. Other diagnoses would be B20 followed by additional diagnosis codes for all reported HIV-related conditions.

(c) Whether the patient is newly diagnosed

Whether the patient is newly diagnosed or has had previous admissions/encounters for HIV conditions is irrelevant to the sequencing decision.

(d) Asymptomatic human immunodeficiency virus

Z21, Asymptomatic human immunodeficiency virus [HIV] infection status, is to be applied when the patient without any documentation of symptoms is listed as being "HIV positive," "known HIV," "HIV test positive," or similar terminology. Do not use this code if the term "AIDS" is used or if the patient is treated for any HIV-related illness or is described as having any condition(s) resulting from his/her HIV positive status; use B20 in these cases.

(e) Patients with inconclusive HIV serology

Patients with inconclusive HIV serology, but no definitive diagnosis or manifestations of the illness, may be assigned code R75, Inconclusive laboratory evidence of human immunodeficiency virus [HIV].

(f) Previously diagnosed HIV-related illness

Patients with any known prior diagnosis of an HIV-related illness should be coded to B20. Once a patient has developed an HIV-related illness, the patient should always be assigned code B20 on every subsequent admission/encounter. Patients previously diagnosed with any HIV illness (B20) should never be assigned to R75 or Z21, Asymptomatic human immunodeficiency virus [HIV] infection status.

(g) HIV Infection in Pregnancy, Childbirth and the Puerperium

During pregnancy, childbirth or the puerperium, a patient admitted (or presenting for a health care encounter) because of an HIV-related illness should receive a principal diagnosis code of O98.7-, Human immunodeficiency [HIV] disease complicating pregnancy, childbirth and the puerperium, followed by B20 and the code(s) for the HIV-related illness(es). Codes from Chapter 15 always take sequencing priority.

Patients with asymptomatic HIV infection status admitted (or presenting for a health care encounter) during pregnancy, childbirth, or the puerperium should receive codes of O98.7- and Z21.

(h) Encounters for testing for HIV

If a patient is being seen to determine his/her HIV status, use code Z11.4, Encounter for screening for human immunodeficiency virus [HIV]. Use additional codes for any associated high risk behavior.

If a patient with signs or symptoms is being seen for HIV testing, code the signs and symptoms. An additional counseling code Z71.7, Human immunodeficiency virus [HIV] counseling, may be used if counseling is provided during the encounter for the test.

When a patient returns to be informed of his/her HIV test results and the test result is negative, use code Z71.7, Human immunodeficiency virus [HIV] counseling.

If the results are positive, see previous guidelines and assign codes as appropriate.

b. Infectious agents as the cause of diseases classified to other chapters

Certain infections are classified in chapters other than Chapter 1 and no organism is identified as part of the infection code. In these instances, it is necessary to use an additional code from Chapter 1 to identify the organism. A code from category B95, Streptococcus, Staphylococcus, and Enterococcus as the cause of diseases classified to other chapters, B96, Other bacterial agents as the cause of diseases classified to other chapters, or B97, Viral agents as the cause of diseases classified to other chapters, is to be used as an additional code to identify the organism. An instructional note will be found at the infection code advising that an additional organism code is required.

c. Infections resistant to antibiotics

Many bacterial infections are resistant to current antibiotics. It is necessary to identify all infections documented as antibiotic resistant. Assign a code from category Z16, Resistance to antimicrobial drugs, following the infection code only if the infection code does not identify drug resistance.

d. Sepsis, Severe Sepsis, and Septic Shock
  1) Coding of Sepsis and Severe Sepsis
    (a) Sepsis

For a diagnosis of sepsis, assign the appropriate code for the underlying systemic infection. If the type of infection or causal organism is not further specified, assign code A41.9, Sepsis, unspecified organism.

A code from subcategory R65.2, Severe sepsis, should not be assigned unless severe sepsis or an associated acute organ dysfunction is documented.

   (i) Negative or inconclusive blood cultures and sepsis

Negative or inconclusive blood cultures do not preclude a diagnosis of sepsis in patients with clinical evidence of the condition; however, the provider should be queried.

   (ii) Urosepsis

The term urosepsis is a nonspecific term. It is not to be considered synonymous with sepsis. It has no default code in the Alphabetic Index. Should a provider use this term, he/she must be queried for clarification.

   (iii) Sepsis with organ dysfunction

If a patient has sepsis and associated acute organ dysfunction or multiple organ dysfunction (MOD), follow the instructions for coding severe sepsis.

   (iv) Acute organ dysfunction that is not clearly associated with the sepsis

If a patient has sepsis and an acute organ dysfunction, but the medical record documentation indicates that the acute organ dysfunction is related to a medical condition other than the sepsis, do not assign a code from subcategory R65.2, Severe sepsis. An acute organ dysfunction must be associated with the sepsis in order to assign the severe sepsis code. If the documentation is not clear as to whether an acute organ dysfunction is related to the sepsis or another medical condition, query the provider.

    (b) Severe sepsis

The coding of severe sepsis requires a minimum of 2 codes: first a code for the underlying systemic infection, followed by a code from subcategory R65.2, Severe sepsis. If the causal organism is not documented, assign code A41.9, Sepsis, unspecified organism, for the infection. Additional code(s) for the associated acute organ dysfunction are also required.

Due to the complex nature of severe sepsis, some cases may require querying the provider prior to assignment of the codes.

  2) Septic shock
    (a) Septic shock generally refers to circulatory failure associated with severe sepsis, and therefore, it represents a type of acute organ dysfunction.

For cases of septic shock, the code for the systemic infection should be sequenced first, followed by code R65.21, Severe sepsis with septic shock or code T81.12, Postprocedural septic shock. Any additional codes for the other acute organ dysfunctions should also be assigned. As noted in the sequencing instructions in the Tabular List, the code for septic shock cannot be assigned as a principal diagnosis.

  3) Sequencing of severe sepsis

If severe sepsis is present on admission, and meets the definition of principal diagnosis, the underlying systemic infection should be assigned as principal diagnosis followed by the appropriate code from subcategory R65.2 as required by the sequencing rules in the Tabular List. A code from subcategory R65.2 can never be assigned as a principal diagnosis.

When severe sepsis develops during an encounter (it was not present on admission), the underlying systemic infection and the appropriate code from subcategory R65.2 should be assigned as secondary diagnoses.

Severe sepsis may be present on admission, but the diagnosis may not be confirmed until sometime after admission. If the documentation is not clear whether severe sepsis was present on admission, the provider should be queried.

  4) Sepsis and severe sepsis with a localized infection

If the reason for admission is both sepsis or severe sepsis and a localized infection, such as pneumonia or cellulitis, a code(s) for the underlying systemic infection should be assigned first and the

code for the localized infection should be assigned as a secondary diagnosis. If the patient has severe sepsis, a code from subcategory R65.2 should also be assigned as a secondary diagnosis. If the patient is admitted with a localized infection, such as pneumonia, and sepsis/severe sepsis doesn't develop until after admission, the localized infection should be assigned first, followed by the appropriate sepsis/severe sepsis codes.

5) Sepsis due to a postprocedural infection

(a) Documentation of causal relationship

As with all postprocedural complications, code assignment is based on the provider's documentation of the relationship between the infection and the procedure.

(b) Sepsis due to a postprocedural infection

For in**fections following a procedure, a code from** T81.**40, to T81.43** Infection following a procedure, or **a code from** O86.**00 to O86.03,** Infection of obstetric surgical wound, **that identifies the site of the infection** should be coded first, **if known. Assign an additional code for sepsis following a procedure (T81.44) or sepsis following an obstetrical procedure (O86.04). Use an additional code to identify the infectious agent.** If the patient has severe sepsis, the appropriate code from subcategory R65.2 should also be assigned with the additional code(s) for any acute organ dysfunction.

For infections following infusion, transfusion, therapeutic injection, or immunization, a code from subcategory T80.2, Infections following infusion, transfusion, and therapeutic injection, or code T88.0-, Infection following immunization, should be coded first, followed by the code for the specific infection. If the patient has severe sepsis, the appropriate code from subcategory R65.2 should also be assigned, with the additional codes(s) for any acute organ dysfunction.

(c) Postprocedural infection and postprocedural septic shock

If a postprocedural infection has resulted in postprocedural septic shock, **assign the codes indicated above for sepsis due to a postprocedural infection, followed by code T81.12-, Postprocedural septic shock. Do not assign code R65.21, Severe sepsis with septic shock. Additional code(s) should be assigned for any acute organ dysfunction.**

6) Sepsis and severe sepsis associated with a noninfectious process (condition)

In some cases a noninfectious process (condition), such as trauma, may lead to an infection which can result in sepsis or severe sepsis. If sepsis or severe sepsis is documented as associated with a noninfectious condition, such as a burn or serious injury, and this condition meets the definition for principal diagnosis, the code for the noninfectious condition should be sequenced first, followed by the code for the resulting infection. If severe sepsis is present, a code from subcategory R65.2 should also be assigned with any associated organ dysfunction(s) codes. It is not necessary to assign a code from subcategory R65.1, Systemic inflammatory response syndrome (SIRS) of non-infectious origin, for these cases.

If the infection meets the definition of principal diagnosis, it should be sequenced before the non-infectious condition. When both the associated non-infectious condition and the infection meet the definition of principal diagnosis, either may be assigned as principal diagnosis.

Only one code from category R65, Symptoms and signs specifically associated with systemic inflammation and infection, should be assigned. Therefore, when a non-infectious condition leads to an infection resulting in severe sepsis, assign the appropriate code from subcategory R65.2, Severe sepsis. Do not additionally assign a code from subcategory R65.1, Systemic inflammatory response syndrome (SIRS) of non-infectious origin.

See Section I.C.18. SIRS due to non-infectious process

7) Sepsis and septic shock complicating abortion, pregnancy, childbirth, and the puerperium

See Section I.C.15. Sepsis and septic shock complicating abortion, pregnancy, childbirth and the puerperium

8) Newborn sepsis

See Section I.C.16. f. Bacterial sepsis of Newborn

e. Methicillin Resistant Staphylococcus aureus (MRSA) Conditions

1) Selection and sequencing of MRSA codes

(a) Combination codes for MRSA infection

When a patient is diagnosed with an infection that is due to methicillin resistant *Staphylococcus aureus* (MRSA), and that infection has a combination code that includes the causal organism (e.g., sepsis, pneumonia) assign the appropriate combination code for the condition (e.g., code A41.02, Sepsis due to Methicillin resistant Staphylococcus aureus or code J15.212, Pneumonia due to Methicillin resistant Staphylococcus aureus). Do not assign code B95.62, Methicillin resistant Staphylococcus aureus infection as the cause of diseases classified elsewhere, as an additional code, because the combination code includes the type of infection and the MRSA organism. Do not assign a code from subcategory Z16.11, Resistance to penicillins, as an additional diagnosis.

See Section C.1. for instructions on coding and sequencing of sepsis and severe sepsis.

(b) Other codes for MRSA infection

When there is documentation of a current infection (e.g., wound infection, stitch abscess, urinary tract infection) due to MRSA, and that infection does not have a combination code that includes the causal organism, assign the appropriate code to identify the condition along with code B95.62, Methicillin resistant Staphylococcus aureus infection as the cause of diseases classified elsewhere for the MRSA infection. Do not assign a code from subcategory Z16.11, Resistance to penicillins.

(c) Methicillin susceptible Staphylococcus aureus (MSSA) and MRSA colonization

The condition or state of being colonized or carrying MSSA or MRSA is called colonization or carriage, while an individual person is described as being colonized or being a carrier. Colonization means that MSSA or MSRA is present on or in the body without necessarily causing illness. A positive MRSA colonization test might be documented by the provider as "MRSA screen positive" or "MRSA nasal swab positive".

Assign code Z22.322, Carrier or suspected carrier of Methicillin resistant Staphylococcus aureus, for patients documented as having MRSA colonization. Assign code Z22.321, Carrier or suspected carrier of Methicillin susceptible Staphylococcus aureus, for patient documented as having MSSA colonization. Colonization is not necessarily indicative of a disease process or as the cause of a specific condition the patient may have unless documented as such by the provider.

(d) MRSA colonization and infection

If a patient is documented as having both MRSA colonization and infection during a hospital admission, code Z22.322, Carrier or suspected carrier of Methicillin resistant Staphylococcus aureus, and a code for the MRSA infection may both be assigned.

f. Zika virus infections

1) Code only confirmed cases

Code only a confirmed diagnosis of Zika virus (A92.5, Zika virus disease) as documented by the provider. This is an exception to the hospital inpatient guideline Section II, H. In this context, "confirmation" does not require documentation of the type of test performed; the physician's diagnostic statement that the condition is confirmed is sufficient. This code should be assigned regardless of the stated mode of transmission.

If the provider documents "suspected", "possible" or "probable" Zika, do not assign code A92.5. Assign a code(s) explaining the reason for encounter (such as fever, rash, or joint pain) or Z20.**821**, Contact with and (suspected) exposure to **Zika virus**.

2. Chapter 2: Neoplasms (C00-D49)

General guidelines

Chapter 2 of the ICD-10-CM contains the codes for most benign and all malignant neoplasms. Certain benign neoplasms, such as prostatic adenomas, may be found in the specific body system chapters. To properly code a neoplasm it is necessary to determine from the record if the neoplasm is benign, in-situ, malignant, or of uncertain histologic behavior. If malignant, any secondary (metastatic) sites should also be determined.

Primary malignant neoplasms overlapping site boundaries

A primary malignant neoplasm that overlaps two or more contiguous (next to each other) sites should be classified to the subcategory/code .8 ('overlapping lesion'), unless the combination is specifically indexed elsewhere. For multiple neoplasms of the same site that are not contiguous such as tumors in different quadrants of the same breast, codes for each site should be assigned.

Malignant neoplasm of ectopic tissue

Malignant neoplasms of ectopic tissue are to be coded to the site of origin mentioned, e.g., ectopic pancreatic malignant neoplasms involving the stomach are coded to malignant neoplasm of pancreas, unspecified (C25.9).

The neoplasm table in the Alphabetic Index should be referenced first. However, if the histological term is documented, that term should be referenced first, rather than going immediately to the Neoplasm Table, in order to determine which column in the Neoplasm Table is appropriate. For example, if the documentation indicates "adenoma," refer to the term in the Alphabetic Index to review the entries under this term and the instructional note to "see also neoplasm, by site, benign." The table provides the proper code based on the type of neoplasm and the site. It is important to select the proper column in the table that corresponds to the type of neoplasm. The Tabular List should then be referenced to verify that the correct code has been selected from the table and that a more specific site code does not exist.

See Section I.C.21. Factors influencing health status and contact with health services, Status, for information regarding Z15.0, codes for genetic susceptibility to cancer.

a. Treatment directed at the malignancy

If the treatment is directed at the malignancy, designate the malignancy as the principal diagnosis.

The only exception to this guideline is if a patient admission/encounter is solely for the administration of chemotherapy, immunotherapy or external beam radiation therapy, assign the appropriate Z51.-- code as the first-listed or principal diagnosis, and the diagnosis or problem for which the service is being performed as a secondary diagnosis.

b. Treatment of secondary site

When a patient is admitted because of a primary neoplasm with metastasis and treatment is directed toward the secondary site only, the secondary neoplasm is designated as the principal diagnosis even though the primary malignancy is still present.

c. Coding and sequencing of complications

Coding and sequencing of complications associated with the malignancies or with the therapy thereof are subject to the following guidelines:

1) **Anemia associated with malignancy**

When admission/encounter is for management of an anemia associated with the malignancy, and the treatment is only for anemia, the appropriate code for the malignancy is sequenced as the principal or first-listed diagnosis followed by the appropriate code for the anemia (such as code D63.0, Anemia in neoplastic disease).

2) **Anemia associated with chemotherapy, immunotherapy and radiation therapy**

When the admission/encounter is for management of an anemia associated with an adverse effect of the administration of chemotherapy or immunotherapy and the only treatment is for the anemia, the anemia code is sequenced first followed by the appropriate codes for the neoplasm and the adverse effect (T45.1X5-, Adverse effect of antineoplastic and immunosuppressive drugs).

When the admission/encounter is for management of an anemia associated with an adverse effect of radiotherapy, the anemia code should be sequenced first, followed by the appropriate neoplasm code and code Y84.2, Radiological procedure and radiotherapy as the cause of abnormal reaction of the patient, or of later complication, without mention of misadventure at the time of the procedure.

3) **Management of dehydration due to the malignancy**

When the admission/encounter is for management of dehydration due to the malignancy and only the dehydration is being treated (intravenous rehydration), the dehydration is sequenced first, followed by the code(s) for the malignancy.

4) **Treatment of a complication resulting from a surgical procedure**

When the admission/encounter is for treatment of a complication resulting from a surgical procedure, designate the complication as the principal or first-listed diagnosis if treatment is directed at resolving the complication.

d. Primary malignancy previously excised

When a primary malignancy has been previously excised or eradicated from its site and there is no further treatment directed to that site and there is no evidence of any existing primary malignancy **at that site**, a code from category Z85, Personal history of malignant neoplasm, should be used to indicate the former site of the malignancy. Any mention of extension, invasion, or metastasis to another site is coded as a secondary malignant neoplasm to that site. The secondary site may be the principal or first-listed with the Z85 code used as a secondary code.

e. Admissions/Encounters involving chemotherapy, immunotherapy and radiation therapy

1) **Episode of care involves surgical removal of neoplasm**

When an episode of care involves the surgical removal of a neoplasm, primary or secondary site, followed by adjunct chemotherapy or radiation treatment during the same episode of care, the code for the neoplasm should be assigned as principal or first-listed diagnosis.

2) **Patient admission/encounter solely for administration of chemotherapy, immunotherapy and radiation therapy**

If a patient admission/encounter is solely for the administration of chemotherapy, immunotherapy or external beam radiation therapy assign code Z51.0, Encounter for antineoplastic radiation therapy, or Z51.11, Encounter for antineoplastic chemotherapy, or Z51.12, Encounter for antineoplastic immunotherapy as the first-listed or principal diagnosis. If a patient receives more than one of these therapies during the same admission more than one of these codes may be assigned, in any sequence.

The malignancy for which the therapy is being administered should be assigned as a secondary diagnosis.

If a patient admission/encounter is for the insertion or implantation of radioactive elements (e.g., brachytherapy) the appropriate code for the malignancy is sequenced as the principal or first-listed diagnosis. Code Z51.0 should not be assigned.

3) **Patient admitted for radiation therapy, chemotherapy or immunotherapy and develops complications**

When a patient is admitted for the purpose of external beam radiotherapy, immunotherapy or chemotherapy and develops complications such as uncontrolled nausea and vomiting or dehydration, the principal or first-listed diagnosis is Z51.0, Encounter for antineoplastic radiation therapy, or Z51.11, Encounter for antineoplastic chemotherapy, or Z51.12, Encounter for antineoplastic immunotherapy followed by any codes for the complications.

When a patient is admitted for the purpose of insertion or implantation of radioactive elements (e.g., brachytherapy)and develops complications such as uncontrolled nausea and vomiting or dehydration, the principal or first-listed diagnosis is the appropriate code for the malignancy followed by any codes for the complications.

f. Admission/encounter to determine extent of malignancy

When the reason for admission/encounter is to determine the extent of the malignancy, or for a procedure such as paracentesis or thoracentesis, the primary malignancy or appropriate metastatic site is designated as the principal or first-listed diagnosis, even though chemotherapy or radiotherapy is administered.

g. Symptoms, signs, and abnormal findings listed in Chapter 18 associated with neoplasms

Symptoms, signs, and ill-defined conditions listed in Chapter 18 characteristic of, or associated with, an existing primary or secondary site malignancy cannot be used to replace the malignancy as principal or first-listed diagnosis, regardless of the number of admissions or encounters for treatment and care of the neoplasm.

See section I.C.21. Factors influencing health status and contact with health services, Encounter for prophylactic organ removal.

h. Admission/encounter for pain control/management

See Section I.C.6. for information on coding admission/encounter for pain control/management.

i. **Malignancy in two or more noncontiguous sites**
A patient may have more than one malignant tumor in the same organ. These tumors may represent different primaries or metastatic disease, depending on the site. Should the documentation be unclear, the provider should be queried as to the status of each tumor so that the correct codes can be assigned.

j. **Disseminated malignant neoplasm, unspecified**
Code C80.0, Disseminated malignant neoplasm, unspecified, is for use only in those cases where the patient has advanced metastatic disease and no known primary or secondary sites are specified. It should not be used in place of assigning codes for the primary site and all known secondary sites.

k. **Malignant neoplasm without specification of site**
Code C80.1, Malignant (primary) neoplasm, unspecified, equates to Cancer, unspecified. This code should only be used when no determination can be made as to the primary site of a malignancy. This code should rarely be used in the inpatient setting.

l. **Sequencing of neoplasm codes**
   1) **Encounter for treatment of primary malignancy**
   If the reason for the encounter is for treatment of a primary malignancy, assign the malignancy as the principal/first-listed diagnosis. The primary site is to be sequenced first, followed by any metastatic sites.

   2) **Encounter for treatment of secondary malignancy**
   When an encounter is for a primary malignancy with metastasis and treatment is directed toward the metastatic (secondary) site(s) only, the metastatic site(s) is designated as the principal/first-listed diagnosis. The primary malignancy is coded as an additional code.

   3) **Malignant neoplasm in a pregnant patient**
   When a pregnant woman has a malignant neoplasm, a code from subcategory O9A.1-, Malignant neoplasm complicating pregnancy, childbirth, and the puerperium, should be sequenced first, followed by the appropriate code from Chapter 2 to indicate the type of neoplasm.

   4) **Encounter for complication associated with a neoplasm**
   When an encounter is for management of a complication associated with a neoplasm, such as dehydration, and the treatment is only for the complication, the complication is coded first, followed by the appropriate code(s) for the neoplasm.

   The exception to this guideline is anemia. When the admission/encounter is for management of an anemia associated with the malignancy, and the treatment is only for anemia, the appropriate code for the malignancy is sequenced as the principal or first-listed diagnosis followed by code D63.0, Anemia in neoplastic disease.

   5) **Complication from surgical procedure for treatment of a neoplasm**
   When an encounter is for treatment of a complication resulting from a surgical procedure performed for the treatment of the neoplasm, designate the complication as the principal/first-listed diagnosis. See guideline regarding the coding of a current malignancy versus personal history to determine if the code for the neoplasm should also be assigned.

   6) **Pathologic fracture due to a neoplasm**
   When an encounter is for a pathological fracture due to a neoplasm, and the focus of treatment is the fracture, a code from subcategory M84.5, Pathological fracture in neoplastic disease, should be sequenced first, followed by the code for the neoplasm.

   If the focus of treatment is the neoplasm with an associated pathological fracture, the neoplasm code should be sequenced first, followed by a code from M84.5 for the pathological fracture.

m. **Current malignancy versus personal history of malignancy**
When a primary malignancy has been excised but further treatment, such as an additional surgery for the malignancy, radiation therapy or chemotherapy is directed to that site, the primary malignancy code should be used until treatment is completed.

When a primary malignancy has been previously excised or eradicated from its site, there is no further treatment (of the malignancy) directed to that site, and there is no evidence of any existing primary malignancy **at that site**, a code from category Z85, Personal history of malignant neoplasm, should be used to indicate the former site of the malignancy.

Subcategories Z85.0 – Z85.7 should only be assigned for the former site of a primary malignancy, not the site of a secondary malignancy. Codes from subcategory Z85.8-, may be assigned for the former site(s) of either a primary or secondary malignancy included in this subcategory.
See Section I.C.21. Factors influencing health status and contact with health services, History (of)

n. **Leukemia, Multiple Myeloma, and Malignant Plasma Cell Neoplasms in remission versus personal history**
The categories for leukemia, and category C90, Multiple myeloma and malignant plasma cell neoplasms, have codes indicating whether or not the leukemia has achieved remission. There are also codes Z85.6, Personal history of leukemia, and Z85.79, Personal history of other malignant neoplasms of lymphoid, hematopoietic and related tissues. If the documentation is unclear as to whether the leukemia has achieved remission, the provider should be queried.

See Section I.C.21. Factors influencing health status and contact with health services, History (of)

o. **Aftercare following surgery for neoplasm**
See Section I.C.21. Factors influencing health status and contact with health services, Aftercare

p. **Follow-up care for completed treatment of a malignancy**
See Section I.C.21. Factors influencing health status and contact with health services, Follow-up

q. **Prophylactic organ removal for prevention of malignancy**
See Section I.C. 21, Factors influencing health status and contact with health services, Prophylactic organ removal

r. **Malignant neoplasm associated with transplanted organ**
A malignant neoplasm of a transplanted organ should be coded as a transplant complication. Assign first the appropriate code from category T86.-, Complications of transplanted organs and tissue, followed by code C80.2, Malignant neoplasm associated with transplanted organ. Use an additional code for the specific malignancy.

3. **Chapter 3: Disease of the blood and blood-forming organs and certain disorders involving the immune mechanism (D50-D89)**
Reserved for future guideline expansion

4. **Chapter 4: Endocrine, Nutritional, and Metabolic Diseases (E00-E89)**
   a. **Diabetes mellitus**
   The diabetes mellitus codes are combination codes that include the type of diabetes mellitus, the body system affected, and the complications affecting that body system. As many codes within a particular category as are necessary to describe all of the complications of the disease may be used. They should be sequenced based on the reason for a particular encounter. Assign as many codes from categories E08 – E13 as needed to identify all of the associated conditions that the patient has.

   1) **Type of diabetes**
   The age of a patient is not the sole determining factor, though most type 1 diabetics develop the condition before reaching puberty. For this reason type 1 diabetes mellitus is also referred to as juvenile diabetes.

   2) **Type of diabetes mellitus not documented**
   If the type of diabetes mellitus is not documented in the medical record the default is E11.-, Type 2 diabetes mellitus.

   3) **Diabetes mellitus and the use of insulin and oral hypoglycemics**
   If the documentation in a medical record does not indicate the type of diabetes but does indicate that the patient uses insulin, code E11-, Type 2 diabetes mellitus, should be assigned. An additional code should be assigned from category Z79 to identify the long-term (current) use of insulin or oral hypoglycemic drugs. If the patient is treated with both oral medications and insulin, only the code for long-term (current) use of insulin should be assigned. Code Z79.4 should not be assigned if insulin is given temporarily to bring a type 2 patient's blood sugar under control during an encounter.

   4) **Diabetes mellitus in pregnancy and gestational diabetes**
   See Section I.C.15. Diabetes mellitus in pregnancy.
   See Section I.C.15. Gestational (pregnancy induced) diabetes

5) Complications due to insulin pump malfunction

(a) Underdose of insulin due to insulin pump failure

An underdose of insulin due to an insulin pump failure should be assigned to a code from subcategory T85.6, Mechanical complication of other specified internal and external prosthetic devices, implants and grafts, that specifies the type of pump malfunction, as the principal or first-listed code, followed by code T38.3X6-, Underdosing of insulin and oral hypoglycemic [antidiabetic] drugs. Additional codes for the type of diabetes mellitus and any associated complications due to the underdosing should also be assigned.

(b) Overdose of insulin due to insulin pump failure

The principal or first-listed code for an encounter due to an insulin pump malfunction resulting in an overdose of insulin, should also be T85.6-, Mechanical complication of other specified internal and external prosthetic devices, implants and grafts, followed by code T38.3X1-, Poisoning by insulin and oral hypoglycemic [antidiabetic] drugs, accidental (unintentional).

6) Secondary diabetes mellitus

Codes under categories E08, Diabetes mellitus due to underlying condition, E09, Drug or chemical induced diabetes mellitus, and E13, Other specified diabetes mellitus, identify complications/manifestations associated with secondary diabetes mellitus. Secondary diabetes is always caused by another condition or event (e.g., cystic fibrosis, malignant neoplasm of pancreas, pancreatectomy, adverse effect of drug, or poisoning).

(a) Secondary diabetes mellitus and the use of insulin or oral hypoglycemic drugs

For patients with secondary diabetes mellitus who routinely use insulin or oral hypoglycemic drugs, an additional code from category Z79 should be assigned to identify the long-term (current) use of insulin or oral hypoglycemic drugs. If the patient is treated with both oral medications and insulin, only the code for long-term (current) use of insulin should be assigned. Code Z79.4 should not be assigned if insulin is given temporarily to bring a secondary diabetic patient's blood sugar under control during an encounter.

(b) Assigning and sequencing secondary diabetes codes and its causes

The sequencing of the secondary diabetes codes in relationship to codes for the cause of the diabetes is based on the Tabular List instructions for categories E08, E09 and E13.

(i) Secondary diabetes mellitus due to pancreatectomy

For postpancreatectomy diabetes mellitus (lack of insulin due to the surgical removal of all or part of the pancreas), assign code E89.1, Postprocedural hypoinsulinemia. Assign a code from category E13 and a code from subcategory Z90.41, Acquired absence of pancreas, as additional codes.

(ii) Secondary diabetes due to drugs

Secondary diabetes may be caused by an adverse effect of correctly administered medications, poisoning or sequela of poisoning.

See section I.C.19.e for coding of adverse effects and poisoning, and section I.C.20 for external cause code reporting.

5. Chapter 5: Mental, Behavioral and Neurodevelopmental disorders (F01–F99)

a. Pain disorders related to psychological factors

Assign code F45.41, for pain that is exclusively related to psychological disorders. As indicated by the Excludes 1 note under category G89, a code from category G89 should not be assigned with code F45.41.

Code F45.42, Pain disorders with related psychological factors, should be used with a code from category G89, Pain, not elsewhere classified, if there is documentation of a psychological component for a patient with acute or chronic pain.

See Section I.C.6. Pain

b. Mental and behavioral disorders due to psychoactive substance use

1) In Remission

Selection of codes for "in remission" for categories F10-F19, Mental and behavioral disorders due to psychoactive substance use (categories F10-F19 with -.11, -.21) requires the provider's clinical judgment. The appropriate codes for "in remission" are assigned only on the basis of provider documentation (as defined in the Official Guidelines for Coding and Reporting), unless otherwise instructed by the classification.

Mild substance use disorders in early or sustained remission are classified to the appropriate codes for substance abuse in remission, and moderate or severe substance use disorders in early or sustained remission are classified to the appropriate codes for substance dependence in remission.

2) Psychoactive Substance Use, Abuse and Dependence

When the provider documentation refers to use, abuse and dependence of the same substance (e.g. alcohol, opioid, cannabis, etc.), only one code should be assigned to identify the pattern of use based on the following hierarchy:

- If both use and abuse are documented, assign only the code for abuse
- If both abuse and dependence are documented, assign only the code for dependence
- If use, abuse and dependence are all documented, assign only the code for dependence
- If both use and dependence are documented, assign only the code for dependence.

3) Psychoactive Substance Use, *Unspecified*

As with all other **unspecified** diagnoses, the codes for **unspecified** psychoactive substance use (F10.9-, F11.9-, F12.9-, F13.9-, F14.9-, F15.9-, F16.9-, **F18.9-, F19.9-**) should only be assigned based on provider documentation and when they meet the definition of a reportable diagnosis (see Section III, Reporting Additional Diagnoses). The**se** codes are to be used only when the psychoactive substance use is associated with a physical, mental or behavioral disorder, and such a relationship is documented by the provider.

c. Factitious Disorder

Factitious disorder imposed on self or Munchausen's syndrome is a disorder in which a person falsely reports or causes his or her own physical or psychological signs or symptoms. For patients with documented factitious disorder on self or Munchausen's syndrome, assign the appropriate code from subcategory F68.1-, Factitious disorder imposed on self.

Munchausen's syndrome by proxy (MSBP) is a disorder in which a caregiver (perpetrator) falsely reports or causes an illness or injury in another person (victim) under his or her care, such as a child, an elderly adult, or a person who has a disability. The condition is also referred to as "factitious disorder imposed on another" or "factitious disorder by proxy." The perpetrator, not the victim, receives this diagnosis. Assign code F68.A, Factitious disorder imposed on another, to the perpetrator's record. For the victim of a patient suffering from MSBP, assign the appropriate code from categories T74, Adult and child abuse, neglect and other maltreatment, confirmed, or T76, Adult and child abuse, neglect and other maltreatment, suspected.

See Section I.C.19.f. Adult and child abuse, neglect and other maltreatment

6. Chapter 6: Diseases of the Nervous System (G00-G99)

a. Dominant/nondominant side

Codes from category G81, Hemiplegia and hemiparesis, and subcategories G83.1, Monoplegia of lower limb, G83.2, Monoplegia of upper limb, and G83.3, Monoplegia, unspecified, identify whether the dominant or nondominant side is affected. Should the affected side be documented, but not specified as dominant or nondominant, and the classification system does not indicate a default, code selection is as follows:

- For ambidextrous patients, the default should be dominant.
- If the left side is affected, the default is non-dominant.
- If the right side is affected, the default is dominant.

b. Pain - Category G89

1) General coding information

Codes in category G89, Pain, not elsewhere classified, may be used in conjunction with codes from other categories and

chapters to provide more detail about acute or chronic pain and neoplasm-related pain, unless otherwise indicated below.

If the pain is not specified as acute or chronic, post-thoracotomy, postprocedural, or neoplasm-related, do not assign codes from category G89.

A code from category G89 should not be assigned if the underlying (definitive) diagnosis is known, unless the reason for the encounter is pain control/ management and not management of the underlying condition.

When an admission or encounter is for a procedure aimed at treating the underlying condition (e.g., spinal fusion, kyphoplasty), a code for the underlying condition (e.g., vertebral fracture, spinal stenosis) should be assigned as the principal diagnosis. No code from category G89 should be assigned.

(a) Category G89 Codes as Principal or First-Listed Diagnosis

Category G89 codes are acceptable as principal diagnosis or the first-listed code:

- When pain control or pain management is the reason for the admission/encounter (e.g., a patient with displaced intervertebral disc, nerve impingement and severe back pain presents for injection of steroid into the spinal canal). The underlying cause of the pain should be reported as an additional diagnosis, if known.

- When a patient is admitted for the insertion of a neurostimulator for pain control, assign the appropriate pain code as the principal or first-listed diagnosis. When an admission or encounter is for a procedure aimed at treating the underlying condition and a neurostimulator is inserted for pain control during the same admission/encounter, a code for the underlying condition should be assigned as the principal diagnosis and the appropriate pain code should be assigned as a secondary diagnosis.

(b) Use of Category G89 Codes in Conjunction with Site Specific Pain Codes

(i) Assigning Category G89 and Site-Specific Pain Codes

Codes from category G89 may be used in conjunction with codes that identify the site of pain (including codes from chapter 18) if the category G89 code provides additional information. For example, if the code describes the site of the pain, but does not fully describe whether the pain is acute or chronic, then both codes should be assigned.

(ii) Sequencing of Category G89 Codes with Site-Specific Pain Codes

The sequencing of category G89 codes with site-specific pain codes (including chapter 18 codes), is dependent on the circumstances of the encounter/admission as follows:

- If the encounter is for pain control or pain management, assign the code from category G89 followed by the code identifying the specific site of pain (e.g., encounter for pain management for acute neck pain from trauma is assigned code G89.11, Acute pain due to trauma, followed by code M54.2, Cervicalgia, to identify the site of pain).

- If the encounter is for any other reason except pain control or pain management, and a related definitive diagnosis has not been established (confirmed) by the provider, assign the code for the specific site of pain first, followed by the appropriate code from category G89.

2) Pain due to devices, implants and grafts
See Section I.C.19. Pain due to medical devices

3) Postoperative Pain
The provider's documentation should be used to guide the coding of postoperative pain, as well as *Section III. Reporting Additional Diagnoses* and *Section IV. Diagnostic Coding and Reporting in the Outpatient Setting.*

The default for post-thoracotomy and other postoperative pain not specified as acute or chronic is the code for the acute form.

Routine or expected postoperative pain immediately after surgery should not be coded.

(a) Postoperative pain not associated with specific postoperative complication
Postoperative pain not associated with a specific postoperative complication is assigned to the appropriate postoperative pain code in category G89.

(b) Postoperative pain associated with specific postoperative complication
Postoperative pain associated with a specific postoperative complication (such as painful wire sutures) is assigned to the appropriate code(s) found in Chapter 19, Injury, poisoning, and certain other consequences of external causes. If appropriate, use additional code(s) from category G89 to identify acute or chronic pain (G89.18 or G89.28).

4) Chronic pain
Chronic pain is classified to subcategory G89.2. There is no time frame defining when pain becomes chronic pain. The provider's documentation should be used to guide use of these codes.

5) Neoplasm Related Pain
Code G89.3 is assigned to pain documented as being related, associated or due to cancer, primary or secondary malignancy, or tumor. This code is assigned regardless of whether the pain is acute or chronic.

This code may be assigned as the principal or first-listed code when the stated reason for the admission/encounter is documented as pain control/pain management. The underlying neoplasm should be reported as an additional diagnosis.

When the reason for the admission/encounter is management of the neoplasm and the pain associated with the neoplasm is also documented, code G89.3 may be assigned as an additional diagnosis. It is not necessary to assign an additional code for the site of the pain.

See Section I.C.2 for instructions on the sequencing of neoplasms for all other stated reasons for the admission/encounter (except for pain control/pain management).

6) Chronic pain syndrome
Central pain syndrome (G89.0) and chronic pain syndrome (G89.4) are different than the term "chronic pain," and therefore codes should only be used when the provider has specifically documented this condition.

See Section I.C.5. Pain disorders related to psychological factors

7. Chapter 7: Diseases of the Eye and Adnexa (H00-H59)
a. Glaucoma
1) Assigning Glaucoma Codes
Assign as many codes from category H40, Glaucoma, as needed to identify the type of glaucoma, the affected eye, and the glaucoma stage.

2) Bilateral glaucoma with same type and stage
When a patient has bilateral glaucoma and both eyes are documented as being the same type and stage, and there is a code for bilateral glaucoma, report only the code for the type of glaucoma, bilateral, with the seventh character for the stage.

When a patient has bilateral glaucoma and both eyes are documented as being the same type and stage, and the classification does not provide a code for bilateral glaucoma (i.e. subcategories H40.10 and H40.20) report only one code for the type of glaucoma with the appropriate seventh character for the stage.

3) Bilateral glaucoma stage with different types or stages
When a patient has bilateral glaucoma and each eye is documented as having a different type or stage, and the classification distinguishes laterality, assign the appropriate code for each eye rather than the code for bilateral glaucoma.

When a patient has bilateral glaucoma and each eye is documented as having a different type, and the classification does not distinguish laterality (i.e. subcategories H40.10 and H40.20), assign one code for each type of glaucoma with the appropriate seventh character for the stage.

When a patient has bilateral glaucoma and each eye is documented as having the same type, but different stage, and the classification does not distinguish laterality (i.e. subcategories H40.10 and H40.20), assign a code for the type of glaucoma for

each eye with the seventh character for the specific glaucoma stage documented for each eye.

4) **Patient admitted with glaucoma and stage evolves during the admission**
If a patient is admitted with glaucoma and the stage progresses during the admission, assign the code for highest stage documented.

5) **Indeterminate stage glaucoma**
Assignment of the seventh character "4" for "indeterminate stage" should be based on the clinical documentation. The seventh character "4" is used for glaucomas whose stage cannot be clinically determined. This seventh character should not be confused with the seventh character "0", unspecified, which should be assigned when there is no documentation regarding the stage of the glaucoma.

b. **Blindness**
If "blindness" or "low vision" of both eyes is documented but the visual impairment category is not documented, assign code H54.3, Unqualified visual loss, both eyes. If "blindness" or "low vision" in one eye is documented but the visual impairment category is not documented, assign a code from H54.6-, Unqualified visual loss, one eye. If "blindness" or "visual loss" is documented without any information about whether one or both eyes are affected, assign code H54.7, Unspecified visual loss.

8. **Chapter 8: Diseases of the Ear and Mastoid Process (H60-H95)**
Reserved for future guideline expansion

9. **Chapter 9: Diseases of the Circulatory System (I00-I99)**

a. **Hypertension**
The classification presumes a causal relationship between hypertension and heart involvement and between hypertension and kidney involvement, as the two conditions are linked by the term "with" in the Alphabetic Index. These conditions should be coded as related even in the absence of provider documentation explicitly linking them, unless the documentation clearly states the conditions are unrelated.

For hypertension and conditions not specifically linked by relational terms such as "with," "associated with" or "due to" in the classification, provider documentation must link the conditions in order to code them as related.

1) **Hypertension with Heart Disease**
Hypertension with heart conditions classified to I50.- or **I51.4-I51.7, I51.89, I51.9**, are assigned to a code from category I11, Hypertensive heart disease. Use additional code(s) from category I50, Heart failure, to identify the type(s) of heart failure in those patients with heart failure.

The same heart conditions (I50.-, **I51.4-I51.7, I51.89, I51.9**) with hypertension are coded separately if the provider has **documented they are unrelated to the hypertension**. Sequence according to the circumstances of the admission/encounter.

2) **Hypertensive Chronic Kidney Disease**
Assign codes from category I12, Hypertensive chronic kidney disease, when both hypertension and a condition classifiable to category N18, Chronic kidney disease (CKD), are present. CKD should not be coded as hypertensive if the **provider indicates the CKD is not related to the hypertension**.

The appropriate code from category N18 should be used as a secondary code with a code from category I12 to identify the stage of chronic kidney disease.

See Section I.C.14. Chronic kidney disease.

If a patient has hypertensive chronic kidney disease and acute renal failure, an additional code for the acute renal failure is required.

3) **Hypertensive Heart and Chronic Kidney Disease**
Assign codes from combination category I13, Hypertensive heart and chronic kidney disease, when there is hypertension with both heart and kidney involvement. If heart failure is present, assign an additional code from category I50 to identify the type of heart failure.

The appropriate code from category N18, Chronic kidney disease, should be used as a secondary code with a code from category I13 to identify the stage of chronic kidney disease.

See Section I.C.14. Chronic kidney disease.

The codes in category I13, Hypertensive heart and chronic kidney disease, are combination codes that include hypertension, heart disease and chronic kidney disease. The Includes note at I13 specifies that the conditions included at I11 and I12 are included together in I13. If a patient has hypertension, heart disease and chronic kidney disease, then a code from I13 should be used, not individual codes for hypertension, heart disease and chronic kidney disease, or codes from I11 or I12.

For patients with both acute renal failure and chronic kidney disease, an additional code for acute renal failure is required.

4) **Hypertensive Cerebrovascular Disease**
For hypertensive cerebrovascular disease, first assign the appropriate code from categories I60-I69, followed by the appropriate hypertension code.

5) **Hypertensive Retinopathy**
Subcategory H35.0, Background retinopathy and retinal vascular changes, should be used with a code from category I10- I15, Hypertensive disease to include the systemic hypertension. The sequencing is based on the reason for the encounter.

6) **Hypertension, Secondary**
Secondary hypertension is due to an underlying condition. Two codes are required: one to identify the underlying etiology and one from category I15 to identify the hypertension. Sequencing of codes is determined by the reason for admission/encounter.

7) **Hypertension, Transient**
Assign code R03.0, Elevated blood pressure reading without diagnosis of hypertension, unless patient has an established diagnosis of hypertension. Assign code O13.-, Gestational [pregnancy-induced] hypertension without significant proteinuria, or O14.-, Pre-eclampsia, for transient hypertension of pregnancy.

8) **Hypertension, Controlled**
This diagnostic statement usually refers to an existing state of hypertension under control by therapy. Assign the appropriate code from categories I10-I15, Hypertensive diseases.

9) **Hypertension, Uncontrolled**
Uncontrolled hypertension may refer to untreated hypertension or hypertension not responding to current therapeutic regimen. In either case, assign the appropriate code from categories I10-I15, Hypertensive diseases.

10) **Hypertensive Crisis**
Assign a code from category I16, Hypertensive crisis, for documented hypertensive urgency, hypertensive emergency or unspecified hypertensive crisis. Code also any identified hypertensive disease (I10-I15). The sequencing is based on the reason for the encounter.

11) **Pulmonary Hypertension**
Pulmonary hypertension is classified to category I27, Other pulmonary heart diseases. For secondary pulmonary hypertension (I27.1, I27.2-), code also any associated conditions or adverse effects of drugs or toxins. The sequencing is based on the reason for the encounter, **except for adverse effects of drugs (See Section I.C.19.e.)**.

b. **Atherosclerotic Coronary Artery Disease and Angina**
ICD-10-CM has combination codes for atherosclerotic heart disease with angina pectoris. The subcategories for these codes are I25.11, Atherosclerotic heart disease of native coronary artery with angina pectoris and I25.7, Atherosclerosis of coronary artery bypass graft(s) and coronary artery of transplanted heart with angina pectoris.

When using one of these combination codes it is not necessary to use an additional code for angina pectoris. A causal relationship can be assumed in a patient with both atherosclerosis and angina pectoris, unless the documentation indicates the angina is due to something other than the atherosclerosis.

If a patient with coronary artery disease is admitted due to an acute myocardial infarction (AMI), the AMI should be sequenced before the coronary artery disease.

See Section I.C.9. Acute myocardial infarction (AMI)

c. **Intraoperative and Postprocedural Cerebrovascular Accident**
Medical record documentation should clearly specify the cause-and-effect relationship between the medical intervention and the cerebrovascular accident in order to assign a code for intraoperative or postprocedural cerebrovascular accident.

Proper code assignment depends on whether it was an infarction or hemorrhage and whether it occurred intraoperatively or postoperatively. If it was a cerebral hemorrhage, code assignment depends on the type of procedure performed.

d. Sequelae of Cerebrovascular Disease

1) Category I69, Sequelae of Cerebrovascular disease

Category I69 is used to indicate conditions classifiable to categories I60-I67 as the causes of sequela (neurologic deficits), themselves classified elsewhere. These "late effects" include neurologic deficits that persist after initial onset of conditions classifiable to categories I60-I67. The neurologic deficits caused by cerebrovascular disease may be present from the onset or may arise at any time after the onset of the condition classifiable to categories I60-I67.

Codes from category I69, Sequelae of cerebrovascular disease, that specify hemiplegia, hemiparesis and monoplegia identify whether the dominant or nondominant side is affected. Should the affected side be documented, but not specified as dominant or nondominant, and the classification system does not indicate a default, code selection is as follows:

- For ambidextrous patients, the default should be dominant.
- If the left side is affected, the default is non-dominant.
- If the right side is affected, the default is dominant.

2) Codes from category I69 with codes from I60-I67

Codes from category I69 may be assigned on a health care record with codes from I60-I67, if the patient has a current cerebrovascular disease and deficits from an old cerebrovascular disease.

3) Codes from category I69 and Personal history of transient ischemic attack (TIA) and cerebral infarction (Z86.73)

Codes from category I69 should not be assigned if the patient does not have neurologic deficits.

See Section I.C.21. 4. History (of) for use of personal history codes

e. Acute myocardial infarction (AMI)

1) Type 1 ST elevation myocardial infarction (STEMI) and non-ST elevation myocardial infarction (NSTEMI)

The ICD-10-CMcodes for type 1 acute myocardial infarction (AMI) identify the site, such as anterolateral wall or true posterior wall. Subcategories I21.0-I21.2 and code I21.3 are used for type 1 ST elevation myocardial infarction (STEMI). Code I21.4, Non-ST elevation (NSTEMI) myocardial infarction, is used for type 1 non ST elevation myocardial infarction (NSTEMI) and nontransmural MIs.

If a type 1 NSTEMI evolves to STEMI, assign the STEMI code. If a type 1 STEMI converts to NSTEMI due to thrombolytic therapy, it is still coded as STEMI.

For encounters occurring while the myocardial infarction is equal to, or less than, four weeks old, including transfers to another acute setting or a postacute setting, and the myocardial infarction meets the definition for "other diagnoses" (see Section III, Reporting Additional Diagnoses), codes from category I21 may continue to be reported. For encounters after the 4 week time frame and the patient is still receiving care related to the myocardial infarction, the appropriate aftercare code should be assigned, rather than a code from category I21. For old or healed myocardial infarctions not requiring further care, code I25.2, Old myocardial infarction, may be assigned.

2) Acute myocardial infarction, unspecified

Code I21.9, Acute myocardial infarction, unspecified, is the default for unspecified acute myocardial infarction or unspecified type. If only type 1 STEMI or transmural MI without the site is documented, assign code I21.3, ST elevation (STEMI) myocardial infarction of unspecified site.

3) AMI documented as nontransmural or subendocardial but site provided

If an AMI is documented as nontransmural or subendocardial, but the site is provided, it is still coded as a subendocardial AMI.

See Section I.C.21.3 for information on coding status post administration of tPA in a different facility within the last 24 hours.

4) Subsequent acute myocardial infarction

A code from category I22, Subsequent ST elevation (STEMI) and non-ST elevation (NSTEMI) myocardial infarction, is to be used when a patient who has suffered a type 1 or unspecified AMI has a new AMI within the 4 week time frame of the initial AMI. A code

from category I22 must be used in conjunction with a code from category I21. The sequencing of the I22 and I21 codes depends on the circumstances of the encounter.

Do not assign code I22 for subsequent myocardial infarctions other than type 1 or unspecified. For subsequent type 2 AMI assign only code I21.A1. For subsequent type 4 or type 5 AMI, assign only code I21.A9.

If a subsequent myocardial infarction of one type occurs within 4 weeks of a myocardial infarction of a different type, assign the appropriate codes from category I21 to identify each type. Do not assign a code from I22. Codes from category I22 should only be assigned if both the initial and subsequent myocardial infarctions are type 1 or unspecified.

5) Other Types of Myocardial Infarction

The ICD-10-CM provides codes for different types of myocardial infarction. Type 1 myocardial infarctions are assigned to codes I21.0-I21.4 **and I21.9**.

Type 2 myocardial infarction (myocardial infarction due to demand ischemia or secondary to ischemic balance), is assigned to code I21.A1, Myocardial infarction type 2 with a code for the underlying cause. Do not assign code I24.8, Other forms of acute ischemic heart disease, for the demand ischemia. Sequencing of type 2 AMI or the underlying cause is dependent on the circumstances of admission. When a type 2 AMI code is described as NSTEMI or STEMI, only assign code I21.A1. Codes I21.01-I21.4 should only be assigned for type 1 AMIs.

Acute myocardial infarctions type 3, 4a, 4b, 4c and 5 are assigned to code I21.A9, Other myocardial infarction type.

The "Code also" and "Code first" notes should be followed related to complications, and for coding of postprocedural myocardial infarctions during or following cardiac surgery.

10. Chapter 10: Diseases of the Respiratory System (J00-J99)

a. Chronic Obstructive Pulmonary Disease [COPD] and Asthma

1) Acute exacerbation of chronic obstructive bronchitis and asthma

The codes in categories J44 and J45 distinguish between uncomplicated cases and those in acute exacerbation. An acute exacerbation is a worsening or a decompensation of a chronic condition. An acute exacerbation is not equivalent to an infection superimposed on a chronic condition, though an exacerbation may be triggered by an infection.

b. Acute Respiratory Failure

1) Acute respiratory failure as principal diagnosis

A code from subcategory J96.0, Acute respiratory failure, or subcategory J96.2, Acute and chronic respiratory failure, may be assigned as a principal diagnosis when it is the condition established after study to be chiefly responsible for occasioning the admission to the hospital, and the selection is supported by the Alphabetic Index and Tabular List. However, chapter-specific coding guidelines (such as obstetrics, poisoning, HIV, newborn) that provide sequencing direction take precedence.

2) Acute respiratory failure as secondary diagnosis

Respiratory failure may be listed as a secondary diagnosis if it occurs after admission, or if it is present on admission, but does not meet the definition of principal diagnosis.

3) Sequencing of acute respiratory failure and another acute condition

When a patient is admitted with respiratory failure and another acute condition, (e.g., myocardial infarction, cerebrovascular accident, aspiration pneumonia), the principal diagnosis will not be the same in every situation. This applies whether the other acute condition is a respiratory or nonrespiratory condition. Selection of the principal diagnosis will be dependent on the circumstances of admission. If both the respiratory failure and the other acute condition are equally responsible for occasioning the admission to the hospital, and there are no chapter-specific sequencing rules, the guideline regarding two or more diagnoses that equally meet the definition for principal diagnosis *(Section II, C.)* may be applied in these situations.

If the documentation is not clear as to whether acute respiratory failure and another condition are equally responsible for occasioning the admission, query the provider for clarification.

c. Influenza due to certain identified influenza viruses

Code only confirmed cases of influenza due to certain identified influenza viruses (category J09), and due to other identified influenza

virus (category J1Ø). This is an exception to the hospital inpatient guideline Section II, H. (Uncertain Diagnosis).

In this context, "confirmation" does not require documentation of positive laboratory testing specific for avian or other novel influenza A or other identified influenza virus. However, coding should be based on the provider's diagnostic statement that the patient has avian influenza, or other novel influenza A, for category JØ9, or has another particular identified strain of influenza, such as H1N1 or H3N2, but not identified as novel or variant, for category J1Ø.

If the provider records "suspected" or "possible" or "probable" avian influenza, or novel influenza, or other identified influenza, then the appropriate influenza code from category J11, Influenza due to unidentified influenza virus, should be assigned. A code from category JØ9, Influenza due to certain identified influenza viruses, should not be assigned nor should a code from category J1Ø, Influenza due to other identified influenza virus.

d. Ventilator associated Pneumonia

1) Documentation of Ventilator associated Pneumonia
As with all procedural or postprocedural complications, code assignment is based on the provider's documentation of the relationship between the condition and the procedure.

Code J95.851, Ventilator associated pneumonia, should be assigned only when the provider has documented ventilator associated pneumonia (VAP). An additional code to identify the organism (e.g., Pseudomonas aeruginosa, code B96.5) should also be assigned. Do not assign an additional code from categories J12-J18 to identify the type of pneumonia.

Code J95.851 should not be assigned for cases where the patient has pneumonia and is on a mechanical ventilator and the provider has not specifically stated that the pneumonia is ventilator-associated pneumonia. If the documentation is unclear as to whether the patient has a pneumonia that is a complication attributable to the mechanical ventilator, query the provider.

2) Ventilator associated Pneumonia Develops after Admission
A patient may be admitted with one type of pneumonia (e.g., code J13, Pneumonia due to Streptococcus pneumonia) and subsequently develop VAP. In this instance, the principal diagnosis would be the appropriate code from categories J12-J18 for the pneumonia diagnosed at the time of admission. Code J95.851, Ventilator associated pneumonia, would be assigned as an additional diagnosis when the provider has also documented the presence of ventilator associated pneumonia.

11. Chapter 11: Diseases of the Digestive System (KØØ-K95)
Reserved for future guideline expansion

12. Chapter 12: Diseases of the Skin and Subcutaneous Tissue (LØØ-L99)
a. Pressure ulcer stage codes
1) Pressure ulcer stages
Codes from category L89, Pressure ulcer, identify the site of the pressure ulcer as well as the stage of the ulcer.

The ICD-10-CM classifies pressure ulcer stages based on severity, which is designated by stages 1-4, unspecified stage and unstageable.

Assign as many codes from category L89 as needed to identify all the pressure ulcers the patient has, if applicable.

See Section I.B.14 for pressure ulcer stage documentation by clinicians other than patient's provider

2) Unstageable pressure ulcers
Assignment of the code for unstageable pressure ulcer (L89.--Ø) should be based on the clinical documentation. These codes are used for pressure ulcers whose stage cannot be clinically determined (e.g., the ulcer is covered by eschar or has been treated with a skin or muscle graft) and pressure ulcers that are documented as deep tissue injury but not documented as due to trauma. This code should not be confused with the codes for unspecified stage (L89.--9). When there is no documentation regarding the stage of the pressure ulcer, assign the appropriate code for unspecified stage (L89.--9).

3) Documented pressure ulcer stage
Assignment of the pressure ulcer stage code should be guided by clinical documentation of the stage or documentation of the terms found in the Alphabetic Index. For clinical terms describing the stage that are not found in the Alphabetic Index, and there is no documentation of the stage, the provider should be queried.

4) Patients admitted with pressure ulcers documented as healed
No code is assigned if the documentation states that the pressure ulcer is completely healed.

5) Patients admitted with pressure ulcers documented as healing
Pressure ulcers described as healing should be assigned the appropriate pressure ulcer stage code based on the documentation in the medical record. If the documentation does not provide information about the stage of the healing pressure ulcer, assign the appropriate code for unspecified stage.

If the documentation is unclear as to whether the patient has a current (new) pressure ulcer or if the patient is being treated for a healing pressure ulcer, query the provider.

For ulcers that were present on admission but healed at the time of discharge, assign the code for the site and stage of the pressure ulcer at the time of admission.

6) Patient admitted with pressure ulcer evolving into another stage during the admission
If a patient is admitted to an inpatient hospital with a pressure ulcer at one stage and it progresses to a higher stage, two separate codes should be assigned: one code for the site and stage of the ulcer on admission and a second code for the same ulcer site and the highest stage reported during the stay.

b. Non-Pressure Chronic Ulcers
1) Patients admitted with non-pressure ulcers documented as healed
No code is assigned if the documentation states that the non-pressure ulcer is completely healed.

2) Patients admitted with non-pressure ulcers documented as healing
Non-pressure ulcers described as healing should be assigned the appropriate non-pressure ulcer code based on the documentation in the medical record. If the documentation does not provide information about the severity of the healing non-pressure ulcer, assign the appropriate code for unspecified severity.

If the documentation is unclear as to whether the patient has a current (new) non-pressure ulcer or if the patient is being treated for a healing non-pressure ulcer, query the provider.

For ulcers that were present on admission but healed at the time of discharge, assign the code for the site and severity of the non-pressure ulcer at the time of admission.

3) Patient admitted with non-pressure ulcer that progresses to another severity level during the admission
If a patient is admitted to an inpatient hospital with a non-pressure ulcer at one severity level and it progresses to a higher severity level, two separate codes should be assigned: one code for the site and severity level of the ulcer on admission and a second code for the same ulcer site and the highest severity level reported during the stay.

See Section I.B.14 for pressure ulcer stage documentation by clinicians other than patient's provider

13. Chapter 13: Diseases of the Musculoskeletal System and Connective Tissue (MØØ-M99)
a. Site and laterality
Most of the codes within Chapter 13 have site and laterality designations. The site represents the bone, joint or the muscle involved. For some conditions where more than one bone, joint or muscle is usually involved, such as osteoarthritis, there is a "multiple sites" code available. For categories where no multiple site code is provided and more than one bone, joint or muscle is involved, multiple codes should be used to indicate the different sites involved.

1) Bone versus joint
For certain conditions, the bone may be affected at the upper or lower end, (e.g., avascular necrosis of bone, M87, Osteoporosis, M8Ø, M81). Though the portion of the bone affected may be at the joint, the site designation will be the bone, not the joint.

b. Acute traumatic versus chronic or recurrent musculoskeletal conditions
Many musculoskeletal conditions are a result of previous injury or trauma to a site, or are recurrent conditions. Bone, joint or muscle conditions that are the result of a healed injury are usually found in chapter 13. Recurrent bone, joint or muscle conditions are also usually

found in chapter 13. Any current, acute injury should be coded to the appropriate injury code from chapter 19. Chronic or recurrent conditions should generally be coded with a code from chapter 13. If it is difficult to determine from the documentation in the record which code is best to describe a condition, query the provider.

c. Coding of Pathologic Fractures

7th character A is for use as long as the patient is receiving active treatment for the fracture. While the patient may be seen by a new or different provider over the course of treatment for a pathological fracture, assignment of the 7th character is based on whether the patient is undergoing active treatment and not whether the provider is seeing the patient for the first time.

7th character D is to be used for encounters after the patient has completed active treatment for the fracture and is receiving routine care for the fracture during the healing or recovery phase. The other 7th characters, listed under each subcategory in the Tabular List, are to be used for subsequent encounters for treatment of problems associated with the healing, such as malunions, nonunions, and sequelae.

Care for complications of surgical treatment for fracture repairs during the healing or recovery phase should be coded with the appropriate complication codes.

See Section I.C.19. Coding of traumatic fractures.

d. Osteoporosis

Osteoporosis is a systemic condition, meaning that all bones of the musculoskeletal system are affected. Therefore, site is not a component of the codes under category M81, Osteoporosis without current pathological fracture. The site codes under category M80, Osteoporosis with current pathological fracture, identify the site of the fracture, not the osteoporosis.

1) Osteoporosis without pathological fracture

Category M81, Osteoporosis without current pathological fracture, is for use for patients with osteoporosis who do not currently have a pathologic fracture due to the osteoporosis, even if they have had a fracture in the past. For patients with a history of osteoporosis fractures, status code Z87.310, Personal history of (healed) osteoporosis fracture, should follow the code from M81.

2) Osteoporosis with current pathological fracture

Category M80, Osteoporosis with current pathological fracture, is for patients who have a current pathologic fracture at the time of an encounter. The codes under M80 identify the site of the fracture. A code from category M80, not a traumatic fracture code, should be used for any patient with known osteoporosis who suffers a fracture, even if the patient had a minor fall or trauma, if that fall or trauma would not usually break a normal, healthy bone.

14. Chapter 14: Diseases of Genitourinary System (N00-N99)

a. Chronic kidney disease

1) Stages of chronic kidney disease (CKD)

The ICD-10-CM classifies CKD based on severity. The severity of CKD is designated by stages 1-5. Stage 2, code N18.2, equates to mild CKD; stage 3, code N18.3, equates to moderate CKD; and stage 4, code N18.4, equates to severe CKD. Code N18.6, End stage renal disease (ESRD), is assigned when the provider has documented end-stage-renal disease (ESRD).

If both a stage of CKD and ESRD are documented, assign code N18.6 only.

2) Chronic kidney disease and kidney transplant status

Patients who have undergone kidney transplant may still have some form of chronic kidney disease (CKD) because the kidney transplant may not fully restore kidney function. Therefore, the presence of CKD alone does not constitute a transplant complication. Assign the appropriate N18 code for the patient's stage of CKD and code Z94.0, Kidney transplant status. If a transplant complication such as failure or rejection or other transplant complication is documented, see section I.C.19.g for information on coding complications of a kidney transplant. If the documentation is unclear as to whether the patient has a complication of the transplant, query the provider.

3) Chronic kidney disease with other conditions

Patients with CKD may also suffer from other serious conditions, most commonly diabetes mellitus and hypertension. The sequencing of the CKD code in relationship to codes for other

contributing conditions is based on the conventions in the Tabular List.

See I.C.9. Hypertensive chronic kidney disease.

See I.C.19. Chronic kidney disease and kidney transplant complications.

15. Chapter 15: Pregnancy, Childbirth, and the Puerperium (O00-O9A)

a. General Rules for Obstetric Cases

1) Codes from chapter 15 and sequencing priority

Obstetric cases require codes from chapter 15, codes in the range O00-O9A, Pregnancy, Childbirth, and the Puerperium. Chapter 15 codes have sequencing priority over codes from other chapters. Additional codes from other chapters may be used in conjunction with chapter 15 codes to further specify conditions. Should the provider document that the pregnancy is incidental to the encounter, then code Z33.1, Pregnant state, incidental, should be used in place of any chapter 15 codes. It is the provider's responsibility to state that the condition being treated is not affecting the pregnancy.

2) Chapter 15 codes used only on the maternal record

Chapter 15 codes are to be used only on the maternal record, never on the record of the newborn.

3) Final character for trimester

The majority of codes in Chapter 15 have a final character indicating the trimester of pregnancy. The timeframes for the trimesters are indicated at the beginning of the chapter. If trimester is not a component of a code, it is because the condition always occurs in a specific trimester, or the concept of trimester of pregnancy is not applicable. Certain codes have characters for only certain trimesters because the condition does not occur in all trimesters, but it may occur in more than just one.

Assignment of the final character for trimester should be based on the provider's documentation of the trimester (or number of weeks) for the current admission/encounter. This applies to the assignment of trimester for pre-existing conditions as well as those that develop during or are due to the pregnancy. The provider's documentation of the number of weeks may be used to assign the appropriate code identifying the trimester.

Whenever delivery occurs during the current admission, and there is an "in childbirth" option for the obstetric complication being coded, the "in childbirth" code should be assigned.

4) Selection of trimester for inpatient admissions that encompass more than one trimester

In instances when a patient is admitted to a hospital for complications of pregnancy during one trimester and remains in the hospital into a subsequent trimester, the trimester character for the antepartum complication code should be assigned on the basis of the trimester when the complication developed, not the trimester of the discharge. If the condition developed prior to the current admission/encounter or represents a pre-existing condition, the trimester character for the trimester at the time of the admission/encounter should be assigned.

5) Unspecified trimester

Each category that includes codes for trimester has a code for "unspecified trimester." The "unspecified trimester" code should rarely be used, such as when the documentation in the record is insufficient to determine the trimester and it is not possible to obtain clarification.

6) 7th character for Fetus Identification

Where applicable, a 7th character is to be assigned for certain categories (O31, O32, O33.3 - O33.6, O35, O36, O40, O41, O60.1, O60.2, O64, and O69) to identify the fetus for which the complication code applies.

Assign 7th character "0":

- For single gestations
- When the documentation in the record is insufficient to determine the fetus affected and it is not possible to obtain clarification.
- When it is not possible to clinically determine which fetus is affected.

b. Selection of OB Principal or First-listed Diagnosis

1) Routine outpatient prenatal visits

For routine outpatient prenatal visits when no complications are present, a code from category Z34, Encounter for supervision of normal pregnancy, should be used as the first-listed diagnosis.

These codes should not be used in conjunction with chapter 15 codes.

2) Supervision of High-Risk Pregnancy
Codes from category O09, Supervision of high-risk pregnancy, are intended for use only during the prenatal period. For complications during the labor or delivery episode as a result of a high-risk pregnancy, assign the applicable complication codes from Chapter 15. If there are no complications during the labor or delivery episode, assign code O80, Encounter for full-term uncomplicated delivery.

For routine prenatal outpatient visits for patients with high-risk pregnancies, a code from category O09, Supervision of high-risk pregnancy, should be used as the first-listed diagnosis. Secondary chapter 15 codes may be used in conjunction with these codes if appropriate.

3) Episodes when no delivery occurs
In episodes when no delivery occurs, the principal diagnosis should correspond to the principal complication of the pregnancy which necessitated the encounter. Should more than one complication exist, all of which are treated or monitored, any of the complications codes may be sequenced first.

4) When a delivery occurs
When an obstetric patient is admitted and delivers during that admission, the condition that prompted the admission should be sequenced as the principal diagnosis. If multiple conditions prompted the admission, sequence the one most related to the delivery as the principal diagnosis. A code for any complication of the delivery should be assigned as an additional diagnosis. In cases of cesarean delivery, if the patient was admitted with a condition that resulted in the performance of a cesarean procedure, that condition should be selected as the principal diagnosis. If the reason for the admission was unrelated to the condition resulting in the cesarean delivery, the condition related to the reason for the admission should be selected as the principal diagnosis.

5) Outcome of delivery
A code from category Z37, Outcome of delivery, should be included on every maternal record when a delivery has occurred. These codes are not to be used on subsequent records or on the newborn record.

c. Pre-existing conditions versus conditions due to the pregnancy
Certain categories in Chapter 15 distinguish between conditions of the mother that existed prior to pregnancy (pre-existing) and those that are a direct result of pregnancy. When assigning codes from Chapter 15, it is important to assess if a condition was pre-existing prior to pregnancy or developed during or due to the pregnancy in order to assign the correct code.

Categories that do not distinguish between pre-existing and pregnancy-related conditions may be used for either. It is acceptable to use codes specifically for the puerperium with codes complicating pregnancy and childbirth if a condition arises postpartum during the delivery encounter.

d. Pre-existing hypertension in pregnancy
Category O10, Pre-existing hypertension complicating pregnancy, childbirth and the puerperium, includes codes for hypertensive heart and hypertensive chronic kidney disease. When assigning one of the O10 codes that includes hypertensive heart disease or hypertensive chronic kidney disease, it is necessary to add a secondary code from the appropriate hypertension category to specify the type of heart failure or chronic kidney disease.

See Section I.C.9. Hypertension.

e. Fetal Conditions Affecting the Management of the Mother
1) Codes from categories O35 and O36
Codes from categories O35, Maternal care for known or suspected fetal abnormality and damage, and O36, Maternal care for other fetal problems, are assigned only when the fetal condition is actually responsible for modifying the management of the mother, i.e., by requiring diagnostic studies, additional observation, special care, or termination of pregnancy. The fact that the fetal condition exists does not justify assigning a code from this series to the mother's record.

2) In utero surgery
In cases when surgery is performed on the fetus, a diagnosis code from category O35, Maternal care for known or suspected fetal abnormality and damage, should be assigned identifying the

fetal condition. Assign the appropriate procedure code for the procedure performed.

No code from Chapter 16, the perinatal codes, should be used on the mother's record to identify fetal conditions. Surgery performed in utero on a fetus is still to be coded as an obstetric encounter.

f. HIV Infection in Pregnancy, Childbirth and the Puerperium
During pregnancy, childbirth or the puerperium, a patient admitted because of an HIV-related illness should receive a principal diagnosis from subcategory O98.7-, Human immunodeficiency [HIV] disease complicating pregnancy, childbirth and the puerperium, followed by the code(s) for the HIV-related illness(es).

Patients with asymptomatic HIV infection status admitted during pregnancy, childbirth, or the puerperium should receive codes of O98.7- and Z21, Asymptomatic human immunodeficiency virus [HIV] infection status.

g. Diabetes mellitus in pregnancy
Diabetes mellitus is a significant complicating factor in pregnancy. Pregnant women who are diabetic should be assigned a code from category O24, Diabetes mellitus in pregnancy, childbirth, and the puerperium, first, followed by the appropriate diabetes code(s) (E08-E13) from Chapter 4.

h. Long term use of insulin and oral hypoglycemics
See section I.C.4.a.3 for information on the long term use of insulin and oral hypoglycemic.

i. Gestational (pregnancy induced) diabetes
Gestational (pregnancy induced) diabetes can occur during the second and third trimester of pregnancy in women who were not diabetic prior to pregnancy. Gestational diabetes can cause complications in the pregnancy similar to those of pre-existing diabetes mellitus. It also puts the woman at greater risk of developing diabetes after the pregnancy. Codes for gestational diabetes are in subcategory O24.4, Gestational diabetes mellitus. No other code from category O24, Diabetes mellitus in pregnancy, childbirth, and the puerperium, should be used with a code from O24.4.

The codes under subcategory O24.4 include diet controlled, insulin controlled, and controlled by oral hypoglycemic drugs. If a patient with gestational diabetes is treated with both diet and insulin, only the code for insulin-controlled is required. If a patient with gestational diabetes is treated with both diet and oral hypoglycemic medications, only the code for "controlled by oral hypoglycemic drugs" is required. Code Z79.4, Long-term (current) use of insulin or code Z79.84, Long-term (current) use of oral hypoglycemic drugs, should not be assigned with codes from subcategory O24.4.

An abnormal glucose tolerance in pregnancy is assigned a code from subcategory O99.81, Abnormal glucose complicating pregnancy, childbirth, and the puerperium.

j. Sepsis and septic shock complicating abortion, pregnancy, childbirth and the puerperium
When assigning a chapter 15 code for sepsis complicating abortion, pregnancy, childbirth, and the puerperium, a code for the specific type of infection should be assigned as an additional diagnosis. If severe sepsis is present, a code from subcategory R65.2, Severe sepsis, and code(s) for associated organ dysfunction(s) should also be assigned as additional diagnoses.

k. Puerperal sepsis
Code O85, Puerperal sepsis, should be assigned with a secondary code to identify the causal organism (e.g., for a bacterial infection, assign a code from category B95-B96, Bacterial infections in conditions classified elsewhere). A code from category A40, Streptococcal sepsis, or A41, Other sepsis, should not be used for puerperal sepsis. If applicable, use additional codes to identify severe sepsis (R65.2-) and any associated acute organ dysfunction.

l. Alcohol, tobacco *and drug* use during pregnancy, childbirth and the puerperium
1) Alcohol use during pregnancy, childbirth and the puerperium
Codes under subcategory O99.31, Alcohol use complicating pregnancy, childbirth, and the puerperium, should be assigned for any pregnancy case when a mother uses alcohol during the pregnancy or postpartum. A secondary code from category F10, Alcohol related disorders, should also be assigned to identify manifestations of the alcohol use.

2) Tobacco use during pregnancy, childbirth and the puerperium

Codes under subcategory O99.33, Smoking (tobacco) complicating pregnancy, childbirth, and the puerperium, should be assigned for any pregnancy case when a mother uses any type of tobacco product during the pregnancy or postpartum. A secondary code from category F17, Nicotine dependence, should also be assigned to identify the type of nicotine dependence.

3) Drug use during pregnancy, childbirth and the puerperium

Codes under subcategory O99.32, Drug use complicating pregnancy, childbirth, and the puerperium, should be assigned for any pregnancy case when a mother uses drugs during the pregnancy or postpartum. This can involve illegal drugs, or inappropriate use or abuse of prescription drugs. Secondary code(s) from categories F11-F16 and F18-F19 should also be assigned to identify manifestations of the drug use.

m. Poisoning, toxic effects, adverse effects and underdosing in a pregnant patient

A code from subcategory O9A.2, Injury, poisoning and certain other consequences of external causes complicating pregnancy, childbirth, and the puerperium, should be sequenced first, followed by the appropriate injury, poisoning, toxic effect, adverse effect or underdosing code, and then the additional code(s) that specifies the condition caused by the poisoning, toxic effect, adverse effect or underdosing.

See Section I.C.19. Adverse effects, poisoning, underdosing and toxic effects.

n. Normal Delivery, Code O80

1) Encounter for full term uncomplicated delivery

Code O80 should be assigned when a woman is admitted for a full-term normal delivery and delivers a single, healthy infant without any complications antepartum, during the delivery, or postpartum during the delivery episode. Code O80 is always a principal diagnosis. It is not to be used if any other code from chapter 15 is needed to describe a current complication of the antenatal, delivery, or perinatal period. Additional codes from other chapters may be used with code O80 if they are not related to or are in any way complicating the pregnancy.

2) Uncomplicated delivery with resolved antepartum complication

Code O80 may be used if the patient had a complication at some point during the pregnancy, but the complication is not present at the time of the admission for delivery.

3) Outcome of delivery for O80

Z37.0, Single live birth, is the only outcome of delivery code appropriate for use with O80.

o. The Peripartum and Postpartum Periods

1) Peripartum and Postpartum periods

The postpartum period begins immediately after delivery and continues for six weeks following delivery. The peripartum period is defined as the last month of pregnancy to five months postpartum.

2) Peripartum and postpartum complication

A postpartum complication is any complication occurring within the six-week period.

3) Pregnancy-related complications after 6 week period

Chapter 15 codes may also be used to describe pregnancy-related complications after the peripartum or postpartum period if the provider documents that a condition is pregnancy related.

4) Admission for routine postpartum care following delivery outside hospital

When the mother delivers outside the hospital prior to admission and is admitted for routine postpartum care and no complications are noted, code Z39.0, Encounter for care and examination of mother immediately after delivery, should be assigned as the principal diagnosis.

5) Pregnancy associated cardiomyopathy

Pregnancy associated cardiomyopathy, code O90.3, is unique in that it may be diagnosed in the third trimester of pregnancy but may continue to progress months after delivery. For this reason, it is referred to as peripartum cardiomyopathy. Code O90.3 is only for use when the cardiomyopathy develops as a result of pregnancy in a woman who did not have pre-existing heart disease.

p. Code O94, Sequelae of complication of pregnancy, childbirth, and the puerperium

1) Code O94

Code O94, Sequelae of complication of pregnancy, childbirth, and the puerperium, is for use in those cases when an initial complication of a pregnancy develops a sequelae requiring care or treatment at a future date.

2) After the initial postpartum period

This code may be used at any time after the initial postpartum period.

3) Sequencing of Code O94

This code, like all sequela codes, is to be sequenced following the code describing the sequelae of the complication.

q. Termination of Pregnancy and Spontaneous abortions

1) Abortion with Liveborn Fetus

When an attempted termination of pregnancy results in a liveborn fetus, assign code Z33.2, Encounter for elective termination of pregnancy and a code from category Z37, Outcome of Delivery.

2) Retained Products of Conception following an abortion

Subsequent encounters for retained products of conception following a spontaneous abortion or elective termination of pregnancy, without complications are assigned O03.4, Incomplete spontaneous abortion without complication, or code O07.4, Failed attempted termination of pregnancy without complication. This advice is appropriate even when the patient was discharged previously with a discharge diagnosis of complete abortion. If the patient has a specific complication associated with the spontaneous abortion or elective termination of pregnancy in addition to retained products of conception, assign the appropriate complication in category O03 or O07 instead of code O03.4 or O07.4

3) Complications leading to abortion

Codes from Chapter 15 may be used as additional codes to identify any documented complications of the pregnancy in conjunction with codes in categories in O04, O07 and O08.

r. Abuse in a pregnant patient

For suspected or confirmed cases of abuse of a pregnant patient, a code(s) from subcategories O9A.3, Physical abuse complicating pregnancy, childbirth, and the puerperium, O9A.4, Sexual abuse complicating pregnancy, childbirth, and the puerperium, and O9A.5, Psychological abuse complicating pregnancy, childbirth, and the puerperium, should be sequenced first, followed by the appropriate codes (if applicable) to identify any associated current injury due to physical abuse, sexual abuse, and the perpetrator of abuse.

See Section I.C.19. Adult and child abuse, neglect and other maltreatment.

16. Chapter 16: Certain Conditions Originating in the Perinatal Period (P00-P96)

For coding and reporting purposes the perinatal period is defined as before birth through the 28th day following birth. The following guidelines are provided for reporting purposes.

a. General Perinatal Rules

1) Use of Chapter 16 Codes

Codes in this chapter are never for use on the maternal record. Codes from Chapter 15, the obstetric chapter, are never permitted on the newborn record. Chapter 16 codes may be used throughout the life of the patient if the condition is still present.

2) Principal Diagnosis for Birth Record

When coding the birth episode in a newborn record, assign a code from category Z38, Liveborn infants according to place of birth and type of delivery, as the principal diagnosis. A code from category Z38 is assigned only once, to a newborn at the time of birth. If a newborn is transferred to another institution, a code from category Z38 should not be used at the receiving hospital.

A code from category Z38 is used only on the newborn record, not on the mother's record.

3) Use of Codes from other Chapters with Codes from Chapter 16

Codes from other chapters may be used with codes from chapter 16 if the codes from the other chapters provide more specific detail. Codes for signs and symptoms may be assigned when a definitive diagnosis has not been established. If the reason for the encounter is a perinatal condition, the code from chapter 16 should be sequenced first.

4) **Use of Chapter 16 Codes after the Perinatal Period**
Should a condition originate in the perinatal period, and continue throughout the life of the patient, the perinatal code should continue to be used regardless of the patient's age.

5) **Birth process or community acquired conditions**
If a newborn has a condition that may be either due to the birth process or community acquired and the documentation does not indicate which it is, the default is due to the birth process and the code from Chapter 16 should be used. If the condition is community-acquired, a code from Chapter 16 should not be assigned.

6) **Code all clinically significant conditions**
All clinically significant conditions noted on routine newborn examination should be coded. A condition is clinically significant if it requires:

- clinical evaluation; or
- therapeutic treatment; or
- diagnostic procedures; or
- extended length of hospital stay; or
- increased nursing care and/or monitoring; or
- has implications for future health care needs

Note: The perinatal guidelines listed above are the same as the general coding guidelines for "additional diagnoses", except for the final point regarding implications for future health care needs. Codes should be assigned for conditions that have been specified by the provider as having implications for future health care needs.

b. **Observation and Evaluation of Newborns for Suspected Conditions not Found**

1) **Use of Z05 codes**
Assign a code from category Z05, Observation and evaluation of newborns and infants for suspected conditions ruled out, to identify those instances when a healthy newborn is evaluated for a suspected condition that is determined after study not to be present. Do not use a code from category Z05 when the patient has identified signs or symptoms of a suspected problem; in such cases code the sign or symptom.

2) **Z05 on Other than the Birth Record**
A code from category Z05 may also be assigned as a principal or first-listed code for readmissions or encounters when the code from category Z38 code no longer applies. Codes from category Z05 are for use only for healthy newborns and infants for which no condition after study is found to be present.

3) **Z05 on a birth record**
A code from category Z05 is to be used as a secondary code after the code from category Z38, Liveborn infants according to place of birth and type of delivery.

c. **Coding Additional Perinatal Diagnoses**

1) **Assigning codes for conditions that require treatment**
Assign codes for conditions that require treatment or further investigation, prolong the length of stay, or require resource utilization.

2) **Codes for conditions specified as having implications for future health care needs**
Assign codes for conditions that have been specified by the provider as having implications for future health care needs.
Note: This guideline should not be used for adult patients.

d. **Prematurity and Fetal Growth Retardation**
Providers utilize different criteria in determining prematurity. A code for prematurity should not be assigned unless it is documented. Assignment of codes in categories P05, Disorders of newborn related to slow fetal growth and fetal malnutrition, and P07, Disorders of newborn related to short gestation and low birth weight, not elsewhere classified, should be based on the recorded birth weight and estimated gestational age.

When both birth weight and gestational age are available, two codes from category P07 should be assigned, with the code for birth weight sequenced before the code for gestational age.

e. **Low birth weight and immaturity status**
Codes from category P07, Disorders of newborn related to short gestation and low birth weight, not elsewhere classified, are for use for a child or adult who was premature or had a low birth weight as a newborn and this is affecting the patient's current health status.

See Section I.C.21. Factors influencing health status and contact with health services, Status.

f. **Bacterial Sepsis of Newborn**
Category P36, Bacterial sepsis of newborn, includes congenital sepsis. If a perinate is documented as having sepsis without documentation of congenital or community acquired, the default is congenital and a code from category P36 should be assigned. If the P36 code includes the causal organism, an additional code from category B95, Streptococcus, Staphylococcus, and Enterococcus as the cause of diseases classified elsewhere, or B96, Other bacterial agents as the cause of diseases classified elsewhere, should not be assigned. If the P36 code does not include the causal organism, assign an additional code from category B96. If applicable, use additional codes to identify severe sepsis (R65.2-) and any associated acute organ dysfunction.

g. **Stillbirth**
Code P95, Stillbirth, is only for use in institutions that maintain separate records for stillbirths. No other code should be used with P95. Code P95 should not be used on the mother's record.

17. **Chapter 17: Congenital malformations, deformations, and chromosomal abnormalities (Q00-Q99)**
Assign an appropriate code(s) from categories Q00-Q99, Congenital malformations, deformations, and chromosomal abnormalities when a malformation/deformation or chromosomal abnormality is documented. A malformation/deformation/or chromosomal abnormality may be the principal/first-listed diagnosis on a record or a secondary diagnosis.

When a malformation/deformation or chromosomal abnormality does not have a unique code assignment, assign additional code(s) for any manifestations that may be present.

When the code assignment specifically identifies the malformation/deformation or chromosomal abnormality, manifestations that are an inherent component of the anomaly should not be coded separately. Additional codes should be assigned for manifestations that are not an inherent component.

Codes from Chapter 17 may be used throughout the life of the patient. If a congenital malformation or deformity has been corrected, a personal history code should be used to identify the history of the malformation or deformity. Although present at birth, malformation/deformation/or chromosomal abnormality may not be identified until later in life. Whenever the condition is diagnosed by the physician, it is appropriate to assign a code from codes Q00-Q99. For the birth admission, the appropriate code from category Z38, Liveborn infants, according to place of birth and type of delivery, should be sequenced as the principal diagnosis, followed by any congenital anomaly codes, Q00-Q99.

18. **Chapter 18: Symptoms, signs, and abnormal clinical and laboratory findings, not elsewhere classified (R00-R99)**
Chapter 18 includes symptoms, signs, abnormal results of clinical or other investigative procedures, and ill-defined conditions regarding which no diagnosis classifiable elsewhere is recorded. Signs and symptoms that point to a specific diagnosis have been assigned to a category in other chapters of the classification.

a. **Use of symptom codes**
Codes that describe symptoms and signs are acceptable for reporting purposes when a related definitive diagnosis has not been established (confirmed) by the provider.

b. **Use of a symptom code with a definitive diagnosis code**
Codes for signs and symptoms may be reported in addition to a related definitive diagnosis when the sign or symptom is not routinely associated with that diagnosis, such as the various signs and symptoms associated with complex syndromes. The definitive diagnosis code should be sequenced before the symptom code.

Signs or symptoms that are associated routinely with a disease process should not be assigned as additional codes, unless otherwise instructed by the classification.

c. **Combination codes that include symptoms**
ICD-10-CM contains a number of combination codes that identify both the definitive diagnosis and common symptoms of that diagnosis.

When using one of these combination codes, an additional code should not be assigned for the symptom.

d. **Repeated falls**
Code R29.6, Repeated falls, is for use for encounters when a patient has recently fallen and the reason for the fall is being investigated.

Code Z91.81, History of falling, is for use when a patient has fallen in the past and is at risk for future falls. When appropriate, both codes R29.6 and Z91.81 may be assigned together.

e. Coma scale

The coma scale codes (R40.2-) can be used in conjunction with traumatic brain injury codes, acute cerebrovascular disease or sequelae of cerebrovascular disease codes. These codes are primarily for use by trauma registries, but they may be used in any setting where this information is collected. The coma scale may also be used to assess the status of the central nervous system for other non-trauma conditions, such as monitoring patients in the intensive care unit regardless of medical condition. The coma scale codes should be sequenced after the diagnosis code(s).

These codes, one from each subcategory, are needed to complete the scale. The 7th character indicates when the scale was recorded. The 7th character should match for all three codes.

At a minimum, report the initial score documented on presentation at your facility. This may be a score from the emergency medicine technician (EMT) or in the emergency department. If desired, a facility may choose to capture multiple coma scale scores.

Assign code R40.24, Glasgow coma scale, total score, when only the total score is documented in the medical record and not the individual score(s).

Do not report codes for individual or total Glasgow coma scale scores for a patient with a medically induced coma or a sedated patient.

See Section I.B.14 for coma scale documentation by clinicians other than patient's provider

f. Functional quadriplegia

GUIDELINE HAS BEEN DELETED EFFECTIVE OCTOBER 1, 2017

g. SIRS due to Non-Infectious Process

The systemic inflammatory response syndrome (SIRS) can develop as a result of certain non-infectious disease processes, such as trauma, malignant neoplasm, or pancreatitis. When SIRS is documented with a noninfectious condition, and no subsequent infection is documented, the code for the underlying condition, such as an injury, should be assigned, followed by code R65.10, Systemic inflammatory response syndrome (SIRS) of non-infectious origin without acute organ dysfunction, or code R65.11, Systemic inflammatory response syndrome (SIRS) of non-infectious origin with acute organ dysfunction. If an associated acute organ dysfunction is documented, the appropriate code(s) for the specific type of organ dysfunction(s) should be assigned in addition to code R65.11. If acute organ dysfunction is documented, but it cannot be determined if the acute organ dysfunction is associated with SIRS or due to another condition (e.g., directly due to the trauma), the provider should be queried.

h. Death NOS

Code R99, Ill-defined and unknown cause of mortality, is only for use in the very limited circumstance when a patient who has already died is brought into an emergency department or other healthcare facility and is pronounced dead upon arrival. It does not represent the discharge disposition of death.

i. NIHSS Stroke Scale

The NIH stroke scale (NIHSS) codes (R29.7- -) can be used in conjunction with acute stroke codes (I63) to identify the patient's neurological status and the severity of the stroke. The stroke scale codes should be sequenced after the acute stroke diagnosis code(s).

At a minimum, report the initial score documented. If desired, a facility may choose to capture multiple stroke scale scores.

See Section I.B.14 for NIHSS stroke scale documentation by clinicians other than patient's provider

19. Chapter 19: Injury, poisoning, and certain other consequences of external causes (S00-T88)

a. Application of 7th Characters in Chapter 19

Most categories in chapter 19 have a 7th character requirement for each applicable code. Most categories in this chapter have three 7th character values (with the exception of fractures): A, initial encounter, D, subsequent encounter and S, sequela. Categories for traumatic fractures have additional 7th character values. While the patient may be seen by a new or different provider over the course of treatment for an injury, assignment of the 7th character is based on whether the patient is undergoing active treatment and not whether the provider is seeing the patient for the first time.

For complication codes, active treatment refers to treatment for the condition described by the code, even though it may be related to an earlier precipitating problem. For example, code T84.50XA, Infection and inflammatory reaction due to unspecified internal joint prosthesis, initial encounter, is used when active treatment is provided for the infection, even though the condition relates to the prosthetic device, implant or graft that was placed at a previous encounter.

7th character "A", initial encounter is used for each encounter where the patient is receiving active treatment for the condition.

7th character "D" subsequent encounter is used for encounters after the patient has completed active treatment of the condition and is receiving routine care for the condition during the healing or recovery phase.

The aftercare Z codes should not be used for aftercare for conditions such as injuries or poisonings, where 7th characters are provided to identify subsequent care. For example, for aftercare of an injury, assign the acute injury code with the 7th character "D" (subsequent encounter).

7th character "S", sequela, is for use for complications or conditions that arise as a direct result of a condition, such as scar formation after a burn. The scars are sequelae of the burn. When using 7th character "S", it is necessary to use both the injury code that precipitated the sequela and the code for the sequela itself. The "S" is added only to the injury code, not the sequela code. The 7th character "S" identifies the injury responsible for the sequela. The specific type of sequela (e.g. scar) is sequenced first, followed by the injury code.

See Section I.B.10 Sequelae, (Late Effects)

b. Coding of Injuries

When coding injuries, assign separate codes for each injury unless a combination code is provided, in which case the combination code is assigned. Codes from category T07, Unspecified multiple injuries should not be assigned in the inpatient setting unless information for a more specific code is not available. Traumatic injury codes (S00-T14.9) are not to be used for normal, healing surgical wounds or to identify complications of surgical wounds.

The code for the most serious injury, as determined by the provider and the focus of treatment, is sequenced first.

1) Superficial injuries

Superficial injuries such as abrasions or contusions are not coded when associated with more severe injuries of the same site.

2) Primary injury with damage to nerves/blood vessels

When a primary injury results in minor damage to peripheral nerves or blood vessels, the primary injury is sequenced first with additional code(s) for injuries to nerves and spinal cord (such as category S04), and/or injury to blood vessels (such as category S15). When the primary injury is to the blood vessels or nerves, that injury should be sequenced first.

c. Coding of Traumatic Fractures

The principles of multiple coding of injuries should be followed in coding fractures. Fractures of specified sites are coded individually by site in accordance with both the provisions within categories S02, S12, S22, S32, S42, S49, S52, S59, S62, S72, S79, S82, S89, S92 and the level of detail furnished by medical record content.

A fracture not indicated as open or closed should be coded to closed. A fracture not indicated whether displaced or not displaced should be coded to displaced.

More specific guidelines are as follows:

1) Initial vs. Subsequent Encounter for Fractures

Traumatic fractures are coded using the appropriate 7th character for initial encounter (A, B, C) for each encounter where the patient is receiving active treatment for the fracture. The appropriate 7th character for initial encounter should also be assigned for a patient who delayed seeking treatment for the fracture or nonunion.

Fractures are coded using the appropriate 7th character for subsequent care for encounters after the patient has completed active treatment of the fracture and is receiving routine care for the fracture during the healing or recovery phase.

Care for complications of surgical treatment for fracture repairs during the healing or recovery phase should be coded with the appropriate complication codes.

Care of complications of fractures, such as malunion and nonunion, should be reported with the appropriate 7th character for subsequent care with nonunion (K, M, N,) or subsequent care with malunion (P, Q, R).

Malunion/nonunion: The appropriate 7th character for initial encounter should also be assigned for a patient who delayed seeking treatment for the fracture or nonunion.

The open fracture designations in the assignment of the 7th character for fractures of the forearm, femur and lower leg, including ankle are based on the Gustilo open fracture classification. When the Gustilo classification type is not specified for an open fracture, the 7th character for open fracture type I or II should be assigned (B, E, H, M, Q).

A code from category M80, not a traumatic fracture code, should be used for any patient with known osteoporosis who suffers a fracture, even if the patient had a minor fall or trauma, if that fall or trauma would not usually break a normal, healthy bone.

See Section I.C.13. Osteoporosis.

The aftercare Z codes should not be used for aftercare for traumatic fractures. For aftercare of a traumatic fracture, assign the acute fracture code with the appropriate 7th character.

2) **Multiple fractures sequencing**
   Multiple fractures are sequenced in accordance with the severity of the fracture.

d. **Coding of Burns and Corrosions**
   The ICD-10-CM makes a distinction between burns and corrosions. The burn codes are for thermal burns, except sunburns, that come from a heat source, such as a fire or hot appliance. The burn codes are also for burns resulting from electricity and radiation. Corrosions are burns due to chemicals. The guidelines are the same for burns and corrosions.

   Current burns (T20-T25) are classified by depth, extent and by agent (X code). Burns are classified by depth as first degree (erythema), second degree (blistering), and third degree (full-thickness involvement). Burns of the eye and internal organs (T26-T28) are classified by site, but not by degree.

   1) **Sequencing of burn and related condition codes**
      Sequence first the code that reflects the highest degree of burn when more than one burn is present.

      a. When the reason for the admission or encounter is for treatment of external multiple burns, sequence first the code that reflects the burn of the highest degree.

      b. When a patient has both internal and external burns, the circumstances of admission govern the selection of the principal diagnosis or first-listed diagnosis.

      c. When a patient is admitted for burn injuries and other related conditions such as smoke inhalation and/or respiratory failure, the circumstances of admission govern the selection of the principal or first-listed diagnosis.

   2) **Burns of the same *anatomic* site**
      Classify burns of the same **anatomic** site **and on the same side** but of different degrees to the subcategory identifying the highest degree recorded in the diagnosis **(e.g., for second and third degree burns of right thigh, assign only code T24.311-).**

   3) **Non-healing burns**
      Non-healing burns are coded as acute burns.
      Necrosis of burned skin should be coded as a non-healed burn.

   4) **Infected Burn**
      For any documented infected burn site, use an additional code for the infection.

   5) **Assign separate codes for each burn site**
      When coding burns, assign separate codes for each burn site. Category T30, Burn and corrosion, body region unspecified is extremely vague and should rarely be used.

      Codes for burns of "multiple sites" should only be assigned when the medical record documentation does not specify the individual sites.

   6) **Burns and Corrosions Classified According to Extent of Body Surface Involved**
      Assign codes from category T31, Burns classified according to extent of body surface involved, or T32, Corrosions classified according to extent of body surface involved, when the site of the burn is not specified or when there is a need for additional data. It is advisable to use category T31 as additional coding when needed to provide data for evaluating burn mortality, such as that needed by burn units. It is also advisable to use category T31 as an additional code for reporting purposes when there is

mention of a third-degree burn involving 20 percent or more of the body surface.

Categories T31 and T32 are based on the classic "rule of nines" in estimating body surface involved: head and neck are assigned nine percent, each arm nine percent, each leg 18 percent, the anterior trunk 18 percent, posterior trunk 18 percent, and genitalia one percent. Providers may change these percentage assignments where necessary to accommodate infants and children who have proportionately larger heads than adults, and patients who have large buttocks, thighs, or abdomen that involve burns.

7) **Encounters for treatment of sequela of burns**
   Encounters for the treatment of the late effects of burns or corrosions (i.e., scars or joint contractures) should be coded with a burn or corrosion code with the 7th character "S" for sequela.

8) **Sequelae with a late effect code and current burn**
   When appropriate, both a code for a current burn or corrosion with 7th character "A" or "D" and a burn or corrosion code with 7th character "S" may be assigned on the same record (when both a current burn and sequelae of an old burn exist). Burns and corrosions do not heal at the same rate and a current healing wound may still exist with sequela of a healed burn or corrosion.
   See Section I.B.10 Sequela (Late Effects)

9) **Use of an external cause code with burns and corrosions**
   An external cause code should be used with burns and corrosions to identify the source and intent of the burn, as well as the place where it occurred.

e. **Adverse Effects, Poisoning, Underdosing and Toxic Effects**
   Codes in categories T36-T65 are combination codes that include the substance that was taken as well as the intent. No additional external cause code is required for poisonings, toxic effects, adverse effects and underdosing codes.

   1) **Do not code directly from the Table of Drugs**
      Do not code directly funderdosinrom the Table of Drugs and Chemicals. Always refer back to the Tabular List.

   2) **Use as many codes as necessary to describe**
      Use as many codes as necessary to describe completely all drugs, medicinal or biological substances.

   3) **If the same code would describe the causative agent**
      If the same code would describe the causative agent for more than one adverse reaction, poisoning, toxic effect or underdosing, assign the code only once.

   4) **If two or more drugs, medicinal or biological substances**
      If two or more drugs, medicinal or biological substances are reported, code each individually unless a combination code is listed in the Table of Drugs and Chemicals.

   5) **The occurrence of drug toxicity is classified in ICD-10-CM as follows:**
      (a) **Adverse Effect**
          When coding an adverse effect of a drug that has been correctly prescribed and properly administered, assign the appropriate code for the nature of the adverse effect followed by the appropriate code for the adverse effect of the drug (T36-T50). The code for the drug should have a 5th or 6th character "5" (for example T36.0X5-) Examples of the nature of an adverse effect are tachycardia, delirium, gastrointestinal hemorrhaging, vomiting, hypokalemia, hepatitis, renal failure, or respiratory failure.

      (b) **Poisoning**
          When coding a poisoning or reaction to the improper use of a medication (e.g., overdose, wrong substance given or taken in error, wrong route of administration), first assign the appropriate code from categories T36-T50. The poisoning codes have an associated intent as their 5th or 6th character (accidental, intentional self-harm, assault and undetermined. If the intent of the poisoning is unknown or unspecified, code the intent as accidental intent. The undetermined intent is only for use if the documentation in the record specifies that the intent cannot be determined. Use additional code(s) for all manifestations of poisonings.

          If there is also a diagnosis of abuse or dependence of the substance, the abuse or dependence is assigned as an additional code.

          Examples of poisoning include:

(i) **Error was made in drug prescription**
Errors made in drug prescription or in the administration of the drug by provider, nurse, patient, or other person.

(ii) **Overdose of a drug intentionally taken**
If an overdose of a drug was intentionally taken or administered and resulted in drug toxicity, it would be coded as a poisoning.

(iii) **Nonprescribed drug taken with correctly prescribed and properly administered drug**
If a nonprescribed drug or medicinal agent was taken in combination with a correctly prescribed and properly administered drug, any drug toxicity or other reaction resulting from the interaction of the two drugs would be classified as a poisoning.

(iv) **Interaction of drug(s) and alcohol**
When a reaction results from the interaction of a drug(s) and alcohol, this would be classified as poisoning.

See Section I.C.4. if poisoning is the result of insulin pump malfunctions.

(c) **Underdosing**
Underdosing refers to taking less of a medication than is prescribed by a provider or a manufacturer's instruction. **Discontinuing the use of a prescribed medication on the patient's own initiative (not directed by the patient's provider) is also classified as an underdosing.** For underdosing, assign the code from categories T36-T50 (fifth or sixth character "6").

Codes for underdosing should never be assigned as principal or first-listed codes. If a patient has a relapse or exacerbation of the medical condition for which the drug is prescribed because of the reduction in dose, then the medical condition itself should be coded.

Noncompliance (Z91.12-, Z91.13- **and Z91.14-**) or complication of care (Y63.6-Y63.9) codes are to be used with an underdosing code to indicate intent, if known.

(d) **Toxic Effects**
When a harmful substance is ingested or comes in contact with a person, this is classified as a toxic effect. The toxic effect codes are in categories T51-T65.

Toxic effect codes have an associated intent: accidental, intentional self-harm, assault and undetermined.

f. **Adult and child abuse, neglect and other maltreatment**
Sequence first the appropriate code from categories T74, Adult and child abuse, neglect and other maltreatment, confirmed) or T76, Adult and child abuse, neglect and other maltreatment, suspected) for abuse, neglect and other maltreatment, followed by any accompanying mental health or injury code(s).

If the documentation in the medical record states abuse or neglect it is coded as confirmed (T74.-). It is coded as suspected if it is documented as suspected (T76.-).

For cases of confirmed abuse or neglect an external cause code from the assault section (X92-Y09) should be added to identify the cause of any physical injuries. A perpetrator code (Y07) should be added when the perpetrator of the abuse is known. For suspected cases of abuse or neglect, do not report external cause or perpetrator code.

If a suspected case of abuse, neglect or mistreatment is ruled out during an encounter code Z04.71, Encounter for examination and observation following alleged physical adult abuse, ruled out, or code Z04.72, Encounter for examination and observation following alleged child physical abuse, ruled out, should be used, not a code from T76.

If a suspected case of alleged rape or sexual abuse is ruled out during an encounter code Z04.41, Encounter for examination and observation following alleged adult rape or code Z04.42, Encounter for examination and observation following alleged child rape, should be used, not a code from T76.

If a suspected case of forced sexual exploitation or forced labor exploitation is ruled out during an encounter, code Z04.81, Encounter for examination and observation of victim following forced sexual exploitation, or code Z04.82, Encounter for examination and observation of victim following forced labor exploitation, should be used, not a code from T76.
See Section I.C.15. Abuse in a pregnant patient.

g. **Complications of care**
1) **General guidelines for complications of care**
   (a) **Documentation of complications of care**
   See Section I.B.16. for information on documentation of complications of care.

2) **Pain due to medical devices**
Pain associated with devices, implants or grafts left in a surgical site (for example painful hip prosthesis) is assigned to the appropriate code(s) found in Chapter 19, Injury, poisoning, and certain other consequences of external causes. Specific codes for pain due to medical devices are found in the T code section of the ICD-10-CM. Use additional code(s) from category G89 to identify acute or chronic pain due to presence of the device, implant or graft (G89.18 or G89.28).

3) **Transplant complications**
   (a) **Transplant complications other than kidney**
   Codes under category T86, Complications of transplanted organs and tissues, are for use for both complications and rejection of transplanted organs. A transplant complication code is only assigned if the complication affects the function of the transplanted organ. Two codes are required to fully describe a transplant complication: the appropriate code from category T86 and a secondary code that identifies the complication.

   Pre-existing conditions or conditions that develop after the transplant are not coded as complications unless they affect the function of the transplanted organs.

   See I.C.21. for transplant organ removal status
   See I.C.2. for malignant neoplasm associated with transplanted organ.

   (b) **Kidney transplant complications**
   Patients who have undergone kidney transplant may still have some form of chronic kidney disease (CKD) because the kidney transplant may not fully restore kidney function. Code T86.1- should be assigned for documented complications of a kidney transplant, such as transplant failure or rejection or other transplant complication. Code T86.1- should not be assigned for post kidney transplant patients who have chronic kidney (CKD) unless a transplant complication such as transplant failure or rejection is documented. If the documentation is unclear as to whether the patient has a complication of the transplant, query the provider.

   Conditions that affect the function of the transplanted kidney, other than CKD, should be assigned a code from subcategory T86.1, Complications of transplanted organ, Kidney, and a secondary code that identifies the complication.

   For patients with CKD following a kidney transplant, but who do not have a complication such as failure or rejection, *see section I.C.14. Chronic kidney disease and kidney transplant status.*

4) **Complication codes that include the external cause**
As with certain other T codes, some of the complications of care codes have the external cause included in the code. The code includes the nature of the complication as well as the type of procedure that caused the complication. No external cause code indicating the type of procedure is necessary for these codes.

5) **Complications of care codes within the body system chapters**
Intraoperative and postprocedural complication codes are found within the body system chapters with codes specific to the organs and structures of that body system. These codes should be sequenced first, followed by a code(s) for the specific complication, if applicable.

20. **Chapter 20: External Causes of Morbidity (V00-Y99)**
The external causes of morbidity codes should never be sequenced as the first-listed or principal diagnosis.

External cause codes are intended to provide data for injury research and evaluation of injury prevention strategies. These codes capture how the injury or health condition happened (cause), the intent (unintentional or accidental; or intentional, such as suicide or assault), the place where the event occurred the activity of the patient at the time of the event, and the person's status (e.g., civilian, military).

There is no national requirement for mandatory ICD-10-CM external cause code reporting. Unless a provider is subject to a state-based external cause code reporting mandate or these codes are required by a particular payer, reporting of ICD-10-CM codes in Chapter 20, External Causes of Morbidity, is not required. In the absence of a mandatory reporting requirement, providers are encouraged to voluntarily report external cause codes, as they provide valuable data for injury research and evaluation of injury prevention strategies.

a. **General External Cause Coding Guidelines**

   1) **Used with any code in the range of A00.0-T88.9 Z00-Z99**
      An external cause code may be used with any code in the range of A00.0-T88.9, Z00-Z99, classification that represents a health condition due to an external cause. Though they are most applicable to injuries, they are also valid for use with such things as infections or diseases due to an external source, and other health conditions, such as a heart attack that occurs during strenuous physical activity.

   2) **External cause code used for length of treatment**
      Assign the external cause code, with the appropriate 7th character (initial encounter, subsequent encounter or sequela) for each encounter for which the injury or condition is being treated.

      Most categories in chapter 20 have a 7th character requirement for each applicable code. Most categories in this chapter have three 7th character values: A, initial encounter, D, subsequent encounter and S, sequela. While the patient may be seen by a new or different provider over the course of treatment for an injury or condition, assignment of the 7th character for external cause should match the 7th character of the code assigned for the associated injury or condition for the encounter.

   3) **Use the full range of external cause codes**
      Use the full range of external cause codes to completely describe the cause, the intent, the place of occurrence, and if applicable, the activity of the patient at the time of the event, and the patient's status, for all injuries, and other health conditions due to an external cause.

   4) **Assign as many external cause codes as necessary**
      Assign as many external cause codes as necessary to fully explain each cause. If only one external code can be recorded, assign the code most related to the principal diagnosis.

   5) **The selection of the appropriate external cause code**
      The selection of the appropriate external cause code is guided by the Alphabetic Index of External Causes and by Inclusion and Exclusion notes in the Tabular List.

   6) **External cause code can never be a principal diagnosis**
      An external cause code can never be a principal (first-listed) diagnosis.

   7) **Combination external cause codes**
      Certain of the external cause codes are combination codes that identify sequential events that result in an injury, such as a fall which results in striking against an object. The injury may be due to either event or both. The combination external cause code used should correspond to the sequence of events regardless of which caused the most serious injury.

   8) **No external cause code needed in certain circumstances**
      No external cause code from Chapter 20 is needed if the external cause and intent are included in a code from another chapter (e.g. T36.0X1- Poisoning by penicillins, accidental (unintentional)).

b. **Place of Occurrence Guideline**
   Codes from category Y92, Place of occurrence of the external cause, are secondary codes for use after other external cause codes to identify the location of the patient at the time of injury or other condition.

   Generally, a place of occurrence code is assigned only once, at the initial encounter for treatment. However, in the rare instance that a new injury occurs during hospitalization, an additional place of occurrence code may be assigned. No 7th characters are used for Y92.

   Do not use place of occurrence code Y92.9 if the place is not stated or is not applicable.

c. **Activity Code**
   Assign a code from category Y93, Activity code, to describe the activity of the patient at the time the injury or other health condition occurred.

An activity code is used only once, at the initial encounter for treatment. Only one code from Y93 should be recorded on a medical record.

The activity codes are not applicable to poisonings, adverse effects, misadventures or sequela.

Do not assign Y93.9, Unspecified activity, if the activity is not stated.

A code from category Y93 is appropriate for use with external cause and intent codes if identifying the activity provides additional information about the event.

d. **Place of Occurrence, Activity, and Status Codes Used with other External Cause Code**
   When applicable, place of occurrence, activity, and external cause status codes are sequenced after the main external cause code(s). Regardless of the number of external cause codes assigned, generally there should be only one place of occurrence code, one activity code, and one external cause status code assigned to an encounter. However, in the rare instance that a new injury occurs during hospitalization, an additional place of occurrence code may be assigned.

e. **If the Reporting Format Limits the Number of External Cause Codes**
   If the reporting format limits the number of external cause codes that can be used in reporting clinical data, report the code for the cause/intent most related to the principal diagnosis. If the format permits capture of additional external cause codes, the cause/intent, including medical misadventures, of the additional events should be reported rather than the codes for place, activity, or external status.

f. **Multiple External Cause Coding Guidelines**
   More than one external cause code is required to fully describe the external cause of an illness or injury. The assignment of external cause codes should be sequenced in the following priority:

   If two or more events cause separate injuries, an external cause code should be assigned for each cause. The first-listed external cause code will be selected in the following order:

   External codes for child and adult abuse take priority over all other external cause codes.
   See Section I.C.19., Child and Adult abuse guidelines.

   External cause codes for terrorism events take priority over all other external cause codes except child and adult abuse.

   External cause codes for cataclysmic events take priority over all other external cause codes except child and adult abuse and terrorism.

   External cause codes for transport accidents take priority over all other external cause codes except cataclysmic events, child and adult abuse and terrorism.

   Activity and external cause status codes are assigned following all causal (intent) external cause codes.

   The first-listed external cause code should correspond to the cause of the most serious diagnosis due to an assault, accident, or self-harm, following the order of hierarchy listed above.

g. **Child and Adult Abuse Guideline**
   Adult and child abuse, neglect and maltreatment are classified as assault. Any of the assault codes may be used to indicate the external cause of any injury resulting from the confirmed abuse.

   For confirmed cases of abuse, neglect and maltreatment, when the perpetrator is known, a code from Y07, Perpetrator of maltreatment and neglect, should accompany any other assault codes.
   See Section I.C.19. Adult and child abuse, neglect and other maltreatment

h. **Unknown or Undetermined Intent Guideline**
   If the intent (accident, self-harm, assault) of the cause of an injury or other condition is unknown or unspecified, code the intent as accidental intent. All transport accident categories assume accidental intent.

   1) **Use of undetermined intent**
      External cause codes for events of undetermined intent are only for use if the documentation in the record specifies that the intent cannot be determined.

i. **Sequelae (Late Effects) of External Cause Guidelines**
   1) **Sequelae external cause codes**
      Sequela are reported using the external cause code with the 7th character "S" for sequela. These codes should be used with any report of a late effect or sequela resulting from a previous injury.
      See Section I.B.10 Sequela (Late Effects)

    2) **Sequela external cause code with a related current injury**
A sequela external cause code should never be used with a related current nature of injury code.

    3) **Use of sequela external cause codes for subsequent visits**
Use a late effect external cause code for subsequent visits when a late effect of the initial injury is being treated. Do not use a late effect external cause code for subsequent visits for follow-up care (e.g., to assess healing, to receive rehabilitative therapy) of the injury when no late effect of the injury has been documented.

  j. Terrorism Guidelines

    1) **Cause of injury identified by the Federal Government (FBI) as terrorism**
When the cause of an injury is identified by the Federal Government (FBI) as terrorism, the first-listed external cause code should be a code from category Y38, Terrorism. The definition of terrorism employed by the FBI is found at the inclusion note at the beginning of category Y38. Use additional code for place of occurrence (Y92.-). More than one Y38 code may be assigned if the injury is the result of more than one mechanism of terrorism.

    2) **Cause of an injury is suspected to be the result of terrorism**
When the cause of an injury is suspected to be the result of terrorism a code from category Y38 should not be assigned. Suspected cases should be classified as assault.

    3) **Code Y38.9, Terrorism, secondary effects**
Assign code Y38.9, Terrorism, secondary effects, for conditions occurring subsequent to the terrorist event. This code should not be assigned for conditions that are due to the initial terrorist act.

    It is acceptable to assign code Y38.9 with another code from Y38 if there is an injury due to the initial terrorist event and an injury that is a subsequent result of the terrorist event.

  k. External cause status
A code from category Y99, External cause status, should be assigned whenever any other external cause code is assigned for an encounter, including an Activity code, except for the events noted below. Assign a code from category Y99, External cause status, to indicate the work status of the person at the time the event occurred. The status code indicates whether the event occurred during military activity, whether a non-military person was at work, whether an individual including a student or volunteer was involved in a non-work activity at the time of the causal event.

A code from Y99, External cause status, should be assigned, when applicable, with other external cause codes, such as transport accidents and falls. The external cause status codes are not applicable to poisonings, adverse effects, misadventures or late effects.

Do not assign a code from category Y99 if no other external cause codes (cause, activity) are applicable for the encounter.

An external cause status code is used only once, at the initial encounter for treatment. Only one code from Y99 should be recorded on a medical record.

Do not assign code Y99.9, Unspecified external cause status, if the status is not stated.

21. Chapter 21: Factors influencing health status and contact with health services (Z00-Z99)
Note: The chapter specific guidelines provide additional information about the use of Z codes for specified encounters.

  a. Use of Z codes in any healthcare setting
Z codes are for use in any healthcare setting. Z codes may be used as either a first-listed (principal diagnosis code in the inpatient setting) or secondary code, depending on the circumstances of the encounter. Certain Z codes may only be used as first-listed or principal diagnosis.

  b. Z Codes indicate a reason for an encounter
Z codes are not procedure codes. A corresponding procedure code must accompany a Z code to describe any procedure performed.

  c. Categories of Z Codes

    1) **Contact/Exposure**
Category Z20 indicates contact with, and suspected exposure to, communicable diseases. These codes are for patients who do not show any sign or symptom of a disease but are suspected to have been exposed to it by close personal contact with an infected individual or are in an area where a disease is epidemic.

Category Z77, Other contact with and (suspected) exposures hazardous to health, indicates contact with and suspected exposures hazardous to health.

Contact/exposure codes may be used as a first-listed code to explain an encounter for testing, or, more commonly, as a secondary code to identify a potential risk.

    2) **Inoculations and vaccinations**
Code Z23 is for encounters for inoculations and vaccinations. It indicates that a patient is being seen to receive a prophylactic inoculation against a disease. Procedure codes are required to identify the actual administration of the injection and the type(s) of immunizations given. Code Z23 may be used as a secondary code if the inoculation is given as a routine part of preventive health care, such as a well-baby visit.

    3) **Status**
Status codes indicate that a patient is either a carrier of a disease or has the sequelae or residual of a past disease or condition. This includes such things as the presence of prosthetic or mechanical devices resulting from past treatment. A status code is informative, because the status may affect the course of treatment and its outcome. A status code is distinct from a history code. The history code indicates that the patient no longer has the condition.

A status code should not be used with a diagnosis code from one of the body system chapters, if the diagnosis code includes the information provided by the status code. For example, code Z94.1, Heart transplant status, should not be used with a code from subcategory T86.2, Complications of heart transplant. The status code does not provide additional information. The complication code indicates that the patient is a heart transplant patient.

For encounters for weaning from a mechanical ventilator, assign a code from subcategory J96.1, Chronic respiratory failure, followed by code Z99.11, Dependence on respirator [ventilator] status.

The status Z codes/categories are:

Z14   Genetic carrier

        Genetic carrier status indicates that a person carries a gene, associated with a particular disease, which may be passed to offspring who may develop that disease. The person does not have the disease and is not at risk of developing the disease.

Z15   Genetic susceptibility to disease

        Genetic susceptibility indicates that a person has a gene that increases the risk of that person developing the disease.

        Codes from category Z15 should not be used as principal or first-listed codes. If the patient has the condition to which he/she is susceptible, and that condition is the reason for the encounter, the code for the current condition should be sequenced first. If the patient is being seen for follow-up after completed treatment for this condition, and the condition no longer exists, a follow-up code should be sequenced first, followed by the appropriate personal history and genetic susceptibility codes. If the purpose of the encounter is genetic counseling associated with procreative management, code Z31.5, Encounter for genetic counseling, should be assigned as the first-listed code, followed by a code from category Z15. Additional codes should be assigned for any applicable family or personal history.

Z16   Resistance to antimicrobial drugs

        This code indicates that a patient has a condition that is resistant to antimicrobial drug treatment. Sequence the infection code first.

Z17   Estrogen receptor status

Z18   Retained foreign body fragments

Z19   Hormone sensitivity malignancy status

Z21   Asymptomatic HIV infection status

        This code indicates that a patient has tested positive for HIV but has manifested no signs or symptoms of the disease.

Z22   Carrier of infectious disease

Carrier status indicates that a person harbors the specific organisms of a disease without manifest symptoms and is capable of transmitting the infection.

Z28.3   Underimmunization status

Z33.1   Pregnant state, incidental

This code is a secondary code only for use when the pregnancy is in no way complicating the reason for visit. Otherwise, a code from the obstetric chapter is required.

Z66   Do not resuscitate

This code may be used when it is documented by the provider that a patient is on do not resuscitate status at any time during the stay.

Z67   Blood type

Z68   Body mass index (BMI)

BMI codes should only be assigned when the associated diagnosis (such as overweight or obesity) meets the definition of a reportable diagnosis (see Section III, Reporting Additional Diagnoses). **Do not assign BMI codes during pregnancy.** *See Section I.B.14 for BMI documentation by clinicians other than the patient's provider.*

Z74.01   Bed confinement status

Z76.82   Awaiting organ transplant status

Z78   Other specified health status

Code Z78.1, Physical restraint status, may be used when it is documented by the provider that a patient has been put in restraints during the current encounter. Please note that this code should not be reported when it is documented by the provider that a patient is temporarily restrained during a procedure.

Z79   Long-term (current) drug therapy

Codes from this category indicate a patient's continuous use of a prescribed drug (including such things as aspirin therapy) for the long-term treatment of a condition or for prophylactic use. It is not for use for patients who have addictions to drugs. This subcategory is not for use of medications for detoxification or maintenance programs to prevent withdrawal symptoms in patients with drug dependence (e.g., methadone maintenance for opiate dependence). Assign the appropriate code for the drug dependence instead.

Assign a code from Z79 if the patient is receiving a medication for an extended period as a prophylactic measure (such as for the prevention of deep vein thrombosis) or as treatment of a chronic condition (such as arthritis) or a disease requiring a lengthy course of treatment (such as cancer). Do not assign a code from category Z79 for medication being administered for a brief period of time to treat an acute illness or injury (such as a course of antibiotics to treat acute bronchitis).

Z88   Allergy status to drugs, medicaments and biological substances

Except: Z88.9, Allergy status to unspecified drugs, medicaments and biological substances status

Z89   Acquired absence of limb

Z90   Acquired absence of organs, not elsewhere classified

Z91.0-   Allergy status, other than to drugs and biological substances

Z92.82   Status post administration of tPA (rtPA) in a different facility within the last 24 hours prior to admission to a current facility

Assign code Z92.82, Status post administration of tPA (rtPA) in a different facility within the last 24 hours prior to admission to current facility, as a secondary diagnosis when a patient is received by transfer into a facility and documentation indicates they were administered tissue plasminogen activator (tPA) within the last 24 hours prior to admission to the current facility.

This guideline applies even if the patient is still receiving the tPA at the time they are received into the current facility.

The appropriate code for the condition for which the tPA was administered (such as cerebrovascular disease or myocardial infarction) should be assigned first.

Code Z92.82 is only applicable to the receiving facility record and not to the transferring facility record.

Z93   Artificial opening status

Z94   Transplanted organ and tissue status

Z95   Presence of cardiac and vascular implants and grafts

Z96   Presence of other functional implants

Z97   Presence of other devices

Z98   Other postprocedural states

Assign code Z98.85, Transplanted organ removal status, to indicate that a transplanted organ has been previously removed. This code should not be assigned for the encounter in which the transplanted organ is removed. The complication necessitating removal of the transplant organ should be assigned for that encounter.

See section I.C19. for information on the coding of organ transplant complications.

Z99   Dependence on enabling machines and devices, not elsewhere classified

Note: Categories Z89-Z90 and Z93-Z99 are for use only if there are no complications or malfunctions of the organ or tissue replaced, the amputation site or the equipment on which the patient is dependent.

4)   **History (of)**

There are two types of history Z codes, personal and family. Personal history codes explain a patient's past medical condition that no longer exists and is not receiving any treatment, but that has the potential for recurrence, and therefore may require continued monitoring.

Family history codes are for use when a patient has a family member(s) who has had a particular disease that causes the patient to be at higher risk of also contracting the disease.

Personal history codes may be used in conjunction with follow-up codes and family history codes may be used in conjunction with screening codes to explain the need for a test or procedure. History codes are also acceptable on any medical record regardless of the reason for visit. A history of an illness, even if no longer present, is important information that may alter the type of treatment ordered.

The history Z code categories are:

Z80   Family history of primary malignant neoplasm

Z81   Family history of mental and behavioral disorders

Z82   Family history of certain disabilities and chronic diseases (leading to disablement)

Z83   Family history of other specific disorders

Z84   Family history of other conditions

Z85   Personal history of malignant neoplasm

Z86   Personal history of certain other diseases

Z87   Personal history of other diseases and conditions

Z91.4-   Personal history of psychological trauma, not elsewhere classified

Z91.5   Personal history of self-harm

Z91.81   History of falling

Z91.82   Personal history of military deployment

Z92   Personal history of medical treatment

Except: Z92.0, Personal history of contraception

Except: Z92.82, Status post administration of tPA (rtPA) in a different facility within the last 24 hours prior to admission to a current facility

5)   **Screening**

Screening is the testing for disease or disease precursors in seemingly well individuals so that early detection and treatment can be provided for those who test positive for the disease (e.g., screening mammogram).

The testing of a person to rule out or confirm a suspected diagnosis because the patient has some sign or symptom is a diagnostic examination, not a screening. In these cases, the sign or symptom is used to explain the reason for the test.

A screening code may be a first-listed code if the reason for the visit is specifically the screening exam. It may also be used as an additional code if the screening is done during an office visit for other health problems. A screening code is not necessary if the screening is inherent to a routine examination, such as a pap smear done during a routine pelvic examination.

Should a condition be discovered during the screening then the code for the condition may be assigned as an additional diagnosis.

The Z code indicates that a screening exam is planned. A procedure code is required to confirm that the screening was performed.

The screening Z codes/categories:

Z11   Encounter for screening for infectious and parasitic diseases

Z12   Encounter for screening for malignant neoplasms

Z13   Encounter for screening for other diseases and disorders

          Except: Z13.9, Encounter for screening, unspecified

Z36   Encounter for antenatal screening for mother

6) Observation

There are three observation Z code categories. They are for use in very limited circumstances when a person is being observed for a suspected condition that is ruled out. The observation codes are not for use if an injury or illness or any signs or symptoms related to the suspected condition are present. In such cases the diagnosis/symptom code is used with the corresponding external cause code.

The observation codes are to be used as principal diagnosis only. The only exception to this is when the principal diagnosis is required to be a code from category Z38, Liveborn infants according to place of birth and type of delivery. Then a code from category Z05, Encounter for observation and evaluation of newborn for suspected diseases and conditions ruled out, is sequenced after the Z38 code. Additional codes may be used in addition to the observation code, but only if they are unrelated to the suspected condition being observed.

Codes from subcategory Z03.7, Encounter for suspected maternal and fetal conditions ruled out, may either be used as a first-listed or as an additional code assignment depending on the case. They are for use in very limited circumstances on a maternal record when an encounter is for a suspected maternal or fetal condition that is ruled out during that encounter (for example, a maternal or fetal condition may be suspected due to an abnormal test result). These codes should not be used when the condition is confirmed. In those cases, the confirmed condition should be coded. In addition, these codes are not for use if an illness or any signs or symptoms related to the suspected condition or problem are present. In such cases the diagnosis/symptom code is used.

Additional codes may be used in addition to the code from subcategory Z03.7, but only if they are unrelated to the suspected condition being evaluated.

Codes from subcategory Z03.7 may not be used for encounters for antenatal screening of mother. *See Section I.C.21. Screening.*

For encounters for suspected fetal condition that are inconclusive following testing and evaluation, assign the appropriate code from category O35, O36, O40 or O41.

The observation Z code categories:

Z03   Encounter for medical observation for suspected diseases and conditions ruled out

Z04   Encounter for examination and observation for other reasons

          Except: Z04.9, Encounter for examination and observation for unspecified reason

Z05   Encounter for observation and evaluation of newborn for suspected diseases and conditions ruled out

7) Aftercare

Aftercare visit codes cover situations when the initial treatment of a disease has been performed and the patient requires continued care during the healing and recovery phase, or for the long-term consequences of the disease. The aftercare Z code should not be used if treatment is directed at a current, acute disease. The diagnosis code is to be used in these cases. Exceptions to this rule are codes Z51.0, Encounter for antineoplastic radiation therapy,

and codes from subcategory Z51.1, Encounter for antineoplastic chemotherapy and immunotherapy. These codes are to be first-listed, followed by the diagnosis code when a patient's encounter is solely to receive radiation therapy, chemotherapy, or immunotherapy for the treatment of a neoplasm. If the reason for the encounter is more than one type of antineoplastic therapy, code Z51.0 and a code from subcategory Z51.1 may be assigned together, in which case one of these codes would be reported as a secondary diagnosis.

The aftercare Z codes should also not be used for aftercare for injuries. For aftercare of an injury, assign the acute injury code with the appropriate 7th character (for subsequent encounter).

The aftercare codes are generally first-listed to explain the specific reason for the encounter. An aftercare code may be used as an additional code when some type of aftercare is provided in addition to the reason for admission and no diagnosis code is applicable. An example of this would be the closure of a colostomy during an encounter for treatment of another condition.

Aftercare codes should be used in conjunction with other aftercare codes or diagnosis codes to provide better detail on the specifics of an aftercare encounter visit, unless otherwise directed by the classification. Should a patient receive multiple types of antineoplastic therapy during the same encounter, code Z51.0, Encounter for antineoplastic radiation therapy, and codes from subcategory Z51.1, Encounter for antineoplastic chemotherapy and immunotherapy, may be used together on a record. The sequencing of multiple aftercare codes depends on the circumstances of the encounter.

Certain aftercare Z code categories need a secondary diagnosis code to describe the resolving condition or sequelae. For others, the condition is included in the code title.

Additional Z code aftercare category terms include fitting and adjustment, and attention to artificial openings.

Status Z codes may be used with aftercare Z codes to indicate the nature of the aftercare. For example code Z95.1, Presence of aortocoronary bypass graft, may be used with code Z48.812, Encounter for surgical aftercare following surgery on the circulatory system, to indicate the surgery for which the aftercare is being performed. A status code should not be used when the aftercare code indicates the type of status, such as using Z43.0, Encounter for attention to tracheostomy, with Z93.0, Tracheostomy status.

The aftercare Z category/codes:

Z42   Encounter for plastic and reconstructive surgery following medical procedure or healed injury

Z43   Encounter for attention to artificial openings

Z44   Encounter for fitting and adjustment of external prosthetic device

Z45   Encounter for adjustment and management of implanted device

Z46   Encounter for fitting and adjustment of other devices

Z47   Orthopedic aftercare

Z48   Encounter for other postprocedural aftercare

Z49   Encounter for care involving renal dialysis

Z51   Encounter for other aftercare and medical care

8) Follow-up

The follow-up codes are used to explain continuing surveillance following completed treatment of a disease, condition, or injury. They imply that the condition has been fully treated and no longer exists. They should not be confused with aftercare codes, or injury codes with a 7th character for subsequent encounter, that explain ongoing care of a healing condition or its sequelae. Follow-up codes may be used in conjunction with history codes to provide the full picture of the healed condition and its treatment. The follow-up code is sequenced first, followed by the history code.

A follow-up code may be used to explain multiple visits. Should a condition be found to have recurred on the follow-up visit, then the diagnosis code for the condition should be assigned in place of the follow-up code.

The follow-up Z code categories:

Z08   Encounter for follow-up examination after completed treatment for malignant neoplasm

Z09   Encounter for follow-up examination after completed treatment for conditions other than malignant neoplasm

Z39   Encounter for maternal postpartum care and examination

9) Donor

Codes in category Z52, Donors of organs and tissues, are used for living individuals who are donating blood or other body tissue. These codes are only for individuals donating for others, not for self-donations. They are not used to identify cadaveric donations.

10) Counseling

Counseling Z codes are used when a patient or family member receives assistance in the aftermath of an illness or injury, or when support is required in coping with family or social problems.

The counseling Z codes/categories:

Z30.0-   Encounter for general counseling and advice on contraception

Z31.5   Encounter for procreative genetic counseling

Z31.6-   Encounter for general counseling and advice on procreation

Z32.2   Encounter for childbirth instruction

Z32.3   Encounter for childcare instruction

Z69   Encounter for mental health services for victim and perpetrator of abuse

Z70   Counseling related to sexual attitude, behavior and orientation

Z71   Persons encountering health services for other counseling and medical advice, not elsewhere classified

Z76.81 Expectant mother prebirth pediatrician visit

11) Encounters for Obstetrical and Reproductive Services

See Section I.C.15. Pregnancy, Childbirth, and the Puerperium, for further instruction on the use of these codes.

Z codes for pregnancy are for use in those circumstances when none of the problems or complications included in the codes from the Obstetrics chapter exist (a routine prenatal visit or postpartum care). Codes in category Z34, Encounter for supervision of normal pregnancy, are always first-listed and are not to be used with any other code from the OB chapter.

Codes in category Z3A, Weeks of gestation, may be assigned to provide additional information about the pregnancy. Category Z3A codes should not be assigned for pregnancies with abortive outcomes (categories O00-O08), elective termination of pregnancy (code Z33.2), nor for postpartum conditions, as category Z3A is not applicable to these conditions. The date of the admission should be used to determine weeks of gestation for inpatient admissions that encompass more than one gestational week.

The outcome of delivery, category Z37, should be included on all maternal delivery records. It is always a secondary code. Codes in category Z37 should not be used on the newborn record.

Z codes for family planning (contraceptive) or procreative management and counseling should be included on an obstetric record either during the pregnancy or the postpartum stage, if applicable.

Z codes/categories for obstetrical and reproductive services:

Z30   Encounter for contraceptive management

Z31   Encounter for procreative management

Z32.2   Encounter for childbirth instruction

Z32.3   Encounter for childcare instruction

Z33   Pregnant state

Z34   Encounter for supervision of normal pregnancy

Z36   Encounter for antenatal screening of mother

Z3A   Weeks of gestation

Z37   Outcome of delivery

Z39   Encounter for maternal postpartum care and examination

Z76.81 Expectant mother prebirth pediatrician visit

12) Newborns and Infants

See Section I.C.16. Newborn (Perinatal) Guidelines, for further instruction on the use of these codes.

Newborn Z codes/categories:

Z76.1   Encounter for health supervision and care of foundling

Z00.1-   Encounter for routine child health examination

Z38   Liveborn infants according to place of birth and type of delivery

13) Routine and administrative examinations

The Z codes allow for the description of encounters for routine examinations, such as, a general check-up, or, examinations for administrative purposes, such as, a pre-employment physical. The codes are not to be used if the examination is for diagnosis of a suspected condition or for treatment purposes. In such cases the diagnosis code is used. During a routine exam, should a diagnosis or condition be discovered, it should be coded as an additional code. Pre-existing and chronic conditions and history codes may also be included as additional codes as long as the examination is for administrative purposes and not focused on any particular condition.

Some of the codes for routine health examinations distinguish between "with" and "without" abnormal findings. Code assignment depends on the information that is known at the time the encounter is being coded. For example, if no abnormal findings were found during the examination, but the encounter is being coded before test results are back, it is acceptable to assign the code for "without abnormal findings." When assigning a code for "with abnormal findings," additional code(s) should be assigned to identify the specific abnormal finding(s).

Pre-operative examination and pre-procedural laboratory examination Z codes are for use only in those situations when a patient is being cleared for a procedure or surgery and no treatment is given.

The Z codes/categories for routine and administrative examinations:

Z00   Encounter for general examination without complaint, suspected or reported diagnosis

Z01   Encounter for other special examination without complaint, suspected or reported diagnosis

Z02   Encounter for administrative examination

Except: Z02.9, Encounter for administrative examinations, unspecified

Z32.0-   Encounter for pregnancy test

14) Miscellaneous Z codes

The miscellaneous Z codes capture a number of other health care encounters that do not fall into one of the other categories. Certain of these codes identify the reason for the encounter; others are for use as additional codes that provide useful information on circumstances that may affect a patient's care and treatment.

Prophylactic Organ Removal

For encounters specifically for prophylactic removal of an organ (such as prophylactic removal of breasts due to a genetic susceptibility to cancer or a family history of cancer), the principal or first-listed code should be a code from category Z40, Encounter for prophylactic surgery, followed by the appropriate codes to identify the associated risk factor (such as genetic susceptibility or family history).

If the patient has a malignancy of one site and is having prophylactic removal at another site to prevent either a new primary malignancy or metastatic disease, a code for the malignancy should also be assigned in addition to a code from subcategory Z40.0, Encounter for prophylactic surgery for risk factors related to malignant neoplasms. A Z40.0 code should not be assigned if the patient is having organ removal for treatment of a malignancy, such as the removal of the testes for the treatment of prostate cancer.

Miscellaneous Z codes/categories:

Z28   Immunization not carried out

Except: Z28.3, Underimmunization status

Z29   Encounter for other prophylactic measures

Z40   Encounter for prophylactic surgery

Z41   Encounter for procedures for purposes other than remedying health state

        Except: Z41.9, Encounter for procedure for purposes other than remedying health state, unspecified

Z53   Persons encountering health services for specific procedures and treatment, not carried out

Z55   Problems related to education and literacy

Z56   Problems related to employment and unemployment

Z57   Occupational exposure to risk factors

Z58   Problems related to physical environment

Z59   Problems related to housing and economic circumstances

Z60   Problems related to social environment

Z62   Problems related to upbringing

Z63   Other problems related to primary support group, including family circumstances

Z64   Problems related to certain psychosocial circumstances

Z65   Problems related to other psychosocial circumstances

Z72   Problems related to lifestyle

        Note: These codes should be assigned only when the documentation specifies that the patient has an associated problem

Z73   Problems related to life management difficulty

Z74   Problems related to care provider dependency

        Except: Z74.01, Bed confinement status

Z75   Problems related to medical facilities and other health care

Z76.0   Encounter for issue of repeat prescription

Z76.3   Healthy person accompanying sick person

Z76.4   Other boarder to healthcare facility

Z76.5   Malingerer [conscious simulation]

Z91.1- Patient's noncompliance with medical treatment and regimen

Z91.83 Wandering in diseases classified elsewhere

Z91.84- Oral health risk factors

Z91.89 Other specified personal risk factors, not elsewhere classified

See Section I.B.14 for Z55-Z65 Persons with potential health hazards related to socioeconomic and psychosocial circumstances, documentation by clinicians other than the patient's provider.

15) **Nonspecific Z codes**

Certain Z codes are so non-specific, or potentially redundant with other codes in the classification, that there can be little justification for their use in the inpatient setting. Their use in the outpatient setting should be limited to those instances when there is no further documentation to permit more precise coding. Otherwise, any sign or symptom or any other reason for visit that is captured in another code should be used.

Nonspecific Z codes/categories:

Z02.9   Encounter for administrative examinations, unspecified

Z04.9   Encounter for examination and observation for unspecified reason

Z13.9   Encounter for screening, unspecified

Z41.9   Encounter for procedure for purposes other than remedying health state, unspecified

Z52.9   Donor of unspecified organ or tissue

Z86.59 Personal history of other mental and behavioral disorders

Z88.9   Allergy status to unspecified drugs, medicaments and biological substances status

Z92.0   Personal history of contraception

16) **Z Codes That May Only be Principal/First-Listed Diagnosis**

The following Z codes/categories may only be reported as the principal/first-listed diagnosis, except when there are multiple encounters on the same day and the medical records for the encounters are combined:

Z00   Encounter for general examination without complaint, suspected or reported diagnosis

        Except: Z00.6

Z01   Encounter for other special examination without complaint, suspected or reported diagnosis

Z02   Encounter for administrative examination

Z03   Encounter for medical observation for suspected diseases and conditions ruled out

Z04   Encounter for examination and observation for other reasons

Z33.2   Encounter for elective termination of pregnancy

Z31.81 Encounter for male factor infertility in female patient

Z31.83 Encounter for assisted reproductive fertility procedure cycle

Z31.84 Encounter for fertility preservation procedure

Z34   Encounter for supervision of normal pregnancy

Z39   Encounter for maternal postpartum care and examination

Z38   Liveborn infants according to place of birth and type of delivery

Z40   Encounter for prophylactic surgery

Z42   Encounter for plastic and reconstructive surgery following medical procedure or healed injury

Z51.0   Encounter for antineoplastic radiation therapy

Z51.1- Encounter for antineoplastic chemotherapy and immunotherapy

Z52   Donors of organs and tissues

        Except: Z52.9, Donor of unspecified organ or tissue

Z76.1   Encounter for health supervision and care of foundling

Z76.2   Encounter for health supervision and care of other healthy infant and child

Z99.12 Encounter for respirator [ventilator] dependence during power failure

Section II. Selection of Principal Diagnosis

The circumstances of inpatient admission always govern the selection of principal diagnosis. The principal diagnosis is defined in the Uniform Hospital Discharge Data Set (UHDDS) as "that condition established after study to be chiefly responsible for occasioning the admission of the patient to the hospital for care."

The UHDDS definitions are used by hospitals to report inpatient data elements in a standardized manner. These data elements and their definitions can be found in the July 31, 1985, Federal Register (Vol. 50, No, 147), pp. 31038-40.

Since that time the application of the UHDDS definitions has been expanded to include all non-outpatient settings (acute care, short term, long term care and psychiatric hospitals; home health agencies; rehab facilities; nursing homes, etc). The UHDDS definitions also apply to hospice services (all levels of care).

In determining principal diagnosis, coding conventions in the ICD-10-CM, the Tabular List and Alphabetic Index take precedence over these official coding guidelines.

(See Section I.A., Conventions for the ICD-10-CM)

The importance of consistent, complete documentation in the medical record cannot be overemphasized. Without such documentation the application of all coding guidelines is a difficult, if not impossible, task.

A. **Codes for symptoms, signs, and ill-defined conditions**

Codes for symptoms, signs, and ill-defined conditions from Chapter 18 are not to be used as principal diagnosis when a related definitive diagnosis has been established.

B. **Two or more interrelated conditions, each potentially meeting the definition for principal diagnosis.**

When there are two or more interrelated conditions (such as diseases in the same ICD-10-CM chapter or manifestations characteristically associated with a certain disease) potentially meeting the definition of principal diagnosis, either condition may be sequenced first, unless the circumstances of the admission, the therapy provided, the Tabular List, or the Alphabetic Index indicate otherwise.

C. **Two or more diagnoses that equally meet the definition for principal diagnosis**

In the unusual instance when two or more diagnoses equally meet the criteria for principal diagnosis as determined by the circumstances of admission, diagnostic workup and/or therapy provided, and the

Alphabetic Index, Tabular List, or another coding guidelines does not provide sequencing direction, any one of the diagnoses may be sequenced first.

D. Two or more comparative or contrasting conditions

In those rare instances when two or more contrasting or comparative diagnoses are documented as "either/or" (or similar terminology), they are coded as if the diagnoses were confirmed and the diagnoses are sequenced according to the circumstances of the admission. If no further determination can be made as to which diagnosis should be principal, either diagnosis may be sequenced first.

E. A symptom(s) followed by contrasting/comparative diagnoses

GUIDELINE HAS BEEN DELETED EFFECTIVE OCTOBER 1, 2014

F. Original treatment plan not carried out

Sequence as the principal diagnosis the condition, which after study occasioned the admission to the hospital, even though treatment may not have been carried out due to unforeseen circumstances.

G. Complications of surgery and other medical care

When the admission is for treatment of a complication resulting from surgery or other medical care, the complication code is sequenced as the principal diagnosis. If the complication is classified to the T80-T88 series and the code lacks the necessary specificity in describing the complication, an additional code for the specific complication should be assigned.

H. Uncertain Diagnosis

If the diagnosis documented at the time of discharge is qualified as "probable", "suspected", "likely", "questionable", "possible", or "still to be ruled out", or other similar terms indicating uncertainty, code the condition as if it existed or was established. The bases for these guidelines are the diagnostic workup, arrangements for further workup or observation, and initial therapeutic approach that correspond most closely with the established diagnosis.

Note: This guideline is applicable only to inpatient admissions to short-term, acute, long-term care and psychiatric hospitals.

I. Admission from Observation Unit

1. Admission Following Medical Observation

When a patient is admitted to an observation unit for a medical condition, which either worsens or does not improve, and is subsequently admitted as an inpatient of the same hospital for this same medical condition, the principal diagnosis would be the medical condition which led to the hospital admission.

2. Admission Following Post-Operative Observation

When a patient is admitted to an observation unit to monitor a condition (or complication) that develops following outpatient surgery, and then is subsequently admitted as an inpatient of the same hospital, hospitals should apply the Uniform Hospital Discharge Data Set (UHDDS) definition of principal diagnosis as "that condition established after study to be chiefly responsible for occasioning the admission of the patient to the hospital for care."

J. Admission from Outpatient Surgery

When a patient receives surgery in the hospital's outpatient surgery department and is subsequently admitted for continuing inpatient care at the same hospital, the following guidelines should be followed in selecting the principal diagnosis for the inpatient admission:

- If the reason for the inpatient admission is a complication, assign the complication as the principal diagnosis.
- If no complication, or other condition, is documented as the reason for the inpatient admission, assign the reason for the outpatient surgery as the principal diagnosis.
- If the reason for the inpatient admission is another condition unrelated to the surgery, assign the unrelated condition as the principal diagnosis.

K. Admissions/Encounters for Rehabilitation

When the purpose for the admission/encounter is rehabilitation, sequence first the code for the condition for which the service is being performed. For example, for an admission/encounter for rehabilitation for right-sided dominant hemiplegia following a cerebrovascular infarction, report code I69.351, Hemiplegia and hemiparesis following cerebral infarction affecting right dominant side, as the first-listed or principal diagnosis.

If the condition for which the rehabilitation service is being provided is no longer present, report the appropriate aftercare code as the first-listed or principal diagnosis, unless the rehabilitation service is being provided following an injury. For rehabilitation services following active treatment of an injury, assign the injury code with the appropriate seventh character for subsequent encounter as the first-listed or principal diagnosis. For example, if a patient with severe degenerative osteoarthritis of the hip,

underwent hip replacement and the current encounter/admission is for rehabilitation, report code Z47.1, Aftercare following joint replacement surgery, as the first-listed or principal diagnosis. If the patient requires rehabilitation post hip replacement for right intertrochanteric femur fracture, report code S72.141D, Displaced intertrochanteric fracture of right femur, subsequent encounter for closed fracture with routine healing, as the first-listed or principal diagnosis.

See Section I.C.21.c.7, Factors influencing health states and contact with health services, Aftercare.

See Section I.C.19.a for additional information about the use of 7th characters for injury codes.

Section III. Reporting Additional Diagnoses

GENERAL RULES FOR OTHER (ADDITIONAL) DIAGNOSES

For reporting purposes the definition for "other diagnoses" is interpreted as additional conditions that affect patient care in terms of requiring:

clinical evaluation; or
therapeutic treatment; or
diagnostic procedures; or
extended length of hospital stay; or
increased nursing care and/or monitoring.

The UHDDS item #11-b defines Other Diagnoses as "all conditions that coexist at the time of admission, that develop subsequently, or that affect the treatment received and/or the length of stay. Diagnoses that relate to an earlier episode which have no bearing on the current hospital stay are to be excluded." UHDDS definitions apply to inpatients in acute care, short-term, long term care and psychiatric hospital setting. The UHDDS definitions are used by acute care short-term hospitals to report inpatient data elements in a standardized manner. These data elements and their definitions can be found in the July 31, 1985, Federal Register (Vol. 50, No, 147), pp. 31038-40.

Since that time the application of the UHDDS definitions has been expanded to include all non-outpatient settings (acute care, short term, long term care and psychiatric hospitals; home health agencies; rehab facilities; nursing homes, etc). The UHDDS definitions also apply to hospice services (all levels of care).

The following guidelines are to be applied in designating "other diagnoses" when neither the Alphabetic Index nor the Tabular List in ICD-10-CM provide direction. The listing of the diagnoses in the patient record is the responsibility of the attending provider.

A. Previous conditions

If the provider has included a diagnosis in the final diagnostic statement, such as the discharge summary or the face sheet, it should ordinarily be coded. Some providers include in the diagnostic statement resolved conditions or diagnoses and status-post procedures from previous admission that have no bearing on the current stay. Such conditions are not to be reported and are coded only if required by hospital policy.

However, history codes (categories Z80-Z87) may be used as secondary codes if the historical condition or family history has an impact on current care or influences treatment.

B. Abnormal findings

Abnormal findings (laboratory, x-ray, pathologic, and other diagnostic results) are not coded and reported unless the provider indicates their clinical significance. If the findings are outside the normal range and the attending provider has ordered other tests to evaluate the condition or prescribed treatment, it is appropriate to ask the provider whether the abnormal finding should be added.

Please note: This differs from the coding practices in the outpatient setting for coding encounters for diagnostic tests that have been interpreted by a provider.

C. Uncertain Diagnosis

If the diagnosis documented at the time of discharge is qualified as "probable", "suspected", "likely", "questionable", "possible", or "still to be ruled out" or other similar terms indicating uncertainty, code the condition as if it existed or was established. The bases for these guidelines are the diagnostic workup, arrangements for further workup or observation, and initial therapeutic approach that correspond most closely with the established diagnosis.

Note: This guideline is applicable only to inpatient admissions to short-term, acute, long-term care and psychiatric hospitals.

Section IV.Diagnostic Coding and Reporting Guidelines for Outpatient Services

These coding guidelines for outpatient diagnoses have been approved for use by hospitals/ providers in coding and reporting hospital-based outpatient services and provider-based office visits. Guidelines in Section I, Conventions, general coding guidelines and chapter-specific guidelines, should also be applied for outpatient services and office visits.

Information about the use of certain abbreviations, punctuation, symbols, and other conventions used in the ICD-10-CM Tabular List (code numbers and titles), can be found in Section IA of these guidelines, under "Conventions Used in the Tabular List." Section I.B. contains general guidelines that apply to the entire classification. Section I.C. contains chapter-specific guidelines that correspond to the chapters as they are arranged in the classification. Information about the correct sequence to use in finding a code is also described in Section I.

The terms encounter and visit are often used interchangeably in describing outpatient service contacts and, therefore, appear together in these guidelines without distinguishing one from the other.

Though the conventions and general guidelines apply to all settings, coding guidelines for outpatient and provider reporting of diagnoses will vary in a number of instances from those for inpatient diagnoses, recognizing that:

The Uniform Hospital Discharge Data Set (UHDDS) definition of principal diagnosis does not apply to hospital-based outpatient services and provider-based office visits.

Coding guidelines for inconclusive diagnoses (probable, suspected, rule out, etc.) were developed for inpatient reporting and do not apply to outpatients.

A. Selection of first-listed condition
In the outpatient setting, the term first-listed diagnosis is used in lieu of principal diagnosis.

In determining the first-listed diagnosis the coding conventions of ICD-10-CM, as well as the general and disease specific guidelines take precedence over the outpatient guidelines.

Diagnoses often are not established at the time of the initial encounter/visit. It may take two or more visits before the diagnosis is confirmed.

The most critical rule involves beginning the search for the correct code assignment through the Alphabetic Index. Never begin searching initially in the Tabular List as this will lead to coding errors.

1. Outpatient Surgery
When a patient presents for outpatient surgery (same day surgery), code the reason for the surgery as the first-listed diagnosis (reason for the encounter), even if the surgery is not performed due to a contraindication.

2. Observation Stay
When a patient is admitted for observation for a medical condition, assign a code for the medical condition as the first-listed diagnosis.

When a patient presents for outpatient surgery and develops complications requiring admission to observation, code the reason for the surgery as the first reported diagnosis (reason for the encounter), followed by codes for the complications as secondary diagnoses.

B. Codes from A00.0 through T88.9, Z00-Z99
The appropriate code(s) from A00.0 through T88.9, Z00-Z99 must be used to identify diagnoses, symptoms, conditions, problems, complaints, or other reason(s) for the encounter/visit.

C. Accurate reporting of ICD-10-CM diagnosis codes
For accurate reporting of ICD-10-CM diagnosis codes, the documentation should describe the patient's condition, using terminology which includes specific diagnoses as well as symptoms, problems, or reasons for the encounter. There are ICD-10-CM codes to describe all of these.

D. Codes that describe symptoms and signs
Codes that describe symptoms and signs, as opposed to diagnoses, are acceptable for reporting purposes when a diagnosis has not been established (confirmed) by the provider. Chapter 18 of ICD-10-CM, Symptoms, Signs, and Abnormal Clinical and Laboratory Findings Not Elsewhere Classified (codes R00-R99) contain many, but not all codes for symptoms.

E. Encounters for circumstances other than a disease or injury
ICD-10-CM provides codes to deal with encounters for circumstances other than a disease or injury. The Factors Influencing Health Status and Contact with Health Services codes (Z00-Z99) are provided to deal with occasions when circumstances other than a disease or injury are recorded as diagnosis or problems.

See Section I.C.21. Factors influencing health status and contact with health services.

F. Level of Detail in Coding
1. ICD-10-CM codes with 3, 4, 5, 6 or 7 characters
ICD-10-CM is composed of codes with 3, 4, 5, 6 or 7 characters. Codes with three characters are included in ICD-10-CM as the heading of a category of codes that may be further subdivided by the use of fourth, fifth, sixth or seventh characters to provide greater specificity.

2. Use of full number of characters required for a code
A three-character code is to be used only if it is not further subdivided. A code is invalid if it has not been coded to the full number of characters required for that code, including the 7th character, if applicable.

G. ICD-10-CM code for the diagnosis, condition, problem, or other reason for encounter/visit
List first the ICD-10-CM code for the diagnosis, condition, problem, or other reason for encounter/visit shown in the medical record to be chiefly responsible for the services provided. List additional codes that describe any coexisting conditions. In some cases the first-listed diagnosis may be a symptom when a diagnosis has not been established (confirmed) by the physician.

H. Uncertain diagnosis
Do not code diagnoses documented as "probable", "suspected," "questionable," "rule out," or "working diagnosis" or other similar terms indicating uncertainty. Rather, code the condition(s) to the highest degree of certainty for that encounter/visit, such as symptoms, signs, abnormal test results, or other reason for the visit.

Please note: This differs from the coding practices used by short-term, acute care, long-term care and psychiatric hospitals.

I. Chronic diseases
Chronic diseases treated on an ongoing basis may be coded and reported as many times as the patient receives treatment and care for the condition(s)

J. Code all documented conditions that coexist
Code all documented conditions that coexist at the time of the encounter/visit, and require or affect patient care treatment or management. Do not code conditions that were previously treated and no longer exist. However, history codes (categories Z80-Z87) may be used as secondary codes if the historical condition or family history has an impact on current care or influences treatment.

K. Patients receiving diagnostic services only
For patients receiving diagnostic services only during an encounter/visit, sequence first the diagnosis, condition, problem, or other reason for encounter/visit shown in the medical record to be chiefly responsible for the outpatient services provided during the encounter/visit. Codes for other diagnoses (e.g., chronic conditions) may be sequenced as additional diagnoses.

For encounters for routine laboratory/radiology testing in the absence of any signs, symptoms, or associated diagnosis, assign Z01.89, Encounter for other specified special examinations. If routine testing is performed during the same encounter as a test to evaluate a sign, symptom, or diagnosis, it is appropriate to assign both the Z code and the code describing the reason for the non-routine test.

For outpatient encounters for diagnostic tests that have been interpreted by a physician, and the final report is available at the time of coding, code any confirmed or definitive diagnosis(es) documented in the interpretation. Do not code related signs and symptoms as additional diagnoses.

Please note: This differs from the coding practice in the hospital inpatient setting regarding abnormal findings on test results.

L. Patients receiving therapeutic services only
For patients receiving therapeutic services only during an encounter/visit, sequence first the diagnosis, condition, problem, or other reason for encounter/visit shown in the medical record to be chiefly responsible for the outpatient services provided during the encounter/visit. Codes for other diagnoses (e.g., chronic conditions) may be sequenced as additional diagnoses.

The only exception to this rule is that when the primary reason for the admission/encounter is chemotherapy or radiation therapy, the appropriate Z code for the service is listed first, and the diagnosis or problem for which the service is being performed listed second.

M. Patients receiving preoperative evaluations only

For patients receiving preoperative evaluations only, sequence first a code from subcategory Z01.81, Encounter for pre-procedural examinations, to describe the pre-op consultations. Assign a code for the condition to describe the reason for the surgery as an additional diagnosis. Code also any findings related to the pre-op evaluation.

N. Ambulatory surgery

For ambulatory surgery, code the diagnosis for which the surgery was performed. If the postoperative diagnosis is known to be different from the preoperative diagnosis at the time the diagnosis is confirmed, select the postoperative diagnosis for coding, since it is the most definitive.

O. Routine outpatient prenatal visits

See Section I.C.15. Routine outpatient prenatal visits.

P. Encounters for general medical examinations with abnormal findings

The subcategories for encounters for general medical examinations, Z00.0- and encounter for routine child health examination, Z00.12-, provide codes for with and without abnormal findings. Should a general medical examination result in an abnormal finding, the code for general medical examination with abnormal finding should be assigned as the first-listed diagnosis. An examination with abnormal findings refers to a condition/diagnosis that is newly identified or a change in severity of a chronic condition (such as uncontrolled hypertension, or an acute exacerbation of chronic obstructive pulmonary disease) during a routine physical examination. A secondary code for the abnormal finding should also be coded.

Q. Encounters for routine health screenings

See Section I.C.21. Factors influencing health status and contact with health services, Screening

Appendix I. Present on Admission Reporting Guidelines

Introduction

These guidelines are to be used as a supplement to the *ICD-10-CM Official Guidelines for Coding and Reporting* to facilitate the assignment of the Present on Admission (POA) indicator for each diagnosis and external cause of injury code reported on claim forms (UB-04 and 837 Institutional).

These guidelines are not intended to replace any guidelines in the main body of the *ICD-10-CM Official Guidelines for Coding and Reporting*. The POA guidelines are not intended to provide guidance on when a condition should be coded, but rather, how to apply the POA indicator to the final set of diagnosis codes that have been assigned in accordance with Sections I, II, and III of the official coding guidelines. Subsequent to the assignment of the ICD-10-CM codes, the POA indicator should then be assigned to those conditions that have been coded.

As stated in the Introduction to the *ICD-10-CM Official Guidelines for Coding and Reporting,* a joint effort between the healthcare provider and the coder is essential to achieve complete and accurate documentation, code assignment, and reporting of diagnoses and procedures. The importance of consistent, complete documentation in the medical record cannot be overemphasized. Medical record documentation from any provider involved in the care and treatment of the patient may be used to support the determination of whether a condition was present on admission or not. In the context of the official coding guidelines, the term "provider" means a physician or any qualified healthcare practitioner who is legally accountable for establishing the patient's diagnosis.

These guidelines are not a substitute for the provider's clinical judgment as to the determination of whether a condition was/was not present on admission. The provider should be queried regarding issues related to the linking of signs/symptoms, timing of test results, and the timing of findings.

Please see the CDC website for the detailed list of ICD-10-CM codes that do not require the use of a POA indicator (https://www.cdc.gov/nchs/icd/icd10cm.htm). The codes and categories on this exempt list are for circumstances regarding the healthcare encounter or factors influencing health status that do not represent a current disease or injury or that describe conditions that are always present on admission.

General Reporting Requirements

All claims involving inpatient admissions to general acute care hospitals or other facilities that are subject to a law or regulation mandating collection of present on admission information.

Present on admission is defined as present at the time the order for inpatient admission occurs -- conditions that develop during an outpatient encounter, including emergency department, observation, or outpatient surgery, are considered as present on admission.

POA indicator is assigned to principal and secondary diagnoses (as defined in Section II of the Official Guidelines for Coding and Reporting) and the external cause of injury codes.

Issues related to inconsistent, missing, conflicting or unclear documentation must still be resolved by the provider.

If a condition would not be coded and reported based on UHDDS definitions and current official coding guidelines, then the POA indicator would not be reported.

Reporting Options

> Y - Yes
>
> N - No
>
> U - Unknown
>
> W – Clinically undetermined
>
> Unreported/Not used – (Exempt from POA reporting)

Reporting Definitions

> Y = present at the time of inpatient admission
>
> N = not present at the time of inpatient admission
>
> U = documentation is insufficient to determine if condition is present on admission
>
> W = provider is unable to clinically determine whether condition was present on admission or not

Timeframe for POA Identification and Documentation

There is no required timeframe as to when a provider (per the definition of "provider" used in these guidelines) must identify or document a condition to be present on admission. In some clinical situations, it may not be possible for a provider to make a definitive diagnosis (or a condition may not be recognized or reported by the patient) for a period of time after admission. In some cases it may be several days before the provider arrives at a definitive diagnosis. This does not mean that the condition was not present on admission. Determination of whether the condition was present on admission or not will be based on the applicable POA guideline as identified in this document, or on the provider's best clinical judgment.

If at the time of code assignment the documentation is unclear as to whether a condition was present on admission or not, it is appropriate to query the provider for clarification.

Assigning the POA Indicator

Condition is on the "Exempt from Reporting" list

> Leave the "present on admission" field blank if the condition is on the list of ICD-10-CM codes for which this field is not applicable. This is the only circumstance in which the field may be left blank.

POA Explicitly Documented

> Assign Y for any condition the provider explicitly documents as being present on admission.
>
> Assign N for any condition the provider explicitly documents as not present at the time of admission.

Conditions diagnosed prior to inpatient admission

> Assign "Y" for conditions that were diagnosed prior to admission (example: hypertension, diabetes mellitus, asthma)

Conditions diagnosed during the admission but clearly present before admission

> Assign "Y" for conditions diagnosed during the admission that were clearly present but not diagnosed until after admission occurred.
>
> Diagnoses subsequently confirmed after admission are considered present on admission if at the time of admission they are documented as suspected, possible, rule out, differential diagnosis, or constitute an underlying cause of a symptom that is present at the time of admission.

Condition develops during outpatient encounter prior to inpatient admission

> Assign Y for any condition that develops during an outpatient encounter prior to a written order for inpatient admission.

Documentation does not indicate whether condition was present on admission

> Assign "U" when the medical record documentation is unclear as to whether the condition was present on admission. "U" should not be routinely assigned and used only in very limited circumstances. Coders are encouraged to query the providers when the documentation is unclear.

Documentation states that it cannot be determined whether the condition was or was not present on admission

> Assign "W" when the medical record documentation indicates that it cannot be clinically determined whether or not the condition was present on admission.

Chronic condition with acute exacerbation during the admission

If a single code identifies both the chronic condition and the acute exacerbation, see POA guidelines pertaining to codes that contain multiple clinical concepts.

If a single code only identifies the chronic condition and not the acute exacerbation (e.g., acute exacerbation of chronic leukemia), assign "Y."

Conditions documented as possible, probable, suspected, or rule out at the time of discharge

If the final diagnosis contains a possible, probable, suspected, or rule out diagnosis, and this diagnosis was based on signs, symptoms or clinical findings suspected at the time of inpatient admission, assign "Y."

If the final diagnosis contains a possible, probable, suspected, or rule out diagnosis, and this diagnosis was based on signs, symptoms or clinical findings that were not present on admission, assign "N".

Conditions documented as impending or threatened at the time of discharge

If the final diagnosis contains an impending or threatened diagnosis, and this diagnosis is based on symptoms or clinical findings that were present on admission, assign "Y".

If the final diagnosis contains an impending or threatened diagnosis, and this diagnosis is based on symptoms or clinical findings that were not present on admission, assign "N".

Acute and Chronic Conditions

Assign "Y" for acute conditions that are present at time of admission and N for acute conditions that are not present at time of admission.

Assign "Y" for chronic conditions, even though the condition may not be diagnosed until after admission.

If a single code identifies both an acute and chronic condition, see the POA guidelines for codes that contain multiple clinical concepts.

Codes That Contain Multiple Clinical Concepts

Assign "N" if at least one of the clinical concepts included in the code was not present on admission (e.g., COPD with acute exacerbation and the exacerbation was not present on admission; gastric ulcer that does not start bleeding until after admission; asthma patient develops status asthmaticus after admission).

Assign "Y" if all of the clinical concepts included in the code were present on admission (e.g., duodenal ulcer that perforates prior to admission).

For infection codes that include the causal organism, assign "Y" if the infection (or signs of the infection) were present on admission, even though the culture results may not be known until after admission (e.g., patient is admitted with pneumonia and the provider documents Pseudomonas as the causal organism a few days later).

Same Diagnosis Code for Two or More Conditions

When the same ICD-10-CM diagnosis code applies to two or more conditions during the same encounter (e.g. two separate conditions classified to the same ICD-10-CM diagnosis code):

Assign "Y" if all conditions represented by the single ICD-10-CM code were present on admission (e.g. bilateral unspecified age-related cataracts).

Assign "N" if any of the conditions represented by the single ICD-10-CM code was not present on admission (e.g. traumatic secondary and recurrent hemorrhage and seroma is assigned to a single code T79.2, but only one of the conditions was present on admission).

Obstetrical conditions

Whether or not the patient delivers during the current hospitalization does not affect assignment of the POA indicator. The determining factor for POA assignment is whether the pregnancy complication or obstetrical condition described by the code was present at the time of admission or not.

If the pregnancy complication or obstetrical condition was present on admission (e.g., patient admitted in preterm labor), assign "Y".

If the pregnancy complication or obstetrical condition was not present on admission (e.g., 2nd degree laceration during delivery, postpartum hemorrhage that occurred during current hospitalization, fetal distress develops after admission), assign "N".

If the obstetrical code includes more than one diagnosis and any of the diagnoses identified by the code were not present on admission assign "N". (e.g., Category O11, Pre-existing hypertension with pre-eclampsia)

Perinatal conditions

Newborns are not considered to be admitted until after birth. Therefore, any condition present at birth or that developed in utero is considered present at admission and should be assigned "Y". This includes conditions that occur during delivery (e.g., injury during delivery, meconium aspiration, exposure to streptococcus B in the vaginal canal).

Congenital conditions and anomalies

Assign "Y" for congenital conditions and anomalies except for categories Q00-Q99, Congenital anomalies, which are on the exempt list. Congenital conditions are always considered present on admission.

External cause of injury codes

Assign "Y" for any external cause code representing an external cause of morbidity that occurred prior to inpatient admission (e.g., patient fell out of bed at home, patient fell out of bed in emergency room prior to admission)

Assign "N" for any external cause code representing an external cause of morbidity that occurred during inpatient hospitalization (e.g., patient fell out of hospital bed during hospital stay, patient experienced an adverse reaction to a medication administered after inpatient admission).

A

Aarskog's syndrome Q87.1
Abandonment — *see* Maltreatment
Abasia (-astasia) (hysterical) F44.4
Abderhalden-Kaufmann-Lignac syndrome (cystinosis) E72.04
Abdomen, abdominal (*see also* condition)
  muscle deficiency syndrome Q79.4
  angina K55.1
  acute R10.0
Abdominalgia — *see* Pain, abdominal
Abduction contracture, hip or other joint — *see* Contraction, joint
Aberrant (congenital) (*see also* Malposition, congenital)
  hepatic duct Q44.5
  endocrine gland NEC Q89.2
  breast Q83.8
  artery (peripheral) Q27.8
    basilar NEC Q28.1
    cerebral Q28.3
    coronary Q24.5
    digestive system Q27.8
    eye Q15.8
    lower limb Q27.8
    precerebral Q28.1
    pulmonary Q25.79
    renal Q27.2
    retina Q14.1
    specified site NEC Q27.8
    subclavian Q27.8
    upper limb Q27.8
    vertebral Q28.1
  adrenal gland Q89.1
  pancreas Q45.3
  parathyroid gland Q89.2
  pituitary gland Q89.2
  sebaceous glands, mucous membrane, mouth, congenital Q38.6
  spleen Q89.09
  subclavian artery Q27.8
  thymus (gland) Q89.2
  thyroid gland Q89.2
  vein (peripheral) NEC Q27.8
    cerebral Q28.3
    digestive system Q27.8
    lower limb Q27.8
    precerebral Q28.1
    specified site NEC Q27.8
    upper limb Q27.8
Aberration
  distantial — *see* Disturbance, visual
  mental F99
Abetalipoproteinemia E78.6
Abiotrophy R68.89
Ablatio, ablation
  retinae — *see* Detachment, retina
Ablepharia, ablepharon Q10.3
Abnormal, abnormality, abnormalities (*see also* Anomaly)
  acid-base balance (mixed) E87.4
  albumin R77.0
  alphafetoprotein R77.2
  alveolar ridge K08.9
  anatomical relationship Q89.9
  apertures, congenital, diaphragm Q79.1
  auditory perception H93.29- ☑
    diplacusis — *see* Diplacusis
    hyperacusis — *see* Hyperacusis
    recruitment — *see* Recruitment, auditory
    threshold shift — *see* Shift, auditory threshold
  autosomes Q99.9
    fragile site Q95.5
  basal metabolic rate R94.8
  biosynthesis, testicular androgen E29.1
  bleeding time R79.1
  blood level (of)
    cobalt R79.0
    copper R79.0
    iron R79.0
    lithium R78.89
    magnesium R79.0

Abnormal, abnormality, abnormalities — *continued*
  blood level — *continued*
    mineral NEC R79.0
    zinc R79.0
  blood pressure
    elevated R03.0
    low reading (nonspecific) R03.1
  blood sugar R73.09
  blood-gas level R79.81
  bowel sounds R19.15
    absent R19.11
    hyperactive R19.12
  brain scan R94.02
  breathing R06.9
  caloric test R94.138
  cerebrospinal fluid R83.9
    cytology R83.6
    drug level R83.2
    enzyme level R83.0
    hormones R83.1
    immunology R83.4
    microbiology R83.5
    nonmedicinal level R83.3
    specified type NEC R83.8
  chemistry, blood R79.9
    C-reactive protein R79.82
    drugs — *see* Findings, abnormal, in blood
    gas level R79.81
    minerals R79.0
    pancytopenia D61.818
    PTT R79.1
    specified NEC R79.89
    toxins — *see* Findings, abnormal, in blood
  chest sounds (friction) (rales) R09.89
  chromosome, chromosomal Q99.9
    with more than three X chromosomes, female Q97.1
    analysis result R89.8
      bronchial washings R84.8
      cerebrospinal fluid R83.8
      cervix uteri NEC R87.89
      nasal secretions R84.8
      nipple discharge R89.8
      peritoneal fluid R85.89
      pleural fluid R84.8
      prostatic secretions R86.8
      saliva R85.89
      seminal fluid R86.8
      sputum R84.8
      synovial fluid R89.8
      throat scrapings R84.8
      vagina R87.89
      vulva R87.89
      wound secretions R89.8
    dicentric replacement Q93.2
    ring replacement Q93.2
    sex Q99.8
      female phenotype Q97.9
        specified NEC Q97.8
      male phenotype Q98.9
        specified NEC Q98.8
      structural male Q98.6
    specified NEC Q99.8
  clinical findings NEC R68.89
  coagulation D68.9
    newborn, transient P61.6
    profile R79.1
    time R79.1
  communication — *see* Fistula
  conjunctiva, vascular H11.41- ☑
  coronary artery Q24.5
  cortisol-binding globulin E27.8
  course, eustachian tube Q17.8
  creatinine clearance R94.4
  cytology
    anus R85.619
      atypical squamous cells cannot exclude high grade squamous intraepithelial lesion (ASC-H) R85.611
      atypical squamous cells of undetermined significance (ASC-US) R85.610
      cytologic evidence of malignancy R85.614

Abnormal, abnormality, abnormalities — *continued*
  cytology — *continued*
    anus — *continued*
      high grade squamous intraepithelial lesion (HGSIL) R85.613
      human papillomavirus (HPV) DNA test
        high risk positive R85.81
        low risk postive R85.82
      inadequate smear R85.615
      low grade squamous intraepithelial lesion (LGSIL) R85.612
      satisfactory anal smear but lacking transformation zone R85.616
      specified NEC R85.618
      unsatisfactory smear R85.615
    female genital organs — *see* Abnormal, Papanicolaou (smear)
  dark adaptation curve H53.61
  dentofacial NEC — *see* Anomaly, dentofacial
  development, developmental Q89.9
    central nervous system Q07.9
  diagnostic imaging
    abdomen, abdominal region NEC R93.5
    biliary tract R93.2
    bladder R93.41
    breast R92.8
    central nervous system NEC R90.89
    cerebrovascular NEC R90.89
    coronary circulation R93.1
    digestive tract NEC R93.3
    gastrointestinal (tract) R93.3
    genitourinary organs R93.89
    head R93.0
    heart R93.1
    intrathoracic organ NEC R93.89
    kidney R93.42- ☑
    limbs R93.6
    liver R93.2
    lung (field) R91.8
    musculoskeletal system NEC R93.7
    renal pelvis R93.41
    retroperitoneum R93.5
    site specified NEC R93.89
    skin and subcutaneous tissue R93.89
    skull R93.0
    testis R93.81- ☑
    ureter R93.41
    urinary organs specified NEC R93.49
  direction, teeth, fully erupted M26.30
  ear ossicles, acquired NEC H74.39- ☑
    ankylosis — *see* Ankylosis, ear ossicles
    discontinuity — *see* Discontinuity, ossicles, ear
    partial loss — *see* Loss, ossicles, ear (partial)
  Ebstein Q22.5
  echocardiogram R93.1
  echoencephalogram R90.81
  echogram — *see* Abnormal, diagnostic imaging
  electrocardiogram [ECG] [EKG] R94.31
  electroencephalogram [EEG] R94.01
  electrolyte — *see* Imbalance, electrolyte
  electromyogram [EMG] R94.131
  electro-oculogram [EOG] R94.110
  electrophysiological intracardiac studies R94.39
  electroretinogram [ERG] R94.111
  erythrocytes
    congenital, with perinatal jaundice D58.9
  feces (color) (contents) (mucus) R19.5
  finding — *see* Findings, abnormal, without diagnosis
  fluid
    amniotic — *see* Abnormal, specimen, specified
    cerebrospinal — *see* Abnormal, cerebrospinal fluid
    peritoneal — *see* Abnormal, specimen, digestive organs
    pleural — *see* Abnormal, specimen, respiratory organs
    synovial — *see* Abnormal, specimen, specified
    thorax (bronchial washings) (pleural fluid) — *see* Abnormal, specimen, respiratory organs
    vaginal — *see* Abnormal, specimen, female genital organs
  form
    teeth K00.2

▽ Subterms under main terms may continue to next column or page   ☑ Additional Character Required — Refer to the Tabular List for Character Selection   1

Aarskog's syndrome — Abnormal, abnormality, abnormalities

Abnormal, abnormality, abnormalities —
continued
form — *continued*
uterus — *see* Anomaly, uterus
function studies
auditory R94.120
bladder R94.8
brain R94.09
cardiovascular R94.30
ear R94.128
endocrine NEC R94.7
eye NEC R94.118
kidney R94.4
liver R94.5
nervous system
central NEC R94.09
peripheral NEC R94.138
pancreas R94.8
placenta R94.8
pulmonary R94.2
special senses NEC R94.128
spleen R94.8
thyroid R94.6
vestibular R94.121
gait — *see* Gait
hysterical F44.4
gastrin secretion E16.4
globulin R77.1
cortisol-binding E27.8
thyroid-binding E07.89
glomerular, minor (*see also* N00-N07 with fourth character .0) N05.0
glucagon secretion E16.3
glucose tolerance (test) (non-fasting) R73.09
gravitational (G) forces or states (effect of) T75.81 ☑
hair (color) (shaft) L67.9
specified NEC L67.8
hard tissue formation in pulp (dental) K04.3
head movement R25.0
heart
rate R00.9
specified NEC R00.8
shadow R93.1
sounds NEC R01.2
hemoglobin (disease) (*see also* Disease, hemoglobin) D58.2
trait — *see* Trait, hemoglobin, abnormal
histology NEC R89.7
immunological findings R89.4
in serum R76.9
specified NEC R76.8
increase in appetite R63.2
involuntary movement — *see* Abnormal, movement, involuntary
jaw closure M26.51
karyotype R89.8
kidney function test R94.4
knee jerk R29.2
leukocyte (cell) (differential) NEC D72.9
liver function test R94.5
loss of
height R29.890
weight R63.4
mammogram NEC R92.8
calcification (calculus) R92.1
microcalcification R92.0
Mantoux test R76.11
movement (disorder) (*see also* Disorder, movement)
head R25.0
involuntary R25.9
fasciculation R25.3
of head R25.0
spasm R25.2
specified type NEC R25.8
tremor R25.1
myoglobin (Aberdeen) (Annapolis) R89.7
neonatal screening P09
oculomotor study R94.113
palmar creases Q82.8
Papanicolaou (smear)
anus R85.619
atypical squamous cells cannot exclude high grade squamous intraepithelial lesion (ASC-H) R85.611
atypical squamous cells of undetermined significance (ASC-US) R85.610
cytologic evidence of malignancy R85.614

Abnormal, abnormality, abnormalities —
continued
Papanicolaou — *continued*
anus — *continued*
high grade squamous intraepithelial lesion (HGSIL) R85.613
human papillomavirus (HPV) DNA test
high risk positive R85.81
low risk postive R85.82
inadequate smear R85.615
low grade squamous intraepithelial lesion (LGSIL) R85.612
satisfactory anal smear but lacking transformation zone R85.616
specified NEC R85.618
unsatisfactory smear R85.615
bronchial washings R84.6
cerebrospinal fluid R83.6
cervix R87.619
atypical squamous cells cannot exclude high grade squamous intraepithelial lesion (ASC-H) R87.611
atypical squamous cells of undetermined significance (ASC-US) R87.610
cytologic evidence of malignancy R87.614
high grade squamous intraepithelial lesion (HGSIL) R87.613
inadequate smear R87.615
low grade squamous intraepithelial lesion (LGSIL) R87.612
non-atypical endometrial cells R87.618
satisfactory cervical smear but lacking transformation zone R87.616
specified NEC R87.618
thin preparaton R87.619
unsatisfactory smear R87.615
nasal secretions R84.6
nipple discharge R89.6
peritoneal fluid R85.69
pleural fluid R84.6
prostatic secretions R86.6
saliva R85.69
seminal fluid R86.6
sites NEC R89.6
sputum R84.6
synovial fluid R89.6
throat scrapings R84.6
vagina R87.629
atypical squamous cells cannot exclude high grade squamous intraepithelial lesion (ASC-H) R87.621
atypical squamous cells of undetermined significance (ASC-US) R87.620
cytologic evidence of malignancy R87.624
high grade squamous intraepithelial lesion (HGSIL) R87.623
inadequate smear R87.625
low grade squamous intraepithelial lesion (LGSIL) R87.622
specified NEC R87.628
thin preparation R87.629
unsatisfactory smear R87.625
vulva R87.69
wound secretions R89.6
partial thromboplastin time (PTT) R79.1
pelvis (bony) — *see* Deformity, pelvis
percussion, chest (tympany) R09.89
periods (grossly) — *see* Menstruation
phonocardiogram R94.39
plantar reflex R29.2
plasma
protein R77.9
specified NEC R77.8
viscosity R70.1
pleural (folds) Q34.0
posture R29.3
product of conception O02.9
specified type NEC O02.89
prothrombin time (PT) R79.1
pulmonary
artery, congenital Q25.79
function, newborn P28.89
test results R94.2
pulsations in neck R00.2
pupillary H21.56- ☑
function (reaction) (reflex) — *see* Anomaly, pupil, function
radiological examination — *see* Abnormal, diagnostic imaging

Abnormal, abnormality, abnormalities —
continued
red blood cell(s) (morphology) (volume) R71.8
reflex — *see* Reflex
renal function test R94.4
response to nerve stimulation R94.130
retinal correspondence H53.31
retinal function study R94.111
rhythm, heart (*see also* Arrhythmia)
saliva — *see* Abnormal, specimen, digestive organs
scan
kidney R94.4
liver R93.2
thyroid R94.6
secretion
gastrin E16.4
glucagon E16.3
semen, seminal fluid — *see* Abnormal, specimen, male genital organs
serum level (of)
acid phosphatase R74.8
alkaline phosphatase R74.8
amylase R74.8
enzymes R74.9
specified NEC R74.8
lipase R74.8
triacylglycerol lipase R74.8
shape
gravid uterus — *see* Anomaly, uterus
sinus venosus Q21.1
size, tooth K00.2
spacing, tooth, teeth, fully erupted M26.30
specimen
digestive organs (peritoneal fluid) (saliva) R85.9
cytology R85.69
drug level R85.2
enzyme level R85.0
histology R85.7
hormones R85.1
immunology R85.4
microbiology R85.5
nonmedicinal level R85.3
specified type NEC R85.89
female genital organs (secretions) (smears) R87.9
cytology R87.69
cervix R87.619
human papillomavirus (HPV) DNA test
high risk positive R87.810
low risk positive R87.820
inadequate (unsatisfactory) smear R87.615
non-atypical endometrial cells R87.618
specified NEC R87.618
vagina R87.629
human papillomavirus (HPV) DNA test
high risk positive R87.811
low risk positive R87.821
inadequate (unsatisfactory) smear R87.625
vulva R87.69
drug level R87.2
enzyme level R87.0
histological R87.7
hormones R87.1
immunology R87.4
microbiology R87.5
nonmedicinal level R87.3
specified type NEC R87.89
male genital organs (prostatic secretions) (semen) R86.9
cytology R86.6
drug level R86.2
enzyme level R86.0
histological R86.7
hormones R86.1
immunology R86.4
microbiology R86.5
nonmedicinal level R86.3
specified type NEC R86.8
nipple discharge — *see* Abnormal, specimen, specified
respiratory organs (bronchial washings) (nasal secretions) (pleural fluid) (sputum) R84.9
cytology R84.6
drug level R84.2
enzyme level R84.0
histology R84.7
hormones R84.1
immunology R84.4

Abnormal, abnormality, abnormalities — *continued*
　specimen — *continued*
　　respiratory organs — *continued*
　　　microbiology R84.5
　　　nonmedicinal level R84.3
　　　specified type NEC R84.8
　　specified organ, system and tissue NOS R89.9
　　　cytology R89.6
　　　drug level R89.2
　　　enzyme level R89.0
　　　histology R89.7
　　　hormones R89.1
　　　immunology R89.4
　　　microbiology R89.5
　　　nonmedicinal level R89.3
　　　specified type NEC R89.8
　　synovial fluid — *see* Abnormal, specimen, specified
　　thorax (bronchial washings) (pleural fluids) — *see* Abnormal, specimen, respiratory organs
　　vagina (secretion) (smear) R87.629
　　vulva (secretion) (smear) R87.69
　　wound secretion — *see* Abnormal, specimen, specified
　spermatozoa — *see* Abnormal, specimen, male genital organs
　sputum (amount) (color) (odor) R09.3
　stool (color) (contents) (mucus) R19.5
　　bloody K92.1
　　guaiac positive R19.5
　synchondrosis Q78.8
　thermography (*see also* Abnormal, diagnostic imaging) R93.89
　thyroid-binding globulin E07.89
　tooth, teeth (form) (size) K00.2
　toxicology (findings) R78.9
　transport protein E88.09
　tumor marker NEC R97.8
　ultrasound results — *see* Abnormal, diagnostic imaging
　umbilical cord complicating delivery O69.9 ☑
　urination NEC R39.198
　urine (constituents) R82.90
　　bile R82.2
　　cytological examination R82.8
　　drugs R82.5
　　fat R82.0
　　glucose R81
　　heavy metals R82.6
　　hemoglobin R82.3
　　histological examination R82.8
　　ketones R82.4
　　microbiological examination (culture) R82.79
　　myoglobin R82.1
　　positive culture R82.79
　　protein — *see* Proteinuria
　　specified substance NEC R82.998
　　　chromoabnormality NEC R82.91
　　substances nonmedical R82.6
　uterine hemorrhage — *see* Hemorrhage, uterus
　vectorcardiogram R94.39
　visually evoked potential (VEP) R94.112
　white blood cells D72.9
　　specified NEC D72.89
　X-ray examination — *see* Abnormal, diagnostic imaging
Abnormity (any organ or part) — *see* Anomaly
Abocclusion M26.29
　hemolytic disease (newborn) P55.1
　incompatibility reaction ABO — *see* Complication(s), transfusion, incompatibility reaction, ABO
Abolition, language R48.8
Aborter, habitual or recurrent — *see* Loss (of), pregnancy, recurrent
Abortion (complete) (spontaneous) O03.9
　with
　　retained products of conception — *see* Abortion, incomplete
　attempted (elective) (failed) O07.4
　　complicated by O07.30
　　　afibrinogenemia O07.1
　　　cardiac arrest O07.36
　　　chemical damage of pelvic organ(s) O07.34
　　　circulatory collapse O07.31
　　　cystitis O07.38
　　　defibrination syndrome O07.1
　　　electrolyte imbalance O07.33
　　　embolism (air) (amniotic fluid) (blood clot) (fat) (pulmonary) (septic) (soap) O07.2
　　　endometritis O07.0

Abortion — *continued*
　attempted — *continued*
　　complicated by — *continued*
　　　genital tract and pelvic infection O07.0
　　　hemolysis O07.1
　　　hemorrhage (delayed) (excessive) O07.1
　　　infection
　　　　genital tract or pelvic O07.0
　　　　urinary tract tract O07.38
　　　intravascular coagulation O07.1
　　　laceration of pelvic organ(s) O07.34
　　　metabolic disorder O07.33
　　　oliguria O07.32
　　　oophoritis O07.0
　　　parametritis O07.0
　　　pelvic peritonitis O07.0
　　　perforation of pelvic organ(s) O07.34
　　　renal failure or shutdown O07.32
　　　salpingitis or salpingo-oophoritis O07.0
　　　sepsis O07.37
　　　shock O07.31
　　　specified condition NEC O07.39
　　　tubular necrosis (renal) O07.32
　　　uremia O07.32
　　　urinary tract infection O07.38
　　　venous complication NEC O07.35
　　　　embolism (air) (amniotic fluid) (blood clot) (fat) (pulmonary) (septic) (soap) O07.2
　complicated (by) (following) O03.80
　　afibrinogenemia O03.6
　　cardiac arrest O03.86
　　chemical damage of pelvic organ(s) O03.84
　　circulatory collapse O03.81
　　cystitis O03.88
　　defibrination syndrome O03.6
　　electrolyte imbalance O03.83
　　embolism (air) (amniotic fluid) (blood clot) (fat) (pulmonary) (septic) (soap) O03.7
　　endometritis O03.5
　　genital tract and pelvic infection O03.5
　　hemolysis O03.6
　　hemorrhage (delayed) (excessive) O03.6
　　infection
　　　genital tract or pelvic O03.5
　　　urinary tract O03.88
　　intravascular coagulation O03.6
　　laceration of pelvic organ(s) O03.84
　　metabolic disorder O03.83
　　oliguria O03.82
　　oophoritis O03.5
　　parametritis O03.5
　　pelvic peritonitis O03.5
　　perforation of pelvic organ(s) O03.84
　　renal failure or shutdown O03.82
　　salpingitis or salpingo-oophoritis O03.5
　　sepsis O03.87
　　shock O03.81
　　specified condition NEC O03.89
　　tubular necrosis (renal) O03.82
　　uremia O03.82
　　urinary tract infection O03.88
　　venous complication NEC O03.85
　　　embolism (air) (amniotic fluid) (blood clot) (fat) (pulmonary) (septic) (soap) O03.7
　failed — *see* Abortion, attempted
　habitual or recurrent N96
　　with current abortion — *see* categories O03-O04
　　without current pregnancy N96
　　care in current pregnancy O26.2- ☑
　incomplete (spontaneous) O03.4
　　complicated (by) (following) O03.30
　　　afibrinogenemia O03.1
　　　cardiac arrest O03.36
　　　chemical damage of pelvic organ(s) O03.34
　　　circulatory collapse O03.31
　　　cystitis O03.38
　　　defibrination syndrome O03.1
　　　electrolyte imbalance O03.33
　　　embolism (air) (amniotic fluid) (blood clot) (fat) (pulmonary) (septic) (soap) O03.2
　　　endometritis O03.0
　　　genital tract and pelvic infection O03.0
　　　hemolysis O03.1
　　　hemorrhage (delayed) (excessive) O03.1
　　　infection
　　　　genital tract or pelvic O03.0
　　　　urinary tract O03.38
　　　intravascular coagulation O03.1
　　　laceration of pelvic organ(s) O03.34

Abortion — *continued*
　incomplete — *continued*
　　complicated — *continued*
　　　metabolic disorder O03.33
　　　oliguria O03.32
　　　oophoritis O03.0
　　　parametritis O03.0
　　　pelvic peritonitis O03.0
　　　perforation of pelvic organ(s) O03.34
　　　renal failure or shutdown O03.32
　　　salpingitis or salpingo-oophoritis O03.0
　　　sepsis O03.37
　　　shock O03.31
　　　specified condition NEC O03.39
　　　tubular necrosis (renal) O03.32
　　　uremia O03.32
　　　urinary infection O03.38
　　　venous complication NEC O03.35
　　　　embolism (air) (amniotic fluid) (blood clot) (fat) (pulmonary) (septic) (soap) O03.2
　induced (encounter for) Z33.2
　　complicated by O04.80
　　　afibrinogenemia O04.6
　　　cardiac arrest O04.86
　　　chemical damage of pelvic organ(s) O04.84
　　　circulatory collapse O04.81
　　　cystitis O04.88
　　　defibrination syndrome O04.6
　　　electrolyte imbalance O04.83
　　　embolism (air) (amniotic fluid) (blood clot) (fat) (pulmonary) (septic) (soap) O04.7
　　　endometritis O04.5
　　　genital tract and pelvic infection O04.5
　　　hemolysis O04.6
　　　hemorrhage (delayed) (excessive) O04.6
　　　infection
　　　　genital tract or pelvic O04.5
　　　　urinary tract O04.88
　　　intravascular coagulation O04.6
　　　laceration of pelvic organ(s) O04.84
　　　metabolic disorder O04.83
　　　oliguria O04.82
　　　oophoritis O04.5
　　　parametritis O04.5
　　　pelvic peritonitis O04.5
　　　perforation of pelvic organ(s) O04.84
　　　renal failure or shutdown O04.82
　　　salpingitis or salpingo-oophoritis O04.5
　　　sepsis O04.87
　　　shock O04.81
　　　specified condition NEC O04.89
　　　tubular necrosis (renal) O04.82
　　　uremia O04.82
　　　urinary tract infection O04.88
　　　venous complication NEC O04.85
　　　　embolism (air) (amniotic fluid) (blood clot) (fat) (pulmonary) (septic) (soap) O04.7
　missed O02.1
　spontaneous — *see* Abortion (complete) (spontaneous)
　　threatened O20.0
　threatened (spontaneous) O20.0
　tubal O00.10- ☑
　　with intrauterine pregnancy O00.11- ☑
Abortus fever A23.1
Aboulomania F60.7
Abrami's disease D59.8
Abramov-Fiedler myocarditis (acute isolated myocarditis) I40.1
Abrasion T14.8 ☑
　abdomen, abdominal (wall) S30.811 ☑
　alveolar process S00.512 ☑
　ankle S90.51- ☑
　antecubital space — *see* Abrasion, elbow
　anus S30.817 ☑
　arm (upper) S40.81- ☑
　auditory canal — *see* Abrasion, ear
　auricle — *see* Abrasion, ear
　axilla — *see* Abrasion, arm
　back, lower S30.810 ☑
　breast S20.11- ☑
　brow S00.81 ☑
　buttock S30.810 ☑
　calf — *see* Abrasion, leg
　canthus — *see* Abrasion, eyelid
　cheek S00.81 ☑
　　internal S00.512 ☑
　chest wall — *see* Abrasion, thorax
　chin S00.81 ☑

Index

Abrasion — Abscess

Abrasion — *continued*
- clitoris S30.814 ☑
- cornea S05.0- ☑
- costal region — *see* Abrasion, thorax
- dental K03.1
- digit(s)
  - foot — *see* Abrasion, toe
  - hand — *see* Abrasion, finger
- ear S00.41- ☑
- elbow S50.31- ☑
- epididymis S30.813 ☑
- epigastric region S30.811 ☑
- epiglottis S10.11 ☑
- esophagus (thoracic) S27.818 ☑
  - cervical S10.11 ☑
- eyebrow — *see* Abrasion, eyelid
- eyelid S00.21- ☑
- face S00.81 ☑
- finger(s) S60.41- ☑
  - index S60.41- ☑
  - little S60.41- ☑
  - middle S60.41- ☑
  - ring S60.41- ☑
- flank S30.811 ☑
- foot (except toe(s) alone) S90.81- ☑
  - toe — *see* Abrasion, toe
- forearm S50.81- ☑
  - elbow only — *see* Abrasion, elbow
- forehead S00.81 ☑
- genital organs, external
  - female S30.816 ☑
  - male S30.815 ☑
- groin S30.811 ☑
- gum S00.512 ☑
- hand S60.51- ☑
- head S00.91 ☑
  - ear — *see* Abrasion, ear
  - eyelid — *see* Abrasion, eyelid
  - lip S00.511 ☑
  - nose S00.31 ☑
  - oral cavity S00.512 ☑
  - scalp S00.01 ☑
  - specified site NEC S00.81 ☑
- heel — *see* Abrasion, foot
- hip S70.21- ☑
- inguinal region S30.811 ☑
- interscapular region S20.419 ☑
- jaw S00.81 ☑
- knee S80.21- ☑
- labium (majus) (minus) S30.814 ☑
- larynx S10.11 ☑
- leg (lower) S80.81- ☑
  - knee — *see* Abrasion, knee
  - upper — *see* Abrasion, thigh
- lip S00.511 ☑
- lower back S30.810 ☑
- lumbar region S30.810 ☑
- malar region S00.81 ☑
- mammary — *see* Abrasion, breast
- mastoid region S00.81 ☑
- mouth S00.512 ☑
- nail
  - finger — *see* Abrasion, finger
  - toe — *see* Abrasion, toe
- nape S10.81 ☑
- nasal S00.31 ☑
- neck S10.91 ☑
  - specified site NEC S10.81 ☑
  - throat S10.11 ☑
- nose S00.31 ☑
- occipital region S00.01 ☑
- oral cavity S00.512 ☑
- orbital region — *see* Abrasion, eyelid
- palate S00.512 ☑
- palm — *see* Abrasion, hand
- parietal region S00.01 ☑
- pelvis S30.810 ☑
- penis S30.812 ☑
- perineum
  - female S30.814 ☑
  - male S30.810 ☑
- periocular area — *see* Abrasion, eyelid
- phalanges
  - finger — *see* Abrasion, finger
  - toe — *see* Abrasion, toe
- pharynx S10.11 ☑

Abrasion — *continued*
- pinna — *see* Abrasion, ear
- popliteal space — *see* Abrasion, knee
- prepuce S30.812 ☑
- pubic region S30.810 ☑
- pudendum
  - female S30.816 ☑
  - male S30.815 ☑
- sacral region S30.810 ☑
- scalp S00.01 ☑
- scapular region — *see* Abrasion, shoulder
- scrotum S30.813 ☑
- shin — *see* Abrasion, leg
- shoulder S40.21- ☑
- skin NEC T14.8 ☑
- sternal region S20.319 ☑
- submaxillary region S00.81 ☑
- submental region S00.81 ☑
- subungual
  - finger(s) — *see* Abrasion, finger
  - toe(s) — *see* Abrasion, toe
- supraclavicular fossa S10.81 ☑
- supraorbital S00.81 ☑
- temple S00.81 ☑
- temporal region S00.81 ☑
- testis S30.813 ☑
- thigh S70.31- ☑
- thorax, thoracic (wall) S20.91 ☑
  - back S20.41- ☑
  - front S20.31- ☑
- throat S10.11 ☑
- thumb S60.31- ☑
- toe(s) (lesser) S90.416 ☑
  - great S90.41- ☑
- tongue S00.512 ☑
- tooth, teeth (dentifrice) (habitual) (hard tissues) (occupational) (ritual) (traditional) K03.1
- trachea S10.11 ☑
- tunica vaginalis S30.813 ☑
- tympanum, tympanic membrane — *see* Abrasion, ear
- uvula S00.512 ☑
- vagina S30.814 ☑
- vocal cords S10.11 ☑
- vulva S30.814 ☑
- wrist S60.81- ☑

Abrism — *see* Poisoning, food, noxious, plant
Abruptio placentae O45.9- ☑
- with
  - afibrinogenemia O45.01- ☑
  - coagulation defect O45.00- ☑
    - specified NEC O45.09- ☑
  - disseminated intravascular coagulation O45.02- ☑
  - hypofibrinogenemia O45.01- ☑
- specified NEC O45.8- ☑
Abruption, placenta — *see* Abruptio placentae
Abscess (connective tissue) (embolic) (fistulous) (infective) (metastatic) (multiple) (pernicious) (pyogenic) (septic) L02.91
- with
  - diverticular disease (intestine) K57.80
    - with bleeding K57.81
    - large intestine K57.20
      - with
        - bleeding K57.21
        - small intestine K57.40
          - with bleeding K57.41
    - small intestine K57.00
      - with
        - bleeding K57.01
        - large intestine K57.40
          - with bleeding K57.41
  - lymphangitis — *code by* site under Abscess
- abdomen, abdominal
  - cavity K65.1
  - wall L02.211
- abdominopelvic K65.1
- accessory sinus — *see* Sinusitis
- adrenal (capsule) (gland) E27.8
- alveolar K04.7
  - with sinus K04.6
- amebic A06.4
  - brain (and liver or lung abscess) A06.6
  - genitourinary tract A06.82
  - liver (without mention of brain or lung abscess) A06.4
  - lung (and liver) (without mention of brain abscess) A06.5

Abscess — *continued*
- amebic — *continued*
  - specified site NEC A06.89
  - spleen A06.89
- anerobic A48.0
- ankle — *see* Abscess, lower limb
- anorectal K61.2
- antecubital space — *see* Abscess, upper limb
- antrum (chronic) (Highmore) — *see* Sinusitis, maxillary
- anus K61.0
- apical (tooth) K04.7
  - with sinus (alveolar) K04.6
- appendix K35.33
- areola (acute) (chronic) (nonpuerperal) N61.1
  - puerperal, postpartum or gestational — *see* Infection, nipple
- arm (any part) — *see* Abscess, upper limb
- artery (wall) I77.89
- atheromatous I77.2
- auricle, ear — *see* Abscess, ear, external
- axilla (region) L02.41- ☑
  - lymph gland or node L04.2
- back (any part, except buttock) L02.212
- Bartholin's gland N75.1
  - with
    - abortion — *see* Abortion, by type complicated by, sepsis
    - ectopic or molar pregnancy O08.0
  - following ectopic or molar pregnancy O08.0
- Bezold's — *see* Mastoiditis, acute
- bilharziasis B65.1
- bladder (wall) — *see* Cystitis, specified type NEC
- bone (subperiosteal) (*see also* Osteomyelitis, specified type NEC)
  - accessory sinus (chronic) — *see* Sinusitis
  - chronic or old — *see* Osteomyelitis, chronic
  - jaw (lower) (upper) M27.2
  - mastoid — *see* Mastoiditis, acute, subperiosteal
  - petrous — *see* Petrositis
  - spinal (tuberculous) A18.01
    - nontuberculous — *see* Osteomyelitis, vertebra
- bowel K63.0
- brain (any part) (cystic) (otogenic) G06.0
  - amebic (with abscess of any other site) A06.6
  - gonococcal A54.82
  - pheomycotic (chromomycotic) B43.1
  - tuberculous A17.81
- breast (acute) (chronic) (nonpuerperal) N61.1
  - newborn P39.0
  - puerperal, postpartum, gestational — *see* Mastitis, obstetric, purulent
- broad ligament N73.2
  - acute N73.0
  - chronic N73.1
- Brodie's (localized) (chronic) M86.8X- ☑
- bronchi J98.09
- buccal cavity K12.2
- bulbourethral gland N34.0
- bursa M71.00
  - ankle M71.07- ☑
  - elbow M71.02- ☑
  - foot M71.07- ☑
  - hand M71.04- ☑
  - hip M71.05- ☑
  - knee M71.06- ☑
  - multiple sites M71.09
  - pharyngeal J39.1
  - shoulder M71.01- ☑
  - specified site NEC M71.08
  - wrist M71.03- ☑
- buttock L02.31
- canthus — *see* Blepharoconjunctivitis
- cartilage — *see* Disorder, cartilage, specified type NEC
- cecum K35.33
- cerebellum, cerebellar G06.0
  - sequelae G09
- cerebral (embolic) G06.0
  - sequelae G09
- cervical (meaning neck) L02.11
  - lymph gland or node L04.0
- cervix (stump) (uteri) — *see* Cervicitis
- cheek (external) L02.01
  - inner K12.2
- chest J86.9
  - with fistula J86.0
  - wall L02.213
- chin L02.01
- choroid — *see* Inflammation, chorioretinal

Abscess — *continued*
- circumtonsillar J36
- cold (lung) (tuberculous) (*see also* Tuberculosis, abscess, lung)
  - articular — *see* Tuberculosis, joint
- colon (wall) K63.0
- colostomy K94.02
- conjunctiva — *see* Conjunctivitis, acute
- cornea H16.31- ☑
- corpus
  - cavernosum N48.21
  - luteum — *see* Oophoritis
- Cowper's gland N34.0
- cranium G06.0
- cul-de-sac (Douglas') (posterior) — *see* Peritonitis, pelvic, female
- cutaneous — *see* Abscess, by site
- dental K04.7
  - with sinus (alveolar) K04.6
- dentoalveolar K04.7
  - with sinus K04.6
- diaphragm, diaphragmatic K65.1
- Douglas' cul-de-sac or pouch — *see* Peritonitis, pelvic, female
- Dubois A50.59
- ear (middle) (*see also* Otitis, media, suppurative)
  - acute — *see* Otitis, media, suppurative, acute
  - external H60.0- ☑
- entamebic — *see* Abscess, amebic
- enterostomy K94.12
- epididymis N45.4
- epidural G06.2
  - brain G06.0
  - spinal cord G06.1
- epiglottis J38.7
- epiploon, epiploic K65.1
- erysipelatous — *see* Erysipelas
- esophagus K20.8
- ethmoid (bone) (chronic) (sinus) J32.2
- external auditory canal — *see* Abscess, ear, external
- extradural G06.2
  - brain G06.0
    - sequelae G09
  - spinal cord G06.1
- extraperitoneal K68.19
- eye — *see* Endophthalmitis, purulent
- eyelid H00.03- ☑
- face (any part, except ear, eye and nose) L02.01
- fallopian tube — *see* Salpingitis
- fascia M72.8
- fauces J39.1
- fecal K63.0
- femoral (region) — *see* Abscess, lower limb
- filaria, filarial — *see* Infestation, filarial
- finger (any) (*see also* Abscess, hand)
  - nail — *see* Cellulitis, finger
- foot L02.61- ☑
- forehead L02.01
- frontal sinus (chronic) J32.1
- gallbladder K81.0
- genital organ or tract
  - female (external) N76.4
  - male N49.9
    - multiple sites N49.8
    - specified NEC N49.8
- gestational mammary O91.11- ☑
- gestational subareolar O91.11- ☑
- gingival — *see* Peridontitis, localized
- gland, glandular (lymph) (acute) — *see* Lymphadenitis, acute
- gluteal (region) L02.31
- gonorrheal — *see* Gonococcus
- groin L02.214
- gum — *see* Peridontitis, localized
- hand L02.51- ☑
- head NEC L02.811
  - face (any part, except ear, eye and nose) L02.01
- heart — *see* Carditis
- heel — *see* Abscess, foot
- helminthic — *see* Infestation, helminth
- hepatic (cholangitic) (hematogenic) (lymphogenic) (pylephlebitic) K75.0
  - amebic A06.4
- hip (region) — *see* Abscess, lower limb
- horseshoe K61.31
- ileocecal K35.33
- ileostomy (bud) K94.12
- iliac (region) L02.214

Abscess — *continued*
- iliac — *continued*
  - fossa K35.33
- infraclavicular (fossa) — *see* Abscess, upper limb
- inguinal (region) L02.214
  - lymph gland or node L04.1
- intersphincteric K61.4
- intestine, intestinal NEC K63.0
  - rectal K61.1
- intra-abdominal (*see also* Abscess, peritoneum) K65.1
  - following procedure T81.43 ☑
    - obstetrical O86.03
  - postprocedural T81.49 ☑
    - retroperitoneal K68.11
- intracranial G06.0
- intramammary — *see* Abscess, breast
- intramuscular, following procedure T81.42 ☑
  - obstetrical O86.02
- intraorbital — *see* Abscess, orbit
- intraperitoneal K65.1
- intrasphincteric (anus) K61.4
- intraspinal G06.1
- intratonsillar J36
- ischiorectal (fossa) (specified NEC) K61.39
- jaw (bone) (lower) (upper) M27.2
- joint — *see* Arthritis, pyogenic or pyemic
  - spine (tuberculous) A18.01
    - nontuberculous — *see* Spondylopathy, infective
- kidney N15.1
  - with calculus N20.0
    - with hydronephrosis N13.6
  - puerperal (postpartum) O86.21
- knee (*see also* Abscess, lower limb)
  - joint M00.9
- labium (majus) (minus) N76.4
- lacrimal
  - caruncle — *see* Inflammation, lacrimal, passages, acute
  - gland — *see* Dacryoadenitis
  - passages (duct) (sac) — *see* Inflammation, lacrimal, passages, acute
- lacunar N34.0
- larynx J38.7
- lateral (alveolar) K04.7
  - with sinus K04.6
- leg (any part) — *see* Abscess, lower limb
- lens H27.8
- lingual K14.0
  - tonsil J36
- lip K13.0
- Littre's gland N34.0
- liver (cholangitic) (hematogenic) (lymphogenic) (pylephlebitic) (pyogenic) K75.0
  - amebic (due to Entamoeba histolytica) (dysenteric) (tropical) A06.4
    - with
      - brain abscess (and liver or lung abscess) A06.6
      - lung abscess A06.5
- loin (region) L02.211
- lower limb L02.41- ☑
- lumbar (tuberculous) A18.01
  - nontuberculous L02.212
- lung (miliary) (putrid) J85.2
  - with pneumonia J85.1
    - due to specified organism (see Pneumonia, in (due to))
  - amebic (with liver abscess) A06.5
    - with
      - brain abscess A06.6
      - pneumonia A06.5
- lymph, lymphatic, gland or node (acute) (*see also* Lymphadenitis, acute)
  - mesentery I88.0
- malar M27.2
- mammary gland — *see* Abscess, breast
- marginal, anus K61.0
- mastoid — *see* Mastoiditis, acute
- maxilla, maxillary M27.2
  - molar (tooth) K04.7
    - with sinus K04.6
  - premolar K04.7
  - sinus (chronic) J32.0
- mediastinum J85.3
- meibomian gland — *see* Hordeolum
- meninges G06.2
- mesentery, mesenteric K65.1
- mesosalpinx — *see* Salpingitis
- mons pubis L02.215

Abscess — *continued*
- mouth (floor) K12.2
- muscle — *see* Myositis, infective
- myocardium I40.0
- nabothian (follicle) — *see* Cervicitis
- nasal J32.9
- nasopharyngeal J39.1
- navel L02.216
  - newborn P38.9
    - with mild hemorrhage P38.1
    - without hemorrhage P38.9
- neck (region) L02.11
  - lymph gland or node L04.0
- nephritic — *see* Abscess, kidney
- nipple N61.1
  - associated with
    - lactation — *see* Pregnancy, complicated by
    - pregnancy — *see* Pregnancy, complicated by
- nose (external) (fossa) (septum) J34.0
  - sinus (chronic) — *see* Sinusitis
- omentum K65.1
- operative wound T81.49 ☑
- orbit, orbital — *see* Cellulitis, orbit
- otogenic G06.0
- ovary, ovarian (corpus luteum) — *see* Oophoritis
- oviduct — *see* Oophoritis
- palate (soft) K12.2
  - hard M27.2
- palmar (space) — *see* Abscess, hand
- pancreas (duct) — *see* Pancreatitis, acute
- parafrenal N48.21
- parametric, parametrium N73.2
  - acute N73.0
  - chronic N73.1
- paranephric N15.1
- parapancreatic — *see* Pancreatitis, acute
- parapharyngeal J39.0
- pararectal K61.1
- parasinus — *see* Sinusitis
- parauterine (*see also* Disease, pelvis, inflammatory) N73.2
- paravaginal — *see* Vaginitis
- parietal region (scalp) L02.811
- parodontal — *see* Peridontitis, aggressive, localized
- parotid (duct) (gland) K11.3
  - region K12.2
- pectoral (region) L02.213
- pelvis, pelvic
  - female — *see* Disease, pelvis, inflammatory
  - male, peritoneal K65.1
- penis N48.21
  - gonococcal (accessory gland) (periurethral) A54.1
- perianal K61.0
- periapical K04.7
  - with sinus (alveolar) K04.6
- periappendicular K35.33
- pericardial I30.1
- pericecal K35.33
- pericemental — *see* Peridontitis, aggressive, localized
- pericholecystic — *see* Cholecystitis, acute
- pericoronal — *see* Peridontitis, aggressive, localized
- peridental — *see* Peridontitis, aggressive, localized
- perimetric (*see also* Disease, pelvis, inflammatory) N73.2
- perinephric, perinephritic — *see* Abscess, kidney
- perineum, perineal (superficial) L02.215
  - urethra N34.0
- periodontal (parietal) — *see* Peridontitis, aggressive, localized
  - apical K04.7
- periosteum, periosteal (*see also* Osteomyelitis, specified type NEC)
  - with osteomyelitis (*see also* Osteomyelitis, specified type NEC)
    - acute — *see* Osteomyelitis, acute
    - chronic — *see* Osteomyelitis, chronic
- peripharyngeal J39.0
- peripleuritic J86.9
  - with fistula J86.0
- periprostatic N41.2
- perirectal K61.1
- perirenal (tissue) — *see* Abscess, kidney
- perisinuous (nose) — *see* Sinusitis
- peritoneum, peritoneal (perforated) (ruptured) K65.1
  - with appendicitis (*see also* Appendicitis) K35.33
  - pelvic
    - female — *see* Peritonitis, pelvic, female
    - male K65.1
  - postoperative T81.49 ☑

Abscess — *continued*
  peritoneum, peritoneal — *continued*
    puerperal, postpartum, childbirth O85
    tuberculous A18.31
  peritonsillar J36
  perityphlic K35.33
  periureteral N28.89
  periurethral N34.0
    gonococcal (accessory gland) (periurethral) A54.1
  periuterine (*see also* Disease, pelvis, inflammatory) N73.2
  perivesical — *see* Cystitis, specified type NEC
  petrous bone — *see* Petrositis
  phagedenic NOS L02.91
    chancroid A57
  pharynx, pharyngeal (lateral) J39.1
  pilonidal L05.01
  pituitary (gland) E23.6
  pleura J86.9
    with fistula J86.0
  popliteal — *see* Abscess, lower limb
  postcecal K35.33
  postlaryngeal J38.7
  postnasal J34.0
  postoperative (any site) (*see also* Infection, postoperative wound) T81.49 ☑
    retroperitoneal K68.11
  postpharyngeal J39.0
  posttonsillar J36
  post-typhoid A01.09
  pouch of Douglas — *see* Peritonitis, pelvic, female
  premammary — *see* Abscess, breast
  prepatellar — *see* Abscess, lower limb
  prostate N41.2
    gonococcal (acute) (chronic) A54.22
  psoas muscle K68.12
  puerperal — *code by* site under Puerperal, abscess
  pulmonary — *see* Abscess, lung
  pulp, pulpal (dental) K04.01
    irreversible K04.02
    reversible K04.01
  rectovaginal septum K63.0
  rectovesical — *see* Cystitis, specified type NEC
  rectum K61.1
  renal — *see* Abscess, kidney
  retina — *see* Inflammation, chorioretinal
  retrobulbar — *see* Abscess, orbit
  retrocecal K65.1
  retrolaryngeal J38.7
  retromammary — *see* Abscess, breast
  retroperitoneal NEC K68.19
    postprocedural K68.11
  retropharyngeal J39.0
  retrouterine — *see* Peritonitis, pelvic, female
  retrovesical — *see* Cystitis, specified type NEC
  root, tooth K04.7
    with sinus (alveolar) K04.6
  round ligament (*see also* Disease, pelvis, inflammatory) N73.2
  rupture (spontaneous) NOS L02.91
  sacrum (tuberculous) A18.01
    nontuberculous M46.28
  salivary (duct) (gland) K11.3
  scalp (any part) L02.811
  scapular — *see* Osteomyelitis, specified type NEC
  sclera — *see* Scleritis
  scrofulous (tuberculous) A18.2
  scrotum N49.2
  seminal vesicle N49.0
  septal, dental K04.7
    with sinus (alveolar) K04.6
  serous — *see* Periostitis
  shoulder (region) — *see* Abscess, upper limb
  sigmoid K63.0
  sinus (accessory) (chronic) (nasal) (*see also* Sinusitis)
    intracranial venous (any) G06.0
  Skene's duct or gland N34.0
  skin — *see* Abscess, by site
  specified site NEC L02.818
  spermatic cord N49.1
  sphenoidal (sinus) (chronic) J32.3
  spinal cord (any part) (staphylococcal) G06.1
    tuberculous A17.81
  spine (column) (tuberculous) A18.01
    epidural G06.1
    nontuberculous — *see* Osteomyelitis, vertebra
  spleen D73.3
    amebic A06.89

Abscess — *continued*
  stitch T81.41 ☑
    following an obstetrical procedure O86.01
  subarachnoid G06.2
    brain G06.0
    spinal cord G06.1
  subareolar — *see* Abscess, breast
  subcecal K35.33
  subcutaneous (*see also* Abscess, by site)
    following procedure T81.41 ☑
      obstetrical O86.01
    pheomycotic (chromomycotic) B43.2
  subdiaphragmatic K65.1
  subdural G06.2
    brain G06.0
      sequelae G09
    spinal cord G06.1
  sub-fascial, following an obstetrical procedure O86.02
  subgaleal L02.811
  subhepatic K65.1
  sublingual K12.2
    gland K11.3
  submammary — *see* Abscess, breast
  submandibular (region) (space) (triangle) K12.2
    gland K11.3
  submaxillary (region) L02.01
    gland K11.3
  submental L02.01
    gland K11.3
  subperiosteal — *see* Osteomyelitis, specified type NEC
  subphrenic K65.1
    following an obstetrical procedure O86.03
    postoperative T81.43 ☑
  suburethral N34.0
  sudoriparous L75.8
  supraclavicular (fossa) — *see* Abscess, upper limb
  supralevator K61.5
  suprapelvic, acute N73.0
  suprarenal (capsule) (gland) E27.8
  sweat gland L74.8
  tear duct — *see* Inflammation, lacrimal, passages, acute
  temple L02.01
  temporal region L02.01
  temporosphenoidal G06.0
  tendon (sheath) M65.00
    ankle M65.07- ☑
    foot M65.07- ☑
    forearm M65.03- ☑
    hand M65.04- ☑
    lower leg M65.06- ☑
    pelvic region M65.05- ☑
    shoulder region M65.01- ☑
    specified site NEC M65.08
    thigh M65.05- ☑
    upper arm M65.02- ☑
  testis N45.4
  thigh — *see* Abscess, lower limb
  thorax J86.9
    with fistula J86.0
  throat J39.1
  thumb (*see also* Abscess, hand)
    nail — *see* Cellulitis, finger
  thymus (gland) E32.1
  thyroid (gland) E06.0
  toe (any) (*see also* Abscess, foot)
    nail — *see* Cellulitis, toe
  tongue (staphylococcal) K14.0
  tonsil(s) (lingual) J36
  tonsillopharyngeal J36
  tooth, teeth (root) K04.7
    with sinus (alveolar) K04.6
    supporting structures NEC — *see* Periodontitis, aggressive, localized
  trachea J39.8
  trunk L02.219
    abdominal wall L02.211
    back L02.212
    chest wall L02.213
    groin L02.214
    perineum L02.215
    umbilicus L02.216
  tubal — *see* Salpingitis
  tuberculous — *see* Tuberculosis, abscess
  tubo-ovarian — *see* Salpingo-oophoritis
  tunica vaginalis N49.1
  umbilicus L02.216
  upper
    limb L02.41- ☑

Abscess — *continued*
  upper — *continued*
    respiratory J39.8
  urethral (gland) N34.0
  urinary N34.0
  uterus, uterine (wall) (*see also* Endometritis)
    ligament (*see also* Disease, pelvis, inflammatory) N73.2
    neck — *see* Cervicitis
  uvula K12.2
  vagina (wall) — *see* Vaginitis
  vaginorectal — *see* Vaginitis
  vas deferens N49.1
  vermiform appendix K35.33
  vertebra (column) (tuberculous) A18.01
    nontuberculous — *see* Osteomyelitis, vertebra
  vesical — *see* Cystitis, specified type NEC
  vesico-uterine pouch — *see* Peritonitis, pelvic, female
  vitreous (humor) — *see* Endophthalmitis, purulent
  vocal cord J38.3
  von Bezold's — *see* Mastoiditis, acute
  vulva N76.4
  vulvovaginal gland N75.1
  web space — *see* Abscess, hand
  wound T81.49 ☑
  wrist — *see* Abscess, upper limb
Absence (of) (organ or part) (complete or partial)
  adrenal (gland) (congenital) Q89.1
    acquired E89.6
  albumin in blood E88.09
  alimentary tract (congenital) Q45.8
    upper Q40.8
  alveolar process (acquired) — *see* Anomaly, alveolar
  ankle (acquired) Z89.44- ☑
  anus (congenital) Q42.3
    with fistula Q42.2
  aorta (congenital) Q25.41
  appendix, congenital Q42.8
  arm (acquired) Z89.20- ☑
    above elbow Z89.22- ☑
      congenital (with hand present) — *see* Agenesis, arm, with hand present
      and hand — *see* Agenesis, forearm, and hand
    below elbow Z89.21- ☑
      congenital (with hand present) — *see* Agenesis, arm, with hand present
      and hand — *see* Agenesis, forearm, and hand
    congenital — *see* Defect, reduction, upper limb
    shoulder (following explantation of shoulder joint prosthesis) (joint) (with or without presence of antibiotic-impregnated cement spacer) Z89.23- ☑
      congenital (with hand present) — *see* Agenesis, arm, with hand present
  artery (congenital) (peripheral) Q27.8
    brain Q28.3
    coronary Q24.5
    pulmonary Q25.79
    specified NEC Q27.8
    umbilical Q27.0
  atrial septum (congenital) Q21.1
  auditory canal (congenital) (external) Q16.1
  auricle (ear), congenital Q16.0
  bile, biliary duct, congenital Q44.5
  bladder (acquired) Z90.6
    congenital Q64.5
  bowel sounds R19.11
  brain Q00.0
    part of Q04.3
  breast(s) (and nipple(s)) (acquired) Z90.1- ☑
    congenital Q83.8
  broad ligament Q50.6
  bronchus (congenital) Q32.4
  canaliculus lacrimalis, congenital Q10.4
  cerebellum (vermis) Q04.3
  cervix (acquired) (with uterus) Z90.710
    with remaining uterus Z90.712
    congenital Q51.5
  chin, congenital Q18.8
  cilia (congenital) Q10.3
    acquired — *see* Madarosis
  clitoris (congenital) Q52.6
  coccyx, congenital Q76.49
  cold sense R20.8
  congenital
    lumen — *see* Atresia
    organ or site NEC — *see* Agenesis
    septum — *see* Imperfect, closure

Absence — *continued*
- corpus callosum Q04.0
- cricoid cartilage, congenital Q31.8
- diaphragm (with hernia), congenital Q79.1
- digestive organ(s) or tract, congenital Q45.8
  - acquired NEC Z90.49
  - upper Q40.8
- ductus arteriosus Q28.8
- duodenum (acquired) Z90.49
  - congenital Q41.0
- ear, congenital Q16.9
  - acquired H93.8- ☑
  - auricle Q16.0
  - external Q16.0
  - inner Q16.5
  - lobe, lobule Q17.8
  - middle, except ossicles Q16.4
    - ossicles Q16.3
  - ossicles Q16.3
- ejaculatory duct (congenital) Q55.4
- endocrine gland (congenital) NEC Q89.2
  - acquired E89.89
- epididymis (congenital) Q55.4
  - acquired Z90.79
- epiglottis, congenital Q31.8
- esophagus (congenital) Q39.8
  - acquired (partial) Z90.49
- eustachian tube (congenital) Q16.2
- extremity (acquired) Z89.9
  - congenital Q73.0
  - knee (following explantation of knee joint prosthesis) (joint) (with or without presence of antibiotic-impregnated cement spacer) Z89.52- ☑
  - lower (above knee) Z89.619
    - below knee Z89.51- ☑
  - upper — *see* Absence, arm
- eye (acquired) Z90.01
  - congenital Q11.1
  - muscle (congenital) Q10.3
- eyeball (acquired) Z90.01
- eyelid (fold) (congenital) Q10.3
  - acquired Z90.01
- face, specified part NEC Q18.8
- fallopian tube(s) (acquired) Z90.79
  - congenital Q50.6
- family member (causing problem in home) NEC (*see also* Disruption, family) Z63.32
- femur, congenital — *see* Defect, reduction, lower limb, longitudinal, femur
- fibrinogen (congenital) D68.2
  - acquired D65
- finger(s) (acquired) Z89.02- ☑
  - congenital — *see* Agenesis, hand
- foot (acquired) Z89.43- ☑
  - congenital — *see* Agenesis, foot
- forearm (acquired) — *see* Absence, arm, below elbow
- gallbladder (acquired) Z90.49
  - congenital Q44.0
- gamma globulin in blood D80.1
  - hereditary D80.0
- genital organs
  - acquired (female) (male) Z90.79
  - female, congenital Q52.8
    - external Q52.71
    - internal NEC Q52.8
  - male, congenital Q55.8
- genitourinary organs, congenital NEC
  - female Q52.8
  - male Q55.8
- globe (acquired) Z90.01
  - congenital Q11.1
- glottis, congenital Q31.8
- hand and wrist (acquired) Z89.11- ☑
  - congenital — *see* Agenesis, hand
- head, part (acquired) NEC Z90.09
- heat sense R20.8
- hip (following explantation of hip joint prosthesis) (joint) (with or without presence of antibiotic-impregnated cement spacer) Z89.62- ☑
- hymen (congenital) Q52.4
- ileum (acquired) Z90.49
  - congenital Q41.2
- immunoglobulin, isolated NEC D80.3
  - IgA D80.2
  - IgG D80.3
  - IgM D80.4
- incus (acquired) — *see* Loss, ossicles, ear
  - congenital Q16.3

Absence — *continued*
- inner ear, congenital Q16.5
- intestine (acquired) (small) Z90.49
  - congenital Q41.9
    - specified NEC Q41.8
  - large Z90.49
    - congenital Q42.9
      - specified NEC Q42.8
- iris, congenital Q13.1
- jejunum (acquired) Z90.49
  - congenital Q41.1
- joint
  - acquired
    - hip (following explantation of hip joint prosthesis) (with or without presence of antibiotic-impregnated cement spacer) Z89.62- ☑
    - knee (following explantation of knee joint prosthesis) (with or without presence of antibiotic-impregnated cement spacer) Z89.52- ☑
    - shoulder (following explantation of shoulder joint prosthesis) (with or without presence of antibiotic-impregnated cement spacer) Z89.23- ☑
    - congenital NEC Q74.8
- kidney(s) (acquired) Z90.5
  - congenital Q60.2
    - bilateral Q60.1
    - unilateral Q60.0
- knee (following explantation of knee joint prosthesis) (joint) (with or without presence of antibiotic-impregnated cement spacer) Z89.52- ☑
- labyrinth, membranous Q16.5
- larynx (congenital) Q31.8
  - acquired Z90.02
- leg (acquired) (above knee) Z89.61- ☑
  - below knee (acquired) Z89.51- ☑
  - congenital — *see* Defect, reduction, lower limb
- lens (acquired) (*see also* Aphakia)
  - congenital Q12.3
  - post cataract extraction Z98.4- ☑
- limb (acquired) — *see* Absence, extremity
- lip Q38.6
- liver (congenital) Q44.7
- lung (fissure) (lobe) (bilateral) (unilateral) (congenital) Q33.3
  - acquired (any part) Z90.2
- menstruation — *see* Amenorrhea
- muscle (congenital) (pectoral) Q79.8
  - ocular Q10.3
- neck, part Q18.8
- neutrophil — *see* Agranulocytosis
- nipple(s) (with breast(s)) (acquired) Z90.1- ☑
  - congenital Q83.2
- nose (congenital) Q30.1
  - acquired Z90.09
- organ
  - of Corti, congenital Q16.5
  - or site, congenital NEC Q89.8
    - acquired NEC Z90.89
- osseous meatus (ear) Q16.4
- ovary (acquired)
  - bilateral Z90.722
  - congenital
    - bilateral Q50.02
    - unilateral Q50.01
  - unilateral Z90.721
- oviduct (acquired)
  - bilateral Z90.722
  - congenital Q50.6
  - unilateral Z90.721
- pancreas (congenital) Q45.0
  - acquired Z90.410
    - complete Z90.410
    - partial Z90.411
    - total Z90.410
- parathyroid gland (acquired) E89.2
  - congenital Q89.2
- patella, congenital Q74.1
- penis (congenital) Q55.5
  - acquired Z90.79
- pericardium (congenital) Q24.8
- pituitary gland (congenital) Q89.2
  - acquired E89.3
- prostate (acquired) Z90.79
  - congenital Q55.4
- pulmonary valve Q22.0
- punctum lacrimale (congenital) Q10.4

Absence — *continued*
- radius, congenital — *see* Defect, reduction, upper limb, longitudinal, radius
- rectum (congenital) Q42.1
  - with fistula Q42.0
  - acquired Z90.49
- respiratory organ NOS Q34.9
- rib (acquired) Z90.89
  - congenital Q76.6
- sacrum, congenital Q76.49
- salivary gland(s), congenital Q38.4
- scrotum, congenital Q55.29
- seminal vesicles (congenital) Q55.4
  - acquired Z90.79
- septum
  - atrial (congenital) Q21.1
  - between aorta and pulmonary artery Q21.4
  - ventricular (congenital) Q20.4
- sex chromosome
  - female phenotype Q97.8
  - male phenotype Q98.8
- skull bone (congenital) Q75.8
  - with
    - anencephaly Q00.0
    - encephalocele — *see* Encephalocele
    - hydrocephalus Q03.9
      - with spina bifida — *see* Spina bifida, by site, with hydrocephalus
    - microcephaly Q02
- spermatic cord, congenital Q55.4
- spine, congenital Q76.49
- spleen (congenital) Q89.01
  - acquired Z90.81
- sternum, congenital Q76.7
- stomach (acquired) (partial) Z90.3
  - congenital Q40.2
- superior vena cava, congenital Q26.8
- teeth, tooth (congenital) K00.0
  - acquired (complete) K08.109
    - class I K08.101
    - class II K08.102
    - class III K08.103
    - class IV K08.104
    - due to
      - caries K08.139
        - class I K08.131
        - class II K08.132
        - class III K08.133
        - class IV K08.134
      - periodontal disease K08.129
        - class I K08.121
        - class II K08.122
        - class III K08.123
        - class IV K08.124
      - specified NEC K08.199
        - class I K08.191
        - class II K08.192
        - class III K08.193
        - class IV K08.194
      - trauma K08.119
        - class I K08.111
        - class II K08.112
        - class III K08.113
        - class IV K08.114
    - partial K08.409
      - class I K08.401
      - class II K08.402
      - class III K08.403
      - class IV K08.404
      - due to
        - caries K08.439
          - class I K08.431
          - class II K08.432
          - class III K08.433
          - class IV K08.434
        - periodontal disease K08.429
          - class I K08.421
          - class II K08.422
          - class III K08.423
          - class IV K08.424
        - specified NEC K08.499
          - class I K08.491
          - class II K08.492
          - class III K08.493
          - class IV K08.494
        - trauma K08.419
          - class I K08.411
          - class II K08.412
          - class III K08.413

Absence — *continued*
  teeth, tooth — *continued*
    acquired — *continued*
      partial — *continued*
        due to — *continued*
          trauma — *continued*
            class IV K08.414
  tendon (congenital) Q79.8
  testis (congenital) Q55.0
    acquired Z90.79
  thumb (acquired) Z89.01- ☑
    congenital — *see* Agenesis, hand
  thymus gland Q89.2
  thyroid (gland) (acquired) E89.0
    cartilage, congenital Q31.8
    congenital E03.1
  toe(s) (acquired) Z89.42- ☑
    with foot — *see* Absence, foot and ankle
    congenital — *see* Agenesis, foot
    great Z89.41- ☑
  tongue, congenital Q38.3
  trachea (cartilage), congenital Q32.1
  transverse aortic arch, congenital Q25.49
  tricuspid valve Q22.4
  umbilical artery, congenital Q27.0
  upper arm and forearm with hand present, congenital — *see* Agenesis, arm, with hand present
  ureter (congenital) Q62.4
    acquired Z90.6
  urethra, congenital Q64.5
  uterus (acquired) Z90.710
    with cervix Z90.710
    with remaining cervical stump Z90.711
    congenital Q51.0
  uvula, congenital Q38.5
  vagina, congenital Q52.0
  vas deferens (congenital) Q55.4
    acquired Z90.79
  vein (peripheral) congenital NEC Q27.8
    cerebral Q28.3
    digestive system Q27.8
    great Q26.8
    lower limb Q27.8
    portal Q26.5
    precerebral Q28.1
    specified site NEC Q27.8
    upper limb Q27.8
  vena cava (inferior) (superior), congenital Q26.8
  ventricular septum Q20.4
  vertebra, congenital Q76.49
  vulva, congenital Q52.71
  wrist (acquired) Z89.12- ☑

Absorbent system disease I87.8
Absorption
  carbohydrate, disturbance K90.49
  chemical — *see* Table of Drugs and Chemicals
    through placenta (newborn) P04.9
      environmental substance P04.6
      nutritional substance P04.5
      obstetric anesthetic or analgesic drug P04.0
  drug NEC — *see* Table of Drugs and Chemicals
    addictive
      through placenta (newborn) (*see also* Newborn, affected by, maternal, use of) P04.40
        cocaine P04.41
        hallucinogens P04.42
        specified drug NEC P04.49
    medicinal
      through placenta (newborn) P04.19
    through placenta (newborn) P04.19
      obstetric anesthetic or analgesic drug P04.0
  fat, disturbance K90.49
    pancreatic K90.3
  noxious substance — *see* Table of Drugs and Chemicals
  protein, disturbance K90.49
  starch, disturbance K90.49
  toxic substance — *see* Table of Drugs and Chemicals
  uremic — *see* Uremia
Abstinence symptoms, syndrome
  alcohol F10.239
    with delirium F10.231
  cocaine F14.23
  neonatal P96.1
  nicotine — *see* Dependence, drug, nicotine, with, withdrawal
  opioid F11.93
    with dependence F11.23
  psychoactive NEC F19.939

Abstinence symptoms, syndrome — *continued*
  psychoactive — *continued*
    with
      delirium F19.931
      dependence F19.239
        with
          delirium F19.231
          perceptual disturbance F19.232
        uncomplicated F19.230
      perceptual disturbance F19.932
    uncomplicated F19.930
  sedative F13.939
    with
      delirium F13.931
      dependence F13.239
        with
          delirium F13.231
          perceptual disturbance F13.232
        uncomplicated F13.230
      perceptual disturbance F13.932
    uncomplicated F13.930
  stimulant NEC F15.93
    with dependence F15.23
Abulia R68.89
Abulomania F60.7
Abuse
  adult — *see* Maltreatment, adult
    as reason for
      couple seeking advice (including offender) Z63.0
  alcohol (non-dependent) F10.10
    with
      anxiety disorder F10.180
      intoxication F10.129
        with delirium F10.121
        uncomplicated F10.120
      mood disorder F10.14
      other specified disorder F10.188
      psychosis F10.159
        delusions F10.150
        hallucinations F10.151
      sexual dysfunction F10.181
      sleep disorder F10.182
      unspecified disorder F10.19
    counseling and surveillance Z71.41
    in remission (early) (sustained) F10.11
  amphetamine (or related substance) — *see* Abuse, drug, stimulant NEC
  analgesics (non-prescribed) (over the counter) F55.8
  antacids F55.0
  antidepressants — *see* Abuse, drug, psychoactive NEC
  anxiolytic — *see* Abuse, drug, sedative
  barbiturates — *see* Abuse, drug, sedative
  caffeine — *see* Abuse, drug, stimulant NEC
  cannabis, cannabinoids — *see* Abuse, drug, cannabis
  child — *see* Maltreatment, child
  cocaine — *see* Abuse, drug, cocaine
  drug NEC (non-dependent) F19.10
    with sleep disorder F19.182
    amphetamine type — *see* Abuse, drug, stimulant NEC
    analgesics (non-prescribed) (over the counter) F55.8
    antacids F55.0
    antidepressants — *see* Abuse, drug, psychoactive NEC
    anxiolytics — *see* Abuse, drug, sedative
    barbiturates — *see* Abuse, drug, sedative
    caffeine — *see* Abuse, drug, stimulant NEC
    cannabis F12.10
      with
        anxiety disorder F12.180
        intoxication F12.129
          with
            delirium F12.121
            perceptual disturbance F12.122
          uncomplicated F12.120
        other specified disorder F12.188
        psychosis F12.159
          delusions F12.150
          hallucinations F12.151
        unspecified disorder F12.19
      in remission (early) (sustained) F12.11
    cocaine F14.10
      with
        anxiety disorder F14.180
        intoxication F14.129
          with
            delirium F14.121
            perceptual disturbance F14.122

Abuse — *continued*
  drug — *continued*
    cocaine — *continued*
      with — *continued*
        intoxication — *continued*
          uncomplicated F14.120
        mood disorder F14.14
        other specified disorder F14.188
        psychosis F14.159
          delusions F14.150
          hallucinations F14.151
        sexual dysfunction F14.181
        sleep disorder F14.182
        unspecified disorder F14.19
      in remission (early) (sustained) F14.11
    counseling and surveillance Z71.51
    hallucinogen F16.10
      with
        anxiety disorder F16.180
        flashbacks F16.183
        intoxication F16.129
          with
            delirium F16.121
            perceptual disturbance F16.122
          uncomplicated F16.120
        mood disorder F16.14
        other specified disorder F16.188
        perception disorder, persisting F16.183
        psychosis F16.159
          delusions F16.150
          hallucinations F16.151
        unspecified disorder F16.19
      in remission (early) (sustained) F16.11
    hashish — *see* Abuse, drug, cannabis
    herbal or folk remedies F55.1
    hormones F55.3
    hypnotics — *see* Abuse, drug, sedative
    in remission (early) (sustained) F19.11
    inhalant F18.10
      with
        anxiety disorder F18.180
        dementia, persisting F18.17
        intoxication F18.129
          with delirium F18.121
          uncomplicated F18.120
        mood disorder F18.14
        other specified disorder F18.188
        psychosis F18.159
          delusions F18.150
          hallucinations F18.151
        unspecified disorder F18.19
      in remission (early) (sustained) F18.11
    laxatives F55.2
    LSD — *see* Abuse, drug, hallucinogen
    marihuana — *see* Abuse, drug, cannabis
    morphine type (opioids) — *see* Abuse, drug, opioid
    opioid F11.10
      with
        intoxication F11.129
          with
            delirium F11.121
            perceptual disturbance F11.122
          uncomplicated F11.120
        mood disorder F11.14
        other specified disorder F11.188
        psychosis F11.159
          delusions F11.150
          hallucinations F11.151
        sexual dysfunction F11.181
        sleep disorder F11.182
        unspecified disorder F11.19
      in remission (early) (sustained) F11.11
    PCP (phencyclidine) (or related substance) — *see* Abuse, drug, hallucinogen
    psychoactive NEC F19.10
      with
        amnestic disorder F19.16
        anxiety disorder F19.180
        dementia F19.17
        intoxication F19.129
          with
            delirium F19.121
            perceptual disturbance F19.122
          uncomplicated F19.120
        mood disorder F19.14
        other specified disorder F19.188
        psychosis F19.159
          delusions F19.150
          hallucinations F19.151

Abuse — continued
  drug — continued
    psychoactive — continued
      with — continued
        sexual dysfunction F19.181
        sleep disorder F19.182
        unspecified disorder F19.19
    sedative, hypnotic or anxiolytic F13.10
      with
        anxiety disorder F13.180
        intoxication F13.129
          with delirium F13.121
          uncomplicated F13.120
        mood disorder F13.14
        other specified disorder F13.188
        psychosis F13.159
          delusions F13.150
          hallucinations F13.151
        sexual dysfunction F13.181
        sleep disorder F13.182
        unspecified disorder F13.19
      in remission (early) (sustained) F13.11
    solvent — see Abuse, drug, inhalant
    steroids F55.3
    stimulant NEC F15.10
      with
        anxiety disorder F15.180
        intoxication F15.129
          with
            delirium F15.121
            perceptual disturbance F15.122
          uncomplicated F15.120
        mood disorder F15.14
        other specified disorder F15.188
        psychosis F15.159
          delusions F15.150
          hallucinations F15.151
        sexual dysfunction F15.181
        sleep disorder F15.182
        unspecified disorder F15.19
      in remission (early) (sustained) F15.11
    tranquilizers — see Abuse, drug, sedative
    vitamins F55.4
  hallucinogens — see Abuse, drug, hallucinogen
  hashish — see Abuse, drug, cannabis
  herbal or folk remedies F55.1
  hormones F55.3
  hypnotic — see Abuse, drug, sedative
  inhalant — see Abuse, drug, inhalant
  laxatives F55.2
  LSD — see Abuse, drug, hallucinogen
  marihuana — see Abuse, drug, cannabis
  morphine type (opioids) — see Abuse, drug, opioid
  non-psychoactive substance NEC F55.8
    antacids F55.0
    folk remedies F55.1
    herbal remedies F55.1
    hormones F55.3
    laxatives F55.2
    steroids F55.3
    vitamins F55.4
  opioids — see Abuse, drug, opioid
  PCP (phencyclidine) (or related substance) — see Abuse, drug, hallucinogen
  physical (adult) (child) — see Maltreatment
  psychoactive substance — see Abuse, drug, psychoactive NEC
  psychological (adult) (child) — see Maltreatment
  sedative — see Abuse, drug, sedative
  sexual — see Maltreatment
  solvent — see Abuse, drug, inhalant
  steroids F55.3
  vitamins F55.4
Acalculia R48.8
  developmental F81.2
Acanthamebiasis (with) B60.10
  conjunctiva B60.12
  keratoconjunctivitis B60.13
  meningoencephalitis B60.11
  other specified B60.19
Acanthocephaliasis B83.8
Acanthocheilonemiasis B74.4
Acanthocytosis E78.6
Acantholysis L11.9
Acanthosis (acquired) (nigricans) L83
  benign Q82.8
  congenital Q82.8
  seborrheic L82.1

Acanthosis — continued
  seborrheic — continued
    inflamed L82.0
    tongue K14.3
Acapnia E87.3
Acarbia E87.2
Acardia, acardius Q89.8
Acardiacus amorphus Q89.8
Acardiotrophia I51.4
Acariasis B88.0
  scabies B86
Acarodermatitis (urticarioides) B88.0
Acarophobia F40.218
Acatalasemia, acatalasia E80.3
Acathisia (drug induced) G25.71
Accelerated atrioventricular conduction I45.6
Accentuation of personality traits (type A) Z73.1
Accessory (congenital)
  adrenal gland Q89.1
  anus Q43.4
  appendix Q43.4
  atrioventricular conduction I45.6
  auditory ossicles Q16.3
  auricle (ear) Q17.0
  biliary duct or passage Q44.5
  bladder Q64.79
  blood vessels NEC Q27.9
    coronary Q24.5
  bone NEC Q79.8
  breast tissue, axilla Q83.1
  carpal bones Q74.0
  cecum Q43.4
  chromosome(s) NEC (nonsex) Q92.9
    with complex rearrangements NEC Q92.5
      seen only at prometaphase Q92.8
    13 — see Trisomy, 13
    18 — see Trisomy, 18
    21 — see Trisomy, 21
    partial Q92.9
    sex
      female phenotype Q97.8
  coronary artery Q24.5
  cusp(s), heart valve NEC Q24.8
    pulmonary Q22.3
  cystic duct Q44.5
  digit(s) Q69.9
  ear (auricle) (lobe) Q17.0
  endocrine gland NEC Q89.2
  eye muscle Q10.3
  eyelid Q10.3
  face bone(s) Q75.8
  fallopian tube (fimbria) (ostium) Q50.6
  finger(s) Q69.0
  foreskin N47.8
  frontonasal process Q75.8
  gallbladder Q44.1
  genital organ(s)
    female Q52.8
      external Q52.79
      internal NEC Q52.8
    male Q55.8
  genitourinary organs NEC Q89.8
    female Q52.8
    male Q55.8
  hallux Q69.2
  heart Q24.8
    valve NEC Q24.8
      pulmonary Q22.3
  hepatic ducts Q44.5
  hymen Q52.4
  intestine (large) (small) Q43.4
  kidney Q63.0
  lacrimal canal Q10.6
  leaflet, heart valve NEC Q24.8
  ligament, broad Q50.6
  liver Q44.7
    duct Q44.5
  lobule (ear) Q17.0
  lung (lobe) Q33.1
  muscle Q79.8
  navicular of carpus Q74.0
  nervous system, part NEC Q07.8
  nipple Q83.3
  nose Q30.8
  organ or site not listed — see Anomaly, by site
  ovary Q50.31
  oviduct Q50.6
  pancreas Q45.3

Accessory — continued
  parathyroid gland Q89.2
  parotid gland (and duct) Q38.4
  pituitary gland Q89.2
  preauricular appendage Q17.0
  prepuce N47.8
  renal arteries (multiple) Q27.2
  rib Q76.6
    cervical Q76.5
  roots (teeth) K00.2
  salivary gland Q38.4
  sesamoid bones Q74.8
    foot Q74.2
    hand Q74.0
  skin tags Q82.8
  spleen Q89.09
  sternum Q76.7
  submaxillary gland Q38.4
  tarsal bones Q74.2
  teeth, tooth K00.1
  tendon Q79.8
  thumb Q69.1
  thymus gland Q89.2
  thyroid gland Q89.2
  toes Q69.2
  tongue Q38.3
  tooth, teeth K00.1
  tragus Q17.0
  ureter Q62.5
  urethra Q64.79
  urinary organ or tract NEC Q64.8
  uterus Q51.28
  vagina Q52.10
  valve, heart NEC Q24.8
    pulmonary Q22.3
  vertebra Q76.49
  vocal cords Q31.8
  vulva Q52.79
Accident
  birth — see Birth, injury
  cardiac — see Infarct, myocardium
  cerebral I63.9
  cerebrovascular (embolic) (ischemic) (thrombotic) I63.9
    aborted I63.9
    hemorrhagic — see Hemorrhage, intracranial, intracerebral
    old (without sequelae) Z86.73
      with sequelae (of) — see Sequelae, infarction, cerebral
  coronary — see Infarct, myocardium
  craniovascular I63.9
  vascular, brain I63.9
Accidental — see condition
Accommodation (disorder) (see also condition)
  hysterical paralysis of F44.89
  insufficiency of H52.4
  paresis — see Paresis, of accommodation
  spasm — see Spasm, of accommodation
Accouchement — see Delivery
Accreta placenta O43.21- ☑
Accretio cordis (nonrheumatic) I31.0
Accretions, tooth, teeth K03.6
Acculturation difficulty Z60.3
Accumulation secretion, prostate N42.89
Acephalia, acephalism, acephalus, acephaly Q00.0
Acephalobrachia monster Q89.8
Acephalochirus monster Q89.8
Acephalogaster Q89.8
Acephalostomus monster Q89.8
Acephalothorax Q89.8
Acerophobia F40.298
Acetonemia R79.89
  in Type 1 diabetes E10.10
    with coma E10.11
Acetonuria R82.4
Achalasia (cardia) (esophagus) K22.0
  congenital Q39.5
  pylorus Q40.0
  sphincteral NEC K59.8
Ache(s) — see Pain
Acheilia Q38.6
Achillobursitis — see Tendinitis, Achilles
Achillodynia — see Tendinitis, Achilles
Achlorhydria, achlorhydric (neurogenic) K31.83
  anemia D50.8
  diarrhea K31.83
  psychogenic F45.8
  secondary to vagotomy K91.1

Achluophobia F40.228
Acholia K82.8
Acholuric jaundice (familial) (splenomegalic) (*see also*
    Spherocytosis)
    acquired D59.8
Achondrogenesis Q77.0
Achondroplasia (osteosclerosis congenita) Q77.4
Achroma, cutis L80
Achromat (ism), achromatopsia (acquired) (congenital)
    H53.51
Achromia, congenital — *see* Albinism
Achromia parasitica B36.0
Achylia gastrica K31.89
    psychogenic F45.8
Acid
    burn — *see* Corrosion
    deficiency
        amide nicotinic E52
        ascorbic E54
        folic E53.8
        nicotinic E52
        pantothenic E53.8
    intoxication E87.2
    peptic disease K30
    phosphatase deficiency E83.39
    stomach K30
        psychogenic F45.8
Acidemia E87.2
    argininosuccinic E72.22
    isovaleric E71.110
    metabolic (newborn) P19.9
        first noted before onset of labor P19.0
        first noted during labor P19.1
        noted at birth P19.2
    methylmalonic E71.120
    pipecolic E72.3
    propionic E71.121
Acidity, gastric (high) K30
    psychogenic F45.8
Acidocytopenia — *see* Agranulocytosis
Acidocytosis D72.1
Acidopenia — *see* Agranulocytosis
Acidosis (lactic) (respiratory) E87.2
    in Type 1 diabetes E10.10
        with coma E10.11
    kidney, tubular N25.89
    lactic E87.2
    metabolic NEC E87.2
        with respiratory acidosis E87.4
        hyperchloremic, of newborn P74.421
        late, of newborn P74.0
    mixed metabolic and respiratory, newborn P84
    newborn P84
    renal (hyperchloremic) (tubular) N25.89
    respiratory E87.2
        complicated by
            metabolic
                acidosis E87.4
                alkalosis E87.4
Aciduria
    4-hydroxybutyric E72.81
    argininosuccinic E72.22
    gamma-hydroxybutyric E72.81
    glutaric (type I) E72.3
        type II E71.313
        type III E71.5- ☑
    orotic (congenital) (hereditary) (pyrimidine deficiency)
        E79.8
        anemia D53.0
Acladiosis (skin) B36.0
Aclasis, diaphyseal Q78.6
Acleistocardia Q21.1
Aclusion — *see* Anomaly, dentofacial, malocclusion
Acne L70.9
    artificialis L70.8
    atrophica L70.2
    cachecticorum (Hebra) L70.8
    conglobata L70.1
    cystic L70.0
    decalvans L66.2
    excoriée (des jeunes filles) L70.5
    frontalis L70.2
    indurata L70.0
    infantile L70.4
    keloid L73.0
    lupoid L70.2
    necrotic, necrotica (miliaris) L70.2
    neonatal L70.4

Acne — *continued*
    nodular L70.0
    occupational L70.8
    picker's L70.5
    pustular L70.0
    rodens L70.2
    rosacea L71.9
    specified NEC L70.8
    tropica L70.3
    varioliformis L70.2
    vulgaris L70.0
Acnitis (primary) A18.4
Acosta's disease T70.29 ☑
Acoustic — *see* condition
Acousticophobia F40.298
Acquired (*see also* condition)
    immunodeficiency syndrome (AIDS) B20
Acrania Q00.0
Acroangiodermatitis I78.9
Acroasphyxia, chronic I73.89
Acrobystitis N47.7
Acrocephalopolysyndactyly Q87.0
Acrocephalosyndactyly Q87.0
Acrocephaly Q75.0
Acrochondrohyperplasia — *see* Syndrome, Marfan's
Acrocyanosis I73.8 ☑
    newborn P28.2
        meaning transient blue hands and feet — *omit code*
Acrodermatitis L30.8
    atrophicans (chronica) L90.4
    continua (Hallopeau) L40.2
    enteropathica (hereditary) E83.2
    Hallopeau's L40.2
    infantile papular L44.4
    perstans L40.2
    pustulosa continua L40.2
    recalcitrant pustular L40.2
Acrodynia — *see* Poisoning, mercury
Acromegaly, acromegalia E22.0
Acromelalgia I73.81
Acromicria, acromikria Q79.8
Acronyx L60.0
Acropachy, thyroid — *see* Thyrotoxicosis
Acroparesthesia (simple) (vasomotor) I73.89
Acropathy, thyroid — *see* Thyrotoxicosis
Acrophobia F40.241
Acroposthitis N47.7
Acroscleriasis, acroscleroderma, acrosclerosis — *see*
    Sclerosis, systemic
Acrosphacelus I96
Acrospiroma, eccrine — *see* Neoplasm, skin, benign
Acrostealgia — *see* Osteochondropathy
Acrotrophodynia — *see* Immersion
ACTH ectopic syndrome E24.3
Actinic — *see* condition
Actinobacillosis, actinobacillus A28.8
    mallei A24.0
    muris A25.1
Actinomyces israelii (infection) — *see* Actinomycosis
Actinomycetoma (foot) B47.1
Actinomycosis, actinomycotic A42.9
    with pneumonia A42.0
    abdominal A42.1
    cervicofacial A42.2
    cutaneous A42.89
    gastrointestinal A42.1
    pulmonary A42.0
    sepsis A42.7
    specified site NEC A42.89
Actinoneuritis G62.82
Action, heart
    disorder I49.9
    irregular I49.9
        psychogenic F45.8
Activated protein C resistance D68.51
Activation
    mast cell (disorder) (syndrome) D89.40
        idiopathic D89.42
        monoclonal D89.41
        secondary D89.43
        specified type NEC D89.49
Active — *see* condition
Acute (*see also* condition)
    abdomen R10.0
    gallbladder — *see* Cholecystitis, acute
Acyanotic heart disease (congenital) Q24.9
Acystia Q64.5

Adair-Dighton syndrome (brittle bones and blue sclera,
    deafness) Q78.0
Adamantinoblastoma — *see* Ameloblastoma
Adamantinoma (*see also* Cyst, calcifying odontogenic)
    long bones C40.90
        lower limb C40.2- ☑
        upper limb C40.0- ☑
    malignant C41.1
        jaw (bone) (lower) C41.1
            upper C41.0
    tibial C40.2- ☑
Adamantoblastoma — *see* Ameloblastoma
Adams-Stokes (-Morgagni) disease or syndrome I45.9
Adaption reaction — *see* Disorder, adjustment
Addiction (*see also* Dependence) F19.20
    alcohol, alcoholic (ethyl) (methyl) (wood) (without re-
        mission) F10.20
        with remission F10.21
    drug — *see* Dependence, drug
    ethyl alcohol (without remission) F10.20
        with remission F10.21
    heroin — *see* Dependence, drug, opioid
    methyl alcohol (without remission) F10.20
        with remission F10.21
    methylated spirit (without remission) F10.20
        with remission F10.21
    morphine (-like substances) — *see* Dependence, drug,
        opioid
    nicotine — *see* Dependence, drug, nicotine
    opium and opioids — *see* Dependence, drug, opioid
    tobacco — *see* Dependence, drug, nicotine
Addison-Biermer anemia (pernicious) D51.0
Addisonian crisis E27.2
Addison's
    anemia (pernicious) D51.0
    disease (bronze) or syndrome E27.1
        tuberculous A18.7
    keloid L94.0
Addison-Schilder complex E71.528
Additional (*see also* Accessory)
    chromosome(s) Q99.8
        21 — *see* Trisomy, 21
    sex — *see* Abnormal, chromosome, sex
Adduction contracture, hip or other joint — *see*
    Contraction, joint
Adenitis (*see also* Lymphadenitis)
    acute, unspecified site L04.9
    axillary I88.9
        acute L04.2
        chronic or subacute I88.1
    Bartholin's gland N75.8
    bulbourethral gland — *see* Urethritis
    cervical I88.9
        acute L04.0
        chronic or subacute I88.1
    chancroid (Hemophilus ducreyi) A57
    chronic, unspecified site I88.1
    Cowper's gland — *see* Urethritis
    due to Pasteurella multocida (P. septica) A28.0
    epidemic, acute B27.09
    gangrenous L04.9
    gonorrheal NEC A54.89
    groin I88.9
        acute L04.1
        chronic or subacute I88.1
    infectious (acute) (epidemic) B27.09
    inguinal I88.9
        acute L04.1
        chronic or subacute I88.1
    lymph gland or node, except mesenteric I88.9
        acute — *see* Lymphadenitis, acute
        chronic or subacute I88.1
    mesenteric (acute) (chronic) (nonspecific) (subacute)
        I88.0
    parotid gland (suppurative) — *see* Sialoadenitis
    salivary gland (any) (suppurative) — *see* Sialoadenitis
    scrofulous (tuberculous) A18.2
    Skene's duct or gland — *see* Urethritis
    strumous, tuberculous A18.2
    subacute, unspecified site I88.1
    sublingual gland (suppurative) — *see* Sialoadenitis
    submandibular gland (suppurative) — *see* Sialoadenitis
    submaxillary gland (suppurative) — *see* Sialoadenitis
    tuberculous — *see* Tuberculosis, lymph gland
    urethral gland — *see* Urethritis
    Wharton's duct (suppurative) — *see* Sialoadenitis
Adenoacanthoma — *see* Neoplasm, malignant, by site

☑ **Additional Character Required** — Refer to the Tabular List for Character Selection   **Subterms under main terms may continue to next column or page**

Adenoameloblastoma — *see* Cyst, calcifying odontogenic

Adenocarcinoid (tumor) — *see* Neoplasm, malignant, by site

Adenocarcinoma (*see also* Neoplasm, malignant, by site)
  acidophil
    specified site — *see* Neoplasm, malignant, by site
    unspecified site C75.1
  adrenal cortical C74.0- ☑
  alveolar — *see* Neoplasm, lung, malignant
  apocrine
    breast — *see* Neoplasm, breast, malignant
    in situ
      breast D05.8- ☑
      specified site NEC — *see* Neoplasm, skin, in situ
      unspecified site D04.9
    specified site NEC — *see* Neoplasm, skin, malignant
    unspecified site C44.99
  basal cell
    specified site — *see* Neoplasm, skin, malignant
    unspecified site C08.9
  basophil
    specified site — *see* Neoplasm, malignant, by site
    unspecified site C75.1
  bile duct type C22.1
    liver C22.1
    specified site NEC — *see* Neoplasm, malignant, by site
    unspecified site C22.1
  bronchiolar — *see* Neoplasm, lung, malignant
  bronchioloalveolar — *see* Neoplasm, lung, malignant
  ceruminous C44.29- ☑
  cervix, in situ (*see also* Carcinoma, cervix uteri, in situ) D06.9
  chromophobe
    specified site — *see* Neoplasm, malignant, by site
    unspecified site C75.1
  diffuse type
    specified site — *see* Neoplasm, malignant, by site
    unspecified site C16.9
  duct
    infiltrating
      with Paget's disease — *see* Neoplasm, breast, malignant
      specified site — *see* Neoplasm, malignant, by site
      unspecified site (female) C50.91- ☑
        male C50.92- ☑
    specified site — *see* Neoplasm, malignant, by site
    unspecified site
      female C56.9
      male C61
  eosinophil
    specified site — *see* Neoplasm, malignant, by site
    unspecified site C75.1
  follicular
    with papillary C73
    moderately differentiated C73
    specified site — *see* Neoplasm, malignant, by site
    trabecular C73
    unspecified site C73
    well differentiated C73
  Hurthle cell C73
  in
    adenomatous
      polyposis coli C18.9
  infiltrating duct
    with Paget's disease — *see* Neoplasm, breast, malignant
    specified site — *see* Neoplasm, by site, malignant
    unspecified site (female) C50.91- ☑
      male C50.92- ☑
  inflammatory
    specified site — *see* Neoplasm, by site, malignant
    unspecified site (female) C50.91- ☑
      male C50.92- ☑
  intestinal type
    specified site — *see* Neoplasm, by site, malignant
    unspecified site C16.9
  intracystic papillary
  intraductal
    breast D05.1- ☑
    noninfiltrating
      breast D05.1- ☑

Adenocarcinoma — *continued*
  intraductal — *continued*
    noninfiltrating — *continued*
      papillary
        with invasion
          specified site — *see* Neoplasm, by site, malignant
          unspecified site (female) C50.91- ☑
            male C50.92- ☑
        breast D05.1- ☑
        specified site NEC — *see* Neoplasm, in situ, by site
        unspecified site D05.1- ☑
      specified site NEC — *see* Neoplasm, in situ, by site
      unspecified site D05.1- ☑
    papillary
      with invasion
        specified site — *see* Neoplasm, malignant, by site
        unspecified site (female) C50.91- ☑
          male C50.92- ☑
      breast D05.1- ☑
      specified site — *see* Neoplasm, in situ, by site
      unspecified site D05.1- ☑
    specified site NEC — *see* Neoplasm, in situ, by site
    unspecified site D05.1- ☑
  islet cell
    with exocrine, mixed
      specified site — *see* Neoplasm, malignant, by site
      unspecified site C25.9
    pancreas C25.4
    specified site NEC — *see* Neoplasm, malignant, by site
    unspecified site C25.4
  lobular
    in situ
      breast D05.0- ☑
      specified site NEC — *see* Neoplasm, in situ, by site
      unspecified site D05.0- ☑
    specified site — *see* Neoplasm, malignant, by site
    unspecified site (female) C50.91- ☑
      male C50.92- ☑
  mucoid (*see also* Neoplasm, malignant, by site)
    cell
      specified site — *see* Neoplasm, malignant, by site
      unspecified site C75.1
  nonencapsulated sclerosing C73
  papillary
    with follicular C73
    follicular variant C73
    intraductal (noninfiltrating)
      with invasion
        specified site — *see* Neoplasm, malignant, by site
        unspecified site (female) C50.91- ☑
          male C50.92- ☑
      breast D05.1- ☑
      specified site NEC — *see* Neoplasm, in situ, by site
      unspecified site D05.1- ☑
    serous
      specified site — *see* Neoplasm, malignant, by site
      unspecified site C56.9
  papillocystic
    specified site — *see* Neoplasm, malignant, by site
    unspecified site C56.9
  pseudomucinous
    specified site — *see* Neoplasm, malignant, by site
    unspecified site C56.9
  renal cell C64- ☑
  sebaceous — *see* Neoplasm, skin, malignant
  serous (*see also* Neoplasm, malignant, by site)
    papillary
      specified site — *see* Neoplasm, malignant, by site
      unspecified site C56.9
  sweat gland — *see* Neoplasm, skin, malignant
  water-clear cell C75.0

Adenocarcinoma-in-situ (*see also* Neoplasm, in situ, by site)
  breast D05.9- ☑

Adenofibroma
  clear cell — *see* Neoplasm, benign, by site
  endometrioid D27.9
    borderline malignancy D39.10
    malignant C56- ☑
  mucinous
    specified site — *see* Neoplasm, benign, by site
    unspecified site D27.9
  papillary
    specified site — *see* Neoplasm, benign, by site
    unspecified site D27.9
  prostate — *see* Enlargement, enlarged, prostate
  serous
    specified site — *see* Neoplasm, benign, by site
    unspecified site D27.9
  specified site — *see* Neoplasm, benign, by site
  unspecified site D27.9

Adenofibrosis
  breast — *see* Fibroadenosis, breast
  endometrioid N80.0

Adenoiditis (chronic) J35.02
  with tonsillitis J35.03
  acute J03.90
    recurrent J03.91
    specified organism NEC J03.80
      recurrent J03.81
    staphylococcal J03.80
      recurrent J03.81
    streptococcal J03.00
      recurrent J03.01

Adenoids — *see* condition

Adenolipoma — *see* Neoplasm, benign, by site

Adenolipomatosis, Launois-Bensaude E88.89

Adenolymphoma
  specified site — *see* Neoplasm, benign, by site
  unspecified site D11.9

Adenoma (*see also* Neoplasm, benign, by site)
  acidophil
    specified site — *see* Neoplasm, benign, by site
    unspecified site D35.2
  acidophil-basophil, mixed
    specified site — *see* Neoplasm, benign, by site
    unspecified site D35.2
  adrenal (cortical) D35.00
    clear cell D35.00
    compact cell D35.00
    glomerulosa cell D35.00
    heavily pigmented variant D35.00
    mixed cell D35.00
  alpha-cell
    pancreas D13.7
    specified site NEC — *see* Neoplasm, benign, by site
    unspecified site D13.7
  alveolar D14.30
  apocrine
    breast D24- ☑
    specified site NEC — *see* Neoplasm, skin, benign, by site
    unspecified site D23.9
  basal cell D11.9
  basophil
    specified site — *see* Neoplasm, benign, by site
    unspecified site D35.2
  basophil-acidophil, mixed
    specified site — *see* Neoplasm, benign, by site
    unspecified site D35.2
  beta-cell
    pancreas D13.7
    specified site NEC — *see* Neoplasm, benign, by site
    unspecified site D13.7
  bile duct D13.4
    common D13.5
    extrahepatic D13.5
    intrahepatic D13.4
    specified site NEC — *see* Neoplasm, benign, by site
    unspecified site D13.4
  black D35.00
  bronchial D38.1
    cylindroid type — *see* Neoplasm, lung, malignant
  ceruminous D23.2- ☑
  chief cell D35.1
  chromophobe
    specified site — *see* Neoplasm, benign, by site
    unspecified site D35.2
  colloid
    specified site — *see* Neoplasm, benign, by site
    unspecified site D34

Adenoma — *continued*
- duct
  - eccrine, papillary — *see* Neoplasm, skin, benign
  - endocrine, multiple
    - single specified site — *see* Neoplasm, uncertain behavior, by site
    - two or more specified sites D44- ☑
    - unspecified site D44.9
  - endometrioid (*see also* Neoplasm, benign)
    - borderline malignancy — *see* Neoplasm, uncertain behavior, by site
  - eosinophil
    - specified site — *see* Neoplasm, benign, by site
    - unspecified site D35.2
  - fetal
    - specified site — *see* Neoplasm, benign, by site
    - unspecified site D34
  - follicular
    - specified site — *see* Neoplasm, benign, by site
    - unspecified site D34
  - hepatocellular D13.4
  - Hurthle cell D34
  - islet cell
    - pancreas D13.7
    - specified site NEC — *see* Neoplasm, benign, by site
    - unspecified site D13.7
  - liver cell D13.4
  - macrofollicular
    - specified site — *see* Neoplasm, benign, by site
    - unspecified site D34
  - malignant, malignum — *see* Neoplasm, malignant, by site
  - microcystic
    - pancreas D13.6
    - specified site NEC — *see* Neoplasm, benign, by site
    - unspecified site D13.6
  - microfollicular
    - specified site — *see* Neoplasm, benign, by site
    - unspecified site D34
  - mucoid cell
    - specified site — *see* Neoplasm, benign, by site
    - unspecified site D35.2
  - multiple endocrine
    - single specified site — *see* Neoplasm, uncertain behavior, by site
    - two or more specified sites D44- ☑
    - unspecified site D44.9
  - nipple D24- ☑
  - papillary (*see also* Neoplasm, benign, by site)
    - eccrine — *see* Neoplasm, skin, benign, by site
  - Pick's tubular
    - specified site — *see* Neoplasm, benign, by site
    - unspecified site
      - female D27.9
      - male D29.20
  - pleomorphic
    - carcinoma in — *see* Neoplasm, salivary gland, malignant
    - specified site — *see* Neoplasm, malignant, by site
    - unspecified site C08.9
  - polypoid (*see also* Neoplasm, benign)
    - adenocarcinoma in — *see* Neoplasm, malignant, by site
    - adenocarcinoma in situ — *see* Neoplasm, in situ, by site
  - prostate — *see* Neoplasm, benign, prostate
  - rete cell D29.20
  - sebaceous — *see* Neoplasm, skin, benign
  - Sertoli cell
    - specified site — *see* Neoplasm, benign, by site
    - unspecified site
      - female D27.9
      - male D29.20
  - skin appendage — *see* Neoplasm, skin, benign
  - sudoriferous gland — *see* Neoplasm, skin, benign
  - sweat gland — *see* Neoplasm, skin, benign
  - testicular
    - specified site — *see* Neoplasm, benign, by site
    - unspecified site
      - female D27.9
      - male D29.20
  - tubular (*see also* Neoplasm, benign, by site)
    - adenocarcinoma in — *see* Neoplasm, malignant, by site
    - adenocarcinoma in situ — *see* Neoplasm, in situ, by site

Adenoma — *continued*
- tubular (*see also* Neoplasm, benign, by site) — *continued*
  - Pick's
    - specified site — *see* Neoplasm, benign, by site
    - unspecified site
      - female D27.9
      - male D29.20
  - tubulovillous (*see also* Neoplasm, benign, by site)
    - adenocarcinoma in — *see* Neoplasm, malignant, by site
    - adenocarcinoma in situ — *see* Neoplasm, in situ, by site
  - villous — *see* Neoplasm, uncertain behavior, by site
    - adenocarcinoma in — *see* Neoplasm, malignant, by site
    - adenocarcinoma in situ — *see* Neoplasm, in situ, by site
  - water-clear cell D35.1
Adenomatosis
- endocrine (multiple) E31.20
  - single specified site — *see* Neoplasm, uncertain behavior, by site
- erosive of nipple D24- ☑
- pluriendocrine — *see* Adenomatosis, endocrine
- pulmonary D38.1
  - malignant — *see* Neoplasm, lung, malignant
- specified site — *see* Neoplasm, benign, by site
- unspecified site D12.6
Adenomatous
- goiter (nontoxic) E04.9
  - with hyperthyroidism — *see* Hyperthyroidism, with, goiter, nodular
  - toxic — *see* Hyperthyroidism, with, goiter, nodular
Adenomyoma (*see also* Neoplasm, benign, by site)
- prostate — *see* Enlarged, prostate
Adenomyometritis N80.0
Adenomyosis N80.0
Adenopathy (lymph gland) R59.9
- generalized R59.1
- inguinal R59.0
- localized R59.0
- mediastinal R59.0
- mesentery R59.0
- syphilitic (secondary) A51.49
- tracheobronchial R59.0
  - tuberculous A15.4
    - primary (progressive) A15.7
- tuberculous (*see also* Tuberculosis, lymph gland)
  - tracheobronchial A15.4
    - primary (progressive) A15.7
Adenosalpingitis — *see* Salpingitis
Adenosarcoma — *see* Neoplasm, malignant, by site
Adenosclerosis I88.8
Adenosis (sclerosing) breast — *see* Fibroadenosis, breast
Adenovirus, as cause of disease classified elsewhere B97.0
Adentia (complete) (partial) — *see* Absence, teeth
Adherent (*see also* Adhesions)
- labia (minora) N90.89
- pericardium (nonrheumatic) I31.0
  - rheumatic I09.2
- placenta (with hemorrhage) O72.0
  - without hemorrhage O73.0
- prepuce, newborn N47.0
- scar (skin) L90.5
- tendon in scar L90.5
Adhesions, adhesive (postinfective) K66.0
- with intestinal obstruction K56.50
  - complete K56.52
  - incomplete K56.51
  - partial K56.51
- abdominal (wall) — *see* Adhesions, peritoneum
- appendix K38.8
- bile duct (common) (hepatic) K83.8
- bladder (sphincter) N32.89
- bowel — *see* Adhesions, peritoneum
- cardiac I31.0
  - rheumatic I09.2
- cecum — *see* Adhesions, peritoneum
- cervicovaginal N88.1
  - congenital Q52.8
  - postpartal O90.89
    - old N88.1
- cervix N88.1
- ciliary body NEC — *see* Adhesions, iris
- clitoris N90.89
- colon — *see* Adhesions, peritoneum

Adhesions, adhesive — *continued*
- common duct K83.8
- congenital (*see also* Anomaly, by site)
  - fingers — *see* Syndactylism, complex, fingers
  - omental, anomalous Q43.3
  - peritoneal Q43.3
  - tongue (to gum or roof of mouth) Q38.3
- conjunctiva (acquired) H11.21- ☑
  - congenital Q15.8
- cystic duct K82.8
- diaphragm — *see* Adhesions, peritoneum
- due to foreign body — *see* Foreign body
- duodenum — *see* Adhesions, peritoneum
- ear
  - middle H74.1- ☑
- epididymis N50.89
- epidural — *see* Adhesions, meninges
- epiglottis J38.7
- eyelid H02.59
- female pelvis N73.6
- gallbladder K82.8
- globe H44.89
- heart I31.0
  - rheumatic I09.2
- ileocecal (coil) — *see* Adhesions, peritoneum
- ileum — *see* Adhesions, peritoneum
- intestine (*see also* Adhesions, peritoneum)
  - with obstruction K56.50
    - complete K56.52
    - incomplete K56.51
    - partial K56.51
- intra-abdominal — *see* Adhesions, peritoneum
- iris H21.50- ☑
  - anterior H21.51- ☑
  - goniosynechiae H21.52- ☑
  - posterior H21.54- ☑
  - to corneal graft T85.898 ☑
- joint — *see* Ankylosis
  - knee M23.8X ☑
  - temporomandibular M26.61- ☑
- labium (majus) (minus), congenital Q52.5
- liver — *see* Adhesions, peritoneum
- lung J98.4
- mediastinum J98.59
- meninges (cerebral) (spinal) G96.12
  - congenital Q07.8
  - tuberculous (cerebral) (spinal) A17.0
- mesenteric — *see* Adhesions, peritoneum
- nasal (septum) (to turbinates) J34.89
- ocular muscle — *see* Strabismus, mechanical
- omentum — *see* Adhesions, peritoneum
- ovary N73.6
  - congenital (to cecum, kidney or omentum) Q50.39
- paraovarian N73.6
- pelvic (peritoneal)
  - female N73.6
    - postprocedural N99.4
  - male — *see* Adhesions, peritoneum
  - postpartal (old) N73.6
  - tuberculous A18.17
- penis to scrotum (congenital) Q55.8
- periappendiceal (*see also* Adhesions, peritoneum)
- pericardium (nonrheumatic) I31.0
  - focal I31.8
  - rheumatic I09.2
  - tuberculous A18.84
- pericholecystic K82.8
- perigastric — *see* Adhesions, peritoneum
- periovarian N73.6
- periprostatic N42.89
- perirectal — *see* Adhesions, peritoneum
- perirenal N28.89
- peritoneum, peritoneal (postinfective)
  - with obstruction (intestinal) K56.50
    - complete K56.52
    - incomplete K56.51
    - partial K56.51
  - congenital Q43.3
  - pelvic, female N73.6
    - postprocedural N99.4
  - postpartal, pelvic N73.6
  - postprocedural K66.0
  - to uterus N73.6
- peritubal N73.6
- periureteral N28.89
- periuterine N73.6
- perivesical N32.89
- perivesicular (seminal vesicle) N50.89

☑ **Additional Character Required** — Refer to the Tabular List for Character Selection   ▽ **Subterms under main terms may continue to next column or page**

Adhesions, adhesive — *continued*
  pleura, pleuritic J94.8
    tuberculous NEC A15.6
  pleuropericardial J94.8
  postoperative (gastrointestinal tract) K66.0
    with obstruction (*see also* Obstruction, intestine, postoperative) K91.30
    due to foreign body accidentally left in wound — *see* Foreign body, accidentally left during a procedure
  pelvic peritoneal N99.4
  urethra — *see* Stricture, urethra, postprocedural
  vagina N99.2
  postpartal, old (vulva or perineum) N90.89
  preputial, prepuce N47.5
  pulmonary J98.4
  pylorus — *see* Adhesions, peritoneum
  sciatic nerve — *see* Lesion, nerve, sciatic
  seminal vesicle N50.89
  shoulder (joint) — *see* Capsulitis, adhesive
  sigmoid flexure — *see* Adhesions, peritoneum
  spermatic cord (acquired) N50.89
    congenital Q55.4
  spinal canal G96.12
  stomach — *see* Adhesions, peritoneum
  subscapular — *see* Capsulitis, adhesive
  temporomandibular M26.61- ☑
  tendinitis (*see also* Tenosynovitis, specified type NEC)
    shoulder — *see* Capsulitis, adhesive
  testis N44.8
  tongue, congenital (to gum or roof of mouth) Q38.3
    acquired K14.8
  trachea J39.8
  tubo-ovarian N73.6
  tunica vaginalis N44.8
  uterus N73.6
    internal N85.6
    to abdominal wall N73.6
  vagina (chronic) N89.5
    postoperative N99.2
  vitreomacular H43.82- ☑
  vitreous H43.89
  vulva N90.89
Adiaspiromycosis B48.8
Adie (-Holmes) **pupil or syndrome** — *see* Anomaly, pupil, function, tonic pupil
Adiponecrosis neonatorum P83.88
Adiposis (*see also* Obesity)
  cerebralis E23.6
  dolorosa E88.2
Adiposity (*see also* Obesity)
  heart — *see* Degeneration, myocardial
  localized E65
Adiposogenital dystrophy E23.6
Adjustment
  disorder — *see* Disorder, adjustment
  implanted device — *see* Encounter (for), adjustment (of)
  prosthesis, external — *see* Fitting
  reaction — *see* Disorder, adjustment
Administration of tPA (rtPA) in a different facility within the last 24 hours prior to admission to current facility Z92.82
Admission (for) (*see also* Encounter (for))
  adjustment (of)
    artificial
      arm Z44.00- ☑
        complete Z44.01- ☑
        partial Z44.02- ☑
      eye Z44.2 ☑
      leg Z44.10- ☑
        complete Z44.11- ☑
        partial Z44.12- ☑
    brain neuropacemaker Z46.2
      implanted Z45.42
    breast
      implant Z45.81 ☑
      prosthesis (external) Z44.3 ☑
    colostomy belt Z46.89
    contact lenses Z46.0
    cystostomy device Z46.6
    dental prosthesis Z46.3
    device NEC
      abdominal Z46.89
      implanted Z45.89
        cardiac Z45.09

Admission — *continued*
  adjustment — *continued*
    device — *continued*
      implanted — *continued*
        cardiac — *continued*
          defibrillator (with synchronous cardiace pacemaker) Z45.02
          pacemaker (cardiac resynchronization therapy (CRT-P)) Z45.018
          pulse generator Z45.010
          resynchronization therapy defibrillator (CRT-D) Z45.02
        hearing device Z45.328
          bone conduction Z45.320
          cochlear Z45.321
        infusion pump Z45.1
        nervous system Z45.49
          CSF drainage Z45.41
          hearing device — *see* Admission, adjustment, device, implanted, hearing device
          neuropacemaker Z45.42
          visual substitution Z45.31
        specified NEC Z45.89
        vascular access Z45.2
        visual substitution Z45.31
      nervous system Z46.2
        implanted — *see* Admission, adjustment, device, implanted, nervous system
    orthodontic Z46.4
    prosthetic Z44.9
      arm — *see* Admission, adjustment, artificial, arm
      breast Z44.3 ☑
      dental Z46.3
      eye Z44.2 ☑
      leg — *see* Admission, adjustment, artificial, leg
      specified type NEC Z44.8
    substitution
      auditory Z46.2
        implanted — *see* Admission, adjustment, device, implanted, hearing device
      nervous system Z46.2
        implanted — *see* Admission, adjustment, device, implanted, nervous system
      visual Z46.2
        implanted Z45.31
    urinary Z46.6
  hearing aid Z46.1
    implanted — *see* Admission, adjustment, device, implanted, hearing device
  ileostomy device Z46.89
  intestinal appliance or device NEC Z46.89
  neuropacemaker (brain) (peripheral nerve) (spinal cord) Z46.2
    implanted Z45.42
  orthodontic device Z46.4
  orthopedic (brace) (cast) (device) (shoes) Z46.89
  pacemaker (cardiac resynchronization therapy (CRT-P))
    cardiac Z45.018
      pulse generator Z45.010
    nervous system Z46.2
      implanted Z45.42
  portacath (port-a-cath) Z45.2
  prosthesis Z44.9
    arm — *see* Admission, adjustment, artificial, arm
    breast Z44.3 ☑
    dental Z46.3
    eye Z44.2 ☑
    leg — *see* Admission, adjustment, artificial, leg
    specified NEC Z44.8
  spectacles Z46.0
  aftercare (*see also* Aftercare) Z51.89
    postpartum
      immediately after delivery Z39.0
      routine follow-up Z39.2
    radiation therapy (antineoplastic) Z51.0
  attention to artificial opening (of) Z43.9
    artificial vagina Z43.7
    colostomy Z43.3
    cystostomy Z43.5
    enterostomy Z43.4
    gastrostomy Z43.1
    ileostomy Z43.2
    jejunostomy Z43.4
    nephrostomy Z43.6

Admission — *continued*
  attention to artificial opening — *continued*
    specified site NEC Z43.8
      intestinal tract Z43.4
      urinary tract Z43.6
    tracheostomy Z43.0
    ureterostomy Z43.6
    urethrostomy Z43.6
  breast augmentation or reduction Z41.1
  breast reconstruction following mastectomy Z42.1
  change of
    dressing (nonsurgical) Z48.00
    neuropacemaker device (brain) (peripheral nerve) (spinal cord) Z46.2
      implanted Z45.42
    surgical dressing Z48.01
  circumcision, ritual or routine (in absence of diagnosis) Z41.2
  clinical research investigation (control) (normal comparison) (participant) Z00.6
  contraceptive management Z30.9
  cosmetic surgery NEC Z41.1
  counseling (*see also* Counseling)
    dietary Z71.3
    gestational carrier Z31.7
    HIV Z71.7
    human immunodeficiency virus Z71.7
    nonattending third party Z71.0
    procreative management NEC Z31.69
  delivery, full-term, uncomplicated O80
    cesarean, without indication O82
  desensitization to allergens Z51.6
  dietary surveillance and counseling Z71.3
  ear piercing Z41.3
  examination at health care facility (adult) (*see also* Examination) Z00.00
    with abnormal findings Z00.01
    clinical research investigation (control) (normal comparison) (participant) Z00.6
    dental Z01.20
      with abnormal findings Z01.21
    donor (potential) Z00.5
    ear Z01.10
      with abnormal findings NEC Z01.118
    eye Z01.00
      with abnormal findings Z01.01
    general, specified reason NEC Z00.8
    hearing Z01.10
      with abnormal findings NEC Z01.118
      infant or child (over 28 days old) Z00.129
        with abnormal findings Z00.121
    postpartum checkup Z39.2
    psychiatric (general) Z00.8
      requested by authority Z04.6
    vision Z01.00
      with abnormal findings Z01.01
      infant or child (over 28 days old) Z00.129
        with abnormal findings Z00.121
  fitting (of)
    artificial
      arm — *see* Admission, adjustment, artificial, arm
      eye Z44.2 ☑
      leg — *see* Admission, adjustment, artificial, leg
    brain neuropacemaker Z46.2
      implanted Z45.42
    breast prosthesis (external) Z44.3 ☑
    colostomy belt Z46.89
    contact lenses Z46.0
    cystostomy device Z46.6
    dental prosthesis Z46.3
    dentures Z46.3
    device NEC
      abdominal Z46.89
      nervous system Z46.2
        implanted — *see* Admission, adjustment, device, implanted, nervous system
      orthodontic Z46.4
      prosthetic Z44.9
        breast Z44.3 ☑
        dental Z46.3
        eye Z44.2 ☑
      substitution
        auditory Z46.2
          implanted — *see* Admission, adjustment, device, implanted, hearing device
        nervous system Z46.2
          implanted — *see* Admission, adjustment, device, implanted, nervous system

Admission — *continued*
  fitting — *continued*
    device — *continued*
      substitution — *continued*
        visual Z46.2
          implanted Z45.31
      hearing aid Z46.1
      ileostomy device Z46.89
      intestinal appliance or device NEC Z46.89
      neuropacemaker (brain) (peripheral nerve) (spinal cord) Z46.2
        implanted Z45.42
      orthodontic device Z46.4
      orthopedic device (brace) (cast) (shoes) Z46.89
      prosthesis Z44.9
        arm — *see* Admission, adjustment, artificial, arm
        breast Z44.3 ☑
        dental Z46.3
        eye Z44.2 ☑
        leg — *see* Admission, adjustment, artificial, leg
        specified type NEC Z44.8
      spectacles Z46.0
  follow-up examination Z09
  intrauterine device management Z30.431
    initial prescription Z30.014
  mental health evaluation Z00.8
    requested by authority Z04.6
  observation — *see* Observation
  Papanicolaou smear, cervix Z12.4
    for suspected malignant neoplasm Z12.4
  plastic and reconstructive surgery following medical procedure or healed injury NEC Z42.8
  plastic surgery, cosmetic NEC Z41.1
  postpartum observation
    immediately after delivery Z39.0
    routine follow-up Z39.2
  poststerilization (for restoration) Z31.0
    aftercare Z31.42
  procreative management Z31.9
  prophylactic (measure) — (*see also* Encounter, prophylactic measures)
    organ removal Z40.00
      breast Z40.01
      fallopian tube(s) Z40.03
        with ovary(s) Z40.02
      ovary(s) Z40.02
      specified organ NEC Z40.09
      testes Z40.09
    vaccination Z23
  psychiatric examination (general) Z00.8
    requested by authority Z04.6
  radiation therapy (antineoplastic) Z51.0
  reconstructive surgery following medical procedure or healed injury NEC Z42.8
  removal of
    cystostomy catheter Z43.5
    drains Z48.03
    dressing (nonsurgical) Z48.00
    implantable subdermal contraceptive Z30.46
    intrauterine contraceptive device Z30.432
    neuropacemaker (brain) (peripheral nerve) (spinal cord) Z46.2
      implanted Z45.42
    staples Z48.02
    surgical dressing Z48.01
    sutures Z48.02
    ureteral stent Z46.6
  respirator [ventilator] use during power failure Z99.12
  restoration of organ continuity (poststerilization) Z31.0
    aftercare Z31.42
  sensitivity test (*see also* Test, skin)
    allergy NEC Z01.82
    Mantoux Z11.1
  tuboplasty following previous sterilization Z31.0
    aftercare Z31.42
  vasoplasty following previous sterilization Z31.0
    aftercare Z31.42
  vision examination Z01.00
    with abnormal findings Z01.01
    infant or child (over 28 days old) Z00.129
      with abnormal findings Z00.121
  waiting period for admission to other facility Z75.1
Adnexitis (suppurative) — *see* Salpingo-oophoritis
Adolescent X-linked adrenoleukodystrophy E71.521
Adrenal (gland) — *see* condition
Adrenalism, tuberculous A18.7
Adrenalitis, adrenitis E27.8
  autoimmune E27.1

Adrenalitis, adrenitis — *continued*
  meningococcal, hemorrhagic A39.1
Adrenarche, premature E27.0
Adrenocortical syndrome — *see* Cushing's, syndrome
Adrenogenital syndrome E25.9
  acquired E25.8
  congenital E25.0
  salt loss E25.0
Adrenogenitalism, congenital E25.0
Adrenoleukodystrophy E71.529
  neonatal E71.511
  X-linked E71.529
    Addison only phenotype E71.528
    Addison-Schilder E71.528
    adolescent E71.521
    adrenomyeloneuropathy E71.522
    childhood cerebral E71.520
    other specified E71.528
Adrenomyeloneuropathy E71.522
Adventitious bursa — *see* Bursopathy, specified type NEC
Adverse effect — *see* Table of Drugs and Chemicals, categories T36-T50, with 6th character 5
Advice — *see* Counseling
Adynamia (episodica) (hereditary) (periodic) G72.3
Aeration lung imperfect, newborn — *see* Atelectasis
Aerobullosis T70.3 ☑
Aerocele — *see* Embolism, air
Aerodermectasia
  subcutaneous (traumatic) T79.7 ☑
Aerodontalgia T70.29 ☑
Aeroembolism T70.3 ☑
Aerogenes capsulatus infection A48.0
Aero-otitis media T70.0 ☑
Aerophagy, aerophagia (psychogenic) F45.8
Aerophobia F40.228
Aerosinusitis T70.1 ☑
Aerotitis T70.0 ☑
Affection — *see* Disease
Afibrinogenemia (*see also* Defect, coagulation) D68.8
  acquired D65
  congenital D68.2
  following ectopic or molar pregnancy O08.1
  in abortion — *see* Abortion, by type, complicated by, afibrinogenemia
  puerperal O72.3
African
  sleeping sickness B56.9
  tick fever A68.1
  trypanosomiasis B56.9
    gambian B56.0
    rhodesian B56.1
Aftercare (*see also* Care) Z51.89
  following surgery (for) (on)
    amputation Z47.81
    attention to
      drains Z48.03
      dressings (nonsurgical) Z48.00
        surgical Z48.01
      sutures Z48.02
    circulatory system Z48.812
    delayed (planned) wound closure Z48.1
    digestive system Z48.815
    explantation of joint prosthesis (staged procedure)
      hip Z47.32
      knee Z47.33
      shoulder Z47.31
    genitourinary system Z48.816
    joint replacement Z47.1
    neoplasm Z48.3
    nervous system Z48.811
    oral cavity Z48.814
    organ transplant
      bone marrow Z48.290
      heart Z48.21
      heart-lung Z48.280
      kidney Z48.22
      liver Z48.23
      lung Z48.24
      multiple organs NEC Z48.288
      specified NEC Z48.298
    orthopedic NEC Z47.89
    planned wound closure Z48.1
    removal of internal fixation device Z47.2
    respiratory system Z48.813
    scoliosis Z47.82
    sense organs Z48.810
    skin and subcutaneous tissue Z48.817

Aftercare — *continued*
  following surgery — *continued*
    specified body system
      circulatory Z48.812
      digestive Z48.815
      genitourinary Z48.816
      nervous Z48.811
      oral cavity Z48.814
      respiratory Z48.813
      sense organs Z48.810
      skin and subcutaneous tissue Z48.817
      teeth Z48.814
    specified NEC Z48.89
    spinal Z47.89
    teeth Z48.814
  fracture — *code to* fracture with seventh character D
  involving
    removal of
      drains Z48.03
      dressings (nonsurgical) Z48.00
      staples Z48.02
      surgical dressings Z48.01
      sutures Z48.02
  neuropacemaker (brain) (peripheral nerve) (spinal cord) Z46.2
    implanted Z45.42
  orthopedic NEC Z47.89
  postprocedural — *see* Aftercare, following surgery
After-cataract — *see* Cataract, secondary
Agalactia (primary) O92.3
  elective, secondary or therapeutic O92.5
Agammaglobulinemia (acquired) (secondary) (nonfamilial) D80.1
  with
    immunoglobulin-bearing B-lymphocytes D80.1
    lymphopenia D81.9
  autosomal recessive (Swiss type) D80.0
  Bruton's X-linked D80.0
  common variable (CVAgamma) D80.1
  congenital sex-linked D80.0
  hereditary D80.0
  lymphopenic D81.9
  Swiss type (autosomal recessive) D80.0
  X-linked (with growth hormone deficiency) (Bruton) D80.0
Aganglionosis (bowel) (colon) Q43.1
Age (old) — *see* Senility
Agenesis
  adrenal (gland) Q89.1
  alimentary tract (complete) (partial) NEC Q45.8
    upper Q40.8
  anus, anal (canal) Q42.3
    with fistula Q42.2
  aorta Q25.41
  appendix Q42.8
  arm (complete) Q71.0- ☑
    with hand present Q71.1- ☑
  artery (peripheral) Q27.9
    brain Q28.3
    coronary Q24.5
    pulmonary Q25.79
    specified NEC Q27.8
    umbilical Q27.0
  auditory (canal) (external) Q16.1
  auricle (ear) Q16.0
  bile duct or passage Q44.5
  bladder Q64.5
  bone Q79.9
  brain Q00.0
    part of Q04.3
  breast (with nipple present) Q83.8
    with absent nipple Q83.0
  bronchus Q32.4
  canaliculus lacrimalis Q10.4
  carpus — *see* Agenesis, hand
  cartilage Q79.9
  cecum Q42.8
  cerebellum Q04.3
  cervix Q51.5
  chin Q18.8
  cilia Q10.3
  circulatory system, part NOS Q28.9
  clavicle Q74.0
  clitoris Q52.6
  coccyx Q76.49
  colon Q42.9
    specified NEC Q42.8
  corpus callosum Q04.0

Agenesis — *continued*
cricoid cartilage Q31.8
diaphragm (with hernia) Q79.1
digestive organ(s) or tract (complete) (partial) NEC
Q45.8
upper Q40.8
ductus arteriosus Q28.8
duodenum Q41.0
ear Q16.9
auricle Q16.0
lobe Q17.8
ejaculatory duct Q55.4
endocrine (gland) NEC Q89.2
epiglottis Q31.8
esophagus Q39.8
eustachian tube Q16.2
eye Q11.1
adnexa Q15.8
eyelid (fold) Q10.3
face
bones NEC Q75.8
specified part NEC Q18.8
fallopian tube Q50.6
femur — *see* Defect, reduction, lower limb, longitudinal, femur
fibula — *see* Defect, reduction, lower limb, longitudinal,
fibula
finger (complete) (partial) — *see* Agenesis, hand
foot (and toes) (complete) (partial) Q72.3- ☑
forearm (with hand present) — *see* Agenesis, arm, with
hand present
and hand Q71.2- ☑
gallbladder Q44.0
gastric Q40.2
genitalia, genital (organ(s))
female Q52.8
external Q52.71
internal NEC Q52.8
male Q55.8
glottis Q31.8
hair Q84.0
hand (and fingers) (complete) (partial) Q71.3- ☑
heart Q24.8
valve NEC Q24.8
pulmonary Q22.0
hepatic Q44.7
humerus — *see* Defect, reduction, upper limb
hymen Q52.4
ileum Q41.2
incus Q16.3
intestine (small) Q41.9
large Q42.9
specified NEC Q42.8
iris (dilator fibers) Q13.1
jaw M26.09
jejunum Q41.1
kidney(s) (partial) Q60.2
bilateral Q60.1
unilateral Q60.0
labium (majus) (minus) Q52.71
labyrinth, membranous Q16.5
lacrimal apparatus Q10.4
larynx Q31.8
leg (complete) Q72.0- ☑
with foot present Q72.1- ☑
lower leg (with foot present) — *see* Agenesis, leg,
with foot present
and foot Q72.2- ☑
lens Q12.3
limb (complete) Q73.0
lower — *see* Agenesis, leg
upper — *see* Agenesis, arm
lip Q38.0
liver Q44.7
lung (fissure) (lobe) (bilateral) (unilateral) Q33.3
mandible, maxilla M26.09
metacarpus — *see* Agenesis, hand
metatarsus — *see* Agenesis, foot
muscle Q79.8
eyelid Q10.3
ocular Q15.8
musculoskeletal system NEC Q79.8
nail(s) Q84.3
neck, part Q18.8
nerve Q07.8
nervous system, part NEC Q07.8
nipple Q83.2
nose Q30.1

Agenesis — *continued*
nuclear Q07.8
organ
of Corti Q16.5
or site not listed — *see* Anomaly, by site
osseous meatus (ear) Q16.1
ovary
bilateral Q50.02
unilateral Q50.01
oviduct Q50.6
pancreas Q45.0
parathyroid (gland) Q89.2
parotid gland(s) Q38.4
patella Q74.1
pelvic girdle (complete) (partial) Q74.2
penis Q55.5
pericardium Q24.8
pituitary (gland) Q89.2
prostate Q55.4
punctum lacrimale Q10.4
radioulnar — *see* Defect, reduction, upper limb
radius — *see* Defect, reduction, upper limb, longitudinal, radius
rectum Q42.1
with fistula Q42.0
renal Q60.2
bilateral Q60.1
unilateral Q60.0
respiratory organ NEC Q34.8
rib Q76.6
roof of orbit Q75.8
round ligament Q52.8
sacrum Q76.49
salivary gland Q38.4
scapula Q74.0
scrotum Q55.29
seminal vesicles Q55.4
septum
atrial Q21.1
between aorta and pulmonary artery Q21.4
ventricular Q20.4
shoulder girdle (complete) (partial) Q74.0
skull (bone) Q75.8
with
anencephaly Q00.0
encephalocele — *see* Encephalocele
hydrocephalus Q03.9
with spina bifida — *see* Spina bifida, by site,
with hydrocephalus
microcephaly Q02
spermatic cord Q55.4
spinal cord Q06.0
spine Q76.49
spleen Q89.01
sternum Q76.7
stomach Q40.2
submaxillary gland(s) (congenital) Q38.4
tarsus — *see* Agenesis, foot
tendon Q79.8
testicle Q55.0
thymus (gland) Q89.2
thyroid (gland) E03.1
cartilage Q31.8
tibia — *see* Defect, reduction, lower limb, longitudinal,
tibia
tibiofibular — *see* Defect, reduction, lower limb, specified type NEC
toe (and foot) (complete) (partial) — *see* Agenesis, foot
tongue Q38.3
trachea (cartilage) Q32.1
ulna — *see* Defect, reduction, upper limb, longitudinal,
ulna
upper limb — *see* Agenesis, arm
ureter Q62.4
urethra Q64.5
urinary tract NEC Q64.8
uterus Q51.0
uvula Q38.5
vagina Q52.0
vas deferens Q55.4
vein(s) (peripheral) Q27.9
brain Q28.3
great NEC Q26.8
portal Q26.5
vena cava (inferior) (superior) Q26.8
vermis of cerebellum Q04.3
vertebra Q76.49
vulva Q52.71

Ageusia R43.2
Agitated — *see* condition
Agitation R45.1
Aglossia (congenital) Q38.3
Aglossia-adactylia syndrome Q87.0
Aglycogenosis E74.00
Agnosia (body image) (other senses) (tactile) R48.1
developmental F88
verbal R48.1
auditory R48.1
developmental F80.2
developmental F80.2
visual (object) R48.3
Agoraphobia F40.00
with panic disorder F40.01
without panic disorder F40.02
Agrammatism R48.8
Agranulocytopenia — *see* Agranulocytosis
Agranulocytosis (chronic) (cyclical) (genetic) (infantile)
(periodic) (pernicious) (*see also* Neutropenia) D70.9
congenital D70.0
cytoreductive cancer chemotherapy sequela D70.1
drug-induced D70.2
due to cytoreductive cancer chemotherapy D70.1
due to infection D70.3
secondary D70.4
drug-induced D70.2
due to cytoreductive cancer chemotherapy D70.1
Agraphia (absolute) R48.8
with alexia R48.0
developmental F81.81
Ague (dumb) — *see* Malaria
Agyria Q04.3
Ahumada-del Castillo syndrome E23.0
Aichomophobia F40.298
AIDS (related complex) (any site) B20
Ailment heart — *see* Disease, heart
Ailurophobia F40.218
AIN — *see* Neoplasia, intraepithelial, anal
Ainhum (disease) L94.6
AIPHI (acute idiopathic pulmonary hemorrhage in infants
(over 28 days old)) R04.81
Air
anterior mediastinum J98.2
compressed, disease T70.3 ☑
conditioner lung or pneumonitis J67.7
embolism (artery) (cerebral) (any site) T79.0 ☑
with ectopic or molar pregnancy O08.2
due to implanted device NEC — *see* Complications,
by site and type, specified NEC
following
abortion — *see* Abortion by type, complicated
by, embolism
ectopic or molar pregnancy O08.2
infusion, therapeutic injection or transfusion
T80.0 ☑
in pregnancy, childbirth or puerperium — *see* Embolism, obstetric
traumatic T79.0 ☑
hunger, psychogenic F45.8
rarefied, effects of — *see* Effect, adverse, high altitude
sickness T75.3 ☑
Airplane sickness T75.3 ☑
Akathisia (drug-induced) (treatment-induced) G25.71
neuroleptic induced (acute) G25.71
tardive G25.71
Akinesia R29.898
Akinetic mutism R41.89
Akureyri's disease G93.3
Alactasia, congenital E73.0
Alagille's syndrome Q44.7
Alastrim B03
Albers-Schönberg syndrome Q78.2
Albert's syndrome — *see* Tendinitis, Achilles
Albinism, albino E70.30
with hematologic abnormality E70.339
Chédiak-Higashi syndrome E70.330
Hermansky-Pudlak syndrome E70.331
other specified E70.338
I E70.320
II E70.321
ocular E70.319
autosomal recessive E70.311
other specified E70.318
X-linked E70.310
oculocutaneous E70.329
other specified E70.328

Albinism, albino — *continued*
  oculocutaneous — *continued*
    tyrosinase (ty) negative E70.320
    tyrosinase (ty) positive E70.321
    other specified E70.39
Albinismus E70.30
Albright (-McCune)(-Sternberg) syndrome Q78.1
Albuminous — *see* condition
Albuminuria, albuminuric (acute) (chronic) (subacute)
    (*see also* Proteinuria) R80.9
  complicating pregnancy — *see* Proteinuria, gestational
    with
      gestational hypertension — *see* Pre-eclampsia
      pre-existing hypertension — *see* Hypertension,
        complicating pregnancy, pre-existing,
        with, pre-eclampsia
  gestational — *see* Proteinuria, gestational
    with
      gestational hypertension — *see* Pre-eclampsia
      pre-existing hypertension — *see* Hypertension,
        complicating pregnancy, pre-existing,
        with, pre-eclampsia
  orthostatic R80.2
  postural R80.2
  pre-eclamptic — *see* Pre-eclampsia
  scarlatinal A38.8
Albuminurophobia F40.298
Alcaptonuria E70.29
Alcohol, alcoholic, alcohol-induced
  addiction (without remission) F10.20
    with remission F10.21
  amnestic disorder, persisting F10.96
    with dependence F10.26
  anxiety disorder F10.980
  bipolar and related disorder F10.94
  brain syndrome, chronic F10.97
    with dependence F10.27
  cardiopathy I42.6
  counseling and surveillance Z71.41
    family member Z71.42
  delirium (acute) (tremens) (withdrawal) F10.231
    with intoxication F10.921
      in
        abuse F10.121
        dependence F10.221
  dementia F10.97
    with dependence F10.27
  depressive disorder F10.94
  deterioration F10.97
    with dependence F10.27
  hallucinosis (acute) F10.951
    in
      abuse F10.151
      dependence F10.251
  insanity F10.959
  intoxication (acute) (without dependence) F10.129
    with
      delirium F10.121
      dependence F10.229
        with delirium F10.221
        uncomplicated F10.220
      uncomplicated F10.120
  jealousy F10.988
  Korsakoff's, Korsakov's, Korsakow's F10.26
  liver K70.9
    acute — *see* Disease, liver, alcoholic, hepatitis
  major neurocognitive disorder, amnestic-confabulatory
    type F10.96
  major neurocognitive disorder, nonamnestic-confabu-
    latory type F10.97
  mania (acute) (chronic) F10.959
  mild neurocognitive disorder F10.988
  paranoia, paranoid (type) psychosis F10.950
  pellagra E52
  poisoning, accidental (acute) NEC — *see* Table of Drugs
    and Chemicals, alcohol, poisoning
  psychosis — *see* Psychosis, alcoholic
  psychotic disorder F10.959
  sexual dysfunction F10.981
  sleep disorder F10.982
  withdrawal (without convulsions) F10.239
    with delirium F10.231
Alcoholism (chronic) (without remission) F10.20
  with
    psychosis — *see* Psychosis, alcoholic
    remission F10.21
  Korsakov's F10.96
    with dependence F10.26

Alder (-Reilly) **anomaly or syndrome** (leukocyte granu-
    lation) D72.0
Aldosteronism E26.9
  familial (type I) E26.02
    glucocorticoid-remediable E26.02
  primary (due to (bilateral) adrenal hyperplasia) E26.09
  primary NEC E26.09
  secondary E26.1
  specified NEC E26.89
Aldosteronoma D44.10
Aldrich (-Wiskott) **syndrome** (eczema-thrombocytope-
    nia) D82.0
Alektorophobia F40.218
Aleppo boil B55.1
Aleukemic — *see* condition
Aleukia
  congenital D70.0
  hemorrhagica D61.9
    congenital D61.09
  splenica D73.1
Alexia R48.0
  developmental F81.0
  secondary to organic lesion R48.0
Algoneurodystrophy M89.00
  ankle M89.07- ☑
  foot M89.07- ☑
  forearm M89.03- ☑
  hand M89.04- ☑
  lower leg M89.06- ☑
  multiple sites M89.0- ☑
  shoulder M89.01- ☑
  specified site NEC M89.08
  thigh M89.05- ☑
  upper arm M89.02- ☑
Algophobia F40.298
Alienation, mental — *see* Psychosis
Alkalemia E87.3
Alkalosis E87.3
  metabolic E87.3
    with respiratory acidosis E87.4
    of newborn P74.41
  respiratory E87.3
Alkaptonuria E70.29
Allen-Masters syndrome N83.8
Allergy, allergic (reaction) (to) T78.40 ☑
  air-borne substance NEC (rhinitis) J30.89
  alveolitis (extrinsic) J67.9
    due to
      Aspergillus clavatus J67.4
      Cryptostroma corticale J67.6
      organisms (fungal, thermophilic actinomycete)
        growing in ventilation (air conditioning)
        systems J67.7
    specified type NEC J67.8
  anaphylactic reaction or shock T78.2 ☑
  angioneurotic edema T78.3 ☑
  animal (dander) (epidermal) (hair) (rhinitis) J30.81
  bee sting (anaphylactic shock) — *see* Toxicity, venom,
    arthropod, bee
  biological — *see* Allergy, drug
  colitis (*see also* Colitis, allergic) K52.29
  dander (animal) (rhinitis) J30.81
  dandruff (rhinitis) J30.81
  dental restorative material (existing) K08.55
  dermatitis — *see* Dermatitis, contact, allergic
  diathesis — *see* History, allergy
  drug, medicament & biological (any) (external) (inter-
    nal) T78.40 ☑
    correct substance properly administered — *see* Ta-
      ble of Drugs and Chemicals, by drug, adverse
      effect
    wrong substance given or taken NEC (by accident)
      — *see* Table of Drugs and Chemicals, by drug,
      poisoning
  due to pollen J30.1
  dust (house) (stock) (rhinitis) J30.89
    with asthma — *see* Asthma, allergic extrinsic
  eczema — *see* Dermatitis, contact, allergic
  epidermal (animal) (rhinitis) J30.81
  feathers (rhinitis) J30.89
  food (any) (ingested) NEC T78.1 ☑
    anaphylactic shock — *see* Shock, anaphylactic, due
      to food
    dermatitis — *see* Dermatitis, due to, food
    dietary counseling and surveillance Z71.3
    in contact with skin L23.6
    rhinitis J30.5

Allergy, allergic — *continued*
  food — *continued*
    status (without reaction) Z91.018
      eggs Z91.012
      milk products Z91.011
      peanuts Z91.010
      seafood Z91.013
      specified NEC Z91.018
  gastrointestinal — *see also* specific type of allergic re-
    action
    meaning colitis (*see also* Colitis, allergic) K52.29
    meaning gastroenteritis (*see also* Gastroenteritis,
      allergic) K52.29
    meaning other adverse food reaction not elsewhere
      classified T78.1 ☑
  grain J30.1
  grass (hay fever) (pollen) J30.1
    asthma — *see* Asthma, allergic extrinsic
  hair (animal) (rhinitis) J30.81
  history (of) — *see* History, allergy
  horse serum — *see* Allergy, serum
  inhalant (rhinitis) J30.89
    pollen J30.1
  kapok (rhinitis) J30.89
  medicine — *see* Allergy, drug
  milk protein (*see also* Allergy, food) Z91.011
    anaphylactic reaction T78.07 ☑
    dermatitis L27.2
    enterocolitis syndrome K52.21
    enteropathy K52.22
    gastroenteritis K52.29
    gastroesophageal reflux (*see also* Reaction, adverse,
      food) K21.9
      with esophagitis K21.0
    proctocolitis K52.82
  nasal, seasonal due to pollen J30.1
  pneumonia J82
  pollen (any) (hay fever) J30.1
    asthma — *see* Asthma, allergic extrinsic
  primrose J30.1
  primula J30.1
  proctocolitis K52.82
  purpura D69.0
  ragweed (hay fever) (pollen) J30.1
    asthma — *see* Asthma, allergic extrinsic
  rose (pollen) J30.1
  seasonal NEC J30.2
  Senecio jacobae (pollen) J30.1
  serum (*see also* Reaction, serum) T80.69 ☑
    anaphylactic shock T80.59 ☑
  shock (anaphylactic) T78.2 ☑
    due to
      administration of blood and blood products
        T80.51 ☑
      adverse effect of correct medicinal substance
        properly administered T88.6 ☑
      immunization T80.52 ☑
      serum NEC T80.59 ☑
      vaccination T80.52 ☑
  specific NEC T78.49 ☑
  tree (any) (hay fever) (pollen) J30.1
    asthma — *see* Asthma, allergic extrinsic
  upper respiratory J30.9
  urticaria L50.0
  vaccine — *see* Allergy, serum
  wheat — *see* Allergy, food
Allescheriasis B48.2
Alligator skin disease Q80.9
Allocheiria, allochiria R20.8
Almeida's disease — *see* Paracoccidioidomycosis
Alopecia (hereditaria) (seborrheica) L65.9
  androgenic L64.9
    drug-induced L64.0
    specified NEC L64.8
  areata L63.9
    ophiasis L63.2
    specified NEC L63.8
    totalis L63.0
    universalis L63.1
  cicatricial L66.9
    specified NEC L66.8
  circumscripta L63.9
  congenital, congenitalis Q84.0
  due to cytotoxic drugs NEC L65.8
  mucinosa L65.2
  postinfective NEC L65.8
  postpartum L65.0
  premature L64.8

☑ **Additional Character Required** — Refer to the Tabular List for Character Selection   ▥ **Subterms under main terms may continue to next column or page**

Alopecia — *continued*
  specific (syphilitic) A51.32
  specified NEC L65.8
  syphilitic (secondary) A51.32
  totalis (capitis) L63.0
  universalis (entire body) L63.1
  X-ray L58.1
Alpers' disease G31.81
Alpine sickness T70.29 ☑
Alport syndrome Q87.81
ALTE (apparent life threatening event) **in newborn and infant** R68.13
Alteration (of), **Altered**
  awareness
    transient R40.4
    unintended under general anesthesia, during procedure T88.53 ☑
  mental status R41.82
  pattern of family relationships affecting child Z62.898
  sensation
    following
      cerebrovascular disease I69.998
        cerebral infarction I69.398
        intracerebral hemorrhage I69.198
        nontraumatic intracranial hemorrhage NEC I69.298
        specified disease NEC I69.898
        subarachnoid hemorrhage I69.098
Alternating — *see* condition
Altitude, high (effects) — *see* Effect, adverse, high altitude
Aluminosis (of lung) J63.0
Alveolitis
  allergic (extrinsic) — *see* Pneumonitis, hypersensitivity
  due to
    Aspergillus clavatus J67.4
    Cryptostroma corticale J67.6
  fibrosing (cryptogenic) (idiopathic) J84.112
  jaw M27.3
  sicca dolorosa M27.3
Alveolus, alveolar — *see* condition
Alymphocytosis D72.810
  thymic (with immunodeficiency) D82.1
Alymphoplasia, thymic D82.1
Alzheimer's disease or sclerosis — *see* Disease, Alzheimer's
Amastia (with nipple present) Q83.8
  with absent nipple Q83.0
Amathophobia F40.228
Amaurosis (acquired) (congenital) (*see also* Blindness)
  fugax G45.3
  hysterical F44.6
  Leber's congenital H35.50
  uremic — *see* Uremia
Amaurotic idiocy (infantile) (juvenile) (late) E75.4
Amaxophobia F40.248
Ambiguous genitalia Q56.4
Amblyopia (congenital) (ex anopsia) (partial) (suppression) H53.00- ☑
  anisometropic — *see* Amblyopia, refractive
  deprivation H53.01- ☑
  hysterical F44.6
  nocturnal (*see also* Blindness, night)
    vitamin A deficiency E50.5
  refractive H53.02- ☑
  strabismic H53.03- ☑
  suspect H53.04- ☑
  tobacco H53.8
  toxic NEC H53.8
  uremic — *see* Uremia
Ameba, amebic (histolytica) (*see also* Amebiasis)
  abscess (liver) A06.4
Amebiasis A06.9
  with abscess — *see* Abscess, amebic
  acute A06.0
  chronic (intestine) A06.1
    with abscess — *see* Abscess, amebic
  cutaneous A06.7
  cutis A06.7
  cystitis A06.81
  genitourinary tract NEC A06.82
  hepatic — *see* Abscess, liver, amebic
  intestine A06.0
  nondysenteric colitis A06.2
  skin A06.7
  specified site NEC A06.89
Ameboma (of intestine) A06.3

Amelia Q73.0
  lower limb — *see* Agenesis, leg
  upper limb — *see* Agenesis, arm
Ameloblastoma (*see also* Cyst, calcifying odontogenic)
  long bones C40.9- ☑
    lower limb C40.2- ☑
    upper limb C40.0- ☑
  malignant C41.1
    jaw (bone) (lower) C41.1
      upper C41.0
  tibial C40.2- ☑
Amelogenesis imperfecta K00.5
  nonhereditaria (segmentalis) K00.4
Amenorrhea N91.2
  hyperhormonal E28.8
  primary N91.0
  secondary N91.1
Amentia — *see* Disability, intellectual
  Meynert's (nonalcoholic) F04
American
  leishmaniasis B55.2
  mountain tick fever A93.2
Ametropia — *see* Disorder, refraction
AMH (asymptomatic microscopic hematuria) R31.21
Amimia R48.8
Amino-acid disorder E72.9
  anemia D53.0
Aminoacidopathy E72.9
Aminoaciduria E72.9
Amnesia R41.3
  anterograde R41.1
  auditory R48.8
  dissociative F44.0
    with dissociative fugue F44.1
  hysterical F44.0
  postictal in epilepsy — *see* Epilepsy
  psychogenic F44.0
  retrograde R41.2
  transient global G45.4
Amnes(t)ic syndrome (post-traumatic) F04
  induced by
    alcohol F10.96
      with dependence F10.26
    psychoactive NEC F19.96
      with
        abuse F19.16
        dependence F19.26
    sedative F13.96
      with dependence F13.26
Amnion, amniotic — *see* condition
Amnionitis — *see* Pregnancy, complicated by
Amok F68.8
Amoral traits F60.89
Amphetamine (or other stimulant) **-induced**
  anxiety disorder F15.980
  bipolar and related disorder F15.94
  delirium F15.921
  depressive disorder F15.94
  obsessive-compulsive and related disorder F15.988
  psychotic disorder F15.959
  sexual dysfunction F15.981
  sleep disorder F15.982
  stimulant withdrawal F15.23
Ampulla
  lower esophagus K22.8
  phrenic K22.8
Amputation (*see also* Absence, by site, acquired)
  neuroma (postoperative) (traumatic) — *see* Complications, amputation stump, neuroma
  stump (surgical)
    abnormal, painful, or with complication (late) — *see* Complications, amputation stump
    healed or old NOS Z89.9
  traumatic (complete) (partial)
    arm (upper) (complete) S48.91- ☑
      at
        elbow S58.01- ☑
          partial S58.02- ☑
        shoulder joint (complete) S48.01- ☑
          partial S48.02- ☑
      between
        elbow and wrist (complete) S58.11- ☑
          partial S58.12- ☑
        shoulder and elbow (complete) S48.11- ☑
          partial S48.12- ☑
    partial S48.92- ☑

Amputation — *continued*
  traumatic — *continued*
    breast (complete) S28.21- ☑
      partial S28.22- ☑
    clitoris (complete) S38.211 ☑
      partial S38.212 ☑
    ear (complete) S08.11- ☑
      partial S08.12- ☑
    finger (complete) (metacarpophalangeal) S68.11- ☑
      index S68.11- ☑
      little S68.11- ☑
      middle S68.11- ☑
      partial S68.12- ☑
        index S68.12- ☑
        little S68.12- ☑
        middle S68.12- ☑
        ring S68.12- ☑
      ring S68.11- ☑
      thumb — *see* Amputation, traumatic, thumb
      transphalangeal (complete) S68.61- ☑
        index S68.61- ☑
        little S68.61- ☑
        middle S68.61- ☑
        partial S68.62- ☑
          index S68.62- ☑
          little S68.62- ☑
          middle S68.62- ☑
          ring S68.62- ☑
        ring S68.61- ☑
    foot (complete) S98.91- ☑
      at ankle level S98.01- ☑
        partial S98.02- ☑
      midfoot S98.31- ☑
        partial S98.32- ☑
      partial S98.92- ☑
    forearm (complete) S58.91- ☑
      at elbow level (complete) S58.01- ☑
        partial S58.02- ☑
      between elbow and wrist (complete) S58.11- ☑
        partial S58.12- ☑
      partial S58.92- ☑
    genital organ(s) (external)
      female (complete) S38.211 ☑
        partial S38.212 ☑
      male
        penis (complete) S38.221 ☑
          partial S38.222 ☑
        scrotum (complete) S38.231 ☑
          partial S38.232 ☑
        testes (complete) S38.231 ☑
          partial S38.232 ☑
    hand (complete) (wrist level) S68.41- ☑
      finger(s) alone — *see* Amputation, traumatic, finger
      partial S68.42- ☑
      thumb alone — *see* Amputation, traumatic, thumb
      transmetacarpal (complete) S68.71- ☑
        partial S68.72- ☑
    head
      ear — *see* Amputation, traumatic, ear
      nose (partial) S08.812 ☑
        complete S08.811 ☑
      part S08.89 ☑
        scalp S08.0 ☑
    hip (and thigh) (complete) S78.91- ☑
      at hip joint (complete) S78.01- ☑
        partial S78.02- ☑
      between hip and knee (complete) S78.11- ☑
        partial S78.12- ☑
      partial S78.92- ☑
    labium (majus) (minus) (complete) S38.21- ☑
      S38.21- ☑
    leg (lower) S88.91- ☑
      at knee level S88.01- ☑
        partial S88.02- ☑
      between knee and ankle S88.11- ☑
        partial S88.12- ☑
      partial S88.92- ☑
    nose (partial) S08.812 ☑
      complete S08.811 ☑
    penis (complete) S38.221 ☑
      partial S38.222 ☑
    scrotum (complete) S38.231 ☑
      partial S38.232 ☑
    shoulder — *see* Amputation, traumatic, arm

Amputation — *continued*
  traumatic — *continued*
    shoulder — *see* Amputation, traumatic, arm —
      continued
      at shoulder joint — *see* Amputation, traumatic,
        arm, at shoulder joint
    testes (complete) S38.231 ☑
      partial S38.232 ☑
    thigh — *see* Amputation, traumatic, hip
    thorax, part of S28.1 ☑
      breast — *see* Amputation, traumatic, breast
    thumb (complete) (metacarpophalangeal)
      S68.01- ☑
      partial S68.02- ☑
      transphalangeal (complete) S68.51- ☑
        partial S68.52- ☑
    toe (lesser) S98.13- ☑
      great S98.11- ☑
        partial S98.12- ☑
      more than one S98.21- ☑
        partial S98.22- ☑
      partial S98.14- ☑
    vulva (complete) S38.211 ☑
      partial S38.212 ☑
Amputee (bilateral) (old) Z89.9
Amsterdam dwarfism Q87.1
Amusia R48.8
  developmental F80.89
Amyelencephalus, amyelencephaly Q00.0
Amyelia Q06.0
Amygdalitis — *see* Tonsillitis
Amygdalolith J35.8
Amyloid heart (disease) E85.4 [I43]
Amyloidosis (generalized) (primary) E85.9
  with lung involvement E85.4 [J99]
  familial E85.2
  genetic E85.2
  heart E85.4 [I43]
  hemodialysis-associated E85.3
  light chain (AL) E85.81
  liver E85.4 [K77]
  localized E85.4
  neuropathic heredofamilial E85.1
  non-neuropathic heredofamilial E85.0
  organ limited E85.4
  Portuguese E85.1
  pulmonary E85.4 [J99]
  secondary systemic E85.3
  senile systemic (SSA) E85.82
  skin (lichen) (macular) E85.4 [L99]
  specified NEC E85.89
  subglottic E85.4 [J99]
  wild-type transthyretin-related (ATTR) E85.82
Amylopectinosis (brancher enzyme deficiency) E74.03
Amylophagia — *see* Pica
Amyoplasia congenita Q79.8
Amyotonia M62.89
  congenita G70.2
Amyotrophia, amyotrophy, amyotrophic G71.8
  congenita Q79.8
  diabetic — *see* Diabetes, amyotrophy
  lateral sclerosis G12.21
  neuralgic G54.5
  spinal progressive G12.25
Anacidity, gastric K31.83
  psychogenic F45.8
Anaerosis of newborn P28.89
Analbuminemia E88.09
Analgesia — *see* Anesthesia
Analphalipoproteinemia E78.6
Anaphylactic
  purpura D69.0
  shock or reaction — *see* Shock, anaphylactic
Anaphylactoid shock or reaction — *see* Shock, anaphylactic
Anaphylactoid syndrome of pregnancy O88.01- ☑
Anaphylaxis — *see* Shock, anaphylactic
Anaplasia cervix (*see also* Dysplasia, cervix) N87.9
Anaplasmosis, human A77.49
Anarthria R47.1
Anasarca R60.1
  cardiac — *see* Failure, heart, congestive
  lung J18.2
  newborn P83.2
  nutritional E43
  pulmonary J18.2
  renal N04.9

Anastomosis
  aneurysmal — *see* Aneurysm
  arteriovenous ruptured brain I60.8
  intestinal K63.89
    complicated NEC K91.89
      involving urinary tract N99.89
  retinal and choroidal vessels (congenital) Q14.8
Anatomical narrow angle H40.03- ☑
Ancylostoma, ancylostomiasis (braziliense) (caninum)
  (ceylanicum) (duodenale) B76.0
  Necator americanus B76.1
Andersen's disease (glycogen storage) E74.09
Anderson-Fabry disease E75.21
Andes disease T70.29 ☑
Andrews' disease (bacterid) L08.89
Androblastoma
  benign
    specified site — *see* Neoplasm, benign, by site
    unspecified site
      female D27.9
      male D29.20
  malignant
    specified site — *see* Neoplasm, malignant, by site
    unspecified site
      female C56.9
      male C62.90
  specified site — *see* Neoplasm, uncertain behavior, by
    site
  tubular
    with lipid storage
      specified site — *see* Neoplasm, benign, by site
      unspecified site
        female D27.9
        male D29.20
    specified site — *see* Neoplasm, benign, by site
    unspecified site
      female D27.9
      male D29.20
  unspecified site
    female D39.10
    male D40.10
Androgen insensitivity syndrome (*see also* Syndrome,
  androgen insensitivity) E34.50
Androgen resistance syndrome (*see also* Syndrome,
  androgen insensitivity) E34.50
Android pelvis Q74.2
  with disproportion (fetopelvic) O33.3 ☑
    causing obstructed labor O65.3
Androphobia F40.290
Anectasis, pulmonary (newborn) — *see* Atelectasis
Anemia (essential) (general) (hemoglobin deficiency)
  (infantile) (primary) (profound) D64.9
  with (due to) (in)
    disorder of
      anaerobic glycolysis D55.2
      pentose phosphate pathway D55.1
    koilonychia D50.9
  achlorhydric D50.8
  achrestic D53.1
  Addison (-Biermer) (pernicious) D51.0
  agranulocytic — *see* Agranulocytosis
  amino-acid-deficiency D53.0
  aplastic D61.9
    congenital D61.09
    drug-induced D61.1
    due to
      drugs D61.1
      external agents NEC D61.2
      infection D61.2
      radiation D61.2
    idiopathic D61.3
    red cell (pure) D60.9
      chronic D60.0
      congenital D61.01
      specified type NEC D60.8
      transient D60.1
    specified type NEC D61.89
    toxic D61.2
  aregenerative
    congenital D61.09
  asiderotic D50.9
  atypical (primary) D64.9
  Baghdad spring D55.0
  Balantidium coli A07.0
  Biermer's (pernicious) D51.0
  blood loss (chronic) D50.0
    acute D62
  bothriocephalus B70.0 [D63.8]

Anemia — *continued*
  brickmaker's B76.9 [D63.8]
  cerebral I67.89
  childhood D58.9
  chlorotic D50.8
  chronic
    blood loss D50.0
    hemolytic D58.9
      idiopathic D59.9
    simple D53.9
  chronica congenita aregenerativa D61.09
  combined system disease NEC D51.0 [G32.0]
    due to dietary vitamin B12 deficiency D51.3 [G32.0]
  complicating pregnancy, childbirth or puerperium —
    see Pregnancy, complicated by (management
    affected by), anemia
  congenital P61.4
    aplastic D61.09
    due to isoimmunization NOS P55.9
    dyserythropoietic, dyshematopoietic D64.4
    following fetal blood loss P61.3
    Heinz body D58.2
    hereditary hemolytic NOS D58.9
    pernicious D51.0
    spherocytic D58.0
  Cooley's (erythroblastic) D56.1
  cytogenic D51.0
  deficiency D53.9
    2, 3 diphosphoglycurate mutase D55.2
    2, 3 PG D55.2
    6 phosphogluconate dehydrogenase D55.1
    6-PGD D55.1
    amino-acid D53.0
    combined B12 and folate D53.1
    enzyme D55.9
      drug-induced (hemolytic) D59.2
      glucose-6-phosphate dehydrogenase (G6PD)
        D55.0
      glycolytic D55.2
      nucleotide metabolism D55.3
      related to hexose monophosphate (HMP) shunt
        pathway NEC D55.1
      specified type NEC D55.8
    erythrocytic glutathione D55.1
    folate D52.9
      dietary D52.0
      drug-induced D52.1
    folic acid D52.9
      dietary D52.0
      drug-induced D52.1
    G SH D55.1
    G6PD D55.0
    GGS-R D55.1
    glucose-6-phosphate dehydrogenase D55.0
    glutathione reductase D55.1
    glyceraldehyde phosphate dehydrogenase D55.2
    hexokinase D55.2
    iron D50.9
      secondary to blood loss (chronic) D50.0
    nutritional D53.9
      with
        poor iron absorption D50.8
        specified deficiency NEC D53.8
    phosphofructo-aldolase D55.2
    phosphoglycerate kinase D55.2
    PK D55.2
    protein D53.0
    pyruvate kinase D55.2
    transcobalamin II D51.2
    triose-phosphate isomerase D55.2
    vitamin B12 NOS D51.9
      dietary D51.3
      due to
        intrinsic factor deficiency D51.0
        selective vitamin B12 malabsorption with
          proteinuria D51.1
      pernicious D51.0
      specified type NEC D51.8
  Diamond-Blackfan (congenital hypoplastic) D61.01
  dibothriocephalus B70.0 [D63.8]
  dimorphic D53.1
  diphasic D53.1
  Diphyllobothrium (Dibothriocephalus) B70.0 [D63.8]
  due to (in) (with)
    antineoplastic chemotherapy D64.81
    blood loss (chronic) D50.0
      acute D62
    chemotherapy, antineoplastic D64.81
    chronic disease classified elsewhere NEC D63.8

Anemia — continued
    due to — continued
        chronic kidney disease D63.1
        deficiency
            amino-acid D53.0
            copper D53.8
            folate (folic acid) D52.9
                dietary D52.0
                drug-induced D52.1
            molybdenum D53.8
            protein D53.0
            zinc D53.8
        dietary vitamin B12 deficiency D51.3
        disorder of
            glutathione metabolism D55.1
            nucleotide metabolism D55.3
        drug — see Anemia, by type (see also Table of Drugs and Chemicals)
        end stage renal disease D63.1
        enzyme disorder D55.9
        fetal blood loss P61.3
        fish tapeworm (D.latum) infestation B70.0 [D63.8]
        hemorrhage (chronic) D50.0
            acute D62
        impaired absorption D50.9
        loss of blood (chronic) D50.0
            acute D62
        myxedema E03.9 [D63.8]
        Necator americanus B76.1 [D63.8]
        prematurity P61.2
        selective vitamin B12 malabsorption with proteinuria D51.1
        transcobalamin II deficiency D51.2
    Dyke-Young type (secondary) (symptomatic) D59.1
    dyserythropoietic (congenital) D64.4
    dyshematopoietic (congenital) D64.4
    Egyptian B76.9 [D63.8]
    elliptocytosis — see Elliptocytosis
    enzyme-deficiency, drug-induced D59.2
    epidemic (see also Ancylostomiasis) B76.9 [D63.8]
    erythroblastic
        familial D56.1
        newborn (see also Disease, hemolytic) P55.9
        of childhood D56.1
    erythrocytic glutathione deficiency D55.1
    erythropoietin-resistant anemia (EPO resistant anemia) D63.1
    Faber's (achlorhydric anemia) D50.9
    factitious (self-induced blood letting) D50.0
    familial erythroblastic D56.1
    Fanconi's (congenital pancytopenia) D61.09
    favism D55.0
    fish tapeworm (D. latum) infestation B70.0 [D63.8]
    folate (folic acid) deficiency D52.9
    glucose-6-phosphate dehydrogenase (G6PD) deficiency D55.0
    glutathione-reductase deficiency D55.1
    goat's milk D52.0
    granulocytic — see Agranulocytosis
    Heinz body, congenital D58.2
    hemolytic D58.9
        acquired D59.9
            with hemoglobinuria NEC D59.6
            autoimmune NEC D59.1
            infectious D59.4
            specified type NEC D59.8
            toxic D59.4
        acute D59.9
            due to enzyme deficiency specified type NEC D55.8
            Lederer's D59.1
        autoimmune D59.1
            drug-induced D59.0
        chronic D58.9
            idiopathic D59.9
        cold type (secondary) (symptomatic) D59.1
        congenital (spherocytic) — see Spherocytosis
        due to
            cardiac conditions D59.4
            drugs (nonautoimmune) D59.2
                autoimmune D59.0
            enzyme disorder D55.9
                drug-induced D59.2
            presence of shunt or other internal prosthetic device D59.4
        familial D58.9
        hereditary D58.9
            due to enzyme disorder D55.9
                specified type NEC D55.8

Anemia — continued
    hemolytic — continued
        hereditary — continued
            specified type NEC D58.8
        idiopathic (chronic) D59.9
        mechanical D59.4
        microangiopathic D59.4
        nonautoimmune D59.4
            drug-induced D59.2
        nonspherocytic
            congenital or hereditary NEC D55.8
                glucose-6-phosphate dehydrogenase deficiency D55.0
                pyruvate kinase deficiency D55.2
                type
                    I D55.1
                    II D55.2
            type
                I D55.1
                II D55.2
        secondary D59.4
            autoimmune D59.1
        specified (hereditary) type NEC D58.8
        Stransky-Regala type (see also Hemoglobinopathy) D58.8
        symptomatic D59.4
            autoimmune D59.1
        toxic D59.4
        warm type (secondary) (symptomatic) D59.1
    hemorrhagic (chronic) D50.0
        acute D62
    Herrick's D57.1
    hexokinase deficiency D55.2
    hookworm B76.9 [D63.8]
    hypochromic (idiopathic) (microcytic) (normoblastic) D50.9
        due to blood loss (chronic) D50.0
            acute D62
        familial sex-linked D64.0
        pyridoxine-responsive D64.3
        sideroblastic, sex-linked D64.0
    hypoplasia, red blood cells D61.9
        congenital or familial D61.01
    hypoplastic (idiopathic) D61.9
        congenital or familial (of childhood) D61.01
    hypoproliferative (refractive) D61.9
    idiopathic D64.9
        aplastic D61.3
        hemolytic, chronic D59.9
    in (due to) (with)
        chronic kidney disease D63.1
        end stage renal disease D63.1
        failure, kidney (renal) D63.1
        neoplastic disease (see also Neoplasm) D63.0
    intertropical (see also Ancylostomiasis) D63.8
    iron deficiency D50.9
        secondary to blood loss (chronic) D50.0
            acute D62
        specified type NEC D50.8
    Joseph-Diamond-Blackfan (congenital hypoplastic) D61.01
    Lederer's (hemolytic) D59.1
    leukoerythroblastic D61.82
    macrocytic D53.9
        nutritional D52.0
        tropical D52.8
    malarial (see also Malaria) B54 [D63.8]
    malignant (progressive) D51.0
    malnutrition D53.9
    marsh (see also Malaria) B54 [D63.8]
    Mediterranean (with other hemoglobinopathy) D56.9
    megaloblastic D53.1
        combined B12 and folate deficiency D53.1
        hereditary D51.1
        nutritional D52.0
        orotic aciduria D53.0
        refractory D53.1
        specified type NEC D53.1
    megalocytic D53.1
    microcytic (hypochromic) D50.9
        due to blood loss (chronic) D50.0
            acute D62
        familial D56.8
    microdrepanocytosis D57.40
    microelliptopoikilocytic (Rietti-Greppi- Micheli) D56.9
    miner's B76.9 [D63.8]
    myelodysplastic D46.9
    myelofibrosis D75.81
    myelogenous D64.89

Anemia — continued
    myelopathic D64.89
    myelophthisic D61.82
    myeloproliferative D47.Z9 (following D47.4)
    newborn P61.4
        due to
            ABO (antibodies, isoimmunization, maternal/fetal incompatibility) P55.1
            Rh (antibodies, isoimmunization, maternal/fetal incompatibility) P55.0
        following fetal blood loss P61.3
        posthemorrhagic (fetal) P61.3
    nonspherocytic hemolytic — see Anemia, hemolytic, nonspherocytic
    normocytic (infectional) D64.9
        due to blood loss (chronic) D50.0
            acute D62
        myelophthisic D61.82
    nutritional (deficiency) D53.9
        with
            poor iron absorption D50.8
            specified deficiency NEC D53.8
        megaloblastic D52.0
    of prematurity P61.2
    orotaciduric (congenital) (hereditary) D53.0
    osteosclerotic D64.89
    ovalocytosis (hereditary) — see Elliptocytosis
    paludal (see also Malaria) B54 [D63.8]
    pernicious (congenital) (malignant) (progressive) D51.0
    pleochromic D64.89
    posthemorrhagic (chronic) D50.0
        acute D62
        newborn P61.3
    postoperative (postprocedural)
        due to (acute) blood loss D62
            chronic blood loss D50.0
        specified NEC D64.9
    postpartum O90.81
    pressure D64.89
    progressive D64.9
        malignant D51.0
        pernicious D51.0
    protein-deficiency D53.0
    pseudoleukemica infantum D64.89
    pure red cell D60.9
        congenital D61.01
    pyridoxine-responsive D64.3
    pyruvate kinase deficiency D55.2
    refractory D46.4
        with
            excess of blasts D46.20
                1 (RAEB 1) D46.21
                2 (RAEB 2) D46.22
                in transformation (RAEB T) — see Leukemia, acute myeloblastic
            hemochromatosis D46.1
            sideroblasts (ring) (RARS) D46.1
        megaloblastic D53.1
        sideroblastic D46.1
        sideropenic D50.9
        without ring sideroblasts, so stated D46.0
        without sideroblasts without excess of blasts D46.0
    Rietti-Greppi-Micheli D56.9
    scorbutic D53.2
    secondary to
        blood loss (chronic) D50.0
            acute D62
        hemorrhage (chronic) D50.0
            acute D62
    semiplastic D61.89
    sickle-cell — see Disease, sickle-cell
    sideroblastic D64.3
        hereditary D64.0
        hypochromic, sex-linked D64.0
        pyridoxine-responsive NEC D64.3
        refractory D46.1
        secondary (due to)
            disease D64.1
            drugs and toxins D64.2
        specified type NEC D64.3
    sideropenic (refractory) D50.9
        due to blood loss (chronic) D50.0
            acute D62
    simple chronic D53.9
    specified type NEC D64.89
    spherocytic (hereditary) — see Spherocytosis
    splenic D64.89
    splenomegalic D64.89

Anemia — *continued*
  stomatocytosis D58.8
  syphilitic (acquired) (late) A52.79 [D63.8]
  target cell D64.89
  thalassemia D56.9
  thrombocytopenic — *see* Thrombocytopenia
  toxic D61.2
  tropical B76.9 [D63.8]
    macrocytic D52.8
  tuberculous A18.89 [D63.8]
  vegan D51.3
  vitamin
    B12 deficiency (dietary) pernicious D51.0
    B6-responsive D64.3
  von Jaksch's D64.89
  Witts' (achlorhydric anemia) D50.8
Anemophobia F40.228
Anencephalus, anencephaly Q00.0
Anergasia — *see* Psychosis, organic
Anesthesia, anesthetic R20.0
  complication or reaction NEC (*see also* Complications, anesthesia) T88.59 ☑
    due to
      correct substance properly administered — *see* Table of Drugs and Chemicals, by drug, adverse effect
      overdose or wrong substance given — *see* Table of Drugs and Chemicals, by drug, poisoning
    unintended awareness under general anesthesia during procedure T88.53 ☑
      personal history of Z92.84
  cornea H18.81- ☑
  dissociative F44.6
  functional (hysterical) F44.6
  hyperesthetic, thalamic G89.0
  hysterical F44.6
  local skin lesion R20.0
  sexual (psychogenic) F52.1
  shock (due to) T88.2 ☑
  skin R20.0
  testicular N50.9
Anetoderma (maculosum) (of) L90.8
  Jadassohn-Pellizzari L90.2
  Schweniger-Buzzi L90.1
Aneurin deficiency E51.9
Aneurysm (anastomotic) (artery) (cirsoid) (diffuse) (false) (fusiform) (multiple) (saccular) I72.9
  abdominal (aorta) I71.4
    ruptured I71.3
    syphilitic A52.01
  aorta, aortic (nonsyphilitic) I71.9
    abdominal I71.4
      ruptured I71.3
    arch I71.2
      ruptured I71.1
    arteriosclerotic I71.9
      ruptured I71.8
    ascending I71.2
      ruptured I71.1
    congenital Q25.43
    descending I71.9
      abdominal I71.4
        ruptured I71.3
      ruptured I71.8
      thoracic I71.2
        ruptured I71.1
    root Q25.43
    ruptured I71.8
    sinus, congenital Q25.43
    syphilitic A52.01
    thoracic I71.2
      ruptured I71.1
    thoracoabdominal I71.6
      ruptured I71.5
    thorax, thoracic (arch) I71.2
      ruptured I71.1
    transverse I71.2
      ruptured I71.1
    valve (heart) (*see also* Endocarditis, aortic) I35.8
  arteriosclerotic I72.9
    cerebral I67.1
      ruptured — *see* Hemorrhage, intracranial, subarachnoid
  arteriovenous (congenital) (*see also* Malformation, arteriovenous)
    acquired I77.0
      brain I67.1

Aneurysm — *continued*
  arteriovenous (*see also* Malformation, arteriovenous) — *continued*
    acquired — *continued*
      coronary I25.41
      pulmonary I28.0
    brain Q28.2
      ruptured I60.8
    peripheral — *see* Malformation, arteriovenous, peripheral
    precerebral vessels Q28.0
    specified site NEC (*see also* Malformation, arteriovenous)
      acquired I77.0
  basal — *see* Aneurysm, brain
  basilar (trunk) I72.5
  berry (congenital) (nonruptured) I67.1
    ruptured I60.7
  brain I67.1
    arteriosclerotic I67.1
      ruptured — *see* Hemorrhage, intracranial, subarachnoid
    arteriovenous (congenital) (nonruptured) Q28.2
      acquired I67.1
        ruptured I60.8
      ruptured I60.8
    berry (congenital) (nonruptured) I67.1
      ruptured (*see also* Hemorrhage, intracranial, subarachnoid) I60.7
    congenital Q28.3
      ruptured I60.7
    meninges I67.1
      ruptured I60.8
    miliary (congenital) (nonruptured) I67.1
      ruptured (*see also* Hemorrhage, intracranial, subarachnoid) I60.7
    mycotic I33.0
    ruptured — *see* Hemorrhage, intracranial, subarachnoid
    syphilitic (hemorrhage) A52.05
  cardiac (false) (*see also* Aneurysm, heart) I25.3
  carotid artery (common) (external) I72.0
    internal (intracranial) I67.1
      extracranial portion I72.0
    ruptured into brain I60.0- ☑
    syphilitic A52.09
      intracranial A52.05
  cavernous sinus I67.1
    arteriovenous (congenital) (nonruptured) Q28.3
      ruptured I60.8
  celiac I72.8
  central nervous system, syphilitic A52.05
  cerebral — *see* Aneurysm, brain
  chest — *see* Aneurysm, thorax
  circle of Willis I67.1
    congenital Q28.3
      ruptured I60.6
    ruptured I60.6
  common iliac artery I72.3
  congenital (peripheral) Q27.8
    aorta (root) (sinus) Q25.43
    brain Q28.3
      ruptured I60.7
    coronary Q24.5
    digestive system Q27.8
    lower limb Q27.8
    pulmonary Q25.79
    retina Q14.1
    specified site NEC Q27.8
    upper limb Q27.8
  conjunctiva — *see* Abnormality, conjunctiva, vascular
  conus arteriosus — *see* Aneurysm, heart
  coronary (arteriosclerotic) (artery) I25.41
    arteriovenous, congenital Q24.5
    congenital Q24.5
    ruptured — *see* Infarct, myocardium
    syphilitic A52.06
    vein I25.89
  cylindroid (aorta) I71.9
    ruptured I71.8
    syphilitic A52.01
  ductus arteriosus Q25.0
  endocardial, infective (any valve) I33.0
  femoral (artery) (ruptured) I72.4
  gastroduodenal I72.8
  gastroepiploic I72.8
  heart (wall) (chronic or with a stated duration of over 4 weeks) I25.3

Aneurysm — *continued*
  heart — *continued*
    valve — *see* Endocarditis
  hepatic I72.8
  iliac (common) (artery) (ruptured) I72.3
  infective I72.9
    endocardial (any valve) I33.0
  innominate (nonsyphilitic) I72.8
    syphilitic A52.09
  interauricular septum — *see* Aneurysm, heart
  interventricular septum — *see* Aneurysm, heart
  intrathoracic (nonsyphilitic) I71.2
    ruptured I71.1
    syphilitic A52.01
  lower limb I72.4
  lung (pulmonary artery) I28.1
  mediastinal (nonsyphilitic) I72.8
    syphilitic A52.09
  miliary (congenital) I67.1
    ruptured — *see* Hemorrhage, intracerebral, subarachnoid, intracranial
  mitral (heart) (valve) I34.8
  mural — *see* Aneurysm, heart
  mycotic I72.9
    endocardial (any valve) I33.0
    ruptured, brain — *see* Hemorrhage, intracerebral, subarachnoid
  myocardium — *see* Aneurysm, heart
  neck I72.0
  pancreaticoduodenal I72.8
  patent ductus arteriosus Q25.0
  peripheral NEC I72.8
    congenital Q27.8
      digestive system Q27.8
      lower limb Q27.8
      specified site NEC Q27.8
      upper limb Q27.8
  popliteal (artery) (ruptured) I72.4
  precerebral
    congenital (nonruptured) Q28.1
    specified site, NEC I72.5
  pulmonary I28.1
    arteriovenous Q25.72
      acquired I28.0
    syphilitic A52.09
    valve (heart) — *see* Endocarditis, pulmonary
  racemose (peripheral) I72.9
    congenital — *see* Aneurysm, congenital
  radial I72.1
  Rasmussen NEC A15.0
  renal (artery) I72.2
  retina (*see also* Disorder, retina, microaneurysms)
    congenital Q14.1
    diabetic — *see* Diabetes, microaneurysms, retinal
  sinus of Valsalva Q25.49
  specified NEC I72.8
  spinal (cord) I72.8
    syphilitic (hemorrhage) A52.09
  splenic I72.8
  subclavian (artery) (ruptured) I72.8
    syphilitic A52.09
  superior mesenteric I72.8
  syphilitic (aorta) A52.01
    central nervous system A52.05
    congenital (late) A50.54 [I79.0]
    spine, spinal A52.09
  thoracoabdominal (aorta) I71.6
    ruptured I71.5
    syphilitic A52.01
  thorax, thoracic (aorta) (arch) (nonsyphilitic) I71.2
    ruptured I71.1
    syphilitic A52.01
  traumatic (complication) (early), specified site — *see* Injury, blood vessel
  tricuspid (heart) (valve) I07.8
  ulnar I72.1
  upper limb (ruptured) I72.1
  valve, valvular — *see* Endocarditis
  venous (*see also* Varix) I86.8
    congenital Q27.8
      digestive system Q27.8
      lower limb Q27.8
      specified site NEC Q27.8
      upper limb Q27.8
  ventricle — *see* Aneurysm, heart
  vertebral artery I72.6
  visceral NEC I72.8
Angelman syndrome Q93.51

☑ Additional Character Required — Refer to the Tabular List for Character Selection   ▽ Subterms under main terms may continue to next column or page

Anger R45.4

Angiectasis, angiectopia I99.8

Angiitis I77.6
  allergic granulomatous M30.1
  hypersensitivity M31.0
  necrotizing M31.9
    specified NEC M31.8
  nervous system, granulomatous I67.7

Angina (attack) (cardiac) (chest) (heart) (pectoris) (syndrome) (vasomotor) I20.9
  with
    atherosclerotic heart disease — see Arteriosclerosis, coronary (artery),
      documented spasm I20.1
  abdominal K55.1
  accelerated — see Angina, unstable
  agranulocytic — see Agranulocytosis
  angiospastic — see Angina, with documented spasm
  aphthous B08.5
  crescendo — see Angina, unstable
  croupous J05.0
  cruris I73.9
  de novo effort — see Angina, unstable
  diphtheritic, membranous A36.0
  equivalent I20.8
  exudative, chronic J37.0
  following acute myocardial infarction I23.7
  gangrenous diphtheritic A36.0
  intestinal K55.1
  Ludovici K12.2
  Ludwig's K12.2
  malignant diphtheritic A36.0
  membranous J05.0
    diphtheritic A36.0
    Vincent's A69.1
  mesenteric K55.1
  monocytic — see Mononucleosis, infectious
  of effort — see Angina, specified NEC
  phlegmonous J36
    diphtheritic A36.0
  post-infarctional I23.7
  pre-infarctional — see Angina, unstable
  Prinzmetal — see Angina, with documented spasm
  progressive — see Angina, unstable
  pseudomembranous A69.1
  pultaceous, diphtheritic A36.0
  spasm-induced — see Angina, with documented spasm
  specified NEC I20.8
  stable I20.8
  stenocardia — see Angina, specified NEC
  stridulous, diphtheritic A36.2
  tonsil J36
  trachealis J05.0
  unstable I20.0
  variant — see Angina, with documented spasm
  Vincent's A69.1
  worsening effort — see Angina, unstable

Angioblastoma — see Neoplasm, connective tissue, uncertain behavior

Angiocholecystitis — see Cholecystitis, acute

Angiocholitis (see also Cholecystitis, acute) K83.09

Angiodysgenesis spinalis G95.19

Angiodysplasia (cecum) (colon) K55.20
  with bleeding K55.21
  duodenum (and stomach) K31.819
    with bleeding K31.811
  stomach (and duodenum) K31.819
    with bleeding K31.811

Angioedema (allergic) (any site) (with urticaria) T78.3 ☑
  hereditary D84.1

Angioendothelioma — see Neoplasm, uncertain behavior, by site
  benign D18.00
    intra-abdominal D18.03
    intracranial D18.02
    skin D18.01
    specified site NEC D18.09
  bone — see Neoplasm, bone, malignant
  Ewing's — see Neoplasm, bone, malignant

Angioendotheliomatosis C85.8- ☑

Angiofibroma (see also Neoplasm, benign, by site)
  juvenile
    specified site — see Neoplasm, benign, by site
    unspecified site D10.6

Angiohemophilia (A) (B) D68.0

Angioid streaks (choroid) (macula) (retina) H35.33

Angiokeratoma — see Neoplasm, skin, benign
  corporis diffusum E75.21

Angioleiomyoma — see Neoplasm, connective tissue, benign

Angiolipoma (see also Lipoma)
  infiltrating — see Lipoma

Angioma (see also Hemangioma, by site)
  capillary I78.1
  hemorrhagicum hereditaria I78.0
  intra-abdominal D18.03
  intracranial D18.02
  malignant — see Neoplasm, connective tissue, malignant
  plexiform D18.00
    intra-abdominal D18.03
    intracranial D18.02
    skin D18.01
    specified site NEC D18.09
  senile I78.1
  serpiginosum L81.7
  skin D18.01
  specified site NEC D18.09
  spider I78.1
  stellate I78.1
  venous Q28.3

Angiomatosis Q82.8
  bacillary A79.89
  encephalotrigeminal Q85.8
  hemorrhagic familial I78.0
  hereditary familial I78.0
  liver K76.4

Angiomyolipoma — see Lipoma

Angiomyoliposarcoma — see Neoplasm, connective tissue, malignant

Angiomyoma — see Neoplasm, connective tissue, benign

Angiomyosarcoma — see Neoplasm, connective tissue, malignant

Angiomyxoma — see Neoplasm, connective tissue, uncertain behavior

Angioneurosis F45.8

Angioneurotic edema (allergic) (any site) (with urticaria) T78.3 ☑
  hereditary D84.1

Angiopathia, angiopathy I99.9
  cerebral I67.9
    amyloid E85.4 [I68.0]
  diabetic (peripheral) — see Diabetes, angiopathy
  peripheral I73.9
    diabetic — see Diabetes, angiopathy
    specified type NEC I73.89
  retinae syphilitica A52.05
  retinalis (juvenilis)
    diabetic — see Diabetes, retinopathy
    proliferative — see Retinopathy, proliferative

Angiosarcoma (see also Neoplasm, connective tissue, malignant)
  liver C22.3

Angiosclerosis — see Arteriosclerosis

Angiospasm (peripheral) (traumatic) (vessel) I73.9
  brachial plexus G54.0
  cerebral G45.9
  cervical plexus G54.2
  nerve
    arm — see Mononeuropathy, upper limb
      axillary G54.0
      median — see Lesion, nerve, median
      ulnar — see Lesion, nerve, ulnar
    axillary G54.0
    leg — see Mononeuropathy, lower limb
    median — see Lesion, nerve, median
    plantar — see Lesion, nerve, plantar
    ulnar — see Lesion, nerve, ulnar

Angiospastic disease or edema I73.9

Angiostrongyliasis
  due to
    Parastrongylus
      cantonensis B83.2
      costaricensis B81.3
    intestinal B81.3

Anguillulosis — see Strongyloidiasis

Angulation
  cecum — see Obstruction, intestine
  coccyx (acquired) (see also subcategory) M43.8 ☑
    congenital NEC Q76.49
  femur (acquired) (see also Deformity, limb, specified type NEC, thigh)
    congenital Q74.2
  intestine (large) (small) — see Obstruction, intestine
  sacrum (acquired) (see also subcategory) M43.8 ☑
    congenital NEC Q76.49

Angulation — continued
  sigmoid (flexure) — see Obstruction, intestine
  spine — see Dorsopathy, deforming, specified NEC
  tibia (acquired) (see also Deformity, limb, specified type NEC, lower leg)
    congenital Q74.2
  ureter N13.5
    with infection N13.6
  wrist (acquired) (see also Deformity, limb, specified type NEC, forearm)
    congenital Q74.0

Angulus infectiosus (lips) K13.0

Anhedonia R45.84
  sexual F52.0

Anhidrosis L74.4

Anhydration E86.0

Anhydremia E86.0

Anidrosis L74.4

Aniridia (congenital) Q13.1

Anisakiasis (infection) (infestation) B81.0

Anisakis larvae infestation B81.0

Aniseikonia H52.32

Anisocoria (pupil) H57.02
  congenital Q13.2

Anisocytosis R71.8

Anisometropia (congenital) H52.31

Ankle — see condition

Ankyloblepharon (eyelid) (acquired) (see also Blepharophimosis)
  filiforme (adnatum) (congenital) Q10.3
  total Q10.3

Ankyloglossia Q38.1

Ankylosis (fibrous) (osseous) (joint) M24.60
  ankle M24.67- ☑
  arthrodesis status Z98.1
  cricoarytenoid (cartilage) (joint) (larynx) J38.7
  dental K03.5
  ear ossicles H74.31- ☑
  elbow M24.62- ☑
  foot M24.67- ☑
  hand M24.64- ☑
  hip M24.65- ☑
  incostapedial joint (infectional) — see Ankylosis, ear ossicles
  jaw (temporomandibular) M26.61- ☑
  knee M24.66- ☑
  lumbosacral (joint) M43.27
  postoperative (status) Z98.1
  produced by surgical fusion, status Z98.1
  sacro-iliac (joint) M43.28
  shoulder M24.61- ☑
  spine (joint) (see also Fusion, spine)
    spondylitic — see Spondylitis, ankylosing
  surgical Z98.1
  temporomandibular M26.61- ☑
  tooth, teeth (hard tissues) K03.5
  wrist M24.63- ☑

Ankylostoma — see Ancylostoma

Ankylostomiasis — see Ancylostomiasis

Ankylurethria — see Stricture, urethra

Annular (see also condition)
  detachment, cervix N88.8
  organ or site, congenital NEC — see Distortion
  pancreas Q45.1

Anodontia (complete) (partial) (vera) K00.0
  acquired K08.10 ☑

Anomaly, anomalous (congenital) (unspecified type) Q89.9
  abdominal wall NEC Q79.59
  acoustic nerve Q07.8
  adrenal (gland) Q89.1
  Alder (-Reilly) (leukocyte granulation) D72.0
  alimentary tract Q45.9
    upper Q40.9
  alveolar M26.70
    hyperplasia M26.79
      mandibular M26.72
      maxillary M26.71
    hypoplasia M26.79
      mandibular M26.74
      maxillary M26.73
    ridge (process) M26.79
    specified NEC M26.79
  ankle (joint) Q74.2
  anus Q43.9
  aorta (arch) NEC Q25.40
    coarctation (preductal) (postductal) Q25.1

Anomaly, anomalous — *continued*
   aortic cusp or valve Q23.9
   appendix Q43.8
   apple peel syndrome Q41.1
   aqueduct of Sylvius Q03.0
      with spina bifida — *see* Spina bifida, with hydro-
         cephalus
   arm Q74.0
   arteriovenous NEC
      coronary Q24.5
      gastrointestinal Q27.33
         acquired — *see* Angiodysplasia
   artery (peripheral) Q27.9
      basilar NEC Q28.1
      cerebral Q28.3
      coronary Q24.5
      digestive system Q27.8
      eye Q15.8
      great Q25.9
         specified NEC Q25.8
      lower limb Q27.8
      peripheral Q27.9
         specified NEC Q27.8
      pulmonary NEC Q25.79
      renal Q27.2
      retina Q14.1
      specified site NEC Q27.8
      subclavian Q27.8
         origin Q25.48
      umbilical Q27.0
      upper limb Q27.8
      vertebral NEC Q28.1
   aryteno-epiglottic folds Q31.8
   atrial
      bands or folds Q20.8
      septa Q21.1
   atrioventricular
      excitation I45.6
      septum Q21.0
   auditory canal Q17.8
   auricle
      ear Q17.8
         causing impairment of hearing Q16.9
      heart Q20.8
   Axenfeld's Q15.0
   back Q89.9
   band
      atrial Q20.8
      heart Q24.8
      ventricular Q24.8
   Bartholin's duct Q38.4
   biliary duct or passage Q44.5
   bladder Q64.70
      absence Q64.5
      diverticulum Q64.6
      exstrophy Q64.10
         cloacal Q64.12
         extroversion Q64.19
         specified type NEC Q64.19
         supravesical fissure Q64.11
      neck obstruction Q64.31
      specified type NEC Q64.79
   bone Q79.9
      arm Q74.0
      face Q75.9
      leg Q74.2
      pelvic girdle Q74.2
      shoulder girdle Q74.0
      skull Q75.9
         with
            anencephaly Q00.0
            encephalocele — *see* Encephalocele
            hydrocephalus Q03.9
               with spina bifida — *see* Spina bifida, by
                  site, with hydrocephalus
            microcephaly Q02
   brain (multiple) Q04.9
      vessel Q28.3
   breast Q83.9
   broad ligament Q50.6
   bronchus Q32.4
   bulbus cordis Q21.9
   bursa Q79.9
   canal of Nuck Q52.4
   canthus Q10.3
   capillary Q27.9
   cardiac Q24.9
      chambers Q20.9
         specified NEC Q20.8

Anomaly, anomalous — *continued*
   cardiac — *continued*
      septal closure Q21.9
         specified NEC Q21.8
      valve NEC Q24.8
         pulmonary Q22.3
   cardiovascular system Q28.8
   carpus Q74.0
   caruncle, lacrimal Q10.6
   cascade stomach Q40.2
   cauda equina Q06.3
   cecum Q43.9
   cerebral Q04.9
      vessels Q28.3
   cervix Q51.9
   Chédiak-Higashi (-Steinbrinck) (congenital gigantism
      of peroxidase granules) E70.330
   cheek Q18.9
   chest wall Q67.8
      bones Q76.9
   chin Q18.9
   chordae tendineae Q24.8
   choroid Q14.3
      plexus Q07.8
   chromosomes, chromosomal Q99.9
      D (1) — *see* condition, chromosome 13
      E (3) — *see* condition, chromosome 18
      G — *see* condition, chromosome 21
      sex
         female phenotype Q97.8
         gonadal dysgenesis (pure) Q99.1
         Klinefelter's Q98.4
         male phenotype Q98.9
         Turner's Q96.9
      specified NEC Q99.8
   cilia Q10.3
   circulatory system Q28.9
   clavicle Q74.0
   clitoris Q52.6
   coccyx Q76.49
   colon Q43.9
   common duct Q44.5
   communication
      coronary artery Q24.5
      left ventricle with right atrium Q21.0
   concha (ear) Q17.3
   connection
      portal vein Q26.5
      pulmonary venous Q26.4
         partial Q26.3
         total Q26.2
      renal artery with kidney Q27.2
   cornea (shape) Q13.4
   coronary artery or vein Q24.5
   cranium — *see* Anomaly, skull
   cricoid cartilage Q31.8
   cystic duct Q44.5
   dental
      alveolar — *see* Anomaly, alveolar
      arch relationship M26.20
         specified NEC M26.29
   dentofacial M26.9
      alveolar — *see* Anomaly, alveolar
      dental arch relationship M26.20
         specified NEC M26.29
      functional M26.50
         specified NEC M26.59
      jaw size M26.00
         macrogenia M26.05
         mandibular
            hyperplasia M26.03
            hypoplasia M26.04
         maxillary
            hyperplasia M26.01
            hypoplasia M26.02
         microgenia M26.06
         specified type NEC M26.09
      jaw-cranial base relationship M26.10
         asymmetry M26.12
            maxillary M26.11
         specified type NEC M26.19
      malocclusion M26.4
         dental arch relationship NEC M26.29
         jaw size — *see* Anomaly, dentofacial, jaw size
         jaw-cranial base relationship — *see* Anomaly,
            dentofacial, jaw-cranial base relationship
      specified type NEC M26.89
      temporomandibular joint M26.60- ☑

Anomaly, anomalous — *continued*
   dentofacial — *continued*
      temporomandibular joint — *continued*
         adhesions M26.61- ☑
         ankylosis M26.61- ☑
         arthralgia M26.62- ☑
         articular disc M26.63- ☑
         specified type NEC M26.69
      tooth position, fully erupted M26.30
         specified NEC M26.39
   dermatoglyphic Q82.8
   diaphragm (apertures) NEC Q79.1
   digestive organ(s) or tract Q45.9
      lower Q43.9
      upper Q40.9
   distance, interarch (excessive) (inadequate) M26.25
   distribution, coronary artery Q24.5
   ductus
      arteriosus Q25.0
      botalli Q25.0
   duodenum Q43.9
   dura (brain) Q04.9
      spinal cord Q06.9
   ear (external) Q17.9
      causing impairment of hearing Q16.9
      inner Q16.5
      middle (causing impairment of hearing) Q16.4
      ossicles Q16.3
   Ebstein's (heart) (tricuspid valve) Q22.5
   ectodermal Q82.9
   Eisenmenger's (ventricular septal defect) Q21.8
   ejaculatory duct Q55.4
   elbow Q74.0
   endocrine gland NEC Q89.2
   epididymis Q55.4
   epiglottis Q31.8
   esophagus Q39.9
   eustachian tube Q17.8
   eye Q15.9
      anterior segment Q13.9
         specified NEC Q13.89
      posterior segment Q14.9
         specified NEC Q14.8
      ptosis (eyelid) Q10.0
      specified NEC Q15.8
   eyebrow Q18.8
   eyelid Q10.3
      ptosis Q10.0
   face Q18.9
      bone(s) Q75.9
   fallopian tube Q50.6
   fascia Q79.9
   femur NEC Q74.2
   fibula NEC Q74.2
   finger Q74.0
   fixation, intestine Q43.3
   flexion (joint) NOS Q74.9
      hip or thigh Q65.89
   foot NEC Q74.2
      varus (congenital) Q66.3
   foramen
      Botalli Q21.1
      ovale Q21.1
   forearm Q74.0
   forehead Q75.8
   form, teeth K00.2
   fovea centralis Q14.1
   frontal bone — *see* Anomaly, skull
   gallbladder (position) (shape) (size) Q44.1
   Gartner's duct Q52.4
   gastrointestinal tract Q45.9
   genitalia, genital organ(s) or system
      female Q52.9
         external Q52.70
         internal NOS Q52.9
      male Q55.9
         hydrocele P83.5
         specified NEC Q55.8
   genitourinary NEC
      female Q52.9
      male Q55.9
   Gerbode Q21.0
   glottis Q31.8
   granulation or granulocyte, genetic (constitutional)
      (leukocyte) D72.0
   gum Q38.6
   gyri Q07.9
   hair Q84.2
   hand Q74.0

Anomaly, anomalous — *continued*
  hard tissue formation in pulp KØ4.3
  head — *see* Anomaly, skull
  heart Q24.9
    auricle Q2Ø.8
    bands or folds Q24.8
    fibroelastosis cordis I42.4
    obstructive NEC Q22.6
    patent ductus arteriosus (Botalli) Q25.Ø
    septum Q21.9
      auricular Q21.1
      interatrial Q21.1
      interventricular Q21.Ø
        with pulmonary stenosis or atresia, dextrapo-
          sition of aorta and hypertrophy of right
          ventricle Q21.3
      specified NEC Q21.8
      ventricular Q21.Ø
        with pulmonary stenosis or atresia, dextrapo-
          sition of aorta and hypertrophy of right
          ventricle Q21.3
    tetralogy of Fallot Q21.3
    valve NEC Q24.8
      aortic
        bicuspid valve Q23.1
        insufficiency Q23.1
        stenosis Q23.Ø
          subaortic Q24.4
      mitral
        insufficiency Q23.3
        stenosis Q23.2
      pulmonary Q22.3
        atresia Q22.Ø
        insufficiency Q22.2
        stenosis Q22.1
          infundibular Q24.3
          subvalvular Q24.3
      tricuspid
        atresia Q22.4
        stenosis Q22.4
    ventricle Q2Ø.8
  heel NEC Q74.2
  Hegglin's D72.Ø
  hemianencephaly QØØ.Ø
  hemicephaly QØØ.Ø
  hemicrania QØØ.Ø
  hepatic duct Q44.5
  hip NEC Q74.2
  hourglass stomach Q4Ø.2
  humerus Q74.Ø
  hydatid of Morgagni
    female Q5Ø.5
    male (epididymal) Q55.4
      testicular Q55.29
  hymen Q52.4
  hypersegmentation of neutrophils, hereditary D72.Ø
  hypophyseal Q89.2
  ileocecal (coil) (valve) Q43.9
  ileum Q43.9
  ilium NEC Q74.2
  integument Q84.9
    specified NEC Q84.8
  interarch distance (excessive) (inadequate) M26.25
  intervertebral cartilage or disc Q76.49
  intestine (large) (small) Q43.9
    with anomalous adhesions, fixation or malrotation
      Q43.3
  iris Q13.2
  ischium NEC Q74.2
  jaw — *see* Anomaly, dentofacial
    alveolar — *see* Anomaly, alveolar
  jaw-cranial base relationship — *see* Anomaly, dentofa-
    cial, jaw-cranial base relationship
  jejunum Q43.8
  joint Q74.9
    specified NEC Q74.8
  Jordan's D72.Ø
  kidney(s) (calyx) (pelvis) Q63.9
    artery Q27.2
    specified NEC Q63.8
  Klippel-Feil (brevicollis) Q76.1
  knee Q74.1
  labium (majus) (minus) Q52.7Ø
  labyrinth, membranous Q16.5
  lacrimal apparatus or duct Q1Ø.6
  larynx, laryngeal (muscle) Q31.9
    web (bed) Q31.Ø
  lens Q12.9
  leukocytes, genetic D72.Ø

Anomaly, anomalous — *continued*
  leukocytes, genetic — *continued*
    granulation (constitutional) D72.Ø
  lid (fold) Q1Ø.3
  ligament Q79.9
    broad Q5Ø.6
    round Q52.8
  limb Q74.9
    lower NEC Q74.2
      reduction deformity — *see* Defect, reduction,
        lower limb
    upper Q74.Ø
  lip Q38.Ø
  liver Q44.7
    duct Q44.5
  lower limb NEC Q74.2
  lumbosacral (joint) (region) Q76.49
    kyphosis — *see* Kyphosis, congenital
    lordosis — *see* Lordosis, congenital
  lung (fissure) (lobe) Q33.9
  mandible — *see* Anomaly, dentofacial
  maxilla — *see* Anomaly, dentofacial
  May (-Hegglin) D72.Ø
  meatus urinarius NEC Q64.79
  meningeal bands or folds QØ7.9
    constriction of QØ7.8
    spinal QØ6.9
  meninges QØ7.9
    cerebral QØ4.8
    spinal QØ6.9
  meningocele QØ5.9
  mesentery Q45.9
  metacarpus Q74.Ø
  metatarsus NEC Q74.2
  middle ear Q16.4
    ossicles Q16.3
  mitral (leaflets) (valve) Q23.9
    insufficiency Q23.3
    specified NEC Q23.8
    stenosis Q23.2
  mouth Q38.6
  Müllerian (*see also* Anomaly, by site)
    uterus NEC Q51.818
  multiple NEC Q89.7
  muscle Q79.9
    eyelid Q1Ø.3
  musculoskeletal system, except limbs Q79.9
  myocardium Q24.8
  nail Q84.6
  narrowness, eyelid Q1Ø.3
  nasal sinus (wall) Q3Ø.8
  neck (any part) Q18.9
  nerve QØ7.9
    acoustic QØ7.8
    optic QØ7.8
  nervous system (central) QØ7.9
  nipple Q83.9
  nose, nasal (bones) (cartilage) (septum) (sinus) Q3Ø.9
    specified NEC Q3Ø.8
  ocular muscle Q15.8
  omphalomesenteric duct Q43.Ø
  opening, pulmonary veins Q26.4
  optic
    disc Q14.2
    nerve QØ7.8
  opticociliary vessels Q13.2
  orbit (eye) Q1Ø.7
  organ Q89.9
    of Corti Q16.5
  origin
    artery
      innominate Q25.8
      pulmonary Q25.79
      renal Q27.2
      subclavian Q25.48
    osseous meatus (ear) Q16.1
  ovary Q5Ø.39
  oviduct Q5Ø.6
  palate (hard) (soft) NEC Q38.5
  pancreas or pancreatic duct Q45.3
  papillary muscles Q24.8
  parathyroid gland Q89.2
  paraurethral ducts Q64.79
  parotid (gland) Q38.4
  patella Q74.1
  Pelger-Huët (hereditary hyposegmentation) D72.Ø
  pelvic girdle NEC Q74.2
  pelvis (bony) NEC Q74.2
    rachitic E64.3

Anomaly, anomalous — *continued*
  penis (glans) Q55.69
  pericardium Q24.8
  peripheral vascular system Q27.9
  Peter's Q13.4
  pharynx Q38.8
  pigmentation L81.9
    congenital Q82.8
  pituitary (gland) Q89.2
  pleural (folds) Q34.Ø
  portal vein Q26.5
    connection Q26.5
  position, tooth, teeth, fully erupted M26.3Ø
    specified NEC M26.39
  precerebral vessel Q28.1
  prepuce Q55.69
  prostate Q55.4
  pulmonary Q33.9
    artery NEC Q25.79
    valve Q22.3
      atresia Q22.Ø
      insufficiency Q22.2
      specified type NEC Q22.3
      stenosis Q22.1
        infundibular Q24.3
        subvalvular Q24.3
    venous connection Q26.4
      partial Q26.3
      total Q26.2
  pupil Q13.2
    function H57.ØØ
      anisocoria H57.Ø2
      Argyll Robertson pupil H57.Ø1
      miosis H57.Ø3
      mydriasis H57.Ø4
      specified type NEC H57.Ø9
      tonic pupil H57.Ø5- ☑
  pylorus Q4Ø.3
  radius Q74.Ø
  rectum Q43.9
  reduction (extremity) (limb)
    femur (longitudinal) — *see* Defect, reduction, lower
      limb, longitudinal, femur
    fibula (longitudinal) — *see* Defect, reduction, lower
      limb, longitudinal, fibula
    lower limb — *see* Defect, reduction, lower limb
    radius (longitudinal) — *see* Defect, reduction, upper
      limb, longitudinal, radius
    tibia (longitudinal) — *see* Defect, reduction, lower
      limb, longitudinal, tibia
    ulna (longitudinal) — *see* Defect, reduction, upper
      limb, longitudinal, ulna
    upper limb — *see* Defect, reduction, upper limb
  refraction — *see* Disorder, refraction
  renal Q63.9
    artery Q27.2
    pelvis Q63.9
      specified NEC Q63.8
  respiratory system Q34.9
    specified NEC Q34.8
  retina Q14.1
  rib Q76.6
    cervical Q76.5
  Rieger's Q13.81
  rotation — *see* Malrotation
    hip or thigh Q65.89
  round ligament Q52.8
  sacroiliac (joint) NEC Q74.2
  sacrum NEC Q76.49
    kyphosis — *see* Kyphosis, congenital
    lordosis — *see* Lordosis, congenital
  saddle nose, syphilitic A5Ø.57
  salivary duct or gland Q38.4
  scapula Q74.Ø
  scrotum — *see* Malformation, testis and scrotum
  sebaceous gland Q82.9
  seminal vesicles Q55.4
  sense organs NEC QØ7.8
  sex chromosomes NEC (*see also* Anomaly, chromo-
    somes)
    female phenotype Q97.8
    male phenotype Q98.9
  shoulder (girdle) (joint) Q74.Ø
  sigmoid (flexure) Q43.9
  simian crease Q82.8
  sinus of Valsalva Q25.49
  skeleton generalized Q78.9
  skin (appendage) Q82.9

Index

Anomaly, anomalous — *continued*
- skull Q75.9
  - with
    - anencephaly Q00.0
    - encephalocele — *see* Encephalocele
    - hydrocephalus Q03.9
      - with spina bifida — *see* Spina bifida, by site, with hydrocephalus
    - microcephaly Q02
- specified organ or site NEC Q89.8
- spermatic cord Q55.4
- spine, spinal NEC Q76.49
  - column NEC Q76.49
    - kyphosis — *see* Kyphosis, congenital
    - lordosis — *see* Lordosis, congenital
  - cord Q06.9
  - nerve root Q07.8
- spleen Q89.09
  - agenesis Q89.01
- stenonian duct Q38.4
- sternum NEC Q76.7
- stomach Q40.3
- submaxillary gland Q38.4
- tarsus NEC Q74.2
- tendon Q79.9
- testis — *see* Malformation, testis and scrotum
- thigh NEC Q74.2
- thorax (wall) Q67.8
  - bony Q76.9
- throat Q38.8
- thumb Q74.0
- thymus gland Q89.2
- thyroid (gland) Q89.2
  - cartilage Q31.8
- tibia NEC Q74.2
  - saber A50.56
- toe Q74.2
- tongue Q38.3
- tooth, teeth K00.9
  - eruption K00.6
  - position, fully erupted M26.30
  - spacing, fully erupted M26.30
- trachea (cartilage) Q32.1
- tragus Q17.9
- tricuspid (leaflet) (valve) Q22.9
  - atresia or stenosis Q22.4
  - Ebstein's Q22.5
- Uhl's (hypoplasia of myocardium, right ventricle) Q24.8
- ulna Q74.0
- umbilical artery Q27.0
- urachus Q64.4
- ureter Q62.8
  - obstructive NEC Q62.39
    - cecoureterocele Q62.32
    - orthotopic ureterocele Q62.31
- urethra Q64.70
  - absence Q64.5
  - double Q64.74
  - fistula to rectum Q64.73
  - obstructive Q64.39
    - stricture Q64.32
  - prolapse Q64.71
  - specified type NEC Q64.79
- urinary tract Q64.9
- uterus Q51.9
  - with only one functioning horn Q51.4
- uvula Q38.5
- vagina Q52.4
- valleculae Q31.8
- valve (heart) NEC Q24.8
  - coronary sinus Q24.5
  - inferior vena cava Q24.8
  - pulmonary Q22.3
  - sinus coronario Q24.5
  - venae cavae inferioris Q24.8
- vas deferens Q55.4
- vascular Q27.9
  - brain Q28.3
  - ring Q25.45
- vein(s) (peripheral) Q27.9
  - brain Q28.3
  - cerebral Q28.3
  - coronary Q24.5
  - developmental Q28.3

Anomaly, anomalous — *continued*
- vein(s) — *continued*
  - great Q26.9
    - specified NEC Q26.8
  - vena cava (inferior) (superior) Q26.9
  - venous — *see* Anomaly, vein(s)
  - venous return Q26.8
  - ventricular
    - bands or folds Q24.8
    - septa Q21.0
  - vertebra Q76.49
    - kyphosis — *see* Kyphosis, congenital
    - lordosis — *see* Lordosis, congenital
  - vesicourethral orifice Q64.79
  - vessel(s) Q27.9
    - optic papilla Q14.2
    - precerebral Q28.1
  - vitelline duct Q43.0
  - vitreous body or humor Q14.0
  - vulva Q52.70
  - wrist (joint) Q74.0

Anomia R48.8
Anonychia (congenital) Q84.3
- acquired L60.8
Anophthalmos, anophthalmus (congenital) (globe) Q11.1
- acquired Z90.01
Anopia, anopsia H53.46- ☑
- quadrant H53.46- ☑
Anorchia, anorchism, anorchidism Q55.0
Anorexia R63.0
- hysterical F44.89
- nervosa F50.00
  - atypical F50.9
  - binge-eating type F50.2
    - with purging F50.02
  - restricting type F50.01
Anorgasmy, psychogenic (female) F52.31
- male F52.32
Anosmia R43.0
- hysterical F44.6
- postinfectional J39.8
Anosognosia R41.89
Anosteoplasia Q78.9
Anovulatory cycle N97.0
Anoxemia R09.02
- newborn P84
Anoxia (pathological) R09.02
- altitude T70.29 ☑
- cerebral G93.1
  - complicating
    - anesthesia (general) (local) or other sedation T88.59 ☑
      - in labor and delivery O74.3
      - in pregnancy O29.21- ☑
      - postpartum, puerperal O89.2
    - delivery (cesarean) (instrumental) O75.4
  - during a procedure G97.81
  - newborn P84
  - resulting from a procedure G97.82
- due to
  - drowning T75.1 ☑
  - high altitude T70.29 ☑
- heart — *see* Insufficiency, coronary
- intrauterine P84
- myocardial — *see* Insufficiency, coronary
- newborn P84
- spinal cord G95.11
- systemic (by suffocation) (low content in atmosphere) — *see* Asphyxia, traumatic
Anteflexion — *see* Anteversion
Antenatal
- care (normal pregnancy) Z34.90
- screening (encounter for) of mother (*see also* Encounter, antenatal screening) Z36.9
Antepartum — *see* condition
Anterior — *see* condition
Antero-occlusion M26.220
Anteversion
- cervix — *see* Anteversion, uterus
- femur (neck), congenital Q65.89
- uterus, uterine (cervix) (postinfectional) (postpartal, old) N85.4
  - congenital Q51.818
  - in pregnancy or childbirth — *see* Pregnancy, complicated by
Anthophobia F40.228
Anthracosilicosis J60

Anthracosis (lung) (occupational) J60
- lingua K14.3
Anthrax A22.9
- with pneumonia A22.1
- cerebral A22.8
- colitis A22.2
- cutaneous A22.0
- gastrointestinal A22.2
- inhalation A22.1
- intestinal A22.2
- meningitis A22.8
- pulmonary A22.1
- respiratory A22.1
- sepsis A22.7
- specified manifestation NEC A22.8
Anthropoid pelvis Q74.2
- with disproportion (fetopelvic) O33.0
Anthropophobia F40.10
- generalized F40.11
Antibodies, maternal (blood group) — *see* Isoimmunization, affecting management of pregnancy
- anti-D — *see* Isoimmunization, affecting management of pregnancy, Rh
- newborn P55.0
Antibody
- anticardiolipin R76.0
  - with
    - hemorrhagic disorder D68.312
    - hypercoagulable state D68.61
- antiphosphatidylglycerol R76.0
  - with
    - hemorrhagic disorder D68.312
    - hypercoagulable state D68.61
- antiphosphatidylinositol R76.0
  - with
    - hemorrhagic disorder D68.312
    - hypercoagulable state D68.61
- antiphosphatidylserine R76.0
  - with
    - hemorrhagic disorder D68.312
    - hypercoagulable state D68.61
- antiphospholipid R76.0
  - with
    - hemorrhagic disorder D68.312
    - hypercoagulable state D68.61
Anticardiolipin syndrome D68.61
Anticoagulant, circulating (intrinsic) (*see also* Disorder, hemorrhagic) D68.318
- drug-induced (extrinsic) (*see also* Disorder, hemorrhagic) D68.32
- iatrogenic D68.32
Antidiuretic hormone syndrome E22.2
Antimonial cholera — *see* Poisoning, antimony
Antiphospholipid
- antibody
  - with hemorrhagic disorder D68.312
  - syndrome D68.61
Antisocial personality F60.2
Antithrombinemia — *see* Circulating anticoagulants
Antithromboplastinemia D68.318
Antithromboplastinogenemia D68.318
Antitoxin complication or reaction — *see* Complications, vaccination
Antlophobia F40.228
Antritis J32.0
- maxilla J32.0
  - acute J01.00
    - recurrent J01.01
- stomach K29.60
  - with bleeding K29.61
Antrum, antral — *see* condition
Anuria R34
- calculous (impacted) (recurrent) (*see also* Calculus, urinary) N20.9
- following
  - abortion — *see* Abortion by type complicated by, renal failure
  - ectopic or molar pregnancy O08.4
- newborn P96.0
- postprocedural N99.0
- postrenal N13.8
- traumatic (following crushing) T79.5 ☑
Anus, anal — *see* condition
Anusitis K62.89
Anxiety F41.9
- depression F41.8
- episodic paroxysmal F41.0
- generalized F41.1

Anxiety — *continued*
hysteria F41.8
neurosis F41.1
panic type F41.0
reaction F41.1
separation, abnormal (of childhood) F93.0
specified NEC F41.8
state F41.1
Aorta, aortic — *see* condition
Aortectasia — *see* Ectasia, aorta
with aneurysm — *see* Aneurysm, aorta
Aortitis (nonsyphilitic) (calcific) I77.6
arteriosclerotic I70.0
Doehle-Heller A52.02
luetic A52.02
rheumatic — *see* Endocarditis, acute, rheumatic
specific (syphilitic) A52.02
syphilitic A52.02
congenital A50.54 [I79.1]
Apathetic thyroid storm — *see* Thyrotoxicosis
Apathy R45.3
Apeirophobia F40.228
Apepsia K30
psychogenic F45.8
Aperistalsis, esophagus K22.0
Apertognathia M26.29
Apert's syndrome Q87.0
Aphagia R13.0
psychogenic F50.9
Aphakia (acquired) (postoperative) H27.0- ☑
congenital Q12.3
Aphasia (amnestic) (global) (nominal) (semantic) (syntactic) R47.01
acquired, with epilepsy (Landau-Kleffner syndrome)
— *see* Epilepsy, specified NEC
auditory (developmental) F80.2
developmental (receptive type) F80.2
expressive type F80.1
Wernicke's F80.2
following
cerebrovascular disease I69.920
cerebral infarction I69.320
intracerebral hemorrhage I69.120
nontraumatic intracranial hemorrhage NEC
I69.220
specified disease NEC I69.820
subarachnoid hemorrhage I69.020
primary progressive G31.01 [F02.80]
with behavioral disturbance G31.01 [F02.81]
progressive isolated G31.01 [F02.80]
with behavioral disturbance G31.01 [F02.81]
sensory F80.2
syphilis, tertiary A52.19
Wernicke's (developmental) F80.2
Aphonia (organic) R49.1
hysterical F44.4
psychogenic F44.4
Aphthae, aphthous (*see also* condition)
Bednar's K12.0
cachectic K14.0
epizootic B08.8
fever B08.8
oral (recurrent) K12.0
stomatitis (major) (minor) K12.0
thrush B37.0
ulcer (oral) (recurrent) K12.0
genital organ(s) NEC
female N76.6
male N50.89
larynx J38.7
Apical — *see* condition
Apiphobia F40.218
Aplasia (*see also* Agenesis)
abdominal muscle syndrome Q79.4
alveolar process (acquired) — *see* Anomaly, alveolar
congenital Q38.6
aorta (congenital) Q25.41
axialis extracorticalis (congenita) E75.29
bone marrow (myeloid) D61.9
congenital D61.01
brain Q00.0
part of Q04.3
bronchus Q32.4
cementum K00.4
cerebellum Q04.3
cervix (congenital) Q51.5
congenital pure red cell D61.01
corpus callosum Q04.0

Aplasia — *continued*
cutis congenita Q84.8
erythrocyte congenital D61.01
extracortical axial E75.29
eye Q11.1
fovea centralis (congenital) Q14.1
gallbladder, congenital Q44.0
iris Q13.1
labyrinth, membranous Q16.5
limb (congenital) Q73.8
lower — *see* Defect, reduction, lower limb
upper — *see* Agenesis, arm
lung, congenital (bilateral) (unilateral) Q33.3
pancreas Q45.0
parathyroid-thymic D82.1
Pelizaeus-Merzbacher E75.29
penis Q55.5
prostate Q55.4
red cell (with thymoma) D60.9
acquired D60.9
due to drugs D60.9
adult D60.9
chronic D60.0
congenital D61.01
constitutional D61.01
due to drugs D60.9
hereditary D61.01
of infants D61.01
primary D61.01
pure D61.01
due to drugs D60.9
specified type NEC D60.8
transient D60.1
round ligament Q52.8
skin Q84.8
spermatic cord Q55.4
spleen Q89.01
testicle Q55.0
thymic, with immunodeficiency D82.1
thyroid (congenital) (with myxedema) E03.1
uterus Q51.0
ventral horn cell Q06.1
Apnea, apneic (of) (spells) R06.81
newborn NEC P28.4
obstructive P28.4
sleep (central) (obstructive) (primary) P28.3
prematurity P28.4
sleep G47.30
central (primary) G47.31
idiopathic G47.31
in conditions classified elsewhere G47.37
obstructive (adult) (pediatric) G47.33
hypopnea G47.33
primary central G47.31
specified NEC G47.39
Apneumatosis, newborn P28.0
Apocrine metaplasia (breast) — *see* Dysplasia, mammary, specified type NEC
Apophysitis (bone) (*see also* Osteochondropathy)
calcaneus M92.8
juvenile M92.9
Apoplectiform convulsions (cerebral ischemia) I67.82
Apoplexia, apoplexy, apoplectic
adrenal A39.1
heart (auricle) (ventricle) — *see* Infarct, myocardium
heat T67.0 ☑
hemorrhagic (stroke) — *see* Hemorrhage, intracranial
meninges, hemorrhagic — *see* Hemorrhage, intracranial, subarachnoid
uremic N18.9 [I68.8]
Appearance
bizarre R46.1
specified NEC R46.89
very low level of personal hygiene R46.0
Appendage
epididymal (organ of Morgagni) Q55.4
intestine (epiploic) Q43.8
preauricular Q17.0
testicular (organ of Morgagni) Q55.29
Appendicitis (pneumococcal) (retrocecal) K37
with
gangrene K35.891
perforation NOS K35.32
peritoneal abscess K35.33
peritonitis NEC K35.33
generalized (with perforation or rupture) K35.20
with abscess K35.21
localized K35.30

Appendicitis — *continued*
with — *continued*
peritonitis — *continued*
localized — *continued*
with
gangrene K35.31
perforation K35.32
and abscess K35.33
rupture (with localized peritonitis) K35.32
acute (catarrhal) (fulminating) (gangrenous) (obstructive) (retrocecal) (suppurative) K35.80
with
gangrene K35.891
peritoneal abscess K35.33
peritonitis NEC K35.33
generalized (with perforation or rupture)
K35.20
with abscess K35.21
localized K35.30
with
gangrene K35.31
perforation K35.32
and abscess K35.33
specified NEC K35.890
with gangrene K35.891
amebic A06.89
chronic (recurrent) K36
exacerbation — *see* Appendicitis, acute
gangrenous — *see* Appendicitis, acute
healed (obliterative) K36
interval K36
neurogenic K36
obstructive K36
recurrent K36
relapsing K36
ruptured NOS (with localized peritonitis) K35.32
subacute (adhesive) K36
subsiding K36
suppurative — *see* Appendicitis, acute
tuberculous A18.32
Appendicopathia oxyurica B80
Appendix, appendicular (*see also* condition)
epididymis Q55.4
Morgagni
female Q50.5
male (epididymal) Q55.4
testicular Q55.29
testis Q55.29
Appetite
depraved — *see* Pica
excessive R63.2
lack or loss (*see also* Anorexia) R63.0
nonorganic origin F50.89
psychogenic F50.89
perverted (hysterical) — *see* Pica
Apple peel syndrome Q41.1
Apprehension state F41.1
Apprehensiveness, abnormal F41.9
Approximal wear K03.0
Apraxia (classic) (ideational) (ideokinetic) (ideomotor)
(motor) (verbal) R48.2
following
cerebrovascular disease I69.990
cerebral infarction I69.390
intracerebral hemorrhage I69.190
nontraumatic intracranial hemorrhage NEC
I69.290
specified disease NEC I69.890
subarachnoid hemorrhage I69.090
oculomotor, congenital H51.8
Aptyalism K11.7
Apudoma — *see* Neoplasm, uncertain behavior, by site
Aqueous misdirection H40.83- ☑
Arabicum elephantiasis — *see* Infestation, filarial
Arachnitis — *see* Meningitis
Arachnodactyly — *see* Syndrome, Marfan's
Arachnoiditis (acute) (adhesive) (basal) (brain) (cerebrospinal) — *see* Meningitis
Arachnophobia F40.210
Arboencephalitis, Australian A83.4
Arborization block (heart) I45.5
ARC (AIDS-related complex) B20
Arch
aortic Q25.49
bovine Q25.49
Arches — *see* condition
Arcuate uterus Q51.810
Arcuatus uterus Q51.810

Arcus (cornea) senilis — *see* Degeneration, cornea, senile
Arc-welder's lung J63.4
Areflexia R29.2
Areola — *see* condition
Argentaffinoma (*see also* Neoplasm, uncertain behavior, by site)
   malignant — *see* Neoplasm, malignant, by site
   syndrome E34.0
Argininemia E72.21
Arginosuccinic aciduria E72.22
Argyll Robertson phenomenon, pupil or syndrome
   (syphilitic) A52.19
   atypical H57.09
   nonsyphilitic H57.09
Argyria, argyriasis
   conjunctival H11.13- ☑
   from drug or medicament — *see* Table of Drugs and Chemicals, by substance
Argyrosis, conjunctival H11.13- ☑
Arhinencephaly Q04.1
Ariboflavinosis E53.0
Arm — *see* condition
Arnold-Chiari disease, obstruction or syndrome (type II) Q07.00
   with
      hydrocephalus Q07.02
         with spina bifida Q07.03
      spina bifida Q07.01
         with hydrocephalus Q07.03
   type III — *see* Encephalocele
   type IV Q04.8
Aromatic amino-acid metabolism disorder E70.9
   specified NEC E70.8
Arousals, confusional G47.51
Arrest, arrested
   cardiac I46.9
      complicating
         abortion — *see* Abortion, by type, complicated by, cardiac arrest
         anesthesia (general) (local) or other sedation — *see* Table of Drugs and Chemicals, by drug
            in labor and delivery O74.2
            in pregnancy O29.11- ☑
               postpartum, puerperal O89.1
         delivery (cesarean) (instrumental) O75.4
      due to
         cardiac condition I46.2
         specified condition NEC I46.8
      intraoperative I97.71- ☑
      newborn P29.81
      personal history, successfully resuscitated Z86.74
      postprocedural I97.12- ☑
         obstetric procedure O75.4
   cardiorespiratory — *see* Arrest, cardiac
   circulatory — *see* Arrest, cardiac
   deep transverse O64.0 ☑
   development or growth
      bone — *see* Disorder, bone, development or growth
      child R62.50
      tracheal rings Q32.1
   epiphyseal
      complete
         femur M89.15- ☑
         humerus M89.12- ☑
         tibia M89.16- ☑
         ulna M89.13- ☑
      forearm M89.13- ☑
         specified NEC M89.13- ☑
         ulna — *see* Arrest, epiphyseal, by type, ulna
      lower leg M89.16- ☑
         specified NEC M89.168
         tibia — *see* Arrest, epiphyseal, by type, tibia
      partial
         femur M89.15- ☑
         humerus M89.12- ☑
         tibia M89.16- ☑
         ulna M89.13- ☑
      specified NEC M89.18
   granulopoiesis — *see* Agranulocytosis
   growth plate — *see* Arrest, epiphyseal
   heart — *see* Arrest, cardiac
   legal, anxiety concerning Z65.3
   physeal — *see* Arrest, epiphyseal
   respiratory R09.2
      newborn P28.81
   sinus I45.5
   spermatogenesis (complete) — *see* Azoospermia

Arrest, arrested — *continued*
   spermatogenesis — *see* Azoospermia — *continued*
      incomplete — *see* Oligospermia
   transverse (deep) O64.0 ☑
Arrhenoblastoma
   benign
      specified site — *see* Neoplasm, benign, by site
      unspecified site
         female D27.9
         male D29.20
   malignant
      specified site — *see* Neoplasm, malignant, by site
      unspecified site
         female C56.9
         male C62.90
   specified site — *see* Neoplasm, uncertain behavior, by site
   unspecified site
      female D39.10
      male D40.10
Arrhythmia (auricle) (cardiac) (juvenile) (nodal) (reflex) (sinus) (supraventricular) (transitory) (ventricle) I49.9
   block I45.9
   extrasystolic I49.49
   newborn
      bradycardia P29.12
      occurring before birth P03.819
         before onset of labor P03.810
         during labor P03.811
      tachycardia P29.11
   psychogenic F45.8
   specified NEC I49.8
   vagal R55
   ventricular re-entry I47.0
Arrillaga-Ayerza syndrome (pulmonary sclerosis with pulmonary hypertension) I27.0
Arsenical pigmentation L81.8
   from drug or medicament — *see* Table of Drugs and Chemicals
Arsenism — *see* Poisoning, arsenic
Arterial — *see* condition
Arteriofibrosis — *see* Arteriosclerosis
Arteriolar sclerosis — *see* Arteriosclerosis
Arteriolith — *see* Arteriosclerosis
Arteriolitis I77.6
   necrotizing, kidney I77.5
   renal — *see* Hypertension, kidney
Arteriolosclerosis — *see* Arteriosclerosis
Arterionephrosclerosis — *see* Hypertension, kidney
Arteriopathy I77.9
   cerebral autosomal dominant, with subcortical infarcts and leukoencephalopathy (CADASIL) I67.850
Arteriosclerosis, arteriosclerotic (diffuse) (obliterans) (of) (senile) (with calcification) I70.90
   aorta I70.0
   arteries of extremities — *see* Arteriosclerosis, extremities
   brain I67.2
   bypass graft
      coronary — *see* Arteriosclerosis, coronary, bypass graft
      extremities — *see* Arteriosclerosis, extremities, bypass graft
   cardiac — *see* Disease, heart, ischemic, atherosclerotic
   cardiopathy — *see* Disease, heart, ischemic, atherosclerotic
   cardiorenal — *see* Hypertension, cardiorenal
   cardiovascular — *see* Disease, heart, ischemic, atherosclerotic
   carotid (*see also* Occlusion, artery, carotid) I65.2- ☑
   central nervous system I67.2
   cerebral I67.2
   cerebrovascular I67.2
   coronary (artery)
      due to
         calcified coronary lesion (severely) I25.84
         lipid rich plaque I25.83
      bypass graft I25.810
         with
            angina pectoris I25.709
               with documented spasm I25.701
               specified type NEC I25.708
               unstable I25.700
            ischemic chest pain I25.709
         autologous artery I25.810
           with
              angina pectoris I25.729
                 with documented spasm I25.721

Arteriosclerosis, arteriosclerotic — *continued*
   coronary — *continued*
      bypass graft — *continued*
         autologous artery — *continued*
           with — *continued*
              angina pectoris — *continued*
                 specified type I25.728
                 unstable I25.720
              ischemic chest pain I25.729
         autologous vein I25.810
           with
              angina pectoris I25.719
                 with documented spasm I25.711
                 specified type I25.718
                 unstable I25.710
              ischemic chest pain I25.719
         nonautologous biological I25.810
           with
              angina pectoris I25.739
                 with documented spasm I25.731
                 specified type I25.738
                 unstable I25.730
              ischemic chest pain I25.739
         specified type NEC I25.810
           with
              angina pectoris I25.799
                 with documented spasm I25.791
                 specified type I25.798
                 unstable I25.790
              ischemic chest pain I25.799
      native vessel
         with
           angina pectoris I25.119
              with documented spasm I25.111
              specified type NEC I25.118
              unstable I25.110
           ischemic chest pain I25.119
      transplanted heart I25.811
         bypass graft I25.812
           with
              angina pectoris I25.769
                 with documented spasm I25.761
                 specified type I25.768
                 unstable I25.760
              ischemic chest pain I25.769
         native coronary artery I25.811
           with
              angina pectoris I25.759
                 with documented spasm I25.751
                 specified type I25.758
                 unstable I25.750
              ischemic chest pain I25.759
   extremities (native arteries) I70.209
      bypass graft I70.309
         autologous vein graft I70.409
           leg I70.409
              with
                 gangrene (and intermittent claudication, rest pain and ulcer) I70.469
                 intermittent claudication I70.419
                 rest pain (and intermittent claudication) I70.429
           bilateral I70.403
              with
                 gangrene (and intermittent claudication, rest pain and ulcer) I70.463
                 intermittent claudication I70.463
                 rest pain (and intermittent claudication) I70.423
                 specified type NEC I70.493
           left I70.402
              with
                 gangrene (and intermittent claudication, rest pain and ulcer) I70.462
                 intermittent claudication I70.412
                 rest pain (and intermittent claudication) I70.422
                 ulceration (and intermittent claudication and rest pain) I70.449
                   ankle I70.443
                   calf I70.442
                   foot site NEC I70.445
                   heel I70.444
                   lower leg NEC I70.448
                   midfoot I70.444
                   thigh I70.441
               specified type NEC I70.492

☑ **Additional Character Required** — Refer to the Tabular List for Character Selection   ▽ **Subterms under main terms may continue to next column or page**

Arteriosclerosis, arteriosclerotic — *continued*
  extremities — *continued*
    bypass graft — *continued*
      autologous vein graft — *continued*
        leg — *continued*
          right I70.401
            with
              gangrene (and intermittent claudication, rest pain and ulcer) I70.461
              intermittent claudication I70.411
              rest pain (and intermittent claudication) I70.421
              ulceration (and intermittent claudication and rest pain) I70.439
                ankle I70.433
                calf I70.432
                foot site NEC I70.435
                heel I70.434
                lower leg NEC I70.438
                midfoot I70.434
                thigh I70.431
              specified type NEC I70.491
          specified type NEC I70.499
        specified NEC I70.408
          with
            gangrene (and intermittent claudication, rest pain and ulcer) I70.468
            intermittent claudication I70.418
            rest pain (and intermittent claudication) I70.428
            ulceration (and intermittent claudication and rest pain) I70.45
          specified type NEC I70.498
      leg I70.309
        with
          gangrene (and intermittent claudication, rest pain and ulcer) I70.369
          intermittent claudication I70.319
          rest pain (and intermittent claudication) I70.329
        bilateral I70.303
          with
            gangrene (and intermittent claudication, rest pain and ulcer) I70.363
            intermittent claudication I70.313
            rest pain (and intermittent claudication) I70.323
          specified type NEC I70.393
        left I70.302
          with
            gangrene (and intermittent claudication, rest pain and ulcer) I70.362
            intermittent claudication I70.312
            rest pain (and intermittent claudication) I70.322
            ulceration (and intermittent claudication and rest pain) I70.349
              ankle I70.343
              calf I70.342
              foot site NEC I70.345
              heel I70.344
              lower leg NEC I70.348
              midfoot I70.344
              thigh I70.341
            specified type NEC I70.392
        right I70.301
          with
            gangrene (and intermittent claudication, rest pain and ulcer) I70.361
            intermittent claudication I70.311
            rest pain (and intermittent claudication) I70.321
            ulceration (and intermittent claudication and rest pain I70.339
              ankle I70.333
              calf I70.332
              foot site NEC I70.335
              heel I70.334
              lower leg NEC I70.338
              midfoot I70.334
              thigh I70.331
            specified type NEC I70.391
        specified type NEC I70.399
      nonautologous biological graft I70.509
        leg I70.509
          with
            gangrene (and intermittent claudication, rest pain and ulcer) I70.569

Arteriosclerosis, arteriosclerotic — *continued*
  extremities — *continued*
    bypass graft — *continued*
      nonautologous biological graft — *continued*
        leg — *continued*
          with — *continued*
            intermittent claudication I70.519
            rest pain (and intermittent claudication) I70.529
        bilateral I70.503
          with
            gangrene (and intermittent claudication, rest pain and ulcer) I70.563
            intermittent claudication I70.513
            rest pain (and intermittent claudication) I70.523
          specified type NEC I70.593
        left I70.502
          with
            gangrene (and intermittent claudication, rest pain and ulcer) I70.562
            intermittent claudication I70.512
            rest pain (and intermittent claudication) I70.522
            ulceration (and intermittent claudication and rest pain) I70.549
              ankle I70.543
              calf I70.542
              foot site NEC I70.545
              heel I70.544
              lower leg NEC I70.548
              midfoot I70.544
              thigh I70.541
          specified type NEC I70.592
        right I70.501
          with
            gangrene (and intermittent claudication, rest pain and ulcer) I70.561
            intermittent claudication I70.511
            rest pain (and intermittent claudication) I70.521
            ulceration (and intermittent claudication and rest pain) I70.539
              ankle I70.533
              calf I70.532
              foot site NEC I70.535
              heel I70.534
              lower leg NEC I70.538
              midfoot I70.534
              thigh I70.531
          specified type NEC I70.591
        specified type NEC I70.599
        specified NEC I70.508
          with
            gangrene (and intermittent claudication, rest pain and ulcer) I70.568
            intermittent claudication I70.518
            rest pain (and intermittent claudication) I70.528
            ulceration (and intermittent claudication and rest pain) I70.55
          specified type NEC I70.598
      nonbiological graft I70.609
        leg I70.609
          with
            gangrene (and intermittent claudication, rest pain and ulcer) I70.669
            intermittent claudication I70.619
            rest pain (and intermittent claudication) I70.629
        bilateral I70.603
          with
            gangrene (and intermittent claudication, rest pain and ulcer) I70.663
            intermittent claudication I70.613
            rest pain (and intermittent claudication) I70.623
          specified type NEC I70.693
        left I70.602
          with
            gangrene (and intermittent claudication, rest pain and ulcer) I70.662
            intermittent claudication I70.612

Arteriosclerosis, arteriosclerotic — *continued*
  extremities — *continued*
    bypass graft — *continued*
      nonbiological graft — *continued*
        leg — *continued*
          left — *continued*
            with — *continued*
              rest pain (and intermittent claudication) I70.622
              ulceration (and intermittent claudication and rest pain) I70.649
                ankle I70.643
                calf I70.642
                foot site NEC I70.645
                heel I70.644
                lower leg NEC I70.648
                midfoot I70.644
                thigh I70.641
          specified type NEC I70.692
        right I70.601
          with
            gangrene (and intermittent claudication, rest pain and ulcer) I70.661
            intermittent claudication I70.611
            rest pain (and intermittent claudication) I70.621
            ulceration (and intermittent claudication and rest pain) I70.639
              ankle I70.633
              calf I70.632
              foot site NEC I70.635
              heel I70.634
              lower leg NEC I70.638
              midfoot I70.634
              thigh I70.631
          specified type NEC I70.691
        specified NEC I70.608
          with
            gangrene (and intermittent claudication, rest pain and ulcer) I70.668
            intermittent claudication I70.618
            rest pain (and intermittent claudication) I70.628
            ulceration (and intermittent claudication and rest pain) I70.65
          specified type NEC I70.698
      specified graft NEC I70.709
        leg I70.709
          with
            gangrene (and intermittent claudication, rest pain and ulcer) I70.769
            intermittent claudication I70.719
            rest pain (and intermittent claudication) I70.729
        bilateral I70.703
          with
            gangrene (and intermittent claudication, rest pain and ulcer) I70.763
            intermittent claudication I70.713
            rest pain (and intermittent claudication) I70.723
          specified type NEC I70.793
        left I70.702
          with
            gangrene (and intermittent claudication, rest pain and ulcer) I70.762
            intermittent claudication I70.712
            rest pain (and intermittent claudication) I70.722
            ulceration (and intermittent claudication and rest pain) I70.749
              ankle I70.743
              calf I70.742
              foot site NEC I70.745
              heel I70.744
              lower leg NEC I70.748
              midfoot I70.744
              thigh I70.741
          specified type NEC I70.792
        right I70.701
          with
            gangrene (and intermittent claudication, rest pain and ulcer) I70.761
            intermittent claudication I70.711

Arthritis, arthritic — *continued*
  in — *continued*
    hyperparathyroidism NEC (*see also* subcategory M14.8-) E21.3
    hypersensitivity reaction NEC T78.49 ☑ [M36.4]
    hypogammaglobulinemia (*see also* subcategory M14.8-) D80.1
    hypothyroidism NEC (*see also* subcategory M14.8-) E03.9
    infection — *see* Arthritis, pyogenic or pyemic
      spine — *see* Spondylopathy, infective
    infectious disease NEC M01 ☑
    leprosy (*see also* category M01) A30.9
    leukemia NEC C95.9- ☑ [M36.1]
    lipoid dermatoarthritis E78.81
    Lyme disease A69.23
    Mediterranean fever, familial (*see also* subcategory M14.8-) M04.1
    Meningococcus A39.83
    metabolic disorder NEC (*see also* subcategory M14.8-) E88.9
    multiple myelomatosis C90.0- ☑ [M36.1]
    mumps B26.85
    mycosis NEC (*see also* category M01) B49
    myelomatosis (multiple) C90.0- ☑ [M36.1]
    neurological disorder NEC G98.0
    ochronosis (*see also* subcategory M14.8-) E70.29
    O'nyong-nyong (*see also* category M01) A92.1
    parasitic disease NEC (*see also* category M01) B89
    paratyphoid fever (*see also* category M01) A01.4
    Pseudomonas — *see* Arthritis, pyogenic, bacterial NEC
    psoriasis L40.50
    pyogenic organism NEC — *see* Arthritis, pyogenic, bacterial NEC
    Reiter's disease — *see* Reiter's disease
    respiratory disorder NEC (*see also* subcategory M14.8-) J98.9
    reticulosis, malignant (*see also* subcategory M14.8-) C86.0
    rubella B06.82
    Salmonella (arizonae) (cholerae-suis) (enteritidis) (typhimurium) A02.23
    sarcoidosis D86.86
    specified bacteria NEC — *see* Arthritis, pyogenic, bacterial NEC
    sporotrichosis B42.82
    syringomyelia G95.0
    thalassemia NEC D56.9 [M36.3]
    tuberculosis — *see* Tuberculosis, arthritis
    typhoid fever A01.04
    urethritis, Reiter's — *see* Reiter's disease
    viral disease NEC (*see also* category M01) B34.9
  infectious or infective (*see also* Arthritis, pyogenic or pyemic)
    spine — *see* Spondylopathy, infective
  juvenile M08.90
    with systemic onset — *see* Still's disease
    ankle M08.97- ☑
    elbow M08.92- ☑
    foot joint M08.97- ☑
    hand joint M08.94- ☑
    hip M08.95- ☑
    knee M08.96- ☑
    multiple site M08.99
    pauciarticular M08.40
      ankle M08.47- ☑
      elbow M08.42- ☑
      foot joint M08.47- ☑
      hand joint M08.44- ☑
      hip M08.45- ☑
      knee M08.46- ☑
      shoulder M08.41- ☑
      vertebrae M08.48
      wrist M08.43- ☑
    psoriatic L40.54
    rheumatoid — *see* Arthritis, rheumatoid, juvenile
    shoulder M08.91- ☑
    specified type NEC M08.80
      ankle M08.87- ☑
      elbow M08.82- ☑
      foot joint M08.87- ☑
      hand joint M08.84- ☑
      hip M08.85- ☑
      knee M08.86- ☑
      multiple site M08.89
      shoulder M08.81- ☑

Arthritis, arthritic — *continued*
  juvenile — *continued*
    specified type — *continued*
      specified joint NEC M08.88
      vertebrae M08.88
      wrist M08.83- ☑
    wrist M08.93- ☑
  meaning osteoarthritis — *see* Osteoarthritis
  meningococcal A39.83
  menopausal (any site) NEC — *see* Arthritis, specified form NEC
  mutilans (psoriatic) L40.52
  mycotic NEC (*see also* category M01) B49
  neuropathic (Charcot) — *see* Arthropathy, neuropathic
    diabetic — *see* Diabetes, arthropathy, neuropathic
    nonsyphilitic NEC G98.0
    syringomyelic G95.0
  ochronotic (*see also* subcategory M14.8-) E70.29
  palindromic (any site) — *see* Rheumatism, palindromic
  pneumococcal M00.10
    ankle M00.17- ☑
    elbow M00.12- ☑
    foot joint — *see* Arthritis, pneumococcal, ankle
    hand joint M00.14- ☑
    hip M00.15- ☑
    knee M00.16- ☑
    multiple site M00.19
    shoulder M00.11- ☑
    vertebra M00.18
    wrist M00.13- ☑
  postdysenteric — *see* Arthropathy, postdysenteric
  postmeningococcal A39.84
  postrheumatic, chronic — *see* Arthropathy, postrheumatic, chronic
  primary progressive (*see also* Arthritis, specified form NEC)
    spine — *see* Spondylitis, ankylosing
  psoriatic L40.50
  purulent (any site except spine) — *see* Arthritis, pyogenic or pyemic
    spine — *see* Spondylopathy, infective
  pyogenic or pyemic (any site except spine) M00.9
    bacterial NEC M00.80
      ankle M00.87- ☑
      elbow M00.82- ☑
      foot joint — *see* Arthritis, pyogenic, bacterial NEC, ankle
      hand joint M00.84- ☑
      hip M00.85- ☑
      knee M00.86- ☑
      multiple site M00.89
      shoulder M00.81- ☑
      vertebra M00.88
      wrist M00.83- ☑
    pneumococcal — *see* Arthritis, pneumococcal
    spine — *see* Spondylopathy, infective
    staphylococcal — *see* Arthritis, staphylococcal
    streptococcal — *see* Arthritis, streptococcal NEC
      pneumococcal — *see* Arthritis, pneumococcal
  reactive — *see* Reiter's disease
  rheumatic (*see also* Arthritis, rheumatoid)
    acute or subacute — *see* Fever, rheumatic
  rheumatoid M06.9
    with
      carditis — *see* Rheumatoid, carditis
      endocarditis — *see* Rheumatoid, carditis
      heart involvement NEC — *see* Rheumatoid, carditis
      lung involvement — *see* Rheumatoid, lung
      myocarditis — *see* Rheumatoid, carditis
      myopathy — *see* Rheumatoid, myopathy
      pericarditis — *see* Rheumatoid, carditis
      polyneuropathy — *see* Rheumatoid, polyneuropathy
      rheumatoid factor — *see* Arthritis, rheumatoid, seropositive
      splenoadenomegaly and leukopenia — *see* Felty's syndrome
      vasculitis — *see* Rheumatoid, vasculitis
      visceral involvement NEC — *see* Rheumatoid, arthritis, with involvement of organs NEC
    juvenile (with or without rheumatoid factor) M08.00
      ankle M08.07- ☑
      elbow M08.02- ☑
      foot joint M08.07- ☑
      hand joint M08.04- ☑
      hip M08.05- ☑

Arthritis, arthritic — *continued*
  rheumatoid — *continued*
    juvenile — *continued*
      knee M08.06- ☑
      multiple site M08.09
      shoulder M08.01- ☑
      vertebra M08.08
      wrist M08.03- ☑
    seronegative M06.00
      ankle M06.07- ☑
      elbow M06.02- ☑
      foot joint M06.07- ☑
      hand joint M06.04- ☑
      hip M06.05- ☑
      knee M06.06- ☑
      multiple site M06.09
      shoulder M06.01- ☑
      vertebra M06.08
      wrist M06.03- ☑
    seropositive M05.9
      specified NEC M05.80
        ankle M05.87- ☑
        elbow M05.82- ☑
        foot joint M05.87- ☑
        hand joint M05.84- ☑
        hip M05.85- ☑
        knee M05.86- ☑
        multiple sites M05.89
        shoulder M05.81- ☑
        vertebra — *see* Spondylitis, ankylosing
        wrist M05.83- ☑
      without organ involvement M05.70
        ankle M05.77- ☑
        elbow M05.72- ☑
        foot joint M05.77- ☑
        hand joint M05.74- ☑
        hip M05.75- ☑
        knee M05.76- ☑
        multiple sites M05.79
        shoulder M05.71- ☑
        vertebra — *see* Spondylitis, ankylosing
        wrist M05.73- ☑
    specified type NEC M06.80
      ankle M06.87- ☑
      elbow M06.82- ☑
      foot joint M06.87- ☑
      hand joint M06.84- ☑
      hip M06.85- ☑
      knee M06.86- ☑
      multiple site M06.89
      shoulder M06.81- ☑
      vertebra M06.88
      wrist M06.83- ☑
    spine — *see* Spondylitis, ankylosing
  rubella B06.82
  scorbutic (*see also* subcategory M14.8-) E54
  senile or senescent — *see* Osteoarthritis
  septic (any site except spine) — *see* Arthritis, pyogenic or pyemic
    spine — *see* Spondylopathy, infective
  serum (nontherapeutic) (therapeutic) — *see* Arthropathy, postimmunization
  specified form NEC M13.80
    ankle M13.87- ☑
    elbow M13.82- ☑
    foot joint M13.87- ☑
    hand joint M13.84- ☑
    hip M13.85- ☑
    knee M13.86- ☑
    multiple site M13.89
    shoulder M13.81- ☑
    specified joint NEC M13.88
    wrist M13.83- ☑
  spine (*see also* Spondylopathy, inflammatory)
    infectious or infective NEC — *see* Spondylopathy, infective
    Marie-Strümpell — *see* Spondylitis, ankylosing
    pyogenic — *see* Spondylopathy, infective
    rheumatoid — *see* Spondylitis, ankylosing
    traumatic (old) — *see* Spondylopathy, traumatic
    tuberculous A18.01
  staphylococcal M00.00
    ankle M00.07- ☑
    elbow M00.02- ☑
    foot joint — *see* Arthritis, staphylococcal, ankle
    hand joint M00.04- ☑

Arthritis, arthritic — *continued*
staphylococcal — *continued*
hip M00.05- ☑
knee M00.06- ☑
multiple site M00.09
shoulder M00.01- ☑
vertebra M00.08
wrist M00.03- ☑
streptococcal NEC M00.20
ankle M00.27- ☑
elbow M00.22- ☑
foot joint — *see* Arthritis, streptococcal, ankle
hand joint M00.24- ☑
hip M00.25- ☑
knee M00.26- ☑
multiple site M00.29
shoulder M00.21- ☑
vertebra M00.28
wrist M00.23- ☑
suppurative — *see* Arthritis, pyogenic or pyemic
syphilitic (late) A52.16
congenital A50.55 [M12.80]
syphilitica deformans (Charcot) A52.16
temporomandibular M26.69
toxic of menopause (any site) — *see* Arthritis, specified
form NEC
transient — *see* Arthropathy, specified form NEC
traumatic (chronic) — *see* Arthropathy, traumatic
tuberculous A18.02
spine A18.01
uratic — *see* Gout
urethritica (Reiter's) — *see* Reiter's disease
vertebral — *see* Spondylopathy, inflammatory
villous (any site) — *see* Arthropathy, specified form
NEC
Arthrocele — *see* Effusion, joint
Arthrodesis status Z98.1
Arthrodynia (*see also* Pain, joint)
Arthrodysplasia Q74.9
Arthrofibrosis, joint — *see* Ankylosis
Arthrogryposis (congenital) Q68.8
multiplex congenita Q74.3
Arthrokatadysis M24.7
Arthropathy (*see also* Arthritis) M12.9
Charcot's — *see* Arthropathy, neuropathic
diabetic — *see* Diabetes, arthropathy, neuropathic
syringomyelic G95.0
cricoarytenoid J38.7
crystal (-induced) — *see* Arthritis, in, crystals
diabetic NEC — *see* Diabetes, arthropathy
distal interphalangeal, psoriatic L40.51
enteropathic M07.60
ankle M07.67- ☑
elbow M07.62- ☑
foot joint M07.67- ☑
hand joint M07.64- ☑
hip M07.65- ☑
knee M07.66- ☑
multiple site M07.69
shoulder M07.61- ☑
vertebra M07.68
wrist M07.63- ☑
following intestinal bypass M02.00
ankle M02.07- ☑
elbow M02.02- ☑
foot joint M02.07- ☑
hand joint M02.04- ☑
hip M02.05- ☑
knee M02.06- ☑
multiple site M02.09
shoulder M02.01- ☑
vertebra M02.08
wrist M02.03- ☑
gouty (*see also* Gout)
in (due to)
Lesch-Nyhan syndrome E79.1 [M14.8-] ☑
sickle-cell disorders D57- ☑ [M14.8-] ☑
hemophilic NEC D66 [M36.2]
in (due to)
hyperparathyroidism NEC E21.3 [M14.8-] ☑
metabolic disease NOS E88.9 [M14.8-] ☑
in (due to)
acromegaly E22.0 [M14.8-] ☑
amyloidosis E85.4 [M14.8-] ☑
blood disorder NOS D75.9 [M36.3]
diabetes — *see* Diabetes, arthropathy
endocrine disease NOS E34.9 [M14.8-] ☑

Arthropathy — *continued*
in — *continued*
erythema
multiforme L51.9 [M14.8-] ☑
nodosum L52 [M14.8-] ☑
hemochromatosis E83.118 [M14.8-] ☑
hemoglobinopathy NEC D58.2 [M36.3]
hemophilia NEC D66 [M36.2]
Henoch-Schönlein purpura D69.0 [M36.4]
hyperthyroidism E05.90 [M14.8-] ☑
hypothyroidism E03.9 [M14.8-] ☑
infective endocarditis I33.0 [M12.80]
leukemia NEC C95.9- ☑ [M36.1]
malignant histiocytosis C96.A [M36.1]
metabolic disease NOS E88.9 [M14.8-] ☑
multiple myeloma C90.0- ☑ [M36.1]
neoplastic disease NOS (*see also* Neoplasm)
D49.9 [M36.1]
nutritional deficiency (*see also* subcategory
M14.8-) E63.9
psoriasis NOS L40.50
sarcoidosis D86.86
syphilis (late) A52.77
congenital A50.55 [M12.80]
thyrotoxicosis (*see also* subcategory M14.8-) E05.90
ulcerative colitis K51.90 [M07.60]
viral hepatitis (postinfection) NEC B19.9 [M12.80]
Whipple's disease (*see also* subcategory M14.8-)
K90.81
Jaccoud — *see* Arthropathy, postrheumatic, chronic
juvenile — *see* Arthritis, juvenile
psoriatic L40.54
mutilans (psoriatic) L40.52
neuropathic (Charcot) M14.60
ankle M14.67- ☑
diabetic — *see* Diabetes, arthropathy, neuropathic
elbow M14.62- ☑
foot joint M14.67- ☑
hand joint M14.64- ☑
hip M14.65- ☑
knee M14.66- ☑
multiple site M14.69
nonsyphilitic NEC G98.0
shoulder M14.61- ☑
syringomyelic G95.0
vertebra M14.68
wrist M14.63- ☑
osteopulmonary — *see* Osteoarthropathy, hypertrophic, specified NEC
postdysenteric M02.10
ankle M02.17- ☑
elbow M02.12- ☑
foot joint M02.17- ☑
hand joint M02.14- ☑
hip M02.15- ☑
knee M02.16- ☑
multiple site M02.19
shoulder M02.11- ☑
vertebra M02.18
wrist M02.13- ☑
postimmunization M02.20
ankle M02.27- ☑
elbow M02.22- ☑
foot joint M02.27- ☑
hand joint M02.24- ☑
hip M02.25- ☑
knee M02.26- ☑
multiple site M02.29
shoulder M02.21- ☑
vertebra M02.28
wrist M02.23- ☑
postinfectious NEC B99 ☑ [M12.80]
in (due to)
enteritis due to Yersinia enterocolitica
A04.6 [M12.80]
syphilis A52.77
viral hepatitis NEC B19.9 [M12.80]
postrheumatic, chronic (Jaccoud) M12.00
ankle M12.07- ☑
elbow M12.02- ☑
foot joint M12.07- ☑
hand joint M12.04- ☑
hip M12.05- ☑
knee M12.06- ☑
multiple site M12.09
shoulder M12.01- ☑
specified joint NEC M12.08

Arthropathy — *continued*
postrheumatic, chronic — *continued*
vertebrae M12.08
wrist M12.03- ☑
psoriatic NEC L40.59
interphalangeal, distal L40.51
reactive M02.9
in (due to)
infective endocarditis I33.0 [M02.9]
specified type NEC M02.80
ankle M02.87- ☑
elbow M02.82- ☑
foot joint M02.87- ☑
hand joint M02.84- ☑
hip M02.85- ☑
knee M02.86- ☑
multiple site M02.89
shoulder M02.81- ☑
vertebra M02.88
wrist M02.83- ☑
specified form NEC M12.80
ankle M12.87- ☑
elbow M12.82- ☑
foot joint M12.87- ☑
hand joint M12.84- ☑
hip M12.85- ☑
knee M12.86- ☑
multiple site M12.89
shoulder M12.81- ☑
specified joint NEC M12.88
vertebrae M12.88
wrist M12.83- ☑
syringomyelic G95.0
tabes dorsalis A52.16
tabetic A52.16
transient — *see* Arthropathy, specified form NEC
traumatic M12.50
ankle M12.57- ☑
elbow M12.52- ☑
foot joint M12.57- ☑
hand joint M12.54- ☑
hip M12.55- ☑
knee M12.56- ☑
multiple site M12.59
shoulder M12.51- ☑
specified joint NEC M12.58
vertebrae M12.58
wrist M12.53- ☑
Arthropyosis — *see* Arthritis, pyogenic or pyemic
Arthrosis (deformans) (degenerative) (localized) (*see also*
Osteoarthritis) M19.90
spine — *see* Spondylosis
Arthus' phenomenon or reaction T78.41 ☑
due to
drug — *see* Table of Drugs and Chemicals, by drug
Articular — *see* condition
Articulation, reverse (teeth) M26.24
Artificial
insemination complication — *see* Complications, artificial, fertilization
opening status (functioning) (without complication)
Z93.9
anus (colostomy) Z93.3
colostomy Z93.3
cystostomy Z93.50
appendico-vesicostomy Z93.52
cutaneous Z93.51
specified NEC Z93.59
enterostomy Z93.4
gastrostomy Z93.1
ileostomy Z93.2
intestinal tract NEC Z93.4
jejunostomy Z93.4
nephrostomy Z93.6
specified site NEC Z93.8
tracheostomy Z93.0
ureterostomy Z93.6
urethrostomy Z93.6
urinary tract NEC Z93.6
vagina Z93.8
vagina status Z93.8
Arytenoid — *see* condition
Asbestosis (occupational) J61
Ascariasis B77.9
with
complications NEC B77.89
intestinal complications B77.0

Ascariasis — *continued*
  with — *continued*
    pneumonia, pneumonitis B77.81
Ascaridosis, ascariasis — *see* Ascariasis
Ascaris (infection) (infestation) (lumbricoides) — *see* Ascariasis
Ascending — *see* condition
ASC-H (atypical squamous cells cannot exclude high grade squamous intraepithelial lesion on cytologic smear)
  anus R85.611
  cervix R87.611
  vagina R87.621
Aschoff's bodies — *see* Myocarditis, rheumatic
Ascites (abdominal) R18.8
  cardiac (*see also* Failure, heart, right) I50.810
  chylous (nonfilarial) I89.8
    filarial — *see* Infestation, filarial
  due to
    cirrhosis, alcoholic K70.31
    hepatitis
      alcoholic K70.11
      chronic active K71.51
      S. japonicum B65.2
  heart (*see also* Failure, heart, right) I50.810
  malignant R18.0
  pseudochylous R18.8
  syphilitic A52.74
  tuberculous A18.31
ASC-US (atypical squamous cells of undetermined significance on cytologic smear)
  anus R85.610
  cervix R87.610
  vagina R87.620
Aseptic — *see* condition
Asherman's syndrome N85.6
Asialia K11.7
Asiatic cholera — *see* Cholera
Asimultagnosia (simultanagnosia) R48.3
Askin's tumor — *see* Neoplasm, connective tissue, malignant
Asocial personality F60.2
Asomatognosia R41.4
Aspartylglucosaminuria E77.1
Asperger's disease or syndrome F84.5
Aspergilloma — *see* Aspergillosis
Aspergillosis (with pneumonia) B44.9
  bronchopulmonary, allergic B44.81
  disseminated B44.7
  generalized B44.7
  pulmonary NEC B44.1
    allergic B44.81
    invasive B44.0
  specified NEC B44.89
  tonsillar B44.2
Aspergillus (flavus) (fumigatus) (infection) (terreus) — *see* Aspergillosis
Aspermatogenesis — *see* Azoospermia
Aspermia (testis) — *see* Azoospermia
Asphyxia, asphyxiation (by) R09.01
  antenatal P84
  birth P84
  bunny bag — *see* Asphyxia, due to, mechanical threat to breathing, trapped in bed clothes
  crushing S28.0 ☑
  drowning T75.1 ☑
  gas, fumes, or vapor — *see* Table of Drugs and Chemicals
  inhalation — *see* Inhalation
  intrauterine P84
  local I73.00
    with gangrene I73.01
  mucus (*see also* Foreign body, respiratory tract, causing asphyxia)
  newborn P84
  pathological R09.01
  postnatal P84
    mechanical — *see* Asphyxia, due to, mechanical threat to breathing
  prenatal P84
  reticularis R23.1
  strangulation — *see* Asphyxia, due to, mechanical threat to breathing
  submersion T75.1 ☑
  traumatic T71.9 ☑
    due to
      crushed chest S28.0 ☑

Asphyxia, asphyxiation — *continued*
  traumatic — *continued*
    due to — *continued*
      foreign body (in) — *see* Foreign body, respiratory tract, causing asphyxia
      low oxygen content of ambient air T71.20 ☑
      due to
        being trapped in
          low oxygen environment T71.29 ☑
          in car trunk T71.221 ☑
            circumstances undetermined T71.224 ☑
            done with intent to harm by
              another person T71.223 ☑
              self T71.222 ☑
          in refrigerator T71.231 ☑
            circumstances undetermined T71.234 ☑
            done with intent to harm by
              another person T71.233 ☑
              self T71.232 ☑
      cave-in T71.21 ☑
      mechanical threat to breathing (accidental) T71.191 ☑
        circumstances undetermined T71.194 ☑
        done with intent to harm by
          another person T71.193 ☑
          self T71.192 ☑
        hanging T71.161 ☑
          circumstances undetermined T71.164 ☑
          done with intent to harm by
            another person T71.163 ☑
            self T71.162 ☑
        plastic bag T71.121 ☑
          circumstances undetermined T71.124 ☑
          done with intent to harm by
            another person T71.123 ☑
            self T71.122 ☑
        smothering
          in furniture T71.151 ☑
            circumstances undetermined T71.154 ☑
            done with intent to harm by
              another person T71.153 ☑
              self T71.152 ☑
          under
            another person's body T71.141 ☑
              circumstances undetermined T71.144 ☑
              done with intent to harm T71.143 ☑
            pillow T71.111 ☑
              circumstances undetermined T71.114 ☑
              done with intent to harm by
                another person T71.113 ☑
                self T71.112 ☑
        trapped in bed clothes T71.131 ☑
          circumstances undetermined T71.134 ☑
          done with intent to harm by
            another person T71.133 ☑
            self T71.132 ☑
  vomiting, vomitus — *see* Foreign body, respiratory tract, causing asphyxia
Aspiration
  amniotic (clear) fluid (newborn) P24.10
    with
      pneumonia (pneumonitis) P24.11
      respiratory symptoms P24.11
  blood
    newborn (without respiratory symptoms) P24.20
      with
        pneumonia (pneumonitis) P24.21
        respiratory symptoms P24.21
      specified age NEC — *see* Foreign body, respiratory tract
  bronchitis J69.0
  food or foreign body (with asphyxiation) — *see* Asphyxia, food
  liquor (amnii) (newborn) P24.10
    with
      pneumonia (pneumonitis) P24.11
      respiratory symptoms P24.11
  meconium (newborn) (without respiratory symptoms) P24.00
    with
      pneumonitis (pneumonitis) P24.01
      respiratory symptoms P24.01

Aspiration — *continued*
  milk (newborn) (without respiratory symptoms) P24.30
    with
      pneumonia (pneumonitis) P24.31
      respiratory symptoms P24.31
    specified age NEC — *see* Foreign body, respiratory tract
  mucus (*see also* Foreign body, by site, causing asphyxia)
    newborn P24.10
      with
        pneumonia (pneumonitis) P24.11
        respiratory symptoms P24.11
  neonatal P24.9
    specific NEC (without respiratory symptoms) P24.80
      with
        pneumonia (pneumonitis) P24.81
        respiratory symptoms P24.81
  newborn P24.9
    specific NEC (without respiratory symptoms) P24.80
      with
        pneumonia (pneumonitis) P24.81
        respiratory symptoms P24.81
  pneumonia J69.0
  pneumonitis J69.0
  syndrome of newborn — *see* Aspiration, by substance, with pneumonia
  vernix caseosa (newborn) P24.80
    with
      pneumonia (pneumonitis) P24.81
      respiratory symptoms P24.81
  vomitus (*see also* Foreign body, respiratory tract)
    newborn (without respiratory symptoms) P24.30
      with
        pneumonia (pneumonitis) P24.31
        respiratory symptoms P24.31
Asplenia (congenital) Q89.01
  postsurgical Z90.81
Assam fever B55.0
Assault, sexual — *see* Maltreatment
Assmann's focus NEC A15.0
Astasia (-abasia) (hysterical) F44.4
Asteatosis cutis L85.3
Astereognosia, astereognosis R48.1
Asterixis R27.8
  in liver disease K71.3
Asteroid hyalitis — *see* Deposit, crystalline
Asthenia, asthenic R53.1
  cardiac (*see also* Failure, heart) I50.9
    psychogenic F45.8
  cardiovascular (*see also* Failure, heart) I50.9
    psychogenic F45.8
  heart (*see also* Failure, heart) I50.9
    psychogenic F45.8
  hysterical F44.4
  myocardial (*see also* Failure, heart) I50.9
    psychogenic F45.8
  nervous F48.8
  neurocirculatory F45.8
  neurotic F48.8
  psychogenic F48.8
  psychoneurotic F48.8
  psychophysiologic F48.8
  reaction (psychophysiologic) F48.8
  senile R54
Asthenopia (*see also* Discomfort, visual)
  hysterical F44.6
  psychogenic F44.6
Asthenospermia — *see* Abnormal, specimen, male genital organs
Asthma, asthmatic (bronchial) (catarrh) (spasmodic) J45.909
  with
    chronic obstructive bronchitis J44.9
      with
        acute lower respiratory infection J44.0
        exacerbation (acute) J44.1
    chronic obstructive pulmonary disease J44.9
      with
        acute lower respiratory infection J44.0
        exacerbation (acute) J44.1
    exacerbation (acute) J45.901
    hay fever — *see* Asthma, allergic extrinsic
    rhinitis, allergic — *see* Asthma, allergic extrinsic
    status asthmaticus J45.902
  allergic extrinsic J45.909
    with
      exacerbation (acute) J45.901
      status asthmaticus J45.902

▽ **Subterms under main terms may continue to next column or page**   ☑ **Additional Character Required — Refer to the Tabular List for Character Selection**   **31**

Ascariasis — Asthma, asthmatic

Asthma, asthmatic — *continued*
- atopic — *see* Asthma, allergic extrinsic
- cardiac — *see* Failure, ventricular, left
- cardiobronchial I50.1
- childhood J45.909
  - with
    - exacerbation (acute) J45.901
    - status asthmaticus J45.902
- chronic obstructive J44.9
  - with
    - acute lower respiratory infection J44.0
    - exacerbation (acute) J44.1
- collier's J60
- cough variant J45.991
- detergent J69.8
- due to
  - detergent J69.8
  - inhalation of fumes J68.3
- eosinophilic J82
- extrinsic, allergic — *see* Asthma, allergic extrinsic
- grinder's J62.8
- hay — *see* Asthma, allergic extrinsic
- heart I50.1
- idiosyncratic — *see* Asthma, nonallergic
- intermittent (mild) J45.20
  - with
    - exacerbation (acute) J45.21
    - status asthmaticus J45.22
- intrinsic, nonallergic — *see* Asthma, nonallergic
- Kopp's E32.8
- late-onset J45.909
  - with
    - exacerbation (acute) J45.901
    - status asthmaticus J45.902
- mild intermittent J45.20
  - with
    - exacerbation (acute) J45.21
    - status asthmaticus J45.22
- mild persistent J45.30
  - with
    - exacerbation (acute) J45.31
    - status asthmaticus J45.32
- Millar's (laryngismus stridulus) J38.5
- miner's J60
- mixed J45.909
  - with
    - exacerbation (acute) J45.901
    - status asthmaticus J45.902
- moderate persistent J45.40
  - with
    - exacerbation (acute) J45.41
    - status asthmaticus J45.42
- nervous — *see* Asthma, nonallergic
- nonallergic (intrinsic) J45.909
  - with
    - exacerbation (acute) J45.901
    - status asthmaticus J45.902
- persistent
  - mild J45.30
    - with
      - exacerbation (acute) J45.31
      - status asthmaticus J45.32
  - moderate J45.40
    - with
      - exacerbation (acute) J45.41
      - status asthmaticus J45.42
  - severe J45.50
    - with
      - exacerbation (acute) J45.51
      - status asthmaticus J45.52
- platinum J45.998
- pneumoconiotic NEC J64
- potter's J62.8
- predominantly allergic J45.909
- psychogenic F54
- pulmonary eosinophilic J82
- red cedar J67.8
- Rostan's I50.1
- sandblaster's J62.8
- sequoiosis J67.8
- severe persistent J45.50
  - with
    - exacerbation (acute) J45.51
    - status asthmaticus J45.52
- specified NEC J45.998
- stonemason's J62.8
- thymic E32.8
- tuberculous — *see* Tuberculosis, pulmonary

Asthma, asthmatic — *continued*
- Wichmann's (laryngismus stridulus) J38.5
- wood J67.8

Astigmatism (compound) (congenital) H52.20- ☑
- irregular H52.21- ☑
- regular H52.22- ☑

Astraphobia F40.220

Astroblastoma
- specified site — *see* Neoplasm, malignant, by site
- unspecified site C71.9

Astrocytoma (cystic)
- anaplastic
  - specified site — *see* Neoplasm, malignant, by site
  - unspecified site C71.9
- fibrillary
  - specified site — *see* Neoplasm, malignant, by site
  - unspecified site C71.9
- fibrous
  - specified site — *see* Neoplasm, malignant, by site
  - unspecified site C71.9
- gemistocytic
  - specified site — *see* Neoplasm, malignant, by site
  - unspecified site C71.9
- juvenile
  - specified site — *see* Neoplasm, malignant, by site
  - unspecified site C71.9
- pilocytic
  - specified site — *see* Neoplasm, malignant, by site
  - unspecified site C71.9
- piloid
  - specified site — *see* Neoplasm, malignant, by site
  - unspecified site C71.9
- protoplasmic
  - specified site — *see* Neoplasm, malignant, by site
  - unspecified site C71.9
- specified site NEC — *see* Neoplasm, malignant, by site
- subependymal D43.2
  - giant cell
    - specified site — *see* Neoplasm, uncertain behavior, by site
    - unspecified site D43.2
  - specified site — *see* Neoplasm, uncertain behavior, by site
  - unspecified site D43.2
- unspecified site C71.9

Astroglioma
- specified site — *see* Neoplasm, malignant, by site
- unspecified site C71.9

Asymbolia R48.8

Asymmetry (*see also* Distortion)
- between native and reconstructed breast N65.1
- face Q67.0
- jaw (lower) — *see* Anomaly, dentofacial, jaw-cranial base relationship, asymmetry

Asynergia, asynergy R27.8
- ventricular I51.89

Asystole (heart) — *see* Arrest, cardiac

At risk
- for
  - dental caries Z91.849
    - high Z91.843
    - low Z91.841
    - moderate Z91.842
  - falling Z91.81

Ataxia, ataxy, ataxic R27.0
- acute R27.8
- brain (hereditary) G11.9
- cerebellar (hereditary) G11.9
  - with defective DNA repair G11.3
  - alcoholic G31.2
  - early-onset G11.1
  - in
    - alcoholism G31.2
    - myxedema E03.9 [G13.2]
    - neoplastic disease (*see also* Neoplasm) D49.9 [G32.81]
    - specified disease NEC G32.81
  - late-onset (Marie's) G11.2
- cerebral (hereditary) G11.9
- congenital nonprogressive G11.0
- family, familial — *see* Ataxia, hereditary
- following
  - cerebrovascular disease I69.993
    - cerebral infarction I69.393
    - intracerebral hemorrhage I69.193
    - nontraumatic intracranial hemorrhage NEC I69.293
    - specified disease NEC I69.893

Ataxia, ataxy, ataxic — *continued*
- following — *continued*
  - cerebrovascular disease — *continued*
    - subarachnoid hemorrhage I69.093
- Friedreich's (heredofamilial) (cerebellar) (spinal) G11.1
- gait R26.0
  - hysterical F44.4
- general R27.8
- gluten M35.9 [G32.81]
  - with celiac disease K90.0 [G32.81]
- hereditary G11.9
  - with neuropathy G60.2
  - cerebellar — *see* Ataxia, cerebellar
  - spastic G11.4
  - specified NEC G11.8
  - spinal (Friedreich's) G11.1
- heredofamilial — *see* Ataxia, hereditary
- Hunt's G11.1
- hysterical F44.4
- locomotor (progressive) (syphilitic) (partial) (spastic) A52.11
  - diabetic — *see* Diabetes, ataxia
- Marie's (cerebellar) (heredofamilial) (late-onset) G11.2
- nonorganic origin F44.4
- nonprogressive, congenital G11.0
- psychogenic F44.4
- Roussy-Lévy G60.0
- Sanger-Brown's (hereditary) G11.2
- spastic hereditary G11.4
- spinal
  - hereditary (Friedreich's) G11.1
  - progressive (syphilitic) A52.11
- spinocerebellar, X-linked recessive G11.1
- telangiectasia (Louis-Bar) G11.3

Ataxia-telangiectasia (Louis-Bar) G11.3

Atelectasis (massive) (partial) (pressure) (pulmonary) J98.11
- newborn P28.10
  - due to resorption P28.11
  - partial P28.19
  - primary P28.0
  - secondary P28.19
- primary (newborn) P28.0
- tuberculous — *see* Tuberculosis, pulmonary

Atelocardia Q24.9

Atelomyelia Q06.1

Atheroembolism
- of
  - extremities
    - lower I75.02- ☑
    - upper I75.01- ☑
  - kidney I75.81
  - specified NEC I75.89

Atheroma, atheromatous (*see also* Arteriosclerosis) I70.90
- aorta, aortic I70.0
  - valve (*see also* Endocarditis, aortic) I35.8
- aorto-iliac I70.0
- artery — *see* Arteriosclerosis
- basilar (artery) I67.2
- carotid (artery) (common) (internal) I67.2
- cerebral (arteries) I67.2
- coronary (artery) I25.10
  - with angina pectoris — *see* Arteriosclerosis, coronary (artery),
- degeneration — *see* Arteriosclerosis
- heart, cardiac — *see* Disease, heart, ischemic, atherosclerotic
- mitral (valve) I34.8
- myocardium, myocardial — *see* Disease, heart, ischemic, atherosclerotic
- pulmonary valve (heart) (*see also* Endocarditis, pulmonary) I37.8
- tricuspid (heart) (valve) I36.8
- valve, valvular — *see* Endocarditis
- vertebral (artery) I67.2

Atheromatosis — *see* Arteriosclerosis

Atherosclerosis (*see also* Arteriosclerosis)
- coronary
  - artery I25.10
    - with angina pectoris — *see* Arteriosclerosis, coronary (artery),
    - due to
      - calcified coronary lesion (severely) I25.84
      - lipid rich plaque I25.83
- transplanted heart I25.811
  - bypass graft I25.812

Atherosclerosis — continued
  transplanted heart — continued
    bypass graft — continued
      with angina pectoris — see Arteriosclerosis,
        coronary (artery),
      native coronary artery I25.811
        with angina pectoris — see Arteriosclerosis,
          coronary (artery),
Athetosis (acquired) R25.8
  bilateral (congenital) G80.3
  congenital (bilateral) (double) G80.3
  double (congenital) G80.3
  unilateral R25.8
Athlete's
  foot B35.3
  heart I51.7
Athrepsia E41
Athyrea (acquired) (see also Hypothyroidism)
  congenital E03.1
Atonia, atony, atonic
  bladder (sphincter) (neurogenic) N31.2
  capillary I78.8
  cecum K59.8
    psychogenic F45.8
  colon — see Atony, intestine
  congenital P94.2
  esophagus K22.8
  intestine K59.8
    psychogenic F45.8
  stomach K31.89
    neurotic or psychogenic F45.8
  uterus (during labor) O62.2
    with hemorrhage (postpartum) O72.1
    postpartum (with hemorrhage) O72.1
      without hemorrhage O75.89
Atopy — see History, allergy
Atransferrinemia, congenital E88.09
Atresia, atretic
  alimentary organ or tract NEC Q45.8
    upper Q40.8
  ani, anus, anal (canal) Q42.3
    with fistula Q42.2
  aorta (ring) Q25.29
  aortic (orifice) (valve) Q23.0
    arch Q25.21
    congenital with hypoplasia of ascending aorta and
      defective development of left ventricle (with
      mitral stenosis) Q23.4
    in hypoplastic left heart syndrome Q23.4
  aqueduct of Sylvius Q03.0
    with spina bifida — see Spina bifida, with hydro-
      cephalus
  artery NEC Q27.8
    cerebral Q28.3
    coronary Q24.5
    digestive system Q27.8
    eye Q15.8
    lower limb Q27.8
    pulmonary Q25.5
    specified site NEC Q27.8
    umbilical Q27.0
    upper limb Q27.8
  auditory canal (external) Q16.1
  bile duct (common) (congenital) (hepatic) Q44.2
    acquired — see Obstruction, bile duct
  bladder (neck) Q64.39
    obstruction Q64.31
  bronchus Q32.4
  cecum Q42.8
  cervix (acquired) N88.2
    congenital Q51.828
    in pregnancy or childbirth — see Anomaly, cervix,
      in pregnancy or childbirth
      causing obstructed labor O65.5
  choana Q30.0
  colon Q42.9
    specified NEC Q42.8
  common duct Q44.2
  cricoid cartilage Q31.8
  cystic duct Q44.2
    acquired K82.8
      with obstruction K82.0
  digestive organs NEC Q45.8
  duodenum Q41.0
  ear canal Q16.1
  ejaculatory duct Q55.4
  epiglottis Q31.8
  esophagus Q39.0

Atresia, atretic — continued
  esophagus — continued
    with tracheoesophageal fistula Q39.1
  eustachian tube Q17.8
  fallopian tube (congenital) Q50.6
    acquired N97.1
  follicular cyst N83.0- ☑
  foramen of
    Luschka Q03.1
      with spina bifida — see Spina bifida, with hydro-
        cephalus
    Magendie Q03.1
      with spina bifida — see Spina bifida, with hydro-
        cephalus
  gallbladder Q44.1
  genital organ
    external
      female Q52.79
      male Q55.8
    internal
      female Q52.8
      male Q55.8
  glottis Q31.8
  gullet Q39.0
    with tracheoesophageal fistula Q39.1
  heart valve NEC Q24.8
    pulmonary Q22.0
    tricuspid Q22.4
  hymen Q52.3
    acquired (postinfective) N89.6
  ileum Q41.2
  intestine (small) Q41.9
    large Q42.9
      specified NEC Q42.8
  iris, filtration angle Q15.0
  jejunum Q41.1
  lacrimal apparatus Q10.4
  larynx Q31.8
  meatus urinarius Q64.33
  mitral valve Q23.2
    in hypoplastic left heart syndrome Q23.4
  nares (anterior) (posterior) Q30.0
  nasopharynx Q34.8
  nose, nostril Q30.0
    acquired J34.89
  organ or site NEC Q89.8
  osseous meatus (ear) Q16.1
  oviduct (congenital) Q50.6
    acquired N97.1
  parotid duct Q38.4
    acquired K11.8
  pulmonary (artery) Q25.5
    valve Q22.0
  pulmonic Q22.0
  pupil Q13.2
  rectum Q42.1
    with fistula Q42.0
  salivary duct Q38.4
    acquired K11.8
  sublingual duct Q38.4
    acquired K11.8
  submandibular duct Q38.4
    acquired K11.8
  submaxillary duct Q38.4
    acquired K11.8
  thyroid cartilage Q31.8
  trachea Q32.1
  tricuspid valve Q22.4
  ureter Q62.10
    pelvic junction Q62.11
    vesical orifice Q62.12
  ureteropelvic junction Q62.11
  ureterovesical orifice Q62.12
  urethra (valvular) Q64.39
    stricture Q64.32
  urinary tract NEC Q64.8
  uterus Q51.818
    acquired N85.8
  vagina (congenital) Q52.4
    acquired (postinfectional) (senile) N89.5
  vas deferens Q55.3
  vascular NEC Q27.8
    cerebral Q28.3
    digestive system Q27.8
    lower limb Q27.8
    specified site NEC Q27.8
    upper limb Q27.8
  vein NEC Q27.8
    digestive system Q27.8

Atresia, atretic — continued
  vein — continued
    great Q26.8
    lower limb Q27.8
    portal Q26.5
    pulmonary Q26.4
      partial Q26.3
      total Q26.2
    specified site NEC Q27.8
    upper limb Q27.8
  vena cava (inferior) (superior) Q26.8
  vesicourethral orifice Q64.31
  vulva Q52.79
    acquired N90.5
Atrichia, atrichosis — see Alopecia
Atrophia (see also Atrophy)
  cutis senilis L90.8
    due to radiation L57.8
  gyrata of choroid and retina H31.23
  senilis R54
    dermatological L90.8
      due to radiation (nonionizing) (solar) L57.8
  unguium L60.3
    congenita Q84.6
Atrophie blanche (en plaque) (de Milian) L95.0
Atrophoderma, atrophodermia (of) L90.9
  diffusum (idiopathic) L90.4
  maculatum L90.8
    et striatum L90.8
      due to syphilis A52.79
    syphilitic A51.39
  neuriticum L90.8
  Pasini and Pierini L90.3
  pigmentosum Q82.1
  reticulatum symmetricum faciei L66.4
  senile L90.8
    due to radiation (nonionizing) (solar) L57.8
  vermiculata (cheeks) L66.4
Atrophy, atrophic (of)
  adrenal (capsule) (gland) E27.49
    primary (autoimmune) E27.1
  alveolar process or ridge (edentulous) K08.20
  anal sphincter (disuse) N81.84
  appendix K38.8
  arteriosclerotic — see Arteriosclerosis
  bile duct (common) (hepatic) K83.8
  bladder N32.89
    neurogenic N31.8
  blanche (en plaque) (of Milian) L95.0
  bone (senile) NEC (see also Disorder, bone, specified
    type NEC)
    due to
      tabes dorsalis (neurogenic) A52.11
  brain (cortex) (progressive) G31.9
    frontotemporal circumscribed G31.01 [F02.80]
      with behavioral disturbance G31.01 [F02.81]
    senile NEC G31.1
  breast N64.2
    obstetric — see Disorder, breast, specified type NEC
  buccal cavity K13.79
  cardiac — see Degeneration, myocardial
  cartilage (infectional) (joint) — see Disorder, cartilage,
    specified NEC
  cerebellar — see Atrophy, brain
  cerebral — see Atrophy, brain
  cervix (mucosa) (senile) (uteri) N88.8
    menopausal N95.8
  Charcot-Marie-Tooth G60.0
  choroid (central) (macular) (myopic) (retina) H31.10- ☑
    diffuse secondary H31.12- ☑
    gyrate H31.23
    senile H31.11- ☑
  ciliary body — see Atrophy, iris
  conjunctiva (senile) H11.89
  corpus cavernosum N48.89
  cortical — see Atrophy, brain
  cystic duct K82.8
  Déjérine-Thomas G23.8
  disuse NEC — see Atrophy, muscle
  Duchenne-Aran G12.21
  ear H93.8- ☑
  edentulous alveolar ridge K08.20
  endometrium (senile) N85.8
    cervix N88.8
  enteric K63.89
  epididymis N50.89
  eyeball — see Disorder, globe, degenerated condition,
    atrophy

Index

Atrophy, atrophic — *continued*
eyelid (senile) — *see* Disorder, eyelid, degenerative
facial (skin) L90.9
fallopian tube (senile) N83.32- ☑
  with ovary N83.33- ☑
fascioscapulohumeral (Landouzy- Déjérine) G71.02
fatty, thymus (gland) E32.8
gallbladder K82.8
gastric K29.40
  with bleeding K29.41
gastrointestinal K63.89
glandular I89.8
globe H44.52- ☑
gum — *see* Recession, gingival
hair L67.8
heart (brown) — *see* Degeneration, myocardial
hemifacial Q67.4
  Romberg G51.8
infantile E41
  paralysis, acute — *see* Poliomyelitis, paralytic
intestine K63.89
iris (essential) (progressive) H21.26- ☑
  specified NEC H21.29
kidney (senile) (terminal) (*see also* Sclerosis, renal) N26.1
  congenital or infantile Q60.5
    bilateral Q60.4
    unilateral Q60.3
  hydronephrotic — *see* Hydronephrosis
lacrimal gland (primary) H04.14- ☑
  secondary H04.15- ☑
Landouzy-Déjérine G71.02
laryngitis, infective J37.0
larynx J38.7
Leber's optic (hereditary) H47.22
lip K13.0
liver (yellow) K72.90
  with coma K72.91
  acute, subacute K72.00
    with coma K72.01
  chronic K72.10
    with coma K72.11
lung (senile) J98.4
macular (dermatological) L90.8
  syphilitic, skin A51.39
    striated A52.79
mandible (edentulous) K08.20
  minimal K08.21
  moderate K08.22
  severe K08.23
maxilla K08.20
  minimal K08.24
  moderate K08.25
  severe K08.26
muscle, muscular (diffuse) (general) (idiopathic) (primary) M62.50
  ankle M62.57- ☑
  Duchenne-Aran G12.21
  foot M62.57- ☑
  forearm M62.53- ☑
  hand M62.54- ☑
  infantile spinal G12.0
  lower leg M62.56- ☑
  multiple sites M62.59
  myelopathic — *see* Atrophy, muscle, spinal
  myotonic G71.11
  neuritic G58.9
  neuropathic (peroneal) (progressive) G60.0
  pelvic (disuse) N81.84
  peroneal G60.0
  progressive (bulbar) G12.21
    adult G12.1
    infantile (spinal) G12.0
    spinal G12.25
      adult G12.1
      infantile G12.0
  pseudohypertrophic G71.02
  shoulder region M62.51- ☑
  specified site NEC M62.58
  spinal G12.9
    adult form G12.1
    Aran-Duchenne G12.21
    childhood form, type II G12.1
    distal G12.1
    hereditary NEC G12.1
    infantile, type I (Werdnig-Hoffmann) G12.0
    juvenile form, type III (Kugelberg- Welander) G12.1

Atrophy, atrophic — *continued*
muscle, muscular — *continued*
  spinal — *continued*
    progressive G12.25
    scapuloperoneal form G12.1
    specified NEC G12.8
  syphilitic A52.78
  thigh M62.55- ☑
  upper arm M62.52- ☑
myocardium — *see* Degeneration, myocardial
myometrium (senile) N85.8
  cervix N88.8
myopathic NEC — *see* Atrophy, muscle
myotonia G71.11
nail L60.3
nasopharynx J31.1
nerve (*see also* Disorder, nerve)
  abducens — *see* Strabismus, paralytic, sixth nerve
  accessory G52.8
  acoustic or auditory H93.3 ☑
  cranial G52.9
    eighth (auditory) H93.3 ☑
    eleventh (accessory) G52.8
    fifth (trigeminal) G50.8
    first (olfactory) G52.0
    fourth (trochlear) — *see* Strabismus, paralytic, fourth nerve
    second (optic) H47.20
    sixth (abducens) — *see* Strabismus, paralytic, sixth nerve
    tenth (pneumogastric) (vagus) G52.2
    third (oculomotor) — *see* Strabismus, paralytic, third nerve
    twelfth (hypoglossal) G52.3
  hypoglossal G52.3
  oculomotor — *see* Strabismus, paralytic, third nerve
  olfactory G52.0
  optic (papillomacular bundle)
    syphilitic (late) A52.15
      congenital A50.44
  pneumogastric G52.2
  trigeminal G50.8
  trochlear — *see* Strabismus, paralytic, fourth nerve
  vagus (pneumogastric) G52.2
neurogenic, bone, tabetic A52.11
nutritional E41
old age R54
olivopontocerebellar G23.8
optic (nerve) H47.20
  glaucomatous H47.23- ☑
  hereditary H47.22
  primary H47.21- ☑
  specified type NEC H47.29- ☑
  syphilitic (late) A52.15
    congenital A50.44
orbit H05.31- ☑
ovary (senile) N83.31- ☑
  with fallopian tube N83.33- ☑
oviduct (senile) — *see* Atrophy, fallopian tube
palsy, diffuse (progressive) G12.22
pancreas (duct) (senile) K86.89
parotid gland K11.0
pelvic muscle N81.84
penis N48.89
pharynx J39.2
pluriglandular E31.8
  autoimmune E31.0
polyarthritis M15.9
prostate N42.89
pseudohypertrophic (muscle) G71.02
renal (*see also* Sclerosis, renal) N26.1
retina, retinal (postinfectional) H35.89
rhinitis J31.0
salivary gland K11.0
scar L90.5
sclerosis, lobar (of brain) G31.09 [F02.80]
  with behavioral disturbance G31.09 [F02.81]
scrotum N50.89
seminal vesicle N50.89
senile R54
  due to radiation (nonionizing) (solar) L57.8
skin (patches) (spots) L90.9
  degenerative (senile) L90.8
  due to radiation (nonionizing) (solar) L57.8
  senile L90.8
spermatic cord N50.89
spinal (acute) (cord) G95.89
  muscular — *see* Atrophy, muscle, spinal

Atrophy, atrophic — *continued*
spinal — *continued*
  paralysis G12.20
    acute — *see* Poliomyelitis, paralytic
    meaning progressive muscular atrophy G12.21
spine (column) — *see* Spondylopathy, specified NEC
spleen (senile) D73.0
stomach K29.40
  with bleeding K29.41
striate (skin) L90.6
  syphilitic A52.79
subcutaneous L90.9
sublingual gland K11.0
submandibular gland K11.0
submaxillary gland K11.0
Sudeck's — *see* Algoneurodystrophy
suprarenal (capsule) (gland) E27.49
  primary E27.1
systemic affecting central nervous system in
    myxedema E03.9 [G13.2]
    neoplastic disease (*see also* Neoplasm) D49.9 [G13.1]
    specified disease NEC G13.8
tarso-orbital fascia, congenital Q10.3
testis N50.0
thenar, partial — *see* Syndrome, carpal tunnel
thymus (fatty) E32.8
thyroid (gland) (acquired) E03.4
  with cretinism E03.1
  congenital (with myxedema) E03.1
tongue (senile) K14.8
  papillae K14.4
trachea J39.8
tunica vaginalis N50.89
turbinate J34.89
tympanic membrane (nonflaccid) H73.82- ☑
  flaccid H73.81- ☑
upper respiratory tract J39.8
uterus, uterine (senile) N85.8
  cervix N88.8
  due to radiation (intended effect) N85.8
    adverse effect or misadventure N99.89
vagina (senile) N95.2
vas deferens N50.89
vascular I99.8
vertebra (senile) — *see* Spondylopathy, specified NEC
vulva (senile) N90.5
Werdnig-Hoffmann G12.0
yellow — *see* Failure, hepatic
Attack, attacks
  with alteration of consciousness (with automatisms) — *see* Epilepsy, localization-related, symptomatic, with complex partial seizures
  Adams-Stokes I45.9
  akinetic — *see* Epilepsy, generalized, specified NEC
  angina — *see* Angina
  atonic — *see* Epilepsy, generalized, specified NEC
  benign shuddering G25.83
  cataleptic — *see* Catalepsy
  coronary — *see* Infarct, myocardium
  cyanotic, newborn P28.2
  drop NEC R55
  epileptic — *see* Epilepsy
  heart — *see* infarct, myocardium
  hysterical F44.9
  jacksonian — *see* Epilepsy, localization-related, symptomatic, with simple partial seizures
  myocardium, myocardial — *see* Infarct, myocardium
  myoclonic — *see* Epilepsy, generalized, specified NEC
  panic F41.0
  psychomotor — *see* Epilepsy, localization-related, symptomatic, with complex partial seizures
  salaam — *see* Epilepsy, spasms
  schizophreniform, brief F23
  shuddering, benign G25.83
  Stokes-Adams I45.9
  syncope R55
  transient ischemic (TIA) G45.9
    specified NEC G45.8
  unconsciousness R55
    hysterical F44.89
  vasomotor R55
  vasovagal (paroxysmal) (idiopathic) R55
  without alteration of consciousness — *see* Epilepsy, localization-related, symptomatic, with simple partial seizures

Atrophy, atrophic — Attack, attacks

Attention (to)
  artificial
    opening (of) Z43.9
      digestive tract NEC Z43.4
        colon Z43.3
        ilium Z43.2
        stomach Z43.1
      specified NEC Z43.8
      trachea Z43.0
      urinary tract NEC Z43.6
        cystostomy Z43.5
        nephrostomy Z43.6
        ureterostomy Z43.6
        urethrostomy Z43.6
      vagina Z43.7
    colostomy Z43.3
    cystostomy Z43.5
  deficit disorder or syndrome F98.8
    with hyperactivity — *see* Disorder, attention-deficit
      hyperactivity
  gastrostomy Z43.1
  ileostomy Z43.2
  jejunostomy Z43.4
  nephrostomy Z43.6
  surgical dressings Z48.01
  sutures Z48.02
  tracheostomy Z43.0
  ureterostomy Z43.6
  urethrostomy Z43.6
Attrition
  gum — *see* Recession, gingival
  tooth, teeth (excessive) (hard tissues) K03.0
Atypical, atypism (*see also* condition)
  cells (on cytolgocial smear) (endocervical) (endometrial)
    (glandular)
    cervix R87.619
    vagina R87.629
  cervical N87.9
  endometrium N85.9
    hyperplasia N85.00
  parenting situation Z62.9
Auditory — *see* condition
Aujeszky's disease B33.8
Aurantiasis, cutis E67.1
Auricle, auricular (*see also* condition)
  cervical Q18.2
Auriculotemporal syndrome G50.8
Austin Flint murmur (aortic insufficiency) I35.1
Australian
  Q fever A78
  X disease A83.4
Autism, autistic (childhood) (infantile) F84.0
  atypical F84.9
  spectrum disorder F84.0
Autodigestion R68.89
Autoerythrocyte sensitization (syndrome) D69.2
Autographism L50.3
Autoimmune
  disease (systemic) M35.9
  inhibitors to clotting factors D68.311
  lymphoproliferative syndrome [ALPS] D89.82
  thyroiditis E06.3
Autointoxication R68.89
Automatism G93.89
  with temporal sclerosis G93.81
  epileptic — *see* Epilepsy, localization-related, symp-
    tomatic, with complex partial seizures
  paroxysmal, idiopathic — *see* Epilepsy, localization-
    related, symptomatic, with complex partial
    seizures
Autonomic, autonomous
  bladder (neurogenic) N31.2
  hysteria seizure F44.5
Autosensitivity, erythrocyte D69.2
Autosensitization, cutaneous L30.2
Autosome — *see* condition by chromosome involved
Autotopagnosia R48.1
Autotoxemia R68.89
Autumn — *see* condition
Avellis' syndrome G46.8
Aversion
  oral R63.3
    newborn P92.- ☑
      nonorganic origin F98.2 ☑
  sexual F52.1
Aviator's
  disease or sickness — *see* Effect, adverse, high altitude
  ear T70.0 ☑

Avitaminosis (multiple) (*see also* Deficiency, vitamin)
  E56.9
  B E53.9
    with
      beriberi E51.11
      pellagra E52
  B2 E53.0
  B6 E53.1
  B12 E53.8
  D E55.9
    with rickets E55.0
  G E53.0
  K E56.1
  nicotinic acid E52
AVNRT (atrioventricular nodal re-entrant tachycardia)
  I47.1
AVRT (atrioventricular nodal re-entrant tachycardia) I47.1
Avulsion (traumatic)
  blood vessel — *see* Injury, blood vessel
  bone — *see* Fracture, by site
  cartilage (*see also* Dislocation, by site)
    symphyseal (inner), complicating delivery O71.6
  external site other than limb — *see* Wound, open, by
    site
  eye S05.7- ☑
  head (intracranial)
    external site NEC S08.89 ☑
    scalp S08.0 ☑
  internal organ or site — *see* Injury, by site
  joint (*see also* Dislocation, by site)
    capsule — *see* Sprain, by site
  kidney S37.06- ☑
  ligament — *see* Sprain, by site
  limb (*see also* Amputation, traumatic, by site)
    skin and subcutaneous tissue — *see* Wound, open,
      by site
  muscle — *see* Injury, muscle
  nerve (root) — *see* Injury, nerve
  scalp S08.0 ☑
  skin and subcutaneous tissue — *see* Wound, open, by
    site
  spleen S36.032 ☑
  symphyseal cartilage (inner), complicating delivery
    O71.6
  tendon — *see* Injury, muscle
  tooth S03.2 ☑
Awareness of heart beat R00.2
Axenfeld's
  anomaly or syndrome Q15.0
  degeneration (calcareous) Q13.4
Axilla, axillary (*see also* condition)
  breast Q83.1
Axonotmesis — *see* Injury, nerve
Ayerza's disease or syndrome (pulmonary artery sclerosis with pulmonary hypertension) I27.0
Azoospermia (organic) N46.01
  due to
    drug therapy N46.021
    efferent duct obstruction N46.023
    infection N46.022
    radiation N46.024
    specified cause NEC N46.029
    systemic disease N46.025
Azotemia R79.89
  meaning uremia N19
Aztec ear Q17.3
Azygos
  continuation inferior vena cava Q26.8
  lobe (lung) Q33.1

B

Baastrup's disease — *see* Kissing spine
Babesiosis B60.0
Babington's disease (familial hemorrhagic telangiecta-
  sia) I78.0
Babinski's syndrome A52.79
Baby
  crying constantly R68.11
  floppy (syndrome) P94.2
Bacillary — *see* condition
Bacilluria R82.71
Bacillus (*see also* Infection, bacillus)
  abortus infection A23.1
  anthracis infection A22.9
  coli infection (*see also* Escherichia coli) B96.20
  Flexner's A03.1

Bacillus — *continued*
  mallei infection A24.0
  Shiga's A03.0
  suipestifer infection — *see* Infection, salmonella
Back — *see* condition
Backache (postural) M54.9
  sacroiliac M53.3
  specified NEC M54.89
Backflow — *see* Reflux
Backward reading (dyslexia) F81.0
Bacteremia R78.81
  with sepsis — *see* Sepsis
Bactericholia — *see* Cholecystitis, acute
Bacterid, bacteride (pustular) L40.3
Bacterium, bacteria, bacterial
  agent NEC, as cause of disease classified elsewhere
    B96.89
  in blood — *see* Bacteremia
  in urine — *see* Bacteriuria
Bacteriuria, bacteruria R82.71
  asymptomatic R82.71
Bacteroides
  fragilis, as cause of disease classified elsewhere B96.6
Bad
  heart — *see* Disease, heart
  trip
    due to drug abuse — *see* Abuse, drug, hallucinogen
    due to drug dependence — *see* Dependence, drug,
      hallucinogen
Baelz's disease (cheilitis glandularis apostematosa) K13.0
Baerensprung's disease (eczema marginatum) B35.6
Bagasse disease or pneumonitis J67.1
Bagassosis J67.1
Baker's cyst — *see* Cyst, Baker's
Bakwin-Krida syndrome (metaphyseal dysplasia) Q78.5
Balancing side interference M26.56
Balanitis (circinata) (erosiva) (gangrenosa) (phagedenic)
  (vulgaris) N48.1
  amebic A06.82
  candidal B37.42
  due to Haemophilus ducreyi A57
  gonococcal (acute) (chronic) A54.23
  xerotica obliterans N48.0
Balanoposthitis N47.6
  gonococcal (acute) (chronic) A54.23
  ulcerative (specific) A63.8
Balanorrhagia — *see* Balanitis
Balantidiasis, balantidiosis A07.0
Bald tongue K14.4
Baldness (*see also* Alopecia)
  male-pattern — *see* Alopecia, androgenic
Balkan grippe A78
Balloon disease — *see* Effect, adverse, high altitude
Balo's disease (concentric sclerosis) G37.5
Bamberger-Marie disease — *see* Osteoarthropathy,
  hypertrophic, specified type NEC
Bancroft's filariasis B74.0
Band(s)
  adhesive — *see* Adhesions, peritoneum
  anomalous or congenital (*see also* Anomaly, by site)
    heart (atrial) (ventricular) Q24.8
    intestine Q43.3
    omentum Q43.3
  cervix N88.1
  constricting, congenital Q79.8
  gallbladder (congenital) Q44.1
  intestinal (adhesive) — *see* Adhesions, peritoneum
  obstructive
    intestine K56.50
      complete K56.52
      incomplete K56.51
      partial K56.51
    peritoneum K56.50
      complete K56.52
      incomplete K56.51
      partial K56.51
  periappendiceal, congenital Q43.3
  peritoneal (adhesive) — *see* Adhesions, peritoneum
  uterus N73.6
    internal N85.6
  vagina N89.5
Bandemia D72.825
Bandl's ring (contraction), complicating delivery O62.4
Bangkok hemorrhagic fever A91
Bang's disease (brucella abortus) A23.1
Bankruptcy, anxiety concerning Z59.8
Bannister's disease T78.3 ☑

Bannister's disease — *continued*
 hereditary D84.1
Banti's disease or syndrome (with cirrhosis) (with portal hypertension) K76.6
Bar, median, prostate — *see* Enlargement, enlarged, prostate
Barcoo disease or rot — *see* Ulcer, skin
Barlow's disease E54
Barodontalgia T70.29 ☑
Baron Münchausen syndrome — *see* Disorder, factitious
Barosinusitis T70.1 ☑
Barotitis T70.0 ☑
Barotrauma T70.29 ☑
 odontalgia T70.29 ☑
 otitic T70.0 ☑
 sinus T70.1 ☑
Barraquer (-Simons) **disease or syndrome** (progressive lipodystrophy) E88.1
Barré-Guillain disease or syndrome G61.0
Barrel chest M95.4
Barré-Liéou syndrome (posterior cervical sympathetic) M53.0
Barrett's
 disease — *see* Barrett's, esophagus
 esophagus K22.70
 with dysplasia K22.719
 high grade K22.711
 low grade K22.710
 without dysplasia K22.70
 syndrome — *see* Barrett's, esophagus
 ulcer K22.10
 with bleeding K22.11
 without bleeding K22.10
Bársony (-Polgár) (-Teschendorf) **syndrome** (corkscrew esophagus) K22.4
Barth syndrome E78.71
Bartholinitis (suppurating) N75.8
 gonococcal (acute) (chronic) (with abscess) A54.1
Bartonellosis A44.9
 cutaneous A44.1
 mucocutaneous A44.1
 specified NEC A44.8
 systemic A44.0
Barton's fracture S52.56- ☑
Bartter's syndrome E26.81
Basal — *see* condition
Basan's (hidrotic) ectodermal dysplasia Q82.4
Baseball finger — *see* Dislocation, finger
Basedow's disease (exophthalmic goiter) — *see* Hyperthyroidism, with, goiter
Basic — *see* condition
Basilar — *see* condition
Bason's (hidrotic) ectodermal dysplasia Q82.4
Basopenia — *see* Agranulocytosis
Basophilia D72.824
Basophilism (cortico-adrenal) (Cushing's) (pituitary) E24.0
Bassen-Kornzweig disease or syndrome E78.6
Bat ear Q17.5
Bateman's
 disease B08.1
 purpura (senile) D69.2
Bathing cramp T75.1 ☑
Bathophobia F40.248
Batten (-Mayou) **disease** E75.4
 retina E75.4 [H36]
Batten-Steinert syndrome G71.11
Battered — *see* Maltreatment
Battey Mycobacterium infection A31.0
Battle exhaustion F43.0
Battledore placenta O43.19- ☑
Baumgarten-Cruveilhier cirrhosis, disease or syndrome K74.69
Bauxite fibrosis (of lung) J63.1
Bayle's disease (general paresis) A52.17
Bazin's disease (primary) (tuberculous) A18.4
Beach ear — *see* Swimmer's, ear
Beaded hair (congenital) Q84.1
Béal conjunctivitis or syndrome B30.2
Beard's disease (neurasthenia) F48.8
Beat(s)
 atrial, premature I49.1
 ectopic I49.49
 elbow — *see* Bursitis, elbow
 escaped, heart I49.49
 hand — *see* Bursitis, hand
 knee — *see* Bursitis, knee

Beat(s) — *continued*
 premature I49.40
 atrial I49.1
 auricular I49.1
 supraventricular I49.1
Beau's
 disease or syndrome — *see* Degeneration, myocardial
 lines (transverse furrows on fingernails) L60.4
Bechterev's syndrome — *see* Spondylitis, ankylosing
Becker's
 cardiomyopathy I42.8
 disease
 idiopathic mural endomyocardial disease I42.3
 myotonia congenita, recessive form G71.12
 dystrophy G71.01
 pigmented hairy nevus D22.5
Beck's syndrome (anterior spinal artery occlusion) I65.8
Beckwith-Wiedemann syndrome Q87.3
Bed confinement status Z74.01
Bed sore — *see* Ulcer, pressure, by site
Bedbug bite(s) — *see* Bite(s), by site, superficial, insect
Bedclothes, asphyxiation or suffocation by — *see* Asphyxia, traumatic, due to, mechanical, trapped
Bednar's
 aphthae K12.0
 tumor — *see* Neoplasm, malignant, by site
Bedridden Z74.01
Bedsore — *see* Ulcer, pressure, by site
Bedwetting — *see* Enuresis
Bee sting (with allergic or anaphylactic shock) — *see* Toxicity, venom, arthropod, bee
Beer drinker's heart (disease) I42.6
Begbie's disease (exophthalmic goiter) — *see* Hyperthyroidism, with, goiter
Behavior
 antisocial
 adult Z72.811
 child or adolescent Z72.810
 disorder, disturbance — *see* Disorder, conduct
 disruptive — *see* Disorder, conduct
 drug seeking Z76.5
 inexplicable R46.2
 marked evasiveness R46.5
 obsessive-compulsive R46.81
 overactivity R46.3
 poor responsiveness R46.4
 self-damaging (life-style) Z72.89
 sleep-incompatible Z72.821
 slowness R46.4
 specified NEC R46.89
 strange (and inexplicable) R46.2
 suspiciousness R46.5
 type A pattern Z73.1
 undue concern or preoccupation with stressful events R46.6
 verbosity and circumstantial detail obscuring reason for contact R46.7
Behçet's disease or syndrome M35.2
Behr's disease — *see* Degeneration, macula
Beigel's disease or morbus (white piedra) B36.2
Bejel A65
Bekhterev's syndrome — *see* Spondylitis, ankylosing
Belching — *see* Eructation
Bell's
 mania F30.8
 palsy, paralysis G51.0
 infant or newborn P11.3
 spasm G51.3- ☑
Bence Jones albuminuria or proteinuria NEC R80.3
Bends T70.3 ☑
Benedikt's paralysis or syndrome G46.3
Benign (*see also* condition)
 prostatic hyperplasia — *see* Hyperplasia, prostate
Bennett's fracture (displaced) S62.21- ☑
Benson's disease — *see* Deposit, crystalline
Bent
 back (hysterical) F44.4
 nose M95.0
 congenital Q67.4
Bereavement (uncomplicated) Z63.4
Bergeron's disease (hysterical chorea) F44.4
Berger's disease — *see* Nephropathy, IgA
Beriberi (dry) E51.11
 heart (disease) E51.12
 polyneuropathy E51.11
 wet E51.12
 involving circulatory system E51.11

Berlin's disease or edema (traumatic) S05.8X- ☑
Berlock (berloque) **dermatitis** L56.2
Bernard-Horner syndrome G90.2
Bernard-Soulier disease or thrombopathia D69.1
Bernhardt (-Roth) **disease** — *see* Mononeuropathy, lower limb, meralgia paresthetica
Bernheim's syndrome — *see* Failure, heart, right
Bertielliasis B71.8
Berylliosis (lung) J63.2
Besnier-Boeck (-Schaumann) **disease** — *see* Sarcoidosis
Besnier's
 lupus pernio D86.3
 prurigo L20.0
Bestiality F65.89
Best's disease H35.50
Betalipoproteinemia, broad or floating E78.2
Beta-mercaptolactate-cysteine disulfiduria E72.09
Betting and gambling Z72.6
 pathological (compulsive) F63.0
Bezoar T18.9 ☑
 intestine T18.3 ☑
 stomach T18.2 ☑
Bezold's abscess — *see* Mastoiditis, acute
Bianchi's syndrome R48.8
Bicornate or bicornis uterus Q51.3
 in pregnancy or childbirth O34.00
 causing obstructed labor O65.5
Bicuspid aortic valve Q23.1
Biedl-Bardet syndrome Q87.89
Bielschowsky (-Jansky) **disease** E75.4
Biermer's (pernicious) anemia or disease D51.0
Biett's disease L93.0
Bifid (congenital)
 apex, heart Q24.8
 clitoris Q52.6
 kidney Q63.8
 nose Q30.2
 patella Q74.1
 scrotum Q55.29
 toe NEC Q74.2
 tongue Q38.3
 ureter Q62.8
 uterus Q51.3
 uvula Q35.7
Biforis uterus (suprasimplex) Q51.3
Bifurcation (congenital)
 gallbladder Q44.1
 kidney pelvis Q63.8
 renal pelvis Q63.8
 rib Q76.6
 tongue, congenital Q38.3
 trachea Q32.1
 ureter Q62.8
 urethra Q64.74
 vertebra Q76.49
Big spleen syndrome D73.1
Bigeminal pulse R00.8
Bilateral — *see* condition
Bile
 duct — *see* condition
 pigments in urine R82.2
Bilharziasis (*see also* Schistosomiasis)
 chyluria B65.0
 cutaneous B65.3
 galacturia B65.0
 hematochyluria B65.0
 intestinal B65.1
 lipemia B65.9
 lipuria B65.0
 oriental B65.2
 piarhemia B65.9
 pulmonary NOS B65.9 [J99]
 pneumonia B65.9 [J17]
 tropical hematuria B65.0
 vesical B65.0
Biliary — *see* condition
Bilirubin metabolism disorder E80.7
 specified NEC E80.6
Bilirubinemia, familial nonhemolytic E80.4
Bilirubinuria R82.2
Biliuria R82.2
Bilocular stomach K31.2
Binswanger's disease I67.3
Biparta, bipartite
 carpal scaphoid Q74.0
 patella Q74.1
 vagina Q52.10

Bird
- face Q75.8
- fancier's disease or lung J67.2

Birth
- complications in mother — see Delivery, complicated
- compression during NOS P15.9
- defect — see Anomaly
- immature (less than 37 completed weeks) — see Preterm, newborn
  - extremely (less than 28 completed weeks) — see Immaturity, extreme
- inattention, at or after — see Maltreatment, child, neglect
- injury NOS P15.9
  - basal ganglia P11.1
  - brachial plexus NEC P14.3
  - brain (compression) (pressure) P11.2
  - central nervous system NOS P11.9
  - cerebellum P11.1
  - cerebral hemorrhage P10.1
  - external genitalia P15.5
  - eye P15.3
  - face P15.4
  - fracture
    - bone P13.9
      - specified NEC P13.8
    - clavicle P13.4
    - femur P13.2
    - humerus P13.3
    - long bone, except femur P13.3
    - radius and ulna P13.3
    - skull P13.0
    - spine P11.5
    - tibia and fibula P13.3
  - intracranial P11.2
    - laceration or hemorrhage P10.9
      - specified NEC P10.8
  - intraventricular hemorrhage P10.2
  - laceration
    - brain P10.1
    - by scalpel P15.8
    - peripheral nerve P14.9
  - liver P15.0
  - meninges
    - brain P11.1
    - spinal cord P11.5
  - nerve
    - brachial plexus P14.3
    - cranial NEC (except facial) P11.4
    - facial P11.3
    - peripheral P14.9
    - phrenic (paralysis) P14.2
  - paralysis
    - facial nerve P11.3
    - spinal P11.5
  - penis P15.5
  - rupture
    - spinal cord P11.5
  - scalp P12.9
  - scalpel wound P15.8
  - scrotum P15.5
  - skull NEC P13.1
    - fracture P13.0
  - specified type NEC P15.8
  - spinal cord P11.5
  - spine P11.5
  - spleen P15.1
  - sternomastoid (hematoma) P15.2
  - subarachnoid hemorrhage P10.3
  - subcutaneous fat necrosis P15.6
  - subdural hemorrhage P10.0
  - tentorial tear P10.4
  - testes P15.5
  - vulva P15.5
- lack of care, at or after — see Maltreatment, child, neglect
- neglect, at or after — see Maltreatment, child, neglect
- palsy or paralysis, newborn, NOS (birth injury) P14.9
- premature (infant) — see Preterm, newborn
- shock, newborn P96.89
- trauma — see Birth, injury
- weight
  - low (2499 grams or less) — see Low, birthweight
    - extremely (999 grams or less) — see Low, birthweight, extreme
  - 4000 grams to 4499 grams P08.1
  - 4500 grams or more P08.0

Birthmark Q82.5

Birt-Hogg-Dube syndrome Q87.89
Bisalbuminemia E88.09
Biskra's button B55.1
Bite(s) (animal) (human)
- abdomen, abdominal
  - wall S31.159 ☑
    - with penetration into peritoneal cavity S31.659 ☑
    - epigastric region S31.152 ☑
      - with penetration into peritoneal cavity S31.652 ☑
    - left
      - lower quadrant S31.154 ☑
        - with penetration into peritoneal cavity S31.654 ☑
      - upper quadrant S31.151 ☑
        - with penetration into peritoneal cavity S31.651 ☑
    - periumbilic region S31.155 ☑
      - with penetration into peritoneal cavity S31.655 ☑
    - right
      - lower quadrant S31.153 ☑
        - with penetration into peritoneal cavity S31.653 ☑
      - upper quadrant S31.150 ☑
        - with penetration into peritoneal cavity S31.650 ☑
    - superficial NEC S30.871 ☑
      - insect S30.861 ☑
- alveolar (process) — see Bite, oral cavity
- amphibian (venomous) — see Venom, bite, amphibian
- animal (see also Bite, by site)
  - venomous — see Venom
- ankle S91.05- ☑
  - superficial NEC S90.57- ☑
    - insect S90.56- ☑
- antecubital space — see Bite, elbow
- anus S31.835 ☑
  - superficial NEC S30.877 ☑
    - insect S30.867 ☑
- arm (upper) S41.15- ☑
  - lower — see Bite, forearm
  - superficial NEC S40.87- ☑
    - insect S40.86- ☑
- arthropod NEC — see Venom, bite, arthropod
- auditory canal (external) (meatus) — see Bite, ear
- auricle, ear — see Bite, ear
- axilla — see Bite, arm
- back (see also Bite, thorax, back)
  - lower S31.050 ☑
    - with penetration into retroperitoneal space S31.051 ☑
  - superficial NEC S30.870 ☑
    - insect S30.860 ☑
- bedbug — see Bite(s), by site, superficial, insect
- breast S21.05- ☑
  - superficial NEC S20.17- ☑
    - insect S20.16- ☑
- brow — see Bite, head, specified site NEC
- buttock S31.805 ☑
  - left S31.825 ☑
  - right S31.815 ☑
  - superficial NEC S30.870 ☑
    - insect S30.860 ☑
- calf — see Bite, leg
- canaliculus lacrimalis — see Bite, eyelid
- canthus, eye — see Bite, eyelid
- centipede — see Toxicity, venom, arthropod, centipede
- cheek (external) S01.45- ☑
  - internal — see Bite, oral cavity
  - superficial NEC S00.87 ☑
    - insect S00.86 ☑
- chest wall — see Bite, thorax
- chigger B88.0
- chin — see Bite, head, specified site NEC
- clitoris — see Bite, vulva
- costal region — see Bite, thorax
- digit(s)
  - hand — see Bite, finger
  - toe — see Bite, toe
- ear (canal) (external) S01.35- ☑
  - superficial NEC S00.47- ☑
    - insect S00.46- ☑
- elbow S51.05- ☑
  - superficial NEC S50.37- ☑

Bite(s) — continued
- elbow — continued
  - superficial — continued
    - insect S50.36- ☑
- epididymis — see Bite, testis
- epigastric region — see Bite, abdomen
- epiglottis — see Bite, neck, specified site NEC
- esophagus, cervical S11.25 ☑
  - superficial NEC S10.17 ☑
    - insect S10.16 ☑
- eyebrow — see Bite, eyelid
- eyelid S01.15- ☑
  - superficial NEC S00.27- ☑
    - insect S00.26- ☑
- face NEC — see Bite, head, specified site NEC
- finger(s) S61.259 ☑
  - with
    - damage to nail S61.359 ☑
  - index S61.258 ☑
    - with
      - damage to nail S61.358 ☑
    - left S61.251 ☑
      - with
        - damage to nail S61.351 ☑
    - right S61.250 ☑
      - with
        - damage to nail S61.350 ☑
    - superficial NEC S60.478 ☑
      - insect S60.46- ☑
  - little S61.25- ☑
    - with
      - damage to nail S61.35- ☑
    - superficial NEC S60.47- ☑
      - insect S60.46- ☑
  - middle S61.25- ☑
    - with
      - damage to nail S61.35- ☑
    - superficial NEC S60.47- ☑
      - insect S60.46- ☑
  - ring S61.25- ☑
    - with
      - damage to nail S61.35- ☑
    - superficial NEC S60.47- ☑
      - insect S60.46- ☑
  - superficial NEC S60.479 ☑
    - insect S60.469 ☑
  - thumb — see Bite, thumb
- flank — see Bite, abdomen, wall
- flea — see Bite, by site, superficial, insect
- foot (except toe(s) alone) S91.35- ☑
  - superficial NEC S90.87- ☑
    - insect S90.86- ☑
  - toe — see Bite, toe
- forearm S51.85- ☑
  - elbow only — see Bite, elbow
  - superficial NEC S50.87- ☑
    - insect S50.86- ☑
- forehead — see Bite, head, specified site NEC
- genital organs, external
  - female S31.552 ☑
    - superficial NEC S30.876 ☑
      - insect S30.866 ☑
    - vagina and vulva — see Bite, vulva
  - male S31.551 ☑
    - penis — see Bite, penis
    - scrotum — see Bite, scrotum
    - superficial NEC S30.875 ☑
      - insect S30.865 ☑
    - testes — see Bite, testis
- groin — see Bite, abdomen, wall
- gum — see Bite, oral cavity
- hand S61.45- ☑
  - finger — see Bite, finger
  - superficial NEC S60.57- ☑
    - insect S60.56- ☑
  - thumb — see Bite, thumb
- head S01.95 ☑
  - cheek — see Bite, cheek
  - ear — see Bite, ear
  - eyelid — see Bite, eyelid
  - lip — see Bite, lip
  - nose — see Bite, nose
  - oral cavity — see Bite, oral cavity
  - scalp — see Bite, scalp
  - specified site NEC S01.85 ☑
    - superficial NEC S00.87 ☑

Bite(s) — *continued*
 head — *continued*
  specified site — *continued*
   superficial — *continued*
    insect S00.86 ☑
   superficial NEC S00.97 ☑
    insect S00.96 ☑
   temporomandibular area — *see* Bite, cheek
 heel — *see* Bite, foot
 hip S71.05- ☑
  superficial NEC S70.27- ☑
   insect S70.26- ☑
 hymen S31.45 ☑
 hypochondrium — *see* Bite, abdomen, wall
 hypogastric region — *see* Bite, abdomen, wall
 inguinal region — *see* Bite, abdomen, wall
 insect — *see* Bite, by site, superficial, insect
 instep — *see* Bite, foot
 interscapular region — *see* Bite, thorax, back
 jaw — *see* Bite, head, specified site NEC
 knee S81.05- ☑
  superficial NEC S80.27- ☑
   insect S80.26- ☑
 labium (majus) (minus) — *see* Bite, vulva
 lacrimal duct — *see* Bite, eyelid
 larynx S11.015 ☑
  superficial NEC S10.17- ☑
   insect S10.16 ☑
 leg (lower) S81.85- ☑
  ankle — *see* Bite, ankle
  foot — *see* Bite, foot
  knee — *see* Bite, knee
  superficial NEC S80.87- ☑
   insect S80.86- ☑
  toe — *see* Bite, toe
  upper — *see* Bite, thigh
 lip S01.551 ☑
  superficial NEC S00.571 ☑
   insect S00.561 ☑
 lizard (venomous) — *see* Venom, bite, reptile
 loin — *see* Bite, abdomen, wall
 lower back — *see* Bite, back, lower
 lumbar region — *see* Bite, back, lower
 malar region — *see* Bite, head, specified site NEC
 mammary — *see* Bite, breast
 marine animals (venomous) — *see* Toxicity, venom, marine animal
 mastoid region — *see* Bite, head, specified site NEC
 mouth — *see* Bite, oral cavity
 nail
  finger — *see* Bite, finger
  toe — *see* Bite, toe
 nape — *see* Bite, neck, specified site NEC
 nasal (septum) (sinus) — *see* Bite, nose
 nasopharynx — *see* Bite, head, specified site NEC
 neck S11.95 ☑
  involving
   cervical esophagus — *see* Bite, esophagus, cervical
   larynx — *see* Bite, larynx
   pharynx — *see* Bite, pharynx
   thyroid gland S11.15 ☑
   trachea — *see* Bite, trachea
  specified site NEC S11.85 ☑
   superficial NEC S10.87 ☑
    insect S10.86 ☑
  superficial NEC S10.97 ☑
   insect S10.96 ☑
  throat S11.85 ☑
   superficial NEC S10.17 ☑
    insect S10.16 ☑
 nose (septum) (sinus) S01.25 ☑
  superficial NEC S00.37 ☑
   insect S00.36 ☑
 occipital region — *see* Bite, scalp
 oral cavity S01.552 ☑
  superficial NEC S00.572 ☑
   insect S00.562 ☑
 orbital region — *see* Bite, eyelid
 palate — *see* Bite, oral cavity
 palm — *see* Bite, hand
 parietal region — *see* Bite, scalp
 pelvis S31.050 ☑
  with penetration into retroperitoneal space S31.051 ☑
  superficial NEC S30.870 ☑

Bite(s) — *continued*
 pelvis — *continued*
  superficial — *continued*
   insect S30.860 ☑
 penis S31.25 ☑
  superficial NEC S30.872 ☑
   insect S30.862 ☑
 perineum
  female — *see* Bite, vulva
  male — *see* Bite, pelvis
 periocular area (with or without lacrimal passages) — *see* Bite, eyelid
 phalanges
  finger — *see* Bite, finger
  toe — *see* Bite, toe
 pharynx S11.25 ☑
  superficial NEC S10.17 ☑
   insect S10.16 ☑
 pinna — *see* Bite, ear
 poisonous — *see* Venom
 popliteal space — *see* Bite, knee
 prepuce — *see* Bite, penis
 pubic region — *see* Bite, abdomen, wall
 rectovaginal septum — *see* Bite, vulva
 red bug B88.0
 reptile NEC (*see also* Venom, bite, reptile)
  nonvenomous — *see* Bite, by site
  snake — *see* Venom, bite, snake
 sacral region — *see* Bite, back, lower
 sacroiliac region — *see* Bite, back, lower
 salivary gland — *see* Bite, oral cavity
 scalp S01.05 ☑
  superficial NEC S00.07 ☑
   insect S00.06 ☑
 scapular region — *see* Bite, shoulder
 scrotum S31.35 ☑
  superficial NEC S30.873 ☑
   insect S30.863 ☑
 sea-snake (venomous) — *see* Toxicity, venom, snake, sea snake
 shin — *see* Bite, leg
 shoulder S41.05- ☑
  superficial NEC S40.27- ☑
   insect S40.26- ☑
 snake (*see also* Venom, bite, snake)
  nonvenomous — *see* Bite, by site
 spermatic cord — *see* Bite, testis
 spider (venomous) — *see* Toxicity, venom, spider
  nonvenomous — *see* Bite, by site, superficial, insect
 sternal region — *see* Bite, thorax, front
 submaxillary region — *see* Bite, head, specified site NEC
 submental region — *see* Bite, head, specified site NEC
 subungual
  finger(s) — *see* Bite, finger
  toe — *see* Bite, toe
 superficial — *see* Bite, by site, superficial
 supraclavicular fossa S11.85 ☑
 supraorbital — *see* Bite, head, specified site NEC
 temple, temporal region — *see* Bite, head, specified site NEC
 temporomandibular area — *see* Bite, cheek
 testis S31.35 ☑
  superficial NEC S30.873 ☑
   insect S30.863 ☑
 thigh S71.15- ☑
  superficial NEC S70.37- ☑
   insect S70.36- ☑
 thorax, thoracic (wall) S21.95 ☑
  back S21.25- ☑
   with penetration into thoracic cavity S21.45- ☑
  breast — *see* Bite, breast
  front S21.15- ☑
   with penetration into thoracic cavity S21.35- ☑
  superficial NEC S20.97 ☑
   back S20.47- ☑
   front S20.37- ☑
   insect S20.96 ☑
    back S20.46- ☑
    front S20.36- ☑
 throat — *see* Bite, neck, throat
 thumb S61.05- ☑
  with
   damage to nail S61.15- ☑
  superficial NEC S60.37- ☑
   insect S60.36- ☑

Bite(s) — *continued*
 thyroid S11.15 ☑
  superficial NEC S10.87 ☑
   insect S10.86 ☑
 toe(s) S91.15- ☑
  with
   damage to nail S91.25- ☑
  great S91.15- ☑
   with
    damage to nail S91.25- ☑
  lesser S91.15- ☑
   with
    damage to nail S91.25- ☑
  superficial NEC S90.47- ☑
   great S90.47- ☑
   insect S90.46- ☑
    great S90.46- ☑
 tongue S01.552 ☑
 trachea S11.025 ☑
  superficial NEC S10.17 ☑
   insect S10.16 ☑
 tunica vaginalis — *see* Bite, testis
 tympanum, tympanic membrane — *see* Bite, ear
 umbilical region S31.155 ☑
 uvula — *see* Bite, oral cavity
 vagina — *see* Bite, vulva
 venomous — *see* Venom
 vocal cords S11.035 ☑
  superficial NEC S10.17 ☑
   insect S10.16 ☑
 vulva S31.45 ☑
  superficial NEC S30.874 ☑
   insect S30.864 ☑
 wrist S61.55- ☑
  superficial NEC S60.87- ☑
   insect S60.86- ☑
Biting, cheek or lip K13.1
Biventricular failure (heart) I50.82
Björck (-Thorson) **syndrome** (malignant carcinoid) E34.0
Black
 death A20.9
 eye S00.1- ☑
 hairy tongue K14.3
 heel (foot) S90.3- ☑
 lung (disease) J60
 palm (hand) S60.22- ☑
Blackfan-Diamond anemia or syndrome (congenital hypoplastic anemia) D61.01
Blackhead L70.0
Blackout R55
Bladder — *see* condition
Blast (air) (hydraulic) (immersion) (underwater)
 blindness S05.8X- ☑
 injury
  abdomen or thorax — *see* Injury, by site
  ear (acoustic nerve trauma) — *see* Injury, nerve, acoustic, specified type NEC
  syndrome NEC T70.8 ☑
Blastoma — *see* Neoplasm, malignant, by site
 pulmonary — *see* Neoplasm, lung, malignant
Blastomycosis, blastomycotic B40.9
 Brazilian — *see* Paracoccidioidomycosis
 cutaneous B40.3
 disseminated B40.7
 European — *see* Cryptococcosis
 generalized B40.7
 keloidal B48.0
 North American B40.9
 primary pulmonary B40.0
 pulmonary B40.2
  acute B40.0
  chronic B40.1
 skin B40.3
 South American — *see* Paracoccidioidomycosis
 specified NEC B40.89
Bleb(s) R23.8
 emphysematous (lung) (solitary) J43.9
 endophthalmitis H59.43
 filtering (vitreous), after glaucoma surgery Z98.83
 inflamed (infected), postprocedural H59.40
  stage 1 H59.41
  stage 2 H59.42
  stage 3 H59.43
 lung (ruptured) J43.9
  congenital — *see* Atelectasis
  newborn P25.8
 subpleural (emphysematous) J43.9

Blebitis, postprocedural H59.40
  stage 1 H59.41
  stage 2 H59.42
  stage 3 H59.43
Bleeder (familial) (hereditary) — *see* Hemophilia
Bleeding (*see also* Hemorrhage)
  anal K62.5
  anovulatory N97.0
  atonic, following delivery O72.1
  capillary I78.8
    puerperal O72.2
  contact (postcoital) N93.0
  due to uterine subinvolution N85.3
  ear — *see* Otorrhagia
  excessive, associated with menopausal onset N92.4
  familial — *see* Defect, coagulation
  following intercourse N93.0
  gastrointestinal K92.2
  hemorrhoids — *see* Hemorrhoids
  intermenstrual (regular) N92.3
    irregular N92.1
  intraoperative — *see* Complication, intraoperative, hemorrhage
  irregular N92.6
  menopausal N92.4
  newborn, intraventricular — *see* Newborn, affected by, hemorrhage, intraventricular
  nipple N64.59
  nose R04.0
  ovulation N92.3
  postclimacteric N95.0
  postcoital N93.0
  postmenopausal N95.0
  postoperative — *see* Complication, postprocedural, hemorrhage
  preclimacteric N92.4
  pre-pubertal vaginal N93.1
  puberty (excessive, with onset of menstrual periods) N92.2
  rectum, rectal K62.5
    newborn P54.2
  tendencies — *see* Defect, coagulation
  throat R04.1
  tooth socket (post-extraction) K91.840
  umbilical stump P51.9
  uterus, uterine NEC N93.9
    climacteric N92.4
    dysfunctional or functional N93.8
    menopausal N92.4
    preclimacteric or premenopausal N92.4
    unrelated to menstrual cycle N93.9
  vagina, vaginal (abnormal) N93.9
    dysfunctional or functional N93.8
    newborn P54.6
    pre-pubertal N93.1
  vicarious N94.89
Blennorrhagia, blennorrhagic — *see* Gonorrhea
Blennorrhea (acute) (chronic) (*see also* Gonorrhea)
  inclusion (neonatal) (newborn) P39.1
  lower genitourinary tract (gonococcal) A54.00
  neonatorum (gonococcal ophthalmia) A54.31
Blepharelosis — *see* Entropion
Blepharitis (angularis) (ciliaris) (eyelid) (marginal) (nonulcerative) H01.009
  herpes zoster B02.39
  left H01.006
    lower H01.005
    upper H01.004
    upper and lower H01.00B
  right H01.003
    lower H01.002
    upper H01.001
    upper and lower H01.00A
  squamous H01.029
    left H01.026
      lower H01.025
      upper H01.024
      upper and lower H01.02B
    right H01.023
      lower H01.022
      upper H01.021
      upper and lower H01.02A
  ulcerative H01.019
    left H01.016
      lower H01.015
      upper H01.014
      upper and lower H01.01B
    right H01.013

Blepharitis — *continued*
  ulcerative — *continued*
    right — *continued*
      lower H01.012
      upper H01.011
      upper and lower H01.01A
Blepharochalasis H02.30
  congenital Q10.0
  left H02.36
    lower H02.35
    upper H02.34
  right H02.33
    lower H02.32
    upper H02.31
Blepharoclonus H02.59
Blepharoconjunctivitis H10.50- ☑
  angular H10.52- ☑
  contact H10.53- ☑
  ligneous H10.51- ☑
Blepharophimosis (eyelid) H02.529
  congenital Q10.3
  left H02.526
    lower H02.525
    upper H02.524
  right H02.523
    lower H02.522
    upper H02.521
Blepharoptosis H02.40- ☑
  congenital Q10.0
  mechanical H02.41- ☑
  myogenic H02.42- ☑
  neurogenic H02.43- ☑
  paralytic H02.43- ☑
Blepharopyorrhea, gonococcal A54.39
Blepharospasm G24.5
  drug induced G24.01
Blighted ovum O02.0
Blind (*see also* Blindness)
  bronchus (congenital) Q32.4
  loop syndrome K90.2
    congenital Q43.8
  sac, fallopian tube (congenital) Q50.6
  spot, enlarged — *see* Defect, visual field, localized, scotoma, blind spot area
  tract or tube, congenital NEC — *see* Atresia, by site
Blindness (acquired) (congenital) (both eyes) H54.0X- ☑
  blast S05.8X- ☑
  color — *see* Deficiency, color vision
  concussion S05.8X- ☑
  cortical H47.619
    left brain H47.612
    right brain H47.611
  day H53.11
  due to injury (current episode) S05.9- ☑
    sequelae — *code to* injury with seventh character S
  eclipse (total) — *see* Retinopathy, solar
  emotional (hysterical) F44.6
  face H53.16
  hysterical F44.6
  legal (both eyes) (USA definition) H54.8
  mind R48.8
  night H53.60
    abnormal dark adaptation curve H53.61
    acquired H53.62
    congenital H53.63
    specified type NEC H53.69
    vitamin A deficiency E50.5
  one eye (other eye normal) H54.40
    left (normal vision on right) H54.42- ☑
      low vision on right H54.12- ☑
    low vision, other eye H54.10
    right (normal vision on left) H54.41- ☑
      low vision on left H54.11- ☑
  psychic R48.8
  river B73.01
  snow — *see* Photokeratitis
  sun, solar — *see* Retinopathy, solar
  transient — *see* Disturbance, vision, subjective, loss, transient
  traumatic (current episode) S05.9- ☑
  word (developmental) F81.0
    acquired R48.0
    secondary to organic lesion R48.0
Blister (nonthermal)
  abdominal wall S30.821 ☑
  alveolar process S00.522 ☑

Blister — *continued*
  ankle S90.52- ☑
  antecubital space — *see* Blister, elbow
  anus S30.827 ☑
  arm (upper) S40.82- ☑
  auditory canal — *see* Blister, ear
  auricle — *see* Blister, ear
  axilla — *see* Blister, arm
  back, lower S30.820 ☑
  beetle dermatitis L24.89
  breast S20.12- ☑
  brow S00.82 ☑
  calf — *see* Blister, leg
  canthus — *see* Blister, eyelid
  cheek S00.82 ☑
    internal S00.522 ☑
  chest wall — *see* Blister, thorax
  chin S00.82 ☑
  costal region — *see* Blister, thorax
  digit(s)
    foot — *see* Blister, toe
    hand — *see* Blister, finger
  due to burn — *see* Burn, by site, second degree
  ear S00.42- ☑
  elbow S50.32- ☑
  epiglottis S10.12 ☑
  esophagus, cervical S10.12 ☑
  eyebrow — *see* Blister, eyelid
  eyelid S00.22- ☑
  face S00.82 ☑
  fever B00.1
  finger(s) S60.429 ☑
    index S60.42- ☑
    little S60.42- ☑
    middle S60.42- ☑
    ring S60.42- ☑
  foot (except toe(s) alone) S90.82- ☑
    toe — *see* Blister, toe
  forearm S50.82- ☑
    elbow only — *see* Blister, elbow
  forehead S00.82 ☑
  fracture — *omit code*
  genital organ
    female S30.826 ☑
    male S30.825 ☑
  gum S00.522 ☑
  hand S60.52- ☑
  head S00.92 ☑
    ear — *see* Blister, ear
    eyelid — *see* Blister, eyelid
    lip S00.521 ☑
    nose S00.32 ☑
    oral cavity S00.522 ☑
    scalp S00.02 ☑
    specified site NEC S00.82 ☑
  heel — *see* Blister, foot
  hip S70.22- ☑
  interscapular region S20.429 ☑
  jaw S00.82 ☑
  knee S80.22- ☑
  larynx S10.12 ☑
  leg (lower) S80.82- ☑
    knee — *see* Blister, knee
    upper — *see* Blister, thigh
  lip S00.521 ☑
  malar region S00.82 ☑
  mammary — *see* Blister, breast
  mastoid region S00.82 ☑
  mouth S00.522 ☑
  multiple, skin, nontraumatic R23.8
  nail
    finger — *see* Blister, finger
    toe — *see* Blister, toe
  nasal S00.32 ☑
  neck S10.92 ☑
    specified site NEC S10.82 ☑
    throat S10.12 ☑
  nose S00.32 ☑
  occipital region S00.02 ☑
  oral cavity S00.522 ☑
  orbital region — *see* Blister, eyelid
  palate S00.522 ☑
  palm — *see* Blister, hand
  parietal region S00.02 ☑
  pelvis S30.820 ☑
  penis S30.822 ☑

Subterms under main terms may continue to next column or page   ☑ Additional Character Required — Refer to the Tabular List for Character Selection   39

Blebitis, postprocedural — Blister

Index

Blister — *continued*
- periocular area — *see* Blister, eyelid
- phalanges
  - finger — *see* Blister, finger
  - toe — *see* Blister, toe
- pharynx S10.12 ☑
- pinna — *see* Blister, ear
- popliteal space — *see* Blister, knee
- scalp S00.02 ☑
- scapular region — *see* Blister, shoulder
- scrotum S30.823 ☑
- shin — *see* Blister, leg
- shoulder S40.22- ☑
- sternal region S20.329 ☑
- submaxillary region S00.82 ☑
- submental region S00.82 ☑
- subungual
  - finger(s) — *see* Blister, finger
  - toe(s) — *see* Blister, toe
- supraclavicular fossa S10.82 ☑
- supraorbital S00.82 ☑
- temple S00.82 ☑
- temporal region S00.82 ☑
- testis S30.823 ☑
- thermal — *see* Burn, second degree, by site
- thigh S70.32- ☑
- thorax, thoracic (wall) S20.92 ☑
  - back S20.42- ☑
  - front S20.32- ☑
- throat S10.12 ☑
- thumb S60.32- ☑
- toe(s) S90.42- ☑
  - great S90.42- ☑
- tongue S00.522 ☑
- trachea S10.12 ☑
- tympanum, tympanic membrane — *see* Blister, ear
- upper arm — *see* Blister, arm (upper)
- uvula S00.522 ☑
- vagina S30.824 ☑
- vocal cords S10.12 ☑
- vulva S30.824 ☑
- wrist S60.82- ☑

Bloating R14.0
Bloch-Sulzberger disease or syndrome Q82.3
Block, blocked
- alveolocapillary J84.10
- arborization (heart) I45.5
- arrhythmic I45.9
- atrioventricular (incomplete) (partial) I44.30
  - with atrioventricular dissociation I44.2
  - complete I44.2
    - congenital Q24.6
  - congenital Q24.6
  - first degree I44.0
  - second degree (types I and II) I44.1
  - specified NEC I44.39
  - third degree I44.2
  - types I and II I44.1
- auriculoventricular — *see* Block, atrioventricular
- bifascicular (cardiac) I45.2
- bundle-branch (complete) (false) (incomplete) I45.4
  - bilateral I45.2
  - left I44.7
    - with right bundle branch block I45.2
    - hemiblock I44.60
      - anterior I44.4
      - posterior I44.5
    - incomplete I44.7
      - with right bundle branch block I45.2
  - right I45.10
    - with
      - left bundle branch block I45.2
      - left fascicular block I45.2
    - specified NEC I45.19
  - Wilson's type I45.19
- cardiac I45.9
- conduction I45.9
  - complete I44.2
- fascicular (left) I44.60
  - anterior I44.4
  - posterior I44.5
  - right I45.0
  - specified NEC I44.69
- foramen Magendie (acquired) G91.1
  - congenital Q03.1
    - with spina bifida — *see* Spina bifida, by site, with hydrocephalus

Block, blocked — *continued*
- heart I45.9
  - bundle branch I45.4
    - bilateral I45.2
  - complete (atrioventricular) I44.2
  - congenital Q24.6
  - first degree (atrioventricular) I44.0
  - second degree (atrioventricular) I44.1
  - specified type NEC I45.5
  - third degree (atrioventricular) I44.2
- hepatic vein I82.0
- intraventricular (nonspecific) I45.4
  - bundle branch
    - bilateral I45.2
- kidney N28.9
  - postcystoscopic or postprocedural N99.0
- Mobitz (types I and II) I44.1
- myocardial — *see* Block, heart
- nodal I45.5
- organ or site, congenital NEC — *see* Atresia, by site
- portal (vein) I81
- second degree (types I and II) I44.1
- sinoatrial I45.5
- sinoauricular I45.5
- third degree I44.2
- trifascicular I45.3
- tubal N97.1
- vein NOS I82.90
- Wenckebach (types I and II) I44.1

Blockage — *see* Obstruction
Blocq's disease F44.4
Blood
- constituents, abnormal R78.9
- disease D75.9
- donor — *see* Donor, blood
- dyscrasia D75.9
  - with
    - abortion — *see* Abortion, by type, complicated by, hemorrhage
    - ectopic pregnancy O08.1
    - molar pregnancy O08.1
  - following ectopic or molar pregnancy O08.1
  - newborn P61.9
  - puerperal, postpartum O72.3
- flukes NEC — *see* Schistosomiasis
- in
  - feces K92.1
    - occult R19.5
  - urine — *see* Hematuria
- mole O02.0
- occult in feces R19.5
- pressure
  - decreased, due to shock following injury T79.4 ☑
  - examination only Z01.30
  - fluctuating I99.8
  - high — *see* Hypertension
    - borderline R03.0
    - incidental reading, without diagnosis of hypertension R03.0
  - low (*see also* Hypotension)
    - incidental reading, without diagnosis of hypotension R03.1
- spitting — *see* Hemoptysis
- staining cornea — *see* Pigmentation, cornea, stromal
- transfusion
  - reaction or complication — *see* Complications, transfusion
- type
  - A (Rh positive) Z67.10
    - Rh negative Z67.11
  - AB (Rh positive) Z67.30
    - Rh negative Z67.31
  - B (Rh positive) Z67.20
    - Rh negative Z67.21
  - O (Rh positive) Z67.40
    - Rh negative Z67.41
  - Rh (positive) Z67.90
    - negative Z67.91
- vessel rupture — *see* Hemorrhage
- vomiting — *see* Hematemesis

Blood-forming organs, disease D75.9
Bloodgood's disease — *see* Mastopathy, cystic
Bloom (-Machacek)(-Torre) **syndrome** Q82.8
Blount's disease or osteochondrosis — *see* Osteochondrosis, juvenile, tibia
Blue
- baby Q24.9
- diaper syndrome E72.09

Blue — *continued*
- dome cyst (breast) — *see* Cyst, breast
- dot cataract Q12.0
- nevus D22.9
- sclera Q13.5
  - with fragility of bone and deafness Q78.0
- toe syndrome I75.02- ☑
Blueness — *see* Cyanosis
Blues, postpartal O90.6
- baby O90.6
Blurring, visual H53.8
Blushing (abnormal) (excessive) R23.2
BMI — *see* Body, mass index
Boarder, hospital NEC Z76.4
- accompanying sick person Z76.3
- healthy infant or child Z76.2
  - foundling Z76.1
Bockhart's impetigo L01.02
Bodechtel-Guttman disease (subacute sclerosing panencephalitis) A81.1
Boder-Sedgwick syndrome (ataxia-telangiectasia) G11.3
Body, bodies
- Aschoff's — *see* Myocarditis, rheumatic
- asteroid, vitreous — *see* Deposit, crystalline
- cytoid (retina) — *see* Occlusion, artery, retina
- drusen (degenerative) (macula) (retinal) (*see also* Degeneration, macula, drusen)
  - optic disc — *see* Drusen, optic disc
- foreign — *see* Foreign body
- loose
  - joint, except knee — *see* Loose, body, joint
    - knee M23.4- ☑
  - sheath, tendon — *see* Disorder, tendon, specified type NEC
- mass index (BMI)
  - adult
    - 19.9 or less Z68.1
    - 20.0-20.9 Z68.20
    - 21.0-21.9 Z68.21
    - 22.0-22.9 Z68.22
    - 23.0-23.9 Z68.23
    - 24.0-24.9 Z68.24
    - 25.0-25.9 Z68.25
    - 26.0-26.9 Z68.26
    - 27.0-27.9 Z68.27
    - 28.0-28.9 Z68.28
    - 29.0-29.9 Z68.29
    - 30.0-30.9 Z68.30
    - 31.0-31.9 Z68.31
    - 32.0-32.9 Z68.32
    - 33.0-33.9 Z68.33
    - 34.0-34.9 Z68.34
    - 35.0-35.9 Z68.35
    - 36.0-36.9 Z68.36
    - 37.0-37.9 Z68.37
    - 38.0-38.9 Z68.38
    - 39.0-39.9 Z68.39
    - 40.0-44.9 Z68.41
    - 45.0-49.9 Z68.42
    - 50.0-59.9 Z68.43
    - 60.0-69.9 Z68.44
    - 70 and over Z68.45
  - pediatric
    - 5th percentile to less than 85th percentile for age Z68.52
    - 85th percentile to less than 95th percentile for age Z68.53
    - greater than or equal to ninety-fifth percentile for age Z68.54
    - less than fifth percentile for age Z68.51
- Mooser's A75.2
- rice (*see also* Loose, body, joint)
  - knee M23.4- ☑
- rocking F98.4
Boeck's
- disease or sarcoid — *see* Sarcoidosis
- lupoid (miliary) D86.3
Boerhaave's syndrome (spontaneous esophageal rupture) K22.3
Boggy
- cervix N88.8
- uterus N85.8
Boil (*see also* Furuncle, by site)
- Aleppo B55.1
- Baghdad B55.1
- Delhi B55.1
- lacrimal
  - gland — *see* Dacryoadenitis

Boil — *continued*
  lacrimal — *continued*
    passages (duct) (sac) — *see* Inflammation, lacrimal, passages, acute
    Natal B55.1
    orbit, orbital — *see* Abscess, orbit
    tropical B55.1
Bold hives — *see* Urticaria
Bombé, iris — *see* Membrane, pupillary
Bone — *see* condition
Bonnevie-Ullrich syndrome (*see also* Turner's syndrome) Q87.1
Bonnier's syndrome H81.8 ☑
Bonvale dam fever T73.3 ☑
Bony block of joint — *see* Ankylosis
BOOP (bronchiolitis obliterans organized pneumonia) J84.89
Borderline
  diabetes mellitus R73.03
  hypertension R03.0
  osteopenia M85.8- ☑
  pelvis, with obstruction during labor O65.1
  personality F60.3
Borna disease A83.9
Bornholm disease B33.0
Boston exanthem A88.0
Botalli, ductus (patent) (persistent) Q25.0
Bothriocephalus latus infestation B70.0
Botulism (foodborne intoxication) A05.1
  infant A48.51
  non-foodborne A48.52
  wound A48.52
Bouba — *see* Yaws
Bouchard's nodes (with arthropathy) M15.2
Bouffée délirante F23
Bouillaud's disease or syndrome (rheumatic heart disease) I01.9
Bourneville's disease Q85.1
Boutonnière deformity (finger) — *see* Deformity, finger, boutonnière
Bouveret (-Hoffmann) **syndrome** (paroxysmal tachycardia) I47.9
Bovine heart — *see* Hypertrophy, cardiac
Bowel — *see* condition
Bowen's
  dermatosis (precancerous) — *see* Neoplasm, skin, in situ
  disease — *see* Neoplasm, skin, in situ
  epithelioma — *see* Neoplasm, skin, in situ
  type
    epidermoid carcinoma-in-situ — *see* Neoplasm, skin, in situ
    intraepidermal squamous cell carcinoma — *see* Neoplasm, skin, in situ
Bowing
  femur (*see also* Deformity, limb, specified type NEC, thigh)
    congenital Q68.3
  fibula (*see also* Deformity, limb, specified type NEC, lower leg)
    congenital Q68.4
  forearm — *see* Deformity, limb, specified type NEC, forearm
  leg(s), long bones, congenital Q68.5
  radius — *see* Deformity, limb, specified type NEC, forearm
  tibia (*see also* Deformity, limb, specified type NEC, lower leg)
    congenital Q68.4
Bowleg(s) (acquired) M21.16- ☑
  congenital Q68.5
  rachitic E64.3
Boyd's dysentery A03.2
Brachial — *see* condition
Brachycardia R00.1
Brachycephaly Q75.0
Bradley's disease A08.19
Bradyarrhythmia, cardiac I49.8
Bradycardia (sinoatrial) (sinus) (vagal) R00.1
  neonatal P29.12
  reflex G90.09
  tachycardia syndrome I49.5
Bradykinesia R25.8
Bradypnea R06.89
Bradytachycardia I49.5
Brailsford's disease or osteochondrosis — *see* Osteochondrosis, juvenile, radius

Brain (*see also* condition)
  death G93.82
  syndrome — *see* Syndrome, brain
Branched-chain amino-acid disorder E71.2
Branchial — *see* condition
  cartilage, congenital Q18.2
Branchiogenic remnant (in neck) Q18.0
Brandt's syndrome (acrodermatitis enteropathica) E83.2
Brash (water) R12
Bravais-jacksonian epilepsy — *see* Epilepsy, localization-related, symptomatic, with simple partial seizures
Braxton Hicks contractions — *see* False, labor
Brazilian leishmaniasis B55.2
BRBPR K62.5
Break, retina (without detachment) H33.30- ☑
  with retinal detachment — *see* Detachment, retina
  horseshoe tear H33.31- ☑
  multiple H33.33- ☑
  round hole H33.32- ☑
Breakdown
  device, graft or implant (*see also* Complications, by site and type, mechanical) T85.618 ☑
    arterial graft NEC — *see* Complication, cardiovascular device, mechanical, vascular
    breast (implant) T85.41 ☑
    catheter NEC T85.618 ☑
      cystostomy T83.010 ☑
      dialysis (renal) T82.41 ☑
        intraperitoneal T85.611 ☑
      Hopkins T83.018 ☑
      ileostomy T83.018 ☑
      infusion NEC T82.514 ☑
        cranial T85.610- ☑
        epidural T85.610 ☑
        intrathecal T85.610 ☑
        spinal T85.610 ☑
        subarachnoid T85.610 ☑
        subdural T85.610 ☑
      nephrostomy T83.012 ☑
      urethral indwelling T83.011 ☑
      urinary NEC T83.018 ☑
      urostomy T83.018 ☑
    electronic (electrode) (pulse generator) (stimulator)
      bone T84.310 ☑
      cardiac T82.119 ☑
        electrode T82.110 ☑
        pulse generator T82.111 ☑
        specified NEC T82.118 ☑
      nervous system — *see* Complication, prosthetic device, mechanical, electronic nervous system stimulator
      urinary — *see* Complication, genitourinary, device, urinary, mechanical
    fixation, internal (orthopedic) NEC — *see* Complication, fixation device, mechanical
    gastrointestinal — *see* Complications, prosthetic device, mechanical, gastrointestinal device
    genital NEC T83.418 ☑
      intrauterine contraceptive device T83.31 ☑
      penile prosthesis (cylinder) (implanted) (pump) (resevoir) T83.410 ☑
      testicular prosthesis T83.411 ☑
    heart NEC — *see* Complication, cardiovascular device, mechanical
    intrathecal infusion pump T85.615 ☑
    joint prosthesis — *see* Complications..., joint prosthesis,internal, mechanical, by site
    nervous system, specified device NEC T85.615 ☑
    ocular NEC — *see* Complications, prosthetic device, mechanical, ocular device
    orthopedic NEC — *see* Complication, orthopedic, device, mechanical
    specified NEC T85.618 ☑
    subcutaneous device pocket
      nervous system prosthetic device, implant, or graft T85.890 ☑
      other internal prosthetic device, implant, or graft T85.898 ☑
    sutures, permanent T85.612 ☑
      used in bone repair — *see* Complications, fixation device, internal (orthopedic), mechanical
    urinary NEC T83.118 ☑
      graft T83.21 ☑
      sphincter, implanted T83.111 ☑
      stent (ileal conduit) (nephroureteral) T83.113 ☑

Breakdown — *continued*
  device, graft or implant (*see also* Complications, by site and type, mechanical) — *continued*
    urinary — *continued*
      stent — *continued*
        ureteral indwelling T83.112 ☑
      vascular NEC — *see* Complication, cardiovascular device, mechanical
      ventricular intracranial shunt T85.01 ☑
  nervous F48.8
  perineum O90.1
  respirator J95.850
    specified NEC J95.859
  ventilator J95.850
    specified NEC J95.859
Breast (*see also* condition)
  buds E30.1
    in newborn P96.89
  dense R92.2
  nodule (*see also* Lump, breast) N63.0
Breath
  foul R19.6
  holder, child R06.89
  holding spell R06.89
  shortness R06.02
Breathing
  labored — *see* Hyperventilation
  mouth R06.5
    causing malocclusion M26.5 ☑
  periodic R06.3
    high altitude G47.32
Breathlessness R06.81
Breda's disease — *see* Yaws
Breech presentation (mother) O32.1 ☑
  causing obstructed labor O64.1 ☑
  footling O32.8 ☑
    causing obstructed labor O64.8 ☑
  incomplete O32.8 ☑
    causing obstructed labor O64.8 ☑
Breisky's disease N90.4
Brennemann's syndrome I88.0
Brenner
  tumor (benign) D27.9
    borderline malignancy D39.1- ☑
    malignant C56 ☑
    proliferating D39.1- ☑
Bretonneau's disease or angina A36.0
Breus' mole O02.0
Brevicollis Q76.49
Brickmakers' anemia B76.9 [D63.8]
Bridge, myocardial Q24.5
Bright red blood per rectum (BRBPR) K62.5
Bright's disease (*see also* Nephritis)
  arteriosclerotic — *see* Hypertension, kidney
Brill (-Zinsser) **disease** (recrudescent typhus) A75.1
  flea-borne A75.2
  louse-borne A75.1
Brill-Symmers' disease C82.90
Brion-Kayser disease — *see* Fever, parathyroid
Briquet's disorder or syndrome F45.0
Brissaud's
  infantilism or dwarfism E23.0
  motor-verbal tic F95.2
Brittle
  bones disease Q78.0
  nails L60.3
    congenital Q84.6
Broad (*see also* condition)
  beta disease E78.2
  ligament laceration syndrome N83.8
Broad- or floating-betalipoproteinemia E78.2
Brock's syndrome (atelectasis due to enlarged lymph nodes) J98.19
Brocq-Duhring disease (dermatitis herpetiformis) L13.0
Brodie's abscess or disease M86.8X- ☑
Broken
  arches (*see also* Deformity, limb, flat foot)
  arm (meaning upper limb) — *see* Fracture, arm
  back — *see* Fracture, vertebra
  bone — *see* Fracture
  implant or internal device — *see* Complications, by site and type, mechanical
  leg (meaning lower limb) — *see* Fracture, leg
  nose S02.2 ☑
  tooth, teeth — *see* Fracture, tooth
Bromhidrosis, bromidrosis L75.0
Bromidism, bromism G92

Bromidism, bromism — *continued*
  due to
    correct substance properly administered — *see* Table of Drugs and Chemicals, by drug, adverse effect
    overdose or wrong substance given or taken — *see* Table of Drugs and Chemicals, by drug, poisoning
  chronic (dependence) F13.20
Bromidrosiphobia F40.298
Bronchi, bronchial — *see* condition
Bronchiectasis (cylindrical) (diffuse) (fusiform) (localized) (saccular) J47.9
  with
    acute
      bronchitis J47.0
      lower respiratory infection J47.0
    exacerbation (acute) J47.1
  congenital Q33.4
  tuberculous NEC — *see* Tuberculosis, pulmonary
Bronchiolectasis — *see* Bronchiectasis
Bronchiolitis (acute) (infective) (subacute) J21.9
  with
    bronchospasm or obstruction J21.9
    influenza, flu or grippe — *see* Influenza, with, respiratory manifestations NEC
  chemical (chronic) J68.4
    acute J68.0
  chronic (fibrosing) (obliterative) J44.9
  due to
    external agent — *see* Bronchitis, acute, due to
    human metapneumovirus J21.1
    respiratory syncytial virus J21.0
    specified organism NEC J21.8
  fibrosa obliterans J44.9
  influenzal — *see* Influenza, with, respiratory manifestations NEC
  obliterans J42
    with organizing pneumonia (BOOP) J84.89
  obliterative (chronic) (subacute) J44.9
    due to fumes or vapors J68.4
    due to chemicals, gases, fumes or vapors (inhalation) J68.4
  respiratory, interstitial lung disease J84.115
Bronchitis (diffuse) (fibrinous) (hypostatic) (infective) (membranous) J40
  with
    influenza, flu or grippe — *see* Influenza, with, respiratory manifestations NEC
    obstruction (airway) (lung) J44.9
    tracheitis (15 years of age and above) J40
      acute or subacute J20.9
      chronic J42
      under 15 years of age J20.9
  acute or subacute (with bronchospasm or obstruction) J20.9
    with
      bronchiectasis J47.0
      chronic obstructive pulmonary disease J44.0
    chemical (due to gases, fumes or vapors) J68.0
    due to
      fumes or vapors J68.0
      Haemophilus influenzae J20.1
      Mycoplasma pneumoniae J20.0
      radiation J70.0
      specified organism NEC J20.8
      Streptococcus J20.2
      virus
        coxsackie J20.3
        echovirus J20.7
        parainfluenzae J20.4
        respiratory syncytial J20.5
        rhinovirus J20.6
    viral NEC J20.8
  allergic (acute) J45.909
    with
      exacerbation (acute) J45.901
      status asthmaticus J45.902
  arachidic T17.528 ☑
  aspiration (due to fumes or vapors) J68.0
  asthmatic J45.9 ☑
    chronic J44.9
      with
        acute lower respiratory infection J44.0
        exacerbation (acute) J44.1
  capillary — *see* Pneumonia, broncho
  caseous (tuberculous) A15.5
  Castellani's A69.8

Bronchitis — *continued*
  catarrhal (15 years of age and above) J40
    acute — *see* Bronchitis, acute
    chronic J41.0
    under 15 years of age J20.9
  chemical (acute) (subacute) J68.0
    chronic J68.4
    due to fumes or vapors J68.0
      chronic J68.4
  chronic J42
    with
      airways obstruction J44.9
      tracheitis (chronic) J42
    asthmatic (obstructive) J44.9
    catarrhal J41.0
    chemical (due to fumes or vapors) J68.4
    due to
      chemicals, gases, fumes or vapors (inhalation) J68.4
      radiation J70.1
      tobacco smoking J41.0
    emphysematous J44.9
    mucopurulent J41.1
    non-obstructive J41.0
    obliterans J44.9
    obstructive J44.9
    purulent J41.1
    simple J41.0
  croupous — *see* Bronchitis, acute
  due to gases, fumes or vapors (chemical) J68.0
  emphysematous (obstructive) J44.9
  exudative — *see* Bronchitis, acute
  fetid J41.1
  grippal — *see* Influenza, with, respiratory manifestations NEC
  in those under 15 years age — *see* Bronchitis, acute
    chronic — *see* Bronchitis, chronic
  influenzal — *see* Influenza, with, respiratory manifestations NEC
  mixed simple and mucopurulent J41.8
  moulder's J62.8
  mucopurulent (chronic) (recurrent) J41.1
    acute or subacute J20.9
    simple (mixed) J41.8
  obliterans (chronic) J44.9
  obstructive (chronic) (diffuse) J44.9
  pituitous J41.1
  pneumococcal, acute or subacute J20.2
  pseudomembranous, acute or subacute — *see* Bronchitis, acute
  purulent (chronic) (recurrent) J41.1
    acute or subacute — *see* Bronchitis, acute
  putrid J41.1
  senile (chronic) J42
  simple and mucopurulent (mixed) J41.8
  smokers' J41.0
  spirochetal NEC A69.8
  subacute — *see* Bronchitis, acute
  suppurative (chronic) J41.1
    acute or subacute — *see* Bronchitis, acute
  tuberculous A15.5
  under 15 years of age — *see* Bronchitis, acute
    chronic — *see* Bronchitis, chronic
  viral NEC, acute or subacute (*see also* Bronchitis, acute) J20.8
Bronchoalveolitis J18.0
Bronchoaspergillosis B44.1
Bronchocele meaning goiter E04.0
Broncholithiasis J98.09
  tuberculous NEC A15.5
Bronchomalacia J98.09
  congenital Q32.2
Bronchomycosis NOS B49 [J99]
  candidal B37.1
Bronchopleuropneumonia — *see* Pneumonia, broncho
Bronchopneumonia — *see* Pneumonia, broncho
Bronchopneumonitis — *see* Pneumonia, broncho
Bronchopulmonary — *see* condition
Bronchopulmonitis — *see* Pneumonia, broncho
Bronchorrhagia (see Hemoptysis)
Bronchorrhea J98.09
  acute J20.9
  chronic (infective) (purulent) J42
Bronchospasm (acute) J98.01
  with
    bronchiolitis, acute J21.9
    bronchitis, acute (conditions in J20) — *see* Bronchitis, acute

Bronchospasm — *continued*
  due to external agent — *see* condition, respiratory, acute, due to
  exercise induced J45.990
Bronchospirochetosis A69.8
  Castellani A69.8
Bronchostenosis J98.09
Bronchus — *see* condition
Brontophobia F40.220
Bronze baby syndrome P83.88
Brooke's tumor — *see* Neoplasm, skin, benign
Brown enamel of teeth (hereditary) K00.5
Brown's sheath syndrome H50.61- ☑
Brown-Séquard disease, paralysis or syndrome G83.81
Bruce sepsis A23.0
Brucellosis (infection) A23.9
  abortus A23.1
  canis A23.3
  dermatitis A23.9
  melitensis A23.0
  mixed A23.8
  sepsis A23.9
    melitensis A23.0
    specified NEC A23.8
  suis A23.2
Bruck-de Lange disease Q87.1
Bruck's disease — *see* Deformity, limb
BRUE (brief resolved unexplained event) R68.13
Brugsch's syndrome Q82.8
Bruise (skin surface intact) (*see also* Contusion)
  with
    open wound — *see* Wound, open
  internal organ — *see* Injury, by site
  newborn P54.5
  scalp, due to birth injury, newborn P12.3
  umbilical cord O69.5 ☑
Bruit (arterial) R09.89
  cardiac R01.1
Brush burn — *see* Abrasion, by site
Bruton's X-linked agammaglobulinemia D80.0
Bruxism
  psychogenic F45.8
  sleep related G47.63
Bubbly lung syndrome P27.0
Bubo I88.8
  blennorrhagic (gonococcal) A54.89
  chancroidal A57
  climatic A55
  due to Haemophilus ducreyi A57
  gonococcal A54.89
  indolent (nonspecific) I88.8
  inguinal (nonspecific) I88.8
    chancroidal A57
    climatic A55
    due to H. ducreyi A57
    infective I88.8
  scrofulous (tuberculous) A18.2
  soft chancre A57
  suppurating — *see* Lymphadenitis, acute
  syphilitic (primary) A51.0
    congenital A50.07
  tropical A55
  virulent (chancroidal) A57
Bubonic plague A20.0
Bubonocele — *see* Hernia, inguinal
Buccal — *see* condition
Buchanan's disease or osteochondrosis M91.0
Buchem's syndrome (hyperostosis corticalis) M85.2
Bucket-handle fracture or tear (semilunar cartilage) — *see* Tear, meniscus
Budd-Chiari syndrome (hepatic vein thrombosis) I82.0
Budgerigar fancier's disease or lung J67.2
Buds
  breast E30.1
    in newborn P96.89
Buerger's disease (thromboangiitis obliterans) I73.1
Bulbar — *see* condition
Bulbus cordis (left ventricle) (persistent) Q21.8
Bulimia (nervosa) F50.2
  atypical F50.9
  normal weight F50.9
Bulky
  stools R19.5
  uterus N85.2
Bulla (e) R23.8
  lung (emphysematous) (solitary) J43.9

☑ **Additional Character Required** — **Refer to the Tabular List for Character Selection**   ▽ **Subterms under main terms may continue to next column or page**

Bromidism, bromism — Bulla
Index

Bulla — *continued*
    lung — *continued*
      newborn P25.8
Bullet wound (*see also* Wound, open)
    fracture — *code as* Fracture, by site
    internal organ — *see* Injury, by site
Bundle
    branch block (complete) (false) (incomplete) — *see* Block, bundle-branch
    of His — *see* condition
Bunion M21.61- ☑
    tailor's M21.62- ☑
Bunionette M21.62- ☑
Buphthalmia, buphthalmos (congenital) Q15.0
Burdwan fever B55.0
Bürger-Grütz disease or syndrome E78.3
Buried
    penis (congenital) Q55.64
      acquired N48.83
    roots K08.3
Burke's syndrome K86.89
Burkitt
    cell leukemia C91.0- ☑
    lymphoma (malignant) C83.7- ☑
      small noncleaved, diffuse C83.7- ☑
      spleen C83.77
      undifferentiated C83.7- ☑
    tumor C83.7- ☑
    type
      acute lymphoblastic leukemia C91.0- ☑
      undifferentiated C83.7- ☑
Burn (electricity) (flame) (hot gas, liquid or hot object) (radiation) (steam) (thermal) T30.0
    abdomen, abdominal (muscle) (wall) T21.02 ☑
      first degree T21.12 ☑
      second degree T21.22 ☑
      third degree T21.32 ☑
    above elbow T22.039 ☑
      first degree T22.139 ☑
      left T22.032 ☑
       first degree T22.132 ☑
       second degree T22.232 ☑
       third degree T22.332 ☑
      right T22.031 ☑
       first degree T22.131 ☑
       second degree T22.231 ☑
       third degree T22.331 ☑
      second degree T22.239 ☑
      third degree T22.339 ☑
    acid (caustic) (external) (internal) — *see* Corrosion, by site
    alimentary tract NEC T28.2 ☑
      esophagus T28.1 ☑
      mouth T28.0 ☑
      pharynx T28.0 ☑
    alkaline (caustic) (external) (internal) — *see* Corrosion, by site
    ankle T25.019 ☑
      first degree T25.119 ☑
      left T25.012 ☑
       first degree T25.112 ☑
       second degree T25.212 ☑
       third degree T25.312 ☑
      multiple with foot — *see* Burn, lower, limb, multiple, ankle and foot
      right T25.011 ☑
       first degree T25.111 ☑
       second degree T25.211 ☑
       third degree T25.311 ☑
      second degree T25.219 ☑
      third degree T25.319 ☑
    anus — *see* Burn, buttock
    arm (lower) (upper) — *see* Burn, upper, limb
    axilla T22.049 ☑
      first degree T22.149 ☑
      left T22.042 ☑
       first degree T22.142 ☑
       second degree T22.242 ☑
       third degree T22.342 ☑
      right T22.041 ☑
       first degree T22.141 ☑
       second degree T22.241 ☑
       third degree T22.341 ☑
      second degree T22.249 ☑
      third degree T22.349 ☑
    back (lower) T21.04 ☑

Burn — *continued*
    back — *continued*
      first degree T21.14 ☑
      second degree T21.24 ☑
      third degree T21.34 ☑
      upper T21.03 ☑
       first degree T21.13 ☑
       second degree T21.23 ☑
       third degree T21.33 ☑
    blisters — *code as* Burn, second degree, by site
    breast(s) — *see* Burn, chest wall
    buttock(s) T21.05 ☑
      first degree T21.15 ☑
      second degree T21.25 ☑
      third degree T21.35 ☑
    calf T24.039 ☑
      first degree T24.139 ☑
      left T24.032 ☑
       first degree T24.132 ☑
       second degree T24.232 ☑
       third degree T24.332 ☑
      right T24.031 ☑
       first degree T24.131 ☑
       second degree T24.231 ☑
       third degree T24.331 ☑
      second degree T24.239 ☑
      third degree T24.339 ☑
    canthus (eye) — *see* Burn, eyelid
    caustic acid or alkaline — *see* Corrosion, by site
    cervix T28.3 ☑
    cheek T20.06 ☑
      first degree T20.16 ☑
      second degree T20.26 ☑
      third degree T20.36 ☑
    chemical (acids) (alkalines) (caustics) (external) (internal) — *see* Corrosion, by site
    chest wall T21.01 ☑
      first degree T21.11 ☑
      second degree T21.21 ☑
      third degree T21.31 ☑
    chin T20.03 ☑
      first degree T20.13 ☑
      second degree T20.23 ☑
      third degree T20.33 ☑
    colon T28.2 ☑
    conjunctiva (and cornea) — *see* Burn, cornea
    cornea (and conjunctiva) T26.1- ☑
      chemical — *see* Corrosion, cornea
    corrosion (external) (internal) — *see* Corrosion, by site
    deep necrosis of underlying tissue — *code as* Burn, third degree, by site
    dorsum of hand T23.069 ☑
      first degree T23.169 ☑
      left T23.062 ☑
       first degree T23.162 ☑
       second degree T23.262 ☑
       third degree T23.362 ☑
      right T23.061 ☑
       first degree T23.161 ☑
       second degree T23.261 ☑
       third degree T23.361 ☑
      second degree T23.269 ☑
      third degree T23.369 ☑
    due to ingested chemical agent — *see* Corrosion, by site
    ear (auricle) (external) (canal) T20.01 ☑
      first degree T20.11 ☑
      second degree T20.21 ☑
      third degree T20.31 ☑
    elbow T22.029 ☑
      first degree T22.129 ☑
      left T22.022 ☑
       first degree T22.122 ☑
       second degree T22.222 ☑
       third degree T22.322 ☑
      right T22.021 ☑
       first degree T22.121 ☑
       second degree T22.221 ☑
       third degree T22.321 ☑
      second degree T22.229 ☑
      third degree T22.329 ☑
    epidermal loss — *code as* Burn, second degree, by site
    erythema, erythematous — *code as* Burn, first degree, by site
    esophagus T28.1 ☑

Burn — *continued*
    extent (percentage of body surface)
      less than 10 percent T31.0
      10-19 percent T31.10
       with 0-9 percent third degree burns T31.10
       with 10-19 percent third degree burns T31.11
      20-29 percent T31.20
       with 0-9 percent third degree burns T31.20
       with 10-19 percent third degree burns T31.21
       with 20-29 percent third degree burns T31.22
      30-39 percent T31.30
       with 0-9 percent third degree burns T31.30
       with 10-19 percent third degree burns T31.31
       with 20-29 percent third degree burns T31.32
       with 30-39 percent third degree burns T31.33
      40-49 percent T31.40
       with 0-9 percent third degree burns T31.40
       with 10-19 percent third degree burns T31.41
       with 20-29 percent third degree burns T31.42
       with 30-39 percent third degree burns T31.43
       with 40-49 percent third degree burns T31.44
      50-59 percent T31.50
       with 0-9 percent third degree burns T31.50
       with 10-19 percent third degree burns T31.51
       with 20-29 percent third degree burns T31.52
       with 30-39 percent third degree burns T31.53
       with 40-49 percent third degree burns T31.54
       with 50-59 percent third degree burns T31.55
      60-69 percent T31.60
       with 0-9 percent third degree burns T31.60
       with 10-19 percent third degree burns T31.61
       with 20-29 percent third degree burns T31.62
       with 30-39 percent third degree burns T31.63
       with 40-49 percent third degree burns T31.64
       with 50-59 percent third degree burns T31.65
       with 60-69 percent third degree burns T31.66
      70-79 percent T31.70
       with 0-9 percent third degree burns T31.70
       with 10-19 percent third degree burns T31.71
       with 20-29 percent third degree burns T31.72
       with 30-39 percent third degree burns T31.73
       with 40-49 percent third degree burns T31.74
       with 50-59 percent third degree burns T31.75
       with 60-69 percent third degree burns T31.76
       with 70-79 percent third degree burns T31.77
      80-89 percent T31.80
       with 0-9 percent third degree burns T31.80
       with 10-19 percent third degree burns T31.81
       with 20-29 percent third degree burns T31.82
       with 30-39 percent third degree burns T31.83
       with 40-49 percent third degree burns T31.84
       with 50-59 percent third degree burns T31.85
       with 60-69 percent third degree burns T31.86
       with 70-79 percent third degree burns T31.87
       with 80-89 percent third degree burns T31.88
      90 percent or more T31.90
       with 0-9 percent third degree burns T31.90
       with 10-19 percent third degree burns T31.91
       with 20-29 percent third degree burns T31.92
       with 30-39 percent third degree burns T31.93
       with 40-49 percent third degree burns T31.94
       with 50-59 percent third degree burns T31.95
       with 60-69 percent third degree burns T31.96
       with 70-79 percent third degree burns T31.97
       with 80-89 percent third degree burns T31.98
       with 90 percent or more third degree burns T31.99
    extremity — *see* Burn, limb
    eye(s) and adnexa T26.4- ☑
      with resulting rupture and destruction of eyeball T26.2- ☑
      conjunctival sac — *see* Burn, cornea
      cornea — *see* Burn, cornea
      lid — *see* Burn, eyelid
      periocular area — *see* Burn, eyelid
      specified site NEC T26.3- ☑
    eyeball — *see* Burn, eye
    eyelid(s) T26.0- ☑
      chemical — *see* Corrosion, eyelid
    face — *see* Burn, head
    finger T23.029 ☑
      first degree T23.129 ☑
      left T23.022 ☑
       first degree T23.122 ☑
       second degree T23.222 ☑
       third degree T23.322 ☑
      multiple sites (without thumb) T23.039 ☑
       with thumb T23.049 ☑

Burn — *continued*
  finger — *continued*
    multiple sites — *continued*
      with thumb — *continued*
        first degree T23.149 ☑
        left T23.042 ☑
          first degree T23.142 ☑
          second degree T23.242 ☑
          third degree T23.342 ☑
        right T23.041 ☑
          first degree T23.141 ☑
          second degree T23.241 ☑
          third degree T23.341 ☑
        second degree T23.249 ☑
        third degree T23.349 ☑
      first degree T23.139 ☑
      left T23.032 ☑
        first degree T23.132 ☑
        second degree T23.232 ☑
        third degree T23.332 ☑
      right T23.031 ☑
        first degree T23.131 ☑
        second degree T23.231 ☑
        third degree T23.331 ☑
      second degree T23.239 ☑
      third degree T23.339 ☑
    right T23.021 ☑
      first degree T23.121 ☑
      second degree T23.221 ☑
      third degree T23.321 ☑
    second degree T23.229 ☑
    third degree T23.329 ☑
  flank — *see* Burn, abdominal wall
  foot T25.029 ☑
    first degree T25.129 ☑
    left T25.022 ☑
      first degree T25.122 ☑
      second degree T25.222 ☑
      third degree T25.322 ☑
    multiple with ankle — *see* Burn, lower, limb, multiple, ankle and foot
    right T25.021 ☑
      first degree T25.121 ☑
      second degree T25.221 ☑
      third degree T25.321 ☑
    second degree T25.229 ☑
    third degree T25.329 ☑
  forearm T22.019 ☑
    first degree T22.119 ☑
    left T22.012 ☑
      first degree T22.112 ☑
      second degree T22.212 ☑
      third degree T22.312 ☑
    right T22.011 ☑
      first degree T22.111 ☑
      second degree T22.211 ☑
      third degree T22.311 ☑
    second degree T22.219 ☑
    third degree T22.319 ☑
  forehead T20.06 ☑
    first degree T20.16 ☑
    second degree T20.26 ☑
    third degree T20.36 ☑
  fourth degree — *code as* Burn, third degree, by site
  friction — *see* Burn, by site
  from swallowing caustic or corrosive substance NEC — *see* Corrosion, by site
  full thickness skin loss — *code as* Burn, third degree, by site
  gastrointestinal tract NEC T28.2
    from swallowing caustic or corrosive substance T28.7 ☑
  genital organs
    external
      female T21.07 ☑
        first degree T21.17 ☑
        second degree T21.27 ☑
        third degree T21.37 ☑
      male T21.06 ☑
        first degree T21.16 ☑
        second degree T21.26 ☑
        third degree T21.36 ☑
    internal T28.3
      from caustic or corrosive substance T28.8 ☑
  groin — *see* Burn, abdominal wall
  hand(s) T23.009 ☑

Burn — *continued*
  hand(s) — *continued*
    back — *see* Burn, dorsum of hand
    finger — *see* Burn, finger
    first degree T23.109 ☑
    left T23.002 ☑
      first degree T23.102 ☑
      second degree T23.202 ☑
      third degree T23.302 ☑
    multiple sites with wrist T23.099 ☑
      first degree T23.199 ☑
      left T23.092 ☑
        first degree T23.192 ☑
        second degree T23.292 ☑
        third degree T23.392 ☑
      right T23.091 ☑
        first degree T23.191 ☑
        second degree T23.291 ☑
        third degree T23.391 ☑
      second degree T23.299 ☑
      third degree T23.399 ☑
    palm — *see* Burn, palm
    right T23.001 ☑
      first degree T23.101 ☑
      second degree T23.201 ☑
      third degree T23.301 ☑
    second degree T23.209 ☑
    third degree T23.309 ☑
    thumb — *see* Burn, thumb
  head (and face) (and neck) T20.00 ☑
    cheek — *see* Burn, cheek
    chin — *see* Burn, chin
    ear — *see* Burn, ear
    eye(s) only — *see* Burn, eye
    first degree T20.10 ☑
    forehead — *see* Burn, forehead
    lip — *see* Burn, lip
    multiple sites T20.09 ☑
      first degree T20.19 ☑
      second degree T20.29 ☑
      third degree T20.39 ☑
    neck — *see* Burn, neck
    nose — *see* Burn, nose
    scalp — *see* Burn, scalp
    second degree T20.20 ☑
    third degree T20.30 ☑
  hip(s) — *see* Burn, thigh
  inhalation — *see* Burn, respiratory tract
    caustic or corrosive substance (fumes) — *see* Corrosion, respiratory tract
  internal organ(s) T28.40 ☑
    alimentary tract T28.2 ☑
      esophagus T28.1 ☑
    eardrum T28.41 ☑
    esophagus T28.1 ☑
    from caustic or corrosive substance (swallowing) NEC — *see* Corrosion, by site
    genitourinary T28.3 ☑
    mouth T28.0 ☑
    pharynx T28.0 ☑
    respiratory tract — *see* Burn, respiratory tract
    specified organ NEC T28.49 ☑
  interscapular region — *see* Burn, back, upper
  intestine (large) (small) T28.2 ☑
  knee T24.029 ☑
    first degree T24.129 ☑
    left T24.022 ☑
      first degree T24.122 ☑
      second degree T24.222 ☑
      third degree T24.322 ☑
    right T24.021 ☑
      first degree T24.121 ☑
      second degree T24.221 ☑
      third degree T24.321 ☑
    second degree T24.229 ☑
    third degree T24.329 ☑
  labium (majus) (minus) — *see* Burn, genital organs, external, female
  lacrimal apparatus, duct, gland or sac — *see* Burn, eye, specified site NEC
  larynx T27.0 ☑
    with lung T27.1 ☑
  leg(s) (lower) (upper) — *see* Burn, lower, limb
  lightning — *see* Burn, by site

Burn — *continued*
  limb(s)
    lower (except ankle or foot alone) — *see* Burn, lower, limb
    upper — *see* Burn, upper limb
  lip(s) T20.02 ☑
    first degree T20.12 ☑
    second degree T20.22 ☑
    third degree T20.32 ☑
  lower
    back — *see* Burn, back
    limb T24.009 ☑
      ankle — *see* Burn, ankle
      calf — *see* Burn, calf
      first degree T24.109 ☑
      foot — *see* Burn, foot
      hip — *see* Burn, thigh
      knee — *see* Burn, knee
      left T24.002 ☑
        first degree T24.102 ☑
        second degree T24.202 ☑
        third degree T24.302 ☑
      multiple sites, except ankle and foot T24.099 ☑
        ankle and foot T25.099 ☑
          first degree T25.199 ☑
          left T25.092 ☑
            first degree T25.192 ☑
            second degree T25.292 ☑
            third degree T25.392 ☑
          right T25.091 ☑
            first degree T25.191 ☑
            second degree T25.291 ☑
            third degree T25.391 ☑
          second degree T25.299 ☑
          third degree T25.399 ☑
        first degree T24.199 ☑
        left T24.092 ☑
          first degree T24.192 ☑
          second degree T24.292 ☑
          third degree T24.392 ☑
        right T24.091 ☑
          first degree T24.191 ☑
          second degree T24.291 ☑
          third degree T24.391 ☑
        second degree T24.299 ☑
        third degree T24.399 ☑
      right T24.001 ☑
        first degree T24.101 ☑
        second degree T24.201 ☑
        third degree T24.301 ☑
      second degree T24.209 ☑
      thigh — *see* Burn, thigh
      third degree T24.309 ☑
      toe — *see* Burn, toe
  lung (with larynx and trachea) T27.1 ☑
  mouth T28.0 ☑
  neck T20.07 ☑
    first degree T20.17 ☑
    second degree T20.27 ☑
    third degree T20.37 ☑
  nose (septum) T20.04 ☑
    first degree T20.14 ☑
    second degree T20.24 ☑
    third degree T20.34 ☑
  ocular adnexa — *see* Burn, eye
  orbit region — *see* Burn, eyelid
  palm T23.059 ☑
    first degree T23.159 ☑
    left T23.052 ☑
      first degree T23.152 ☑
      second degree T23.252 ☑
      third degree T23.352 ☑
    right T23.051 ☑
      first degree T23.151 ☑
      second degree T23.251 ☑
      third degree T23.351 ☑
    second degree T23.259 ☑
    third degree T23.359 ☑
  partial thickness — *code as* Burn, unspecified degree, by site
  pelvis — *see* Burn, trunk
  penis — *see* Burn, genital organs, external, male
  perineum
    female — *see* Burn, genital organs, external, female
    male — *see* Burn, genital organs, external, male
  periocular area — *see* Burn, eyelid

Burns' disease or osteochondrosis — *see* Osteochondrosis, juvenile, ulna
Bursa — *see* condition
Bursitis M71.9
   Achilles — *see* Tendinitis, Achilles
   adhesive — *see* Bursitis, specified NEC
   ankle — *see* Enthesopathy, lower limb, ankle, specified type NEC
   calcaneal — *see* Enthesopathy, foot, specified type NEC
   collateral ligament, tibial — *see* Bursitis, tibial collateral
   due to use, overuse, pressure (*see also* Disorder, soft tissue, due to use, specified type NEC)
      specified NEC — *see* Disorder, soft tissue, due to use, specified NEC
   Duplay's M75.0 ☑
   elbow NEC M70.3- ☑
      olecranon M70.2- ☑
   finger — *see* Disorder, soft tissue, due to use, specified type NEC, hand
   foot — *see* Enthesopathy, foot, specified type NEC
   gonococcal A54.49
   gouty — *see* Gout
   hand M70.1- ☑
   hip NEC M70.7- ☑
      trochanteric M70.6- ☑
   infective NEC M71.10
      abscess — *see* Abscess, bursa
      ankle M71.17- ☑
      elbow M71.12- ☑
      foot M71.17- ☑
      hand M71.14- ☑
      hip M71.15- ☑
      knee M71.16- ☑
      multiple sites M71.19
      shoulder M71.11- ☑
      specified site NEC M71.18
      wrist M71.13- ☑
   ischial — *see* Bursitis, hip
   knee NEC M70.5- ☑
      prepatellar M70.4- ☑
   occupational NEC (*see also* Disorder, soft tissue, due to, use)
   olecranon — *see* Bursitis, elbow, olecranon
   pharyngeal J39.1
   popliteal — *see* Bursitis, knee
   prepatellar M70.4- ☑
   radiohumeral M77.8
   rheumatoid M06.20
      ankle M06.27- ☑
      elbow M06.22- ☑
      foot joint M06.27- ☑
      hand joint M06.24- ☑
      hip M06.25- ☑
      knee M06.26- ☑
      multiple site M06.29
      shoulder M06.21- ☑
      vertebra M06.28
      wrist M06.23- ☑
   scapulohumeral — *see* Bursitis, shoulder
   semimembranous muscle (knee) — *see* Bursitis, knee
   shoulder M75.5- ☑
      adhesive — *see* Capsulitis, adhesive
   specified NEC M71.50
      ankle M71.57- ☑
      due to use, overuse or pressure — *see* Disorder, soft tissue, due to, use
      elbow M71.52- ☑
      foot M71.57- ☑
      hand M71.54- ☑
      hip M71.55- ☑
      knee M71.56- ☑
      shoulder — *see* Bursitis, shoulder
      specified site NEC M71.58
      tibial collateral M76.4- ☑
      wrist M71.53- ☑
   subacromial — *see* Bursitis, shoulder
   subcoracoid — *see* Bursitis, shoulder
   subdeltoid — *see* Bursitis, shoulder
   syphilitic A52.78
   Thornwaldt, Tornwaldt J39.2
   tibial collateral M76.4- ☑
   toe — *see* Enthesopathy, foot, specified type NEC
   trochanteric (area) — *see* Bursitis, hip, trochanteric
   wrist — *see* Bursitis, hand
Bursopathy M71.9
   specified type NEC M71.80

Bursopathy — *continued*
   specified type — *continued*
      ankle M71.87- ☑
      elbow M71.82- ☑
      foot M71.87- ☑
      hand M71.84- ☑
      hip M71.85- ☑
      knee M71.86- ☑
      multiple sites M71.89
      shoulder M71.81- ☑
      specified site NEC M71.88
      wrist M71.83- ☑
Burst stitches or sutures (complication of surgery) T81.31
   external operation wound T81.31 ☑
   internal operation wound T81.32 ☑
Buruli ulcer A31.1
Bury's disease L95.1
Buschke's
   disease B45.3
   scleredema — *see* Sclerosis, systemic
Busse-Buschke disease B45.3
Buttock — *see* condition
Button
   Biskra B55.1
   Delhi B55.1
   oriental B55.1
Buttonhole deformity (finger) — *see* Deformity, finger, boutonniere
Bwamba fever A92.8
Byssinosis J66.0
Bywaters' syndrome T79.5 ☑

C

Cachexia R64
   cancerous R64
   cardiac — *see* Disease, heart
   dehydration E86.0
   due to malnutrition R64
   exophthalmic — *see* Hyperthyroidism
   heart — *see* Disease, heart
   hypophyseal E23.0
   hypopituitary E23.0
   lead — *see* Poisoning, lead
   malignant R64
   marsh — *see* Malaria
   nervous F48.8
   old age R54
   paludal — *see* Malaria
   pituitary E23.0
   renal N28.9
   saturnine — *see* Poisoning, lead
   senile R54
   Simmonds' E23.0
   splenica D73.0
   strumipriva E03.4
   tuberculous NEC — *see* Tuberculosis
CADASIL (cerebral autosomal dominant arteriopathy with subcortical infarcts and leukoencephalopathy) I67.850
Café, au lait spots L81.3
Caffeine-induced
   anxiety disorder F15.980
   sleep disorder F15.982
Caffey's syndrome Q78.8
Caisson disease T70.3 ☑
Cake kidney Q63.1
Caked breast (puerperal, postpartum) O92.79
Calabar swelling B74.3
Calcaneal spur — *see* Spur, bone, calcaneal
Calcaneo-apophysitis M92.8
Calcareous — *see* condition
Calcicosis J62.8
Calciferol (vitamin D) deficiency E55.9
   with rickets E55.0
Calcification
   adrenal (capsule) (gland) E27.49
      tuberculous E35 [B90.8]
   aorta I70.0
   artery (annular) — *see* Arteriosclerosis
   auricle (ear) — *see* Disorder, pinna, specified type NEC
   basal ganglia G23.8
   bladder N32.89
      due to Schistosoma hematobium B65.0
   brain (cortex) — *see* Calcification, cerebral
   bronchus J98.09

Calcification — *continued*
   bursa M71.40
      ankle M71.47- ☑
      elbow M71.42- ☑
      foot M71.47- ☑
      hand M71.44- ☑
      hip M71.45- ☑
      knee M71.46- ☑
      multiple sites M71.49
      shoulder M75.3- ☑
      specified site NEC M71.48
      wrist M71.43- ☑
   cardiac — *see* Degeneration, myocardial
   cerebral (cortex) G93.89
      artery I67.2
   cervix (uteri) N88.8
   choroid plexus G93.89
   conjunctiva — *see* Concretion, conjunctiva
   corpora cavernosa (penis) N48.89
   cortex (brain) — *see* Calcification, cerebral
   dental pulp (nodular) K04.2
   dentinal papilla K00.4
   fallopian tube N83.8
   falx cerebri G96.19
   gallbladder K82.8
   general E83.59
   heart (*see also* Degeneration, myocardial)
      valve — *see* Endocarditis
   idiopathic infantile arterial (IIAC) Q28.8
   intervertebral cartilage or disc (postinfective) — *see* Disorder, disc, specified NEC
   intracranial — *see* Calcification, cerebral
   joint — *see* Disorder, joint, specified type NEC
   kidney N28.89
      tuberculous N29 [B90.1]
   larynx (senile) J38.7
   lens — *see* Cataract, specified NEC
   lung (active) (postinfectional) J98.4
      tuberculous B90.9
   lymph gland or node (postinfectional) I89.8
      tuberculous (*see also* Tuberculosis, lymph gland) B90.8
   mammographic R92.1
   massive (paraplegic) — *see* Myositis, ossificans, in, quadriplegia
   medial — *see* Arteriosclerosis, extremities
   meninges (cerebral) (spinal) G96.19
   metastatic E83.59
   Mönckeberg's — *see* Arteriosclerosis, extremities
   muscle M61.9
      due to burns — *see* Myositis, ossificans, in, burns
      paralytic — *see* Myositis, ossificans, in, quadriplegia
      specified type NEC M61.40
         ankle M61.47- ☑
         foot M61.47- ☑
         forearm M61.43- ☑
         hand M61.44- ☑
         lower leg M61.46- ☑
         multiple sites M61.49
         pelvic region M61.45- ☑
         shoulder region M61.41- ☑
         specified site NEC M61.48
         thigh M61.45- ☑
         upper arm M61.42- ☑
   myocardium, myocardial — *see* Degeneration, myocardial
   ovary N83.8
   pancreas K86.89
   penis N48.89
   periarticular — *see* Disorder, joint, specified type NEC
   pericardium (*see also* Pericarditis) I31.1
   pineal gland E34.8
   pleura J94.8
      postinfectional J94.8
      tuberculous NEC B90.9
   pulpal (dental) (nodular) K04.2
   sclera H15.89
   spleen D73.89
   subcutaneous L94.2
   suprarenal (capsule) (gland) E27.49
   tendon (sheath) (*see also* Tenosynovitis, specified type NEC)
      with bursitis, synovitis or tenosynovitis — *see* Tendinitis, calcific
   trachea J39.8
   ureter N28.89
   uterus N85.8

☑ **Additional Character Required** — Refer to the Tabular List for Character Selection   📑 **Subterms under main terms may continue to next column or page**

Calcification — *continued*
  vitreous — *see* Deposit, crystalline
Calcified — *see* Calcification
Calcinosis (interstitial) (tumoral) (universalis) E83.59
  with Raynaud's phenomenon, esophageal dysfunction, sclerodactyly, telangiectasia (CREST syndrome) M34.1
  circumscripta (skin) L94.2
  cutis L94.2
Calciphylaxis (*see also* Calcification, by site) E83.59
Calcium
  deposits — *see* Calcification, by site
  metabolism disorder E83.50
  salts or soaps in vitreous — *see* Deposit, crystalline
Calciuria R82.994
Calculi — *see* Calculus
Calculosis, intrahepatic — *see* Calculus, bile duct
Calculus, calculi, calculous
  ampulla of Vater — *see* Calculus, bile duct
  anuria (impacted) (recurrent) (*see also* Calculus, urinary) N20.9
  appendix K38.1
  bile duct (common) (hepatic) K80.50
    with
      calculus of gallbladder — *see* Calculus, gallbladder and bile duct
      cholangitis K80.30
        with
          cholecystitis — *see* Calculus, bile duct, with cholecystitis
          obstruction K80.31
        acute K80.32
          with
            chronic cholangitis K80.36
              with obstruction K80.37
            obstruction K80.33
        chronic K80.34
          with
            acute cholangitis K80.36
              with obstruction K80.37
            obstruction K80.35
      cholecystitis (with cholangitis) K80.40
        with obstruction K80.41
        acute K80.42
          with
            chronic cholecystitis K80.46
              with obstruction K80.47
            obstruction K80.43
        chronic K80.44
          with
            acute cholecystitis K80.46
              with obstruction K80.47
            obstruction K80.45
  biliary (*see also* Calculus, gallbladder)
    specified NEC K80.80
      with obstruction K80.81
  bilirubin, multiple — *see* Calculus, gallbladder
  bladder (encysted) (impacted) (urinary) (diverticulum) N21.0
  bronchus J98.09
  calyx (kidney) (renal) — *see* Calculus, kidney
  cholesterol (pure) (solitary) — *see* Calculus, gallbladder
  common duct (bile) — *see* Calculus, bile duct
  conjunctiva — *see* Concretion, conjunctiva
  cystic N21.0
    duct — *see* Calculus, gallbladder
  dental (subgingival) (supragingival) K03.6
  diverticulum
    bladder N21.0
    kidney N20.0
  epididymis N50.89
  gallbladder K80.20
    with
      bile duct calculus — *see* Calculus, gallbladder and bile duct
      cholecystitis K80.10
        with obstruction K80.11
        acute K80.00
          with
            chronic cholecystitis K80.12
              with obstruction K80.13
            obstruction K80.01
        chronic K80.10
          with
            acute cholecystitis K80.12
              with obstruction K80.13
            obstruction K80.11
      specified NEC K80.18

Calculus, calculi, calculous — *continued*
  gallbladder — *continued*
    with — *continued*
      cholecystitis — *continued*
        specified — *continued*
          with obstruction K80.19
        obstruction K80.21
  gallbladder and bile duct K80.70
    with
      cholecystitis K80.60
        with obstruction K80.61
        acute K80.62
          with
            chronic cholecystitis K80.66
              with obstruction K80.67
            obstruction K80.63
        chronic K80.64
          with
            acute cholecystitis K80.66
              with obstruction K80.67
            obstruction K80.65
        obstruction K80.71
  hepatic (duct) — *see* Calculus, bile duct
  ileal conduit N21.8
  intestinal (impaction) (obstruction) K56.49
  kidney (impacted) (multiple) (pelvis) (recurrent) (staghorn) N20.0
    with calculus, ureter N20.2
    congenital Q63.8
  lacrimal passages — *see* Dacryolith
  liver (impacted) — *see* Calculus, bile duct
  lung J98.4
  mammographic R92.1
  nephritic (impacted) (recurrent) — *see* Calculus, kidney
  nose J34.89
  pancreas (duct) K86.89
  parotid duct or gland K11.5
  pelvis, encysted — *see* Calculus, kidney
  prostate N42.0
  pulmonary J98.4
  pyelitis (impacted) (recurrent) N20.0
    with hydronephrosis N13.2
  pyelonephritis (impacted) (recurrent) N20 ☑
    with hydronephrosis N13.2
  renal (impacted) (recurrent) — *see* Calculus, kidney
  salivary (duct) (gland) K11.5
  seminal vesicle N50.89
  staghorn — *see* Calculus, kidney
  Stensen's duct K11.5
  stomach K31.89
  sublingual duct or gland K11.5
    congenital Q38.4
  submandibular duct, gland or region K11.5
  submaxillary duct, gland or region K11.5
  suburethral N21.8
  tonsil J35.8
  tooth, teeth (subgingival) (supragingival) K03.6
  tunica vaginalis N50.89
  ureter (impacted) (recurrent) N20.1
    with calculus, kidney N20.2
      with hydronephrosis N13.2
        with infection N13.6
  urethra (impacted) N21.1
  urinary (duct) (impacted) (passage) (tract) N20.9
    with hydronephrosis N13.2
      with infection N13.6
    in (due to)
    lower N21.9
      specified NEC N21.8
  vagina N89.8
  vesical (impacted) N21.0
  Wharton's duct K11.5
  xanthine E79.8 [N22]
Calicectasis N28.89
Caliectasis N28.89
California
  disease B38.9
  encephalitis A83.5
Caligo cornea — *see* Opacity, cornea, central
Callositas, callosity (infected) L84
Callus (infected) L84
  bone — *see* Osteophyte
    excessive, following fracture — *code as* Sequelae of fracture
CALME (childhood asymmetric labium majus enlargement) N90.61
Calorie deficiency or malnutrition (*see also* Malnutrition) E46

Calvé-Perthes disease — *see* Legg-Calvé-Perthes disease
Calvé's disease — *see* Osteochondrosis, juvenile, spine
Calvities — *see* Alopecia, androgenic
Cameroon fever — *see* Malaria
Camptocormia (hysterical) F44.4
Camurati-Engelmann syndrome Q78.3
Canal (*see also* condition)
  atrioventricular common Q21.2
Canaliculitis (lacrimal) (acute) (subacute) H04.33- ☑
  Actinomyces A42.89
  chronic H04.42- ☑
Canavan's disease E75.29
Canceled procedure (surgical) Z53.9
  because of
    contraindication Z53.09
      smoking Z53.01
    left against medical advice (AMA) Z53.21
    patient's decision Z53.20
      for reasons of belief or group pressure Z53.1
      specified reason NEC Z53.29
    specified reason NEC Z53.8
Cancer (*see also* Neoplasm, by site, malignant)
  bile duct type liver C22.1
  blood — *see* Leukemia
  breast (*see also* Neoplasm, breast, malignant) C50.91- ☑
  hepatocellular C22.0
  lung (*see also* Neoplasm, lung, malignant) C34.90
  ovarian (*see also* Neoplasm ovary, malignant) C56.9
  unspecified site (primary) C80.1
Cancer (o)phobia F45.29
Cancerous — *see* Neoplasm, malignant, by site
Cancrum oris A69.0
Candidiasis, candidal B37.9
  balanitis B37.42
  bronchitis B37.1
  cheilitis B37.83
  congenital P37.5
  cystitis B37.41
  disseminated B37.7
  endocarditis B37.6
  enteritis B37.82
  esophagitis B37.81
  intertrigo B37.2
  lung B37.1
  meningitis B37.5
  mouth B37.0
  nails B37.2
  neonatal P37.5
  onychia B37.2
  oral B37.0
  osteomyelitis B37.89
  otitis externa B37.84
  paronychia B37.2
  perionyxis B37.2
  pneumonia B37.1
  proctitis B37.82
  pulmonary B37.1
  pyelonephritis B37.49
  sepsis B37.7
  skin B37.2
  specified site NEC B37.89
  stomatitis B37.0
  systemic B37.7
  urethritis B37.41
  urogenital site NEC B37.49
  vagina B37.3
  vulva B37.3
  vulvovaginitis B37.3
Candidid L30.2
Candidosis — *see* Candidiasis
Candiru infection or infestation B88.8
Canities (premature) L67.1
  congenital Q84.2
Canker (mouth) (sore) K12.0
  rash A38.9
Cannabinosis J66.2
Cannabis induced
  anxiety disorder F12.980
  psychotic disorder F12.959
  sleep disorder F12.988
Canton fever A75.9
Cantrell's syndrome Q87.89
Capillariasis (intestinal) B81.1
  hepatic B83.8
Capillary — *see* condition
Caplan's syndrome — *see* Rheumatoid, lung

Capsule — *see* condition
Capsulitis (joint) (*see also* Enthesopathy)
  adhesive (shoulder) M75.0- ☑
  hepatic K65.8
  labyrinthine — *see* Otosclerosis, specified NEC
  thyroid E06.9
Caput
  crepitus Q75.8
  medusae I86.8
  succedaneum P12.81
Car sickness T75.3 ☑
Carapata (disease) A68.0
Carate — *see* Pinta
Carbon lung J60
Carbuncle L02.93
  abdominal wall L02.231
  anus K61.0
  auditory canal, external — *see* Abscess, ear, external
  auricle ear — *see* Abscess, ear, external
  axilla L02.43- ☑
  back (any part) L02.232
  breast N61.1
  buttock L02.33
  cheek (external) L02.03
  chest wall L02.233
  chin L02.03
  corpus cavernosum N48.21
  ear (any part) (external) (middle) — *see* Abscess, ear, external
  external auditory canal — *see* Abscess, ear, external
  eyelid — *see* Abscess, eyelid
  face NEC L02.03
  femoral (region) — *see* Carbuncle, lower limb
  finger — *see* Carbuncle, hand
  flank L02.231
  foot L02.63- ☑
  forehead L02.03
  genital — *see* Abscess, genital
  gluteal (region) L02.33
  groin L02.234
  hand L02.53- ☑
  head NEC L02.831
  heel — *see* Carbuncle, foot
  hip — *see* Carbuncle, lower limb
  kidney — *see* Abscess, kidney
  knee — *see* Carbuncle, lower limb
  labium (majus) (minus) N76.4
  lacrimal
    gland — *see* Dacryoadenitis
    passages (duct) (sac) — *see* Inflammation, lacrimal, passages, acute
  leg — *see* Carbuncle, lower limb
  lower limb L02.43- ☑
  malignant A22.0
  navel L02.236
  neck L02.13
  nose (external) (septum) J34.0
  orbit, orbital — *see* Abscess, orbit
  palmar (space) — *see* Carbuncle, hand
  partes posteriores L02.33
  pectoral region L02.233
  penis N48.21
  perineum L02.235
  pinna — *see* Abscess, ear, external
  popliteal — *see* Carbuncle, lower limb
  scalp L02.831
  seminal vesicle N49.0
  shoulder — *see* Carbuncle, upper limb
  specified site NEC L02.838
  temple (region) L02.03
  thumb — *see* Carbuncle, hand
  toe — *see* Carbuncle, foot
  trunk L02.239
    abdominal wall L02.231
    back L02.232
    chest wall L02.233
    groin L02.234
    perineum L02.235
    umbilicus L02.236
  umbilicus L02.236
  upper limb L02.43- ☑
  urethra N34.0
  vulva N76.4
Carbunculus — *see* Carbuncle
Carcinoid (tumor) — *see* Tumor, carcinoid
Carcinoidosis E34.0

Carcinoma (malignant) (*see also* Neoplasm, by site, malignant)
  acidophil
    specified site — *see* Neoplasm, malignant, by site
    unspecified site C75.1
  acidophil-basophil, mixed
    specified site — *see* Neoplasm, malignant, by site
    unspecified site C75.1
  adnexal (skin) — *see* Neoplasm, skin, malignant
  adrenal cortical C74.0- ☑
  alveolar — *see* Neoplasm, lung, malignant
    cell — *see* Neoplasm, lung, malignant
  ameloblastic C41.1
    upper jaw (bone) C41.0
  apocrine
    breast — *see* Neoplasm, breast, malignant
    specified site NEC — *see* Neoplasm, skin, malignant
    unspecified site C44.99
  basal cell (pigmented) (*see also* Neoplasm, skin, malignant) C44.91
    fibro-epithelial — *see* Neoplasm, skin, malignant
    morphea — *see* Neoplasm, skin, malignant
    multicentric — *see* Neoplasm, skin, malignant
  basaloid
  basal-squamous cell, mixed — *see* Neoplasm, skin, malignant
  basophil
    specified site — *see* Neoplasm, malignant, by site
    unspecified site C75.1
  basophil-acidophil, mixed
    specified site — *see* Neoplasm, malignant, by site
    unspecified site C75.1
  basosquamous — *see* Neoplasm, skin, malignant
  bile duct
    with hepatocellular, mixed C22.0
    liver C22.1
    specified site NEC — *see* Neoplasm, malignant, by site
    unspecified site C22.1
  branchial or branchiogenic C10.4
  bronchial or bronchogenic — *see* Neoplasm, lung, malignant
  bronchiolar — *see* Neoplasm, lung, malignant
  bronchioloalveolar — *see* Neoplasm, lung, malignant
  C cell
    specified site — *see* Neoplasm, malignant, by site
    unspecified site C73
  ceruminous C44.29- ☑
  cervix uteri
    in situ D06.9
      endocervix D06.0
      exocervix D06.1
      specified site NEC D06.7
  chorionic
    specified site — *see* Neoplasm, malignant, by site
    unspecified site
      female C58
      male C62.90
  chromophobe
    specified site — *see* Neoplasm, malignant, by site
    unspecified site C75.1
  cloacogenic
    specified site — *see* Neoplasm, malignant, by site
    unspecified site C21.2
  diffuse type
    specified site — *see* Neoplasm, malignant, by site
    unspecified site C16.9
  duct (cell)
    with Paget's disease — *see* Neoplasm, breast, malignant
    infiltrating
      with lobular carcinoma (in situ)
        specified site — *see* Neoplasm, malignant, by site
        unspecified site (female) C50.91- ☑
          male C50.92- ☑
      specified site — *see* Neoplasm, malignant, by site
      unspecified site (female) C50.91- ☑
        male C50.92- ☑
  ductal
    with lobular
      specified site — *see* Neoplasm, malignant, by site
      unspecified site (female) C50.91- ☑
        male C50.92- ☑

Carcinoma — *continued*
  ductular, infiltrating
    specified site — *see* Neoplasm, malignant, by site
    unspecified site (female) C50.91- ☑
      male C50.92- ☑
  embryonal
    liver C22.7
  endometrioid
    specified site — *see* Neoplasm, malignant, by site
    unspecified site
      female C56.9
      male C61
  eosinophil
    specified site — *see* Neoplasm, malignant, by site
    unspecified site C75.1
  epidermoid (*see also* Neoplasm, skin, malignant)
    in situ, Bowen's type — *see* Neoplasm, skin, in situ
  fibroepithelial, basal cell — *see* Neoplasm, skin, malignant
  follicular
    with papillary (mixed) C73
    moderately differentiated C73
    pure follicle C73
    specified site — *see* Neoplasm, malignant, by site
    trabecular C73
    unspecified site C73
    well differentiated C73
  generalized, with unspecified primary site C80.0
  glycogen-rich — *see* Neoplasm, breast, malignant
  granulosa cell C56- ☑
  hepatic cell C22.0
  hepatocellular C22.0
    with bile duct, mixed C22.0
    fibrolamellar C22.0
  hepatocholangiolitic C22.0
  Hurthle cell C73
  in
    adenomatous
      polyposis coli C18.9
    pleomorphic adenoma — *see* Neoplasm, salivary glands, malignant
    situ — *see* Carcinoma-in-situ
  infiltrating
    duct
      with lobular
        specified site — *see* Neoplasm, malignant, by site
        unspecified site (female) C50.91- ☑
          male C50.92- ☑
        with Paget's disease — *see* Neoplasm, breast, malignant
      specified site — *see* Neoplasm, malignant
      unspecified site (female) C50.91- ☑
        male C50.92- ☑
    ductular
      specified site — *see* Neoplasm, malignant
      unspecified site (female) C50.91- ☑
        male C50.92- ☑
    lobular
      specified site — *see* Neoplasm, malignant
      unspecified site (female) C50.91- ☑
        male C50.92- ☑
  inflammatory
    specified site — *see* Neoplasm, malignant
    unspecified site (female) C50.91- ☑
      male C50.92- ☑
  intestinal type
    specified site — *see* Neoplasm, malignant, by site
    unspecified site C16.9
  intracystic
    noninfiltrating — *see* Neoplasm, in situ, by site
  intraductal (noninfiltrating)
    with Paget's disease — *see* Neoplasm, breast, malignant
    breast D05.1- ☑
    papillary
      with invasion
        specified site — *see* Neoplasm, malignant, by site
        unspecified site (female) C50.91- ☑
          male C50.92- ☑
      breast D05.1- ☑
      specified site NEC — *see* Neoplasm, in situ, by site
      unspecified site (female) D05.1- ☑
    specified site NEC — *see* Neoplasm, in situ, by site
    unspecified site (female) D05.1- ☑

☑ **Additional Character Required** — **Refer to the Tabular List for Character Selection**   🔄 **Subterms under main terms may continue to next column or page**

Carcinoma — *continued*
  intraepidermal — *see* Neoplasm, in situ
    squamous cell, Bowen's type — *see* Neoplasm, skin, in situ
  intraepithelial — *see* Neoplasm, in situ, by site
    squamous cell — *see* Neoplasm, in situ, by site
  intraosseous C41.1
    upper jaw (bone) C41.0
  islet cell
    with exocrine, mixed
      specified site — *see* Neoplasm, malignant, by site
      unspecified site C25.9
    pancreas C25.4
    specified site NEC — *see* Neoplasm, malignant, by site
    unspecified site C25.4
  juvenile, breast — *see* Neoplasm, breast, malignant
  large cell
    small cell
      specified site — *see* Neoplasm, malignant, by site
      unspecified site C34.90
  Leydig cell (testis)
    specified site — *see* Neoplasm, malignant, by site
    unspecified site
      female C56.9
      male C62.90
  lipid-rich (female) C50.91- ☑
    male C50.92- ☑
  liver cell C22.0
  liver NEC C22.7
  lobular (infiltrating)
    with intraductal
      specified site — *see* Neoplasm, malignant, by site
      unspecified site (female) C50.91- ☑
        male C50.92- ☑
    noninfiltrating
      breast D05.0- ☑
      specified site NEC — *see* Neoplasm, in situ, by site
      unspecified site D05.0- ☑
    specified site — *see* Neoplasm, malignant, by site
    unspecified site (female) C50.91- ☑
      male C50.92- ☑
  medullary
    with
      amyloid stroma
        specified site — *see* Neoplasm, malignant, by site
        unspecified site C73
      lymphoid stroma
        specified site — *see* Neoplasm, malignant, by site
        unspecified site (female) C50.91- ☑
          male C50.92- ☑
  Merkel cell C4A.9 (*following* C43)
    anal margin C4A.51 (*following* C43)
    anal skin C4A.51 (*following* C43)
    canthus C4A.1- ☑ (*following* C43)
    ear and external auricular canal C4A.2- ☑ (*following* C43)
    external auricular canal C4A.2- ☑ (*following* C43)
    eyelid, including canthus C4A.1- ☑ (*following* C43)
    face C4A.30 (*following* C43)
      specified NEC C4A.39 (*following* C43)
    hip C4A.7- ☑ (*following* C43)
    lip C4A.0 (*following* C43)
    lower limb, including hip C4A.7- ☑ (*following* C43)
    neck C4A.4 (*following* C43)
    nodal presentation C7B.1 (*following* C75)
    nose C4A.31 (*following* C43)
    overlapping sites C4A.8 (*following* C43)
    perianal skin C4A.51 (*following* C43)
    scalp C4A.4 (*following* C43)
    secondary C7B.1 (*following* C75)
    shoulder C4A.6- ☑ (*following* C43)
    skin of breast C4A.52 (*following* C43)
    trunk NEC C4A.59 (*following* C43)
    upper limb, including shoulder C4A.6- ☑ (*following* C43)
    visceral metastatic C7B.1 (*following* C75)
  metastatic — *see* Neoplasm, secondary, by site
  metatypical — *see* Neoplasm, skin, malignant
  morphea, basal cell — *see* Neoplasm, skin, malignant

Carcinoma — *continued*
  mucoid
    cell
      specified site — *see* Neoplasm, malignant, by site
      unspecified site C75.1
  neuroendocrine (*see also* Tumor, neuroendocrine)
    high grade, any site C7A.1 (*following* C75)
    poorly differentiated, any site C7A.1 (*following* C75)
  nonencapsulated sclerosing C73
  noninfiltrating
    intracystic — *see* Neoplasm, in situ, by site
    intraductal
      breast D05.1- ☑
      papillary
        breast D05.1- ☑
        specified site NEC — *see* Neoplasm, in situ, by site
        unspecified site D05.1- ☑
      specified site — *see* Neoplasm, in situ, by site
      unspecified site D05.1- ☑
    lobular
      breast D05.0- ☑
      specified site NEC — *see* Neoplasm, in situ, by site
      unspecified site (female) D05.0- ☑
  oat cell
    specified site — *see* Neoplasm, malignant, by site
    unspecified site C34.90
  odontogenic C41.1
    upper jaw (bone) C41.0
  papillary
    with follicular (mixed) C73
    follicular variant C73
    intraductal (noninfiltrating)
      with invasion
        specified site — *see* Neoplasm, malignant, by site
        unspecified site (female) C50.91- ☑
          male C50.92- ☑
      breast D05.1- ☑
      specified site NEC — *see* Neoplasm, in situ, by site
      unspecified site D05.1- ☑
    serous
      specified site — *see* Neoplasm, malignant, by site
      surface
        specified site — *see* Neoplasm, malignant, by site
        unspecified site C56.9
      unspecified site C56.9
  papillocystic
    specified site — *see* Neoplasm, malignant, by site
    unspecified site C56.9
  parafollicular cell
    specified site — *see* Neoplasm, malignant, by site
    unspecified site C73
  pilomatrix — *see* Neoplasm, skin, malignant
  pseudomucinous
    specified site — *see* Neoplasm, malignant, by site
    unspecified site C56.9
  renal cell C64- ☑
  Schmincke — *see* Neoplasm, nasopharynx, malignant
  Schneiderian
    specified site — *see* Neoplasm, malignant, by site
    unspecified site C30.0
  sebaceous — *see* Neoplasm, skin, malignant
  secondary (*see also* Neoplasm, secondary, by site)
    Merkel cell C7B.1 (*following* C75)
  secretory, breast — *see* Neoplasm, breast, malignant
  serous
    papillary
      specified site — *see* Neoplasm, malignant, by site
      unspecified site C56.9
    surface, papillary
      specified site — *see* Neoplasm, malignant, by site
      unspecified site C56.9
  Sertoli cell
    specified site — *see* Neoplasm, malignant, by site
    unspecified site C62.90
      female C56.9
      male C62.90
  skin appendage — *see* Neoplasm, skin, malignant

Carcinoma — *continued*
  small cell
    fusiform cell
      specified site — *see* Neoplasm, malignant, by site
      unspecified site C34.90
    intermediate cell
      specified site — *see* Neoplasm, malignant, by site
      unspecified site C34.90
    large cell
      specified site — *see* Neoplasm, malignant, by site
      unspecified site C34.90
  solid
    with amyloid stroma
      specified site — *see* Neoplasm, malignant, by site
      unspecified site C73
    microinvasive
      specified site — *see* Neoplasm, malignant, by site
      unspecified site C53.9
  sweat gland — *see* Neoplasm, skin, malignant
  theca cell C56.- ☑
  thymic C37
  unspecified site (primary) C80.1
  water-clear cell C75.0
Carcinoma-in-situ (*see also* Neoplasm, in situ, by site)
  breast NOS D05.9- ☑
    specified type NEC D05.8- ☑
  epidermoid (*see also* Neoplasm, in situ, by site)
    with questionable stromal invasion
      cervix D06.9
      specified site NEC — *see* Neoplasm, in situ, by site
      unspecified site D06.9
    Bowen's type — *see* Neoplasm, skin, in situ
  intraductal
    breast D05.1- ☑
    specified site NEC — *see* Neoplasm, in situ, by site
    unspecified site D05.1- ☑
  lobular
    with
      infiltrating duct
        breast (female) C50.91- ☑
          male C50.92- ☑
        specified site NEC — *see* Neoplasm, malignant
        unspecified site (female) C50.91- ☑
          male C50.92- ☑
      intraductal
        breast D05.8- ☑
        specified site NEC — *see* Neoplasm, in situ, by site
        unspecified site (female) D05.8- ☑
    breast D05.0- ☑
    specified site NEC — *see* Neoplasm, in situ, by site
    unspecified site D05.0- ☑
  squamous cell (*see also* Neoplasm, in situ, by site)
    with questionable stromal invasion
      cervix D06.9
      specified site NEC — *see* Neoplasm, in situ, by site
      unspecified site D06.9
Carcinomaphobia F45.29
Carcinomatosis C80.0
  peritonei C78.6
  unspecified site (primary) (secondary) C80.0
Carcinosarcoma — *see* Neoplasm, malignant, by site
  embryonal — *see* Neoplasm, malignant, by site
Cardia, cardial — *see* condition
Cardiac (*see also* condition)
  death, sudden — *see* Arrest, cardiac
  pacemaker
    in situ Z95.0
    management or adjustment Z45.018
  tamponade I31.4
Cardialgia — *see* Pain, precordial
Cardiectasis — *see* Hypertrophy, cardiac
Cardiochalasia K21.9
Cardiomalacia I51.5
Cardiomegalia glycogenica diffusa E74.02 [I43]
Cardiomegaly (*see also* Hypertrophy, cardiac)
  congenital Q24.8
  glycogen E74.02 [I43]
  idiopathic I51.7
Cardiomyoliposis I51.5

▽ Subterms under main terms may continue to next column or page   ☑ Additional Character Required — Refer to the Tabular List for Character Selection   49

Carcinoma — Cardiomyoliposis

Cardiomyopathy (familial) (idiopathic) I42.9
  alcoholic I42.6
  amyloid E85.4 [I43]
    transthyretin-related (ATTR) familial E85.4
  arteriosclerotic — see Disease, heart, ischemic,
    atherosclerotic
  beriberi E51.12
  cobalt-beer I42.6
  congenital I42.4
  congestive I42.0
  constrictive NOS I42.5
  dilated I42.0
  due to
    alcohol I42.6
    beriberi E51.12
    cardiac glycogenosis E74.02 [I43]
    drugs I42.7
    external agents NEC I42.7
    Friedreich's ataxia G11.1
    myotonia atrophica G71.11 [I43]
    progressive muscular dystrophy G71.09 [I43]
  glycogen storage E74.02 [I43]
  hypertensive — see Hypertension, heart
  hypertrophic (nonobstructive) I42.2
    obstructive I42.1
      congenital Q24.8
  in
    Chagas' disease (chronic) B57.2
      acute B57.0
    sarcoidosis D86.85
  ischemic I25.5
  metabolic E88.9 [I43]
    thyrotoxic E05.90 [I43]
      with thyroid storm E05.91 [I43]
  newborn I42.8
    congenital I42.4
  nutritional E63.9 [I43]
    beriberi E51.12
  obscure of Africa I42.8
  peripartum O90.3
  postpartum O90.3
  restrictive NEC I42.5
  rheumatic I09.0
  secondary I42.9
  stress induced I51.81
  takotsubo I51.81
  thyrotoxic E05.90 [I43]
    with thyroid storm E05.91 [I43]
  toxic NEC I42.7
  transthyretin-related (ATTR) familial amyloid E85.4
  tuberculous A18.84
  viral B33.24
Cardionephritis — see Hypertension, cardiorenal
Cardionephropathy — see Hypertension, cardiorenal
Cardionephrosis — see Hypertension, cardiorenal
Cardiopathia nigra I27.0
Cardiopathy (see also Disease, heart) I51.9
  idiopathic I42.9
  mucopolysaccharidosis E76.3 [I52]
Cardiopericarditis — see Pericarditis
Cardiophobia F45.29
Cardiorenal — see condition
Cardiorrhexis — see Infarct, myocardium
Cardiosclerosis — see Disease, heart, ischemic,
  atherosclerotic
Cardiosis — see Disease, heart
Cardiospasm (esophagus) (reflex) (stomach) K22.0
  congenital Q39.5
    with megaesophagus Q39.5
Cardiostenosis — see Disease, heart
Cardiosymphysis I31.0
Cardiovascular — see condition
Carditis (acute) (bacterial) (chronic) (subacute) I51.89
  meningococcal A39.50
  rheumatic — see Disease, heart, rheumatic
  rheumatoid — see Rheumatoid, carditis
  viral B33.20
Care (of) (for) (following)
  child (routine) Z76.2
  family member (handicapped) (sick)
    creating problem for family Z63.6
    provided away from home for holiday relief Z75.5
    unavailable, due to
      absence (person rendering care) (sufferer) Z74.2
      inability (any reason) of person rendering care
        Z74.2
  foundling Z76.1
  holiday relief Z75.5

Care — continued
  improper — see Maltreatment
  lack of (at or after birth) (infant) — see Maltreatment,
    child, neglect
  lactating mother Z39.1
  palliative Z51.5
  postpartum
    immediately after delivery Z39.0
    routine follow-up Z39.2
  respite Z75.5
  unavailable, due to
    absence of person rendering care Z74.2
    inability (any reason) of person rendering care Z74.2
  well-baby Z76.2
Caries
  bone NEC A18.03
  dental (dentino enamel junction) (early childhood) (of
    dentine) (pre-eruptive) (recurrent) (to the pulp)
    K02.9
    arrested (coronal) (root) K02.3
    chewing surface
      limited to enamel K02.51
      penetrating into dentin K02.52
      penetrating into pulp K02.53
    coronal surface
      chewing surface
        limited to enamel K02.51
        penetrating into dentin K02.52
        penetrating into pulp K02.53
      pit and fissure surface
        limited to enamel K02.51
        penetrating into dentin K02.52
        penetrating into pulp K02.53
      smooth surface
        limited to enamel K02.61
        penetrating into dentin K02.62
        penetrating into pulp K02.63
    pit and fissure surface
      limited to enamel K02.51
      penetrating into dentin K02.52
      penetrating into pulp K02.53
    primary, cervical origin K02.52
    root K02.7
    smooth surface
      limited to enamel K02.61
      penetrating into dentin K02.62
      penetrating into pulp K02.63
  external meatus — see Disorder, ear, external, specified
    type NEC
  hip (tuberculous) A18.02
  initial (tooth)
    chewing surface K02.51
    pit and fissure surface K02.51
    smooth surface K02.61
  knee (tuberculous) A18.02
  labyrinth H83.8 ☑
  limb NEC (tuberculous) A18.03
  mastoid process (chronic) — see Mastoiditis, chronic
    tuberculous A18.03
  middle ear H74.8 ☑
  nose (tuberculous) A18.03
  orbit (tuberculous) A18.03
  ossicles, ear — see Abnormal, ear ossicles
  petrous bone — see Petrositis
  root (dental) (tooth) K02.7
  sacrum (tuberculous) A18.01
  spine, spinal (column) (tuberculous) A18.01
  syphilitic A52.77
    congenital (early) A50.02 [M90.80]
  tooth, teeth — see Caries, dental
  tuberculous A18.01
  vertebra (column) (tuberculous) A18.01
Carious teeth — see Caries, dental
Carneous mole O02.0
Carnitine insufficiency E71.40
Carotenemia (dietary) E67.1
Carotenosis (cutis) (skin) E67.1
Carotid body or sinus syndrome G90.01
Carotidynia G90.01
Carpal tunnel syndrome — see Syndrome, carpal tunnel
Carpenter's syndrome Q87.0
Carpopedal spasm — see Tetany
Carr-Barr-Plunkett syndrome Q97.1
Carrier (suspected) of
  amebiasis Z22.1
  bacterial disease NEC Z22.39
    diphtheria Z22.2
    intestinal infectious NEC Z22.1

Carrier of — continued
  bacterial disease — continued
    intestinal infectious — continued
      typhoid Z22.0
    meningococcal Z22.31
    sexually transmitted Z22.4
    specified NEC Z22.39
    staphylococcal (Methicillin susceptible) Z22.321
      Methicillin resistant Z22.322
    streptococcal Z22.338
      group B Z22.330
        complicating pregnancy or delivery
          O99.82- ☑
    typhoid Z22.0
  cholera Z22.1
  diphtheria Z22.2
  gastrointestinal pathogens NEC Z22.1
  genetic Z14.8
    cystic fibrosis Z14.1
    hemophilia A (asymptomatic) Z14.01
      symptomatic Z14.02
  gestational, pregnant Z33.1
  gonorrhea Z22.4
  HAA (hepatitis Australian-antigen) B18.8
  HB (c)(s)-AG B18.1
  hepatitis (viral) B18.9
    Australia-antigen (HAA) B18.8
    B surface antigen (HBsAg) B18.1
      with acute delta- (super)infection B17.0
    C B18.2
    specified NEC B18.8
  human T-cell lymphotropic virus type-1 (HTLV-1) infec-
    tion Z22.6
  infectious organism Z22.9
    specified NEC Z22.8
  meningococci Z22.31
  Salmonella typhosa Z22.0
  serum hepatitis — see Carrier, hepatitis
  staphylococci (Methicillin susceptible) Z22.321
    Methicillin resistant Z22.322
  streptococci Z22.338
    group B Z22.330
      complicating pregnancy or delivery O99.82- ☑
  syphilis Z22.4
  typhoid Z22.0
  venereal disease NEC Z22.4
Carrion's disease A44.0
Carter's relapsing fever (Asiatic) A68.1
Cartilage — see condition
Caruncle (inflamed)
  conjunctiva (acute) — see Conjunctivitis, acute
  labium (majus) (minus) N90.89
  lacrimal — see Inflammation, lacrimal, passages
  myrtiform N89.8
  urethral (benign) N36.2
Cascade stomach K31.2
Caseation lymphatic gland (tuberculous) A18.2
Cassidy (-Scholte) syndrome (malignant carcinoid) E34.0
Castellani's disease A69.8
Castration, traumatic, male S38.231 ☑
Casts in urine R82.998
Cat
  cry syndrome Q93.4
  ear Q17.3
  eye syndrome Q92.8
Catabolism, senile R54
Catalepsy (hysterical) F44.2
  schizophrenic F20.2
Cataplexy (idiopathic) — see Narcolepsy
Cataract (cortical) (immature) (incipient) H26.9
  with
    neovascularization — see Cataract, complicated
  age-related — see Cataract, senile
  anterior
    and posterior axial embryonal Q12.0
    pyramidal Q12.0
  associated with
    galactosemia E74.21 [H28]
    myotonic disorders G71.19 [H28]
  blue Q12.0
  central Q12.0
  cerulean Q12.0
  complicated H26.20
    with
      neovascularization H26.21- ☑
      ocular disorder H26.22- ☑
    glaucomatous flecks H26.23- ☑
  congenital Q12.0

Cataract — *continued*
- coraliform Q12.0
- coronary Q12.0
- crystalline Q12.0
- diabetic — *see* Diabetes, cataract
- drug-induced H26.3- ☑
- due to
  - ocular disorder — *see* Cataract, complicated
  - radiation H26.8
- electric H26.8
- extraction status Z98.4- ☑
- glass-blower's H26.8
- heat ray H26.8
- heterochromic — *see* Cataract, complicated
- hypermature — *see* Cataract, senile, morgagnian type
- in (due to)
  - chronic iridocyclitis — *see* Cataract, complicated
  - diabetes — *see* Diabetes, cataract
  - endocrine disease E34.9 [H28]
  - eye disease — *see* Cataract, complicated
  - hypoparathyroidism E20.9 [H28]
  - malnutrition-dehydration E46 [H28]
  - metabolic disease E88.9 [H28]
  - myotonic disorders G71.19 [H28]
  - nutritional disease E63.9 [H28]
- infantile — *see* Cataract, presenile
- irradiational — *see* Cataract, specified NEC
- juvenile — *see* Cataract, presenile
- malnutrition-dehydration E46 [H28]
- morgagnian — *see* Cataract, senile, morgagnian type
- myotonic G71.19 [H28]
- myxedema E03.9 [H28]
- nuclear
  - embryonal Q12.0
  - sclerosis — *see* Cataract, senile, nuclear
- presenile H26.00- ☑
  - combined forms H26.06- ☑
  - cortical H26.01- ☑
  - lamellar — *see* Cataract, presenile, cortical
  - nuclear H26.03- ☑
  - specified NEC H26.09
  - subcapsular polar (anterior) H26.04- ☑
    - posterior H26.05- ☑
  - zonular — *see* Cataract, presenile, cortical
- secondary H26.40
  - Soemmering's ring H26.41- ☑
  - specified NEC H26.49- ☑
  - to eye disease — *see* Cataract, complicated
- senile H25.9
  - brunescens — *see* Cataract, senile, nuclear
  - combined forms H25.81- ☑
  - coronary — *see* Cataract, senile, incipient
  - cortical H25.01- ☑
  - hypermature — *see* Cataract, senile, morgagnian type
  - incipient (mature) (total) H25.09- ☑
    - cortical — *see* Cataract, senile, cortical
    - subcapsular — *see* Cataract, senile, subcapsular
  - morgagnian type (hypermature) H25.2- ☑
  - nuclear (sclerosis) H25.1- ☑
  - polar subcapsular (anterior) (posterior) — *see* Cataract, senile, incipient
  - punctate — *see* Cataract, senile, incipient
  - specified NEC H25.89
  - subcapsular polar (anterior) H25.03- ☑
    - posterior H25.04- ☑
- snowflake — *see* Diabetes, cataract
- specified NEC H26.8
- toxic — *see* Cataract, drug-induced
- traumatic H26.10- ☑
  - localized H26.11- ☑
  - partially resolved H26.12- ☑
  - total H26.13- ☑
- zonular (perinuclear) Q12.0

Cataracta (*see also* Cataract)
- brunescens — *see* Cataract, senile, nuclear
- centralis pulverulenta Q12.0
- cerulea Q12.0
- complicata — *see* Cataract, complicated
- congenita Q12.0
- coralliformis Q12.0
- coronaria Q12.0
- diabetic — *see* Diabetes, cataract
- membranacea
  - accreta — *see* Cataract, secondary
  - congenita Q12.0
- nigra — *see* Cataract, senile, nuclear

Cataracta — *continued*
- sunflower — *see* Cataract, complicated

Catarrh, catarrhal (acute) (febrile) (infectious) (inflammation) (*see also* condition) J00
- bronchial — *see* Bronchitis
- chest — *see* Bronchitis
- chronic J31.0
- due to congenital syphilis A50.03
- enteric — *see* Enteritis
- eustachian H68.009
- fauces — *see* Pharyngitis
- gastrointestinal — *see* Enteritis
- gingivitis K05.00
  - nonplaque induced K05.01
  - plaque induced K05.00
- hay — *see* Fever, hay
- intestinal — *see* Enteritis
- larynx, chronic J37.0
- liver B15.9
  - with hepatic coma B15.0
- lung — *see* Bronchitis
- middle ear, chronic — *see* Otitis, media, nonsuppurative, chronic, serous
- mouth K12.1
- nasal (chronic) — *see* Rhinitis
- nasobronchial J31.1
- nasopharyngeal (chronic) J31.1
  - acute J00
- pulmonary — *see* Bronchitis
- spring (eye) (vernal) — *see* Conjunctivitis, acute, atopic
- summer (hay) — *see* Fever, hay
- throat J31.2
- tubotympanal (*see also* Otitis, media, nonsuppurative)
  - chronic — *see* Otitis, media, nonsuppurative, chronic, serous

Catatonia (schizophrenic) F20.2
Catatonic
- disorder due to known physiologic condition F06.1
- schizophrenia F20.2
- stupor R40.1
Cat-scratch (*see also* Abrasion)
- disease or fever A28.1
Cauliflower ear M95.1- ☑
Causalgia (upper limb) G56.4- ☑
- lower limb G57.7- ☑
Cause
- external, general effects T75.89 ☑
Caustic burn — *see* Corrosion, by site
Cavare's disease (familial periodic paralysis) G72.3
Cave-in, injury
- crushing (severe) — *see* Crush
- suffocation — *see* Asphyxia, traumatic, due to low oxygen, due to cave-in
Cavernitis (penis) N48.29
Cavernositis N48.29
Cavernous — *see* condition
Cavitation of lung (*see also* Tuberculosis, pulmonary) J98.4
- nontuberculous J98.4
Cavities, dental — *see* Caries, dental
Cavity
- lung — *see* Cavitation of lung
- optic papilla Q14.2
- pulmonary — *see* Cavitation of lung
Cavovarus foot, congenital Q66.1
Cavus foot (congenital) Q66.7
- acquired (*see also* Deformity, limb, foot, specified NEC
Cazenave's disease L10.2
Cecitis K52.9
- with perforation, peritonitis, or rupture K65.8
Cecum — *see* condition
Celiac
- artery compression syndrome I77.4
- disease (with steatorrhea) K90.0
- infantilism K90.0
Cell(s), **cellular** (*see also* condition)
- in urine R82.998
Cellulitis (diffuse) (phlegmonous) (septic) (suppurative) L03.90
- abdominal wall L03.311
- anaerobic A48.0
- ankle — *see* Cellulitis, lower limb
- anus K61.0
- arm — *see* Cellulitis, upper limb
- auricle (ear) — *see* Cellulitis, ear
- axilla L03.11- ☑
- back (any part) L03.312

Cellulitis — *continued*
- breast (acute) (nonpuerperal) (subacute) N61.0
  - nipple N61.0
- broad ligament
  - acute N73.0
- buttock L03.317
- cervical (meaning neck) L03.221
- cervix (uteri) — *see* Cervicitis
- cheek (external) L03.211
  - internal K12.2
- chest wall L03.313
- chronic L03.90
- clostridial A48.0
- corpus cavernosum N48.22
- digit
  - finger — *see* Cellulitis, finger
  - toe — *see* Cellulitis, toe
- Douglas' cul-de-sac or pouch
  - acute N73.0
- drainage site (following operation) T81.49 ☑
- ear (external) H60.1- ☑
- eosinophilic (granulomatous) L98.3
- erysipelatous — *see* Erysipelas
- external auditory canal — *see* Cellulitis, ear
- eyelid — *see* Abscess, eyelid
- face NEC L03.211
- finger (intrathecal) (periosteal) (subcutaneous) (subcuticular) L03.01- ☑
- foot — *see* Cellulitis, lower limb
- gangrenous — *see* Gangrene
- genital organ NEC
  - female (external) N76.4
  - male N49.9
    - multiple sites N49.8
    - specified NEC N49.8
- gluteal (region) L03.317
- gonococcal A54.89
- groin L03.314
- hand — *see* Cellulitis, upper limb
- head NEC L03.811
  - face (any part, except ear, eye and nose) L03.211
- heel — *see* Cellulitis, lower limb
- hip — *see* Cellulitis, lower limb
- jaw (region) L03.211
- knee — *see* Cellulitis, lower limb
- labium (majus) (minus) — *see* Vulvitis
- lacrimal passages — *see* Inflammation, lacrimal, passages
- larynx J38.7
- leg — *see* Cellulitis, lower limb
- lip K13.0
- lower limb L03.11- ☑
  - toe — *see* Cellulitis, toe
- mouth (floor) K12.2
- multiple sites, so stated L03.90
- nasopharynx J39.1
- navel L03.316
  - newborn P38.9
    - with mild hemorrhage P38.1
    - without hemorrhage P38.9
- neck (region) L03.221
- nipple (acute) (nonpuerperal) (subacute) N61.0
- nose (septum) (external) J34.0
- orbit, orbital H05.01- ☑
- palate (soft) K12.2
- pectoral (region) L03.313
- pelvis, pelvic (chronic)
  - female (*see also* Disease, pelvis, inflammatory) N73.2
    - acute N73.0
    - following ectopic or molar pregnancy O08.0
  - male K65.0
- penis N48.22
- perineal, perineum L03.315
- periorbital L03.213
- perirectal K61.1
- peritonsillar J36
- periurethral N34.0
- periuterine (*see also* Disease, pelvis, inflammatory) N73.2
  - acute N73.0
- pharynx J39.1
- preseptal L03.213
- rectum K61.1
- retroperitoneal K68.9
- round ligament
  - acute N73.0
- scalp (any part) L03.811
- scrotum N49.2

Cellulitis — *continued*
- seminal vesicle N49.0
- shoulder — *see* Cellulitis, upper limb
- specified site NEC L03.818
- submandibular (region) (space) (triangle) K12.2
  - gland K11.3
- submaxillary (region) K12.2
  - gland K11.3
- thigh — *see* Cellulitis, lower limb
- thumb (intrathecal) (periosteal) (subcutaneous) (sub-cuticular) — *see* Cellulitis, finger
- toe (intrathecal) (periosteal) (subcutaneous) (subcuticular) L03.03- ☑
- tonsil J36
- trunk L03.319
  - abdominal wall L03.311
  - back (any part) L03.312
  - buttock L03.317
  - chest wall L03.313
  - groin L03.314
  - perineal, perineum L03.315
  - umbilicus L03.316
- tuberculous (primary) A18.4
- umbilicus L03.316
- upper limb L03.11- ☑
  - axilla — *see* Cellulitis, axilla
  - finger — *see* Cellulitis, finger
  - thumb — *see* Cellulitis, finger
- vaccinal T88.0 ☑
- vocal cord J38.3
- vulva — *see* Vulvitis
- wrist — *see* Cellulitis, upper limb

Cementoblastoma, benign — *see* Cyst, calcifying odontogenic
Cementoma — *see* Cyst, calcifying odontogenic
Cementoperiostitis — *see* Periodontitis
Cementosis K03.4
Central auditory processing disorder H93.25
Central pain syndrome G89.0
Cephalematocele, cephal (o)hematocele
- newborn P52.8
  - birth injury P10.8
- traumatic — *see* Hematoma, brain
Cephalematoma, cephalhematoma (calcified)
- newborn (birth injury) P12.0
- traumatic — *see* Hematoma, brain
Cephalgia, cephalalgia (*see also* Headache)
- histamine G44.009
  - intractable G44.001
  - not intractable G44.009
- trigeminal autonomic (TAC) NEC G44.099
  - intractable G44.091
  - not intractable G44.099
Cephalic — *see* condition
Cephalitis — *see* Encephalitis
Cephalocele — *see* Encephalocele
Cephalomenia N94.89
Cephalopelvic — *see* condition
Cerclage (with cervical incompetence) in pregnancy — *see* Incompetence, cervix, in pregnancy
Cerebellitis — *see* Encephalitis
Cerebellum, cerebellar — *see* condition
Cerebral — *see* condition
Cerebritis — *see* Encephalitis
Cerebro-hepato-renal syndrome Q87.89
Cerebromalacia — *see* Softening, brain
- sequelae of cerebrovascular disease I69.398
Cerebroside lipidosis E75.22
Cerebrospasticity (congenital) G80.1
Cerebrospinal — *see* condition
Cerebrum — *see* condition
Ceroid-lipofuscinosis, neuronal E75.4
Cerumen (accumulation) (impacted) H61.2- ☑
Cervical (*see also* condition)
- auricle Q18.2
- dysplasia in pregnancy — *see* Abnormal, cervix, in pregnancy or childbirth
- erosion in pregnancy — *see* Abnormal, cervix, in pregnancy or childbirth
- fibrosis in pregnancy — *see* Abnormal, cervix, in pregnancy or childbirth
- fusion syndrome Q76.1
- rib Q76.5
- shortening (complicating pregnancy) O26.87- ☑
Cervicalgia M54.2
Cervicitis (acute) (chronic) (nonvenereal) (senile (atrophic)) (subacute) (with ulceration) N72

Cervicitis — *continued*
- with
  - abortion — *see* Abortion, by type complicated by genital tract and pelvic infection
  - ectopic pregnancy O08.0
  - molar pregnancy O08.0
- chlamydial A56.09
- gonococcal A54.03
- herpesviral A60.03
- puerperal (postpartum) O86.11
- syphilitic A52.76
- trichomonal A59.09
- tuberculous A18.16
Cervicocolpitis (emphysematosa) (*see also* Cervicitis) N72
Cervix — *see* condition
Cesarean delivery, previous, affecting management of pregnancy O34.219
- classical (vertical) scar O34.212
- low transverse scar O34.211
Céstan (-Chenais) paralysis or syndrome G46.3
Céstan-Raymond syndrome I65.8
Cestode infestation B71.9
- specified type NEC B71.8
Cestodiasis B71.9
Chabert's disease A22.9
Chacaleh E53.8
Chafing L30.4
Chagas' (-Mazza) disease (chronic) B57.2
- with
  - cardiovascular involvement NEC B57.2
  - digestive system involvement B57.30
    - megacolon B57.32
    - megaesophagus B57.31
    - other specified B57.39
  - megacolon B57.32
  - megaesophagus B57.31
  - myocarditis B57.2
  - nervous system involvement B57.40
    - meningitis B57.41
    - meningoencephalitis B57.42
    - other specified B57.49
  - specified organ involvement NEC B57.5
- acute (with) B57.1
  - cardiovascular NEC B57.0
  - myocarditis B57.0
Chagres fever B50.9
Chairridden Z74.09
Chalasia (cardiac sphincter) K21.9
Chalazion H00.19
- left H00.16
  - lower H00.15
  - upper H00.14
- right H00.13
  - lower H00.12
  - upper H00.11
Chalcosis (*see also* Disorder, globe, degenerative, chalcosis)
- cornea — *see* Deposit, cornea
- crystalline lens — *see* Cataract, complicated
- retina H35.89
Chalicosis (pulmonum) J62.8
Chancre (any genital site) (hard) (hunterian) (mixed) (primary) (seronegative) (seropositive) (syphilitic) A51.0
- congenital A50.07
- conjunctiva NEC A51.2
- Ducrey's A57
- extragenital A51.2
- eyelid A51.2
- lip A51.2
- nipple A51.2
- Nisbet's A57
- of
  - carate A67.0
  - pinta A67.0
  - yaws A66.0
- palate, soft A51.2
- phagedenic A57
- simple A57
- soft A57
  - bubo A57
  - palate A51.2
- urethra A51.2
- yaws A66.0
Chancroid (anus) (genital) (penis) (perineum) (rectum) (urethra) (vulva) A57

Chandler's disease (osteochondritis dissecans, hip) — *see* Osteochondritis, dissecans, hip
Change(s) (in) (of) (*see also* Removal)
- arteriosclerotic — *see* Arteriosclerosis
- bone (*see also* Disorder, bone)
  - diabetic — *see* Diabetes, bone change
- bowel habit R19.4
- cardiorenal (vascular) — *see* Hypertension, cardiorenal
- cardiovascular — *see* Disease, cardiovascular
- circulatory I99.9
- cognitive (mild) (organic) R41.89
- color, tooth, teeth
  - during formation K00.8
  - posteruptive K03.7
- contraceptive device Z30.433
- corneal membrane H18.30
  - Bowman's membrane fold or rupture H18.31- ☑
  - Descemet's membrane
    - fold H18.32- ☑
    - rupture H18.33- ☑
- coronary — *see* Disease, heart, ischemic
- degenerative, spine or vertebra — *see* Spondylosis
- dental pulp, regressive K04.2
- dressing (nonsurgical) Z48.00
  - surgical Z48.01
- heart — *see* Disease, heart
- hip joint — *see* Derangement, joint, hip
- hyperplastic larynx J38.7
- hypertrophic
  - nasal sinus J34.89
  - turbinate, nasal J34.3
  - upper respiratory tract J39.8
- indwelling catheter Z46.6
- inflammatory (*see also* Inflammation)
  - sacroiliac M46.1
- job, anxiety concerning Z56.1
- joint — *see* Derangement, joint
- life — *see* Menopause
- mental status R41.82
- minimal (glomerular) (*see also* N00-N07 with fourth character .0) N05.0
- myocardium, myocardial — *see* Degeneration, myocardial
- of life — *see* Menopause
- pacemaker Z45.018
  - pulse generator Z45.010
- personality (enduring) F68.8
  - due to (secondary to)
    - general medical condition F07.0
  - secondary (nonspecific) F60.89
- regressive, dental pulp K04.2
- renal — *see* Disease, renal
- retina H35.9
  - myopic (*see also* Myopia, degenerative) H44.2- ☑
- sacroiliac joint M53.3
- senile (*see also* condition) R54
- sensory R20.8
- skin R23.9
  - acute, due to ultraviolet radiation L56.9
    - specified NEC L56.8
  - chronic, due to nonionizing radiation L57.9
    - specified NEC L57.8
  - cyanosis R23.0
  - flushing R23.2
  - pallor R23.1
  - petechiae R23.3
  - specified change NEC R23.8
  - swelling — *see* Mass, localized
  - texture R23.4
- trophic
  - arm — *see* Mononeuropathy, upper limb
  - leg — *see* Mononeuropathy, lower limb
- vascular I99.9
- vasomotor I73.9
- voice R49.9
  - psychogenic F44.4
  - specified NEC R49.8
Changing sleep-work schedule, affecting sleep G47.26
Changuinola fever A93.1
Chapping skin T69.8 ☑
Charcot-Marie-Tooth disease, paralysis or syndrome G60.0
Charcot's
- arthropathy — *see* Arthropathy, neuropathic
- cirrhosis K74.3
- disease (tabetic arthropathy) A52.16
- joint (disease) (tabetic) A52.16

Charcot's — continued
  joint — continued
    diabetic — see Diabetes, with, arthropathy
    syringomyelic G95.0
    syndrome (intermittent claudication) I73.9
CHARGE association Q89.8
Charley-horse (quadriceps) M62.831
  traumatic (quadriceps) S76.11- ☑
Charlouis' disease — see Yaws
Cheadle's disease E54
Checking (of)
  cardiac pacemaker (battery) (electrode(s)) Z45.018
    pulse generator Z45.010
  implantable subdermal contraceptive Z30.46
  intrauterine contraceptive device Z30.431
  wound Z48.0- ☑
    due to injury — code to Injury, by site, using appro-
      priate seventh character for subsequent en-
      counter
Check-up — see Examination
Chédiak-Higashi (-Steinbrinck) **syndrome** (congenital
  gigantism of peroxidase granules) E70.330
Cheek — see condition
Cheese itch B88.0
Cheese-washer's lung J67.8
Cheese-worker's lung J67.8
Cheilitis (acute) (angular) (catarrhal) (chronic) (exfoliative)
  (gangrenous) (glandular) (infectional) (suppurative)
  (ulcerative) (vesicular) K13.0
  actinic (due to sun) L56.8
    other than from sun L59.8
  candidal B37.83
Cheilodynia K13.0
Cheiloschisis — see Cleft, lip
Cheilosis (angular) K13.0
  with pellagra E52
  due to
    vitamin B2 (riboflavin) deficiency E53.0
Cheiromegaly M79.89
Cheiropompholyx L30.1
Cheloid — see Keloid
Chemical burn — see Corrosion, by site
Chemodectoma — see Paraganglioma, nonchromaffin
Chemosis, conjunctiva — see Edema, conjunctiva
Chemotherapy (session) (for)
  cancer Z51.11
  neoplasm Z51.11
Cherubism M27.8
Chest — see condition
Cheyne-Stokes breathing (respiration) R06.3
Chiari's
  disease or syndrome (hepatic vein thrombosis) I82.0
  malformation
    type I G93.5
    type II — see Spina bifida
    net Q24.8
Chicago disease B40.9
Chickenpox — see Varicella
Chiclero ulcer or sore B55.1
Chigger (infestation) B88.0
Chignon (disease) B36.8
  newborn (from vacuum extraction) (birth injury) P12.1
Chilaiditi's syndrome (subphrenic displacement, colon)
  Q43.3
Chilblain(s) (lupus) T69.1 ☑
Child
  custody dispute Z65.3
Childbirth — see Delivery
Childhood
  cerebral X-linked adrenoleukodystrophy E71.520
  period of rapid growth Z00.2
Chill(s) R68.83
  with fever R50.9
  congestive in malarial regions B54
  without fever R68.83
Chilomastigiasis A07.8
Chimera 46,XX/46,XY Q99.0
Chin — see condition
Chinese dysentery A03.9
Chionophobia F40.228
Chitral fever A93.1
Chlamydia, chlamydial A74.9
  cervicitis A56.09
  conjunctivitis A74.0
  cystitis A56.01
  endometritis A56.11
  epididymitis A56.19

Chlamydia, chlamydial — continued
  female
    pelvic inflammatory disease A56.11
      pelviperitonitis A56.11
  orchitis A56.19
  peritonitis A74.81
  pharyngitis A56.4
  proctitis A56.3
  psittaci (infection) A70
  salpingitis A56.11
  sexually-transmitted infection NEC A56.8
  specified NEC A74.89
  urethritis A56.01
  vulvovaginitis A56.02
Chlamydiosis — see Chlamydia
Chloasma (skin) (idiopathic) (symptomatic) L81.1
  eyelid H02.719
    hyperthyroid E05.90 [H02.719]
      with thyroid storm E05.91 [H02.719]
    left H02.716
      lower H02.715
      upper H02.714
    right H02.713
      lower H02.712
      upper H02.711
Chloroma C92.3- ☑
Chlorosis D50.9
  Egyptian B76.9 [D63.8]
  miner's B76.9 [D63.8]
Chlorotic anemia D50.8
Chocolate cyst (ovary) N80.1
Choked
  disc or disk — see Papilledema
  on food, phlegm, or vomitus NOS — see Foreign body,
    by site
  while vomiting NOS — see Foreign body, by site
Chokes (resulting from bends) T70.3 ☑
Choking sensation R09.89
Cholangiectasis K83.8
Cholangiocarcinoma
  with hepatocellular carcinoma, combined C22.0
  liver C22.1
  specified site NEC — see Neoplasm, malignant, by site
  unspecified site C22.1
Cholangiohepatitis K83.8
  due to fluke infestation B66.1
Cholangiohepatoma C22.0
Cholangiolitis (acute) (chronic) (extrahepatic) (gangrenous) (intrahepatic) K83.09
  paratyphoidal — see Fever, paratyphoid
  typhoidal A01.09
Cholangioma D13.4
  malignant — see Cholangiocarcinoma
Cholangitis (ascending) (recurrent) (secondary) (stenos-
  ing) (suppurative) K83.09
  with calculus, bile duct — see Calculus, bile duct, with
    cholangitis
  chronic nonsuppurative destructive K74.3
  primary K83.09
    sclerosing K83.01
  sclerosing K83.09
Cholecystasia K82.8
Cholecystitis K81.9
  with
    calculus, stones in
      bile duct (common) (hepatic) — see Calculus,
        bile duct, with cholecystitis
      cystic duct — see Calculus, gallbladder, with
        cholecystitis
      gallbladder — see Calculus, gallbladder, with
        cholecystitis
      choledocholithiasis — see Calculus, bile duct, with
        cholecystitis
      cholelithiasis — see Calculus, gallbladder, with
        cholecystitis
    gangrene of gallbladder K82.A1
    perforation of gallbladder K82.A2
  acute (emphysematous) (gangrenous) (suppurative)
    K81.0
    with
      calculus, stones in
        cystic duct — see Calculus, gallbladder, with
          cholecystitis, acute
        gallbladder — see Calculus, gallbladder, with
          cholecystitis, acute
        choledocholithiasis — see Calculus, bile duct,
          with cholecystitis, acute

Cholecystitis — continued
  acute — continued
    with — continued
      cholelithiasis — see Calculus, gallbladder, with
        cholecystitis, acute
    chronic cholecystitis K81.2
      with gallbladder calculus K80.12
        with obstruction K80.13
  chronic K81.1
    with acute cholecystitis K81.2
      with gallbladder calculus K80.12
        with obstruction K80.13
  emphysematous (acute) — see Cholecystitis, acute
  gangrenous — see Cholecystitis, acute
  paratyphoidal, current A01.4
  suppurative — see Cholecystitis, acute
  typhoidal A01.09
Cholecystolithiasis — see Calculus, gallbladder
Choledochitis (suppurative) K83.09
Choledocholith — see Calculus, bile duct
Choledocholithiasis (common duct) (hepatic duct) —
  see Calculus, bile duct
  cystic — see Calculus, gallbladder
  typhoidal A01.09
Cholelithiasis (cystic duct) (gallbladder) (impacted)
  (multiple) — see Calculus, gallbladder
  bile duct (common) (hepatic) — see Calculus, bile duct
  hepatic duct — see Calculus, bile duct
  specified NEC K80.80
    with obstruction K80.81
Cholemia (see also Jaundice)
  familial (simple) (congenital) E80.4
  Gilbert's E80.4
Choleperitoneum, choleperitonitis K65.3
Cholera (Asiatic) (epidemic) (malignant) A00.9
  antimonial — see Poisoning, antimony
  classical A00.0
  due to Vibrio cholerae 01 A00.9
    biovar cholerae A00.0
    biovar eltor A00.1
    el tor A00.1
  el tor A00.1
Cholerine — see Cholera
Cholestasis NEC K83.1
  with hepatocyte injury K71.0
  due to total parenteral nutrition (TPN) K76.89
  pure K71.0
Cholesteatoma (ear) (middle) (with reaction) H71.9- ☑
  attic H71.0- ☑
  external ear (canal) H60.4- ☑
  mastoid H71.2- ☑
  postmastoidectomy cavity (recurrent) — see Complica-
    tions, postmastoidectomy, recurrent
    cholesteatoma
  recurrent (postmastoidectomy) — see Complications,
    postmastoidectomy, recurrent cholesteatoma
  tympanum H71.1- ☑
Cholesteatosis, diffuse H71.3- ☑
Cholesteremia E78.00
Cholesterin in vitreous — see Deposit, crystalline
Cholesterol
  deposit
    retina H35.89
    vitreous — see Deposit, crystalline
  elevated (high) E78.00
    with elevated (high) triglycerides E78.2
    screening for Z13.220
  imbibition of gallbladder K82.4
Cholesterolemia (essential) (pure) E78.00
  familial E78.01
  hereditary E78.01
Cholesterolosis, cholesterosis (gallbladder) K82.4
  cerebrotendinous E75.5
Cholocolic fistula K82.3
Choluria R82.2
Chondritis M94.8X9
  aurical H61.03- ☑
  costal (Tietze's) M94.0
  external ear H61.03- ☑
  patella, posttraumatic — see Chondromalacia, patella
  pinna H61.03- ☑
  purulent M94.8X- ☑
  tuberculous NEC A18.02
    intervertebral A18.01
Chondroblastoma (see also Neoplasm, bone, benign)
  malignant — see Neoplasm, bone, malignant
Chondrocalcinosis M11.20

☟ Subterms under main terms may continue to next column or page   ☑ Additional Character Required — Refer to the Tabular List for Character Selection   53

Charcot's — Chondrocalcinosis

Chondrocalcinosis — *continued*
ankle M11.27- ☑
elbow M11.22- ☑
familial M11.10
  ankle M11.17- ☑
  elbow M11.12- ☑
  foot joint M11.17- ☑
  hand joint M11.14- ☑
  hip M11.15- ☑
  knee M11.16- ☑
  multiple site M11.19
  shoulder M11.11- ☑
  vertebrae M11.18
  wrist M11.13- ☑
foot joint M11.27- ☑
hand joint M11.24- ☑
hip M11.25- ☑
knee M11.26- ☑
multiple site M11.29
shoulder M11.21- ☑
specified type NEC M11.20
  ankle M11.27- ☑
  elbow M11.22- ☑
  foot joint M11.27- ☑
  hand joint M11.24- ☑
  hip M11.25- ☑
  knee M11.26- ☑
  multiple site M11.29
  shoulder M11.21- ☑
  vertebrae M11.28
  wrist M11.23- ☑
vertebrae M11.28
wrist M11.23- ☑
Chondrodermatitis nodularis helicis or anthelicis — *see* Perichondritis, ear
Chondrodysplasia Q78.9
with hemangioma Q78.4
calcificans congenita Q77.3
fetalis Q77.4
metaphyseal (Jansen's) (McKusick's) (Schmid's) Q78.8
punctata Q77.3
Chondrodystrophy, chondrodystrophia (familial) (fetalis) (hypoplastic) Q78.9
calcificans congenita Q77.3
myotonic (congenital) G71.13
punctata Q77.3
Chondroectodermal dysplasia Q77.6
Chondrogenesis imperfecta Q77.4
Chondrolysis M94.35- ☑
Chondroma (*see also* Neoplasm, cartilage, benign)
juxtacortical — *see* Neoplasm, bone, benign
periosteal — *see* Neoplasm, bone, benign
Chondromalacia (systemic) M94.20
acromioclavicular joint M94.21- ☑
ankle M94.27- ☑
elbow M94.22- ☑
foot joint M94.27- ☑
glenohumeral joint M94.21- ☑
hand joint M94.24- ☑
hip M94.25- ☑
knee M94.26- ☑
  patella M22.4- ☑
multiple sites M94.29
patella M22.4- ☑
rib M94.28
sacroiliac joint M94.259
shoulder M94.21- ☑
sternoclavicular joint M94.21- ☑
vertebral joint M94.28
wrist M94.23- ☑
Chondromatosis (*see also* Neoplasm, cartilage, uncertain behavior)
internal Q78.4
Chondromyxosarcoma — *see* Neoplasm, cartilage, malignant
Chondro-osteodysplasia (Morquio-Brailsford type) E76.219
Chondro-osteodystrophy E76.29
Chondro-osteoma — *see* Neoplasm, bone, benign
Chondropathia tuberosa M94.0
Chondrosarcoma — *see* Neoplasm, cartilage, malignant
juxtacortical — *see* Neoplasm, bone, malignant
mesenchymal — *see* Neoplasm, connective tissue, malignant
myxoid — *see* Neoplasm, cartilage, malignant
Chordee (nonvenereal) N48.89
congenital Q54.4

Chordee — *continued*
gonococcal A54.09
Chorditis (fibrinous) (nodosa) (tuberosa) J38.2
Chordoma — *see* Neoplasm, vertebral (column), malignant
Chorea (chronic) (gravis) (posthemiplegic) (senile) (spasmodic) G25.5
with
  heart involvement I02.0
    active or acute (conditions in I01-) I02.0
    rheumatic I02.9
      with valvular disorder I02.0
    rheumatic heart disease (chronic) (inactive)(quiescent) — *code to* rheumatic heart condition involved
drug-induced G25.4
habit F95.8
hereditary G10
Huntington's G10
hysterical F44.4
minor I02.9
  with heart involvement I02.0
progressive G25.5
  hereditary G10
rheumatic (chronic) I02.9
  with heart involvement I02.0
Sydenham's I02.9
  with heart involvement — *see* Chorea, with rheumatic heart disease
  nonrheumatic G25.5
Choreoathetosis (paroxysmal) G25.5
Chorioadenoma (destruens) D39.2
Chorioamnionitis O41.12- ☑
Chorioangioma D26.7
Choriocarcinoma — *see* Neoplasm, malignant, by site
combined with
  embryonal carcinoma — *see* Neoplasm, malignant, by site
  other germ cell elements — *see* Neoplasm, malignant, by site
  teratoma — *see* Neoplasm, malignant, by site
specified site — *see* Neoplasm, malignant, by site
unspecified site
  female C58
  male C62.90
Chorioencephalitis (acute) (lymphocytic) (serous) A87.2
Chorioepithelioma — *see* Choriocarcinoma
Choriomeningitis (acute) (lymphocytic) (serous) A87.2
Chorionepithelioma — *see* Choriocarcinoma
Chorioretinitis (*see also* Inflammation, chorioretinal)
disseminated (*see also* Inflammation, chorioretinal, disseminated)
  in neurosyphilis A52.19
Egyptian B76.9 [D63.8]
focal (*see also* Inflammation, chorioretinal, focal)
histoplasmic B39.9 [H32]
in (due to)
  histoplasmosis B39.9 [H32]
  syphilis (secondary) A51.43
    late A52.71
  toxoplasmosis (acquired) B58.01
    congenital (active) P37.1 [H32]
  tuberculosis A18.53
juxtapapillary, juxtapapillaris — *see* Inflammation, chorioretinal, focal, juxtapapillary
leprous A30.9 [H32]
miner's B76.9 [D63.8]
progressive myopia (degeneration) (*see also* Myopia, degenerative) H44.2- ☑
syphilitic (secondary) A51.43
  congenital (early) A50.01 [H32]
    late A50.32
  late A52.71
tuberculous A18.53
Chorioretinopathy, central serous H35.71- ☑
Choroid — *see* condition
Choroideremia H31.21
Choroiditis — *see* Chorioretinitis
Choroidopathy — *see* Disorder, choroid
Choroidoretinitis — *see* Chorioretinitis
Choroidoretinopathy, central serous — *see* Chorioretinopathy, central serous
Christian-Weber disease M35.6
Christmas disease D67
Chromaffinoma (*see also* Neoplasm, benign, by site)
malignant — *see* Neoplasm, malignant, by site
Chromatopsia — *see* Deficiency, color vision
Chromhidrosis, chromidrosis L75.1

Chromoblastomycosis — *see* Chromomycosis
Chromoconversion R82.91
Chromomycosis B43.9
brain abscess B43.1
cerebral B43.1
cutaneous B43.0
skin B43.0
specified NEC B43.8
subcutaneous abscess or cyst B43.2
Chromophytosis B36.0
Chromosome — *see* Anomaly, by chromosome involved
D (1) — *see* Anomaly, chromosome 13
E (3) — *see* Anomaly, chromosome 18
G — *see* Anomaly, chromosome 21
Chromotrichomycosis B36.8
Chronic — *see* condition
fracture — *see* Fracture, pathological
Churg-Strauss syndrome M30.1
Chyle cyst, mesentery I89.8
Chylocele (nonfilarial) I89.8
filarial (*see also* Infestation, filarial) B74.9 [N51]
tunica vaginalis N50.89
  filarial (*see also* Infestation, filarial) B74.9 [N51]
Chylomicronemia (fasting) (with hyperprebetalipoproteinemia) E78.3
Chylopericardium I31.3
acute I30.9
Chylothorax (nonfilarial) I89.8
filarial (*see also* Infestation, filarial) B74.9 [J91.8]
Chylous — *see* condition
Chyluria (nonfilarial) R82.0
due to
  bilharziasis B65.0
  Brugia (malayi) B74.1
    timori B74.2
  schistosomiasis (bilharziasis) B65.0
  Wuchereria (bancrofti) B74.0
filarial — *see* Infestation, filarial
Cicatricial (deformity) — *see* Cicatrix
Cicatrix (adherent) (contracted) (painful) (vicious) (*see also* Scar) L90.5
adenoid (and tonsil) J35.8
alveolar process M26.79
anus K62.89
auricle — *see* Disorder, pinna, specified type NEC
bile duct (common) (hepatic) K83.8
bladder N32.89
bone — *see* Disorder, bone, specified type NEC
brain G93.89
cervix (postoperative) (postpartal) N88.1
common duct K83.8
cornea H17.9
  tuberculous A18.59
duodenum (bulb), obstructive K31.5
esophagus K22.2
eyelid — *see* Disorder, eyelid function
hypopharynx J39.2
lacrimal passages — *see* Obstruction, lacrimal
larynx J38.7
lung J98.4
middle ear H74.8 ☑
mouth K13.79
muscle M62.89
  with contracture — *see* Contraction, muscle NEC
nasopharynx J39.2
palate (soft) K13.79
penis N48.89
pharynx J39.2
prostate N42.89
rectum K62.89
retina — *see* Scar, chorioretinal
semilunar cartilage — *see* Derangement, meniscus
seminal vesicle N50.89
skin L90.5
  infected L08.89
  postinfective L90.5
  tuberculous B90.8
specified site NEC L90.5
throat J39.2
tongue K14.8
tonsil (and adenoid) J35.8
trachea J39.8
tuberculous NEC B90.9
urethra N36.8
uterus N85.8
vagina N89.8
  postoperative N99.2
vocal cord J38.3

☑ **Additional Character Required** — Refer to the Tabular List for Character Selection   ▽ Subterms under main terms may continue to next column or page

Cicatrix — *continued*
wrist, constricting (annular) L90.5
CIDP (chronic inflammatory demyelinating polyneuropathy) G61.81
CIN — *see* Neoplasia, intraepithelial, cervix
CINCA (chronic infantile neurological, cutaneous and articular syndrome) M04.2
Cinchonism — *see* Deafness, ototoxic
correct substance properly administered — *see* Table of Drugs and Chemicals, by drug, adverse effect
overdose or wrong substance given or taken — *see* Table of Drugs and Chemicals, by drug, poisoning
Circle of Willis — *see* condition
Circular — *see* condition
Circulating anticoagulants (*see also* Disorder, hemorrhagic) D68.318
due to drugs (*see also* Disorder, hemorrhagic) D68.32
following childbirth O72.3
Circulation
collateral, any site I99.8
defective (lower extremity) I99.9
congenital Q28.9
embryonic Q28.9
failure (peripheral) R57.9
newborn P29.89
fetal, persistent P29.38
heart, incomplete Q28.9
Circulatory system — *see* condition
Circulus senilis (cornea) — *see* Degeneration, cornea, senile
Circumcision (in absence of medical indication) (ritual) (routine) Z41.2
Circumscribed — *see* condition
Circumvallate placenta O43.11- ☑
Cirrhosis, cirrhotic (hepatic) (liver) K74.60
alcoholic K70.30
with ascites K70.31
atrophic — *see* Cirrhosis, liver
Baumgarten-Cruveilhier K74.69
biliary (cholangiolitic) (cholangitic) (hypertrophic) (obstructive) (pericholangiolitic) K74.5
due to
Clonorchiasis B66.1
flukes B66.3
primary K74.3
secondary K74.4
cardiac (of liver) K76.1
Charcot's K74.3
cholangiolitic, cholangitic, cholostatic (primary) K74.3
congestive K76.1
Cruveilhier-Baumgarten K74.69
cryptogenic (liver) K74.69
due to
hepatolenticular degeneration E83.01
Wilson's disease E83.01
xanthomatosis E78.2
fatty K76.0
alcoholic K70.0
Hanot's (hypertrophic) K74.3
hepatic — *see* Cirrhosis, liver
hypertrophic K74.3
Indian childhood K74.69
kidney — *see* Sclerosis, renal
Laennec's K70.30
with ascites K70.31
alcoholic K70.30
with ascites K70.31
nonalcoholic K74.69
liver K74.60
alcoholic K70.30
with ascites K70.31
fatty K70.0
congenital P78.81
syphilitic A52.74
lung (chronic) J84.10
macronodular K74.69
alcoholic K70.30
with ascites K70.31
micronodular K74.69
alcoholic K70.30
with ascites K70.31
mixed type K74.69
monolobular K74.3
nephritis — *see* Sclerosis, renal
nutritional K74.69
alcoholic K70.30
with ascites K70.31
obstructive — *see* Cirrhosis, biliary

Cirrhosis, cirrhotic — *continued*
ovarian N83.8
pancreas (duct) K86.89
pigmentary E83.110
portal K74.69
alcoholic K70.30
with ascites K70.31
postnecrotic K74.69
alcoholic K70.30
with ascites K70.31
pulmonary J84.10
renal — *see* Sclerosis, renal
spleen D73.2
stasis K76.1
Todd's K74.3
unilobar K74.3
xanthomatous (biliary) K74.5
due to xanthomatosis (familial) (metabolic) (primary) E78.2
Cistern, subarachnoid R93.0
Citrullinemia E72.23
Citrullinuria E72.23
Civatte's disease or poikiloderma L57.3
Clam digger's itch B65.3
Clammy skin R23.1
Clap — *see* Gonorrhea
Clarke-Hadfield syndrome (pancreatic infantilism) K86.89
Clark's paralysis G80.9
Clastothrix L67.8
Claude Bernard-Horner syndrome G90.2
traumatic — *see* Injury, nerve, cervical sympathetic
Claude's disease or syndrome G46.3
Claudicatio venosa intermittens I87.8
Claudication (intermittent) I73.9
cerebral (artery) G45.9
spinal cord (arteriosclerotic) G95.19
syphilitic A52.09
venous (axillary) I87.8
Claustrophobia F40.240
Clavus (infected) L84
Clawfoot (congenital) Q66.89
acquired — *see* Deformity, limb, clawfoot
Clawhand (acquired) (*see also* Deformity, limb, clawhand)
congenital Q68.1
Clawtoe (congenital) Q66.89
acquired — *see* Deformity, toe, specified NEC
Clay eating — *see* Pica
Cleansing of artificial opening — *see* Attention to, artificial, opening
Cleft (congenital) — *see also* Imperfect, closure
alveolar process M26.79
branchial (persistent) Q18.2
cyst Q18.0
fistula Q18.0
sinus Q18.0
cricoid cartilage, posterior Q31.8
cyst Q18.0
fistula Q18.0
sinus Q18.0
foot Q72.7 ☑
hand Q71.6 ☑
lip (unilateral) Q36.9
with cleft palate Q37.9
hard Q37.1
with soft Q37.5
soft Q37.3
with hard Q37.5
bilateral Q36.9
with cleft palate Q37.8
hard Q37.0
with soft Q37.4
soft Q37.2
with hard Q37.4
median Q36.1
nose Q30.2
palate Q35.9
with cleft lip (unilateral) Q37.9
bilateral Q37.8
hard Q35.1
with
cleft lip (unilateral) Q37.1
bilateral Q37.0
soft Q35.5
with cleft lip (unilateral) Q37.5
bilateral Q37.4
medial Q35.5
soft Q35.3

Cleft — *continued*
palate — *continued*
soft — *continued*
with
cleft lip (unilateral) Q37.3
bilateral Q37.2
hard Q35.5
with cleft lip (unilateral) Q37.5
bilateral Q37.4
penis Q55.69
scrotum Q55.29
thyroid cartilage Q31.8
uvula Q35.7
Cleidocranial dysostosis Q74.0
Cleptomania F63.2
Clicking hip (newborn) R29.4
Climacteric (female) (*see also* Menopause)
arthritis (any site) NEC — *see* Arthritis, specified form NEC
depression (single episode) F32.89
recurrent episode F33.8
male (symptoms) (syndrome) NEC N50.89
melancholia (single episode) F32.89
recurrent episode F33.8
paranoid state F22
polyarthritis NEC — *see* Arthritis, specified form NEC
symptoms (female) N95.1
Clinical research investigation (clinical trial) (control subject) (normal comparison) (participant) Z00.6
Clitoris — *see* condition
Cloaca (persistent) Q43.7
Clonorchiasis, clonorchis infection (liver) B66.1
Clonus R25.8
Closed bite M26.29
Clostridium (C.) **perfringens, as cause of disease classified elsewhere** B96.7
Closure
congenital, nose Q30.0
cranial sutures, premature Q75.0
defective or imperfect NEC — *see* Imperfect, closure
fistula, delayed — *see* Fistula
foramen ovale, imperfect Q21.1
hymen N89.6
interauricular septum, defective Q21.1
interventricular septum, defective Q21.0
lacrimal duct (*see also* Stenosis, lacrimal, duct)
congenital Q10.5
nose (congenital) Q30.0
acquired M95.0
of artificial opening — *see* Attention to, artificial, opening
vagina N89.5
valve — *see* Endocarditis
vulva N90.5
Clot (blood) (*see also* Embolism)
artery (obstruction) (occlusion) — *see* Embolism
bladder N32.89
brain (intradural or extradural) — *see* Occlusion, artery, cerebral
circulation I74.9
heart (*see also* Infarct, myocardium)
not resulting in infarction I51.3
vein — *see* Thrombosis
Clouded state R40.1
epileptic — *see* Epilepsy, specified NEC
paroxysmal — *see* Epilepsy, specified NEC
Cloudy antrum, antra J32.0
Clouston's (hidrotic) **ectodermal dysplasia** Q82.4
Clubbed nail pachydermoperiostosis M89.40 [L62]
Clubbing of finger(s) (nails) R68.3
Clubfinger R68.3
congenital Q68.1
Clubfoot (congenital) Q66.89
acquired — *see* Deformity, limb, clubfoot
equinovarus Q66.0
paralytic — *see* Deformity, limb, clubfoot
Clubhand (congenital) (radial) Q71.4- ☑
acquired — *see* Deformity, limb, clubhand
Clubnail R68.3
congenital Q84.6
Clump, kidney Q63.1
Clumsiness, clumsy child syndrome F82
Cluttering F80.81
Clutton's joints A50.51 [M12.80]
Coagulation, intravascular (diffuse) (disseminated) (*see also* Defibrination syndrome)

Coagulation, intravascular — *continued*
  complicating abortion — *see* Abortion, by type, complicated by, intravascular coagulation
  following ectopic or molar pregnancy O08.1
Coagulopathy (*see also* Defect, coagulation)
  consumption D65
  intravascular D65
    newborn P60
Coalition
  calcaneo-scaphoid Q66.89
  tarsal Q66.89
Coalminer's
  elbow — *see* Bursitis, elbow, olecranon
  lung or pneumoconiosis J60
Coalworker's lung or pneumoconiosis J60
Coarctation
  aorta (preductal) (postductal) Q25.1
  pulmonary artery Q25.71
Coated tongue K14.3
Coats' disease (exudative retinopathy) — *see* Retinopathy, exudative
Cocaine-induced
  anxiety disorder F14.980
  bipolar and related disorder F14.94
  depressive disorder F14.94
  obsessive-compulsive and related disorder F14.988
  psychotic disorder F14.959
  sexual dysfunction F14.981
  sleep disorder F14.982
Cocainism — *see* Disorder, cocaine use
Coccidioidomycosis B38.9
  cutaneous B38.3
  disseminated B38.7
  generalized B38.7
  meninges B38.4
  prostate B38.81
  pulmonary B38.2
    acute B38.0
    chronic B38.1
  skin B38.3
  specified NEC B38.89
Coccidioidosis — *see* Coccidioidomycosis
Coccidiosis (intestinal) A07.3
Coccydynia, coccygodynia M53.3
Coccyx — *see* condition
Cochin-China diarrhea K90.1
Cockayne's syndrome Q87.1
Cocked up toe — *see* Deformity, toe, specified NEC
Cock's peculiar tumor L72.3
Codman's tumor — *see* Neoplasm, bone, benign
Coenurosis B71.8
Coffee-worker's lung J67.8
Cogan's syndrome H16.32- ☑
  oculomotor apraxia H51.8
Coitus, painful (female) N94.10
  male N53.12
  psychogenic F52.6
Cold J00
  with influenza, flu, or grippe — *see* Influenza, with, respiratory manifestations NEC
  agglutinin disease or hemoglobinuria (chronic) D59.1
  bronchial — *see* Bronchitis
  chest — *see* Bronchitis
  common (head) J00
  effects of T69.9 ☑
    specified effect NEC T69.8 ☑
  excessive, effects of T69.9 ☑
    specified effect NEC T69.8 ☑
  exhaustion from T69.8 ☑
  exposure to T69.9 ☑
    specified effect NEC T69.8 ☑
  head J00
  injury syndrome (newborn) P80.0
  on lung — *see* Bronchitis
  rose J30.1
  sensitivity, auto-immune D59.1
  symptoms J00
  virus J00
Coldsore B00.1
Colibacillosis A49.8
  as the cause of other disease (*see also* Escherichia coli) B96.20
  generalized A41.50
Colic (bilious) (infantile) (intestinal) (recurrent) (spasmodic) R10.83
  abdomen R10.83
    psychogenic F45.8

Colic — *continued*
  appendix, appendicular K38.8
  bile duct — *see* Calculus, bile duct
  biliary — *see* Calculus, bile duct
  common duct — *see* Calculus, bile duct
  cystic duct — *see* Calculus, gallbladder
  Devonshire NEC — *see* Poisoning, lead
  gallbladder — *see* Calculus, gallbladder
  gallstone — *see* Calculus, gallbladder
    gallbladder or cystic duct — *see* Calculus, gallbladder
  hepatic (duct) — *see* Calculus, bile duct
  hysterical F45.8
  kidney N23
  lead NEC — *see* Poisoning, lead
  mucous K58.9
    with diarrhea K58.0
    psychogenic F54
  nephritic N23
  painter's NEC — *see* Poisoning, lead
  pancreas K86.89
  psychogenic F45.8
  renal N23
  saturnine NEC — *see* Poisoning, lead
  ureter N23
  urethral N36.8
    due to calculus N21.1
  uterus NEC N94.89
    menstrual — *see* Dysmenorrhea
  worm NOS B83.9
Colicystitis — *see* Cystitis
Colitis (acute) (catarrhal) (chronic) (noninfective) (hemorrhagic) (*see also* Enteritis) K52.9
  allergic K52.29
    with
      food protein-induced enterocolitis syndrome K52.21
      proctocolitis K52.82
  amebic (acute) (*see also* Amebiasis) A06.0
    nondysenteric A06.2
  anthrax A22.2
  bacillary — *see* Infection, Shigella
  balantidial A07.0
  Clostridium difficile
    not specified as recurrent A04.72
    recurrent A04.71
  coccidial A07.3
  collagenous K52.831
  cystica superficialis K52.89
  dietary counseling and surveillance (for) Z71.3
  dietetic (*see also* Colitis, allergic) K52.29
  drug-induced K52.1
  due to radiation K52.0
  eosinophilic K52.82
  food hypersensitivity (*see also* Colitis, allergic) K52.29
  giardial A07.1
  granulomatous — *see* Enteritis, regional, large intestine
  indeterminate, so stated K52.3
  infectious — *see* Enteritis, infectious
  ischemic K55.9
    acute (subacute) (*see also* Ischemia, intestine, acute) K55.039
    chronic K55.1
    due to mesenteric artery insufficiency K55.1
    fulminant (acute) (*see also* Ischemia, intestine, acute) K55.039
  left sided K51.50
    with
      abscess K51.514
      complication K51.519
        specified NEC K51.518
      fistula K51.513
      obstruction K51.512
      rectal bleeding K51.511
  lymphocytic K52.832
  membranous
    psychogenic F54
  microscopic K52.839
    specified NEC K52.838
  mucous — *see* Syndrome, irritable, bowel
    psychogenic F54
  noninfective K52.9
    specified NEC K52.89
  polyposa — *see* Polyp, colon, inflammatory
  protozoal A07.9
  pseudomembranous
    not specified as recurrent A04.72
    recurrent A04.71

Colitis — *continued*
  pseudomucinous — *see* Syndrome, irritable, bowel
  regional — *see* Enteritis, regional, large intestine
    infectious A09
  segmental — *see* Enteritis, regional, large intestine
  septic — *see* Enteritis, infectious
  spastic K58.9
    with diarrhea K58.0
    psychogenic F54
  staphylococcal A04.8
    foodborne A05.0
  subacute ischemic (*see also* Ischemia, intestine, acute) K55.039
  thromboulcerative (*see also* Ischemia, intestine, acute) K55.039
  toxic NEC K52.1
    due to Clostridium difficile
      not specified as recurrent A04.72
      recurrent A04.71
  transmural — *see* Enteritis, regional, large intestine
  trichomonal A07.8
  tuberculous (ulcerative) A18.32
  ulcerative (chronic) K51.90
    with
      complication K51.919
        abscess K51.914
        fistula K51.913
        obstruction K51.912
        rectal bleeding K51.911
        specified complication NEC K51.918
    enterocolitis — *see* Enterocolitis, ulcerative
    ileocolitis — *see* Ileocolitis, ulcerative
    mucosal proctocolitis — *see* Proctocolitis, mucosal
    proctitis — *see* Proctitis, ulcerative
    pseudopolyposis — *see* Polyp, colon, inflammatory
    psychogenic F54
    rectosigmoiditis — *see* Rectosigmoiditis, ulcerative
    specified type NEC K51.80
      with
        complication K51.819
          abscess K51.814
          fistula K51.813
          obstruction K51.812
          rectal bleeding K51.811
          specified complication NEC K51.818
Collagenosis, collagen disease (nonvascular) (vascular) M35.9
  cardiovascular I42.8
  reactive perforating L87.1
  specified NEC M35.8
Collapse R55
  adrenal E27.2
  cardiorespiratory R57.0
  cardiovascular R57.0
    newborn P29.89
  circulatory (peripheral) R57.9
    during or after labor and delivery O75.1
    following ectopic or molar pregnancy O08.3
    newborn P29.89
  during or
    after labor and delivery O75.1
    resulting from a procedure, not elsewhere classified T81.10 ☑
  external ear canal — *see* Stenosis, external ear canal
  general R55
  heart — *see* Disease, heart
  heat T67.1 ☑
  hysterical F44.89
  labyrinth, membranous (congenital) Q16.5
  lung (massive) (*see also* Atelectasis) J98.19
    pressure due to anesthesia (general) (local) or other sedation T88.2 ☑
      during labor and delivery O74.1
      in pregnancy O29.02- ☑
      postpartum, puerperal O89.09
  myocardial — *see* Disease, heart
  nervous F48.8
  neurocirculatory F45.8
  nose M95.0
  postoperative T81.10 ☑
  pulmonary (*see also* Atelectasis) J98.19
    newborn — *see* Atelectasis
  trachea J39.8
  tracheobronchial J98.09
  valvular — *see* Endocarditis
  vascular (peripheral) R57.9
    during or after labor and delivery O75.1
    following ectopic or molar pregnancy O08.3

Collapse — *continued*
  vascular — *continued*
    newborn P29.89
  vertebra M48.50- ☑
    cervical region M48.52- ☑
    cervicothoracic region M48.53- ☑
    in (due to)
      metastasis — *see* Collapse, vertebra, in, specified disease NEC
      osteoporosis (*see also* Osteoporosis) M80.88 ☑
        cervical region M80.88 ☑
        cervicothoracic region M80.88 ☑
        lumbar region M80.88 ☑
        lumbosacral region M80.88 ☑
        multiple sites M80.88 ☑
        occipito-atlanto-axial region M80.88 ☑
        sacrococcygeal region M80.88 ☑
        thoracic region M80.88 ☑
        thoracolumbar region M80.88 ☑
      specified disease NEC M48.50- ☑
        cervical region M48.52- ☑
        cervicothoracic region M48.53- ☑
        lumbar region M48.56- ☑
        lumbosacral region M48.57- ☑
        occipito-atlanto-axial region M48.51- ☑
        sacrococcygeal region M48.58- ☑
        thoracic region M48.54- ☑
        thoracolumbar region M48.55- ☑
    lumbar region M48.56- ☑
    lumbosacral region M48.57- ☑
    occipito-atlanto-axial region M48.51- ☑
    sacrococcygeal region M48.58- ☑
    thoracic region M48.54- ☑
    thoracolumbar region M48.55- ☑
Collateral (*see also* condition)
  circulation (venous) I87.8
  dilation, veins I87.8
Colles' fracture S52.53- ☑
Collet (-Sicard) syndrome G52.7
Collier's asthma or lung J60
Collodion baby Q80.2
Colloid nodule (of thyroid) (cystic) E04.1
Coloboma (iris) Q13.0
  eyelid Q10.3
  fundus Q14.8
  lens Q12.2
  optic disc (congenital) Q14.2
    acquired H47.31- ☑
Coloenteritis — *see* Enteritis
Colon — *see* condition
Colonization
  MRSA (Methicillin resistant Staphylococcus aureus) Z22.322
  MSSA (Methicillin susceptible Staphylococcus aureus) Z22.321
  status — *see* Carrier (suspected) of
Coloptosis K63.4
Color blindness — *see* Deficiency, color vision
Colostomy
  attention to Z43.3
  fitting or adjustment Z46.89
  malfunctioning K94.03
  status Z93.3
Colpitis (acute) — *see* Vaginitis
Colpocele N81.5
Colpocystitis — *see* Vaginitis
Colpospasm N94.2
Column, spinal, vertebral — *see* condition
Coma R40.20
  with
    motor response (none) R40.231 ☑
      abnormal extensor posturing to pain or noxious stimuli (< 2 years of age) R40.232 ☑
      abnormal flexure posturing to pain or noxious stimuli (0-5 years of age) R40.233 ☑
      extensor posturing to pain or noxious stimuli (2-5 years of age) R40.232 ☑
      flexion/decorticate posturing (< 2 years of age) R40.233 ☑
      localizes pain (2-5 years of age) R40.235 ☑
      normal or spontaneous movement (< 2 years of age) R40.236 ☑
      obeys commands (2-5 years of age) R40.236 ☑
      score of
        1 R40.231 ☑
        2 R40.232 ☑

  with — *continued*
    motor response — *continued*
      score of — *continued*
        3 R40.233 ☑
        4 R40.234 ☑
        5 R40.235 ☑
        6 R40.236 ☑
      withdraws from pain or noxious stimuli (0-5 years of age) R40.234 ☑
      withdraws to touch (< 2 years of age) R40.235 ☑
    opening of eyes (never) R40.211 ☑
      in response to
        pain R40.212 ☑
        sound R40.213 ☑
      score of
        1 R40.211 ☑
        2 R40.212 ☑
        3 R40.213 ☑
        4 R40.214 ☑
      spontaneous R40.214 ☑
    verbal response (none) R40.221 ☑
      confused conversation R40.224 ☑
      cooing or babbling or crying appropriately (<2 years of age) R40.225 ☑
      inappropriate crying or screaming (< 2 years of age) R40.223 ☑
      inappropriate words (2-5 years of age) R40.224 ☑
      incomprehensible sounds (2-5 years of age) R40.222 ☑
      incomprehensible words R40.222 ☑
      irritable cries (< 2 years of age) R40.224 ☑
      moans/grunts to pain; restless (< 2 years old) R40.222 ☑
      oriented R40.225 ☑
      score of
        1 R40.221 ☑
        2 R40.222 ☑
        3 R40.223 ☑
        4 R40.224 ☑
        5 R40.225 ☑
      screaming (2-5 years of age) R40.223 ☑
      uses appropriate words (2-5 years of age) R40.225 ☑
  eclamptic — *see* Eclampsia
  epileptic — *see* Epilepsy
  Glasgow, scale score — *see* Glasgow coma scale
  hepatic — *see* Failure, hepatic, by type, with coma
  hyperglycemic (diabetic) — *see* Diabetes, by type, with hyperosmolarity, with coma
  hyperosmolar (diabetic) — *see* Diabetes, by type, with hyperosmolarity, with coma
  hypoglycemic (diabetic) — *see* Diabetes, by type, with hypoglycemia, with coma
    nondiabetic E15
  in diabetes — *see* Diabetes, coma
  insulin-induced — *see* Coma, hypoglycemic
  ketoacidotic (diabetic) — *see* Diabetes, by type, with ketoacidosis, with coma
  myxedematous E03.5
  newborn P91.5
  persistent vegetative state R40.3
  specified NEC, without documented Glasgow coma scale score, or with partial Glasgow coma scale score reported R40.244 ☑
Comatose — *see* Coma
Combat fatigue F43.0
Combined — *see* condition
Comedo, comedones (giant) L70.0
Comedocarcinoma (*see also* Neoplasm, breast, malignant)
  noninfiltrating
    breast D05.8- ☑
    specified site — *see* Neoplasm, in situ, by site
    unspecified site D05.8- ☑
Comedomastitis — *see* Ectasia, mammary duct
Comminuted fracture — *code as* Fracture, closed
Common
  arterial trunk Q20.0
  atrioventricular canal Q21.2
  atrium Q21.1
  cold (head) J00
  truncus (arteriosus) Q20.0
  variable immunodeficiency — *see* Immunodeficiency, common variable
  ventricle Q20.4

Commotio, commotion (current)
  brain — *see* Injury, intracranial, concussion
  cerebri — *see* Injury, intracranial, concussion
  retinae S05.8X- ☑
  spinal cord — *see* Injury, spinal cord, by region
  spinalis — *see* Injury, spinal cord, by region
Communication
  between
    base of aorta and pulmonary artery Q21.4
    left ventricle and right atrium Q20.5
    pericardial sac and pleural sac Q34.8
    pulmonary artery and pulmonary vein, congenital Q25.72
  congenital between uterus and digestive or urinary tract Q51.7
Compartment syndrome (deep) (posterior) (traumatic) T79.A0 ☑ (*following* T79.7)
  abdomen T79.A3 ☑ (*following* T79.7)
  lower extremity (hip, buttock, thigh, leg, foot, toes) T79.A2 ☑ (*following* T79.7)
  nontraumatic
    abdomen M79.A3 (*following* M79.7)
    lower extremity (hip, buttock, thigh, leg, foot, toes) M79.A2- ☑ (*following* M79.7)
    specified site NEC M79.A9 (*following* M79.7)
    upper extremity (shoulder, arm, forearm, wrist, hand, fingers) M79.A1- ☑ (*following* M79.7)
  specified site NEC T79.A9 ☑ (*following* T79.7)
  upper extremity (shoulder, arm, forearm, wrist, hand, fingers) T79.A1- ☑ (*following* T79.7)
Compensation
  failure — *see* Disease, heart
  neurosis, psychoneurosis — *see* Disorder, factitious
Complaint (*see also* Disease)
  bowel, functional K59.9
    psychogenic F45.8
  intestine, functional K59.9
    psychogenic F45.8
  kidney — *see* Disease, renal
  miners' J60
Complete — *see* condition
Complex
  Addison-Schilder E71.528
  cardiorenal — *see* Hypertension, cardiorenal
  Costen's M26.69
  disseminated mycobacterium avium- intracellulare (DMAC) A31.2
  Eisenmenger's (ventricular septal defect) I27.83
  hypersexual F52.8
  jumped process, spine — *see* Dislocation, vertebra
  primary, tuberculous A15.7
  Schilder-Addison E71.528
  subluxation (vertebral) M99.19
    abdomen M99.19
    acromioclavicular M99.17
    cervical region M99.11
    cervicothoracic M99.11
    costochondral M99.18
    costovertebral M99.18
    head region M99.10
    hip M99.15
    lower extremity M99.16
    lumbar region M99.13
    lumbosacral M99.13
    occipitocervical M99.10
    pelvic region M99.15
    pubic M99.15
    rib cage M99.18
    sacral region M99.14
    sacrococcygeal M99.14
    sacroiliac M99.14
    specified NEC M99.19
    sternochondral M99.18
    sternoclavicular M99.17
    thoracic region M99.12
    thoracolumbar M99.12
    upper extremity M99.17
  Taussig-Bing (transposition, aorta and overriding pulmonary artery) Q20.1
Complication(s) (from) (of)
  accidental puncture or laceration during a procedure (of) — *see* Complications, intraoperative (intraprocedural), puncture or laceration
  amputation stump (surgical) (late) NEC T87.9
    dehiscence T87.81
    infection or inflammation T87.40
      lower limb T87.4- ☑
      upper limb T87.4- ☑

▽ Subterms under main terms may continue to next column or page   ☑ Additional Character Required — Refer to the Tabular List for Character Selection   57

Collapse — Complication

Complication(s) — *continued*
  amputation stump — *continued*
    necrosis T87.5Ø
      lower limb T87.5- ☑
      upper limb T87.5- ☑
    neuroma T87.3Ø
      lower limb T87.3- ☑
      upper limb T87.3- ☑
    specified type NEC T87.89
  anastomosis (and bypass) (*see also* Complications, prosthetic device or implant)
    intestinal (internal) NEC K91.89
      involving urinary tract N99.89
    urinary tract (involving intestinal tract) N99.89
    vascular — *see* Complications, cardiovascular device or implant
  anesthesia, anesthetic (*see also* Anesthesia, complication) T88.59 ☑
    brain, postpartum, puerperal O89.2
    cardiac
      in
        labor and delivery O74.2
        pregnancy O29.19- ☑
      postpartum, puerperal O89.1
    central nervous system
      in
        labor and delivery O74.3
        pregnancy O29.29- ☑
      postpartum, puerperal O89.2
    difficult or failed intubation T88.4 ☑
      in pregnancy O29.6- ☑
    failed sedation (conscious) (moderate) during procedure T88.52 ☑
    general, unintended awareness during procedure T88.53 ☑
    hyperthermia, malignant T88.3 ☑
    hypothermia T88.51 ☑
    intubation failure T88.4 ☑
    malignant hyperthermia T88.3 ☑
    pulmonary
      in
        labor and delivery O74.1
        pregnancy NEC O29.Ø9- ☑
      postpartum, puerperal O89.Ø9
    shock T88.2 ☑
    spinal and epidural
      in
        labor and delivery NEC O74.6
          headache O74.5
        pregnancy NEC O29.5X- ☑
      postpartum, puerperal NEC O89.5
        headache O89.4
    unintended awareness under general anesthesia during procedure T88.53 ☑
  anti-reflux device — *see* Complications, esophageal anti-reflux device
  aortic (bifurcation) graft — *see* Complications, graft, vascular
  aortocoronary (bypass) graft — *see* Complications, coronary artery (bypass) graft
  aortofemoral (bypass) graft — *see* Complications, extremity artery (bypass) graft
  arteriovenous
    fistula, surgically created T82.9 ☑
      embolism T82.818 ☑
      fibrosis T82.828 ☑
      hemorrhage T82.838 ☑
      infection or inflammation T82.7 ☑
      mechanical
        breakdown T82.51Ø ☑
        displacement T82.52Ø ☑
        leakage T82.53Ø ☑
        malposition T82.52Ø ☑
        obstruction T82.59Ø ☑
        perforation T82.59Ø ☑
        protrusion T82.59Ø ☑
      pain T82.848 ☑
      specified type NEC T82.898 ☑
      stenosis T82.858 ☑
      thrombosis T82.868 ☑
    shunt, surgically created T82.9 ☑
      embolism T82.818 ☑
      fibrosis T82.828 ☑
      hemorrhage T82.838 ☑
      infection or inflammation T82.7 ☑
      mechanical
        breakdown T82.511 ☑

Complication(s) — *continued*
  arteriovenous — *continued*
    shunt, surgically created — *continued*
      mechanical — *continued*
        displacement T82.521 ☑
        leakage T82.531 ☑
        malposition T82.521 ☑
        obstruction T82.591 ☑
        perforation T82.591 ☑
        protrusion T82.591 ☑
      pain T82.848 ☑
      specified type NEC T82.898 ☑
      stenosis T82.858 ☑
      thrombosis T82.868 ☑
  arthroplasty — *see* Complications, joint prosthesis
  artificial
    fertilization or insemination N98.9
      attempted introduction (of)
        embryo in embryo transfer N98.3
        ovum following in vitro fertilization N98.2
      hyperstimulation of ovaries N98.1
      infection N98.Ø
      specified NEC N98.8
    heart T82.9 ☑
      embolism T82.817 ☑
      fibrosis T82.827 ☑
      hemorrhage T82.837 ☑
      infection or inflammation T82.7 ☑
      mechanical
        breakdown T82.512 ☑
        displacement T82.522 ☑
        leakage T82.532 ☑
        malposition T82.522 ☑
        obstruction T82.592 ☑
        perforation T82.592 ☑
        protrusion T82.592 ☑
      pain T82.847 ☑
      specified type NEC T82.897 ☑
      stenosis T82.857 ☑
      thrombosis T82.867 ☑
    opening
      cecostomy — *see* Complications, colostomy
      colostomy — *see* Complications, colostomy
      cystostomy — *see* Complications, cystostomy
      enterostomy — *see* Complications, enterostomy
      gastrostomy — *see* Complications, gastrostomy
      ileostomy — *see* Complications, enterostomy
      jejunostomy — *see* Complications, enterostomy
      nephrostomy — *see* Complications, stoma, urinary tract
      tracheostomy — *see* Complications, tracheostomy
      ureterostomy — *see* Complications, stoma, urinary tract
      urethrostomy — *see* Complications, stoma, urinary tract
  balloon implant or device
    gastrointestinal T85.9 ☑
      embolism T85.818 ☑
      fibrosis T85.828 ☑
      hemorrhage T85.838 ☑
      infection and inflammation T85.79 ☑
      pain T85.848 ☑
      specified type NEC T85.898 ☑
      stenosis T85.858 ☑
      thrombosis T85.868 ☑
    vascular (counterpulsation) T82.9 ☑
      embolism T82.818 ☑
      fibrosis T82.828 ☑
      hemorrhage T82.838 ☑
      infection or inflammation T82.7 ☑
      mechanical
        breakdown T82.513 ☑
        displacement T82.523 ☑
        leakage T82.533 ☑
        malposition T82.523 ☑
        obstruction T82.593 ☑
        perforation T82.593 ☑
        protrusion T82.593 ☑
      pain T82.848 ☑
      specified type NEC T82.898 ☑
      stenosis T82.858 ☑
      thrombosis T82.868 ☑
  bariatric procedure
    gastric band procedure K95.Ø9
      infection K95.Ø1

Complication(s) — *continued*
  bariatric procedure — *continued*
    specified procedure NEC K95.89
      infection K95.81
  bile duct implant (prosthetic) T85.9 ☑
    embolism T85.818 ☑
    fibrosis T85.828 ☑
    hemorrhage T85.838 ☑
    infection and inflammation T85.79 ☑
    mechanical
      breakdown T85.51Ø ☑
      displacement T85.52Ø ☑
      malfunction T85.51Ø ☑
      malposition T85.52Ø ☑
      obstruction T85.59Ø ☑
      perforation T85.59Ø ☑
      protrusion T85.59Ø ☑
      specified NEC T85.59Ø ☑
    pain T85.848 ☑
    specified type NEC T85.898 ☑
    stenosis T85.858 ☑
    thrombosis T85.868 ☑
  bladder device (auxiliary) — *see* Complications, genitourinary, device or implant, urinary system
  bleeding (postoperative) — *see* Complication, postoperative, hemorrhage
    intraoperative — *see* Complication, intraoperative, hemorrhage
  blood vessel graft — *see* Complications, graft, vascular
  bone
    device NEC T84.9 ☑
      embolism T84.81 ☑
      fibrosis T84.82 ☑
      hemorrhage T84.83 ☑
      infection or inflammation T84.7 ☑
      mechanical
        breakdown T84.318 ☑
        displacement T84.328 ☑
        malposition T84.328 ☑
        obstruction T84.398 ☑
        perforation T84.398 ☑
        protrusion T84.398 ☑
      pain T84.84 ☑
      specified type NEC T84.89 ☑
      stenosis T84.85 ☑
      thrombosis T84.86 ☑
    graft — *see* Complications, graft, bone
    growth stimulator (electrode) — *see* Complications, electronic stimulator device, bone
    marrow transplant — *see* Complications, transplant, bone, marrow
  brain neurostimulator (electrode) — *see* Complications, electronic stimulator device, brain
  breast implant (prosthetic) T85.9 ☑
    capsular contracture T85.44 ☑
    embolism T85.818 ☑
    fibrosis T85.828 ☑
    hemorrhage T85.838 ☑
    infection and inflammation T85.79 ☑
    mechanical
      breakdown T85.41 ☑
      displacement T85.42 ☑
      leakage T85.43 ☑
      malposition T85.42 ☑
      obstruction T85.49 ☑
      perforation T85.49 ☑
      protrusion T85.49 ☑
      specified NEC T85.49 ☑
    pain T85.848 ☑
    specified type NEC T85.898 ☑
    stenosis T85.858 ☑
    thrombosis T85.868 ☑
  bypass (*see also* Complications, prosthetic device or implant)
    aortocoronary — *see* Complications, coronary artery (bypass) graft
    arterial (*see also* Complications, graft, vascular)
      extremity — *see* Complications, extremity artery (bypass) graft
  cardiac (*see also* Disease, heart)
    device, implant or graft T82.9 ☑
      embolism T82.817 ☑
      fibrosis T82.827 ☑
      hemorrhage T82.837 ☑
      infection or inflammation T82.7 ☑
        valve prosthesis T82.6 ☑

Complication(s) — *continued*
  cardiac (*see also* Disease, heart) — *continued*
    device, implant or graft — *continued*
      mechanical
        breakdown T82.519 ☑
          specified device NEC T82.518 ☑
        displacement T82.529 ☑
          specified device NEC T82.528 ☑
        leakage T82.539 ☑
          specified device NEC T82.538 ☑
        malposition T82.529 ☑
          specified device NEC T82.528 ☑
        obstruction T82.599 ☑
          specified device NEC T82.598 ☑
        perforation T82.599 ☑
          specified device NEC T82.598 ☑
        protrusion T82.599 ☑
          specified device NEC T82.598 ☑
      pain T82.847 ☑
      specified type NEC T82.897 ☑
      stenosis T82.857 ☑
      thrombosis T82.867 ☑
  cardiovascular device, graft or implant T82.9 ☑
    aortic graft — *see* Complications, graft, vascular
    arteriovenous
      fistula, artificial — *see* Complication, arteriove-
        nous, fistula, surgically created
      shunt — *see* Complication, arteriovenous, shunt,
        surgically created
    artificial heart — *see* Complication, artificial, heart
    balloon (counterpulsation) device — *see* Complica-
      tion, balloon implant, vascular
    carotid artery graft — *see* Complications, graft,
      vascular
    coronary bypass graft — *see* Complication, coronary
      artery (bypass) graft
    dialysis catheter (vascular) — *see* Complication,
      catheter, dialysis
    electronic T82.9 ☑
      electrode T82.9 ☑
        embolism T82.817 ☑
        fibrosis T82.827 ☑
        hemorrhage T82.837 ☑
        infection T82.7 ☑
        mechanical
          breakdown T82.110 ☑
          displacement T82.120 ☑
          leakage T82.190 ☑
          obstruction T82.190 ☑
          perforation T82.190 ☑
          protrusion T82.190 ☑
          specified type NEC T82.190 ☑
        pain T82.847 ☑
        specified NEC T82.897 ☑
        stenosis T82.857 ☑
        thrombosis T82.867 ☑
      embolism T82.817 ☑
      fibrosis T82.827 ☑
      hemorrhage T82.837 ☑
      infection T82.7 ☑
      mechanical
        breakdown T82.119 ☑
        displacement T82.129 ☑
        leakage T82.199 ☑
        obstruction T82.199 ☑
        perforation T82.199 ☑
        protrusion T82.199 ☑
        specified type NEC T82.199 ☑
      pain T82.847 ☑
      pulse generator T82.9 ☑
        embolism T82.817 ☑
        fibrosis T82.827 ☑
        hemorrhage T82.837 ☑
        infection T82.7 ☑
        mechanical
          breakdown T82.111 ☑
          displacement T82.121 ☑
          leakage T82.191 ☑
          obstruction T82.191 ☑
          perforation T82.191 ☑
          protrusion T82.191 ☑
          specified type NEC T82.191 ☑
        pain T82.847 ☑
        specified NEC T82.897 ☑
        stenosis T82.857 ☑
        thrombosis T82.867 ☑

Complication(s) — *continued*
  cardiovascular device, graft or implant — *continued*
    electronic — *continued*
      specified condition NEC T82.897 ☑
      specified device NEC T82.9 ☑
        embolism T82.817 ☑
        fibrosis T82.827 ☑
        hemorrhage T82.837 ☑
        infection T82.7 ☑
        mechanical
          breakdown T82.118 ☑
          displacement T82.128 ☑
          leakage T82.198 ☑
          obstruction T82.198 ☑
          perforation T82.198 ☑
          protrusion T82.198 ☑
          specified type NEC T82.198 ☑
        pain T82.847 ☑
        specified NEC T82.897 ☑
        stenosis T82.857 ☑
        thrombosis T82.867 ☑
      stenosis T82.857 ☑
      thrombosis T82.867 ☑
    extremity artery graft — *see* Complication, extrem-
      ity artery (bypass) graft
    femoral artery graft — *see* Complication, extremity
      artery (bypass) graft
    heart
      transplant — *see* Complication, transplant, heart
      valve — *see* Complication, prosthetic device,
        heart valve
        graft — *see* Complication, heart, valve, graft
    heart-lung transplant — *see* Complication, trans-
      plant, heart, with lung
    infection or inflammation T82.7 ☑
    umbrella device — *see* Complication, umbrella de-
      vice, vascular
    vascular graft (or anastomosis) — *see* Complication,
      graft, vascular
  carotid artery (bypass) graft — *see* Complications, graft,
    vascular
  catheter (device) NEC (*see also* Complications, prosthet-
    ic device or implant)
    cranial infusion
      infection and inflammation T85.735 ☑
      mechanical
        breakdown T85.610 ☑
        displacement T85.620 ☑
        leakage T85.630 ☑
        malfunction T85.690 ☑
        malposition T85.620 ☑
        obstruction T85.690 ☑
        perforation T85.690 ☑
        protrusion T85.690 ☑
        specified NEC T85.690 ☑
    cystostomy T83.9 ☑
      embolism T83.81 ☑
      fibrosis T83.82 ☑
      hemorrhage T83.83 ☑
      infection and inflammation T83.510 ☑
      mechanical
        breakdown T83.010 ☑
        displacement T83.020 ☑
        leakage T83.030 ☑
        malposition T83.020 ☑
        obstruction T83.090 ☑
        perforation T83.090 ☑
        protrusion T83.090 ☑
        specified NEC T83.090 ☑
      pain T83.84 ☑
      specified type NEC T83.89 ☑
      stenosis T83.85 ☑
      thrombosis T83.86 ☑
    dialysis (vascular) T82.9 ☑
      embolism T82.818 ☑
      fibrosis T82.828 ☑
      hemorrhage T82.838 ☑
      infection and inflammation T82.7 ☑
      intraperitoneal — *see* Complications, catheter,
        intraperitoneal
      mechanical
        breakdown T82.41 ☑
        displacement T82.42 ☑
        leakage T82.43 ☑
        malposition T82.42 ☑
        obstruction T82.49 ☑

Complication(s) — *continued*
  catheter (*see also* Complications, prosthetic device or
    implant) — *continued*
    dialysis — *continued*
      mechanical — *continued*
        perforation T82.49 ☑
        protrusion T82.49 ☑
      pain T82.848 ☑
      specified type NEC T82.898 ☑
      stenosis T82.858 ☑
      thrombosis T82.868 ☑
    epidural infusion T85.9 ☑
      embolism T85.810 ☑
      fibrosis T85.820 ☑
      hemorrhage T85.830 ☑
      infection and inflammation T85.735 ☑
      mechanical
        breakdown T85.610 ☑
        displacement T85.620 ☑
        leakage T85.630 ☑
        malfunction T85.610 ☑
        malposition T85.620 ☑
        obstruction T85.690 ☑
        perforation T85.690 ☑
        protrusion T85.690 ☑
        specified NEC T85.690 ☑
      pain T85.840 ☑
      specified type NEC T85.890 ☑
      stenosis T85.850 ☑
      thrombosis T85.860 ☑
    intraperitoneal dialysis T85.9 ☑
      embolism T85.818 ☑
      fibrosis T85.828 ☑
      hemorrhage T85.838 ☑
      infection and inflammation T85.71 ☑
      mechanical
        breakdown T85.611 ☑
        displacement T85.621 ☑
        leakage T85.631 ☑
        malfunction T85.611 ☑
        malposition T85.621 ☑
        obstruction T85.691 ☑
        perforation T85.691 ☑
        protrusion T85.691 ☑
        specified NEC T85.691 ☑
      pain T85.848 ☑
      specified type NEC T85.898 ☑
      stenosis T85.858 ☑
      thrombosis T85.868 ☑
    intrathecal infusion
      infection and inflammation T85.735 ☑
      mechanical
        breakdown T85.610 ☑
        displacement T85.620 ☑
        leakage T85.630 ☑
        malfunction T85.690 ☑
        malposition T85.620 ☑
        obstruction T85.690 ☑
        perforation T85.690 ☑
        protrusion T85.690 ☑
        specified NEC T85.690 ☑
    intravenous infusion T82.9 ☑
      embolism T82.818 ☑
      fibrosis T82.828 ☑
      hemorrhage T82.838 ☑
      infection or inflammation T82.7 ☑
      mechanical
        breakdown T82.514 ☑
        displacement T82.524 ☑
        leakage T82.534 ☑
        malposition T82.524 ☑
        obstruction T82.594 ☑
        perforation T82.594 ☑
        protrusion T82.594 ☑
      pain T82.848 ☑
      specified type NEC T82.898 ☑
      stenosis T82.858 ☑
      thrombosis T82.868 ☑
    spinal infusion
      infection and inflammation T85.735 ☑
      mechanical
        breakdown T85.610 ☑
        displacement T85.620 ☑
        leakage T85.630 ☑
        malfunction T85.690 ☑
        malposition T85.620 ☑

Index

Complication — Complication

Complication(s) — *continued*
  catheter (*see also* Complications, prosthetic device or implant) — *continued*
    spinal infusion — *continued*
      mechanical — *continued*
        obstruction T85.690 ☑
        perforation T85.690 ☑
        protrusion T85.690 ☑
        specified NEC T85.690 ☑
    subarachnoid infusion
      infection and inflammation T85.735 ☑
      mechanical
        breakdown T85.610 ☑
        displacement T85.620 ☑
        leakage T85.630 ☑
        malfunction T85.690 ☑
        malposition T85.620 ☑
        obstruction T85.690 ☑
        perforation T85.690 ☑
        protrusion T85.690 ☑
        specified NEC T85.690 ☑
    subdural infusion T85.9 ☑
      embolism T85.810 ☑
      fibrosis T85.820 ☑
      hemorrhage T85.830 ☑
      infection and inflammation T85.735 ☑
      mechanical
        breakdown T85.610 ☑
        displacement T85.620 ☑
        leakage T85.630 ☑
        malfunction T85.610 ☑
        malposition T85.620 ☑
        obstruction T85.690 ☑
        perforation T85.690 ☑
        protrusion T85.690 ☑
        specified NEC T85.690 ☑
      pain T85.840 ☑
      specified type NEC T85.890 ☑
      stenosis T85.850 ☑
      thrombosis T85.860 ☑
    urethral T83.9 ☑
      displacement T83.028 ☑
      embolism T83.81 ☑
      fibrosis T83.82 ☑
      hemorrhage T83.83 ☑
      indwelling
        breakdown T83.011 ☑
        displacement T83.021 ☑
        infection and inflammation T83.511 ☑
        leakage T83.031 ☑
        specified complication NEC T83.091 ☑
      infection and inflammation T83.511 ☑
      leakage T83.038 ☑
      malposition T83.028 ☑
      mechanical
        breakdown T83.011 ☑
      obstruction (mechanical) T83.091 ☑
      pain T83.84 ☑
      perforation T83.091 ☑
      protrusion T83.091 ☑
      specified type NEC T83.091 ☑
      stenosis T83.85 ☑
      thrombosis T83.86 ☑
    urinary NEC
      breakdown T83.018 ☑
      displacement T83.028 ☑
      infection and inflammation T83.518 ☑
      leakage T83.038 ☑
      specified complication NEC T83.098 ☑
  cecostomy (stoma) — *see* Complications, colostomy
  cesarean delivery wound NEC O90.89
    disruption O90.0
    hematoma O90.2
    infection (following delivery) O86.00
  chemotherapy (antineoplastic) NEC T88.7 ☑
  chin implant (prosthetic) — *see* Complication, prosthetic device or implant, specified NEC
  circulatory system I99.8
    intraoperative I97.88
    postprocedural I97.89
      following cardiac surgery (*see also* Infarct, myocardium, associated with revascularization procedure) I97.19- ☑
        postcardiotomy syndrome I97.0
      hypertension I97.3
      lymphedema after mastectomy I97.2

Complication(s) — *continued*
  circulatory system — *continued*
    postprocedural — *continued*
      postcardiotomy syndrome I97.0
      specified NEC I97.89
  colostomy (stoma) K94.00
    hemorrhage K94.01
    infection K94.02
    malfunction K94.03
    mechanical K94.03
    specified complication NEC K94.09
  contraceptive device, intrauterine — *see* Complications, intrauterine, contraceptive device
  cord (umbilical) — *see* Complications, umbilical cord
  corneal graft — *see* Complications, graft, cornea
  coronary artery (bypass) graft T82.9 ☑
    atherosclerosis — *see* Arteriosclerosis, coronary (artery),
    embolism T82.818 ☑
    fibrosis T82.828 ☑
    hemorrhage T82.838 ☑
    infection and inflammation T82.7 ☑
    mechanical
      breakdown T82.211 ☑
      displacement T82.212 ☑
      leakage T82.213 ☑
      malposition T82.212 ☑
      obstruction T82.218 ☑
      perforation T82.218 ☑
      protrusion T82.218 ☑
      specified NEC T82.218 ☑
    pain T82.848 ☑
    specified type NEC T82.898 ☑
    stenosis T82.858 ☑
    thrombosis T82.868 ☑
  counterpulsation device (balloon), intra- aortic — *see* Complications, balloon implant, vascular
  cystostomy (stoma) N99.518
    catheter — *see* Complications, catheter, cystostomy
    hemorrhage N99.510
    infection N99.511
    malfunction N99.512
    specified type NEC N99.518
  delivery (*see also* Complications, obstetric) O75.9
    procedure (instrumental) (manual) (surgical) O75.4
    specified NEC O75.89
  dialysis (peritoneal) (renal) (*see also* Complications, infusion)
    catheter (vascular) — *see* Complication, catheter, dialysis
      peritoneal, intraperitoneal — *see* Complications, catheter, intraperitoneal
  dorsal column (spinal) neurostimulator — *see* Complications, electronic stimulator device, spinal cord
  drug NEC T88.7 ☑
  ear procedure (*see also* Disorder, ear)
    intraoperative H95.88
      hematoma — *see* Complications, intraoperative, hemorrhage (hematoma) (of), ear
      hemorrhage — *see* Complications, intraoperative, hemorrhage (hematoma) (of), ear
      laceration — *see* Complications, intraoperative, puncture or laceration..., ear
      specified NEC H95.88
    postoperative H95.89
      external ear canal stenosis H95.81- ☑
      hematoma — *see* Complications, postprocedural, hematoma (of), ear
      hemorrhage — *see* Complications, postprocedural, hemorrhage (of), ear
      postmastoidectomy — *see* Complications, postmastoidectomy
      seroma — *see* Complications, postprocedural, seroma (of), mastoid process
      specified NEC H95.89
  ectopic pregnancy O08.9
    damage to pelvic organs O08.6
    embolism O08.2
    genital infection O08.0
    hemorrhage (delayed) (excessive) O08.1
    metabolic disorder O08.5
    renal failure O08.4
    shock O08.3
    specified type NEC O08.0
    venous complication NEC O08.7

Complication(s) — *continued*
  electronic stimulator device
    bladder (urinary) — *see* Complications, electronic stimulator device, urinary
    bone T84.9 ☑
      breakdown T84.310 ☑
      displacement T84.320 ☑
      embolism T84.81 ☑
      fibrosis T84.82 ☑
      hemorrhage T84.83 ☑
      infection or inflammation T84.7 ☑
      malfunction T84.310 ☑
      malposition T84.320 ☑
      mechanical NEC T84.390 ☑
      obstruction T84.390 ☑
      pain T84.84 ☑
      perforation T84.390 ☑
      protrusion T84.390 ☑
      specified type NEC T84.89 ☑
      stenosis T84.85 ☑
      thrombosis T84.86 ☑
    brain T85.9 ☑
      embolism T85.810 ☑
      fibrosis T85.820 ☑
      hemorrhage T85.830 ☑
      infection and inflammation T85.731 ☑
      mechanical
        breakdown T85.110 ☑
        displacement T85.120 ☑
        leakage T85.190 ☑
        malposition T85.120 ☑
        obstruction T85.190 ☑
        perforation T85.190 ☑
        protrusion T85.190 ☑
        specified NEC T85.190 ☑
      pain T85.840 ☑
      specified type NEC T85.890 ☑
      stenosis T85.850 ☑
      thrombosis T85.860 ☑
    cardiac (defibrillator) (pacemaker) — *see* Complications, cardiovascular device or implant, electronic
    generator (brain) (gastric) (peripheral) (sacral) (spinal)
      breakdown T85.113 ☑
      displacement T85.123 ☑
      leakage T85.193 ☑
      malposition T85.123 ☑
      obstruction T85.193 ☑
      perforation T85.193 ☑
      protrusion T85.193 ☑
      specified type NEC T85.193 ☑
    muscle T84.9 ☑
      breakdown T84.418 ☑
      displacement T84.428 ☑
      embolism T84.81 ☑
      fibrosis T84.82 ☑
      hemorrhage T84.83 ☑
      infection or inflammation T84.7 ☑
      mechanical NEC T84.498 ☑
      pain T84.84 ☑
      specified type NEC T84.89 ☑
      stenosis T84.85 ☑
      thrombosis T84.86 ☑
    nervous system T85.9 ☑
      brain — *see* Complications, electronic stimulator device, brain
      cranial nerve — *see* Complications, electronic stimulator device, peripheral nerve
      embolism T85.810 ☑
      fibrosis T85.820 ☑
      gastric nerve — *see* Complications, electronic stimulator device, peripheral nerve
      hemorrhage T85.830 ☑
      infection and inflammation T85.738 ☑
      mechanical
        breakdown T85.118 ☑
        displacement T85.128 ☑
        leakage T85.199 ☑
        malposition T85.128 ☑
        obstruction T85.199 ☑
        perforation T85.199 ☑
        protrusion T85.199 ☑
        specified NEC T85.199 ☑
      pain T85.840 ☑

☑ **Additional Character Required** — Refer to the Tabular List for Character Selection   ⑭ **Subterms under main terms may continue to next column or page**

Complication(s) — *continued*
  electronic stimulator device — *continued*
    nervous system — *continued*
      peripheral nerve — *see* Complications, electronic
          stimulator device, peripheral nerve
      sacral nerve — *see* Complications, electronic
          stimulator device, peripheral nerve
      specified type NEC T85.890 ☑
      spinal cord — *see* Complications, electronic
          stimulator device, spinal cord
      stenosis T85.850 ☑
      thrombosis T85.860 ☑
      vagal nerve — *see* Complications, electronic
          stimulator device, peripheral nerve
    peripheral nerve T85.9 ☑
      embolism T85.810 ☑
      fibrosis T85.820 ☑
      hemorrhage T85.830 ☑
      infection and inflammation T85.732 ☑
      mechanical
        breakdown T85.111 ☑
        displacement T85.121 ☑
        leakage T85.191 ☑
        malposition T85.121 ☑
        obstruction T85.191 ☑
        perforation T85.191 ☑
        protrusion T85.191 ☑
        specified NEC T85.191 ☑
      pain T85.840 ☑
      specified type NEC T85.890 ☑
      stenosis T85.850 ☑
      thrombosis T85.860 ☑
    spinal cord T85.9 ☑
      embolism T85.810 ☑
      fibrosis T85.820 ☑
      hemorrhage T85.830 ☑
      infection and inflammation T85.733 ☑
      mechanical
        breakdown T85.112 ☑
        displacement T85.122 ☑
        leakage T85.192 ☑
        malposition T85.122 ☑
        obstruction T85.192 ☑
        perforation T85.192 ☑
        protrusion T85.192 ☑
        specified NEC T85.192 ☑
      pain T85.840 ☑
      specified type NEC T85.890 ☑
      stenosis T85.850 ☑
      thrombosis T85.860 ☑
    urinary T83.9 ☑
      embolism T83.81 ☑
      fibrosis T83.82 ☑
      hemorrhage T83.83 ☑
      infection and inflammation T83.598 ☑
      mechanical
        breakdown T83.110 ☑
        displacement T83.120 ☑
        malposition T83.120 ☑
        perforation T83.190 ☑
        protrusion T83.190 ☑
        specified NEC T83.190 ☑
      pain T83.84 ☑
      specified type NEC T83.89 ☑
      stenosis T83.85 ☑
      thrombosis T83.86 ☑
  electroshock therapy T88.9 ☑
    specified NEC T88.8 ☑
  endocrine E34.9
    postprocedural
      adrenal hypofunction E89.6
      hypoinsulinemia E89.1
      hypoparathyroidism E89.2
      hypopituitarism E89.3
      hypothyroidism E89.0
      ovarian failure E89.40
        asymptomatic E89.40
        symptomatic E89.41
      specified NEC E89.89
      testicular hypofunction E89.5
  endodontic treatment NEC M27.59
  enterostomy (stoma) K94.10
    hemorrhage K94.11
    infection K94.12
    malfunction K94.13
    mechanical K94.13

Complication(s) — *continued*
  enterostomy — *continued*
    specified complication NEC K94.19
  episiotomy, disruption O90.1
  esophageal anti-reflux device T85.9 ☑
    embolism T85.818 ☑
    fibrosis T85.828 ☑
    hemorrhage T85.838 ☑
    infection and inflammation T85.79 ☑
    mechanical
      breakdown T85.511 ☑
      displacement T85.521 ☑
      malfunction T85.511 ☑
      malposition T85.521 ☑
      obstruction T85.591 ☑
      perforation T85.591 ☑
      protrusion T85.591 ☑
      specified NEC T85.591 ☑
    pain T85.848 ☑
    specified type NEC T85.898 ☑
    stenosis T85.858 ☑
    thrombosis T85.868 ☑
  esophagostomy K94.30
    hemorrhage K94.31
    infection K94.32
    malfunction K94.33
    mechanical K94.33
    specified complication NEC K94.39
  extracorporeal circulation T80.90 ☑
  extremity artery (bypass) graft T82.9 ☑
    arteriosclerosis — *see* Arteriosclerosis, extremities,
        bypass graft
    embolism T82.818 ☑
    fibrosis T82.828 ☑
    hemorrhage T82.838 ☑
    infection and inflammation T82.7 ☑
    mechanical
      breakdown T82.318 ☑
        femoral artery T82.312 ☑
      displacement T82.328 ☑
        femoral artery T82.322 ☑
      leakage T82.338 ☑
        femoral artery T82.332 ☑
      malposition T82.328 ☑
        femoral artery T82.322 ☑
      obstruction T82.398 ☑
        femoral artery T82.392 ☑
      perforation T82.398 ☑
        femoral artery T82.392 ☑
      protrusion T82.398 ☑
        femoral artery T82.392 ☑
    pain T82.848 ☑
    specified type NEC T82.898 ☑
    stenosis T82.858 ☑
    thrombosis T82.868 ☑
  eye H57.9
    corneal graft — *see* Complications, graft, cornea
    implant (prosthetic) T85.9 ☑
      embolism T85.818 ☑
      fibrosis T85.828 ☑
      hemorrhage T85.838 ☑
      infection and inflammation T85.79 ☑
      mechanical
        breakdown T85.318 ☑
        displacement T85.328 ☑
        leakage T85.398 ☑
        malposition T85.328 ☑
        obstruction T85.398 ☑
        perforation T85.398 ☑
        protrusion T85.398 ☑
        specified NEC T85.398 ☑
      pain T85.848 ☑
      specified type NEC T85.898 ☑
      stenosis T85.858 ☑
      thrombosis T85.868 ☑
    intraocular lens — *see* Complications, intraocular
        lens
    orbital prosthesis — *see* Complications, orbital
        prosthesis
  female genital N94.9
    device, implant or graft NEC — *see* Complications,
        genitourinary, device or implant, genital tract
  femoral artery (bypass) graft — *see* Complication, ex-
      tremity artery (bypass) graft
  fixation device, internal (orthopedic) T84.9 ☑
    infection and inflammation T84.60 ☑

Complication(s) — *continued*
  fixation device, internal — *continued*
    infection and inflammation — *continued*
      arm T84.61- ☑
        humerus T84.61- ☑
        radius T84.61- ☑
        ulna T84.61- ☑
      leg T84.629 ☑
        femur T84.62- ☑
        fibula T84.62- ☑
        tibia T84.62- ☑
      specified site NEC T84.89 ☑
      spine T84.63 ☑
    mechanical
      breakdown
        limb T84.119 ☑
          carpal T84.210 ☑
          femur T84.11- ☑
          fibula T84.11- ☑
          humerus T84.11- ☑
          metacarpal T84.210 ☑
          metatarsal T84.213 ☑
          phalanx
            foot T84.213 ☑
            hand T84.210 ☑
          radius T84.11- ☑
          tarsal T84.213 ☑
          tibia T84.11- ☑
          ulna T84.11- ☑
        specified bone NEC T84.218 ☑
        spine T84.216 ☑
      displacement
        limb T84.129 ☑
          carpal T84.220 ☑
          femur T84.12- ☑
          fibula T84.12- ☑
          humerus T84.12- ☑
          metacarpal T84.220 ☑
          metatarsal T84.223 ☑
          phalanx
            foot T84.223 ☑
            hand T84.220 ☑
          radius T84.12- ☑
          tarsal T84.223 ☑
          tibia T84.12- ☑
          ulna T84.12- ☑
        specified bone NEC T84.228 ☑
        spine T84.226 ☑
      malposition — *see* Complications, fixation de-
          vice, internal, mechanical, displacement
      obstruction — *see* Complications, fixation device,
          internal, mechanical, specified type NEC
      perforation — *see* Complications, fixation device,
          internal, mechanical, specified type NEC
      protrusion — *see* Complications, fixation device,
          internal, mechanical, specified type NEC
      specified type NEC
        limb T84.199 ☑
          carpal T84.290 ☑
          femur T84.19- ☑
          fibula T84.19- ☑
          humerus T84.19- ☑
          metacarpal T84.290 ☑
          metatarsal T84.293 ☑
          phalanx
            foot T84.293 ☑
            hand T84.290 ☑
          radius T84.19- ☑
          tarsal T84.293 ☑
          tibia T84.19- ☑
          ulna T84.19- ☑
        specified bone NEC T84.298 ☑
        vertebra T84.296 ☑
    specified type NEC T84.89 ☑
      embolism T84.81 ☑
      fibrosis T84.82 ☑
      hemorrhage T84.83 ☑
      pain T84.84 ☑
      specified complication NEC T84.89 ☑
      stenosis T84.85 ☑
      thrombosis T84.86 ☑
  following
    acute myocardial infarction NEC I23.8
      aneurysm (false) (of cardiac wall) (of heart wall)
          (ruptured) I23.3
      angina I23.7

Complication(s) — *continued*
  following — *continued*
    acute myocardial infarction — *continued*
      atrial
        septal defect I23.1
        thrombosis I23.6
      cardiac wall rupture I23.3
      chordae tendinae rupture I23.4
      defect
        septal
          atrial (heart) I23.1
          ventricular (heart) I23.2
      hemopericardium I23.0
      papillary muscle rupture I23.5
      rupture
        cardiac wall I23.3
          with hemopericardium I23.0
        chordae tendineae I23.4
        papillary muscle I23.5
      specified NEC I23.8
      thrombosis
        atrium I23.6
        auricular appendage I23.6
        ventricle (heart) I23.6
      ventricular
        septal defect I23.2
        thrombosis I23.6
    ectopic or molar pregnancy O08.9
      cardiac arrest O08.81
      sepsis O08.82
      specified type NEC O08.89
      urinary tract infection O08.83
    termination of pregnancy — *see* Abortion
  gastrointestinal K92.9
    bile duct prosthesis — *see* Complications, bile duct implant
    esophageal anti-reflux device — *see* Complications, esophageal anti-reflux device
    postoperative
      colostomy — *see* Complications, colostomy
      dumping syndrome K91.1
      enterostomy — *see* Complications, enterostomy
      gastrostomy — *see* Complications, gastrostomy
      malabsorption NEC K91.2
      obstruction (*see also* Obstruction, intestine, postoperative) K91.30
      postcholecystectomy syndrome K91.5
      specified NEC K91.89
      vomiting after GI surgery K91.0
    prosthetic device or implant
      bile duct prosthesis — *see* Complications, bile duct implant
      esophageal anti-reflux device — *see* Complications, esophageal anti-reflux device
      specified type NEC
        embolism T85.818 ☑
        fibrosis T85.828 ☑
        hemorrhage T85.838 ☑
        mechanical
          breakdown T85.518 ☑
          displacement T85.528 ☑
          malfunction T85.518 ☑
          malposition T85.528 ☑
          obstruction T85.598 ☑
          perforation T85.598 ☑
          protrusion T85.598 ☑
          specified NEC T85.598 ☑
        pain T85.848 ☑
        specified complication NEC T85.898 ☑
        stenosis T85.858 ☑
        thrombosis T85.868 ☑
  gastrostomy (stoma) K94.20
    hemorrhage K94.21
    infection K94.22
    malfunction K94.23
    mechanical K94.23
    specified complication NEC K94.29
  genitourinary
    device or implant T83.9 ☑
      genital tract T83.9 ☑
        infection or inflammation T83.69 ☑
        intrauterine contraceptive device — *see* Complications, intrauterine, contraceptive device
        mechanical — *see* Complications, by device, mechanical
        mesh — *see* Complications, mesh

Complication(s) — *continued*
  genitourinary — *continued*
    device or implant — *continued*
      genital tract — *continued*
        penile prosthesis — *see* Complications, prosthetic device, penile
        specified type NEC T83.89 ☑
          embolism T83.81 ☑
          fibrosis T83.82 ☑
          hemorrhage T83.83 ☑
          pain T83.84 ☑
          specified complication NEC T83.89 ☑
          stenosis T83.85 ☑
          thrombosis T83.86 ☑
        vaginal mesh — *see* Complications, mesh
      urinary system T83.9 ☑
        cystostomy catheter — *see* Complication, catheter, cystostomy
        electronic stimulator — *see* Complications, electronic stimulator device, urinary
        indwelling urethral catheter — *see* Complications, catheter, urethral, indwelling
        infection or inflammation T83.598 ☑
          indwelling urethral catheter T83.511 ☑
        kidney transplant — *see* Complication, transplant, kidney
        organ graft — *see* Complication, graft, urinary organ
        specified type NEC T83.89 ☑
          embolism T83.81 ☑
          fibrosis T83.82 ☑
          hemorrhage T83.83 ☑
          mechanical T83.198 ☑
            breakdown T83.118 ☑
            displacement T83.128 ☑
            malfunction T83.118 ☑
            malposition T83.128 ☑
            obstruction T83.198 ☑
            perforation T83.198 ☑
            protrusion T83.198 ☑
            specified NEC T83.198 ☑
        sphincter implant — *see* Complications, implant, urinary sphincter
        sphincter, implanted T83.191 ☑
        stent (ileal conduit) (nephroureteral) T83.193 ☑
          pain T83.84 ☑
          specified complication NEC T83.89 ☑
          stenosis T83.85 ☑
          thrombosis T83.86 ☑
          ureteral indwelling T83.192 ☑
    postprocedural
      pelvic peritoneal adhesions N99.4
      renal failure N99.0
      specified NEC N99.89
      stoma — *see* Complications, stoma, urinary tract
      urethral stricture — *see* Stricture, urethra, postprocedural
      vaginal
        adhesions N99.2
        vault prolapse N99.3
  graft (bypass) (patch) (*see also* Complications, prosthetic device or implant)
    aorta — *see* Complications, graft, vascular
    arterial — *see* Complication, graft, vascular
    bone T86.839
      failure T86.831
      infection T86.832
      mechanical T84.318 ☑
        breakdown T84.318 ☑
        displacement T84.328 ☑
        protrusion T84.398 ☑
        specified type NEC T84.398 ☑
      rejection T86.830
      specified type NEC T86.838
    carotid artery — *see* Complications, graft, vascular
    cornea T86.849
      failure T86.841
      infection T86.842
      mechanical T85.398 ☑
        breakdown T85.318 ☑
        displacement T85.328 ☑
        protrusion T85.398 ☑
        specified type NEC T85.398 ☑
      rejection T86.840
      retroprosthetic membrane T85.398 ☑
      specified type NEC T86.848

Complication(s) — *continued*
  graft (*see also* Complications, prosthetic device or implant) — *continued*
    femoral artery (bypass) — *see* Complication, extremity artery (bypass) graft
    genital organ or tract — *see* Complications, genitourinary, device or implant, genital tract
    muscle T84.9 ☑
      breakdown T84.410 ☑
      displacement T84.420 ☑
      embolism T84.81 ☑
      fibrosis T84.82 ☑
      hemorrhage T84.83 ☑
      infection and inflammation T84.7 ☑
      mechanical NEC T84.490 ☑
      pain T84.84 ☑
      specified type NEC T84.89 ☑
      stenosis T84.85 ☑
      thrombosis T84.86 ☑
    nerve — *see* Complication, prosthetic device or implant, specified NEC
    skin — *see* Complications, prosthetic device or implant, skin graft
    tendon T84.9 ☑
      breakdown T84.410 ☑
      displacement T84.420 ☑
      embolism T84.81 ☑
      fibrosis T84.82 ☑
      hemorrhage T84.83 ☑
      infection and inflammation T84.7 ☑
      mechanical NEC T84.490 ☑
      pain T84.84 ☑
      specified type NEC T84.89 ☑
      stenosis T84.85 ☑
      thrombosis T84.86 ☑
    urinary organ T83.9 ☑
      embolism T83.81 ☑
      fibrosis T83.82 ☑
      hemorrhage T83.83 ☑
      infection and inflammation T83.598 ☑
        indwelling urethral catheter T83.511 ☑
      mechanical
        breakdown T83.21 ☑
        displacement T83.22 ☑
        erosion T83.24 ☑
        exposure T83.25 ☑
        leakage T83.23 ☑
        malposition T83.22 ☑
        obstruction T83.29 ☑
        perforation T83.29 ☑
        protrusion T83.29 ☑
        specified NEC T83.29 ☑
      pain T83.84 ☑
      specified type NEC T83.89 ☑
      stenosis T83.85 ☑
      thrombosis T83.86 ☑
    vascular T82.9 ☑
      embolism T82.818 ☑
      femoral artery — *see* Complication, extremity artery (bypass) graft
      fibrosis T82.828 ☑
      hemorrhage T82.838 ☑
      mechanical
        breakdown T82.319 ☑
          aorta (bifurcation) T82.310 ☑
          carotid artery T82.311 ☑
          specified vessel NEC T82.318 ☑
        displacement T82.329 ☑
          aorta (bifurcation) T82.320 ☑
          carotid artery T82.321 ☑
          specified vessel NEC T82.328 ☑
        leakage T82.339 ☑
          aorta (bifurcation) T82.330 ☑
          carotid artery T82.331 ☑
          specified vessel NEC T82.338 ☑
        malposition T82.329 ☑
          aorta (bifurcation) T82.320 ☑
          carotid artery T82.321 ☑
          specified vessel NEC T82.328 ☑
        obstruction T82.399 ☑
          aorta (bifurcation) T82.390 ☑
          carotid artery T82.391 ☑
          specified vessel NEC T82.398 ☑
        perforation T82.399 ☑
          aorta (bifurcation) T82.390 ☑
          carotid artery T82.391 ☑

Complication(s) — *continued*
graft (*see also* Complications, prosthetic device or implant) — *continued*
  vascular — *continued*
    mechanical — *continued*
      perforation — *continued*
        specified vessel NEC T82.398 ☑
      protrusion T82.399 ☑
        aorta (bifurcation) T82.390 ☑
        carotid artery T82.391 ☑
        specified vessel NEC T82.398 ☑
      pain T82.848 ☑
      specified complication NEC T82.898 ☑
      stenosis T82.858 ☑
      thrombosis T82.868 ☑
heart I51.9
  assist device
    infection and inflammation T82.7 ☑
  following acute myocardial infarction — *see* Complications, following, acute myocardial infarction
  postoperative — *see* Complications, circulatory system
  transplant — *see* Complication, transplant, heart and lung(s) — *see* Complications, transplant, heart, with lung
  valve
    graft (biological) T82.9 ☑
      embolism T82.817 ☑
      fibrosis T82.827 ☑
      hemorrhage T82.837 ☑
      infection and inflammation T82.7 ☑
      mechanical T82.228 ☑
        breakdown T82.221 ☑
        displacement T82.222 ☑
        leakage T82.223 ☑
        malposition T82.222 ☑
        obstruction T82.228 ☑
        perforation T82.228 ☑
        protrusion T82.228 ☑
      pain T82.847 ☑
      specified type NEC T82.897 ☑
      stenosis T82.857 ☑
      thrombosis T82.867 ☑
    prosthesis T82.9 ☑
      embolism T82.817 ☑
      fibrosis T82.827 ☑
      hemorrhage T82.837 ☑
      infection or inflammation T82.6 ☑
      mechanical T82.09 ☑
        breakdown T82.01 ☑
        displacement T82.02 ☑
        leakage T82.03 ☑
        malposition T82.02 ☑
        obstruction T82.09 ☑
        perforation T82.09 ☑
        protrusion T82.09 ☑
      pain T82.847 ☑
      specified type NEC T82.897 ☑
        mechanical T82.09 ☑
      stenosis T82.857 ☑
      thrombosis T82.867 ☑
hematoma
  intraoperative — *see* Complication, intraoperative, hemorrhage
  postprocedural — *see* Complication, postprocedural, hematoma
hemodialysis — *see* Complications, dialysis
hemorrhage
  intraoperative — *see* Complication, intraoperative, hemorrhage
  postprocedural — *see* Complication, postprocedural, hemorrhage
ileostomy (stoma) — *see* Complications, enterostomy
immunization (procedure) — *see* Complications, vaccination
implant (*see also* Complications, by site and type)
  urinary sphincter T83.9 ☑
    embolism T83.81 ☑
    fibrosis T83.82 ☑
    hemorrhage T83.83 ☑
    infection and inflammation T83.591 ☑
    mechanical
      breakdown T83.111 ☑
      displacement T83.121 ☑
      leakage T83.191 ☑

Complication(s) — *continued*
implant (*see also* Complications, by site and type) — *continued*
  urinary sphincter — *continued*
    mechanical — *continued*
      malposition T83.121 ☑
      obstruction T83.191 ☑
      perforation T83.191 ☑
      protrusion T83.191 ☑
      specified NEC T83.191 ☑
    pain T83.84 ☑
    specified type NEC T83.89 ☑
    stenosis T83.85 ☑
    thrombosis T83.86 ☑
infusion (procedure) T80.90 ☑
  air embolism T80.0 ☑
  blood — *see* Complications, transfusion
  catheter — *see* Complications, catheter
  infection T80.29 ☑
  pump — *see* Complications, cardiovascular, device or implant
  sepsis T80.29 ☑
  serum reaction (*see also* Reaction, serum) T80.69 ☑
    anaphylactic shock (*see also* Shock, anaphylactic) T80.59 ☑
  specified type NEC T80.89 ☑
inhalation therapy NEC T81.81 ☑
injection (procedure) T80.90 ☑
  drug reaction — *see* Reaction, drug
  infection T80.29 ☑
  sepsis T80.29 ☑
  serum (prophylactic) (therapeutic) — *see* Complications, vaccination
  specified type NEC T80.89 ☑
  vaccine (any) — *see* Complications, vaccination
inoculation (any) — *see* Complications, vaccination
insulin pump
  infection and inflammation T85.72 ☑
  mechanical
    breakdown T85.614 ☑
    displacement T85.624 ☑
    leakage T85.633 ☑
    malposition T85.624 ☑
    obstruction T85.694 ☑
    perforation T85.694 ☑
    protrusion T85.694 ☑
    specified NEC T85.694 ☑
intestinal pouch NEC K91.858
intraocular lens (prosthetic) T85.9 ☑
  embolism T85.818 ☑
  fibrosis T85.828 ☑
  hemorrhage T85.838 ☑
  infection and inflammation T85.79 ☑
  mechanical
    breakdown T85.21 ☑
    displacement T85.22 ☑
    malposition T85.22 ☑
    obstruction T85.29 ☑
    perforation T85.29 ☑
    protrusion T85.29 ☑
    specified NEC T85.29 ☑
  pain T85.848 ☑
  specified type NEC T85.898 ☑
  stenosis T85.858 ☑
  thrombosis T85.868 ☑
intraoperative (intraprocedural)
  cardiac arrest (*see also* Infarct, myocardium, associated with revascularization procedure)
    during cardiac surgery I97.710
    during other surgery I97.711
  cardiac functional disturbance NEC (*see also* Infarct, myocardium, associated with revascularization procedure)
    during cardiac surgery I97.790
    during other surgery I97.791
  hemorrhage (hematoma) (of)
    circulatory system organ or structure
      during cardiac bypass I97.411
      during cardiac catheterization I97.410
      during other circulatory system procedure I97.418
      during other procedure I97.42
    digestive system organ
      during procedure on digestive system K91.61
      during procedure on other organ K91.62

Complication(s) — *continued*
intraoperative — *continued*
  hemorrhage — *continued*
    ear
      during procedure on ear and mastoid process H95.21
      during procedure on other organ H95.22
    endocrine system organ or structure
      during procedure on endocrine system organ or structure E36.01
      during procedure on other organ E36.02
    eye and adnexa
      during ophthalmic procedure H59.11- ☑
      during other procedure H59.12- ☑
    genitourinary organ or structure
      during procedure on genitourinary organ or structure N99.61
      during procedure on other organ N99.62
    mastoid process
      during procedure on ear and mastoid process H95.21
      during procedure on other organ H95.22
    musculoskeletal structure
      during musculoskeletal surgery M96.810
      during non-orthopedic surgery M96.811
      during orthopedic surgery M96.810
    nervous system
      during a nervous system procedure G97.31
      during other procedure G97.32
    respiratory system
      during other procedure J95.62
      during procedure on respiratory system organ or structure J95.61
    skin and subcutaneous tissue
      during a dermatologic procedure L76.01
      during a procedure on other organ L76.02
    spleen
      during a procedure on other organ D78.02
      during a procedure on the spleen D78.01
  puncture or laceration (accidental) (unintentional) (of)
    brain
      during a nervous system procedure G97.48
      during other procedure G97.49
    circulatory system organ or structure
      during circulatory system procedure I97.51
      during other procedure I97.52
    digestive system
      during procedure on digestive system K91.71
      during procedure on other organ K91.72
    ear
      during procedure on ear and mastoid process H95.31
      during procedure on other organ H95.32
    endocrine system organ or structure
      during procedure on endocrine system organ or structure E36.11
      during procedure on other organ E36.12
    eye and adnexa
      during ophthalmic procedure H59.21- ☑
      during other procedure H59.22- ☑
    genitourinary organ or structure
      during procedure on genitourinary organ or structure N99.71
      during procedure on other organ N99.72
    mastoid process
      during procedure on ear and mastoid process H95.31
      during procedure on other organ H95.32
    musculoskeletal structure
      during musculoskeletal surgery M96.820
      during non-orthopedic surgery M96.821
      during orthopedic surgery M96.820
    nervous system
      during a nervous system procedure G97.48
      during other procedure G97.49
    respiratory system
      during other procedure J95.72
      during procedure on respiratory system organ or structure J95.71
    skin and subcutaneous tissue
      during a dermatologic procedure L76.11
      during a procedure on other organ L76.12
    spleen
      during a procedure on other organ D78.12
      during a procedure on the spleen D78.11
  specified NEC
    circulatory system I97.88
    digestive system K91.81

Complication(s) — *continued*
intraoperative — *continued*
    specified — *continued*
        ear H95.88
        endocrine system E36.8
        eye and adnexa H59.88
        genitourinary system N99.81
        mastoid process H95.88
        musculoskeletal structure M96.89
        nervous system G97.81
        respiratory system J95.88
        skin and subcutaneous tissue L76.81
        spleen D78.81
intraperitoneal catheter (dialysis) (infusion) — *see* Complications, catheter, intraperitoneal
intrathecal infusion pump
    infection and inflammation T85.738 ☑
    mechanical
        breakdown T85.615 ☑
        displacement T85.625 ☑
        leakage T85.635 ☑
        malfunction T85.695 ☑
        malposition T85.625 ☑
        obstruction T85.695 ☑
        perforation T85.695 ☑
        protrusion T85.695 ☑
        specified NEC T85.695 ☑
intrauterine
    contraceptive device
        embolism T83.81 ☑
        fibrosis T83.82 ☑
        hemorrhage T83.83 ☑
        infection and inflammation T83.69 ☑
        mechanical
            breakdown T83.31 ☑
            displacement T83.32 ☑
            malposition T83.32 ☑
            obstruction T83.39 ☑
            perforation T83.39 ☑
            protrusion T83.39 ☑
            specified NEC T83.39 ☑
        pain T83.84 ☑
        specified type NEC T83.89 ☑
        stenosis T83.85 ☑
        thrombosis T83.86 ☑
    procedure (fetal), to newborn P96.5
jejunostomy (stoma) — *see* Complications, enterostomy
joint prosthesis, internal T84.9 ☑
    breakage (fracture) T84.01- ☑
    dislocation T84.02- ☑
    fracture T84.01- ☑
    infection or inflammation T84.50 ☑
        hip T84.5- ☑
        knee T84.5- ☑
        specified joint NEC T84.59 ☑
    instability T84.02- ☑
    malposition — *see* Complications, joint prosthesis, mechanical, displacement
    mechanical
        breakage, broken T84.01- ☑
        dislocation T84.02- ☑
        fracture T84.01- ☑
        instability T84.02- ☑
        leakage — *see* Complications, joint prosthesis, mechanical, specified NEC
        loosening T84.039 ☑
            hip T84.03- ☑
            knee T84.03- ☑
            specified joint NEC T84.038 ☑
        obstruction — *see* Complications, joint prosthesis, mechanical, specified NEC
        perforation — *see* Complications, joint prosthesis, mechanical, specified NEC
        osteolysis T84.059 ☑
            hip T84.05- ☑
            knee T84.05- ☑
            other specified joint T84.058 ☑
        protrusion — *see* Complications, joint prosthesis, mechanical, specified NEC
        specified complication NEC T84.099 ☑
            hip T84.09- ☑
            knee T84.09- ☑
            other specified joint T84.098 ☑
        subluxation T84.02- ☑
        wear of articular bearing surface T84.069 ☑

Complication(s) — *continued*
joint prosthesis, internal — *continued*
    mechanical — *continued*
        wear of articular bearing surface — *continued*
            hip T84.06- ☑
            knee T84.06- ☑
            other specified joint T84.068 ☑
    specified joint NEC T84.89 ☑
        embolism T84.81 ☑
        fibrosis T84.82 ☑
        hemorrhage T84.83 ☑
        pain T84.84 ☑
        specified complication NEC T84.89 ☑
        stenosis T84.85 ☑
        thrombosis T84.86 ☑
        subluxation T84.02- ☑
kidney transplant — *see* Complications, transplant, kidney
labor O75.9
    specified NEC O75.89
liver transplant (immune or nonimmune) — *see* Complications, transplant, liver
lumbar puncture G97.1
    cerebrospinal fluid leak G97.0
    headache or reaction G97.1
lung transplant — *see* Complications, transplant, lung
    and heart — *see* Complications, transplant, lung, with heart
male genital N50.9
    device, implant or graft — *see* Complications, genitourinary, device or implant, genital tract
    postprocedural or postoperative — *see* Complications, genitourinary, postprocedural
    specified NEC N99.89
mastoid (process) procedure
    intraoperative H95.88
        hematoma — *see* Complications, intraoperative, hemorrhage (hematoma) (of), mastoid process
        hemorrhage — *see* Complications, intraoperative, hemorrhage (hematoma) (of), mastoid process
        laceration — *see* Complications, intraoperative, puncture or laceration, mastoid process
        specified NEC H95.88
    postmastoidectomy — *see* Complications, postmastoidectomy
    postoperative H95.89
        external ear canal stenosis H95.81 ☑
        hematoma — *see* Complications, postprocedural, hematoma (of), mastoid process
        hemorrhage — *see* Complications, postprocedural, hemorrhage (of), mastoid process
        postmastoidectomy — *see* Complications, postmastoidectomy
        seroma — *see* Complications, postprocedural, seroma (of), mastoid process
        specified NEC H95.89
mastoidectomy cavity — *see* Complications, postmastoidectomy
mechanical — *see* Complications, by site and type, mechanical
medical procedures (*see also* Complication(s), intraoperative) T88.9 ☑
metabolic E88.9
    postoperative E89.89
        specified NEC E89.89
molar pregnancy NOS O08.9
    damage to pelvic organs O08.6
    embolism O08.2
    genital infection O08.0
    hemorrhage (delayed) (excessive) O08.1
    metabolic disorder O08.5
    renal failure O08.4
    shock O08.3
    specified type NEC O08.0
    venous complication NEC O08.7
musculoskeletal system (*see also* Complication, intraoperative (intraprocedural), by site)
    device, implant or graft NEC — *see* Complications, orthopedic, device or implant
    internal fixation (nail) (plate) (rod) — *see* Complications, fixation device, internal
    joint prosthesis — *see* Complications, joint prosthesis
    post radiation M96.89
        kyphosis M96.2

Complication(s) — *continued*
musculoskeletal system (*see also* Complication, intraoperative, by site) — *continued*
    post radiation — *continued*
        scoliosis M96.5
        specified complication NEC M96.89
    postoperative (postprocedural) M96.89
        with osteoporosis — *see* Osteoporosis
        fracture following insertion of device — *see* Fracture, following insertion of orthopedic implant, joint prosthesis or bone plate
        joint instability after prosthesis removal M96.89
        lordosis M96.4
        postlaminectomy syndrome NEC M96.1
            kyphosis M96.3
        pseudarthrosis M96.0
        specified complication NEC M96.89
nephrostomy (stoma) — *see* Complications, stoma, urinary tract, external NEC
nervous system G98.8
    central G96.9
    device, implant or graft (*see also* Complication, prosthetic device or implant, specified NEC)
        electronic stimulator (electrode(s)) — *see* Complications, electronic stimulator device
        specified NEC
            infection and inflammation T85.738 ☑
            mechanical T85.695 ☑
                breakdown T85.615 ☑
                displacement T85.625 ☑
                leakage T85.635 ☑
                malfunction T85.695 ☑
                malposition T85.625 ☑
                obstruction T85.695 ☑
                perforation T85.695 ☑
                protrusion T85.695 ☑
                specified NEC T85.695 ☑
        ventricular shunt — *see* Complications, ventricular shunt
    electronic stimulator (electrode(s)) — *see* Complications, electronic stimulator device
    postprocedural G97.82
        intracranial hypotension G97.2
        specified NEC G97.82
        spinal fluid leak G97.0
newborn, due to intrauterine (fetal) procedure P96.5
nonabsorbable (permanent) sutures — *see* Complication, sutures, permanent
obstetric O75.9
    procedure (instrumental) (manual) (surgical) specified NEC O75.4
    specified NEC O75.89
    surgical wound NEC O90.89
        hematoma O90.2
        infection O86.00
ocular lens implant — *see* Complications, intraocular lens
ophthalmologic
    postprocedural bleb — *see* Blebitis
orbital prosthesis T85.9 ☑
    embolism T85.818 ☑
    fibrosis T85.828 ☑
    hemorrhage T85.838 ☑
    infection and inflammation T85.79 ☑
    mechanical
        breakdown T85.31- ☑
        displacement T85.32- ☑
        malposition T85.32- ☑
        obstruction T85.39- ☑
        perforation T85.39- ☑
        protrusion T85.39- ☑
        specified NEC T85.39- ☑
    pain T85.848 ☑
    specified type NEC T85.898 ☑
    stenosis T85.858 ☑
    thrombosis T85.868 ☑
organ or tissue transplant (partial) (total) — *see* Complications, transplant
orthopedic (*see also* Disorder, soft tissue)
    device or implant T84.9 ☑
        bone
            device or implant — *see* Complication, bone, device NEC
            graft — *see* Complication, graft, bone
            breakdown T84.418 ☑
            displacement T84.428 ☑

Complication(s) — *continued*
  orthopedic (*see also* Disorder, soft tissue) — *continued*
    device or implant — *continued*
      electronic bone stimulator — *see* Complications, electronic stimulator device, bone
      embolism T84.81 ☑
      fibrosis T84.82 ☑
      fixation device — *see* Complication, fixation device, internal
      hemorrhage T84.83 ☑
      infection or inflammation T84.7 ☑
      joint prosthesis — *see* Complication, joint prosthesis, internal
      malfunction T84.418 ☑
      malposition T84.428 ☑
      mechanical NEC T84.498 ☑
      muscle graft — *see* Complications, graft, muscle
      obstruction T84.498 ☑
      pain T84.84 ☑
      perforation T84.498 ☑
      protrusion T84.498 ☑
      specified complication NEC T84.89 ☑
      stenosis T84.85 ☑
      tendon graft — *see* Complications, graft, tendon
      thrombosis T84.86 ☑
    fracture (following insertion of device) — *see* Fracture, following insertion of orthopedic implant, joint prosthesis or bone plate
    postprocedural M96.89
      fracture — *see* Fracture, following insertion of orthopedic implant, joint prosthesis or bone plate
      postlaminectomy syndrome NEC M96.1
        kyphosis M96.3
        lordosis M96.4
      postradiation
        kyphosis M96.2
        scoliosis M96.5
      pseudarthrosis post-fusion M96.0
      specified type NEC M96.89
  pacemaker (cardiac) — *see* Complications, cardiovascular device or implant, electronic
  pancreas transplant — *see* Complications, transplant, pancreas
  penile prosthesis (implant) — *see* Complications, prosthetic device, penile
  perfusion NEC T80.90 ☑
  perineal repair (obstetrical) NEC O90.89
    disruption O90.1
    hematoma O90.2
    infection (following delivery) O86.09
  phototherapy T88.9 ☑
    specified NEC T88.8 ☑
  postmastoidectomy NEC H95.19- ☑
    cyst, mucosal H95.13- ☑
    granulation H95.12- ☑
    inflammation, chronic H95.11- ☑
    recurrent cholesteatoma H95.0- ☑
  postoperative — *see* Complications, postprocedural
    circulatory — *see* Complications, circulatory system
    ear — *see* Complications, ear
    endocrine — *see* Complications, endocrine
    eye — *see* Complications, eye
    lumbar puncture G97.1
      cerebrospinal fluid leak G97.0
    nervous system (central) (peripheral) — *see* Complications, nervous system
    respiratory system — *see* Complications, respiratory system
  postprocedural (*see also* Complications, surgical procedure)
    cardiac arrest (*see also* Infarct, myocardium, associated with revascularization procedure)
      following cardiac surgery I97.120
      following other surgery I97.121
    cardiac functional disturbance NEC (*see also* Infarct, myocardium, associated with revascularization procedure)
      following cardiac surgery I97.190
      following other surgery I97.191
    cardiac insufficiency
      following cardiac surgery I97.110
      following other surgery I97.111
    chorioretinal scars following retinal surgery H59.81- ☑

Complication(s) — *continued*
  postprocedural (*see also* Complications, surgical procedure) — *continued*
    following cataract surgery
      cataract (lens) fragments H59.02- ☑
      cystoid macular edema H59.03- ☑
      specified NEC H59.09- ☑
      vitreous (touch) syndrome H59.01- ☑
    heart failure
      following cardiac surgery I97.130
      following other surgery I97.131
    hematoma (of)
      circulatory system organ or structure
        following cardiac bypass I97.631
        following cardiac catheterization I97.630
        following other circulatory system procedure I97.638
        following other procedure I97.621
      digestive system
        following procedure on digestive system K91.870
        following procedure on other organ K91.871
      ear
        following other procedure H95.52
        following procedure on ear and mastoid process H95.51
      endocrine system
        following endocrine system procedure E89.820
        following other procedure E89.821
      eye and adnexa
        following ophthalmic procedure H59.33- ☑
        following other procedure H59.34- ☑
      genitourinary organ or structure
        following procedure on genitourinary organ or structure N99.840
        following procedure on other organ N99.841
      mastoid process
        following other procedure H95.52
        following procedure on ear and mastoid process H95.51
      musculoskeletal structure
        following musculoskeletal surgery M96.840
        following non-orthopedic surgery M96.841
        following orthopedic surgery M96.840
      nervous system
        following nervous system procedure G97.61
        following other procedure G97.62
      respiratory system
        following other procedure J95.861
        following procedure on respiratory system organ or structure J95.860
      skin and subcutaneous tissue
        following dermatologic procedure L76.31
        following procedure on other organ L76.32
      spleen
        following procedure on other organ D78.32
        following procedure on the spleen D78.31
    hemorrhage (of)
      circulatory system organ or structure
        following cardiac bypass I97.611
        following cardiac catheterization I97.610
        following other circulatory system procedure I97.618
        following other procedure I97.620
      digestive system
        following procedure on digestive system K91.840
        following procedure on other organ K91.841
      ear
        following other procedure H95.42
        following procedure on ear and mastoid process H95.41
      endocrine system
        following endocrine system procedure E89.810
        following other procedure E89.811
      eye and adnexa
        following ophthalmic procedure H59.31- ☑
        following other procedure H59.32- ☑
      genitourinary organ or structure
        following procedure on genitourinary organ or structure N99.820
        following procedure on other organ N99.821
      mastoid process
        following other procedure H95.42
        following procedure on ear and mastoid process H95.41

Complication(s) — *continued*
  postprocedural (*see also* Complications, surgical procedure) — *continued*
    hemorrhage — *continued*
      musculoskeletal structure
        following musculoskeletal surgery M96.830
        following non-orthopedic surgery M96.831
        following orthopedic surgery M96.830
      nervous system
        following nervous system procedure G97.51
        following other procedure G97.52
      respiratory system
        following a respiratory system procedure J95.830
        following other procedure J95.831
      skin and subcutaneous tissue
        following a procedure on other organ L76.22
        following dermatologic procedure L76.21
      spleen
        following procedure on other organ D78.22
        following procedure on the spleen D78.21
    seroma (of)
      circulatory system organ or structure
        following cardiac bypass I97.641
        following cardiac catheterization I97.640
        following other circulatory system procedure I97.648
        following other procedure I97.622
      digestive system
        following procedure on digestive system K91.872
        following procedure on other organ K91.873
      ear
        following other procedure H95.54
        following procedure on ear and mastoid process H95.53
      endocrine system
        following endocrine system procedure E89.822
        following other procedure E89.823
      eye and adnexa
        following ophthalmic procedure H59.35- ☑
        following other procedure H59.36- ☑
      genitourinary organ or structure
        following procedure on genitourinary organ or structure N99.842
        following procedure on other organ N99.843
      mastoid process
        following other procedure H95.54
        following procedure on ear and mastoid process H95.53
      musculoskeletal structure
        following musculoskeletal surgery M96.842
        following non-orthopedic surgery M96.843
        following orthopedic surgery M96.842
      nervous system
        following nervous system procedure G97.63
        following other procedure G97.64
      respiratory system
        following other procedure J95.863
        following procedure on respiratory system organ or structure J95.862
      skin and subcutaneous tissue
        following dermatologic procedure L76.33
        following procedure on other organ L76.34
      spleen
        following procedure on other organ D78.34
        following procedure on the spleen D78.33
    specified NEC
      circulatory system I97.89
      digestive K91.89
      ear H95.89
      endocrine E89.89
      eye and adnexa H59.89
      genitourinary N99.89
      mastoid process H95.89
      metabolic E89.89
      musculoskeletal structure M96.89
      nervous system G97.82
      respiratory system J95.89
      skin and subcutaneous tissue L76.82
      spleen D78.89
  pregnancy NEC — *see* Pregnancy, complicated by
  prosthetic device or implant T85.9 ☑
    bile duct — *see* Complications, bile duct implant
    breast — *see* Complications, breast implant

Index

Complication — Complication

Complication(s) — *continued*
  prosthetic device or implant — *continued*
    bulking agent
      ureteral
        erosion T83.714 ☑
        exposure T83.724 ☑
      urethral
        erosion T83.713 ☑
        exposure T83.723 ☑
    cardiac and vascular NEC — *see* Complications, cardiovascular device or implant
    corneal transplant — *see* Complications, graft, cornea
    electronic nervous system stimulator — *see* Complications, electronic stimulator device
    epidural infusion catheter — *see* Complications, catheter, epidural
    esophageal anti-reflux device — *see* Complications, esophageal anti-reflux device
    genital organ or tract — *see* Complications, genitourinary, device or implant, genital tract
    specified NEC T83.79- ☑
    heart valve — *see* Complications, heart, valve, prosthesis
    infection or inflammation T85.79 ☑
      intestine transplant T86.892
      liver transplant T86.43
      lung transplant T86.812
      pancreas transplant T86.892
      skin graft T86.822
    intraocular lens — *see* Complications, intraocular lens
    intraperitoneal (dialysis) catheter — *see* Complications, catheter, intraperitoneal
    joint — *see* Complications, joint prosthesis, internal
    mechanical NEC T85.698 ☑
      dialysis catheter (vascular) (*see also* Complication, catheter, dialysis, mechanical)
      peritoneal — *see* Complication, catheter, intraperitoneal, mechanical
      gastrointestinal device T85.598 ☑
      ocular device T85.398 ☑
      subdural (infusion) catheter T85.690 ☑
      suture, permanent T85.692 ☑
        that for bone repair — *see* Complications, fixation device, internal (orthopedic), mechanical
      ventricular shunt
        breakdown T85.01 ☑
        displacement T85.02 ☑
        leakage T85.03 ☑
        malposition T85.02 ☑
        obstruction T85.09 ☑
        perforation T85.09 ☑
        protrusion T85.09 ☑
        specified NEC T85.09 ☑
    mesh
      erosion (to surrounding organ or tissue) T83.718 ☑
        urethral (into pelvic floor muscles) T83.712 ☑
        vaginal (into pelvic floor muscles) T83.711 ☑
      exposure (into surrounding organ or tissue) T83.728 ☑
        urethral (through urethral wall) T83.722 ☑
        vaginal (into vagina) (through vaginal wall) T83.721 ☑
    orbital — *see* Complications, orbital prosthesis
    penile T83.9 ☑
      embolism T83.81 ☑
      fibrosis T83.82 ☑
      hemorrhage T83.83 ☑
      infection and inflammation T83.61 ☑
      mechanical
        breakdown T83.410 ☑
        displacement T83.420 ☑
        leakage T83.490 ☑
        malposition T83.420 ☑
        obstruction T83.490 ☑
        perforation T83.490 ☑
        protrusion T83.490 ☑
        specified NEC T83.490 ☑
      pain T83.84 ☑
      specified type NEC T83.89 ☑
      stenosis T83.85 ☑
      thrombosis T83.86 ☑

Complication(s) — *continued*
  prosthetic device or implant — *continued*
    prosthetic materials NEC
      erosion (to surrounding organ or tissue) T83.718 ☑
      exposure (into surrounding organ or tissue) T83.728 ☑
    skin graft T86.829
      artificial skin or decellularized allodermis
        embolism T85.818 ☑
        fibrosis T85.828 ☑
        hemorrhage T85.838 ☑
        infection and inflammation T85.79 ☑
        mechanical
          breakdown T85.613 ☑
          displacement T85.623 ☑
          malfunction T85.613 ☑
          malposition T85.623 ☑
          obstruction T85.693 ☑
          perforation T85.693 ☑
          protrusion T85.693 ☑
          specified NEC T85.693 ☑
        pain T85.848 ☑
        specified type NEC T85.898 ☑
        stenosis T85.858 ☑
        thrombosis T85.868 ☑
      failure T86.821
      infection T86.822
      rejection T86.820
      specified NEC T86.828
    sling
      urethral (female) (male)
        erosion T83.712 ☑
        exposure T83.722 ☑
    specified NEC T85.9 ☑
      embolism T85.818 ☑
      fibrosis T85.828 ☑
      hemorrhage T85.838 ☑
      infection and inflammation T85.79 ☑
      mechanical
        breakdown T85.618 ☑
        displacement T85.628 ☑
        leakage T85.638 ☑
        malfunction T85.618 ☑
        malposition T85.628 ☑
        obstruction T85.698 ☑
        perforation T85.698 ☑
        protrusion T85.698 ☑
        specified NEC T85.698 ☑
      pain T85.848 ☑
      specified type NEC T85.898 ☑
      stenosis T85.858 ☑
      thrombosis T85.868 ☑
    subdural infusion catheter — *see* Complications, catheter, subdural
    sutures — *see* Complications, sutures
    urinary organ or tract NEC — *see* Complications, genitourinary, device or implant, urinary system
    vascular — *see* Complications, cardiovascular device or implant
    ventricular shunt — *see* Complications, ventricular shunt (device)
  puerperium — *see* Puerperal
  puncture, spinal G97.1
    cerebrospinal fluid leak G97.0
    headache or reaction G97.1
  pyelogram N99.89
  radiation
    kyphosis M96.2
    scoliosis M96.5
  reattached
    extremity (infection) (rejection)
      lower T87.1X- ☑
      upper T87.0X- ☑
    specified body part NEC T87.2
  reconstructed breast
    asymmetry between native and reconstructed breast N65.1
    deformity N65.0
    disproportion between native and reconstructed breast N65.1
    excess tissue N65.0
    misshappen N65.0
  reimplant NEC (*see also* Complications, prosthetic device or implant)

Complication(s) — *continued*
  reimplant (*see also* Complications, prosthetic device or implant) — *continued*
    limb (infection) (rejection) — *see* Complications, reattached, extremity
    organ (partial) (total) — *see* Complications, transplant
    prosthetic device NEC — *see* Complications, prosthetic device
  renal N28.9
    allograft — *see* Complications, transplant, kidney
    dialysis — *see* Complications, dialysis
  respirator
    mechanical J95.850
    specified NEC J95.859
  respiratory system J98.9
    device, implant or graft — *see* Complication, prosthetic device or implant, specified NEC
    lung transplant — *see* Complications, prosthetic device or implant, lung transplant
    postoperative J95.89
      air leak J95.812
      Mendelson's syndrome (chemical pneumonitis) J95.4
      pneumothorax J95.811
      pulmonary insufficiency (acute) (after nonthoracic surgery) J95.2
        chronic J95.3
        following thoracic surgery J95.1
      respiratory failure (acute) J95.821
        acute and chronic J95.822
      specified NEC J95.89
      subglottic stenosis J95.5
      tracheostomy complication — *see* Complications, tracheostomy
    therapy T81.89
  sedation during labor and delivery O74.9
    cardiac O74.2
    central nervous system O74.3
    pulmonary NEC O74.1
  shunt (*see also* Complications, prosthetic device or implant)
    arteriovenous — *see* Complications, arteriovenous, shunt
    ventricular (communicating) — *see* Complications, ventricular shunt
  skin
    graft T86.829
      failure T86.821
      infection T86.822
      rejection T86.820
      specified type NEC T86.828
  spinal
    anesthesia — *see* Complications, anesthesia, spinal
    catheter (epidural) (subdural) — *see* Complications, catheter
    puncture or tap G97.1
      cerebrospinal fluid leak G97.0
      headache or reaction G97.1
  stent
    bile duct — *see* Complications, bile duct prosthesis
    ureteral indwelling
      breakdown T83.112 ☑
      displacement T83.122 ☑
      leakage T83.192 ☑
      malposition T83.122 ☑
      obstruction T83.192 ☑
      perforation T83.192 ☑
      protrusion T83.192 ☑
      specified NEC T83.192 ☑
    urinary NEC (ileal conduit) (nephroureteral) T83.193 ☑
      embolism T83.81 ☑
      fibrosis T83.82 ☑
      hemorrhage T83.83 ☑
      infection and inflammation T83.593 ☑
      mechanical
        breakdown T83.113 ☑
        displacement T83.123 ☑
        leakage T83.193 ☑
        malposition T83.123 ☑
        obstruction T83.193 ☑
        perforation T83.193 ☑
        protrusion T83.193 ☑
        specified NEC T83.193 ☑
      pain T83.84 ☑
      specified type NEC T83.89 ☑

Complication(s) — continued
  stent — continued
    urinary — continued
      stenosis T83.85 ☑
      thrombosis T83.86 ☑
    vascular
      end stent stenosis — see Restenosis, stent
      in stent stenosis — see Restenosis, stent
  stoma
    digestive tract
      colostomy — see Complications, colostomy
      enterostomy — see Complications, enterostomy
      esophagostomy — see Complications,
        esophagostomy
      gastrostomy — see Complications, gastrostomy
    urinary tract N99.528
      continent N99.538
        hemorrhage N99.530
        herniation N99.533
        infection N99.531
        malfunction N99.532
        specified type NEC N99.538
        stenosis N99.534
      cystostomy — see Complications, cystostomy
      external NOS N99.528
      hemorrhage N99.520
      herniation N99.523
      incontinent N99.528
        hemorrhage N99.520
        herniation N99.523
        infection N99.521
        malfunction N99.522
        specified type NEC N99.528
        stenosis N99.524
      infection N99.521
      malfunction N99.522
      specified type NEC N99.528
      stenosis N99.524
  stomach banding — see Complication(s), bariatric
    procedure
  stomach stapling — see Complication(s), bariatric
    procedure
  surgical material, nonabsorbable — see Complication,
    suture, permanent
  surgical procedure (on) T81.9 ☑
    amputation stump (late) — see Complications,
      amputation stump
    cardiac — see Complications, circulatory system
    cholesteatoma, recurrent — see Complications,
      postmastoidectomy, recurrent cholesteatoma
    circulatory (early) — see Complications, circulatory
      system
    digestive system — see Complications, gastrointesti-
      nal
    dumping syndrome (postgastrectomy) K91.1
    ear — see Complications, ear
    elephantiasis or lymphedema I97.89
      postmastectomy I97.2
    emphysema (surgical) T81.82 ☑
    endocrine — see Complications, endocrine
    eye — see Complications, eye
    fistula (persistent postoperative) T81.83 ☑
    foreign body inadvertently left in wound (sponge)
      (suture) (swab) — see Foreign body, acciden-
      tally left during a procedure
    gastrointestinal — see Complications, gastrointesti-
      nal
    genitourinary NEC N99.89
    hematoma
      intraoperative — see Complication, intraopera-
        tive, hemorrhage
      postprocedural — see Complication, postproce-
        dural, hematoma
    hemorrhage
      intraoperative — see Complication, intraopera-
        tive, hemorrhage
      postprocedural — see Complication, postproce-
        dural, hemorrhage
    hepatic failure K91.82
    hyperglycemia (postpancreatectomy) E89.1
    hypoinsulinemia (postpancreatectomy) E89.1
    hypoparathyroidism (postparathyroidectomy) E89.2
    hypopituitarism (posthypophysectomy) E89.3
    hypothyroidism (post-thyroidectomy) E89.0
    intestinal obstruction (see also Obstruction, intes-
      tine, postoperative) K91.30
    intracranial hypotension following ventricular
      shunting (ventriculostomy) G97.2

Complication(s) — continued
  surgical procedure — continued
    lymphedema I97.89
      postmastectomy I97.2
    malabsorption (postsurgical) NEC K91.2
      osteoporosis — see Osteoporosis, postsurgical
        malabsorption
    mastoidectomy cavity NEC — see Complications,
      postmastoidectomy
    metabolic E89.89
      specified NEC E89.89
    musculoskeletal — see Complications, musculoskele-
      tal system
    nervous system (central) (peripheral) — see Compli-
      cations, nervous system
    ovarian failure E89.40
      asymptomatic E89.40
      symptomatic E89.41
    peripheral vascular — see Complications, surgical
      procedure, vascular
    postcardiotomy syndrome I97.0
    postcholecystectomy syndrome K91.5
    postcommissurotomy syndrome I97.0
    postgastrectomy dumping syndrome K91.1
    postlaminectomy syndrome NEC M96.1
      kyphosis M96.3
    postmastectomy lymphedema syndrome I97.2
    postmastoidectomy cholesteatoma — see Compli-
      cations, postmastoidectomy, recurrent
      cholesteatoma
    postvagotomy syndrome K91.1
    postvalvulotomy syndrome I97.0
    pulmonary insufficiency (acute) J95.2
      chronic J95.3
      following thoracic surgery J95.1
    reattached body part — see Complications, reat-
      tached
    respiratory — see Complications, respiratory system
    shock (hypovolemic) T81.19 ☑
    spleen (postoperative) D78.89
      intraoperative D78.81
    stitch abscess T81.41 ☑
    subglottic stenosis (postsurgical) J95.5
    testicular hypofunction E89.5
    transplant — see Complications, organ or tissue
      transplant
    urinary NEC N99.89
    vaginal vault prolapse (posthysterectomy) N99.3
    vascular (peripheral)
      artery T81.719 ☑
        mesenteric T81.710 ☑
        renal T81.711 ☑
        specified NEC T81.718 ☑
      vein T81.72 ☑
    wound infection T81.49 ☑
  suture, permanent (wire) NEC T85.9 ☑
    with repair of bone — see Complications, fixation
      device, internal
    embolism T85.818 ☑
    fibrosis T85.828 ☑
    hemorrhage T85.838 ☑
    infection and inflammation T85.79 ☑
    mechanical
      breakdown T85.612 ☑
      displacement T85.622 ☑
      malfunction T85.612 ☑
      malposition T85.622 ☑
      obstruction T85.692 ☑
      perforation T85.692 ☑
      protrusion T85.692 ☑
      specified NEC T85.692 ☑
    pain T85.848 ☑
    specified type NEC T85.898 ☑
    stenosis T85.858 ☑
    thrombosis T85.868 ☑
  tracheostomy J95.00
    granuloma J95.09
    hemorrhage J95.01
    infection J95.02
    malfunction J95.03
    mechanical J95.03
    obstruction J95.03
    specified type NEC J95.09
    tracheo-esophageal fistula J95.04
  transfusion (blood) (lymphocytes) (plasma) T80.92 ☑
    air embolism T80.0 ☑
    circulatory overload E87.71

Complication(s) — continued
  transfusion — continued
    febrile nonhemolytic transfusion reaction R50.84
    hemochromatosis E83.111
    hemolysis T80.89 ☑
    hemolytic reaction (antigen unspecified) T80.919 ☑
    incompatibility reaction (antigen unspecified)
      T80.919 ☑
      ABO T80.30 ☑
        delayed serologic (DSTR) T80.39 ☑
        hemolytic transfusion reaction (HTR) (unspec-
          ified time after transfusion) T80.319 ☑
          acute (AHTR) (less than 24 hours after
            transfusion) T80.310 ☑
          delayed (DHTR) (24 hours or more after
            transfusion) T80.311 ☑
        specified NEC T80.39 ☑
      acute (antigen unspecified) T80.910 ☑
      delayed (antigen unspecified) T80.911 ☑
      delayed serologic (DSTR) T80.89 ☑
      non-ABO (minor antigens (Duffy) (K) (Kell) (Kidd)
        (Lewis) (M) (N) (P) (S)) T80.A0 ☑ (following
        T80.4)
        delayed serologic (DSTR) T80.A9 ☑ (following
          T80.4)
        hemolytic transfusion reaction (HTR) (unspec-
          ified time after transfusion) T80.A19 ☑
          (following T80.4)
          acute (AHTR) (less than 24 hours after
            transfusion) T80.A10 ☑ (following
            T80.4)
          delayed (DHTR) (24 hours or more after
            transfusion) T80.A11 ☑ (following
            T80.4)
        specified NEC T80.A9 ☑ (following T80.4)
      Rh (antigens (C) (c) (D) (E) (e)) (factor) T80.40 ☑
        delayed serologic (DSTR) T80.49 ☑
        hemolytic transfusion reaction (HTR) (unspec-
          ified time after transfusion) T80.419 ☑
          acute (AHTR) (less than 24 hours after
            transfusion) T80.410 ☑
          delayed (DHTR) (24 hours or more after
            transfusion) T80.411 ☑
        specified NEC T80.49 ☑
    infection T80.29 ☑
      acute T80.22- ☑
    reaction NEC T80.89 ☑
    sepsis T80.29 ☑
    shock T80.89 ☑
  transplant T86.90
    bone T86.839
      failure T86.831
      infection T86.832
      rejection T86.830
      specified type NEC T86.838
    bone marrow T86.00
      failure T86.02
      infection T86.03
      rejection T86.01
      specified type NEC T86.09
    cornea T86.849
      failure T86.841
      infection T86.842
      rejection T86.840
      specified type NEC T86.848
    failure T86.92
    heart T86.20
      with lung T86.30
      cardiac allograft vasculopathy T86.290
        failure T86.32
        infection T86.33
        rejection T86.31
        specified type NEC T86.39
      failure T86.22
      infection T86.23
      rejection T86.21
      specified type NEC T86.298
    infection T86.93
    intestine T86.859
      failure T86.851
      infection T86.852
      rejection T86.850
      specified type NEC T86.858
    kidney T86.10
      failure T86.12
      infection T86.13
      rejection T86.11
      specified type NEC T86.19

Complication — Compression

Complication(s) — *continued*
transplant — *continued*
liver T86.40
failure T86.42
infection T86.43
rejection T86.41
specified type NEC T86.49
lung T86.819
with heart T86.30
failure T86.32
infection T86.33
rejection T86.31
specified type NEC T86.39
failure T86.811
infection T86.812
rejection T86.810
specified type NEC T86.818
malignant neoplasm C80.2
pancreas T86.899
failure T86.891
infection T86.892
rejection T86.890
specified type NEC T86.898
peripheral blood stem cells T86.5
post-transplant lymphoproliferative disorder (PTLD) D47.Z1 (*following* D47.4)
rejection T86.91
skin T86.829
failure T86.821
infection T86.822
rejection T86.820
specified type NEC T86.828
specified
tissue T86.899
failure T86.891
infection T86.892
rejection T86.890
specified type NEC T86.898
type NEC T86.99
stem cell (from peripheral blood) (from umbilical cord) T86.5
umbilical cord stem cells T86.5
trauma (early) T79.9 ☑
specified NEC T79.8 ☑
ultrasound therapy NEC T88.9 ☑
umbilical cord NEC
complicating delivery O69.9 ☑
specified NEC O69.89 ☑
umbrella device, vascular T82.9 ☑
embolism T82.818 ☑
fibrosis T82.828 ☑
hemorrhage T82.838 ☑
infection or inflammation T82.7 ☑
mechanical
breakdown T82.515 ☑
displacement T82.525 ☑
leakage T82.535 ☑
malposition T82.525 ☑
obstruction T82.595 ☑
perforation T82.595 ☑
protrusion T82.595 ☑
pain T82.848 ☑
specified type NEC T82.898 ☑
stenosis T82.858 ☑
thrombosis T82.868 ☑
urethral catheter — *see* Complications, catheter, urethral, indwelling
vaccination T88.1 ☑
anaphylaxis NEC T80.52 ☑
arthropathy — *see* Arthropathy, postimmunization
cellulitis T88.0 ☑
encephalitis or encephalomyelitis G04.02
infection (general) (local) NEC T88.0 ☑
meningitis G03.8
myelitis G04.02
protein sickness T80.62 ☑
rash T88.1 ☑
reaction (allergic) T88.1 ☑
serum T80.62 ☑
sepsis T88.0 ☑
serum intoxication, sickness, rash, or other serum reaction NEC T80.62 ☑
anaphylactic shock T80.52 ☑
shock (allergic) (anaphylactic) T80.52 ☑
vaccinia (generalized) (localized) T88.1 ☑
vas deferens device or implant — *see* Complications, genitourinary, device or implant, genital tract

Complication(s) — *continued*
vascular I99.9
device or implant T82.9 ☑
embolism T82.818 ☑
fibrosis T82.828 ☑
hemorrhage T82.838 ☑
infection or inflammation T82.7 ☑
mechanical
breakdown T82.519 ☑
specified device NEC T82.518 ☑
displacement T82.529 ☑
specified device NEC T82.528 ☑
leakage T82.539 ☑
specified device NEC T82.538 ☑
malposition T82.529 ☑
specified device NEC T82.528 ☑
obstruction T82.599 ☑
specified device NEC T82.598 ☑
perforation T82.599 ☑
specified device NEC T82.598 ☑
protrusion T82.599 ☑
specified device NEC T82.598 ☑
pain T82.848 ☑
specified type NEC T82.898 ☑
stenosis T82.858 ☑
thrombosis T82.868 ☑
dialysis catheter — *see* Complication, catheter, dialysis
following infusion, therapeutic injection or transfusion T80.1 ☑
graft T82.9 ☑
embolism T82.818 ☑
fibrosis T82.828 ☑
hemorrhage T82.838 ☑
mechanical
breakdown T82.319 ☑
aorta (bifurcation) T82.310 ☑
carotid artery T82.311 ☑
specified vessel NEC T82.318 ☑
displacement T82.329 ☑
aorta (bifurcation) T82.320 ☑
carotid artery T82.321 ☑
specified vessel NEC T82.328 ☑
leakage T82.339 ☑
aorta (bifurcation) T82.330 ☑
carotid artery T82.331 ☑
specified vessel NEC T82.338 ☑
malposition T82.329 ☑
aorta (bifurcation) T82.320 ☑
carotid artery T82.321 ☑
specified vessel NEC T82.328 ☑
obstruction T82.399 ☑
aorta (bifurcation) T82.390 ☑
carotid artery T82.391 ☑
specified vessel NEC T82.398 ☑
perforation T82.399 ☑
aorta (bifurcation) T82.390 ☑
carotid artery T82.391 ☑
specified vessel NEC T82.398 ☑
protrusion T82.399 ☑
aorta (bifurcation) T82.390 ☑
carotid artery T82.391 ☑
specified vessel NEC T82.398 ☑
pain T82.848 ☑
specified complication NEC T82.898 ☑
stenosis T82.858 ☑
thrombosis T82.868 ☑
postoperative — *see* Complications, postoperative, circulatory
vena cava device (filter) (sieve) (umbrella) — *see* Complications, umbrella device, vascular
ventilation therapy NEC T81.81 ☑
ventilator
mechanical J95.850
specified NEC J95.859
ventricular (communicating) shunt (device) T85.9 ☑
embolism T85.810 ☑
fibrosis T85.820 ☑
hemorrhage T85.830 ☑
infection and inflammation T85.730 ☑
mechanical
breakdown T85.01 ☑
displacement T85.02 ☑
leakage T85.03 ☑
malposition T85.02 ☑
obstruction T85.09 ☑

Complication(s) — *continued*
ventricular shunt — *continued*
mechanical — *continued*
perforation T85.09 ☑
protrusion T85.09 ☑
specified NEC T85.09 ☑
pain T85.840 ☑
specified type NEC T85.890 ☑
stenosis T85.850 ☑
thrombosis T85.860 ☑
wire suture, permanent (implanted) — *see* Complications, suture, permanent
Compressed air disease T70.3 ☑
Compression
with injury — *code by* Nature of injury
artery I77.1
celiac, syndrome I77.4
brachial plexus G54.0
brain (stem) G93.5
due to
contusion (diffuse) — *see* Injury, intracranial, diffuse
focal — *see* Injury, intracranial, focal
injury NEC — *see* Injury, intracranial, diffuse
traumatic — *see* Injury, intracranial, diffuse
bronchus J98.09
cauda equina G83.4
celiac (artery) (axis) I77.4
cerebral — *see* Compression, brain
cervical plexus G54.2
cord
spinal — *see* Compression, spinal
umbilical — *see* Compression, umbilical cord
cranial nerve G52.9
eighth H93.3 ☑
eleventh G52.8
fifth G50.8
first G52.0
fourth — *see* Strabismus, paralytic, fourth nerve
ninth G52.1
second — *see* Disorder, nerve, optic
seventh G51.8
sixth — *see* Strabismus, paralytic, sixth nerve
tenth G52.2
third — *see* Strabismus, paralytic, third nerve
twelfth G52.3
diver's squeeze T70.3 ☑
during birth (newborn) P15.9
esophagus K22.2
eustachian tube — *see* Obstruction, eustachian tube, cartilaginous
facies Q67.1
fracture
nontraumatic NOS — *see* Collapse, vertebra
pathological — *see* Fracture, pathological
traumatic — *see* Fracture, traumatic
heart — *see* Disease, heart
intestine — *see* Obstruction, intestine
laryngeal nerve, recurrent G52.2
with paralysis of vocal cords and larynx J38.00
bilateral J38.02
unilateral J38.01
lumbosacral plexus G54.1
lung J98.4
lymphatic vessel I89.0
medulla — *see* Compression, brain
nerve (*see also* Disorder, nerve) G58.9
arm NEC — *see* Mononeuropathy, upper limb
axillary G54.0
cranial — *see* Compression, cranial nerve
leg NEC — *see* Mononeuropathy, lower limb
median (in carpal tunnel) — *see* Syndrome, carpal tunnel
optic — *see* Disorder, nerve, optic
plantar — *see* Lesion, nerve, plantar
posterior tibial (in tarsal tunnel) — *see* Syndrome, tarsal tunnel
root or plexus NOS (in) G54.9
intervertebral disc disorder NEC — *see* Disorder, disc, with, radiculopathy
with myelopathy — *see* Disorder, disc, with, myelopathy
neoplastic disease (*see also* Neoplasm) D49.9 [G55]
spondylosis — *see* Spondylosis, with radiculopathy
sciatic (acute) — *see* Lesion, nerve, sciatic

Compression — continued
- nerve (see also Disorder, nerve) — continued
  - sympathetic G90.8
  - traumatic — see Injury, nerve
  - ulnar — see Lesion, nerve, ulnar
  - upper extremity NEC — see Mononeuropathy, upper limb
  - spinal (cord) G95.20
    - by displacement of intervertebral disc NEC (see also Disorder, disc, with, myelopathy)
  - nerve root NOS G54.9
    - due to displacement of intervertebral disc NEC — see Disorder, disc, with, radiculopathy
    - with myelopathy — see Disorder, disc, with, myelopathy
    - specified NEC G95.29
    - spondylogenic (cervical) (lumbar, lumbosacral) (thoracic) — see Spondylosis, with myelopathy NEC
      - anterior — see Syndrome, anterior, spinal artery, compression
    - traumatic — see Injury, spinal cord, by region
  - subcostal nerve (syndrome) — see Mononeuropathy, upper limb, specified NEC
  - sympathetic nerve NEC G90.8
  - syndrome T79.5 ☑
  - trachea J39.8
  - ulnar nerve (by scar tissue) — see Lesion, nerve, ulnar
  - umbilical cord
    - complicating delivery O69.2 ☑
      - cord around neck O69.1 ☑
      - prolapse O69.0 ☑
      - specified NEC O69.2 ☑
  - ureter N13.5
  - vein I87.1
  - vena cava (inferior) (superior) I87.1

Compulsion, compulsive
- gambling F63.0
- neurosis F42.8
- personality F60.5
- states F42.8
- swearing F42.8
  - in Gilles de la Tourette's syndrome F95.2
- tics and spasms F95.9

Concato's disease (pericardial polyserositis) A19.9
- nontubercular I31.1
- pleural — see Pleurisy, with effusion

Concavity chest wall M95.4
Concealed penis Q55.64
Concern (normal) **about sick person in family** Z63.6
Concrescence (teeth) K00.2
Concretio cordis I31.1
- rheumatic I09.2
Concretion (see also Calculus)
- appendicular K38.1
- canaliculus — see Dacryolith
- clitoris N90.89
- conjunctiva H11.12- ☑
- eyelid — see Disorder, eyelid, specified type NEC
- lacrimal passages — see Dacryolith
- prepuce (male) N47.8
- salivary gland (any) K11.5
- seminal vesicle N50.89
- tonsil J35.8
Concussion (brain) (cerebral) (current) S06.0X9 ☑
- with
  - loss of consciousness of 30 minutes or less S06.0X1 ☑
  - loss of consciousness of unspecified duration S06.0X9 ☑
- blast (air) (hydraulic) (immersion) (underwater)
  - abdomen or thorax — see Injury, blast, by site
  - ear with acoustic nerve injury — see Injury, nerve, acoustic, specified type NEC
- cauda equina S34.3 ☑
- conus medullaris S34.02 ☑
- ocular S05.8X- ☑
- spinal (cord)
  - cervical S14.0 ☑
  - lumbar S34.01 ☑
  - sacral S34.02 ☑
  - thoracic S24.0 ☑
  - syndrome F07.81
- without loss of consciousness S06.0X0 ☑
Condition — see Disease
Conditions arising in the perinatal period — see Newborn, affected by

Conduct disorder — see Disorder, conduct
Condyloma A63.0
- acuminatum A63.0
- gonorrheal A54.09
- latum A51.31
- syphilitic A51.31
  - congenital A50.07
- venereal, syphilitic A51.31
Conflagration (see also Burn)
- asphyxia (by inhalation of gases, fumes or vapors) (see also Table of Drugs and Chemicals) T59.9- ☑
Conflict (with) (see also Discord)
- family Z73.9
- marital Z63.0
  - involving divorce or estrangement Z63.5
- parent-child Z62.820
  - parent-adopted child Z62.821
  - parent-biological child Z62.820
  - parent-foster child Z62.822
- social role NEC Z73.5
Confluent — see condition
Confusion, confused R41.0
- epileptic F05
- mental state (psychogenic) F44.89
- psychogenic F44.89
- reactive (from emotional stress, psychological trauma) F44.89
Confusional arousals G47.51
Congelation T69.9 ☑
Congenital (see also condition)
- aortic septum Q25.49
- intrinsic factor deficiency D51.0
- malformation — see Anomaly
Congestion, congestive
- bladder N32.89
- bowel K63.89
- brain G93.89
- breast N64.59
- bronchial J98.09
- catarrhal J31.0
- chest R09.89
- chill, malarial — see Malaria
- circulatory NEC I99.8
- duodenum K31.89
- eye — see Hyperemia, conjunctiva
- facial, due to birth injury P15.4
- general R68.89
- glottis J37.0
- heart — see Failure, heart, congestive
- hepatic K76.1
- hypostatic (lung) — see Edema, lung
- intestine K63.89
- kidney N28.89
- labyrinth H83.8 ☑
- larynx J37.0
- liver K76.1
- lung R09.89
  - active or acute — see Pneumonia
- malaria, malarial — see Malaria
- nasal R09.81
- nose R09.81
- orbit, orbital (see also Exophthalmos)
  - inflammatory (chronic) — see Inflammation, orbit
- ovary N83.8
- pancreas K86.89
- pelvic, female N94.89
- pleural J94.8
- prostate (active) N42.1
- pulmonary — see Congestion, lung
- renal N28.89
- retina H35.81
- seminal vesicle N50.1
- spinal cord G95.19
- spleen (chronic) D73.2
- stomach K31.89
- trachea — see Tracheitis
- urethra N36.8
- uterus N85.8
  - with subinvolution N85.3
- venous (passive) I87.8
- viscera R68.89
Congestive — see Congestion
Conical
- cervix (hypertrophic elongation) N88.4
- cornea — see Keratoconus
- teeth K00.2
Conjoined twins Q89.4
Conjugal maladjustment Z63.0

Conduct disorder — see Disorder, conduct

Conjugal maladjustment — continued
- involving divorce or estrangement Z63.5
Conjunctiva — see condition
Conjunctivitis (staphylococcal) (streptococcal) NOS H10.9
- Acanthamoeba B60.12
- acute H10.3- ☑
  - atopic H10.1- ☑
  - chemical (see also Corrosion, cornea) H10.21- ☑
  - mucopurulent H10.02- ☑
    - follicular H10.01- ☑
  - pseudomembranous H10.22- ☑
  - serous except viral H10.23- ☑
    - viral — see Conjunctivitis, viral
  - toxic H10.21- ☑
- adenoviral (acute) (follicular) B30.1
- allergic (acute) — see Conjunctivitis, acute, atopic
  - chronic H10.45
  - vernal H10.44
- anaphylactic — see Conjunctivitis, acute, atopic
- Apollo B30.3
- atopic (acute) — see Conjunctivitis, acute, atopic
- Béal's B30.2
- blennorrhagic (gonococcal) (neonatorum) A54.31
- chemical (acute) (see also Corrosion, cornea) H10.21- ☑
- chlamydial A74.0
  - due to trachoma A71.1
  - neonatal P39.1
- chronic (nodosa) (petrificans) (phlyctenular) H10.40- ☑
  - allergic H10.45
    - vernal H10.44
  - follicular H10.43- ☑
  - giant papillary H10.41- ☑
  - simple H10.42- ☑
  - vernal H10.44
- coxsackievirus 24 B30.3
- diphtheritic A36.86
- due to
  - dust — see Conjunctivitis, acute, atopic
  - filariasis B74.9
  - mucocutaneous leishmaniasis B55.2
- enterovirus type 70 (hemorrhagic) B30.3
- epidemic (viral) B30.9
  - hemorrhagic B30.3
- gonococcal (neonatorum) A54.31
- granular (trachomatous) A71.1
  - sequelae (late effect) B94.0
- hemorrhagic (acute) (epidemic) B30.3
- herpes zoster B02.31
- in (due to)
  - Acanthamoeba B60.12
  - adenovirus (acute) (follicular) B30.1
  - Chlamydia A74.0
  - coxsackievirus 24 B30.3
  - diphtheria A36.86
  - enterovirus type 70 (hemorrhagic) B30.3
  - filariasis B74.9
  - gonococci A54.31
  - herpes (simplex) virus B00.53
    - zoster B02.31
  - infectious disease NEC B99 ☑
  - meningococci A39.89
  - mucocutaneous leishmaniasis B55.2
  - rosacea H10.82- ☑
  - syphilis (late) A52.71
  - zoster B02.31
- inclusion A74.0
- infantile P39.1
  - gonococcal A54.31
- Koch-Weeks' — see Conjunctivitis, acute, mucopurulent
- light — see Conjunctivitis, acute, atopic
- ligneous — see Blepharoconjunctivitis, ligneous
- meningococcal A39.89
- mucopurulent — see Conjunctivitis, acute, mucopurulent
- neonatal P39.1
  - gonococcal A54.31
- Newcastle B30.8
- of Béal B30.2
- parasitic
  - filariasis B74.9
  - mucocutaneous leishmaniasis B55.2
- Parinaud's H10.89
- petrificans H10.89
- rosacea H10.82- ☑
- specified NEC H10.89
- swimming-pool B30.1
- trachomatous A71.1
  - acute A71.0

Conjunctivitis — *continued*
  trachomatous — *continued*
    sequelae (late effect) B94.0
  traumatic NEC H10.89
  tuberculous A18.59
  tularemic A21.1
  tularensis A21.1
  viral B30.9
    due to
      adenovirus B30.1
      enterovirus B30.3
    specified NEC B30.8
Conjunctivochalasis H11.82- ☑
Connective tissue — *see* condition
Conn's syndrome E26.01
Conradi (-Hunermann) **disease** Q77.3
Consanguinity Z84.3
  counseling Z71.89
Conscious simulation (of illness) Z76.5
Consecutive — *see* condition
Consolidation lung (base) — *see* Pneumonia, lobar
Constipation (atonic) (neurogenic) (simple) (spastic)
  K59.00
  chronic K59.09
    idiopathic K59.04
  drug-induced K59.03
  functional K59.04
  outlet dysfunction K59.02
  psychogenic F45.8
  slow transit K59.01
  specified NEC K59.09
Constitutional (*see also* condition)
  substandard F60.7
Constitutionally substandard F60.7
Constriction (*see also* Stricture)
  auditory canal — *see* Stenosis, external ear canal
  bronchial J98.09
  duodenum K31.5
  esophagus K22.2
  external
    abdomen, abdominal (wall) S30.841 ☑
    alveolar process S00.542 ☑
    ankle S90.54- ☑
    antecubital space — *see* Constriction, external, forearm
    arm (upper) S40.84- ☑
    auricle — *see* Constriction, external, ear
    axilla — *see* Constriction, external, arm
    back, lower S30.840 ☑
    breast S20.14- ☑
    brow S00.84 ☑
    buttock S30.840 ☑
    calf — *see* Constriction, external, leg
    canthus — *see* Constriction, external, eyelid
    cheek S00.84 ☑
      internal S00.542 ☑
    chest wall — *see* Constriction, external, thorax
    chin S00.84 ☑
    clitoris S30.844 ☑
    costal region — *see* Constriction, external, thorax
    digit(s)
      foot — *see* Constriction, external, toe
      hand — *see* Constriction, external, finger
    ear S00.44- ☑
    elbow S50.34- ☑
    epididymis S30.843 ☑
    epigastric region S30.841 ☑
    esophagus, cervical S10.14 ☑
    eyebrow — *see* Constriction, external, eyelid
    eyelid S00.24- ☑
    face S00.84 ☑
    finger(s) S60.44- ☑
      index S60.44- ☑
      little S60.44- ☑
      middle S60.44- ☑
      ring S60.44- ☑
    flank S30.841 ☑
    foot (except toe(s) alone) S90.84- ☑
      toe — *see* Constriction, external, toe
    forearm S50.84- ☑
      elbow only — *see* Constriction, external, elbow
    forehead S00.84 ☑
    genital organs, external
      female S30.846 ☑
      male S30.845 ☑
    groin S30.841 ☑
    gum S00.542 ☑

Constriction — *continued*
  external — *continued*
    hand S60.54- ☑
    head S00.94 ☑
      ear — *see* Constriction, external, ear
      eyelid — *see* Constriction, external, eyelid
      lip S00.541 ☑
      nose S00.34 ☑
      oral cavity S00.542 ☑
      scalp S00.04 ☑
      specified site NEC S00.84 ☑
    heel — *see* Constriction, external, foot
    hip S70.24- ☑
    inguinal region S30.841 ☑
    interscapular region S20.449 ☑
    jaw S00.84 ☑
    knee S80.24- ☑
    labium (majus) (minus) S30.844 ☑
    larynx S10.14 ☑
    leg (lower) S80.84- ☑
      knee — *see* Constriction, external, knee
      upper — *see* Constriction, external, thigh
    lip S00.541 ☑
    lower back S30.840 ☑
    lumbar region S30.840 ☑
    malar region S00.84 ☑
    mammary — *see* Constriction, external, breast
    mastoid region S00.84 ☑
    mouth S00.542 ☑
    nail
      finger — *see* Constriction, external, finger
      toe — *see* Constriction, external, toe
    nasal S00.34 ☑
    neck S10.94 ☑
      specified site NEC S10.84 ☑
      throat S10.14 ☑
    nose S00.34 ☑
    occipital region S00.04 ☑
    oral cavity S00.542 ☑
    orbital region — *see* Constriction, external, eyelid
    palate S00.542 ☑
    palm — *see* Constriction, external, hand
    parietal region S00.04 ☑
    pelvis S30.840 ☑
    penis S30.842 ☑
    perineum
      female S30.844 ☑
      male S30.840 ☑
    periocular area — *see* Constriction, external, eyelid
    phalanges
      finger — *see* Constriction, external, finger
      toe — *see* Constriction, external, toe
    pharynx S10.14 ☑
    pinna — *see* Constriction, external, ear
    popliteal space — *see* Constriction, external, knee
    prepuce S30.842 ☑
    pubic region S30.840 ☑
    pudendum
      female S30.846 ☑
      male S30.845 ☑
    sacral region S30.840 ☑
    scalp S00.04 ☑
    scapular region — *see* Constriction, external, shoulder
    scrotum S30.843 ☑
    shin — *see* Constriction, external, leg
    shoulder S40.24- ☑
    sternal region S20.349 ☑
    submaxillary region S00.84 ☑
    submental region S00.84 ☑
    subungual
      finger(s) — *see* Constriction, external, finger
      toe(s) — *see* Constriction, external, toe
    supraclavicular fossa S10.84 ☑
    supraorbital S00.84 ☑
    temple S00.84 ☑
    temporal region S00.84 ☑
    testis S30.843 ☑
    thigh S70.34- ☑
    thorax, thoracic (wall) S20.94 ☑
      back S20.44- ☑
      front S20.34- ☑
    throat S10.14 ☑
    thumb S60.34- ☑
    toe(s) (lesser) S90.44- ☑
      great S90.44- ☑

Constriction — *continued*
  external — *continued*
    tongue S00.542 ☑
    trachea S10.14 ☑
    tunica vaginalis S30.843 ☑
    uvula S00.542 ☑
    vagina S30.844 ☑
    vulva S30.844 ☑
    wrist S60.84- ☑
  gallbladder — *see* Obstruction, gallbladder
  intestine — *see* Obstruction, intestine
  larynx J38.6
    congenital Q31.8
      specified NEC Q31.8
      subglottic Q31.1
  organ or site, congenital NEC — *see* Atresia, by site
  prepuce (acquired) (congenital) N47.1
  pylorus (adult hypertrophic) K31.1
    congenital or infantile Q40.0
    newborn Q40.0
  ring dystocia (uterus) O62.4
  spastic (*see also* Spasm)
    ureter N13.5
  ureter N13.5
    with infection N13.6
  urethra — *see* Stricture, urethra
  visual field (peripheral) (functional) — *see* Defect, visual field
Constrictive — *see* condition
Consultation
  medical — *see* Counseling, medical
  religious Z71.81
  specified reason NEC Z71.89
  spiritual Z71.81
  without complaint or sickness Z71.9
    feared complaint unfounded Z71.1
    specified reason NEC Z71.89
Consumption — *see* Tuberculosis
Contact (with) (*see also* Exposure (to))
  acariasis Z20.7
  AIDS virus Z20.6
  air pollution Z77.110
  algae and algae toxins Z77.121
  algae bloom Z77.121
  anthrax Z20.810
  aromatic amines Z77.020
  aromatic (hazardous) compounds NEC Z77.028
  aromatic dyes NOS Z77.028
  arsenic Z77.010
  asbestos Z77.090
  bacterial disease NEC Z20.818
  benzene Z77.021
  blue-green algae bloom Z77.121
  body fluids (potentially hazardous) Z77.21
  brown tide Z77.121
  chemicals (chiefly nonmedicinal) (hazardous) NEC Z77.098
  cholera Z20.09
  chromium compounds Z77.018
  communicable disease Z20.9
    bacterial NEC Z20.818
    specified NEC Z20.89
    viral NEC Z20.828
    Zika virus Z20.821
  cyanobacteria bloom Z77.121
  dyes Z77.098
  Escherichia coli (E. coli) Z20.01
  fiberglass — *see* Table of Drugs and Chemicals, fiberglass
  German measles Z20.4
  gonorrhea Z20.2
  hazardous metals NEC Z77.018
  hazardous substances NEC Z77.29
  hazards in the physical environment NEC Z77.128
  hazards to health NEC Z77.9
  HIV Z20.6
  HTLV-III/LAV Z20.6
  human immunodeficiency virus (HIV) Z20.6
  infection Z20.9
    specified NEC Z20.89
  infestation (parasitic) NEC Z20.7
  intestinal infectious disease NEC Z20.09
    Escherichia coli (E. coli) Z20.01
  lead Z77.011
  meningococcus Z20.811
  mold (toxic) Z77.120
  nickel dust Z77.018
  noise Z77.122

Contact — *continued*
- parasitic disease Z20.7
- pediculosis Z20.7
- pfiesteria piscicida Z77.121
- poliomyelitis Z20.89
- pollution
  - air Z77.110
    - environmental NEC Z77.118
    - soil Z77.112
    - water Z77.111
  - polycyclic aromatic hydrocarbons Z77.028
- rabies Z20.3
- radiation, naturally occurring NEC Z77.123
- radon Z77.123
- red tide (Florida) Z77.121
- rubella Z20.4
- sexually-transmitted disease Z20.2
- smallpox (laboratory) Z20.89
- syphilis Z20.2
- tuberculosis Z20.1
- uranium Z77.012
- varicella Z20.820
- venereal disease Z20.2
- viral disease NEC Z20.828
- viral hepatitis Z20.5
- water pollution Z77.111
- Zika virus Z20.821

Contamination, food — *see* Intoxication, foodborne

Contraception, contraceptive
- advice Z30.09
- counseling Z30.09
- device (intrauterine) (in situ) Z97.5
  - causing menorrhagia T83.83 ☑
  - checking Z30.431
  - complications — *see* Complications, intrauterine, contraceptive device
  - in place Z97.5
  - initial prescription Z30.014
  - reinsertion Z30.433
  - removal Z30.432
  - replacement Z30.433
- emergency (postcoital) Z30.012
- initial prescription Z30.019
  - barrier Z30.018
  - diaphragm Z30.018
  - injectable Z30.013
  - intrauterine device Z30.014
  - pills Z30.011
  - postcoital (emergency) Z30.012
  - specified type NEC Z30.018
  - subdermal implantable Z30.017
  - transdermal patch hormonal Z30.016
  - vaginal ring hormonal Z30.015
- maintenance Z30.40
  - barrier Z30.49
  - diaphragm Z30.49
  - examination Z30.8
  - injectable Z30.42
  - intrauterine device Z30.431
  - pills Z30.41
  - specified type NEC Z30.49
  - subdermal implantable Z30.46
  - transdermal patch hormonal Z30.45
  - vaginal ring hormonal Z30.44
- management Z30.9
  - specified NEC Z30.8
- postcoital (emergency) Z30.012
- prescription Z30.019
  - repeat Z30.40
- sterilization Z30.2
- surveillance (drug) — *see* Contraception, maintenance

Contraction(s), contracture, contracted
- Achilles tendon (*see also* Short, tendon, Achilles)
  - congenital Q66.89
- amputation stump (surgical) (flexion) (late) (next proximal joint) T87.89
- anus K59.8
- bile duct (common) (hepatic) K83.8
- bladder N32.89
  - neck or sphincter N32.0
- bowel, cecum, colon or intestine, any part — *see* Obstruction, intestine
- Braxton Hicks — *see* False, labor
- breast implant, capsular T85.44 ☑
- bronchial J98.09
- burn (old) — *see* Cicatrix
- cervix — *see* Stricture, cervix
- cicatricial — *see* Cicatrix

Contraction(s), contracture, contracted — *continued*
- conjunctiva, trachomatous, active A71.1
  - sequelae (late effect) B94.0
- Dupuytren's M72.0
- eyelid — *see* Disorder, eyelid function
- fascia (lata) (postural) M72.8
  - Dupuytren's M72.0
  - palmar M72.0
  - plantar M72.2
- finger NEC (*see also* Deformity, finger)
  - congenital Q68.1
  - joint — *see* Contraction, joint, hand
- flaccid — *see* Contraction, paralytic
- gallbladder K82.0
- heart valve — *see* Endocarditis
- hip — *see* Contraction, joint, hip
- hourglass
  - bladder N32.89
    - congenital Q64.79
  - gallbladder K82.0
    - congenital Q44.1
  - stomach K31.89
    - congenital Q40.2
    - psychogenic F45.8
  - uterus (complicating delivery) O62.4
- hysterical F44.4
- internal os — *see* Stricture, cervix
- joint (abduction) (acquired) (adduction) (flexion) (rotation) M24.50
  - ankle M24.57- ☑
  - congenital NEC Q68.8
    - hip Q65.89
  - elbow M24.52- ☑
  - foot joint M24.57- ☑
  - hand joint M24.54- ☑
  - hip M24.55- ☑
    - congenital Q65.89
  - hysterical F44.4
  - knee M24.56- ☑
  - shoulder M24.51- ☑
  - wrist M24.53- ☑
- kidney (granular) (secondary) N26.9
  - congenital Q63.8
  - hydronephritic — *see* Hydronephrosis
  - Page N26.2
  - pyelonephritic — *see* Pyelitis, chronic
  - tuberculous A18.11
- ligament (*see also* Disorder, ligament)
  - congenital Q79.8
- muscle (postinfective) (postural) NEC M62.40
  - with contracture of joint — *see* Contraction, joint
  - ankle M62.47- ☑
  - congenital Q79.8
    - sternocleidomastoid Q68.0
  - extraocular — *see* Strabismus
  - eye (extrinsic) — *see* Strabismus
  - foot M62.47- ☑
  - forearm M62.43- ☑
  - hand M62.44- ☑
  - hysterical F44.4
  - ischemic (Volkmann's) T79.6 ☑
  - lower leg M62.46- ☑
  - multiple sites M62.49
  - pelvic region M62.45- ☑
  - posttraumatic — *see* Strabismus, paralytic
  - psychogenic F45.8
    - conversion reaction F44.4
  - shoulder region M62.41- ☑
  - specified site NEC M62.48
  - thigh M62.45- ☑
  - upper arm M62.42- ☑
- neck — *see* Torticollis
- ocular muscle — *see* Strabismus
- organ or site, congenital NEC — *see* Atresia, by site
- outlet (pelvis) — *see* Contraction, pelvis
- palmar fascia M72.0
- paralytic
  - joint — *see* Contraction, joint
  - muscle (*see also* Contraction, muscle NEC)
    - ocular — *see* Strabismus, paralytic
- pelvis (acquired) (general) M95.5
  - with disproportion (fetopelvic) O33.1
    - causing obstructed labor O65.1
  - inlet O33.2
  - mid-cavity O33.3 ☑
  - outlet O33.3 ☑

Contraction(s), contracture, contracted — *continued*
- plantar fascia M72.2
- premature
  - atrium I49.1
    - auriculoventricular I49.49
  - heart I49.49
  - junctional I49.2
  - supraventricular I49.1
  - ventricular I49.3
- prostate N42.89
- pylorus NEC (*see also* Pylorospasm)
  - psychogenic F45.8
- rectum, rectal (sphincter) K59.8
- ring (Bandl's) (complicating delivery) O62.4
- scar — *see* Cicatrix
- spine — *see* Dorsopathy, deforming
- sternocleidomastoid (muscle), congenital Q68.0
- stomach K31.89
  - hourglass K31.89
    - congenital Q40.2
    - psychogenic F45.8
  - psychogenic F45.8
- tendon (sheath) M62.40
  - with contracture of joint — *see* Contraction, joint
  - Achilles — *see* Short, tendon, Achilles
  - ankle M62.47- ☑
    - Achilles — *see* Short, tendon, Achilles
  - foot M62.47- ☑
  - forearm M62.43- ☑
  - hand M62.44- ☑
  - lower leg M62.46- ☑
  - multiple sites M62.49
  - neck M62.48
  - pelvic region M62.45- ☑
  - shoulder region M62.41- ☑
  - specified site NEC M62.48
  - thigh M62.45- ☑
  - thorax M62.48
  - trunk M62.48
  - upper arm M62.42- ☑
- toe — *see* Deformity, toe, specified NEC
- ureterovesical orifice (postinfectional) N13.5
  - with infection N13.6
- urethra (*see also* Stricture, urethra)
  - orifice N32.0
- uterus N85.8
  - abnormal NEC O62.9
  - clonic (complicating delivery) O62.4
  - dyscoordinate (complicating delivery) O62.4
  - hourglass (complicating delivery) O62.4
  - hypertonic O62.4
  - hypotonic NEC O62.2
  - inadequate
    - primary O62.0
    - secondary O62.1
  - incoordinate (complicating delivery) O62.4
  - poor O62.2
  - tetanic (complicating delivery) O62.4
- vagina (outlet) N89.5
- vesical N32.89
  - neck or urethral orifice N32.0
- visual field — *see* Defect, visual field, generalized
- Volkmann's (ischemic) T79.6 ☑

Contusion (skin surface intact) T14.8 ☑
- abdomen, abdominal (muscle) (wall) S30.1 ☑
- adnexa, eye NEC S05.8X- ☑
- adrenal gland S37.812 ☑
- alveolar process S00.532 ☑
- ankle S90.0- ☑
- antecubital space — *see* Contusion, forearm
- anus S30.3 ☑
- arm (upper) S40.02- ☑
  - lower (with elbow) — *see* Contusion, forearm
- auditory canal — *see* Contusion, ear
- auricle — *see* Contusion, ear
- axilla — *see* Contusion, arm, upper
- back (*see also* Contusion, thorax, back)
  - lower S30.0 ☑
- bile duct S36.13 ☑
- bladder S37.22 ☑
- bone NEC T14.8 ☑
- brain (diffuse) — *see* Injury, intracranial, diffuse
  - focal — *see* Injury, intracranial, focal
- brainstem S06.38- ☑
- breast S20.0- ☑
- broad ligament S37.892 ☑

Contusion — *continued*
- brow S00.83 ☑
- buttock S30.0 ☑
- canthus, eye S00.1- ☑
- cauda equina S34.3 ☑
- cerebellar, traumatic S06.37- ☑
- cerebral S06.33- ☑
  - left side S06.32- ☑
  - right side S06.31- ☑
- cheek S00.83 ☑
  - internal S00.532 ☑
- chest (wall) — *see* Contusion, thorax
- chin S00.83 ☑
- clitoris S30.23 ☑
- colon — *see* Injury, intestine, large, contusion
- common bile duct S36.13 ☑
- conjunctiva S05.1- ☑
  - with foreign body (in conjunctival sac) — *see* Foreign body, conjunctival sac
- conus medullaris (spine) S34.139 ☑
- cornea — *see* Contusion, eyeball
  - with foreign body — *see* Foreign body, cornea
- corpus cavernosum S30.21 ☑
- cortex (brain) (cerebral) — *see* Injury, intracranial, diffuse
  - focal — *see* Injury, intracranial, focal
- costal region — *see* Contusion, thorax
- cystic duct S36.13 ☑
- diaphragm S27.802 ☑
- duodenum S36.420 ☑
- ear S00.43- ☑
- elbow S50.0- ☑
  - with forearm — *see* Contusion, forearm
- epididymis S30.22 ☑
- epigastric region S30.1 ☑
- epiglottis S10.0 ☑
- esophagus (thoracic) S27.812 ☑
  - cervical S10.0 ☑
- eyeball S05.1- ☑
- eyebrow S00.1- ☑
- eyelid (and periocular area) S00.1- ☑
- face NEC S00.83 ☑
- fallopian tube S37.529 ☑
  - bilateral S37.522 ☑
  - unilateral S37.521 ☑
- femoral triangle S30.1 ☑
- finger(s) S60.00 ☑
  - with damage to nail (matrix) S60.10 ☑
  - index S60.02- ☑
    - with damage to nail S60.12- ☑
  - little S60.05- ☑
    - with damage to nail S60.15- ☑
  - middle S60.03- ☑
    - with damage to nail S60.13- ☑
  - ring S60.04- ☑
    - with damage to nail S60.14- ☑
  - thumb — *see* Contusion, thumb
- flank S30.1 ☑
- foot (except toe(s) alone) S90.3- ☑
  - toe — *see* Contusion, toe
- forearm S50.1- ☑
  - elbow only — *see* Contusion, elbow
- forehead S00.83 ☑
- gallbladder S36.122 ☑
- genital organs, external
  - female S30.202 ☑
  - male S30.201 ☑
- globe (eye) — *see* Contusion, eyeball
- groin S30.1 ☑
- gum S00.532 ☑
- hand S60.22- ☑
  - finger(s) — *see* Contusion, finger
  - wrist — *see* Contusion, wrist
- head S00.93 ☑
  - ear — *see* Contusion, ear
  - eyelid — *see* Contusion, eyelid
  - lip S00.531 ☑
  - nose S00.33 ☑
  - oral cavity S00.532 ☑
  - scalp S00.03 ☑
  - specified part NEC S00.83 ☑
- heart (*see also* Injury, heart) S26.91 ☑
- heel — *see* Contusion, foot
- hepatic duct S36.13 ☑
- hip S70.0- ☑
- ileum S36.428 ☑

Contusion — *continued*
- iliac region S30.1 ☑
- inguinal region S30.1 ☑
- interscapular region S20.229 ☑
- intra-abdominal organ S36.92 ☑
  - colon — *see* Injury, intestine, large, contusion
  - liver S36.112 ☑
  - pancreas — *see* Contusion, pancreas
  - rectum S36.62 ☑
  - small intestine — *see* Injury, intestine, small, contusion
  - specified organ NEC S36.892 ☑
  - spleen — *see* Contusion, spleen
  - stomach S36.32 ☑
- iris (eye) — *see* Contusion, eyeball
- jaw S00.83 ☑
- jejunum S36.428 ☑
- kidney S37.01- ☑
  - major (greater than 2 cm) S37.02- ☑
  - minor (less than 2 cm) S37.01- ☑
- knee S80.0- ☑
- labium (majus) (minus) S30.23 ☑
- lacrimal apparatus, gland or sac S05.8X- ☑
- larynx S10.0 ☑
- leg (lower) S80.1- ☑
  - knee — *see* Contusion, knee
- lens — *see* Contusion, eyeball
- lip S00.531 ☑
- liver S36.112 ☑
- lower back S30.0 ☑
- lumbar region S30.0 ☑
- lung S27.329 ☑
  - bilateral S27.322 ☑
  - unilateral S27.321 ☑
- malar region S00.83 ☑
- mastoid region S00.83 ☑
- membrane, brain — *see* Injury, intracranial, diffuse
  - focal — *see* Injury, intracranial, focal
- mesentery S36.892 ☑
- mesosalpinx S37.892 ☑
- mouth S00.532 ☑
- muscle — *see* Contusion, by site
- nail
  - finger — *see* Contusion, finger, with damage to nail
  - toe — *see* Contusion, toe, with damage to nail
- nasal S00.33 ☑
- neck S10.93 ☑
  - specified site NEC S10.83 ☑
  - throat S10.0 ☑
- nerve — *see* Injury, nerve
- newborn P54.5
- nose S00.33 ☑
- occipital
  - lobe (brain) — *see* Injury, intracranial, diffuse
    - focal — *see* Injury, intracranial, focal
  - region (scalp) S00.03 ☑
- orbit (region) (tissues) S05.1- ☑
- ovary S37.429 ☑
  - bilateral S37.422 ☑
  - unilateral S37.421 ☑
- palate S00.532 ☑
- pancreas S36.229 ☑
  - body S36.221 ☑
  - head S36.220 ☑
  - tail S36.222 ☑
- parietal
  - lobe (brain) — *see* Injury, intracranial, diffuse
    - focal — *see* Injury, intracranial, focal
  - region (scalp) S00.03 ☑
- pelvic organ S37.92 ☑
  - adrenal gland S37.812 ☑
  - bladder S37.22 ☑
  - fallopian tube — *see* Contusion, fallopian tube
  - kidney — *see* Contusion, kidney
  - ovary — *see* Contusion, ovary
  - prostate S37.822 ☑
  - specified organ NEC S37.892 ☑
  - ureter S37.12 ☑
  - urethra S37.32 ☑
  - uterus S37.62 ☑
- pelvis S30.0 ☑
- penis S30.21 ☑
- perineum
  - female S30.23 ☑
  - male S30.0 ☑
- periocular area S00.1- ☑

Contusion — *continued*
- peritoneum S36.81 ☑
- periurethral tissue — *see* Contusion, urethra
- pharynx S10.0 ☑
- pinna — *see* Contusion, ear
- popliteal space — *see* Contusion, knee
- prepuce S30.21 ☑
- prostate S37.822 ☑
- pubic region S30.1 ☑
- pudendum
  - female S30.202 ☑
  - male S30.201 ☑
- quadriceps femoris — *see* Contusion, thigh
- rectum S36.62 ☑
- retroperitoneum S36.892 ☑
- round ligament S37.892 ☑
- sacral region S30.0 ☑
- scalp S00.03 ☑
  - due to birth injury P12.3
- scapular region — *see* Contusion, shoulder
- sclera — *see* Contusion, eyeball
- scrotum S30.22 ☑
- seminal vesicle S37.892 ☑
- shoulder S40.01- ☑
- skin NEC T14.8 ☑
- small intestine — *see* Injury, intestine, small, contusion
- spermatic cord S30.22 ☑
- spinal cord — *see* Injury, spinal cord, by region
  - cauda equina S34.3 ☑
  - conus medullaris S34.139 ☑
- spleen S36.029 ☑
  - major S36.021 ☑
  - minor S36.020 ☑
- sternal region S20.219 ☑
- stomach S36.32 ☑
- subconjunctival S05.1- ☑
- subcutaneous NEC T14.8 ☑
- submaxillary region S00.83 ☑
- submental region S00.83 ☑
- subperiosteal NEC T14.8 ☑
- subungual
  - finger — *see* Contusion, finger, with damage to nail
  - toe — *see* Contusion, toe, with damage to nail
- supraclavicular fossa S10.83 ☑
- supraorbital S00.83 ☑
- suprarenal gland S37.812 ☑
- temple (region) S00.83 ☑
- temporal
  - lobe (brain) — *see* Injury, intracranial, diffuse
    - focal — *see* Injury, intracranial, focal
  - region S00.83 ☑
- testis S30.22 ☑
- thigh S70.1- ☑
- thorax (wall) S20.20 ☑
  - back S20.22- ☑
  - front S20.21- ☑
- throat S10.0 ☑
- thumb S60.01- ☑
  - with damage to nail S60.11- ☑
- toe(s) (lesser) S90.12- ☑
  - with damage to nail S90.22- ☑
  - great S90.11- ☑
    - with damage to nail S90.21- ☑
- tongue S00.532 ☑
- trachea (cervical) S10.0 ☑
  - thoracic S27.52 ☑
- tunica vaginalis S30.22 ☑
- tympanum, tympanic membrane — *see* Contusion, ear
- ureter S37.12 ☑
- urethra S37.32 ☑
- urinary organ NEC S37.892 ☑
- uterus S37.62 ☑
- uvula S00.532 ☑
- vagina S30.23 ☑
- vas deferens S37.892 ☑
- vesical S37.22 ☑
- vocal cord(s) S10.0 ☑
- vulva S30.23 ☑
- wrist S60.21- ☑

Conus (congenital) (any type) Q14.8
- cornea — *see* Keratoconus
- medullaris syndrome G95.81

Conversion hysteria, neurosis or reaction F44.9
Converter, tuberculosis (test reaction) R76.11
Conviction (legal), **anxiety concerning** Z65.0

☑ **Additional Character Required** — Refer to the Tabular List for Character Selection   ▽ **Subterms under main terms may continue to next column or page**

Conviction (legal), **anxiety concerning** — *continued*
  with imprisonment Z65.1
Convulsions (idiopathic) (*see also* Seizure(s)) R56.9
  apoplectiform (cerebral ischemia) I67.82
  dissociative F44.5
  epileptic — *see* Epilepsy
  epileptiform, epileptoid — *see* Seizure, epileptiform
  ether (anesthetic) — *see* Table of Drugs and Chemicals,
    by drug
  febrile R56.00
    with status epilepticus G40.901
    complex R56.01
      with status epilepticus G40.901
    simple R56.00
  hysterical F44.5
  infantile P90
    epilepsy — *see* Epilepsy
  jacksonian — *see* Epilepsy, localization-related, symp-
    tomatic, with simple partial seizures
  myoclonic G25.3
  newborn P90
  obstetrical (nephritic) (uremic) — *see* Eclampsia
  paretic A52.17
  post traumatic R56.1
  psychomotor — *see* Epilepsy, localization-related,
    symptomatic, with complex partial seizures
  recurrent R56.9
  reflex R25.8
  scarlatinal A38.8
  tetanus, tetanic — *see* Tetanus
  thymic E32.8
Convulsive (*see also* Convulsions)
Cooley's anemia D56.1
Coolie itch B76.9
Cooper's
  disease — *see* Mastopathy, cystic
  hernia — *see* Hernia, abdomen, specified site NEC
Copra itch B88.0
Coprophagy F50.89
Coprophobia F40.298
Coproporphyria, hereditary E80.29
Cor
  biloculare Q20.8
  bovis, bovinum — *see* Hypertrophy, cardiac
  pulmonale (chronic) I27.81
    acute I26.09
  triatriatum, triatrium Q24.2
  triloculare Q20.8
    biatrium Q20.4
    biventriculare Q21.1
Corbus' disease (gangrenous balanitis) N48.1
Cord (*see also* condition)
  around neck
    complicating delivery O69.81 ☑
      with compression O69.1 ☑
  bladder G95.89
    tabetic A52.19
Cordis ectopia Q24.8
Corditis (spermatic) N49.1
Corectopia Q13.2
Cori's disease (glycogen storage) E74.03
Corkhandler's disease or lung J67.3
Corkscrew esophagus K22.4
Corkworker's disease or lung J67.3
Corn (infected) L84
Cornea (*see also* condition)
  donor Z52.5
  plana Q13.4
Cornelia de Lange syndrome Q87.1
Cornu cutaneum L85.8
Cornual gestation or pregnancy O00.80
  with intrauterine pregnancy O00.81
Coronary (artery) — *see* condition
Coronavirus, as cause of disease classified elsewhere
  B97.29
  SARS-associated B97.21
Corpora (*see also* condition)
  amylacea, prostate N42.89
  cavernosa — *see* condition
Corpulence — *see* Obesity
Corpus — *see* condition
Corrected transposition Q20.5
Corrosion (injury) (acid) (caustic) (chemical) (lime) (exter-
  nal) (internal) T30.4
  abdomen, abdominal (muscle) (wall) T21.42 ☑
    first degree T21.52 ☑
    second degree T21.62 ☑

Corrosion — *continued*
  abdomen, abdominal — *continued*
    third degree T21.72 ☑
  above elbow T22.439 ☑
    first degree T22.539 ☑
    left T22.432 ☑
      first degree T22.532 ☑
      second degree T22.632 ☑
      third degree T22.732 ☑
    right T22.431 ☑
      first degree T22.531 ☑
      second degree T22.631 ☑
      third degree T22.731 ☑
    second degree T22.639 ☑
    third degree T22.739 ☑
  alimentary tract NEC T28.7
  ankle T25.419 ☑
    first degree T25.519 ☑
    left T25.412 ☑
      first degree T25.512 ☑
      second degree T25.612 ☑
      third degree T25.712 ☑
    multiple with foot — *see* Corrosion, lower, limb,
      multiple, ankle and foot
    right T25.411 ☑
      first degree T25.511 ☑
      second degree T25.611 ☑
      third degree T25.711 ☑
    second degree T25.619 ☑
    third degree T25.719 ☑
  anus — *see* Corrosion, buttock
  arm(s) (meaning upper limb(s)) — *see* Corrosion, upper
    limb
  axilla T22.449 ☑
    first degree T22.549 ☑
    left T22.442 ☑
      first degree T22.542 ☑
      second degree T22.642 ☑
      third degree T22.742 ☑
    right T22.441 ☑
      first degree T22.541 ☑
      second degree T22.641 ☑
      third degree T22.741 ☑
    second degree T22.649 ☑
    third degree T22.749 ☑
  back (lower) T21.44 ☑
    first degree T21.54 ☑
    second degree T21.64 ☑
    third degree T21.74 ☑
    upper T21.43 ☑
      first degree T21.53 ☑
      second degree T21.63 ☑
      third degree T21.73 ☑
  blisters — *code as* Corrosion, second degree, by site
  breast(s) — *see* Corrosion, chest wall
  buttock(s) T21.45 ☑
    first degree T21.55 ☑
    second degree T21.65 ☑
    third degree T21.75 ☑
  calf T24.439 ☑
    first degree T24.539 ☑
    left T24.432 ☑
      first degree T24.532 ☑
      second degree T24.632 ☑
      third degree T24.732 ☑
    right T24.431 ☑
      first degree T24.531 ☑
      second degree T24.631 ☑
      third degree T24.731 ☑
    second degree T24.639 ☑
    third degree T24.739 ☑
  canthus (eye) — *see* Corrosion, eyelid
  cervix T28.8 ☑
  cheek T20.46 ☑
    first degree T20.56 ☑
    second degree T20.66 ☑
    third degree T20.76 ☑
  chest wall T21.41 ☑
    first degree T21.51 ☑
    second degree T21.61 ☑
    third degree T21.71 ☑
  chin T20.43 ☑
    first degree T20.53 ☑
    second degree T20.63 ☑
    third degree T20.73 ☑
  colon T28.7 ☑

Corrosion — *continued*
  conjunctiva (and cornea) — *see* Corrosion, cornea
  cornea (and conjunctiva) T26.6-
  deep necrosis of underlying tissue — *code as* Corrosion,
    third degree, by site
  dorsum of hand T23.469 ☑
    first degree T23.569 ☑
    left T23.462 ☑
      first degree T23.562 ☑
      second degree T23.662 ☑
      third degree T23.762 ☑
    right T23.461 ☑
      first degree T23.561 ☑
      second degree T23.661 ☑
      third degree T23.761 ☑
    second degree T23.669 ☑
    third degree T23.769 ☑
  ear (auricle) (external) (canal) T20.41 ☑
    drum T28.91 ☑
    first degree T20.51 ☑
    second degree T20.61 ☑
    third degree T20.71 ☑
  elbow T22.429 ☑
    first degree T22.529 ☑
    left T22.422 ☑
      first degree T22.522 ☑
      second degree T22.622 ☑
      third degree T22.722 ☑
    right T22.421 ☑
      first degree T22.521 ☑
      second degree T22.621 ☑
      third degree T22.721 ☑
    second degree T22.629 ☑
    third degree T22.729 ☑
  entire body — *see* Corrosion, multiple body regions
  epidermal loss — *code as* Corrosion, second degree,
    by site
  epiglottis T27.4 ☑
  erythema, erythematous — *code as* Corrosion, first
    degree, by site
  esophagus T28.6 ☑
  extent (percentage of body surface)
    less than 10 percent T32.0
    10-19 percent (0-9 percent third degree) T32.10
      with 10-19 percent third degree T32.11
    20-29 percent (0-9 percent third degree) T32.20
      with
        10-19 percent third degree T32.21
        20-29 percent third degree T32.22
    30-39 percent (0-9 percent third degree) T32.30
      with
        10-19 percent third degree T32.31
        20-29 percent third degree T32.32
        30-39 percent third degree T32.33
    40-49 percent (0-9 percent third degree) T32.40
      with
        10-19 percent third degree T32.41
        20-29 percent third degree T32.42
        30-39 percent third degree T32.43
        40-49 percent third degree T32.44
    50-59 percent (0-9 percent third degree) T32.50
      with
        10-19 percent third degree T32.51
        20-29 percent third degree T32.52
        30-39 percent third degree T32.53
        40-49 percent third degree T32.54
        50-59 percent third degree T32.55
    60-69 percent (0-9 percent third degree) T32.60
      with
        10-19 percent third degree T32.61
        20-29 percent third degree T32.62
        30-39 percent third degree T32.63
        40-49 percent third degree T32.64
        50-59 percent third degree T32.65
        60-69 percent third degree T32.66
    70-79 percent (0-9 percent third degree) T32.70
      with
        10-19 percent third degree T32.71
        20-29 percent third degree T32.72
        30-39 percent third degree T32.73
        40-49 percent third degree T32.74
        50-59 percent third degree T32.75
        60-69 percent third degree T32.76
        70-79 percent third degree T32.77
    80-89 percent (0-9 percent third degree) T32.80
      with
        10-19 percent third degree T32.81

☒ **Subterms under main terms may continue to next column or page**   ☑ **Additional Character Required — Refer to the Tabular List for Character Selection**   **73**

Conviction — Corrosion

Index

Corrosion — Corrosion

Corrosion — *continued*
- nose — *continued*
  - second degree T20.64 ☑
  - third degree T20.74 ☑
- ocular adnexa — *see* Corrosion, eye
- orbit region — *see* Corrosion, eyelid
- palm T23.459 ☑
  - first degree T23.559 ☑
  - left T23.452 ☑
    - first degree T23.552 ☑
    - second degree T23.652 ☑
    - third degree T23.752 ☑
  - right T23.451 ☑
    - first degree T23.551 ☑
    - second degree T23.651 ☑
    - third degree T23.751 ☑
  - second degree T23.659 ☑
  - third degree T23.759 ☑
- partial thickness — *code as* Corrosion, unspecified degree, by site
- pelvis — *see* Corrosion, trunk
- penis — *see* Corrosion, genital organs, external, male
- perineum
  - female — *see* Corrosion, genital organs, external, female
  - male — *see* Corrosion, genital organs, external, male
- periocular area — *see* Corrosion, eyelid
- pharynx T28.5 ☑
- rectum T28.7 ☑
- respiratory tract T27.7 ☑
  - larynx — *see* Corrosion, larynx
  - specified part NEC T27.6 ☑
  - trachea — *see* Corrosion, larynx
- sac, lacrimal — *see* Corrosion, eye, specified site NEC
- scalp T20.45 ☑
  - first degree T20.55 ☑
  - second degree T20.65 ☑
  - third degree T20.75 ☑
- scapular region T22.469 ☑
  - first degree T22.569 ☑
  - left T22.462 ☑
    - first degree T22.562 ☑
    - second degree T22.662 ☑
    - third degree T22.762 ☑
  - right T22.461 ☑
    - first degree T22.561 ☑
    - second degree T22.661 ☑
    - third degree T22.761 ☑
  - second degree T22.669 ☑
  - third degree T22.769 ☑
- sclera — *see* Corrosion, eye, specified site NEC
- scrotum — *see* Corrosion, genital organs, external, male
- shoulder T22.459 ☑
  - first degree T22.559 ☑
  - left T22.452 ☑
    - first degree T22.552 ☑
    - second degree T22.652 ☑
    - third degree T22.752 ☑
  - right T22.451 ☑
    - first degree T22.551 ☑
    - second degree T22.651 ☑
    - third degree T22.751 ☑
  - second degree T22.659 ☑
  - third degree T22.759 ☑
- stomach T28.7 ☑
- temple — *see* Corrosion, head
- testis — *see* Corrosion, genital organs, external, male
- thigh T24.419 ☑
  - first degree T24.519 ☑
  - left T24.412 ☑
    - first degree T24.512 ☑
    - second degree T24.612 ☑
    - third degree T24.712 ☑
  - right T24.411 ☑
    - first degree T24.511 ☑
    - second degree T24.611 ☑
    - third degree T24.711 ☑
  - second degree T24.619 ☑
  - third degree T24.719 ☑
- thorax (external) — *see* Corrosion, trunk
- throat (meaning pharynx) T28.5 ☑
- thumb(s) T23.419 ☑
  - first degree T23.519 ☑
  - left T23.412 ☑
    - first degree T23.512 ☑

Corrosion — *continued*
- thumb(s) — *continued*
  - left — *continued*
    - second degree T23.612 ☑
    - third degree T23.712 ☑
  - multiple sites with fingers T23.449 ☑
    - first degree T23.549 ☑
    - left T23.442 ☑
      - first degree T23.542 ☑
      - second degree T23.642 ☑
      - third degree T23.742 ☑
    - right T23.441 ☑
      - first degree T23.541 ☑
      - second degree T23.641 ☑
      - third degree T23.741 ☑
    - second degree T23.649 ☑
    - third degree T23.749 ☑
  - right T23.411 ☑
    - first degree T23.511 ☑
    - second degree T23.611 ☑
    - third degree T23.711 ☑
  - second degree T23.619 ☑
  - third degree T23.719 ☑
- toe T25.439 ☑
  - first degree T25.539 ☑
  - left T25.432 ☑
    - first degree T25.532 ☑
    - second degree T25.632 ☑
    - third degree T25.732 ☑
  - right T25.431 ☑
    - first degree T25.531 ☑
    - second degree T25.631 ☑
    - third degree T25.731 ☑
  - second degree T25.639 ☑
  - third degree T25.739 ☑
- tongue T28.5 ☑
- tonsil(s) T28.5 ☑
- total body — *see* Corrosion, multiple body regions
- trachea T27.4 ☑
  - with lung T27.5 ☑
- trunk T21.40 ☑
  - abdominal wall — *see* Corrosion, abdominal wall
  - anus — *see* Corrosion, buttock
  - axilla — *see* Corrosion, upper limb
  - back — *see* Corrosion, back
  - breast — *see* Corrosion, chest wall
  - buttock — *see* Corrosion, buttock
  - chest wall — *see* Corrosion, chest wall
  - first degree T21.50 ☑
  - flank — *see* Corrosion, abdominal wall
  - genital
    - female — *see* Corrosion, genital organs, external, female
    - male — *see* Corrosion, genital organs, external, male
  - groin — *see* Corrosion, abdominal wall
  - interscapular region — *see* Corrosion, back, upper
  - labia — *see* Corrosion, genital organs, external, female
  - lower back — *see* Corrosion, back
  - penis — *see* Corrosion, genital organs, external, male
  - perineum
    - female — *see* Corrosion, genital organs, external, female
    - male — *see* Corrosion, genital organs, external, male
  - scapular region — *see* Corrosion, upper limb
  - scrotum — *see* Corrosion, genital organs, external, male
  - second degree T21.60 ☑
  - shoulder — *see* Corrosion, upper limb
  - specified site NEC T21.49 ☑
    - first degree T21.59 ☑
    - second degree T21.69 ☑
    - third degree T21.79 ☑
  - testes — *see* Corrosion, genital organs, external, male
  - third degree T21.70 ☑
  - upper back — *see* Corrosion, back, upper
  - vagina T28.8 ☑
  - vulva — *see* Corrosion, genital organs, external, female
- unspecified site with extent of body surface involved specified
  - less than 10 percent T32.0

Corrosion — *continued*
- unspecified site with extent of body surface involved specified — *continued*
  - 10-19 percent (0-9 percent third degree) T32.10
    - with 10-19 percent third degree T32.11
  - 20-29 percent (0-9 percent third degree) T32.20
    - with
      - 10-19 percent third degree T32.21
      - 20-29 percent third degree T32.22
  - 30-39 percent (0-9 percent third degree) T32.30
    - with
      - 10-19 percent third degree T32.31
      - 20-29 percent third degree T32.32
      - 30-39 percent third degree T32.33
  - 40-49 percent (0-9 percent third degree) T32.40
    - with
      - 10-19 percent third degree T32.41
      - 20-29 percent third degree T32.42
      - 30-39 percent third degree T32.43
      - 40-49 percent third degree T32.44
  - 50-59 percent (0-9 percent third degree) T32.50
    - with
      - 10-19 percent third degree T32.51
      - 20-29 percent third degree T32.52
      - 30-39 percent third degree T32.53
      - 40-49 percent third degree T32.54
      - 50-59 percent third degree T32.55
  - 60-69 percent (0-9 percent third degree) T32.60
    - with
      - 10-19 percent third degree T32.61
      - 20-29 percent third degree T32.62
      - 30-39 percent third degree T32.63
      - 40-49 percent third degree T32.64
      - 50-59 percent third degree T32.65
      - 60-69 percent third degree T32.66
  - 70-79 percent (0-9 percent third degree) T32.70
    - with
      - 10-19 percent third degree T32.71
      - 20-29 percent third degree T32.72
      - 30-39 percent third degree T32.73
      - 40-49 percent third degree T32.74
      - 50-59 percent third degree T32.75
      - 60-69 percent third degree T32.76
      - 70-79 percent third degree T32.77
  - 80-89 percent (0-9 percent third degree) T32.80
    - with
      - 10-19 percent third degree T32.81
      - 20-29 percent third degree T32.82
      - 30-39 percent third degree T32.83
      - 40-49 percent third degree T32.84
      - 50-59 percent third degree T32.85
      - 60-69 percent third degree T32.86
      - 70-79 percent third degree T32.87
      - 80-89 percent third degree T32.88
  - 90 percent or more (0-9 percent third degree) T32.90
    - with
      - 10-19 percent third degree T32.91
      - 20-29 percent third degree T32.92
      - 30-39 percent third degree T32.93
      - 40-49 percent third degree T32.94
      - 50-59 percent third degree T32.95
      - 60-69 percent third degree T32.96
      - 70-79 percent third degree T32.97
      - 80-89 percent third degree T32.98
      - 90-99 percent third degree T32.99
- upper limb (axilla) (scapular region) T22.40 ☑
  - above elbow — *see* Corrosion, above elbow
  - axilla — *see* Corrosion, axilla
  - elbow — *see* Corrosion, elbow
  - first degree T22.50 ☑
  - forearm — *see* Corrosion, forearm
  - hand — *see* Corrosion, hand
  - interscapular region — *see* Corrosion, back, upper
  - multiple sites T22.499 ☑
    - first degree T22.599 ☑
    - left T22.492 ☑
      - first degree T22.592 ☑
      - second degree T22.692 ☑
      - third degree T22.792 ☑
    - right T22.491 ☑
      - first degree T22.591 ☑
      - second degree T22.691 ☑
      - third degree T22.791 ☑
    - second degree T22.699 ☑
    - third degree T22.799 ☑
  - scapular region — *see* Corrosion, scapular region
  - second degree T22.60 ☑
  - shoulder — *see* Corrosion, shoulder

▽ Subterms under main terms may continue to next column or page   ☑ Additional Character Required — Refer to the Tabular List for Character Selection   75

Corrosion — Corrosion

Corrosion — *continued*
  upper limb — *continued*
    third degree T22.70 ☑
    wrist — *see* Corrosion, hand
  uterus T28.8 ☑
  vagina T28.8 ☑
  vulva — *see* Corrosion, genital organs, external, female
  wrist T23.479 ☑
    first degree T23.579 ☑
    left T23.472 ☑
      first degree T23.572 ☑
      second degree T23.672 ☑
      third degree T23.772 ☑
    multiple sites with hand T23.499 ☑
      first degree T23.599 ☑
      left T23.492 ☑
        first degree T23.592 ☑
        second degree T23.692 ☑
        third degree T23.792 ☑
      right T23.491 ☑
        first degree T23.591 ☑
        second degree T23.691 ☑
        third degree T23.791 ☑
      second degree T23.699 ☑
      third degree T23.799 ☑
    right T23.471 ☑
      first degree T23.571 ☑
      second degree T23.671 ☑
      third degree T23.771 ☑
    second degree T23.679 ☑
    third degree T23.779 ☑
Corrosive burn — *see* Corrosion
Corsican fever — *see* Malaria
Cortical — *see* condition
Cortico-adrenal — *see* condition
Coryza (acute) J00
  with grippe or influenza — *see* Influenza, with, respiratory manifestations NEC
  syphilitic
    congenital (chronic) A50.05
Costen's syndrome or complex M26.69
Costiveness — *see* Constipation
Costochondritis M94.0
Cot death R99
Cotard's syndrome F22
Cotia virus B08.8
Cotton wool spots (retinal) H35.81
Cotungo's disease — *see* Sciatica
Cough (affected) (chronic) (epidemic) (nervous) R05
  with hemorrhage — *see* Hemoptysis
  bronchial R05
    with grippe or influenza — *see* Influenza, with, respiratory manifestations NEC
  functional F45.8
  hysterical F45.8
  laryngeal, spasmodic R05
  psychogenic F45.8
  smokers' J41.0
  tea taster's B49
Counseling (for) Z71.9
  abuse NEC
    perpetrator Z69.82
    victim Z69.81
  alcohol abuser Z71.41
    family Z71.42
  child abuse
    nonparental
      perpetrator Z69.021
      victim Z69.020
    parental
      perpetrator Z69.011
      victim Z69.010
  consanguinity Z71.89
  contraceptive Z30.09
  dietary Z71.3
  drug abuser Z71.51
    family member Z71.52
  exercise Z71.82
  family Z71.89
  fertility preservation (prior to cancer therapy) (prior to removal of gonads) Z31.62
  for non-attending third party Z71.0
    related to sexual behavior or orientation Z70.2
  genetic
    nonprocreative Z71.83
    procreative NEC Z31.5
  gestational carrier Z31.7

Counseling — *continued*
  health (advice) (education) (instruction) — *see* Counseling, medical
  human immunodeficiency virus (HIV) Z71.7
  impotence Z70.1
  insulin pump use Z46.81
  medical (for) Z71.9
    boarding school resident Z59.3
    consanguinity Z71.89
    feared complaint and no disease found Z71.1
    human immunodeficiency virus (HIV) Z71.7
    institutional resident Z59.3
    on behalf of another Z71.0
      related to sexual behavior or orientation Z70.2
    person living alone Z60.2
    specified reason NEC Z71.89
  natural family planning
    procreative Z31.61
    to avoid pregnancy Z30.02
  perpetrator (of)
    abuse NEC Z69.82
    child abuse
      non-parental Z69.021
      parental Z69.011
    rape NEC Z69.82
    spousal abuse Z69.12
  procreative NEC Z31.69
    fertility preservation (prior to cancer therapy) (prior to removal of gonads) Z31.62
    using natural family planning Z31.61
  promiscuity Z70.1
  rape victim Z69.81
  religious Z71.81
  sex, sexual (related to) Z70.9
    attitude(s) Z70.0
    behavior or orientation Z70.1
    combined concerns Z70.3
    non-responsiveness Z70.1
    on behalf of third party Z70.2
    specified reason NEC Z70.8
  specified reason NEC Z71.89
  spiritual Z71.81
  spousal abuse (perpetrator) Z69.12
    victim Z69.11
  substance abuse Z71.89
    alcohol Z71.41
    drug Z71.51
    tobacco Z71.6
  tobacco use Z71.6
  use (of)
    insulin pump Z46.81
  victim (of)
    abuse Z69.81
    child abuse
      by parent Z69.010
      non-parental Z69.020
    rape NEC Z69.81
Coupled rhythm R00.8
Couvelaire syndrome or uterus (complicating delivery) O45.8X- ☑
Cowperitis — *see* Urethritis
Cowper's gland — *see* condition
Cowpox B08.010
  due to vaccination T88.1 ☑
Coxa
  magna M91.4- ☑
  plana M91.2- ☑
  valga (acquired) (*see also* Deformity, limb, specified type NEC, thigh)
    congenital Q65.81
    sequelae (late effect) of rickets E64.3
  vara (acquired) (*see also* Deformity, limb, specified type NEC, thigh)
    congenital Q65.82
    sequelae (late effect) of rickets E64.3
Coxalgia, coxalgic (nontuberculous) (*see also* Pain, joint, hip)
  tuberculous A18.02
Coxitis — *see* Monoarthritis, hip
Coxsackie (virus) (infection) B34.1
  as cause of disease classified elsewhere B97.11
  carditis B33.20
  central nervous system NEC A88.8
  endocarditis B33.21
  enteritis A08.39
  meningitis (aseptic) A87.0
  myocarditis B33.22
  pericarditis B33.23

Coxsackie — *continued*
  pharyngitis B08.5
  pleurodynia B33.0
  specific disease NEC B33.8
Crabs, meaning pubic lice B85.3
Crack baby P04.41
Cracked nipple N64.0
  associated with
    lactation O92.13
    pregnancy O92.11- ☑
    puerperium O92.12
Cracked tooth K03.81
Cradle cap L21.0
Craft neurosis F48.8
Cramp(s) R25.2
  abdominal — *see* Pain, abdominal
  bathing T75.1 ☑
  colic R10.83
    psychogenic F45.8
  due to immersion T75.1 ☑
  fireman T67.2 ☑
  heat T67.2 ☑
  immersion T75.1 ☑
  intestinal — *see* Pain, abdominal
    psychogenic F45.8
  leg, sleep related G47.62
  limb (lower) (upper) NEC R25.2
    sleep related G47.62
  linotypist's F48.8
    organic G25.89
  muscle (limb) (general) R25.2
    due to immersion T75.1 ☑
    psychogenic F45.8
  occupational (hand) F48.8
    organic G25.89
  salt-depletion E87.1
  sleep related, leg G47.62
  stoker's T67.2 ☑
  swimmer's T75.1 ☑
  telegrapher's F48.8
    organic G25.89
  typist's F48.8
    organic G25.89
  uterus N94.89
    menstrual — *see* Dysmenorrhea
  writer's F48.8
    organic G25.89
Cranial — *see* condition
Craniocleidodysostosis Q74.0
Craniofenestria (skull) Q75.8
Craniolacunia (skull) Q75.8
Craniopagus Q89.4
Craniopathy, metabolic M85.2
Craniopharyngeal — *see* condition
Craniopharyngioma D44.4
Craniorachischisis (totalis) Q00.1
Cranioschisis Q75.8
Craniostenosis Q75.0
Craniosynostosis Q75.0
Craniotabes (cause unknown) M83.8
  neonatal P96.3
  rachitic E64.3
  syphilitic A50.56
Cranium — *see* condition
Craw-craw — *see* Onchocerciasis
Creaking joint — *see* Derangement, joint, specified type NEC
Creeping
  eruption B76.9
  palsy or paralysis G12.22
Crenated tongue K14.8
Creotoxism A05.9
Crepitus
  caput Q75.8
  joint — *see* Derangement, joint, specified type NEC
Crescent or conus choroid, congenital Q14.3
CREST syndrome M34.1
Cretin, cretinism (congenital) (endemic) (nongoitrous) (sporadic) E00.9
  pelvis
    with disproportion (fetopelvic) O33.0
      causing obstructed labor O65.0
  type
    hypothyroid E00.1
    mixed E00.2
    myxedematous E00.1
    neurological E00.0

☑ **Additional Character Required** — Refer to the Tabular List for Character Selection   ▽ **Subterms under main terms may continue to next column or page**

Creutzfeldt-Jakob disease or syndrome (with dementia) A81.00
  familial A81.09
  iatrogenic A81.09
  specified NEC A81.09
  sporadic A81.09
  variant (vCJD) A81.01
Crib death R99
Cribriform hymen Q52.3
Cri-du-chat syndrome Q93.4
Crigler-Najjar disease or syndrome E80.5
Crime, victim of Z65.4
Crimean hemorrhagic fever A98.0
Criminalism F60.2
Crisis
  abdomen R10.0
  acute reaction F43.0
  addisonian E27.2
  adrenal (cortical) E27.2
  celiac K90.0
  Dietl's N13.8
  emotional (see also Disorder, adjustment)
    acute reaction to stress F43.0
    specific to childhood and adolescence F93.8
  glaucomatocyclitic — see Glaucoma, secondary, inflammation
  heart — see Failure, heart
  nitritoid I95.2
    correct substance properly administered — see Table of Drugs and Chemicals, by drug, adverse effect
    overdose or wrong substance given or taken — see Table of Drugs and Chemicals, by drug, poisoning
  oculogyric H51.8
    psychogenic F45.8
  Pel's (tabetic) A52.11
  psychosexual identity F64.2
  renal N28.0
  sickle-cell D57.00
    with
      acute chest syndrome D57.01
      splenic sequestration D57.02
  state (acute reaction) F43.0
  tabetic A52.11
  thyroid — see Thyrotoxicosis with thyroid storm
  thyrotoxic — see Thyrotoxicosis with thyroid storm
Crocq's disease (acrocyanosis) I73.89
Crohn's disease — see Enteritis, regional
Crooked septum, nasal J34.2
Cross syndrome E70.328
Crossbite (anterior) (posterior) M26.24
Cross-eye — see Strabismus, convergent concomitant
Croup, croupous (catarrhal) (infectious) (inflammatory) (nondiphtheritic) J05.0
  bronchial J20.9
  diphtheritic A36.2
  false J38.5
  spasmodic J38.5
    diphtheritic A36.2
  stridulous J38.5
    diphtheritic A36.2
Crouzon's disease Q75.1
Crowding, tooth, teeth, fully erupted M26.31
CRST syndrome M34.1
Cruchet's disease A85.8
Cruelty in children (see also Disorder, conduct)
Crural ulcer — see Ulcer, lower limb
Crush, crushed, crushing T14.8 ☑
  abdomen S38.1 ☑
  ankle S97.0- ☑
  arm (upper) (and shoulder) S47.- ☑
  axilla — see Crush, arm
  back, lower S38.1 ☑
  buttock S38.1 ☑
  cheek S07.0 ☑
  chest S28.0 ☑
  cranium S07.1 ☑
  ear S07.0 ☑
  elbow S57.0- ☑
  extremity
    lower
      ankle — see Crush, ankle
      below knee — see Crush, leg
      foot — see Crush, foot
      hip — see Crush, hip
      knee — see Crush, knee

Crush, crushed, crushing — continued
  extremity — continued
    lower — continued
      thigh — see Crush, thigh
      toe — see Crush, toe
    upper
      below elbow S67.9- ☑
      elbow — see Crush, elbow
      finger — see Crush, finger
      forearm — see Crush, forearm
      hand — see Crush, hand
      thumb — see Crush, thumb
      upper arm — see Crush, arm
      wrist — see Crush, wrist
  face S07.0 ☑
  finger(s) S67.1- ☑
    with hand (and wrist) — see Crush, hand, specified site NEC
    index S67.19- ☑
    little S67.19- ☑
    middle S67.19- ☑
    ring S67.19- ☑
    thumb — see Crush, thumb
  foot S97.8- ☑
    toe — see Crush, toe
  forearm S57.8- ☑
  genitalia, external
    female S38.002 ☑
      vagina S38.03 ☑
      vulva S38.03 ☑
    male S38.001 ☑
      penis S38.01 ☑
      scrotum S38.02 ☑
      testis S38.02 ☑
  hand (except fingers alone) S67.2- ☑
    with wrist S67.4- ☑
  head S07.9 ☑
    specified NEC S07.8 ☑
  heel — see Crush, foot
  hip S77.0- ☑
    with thigh S77.2- ☑
  internal organ (abdomen, chest, or pelvis) NEC T14.8 ☑
  knee S87.0- ☑
  labium (majus) (minus) S38.03 ☑
  larynx S17.0 ☑
  leg (lower) S87.8- ☑
    knee — see Crush, knee
  lip S07.0 ☑
  lower
    back S38.1 ☑
    leg — see Crush, leg
  neck S17.9 ☑
  nerve — see Injury, nerve
  nose S07.0 ☑
  pelvis S38.1 ☑
  penis S38.01 ☑
  scalp S07.8 ☑
  scapular region — see Crush, arm
  scrotum S38.02 ☑
  severe, unspecified site T14.8 ☑
  shoulder (and upper arm) — see Crush, arm
  skull S07.1 ☑
  syndrome (complication of trauma) T79.5 ☑
  testis S38.02 ☑
  thigh S77.1- ☑
    with hip S77.2- ☑
  throat S17.8 ☑
  thumb S67.0- ☑
    with hand (and wrist) — see Crush, hand, specified site NEC
  toe(s) S97.10- ☑
    great S97.11- ☑
    lesser S97.12- ☑
  trachea S17.0 ☑
  vagina S38.03 ☑
  vulva S38.03 ☑
  wrist S67.3- ☑
    with hand S67.4- ☑
Crusta lactea L21.0
Crusts R23.4
Crutch paralysis — see Injury, brachial plexus
Cruveilhier-Baumgarten cirrhosis, disease or syndrome K74.69
Cruveilhier's atrophy or disease G12.8
Crying (constant) (continuous) (excessive)
  child, adolescent, or adult R45.83

Crying — continued
  infant (baby) (newborn) R68.11
Cryofibrinogenemia D89.2
Cryoglobulinemia (essential) (idiopathic) (mixed) (primary) (purpura) (secondary) (vasculitis) D89.1
  with lung involvement D89.1 [J99]
Cryptitis (anal) (rectal) K62.89
Cryptococcosis, cryptococcus (infection) (neoformans) B45.9
  bone B45.3
  cerebral B45.1
  cutaneous B45.2
  disseminated B45.7
  generalized B45.7
  meningitis B45.1
  meningocerebralis B45.1
  osseous B45.3
  pulmonary B45.0
  skin B45.2
  specified NEC B45.8
Cryptopapillitis (anus) K62.89
Cryptophthalmos Q11.2
  syndrome Q87.0
Cryptorchid, cryptorchism, cryptorchidism Q53.9
  bilateral Q53.20
    abdominal Q53.211
    perineal Q53.22
  unilateral Q53.10
    abdominal Q53.111
    perineal Q53.12
Cryptosporidiosis A07.2
  hepatobiliary B88.8
  respiratory B88.8
Cryptostromosis J67.6
Crystalluria R82.998
Cubitus
  congenital Q68.8
  valgus (acquired) M21.0- ☑
    congenital Q68.8
    sequelae (late effect) of rickets E64.3
  varus (acquired) M21.1- ☑
    congenital Q68.8
    sequelae (late effect) of rickets E64.3
Cultural deprivation or shock Z60.3
Curling esophagus K22.4
Curling's ulcer — see Ulcer, peptic, acute
Curschmann (-Batten) (-Steinert) **disease or syndrome** G71.11
Curse, Ondine's — see Apnea, sleep
Curvature
  organ or site, congenital NEC — see Distortion
  penis (lateral) Q55.61
  Pott's (spinal) A18.01
  radius, idiopathic, progressive (congenital) Q74.0
  spine (acquired) (angular) (idiopathic) (incorrect) (postural) — see Dorsopathy, deforming
    congenital Q67.5
    due to or associated with
      Charcot-Marie-Tooth disease (see also subcategory M49.8) G60.0
      osteitis
        deformans M88.88
        fibrosa cystica (see also subcategory M49.8) E21.0
      tuberculosis (Pott's curvature) A18.01
    sequelae (late effect) of rickets E64.3
    tuberculous A18.01
Cushingoid due to steroid therapy E24.2
  correct substance properly administered — see Table of Drugs and Chemicals, by drug, adverse effect
  overdose or wrong substance given or taken — see Table of Drugs and Chemicals, by drug, poisoning
Cushing's
  syndrome or disease E24.9
    drug-induced E24.2
    iatrogenic E24.2
    pituitary-dependent E24.0
    specified NEC E24.8
  ulcer — see Ulcer, peptic, acute
Cusp, Carabelli — omit code
Cut (external) (see also Laceration)
  muscle — see Injury, muscle
Cutaneous (see also condition)
  hemorrhage R23.3
  larva migrans B76.9
Cutis (see also condition)
  hyperelastica Q82.8
    acquired L57.4

Cutis — *continued*
  laxa (hyperelastica) — *see* Dermatolysis
  marmorata R23.8
  osteosis L94.2
  pendula — *see* Dermatolysis
  rhomboidalis nuchae L57.2
  verticis gyrata Q82.8
    acquired L91.8
Cyanosis R23.0
  due to
    patent foramen botalli Q21.1
    persistent foramen ovale Q21.1
  enterogenous D74.8
  paroxysmal digital — *see* Raynaud's disease
    with gangrene I73.01
  retina, retinal H35.89
Cyanotic heart disease I24.9
  congenital Q24.9
Cycle
  anovulatory N97.0
  menstrual, irregular N92.6
Cyclencephaly Q04.9
Cyclical vomiting (*see also* Vomiting, cyclical) G43.A0
  (*following* G43.7)
  psychogenic F50.89
Cyclitis (*see also* Iridocyclitis) H20.9
  chronic — *see* Iridocyclitis, chronic
  Fuchs' heterochromic H20.81- ☑
  granulomatous — *see* Iridocyclitis, chronic
  lens-induced — *see* Iridocyclitis, lens-induced
  posterior H30.2- ☑
Cycloid personality F34.0
Cyclophoria H50.54
Cyclopia, cyclops Q87.0
Cyclopism Q87.0
Cyclosporiasis A07.4
Cyclothymia F34.0
Cyclothymic personality F34.0
Cyclotropia H50.41- ☑
Cylindroma (*see also* Neoplasm, malignant, by site)
  eccrine dermal — *see* Neoplasm, skin, benign
  skin — *see* Neoplasm, skin, benign
Cylindruria R82.998
Cynanche
  diphtheritic A36.2
  tonsillaris J36
Cynophobia F40.218
Cynorexia R63.2
Cyphosis — *see* Kyphosis
Cyprus fever — *see* Brucellosis
Cyst (colloid) (mucous) (simple) (retention)
  adenoid (infected) J35.8
  adrenal gland E27.8
    congenital Q89.1
  air, lung J98.4
  allantoic Q64.4
  alveolar process (jaw bone) M27.40
  amnion, amniotic O41.8X- ☑
  aneurysmal M27.49
  anterior
    chamber (eye) — *see* Cyst, iris
    nasopalatine K09.1
  antrum J34.1
  anus K62.89
  apical (tooth) (periodontal) K04.8
  appendix K38.8
  arachnoid, brain (acquired) G93.0
    congenital Q04.6
  arytenoid J38.7
  Baker's M71.2- ☑
    ruptured M66.0
    tuberculous A18.02
  Bartholin's gland N75.0
  bile duct (common) (hepatic) K83.5
  bladder (multiple) (trigone) N32.89
  blue dome (breast) — *see* Cyst, breast
  bone (local) NEC M85.60
    aneurysmal M85.50
      ankle M85.57- ☑
      foot M85.57- ☑
      forearm M85.53- ☑
      hand M85.54- ☑
      jaw M27.49
      lower leg M85.56- ☑
      multiple site M85.59
      neck M85.58
      rib M85.58

Cyst — *continued*
  bone — *continued*
    aneurysmal — *continued*
      shoulder M85.51- ☑
      skull M85.58
      specified site NEC M85.58
      thigh M85.55- ☑
      toe M85.57- ☑
      upper arm M85.52- ☑
      vertebra M85.58
    solitary M85.40
      ankle M85.47- ☑
      fibula M85.46- ☑
      foot M85.47- ☑
      hand M85.44- ☑
      humerus M85.42- ☑
      jaw M27.49
      neck M85.48
      pelvis M85.45- ☑
      radius M85.43- ☑
      rib M85.48
      shoulder M85.41- ☑
      skull M85.48
      specified site NEC M85.48
      tibia M85.46- ☑
      toe M85.47- ☑
      ulna M85.43- ☑
      vertebra M85.48
    specified type NEC M85.60
      ankle M85.67- ☑
      foot M85.67- ☑
      forearm M85.63- ☑
      hand M85.64- ☑
      jaw M27.40
        developmental (nonodontogenic) K09.1
          odontogenic K09.0
        latent M27.0
      lower leg M85.66- ☑
      multiple site M85.69
      neck M85.68
      rib M85.68
      shoulder M85.61- ☑
      skull M85.68
      specified site NEC M85.68
      thigh M85.65- ☑
      toe M85.67- ☑
      upper arm M85.62- ☑
      vertebra M85.68
  brain (acquired) G93.0
    congenital Q04.6
    hydatid B67.99 [G94]
    third ventricle (colloid), congenital Q04.6
  branchial (cleft) Q18.0
  branchiogenic Q18.0
  breast (benign) (blue dome) (pedunculated) (solitary) N60.0- ☑
    involution — *see* Dysplasia, mammary, specified type NEC
    sebaceous — *see* Dysplasia, mammary, specified type NEC
  broad ligament (benign) N83.8
  bronchogenic (mediastinal) (sequestration) J98.4
    congenital Q33.0
  buccal K09.8
  bulbourethral gland N36.8
  bursa, bursal NEC M71.30
    with rupture — *see* Rupture, synovium
    ankle M71.37- ☑
    elbow M71.32- ☑
    foot M71.37- ☑
    hand M71.34- ☑
    hip M71.35- ☑
    multiple sites M71.39
    pharyngeal J39.2
    popliteal space — *see* Cyst, Baker's
    shoulder M71.31- ☑
    specified site NEC M71.38
    wrist M71.33- ☑
  calcifying odontogenic D16.5
    upper jaw (bone) (maxilla) D16.4
  canal of Nuck (female) N94.89
    congenital Q52.4
  canthus — *see* Cyst, conjunctiva
  carcinomatous — *see* Neoplasm, malignant, by site
  cauda equina G95.89
  cavum septi pellucidi — *see* Cyst, brain
  celomic (pericardium) Q24.8

Cyst — *continued*
  cerebellopontine (angle) — *see* Cyst, brain
  cerebellum — *see* Cyst, brain
  cerebral — *see* Cyst, brain
  cervical lateral Q18.0
  cervix NEC N88.8
    embryonic Q51.6
    nabothian N88.8
  chiasmal optic NEC — *see* Disorder, optic, chiasm
  chocolate (ovary) N80.1
  choledochus, congenital Q44.4
  chorion O41.8X- ☑
  choroid plexus G93.0
  ciliary body — *see* Cyst, iris
  clitoris N90.7
  colon K63.89
  common (bile) duct K83.5
  congenital NEC Q89.8
    adrenal gland Q89.1
    epiglottis Q31.8
    esophagus Q39.8
    fallopian tube Q50.4
    kidney Q61.00
      more than one (multiple) Q61.02
        specified as polycystic Q61.3
          adult type Q61.2
          infantile type NEC Q61.19
            collecting duct dilation Q61.11
      solitary Q61.01
    larynx Q31.8
    liver Q44.6
    lung Q33.0
    mediastinum Q34.1
    ovary Q50.1
    oviduct Q50.4
    periurethral (tissue) Q64.79
    prepuce Q55.69
    salivary gland (any) Q38.4
    sublingual Q38.6
    submaxillary gland Q38.6
    thymus (gland) Q89.2
    tongue Q38.3
    ureterovesical orifice Q62.8
    vulva Q52.79
  conjunctiva H11.44- ☑
  cornea H18.89- ☑
  corpora quadrigemina G93.0
  corpus
    albicans N83.29- ☑
    luteum (hemorrhagic) (ruptured) N83.1- ☑
  Cowper's gland (benign) (infected) N36.8
  cranial meninges G93.0
  craniobuccal pouch E23.6
  craniopharyngeal pouch E23.6
  cystic duct K82.8
  Cysticercus — *see* Cysticercosis
  Dandy-Walker Q03.1
    with spina bifida — *see* Spina bifida
  dental (root) K04.8
    developmental K09.0
    eruption K09.0
    primordial K09.0
  dentigerous (mandible) (maxilla) K09.0
  dermoid — *see* Neoplasm, benign, by site
    with malignant transformation C56.- ☑
    implantation
      external area or site (skin) NEC L72.0
      iris — *see* Cyst, iris, implantation
      vagina N89.8
      vulva N90.7
    mouth K09.8
    oral soft tissue K09.8
    sacrococcygeal — *see* Cyst, pilonidal
  developmental K09.1
    odontogenic K09.0
    oral region (nonodontogenic) K09.1
    ovary, ovarian Q50.1
  dura (cerebral) G93.0
    spinal G96.19
  ear (external) Q18.1
  echinococcal — *see* Echinococcus
  embryonic
    cervix uteri Q51.6
    fallopian tube Q50.4
    vagina Q52.4
  endometrium, endometrial (uterus) N85.8
    ectopic — *see* Endometriosis
  enterogenous Q43.8

Cyst — *continued*
　　epidermal, epidermoid (inclusion) (*see also* Cyst, skin) L72.0
　　　　mouth K09.8
　　　　oral soft tissue K09.8
　　epididymis N50.3
　　epiglottis J38.7
　　epiphysis cerebri E34.8
　　epithelial (inclusion) L72.0
　　epoophoron Q50.5
　　eruption K09.0
　　esophagus K22.8
　　ethmoid sinus J34.1
　　external female genital organs NEC N90.7
　　eyelid (sebaceous) H02.829
　　　　infected — *see* Hordeolum
　　　　left H02.826
　　　　　　lower H02.825
　　　　　　upper H02.824
　　　　right H02.823
　　　　　　lower H02.822
　　　　　　upper H02.821
　　eye NEC H57.89
　　　　congenital Q15.8
　　fallopian tube N83.8
　　　　congenital Q50.4
　　fimbrial (twisted) Q50.4
　　follicle (graafian) (hemorrhagic) N83.0- ☑
　　　　nabothian N88.8
　　follicular (atretic) (hemorrhagic) (ovarian) N83.0- ☑
　　　　dentigerous K09.0
　　　　odontogenic K09.0
　　　　skin L72.9
　　　　　　specified NEC L72.8
　　frontal sinus J34.1
　　gallbladder K82.8
　　ganglion — *see* Ganglion
　　Gartner's duct Q52.4
　　gingiva K09.0
　　gland of Moll — *see* Cyst, eyelid
　　globulomaxillary K09.1
　　graafian follicle (hemorrhagic) N83.0- ☑
　　granulosal lutein (hemorrhagic) N83.1- ☑
　　hemangiomatous D18.00
　　　　intra-abdominal D18.03
　　　　intracranial D18.02
　　　　skin D18.01
　　　　specified site NEC D18.09
　　hemorrhagic M27.49
　　hydatid (*see also* Echinococcus) B67.90
　　　　brain B67.99 [G94]
　　　　liver (*see also* Cyst, liver, hydatid) B67.8
　　　　lung NEC B67.99 [J99]
　　　　Morgagni
　　　　　　female Q50.5
　　　　　　male (epididymal) Q55.4
　　　　　　　　testicular Q55.29
　　　　specified site NEC B67.99
　　hymen N89.8
　　　　embryonic Q52.4
　　hypopharynx J39.2
　　hypophysis, hypophyseal (duct) (recurrent) E23.6
　　　　cerebri E23.6
　　implantation (dermoid)
　　　　external area or site (skin) NEC L72.0
　　　　iris — *see* Cyst, iris, implantation
　　　　vagina N89.8
　　　　vulva N90.7
　　incisive canal K09.1
　　inclusion (epidermal) (epithelial) (epidermoid) (squamous) L72.0
　　　　not of skin — *code under* Cyst, by site
　　intestine (large) (small) K63.89
　　intracranial — *see* Cyst, brain
　　intraligamentous (*see also* Disorder, ligament)
　　　　knee — *see* Derangement, knee
　　intrasellar E23.6
　　iris H21.309
　　　　exudative H21.31- ☑
　　　　idiopathic H21.30- ☑
　　　　implantation H21.32- ☑
　　　　parasitic H21.33- ☑
　　　　pars plana (primary) H21.34- ☑
　　　　　　exudative H21.35- ☑
　　jaw (bone) M27.40
　　　　aneurysmal M27.49
　　　　developmental (odontogenic) K09.0

Cyst — *continued*
　　jaw — *continued*
　　　　fissural K09.1
　　　　hemorrhagic M27.49
　　　　traumatic M27.49
　　joint NEC — *see* Disorder, joint, specified type NEC
　　kidney (acquired) N28.1
　　　　calyceal — *see* Hydronephrosis
　　　　congenital Q61.00
　　　　more than one (multiple) Q61.02
　　　　　　specified as polycystic Q61.3
　　　　　　　　adult type (autosomal dominant) Q61.2
　　　　　　　　infantile type (autosomal recessive) NEC Q61.19
　　　　　　　　　　collecting duct dilation Q61.11
　　　　pyelogenic — *see* Hydronephrosis
　　　　simple N28.1
　　　　solitary (single) Q61.01
　　　　　　acquired N28.1
　　labium (majus) (minus) N90.7
　　　　sebaceous N90.7
　　lacrimal (*see also* Disorder, lacrimal system, specified NEC)
　　　　gland H04.13- ☑
　　　　passages or sac — *see* Disorder, lacrimal system, specified NEC
　　larynx J38.7
　　lateral periodontal K09.0
　　lens H27.8
　　　　congenital Q12.8
　　lip (gland) K13.0
　　liver (idiopathic) (simple) K76.89
　　　　congenital Q44.6
　　　　hydatid B67.8
　　　　　　granulosus B67.0
　　　　　　multilocularis B67.5
　　lung J98.4
　　　　congenital Q33.0
　　　　giant bullous J43.9
　　lutein N83.1- ☑
　　lymphangiomatous D18.1
　　lymphoepithelial, oral soft tissue K09.8
　　macula — *see* Degeneration, macula, hole
　　malignant — *see* Neoplasm, malignant, by site
　　mammary gland — *see* Cyst, breast
　　mandible M27.40
　　　　dentigerous K09.0
　　　　radicular K04.8
　　maxilla M27.40
　　　　dentigerous K09.0
　　　　radicular K04.8
　　medial, face and neck Q18.8
　　median
　　　　anterior maxillary K09.1
　　　　palatal K09.1
　　mediastinum, congenital Q34.1
　　meibomian (gland) — *see* Chalazion
　　　　infected — *see* Hordeolum
　　membrane, brain G93.0
　　meninges (cerebral) G93.0
　　　　spinal G96.19
　　meniscus, knee — *see* Derangement, knee, meniscus, cystic
　　mesentery, mesenteric K66.8
　　　　chyle I89.8
　　mesonephric duct
　　　　female Q50.5
　　　　male Q55.4
　　milk N64.89
　　Morgagni (hydatid)
　　　　female Q50.5
　　　　male (epididymal) Q55.4
　　　　　　testicular Q55.29
　　mouth K09.8
　　Müllerian duct Q50.4
　　　　appendix testis Q55.29
　　　　cervix Q51.6
　　　　fallopian tube Q50.4
　　　　female Q50.4
　　　　male Q55.29
　　　　prostatic utricle Q55.4
　　　　vagina (embryonal) Q52.4
　　multilocular (ovary) D39.10
　　　　benign — *see* Neoplasm, benign, by site
　　myometrium N85.8
　　nabothian (follicle) (ruptured) N88.8
　　nasoalveolar K09.1
　　nasolabial K09.1

Cyst — *continued*
　　nasopalatine (anterior) (duct) K09.1
　　nasopharynx J39.2
　　neoplastic — *see* Neoplasm, uncertain behavior, by site
　　　　benign — *see* Neoplasm, benign, by site
　　nervous system NEC G96.8
　　neuroenteric (congenital) Q06.8
　　nipple — *see* Cyst, breast
　　nose (turbinates) J34.1
　　　　sinus J34.1
　　odontogenic, developmental K09.0
　　omentum (lesser) K66.8
　　　　congenital Q45.8
　　ora serrata — *see* Cyst, retina, ora serrata
　　oral
　　　　region K09.9
　　　　　　developmental (nonodontogenic) K09.1
　　　　　　　　specified NEC K09.8
　　　　soft tissue K09.9
　　　　　　specified NEC K09.8
　　orbit H05.81- ☑
　　ovary, ovarian (twisted) N83.20- ☑
　　　　adherent N83.20- ☑
　　　　chocolate N80.1
　　　　corpus
　　　　　　albicans N83.29- ☑
　　　　　　luteum (hemorrhagic) N83.1- ☑
　　　　dermoid D27.9
　　　　developmental Q50.1
　　　　due to failure of involution NEC N83.20- ☑
　　　　endometrial N80.1
　　　　follicular (graafian) (hemorrhagic) N83.0- ☑
　　　　hemorrhagic N83.20- ☑
　　　　in pregnancy or childbirth O34.8- ☑
　　　　　　with obstructed labor O65.5
　　　　multilocular D39.10
　　　　pseudomucinous D27.9
　　　　retention N83.29- ☑
　　　　serous N83.20- ☑
　　　　specified NEC N83.29- ☑
　　　　theca lutein (hemorrhagic) N83.1- ☑
　　　　tuberculous A18.18
　　oviduct N83.8
　　palate (median) (fissural) K09.1
　　palatine papilla (jaw) K09.1
　　pancreas, pancreatic (hemorrhagic) (true) K86.2
　　　　congenital Q45.2
　　　　false K86.3
　　paralabral
　　　　hip M24.85- ☑
　　　　shoulder S43.43- ☑
　　paramesonephric duct Q50.4
　　　　female Q50.4
　　　　male Q55.29
　　paranephric N28.1
　　paraphysis, cerebri, congenital Q04.6
　　parasitic B89
　　parathyroid (gland) E21.4
　　paratubal N83.8
　　paraurethral duct N36.8
　　paroophoron Q50.5
　　parotid gland K11.6
　　parovarian Q50.5
　　pelvis, female N94.89
　　　　in pregnancy or childbirth O34.8- ☑
　　　　　　causing obstructed labor O65.5
　　penis (sebaceous) N48.89
　　periapical K04.8
　　pericardial (congenital) Q24.8
　　　　acquired (secondary) I31.8
　　pericoronal K09.0
　　periodontal K04.8
　　　　lateral K09.0
　　peripelvic (lymphatic) N28.1
　　periventricular, acquired, newborn P91.1
　　peritoneum K66.8
　　　　chylous I89.8
　　periventricular, acquired, newborn P91.1
　　pharynx (wall) J39.2
　　pilar L72.11
　　pilonidal (infected) (rectum) L05.91
　　　　with abscess L05.01
　　　　malignant C44.59- ☑
　　pituitary (duct) (gland) E23.6
　　placenta O43.19- ☑
　　pleura J94.8
　　popliteal — *see* Cyst, Baker's
　　porencephalic Q04.6

Cyst — Cyst

Cyst — *continued*
porencephalic — *continued*
acquired G93.0
postanal (infected) — *see* Cyst, pilonidal
postmastoidectomy cavity (mucosal) — *see* Complications, postmastoidectomy, cyst
preauricular Q18.1
prepuce N47.4
congenital Q55.69
primordial (jaw) K09.0
prostate N42.83
pseudomucinous (ovary) D27.9
pupillary, miotic H21.27- ☑
radicular (residual) K04.8
radiculodental K04.8
ranular K11.8
Rathke's pouch E23.6
rectum (epithelium) (mucous) K62.89
renal — *see* Cyst, kidney
residual (radicular) K04.8
retention (ovary) N83.29- ☑
salivary gland K11.6
retina H33.19- ☑
ora serrata H33.11- ☑
parasitic H33.12- ☑
retroperitoneal K68.9
sacrococcygeal (dermoid) — *see* Cyst, pilonidal
salivary gland or duct (mucous extravasation or retention) K11.6
Sampson's N80.1
sclera H15.89
scrotum L72.9
sebaceous L72.3
sebaceous (duct) (gland) L72.3
breast — *see* Dysplasia, mammary, specified type NEC
eyelid — *see* Cyst, eyelid
genital organ NEC
female N94.89
male N50.89
scrotum L72.3
semilunar cartilage (knee) (multiple) — *see* Derangement, knee, meniscus, cystic
seminal vesicle N50.89
serous (ovary) N83.20- ☑
sinus (accessory) (nasal) J34.1
Skene's gland N36.8
skin L72.9
breast — *see* Dysplasia, mammary, specified type NEC
epidermal, epidermoid L72.0
epithelial L72.0
eyelid — *see* Cyst, eyelid
genital organ NEC
female N90.7
male N50.89
inclusion L72.0
scrotum L72.9
sebaceous L72.3
sweat gland or duct L74.8
solitary
bone — *see* Cyst, bone, solitary
jaw M27.40
kidney N28.1
spermatic cord N50.89
sphenoid sinus J34.1
spinal meninges G96.19
spleen NEC D73.4
congenital Q89.09
hydatid (*see also* Echinococcus) B67.99 [D77]
Stafne's M27.0
subarachnoid intrasellar R93.0
subcutaneous, pheomycotic (chromomycotic) B43.2
subdural (cerebral) G93.0
spinal cord G96.19
sublingual gland K11.6
submandibular gland K11.6
submaxillary gland K11.6
suburethral N36.8
suprarenal gland E27.8
suprasellar — *see* Cyst, brain
sweat gland or duct L74.8
synovial (*see also* Cyst, bursa)
ruptured — *see* Rupture, synovium
tarsal — *see* Chalazion
tendon (sheath) — *see* Disorder, tendon, specified type NEC
testis N44.2

Cyst — *continued*
testis — *continued*
tunica albuginea N44.1
theca lutein (ovary) N83.1- ☑
Thornwaldt's J39.2
thymus (gland) E32.8
thyroglossal duct (infected) (persistent) Q89.2
thyroid (gland) E04.1
thyrolingual duct (infected) (persistent) Q89.2
tongue K14.8
tonsil J35.8
tooth — *see* Cyst, dental
Tornwaldt's J39.2
trichilemmal (proliferating) L72.12
trichodermal L72.12
tubal (fallopian) N83.8
inflammatory — *see* Salpingitis, chronic
tubo-ovarian N83.8
inflammatory N70.13
tunica
albuginea testis N44.1
vaginalis N50.89
turbinate (nose) J34.1
Tyson's gland N48.89
urachus, congenital Q64.4
ureter N28.89
ureterovesical orifice N28.89
urethra, urethral (gland) N36.8
uterine ligament N83.8
uterus (body) (corpus) (recurrent) N85.8
embryonic Q51.818
cervix Q51.6
vagina, vaginal (implantation) (inclusion) (squamous cell) (wall) N89.8
embryonic Q52.4
vallecula, vallecular (epiglottis) J38.7
vesical (orifice) N32.89
vitreous body H43.89
vulva (implantation) (inclusion) N90.7
congenital Q52.79
sebaceous gland N90.7
vulvovaginal gland N90.7
wolffian
female Q50.5
male Q55.4
Cystadenocarcinoma — *see* Neoplasm, malignant, by site
bile duct C22.1
endometrioid — *see* Neoplasm, malignant, by site
specified site — *see* Neoplasm, malignant, by site
unspecified site
female C56.9
male C61
mucinous
papillary
specified site — *see* Neoplasm, malignant, by site
unspecified site C56.9
specified site — *see* Neoplasm, malignant, by site
unspecified site C56.9
papillary
mucinous
specified site — *see* Neoplasm, malignant, by site
unspecified site C56.9
pseudomucinous
specified site — *see* Neoplasm, malignant, by site
unspecified site C56.9
serous
specified site — *see* Neoplasm, malignant, by site
unspecified site C56.9
specified site — *see* Neoplasm, malignant, by site
unspecified site C56.9
pseudomucinous
papillary
specified site — *see* Neoplasm, malignant, by site
unspecified site C56.9
specified site — *see* Neoplasm, malignant, by site
unspecified site C56.9
serous
papillary
specified site — *see* Neoplasm, malignant, by site
unspecified site C56.9
specified site — *see* Neoplasm, malignant, by

Cystadenocarcinoma — *continued*
serous — *continued*
unspecified site C56.9
Cystadenofibroma
clear cell — *see* Neoplasm, benign, by site
endometrioid D27.9
borderline malignancy D39.1- ☑
malignant C56.- ☑
mucinous
specified site — *see* Neoplasm, benign, by site
unspecified site D27.9
serous
specified site — *see* Neoplasm, benign, by site
unspecified site D27.9
specified site — *see* Neoplasm, benign, by site
unspecified site D27.9
Cystadenoma (*see also* Neoplasm, benign, by site)
bile duct D13.4
endometrioid — *see* Neoplasm, benign, by site
borderline malignancy — *see* Neoplasm, uncertain behavior, by site
malignant — *see* Neoplasm, malignant, by site
mucinous
borderline malignancy
ovary C56.- ☑
specified site NEC — *see* Neoplasm, uncertain behavior, by site
unspecified site C56.9
papillary
borderline malignancy
ovary C56.- ☑
specified site NEC — *see* Neoplasm, uncertain behavior, by site
unspecified site C56.9
specified site — *see* Neoplasm, benign, by site
unspecified site D27.9
specified site — *see* Neoplasm, benign, by site
unspecified site D27.9
papillary
borderline malignancy
ovary C56.- ☑
specified site NEC — *see* Neoplasm, uncertain behavior, by site
unspecified site C56.9
lymphomatosum
specified site — *see* Neoplasm, benign, by site
unspecified site D11.9
mucinous
borderline malignancy
ovary C56.- ☑
specified site NEC — *see* Neoplasm, uncertain behavior, by site
unspecified site C56.9
specified site — *see* Neoplasm, benign, by site
unspecified site D27.9
pseudomucinous
borderline malignancy
ovary C56.- ☑
specified site NEC — *see* Neoplasm, uncertain behavior, by site
unspecified site C56.9
specified site — *see* Neoplasm, benign, by site
unspecified site D27.9
serous
borderline malignancy
ovary C56.- ☑
specified site NEC — *see* Neoplasm, uncertain behavior, by site
unspecified site C56.9
specified site — *see* Neoplasm, benign, by site
unspecified site D27.9
specified site — *see* Neoplasm, benign, by site
unspecified site D27.9
pseudomucinous
borderline malignancy
ovary C56.- ☑
specified site NEC — *see* Neoplasm, uncertain behavior, by site
unspecified site C56.9
papillary
borderline malignancy
ovary C56.- ☑
specified site NEC — *see* Neoplasm, uncertain behavior, by site
unspecified site C56.9
specified site — *see* Neoplasm, benign, by site
unspecified site D27.9
specified site — *see* Neoplasm, benign, by site

☑ **Additional Character Required** — **Refer to the Tabular List for Character Selection**   ▼ **Subterms under main terms may continue to next column or page**

Cystadenoma — *continued*
　pseudomucinous — *continued*
　　unspecified site D27.9
　serous
　　borderline malignancy
　　　ovary C56.- ☑
　　　specified site NEC — *see* Neoplasm, uncertain
　　　　　　behavior, by site
　　　unspecified site C56.9
　　papillary
　　　borderline malignancy
　　　　ovary C56.- ☑
　　　　specified site NEC — *see* Neoplasm, uncertain
　　　　　　behavior, by site
　　　　unspecified site C56.9
　　　specified site — *see* Neoplasm, benign, by site
　　　unspecified site D27.9
　　specified site — *see* Neoplasm, benign, by site
　　unspecified site D27.9
Cystathionine synthase deficiency E72.11
Cystathioninemia E72.19
Cystathioninuria E72.19
Cystic (*see also* condition)
　breast (chronic) — *see* Mastopathy, cystic
　corpora lutea (hemorrhagic) N83.1- ☑
　duct — *see* condition
　eyeball (congenital) Q11.0
　fibrosis — *see* Fibrosis, cystic
　kidney (congenital) Q61.9
　　adult type Q61.2
　　infantile type NEC Q61.19
　　　collecting duct dilatation Q61.11
　　medullary Q61.5
　liver, congenital Q44.6
　lung disease J98.4
　　congenital Q33.0
　mastitis, chronic — *see* Mastopathy, cystic
　medullary, kidney Q61.5
　meniscus — *see* Derangement, knee, meniscus, cystic
　ovary N83.20- ☑
Cysticercosis, cysticerciasis B69.9
　with
　　epileptiform fits B69.0
　　myositis B69.81
　brain B69.0
　central nervous system B69.0
　cerebral B69.0
　ocular B69.1
　specified NEC B69.89
Cysticercus cellulose infestation — *see* Cysticercosis
Cystinosis (malignant) E72.04
Cystinuria E72.01
Cystitis (exudative) (hemorrhagic) (septic) (suppurative)
　　N30.90
　with
　　fibrosis — *see* Cystitis, chronic, interstitial

Cystitis — *continued*
　with — *continued*
　　hematuria N30.91
　　leukoplakia — *see* Cystitis, chronic, interstitial
　　malakoplakia — *see* Cystitis, chronic, interstitial
　　metaplasia — *see* Cystitis, chronic, interstitial
　　prostatitis N41.3
　acute N30.00
　　with hematuria N30.01
　　of trigone N30.30
　　　with hematuria N30.31
　allergic — *see* Cystitis, specified type NEC
　amebic A06.81
　bilharzial B65.9 [N33]
　blennorrhagic (gonococcal) A54.01
　bullous — *see* Cystitis, specified type NEC
　calculous N21.0
　chlamydial A56.01
　chronic N30.20
　　with hematuria N30.21
　　interstitial N30.10
　　　with hematuria N30.11
　　of trigone N30.30
　　　with hematuria N30.31
　　specified NEC N30.20
　　　with hematuria N30.21
　cystic (a) — *see* Cystitis, specified type NEC
　diphtheritic A36.85
　echinococcal
　　granulosus B67.39
　　multilocularis B67.69
　emphysematous — *see* Cystitis, specified type NEC
　encysted — *see* Cystitis, specified type NEC
　eosinophilic — *see* Cystitis, specified type NEC
　follicular — *see* Cystitis, of trigone
　gangrenous — *see* Cystitis, specified type NEC
　glandularis — *see* Cystitis, specified type NEC
　gonococcal A54.01
　incrusted — *see* Cystitis, specified type NEC
　interstitial (chronic) — *see* Cystitis, chronic, interstitial
　irradiation N30.40
　　with hematuria N30.41
　irritation —·*see* Cystitis, specified type NEC
　malignant — *see* Cystitis, specified type NEC
　of trigone N30.30
　　with hematuria N30.31
　panmural — *see* Cystitis, chronic, interstitial
　polyposa — *see* Cystitis, specified type NEC
　prostatic N41.3
　puerperal (postpartum) O86.22
　radiation — *see* Cystitis, irradiation
　specified type NEC N30.80
　　with hematuria N30.81
　subacute — *see* Cystitis, chronic
　submucous — *see* Cystitis, chronic, interstitial
　syphilitic (late) A52.76

Cystitis — *continued*
　trichomonal A59.03
　tuberculous A18.12
　ulcerative — *see* Cystitis, chronic, interstitial
Cystocele (-urethrocele)
　female N81.10
　　with prolapse of uterus — *see* Prolapse, uterus
　　lateral N81.12
　　midline N81.11
　　paravaginal N81.12
　in pregnancy or childbirth O34.8- ☑
　　causing obstructed labor O65.5
　male N32.89
Cystolithiasis N21.0
Cystoma (*see also* Neoplasm, benign, by site)
　endometrial, ovary N80.1
　mucinous
　　specified site — *see* Neoplasm, benign, by site
　　unspecified site D27.9
　serous
　　specified site — *see* Neoplasm, benign, by site
　　unspecified site D27.9
　simple (ovary) N83.29- ☑
Cystoplegia N31.2
Cystoptosis N32.89
Cystopyelitis — *see* Pyelonephritis
Cystorrhagia N32.89
Cystosarcoma phyllodes D48.6- ☑
　benign D24- ☑
　malignant — *see* Neoplasm, breast, malignant
Cystostomy
　attention to Z43.5
　complication — *see* Complications, cystostomy
　status Z93.50
　　appendico-vesicostomy Z93.52
　　cutaneous Z93.51
　　specified NEC Z93.59
Cystourethritis — *see* Urethritis
Cystourethrocele (*see also* Cystocele)
　female N81.10
　　with uterine prolapse — *see* Prolapse, uterus
　　lateral N81.12
　　midline N81.11
　　paravaginal N81.12
　male N32.89
Cytomegalic inclusion disease
　congenital P35.1
Cytomegalovirus infection B25.9
Cytomycosis (reticuloendothelial) B39.4
Cytopenia D75.9
　refractory
　　with multilineage dysplasia D46.A (*following* D46.2)
　　　and ring sideroblasts (RCMD RS) D46.B (*following*
　　　　D46.2)
Czerny's disease (periodic hydrarthrosis of the knee) —
　　see Effusion, joint, knee

D

Da Costa's syndrome F45.8
Daae (-Finsen) **disease** (epidemic pleurodynia) B33.0
Dabney's grip B33.0
Dacryoadenitis, dacryadenitis H04.00- ☑
　　acute H04.01- ☑
　　chronic H04.02- ☑
Dacryocystitis H04.30- ☑
　　acute H04.32- ☑
　　chronic H04.41- ☑
　　neonatal P39.1
　　phlegmonous H04.31- ☑
　　syphilitic A52.71
　　　· congenital (early) A50.01
　　trachomatous, active A71.1
　　　sequelae (late effect) B94.0
Dacryocystoblenorrhea — *see* Inflammation, lacrimal, passages, chronic
Dacryocystocele — *see* Disorder, lacrimal system, changes
Dacryolith, dacryolithiasis H04.51- ☑
Dacryoma — *see* Disorder, lacrimal system, changes
Dacryopericystitis — *see* Dacryocystitis
Dacryops H04.11- ☑
Dacryostenosis (*see also* Stenosis, lacrimal)
　　congenital Q10.5
Dactylitis
　　bone — *see* Osteomyelitis
　　sickle-cell D57.00
　　　Hb C D57.219
　　　Hb SS D57.00
　　　specified NEC D57.819
　　skin L08.9
　　syphilitic A52.77
　　tuberculous A18.03
Dactylolysis spontanea (ainhum) L94.6
Dactylosymphysis Q70.9
　　fingers — *see* Syndactylism, complex, fingers
　　toes — *see* Syndactylism, complex, toes
Damage
　　arteriosclerotic — *see* Arteriosclerosis
　　brain (nontraumatic) G93.9
　　　anoxic, hypoxic G93.1
　　　　resulting from a procedure G97.82
　　　child NEC G80.9
　　　due to birth injury P11.2
　　cardiorenal (vascular) — *see* Hypertension, cardiorenal
　　cerebral NEC — *see* Damage, brain
　　coccyx, complicating delivery O71.6
　　coronary — *see* Disease, heart, ischemic
　　eye, birth injury P15.3
　　liver (nontraumatic) K76.9
　　　alcoholic K70.9
　　　due to drugs — *see* Disease, liver, toxic
　　　toxic — *see* Disease, liver, toxic
　　medication T88.7 ☑
　　pelvic
　　　joint or ligament, during delivery O71.6
　　　organ NEC
　　　　during delivery O71.5
　　　　following ectopic or molar pregnancy O08.6
　　renal — *see* Disease, renal
　　subendocardium, subendocardial — *see* Degeneration, myocardial
　　vascular I99.9
Dana-Putnam syndrome (subacute combined sclerosis with pernicious anemia) — *see* Degeneration, combined
Danbolt (-Cross) **syndrome** (acrodermatitis enteropathica) E83.2
Dandruff L21.0
Dandy-Walker syndrome Q03.1
　　with spina bifida — *see* Spina bifida
Danlos' syndrome Q79.6
Darier (-White) **disease** (congenital) Q82.8
　　meaning erythema annulare centrifugum L53.1
Darier-Roussy sarcoid D86.3
Darling's disease or histoplasmosis B39.4
Darwin's tubercle Q17.8
Dawson's (inclusion body) **encephalitis** A81.1

De Beurmann (-Gougerot) **disease** B42.1
De la Tourette's syndrome F95.2
De Lange's syndrome Q87.1
De Morgan's spots (senile angiomas) I78.1
De Quervain's
　　disease (tendon sheath) M65.4
　　syndrome E34.51
　　thyroiditis (subacute granulomatous thyroiditis) E06.1
De Toni-Fanconi (-Debré) **syndrome** E72.09
　　with cystinosis E72.04
Dead
　　fetus, retained (mother) O36.4 ☑
　　　early pregnancy O02.1
　　labyrinth H83.2 ☑
　　ovum, retained O02.0
Deaf nonspeaking NEC H91.3
Deafmutism (acquired) (congenital) NEC H91.3
　　hysterical F44.6
　　syphilitic, congenital (*see also* subcategory) H94.8 A50.09
Deafness (acquired) (complete) (hereditary) (partial) H91.9- ☑
　　with blue sclera and fragility of bone Q78.0
　　auditory fatigue — *see* Deafness, specified type NEC
　　aviation T70.0 ☑
　　　nerve injury — *see* Injury, nerve, acoustic, specified type NEC
　　boilermaker's H83.3 ☑
　　central — *see* Deafness, sensorineural
　　conductive H90.2
　　　and sensorineural
　　　　mixed H90.8
　　　　　bilateral H90.6
　　　　bilateral H90.0
　　　　unilateral H90.1- ☑
　　　　　with restricted hearing on the contralateral side H90.A- ☑
　　congenital H90.5
　　　with blue sclera and fragility of bone Q78.0
　　due to toxic agents — *see* Deafness, ototoxic
　　emotional (hysterical) F44.6
　　functional (hysterical) F44.6
　　high frequency H91.9- ☑
　　hysterical F44.6
　　low frequency H91.9- ☑
　　mental R48.8
　　mixed conductive and sensorineural H90.8
　　　bilateral H90.6
　　　unilateral H90.7- ☑
　　nerve — *see* Deafness, sensorineural
　　neural — *see* Deafness, sensorineural
　　noise-induced (*see also* subcategory) H83.3 ☑
　　　nerve injury — *see* Injury, nerve, acoustic, specified type NEC
　　nonspeaking H91.3
　　ototoxic H91.0 ☑
　　perceptive — *see* Deafness, sensorineural
　　psychogenic (hysterical) F44.6
　　sensorineural H90.5
　　　and conductive
　　　　bilateral H90.6
　　　　mixed H90.8
　　　　　bilateral H90.6
　　　bilateral H90.3
　　　unilateral H90.4- ☑
　　　　with restricted hearing on the contralateral side H90.A- ☑
　　sensory — *see* Deafness, sensorineural
　　specified type NEC H91.8 ☑
　　sudden (idiopathic) H91.2- ☑
　　syphilitic A52.15
　　transient ischemic H93.01- ☑
　　traumatic — *see* Injury, nerve, acoustic, specified type NEC
　　word (developmental) H93.25
Death (cause unknown) (of) (unexplained) (unspecified cause) R99
　　brain G93.9
　　brain G93.82
　　cardiac (sudden) (with successful resuscitation) — *code to* underlying disease
　　　family history of Z82.41
　　　personal history of Z86.74

Death — *continued*
　　family member (assumed) Z63.4
Debility (chronic) (general) (nervous) R53.81
　　congenital or neonatal NOS P96.9
　　nervous R53.81
　　old age R54
　　senile R54
Débove's disease (splenomegaly) R16.1
Decalcification
　　bone — *see* Osteoporosis
　　teeth K03.89
Decapsulation, kidney N28.89
Decay
　　dental — *see* Caries, dental
　　senile R54
　　tooth, teeth — *see* Caries, dental
Deciduitis (acute)
　　following ectopic or molar pregnancy O08.0
Decline (general) — *see* Debility
　　cognitive, age-associated R41.81
Decompensation
　　cardiac (acute) (chronic) — *see* Disease, heart
　　cardiovascular — *see* Disease, cardiovascular
　　heart — *see* Disease, heart
　　hepatic — *see* Failure, hepatic
　　myocardial (acute) (chronic) — *see* Disease, heart
　　respiratory J98.8
Decompression sickness T70.3 ☑
Decrease (d)
　　absolute neutrophile count — *see* Neutropenia
　　blood
　　　platelets — *see* Thrombocytopenia
　　　pressure R03.1
　　　　due to shock following
　　　　　injury T79.4 ☑
　　　　　operation T81.19 ☑
　　estrogen E28.39
　　　postablative E89.40
　　　　asymptomatic E89.40
　　　　symptomatic E89.41
　　fragility of erythrocytes D58.8
　　function
　　　lipase (pancreatic) K90.3
　　　ovary in hypopituitarism E23.0
　　　parenchyma of pancreas K86.89
　　　pituitary (gland) (anterior) (lobe) E23.0
　　　　posterior (lobe) E23.0
　　functional activity R68.89
　　glucose R73.09
　　hematocrit R71.0
　　hemoglobin R71.0
　　leukocytes D72.819
　　　specified NEC D72.818
　　libido R68.82
　　lymphocytes D72.810
　　platelets D69.6
　　respiration, due to shock following injury T79.4 ☑
　　sexual desire R68.82
　　tear secretion NEC — *see* Syndrome, dry eye
　　tolerance
　　　fat K90.49
　　　glucose R73.09
　　　pancreatic K90.3
　　　salt and water E87.8
　　vision NEC H54.7
　　white blood cell count D72.819
　　　specified NEC D72.818
Decubitus (ulcer) — *see* Ulcer, pressure, by site
　　cervix N86
Deepening acetabulum — *see* Derangement, joint, specified type NEC, hip
Defect, defective Q89.9
　　3-beta-hydroxysteroid dehydrogenase E25.0
　　11-hydroxylase E25.0
　　21-hydroxylase E25.0
　　abdominal wall, congenital Q79.59
　　antibody immunodeficiency D80.9
　　aorticopulmonary septum Q21.4
　　atrial septal (ostium secundum type) Q21.1
　　　following acute myocardial infarction (current complication) I23.1
　　　ostium primum type Q21.2

☑ Additional Character Required — Refer to the Tabular List for Character Selection　　　🔻 Subterms under main terms may continue to next column or page

Defect, defective — *continued*
  atrioventricular
    canal Q21.2
    septum Q21.2
  auricular septal Q21.1
  bilirubin excretion NEC E80.6
  biosynthesis, androgen (testicular) E29.1
  bulbar septum Q21.0
  catalase E80.3
  cell membrane receptor complex (CR3) D71
  circulation I99.9
    congenital Q28.9
    newborn Q28.9
  coagulation (factor) (*see also* Deficiency, factor) D68.9
    with
      ectopic pregnancy O08.1
      molar pregnancy O08.1
    acquired D68.4
    antepartum with hemorrhage — *see* Hemorrhage, antepartum, with coagulation defect
    due to
      liver disease D68.4
      vitamin K deficiency D68.4
    hereditary NEC D68.2
    intrapartum O67.0
    newborn, transient P61.6
    postpartum O99.13
      with hemorrhage O72.3
    specified type NEC D68.8
  complement system D84.1
  conduction (heart) I45.9
    bone — *see* Deafness, conductive
  congenital, organ or site not listed — *see* Anomaly, by site
  coronary sinus Q21.1
  cushion, endocardial Q21.2
  degradation, glycoprotein E77.1
  dental bridge, crown, fillings — *see* Defect, dental restoration
  dental restoration K08.50
    specified NEC K08.59
  dentin (hereditary) K00.5
  Descemet's membrane, congenital Q13.89
  developmental (*see also* Anomaly)
    cauda equina Q06.3
  diaphragm
    with elevation, eventration or hernia — *see* Hernia, diaphragm
    congenital Q79.1
      with hernia Q79.0
      gross (with hernia) Q79.0
  ectodermal, congenital Q82.9
  Eisenmenger's Q21.8
  enzyme
    catalase E80.3
    peroxidase E80.3
  esophagus, congenital Q39.9
  extensor retinaculum M62.89
  fibrin polymerization D68.2
  filling
    bladder R93.41
    kidney R93.42- ☑
    renal pelvis R93.41
    stomach R93.3
    ureter R93.41
    urinary organs, specified NEC R93.49
  GABA (gamma aminobutyric acid) metabolic E72.81
  Gerbode Q21.0
  glycoprotein degradation E77.1
  Hageman (factor) D68.2
  hearing — *see* Deafness
  high grade F70
  interatrial septal Q21.1
  interauricular septal Q21.1
  interventricular septal Q21.0
    with dextroposition of aorta, pulmonary stenosis and hypertrophy of right ventricle Q21.3
    in tetralogy of Fallot Q21.3
  learning (specific) — *see* Disorder, learning
  lymphocyte function antigen-1 (LFA-1) D84.0
  lysosomal enzyme, post-translational modification E77.0
  major osseous M89.70
    ankle M89.77- ☑
    carpus M89.74- ☑
    clavicle M89.71- ☑
    femur M89.75- ☑
    fibula M89.76- ☑

Defect, defective — *continued*
  major osseous — *continued*
    fingers M89.74- ☑
    foot M89.77- ☑
    forearm M89.73- ☑
    hand M89.74- ☑
    humerus M89.72- ☑
    lower leg M89.76- ☑
    metacarpus M89.74- ☑
    metatarsus M89.77- ☑
    multiple sites M89.79
    pelvic region M89.75- ☑
    pelvis M89.75- ☑
    radius M89.73- ☑
    scapula M89.71- ☑
    shoulder region M89.71- ☑
    specified NEC M89.78
    tarsus M89.77- ☑
    thigh M89.75- ☑
    tibia M89.76- ☑
    toes M89.77- ☑
    ulna M89.73- ☑
  mental — *see* Disability, intellectual
  modification, lysosomal enzymes, post-translational E77.0
  obstructive, congenital
    renal pelvis Q62.39
    ureter Q62.39
      atresia — *see* Atresia, ureter
      cecoureterocele Q62.32
      megaureter Q62.2
      orthotopic ureterocele Q62.31
  osseous, major M89.70
    ankle M89.77- ☑
    carpus M89.74- ☑
    clavicle M89.71- ☑
    femur M89.75- ☑
    fibula M89.76- ☑
    fingers M89.74- ☑
    foot M89.77- ☑
    forearm M89.73- ☑
    hand M89.74- ☑
    humerus M89.72- ☑
    lower leg M89.76- ☑
    metacarpus M89.74- ☑
    metatarsus M89.77- ☑
    multiple sites M89.9
    pelvic region M89.75- ☑
    pelvis M89.75- ☑
    radius M89.73- ☑
    scapula M89.71- ☑
    shoulder region M89.71- ☑
    specified NEC M89.78
    tarsus M89.77- ☑
    thigh M89.75- ☑
    tibia M89.76- ☑
    toes M89.77- ☑
    ulna M89.73- ☑
  osteochondral NEC (*see also* Deformity) M95.8
  ostium
    primum Q21.2
    secundum Q21.1
  peroxidase E80.3
  placental blood supply — *see* Insufficiency, placental
  platelets, qualitative D69.1
    constitutional D68.0
  postural NEC, spine — *see* Dorsopathy, deforming
  reduction
    limb Q73.8
      lower Q72.9- ☑
        absence — *see* Agenesis, leg
          foot — *see* Agenesis, foot
        longitudinal
          femur Q72.4- ☑
          fibula Q72.6- ☑
          tibia Q72.5- ☑
        specified type NEC Q72.89- ☑
        split foot Q72.7- ☑
      specified type NEC Q73.8
      upper Q71.9- ☑
        absence — *see* Agenesis, arm
          forearm — *see* Agenesis, forearm
          hand — *see* Agenesis, hand
        lobster-claw hand Q71.6- ☑
        longitudinal
          radius Q71.4- ☑

Defect, defective — *continued*
  reduction — *continued*
    limb — *continued*
      upper — *continued*
        longitudinal — *continued*
          ulna Q71.5- ☑
        specified type NEC Q71.89- ☑
  renal pelvis Q63.8
    obstructive Q62.39
  respiratory system, congenital Q34.9
  restoration, dental K08.50
    specified NEC K08.59
  retinal nerve bundle fibers H35.89
  septal (heart) NOS Q21.9
    acquired (atrial) (auricular) (ventricular) (old) I51.0
    atrial Q21.1
      concurrent with acute myocardial infarction — *see* Infarct, myocardial
      following acute myocardial infarction (current complication) I23.1
    ventricular (*see also* Defect, ventricular septal) Q21.0
  sinus venosus Q21.1
  speech R47.9
    developmental F80.9
    specified NEC R47.89
  Taussig-Bing (aortic transposition and overriding pulmonary artery) Q20.1
  teeth, wedge K03.1
  vascular (local) I99.9
    congenital Q27.9
  ventricular septal Q21.0
    concurrent with acute myocardial infarction — *see* Infarct, myocardium
    following acute myocardial infarction (current complication) I23.2
    in tetralogy of Fallot Q21.3
  vision NEC H54.7
  visual field H53.40
    bilateral
      heteronymous H53.47
      homonymous H53.46- ☑
    generalized contraction H53.48- ☑
    localized
      arcuate H53.43- ☑
      scotoma (central area) H53.41- ☑
        blind spot area H53.42- ☑
      sector H53.43- ☑
      specified type NEC H53.45- ☑
  voice R49.9
    specified NEC R49.8
  wedge, tooth, teeth (abrasion) K03.1

Deferentitis N49.1
  gonorrheal (acute) (chronic) A54.23

Defibrination (syndrome) D65
  antepartum — *see* Hemorrhage, antepartum, with coagulation defect, disseminated intravascular coagulation
  following ectopic or molar pregnancy O08.1
  intrapartum O67.0
  newborn P60
  postpartum O72.3

Deficiency, deficient
  3-beta hydroxysteroid dehydrogenase E25.0
  5-alpha reductase (with male pseudohermaphroditism) E29.1
  11-hydroxylase E25.0
  21-hydroxylase E25.0
  abdominal muscle syndrome Q79.4
  AC globulin (congenital) (hereditary) D68.2
    acquired D68.4
  accelerator globulin (Ac G) (blood) D68.2
  acid phosphatase E83.39
  activating factor (blood) D68.2
  adenosine deaminase (ADA) D81.3
  aldolase (hereditary) E74.19
  alpha-1-antitrypsin E88.01
  amino-acids E72.9
  anemia — *see* Anemia
  aneurin E51.9
  antibody with
    hyperimmunoglobulinemia D80.6
    near-normal immunoglobins D80.6
  antidiuretic hormone E23.2
  anti-hemophilic
    factor (A) D66
      B D67
      C D68.1
    globulin (AHG) NEC D66

Deficiency, deficient — *continued*
- antithrombin (antithrombin III) D68.59
- ascorbic acid E54
- attention (disorder) (syndrome) F98.8
  - with hyperactivity — *see* Disorder, attention-deficit hyperactivity
- autoprothrombin
  - C D68.2
  - I D68.2
  - II D67
- beta-glucuronidase E76.29
- biotin E53.8
- biotin-dependent carboxylase D81.819
- biotinidase D81.810
- brancher enzyme (amylopectinosis) E74.03
- C1 esterase inhibitor (C1-INH) D84.1
- calciferol E55.9
  - with
    - adult osteomalacia M83.8
    - rickets — *see* Rickets
- calcium (dietary) E58
- calorie, severe E43
  - with marasmus E41
    - and kwashiorkor E42
- cardiac — *see* Insufficiency, myocardial
- carnitine E71.40
  - due to
    - hemodialysis E71.43
    - inborn errors of metabolism E71.42
    - Valproic acid therapy E71.43
  - iatrogenic E71.43
  - muscle palmityltransferase E71.314
  - primary E71.41
  - secondary E71.448
- carotene E50.9
- central nervous system G96.8
- ceruloplasmin (Wilson) E83.01
- choline E53.8
- Christmas factor D67
- chromium E61.4
- clotting (blood) (*see also* Deficiency, coagulation factor) D68.9
- clotting factor NEC (hereditary) (*see also* Deficiency, factor) D68.2
- coagulation NOS D68.9
  - with
    - ectopic pregnancy O08.1
    - molar pregnancy O08.1
  - acquired (any) D68.4
  - antepartum hemorrhage — *see* Hemorrhage, antepartum, with coagulation defect
  - clotting factor NEC (*see also* Deficiency, factor) D68.2
  - due to
    - hyperprothrombinemia D68.4
    - liver disease D68.4
    - vitamin K deficiency D68.4
  - newborn, transient P61.6
  - postpartum O72.3
  - specified NEC D68.8
- cognitive F09
- color vision H53.50
  - achromatopsia H53.51
  - acquired H53.52
  - deuteranomaly H53.53
  - protanomaly H53.54
  - specified NEC H53.59
  - tritanomaly H53.55
- combined glucocorticoid and mineralocorticoid E27.49
- contact factor D68.2
- copper (nutritional) E61.0
- corticoadrenal E27.40
  - primary E27.1
- craniofacial axis Q75.0
- cyanocobalamin E53.8
- debrancher enzyme (limit dextrinosis) E74.03
- dehydrogenase
  - long chain/very long chain acyl CoA E71.310
  - medium chain acyl CoA E71.311
  - short chain acyl CoA E71.312
- diet E63.9
- dihydropyrimidine dehydrogenase (DPD) E88.89
- disaccharidase E73.9
- edema — *see* Malnutrition, severe
- endocrine E34.9
- energy-supply — *see* Malnutrition
- enzymes, circulating NEC E88.09
- ergosterol E55.9

Deficiency, deficient — *continued*
- ergosterol — *continued*
  - with
    - adult osteomalacia M83.8
    - rickets — *see* Rickets
  - essential fatty acid (EFA) E63.0
- factor (*see also* Deficiency, coagulation)
  - Hageman D68.2
  - I (congenital) (hereditary) D68.2
  - II (congenital) (hereditary) D68.2
  - IX (congenital) (functional) (hereditary) (with functional defect) D67
  - multiple (congenital) D68.8
    - acquired D68.4
  - V (congenital) (hereditary) D68.2
  - VII (congenital) (hereditary) D68.2
  - VIII (congenital) (functional) (hereditary) (with functional defect) D66
    - with vascular defect D68.0
  - X (congenital) (hereditary) D68.2
  - XI (congenital) (hereditary) D68.1
  - XII (congenital) (hereditary) D68.2
  - XIII (congenital) (hereditary) D68.2
- femoral, proximal focal (congenital) — *see* Defect, reduction, lower limb, longitudinal, femur
- fibrinase D68.2
- fibrinogen (congenital) (hereditary) D68.2
  - acquired D65
- fibrin-stabilizing factor (congenital) (hereditary) D68.2
  - acquired D68.4
- folate E53.8
- folic acid E53.8
- foreskin N47.3
- fructokinase E74.11
- fructose 1,6-diphosphatase E74.19
- fructose-1-phosphate aldolase E74.19
- GABA (gamma aminobutyric acid) transaminase E72.81
- GABA-T (gamma aminobutyric acid transaminase) E72.81
- galactokinase E74.29
- galactose-1-phosphate uridyl transferase E74.29
- gammaglobulin in blood D80.1
  - hereditary D80.0
- glass factor D68.2
- glucocorticoid E27.49
  - mineralocorticoid E27.49
- glucose-6-phosphatase E74.01
- glucose-6-phosphate dehydrogenase anemia D55.0
- glucuronyl transferase E80.5
- glycogen synthetase E74.09
- gonadotropin (isolated) E23.0
- growth hormone (idiopathic) (isolated) E23.0
- Hageman factor D68.2
- hemoglobin D64.9
- hepatophosphorylase E74.09
- homogentisate 1,2-dioxygenase E70.29
- hormone
  - anterior pituitary (partial) NEC E23.0
    - growth E23.0
  - growth (isolated) E23.0
  - pituitary E23.0
  - testicular E29.1
- hypoxanthine- (guanine)-phosphoribosyltransferase (HG- PRT) (total H-PRT) E79.1
- immunity D84.9
  - cell-mediated D84.8
    - with thrombocytopenia and eczema D82.0
  - combined D81.9
  - humoral D80.9
  - IgA (secretory) D80.2
  - IgG D80.3
  - IgM D80.4
- immuno — *see* Immunodeficiency
- immunoglobulin, selective
  - A (IgA) D80.2
  - G (IgG) (subclasses) D80.3
  - M (IgM) D80.4
- inositol (B complex) E53.8
- intrinsic
  - factor (congenital) D51.0
  - sphincter N36.42
    - with urethral hypermobility N36.43
- iodine E61.8
  - congenital syndrome — *see* Syndrome, iodine-deficiency, congenital
- iron E61.1
  - anemia D50.9
- kalium E87.6
- kappa-light chain D80.8

Deficiency, deficient — *continued*
- labile factor (congenital) (hereditary) D68.2
  - acquired D68.4
- lacrimal fluid (acquired) (*see also* Syndrome, dry eye)
  - congenital Q10.6
- lactase
  - congenital E73.0
  - secondary E73.1
- Laki-Lorand factor D68.2
- lecithin cholesterol acyltransferase E78.6
- lipocaic K86.89
- lipoprotein (familial) (high density) E78.6
- liver phosphorylase E74.09
- lysosomal alpha-1, 4 glucosidase E74.02
- magnesium E61.2
- major histocompatibility complex
  - class I D81.6
  - class II D81.7
- manganese E61.3
- menadione (vitamin K) E56.1
  - newborn P53
- mental (familial) (hereditary) — *see* Disability, intellectual
- methylenetetrahydrofolate reductase (MTHFR) E72.12
- mevalonate kinase M04.1
- mineralocorticoid E27.49
  - with glucocorticoid E27.49
- mineral NEC E61.8
- molybdenum (nutritional) E61.5
- moral F60.2
- multiple nutrient elements E61.7
- multiple sulfatase (MSD) E75.26
- muscle
  - carnitine (palmityltransferase) E71.314
  - phosphofructokinase E74.09
- myoadenylate deaminase E79.2
- myocardial — *see* Insufficiency, myocardial
- myophosphorylase E74.04
- NADH diaphorase or reductase (congenital) D74.0
- NADH-methemoglobin reductase (congenital) D74.0
- natrium E87.1
- niacin (amide) (-tryptophan) E52
- nicotinamide E52
- nicotinic acid E52
- number of teeth — *see* Anodontia
- nutrient element E61.9
  - multiple E61.7
  - specified NEC E61.8
- nutrition, nutritional E63.9
  - sequelae — *see* Sequelae, nutritional deficiency
  - specified NEC E63.8
- of interleukin 1 receptor antagonist [DIRA] M04.8
- ornithine transcarbamylase E72.4
- ovarian E28.39
- oxygen — *see* Anoxia
- pantothenic acid E53.8
- parathyroid (gland) E20.9
- perineum (female) N81.89
- phenylalanine hydroxylase E70.1
- phosphoenolpyruvate carboxykinase E74.4
- phosphofructokinase E74.19
- phosphomannomutase E74.8
- phosphomannose isomerase E74.8
- phosphomannosyl mutase E74.8
- phosphorylase kinase, liver E74.09
- pituitary hormone (isolated) E23.0
- plasma thromboplastin
  - antecedent (PTA) D68.1
  - component (PTC) D67
- plasminogen (type 1) (type 2) E88.02
- platelet NEC D69.1
  - constitutional D68.0
- polyglandular E31.8
  - autoimmune E31.0
- potassium (K) E87.6
- prepuce N47.3
- proaccelerin (congenital) (hereditary) D68.2
  - acquired D68.4
- proconvertin factor (congenital) (hereditary) D68.2
  - acquired D68.4
- protein (*see also* Malnutrition) E46
  - anemia D53.0
  - C D68.59
  - S D68.59
- prothrombin (congenital) (hereditary) D68.2
  - acquired D68.4
- Prower factor D68.2
- pseudocholinesterase E88.09

Deficiency, deficient — *continued*
    PTA (plasma thromboplastin antecedent) D68.1
    PTC (plasma thromboplastin component) D67
    purine nucleoside phosphorylase (PNP) D81.5
    pyracin (alpha) (beta) E53.1
    pyridoxal E53.1
    pyridoxamine E53.1
    pyridoxine (derivatives) E53.1
    pyruvate
        carboxylase E74.4
        dehydrogenase E74.4
    riboflavin (vitamin B2) E53.0
    salt E87.1
    secretion
        ovary E28.39
        salivary gland (any) K11.7
        urine R34
    selenium (dietary) E59
    serum antitrypsin, familial E88.01
    short stature homeobox gene (SHOX)
        with
            dyschondrosteosis Q78.8
            short stature (idiopathic) E34.3
            Turner's syndrome Q96.9
    sodium (Na) E87.1
    SPCA (factor VII) D68.2
    sphincter, intrinsic N36.42
        with urethral hypermobility N36.43
    stable factor (congenital) (hereditary) D68.2
        acquired D68.4
    Stuart-Prower (factor X) D68.2
    succinic semialdehyde dehydrogenase E72.81
    sucrase E74.39
    sulfatase E75.26
    sulfite oxidase E72.19
    thiamin, thiaminic (chloride) E51.9
        beriberi (dry) E51.11
            wet E51.12
    thrombokinase D68.2
        newborn P53
    thyroid (gland) — *see* Hypothyroidism
    tocopherol E56.0
    tooth bud K00.0
    transcobalamine II (anemia) D51.2
    vanadium E61.6
    vascular I99.9
    vasopressin E23.2
    vertical ridge K06.8
    viosterol — *see* Deficiency, calciferol
    vitamin (multiple) NOS E56.9
        A E50.9
            with
                Bitot's spot (corneal) E50.1
                follicular keratosis E50.8
                keratomalacia E50.4
                manifestations NEC E50.8
                night blindness E50.5
                scar of cornea, xerophthalmic E50.6
                xeroderma E50.8
                xerophthalmia E50.7
                xerosis
                    conjunctival E50.0
                        and Bitot's spot E50.1
                    cornea E50.2
                        and ulceration E50.3
            sequelae E64.1
        B (complex) NOS E53.9
            with
                beriberi (dry) E51.11
                    wet E51.12
                pellagra E52
        B1 NOS E51.9
            beriberi (dry) E51.11
                with circulatory system manifestations E51.11
                wet E51.12
        B12 E53.8
        B2 (riboflavin) E53.0
        B6 E53.1
        C E54
            sequelae E64.2
        D E55.9
            with
                adult osteomalacia M83.8
                rickets — *see* Rickets
            25-hydroxylase E83.32
        E E56.0
        folic acid E53.8
        G E53.0
        group B E53.9

Deficiency, deficient — *continued*
    vitamin — *continued*
        group B — *continued*
            specified NEC E53.8
        H (biotin) E53.8
        K E56.1
            of newborn P53
        nicotinic E52
        P E56.8
        PP (pellagra-preventing) E52
        specified NEC E56.8
        thiamin E51.9
            beriberi — *see* Beriberi
    zinc, dietary E60
Deficit (*see also* Deficiency)
    attention and concentration R41.840
        disorder — *see* Attention, deficit
        following
            cerebral infarction I69.310
            cerebrovascular disease I69.910
                specified disease NEC I69.810
            nontraumatic
                intracerebral hemorrhage I69.110
                specified intracranial hemorrhage NEC I69.210
                subarachnoid hemorrhage I69.010
    cognitive
        communication R41.841
        emotional
            following
                cerebral infarction I69.315
                cerebrovascular disease I69.915
                    specified disease NEC I69.815
                nontraumatic
                    intracerebral hemorrhage I69.115
                    specified intracranial hemorrhage NEC
                        I69.215
                    subarachnoid hemorrhage I69.015
        following
            cerebral infarction I69.319
            cerebrovascular disease I69.919
                specified disease NEC I69.819
            nontraumatic
                intracerebral hemorrhage I69.119
                specified intracranial hemorrhage NEC I69.219
                subarachnoid hemorrhage I69.019
        social
            following
                cerebral infarction I69.315
                cerebrovascular disease I69.915
                    specified disease NEC I69.815
                nontraumatic
                    intracerebral hemorrhage I69.115
                    specified intracranial hemorrhage NEC
                        I69.215
                    subarachnoid hemorrhage I69.015
    cognitive NEC R41.89
        following
            cerebral infarction I69.318
            cerebrovascular disease I69.918
                specified disease NEC I69.818
            nontraumatic
                intracerebral hemorrhage I69.118
                specified intracranial hemorrhage NEC I69.218
                subarachnoid hemorrhage I69.018
    concentration R41.840
    executive function R41.844
        following
            cerebral infarction I69.314
            cerebrovascular disease I69.914
                specified disease NEC I69.814
            nontraumatic
                intracerebral hemorrhage I69.114
                specified intracranial hemorrhage NEC I69.214
                subarachnoid hemorrhage I69.014
    frontal lobe R41.844
        following
            cerebral infarction I69.314
            cerebrovascular disease I69.914
                specified disease NEC I69.814
            nontraumatic
                intracerebral hemorrhage I69.114
                specified intracranial hemorrhage NEC I69.214
                subarachnoid hemorrhage I69.014
    memory
        following
            cerebral infarction I69.311
            cerebrovascular disease I69.911
                specified disease NEC I69.811

Deficit — *continued*
    memory — *continued*
        following — *continued*
            nontraumatic
                intracerebral hemorrhage I69.111
                specified intracranial hemorrhage NEC I69.211
                subarachnoid hemorrhage I69.011
    neurologic NEC R29.818
        ischemic
            reversible (RIND) I63.9
                prolonged (PRIND) I63.9
    oxygen R09.02
    prolonged reversible ischemic neurologic (PRIND) I63.9
    psychomotor R41.843
        following
            cerebral infarction I69.313
            cerebrovascular disease I69.913
                specified disease NEC I69.813
            nontraumatic
                intracerebral hemorrhage I69.113
                specified intracranial hemorrhage NEC I69.213
                subarachnoid hemorrhage I69.013
    visuospatial R41.842
        following
            cerebral infarction I69.312
            cerebrovascular disease I69.912
                specified disease NEC I69.812
            nontraumatic
                intracerebral hemorrhage I69.112
                specified intracranial hemorrhage NEC I69.212
                subarachnoid hemorrhage I69.012
Deflection
    radius — *see* Deformity, limb, specified type NEC,
        forearm
    septum (acquired) (nasal) (nose) J34.2
    spine — *see* Curvature, spine
    turbinate (nose) J34.2
Defluvium
    capillorum — *see* Alopecia
    ciliorum — *see* Madarosis
    unguium L60.8
Deformity Q89.9
    abdomen, congenital Q89.9
    abdominal wall
        acquired M95.8
        congenital Q79.59
    acquired (unspecified site) M95.9
    adrenal gland Q89.1
    alimentary tract, congenital Q45.9
        upper Q40.9
    ankle (joint) (acquired) (*see also* Deformity, limb, lower
        leg)
        abduction — *see* Contraction, joint, ankle
        congenital Q68.8
        contraction — *see* Contraction, joint, ankle
        specified type NEC — *see* Deformity, limb, foot,
            specified NEC
    anus (acquired) K62.89
        congenital Q43.9
    aorta (arch) (congenital) Q25.40
        acquired I77.89
    aortic
        arch, acquired I77.89
        cusp or valve (congenital) Q23.8
            acquired (*see also* Endocarditis, aortic) I35.8
    arm (acquired) (upper) (*see also* Deformity, limb, upper
        arm)
        congenital Q68.8
        forearm — *see* Deformity, limb, forearm
    artery (congenital) (peripheral) NOS Q27.9
        acquired I77.89
        coronary (acquired) I25.9
            congenital Q24.5
        umbilical Q27.0
    atrial septal Q21.1
    auditory canal (external) (congenital) (*see also* Malfor-
        mation, ear, external)
        acquired — *see* Disorder, ear, external, specified
            type NEC
    auricle
        ear (congenital) (*see also* Malformation, ear, exter-
            nal)
        acquired — *see* Disorder, pinna, deformity
    back — *see* Dorsopathy, deforming
    bile duct (common) (congenital) (hepatic) Q44.5
        acquired K83.8
    biliary duct or passage (congenital) Q44.5
        acquired K83.8

Deformity — *continued*
- bladder (neck) (trigone) (sphincter) (acquired) N32.89
  - congenital Q64.79
- bone (acquired) NOS M95.9
  - congenital Q79.9
  - turbinate M95.0
- brain (congenital) Q04.9
  - acquired G93.89
  - reduction Q04.3
- breast (acquired) N64.89
  - congenital Q83.9
  - reconstructed N65.0
- bronchus (congenital) Q32.4
  - acquired NEC J98.09
- bursa, congenital Q79.9
- canaliculi (lacrimalis) (acquired) (*see also* Disorder, lacrimal system, changes)
  - congenital Q10.6
- canthus, acquired — *see* Disorder, eyelid, specified type NEC
- capillary (acquired) I78.8
- cardiovascular system, congenital Q28.9
- caruncle, lacrimal (acquired) (*see also* Disorder, lacrimal system, changes)
  - congenital Q10.6
- cascade, stomach K31.2
- cecum (congenital) Q43.9
  - acquired K63.89
- cerebral, acquired G93.89
  - congenital Q04.9
- cervix (uterus) (acquired) NEC N88.8
  - congenital Q51.9
- cheek (acquired) M95.2
  - congenital Q18.9
- chest (acquired) (wall) M95.4
  - congenital Q67.8
  - sequelae (late effect) of rickets E64.3
- chin (acquired) M95.2
  - congenital Q18.9
- choroid (congenital) Q14.3
  - acquired H31.8
  - plexus Q07.8
    - acquired G96.19
- cicatricial — *see* Cicatrix
- cilia, acquired — *see* Disorder, eyelid, specified type NEC
- clavicle (acquired) M95.8
  - congenital Q68.8
- clitoris (congenital) Q52.6
  - acquired N90.89
- clubfoot — *see* Clubfoot
- coccyx (acquired) — *see* subcategory M43.8 ☑
- colon (congenital) Q43.9
  - acquired K63.89
- concha (ear), congenital (*see also* Malformation, ear, external)
  - acquired — *see* Disorder, pinna, deformity
- cornea (acquired) H18.70
  - congenital Q13.4
  - descemetocele — *see* Descemetocele
  - ectasia — *see* Ectasia, cornea
  - specified NEC H18.79- ☑
  - staphyloma — *see* Staphyloma, cornea
- coronary artery (acquired) I25.9
  - congenital Q24.5
- cranium (acquired) — *see* Deformity, skull
- cricoid cartilage (congenital) Q31.8
  - acquired J38.7
- cystic duct (congenital) Q44.5
  - acquired K82.8
- Dandy-Walker Q03.1
  - with spina bifida — *see* Spina bifida
- diaphragm (congenital) Q79.1
  - acquired J98.6
- digestive organ NOS Q45.9
- ductus arteriosus Q25.0
- duodenal bulb K31.89
- duodenum (congenital) Q43.9
  - acquired K31.89
- dura — *see* Deformity, meninges
- ear (acquired) (*see also* Disorder, pinna, deformity)
  - congenital (external) Q17.9
    - internal Q16.5
    - middle Q16.4
      - ossicles Q16.3
    - ossicles Q16.3
- ectodermal (congenital) NEC Q84.9
- ejaculatory duct (congenital) Q55.4

Deformity — *continued*
- ejaculatory duct — *continued*
  - acquired N50.79
- elbow (joint) (acquired) (*see also* Deformity, limb, upper arm)
  - congenital Q68.8
  - contraction — *see* Contraction, joint, elbow
- endocrine gland NEC Q89.2
- epididymis (congenital) Q55.4
  - acquired N50.89
- epiglottis (congenital) Q31.8
  - acquired J38.7
- esophagus (congenital) Q39.9
  - acquired K22.8
- eustachian tube (congenital) NEC Q17.8
- eye, congenital Q15.9
- eyebrow (congenital) Q18.8
- eyelid (acquired) (*see also* Disorder, eyelid, specified type NEC)
  - congenital Q10.3
- face (acquired) M95.2
  - congenital Q18.9
- fallopian tube, acquired N83.8
- femur (acquired) — *see* Deformity, limb, specified type NEC, thigh
- fetal
  - with fetopelvic disproportion O33.7 ☑
  - causing obstructed labor O66.3
- finger (acquired) M20.00- ☑
  - boutonniere M20.02- ☑
  - congenital Q68.1
  - flexion contracture — *see* Contraction, joint, hand
  - mallet finger M20.01- ☑
  - specified NEC M20.09- ☑
  - swan-neck M20.03- ☑
- flexion (joint) (acquired) (*see also* Deformity, limb, flexion) M21.20
  - congenital NOS Q74.9
    - hip Q65.89
- foot (acquired) (*see also* Deformity, limb, lower leg) M21.
  - cavovarus (congenital) Q66.1
  - congenital NOS Q66.9
    - specified type NEC Q66.89
  - specified type NEC — *see* Deformity, limb, foot, specified NEC
  - valgus (congenital) Q66.6
    - acquired — *see* Deformity, valgus, ankle
  - varus (congenital) NEC Q66.3
    - acquired — *see* Deformity, varus, ankle
- forearm (acquired) (*see also* Deformity, limb, forearm)
  - congenital Q68.8
- forehead (acquired) M95.2
  - congenital Q75.8
- frontal bone (acquired) M95.2
  - congenital Q75.8
- gallbladder (congenital) Q44.1
  - acquired K82.8
- gastrointestinal tract (congenital) NOS Q45.9
  - acquired K63.89
- genitalia, genital organ(s) or system NEC
  - female (congenital) Q52.9
    - acquired N94.89
    - external Q52.70
  - male (congenital) Q55.9
    - acquired N50.89
- globe (eye) (congenital) Q15.8
  - acquired H44.89
- gum, acquired NEC K06.8
- hand (acquired) — *see* Deformity, limb, hand
  - congenital Q68.1
- head (acquired) M95.2
  - congenital Q75.8
- heart (congenital) Q24.9
  - septum Q21.9
    - auricular Q21.1
    - ventricular Q21.0
  - valve (congenital) NEC Q24.8
    - acquired — *see* Endocarditis
- heel (acquired) — *see* Deformity, foot
- hepatic duct (congenital) Q44.5
  - acquired K83.8
- hip (joint) (acquired) (*see also* Deformity, limb, thigh)
  - congenital Q65.9
  - due to (previous) juvenile osteochondrosis — *see* Coxa, plana
  - flexion — *see* Contraction, joint, hip
- hourglass — *see* Contraction, hourglass
- humerus (acquired) M21.82- ☑

Deformity — *continued*
- humerus — *continued*
  - congenital Q74.0
- hypophyseal (congenital) Q89.2
- ileocecal (coil) (valve) (acquired) K63.89
  - congenital Q43.9
- ileum (congenital) Q43.9
  - acquired K63.89
- ilium (acquired) M95.5
  - congenital Q74.2
- integument (congenital) Q84.9
- intervertebral cartilage or disc (acquired) — *see* Disorder, disc, specified NEC
- intestine (large) (small) (congenital) NOS Q43.9
  - acquired K63.89
- intrinsic minus or plus (hand) — *see* Deformity, limb, specified type NEC, forearm
- iris (acquired) H21.89
  - congenital Q13.2
- ischium (acquired) M95.5
  - congenital Q74.2
- jaw (acquired) (congenital) M26.9
- joint (acquired) NEC M21.90
  - congenital Q68.8
  - elbow M21.92- ☑
  - hand M21.94- ☑
  - hip M21.95- ☑
  - knee M21.96- ☑
  - shoulder M21.92- ☑
  - wrist M21.93- ☑
- kidney(s) (calyx) (pelvis) (congenital) Q63.9
  - acquired N28.89
  - artery (congenital) Q27.2
    - acquired I77.89
- Klippel-Feil (brevicollis) Q76.1
- knee (acquired) NEC (*see also* Deformity, limb, lower leg)
  - congenital Q68.2
- labium (majus) (minus) (congenital) Q52.79
  - acquired N90.89
- lacrimal passages or duct (congenital) NEC Q10.6
  - acquired — *see* Disorder, lacrimal system, changes
- larynx (muscle) (congenital) Q31.8
  - acquired J38.7
  - web (glottic) Q31.0
- leg (upper) (acquired) NEC (*see also* Deformity, limb, thigh)
  - congenital Q68.8
  - lower leg — *see* Deformity, limb, lower leg
- lens (acquired) H27.8
  - congenital Q12.9
- lid (fold) (acquired) (*see also* Disorder, eyelid, specified type NEC)
  - congenital Q10.3
- ligament (acquired) — *see* Disorder, ligament
  - congenital Q79.9
- limb (acquired) M21.90
  - clawfoot M21.53- ☑
  - clawhand M21.51- ☑
  - clubfoot M21.54- ☑
  - clubhand M21.52- ☑
  - congenital, except reduction deformity Q74.9
  - flat foot M21.4- ☑
  - flexion M21.20
    - ankle M21.27- ☑
    - elbow M21.22- ☑
    - finger M21.24- ☑
    - hip M21.25- ☑
    - knee M21.26- ☑
    - shoulder M21.21- ☑
    - toe M21.27- ☑
    - wrist M21.23- ☑
  - foot
    - claw — *see* Deformity, limb, clawfoot
    - club — *see* Deformity, limb, clubfoot
    - drop M21.37- ☑
    - flat — *see* Deformity, limb, flat foot
    - specified NEC M21.6X- ☑
  - forearm M21.93- ☑
  - hand M21.94- ☑
  - lower leg M21.96- ☑
  - specified type NEC M21.80
    - forearm M21.83- ☑
    - lower leg M21.86- ☑
    - thigh M21.85- ☑
    - upper arm M21.82- ☑
  - thigh M21.95- ☑

Deformity — *continued*
- limb — *continued*
  - unequal length M21.70
    - short site is
      - femur M21.75- ☑
      - fibula M21.76- ☑
      - humerus M21.72- ☑
      - radius M21.73- ☑
      - tibia M21.76- ☑
      - ulna M21.73- ☑
    - upper arm M21.92- ☑
  - valgus — *see* Deformity, valgus
  - varus — *see* Deformity, varus
  - wrist drop M21.33- ☑
- lip (acquired) NEC K13.0
  - congenital Q38.0
- liver (congenital) Q44.7
  - acquired K76.89
- lumbosacral (congenital) (joint) (region) Q76.49
  - acquired — *see* subcategory M43.8 ☑
  - kyphosis — *see* Kyphosis, congenital
  - lordosis — *see* Lordosis, congenital
- lung (congenital) Q33.9
  - acquired J98.4
- lymphatic system, congenital Q89.9
- Madelung's (radius) Q74.0
- mandible (acquired) (congenital) M26.9
- maxilla (acquired) (congenital) M26.9
- meninges or membrane (congenital) Q07.9
  - cerebral Q04.8
    - acquired G96.19
  - spinal cord (congenital) G96.19
    - acquired G96.19
- metacarpus (acquired) — *see* Deformity, limb, forearm
  - congenital Q74.0
- metatarsus (acquired) — *see* Deformity, foot
  - congenital Q66.9
- middle ear (congenital) Q16.4
  - ossicles Q16.3
- mitral (leaflets) (valve) I05.8
  - parachute Q23.2
  - stenosis, congenital Q23.2
- mouth (acquired) K13.79
  - congenital Q38.6
- multiple, congenital NEC Q89.7
- muscle (acquired) M62.89
  - congenital Q79.9
    - sternocleidomastoid Q68.0
- musculoskeletal system (acquired) M95.9
  - congenital Q79.9
  - specified NEC M95.8
- nail (acquired) L60.8
  - congenital Q84.6
- nasal — *see* Deformity, nose
- neck (acquired) M95.3
  - congenital Q18.9
    - sternocleidomastoid Q68.0
- nervous system (congenital) Q07.9
- nipple (congenital) Q83.9
  - acquired N64.89
- nose (acquired) (cartilage) M95.0
  - bone (turbinate) M95.0
  - congenital Q30.9
    - bent or squashed Q67.4
  - saddle M95.0
    - syphilitic A50.57
  - septum (acquired) J34.2
    - congenital Q30.8
  - sinus (wall) (congenital) Q30.8
    - acquired M95.0
  - syphilitic (congenital) A50.57
    - late A52.73
- ocular muscle (congenital) Q10.3
  - acquired — *see* Strabismus, mechanical
- opticociliary vessels (congenital) Q13.2
- orbit (eye) (acquired) H05.30
  - atrophy — *see* Atrophy, orbit
  - congenital Q10.7
  - due to
    - bone disease NEC H05.32- ☑
    - trauma or surgery H05.33- ☑
  - enlargement — *see* Enlargement, orbit
  - exostosis — *see* Exostosis, orbit
- organ of Corti (congenital) Q16.5
- ovary (congenital) Q50.39
  - acquired N83.8
- oviduct, acquired N83.8
- palate (congenital) Q38.5

Deformity — *continued*
- palate — *continued*
  - acquired M27.8
  - cleft (congenital) — *see* Cleft, palate
- pancreas (congenital) Q45.3
  - acquired K86.89
- parathyroid (gland) Q89.2
- parotid (gland) (congenital) Q38.4
  - acquired K11.8
- patella (acquired) — *see* Disorder, patella, specified NEC
- pelvis, pelvic (acquired) (bony) M95.5
  - with disproportion (fetopelvic) O33.0
    - causing obstructed labor O65.0
  - congenital Q74.2
  - rachitic sequelae (late effect) E64.3
- penis (glans) (congenital) Q55.69
  - acquired N48.89
- pericardium (congenital) Q24.8
  - acquired — *see* Pericarditis
- pharynx (congenital) Q38.8
  - acquired J39.2
- pinna, acquired (*see also* Disorder, pinna, deformity)
  - congenital Q17.9
- pituitary (congenital) Q89.2
- posture — *see* Dorsopathy, deforming
- prepuce (congenital) Q55.69
  - acquired N47.8
- prostate (congenital) Q55.4
  - acquired N42.89
- pupil (congenital) Q13.2
  - acquired — *see* Abnormality, pupillary
- pylorus (congenital) Q40.3
  - acquired K31.89
- rachitic (acquired), old or healed E64.3
- radius (acquired) (*see also* Deformity, limb, forearm)
  - congenital Q68.8
- rectum (congenital) Q43.9
  - acquired K62.89
- reduction (extremity) (limb), congenital (*see also* condition and site) Q73.8
  - brain Q04.3
  - lower — *see* Defect, reduction, lower limb
  - upper — *see* Defect, reduction, upper limb
- renal — *see* Deformity, kidney
- respiratory system (congenital) Q34.9
- rib (acquired) M95.4
  - congenital Q76.6
    - cervical Q76.5
- rotation (joint) (acquired) — *see* Deformity, limb, specified site NEC
  - congenital Q74.9
  - hip — *see* Deformity, limb, specified type NEC, thigh
    - congenital Q65.89
- sacroiliac joint (congenital) — *see* subcategory Q74.2
  - acquired — *see* subcategory M43.8 ☑
- sacrum (acquired) — *see* subcategory M43.8 ☑
- saddle
  - back — *see* Lordosis
  - nose M95.0
    - syphilitic A50.57
- salivary gland or duct (congenital) Q38.4
  - acquired K11.8
- scapula (acquired) M95.8
  - congenital Q68.8
- scrotum (congenital) (*see also* Malformation, testis and scrotum)
  - acquired N50.89
- seminal vesicles (congenital) Q55.4
  - acquired N50.89
- septum, nasal (acquired) J34.2
- shoulder (joint) (acquired) — *see* Deformity, limb, upper arm
  - congenital Q74.0
  - contraction — *see* Contraction, joint, shoulder
- sigmoid (flexure) (congenital) Q43.9
  - acquired K63.89
- skin (congenital) Q82.9
- skull (acquired) M95.2
  - congenital Q75.8
    - with
      - anencephaly Q00.0
      - encephalocele — *see* Encephalocele
      - hydrocephalus Q03.9
        - with spina bifida — *see* Spina bifida, by site, with hydrocephalus
      - microcephaly Q02

Deformity — *continued*
- soft parts, organs or tissues (of pelvis)
  - in pregnancy or childbirth NEC O34.8- ☑
    - causing obstructed labor O65.5
- spermatic cord (congenital) Q55.4
  - acquired N50.89
    - torsion — *see* Torsion, spermatic cord
- spinal — *see* Dorsopathy, deforming
  - column (acquired) — *see* Dorsopathy, deforming
  - congenital Q67.5
  - cord (congenital) Q06.9
    - acquired G95.89
  - nerve root (congenital) Q07.9
- spine (acquired) (*see also* Dorsopathy, deforming)
  - congenital Q67.5
  - rachitic E64.3
  - specified NEC — *see* Dorsopathy, deforming, specified NEC
- spleen
  - acquired D73.89
  - congenital Q89.09
- Sprengel's (congenital) Q74.0
- sternocleidomastoid (muscle), congenital Q68.0
- sternum (acquired) M95.4
  - congenital NEC Q76.7
- stomach (congenital) Q40.3
  - acquired K31.89
- submandibular gland (congenital) Q38.4
- submaxillary gland (congenital) Q38.4
  - acquired K11.8
- talipes — *see* Talipes
- testis (congenital) (*see also* Malformation, testis and scrotum)
  - acquired N44.8
  - torsion — *see* Torsion, testis
- thigh (acquired) (*see also* Deformity, limb, thigh)
  - congenital NEC Q68.8
- thorax (acquired) (wall) M95.4
  - congenital Q67.8
  - sequelae of rickets E64.3
- thumb (acquired) (*see also* Deformity, finger)
  - congenital NEC Q68.1
- thymus (tissue) (congenital) Q89.2
- thyroid (gland) (congenital) Q89.2
  - cartilage Q31.8
    - acquired J38.7
- tibia (acquired) (*see also* Deformity, limb, specified type NEC, lower leg)
  - congenital NEC Q68.8
  - saber (syphilitic) A50.56
- toe (acquired) M20.6- ☑
  - congenital Q66.9
  - hallux rigidus M20.2- ☑
  - hallux valgus M20.1- ☑
  - hallux varus M20.3- ☑
  - hammer toe M20.4- ☑
  - specified NEC M20.5X- ☑
- tongue (congenital) Q38.3
  - acquired K14.8
- tooth, teeth K00.2
- trachea (rings) (congenital) Q32.1
  - acquired J39.8
- transverse aortic arch (congenital) Q25.49
- tricuspid (leaflets) (valve) I07.8
  - atresia or stenosis Q22.4
  - Ebstein's Q22.5
- trunk (acquired) M95.8
  - congenital Q89.9
- ulna (acquired) (*see also* Deformity, limb, forearm)
  - congenital NEC Q68.8
- urachus, congenital Q64.4
- ureter (opening) (congenital) Q62.8
  - acquired N28.89
- urethra (congenital) Q64.79
  - acquired N36.8
- urinary tract (congenital) Q64.9
  - urachus Q64.4
- uterus (congenital) Q51.9
  - acquired N85.8
- uvula (congenital) Q38.5
- vagina (acquired) N89.8
  - congenital Q52.4
- valgus NEC M21.00
  - ankle M21.07- ☑
  - elbow M21.02- ☑
  - hip M21.05- ☑
  - knee M21.06- ☑
- valve, valvular (congenital) (heart) Q24.8

Deformity — *continued*
 valve, valvular — *continued*
  acquired — *see* Endocarditis
 varus NEC M21.10
  ankle M21.17- ☑
  elbow M21.12- ☑
  hip M21.15 ☑
  knee M21.16- ☑
  tibia — *see* Osteochondrosis, juvenile, tibia
 vas deferens (congenital) Q55.4
  acquired N50.89
 vein (congenital) Q27.9
  great Q26.9
 vertebra — *see* Dorsopathy, deforming
 vertical talus (congenital) Q66.80
  left foot Q66.82
  right foot Q66.81
 vesicourethral orifice (acquired) N32.89
  congenital NEC Q64.79
 vessels of optic papilla (congenital) Q14.2
 visual field (contraction) — *see* Defect, visual field
 vitreous body, acquired H43.89
 vulva (congenital) Q52.79
  acquired N90.89
 wrist (joint) (acquired) (*see also* Deformity, limb, fore-arm)
  congenital Q68.8
  contraction — *see* Contraction, joint, wrist

Degeneration, degenerative
 adrenal (capsule) (fatty) (gland) (hyaline) (infectional) E27.8
 amyloid (*see also* Amyloidosis) E85.9
 anterior cornua, spinal cord G12.29
 anterior labral S43.49- ☑
 aorta, aortic I70.0
  fatty I77.89
 aortic valve (heart) — *see* Endocarditis, aortic
 arteriovascular — *see* Arteriosclerosis
 artery, arterial (atheromatous) (calcareous) (*see also* Arteriosclerosis)
  cerebral, amyloid E85.4 [I68.0]
  medial — *see* Arteriosclerosis, extremities
 articular cartilage NEC — *see* Derangement, joint, articular cartilage, by site
 atheromatous — *see* Arteriosclerosis
 basal nuclei or ganglia G23.9
  specified NEC G23.8
 bone NEC — *see* Disorder, bone, specified type NEC
 brachial plexus G54.0
 brain (cortical) (progressive) G31.9
  alcoholic G31.2
  arteriosclerotic I67.2
  childhood G31.9
   specified NEC G31.89
  cystic G31.89
   congenital Q04.6
  in
   alcoholism G31.2
   beriberi E51.2
   cerebrovascular disease I67.9
   congenital hydrocephalus Q03.9
    with spina bifida (*see also* Spina bifida)
   Fabry-Anderson disease E75.21
   Gaucher's disease E75.22
   Hunter's syndrome E76.1
   lipidosis
    cerebral E75.4
    generalized E75.6
   mucopolysaccharidosis — *see* Mucopolysaccharidosis
   myxedema E03.9 [G32.89]
   neoplastic disease (*see also* Neoplasm) D49.6 [G32.89]
   Niemann-Pick disease E75.249 [G32.89]
   sphingolipidosis E75.3 [G32.89]
   vitamin B12 deficiency E53.8 [G32.89]
  senile NEC G31.1
 breast N64.89
 Bruch's membrane — *see* Degeneration, choroid
 capillaries (fatty) I78.8
  amyloid E85.89 [I79.8]
 cardiac (*see also* Degeneration, myocardial)
  valve, valvular — *see* Endocarditis
 cardiorenal — *see* Hypertension, cardiorenal
 cardiovascular (*see also* Disease, cardiovascular)
  renal — *see* Hypertension, cardiorenal
 cerebellar NOS G31.9
  alcoholic G31.2

Degeneration, degenerative — *continued*
 cerebellar — *continued*
  primary (hereditary) (sporadic) G11.9
 cerebral — *see* Degeneration, brain
 cerebrovascular I67.9
  due to hypertension I67.4
 cervical plexus G54.2
 cervix N88.8
  due to radiation (intended effect) N88.8
   adverse effect or misadventure N99.89
 chamber angle H21.21- ☑
 changes, spine or vertebra — *see* Spondylosis
 chorioretinal (*see also* Degeneration, choroid)
  hereditary H31.20
 choroid (colloid) (drusen) H31.10- ☑
  atrophy — *see* Atrophy, choroidal
  hereditary — *see* Dystrophy, choroidal, hereditary
 ciliary body H21.22- ☑
 cochlear — *see* subcategory H83.8 ☑
 combined (spinal cord) (subacute) E53.8 [G32.0]
  with anemia (pernicious) D51.0 [G32.0]
   due to dietary vitamin B12 deficiency D51.3 [G32.0]
  in (due to)
   vitamin B12 deficiency E53.8 [G32.0]
    anemia D51.9 [G32.0]
 conjunctiva H11.10
  concretions — *see* Concretion, conjunctiva
  deposits — *see* Deposit, conjunctiva
  pigmentations — *see* Pigmentation, conjunctiva
  pinguecula — *see* Pinguecula
  xerosis — *see* Xerosis, conjunctiva
 cornea H18.40
  calcerous H18.43
   band keratopathy H18.42- ☑
  familial, hereditary — *see* Dystrophy, cornea
  hyaline (of old scars) H18.49
  keratomalacia — *see* Keratomalacia
  nodular H18.45- ☑
  peripheral H18.46- ☑
  senile H18.41- ☑
  specified type NEC H18.49
 cortical (cerebellar) (parenchymatous) G31.89
  alcoholic G31.2
  diffuse, due to arteriopathy I67.2
 corticobasal G31.85
 cutis L98.8
  amyloid E85.4 [L99]
 dental pulp K04.2
 disc disease — *see* Degeneration, intervertebral disc NEC
 dorsolateral (spinal cord) — *see* Degeneration, combined
 extrapyramidal G25.9
 eye, macular (*see also* Degeneration, macula)
  congenital or hereditary — *see* Dystrophy, retina
 facet joints — *see* Spondylosis
 fatty
  liver NEC K76.0
   alcoholic K70.0
 grey matter (brain) (Alpers') G31.81
 heart (*see also* Degeneration, myocardial)
  amyloid E85.4 [I43]
  atheromatous — *see* Disease, heart, ischemic, atherosclerotic
  ischemic — *see* Disease, heart, ischemic
 hepatolenticular (Wilson's) E83.01
 hepatorenal K76.7
 hyaline (diffuse) (generalized)
  localized — *see* Degeneration, by site
 infrapatellar fat pad M79.4
 intervertebral disc NOS
  with
   myelopathy — *see* Disorder, disc, with, myelopathy
   radiculitis or radiculopathy — *see* Disorder, disc, with, radiculopathy
  cervical, cervicothoracic — *see* Disorder, disc, cervical, degeneration
   with
    myelopathy — *see* Disorder, disc, cervical, with myelopathy
    neuritis, radiculitis or radiculopathy — *see* Disorder, disc, cervical, with neuritis
  lumbar region M51.36
   with
    myelopathy M51.06

Degeneration, degenerative — *continued*
 intervertebral disc — *continued*
  lumbar region — *continued*
   with — *continued*
    neuritis, radiculitis, radiculopathy or sciatica M51.16
  lumbosacral region M51.37
   with
    neuritis, radiculitis, radiculopathy or sciatica M51.17
  sacrococcygeal region M53.3
  thoracic region M51.34
   with
    myelopathy M51.04
    neuritis, radiculitis, radiculopathy M51.14
  thoracolumbar region M51.35
   with
    myelopathy M51.05
    neuritis, radiculitis, radiculopathy M51.15
 intestine, amyloid E85.4
 iris (pigmentary) H21.23- ☑
 ischemic — *see* Ischemia
 joint disease — *see* Osteoarthritis
 kidney N28.89
  amyloid E85.4 [N29]
  cystic, congenital Q61.9
  fatty N28.89
  polycystic Q61.3
   adult type (autosomal dominant) Q61.2
   infantile type (autosomal recessive) NEC Q61.19
    collecting duct dilatation Q61.11
 Kuhnt-Junius (*see also* Degeneration, macula) H35.32- ☑
 lens — *see* Cataract
 lenticular (familial) (progressive) (Wilson's) (with cirrhosis of liver) E83.01
 liver (diffuse) NEC K76.89
  amyloid E85.4 [K77]
  cystic K76.89
   congenital Q44.6
  fatty NEC K76.0
   alcoholic K70.0
  hypertrophic K76.89
  parenchymatous, acute or subacute K72.00
   with coma K72.01
  pigmentary K76.89
  toxic (acute) K71.9
 lung J98.4
 lymph gland I89.8
  hyaline I89.8
 macula, macular (acquired) (age-related) (senile) H35.30
  angioid streaks H35.33
  atrophic age-related H35.31- ☑
  congenital or hereditary — *see* Dystrophy, retina
  cystoid H35.35- ☑
  drusen H35.36- ☑
  dry age-related H35.31- ☑
  exudative H35.32- ☑
  hole H35.34- ☑
  nonexudative H35.31- ☑
  puckering H35.37- ☑
  toxic H35.38- ☑
  wet age-related H35.32- ☑
 membranous labyrinth, congenital (causing impairment of hearing) Q16.5
 meniscus — *see* Derangement, meniscus
 mitral — *see* Insufficiency, mitral
 Mönckeberg's — *see* Arteriosclerosis, extremities
 motor centers, senile G31.1
 multi-system G90.3
 mural — *see* Degeneration, myocardial
 muscle (fatty) (fibrous) (hyaline) (progressive) M62.89
  heart — *see* Degeneration, myocardial
 myelin, central nervous system G37.9
 myocardial, myocardium (fatty) (hyaline) (senile) I51.5
  with rheumatic fever (conditions in I00) I09.0
   active, acute or subacute I01.2
    with chorea I02.0
   inactive or quiescent (with chorea) I09.0
  hypertensive — *see* Hypertension, heart
  rheumatic — *see* Degeneration, myocardial, with rheumatic fever
 syphilitic A52.06
 nasal sinus (mucosa) J32.9
  frontal J32.1
  maxillary J32.0
 nerve — *see* Disorder, nerve

Degeneration, degenerative — continued
  nervous system G31.9
    alcoholic G31.2
    amyloid E85.4 [G99.8]
    autonomic G90.9
    fatty G31.89
    specified NEC G31.89
  nipple N64.89
  olivopontocerebellar (hereditary) (familial) G23.8
  osseous labyrinth — see subcategory H83.8 ☑
  ovary N83.8
    cystic N83.20- ☑
    microcystic N83.20- ☑
  pallidal pigmentary (progressive) G23.0
  pancreas K86.89
    tuberculous A18.83
  penis N48.89
  pigmentary (diffuse) (general)
    localized — see Degeneration, by site
    pallidal (progressive) G23.0
  pineal gland E34.8
  pituitary (gland) E23.6
  popliteal fat pad M79.4
  posterolateral (spinal cord) — see Degeneration, combined
  pulmonary valve (heart) I37.8
  pulp (tooth) K04.2
  pupillary margin H21.24- ☑
  renal — see Degeneration, kidney
  retina H35.9
    hereditary (cerebroretinal) (congenital) (juvenile) (macula) (peripheral) (pigmentary) — see Dystrophy, retina
    Kuhnt-Junius (see also Degeneration, macula) H35.32- ☑
    macula (cystic) (exudative) (hole) (nonexudative) (pseudohole) (senile) (toxic) — see Degeneration, macula
    peripheral H35.40
      lattice H35.41- ☑
      microcystoid H35.42- ☑
      paving stone H35.43- ☑
      secondary
        pigmentary H35.45- ☑
        vitreoretinal H35.46- ☑
      senile reticular H35.44- ☑
    pigmentary (primary) (see also Dystrophy, retina)
      secondary — see Degeneration, retina, peripheral, secondary
    posterior pole — see Degeneration, macula
  saccule, congenital (causing impairment of hearing) Q16.5
  senile R54
    brain G31.1
    cardiac, heart or myocardium — see Degeneration, myocardial
    motor centers G31.1
    vascular — see Arteriosclerosis
  sinus (cystic) (see also Sinusitis)
    polypoid J33.1
  skin L98.8
    amyloid E85.4 [L99]
    colloid L98.8
  spinal (cord) G31.89
    amyloid E85.4 [G32.89]
    combined (subacute) — see Degeneration, combined
    dorsolateral — see Degeneration, combined
    familial NEC G31.89
    fatty G31.89
    funicular — see Degeneration, combined
    posterolateral — see Degeneration, combined
    subacute combined — see Degeneration, combined
    tuberculous A17.81
  spleen D73.0
    amyloid E85.4 [D77]
  stomach K31.89
  striatonigral G23.2
  suprarenal (capsule) (gland) E27.8
  synovial membrane (pulpy) — see Disorder, synovium, specified type NEC
  tapetoretinal — see Dystrophy, retina
  thymus (gland) E32.8
    fatty E32.8
  thyroid (gland) E07.89
  tricuspid (heart) (valve) I07.9
  tuberculous NEC — see Tuberculosis
  turbinate J34.89

Degeneration, degenerative — continued
  uterus (cystic) N85.8
  vascular (senile) — see Arteriosclerosis
    hypertensive — see Hypertension
  vitreoretinal, secondary — see Degeneration, retina, peripheral, secondary, vitreoretinal
  vitreous (body) H43.81- ☑
  Wallerian — see Disorder, nerve
  Wilson's hepatolenticular E83.01
Deglutition
  paralysis R13.0
    hysterical F44.4
  pneumonia J69.0
Degos' disease I77.89
Dehiscence (of)
  amputation stump T87.81
  cesarean wound O90.0
  closure of
    cornea T81.31 ☑
    craniotomy T81.32 ☑
    fascia (muscular) (superficial) T81.32 ☑
    internal organ or tissue T81.32 ☑
    laceration (external) (internal) T81.33 ☑
    ligament T81.32 ☑
    mucosa T81.31 ☑
    muscle or muscle flap T81.32 ☑
    ribs or rib cage T81.32 ☑
    skin and subcutaneous tissue (full-thickness) (superficial) T81.31 ☑
    skull T81.32 ☑
    sternum (sternotomy) T81.32 ☑
    tendon T81.32 ☑
    traumatic laceration (external) (internal) T81.33 ☑
  episiotomy O90.1
  operation wound NEC T81.31 ☑
    external operation wound (superficial) T81.31 ☑
    internal operation wound (deep) T81.32 ☑
  perineal wound (postpartum) O90.1
  traumatic injury wound repair T81.33 ☑
  wound T81.30 ☑
    traumatic repair T81.33 ☑
Dehydration E86.0
  newborn P74.1
Déjérine-Roussy syndrome G89.0
Déjérine-Sottas disease or neuropathy (hypertrophic) G60.0
Déjérine-Thomas atrophy G23.8
Delay, delayed
  any plane in pelvis
    complicating delivery O66.9
  birth or delivery NOS O63.9
  closure, ductus arteriosus (Botalli) P29.38
  coagulation — see Defect, coagulation
  conduction (cardiac) (ventricular) I45.9
  delivery, second twin, triplet, etc O63.2
  development R62.50
    global F88
    intellectual (specific) F81.9
    language F80.9
      due to hearing loss F80.4
    learning F81.9
    pervasive F84.9
    physiological R62.50
      specified stage NEC R62.0
    reading F81.0
    sexual E30.0
    speech F80.9
      due to hearing loss F80.4
    spelling F81.81
  ejaculation F52.32
  gastric emptying K30
  menarche E30.0
  menstruation (cause unknown) N91.0
  milestone R62.0
  passage of meconium (newborn) P76.0
  primary respiration P28.9
  puberty (constitutional) E30.0
  separation of umbilical cord P96.82
  sexual maturation, female E30.0
  sleep phase syndrome G47.21
  union, fracture — see Fracture, by site
  vaccination Z28.9
Deletion(s)
  autosome Q93.9
    identified by fluorescence in situ hybridization (FISH) Q93.89
    identified by in situ hybridization (ISH) Q93.89

Deletion(s) — continued
  chromosome
    with complex rearrangements NEC Q93.7
    part of NEC Q93.59
    seen only at prometaphase Q93.89
    short arm
      22q11.2 Q93.81
      4 Q93.3
      5p Q93.4
    specified NEC Q93.89
  long arm chromosome 18 or 21 Q93.89
    with complex rearrangements NEC Q93.7
  microdeletions NEC Q93.88
Delhi boil or button B55.1
Delinquency (juvenile) (neurotic) F91.8
  group Z72.810
Delinquent immunization status Z28.3
Delirium, delirious (acute or subacute) (not alcohol- or drug-induced) (with dementia) R41.0
  alcoholic (acute) (tremens) (withdrawal) F10.921
    with intoxication F10.921
      in
        abuse F10.121
        dependence F10.221
  due to (secondary to)
    alcohol
      intoxication F10.921
        in
          abuse F10.121
          dependence F10.221
      withdrawal F10.231
    amphetamine intoxication F15.921
      in
        abuse F15.121
        dependence F15.221
    anxiolytic
      intoxication F13.921
        in
          abuse F13.121
          dependence F13.221
      withdrawal F13.231
    cannabis intoxication (acute) F12.921
      in
        abuse F12.121
        dependence F12.221
    cocaine intoxication (acute) F14.921
      in
        abuse F14.121
        dependence F14.221
    general medical condition F05
    hallucinogen intoxication F16.921
      in
        abuse F16.121
        dependence F16.221
    hypnotic
      intoxication F13.921
        in
          abuse F13.121
          dependence F13.221
      withdrawal F13.231
    inhalant intoxication (acute) F18.921
      in
        abuse F18.121
        dependence F18.221
    multiple etiologies F05
    opioid intoxication (acute) F11.921
      in
        abuse F11.121
        dependence F11.221
    other (or unknown) substance F19.921
    phencyclidine intoxication (acute) F16.921
      in
        abuse F16.121
        dependence F16.221
    psychoactive substance NEC intoxication (acute) F19.921
      in
        abuse F19.121
        dependence F19.221
    sedative
      intoxication F13.921
        in
          abuse F13.121
          dependence F13.221
      withdrawal F13.231
    unknown etiology F05
  exhaustion F43.0
  hysterical F44.89
  postprocedural (postoperative) F05

Delirium, delirious — *continued*
  puerperal FØ5
  thyroid — *see* Thyrotoxicosis with thyroid storm
  traumatic — *see* Injury, intracranial
  tremens (alcohol-induced) F1Ø.231
    sedative-induced F13.231
Delivery (childbirth) (labor)
  arrested active phase O62.1
  cesarean (for)
    abnormal
      pelvis (bony) (deformity) (major) NEC with dispro-
          portion (fetopelvic) O33.Ø
        with obstructed labor O65.Ø
      presentation or position O32.9 ☑
    abruptio placentae (*see also* Abruptio placentae)
        O45.9- ☑
    acromion presentation O32.2 ☑
    atony, uterus O62.2
    breech presentation O32.1 ☑
      incomplete O32.8 ☑
    brow presentation O32.3 ☑
    cephalopelvic disproportion O33.9
    cerclage O34.3- ☑
    chin presentation O32.3 ☑
    cicatrix of cervix O34.4- ☑
    contracted pelvis (general)
      inlet O33.2
      outlet O33.3 ☑
    cord presentation or prolapse O69.Ø ☑
    cystocele O34.8- ☑
    deformity (acquired) (congenital)
      pelvic organs or tissues NEC O34.8- ☑
      pelvis (bony) NEC O33.Ø
    disproportion NOS O33.9
    eclampsia — *see* Eclampsia
    face presentation O32.3 ☑
    failed
      forceps O66.5
      induction of labor O61.9
        instrumental O61.1
        mechanical O61.1
        medical O61.Ø
        specified NEC O61.8
        surgical O61.1
      trial of labor NOS O66.4Ø
        following previous cesarean delivery O66.41
      vacuum extraction O66.5
      ventouse O66.5
    fetal-maternal hemorrhage O43.Ø1- ☑
    hemorrhage (intrapartum) O67.9
      with coagulation defect O67.Ø
      specified cause NEC O67.8
    high head at term O32.4 ☑
    hydrocephalic fetus O33.6 ☑
    incarceration of uterus O34.51- ☑
    incoordinate uterine action O62.4
    increased size, fetus O33.5 ☑
    inertia, uterus O62.2
      primary O62.Ø
      secondary O62.1
    lateroversion, uterus O34.59- ☑
    mal lie O32.9 ☑
    malposition
      fetus O32.9 ☑
      pelvic organs or tissues NEC O34.8- ☑
      uterus NEC O34.59- ☑
    malpresentation NOS O32.9 ☑
    oblique presentation O32.2 ☑
    occurring after 37 completed weeks of gestation
        but before 39 completed weeks gestation due
        to (spontaneous) onset of labor O75.82
    oversize fetus O33.5 ☑
    pelvic tumor NEC O34.8- ☑
    placenta previa O44.Ø- ☑
      complete O44.Ø- ☑
        with hemorrhage O44.1- ☑
    placental insufficiency O36.51- ☑
    planned, occurring after 37 completed weeks of
        gestation but before 39 completed weeks
        gestation due to (spontaneous) onset of labor
        O75.82
    polyp, cervix O34.4- ☑
      causing obstructed labor O65.5
    poor dilatation, cervix O62.Ø
    pre-eclampsia O14.94
      mild O14.Ø4
      moderate O14.Ø4

Delivery — *continued*
  cesarean — *continued*
    pre-eclampsia — *continued*
      severe O14.14
        with hemolysis, elevated liver enzymes and
            low platelet count (HELLP) O14.24
    previous
      cesarean delivery O34.219
        classical (vertical) scar O34.212
        low transverse scar O34.211
      surgery (to)
        cervix O34.4- ☑
        gynecological NEC O34.8- ☑
        rectum O34.7- ☑
        uterus O34.29
        vagina O34.6- ☑
    prolapse
      arm or hand O32.2 ☑
      uterus O34.52- ☑
    prolonged labor NOS O63.9
    rectocele O34.8- ☑
    retroversion
      uterus O34.53- ☑
    rigid
      cervix O34.4- ☑
      pelvic floor O34.8- ☑
      perineum O34.7- ☑
      vagina O34.6- ☑
      vulva O34.7- ☑
    sacculation, pregnant uterus O34.59- ☑
    scar(s)
      cervix O34.4- ☑
      cesarean delivery O34.219
        classical (vertical) O34.212
        low transverse O34.211
      transmural uterine O34.29
      uterus O34.29
    Shirodkar suture in situ O34.3- ☑
    shoulder presentation O32.2 ☑
    stenosis or stricture, cervix O34.4- ☑
    streptococcus group B (GBS) carrier state O99.824
    transmural uterine scar O34.29
    transverse presentation or lie O32.2 ☑
    tumor, pelvic organs or tissues NEC O34.8- ☑
      cervix O34.4- ☑
    umbilical cord presentation or prolapse O69.Ø ☑
    without indication O82
  completely normal case O8Ø
  complicated O75.9
    by
      abnormal, abnormality (of)
        forces of labor O62.9
          specified type NEC O62.8
        glucose O99.814
        uterine contractions NOS O62.9
      abruptio placentae (*see also* Abruptio placentae)
          O45.9- ☑
      abuse
        physical O9A.32 (*following* O99)
        psychological O9A.52 (*following* O99)
        sexual O9A.42 (*following* O99)
      adherent placenta O72.Ø
        without hemorrhage O73.Ø
      alcohol use O99.314
      anemia (pre-existing) O99.Ø2
      anesthetic death O74.8
      annular detachment of cervix O71.3
      atony, uterus O62.2
      attempted vacuum extraction and forceps O66.5
      Bandl's ring O62.4
      bariatric surgery status O99.844
      biliary tract disorder O26.62
      bleeding — *see* Delivery, complicated by, hem-
          orrhage
      blood disorder NEC O99.12
      cervical dystocia (hypotonic) O62.2
        primary O62.Ø
        secondary O62.1
      circulatory system disorder O99.42
      compression of cord (umbilical) NEC O69.2 ☑
      condition NEC O99.89
      contraction, contracted ring O62.4
      cord (umbilical)
        around neck
          with compression O69.1 ☑
          without compression O69.81 ☑
        bruising O69.5 ☑
        complication O69.9 ☑

Delivery — *continued*
  complicated — *continued*
    by — *continued*
      cord — *continued*
        complication — *continued*
          specified NEC O69.89 ☑
          compression NEC O69.2 ☑
          entanglement O69.2 ☑
            without compression O69.82 ☑
          hematoma O69.5 ☑
          presentation O69.Ø ☑
          prolapse O69.Ø ☑
          short O69.3 ☑
          thrombosis (vessels) O69.5 ☑
          vascular lesion O69.5 ☑
      Couvelaire uterus O45.8X- ☑
      damage to (injury to) NEC
        perineum O71.82
        periurethral tissue O71.82
        vulva O71.82
      delay following rupture of membranes (sponta-
          neous) — *see* Pregnancy, complicated by,
          premature rupture of membranes
      depressed fetal heart tones O76
      diabetes O24.92
        gestational O24.429
          diet controlled O24.42Ø
          insulin controlled O24.424
          oral drug controlled (antidiabetic) (hypo-
              glycemic) O24.425
        pre-existing O24.32
          specified NEC O24.82
          type 1 O24.Ø2
          type 2 O24.12
      diastasis recti (abdominis) O71.89
      dilatation
        bladder O66.8
        cervix incomplete, poor or slow O62.Ø
      disease NEC O99.89
      disruptio uteri — *see* Delivery, complicated by,
          rupture, uterus
      drug use O99.324
      dysfunction, uterus NOS O62.9
        hypertonic O62.4
        hypotonic O62.2
          primary O62.Ø
          secondary O62.1
        incoordinate O62.4
      eclampsia O15.1
      embolism (pulmonary) — *see* Embolism, obstet-
          ric
      endocrine, nutritional or metabolic disease NEC
          O99.284
      failed
        attempted vaginal birth after previous cesare-
            an delivery O66.41
        induction of labor O61.9
          instrumental O61.1
          mechanical O61.1
          medical O61.Ø
          specified NEC O61.8
          surgical O61.1
        trial of labor O66.4Ø
      female genital mutilation O65.5
      fetal
        abnormal acid-base balance O68
        acidemia O68
        acidosis O68
        alkalosis O68
        death, early OØ2.1
        deformity O66.3
        heart rate or rhythm (abnormal) (non-reassur-
            ing) O76
        hypoxia O77.8
        stress O77.9
          due to drug administration O77.1
          electrocardiographic evidence of O77.8
          specified NEC O77.8
          ultrasound evidence of O77.8
      fever during labor O75.2
      gastric banding status O99.844
      gastric bypass status O99.844
      gastrointestinal disease NEC O99.62
      gestational
        diabetes O24.429
          diet controlled O24.42Ø
          insulin (and diet) controlled O24.424

☑ **Additional Character Required** — Refer to the Tabular List for Character Selection   ⤵ **Subterms under main terms may continue to next column or page**

Delivery — *continued*
  complicated — *continued*
    by — *continued*
      gestational — *continued*
        diabetes — *continued*
          oral drug controlled (antidiabetic) (hypo-glycemic) O24.425
        edema O12.04
          with proteinuria O12.24
        proteinuria O12.14
      gonorrhea O98.22
      hematoma O71.7
        ischial spine O71.7
        pelvic O71.7
        vagina O71.7
        vulva or perineum O71.7
      hemorrhage (uterine) O67.9
        associated with
          afibrinogenemia O67.0
          coagulation defect O67.0
          hyperfibrinolysis O67.0
          hypofibrinogenemia O67.0
        due to
          low implantation of placenta O44.5- ☑
          low-lying placenta O44.5- ☑
          placenta previa O44.1- ☑
            marginal O44.3- ☑
            partial O44.3- ☑
          premature separation of placenta (normally implanted) (*see also* Abruptio placentae) O45.9- ☑
          retained placenta O72.0
          uterine leiomyoma O67.8
        placenta NEC O67.8
        postpartum NEC (atonic) (immediate) O72.1
          with retained or trapped placenta O72.0
         delayed O72.2
        secondary O72.2
        third stage O72.0
      hourglass contraction, uterus O62.4
      hypertension, hypertensive (pre-existing) — *see* Hypertension, complicated by, childbirth (labor)
      hypotension O26.5- ☑
      incomplete dilatation (cervix) O62.0
      incoordinate uterus contractions O62.4
      inertia, uterus O62.2
        during latent phase of labor O62.0
        primary O62.0
        secondary O62.1
      infection (maternal) O98.92
        carrier state NEC O99.834
        gonorrhea O98.22
        human immunodeficiency virus (HIV) O98.72
        sexually transmitted NEC O98.32
        specified NEC O98.82
        syphilis O98.12
        tuberculosis O98.02
        viral hepatitis O98.42
        viral NEC O98.52
      injury (to mother) (*see also* Delivery, complicated, by, damage to) O71.9
        nonobstetric O9A.22 (*following* O99)
          caused by abuse — *see* Delivery, complicated by, abuse
      intrauterine fetal death, early O02.1
      inversion, uterus O71.2
      laceration (perineal) O70.9
        anus (sphincter) O70.4
          with third degree laceration (*see also* Delivery, complicated, by, laceration, perineum, third degree) O70.20
            with mucosa O70.3
          without third degree laceration O70.2 ☑
        bladder (urinary) O71.5
        bowel O71.5
        cervix (uteri) O71.3
        fourchette O70.0
        hymen O70.0
        labia O70.0
        pelvic
          floor O70.1
          organ NEC O71.5
        perineum, perineal O70.9
          first degree O70.0
          fourth degree O70.3
          muscles O70.1

Delivery — *continued*
  complicated — *continued*
    by — *continued*
      laceration — *continued*
        perineum, perineal — *continued*
          second degree O70.1
          skin O70.0
          slight O70.0
          third degree O70.20
            with
              both external anal sphincter (EAS) and internal anal sphincter (IAS) torn (IIIc) O70.23
              less than 50% of external anal sphincter (EAS) thickness torn (IIIa) O70.21
              more than 50% external anal sphincter (EAS) thickness torn (IIIb) O70.22
            IIIa O70.21
            IIIb O70.22
            IIIc O70.23
        peritoneum (pelvic) O71.5
        rectovaginal (septum) (without perineal laceration) O71.4
          with perineum (*see also* Delivery, complicated, by, laceration, perineum, third degree) O70.20
          with anal or rectal mucosa O70.3
        specified NEC O71.89
        sphincter ani — *see* Delivery, complicated, by, laceration, anus (sphincter)
        urethra O71.5
        uterus O71.81
          before labor O71.81
        vagina, vaginal (deep) (high) (without perineal laceration) O71.4
          with perineum O70.0
          muscles, with perineum O70.1
        vulva O70.0
      liver disorder O26.62
      malignancy O9A.12 (*following* O99)
      malnutrition O25.2
      malposition, malpresentation
        uterus or cervix O65.5
        placenta O44.0- ☑
          with hemorrhage O44.1- ☑
        without obstruction (*see also* Delivery, complicated by, obstruction) O32.9
          breech O32.1 ☑
          compound O32.6 ☑
          face (brow) (chin) O32.3 ☑
          footling O32.8 ☑
          high head O32.4 ☑
          oblique O32.2 ☑
          specified NEC O32.8 ☑
          transverse O32.2 ☑
          unstable lie O32.0 ☑
      meconium in amniotic fluid O77.0
      mental disorder NEC O99.344
      metrorrhexis — *see* Delivery, complicated by, rupture, uterus
      nervous system disorder O99.354
      obesity (pre-existing) O99.214
      obesity surgery status O99.844
      obstetric trauma O71.9
        specified NEC O71.89
      obstructed labor
        due to
          breech (complete) (frank) presentation O64.1 ☑
            incomplete O64.8 ☑
          brow presentation O64.3 ☑
          buttock presentation O64.1 ☑
          chin presentation O64.2 ☑
          compound presentation O64.5 ☑
          contracted pelvis O65.1
          deep transverse arrest O64.0 ☑
          deformed pelvis O65.0
          dystocia (fetal) O66.9
            due to
              conjoined twins O66.3
              fetal
                abnormality NEC O66.3
                ascites O66.3
                hydrops O66.3
                meningomyelocele O66.3
                sacral teratoma O66.3

Delivery — *continued*
  complicated — *continued*
    by — *continued*
      obstructed labor — *continued*
        due to — *continued*
          dystocia — *continued*
            due to — *continued*
              fetal — *continued*
                tumor O66.3
              hydrocephalic fetus O66.3
              shoulder O66.0
          face presentation O64.2 ☑
          fetopelvic disproportion O65.4
          footling presentation O64.8 ☑
          impacted shoulders O66.0
          incomplete rotation of fetal head O64.0 ☑
          large fetus O66.2
          locked twins O66.1
          malposition O64.9 ☑
            specified NEC O64.8 ☑
          malpresentation O64.9 ☑
            specified NEC O64.8 ☑
          multiple fetuses NEC O66.6
          pelvic
            abnormality (maternal) O65.9
              organ O65.5
              specified NEC O65.8
            contraction
              inlet O65.2
              mid-cavity O65.3
              outlet O65.3
          persistent (position)
            occipitoiliac O64.0 ☑
            occipitoposterior O64.0 ☑
            occipitosacral O64.0 ☑
            occipitotransverse O64.0 ☑
          prolapsed arm O64.4 ☑
          shoulder presentation O64.4 ☑
        specified NEC O66.8
      pathological retraction ring, uterus O62.4
      penetration, pregnant uterus by instrument O71.1
      perforation — *see* Delivery, complicated by, laceration
      placenta, placental
        ablatio (*see also* Abruptio placentae) O45.9- ☑
        abnormality O43.9- ☑
          specified NEC O43.89- ☑
        abruptio (*see also* Abruptio placentae) O45.9- ☑
        accreta O43.21- ☑
        adherent (with hemorrhage) O72.0
          without hemorrhage O73.0
        detachment (premature) (*see also* Abruptio placentae) O45.9- ☑
        disorder O43.9- ☑
          specified NEC O43.89- ☑
        hemorrhage NEC O67.8
        increta O43.22- ☑
        low (implantation) (lying) O44.4- ☑
          with hemorrhage O44.5- ☑
        malformation O43.10- ☑
        malposition O44.0- ☑
          without hemorrhage O44.1- ☑
        percreta O43.23- ☑
        previa (central) (complete) (lateral) (total) O44.0- ☑
          with hemorrhage O44.1- ☑
          marginal O44.2- ☑
            with hemorrhage O44.3- ☑
          partial O44.2- ☑
            with hemorrhage O44.3- ☑
        retained (with hemorrhage) O72.0
          without hemorrhage O73.0
        separation (premature) O45.9- ☑
          specified NEC O45.8X- ☑
        vicious insertion O44.1- ☑
      precipitate labor O62.3
      premature rupture, membranes (*see also* Pregnancy, complicated by, premature rupture of membranes) O42.90
      prolapse
        arm or hand O32.2 ☑
        cord (umbilical) O69.0 ☑
        foot or leg O32.8 ☑

⬛ Subterms under main terms may continue to next column or page   ☑ **Additional Character Required — Refer to the Tabular List for Character Selection**   **91**

Delivery — Delivery

Delivery — *continued*
　complicated — *continued*
　　by — *continued*
　　　prolapse — *continued*
　　　　uterus O34.52- ☑
　　　prolonged labor O63.9
　　　　first stage O63.0
　　　　second stage O63.1
　　　protozoal disease (maternal) O98.62
　　　respiratory disease NEC O99.52
　　　retained membranes or portions of placenta
　　　　　O72.2
　　　　without hemorrhage O73.1
　　　retarded birth O63.9
　　　retention of secundines (with hemorrhage) O72.0
　　　　without hemorrhage O73.0
　　　　partial O72.2
　　　　　without hemorrhage O73.1
　　　rupture
　　　　bladder (urinary) O71.5
　　　　cervix O71.3
　　　　pelvic organ NEC O71.5
　　　　urethra O71.5
　　　　uterus (during or after labor) O71.1
　　　　　before labor O71.0- ☑
　　　separation, pubic bone (symphysis pubis) O71.6
　　　shock O75.1
　　　shoulder presentation O64.4 ☑
　　　skin disorder NEC O99.72
　　　spasm, cervix O62.4
　　　stenosis or stricture, cervix O65.5
　　　streptococcus group B (GBS) carrier state O99.824
　　　subluxation of symphysis (pubis) O26.72
　　　syphilis (maternal) O98.12
　　　tear — *see* Delivery, complicated by, laceration
　　　tetanic uterus O62.4
　　　trauma (obstetrical) (*see also* Delivery, complicat-
　　　　　ed, by, damage to) O71.9
　　　　non-obstetric O9A.22 (*following* O99)
　　　　periurethral O71.82
　　　　specified NEC O71.89
　　　tuberculosis (maternal) O98.02
　　　tumor, pelvic organs or tissues NEC O65.5
　　　umbilical cord around neck
　　　　with compression O69.1 ☑
　　　　without compression O69.81 ☑
　　　uterine inertia O62.2
　　　　during latent phase of labor O62.0
　　　　primary O62.0
　　　　secondary O62.1
　　　vasa previa O69.4 ☑
　　　velamentous insertion of cord O43.12- ☑
　　specified complication NEC O75.89
　delayed NOS O63.9
　　following rupture of membranes
　　　artificial O75.5
　　second twin, triplet, etc. O63.2
　forceps, low following failed vacuum extraction O66.5
　missed (at or near term) O36.4 ☑
　normal O80
　obstructed — *see* Delivery, complicated by, obstructed
　　labor
　precipitate O62.3
　preterm (*see also* Pregnancy, complicated by, preterm
　　labor) O60.10 ☑
　spontaneous O80
　term pregnancy NOS O80
　uncomplicated O80
　vaginal, following previous cesarean delivery O34.219
　　classical (vertical) scar O34.212
　　low transverse scar O34.211
Delusions (paranoid) — *see* Disorder, delusional
Dementia (degenerative (primary)) (old age) (persisting)
　　F03.90
　with
　　aggressive behavior F03.91
　　behavioral disturbance F03.91
　　combative behavior F03.91
　　Lewy bodies G31.83 [F02.80]
　　　with behavioral disturbance G31.83 [F02.81]
　　Parkinsonism G31.83 [F02.80]
　　　with behavioral disturbance G31.83 [F02.81]
　　Parkinson's disease G20 [F02.80]
　　　with behavioral disturbance G20 [F02.81]
　　violent behavior F03.91
　alcoholic F10.97
　　with dependence F10.27
　Alzheimer's type — *see* Disease, Alzheimer's

Dementia — *continued*
　arteriosclerotic — *see* Dementia, vascular
　atypical, Alzheimer's type — *see* Disease, Alzheimer's,
　　specified NEC
　congenital — *see* Disability, intellectual
　frontal (lobe) G31.09 [F02.80]
　　with behavioral disturbance G31.09 [F02.81]
　frontotemporal G31.09 [F02.80]
　　with behavioral disturbance G31.09 [F02.81]
　　specified NEC G31.09 [F02.80]
　　　with behavioral disturbance G31.09 [F02.81]
　Huntington's disease or chorea G10
　　with dementia G10 [F02.80]
　in (due to)
　　with behavioral disturbance G31.83 [F02.81]
　　alcohol F10.97
　　　with dependence F10.27
　　Alzheimer's disease — *see* Disease, Alzheimer's
　　arteriosclerotic brain disease — *see* Dementia, vas-
　　　cular
　　cerebral lipidoses E75.- ☑ [F02.80]
　　　with behavioral disturbance E75.- ☑ [F02.81]
　　Creutzfeldt-Jakob disease (*see also* Creutzfeldt-
　　　Jakob disease or syndrome (with dementia))
　　　A81.00
　　epilepsy G40.- ☑ [F02.80]
　　　with behavioral disturbance G40.- ☑ [F02.81]
　　hepatolenticular degeneration E83.01 [F02.80]
　　　with behavioral disturbance E83.01 [F02.81]
　　human immunodeficiency virus (HIV) disease
　　　B20 [F02.80]
　　　with behavioral disturbance B20 [F02.81]
　　Huntington's disease or chorea G10 [F02.80]
　　　with behavioral disturbance G10 [F02.81]
　　hypercalcemia E83.52 [F02.80]
　　　with behavioral disturbance E83.52 [F02.81]
　　hypothyroidism, acquired E03.9 [F02.80]
　　　with behavioral disturbance E03.9 [F02.81]
　　　due to iodine deficiency E01.8 [F02.80]
　　　　with behavioral disturbance E01.8 [F02.81]
　　inhalants F18.97
　　　with dependence F18.27
　　multiple
　　　etiologies F03 ☑
　　　sclerosis G35 [F02.80]
　　　　with behavioral disturbance G35 [F02.81]
　　neurosyphilis A52.17 [F02.80]
　　　with behavioral disturbance A52.17 [F02.81]
　　　juvenile A50.49 [F02.80]
　　　　with behavioral disturbance A50.49 [F02.81]
　　niacin deficiency E52 [F02.80]
　　　with behavioral disturbance E52 [F02.81]
　　paralysis agitans G20 [F02.80]
　　　with behavioral disturbance G20 [F02.81]
　　Parkinson's disease G20 [F02.80]
　　pellagra E52 [F02.80]
　　　with behavioral disturbance E52 [F02.81]
　　Pick's G31.01 [F02.80]
　　　with behavioral disturbance G31.01 [F02.81]
　　polyarteritis nodosa M30.0 [F02.80]
　　　with behavioral disturbance M30.0 [F02.81]
　　psychoactive drug F19.97
　　　with dependence F19.27
　　　inhalants F18.97
　　　　with dependence F18.27
　　　sedatives, hypnotics or anxiolytics F13.97
　　　　with dependence F13.27
　　sedatives, hypnotics or anxiolytics F13.97
　　　with dependence F13.27
　　systemic lupus erythematosus M32.- ☑ [F02.80]
　　　with behavioral disturbance M32.- ☑ [F02.81]
　　trypanosomiasis
　　　African B56.9 [F02.80]
　　　　with behavioral disturbance B56.9 [F02.81]
　　unknown etiology F03 ☑
　　vitamin B12 deficiency E53.8 [F02.80]
　　　with behavioral disturbance E53.8 [F02.81]
　　volatile solvents F18.97
　　　with dependence F18.27
　infantile, infantilis F84.3
　Lewy body G31.83 [F02.80]
　　with behavioral disturbance G31.83 [F02.81]
　multi-infarct — *see* Dementia, vascular
　paralytica, paralytic (syphilitic) A52.17 [F02.80]
　　with behavioral disturbance A52.17 [F02.81]
　　juvenilis A50.45
　paretic A52.17
　praecox — *see* Schizophrenia

Dementia — *continued*
　presenile F03 ☑
　　Alzheimer's type — *see* Disease, Alzheimer's, early
　　　onset
　primary degenerative F03 ☑
　progressive, syphilitic A52.17
　senile F03 ☑
　　with acute confusional state F05
　　Alzheimer's type — *see* Disease, Alzheimer's, late
　　　onset
　　depressed or paranoid type F03 ☑
　vascular (acute onset) (mixed) (multi-infarct) (subcorti-
　　cal) F01.50
　　with behavioral disturbance F01.51
Demineralization, bone — *see* Osteoporosis
Demodex folliculorum (infestation) B88.0
Demophobia F40.248
Demoralization R45.3
Demyelination, demyelinization
　central nervous system G37.9
　　specified NEC G37.8
　corpus callosum (central) G37.1
　disseminated, acute G36.9
　　specified NEC G36.8
　global G35
　in optic neuritis G36.0
Dengue (classical) (fever) A90
　hemorrhagic A91
　sandfly A93.1
Dennie-Marfan syphilitic syndrome A50.45
Dens evaginatus, in dente or invaginatus K00.2
Dense breasts R92.2
Density
　increased, bone (disseminated) (generalized) (spotted)
　　— *see* Disorder, bone, density and structure,
　　specified type NEC
　lung (nodular) J98.4
Dental (*see also* condition)
　examination Z01.20
　　with abnormal findings Z01.21
　restoration
　　aesthetically inadequate or displeasing K08.56
　　defective K08.50
　　　specified NEC K08.59
　　failure of marginal integrity K08.51
　　failure of periodontal anatomical integrity K08.54
Dentia praecox K00.6
Denticles (pulp) K04.2
Dentigerous cyst K09.0
Dentin
　irregular (in pulp) K04.3
　opalescent K00.5
　secondary (in pulp) K04.3
　sensitive K03.89
Dentinogenesis imperfecta K00.5
Dentinoma — *see* Cyst, calcifying odontogenic
Dentition (syndrome) K00.7
　delayed K00.6
　difficult K00.7
　precocious K00.6
　premature K00.6
　retarded K00.6
Dependence (on) (syndrome) F19.20
　with remission F19.21
　alcohol (ethyl) (methyl) (without remission) F10.20
　　with
　　　amnestic disorder, persisting F10.26
　　　anxiety disorder F10.280
　　　dementia, persisting F10.27
　　　intoxication F10.229
　　　　with delirium F10.221
　　　　uncomplicated F10.220
　　　mood disorder F10.24
　　　psychotic disorder F10.259
　　　　with
　　　　　delusions F10.250
　　　　　hallucinations F10.251
　　　remission F10.21
　　　sexual dysfunction F10.281
　　　sleep disorder F10.282
　　　specified disorder NEC F10.288
　　　withdrawal F10.239
　　　　with
　　　　　delirium F10.231
　　　　　perceptual disturbance F10.232
　　　　uncomplicated F10.230
　　counseling and surveillance Z71.41
　amobarbital — *see* Dependence, drug, sedative

☑ **Additional Character Required** — **Refer to the Tabular List for Character Selection**　　☒ **Subterms under main terms may continue to next column or page**

Dependence — *continued*
amphetamine(s) (type) — *see* Dependence, drug, stimulant NEC
amytal (sodium) — *see* Dependence, drug, sedative
analgesic NEC F55.8
anesthetic (agent) (gas) (general) (local) NEC — *see* Dependence, drug, psychoactive NEC
anxiolytic NEC — *see* Dependence, drug, sedative
barbital(s) — *see* Dependence, drug, sedative
barbiturate(s) (compounds) (drugs classifiable to T42) — *see* Dependence, drug, sedative
benzedrine — *see* Dependence, drug, stimulant NEC
bhang — *see* Dependence, drug, cannabis
bromide(s) NEC — *see* Dependence, drug, sedative
caffeine — *see* Dependence, drug, stimulant NEC
cannabis (sativa) (indica) (resin) (derivatives) (type) — *see* Dependence, drug, cannabis
chloral (betaine) (hydrate) — *see* Dependence, drug, sedative
chlordiazepoxide — *see* Dependence, drug, sedative
coca (leaf) (derivatives) — *see* Dependence, drug, cocaine
cocaine — *see* Dependence, drug, cocaine
codeine — *see* Dependence, drug, opioid
combinations of drugs F19.20
dagga — *see* Dependence, drug, cannabis
demerol — *see* Dependence, drug, opioid
dexamphetamine — *see* Dependence, drug, stimulant NEC
dexedrine — *see* Dependence, drug, stimulant NEC
dextromethorphan — *see* Dependence, drug, opioid
dextromoramide — *see* Dependence, drug, opioid
dextro-nor-pseudo-ephedrine — *see* Dependence, drug, stimulant NEC
dextrorphan — *see* Dependence, drug, opioid
diazepam — *see* Dependence, drug, sedative
dilaudid — *see* Dependence, drug, opioid
D-lysergic acid diethylamide — *see* Dependence, drug, hallucinogen
drug NEC F19.20
  with sleep disorder F19.282
  cannabis F12.20
    with
      anxiety disorder F12.280
      intoxication F12.229
        with
          delirium F12.221
          perceptual disturbance F12.222
        uncomplicated F12.220
      other specified disorder F12.288
      psychosis F12.259
        delusions F12.250
        hallucinations F12.251
      unspecified disorder F12.29
      withdrawal F12.23
    in remission F12.21
  cocaine F14.20
    with
      anxiety disorder F14.280
      intoxication F14.229
        with
          delirium F14.221
          perceptual disturbance F14.222
        uncomplicated F14.220
      mood disorder F14.24
      other specified disorder F14.288
      psychosis F14.259
        delusions F14.250
        hallucinations F14.251
      sexual dysfunction F14.281
      sleep disorder F14.282
      unspecified disorder F14.29
      withdrawal F14.23
    in remission F14.21
    withdrawal symptoms in newborn P96.1
  counseling and surveillance Z71.51
  hallucinogen F16.20
    with
      anxiety disorder F16.280
      flashbacks F16.283
      intoxication F16.229
        with delirium F16.221
        uncomplicated F16.220
      mood disorder F16.24
      other specified disorder F16.288
      perception disorder, persisting F16.283
      psychosis F16.259
        delusions F16.250

Dependence — *continued*
drug — *continued*
  hallucinogen — *continued*
    with — *continued*
      psychosis — *continued*
        hallucinations F16.251
      unspecified disorder F16.29
    in remission F16.21
  in remission F19.21
  inhalant F18.20
    with
      anxiety disorder F18.280
      dementia, persisting F18.27
      intoxication F18.229
        with delirium F18.221
        uncomplicated F18.220
      mood disorder F18.24
      other specified disorder F18.288
      psychosis F18.259
        delusions F18.250
        hallucinations F18.251
      unspecified disorder F18.29
    in remission F18.21
  nicotine F17.200
    with disorder F17.209
      in remission F17.201
      specified disorder NEC F17.208
      withdrawal F17.203
    chewing tobacco F17.220
      with disorder F17.229
        in remission F17.221
        specified disorder NEC F17.228
        withdrawal F17.223
    cigarettes F17.210
      with disorder F17.219
        in remission F17.211
        specified disorder NEC F17.218
        withdrawal F17.213
    specified product NEC F17.290
      with disorder F17.299
        remission F17.291
        specified disorder NEC F17.298
        withdrawal F17.293
  opioid F11.20
    with
      intoxication F11.229
        with
          delirium F11.221
          perceptual disturbance F11.222
        uncomplicated F11.220
      mood disorder F11.24
      other specified disorder F11.288
      psychosis F11.259
        delusions F11.250
        hallucinations F11.251
      sexual dysfunction F11.281
      sleep disorder F11.282
      unspecified disorder F11.29
      withdrawal F11.23
    in remission F11.21
  psychoactive NEC F19.20
    with
      amnestic disorder F19.26
      anxiety disorder F19.280
      dementia F19.27
      intoxication F19.229
        with
          delirium F19.221
          perceptual disturbance F19.222
        uncomplicated F19.220
      mood disorder F19.24
      other specified disorder F19.288
      psychosis F19.259
        delusions F19.250
        hallucinations F19.251
      sexual dysfunction F19.281
      sleep disorder F19.282
      unspecified disorder F19.29
      withdrawal F19.239
        with
          delirium F19.231
          perceptual disturbance F19.232
        uncomplicated F19.230
  sedative, hypnotic or anxiolytic F13.20
    with
      amnestic disorder F13.26
      anxiety disorder F13.280
      dementia, persisting F13.27
      intoxication F13.229

Dependence — *continued*
drug — *continued*
  sedative, hypnotic or anxiolytic — *continued*
    with — *continued*
      intoxication — *continued*
        with delirium F13.221
        uncomplicated F13.220
      mood disorder F13.24
      other specified disorder F13.288
      psychosis F13.259
        delusions F13.250
        hallucinations F13.251
      sexual dysfunction F13.281
      sleep disorder F13.282
      unspecified disorder F13.29
      withdrawal F13.239
        with
          delirium F13.231
          perceptual disturbance F13.232
        uncomplicated F13.230
    in remission F13.21
  stimulant NEC F15.20
    with
      anxiety disorder F15.280
      intoxication F15.229
        with
          delirium F15.221
          perceptual disturbance F15.222
        uncomplicated F15.220
      mood disorder F15.24
      other specified disorder F15.288
      psychosis F15.259
        delusions F15.250
        hallucinations F15.251
      sexual dysfunction F15.281
      sleep disorder F15.282
      unspecified disorder F15.29
      withdrawal F15.23
    in remission F15.21
ethyl
  alcohol (without remission) F10.20
    with remission F10.21
  bromide — *see* Dependence, drug, sedative
  carbamate F19.20
  chloride F19.20
  morphine — *see* Dependence, drug, opioid
ganja — *see* Dependence, drug, cannabis
glue (airplane) (sniffing) — *see* Dependence, drug, inhalant
glutethimide — *see* Dependence, drug, sedative
hallucinogenics — *see* Dependence, drug, hallucinogen
hashish — *see* Dependence, drug, cannabis
hemp — *see* Dependence, drug, cannabis
heroin (salt) (any) — *see* Dependence, drug, opioid
hypnotic NEC — *see* Dependence, drug, sedative
Indian hemp — *see* Dependence, drug, cannabis
inhalants — *see* Dependence, drug, inhalant
khat — *see* Dependence, drug, stimulant NEC
laudanum — *see* Dependence, drug, opioid
LSD (-25) (derivatives) — *see* Dependence, drug, hallucinogen
luminal — *see* Dependence, drug, sedative
lysergic acid — *see* Dependence, drug, hallucinogen
maconha — *see* Dependence, drug, cannabis
marihuana — *see* Dependence, drug, cannabis
meprobamate — *see* Dependence, drug, sedative
mescaline — *see* Dependence, drug, hallucinogen
methadone — *see* Dependence, drug, opioid
methamphetamine(s) — *see* Dependence, drug, stimulant NEC
methaqualone — *see* Dependence, drug, sedative
methyl
  alcohol (without remission) F10.20
    with remission F10.21
  bromide — *see* Dependence, drug, sedative
  morphine — *see* Dependence, drug, opioid
  phenidate — *see* Dependence, drug, stimulant NEC
  sulfonal — *see* Dependence, drug, sedative
morphine (sulfate) (sulfite) (type) — *see* Dependence, drug, opioid
narcotic (drug) NEC — *see* Dependence, drug, opioid
nembutal — *see* Dependence, drug, sedative
neraval — *see* Dependence, drug, sedative
neravan — *see* Dependence, drug, sedative
neurobarb — *see* Dependence, drug, sedative
nicotine — *see* Dependence, drug, nicotine
nitrous oxide F19.20

⛟ **Subterms under main terms may continue to next column or page**   ☑ **Additional Character Required** — Refer to the Tabular List for Character Selection   **93**

Dependence — Dependence

Dependence — *continued*
nonbarbiturate sedatives and tranquilizers with similar
effect — *see* Dependence, drug, sedative
on
artificial heart (fully implantable) (mechanical)
Z95.812
aspirator Z99.0
care provider (because of) Z74.9
impaired mobility Z74.09
need for
assistance with personal care Z74.1
continuous supervision Z74.3
no other household member able to render care
Z74.2
specified reason NEC Z74.8
machine Z99.89
enabling NEC Z99.89
specified type NEC Z99.89
renal dialysis (hemodialysis) (peritoneal) Z99.2
respirator Z99.11
ventilator Z99.11
wheelchair Z99.3
opiate — *see* Dependence, drug, opioid
opioids — *see* Dependence, drug, opioid
opium (alkaloids) (derivatives) (tincture) — *see* Dependence, drug, opioid
oxygen (long-term) (supplemental) Z99.81
paraldehyde — *see* Dependence, drug, sedative
paregoric — *see* Dependence, drug, opioid
PCP (phencyclidine) (or related substance) — *see* Dependence, drug, hallucinogen
pentobarbital — *see* Dependence, drug, sedative
pentobarbitone (sodium) — *see* Dependence, drug, sedative
pentothal — *see* Dependence, drug, sedative
peyote — *see* Dependence, drug, hallucinogen
phencyclidine (PCP) (or related substance) — *see* Dependence, drug, hallucinogen
phenmetrazine — *see* Dependence, drug, stimulant NEC
phenobarbital — *see* Dependence, drug, sedative
polysubstance F19.20
psilocibin, psilocin, psilocyn, psilocyline — *see* Dependence, drug, hallucinogen
psychostimulant NEC — *see* Dependence, drug, stimulant NEC
secobarbital — *see* Dependence, drug, sedative
seconal — *see* Dependence, drug, sedative
sedative NEC — *see* Dependence, drug, sedative
specified drug NEC — *see* Dependence, drug
stimulant NEC — *see* Dependence, drug, stimulant NEC
substance NEC — *see* Dependence, drug
supplemental oxygen Z99.81
tobacco — *see* Dependence, drug, nicotine
counseling and surveillance Z71.6
tranquilizer NEC — *see* Dependence, drug, sedative
vitamin B6 E53.1
volatile solvents — *see* Dependence, drug, inhalant

Dependency
care-provider Z74.9
passive F60.7
reactions (persistent) F60.7

Depersonalization (in neurotic state) (neurotic) (syndrome) F48.1

Depletion
extracellular fluid E86.9
plasma E86.1
potassium E87.6
nephropathy N25.89
salt or sodium E87.1
causing heat exhaustion or prostration T67.4 ☑
nephropathy N28.9
volume NOS E86.9

Deployment (current) (military) status Z56.82
in theater or in support of military war, peacekeeping
and humanitarian operations Z56.82
personal history of Z91.82
military war, peacekeeping and humanitarian deployment (current or past conflict) Z91.82
returned from Z91.82

Depolarization, premature I49.40
atrial I49.1
junctional I49.2
specified NEC I49.49
ventricular I49.3

Deposit
bone in Boeck's sarcoid D86.89
calcareous, calcium — *see* Calcification

Deposit — *continued*
cholesterol
retina H35.89
vitreous (body) (humor) — *see* Deposit, crystalline
conjunctiva H11.11- ☑
cornea H18.00- ☑
argentous H18.02- ☑
due to metabolic disorder H18.03- ☑
Kayser-Fleischer ring H18.04- ☑
pigmentation — *see* Pigmentation, cornea
crystalline, vitreous (body) (humor) H43.2- ☑
hemosiderin in old scars of cornea — *see* Pigmentation, cornea, stromal
metallic in lens — *see* Cataract, specified NEC
skin R23.8
tooth, teeth (betel) (black) (green) (materia alba) (orange) (tobacco) K03.6
urate, kidney — *see* Calculus, kidney

Depraved appetite — *see* Pica

Depressed
HDL cholesterol E78.6

Depression (acute) (mental) F32.9
agitated (single episode) F32.2
anaclitic — *see* Disorder, adjustment
anxiety F41.8
persistent F34.1
arches (*see also* Deformity, limb, flat foot)
atypical (single episode) F32.89
recurrent episode F33.8
basal metabolic rate R94.8
bone marrow D75.89
central nervous system R09.2
cerebral R29.818
newborn P91.4
cerebrovascular I67.9
chest wall M95.4
climacteric (single episode) F32.89
recurrent episode F33.8
endogenous (without psychotic symptoms) F33.2
with psychotic symptoms F33.3
functional activity R68.89
hysterical F44.89
involutional (single episode) F32.89
recurrent episode F33.8
major F32.9
with psychotic symptoms F32.3
recurrent — *see* Disorder, depressive, recurrent
manic-depressive — *see* Disorder, depressive, recurrent
masked (single episode) F32.89
medullary G93.89
menopausal (single episode) F32.89
recurrent episode F33.8
metatarsus — *see* Depression, arches
monopolar F33.9
nervous F34.1
neurotic F34.1
nose M95.0
postnatal (NOS) F53.0
postpartum (NOS) F53.0
post-psychotic of schizophrenia F32.89
post-schizophrenic F32.89
psychogenic (reactive) (single episode) F32.9
psychoneurotic F34.1
psychotic (single episode) F32.3
recurrent F33.3
reactive (psychogenic) (single episode) F32.9
psychotic (single episode) F32.3
recurrent — *see* Disorder, depressive, recurrent
respiratory center G93.89
seasonal — *see* Disorder, depressive, recurrent
senile F03 ☑
severe, single episode F32.2
situational F43.21
skull Q67.4
specified NEC (single episode) F32.89
sternum M95.4
visual field — *see* Defect, visual field
vital (recurrent) (without psychotic symptoms) F33.2
with psychotic symptoms F33.3
single episode F32.2

Deprivation
cultural Z60.3
effects NOS T73.9 ☑
specified NEC T73.8 ☑
emotional NEC Z65.8
affecting infant or child — *see* Maltreatment, child, psychological
food T73.0 ☑

Deprivation — *continued*
protein — *see* Malnutrition
sleep Z72.820
social Z60.4
affecting infant or child — *see* Maltreatment, child, psychological
specified NEC T73.8 ☑
vitamins — *see* Deficiency, vitamin
water T73.1 ☑

Derangement
ankle (internal) — *see* Derangement, joint, ankle
cartilage (articular) NEC — *see* Derangement, joint, articular cartilage, by site
recurrent — *see* Dislocation, recurrent
cruciate ligament, anterior, current injury — *see* Sprain, knee, cruciate, anterior
elbow (internal) — *see* Derangement, joint, elbow
hip (joint) (internal) (old) — *see* Derangement, joint, hip
joint (internal) M24.9
ankylosis — *see* Ankylosis
articular cartilage M24.10
ankle M24.17- ☑
elbow M24.12- ☑
foot M24.17- ☑
hand M24.14- ☑
hip M24.15- ☑
knee NEC M23.9- ☑
loose body — *see* Loose, body
shoulder M24.11- ☑
wrist M24.13- ☑
contracture — *see* Contraction, joint
current injury (*see also* Dislocation)
knee, meniscus or cartilage — *see* Tear, meniscus
dislocation
pathological — *see* Dislocation, pathological
recurrent — *see* Dislocation, recurrent
knee — *see* Derangement, knee
ligament — *see* Disorder, ligament
loose body — *see* Loose, body
recurrent — *see* Dislocation, recurrent
specified type NEC M24.80
ankle M24.87- ☑
elbow M24.82- ☑
foot joint M24.87- ☑
hand joint M24.84- ☑
hip M24.85- ☑
shoulder M24.81- ☑
wrist M24.83- ☑
temporomandibular M26.69
knee (recurrent) M23.9- ☑
ligament disruption, spontaneous M23.60- ☑
anterior cruciate M23.61- ☑
capsular M23.67- ☑
instability, chronic M23.5- ☑
lateral collateral M23.64- ☑
medial collateral M23.63- ☑
posterior cruciate M23.62- ☑
loose body M23.4- ☑
meniscus M23.30- ☑
cystic M23.00- ☑
lateral M23.002
anterior horn M23.04- ☑
posterior horn M23.05- ☑
specified NEC M23.06- ☑
medial M23.005
anterior horn M23.01- ☑
posterior horn M23.02- ☑
specified NEC M23.03- ☑
degenerate — *see* Derangement, knee, meniscus, specified NEC
detached — *see* Derangement, knee, meniscus, specified NEC
due to old tear or injury M23.20- ☑
lateral M23.20- ☑
anterior horn M23.24- ☑
posterior horn M23.25- ☑
specified NEC M23.26- ☑
medial M23.20- ☑
anterior horn M23.21- ☑
posterior horn M23.22- ☑
specified NEC M23.23- ☑
retained — *see* Derangement, knee, meniscus, specified NEC
specified NEC M23.30- ☑
lateral M23.30- ☑

☑ **Additional Character Required** — Refer to the Tabular List for Character Selection ▽ **Subterms under main terms may continue to next column or page**

Derangement — *continued*
  knee — *continued*
    meniscus — *continued*
      specified — *continued*
        lateral — *continued*
          anterior horn M23.34- ☑
          posterior horn M23.35- ☑
          specified NEC M23.36- ☑
        medial M23.30- ☑
          anterior horn M23.31- ☑
          posterior horn M23.32- ☑
          specified NEC M23.33- ☑
      old M23.8X- ☑
      specified NEC — *see* subcategory M23.8 ☑
  low back NEC — *see* Dorsopathy, specified NEC
  meniscus — *see* Derangement, knee, meniscus
  mental — *see* Psychosis
  patella, specified NEC — *see* Disorder, patella, derangement NEC
  semilunar cartilage (knee) — *see* Derangement, knee, meniscus, specified NEC
  shoulder (internal) — *see* Derangement, joint, shoulder
Dercum's disease E88.2
Derealization (neurotic) F48.1
Dermal — *see* condition
Dermaphytid — *see* Dermatophytosis
Dermatitis (eczematous) L30.9
  ab igne L59.0
  acarine B88.0
  actinic (due to sun) L57.8
    other than from sun L59.8
  allergic — *see* Dermatitis, contact, allergic
  ambustionis, due to burn or scald — *see* Burn
  amebic A06.7
  ammonia L22
  arsenical (ingested) L27.8
  artefacta L98.1
    psychogenic F54
  atopic L20.9
    psychogenic F54
    specified NEC L20.89
  autoimmune progesterone L30.8
  berlock, berloque L56.2
  blastomycotic B40.3
  blister beetle L24.89
  bullous, bullosa L13.9
    mucosynechial, atrophic L12.1
    seasonal L30.8
    specified NEC L13.8
  calorica L59.0
    due to burn or scald — *see* Burn
  caterpillar L24.89
  cercarial B65.3
  combustionis L59.0
    due to burn or scald — *see* Burn
  congelationis T69.1 ☑
  contact (occupational) L25.9
    allergic L23.9
      due to
        adhesives L23.1
        cement L23.5
        chemical products NEC L23.5
        chromium L23.0
        cosmetics L23.2
        dander (cat) (dog) L23.81
        drugs in contact with skin L23.3
        dyes L23.4
        food in contact with skin L23.6
        hair (cat) (dog) L23.81
        insecticide L23.5
        metals L23.0
        nickel L23.0
        plants, non-food L23.7
        plastic L23.5
        rubber L23.5
        specified agent NEC L23.89
    due to
      cement L25.3
      chemical products NEC L25.3
      cosmetics L25.0
      dander (cat) (dog) L23.81
      drugs in contact with skin L25.1
      dyes L25.2
      food in contact with skin L25.4
      hair (cat) (dog) L23.81
      plants, non-food L25.5
      specified agent NEC L25.8
    irritant L24.9

Dermatitis — *continued*
  contact — *continued*
    irritant — *continued*
      due to
        cement L24.5
        chemical products NEC L24.5
        cosmetics L24.3
        detergents L24.0
        drugs in contact with skin L24.4
        food in contact with skin L24.6
        oils and greases L24.1
        plants, non-food L24.7
        solvents L24.2
        specified agent NEC L24.89
  contusiformis L52
  diabetic — *see* E08-E13 with .620
  diaper L22
  diphtheritica A36.3
  dry skin L85.3
  due to
    acetone (contact) (irritant) L24.2
    acids (contact) (irritant) L24.5
    adhesive(s) (allergic) (contact) (plaster) L23.1
      irritant L24.5
    alcohol (irritant) (skin contact) (substances in category T51) L24.2
      taken internally L27.8
    alkalis (contact) (irritant) L24.5
    arsenic (ingested) L27.8
    carbon disulfide (contact) (irritant) L24.2
    caustics (contact) (irritant) L24.5
    cement (contact) L25.3
    cereal (ingested) L27.2
    chemical(s) NEC L25.3
      taken internally L27.8
    chlorocompounds L24.2
    chromium (contact) (irritant) L24.81
    coffee (ingested) L27.2
    cold weather L30.8
    cosmetics (contact) L25.0
      allergic L23.2
      irritant L24.3
    cyclohexanes L24.2
    dander (cat) (dog) L23.81
    Demodex species B88.0
    Dermanyssus gallinae B88.0
    detergents (contact) (irritant) L24.0
    dichromate L24.81
    drugs and medicaments (generalized) (internal use) L27.0
      external — *see* Dermatitis, due to, drugs, in contact with skin
      in contact with skin L25.1
        allergic L23.3
        irritant L24.4
      localized skin eruption L27.1
      specified substance — *see* Table of Drugs and Chemicals
    dyes (contact) L25.2
      allergic L23.4
      irritant L24.89
    epidermophytosis — *see* Dermatophytosis
    esters L24.2
    external irritant NEC L24.9
    fish (ingested) L27.2
    flour (ingested) L27.2
    food (ingested) L27.2
      in contact with skin L25.4
    fruit (ingested) L27.2
    furs (allergic) (contact) L23.81
    glues — *see* Dermatitis, due to, adhesives
    glycols L24.2
    greases NEC (contact) (irritant) L24.1
    hair (cat) (dog) L23.81
    hot
      objects and materials — *see* Burn
      weather or places L59.0
    hydrocarbons L24.2
    infrared rays L59.8
    ingestion, ingested substance L27.9
      chemical NEC L27.8
      drugs and medicaments — *see* Dermatitis, due to, drugs
      food L27.2
      specified NEC L27.8
    insecticide in contact with skin L24.5
    internal agent L27.9

Dermatitis — *continued*
  due to — *continued*
    internal agent — *continued*
      drugs and medicaments (generalized) — *see* Dermatitis, due to, drugs
      food L27.2
      irradiation — *see* Dermatitis, due to, radioactive substance
      ketones L24.2
      lacquer tree (allergic) (contact) L23.7
      light (sun) NEC L57.8
        acute L56.8
        other L59.8
      Liponyssoides sanguineus B88.0
      low temperature L30.8
      meat (ingested) L27.2
      metals, metal salts (contact) (irritant) L24.81
      milk (ingested) L27.2
      nickel (contact) (irritant) L24.81
      nylon (contact) (irritant) L24.5
      oils NEC (contact) (irritant) L24.1
      paint solvent (contact) (irritant) L24.2
      petroleum products (contact) (irritant) (substances in T52.0) L24.2
      plants NEC (contact) L25.5
        allergic L23.7
        irritant L24.7
      plasters (adhesive) (any) (allergic) (contact) L23.1
        irritant L24.5
      plastic (contact) L25.3
      preservatives (contact) — *see* Dermatitis, due to, chemical, in contact with skin
      primrose (allergic) (contact) L23.7
      primula (allergic) (contact) L23.7
      radiation L59.8
        nonionizing (chronic exposure) L57.8
        sun NEC L57.8
          acute L56.8
      radioactive substance L58.9
        acute L58.0
        chronic L58.1
      radium L58.9
        acute L58.0
        chronic L58.1
      ragweed (allergic) (contact) L23.7
      Rhus (allergic) (contact) (diversiloba) (radicans) (toxicodendron) (venenata) (verniciflua) L23.7
      rubber (contact) L24.5
      Senecio jacobaea (allergic) (contact) L23.7
      solvents (contact) (irritant) (substances in category T52) L24.2
      specified agent NEC (contact) L25.8
        allergic L23.89
        irritant L24.89
      sunshine NEC L57.8
        acute L56.8
      tetrachlorethylene (contact) (irritant) L24.2
      toluene (contact) (irritant) L24.2
      turpentine (contact) L24.2
      ultraviolet rays (sun NEC) (chronic exposure) L57.8
        acute L56.8
      vaccine or vaccination L27.0
        specified substance — *see* Table of Drugs and Chemicals
      varicose veins — *see* Varix, leg, with, inflammation
      X-rays L58.9
        acute L58.0
        chronic L58.1
  dyshydrotic L30.1
  dysmenorrheica N94.6
  escharotica — *see* Burn
  exfoliative, exfoliativa (generalized) L26
    neonatorum L00
  eyelid (*see also* Dermatosis, eyelid)
    allergic H01.119
      left H01.116
        lower H01.115
        upper H01.114
      right H01.113
        lower H01.112
        upper H01.111
    contact — *see* Dermatitis, eyelid, allergic
    due to
      Demodex species B88.0
      herpes (zoster) B02.39
        simplex B00.59
    eczematous H01.139
      left H01.136

🔻 **Subterms under main terms may continue to next column or page**

Index

Derangement — Dermatitis

Dermatitis — *continued*
eyelid (*see also* Dermatosis, eyelid) — *continued*
eczematous — *continued*
left — *continued*
lower H01.135
upper H01.134
right H01.133
lower H01.132
upper H01.131
facta, factitia, factitial L98.1
psychogenic F54
flexural NEC L20.82
friction L30.4
fungus B36.9
specified type NEC B36.8
gangrenosa, gangrenous infantum L08.0
harvest mite B88.0
heat L59.0
herpesviral, vesicular (ear) (lip) B00.1
herpetiformis (bullous) (erythematous) (pustular)
(vesicular) L13.0
juvenile L12.2
senile L12.0
hiemalis L30.8
hypostatic, hypostatica — *see* Varix, leg, with, inflammation
infectious eczematoid L30.3
infective L30.3
irritant — *see* Dermatitis, contact, irritant
Jacquet's (diaper dermatitis) L22
Leptus B88.0
lichenified NEC L28.0
medicamentosa (generalized) (internal use) — *see* Dermatitis, due to drugs
mite B88.0
multiformis L13.0
juvenile L12.2
napkin L22
neurotica L13.0
nummular L30.0
papillaris capillitii L73.0
pellagrous E52
perioral L71.0
photocontact L56.2
polymorpha dolorosa L13.0
pruriginosa L13.0
pruritic NEC L30.8
psychogenic F54
purulent L08.0
pustular
contagious B08.02
subcorneal L13.1
pyococcal L08.0
pyogenica L08.0
repens L40.2
Ritter's (exfoliativa) L00
Schamberg's L81.7
schistosome B65.3
seasonal bullous L30.8
seborrheic L21.9
infantile L21.1
specified NEC L21.8
sensitization NOS L23.9
septic L08.0
solare L57.8
specified NEC L30.8
stasis I87.2
with
varicose ulcer — *see* Varix, leg, with ulcer, with inflammation
varicose veins — *see* Varix, leg, with, inflammation
due to postthrombotic syndrome — *see* Syndrome, postthrombotic
suppurative L08.0
traumatic NEC L30.4
trophoneurotica L13.0
ultraviolet (sun) (chronic exposure) L57.8
acute L56.8
varicose — *see* Varix, leg, with, inflammation
vegetans L10.1
verrucosa B43.0
vesicular, herpesviral B00.1
Dermatoarthritis, lipoid E78.81
Dermatochalasis, eyelid H02.839
left H02.836
lower H02.835
upper H02.834

Dermatochalasis, eyelid — *continued*
right H02.833
lower H02.832
upper H02.831
Dermatofibroma (lenticulare) — *see* Neoplasm, skin, benign
protuberans — *see* Neoplasm, skin, uncertain behavior
Dermatofibrosarcoma (pigmented) (protuberans) — *see* Neoplasm, skin, malignant
Dermatographia L50.3
Dermatolysis (exfoliativa) (congenital) Q82.8
acquired L57.4
eyelids — *see* Blepharochalasis
palpebrarum — *see* Blepharochalasis
senile L57.4
Dermatomegaly NEC Q82.8
Dermatomucosomyositis M33.10
with
myopathy M33.12
respiratory involvement M33.11
specified organ involvement NEC M33.19
Dermatomycosis B36.9
furfuracea B36.0
specified type NEC B36.8
Dermatomyositis (acute) (chronic) (*see also* Dermatopolymyositis)
adult (*see also* Dermatomyositis, specified NEC) M33.10
in (due to) neoplastic disease (*see also* Neoplasm) D49.9 [M36.0]
juvenile M33.00
with
myopathy M33.02
respiratory involvement M33.01
specified organ involvement NEC M33.09
without myopathy M33.03
specified NEC M33.10
with
myopathy M33.12
respiratory involvement M33.11
specified organ involvement NEC M33.19
without myopathy M33.13
Dermatoneuritis of children — *see* Poisoning, mercury
Dermatophilosis A48.8
Dermatophytid L30.2
Dermatophytide — *see* Dermatophytosis
Dermatophytosis (epidermophyton) (infection) (Microsporum) (tinea) (Trichophyton) B35.9
beard B35.0
body B35.4
capitis B35.0
corporis B35.4
deep-seated B35.8
disseminated B35.8
foot B35.3
granulomatous B35.8
groin B35.6
hand B35.2
nail B35.1
perianal (area) B35.6
scalp B35.0
specified NEC B35.8
Dermatopolymyositis M33.90
with
myopathy M33.92
respiratory involvement M33.91
specified organ involvement NEC M33.99
in neoplastic disease (*see also* Neoplasm) D49.9 [M36.0]
juvenile M33.00
with
myopathy M33.02
respiratory involvement M33.01
specified organ involvement NEC M33.09
specified NEC M33.10
myopathy M33.12
respiratory involvement M33.11
specified organ involvement NEC M33.19
without myopathy M33.93
Dermatopolyneuritis — *see* Poisoning, mercury
Dermatorrhexis Q79.6
acquired L57.4
Dermatosclerosis (*see also* Scleroderma)
localized L94.0
Dermatosis L98.9
Andrews' L08.89
Bowen's — *see* Neoplasm, skin, in situ
bullous L13.9
specified NEC L13.8
exfoliativa L26

Dermatosis — *continued*
eyelid (noninfectious)
dermatitis — *see* Dermatitis, eyelid
discoid lupus erythematosus — *see* Lupus, erythematosus, eyelid
xeroderma — *see* Xeroderma, acquired, eyelid
factitial L98.1
febrile neutrophilic L98.2
gonococcal A54.89
herpetiformis L13.0
juvenile L12.2
linear IgA L13.8
menstrual NEC L98.8
neutrophilic, febrile L98.2
occupational — *see* Dermatitis, contact
papulosa nigra L82.1
pigmentary L81.9
progressive L81.7
Schamberg's L81.7
psychogenic F54
purpuric, pigmented L81.7
pustular, subcorneal L13.1
transient acantholytic L11.1
Dermographia, dermographism L50.3
Dermoid (cyst) (*see also* Neoplasm, benign, by site)
with malignant transformation C56- ☑
due to radiation (nonionizing) L57.8
Dermopathy
infiltrative with thyrotoxicosis — *see* Thyrotoxicosis
nephrogenic fibrosing L90.8
Dermophytosis — *see* Dermatophytosis
Descemetocele H18.73- ☑
Descemet's membrane — *see* condition
Descending — *see* condition
Descensus uteri — *see* Prolapse, uterus
Desert
rheumatism B38.0
sore — *see* Ulcer, skin
Desertion (newborn) — *see* Maltreatment
Desmoid (extra-abdominal) (tumor) — *see* Neoplasm, connective tissue, uncertain behavior
abdominal D48.1
Despondency F32.9
Desquamation, skin R23.4
Destruction, destructive (*see also* Damage)
articular facet (*see also* Derangement, joint, specified type NEC)
knee M23.8X- ☑
vertebra — *see* Spondylosis
bone (*see also* Disorder, bone, specified type NEC)
syphilitic A52.77
joint (*see also* Derangement, joint, specified type NEC)
sacroiliac M53.3
rectal sphincter K62.89
septum (nasal) J34.89
tuberculous NEC — *see* Tuberculosis
tympanum, tympanic membrane (nontraumatic) — *see* Disorder, tympanic membrane, specified NEC
vertebral disc — *see* Degeneration, intervertebral disc
Destructiveness (*see also* Disorder, conduct)
adjustment reaction — *see* Disorder, adjustment
Desultory labor O62.2
Detachment
cartilage — *see* Sprain
cervix, annular N88.8
complicating delivery O71.3
choroid (old) (postinfectional) (simple) (spontaneous) H31.40- ☑
hemorrhagic H31.41- ☑
serous H31.42- ☑
ligament — *see* Sprain
meniscus (knee) (*see also* Derangement, knee, meniscus, specified NEC)
current injury — *see* Tear, meniscus
due to old tear or injury — *see* Derangement, knee, meniscus, due to old tear
retina (without retinal break) (serous) H33.2- ☑
with retinal:
break H33.00- ☑
giant H33.03- ☑
multiple H33.02- ☑
single H33.01- ☑
dialysis H33.04- ☑
pigment epithelium — *see* Degeneration, retina, separation of layers, pigment epithelium detachment

☑ **Additional Character Required — Refer to the Tabular List for Character Selection**   ▽ **Subterms under main terms may continue to next column or page**

Detachment — *continued*
  retina — *continued*
    rhegmatogenous — *see* Detachment, retina, with
      retinal, break
    specified NEC H33.8
    total H33.05- ☑
    traction H33.4- ☑
  vitreous (body) H43.81 ☑
Detergent asthma J69.8
Deterioration
  epileptic F06.8
  general physical R53.81
  heart, cardiac — *see* Degeneration, myocardial
  mental — *see* Psychosis
  myocardial, myocardium — *see* Degeneration, myocar-
    dial
  senile (simple) R54
Deuteranomaly (anomalous trichromat) H53.53
Deuteranopia (complete) (incomplete) H53.53
Development
  abnormal, bone Q79.9
  arrested R62.50
    bone — *see* Arrest, development or growth, bone
    child R62.50
    due to malnutrition E45
  defective, congenital (*see also* Anomaly, by site)
    cauda equina Q06.3
    left ventricle Q24.8
      in hypoplastic left heart syndrome Q23.4
    valve Q24.8
      pulmonary Q22.3
  delayed (*see also* Delay, development) R62.50
    arithmetical skills F81.2
    language (skills) (expressive) F80.1
    learning skill F81.9
    mixed skills F88
    motor coordination F82
    reading F81.0
    specified learning skill NEC F81.89
    speech F80.9
    spelling F81.81
    written expression F81.81
  imperfect, congenital (*see also* Anomaly, by site)
    heart Q24.9
    lungs Q33.6
  incomplete
    bronchial tree Q32.4
    organ or site not listed — *see* Hypoplasia, by site
    respiratory system Q34.9
    sexual, precocious NEC E30.1
  tardy, mental (*see also* Disability, intellectual) F79
Developmental — *see* condition
  testing, infant or child — *see* Examination, child
Devergie's disease (pityriasis rubra pilaris) L44.0
Deviation (in)
  conjugate palsy (eye) (spastic) H51.0
  esophagus (acquired) K22.8
  eye, skew H51.8
  midline (jaw) (teeth) (dental arch) M26.29
    specified site NEC — *see* Malposition
  nasal septum J34.2
    congenital Q67.4
  opening and closing of the mandible M26.53
  organ or site, congenital NEC — *see* Malposition, con-
    genital
  septum (nasal) (acquired) J34.2
    congenital Q67.4
  sexual F65.9
    bestiality F65.89
    erotomania F52.8
    exhibitionism F65.2
    fetishism, fetishistic F65.0
      transvestism F65.1
    frotteurism F65.81
    masochism F65.51
    multiple F65.89
    necrophilia F65.89
    nymphomania F52.8
    pederosis F65.4
    pedophilia F65.4
    sadism, sadomasochism F65.52
    satyriasis F52.8
    specified type NEC F65.89
    transvestism F64.1
    voyeurism F65.3
  teeth, midline M26.29
  trachea J39.8
  ureter, congenital Q62.61

Device
  cerebral ventricle (communicating) in situ Z98.2
  contraceptive — *see* Contraceptive, device
  drainage, cerebrospinal fluid, in situ Z98.2
Devic's disease G36.0
Devil's
  grip B33.0
  pinches (purpura simplex) D69.2
Devitalized tooth K04.99
Devonshire colic — *see* Poisoning, lead
Dextraposition, aorta Q20.3
  in tetralogy of Fallot Q21.3
Dextrinosis, limit (debrancher enzyme deficiency) E74.03
Dextrocardia (true) Q24.0
  with
    complete transposition of viscera Q89.3
    situs inversus Q89.3
Dextrotransposition, aorta Q20.3
d-glycericacidemia E72.59
Dhat syndrome F48.8
Dhobi itch B35.6
Di George's syndrome D82.1
Di Guglielmo's disease C94.0- ☑
Diabetes, diabetic (mellitus) (sugar) E11.9
  with
    amyotrophy E11.44
    arthropathy NEC E11.618
    autonomic (poly)neuropathy E11.43
    cataract E11.36
    Charcot's joints E11.610
    chronic kidney disease E11.22
    circulatory complication NEC E11.59
    complication E11.8
      specified NEC E11.69
    dermatitis E11.620
    foot ulcer E11.621
    gangrene E11.52
    gastroparalysis E11.43
    gastroparesis E11.43
    glomerulonephrosis, intracapillary E11.21
    glomerulosclerosis, intercapillary E11.21
    hyperglycemia E11.65
    hyperosmolarity E11.00
      with coma E11.01
    hypoglycemia E11.649
      with coma E11.641
    ketoacidosis E11.10
      with coma E11.11
    kidney complications NEC E11.29
    Kimmelstiel-Wilson disease E11.21
    loss of protective sensation (LOPS) — *see* Diabetes,
      by type, with neuropathy
    mononeuropathy E11.41
    myasthenia E11.44
    necrobiosis lipoidica E11.620
    nephropathy E11.21
    neuralgia E11.42
    neurologic complication NEC E11.49
    neuropathic arthropathy E11.610
    neuropathy E11.40
    ophthalmic complication NEC E11.39
    oral complication NEC E11.638
    osteomyelitis E11.69
    periodontal disease E11.630
    peripheral angiopathy E11.51
      with gangrene E11.52
    polyneuropathy E11.42
    renal complication NEC E11.29
    renal tubular degeneration E11.29
    retinopathy E11.319
      with macular edema E11.311
        resolved following treatment E11.37 ☑
      nonproliferative E11.329 ☑
        with macular edema E11.321 ☑
        mild E11.329 ☑
          with macular edema E11.321 ☑
        moderate E11.339 ☑
          with macular edema E11.331 ☑
        severe E11.349 ☑
          with macular edema E11.341 ☑
      proliferative E11.359 ☑
        with
          combined traction retinal detachment
            and rhegmatogenous retinal de-
            tachment E11.354 ☑
          macular edema E11.351 ☑
          stable proliferative diabetic retinopathy
            E11.355 ☑

Diabetes, diabetic — *continued*
  with — *continued*
    retinopathy — *continued*
      proliferative — *continued*
        with — *continued*
          traction retinal detachment involving the
            macula E11.352 ☑
          traction retinal detachment not involving
            the macula E11.353 ☑
      resolved following treatment E09.37 ☑
    skin complication NEC E11.628
    skin ulcer NEC E11.622
  brittle — *see* Diabetes, type 1
  bronzed E83.110
  complicating pregnancy — *see* Pregnancy, complicated
    by, diabetes
  dietary counseling and surveillance Z71.3
  due to
    autoimmune process — *see* Diabetes, type 1
    immune mediated pancreatic islet beta-cell destruc-
      tion — *see* Diabetes, type 1
  due to drug or chemical E09.9
    with
      amyotrophy E09.44
      arthropathy NEC E09.618
      autonomic (poly)neuropathy E09.43
      cataract E09.36
      Charcot's joints E09.610
      chronic kidney disease E09.22
      circulatory complication NEC E09.59
      complication E09.8
        specified NEC E09.69
      dermatitis E09.620
      foot ulcer E09.621
      gangrene E09.52
      gastroparalysis E09.43
      gastroparesis E09.43
      glomerulonephrosis, intracapillary E09.21
      glomerulosclerosis, intercapillary E09.21
      hyperglycemia E09.65
      hyperosmolarity E09.00
        with coma E09.01
      hypoglycemia E09.649
        with coma E09.641
      ketoacidosis E09.10
        with coma E09.11
      kidney complications NEC E09.29
      Kimmelsteil-Wilson disease E09.21
      mononeuropathy E09.41
      myasthenia E09.44
      necrobiosis lipoidica E09.620
      nephropathy E09.21
      neuralgia E09.42
      neurologic complication NEC E09.49
      neuropathic arthropathy E09.610
      neuropathy E09.40
      ophthalmic complication NEC E09.39
      oral complication NEC E09.638
      periodontal disease E09.630
      peripheral angiopathy E09.51
        with gangrene E09.52
      polyneuropathy E09.42
      renal complication NEC E09.29
      renal tubular degeneration E09.29
      retinopathy E09.319
        with macular edema E09.311
        resolved following treatment E09.37 ☑
        nonproliferative E09.329 ☑
          with macular edema E09.321 ☑
          mild E09.329 ☑
            with macular edema E09.321 ☑
          moderate E09.339 ☑
            with macular edema E09.331 ☑
          severe E09.349 ☑
            with macular edema E09.341 ☑
        proliferative E09.359 ☑
          with
            combined traction retinal detachment
              and rhegmatogenous retinal
              detachment E09.354 ☑
            macular edema E09.351 ☑
            stable proliferative diabetic retinopa-
              thy E09.355 ☑
            traction retinal detachment involving
              the macula E09.352 ☑
            traction retinal detachment not involv-
              ing the macula E09.353 ☑
    skin complication NEC E09.628

Diabetes, diabetic — *continued*
  due to drug or chemical — *continued*
    with — *continued*
      skin ulcer NEC E09.622
  due to underlying condition E08.9
    with
      amyotrophy E08.44
      arthropathy NEC E08.618
      autonomic (poly)neuropathy E08.43
      cataract E08.36
      Charcot's joints E08.610
      chronic kidney disease E08.22
      circulatory complication NEC E08.59
      complication E08.8
        specified NEC E08.69
      dermatitis E08.620
      foot ulcer E08.621
      gangrene E08.52
      gastroparalysis E08.43
      gastroparesis E08.43
      glomerulonephrosis, intracapillary E08.21
      glomerulosclerosis, intercapillary E08.21
      hyperglycemia E08.65
      hyperosmolarity E08.00
        with coma E08.01
      hypoglycemia E08.649
        with coma E08.641
      ketoacidosis E08.10
        with coma E08.11
      kidney complications NEC E08.29
      Kimmelstiel-Wilson disease E08.21
      mononeuropathy E08.41
      myasthenia E08.44
      necrobiosis lipoidica E08.620
      nephropathy E08.21
      neuralgia E08.42
      neurologic complication NEC E08.49
      neuropathic arthropathy E08.610
      neuropathy E08.40
      ophthalmic complication NEC E08.39
      oral complication NEC E08.638
      periodontal disease E08.630
      peripheral angiopathy E08.51
        with gangrene E08.52
      polyneuropathy E08.42
      renal complication NEC E08.29
      renal tubular degeneration E08.29
      retinopathy E08.319
        with macular edema E08.311
          resolved following treatment E08.37 ☑
        nonproliferative E08.329 ☑
          with macular edema E08.321 ☑
          mild E08.329 ☑
            with macular edema E08.321 ☑
          moderate E08.339 ☑
            with macular edema E08.331 ☑
          severe E08.349 ☑
            with macular edema E08.341 ☑
        proliferative E08.359 ☑
          with
            combined traction retinal detachment and rhegmatogenous retinal detachment E08.354 ☑
            macular edema E08.351 ☑
            stable proliferative diabetic retinopathy E08.355 ☑
            traction retinal detachment involving the macula E08.352 ☑
            traction retinal detachment not involving the macula E08.353 ☑
      skin complication NEC E08.628
      skin ulcer NEC E08.622
  gestational (in pregnancy) O24.419
    affecting newborn P70.0
    diet controlled O24.410
    in childbirth O24.429
      diet controlled O24.420
      insulin (and diet) controlled O24.424
      oral drug controlled (antidiabetic) (hypoglycemic) O24.425
    insulin (and diet) controlled O24.414
    oral drug controlled (antidiabetic) (hypoglycemic) O24.415
    puerperal O24.439
      diet controlled O24.430
      insulin (and diet) controlled O24.434
      oral drug controlled (antidiabetic) (hypoglycemic) O24.435

Diabetes, diabetic — *continued*
  hepatogenous E13.9
  idiopathic — *see* Diabetes, type 1
  inadequately controlled — *code to* Diabetes, by type, with hyperglycemia
  insipidus E23.2
    nephrogenic N25.1
    pituitary E23.2
    vasopressin resistant N25.1
  insulin dependent — *code to* type of diabetes
  juvenile-onset — *see* Diabetes, type 1
  ketosis-prone — *see* Diabetes, type 1
  latent R73.03
  neonatal (transient) P70.2
  non-insulin dependent — *code to* type of diabetes
  out of control — *code to* Diabetes, by type, with hyperglycemia
  phosphate E83.39
  poorly controlled — *code to* Diabetes, by type, with hyperglycemia
  postpancreatectomy — *see* Diabetes, specified type NEC
  postprocedural — *see* Diabetes, specified type NEC
  secondary diabetes mellitus NEC — *see* Diabetes, specified type NEC
  specified type NEC E13.9
    with
      amyotrophy E13.44
      arthropathy NEC E13.618
      autonomic (poly)neuropathy E13.43
      cataract E13.36
      Charcot's joints E13.610
      chronic kidney disease E13.22
      circulatory complication NEC E13.59
      complication E13.8
        specified NEC E13.69
      dermatitis E13.620
      foot ulcer E13.621
      gangrene E13.52
      gastroparalysis E13.43
      gastroparesis E13.43
      glomerulonephrosis, intracapillary E13.21
      glomerulosclerosis, intercapillary E13.21
      hyperglycemia E13.65
      hyperosmolarity E13.00
        with coma E13.01
      hypoglycemia E13.649
        with coma E13.641
      ketoacidosis E13.10
        with coma E13.11
      kidney complications NEC E13.29
      Kimmelstiel-Wilson disease E13.21
      mononeuropathy E13.41
      myasthenia E13.44
      necrobiosis lipoidica E13.620
      nephropathy E13.21
      neuralgia E13.42
      neurologic complication NEC E13.49
      neuropathic arthropathy E13.610
      neuropathy E13.40
      ophthalmic complication NEC E13.39
      oral complication NEC E13.638
      periodontal disease E13.630
      peripheral angiopathy E13.51
        with gangrene E13.52
      polyneuropathy E13.42
      renal complication NEC E13.29
      renal tubular degeneration E13.29
      retinopathy E13.319
        with macular edema E13.311
          resolved following treatment E13.37 ☑
        nonproliferative E13.329 ☑
          with macular edema E13.321 ☑
          mild E13.329 ☑
            with macular edema E13.321 ☑
          moderate E13.339 ☑
            with macular edema E13.331 ☑
          severe E13.349 ☑
            with macular edema E13.341 ☑
        proliferative E13.359 ☑
          with
            combined traction retinal detachment and rhegmatogenous retinal detachment E13.354 ☑
            macular edema E13.351 ☑
            stable proliferative diabetic retinopathy E13.355 ☑

Diabetes, diabetic — *continued*
  specified type — *continued*
    with — *continued*
      retinopathy — *continued*
        proliferative — *continued*
          with — *continued*
            traction retinal detachment involving the macula E13.352 ☑
            traction retinal detachment not involving the macula E13.353 ☑
      skin complication NEC E13.628
      skin ulcer NEC E13.622
  steroid-induced — *see* Diabetes, due to, drug or chemical
  type 1 E10.9
    with
      amyotrophy E10.44
      arthropathy NEC E10.618
      autonomic (poly)neuropathy E10.43
      cataract E10.36
      Charcot's joints E10.610
      chronic kidney disease E10.22
      circulatory complication NEC E10.59
      complication E10.8
        specified NEC E10.69
      dermatitis E10.620
      foot ulcer E10.621
      gangrene E10.52
      gastroparalysis E10.43
      gastroparesis E10.43
      glomerulonephrosis, intracapillary E10.21
      glomerulosclerosis, intercapillary E10.21
      hyperglycemia E10.65
      hypoglycemia E10.649
        with coma E10.641
      ketoacidosis E10.10
        with coma E10.11
      kidney complications NEC E10.29
      Kimmelstiel-Wilson disease E10.21
      mononeuropathy E10.41
      myasthenia E10.44
      necrobiosis lipoidica E10.620
      nephropathy E10.21
      neuralgia E10.42
      neurologic complication NEC E10.49
      neuropathic arthropathy E10.610
      neuropathy E10.40
      ophthalmic complication NEC E10.39
      oral complication NEC E10.638
      osteomyelitis E10.69
      periodontal disease E10.630
      peripheral angiopathy E10.51
        with gangrene E10.52
      polyneuropathy E10.42
      renal complication NEC E10.29
      renal tubular degeneration E10.29
      retinopathy E10.319
        with macular edema E10.311
          resolved following treatment E10.37 ☑
        nonproliferative E10.329 ☑
          with macular edema E10.321 ☑
          mild E10.329 ☑
            with macular edema E10.321 ☑
          moderate E10.339 ☑
            with macular edema E10.331 ☑
          severe E10.349 ☑
            with macular edema E10.341 ☑
        proliferative E10.359 ☑
          with
            combined traction retinal detachment and rhegmatogenous retinal detachment E10.354 ☑
            macular edema E10.351 ☑
            stable proliferative diabetic retinopathy E10.355 ☑
            traction retinal detachment involving the macula E10.352 ☑
            traction retinal detachment not involving the macula E10.353 ☑
      skin complication NEC E10.628
      skin ulcer NEC E10.622
  type 2 E11.9
    with
      amyotrophy E11.44
      arthropathy NEC E11.618
      autonomic (poly)neuropathy E11.43
      cataract E11.36
      Charcot's joints E11.610

Diabetes, diabetic — *continued*
  type 2 — *continued*
    with — *continued*
      chronic kidney disease E11.22
      circulatory complication NEC E11.59
      complication E11.8
        specified NEC E11.69
      dermatitis E11.620
      foot ulcer E11.621
      gangrene E11.52
      gastroparalysis E11.43
      gastroparesis E11.43
      glomerulonephrosis, intracapillary E11.21
      glomerulosclerosis, intercapillary E11.21
      hyperglycemia E11.65
      hyperosmolarity E11.00
        with coma E11.01
      hypoglycemia E11.649
        with coma E11.641
      ketoacidosis E11.10
        with coma E11.11
      kidney complications NEC E11.29
      Kimmelstiel-Wilson disease E11.21
      mononeuropathy E11.41
      myasthenia E11.44
      necrobiosis lipoidica E11.620
      nephropathy E11.21
      neuralgia E11.42
      neurologic complication NEC E11.49
      neuropathic arthropathy E11.610
      neuropathy E11.40
      ophthalmic complication NEC E11.39
      oral complication NEC E11.638
      osteomyelitis E11.69
      periodontal disease E11.630
      peripheral angiopathy E11.51
        with gangrene E11.52
      polyneuropathy E11.42
      renal complication NEC E11.29
      renal tubular degeneration E11.29
      retinopathy E11.319
        with macular edema E11.311
        resolved following treatment E11.37 ☑
        nonproliferative E11.329 ☑
          with macular edema E11.321 ☑
          mild E11.329 ☑
            with macular edema E11.321 ☑
          moderate E11.339 ☑
            with macular edema E11.331 ☑
          severe E11.349 ☑
            with macular edema E11.341 ☑
        proliferative E11.359 ☑
          with
            combined traction retinal detachment
              and rhegmatogenous retinal
              detachment E11.354 ☑
            macular edema E11.351 ☑
            stable proliferative diabetic retinopa-
              thy E11.355 ☑
            traction retinal detachment involving
              the macula E11.352 ☑
            traction retinal detachment not involv-
              ing the macula E11.353 ☑
      skin complication NEC E11.628
      skin ulcer NEC E11.622
  uncontrolled
    meaning
      hyperglycemia — *see* Diabetes, by type, with,
        hyperglycemia
      hypoglycemia — *see* Diabetes, by type, with,
        hypoglycemia
Diacyclothrombopathia D69.1
Diagnosis deferred R69
Dialysis (intermittent) (treatment)
  noncompliance (with) Z91.15
  renal (hemodialysis) (peritoneal), status Z99.2
  retina, retinal — *see* Detachment, retina, with retinal,
    dialysis
Diamond-Blackfan anemia (congenital hypoplastic)
  D61.01
Diamond-Gardener syndrome (autoerythrocyte sensi-
  tization) D69.2
Diaper rash L22
Diaphoresis (excessive) R61
Diaphragm — *see* condition
Diaphragmalgia R07.1
Diaphragmatitis, diaphragmitis J98.6
Diaphysial aclasis Q78.6

Diaphysitis — *see* Osteomyelitis, specified type NEC
Diarrhea, diarrheal (disease) (infantile) (inflammatory)
  R19.7
  achlorhydric K31.83
  allergic K52.29
    due to
      colitis — *see* Colitis, allergic
      enteritis — *see* Enteritis, allergic
  amebic (*see also* Amebiasis) A06.0
    with abscess — *see* Abscess, amebic
    acute A06.0
    chronic A06.1
    nondysenteric A06.2
  bacillary — *see* Dysentery, bacillary
  balantidial A07.0
  cachectic NEC K52.89
  Chilomastix A07.8
  choleriformis A00.1
  chronic (noninfectious) K52.9
  coccidial A07.3
  Cochin-China K90.1
    strongyloidiasis B78.0
  Dientamoeba A07.8
  dietetic (*see also* Diarrhea, allergic) K52.29
  drug-induced K52.1
  due to
    bacteria A04.9
      specified NEC A04.8
    Campylobacter A04.5
    Capillaria philippinensis B81.1
    Clostridium difficile
      not specified as recurrent A04.72
      recurrent A04.71
    Clostridium perfringens (C) (F) A04.8
    Cryptosporidium A07.2
    drugs K52.1
    Escherichia coli A04.4
      enteroaggregative A04.4
      enterohemorrhagic A04.3
      enteroinvasive A04.2
      enteropathogenic A04.0
      enterotoxigenic A04.1
      specified NEC A04.4
    food hypersensitivity (*see also* Diarrhea, allergic)
      K52.29
    Necator americanus B76.1
    S. japonicum B65.2
    specified organism NEC A08.8
      bacterial A04.8
      viral A08.39
    Staphylococcus A04.8
    Trichuris trichiuria B79
    virus — *see* Enteritis, viral
    Yersinia enterocolitica A04.6
  dysenteric A09
  endemic A09
  epidemic A09
  flagellate A07.9
  Flexner's (ulcerative) A03.1
  functional K59.1
    following gastrointestinal surgery K91.89
    psychogenic F45.8
  Giardia lamblia A07.1
  giardial A07.1
  hill K90.1
  infectious A09
  malarial — *see* Malaria
  mite B88.0
  mycotic NEC B49
  neonatal (noninfectious) P78.3
  nervous F45.8
  neurogenic K59.1
  noninfectious K52.9
  postgastrectomy K91.1
  postvagotomy K91.1
  protozoal A07.9
    specified NEC A07.8
  psychogenic F45.8
  specified
    bacterium NEC A04.8
    virus NEC A08.39
  strongyloidiasis B78.0
  toxic K52.1
  trichomonal A07.8
  tropical K90.1
  tuberculous A18.32
  viral — *see* Enteritis, viral

Diastasis
  cranial bones M84.88
    congenital NEC Q75.8
  joint (traumatic) — *see* Dislocation
  muscle M62.00
    ankle M62.07- ☑
    congenital Q79.8
    foot M62.07- ☑
    forearm M62.03- ☑
    hand M62.04- ☑
    lower leg M62.06- ☑
    pelvic region M62.05- ☑
    shoulder region M62.01- ☑
    specified site NEC M62.08
    thigh M62.05- ☑
    upper arm M62.02- ☑
  recti (abdomen)
    complicating delivery O71.89
    congenital Q79.59
Diastema, tooth, teeth, fully erupted M26.32
Diastematomyelia Q06.2
Diataxia, cerebral G80.4
Diathesis
  allergic — *see* History, allergy
  bleeding (familial) D69.9
  cystine (familial) E72.00
  gouty — *see* Gout
  hemorrhagic (familial) D69.9
    newborn NEC P53
  spasmophilic R29.0
Diaz's disease or osteochondrosis (juvenile) (talus) —
  see Osteochondrosis, juvenile, tarsus
Dibothriocephalus, dibothriocephaliasis (latus) (infection) (infestation) B70.0
  larval B70.1
Dicephalus, dicephaly Q89.4
Dichotomy, teeth K00.2
Dichromat, dichromatopsia (congenital) — *see* Deficiency, color vision
Dichuchwa A65
Dicroceliasis B66.2
Didelphia, didelphys — *see* Double uterus
Didymytis N45.1
  with orchitis N45.3
Dietary
  inadequacy or deficiency E63.9
  surveillance and counseling Z71.3
Dietl's crisis N13.8
Dieulafoy lesion (hemorrhagic)
  duodenum K31.82
  esophagus K22.8
  intestine (colon) K63.81
  stomach K31.82
Difficult, difficulty (in)
  acculturation Z60.3
  feeding R63.3
    newborn P92.9
      breast P92.5
      specified NEC P92.8
    nonorganic (infant or child) F98.29
  intubation, in anesthesia T88.4 ☑
  mechanical, gastroduodenal stoma K91.89
    causing obstruction (*see also* Obstruction, intestine,
      postoperative) K91.30
  micturition
    need to immediately re-void R39.191
    position dependent R39.192
    specified NEC R39.198
  reading (developmental) F81.0
    secondary to emotional disorders F93.9
  spelling (specific) F81.81
    with reading disorder F81.89
    due to inadequate teaching Z55.8
  swallowing — *see* Dysphagia
  walking R26.2
  work
    conditions NEC Z56.5
    schedule Z56.3
Diffuse — *see* condition
Digestive — *see* condition
Dihydropyrimidine dehydrogenase disease (DPD)
  E88.89
Diktyoma — *see* Neoplasm, malignant, by site
Dilaceration, tooth K00.4
Dilatation
  anus K59.8
    venule — *see* Hemorrhoids

Dilatation — *continued*
aorta (focal) (general) — *see* Ectasia, aorta
  with aneuysm — *see* Aneurysm, aorta
  congenital Q25.44
artery — *see* Aneurysm
bladder (sphincter) N32.89
  congenital Q64.79
blood vessel I99.8
bronchial J47.9
  with
    exacerbation (acute) J47.1
    lower respiratory infection J47.0
calyx (due to obstruction) — *see* Hydronephrosis
capillaries I78.8
cardiac (acute) (chronic) (*see also* Hypertrophy, cardiac)
  congenital Q24.8
    valve NEC Q24.8
    pulmonary Q22.3
  valve — *see* Endocarditis
cavum septi pellucidi Q06.8
cervix (uteri) (*see also* Incompetency, cervix)
  incomplete, poor, slow complicating delivery O62.0
colon K59.39
  congenital Q43.1
  psychogenic F45.8
  toxic K59.31
common duct (acquired) K83.8
  congenital Q44.5
cystic duct (acquired) K82.8
  congenital Q44.5
duct, mammary — *see* Ectasia, mammary duct
duodenum K59.8
esophagus K22.8
  congenital Q39.5
  due to achalasia K22.0
eustachian tube, congenital Q17.8
gallbladder K82.8
gastric — *see* Dilatation, stomach
heart (acute) (chronic) (*see also* Hypertrophy, cardiac)
  congenital Q24.8
  valve — *see* Endocarditis
ileum K59.8
  psychogenic F45.8
jejunum K59.8
  psychogenic F45.8
kidney (calyx) (collecting structures) (cystic)
  (parenchyma) (pelvis) (idiopathic) N28.89
lacrimal passages or duct — *see* Disorder, lacrimal
  system, changes
lymphatic vessel I89.0
mammary duct — *see* Ectasia, mammary duct
Meckel's diverticulum (congenital) Q43.0
  malignant — *see* Table of Neoplasms, small intes-
    tine, malignant
myocardium (acute) (chronic) — *see* Hypertrophy,
  cardiac
organ or site, congenital NEC — *see* Distortion
pancreatic duct K86.89
pericardium — *see* Pericarditis
pharynx J39.2
prostate N42.89
pulmonary
  artery (idiopathic) I28.8
  valve, congenital Q22.3
pupil H57.04
rectum K59.39
saccule, congenital Q16.5
salivary gland (duct) K11.8
sphincter ani K62.89
stomach K31.89
  acute K31.0
  psychogenic F45.8
submaxillary duct K11.8
trachea, congenital Q32.1
ureter (idiopathic) N28.82
  congenital Q62.2
  due to obstruction N13.4
urethra (acquired) N36.8
vasomotor I73.9
vein I86.8
ventricular, ventricle (acute) (chronic) (*see also* Hypertrophy, cardiac)
  cerebral, congenital Q04.8
venule NEC I86.8
vesical orifice N32.89
Dilated, dilation — *see* Dilatation
Diminished, diminution
hearing (acuity) — *see* Deafness

Diminished, diminution — *continued*
sense or sensation (cold) (heat) (tactile) (vibratory)
  R20.8
vision NEC H54.7
vital capacity R94.2
Diminuta taenia B71.0
Dimitri-Sturge-Weber disease Q85.8
Dimple
congenital sacral Q82.6
parasacral Q82.6
pilonidal or postanal — *see* Cyst, pilonidal
Dioctophyme renalis (infection) (infestation) B83.8
Dipetalonemiasis B74.4
Diphallus Q55.69
Diphtheria, diphtheritic (gangrenous) (hemorrhagic)
  A36.9
carrier (suspected) Z22.2
cutaneous A36.3
faucial A36.0
infection of wound A36.3
laryngeal A36.2
myocarditis A36.81
nasal, anterior A36.89
nasopharyngeal A36.1
neurological complication A36.89
pharyngeal A36.0
specified site NEC A36.89
tonsillar A36.0
Diphyllobothriasis (intestine) B70.0
larval B70.1
Diplacusis H93.22- ☑
Diplegia (upper limbs) G83.0
congenital (cerebral) G80.8
facial G51.0
lower limbs G82.20
spastic G80.1
Diplococcus, diplococcal — *see* condition
Diplopia H53.2
Dipsomania F10.20
  with
    psychosis — *see* Psychosis, alcoholic
    remission F10.21
Dipylidiasis B71.1
DIRA (deficiency of interleukin 1 receptor antagonist)
  M04.8
Direction, teeth, abnormal, fully erupted M26.30
Dirofilariasis B74.8
Dirt-eating child F98.3
Disability, disabilities
heart — *see* Disease, heart
intellectual F79
  with
    autistic features F84.9
  mild (I.Q. 50-69) F70
  moderate (I.Q. 35-49) F71
  profound (I.Q. under 20) F73
  severe (I.Q. 20-34) F72
  specified level NEC F78
knowledge acquisition F81.9
learning F81.9
limiting activities Z73.6
spelling, specific F81.81
Disappearance of family member Z63.4
Disarticulation — *see* Amputation
meaning traumatic amputation — *see* Amputation,
  traumatic
Discharge (from)
abnormal finding in — *see* Abnormal, specimen
breast (female) (male) N64.52
diencephalic autonomic idiopathic — *see* Epilepsy,
  specified NEC
ear (*see also* Otorrhea)
  blood — *see* Otorrhagia
excessive urine R35.8
nipple N64.52
penile R36.9
postnasal R09.82
prison, anxiety concerning Z65.2
urethral R36.9
  without blood R36.0
  hematospermia R36.1
vaginal N89.8
Discitis, diskitis M46.40
cervical region M46.42
cervicothoracic region M46.43
lumbar region M46.46
lumbosacral region M46.47
multiple sites M46.49

Discitis, diskitis — *continued*
occipito-atlanto-axial region M46.41
pyogenic — *see* Infection, intervertebral disc, pyogenic
sacrococcygeal region M46.48
thoracic region M46.44
thoracolumbar region M46.45
Discoid
meniscus (congenital) Q68.6
semilunar cartilage (congenital) — *see* Derangement,
  knee, meniscus, specified NEC
Discoloration
nails L60.8
teeth (posteruptive) K03.7
  during formation K00.8
Discomfort
chest R07.89
visual H53.14- ☑
Discontinuity, ossicles, ear H74.2- ☑
Discord (with)
boss Z56.4
classmates Z55.4
counselor Z64.4
employer Z56.4
family Z63.8
fellow employees Z56.4
in-laws Z63.1
landlord Z59.2
lodgers Z59.2
neighbors Z59.2
probation officer Z64.4
social worker Z64.4
teachers Z55.4
workmates Z56.4
Discordant connection
atrioventricular (congenital) Q20.5
ventriculoarterial Q20.3
Discrepancy
centric occlusion maximum intercuspation M26.55
leg length (acquired) — *see* Deformity, limb, unequal
  length
  congenital — *see* Defect, reduction, lower limb
uterine size date O26.84- ☑
Discrimination
ethnic Z60.5
political Z60.5
racial Z60.5
religious Z60.5
sex Z60.5
Disease, diseased (*see also* Syndrome)
absorbent system I87.8
acid-peptic K30
Acosta's T70.29 ☑
Adams-Stokes (-Morgagni) (syncope with heart block)
  I45.9
Addison's anemia (pernicious) D51.0
adenoids (and tonsils) J35.9
adrenal (capsule) (cortex) (gland) (medullary) E27.9
  hyperfunction E27.0
  specified NEC E27.8
ainhum L94.6
airway
  obstructive, chronic J44.9
    due to
      cotton dust J66.0
      specific organic dusts NEC J66.8
  reactive — *see* Asthma
akamushi (scrub typhus) A75.3
Albers-Schönberg (marble bones) Q78.2
Albert's — *see* Tendinitis, Achilles
alimentary canal K63.9
alligator-skin Q80.9
  acquired L85.0
alpha heavy chain C88.3
alpine T70.29 ☑
altitude T70.20 ☑
alveolar ridge
  edentulous K06.9
    specified NEC K06.8
alveoli, teeth K08.9
Alzheimer's G30.9 [F02.80]
  with behavioral disturbance G30.9 [F02.81]
  early onset G30.0 [F02.80]
    with behavioral disturbance G30.0 [F02.81]
  late onset G30.1 [F02.80]
    with behavioral disturbance G30.1 [F02.81]
  specified NEC G30.8 [F02.80]
    with behavioral disturbance G30.8 [F02.81]
amyloid — *see* Amyloidosis

☑ **Additional Character Required** — Refer to the Tabular List for Character Selection   ▽ **Subterms under main terms may continue to next column or page**

Disease, diseased — *continued*
- Andersen's (glycogenosis IV) E74.09
- Andes T70.29 ☑
- Andrews' (bacterid) L08.89
- angiospastic I73.9
  - cerebral G45.9
  - vein I87.8
- anterior
  - chamber H21.9
  - horn cell G12.29
- antiglomerular basement membrane (anti- GBM) antibody M31.0
  - tubulo-interstitial nephritis N12
- antral — *see* Sinusitis, maxillary
- anus K62.9
  - specified NEC K62.89
- aorta (nonsyphilitic) I77.9
  - syphilitic NEC A52.02
- aortic (heart) (valve) I35.9
  - rheumatic I06.9
- Apollo B30.3
- aponeuroses — *see* Enthesopathy
- appendix K38.9
  - specified NEC K38.8
- aqueous (chamber) H21.9
- Arnold-Chiari — *see* Arnold-Chiari disease
- arterial I77.9
  - occlusive — *see* Occlusion, by site
    - due to stricture or stenosis I77.1
- arteriocardiorenal — *see* Hypertension, cardiorenal
- arteriolar (generalized) (obliterative) I77.9
- arteriorenal — *see* Hypertension, kidney
- arteriosclerotic (*see also* Arteriosclerosis)
  - cardiovascular — *see* Disease, heart, ischemic, atherosclerotic
  - coronary (artery) — *see* Disease, heart, ischemic, atherosclerotic
  - heart — *see* Disease, heart, ischemic, atherosclerotic
- artery I77.9
  - cerebral I67.9
  - coronary I25.10
    - with angina pectoris — *see* Arteriosclerosis, coronary (artery)
- arthropod-borne NOS (viral) A94
  - specified type NEC A93.8
- atticoantral, chronic H66.20
  - left H66.22
    - with right H66.23
  - right H66.21
    - with left H66.23
- auditory canal — *see* Disorder, ear, external
- auricle, ear NEC — *see* Disorder, pinna
- Australian X A83.4
- autoimmune (systemic) NOS M35.9
  - hemolytic (cold type) (warm type) D59.1
    - drug-induced D59.0
  - thyroid E06.3
- autoinflammatory M04.9
  - NOD2-associated M04.8
  - specified type NEC M04.8
- aviator's — *see* Effect, adverse, high altitude
- Ayerza's (pulmonary artery sclerosis with pulmonary hypertension) I27.0
- Babington's (familial hemorrhagic telangiectasia) I78.0
- bacterial A49.9
  - specified NEC A48.8
  - zoonotic A28.9
    - specified type NEC A28.8
- Baelz's (cheilitis glandularis apostematosa) K13.0
- bagasse J67.1
- balloon — *see* Effect, adverse, high altitude
- Bang's (brucella abortus) A23.1
- Bannister's T78.3 ☑
- barometer makers' — *see* Poisoning, mercury
- Barraquer (-Simons') (progressive lipodystrophy) E88.1
- Barrett's — *see* Barrett's, esophagus
- Bartholin's gland N75.9
- basal ganglia G25.9
  - degenerative G23.9
    - specified NEC G23.8
  - specified NEC G25.89
- Basedow's (exophthalmic goiter) — *see* Hyperthyroidism, with, goiter (diffuse)
- Bateman's B08.1
- Batten-Steinert G71.11
- Battey A31.0
- Beard's (neurasthenia) F48.8

Disease, diseased — *continued*
- Becker
  - idiopathic mural endomyocardial I42.3
  - myotonia congenita G71.12
- Begbie's (exophthalmic goiter) — *see* Hyperthyroidism, with, goiter (diffuse)
- behavioral, organic F07.9
- Beigel's (white piedra) B36.2
- Benson's — *see* Deposit, crystalline
- Bernard-Soulier (thrombopathy) D69.1
- Bernhardt (-Roth) — *see* Mononeuropathy, lower limb, meralgia paresthetica
- Biermer's (pernicious anemia) D51.0
- bile duct (common) (hepatic) K83.9
  - with calculus, stones — *see* Calculus, bile duct
  - specified NEC K83.8
- biliary (tract) K83.9
  - specified NEC K83.8
- Billroth's — *see* Spina bifida
- bird fancier's J67.2
- black lung J60
- bladder N32.9
  - in (due to)
    - schistosomiasis (bilharziasis) B65.0 [N33]
  - specified NEC N32.89
- bleeder's D66
- blood D75.9
  - forming organs D75.9
  - vessel I99.9
- Bloodgood's — *see* Mastopathy, cystic
- Bodechtel-Guttmann (subacute sclerosing panencephalitis) A81.1
- bone (*see also* Disorder, bone)
  - aluminum M83.4
  - fibrocystic NEC
    - jaw M27.49
- bone-marrow D75.9
- Borna A83.9
- Bornholm (epidemic pleurodynia) B33.0
- Bouchard's (myopathic dilatation of the stomach) K31.0
- Bouillaud's (rheumatic heart disease) I01.9
- Bourneville (-Brissaud) (tuberous sclerosis) Q85.1
- Bouveret (-Hoffmann) (paroxysmal tachycardia) I47.9
- bowel K63.9
  - functional K59.9
    - psychogenic F45.8
- brain G93.9
  - arterial, artery I67.9
  - arteriosclerotic I67.2
  - congenital Q04.9
  - degenerative — *see* Degeneration, brain
  - inflammatory — *see* Encephalitis
  - organic G93.9
    - arteriosclerotic I67.2
  - parasitic NEC B71.9 [G94]
  - senile NEC G31.1
  - specified NEC G93.89
- breast (*see also* Disorder, breast) N64.9
  - cystic (chronic) — *see* Mastopathy, cystic
  - fibrocystic — *see* Mastopathy, cystic
  - Paget's
    - female, unspecified side C50.91- ☑
    - male, unspecified side C50.92- ☑
  - specified NEC N64.89
- Breda's — *see* Yaws
- Bretonneau's (diphtheritic malignant angina) A36.0
- Bright's — *see* Nephritis
  - arteriosclerotic — *see* Hypertension, kidney
- Brill's (recrudescent typhus) A75.1
- Brill-Zinsser (recrudescent typhus) A75.1
- Brion-Kayser — *see* Fever, paratyphoid
- broad
  - beta E78.2
  - ligament (noninflammatory) N83.9
    - inflammatory — *see* Disease, pelvis, inflammatory
    - specified NEC N83.8
- Brocq-Duhring (dermatitis herpetiformis) L13.0
- Brocq's
  - meaning
    - dermatitis herpetiformis L13.0
    - prurigo L28.2
- bronchopulmonary J98.4
- bronchus NEC J98.09
- bronze Addison's E27.1
  - tuberculous A18.7
- budgerigar fancier's J67.2
- Buerger's (thromboangiitis obliterans) I73.1

Disease, diseased — *continued*
- bullous L13.9
  - chronic of childhood L12.2
  - specified NEC L13.8
- Bürger-Grütz (essential familial hyperlipemia) E78.3
- bursa — *see* Bursopathy
- caisson T70.3 ☑
- California — *see* Coccidioidomycosis
- capillaries I78.9
  - specified NEC I78.8
- Carapata A68.0
- cardiac — *see* Disease, heart
- cardiopulmonary, chronic I27.9
- cardiorenal (hepatic) (hypertensive) (vascular) — *see* Hypertension, cardiorenal
- cardiovascular (atherosclerotic) I25.10
  - with angina pectoris — *see* Arteriosclerosis, coronary (artery),
  - congenital Q28.9
  - hypertensive — *see* Hypertension, heart
  - newborn P29.9
    - specified NEC P29.89
  - renal (hypertensive) — *see* Hypertension, cardiorenal
  - syphilitic (asymptomatic) A52.00
- cartilage — *see* Disorder, cartilage
- Castellani's A69.8
- Castleman (unicentric) (multicentric) D47.Z2
  - HHV-8-associated (*see also* Herpesvirus, human, 8) D47.Z2
- cat-scratch A28.1
- Cavare's (familial periodic paralysis) G72.3
- cecum K63.9
- celiac (adult) (infantile) (with steatorrhea) K90.0
- cellular tissue L98.9
- central core G71.2
- cerebellar, cerebellum — *see* Disease, brain
- cerebral (*see also* Disease, brain)
  - degenerative — *see* Degeneration, brain
- cerebrospinal G96.9
- cerebrovascular I67.9
  - acute I67.89
    - embolic I63.4- ☑
    - thrombotic I63.3- ☑
  - arteriosclerotic I67.2
  - hereditary NEC I67.858
  - specified NEC I67.89
- cervix (uteri) (noninflammatory) N88.9
  - inflammatory — *see* Cervicitis
  - specified NEC N88.8
- Chabert's A22.9
- Chandler's (osteochondritis dissecans, hip) — *see* Osteochondritis, dissecans, hip
- Charlouis — *see* Yaws
- Chédiak-Steinbrinck (-Higashi) (congenital gigantism of peroxidase granules) E70.330
- chest J98.9
- Chiari's (hepatic vein thrombosis) I82.0
- Chicago B40.9
- Chignon B36.8
- chigo, chigoe B88.1
- childhood granulomatous D71
- Chinese liver fluke B66.1
- chlamydial A74.9
  - specified NEC A74.89
- cholecystic K82.9
- choroid H31.9
  - specified NEC H31.8
- Christmas D67
- chronic bullous of childhood L12.2
- chylomicron retention E78.3
- ciliary body H21.9
  - specified NEC H21.89
- circulatory (system) NEC I99.8
  - newborn P29.9
  - syphilitic A52.00
    - congenital A50.54
- coagulation factor deficiency (congenital) — *see* Defect, coagulation
- coccidioidal — *see* Coccidioidomycosis
- cold
  - agglutinin or hemoglobinuria D59.1
    - paroxysmal D59.6
  - hemagglutinin (chronic) D59.1
- collagen NOS (nonvascular) (vascular) M35.9
  - specified NEC M35.9
- colon K63.9
  - functional K59.9

Disease, diseased — *continued*

colon — *continued*
  functional — *continued*
    congenital Q43.2
    ischemic (*see also* Ischemia, intestine, acute) K55.Ø39
  colonic inflammatory bowel, unclassified (IBDU) K52.3
combined system — *see* Degeneration, combined
compressed air T7Ø.3 ☑
Concato's (pericardial polyserositis) A19.9
  nontubercular I31.1
  pleural — *see* Pleurisy, with effusion
conjunctiva H11.9
  chlamydial A74.Ø
  specified NEC H11.89
  viral B3Ø.9
    specified NEC B3Ø.8
connective tissue, systemic (diffuse) M35.9
  in (due to)
    hypogammaglobulinemia D8Ø.1 [M36.8]
    ochronosis E7Ø.29 [M36.8]
  specified NEC M35.8
Conor and Bruch's (boutonneuse fever) A77.1
Cooper's — *see* Mastopathy, cystic
Cori's (glycogenosis III) E74.Ø3
corkhandler's or corkworker's J67.3
cornea H18.9
  specified NEC H18.89- ☑
coronary (artery) — *see* Disease, heart, ischemic, atherosclerotic
  congenital Q24.5
  ostial, syphilitic (aortic) (mitral) (pulmonary) A52.Ø3
corpus cavernosum N48.9
  specified NEC N48.89
Cotugno's — *see* Sciatica
coxsackie (virus) NEC B34.1
cranial nerve NOS G52.9
Creutzfeldt-Jakob — *see* Creutzfeldt-Jakob disease or syndrome
Crocq's (acrocyanosis) I73.89
Crohn's — *see* Enteritis, regional
Curschmann G71.11
cystic
  breast (chronic) — *see* Mastopathy, cystic
  kidney, congenital Q61.9
  liver, congenital Q44.6
  lung J98.4
    congenital Q33.Ø
cytomegalic inclusion (generalized) B25.9
  with pneumonia B25.Ø
  congenital P35.1
cytomegaloviral B25.9
  specified NEC B25.8
Czerny's (periodic hydrarthrosis of the knee) — *see* Effusion, joint, knee
Daae (-Finsen) (epidemic pleurodynia) B33.Ø
Darling's — *see* Histoplasmosis capsulati
de Quervain's (tendon sheath) M65.4
  thyroid (subacute granulomatous thyroiditis) EØ6.1
Débove's (splenomegaly) R16.1
deer fly — *see* Tularemia
Degos' I77.89
demyelinating, demyelinizating (nervous system) G37.9
  multiple sclerosis G35
  specified NEC G37.8
dense deposit (*see also* NØØ-NØ7 with fourth character .6) NØ5.6
deposition, hydroxyapatite — *see* Disease, hydroxyapatite deposition
Devergie's (pityriasis rubra pilaris) L44.Ø
Devic's G36.Ø
diaphorase deficiency D74.Ø
diaphragm J98.6
diarrheal, infectious NEC AØ9
digestive system K92.9
  specified NEC K92.89
disc, degenerative — *see* Degeneration, intervertebral disc
discogenic (*see also* Displacement, intervertebral disc NEC)
  with myelopathy — *see* Disorder, disc, with, myelopathy
diverticular — *see* Diverticula
Dubois (thymus) A5Ø.59 [E35]
Duchenne-Griesinger G71.Ø1
Duchenne's
  muscular dystrophy G71.Ø1
  pseudohypertrophy, muscles G71.Ø1
ductless glands E34.9

Disease, diseased — *continued*

Duhring's (dermatitis herpetiformis) L13.Ø
duodenum K31.9
  specified NEC K31.89
Dupré's (meningism) R29.1
Dupuytren's (muscle contracture) M72.Ø
Durand-Nicholas-Favre (climatic bubo) A55
Duroziez's (congenital mitral stenosis) Q23.2
ear — *see* Disorder, ear
Eberth's — *see* Fever, typhoid
Ebola (virus) A98.4
Ebstein's heart Q22.5
Echinococcus — *see* Echinococcus
echovirus NEC B34.1
Eddowes' (brittle bones and blue sclera) Q78.Ø
edentulous (alveolar) ridge KØ6.9
  specified NEC KØ6.8
Edsall's T67.2 ☑
Eichstedt's (pityriasis versicolor) B36.Ø
Eisenmenger's (irreversible) I27.83
Ellis-van Creveld (chondroectodermal dysplasia) Q77.6
end stage renal (ESRD) N18.6
  due to hypertension I12.Ø
endocrine glands or system NEC E34.9
endomyocardial (eosinophilic) I42.3
English (rickets) E55.Ø
enteroviral, enterovirus NEC B34.1
  central nervous system NEC A88.8
epidemic B99.9
  specified NEC B99.8
epididymis N5Ø.9
Erb (-Landouzy) G71.Ø2
Erdheim-Chester (ECD) E88.89
esophagus K22.9
  functional K22.4
  psychogenic F45.8
  specified NEC K22.8
Eulenburg's (congenital paramyotonia) G71.19
eustachian tube — *see* Disorder, eustachian tube
external
  auditory canal — *see* Disorder, ear, external
  ear — *see* Disorder, ear, external
extrapyramidal G25.9
  specified NEC G25.89
eye H57.9
  anterior chamber H21.9
  inflammatory NEC H57.89
  muscle (external) — *see* Strabismus
  specified NEC H57.89
  syphilitic — *see* Oculopathy, syphilitic
eyeball H44.9
  specified NEC H44.89
eyelid — *see* Disorder, eyelid
  specified NEC — *see* Disorder, eyelid, specified type NEC
eyeworm of Africa B74.3
facial nerve (seventh) G51.9
  newborn (birth injury) P11.3
Fahr (of brain) G23.8
Fahr Volhard (of kidney) I12.- ☑
fallopian tube (noninflammatory) N83.9
  inflammatory — *see* Salpingo-oophoritis
  specified NEC N83.8
familial periodic paralysis G72.3
Fanconi's (congenital pancytopenia) D61.Ø9
fascia NEC (*see also* Disorder, muscle)
  inflammatory — *see* Myositis
  specified NEC M62.89
Fauchard's (periodontitis) — *see* Periodontitis
Favre-Durand-Nicolas (climatic bubo) A55
Fede's K14.Ø
Feer's — *see* Poisoning, mercury
female pelvic inflammatory (*see also* Disease, pelvis, inflammatory) N73.9
  syphilitic (secondary) A51.42
  tuberculous A18.17
Fernels' (aortic aneurysm) I71.9
fibrocaseous of lung — *see* Tuberculosis, pulmonary
fibrocystic — *see* Fibrocystic disease
Fiedler's (leptospiral jaundice) A27.Ø
fifth BØ8.3
file-cutter's — *see* Poisoning, lead
fish-skin Q8Ø.9
  acquired L85.Ø
Flajani (-Basedow) (exophthalmic goiter) — *see* Hyperthyroidism, with, goiter (diffuse)
flax-dresser's J66.1
fluke — *see* Infestation, fluke

Disease, diseased — *continued*

foot and mouth BØ8.8
foot process NØ4.9
Forbes' (glycogenosis III) E74.Ø3
Fordyce-Fox (apocrine miliaria) L75.2
Fordyce's (ectopic sebaceous glands) (mouth) Q38.6
Forestier's (rhizomelic pseudopolyarthritis) M35.3
  meaning ankylosing hyperostosis — *see* Hyperostosis, ankylosing
Fothergill's
  neuralgia — *see* Neuralgia, trigeminal
  scarlatina anginosa A38.9
Fournier (gangrene) N49.3
  female N76.89
fourth BØ8.8
Fox (-Fordyce) (apocrine miliaria) L75.2
Francis' — *see* Tularemia
Franklin C88.2
Frei's (climatic bubo) A55
Friedreich's
  combined systemic or ataxia G11.1
  myoclonia G25.3
frontal sinus — *see* Sinusitis, frontal
fungus NEC B49
Gaisböck's (polycythemia hypertonica) D75.1
gallbladder K82.9
  calculus — *see* Calculus, gallbladder
  cholecystitis — *see* Cholecystitis
  cholesterolosis K82.4
  fistula — *see* Fistula, gallbladder
  hydrops K82.1
  obstruction — *see* Obstruction, gallbladder
  perforation K82.2
  specified NEC K82.8
gamma heavy chain C88.2
Gamna's (siderotic splenomegaly) D73.2
Gamstorp's (adynamia episodica hereditaria) G72.3
Gandy-Nanta (siderotic splenomegaly) D73.2
ganister J62.8
gastric — *see* Disease, stomach
gastroesophageal reflux (GERD) K21.9
  with esophagitis K21.Ø
gastrointestinal (tract) K92.9
  amyloid E85.4
  functional K59.9
    psychogenic F45.8
  specified NEC K92.89
Gee (-Herter) (-Heubner) (-Thaysen) (nontropical sprue) K9Ø.Ø
genital organs
  female N94.9
  male N5Ø.9
Gerhardt's (erythromelalgia) I73.81
Gibert's (pityriasis rosea) L42
Gierke's (glycogenosis I) E74.Ø1
Gilles de la Tourette's (motor-verbal tic) F95.2
gingiva KØ6.9
  plaque induced KØ5.ØØ
  specified NEC KØ6.8
gland (lymph) I89.9
Glanzmann's (hereditary hemorrhagic thrombasthenia) D69.1
glass-blower's (cataract) — *see* Cataract, specified NEC
  salivary gland hypertrophy K11.1
Glisson's — *see* Rickets
globe H44.9
  specified NEC H44.89
glomerular (*see also* Glomerulonephritis)
  with edema — *see* Nephrosis
  acute — *see* Nephritis, acute
  chronic — *see* Nephritis, chronic
  minimal change NØ5.Ø
  rapidly progressive NØ1.9
glycogen storage E74.ØØ
  Andersen's E74.Ø9
  Cori's E74.Ø3
  Forbes' E74.Ø3
  generalized E74.ØØ
  glucose-6-phosphatase deficiency E74.Ø1
  heart E74.Ø2 [I43]
  hepatorenal E74.Ø9
  Hers' E74.Ø9
  liver and kidney E74.Ø9
  McArdle's E74.Ø4
  muscle phosphofructokinase E74.Ø9
  myocardium E74.Ø2 [I43]
  Pompe's E74.Ø2
  Tauri's E74.Ø9

☑ **Additional Character Required** — Refer to the Tabular List for Character Selection   ▽ Subterms under main terms may continue to next column or page

Disease, diseased — continued
  glycogen storage — continued
    type Ø E74.Ø9
    type I E74.Ø1
    type II E74.Ø2
    type III E74.Ø3
    type IV E74.Ø9
    type V E74.Ø4
    type VI-XI E74.Ø9
    Von Gierke's E74.Ø1
  Goldstein's (familial hemorrhagic telangiectasia) I78.Ø
  gonococcal NOS A54.9
  graft-versus-host (GVH) D89.813
    acute D89.81Ø
    acute on chronic D89.812
    chronic D89.811
  grainhandler's J67.8
  granulomatous (childhood) (chronic) D71
  Graves' (exophthalmic goiter) — see Hyperthyroidism, with, goiter (diffuse)
  Griesinger's — see Ancylostomiasis
  Grisel's M43.6
  Gruby's (tinea tonsurans) B35.Ø
  Guillain-Barré G61.Ø
  Guinon's (motor-verbal tic) F95.2
  gum KØ6.9
  gynecological N94.9
  H (Hartnup's) E72.Ø2
  Haff — see Poisoning, mercury
  Hageman (congenital factor XII deficiency) D68.2
  hair (color) (shaft) L67.9
    follicles L73.9
      specified NEC L73.8
  Hamman's (spontaneous mediastinal emphysema) J98.2
  hand, foot and mouth BØ8.4
  Hansen's — see Leprosy
  Hantavirus, with pulmonary manifestations B33.4
    with renal manifestations A98.5
  Harada's H3Ø.81- ☑
  Hartnup (pellagra-cerebellar ataxia-renal aminoaciduria) E72.Ø2
  Hart's (pellagra-cerebellar ataxia-renal aminoaciduria) E72.Ø2
  Hashimoto's (struma lymphomatosa) EØ6.3
  Hb — see Disease, hemoglobin
  heart (organic) I51.9
    with
      pulmonary edema (acute) (see also Failure, ventricular, left) I5Ø.1
      rheumatic fever (conditions in IØØ)
        active IØ1.9
          with chorea IØ2.Ø
          specified NEC IØ1.8
        inactive or quiescent (with chorea) IØ9.9
          specified NEC IØ9.89
    amyloid E85.4 [I43]
    aortic (valve) I35.9
    arteriosclerotic or sclerotic (senile) — see Disease, heart, ischemic, atherosclerotic
    artery, arterial — see Disease, heart, ischemic, atherosclerotic
    beer drinkers' I42.6
    beriberi (wet) E51.12
    black I27.Ø
    congenital Q24.9
      cyanotic Q24.9
      specified NEC Q24.8
    coronary — see Disease, heart, ischemic
    cryptogenic I51.9
    fibroid — see Myocarditis
    functional I51.89
      psychogenic F45.8
    glycogen storage E74.Ø2 [I43]
    gonococcal A54.83
    hypertensive — see Hypertension, heart
    hyperthyroid (see also Hyperthyroidism) EØ5.9Ø [I43]
      with thyroid storm EØ5.91 [I43]
    ischemic (chronic or with a stated duration of over 4 weeks) I25.9
      atherosclerotic (of) I25.1Ø
        with angina pectoris — see Arteriosclerosis, coronary (artery)
        coronary artery bypass graft — see Arteriosclerosis, coronary (artery), cardiomyopathy I25.5

Disease, diseased — continued
  heart — continued
    ischemic — continued
      diagnosed on ECG or other special investigation, but currently presenting no symptoms I25.6
      silent I25.6
      specified form NEC I25.89
    kyphoscoliotic I27.1
    meningococcal A39.5Ø
      endocarditis A39.51
      myocarditis A39.52
      pericarditis A39.53
    mitral IØ5.9
      specified NEC IØ5.8
    muscular — see Degeneration, myocardial
    psychogenic (functional) F45.8
    pulmonary (chronic) I27.9
      in schistosomiasis B65.9 [I52]
      specified NEC I27.89
    rheumatic (chronic) (inactive) (old) (quiescent) (with chorea) IØ9.9
      active or acute IØ1.9
        with chorea (acute) (rheumatic) (Sydenham's) IØ2.Ø
      specified NEC IØ9.89
    senile — see Myocarditis
    syphilitic A52.Ø6
      aortic A52.Ø3
        aneurysm A52.Ø1
      congenital A5Ø.54 [I52]
    thyrotoxic (see also Thyrotoxicosis) EØ5.9Ø [I43]
      with thyroid storm EØ5.91 [I43]
    valve, valvular (obstructive) (regurgitant) (see also Endocarditis)
      congenital NEC Q24.8
      pulmonary Q22.3
    vascular — see Disease, cardiovascular
  heavy chain NEC C88.2
    alpha C88.3
    gamma C88.2
    mu C88.2
  Hebra's
    pityriasis
      maculata et circinata L42
      rubra pilaris L44.Ø
    prurigo L28.2
  hematopoietic organs D75.9
  hemoglobin or Hb
    abnormal (mixed) NEC D58.2
      with thalassemia D56.9
    AS genotype D57.3
    Bart's D56.Ø
    C (Hb-C) D58.2
      with other abnormal hemoglobin NEC D58.2
      elliptocytosis D58.1
      Hb-S D57.2- ☑
      sickle-cell D57.2- ☑
      thalassemia D56.8
    Constant Spring D58.2
    D (Hb-D) D58.2
    E (Hb-E) D58.2
    E-beta thalassemia D56.5
    elliptocytosis D58.1
    H (Hb-H) (thalassemia) D56.Ø
      with other abnormal hemoglobin NEC D56.9
      Constant Spring D56.Ø
    I thalassemia D56.9
    M D74.Ø
    S or SS D57.1
    SC D57.2- ☑
    SD D57.8- ☑
    SE D57.8- ☑
    spherocytosis D58.Ø
    unstable, hemolytic D58.2
  hemolytic (newborn) P55.9
    autoimmune (cold type) (warm type) D59.1
    drug-induced D59.Ø
    due to or with
      incompatibility
        ABO (blood group) P55.1
        blood (group) (Duffy) (K) (Kell) (Kidd) (Lewis) (M) (S) NEC P55.8
        Rh (blood group) (factor) P55.Ø
      Rh negative mother P55.Ø
    specified type NEC P55.8
    unstable hemoglobin D58.2
  hemorrhagic D69.9

Disease, diseased — continued
  hemorrhagic — continued
    newborn P53
  Henoch (-Schönlein) (purpura nervosa) D69.Ø
  hepatic — see Disease, liver
  hepatolenticular E83.Ø1
  heredodegenerative NEC
    spinal cord G95.89
  herpesviral, disseminated BØØ.7
  Hers' (glycogenosis VI) E74.Ø9
  Herter (-Gee) (-Heubner) (nontropical sprue) K9Ø.Ø
  Heubner-Herter (nontropical sprue) K9Ø.Ø
  high fetal gene or hemoglobin thalassemia D56.9
  Hildenbrand's — see Typhus
  hip (joint) M25.9
    congenital Q65.89
    suppurative MØØ.9
    tuberculous A18.Ø2
  His (-Werner) (trench fever) A79.Ø
  Hodgson's I71.2
    ruptured I71.1
  Holla — see Spherocytosis
  hookworm B76.9
    specified NEC B76.8
  host-versus-graft D89.813
    acute D89.81Ø
    acute on chronic D89.812
    chronic D89.811
  human immunodeficiency virus (HIV) B2Ø
  Huntington's G1Ø
    with dementia G1Ø [FØ2.8Ø]
  Hutchinson's (cheiropompholyx) — see Hutchinson's disease
  hyaline (diffuse) (generalized)
    membrane (lung) (newborn) P22.Ø
      adult J8Ø
  hydatid — see Echinococcus
  hydroxyapatite deposition M11.ØØ
    ankle M11.Ø7- ☑
    elbow M11.Ø2- ☑
    foot joint M11.Ø7- ☑
    hand joint M11.Ø4- ☑
    hip M11.Ø5- ☑
    knee M11.Ø6- ☑
    multiple site M11.Ø9
    shoulder M11.Ø1- ☑
    vertebra M11.Ø8
    wrist M11.Ø3- ☑
  hyperkinetic — see Hyperkinesia
  hypertensive — see Hypertension
  hypophysis E23.7
  Iceland G93.3
  I-cell E77.Ø
  immune D89.9
  immunoproliferative (malignant) C88.9
    small intestinal C88.3
    specified NEC C88.8
  inclusion B25.9
    salivary gland B25.9
  infectious, infective B99.9
    congenital P37.9
      specified NEC P37.8
      viral P35.9
        specified type NEC P35.8
    specified NEC B99.8
  inflammatory
    penis N48.29
      abscess N48.21
      cellulitis N48.22
    prepuce N47.7
      balanoposthitis N47.6
    tubo-ovarian — see Salpingo-oophoritis
  intervertebral disc (see also Disorder, disc)
    with myelopathy — see Disorder, disc, with, myelopathy
    cervical, cervicothoracic — see Disorder, disc, cervical
    with
      myelopathy — see Disorder, disc, cervical, with myelopathy
      neuritis, radiculitis or radiculopathy — see Disorder, disc, cervical, with neuritis
      specified NEC — see Disorder, disc, cervical, specified type NEC
    lumbar (with)
      myelopathy M51.Ø6
      neuritis, radiculitis, radiculopathy or sciatica M51.16

Disease, diseased — *continued*

  intervertebral disc (*see also* Disorder, disc) — *continued*
    lumbar — *continued*
      specified NEC M51.86
    lumbosacral (with)
      neuritis, radiculitis, radiculopathy or sciatica M51.17
      specified NEC M51.87
    specified NEC — *see* Disorder, disc, specified NEC
    thoracic (with)
      myelopathy M51.04
      neuritis, radiculitis or radiculopathy M51.14
      specified NEC M51.84
    thoracolumbar (with)
      myelopathy M51.05
      neuritis, radiculitis or radiculopathy M51.15
      specified NEC M51.85
  intestine K63.9
    functional K59.9
      psychogenic F45.8
      specified NEC K59.8
    organic K63.9
    protozoal A07.9
    specified NEC K63.89
  iris H21.9
    specified NEC H21.89
  iron metabolism or storage E83.10
  island (scrub typhus) A75.3
  itai-itai — *see* Poisoning, cadmium
  Jakob-Creutzfeldt — *see* Creutzfeldt-Jakob disease or syndrome
  jaw M27.9
    fibrocystic M27.49
    specified NEC M27.8
  jigger B88.1
  joint (*see also* Disorder, joint)
    Charcot's — *see* Arthropathy, neuropathic (Charcot)
    degenerative — *see* Osteoarthritis
      multiple M15.9
      spine — *see* Spondylosis
    hypertrophic — *see* Osteoarthritis
    sacroiliac M53.3
    specified NEC — *see* Disorder, joint, specified type NEC
    spine NEC — *see* Dorsopathy
    suppurative — *see* Arthritis, pyogenic or pyemic
  Jourdain's (acute gingivitis) K05.00
    nonplaque induced K05.01
    plaque induced K05.00
  Kaschin-Beck (endemic polyarthritis) M12.10
    ankle M12.17- ☑
    elbow M12.12- ☑
    foot joint M12.17- ☑
    hand joint M12.14- ☑
    hip M12.15- ☑
    knee M12.16- ☑
    multiple site M12.19
    shoulder M12.11- ☑
    vertebra M12.18
    wrist M12.13- ☑
  Katayama B65.2
  Kedani (scrub typhus) A75.3
  Keshan E59
  kidney (functional) (pelvis) N28.9
    chronic N18.9
      hypertensive — *see* Hypertension, kidney
      stage 1 N18.1
      stage 2 (mild) N18.2
      stage 3 (moderate) N18.3
      stage 4 (severe) N18.4
      stage 5 N18.5
    complicating pregnancy — *see* Pregnancy, complicated by, renal disease
    cystic (congenital) Q61.9
    fibrocystic (congenital) Q61.8
    hypertensive — *see* Hypertension, kidney
    in (due to)
      schistosomiasis (bilharziasis) B65.9 [N29]
    multicystic Q61.4
    polycystic Q61.3
      adult type Q61.2
      childhood type NEC Q61.19
        collecting duct dilatation Q61.11
  Kimmelstiel (-Wilson) (intercapillary polycystic (congenital) glomerulosclerosis) — *see* E08-E13 with .21
  Kinnier Wilson's (hepatolenticular degeneration) E83.01
  kissing — *see* Mononucleosis, infectious

Disease, diseased — *continued*

  Klebs' (*see also* Glomerulonephritis) N05- ☑
  Klippel-Feil (brevicollis) Q76.1
  Köhler-Pellegrini-Stieda (calcification, knee joint) — *see* Bursitis, tibial collateral
  Kok Q89.8
  König's (osteochondritis dissecans) — *see* Osteochondritis, dissecans
  Korsakoff's (nonalcoholic) F04
    alcoholic F10.96
      with dependence F10.26
  Kostmann's (infantile genetic agranulocytosis) D70.0
  kuru A81.81
  Kyasanur Forest A98.2
  labyrinth, ear — *see* Disorder, ear, inner
  lacrimal system — *see* Disorder, lacrimal system
  Lafora's — *see* Epilepsy, generalized, idiopathic
  Lancereaux-Mathieu (leptospiral jaundice) A27.0
  Landry's G61.0
  Larrey-Weil (leptospiral jaundice) A27.0
  larynx J38.7
  legionnaires' A48.1
    nonpneumonic A48.2
  Lenegre's I44.2
  lens H27.9
    specified NEC H27.8
  Lev's (acquired complete heart block) I44.2
  Lewy body (dementia) G31.83 [F02.80]
    with behavioral disturbance G31.83 [F02.81]
  Lichtheim's (subacute combined sclerosis with pernicious anemia) D51.0
  Lightwood's (renal tubular acidosis) N25.89
  Lignac's (cystinosis) E72.04
  lip K13.0
  lipid-storage E75.6
    specified NEC E75.5
  Lipschütz's N76.6
  liver (chronic) (organic) K76.9
    alcoholic (chronic) K70.9
      acute — *see* Disease, liver, alcoholic, hepatitis
      cirrhosis K70.30
        with ascites K70.31
      failure K70.40
        with coma K70.41
      fatty liver K70.0
      fibrosis K70.2
      hepatitis K70.10
        with ascites K70.11
      sclerosis K70.2
    cystic, congenital Q44.6
    drug-induced (idiosyncratic) (toxic) (predictable) (unpredictable) — *see* Disease, liver, toxic
    end stage K72.90
      due to hepatitis — *see* Hepatitis
    fatty, nonalcoholic (NAFLD) K76.0
      alcoholic K70.0
    fibrocystic (congenital) Q44.6
    fluke
      Chinese B66.1
      oriental B66.1
      sheep B66.3
    gestational alloimmune (GALD) P78.84
    glycogen storage E74.09 [K77]
    in (due to)
      schistosomiasis (bilharziasis) B65.9 [K77]
    inflammatory K75.9
      alcoholic K70.1 ☑
      specified NEC K75.89
    polycystic (congenital) Q44.6
    toxic K71.9
      with
        cholestasis K71.0
        cirrhosis (liver) K71.7
        fibrosis (liver) K71.7
        focal nodular hyperplasia K71.8
        hepatic granuloma K71.8
        hepatic necrosis K71.10
          with coma K71.11
        hepatitis NEC K71.6
          acute K71.2
          chronic
            active K71.50
              with ascites K71.51
            lobular K71.4
            persistent K71.3
        lupoid K71.50
          with ascites K71.51
      peliosis hepatis K71.8

Disease, diseased — *continued*

  liver — *continued*
    toxic — *continued*
      with — *continued*
        veno-occlusive disease (VOD) of liver K71.8
      veno-occlusive K76.5
  Lobo's (keloid blastomycosis) B48.0
  Lobstein's (brittle bones and blue sclera) Q78.0
  Ludwig's (submaxillary cellulitis) K12.2
  lumbosacral region M53.87
  lung J98.4
    black J60
    congenital Q33.9
    cystic J98.4
      congenital Q33.0
    fibroid (chronic) — *see* Fibrosis, lung
    fluke B66.4
      oriental B66.4
    in
      amyloidosis E85.4 [J99]
      sarcoidosis D86.0
      Sjögren's syndrome M35.02
      systemic
        lupus erythematosus M32.13
        sclerosis M34.81
    interstitial J84.9
      of childhood, specified NEC J84.848
      respiratory bronchiolitis J84.115
      specified NEC J84.89
    obstructive (chronic) J44.9
      with
        acute
          bronchitis J44.0
          exacerbation NEC J44.1
          lower respiratory infection J44.0
        alveolitis, allergic J67.9
        asthma J44.9
        bronchiectasis J47.9
          with
            exacerbation (acute) J47.1
            lower respiratory infection J47.0
        bronchitis J44.9
          with
            exacerbation (acute) J44.1
            lower respiratory infection J44.0
        emphysema J43.9
        hypersensitivity pneumonitis J67.9
      decompensated J44.1
        with
          exacerbation (acute) J44.1
    polycystic J98.4
      congenital Q33.0
    rheumatoid (diffuse) (interstitial) — *see* Rheumatoid, lung
  Lutembacher's (atrial septal defect with mitral stenosis) Q21.1
  Lyme A69.20
  lymphatic (gland) (system) (channel) (vessel) I89.9
  lymphoproliferative D47.9
    specified NEC D47.Z9 (*following* D47.4)
    T-gamma D47.Z9 (*following* D47.4)
    X-linked D82.3
  Magitot's M27.2
  malarial — *see* Malaria
  malignant (*see also* Neoplasm, malignant, by site)
  Manson's B65.1
  maple bark J67.6
  maple-syrup-urine E71.0
  Marburg (virus) A98.3
  Marion's (bladder neck obstruction) N32.0
  Marsh's (exophthalmic goiter) — *see* Hyperthyroidism, with, goiter (diffuse)
  mastoid (process) — *see* Disorder, ear, middle
  Mathieu's (leptospiral jaundice) A27.0
  Maxcy's A75.2
  McArdle (-Schmid-Pearson) (glycogenosis V) E74.04
  mediastinum J98.59
  medullary center (idiopathic) (respiratory) G93.89
  Meige's (chronic hereditary edema) Q82.0
  meningococcal — *see* Infection, meningococcal
  mental F99
    organic F09
  mesenchymal M35.9
  mesenteric embolic (*see also* Ischemia, intestine, acute) K55.039
  metabolic, metabolism E88.9
    bilirubin E80.7
  metal-polisher's J62.8

Disease, diseased — continued

metastatic (see also Neoplasm, secondary, by site) C79.9
microvascular - code to condition
microvillus
  atrophy Q43.8
  inclusion (MVD) Q43.8
middle ear — see Disorder, ear, middle
Mikulicz' (dryness of mouth, absent or decreased
    lacrimation) K11.8
Milroy's (chronic hereditary edema) Q82.0
Minamata — see Poisoning, mercury
minicore G71.2
Minor's G95.19
Minot's (hemorrhagic disease, newborn) P53
Minot-von Willebrand-Jürgens (angiohemophilia) D68.0
Mitchell's (erythromelalgia) I73.81
mitral (valve) I05.9
  nonrheumatic I34.9
mixed connective tissue M35.1
moldy hay J67.0
Monge's T70.29 ☑
Morgagni-Adams-Stokes (syncope with heart block)
    I45.9
Morgagni's (syndrome) (hyperostosis frontalis interna)
    M85.2
Morton's (with metatarsalgia) — see Lesion, nerve,
    plantar
Morvan's G60.8
motor neuron (bulbar) (mixed type) (spinal) G12.20
  amyotrophic lateral sclerosis G12.21
  familial G12.24
  progressive bulbar palsy G12.22
  specified NEC G12.29
moyamoya I67.5
mu heavy chain disease C88.2
multicore G71.2
muscle (see also Disorder, muscle)
  inflammatory — see Myositis
  ocular (external) — see Strabismus
musculoskeletal system, soft tissue — see also Disorder,
    soft tissue
  specified NEC — see Disorder, soft tissue, specified
    type NEC
mushroom workers' J67.5
mycotic B49
myelodysplastic, not classified C94.6
myeloproliferative, not classified C94.6
  chronic D47.1
myocardium, myocardial (see also Degeneration, my-
    ocardial) I51.5
  primary (idiopathic) I42.9
myoneural G70.9
Naegeli's D69.1
nails L60.9
  specified NEC L60.8
Nairobi (sheep virus) A93.8
nasal J34.9
nemaline body G71.2
nerve — see Disorder, nerve
nervous system G98.8
  autonomic G90.9
  central G96.9
    specified NEC G96.8
  congenital Q07.9
  parasympathetic G90.9
  specified NEC G98.8
  sympathetic G90.9
  vegetative G90.9
neuromuscular system G70.9
Newcastle B30.8
Nicolas (-Durand)-Favre (climatic bubo) A55
nipple N64.9
  Paget's C50.01- ☑
    female C50.01- ☑
    male C50.02- ☑
Nishimoto (-Takeuchi) I67.5
nonarthropod-borne NOS (viral) B34.9
  enterovirus NEC B34.1
nonautoimmune hemolytic D59.4
  drug-induced D59.2
Nonne-Milroy-Meige (chronic hereditary edema) Q82.0
nose J34.9
nucleus pulposus — see Disorder, disc
nutritional E63.9
oast-house-urine E72.19
  ocular
    herpesviral B00.50
    zoster B02.30

Disease, diseased — continued

obliterative vascular I77.1
Ohara's — see Tularemia
Opitz's (congestive splenomegaly) D73.2
Oppenheim-Urbach (necrobiosis lipoidica diabetico-
    rum) — see E08-E13 with .620
optic nerve NEC — see Disorder, nerve, optic
orbit — see Disorder, orbit
Oriental liver fluke B66.1
Oriental lung fluke B66.4
Ormond's N13.5
Oropouche virus A93.0
Osler-Rendu (familial hemorrhagic telangiectasia) I78.0
osteofibrocystic E21.0
Otto's M24.7
outer ear — see Disorder, ear, external
ovary (noninflammatory) N83.9
  cystic N83.20- ☑
  inflammatory — see Salpingo-oophoritis
  polycystic E28.2
  specified NEC N83.8
Owren's (congenital) — see Defect, coagulation
pancreas K86.9
  cystic K86.2
  fibrocystic E84.9
  specified NEC K86.89
panvalvular I08.9
  specified NEC I08.8
parametrium (noninflammatory) N83.9
parasitic B89
  cerebral NEC B71.9 [G94]
  intestinal NOS B82.9
  mouth B37.0
  skin NOS B88.9
  specified type — see Infestation
  tongue B37.0
parathyroid (gland) E21.5
  specified NEC E21.4
Parkinson's G20
parodontal K05.6
Parrot's (syphilitic osteochondritis) A50.02
Parry's (exophthalmic goiter) — see Hyperthyroidism,
    with, goiter (diffuse)
Parson's (exophthalmic goiter) — see Hyperthyroidism,
    with, goiter (diffuse)
Paxton's (white piedra) B36.2
pearl-worker's — see Osteomyelitis, specified type NEC
Pellegrini-Stieda (calcification, knee joint) — see Bursi-
    tis, tibial collateral
pelvis, pelvic
  female NOS N94.9
    specified NEC N94.89
  gonococcal (acute) (chronic) A54.24
  inflammatory (female) N73.9
    acute N73.0
    chlamydial A56.11
    chronic N73.1
    specified NEC N73.8
    syphilitic (secondary) A51.42
      late A52.76
    tuberculous A18.17
  organ, female N94.9
  peritoneum, female NEC N94.89
penis N48.9
  inflammatory N48.29
    abscess N48.21
    cellulitis N48.22
  specified NEC N48.89
periapical tissues NOS K04.90
periodontal K05.6
  specified NEC K05.5
periosteum — see Disorder, bone, specified type NEC
peripheral
  arterial I73.9
  autonomic nervous system G90.9
  nerves — see Polyneuropathy
  vascular NOS I73.9
peritoneum K66.9
  pelvic, female NEC N94.89
  specified NEC K66.8
persistent mucosal (middle ear) H66.20
  left H66.22
    with right H66.23
  right H66.21
    with left H66.23
Petit's — see Hernia, abdomen, specified site NEC
pharynx J39.2
  specified NEC J39.2

Disease, diseased — continued

Phocas' — see Mastopathy, cystic
photochromogenic (acid-fast bacilli) (pulmonary) A31.0
  nonpulmonary A31.9
Pick's G31.01 [F02.80]
  with behavioral disturbance G31.01 [F02.81]
    brain G31.01 [F02.80]
      with behavioral disturbance G31.01 [F02.81]
  of pericardium (pericardial pseudocirrhosis of liver)
    I31.1
pigeon fancier's J67.2
pineal gland E34.8
pink — see Poisoning, mercury
Pinkus' (lichen nitidus) L44.1
pinworm B80
Piry virus A93.8
pituitary (gland) E23.7
pituitary-snuff-taker's J67.8
pleura (cavity) J94.9
  specified NEC J94.8
pneumatic drill (hammer) T75.21 ☑
Pollitzer's (hidradenitis suppurativa) L73.2
polycystic
  kidney or renal Q61.3
    adult type Q61.2
    childhood type NEC Q61.19
      collecting duct dilatation Q61.11
  liver or hepatic Q44.6
  lung or pulmonary J98.4
    congenital Q33.0
  ovary, ovaries E28.2
  spleen Q89.09
polyethylene T84.05- ☑
Pompe's (glycogenosis II) E74.02
Posadas-Wernicke B38.9
Potain's (pulmonary edema) — see Edema, lung
prepuce N47.8
  inflammatory N47.7
    balanoposthitis N47.6
Pringle's (tuberous sclerosis) Q85.1
prion, central nervous system A81.9
  specified NEC A81.89
prostate N42.9
  specified NEC N42.89
protozoal B64
  acanthamebiasis — see Acanthamebiasis
  African trypanosomiasis — see African trypanosomi-
    asis
  babesiosis B60.0
  Chagas disease — see Chagas disease
  intestine, intestinal A07.9
  leishmaniasis — see Leishmaniasis
  malaria — see Malaria
  naegleriasis B60.2
  pneumocystosis B59
  specified organism NEC B60.8
  toxoplasmosis — see Toxoplasmosis
pseudo-Hurler's E77.0
psychiatric F99
psychotic — see Psychosis
Puente's (simple glandular cheilitis) K13.0
puerperal (see also Puerperal) O90.89
pulmonary (see also Disease, lung)
  artery I28.9
  chronic obstructive J44.9
    with
      acute bronchitis J44.0
      exacerbation (acute) J44.1
      lower respiratory infection (acute) J44.0
    decompensated J44.1
      with
        exacerbation (acute) J44.1
  heart I27.9
    specified NEC I27.89
  hypertensive (vascular) (see also Hypertension,
    pulmonary) I27.20
  NEC I27.2 ☑
    primary (idiopathic) I27.0
  valve I37.9
    rheumatic I09.89
pulp (dental) NOS K04.90
pulseless M31.4
Putnam's (subacute combined sclerosis with pernicious
    anemia) D51.0
Pyle (-Cohn) (metaphyseal dysplasia) Q78.5
ragpicker's or ragsorter's A22.1
Raynaud's — see Raynaud's disease
reactive airway — see Asthma

Disease, diseased — *continued*
- Reclus' (cystic) — *see* Mastopathy, cystic
- rectum K62.9
  - specified NEC K62.89
- Refsum's (heredopathia atactica polyneuritiformis) G60.1
- renal (functional) (pelvis) (*see also* Disease, kidney) N28.9
  - with
    - edema — *see* Nephrosis
    - glomerular lesion — *see* Glomerulonephritis
      - with edema — *see* Nephrosis
    - interstitial nephritis N12
  - acute N28.9
  - chronic (*see also* Disease, kidney, chronic) N18.9
  - cystic, congenital Q61.9
  - diabetic — *see* E08-E13 with .22
  - end-stage (failure) N18.6
    - due to hypertension I12.0
  - fibrocystic (congenital) Q61.8
  - hypertensive — *see* Hypertension, kidney
  - lupus M32.14
  - phosphate-losing (tubular) N25.0
  - polycystic (congenital) Q61.3
    - adult type Q61.2
    - childhood type NEC Q61.19
      - collecting duct dilatation Q61.11
  - rapidly progressive N01.9
  - subacute N01.9
- Rendu-Osler-Weber (familial hemorrhagic telangiectasia) I78.0
- renovascular (arteriosclerotic) — *see* Hypertension, kidney
- respiratory (tract) J98.9
  - acute or subacute NOS J06.9
    - due to
      - chemicals, gases, fumes or vapors (inhalation) J68.3
      - external agent J70.9
        - specified NEC J70.8
      - radiation J70.0
      - smoke inhalation J70.5
    - noninfectious J39.8
  - chronic NOS J98.9
    - due to
      - chemicals, gases, fumes or vapors J68.4
      - external agent J70.9
        - specified NEC J70.8
      - radiation J70.1
    - newborn P27.9
      - specified NEC P27.8
  - due to
    - chemicals, gases, fumes or vapors J68.9
      - acute or subacute NEC J68.3
      - chronic J68.4
    - external agent J70.9
      - specified NEC J70.8
  - newborn P28.9
    - specified type NEC P28.89
  - upper J39.9
    - acute or subacute J06.9
    - noninfectious NEC J39.8
    - specified NEC J39.8
    - streptococcal J06.9
- retina, retinal H35.9
  - Batten's or Batten-Mayou E75.4 [H36]
  - specified NEC H35.89
- rheumatoid — *see* Arthritis, rheumatoid
- rickettsial NOS A79.9
  - specified type NEC A79.89
- Riga (-Fede) (cachectic aphthae) K14.0
- Riggs' (compound periodontitis) — *see* Periodontitis
- Ritter's L00
- Rivalta's (cervicofacial actinomycosis) A42.2
- Robles' (onchocerciasis) B73.01
- Roger's (congenital interventricular septal defect) Q21.0
- Rosenthal's (factor XI deficiency) D68.1
- Ross River B33.1
- Rossbach's (hyperchlorhydria) K30
- Rotes Quérol — *see* Hyperostosis, ankylosing
- Roth (-Bernhardt) — *see* Mononeuropathy, lower limb, meralgia paresthetica
- Runeberg's (progressive pernicious anemia) D51.0
- sacroiliac NEC M53.3
- salivary gland or duct K11.9
  - inclusion B25.9
  - specified NEC K11.8
  - virus B25.9

Disease, diseased — *continued*
- sandworm B76.9
- Schimmelbusch's — *see* Mastopathy, cystic
- Schmorl's — *see* Schmorl's disease or nodes
- Schönlein (-Henoch) (purpura rheumatica) D69.0
- Schottmüller's — *see* Fever, paratyphoid
- Schultz's (agranulocytosis) — *see* Agranulocytosis
- Schwalbe-Ziehen-Oppenheim G24.1
- Schwartz-Jampel G71.13
- sclera H15.9
  - specified NEC H15.89
- scrofulous (tuberculous) A18.2
- scrotum N50.9
- sebaceous glands L73.9
- semilunar cartilage, cystic (*see also* Derangement, knee, meniscus, cystic)
- seminal vesicle N50.9
- serum NEC (*see also* Reaction, serum) T80.69 ☑
- sexually transmitted A64
  - anogenital
    - herpesviral infection — *see* Herpes, anogenital
    - warts A63.0
  - chancroid A57
  - chlamydial infection — *see* Chlamydia
  - gonorrhea — *see* Gonorrhea
  - granuloma inguinale A58
  - specified organism NEC A63.8
  - syphilis — *see* Syphilis
  - trichomoniasis — *see* Trichomoniasis
- Sézary C84.1- ☑
- shimamushi (scrub typhus) A75.3
- shipyard B30.0
- sickle-cell D57.1
  - with crisis (vasoocclusive pain) D57.00
    - with
      - acute chest syndrome D57.01
      - splenic sequestration D57.02
  - elliptocytosis D57.8- ☑
  - Hb-C D57.20
    - with crisis (vasoocclusive pain) D57.219
      - with
        - acute chest syndrome D57.211
        - splenic sequestration D57.212
    - without crisis D57.20
  - Hb-SD D57.80
    - with crisis D57.819
      - with
        - acute chest syndrome D57.811
        - splenic sequestration D57.812
  - Hb-SE D57.80
    - with crisis D57.819
      - with
        - acute chest syndrome D57.811
        - splenic sequestration D57.812
  - specified NEC D57.80
    - with crisis D57.819
      - with
        - acute chest syndrome D57.811
        - splenic sequestration D57.812
  - spherocytosis D57.80
    - with crisis D57.819
      - with
        - acute chest syndrome D57.811
        - splenic sequestration D57.812
  - thalassemia D57.40
    - with crisis (vasoocclusive pain) D57.419
      - with
        - acute chest syndrome D57.411
        - splenic sequestration D57.412
    - without crisis D57.40
- silo-filler's J68.8
  - bronchitis J68.0
  - pneumonitis J68.0
  - pulmonary edema J68.1
- simian B B00.4
- Simons' (progressive lipodystrophy) E88.1
- sin nombre virus B33.4
- sinus — *see* Sinusitis
- Sirkari's B55.0
- sixth B08.20
  - due to human herpesvirus 6 B08.21
  - due to human herpesvirus 7 B08.22
- skin L98.9
  - due to metabolic disorder NEC E88.9 [L99]
  - specified NEC L98.8
- slim (HIV) B20
- small vessel I73.9

Disease, diseased — *continued*
- Sneddon-Wilkinson (subcorneal pustular dermatosis) L13.1
- South African creeping B88.0
- spinal (cord) G95.9
  - congenital Q06.9
  - specified NEC G95.89
- spine (*see also* Spondylopathy)
  - joint — *see* Dorsopathy
  - tuberculous A18.01
- spinocerebellar (hereditary) G11.9
  - specified NEC G11.8
- spleen D73.9
  - amyloid E85.4 [D77]
  - organic D73.9
  - polycystic Q89.09
  - postinfectional D73.89
- sponge-diver's — *see* Toxicity, venom, marine animal, sea anemone
- Startle Q89.8
- Steinert's G71.11
- Sticker's (erythema infectiosum) B08.3
- Stieda's (calcification, knee joint) — *see* Bursitis, tibial collateral
- Stokes' (exophthalmic goiter) — *see* Hyperthyroidism, with, goiter (diffuse)
- Stokes-Adams (syncope with heart block) I45.9
- stomach K31.9
  - functional, psychogenic F45.8
  - specified NEC K31.89
- stonemason's J62.8
- storage
  - glycogen — *see* Disease, glycogen storage
  - mucopolysaccharide — *see* Mucopolysaccharidosis
- striatopallidal system NEC G25.89
- Stuart-Prower (congenital factor X deficiency) D68.2
- Stuart's (congenital factor X deficiency) D68.2
- subcutaneous tissue — *see* Disease, skin
- supporting structures of teeth K08.9
  - specified NEC K08.89
- suprarenal (capsule) (gland) E27.9
  - hyperfunction E27.0
  - specified NEC E27.8
- sweat glands L74.9
  - specified NEC L74.8
- Sweeley-Klionsky E75.21
- Swift (-Feer) — *see* Poisoning, mercury
- swimming-pool granuloma A31.1
- Sylvest's (epidemic pleurodynia) B33.0
- sympathetic nervous system G90.9
- synovium — *see* Disorder, synovium
- syphilitic — *see* Syphilis
- systemic tissue mast cell C96.20
- tanapox (virus) B08.71
- Tangier E78.6
- Tarral-Besnier (pityriasis rubra pilaris) L44.0
- Tauri's E74.09
- tear duct — *see* Disorder, lacrimal system
- tendon, tendinous (*see also* Disorder, tendon)
  - nodular — *see* Trigger finger
- terminal vessel I73.9
- testis N50.9
- thalassemia Hb-S — *see* Disease, sickle-cell, thalassemia
- Thaysen-Gee (nontropical sprue) K90.0
- Thomsen G71.12
- throat J39.2
  - septic J02.0
- thromboembolic — *see* Embolism
- thymus (gland) E32.9
  - specified NEC E32.8
- thyroid (gland) E07.9
  - heart (*see also* Hyperthyroidism) E05.90 [I43]
    - with thyroid storm E05.91 [I43]
  - specified NEC E07.89
- Tietze's M94.0
- tongue K14.9
  - specified NEC K14.8
- tonsils, tonsillar (and adenoids) J35.9
- tooth, teeth K08.9
  - hard tissues K03.9
    - specified NEC K03.89
  - pulp NEC K04.99
  - specified NEC K08.89
- Tourette's F95.2
- trachea NEC J39.8
- tricuspid I07.9
  - nonrheumatic I36.9
- triglyceride-storage E75.5

☑ **Additional Character Required** — Refer to the Tabular List for Character Selection   **Subterms under main terms may continue to next column or page**

Disease, diseased — *continued*
- trophoblastic — *see* Mole, hydatidiform
- tsutsugamushi A75.3
- tube (fallopian) (noninflammatory) N83.9
  - inflammatory — *see* Salpingitis
  - specified NEC N83.8
- tuberculous NEC — *see* Tuberculosis
- tubo-ovarian (noninflammatory) N83.9
  - inflammatory — *see* Salpingo-oophoritis
  - specified NEC N83.8
- tubotympanic, chronic — *see* Otitis, media, suppurative, chronic, tubotympanic
- tubulo-interstitial N15.9
  - specified NEC N15.8
- tympanum — *see* Disorder, tympanic membrane
- Uhl's Q24.8
- Underwood's (sclerema neonatorum) P83.0
- Unverricht (-Lundborg) — *see* Epilepsy, generalized, idiopathic
- Urbach-Oppenheim (necrobiosis lipoidica diabeticorum) — *see* E08-E13 with .620
- ureter N28.9
  - in (due to)
    - schistosomiasis (bilharziasis) B65.0 [N29]
- urethra N36.9
  - specified NEC N36.8
- urinary (tract) N39.9
  - bladder N32.9
    - specified NEC N32.89
  - specified NEC N39.8
- uterus (noninflammatory) N85.9
  - infective — *see* Endometritis
  - inflammatory — *see* Endometritis
  - specified NEC N85.8
- uveal tract (anterior) H21.9
  - posterior H31.9
- vagabond's B85.1
- vagina, vaginal (noninflammatory) N89.9
  - inflammatory NEC N76.89
  - specified NEC N89.8
- valve, valvular I38
  - multiple I08.9
    - specified NEC I08.8
- van Creveld-von Gierke (glycogenosis I) E74.01
- vas deferens N50.9
- vascular I99.9
  - arteriosclerotic — *see* Arteriosclerosis
  - ciliary body NEC — *see* Disorder, iris, vascular
  - hypertensive — *see* Hypertension
  - iris NEC — *see* Disorder, iris, vascular
  - obliterative I77.1
    - peripheral I73.9
  - occlusive I99.8
  - peripheral (occlusive) I73.9
    - in diabetes mellitus — *see* E08-E13 with .51
- vasomotor I73.9
- vasospastic I73.9
- vein I87.9
- venereal (*see also* Disease, sexually transmitted) A64
  - chlamydial NEC A56.8
    - anus A56.3
    - genitourinary NOS A56.2
    - pharynx A56.4
    - rectum A56.3
  - fifth A55
  - sixth A55
  - specified nature or type NEC A63.8
- vertebra, vertebral (*see also* Spondylopathy)
  - disc — *see* Disorder, disc
- vibration — *see* Vibration, adverse effects
- viral, virus (*see also* Disease, by type of virus) B34.9
  - arbovirus NOS A94
  - arthropod-borne NOS A94
  - congenital P35.9
    - specified NEC P35.8
  - Hanta (with renal manifestations) (Dobrava) (Puumala) (Seoul) A98.5
    - with pulmonary manifestations (Andes) (Bayou) (Bermejo) (Black Creek Canal) (Choclo) (Juquitiba) (Laguna negra) (Lechiguanas) (New York) (Oran) (Sin nombre) B33.4
  - Hantaan (Korean hemorrhagic fever) A98.5
  - human immunodeficiency (HIV) B20
  - Kunjin A83.4
  - nonarthropod-borne NOS B34.9
  - Powassan A84.8
  - Rocio (encephalitis) A83.6

Disease, diseased — *continued*
- viral, virus (*see also* Disease, by type of virus) — *continued*
  - Sin nombre (Hantavirus) (cardio)-pulmonary syndrome) B33.4
  - Tahyna B33.8
  - vesicular stomatitis A93.8
- vitreous H43.9
  - specified NEC H43.89
- vocal cord J38.3
- Volkmann's, acquired T79.6 ☑
- von Eulenburg's (congenital paramyotonia) G71.19
- von Gierke's (glycogenosis I) E74.01
- von Graefe's — *see* Strabismus, paralytic, ophthalmoplegia, progressive
- von Willebrand (-Jürgens) (angiohemophilia) D68.0
- Vrolik's (osteogenesis imperfecta) Q78.0
- vulva (noninflammatory) N90.9
  - inflammatory NEC N76.89
  - specified NEC N90.89
- Wallgren's (obstruction of splenic vein with collateral circulation) I87.8
- Wassilieff's (leptospiral jaundice) A27.0
- wasting NEC R64
  - due to malnutrition E41
- Waterhouse-Friderichsen A39.1
- Wegner's (syphilitic osteochondritis) A50.02
- Weil's (leptospiral jaundice of lung) A27.0
- Weir Mitchell's (erythromelalgia) I73.81
- Werdnig-Hoffmann G12.0
- Wermer's E31.21
- Werner-His (trench fever) A79.0
- Werner-Schultz (neutropenic splenomegaly) D73.81
- Wernicke-Posadas B38.9
- whipworm B79
- white blood cells D72.9
  - specified NEC D72.89
- white matter R90.82
- white-spot, meaning lichen sclerosus et atrophicus L90.0
  - penis N48.0
  - vulva N90.4
- Wilkie's K55.1
- Wilkinson-Sneddon (subcorneal pustular dermatosis) L13.1
- Willis' — *see* Diabetes
- Wilson's (hepatolenticular degeneration) E83.01
- woolsorter's A22.1
- yaba monkey tumor B08.72
- yaba pox (virus) B08.72
- Zika virus A92.5
  - congenital P35.4
- zoonotic, bacterial A28.9
  - specified type NEC A28.8

Disfigurement (due to scar) L90.5
Disgerminoma — *see* Dysgerminoma
DISH (diffuse idiopathic skeletal hyperostosis) — *see* Hyperostosis, ankylosing
Disinsertion, retina — *see* Detachment, retina
Dislocatable hip, congenital Q65.6
Dislocation (articular)
- with fracture — *see* Fracture
- acromioclavicular (joint) S43.10- ☑
  - with displacement
    - 100%-200% S43.12- ☑
    - more than 200% S43.13- ☑
  - inferior S43.14- ☑
  - posterior S43.15- ☑
- ankle S93.0- ☑
- astragalus — *see* Dislocation, ankle
- atlantoaxial S13.121 ☑
- atlantooccipital S13.111 ☑
- atloidooccipital S13.111 ☑
- breast bone S23.29 ☑
- capsule, joint — *code by* site under Dislocation
- carpal (bone) — *see* Dislocation, wrist
- carpometacarpal (joint) NEC S63.05- ☑
  - thumb S63.04- ☑
- cartilage (joint) — *code by* site under Dislocation
- cervical spine (vertebra) — *see* Dislocation, vertebra, cervical
- chronic — *see* Dislocation, recurrent
- clavicle — *see* Dislocation, acromioclavicular joint
- coccyx S33.2 ☑
- congenital NEC Q68.8
- coracoid — *see* Dislocation, shoulder
- costal cartilage S23.29 ☑
- costochondral S23.29 ☑

Dislocation — *continued*
- cricoarytenoid articulation S13.29 ☑
- cricothyroid articulation S13.29 ☑
- dorsal vertebra — *see* Dislocation, vertebra, thoracic
- ear ossicle — *see* Discontinuity, ossicles, ear
- elbow S53.10- ☑
  - congenital Q68.8
  - pathological — *see* Dislocation, pathological NEC, elbow
  - radial head alone — *see* Dislocation, radial head
  - recurrent — *see* Dislocation, recurrent, elbow
  - traumatic S53.10- ☑
    - anterior S53.11- ☑
    - lateral S53.14- ☑
    - medial S53.13- ☑
    - posterior S53.12- ☑
    - specified type NEC S53.19- ☑
- eye, nontraumatic — *see* Luxation, globe
- eyeball, nontraumatic — *see* Luxation, globe
- femur
  - distal end — *see* Dislocation, knee
  - proximal end — *see* Dislocation, hip
- fibula
  - distal end — *see* Dislocation, ankle
  - proximal end — *see* Dislocation, knee
- finger S63.25- ☑
  - index S63.25- ☑
  - interphalangeal S63.27- ☑
    - distal S63.29- ☑
      - index S63.29- ☑
      - little S63.29- ☑
      - middle S63.29- ☑
      - ring S63.29- ☑
    - index S63.27- ☑
    - little S63.27- ☑
    - middle S63.27- ☑
    - proximal S63.28- ☑
      - index S63.28- ☑
      - little S63.28- ☑
      - middle S63.28- ☑
      - ring S63.28- ☑
    - ring S63.27- ☑
  - little S63.25- ☑
  - metacarpophalangeal S63.26- ☑
    - index S63.26- ☑
    - little S63.26- ☑
    - middle S63.26- ☑
    - ring S63.26- ☑
  - middle S63.25- ☑
  - recurrent — *see* Dislocation, recurrent, finger
  - ring S63.25- ☑
  - thumb — *see* Dislocation, thumb
- foot S93.30- ☑
  - recurrent — *see* Dislocation, recurrent, foot
  - specified site NEC S93.33- ☑
  - tarsal joint S93.31- ☑
  - tarsometatarsal joint S93.32- ☑
  - toe — *see* Dislocation, toe
- fracture — *see* Fracture
- glenohumeral (joint) — *see* Dislocation, shoulder
- glenoid — *see* Dislocation, shoulder
- habitual — *see* Dislocation, recurrent
- hip S73.00- ☑
  - anterior S73.03- ☑
    - obturator S73.02- ☑
  - central S73.04- ☑
  - congenital (total) Q65.2
    - bilateral Q65.1
    - partial Q65.5
      - bilateral Q65.4
        - unilateral Q65.3- ☑
      - unilateral Q65.0- ☑
  - developmental M24.85- ☑
  - pathological — *see* Dislocation, pathological NEC, hip
  - posterior S73.01- ☑
  - recurrent — *see* Dislocation, recurrent, hip
- humerus, proximal end — *see* Dislocation, shoulder
- incomplete — *see* Subluxation, by site
- incus — *see* Discontinuity, ossicles, ear
- infracoracoid — *see* Dislocation, shoulder
- innominate (pubic junction) (sacral junction) S33.39 ☑
  - acetabulum — *see* Dislocation, hip
- interphalangeal (joint(s))
  - finger S63.279 ☑
    - distal S63.29- ☑

Dislocation — *continued*
- interphalangeal(s) — *continued*
  - finger — *continued*
    - distal — *continued*
      - index S63.29- ☑
      - little S63.29- ☑
      - middle S63.29- ☑
      - ring S63.29- ☑
    - index S63.27- ☑
    - little S63.27- ☑
    - middle S63.27- ☑
    - proximal S63.28- ☑
      - index S63.28- ☑
      - little S63.28- ☑
      - middle S63.28- ☑
      - ring S63.28- ☑
    - ring S63.27- ☑
    - foot or toe — *see* Dislocation, toe
    - thumb S63.12- ☑
- jaw (cartilage) (meniscus) S03.0- ☑
- joint prosthesis — *see* Complications, joint prosthesis, mechanical, displacement, by site
- knee S83.106 ☑
  - cap — *see* Dislocation, patella
  - congenital Q68.2
  - old M23.8X- ☑
  - patella — *see* Dislocation, patella
  - pathological — *see* Dislocation, pathological NEC, knee
  - proximal tibia
    - anteriorly S83.11- ☑
    - laterally S83.14- ☑
    - medially S83.13- ☑
    - posteriorly S83.12- ☑
  - recurrent (*see also* Derangement, knee, specified NEC)
  - specified type NEC S83.19- ☑
- lacrimal gland H04.16- ☑
- lens (complete) H27.10
  - anterior H27.12- ☑
  - congenital Q12.1
  - ocular implant — *see* Complications, intraocular lens
  - partial H27.11- ☑
  - posterior H27.13- ☑
  - traumatic S05.8X- ☑
- ligament — *code by* site under Dislocation
- lumbar (vertebra) — *see* Dislocation, vertebra, lumbar
- lumbosacral (vertebra) (*see also* Dislocation, vertebra, lumbar)
  - congenital Q76.49
- mandible S03.0- ☑
- meniscus (knee) — *see* Tear, meniscus
  - other sites - code by site under Dislocation
- metacarpal (bone)
  - distal end — *see* Dislocation, finger
  - proximal end S63.06- ☑
- metacarpophalangeal (joint)
  - finger S63.26- ☑
    - index S63.26- ☑
    - little S63.26- ☑
    - middle S63.26- ☑
    - ring S63.26- ☑
  - thumb S63.11- ☑
- metatarsal (bone) — *see* Dislocation, foot
- metatarsophalangeal (joint(s)) — *see* Dislocation, toe
- midcarpal (joint) S63.03- ☑
- midtarsal (joint) — *see* Dislocation, foot
- neck S13.20 ☑
  - specified site NEC S13.29 ☑
  - vertebra — *see* Dislocation, vertebra, cervical
- nose (septal cartilage) S03.1 ☑
- occipitoatloid S13.111 ☑
- old — *see* Derangement, joint, specified type NEC
- ossicles, ear — *see* Discontinuity, ossicles, ear
- partial — *see* Subluxation, by site
- patella S83.006 ☑
  - congenital Q74.1
  - lateral S83.01- ☑
  - recurrent (nontraumatic) M22.0- ☑
    - incomplete M22.1- ☑
  - specified type NEC S83.09- ☑
- pathological NEC M24.30
  - ankle M24.37- ☑
  - elbow M24.32- ☑
  - foot joint M24.37- ☑

Dislocation — *continued*
- pathological — *continued*
  - hand joint M24.34- ☑
  - hip M24.35- ☑
  - knee M24.36- ☑
  - lumbosacral joint — *see* subcategory M53.2 ☑
  - pelvic region — *see* Dislocation, pathological, hip
  - sacroiliac — *see* subcategory M53.2 ☑
  - shoulder M24.31- ☑
  - wrist M24.33- ☑
- pelvis NEC S33.30 ☑
  - specified NEC S33.39 ☑
- phalanx
  - finger or hand — *see* Dislocation, finger
  - foot or toe — *see* Dislocation, toe
- prosthesis, internal — *see* Complications, prosthetic device, by site, mechanical
- radial head S53.006 ☑
  - anterior S53.01- ☑
  - posterior S53.02- ☑
  - specified type NEC S53.09- ☑
- radiocarpal (joint) S63.02- ☑
- radiohumeral (joint) — *see* Dislocation, radial head
- radioulnar (joint)
  - distal S63.01- ☑
  - proximal — *see* Dislocation, elbow
- radius
  - distal end — *see* Dislocation, wrist
  - proximal end — *see* Dislocation, radial head
- recurrent M24.40
  - ankle M24.47- ☑
  - elbow M24.42- ☑
  - finger M24.44- ☑
  - foot joint M24.47- ☑
  - hand joint M24.44- ☑
  - hip M24.45- ☑
  - knee M24.46- ☑
    - patella — *see* Dislocation, patella, recurrent
  - patella — *see* Dislocation, patella, recurrent
  - sacroiliac — *see* subcategory M53.2 ☑
  - shoulder M24.41- ☑
  - toe M24.47- ☑
  - vertebra (*see also* subcategory) M43.5 ☑
    - atlantoaxial M43.4
      - with myelopathy M43.3
  - wrist M24.43- ☑
- rib (cartilage) S23.29 ☑
- sacrococcygeal S33.2 ☑
- sacroiliac (joint) (ligament) S33.2 ☑
  - congenital Q74.2
  - recurrent — *see* subcategory M53.2 ☑
- sacrum S33.2 ☑
- scaphoid (bone) (hand) (wrist) — *see* Dislocation, wrist
  - foot — *see* Dislocation, foot
- scapula — *see* Dislocation, shoulder, girdle, scapula
- semilunar cartilage, knee — *see* Tear, meniscus
- septal cartilage (nose) S03.1 ☑
- septum (nasal) (old) J34.2
- sesamoid bone — *code by* site under Dislocation
- shoulder (blade) (ligament) (joint) (traumatic)
  - S43.006 ☑
  - acromioclavicular — *see* Dislocation, acromioclavicular
  - chronic — *see* Dislocation, recurrent, shoulder
  - congenital Q68.8
  - girdle S43.30- ☑
    - scapula S43.31- ☑
    - specified site NEC S43.39- ☑
  - humerus S43.00- ☑
    - anterior S43.01- ☑
    - inferior S43.03- ☑
    - posterior S43.02- ☑
  - pathological — *see* Dislocation, pathological NEC, shoulder
  - recurrent — *see* Dislocation, recurrent, shoulder
  - specified type NEC S43.08- ☑
- spine
  - cervical — *see* Dislocation, vertebra, cervical
  - congenital Q76.49
  - due to birth trauma P11.5
  - lumbar — *see* Dislocation, vertebra, lumbar
  - thoracic — *see* Dislocation, vertebra, thoracic
- spontaneous — *see* Dislocation, pathological
- sternoclavicular (joint) S43.206 ☑
  - anterior S43.21- ☑
  - posterior S43.22- ☑

Dislocation — *continued*
- sternum S23.29 ☑
- subglenoid — *see* Dislocation, shoulder
- symphysis pubis S33.4 ☑
- talus — *see* Dislocation, ankle
- tarsal (bone(s)) (joint(s)) — *see* Dislocation, foot
- tarsometatarsal (joint(s)) — *see* Dislocation, foot
- temporomandibular (joint) S03.0- ☑
- thigh, proximal end — *see* Dislocation, hip
- thorax S23.20 ☑
  - specified site NEC S23.29 ☑
  - vertebra — *see* Dislocation, vertebra
- thumb S63.10- ☑
  - interphalangeal joint — *see* Dislocation, interphalangeal (joint), thumb
  - metacarpophalangeal joint — *see* Dislocation, metacarpophalangeal (joint), thumb
- thyroid cartilage S13.29 ☑
- tibia
  - distal end — *see* Dislocation, ankle
  - proximal end — *see* Dislocation, knee
- tibiofibular (joint)
  - distal — *see* Dislocation, ankle
  - superior — *see* Dislocation, knee
- toe(s) S93.106 ☑
  - great S93.10- ☑
    - interphalangeal joint S93.11- ☑
    - metatarsophalangeal joint S93.12- ☑
  - interphalangeal joint S93.119 ☑
  - lesser S93.106 ☑
    - interphalangeal joint S93.11- ☑
    - metatarsophalangeal joint S93.12- ☑
  - metatarsophalangeal joint S93.12- ☑
- tooth S03.2 ☑
- trachea S23.29 ☑
- ulna
  - distal end S63.07- ☑
  - proximal end — *see* Dislocation, elbow
- ulnohumeral (joint) — *see* Dislocation, elbow
- vertebra (articular process) (body) (traumatic)
  - cervical S13.101 ☑
    - atlantoaxial joint S13.121 ☑
    - atlantooccipital joint S13.111 ☑
    - atloidooccipital joint S13.111 ☑
    - joint between
      - C0 and C1 S13.111 ☑
      - C1 and C2 S13.121 ☑
      - C2 and C3 S13.131 ☑
      - C3 and C4 S13.141 ☑
      - C4 and C5 S13.151 ☑
      - C5 and C6 S13.161 ☑
      - C6 and C7 S13.171 ☑
      - C7 and T1 S13.181 ☑
    - occipitoatloid joint S13.111 ☑
  - congenital Q76.49
  - lumbar S33.101 ☑
    - joint between
      - L1 and L2 S33.111 ☑
      - L2 and L3 S33.121 ☑
      - L3 and L4 S33.131 ☑
      - L4 and L5 S33.141 ☑
  - nontraumatic — *see* Displacement, intervertebral disc
  - partial — *see* Subluxation, by site
  - recurrent NEC — *see* subcategory M43.5 ☑
  - thoracic S23.101 ☑
    - joint between
      - T1 and T2 S23.111 ☑
      - T2 and T3 S23.121 ☑
      - T3 and T4 S23.123 ☑
      - T4 and T5 S23.131 ☑
      - T5 and T6 S23.133 ☑
      - T6 and T7 S23.141 ☑
      - T7 and T8 S23.143 ☑
      - T8 and T9 S23.151 ☑
      - T9 and T10 S23.153 ☑
      - T10 and T11 S23.161 ☑
      - T11 and T12 S23.163 ☑
      - T12 and L1 S23.171 ☑
- wrist (carpal bone) S63.006 ☑
  - carpometacarpal joint — *see* Dislocation, carpometacarpal (joint)
  - distal radioulnar joint — *see* Dislocation, radioulnar (joint), distal
  - metacarpal bone, proximal — *see* Dislocation, metacarpal (bone), proximal end

☑ **Additional Character Required — Refer to the Tabular List for Character Selection**   ▽ **Subterms under main terms may continue to next column or page**

Dislocation — continued
  wrist — continued
    midcarpal — see Dislocation, midcarpal (joint)
    radiocarpal joint — see Dislocation, radiocarpal (joint)
    recurrent — see Dislocation, recurrent, wrist
    specified site NEC S63.09- ☑
    ulna — see Dislocation, ulna, distal end
  xiphoid cartilage S23.29 ☑
Disorder (of) (see also Disease)
  acantholytic L11.9
    specified NEC L11.8
  acute
    psychotic — see Psychosis, acute
    stress F43.0
  adjustment (grief) F43.20
    with
      anxiety F43.22
        with depressed mood F43.23
      conduct disturbance F43.24
        with emotional disturbance F43.25
      depressed mood F43.21
        with anxiety F43.23
      other specified symptom F43.29
  adrenal (capsule) (gland) (medullary) E27.9
    specified NEC E27.8
  adrenogenital E25.9
    drug-induced E25.8
    iatrogenic E25.8
    idiopathic E25.8
  adult personality (and behavior) F69
    specified NEC F68.8
  affective (mood) — see Disorder, mood
  aggressive, unsocialized F91.1
  alcohol use
    mild F10.10
      with
        alcohol intoxication F10.129
          delirium F10.121
        alcohol-induced
          anxiety disorder F10.180
          bipolar and related disorder F10.14
          depressive disorder F10.14
          psychotic disorder F10.159
          sexual dysfunction F10.181
          sleep disorder F10.182
        in remission (early) (sustained) F10.11
    moderate or severe F10.20
      with
        alcohol intoxication F10.229
          delirium F10.221
        alcohol-induced
          anxiety disorder F10.280
          bipolar and related disorder F10.24
          depressive disorder F10.24
          major neurocognitive disorder, amnestic-confabulatory type F10.26
          major neurocognitive disorder, non-amnestic-confabulatory type F10.27
          mild neurocognitive disorder F10.288
          psychotic disorder F10.259
          sexual dysfunction F10.281
          sleep disorder F10.282
        in remission (early) (sustained) F10.21
  alcohol-related F10.99
    with
      amnestic disorder, persisting F10.96
      anxiety disorder F10.980
      dementia, persisting F10.97
      intoxication F10.929
        with delirium F10.921
        uncomplicated F10.920
      mood disorder F10.94
      other specified F10.988
      psychotic disorder F10.959
        with
          delusions F10.950
          hallucinations F10.951
      sexual dysfunction F10.981
      sleep disorder F10.982
  allergic — see Allergy
  alveolar NEC J84.09
  amino-acid
    cystathioninuria E72.19
    cystinosis E72.04
    cystinuria E72.01
    glycinuria E72.09

Disorder — continued
  amino-acid — continued
    homocystinuria E72.11
    metabolism — see Disturbance, metabolism, amino-acid
    specified NEC E72.89
    neonatal, transitory P74.8
    renal transport NEC E72.09
    transport NEC E72.09
  amnesic, amnestic
    alcohol-induced F10.96
      with dependence F10.26
    due to (secondary to) general medical condition F04
    psychoactive NEC-induced F19.96
      with
        abuse F19.16
        dependence F19.26
    sedative, hypnotic or anxiolytic-induced F13.96
      with dependence F13.26
  amphetamine (or other stimulant) use
    mild
      with
        amphetamine, cocaine, or other stimulant intoxication
          with perceptual disturbances F15.122
          without perceptual disturbances F15.129
        amphetamine (or other stimulant) -induced
          anxiety disorder F15.180
          bipolar and related disorder F15.14
          depressive disorder F15.14
          obsessive-compulsive and related disorder F15.188
          psychotic disorder F15.159
          sexual dysfunction F15.181
        intoxication delirium F15.121
    moderate or severe
      with
        amphetamine, cocaine, or other stimulant intoxication
          with perceptual disturbances F15.222
          without perceptual disturbances F15.229
        amphetamine (or other stimulant) -induced
          anxiety disorder F15.280
          bipolar and related disorder F15.24
          depressive disorder F15.24
          obsessive-compulsive and related disorder F15.288
          psychotic disorder F15.259
          sexual dysfunction F15.281
        intoxication delirium F15.221
  amphetamine-type substance use
    mild F15.10
      in remission (early) (sustained) F15.11
    moderate F15.20
      in remission (early) (sustained) F15.21
    severe F15.20
      in remission (early) (sustained) F15.21
  anaerobic glycolysis with anemia D55.2
  anxiety F41.9
    due to (secondary to)
      alcohol F10.980
        in
          abuse F10.180
          dependence F10.280
      amphetamine F15.980
        in
          abuse F15.180
          dependence F15.280
      anxiolytic F13.980
        in
          abuse F13.180
          dependence F13.280
      caffeine F15.980
        in
          abuse F15.180
          dependence F15.280
      cannabis F12.980
        in
          abuse F12.180
          dependence F12.280
      cocaine F14.980
        in
          abuse F14.180
          dependence F14.180
      general medical condition F06.4
      hallucinogen F16.980
        in
          abuse F16.180
          dependence F16.280

Disorder — continued
  anxiety — continued
    due to — continued
      hypnotic F13.980
        in
          abuse F13.180
          dependence F13.280
      inhalant F18.980
        in
          abuse F18.180
          dependence F18.280
      phencyclidine F16.980
        in
          abuse F16.180
          dependence F16.280
      psychoactive substance NEC F19.980
        in
          abuse F19.180
          dependence F19.280
      sedative F13.980
        in
          abuse F13.180
          dependence F13.280
      volatile solvents F18.980
        in
          abuse F18.180
          dependence F18.280
    generalized F41.1
    illness F45.21
    mixed
      with depression (mild) F41.8
      specified NEC F41.3
    organic F06.4
    phobic F40.9
      of childhood F40.8
    specified NEC F41.8
  aortic valve — see Endocarditis, aortic
  aromatic amino-acid metabolism E70.9
    specified NEC E70.8
  arteriole NEC I77.89
  artery NEC I77.89
  articulation — see Disorder, joint
  attachment (childhood)
    disinhibited F94.2
    reactive F94.1
  attention-deficit hyperactivity (adolescent) (adult) (child) F90.9
    combined
      presentation F90.2
      type F90.2
    hyperactive
      impulsive presentation F90.1
      type F90.1
    inattentive
      presentation F90.0
      type F90.0
    specified type NEC F90.8
  attention-deficit without hyperactivity (adolescent) (adult) (child) F98.8
  auditory processing (central) H93.25
  autism spectrum F84.0
  autistic F84.0
  autoimmune D89.89
  autonomic nervous system G90.9
    specified NEC G90.8
  avoidant
    child or adolescent F40.10
    restrictive food intake F50.82
  balance
    acid-base E87.8
      mixed E87.4
    electrolyte E87.8
    fluid NEC E87.8
  behavioral (disruptive) — see Disorder, conduct
  beta-amino-acid metabolism E72.89
  bile acid and cholesterol metabolism E78.70
    Barth syndrome E78.71
    other specified E78.79
    Smith-Lemli-Opitz syndrome E78.72
  bilirubin excretion E80.6
  binge eating F50.81
  binocular
    movement H51.9
      convergence
        excess H51.12
        insufficiency H51.11
      internuclear ophthalmoplegia — see Ophthalmoplegia, internuclear
      palsy of conjugate gaze H51.0

Disorder — *continued*
  binocular — *continued*
    movement — *continued*
      specified type NEC H51.8
    vision NEC — *see* Disorder, vision, binocular
  bipolar (I) (type I) F31.9
    and related due to a known physiological condition
      with
        manic features F06.33
        manic- or hypomanic-like episodes F06.33
        mixed features F06.34
    current (or most recent) episode
      depressed F31.9
        with psychotic features F31.5
        without psychotic features F31.30
          mild F31.31
          moderate F31.32
          severe (without psychotic features) F31.4
            with psychotic features F31.5
      hypomanic F31.0
      manic F31.9
        with psychotic features F31.2
        without psychotic features F31.10
          mild F31.11
          moderate F31.12
          severe (without psychotic features)
            F31.13
            with psychotic features F31.2
      mixed F31.60
        mild F31.61
        moderate F31.62
        severe (without psychotic features) F31.63
          with psychotic features F31.64
        severe depression (without psychotic features)
          F31.4
          with psychotic features F31.5
    in remission (currently) F31.70
      in full remission
        most recent episode
          depressed F31.76
          hypomanic F31.72
          manic F31.74
          mixed F31.78
      in partial remission
        most recent episode
          depressed F31.75
          hypomanic F31.71
          manic F31.73
          mixed F31.77
    organic F06.30
    single manic episode F30.9
      mild F30.11
      moderate F30.12
      severe (without psychotic symptoms) F30.13
        with psychotic symptoms F30.2
    specified NEC F31.89
  bipolar II (type 2) F31.81
  bladder N32.9
    functional NEC N31.9
    in schistosomiasis B65.0 [N33]
    specified NEC N32.89
  bleeding D68.9
  blood D75.9
    in congenital early syphilis A50.09 [D77]
  body dysmorphic F45.22
  bone M89.9
    continuity M84.9
      specified type NEC M84.80
        ankle M84.87- ☑
        fibula M84.86- ☑
        foot M84.87- ☑
        hand M84.84- ☑
        humerus M84.82- ☑
        neck M84.88
        pelvis M84.859
        radius M84.83- ☑
        rib M84.88
        shoulder M84.81- ☑
        skull M84.88
        thigh M84.85- ☑
        tibia M84.86- ☑
        ulna M84.83- ☑
        vertebra M84.88
    density and structure M85.9
      cyst (*see also* Cyst, bone, specified type NEC)
        aneurysmal — *see* Cyst, bone, aneurysmal
        solitary — *see* Cyst, bone, solitary

Disorder — *continued*
  bone — *continued*
    density and structure — *continued*
      diffuse idiopathic skeletal hyperostosis — *see*
        Hyperostosis, ankylosing
      fibrous dysplasia (monostotic) — *see* Dysplasia,
        fibrous, bone
      fluorosis — *see* Fluorosis, skeletal
      hyperostosis of skull M85.2
      osteitis condensans — *see* Osteitis, condensans
      specified type NEC M85.8- ☑
        ankle M85.87- ☑
        foot M85.87- ☑
        forearm M85.83- ☑
        hand M85.84- ☑
        lower leg M85.86- ☑
        multiple sites M85.89
        neck M85.88
        rib M85.88
        shoulder M85.81- ☑
        skull M85.88
        thigh M85.85- ☑
        upper arm M85.82- ☑
        vertebra M85.88
    development and growth NEC M89.20
      carpus M89.24- ☑
      clavicle M89.21- ☑
      femur M89.25- ☑
      fibula M89.26- ☑
      finger M89.24- ☑
      humerus M89.22- ☑
      ilium M89.259
      ischium M89.259
      metacarpus M89.24- ☑
      metatarsus M89.27- ☑
      multiple sites M89.29
      neck M89.28
      radius M89.23- ☑
      rib M89.28
      scapula M89.21- ☑
      skull M89.28
      tarsus M89.27- ☑
      tibia M89.26- ☑
      toe M89.27- ☑
      ulna M89.23- ☑
      vertebra M89.28
    specified type NEC M89.8X- ☑
  brachial plexus G54.0
  branched-chain amino-acid metabolism E71.2
    specified NEC E71.19
  breast N64.9
    agalactia — *see* Agalactia
    associated with
      lactation O92.70
        specified NEC O92.79
      pregnancy O92.20
        specified NEC O92.29
      puerperium O92.20
        specified NEC O92.29
    cracked nipple — *see* Cracked nipple
    galactorrhea — *see* Galactorrhea
    hypogalactia O92.4
    lactation disorder NEC O92.79
    mastitis — *see* Mastitis
    nipple infection — *see* Infection, nipple
    retracted nipple — *see* Retraction, nipple
    specified type NEC N64.89
  Briquet's F45.0
  bullous, in diseases classified elsewhere L14
  caffeine use
    mild
      with
        caffeine-induced
          anxiety disorder F15.180
          sleep disorder F15.182
    moderate or severe
      with
        caffeine-induced
          anxiety disorder F15.280
          sleep disorder F15.282
  cannabis use
    mild F12.10
      with
        cannabis intoxication delirium F12.121
          with perceptual disturbances F12.122
          without perceptual disturbances F12.129

Disorder — *continued*
  cannabis use — *continued*
    mild — *continued*
      with — *continued*
        cannabis-induced
          anxiety disorder F12.180
          psychotic disorder F12.159
          sleep disorder F12.188
      in remission (early) (sustained) F12.11
    moderate or severe F12.20
      with
        cannabis intoxication
          with perceptual disturbances F12.222
          without perceptual disturbances F12.229
        cannabis-induced
          anxiety disorder F12.280
          psychotic disorder F12.259
          sleep disorder F12.288
        delirium F12.221
      in remission (early) (sustained) F12.21
  carbohydrate
    absorption, intestinal NEC E74.39
    metabolism (congenital) E74.9
      specified NEC E74.8
  cardiac, functional I51.89
  carnitine metabolism E71.40
  cartilage M94.9
    articular NEC — *see* Derangement, joint, articular
      cartilage
    chondrocalcinosis — *see* Chondrocalcinosis
    specified type NEC M94.8X- ☑
      articular — *see* Derangement, joint, articular
        cartilage
      multiple sites M94.8X0
  catatonia (due to known physiological condition) (with
    another mental disorder) F06.1
  catatonic
    due to (secondary to) known physiological condition
      F06.1
    organic F06.1
  central auditory processing H93.25
  cervical
    region NEC M53.82
    root (nerve) NEC G54.2
  character NOS F60.9
  childhood disintegrative NEC F84.3
  cholesterol and bile acid metabolism E78.70
    Barth syndrome E78.71
    other specified E78.79
    Smith-Lemli-Opitz syndrome E78.72
  choroid H31.9
    atrophy — *see* Atrophy, choroid
    degeneration — *see* Degeneration, choroid
    detachment — *see* Detachment, choroid
    dystrophy — *see* Dystrophy, choroid
    hemorrhage — *see* Hemorrhage, choroid
    rupture — *see* Rupture, choroid
    scar — *see* Scar, chorioretinal
    solar retinopathy — *see* Retinopathy, solar
    specified type NEC H31.8
  ciliary body — *see* Disorder, iris
    degeneration — *see* Degeneration, ciliary body
  coagulation (factor) (*see also* Defect, coagulation) D68.9
    newborn, transient P61.6
  cocaine use
    mild F14.10
      with
        amphetamine, cocaine, or other stimulant
          intoxication
          with perceptual disturbances F14.122
          without perceptual disturbances F14.129
        cocaine intoxication delirium F14.121
        cocaine-induced
          anxiety disorder F14.180
          bipolar and related disorder F14.14
          depressive disorder F14.14
          obsessive-compulsive and related disor-
            der F14.188
          psychotic disorder F14.159
          sexual dysfunction F14.181
          sleep disorder F14.182
      in remission (early) (sustained) F14.11
    moderate or severe F14.20
      with
        amphetamine, cocaine, or other stimulant
          intoxication
          with perceptual disturbances F14.222
          without perceptual disturbances F14.229

☑ **Additional Character Required** — Refer to the Tabular List for Character Selection   ▽ **Subterms under main terms may continue to next column or page**

Disorder — *continued*
  cocaine use — *continued*
    moderate or severe — *continued*
      with — *continued*
        cocaine intoxication delirium F14.221
        cocaine-induced
          anxiety disorder F14.280
          bipolar and related disorder F14.24
          depressive disorder F14.24
          obsessive-compulsive and related disor-
            der F14.288
          psychotic disorder F14.259
          sexual dysfunction F14.281
          sleep disorder F14.282
      in remission (early) (sustained) F14.21
  coccyx NEC M53.3
  cognitive F09
    due to (secondary to) general medical condition F09
    persisting R41.89
      due to
        alcohol F10.97
          with dependence F10.27
        anxiolytics F13.97
          with dependence F13.27
        hypnotics F13.97
          with dependence F13.27
        sedatives F13.97
          with dependence F13.27
        specified substance NEC F19.97
          with
            abuse F19.17
            dependence F19.27
  communication F80.9
    social pragmatic F80.82
  conduct (childhood) F91.9
    adjustment reaction — *see* Disorder, adjustment
    adolescent onset type F91.2
    childhood onset type F91.1
    compulsive F63.9
    confined to family context F91.0
    depressive F91.8
    group type F91.2
    hyperkinetic — *see* Disorder, attention-deficit hy-
      peractivity
    oppositional defiance F91.3
    socialized F91.2
    solitary aggressive type F91.1
    specified NEC F91.8
    unsocialized (aggressive) F91.1
  conduction, heart I45.9
  congenital glycosylation (CDG) E74.8
  conjunctiva H11.9
    infection — *see* Conjunctivitis
  connective tissue, localized L94.9
    specified NEC L94.8
  conversion (functional neurological symptom disorder)
    with
      abnormal movement F44.4
      anesthesia or sensory loss F44.6
      attacks or seizures F44.5
      mixed symptoms F44.7
      special sensory symptoms F44.6
      speech symptoms F44.4
      swallowing symptoms F44.4
      weakness or paralysis F44.4
  convulsive (secondary) — *see* Convulsions
  cornea H18.9
    deformity — *see* Deformity, cornea
    degeneration — *see* Degeneration, cornea
    deposits — *see* Deposit, cornea
    due to contact lens H18.82- ☑
      specified as edema — *see* Edema, cornea
    edema — *see* Edema, cornea
    keratitis — *see* Keratitis
    keratoconjunctivitis — *see* Keratoconjunctivitis
    membrane change — *see* Change, corneal mem-
      brane
    neovascularization — *see* Neovascularization,
      cornea
    scar — *see* Opacity, cornea
    specified type NEC H18.89- ☑
    ulcer — *see* Ulcer, cornea
  corpus cavernosum N48.9
  cranial nerve — *see* Disorder, nerve, cranial
  cyclothymic F34.0
  defiant oppositional F91.3
  delusional (persistent) (systematized) F22
    induced F24

Disorder — *continued*
  depersonalization F48.1
  depressive F32.9
    due to known physiological condition
      with
        depressive features F06.31
        major depressive-like episode F06.32
        mixed features F06.34
    major F32.9
      with psychotic symptoms F32.3
      in remission (full) F32.5
        partial F32.4
      recurrent F33.9
        with psychotic features F33.3
      single episode F32.9
        mild F32.0
        moderate F32.1
        severe (without psychotic symptoms) F32.2
          with psychotic symptoms F32.3
    organic F06.31
    persistent F34.1
    recurrent F33.9
      current episode
        mild F33.0
        moderate F33.1
        severe (without psychotic symptoms) F33.2
          with psychotic symptoms F33.3
      in remission F33.40
        full F33.42
        partial F33.41
      specified NEC F33.8
    single episode — *see* Episode, depressive
    specified NEC F32.89
  developmental F89
    arithmetical skills F81.2
    coordination (motor) F82
    expressive writing F81.81
    language F80.9
      expressive F80.1
      mixed receptive and expressive F80.2
      receptive type F80.2
      specified NEC F80.89
    learning F81.9
      arithmetical F81.2
      reading F81.0
    mixed F88
    motor coordination or function F82
    pervasive F84.9
      specified NEC F84.8
    phonological F80.0
    reading F81.0
    scholastic skills (*see also* Disorder, learning)
      mixed F81.89
    specified NEC F88
    speech F80.9
      articulation F80.0
      specified NEC F80.89
    written expression F81.81
  diaphragm J98.6
  digestive (system) K92.9
    newborn P78.9
      specified NEC P78.89
    postprocedural — *see* Complication, gastrointestinal
    psychogenic F45.8
  disc (intervertebral) M51.9
    with
      myelopathy
        cervical region M50.00
        cervicothoracic region M50.03
        high cervical region M50.01
        lumbar region M51.06
        mid-cervical region M50.020
        sacrococcygeal region M53.3
        thoracic region M51.04
        thoracolumbar region M51.05
      radiculopathy
        cervical region M50.10
        cervicothoracic region M50.13
        high cervical region M50.11
        lumbar region M51.16
        lumbosacral region M51.17
        mid-cervical region M50.120
        sacrococcygeal region M53.3
        thoracic region M51.14
        thoracolumbar region M51.15
    cervical M50.90
      with
        myelopathy M50.00
          C2-C3 M50.01

Disorder — *continued*
  disc — *continued*
    cervical — *continued*
      with — *continued*
        myelopathy — *continued*
          C3-C4 M50.01
          C4-C5 M50.021
          C5-C6 M50.022
          C6-C7 M50.023
          C7-T1 M50.03
          cervicothoracic region M50.03
          high cervical region M50.01
          mid-cervical region M50.020
        neuritis, radiculitis or radiculopathy M50.10
          C2-C3 M50.11
          C3-C4 M50.11
          C4-C5 M50.121
          C5-C6 M50.122
          C6-C7 M50.123
          C7-T1 M50.13
          cervicothoracic region M50.13
          high cervical region M50.11
          mid-cervical region M50.120
        C2-C3 M50.91
        C3-C4 M50.91
        C4-C5 M50.921
        C5-C6 M50.922
        C6-C7 M50.923
        C7-T1 M50.93
        cervicothoracic region M50.93
        degeneration M50.30
          C2-C3 M50.31
          C3-C4 M50.31
          C4-C5 M50.321
          C5-C6 M50.322
          C6-C7 M50.323
          C7-T1 M50.33
          cervicothoracic region M50.33
          high cervical region M50.31
          mid-cervical region M50.320
        displacement M50.20
          C2-C3 M50.21
          C3-C4 M50.21
          C4-C5 M50.221
          C5-C6 M50.222
          C6-C7 M50.223
          C7-T1 M50.23
          cervicothoracic region M50.23
          high cervical region M50.21
          mid-cervical region M50.220
        high cervical region M50.91
        mid-cervical region M50.920
        specified type NEC M50.80
          C2-C3 M50.81
          C3-C4 M50.81
          C4-C5 M50.821
          C5-C6 M50.822
          C6-C7 M50.823
          C7-T1 M50.83
          cervicothoracic region M50.83
          high cervical region M50.81
          mid-cervical region M50.820
      specified NEC
        lumbar region M51.86
        lumbosacral region M51.87
        sacrococcygeal region M53.3
        thoracic region M51.84
        thoracolumbar region M51.85
    disinhibited attachment (childhood) F94.2
    disintegrative, childhood NEC F84.3
    disruptive F91.9
      mood dysregulation F34.81
      specified NEC F91.8
    disruptive behavior — *see* Disorder, conduct
    dissocial personality F60.2
    dissociative F44.9
      affecting
        motor function F44.4
          and sensation F44.7
        sensation F44.6
          and motor function F44.7
      brief reactive F43.0
      due to (secondary to) general medical condition
        F06.8
      mixed F44.7
      organic F06.8
      other specified NEC F44.89
    double heterozygous sickling — *see* Disease, sickle-cell
    dream anxiety F51.5

Disorder — *continued*
 drug induced hemorrhagic D68.32
 drug related F19.99
  abuse — *see* Abuse, drug
  dependence — *see* Dependence, drug
 dysmorphic body F45.22
 dysthymic F34.1
 ear H93.9- ☑
  bleeding — *see* Otorrhagia
  deafness — *see* Deafness
  degenerative H93.09- ☑
  discharge — *see* Otorrhea
  external H61.9- ☑
   auditory canal stenosis — *see* Stenosis, external ear canal
   exostosis — *see* Exostosis, external ear canal
   impacted cerumen — *see* Impaction, cerumen
   otitis — *see* Otitis, externa
   perichondritis — *see* Perichondritis, ear
   pinna — *see* Disorder, pinna
   specified type NEC H61.89- ☑
  inner H83.9- ☑
   vestibular dysfunction — *see* Disorder, vestibular function
  middle H74.9- ☑
   adhesive H74.1- ☑
   ossicle — *see* Abnormal, ear ossicles
   polyp — *see* Polyp, ear (middle)
   specified NEC, in diseases classified elsewhere H75.8- ☑
  postprocedural — *see* Complications, ear, procedure
  specified NEC, in diseases classified elsewhere H94.8- ☑
 eating (adult) (psychogenic) F50.9
  anorexia — *see* Anorexia
  binge F50.81
  bulimia F50.2
  child F98.29
   pica F98.3
   rumination disorder F98.21
  pica F50.89
   childhood F98.3
 electrolyte (balance) NEC E87.8
  with
   abortion — *see* Abortion by type complicated by specified condition NEC
   ectopic pregnancy O08.5
   molar pregnancy O08.5
  acidosis (metabolic) (respiratory) E87.2
  alkalosis (metabolic) (respiratory) E87.3
 elimination, transepidermal L87.9
  specified NEC L87.8
 emotional (persistent) F34.9
  of childhood F93.9
   specified NEC F93.8
 endocrine E34.9
  postprocedural E89.89
  specified NEC E89.89
 erectile (male) (organic) (*see also* Dysfunction, sexual, male, erectile) N52.9
  nonorganic F52.21
 erythematous — *see* Erythema
 esophagus K22.9
  functional K22.4
  psychogenic F45.8
 eustachian tube H69.9- ☑
  infection — *see* Salpingitis, eustachian
  obstruction — *see* Obstruction, eustachian tube
  patulous — *see* Patulous, eustachian tube
  specified NEC H69.8- ☑
 exhibitionistic F65.2
 extrapyramidal G25.9
  in deseases classified elsewhere — *see* category G26
  specified type NEC G25.89
 eye H57.9
  postprocedural — *see* Complication, postprocedural, eye
 eyelid H02.9
  cyst — *see* Cyst, eyelid
  degenerative H02.70
   chloasma — *see* Chloasma, eyelid
   madarosis — *see* Madarosis
   specified type NEC H02.79
   vitiligo — *see* Vitiligo, eyelid
   xanthelasma — *see* Xanthelasma
  dermatochalasis — *see* Dermatochalasis

Disorder — *continued*
 eyelid — *continued*
  edema — *see* Edema, eyelid
  elephantiasis — *see* Elephantiasis, eyelid
  foreign body, retained — *see* Foreign body, retained, eyelid
  function H02.59
   abnormal innervation syndrome — *see* Syndrome, abnormal innervation
   blepharochalasis — *see* Blepharochalasis
   blepharoclonus — *see* Blepharoclonus
   blepharophimosis — *see* Blepharophimosis
   blepharoptosis — *see* Blepharoptosis
   lagophthalmos — *see* Lagophthalmos
   lid retraction — *see* Retraction, lid
  hypertrichosis — *see* Hypertrichosis, eyelid
  specified type NEC H02.89
  vascular H02.879
   left H02.876
    lower H02.875
    upper H02.874
   right H02.873
    lower H02.872
    upper H02.871
 factitious
  by proxy F68.A
  imposed on another F68.A
  imposed on self F68.10
   with predominantly
    psychological symptoms F68.11
     with physical symptoms F68.13
    physical symptoms F68.12
     with psychological symptoms F68.13
 factor, coagulation — *see* Defect, coagulation
 fatty acid
  metabolism E71.30
   specified NEC E71.39
  oxidation
   LCAD E71.310
   MCAD E71.311
   SCAD E71.312
   specified deficiency NEC E71.318
 feeding (infant or child) (*see also* Disorder, eating) R63.3
  or eating disorder F50.9
  specified NEC F50.9
 feigned (with obvious motivation) Z76.5
  without obvious motivation — *see* Disorder, factitious
 female
  hypoactive sexual desire F52.0
  orgasmic F52.31
  sexual interest/arousal F52.22
 fetishistic F65.0
 fibroblastic M72.9
  specified NEC M72.8
 fluency
  adult onset F98.5
  childhood onset F80.81
  following
   cerebral infarction I69.323
   cerebrovascular disease I69.923
    specified disease NEC I69.823
   intracerebral hemorrhage I69.123
   nontraumatic intracranial hemorrhage NEC I69.223
   subarachnoid hemorrhage I69.023
  in conditions classified elsewhere R47.82
 fluid balance E87.8
 follicular (skin) L73.9
  specified NEC L73.8
 frotteuristic F65.81
 fructose metabolism E74.10
  essential fructosuria E74.11
  fructokinase deficiency E74.11
  fructose-1, 6-diphosphatase deficiency E74.19
  hereditary fructose intolerance E74.12
  other specified E74.19
 functional polymorphonuclear neutrophils D71
 gallbladder, biliary tract and pancreas in diseases classified elsewhere K87
 gambling F63.0
 gamma aminobutyric acid (GABA) metabolism E72.81
 gamma-glutamyl cycle E72.89
 gastric (functional) K31.9
  motility K30
  psychogenic F45.8
  secretion K30
 gastrointestinal (functional) NOS K92.9

Disorder — *continued*
 gastrointestinal — *continued*
  newborn P78.9
  psychogenic F45.8
 gender-identity or -role F64.9
  childhood F64.2
  effect on relationship F66
  of adolescence or adulthood F64.0
   nontranssexual F64.8
  specified NEC F64.8
  uncertainty F66
 genito-pelvic pain penetration F52.6
 genitourinary system
  female N94.9
  male N50.9
  psychogenic F45.8
 globe H44.9
  degenerated condition H44.50
   absolute glaucoma H44.51- ☑
   atrophy H44.52- ☑
   leucocoria H44.53- ☑
  degenerative H44.30
   chalcosis H44.31- ☑
   myopia (*see also* Myopia, degenerative) H44.2- ☑
   siderosis H44.32- ☑
   specified type NEC H44.39- ☑
  endophthalmitis — *see* Endophthalmitis
  foreign body, retained — *see* Foreign body, intraocular, old, retained
  hemophthalmos — *see* Hemophthalmos
  hypotony H44.40
   due to
    ocular fistula H44.42- ☑
    specified disorder NEC H44.43- ☑
   flat anterior chamber H44.41- ☑
   primary H44.44- ☑
  luxation — *see* Luxation, globe
  specified type NEC H44.89
 glomerular (in) N05.9
  amyloidosis E85.4 [N08]
  cryoglobulinemia D89.1 [N08]
  disseminated intravascular coagulation D65 [N08]
  Fabry's disease E75.21 [N08]
  familial lecithin cholesterol acyltransferase deficiency E78.6 [N08]
  Goodpasture's syndrome M31.0
  hemolytic-uremic syndrome D59.3
  Henoch (-Schönlein) purpura D69.0 [N08]
  malariae malaria B52.0
  microscopic polyangiitis M31.7 [N08]
  multiple myeloma C90.0- ☑ [N08]
  mumps B26.83
  schistosomiasis B65.9 [N08]
  sepsis NEC A41.- ☑ [N08]
   streptococcal A40.- ☑ [N08]
  sickle-cell disorders D57.- ☑ [N08]
  strongyloidiasis B78.9 [N08]
  subacute bacterial endocarditis I33.0 [N08]
  syphilis A52.75
  systemic lupus erythematosus M32.14
  thrombotic thrombocytopenic purpura M31.1 [N08]
  Waldenström macroglobulinemia C88.0 [N08]
  Wegener's granulomatosis M31.31
 gluconeogenesis E74.4
 glucosaminoglycan metabolism — *see* Disorder, metabolism, glucosaminoglycan
 glycine metabolism E72.50
  d-glycericacidemia E72.59
  hyperhydroxyprolinemia E72.59
  hyperoxaluria R82.992
   primary E72.53
  hyperprolinemia E72.59
  non-ketotic hyperglycinemia E72.51
  oxalosis E72.53
  oxaluria E72.53
  sarcosinemia E72.59
  trimethylaminuria E72.52
 glycoprotein metabolism E77.9
  specified NEC E77.8
 habit (and impulse) F63.9
  involving sexual behavior NEC F65.9
  specified NEC F63.89
 hallucinogen use
  mild F16.10
   with
    hallucinogen intoxication delirium F16.121

☑ **Additional Character Required** — Refer to the Tabular List for Character Selection ᵛᵉᵍ **Subterms under main terms may continue to next column or page**

Disorder — continued
　hallucinogen use — continued
　　mild — continued
　　　with — continued
　　　　hallucinogen-induced
　　　　　anxiety disorder F16.180
　　　　　bipolar and related disorder F16.14
　　　　　depressive disorder F16.14
　　　　　psychotic disorder F16.159
　　　　other hallucinogen intoxication F16.129
　　　　in remission (early) (sustained) F16.11
　　　moderate or severe F16.20
　　　　with
　　　　　hallucinogen intoxication delirium F16.221
　　　　　hallucinogen-induced
　　　　　　anxiety disorder F16.280
　　　　　　bipolar and related disorder F16.24
　　　　　　depressive disorder F16.24
　　　　　　psychotic disorder F16.259
　　　　　other hallucinogen intoxication F16.229
　　　　　in remission (early) (sustained) F16.21
　heart action I49.9
　hematological D75.9
　　newborn (transient) P61.9
　　specified NEC P61.8
　hematopoietic organs D75.9
　hemorrhagic NEC D69.9
　　drug-induced D68.32
　　due to
　　　extrinsic circulating anticoagulants D68.32
　　　increase in
　　　　anti-IIa D68.32
　　　　anti-Xa D68.32
　　　intrinsic
　　　　circulating anticoagulants D68.318
　　　　increase in
　　　　　anti-IXa D68.318
　　　　　antithrombin D68.318
　　　　　anti-VIIIa D68.318
　　　　　anti-XIa D68.318
　　　following childbirth O72.3
　hemostasis — see Defect, coagulation
　histidine metabolism E70.40
　　histidinemia E70.41
　　other specified E70.49
　hoarding F42.3
　hyperkinetic — see Disorder, attention-deficit hyperactivity
　hyperleucine-isoleucinemia E71.19
　hypervalinemia E71.19
　hypoactive sexual desire F52.0
　hypochondriacal F45.20
　　body dysmorphic F45.22
　　neurosis F45.21
　　other specified F45.29
　identity
　　dissociative F44.81
　　illness anxiety F45.21
　　of childhood F93.8
　immune mechanism (immunity) D89.9
　　specified type NEC D89.89
　impaired renal tubular function N25.9
　　specified NEC N25.89
　impulse (control) F63.9
　inflammatory
　　pelvic, in diseases classified elsewhere — see category N74
　　penis N48.29
　　　abscess N48.21
　　　cellulitis N48.22
　inhalant use
　　mild F18.10
　　　with
　　　　inhalant intoxication F18.129
　　　　inhalant intoxication delirium F18.121
　　　　inhalant-induced
　　　　　anxiety disorder F18.180
　　　　　depressive disorder F18.14
　　　　　major neurocognitive disorder F18.17
　　　　　mild neurocognitive disorder F18.188
　　　　　psychotic disorder F18.159
　　　　in remission (early) (sustained) F18.11
　　　moderate or severe F18.20
　　　　with
　　　　　inhalant intoxication F18.229
　　　　　inhalant intoxication delirium F18.221
　　　　　inhalant-induced
　　　　　　anxiety disorder F18.280
　　　　　　depressive disorder F18.24

Disorder — continued
　inhalant use — continued
　　moderate or severe — continued
　　　with — continued
　　　　inhalant-induced — continued
　　　　　major neurocognitive disorder F18.27
　　　　　mild neurocognitive disorder F18.288
　　　　　psychotic disorder F18.259
　　　　in remission (early) (sustained) F18.21
　integument, newborn P83.9
　　specified NEC P83.88
　intermittent explosive F63.81
　internal secretion pancreas — see Increased, secretion, pancreas, endocrine
　intestine, intestinal
　　carbohydrate absorption NEC E74.39
　　　postoperative K91.2
　　functional NEC K59.9
　　　postoperative K91.89
　　psychogenic F45.8
　　vascular K55.9
　　　chronic K55.1
　　　specified NEC K55.8
　intraoperative (intraprocedural) — see Complications, intraoperative
　involuntary emotional expression (IEED) F07.89
　iris H21.9
　　adhesions — see Adhesions, iris
　　atrophy — see Atrophy, iris
　　chamber angle recession — see Recession, chamber angle
　　cyst — see Cyst, iris
　　degeneration — see Degeneration, iris
　　in diseases classified elsewhere H22
　　iridodialysis — see Iridodialysis
　　iridoschisis — see Iridoschisis
　　miotic pupillary cyst — see Cyst, pupillary
　　pupillary
　　　abnormality — see Abnormality, pupillary
　　　membrane — see Membrane, pupillary
　　specified type NEC H21.89
　　vascular NEC H21.1X- ☑
　iron metabolism E83.10
　　specified NEC E83.19
　isovaleric acidemia E71.110
　jaw, developmental M27.0
　　temporomandibular (see also Anomaly, dentofacial, temporomandibular joint) M26.60- ☑
　joint M25.9
　　derangement — see Derangement, joint
　　effusion — see Effusion, joint
　　fistula — see Fistula, joint
　　hemarthrosis — see Hemarthrosis
　　instability — see Instability, joint
　　osteophyte — see Osteophyte
　　pain — see Pain, joint
　　psychogenic F45.8
　　specified type NEC M25.80
　　　ankle M25.87- ☑
　　　elbow M25.82- ☑
　　　foot joint M25.87- ☑
　　　hand joint M25.84- ☑
　　　hip M25.85- ☑
　　　knee M25.86- ☑
　　　shoulder M25.81- ☑
　　　wrist M25.83- ☑
　　stiffness — see Stiffness, joint
　ketone metabolism E71.32
　kidney N28.9
　　functional (tubular) N25.9
　　in
　　　schistosomiasis B65.9 [N29]
　　tubular function N25.9
　　　specified NEC N25.89
　lacrimal system H04.9
　　changes H04.69
　　fistula — see Fistula, lacrimal
　　gland H04.19
　　　atrophy — see Atrophy, lacrimal gland
　　　cyst — see Cyst, lacrimal, gland
　　　dacryops — see Dacryops
　　　dislocation — see Dislocation, lacrimal gland
　　　dry eye syndrome — see Syndrome, dry eye
　　　infection — see Dacryoadenitis
　　granuloma — see Granuloma, lacrimal
　　inflammation — see Inflammation, lacrimal
　　obstruction — see Obstruction, lacrimal

Disorder — continued
　lacrimal system — continued
　　specified NEC H04.89
　lactation NEC O92.79
　language (developmental) F80.9
　　expressive F80.1
　　mixed receptive and expressive F80.2
　　receptive F80.2
　late luteal phase dysphoric N94.89
　learning (specific) F81.9
　　acalculia R48.8
　　alexia R48.0
　　mathematics F81.2
　　reading F81.0
　　specified
　　　with impairment in
　　　　mathematics F81.2
　　　　reading F81.0
　　　　written expression F81.81
　　specified NEC F81.89
　　spelling F81.81
　　written expression F81.81
　lens H27.9
　　aphakia — see Aphakia
　　cataract — see Cataract
　　dislocation — see Dislocation, lens
　　specified type NEC H27.8
　ligament M24.20
　　ankle M24.27- ☑
　　attachment, spine — see Enthesopathy, spinal
　　elbow M24.22- ☑
　　foot joint M24.27- ☑
　　hand joint M24.24- ☑
　　hip M24.25- ☑
　　knee — see Derangement, knee, specified NEC
　　shoulder M24.21- ☑
　　vertebra M24.28
　　wrist M24.23- ☑
　ligamentous attachments (see also Enthesopathy)
　　spine — see Enthesopathy, spinal
　lipid
　　metabolism, congenital E78.9
　　storage E75.6
　　　specified NEC E75.5
　lipoprotein
　　deficiency (familial) E78.6
　　metabolism E78.9
　　　specified NEC E78.89
　liver K76.9
　　malarial B54 [K77]
　low back (see also Dorsopathy, specified NEC)
　lumbosacral
　　plexus G54.1
　　root (nerve) NEC G54.4
　lung, interstitial, drug-induced J70.4
　　acute J70.2
　　chronic J70.3
　lymphoproliferative, post-transplant (PTLD) D47.Z1
　　(following D47.4)
　lysine and hydroxylysine metabolism E72.3
　major neurocognitive — see Dementia, in (due to)
　male
　　erectile (organic) (see also Dysfunction, sexual, male, erectile) N52.9
　　　nonorganic F52.21
　　hypoactive sexual desire F52.0
　　orgasmic F52.32
　manic F30.9
　　organic F06.33
　mast cell activation — see Activation, mast cell
　mastoid (see also Disorder, ear, middle)
　　postprocedural — see Complications, ear, procedure
　meniscus — see Derangement, knee, meniscus
　menopausal N95.9
　　specified NEC N95.8
　menstrual N92.6
　　psychogenic F45.8
　　specified NEC N92.5
　mental (or behavioral) (nonpsychotic) F99
　　due to (secondary to)
　　　amphetamine
　　　　due to drug abuse — see Abuse, drug, stimulant
　　　　due to drug dependence — see Dependence, drug, stimulant
　　　brain disease, damage and dysfunction F09
　　　caffeine use

Disorder — *continued*
  mental — *continued*
    due to — *continued*
      caffeine use — *continued*
        due to drug abuse — *see* Abuse, drug, stimulant
        due to drug dependence — *see* Dependence, drug, stimulant
      cannabis use
        due to drug abuse — *see* Abuse, drug, cannabis
        due to drug dependence — *see* Dependence, drug, cannabis
      general medical condition F09
      sedative or hypnotic use
        due to drug abuse — *see* Abuse, drug, sedative
        due to drug dependence — *see* Dependence, drug, sedative
      tobacco (nicotine) use — *see* Dependence, drug, nicotine
    following organic brain damage F07.9
      frontal lobe syndrome F07.0
      personality change F07.0
      postconcussional syndrome F07.81
      specified NEC F07.89
    infancy, childhood or adolescence F98.9
    neurotic — *see* Neurosis
    organic or symptomatic F09
    presenile, psychotic F03 ☑
    problem NEC
    psychoneurotic — *see* Neurosis
    psychotic — *see* Psychosis
    puerperal F53.0
    senile, psychotic NEC F03 ☑
  metabolic, amino acid, transitory, newborn P74.8
  metabolism NOS E88.9
    amino-acid E72.9
      aromatic E70.9
        albinism — *see* Albinism
        histidine E70.40
          histidinemia E70.41
          other specified E70.49
        hyperphenylalaninemia E70.1
          classical phenylketonuria E70.0
        other specified E70.8
        tryptophan E70.5
        tyrosine E70.20
          hypertyrosinemia E70.21
          other specified E70.29
      branched chain E71.2
        3-methylglutaconic aciduria E71.111
        hyperleucine-isoleucinemia E71.19
        hypervalinemia E71.19
        isovaleric acidemia E71.110
        maple syrup urine disease E71.0
        methylmalonic acidemia E71.120
        organic aciduria NEC E71.118
        other specified E71.19
        proprionate NEC E71.128
        proprionic acidemia E71.121
      glycine E72.50
        d-glycericacidemia E72.59
        hyperhydroxyprolinemia E72.59
        hyperoxaluria R82.992
          primary E72.53
        hyperprolinemia E72.59
        non-ketotic hyperglycinemia E72.51
        other specified E72.59
        sarcosinemia E72.59
        trimethylaminuria E72.52
      hydroxylysine E72.3
      lysine E72.3
      ornithine E72.4
      other specified E72.89
        beta-amino acid E72.89
        gamma-glutamyl cycle E72.89
      straight-chain E72.89
      sulfur-bearing E72.10
        homocystinuria E72.11
        methylenetetrahydrofolate reductase deficiency E72.12
        other specified E72.19
    bile acid and cholesterol metabolism E78.70
    bilirubin E80.7
      specified NEC E80.6
    calcium E83.50
      hypercalcemia E83.52

Disorder — *continued*
  metabolism — *continued*
    calcium — *continued*
      hypocalcemia E83.51
      other specified E83.59
    carbohydrate E74.9
      specified NEC E74.8
    cholesterol and bile acid metabolism E78.70
    congenital E88.9
    copper E83.00
      specified type NEC E83.09
      Wilson's disease E83.01
    cystinuria E72.01
    fructose E74.10
    galactose E74.20
    glucosaminoglycan E76.9
      mucopolysaccharidosis — *see* Mucopolysaccharidosis
      specified NEC E76.8
    glutamine E72.89
    glycine E72.50
    glycogen storage (hepatorenal) E74.09
    glycoprotein E77.9
      specified NEC E77.8
    glycosaminoglycan E76.9
      specified NEC E76.8
    in labor and delivery O75.89
    iron E83.10
    isoleucine E71.19
    leucine E71.19
    lipoid E78.9
    lipoprotein E78.9
      specified NEC E78.89
    magnesium E83.40
      hypermagnesemia E83.41
      hypomagnesemia E83.42
      other specified E83.49
    mineral E83.9
      specified NEC E83.89
    mitochondrial E88.40
      MELAS syndrome E88.41
      MERRF syndrome (myoclonic epilepsy associated with ragged-red fibers) E88.42
      other specified E88.49
    ornithine E72.4
    phosphatases E83.30
    phosphorus E83.30
      acid phosphatase deficiency E83.39
      hypophosphatasia E83.39
      hypophosphatemia E83.39
        familial E83.31
      other specified E83.39
      pseudovitamin D deficiency E83.32
    plasma protein NEC E88.09
    porphyrin — *see* Porphyria
    postprocedural E89.89
      specified NEC E89.89
    purine E79.9
      specified NEC E79.8
    pyrimidine E79.9
      specified NEC E79.8
    pyruvate E74.4
    serine E72.89
    sodium E87.8
    specified NEC E88.89
    threonine E72.89
    valine E71.19
    zinc E83.2
  methylmalonic acidemia E71.120
  micturition NEC (*see also* Difficulty, micturition) R39.198
    feeling of incomplete emptying R39.14
    hesitancy R39.11
    poor stream R39.12
    psychogenic F45.8
    split stream R39.13
    straining R39.16
    urgency R39.15
  mild neurocognitive G31.84
  mitochondrial metabolism E88.40
  mitral (valve) — *see* Endocarditis, mitral
  mixed
    anxiety and depressive F41.8
    of scholastic skills (developmental) F81.89
    receptive expressive language F80.2
  mood F39
    bipolar — *see* Disorder, bipolar
    depressive — *see* Disorder, depressive
    due to (secondary to)
      alcohol F10.94

Disorder — *continued*
  mood — *continued*
    due to — *continued*
      amphetamine F15.94
        in
          abuse F15.14
          dependence F15.24
      anxiolytic F13.94
        in
          abuse F13.14
          dependence F13.24
      cocaine F14.94
        in
          abuse F14.14
          dependence F14.24
      general medical condition F06.30
      hallucinogen F16.94
        in
          abuse F16.14
          dependence F16.24
      hypnotic F13.94
        in
          abuse F13.14
          dependence F13.24
      inhalant F18.94
        in
          abuse F18.14
          dependence F18.24
      opioid F11.94
        in
          abuse F11.14
          dependence F11.24
      phencyclidine (PCP) F16.94
        in
          abuse F16.14
          dependence F16.24
      physiological condition F06.30
        with
          depressive features F06.31
          major depressive-like episode F06.32
          manic features F06.33
          mixed features F06.34
      psychoactive substance NEC F19.94
        in
          abuse F19.14
          dependence F19.24
      sedative F13.94
        in
          abuse F13.14
          dependence F13.24
      volatile solvents F18.94
        in
          abuse F18.14
          dependence F18.24
    manic episode F30.9
      with psychotic symptoms F30.2
      in remission (full) F30.4
        partial F30.3
      specified type NEC F30.8
      without psychotic symptoms F30.10
        mild F30.11
        moderate F30.12
        severe F30.13
    organic F06.30
      right hemisphere F07.89
    persistent F34.9
      cyclothymia F34.0
      dysthymia F34.1
      specified type NEC F34.89
    recurrent F39
    right hemisphere organic F07.89
  movement G25.9
    drug-induced G25.70
      akathisia G25.71
      specified NEC G25.79
    hysterical F44.4
    in diseases classified elsewhere — *see* category G26
    periodic limb G47.61
      sleep related G47.61
    sleep related NEC G47.69
    specified NEC G25.89
    stereotyped F98.4
    treatment-induced G25.9
  multiple personality F44.81
  muscle M62.9
    attachment, spine — *see* Enthesopathy, spinal
    in trichinellosis — *see* Trichinellosis, with muscle disorder
    psychogenic F45.8

☑ **Additional Character Required** — **Refer to the Tabular List for Character Selection**   ⬇ Subterms under main terms may continue to next column or page

Disorder — *continued*
  muscle — *continued*
    specified type NEC M62.89
    tone, newborn P94.9
      specified NEC P94.8
  muscular
    attachments (*see also* Enthesopathy)
      spine — *see* Enthesopathy, spinal
    urethra N36.44
  musculoskeletal system, soft tissue — *see* Disorder, soft tissue
    postprocedural M96.89
    psychogenic F45.8
  myoneural G70.9
    due to lead G70.1
    specified NEC G70.89
    toxic G70.1
  myotonic NEC G71.19
  nail, in diseases classified elsewhere L62
  neck region NEC — *see* Dorsopathy, specified NEC
  neonatal onset multisystemic inflammatory (NOMID) M04.2
  nerve G58.9
    abducent NEC — *see* Strabismus, paralytic, sixth nerve
    accessory G52.8
    acoustic — *see* subcategory H93.3 ☑
    auditory — *see* subcategory H93.3 ☑
    auriculotemporal G50.8
    axillary G54.0
    cerebral — *see* Disorder, nerve, cranial
    cranial G52.9
      eighth — *see* subcategory H93.3 ☑
      eleventh G52.8
      fifth G50.9
      first G52.0
      fourth NEC — *see* Strabismus, paralytic, fourth nerve
      multiple G52.7
      ninth G52.1
      second NEC — *see* Disorder, nerve, optic
      seventh NEC G51.8
      sixth NEC — *see* Strabismus, paralytic, sixth nerve
      specified NEC G52.8
      tenth G52.2
      third NEC — *see* Strabismus, paralytic, third nerve
      twelfth G52.3
    entrapment — *see* Neuropathy, entrapment
    facial G51.9
      specified NEC G51.8
    femoral — *see* Lesion, nerve, femoral
    glossopharyngeal NEC G52.1
    hypoglossal G52.3
    intercostal G58.0
    lateral
      cutaneous of thigh — *see* Mononeuropathy, lower limb, meralgia paresthetica
      popliteal — *see* Lesion, nerve, popliteal
    lower limb — *see* Mononeuropathy, lower limb
    medial popliteal — *see* Lesion, nerve, popliteal, medial
    median NEC — *see* Lesion, nerve, median
    multiple G58.7
    oculomotor NEC — *see* Strabismus, paralytic, third nerve
    olfactory G52.0
    optic NEC H47.09- ☑
      hemorrhage into sheath — *see* Hemorrhage, optic nerve
      ischemic H47.01- ☑
    peroneal — *see* Lesion, nerve, popliteal
    phrenic G58.8
    plantar — *see* Lesion, nerve, plantar
    pneumogastric G52.2
    posterior tibial — *see* Syndrome, tarsal tunnel
    radial — *see* Lesion, nerve, radial
    recurrent laryngeal G52.2
    root G54.9
      cervical G54.2
      lumbosacral G54.1
      specified NEC G54.8
      thoracic G54.3
    sciatic NEC — *see* Lesion, nerve, sciatic
    specified NEC G58.8
      lower limb — *see* Mononeuropathy, lower limb, specified NEC
      upper limb — *see* Mononeuropathy, upper limb, specified NEC

Disorder — *continued*
  nerve — *continued*
    sympathetic G90.9
    tibial — *see* Lesion, nerve, popliteal, medial
    trigeminal G50.9
      specified NEC G50.8
    trochlear NEC — *see* Strabismus, paralytic, fourth nerve
    ulnar — *see* Lesion, nerve, ulnar
    upper limb — *see* Mononeuropathy, upper limb
    vagus G52.2
  nervous system G98.8
    autonomic (peripheral) G90.9
      specified NEC G90.8
    central G96.9
      specified NEC G96.8
    parasympathetic G90.9
    specified NEC G98.8
    sympathetic G90.9
    vegetative G90.9
  neurocognitive R41.9
    major
      with
        aggressive behavior F01.51
        combative behavior F01.51
        violent behavior F01.51
      due to vascular disease, with behavioral disturbance F01.51
      in (due to) (other diseases classified elsewhere) (*see also* Dementia, in (due to)) F02.80
        with
          aggressive behavior F02.81
          combative behavior F02.81
          violent behavior F02.81
        without behavioral disturbance F01.50
    mild G31.84
  neurodevelopmental F89
    specified NEC F88
  neurohypophysis NEC E23.3
  neurological NEC R29.818
  neuromuscular G70.9
    hereditary NEC G71.9
    specified NEC G70.89
    toxic G70.1
  neurotic F48.9
    specified NEC F48.8
  neutrophil, polymorphonuclear D71
  nicotine use — *see* Dependence, drug, nicotine
  nightmare F51.5
  non-rapid eye movement sleep arousal
    sleep terror type F51.4
    sleepwalking type F51.3
  nose J34.9
    specified NEC J34.89
  obsessive-compulsive F42.9
    and related disorder due to a known physiological condition F06.8
  odontogenesis NOS K00.9
  opioid use
    with
      opioid-induced psychotic disorder F11.959
        with
          delusions F11.950
          hallucinations F11.951
      due to drug abuse — *see* Abuse, drug, opioid
      due to drug dependence — *see* Dependence, drug, opioid
    mild F11.10
      with
        opioid-induced
          anxiety disorder F11.188
          depressive disorder F11.14
          sexual dysfunction F11.181
        opioid intoxication
          with perceptual disturbances F11.122
          delirium F11.121
          without perceptual disturbances F11.129
        in remission (early) (sustained) F11.11
    moderate or severe F11.20
      with
        opioid-induced
          anxiety disorder F11.288
          anxiety disorder F11.988
          depressive disorder F11.24
          depressive disorder F11.94
          sexual dysfunction F11.281
          sexual dysfunction F11.981

Disorder — *continued*
  opioid use — *continued*
    moderate or severe — *continued*
      with — *continued*
        opioid intoxication
          with perceptual disturbances F11.222
          delirium F11.221
          without perceptual disturbances F11.229
        in remission (early) (sustained) F11.21
  oppositional defiant F91.3
  optic
    chiasm H47.49
      due to
        inflammatory disorder H47.41
        neoplasm H47.42
        vascular disorder H47.43
    disc H47.39- ☑
      coloboma — *see* Coloboma, optic disc
      drusen — *see* Drusen, optic disc
      pseudopapilledema — *see* Pseudopapilledema
    radiations — *see* Disorder, visual, pathway
    tracts — *see* Disorder, visual, pathway
  orbit H05.9
    cyst — *see* Cyst, orbit
    deformity — *see* Deformity, orbit
    edema — *see* Edema, orbit
    enophthalmos — *see* Enophthalmos
    exophthalmos — *see* Exophthalmos
    hemorrhage — *see* Hemorrhage, orbit
    inflammation — *see* Inflammation, orbit
    myopathy — *see* Myopathy, extraocular muscles
    retained foreign body — *see* Foreign body, orbit, old
    specified type NEC H05.89
  organic
    anxiety F06.4
    catatonic F06.1
    delusional F06.2
    dissociative F06.8
    emotionally labile (asthenic) F06.8
    mood (affective) F06.30
    schizophrenia-like F06.2
  orgasmic (female) F52.31
    male F52.32
  ornithine metabolism E72.4
  overanxious F41.1
    of childhood F93.8
  pain
    with related psychological factors F45.42
    exclusively related to psychological factors F45.41
    genito-pelvic penetration disorder F52.6
  pancreatic internal secretion E16.9
    specified NEC E16.8
  panic F41.0
    with agoraphobia F40.01
  papulosquamous L44.9
    in diseases classified elsewhere L45
    specified NEC L44.8
  paranoid F22
    induced F24
    shared F24
  paraphilic F65.9
    specified NEC F65.89
  parathyroid (gland) E21.5
    specified NEC E21.4
  parietoalveolar NEC J84.09
  paroxysmal, mixed R56.9
  patella M22.9- ☑
    chondromalacia — *see* Chondromalacia, patella
    derangement NEC M22.3X- ☑
    recurrent
      dislocation — *see* Dislocation, patella, recurrent
      subluxation — *see* Dislocation, patella, recurrent, incomplete
    specified NEC M22.8X- ☑
  patellofemoral M22.2X- ☑
  pedophilic F65.4
  pentose phosphate pathway with anemia D55.1
  perception, due to hallucinogens F16.983
    in
      abuse F16.183
      dependence F16.283
  peripheral nervous system NEC G64
  peroxisomal E71.50
    biogenesis
      neonatal adrenoleukodystrophy E71.511
      specified disorder NEC E71.518
      Zellweger syndrome E71.510

Disorder — continued

peroxisomal — continued
rhizomelic chondrodysplasia punctata E71.54Ø
specified form NEC E71.548
group 1 E71.518
group 2 E71.53
group 3 E71.542
X-linked adrenoleukodystrophy E71.529
adolescent E71.521
adrenomyeloneuropathy E71.522
childhood E71.52Ø
specified form NEC E71.528
Zellweger-like syndrome E71.541
persistent
(somatoform) pain F45.41
affective (mood) F34.9
personality (see also Personality) F6Ø.9
affective F34.Ø
aggressive F6Ø.3
amoral F6Ø.2
anankastic F6Ø.5
antisocial F6Ø.2
anxious F6Ø.6
asocial F6Ø.2
asthenic F6Ø.7
avoidant F6Ø.6
borderline F6Ø.3
change (secondary) due to general medical condition F07.0
compulsive F6Ø.5
cyclothymic F34.Ø
dependent (passive) F6Ø.7
depressive F34.1
dissocial F6Ø.2
emotional instability F6Ø.3
expansive paranoid F6Ø.Ø
explosive F6Ø.3
following organic brain damage F07.9
histrionic F6Ø.4
hyperthymic F34.Ø
hypothymic F34.1
hysterical F6Ø.4
immature F6Ø.89
inadequate F6Ø.7
labile F6Ø.3
mixed (nonspecific) F6Ø.89
moral deficiency F6Ø.2
narcissistic F6Ø.81
negativistic F6Ø.89
obsessional F6Ø.5
obsessive (-compulsive) F6Ø.5
organic F07.9
overconscientious F6Ø.5
paranoid F6Ø.Ø
passive (-dependent) F6Ø.7
passive-aggressive F6Ø.89
pathological NEC F6Ø.9
pseudosocial F6Ø.2
psychopathic F6Ø.2
schizoid F6Ø.1
schizotypal F21
self-defeating F6Ø.7
specified NEC F6Ø.89
type A F6Ø.5
unstable (emotional) F6Ø.3
pervasive, developmental F84.9
phencyclidine use
mild F16.1Ø
with
phencyclidine intoxication F16.129
phencyclidine intoxication delirium F16.121
phencyclidine-induced
anxiety disorder F16.18Ø
bipolar and related disorder F16.14
depressive disorder F16.14
psychotic disorder F16.159
in remission (early) (sustained) F16.11
moderate or severe F16.2Ø
with
phencyclidine intoxication F16.229
phencyclidine intoxication delirium F16.221
phencyclidine-induced
anxiety disorder F16.28Ø
bipolar and related disorder F16.14
depressive disorder F16.24
psychotic disorder F16.259
in remission (early) (sustained) F16.21
phobic anxiety, childhood F4Ø.8
phosphate-losing tubular N25.Ø

Disorder — continued

pigmentation L81.9
choroid, congenital Q14.3
diminished melanin formation L81.6
iron L81.8
specified NEC L81.8
pinna (noninfective) H61.1Ø- ☑
deformity, acquired H61.11- ☑
hematoma H61.12- ☑
perichondritis — see Perichondritis, ear
specified type NEC H61.19- ☑
pituitary gland E23.7
iatrogenic (postprocedural) E89.3
specified NEC E23.6
platelets D69.1
plexus G54.9
specified NEC G54.8
polymorphonuclear neutrophils D71
porphyrin metabolism — see Porphyria
postconcussional F07.81
posthallucinogen perception F16.983
in
abuse F16.183
dependence F16.283
postmenopausal N95.9
specified NEC N95.8
postprocedural (postoperative) — see Complications, postprocedural
post-transplant lymphoproliferative D47.Z1 (following D47.4)
post-traumatic stress (PTSD) F43.1Ø
acute F43.11
chronic F43.12
premenstrual dysphoric (PMDD) F32.81
prepuce N47.8
propionic acidemia E71.121
prostate N42.9
specified NEC N42.89
psychogenic NOS (see also condition) F45.9
anxiety F41.8
appetite F5Ø.9
asthenic F48.8
cardiovascular (system) F45.8
compulsive F42.8
cutaneous F54
depressive F32.9
digestive (system) F45.8
dysmenorrheic F45.8
dyspneic F45.8
endocrine (system) F54
eye NEC F45.8
feeding — see Disorder, eating
functional NEC F45.8
gastric F45.8
gastrointestinal (system) F45.8
genitourinary (system) F45.8
heart (function) (rhythm) F45.8
hyperventilatory F45.8
hypochondriacal — see Disorder, hypochondriacal
intestinal F45.8
joint F45.8
learning F81.9
limb F45.8
lymphatic (system) F45.8
menstrual F45.8
micturition F45.8
monoplegic NEC F44.4
motor F44.4
muscle F45.8
musculoskeletal F45.8
neurocirculatory F45.8
obsessive F42.8
occupational F48.8
organ or part of body NEC F45.8
paralytic NEC F44.4
phobic F4Ø.9
physical NEC F45.8
rectal F45.8
respiratory (system) F45.8
rheumatic F45.8
sexual (function) F52.9
skin (allergic) (eczematous) F54
sleep F51.9
specified part of body NEC F45.8
stomach F45.8
psychological F99
associated with
disease classified elsewhere F54

Disorder — continued

psychological — continued
associated with — continued
sexual
development F66
relationship F66
uncertainty about gender identity F64.9
psychomotor NEC F44.4
hysterical F44.4
psychoneurotic (see also Neurosis)
mixed NEC F48.8
psychophysiologic — see Disorder, somatoform
psychosexual F65.9
development F66
identity of childhood F64.2
psychosomatic NOS — see Disorder, somatoform
multiple F45.Ø
undifferentiated F45.1
psychotic — see Psychosis
transient (acute) F23
puberty E3Ø.9
specified NEC E3Ø.8
pulmonary (valve) — see Endocarditis, pulmonary
purine metabolism E79.9
pyrimidine metabolism E79.9
pyruvate metabolism E74.4
reactive attachment (childhood) F94.1
reading R48.Ø
developmental (specific) F81.Ø
receptive language F8Ø.2
receptor, hormonal, peripheral (see also Syndrome, androgen insensitivity) E34.5Ø
recurrent brief depressive F33.8
reflex R29.2
refraction H52.7
aniseikonia H52.32
anisometropia H52.31
astigmatism — see Astigmatism
hypermetropia — see Hypermetropia
myopia — see Myopia
presbyopia H52.4
specified NEC H52.6
relationship F68.8
due to sexual orientation F66
REM sleep behavior G47.52
renal function, impaired (tubular) N25.9
resonance R49.9
specified NEC R49.8
respiratory function, impaired (see also Failure, respiration)
postprocedural — see Complication, postoperative, respiratory system
psychogenic F45.8
retina H35.9
angioid streaks H35.33
changes in vascular appearance H35.Ø1- ☑
degeneration — see Degeneration, retina
dystrophy (hereditary) — see Dystrophy, retina
edema H35.81
hemorrhage — see Hemorrhage, retina
ischemia H35.82
macular degeneration — see Degeneration, macula
microaneurysms H35.Ø4- ☑
microvascular abnormality NEC H35.Ø9
neovascularization — see Neovascularization, retina
retinopathy — see Retinopathy
separation of layers H35.7Ø
central serous chorioretinopathy H35.71- ☑
pigment epithelium detachment (serous) H35.72- ☑
hemorrhagic H35.73- ☑
specified type NEC H35.89
telangiectasis — see Telangiectasis, retina
vasculitis — see Vasculitis, retina
retroperitoneal K68.9
right hemisphere organic affective FØ7.89
rumination (infant or child) F98.21
sacrum, sacrococcygeal NEC M53.3
schizoaffective F25.9
bipolar type F25.Ø
depressive type F25.1
manic type F25.Ø
mixed type F25.Ø
specified NEC F25.8
schizoid of childhood F84.5
schizophrenia spectrum and other psychotic disorder F29
specified NEC F28

☑ **Additional Character Required** — Refer to the Tabular List for Character Selection   ◥ᴺᴱᶜ **Subterms under main terms may continue to next column or page**

Disorder — *continued*
- schizophreniform F20.81
  - brief F23
- schizotypal (personality) F21
- secretion, thyrocalcitonin E07.0
- sedative, hypnotic, or anxiolytic use
  - mild F13.10
    - with
      - sedative, hypnotic, or anxiolytic intoxication F13.129
      - sedative, hypnotic, or anxiolytic intoxication delirium F13.121
      - sedative, hypnotic, or anxiolytic-induced
        - anxiety disorder F13.180
        - bipolar and related disorder F13.14
        - depressive disorder F13.14
        - psychotic disorder F13.159
        - sexual dysfunction F13.181
      - in remission (early) (sustained) F13.11
  - moderate or severe F13.20
    - with
      - sedative, hypnotic, or anxiolytic intoxication F13.229
      - sedative, hypnotic, or anxiolytic intoxication delirium F13.221
      - sedative, hypnotic, or anxiolytic-induced
        - anxiety disorder F13.280
        - bipolar and related disorder F13.24
        - depressive disorder F13.24
        - major neurocognitive disorder F13.27
        - mild neurocognitive disorder F13.288
        - psychotic disorder F13.259
        - sexual dysfunction F13.281
      - in remission (early) (sustained) F13.21
- seizure (*see also* Epilepsy) G40.909
  - intractable G40.919
    - with status epilepticus G40.911
- semantic pragmatic F80.89
  - with autism F84.0
- sense of smell R43.1
  - psychogenic F45.8
- separation anxiety, of childhood F93.0
- sexual
  - aversion F52.1
  - function, psychogenic F52.9
  - interest/arousal, female F52.22
  - masochism F65.51
  - maturation F66
  - nonorganic F52.9
  - preference (*see also* Deviation, sexual) F65.9
    - fetishistic transvestism F65.1
  - relationship F66
  - sadism F65.52
- shyness, of childhood and adolescence F40.10
- sibling rivalry F93.8
- sickle-cell (sickling) (homozygous) — *see* Disease, sickle-cell
  - heterozygous D57.3
  - specified type NEC D57.8- ☑
  - trait D57.3
- sinus (nasal) J34.9
  - specified NEC J34.89
- skin L98.9
  - atrophic L90.9
    - specified NEC L90.8
  - granulomatous L92.9
    - specified NEC L92.8
  - hypertrophic L91.9
    - specified NEC L91.8
  - infiltrative NEC L98.6
  - newborn P83.9
    - specified NEC P83.88
  - picking F42.4
  - psychogenic (allergic) (eczematous) F54
- sleep G47.9
  - breathing-related — *see* Apnea, sleep
  - circadian rhythm G47.20
    - advance sleep phase type G47.22
    - delayed sleep phase type G47.21
    - due to
      - alcohol
        - abuse F10.182
        - dependence F10.282
        - use F10.982
      - amphetamines
        - abuse F15.182
        - dependence F15.282
        - use F15.982

Disorder — *continued*
- sleep — *continued*
  - circadian rhythm — *continued*
    - due to — *continued*
      - caffeine
        - abuse F15.182
        - dependence F15.282
        - use F15.982
      - cocaine
        - abuse F14.182
        - dependence F14.282
        - use F14.982
      - drug NEC
        - abuse F19.182
        - dependence F19.282
        - use F19.982
      - opioid
        - abuse F11.182
        - dependence F11.282
        - use F11.982
      - psychoactive substance NEC
        - abuse F19.182
        - dependence F19.282
        - use F19.982
      - sedative, hypnotic, or anxiolytic
        - abuse F13.182
        - dependence F13.282
        - use F13.982
      - stimulant NEC
        - abuse F15.182
        - dependence F15.282
        - use F15.982
    - free running type G47.24
    - in conditions classified elsewhere G47.27
    - irregular sleep wake type G47.23
    - jet lag type G47.25
    - non-24-hour sleep-wake type G47.24
    - shift work type G47.26
    - specified NEC G47.29
  - due to
    - alcohol
      - abuse F10.182
      - dependence F10.282
      - use F10.982
    - amphetamine
      - abuse F15.182
      - dependence F15.282
      - use F15.982
    - anxiolytic
      - abuse F13.182
      - dependence F13.282
      - use F13.982
    - caffeine
      - abuse F15.182
      - dependence F15.282
      - use F15.982
    - cocaine
      - abuse F14.182
      - dependence F14.282
      - use F14.982
    - drug NEC
      - abuse F19.182
      - dependence F19.282
      - use F19.982
    - hypnotic
      - abuse F13.182
      - dependence F13.282
      - use F13.982
    - opioid
      - abuse F11.182
      - dependence F11.282
      - use F11.982
    - psychoactive substance NEC
      - abuse F19.182
      - dependence F19.282
      - use F19.982
    - sedative
      - abuse F13.182
      - dependence F13.282
      - use F13.982
    - stimulant NEC
      - abuse F15.182
      - dependence F15.282
      - use F15.982
  - emotional F51.9
  - excessive somnolence — *see* Hypersomnia
  - hypersomnia type — *see* Hypersomnia
  - initiating or maintaining — *see* Insomnia
  - nightmares F51.5

Disorder — *continued*
- sleep — *continued*
  - nonorganic F51.9
    - specified NEC F51.8
  - parasomnia type G47.50
    - specified NEC G47.8
  - terrors F51.4
  - walking F51.3
- sleep-wake pattern or schedule (*see also* Disorder, sleep, circadian rhythm) G47.9
  - specified NEC G47.8
- social
  - anxiety (of childhood) F40.10
    - generalized F40.11
  - functioning in childhood F94.9
    - specified NEC F94.8
  - pragmatic F80.82
- soft tissue M79.9
  - ankle M79.9
  - due to use, overuse and pressure M70.90
    - ankle M70.97- ☑
    - bursitis — *see* Bursitis
    - foot M70.97- ☑
    - forearm M70.93- ☑
    - hand M70.94- ☑
    - lower leg M70.96- ☑
    - multiple sites M70.99
    - pelvic region M70.95- ☑
    - shoulder region M70.91- ☑
    - specified site NEC M70.98
    - specified type NEC M70.80
      - ankle M70.87- ☑
      - foot M70.87- ☑
      - forearm M70.83- ☑
      - hand M70.84- ☑
      - lower leg M70.86- ☑
      - multiple sites M70.89
      - pelvic region M70.85- ☑
      - shoulder region M70.81- ☑
      - specified site NEC M70.88
      - thigh M70.85- ☑
      - upper arm M70.82- ☑
    - thigh M70.95- ☑
    - upper arm M70.92- ☑
  - foot M79.9
  - forearm M79.9
  - hand M79.9
  - lower leg M79.9
  - multiple sites M79.9
  - occupational — *see* Disorder, soft tissue, due to use, overuse and pressure
  - pelvic region M79.9
  - shoulder region M79.9
  - specified type NEC M79.89
  - thigh M79.9
  - upper arm M79.9
- somatic symptom F45.1
- somatization F45.0
- somatoform F45.9
  - pain (persistent) F45.41
  - somatization (multiple) (long-lasting) F45.0
  - specified NEC F45.8
  - undifferentiated F45.1
- somnolence, excessive — *see* Hypersomnia
- specific
  - arithmetical F81.2
  - developmental, of motor F82
  - reading F81.0
  - speech and language F80.9
  - spelling F81.81
  - written expression F81.81
- speech R47.9
  - articulation (functional) (specific) F80.0
  - developmental F80.9
  - specified NEC R47.89
- speech-sound F80.0
- spelling (specific) F81.81
- spine (*see also* Dorsopathy)
  - ligamentous or muscular attachments, peripheral — *see* Enthesopathy, spinal
  - specified NEC — *see* Dorsopathy, specified NEC
- stereotyped, habit or movement F98.4
- stimulant use (other) (unspecified)
  - mild F15.10
    - in remission (early) (sustained) F15.11
  - moderate or severe F15.20
    - in remission (early) (sustained) F15.21
- stomach (functional) — *see* Disorder, gastric

Disorder — *continued*
  stress F43.9
    acute F43.0
    post-traumatic F43.10
      acute F43.11
      chronic F43.12
  substance use (other) (unknown)
    mild F19.10
      with substance-induced
        anxiety disorder F19.180
        bipolar and related disorder F19.14
        depressive disorder F19.14
        major neurocognitive disorder F19.17
        mild neurocognitive disorder F19.188
        obsessive-compulsive and related disorder F19.188
        sexual dysfunction F19.181
      substance intoxication F19.129
      substance intoxication delirium F19.121
    moderate or severe F19.20
      with substance-induced
        anxiety disorder F19.280
        bipolar and related disorder F19.24
        depressive disorder F19.24
        major neurocognitive disorder F19.27
        mild neurocognitive disorder F19.288
        obsessive-compulsive and related disorder F19.288
        sexual dysfunction F19.281
      in remission (early) (sustained) F19.21
      substance intoxication F19.229
      substance intoxication delirium F19.221
  sulfur-bearing amino-acid metabolism E72.10
  sweat gland (eccrine) L74.9
    apocrine L75.9
      specified NEC L75.8
    specified NEC L74.8
  synovium M67.90
    acromioclavicular M67.91- ☑
    ankle M67.97- ☑
    elbow M67.92- ☑
    foot M67.97- ☑
    forearm M67.93- ☑
    hand M67.94- ☑
    hip M67.95- ☑
    knee M67.96- ☑
    multiple sites M67.99
    rupture — *see* Rupture, synovium
    shoulder M67.91- ☑
    specified type NEC M67.80
      acromioclavicular M67.81- ☑
      ankle M67.87- ☑
      elbow M67.82- ☑
      foot M67.87- ☑
      hand M67.84- ☑
      hip M67.85- ☑
      knee M67.86- ☑
      multiple sites M67.89
      wrist M67.83- ☑
    synovitis — *see* Synovitis
    upper arm M67.92- ☑
    wrist M67.93- ☑
  temperature regulation, newborn P81.9
    specified NEC P81.8
  temporomandibular joint M26.60- ☑
  tendon M67.90
    acromioclavicular M67.91- ☑
    ankle M67.97- ☑
    contracture — *see* Contracture, tendon
    elbow M67.92- ☑
    foot M67.97- ☑
    forearm M67.93- ☑
    hand M67.94- ☑
    hip M67.95- ☑
    knee M67.96- ☑
    multiple sites M67.99
    rupture — *see* Rupture, tendon
    shoulder M67.91- ☑
    specified type NEC M67.80
      acromioclavicular M67.81- ☑
      ankle M67.87- ☑
      elbow M67.82- ☑
      foot M67.87- ☑
      hand M67.84- ☑
      hip M67.85- ☑
      knee M67.86- ☑
      multiple sites M67.89

Disorder — *continued*
  tendon — *continued*
    specified type — *continued*
      trunk M67.88
      wrist M67.83- ☑
    synovitis — *see* Synovitis
    tendinitis — *see* Tendinitis
    tenosynovitis — *see* Tenosynovitis
    trunk M67.98
    upper arm M67.92- ☑
    wrist M67.93- ☑
  thoracic root (nerve) NEC G54.3
  thyrocalcitonin hypersecretion E07.0
  thyroid (gland) E07.9
    function NEC, neonatal, transitory P72.2
    iodine-deficiency related E01.8
    specified NEC E07.89
  tic — *see* Tic
  tobacco use
    chewing tobacco (mild) (moderate) (severe)
      in remission (early) (sustained) F17.221
    cigarettes (mild) (moderate) (severe)
      in remission (early) (sustained) F17.211
    mild Z72.0
      in remission (early) (sustained) F17.201
    moderate F17.200
      in remission (early) (sustained) F17.201
    severe F17.200
      in remission (early) (sustained) F17.201
    specified product NEC (mild) (moderate) (severe)
      in remission (early) (sustained) F17.291
  tooth K08.9
    development K00.9
      specified NEC K00.8
    eruption K00.6
  Tourette's F95.2
  trance and possession F44.89
  transvestic F65.1
  trauma and stressor-related F43.9
    other specified F43.8
  tricuspid (valve) — *see* Endocarditis, tricuspid
  tryptophan metabolism E70.5
  tubular, phosphate-losing N25.0
  tubulo-interstitial (in)
    brucellosis A23.9 [N16]
    cystinosis E72.04
    diphtheria A36.84
    glycogen storage disease E74.00 [N16]
    leukemia NEC C95.9- ☑ [N16]
    lymphoma NEC C85.9- ☑ [N16]
    mixed cryoglobulinemia D89.1 [N16]
    multiple myeloma C90.0- ☑ [N16]
    Salmonella infection A02.25
    sarcoidosis D86.84
    sepsis A41.9 [N16]
      streptococcal A40.9 [N16]
    systemic lupus erythematosus M32.15
    toxoplasmosis B58.83
    transplant rejection T86.91 [N16]
    Wilson's disease E83.01 [N16]
  tubulo-renal function, impaired N25.9
    specified NEC N25.89
  tympanic membrane H73.9- ☑
    atrophy — *see* Atrophy, tympanic membrane
    infection — *see* Myringitis
    perforation — *see* Perforation, tympanum
    specified NEC H73.89- ☑
  unsocialized aggressive F91.1
  urea cycle metabolism E72.20
    argininemia E72.21
    arginosuccinic aciduria E72.22
    citrullinemia E72.23
    ornithine transcarbamylase deficiency E72.4
    other specified E72.29
  ureter (in) N28.9
    schistosomiasis B65.0 [N29]
    tuberculosis A18.11
  urethra N36.9
    specified NEC N36.8
  urinary system N39.9
    specified NEC N39.8
  valve, heart
    aortic — *see* Endocarditis, aortic
    mitral — *see* Endocarditis, mitral
    pulmonary — *see* Endocarditis, pulmonary
    rheumatic
      aortic — *see* Endocarditis, aortic, rheumatic
      mitral — *see* Endocarditis, mitral

Disorder — *continued*
  valve, heart — *continued*
    rheumatic — *continued*
      pulmonary — *see* Endocarditis, pulmonary, rheumatic
      tricuspid — *see* Endocarditis, tricuspid
    tricuspid — *see* Endocarditis, tricuspid
  vestibular function H81.9- ☑
    specified NEC — *see* subcategory H81.8 ☑
    in diseases classified elsewhere H82.- ☑
    vertigo — *see* Vertigo
  vision, binocular H53.30
    abnormal retinal correspondence H53.31
    diplopia H53.2
    fusion with defective stereopsis H53.32
    simultaneous perception H53.33
    suppression H53.34
  visual
    cortex
      blindness H47.619
        left brain H47.612
        right brain H47.611
      due to
        inflammatory disorder H47.629
          left brain H47.622
          right brain H47.621
        neoplasm H47.639
          left brain H47.632
          right brain H47.631
        vascular disorder H47.649
          left brain H47.642
          right brain H47.641
    pathway H47.9
      due to
        inflammatory disorder H47.51- ☑
        neoplasm H47.52- ☑
        vascular disorder H47.53- ☑
    optic chiasm — *see* Disorder, optic, chiasm
  vitreous body H43.9
    crystalline deposits — *see* Deposit, crystalline
    degeneration — *see* Degeneration, vitreous
    hemorrhage — *see* Hemorrhage, vitreous
    opacities — *see* Opacity, vitreous
    prolapse — *see* Prolapse, vitreous
    specified type NEC H43.89
  voice R49.9
    specified type NEC R49.8
  volatile solvent use
    due to drug abuse — *see* Abuse, drug, inhalant
    due to drug dependence — *see* Dependence, drug, inhalant
  voyeuristic F65.3
  white blood cells D72.9
    specified NEC D72.89
  withdrawing, child or adolescent F40.10
Disorientation R41.0
Displacement, displaced
  acquired traumatic of bone, cartilage, joint, tendon NEC — *see* Dislocation
  adrenal gland (congenital) Q89.1
  appendix, retrocecal (congenital) Q43.8
  auricle (congenital) Q17.4
  bladder (acquired) N32.89
    congenital Q64.19
  brachial plexus (congenital) Q07.8
  brain stem, caudal (congenital) Q04.8
  canaliculus (lacrimalis), congenital Q10.6
  cardia through esophageal hiatus (congenital) Q40.1
  cerebellum, caudal (congenital) Q04.8
  cervix — *see* Malposition, uterus
  colon (congenital) Q43.3
  device, implant or graft (*see also* Complications, by site and type, mechanical) T85.628 ☑
    arterial graft NEC — *see* Complication, cardiovascular device, mechanical, vascular
    breast (implant) T85.42 ☑
    catheter NEC T85.628 ☑
      dialysis (renal) T82.42 ☑
        intraperitoneal T85.621 ☑
      infusion NEC T82.524 ☑
        spinal (epidural) (subdural) T85.620 ☑
      urinary
        cystostomy T83.020 ☑
        Hopkins T83.028 ☑
        ileostomy T83.028 ☑
        indwelling T83.021 ☑
        nephrostomy T83.022 ☑

Displacement, displaced — *continued*
  device, implant or graft (*see also* Complications, by site and type, mechanical) — *continued*
    catheter — *continued*
      urinary — *continued*
        specified NEC T83.028 ☑
        urostomy T83.028 ☑
    electronic (electrode) (pulse generator) (stimulator) — *see* Complication, electronic stimulator
    fixation, internal (orthopedic) NEC — *see* Complication, fixation device, mechanical
    gastrointestinal — *see* Complications, prosthetic device, mechanical, gastrointestinal device
    genital NEC T83.428 ☑
      intrauterine contraceptive device (string) T83.32 ☑
      penile prosthesis (cylinder) (implanted) (pump) (reservoir) T83.420 ☑
      testicular prosthesis T83.421 ☑
    heart NEC — *see* Complication, cardiovascular device, mechanical
    joint prosthesis — *see* Complications, joint prosthesis, mechanical
    ocular — *see* Complications, prosthetic device, mechanical, ocular device
    orthopedic NEC — *see* Complication, orthopedic, device or graft, mechanical
    specified NEC T85.628 ☑
    urinary NEC T83.128 ☑
      graft T83.22 ☑
      sphincter, implanted T83.121 ☑
      stent (ileal conduit) (nephroureteral) T83.123 ☑
        ureteral indwelling T83.122 ☑
    vascular NEC — *see* Complication, cardiovascular device, mechanical
    ventricular intracranial shunt T85.02 ☑
  electronic stimulator
    bone T84.320 ☑
    cardiac — *see* Complications, cardiac device, electronic
    nervous system — *see* Complication, prosthetic device, mechanical, electronic nervous system stimulator
    urinary — *see* Complications, electronic stimulator, urinary
  esophageal mucosa into cardia of stomach, congenital Q39.8
  esophagus (acquired) K22.8
    congenital Q39.8
  eyeball (acquired) (lateral) (old) — *see* Displacement, globe
    congenital Q15.8
    current — *see* Avulsion, eye
  fallopian tube (acquired) N83.4- ☑
    congenital Q50.6
    opening (congenital) Q50.6
  gallbladder (congenital) Q44.1
  gastric mucosa (congenital) Q40.2
  globe (acquired) (old) (lateral) H05.21- ☑
    current — *see* Avulsion, eye
  heart (congenital) Q24.8
    acquired I51.89
  hymen (upward) (congenital) Q52.4
  intervertebral disc NEC
    with myelopathy — *see* Disorder, disc, with, myelopathy
    cervical, cervicothoracic (with) M50.20
      myelopathy — *see* Disorder, disc, cervical, with myelopathy
      neuritis, radiculitis or radiculopathy — *see* Disorder, disc, cervical, with neuritis
    due to trauma — *see* Dislocation, vertebra
    lumbar region M51.26
      with
        myelopathy M51.06
        neuritis, radiculitis, radiculopathy or sciatica M51.16
    lumbosacral region M51.27
      with
        neuritis, radiculitis, radiculopathy or sciatica M51.17
    sacrococcygeal region M53.3
    thoracic region M51.24
      with
        myelopathy M51.04
        neuritis, radiculitis, radiculopathy M51.14
    thoracolumbar region M51.25

Displacement, displaced — *continued*
  intervertebral disc — *continued*
    thoracolumbar region — *continued*
      with
        myelopathy M51.05
        neuritis, radiculitis, radiculopathy M51.15
  intrauterine device (string) T83.32 ☑
  kidney (acquired) N28.83
    congenital Q63.2
  lachrymal, lacrimal apparatus or duct (congenital) Q10.6
  lens, congenital Q12.1
  macula (congenital) Q14.1
  Meckel's diverticulum Q43.0
    malignant — *see* Table of Neoplasms, small intestine, malignant
  nail (congenital) Q84.6
    acquired L60.8
  opening of Wharton's duct in mouth Q38.4
  organ or site, congenital NEC — *see* Malposition, congenital
  ovary (acquired) N83.4- ☑
    congenital Q50.39
    free in peritoneal cavity (congenital) Q50.39
    into hernial sac N83.4- ☑
  oviduct (acquired) N83.4- ☑
    congenital Q50.6
  parathyroid (gland) E21.4
  parotid gland (congenital) Q38.4
  punctum lacrimale (congenital) Q10.6
  sacro-iliac (joint) (congenital) Q74.2
    current injury S33.2 ☑
    old — *see* subcategory M53.2 ☑
  salivary gland (any) (congenital) Q38.4
  spleen (congenital) Q89.09
  stomach, congenital Q40.2
  sublingual duct Q38.4
  tongue (downward) (congenital) Q38.3
  tooth, teeth, fully erupted M26.30
    horizontal M26.33
    vertical M26.34
  trachea (congenital) Q32.1
  ureter or ureteric opening or orifice (congenital) Q62.62
  uterine opening of oviducts or fallopian tubes Q50.6
  uterus, uterine — *see* Malposition, uterus
  ventricular septum Q21.0
    with rudimentary ventricle Q20.4

Disproportion
  between native and reconstructed breast N65.1
  fiber-type G71.2

Disruptio uteri — *see* Rupture, uterus
Disruption (of)
  ciliary body NEC H21.89
  closure of
    cornea T81.31 ☑
    craniotomy T81.32 ☑
    fascia (muscular) (superficial) T81.32 ☑
    internal organ or tissue T81.32 ☑
    laceration (external) (internal) T81.33 ☑
    ligament T81.32 ☑
    mucosa T81.31 ☑
    muscle or muscle flap T81.32 ☑
    ribs or rib cage T81.32 ☑
    skin and subcutaneous tissue (full-thickness) (superficial) T81.31 ☑
    skull T81.32 ☑
    sternum (sternotomy) T81.32 ☑
    tendon T81.32 ☑
    traumatic laceration (external) (internal) T81.33 ☑
  family Z63.8
    due to
      absence of family member due to military deployment Z63.31
      absence of family member NEC Z63.32
      alcoholism and drug addiction in family Z63.72
      bereavement Z63.4
      death (assumed) or disappearance of family member Z63.4
      divorce or separation Z63.5
      drug addiction in family Z63.72
      return of family member from military deployment (current or past conflict) Z63.71
      stressful life events NEC Z63.79
  iris NEC H21.89
  ligament(s) (*see also* Sprain)
    knee
      current injury — *see* Dislocation, knee
      old (chronic) — *see* Derangement, knee, instability

Disruption — *continued*
  ligament(s) (*see also* Sprain) — *continued*
    knee — *continued*
      spontaneous NEC — *see* Derangement, knee, disruption ligament
    ossicular chain — *see* Discontinuity, ossicles, ear
    pelvic ring (stable) S32.810 ☑
      unstable S32.811 ☑
    traumatic injury wound repair T81.33 ☑
  wound T81.30 ☑
    episiotomy O90.1
    operation T81.31 ☑
      cesarean O90.0
      external operation wound (superficial) T81.31 ☑
      internal operation wound (deep) T81.32 ☑
    perineal (obstetric) O90.1
    traumatic injury repair T81.33 ☑

Dissatisfaction with
  employment Z56.9
  school environment Z55.4
Dissecting — *see* condition
Dissection
  aorta I71.00
    abdominal I71.02
    thoracic I71.01
    thoracoabdominal I71.03
  artery I77.70
    basilar (trunk) I77.75
    carotid I77.71
    cerebral (nonruptured) I67.0
      ruptured — *see* Hemorrhage, intracranial, subarachnoid
    coronary I25.42
    extremity
      lower I77.77
      upper I77.76
    iliac I77.72
    precerebral
      congenital (nonruptured) Q28.1
      specified site NEC I77.75
    renal I77.73
    specified NEC I77.79
    vertebral I77.74
  precerebral artery, congenital (nonruptured) Q28.1
  Heartland A93.8
  traumatic — *see* Wound, open, by site
  vascular I99.8
  wound — *see* Wound, open
Disseminated — *see* condition
Dissociation
  auriculoventricular or atrioventricular (AV) (any degree) (isorhythmic) I45.89
    with heart block I44.2
  interference I45.89
Dissociative reaction, state F44.9
Dissolution, vertebra — *see* Osteoporosis
Distension, distention
  abdomen R14.0
  bladder N32.89
  cecum K63.89
  colon K63.89
  gallbladder K82.8
  intestine K63.89
  kidney N28.89
  liver K76.89
  seminal vesicle N50.89
  stomach K31.89
    acute K31.0
    psychogenic F45.8
  ureter — *see* Dilatation, ureter
  uterus N85.8
Distoma hepaticum infestation B66.3
Distomiasis B66.9
  bile passages B66.3
  hemic B65.9
  hepatic B66.3
    due to Clonorchis sinensis B66.1
  intestinal B66.5
  liver B66.3
    due to Clonorchis sinensis B66.1
  lung B66.4
  pulmonary B66.4
Distomolar (fourth molar) K00.1
Disto-occlusion (Division I) (Division II) M26.212
Distortion(s) (congenital)
  adrenal (gland) Q89.1
  arm NEC Q68.8
  bile duct or passage Q44.5

Distortion(s) — *continued*
  bladder Q64.79
  brain Q04.9
  cervix (uteri) Q51.9
  chest (wall) Q67.8
    bones Q76.8
  clavicle Q74.0
  clitoris Q52.6
  coccyx Q76.49
  common duct Q44.5
  coronary Q24.5
  cystic duct Q44.5
  ear (auricle) (external) Q17.3
    inner Q16.5
    middle Q16.4
      ossicles Q16.3
  endocrine NEC Q89.2
  eustachian tube Q17.8
  eye (adnexa) Q15.8
  face bone(s) NEC Q75.8
  fallopian tube Q50.6
  femur NEC Q68.8
  fibula NEC Q68.8
  finger(s) Q68.1
  foot Q66.9
  genitalia, genital organ(s)
    female Q52.8
      external Q52.79
      internal NEC Q52.8
  gyri Q04.8
  hand bone(s) Q68.1
  heart (auricle) (ventricle) Q24.8
    valve (cusp) Q24.8
  hepatic duct Q44.5
  humerus NEC Q68.8
  hymen Q52.4
  intrafamilial communications Z63.8
  jaw NEC M26.89
  labium (majus) (minus) Q52.79
  leg NEC Q68.8
  lens Q12.8
  liver Q44.7
  lumbar spine Q76.49
    with disproportion O33.8
      causing obstructed labor O65.0
  lumbosacral (joint) (region) Q76.49
    kyphosis — *see* Kyphosis, congenital
    lordosis — *see* Lordosis, congenital
  nerve Q07.8
  nose Q30.8
  organ
    of Corti Q16.5
    or site not listed — *see* Anomaly, by site
  ossicles, ear Q16.3
  oviduct Q50.6
  pancreas Q45.3
  parathyroid (gland) Q89.2
  pituitary (gland) Q89.2
  radius NEC Q68.8
  sacroiliac joint Q74.2
  sacrum Q76.49
  scapula Q74.0
  shoulder girdle Q74.0
  skull bone(s) NEC Q75.8
    with
      anencephalus Q00.0
      encephalocele — *see* Encephalocele
      hydrocephalus Q03.9
        with spina bifida — *see* Spina bifida, with hydrocephalus
      microcephaly Q02
  spinal cord Q06.8
  spine Q76.49
    kyphosis — *see* Kyphosis, congenital
    lordosis — *see* Lordosis, congenital
  spleen Q89.09
  sternum NEC Q76.7
  thorax (wall) Q67.8
    bony Q76.8
  thymus (gland) Q89.2
  thyroid (gland) Q89.2
  tibia NEC Q68.8
  toe(s) Q66.9
  tongue Q38.3
  trachea (cartilage) Q32.1
  ulna NEC Q68.8
  ureter Q62.8
  urethra Q64.79

Distortion(s) — *continued*
  urethra — *continued*
    causing obstruction Q64.39
  uterus Q51.9
  vagina Q52.4
  vertebra Q76.49
    kyphosis — *see* Kyphosis, congenital
    lordosis — *see* Lordosis, congenital
  visual (*see also* Disturbance, vision)
    shape and size H53.15
  vulva Q52.79
  wrist (bones) (joint) Q68.8
Distress
  abdomen — *see* Pain, abdominal
  acute respiratory R06.03
    syndrome (adult) (child) J80
  epigastric R10.13
  fetal P84
    complicating pregnancy — *see* Stress, fetal
  gastrointestinal (functional) K30
    psychogenic F45.8
  intestinal (functional) NOS K59.9
    psychogenic F45.8
  maternal, during labor and delivery O75.0
  relationship, with spouse or intimate partner Z63.0
  respiratory (adult) (child) R06.03
    newborn P22.9
      specified NEC P22.8
    orthopnea R06.01
    psychogenic F45.8
    shortness of breath R06.02
    specified type NEC R06.09
Distribution vessel, atypical Q27.9
  coronary artery Q24.5
  precerebral Q28.1
Distichiasis L68.8
Disturbance(s) (*see also* Disease)
  absorption K90.9
    calcium E58
    carbohydrate K90.49
    fat K90.49
      pancreatic K90.3
    protein K90.49
    starch K90.49
    vitamin — *see* Deficiency, vitamin
  acid-base equilibrium E87.8
    mixed E87.4
  activity and attention (with hyperkinesis) — *see* Disorder, attention-deficit hyperactivity
  amino acid transport E72.00
  assimilation, food K90.9
  auditory nerve, except deafness — *see* subcategory H93.3 ☑
  behavior — *see* Disorder, conduct
  blood clotting (mechanism) (*see also* Defect, coagulation) D68.9
  cerebral
    nerve — *see* Disorder, nerve, cranial
    status, newborn P91.9
      specified NEC P91.88
  circulatory I99.9
  conduct (*see also* Disorder, conduct) F91.9
    adjustment reaction — *see* Disorder, adjustment
    compulsive F63.9
    disruptive F91.9
    hyperkinetic — *see* Disorder, attention-deficit hyperactivity
    socialized F91.2
    specified NEC F91.8
    unsocialized F91.1
  coordination R27.8
  cranial nerve — *see* Disorder, nerve, cranial
  deep sensibility — *see* Disturbance, sensation
  digestive K30
    psychogenic F45.8
  electrolyte (*see also* Imbalance, electrolyte)
    newborn, transitory P74.49
      hyperammonemia P74.6
      hyperchloremia P74.421
      hyperchloremic metabolic acidosis P74.421
      hypochloremia P74.422
      potassium balance
        hyperkalemia P74.31
        hypokalemia P74.32
      sodium balance
        hypernatremia P74.21
        hyponatremia P74.22
      specified type NEC P74.49

Disturbance(s) — *continued*
  emotions specific to childhood and adolescence F93.9
    with
      anxiety and fearfulness NEC F93.8
      elective mutism F94.0
      oppositional disorder F91.3
      sensitivity (withdrawal) F40.10
      shyness F40.10
      social withdrawal F40.10
    involving relationship problems F93.8
    mixed F93.8
    specified NEC F93.8
  endocrine (gland) E34.9
    neonatal, transitory P72.9
      specified NEC P72.8
  equilibrium R42
  fructose metabolism E74.10
  gait — *see* Gait
    hysterical F44.4
    psychogenic F44.4
  gastrointestinal (functional) K30
    psychogenic F45.8
  habit, child F98.9
  hearing, except deafness and tinnitus — *see* Abnormal, auditory perception
  heart, functional (conditions in I44-I50)
    due to presence of (cardiac) prosthesis I97.19- ☑
    postoperative I97.89
      cardiac surgery (*see also* Infarct, myocardium, associated with revascularization procedure) I97.19- ☑
  hormones E34.9
  innervation uterus (parasympathetic) (sympathetic) N85.8
  keratinization NEC
    gingiva K05.10
      nonplaque induced K05.11
      plaque induced K05.10
    lip K13.0
    oral (mucosa) (soft tissue) K13.29
    tongue K13.29
  learning (specific) — *see* Disorder, learning
  memory — *see* Amnesia
    mild, following organic brain damage F06.8
  mental F99
    associated with diseases classified elsewhere F54
  metabolism E88.9
    with
      abortion — *see* Abortion, by type with other specified complication
      ectopic pregnancy O08.5
      molar pregnancy O08.5
    amino-acid E72.9
      aromatic E70.9
      branched-chain E71.2
      straight-chain E72.89
      sulfur-bearing E72.10
    ammonia E72.20
    arginine E72.21
    arginosuccinic acid E72.22
    carbohydrate E74.9
    cholesterol E78.9
    citrulline E72.23
    cystathionine E72.19
    general E88.9
    glutamine E72.89
    histidine E70.40
    homocystine E72.19
    hydroxylysine E72.3
    in labor or delivery O75.89
    iron E83.10
    lipoid E78.9
    lysine E72.3
    methionine E72.19
    neonatal, transitory P74.9
      calcium and magnesium P71.9
        specified type NEC P71.8
      carbohydrate metabolism P70.9
        specified type NEC P70.8
      specified NEC P74.8
    ornithine E72.4
    phosphate E83.39
    sodium NEC E87.8
    threonine E72.89
    tryptophan E70.5
    tyrosine E70.20
    urea cycle E72.20
  motor R29.2

☑ **Additional Character Required** — Refer to the Tabular List for Character Selection   ▽ **Subterms under main terms may continue to next column or page**

Disturbance(s) — continued
  nervous, functional R45.0
  neuromuscular mechanism (eye), due to syphilis A52.15
  nutritional E63.9
    nail L60.3
  ocular motion H51.9
    psychogenic F45.8
  oculogyric H51.8
    psychogenic F45.8
  oculomotor H51.9
    psychogenic F45.8
  olfactory nerve R43.1
  optic nerve NEC — see Disorder, nerve, optic
  oral epithelium, including tongue NEC K13.29
  perceptual due to
    alcohol withdrawal F10.232
    amphetamine intoxication F15.922
      in
        abuse F15.122
        dependence F15.222
    anxiolytic withdrawal F13.232
    cannabis intoxication (acute) F12.922
      in
        abuse F12.122
        dependence F12.222
    cocaine intoxication (acute) F14.922
      in
        abuse F14.122
        dependence F14.222
    hypnotic withdrawal F13.232
    opioid intoxication (acute) F11.922
      in
        abuse F11.122
        dependence F11.222
    phencyclidine intoxication (acute) F16.122
    sedative withdrawal F13.232
  personality (pattern) (trait) (see also Disorder, personality) F60.9
    following organic brain damage F07.9
  polyglandular E31.9
    specified NEC E31.8
  potassium balance, newborn
    hyperkalemia P74.31
    hypokalemia P74.32
  psychogenic F45.9
  psychomotor F44.4
  psychophysical visual H53.16
  pupillary — see Anomaly, pupil, function
  reflex R29.2
  rhythm, heart I49.9
  salivary secretion K11.7
  sensation (cold) (heat) (localization) (tactile discrimination) (texture) (vibratory) NEC R20.9
    hysterical F44.6
    skin R20.9
      anesthesia R20.0
      hyperesthesia R20.3
      hypoesthesia R20.1
      paresthesia R20.2
      specified type NEC R20.8
    smell R43.9
      and taste (mixed) R43.8
      anosmia R43.0
      parosmia R43.1
      specified NEC R43.8
    taste R43.9
      and smell (mixed) R43.8
      parageusia R43.2
      specified NEC R43.8
  sensory — see Disturbance, sensation
  situational (transient) (see also Disorder, adjustment)
    acute F43.0
  sleep G47.9
    nonorganic origin F51.9
  smell — see Disturbance, sensation, smell
  sociopathic F60.2
  sodium balance, newborn
    hypernatremia P74.21
    hyponatremia P74.22
  speech R47.9
    developmental F80.9
    specified NEC R47.89
  stomach (functional) K31.9
  sympathetic (nerve) G90.9
  taste — see Disturbance, sensation, taste
  temperature
    regulation, newborn P81.9
      specified NEC P81.8
    sense R20.8

Disturbance(s) — continued
  temperature — continued
    sense — continued
      hysterical F44.6
  tooth
    eruption K00.6
    formation K00.4
    structure, hereditary NEC K00.5
  touch — see Disturbance, sensation
  vascular I99.9
    arteriosclerotic — see Arteriosclerosis
  vasomotor I73.9
  vasospastic I73.9
  vision, visual H53.9
    following
      cerebral infarction I69.398
      cerebrovascular disease I69.998
        specified NEC I69.898
      intracerebral hemorrhage I69.198
      nontraumatic intracranial hemorrhage NEC I69.298
      specified disease NEC I69.898
      subarachnoid hemorrhage I69.098
    psychophysical H53.16
    specified NEC H53.8
    subjective H53.10
      day blindness H53.11
      discomfort H53.14- ☑
      distortions of shape and size H53.15
      loss
        sudden H53.13- ☑
        transient H53.12- ☑
      specified type NEC H53.19
  voice R49.9
    psychogenic F44.4
    specified NEC R49.8
Diuresis R35.8
Diver's palsy, paralysis or squeeze T70.3 ☑
Diverticulitis (acute) K57.92
  bladder — see Cystitis
  ileum — see Diverticulitis, intestine, small
  intestine K57.92
    with
      abscess, perforation or peritonitis K57.80
        with bleeding K57.81
      bleeding K57.93
    congenital Q43.8
    large K57.32
      with
        abscess, perforation or peritonitis K57.20
          with bleeding K57.21
        bleeding K57.33
        small intestine K57.52
          with
            abscess, perforation or peritonitis K57.40
              with bleeding K57.41
            bleeding K57.53
    small K57.12
      with
        abscess, perforation or peritonitis K57.00
          with bleeding K57.01
        bleeding K57.13
        large intestine K57.52
          with
            abscess, perforation or peritonitis K57.40
              with bleeding K57.41
            bleeding K57.53
Diverticulosis K57.90
  with bleeding K57.91
  large intestine K57.30
    with
      bleeding K57.31
      small intestine K57.50
        with bleeding K57.51
  small intestine K57.10
    with
      bleeding K57.11
      large intestine K57.50
        with bleeding K57.51
Diverticulum, diverticula (multiple) K57.90
  appendix (noninflammatory) K38.2
  bladder (sphincter) N32.3
    congenital Q64.6
  bronchus (congenital) Q32.4
    acquired J98.09
  calyx, calyceal (kidney) N28.89

Diverticulum, diverticula — continued
  cardia (stomach) K31.4
  cecum — see Diverticulosis, intestine, large
    congenital Q43.8
  colon — see Diverticulosis, intestine, large
    congenital Q43.8
  duodenum — see Diverticulosis, intestine, small
    congenital Q43.8
  epiphrenic (esophagus) K22.5
  esophagus (congenital) Q39.6
    acquired (epiphrenic) (pulsion) (traction) K22.5
  eustachian tube — see Disorder, eustachian tube, specified NEC
  fallopian tube N83.8
  gastric K31.4
  heart (congenital) Q24.8
  ileum — see Diverticulosis, intestine, small
  jejunum — see Diverticulosis, intestine, small
  kidney (pelvis) (calyces) N28.89
    with calculus — see Calculus, kidney
  Meckel's (displaced) (hypertrophic) Q43.0
    malignant — see Table of Neoplasms, small intestine, malignant
  midthoracic K22.5
  organ or site, congenital NEC — see Distortion
  pericardium (congenital) (cyst) Q24.8
    acquired I31.8
  pharyngoesophageal (congenital) Q39.6
    acquired K22.5
  pharynx (congenital) Q38.7
  rectosigmoid — see Diverticulosis, intestine, large
    congenital Q43.8
  rectum — see Diverticulosis, intestine, large
  Rokitansky's K22.5
  seminal vesicle N50.89
  sigmoid — see Diverticulosis, intestine, large
    congenital Q43.8
  stomach (acquired) K31.4
    congenital Q40.2
  trachea (acquired) J39.8
  ureter (acquired) N28.89
    congenital Q62.8
  ureterovesical orifice N28.89
  urethra (acquired) N36.1
    congenital Q64.79
  ventricle, left (congenital) Q24.8
  vesical N32.3
    congenital Q64.6
  Zenker's (esophagus) K22.5
Division
  cervix uteri (acquired) N88.8
  glans penis Q55.69
  labia minora (congenital) Q52.79
  ligament (partial or complete) (current) (see also Sprain)
    with open wound — see Wound, open
  muscle (partial or complete) (current) (see also Injury, muscle)
    with open wound — see Wound, open
  nerve (traumatic) — see Injury, nerve
  spinal cord — see Injury, spinal cord, by region
  vein I87.8
Divorce, causing family disruption Z63.5
Dix-Hallpike neurolabyrinthitis — see Neuronitis, vestibular
Dizziness R42
  hysterical F44.89
  psychogenic F45.8
DMAC (disseminated mycobacterium avium- intracellulare complex) A31.2
DNR (do not resuscitate) Z66
Doan-Wiseman syndrome (primary splenic neutropenia) — see Agranulocytosis
Doehle-Heller aortitis A52.02
Dog bite — see Bite
Dohle body panmyelopathic syndrome D72.0
Dolichocephaly Q67.2
Dolichocolon Q43.8
Dolichostenomelia — see Syndrome, Marfan's
Donohue's syndrome E34.8
Donor (organ or tissue) Z52.9
  blood (whole) Z52.000
    autologous Z52.010
    specified component (lymphocytes) (platelets) NEC Z52.008
      autologous Z52.018
      specified donor NEC Z52.098
    specified donor NEC Z52.090
  stem cells Z52.001

Donor — *continued*
  blood — *continued*
    stem cells — *continued*
      autologous Z52.011
      specified donor NEC Z52.091
  bone Z52.20
    autologous Z52.21
    marrow Z52.3
    specified type NEC Z52.29
  cornea Z52.5
  egg (Oocyte) Z52.819
    age 35 and over Z52.812
      anonymous recipient Z52.812
      designated recipient Z52.813
    under age 35 Z52.810
      anonymous recipient Z52.810
      designated recipient Z52.811
  kidney Z52.4
  liver Z52.6
  lung Z52.89
  lymphocyte — *see* Donor, blood, specified components NEC
  Oocyte — *see* Donor, egg
  platelets Z52.008
  potential, examination of Z00.5
  semen Z52.89
  skin Z52.10
    autologous Z52.11
    specified type NEC Z52.19
  specified organ or tissue NEC Z52.89
  sperm Z52.89
Donovanosis A58
Dorsalgia M54.9
  psychogenic F45.41
  specified NEC M54.89
Dorsopathy M53.9
  deforming M43.9
    specified NEC — *see* subcategory M43.8 ☑
  specified NEC M53.80
    cervical region M53.82
    cervicothoracic region M53.83
    lumbar region M53.86
    lumbosacral region M53.87
    occipito-atlanto-axial region M53.81
    sacrococcygeal region M53.88
    thoracic region M53.84
    thoracolumbar region M53.85
Double
  albumin E88.09
  aortic arch Q25.45
  auditory canal Q17.8
  auricle (heart) Q20.8
  bladder Q64.79
  cervix Q51.820
    with doubling of uterus (and vagina) Q51.10
      with obstruction Q51.11
  inlet ventricle Q20.4
  kidney with double pelvis (renal) Q63.0
  meatus urinarius Q64.75
  monster Q89.4
  outlet
    left ventricle Q20.2
    right ventricle Q20.1
  pelvis (renal) with double ureter Q62.5
  tongue Q38.3
  ureter (one or both sides) Q62.5
    with double pelvis (renal) Q62.5
  urethra Q64.74
  urinary meatus Q64.75
  uterus Q51.20
    with
      doubling of cervix (and vagina) Q51.10
        with obstruction Q51.11
    complete Q51.21
    in pregnancy or childbirth O34.59- ☑
      causing obstructed labor O65.5
    partial Q51.22
    specified NEC Q51.28
  vagina Q52.10
    with doubling of uterus (and cervix) Q51.10
      with obstruction Q51.11
  vision H53.2
  vulva Q52.79
Douglas' pouch, cul-de-sac — *see* condition
Down syndrome Q90.9
  meiotic nondisjunction Q90.0
  mitotic nondisjunction Q90.1
  mosaicism Q90.1

Down syndrome — *continued*
  translocation Q90.2
DPD (dihydropyrimidine dehydrogenase deficiency) E88.89
Dracontiasis B72
Dracunculiasis, dracunculosis B72
Dream state, hysterical F44.89
Drepanocytic anemia — *see* Disease, sickle-cell
Dresbach's syndrome (elliptocytosis) D58.1
Dreschlera (hawaiiensis) (infection) B43.8
Dressler's syndrome I24.1
Drift, ulnar — *see* Deformity, limb, specified type NEC, forearm
Drinking (alcohol)
  excessive, to excess NEC (without dependence) F10.10
    habitual (continual) (without remission) F10.20
      with remission F10.21
Drip, postnasal (chronic) R09.82
  due to
    allergic rhinitis — *see* Rhinitis, allergic
    common cold J00
    gastroesophageal reflux — *see* Reflux, gastroesophageal
    nasopharyngitis — *see* Nasopharyngitis
    other known condition — *code to* condition
    sinusitis — *see* Sinusitis
Droop
  facial R29.810
    cerebrovascular disease I69.992
      cerebral infarction I69.392
      intracerebral hemorrhage I69.192
      nontraumatic intracranial hemorrhage NEC I69.292
      specified disease NEC I69.892
      subarachnoid hemorrhage I69.092
Drop (in)
  attack NEC R55
  finger — *see* Deformity, finger
  foot — *see* Deformity, limb, foot, drop
  hematocrit (precipitous) R71.0
  hemoglobin R71.0
  toe — *see* Deformity, toe, specified NEC
  wrist — *see* Deformity, limb, wrist drop
Dropped heart beats I45.9
Dropsy, dropsical (*see also* Hydrops)
  abdomen R18.8
  brain — *see* Hydrocephalus
  cardiac, heart — *see* Failure, heart, congestive
  gangrenous — *see* Gangrene
  heart — *see* Failure, heart, congestive
  kidney — *see* Nephrosis
  lung — *see* Edema, lung
  newborn due to isoimmunization P56.0
  pericardium — *see* Pericarditis
Drowned, drowning (near) T75.1 ☑
Drowsiness R40.0
Drug
  abuse counseling and surveillance Z71.51
  addiction — *see* Dependence
  dependence — *see* Dependence
  habit — *see* Dependence
  harmful use — *see* Abuse, drug
  induced fever R50.2
  overdose — *see* Table of Drugs and Chemicals, by drug, poisoning
  poisoning — *see* Table of Drugs and Chemicals, by drug, poisoning
  resistant organism infection (*see also* Resistant, organism, to, drug) Z16.30
  therapy
    long term (current) (prophylactic) — *see* Therapy, drug long-term (current) (prophylactic)
    short term — *omit code*
  wrong substance given or taken in error — *see* Table of Drugs and Chemicals, by drug, poisoning
Drunkenness (without dependence) F10.129
  acute in alcoholism F10.229
  chronic (without remission) F10.20
    with remission F10.21
  pathological (without dependence) F10.129
    with dependence F10.229
  sleep F51.9
Drusen
  macula (degenerative) (retina) — *see* Degeneration, macula, drusen
  optic disc H47.32- ☑
Dry, dryness (*see also* condition)

Dry, dryness — *continued*
  larynx J38.7
  mouth R68.2
    due to dehydration E86.0
  nose J34.89
  socket (teeth) M27.3
  throat J39.2
DSAP L56.5
Duane's syndrome H50.81- ☑
Dubin-Johnson disease or syndrome E80.6
Dubois' disease (thymus gland) A50.59 [E35]
Dubowitz' syndrome Q87.1
Duchenne-Aran muscular atrophy G12.21
Duchenne-Griesinger disease G71.01
Duchenne's
  disease or syndrome
    motor neuron disease G12.22
    muscular dystrophy G71.01
  locomotor ataxia (syphilitic) A52.11
  paralysis
    birth injury P14.0
    due to or associated with
      motor neuron disease G12.22
      muscular dystrophy G71.01
Ducrey's chancre A57
Duct, ductus — *see* condition
Duhring's disease (dermatitis herpetiformis) L13.0
Dullness, cardiac (decreased) (increased) R01.2
Dumb ague — *see* Malaria
Dumbness — *see* Aphasia
Dumdum fever B55.0
Dumping syndrome (postgastrectomy) K91.1
Duodenitis (nonspecific) (peptic) K29.80
  with bleeding K29.81
Duodenocholangitis — *see* Cholangitis
Duodenum, duodenal — *see* condition
Duplay's bursitis or periarthritis — *see* Tendinitis, calcific, shoulder
Duplication, duplex (*see also* Accessory)
  alimentary tract Q45.8
  anus Q43.4
  appendix (and cecum) Q43.4
  biliary duct (any) Q44.5
  bladder Q64.79
  cecum (and appendix) Q43.4
  cervix Q51.820
  chromosome NEC
    with complex rearrangements NEC Q92.5
    seen only at prometaphase Q92.8
  cystic duct Q44.5
  digestive organs Q45.8
  esophagus Q39.8
  frontonasal process Q75.8
  intestine (large) (small) Q43.4
  kidney Q63.0
  liver Q44.7
  pancreas Q45.3
  penis Q55.69
  respiratory organs NEC Q34.8
  salivary duct Q38.4
  spinal cord (incomplete) Q06.2
  stomach Q40.2
Dupré's disease (meningism) R29.1
Dupuytren's contraction or disease M72.0
Durand-Nicolas-Favre disease A55
Durotomy (inadvertent) (incidental) G97.41
Duroziez's disease (congenital mitral stenosis) Q23.2
Dutton's relapsing fever (West African) A68.1
Dwarfism E34.3
  achondroplastic Q77.4
  congenital E34.3
  constitutional E34.3
  hypochondroplastic Q77.4
  hypophyseal E23.0
  infantile E34.3
  Laron-type E34.3
  Lorain (-Levi) type E23.0
  metatropic Q77.8
  nephrotic-glycosuric (with hypophosphatemic rickets) E72.09
  nutritional E45
  pancreatic K86.89
  pituitary E23.0
  renal N25.0
  thanatophoric Q77.1
Dyke-Young anemia (secondary) (symptomatic) D59.1
Dysacusis — *see* Abnormal, auditory perception
Dysadrenocortism E27.9

Dysadrenocortism — *continued*
  hyperfunction E27.Ø
Dysarthria R47.1
  following
    cerebral infarction I69.322
    cerebrovascular disease I69.922
      specified disease NEC I69.822
    intracerebral hemorrhage I69.122
    nontraumatic intracranial hemorrhage NEC I69.222
    subarachnoid hemorrhage I69.Ø22
Dysautonomia (familial) G9Ø.1
Dysbarism T7Ø.3 ☑
Dysbasia R26.2
  angiosclerotica intermittens I73.9
  hysterical F44.4
  lordotica (progressiva) G24.1
  nonorganic origin F44.4
  psychogenic F44.4
Dysbetalipoproteinemia (familial) E78.2
Dyscalculia R48.8
  developmental F81.2
Dyschezia K59.ØØ
Dyschondroplasia (with hemangiomata) Q78.4
Dyschromia (skin) L81.9
Dyscollagenosis M35.9
Dyscranio-pygo-phalangy Q87.Ø
Dyscrasia
  blood (with) D75.9
    antepartum hemorrhage — *see* Hemorrhage, antepartum, with coagulation defect
    intrapartum hemorrhage O67.Ø
    newborn P61.9
      specified type NEC P61.8
    puerperal, postpartum O72.3
  polyglandular, pluriglandular E31.9
Dysendocrinism E34.9
Dysentery, dysenteric (catarrhal) (diarrhea) (epidemic) (hemorrhagic) (infectious) (sporadic) (tropical) AØ9
  abscess, liver AØ6.4
  amebic (*see also* Amebiasis) AØ6.Ø
    with abscess — *see* Abscess, amebic
    acute AØ6.Ø
    chronic AØ6.1
  arthritis (*see also* category MØ1) AØ9
    bacillary (*see also* category MØ1) AØ3.9
  bacillary AØ3.9
    arthritis (*see also* category MØ1) AØ3.9
    Boyd AØ3.2
    Flexner AØ3.1
    Schmitz (-Stutzer) AØ3.Ø
    Shiga (-Kruse) AØ3.Ø
    Shigella AØ3.9
      boydii AØ3.2
      dysenteriae AØ3.Ø
      flexneri AØ3.1
      group A AØ3.Ø
      group B AØ3.1
      group C AØ3.2
      group D AØ3.3
      sonnei AØ3.3
      specified type NEC AØ3.8
    Sonne AØ3.3
    specified type NEC AØ3.8
  balantidial AØ7.Ø
  Balantidium coli AØ7.Ø
  Boyd's AØ3.2
  candidal B37.82
  Chilomastix AØ7.8
  Chinese AØ3.9
  coccidial AØ7.3
  Dientamoeba (fragilis) AØ7.8
  Embadomonas AØ7.8
  Entamoeba, entamebic — *see* Dysentery, amebic
  Flexner-Boyd AØ3.2
  Flexner's AØ3.1
  Giardia lamblia AØ7.1
  Hiss-Russell AØ3.1
  Lamblia AØ7.1
  leishmanial B55.Ø
  malarial — *see* Malaria
  metazoal B82.Ø
  monilial B37.82
  protozoal AØ7.9
  Salmonella AØ2.Ø
  schistosomal B65.1
  Schmitz (-Stutzer) AØ3.Ø
  Shiga (-Kruse) AØ3.Ø
  Shigella NOS — *see* Dysentery, bacillary

Dysentery, dysenteric — *continued*
  Sonne AØ3.3
  strongyloidiasis B78.Ø
  trichomonal AØ7.8
  viral (*see also* Enteritis, viral) AØ8.4
Dysequilibrium R42
Dysesthesia R2Ø.8
  hysterical F44.6
Dysfibrinogenemia (congenital) D68.2
Dysfunction
  adrenal E27.9
    hyperfunction E27.Ø
  autonomic
    due to alcohol G31.2
    somatoform F45.8
  bladder N31.9
    neurogenic NOS — *see* Dysfunction, bladder, neuromuscular
    neuromuscular NOS N31.9
      atonic (motor) (sensory) N31.2
      autonomous N31.2
      flaccid N31.2
      nonreflex N31.2
      reflex N31.1
      specified NEC N31.8
      uninhibited N31.Ø
  bleeding, uterus N93.8
  cerebral G93.89
  colon K59.9
    psychogenic F45.8
  colostomy K94.Ø3
  cystic duct K82.8
  cystostomy (stoma) — *see* Complications, cystostomy
  ejaculatory N53.19
    anejaculatory orgasm N53.13
    painful N53.12
    premature F52.4
    retarded N53.11
  endocrine NOS E34.9
  endometrium N85.8
  enterostomy K94.13
  erectile — *see* Dysfunction, sexual, male, erectile
  gallbladder K82.8
  gastrostomy (stoma) K94.23
  gland, glandular NOS E34.9
    meibomian, of eyelid — *see* Dysfunction, meibomian gland
  heart I51.89
  hemoglobin D75.89
  hepatic K76.89
  hypophysis E23.7
  hypothalamic NEC E23.3
  ileostomy (stoma) K94.13
  jejunostomy (stoma) K94.13
  kidney — *see* Disease, renal
  labyrinthine — *see* subcategory H83.2 ☑
  left ventricular, following sudden emotional stress I51.81
  liver K76.89
  male — *see* Dysfunction, sexual, male
  meibomian gland, of eyelid H02.889
    left H02.886
      lower H02.885
      upper H02.884
      upper and lower eyelids H02.88B
    right H02.883
      lower H02.882
      upper H02.881
      upper and lower eyelids H02.88A
  orgasmic (female) F52.31
    male F52.32
  ovary E28.9
    specified NEC E28.8
  papillary muscle I51.89
  parathyroid E21.4
  physiological NEC R68.89
    psychogenic F59
  pineal gland E34.8
  pituitary (gland) E23.3
  platelets D69.1
  polyglandular E31.9
    specified NEC E31.8
  psychophysiologic F59
  psychosexual F52.9
    with
      dyspareunia F52.6
      premature ejaculation F52.4
      vaginismus F52.5

Dysfunction — *continued*
  pylorus K31.9
  rectum K59.9
    psychogenic F45.8
  reflex (sympathetic) — *see* Syndrome, pain, complex regional I
  segmental — *see* Dysfunction, somatic
  senile R54
  sexual (due to) R37
    alcohol F1Ø.981
    amphetamine F15.981
      in
        abuse F15.181
        dependence F15.281
    anxiolytic F13.981
      in
        abuse F13.181
        dependence F13.281
    cocaine F14.981
      in
        abuse F14.181
        dependence F14.281
    excessive sexual drive F52.8
    failure of genital response (male) F52.21
      female F52.22
    female N94.9
      aversion F52.1
      dyspareunia N94.1Ø
        psychogenic F52.6
      frigidity F52.22
      nymphomania F52.8
      orgasmic F52.31
      psychogenic F52.9
        aversion F52.1
        dyspareunia F52.6
        frigidity F52.22
        nymphomania F52.8
        orgasmic F52.31
        vaginismus F52.5
      vaginismus N94.2
        psychogenic F52.5
    hypnotic F13.981
      in
        abuse F13.181
        dependence F13.281
    inhibited orgasm (female) F52.31
      male F52.32
    lack
      of sexual enjoyment F52.1
      or loss of sexual desire F52.Ø
    male N53.9
      anejaculatory orgasm N53.13
      ejaculatory N53.19
        painful N53.12
        premature F52.4
        retarded N53.11
      erectile N52.9
        drug induced N52.2
        due to
          disease classified elsewhere N52.1
          drug N52.2
        postoperative (postprocedural) N52.39
          following
            cryotherapy N52.37
            interstitial seed therapy N52.36
            prostate ablative therapy N52.37
            prostatectomy N52.34
              radical N52.31
            radiation therapy N52.35
            radical cystectomy N52.32
            ultrasound ablative therapy N52.37
            urethral surgery N52.33
        psychogenic F52.21
        specified cause NEC N52.8
        vasculogenic
          arterial insufficiency N52.Ø1
            with corporo-venous occlusive N52.Ø3
          corporo-venous occlusive N52.Ø2
            with arterial insufficiency N52.Ø3
      impotence — *see* Dysfunction, sexual, male, erectile
      psychogenic F52.9
        aversion F52.1
        erectile F52.21
        orgasmic F52.32
        premature ejaculation F52.4
        satyriasis F52.8
        specified type NEC F52.8
      specified type NEC N53.8

Dysfunction — continued
  sexual — continued
    nonorganic F52.9
      specified NEC F52.8
    opioid F11.981
      in
        abuse F11.181
        dependence F11.281
    orgasmic dysfunction (female) F52.31
      male F52.32
    premature ejaculation F52.4
    psychoactive substances NEC F19.981
      in
        abuse F19.181
        dependence F19.281
    psychogenic F52.9
    sedative F13.981
      in
        abuse F13.181
        dependence F13.281
    sexual aversion F52.1
    vaginismus (nonorganic) (psychogenic) F52.5
  sinoatrial node I49.5
  somatic M99.09
    abdomen M99.09
    acromioclavicular M99.07
    cervical region M99.01
    cervicothoracic M99.01
    costochondral M99.08
    costovertebral M99.08
    head region M99.00
    hip M99.05
    lower extremity M99.06
    lumbar region M99.03
    lumbosacral M99.03
    occipitocervical M99.00
    pelvic region M99.05
    pubic M99.05
    rib cage M99.08
    sacral region M99.04
    sacrococcygeal M99.04
    sacroiliac M99.04
    specified NEC M99.09
    sternochondral M99.08
    sternoclavicular M99.07
    thoracic region M99.02
    thoracolumbar M99.02
    upper extremity M99.07
  somatoform autonomic F45.8
  stomach K31.89
    psychogenic F45.8
  suprarenal E27.9
    hyperfunction E27.0
  symbolic R48.9
    specified type NEC R48.8
  temporomandibular (joint) M26.69
    joint-pain syndrome M26.62- ☑
  testicular (endocrine) E29.9
    specified NEC E29.8
  thymus E32.9
  thyroid E07.9
  ureterostomy (stoma) — see Complications, stoma, urinary tract
  urethrostomy (stoma) — see Complications, stoma, urinary tract
  uterus, complicating delivery O62.9
    hypertonic O62.4
    hypotonic O62.2
      primary O62.0
      secondary O62.1
  ventricular I51.9
    with congestive heart failure (see also Failure, heart) I50.9
    left, reversible, following sudden emotional stress I51.81

Dysgenesis
  gonadal (due to chromosomal anomaly) Q96.9
    pure Q99.1
  renal Q60.5
    bilateral Q60.4
    unilateral Q60.3
  reticular D72.0
  tidal platelet D69.3

Dysgerminoma
  specified site — see Neoplasm, malignant, by site
  unspecified site
    female C56.9
    male C62.90

Dysgeusia R43.2
Dysgraphia R27.8
Dyshidrosis, dysidrosis L30.1
Dyskaryotic cervical smear R87.619
Dyskeratosis L85.8
  cervix — see Dysplasia, cervix
  congenital Q82.8
  uterus NEC N85.8
Dyskinesia G24.9
  biliary (cystic duct or gallbladder) K82.8
  drug induced
    orofacial G24.01
  esophagus K22.4
  hysterical F44.4
  intestinal K59.8
  nonorganic origin F44.4
  orofacial (idiopathic) G24.4
    drug induced G24.01
  psychogenic F44.4
  subacute, drug induced G24.01
  tardive G24.01
    neuroleptic induced G24.01
  trachea J39.8
  tracheobronchial J98.09
Dyslalia (developmental) F80.0
Dyslexia R48.0
  developmental F81.0
Dyslipidemia E78.5
  depressed HDL cholesterol E78.6
  elevated fasting triglycerides E78.1
Dysmaturity (see also Light for dates)
  pulmonary (newborn) (Wilson-Mikity) P27.0
Dysmenorrhea (essential) (exfoliative) N94.6
  congestive (syndrome) N94.6
  primary N94.4
  psychogenic F45.8
  secondary N94.5
Dysmetabolic syndrome X E88.81
Dysmetria R27.8
Dysmorphism (due to)
  alcohol Q86.0
  exogenous cause NEC Q86.8
  hydantoin Q86.1
  warfarin Q86.2
Dysmorphophobia (nondelusional) F45.22
  delusional F22
Dysnomia R47.01
Dysorexia R63.0
  psychogenic F50.89
Dysostosis
  cleidocranial, cleidocranialis Q74.0
  craniofacial Q75.1
  Fairbank's (idiopathic familial generalized osteophytosis) Q78.9
  mandibulofacial (incomplete) Q75.4
  multiplex E76.01
  oculomandibular Q75.5
Dyspareunia (female) N94.10
  deep N94.12
  male N53.12
  nonorganic F52.6
  psychogenic F52.6
  secondary N94.19
  specified NEC N94.19
  superficial (introital) N94.11
Dyspepsia R10.13
  atonic K30
  functional (allergic) (congenital) (gastrointestinal) (occupational) (reflex) K30
  intestinal K59.8
  nervous F45.8
  neurotic F45.8
  psychogenic F45.8
Dysphagia R13.10
  cervical R13.19
  following
    cerebral infarction I69.391
    cerebrovascular disease I69.991
      specified NEC I69.891
    intracerebral hemorrhage I69.191
    nontraumatic intracranial hemorrhage NEC I69.291
    specified disease NEC I69.891
    subarachnoid hemorrhage I69.091
  functional (hysterical) F45.8
  hysterical F45.8
  nervous (hysterical) F45.8
  neurogenic R13.19
  oral phase R13.11

Dysphagia — continued
  oropharyngeal phase R13.12
  pharyngeal phase R13.13
  pharyngoesophageal phase R13.14
  psychogenic F45.8
  sideropenic D50.1
  spastica K22.4
  specified NEC R13.19
Dysphagocytosis, congenital D71
Dysphasia R47.02
  developmental
    expressive type F80.1
    receptive type F80.2
  following
    cerebrovascular disease I69.921
      cerebral infarction I69.321
      intracerebral hemorrhage I69.121
      nontraumatic intracranial hemorrhage NEC I69.221
      specified disease NEC I69.821
      subarachnoid hemorrhage I69.021
Dysphonia R49.0
  functional F44.4
  hysterical F44.4
  psychogenic F44.4
  spastica J38.3
Dysphoria
  gender F64.9
    in
      adolescence and adulthood F64.0
      children F64.2
    specified NEC F64.8
  postpartal O90.6
Dyspituitarism E23.3
Dysplasia (see also Anomaly)
  acetabular, congenital Q65.89
  alveolar capillary, with vein misalignment J84.843
  anus (histologically confirmed) (mild) (moderate) K62.82
    severe D01.3
  arrhythmogenic right ventricular I42.8
  arterial, fibromuscular I77.3
  asphyxiating thoracic (congenital) Q77.2
  brain Q07.9
  bronchopulmonary, perinatal P27.1
  cervix (uteri) N87.9
    mild N87.0
    moderate N87.1
    severe D06.9
  chondroectodermal Q77.6
  colon D12.6
  craniometaphyseal Q78.8
  dentinal K00.5
  diaphyseal, progressive Q78.3
  dystrophic Q77.5
  ectodermal (anhidrotic) (congenital) (hereditary) Q82.4
    hydrotic Q82.8
  epithelial, uterine cervix — see Dysplasia, cervix
  eye (congenital) Q11.2
  fibrous
    bone NEC (monostotic) M85.00
      ankle M85.07- ☑
      foot M85.07- ☑
      forearm M85.03- ☑
      hand M85.04- ☑
      lower leg M85.06- ☑
      multiple site M85.09
      neck M85.08
      rib M85.08
      shoulder M85.01- ☑
      skull M85.08
      specified site NEC M85.08
      thigh M85.05- ☑
      toe M85.07- ☑
      upper arm M85.02- ☑
      vertebra M85.08
  diaphyseal, progressive Q78.3
  jaw M27.8
  polyostotic Q78.1
  florid osseous (see also Cyst, calcifying odontogenic)
  high grade, focal D12.6
  hip, congenital Q65.89
  joint, congenital Q74.8
  kidney Q61.4
    multicystic Q61.4
  leg Q74.2
  lung, congenital (not associated with short gestation) Q33.6

☑ **Additional Character Required** — Refer to the Tabular List for Character Selection   ▽ **Subterms under main terms may continue to next column or page**

Dysplasia — *continued*
  mammary (gland) (benign) N60.9- ☑
    cyst (solitary) — *see* Cyst, breast
    cystic — *see* Mastopathy, cystic
    duct ectasia — *see* Ectasia, mammary duct
    fibroadenosis — *see* Fibroadenosis, breast
    fibrosclerosis — *see* Fibrosclerosis, breast
    specified type NEC N60.8- ☑
  metaphyseal Q78.5
  muscle Q79.8
  oculodentodigital Q87.0
  periapical (cemental) (cemento-osseous) — *see* Cyst,
     calcifying odontogenic
  periosteum — *see* Disorder, bone, specified type NEC
  polyostotic fibrous Q78.1
  prostate (*see also* Neoplasia, intraepithelial, prostate)
     N42.30
    severe D07.5
    specified NEC N42.39
  renal Q61.4
    multicystic Q61.4
  retinal, congenital Q14.1
  right ventricular, arrhythmogenic I42.8
  septo-optic Q04.4
  skin L98.8
  spinal cord Q06.1
  spondyloepiphyseal Q77.7
  thymic, with immunodeficiency D82.1
  vagina N89.3
    mild N89.0
    moderate N89.1
    severe NEC D07.2
  vulva N90.3
    mild N90.0
    moderate N90.1
    severe NEC D07.1
Dysplasminogenemia E88.02
Dyspnea (nocturnal) (paroxysmal) R06.00
  asthmatic (bronchial) J45.909
    with
      bronchitis J45.909
        with
          exacerbation (acute) J45.901
          status asthmaticus J45.902
        chronic J44.9
      exacerbation (acute) J45.901
      status asthmaticus J45.902
  cardiac — *see* Failure, ventricular, left
  cardiac — *see* Failure, ventricular, left
  functional F45.8
  hyperventilation R06.4
  hysterical F45.8
  newborn P28.89
  orthopnea R06.01
  psychogenic F45.8
  shortness of breath R06.02
  specified type NEC R06.09
Dyspraxia R27.8
  developmental (syndrome) F82
Dysproteinemia E88.09
Dysreflexia, autonomic G90.4
Dysrhythmia
  cardiac I49.9
    newborn
      bradycardia P29.12
      occurring before birth P03.819
        before onset of labor P03.810
        during labor P03.811
      tachycardia P29.11
    postoperative I97.89
  cerebral or cortical — *see* Epilepsy
Dyssomnia — *see* Disorder, sleep
Dyssynergia
  biliary K83.8
  bladder sphincter N36.44
  cerebellaris myoclonica (Hunt's ataxia) G11.1
Dysthymia F34.1
Dysthyroidism E07.9
Dystocia O66.9
  affecting newborn P03.1
  cervical (hypotonic) O62.2
    affecting newborn P03.6
    primary O62.0
    secondary O62.1
  contraction ring O62.4
  fetal O66.9
    abnormality NEC O66.3
    conjoined twins O66.3

Dystocia — *continued*
  fetal — *continued*
    oversize O66.2
  maternal O66.9
  positional O64.9 ☑
  shoulder (girdle) O66.0
    causing obstructed labor O66.0
  uterine NEC O62.4
Dystonia G24.9
  cervical G24.3
  deformans progressiva G24.1
  drug induced NEC G24.09
    acute G24.02
    specified NEC G24.09
  familial G24.1
  idiopathic G24.1
    familial G24.1
    nonfamilial G24.2
    orofacial G24.4
  lenticularis G24.8
  musculorum deformans G24.1
  neuroleptic induced (acute) G24.02
  orofacial (idiopathic) G24.4
  oromandibular G24.4
    due to drug G24.01
  specified NEC G24.8
  torsion (familial) (idiopathic) G24.1
    acquired G24.8
    genetic G24.1
    symptomatic (nonfamilial) G24.2
Dystonic movements R25.8
Dystrophy, dystrophia
  adiposogenital E23.6
  autosomal recessive, childhood type, muscular dystro-
     phy resembling Duchenne or Becker G71.01
  Becker's type G71.01
  cervical sympathetic G90.2
  choroid (hereditary) H31.20
    central areolar H31.22
    choroideremia H31.21
    gyrate atrophy H31.23
    specified type NEC H31.29
  cornea (hereditary) H18.50
    endothelial H18.51
    epithelial H18.52
    granular H18.53
    lattice H18.54
    macular H18.55
    specified type NEC H18.59
  Duchenne's type G71.01
  due to malnutrition E45
  Erb's G71.02
  Fuchs' H18.51
  Gower's muscular G71.01
  hair L67.8
  infantile neuraxonal G31.89
  Landouzy-Déjérine G71.02
  Leyden-Möbius G71.09
  muscular G71.00
    autosomal recessive, childhood type, muscular
      dystrophy resembling Duchenne or Becker
      G71.01
    benign (Becker type) G71.01
      scapuloperoneal with early contractures [Emery-
        Dreifuss] G71.09
    congenital (hereditary) (progressive) (with specific
      morphological abnormalities of the muscle
      fiber) G71.09
      myotonic G71.11
    distal G71.09
    Duchenne type G71.01
    Emery-Dreifuss G71.09
    Erb type G71.02
    facioscapulohumeral G71.02
    Gower's G71.01
    hereditary (progressive) G71.09
    Landouzy-Déjérine type G71.02
    limb-girdle G71.09
    myotonic G71.11
    progressive (hereditary) G71.09
      Charcot-Marie (-Tooth) type G60.0
    pseudohypertrophic (infantile) G71.01
    scapulohumeral G71.02
    scapuloperoneal G71.09
    severe (Duchenne type) G71.01
    specified type NEC G71.09
  myocardium, myocardial — *see* Degeneration, myocar-
     dial
  nail L60.3

Dystrophy, dystrophia — *continued*
  nail — *continued*
    congenital Q84.6
  nutritional E45
  ocular G71.09
  oculocerebrorenal E72.03
  oculopharyngeal G71.09
  ovarian N83.8
  polyglandular E31.8
  reflex (neuromuscular) (sympathetic) — *see* Syndrome,
     pain, complex regional I
  retinal (hereditary) H35.50
    in
      lipid storage disorders E75.6 [H36]
      systemic lipidoses E75.6 [H36]
    involving
      pigment epithelium H35.54
      sensory area H35.53
    pigmentary H35.52
    vitreoretinal H35.51
  Salzmann's nodular — *see* Degeneration, cornea,
     nodular
  scapuloperoneal G71.09
  skin NEC L98.8
  sympathetic (reflex) — *see* Syndrome, pain, complex
     regional I
    cervical G90.2
  tapetoretinal H35.54
  thoracic, asphyxiating Q77.2
  unguium L60.3
    congenital Q84.6
  vitreoretinal H35.51
  vulva N90.4
  yellow (liver) — *see* Failure, hepatic
Dysuria R30.0
  psychogenic F45.8

E

Eales' disease H35.06- ☑
Ear (*see also* condition)
  piercing Z41.3
  tropical NEC B36.9 [H62.40]
    in
      aspergillosis B44.89
      candidiasis B37.84
      moniliasis B37.84
  wax (impacted) H61.20
    left H61.22
      with right H61.23
    right H61.21
      with left H61.23
Earache — *see* subcategory H92.0 ☑
Early satiety R68.81
Eaton-Lambert syndrome — *see* Syndrome, Lambert-
    Eaton
Eberth's disease (typhoid fever) A01.00
Ebola virus disease A98.4
Ebstein's anomaly or syndrome (heart) Q22.5
Eccentro-osteochondrodysplasia E76.29
Ecchondroma — *see* Neoplasm, bone, benign
Ecchondrosis D48.0
Ecchymosis R58
  conjunctiva — *see* Hemorrhage, conjunctiva
  eye (traumatic) — *see* Contusion, eyeball
  eyelid (traumatic) — *see* Contusion, eyelid
  newborn P54.5
  spontaneous R23.3
  traumatic — *see* Contusion
Echinococciasis — *see* Echinococcus
Echinococcosis — *see* Echinococcus
Echinococcus (infection) B67.90
  granulosus B67.4
    bone B67.2
    liver B67.0
    lung B67.1
    multiple sites B67.32
    specified site NEC B67.39
    thyroid B67.31
  liver NOS B67.8
    granulosus B67.0
    multilocularis B67.5
  lung NEC B67.99
    granulosus B67.1
    multilocularis B67.69
  multilocularis B67.7
    liver B67.5
    multiple sites B67.61

Echinococcus — *continued*
  multilocularis — *continued*
    specified site NEC B67.69
  specified site NEC B67.99
    granulosus B67.39
    multilocularis B67.69
  thyroid NEC B67.99
    granulosus B67.31
    multilocularis B67.69 [E35]
Echinorhynchiasis B83.8
Echinostomiasis B66.8
Echolalia R48.8
Echovirus, as cause of disease classified elsewhere
  B97.12
Eclampsia, eclamptic (coma) (convulsions) (delirium)
  (with hypertension) NEC O15.9
  complicating
    labor and delivery O15.1
    postpartum O15.2
    pregnancy O15.0- ☑
    puerperium O15.2
Economic circumstances affecting care Z59.9
Economo's disease A85.8
Ectasia, ectasis
  annuloaortic I35.8
  aorta I77.819
    with aneurysm — *see* Aneurysm, aorta
    abdominal I77.811
    thoracic I77.810
    thoracoabdominal I77.812
  breast — *see* Ectasia, mammary duct
  capillary I78.8
  cornea H18.71- ☑
  gastric antral vascular (GAVE) K31.819
    with hemorrhage K31.811
    without hemorrhage K31.819
  mammary duct N60.4- ☑
  salivary gland (duct) K11.8
  sclera — *see* Sclerectasia
Ecthyma L08.0
  contagiosum B08.02
  gangrenosum L08.0
  infectiosum B08.02
Ectocardia Q24.8
Ectodermal dysplasia (anhidrotic) Q82.4
Ectodermosis erosiva pluriorificialis L51.1
Ectopic, ectopia (congenital)
  abdominal viscera Q45.8
    due to defect in anterior abdominal wall Q79.59
  ACTH syndrome E24.3
  adrenal gland Q89.1
  anus Q43.5
  atrial beats I49.1
  beats I49.49
    atrial I49.1
    ventricular I49.3
  bladder Q64.10
  bone and cartilage in lung Q33.5
  brain Q04.8
  breast tissue Q83.8
  cardiac Q24.8
  cerebral Q04.8
  cordis Q24.8
  endometrium — *see* Endometriosis
  gastric mucosa Q40.2
  gestation — *see* Pregnancy, by site
  heart Q24.8
  hormone secretion NEC E34.2
  kidney (crossed) (pelvis) Q63.2
  lens, lentis Q12.1
  mole — *see* Pregnancy, by site
  organ or site NEC — *see* Malposition, congenital
  pancreas Q45.3
  pregnancy — *see* Pregnancy, ectopic
  pupil — *see* Abnormality, pupillary
  renal Q63.2
  sebaceous glands of mouth Q38.6
  spleen Q89.09
  testis Q53.00
    bilateral Q53.02
    unilateral Q53.01
  thyroid Q89.2
  tissue in lung Q33.5
  ureter Q62.63
  ventricular beats I49.3
  vesicae Q64.10
Ectromelia Q73.8

Ectromelia — *continued*
  lower limb — *see* Defect, reduction, limb, lower, specified type NEC
  upper limb — *see* Defect, reduction, limb, upper, specified type NEC
Ectropion H02.109
  cervix N86
    with cervicitis N72
  congenital Q10.1
  eyelid H02.109
    cicatricial H02.119
      left H02.116
        lower H02.115
        upper H02.114
      right H02.113
        lower H02.112
        upper H02.111
    congenital Q10.1
    left H02.106
      lower H02.105
      upper H02.104
    mechanical H02.129
      left H02.126
        lower H02.125
        upper H02.124
      right H02.123
        lower H02.122
        upper H02.121
    paralytic H02.159
      left H02.156
        lower H02.155
        upper H02.154
      right H02.153
        lower H02.152
        upper H02.151
    right H02.103
      lower H02.102
      upper H02.101
    senile H02.139
      left H02.136
        lower H02.135
        upper H02.134
      right H02.133
        lower H02.132
        upper H02.131
    spastic H02.149
      left H02.146
        lower H02.145
        upper H02.144
      right H02.143
        lower H02.142
        upper H02.141
  iris H21.89
  lip (acquired) K13.0
    congenital Q38.0
  urethra N36.8
  uvea H21.89
Eczema (acute) (chronic) (erythematous) (fissum) (rubrum) (squamous) (*see also* Dermatitis) L30.9
  contact — *see* Dermatitis, contact
  dyshydrotic L30.1
  external ear — *see* Otitis, externa, acute, eczematoid
  flexural L20.82
  herpeticum B00.0
  hypertrophicum L28.0
  hypostatic — *see* Varix, leg, with, inflammation
  impetiginous L01.1
  infantile (due to any substance) L20.83
    intertriginous L21.1
    seborrheic L21.1
  intertriginous NEC L30.4
    infantile L21.1
  intrinsic (allergic) L20.84
  lichenified NEC L28.0
  marginatum (hebrae) B35.6
  pustular L30.3
  stasis I87.2
    with varicose veins — *see* Varix, leg, with, inflammation
  vaccination, vaccinatum T88.1 ☑
  varicose — *see* Varix, leg, with, inflammation
Eczematid L30.2
Eddowes (-Spurway) **syndrome** Q78.0
Edema, edematous (infectious) (pitting) (toxic) R60.9
  with nephritis — *see* Nephrosis
  allergic T78.3 ☑
  amputation stump (surgical) (sequelae (late effect)) T87.89

Edema, edematous — *continued*
  angioneurotic (allergic) (any site) (with urticaria)
    T78.3 ☑
    hereditary D84.1
  angiospastic I73.9
  Berlin's (traumatic) S05.8X- ☑
  brain (cytotoxic) (vasogenic) G93.6
    due to birth injury P11.0
    newborn (anoxia or hypoxia) P52.4
      birth injury P11.0
    traumatic — *see* Injury, intracranial, cerebral edema
  cardiac — *see* Failure, heart, congestive
  cardiovascular — *see* Failure, heart, congestive
  cerebral — *see* Edema, brain
  cerebrospinal — *see* Edema, brain
  cervix (uteri) (acute) N88.8
    puerperal, postpartum O90.89
  chronic hereditary Q82.0
  circumscribed, acute T78.3 ☑
    hereditary D84.1
  conjunctiva H11.42- ☑
  cornea H18.2- ☑
    idiopathic H18.22- ☑
    secondary H18.23- ☑
      due to contact lens H18.21- ☑
  due to
    lymphatic obstruction I89.0
    salt retention E87.0
  epiglottis — *see* Edema, glottis
  essential, acute T78.3 ☑
    hereditary D84.1
  extremities, lower — *see* Edema, legs
  eyelid NEC H02.849
    left H02.846
      lower H02.845
      upper H02.844
    right H02.843
      lower H02.842
      upper H02.841
  familial, hereditary Q82.0
  famine — *see* Malnutrition, severe
  generalized R60.1
  glottis, glottic, glottidis (obstructive) (passive) J38.4
    allergic T78.3 ☑
      hereditary D84.1
  heart — *see* Failure, heart, congestive
  heat T67.7 ☑
  hereditary Q82.0
  inanition — *see* Malnutrition, severe
  intracranial G93.6
  iris H21.89
  joint — *see* Effusion, joint
  larynx — *see* Edema, glottis
  legs R60.0
    due to venous obstruction I87.1
    hereditary Q82.0
  localized R60.0
    due to venous obstruction I87.1
  lower limbs — *see* Edema, legs
  lung J81.1
    with heart condition or failure — *see* Failure, ventricular, left
    acute J81.0
    chemical (acute) J68.1
      chronic J68.1
    chronic J81.1
      due to
        chemicals, gases, fumes or vapors (inhalation) J68.1
        external agent J70.9
          specified NEC J70.8
        radiation J70.1
    due to
      chemicals, fumes or vapors (inhalation) J68.1
      external agent J70.9
        specified NEC J70.8
      high altitude T70.29 ☑
      near drowning T75.1 ☑
      radiation J70.0
    meaning failure, left ventricle I50.1
  lymphatic I89.0
    due to mastectomy I97.2
  macula H35.81
    cystoid, following cataract surgery — *see* Complications, postprocedural, following cataract surgery
    diabetic — *see* Diabetes, by type, with, retinopathy, with macular edema

☑ **Additional Character Required** — Refer to the Tabular List for Character Selection   ▽ **Subterms under main terms may continue to next column or page**

Edema, edematous — *continued*
- malignant — *see* Gangrene, gas
- Milroy's Q82.0
- nasopharynx J39.2
- newborn P83.30
  - hydrops fetalis — *see* Hydrops, fetalis
  - specified NEC P83.39
- nutritional (*see also* Malnutrition, severe)
  - with dyspigmentation, skin and hair E40
- optic disc or nerve — *see* Papilledema
- orbit H05.22-
- pancreas K86.89
- papilla, optic — *see* Papilledema
- penis N48.89
- periodic T78.3 ☑
  - hereditary D84.1
- pharynx J39.2
- pulmonary — *see* Edema, lung
- Quincke's T78.3 ☑
  - hereditary D84.1
- renal — *see* Nephrosis
- retina H35.81
  - diabetic — *see* Diabetes, by type, with, retinopathy, with macular edema
- salt E87.0
- scrotum N50.89
- seminal vesicle N50.89
- spermatic cord N50.89
- spinal (cord) (vascular) (nontraumatic) G95.19
- starvation — *see* Malnutrition, severe
- stasis — *see* Hypertension, venous, (chronic)
- subglottic — *see* Edema, glottis
- supraglottic — *see* Edema, glottis
- testis N44.8
- tunica vaginalis N50.89
- vas deferens N50.89
- vulva (acute) N90.89

Edentulism — *see* Absence, teeth, acquired
Edsall's disease T67.2 ☑
Educational handicap Z55.9
- specified NEC Z55.8
Edward's syndrome — *see* Trisomy, 18
Effect(s) (of) (from) — *see* Effect, adverse NEC
Effect, adverse
- abnormal gravitational (G) forces or states T75.81 ☑
- abuse — *see* Maltreatment
- air pressure T70.9 ☑
  - specified NEC T70.8 ☑
- altitude (high) — *see* Effect, adverse, high altitude
- anesthesia (*see also* Anesthesia) T88.59 ☑
  - in labor and delivery O74.9
  - local, toxic
    - in labor and delivery O74.4
    - in pregnancy NEC O29.3- ☑
    - postpartum, puerperal O89.3
  - postpartum, puerperal O89.9
  - specified NEC T88.59 ☑
    - in labor and delivery O74.8
    - postpartum, puerperal O89.8
  - spinal and epidural T88.59 ☑
    - headache T88.59 ☑
      - in labor and delivery O74.5
      - postpartum, puerperal O89.4
    - specified NEC
      - in labor and delivery O74.6
      - postpartum, puerperal O89.5
- antitoxin — *see* Complications, vaccination
- atmospheric pressure T70.9 ☑
  - due to explosion T70.8 ☑
  - high T70.3 ☑
  - low — *see* Effect, adverse, high altitude
  - specified effect NEC T70.8 ☑
- biological, correct substance properly administered — *see* Effect, adverse, drug
- blood (derivatives) (serum) (transfusion) — *see* Complications, transfusion
- chemical substance — *see* Table of Drugs and Chemicals
- cold (temperature) (weather) T69.9 ☑
  - chilblains T69.1 ☑
  - frostbite — *see* Frostbite
  - specified effect NEC T69.8 ☑
- drugs and medicaments T88.7 ☑
  - specified drug — *see* Table of Drugs and Chemicals, by drug, adverse effect
  - specified effect — *code to* condition
- electric current, electricity (shock) T75.4 ☑

Effect, adverse — *continued*
- electric current, electricity — *continued*
  - burn — *see* Burn
- exertion (excessive) T73.3 ☑
- exposure — *see* Exposure
- external cause NEC T75.89 ☑
- foodstuffs T78.1 ☑
  - allergic reaction — *see* Allergy, food
    - causing anaphylaxis — *see* Shock, anaphylactic, due to food
  - noxious — *see* Poisoning, food, noxious
- gases, fumes, or vapors T59.9- ☑
  - specified agent — *see* Table of Drugs and Chemicals
- glue (airplane) sniffing
  - due to drug abuse — *see* Abuse, drug, inhalant
  - due to drug dependence — *see* Dependence, drug, inhalant
- heat — *see* Heat
- high altitude NEC T70.29 ☑
  - anoxia T70.29 ☑
  - on
    - ears T70.0 ☑
    - sinuses T70.1 ☑
  - polycythemia D75.1
- high pressure fluids T70.4 ☑
- hot weather — *see* Heat
- hunger T73.0 ☑
- immersion, foot — *see* Immersion
- immunization — *see* Complications, vaccination
- immunological agents — *see* Complications, vaccination
- infrared (radiation) (rays) NOS T66 ☑
  - dermatitis or eczema L59.8
- infusion — *see* Complications, infusion
- lack of care of infants — *see* Maltreatment, child
- lightning — *see* Lightning
- medical care T88.9 ☑
  - specified NEC T88.8 ☑
- medicinal substance, correct, properly administered — *see* Effect, adverse, drug
- motion T75.3 ☑
- noise, on inner ear — *see* subcategory H83.3 ☑
- overheated places — *see* Heat
- psychosocial, of work environment Z56.5
- radiation (diagnostic) (infrared) (natural source) (therapeutic) (ultraviolet) (X-ray) NOS T66 ☑
  - dermatitis or eczema — *see* Dermatitis, due to, radiation
  - fibrosis of lung J70.1
  - pneumonitis J70.0
  - pulmonary manifestations
    - acute J70.0
    - chronic J70.1
  - skin L59.9
- radioactive substance NOS
  - dermatitis or eczema — *see* Radiodermatitis
- reduced temperature T69.9 ☑
  - immersion foot or hand — *see* Immersion
  - specified effect NEC T69.8 ☑
- serum NEC (*see also* Reaction, serum) T80.69 ☑
- specified NEC T78.8 ☑
  - external cause NEC T75.89 ☑
- strangulation — *see* Asphyxia, traumatic
- submersion T75.1 ☑
- thirst T73.1 ☑
- toxic — *see* Toxicity
- transfusion — *see* Complications, transfusion
- ultraviolet (radiation) (rays) NOS T66 ☑
  - burn — *see* Burn
  - dermatitis or eczema — *see* Dermatitis, due to, ultraviolet rays
    - acute L56.8
- vaccine (any) — *see* Complications, vaccination
- vibration — *see* Vibration, adverse effects
- water pressure NEC T70.9 ☑
  - specified NEC T70.8 ☑
- weightlessness T75.82 ☑
- whole blood — *see* Complications, transfusion
- work environment Z56.5

Effects, late — *see* Sequelae
Effluvium
- anagen L65.1
- telogen L65.0
Effort syndrome (psychogenic) F45.8
Effusion
- amniotic fluid — *see* Pregnancy, complicated by, premature rupture of membranes

Effusion — *continued*
- brain (serous) G93.6
- bronchial — *see* Bronchitis
- cerebral G93.6
- cerebrospinal (*see also* Meningitis)
  - vessel G93.6
- chest — *see* Effusion, pleura
- chylous, chyliform (pleura) J94.0
- intracranial G93.6
- joint M25.40
  - ankle M25.47- ☑
  - elbow M25.42- ☑
  - foot joint M25.47- ☑
  - hand joint M25.44- ☑
  - hip M25.45- ☑
  - knee M25.46- ☑
  - shoulder M25.41- ☑
  - specified joint NEC M25.48
  - wrist M25.43- ☑
- malignant pleural J91.0
- meninges — *see* Meningitis
- pericardium, pericardial (noninflammatory) I31.3
  - acute — *see* Pericarditis, acute
- peritoneal (chronic) R18.8
- pleura, pleurisy, pleuritic, pleuropericardial J90
  - chylous, chyliform J94.0
  - due to systemic lupus erythematosis M32.13
  - in conditions classified elsewhere J91.8
  - influenzal — *see* Influenza, with, respiratory manifestations NEC
  - malignant J91.0
  - newborn P28.89
  - tuberculous NEC A15.6
    - primary (progressive) A15.7
- spinal — *see* Meningitis
- thorax, thoracic — *see* Effusion, pleura

Egg shell nails L60.3
- congenital Q84.6
Egyptian splenomegaly B65.1
Ehlers-Danlos syndrome Q79.6
Ehrlichiosis A77.40
- due to
  - E. chafeensis A77.41
  - E. sennetsu A79.81
  - specified organism NEC A77.49
Eichstedt's disease B36.0
Eisenmenger's
- complex or syndrome I27.83
- defect Q21.8
Ejaculation
- delayed F52.32
- painful N53.12
- premature F52.4
- retarded N53.11
- retrograde N53.14
- semen, painful N53.12
- psychogenic F52.6
Ekbom's syndrome (restless legs) G25.81
Ekman's syndrome (brittle bones and blue sclera) Q78.0
Elastic skin Q82.8
- acquired L57.4
Elastofibroma — *see* Neoplasm, connective tissue, benign
Elastoma (juvenile) Q82.8
- Miescher's L87.2
Elastomyofibrosis I42.4
Elastosis
- actinic, solar L57.8
- atrophicans (senile) L57.4
- perforans serpiginosa L87.2
- senilis L57.4
Elbow — *see* condition
Electric current, electricity, effects (concussion) (fatal) (nonfatal) (shock) T75.4 ☑
- burn — *see* Burn
Electric feet syndrome E53.8
Electrocution T75.4 ☑
- from electroshock gun (taser) T75.4 ☑
Electrolyte imbalance E87.8
- with
  - abortion — *see* Abortion by type, complicated by, electrolyte imbalance
  - ectopic pregnancy O08.5
  - molar pregnancy O08.5
Elephantiasis (nonfilarial) I89.0
- arabicum — *see* Infestation, filarial
- bancroftian B74.0

◭ **Subterms under main terms may continue to next column or page**   ☑ **Additional Character Required — Refer to the Tabular List for Character Selection**   **127**

Edema, edematous — Elephantiasis

Elephantiasis — *continued*
congenital (any site) (hereditary) Q82.0
due to
Brugia (malayi) B74.1
timori B74.2
mastectomy I97.2
Wuchereria (bancrofti) B74.0
eyelid H02.859
left H02.856
lower H02.855
upper H02.854
right H02.853
lower H02.852
upper H02.851
filarial, filariensis — *see* Infestation, filarial
glandular I89.0
graecorum A30.9
lymphangiectatic I89.0
lymphatic vessel I89.0
due to mastectomy I97.2
scrotum (nonfilarial) I89.0
streptococcal I89.0
surgical I97.89
postmastectomy I97.2
telangiectodes I89.0
vulva (nonfilarial) N90.89
Elevated, elevation
antibody titer R76.0
basal metabolic rate R94.8
blood pressure (*see also* Hypertension)
reading (incidental) (isolated) (nonspecific), no diagnosis of hypertension R03.0
blood sugar R73.9
body temperature (of unknown origin) R50.9
cancer antigen 125 [CA 125] R97.1
carcinoembryonic antigen [CEA] R97.0
cholesterol E78.00
with high triglycerides E78.2
conjugate, eye H51.0
C-reactive protein (CRP) R79.82
diaphragm, congenital Q79.1
erythrocyte sedimentation rate R70.0
fasting glucose R73.01
fasting triglycerides E78.1
finding on laboratory examination — *see* Findings, abnormal, inconclusive, without diagnosis, by type of exam
GFR (glomerular filtration rate) — *see* Findings, abnormal, inconclusive, without diagnosis, by type of exam
glucose tolerance (oral) R73.02
immunoglobulin level R76.8
indoleacetic acid R82.5
lactic acid dehydrogenase (LDH) level R74.0
leukocytes D72.829
lipoprotein a (Lp(a)) level E78.41
liver function
study R94.5
test R79.89
alkaline phosphatase R74.8
aminotransferase R74.0
bilirubin R17
hepatic enzyme R74.8
lactate dehydrogenase R74.0
Lp(a) (lipoprotein(a)) E78.41
lymphocytes D72.820
prostate specific antigen [PSA] R97.20
Rh titer — *see* Complication(s), transfusion, incompatibility reaction, Rh (factor)
scapula, congenital Q74.0
sedimentation rate R70.0
SGOT R74.0
SGPT R74.0
transaminase level R74.0
triglycerides E78.1
with high cholesterol E78.2
tumor associated antigens [TAA] NEC R97.8
tumor specific antigens [TSA] NEC R97.8
urine level of
17-ketosteroids R82.5
catecholamine R82.5
indoleacetic acid R82.5
steroids R82.5
vanillylmandelic acid (VMA) R82.5
venous pressure I87.8
white blood cell count D72.829
specified NEC D72.828
Elliptocytosis (congenital) (hereditary) D58.1

Elliptocytosis — *continued*
Hb C (disease) D58.1
hemoglobin disease D58.1
sickle-cell (disease) D57.8- ☑
trait D57.3
Ellison-Zollinger syndrome E16.4
Ellis-van Creveld syndrome (chondroectodermal dysplasia) Q77.6
Elongated, elongation (congenital) (*see also* Distortion)
bone Q79.9
cervix (uteri) Q51.828
acquired N88.4
hypertrophic N88.4
colon Q43.8
common bile duct Q44.5
cystic duct Q44.5
frenulum, penis Q55.69
labia minora (acquired) N90.69
ligamentum patellae Q74.1
petiolus (epiglottidis) Q31.8
tooth, teeth K00.2
uvula Q38.6
Eltor cholera A00.1
Emaciation (due to malnutrition) E41
Embadomoniasis A07.8
Embedded tooth, teeth K01.0
root only K08.3
Embolic — *see* condition
Embolism (multiple) (paradoxical) I74.9
air (any site) (traumatic) T79.0 ☑
following
abortion — *see* Abortion by type complicated by embolism
ectopic pregnancy O08.2
infusion, therapeutic injection or transfusion T80.0 ☑
molar pregnancy O08.2
procedure NEC
artery T81.719 ☑
mesenteric T81.710 ☑
renal T81.711 ☑
specified NEC T81.718 ☑
vein T81.72 ☑
in pregnancy, childbirth or puerperium — *see* Embolism, obstetric
amniotic fluid (pulmonary) (*see also* Embolism, obstetric)
following
abortion — *see* Abortion by type complicated by embolism
ectopic pregnancy O08.2
molar pregnancy O08.2
aorta, aortic I74.10
abdominal I74.09
saddle I74.01
bifurcation I74.09
saddle I74.01
thoracic I74.11
artery I74.9
auditory, internal I65.8
basilar — *see* Occlusion, artery, basilar
carotid (common) (internal) — *see* Occlusion, artery, carotid
cerebellar (anterior inferior) (posterior inferior) (superior) I66.3
cerebral — *see* Occlusion, artery, cerebral
choroidal (anterior) I65.8
communicating posterior I65.8
coronary (*see also* Infarct, myocardium)
not resulting in infarction I24.0
extremity I74.4
lower I74.3
upper I74.2
hypophyseal I65.8
iliac I74.5
limb I74.4
lower I74.3
upper I74.2
mesenteric (with gangrene) (*see also* Ischemia, intestine, acute) K55.059
ophthalmic — *see* Occlusion, artery, retina
peripheral I74.4
pontine I65.8
precerebral — *see* Occlusion, artery, precerebral
pulmonary — *see* Embolism, pulmonary
renal N28.0
retinal — *see* Occlusion, artery, retina
septic I76

Embolism — *continued*
artery — *continued*
specified NEC I74.8
vertebral — *see* Occlusion, artery, vertebral
basilar (artery) I65.1
blood clot
following
abortion — *see* Abortion by type complicated by embolism
ectopic or molar pregnancy O08.2
in pregnancy, childbirth or puerperium — *see* Embolism, obstetric
brain (*see also* Occlusion, artery, cerebral)
following
abortion — *see* Abortion by type complicated by embolism
ectopic or molar pregnancy O08.2
puerperal, postpartum, childbirth — *see* Embolism, obstetric
capillary I78.8
cardiac (*see also* Infarct, myocardium)
not resulting in infarction I51.3
carotid (artery) (common) (internal) — *see* Occlusion, artery, carotid
cavernous sinus (venous) — *see* Embolism, intracranial venous sinus
cerebral — *see* Occlusion, artery, cerebral
cholesterol — *see* Atheroembolism
coronary (artery or vein) (systemic) — *see* Occlusion, coronary
due to device, implant or graft (*see also* Complications, by site and type, specified NEC)
arterial graft NEC T82.818 ☑
breast (implant) T85.818 ☑
catheter NEC T85.818 ☑
dialysis (renal) T82.818 ☑
intraperitoneal T85.818 ☑
infusion NEC T82.818 ☑
spinal (epidural) (subdural) T85.810 ☑
urinary (indwelling) T83.81 ☑
electronic (electrode) (pulse generator) (stimulator)
bone T84.81 ☑
cardiac T82.817 ☑
nervous system (brain) (peripheral nerve) (spinal) T85.810 ☑
urinary T83.81 ☑
fixation, internal (orthopedic) NEC T84.81 ☑
gastrointestinal (bile duct) (esophagus) T85.818 ☑
genital NEC T83.81 ☑
heart (graft) (valve) T82.817 ☑
joint prosthesis T84.81 ☑
ocular (corneal graft) (orbital implant) T85.818 ☑
orthopedic (bone graft) NEC T86.838
specified NEC T85.818 ☑
urinary (graft) NEC T83.81 ☑
vascular NEC T82.818 ☑
ventricular intracranial shunt T85.810 ☑
extremities
lower — *see* Embolism, vein, lower extremity
arterial I74.3
upper I74.2
eye H34.9
fat (cerebral) (pulmonary) (systemic) T79.1 ☑
complicating delivery — *see* Embolism, obstetric
following
abortion — *see* Abortion by type complicated by embolism
ectopic or molar pregnancy O08.2
following
abortion — *see* Abortion by type complicated by embolism
ectopic or molar pregnancy O08.2
infusion, therapeutic injection or transfusion air T80.0 ☑
heart (fatty) (*see also* Infarct, myocardium)
not resulting in infarction I51.3
hepatic (vein) I82.0
in pregnancy, childbirth or puerperium — *see* Embolism, obstetric
intestine (artery) (vein) (with gangrene) (*see also* Ischemia, intestine, acute) K55.039
intracranial (*see also* Occlusion, artery, cerebral)
venous sinus (any) G08
nonpyogenic I67.6
intraspinal venous sinuses or veins G08
nonpyogenic G95.19
kidney (artery) N28.0

☑ **Additional Character Required** — Refer to the Tabular List for Character Selection

▽ **Subterms under main terms may continue to next column or page**

Embolism — *continued*
- lateral sinus (venous) — *see* Embolism, intracranial, venous sinus
- leg — *see* Embolism, vein, lower extremity
  - arterial I74.3
- longitudinal sinus (venous) — *see* Embolism, intracranial, venous sinus
- lung (massive) — *see* Embolism, pulmonary
- meninges I66.8
- mesenteric (artery) (vein) (with gangrene) (*see also* Ischemia, intestine, acute) K55.059
- obstetric (in) (pulmonary)
  - childbirth O88.22
    - air O88.02
    - amniotic fluid O88.12
    - blood clot O88.22
    - fat O88.82
    - pyemic O88.32
    - septic O88.32
    - specified type NEC O88.82
  - pregnancy O88.21- ☑
    - air O88.01-
    - amniotic fluid O88.11- ☑
    - blood clot O88.21- ☑
    - fat O88.81- ☑
    - pyemic O88.31- ☑
    - septic O88.31- ☑
    - specified type NEC O88.81- ☑
  - puerperal O88.23
    - air O88.03
    - amniotic fluid O88.13
    - blood clot O88.23
    - fat O88.83
    - pyemic O88.33
    - septic O88.33
    - specified type NEC O88.83
- ophthalmic — *see* Occlusion, artery, retina
- penis N48.81
- peripheral artery NOS I74.4
- pituitary E23.6
- popliteal (artery) I74.3
- portal (vein) I81
- postoperative, postprocedural
  - artery T81.719 ☑
    - mesenteric T81.710 ☑
    - renal T81.711 ☑
    - specified NEC T81.718 ☑
  - vein T81.72 ☑
- precerebral artery — *see* Occlusion, artery, precerebral
- puerperal — *see* Embolism, obstetric
- pulmonary (acute) (artery) (vein) I26.99
  - with acute cor pulmonale I26.09
  - chronic I27.82
  - following
    - abortion — *see* Abortion by type complicated by embolism
    - ectopic or molar pregnancy O08.2
  - healed or old Z86.711
  - in pregnancy, childbirth or puerperium — *see* Embolism, obstetric
  - personal history of Z86.711
  - saddle I26.92
    - with acute cor pulmonale I26.02
  - septic I26.90
    - with acute cor pulmonale I26.01
- pyemic (multiple) I76
  - following
    - abortion — *see* Abortion by type complicated by embolism
    - ectopic or molar pregnancy O08.2
  - Hemophilus influenzae A41.3
  - pneumococcal A40.3
    - with pneumonia J13
  - puerperal, postpartum, childbirth (any organism) — *see* Embolism, obstetric
  - specified organism NEC A41.89
  - staphylococcal A41.2
  - streptococcal A40.9
- renal (artery) N28.0
  - vein I82.3
- retina, retinal — *see* Occlusion, artery, retina
- saddle
  - abdominal aorta I74.01
  - pulmonary artery I26.92
    - with acute cor pulmonale I26.02
- septic (arterial) I76
  - complicating abortion — *see* Abortion, by type, complicated by, embolism

Embolism — *continued*
- sinus — *see* Embolism, intracranial, venous sinus
- soap complicating abortion — *see* Abortion, by type, complicated by, embolism
- spinal cord G95.19
  - pyogenic origin G06.1
- spleen, splenic (artery) I74.8
- upper extremity I74.2
- vein (acute) I82.90
  - antecubital I82.61- ☑
    - chronic I82.71- ☑
  - axillary I82.A1- ☑ (*following* I82.7)
    - chronic I82.A2- ☑ (*following* I82.7)
  - basilic I82.61- ☑
    - chronic I82.71- ☑
  - brachial I82.62- ☑
    - chronic I82.72- ☑
  - brachiocephalic (innominate) I82.290
    - chronic I82.291
  - cephalic I82.61- ☑
    - chronic I82.71- ☑
  - chronic I82.91
  - deep (DVT) I82.40- ☑
    - calf I82.4Z- ☑
      - chronic I82.5Z- ☑
    - lower leg I82.4Z- ☑
      - chronic I82.5Z- ☑
    - thigh I82.4Y- ☑
      - chronic I82.5Y- ☑
    - upper leg I82.4Y ☑
      - chronic I82.5Y-
  - femoral I82.41- ☑
    - chronic I82.51- ☑
  - iliac (iliofemoral) I82.42- ☑
    - chronic I82.52- ☑
  - innominate I82.290
    - chronic I82.291
  - internal jugular I82.C1- ☑ (*following* I82.7)
    - chronic I82.C2- ☑ (*following* I82.7)
  - lower extremity
    - deep I82.40- ☑
      - chronic I82.50- ☑
      - specified NEC I82.49- ☑
        - chronic NEC I82.59- ☑
    - distal
      - deep I82.4Z- ☑
    - proximal
      - deep I82.4Y- ☑
        - chronic I82.5Y- ☑
    - superficial I82.81- ☑
  - popliteal I82.43- ☑
    - chronic I82.53- ☑
  - radial I82.62- ☑
    - chronic I82.72- ☑
  - renal I82.3
  - saphenous (greater) (lesser) I82.81- ☑
  - specified NEC I82.890
    - chronic NEC I82.891
  - subclavian I82.B1- ☑ (*following* I82.7)
    - chronic I82.B2- ☑ (*following* I82.7)
  - thoracic NEC I82.290
    - chronic I82.291
  - tibial I82.44- ☑
    - chronic I82.54- ☑
  - ulnar I82.62- ☑
    - chronic I82.72- ☑
  - upper extremity I82.60- ☑
    - chronic I82.70- ☑
    - deep I82.62- ☑
      - chronic I82.72- ☑
    - superficial I82.61- ☑
      - chronic I82.71- ☑
  - vena cava
    - inferior (acute) I82.220
      - chronic I82.221
    - superior (acute) I82.210
      - chronic I82.211
  - venous sinus G08
  - vessels of brain — *see* Occlusion, artery, cerebral
- **Embolus** — *see* Embolism
- **Embryoma** (*see also* Neoplasm, uncertain behavior, by site)
  - benign — *see* Neoplasm, benign, by site
  - kidney C64.- ☑
  - liver C22.0
  - malignant (*see also* Neoplasm, malignant, by site)

Embryoma — *continued*
- malignant (*see also* Neoplasm, malignant, by site) — *continued*
  - kidney C64.- ☑
  - liver C22.0
  - testis C62.9- ☑
    - descended (scrotal) C62.1- ☑
    - undescended C62.0- ☑
- testis C62.9- ☑
  - descended (scrotal) C62.1- ☑
  - undescended C62.0- ☑
Embryonic
- circulation Q28.9
- heart Q28.9
- vas deferens Q55.4
Embryopathia NOS Q89.9
Embryotoxon Q13.4
Emesis — *see* Vomiting
Emotional lability R45.86
Emotionality, pathological F60.3
Emotogenic disease — *see* Disorder, psychogenic
Emphysema (atrophic) (bullous) (chronic) (interlobular) (lung) (obstructive) (pulmonary) (senile) (vesicular) J43.9
- cellular tissue (traumatic) T79.7 ☑
  - surgical T81.82 ☑
- centrilobular J43.2
- compensatory J98.3
- congenital (interstitial) P25.0
- conjunctiva H11.89
- connective tissue (traumatic) T79.7 ☑
  - surgical T81.82 ☑
- due to chemicals, gases, fumes or vapors J68.4
- eyelid(s) — *see* Disorder, eyelid, specified type NEC
  - surgical T81.82 ☑
  - traumatic T79.7 ☑
- interstitial J98.2
  - congenital P25.0
  - perinatal period P25.0
- laminated tissue T79.7 ☑
  - surgical T81.82 ☑
- mediastinal J98.2
  - newborn P25.2
- orbit, orbital — *see* Disorder, orbit, specified type NEC
- panacinar J43.1
- panlobular J43.1
- specified NEC J43.8
- subcutaneous (traumatic) T79.7 ☑
  - nontraumatic J98.2
  - postprocedural T81.82 ☑
  - surgical T81.82 ☑
- surgical T81.82 ☑
- thymus (gland) (congenital) E32.8
- traumatic (subcutaneous) T79.7 ☑
- unilateral J43.0
Empty nest syndrome Z60.0
Empyema (acute) (chest) (double) (pleura) (supradiaphragmatic) (thorax) J86.9
- with fistula J86.0
- accessory sinus (chronic) — *see* Sinusitis
- antrum (chronic) — *see* Sinusitis, maxillary
- brain (any part) — *see* Abscess, brain
- ethmoidal (chronic) (sinus) — *see* Sinusitis, ethmoidal
- extradural — *see* Abscess, extradural
- frontal (chronic) (sinus) — *see* Sinusitis, frontal
- gallbladder K81.0
- mastoid (process) (acute) — *see* Mastoiditis, acute
- maxilla, maxillary M27.2
  - sinus (chronic) — *see* Sinusitis, maxillary
- nasal sinus (chronic) — *see* Sinusitis
- sinus (accessory) (chronic) (nasal) — *see* Sinusitis
- sphenoidal (sinus) (chronic) — *see* Sinusitis, sphenoidal
- subarachnoid — *see* Abscess, extradural
- subdural — *see* Abscess, subdural
- tuberculous A15.6
- ureter — *see* Ureteritis
- ventricular — *see* Abscess, brain
En coup de sabre lesion L94.1
Enamel pearls K00.2
Enameloma K00.2
Enanthema, viral B09
Encephalitis (chronic) (hemorrhagic) (idiopathic) (nonepidemic) (spurious) (subacute) G04.90
- acute (*see also* Encephalitis, viral) A86
  - disseminated G04.00
    - infectious G04.01
    - noninfectious G04.81

Encephalitis — *continued*
  acute (*see also* Encephalitis, viral) — *continued*
    disseminated — *continued*
      postimmunization (postvaccination) G04.02
      postinfectious G04.01
    inclusion body A85.8
    necrotizing hemorrhagic G04.30
      postimmunization G04.32
      postinfectious G04.31
      specified NEC G04.39
  arboviral, arbovirus NEC A85.2
  arthropod-borne NEC (viral) A85.2
  Australian A83.4
  California (virus) A83.5
  Central European (tick-borne) A84.1
  Czechoslovakian A84.1
  Dawson's (inclusion body) A81.1
  diffuse sclerosing A81.1
  disseminated, acute G04.00
  due to
    cat scratch disease A28.1
    human immunodeficiency virus (HIV) disease
      B20 [G05.3]
    malaria — *see* Malaria
    rickettsiosis — *see* Rickettsiosis
    smallpox inoculation G04.02
    typhus — *see* Typhus
  Eastern equine A83.2
  endemic (viral) A86
  epidemic NEC (viral) A86
  equine (acute) (infectious) (viral) A83.9
    Eastern A83.2
    Venezuelan A92.2
    Western A83.1
  Far Eastern (tick-borne) A84.0
  following vaccination or other immunization procedure
    G04.02
  herpes zoster B02.0
  herpesviral B00.4
    due to herpesvirus 6 B10.01
    due to herpesvirus 7 B10.09
    specified NEC B10.09
  Ilheus (virus) A83.8
  in (due to)
    actinomycosis A42.82
    adenovirus A85.1
    African trypanosomiasis B56.9 [G05.3]
    Chagas' disease (chronic) B57.42
    cytomegalovirus B25.8
    enterovirus A85.0
    herpes (simplex) virus B00.4
      due to herpesvirus 6 B10.01
      due to herpesvirus 7 B10.09
      specified NEC B10.09
    infectious disease NEC B99 ☑ [G05.3]
    influenza — *see* Influenza, with, encephalopathy
    listeriosis A32.12
    measles B05.0
    mumps B26.2
    naegleriasis B60.2
    parasitic disease NEC B89 [G05.3]
    poliovirus A80.9 [G05.3]
    rubella B06.01
    syphilis
      congenital A50.42
      late A52.14
    systemic lupus erythematosus M32.19
    toxoplasmosis (acquired) B58.2
      congenital P37.1
    tuberculosis A17.82
    zoster B02.0
  inclusion body A81.1
  infectious (acute) (virus) NEC A86
  Japanese (B type) A83.0
  La Crosse A83.5
  lead — *see* Poisoning, lead
  lethargica (acute) (infectious) A85.8
  louping ill A84.8
  lupus erythematosus, systemic M32.19
  lymphatica A87.2
  Mengo A85.8
  meningococcal A39.81
  Murray Valley A83.4
  otitic NEC H66.40 [G05.3]
  parasitic NOS B71.9
  periaxial G37.0
  periaxialis (concentrica) (diffuse) G37.5
  postchickenpox B01.11

Encephalitis — *continued*
  postexanthematous NEC B09
  postimmunization G04.02
  postinfectious NEC G04.01
  postmeasles B05.0
  postvaccinal G04.02
  postvaricella B01.11
  postviral NEC A86
  Powassan A84.8
  Rasmussen G04.81
  Rio Bravo A85.8
  Russian
    autumnal A83.0
    spring-summer (taiga) A84.0
  saturnine — *see* Poisoning, lead
  specified NEC G04.81
  St. Louis A83.3
  subacute sclerosing A81.1
  summer A83.0
  suppurative G04.81
  tick-borne A84.9
  Torula, torular (cryptococcal) B45.1
  toxic NEC G92
  trichinosis B75 [G05.3]
  type
    B A83.0
    C A83.3
  van Bogaert's A81.1
  Venezuelan equine A92.2
  Vienna A85.8
  viral, virus A86
    arthropod-borne NEC A85.2
    mosquito-borne A83.9
      Australian X disease A83.4
      California virus A83.5
      Eastern equine A83.2
      Japanese (B type) A83.0
      Murray Valley A83.4
      specified NEC A83.8
      St. Louis A83.3
      type B A83.0
      type C A83.3
      Western equine A83.1
    tick-borne A84.9
      biundulant A84.1
      central European A84.1
      Czechoslovakian A84.1
      diphasic meningoencephalitis A84.1
      Far Eastern A84.0
      Russian spring-summer (taiga) A84.0
      specified NEC A84.8
    specified type NEC A85.8
  Western equine A83.1
Encephalocele Q01.9
  frontal Q01.0
  nasofrontal Q01.1
  occipital Q01.2
  specified NEC Q01.8
Encephalocystocele — *see* Encephalocele
Encephaloduroarteriomyosynangiosis (EDAMS) I67.5
Encephalomalacia (brain) (cerebellar) (cerebral) — *see*
  Softening, brain
Encephalomeningitis — *see* Meningoencephalitis
Encephalomeningocele — *see* Encephalocele
Encephalomeningomyelitis — *see* Meningoencephalitis
Encephalomyelitis (*see also* Encephalitis) G04.90
  acute disseminated G04.00
    infectious G04.01
    noninfectious G04.81
    postimmunization G04.02
    postinfectious G04.01
  acute necrotizing hemorrhagic G04.30
    postimmunization G04.32
    postinfectious G04.31
    specified NEC G04.39
  benign myalgic G93.3
  equine A83.9
    Eastern A83.2
    Venezuelan A92.2
    Western A83.1
  in diseases classified elsewhere G05.3
  myalgic, benign G93.3
  postchickenpox B01.11
  postinfectious NEC G04.01
  postmeasles B05.0
  postvaccinal G04.02
  postvaricella B01.11
  rubella B06.01

Encephalomyelitis — *continued*
  specified NEC G04.81
  Venezuelan equine A92.2
Encephalomyelocele — *see* Encephalocele
Encephalomyelomeningitis — *see* Meningoencephalitis
Encephalomyelopathy G96.9
Encephalomyeloradiculitis (acute) G61.0
Encephalomyeloradiculoneuritis (acute) (Guillain-
  Barré) G61.0
Encephalomyeloradiculopathy G96.9
Encephalopathia hyperbilirubinemica, newborn
  P57.9
  due to isoimmunization (conditions in P55) P57.0
Encephalopathy (acute) G93.40
  acute necrotizing hemorrhagic G04.30
    postimmunization G04.32
    postinfectious G04.31
    specified NEC G04.39
  alcoholic G31.2
  anoxic — *see* Damage, brain, anoxic
  arteriosclerotic I67.2
  centrolobar progressive (Schilder) G37.0
  congenital Q07.9
  degenerative, in specified disease NEC G32.89
  demyelinating callosal G37.1
  due to
    drugs (*see also* Table of Drugs and Chemicals) G92
  hepatic — *see* Failure, hepatic
  hyperbilirubinemic, newborn P57.9
    due to isoimmunization (conditions in P55) P57.0
  hypertensive I67.4
  hypoglycemic E16.2
  hypoxic — *see* Damage, brain, anoxic
  hypoxic ischemic P91.60
    mild P91.61
    moderate P91.62
    severe P91.63
  in (due to) (with)
    birth injury P11.1
    hyperinsulinism E16.1 [G94]
    influenza — *see* Influenza, with, encephalopathy
    lack of vitamin (*see also* Deficiency, vitamin)
      E56.9 [G32.89]
    neoplastic disease (*see also* Neoplasm) D49.9 [G13.1]
    serum (*see also* Reaction, serum) T80.69 ☑
    syphilis A52.17
    trauma (postconcussional) F07.81
      current injury — *see* Injury, intracranial
    vaccination G04.02
  lead — *see* Poisoning, lead
  metabolic G93.41
    drug induced G92
    toxic G92
  myoclonic, early, symptomatic — *see* Epilepsy, gener-
    alized, specified NEC
  necrotizing, subacute (Leigh) G31.82
  neonatal P91.819
    in diseases classified elsewhere P91.811
  pellagrous E52 [G32.89]
  portosystemic — *see* Failure, hepatic
  postcontusional F07.81
    current injury — *see* Injury, intracranial, diffuse
  posthypoglycemic (coma) E16.1 [G94]
  postradiation G93.89
  saturnine — *see* Poisoning, lead
  septic G93.41
  specified NEC G93.49
  spongiform, subacute (viral) A81.09
  toxic G92
    metabolic G92
  traumatic (postconcussional) F07.81
    current injury — *see* Injury, intracranial
  vitamin B deficiency NEC E53.9 [G32.89]
    vitamin B1 E51.2
  Wernicke's E51.2
Encephalorrhagia — *see* Hemorrhage, intracranial, intracerebral
Encephalosis, posttraumatic F07.81
Enchondroma (*see also* Neoplasm, bone, benign)
Enchondromatosis (cartilaginous) (multiple) Q78.4
Encopresis R15.9
  functional F98.1
  nonorganic origin F98.1
  psychogenic F98.1
Encounter (with health service) (for) Z76.89
  adjustment and management (of)
    breast implant Z45.81 ☑
    implanted device NEC Z45.89

☑ Additional Character Required — Refer to the Tabular List for Character Selection ▽ Subterms under main terms may continue to next column or page

Encounter — *continued*
  adjustment and management — *continued*
    myringotomy device (stent) (tube) Z45.82
  administrative purpose only Z02.9
    examination for
      adoption Z02.82
      armed forces Z02.3
      disability determination Z02.71
      driving license Z02.4
      employment Z02.1
      insurance Z02.6
      medical certificate NEC Z02.79
      paternity testing Z02.81
      residential institution admission Z02.2
      school admission Z02.0
      sports Z02.5
      specified reason NEC Z02.89
  aftercare — *see* Aftercare
  antenatal screening Z36.9
    cervical length Z36.86
    chromosomal anomalies Z36.0
    congenital cardiac abnormalities Z36.83
    elevated maternal serum alphafetoprotein Z36.1
    fetal growth retardation Z36.4
    fetal lung maturity Z36.84
    fetal macrosomia Z36.88
    hydrops fetalis Z36.81
    intrauterine growth restriction (IUGR) /small-for-
        dates Z36.4
    isoimmunization Z36.5
    large-for-dates Z36.88
    malformations Z36.3
    non-visualized anatomy on a previous scan Z36.2
    nuchal translucency Z36.82
    raised alphafetoprotein level Z36.1
    risk of pre-term labor Z36.86
    specified follow-up NEC Z36.2
    specified genetic defects NEC Z36.8A
    specified type NEC Z36.89
    Streptococcus B Z36.85
    suspected anomaly Z36.3
    uncertain dates Z36.87
  assisted reproductive fertility procedure cycle Z31.83
  blood typing Z01.83
    Rh typing Z01.83
  breast augmentation or reduction Z41.1
  breast implant exchange (different material) (different size) Z45.81 ☑
  breast reconstruction following mastectomy Z42.1
  check-up — *see* Examination
  chemotherapy for neoplasm Z51.11
  colonoscopy, screening Z12.11
  counseling — *see* Counseling
  delivery, full-term, uncomplicated O80
    cesarean, without indication O82
  desensitization to allergens Z51.6
  ear piercing Z41.3
  examination — *see* Examination
  expectant parent(s) (adoptive) pre-birth pediatrician visit Z76.81
  fertility preservation procedure (prior to cancer therapy) (prior to removal of gonads) Z31.84
  fitting (of) — *see* Fitting (and adjustment) (of)
  genetic
    counseling
      nonprocreative Z71.83
      procreative Z31.5
    testing — *see* Test, genetic
  hearing conservation and treatment Z01.12
  immunotherapy for neoplasm Z51.12
  in vitro fertilization cycle Z31.83
  instruction (in)
    child care (postpartal) (prenatal) Z32.3
    childbirth Z32.2
    natural family planning
      procreative Z31.61
      to avoid pregnancy Z30.02
  insulin pump titration Z46.81
  joint prosthesis insertion following prior explantation of joint prosthesis (staged procedure)
    hip Z47.32
    knee Z47.33
    shoulder Z47.31
  laboratory (as part of a general medical examination) Z00.00
    with abnormal findings Z00.01
  mental health services (for)
    abuse NEC

Encounter — *continued*
  mental health services — *continued*
    abuse — *continued*
      perpetrator Z69.82
      victim Z69.81
    child abuse
      nonparental
        perpetrator Z69.021
        victim Z69.020
      parental
        perpetrator Z69.011
        victim Z69.010
    child neglect
      nonparental
        perpetrator Z69.021
        victim Z69.020
      parental
        perpetrator Z69.011
        victim Z69.010
    child psychological abuse
      nonparental
        perpetrator Z69.021
        victim Z69.020
      parental
        perpetrator Z69.011
        victim Z69.010
    child sexual abuse
      nonparental
        perpetrator Z69.021
        victim Z69.020
      parental
        perpetrator Z69.011
        victim Z69.010
    non-spousal adult abuse (perpetrator) (victim) Z69.81
    spousal or partner
      abuse
        perpetrator Z69.12
        victim Z69.11
      neglect
        perpetrator Z69.12
        victim Z69.11
      psychological abuse
        perpetrator Z69.12
        victim Z69.11
      violence
        perpetrator (physical) (sexual) Z69.12
        victim (physical) Z69.11
          sexual Z69.81
  observation (for) (ruled out)
    exposure to (suspected)
      anthrax Z03.810
      biological agent NEC Z03.818
  pediatrician visit, by expectant parent(s) (adoptive) Z76.81
  placental sample (taken vaginally) (*see also* Encounter, antenatal screening) Z36.9
  plastic and reconstructive surgery following medical procedure or healed injury NEC Z42.8
  pregnancy
    supervision of — *see* Pregnancy, supervision of
    test Z32.00
      result negative Z32.02
      result positive Z32.01
  procreative management and counseling for gestational carrier Z31.7
  prophylactic measures Z29.9
    antivenin Z29.12
    fluoride administration Z29.3
    immunotherapy for respiratory syncytial virus (RSV) Z29.11
    rabies immune globin Z29.14
    Rho (D) immune globulin Z29.13
    specified NEC Z29.8
  radiation therapy (antineoplastic) Z51.0
  radiological (as part of a general medical examination) Z00.00
    with abnormal findings Z00.01
  reconstructive surgery following medical procedure or healed injury NEC Z42.8
  removal (of) (*see also* Removal)
    artificial
      arm Z44.00- ☑
        complete Z44.01- ☑
        partial Z44.02- ☑
      eye Z44.2- ☑
      leg Z44.10- ☑
        complete Z44.11- ☑

Encounter — *continued*
  removal (*see also* Removal) — *continued*
    artificial — *continued*
      leg — *continued*
        partial Z44.12- ☑
    breast implant Z45.81 ☑
      tissue expander (without synchronous insertion of permanent implant) Z45.81 ☑
    device Z46.9
      specified NEC Z46.89
    external
      fixation device — *code to* fracture with seventh character D
      prosthesis, prosthetic device Z44.9
        breast Z44.3- ☑
        specified NEC Z44.8
    implanted device NEC Z45.89
    insulin pump Z46.81
    internal fixation device Z47.2
    myringotomy device (stent) (tube) Z45.82
    nervous system device NEC Z46.2
      brain neuropacemaker Z46.2
      visual substitution device Z46.2
        implanted Z45.31
    non-vascular catheter Z46.82
    orthodontic device Z46.4
    stent
      ureteral Z46.6
    urinary device Z46.6
  repeat cervical smear to confirm findings of recent normal smear following initial abnormal smear Z01.42
  respirator [ventilator] use during power failure Z99.12
  Rh typing Z01.83
  screening — *see* Screening
  specified NEC Z76.89
  sterilization Z30.2
  suspected condition, ruled out
    amniotic cavity and membrane Z03.71
    cervical shortening Z03.75
    fetal anomaly Z03.73
    fetal growth Z03.74
    maternal and fetal conditions NEC Z03.79
    oligohydramnios Z03.71
    placental problem Z03.72
    polyhydramnios Z03.71
  suspected exposure (to), ruled out
    anthrax Z03.810
    biological agents NEC Z03.818
  termination of pregnancy, elective Z33.2
  testing — *see* Test
  therapeutic drug level monitoring Z51.81
  titration, insulin pump Z46.81
  to determine fetal viability of pregnancy O36.80 ☑
  training
    insulin pump Z46.81
  X-ray of chest (as part of a general medical examination) Z00.00
    with abnormal findings Z00.01
Encystment — *see* Cyst
Endarteritis (bacterial, subacute) (infective) I77.6
  brain I67.7
  cerebral or cerebrospinal I67.7
  deformans — *see* Arteriosclerosis
  embolic — *see* Embolism
  obliterans (*see also* Arteriosclerosis)
    pulmonary I28.8
  pulmonary I28.8
  retina — *see* Vasculitis, retina
  senile — *see* Arteriosclerosis
  syphilitic A52.09
    brain or cerebral A52.04
    congenital A50.54 [I79.8]
  tuberculous A18.89
Endemic — *see* condition
Endocarditis (chronic) (marantic) (nonbacterial) (thrombotic) (valvular) I38
  with rheumatic fever (conditions in I00)
    active — *see* Endocarditis, acute, rheumatic
    inactive or quiescent (with chorea) I09.1
  acute or subacute I33.9
    infective I33.0
    rheumatic (aortic) (mitral) (pulmonary) (tricuspid) I01.1
      with chorea (acute) (rheumatic) (Sydenham's) I02.0
  aortic (heart) (nonrheumatic) (valve) I35.8

▽ Subterms under main terms may continue to next column or page   ☑ Additional Character Required — Refer to the Tabular List for Character Selection   **131**

Encounter — Endocarditis

Endocarditis — continued
  aortic — continued
    with
      mitral disease I08.0
        with tricuspid (valve) disease I08.3
          active or acute I01.1
            with chorea (acute) (rheumatic) (Sydenham's) I02.0
        rheumatic fever (conditions in I00)
          active — see Endocarditis, acute, rheumatic
          inactive or quiescent (with chorea) I06.9
        tricuspid (valve) disease I08.2
          with mitral (valve) disease I08.3
  acute or subacute I33.9
  arteriosclerotic I35.8
  rheumatic I06.9
    with mitral disease I08.0
      with tricuspid (valve) disease I08.3
        active or acute I01.1
          with chorea (acute) (rheumatic) (Sydenham's) I02.0
      active or acute I01.1
        with chorea (acute) (rheumatic) (Sydenham's) I02.0
    specified NEC I06.8
  specified cause NEC I35.8
  syphilitic A52.03
  arteriosclerotic I38
  atypical verrucous (Libman-Sacks) M32.11
  bacterial (acute) (any valve) (subacute) I33.0
  candidal B37.6
  congenital Q24.8
  constrictive I33.0
  Coxiella burnetii A78 [I39]
  Coxsackie B33.21
  due to
    prosthetic cardiac valve T82.6 ☑
    Q fever A78 [I39]
    Serratia marcescens I33.0
    typhoid (fever) A01.02
  gonococcal A54.83
  infectious or infective (acute) (any valve) (subacute) I33.0
  lenta (acute) (any valve) (subacute) I33.0
  Libman-Sacks M32.11
  listerial A32.82
  Löffler's I42.3
  malignant (acute) (any valve) (subacute) I33.0
  meningococcal A39.51
  mitral (chronic) (double) (fibroid) (heart) (inactive) (valve) (with chorea) I05.9
    with
      aortic (valve) disease I08.0
        with tricuspid (valve) disease I08.3
          active or acute I01.1
            with chorea (acute) (rheumatic) (Sydenham's) I02.0
        rheumatic fever (conditions in I00)
          active — see Endocarditis, acute, rheumatic
          inactive or quiescent (with chorea) I05.9
      tricuspid (valve) disease I08.1
        with aortic (valve) disease I08.3
    active or acute I01.1
      with chorea (acute) (rheumatic) (Sydenham's) I02.0
    bacterial I33.0
    arteriosclerotic I34.8
    nonrheumatic I34.8
      acute or subacute I33.9
    specified NEC I05.8
  monilial B37.6
  multiple valves I08.9
    specified disorders I08.8
  mycotic (acute) (any valve) (subacute) I33.0
  pneumococcal (acute) (any valve) (subacute) I33.0
  pulmonary (chronic) (heart) (valve) I37.8
    with rheumatic fever (conditions in I00)
      active — see Endocarditis, acute, rheumatic
      inactive or quiescent (with chorea) I09.89
        with aortic, mitral or tricuspid disease I08.8
    acute or subacute I33.9
      rheumatic I01.1
        with chorea (acute) (rheumatic) (Sydenham's) I02.0
    arteriosclerotic I37.8
    congenital Q22.2
    rheumatic (chronic) (inactive) (with chorea) I09.89
      active or acute I01.1

Endocarditis — continued
  pulmonary — continued
    rheumatic — continued
      active or acute — continued
        with chorea (acute) (rheumatic) (Sydenham's) I02.0
      syphilitic A52.03
  purulent (acute) (any valve) (subacute) I33.0
  Q fever A78 [I39]
  rheumatic (chronic) (inactive) (with chorea) I09.1
    active or acute (aortic) (mitral) (pulmonary) (tricuspid) I01.1
      with chorea (acute) (rheumatic) (Sydenham's) I02.0
  rheumatoid — see Rheumatoid, carditis
  septic (acute) (any valve) (subacute) I33.0
  streptococcal (acute) (any valve) (subacute) I33.0
  subacute — see Endocarditis, acute
  suppurative (acute) (any valve) (subacute) I33.0
  syphilitic A52.03
  toxic I33.9
  tricuspid (chronic) (heart) (inactive) (rheumatic) (valve) (with chorea) I07.9
    with
      aortic (valve) disease I08.2
        mitral (valve) disease I08.3
      mitral (valve) disease I08.1
        aortic (valve) disease I08.3
      rheumatic fever (conditions in I00)
        active — see Endocarditis, acute, rheumatic
        inactive or quiescent (with chorea) I07.8
    active or acute I01.1
      with chorea (acute) (rheumatic) (Sydenham's) I02.0
    arteriosclerotic I36.8
    nonrheumatic I36.8
      acute or subacute I33.9
    specified cause, except rheumatic I36.8
  tuberculous — see Tuberculosis, endocarditis
  typhoid A01.02
  ulcerative (acute) (any valve) (subacute) I33.0
  vegetative (acute) (any valve) (subacute) I33.0
  verrucous (atypical) (nonbacterial) (nonrheumatic) M32.11

Endocardium, endocardial (see also condition)
  cushion defect Q21.2
Endocervicitis (see also Cervicitis)
  due to intrauterine (contraceptive) device T83.69 ☑
  hyperplastic N72
Endocrine — see condition
Endocrinopathy, pluriglandular E31.9
Endodontic
  overfill M27.52
  underfill M27.53
Endodontitis K04.01
  irreversible K04.02
  reversible K04.01
Endomastoiditis — see Mastoiditis
Endometrioma N80.9
Endometriosis N80.9
  appendix N80.5
  bladder N80.8
  bowel N80.5
  broad ligament N80.3
  cervix N80.0
  colon N80.5
  cul-de-sac (Douglas') N80.3
  exocervix N80.0
  fallopian tube N80.2
  female genital organ NEC N80.8
  gallbladder N80.8
  in scar of skin N80.6
  internal N80.0
  intestine N80.5
  lung N80.8
  myometrium N80.0
  ovary N80.1
  parametrium N80.3
  pelvic peritoneum N80.3
  peritoneal (pelvic) N80.3
  rectovaginal septum N80.4
  rectum N80.5
  round ligament N80.3
  skin (scar) N80.6
  specified site NEC N80.8
  stromal D39.0
  thorax N80.8
  umbilicus N80.8

Endometriosis — continued
  uterus (internal) N80.0
  vagina N80.4
  vulva N80.8
Endometritis (decidual) (nonspecific) (purulent) (senile) (atrophic) (suppurative) N71.9
  with ectopic pregnancy O08.0
  acute N71.0
  blenorrhagic (gonococcal) (acute) (chronic) A54.24
  cervix, cervical (with erosion or ectropion) (see also Cervicitis)
    hyperplastic N72
  chlamydial A56.11
  chronic N71.1
  following
    abortion — see Abortion by type complicated by genital infection
    ectopic or molar pregnancy O08.0
  gonococcal, gonorrheal (acute) (chronic) A54.24
  hyperplastic (see also Hyperplasia, endometrial) N85.00
    cervix N72
  puerperal, postpartum, childbirth O86.12
  subacute N71.0
  tuberculous A18.17
Endometrium — see condition
Endomyocardiopathy, South African I42.3
Endomyocarditis — see Endocarditis
Endomyofibrosis I42.3
Endomyometritis — see Endometritis
Endopericarditis — see Endocarditis
Endoperineuritis — see Disorder, nerve
Endophlebitis — see Phlebitis
Endophthalmia — see Endophthalmitis, purulent
Endophthalmitis (acute) (infective) (metastatic) (subacute) H44.009
  bleb associated (see also Bleb, inflamed (infected), postprocedural H59.4 ☑
  gonorrheal A54.39
  in (due to)
    cysticercosis B69.1
    onchocerciasis B73.01
    toxocariasis B83.0
  panuveitis — see Panuveitis
  parasitic H44.12- ☑
  purulent H44.00- ☑
    panophthalmitis — see Panophthalmitis
    vitreous abscess H44.02- ☑
  specified NEC H44.19
  sympathetic — see Uveitis, sympathetic
Endosalpingioma D28.2
Endosalpingiosis N94.89
Endosteitis — see Osteomyelitis
Endothelioma, bone — see Neoplasm, bone, malignant
Endotheliosis (hemorrhagic infectional) D69.8
Endotoxemia — code to condition
Endotrachelitis — see Cervicitis
Engelmann (-Camurati) **syndrome** Q78.3
English disease — see Rickets
Engman's disease L30.3
Engorgement
  breast N64.59
    newborn P83.4
    puerperal, postpartum O92.79
  lung (passive) — see Edema, lung
  pulmonary (passive) — see Edema, lung
  stomach K31.89
  venous, retina — see Occlusion, retina, vein, engorgement
Enlargement, enlarged (see also Hypertrophy)
  adenoids J35.2
    with tonsils J35.3
  alveolar ridge K08.89
    congenital — see Anomaly, alveolar
  apertures of diaphragm (congenital) Q79.1
  gingival K06.1
  heart, cardiac — see Hypertrophy, cardiac
  labium majus, childhood asymmetric (CALME) N90.61
  lacrimal gland, chronic H04.03- ☑
  liver — see Hypertrophy, liver
  lymph gland or node R59.9
    generalized R59.1
    localized R59.0
  orbit H05.34- ☑
  organ or site, congenital NEC — see Anomaly, by site
  parathyroid (gland) E21.0
  pituitary fossa R93.0
  prostate N40.0

Enlargement, enlarged — *continued*
  prostate — *continued*
    with lower urinary tract symptoms (LUTS) N40.1
    without lower urinary tract symtpoms (LUTS) N40.0
  sella turcica R93.0
  spleen — *see* Splenomegaly
  thymus (gland) (congenital) E32.0
  thyroid (gland) — *see* Goiter
  tongue K14.8
  tonsils J35.1
    with adenoids J35.3
  uterus N85.2
  vestibular aqueduct Q16.5
Enophthalmos H05.40- ☑
  due to
    orbital tissue atrophy H05.41- ☑
    trauma or surgery H05.42- ☑
Enostosis M27.8
Entamebic, entamebiasis — *see* Amebiasis
Entanglement
  umbilical cord(s) O69.82 ☑
    with compression O69.2 ☑
    around neck (with compression) O69.81 ☑
      with compression O69.1 ☑
      without compression O69.81 ☑
    of twins in monoamniotic sac O69.2 ☑
    without compression O69.82 ☑
Enteralgia — *see* Pain, abdominal
Enteric — *see* condition
Enteritis (acute) (diarrheal) (hemorrhagic) (noninfective) K52.9
  adenovirus A08.2
  aertrycke infection A02.0
  allergic K52.29
    with
      eosinophilic gastritis or gastroenteritis K52.81
      food protein-induced enterocolitis syndrome K52.21
      food protein-induced enteropathy K52.22
      FPIES K52.21
  amebic (acute) A06.0
    with abscess — *see* Abscess, amebic
    chronic A06.1
      with abscess — *see* Abscess, amebic
      nondysenteric A06.2
    nondysenteric A06.2
  astrovirus A08.32
  bacillary NOS A03.9
  bacterial A04.9
    specified NEC A04.8
  calicivirus A08.31
  candidal B37.82
  Chilomastix A07.8
  choleriformis A00.1
  chronic (noninfectious) K52.9
    ulcerative — *see* Colitis, ulcerative
  cicatrizing (chronic) — *see* Enteritis, regional, small intestine
  Clostridium
    botulinum (food poisoning) A05.1
    difficile
      not specified as recurrent A04.72
      recurrent A04.71
  coccidial A07.3
  coxsackie virus A08.39
  dietetic (*see also* Enteritis, allergic) K52.29
  drug-induced K52.1
  due to
    astrovirus A08.32
    calicivirus A08.31
    coxsackie virus A08.39
    drugs K52.1
    echovirus A08.39
    enterovirus NEC A08.39
    food hypersensitivity (*see also* Enteritis, allergic) K52.29
    infectious organism (bacterial) (viral) — *see* Enteritis, infectious
    torovirus A08.39
    Yersinia enterocolitica A04.6
  echovirus A08.39
  eltor A00.1
  enterovirus NEC A08.39
  eosinophilic K52.81
  epidemic (infectious) A09
  fulminant (*see also* Ischemia, intestine, acute) K55.019
  gangrenous — *see* Enteritis, infectious
  giardial A07.1

Enteritis — *continued*
  infectious NOS A09
    due to
      adenovirus A08.2
      Aerobacter aerogenes A04.8
      Arizona (bacillus) A02.0
      bacteria NOS A04.9
        specified NEC A04.8
      Campylobacter A04.5
      Clostridium difficile
        not specified as recurrent A04.72
        recurrent A04.71
      Clostridium perfringens A04.8
      Enterobacter aerogenes A04.8
      enterovirus A08.39
      Escherichia coli A04.4
        enteroaggregative A04.4
        enterohemorrhagic A04.3
        enteroinvasive A04.2
        enteropathogenic A04.0
        enterotoxigenic A04.1
        specified NEC A04.4
      specified
        bacteria NEC A04.8
        virus NEC A08.39
      Staphylococcus A04.8
      virus NEC A08.4
        specified type NEC A08.39
      Yersinia enterocolitica A04.6
    specified organism NEC A08.8
  influenzal — *see* Influenza, with, digestive manifestations
  ischemic K55.9
    acute (*see also* Ischemia, intestine, acute) K55.019
    chronic K55.1
  microsporidial A07.8
  mucomembranous, myxomembranous — *see* Syndrome, irritable bowel
  mucous — *see* Syndrome, irritable bowel
  necroticans A05.2
  necrotizing of newborn — *see* Enterocolitis, necrotizing, in newborn
  neurogenic — *see* Syndrome, irritable bowel
  newborn necrotizing — *see* Enterocolitis, necrotizing, in newborn
  noninfectious K52.9
  norovirus A08.11
  parasitic NEC B82.9
  paratyphoid (fever) — *see* Fever, paratyphoid
  protozoal A07.9
    specified NEC A07.8
  radiation K52.0
  regional (of) K50.90
    with
      complication K50.919
        abscess K50.914
        fistula K50.913
        intestinal obstruction K50.912
        rectal bleeding K50.911
        specified complication NEC K50.918
    colon — *see* Enteritis, regional, large intestine
    duodenum — *see* Enteritis, regional, small intestine
    ileum — *see* Enteritis, regional, small intestine
    jejunum — *see* Enteritis, regional, small intestine
    large bowel — *see* Enteritis, regional, large intestine
    large intestine (colon) (rectum) K50.10
      with
        complication K50.119
          abscess K50.114
          fistula K50.113
          intestinal obstruction K50.112
          rectal bleeding K50.111
          small intestine (duodenum) (ileum) (jejunum) involvement K50.80
            with
              complication K50.819
                abscess K50.814
                fistula K50.813
                intestinal obstruction K50.812
                rectal bleeding K50.811
                specified complication NEC K50.818
          specified complication NEC K50.118
    rectum — *see* Enteritis, regional, large intestine
    small intestine (duodenum) (ileum) (jejunum) K50.00
      with
        complication K50.019
          abscess K50.014

Enteritis — *continued*
  regional — *continued*
    small intestine — *continued*
      with — *continued*
        complication — *continued*
          fistula K50.013
          intestinal obstruction K50.012
          large intestine (colon) (rectum) involvement K50.80
            with
              complication K50.819
                abscess K50.814
                fistula K50.813
                intestinal obstruction K50.812
                rectal bleeding K50.811
                specified complication NEC K50.818
          rectal bleeding K50.011
          specified complication NEC K50.018
  rotaviral A08.0
  Salmonella, salmonellosis (arizonae) (cholerae-suis) (enteritidis) (typhimurium) A02.0
  segmental — *see* Enteritis, regional
  septic A09
  Shigella — *see* Infection, Shigella
  small round structured NEC A08.19
  spasmodic, spastic — *see* Syndrome, irritable bowel
  staphylococcal A04.8
    due to food A05.0
  torovirus A08.39
  toxic NEC K52.1
    due to Clostridium difficile
      not specified as recurrent A04.72
      recurrent A04.71
  trichomonal A07.8
  tuberculous A18.32
  typhosa A01.00
  ulcerative (chronic) — *see* Colitis, ulcerative
  viral A08.4
    adenovirus A08.2
    enterovirus A08.39
    Rotavirus A08.0
    small round structured NEC A08.19
    specified NEC A08.39
    virus specified NEC A08.39
Enterobiasis B80
Enterobius vermicularis (infection) (infestation) B80
Enterocele (*see also* Hernia, abdomen)
  pelvic, pelvis (acquired) (congenital) N81.5
  vagina, vaginal (acquired) (congenital) NEC N81.5
Enterocolitis (*see also* Enteritis) K52.9
  due to Clostridium difficile
    not specified as recurrent A04.72
    recurrent A04.71
  fulminant ischemic (*see also* Ischemia, intestine, acute) K55.059
  granulomatous — *see* Enteritis, regional
  hemorrhagic (acute) (*see also* Ischemia, intestine, acute) K55.059
    chronic K55.1
  infectious NEC A09
  ischemic K55.9
  necrotizing K55.30
    with
      perforation K55.33
      pneumatosis K55.32
        and perforation K55.33
    due to Clostridium difficile
      not specified as recurrent A04.72
      recurrent A04.71
    in non-newborn K55.30
      stage 1 (without pneumatosis, without perforation) K55.31
      stage 2 (with pneumatosis, without perforation) K55.32
      stage 3 (with pneumatosis, with perforation) K55.33
    in newborn P77.9
      stage 1 (without pneumatosis, without perforation) P77.1
      stage 2 (with pneumatosis, without perforation) P77.2
      stage 3 (with pneumatosis, with perforation) P77.3
    without pneumatosis or perforation K55.31
  noninfectious K52.9
    newborn — *see* Enterocolitis, necrotizing, in newborn

Enterocolitis — *continued*
pseudomembranous (newborn)
not specified as recurrent A04.72
recurrent A04.71
radiation K52.0
newborn — *see* Enterocolitis, necrotizing, in newborn
ulcerative (chronic) — *see* Pancolitis, ulcerative
(chronic)
Enterogastritis — *see* Enteritis
Enteropathy K63.9
celiac-gluten-sensitive K90.0
non-celiac K90.41
food protein-induced enterocolitis (FPIES) K52.22
hemorrhagic, terminal (*see also* Ischemia, intestine,
acute) K55.059
protein-losing K90.49
Enteroperitonitis — *see* Peritonitis
Enteroptosis K63.4
Enterorrhagia K92.2
Enterospasm (*see also* Syndrome, irritable, bowel)
psychogenic F45.8
Enterostenosis (*see also* Obstruction, intestine, specified
NEC) K56.699
Enterostomy
complication — *see* Complication, enterostomy
status Z93.4
Enterovirus, as cause of disease classified elsewhere
B97.10
coxsackievirus B97.11
echovirus B97.12
other specified B97.19
Enthesopathy (peripheral) M77.9
Achilles tendinitis — *see* Tendinitis, Achilles
ankle and tarsus M77.9
specified type NEC — *see* Enthesopathy, foot,
specified type NEC
anterior tibial syndrome M76.81- ☑
calcaneal spur — *see* Spur, bone, calcaneal
elbow region M77.8
lateral epicondylitis — *see* Epicondylitis, lateral
medial epicondylitis — *see* Epicondylitis, medial
foot NEC M77.9
metatarsalgia — *see* Metatarsalgia
specified type NEC M77.5- ☑
forearm M77.9
gluteal tendinitis — *see* Tendinitis, gluteal
hand M77.9
hip — *see* Enthesopathy, lower limb, specified type
NEC
iliac crest spur — *see* Spur, bone, iliac crest
iliotibial band syndrome — *see* Syndrome, iliotibial
band
knee — *see* Enthesopathy, lower limb, lower leg,
specified type NEC
lateral epicondylitis — *see* Epicondylitis, lateral
lower limb (excluding foot) M76.9
Achilles tendinitis — *see* Tendinitis, Achilles
anterior tibial syndrome M76.81- ☑
gluteal tendinitis — *see* Tendinitis, gluteal
iliac crest spur — *see* Spur, bone, iliac crest
iliotibial band syndrome — *see* Syndrome, iliotibial
band
patellar tendinitis — *see* Tendinitis, patellar
pelvic region — *see* Enthesopathy, lower limb,
specified type NEC
peroneal tendinitis — *see* Tendinitis, peroneal
posterior tibial syndrome M76.82- ☑
psoas tendinitis — *see* Tendinitis, psoas
shoulder M77.9
specified type NEC M76.89- ☑
tibial collateral bursitis — *see* Bursitis, tibial collateral
medial epicondylitis — *see* Epicondylitis, medial
metatarsalgia — *see* Metatarsalgia
multiple sites M77.9
patellar tendinitis — *see* Tendinitis, patellar
pelvis M77.9
periarthritis of wrist — *see* Periarthritis, wrist
peroneal tendinitis — *see* Tendinitis, peroneal
posterior tibial syndrome M76.82- ☑
psoas tendinitis — *see* Tendinitis, psoas
shoulder region — *see* Lesion, shoulder
specified site NEC M77.9
specified type NEC M77.8
spinal M46.00
cervical region M46.02

Enthesopathy — *continued*
spinal — *continued*
cervicothoracic region M46.03
lumbar region M46.06
lumbosacral region M46.07
multiple sites M46.09
occipito-atlanto-axial region M46.01
sacrococcygeal region M46.08
thoracic region M46.04
thoracolumbar region M46.05
tibial collateral bursitis — *see* Bursitis, tibial collateral
upper arm M77.9
wrist and carpus NEC M77.8
calcaneal spur — *see* Spur, bone, calcaneal
periarthritis of wrist — *see* Periarthritis, wrist
Entomophobia F40.218
Entomophthoromycosis B46.8
Entrance, air into vein — *see* Embolism, air
Entrapment, nerve — *see* Neuropathy, entrapment
Entropion (eyelid) (paralytic) H02.009
cicatricial H02.019
left H02.016
lower H02.015
upper H02.014
right H02.013
lower H02.012
upper H02.011
congenital Q10.2
left H02.006
lower H02.005
upper H02.004
mechanical H02.029
left H02.026
lower H02.025
upper H02.024
right H02.023
lower H02.022
upper H02.021
right H02.003
lower H02.002
upper H02.001
senile H02.039
left H02.036
lower H02.035
upper H02.034
right H02.033
lower H02.032
upper H02.031
spastic H02.049
left H02.046
lower H02.045
upper H02.044
right H02.043
lower H02.042
upper H02.041
Enucleated eye (traumatic, current) S05.7- ☑
Enuresis R32
functional F98.0
habit disturbance F98.0
nocturnal N39.44
psychogenic F98.0
nonorganic origin F98.0
psychogenic F98.0
Eosinopenia — *see* Agranulocytosis
Eosinophilia (allergic) (hereditary) (idiopathic) (secondary) D72.1
with
angiolymphoid hyperplasia (ALHE) D18.01
infiltrative J82
Löffler's J82
peritoneal — *see* Peritonitis, eosinophilic
pulmonary NEC J82
tropical (pulmonary) J82
Eosinophilia-myalgia syndrome M35.8
Ependymitis (acute) (cerebral) (chronic) (granular) —
see Encephalomyelitis
Ependymoblastoma
specified site — *see* Neoplasm, malignant, by site
unspecified site C71.9
Ependymoma (epithelial) (malignant)
anaplastic
specified site — *see* Neoplasm, malignant, by site
unspecified site C71.9
benign
specified site — *see* Neoplasm, benign, by site
unspecified site D33.2
myxopapillary D43.2

Ependymoma — *continued*
myxopapillary — *continued*
specified site — *see* Neoplasm, uncertain behavior,
by site
unspecified site D43.2
papillary D43.2
specified site — *see* Neoplasm, uncertain behavior,
by site
unspecified site D43.2
specified site — *see* Neoplasm, malignant, by site
unspecified site C71.9
Ependymopathy G93.89
Ephelis, ephelides L81.2
Epiblepharon (congenital) Q10.3
Epicanthus, epicanthic fold (eyelid) (congenital) Q10.3
Epicondylitis (elbow)
lateral M77.1- ☑
medial M77.0- ☑
Epicystitis — *see* Cystitis
Epidemic — *see* condition
Epidermidalization, cervix — *see* Dysplasia, cervix
Epidermis, epidermal — *see* condition
Epidermodysplasia verruciformis B07.8
Epidermolysis
bullosa (congenital) Q81.9
acquired L12.30
drug-induced L12.31
specified cause NEC L12.35
dystrophica Q81.2
letalis Q81.1
simplex Q81.0
specified NEC Q81.8
necroticans combustiformis L51.2
due to drug — *see* Table of Drugs and Chemicals,
by drug
Epidermophytid — *see* Dermatophytosis
Epidermophytosis (infected) — *see* Dermatophytosis
Epididymis — *see* condition
Epididymitis (acute) (nonvenereal) (recurrent) (residual)
N45.1
with orchitis N45.3
blennorrhagic (gonococcal) A54.23
caseous (tuberculous) A18.15
chlamydial A56.19
filarial (*see also* Infestation, filarial) B74.9 [N51]
gonococcal A54.23
syphilitic A52.76
tuberculous A18.15
Epididymo-orchitis (*see also* Epididymitis) N45.3
Epidural — *see* condition
Epigastrium, epigastric — *see* condition
Epigastrocele — *see* Hernia, ventral
Epiglottis — *see* condition
Epiglottitis, epiglottiditis (acute) J05.10
with obstruction J05.11
chronic J37.0
Epignathus Q89.4
Epilepsia partialis continua (*see also* Kozhevnikof's
epilepsy) G40.1- ☑
Epilepsy, epileptic, epilepsia (attack) (cerebral) (convul-
sion) (fit) (seizure) G40.909

> *Note: the following terms are to be considered
> equivalent to intractable: pharmacoresistant
> (pharmacologically resistant), treatment resistant,
> refractory (medically) and poorly controlled*

with
complex partial seizures — *see* Epilepsy, localization-related, symptomatic, with complex
partial seizures
grand mal seizures on awakening — *see* Epilepsy,
generalized, specified NEC
myoclonic absences — *see* Epilepsy, generalized,
specified NEC
myoclonic-astatic seizures — *see* Epilepsy, generalized, specified NEC
simple partial seizures — *see* Epilepsy, localization-
related, symptomatic, with simple partial
seizures
akinetic — *see* Epilepsy, generalized, specified NEC
benign childhood with centrotemporal EEG spikes —
see Epilepsy, localization-related, idiopathic
benign myoclonic in infancy G40.80- ☑
Bravais-jacksonian — *see* Epilepsy, localization-related,
symptomatic, with simple partial seizures

Epilepsy, epileptic, epilepsia — *continued*
childhood
with occipital EEG paroxysms — *see* Epilepsy, localization-related, idiopathic
absence G40.A09 (*following* G40.3)
intractable G40.A19 (*following* G40.3)
with status epilepticus G40.A11 (*following* G40.3)
without status epilepticus G40.A19 (*following* G40.3)
not intractable G40.A09 (*following* G40.3)
with status epilepticus G40.A01 (*following* G40.3)
without status epilepticus G40.A09 (*following* G40.3)
climacteric — *see* Epilepsy, specified NEC
cysticercosis B69.0
deterioration (mental) F06.8
due to syphilis A52.19
focal — *see* Epilepsy, localization-related, symptomatic, with simple partial seizures
generalized
idiopathic G40.309
intractable G40.319
with status epilepticus G40.311
without status epilepticus G40.319
not intractable G40.309
with status epilepticus G40.301
without status epilepticus G40.309
specified NEC G40.409
intractable G40.419
with status epilepticus G40.411
without status epilepticus G40.419
not intractable G40.409
with status epilepticus G40.401
without status epilepticus G40.409
impulsive petit mal — *see* Epilepsy, juvenile myoclonic
intractable G40.919
with status epilepticus G40.911
without status epilepticus G40.919
juvenile absence G40.A09 (*following* G40.3)
intractable G40.A19 (*following* G40.3)
with status epilepticus G40.A11 (*following* G40.3)
without status epilepticus G40.A19 (*following* G40.3)
not intractable G40.A09 (*following* G40.3)
with status epilepticus G40.A01 (*following* G40.3)
without status epilepticus G40.A09 (*following* G40.3)
juvenile myoclonic G40.B09 (*following* G40.3)
intractable G40.B19 (*following* G40.3)
with status epilepticus G40.B11 (*following* G40.3)
without status epilepticus G40.B19 (*following* G40.3)
not intractable G40.B09 (*following* G40.3)
with status epilepticus G40.B01 (*following* G40.3)
without status epilepticus G40.B09 (*following* G40.3)
localization-related (focal) (partial)
idiopathic G40.009
with seizures of localized onset G40.009
intractable G40.019
with status epilepticus G40.011
without status epilepticus G40.019
not intractable G40.009
with status epilepticus G40.001
without status epilepticus G40.009
symptomatic
with complex partial seizures G40.209
intractable G40.219
with status epilepticus G40.211
without status epilepticus G40.219
not intractable G40.209
with status epilepticus G40.201
without status epilepticus G40.209
with simple partial seizures G40.109
intractable G40.119
with status epilepticus G40.111
without status epilepticus G40.119
not intractable G40.109
with status epilepticus G40.101
without status epilepticus G40.109
myoclonus, myoclonic — *see* Epilepsy, generalized, specified NEC
progressive — *see* Epilepsy, generalized, idiopathic
not intractable G40.909
with status epilepticus G40.901
without status epilepticus G40.909

Epilepsy, epileptic, epilepsia — *continued*
on awakening — *see* Epilepsy, generalized, specified NEC
parasitic NOS B71.9 [G94]
partialis continua (*see also* Kozhevnikof's epilepsy) G40.1- ☑
peripheral — *see* Epilepsy, specified NEC
procursiva — *see* Epilepsy, localization-related, symptomatic, with simple partial seizures
progressive (familial) myoclonic — *see* Epilepsy, generalized, idiopathic
reflex — *see* Epilepsy, specified NEC
related to
alcohol G40.509
not intractable G40.509
with status epilepticus G40.501
without status epliepticus G40.509
drugs G40.509
not intractable G40.509
with status epilepticus G40.501
without status epliepticus G40.509
external causes G40.509
not intractable G40.509
with status epilepticus G40.501
without status epliepticus G40.509
hormonal changes G40.509
not intractable G40.509
with status epilepticus G40.501
without status epliepticus G40.509
sleep deprivation G40.509
not intractable G40.509
with status epilepticus G40.501
without status epliepticus G40.509
stress G40.509
not intractable G40.509
with status epilepticus G40.501
without status epliepticus G40.509
somatomotor — *see* Epilepsy, localization-related, symptomatic, with simple partial seizures
somatosensory — *see* Epilepsy, localization-related, symptomatic, with simple partial seizures
spasms G40.822
intractable G40.824
with status epilepticus G40.823
without status epilepticus G40.824
not intractable G40.822
with status epilepticus G40.821
without status epilepticus G40.822
specified NEC G40.802
intractable G40.804
with status epilepticus G40.803
without status epilepticus G40.804
not intractable G40.802
with status epilepticus G40.801
without status epilepticus G40.802
syndromes
generalized
idiopathic G40.309
intractable G40.319
with status epilepticus G40.311
without status epilepticus G40.319
not intractable G40.309
with status epilepticus G40.301
without status epilepticus G40.309
specified NEC G40.409
intractable G40.419
with status epilepticus G40.411
without status epilepticus G40.419
not intractable G40.409
with status epilepticus G40.401
without status epilepticus G40.409
localization-related (focal) (partial)
idiopathic G40.009
with seizures of localized onset G40.009
intractable G40.019
with status epilepticus G40.011
without status epilepticus G40.019
not intractable G40.009
with status epilepticus G40.001
without status epilepticus G40.009
symptomatic
with complex partial seizures G40.209
intractable G40.219
with status epilepticus G40.211
without status epilepticus G40.219
not intractable G40.209
with status epilepticus G40.201
without status epilepticus G40.209

Epilepsy, epileptic, epilepsia — *continued*
syndromes — *continued*
localization-related — *continued*
symptomatic — *continued*
with simple partial seizures G40.109
intractable G40.119
with status epilepticus G40.111
without status epilepticus G40.119
not intractable G40.109
with status epilepticus G40.101
without status epilepticus G40.109
specified NEC G40.802
intractable G40.804
with status epilepticus G40.803
without status epilepticus G40.804
not intractable G40.802
with status epilepticus G40.801
without status epilepticus G40.802
tonic (-clonic) — *see* Epilepsy, generalized, specified NEC
twilight F05
uncinate (gyrus) — *see* Epilepsy, localization-related, symptomatic, with complex partial seizures
Unverricht (-Lundborg) (familial myoclonic) — *see* Epilepsy, generalized, idiopathic
visceral — *see* Epilepsy, specified NEC
visual — *see* Epilepsy, specified NEC
Epiloia Q85.1
Epimenorrhea N92.0
Epipharyngitis — *see* Nasopharyngitis
Epiphora H04.20- ☑
due to
excess lacrimation H04.21- ☑
insufficient drainage H04.22- ☑
Epiphyseal arrest — *see* Arrest, epiphyseal
Epiphyseolysis, epiphysiolysis — *see* Osteochondropathy
Epiphysitis (*see also* Osteochondropathy)
juvenile M92.9
syphilitic (congenital) A50.02
Epiplocele — *see* Hernia, abdomen
Epiploitis — *see* Peritonitis
Epiplosarcomphalocele — *see* Hernia, umbilicus
Episcleritis (suppurative) H15.10- ☑
in (due to)
syphilis A52.71
tuberculosis A18.51
nodular H15.12- ☑
periodica fugax H15.11- ☑
angioneurotic — *see* Edema, angioneurotic
syphilitic (late) A52.71
tuberculous A18.51
Episode
affective, mixed F39
depersonalization (in neurotic state) F48.1
depressive F32.9
major F32.9
mild F32.0
moderate F32.1
severe (without psychotic symptoms) F32.2
with psychotic symptoms F32.3
recurrent F33.9
brief F33.8
specified NEC F32.89
hypomanic F30.8
manic F30.9
with
psychotic symptoms F30.2
remission (full) F30.4
partial F30.3
other specified F30.8
recurrent F31.89
without psychotic symptoms F30.10
mild F30.11
moderate F30.12
severe (without psychotic symptoms) F30.13
with psychotic symptoms F30.2
psychotic F23
organic F06.8
schizophrenic (acute) NEC, brief F23
Epispadias (female) (male) Q64.0
Episplenitis D73.89
Epistaxis (multiple) R04.0
hereditary I78.0
vicarious menstruation N94.89
Epithelioma (malignant) (*see also* Neoplasm, malignant, by site)
adenoides cysticum — *see* Neoplasm, skin, benign

Epithelioma — *continued*
  basal cell — *see* Neoplasm, skin, malignant
  benign — *see* Neoplasm, benign, by site
  Bowen's — *see* Neoplasm, skin, in situ
  calcifying, of Malherbe — *see* Neoplasm, skin, benign
  external site — *see* Neoplasm, skin, malignant
  intraepidermal, Jadassohn — *see* Neoplasm, skin, benign
  squamous cell — *see* Neoplasm, malignant, by site
Epitheliomatosis pigmented Q82.1
Epitheliopathy, multifocal placoid pigment H30.14- ☑
Epithelium, epithelial — *see* condition
Epituberculosis (with atelectasis) (allergic) A15.7
Eponychia Q84.6
Epstein's
  nephrosis or syndrome — *see* Nephrosis
  pearl K09.8
Epulis (gingiva) (fibrous) (giant cell) K06.8
Equinia A24.0
Equinovarus (congenital) (talipes) Q66.0
  acquired — *see* Deformity, limb, clubfoot
Equivalent
  convulsive (abdominal) — *see* Epilepsy, specified NEC
  epileptic (psychic) — *see* Epilepsy, localization-related, symptomatic, with complex partial seizures
Erb (-Duchenne) **paralysis** (birth injury) (newborn) P14.0
Erb-Goldflam disease or syndrome G70.00
  with exacerbation (acute) G70.01
  in crisis G70.01
Erb's
  disease G71.02
  palsy, paralysis (brachial) (birth) (newborn) P14.0
    spinal (spastic) syphilitic A52.17
  pseudohypertrophic muscular dystrophy G71.02
Erdheim's syndrome (acromegalic macrospondylitis) E22.0
Erection, painful (persistent) — *see* Priapism
Ergosterol deficiency (vitamin D) E55.9
  with
    adult osteomalacia M83.8
    rickets — *see* Rickets
Ergotism (*see also* Poisoning, food, noxious, plant)
  from ergot used as drug (migraine therapy) — *see* Table of Drugs and Chemicals
Erosio interdigitalis blastomycetica B37.2
Erosion
  artery I77.2
    without rupture I77.89
  bone — *see* Disorder, bone, density and structure, specified NEC
  bronchus J98.09
  cartilage (joint) — *see* Disorder, cartilage, specified type NEC
  cervix (uteri) (acquired) (chronic) (congenital) N86
    with cervicitis N72
  cornea (nontraumatic) — *see* Ulcer, cornea
    recurrent H18.83- ☑
    traumatic — *see* Abrasion, cornea
  dental (idiopathic) (occupational) (due to diet, drugs or vomiting) K03.2
  duodenum, postpyloric — *see* Ulcer, duodenum
  esophagus K22.10
    with bleeding K22.11
  gastric — *see* Ulcer, stomach
  gastrojejunal — *see* Ulcer, gastrojejunal
  implanted mesh — *see* Complications, mesh
  intestine K63.3
  lymphatic vessel I89.8
  pylorus, pyloric (ulcer) — *see* Ulcer, stomach
  spine, aneurysmal A52.09
  stomach — *see* Ulcer, stomach
  subcutaneous device pocket
    nervous system prosthetic device, implant, or graft T85.890 ☑
    other internal prosthetic device, implant, or graft T85.898 ☑
  teeth (idiopathic) (occupational) (due to diet, drugs or vomiting) K03.2
  urethra N36.8
  uterus N85.8
Erotomania F52.8
Error
  metabolism, inborn — *see* Disorder, metabolism
  refractive — *see* Disorder, refraction
Eructation R14.2
  nervous or psychogenic F45.8

Eruption
  creeping B76.9
  drug (generalized) (taken internally) L27.0
    fixed L27.1
    in contact with skin — *see* Dermatitis, due to drugs
    localized L27.1
  Hutchinson, summer L56.4
  Kaposi's varicelliform B00.0
  napkin L22
  polymorphous light (sun) L56.4
  recalcitrant pustular L13.8
  ringed R23.8
  skin (nonspecific) R21
    creeping (meaning hookworm) B76.9
    due to inoculation/vaccination (generalized) (*see also* Dermatitis, due to, vaccine) L27.0
      localized L27.1
    erysipeloid A26.0
    feigned L98.1
    Kaposi's varicelliform B00.0
    lichenoid L28.0
    meaning dermatitis — *see* Dermatitis
    toxic NEC L53.0
  tooth, teeth, abnormal (incomplete) (late) (premature) (sequence) K00.6
  vesicular R23.8
Erysipelas (gangrenous) (infantile) (newborn) (phlegmonous) (suppurative) A46
  external ear A46 [H62.40]
  puerperal, postpartum O86.89
Erysipeloid A26.9
  cutaneous (Rosenbach's) A26.0
  disseminated A26.8
  sepsis A26.7
  specified NEC A26.8
Erythema, erythematous (infectional) (inflammation) L53.9
  ab igne L59.0
  annulare (centrifugum) (rheumaticum) L53.1
  arthriticum epidemicum A25.1
  brucellum — *see* Brucellosis
  chronic figurate NEC L53.3
  chronicum migrans (Borrelia burgdorferi) A69.20
  diaper L22
  due to
    chemical NEC L53.0
      in contact with skin L24.5
    drug (internal use) — *see* Dermatitis, due to, drugs
  elevatum diutinum L95.1
  endemic E52
  epidemic, arthritic A25.1
  figuratum perstans L53.3
  gluteal L22
  heat — *code by site under* Burn, first degree
  ichthyosiforme congenitum bullous Q80.3
  in diseases classified elsewhere L54
  induratum (nontuberculous) L52
    tuberculous A18.4
  infectiosum B08.3
  intertrigo L30.4
  iris L51.9
  marginatum L53.2
    in (due to) acute rheumatic fever I00
  medicamentosum — *see* Dermatitis, due to, drugs
  migrans A26.0
    chronicum A69.20
    tongue K14.1
  multiforme (major) (minor) L51.9
    bullous, bullosum L51.1
    conjunctiva L51.1
    nonbullous L51.0
    pemphigoides L12.0
    specified NEC L51.8
  napkin L22
  neonatorum P83.88
    toxic P83.1
  nodosum L52
    tuberculous A18.4
  palmar L53.8
  pernio T69.1 ☑
  rash, newborn P83.88
  scarlatiniform (recurrent) (exfoliative) L53.8
  solare L55.0
  specified NEC L53.8
  toxic, toxicum NEC L53.0
    newborn P83.1
  tuberculous (primary) A18.4
Erythematous, erythematosus — *see* condition

Erythermalgia (primary) I73.81
Erythralgia I73.81
Erythrasma L08.1
Erythredema (polyneuropathy) — *see* Poisoning, mercury
Erythremia (acute) C94.0- ☑
  chronic D45
  secondary D75.1
Erythroblastopenia (*see also* Aplasia, red cell) D60.9
  congenital D61.01
Erythroblastophthisis D61.09
Erythroblastosis (fetalis) (newborn) P55.9
  due to
    ABO (antibodies) (incompatibility) (isoimmunization) P55.1
    Rh (antibodies) (incompatibility) (isoimmunization) P55.0
Erythrocyanosis (crurum) I73.89
Erythrocythemia — *see* Erythremia
Erythrocytosis (megalosplenic) (secondary) D75.1
  familial D75.0
  oval, hereditary — *see* Elliptocytosis
  secondary D75.1
  stress D75.1
Erythroderma (secondary) (*see also* Erythema) L53.9
  bullous ichthyosiform, congenital Q80.3
  desquamativum L21.1
  ichthyosiform, congenital (bullous) Q80.3
  neonatorum P83.88
  psoriaticum L40.8
Erythrodysesthesia, palmar plantar (PPE) L27.1
Erythrogenesis imperfecta D61.09
Erythroleukemia C94.0- ☑
Erythromelalgia I73.81
Erythrophagocytosis D75.89
Erythrophobia F40.298
Erythroplakia, oral epithelium, and tongue K13.29
Erythroplasia (Queyrat) D07.4
  specified site — *see* Neoplasm, skin, in situ
  unspecified site D07.4
Escherichia coli (E. coli), **as cause of disease classified elsewhere** B96.20
  non-O157 Shiga toxin-producing (with known O group) B96.22
  non-Shiga toxin-producing B96.29
  O157 with confirmation of Shiga toxin when H antigen is unknown, or is not H7 B96.21
  O157:H- (nonmotile) with confirmation of Shiga toxin B96.21
  O157:H7 with or without confirmation of Shiga toxin-production B96.21
    specified NEC B96.22-
  Shiga toxin-producing (with unspecified O group) (STEC) B96.23
  O157 B96.21
  specified NEC B96.29
Esophagismus K22.4
Esophagitis (acute) (alkaline) (chemical) (chronic) (infectional) (necrotic) (peptic) (postoperative) K20.9
  candidal B37.81
  due to gastrointestinal reflux disease K21.0
  eosinophilic K20.0
  reflux K21.0
  specified NEC K20.8
  tuberculous A18.83
  ulcerative K22.10
    with bleeding K22.11
Esophagocele K22.5
Esophagomalacia K22.8
Esophagospasm K22.4
Esophagostenosis K22.2
Esophagostomiasis B81.8
Esophagotracheal — *see* condition
Esophagus — *see* condition
Esophoria H50.51
  convergence, excess H51.12
  divergence, insufficiency H51.8
Esotropia — *see* Strabismus, convergent concomitant
Espundia B55.2
Essential — *see* condition
Esthesioneuroblastoma C30.0
Esthesioneurocytoma C30.0
Esthesioneuroepithelioma C30.0
Esthiomene A55
Estivo-autumnal malaria (fever) B50.9
Estrangement (marital) Z63.5
  parent-child NEC Z62.890

Estriasis — *see* Myiasis
Ethanolism — *see* Alcoholism
Etherism — *see* Dependence, drug, inhalant
Ethmoid, ethmoidal — *see* condition
Ethmoiditis (chronic) (nonpurulent) (purulent) (*see also* Sinusitis, ethmoidal)
 influenzal — *see* Influenza, with, respiratory manifestations NEC
 Woakes' J33.1
Ethylism — *see* Alcoholism
Eulenburg's disease (congenital paramyotonia) G71.19
Eumycetoma B47.0
Eunuchoidism E29.1
 hypogonadotropic E23.0
European blastomycosis — *see* Cryptococcosis
Eustachian — *see* condition
Evaluation (for) (of)
 development state
  adolescent Z00.3
  period of
   delayed growth in childhood Z00.70
    with abnormal findings Z00.71
   rapid growth in childhood Z00.2
   puberty Z00.3
 growth and developmental state (period of rapid growth) Z00.2
  delayed growth Z00.70
   with abnormal findings Z00.71
 mental health (status) Z00.8
  requested by authority Z04.6
 period of
  delayed growth in childhood Z00.70
   with abnormal findings Z00.71
  rapid growth in childhood Z00.2
 suspected condition — *see* Observation
Evans syndrome D69.41
Event
 apparent life threatening in newborn and infant (ALTE) R68.13
 brief resolved unexplained event (BRUE) R68.13
Eventration (*see also* Hernia, ventral)
 colon into chest — *see* Hernia, diaphragm
 diaphragm (congenital) Q79.1
Eversion
 bladder N32.89
 cervix (uteri) N86
  with cervicitis N72
 foot NEC (*see also* Deformity, valgus, ankle)
  congenital Q66.6
 punctum lacrimale (postinfectional) (senile) H04.52- ☑
 ureter (meatus) N28.89
 urethra (meatus) N36.8
 uterus N81.4
Evidence
 cytologic
  of malignancy on anal smear R85.614
  of malignancy on cervical smear R87.614
  of malignancy on vaginal smear R87.624
Evisceration
 birth injury P15.8
 traumatic NEC
  eye — *see* Enucleated eye
Evulsion — *see* Avulsion
Ewing's sarcoma or tumor — *see* Neoplasm, bone, malignant
Examination (for) (following) (general) (of) (routine) Z00.00
 with abnormal findings Z00.01
 abuse, physical (alleged), ruled out
  adult Z04.71
  child Z04.72
 adolescent (development state) Z00.3
 alleged rape or sexual assault (victim), ruled out
  adult Z04.41
  child Z04.42
 allergy Z01.82
 annual (adult) (periodic) (physical) Z00.00
  with abnormal findings Z00.01
  gynecological Z01.419
   with abnormal findings Z01.411
 antibody response Z01.84
 blood — *see* Examination, laboratory
 blood pressure Z01.30
  with abnormal findings Z01.31
 cancer staging — *see* Neoplasm, malignant, by site
 cervical Papanicolaou smear Z12.4
  as part of routine gynecological examination Z01.419

Examination — *continued*
 cervical Papanicolaou smear — *continued*
  as part of routine gynecological examination — *continued*
   with abnormal findings Z01.411
 child (over 28 days old) Z00.129
  with abnormal findings Z00.121
  under 28 days old — *see* Newborn, examination
 clinical research control or normal comparison (control) (participant) Z00.6
 contraceptive (drug) maintenance (routine) Z30.8
  device (intrauterine) Z30.431
 dental Z01.20
  with abnormal findings Z01.21
 developmental — *see* Examination, child
 donor (potential) Z00.5
 ear Z01.10
  with abnormal findings NEC Z01.118
 eye Z01.00
  with abnormal findings Z01.01
 follow-up (routine) (following) Z09
  chemotherapy NEC Z09
   malignant neoplasm Z08
  fracture Z09
  malignant neoplasm Z08
  postpartum Z39.2
  psychotherapy Z09
  radiotherapy NEC Z09
   malignant neoplasm Z08
  surgery NEC Z09
   malignant neoplasm Z08
 following
  accident NEC Z04.3
   transport Z04.1
   work Z04.2
  assault, alleged, ruled out
   adult Z04.71
   child Z04.72
  motor vehicle accident Z04.1
  treatment (for) Z09
   combined NEC Z09
    fracture Z09
    malignant neoplasm Z08
   malignant neoplasm Z08
   mental disorder Z09
   specified condition NEC Z09
 forced sexual exploitation Z04.81
 forced labor exploitation Z04.82
 gynecological Z01.419
  with abnormal findings Z01.411
  for contraceptive maintenance Z30.8
 health — *see* Examination, medical
 hearing Z01.10
  with abnormal findings NEC Z01.118
  following failed hearing screening Z01.110
  infant or child (over 28 days old) Z00.129
   with abnormal findings Z00.121
 immunity status testing Z01.84
 laboratory (as part of a general medical examination) Z00.00
  with abnormal findings Z00.01
  preprocedural Z01.812
 lactating mother Z39.1
 medical (adult) (for) (of) Z00.00
  with abnormal findings Z00.01
  administrative purpose only Z02.9
   specified NEC Z02.89
  admission to
   armed forces Z02.3
   old age home Z02.2
   prison Z02.89
   residential institution Z02.2
   school Z02.0
    following illness or medical treatment Z02.0
   summer camp Z02.89
  adoption Z02.82
  blood alcohol or drug level Z02.83
  camp (summer) Z02.89
  clinical research, normal subject (control) (participant) Z00.6
  control subject in clinical research (normal comparison) (participant) Z00.6
  donor (potential) Z00.5
  driving license Z02.4
  general (adult) Z00.00
   with abnormal findings Z00.01
  immigration Z02.89
  insurance purposes Z02.6
  marriage Z02.89

Examination — *continued*
 medical — *continued*
  medicolegal reasons NEC Z04.89
  naturalization Z02.89
  participation in sport Z02.5
  paternity testing Z02.81
  population survey Z00.8
  pre-employment Z02.1
  pre-operative — *see* Examination, pre-procedural
  pre-procedural
   cardiovascular Z01.810
   respiratory Z01.811
   specified NEC Z01.818
  preschool children
   for admission to school Z02.0
  prisoners
   for entrance into prison Z02.89
  recruitment for armed forces Z02.3
  specified NEC Z00.8
  sport competition Z02.5
 medicolegal reason NEC Z04.89
  following
   forced sexual exploitation Z04.81
   forced labor exploitation Z04.82
 newborn — *see* Newborn, examination
 pelvic (annual) (periodic) Z01.419
  with abnormal findings Z01.411
 period of rapid growth in childhood Z00.2
 periodic (adult) (annual) (routine) Z00.00
  with abnormal findings Z00.01
 physical (adult) (*see also* Examination, medical) Z00.00
  sports Z02.5
 postpartum
  immediately after delivery Z39.0
  routine follow-up Z39.2
 pre-chemotherapy (antineoplastic) Z01.818
 prenatal (normal pregnancy) (*see also* Pregnancy, normal) Z34.9- ☑
 pre-procedural (pre-operative)
  cardiovascular Z01.810
  laboratory Z01.812
  respiratory Z01.811
  specified NEC Z01.818
 prior to chemotherapy (antineoplastic) Z01.818
 psychiatric NEC Z00.8
  follow-up not needing further care Z09
  requested by authority Z04.6
 radiological (as part of a general medical examination) Z00.00
  with abnormal findings Z00.01
 repeat cervical smear to confirm findings of recent normal smear following initial abnormal smear Z01.42
 skin (hypersensitivity) Z01.82
 special (*see also* Examination, by type) Z01.89
  specified type NEC Z01.89
 specified type or reason NEC Z04.89
 teeth Z01.20
  with abnormal findings Z01.21
 urine — *see* Examination, laboratory
 vision Z01.00
  with abnormal findings Z01.01
  infant or child (over 28 days old) Z00.129
   with abnormal findings Z00.121
Exanthem, exanthema (*see also* Rash)
 with enteroviral vesicular stomatitis B08.4
 Boston A88.0
 epidemic with meningitis A88.0 [G02]
 subitum B08.20
  due to human herpesvirus 6 B08.21
  due to human herpesvirus 7 B08.22
 viral, virus B09
  specified type NEC B08.8
Excess, excessive, excessively
 alcohol level in blood R78.0
 androgen (ovarian) E28.1
 attrition, tooth, teeth K03.0
 carotene, carotin (dietary) E67.1
 cold, effects of T69.9 ☑
  specified effect NEC T69.8 ☑
 convergence H51.12
 crying
  in child, adolescent, or adult R45.83
  in infant R68.11
 development, breast N62
 divergence H51.8
 drinking (alcohol) NEC (without dependence) F10.10
  habitual (continual) (without remission) F10.20

Excess, excessive, excessively — *continued*
eating R63.2
estrogen E28.0
fat (*see also* Obesity)
  in heart — *see* Degeneration, myocardial
  localized E65
foreskin N47.8
gas R14.0
glucagon E16.3
heat — *see* Heat
intermaxillary vertical dimension of fully erupted teeth M26.37
interocclusal distance of fully erupted teeth M26.37
kalium E87.5
large
  colon K59.39
    congenital Q43.8
  infant P08.0
  organ or site, congenital NEC — *see* Anomaly, by site
long
  organ or site, congenital NEC — *see* Anomaly, by site
menstruation (with regular cycle) N92.0
  with irregular cycle N92.1
napping Z72.821
natrium E87.0
number of teeth K00.1
nutrient (dietary) NEC R63.2
potassium (K) E87.5
salivation K11.7
secretion (*see also* Hypersecretion)
  milk O92.6
  sputum R09.3
  sweat R61
sexual drive F52.8
short
  organ or site, congenital NEC — *see* Anomaly, by site
  umbilical cord in labor or delivery O69.3 ☑
skin L98.7
  and subcutaneous tissue L98.7
  eyelid (acquired) — *see* Blepharochalasis
    congenital Q10.3
sodium (Na) E87.0
spacing of fully erupted teeth M26.32
sputum R09.3
sweating R61
thirst R63.1
  due to deprivation of water T73.1 ☑
tuberosity of jaw M26.07
vitamin
  A (dietary) E67.0
    administered as drug (prolonged intake) — *see* Table of Drugs and Chemicals, vitamins, adverse effect
    overdose or wrong substance given or taken — *see* Table of Drugs and Chemicals, vitamins, poisoning
  D (dietary) E67.3
    administered as drug (prolonged intake) — *see* Table of Drugs and Chemicals, vitamins, adverse effect
    overdose or wrong substance given or taken — *see* Table of Drugs and Chemicals, vitamins, poisoning
weight
  gain R63.5
  loss R63.4

Excitability, abnormal, under minor stress (personality disorder) F60.3

Excitation
anomalous atrioventricular I45.6
psychogenic F30.8
reactive (from emotional stress, psychological trauma) F30.8

Excitement
hypomanic F30.8
manic F30.9
mental, reactive (from emotional stress, psychological trauma) F30.8
state, reactive (from emotional stress, psychological trauma) F30.8

Excoriation (traumatic) (*see also* Abrasion)
neurotic L98.1
skin picking disorder F42.4

Exfoliation
due to erythematous conditions according to extent of body surface involved L49.0
  10-19 percent of body surface L49.1
  20-29 percent of body surface L49.2
  30-39 percent of body surface L49.3
  40-49 percent of body surface L49.4
  50-59 percent of body surface L49.5
  60-69 percent of body surface L49.6
  70-79 percent of body surface L49.7
  80-89 percent of body surface L49.8
  90-99 percent of body surface L49.9
  less than 10 percent of body surface L49.0
teeth, due to systemic causes K08.0

Exfoliative — *see* condition

Exhaustion, exhaustive (physical NEC) R53.83
battle F43.0
cardiac — *see* Failure, heart
delirium F43.0
due to
  cold T69.8 ☑
  excessive exertion T73.3 ☑
  exposure T73.2 ☑
  neurasthenia F48.8
heart — *see* Failure, heart
heat (*see also* Heat, exhaustion) T67.5 ☑
  due to
    salt depletion T67.4 ☑
    water depletion T67.3 ☑
maternal, complicating delivery O75.81
mental F48.8
myocardium, myocardial — *see* Failure, heart
nervous F48.8
old age R54
psychogenic F48.8
psychosis F43.0
senile R54
vital NEC Z73.0

Exhibitionism F65.2

Exocervicitis — *see* Cervicitis

Exomphalos Q79.2
meaning hernia — *see* Hernia, umbilicus

Exophoria H50.52
convergence, insufficiency H51.11
divergence, excess H51.8

Exophthalmos H05.2- ☑
congenital Q15.8
constant NEC H05.24- ☑
displacement, globe — *see* Displacement, globe
due to thyrotoxicosis (hyperthyroidism) — *see* Hyperthyroidism, with, goiter (diffuse)
dysthyroid — *see* Hyperthyroidism, with, goiter (diffuse)
goiter — *see* Hyperthyroidism, with, goiter (diffuse)
intermittent NEC H05.25- ☑
malignant — *see* Hyperthyroidism, with, goiter (diffuse)
orbital
  edema — *see* Edema, orbit
  hemorrhage — *see* Hemorrhage, orbit
pulsating NEC H05.26- ☑
thyrotoxic, thyrotropic — *see* Hyperthyroidism, with, goiter (diffuse)

Exostosis (*see also* Disorder, bone)
cartilaginous — *see* Neoplasm, bone, benign
congenital (multiple) Q78.6
external ear canal H61.81- ☑
gonococcal A54.49
jaw (bone) M27.8
multiple, congenital Q78.6
orbit H05.35- ☑
osteocartilaginous — *see* Neoplasm, bone, benign
syphilitic A52.77

Exotropia — *see* Strabismus, divergent concomitant

Explanation of
investigation finding Z71.2
medication Z71.89

Exposure (to) (*see also* Contact, with) T75.89 ☑
acariasis Z20.7
AIDS virus Z20.6
air pollution Z77.110
algae and algae toxins Z77.121
algae bloom Z77.121
anthrax Z20.810
aromatic amines Z77.020
aromatic (hazardous) compounds NEC Z77.028
aromatic dyes NOS Z77.028
arsenic Z77.010

Exposure — *continued*
asbestos Z77.090
bacterial disease NEC Z20.818
benzene Z77.021
blue-green algae bloom Z77.121
body fluids (potentially hazardous) Z77.21
brown tide Z77.121
chemicals (chiefly nonmedicinal) (hazardous) NEC Z77.098
cholera Z20.09
chromium compounds Z77.018
cold, effects of T69.9 ☑
  specified effect NEC T69.8 ☑
communicable disease Z20.9
  bacterial NEC Z20.818
  specified NEC Z20.89
  viral NEC Z20.828
  Zika virus Z20.821
cyanobacteria bloom Z77.121
disaster Z65.5
discrimination Z60.5
dyes Z77.098
effects of T73.9 ☑
environmental tobacco smoke (acute) (chronic) Z77.22
Escherichia coli (E. coli) Z20.01
exhaustion due to T73.2 ☑
fiberglass — *see* Table of Drugs and Chemicals, fiberglass
German measles Z20.4
gonorrhea Z20.2
hazardous metals NEC Z77.018
hazardous substances NEC Z77.29
hazards in the physical environment NEC Z77.128
hazards to health NEC Z77.9
human immunodeficiency virus (HIV) Z20.6
human T-lymphotropic virus type-1 (HTLV-1) Z20.89
implanted
  mesh — *see* Complications, mesh
  prosthetic materials NEC — *see* Complications, prosthetic materials NEC
infestation (parasitic) NEC Z20.7
intestinal infectious disease NEC Z20.09
  Escherichia coli (E. coli) Z20.01
lead Z77.011
meningococcus Z20.811
mold (toxic) Z77.120
nickel dust Z77.018
noise Z77.122
occupational
  air contaminants NEC Z57.39
  dust Z57.2
  environmental tobacco smoke Z57.31
  extreme temperature Z57.6
  noise Z57.0
  radiation Z57.1
  risk factors Z57.9
    specified NEC Z57.8
  toxic agents (gases) (liquids) (solids) (vapors) in agriculture Z57.4
  toxic agents (gases) (liquids) (solids) (vapors) in industry NEC Z57.5
  vibration Z57.7
parasitic disease NEC Z20.7
pediculosis Z20.7
persecution Z60.5
pfiesteria piscicida Z77.121
poliomyelitis Z20.89
pollution
  air Z77.110
  environmental NEC Z77.118
  soil Z77.112
  water Z77.111
polycyclic aromatic hydrocarbons Z77.028
prenatal (drugs) (toxic chemicals) — *see* Newborn, affected by, noxious substances transmitted via placenta or breast milk
rabies Z20.3
radiation, naturally occurring NEC Z77.123
radon Z77.123
red tide (Florida) Z77.121
rubella Z20.4
second hand tobacco smoke (acute) (chronic) Z77.22
  in the perinatal period P96.81
sexually-transmitted disease Z20.2
smallpox (laboratory) Z20.89
syphilis Z20.2
terrorism Z65.4
torture Z65.4

Exposure — continued
tuberculosis Z20.1
uranium Z77.012
varicella Z20.820
venereal disease Z20.2
viral disease NEC Z20.828
war Z65.5
water pollution Z77.111
Zika virus Z20.821

Exsanguination — *see* Hemorrhage

Exstrophy
abdominal contents Q45.8
bladder Q64.10
cloacal Q64.12
specified type NEC Q64.19
supravesical fissure Q64.11

Extensive — *see* condition

Extra (*see also* Accessory)
marker chromosomes (normal individual) Q92.61
in abnormal individual Q92.62
rib Q76.6
cervical Q76.5

Extrasystoles (supraventricular) I49.49
atrial I49.1
auricular I49.1
junctional I49.2
ventricular I49.3

Extrauterine gestation or pregnancy — *see* Pregnancy, by site

Extravasation
blood R58
chyle into mesentery I89.8
pelvicalyceal N13.8
pyelosinus N13.8
urine (from ureter) R39.0
vesicant agent
antineoplastic chemotherapy T80.810 ☑
other agent NEC T80.818 ☑

Extremity — *see* condition, limb

Extrophy — *see* Exstrophy

Extroversion
bladder Q64.19
uterus N81.4
complicating delivery O71.2
postpartal (old) N81.4

Extruded tooth (teeth) M26.34

Extrusion
breast implant (prosthetic) T85.42 ☑
eye implant (globe) (ball) T85.328 ☑
intervertebral disc — *see* Displacement, intervertebral disc
ocular lens implant (prosthetic) — *see* Complications, intraocular lens
vitreous — *see* Prolapse, vitreous

Exudate
pleural — *see* Effusion, pleura
retina H35.89

Exudative — *see* condition

Eye, eyeball, eyelid — *see* condition

Eyestrain — *see* Disturbance, vision, subjective

Eyeworm disease of Africa B74.3

F

Faber's syndrome (achlorhydric anemia) D50.9
Fabry (-Anderson) **disease** E75.21
Faciocephalalgia, autonomic (*see also* Neuropathy, peripheral, autonomic) G90.09
Factor(s)
psychic, associated with diseases classified elsewhere F54
psychological
affecting physical conditions F54
or behavioral
affecting general medical condition F54
associated with disorders or diseases classified elsewhere F54

Fahr disease (of brain) G23.8
Fahr Volhard disease (of kidney) I12.- ☑

Failure, failed
abortion — *see* Abortion, attempted
aortic (valve) I35.8
rheumatic I06.8
attempted abortion — *see* Abortion, attempted
biventricular I50.82
due to left heart failure I50.814
bone marrow — *see* Anemia, aplastic

Failure, failed — *continued*
cardiac — *see* Failure, heart
cardiorenal (chronic) (*see also* Failure, renal, and Failure, heart) I50.9
hypertensive I13.2
cardiorespiratory (*see also* Failure, heart) R09.2
cardiovascular (chronic) — *see* Failure, heart
cerebrovascular I67.9
cervical dilatation in labor O62.0
circulation, circulatory (peripheral) R57.9
newborn P29.89
compensation — *see* Disease, heart
compliance with medical treatment or regimen — *see* Noncompliance
congestive — *see* Failure, heart, congestive
dental implant (endosseous) M27.69
due to
failure of dental prosthesis M27.63
lack of attached gingiva M27.62
occlusal trauma (poor prosthetic design) M27.62
parafunctional habits M27.62
periodontal infection (peri-implantitis) M27.62
poor oral hygiene M27.62
osseointegration M27.61
due to
complications of systemic disease M27.61
poor bone quality M27.61
iatrogenic M27.61
post-osseointegration
biological M27.62
due to complications of systemic disease M27.62
iatrogenic M27.62
mechanical M27.63
pre-integration M27.61
pre-osseointegration M27.61
specified NEC M27.69
descent of head (at term) of pregnancy (mother) O32.4 ☑
endosseous dental implant — *see* Failure, dental implant
engagement of head (term of pregnancy) (mother) O32.4 ☑
erection (penile) (*see also* Dysfunction, sexual, male, erectile) N52.9
nonorganic F52.21
examination(s), anxiety concerning Z55.2
expansion terminal respiratory units (newborn) (primary) P28.0
forceps NOS (with subsequent cesarean delivery) O66.5
gain weight (child over 28 days old) R62.51
adult R62.7
newborn P92.6
genital response (male) F52.21
female F52.22
heart (acute) (senile) (sudden) I50.9
with
acute pulmonary edema — *see* Failure, ventricular, left
decompensation (*see also* Failure, heart, by type as diastolic or systolic, acute and chronic) I50.9
dilatation — *see* Disease, heart
normal ejection fraction — *see* Failure, heart, diastolic
preserved ejection fraction — *see* Failure, heart, diastolic
reduced ejection fraction — *see* Failure, heart, systolic
arteriosclerotic I70.90
biventricular I50.82
due to left heart failure I50.814
combined left-right sided I50.82
due to left heart failure I50.814
compensated (*see also* Failure, heart, by type as diastolic or systolic, chronic) I50.9
complicating
anesthesia (general) (local) or other sedation
in labor and delivery O74.2
in pregnancy O29.12- ☑
postpartum, puerperal O89.1
delivery (cesarean) (instrumental) O75.4
congestive I50.9
with rheumatic fever (conditions in I00)
active I01.8
inactive or quiescent (with chorea) I09.81
newborn P29.0
rheumatic (chronic) (inactive) (with chorea) I09.81

Failure, failed — *continued*
heart — *continued*
congestive — *continued*
rheumatic — *continued*
active or acute I01.8
with chorea I02.0
decompensated (*see also* Failure, heart, by type as diastolic or systolic, acute and chronic) I50.9
degenerative — *see* Degeneration, myocardial
diastolic (congestive) (left ventricular) I50.30
acute (congestive) I50.31
and (on) chronic (congestive) I50.33
chronic (congestive) I50.32
and (on) acute (congestive) I50.33
combined with systolic (congestive) I50.40
acute (congestive) I50.41
and (on) chronic (congestive) I50.43
chronic (congestive) I50.42
and (on) acute (congestive) I50.43
due to presence of cardiac prosthesis I97.13- ☑
end stage (*see also* Failure, heart, by type as diastolic or systolic, chronic) I50.84
following cardiac surgery I97.13- ☑
high output NOS I50.83
hypertensive — *see* Hypertension, heart
left (ventricular) (*see also* Failure, ventricular, left)
combined diastolic and systolic — *see* Failure, heart, diastolic, combined with systolic
diastolic — *see* Failure, heart, diastolic
systolic — *see* Failure, heart, systolic
low output (syndrome) NOS I50.9
newborn P29.0
organic — *see* Disease, heart
peripartum O90.3
postprocedural I97.13- ☑
rheumatic (chronic) (inactive) I09.9
right (isolated) (ventricular) I50.810
acute I50.811
and (on) chronic I50.813
chronic I50.812
and acute I50.813
secondary to left heart failure I50.814
specified NEC I50.89

> *Note: heart failure stages A, B, C, and D are based on the American College of Cardiology and American Heart Association stages of heart failure, which complement and should not be confused with the New York Heart Association Classification of Heart Failure, into Class I, Class II, Class III, and Class IV*

stage A Z91.89
stage B (*see also* Failure, heart, by type as diastolic or systolic) I50.9
stage C (*see also* Failure, heart, by type as diastolic or systolic) I50.9
stage D (*see also* Failure, heart, by type as diastolic or systolic, chronic) I50.84
systolic (congestive) (left ventricular) I50.20
acute (congestive) I50.21
and (on) chronic (congestive) I50.23
chronic (congestive) I50.22
and (on) acute (congestive) I50.23
combined with diastolic (congestive) I50.40
acute (congestive) I50.41
and (on) chronic (congestive) I50.43
chronic (congestive) I50.42
and (on) acute (congestive) I50.43
thyrotoxic (*see also* Thyrotoxicosis) E05.90 [I43]
with
high output (*see also* Thyrotoxicosis) I50.83
thyroid storm E05.91 [I43]
high output (*see also* Thyrotoxicosis) I50.83
valvular — *see* Endocarditis
hepatic K72.90
with coma K72.91
acute or subacute K72.00
with coma K72.01
due to drugs K71.10
with coma K71.11
alcoholic (acute) (chronic) (subacute) K70.40
with coma K70.41
chronic K72.10
with coma K72.11
due to drugs (acute) (subacute) (chronic) K71.10
with coma K71.11
due to drugs (acute) (subacute) (chronic) K71.10
with coma K71.11

Failure, failed — *continued*
  hepatic — *continued*
    postprocedural K91.82
  hepatorenal K76.7
  induction (of labor) O61.9
    abortion — *see* Abortion, attempted
    by
      oxytocic drugs O61.0
      prostaglandins O61.0
    instrumental O61.1
    mechanical O61.1
    medical O61.0
    specified NEC O61.8
    surgical O61.1
  intubation during anesthesia T88.4 ☑
    in pregnancy O29.6- ☑
    labor and delivery O74.7
    postpartum, puerperal O89.6
  involution, thymus (gland) E32.0
  kidney (*see also* Disease, kidney, chronic) N19
    acute (*see also* Failure, renal, acute) N17.9
  lactation (complete) O92.3
    partial O92.4
  Leydig's cell, adult E29.1
  liver — *see* Failure, hepatic
  menstruation at puberty N91.0
  mitral I05.8
  myocardial, myocardium (*see also* Failure, heart) I50.9
    chronic (*see also* Failure, heart, congestive) I50.9
    congestive (*see also* Failure, heart, congestive) I50.9
  orgasm (female) (psychogenic) F52.31
    male F52.32
  ovarian (primary) E28.39
    iatrogenic E89.40
      asymptomatic E89.40
      symptomatic E89.41
    postprocedural (postablative) (postirradiation)
      (postsurgical) E89.40
      asymptomatic E89.40
      symptomatic E89.41
  ovulation causing infertility N97.0
  polyglandular, autoimmune E31.0
  prosthetic joint implant — *see* Complications, joint
    prosthesis, mechanical, breakdown, by site
  renal N19
    with
      tubular necrosis (acute) N17.0
    acute N17.9
      with
        cortical necrosis N17.1
        medullary necrosis N17.2
        tubular necrosis N17.0
      specified NEC N17.8
    chronic N18.9
      hypertensive — *see* Hypertension, kidney
    congenital P96.0
    end stage (chronic) N18.6
      due to hypertension I12.0
    following
      abortion — *see* Abortion by type complicated
        by specified condition NEC
      crushing T79.5 ☑
      ectopic or molar pregnancy O08.4
      labor and delivery (acute) O90.4
    hypertensive — *see* Hypertension, kidney
    postprocedural N99.0
  respiration, respiratory J96.90
    with
      hypercapnia J96.92
      hypercarbia J96.02
      hypoxia J96.91
    acute J96.00
      with
        hypercapnia J96.02
        hypercarbia J96.02
        hypoxia J96.01
    center G93.89
    acute and (on) chronic J96.20
      with
        hypercapnia J96.22
        hypercarbia J96.22
        hypoxia J96.21
    chronic J96.10
      with
        hypercapnia J96.12
        hypercarbia J96.12
        hypoxia J96.11
    newborn P28.5

Failure, failed — *continued*
  respiration, respiratory — *continued*
    postprocedural (acute) J95.821
      acute and chronic J95.822
  rotation
    cecum Q43.3
    colon Q43.3
    intestine Q43.3
    kidney Q63.2
  sedation (conscious) (moderate) during procedure
    T88.52 ☑
    history of Z92.83
  segmentation (*see also* Fusion)
    fingers — *see* Syndactylism, complex, fingers
    vertebra Q76.49
      with scoliosis Q76.3
  seminiferous tubule, adult E29.1
  senile (general) R54
  sexual arousal (male) F52.21
    female F52.22
  testicular endocrine function E29.1
  to thrive (child over 28 days old) R62.51
    adult R62.7
    newborn P92.6
  transplant T86.92
    bone T86.831
      marrow T86.02
    cornea T86.841
    heart T86.22
      with lung(s) T86.32
    intestine T86.851
    kidney T86.12
    liver T86.42
    lung(s) T86.811
      with heart T86.32
    pancreas T86.891
    skin (allograft) (autograft) T86.821
    specified organ or tissue NEC T86.891
    stem cell (peripheral blood) (umbilical cord) T86.5
  trial of labor (with subsequent cesarean delivery)
    O66.40
    following previous cesarean delivery O66.41
  tubal ligation N99.89
  urinary — *see* Disease, kidney, chronic
  vacuum extraction NOS (with subsequent cesarean
    delivery) O66.5
  vasectomy N99.89
  ventouse NOS (with subsequent cesarean delivery)
    O66.5
  ventricular (*see also* Failure, heart) I50.9
    left (*see also* Failure, heart, left) I50.1
      with rheumatic fever (conditions in I00)
        active I01.8
          with chorea I02.0
        inactive or quiescent (with chorea) I09.81
      rheumatic (chronic) (inactive) (with chorea)
        I09.81
        active or acute I01.8
          with chorea I02.0
    right — *see* Failure, heart, right
  vital centers, newborn P91.88
Fainting (fit) R55
Fallen arches — *see* Deformity, limb, flat foot
Falling, falls (repeated) R29.6
  any organ or part — *see* Prolapse
Fallopian
  insufflation Z31.41
  tube — *see* condition
Fallot's
  pentalogy Q21.8
  tetrad or tetralogy Q21.3
  triad or trilogy Q22.3
False (*see also* condition)
  croup J38.5
  joint — *see* Nonunion, fracture
  labor (pains) O47.9
    at or after 37 completed weeks of gestation O47.1
    before 37 completed weeks of gestation O47.0- ☑
  passage, urethra (prostatic) N36.5
  pregnancy F45.8
Family, familial (*see also* condition)
  disruption Z63.8
    involving divorce or separation Z63.5
  Li-Fraumeni (syndrome) Z15.01
  planning advice Z30.09
  problem Z63.9
    specified NEC Z63.8
  retinoblastoma C69.2- ☑

Famine (effects of) T73.0 ☑
  edema — *see* Malnutrition, severe
Fanconi (-de Toni)(-Debré) **syndrome** E72.09
  with cystinosis E72.04
Fanconi's anemia (congenital pancytopenia) D61.09
Farber's disease or syndrome E75.29
Farcy A24.0
Farmer's
  lung J67.0
  skin L57.8
Farsightedness — *see* Hypermetropia
Fascia — *see* condition
Fasciculation R25.3
Fasciitis M72.9
  diffuse (eosinophilic) M35.4
  infective M72.8
    necrotizing M72.6
  necrotizing M72.6
  nodular M72.4
  perirenal (with ureteral obstruction) N13.5
    with infection N13.6
  plantar M72.2
  specified NEC M72.8
  traumatic (old) M72.8
    current — *code by* site under Sprain
Fascioliasis B66.3
Fasciolopsis, fasciolopsiasis (intestinal) B66.5
Fascioscapulohumeral myopathy G71.02
Fast pulse R00.0
Fat
  embolism — *see* Embolism, fat
  excessive (*see also* Obesity)
    in heart — *see* Degeneration, myocardial
  in stool R19.5
  localized (pad) E65
    heart — *see* Degeneration, myocardial
    knee M79.4
    retropatellar M79.4
  necrosis
    breast N64.1
    mesentery K65.4
    omentum K65.4
  pad E65
    knee M79.4
Fatigue R53.83
  auditory deafness — *see* Deafness
  chronic R53.82
  combat F43.0
  general R53.83
    psychogenic F48.8
  heat (transient) T67.6 ☑
  muscle M62.89
  myocardium — *see* Failure, heart
  neoplasm-related R53.0
  nervous, neurosis F48.8
  operational F48.8
  psychogenic (general) F48.8
  senile R54
  voice R49.8
Fatness — *see* Obesity
Fatty (*see also* condition)
  apron E65
  degeneration — *see* Degeneration, fatty
  heart (enlarged) — *see* Degeneration, myocardial
  liver NEC K76.0
    alcoholic K70.0
    nonalcoholic K76.0
  necrosis — *see* Degeneration, fatty
Fauces — *see* condition
Fauchard's disease (periodontitis) — *see* Periodontitis
Faucitis J02.9
Favism (anemia) D55.0
Favus — *see* Dermatophytosis
Fazio-Londe disease or syndrome G12.1
Fear complex or reaction F40.9
Fear of — *see* Phobia
Feared complaint unfounded Z71.1
Febris, febrile (*see also* Fever)
  flava (*see also* Fever, yellow) A95.9
  melitensis A23.0
  pestis — *see* Plague
  recurrens — *see* Fever, relapsing
  rubra A38.9
Fecal
  incontinence R15.9
  smearing R15.1
  soiling R15.1

Fecal — *continued*
    urgency R15.2
Fecalith (impaction) K56.41
    appendix K38.1
    congenital P76.8
Fede's disease K14.0
Feeble rapid pulse due to shock following injury
    T79.4 ☑
Feeble-minded F70
Feeding
    difficulties R63.3
    problem R63.3
        newborn P92.9
            specified NEC P92.8
        nonorganic (adult) — *see* Disorder, eating
Feeling (of)
    foreign body in throat R09.89
Feer's disease — *see* Poisoning, mercury
Feet — *see* condition
Feigned illness Z76.5
Feil-Klippel syndrome (brevicollis) Q76.1
Feinmesser's (hidrotic) **ectodermal dysplasia** Q82.4
Felinophobia F40.218
Felon (*see also* Cellulitis, digit)
    with lymphangitis — *see* Lymphangitis, acute, digit
Felty's syndrome M05.00
    ankle M05.07- ☑
    elbow M05.02- ☑
    foot joint M05.07- ☑
    hand joint M05.04- ☑
    hip M05.05- ☑
    knee M05.06- ☑
    multiple site M05.09
    shoulder M05.01- ☑
    vertebra — *see* Spondylitis, ankylosing
    wrist M05.03- ☑
Female genital cutting status — *see* Female genital
    mutilation status (FGM)
Female genital mutilation status (FGM) N90.810
    specified NEC N90.818
    type I (clitorectomy status) N90.811
    type II (clitorectomy with excision of labia minora sta-
        tus) N90.812
    type III (infibulation status) N90.813
    type IV N90.818
Femur, femoral — *see* condition
Fenestration, fenestrated (*see also* Imperfect, closure)
    aortico-pulmonary Q21.4
    cusps, heart valve NEC Q24.8
        pulmonary Q22.3
    pulmonic cusps Q22.3
Fernell's disease (aortic aneurysm) I71.9
Fertile eunuch syndrome E23.0
Fetid
    breath R19.6
    sweat L75.0
Fetishism F65.0
    transvestic F65.1
Fetus, fetal (*see also* condition)
    alcohol syndrome (dysmorphic) Q86.0
    compressus O31.0- ☑
    hydantoin syndrome Q86.1
    lung tissue P28.0
    papyraceous O31.0- ☑
Fever (inanition) (of unknown origin) (persistent) (with
    chills) (with rigor) R50.9
    abortus A23.1
    Aden (dengue) A90
    African tick-borne A68.1
    American
        mountain (tick) A93.2
        spotted A77.0
    aphthous B08.8
    arbovirus, arboviral A94
        hemorrhagic A94
        specified NEC A93.8
    Argentinian hemorrhagic A96.0
    Assam B55.0
    Australian Q A78
    Bangkok hemorrhagic A91
    Barmah forest A92.8
    Bartonella A44.0
    bilious, hemoglobinuric B50.8
    blackwater B50.8
    blister B00.1
    Bolivian hemorrhagic A96.1
    Bonvale dam T73.3 ☑

Fever — *continued*
    boutonneuse A77.1
    brain — *see* Encephalitis
    Brazilian purpuric A48.4
    breakbone A90
    Bullis A77.0
    Bunyamwera A92.8
    Burdwan B55.0
    Bwamba A92.8
    Cameroon — *see* Malaria
    Canton A75.9
    catarrhal (acute) J00
        chronic J31.0
    cat-scratch A28.1
    Central Asian hemorrhagic A98.0
    cerebral — *see* Encephalitis
    cerebrospinal meningococcal A39.0
    Chagres B50.9
    Chandipura A92.8
    Changuinola A93.1
    Charcot's (biliary) (hepatic) (intermittent) — *see* Calcu-
        lus, bile duct
    Chikungunya (viral) (hemorrhagic) A92.0
    Chitral A93.1
    Colombo — *see* Fever, paratyphoid
    Colorado tick (virus) A93.2
    congestive (remittent) — *see* Malaria
    Congo virus A98.0
    continued malarial B50.9
    Corsican — *see* Malaria
    Crimean-Congo hemorrhagic A98.0
    Cyprus — *see* Brucellosis
    dandy A90
    deer fly — *see* Tularemia
    dengue (virus) A90
        hemorrhagic A91
        sandfly A93.1
    desert B38.0
    drug induced R50.2
    due to
        conditions classified elsewhere R50.81
        heat T67.0 ☑
    enteric A01.00
    enteroviral exanthematous (Boston exanthem) A88.0
    ephemeral (of unknown origin) R50.9
    epidemic hemorrhagic A98.5
    erysipelatous — *see* Erysipelas
    estivo-autumnal (malarial) B50.9
    famine A75.0
    five day A79.0
    following delivery O86.4
    Fort Bragg A27.89
    gastroenteric A01.00
    gastromalarial — *see* Malaria
    Gibraltar — *see* Brucellosis
    glandular — *see* Mononucleosis, infectious
    Guama (viral) A92.8
    Haverhill A25.1
    hay (allergic) J30.1
        with asthma (bronchial) J45.909
            with
                exacerbation (acute) J45.901
                status asthmaticus J45.902
        due to
            allergen other than pollen J30.89
            pollen, any plant or tree J30.1
    heat (effects) T67.0 ☑
    hematuric, bilious B50.8
    hemoglobinuric (malarial) (bilious) B50.8
    hemorrhagic (arthropod-borne) NOS A94
        with renal syndrome A98.5
        arenaviral A96.9
            specified NEC A96.8
        Argentinian A96.0
        Bangkok A91
        Bolivian A96.1
        Central Asian A98.0
        Chikungunya A92.0
        Crimean-Congo A98.0
        dengue (virus) A91
        epidemic A98.5
        Junin (virus) A96.0
        Korean A98.5
        Kyasanur forest A98.2
        Machupo (virus) A96.1
        mite-borne A93.8
        mosquito-borne A92.8
        Omsk A98.1

Fever — *continued*
    hemorrhagic — *continued*
        Philippine A91
        Russian A98.5
        Singapore A91
        Southeast Asia A91
        Thailand A91
        tick-borne NEC A93.8
        viral A99
            specified NEC A98.8
    hepatic — *see* Cholecystitis
    herpetic — *see* Herpes
    icterohemorrhagic A27.0
    Indiana A93.8
    infective B99.9
        specified NEC B99.8
    intermittent (bilious) (*see also* Malaria)
        of unknown origin R50.9
        pernicious B50.9
    iodide R50.2
    Japanese river A75.3
    jungle (*see also* Malaria)
        yellow A95.0
    Junin (virus) hemorrhagic A96.0
    Katayama B65.2
    kedani A75.3
    Kenya (tick) A77.1
    Kew Garden A79.1
    Korean hemorrhagic A98.5
    Lassa A96.2
    Lone Star A77.0
    Machupo (virus) hemorrhagic A96.1
    malaria, malarial — *see* Malaria
    Malta A23.9
    Marseilles A77.1
    marsh — *see* Malaria
    Mayaro (viral) A92.8
    Mediterranean (*see also* Brucellosis) A23.9
        familial M04.1
        tick A77.1
    meningeal — *see* Meningitis
    Meuse A79.0
    Mexican A75.2
    mianeh A68.1
    miasmatic — *see* Malaria
    mosquito-borne (viral) A92.9
        hemorrhagic A92.8
    mountain (*see also* Brucellosis)
        meaning Rocky Mountain spotted fever A77.0
        tick (American) (Colorado) (viral) A93.2
    Mucambo (viral) A92.8
    mud A27.9
    Neapolitan — *see* Brucellosis
    neutropenic D70.9
    newborn P81.9
        environmental P81.0
    Nine-Mile A78
    non-exanthematous tick A93.2
    North Asian tick-borne A77.2
    Omsk hemorrhagic A98.1
    O'nyong-nyong (viral) A92.1
    Oropouche (viral) A93.0
    Oroya A44.0
    paludal — *see* Malaria
    Panama (malarial) B50.9
    Pappataci A93.1
    paratyphoid A01.4
        A A01.1
        B A01.2
        C A01.3
    parrot A70
    periodic (Mediterranean) M04.1
    persistent (of unknown origin) R50.9
    petechial A39.0
    pharyngoconjunctival B30.2
    Philippine hemorrhagic A91
    phlebotomus A93.1
    Piry (virus) A93.8
    Pixuna (viral) A92.8
    Plasmodium ovale B53.0
    polioviral (nonparalytic) A80.4
    Pontiac A48.2
    postimmunization R50.83
    postoperative R50.82
        due to infection T81.40 ☑
    posttransfusion R50.84
    postvaccination R50.83
    presenting with conditions classified elsewhere R50.81

Fever — *continued*
  pretibial A27.89
  puerperal O86.4
  Q A78
  quadrilateral A78
  quartan (malaria) B52.9
  Queensland (coastal) (tick) A77.3
  quintan A79.0
  rabbit — *see* Tularemia
  rat-bite A25.9
    due to
      Spirillum A25.0
      Streptobacillus moniliformis A25.1
  recurrent — *see* Fever, relapsing
  relapsing (Borrelia) A68.9
    Carter's (Asiatic) A68.1
    Dutton's (West African) A68.1
    Koch's A68.9
    louse-borne A68.0
    Novy's
      louse-borne A68.0
      tick-borne A68.1
    Obermeyer's (European) A68.0
    tick-borne A68.1
  remittent (bilious) (congestive) (gastric) — *see* Malaria
  rheumatic (active) (acute) (chronic) (subacute) I00
    with central nervous system involvement I02.9
    active with heart involvement — *see* category I01 ☑
    inactive or quiescent with
      cardiac hypertrophy I09.89
      carditis I09.9
      endocarditis I09.1
        aortic (valve) I06.9
          with mitral (valve) disease I08.0
        mitral (valve) I05.9
          with aortic (valve) disease I08.0
        pulmonary (valve) I09.89
        tricuspid (valve) I07.8
      heart disease NEC I09.89
      heart failure (congestive) (conditions in category I50.) I09.81
      left ventricular failure (conditions in I50.1- I50.4-) I09.81
      myocarditis, myocardial degeneration (conditions in I51.4) I09.0
      pancarditis I09.9
      pericarditis I09.2
  Rift Valley (viral) A92.4
  Rocky Mountain spotted A77.0
  rose J30.1
  Ross River B33.1
  Russian hemorrhagic A98.5
  San Joaquin (Valley) B38.0
  sandfly A93.1
  Sao Paulo A77.0
  scarlet A38.9
  seven day (leptospirosis) (autumnal) (Japanese) A27.89
    dengue A90
  shin-bone A79.0
  Singapore hemorrhagic A91
  solar A90
  Songo A98.5
  sore B00.1
  South African tick-bite A68.1
  Southeast Asia hemorrhagic A91
  spinal — *see* Meningitis
  spirillary A25.0
  splenic — *see* Anthrax
  spotted A77.9
    American A77.0
    Brazilian A77.0
    cerebrospinal meningitis A39.0
    Colombian A77.0
    due to Rickettsia
      australis A77.3
      conorii A77.1
      rickettsii A77.0
      sibirica A77.2
      specified type NEC A77.8
    Ehrlichiosis A77.40
      due to
        E. chafeensis A77.41
        specified organism NEC A77.49
    Rocky Mountain A77.0
  steroid R50.2
  streptobacillary A25.1
  subtertian B50.9
  Sumatran mite A75.3

Fever — *continued*
  sun A90
  swamp A27.9
  swine A02.8
  sylvatic, yellow A95.0
  Tahyna B33.8
  tertian — *see* Malaria, tertian
  Thailand hemorrhagic A91
  thermic T67.0 ☑
  three-day A93.1
  tick
    American mountain A93.2
    Colorado A93.2
    Kemerovo A93.8
    Mediterranean A77.1
    mountain A93.2
    nonexanthematous A93.2
    Quaranfil A93.8
  tick-bite NEC A93.8
  tick-borne (hemorrhagic) NEC A93.8
  trench A79.0
  tsutsugamushi A75.3
  typhogastric A01.00
  typhoid (abortive) (hemorrhagic) (intermittent) (malignant) A01.00
    complicated by
      arthritis A01.04
      heart involvement A01.02
      meningitis A01.01
      osteomyelitis A01.05
      pneumonia A01.03
      specified NEC A01.09
  typhomalarial — *see* Malaria
  typhus — *see* Typhus (fever)
  undulant — *see* Brucellosis
  unknown origin R50.9
  uveoparotid D86.89
  valley B38.0
  Venezuelan equine A92.2
  vesicular stomatitis A93.8
  viral hemorrhagic — *see* Fever, hemorrhagic, by type of virus
  Volhynian A79.0
  Wesselsbron (viral) A92.8
  West
    African B50.8
    Nile (viral) A92.30
      with
        complications NEC A92.39
        cranial nerve disorders A92.32
        encephalitis A92.31
        encephalomyelitis A92.31
        neurologic manifestation NEC A92.32
        optic neuritis A92.32
        polyradiculitis A92.32
  Whitmore's — *see* Melioidosis
  Wolhynian A79.0
  worm B83.9
  yellow A95.9
    jungle A95.0
    sylvatic A95.0
    urban A95.1
  Zika virus A92.5
Fibrillation
  atrial or auricular (established) I48.91
    chronic I48.2
    paroxysmal I48.0
    permanent I48.2
    persistent I48.1
  cardiac I49.8
  heart I49.8
  muscular M62.89
  ventricular I49.01
Fibrin
  ball or bodies, pleural (sac) J94.1
  chamber, anterior (eye) (gelatinous exudate) — *see* Iridocyclitis, acute
Fibrinogenolysis — *see* Fibrinolysis
Fibrinogenopenia D68.8
  acquired D65
  congenital D68.2
Fibrinolysis (hemorrhagic) (acquired) D65
  antepartum hemorrhage — *see* Hemorrhage, antepartum, with coagulation defect
  following
    abortion — *see* Abortion by type complicated by hemorrhage
    ectopic or molar pregnancy O08.1

Fibrinolysis — *continued*
    intrapartum O67.0
    newborn, transient P60
    postpartum O72.3
Fibrinopenia (hereditary) D68.2
  acquired D68.4
Fibrinopurulent — *see* condition
Fibrinous — *see* condition
Fibroadenoma
  cellular intracanalicular D24- ☑
  giant D24- ☑
  intracanalicular
    cellular D24- ☑
    giant D24- ☑
    specified site — *see* Neoplasm, benign, by site
    unspecified site D24- ☑
  juvenile D24- ☑
  pericanalicular
    specified site — *see* Neoplasm, benign, by site
    unspecified site D24- ☑
  phyllodes D24- ☑
  prostate D29.1
  specified site NEC — *see* Neoplasm, benign, by site
  unspecified site D24- ☑
Fibroadenosis, breast (chronic) (cystic) (diffuse) (periodic) (segmental) N60.2- ☑
Fibroangioma (*see also* Neoplasm, benign, by site)
  juvenile
    specified site — *see* Neoplasm, benign, by site
    unspecified site D10.6
Fibrochondrosarcoma — *see* Neoplasm, cartilage, malignant
Fibrocystic
  disease (*see also* Fibrosis, cystic)
    breast — *see* Mastopathy, cystic
    jaw M27.49
    kidney (congenital) Q61.8
    liver Q44.6
    pancreas E84.9
  kidney (congenital) Q61.8
Fibrodysplasia ossificans progressiva — *see* Myositis, ossificans, progressiva
Fibroelastosis (cordis) (endocardial) (endomyocardial) I42.4
Fibroid (tumor) (*see also* Neoplasm, connective tissue, benign)
  disease, lung (chronic) — *see* Fibrosis, lung
  heart (disease) — *see* Myocarditis
  in pregnancy or childbirth O34.1- ☑
    causing obstructed labor O65.5
  induration, lung (chronic) — *see* Fibrosis, lung
  lung — *see* Fibrosis, lung
  pneumonia (chronic) — *see* Fibrosis, lung
  uterus (*see also* Leiomyoma, uterus) D25.9
Fibrolipoma — *see* Lipoma
Fibroliposarcoma — *see* Neoplasm, connective tissue, malignant
Fibroma (*see also* Neoplasm, connective tissue, benign)
  ameloblastic — *see* Cyst, calcifying odontogenic
  bone (nonossifying) — *see* Disorder, bone, specified type NEC
    ossifying — *see* Neoplasm, bone, benign
  cementifying — *see* Neoplasm, bone, benign
  chondromyxoid — *see* Neoplasm, bone, benign
  desmoplastic — *see* Neoplasm, connective tissue, uncertain behavior
  durum — *see* Neoplasm, connective tissue, benign
  fascial — *see* Neoplasm, connective tissue, benign
  invasive — *see* Neoplasm, connective tissue, uncertain behavior
  molle — *see* Lipoma
  myxoid — *see* Neoplasm, connective tissue, benign
  nasopharynx, nasopharyngeal (juvenile) D10.6
  nonosteogenic (nonossifying) — *see* Dysplasia, fibrous
  odontogenic (central) — *see* Cyst, calcifying odontogenic
  ossifying — *see* Neoplasm, bone, benign
  periosteal — *see* Neoplasm, bone, benign
  soft — *see* Lipoma
Fibromatosis M72.9
  abdominal — *see* Neoplasm, connective tissue, uncertain behavior
  aggressive — *see* Neoplasm, connective tissue, uncertain behavior
  congenital generalized — *see* Neoplasm, connective tissue, uncertain behavior
  Dupuytren's M72.0

Fibromatosis — *continued*
  gingival K06.1
  palmar (fascial) M72.0
  plantar (fascial) M72.2
  pseudosarcomatous (proliferative) (subcutaneous) M72.4
  retroperitoneal D48.3
  specified NEC M72.8
Fibromyalgia M79.7
Fibromyoma (*see also* Neoplasm, connective tissue, benign)
  uterus (corpus) (*see also* Leiomyoma, uterus)
    in pregnancy or childbirth — *see* Fibroid, in pregnancy or childbirth
      causing obstructed labor O65.5
Fibromyositis M79.7
Fibromyxolipoma D17.9
Fibromyxoma — *see* Neoplasm, connective tissue, benign
Fibromyxosarcoma — *see* Neoplasm, connective tissue, malignant
Fibro-odontoma, ameloblastic — *see* Cyst, calcifying odontogenic
Fibro-osteoma — *see* Neoplasm, bone, benign
Fibroplasia, retrolental H35.17- ☑
Fibropurulent — *see* condition
Fibrosarcoma (*see also* Neoplasm, connective tissue, malignant)
  ameloblastic C41.1
    upper jaw (bone) C41.0
  congenital — *see* Neoplasm, connective tissue, malignant
  fascial — *see* Neoplasm, connective tissue, malignant
  infantile — *see* Neoplasm, connective tissue, malignant
  odontogenic C41.1
    upper jaw (bone) C41.0
  periosteal — *see* Neoplasm, bone, malignant
Fibrosclerosis
  breast N60.3- ☑
  multifocal M35.5
  penis (corpora cavernosa) N48.6
Fibrosis, fibrotic
  adrenal (gland) E27.8
  amnion O41.8X- ☑
  anal papillae K62.89
  arteriocapillary — *see* Arteriosclerosis
  bladder N32.89
    interstitial — *see* Cystitis, chronic, interstitial
    localized submucosal — *see* Cystitis, chronic, interstitial
    panmural — *see* Cystitis, chronic, interstitial
  breast — *see* Fibrosclerosis, breast
  capillary (*see also* Arteriosclerosis) I70.90
    lung (chronic) — *see* Fibrosis, lung
  cardiac — *see* Myocarditis
  cervix N88.8
  chorion O41.8X- ☑
  corpus cavernosum (sclerosing) N48.6
  cystic (of pancreas) E84.9
    with
      distal intestinal obstruction syndrome E84.19
      fecal impaction E84.19
      intestinal manifestations NEC E84.19
      pulmonary manifestations E84.0
      specified manifestations NEC E84.8
    due to device, implant or graft (*see also* Complications, by site and type, specified NEC) T85.828 ☑
      arterial graft NEC T82.828 ☑
      breast (implant) T85.828 ☑
      catheter NEC T85.828 ☑
        dialysis (renal) T82.828 ☑
          intraperitoneal T85.828 ☑
        infusion NEC T82.828 ☑
          spinal (epidural) (subdural) T85.820 ☑
        urinary (indwelling) T83.82 ☑
      electronic (electrode) (pulse generator) (stimulator)
        bone T84.82 ☑
        cardiac T82.827 ☑
        nervous system (brain) (peripheral nerve) (spinal) T85.820 ☑
        urinary T83.82 ☑
      fixation, internal (orthopedic) NEC T84.82 ☑
      gastrointestinal (bile duct) (esophagus) T85.828 ☑
      genital NEC T83.82 ☑
      heart NEC T82.827 ☑
      joint prosthesis T84.82 ☑

Fibrosis, fibrotic — *continued*
  due to device, implant or graft (*see also* Complications, by site and type, specified) — *continued*
    ocular (corneal graft) (orbital implant) NEC T85.828 ☑
    orthopedic NEC T84.82 ☑
    specified NEC T85.828 ☑
    urinary NEC T83.82 ☑
    vascular NEC T82.828 ☑
    ventricular intracranial shunt T85.820 ☑
  ejaculatory duct N50.89
  endocardium — *see* Endocarditis
  endomyocardial (tropical) I42.3
  epididymis N50.89
  eye muscle — *see* Strabismus, mechanical
  heart — *see* Myocarditis
  hepatic — *see* Fibrosis, liver
  hepatolienal (portal hypertension) K76.6
  hepatosplenic (portal hypertension) K76.6
  infrapatellar fat pad M79.4
  intrascrotal N50.89
  kidney N26.9
  liver K74.0
    with sclerosis K74.2
    alcoholic K70.2
  lung (atrophic) (chronic) (confluent) (massive) (perialveolar) (peribronchial) J84.10
    with
      anthracosilicosis J60
      anthracosis J60
      asbestosis J61
      bagassosis J67.1
      bauxite J63.1
      berylliosis J63.2
      byssinosis J66.0
      calcicosis J62.8
      chalicosis J62.8
      dust reticulation J64
      farmer's lung J67.0
      ganister disease J62.8
      graphite J63.3
      pneumoconiosis NOS J64
      siderosis J63.4
      silicosis J62.8
    capillary J84.10
    congenital P27.8
    diffuse (idiopathic) J84.10
      chemicals, gases, fumes or vapors (inhalation) J68.4
      interstitial J84.10
        acute J84.114
      talc J62.0
    following radiation J70.1
    idiopathic J84.112
    postinflammatory J84.10
    silicotic J62.8
    tuberculous — *see* Tuberculosis, pulmonary
  lymphatic gland I89.8
  median bar — *see* Hyperplasia, prostate
  mediastinum (idiopathic) J98.59
  meninges G96.19
  myocardium, myocardial — *see* Myocarditis
  ovary N83.8
  oviduct N83.8
  pancreas K86.89
  penis NEC N48.6
  pericardium I31.0
  perineum, in pregnancy or childbirth O34.7- ☑
    causing obstructed labor O65.5
  pleura J94.1
  popliteal fat pad M79.4
  prostate (chronic) — *see* Hyperplasia, prostate
  pulmonary (*see also* Fibrosis, lung) J84.10
    congenital P27.8
    idiopathic J84.112
  rectal sphincter K62.89
  retroperitoneal, idiopathic (with ureteral obstruction) N13.5
    with infection N13.6
  sclerosing mesenteric (idiopathic) K65.4
  scrotum N50.89
  seminal vesicle N50.89
  senile R54
  skin L90.5
  spermatic cord N50.89
  spleen D73.89
    in schistosomiasis (bilharziasis) B65.9 [D77]
  subepidermal nodular — *see* Neoplasm, skin, benign

Fibrosis, fibrotic — *continued*
  submucous (oral) (tongue) K13.5
  testis N44.8
    chronic, due to syphilis A52.76
  thymus (gland) E32.8
  tongue, submucous K13.5
  tunica vaginalis N50.89
  uterus (non-neoplastic) N85.8
  vagina N89.8
  valve, heart — *see* Endocarditis
  vas deferens N50.89
  vein I87.8
Fibrositis (periarticular) M79.7
  nodular, chronic (Jaccoud's) (rheumatoid) — *see* Arthropathy, postrheumatic, chronic
Fibrothorax J94.1
Fibrotic — *see* Fibrosis
Fibrous — *see* condition
Fibroxanthoma (*see also* Neoplasm, connective tissue, benign)
  atypical — *see* Neoplasm, connective tissue, uncertain behavior
  malignant — *see* Neoplasm, connective tissue, malignant
Fibroxanthosarcoma — *see* Neoplasm, connective tissue, malignant
Fiedler's
  disease (icterohemorrhagic leptospirosis) A27.0
  myocarditis (acute) I40.1
Fifth disease B08.3
  venereal A55
Filaria, filarial, filariasis — *see* Infestation, filarial
Filatov's disease — *see* Mononucleosis, infectious
File-cutter's disease — *see* Poisoning, lead
Filling defect
  biliary tract R93.2
  bladder R93.41
  duodenum R93.3
  gallbladder R93.2
  gastrointestinal tract R93.3
  intestine R93.3
  kidney R93.42- ☑
  stomach R93.3
  ureter R93.41
  urinary organs, specified NEC R93.49
Fimbrial cyst Q50.4
Financial problem affecting care NOS Z59.9
  bankruptcy Z59.8
  foreclosure on loan Z59.8
Findings, abnormal, inconclusive, without diagnosis
    (*see also* Abnormal)
  17-ketosteroids, elevated R82.5
  acetonuria R82.4
  alcohol in blood R78.0
  anisocytosis R71.8
  antenatal screening of mother O28.9
    biochemical O28.1
    chromosomal O28.5
    cytological O28.2
    genetic O28.5
    hematological O28.0
    radiological O28.4
    specified NEC O28.8
    ultrasonic O28.3
  antibody titer, elevated R76.0
  anticardiolipin antibody R76.0
  antiphosphatidylglycerol antibody R76.0
  antiphosphatidylinositol antibody R76.0
  antiphosphatidylserine antibody R76.0
  antiphospholipid antibody R76.0
  bacteriuria R82.71
  bicarbonate E87.8
  bile in urine R82.2
  blood sugar R73.09
    high R73.9
    low (transient) E16.2
  body fluid or substance, specified NEC R88.8
  casts, urine R82.998
  catecholamines R82.5
  cells, urine R82.998
  chloride E87.8
  cholesterol E78.9
    high E78.00
      with high triglycerides E78.2
  chyluria R82.0
  cloudy
    dialysis effluent R88.0
    urine R82.90

Findings, abnormal, inconclusive, without diagnosis
— *continued*
- creatinine clearance R94.4
- crystals, urine R82.998
- culture
  - blood R78.81
    - positive — *see* Positive, culture
- echocardiogram R93.1
- electrolyte level, urinary R82.998
- function study NEC R94.8
  - bladder R94.8
  - endocrine NEC R94.7
    - thyroid R94.6
  - kidney R94.4
  - liver R94.5
  - pancreas R94.8
  - placenta R94.8
  - pulmonary R94.2
  - spleen R94.8
- gallbladder, nonvisualization R93.2
- glucose (tolerance test) (non-fasting) R73.09
- glycosuria R81
- heart
  - shadow R93.1
  - sounds R01.2
- hematinuria R82.3
- hematocrit drop (precipitous) R71.0
- hemoglobinuria R82.3
- human papillomavirus (HPV) DNA test positive
  - cervix
    - high risk R87.810
    - low risk R87.820
  - vagina
    - high risk R87.811
    - low risk R87.821
- in blood (of substance not normally found in blood) R78.9
  - addictive drug NEC R78.4
  - alcohol (excessive level) R78.0
  - cocaine R78.2
  - hallucinogen R78.3
  - heavy metals (abnormal level) R78.79
  - lead R78.71
  - lithium (abnormal level) R78.89
  - opiate drug R78.1
  - psychotropic drug R78.5
  - specified substance NEC R78.89
  - steroid agent R78.6
- indoleacetic acid, elevated R82.5
- ketonuria R82.4
- lactic acid dehydrogenase (LDH) R74.0
- liver function test R79.89
- mammogram NEC R92.8
  - calcification (calculus) R92.1
  - inconclusive result (due to dense breasts) R92.2
  - microcalcification R92.0
- mediastinal shift R93.89
- melanin, urine R82.998
- myoglobinuria R82.1
- neonatal screening P09
- nonvisualization of gallbladder R93.2
- odor of urine NOS R82.90
- Papanicolaou cervix R87.619
  - non-atypical endometrial cells R87.618
- pneumoencephalogram R93.0
- poikilocytosis R71.8
- potassium (deficiency) E87.6
  - excess E87.5
- PPD R76.11
- radiologic (X-ray) R93.89
  - abdomen R93.5
  - biliary tract R93.2
  - breast R92.8
  - gastrointestinal tract R93.3
  - genitourinary organs R93.89
  - head R93.0
  - inconclusive due to excess body fat of patient R93.9
  - intrathoracic organs NEC R93.1
  - placenta R93.89
  - retroperitoneum R93.5
  - skin R93.89
  - skull R93.0
  - subcutaneous tissue R93.89
  - testis R93.81- ☑
- red blood cell (count) (morphology) (sickling) (volume) R71.8
- scan NEC R94.8
  - bladder R94.8
  - bone R94.8

Findings, abnormal, inconclusive, without diagnosis
— *continued*
- scan — *continued*
  - kidney R94.4
  - liver R93.2
  - lung R94.2
  - pancreas R94.8
  - placental R94.8
  - spleen R94.8
  - thyroid R94.6
- sedimentation rate, elevated R70.0
- SGOT R74.0
- SGPT R74.0
- sodium (deficiency) E87.1
  - excess E87.0
- specified body fluid NEC R88.8
- stress test R94.39
- testis R93.81- ☑
- thyroid (function) (metabolic rate) (scan) (uptake) R94.6
- transaminase (level) R74.0
- triglycerides E78.9
  - high E78.1
    - with high cholesterol E78.2
- tuberculin skin test (without active tuberculosis) R76.11
- urine R82.90
  - acetone R82.4
  - bacteria R82.71
  - bile R82.2
  - casts or cells R82.998
  - chyle R82.0
  - culture positive R82.79
  - glucose R81
  - hemoglobin R82.3
  - ketone R82.4
  - sugar R81
- vanillylmandelic acid (VMA), elevated R82.5
- vectorcardiogram (VCG) R94.39
- ventriculogram R93.0
- white blood cell (count) (differential) (morphology) D72.9
- xerography R92.8

Finger — *see* condition
Fire, Saint Anthony's — *see* Erysipelas
Fire-setting
- pathological (compulsive) F63.1
Fish hook stomach K31.89
Fishmeal-worker's lung J67.8
Fissure, fissured
- anus, anal K60.2
  - acute K60.0
  - chronic K60.1
  - congenital Q43.8
- ear, lobule, congenital Q17.8
- epiglottis (congenital) Q31.8
- larynx J38.7
  - congenital Q31.8
- lip K13.0
  - congenital — *see* Cleft, lip
- nipple N64.0
  - associated with
    - lactation O92.13
    - pregnancy O92.11- ☑
    - puerperium O92.12
- nose Q30.2
- palate (congenital) — *see* Cleft, palate
- skin R23.4
- spine (congenital) (*see also* Spina bifida)
  - with hydrocephalus — *see* Spina bifida, by site, with hydrocephalus
- tongue (acquired) K14.5
  - congenital Q38.3
Fistula (cutaneous) L98.8
- abdomen (wall) K63.2
  - bladder N32.2
  - intestine NEC K63.2
  - ureter N28.89
  - uterus N82.5
- abdominorectal K63.2
- abdominosigmoidal K63.2
- abdominothoracic J86.0
- abdominouterine N82.5
  - congenital Q51.7
- abdominovesical N32.2
- accessory sinuses — *see* Sinusitis
- actinomycotic — *see* Actinomycosis
- alveolar antrum — *see* Sinusitis, maxillary
- alveolar process K04.6
- anorectal K60.5

Fistula — *continued*
- antrobuccal — *see* Sinusitis, maxillary
- antrum — *see* Sinusitis, maxillary
- anus, anal (recurrent) (infectional) K60.3
  - congenital Q43.6
    - with absence, atresia and stenosis Q42.2
  - tuberculous A18.32
- aorta-duodenal I77.2
- appendix, appendicular K38.3
- arteriovenous (acquired) (nonruptured) I77.0
  - brain I67.1
    - congenital Q28.2
      - ruptured I60.8
    - ruptured I60.8
  - cerebral — *see* Fistula, arteriovenous, brain
  - congenital (peripheral) (*see also* Malformation, arteriovenous)
    - brain Q28.2
      - ruptured I60.8
    - coronary Q24.5
    - pulmonary Q25.72
  - coronary I25.41
    - congenital Q24.5
  - pulmonary I28.0
    - congenital Q25.72
  - surgically created (for dialysis) Z99.2
    - complication — *see* Complication, arteriovenous, fistula, surgically created
  - traumatic — *see* Injury, blood vessel
- artery I77.2
- aural (mastoid) — *see* Mastoiditis, chronic
- auricle (*see also* Disorder, pinna, specified type NEC)
  - congenital Q18.1
- Bartholin's gland N82.8
- bile duct (common) (hepatic) K83.3
  - with calculus, stones — *see* Calculus, bile duct
- biliary (tract) — *see* Fistula, bile duct
- bladder (sphincter) NEC (*see also* Fistula, vesico-) N32.2
  - into seminal vesicle N32.2
- bone (*see also* Disorder, bone, specified type NEC)
  - with osteomyelitis, chronic — *see* Osteomyelitis, chronic, with draining sinus
- brain G93.89
  - arteriovenous (acquired) I67.1
    - congenital Q28.2
- branchial (cleft) Q18.0
- branchiogenous Q18.0
- breast N61.0
  - puerperal, postpartum or gestational, due to mastitis (purulent) — *see* Mastitis, obstetric, purulent
- bronchial J86.0
- bronchocutaneous, bronchomediastinal, bronchopleural, bronchopleuromediastinal (infective) J86.0
  - tuberculous NEC A15.5
- bronchoesophageal J86.0
  - congenital Q39.2
    - with atresia of esophagus Q39.1
- bronchovisceral J86.0
- buccal cavity (infective) K12.2
- cecosigmoidal K63.2
- cecum K63.2
- cerebrospinal (fluid) G96.0
- cervical, lateral Q18.1
- cervicoaural Q18.1
- cervicosigmoidal N82.4
- cervicovesical N82.1
- cervix N82.8
- chest (wall) J86.0
- cholecystenteric — *see* Fistula, gallbladder
- cholecystocolic — *see* Fistula, gallbladder
- cholecystocolonic — *see* Fistula, gallbladder
- cholecystoduodenal — *see* Fistula, gallbladder
- cholecystogastric — *see* Fistula, gallbladder
- cholecystointestinal — *see* Fistula, gallbladder
- choledochoduodenal — *see* Fistula, bile duct
- cholocolic K82.3
- coccyx — *see* Sinus, pilonidal
- colon K63.2
- colostomy K94.09
- common duct — *see* Fistula, bile duct
- congenital, site not listed — *see* Anomaly, by site
- coronary, arteriovenous I25.41
  - congenital Q24.5
- costal region J86.0
- cul-de-sac, Douglas' N82.8
- cystic duct (*see also* Fistula, gallbladder)
  - congenital Q44.5
- dental K04.6

Fistula — continued

diaphragm J86.Ø
duodenum K31.6
ear (external) (canal) — see Disorder, ear, external,
    specified type NEC
enterocolic K63.2
enterocutaneous K63.2
enterouterine N82.4
    congenital Q51.7
enterovaginal N82.4
    congenital Q52.2
    large intestine N82.3
    small intestine N82.2
enterovesical N32.1
epididymis N5Ø.89
    tuberculous A18.15
esophagobronchial J86.Ø
    congenital Q39.2
        with atresia of esophagus Q39.1
esophagocutaneous K22.8
esophagopleural-cutaneous J86.Ø
esophagotracheal J86.Ø
    congenital Q39.2
        with atresia of esophagus Q39.1
esophagus K22.8
    congenital Q39.2
        with atresia of esophagus Q39.1
ethmoid — see Sinusitis, ethmoidal
eyeball (cornea) (sclera) — see Disorder, globe, hy-
    potony
eyelid HØ1.8
fallopian tube, external N82.5
fecal K63.2
    congenital Q43.6
from periapical abscess KØ4.6
frontal sinus — see Sinusitis, frontal
gallbladder K82.3
    with calculus, cholelithiasis, stones — see Calculus,
        gallbladder
gastric K31.6
gastrocolic K31.6
    congenital Q4Ø.2
    tuberculous A18.32
gastroenterocolic K31.6
gastroesophageal K31.6
gastrojejunal K31.6
gastrojejunocolic K31.6
genital tract (female) N82.9
    specified NEC N82.8
    to intestine NEC N82.4
    to skin N82.5
hepatic artery-portal vein, congenital Q26.6
hepatopleural J86.Ø
hepatopulmonary J86.Ø
ileorectal or ileosigmoidal K63.2
ileovaginal N82.2
ileovesical N32.1
ileum K63.2
in ano K6Ø.3
    tuberculous A18.32
inner ear (labyrinth) — see subcategory H83.1 ☑
intestine NEC K63.2
intestinocolonic (abdominal) K63.2
intestinoureteral N28.89
intestinouterine N82.4
intestinovaginal N82.4
    large intestine N82.3
    small intestine N82.2
intestinovesical N32.1
ischiorectal (fossa) K61.39
jejunum K63.2
joint M25.1Ø
    ankle M25.17- ☑
    elbow M25.12- ☑
    foot joint M25.17- ☑
    hand joint M25.14- ☑
    hip M25.15- ☑
    knee M25.16- ☑
    shoulder M25.11- ☑
    specified joint NEC M25.18
    tuberculous — see Tuberculosis, joint
    vertebrae M25.18
    wrist M25.13- ☑
kidney N28.89
labium (majus) (minus) N82.8
labyrinth — see subcategory H83.1 ☑
lacrimal (gland) (sac) HØ4.61- ☑
lacrimonasal duct — see Fistula, lacrimal

Fistula — continued

laryngotracheal, congenital Q34.8
larynx J38.7
lip K13.Ø
    congenital Q38.Ø
lumbar, tuberculous A18.Ø1
lung J86.Ø
lymphatic I89.8
mammary (gland) N61.Ø
mastoid (process) (region) — see Mastoiditis, chronic
maxillary J32.Ø
medial, face and neck Q18.8
mediastinal J86.Ø
mediastinobronchial J86.Ø
mediastinocutaneous J86.Ø
middle ear — see subcategory H74.8 ☑
mouth K12.2
nasal J34.89
    sinus — see Sinusitis
nasopharynx J39.2
nipple N64.Ø
nose J34.89
oral (cutaneous) K12.2
    maxillary J32.Ø
    nasal (with cleft palate) — see Cleft, palate
orbit, orbital — see Disorder, orbit, specified type NEC
oroantral J32.Ø
oviduct, external N82.5
palate (hard) M27.8
pancreatic K86.89
pancreaticoduodenal K86.89
parotid (gland) K11.4
    region K12.2
penis N48.89
perianal K6Ø.3
pericardium (pleura) (sac) — see Pericarditis
pericecal K63.2
perineorectal K6Ø.4
perineosigmoidal K63.2
perineum, perineal (with urethral involvement) NEC
    N36.Ø
    tuberculous A18.13
    ureter N28.89
perirectal K6Ø.4
    tuberculous A18.32
peritoneum K65.9
pharyngoesophageal J39.2
pharynx J39.2
    branchial cleft (congenital) Q18.Ø
pilonidal (infected) (rectum) — see Sinus, pilonidal
pleura, pleural, pleurocutaneous, pleuroperitoneal
    J86.Ø
    tuberculous NEC A15.6
pleuropericardial I31.8
portal vein-hepatic artery, congenital Q26.6
postauricular H7Ø.81- ☑
postoperative, persistent T81.83 ☑
    specified site — see Fistula, by site
preauricular (congenital) Q18.1
prostate N42.89
pulmonary J86.Ø
    arteriovenous I28.Ø
        congenital Q25.72
    tuberculous — see Tuberculosis, pulmonary
pulmonoperitoneal J86.Ø
rectolabial N82.4
rectosigmoid (intercommunicating) K63.2
rectoureteral N28.89
rectourethral N36.Ø
    congenital Q64.73
rectouterine N82.4
    congenital Q51.7
rectovaginal N82.3
    congenital Q52.2
    tuberculous A18.18
rectovesical N32.1
    congenital Q64.79
rectovesicovaginal N82.3
rectovulval N82.4
    congenital Q52.79
rectum (to skin) K6Ø.4
    congenital Q43.6
        with absence, atresia and stenosis Q42.Ø
    tuberculous A18.32
renal N28.89
retroauricular — see Fistula, postauricular
salivary duct or gland (any) K11.4
    congenital Q38.4

Fistula — continued

scrotum (urinary) N5Ø.89
    tuberculous A18.15
semicircular canals — see subcategory H83.1 ☑
sigmoid K63.2
    to bladder N32.1
sinus — see Sinusitis
skin L98.8
    to genital tract (female) N82.5
splenocolic D73.89
stercoral K63.2
stomach K31.6
sublingual gland K11.4
submandibular gland K11.4
submaxillary (gland) K11.4
    region K12.2
thoracic J86.Ø
    duct I89.8
thoracoabdominal J86.Ø
thoracogastric J86.Ø
thoracointestinal J86.Ø
thorax J86.Ø
thyroglossal duct Q89.2
thyroid EØ7.89
trachea, congenital (external) (internal) Q32.1
tracheoesophageal J86.Ø
    congenital Q39.2
        with atresia of esophagus Q39.1
    following tracheostomy J95.Ø4
traumatic arteriovenous — see Injury, blood vessel, by
    site
tuberculous — code by site under Tuberculosis
typhoid AØ1.Ø9
umbilicourinary Q64.8
urachus, congenital Q64.4
ureter (persistent) N28.89
ureteroabdominal N28.89
ureterorectal N28.89
ureterosigmoido-abdominal N28.89
ureterovaginal N82.1
ureterovesical N32.2
urethra N36.Ø
    congenital Q64.79
    tuberculous A18.13
urethroperineal N36.Ø
urethroperineovesical N32.2
urethrorectal N36.Ø
    congenital Q64.73
urethroscrotal N5Ø.89
urethrovaginal N82.1
urethrovesical N32.2
urinary (tract) (persistent) (recurrent) N36.Ø
uteroabdominal N82.5
    congenital Q51.7
uteroenteric, uterointestinal N82.4
    congenital Q51.7
uterorectal N82.4
    congenital Q51.7
uteroureteric N82.1
uterourethral Q51.7
uterovaginal N82.8
uterovesical N82.1
    congenital Q51.7
uterus N82.8
vagina (postpartal) (wall) N82.8
vaginocutaneous (postpartal) N82.5
vaginointestinal NEC N82.4
    large intestine N82.3
    small intestine N82.2
vaginoperineal N82.5
vasocutaneous, congenital Q55.7
vesical NEC N32.2
vesicoabdominal N32.2
vesicocervicovaginal N82.1
vesicocolic N32.1
vesicocutaneous N32.2
vesicoenteric N32.1
vesicointestinal N32.1
vesicometrorectal N82.4
vesicoperineal N32.2
vesicorectal N32.1
    congenital Q64.79
vesicosigmoidal N32.1
vesicosigmoidovaginal N82.3
vesicoureteral N32.2
vesicoureterovaginal N82.1
vesicourethral N32.2
vesicourethrorectal N32.1
vesicouterine N82.1

▽ Subterms under main terms may continue to next column or page   ☑ Additional Character Required — Refer to the Tabular List for Character Selection   145

Fistula — Fistula

Index

Fistula — continued
vesicouterine — continued
congenital Q51.7
vesicovaginal N82.0
vulvorectal N82.4
congenital Q52.79
Fit R56.9
epileptic — see Epilepsy
fainting R55
hysterical F44.5
newborn P90
Fitting (and adjustment) (of)
artificial
arm — see Admission, adjustment, artificial, arm
breast Z44.3 ☑
eye Z44.2 ☑
leg — see Admission, adjustment, artificial, leg
automatic implantable cardiac defibrillator (with synchronous cardiac pacemaker) Z45.02
brain neuropacemaker Z46.2
implanted Z45.42
cardiac defibrillator — see Fitting (and adjustment) (of), automatic implantable cardiac defibrillator
catheter, non-vascular Z46.82
colostomy belt Z46.89
contact lenses Z46.0
CRT-D (resynchronization therapy defibrillator) Z45.02
CRT-P (cardiac resynchronization therapy pacemaker) Z45.018
pulse generator Z45.010
cystostomy device Z46.6
defibrillator, cardiac — see Fitting (and adjustment) (of), automatic implantable cardiac defibrillator
dentures Z46.3
device NOS Z46.9
abdominal Z46.89
gastrointestinal NEC Z46.59
implanted NEC Z45.89
nervous system Z46.2
implanted — see Admission, adjustment, device, implanted, nervous system
orthodontic Z46.4
orthoptic Z46.0
orthotic Z46.89
prosthetic (external) Z44.9
breast Z44.3 ☑
dental Z46.3
eye Z44.2 ☑
specified NEC Z44.8
specified NEC Z46.89
substitution
auditory Z46.2
implanted — see Admission, adjustment, device, implanted, hearing device
nervous system Z46.2
implanted — see Admission, adjustment, device, implanted, nervous system
visual Z46.2
implanted Z45.31
urinary Z46.6
gastric lap band Z46.51
gastrointestinal appliance NEC Z46.59
glasses (reading) Z46.0
hearing aid Z46.1
ileostomy device Z46.89
insulin pump Z46.81
intestinal appliance NEC Z46.89
myringotomy device (stent) (tube) Z45.82
neuropacemaker Z46.2
implanted Z45.42
non-vascular catheter Z46.82
orthodontic device Z46.4
orthopedic device (brace) (cast) (corset) (shoes) Z46.89
pacemaker (cardiac) (cardiac resynchronization therapy (CRT-P)) Z45.018
nervous system (brain) (peripheral nerve) (spinal cord) Z46.2
implanted Z45.42
pulse generator Z45.010
portacath (port-a-cath) Z45.2
prosthesis (external) Z44.9
arm — see Admission, adjustment, artificial, arm
breast Z44.3 ☑
dental Z46.3
eye Z44.2 ☑
leg — see Admission, adjustment, artificial, leg
specified NEC Z44.8
spectacles Z46.0

Fitting — continued
wheelchair Z46.89
Fitzhugh-Curtis syndrome
due to
Chlamydia trachomatis A74.81
Neisseria gonorrhorea (gonococcal peritonitis) A54.85
Fitz's syndrome (acute hemorrhagic pancreatitis) (see also Pancreatitis, acute) K85.80
Fixation
joint — see Ankylosis
larynx J38.7
stapes — see Ankylosis, ear ossicles
deafness — see Deafness, conductive
uterus (acquired) — see Malposition, uterus
vocal cord J38.3
Flabby ridge K06.8
Flaccid (see also condition)
palate, congenital Q38.5
Flail
chest S22.5 ☑
newborn (birth injury) P13.8
joint (paralytic) M25.20
ankle M25.27- ☑
elbow M25.22- ☑
foot joint M25.27- ☑
hand joint M25.24- ☑
hip M25.25- ☑
knee M25.26- ☑
shoulder M25.21- ☑
specified joint NEC M25.28
wrist M25.23- ☑
Flajani's disease — see Hyperthyroidism, with, goiter (diffuse)
Flap, liver K71.3
Flashbacks (residual to hallucinogen use) F16.283
Flat
chamber (eye) — see Disorder, globe, hypotony, flat anterior chamber
chest, congenital Q67.8
foot (acquired) (fixed type) (painful) (postural) (see also Deformity, limb, flat foot)
congenital (rigid) (spastic (everted)) Q66.5- ☑
rachitic sequelae (late effect) E64.3
organ or site, congenital NEC — see Anomaly, by site
pelvis M95.5
with disproportion (fetopelvic) O33.0
causing obstructed labor O65.0
congenital Q74.2
Flatau-Schilder disease G37.0
Flatback syndrome M40.30
lumbar region M40.36
lumbosacral region M40.37
thoracolumbar region M40.35
Flattening
head, femur M89.8X5
hip — see Coxa, plana
lip (congenital) Q18.8
nose (congenital) Q67.4
acquired M95.0
Flatulence R14.3
psychogenic F45.8
Flatus R14.3
vaginalis N89.8
Flax-dresser's disease J66.1
Flea bite — see Injury, bite, by site, superficial, insect
Flecks, glaucomatous (subcapsular) — see Cataract, complicated
Fleischer (-Kayser) **ring** (cornea) H18.04- ☑
Fleshy mole O02.0
Flexibilitas cerea — see Catalepsy
Flexion
amputation stump (surgical) T87.89
cervix — see Malposition, uterus
contracture, joint — see Contraction, joint
deformity, joint (see also Deformity, limb, flexion) M21.20
hip, congenital Q65.89
uterus (see also Malposition, uterus)
lateral — see Lateroversion, uterus
Flexner-Boyd dysentery A03.2
Flexner's dysentery A03.1
Flexure — see Flexion
Flint murmur (aortic insufficiency) I35.1
Floater, vitreous — see Opacity, vitreous
Floating
cartilage (joint) (see also Loose, body, joint)

Floating — continued
cartilage (see also Loose, body, joint) — continued
knee — see Derangement, knee, loose body
gallbladder, congenital Q44.1
kidney N28.89
congenital Q63.8
spleen D73.89
Flooding N92.0
Floor — see condition
Floppy
baby syndrome (nonspecific) P94.2
iris syndrome (intraoperative) (IFIS) H21.81
nonrheumatic mitral valve syndrome I34.1
Flu (see also Influenza)
avian (see also Influenza, due to, identified novel influenza A virus) J09.X2
bird (see also Influenza, due to, identified novel influenza A virus) J09.X2
intestinal NEC A08.4
swine (viruses that normally cause infections in pigs) (see also Influenza, due to, identified novel influenza A virus) J09.X2
Fluctuating blood pressure I99.8
Fluid
abdomen R18.8
chest J94.8
heart — see Failure, heart, congestive
joint — see Effusion, joint
loss (acute) E86.9
lung — see Edema, lung
overload E87.70
specified NEC E87.79
peritoneal cavity R18.8
pleural cavity J94.8
retention R60.9
Flukes NEC (see also Infestation, fluke)
blood NEC — see Schistosomiasis
liver B66.3
Fluor (vaginalis) N89.8
trichomonal or due to Trichomonas (vaginalis) A59.00
Fluorosis
dental K00.3
skeletal M85.10
ankle M85.17- ☑
foot M85.17- ☑
forearm M85.13- ☑
hand M85.14- ☑
lower leg M85.16- ☑
multiple site M85.19
neck M85.18
rib M85.18
shoulder M85.11- ☑
skull M85.18
specified site NEC M85.18
thigh M85.15- ☑
toe M85.17- ☑
upper arm M85.12- ☑
vertebra M85.18
Flush syndrome E34.0
Flushing R23.2
menopausal N95.1
Flutter
atrial or auricular I48.92
atypical I48.4
type I I48.3
type II I48.4
typical I48.3
heart I49.8
atrial or auricular I48.92
atypical I48.4
type I I48.3
type II I48.4
typical I48.3
ventricular I49.02
ventricular I49.02
FNHTR (febrile nonhemolytic transfusion reaction) R50.84
Fochier's abscess — code by site under Abscess
Focus, Assmann's — see Tuberculosis, pulmonary
Fogo selvagem L10.3
Foix-Alajouanine syndrome G95.19
Fold, folds (anomalous) (see also Anomaly, by site)
Descemet's membrane — see Change, corneal membrane, Descemet's, fold
epicanthic Q10.3
heart Q24.8
Folie à deux F24

☑ **Additional Character Required** — Refer to the Tabular List for Character Selection ▽ **Subterms under main terms may continue to next column or page**

Follicle
  cervix (nabothian) (ruptured) N88.8
  graafian, ruptured, with hemorrhage N83.0- ☑
  nabothian N88.8
Follicular — see condition
Folliculitis (superficial) L73.9
  abscedens et suffodiens L66.3
  cyst N83.0-
  decalvans L66.2
  deep — see Furuncle, by site
  gonococcal (acute) (chronic) A54.01
  keloid, keloidalis L73.0
  pustular L01.02
  ulerythematosa reticulata L66.4
Folliculome lipidique
  specified site — see Neoplasm, benign, by site
  unspecified site
    female D27.9
    male D29.20
Følling's disease E70.0
Follow-up — see Examination, follow-up
Fong's syndrome (hereditary osteo-onychodysplasia) Q87.2
Food
  allergy L27.2
  asphyxia (from aspiration or inhalation) — see Foreign body, by site
  choked on — see Foreign body, by site
  deprivation T73.0 ☑
    specified kind of food NEC E63.8
  intoxication — see Poisoning, food
  lack of T73.0 ☑
  poisoning — see Poisoning, food
  rejection NEC — see Disorder, eating
  strangulation or suffocation — see Foreign body, by site
  toxemia — see Poisoning, food
Foot — see condition
Foramen ovale (nonclosure) (patent) (persistent) Q21.1
Forbes' glycogen storage disease E74.03
Fordyce-Fox disease L75.2
Fordyce's disease (mouth) Q38.6
Forearm — see condition
Foreign body
  with
    laceration — see Laceration, by site, with foreign body
    puncture wound — see Puncture, by site, with foreign body
  accidentally left following a procedure T81.509 ☑
    aspiration T81.506 ☑
      resulting in
        adhesions T81.516 ☑
        obstruction T81.526 ☑
        perforation T81.536 ☑
        specified complication NEC T81.596 ☑
    cardiac catheterization T81.505 ☑
      resulting in
        acute reaction T81.60 ☑
          aseptic peritonitis T81.61 ☑
          specified NEC T81.69 ☑
        adhesions T81.515 ☑
        obstruction T81.525 ☑
        perforation T81.535 ☑
        specified complication NEC T81.595 ☑
      causing
        acute reaction T81.60 ☑
          aseptic peritonitis T81.61 ☑
          specified complication NEC T81.69 ☑
        adhesions T81.519 ☑
        aseptic peritonitis T81.61 ☑
        obstruction T81.529 ☑
        perforation T81.539 ☑
        specified complication NEC T81.599 ☑
    endoscopy T81.504 ☑
      resulting in
        adhesions T81.514 ☑
        obstruction T81.524 ☑
        perforation T81.534 ☑
        specified complication NEC T81.594 ☑
    immunization T81.503 ☑
      resulting in
        adhesions T81.513 ☑
        obstruction T81.523 ☑
        perforation T81.533 ☑
        specified complication NEC T81.593 ☑

Foreign body — continued
  accidentally left following a procedure — continued
    infusion T81.501 ☑
      resulting in
        adhesions T81.511 ☑
        obstruction T81.521 ☑
        perforation T81.531 ☑
        specified complication NEC T81.591 ☑
    injection T81.503 ☑
      resulting in
        adhesions T81.513 ☑
        obstruction T81.523 ☑
        perforation T81.533 ☑
        specified complication NEC T81.593 ☑
    kidney dialysis T81.502 ☑
      resulting in
        adhesions T81.512 ☑
        obstruction T81.522 ☑
        perforation T81.532 ☑
        specified complication NEC T81.592 ☑
    packing removal T81.507 ☑
      resulting in
        acute reaction T81.60 ☑
          aseptic peritonitis T81.61 ☑
          specified NEC T81.69 ☑
        adhesions T81.517 ☑
        obstruction T81.527 ☑
        perforation T81.537 ☑
        specified complication NEC T81.597 ☑
    puncture T81.506 ☑
      resulting in
        adhesions T81.516 ☑
        obstruction T81.526 ☑
        perforation T81.536 ☑
        specified complication NEC T81.596 ☑
    specified procedure NEC T81.508 ☑
      resulting in
        acute reaction T81.60 ☑
          aseptic peritonitis T81.61 ☑
          specified NEC T81.69 ☑
        adhesions T81.518 ☑
        obstruction T81.528 ☑
        perforation T81.538 ☑
        specified complication NEC T81.598 ☑
    surgical operation T81.500 ☑
      resulting in
        acute reaction T81.60 ☑
          aseptic peritonitis T81.61 ☑
          specified NEC T81.69 ☑
        adhesions T81.510 ☑
        obstruction T81.520 ☑
        perforation T81.530 ☑
        specified complication NEC T81.590 ☑
    transfusion T81.501 ☑
      resulting in
        adhesions T81.511 ☑
        obstruction T81.521 ☑
        perforation T81.531 ☑
        specified complication NEC T81.591 ☑
  alimentary tract T18.9 ☑
    anus T18.5 ☑
    colon T18.4 ☑
    esophagus — see Foreign body, esophagus
    mouth T18.0 ☑
    multiple sites T18.8 ☑
    rectosigmoid (junction) T18.5 ☑
    rectum T18.5 ☑
    small intestine T18.3 ☑
    specified site NEC T18.8 ☑
    stomach T18.2 ☑
  anterior chamber (eye) S05.5-
  auditory canal — see Foreign body, entering through orifice, ear
  bronchus T17.508 ☑
    causing
      asphyxiation T17.500 ☑
        food (bone) (seed) T17.520 ☑
        gastric contents (vomitus) T17.510 ☑
        specified type NEC T17.590 ☑
      injury NEC T17.508 ☑
        food (bone) (seed) T17.528 ☑
        gastric contents (vomitus) T17.518 ☑
        specified type NEC T17.598 ☑
  canthus — see Foreign body, conjunctival sac
  ciliary body (eye) S05.5-
  conjunctival sac T15.1-

Foreign body — continued
  cornea T15.0- ☑
  entering through orifice
    accessory sinus T17.0 ☑
    alimentary canal T18.9 ☑
      multiple parts T18.8 ☑
      specified part NEC T18.8 ☑
    alveolar process T18.0 ☑
    antrum (Highmore's) T17.0 ☑
    anus T18.5 ☑
    appendix T18.4 ☑
    auditory canal — see Foreign body, entering through orifice, ear
    auricle — see Foreign body, entering through orifice, ear
    bladder T19.1 ☑
    bronchioles — see Foreign body, respiratory tract, specified site NEC
    bronchus (main) — see Foreign body, bronchus
    buccal cavity T18.0 ☑
    canthus (inner) — see Foreign body, conjunctival sac
    cecum T18.4 ☑
    cervix (canal) (uteri) T19.3 ☑
    colon T18.4 ☑
    conjunctival sac — see Foreign body, conjunctival sac
    cornea — see Foreign body, cornea
    digestive organ or tract NOS T18.9 ☑
      multiple parts T18.8 ☑
      specified part NEC T18.8 ☑
    duodenum T18.3 ☑
    ear (external) T16.- ☑
    esophagus — see Foreign body, esophagus
    eye (external) NOS T15.9- ☑
      conjunctival sac — see Foreign body, conjunctival sac
      cornea — see Foreign body, cornea
      specified part NEC T15.8- ☑
    eyeball (see also Foreign body, entering through orifice, eye, specified part NEC)
      with penetrating wound — see Puncture, eyeball
    eyelid (see also Foreign body, conjunctival sac)
      with
        laceration — see Laceration, eyelid, with foreign body
        puncture — see Puncture, eyelid, with foreign body
        superficial injury — see Foreign body, superficial, eyelid
    gastrointestinal tract T18.9 ☑
      multiple parts T18.8 ☑
      specified part NEC T18.8 ☑
    genitourinary tract T19.9 ☑
      multiple parts T19.8 ☑
      specified part NEC T19.8 ☑
    globe — see Foreign body, entering through orifice, eyeball
    gum T18.0 ☑
    Highmore's antrum T17.0 ☑
    hypopharynx — see Foreign body, pharynx
    ileum T18.3 ☑
    intestine (small) T18.3 ☑
      large T18.4 ☑
    lacrimal apparatus (punctum) — see Foreign body, entering through orifice, eye, specified part NEC
    large intestine T18.4 ☑
    larynx — see Foreign body, larynx
    lung — see Foreign body, respiratory tract, specified site NEC
    maxillary sinus T17.0 ☑
    mouth T18.0 ☑
    nasal sinus T17.0 ☑
    nasopharynx — see Foreign body, pharynx
    nose (passage) T17.1 ☑
    nostril T17.1 ☑
    oral cavity T18.0 ☑
    palate T18.0 ☑
    penis T19.4 ☑
    pharynx — see Foreign body, pharynx
    piriform sinus — see Foreign body, pharynx
    rectosigmoid (junction) T18.5 ☑
    rectum T18.5 ☑
    respiratory tract — see Foreign body, respiratory tract

Foreign body — *continued*
  entering through orifice — *continued*
    sinus (accessory) (frontal) (maxillary) (nasal) T17.0 ☑
      piriform — *see* Foreign body, pharynx
    small intestine T18.3 ☑
    stomach T18.2 ☑
    suffocation by — *see* Foreign body, by site
    tear ducts or glands — *see* Foreign body, entering
      through orifice, eye, specified part NEC
    throat — *see* Foreign body, pharynx
    tongue T18.0 ☑
    tonsil, tonsillar (fossa) — *see* Foreign body, pharynx
    trachea — *see* Foreign body, trachea
    ureter T19.8 ☑
    urethra T19.0 ☑
    uterus (any part) T19.3 ☑
    vagina T19.2 ☑
    vulva T19.2 ☑
  esophagus T18.108 ☑
    causing
      injury NEC T18.108 ☑
        food (bone) (seed) T18.128 ☑
        gastric contents (vomitus) T18.118 ☑
        specified type NEC T18.198 ☑
      tracheal compression T18.100 ☑
        food (bone) (seed) T18.120 ☑
        gastric contents (vomitus) T18.110 ☑
        specified type NEC T18.190 ☑
  feeling of, in throat R09.89
  fragment — *see* Retained, foreign body fragments
    (type of)
  genitourinary tract T19.9 ☑
    bladder T19.1 ☑
    multiple parts T19.8 ☑
    penis T19.4 ☑
    specified site NEC T19.8 ☑
    urethra T19.0 ☑
    uterus T19.3 ☑
      IUD Z97.5
    vagina T19.2 ☑
      contraceptive device Z97.5
    vulva T19.2 ☑
  granuloma (old) (soft tissue) (*see also* Granuloma, foreign body)
    skin L92.3
  in
    laceration — *see* Laceration, by site, with foreign body
    puncture wound — *see* Puncture, by site, with foreign body
    soft tissue (residual) M79.5
  inadvertently left in operation wound — *see* Foreign body, accidentally left during a procedure
  ingestion, ingested NOS T18.9 ☑
  inhalation or inspiration — *see* Foreign body, by site
  internal organ, not entering through a natural orifice — code as specific injury with foreign body
  intraocular S05.5- ☑
    old, retained (nonmagnetic) H44.70- ☑
      anterior chamber H44.71- ☑
      ciliary body H44.72- ☑
      iris H44.72- ☑
      lens H44.73- ☑
      magnetic H44.60- ☑
        anterior chamber H44.61- ☑
        ciliary body H44.62- ☑
        iris H44.62- ☑
        lens H44.63- ☑
        posterior wall H44.64- ☑
        specified site NEC H44.69- ☑
        vitreous body H44.65- ☑
      posterior wall H44.74- ☑
      specified site NEC H44.79- ☑
      vitreous body H44.75- ☑
  iris — *see* Foreign body, intraocular
  lacrimal punctum — *see* Foreign body, entering through orifice, eye, specified part NEC
  larynx T17.308 ☑
    causing
      asphyxiation T17.300 ☑
        food (bone) (seed) T17.320 ☑
        gastric contents (vomitus) T17.310 ☑
        specified type NEC T17.390 ☑
      injury NEC T17.308 ☑
        food (bone) (seed) T17.328 ☑
        gastric contents (vomitus) T17.318 ☑

Foreign body — *continued*
  larynx — *continued*
    causing — *continued*
      injury — *continued*
        specified type NEC T17.398 ☑
  lens — *see* Foreign body, intraocular
  ocular muscle S05.4- ☑
    old, retained — *see* Foreign body, orbit, old
  old or residual
    soft tissue (residual) M79.5
  operation wound, left accidentally — *see* Foreign body, accidentally left during a procedure
  orbit S05.4- ☑
    old, retained H05.5- ☑
  pharynx T17.208 ☑
    causing
      asphyxiation T17.200 ☑
        food (bone) (seed) T17.220 ☑
        gastric contents (vomitus) T17.210 ☑
        specified type NEC T17.290 ☑
      injury NEC T17.208 ☑
        food (bone) (seed) T17.228 ☑
        gastric contents (vomitus) T17.218 ☑
        specified type NEC T17.298 ☑
  respiratory tract T17.908 ☑
    bronchioles — *see* Foreign body, respiratory tract, specified site NEC
    bronchus — *see* Foreign body, bronchus
    causing
      asphyxiation T17.900 ☑
        food (bone) (seed) T17.920 ☑
        gastric contents (vomitus) T17.910 ☑
        specified type NEC T17.990 ☑
      injury NEC T17.908 ☑
        food (bone) (seed) T17.928 ☑
        gastric contents (vomitus) T17.918 ☑
        specified type NEC T17.998 ☑
    larynx — *see* Foreign body, larynx
    lung — *see* Foreign body, respiratory tract, specified site NEC
    multiple parts — *see* Foreign body, respiratory tract, specified site NEC
    nasal sinus T17.0 ☑
    nasopharynx — *see* Foreign body, pharynx
    nose T17.1 ☑
    nostril T17.1 ☑
    pharynx — *see* Foreign body, pharynx
    specified site NEC T17.808 ☑
      causing
        asphyxiation T17.800 ☑
          food (bone) (seed) T17.820 ☑
          gastric contents (vomitus) T17.810 ☑
          specified type NEC T17.890 ☑
        injury NEC T17.808 ☑
          food (bone) (seed) T17.828 ☑
          gastric contents (vomitus) T17.818 ☑
          specified type NEC T17.898 ☑
    throat — *see* Foreign body, pharynx
    trachea — *see* Foreign body, trachea
  retained (old) (nonmagnetic) (in)
    anterior chamber (eye) — *see* Foreign body, intraocular, old, retained, anterior chamber
      magnetic — *see* Foreign body, intraocular, old, retained, magnetic, anterior chamber
    ciliary body — *see* Foreign body, intraocular, old, retained, ciliary body
      magnetic — *see* Foreign body, intraocular, old, retained, magnetic, ciliary body
    eyelid H02.819
      left H02.816
        lower H02.815
        upper H02.814
      right H02.813
        lower H02.812
        upper H02.811
    fragments — *see* Retained, foreign body fragments (type of)
    globe — *see* Foreign body, intraocular, old, retained
      magnetic — *see* Foreign body, intraocular, old, retained, magnetic
    intraocular — *see* Foreign body, intraocular, old, retained
      magnetic — *see* Foreign body, intraocular, old, retained, magnetic
    iris — *see* Foreign body, intraocular, old, retained, iris

Foreign body — *continued*
  retained — *continued*
    iris — *see* Foreign body, intraocular, old, retained, iris — *continued*
      magnetic — *see* Foreign body, intraocular, old, retained, magnetic, iris
    lens — *see* Foreign body, intraocular, old, retained, lens
      magnetic — *see* Foreign body, intraocular, old, retained, magnetic, lens
    muscle — *see* Foreign body, retained, soft tissue
    orbit — *see* Foreign body, orbit, old
    posterior wall of globe — *see* Foreign body, intraocular, old, retained, posterior wall
      magnetic — *see* Foreign body, intraocular, old, retained, magnetic, posterior wall
    retrobulbar — *see* Foreign body, orbit, old, retrobulbar
    soft tissue M79.5
    vitreous — *see* Foreign body, intraocular, old, retained, vitreous body
      magnetic — *see* Foreign body, intraocular, old, retained, magnetic, vitreous body
  retina S05.5- ☑
  superficial, without open wound
    abdomen, abdominal (wall) S30.851 ☑
    alveolar process S00.552 ☑
    ankle S90.55- ☑
    antecubital space — *see* Foreign body, superficial, forearm
    anus S30.857 ☑
    arm (upper) S40.85- ☑
    auditory canal — *see* Foreign body, superficial, ear
    auricle — *see* Foreign body, superficial, ear
    axilla — *see* Foreign body, superficial, arm
    back, lower S30.850 ☑
    breast S20.15- ☑
    brow S00.85 ☑
    buttock S30.850 ☑
    calf — *see* Foreign body, superficial, leg
    canthus — *see* Foreign body, superficial, eyelid
    cheek S00.85 ☑
      internal S00.552 ☑
    chest wall — *see* Foreign body, superficial, thorax
    chin S00.85 ☑
    clitoris S30.854 ☑
    costal region — *see* Foreign body, superficial, thorax
    digit(s)
      foot — *see* Foreign body, superficial, toe
      hand — *see* Foreign body, superficial, finger
    ear S00.45- ☑
    elbow S50.35- ☑
    epididymis S30.853 ☑
    epigastric region S30.851 ☑
    epiglottis S10.15 ☑
    esophagus, cervical S10.15 ☑
    eyebrow — *see* Foreign body, superficial, eyelid
    eyelid S00.25- ☑
    face S00.85 ☑
    finger(s) S60.459 ☑
      index S60.45- ☑
      little S60.45- ☑
      middle S60.45- ☑
      ring S60.45- ☑
    flank S30.851 ☑
    foot (except toe(s) alone) S90.85- ☑
      toe — *see* Foreign body, superficial, toe
    forearm S50.85- ☑
      elbow only — *see* Foreign body, superficial, elbow
    forehead S00.85 ☑
    genital organs, external
      female S30.856 ☑
      male S30.855 ☑
    groin S30.851 ☑
    gum S00.552 ☑
    hand S60.55- ☑
    head S00.95 ☑
      ear — *see* Foreign body, superficial, ear
      eyelid — *see* Foreign body, superficial, eyelid
      lip S00.551 ☑
      nose S00.35 ☑
      oral cavity S00.552 ☑
      scalp S00.05 ☑
      specified site NEC S00.85 ☑
    heel — *see* Foreign body, superficial, foot

Foreign body — *continued*

superficial, without open wound — *continued*

hip S70.25- ☑
inguinal region S30.851 ☑
interscapular region S20.459 ☑
jaw S00.85 ☑
knee S80.25- ☑
labium (majus) (minus) S30.854 ☑
larynx S10.15 ☑
leg (lower) S80.85- ☑
  knee — *see* Foreign body, superficial, knee
  upper — *see* Foreign body, superficial, thigh
lip S00.551 ☑
lower back S30.850 ☑
lumbar region S30.850 ☑
malar region S00.85 ☑
mammary — *see* Foreign body, superficial, breast
mastoid region S00.85 ☑
mouth S00.552 ☑
nail
  finger — *see* Foreign body, superficial, finger
  toe — *see* Foreign body, superficial, toe
nape S10.85 ☑
nasal S00.35 ☑
neck S10.95 ☑
  specified site NEC S10.85 ☑
  throat S10.15 ☑
nose S00.35 ☑
occipital region S00.05 ☑
oral cavity S00.552 ☑
orbital region — *see* Foreign body, superficial, eyelid
palate S00.552 ☑
palm — *see* Foreign body, superficial, hand
parietal region S00.05 ☑
pelvis S30.850 ☑
penis S30.852 ☑
perineum
  female S30.854 ☑
  male S30.850 ☑
periocular area — *see* Foreign body, superficial, eyelid
phalanges
  finger — *see* Foreign body, superficial, finger
  toe — *see* Foreign body, superficial, toe
pharynx S10.15 ☑
pinna — *see* Foreign body, superficial, ear
popliteal space — *see* Foreign body, superficial, knee
prepuce S30.852 ☑
pubic region S30.850 ☑
pudendum
  female S30.856 ☑
  male S30.855 ☑
sacral region S30.850 ☑
scalp S00.05 ☑
scapular region — *see* Foreign body, superficial, shoulder
scrotum S30.853 ☑
shin — *see* Foreign body, superficial, leg
shoulder S40.25- ☑
sternal region S20.359 ☑
submaxillary region S00.85 ☑
submental region S00.85 ☑
subungual
  finger(s) — *see* Foreign body, superficial, finger
  toe(s) — *see* Foreign body, superficial, toe
supraclavicular fossa S10.85 ☑
supraorbital S00.85 ☑
temple S00.85 ☑
temporal region S00.85 ☑
testis S30.853 ☑
thigh S70.35- ☑
thorax, thoracic (wall) S20.95 ☑
  back S20.45- ☑
  front S20.35- ☑
throat S10.15 ☑
thumb S60.35- ☑
toe(s) (lesser) S90.456 ☑
  great S90.45- ☑
tongue S00.552 ☑
trachea S10.15 ☑
tunica vaginalis S30.853 ☑
tympanum, tympanic membrane — *see* Foreign body, superficial, ear
uvula S00.552 ☑
vagina S30.854 ☑

Foreign body — *continued*

superficial, without open wound — *continued*

vocal cords S10.15 ☑
vulva S30.854 ☑
wrist S60.85- ☑
swallowed T18.9 ☑
trachea T17.408 ☑
causing
  asphyxiation T17.400 ☑
   food (bone) (seed) T17.420 ☑
   gastric contents (vomitus) T17.410 ☑
   specified type NEC T17.490 ☑
  injury NEC T17.408 ☑
   food (bone) (seed) T17.428 ☑
   gastric contents (vomitus) T17.418 ☑
   specified type NEC T17.498 ☑
type of fragment — *see* Retained, foreign body fragments (type of)
vitreous (humor) S05.5- ☑

Forestier's disease (rhizomelic pseudopolyarthritis) M35.3
meaning ankylosing hyperostosis — *see* Hyperostosis, ankylosing

Formation
hyalin in cornea — *see* Degeneration, cornea
sequestrum in bone (due to infection) — *see* Osteomyelitis, chronic
valve
  colon, congenital Q43.8
  ureter (congenital) Q62.39

Formication R20.2
Fort Bragg fever A27.89
Fossa (*see also* condition)
pyriform — *see* condition
Foster-Kennedy syndrome H47.14- ☑
Fothergill's
disease (trigeminal neuralgia) (*see also* Neuralgia, trigeminal)
  scarlatina anginosa A38.9
Foul breath R19.6
Foundling Z76.1
Fournier disease or gangrene N49.3
female N76.89
Fourth
cranial nerve — *see* condition
molar K00.1
Foville's (peduncular) **disease or syndrome** G46.3
Fox (-Fordyce) disease (apocrine miliaria) L75.2
FPIES (food protein-induced enteropathy syndrome) K52.21
Fracture, burst — *see* Fracture, traumatic, by site
Fracture, chronic — *see* Fracture, pathological, by site
Fracture, insufficiency — *see* Fracture, pathological, by site
Fracture, nontraumatic, NEC
atypical
  femur M84.750- ☑
  complete
   oblique M84.759 ☑
    left side M84.758 ☑
    right side M84.757 ☑
   transverse M84.756 ☑
    left side M84.755 ☑
    right side M84.754 ☑
  incomplete M84.753 ☑
   left side M84.752 ☑
   right side M84.751 ☑
Fracture, pathological (pathologic) (*see also* Fracture, traumatic) M84.40 ☑
ankle M84.47- ☑
carpus M84.44- ☑
clavicle M84.41- ☑
compression (not due to trauma) (*see also* Collapse, vertebra) M48.50- ☑
dental implant M27.63
dental restorative material K08.539
  with loss of material K08.531
  without loss of material K08.530
due to
  neoplastic disease NEC (*see also* Neoplasm) M84.50
   ankle M84.57- ☑
   carpus M84.54- ☑
   clavicle M84.51- ☑
   femur M84.55- ☑
   fibula M84.56- ☑

Fracture, pathological — *continued*
due to — *continued*
  neoplastic disease (*see also* Neoplasm) — *continued*
   finger M84.54- ☑
   hip M84.559 ☑
   humerus M84.52- ☑
   ilium M84.550 ☑
   ischium M84.550 ☑
   metacarpus M84.54- ☑
   metatarsus M84.57- ☑
   neck M84.58 ☑
   pelvis M84.550 ☑
   radius M84.53- ☑
   rib M84.58 ☑
   scapula M84.51- ☑
   skull M84.58 ☑
   specified site NEC M84.58 ☑
   tarsus M84.57- ☑
   tibia M84.56- ☑
   toe M84.57- ☑
   ulna M84.53- ☑
   vertebra M84.58 ☑
  osteoporosis M80.00 ☑
   disuse — *see* Osteoporosis, specified type NEC, with pathological fracture
   drug-induced — *see* Osteoporosis, drug induced, with pathological fracture
   idiopathic — *see* Osteoporosis, specified type NEC, with pathological fracture
   postmenopausal — *see* Osteoporosis, postmenopausal, with pathological fracture
   postoophorectomy — *see* Osteoporosis, postoophorectomy, with pathological fracture
   postsurgical malabsorption — *see* Osteoporosis, specified type NEC, with pathological fracture
   specified cause NEC — *see* Osteoporosis, specified type NEC, with pathological fracture
  specified disease NEC M84.60 ☑
   ankle M84.67- ☑
   carpus M84.64- ☑
   clavicle M84.61- ☑
   femur M84.65- ☑
   fibula M84.66- ☑
   finger M84.64- ☑
   hip M84.65- ☑
   humerus M84.62- ☑
   ilium M84.650 ☑
   ischium M84.650 ☑
   metacarpus M84.64- ☑
   metatarsus M84.67- ☑
   neck M84.68 ☑
   radius M84.63- ☑
   rib M84.68 ☑
   scapula M84.61- ☑
   skull M84.68 ☑
   tarsus M84.67- ☑
   tibia M84.66- ☑
   toe M84.67- ☑
   ulna M84.63- ☑
   vertebra M84.68 ☑
femur M84.45- ☑
fibula M84.46- ☑
finger M84.44- ☑
hip M84.459 ☑
humerus M84.42- ☑
ilium M84.454 ☑
ischium M84.454 ☑
joint prosthesis — *see* Complications, joint prosthesis, mechanical, breakdown, by site
  periprosthetic — *see* Fracture, pathological, periprosthetic
metacarpus M84.44- ☑
metatarsus M84.47- ☑
neck M84.48 ☑
pelvis M84.454 ☑
periprosthetic M97.9 ☑
  ankle M97.2- ☑
  elbow M97.4- ☑
  finger M97.8 ☑
  hip M97.0- ☑
  knee M97.1- ☑
  other specified joint M97.8 ☑
  shoulder M97.3- ☑
  spinal joint M97.8 ☑

Fracture, pathological — *continued*
  periprosthetic — *continued*
    toe joint M97.8 ☑
    wrist joint M97.8 ☑
  radius M84.43-
  restorative material (dental) K08.539
    with loss of material K08.531
    without loss of material K08.530
  rib M84.48 ☑
  scapula M84.41- ☑
  skull M84.48 ☑
  tarsus M84.47- ☑
  tibia M84.46- ☑
  toe M84.47- ☑
  ulna M84.43- ☑
  vertebra M84.48 ☑
Fracture, traumatic (abduction) (adduction) (separation)
    (*see also* Fracture, pathological) T14.8 ☑
  acetabulum S32.40- ☑
    column
      anterior (displaced) (iliopubic) S32.43- ☑
        nondisplaced S32.436 ☑
      posterior (displaced) (ilioischial) S32.443 ☑
        nondisplaced S32.44- ☑
    dome (displaced) S32.48- ☑
      nondisplaced S32.48 ☑
    specified NEC S32.49- ☑
    transverse (displaced) S32.45- ☑
      with associated posterior wall fracture (displaced)
        S32.46- ☑
      nondisplaced S32.46- ☑
      nondisplaced S32.45- ☑
    wall
      anterior (displaced) S32.41- ☑
        nondisplaced S32.41- ☑
      medial (displaced) S32.47- ☑
        nondisplaced S32.47- ☑
      posterior (displaced) S32.42- ☑
        with associated transverse fracture (displaced)
          S32.46- ☑
        nondisplaced S32.46- ☑
        nondisplaced S32.42- ☑
  acromion — *see* Fracture, scapula, acromial process
  ankle S82.899 ☑
    bimalleolar (displaced) S82.84- ☑
      nondisplaced S82.84- ☑
    lateral malleolus only (displaced) S82.6- ☑
      nondisplaced S82.6- ☑
    medial malleolus (displaced) S82.5- ☑
      associated with Maisonneuve's fracture — *see*
        Fracture, Maisonneuve's
      nondisplaced S82.5- ☑
    talus — *see* Fracture, tarsal, talus
    trimalleolar (displaced) S82.85- ☑
      nondisplaced S82.85- ☑
  arm (upper) (*see also* Fracture, humerus, shaft)
    humerus — *see* Fracture, humerus
    radius — *see* Fracture, radius
    ulna — *see* Fracture, ulna
  astragalus — *see* Fracture, tarsal, talus
  atlas — *see* Fracture, neck, cervical vertebra, first
  axis — *see* Fracture, neck, cervical vertebra, second
  back — *see* Fracture, vertebra
  Barton's — *see* Barton's fracture
  base of skull — *see* Fracture, skull, base
  basicervical (basal) (femoral) S72.0 ☑
  Bennett's — *see* Bennett's fracture
  bimalleolar — *see* Fracture, ankle, bimalleolar
  blow-out S02.3- ☑
  bone NEC T14.8 ☑
    birth injury P13.9
    following insertion of orthopedic implant, joint
        prosthesis or bone plate — *see* Fracture, fol-
        lowing insertion of orthopedic implant, joint
        prosthesis or bone plate
    in (due to) neoplastic disease NEC — *see* Fracture,
        pathological, due to, neoplastic disease
    pathological (cause unknown) — *see* Fracture,
        pathological
  breast bone — *see* Fracture, sternum
  bucket handle (semilunar cartilage) — *see* Tear,
      meniscus
  burst — *see* Fracture, traumatic, by site
  calcaneus — *see* Fracture, tarsal, calcaneus
  carpal bone(s) S62.10- ☑
    capitate (displaced) S62.13- ☑

Fracture, traumatic — *continued*
  carpal bone(s) — *continued*
    capitate — *continued*
      nondisplaced S62.13- ☑
    cuneiform — *see* Fracture, carpal bone, triquetrum
    hamate (body) (displaced) S62.143 ☑
      hook process (displaced) S62.15- ☑
        nondisplaced S62.15- ☑
        nondisplaced S62.14- ☑
    larger multangular — *see* Fracture, carpal bones,
        trapezium
    lunate (displaced) S62.12- ☑
      nondisplaced S62.12- ☑
    navicular S62.00- ☑
      distal pole (displaced) S62.01- ☑
        nondisplaced S62.01- ☑
      middle third (displaced) S62.02- ☑
        nondisplaced S62.02- ☑
      proximal third (displaced) S62.03- ☑
        nondisplaced S62.03- ☑
      volar tuberosity — *see* Fracture, carpal bones,
          navicular, distal pole
    os magnum — *see* Fracture, carpal bones, capitate
    pisiform (displaced) S62.16- ☑
      nondisplaced S62.16- ☑
    semilunar — *see* Fracture, carpal bones, lunate
    smaller multangular — *see* Fracture, carpal bones,
        trapezoid
    trapezium (displaced) S62.17- ☑
      nondisplaced S62.17- ☑
    trapezoid (displaced) S62.18- ☑
      nondisplaced S62.18- ☑
    triquetrum (displaced) S62.11- ☑
      nondisplaced S62.11- ☑
    unciform — *see* Fracture, carpal bones, hamate
  cervical — *see* Fracture, vertebra, cervical
  clavicle S42.00- ☑
    acromial end (displaced) S42.03- ☑
      nondisplaced S42.03- ☑
    birth injury P13.4
    lateral end — *see* Fracture, clavicle, acromial end
    shaft (displaced) S42.02- ☑
      nondisplaced S42.02- ☑
    sternal end (anterior) (displaced) S42.01- ☑
      nondisplaced S42.01- ☑
      posterior S42.01- ☑
  coccyx S32.2 ☑
  collapsed — *see* Collapse, vertebra
  collar bone — *see* Fracture, clavicle
  Colles' — *see* Colles' fracture
  coronoid process — *see* Fracture, ulna, upper end,
      coronoid process
  corpus cavernosum penis S39.840 ☑
  costochondral cartilage S23.41 ☑
  costochondral, costosternal junction — *see* Fracture,
      rib
  cranium — *see* Fracture, skull
  cricoid cartilage S12.8 ☑
  cuboid (ankle) — *see* Fracture, tarsal, cuboid
  cuneiform
    foot — *see* Fracture, tarsal, cuneiform
    wrist — *see* Fracture, carpal, triquetrum
  delayed union — *see* Delay, union, fracture
  dental restorative material K08.539
    with loss of material K08.531
    without loss of material K08.530
  due to
    birth injury — *see* Birth, injury, fracture
    osteoporosis — *see* Osteoporosis, with fracture
  Dupuytren's — *see* Fracture, ankle, lateral malleolus
  elbow S42.40- ☑
  ethmoid (bone) (sinus) — *see* Fracture, skull, base
  face bone S02.92 ☑
  fatigue (*see also* Fracture, stress)
    vertebra M48.40 ☑
      cervical region M48.42 ☑
      cervicothoracic region M48.43 ☑
      lumbar region M48.46 ☑
      lumbosacral region M48.47 ☑
      occipito-atlanto-axial region M48.41 ☑
      sacrococcygeal region M48.48 ☑
      thoracic region M48.44 ☑
      thoracolumbar region M48.45 ☑
  femur, femoral S72.9- ☑
    basicervical (basal) S72.0 ☑
    birth injury P13.2

Fracture, traumatic — *continued*
  femur, femoral — *continued*
    capital epiphyseal S79.01- ☑
    condyles, epicondyles — *see* Fracture, femur, lower
        end
    distal end — *see* Fracture, femur, lower end
    epiphysis
      head — *see* Fracture, femur, upper end, epiphysis
      lower — *see* Fracture, femur, lower end, epiph-
          ysis
      upper — *see* Fracture, femur, upper end, epiph-
          ysis
    following insertion of implant, prosthesis or plate
        M96.66- ☑
    head — *see* Fracture, femur, upper end, head
    intertrochanteric — *see* Fracture, femur,
        trochanteric
    intratrochanteric — *see* Fracture, femur,
        trochanteric
    lower end S72.40- ☑
      condyle (displaced) S72.41- ☑
        lateral (displaced) S72.42- ☑
          nondisplaced S72.42- ☑
        medial (displaced) S72.43- ☑
          nondisplaced S72.43- ☑
        nondisplaced S72.41- ☑
      epiphysis (displaced) S72.44- ☑
        nondisplaced S72.44- ☑
      physeal S79.10- ☑
        Salter-Harris
          Type I S79.11- ☑
          Type II S79.12- ☑
          Type III S79.13- ☑
          Type IV S79.14- ☑
        specified NEC S79.19- ☑
      specified NEC S72.49- ☑
      supracondylar (displaced) S72.45- ☑
        with intracondylar extension (displaced)
            S72.46- ☑
          nondisplaced S72.46- ☑
        nondisplaced S72.45- ☑
      torus S72.47- ☑
    neck — *see* Fracture, femur, upper end, neck
    pertrochanteric — *see* Fracture, femur, trochanteric
    shaft (lower third) (middle third) (upper third)
        S72.30- ☑
      comminuted (displaced) S72.35- ☑
        nondisplaced S72.35- ☑
      oblique (displaced) S72.33- ☑
        nondisplaced S72.33- ☑
      segmental (displaced) S72.36- ☑
        nondisplaced S72.36- ☑
      specified NEC S72.39- ☑
      spiral (displaced) S72.34- ☑
        nondisplaced S72.34- ☑
      transverse (displaced) S72.32- ☑
        nondisplaced S72.32- ☑
    specified site NEC — *see* subcategory S72.8 ☑
    subcapital (displaced) S72.01- ☑
    subtrochanteric (region) (section) (displaced)
        S72.2- ☑
      nondisplaced S72.2- ☑
    transcervical — *see* Fracture, femur, upper end, neck
    transtrochanteric — *see* Fracture, femur,
        trochanteric
    trochanteric S72.10- ☑
      apophyseal (displaced) S72.13- ☑
        nondisplaced S72.13- ☑
      greater trochanter (displaced) S72.11- ☑
        nondisplaced S72.11- ☑
      intertrochanteric (displaced) S72.14- ☑
        nondisplaced S72.14- ☑
      lesser trochanter (displaced) S72.12- ☑
        nondisplaced S72.12- ☑
    upper end S72.00- ☑
      apophyseal (displaced) S72.13- ☑
        nondisplaced S72.13- ☑
      cervicotrochanteric — *see* Fracture, femur, upper
          end, neck, base
      epiphysis (displaced) S72.02- ☑
        nondisplaced S72.02- ☑
      head S72.05- ☑
        articular (displaced) S72.06- ☑
          nondisplaced S72.06- ☑
        specified NEC S72.09- ☑
      intertrochanteric (displaced) S72.14- ☑

☑ **Additional Character Required** — **Refer to the Tabular List for Character Selection**   ⬇ **Subterms under main terms may continue to next column or page**

Fracture, traumatic — *continued*
  femur, femoral — *continued*
    upper end — *continued*
      intertrochanteric — *continued*
        nondisplaced S72.14- ☑
      intracapsular S72.01- ☑
      midcervical (displaced) S72.03- ☑
        nondisplaced S72.03- ☑
      neck S72.00- ☑
        base (displaced) S72.04- ☑
          nondisplaced S72.04- ☑
        specified NEC S72.09- ☑
      pertrochanteric — *see* Fracture, femur, upper
        end, trochanteric
      physeal S79.00- ☑
        Salter-Harris type I S79.01- ☑
        specified NEC S79.09- ☑
      subcapital (displaced) S72.01- ☑
      subtrochanteric (displaced) S72.2- ☑
        nondisplaced S72.2- ☑
      transcervical — *see* Fracture, femur, upper end,
        midcervical
      trochanteric S72.10- ☑
        greater (displaced) S72.11- ☑
          nondisplaced S72.11- ☑
        lesser (displaced) S72.12- ☑
          nondisplaced S72.12- ☑
  fibula (shaft) (styloid) S82.40- ☑
    comminuted (displaced) S82.45- ☑
      nondisplaced S82.45- ☑
    following insertion of implant, prosthesis or plate
      M96.67- ☑
    involving ankle or malleolus — *see* Fracture, fibula,
      lateral malleolus
    lateral malleolus (displaced) S82.6- ☑
      nondisplaced S82.6- ☑
    lower end
      physeal S89.30- ☑
        Salter-Harris
          Type I S89.31- ☑
          Type II S89.32- ☑
        specified NEC S89.39- ☑
      specified NEC S82.83- ☑
      torus S82.82- ☑
    oblique (displaced) S82.43- ☑
      nondisplaced S82.43- ☑
    segmental (displaced) S82.46- ☑
      nondisplaced S82.46- ☑
    specified NEC S82.49- ☑
    spiral (displaced) S82.44- ☑
      nondisplaced S82.44- ☑
    transverse (displaced) S82.42- ☑
      nondisplaced S82.42- ☑
    upper end
      physeal S89.20- ☑
        Salter-Harris
          Type I S89.21- ☑
          Type II S89.22- ☑
        specified NEC S89.29- ☑
      specified NEC S82.83- ☑
      torus S82.81- ☑
  finger (except thumb) S62.60- ☑
    distal phalanx (displaced) S62.63- ☑
      nondisplaced S62.66- ☑
    index S62.60- ☑
      distal phalanx (displaced) S62.63- ☑
        nondisplaced S62.66- ☑
      middle phalanx (displaced) S62.62- ☑
        nondisplaced S62.65- ☑
      proximal phalanx (displaced) S62.61- ☑
        nondisplaced S62.64- ☑
    little S62.60- ☑
      distal phalanx (displaced) S62.63- ☑
        nondisplaced S62.66- ☑
      middle phalanx (displaced) S62.62- ☑
        nondisplaced S62.65- ☑
      proximal phalanx (displaced) S62.61- ☑
        nondisplaced S62.64- ☑
    middle S62.60- ☑
      distal phalanx (displaced) S62.63- ☑
        nondisplaced S62.66- ☑
      middle phalanx (displaced) S62.62- ☑
        nondisplaced S62.65- ☑
      proximal phalanx (displaced) S62.61- ☑
        nondisplaced S62.64- ☑
      middle phalanx (displaced) S62.62- ☑

Fracture, traumatic — *continued*
  finger — *continued*
    middle phalanx — *continued*
      nondisplaced S62.65- ☑
      proximal phalanx (displaced) S62.61- ☑
        nondisplaced S62.64- ☑
    ring S62.60- ☑
      distal phalanx (displaced) S62.63- ☑
        nondisplaced S62.66- ☑
      middle phalanx (displaced) S62.62- ☑
        nondisplaced S62.65- ☑
      proximal phalanx (displaced) S62.61- ☑
        nondisplaced S62.64- ☑
    thumb — *see* Fracture, thumb
  following insertion (intraoperative) (postoperative) of
    orthopedic implant, joint prosthesis or bone
    plate M96.69
    femur M96.66- ☑
    fibula M96.67- ☑
    humerus M96.62- ☑
    pelvis M96.65
    radius M96.63- ☑
    specified bone NEC M96.69
    tibia M96.67- ☑
    ulna M96.63- ☑
  foot S92.90- ☑
    astragalus — *see* Fracture, tarsal, talus
    calcaneus — *see* Fracture, tarsal, calcaneus
    cuboid — *see* Fracture, tarsal, cuboid
    cuneiform — *see* Fracture, tarsal, cuneiform
    metatarsal — *see* Fracture, metatarsal
    navicular — *see* Fracture, tarsal, navicular
    sesamoid S92.81- ☑
    specified NEC S92.81- ☑
    talus — *see* Fracture, tarsal, talus
    tarsal — *see* Fracture, tarsal
    toe — *see* Fracture, toe
  forearm S52.9- ☑
    radius — *see* Fracture, radius
    ulna — *see* Fracture, ulna
  fossa (anterior) (middle) (posterior) S02.19 ☑
  frontal (bone) (skull) S02.0 ☑
    sinus S02.19 ☑
  glenoid (cavity) (scapula) — *see* Fracture, scapula,
    glenoid cavity
  greenstick — *see* Fracture, by site
  hallux — *see* Fracture, toe, great
  hand S62.9- ☑
    carpal — *see* Fracture, carpal bone
    finger (except thumb) — *see* Fracture, finger
    metacarpal — *see* Fracture, metacarpal
    navicular (scaphoid) (hand) — *see* Fracture, carpal
      bone, navicular
    thumb — *see* Fracture, thumb
  healed or old
    with complications — *code by* Nature of the compli-
      cation
  heel bone — *see* Fracture, tarsal, calcaneus
  Hill-Sachs S42.29- ☑
  hip — *see* Fracture, femur, neck
  humerus S42.30- ☑
    anatomical neck — *see* Fracture, humerus, upper
      end
    articular process — *see* Fracture, humerus, lower
      end
    capitellum — *see* Fracture, humerus, lower end,
      condyle, lateral
    distal end — *see* Fracture, humerus, lower end
    epiphysis
      lower — *see* Fracture, humerus, lower end, phy-
        seal
      upper — *see* Fracture, humerus, upper end,
        physeal
    external condyle — *see* Fracture, humerus, lower
      end, condyle, lateral
    following insertion of implant, prosthesis or plate
      M96.62- ☑
    great tuberosity — *see* Fracture, humerus, upper
      end, greater tuberosity
    intercondylar — *see* Fracture, humerus, lower end
    internal epicondyle — *see* Fracture, humerus, lower
      end, epicondyle, medial
    lesser tuberosity — *see* Fracture, humerus, upper
      end, lesser tuberosity
    lower end S42.40- ☑
      condyle
        lateral (displaced) S42.45- ☑

Fracture, traumatic — *continued*
  humerus — *continued*
    lower end — *continued*
      condyle — *continued*
        lateral — *continued*
          nondisplaced S42.45- ☑
        medial (displaced) S42.46- ☑
          nondisplaced S42.46- ☑
      epicondyle
        lateral (displaced) S42.43- ☑
          nondisplaced S42.43- ☑
        medial (displaced) S42.44- ☑
          incarcerated S42.44- ☑
          nondisplaced S42.44- ☑
      physeal S49.10- ☑
        Salter-Harris
          Type I S49.11- ☑
          Type II S49.12- ☑
          Type III S49.13- ☑
          Type IV S49.14- ☑
        specified NEC S49.19- ☑
      specified NEC (displaced) S42.49- ☑
        nondisplaced S42.49- ☑
      supracondylar (simple) (displaced) S42.41- ☑
        with intercondylar fracture — *see* Fracture,
          humerus, lower end
        comminuted (displaced) S42.42- ☑
          nondisplaced S42.42- ☑
        nondisplaced S42.41- ☑
      torus S42.48- ☑
      transcondylar (displaced) S42.47- ☑
        nondisplaced S42.47- ☑
    proximal end — *see* Fracture, humerus, upper end
    shaft S42.30- ☑
      comminuted (displaced) S42.35- ☑
        nondisplaced S42.35- ☑
      greenstick S42.31- ☑
      oblique (displaced) S42.33- ☑
        nondisplaced S42.33- ☑
      segmental (displaced) S42.36- ☑
        nondisplaced S42.36- ☑
      specified NEC S42.39- ☑
      spiral (displaced) S42.34- ☑
        nondisplaced S42.34- ☑
      transverse (displaced) S42.32- ☑
        nondisplaced S42.32- ☑
    supracondylar — *see* Fracture, humerus, lower end
    surgical neck — *see* Fracture, humerus, upper end,
      surgical neck
    trochlea — *see* Fracture, humerus, lower end,
      condyle, medial
    tuberosity — *see* Fracture, humerus, upper end
    upper end S42.20- ☑
      anatomical neck — *see* Fracture, humerus, upper
        end, specified NEC
      articular head — *see* Fracture, humerus, upper
        end, specified NEC
      epiphysis — *see* Fracture, humerus, upper end,
        physeal
      greater tuberosity (displaced) S42.25- ☑
        nondisplaced S42.25- ☑
      lesser tuberosity (displaced) S42.26- ☑
        nondisplaced S42.26- ☑
      physeal S49.00- ☑
        Salter-Harris
          Type I S49.01- ☑
          Type II S49.02- ☑
          Type III S49.03- ☑
          Type IV S49.04- ☑
        specified NEC S49.09- ☑
      specified NEC (displaced) S42.29- ☑
        nondisplaced S42.29- ☑
      surgical neck (displaced) S42.21- ☑
        four-part S42.24- ☑
        nondisplaced S42.21- ☑
        three-part S42.23- ☑
        two-part (displaced) S42.22- ☑
          nondisplaced S42.22- ☑
      torus S42.27- ☑
      transepiphyseal — *see* Fracture, humerus, upper
        end, physeal
  hyoid bone S12.8 ☑
  ilium S32.30- ☑
    with disruption of pelvic ring — *see* Disruption,
      pelvic ring
    avulsion (displaced) S32.31- ☑

Fracture, traumatic — *continued*
  ilium — *continued*
    avulsion — *continued*
      nondisplaced S32.31- ☑
      specified NEC S32.39- ☑
  impaction, impacted — *code as* Fracture, by site
  innominate bone — *see* Fracture, ilium
  instep — *see* Fracture, foot
  ischium S32.60- ☑
    with disruption of pelvic ring — *see* Disruption, pelvic ring
    avulsion (displaced) S32.61- ☑
      nondisplaced S32.61- ☑
    specified NEC S32.69- ☑
  jaw (bone) (lower) — *see* Fracture, mandible
    upper — *see* Fracture, maxilla
  joint prosthesis — *see* Complications, joint prosthesis, mechanical, breakdown, by site
    periprosthetic — *see* Fracture, traumatic, periprosthetic
  knee cap — *see* Fracture, patella
  larynx S12.8 ☑
  late effects — *see* Sequelae, fracture
  leg (lower) S82.9- ☑
    ankle — *see* Fracture, ankle
    femur — *see* Fracture, femur
    fibula — *see* Fracture, fibula
    malleolus — *see* Fracture, ankle
    patella — *see* Fracture, patella
    specified site NEC S82.89- ☑
    tibia — *see* Fracture, tibia
  lumbar spine — *see* Fracture, vertebra, lumbar
  lumbosacral spine S32.9 ☑
  Maisonneuve's (displaced) S82.86- ☑
    nondisplaced S82.86- ☑
  malar bone (*see also* Fracture, maxilla) S02.400 ☑
    left side S02.40B ☑
    right side S02.40A ☑
  malleolus — *see* Fracture, ankle
  malunion — *see* Fracture, by site
  mandible (lower jaw (bone)) S02.609 ☑
    alveolus S02.67- ☑
    angle (of jaw) S02.65- ☑
    body, unspecified S02.600 ☑
      left side S02.602 ☑
      right side S02.601 ☑
    condylar process S02.61- ☑
    coronoid process S02.63- ☑
    ramus, unspecified S02.64- ☑
    specified site NEC S02.69- ☑
    subcondylar process S02.62- ☑
    symphysis S02.66 ☑
  manubrium (sterni) S22.21 ☑
    dissociation from sternum S22.23 ☑
  march — *see* Fracture, traumatic, stress, by site
  maxilla, maxillary (bone) (sinus) (superior) (upper jaw) S02.401 ☑
    alveolus S02.42 ☑
    inferior — *see* Fracture, mandible
    LeFort I S02.411 ☑
    LeFort II S02.412 ☑
    LeFort III S02.413 ☑
    left side S02.40D ☑
    right side S02.40C ☑
  metacarpal S62.309 ☑
    base (displaced) S62.319 ☑
      nondisplaced S62.349 ☑
    fifth S62.30- ☑
      base (displaced) S62.31- ☑
        nondisplaced S62.34- ☑
      neck (displaced) S62.33- ☑
        nondisplaced S62.36- ☑
      shaft (displaced) S62.32- ☑
        nondisplaced S62.35- ☑
      specified NEC S62.398 ☑
    first S62.20- ☑
      base NEC (displaced) S62.23- ☑
        nondisplaced S62.23- ☑
      Bennett's — *see* Bennett's fracture
      neck (displaced) S62.25- ☑
        nondisplaced S62.25- ☑
      shaft (displaced) S62.24- ☑
        nondisplaced S62.24- ☑
      specified NEC S62.29- ☑
    fourth S62.30- ☑
      base (displaced) S62.31- ☑

Fracture, traumatic — *continued*
  metacarpal — *continued*
    fourth — *continued*
      base — *continued*
        nondisplaced S62.34- ☑
      neck (displaced) S62.33- ☑
        nondisplaced S62.36- ☑
      shaft (displaced) S62.32- ☑
        nondisplaced S62.35- ☑
      specified NEC S62.39- ☑
    neck (displaced) S62.33- ☑
      nondisplaced S62.36- ☑
    Rolando's — *see* Rolando's fracture
    second S62.30- ☑
      base (displaced) S62.31- ☑
        nondisplaced S62.34- ☑
      neck (displaced) S62.33- ☑
        nondisplaced S62.36- ☑
      shaft (displaced) S62.32- ☑
        nondisplaced S62.35- ☑
      specified NEC S62.39- ☑
    shaft (displaced) S62.32- ☑
      nondisplaced S62.35- ☑
    specified NEC S62.399 ☑
    third S62.30- ☑
      base (displaced) S62.31- ☑
        nondisplaced S62.34- ☑
      neck (displaced) S62.33- ☑
        nondisplaced S62.36- ☑
      shaft (displaced) S62.32- ☑
        nondisplaced S62.35- ☑
      specified NEC S62.39- ☑
  metastatic — *see* Fracture, pathological, due to, neoplastic disease (*see also* Neoplasm)
  metatarsal bone S92.30- ☑
    fifth (displaced) S92.35- ☑
      nondisplaced S92.35- ☑
    first (displaced) S92.31- ☑
      nondisplaced S92.31- ☑
    fourth (displaced) S92.34- ☑
      nondisplaced S92.34- ☑
    physeal S99.10- ☑
      Salter-Harris
        Type I S99.11- ☑
        Type II S99.12- ☑
        Type III S99.13- ☑
        Type IV S99.14- ☑
      specified NEC S99.19- ☑
    second (displaced) S92.32- ☑
      nondisplaced S92.32- ☑
    third (displaced) S92.33- ☑
      nondisplaced S92.33- ☑
  Monteggia's — *see* Monteggia's fracture
  multiple
    hand (and wrist) NEC — *see* Fracture, by site
    ribs — *see* Fracture, rib, multiple
  nasal (bone(s)) S02.2 ☑
  navicular (scaphoid) (foot) (*see also* Fracture, tarsal, navicular)
    hand — *see* Fracture, carpal, navicular
  neck S12.9 ☑
    cervical vertebra S12.9 ☑
      fifth (displaced) S12.400 ☑
        nondisplaced S12.401 ☑
        specified type NEC (displaced) S12.490 ☑
          nondisplaced S12.491 ☑
      first (displaced) S12.000 ☑
        burst (stable) S12.01 ☑
          unstable S12.02 ☑
        lateral mass (displaced) S12.040 ☑
          nondisplaced S12.041 ☑
        nondisplaced S12.001 ☑
        posterior arch (displaced) S12.030 ☑
          nondisplaced S12.031 ☑
        specified type NEC (displaced) S12.090 ☑
          nondisplaced S12.091 ☑
      fourth (displaced) S12.300 ☑
        nondisplaced S12.301 ☑
        specified type NEC (displaced) S12.390 ☑
          nondisplaced S12.391 ☑
      second (displaced) S12.100 ☑
        dens (anterior) (displaced) (type II) S12.110 ☑
          nondisplaced S12.112 ☑
          posterior S12.111 ☑
        specified type NEC (displaced) S12.120 ☑
          nondisplaced S12.121 ☑

Fracture, traumatic — *continued*
  neck — *continued*
    cervical vertebra — *continued*
      second — *continued*
        nondisplaced S12.101 ☑
        specified type NEC (displaced) S12.190 ☑
          nondisplaced S12.191 ☑
      seventh (displaced) S12.600 ☑
        nondisplaced S12.601 ☑
        specified type NEC (displaced) S12.690 ☑
          nondisplaced S12.691 ☑
      sixth (displaced) S12.500 ☑
        nondisplaced S12.501 ☑
        specified type NEC (displaced) S12.590 ☑
          nondisplaced S12.591 ☑
      third (displaced) S12.200 ☑
        nondisplaced S12.201 ☑
        specified type NEC (displaced) S12.290 ☑
          nondisplaced S12.291 ☑
    hyoid bone S12.8 ☑
    larynx S12.8 ☑
    specified site NEC S12.8 ☑
    thyroid cartilage S12.8 ☑
    trachea S12.8 ☑
  neoplastic NEC — *see* Fracture, pathological, due to, neoplastic disease
  neural arch — *see* Fracture, vertebra
  newborn — *see* Birth, injury, fracture
  nontraumatic — *see* Fracture, pathological
  nonunion — *see* Nonunion, fracture
  nose, nasal (bone) (septum) S02.2 ☑
  occiput — *see* Fracture, skull, base, occiput
  odontoid process — *see* Fracture, neck, cervical vertebra, second
  olecranon (process) (ulna) — *see* Fracture, ulna, upper end, olecranon process
  orbit, orbital (bone) (region) S02.8- ☑
    floor (blow-out) S02.3- ☑
    roof S02.19 ☑
  os
    calcis — *see* Fracture, tarsal, calcaneus
    magnum — *see* Fracture, carpal, capitate
    pubis — *see* Fracture, pubis
  palate S02.8- ☑
  parietal bone (skull) S02.0 ☑
  patella S82.00- ☑
    comminuted (displaced) S82.04- ☑
      nondisplaced S82.04- ☑
    longitudinal (displaced) S82.02- ☑
      nondisplaced S82.02- ☑
    osteochondral (displaced) S82.01- ☑
      nondisplaced S82.01- ☑
    specified NEC S82.09- ☑
    transverse (displaced) S82.03- ☑
      nondisplaced S82.03- ☑
  pedicle (of vertebral arch) — *see* Fracture, vertebra
  pelvis, pelvic (bone) S32.9 ☑
    acetabulum — *see* Fracture, acetabulum
    circle — *see* Disruption, pelvic ring
    following insertion of implant, prosthesis or plate M96.65
    ilium — *see* Fracture, ilium
    ischium — *see* Fracture, ischium
    multiple
      with disruption of pelvic ring (circle) — *see* Disruption, pelvic ring
      without disruption of pelvic ring (circle) S32.82 ☑
    pubis — *see* Fracture, pubis
    sacrum — *see* Fracture, sacrum
    specified site NEC S32.89 ☑
  periprosthetic, around internal prosthetic joint M97.9 ☑
    ankle M97.2- ☑
    elbow M97.4- ☑
    finger M97.8 ☑
    hip M97.0- ☑
    knee M97.1- ☑
    shoulder M97.3- ☑
    specified joint NEC M97.8 ☑
    spine M97.8 ☑
    toe M97.8 ☑
    wrist M97.8 ☑
  phalanx
    foot — *see* Fracture, toe
    hand — *see* Fracture, finger

☑ **Additional Character Required** — Refer to the Tabular List for Character Selection   ▽ Subterms under main terms may continue to next column or page

Fracture, traumatic — *continued*
- pisiform — *see* Fracture, carpal, pisiform
- pond — *see* Fracture, skull
- prosthetic device, internal — *see* Complications, prosthetic device, by site, mechanical
- pubis S32.5Ø- ✓
  - with disruption of pelvic ring — *see* Disruption, pelvic ring
  - specified site NEC S32.59- ✓
  - superior rim S32.51- ✓
- radius S52.9-
  - distal end — *see* Fracture, radius, lower end
  - following insertion of implant, prosthesis or plate M96.63- ✓
  - head — *see* Fracture, radius, upper end, head
  - lower end S52.5Ø-
    - Barton's — *see* Barton's fracture
    - Colles' — *see* Colles' fracture
    - extraarticular NEC S52.55- ✓
    - intraarticular NEC S52.57- ✓
    - physeal S59.2Ø- ✓
      - Salter-Harris
        - Type I S59.21- ✓
        - Type II S59.22- ✓
        - Type III S59.23- ✓
        - Type IV S59.24- ✓
      - specified NEC S59.29- ✓
    - Smith's — *see* Smith's fracture
    - specified NEC S52.59- ✓
    - styloid process (displaced) S52.51- ✓
      - nondisplaced S52.51- ✓
    - torus S52.52- ✓
  - neck — *see* Fracture, radius, upper end
  - proximal end — *see* Fracture, radius, upper end
  - shaft S52.3Ø- ✓
    - bent bone S52.38- ✓
    - comminuted (displaced) S52.35- ✓
      - nondisplaced S52.35- ✓
    - Galeazzi's — *see* Galeazzi's fracture
    - greenstick S52.31- ✓
    - oblique (displaced) S52.33- ✓
      - nondisplaced S52.33- ✓
    - segmental (displaced) S52.36- ✓
      - nondisplaced S52.36- ✓
    - specified NEC S52.39- ✓
    - spiral (displaced) S52.34- ✓
      - nondisplaced S52.34- ✓
    - transverse (displaced) S52.32- ✓
      - nondisplaced S52.32- ✓
  - upper end S52.1Ø- ✓
    - head (displaced) S52.12- ✓
      - nondisplaced S52.12- ✓
    - neck (displaced) S52.13- ✓
      - nondisplaced S52.13- ✓
    - physeal S59.1Ø- ✓
      - Salter-Harris
        - Type I S59.11- ✓
        - Type II S59.12- ✓
        - Type III S59.13- ✓
        - Type IV S59.14- ✓
      - specified NEC S59.19- ✓
    - specified NEC S52.18- ✓
    - torus S52.11- ✓
- ramus
  - inferior or superior, pubis — *see* Fracture, pubis
  - mandible — *see* Fracture, mandible
- restorative material (dental) KØ8.539
  - with loss of material KØ8.531
  - without loss of material KØ8.53Ø
- rib S22.3- ✓
  - with flail chest — *see* Flail, chest
  - multiple S22.4- ✓
    - with flail chest — *see* Flail, chest
- root, tooth — *see* Fracture, tooth
- sacrum S32.1Ø ✓
  - specified NEC S32.19 ✓
  - Type
    - 1 S32.14 ✓
    - 2 S32.15 ✓
    - 3 S32.16 ✓
    - 4 S32.17 ✓
  - Zone
    - I S32.119 ✓
      - displaced (minimally) S32.111 ✓
        - severely S32.112 ✓
      - nondisplaced S32.11Ø ✓

Fracture, traumatic — *continued*
- sacrum — *continued*
  - Zone — *continued*
    - II S32.129 ✓
      - displaced (minimally) S32.121 ✓
        - severely S32.122 ✓
      - nondisplaced S32.12Ø ✓
    - III S32.139 ✓
      - displaced (minimally) S32.131 ✓
        - severely S32.132 ✓
      - nondisplaced S32.13Ø ✓
- scaphoid (hand) (*see also* Fracture, carpal, navicular)
  - foot — *see* Fracture, tarsal, navicular
- scapula S42.1Ø- ✓
  - acromial process (displaced) S42.12- ✓
    - nondisplaced S42.12- ✓
  - body (displaced) S42.11- ✓
    - nondisplaced S42.11- ✓
  - coracoid process (displaced) S42.13- ✓
    - nondisplaced S42.13- ✓
  - glenoid cavity (displaced) S42.14- ✓
    - nondisplaced S42.14- ✓
  - neck (displaced) S42.15- ✓
    - nondisplaced S42.15- ✓
  - specified NEC S42.19- ✓
- semilunar bone, wrist — *see* Fracture, carpal, lunate
- sequelae — *see* Sequelae, fracture
- sesamoid bone
  - foot S92.81- ✓
  - hand — *see* Fracture, carpal
  - other — *see* Fracture, traumatic, by site
- shepherd's — *see* Fracture, tarsal, talus
- shoulder (girdle) S42.9- ✓
  - blade — *see* Fracture, scapula
- sinus (ethmoid) (frontal) SØ2.19 ✓
- skull SØ2.91 ✓
  - base SØ2.1Ø- ✓
    - occiput SØ2.119 ✓
      - condyle SØ2.113 ✓
        - specified NEC SØ2.118 ✓
          - left side SØ2.11H ✓
          - right side SØ2.11G ✓
        - type I SØ2.11Ø ✓
          - left side SØ2.11B ✓
          - right side SØ2.11A ✓
        - type II SØ2.111 ✓
          - left side SØ2.11D ✓
          - right side SØ2.11C ✓
        - type III SØ2.112 ✓
          - left side SØ2.11F ✓
          - right side SØ2.11E ✓
      - specified NEC SØ2.19 ✓
    - birth injury P13.Ø
    - frontal bone SØ2.Ø ✓
    - parietal bone SØ2.Ø ✓
    - specified site NEC SØ2.8- ✓
    - temporal bone SØ2.19 ✓
    - vault SØ2.Ø ✓
- Smith's — *see* Smith's fracture
- sphenoid (bone) (sinus) SØ2.19 ✓
- spine — *see* Fracture, vertebra
- spinous process — *see* Fracture, vertebra
- spontaneous (cause unknown) — *see* Fracture, pathological
- stave (of thumb) — *see* Fracture, metacarpal, first
- sternum S22.2Ø ✓
  - with flail chest — *see* Flail, chest
  - body S22.22 ✓
  - manubrium S22.21 ✓
  - xiphoid (process) S22.24 ✓
- stress M84.3Ø ✓
  - ankle M84.37- ✓
  - carpus M84.34- ✓
  - clavicle M84.31- ✓
  - femoral neck M84.359 ✓
  - femur M84.35- ✓
  - fibula M84.36- ✓
  - finger M84.34- ✓
  - hip M84.359 ✓
  - humerus M84.32- ✓
  - ilium M84.35Ø ✓
  - ischium M84.35Ø ✓
  - metacarpus M84.34- ✓
  - metatarsus M84.37- ✓
  - neck — *see* Fracture, fatigue, vertebra
  - pelvis M84.35Ø ✓

Fracture, traumatic — *continued*
- stress — *continued*
  - radius M84.33- ✓
  - rib M84.38 ✓
  - scapula M84.31- ✓
  - skull M84.38 ✓
  - tarsus M84.37- ✓
  - tibia M84.36- ✓
  - toe M84.37- ✓
  - ulna M84.33- ✓
  - vertebra — *see* Fracture, fatigue, vertebra
- supracondylar, elbow — *see* Fracture, humerus, lower end, supracondylar
- symphysis pubis — *see* Fracture, pubis
- talus (ankle bone) — *see* Fracture, tarsal, talus
- tarsal bone(s) S92.2Ø- ✓
  - astragalus — *see* Fracture, tarsal, talus
  - calcaneus S92.ØØ- ✓
    - anterior process (displaced) S92.Ø2- ✓
      - nondisplaced S92.Ø2- ✓
    - body (displaced) S92.Ø1- ✓
      - nondisplaced S92.Ø1- ✓
    - extraarticular NEC S92.Ø5- ✓
      - nondisplaced S92.Ø5- ✓
    - intraarticular (displaced) S92.Ø6- ✓
      - nondisplaced S92.Ø6- ✓
    - physeal S99.ØØ- ✓
      - Salter-Harris
        - Type I S99.Ø1- ✓
        - Type II S99.Ø2- ✓
        - Type III S99.Ø3- ✓
        - Type IV S99.Ø4- ✓
      - specified NEC S99.Ø9- ✓
    - tuberosity (displaced) S92.Ø4- ✓
      - avulsion (displaced) S92.Ø3- ✓
        - nondisplaced S92.Ø3- ✓
      - nondisplaced S92.Ø4- ✓
  - cuboid (displaced) S92.21- ✓
    - nondisplaced S92.21- ✓
  - cuneiform
    - intermediate (displaced) S92.23- ✓
      - nondisplaced S92.23- ✓
    - lateral (displaced) S92.22- ✓
      - nondisplaced S92.22- ✓
    - medial (displaced) S92.24- ✓
      - nondisplaced S92.24- ✓
  - navicular (displaced) S92.25- ✓
    - nondisplaced S92.25- ✓
  - scaphoid — *see* Fracture, tarsal, navicular
  - talus S92.1Ø- ✓
    - avulsion (displaced) S92.15- ✓
      - nondisplaced S92.15- ✓
    - body (displaced) S92.12- ✓
      - nondisplaced S92.12- ✓
    - dome (displaced) S92.14- ✓
      - nondisplaced S92.14- ✓
    - head (displaced) S92.12- ✓
      - nondisplaced S92.12- ✓
    - lateral process (displaced) S92.14- ✓
      - nondisplaced S92.14- ✓
    - neck (displaced) S92.11- ✓
      - nondisplaced S92.11- ✓
    - posterior process (displaced) S92.13- ✓
      - nondisplaced S92.13- ✓
    - specified NEC S92.19- ✓
- temporal bone (styloid) SØ2.19 ✓
- thorax (bony) S22.9 ✓
  - with flail chest — *see* Flail, chest
  - rib S22.3- ✓
    - multiple S22.4- ✓
      - with flail chest — *see* Flail, chest
  - sternum S22.2Ø ✓
    - body S22.22 ✓
    - manubrium S22.21 ✓
    - xiphoid process S22.24 ✓
  - vertebra (displaced) S22.ØØ9 ✓
    - burst (stable) S22.ØØ1 ✓
      - unstable S22.ØØ2 ✓
    - eighth S22.Ø69 ✓
      - burst (stable) S22.Ø61 ✓
        - unstable S22.Ø62 ✓
      - specified type NEC S22.Ø68 ✓
      - wedge compression S22.Ø6Ø ✓
    - eleventh S22.Ø89 ✓
      - burst (stable) S22.Ø81 ✓
        - unstable S22.Ø82 ✓

◤ Subterms under main terms may continue to next column or page   ✓ Additional Character Required — Refer to the Tabular List for Character Selection   153

Fracture, traumatic — Fracture, traumatic

Fracture, traumatic — *continued*
thorax — *continued*
vertebra — *continued*
eleventh — *continued*
specified type NEC S22.088 ☑
wedge compression S22.080 ☑
fifth S22.059 ☑
burst (stable) S22.051 ☑
unstable S22.052 ☑
specified type NEC S22.058 ☑
wedge compression S22.050 ☑
first S22.019 ☑
burst (stable) S22.011 ☑
unstable S22.012 ☑
specified type NEC S22.018 ☑
wedge compression S22.010 ☑
fourth S22.049 ☑
burst (stable) S22.041 ☑
unstable S22.042 ☑
specified type NEC S22.048 ☑
wedge compression S22.040 ☑
ninth S22.079 ☑
burst (stable) S22.071 ☑
unstable S22.072 ☑
specified type NEC S22.078 ☑
wedge compression S22.070 ☑
nondisplaced S22.001 ☑
second S22.029 ☑
burst (stable) S22.021 ☑
unstable S22.022 ☑
specified type NEC S22.028 ☑
wedge compression S22.020 ☑
seventh S22.069 ☑
burst (stable) S22.061 ☑
unstable S22.062 ☑
specified type NEC S22.068 ☑
wedge compression S22.060 ☑
sixth S22.059 ☑
burst (stable) S22.051 ☑
unstable S22.052 ☑
specified type NEC S22.058 ☑
wedge compression S22.050 ☑
specified type NEC S22.008 ☑
tenth S22.079 ☑
burst (stable) S22.071 ☑
unstable S22.072 ☑
specified type NEC S22.078 ☑
wedge compression S22.070 ☑
third S22.039 ☑
burst (stable) S22.031 ☑
unstable S22.032 ☑
specified type NEC S22.038 ☑
wedge compression S22.030 ☑
twelfth S22.089 ☑
burst (stable) S22.081 ☑
unstable S22.082 ☑
specified type NEC S22.088 ☑
wedge compression S22.080 ☑
wedge compression S22.000 ☑
thumb S62.50- ☑
distal phalanx (displaced) S62.52- ☑
nondisplaced S62.52- ☑
proximal phalanx (displaced) S62.51- ☑
nondisplaced S62.51- ☑
thyroid cartilage S12.8 ☑
tibia (shaft) S82.20- ☑
comminuted (displaced) S82.25- ☑
nondisplaced S82.25- ☑
condyles — *see* Fracture, tibia, upper end
distal end — *see* Fracture, tibia, lower end
epiphysis
lower — *see* Fracture, tibia, lower end
upper — *see* Fracture, tibia, upper end
following insertion of implant, prosthesis or plate
M96.67- ☑
head (involving knee joint) — *see* Fracture, tibia, upper end
intercondyloid eminence — *see* Fracture, tibia, upper end
involving ankle or malleolus — *see* Fracture, ankle, medial malleolus
lower end S82.30- ☑
physeal S89.10- ☑
Salter-Harris
Type I S89.11- ☑
Type II S89.12- ☑

Fracture, traumatic — *continued*
tibia — *continued*
lower end — *continued*
physeal — *continued*
Salter-Harris — *continued*
Type III S89.13- ☑
Type IV S89.14- ☑
specified NEC S89.19- ☑
pilon (displaced) S82.87- ☑
nondisplaced S82.87- ☑
specified NEC S82.39- ☑
torus S82.31- ☑
malleolus — *see* Fracture, ankle, medial malleolus
oblique (displaced) S82.23- ☑
nondisplaced S82.23- ☑
pilon — *see* Fracture, tibia, lower end, pilon
proximal end — *see* Fracture, tibia, upper end
segmental (displaced) S82.26- ☑
nondisplaced S82.26- ☑
specified NEC S82.29- ☑
spine — *see* Fracture, tibia, upper end, spine
spiral (displaced) S82.24- ☑
nondisplaced S82.24- ☑
transverse (displaced) S82.22- ☑
nondisplaced S82.22- ☑
tuberosity — *see* Fracture, tibia, upper end, tuberosity
upper end S82.10- ☑
bicondylar (displaced) S82.14- ☑
nondisplaced S82.14- ☑
lateral condyle (displaced) S82.12- ☑
nondisplaced S82.12- ☑
medial condyle (displaced) S82.13- ☑
nondisplaced S82.13- ☑
physeal S89.00- ☑
Salter-Harris
Type I S89.01- ☑
Type II S89.02- ☑
Type III S89.03- ☑
Type IV S89.04- ☑
specified NEC S89.09- ☑
plateau — *see* Fracture, tibia, upper end, bicondylar
specified NEC S82.19- ☑
spine (displaced) S82.11- ☑
nondisplaced S82.11- ☑
torus S82.16- ☑
tuberosity (displaced) S82.15- ☑
nondisplaced S82.15- ☑
toe S92.91- ☑
great (displaced) S92.40- ☑
distal phalanx (displaced) S92.42- ☑
nondisplaced S92.42- ☑
nondisplaced S92.40- ☑
proximal phalanx (displaced) S92.41- ☑
nondisplaced S92.41- ☑
specified NEC S92.49- ☑
lesser (displaced) S92.50- ☑
distal phalanx (displaced) S92.53- ☑
nondisplaced S92.53- ☑
medial phalanx (displaced) S92.52- ☑
nondisplaced S92.52- ☑
nondisplaced S92.50- ☑
proximal phalanx (displaced) S92.51- ☑
nondisplaced S92.51- ☑
specified NEC S92.59- ☑
physeal
phalanx S99.20- ☑
Salter-Harris
Type I S99.21- ☑
Type II S99.22- ☑
Type III S99.23- ☑
Type IV S99.24- ☑
specified NEC S99.29- ☑
tooth (root) S02.5 ☑
trachea (cartilage) S12.8 ☑
transverse process — *see* Fracture, vertebra
trapezium or trapezoid bone — *see* Fracture, carpal
trimalleolar — *see* Fracture, ankle, trimalleolar
triquetrum (cuneiform of carpus) — *see* Fracture, carpal, triquetrum
trochanter — *see* Fracture, femur, trochanteric
tuberosity (external) — *see* Fracture, traumatic, by site
ulna (shaft) S52.20- ☑
bent bone S52.28- ☑

Fracture, traumatic — *continued*
ulna — *continued*
coronoid process — *see* Fracture, ulna, upper end, coronoid process
distal end — *see* Fracture, ulna, lower end
following insertion of implant, prosthesis or plate M96.63- ☑
head S52.60- ☑
lower end S52.60- ☑
physeal S59.00- ☑
Salter-Harris
Type I S59.01- ☑
Type II S59.02- ☑
Type III S59.03- ☑
Type IV S59.04- ☑
specified NEC S59.09- ☑
specified NEC S52.69- ☑
styloid process (displaced) S52.61- ☑
nondisplaced S52.61- ☑
torus S52.62- ☑
proximal end — *see* Fracture, ulna, upper end
shaft S52.20- ☑
comminuted (displaced) S52.25- ☑
nondisplaced S52.25- ☑
greenstick S52.21- ☑
Monteggia's — *see* Monteggia's fracture
oblique (displaced) S52.23- ☑
nondisplaced S52.23- ☑
segmental (displaced) S52.26- ☑
nondisplaced S52.26- ☑
specified NEC S52.29- ☑
spiral (displaced) S52.24- ☑
nondisplaced S52.24- ☑
transverse (displaced) S52.22- ☑
nondisplaced S52.22- ☑
upper end S52.00- ☑
coronoid process (displaced) S52.04- ☑
nondisplaced S52.04- ☑
olecranon process (displaced) S52.02- ☑
with intraarticular extension S52.03- ☑
nondisplaced S52.02- ☑
with intraarticular extension S52.03- ☑
specified NEC S52.09- ☑
torus S52.01- ☑
unciform — *see* Fracture, carpal, hamate
vault of skull S02.0 ☑
vertebra, vertebral (arch) (body) (column) (neural arch) (pedicle) (spinous process) (transverse process)
atlas — *see* Fracture, neck, cervical vertebra, first
axis — *see* Fracture, neck, cervical vertebra, second
cervical (teardrop) S12.9 ☑
axis — *see* Fracture, neck, cervical vertebra, second
first (atlas) — *see* Fracture, neck, cervical vertebra, first
second (axis) — *see* Fracture, neck, cervical vertebra, second
chronic M84.48 ☑
coccyx S32.2 ☑
dorsal — *see* Fracture, thorax, vertebra
lumbar S32.009 ☑
burst (stable) S32.001 ☑
unstable S32.002 ☑
fifth S32.059 ☑
burst (stable) S32.051 ☑
unstable S32.052 ☑
specified type NEC S32.058 ☑
wedge compression S32.050 ☑
first S32.019 ☑
burst (stable) S32.011 ☑
unstable S32.012 ☑
specified type NEC S32.018 ☑
wedge compression S32.010 ☑
fourth S32.049 ☑
burst (stable) S32.041 ☑
unstable S32.042 ☑
specified type NEC S32.048 ☑
wedge compression S32.040 ☑
second S32.029 ☑
burst (stable) S32.021 ☑
unstable S32.022 ☑
specified type NEC S32.028 ☑
wedge compression S32.020 ☑
specified type NEC S32.008 ☑
third S32.039 ☑
burst (stable) S32.031 ☑

☑ Additional Character Required — Refer to the Tabular List for Character Selection   Subterms under main terms may continue to next column or page

Fracture, traumatic — *continued*
  vertebra, vertebral — *continued*
    lumbar — *continued*
      third — *continued*
        burst — *continued*
          unstable S32.032 ☑
        specified type NEC S32.038 ☑
        wedge compression S32.030 ☑
      wedge compression S32.000 ☑
    metastatic — *see* Collapse, vertebra, in, specified
      disease NEC (*see also* Neoplasm)
    newborn (birth injury) P11.5
    sacrum S32.10 ☑
      specified NEC S32.19 ☑
      Type
        1 S32.14 ☑
        2 S32.15 ☑
        3 S32.16 ☑
        4 S32.17 ☑
      Zone
        I S32.119 ☑
          displaced (minimally) S32.111 ☑
            severely S32.112 ☑
          nondisplaced S32.110 ☑
        II S32.129 ☑
          displaced (minimally) S32.121 ☑
            severely S32.122 ☑
          nondisplaced S32.120 ☑
        III S32.139 ☑
          displaced (minimally) S32.131 ☑
            severely S32.132 ☑
          nondisplaced S32.130 ☑
    thoracic — *see* Fracture, thorax, vertebra
  vertex S02.0 ☑
  vomer (bone) S02.2 ☑
  wrist S62.10- ☑
    carpal — *see* Fracture, carpal bone
    navicular (scaphoid) (hand) — *see* Fracture, carpal,
      navicular
  xiphisternum, xiphoid (process) S22.24 ☑
  zygoma S02.402 ☑
    left side S02.40F ☑
    right side S02.40E ☑
Fragile, fragility
  autosomal site Q95.5
  bone, congenital (with blue sclera) Q78.0
  capillary (hereditary) D69.8
  hair L67.8
  nails L60.3
  non-sex chromosome site Q95.5
  X chromosome Q99.2
Fragilitas
  crinium L67.8
  ossium (with blue sclerae) (hereditary) Q78.0
  unguium L60.3
    congenital Q84.6
Fragments, cataract (lens), **following cataract surgery**
  H59.02- ☑
  retained foreign body — *see* Retained, foreign body
    fragments (type of)
Frailty (frail) R54
  mental R41.81
Frambesia, frambesial (tropica) (*see also* Yaws)
  initial lesion or ulcer A66.0
  primary A66.0
Frambeside
  gummatous A66.4
  of early yaws A66.2
Frambesioma A66.1
Franceschetti-Klein (-Wildervanck) **disease or syn-
  drome** Q75.4
Francis' disease — *see* Tularemia
Franklin disease C88.2
Frank's essential thrombocytopenia D69.3
Fraser's syndrome Q87.0
Freckle(s) L81.2
  malignant melanoma in — *see* Melanoma
  melanotic (Hutchinson's) — *see* Melanoma, in situ
  retinal D49.81
Frederickson's hyperlipoproteinemia, type
  I and V E78.3
  IIA E78.00
  IIB and III E78.2
  IV E78.1
Freeman Sheldon syndrome Q87.0
Freezing (*see also* Effect, adverse, cold) T69.9 ☑

Freiberg's disease (infraction of metatarsal head or osteochondrosis) — *see* Osteochondrosis, juvenile,
  metatarsus
Frei's disease A55
Fremitus, friction, cardiac R01.2
Frenum, frenulum
  external os Q51.828
  tongue (shortening) (congenital) Q38.1
Frequency micturition (nocturnal) R35.0
  psychogenic F45.8
Frey's syndrome
  auriculotemporal G50.8
  hyperhidrosis L74.52
Friction
  burn — *see* Burn, by site
  fremitus, cardiac R01.2
  precordial R01.2
  sounds, chest R09.89
Friderichsen-Waterhouse syndrome or disease A39.1
Friedländer's B (bacillus) **NEC** (*see also* condition) A49.8
Friedreich's
  ataxia G11.1
  combined systemic disease G11.1
  facial hemihypertrophy Q67.4
  sclerosis (cerebellum) (spinal cord) G11.1
Frigidity F52.22
Fröhlich's syndrome E23.6
Frontal (*see also* condition)
  lobe syndrome F07.0
Frostbite (superficial) T33.90 ☑
  with
    partial thickness skin loss — *see* Frostbite (superfi-
      cial), by site
    tissue necrosis T34.90 ☑
  abdominal wall T33.3 ☑
    with tissue necrosis T34.3 ☑
  ankle T33.81- ☑
    with tissue necrosis T34.81- ☑
  arm T33.4- ☑
    with tissue necrosis T34.4- ☑
    finger(s) — *see* Frostbite, finger
    hand — *see* Frostbite, hand
    wrist — *see* Frostbite, wrist
  ear T33.01- ☑
    with tissue necrosis T34.01- ☑
  face T33.09 ☑
    with tissue necrosis T34.09 ☑
  finger T33.53- ☑
    with tissue necrosis T34.53- ☑
  foot T33.82- ☑
    with tissue necrosis T34.82- ☑
  hand T33.52- ☑
    with tissue necrosis T34.52- ☑
  head T33.09 ☑
    with tissue necrosis T34.09 ☑
    ear — *see* Frostbite, ear
    nose — *see* Frostbite, nose
  hip (and thigh) T33.6- ☑
    with tissue necrosis T34.6- ☑
  knee T33.7- ☑
    with tissue necrosis T34.7- ☑
  leg T33.9- ☑
    with tissue necrosis T34.9- ☑
    ankle — *see* Frostbite, ankle
    foot — *see* Frostbite, foot
    knee — *see* Frostbite, knee
    lower T33.7- ☑
      with tissue necrosis T34.7- ☑
    thigh — *see* Frostbite, hip
    toe — *see* Frostbite, toe
  limb
    lower T33.99 ☑
      with tissue necrosis T34.99 ☑
    upper — *see* Frostbite, arm
  neck T33.1 ☑
    with tissue necrosis T34.1 ☑
  nose T33.02 ☑
    with tissue necrosis T34.02 ☑
  pelvis T33.3 ☑
    with tissue necrosis T34.3 ☑
  specified site NEC T33.99 ☑
    with tissue necrosis T34.99 ☑
  thigh — *see* Frostbite, hip
  thorax T33.2 ☑
    with tissue necrosis T34.2 ☑
  toes T33.83- ☑

Frostbite — *continued*
  toes — *continued*
    with tissue necrosis T34.83- ☑
  trunk T33.99 ☑
    with tissue necrosis T34.99 ☑
  wrist T33.51- ☑
    with tissue necrosis T34.51- ☑
Frotteurism F65.81
Frozen (*see also* Effect, adverse, cold) T69.9 ☑
  pelvis (female) N94.89
    male K66.8
  shoulder — *see* Capsulitis, adhesive
Fructokinase deficiency E74.11
Fructose 1,6 diphosphatase deficiency E74.19
Fructosemia (benign) (essential) E74.12
Fructosuria (benign) (essential) E74.11
Fuchs'
  black spot (myopic) (*see also* Myopia, degenerative)
    H44.2- ☑
  dystrophy (corneal endothelium) H18.51
  heterochromic cyclitis — *see* Cyclitis, Fuchs' hete-
    rochromic
Fucosidosis E77.1
Fugue R68.89
  dissociative F44.1
  hysterical (dissociative) F44.1
  postictal in epilepsy — *see* Epilepsy
  reaction to exceptional stress (transient) F43.0
Fulminant, fulminating — *see* condition
Functional (*see also* condition)
  bleeding (uterus) N93.8
Functioning, intellectual, borderline R41.83
Fundus — *see* condition
Fungemia NOS B49
Fungus, fungous
  cerebral G93.89
  disease NOS B49
  infection — *see* Infection, fungus
Funiculitis (acute) (chronic) (endemic) N49.1
  gonococcal (acute) (chronic) A54.23
  tuberculous A18.15
Funnel
  breast (acquired) M95.4
    congenital Q67.6
    sequelae (late effect) of rickets E64.3
  chest (acquired) M95.4
    congenital Q67.6
    sequelae (late effect) of rickets E64.3
  pelvis (acquired) M95.5
    with disproportion (fetopelvic) O33.3 ☑
      causing obstructed labor O65.3
    congenital Q74.2
FUO (fever of unknown origin) R50.9
Furfur L21.0
  microsporon B36.0
Furrier's lung J67.8
Furrowed K14.5
  nail(s) (transverse) L60.4
    congenital Q84.6
  tongue K14.5
    congenital Q38.3
Furuncle L02.92
  abdominal wall L02.221
  ankle — *see* Furuncle, lower limb
  antecubital space — *see* Furuncle, upper limb
  anus K61.0
  arm — *see* Furuncle, upper limb
  auditory canal, external — *see* Abscess, ear, external
  auricle (ear) — *see* Abscess, ear, external
  axilla (region) L02.42- ☑
  back (any part) L02.222
  breast N61.1
  buttock L02.32
  cheek (external) L02.02
  chest wall L02.223
  chin L02.02
  corpus cavernosum N48.21
  ear, external — *see* Abscess, ear, external
  external auditory canal — *see* Abscess, ear, external
  eyelid — *see* Abscess, eyelid
  face L02.02
  femoral (region) — *see* Furuncle, lower limb
  finger — *see* Furuncle, hand
  flank L02.221
  foot L02.62- ☑
  forehead L02.02
  gluteal (region) L02.32

Furuncle — *continued*
  groin L02.224
  hand L02.52- ☑
  head L02.821
    face L02.02
  hip — *see* Furuncle, lower limb
  kidney — *see* Abscess, kidney
  knee — *see* Furuncle, lower limb
  labium (majus) (minus) N76.4
  lacrimal
    gland — *see* Dacryoadenitis
    passages (duct) (sac) — *see* Inflammation, lacrimal,
        passages, acute
  leg (any part) — *see* Furuncle, lower limb
  lower limb L02.42- ☑
  malignant A22.0
  mouth K12.2
  navel L02.226
  neck L02.12
  nose J34.0
  orbit, orbital — *see* Abscess, orbit
  palmar (space) — *see* Furuncle, hand
  partes posteriores L02.32
  pectoral region L02.223
  penis N48.21
  perineum L02.225
  pinna — *see* Abscess, ear, external
  popliteal — *see* Furuncle, lower limb
  prepatellar — *see* Furuncle, lower limb
  scalp L02.821
  seminal vesicle N49.0
  shoulder — *see* Furuncle, upper limb
  specified site NEC L02.828
  submandibular K12.2
  temple (region) L02.02
  thumb — *see* Furuncle, hand
  toe — *see* Furuncle, foot
  trunk L02.229
    abdominal wall L02.221
    back L02.222

Furuncle — *continued*
  trunk — *continued*
    chest wall L02.223
    groin L02.224
    perineum L02.225
    umbilicus L02.226
  umbilicus L02.226
  upper limb L02.42- ☑
  vulva N76.4
Furunculosis — *see* Furuncle
Fused — *see* Fusion, fused
Fusion, fused (congenital)
  astragaloscaphoid Q74.2
  atria Q21.1
  auditory canal Q16.1
  auricles, heart Q21.1
  binocular with defective stereopsis H53.32
  bone Q79.8
  cervical spine M43.22
  choanal Q30.0
  commissure, mitral valve Q23.2
  cusps, heart valve NEC Q24.8
    mitral Q23.2
    pulmonary Q22.1
    tricuspid Q22.4
  ear ossicles Q16.3
  fingers Q70.0 ☑
  hymen Q52.3
  joint (acquired) (*see also* Ankylosis)
    congenital Q74.8
  kidneys (incomplete) Q63.1
  labium (majus) (minus) Q52.5
  larynx and trachea Q34.8
  limb, congenital Q74.8
    lower Q74.2
    upper Q74.0
  lobes, lung Q33.8
  lumbosacral (acquired) M43.27
    arthrodesis status Z98.1
    congenital Q76.49

Fusion, fused — *continued*
  lumbosacral — *continued*
    postprocedural status Z98.1
  nares, nose, nasal, nostril(s) Q30.0
  organ or site not listed — *see* Anomaly, by site
  ossicles Q79.9
    auditory Q16.3
  pulmonic cusps Q22.1
  ribs Q76.6
  sacroiliac (joint) (acquired) M43.28
    arthrodesis status Z98.1
    congenital Q74.2
    postprocedural status Z98.1
  spine (acquired) NEC M43.20
    arthrodesis status Z98.1
    cervical region M43.22
    cervicothoracic region M43.23
    congenital Q76.49
    lumbar M43.26
    lumbosacral region M43.27
    occipito-atlanto-axial region M43.21
    postoperative status Z98.1
    sacrococcygeal region M43.28
    thoracic region M43.24
    thoracolumbar region M43.25
  sublingual duct with submaxillary duct at opening in
      mouth Q38.4
  testes Q55.1
  toes Q70.2- ☑
  tooth, teeth K00.2
  trachea and esophagus Q39.8
  twins Q89.4
  vagina Q52.4
  ventricles, heart Q21.0
  vertebra (arch) — *see* Fusion, spine
  vulva Q52.5
Fusospirillosis (mouth) (tongue) (tonsil) A69.1
Fussy baby R68.12

G

Gain in weight (abnormal) (excessive) (*see also* Weight, gain)
Gaisböck's disease (polycythemia hypertonica) D75.1
Gait abnormality R26.9
  ataxic R26.0
  falling R29.6
  hysterical (ataxic) (staggering) F44.4
  paralytic R26.1
  spastic R26.1
  specified type NEC R26.89
  staggering R26.0
  unsteadiness R26.81
  walking difficulty NEC R26.2
Galactocele (breast) N64.89
  puerperal, postpartum O92.79
Galactokinase deficiency E74.29
Galactophoritis N61.0
  gestational, puerperal, postpartum O91.2- ☑
Galactorrhea O92.6
  not associated with childbirth N64.3
Galactosemia (classic) (congenital) E74.21
Galactosuria E74.29
Galacturia R82.0
  schistosomiasis (bilharziasis) B65.0
GALD (gestational alloimmune liver disease) P78.84
Galeazzi's fracture S52.37- ☑
Galen's vein — *see* condition
Galeophobia F40.218
Gall duct — *see* condition
Gallbladder (*see also* condition)
  acute K81.0
Gallop rhythm R00.8
Gallstone (colic) (cystic duct) (gallbladder) (impacted) (multiple) (*see also* Calculus, gallbladder)
  with
    cholecystitis — *see* Calculus, gallbladder, with cholecystitis
  bile duct (common) (hepatic) — *see* Calculus, bile duct
  causing intestinal obstruction K56.3
  specified NEC K80.80
    with obstruction K80.81
Gambling Z72.6
  pathological (compulsive) F63.0
Gammopathy (of undetermined significance [MGUS]) D47.2
  associated with lymphoplasmacytic dyscrasia D47.2
  monoclonal D47.2
  polyclonal D89.0
Gamna's disease (siderotic splenomegaly) D73.1
Gamophobia F40.298
Gampsodactylia (congenital) Q66.7
Gamstorp's disease (adynamia episodica hereditaria) G72.3
Gandy-Nanta disease (siderotic splenomegaly) D73.1
Gang
  membership offenses Z72.810
Gangliocytoma D36.10
Ganglioglioma — *see* Neoplasm, uncertain behavior, by site
Ganglion (compound) (diffuse) (joint) (tendon (sheath)) M67.40
  ankle M67.47- ☑
  foot M67.47- ☑
  forearm M67.43- ☑
  hand M67.44- ☑
  lower leg M67.46- ☑
  multiple sites M67.49
  of yaws (early) (late) A66.6
  pelvic region M67.45- ☑
  periosteal — *see* Periostitis
  shoulder region M67.41- ☑
  specified site NEC M67.48
  thigh region M67.45- ☑
  tuberculous A18.09
  upper arm M67.42- ☑
  wrist M67.43- ☑
Ganglioneuroblastoma — *see* Neoplasm, nerve, malignant
Ganglioneuroma D36.10
  malignant — *see* Neoplasm, nerve, malignant
Ganglioneuromatosis D36.10
Ganglionitis
  fifth nerve — *see* Neuralgia, trigeminal
  gasserian (postherpetic) (postzoster) B02.21

Ganglionitis — *continued*
  geniculate G51.1
    newborn (birth injury) P11.3
    postherpetic, postzoster B02.21
  herpes zoster B02.21
  postherpetic geniculate B02.21
Gangliosidosis E75.10
  GM1 E75.19
  GM2 E75.00
    other specified E75.09
    Sandhoff disease E75.01
    Tay-Sachs disease E75.02
  GM3 E75.19
  mucolipidosis IV E75.11
Gangosa A66.5
Gangrene, gangrenous (connective tissue) (dropsical) (dry) (moist) (skin) (ulcer) (*see also* Necrosis) I96
  with diabetes (mellitus) — *see* Diabetes, gangrene
  abdomen (wall) I96
  alveolar M27.3
  appendix K35.80
    with
      peritonitis, localized (*see also* Appendicitis) K35.31
  arteriosclerotic (general) (senile) — *see* Arteriosclerosis, extremities, with, gangrene
  auricle I96
  Bacillus welchii A48.0
  bladder (infectious) — *see* Cystitis, specified type NEC
  bowel, cecum, or colon — *see* Gangrene, intestine
  Clostridium perfringens or welchii A48.0
  cornea H18.89- ☑
  corpora cavernosa N48.29
    noninfective N48.89
  cutaneous, spreading I96
  decubital — *see* Ulcer, pressure, by site
  diabetic (any site) — *see* Diabetes, gangrene
  emphysematous — *see* Gangrene, gas
  epidemic — *see* Poisoning, food, noxious, plant
  epididymis (infectional) N45.1
  erysipelas — *see* Erysipelas
  extremity (lower) (upper) I96
  Fournier N49.3
    female N76.89
  fusospirochetal A69.0
  gallbladder — *see* Cholecystitis, acute
  gas (bacillus) A48.0
    following
      abortion — *see* Abortion by type complicated by infection
      ectopic or molar pregnancy O08.0
  glossitis K14.0
  hernia — *see* Hernia, by site, with gangrene
  intestine, intestinal (hemorrhagic) (massive) (*see also* Infarct, intestine) K55.069
    with
      mesenteric embolism (*see also* Infarct, intestine) K55.069
      obstruction — *see* Obstruction, intestine
  laryngitis J04.0
  limb (lower) (upper) I96
  lung J85.0
    spirochetal A69.8
  lymphangitis I89.1
  Meleney's (synergistic) — *see* Ulcer, skin
  mesentery (*see also* Infarct, intestine) K55.069
    with
      embolism (*see also* Infarct, intestine) K55.069
      intestinal obstruction — *see* Obstruction, intestine
  mouth A69.0
  ovary — *see* Oophoritis
  pancreas — *see* Pancreatitis, acute
  penis N48.29
    noninfective N48.89
  perineum I96
  pharynx (*see also* Pharyngitis)
    Vincent's A69.1
  presenile I73.1
  progressive synergistic — *see* Ulcer, skin
  pulmonary J85.0
  pulpal (dental) K04.1
  quinsy J36
  Raynaud's (symmetric gangrene) I73.01
  retropharyngeal J39.2
  scrotum N49.3
    noninfective N50.89

Gangrene, gangrenous — *continued*
  senile (atherosclerotic) — *see* Arteriosclerosis, extremities, with, gangrene
  spermatic cord N49.1
    noninfective N50.89
  spine I96
  spirochetal NEC A69.8
  spreading cutaneous I96
  stomatitis A69.0
  symmetrical I73.01
  testis (infectional) N45.2
    noninfective N44.8
  throat (*see also* Pharyngitis)
    diphtheritic A36.0
    Vincent's A69.1
  thyroid (gland) E07.89
  tooth (pulp) K04.1
  tuberculous NEC — *see* Tuberculosis
  tunica vaginalis N49.1
    noninfective N50.89
  umbilicus I96
  uterus — *see* Endometritis
  uvulitis K12.2
  vas deferens N49.1
    noninfective N50.89
  vulva N76.89
Ganister disease J62.8
Ganser's syndrome (hysterical) F44.89
Gardner-Diamond syndrome (autoerythrocyte sensitization) D69.2
Gargoylism E76.01
Garré's disease, osteitis (sclerosing), osteomyelitis — *see* Osteomyelitis, specified type NEC
Garrod's pad, knuckle M72.1
Gartner's duct
  cyst Q52.4
  persistent Q50.6
Gas R14.3
  asphyxiation, inhalation, poisoning, suffocation NEC — *see* Table of Drugs and Chemicals
  excessive R14.0
  gangrene A48.0
    following
      abortion — *see* Abortion by type complicated by infection
      ectopic or molar pregnancy O08.0
  on stomach R14.0
  pains R14.1
Gastralgia (*see also* Pain, abdominal)
Gastrectasis K31.0
  psychogenic F45.8
Gastric — *see* condition
Gastrinoma
  malignant
    pancreas C25.4
    specified site NEC — *see* Neoplasm, malignant, by site
    unspecified site C25.4
  specified site — *see* Neoplasm, uncertain behavior
  unspecified site D37.9
Gastritis (simple) K29.70
  with bleeding K29.71
  acute (erosive) K29.00
    with bleeding K29.01
  alcoholic K29.20
    with bleeding K29.21
  allergic K29.60
    with bleeding K29.61
  atrophic (chronic) K29.40
    with bleeding K29.41
  chronic (antral) (fundal) K29.50
    with bleeding K29.51
    atrophic K29.40
      with bleeding K29.41
    superficial K29.30
      with bleeding K29.31
  dietary counseling and surveillance Z71.3
  due to diet deficiency E63.9
  eosinophilic K52.81
  giant hypertrophic K29.60
    with bleeding K29.61
  granulomatous K29.60
    with bleeding K29.61
  hypertrophic (mucosa) K29.60
    with bleeding K29.61
  nervous F54
  spastic K29.60
    with bleeding K29.61

▽ Subterms under main terms may continue to next column or page   ☑ **Additional Character Required** — Refer to the Tabular List for Character Selection   **157**

Gain in weight — Gastritis

Gastritis — continued
specified NEC K29.60
   with bleeding K29.61
superficial chronic K29.30
   with bleeding K29.31
tuberculous A18.83
viral NEC A08.4
Gastrocarcinoma — see Neoplasm, malignant, stomach
Gastrocolic — see condition
Gastrodisciasis, gastrodiscoidiasis B66.8
Gastroduodenitis K29.90
with bleeding K29.91
virus, viral A08.4
   specified type NEC A08.39
Gastrodynia — see Pain, abdominal
Gastroenteritis (acute) (chronic) (noninfectious) (see also Enteritis) K52.9
allergic K52.29
  with
     eosinophilic gastritis or gastroenteritis K52.81
     food protein-induced enterocolitis syndrome K52.21
     food protein-induced enteropathy K52.22
dietetic (see also Gastroenteritis, allergic) K52.29
drug-induced K52.1
due to
   Cryptosporidium A07.2
   drugs K52.1
   food poisoning — see Intoxication, foodborne
   radiation K52.0
eosinophilic K52.81
epidemic (infectious) A09
food hypersensitivity (see also Gastroenteritis, allergic) K52.29
infectious — see Enteritis, infectious
influenzal — see Influenza, with gastroenteritis
noninfectious K52.9
   specified NEC K52.89
rotaviral A08.0
Salmonella A02.0
toxic K52.1
viral NEC A08.4
   acute infectious A08.39
     type Norwalk A08.11
   infantile (acute) A08.39
   Norwalk agent A08.11
   rotaviral A08.0
   severe of infants A08.39
   specified type NEC A08.39
Gastroenteropathy (see also Gastroenteritis) K52.9
acute, due to Norovirus A08.11
acute, due to Norwalk agent A08.11
infectious A09
Gastroenteroptosis K63.4
Gastroesophageal laceration- hemorrhage syndrome K22.6
Gastrointestinal — see condition
Gastrojejunal — see condition
Gastrojejunitis (see also Enteritis) K52.9
Gastrojejunocolic — see condition
Gastroliths K31.89
Gastromalacia K31.89
Gastroparalysis K31.84
diabetic — see Diabetes, gastroparalysis
Gastroparesis K31.84
diabetic — see Diabetes, by type, with gastroparesis
Gastropathy K31.9
congestive portal K31.89
erythematous K29.70
exudative K90.89
portal hypertensive K31.89
Gastroptosis K31.89
Gastrorrhagia K92.2
psychogenic F45.8
Gastroschisis (congenital) Q79.3
Gastrospasm (neurogenic) (reflex) K31.89
neurotic F45.8
psychogenic F45.8
Gastrostaxis — see Gastritis, with bleeding
Gastrostenosis K31.89
Gastrostomy
attention to Z43.1
status Z93.1
Gastrosuccorrhea (continuous) (intermittent) K31.89
neurotic F45.8
psychogenic F45.8
Gatophobia F40.218

Gaucher's disease or splenomegaly (adult) (infantile) E75.22
Gee (-Herter)(-Thaysen) **disease** (nontropical sprue) K90.0
Gélineau's syndrome G47.419
with cataplexy G47.411
Gemination, tooth, teeth K00.2
Gemistocytoma
specified site — see Neoplasm, malignant, by site
unspecified site C71.9
General, generalized — see condition
Genetic
carrier (status)
   cystic fibrosis Z14.1
   hemophilia A (asymptomatic) Z14.01
     symptomatic Z14.02
   specified NEC Z14.8
susceptibility to disease NEC Z15.89
   malignant neoplasm Z15.09
     breast Z15.01
     endometrium Z15.04
     ovary Z15.02
     prostate Z15.03
     specified NEC Z15.09
   multiple endocrine neoplasia Z15.81
Genital — see condition
Genito-anorectal syndrome A55
Genitourinary system — see condition
Genu
congenital Q74.1
extrorsum (acquired) (see also Deformity, varus, knee)
   congenital Q74.1
   sequelae (late effect) of rickets E64.3
introrsum (acquired) (see also Deformity, valgus, knee)
   congenital Q74.1
   sequelae (late effect) of rickets E64.3
rachitic (old) E64.3
recurvatum (acquired) (see also Deformity, limb, specified type NEC, lower leg)
   congenital Q68.2
   sequelae (late effect) of rickets E64.3
valgum (acquired) (knock-knee) M21.06- ☑
   congenital Q74.1
   sequelae (late effect) of rickets E64.3
varum (acquired) (bowleg) M21.16- ☑
   congenital Q74.1
   sequelae (late effect) of rickets E64.3
Geographic tongue K14.1
Geophagia — see Pica
Geotrichosis B48.3
stomatitis B48.3
Gephyrophobia F40.242
Gerbode defect Q21.0
GERD (gastroesophageal reflux disease) K21.9
Gerhardt's
disease (erythromelalgia) I73.81
syndrome (vocal cord paralysis) J38.00
   bilateral J38.02
   unilateral J38.01
German measles (see also Rubella)
exposure to Z20.4
Germinoblastoma (diffuse) C85.9- ☑
follicular C82.9- ☑
Germinoma — see Neoplasm, malignant, by site
Gerontoxon — see Degeneration, cornea, senile
Gerstmann's syndrome R48.8
developmental F81.2
Gerstmann-Sträussler-Scheinker syndrome (GSS) A81.82
Gestation (period) (see also Pregnancy)
ectopic — see Pregnancy, by site
multiple O30.9- ☑
   greater than quadruplets — see Pregnancy, multiple (gestation), specified NEC
   specified NEC — see Pregnancy, multiple (gestation), specified NEC
Gestational
mammary abscess O91.11- ☑
purulent mastitis O91.11- ☑
subareolar abscess O91.11- ☑
Ghon tubercle, primary infection A15.7
Ghost
teeth K00.4
vessels (cornea) H16.41- ☑
Ghoul hand A66.3
Gianotti-Crosti disease L44.4

Giant
cell
   epulis K06.8
   peripheral granuloma K06.8
esophagus, congenital Q39.5
kidney, congenital Q63.3
urticaria T78.3 ☑
   hereditary D84.1
Giardiasis A07.1
Gibert's disease or pityriasis L42
Giddiness R42
hysterical F44.89
psychogenic F45.8
Gierke's disease (glycogenosis I) E74.01
Gigantism (cerebral) (hypophyseal) (pituitary) E22.0
constitutional E34.4
Gilbert's disease or syndrome E80.4
Gilchrist's disease B40.9
Gilford-Hutchinson disease E34.8
Gilles de la Tourette's disease or syndrome (motor-verbal tic) F95.2
Gingivitis K05.10
acute (catarrhal) K05.00
   necrotizing A69.1
   nonplaque induced K05.01
   plaque induced K05.00
chronic (desquamative) (hyperplastic) (simple marginal) (pregnancy associated) (ulcerative) K05.10
   nonplaque induced K05.11
   plaque induced K05.10
expulsiva — see Periodontitis
necrotizing ulcerative (acute) A69.1
pellagrous E52
   acute necrotizing A69.1
Vincent's A69.1
Gingivoglossitis K14.0
Gingivopericementitis — see Periodontitis
Gingivosis — see Gingivitis, chronic
Gingivostomatitis K05.10
herpesviral B00.2
necrotizing ulcerative (acute) A69.1
Gland, glandular — see condition
Glanders A24.0
Glanzmann (-Naegeli) **disease or thrombasthenia** D69.1
Glasgow coma scale
total score
   13-15 R40.241 ☑
   3-8 R40.243 ☑
   9-12 R40.242 ☑
Glass-blower's disease (cataract) — see Cataract, specified NEC
Glaucoma H40.9
with
   increased episcleral venous pressure H40.81- ☑
   pseudoexfoliation of lens — see Glaucoma, open angle, primary, capsular
absolute H44.51- ☑
angle-closure (primary) H40.20- ☑
   acute (attack) (crisis) H40.21- ☑
   chronic H40.22- ☑
   intermittent H40.23- ☑
   residual stage H40.24- ☑
borderline H40.00- ☑
capsular (with pseudoexfoliation of lens) — see Glaucoma, open angle, primary, capsular
childhood Q15.0
closed angle — see Glaucoma, angle-closure
congenital Q15.0
corticosteroid-induced — see Glaucoma, secondary, drugs
hypersecretion H40.82- ☑
in (due to)
   amyloidosis E85.4 [H42]
   aniridia Q13.1 [H42]
   concussion of globe — see Glaucoma, secondary, trauma
   dislocation of lens — see Glaucoma, secondary
   disorder of lens NEC — see Glaucoma, secondary
   drugs — see Glaucoma, secondary, drugs
   endocrine disease NOS E34.9 [H42]
   eye
     inflammation — see Glaucoma, secondary, inflammation
     trauma — see Glaucoma, secondary, trauma
   hypermature cataract — see Glaucoma, secondary

ICD-10-CM 2019 — Glycogenosis

Index

Glaucoma — *continued*
  in — *continued*
    iridocyclitis — *see* Glaucoma, secondary, inflammation
    lens disorder — *see* Glaucoma, secondary
    Lowe's syndrome E72.03 [H42]
    metabolic disease NOS E88.9 [H42]
    ocular disorders NEC — *see* Glaucoma, secondary
    onchocerciasis B73.02
    pupillary block — *see* Glaucoma, secondary
    retinal vein occlusion — *see* Glaucoma, secondary
    Rieger's anomaly Q13.81 [H42]
    rubeosis of iris — *see* Glaucoma, secondary
    tumor of globe — *see* Glaucoma, secondary
  infantile Q15.0
  low tension — *see* Glaucoma, open angle, primary, low-tension
  malignant H40.83- ☑
  narrow angle — *see* Glaucoma, angle-closure
  newborn Q15.0
  noncongestive (chronic) — *see* Glaucoma, open angle
  nonobstructive — *see* Glaucoma, open angle
  obstructive (*see also* Glaucoma, angle-closure)
    due to lens changes — *see* Glaucoma, secondary
  open angle H40.10- ☑
    primary H40.11- ☑
      capsular (with pseudoexfoliation of lens) H40.14- ☑
      low-tension H40.12- ☑
      pigmentary H40.13- ☑
      residual stage H40.15- ☑
  phacolytic — *see* Glaucoma, secondary
  pigmentary — *see* Glaucoma, open angle, primary, pigmentary
  postinfectious — *see* Glaucoma, secondary, inflammation
  secondary (to) H40.5- ☑
    drugs H40.6- ☑
    inflammation H40.4- ☑
    trauma H40.3- ☑
  simple (chronic) H40.11- ☑
  simplex H40.11- ☑
  specified type NEC H40.89
  suspect H40.00- ☑
  syphilitic A52.71
  traumatic (*see also* Glaucoma, secondary, trauma)
    newborn (birth injury) P15.3
  tuberculous A18.59
Glaucomatous flecks (subcapsular) — *see* Cataract, complicated
Glazed tongue K14.4
Gleet (gonococcal) A54.01
Glénard's disease K63.4
Glioblastoma (multiforme)
  with sarcomatous component
    specified site — *see* Neoplasm, malignant, by site
    unspecified site C71.9
  giant cell
    specified site — *see* Neoplasm, malignant, by site
    unspecified site C71.9
  specified site — *see* Neoplasm, malignant, by site
  unspecified site C71.9
Glioma (malignant)
  astrocytic
    specified site — *see* Neoplasm, malignant, by site
    unspecified site C71.9
  mixed
    specified site — *see* Neoplasm, malignant, by site
    unspecified site C71.9
  nose Q30.8
  specified site NEC — *see* Neoplasm, malignant, by site
  subependymal D43.2
    specified site — *see* Neoplasm, uncertain behavior, by site
    unspecified site D43.2
  unspecified site C71.9
Gliomatosis cerebri C71.0
Glioneuroma — *see* Neoplasm, uncertain behavior, by site
Gliosarcoma
  specified site — *see* Neoplasm, malignant, by site
  unspecified site C71.9
Gliosis (cerebral) G93.89
  spinal G95.89
Glisson's disease — *see* Rickets
Globinuria R82.3
Globus (hystericus) F45.8

Glomangioma D18.00
  intra-abdominal D18.03
  intracranial D18.02
  skin D18.01
  specified site NEC D18.09
Glomangiomyoma D18.00
  intra-abdominal D18.03
  intracranial D18.02
  skin D18.01
  specified site NEC D18.09
Glomangiosarcoma — *see* Neoplasm, connective tissue, malignant
Glomerular
  disease in syphilis A52.75
  nephritis — *see* Glomerulonephritis
Glomerulitis — *see* Glomerulonephritis
Glomerulonephritis (*see also* Nephritis) N05.9
  with
    edema — *see* Nephrosis
    minimal change N05.0
    minor glomerular abnormality N05.0
  acute N00.9
  chronic N03.9
  crescentic (diffuse) NEC (*see also* N00-N07 with fourth character .7) N05.7
  dense deposit (*see also* N00-N07 with fourth character .6) N05.6
  diffuse
    crescentic (*see also* N00-N07 with fourth character .7) N05.7
    endocapillary proliferative (*see also* N00-N07 with fourth character .4) N05.4
    membranous (*see also* N00-N07 with fourth character .2) N05.2
    mesangial proliferative (*see also* N00-N07 with fourth character .3) N05.3
    mesangiocapillary (*see also* N00-N07 with fourth character .5) N05.5
    sclerosing N18.9
  endocapillary proliferative (diffuse) NEC (*see also* N00-N07 with fourth character .4) N05.4
  extracapillary NEC (*see also* N00-N07 with fourth character .7) N05.7
  focal (and segmental) (*see also* N00-N07 with fourth character .1) N05.1
  hypocomplementemic — *see* Glomerulonephritis, membranoproliferative
  IgA — *see* Nephropathy, IgA
  immune complex (circulating) NEC N05.8
  in (due to)
    amyloidosis E85.4 [N08]
    bilharziasis B65.9 [N08]
    cryoglobulinemia D89.1 [N08]
    defibrination syndrome D65 [N08]
    diabetes mellitus — *see* Diabetes, glomerulosclerosis
    disseminated intravascular coagulation D65 [N08]
    Fabry (-Anderson) disease E75.21 [N08]
    Goodpasture's syndrome M31.0
    hemolytic-uremic syndrome D59.3
    Henoch (-Schönlein) purpura D69.0 [N08]
    lecithin cholesterol acyltransferase deficiency E78.6 [N08]
    microscopic polyangiitis M31.7 [N08]
    multiple myeloma C90.0- ☑ [N08]
    Plasmodium malariae B52.0
    schistosomiasis B65.9 [N08]
    sepsis A41.9 [N08]
      streptococcal A40- ☑ [N08]
    sickle-cell disorders D57.- ☑ [N08]
    strongyloidiasis B78.9 [N08]
    subacute bacterial endocarditis I33.0 [N08]
    syphilis (late) congenital A50.59 [N08]
    systemic lupus erythematosus M32.14
    thrombotic thrombocytopenic purpura M31.1 [N08]
    typhoid fever A01.09
    Waldenström macroglobulinemia C88.0 [N08]
    Wegener's granulomatosis M31.31
  latent or quiescent N03.9
  lobular, lobulonodular — *see* Glomerulonephritis, membranoproliferative
  membranoproliferative (diffuse)(type 1 or 3) (*see also* N00-N07 with fourth character .5) N05.5
    dense deposit (type 2) NEC (*see also* N00-N07 with fourth character .6) N05.6
  membranous (diffuse) NEC (*see also* N00-N07 with fourth character .2) N05.2

Glomerulonephritis — *continued*
  mesangial
    IgA/IgG — *see* Nephropathy, IgA
    proliferative (diffuse) NEC (*see also* N00-N07 with fourth character .3) N05.3
    mesangiocapillary (diffuse) NEC (*see also* N00-N07 with fourth character .5) N05.5
  necrotic, necrotizing NEC (*see also* N00- N07 with fourth character .8) N05.8
  nodular — *see* Glomerulonephritis, membranoproliferative
  poststreptococcal NEC N05.9
    acute N00.9
    chronic N03.9
    rapidly progressive N01.9
  proliferative NEC (*see also* N00-N07 with fourth character .8) N05.8
    diffuse (lupus) M32.14
  rapidly progressive N01.9
  sclerosing, diffuse N18.9
  specified pathology NEC (*see also* N00- N07 with fourth character .8) N05.8
  subacute N01.9
Glomerulopathy — *see* Glomerulonephritis
Glomerulosclerosis (*see also* Sclerosis, renal)
  intercapillary (nodular) (with diabetes) — *see* Diabetes, glomerulosclerosis
  intracapillary — *see* Diabetes, glomerulosclerosis
Glossagra K14.6
Glossalgia K14.6
Glossitis (chronic superficial) (gangrenous) (Moeller's) K14.0
  areata exfoliativa K14.1
  atrophic K14.4
  benign migratory K14.1
  cortical superficial, sclerotic K14.0
  Hunter's D51.0
  interstitial, sclerous K14.0
  median rhomboid K14.2
  pellagrous E52
  superficial, chronic K14.0
Glossocele K14.8
Glossodynia K14.6
  exfoliativa K14.4
Glossoncus K14.8
Glossopathy K14.9
Glossophytia K14.3
Glossoplegia K14.8
Glossoptosis K14.8
Glossopyrosis K14.6
Glossotrichia K14.3
Glossy skin L90.8
Glottis — *see* condition
Glottitis (*see also* Laryngitis) J04.0
Glucagonoma
  pancreas
    benign D13.7
    malignant C25.4
    uncertain behavior D37.8
  specified site NEC
    benign — *see* Neoplasm, benign, by site
    malignant — *see* Neoplasm, malignant, by site
    uncertain behavior — *see* Neoplasm, uncertain behavior, by site
  unspecified site
    benign D13.7
    malignant C25.4
    uncertain behavior D37.8
Glucoglycinuria E72.51
Glucose-galactose malabsorption E74.39
Glue
  ear — *see* Otitis, media, nonsuppurative, chronic, mucoid
  sniffing (airplane) — *see* Abuse, drug, inhalant
    dependence — *see* Dependence, drug, inhalant
Glutaric aciduria E72.3
Glycinemia E72.51
Glycinuria (renal) (with ketosis) E72.09
Glycogen
  infiltration — *see* Disease, glycogen storage
  storage disease — *see* Disease, glycogen storage
Glycogenosis (diffuse) (generalized) (*see also* Disease, glycogen storage)
  cardiac E74.02 [I43]
  diabetic, secondary — *see* Diabetes, glycogenosis, secondary
  pulmonary interstitial J84.842

Glycopenia E16.2
Glycosuria R81
  renal E74.8
Gnathostoma spinigerum (infection) (infestation), **gnathostomiasis** (wandering swelling) B83.1
Goiter (plunging) (substernal) E04.9
  with
    hyperthyroidism (recurrent) — *see* Hyperthyroidism, with, goiter
    thyrotoxicosis — *see* Hyperthyroidism, with, goiter
  adenomatous — *see* Goiter, nodular
  cancerous C73
  congenital (nontoxic) E03.0
    diffuse E03.0
    parenchymatous E03.0
    transitory, with normal functioning P72.0
  cystic E04.2
    due to iodine-deficiency E01.1
  due to
    enzyme defect in synthesis of thyroid hormone E07.1
    iodine-deficiency (endemic) E01.2
  dyshormonogenetic (familial) E07.1
  endemic (iodine-deficiency) E01.2
    diffuse E01.0
    multinodular E01.1
  exophthalmic — *see* Hyperthyroidism, with, goiter
  iodine-deficiency (endemic) E01.2
    diffuse E01.0
    multinodular E01.1
    nodular E01.1
  lingual Q89.2
  lymphadenoid E06.3
  malignant C73
  multinodular (cystic) (nontoxic) E04.2
    toxic or with hyperthyroidism E05.20
      with thyroid storm E05.21
  neonatal NEC P72.0
  nodular (nontoxic) (due to) E04.9
    with
      hyperthyroidism E05.20
        with thyroid storm E05.21
      thyrotoxicosis E05.20
        with thyroid storm E05.21
    endemic E01.1
    iodine-deficiency E01.1
    sporadic E04.9
    toxic E05.20
      with thyroid storm E05.21
  nontoxic E04.9
    diffuse (colloid) E04.0
    multinodular E04.2
    simple E04.0
    specified NEC E04.8
    uninodular E04.1
  simple E04.0
  toxic — *see* Hyperthyroidism, with, goiter
  uninodular (nontoxic) E04.1
    toxic or with hyperthyroidism E05.10
      with thyroid storm E05.11
Goiter-deafness syndrome E07.1
Goldberg syndrome Q89.8
Goldberg-Maxwell syndrome E34.51
Goldblatt's hypertension or kidney I70.1
Goldenhar (-Gorlin) **syndrome** Q87.0
Goldflam-Erb disease or syndrome G70.00
  with exacerbation (acute) G70.01
  in crisis G70.01
Goldscheider's disease Q81.8
Goldstein's disease (familial hemorrhagic telangiectasia) I78.0
Golfer's elbow — *see* Epicondylitis, medial
Gonadoblastoma
  specified site — *see* Neoplasm, uncertain behavior, by site
  unspecified site
    female D39.10
    male D40.10
Gonecystitis — *see* Vesiculitis
Gongylonemiasis B83.8
Goniosynechiae — *see* Adhesions, iris, goniosynechiae
Gonococcemia A54.86
Gonococcus, gonococcal (disease) (infection) (*see also* condition) A54.9
  anus A54.6
  bursa, bursitis A54.49
  conjunctiva, conjunctivitis (neonatorum) A54.31
  endocardium A54.83

Gonococcus, gonococcal — *continued*
  eye A54.30
    conjunctivitis A54.31
    iridocyclitis A54.32
    keratitis A54.33
    newborn A54.31
    other specified A54.39
  fallopian tubes (acute) (chronic) A54.24
  genitourinary (organ) (system) (tract) (acute) A54.00
    lower A54.00
      with abscess (accessory gland) (periurethral) A54.1
    upper (*see also* condition) A54.29
  heart A54.83
  iridocyclitis A54.32
  joint A54.42
  lymphatic (gland) (node) A54.89
  meninges, meningitis A54.81
  musculoskeletal A54.40
    arthritis A54.42
    osteomyelitis A54.43
    other specified A54.49
    spondylopathy A54.41
  pelviperitonitis A54.24
  pelvis (acute) (chronic) A54.24
  pharynx A54.5
  proctitis A54.6
  pyosalpinx (acute) (chronic) A54.24
  rectum A54.6
  skin A54.89
  specified site NEC A54.89
  tendon sheath A54.49
  throat A54.5
  urethra (acute) (chronic) A54.01
    with abscess (accessory gland) (periurethral) A54.1
  vulva (acute) (chronic) A54.02
Gonocytoma
  specified site — *see* Neoplasm, uncertain behavior, by site
  unspecified site
    female D39.10
    male D40.10
Gonorrhea (acute) (chronic) A54.9
  Bartholin's gland (acute) (chronic) (purulent) A54.02
    with abscess (accessory gland) (periurethral) A54.1
  bladder A54.01
  cervix A54.03
  conjunctiva, conjunctivitis (neonatorum) A54.31
  contact Z20.2
  Cowper's gland (with abscess) A54.1
  exposure to Z20.2
  fallopian tube (acute) (chronic) A54.24
  kidney (acute) (chronic) A54.21
  lower genitourinary tract A54.00
    with abscess (accessory gland) (periurethral) A54.1
  ovary (acute) (chronic) A54.24
  pelvis (acute) (chronic) A54.24
    female pelvic inflammatory disease A54.24
  penis A54.09
  prostate (acute) (chronic) A54.22
  seminal vesicle (acute) (chronic) A54.23
  specified site not listed (*see also* Gonococcus) A54.89
  spermatic cord (acute) (chronic) A54.23
  urethra A54.01
    with abscess (accessory gland) (periurethral) A54.1
  vagina A54.02
  vas deferens (acute) (chronic) A54.23
  vulva A54.02
Goodall's disease A08.19
Goodpasture's syndrome M31.0
Gopalan's syndrome (burning feet) E53.0
Gorlin-Chaudry-Moss syndrome Q87.0
Gottron's papules L94.4
Gougerot-Blum syndrome (pigmented purpuric lichenoid dermatitis) L81.7
Gougerot-Carteaud disease or syndrome (confluent reticulate papillomatosis) L83
Gougerot's syndrome (trisymptomatic) L81.7
Gouley's syndrome (constrictive pericarditis) I31.1
Goundou A66.6
Gout, chronic (*see also* Gout, gouty) M1A.9 ☑ (*following* M08)
  drug-induced M1A.20 ☑ (*following* M08)
    ankle M1A.27- ☑ (*following* M08)
    elbow M1A.22- ☑ (*following* M08)
    foot joint M1A.27- ☑ (*following* M08)
    hand joint M1A.24- ☑ (*following* M08)
    hip M1A.25- ☑ (*following* M08)

Gout, chronic — *continued*
  drug-induced — *continued*
    knee M1A.26- ☑ (*following* M08)
    multiple site M1A.29- ☑ (*following* M08)
    shoulder M1A.21- ☑ (*following* M08)
    vertebrae M1A.28 ☑ (*following* M08)
    wrist M1A.23- ☑ (*following* M08)
  idiopathic M1A.00 ☑ (*following* M08)
    ankle M1A.07- ☑ (*following* M08)
    elbow M1A.02- ☑ (*following* M08)
    foot joint M1A.07- ☑ (*following* M08)
    hand joint M1A.04- ☑ (*following* M08)
    hip M1A.05- ☑ (*following* M08)
    knee M1A.06- ☑ (*following* M08)
    multiple site M1A.09 ☑ (*following* M08)
    shoulder M1A.01- ☑ (*following* M08)
    vertebrae M1A.08 ☑ (*following* M08)
    wrist M1A.03- ☑ (*following* M08)
  in (due to) renal impairment M1A.30 ☑ (*following* M08)
    ankle M1A.37- ☑ (*following* M08)
    elbow M1A.32- ☑ (*following* M08)
    foot joint M1A.37- ☑ (*following* M08)
    hand joint M1A.34- ☑ (*following* M08)
    hip M1A.35- ☑ (*following* M08)
    knee M1A.36- ☑ (*following* M08)
    multiple site M1A.39 ☑ (*following* M08)
    shoulder M1A.31- ☑ (*following* M08)
    vertebrae M1A.38 ☑ (*following* M08)
    wrist M1A.33- ☑ (*following* M08)
  lead-induced M1A.10 ☑ (*following* M08)
    ankle M1A.17- ☑ (*following* M08)
    elbow M1A.12- ☑ (*following* M08)
    foot joint M1A.17- ☑ (*following* M08)
    hand joint M1A.14- ☑ (*following* M08)
    hip M1A.15- ☑ (*following* M08)
    knee M1A.16- ☑ (*following* M08)
    multiple site M1A.19 ☑ (*following* M08)
    shoulder M1A.11- ☑ (*following* M08)
    vertebrae M1A.18 ☑ (*following* M08)
    wrist M1A.13- ☑ (*following* M08)
  primary — *see* Gout, chronic, idiopathic
  saturnine — *see* Gout, chronic, lead-induced
  secondary NEC M1A.40 ☑ (*following* M08)
    ankle M1A.47- ☑ (*following* M08)
    elbow M1A.42- ☑ (*following* M08)
    foot joint M1A.47- ☑ (*following* M08)
    hand joint M1A.44- ☑ (*following* M08)
    hip M1A.45- ☑ (*following* M08)
    knee M1A.46- ☑ (*following* M08)
    multiple site M1A.49 ☑ (*following* M08)
    shoulder M1A.41- ☑ (*following* M08)
    vertebrae M1A.48 ☑ (*following* M08)
    wrist M1A.43- ☑ (*following* M08)
  syphilitic (*see also* subcategory M14.8-) A52.77
  tophi M1A.9 ☑ (*following* M08)
Gout, gouty (acute) (attack) (flare) (*see also* Gout, chronic) M10.9
  drug-induced M10.20
    ankle M10.27- ☑
    elbow M10.22- ☑
    foot joint M10.27- ☑
    hand joint M10.24- ☑
    hip M10.25- ☑
    knee M10.26- ☑
    multiple site M10.29
    shoulder M10.21- ☑
    vertebrae M10.28
    wrist M10.23- ☑
  idiopathic M10.00
    ankle M10.07- ☑
    elbow M10.02- ☑
    foot joint M10.07- ☑
    hand joint M10.04- ☑
    hip M10.05- ☑
    knee M10.06- ☑
    multiple site M10.09
    shoulder M10.01- ☑
    vertebrae M10.08
    wrist M10.03- ☑
  in (due to) renal impairment M10.30
    ankle M10.37- ☑
    elbow M10.32- ☑
    foot joint M10.37- ☑
    hand joint M10.34- ☑
    hip M10.35- ☑
    knee M10.36- ☑

Gout, gouty — *continued*
  in renal impairment — *continued*
    multiple site M10.39
    shoulder M10.31- ☑
    vertebrae M10.38
    wrist M10.33- ☑
  lead-induced M10.10
    ankle M10.17- ☑
    elbow M10.12- ☑
    foot joint M10.17- ☑
    hand joint M10.14- ☑
    hip M10.15- ☑
    knee M10.16- ☑
    multiple site M10.19
    shoulder M10.11- ☑
    vertebrae M10.18
    wrist M10.13- ☑
  primary — *see* Gout, idiopathic
  saturnine — *see* Gout, lead-induced
  secondary NEC M10.40
    ankle M10.47- ☑
    elbow M10.42- ☑
    foot joint M10.47- ☑
    hand joint M10.44- ☑
    hip M10.45- ☑
    knee M10.46- ☑
    multiple site M10.49
    shoulder M10.41- ☑
    vertebrae M10.48
    wrist M10.43- ☑
  syphilitic (*see also* subcategory M14.8-) A52.77
  tophi — *see* Gout, chronic
Gower's
  muscular dystrophy G71.01
  syndrome (vasovagal attack) R55
Gradenigo's syndrome — *see* Otitis, media, suppurative, acute
Graefe's disease — *see* Strabismus, paralytic, ophthalmoplegia, progressive
Graft-versus-host disease D89.813
  acute D89.810
  acute on chronic D89.812
  chronic D89.811
Grain mite (itch) B88.0
Grainhandler's disease or lung J67.8
Grand mal — *see* Epilepsy, generalized, specified NEC
Grand multipara status only (not pregnant) Z64.1
  pregnant — *see* Pregnancy, complicated by, grand multiparity
Granite worker's lung J62.8
Granular (*see also* condition)
  inflammation, pharynx J31.2
  kidney (contracting) — *see* Sclerosis, renal
  liver K74.69
Granulation tissue (abnormal) (excessive) L92.9
  postmastoidectomy cavity — *see* Complications, postmastoidectomy, granulation
Granulocytopenia (primary) (malignant) — *see* Agranulocytosis
Granuloma L92.9
  abdomen K66.8
    from residual foreign body L92.3
    pyogenicum L98.0
  actinic L57.5
  annulare (perforating) L92.0
  apical K04.5
  aural — *see* Otitis, externa, specified NEC
  beryllium (skin) L92.3
  bone
    eosinophilic C96.6
    from residual foreign body — *see* Osteomyelitis, specified type NEC
    lung C96.6
  brain (any site) G06.0
    schistosomiasis B65.9 [G07]
  canaliculus lacrimalis — *see* Granuloma, lacrimal
  candidal (cutaneous) B37.2
  cerebral (any site) G06.0
  coccidioidal (primary) (progressive) B38.7
    lung B38.1
    meninges B38.4
  colon K63.89
  conjunctiva H11.22- ☑
  dental K04.5
  ear, middle — *see* Cholesteatoma
  eosinophilic C96.6
    bone C96.6

Granuloma — *continued*
  eosinophilic — *continued*
    lung C96.6
    oral mucosa K13.4
    skin L92.2
  eyelid H01.8
  facial (e) L92.2
  foreign body (in soft tissue) NEC M60.20
    ankle M60.27- ☑
    foot M60.27- ☑
    forearm M60.23- ☑
    hand M60.24- ☑
    in operation wound — *see* Foreign body, accidentally left during a procedure
    lower leg M60.26- ☑
    pelvic region M60.25- ☑
    shoulder region M60.21- ☑
    skin L92.3
    specified site NEC M60.28
    subcutaneous tissue L92.3
    thigh M60.25- ☑
    upper arm M60.22- ☑
  gangraenescens M31.2
  genito-inguinale A58
  giant cell (central) (reparative) (jaw) M27.1
    gingiva (peripheral) K06.8
  gland (lymph) I88.8
  hepatic NEC K75.3
    in (due to)
      berylliosis J63.2 [K77]
      sarcoidosis D86.89
  Hodgkin C81.9 ☑
  ileum K63.89
  infectious B99.9
    specified NEC B99.8
  inguinale (Donovan) (venereal) A58
  intestine NEC K63.89
  intracranial (any site) G06.0
  intraspinal (any part) G06.1
  iridocyclitis — *see* Iridocyclitis, chronic
  jaw (bone) (central) M27.1
    reparative giant cell M27.1
  kidney (*see also* Infection, kidney) N15.8
  lacrimal H04.81- ☑
  larynx J38.7
  lethal midline (faciale(e)) M31.2
  liver NEC — *see* Granuloma, hepatic
  lung (infectious) (*see also* Fibrosis, lung)
    coccidioidal B38.1
    eosinophilic C96.6
  Majocchi's B35.8
  malignant (facial(e)) M31.2
  mandible (central) M27.1
  midline (lethal) M31.2
  monilial (cutaneous) B37.2
  nasal sinus — *see* Sinusitis
  operation wound T81.89 ☑
    foreign body — *see* Foreign body, accidentally left during a procedure
    stitch T81.89 ☑
    talc — *see* Foreign body, accidentally left during a procedure
  oral mucosa K13.4
  orbit, orbital H05.11- ☑
  paracoccidioidal B41.8
  penis, venereal A58
  periapical K04.5
  peritoneum K66.8
    due to ova of helminths NOS (*see also* Helminthiasis) B83.9 [K67]
  postmastoidectomy cavity — *see* Complications, postmastoidectomy, recurrent cholesteatoma
  prostate N42.89
  pudendi (ulcerating) A58
  pulp, internal (tooth) K03.3
  pyogenic, pyogenicum (of) (skin) L98.0
    gingiva K06.8
    maxillary alveolar ridge K04.5
    oral mucosa K13.4
  rectum K62.89
  reticulohistiocytic D76.3
  rubrum nasi L74.8
  Schistosoma — *see* Schistosomiasis
  septic (skin) L98.0
  silica (skin) L92.3
  sinus (accessory) (infective) (nasal) — *see* Sinusitis
  skin L92.9
    from residual foreign body L92.3

Granuloma — *continued*
  skin — *continued*
    pyogenicum L98.0
  spine
    syphilitic (epidural) A52.19
    tuberculous A18.01
  stitch (postoperative) T81.89 ☑
  suppurative (skin) L98.0
  swimming pool A31.1
  talc (*see also* Granuloma, foreign body)
    in operation wound — *see* Foreign body, accidentally left during a procedure
  telangiectaticum (skin) L98.0
  tracheostomy J95.09
  trichophyticum B35.8
  tropicum A66.4
  umbilical P83.81
  umbilicus P83.81
  urethra N36.8
  uveitis — *see* Iridocyclitis, chronic
  vagina A58
  venereum A58
  vocal cord J38.3
Granulomatosis L92.9
  lymphoid C83.8- ☑
  miliary (listerial) A32.89
  necrotizing, respiratory M31.30
  progressive septic D71
  specified NEC L92.8
  Wegener's M31.30
    with renal involvement M31.31
Granulomatous tissue (abnormal) (excessive) L92.9
Granulosis rubra nasi L74.8
Graphite fibrosis (of lung) J63.3
Graphospasm F48.8
  organic G25.89
Grating scapula M89.8X1
Gravel (urinary) — *see* Calculus, urinary
Graves' disease — *see* Hyperthyroidism, with, goiter
Gravis — *see* condition
Grawitz tumor C64.- ☑
Gray syndrome (newborn) P93.0
Grayness, hair (premature) L67.1
  congenital Q84.2
Green sickness D50.8
Greenfield's disease
  meaning
    concentric sclerosis (encephalitis periaxialis concentrica) G37.5
    metachromatic leukodystrophy E75.25
Greenstick fracture — *code as* Fracture, by site
Grey syndrome (newborn) P93.0
Grief F43.21
  prolonged F43.29
  reaction (*see also* Disorder, adjustment) F43.20
Griesinger's disease B76.9
Grinder's lung or pneumoconiosis J62.8
Grinding, teeth
  psychogenic F45.8
  sleep related G47.63
Grip
  Dabney's B33.0
  devil's B33.0
Grippe, grippal (*see also* Influenza)
  Balkan A78
  summer, of Italy A93.1
Grisel's disease M43.6
Groin — *see* condition
Grooved tongue K14.5
Grover's disease or syndrome L11.1
Growing pains, children R29.898
Growth (fungoid) (neoplastic) (new) (*see also* Neoplasm)
  adenoid (vegetative) J35.8
  benign — *see* Neoplasm, benign, by site
  malignant — *see* Neoplasm, malignant, by site
  rapid, childhood Z00.2
  secondary — *see* Neoplasm, secondary, by site
Gruby's disease B35.0
Gubler-Millard paralysis or syndrome G46.3
Guerin-Stern syndrome Q74.3
Guidance, insufficient anterior (occlusal) M26.54
Guillain-Barré disease or syndrome G61.0
  sequelae G65.0
Guinea worms (infection) (infestation) B72
Guinon's disease (motor-verbal tic) F95.2
Gull's disease E03.4

Gum — see condition
Gumboil K04.7
  with sinus K04.6
Gumma (syphilitic) A52.79
  artery A52.09
    cerebral A52.04
  bone A52.77
    of yaws (late) A66.6
  brain A52.19
  cauda equina A52.19
  central nervous system A52.3
  ciliary body A52.71
  congenital A50.59
  eyelid A52.71
  heart A52.06
  intracranial A52.19
  iris A52.71
  kidney A52.75
  larynx A52.73
  leptomeninges A52.19
  liver A52.74
  meninges A52.19
  myocardium A52.06
  nasopharynx A52.73
  neurosyphilitic A52.3
  nose A52.73
  orbit A52.71
  palate (soft) A52.79
  penis A52.76
  pericardium A52.06
  pharynx A52.73
  pituitary A52.79
  scrofulous (tuberculous) A18.4
  skin A52.79
  specified site NEC A52.79
  spinal cord A52.19
  tongue A52.79
  tonsil A52.73
  trachea A52.73
  tuberculous A18.4
  ulcerative due to yaws A66.4
  ureter A52.75
  yaws A66.4
    bone A66.6
Gunn's syndrome Q07.8
Gunshot wound (see also Wound, open)
  fracture — code as Fracture, by site
  internal organs — see Injury, by site
Gynandrism Q56.0
Gynandroblastoma
  specified site — see Neoplasm, uncertain behavior, by
    site
  unspecified site
    female D39.10
    male D40.10
Gynecological examination (periodic) (routine) Z01.419
  with abnormal findings Z01.411
Gynecomastia N62
Gynephobia F40.291
Gyrate scalp Q82.8

H

H (Hartnup's) **disease** E72.02
Haas' disease or osteochondrosis (juvenile) (head of
  humerus) — see Osteochondrosis, juvenile, humerus
Habit, habituation
  bad sleep Z72.821
  chorea F95.8
  disturbance, child F98.9
  drug — see Dependence, drug
  irregular sleep Z72.821
  laxative F55.2
  spasm — see Tic
  tic — see Tic
Haemophilus (H.) **influenzae, as cause of disease**
  classified elsewhere B96.3
Haff disease — see Poisoning, mercury
Hageman's factor defect, deficiency or disease D68.2
Haglund's disease or osteochondrosis (juvenile) (os
  tibiale externum) — see Osteochondrosis, juvenile,
  tarsus
Hailey-Hailey disease Q82.8
Hair (see also condition)
  plucking F63.3
    in stereotyped movement disorder F98.4
  tourniquet syndrome (see also Constriction, external,
    by site)

Hair — continued
  tourniquet syndrome (see also Constriction, external,
    by site) — continued
    finger S60.44- ☑
    penis S30.842 ☑
    thumb S60.34- ☑
    toe S90.44- ☑
Hairball in stomach T18.2 ☑
Hair-pulling, pathological (compulsive) F63.3
Hairy black tongue K14.3
Half vertebra Q76.49
Halitosis R19.6
Hallerman-Streiff syndrome Q87.0
Hallervorden-Spatz disease G23.0
Hallopeau's acrodermatitis or disease L40.2
Hallucination R44.3
  auditory R44.0
  gustatory R44.2
  olfactory R44.2
  specified NEC R44.2
  tactile R44.2
  visual R44.1
Hallucinosis (chronic) F28
  alcoholic (acute) F10.951
    in
      abuse F10.151
      dependence F10.251
  drug-induced F19.951
    cannabis F12.951
    cocaine F14.951
    hallucinogen F16.151
    in
      abuse F19.151
        cannabis F12.151
        cocaine F14.151
        hallucinogen F16.151
        inhalant F18.151
        opioid F11.151
        sedative, anxiolytic or hypnotic F13.151
        stimulant NEC F15.151
      dependence F19.251
        cannabis F12.251
        cocaine F14.251
        hallucinogen F16.251
        inhalant F18.251
        opioid F11.251 ·
        sedative, anxiolytic or hypnotic F13.251
        stimulant NEC F15.251
    inhalant F18.951
    opioid F11.951
    sedative, anxiolytic or hypnotic F13.951
    stimulant NEC F15.951
  organic F06.0
Hallux
  deformity (acquired) NEC M20.5X- ☑
  limitus M20.5X- ☑
  malleus (acquired) NEC M20.3- ☑
  rigidus (acquired) M20.2- ☑
    congenital Q74.2
    sequelae (late effect) of rickets E64.3
  valgus (acquired) M20.1- ☑
    congenital Q66.6
  varus (acquired) M20.3- ☑
    congenital Q66.3
Halo, visual H53.19
Hamartoma, hamartoblastoma Q85.9
  epithelial (gingival), odontogenic, central or peripheral
    — see Cyst, calcifying odontogenic
Hamartosis Q85.9
Hamman-Rich syndrome J84.114
Hammer toe (acquired) NEC (see also Deformity, toe,
  hammer toe)
  congenital Q66.89
  sequelae (late effect) of rickets E64.3
Hand — see condition
Hand-foot syndrome L27.1
Handicap, handicapped
  educational Z55.9
    specified NEC Z55.8
Hand-Schüller-Christian disease or syndrome C96.5
Hanging (asphyxia) (strangulation) (suffocation) — see
  Asphyxia, traumatic, due to mechanical threat
Hangnail (see also Cellulitis, digit)
  with lymphangitis — see Lymphangitis, acute, digit
Hangover (alcohol) F10.129
Hanhart's syndrome Q87.0
Hanot-Chauffard (-Troisier) **syndrome** E83.19

Hanot's cirrhosis or disease K74.3
Hansen's disease — see Leprosy
Hantaan virus disease (Korean hemorrhagic fever) A98.5
Hantavirus disease (with renal manifestations) (Dobrava)
  (Puumala) (Seoul) A98.5
  with pulmonary manifestations (Andes) (Bayou)
    (Bermejo) (Black Creek Canal) (Choclo) (Juquitiba)
    (Laguna negra) (Lechiguanas) (New York) (Oran)
    (Sin nombre) B33.4
Happy puppet syndrome Q93.51
Harada's disease or syndrome H30.81- ☑
Hardening
  artery — see Arteriosclerosis
  brain G93.89
Harelip (complete) (incomplete) — see Cleft, lip
Harlequin (newborn) Q80.4
Harley's disease D59.6
Harmful use (of)
  alcohol F10.10
  anxiolytics — see Abuse, drug, sedative
  cannabinoids — see Abuse, drug, cannabis
  cocaine — see Abuse, drug, cocaine
  drug — see Abuse, drug
  hallucinogens — see Abuse, drug, hallucinogen
  hypnotics — see Abuse, drug, sedative
  opioids — see Abuse, drug, opioid
  PCP (phencyclidine) — see Abuse, drug, hallucinogen
  sedatives — see Abuse, drug, sedative
  stimulants NEC — see Abuse, drug, stimulant
Harris' lines — see Arrest, epiphyseal
Hartnup's disease E72.02
Harvester's lung J67.0
Harvesting ovum for in vitro fertilization Z31.83
Hashimoto's disease or thyroiditis E06.3
Hashitoxicosis (transient) E06.3
Hassal-Henle bodies or warts (cornea) H18.49
Haut mal — see Epilepsy, generalized, specified NEC
Haverhill fever A25.1
Hay fever (see also Fever, hay) J30.1
Hayem-Widal syndrome D59.8
Haygarth's nodes M15.8
Haymaker's lung J67.0
Hb (abnormal)
  Bart's disease D56.0
  disease — see Disease, hemoglobin
  trait — see Trait
Head — see condition
Headache R51
  allergic NEC G44.89
  associated with sexual activity G44.82
  chronic daily R51
  cluster G44.009
    chronic G44.029
      intractable G44.021
      not intractable G44.029
    episodic G44.019
      intractable G44.011
      not intractable G44.019
    intractable G44.001
    not intractable G44.009
  cough (primary) G44.83
  daily chronic R51
  drug-induced NEC G44.40
    intractable G44.41
    not intractable G44.40
  exertional (primary) G44.84
  histamine G44.009
    intractable G44.001
    not intractable G44.009
  hypnic G44.81
  lumbar puncture G97.1
  medication overuse G44.40
    intractable G44.41
    not intractable G44.40
  menstrual — see Migraine, menstrual
  migraine (type) (see also Migraine) G43.909
  nasal septum R51
  neuralgiform, short lasting unilateral, with conjunctival
    injection and tearing (SUNCT) G44.059
    intractable G44.051
    not intractable G44.059
  new daily persistent (NDPH) G44.52
  orgasmic G44.82
  periodic syndromes in adults and children G43.C0 (fol-
    lowing G43.7)
    with refractory migraine G43.C1 (following G43.7)
    intractable G43.C1 (following G43.7)

☑ **Additional Character Required** — Refer to the Tabular List for Character Selection   ⓥ **Subterms under main terms may continue to next column or page**

Headache — *continued*
  periodic syndromes in adults and children — *continued*
    not intractable G43.C0 (*following* G43.7)
    without refractory migraine G43.C0 (*following* G43.7)
  postspinal puncture G97.1
  post-traumatic G44.309
    acute G44.319
      intractable G44.311
      not intractable G44.319
    chronic G44.329
      intractable G44.321
      not intractable G44.329
    intractable G44.301
    not intractable G44.309
  pre-menstrual — *see* Migraine, menstrual
  preorgasmic G44.82
  primary
    cough G44.83
    exertional G44.84
    stabbing G44.85
    thunderclap G44.53
  rebound G44.40
    intractable G44.41
    not intractable G44.40
  short lasting unilateral neuralgiform, with conjunctival
    injection and tearing (SUNCT) G44.059
    intractable G44.051
    not intractable G44.059
  specified syndrome NEC G44.89
  spinal and epidural anesthesia - induced T88.59 ☑
    in labor and delivery O74.5
    in pregnancy O29.4- ☑
    postpartum, puerperal O89.4
  spinal fluid loss (from puncture) G97.1
  stabbing (primary) G44.85
  tension (-type) G44.209
    chronic G44.229
      intractable G44.221
      not intractable G44.229
    episodic G44.219
      intractable G44.211
      not intractable G44.219
    intractable G44.201
    not intractable G44.209
  thunderclap (primary) G44.53
  vascular NEC G44.1
Healthy
  infant
    accompanying sick mother Z76.3
    receiving care Z76.2
  person accompanying sick person Z76.3
Hearing examination Z01.10
  with abnormal findings NEC Z01.118
  following failed hearing screening Z01.110
  for hearing conservation and treatment Z01.12
  infant or child (over 28 days old) Z00.129
    with abnormal findings Z00.121
Heart — *see* condition
Heart beat
  abnormality R00.9
    specified NEC R00.8
  awareness R00.2
  rapid R00.0
  slow R00.1
Heartburn R12
  psychogenic F45.8
Heartland virus disease A93.8
Heat (effects) T67.9 ☑
  apoplexy T67.0 ☑
  burn (*see also* Burn) L55.9
  collapse T67.1 ☑
  cramps T67.2 ☑
  dermatitis or eczema L59.0
  edema T67.7 ☑
  erythema — *code by site under* Burn, first degree
  excessive T67.9 ☑
    specified effect NEC T67.8 ☑
  exhaustion T67.5 ☑
    anhydrotic T67.3 ☑
    due to
      salt (and water) depletion T67.4 ☑
      water depletion T67.3 ☑
        with salt depletion T67.4 ☑
  fatigue (transient) T67.6 ☑
  fever T67.0 ☑
  hyperpyrexia T67.0 ☑
  prickly L74.0

Heat — *continued*
  prostration — *see* Heat, exhaustion
  pyrexia T67.0 ☑
  rash L74.0
  specified effect NEC T67.8 ☑
  stroke T67.0 ☑
  sunburn — *see* Sunburn
  syncope T67.1 ☑
Heavy-for-dates NEC (infant) (4000g to 4499g) P08.1
  exceptionally (4500g or more) P08.0
Hebephrenia, hebephrenic (schizophrenia) F20.1
Heberden's disease or nodes (with arthropathy) M15.1
Hebra's
  pityriasis L26
  prurigo L28.2
Heel — *see* condition
Heerfordt's disease D86.89
Hegglin's anomaly or syndrome D72.0
Heilmeyer-Schoner disease D45
Heine-Medin disease A80.9
Heinz body anemia, congenital D58.2
Heliophobia F40.228
Heller's disease or syndrome F84.3
HELLP syndrome (hemolysis, elevated liver enzymes and
    low platelet count) O14.2- ☑
  complicating
    childbirth O14.24
    puerperium O14.25
Helminthiasis (*see also* Infestation, helminth)
  Ancylostoma B76.0
  intestinal B82.0
    mixed types (types classifiable to more than one of
      the titles B65.0-B81.3 and B81.8) B81.4
    specified type NEC B81.8
  mixed types (intestinal) (types classifiable to more than
    one of the titles B65.0-B81.3 and B81.8) B81.4
  Necator (americanus) B76.1
  specified type NEC B83.8
Heloma L84
Hemangioblastoma — *see* Neoplasm, connective tissue,
    uncertain behavior
  malignant — *see* Neoplasm, connective tissue, malig-
    nant
Hemangioendothelioma (*see also* Neoplasm, uncertain
    behavior, by site)
  benign D18.00
    intra-abdominal D18.03
    intracranial D18.02
    skin D18.01
    specified site NEC D18.09
  bone (diffuse) — *see* Neoplasm, bone, malignant
  epithelioid (*see also* Neoplasm, uncertain behavior, by
    site)
    malignant — *see* Neoplasm, malignant, by site
  malignant — *see* Neoplasm, connective tissue, malig-
    nant
Hemangiofibroma — *see* Neoplasm, benign, by site
Hemangiolipoma — *see* Lipoma
Hemangioma D18.00
  arteriovenous D18.00
    intra-abdominal D18.03
    intracranial D18.02
    skin D18.01
    specified site NEC D18.09
  capillary D18.00
    intra-abdominal D18.03
    intracranial D18.02
    skin D18.01
    specified site NEC D18.09
  cavernous D18.00
    intra-abdominal D18.03
    intracranial D18.02
    skin D18.01
    specified site NEC D18.09
  epithelioid D18.00
    intra-abdominal D18.03
    intracranial D18.02
    skin D18.01
    specified site NEC D18.09
  histiocytoid D18.00
    intra-abdominal D18.03
    intracranial D18.02
    skin D18.01
    specified site NEC D18.09
  infantile D18.00
    intra-abdominal D18.03
    intracranial D18.02
    skin D18.01

Hemangioma — *continued*
  infantile — *continued*
    specified site NEC D18.09
  intra-abdominal D18.03
  intracranial D18.02
  intramuscular D18.00
    intra-abdominal D18.03
    intracranial D18.02
    skin D18.01
    specified site NEC D18.09
  intrathoracic structures D18.09
  juvenile D18.00
  malignant — *see* Neoplasm,connective tissue, malig-
    nant
  plexiform D18.00
    intra-abdominal D18.03
    intracranial D18.02
    skin D18.01
    specified site NEC D18.09
  racemose D18.00
    intra-abdominal D18.03
    intracranial D18.02
    skin D18.01
    specified site NEC D18.09
  sclerosing — *see* Neoplasm, skin, benign
  simplex D18.00
    intra-abdominal D18.03
    intracranial D18.02
    skin D18.01
    specified site NEC D18.09
  skin D18.01
  specified site NEC D18.09
  venous D18.00
    intra-abdominal D18.03
    intracranial D18.02
    skin D18.01
    specified site NEC D18.09
  verrucous keratotic D18.00
    intra-abdominal D18.03
    intracranial D18.02
    skin D18.01
    specified site NEC D18.09
Hemangiomatosis (systemic) I78.8
  involving single site — *see* Hemangioma
Hemangiopericytoma (*see also* Neoplasm, connective
    tissue, uncertain behavior)
  benign — *see* Neoplasm, connective tissue, benign
  malignant — *see* Neoplasm, connective tissue, malig-
    nant
Hemangiosarcoma — *see* Neoplasm, connective tissue,
    malignant
Hemarthrosis (nontraumatic) M25.00
  ankle M25.07- ☑
  elbow M25.02- ☑
  foot joint M25.07- ☑
  hand joint M25.04- ☑
  hip M25.05- ☑
  in hemophilic arthropathy — *see* Arthropathy,
    hemophilic
  knee M25.06- ☑
  shoulder M25.01- ☑
  specified joint NEC M25.08
  traumatic — *see* Sprain, by site
  vertebrae M25.08
  wrist M25.03- ☑
Hematemesis K92.0
  with ulcer — *code by site under* Ulcer, with hemorrhage
    K27.4
  newborn, neonatal P54.0
    due to swallowed maternal blood P78.2
Hematidrosis L74.8
Hematinuria (*see also* Hemoglobinuria)
  malarial B50.8
Hematobilia K83.8
Hematocele
  female NEC N94.89
    with ectopic pregnancy O00.90
      with intrauterine pregnancy O00.91
    ovary N83.8
  male N50.1
Hematochezia (*see also* Melena) K92.1
Hematochyluria (*see also* Infestation, filarial)
  schistosomiasis (bilharziasis) B65.0
Hematocolpos (with hematometra or hematosalpinx)
    N89.7
Hematocornea — *see* Pigmentation, cornea, stromal
Hematogenous — *see* condition

Hematoma (traumatic) (skin surface intact) (*see also* Contusion)
  with
    injury of internal organs — *see* Injury, by site
    open wound — *see* Wound, open
  amputation stump (surgical) (late) T87.89
  aorta, dissecting I71.00
    abdominal I71.02
    thoracic I71.01
    thoracoabdominal I71.03
  aortic intramural — *see* Dissection, aorta
  arterial (complicating trauma) — *see* Injury, blood vessel, by site
  auricle — *see* Contusion, ear
    nontraumatic — *see* Disorder, pinna, hematoma
  birth injury NEC P15.8
  brain (traumatic)
    with
      cerebral laceration or contusion (diffuse) — *see* Injury, intracranial, diffuse
      focal — *see* Injury, intracranial, focal
    cerebellar, traumatic S06.37- ☑
    intracerebral, traumatic — *see* Injury, intracranial, intracerebral hemorrhage
    newborn NEC P52.4
      birth injury P10.1
    nontraumatic — *see* Hemorrhage, intracranial
    subarachnoid, arachnoid, traumatic — *see* Injury, intracranial, subarachnoid hemorrhage
    subdural, traumatic — *see* Injury, intracranial, subdural hemorrhage
  breast (nontraumatic) N64.89
  broad ligament (nontraumatic) N83.7
    traumatic S37.892 ☑
  cerebellar, traumatic S06.37- ☑
  cerebral — *see* Hematoma, brain
  cerebrum S06.36- ☑
    left S06.35- ☑
    right S06.34- ☑
  cesarean delivery wound O90.2
  complicating delivery (perineal) (pelvic) (vagina) (vulva) O71.7
  corpus cavernosum (nontraumatic) N48.89
  epididymis (nontraumatic) N50.1
  epidural (traumatic) — *see* Injury, intracranial, epidural hemorrhage
    spinal — *see* Injury, spinal cord, by region
  episiotomy O90.2
  face, birth injury P15.4
  genital organ NEC (nontraumatic)
    female (nonobstetric) N94.89
      traumatic S30.202 ☑
    male N50.1
      traumatic S30.201 ☑
  internal organs — *see* Injury, by site
  intracerebral, traumatic — *see* Injury, intracranial, intracerebral hemorrhage
  intraoperative — *see* Complications, intraoperative, hemorrhage
  labia (nontraumatic) (nonobstetric) N90.89
  liver (subcapsular) (nontraumatic) K76.89
    birth injury P15.0
  mediastinum — *see* Injury, intrathoracic
  mesosalpinx (nontraumatic) N83.7
    traumatic S37.898 ☑
  muscle — code by site under Contusion
  nontraumatic
    muscle M79.81
    soft tissue M79.81
  obstetrical surgical wound O90.2
  orbit, orbital (nontraumatic) (*see also* Hemorrhage, orbit)
    traumatic — *see* Contusion, orbit
  pelvis (female) (nontraumatic) (nonobstetric) N94.89
    obstetric O71.7
    traumatic — *see* Injury, by site
  penis (nontraumatic) N48.89
    birth injury P15.5
  perianal (nontraumatic) K64.5
  perineal S30.23 ☑
    complicating delivery O71.7
  perirenal — *see* Injury, kidney
  pinna — *see* Contusion, ear
    nontraumatic — *see* Disorder, pinna, hematoma
  placenta O43.89-
  postoperative (postprocedural) — *see* Complication, postprocedural, hematoma

Hematoma — *continued*
  retroperitoneal (nontraumatic) K66.1
    traumatic S36.892 ☑
  scrotum, superficial S30.22 ☑
    birth injury P15.5
  seminal vesicle (nontraumatic) N50.1
    traumatic S37.892 ☑
  spermatic cord (traumatic) S37.892 ☑
    nontraumatic N50.1
  spinal (cord) (meninges) (*see also* Injury, spinal cord, by region)
    newborn (birth injury) P11.5
  spleen D73.5
    intraoperative — *see* Complications, intraoperative, hemorrhage, spleen
    postprocedural (postoperative) — *see* Complications, postprocedural, hemorrhage, spleen
  sternocleidomastoid, birth injury P15.2
  sternomastoid, birth injury P15.2
  subarachnoid (traumatic) — *see* Injury, intracranial, subarachnoid hemorrhage
    newborn (nontraumatic) P52.5
      due to birth injury P10.3
    nontraumatic — *see* Hemorrhage, intracranial, subarachnoid
  subdural (traumatic) — *see* Injury, intracranial, subdural hemorrhage
    newborn (localized) P52.8
      birth injury P10.0
    nontraumatic — *see* Hemorrhage, intracranial, subdural
  superficial, newborn P54.5
  testis (nontraumatic) N50.1
    birth injury P15.5
  tunica vaginalis (nontraumatic) N50.1
  umbilical cord, complicating delivery O69.5 ☑
  uterine ligament (broad) (nontraumatic) N83.7
    traumatic S37.892 ☑
  vagina (ruptured) (nontraumatic) N89.8
    complicating delivery O71.7
  vas deferens (nontraumatic) N50.1
    traumatic S37.892 ☑
  vitreous — *see* Hemorrhage, vitreous
  vulva (nontraumatic) (nonobstetric) N90.89
    complicating delivery O71.7
    newborn (birth injury) P15.5
Hematometra N85.7
  with hematocolpos N89.7
Hematomyelia (central) G95.19
  newborn (birth injury) P11.5
  traumatic T14.8 ☑
Hematomyelitis G04.90
Hematoperitoneum — *see* Hemoperitoneum
Hematophobia F40.230
Hematopneumothorax (see Hemothorax)
Hematopoiesis, cyclic D70.4
Hematoporphyria — *see* Porphyria
Hematorachis, hematorrhachis G95.19
  newborn (birth injury) P11.5
Hematosalpinx N83.6
  with
    hematocolpos N89.7
    hematometra N85.7
      with hematocolpos N89.7
  infectional — *see* Salpingitis
Hematospermia R36.1
Hematothorax (see Hemothorax)
Hematuria R31.9
  benign (familial) (of childhood) (*see also* Hematuria, idiopathic)
    essential microscopic R31.1
  due to sulphonamide, sulfonamide — *see* Table of Drugs and Chemicals, by drug
  endemic (*see also* Schistosomiasis) B65.0
  gross R31.0
  idiopathic N02.9
    with glomerular lesion
      crescentic (diffuse) glomerulonephritis N02.7
      dense deposit disease N02.6
      endocapillary proliferative glomerulonephritis N02.4
      focal and segmental hyalinosis or sclerosis N02.1
      membranoproliferative (diffuse) N02.5
      membranous (diffuse) N02.2
      mesangial proliferative (diffuse) N02.3
      mesangiocapillary (diffuse) N02.5
      minor abnormality N02.0
      proliferative NEC N02.8

Hematuria — *continued*
  idiopathic — *continued*
    with glomerular lesion — *continued*
      specified pathology NEC N02.8
  intermittent — *see* Hematuria, idiopathic
  malarial B50.8
  microscopic NEC (with symptoms) R31.29
    asymptomatic R31.21
    benign essential R31.1
  paroxysmal (*see also* Hematuria, idiopathic)
    nocturnal D59.5
  persistent — *see* Hematuria, idiopathic
  recurrent — *see* Hematuria, idiopathic
  tropical (*see also* Schistosomiasis) B65.0
  tuberculous A18.13
Hemeralopia (day blindness) H53.11
  vitamin A deficiency E50.5
Hemi-akinesia R41.4
Hemianalgesia R20.0
Hemianencephaly Q00.0
Hemianesthesia R20.0
Hemianopia, hemianopsia (heteronymous) H53.47
  homonymous H53.46- ☑
  syphilitic A52.71
Hemiathetosis R25.8
Hemiatrophy R68.89
  cerebellar G31.9
  face, facial, progressive (Romberg) G51.8
  tongue K14.8
Hemiballism (us) G25.5
Hemicardia Q24.8
Hemicephalus, hemicephaly Q00.0
Hemichorea G25.5
Hemicolitis, left — *see* Colitis, left sided
Hemicrania
  congenital malformation Q00.0
  continua G44.51
  meaning migraine (*see also* Migraine) G43.909
  paroxysmal G44.039
    chronic G44.049
      intractable G44.041
      not intractable G44.049
    episodic G44.039
      intractable G44.031
      not intractable G44.039
    intractable G44.031
    not intractable G44.039
Hemidystrophy — *see* Hemiatrophy
Hemiectromelia Q73.8
Hemihypalgesia R20.8
Hemihypesthesia R20.1
Hemi-inattention R41.4
Hemimelia Q73.8
  lower limb — *see* Defect, reduction, lower limb, specified type NEC
  upper limb — *see* Defect, reduction, upper limb, specified type NEC
Hemiparalysis — *see* Hemiplegia
Hemiparesis — *see* Hemiplegia
Hemiparesthesia R20.2
Hemiparkinsonism G20
Hemiplegia G81.9- ☑
  alternans facialis G83.89
  ascending NEC G81.90
    spinal G95.89
  congenital (cerebral) G80.8
    spastic G80.2
  embolic (current episode) I63.4- ☑
  flaccid G81.0- ☑
  following
    cerebrovascular disease I69.959
      cerebral infarction I69.35- ☑
      intracerebral hemorrhage I69.15- ☑
      nontraumatic intracranial hemorrhage NEC I69.25- ☑
      specified disease NEC I69.85- ☑
      stroke NOS I69.35- ☑
      subarachnoid hemorrhage I69.05- ☑
  hysterical F44.4
  newborn NEC P91.88
    birth injury P11.9
  spastic G81.1- ☑
    congenital G80.2
  thrombotic (current episode) I63.3- ☑
Hemisection, spinal cord — *see* Injury, spinal cord, by region
Hemispasm (facial) R25.2

Hemisporosis B48.8
Hemitremor R25.1
Hemivertebra Q76.49
  failure of segmentation with scoliosis Q76.3
  fusion with scoliosis Q76.3
Hemochromatosis E83.119
  with refractory anemia D46.1
  due to repeated red blood cell transfusion E83.111
  hereditary (primary) E83.110
  neonatal P78.84
  primary E83.110
  specified NEC E83.118
Hemoglobin (see also condition)
  abnormal (disease) — see Disease, hemoglobin
  AS genotype D57.3
  Constant Spring D58.2
  E-beta thalassemia D56.5
  fetal, hereditary persistence (HPFH) D56.4
  H Constant Spring D56.0
  low NOS D64.9
  S (Hb S), heterozygous D57.3
Hemoglobinemia D59.9
  due to blood transfusion T80.89 ☑
  paroxysmal D59.6
    nocturnal D59.5
Hemoglobinopathy (mixed) D58.2
  with thalassemia D56.8
  sickle-cell D57.1
    with thalassemia D57.40
      with crisis (vasoocclusive pain) D57.419
        with
          acute chest syndrome D57.411
          splenic sequestration D57.412
      without crisis D57.40
Hemoglobinuria R82.3
  with anemia, hemolytic, acquired (chronic) NEC D59.6
  cold (agglutinin) (paroxysmal) (with Raynaud's syn-
    drome) D59.6
  due to exertion or hemolysis NEC D59.6
  intermittent D59.6
  malarial B50.8
  march D59.6
  nocturnal (paroxysmal) D59.5
  paroxysmal (cold) D59.6
    nocturnal D59.5
Hemolymphangioma D18.1
Hemolysis
  intravascular
    with
      abortion — see Abortion, by type, complicated
        by, hemorrhage
      ectopic or molar pregnancy O08.1
      hemorrhage
        antepartum — see Hemorrhage, antepartum,
          with coagulation defect
        intrapartum (see also Hemorrhage, complicat-
          ing, delivery) O67.0
    postpartum O72.3
  neonatal (excessive) P58.9
    specified NEC P58.8
Hemolytic — see condition
Hemopericardium I31.2
  following acute myocardial infarction (current compli-
    cation) I23.0
  newborn P54.8
  traumatic — see Injury, heart, with hemopericardium
Hemoperitoneum K66.1
  infectional K65.9
  traumatic S36.899 ☑
    with open wound — see Wound, open, with pene-
      tration into peritoneal cavity
Hemophilia (classical) (familial) (hereditary) D66
  A D66
  acquired D68.311
  autoimmune D68.311
  B D67
  C D68.1
  calcipriva (see also Defect, coagulation) D68.4
  nonfamilial (see also Defect, coagulation) D68.4
  secondary D68.311
  vascular D68.0
Hemophthalmos H44.81- ☑
Hemopneumothorax (see also Hemothorax)
  traumatic S27.2 ☑
Hemoptysis R04.2
  newborn P26.9
  tuberculous — see Tuberculosis, pulmonary
Hemorrhage, hemorrhagic (concealed) R58

Hemorrhage, hemorrhagic — continued
  abdomen R58
  accidental antepartum — see Hemorrhage, antepartum
  acute idiopathic pulmonary, in infants R04.81
  adenoid J35.8
  adrenal (capsule) (gland) E27.49
    medulla E27.8
    newborn P54.4
  after delivery — see Hemorrhage, postpartum
  alveolar
    lung, newborn P26.8
    process K08.89
  alveolus K08.89
  amputation stump (surgical) T87.89
  anemia (chronic) D50.0
    acute D62
  antepartum (with) O46.90
    with coagulation defect O46.00- ☑
      afibrinogenemia O46.01- ☑
      disseminated intravascular coagulation
        O46.02- ☑
      hypofibrinogenemia O46.01- ☑
      specified defect NEC O46.09- ☑
    before 20 weeks gestation O20.9
      specified type NEC O20.8
      threatened abortion O20.0
    due to
      abruptio placenta (see also Abruptio placentae)
        O45.9- ☑
      leiomyoma, uterus — see Hemorrhage, antepar-
        tum, specified cause NEC
      placenta previa O44.1- ☑
    specified cause NEC — see subcategory O46.8X- ☑
  anus (sphincter) K62.5
  apoplexy (stroke) — see Hemorrhage, intracranial, in-
    tracerebral
  arachnoid — see Hemorrhage, intracranial, subarach-
    noid
  artery R58
    brain — see Hemorrhage, intracranial, intracerebral
  basilar (ganglion) I61.0
  bladder N32.89
  bowel K92.2
    newborn P54.3
  brain (miliary) (nontraumatic) — see Hemorrhage, in-
    tracranial, intracerebral
    due to
      birth injury P10.1
      syphilis A52.05
    epidural or extradural (traumatic) — see Injury, in-
      tracranial, epidural hemorrhage
    newborn P52.4
      birth injury P10.1
    subarachnoid — see Hemorrhage, intracranial,
      subarachnoid
    subdural — see Hemorrhage, intracranial, subdural
  brainstem (nontraumatic) I61.3
    traumatic S06.38- ☑
  breast N64.59
  bronchial tube — see Hemorrhage, lung
  bronchopulmonary — see Hemorrhage, lung
  bronchus — see Hemorrhage, lung
  bulbar I61.5
  capillary I78.8
    primary D69.8
  cecum K92.2
  cerebellar, cerebellum (nontraumatic) I61.4
    newborn P52.6
    traumatic S06.37- ☑
  cerebral, cerebrum (see also Hemorrhage, intracranial,
    intracerebral)
    lobe I61.1
    newborn (anoxic) P52.4
      birth injury P10.1
  cerebromeningeal I61.8
  cerebrospinal — see Hemorrhage, intracranial, intrac-
    erebral
  cervix (uteri) (stump) NEC N88.8
  chamber, anterior (eye) — see Hyphema
  childbirth — see Hemorrhage, complicating, delivery
  choroid H31.30- ☑
    expulsive H31.31- ☑
  ciliary body — see Hyphema
  cochlea — see subcategory H83.8 ☑
  colon K92.2
  complicating
    abortion — see Abortion, by type, complicated by,
      hemorrhage

Hemorrhage, hemorrhagic — continued
  complicating — continued
    delivery O67.9
      associated with coagulation defect (afibrinogen-
        emia) (DIC) (hyperfibrinolysis) O67.0
      specified cause NEC O67.8
      surgical procedure — see Hemorrhage, intraopera-
        tive
  conjunctiva H11.3- ☑
    newborn P54.8
  cord, newborn (stump) P51.9
  corpus luteum (ruptured) cyst N83.1- ☑
  cortical (brain) I61.1
  cranial — see Hemorrhage, intracranial
  cutaneous R23.3
    due to autosensitivity, erythrocyte D69.2
    newborn P54.5
  delayed
    following ectopic or molar pregnancy O08.1
    postpartum O72.2
  diathesis (familial) D69.9
  disease D69.9
    newborn P53
    specified type NEC D69.8
  due to or associated with
    afibrinogenemia or other coagulation defect (condi-
      tions in categories D65- D69)
      antepartum — see Hemorrhage, antepartum,
        with coagulation defect
      intrapartum O67.0
    dental implant M27.61
    device, implant or graft (see also Complications, by
      site and type, specified NEC) T85.838 ☑
      arterial graft NEC T82.838 ☑
      breast T85.838 ☑
      catheter NEC T85.838 ☑
        dialysis (renal) T82.838 ☑
          intraperitoneal T85.838 ☑
        infusion NEC T82.838 ☑
          spinal (epidural) (subdural) T85.830 ☑
        urinary (indwelling) T83.83 ☑
      electronic (electrode) (pulse generator) (stimula-
        tor)
        bone T84.83 ☑
        cardiac T82.837 ☑
        nervous system (brain) (peripheral nerve)
          (spinal) T85.830 ☑
        urinary T83.83 ☑
      fixation, internal (orthopedic) NEC T84.83 ☑
      gastrointestinal (bile duct) (esophagus)
        T85.838 ☑
      genital NEC T83.83 ☑
      heart NEC T82.837 ☑
      joint prosthesis T84.83 ☑
      ocular (corneal graft) (orbital implant) NEC
        T85.838 ☑
      orthopedic NEC T84.83 ☑
        bone graft T86.838
      specified NEC T85.838 ☑
      urinary NEC T83.83 ☑
      vascular NEC T82.838 ☑
      ventricular intracranial shunt T85.830 ☑
  duodenum, duodenal K92.2
    ulcer — see Ulcer, duodenum, with hemorrhage
  dura mater — see Hemorrhage, intracranial, subdural
  endotracheal — see Hemorrhage, lung
  epicranial subaponeurotic (massive), birth injury P12.2
  epidural (traumatic) (see also Injury, intracranial,
    epidural hemorrhage)
    nontraumatic I62.1
  esophagus K22.8
    varix I85.01
      secondary I85.11
  excessive, following ectopic gestation (subsequent
    episode) O08.1
  extradural (traumatic) — see Injury, intracranial,
    epidural hemorrhage
    birth injury P10.8
    newborn (anoxic) (nontraumatic) P52.8
    nontraumatic I62.1
  eye NEC H57.89
    fundus — see Hemorrhage, retina
    lid — see Disorder, eyelid, specified type NEC
  fallopian tube N83.6
  fibrinogenolysis — see Fibrinolysis
  fibrinolytic (acquired) — see Fibrinolysis

Hemorrhage, hemorrhagic — *continued*
- from
  - ear (nontraumatic) — *see* Otorrhagia
  - tracheostomy stoma J95.01
- fundus, eye — *see* Hemorrhage, retina
- funis — *see* Hemorrhage, umbilicus, cord
- gastric — *see* Hemorrhage, stomach
- gastroenteric K92.2
  - newborn P54.3
- gastrointestinal (tract) K92.2
  - newborn P54.3
- genital organ, male N50.1
- genitourinary (tract) NOS R31.9
- gingiva K06.8
- globe (eye) — *see* Hemophthalmos
- graafian follicle cyst (ruptured) N83.0- ☑
- gum K06.8
- heart I51.89
- hypopharyngeal (throat) R04.1
- intermenstrual (regular) N92.3
  - irregular N92.1
- internal (organs) NEC R58
  - capsule I61.0
  - ear — *see* subcategory H83.8 ☑
  - newborn P54.8
- intestine K92.2
  - newborn P54.3
- intra-abdominal R58
- intra-alveolar (lung), newborn P26.8
- intracerebral (nontraumatic) — *see* Hemorrhage, intracranial, intracerebral
- intracranial (nontraumatic) I62.9
  - birth injury P10.9
  - epidural, nontraumatic I62.1
  - extradural, nontraumatic I62.1
  - intracerebral (nontraumatic) (in) I61.9
    - brain stem I61.3
    - cerebellum I61.4
    - hemisphere I61.2
      - cortical (superficial) I61.1
      - subcortical (deep) I61.0
    - intraoperative
      - during a nervous system procedure G97.31
      - during other procedure G97.32
    - intraventricular I61.5
    - multiple localized I61.6
    - newborn P52.4
      - birth injury P10.1
    - postprocedural
      - following a nervous system procedure G97.51
      - following other procedure G97.52
    - specified NEC I61.8
    - superficial I61.1
    - traumatic (diffuse) — *see* Injury, intracranial, diffuse
      - focal — *see* Injury, intracranial, focal
  - newborn P52.9
    - specified NEC P52.8
  - subarachnoid (nontraumatic) (from) I60.9
    - intracranial (cerebral) artery I60.7
      - anterior communicating I60.2
      - basilar I60.4
      - carotid siphon and bifurcation I60.0- ☑
      - communicating I60.7
        - anterior I60.2
        - posterior I60.3- ☑
      - middle cerebral I60.1- ☑
      - posterior communicating I60.3- ☑
      - specified artery NEC I60.6
      - vertebral I60.5- ☑
    - newborn P52.5
      - birth injury P10.3
    - specified NEC I60.8
    - traumatic S06.6X- ☑
  - subdural (nontraumatic) I62.00
    - acute I62.01
    - birth injury P10.0
    - chronic I62.03
    - newborn (anoxic) (hypoxic) P52.8
      - birth injury P10.0
    - spinal G95.19
    - subacute I62.02
    - traumatic — *see* Injury, intracranial, subdural hemorrhage
  - traumatic — *see* Injury, intracranial, focal brain injury
- intramedullary NEC G95.19
- intraocular — *see* Hemophthalmos

Hemorrhage, hemorrhagic — *continued*
- intraoperative, intraprocedural — *see* Complication, hemorrhage (hematoma), intraoperative (intraprocedural), by site
- intrapartum — *see* Hemorrhage, complicating, delivery
- intrapelvic
  - female N94.89
  - male K66.1
- intraperitoneal K66.1
- intrapontine I61.3
- intraprocedural — *see* Complication, hemorrhage (hematoma), intraoperative (intraprocedural), by site
- intrauterine N85.7
  - complicating delivery (*see also* Hemorrhage, complicating, delivery) O67.9
  - postpartum — *see* Hemorrhage, postpartum
- intraventricular I61.5
  - newborn (nontraumatic) (*see also* Newborn, affected by, hemorrhage) P52.3
    - due to birth injury P10.2
    - grade
      - 1 P52.0
      - 2 P52.1
      - 3 P52.21
      - 4 P52.22
- intravesical N32.89
- iris (postinfectional) (postinflammatory) (toxic) — *see* Hyphema
- joint (nontraumatic) — *see* Hemarthrosis
- kidney N28.89
- knee (joint) (nontraumatic) — *see* Hemarthrosis, knee
- labyrinth — *see* subcategory H83.8 ☑
- lenticular striate artery I61.0
- ligature, vessel — *see* Hemorrhage, postoperative
- liver K76.89
- lung R04.89
  - newborn P26.9
    - massive P26.1
    - specified NEC P26.8
  - tuberculous — *see* Tuberculosis, pulmonary
- massive umbilical, newborn P51.0
- mediastinum — *see* Hemorrhage, lung
- medulla I61.3
- membrane (brain) I60.8
  - spinal cord — *see* Hemorrhage, spinal cord
- meninges, meningeal (brain) (middle) I60.8
  - spinal cord — *see* Hemorrhage, spinal cord
- mesentery K66.1
- metritis — *see* Endometritis
- mouth K13.79
- mucous membrane NEC R58
  - newborn P54.8
- muscle M62.89
- nail (subungual) L60.8
- nasal turbinate R04.0
  - newborn P54.8
- navel, newborn P51.9
- newborn P54.9
  - specified NEC P54.8
- nipple N64.59
- nose R04.0
  - newborn P54.8
- omentum K66.1
- optic nerve (sheath) H47.02- ☑
- orbit, orbital H05.23- ☑
- ovary NEC N83.8
- oviduct N83.6
- pancreas K86.89
- parathyroid (gland) (spontaneous) E21.4
- parturition — *see* Hemorrhage, complicating, delivery
- penis N48.89
- pericardium, pericarditis I31.2
- peritoneum, peritoneal K66.1
- peritonsillar tissue J35.8
  - due to infection J36
- petechial R23.3
  - due to autosensitivity, erythrocyte D69.2
- pituitary (gland) E23.6
- pleura — *see* Hemorrhage, lung
- polioencephalitis, superior E51.2
- polymyositis — *see* Polymyositis
- pons, pontine I61.3
- posterior fossa (nontraumatic) I61.8
  - newborn P52.6
- postmenopausal N95.0
- postnasal R04.0

Hemorrhage, hemorrhagic — *continued*
- postoperative — *see* Complications, postprocedural, hemorrhage, by site
- postpartum NEC (following delivery of placenta) O72.1
  - delayed or secondary O72.2
  - retained placenta O72.0
  - third stage O72.0
- pregnancy — *see* Hemorrhage, antepartum
- preretinal — *see* Hemorrhage, retina
- prostate N42.1
- puerperal — *see* Hemorrhage, postpartum
  - delayed or secondary O72.2
- pulmonary R04.89
  - newborn P26.9
    - massive P26.1
    - specified NEC P26.8
  - tuberculous — *see* Tuberculosis, pulmonary
- purpura (primary) D69.3
- rectum (sphincter) K62.5
  - newborn P54.2
- recurring, following initial hemorrhage at time of injury T79.2 ☑
- renal N28.89
- respiratory passage or tract R04.9
  - specified NEC R04.89
- retina, retinal (vessels) H35.6- ☑
  - diabetic — *see* Diabetes, retinal, hemorrhage
- retroperitoneal R58
- scalp R58
- scrotum N50.1
- secondary (nontraumatic) R58
  - following initial hemorrhage at time of injury T79.2 ☑
- seminal vesicle N50.1
- skin R23.3
  - newborn P54.5
- slipped umbilical ligature P51.8
- spermatic cord N50.1
- spinal (cord) G95.19
  - newborn (birth injury) P11.5
- spleen D73.5
  - intraoperative — *see* Complications, intraoperative, hemorrhage, spleen
  - postprocedural — *see* Complications, postprocedural, hemorrhage, spleen
- stomach K92.2
  - newborn P54.3
  - ulcer — *see* Ulcer, stomach, with hemorrhage
- subarachnoid (nontraumatic) — *see* Hemorrhage, intracranial, subarachnoid
- subconjunctival (*see also* Hemorrhage, conjunctiva)
  - birth injury P15.3
- subcortical (brain) I61.0
- subcutaneous R23.3
- subdiaphragmatic R58
- subdural (acute) (nontraumatic) — *see* Hemorrhage, intracranial, subdural
- subependymal
  - newborn P52.0
    - with intraventricular extension P52.1
      - and intracerebral extension P52.22
- subgaleal P12.2
- subhyaloid — *see* Hemorrhage, retina
- subperiosteal — *see* Disorder, bone, specified type NEC
- subretinal — *see* Hemorrhage, retina
- subtentorial — *see* Hemorrhage, intracranial, subdural
- subungual L60.8
- suprarenal (capsule) (gland) E27.49
  - newborn P54.4
- tentorium (traumatic) NEC — *see* Hemorrhage, brain
  - newborn (birth injury) P10.4
- testis N50.1
- third stage (postpartum) O72.0
- thorax — *see* Hemorrhage, lung
- throat R04.1
- thymus (gland) E32.8
- thyroid (cyst) (gland) E07.89
- tongue K14.8
- tonsil J35.8
- trachea — *see* Hemorrhage, lung
- tracheobronchial R04.89
  - newborn P26.0
- traumatic — *code to* specific injury
  - cerebellar — *see* Hemorrhage, brain
  - intracranial — *see* Hemorrhage, brain
    - recurring or secondary (following initial hemorrhage at time of injury) T79.2 ☑

Hemorrhage, hemorrhagic — *continued*
  tuberculous NEC (*see also* Tuberculosis, pulmonary)
    A15.Ø
  tunica vaginalis N5Ø.1
  ulcer — *code by* site under Ulcer, with hemorrhage
    K27.4
  umbilicus, umbilical
    cord
      after birth, newborn P51.9
      complicating delivery O69.5 ☑
    newborn P51.9
      massive P51.Ø
      slipped ligature P51.8
    stump P51.9
  urethra (idiopathic) N36.8
  uterus, uterine (abnormal) N93.9
    climacteric N92.4
    complicating delivery — *see* Hemorrhage, compli-
      cating, delivery
    dysfunctional or functional N93.8
    intermenstrual (regular) N92.3
      irregular N92.1
    postmenopausal N95.Ø
    postpartum — *see* Hemorrhage, postpartum
    preclimacteric or premenopausal N92.4
    prepubertal N93.8
    pubertal N92.2
  vagina (abnormal) N93.9
    newborn P54.6
  vas deferens N5Ø.1
  vasa previa O69.4 ☑
  ventricular I61.5
  vesical N32.89
  viscera NEC R58
    newborn P54.8
  vitreous (humor) (intraocular) H43.1- ☑
  vulva N9Ø.89
Hemorrhoids (bleeding) (without mention of degree)
    K64.9
  1st degree (grade/stage I) (without prolapse outside
    of anal canal) K64.Ø
  2nd degree (grade/stage II) (that prolapse with strain-
    ing but retract spontaneously) K64.1
  3rd degree (grade/stage III) (that prolapse with strain-
    ing and require manual replacement back inside
    anal canal) K64.2
  4th degree (grade/stage IV) (with prolapsed tissue that
    cannot be manually replaced) K64.3
  complicating
    pregnancy O22.4 ☑
    puerperium O87.2
  external K64.4
    with
      thrombosis K64.5
  internal (without mention of degree) K64.8
  prolapsed K64.8
  skin tags
    anus K64.4
    residual K64.4
  specified NEC K64.8
  strangulated (*see also* Hemorrhoids, by degree) K64.8
  thrombosed (*see also* Hemorrhoids, by degree) K64.5
  ulcerated (*see also* Hemorrhoids, by degree) K64.8
Hemosalpinx N83.6
  with
    hematocolpos N89.7
    hematometra N85.7
      with hematocolpos N89.7
Hemosiderosis (dietary) E83.19
  pulmonary, idiopathic E83.1- ☑ [J84.Ø3]
  transfusion T8Ø.89 ☑
Hemothorax (bacterial) (nontuberculous) J94.2
  newborn P54.8
  traumatic S27.1 ☑
    with pneumothorax S27.2 ☑
  tuberculous NEC A15.6
Henoch (-Schönlein) **disease or syndrome** (purpura)
    D69.Ø
Henpue, henpuye A66.6
Hepar lobatum (syphilitic) A52.74
Hepatalgia K76.89
Hepatitis K75.9
  acute B17.9
    with coma K72.Ø1
    with hepatic failure — *see* Failure, hepatic
    alcoholic — *see* Hepatitis, alcoholic
    infectious B17.9
    non-viral K72.Ø ☑

Hepatitis — *continued*
  acute — *continued*
    viral B17.9
  alcoholic (acute) (chronic) K7Ø.1Ø
    with ascites K7Ø.11
  amebic — *see* Abscess, liver, amebic
  anicteric, (viral) — *see* Hepatitis, viral
  antigen-associated (HAA) — *see* Hepatitis, B
  Australia-antigen (positive) — *see* Hepatitis, B
  autoimmune K75.4
  B B19.1Ø
    with hepatic coma B19.11
    acute B16.9
      with
        delta-agent (coinfection) (without hepatic
          coma) B16.1
          with hepatic coma B16.Ø
        hepatic coma (without delta-agent coinfec-
          tion) B16.2
    chronic B18.1
      with delta-agent B18.Ø
  bacterial NEC K75.89
  C (viral) B19.2Ø
    with hepatic coma B19.21
    acute B17.1Ø
      with hepatic coma B17.11
    chronic B18.2
  catarrhal (acute) B15.9
    with hepatic coma B15.Ø
  cholangiolitic K75.89
  cholestatic K75.89
  chronic K73.9
    active NEC K73.2
    lobular NEC K73.1
    persistent NEC K73.Ø
    specified NEC K73.8
  cytomegaloviral B25.1
  due to ethanol (acute) (chronic) — *see* Hepatitis, alco-
    holic
  epidemic B15.9
    with hepatic coma B15.Ø
  fulminant NEC (viral) — *see* Hepatitis, viral
  granulomatous NEC K75.3
  herpesviral BØØ.81
  history of
    B Z86.19
    C Z86.19
  homologous serum — *see* Hepatitis, viral, type B
  in (due to)
    mumps B26.81
    toxoplasmosis (acquired) B58.1
      congenital (active) P37.1 [K77]
  infectious, infective B15.9
    acute (subacute) B17.9
    chronic B18.9
  inoculation — *see* Hepatitis, viral, type B
  interstitial (chronic) K74.69
  lupoid NEC K75.4
  malignant NEC (with hepatic failure) K72.9Ø
    with coma K72.91
  neonatal (idiopathic) (toxic) P59.29
  neonatal giant cell P59.29
  newborn P59.29
  non-viral K72.Ø ☑
  postimmunization — *see* Hepatitis, viral, type B
  post-transfusion — *see* Hepatitis, viral, type B
  reactive, nonspecific K75.2
  serum — *see* Hepatitis, viral, type B
  specified type NEC
    with hepatic failure — *see* Failure, hepatic
  syphilitic (late) A52.74
    congenital (early) A5Ø.Ø8 [K77]
      late A5Ø.59 [K77]
    secondary A51.45
  toxic (*see also* Disease, liver, toxic) K71.6
  tuberculous A18.83
  viral, virus B19.9
    with hepatic coma B19.Ø
    acute B17.9
    chronic B18.9
      specified NEC B18.8
      type
        B B18.1
          with delta-agent B18.Ø
        C B18.2
    congenital P35.3
    coxsackie B33.8 [K77]
    cytomegalic inclusion B25.1

Hepatitis — *continued*
  viral, virus — *continued*
    in remission, any type — *code to* Hepatitis, chronic,
      by type
    non-A, non-B B17.8
    specified type NEC (with or without coma) B17.8
    type
      A B15.9
        with hepatic coma B15.Ø
      B B19.1Ø
        with hepatic coma B19.11
        acute B16.9
          with
            delta-agent (coinfection) (without
              hepatic coma) B16.1
              with hepatic coma B16.Ø
            hepatic coma (without delta-agent
              coinfection) B16.2
        chronic B18.1
          with delta-agent B18.Ø
      C B19.2Ø
        with hepatic coma B19.21
        acute B17.1Ø
          with hepatic coma B17.11
        chronic B18.2
      E B17.2
      non-A, non-B B17.8
Hepatization lung (acute) — *see* Pneumonia, lobar
Hepatoblastoma C22.2
Hepatocarcinoma C22.Ø
Hepatocholangiocarcinoma C22.Ø
Hepatocholangioma, benign D13.4
Hepatocholangitis K75.89
Hepatolenticular degeneration E83.Ø1
Hepatoma (malignant) C22.Ø
  benign D13.4
  embryonal C22.Ø
Hepatomegaly (*see also* Hypertrophy, liver)
  with splenomegaly R16.2
  congenital Q44.7
  in mononucleosis
    gammaherpesviral B27.Ø9
    infectious specified NEC B27.89
Hepatoptosis K76.89
Hepatorenal syndrome following labor and delivery
    O9Ø.4
Hepatosis K76.89
Hepatosplenomegaly R16.2
  hyperlipemic (Bürger-Grütz type) E78.3 [K77]
Hereditary — *see* condition
Heredodegeneration, macular — *see* Dystrophy, retina
Heredopathia atactica polyneuritiformis G6Ø.1
Heredosyphilis — *see* Syphilis, congenital
Herlitz' syndrome Q81.1
Hermansky-Pudlak syndrome E7Ø.331
Hermaphrodite, hermaphroditism (true) Q56.Ø
  46,XX with streak gonads Q99.1
  46,XX/46,XY Q99.Ø
  46,XY with streak gonads Q99.1
  chimera 46,XX/46,XY Q99.Ø
Hernia, hernial (acquired) (recurrent) K46.9
  with
    gangrene — *see* Hernia, by site, with, gangrene
    incarceration — *see* Hernia, by site, with, obstruction
    irreducible — *see* Hernia, by site, with, obstruction
    obstruction — *see* Hernia, by site, with, obstruction
    strangulation — *see* Hernia, by site, with, obstruc-
      tion
  abdomen, abdominal K46.9
    with
      gangrene (and obstruction) K46.1
      obstruction K46.Ø
    femoral — *see* Hernia, femoral
    incisional — *see* Hernia, incisional
    inguinal — *see* Hernia, inguinal
    specified site NEC K45.8
      with
        gangrene (and obstruction) K45.1
        obstruction K45.Ø
    umbilical — *see* Hernia, umbilical
    wall — *see* Hernia, ventral
  appendix — *see* Hernia, abdomen
  bladder (mucosa) (sphincter)
    congenital (female) (male) Q79.51
    female — *see* Cystocele
    male N32.89
  brain, congenital — *see* Encephalocele

Hernia, hernial — *continued*
cartilage, vertebra — *see* Displacement, intervertebral disc
cerebral, congenital (*see also* Encephalocele)
  endaural Q01.8
ciliary body (traumatic) S05.2- ☑
colon — *see* Hernia, abdomen
Cooper's — *see* Hernia, abdomen, specified site NEC
crural — *see* Hernia, femoral
diaphragm, diaphragmatic K44.9
  with
    gangrene (and obstruction) K44.1
    obstruction K44.0
  congenital Q79.0
direct (inguinal) — *see* Hernia, inguinal
diverticulum, intestine — *see* Hernia, abdomen
double (inguinal) — *see* Hernia, inguinal, bilateral
due to adhesions (with obstruction) K56.50
epigastric (*see also* Hernia, ventral) K43.9
esophageal hiatus — *see* Hernia, hiatal
external (inguinal) — *see* Hernia, inguinal
fallopian tube N83.4- ☑
fascia M62.89
femoral K41.90
  with
    gangrene (and obstruction) K41.40
      not specified as recurrent K41.40
      recurrent K41.41
    obstruction K41.30
      not specified as recurrent K41.30
      recurrent K41.31
    not specified as recurrent K41.90
    recurrent K41.91
  bilateral K41.20
    with
      gangrene (and obstruction) K41.10
        not specified as recurrent K41.10
        recurrent K41.11
      obstruction K41.00
        not specified as recurrent K41.00
        recurrent K41.01
    not specified as recurrent K41.20
    recurrent K41.21
  unilateral K41.90
    with
      gangrene (and obstruction) K41.40
        not specified as recurrent K41.40
        recurrent K41.41
      obstruction K41.30
        not specified as recurrent K41.30
        recurrent K41.31
    not specified as recurrent K41.90
    recurrent K41.91
foramen magnum G93.5
  congenital Q01.8
funicular (umbilical) (*see also* Hernia, umbilicus)
  spermatic (cord) — *see* Hernia, inguinal
gastrointestinal tract — *see* Hernia, abdomen
Hesselbach's — *see* Hernia, femoral, specified site NEC
hiatal (esophageal) (sliding) K44.9
  with
    gangrene (and obstruction) K44.1
    obstruction K44.0
  congenital Q40.1
hypogastric — *see* Hernia, ventral
incarcerated (*see also* Hernia, by site, with obstruction)
  with gangrene — *see* Hernia, by site, with gangrene
incisional K43.2
  with
    gangrene (and obstruction) K43.1
    obstruction K43.0
indirect (inguinal) — *see* Hernia, inguinal
inguinal (direct) (external) (funicular) (indirect) (internal) (oblique) (scrotal) (sliding) K40.90
  with
    gangrene (and obstruction) K40.40
      not specified as recurrent K40.40
      recurrent K40.41
    obstruction K40.30
      not specified as recurrent K40.30
      recurrent K40.31
    not specified as recurrent K40.90
    recurrent K40.91
  bilateral K40.20
    with
      gangrene (and obstruction) K40.10
        not specified as recurrent K40.10
        recurrent K40.11

Hernia, hernial — *continued*
inguinal — *continued*
  bilateral — *continued*
    with — *continued*
      obstruction K40.00
        not specified as recurrent K40.00
        recurrent K40.01
    not specified as recurrent K40.20
    recurrent K40.21
  unilateral K40.90
    with
      gangrene (and obstruction) K40.40
        not specified as recurrent K40.40
        recurrent K40.41
      obstruction K40.30
        not specified as recurrent K40.30
        recurrent K40.31
    not specified as recurrent K40.90
    recurrent K40.91
internal (*see also* Hernia, abdomen)
  inguinal — *see* Hernia, inguinal
interstitial — *see* Hernia, abdomen
intervertebral cartilage or disc — *see* Displacement, intervertebral disc
intestine, intestinal — *see* Hernia, by site
intra-abdominal — *see* Hernia, abdomen
iris (traumatic) S05.2- ☑
irreducible (*see also* Hernia, by site, with obstruction)
  with gangrene — *see* Hernia, by site, with gangrene
ischiatic — *see* Hernia, abdomen, specified site NEC
ischiorectal — *see* Hernia, abdomen, specified site NEC
lens (traumatic) S05.2- ☑
linea (alba) (semilunaris) — *see* Hernia, ventral
Littre's — *see* Hernia, abdomen
lumbar — *see* Hernia, abdomen, specified site NEC
lung (subcutaneous) J98.4
mediastinum J98.59
mesenteric (internal) — *see* Hernia, abdomen
midline — *see* Hernia, ventral
muscle (sheath) M62.89
nucleus pulposus — *see* Displacement, intervertebral disc
oblique (inguinal) — *see* Hernia, inguinal
obstructive (*see also* Hernia, by site, with obstruction)
  with gangrene — *see* Hernia, by site, with gangrene
obturator — *see* Hernia, abdomen, specified site NEC
omental — *see* Hernia, abdomen
ovary N83.4- ☑
oviduct N83.4- ☑
paraesophageal (*see also* Hernia, diaphragm)
  congenital Q40.1
parastomal K43.5
  with
    gangrene (and obstruction) K43.4
    obstruction K43.3
paraumbilical — *see* Hernia, umbilicus
perineal — *see* Hernia, abdomen, specified site NEC
Petit's — *see* Hernia, abdomen, specified site NEC
postoperative — *see* Hernia, incisional
pregnant uterus — *see* Abnormal, uterus in pregnancy or childbirth
prevesical N32.89
properitoneal — *see* Hernia, abdomen, specified site NEC
pudendal — *see* Hernia, abdomen, specified site NEC
rectovaginal N81.6
retroperitoneal — *see* Hernia, abdomen, specified site NEC
Richter's — *see* Hernia, abdomen, with obstruction
Rieux's, Riex's — *see* Hernia, abdomen, specified site NEC
sac condition (adhesion) (dropsy) (inflammation) (laceration) (suppuration) — *code by site under* Hernia
sciatic — *see* Hernia, abdomen, specified site NEC
scrotum, scrotal — *see* Hernia, inguinal
sliding (inguinal) (*see also* Hernia, inguinal)
  hiatus — *see* Hernia, hiatal
spigelian — *see* Hernia, ventral
spinal — *see* Spina bifida
strangulated (*see also* Hernia, by site, with obstruction)
  with gangrene — *see* Hernia, by site, with gangrene
subxiphoid — *see* Hernia, ventral
supra-umbilicus — *see* Hernia, ventral
tendon — *see* Disorder, tendon, specified type NEC
Treitz's (fossa) — *see* Hernia, abdomen, specified site NEC

Hernia, hernial — *continued*
tunica vaginalis Q55.29
umbilicus, umbilical K42.9
  with
    gangrene (and obstruction) K42.1
    obstruction K42.0
ureter N28.89
urethra, congenital Q64.79
urinary meatus, congenital Q64.79
uterus N81.4
  pregnant — *see* Abnormal, uterus in pregnancy or childbirth
vaginal (anterior) (wall) — *see* Cystocele
Velpeau's — *see* Hernia, femoral
ventral K43.9
  with
    gangrene (and obstruction) K43.7
    obstruction K43.6
  incisional K43.2
    with
      gangrene (and obstruction) K43.1
      obstruction K43.0
    recurrent — *see* Hernia, incisional
  specified NEC K43.9
    with
      gangrene (and obstruction) K43.7
      obstruction K43.6
vesical
  congenital (female) (male) Q79.51
  female — *see* Cystocele
  male N32.89
vitreous (into wound) S05.2- ☑
  into anterior chamber — *see* Prolapse, vitreous
Herniation (*see also* Hernia)
brain (stem) G93.5
cerebral G93.5
mediastinum J98.59
nucleus pulposus — *see* Displacement, intervertebral disc
Herpangina B08.5
Herpes, herpesvirus, herpetic B00.9
anogenital A60.9
  perianal skin A60.1
  rectum A60.1
  urogenital tract A60.00
    cervix A60.03
    male genital organ NEC A60.02
    penis A60.01
    specified site NEC A60.09
    vagina A60.04
    vulva A60.04
blepharitis (zoster) B02.39
  simplex B00.59
circinatus B35.4
  bullosus L12.0
conjunctivitis (simplex) B00.53
  zoster B02.31
cornea B02.33
encephalitis B00.4
  due to herpesvirus 6 B10.01
  due to herpesvirus 7 B10.09
  specified NEC B10.09
eye (zoster) B02.30
  simplex B00.50
eyelid (zoster) B02.39
  simplex B00.59
facialis B00.1
febrilis B00.1
geniculate ganglionitis B02.21
genital, genitalis A60.00
  female A60.09
  male A60.02
gestational, gestationis O26.4- ☑
gingivostomatitis B00.2
human B00.9
  1 — *see* Herpes, simplex
  2 — *see* Herpes, simplex
  3 — *see* Varicella
  4 — *see* Mononucleosis, Epstein-Barr (virus)
  5 — *see* Disease, cytomegalic inclusion (generalized)
  6
    encephalitis B10.01
    specified NEC B10.81
  7
    encephalitis B10.09
    specified NEC B10.82
  8 B10.89
infection NEC B10.89

☑ **Additional Character Required** — Refer to the Tabular List for Character Selection   ▽ **Subterms under main terms may continue to next column or page**

Herpes, herpesvirus, herpetic — *continued*
  infection — *continued*
    Kaposi's sarcoma associated B10.89
    iridocyclitis (simplex) B00.51
      zoster B02.32
    iris (vesicular erythema multiforme) L51.9
    iritis (simplex) B00.51
    Kaposi's sarcoma associated B10.89
    keratitis (simplex) (dendritic) (disciform) (interstitial)
        B00.52
      zoster (interstitial) B02.33
    keratoconjunctivitis (simplex) B00.52
      zoster B02.33
    labialis B00.1
    lip B00.1
    meningitis (simplex) B00.3
      zoster B02.1
    ophthalmicus (zoster) NEC B02.30
      simplex B00.50
    penis A60.01
    perianal skin A60.1
    pharyngitis, pharyngotonsillitis B00.2
    rectum A60.1
    scrotum A60.02
    sepsis B00.7
    simplex B00.9
      complicated NEC B00.89
      congenital P35.2
      conjunctivitis B00.53
      external ear B00.1
      eyelid B00.59
      hepatitis B00.81
      keratitis (interstitial) B00.52
      myeitis B00.82
      specified complication NEC B00.89
      visceral B00.89
    stomatitis B00.2
    tonsurans B35.0
    visceral B00.89
    vulva A60.04
    whitlow B00.89
    zoster (*see also* condition) B02.9
      auricularis B02.21
      complicated NEC B02.8
      conjunctivitis B02.31
      disseminated B02.7
      encephalitis B02.0
      eye (lid) B02.39
      geniculate ganglionitis B02.21
      keratitis (interstitial) B02.33
      meningitis B02.1
      myelitis B02.24
      neuritis, neuralgia B02.29
      ophthalmicus NEC B02.30
      oticus B02.21
      polyneuropathy B02.23
      specified complication NEC B02.8
      trigeminal neuralgia B02.22
Herpesvirus (human) — *see* Herpes
Herpetophobia F40.218
Herrick's anemia — *see* Disease, sickle-cell
Hers' disease E74.09
Herter-Gee syndrome K90.0
Herxheimer's reaction R68.89
Hesitancy
  of micturition R39.11
  urinary R39.11
Hesselbach's hernia — *see* Hernia, femoral, specified
    site NEC
Heterochromia (congenital) Q13.2
  cataract — *see* Cataract, complicated
  cyclitis (Fuchs) — *see* Cyclitis, Fuchs' heterochromic
    hair L67.1
  iritis — *see* Cyclitis, Fuchs' heterochromic
  retained metallic foreign body (nonmagnetic) — *see*
      Foreign body, intraocular, old, retained
    magnetic — *see* Foreign body, intraocular, old, re-
        tained, magnetic
  uveitis — *see* Cyclitis, Fuchs' heterochromic
Heterophoria — *see* Strabismus, heterophoria
Heterophyes, heterophyiasis (small intestine) B66.8
Heterotopia, heterotopic (*see also* Malposition, congen-
    ital)
  cerebralis Q04.8
Heterotropia — *see* Strabismus
Heubner-Herter disease K90.0
Hexadactylism Q69.9

HGSIL (cytology finding) (high grade squamous intraep-
    ithelial lesion on cytologic smear) (Pap smear find-
    ing)
  anus R85.613
  cervix R87.613
    biopsy (histology) finding — *see* Neoplasia, intraep-
        ithelial, cervix, grade II or grade III
  vagina R87.623
    biopsy (histology) finding — *see* Neoplasia, intraep-
        ithelial, cervix, grade II or grade III
Hibernoma — *see* Lipoma
Hiccup, hiccough R06.6
  epidemic B33.0
  psychogenic F45.8
Hidden penis (congenital) Q55.64
  acquired N48.83
Hidradenitis (axillaris) (suppurative) L73.2
Hidradenoma (nodular) (*see also* Neoplasm, skin, benign)
  clear cell — *see* Neoplasm, skin, benign
  papillary — *see* Neoplasm, skin, benign
Hidrocystoma — *see* Neoplasm, skin, benign
High
  altitude effects T70.20 ☑
    anoxia T70.29 ☑
    on
      ears T70.0 ☑
      sinuses T70.1 ☑
    polycythemia D75.1
  arch
    foot Q66.7
    palate, congenital Q38.5
  arterial tension — *see* Hypertension
  basal metabolic rate R94.8
  blood pressure (*see also* Hypertension)
    borderline R03.0
    reading (incidental) (isolated) (nonspecific), without
        diagnosis of hypertension R03.0
  cholesterol E78.00
    with high triglycerides E78.2
  diaphragm (congenital) Q79.1
  expressed emotional level within family Z63.8
  head at term O32.4 ☑
  palate, congenital Q38.5
  risk
    infant NEC Z76.2
    sexual behavior (heterosexual) Z72.51
      bisexual Z72.53
      homosexual Z72.52
  scrotal testis, testes
    bilateral Q53.23
    unilateral Q53.13
  temperature (of unknown origin) R50.9
  thoracic rib Q76.6
  triglycerides E78.1
    with high cholesterol E78.2
Hildenbrand's disease A75.0
Hilum — *see* condition
Hip — *see* condition
Hippel's disease Q85.8
Hippophobia F40.218
Hippus H57.09
Hirschsprung's disease or megacolon Q43.1
Hirsutism, hirsuties L68.0
Hirudiniasis
  external B88.3
  internal B83.4
Hiss-Russell dysentery A03.1
Histidinemia, histidinuria E70.41
Histiocytoma (*see also* Neoplasm, skin, benign)
  fibrous (*see also* Neoplasm, skin, benign)
    atypical — *see* Neoplasm, connective tissue, uncer-
        tain behavior
    malignant — *see* Neoplasm, connective tissue, ma-
        lignant
Histiocytosis D76.3
  acute differentiated progressive C96.0
  Langerhans' cell NEC C96.6
    multifocal X
      multisystemic (disseminated) C96.0
      unisystemic C96.5
    pulmonary, adult (adult PLCH) J84.82
    unifocal (X) C96.6
  lipid, lipoid D76.3
    essential E75.29
  malignant C96.A (*following* C96.6)
  mononuclear phagocytes NEC D76.1
    Langerhans' cells C96.6
  non-Langerhans cell D76.3

Histiocytosis — *continued*
  polyostotic sclerosing D76.3
  sinus, with massive lymphadenopathy D76.3
  syndrome NEC D76.3
  X NEC C96.6
    acute (progressive) C96.0
    chronic C96.6
    multifocal C96.5
    multisystemic C96.0
    unifocal C96.6
Histoplasmosis B39.9
  with pneumonia NEC B39.2
  African B39.5
  American — *see* Histoplasmosis, capsulati
  capsulati B39.4
    disseminated B39.3
    generalized B39.3
    pulmonary B39.2
      acute B39.0
      chronic B39.1
  Darling's B39.4
  duboisii B39.5
  lung NEC B39.2
History
  family (of) (*see also* History, personal (of))
    alcohol abuse Z81.1
    allergy NEC Z84.89
    anemia Z83.2
    arthritis Z82.61
    asthma Z82.5
    blindness Z82.1
    cardiac death (sudden) Z82.41
    carrier of genetic disease Z84.81
    chromosomal anomaly Z82.79
    chronic
      disabling disease NEC Z82.8
      lower respiratory disease Z82.5
    colonic polyps Z83.71
    congenital malformations and deformations Z82.79
      polycystic kidney Z82.71
    consanguinity Z84.3
    deafness Z82.2
    diabetes mellitus Z83.3
    disability NEC Z82.8
    disease or disorder (of)
      allergic NEC Z84.89
      behavioral NEC Z81.8
      blood and blood-forming organs Z83.2
      cardiovascular NEC Z82.49
      chronic disabling NEC Z82.8
      digestive Z83.79
      ear NEC Z83.52
      elevated lipoprotein(a) (Lp(a)) Z83.430
      endocrine NEC Z83.49
      eye NEC Z83.518
        glaucoma Z83.511
      familial hypercholesterolemia Z83.42
      genitourinary NEC Z84.2
      glaucoma Z83.511
      hematological Z83.2
      immune mechanism Z83.2
      infectious NEC Z83.1
      ischemic heart Z82.49
      kidney Z84.1
      lipoprotein metabolism Z83.438
      mental NEC Z81.8
      metabolic Z83.49
      musculoskeletal NEC Z82.69
      neurological NEC Z82.0
      nutritional Z83.49
      parasitic NEC Z83.1
      psychiatric NEC Z81.8
      respiratory NEC Z83.6
      skin and subcutaneous tissue NEC Z84.0
      specified NEC Z84.89
    drug abuse NEC Z81.3
    elevated lipoprotein(a) (Lp(a)) Z83.430
    epilepsy Z82.0
    familial hypercholesterolemia Z83.42
    genetic disease carrier Z84.81
    glaucoma Z83.511
    hearing loss Z82.2
    human immunodeficiency virus (HIV) infection Z83.0
    Huntington's chorea Z82.0
    hyperlipidemia, familial combined Z83.438
    intellectual disability Z81.0
    leukemia Z80.6
    lipidemia NEC Z83.438
    malignant neoplasm (of) NOS Z80.9

History — *continued*
 family (*see also* History, personal) — *continued*
  malignant neoplasm — *continued*
   bladder Z80.52
   breast Z80.3
   bronchus Z80.1
   digestive organ Z80.0
   gastrointestinal tract Z80.0
   genital organ Z80.49
    ovary Z80.41
    prostate Z80.42
    specified organ NEC Z80.49
    testis Z80.43
   hematopoietic NEC Z80.7
   intrathoracic organ NEC Z80.2
   kidney Z80.51
   lung Z80.1
   lymphatic NEC Z80.7
   ovary Z80.41
   prostate Z80.42
   respiratory organ NEC Z80.2
   specified site NEC Z80.8
   testis Z80.43
   trachea Z80.1
   urinary organ or tract Z80.59
    bladder Z80.52
    kidney Z80.51
  mental
   disorder NEC Z81.8
  multiple endocrine neoplasia (MEN) syndrome
    Z83.41
  osteoporosis Z82.62
  polycystic kidney Z82.71
  polyps (colon) Z83.71
  psychiatric disorder Z81.8
  psychoactive substance abuse NEC Z81.3
  respiratory condition NEC Z83.6
   asthma and other lower respiratory conditions
    Z82.5
  self-harmful behavior Z81.8
  SIDS (sudden infant death syndrome) Z84.82
  skin condition Z84.0
  specified condition NEC Z84.89
  stroke (cerebrovascular) Z82.3
  substance abuse NEC Z81.4
   alcohol Z81.1
   drug NEC Z81.3
   psychoactive NEC Z81.3
   tobacco Z81.2
  sudden
   cardiac death Z82.41
   infant death syndrome (SIDS) Z84.82
  tobacco abuse Z81.2
  violence, violent behavior Z81.8
  visual loss Z82.1
 personal (of) (*see also* History, family (of))
  abuse
   adult Z91.419
    forced labor or sexual exploitation Z91.42
    physical and sexual Z91.410
    psychological Z91.411
   childhood Z62.819
    forced labor or sexual exploitation in child-
     hood Z62.813
    physical Z62.810
    psychological Z62.811
    sexual Z62.810
  alcohol dependence F10.21
  allergy (to) Z88.9
   analgesic agent NEC Z88.6
   anesthetic Z88.4
   antibiotic agent NEC Z88.1
   anti-infective agent NEC Z88.3
   contrast media Z91.041
   drugs, medicaments and biological substances
     Z88.9
    specified NEC Z88.8
   food Z91.018
    additives Z91.02
    eggs Z91.012
    milk products Z91.011
    peanuts Z91.010
    seafood Z91.013
    specified food NEC Z91.018
   insect Z91.038
    bee Z91.030
   latex Z91.040
   medicinal agents Z88.9
    specified NEC Z88.8

History — *continued*
 personal (*see also* History, family) — *continued*
  allergy — *continued*
   narcotic agent NEC Z88.5
   nonmedicinal agents Z91.048
   penicillin Z88.0
   serum Z88.7
   specified NEC Z91.09
   sulfonamides Z88.2
   vaccine Z88.7
  anaphylactic shock Z87.892
  anaphylaxis Z87.892
  behavioral disorders Z86.59
  benign carcinoid tumor Z86.012
  benign neoplasm Z86.018
   brain Z86.011
   carcinoid Z86.012
   colonic polyps Z86.010
  brain injury (traumatic) Z87.820
  breast implant removal Z98.86
  calculi, renal Z87.442
  cancer — *see* History, personal (of), malignant
    neoplasm (of)
  cardiac arrest (death), successfully resuscitated
    Z86.74
  cerebral infarction without residual deficit Z86.73
  cervical dysplasia Z87.410
  chemotherapy for neoplastic condition Z92.21
  childhood abuse — *see* History, personal (of), abuse
  cleft lip (corrected) Z87.730
  cleft palate (corrected) Z87.730
  collapsed vertebra (healed) Z87.311
   due to osteoporosis Z87.310
  combat and operational stress reaction Z86.51
  congenital malformation (corrected) Z87.798
   circulatory system (corrected) Z87.74
   digestive system (corrected) NEC Z87.738
   ear (corrected) Z87.721
   eye (corrected) Z87.720
   face and neck (corrected) Z87.790
   genitourinary system (corrected) NEC Z87.718
   heart (corrected) Z87.74
   integument (corrected) Z87.76
   limb(s) (corrected) Z87.76
   musculoskeletal system (corrected) Z87.76
   neck (corrected) Z87.790
   nervous system (corrected) NEC Z87.728
   respiratory system (corrected) Z87.75
   sense organs (corrected) NEC Z87.728
   specified NEC Z87.798
  contraception Z92.0
  deployment (military) Z91.82
  diabetic foot ulcer Z86.31
  disease or disorder (of) Z87.898
   anaphylaxis Z87.892
   blood and blood-forming organs Z86.2
   circulatory system Z86.79
    specified condition NEC Z86.79
   connective tissue Z87.39
   digestive system Z87.19
    colonic polyp Z86.010
    peptic ulcer disease Z87.11
    specified condition NEC Z87.19
   ear Z86.69
   endocrine Z86.39
    diabetic foot ulcer Z86.31
    gestational diabetes Z86.32
    specified type NEC Z86.39
   eye Z86.69
   genital (track) system NEC
    female Z87.42
    male Z87.438
   hematological Z86.2
   Hodgkin Z85.71
   immune mechanism Z86.2
   infectious Z86.19
    malaria Z86.13
    Methicillin resistant Staphylococcus aureus
     (MRSA) Z86.14
    poliomyelitis Z86.12
    specified NEC Z86.19
    tuberculosis Z86.11
   mental NEC Z86.59
   metabolic Z86.39
    diabetic foot ulcer Z86.31
    gestational diabetes Z86.32
    specified type NEC Z86.39
   musculoskeletal NEC Z87.39
   nervous system Z86.69

History — *continued*
 personal (*see also* History, family) — *continued*
  disease or disorder — *continued*
   nutritional Z86.39
   parasitic Z86.19
   respiratory system NEC Z87.09
   sense organs Z86.69
   skin Z87.2
   specified site or type NEC Z87.898
   subcutaneous tissue Z87.2
   trophoblastic Z87.59
   urinary system NEC Z87.448
  drug dependence — *see* Dependence, drug, by
    type, in remission
  drug therapy
   antineoplastic chemotherapy Z92.21
   estrogen Z92.23
   immunosupression Z92.25
   inhaled steroids Z92.240
   monoclonal drug Z92.22
   specified NEC Z92.29
   steroid Z92.241
   systemic steroids Z92.241
  dysplasia
   cervical (mild) (moderate) Z87.410
    severe (grade III) Z86.001
   prostatic Z87.430
   vaginal (mild) (moderate) Z87.411
    severe (grade III) Z86.008
   vulvar (mild) (moderate) Z87.412
    severe (grade III) Z86.008
  embolism (venous) Z86.718
   pulmonary Z86.711
  encephalitis Z86.61
  estrogen therapy Z92.23
  extracorporeal membrane oxygenation (ECMO)
    Z92.81
  failed conscious sedation Z92.83
  failed moderate sedation Z92.83
  fall, falling Z91.81
  forced labor or sexual exploitation Z91.42
   in childhood Z62.813
  fracture (healed)
   fatigue Z87.312
   fragility Z87.310
   osteoporosis Z87.310
   pathological NEC Z87.311
   stress Z87.312
   traumatic Z87.81
  gestational diabetes Z86.32
  hepatitis
   B Z86.19
   C Z86.19
  Hodgkin disease Z85.71
  hyperthermia, malignant Z88.4
  hypospadias (corrected) Z87.710
  hysterectomy Z90.710
  immunosupression therapy Z92.25
  in situ neoplasm
   breast Z86.000
   cervix uteri Z86.001
   specified NEC Z86.008
  in utero procedure during pregnancy Z98.870
  in utero procedure while a fetus Z98.871
  infection NEC Z86.19
   central nervous system Z86.61
   Methicillin resistant Staphylococcus aureus
    (MRSA) Z86.14
   urinary (recurrent) (tract) Z87.440
  injury NEC Z87.828
  irradiation Z92.3
  kidney stones Z87.442
  leukemia Z85.6
  lymphoma (non-Hodgkin) Z85.72
  malignant melanoma (skin) Z85.820
  malignant neoplasm (of) Z85.9
   accessory sinuses Z85.22
   anus NEC Z85.048
    carcinoid Z85.040
   bladder Z85.51
   bone Z85.830
   brain Z85.841
   breast Z85.3
   bronchus NEC Z85.118
    carcinoid Z85.110
   carcinoid — *see* History, personal (of), malignant
     neoplasm, by site, carcinioid
   cervix Z85.41
   colon NEC Z85.038

☑ **Additional Character Required** — Refer to the Tabular List for Character Selection   ▽ **Subterms under main terms may continue to next column or page**

History — continued
  personal (see also History, family) — continued
    malignant neoplasm — continued
      colon — continued
        carcinoid Z85.030
      digestive organ Z85.00
        specified NEC Z85.09
      endocrine gland NEC Z85.858
      epididymis Z85.48
      esophagus Z85.01
      eye Z85.840
      gastrointestinal tract — see History, malignant
          neoplasm, digestive organ
      genital organ
        female Z85.40
          specified NEC Z85.44
        male Z85.45
          specified NEC Z85.49
      hematopoietic NEC Z85.79
      intrathoracic organ Z85.20
      kidney NEC Z85.528
        carcinoid Z85.520
      large intestine NEC Z85.038
        carcinoid Z85.030
      larynx Z85.21
      liver Z85.05
      lung NEC Z85.118
        carcinoid Z85.110
      mediastinum Z85.29
      Merkel cell Z85.821
      middle ear Z85.22
      nasal cavities Z85.22
      nervous system NEC Z85.848
      oral cavity Z85.819
        specified site NEC Z85.818
      ovary Z85.43
      pancreas Z85.07
      pelvis Z85.53
      pharynx Z85.819
        specified site NEC Z85.818
      pleura Z85.29
      prostate Z85.46
      rectosigmoid junction NEC Z85.048
        carcinoid Z85.040
      rectum NEC Z85.048
        carcinoid Z85.040
      respiratory organ Z85.20
      sinuses, accessory Z85.22
      skin NEC Z85.828
        melanoma Z85.820
        Merkel cell Z85.821
      small intestine NEC Z85.068
        carcinoid Z85.060
      soft tissue Z85.831
      specified site NEC Z85.89
      stomach NEC Z85.028
        carcinoid Z85.020
      testis Z85.47
      thymus NEC Z85.238
        carcinoid Z85.230
      thyroid Z85.850
      tongue Z85.810
      trachea Z85.12
      urinary organ or tract Z85.50
        specified NEC Z85.59
      uterus Z85.42
    maltreatment Z91.89
    medical treatment NEC Z92.89
    melanoma (malignant) (skin) Z85.820
    meningitis Z86.61
    mental disorder Z86.59
    Merkel cell carcinoma (skin) Z85.821
    Methicillin resistant Staphylococcus aureus (MRSA)
        Z86.14
    military deployment Z91.82
    military war, peacekeeping and humanitarian de-
        ployment (current or past conflict) Z91.82
    myocardial infarction (old) I25.2
    neglect (in)
      adult Z91.412
      childhood Z62.812
    neoplasm
      benign Z86.018
        brain Z86.011
        colon polyp Z86.010
      in situ
        breast Z86.000
        cervix uteri Z86.001
        specified NEC Z86.008

History — continued
  personal (see also History, family) — continued
    neoplasm — continued
      malignant — see History of, malignant neoplasm
      uncertain behavior Z86.03
    nephrotic syndrome Z87.441
    nicotine dependence Z87.891
    noncompliance with medical treatment or regimen
        — see Noncompliance
    nutritional deficiency Z86.39
    obstetric complications Z87.59
      childbirth Z87.59
      pregnancy Z87.59
      pre-term labor Z87.51
      puerperium Z87.59
    osteoporosis fractures Z87.31 ☑
    parasuicide (attempt) Z91.5
    physical trauma NEC Z87.828
      self-harm or suicide attempt Z91.5
    pneumonia (recurrent) Z87.01
    poisoning NEC Z91.89
      self-harm or suicide attempt Z91.5
    poor personal hygiene Z91.89
    preterm labor Z87.51
    procedure during pregnancy Z98.870
    procedure while a fetus Z98.871
    prolonged reversible ischemic neurologic deficit
        (PRIND) Z86.73
    prostatic dysplasia Z87.430
    psychological
      abuse
        adult Z91.411
        child Z62.811
      trauma, specified NEC Z91.49
    radiation therapy Z92.3
    removal
      implant
        breast Z98.86
    renal calculi Z87.442
    respiratory condition NEC Z87.09
    retained foreign body fully removed Z87.821
    risk factors NEC Z91.89
    self-harm Z91.5
    self-poisoning attempt Z91.5
    sex reassignment Z87.890
    sleep-wake cycle problem Z72.821
    specified NEC Z87.898
    steroid therapy (systemic) Z92.241
      inhaled Z92.240
    stroke without residual deficits Z86.73
    substance abuse NEC F10-F19
    sudden cardiac arrest Z86.74
    sudden cardiac death successfully resuscitated
        Z86.74
    suicide attempt Z91.5
    surgery NEC Z98.890
      with uterine scar Z98.891
      sex reassignment Z87.890
      transplant — see Transplant
    thrombophlebitis Z86.72
    thrombosis (venous) Z86.718
      pulmonary Z86.711
    tobacco dependence Z87.891
    transient ischemic attack (TIA) without residual
        deficits Z86.73
    trauma (physical) NEC Z87.828
      psychological NEC Z91.49
      self-harm Z91.5
    traumatic brain injury Z87.820
    unhealthy sleep-wake cycle Z72.821
    unintended awareness under general anesthesia
        Z92.84
    urinary calculi Z87.442
    urinary (recurrent) (tract) infection(s) Z87.440
    uterine scar from previous surgery Z98.891
    vaginal dysplasia Z87.411
    venous thrombosis or embolism Z86.718
      pulmonary Z86.711
    vulvar dysplasia Z87.412
His-Werner disease A79.0
HIV (see also Human, immunodeficiency virus) B20
  laboratory evidence (nonconclusive) R75
  nonconclusive test (in infants) R75
  positive, seropositive B20
Hives (bold) — see Urticaria
Hoarseness R49.0
Hobo Z59.0
Hodgkin disease — see Lymphoma, Hodgkin

Hodgson's disease I71.2
  ruptured I71.1
Hoffa-Kastert disease E88.89
Hoffa's disease E88.89
Hoffmann-Bouveret syndrome I47.9
Hoffmann's syndrome E03.9 [G73.7]
Hole (round)
  macula H35.34- ☑
  retina (without detachment) — see Break, retina, round
      hole
    with detachment — see Detachment, retina, with
        retinal, break
Holiday relief care Z75.5
Hollenhorst's plaque — see Occlusion, artery, retina
Hollow foot (congenital) Q66.7
  acquired — see Deformity, limb, foot, specified NEC
Holoprosencephaly Q04.2
Holt-Oram syndrome Q87.2
Homelessness Z59.0
Homesickness — see Disorder, adjustment
Homocystinemia, homocystinuria E72.11
Homogentisate 1,2-dioxygenase deficiency E70.29
Homologous serum hepatitis (prophylactic) (therapeu-
    tic) — see Hepatitis, viral, type B
Honeycomb lung J98.4
  congenital Q33.0
Hooded
  clitoris Q52.6
  penis Q55.69
Hookworm (anemia) (disease) (infection) (infestation)
    B76.9
  specified NEC B76.8
Hordeolum (eyelid) (externum) (recurrent) H00.019
  internum H00.029
    left H00.026
      lower H00.025
      upper H00.024
    right H00.023
      lower H00.022
      upper H00.021
  left H00.016
    lower H00.015
    upper H00.014
  right H00.013
    lower H00.012
    upper H00.011
Horn
  cutaneous L85.8
  nail L60.2
    congenital Q84.6
Horner (-Claude Bernard) **syndrome** G90.2
  traumatic — see Injury, nerve, cervical sympathetic
Horseshoe kidney (congenital) Q63.1
Horton's headache or neuralgia G44.099
  intractable G44.091
  not intractable G44.099
Hospital hopper syndrome — see Disorder, factitious
Hospitalism in children — see Disorder, adjustment
Hostility R45.5
  towards child Z62.3
Hot flashes
  menopausal N95.1
Hourglass (contracture) (see also Contraction, hourglass)
  stomach K31.89
    congenital Q40.2
    stricture K31.2
Household, housing circumstance affecting care
    Z59.9
  specified NEC Z59.8
Housemaid's knee — see Bursitis, prepatellar
Hudson (-Stähli) **line** (cornea) — see Pigmentation,
    cornea, anterior
Human
  bite (open wound) (see also Bite)
    intact skin surface — see Bite, superficial
  herpesvirus — see Herpes
  immunodeficiency virus (HIV) disease (infection) B20
    asymptomatic status Z21
    contact Z20.6
    counseling Z71.7
    dementia B20 [F02.80]
      with behavioral disturbance B20 [F02.81]
    exposure to Z20.6
    laboratory evidence R75
    type-2 (HIV 2) as cause of disease classified else-
        where B97.35

Human — *continued*
  papillomavirus (HPV)
    DNA test positive
      high risk
        cervix R87.810
        vagina R87.811
      low risk
        cervix R87.820
        vagina R87.821
    screening for Z11.51
  T-cell lymphotropic virus
    type-1 (HTLV-I) infection B33.3
      as cause of disease classified elsewhere B97.33
      carrier Z22.6
    type-2 (HTLV-II) as cause of disease classified else-
      where B97.34
Humidifier lung or pneumonitis J67.7
Humiliation (experience) **in childhood** Z62.898
Humpback (acquired) — *see* Kyphosis
Hunchback (acquired) — *see* Kyphosis
Hunger T73.0 ☑
  air, psychogenic F45.8
Hungry bone syndrome E83.81
Hunner's ulcer — *see* Cystitis, chronic, interstitial
Hunter's
  glossitis D51.0
  syndrome E76.1
Huntington's disease or chorea G10
  with dementia G10 [F02.80]
    with behavioral disturbance G10 [F02.81]
Hunt's
  disease or syndrome (herpetic geniculate ganglionitis)
    B02.21
    dyssynergia cerebellaris myoclonica G11.1
  neuralgia B02.21
Hurler (-Scheie) **disease or syndrome** E76.02
Hurst's disease G36.1
Hurthle cell
  adenocarcinoma C73
  adenoma D34
  carcinoma C73
  tumor D34
Hutchinson-Boeck disease or syndrome — *see* Sarcoidosis
Hutchinson-Gilford disease or syndrome E34.8
Hutchinson's
  disease, meaning
    angioma serpiginosum L81.7
    pompholyx (cheiropompholyx) L30.1
    prurigo estivalis L56.4
    summer eruption or summer prurigo L56.4
  melanotic freckle — *see* Melanoma, in situ
    malignant melanoma in — *see* Melanoma
  teeth or incisors (congenital syphilis) A50.52
  triad (congenital syphilis) A50.53
Hyalin plaque, sclera, senile H15.89
Hyaline membrane (disease) (lung) (pulmonary) (newborn) P22.0
Hyalinosis
  cutis (et mucosae) E78.89
  focal and segmental (glomerular) (*see also* N00-N07
    with fourth character .1) N05.1
Hyalitis, hyalosis, asteroid (*see also* Deposit, crystalline)
  syphilitic (late) A52.71
Hydatid
  cyst or tumor — *see* Echinococcus
  mole — *see* Hydatidiform mole
  Morgagni
    female Q50.5
    male (epididymal) Q55.4
    testicular Q55.29
Hydatidiform mole (benign) (complicating pregnancy)
  (delivered) (undelivered) O01.9
  classical O01.0
  complete O01.0
  incomplete O01.1
  invasive D39.2
  malignant D39.2
  partial O01.1
Hydatidosis — *see* Echinococcus
Hydradenitis (axillaris) (suppurative) L73.2
Hydradenoma — *see* Hidradenoma
Hydramnios O40.- ☑
Hydrancephaly, hydranencephaly Q04.3
  with spina bifida — *see* Spina bifida, with hydro-
    cephalus
Hydrargyrism NEC — *see* Poisoning, mercury
Hydrarthrosis (*see also* Effusion, joint)

Hydrarthrosis — *continued*
  gonococcal A54.42
  intermittent M12.40
    ankle M12.47- ☑
    elbow M12.42- ☑
    foot joint M12.47- ☑
    hand joint M12.44- ☑
    hip M12.45- ☑
    knee M12.46- ☑
    multiple site M12.49
    shoulder M12.41- ☑
    specified joint NEC M12.48
    wrist M12.43- ☑
  of yaws (early) (late) (*see also* subcategory M14.8-)
    A66.6
  syphilitic (late) A52.77
    congenital A50.55 [M12.80]
Hydremia D64.89
Hydrencephalocele (congenital) — *see* Encephalocele
Hydrencephalomeningocele (congenital) — *see* Encephalocele
Hydroa R23.8
  aestivale L56.4
  vacciniforme L56.4
Hydroadenitis (axillaris) (suppurative) L73.2
Hydrocalycosis — *see* Hydronephrosis
Hydrocele (spermatic cord) (testis) (tunica vaginalis)
  N43.3
  canal of Nuck N94.89
  communicating N43.2
    congenital P83.5
  congenital P83.5
  encysted N43.0
  female NEC N94.89
  infected N43.1
  newborn P83.5
  round ligament N94.89
  specified NEC N43.2
  spinalis — *see* Spina bifida
  vulva N90.89
Hydrocephalus (acquired) (external) (internal) (malignant) (recurrent) G91.9
  aqueduct Sylvius stricture Q03.0
  causing disproportion O33.6 ☑
    with obstructed labor O66.3
  communicating G91.0
  congenital (external) (internal) Q03.9
    with spina bifida Q05.4
      cervical Q05.0
      dorsal Q05.1
      lumbar Q05.2
      lumbosacral Q05.2
      sacral Q05.3
      thoracic Q05.1
      thoracolumbar Q05.1
    specified NEC Q03.8
  due to toxoplasmosis (congenital) P37.1
  foramen Magendie block (acquired) G91.1
    congenital (*see also* Hydrocephalus, congenital)
      Q03.1
  in (due to)
    infectious disease NEC B89 [G91.4]
    neoplastic disease NEC (*see also* Neoplasm) G91.4
    parasitic disease B89 [G91.4]
  newborn Q03.9
    with spina bifida — *see* Spina bifida, with hydro-
      cephalus
  noncommunicating G91.1
  normal pressure G91.2
    secondary G91.0
  obstructive G91.1
  otitic G93.2
  post-traumatic NEC G91.3
  secondary G91.4
    post-traumatic G91.3
  specified NEC G91.8
  syphilitic, congenital A50.49
Hydrocolpos (congenital) N89.8
Hydrocystoma — *see* Neoplasm, skin, benign
Hydroencephalocele (congenital) — *see* Encephalocele
Hydroencephalomeningocele (congenital) — *see* Encephalocele
Hydrohematopneumothorax — *see* Hemothorax
Hydromeningitis — *see* Meningitis
Hydromeningocele (spinal) (*see also* Spina bifida)
  cranial — *see* Encephalocele
Hydrometra N85.8
Hydrometrocolpos N89.8

Hydromicrocephaly Q02
Hydromphalos (since birth) Q45.8
Hydromyelia Q06.4
Hydromyelocele — *see* Spina bifida
Hydronephrosis (atrophic) (early) (functionless) (intermittent) (primary) (secondary) NEC N13.30
  with
    infection N13.6
    obstruction (by) (of)
      renal calculus N13.2
        with infection N13.6
      ureteral NEC N13.1
        with infection N13.6
        calculus N13.2
          with infection N13.6
      ureteropelvic junction (congenital) Q62.11
        acquired N13.0
          with infection N13.6
    ureteral stricture NEC N13.1
      with infection N13.6
  congenital Q62.0
  due to acquired occlusion of ureteropelvic junction
    N13.0
  specified type NEC N13.39
  tuberculous A18.11
Hydropericarditis — *see* Pericarditis
Hydropericardium — *see* Pericarditis
Hydroperitoneum R18.8
Hydrophobia — *see* Rabies
Hydrophthalmos Q15.0
Hydropneumohemothorax — *see* Hemothorax
Hydropneumopericarditis — *see* Pericarditis
Hydropneumopericardium — *see* Pericarditis
Hydropneumothorax J94.8
  traumatic — *see* Injury, intrathoracic, lung
  tuberculous NEC A15.6
Hydrops R60.9
  abdominis R18.8
  articulorum intermittens — *see* Hydrarthrosis, intermit-
    tent
  cardiac — *see* Failure, heart, congestive
  causing obstructed labor (mother) O66.3
  endolymphatic H81.0- ☑
  fetal — *see* Pregnancy, complicated by, hydrops, fetalis
  fetalis P83.2
    due to
      ABO isoimmunization P56.0
      alpha thalassemia D56.0
      hemolytic disease P56.90
        specified NEC P56.99
      isoimmunization (ABO) (Rh) P56.0
      other specified nonhemolytic disease NEC P83.2
      Rh incompatibility P56.0
    during pregnancy — *see* Pregnancy, complicated
      by, hydrops, fetalis
  gallbladder K82.1
  joint — *see* Effusion, joint
  labyrinth H81.0- ☑
  newborn (idiopathic) P83.2
    due to
      ABO isoimmunization P56.0
      alpha thalassemia D56.0
      hemolytic disease P56.90
        specified NEC P56.99
      isoimmunization (ABO) (Rh) P56.0
      Rh incompatibility P56.0
  nutritional — *see* Malnutrition, severe
  pericardium — *see* Pericarditis
  pleura — *see* Hydrothorax
  spermatic cord — *see* Hydrocele
Hydropyonephrosis N13.6
Hydrorachis Q06.4
Hydrorrhea (nasal) J34.89
  pregnancy — *see* Rupture, membranes, premature
Hydrosadenitis (axillaris) (suppurative) L73.2
Hydrosalpinx (fallopian tube) (follicularis) N70.11
Hydrothorax (double) (pleura) J94.8
  chylous (nonfilarial) I89.8
    filarial (*see also* Infestation, filarial) B74.9 [J91.8]
  traumatic — *see* Injury, intrathoracic
  tuberculous NEC (non primary) A15.6
Hydroureter (*see also* Hydronephrosis) N13.4
  with infection N13.6
  congenital Q62.39
Hydroureteronephrosis — *see* Hydronephrosis
Hydrourethra N36.8
Hydroxykynureninuria E70.8

☑ **Additional Character Required — Refer to the Tabular List for Character Selection**   ▿ Subterms under main terms may continue to next column or page

Hydroxylysinemia E72.3
Hydroxyprolinemia E72.59
Hygiene, sleep
  abuse Z72.821
  inadequate Z72.821
  poor Z72.821
Hygroma (congenital) (cystic) D18.1
  praepatellare, prepatellar — *see* Bursitis, prepatellar
Hymen — *see* condition
Hymenolepis, hymenolepiasis (diminuta) (infection) (infestation) (nana) B71.0
Hypalgesia R20.8
Hyperacidity (gastric) K31.89
  psychogenic F45.8
Hyperactive, hyperactivity F90.9
  basal cell, uterine cervix — *see* Dysplasia, cervix
  bowel sounds R19.12
  cervix epithelial (basal) — *see* Dysplasia, cervix
  child F90.9
    attention deficit — *see* Disorder, attention-deficit hyperactivity
  detrusor muscle N32.81
  gastrointestinal K31.89
    psychogenic F45.8
  nasal mucous membrane J34.3
  stomach K31.89
  thyroid (gland) — *see* Hyperthyroidism
Hyperacusis H93.23- ☑
Hyperadrenalism E27.5
Hyperadrenocorticism E24.9
  congenital E25.0
  iatrogenic E24.2
    correct substance properly administered — *see* Table of Drugs and Chemicals, by drug, adverse effect
    overdose or wrong substance given or taken — *see* Table of Drugs and Chemicals, by drug, poisoning
  not associated with Cushing's syndrome E27.0
  pituitary-dependent E24.0
Hyperaldosteronism E26.9
  familial (type I) E26.02
  glucocorticoid-remediable E26.02
  primary (due to (bilateral) adrenal hyperplasia) E26.09
  primary NEC E26.09
  secondary E26.1
  specified NEC E26.89
Hyperalgesia R20.8
Hyperalimentation R63.2
  carotene, carotin E67.1
  specified NEC E67.8
  vitamin
    A E67.0
    D E67.3
Hyperaminoaciduria
  arginine E72.21
  cystine E72.01
  lysine E72.3
  ornithine E72.4
Hyperammonemia (congenital) E72.20
Hyperazotemia — *see* Uremia
Hyperbetalipoproteinemia (familial) E78.00
  with prebetalipoproteinemia E78.2
Hyperbicarbonatemia P74.41
Hyperbilirubinemia
  constitutional E80.6
  familial conjugated E80.6
  neonatal (transient) — *see* Jaundice, newborn
Hypercalcemia, hypocalciuric, familial E83.52
Hypercalciuria, idiopathic R82.994
Hypercapnia R06.89
  newborn P84
Hypercarotenemia (dietary) E67.1
Hypercementosis K03.4
Hyperchloremia E87.8
Hyperchlorhydria K31.89
  neurotic F45.8
  psychogenic F45.8
Hypercholesterinemia — *see* Hypercholesterolemia
Hypercholesterolemia (essential) (primary) (pure) E78.00
  with hyperglyceridemia, endogenous E78.2
  dietary counseling and surveillance Z71.3
  familial E78.01
  hereditary E78.01
Hyperchylia gastrica, psychogenic F45.8
Hyperchylomicronemia (familial) (primary) E78.3
  with hyperbetalipoproteinemia E78.3

Hypercoagulable (state) D68.59
  activated protein C resistance D68.51
  antithrombin (III) deficiency D68.59
  factor V Leiden mutation D68.51
  primary NEC D68.59
  protein C deficiency D68.59
  protein S deficiency D68.59
  prothrombin gene mutation D68.52
  secondary D68.69
  specified NEC D68.69
Hypercoagulation (state) D68.59
Hypercorticalism, pituitary-dependent E24.0
Hypercorticosolism — *see* Cushing's, syndrome
Hypercorticosteronism E24.2
  correct substance properly administered — *see* Table of Drugs and Chemicals, by drug, adverse effect
  overdose or wrong substance given or taken — *see* Table of Drugs and Chemicals, by drug, poisoning
Hypercortisonism E24.2
  correct substance properly administered — *see* Table of Drugs and Chemicals, by drug, adverse effect
  overdose or wrong substance given or taken — *see* Table of Drugs and Chemicals, by drug, poisoning
Hyperekplexia Q89.8
Hyperelectrolytemia E87.8
Hyperemesis R11.10
  with nausea R11.2
  gravidarum (mild) O21.0
    with
      carbohydrate depletion O21.1
      dehydration O21.1
      electrolyte imbalance O21.1
      metabolic disturbance O21.1
     severe (with metabolic disturbance) O21.1
  projectile R11.12
  psychogenic F45.8
Hyperemia (acute) (passive) R68.89
  anal mucosa K62.89
  bladder N32.89
  cerebral I67.89
  conjunctiva H11.43- ☑
  ear internal, acute — *see* subcategory H83.0 ☑
  enteric K59.8
  eye — *see* Hyperemia, conjunctiva
  eyelid (active) (passive) — *see* Disorder, eyelid, specified type NEC
  intestine K59.8
  iris — *see* Disorder, iris, vascular
  kidney N28.89
  labyrinth — *see* subcategory H83.0 ☑
  liver (active) K76.89
  lung (passive) — *see* Edema, lung
  pulmonary (passive) — *see* Edema, lung
  renal N28.89
  retina H35.89
  stomach K31.89
Hyperesthesia (body surface) R20.3
  larynx (reflex) J38.7
    hysterical F44.89
  pharynx (reflex) J39.2
    hysterical F44.89
Hyperestrogenism (drug-induced) (iatrogenic) E28.0
Hyperexplexia Q89.8
Hyperfibrinolysis — *see* Fibrinolysis
Hyperfructosemia E74.19
Hyperfunction
  adrenal cortex, not associated with Cushing's syndrome E27.0
    medulla E27.5
      adrenomedullary E27.5
    virilism E25.9
      congenital E25.0
  ovarian E28.8
  pancreas K86.89
  parathyroid (gland) E21.3
  pituitary (gland) (anterior) E22.9
    specified NEC E22.8
  polyglandular E31.1
  testicular E29.0
Hypergammaglobulinemia D89.2
  polyclonal D89.0
  Waldenström D89.0
Hypergastrinemia E16.4
Hyperglobulinemia R77.1
Hyperglycemia, hyperglycemic (transient) R73.9
  coma — *see* Diabetes, by type, with coma
  postpancreatectomy E89.1

Hyperglyceridemia (endogenous) (essential) (familial) (hereditary) (pure) E78.1
  mixed E78.3
Hyperglycinemia (non-ketotic) E72.51
Hypergonadism
  ovarian E28.8
  testicular (primary) (infantile) E29.0
Hyperheparinemia D68.32
Hyperhidrosis, hyperidrosis R61
  focal
    primary L74.519
      axilla L74.510
      face L74.511
      palms L74.512
      soles L74.513
    secondary L74.52
  generalized R61
  localized
    primary L74.519
      axilla L74.510
      face L74.511
      palms L74.512
      soles L74.513
    secondary L74.52
  psychogenic F45.8
  secondary R61
    focal L74.52
Hyperhistidinemia E70.41
Hyperhomocysteinemia E72.11
Hyperhydroxyprolinemia E72.59
Hyperinsulinism (functional) E16.1
  with
    coma (hypoglycemic) E15
    encephalopathy E16.1 [G94]
  ectopic E16.1
  therapeutic misadventure (from administration of insulin) — *see* subcategory T38.3 ☑
Hyperkalemia E87.5
Hyperkeratosis (*see also* Keratosis) L85.9
  cervix N88.0
  due to yaws (early) (late) (palmar or plantar) A66.3
  follicularis Q82.8
    penetrans (in cutem) L87.0
  palmoplantaris climacterica L85.1
  pinta A67.1
  senile (with pruritus) L57.0
  universalis congenita Q80.8
  vocal cord J38.3
  vulva N90.4
Hyperkinesia, hyperkinetic (disease) (reaction) (syndrome) (childhood) (adolescence) (*see also* Disorder, attention-deficit hyperactivity)
  heart I51.89
Hyperleucine-isoleucinemia E71.19
Hyperlipemia, hyperlipidemia E78.5
  combined E78.2
    familial E78.49
  group
    A E78.00
    B E78.1
    C E78.2
    D E78.3
  mixed E78.2
  specified NEC E78.49
Hyperlipidosis E75.6
  hereditary NEC E75.5
Hyperlipoproteinemia E78.5
  Fredrickson's type
    I E78.3
    IIa E78.00
    IIb E78.2
    III E78.2
    IV E78.1
    V E78.3
  low-density-lipoprotein-type (LDL) E78.00
  very-low-density-lipoprotein-type (VLDL) E78.1
Hyperlucent lung, unilateral J43.0
Hyperlysinemia E72.3
Hypermagnesemia E83.41
  neonatal P71.8
Hypermenorrhea N92.0
Hypermethioninemia E72.19
Hypermetropia (congenital) H52.0- ☑
Hypermobility, hypermotility
  cecum — *see* Syndrome, irritable bowel
  coccyx — *see* subcategory M53.2 ☑
  colon — *see* Syndrome, irritable bowel
    psychogenic F45.8

Hypermobility, hypermotility — *continued*
  ileum K58.9
  intestine (*see also* Syndrome, irritable bowel) K58.9
    psychogenic F45.8
  meniscus (knee) — *see* Derangement, knee, meniscus
  scapula — *see* Instability, joint, shoulder
  stomach K31.89
    psychogenic F45.8
  syndrome M35.7
  urethra N36.41
    with intrinsic sphincter deficiency N36.43
Hypernasality R49.21
Hypernatremia E87.0
Hypernephroma C64.- ☑
Hyperopia — *see* Hypermetropia
Hyperorexia nervosa F50.2
Hyperornithinemia E72.4
Hyperosmia R43.1
Hyperosmolality E87.0
Hyperostosis (monomelic) (*see also* Disorder, bone, density and structure, specified NEC)
  ankylosing (spine) M48.10
    cervical region M48.12
    cervicothoracic region M48.13
    lumbar region M48.16
    lumbosacral region M48.17
    multiple sites M48.19
    occipito-atlanto-axial region M48.11
    sacrococcygeal region M48.18
    thoracic region M48.14
    thoracolumbar region M48.15
  cortical (skull) M85.2
    infantile M89.8X- ☑
  frontal, internal of skull M85.2
  interna frontalis M85.2
  skeletal, diffuse idiopathic — *see* Hyperostosis, ankylosing
  skull M85.2
    congenital Q75.8
  vertebral, ankylosing — *see* Hyperostosis, ankylosing
Hyperovarism E28.8
Hyperoxaluria R82.992
  primary E72.53
Hyperparathyroidism E21.3
  primary E21.0
  secondary (renal) N25.81
    non-renal E21.1
  specified NEC E21.2
  tertiary E21.2
Hyperpathia R20.8
Hyperperistalsis R19.2
  psychogenic F45.8
Hyperpermeability, capillary I78.8
Hyperphagia R63.2
Hyperphenylalaninemia NEC E70.1
Hyperphoria (alternating) H50.53
Hyperphosphatemia E83.39
Hyperpiesis, hyperpiesia — *see* Hypertension
Hyperpigmentation (*see also* Pigmentation)
  melanin NEC L81.4
  postinflammatory L81.0
Hyperpinealism E34.8
Hyperpituitarism E22.9
Hyperplasia, hyperplastic
  adenoids J35.2
  adrenal (capsule) (cortex) (gland) E27.8
    with
      sexual precocity (male) E25.9
        congenital E25.0
      virilism, adrenal E25.9
        congenital E25.0
      virilization (female) E25.9
        congenital E25.0
    congenital E25.0
      salt-losing E25.0
  adrenomedullary E27.5
  angiolymphoid, eosinophilia (ALHE) D18.01
  appendix (lymphoid) K38.0
  artery, fibromuscular I77.3
  bone (*see also* Hypertrophy, bone)
    marrow D75.89
  breast (*see also* Hypertrophy, breast)
    ductal (atypical) N60.9- ☑
  C-cell, thyroid E07.0
  cementation (tooth) (teeth) K03.4
  cervical gland R59.0
  cervix (uteri) (basal cell) (endometrium) (polypoid) (*see also* Dysplasia, cervix)

Hyperplasia, hyperplastic — *continued*
  cervix (*see also* Dysplasia, cervix) — *continued*
    congenital Q51.828
    clitoris, congenital Q52.6
  denture K06.2
  endocervicitis N72
  endometrium, endometrial (adenomatous) (benign) (cystic) (glandular) (glandular-cystic) (polypoid) N85.00
    with atypia N85.02
    cervix — *see* Dysplasia, cervix
    complex (without atypia) N85.01
    simple (without atypia) N85.01
  epithelial L85.9
    focal, oral, including tongue K13.29
    nipple N62
    skin L85.9
    tongue K13.29
    vaginal wall N89.3
  erythroid D75.89
  fibromuscular of artery (carotid) (renal) I77.3
  genital
    female NEC N94.89
    male N50.89
  gingiva K06.1
  glandularis cystica uteri (interstitialis) (*see also* Hyperplasia, endometrial) N85.00
  gum K06.1
  hymen, congenital Q52.4
  irritative, edentulous (alveolar) K06.2
  jaw M26.09
    alveolar M26.79
    lower M26.03
      alveolar M26.72
    upper M26.01
      alveolar M26.71
  kidney (congenital) Q63.3
  labia N90.69
    epithelial N90.3
  liver (congenital) Q44.7
    nodular, focal K76.89
  lymph gland or node R59.9
  mandible, mandibular M26.03
    alveolar M26.72
    unilateral condylar M27.8
  maxilla, maxillary M26.01
    alveolar M26.71
  myometrium, myometrial N85.2
  neuroendocrine cell, of infancy J84.841
  nose
    lymphoid J34.89
    polypoid J33.9
  oral mucosa (irritative) K13.6
  organ or site, congenital NEC — *see* Anomaly, by site
  ovary N83.8
  palate, papillary (irritative) K13.6
  pancreatic islet cells E16.9
    alpha E16.8
      with excess
        gastrin E16.4
        glucagon E16.3
    beta E16.1
  parathyroid (gland) E21.0
  pharynx (lymphoid) J39.2
  prostate (adenofibromatous) (nodular) N40.0
    with lower urinary tract symptoms (LUTS) N40.1
    without lower urinary tract symtpoms (LUTS) N40.0
  renal artery I77.89
  reticulo-endothelial (cell) D75.89
  salivary gland (any) K11.1
  Schimmelbusch's — *see* Mastopathy, cystic
  suprarenal capsule (gland) E27.8
  thymus (gland) (persistent) E32.0
  thyroid (gland) — *see* Goiter
  tonsils (faucial) (infective) (lingual) (lymphoid) J35.1
    with adenoids J35.3
  unilateral condylar M27.8
  uterus, uterine N85.2
    endometrium (glandular) (*see also* Hyperplasia, endometrial) N85.00
  vulva N90.69
    epithelial N90.3
Hyperpnea — *see* Hyperventilation
Hyperpotassemia E87.5
Hyperprebetalipoproteinemia (familial) E78.1
Hyperprolactinemia E22.1
Hyperprolinemia (type I) (type II) E72.59
Hyperproteinemia E88.09

Hyperprothrombinemia, causing coagulation factor deficiency D68.4
Hyperpyrexia R50.9
  heat (effects) T67.0 ☑
  malignant, due to anesthetic T88.3 ☑
  rheumatic — *see* Fever, rheumatic
  unknown origin R50.9
Hyper-reflexia R29.2
Hypersalivation K11.7
Hypersecretion
  ACTH (not associated with Cushing's syndrome) E27.0
    pituitary E24.0
  adrenaline E27.5
  adrenomedullary E27.5
  androgen (testicular) E29.0
    ovarian (drug-induced) (iatrogenic) E28.1
  calcitonin E07.0
  catecholamine E27.5
  corticoadrenal E24.9
  cortisol E24.9
  epinephrine E27.5
  estrogen E28.0
  gastric K31.89
    psychogenic F45.8
  gastrin E16.4
  glucagon E16.3
  hormone(s)
    ACTH (not associated with Cushing's syndrome) E27.0
      pituitary E24.0
    antidiuretic E22.2
    growth E22.0
    intestinal NEC E34.1
    ovarian androgen E28.1
    pituitary E22.9
    testicular E29.0
    thyroid stimulating E05.80
      with thyroid storm E05.81
  insulin — *see* Hyperinsulinism
  lacrimal glands — *see* Epiphora
  medulloadrenal E27.5
  milk O92.6
  ovarian androgens E28.1
  salivary gland (any) K11.7
  thyrocalcitonin E07.0
  upper respiratory J39.8
Hypersegmentation, leukocytic, hereditary D72.0
Hypersensitive, hypersensitiveness, hypersensitivity (*see also* Allergy)
  carotid sinus G90.01
  colon — *see* Irritable, colon
  drug T88.7 ☑
  gastrointestinal K52.29
    immediate K52.29
    psychogenic F45.8
  labyrinth — *see* subcategory H83.2 ☑
  pain R20.8
  pneumonitis — *see* Pneumonitis, allergic
  reaction T78.40 ☑
    upper respiratory tract NEC J39.3
Hypersomnia (organic) G47.10
  due to
    alcohol
      abuse F10.182
      dependence F10.282
      use F10.982
    amphetamines
      abuse F15.182
      dependence F15.282
      use F15.982
    caffeine
      abuse F15.182
      dependence F15.282
      use F15.982
    cocaine
      abuse F14.182
      dependence F14.282
      use F14.982
    drug NEC
      abuse F19.182
      dependence F19.282
      use F19.982
    medical condition G47.14
    mental disorder F51.13
    opioid
      abuse F11.182
      dependence F11.282
      use F11.982

☑ **Additional Character Required** — **Refer to the Tabular List for Character Selection**   ▽ **Subterms under main terms may continue to next column or page**

Hypersomnia — continued
- due to — continued
  - psychoactive substance NEC
    - abuse F19.182
    - dependence F19.282
    - use F19.982
  - sedative, hypnotic, or anxiolytic
    - abuse F13.182
    - dependence F13.282
    - use F13.982
  - stimulant NEC
    - abuse F15.182
    - dependence F15.282
    - use F15.982
- idiopathic G47.11
  - with long sleep time G47.11
  - without long sleep time G47.12
- menstrual related G47.13
- nonorganic origin F51.11
  - specified NEC F51.19
- not due to a substance or known physiological condition F51.11
  - specified NEC F51.19
- primary F51.11
- recurrent G47.13
- specified NEC G47.19

Hypersplenia, hypersplenism D73.1
Hyperstimulation, ovaries (associated with induced ovulation) N98.1
Hypersusceptibility — see Allergy
Hypertelorism (ocular) (orbital) Q75.2
Hypertension, hypertensive (accelerated) (benign) (essential) (idiopathic) (malignant) (systemic) I10
- with
  - heart failure (congestive) I11.0
  - heart involvement (conditions in I50.-, I51.4-I51.9 due to hypertension) — see Hypertension, heart
  - kidney involvement — see Hypertension, kidney
- benign, intracranial G93.2
- borderline R03.0
- cardiorenal (disease) I13.10
  - with heart failure I13.0
    - with stage 1 through stage 4 chronic kidney disease I13.0
    - with stage 5 or end stage renal disease I13.2
  - without heart failure I13.10
    - with stage 1 through stage 4 chronic kidney disease I13.10
    - with stage 5 or end stage renal disease I13.11
- cardiovascular
  - disease (arteriosclerotic) (sclerotic) — see Hypertension, heart
  - renal (disease) — see Hypertension, cardiorenal
- chronic venous — see Hypertension, venous (chronic)
- complicating
  - childbirth (labor) O16.4
  - pre-existing O10.92
    - with
      - heart disease O10.12
        - with renal disease O10.32
      - pre-eclampsia O11.4
      - renal disease O10.22
        - with heart disease O10.32
      - essential O10.02
      - secondary O10.42
  - pregnancy O16.- ☑
    - with edema (see also Pre-eclampsia) O14.9- ☑
    - gestational (pregnancy induced) (without proteinuria) O13.- ☑
      - with proteinuria O14.9- ☑
        - mild pre-eclampsia O14.0- ☑
        - moderate pre-eclampsia O14.0- ☑
        - severe pre-eclampsia O14.1- ☑
          - with hemolysis, elevated liver enzymes and low platelet count (HELLP) O14.2- ☑
    - pre-existing O10.91- ☑
      - with
        - heart disease O10.11- ☑
          - with renal disease O10.31- ☑
        - pre-eclampsia — see category O11
        - renal disease O10.21- ☑
          - with heart disease O10.31- ☑
        - essential O10.01- ☑
        - secondary O10.41- ☑
    - transient O13- ☑
  - puerperium, pre-existing O16.5

Hypertension, hypertensive — continued
- complicating — continued
  - puerperium, pre-existing — continued
    - pre-existing
      - with
        - heart disease O10.13
          - with renal disease O10.33
        - pre-eclampsia O11.5
        - renal disease O10.23
          - with heart disease O10.33
      - essential O10.03
    - pregnancy-induced O13.9
    - secondary O10.43
- crisis I16.9
- due to
  - endocrine disorders I15.2
  - pheochromocytoma I15.2
  - renal disorders NEC I15.1
    - arterial I15.0
  - renovascular disorders I15.0
  - specified disease NEC I15.8
- emergency I16.1
- encephalopathy I67.4
- gestational (without significant proteinuria) (pregnancy-induced) (transient) O13.- ☑
  - with significant proteinuria — see Pre-eclampsia
- complicating
  - delivery O13.4
  - puerperium O13.5
- Goldblatt's I70.1
- heart (disease) (conditions in I51.4-I51.9 due to hypertension) I11.9
  - with
    - heart failure (congestive) I11.0
    - kidney disease (chronic) — see Hypertension, cardiorenal
- intracranial (benign) G93.2
- kidney I12.9
  - with
    - heart disease — see Hypertension, cardiorenal
    - stage 1 through stage 4 chronic kidney disease I12.9
    - stage 5 chronic kidney disease (CKD) or end stage renal disease (ESRD) I12.0
- lesser circulation I27.0
- maternal O16- ☑
- newborn P29.2
  - pulmonary (persistent) P29.30
- ocular H40.05- ☑
- pancreatic duct — code to underlying condition
  - with chronic pancreatitis K86.1
- portal (due to chronic liver disease) (idiopathic) K76.6
  - gastropathy K31.89
  - in (due to) schistosomiasis (bilharziasis) B65.9 [K77]
- postoperative I97.3
- psychogenic F45.8
- pulmonary I27.20
  - with
    - cor pulmonale (chronic) I27.29
      - acute I26.09
    - right heart ventricular strain/failure I27.29
      - acute I26.09
    - right to left shunt related to congenital heart disease I27.83
    - unclear multifactorial mechanisms I27.29
  - arterial (associated) (drug-induced) (toxin-induced) I27.21
  - chronic thromboembolic I27.24
  - due to
    - hematologic disorders I27.29
    - left heart disease I27.22
    - lung diseases and hypoxia I27.23
    - metabolic disorders I27.29
    - specified systemic disorders I27.29
  - group 1 (associated) (drug-induced) (toxin-induced) I27.21
  - group 2 I27.22
  - group 3 I27.23
  - group 4 I27.24
  - group 5 I27.29
  - of newborn (persistent) P29.30
  - primary (idiopathic) I27.0
  - secondary
    - arterial I27.21
    - specified NEC I27.29
- renal — see Hypertension, kidney
- renovascular I15.0
- secondary NEC I15.9

Hypertension, hypertensive — continued
- secondary — continued
  - due to
    - endocrine disorders I15.2
    - pheochromocytoma I15.2
    - renal disorders NEC I15.1
      - arterial I15.0
    - renovascular disorders I15.0
  - specified NEC I15.8
- transient R03.0
  - of pregnancy O13.- ☑
- urgency I16.0
- venous (chronic)
  - due to
    - deep vein thrombosis — see Syndrome, post-thrombotic
  - idiopathic I87.309
    - with
      - inflammation I87.32- ☑
        - with ulcer I87.33- ☑
      - specified complication NEC I87.39- ☑
      - ulcer I87.31- ☑
        - with inflammation I87.33- ☑
    - asymptomatic I87.30- ☑

Hypertensive urgency — see Hypertension
Hyperthecosis ovary E28.8
Hyperthermia (of unknown origin) (see also Hyperpyrexia)
- malignant, due to anesthesia T88.3 ☑
- newborn P81.9
  - environmental P81.0
Hyperthyroid (recurrent) — see Hyperthyroidism
Hyperthyroidism (latent) (pre-adult) (recurrent) E05.90
- with
  - goiter (diffuse) E05.00
    - with thyroid storm E05.01
    - nodular (multinodular) E05.20
      - with thyroid storm E05.21
      - uninodular E05.10
        - with thyroid storm E05.11
  - storm E05.91
- due to ectopic thyroid tissue E05.30
  - with thyroid storm E05.31
- neonatal, transitory P72.1
- specified NEC E05.80
  - with thyroid storm E05.81
Hypertony, hypertonia, hypertonicity
- bladder N31.8
- congenital P94.1
- stomach K31.89
  - psychogenic F45.8
- uterus, uterine (contractions) (complicating delivery) O62.4
Hypertrichosis L68.9
- congenital Q84.2
- eyelid H02.869
  - left H02.866
    - lower H02.865
    - upper H02.864
  - right H02.863
    - lower H02.862
    - upper H02.861
- lanuginosa Q84.2
  - acquired L68.1
- localized L68.2
- specified NEC L68.8
Hypertriglyceridemia, essential E78.1
Hypertrophy, hypertrophic
- adenofibromatous, prostate — see Enlargement, enlarged, prostate
- adenoids (infective) J35.2
  - with tonsils J35.3
- adrenal cortex E27.8
- alveolar process or ridge — see Anomaly, alveolar
- anal papillae K62.89
- artery I77.89
  - congenital NEC Q27.8
    - digestive system Q27.8
    - lower limb Q27.8
    - specified site NEC Q27.8
    - upper limb Q27.8
- auricular — see Hypertrophy, cardiac
- Bartholin's gland N75.8
- bile duct (common) (hepatic) K83.8
- bladder (sphincter) (trigone) N32.89
- bone M89.30
  - carpus M89.34- ☑
  - clavicle M89.31- ☑

Hypertrophy, hypertrophic — *continued*
  bone — *continued*
    femur M89.35- ☑
    fibula M89.36- ☑
    finger M89.34- ☑
    humerus M89.32- ☑
    ilium M89.359
    ischium M89.359
    metacarpus M89.34- ☑
    metatarsus M89.37- ☑
    multiple sites M89.39
    neck M89.38
    radius M89.33- ☑
    rib M89.38
    scapula M89.31- ☑
    skull M89.38
    tarsus M89.37- ☑
    tibia M89.36- ☑
    toe M89.37- ☑
    ulna M89.33- ☑
    vertebra M89.38
  brain G93.89
  breast N62
    cystic — *see* Mastopathy, cystic
    newborn P83.4
    pubertal, massive N62
    puerperal, postpartum — *see* Disorder, breast,
      specified type NEC
    senile (parenchymatous) N62
  cardiac (chronic) (idiopathic) I51.7
    with rheumatic fever (conditions in I00)
      active I01.8
      inactive or quiescent (with chorea) I09.89
    congenital NEC Q24.8
    fatty — *see* Degeneration, myocardial
    hypertensive — *see* Hypertension, heart
    rheumatic (with chorea) I09.89
      active or acute I01.8
        with chorea I02.0
    valve — *see* Endocarditis
  cartilage — *see* Disorder, cartilage, specified type NEC
  cecum — *see* Megacolon
  cervix (uteri) N88.8
    congenital Q51.828
    elongation N88.4
  clitoris (cirrhotic) N90.89
    congenital Q52.6
  colon (*see also* Megacolon)
    congenital Q43.2
  conjunctiva, lymphoid H11.89
  corpora cavernosa N48.89
  cystic duct K82.8
  duodenum K31.89
  endometrium (glandular) (*see also* Hyperplasia, en-
      dometrial) N85.00
    cervix N88.8
  epididymis N50.89
  esophageal hiatus (congenital) Q79.1
    with hernia — *see* Hernia, hiatal
  eyelid — *see* Disorder, eyelid, specified type NEC
  fat pad E65
    knee (infrapatellar) (popliteal) (prepatellar)
      (retropatellar) M79.4
  foot (congenital) Q74.2
  frenulum, frenum (tongue) K14.8
    lip K13.0
  gallbladder K82.8
  gastric mucosa K29.60
    with bleeding K29.61
  gland, glandular R59.9
    generalized R59.1
    localized R59.0
  gum (mucous membrane) K06.1
  heart (idiopathic) (*see also* Hypertrophy, cardiac)
    valve (*see also* Endocarditis) I38
  hemifacial Q67.4
  hepatic — *see* Hypertrophy, liver
  hiatus (esophageal) Q79.1
  hilus gland R59.0
  hymen, congenital Q52.4
  ileum K63.89
  intestine NEC K63.89
  jejunum K63.89
  kidney (compensatory) N28.81
    congenital Q63.3
  labium (majus) (minus) N90.60
  ligament — *see* Disorder, ligament
  lingual tonsil (infective) J35.1

Hypertrophy, hypertrophic — *continued*
  lingual tonsil — *continued*
    with adenoids J35.3
  lip K13.0
    congenital Q18.6
  liver R16.0
    acute K76.89
    cirrhotic — *see* Cirrhosis, liver
    congenital Q44.7
    fatty — *see* Fatty, liver
  lymph, lymphatic gland R59.9
    generalized R59.1
    localized R59.0
    tuberculous — *see* Tuberculosis, lymph gland
  mammary gland — *see* Hypertrophy, breast
  Meckel's diverticulum (congenital) Q43.0
    malignant — *see* Table of Neoplasms, small intes-
      tine, malignant
  median bar — *see* Hyperplasia, prostate
  meibomian gland — *see* Chalazion
  meniscus, knee, congenital Q74.1
  metatarsal head — *see* Hypertrophy, bone, metatarsus
  metatarsus — *see* Hypertrophy, bone, metatarsus
  mucous membrane
    alveolar ridge K06.2
    gum K06.1
    nose (turbinate) J34.3
  muscle M62.89
  muscular coat, artery I77.89
  myocardium (*see also* Hypertrophy, cardiac)
    idiopathic I42.2
  myometrium N85.2
  nail L60.2
    congenital Q84.5
  nasal J34.89
    alae J34.89
    bone J34.89
    cartilage J34.89
    mucous membrane (septum) J34.3
    sinus J34.89
    turbinate J34.3
  nasopharynx, lymphoid (infectional) (tissue) (wall) J35.2
  nipple N62
  organ or site, congenital NEC — *see* Anomaly, by site
  ovary N83.8
  palate (hard) M27.8
    soft K13.79
  pancreas, congenital Q45.3
  parathyroid (gland) E21.0
  parotid gland K11.1
  penis N48.89
  pharyngeal tonsil J35.2
  pharynx J39.2
    lymphoid (infectional) (tissue) (wall) J35.2
  pituitary (anterior) (fossa) (gland) E23.6
  prepuce (congenital) N47.8
    female N90.89
  prostate — *see* Enlargement, enlarged, prostate
    congenital Q55.4
  pseudomuscular G71.09
  pylorus (adult) (muscle) (sphincter) K31.1
    congenital or infantile Q40.0
  rectal, rectum (sphincter) K62.89
  rhinitis (turbinate) J31.0
  salivary gland (any) K11.1
    congenital Q38.4
  scaphoid (tarsal) — *see* Hypertrophy, bone, tarsus
  scar L91.0
  scrotum N50.89
  seminal vesicle N50.89
  sigmoid — *see* Megacolon
  skin L91.9
    specified NEC L91.8
  spermatic cord N50.89
  spleen — *see* Splenomegaly
  spondylitis — *see* Spondylosis
  stomach K31.89
  sublingual gland K11.1
  submandibular gland K11.1
  suprarenal cortex (gland) E27.8
  synovial NEC M67.20
    acromioclavicular M67.21- ☑
    ankle M67.27- ☑
    elbow M67.22- ☑
    foot M67.27- ☑
    hand M67.24- ☑
    hip M67.25- ☑
    knee M67.26- ☑

Hypertrophy, hypertrophic — *continued*
  synovial — *continued*
    multiple sites M67.29
    specified site NEC M67.28
    wrist M67.23- ☑
  tendon — *see* Disorder, tendon, specified type NEC
  testis N44.8
    congenital Q55.29
  thymic, thymus (gland) (congenital) E32.0
  thyroid (gland) — *see* Goiter
  toe (congenital) Q74.2
    acquired (*see also* Deformity, toe, specified NEC)
  tongue K14.8
    congenital Q38.2
    papillae (foliate) K14.3
  tonsils (faucial) (infective) (lingual) (lymphoid) J35.1
    with adenoids J35.3
  tunica vaginalis N50.89
  ureter N28.89
  urethra N36.8
  uterus N85.2
    neck (with elongation) N88.4
    puerperal O90.89
  uvula K13.79
  vagina N89.8
  vas deferens N50.89
  vein I87.8
  ventricle, ventricular (heart) (*see also* Hypertrophy,
      cardiac)
    congenital Q24.8
    in tetralogy of Fallot Q21.3
  verumontanum N36.8
  vocal cord J38.3
  vulva N90.60
    stasis (nonfilarial) N90.69
Hypertropia H50.2- ☑
Hypertyrosinemia E70.21
Hyperuricemia (asymptomatic) E79.0
Hyperuricosuria R82.993
Hypervalinemia E71.19
Hyperventilation (tetany) R06.4
  hysterical F45.8
  psychogenic F45.8
  syndrome F45.8
Hypervitaminosis (dietary) NEC E67.8
  A E67.0
    administered as drug (prolonged intake) — *see* Ta-
      ble of Drugs and Chemicals, vitamins, adverse
      effect
    overdose or wrong substance given or taken — *see*
      Table of Drugs and Chemicals, vitamins, poi-
      soning
  B6 E67.2
  D E67.3
    administered as drug (prolonged intake) — *see* Ta-
      ble of Drugs and Chemicals, vitamins, adverse
      effect
    overdose or wrong substance given or taken — *see*
      Table of Drugs and Chemicals, vitamins, poi-
      soning
  K E67.8
    administered as drug (prolonged intake) — *see* Ta-
      ble of Drugs and Chemicals, vitamins, adverse
      effect
    overdose or wrong substance given or taken — *see*
      Table of Drugs and Chemicals, vitamins, poi-
      soning
Hypervolemia E87.70
  specified NEC E87.79
Hypesthesia R20.1
  cornea — *see* Anesthesia, cornea
Hyphema H21.0- ☑
  traumatic S05.1- ☑
Hypoacidity, gastric K31.89
  psychogenic F45.8
Hypoadrenalism, hypoadrenia E27.40
  primary E27.1
  tuberculous A18.7
Hypoadrenocorticism E27.40
  pituitary E23.0
  primary E27.1
Hypoalbuminemia E88.09
Hypoaldosteronism E27.40
Hypoalphalipoproteinemia E78.6
Hypobarism T70.29 ☑
Hypobaropathy T70.29 ☑
Hypobetalipoproteinemia (familial) E78.6
Hypocalcemia E83.51

☑ **Additional Character Required** — Refer to the Tabular List for Character Selection   ⬇ **Subterms under main terms may continue to next column or page**

Hypocalcemia — *continued*
  dietary E58
  neonatal P71.1
    due to cow's milk P71.0
  phosphate-loading (newborn) P71.1
Hypochloremia E87.8
Hypochlorhydria K31.89
  neurotic F45.8
  psychogenic F45.8
Hypochondria, hypochondriac, hypochondriasis
  (reaction) F45.21
  sleep F51.03
Hypochondrogenesis Q77.0
Hypochondroplasia Q77.4
Hypochromasia, blood cells D50.8
Hypocitraturia R82.991
Hypodontia — *see* Anodontia
Hypoeosinophilia D72.89
Hypoesthesia R20.1
Hypofibrinogenemia D68.8
  acquired D65
  congenital (hereditary) D68.2
Hypofunction
  adrenocortical E27.40
    drug-induced E27.3
    postprocedural E89.6
    primary E27.1
  adrenomedullary, postprocedural E89.6
  cerebral R29.818
  corticoadrenal NEC E27.40
  intestinal K59.8
  labyrinth — *see* subcategory H83.2 ☑
  ovary E28.39
  pituitary (gland) (anterior) E23.0
  testicular E29.1
    postprocedural (postsurgical) (postirradiation) (iatrogenic) E89.5
Hypogalactia O92.4
Hypogammaglobulinemia (*see also* Agammaglobulinemia) D80.1
  hereditary D80.0
  nonfamilial D80.1
  transient, of infancy D80.7
Hypogenitalism (congenital) — *see* Hypogonadism
Hypoglossia Q38.3
Hypoglycemia (spontaneous) E16.2
  coma E15
    diabetic — *see* Diabetes, by type, with hypoglycemia, with coma
  diabetic — *see* Diabetes, hypoglycemia
  dietary counseling and surveillance Z71.3
  drug-induced E16.0
    with coma (nondiabetic) E15
  due to insulin E16.0
    with coma (nondiabetic) E15
    therapeutic misadventure — *see* subcategory T38.3 ☑
  functional, nonhyperinsulinemic E16.1
  iatrogenic E16.0
    with coma (nondiabetic) E15
  in infant of diabetic mother P70.1
    gestational diabetes P70.0
  infantile E16.1
  leucine-induced E71.19
  neonatal (transitory) P70.4
    iatrogenic P70.3
  reactive (not drug-induced) E16.1
  transitory neonatal P70.4
Hypogonadism
  female E28.39
  hypogonadotropic E23.0
  male E29.1
  ovarian (primary) E28.39
  pituitary E23.0
  testicular (primary) E29.1
Hypohidrosis, hypoidrosis L74.4
Hypoinsulinemia, postprocedural E89.1
Hypokalemia E87.6
Hypoleukocytosis — *see* Agranulocytosis
Hypolipoproteinemia (alpha) (beta) E78.6
Hypomagnesemia E83.42
  neonatal P71.2
Hypomania, hypomanic reaction F30.8
Hypomenorrhea — *see* Oligomenorrhea
Hypometabolism R63.8
Hypomotility
  gastrointestinal (tract) K31.89
    psychogenic F45.8

Hypomotility — *continued*
  intestine K59.8
    psychogenic F45.8
  stomach K31.89
    psychogenic F45.8
Hyponasality R49.22
Hyponatremia E87.1
Hypo-osmolality E87.1
Hypo-ovarianism, hypo-ovarism E28.39
Hypoparathyroidism E20.9
  familial E20.8
  idiopathic E20.0
  neonatal, transitory P71.4
  postprocedural E89.2
  specified NEC E20.8
Hypoperfusion (in)
  newborn P96.89
Hypopharyngitis — *see* Laryngopharyngitis
Hypophoria H50.53
Hypophosphatemia, hypophosphatasia (acquired) (congenital) (renal) E83.39
  familial E83.31
Hypophyseal, hypophysis (*see also* condition)
  dwarfism E23.0
  gigantism E22.0
Hypopiesis — *see* Hypotension
Hypopinealism E34.8
Hypopituitarism (juvenile) E23.0
  drug-induced E23.1
  due to
    hypophysectomy E89.3
    radiotherapy E89.3
  iatrogenic NEC E23.1
  postirradiation E89.3
  postpartum O99.285
  postprocedural E89.3
Hypoplasia, hypoplastic
  adrenal (gland), congenital Q89.1
  alimentary tract, congenital Q45.8
    upper Q40.8
  anus, anal (canal) Q42.3
    with fistula Q42.2
  aorta, aortic Q25.42
    ascending, in hypoplastic left heart syndrome Q23.4
    valve Q23.1
      in hypoplastic left heart syndrome Q23.4
  areola, congenital Q83.8
  arm (congenital) — *see* Defect, reduction, upper limb
  artery (peripheral) Q27.8
    brain (congenital) Q28.3
    coronary Q24.5
    digestive system Q27.8
    lower limb Q27.8
    pulmonary Q25.79
      functional, unilateral J43.0
    retinal (congenital) Q14.1
    specified site NEC Q27.8
    umbilical Q27.0
    upper limb Q27.8
  auditory canal Q17.8
    causing impairment of hearing Q16.9
  biliary duct or passage Q44.5
  bone NOS Q79.9
    face Q75.8
    marrow D61.9
      megakaryocytic D69.49
    skull — *see* Hypoplasia, skull
  brain Q02
    gyri Q04.3
    part of Q04.3
  breast (areola) N64.82
  bronchus Q32.4
  cardiac Q24.8
  carpus — *see* Defect, reduction, upper limb, specified type NEC
  cartilage hair Q78.8
  cecum Q42.8
  cementum K00.4
  cephalic Q02
  cerebellum Q04.3
  cervix (uteri), congenital Q51.821
  clavicle (congenital) Q74.0
  coccyx Q76.49
  colon Q42.9
    specified NEC Q42.8
  corpus callosum Q04.0
  cricoid cartilage Q31.2
  digestive organ(s) or tract NEC Q45.8

Hypoplasia, hypoplastic — *continued*
  digestive organ(s) or tract — *continued*
    upper (congenital) Q40.8
  ear (auricle) (lobe) Q17.2
    middle Q16.4
  enamel of teeth (neonatal) (postnatal) (prenatal) K00.4
  endocrine (gland) NEC Q89.2
  endometrium N85.8
  epididymis (congenital) Q55.4
  epiglottis Q31.2
  erythroid, congenital D61.01
  esophagus (congenital) Q39.8
  eustachian tube Q17.8
  eye Q11.2
  eyelid (congenital) Q10.3
  face Q18.8
    bone(s) Q75.8
  femur (congenital) — *see* Defect, reduction, lower limb, specified type NEC
  fibula (congenital) — *see* Defect, reduction, lower limb, specified type NEC
  finger (congenital) — *see* Defect, reduction, upper limb, specified type NEC
  focal dermal Q82.8
  foot — *see* Defect, reduction, lower limb, specified type NEC
  gallbladder Q44.0
  genitalia, genital organ(s)
    female, congenital Q52.8
      external Q52.79
      internal NEC Q52.8
    in adiposogenital dystrophy E23.6
  glottis Q31.2
  hair Q84.2
  hand (congenital) — *see* Defect, reduction, upper limb, specified type NEC
  heart Q24.8
  humerus (congenital) — *see* Defect, reduction, upper limb, specified type NEC
  intestine (small) Q41.9
    large Q42.9
      specified NEC Q42.8
  jaw M26.09
    alveolar M26.79
    lower M26.04
      alveolar M26.74
    upper M26.02
      alveolar M26.73
  kidney(s) Q60.5
    bilateral Q60.4
    unilateral Q60.3
  labium (majus) (minus), congenital Q52.79
  larynx Q31.2
  left heart syndrome Q23.4
  leg (congenital) — *see* Defect, reduction, lower limb
  limb Q73.8
    lower (congenital) — *see* Defect, reduction, lower limb
    upper (congenital) — *see* Defect, reduction, upper limb
  liver Q44.7
  lung (lobe) (not associated with short gestation) Q33.6
    associated with immaturity, low birth weight, prematurity, or short gestation P28.0
  mammary (areola), congenital Q83.8
  mandible, mandibular M26.04
    alveolar M26.74
    unilateral condylar M27.8
  maxillary M26.02
    alveolar M26.73
  medullary D61.9
  megakaryocytic D69.49
  metacarpus — *see* Defect, reduction, upper limb, specified type NEC
  metatarsus — *see* Defect, reduction, lower limb, specified type NEC
  muscle Q79.8
  nail(s) Q84.6
  nose, nasal Q30.1
  optic nerve H47.03- ☑
  osseous meatus (ear) Q17.8
  ovary, congenital Q50.39
  pancreas Q45.0
  parathyroid (gland) Q89.2
  parotid gland Q38.4
  patella Q74.1
  pelvis, pelvic girdle Q74.2
  penis (congenital) Q55.62

⬇ Subterms under main terms may continue to next column or page   ☑ Additional Character Required — Refer to the Tabular List for Character Selection   177

Hypocalcemia — Hypoplasia, hypoplastic

Hypoplasia, hypoplastic — *continued*
  peripheral vascular system Q27.8
    digestive system Q27.8
    lower limb Q27.8
    specified site NEC Q27.8
    upper limb Q27.8
  pituitary (gland) (congenital) Q89.2
  pulmonary (not associated with short gestation) Q33.6
    artery, functional J43.0
    associated with short gestation P28.0
  radioulnar — *see* Defect, reduction, upper limb, specified type NEC
  radius — *see* Defect, reduction, upper limb
  rectum Q42.1
    with fistula Q42.0
  respiratory system NEC Q34.8
  rib Q76.6
  right heart syndrome Q22.6
  sacrum Q76.49
  scapula Q74.0
  scrotum Q55.1
  shoulder girdle Q74.0
  skin Q82.8
  skull (bone) Q75.8
    with
      anencephaly Q00.0
      encephalocele — *see* Encephalocele
      hydrocephalus Q03.9
        with spina bifida — *see* Spina bifida, by site, with hydrocephalus
      microcephaly Q02
  spinal (cord) (ventral horn cell) Q06.1
  spine Q76.49
  sternum Q76.7
  tarsus — *see* Defect, reduction, lower limb, specified type NEC
  testis Q55.1
  thymic, with immunodeficiency D82.1
  thymus (gland) Q89.2
    with immunodeficiency D82.1
  thyroid (gland) E03.1
    cartilage Q31.2
  tibiofibular (congenital) — *see* Defect, reduction, lower limb, specified type NEC
  toe — *see* Defect, reduction, lower limb, specified type NEC
  tongue Q38.3
  Turner's K00.4
  ulna (congenital) — *see* Defect, reduction, upper limb
  umbilical artery Q27.0
  unilateral condylar M27.8
  ureter Q62.8
  uterus, congenital Q51.811
  vagina Q52.4
  vascular NEC peripheral Q27.8
    brain Q28.3
    digestive system Q27.8
    lower limb Q27.8
    specified site NEC Q27.8
    upper limb Q27.8
  vein(s) (peripheral) Q27.8
    brain Q28.3
    digestive system Q27.8
    great Q26.8
    lower limb Q27.8
    specified site NEC Q27.8
    upper limb Q27.8
  vena cava (inferior) (superior) Q26.8
  vertebra Q76.49
  vulva, congenital Q52.79
  zonule (ciliary) Q12.8
Hypoplasminogenemia E88.02
Hypopnea, obstructive sleep apnea G47.33
Hypopotassemia E87.6
Hypoproconvertinemia, congenital (hereditary) D68.2
Hypoproteinemia E77.8
Hypoprothrombinemia (congenital) (hereditary) (idiopathic) D68.2
  acquired D68.4
  newborn, transient P61.6
Hypoptyalism K11.7
Hypopyon (eye) (anterior chamber) — *see* Iridocyclitis, acute, hypopyon
Hypopyrexia R68.0
Hyporeflexia R29.2
Hyposecretion
  ACTH E23.0
  antidiuretic hormone E23.2

Hyposecretion — *continued*
  ovary E28.39
  salivary gland (any) K11.7
  vasopressin E23.2
Hyposegmentation, leukocytic, hereditary D72.0
Hyposiderinemia D50.9
Hypospadias Q54.9
  balanic Q54.0
  coronal Q54.0
  glandular Q54.0
  penile Q54.1
  penoscrotal Q54.2
  perineal Q54.3
  specified NEC Q54.8
Hypospermatogenesis — *see* Oligospermia
Hyposplenism D73.0
Hypostasis pulmonary, passive — *see* Edema, lung
Hypostatic — *see* condition
Hyposthenuria N28.89
Hypotension (arterial) (constitutional) I95.9
  chronic I95.89
  due to (of) hemodialysis I95.3
  drug-induced I95.2
  iatrogenic I95.89
  idiopathic (permanent) I95.0
  intracranial, following ventricular shunting (ventriculostomy) G97.2
  intra-dialytic I95.3
  maternal, syndrome (following labor and delivery) O26.5- ☑
  neurogenic, orthostatic G90.3
  orthostatic (chronic) I95.1
    due to drugs I95.2
    neurogenic G90.3
  postoperative I95.81
  postural I95.1
  specified NEC I95.89
Hypothermia (accidental) T68 ☑
  due to anesthesia, anesthetic T88.51 ☑
  low environmental temperature T68 ☑
  neonatal P80.9
    environmental (mild) NEC P80.8
    mild P80.8
    severe (chronic) (cold injury syndrome) P80.0
    specified NEC P80.8
  not associated with low environmental temperature R68.0
Hypothyroidism (acquired) E03.9
  autoimmune — *see* Thyroiditis, autoimmune
  congenital (without goiter) E03.1
    with goiter (diffuse) E03.0
  due to
    exogenous substance NEC E03.2
    iodine-deficiency, acquired E01.8
      subclinical E02
    irradiation therapy E89.0
    medicament NEC E03.2
    P-aminosalicylic acid (PAS) E03.2
    phenylbutazone E03.2
    resorcinol E03.2
    sulfonamide E03.2
    surgery E89.0
    thiourea group drugs E03.2
  iatrogenic NEC E03.2
  iodine-deficiency (acquired) E01.8
    congenital — *see* Syndrome, iodine- deficiency, congenital
    subclinical E02
  neonatal, transitory P72.2
  postinfectious E03.3
  postirradiation E89.0
  postprocedural E89.0
  postsurgical E89.0
  specified NEC E03.8
  subclinical, iodine-deficiency related E02
Hypotonia, hypotonicity, hypotony
  bladder N31.2
  congenital (benign) P94.2
  eye — *see* Disorder, globe, hypotony
Hypotrichosis — *see* Alopecia
Hypotropia H50.2- ☑
Hypoventilation R06.89
  congenital central alveolar G47.35
  sleep related
    idiopathic nonobstructive alveolar G47.34
    in conditions classified elsewhere G47.36
Hypovitaminosis — *see* Deficiency, vitamin
Hypovolemia E86.1

Hypovolemia — *continued*
  surgical shock T81.19 ☑
  traumatic (shock) T79.4 ☑
Hypoxemia R09.02
  newborn P84
  sleep related, in conditions classified elsewhere G47.36
Hypoxia (*see also* Anoxia) R09.02
  cerebral, during a procedure NEC G97.81
    postprocedural NEC G97.82
  intrauterine P84
  myocardial — *see* Insufficiency, coronary
  newborn P84
  sleep-related G47.34
Hypsarhythmia — *see* Epilepsy, generalized, specified NEC
Hysteralgia, pregnant uterus O26.89- ☑
Hysteria, hysterical (conversion) (dissociative state) F44.9
  anxiety F41.8
  convulsions F44.5
  psychosis, acute F44.9
Hysteroepilepsy F44.5

I

IBDU (colonic inflammatory bowel dissease unclassified) K52.3
Ichthyoparasitism due to Vandellia cirrhosa B88.8
Ichthyosis (congenital) Q80.9
  acquired L85.0
  fetalis Q80.4
  hystrix Q80.8
  lamellar Q80.2
  lingual K13.29
  palmaris and plantaris Q82.8
  simplex Q80.0
  vera Q80.8
  vulgaris Q80.0
  X-linked Q80.1
Ichthyotoxism — *see* Poisoning, fish
  bacterial — *see* Intoxication, foodborne
Icteroanemia, hemolytic (acquired) D59.9
  congenital — *see* Spherocytosis
Icterus (*see also* Jaundice)
  conjunctiva R17
  gravis, newborn P55.0
  hematogenous (acquired) D59.9
  hemolytic (acquired) D59.9
    congenital — *see* Spherocytosis
  hemorrhagic (acute) (leptospiral) (spirochetal) A27.0
    newborn P53
  infectious B15.9
    with hepatic coma B15.0
    leptospiral A27.0
    spirochetal A27.0
  neonatorum — *see* Jaundice, newborn
  newborn P59.9
  spirochetal A27.0
Ictus solaris, solis T67.0 ☑
Id reaction (due to bacteria) L30.2
Ideation
  homicidal R45.850
  suicidal R45.851
Identity disorder (child) F64.9
  gender role F64.2
  psychosexual F64.2
Idioglossia F80.0
Idiopathic — *see* condition
Idiot, idiocy (congenital) F73
  amaurotic (Bielschowsky(-Jansky)) (family) (infantile (late)) (juvenile (late)) (Vogt-Spielmeyer) E75.4
  microcephalic Q02
IgE asthma J45.909
IIAC (idiopathic infantile arterial calcification) Q28.8
Ileitis (chronic) (noninfectious) (*see also* Enteritis) K52.9
  backwash — *see* Pancolitis, ulcerative (chronic)
  infectious A09
  regional (ulcerative) — *see* Enteritis, regional, small intestine
  segmental — *see* Enteritis, regional
  terminal (ulcerative) — *see* Enteritis, regional, small intestine
Ileocolitis (*see also* Enteritis) K52.9
  infectious A09
  regional — *see* Enteritis, regional
  ulcerative K51.0- ☑

Ileostomy
  attention to Z43.2
  malfunctioning K94.13
  status Z93.2
    with complication — *see* Complications, enterostomy
Ileotyphus — *see* Typhoid
Ileum — *see* condition
Ileus (bowel) (colon) (inhibitory) (intestine) K56.7
  adynamic K56.0
  due to gallstone (in intestine) K56.3
  duodenal (chronic) K31.5
  gallstone K56.3
  mechanical NEC (*see also* Obstruction, intestine, specified NEC) K56.699
  meconium P76.0
    in cystic fibrosis E84.11
    meaning meconium plug (without cystic fibrosis) P76.0
  myxedema K59.8
  neurogenic K56.0
    Hirschsprung's disease or megacolon Q43.1
  newborn
    due to meconium P76.0
      in cystic fibrosis E84.11
      meaning meconium plug (without cystic fibrosis) P76.0
    transitory P76.1
  obstructive (*see also* Obstruction, intestine, specified NEC) K56.699
  paralytic K56.0
  postoperative K91.89
Iliac — *see* condition
Iliotibial band syndrome M76.3- ☑
Illiteracy Z55.0
Illness (*see also* Disease) R69
  manic-depressive — *see* Disorder, bipolar
Imbalance R26.89
  autonomic G90.8
  constituents of food intake E63.1
  electrolyte E87.8
    with
      abortion — *see* Abortion by type, complicated by, electrolyte imbalance
      molar pregnancy O08.5
    due to hyperemesis gravidarum O21.1
    following ectopic or molar pregnancy O08.5
    neonatal, transitory NEC P74.49
      potassium
        hyperkalemia P74.31
        hypokalemia P74.32
      sodium
        hypernatremia P74.21
        hyponatremia P74.22
  endocrine E34.9
  eye muscle NOS H50.9
  hormone E34.9
  hysterical F44.4
  labyrinth — *see* subcategory H83.2 ☑
  posture R29.3
  protein-energy — *see* Malnutrition
  sympathetic G90.8
Imbecile, imbecility (I.Q. 35-49) F71
Imbedding, intrauterine device T83.39 ☑
Imbibition, cholesterol (gallbladder) K82.4
Imbrication, teeth,, fully erupted M26.30
Imerslund (-Gräsbeck) **syndrome** D51.1
Immature (*see also* Immaturity)
  birth (less than 37 completed weeks) — *see* Preterm, newborn
    extremely (less than 28 completed weeks) — *see* Immaturity, extreme
  personality F60.89
Immaturity (less than 37 completed weeks) (*see also* Preterm, newborn)
  extreme of newborn (less than 28 completed weeks of gestation) (less than 196 completed days of gestation) (unspecified weeks of gestation) P07.20
    gestational age
      23 completed weeks (23 weeks, 0 days through 23 weeks, 6 days) P07.22
      24 completed weeks (24 weeks, 0 days through 24 weeks, 6 days) P07.23
      25 completed weeks (25 weeks, 0 days through 25 weeks, 6 days) P07.24
      26 completed weeks (26 weeks, 0 days through 26 weeks, 6 days) P07.25

Immaturity — *continued*
  extreme of newborn — *continued*
    gestational age — *continued*
      27 completed weeks (27 weeks, 0 days through 27 weeks, 6 days) P07.26
      less than 23 completed weeks P07.21
  fetus or infant light-for-dates — *see* Light-for-dates
  lung, newborn P28.0
  organ or site NEC — *see* Hypoplasia
  pulmonary, newborn P28.0
  reaction F60.89
  sexual (female) (male), after puberty E30.0
Immersion T75.1 ☑
  foot T69.02- ☑
  hand T69.01- ☑
Immobile, immobility
  complete, due to severe physical disability or frailty R53.2
  intestine K59.8
  syndrome (paraplegic) M62.3
Immune reconstitution (inflammatory) syndrome [IRIS] D89.3
Immunization (*see also* Vaccination)
  ABO — *see* Incompatibility, ABO
    in newborn P55.1
  appropriate for age
    child (over 28 days old) Z00.129
      with abnormal findings Z00.121
  complication — *see* Complications, vaccination
  encounter for Z23
  not done (not carried out) Z28.9
    because (of)
      acute illness of patient Z28.01
      allergy to vaccine (or component) Z28.04
      caregiver refusal Z28.82
      chronic illness of patient Z28.02
      contraindication NEC Z28.09
      delay in delivery of vaccine Z28.83
      group pressure Z28.1
      guardian refusal Z28.82
      immune compromised state of patient Z28.03
      lack of availability of vaccine Z28.83
      manufacturer delay of vaccine Z28.83
      parent refusal Z28.82
      patient had disease being vaccinated against Z28.81
      patient refusal Z28.21
      patient's belief Z28.1
      religious beliefs of patient Z28.1
      specified reason NEC Z28.89
        of patient Z28.29
      unavailability of vaccine Z28.83
      unspecified patient reason Z28.20
    Rh factor
      affecting management of pregnancy NEC O36.09- ☑
        anti-D antibody O36.01- ☑
      from transfusion — *see* Complication(s), transfusion, incompatibility reaction, Rh (factor)
Immunocytoma C83.0- ☑
Immunodeficiency D84.9
  with
    adenosine-deaminase deficiency D81.3
    antibody defects D80.9
      specified type NEC D80.8
    hyperimmunoglobulinemia D80.6
    increased immunoglobulin M (IgM) D80.5
    major defect D82.9
      specified type NEC D82.8
    partial albinism D82.8
    short-limbed stature D82.2
    thrombocytopenia and eczema D82.0
  antibody with
    hyperimmunoglobulinemia D80.6
    near-normal immunoglobulins D80.6
  autosomal recessive, Swiss type D80.0
  combined D81.9
    biotin-dependent carboxylase D81.819
      biotinidase D81.810
      holocarboxylase synthetase D81.818
      specified type NEC D81.818
    severe (SCID) D81.9
      with
        low or normal B-cell numbers D81.2
        low T- and B-cell numbers D81.1
        reticular dysgenesis D81.0
    specified type NEC D81.89
  common variable D83.9

Immunodeficiency — *continued*
  common variable — *continued*
    with
      abnormalities of B-cell numbers and function D83.0
      autoantibodies to B- or T-cells D83.2
      immunoregulatory T-cell disorders D83.1
      specified type NEC D83.8
  following hereditary defective response to Epstein-Barr virus (EBV) D82.3
  selective, immunoglobulin
    A (IgA) D80.2
    G (IgG) (subclasses) D80.3
    M (IgM) D80.4
  severe combined (SCID) D81.9
  specified type NEC D84.8
  X-linked, with increased IgM D80.5
Immunotherapy (encounter for)
  antineoplastic Z51.12
Impaction, impacted
  bowel, colon, rectum (*see also* Impaction, fecal) K56.49
    by gallstone K56.3
  calculus — *see* Calculus
  cerumen (ear) (external) H61.2- ☑
  cuspid — *see* Impaction, tooth
  dental (same or adjacent tooth) K01.1
  fecal, feces K56.41
  fracture — *see* Fracture, by site
  gallbladder — *see* Calculus, gallbladder
  gallstone(s) — *see* Calculus, gallbladder
    bile duct (common) (hepatic) — *see* Calculus, bile duct
    cystic duct — *see* Calculus, gallbladder
    in intestine, with obstruction (any part) K56.3
  intestine (calculous) NEC (*see also* Impaction, fecal) K56.49
    gallstone, with ileus K56.3
  intrauterine device (IUD) T83.39 ☑
  molar — *see* Impaction, tooth
  shoulder, causing obstructed labor O66.0
  tooth, teeth K01.1
  turbinate J34.89
Impaired, impairment (function)
  auditory discrimination — *see* Abnormal, auditory perception
  cognitive, mild, so stated G31.84
  dual sensory Z73.82
  fasting glucose R73.01
  glucose tolerance (oral) R73.02
  hearing — *see* Deafness
  heart — *see* Disease, heart
  kidney N28.9
    disorder resulting from N25.9
      specified NEC N25.89
  liver K72.90
    with coma K72.91
  mastication K08.89
  mild cognitive, so stated G31.84
  mobility
    ear ossicles — *see* Ankylosis, ear ossicles
    requiring care provider Z74.09
  myocardium, myocardial — *see* Insufficiency, myocardial
  rectal sphincter R19.8
  renal (acute) (chronic) N28.9
    disorder resulting from N25.9
      specified NEC N25.89
  vision NEC H54.7
    both eyes H54.3
Impediment, speech R47.9
  psychogenic (childhood) F98.8
  slurring R47.81
  specified NEC R47.89
Impending
  coronary syndrome I20.0
  delirium tremens F10.239
  myocardial infarction I20.0
Imperception auditory (acquired) (*see also* Deafness)
  congenital H93.25
Imperfect
  aeration, lung (newborn) NEC — *see* Atelectasis
  closure (congenital)
    alimentary tract NEC Q45.8
      lower Q43.8
      upper Q40.8
    atrioventricular ostium Q21.2
    atrium (secundum) Q21.1
    branchial cleft NOS Q18.2

Imperfect — continued
  closure — continued
    branchial cleft — continued
      cyst Q18.0
      fistula Q18.0
      sinus Q18.0
    choroid Q14.3
    cricoid cartilage Q31.8
    cusps, heart valve NEC Q24.8
      pulmonary Q22.3
    ductus
      arteriosus Q25.0
      Botalli Q25.0
    ear drum (causing impairment of hearing) Q16.4
    esophagus with communication to bronchus or trachea Q39.1
    eyelid Q10.3
    foramen
      botalli Q21.1
      ovale Q21.1
    genitalia, genital organ(s) or system
      female Q52.8
        external Q52.79
        internal NEC Q52.8
      male Q55.8
    glottis Q31.8
    interatrial ostium or septum Q21.1
    interauricular ostium or septum Q21.1
    interventricular ostium or septum Q21.0
    larynx Q31.8
    lip — see Cleft, lip
    nasal septum Q30.3
    nose Q30.2
    omphalomesenteric duct Q43.0
    optic nerve entry Q14.2
    organ or site not listed — see Anomaly, by site
    ostium
      interatrial Q21.1
      interauricular Q21.1
      interventricular Q21.0
    palate — see Cleft, palate
    preauricular sinus Q18.1
    retina Q14.1
    roof of orbit Q75.8
    sclera Q13.5
    septum
      aorticopulmonary Q21.4
      atrial (secundum) Q21.1
      between aorta and pulmonary artery Q21.4
      heart Q21.9
      interatrial (secundum) Q21.1
      interauricular (secundum) Q21.1
      interventricular Q21.0
        in tetralogy of Fallot Q21.3
      nasal Q30.3
      ventricular Q21.0
        with pulmonary stenosis or atresia, dextraposition of aorta, and hypertrophy of right ventricle Q21.3
        in tetralogy of Fallot Q21.3
    skull Q75.0
      with
        anencephaly Q00.0
        encephalocele — see Encephalocele
        hydrocephalus Q03.9
          with spina bifida — see Spina bifida, by site, with hydrocephalus
        microcephaly Q02
    spine (with meningocele) — see Spina bifida
    trachea Q32.1
    tympanic membrane (causing impairment of hearing) Q16.4
    uterus Q51.818
    vitelline duct Q43.0
  erection — see Dysfunction, sexual, male, erectile
  fusion — see Imperfect, closure
  inflation, lung (newborn) — see Atelectasis
  posture R29.3
  rotation, intestine Q43.3
  septum, ventricular Q21.0
Imperfectly descended testis — see Cryptorchid
Imperforate (congenital) (see also Atresia)
  anus Q42.3
    with fistula Q42.2
  cervix (uteri) Q51.828
  esophagus Q39.0
    with tracheoesophageal fistula Q39.1
  hymen Q52.3

Imperforate — continued
  jejunum Q41.1
  pharynx Q38.8
  rectum Q42.1
    with fistula Q42.0
  urethra Q64.39
  vagina Q52.4
Impervious (congenital) (see also Atresia)
  anus Q42.3
    with fistula Q42.2
  bile duct Q44.2
  esophagus Q39.0
    with tracheoesophageal fistula Q39.1
  intestine (small) Q41.9
    large Q42.9
      specified NEC Q42.8
  rectum Q42.1
    with fistula Q42.0
  ureter — see Atresia, ureter
  urethra Q64.39
Impetiginization of dermatoses L01.1
Impetigo (any organism) (any site) (circinate) (contagiosa) (simplex) (vulgaris) L01.00
  Bockhart's L01.02
  bullous, bullosa L01.03
  external ear L01.00 [H62.40]
  follicularis L01.02
  furfuracea L30.5
  herpetiformis L40.1
    nonobstetrical L40.1
  neonatorum L01.03
  nonbullous L01.01
  specified type NEC L01.09
  ulcerative L01.09
Impingement (on teeth)
  soft tissue
    anterior M26.81
    posterior M26.82
Implant, endometrial N80.9
Implantation
  anomalous — see Anomaly, by site
    ureter Q62.63
  cyst
    external area or site (skin) NEC L72.0
    iris — see Cyst, iris, implantation
    vagina N89.8
    vulva N90.7
  dermoid (cyst) — see Implantation, cyst
Impotence (sexual) N52.9
  counseling Z70.1
  organic origin (see also Dysfunction, sexual, male, erectile) N52.9
  psychogenic F52.21
Impression, basilar Q75.8
Imprisonment, anxiety concerning Z65.1
Improper care (child) (newborn) — see Maltreatment
Improperly tied umbilical cord (causing hemorrhage) P51.8
Impulsiveness (impulsive) R45.87
Inability to swallow — see Aphagia
Inaccessible, inaccessibility
  health care NEC Z75.3
    due to
      waiting period Z75.2
        for admission to facility elsewhere Z75.1
    other helping agencies Z75.4
Inactive — see condition
Inadequate, inadequacy
  aesthetics of dental restoration K08.56
  biologic, constitutional, functional, or social F60.7
  development
    child R62.50
    genitalia
      after puberty NEC E30.0
      congenital
        female Q52.8
          external Q52.79
          internal Q52.8
        male Q55.8
    lungs Q33.6
      associated with short gestation P28.0
    organ or site not listed — see Anomaly, by site
  diet (causing nutritional deficiency) E63.9
  eating habits Z72.4
  environment, household Z59.1
  family support Z63.8
  food (supply) NEC Z59.4
    hunger effects T73.0 ☑

Inadequate, inadequacy — continued
  functional F60.7
  household care, due to
    family member
      handicapped or ill Z74.2
      on vacation Z75.5
      temporarily away from home Z74.2
    technical defects in home Z59.1
    temporary absence from home of person rendering care Z74.2
  housing (heating) (space) Z59.1
  income (financial) Z59.6
  intrafamilial communication Z63.8
  material resources Z59.9
  mental — see Disability, intellectual
  parental supervision or control of child Z62.0
  personality F60.7
  pulmonary
    function R06.89
      newborn P28.5
    ventilation, newborn P28.5
  sample of cytologic smear
    anus R85.615
    cervix R87.615
    vagina R87.625
  social F60.7
    insurance Z59.7
    skills NEC Z73.4
  supervision of child by parent Z62.0
  teaching affecting education Z55.8
  welfare support Z59.7
Inanition R64
  with edema — see Malnutrition, severe
  due to
    deprivation of food T73.0 ☑
    malnutrition — see Malnutrition
  fever R50.9
Inappropriate
  change in quantitative human chorionic gonadotropin (hCG) in early pregnancy O02.81
  diet or eating habits Z72.4
  level of quantitative human chorionic gonadotropin (hCG) for gestational age in early pregnancy O02.81
  secretion
    antidiuretic hormone (ADH) (excessive) E22.2
      deficiency E23.2
    pituitary (posterior) E22.2
Inattention at or after birth — see Neglect
Incarceration, incarcerated
  enterocele K46.0
    gangrenous K46.1
  epiplocele K46.0
    gangrenous K46.1
  exomphalos K42.0
    gangrenous K42.1
  hernia (see also Hernia, by site, with obstruction)
    with gangrene — see Hernia, by site, with gangrene
  iris, in wound — see Injury, eye, laceration, with prolapse
  lens, in wound — see Injury, eye, laceration, with prolapse
  omphalocele K42.0
  prison, anxiety concerning Z65.1
  rupture — see Hernia, by site
  sarcoepiplocele K46.0
    gangrenous K46.1
  sarcoepiplomphalocele K42.0
    with gangrene K42.1
  uterus N85.8
    gravid O34.51- ☑
      causing obstructed labor O65.5
Incised wound
  external — see Laceration
  internal organs — see Injury, by site
Incision, incisional
  hernia K43.2
    with
      gangrene (and obstruction) K43.1
      obstruction K43.0
  surgical, complication — see Complications, surgical procedure
  traumatic
    external — see Laceration
    internal organs — see Injury, by site
Inclusion
  azurophilic leukocytic D72.0
  blennorrhea (neonatal) (newborn) P39.1

☑ Additional Character Required — Refer to the Tabular List for Character Selection　　　　☝ Subterms under main terms may continue to next column or page

Inclusion — *continued*
 gallbladder in liver (congenital) Q44.1
Incompatibility
 ABO
  affecting management of pregnancy O36.11- ☑
   anti-A sensitization O36.11- ☑
   anti-B sensitization O36.19- ☑
   specified NEC O36.19- ☑
  infusion or transfusion reaction — *see* Complication(s), transfusion, incompatibility reaction, ABO
  newborn P55.1
 blood (group) (Duffy) (K) (Kell) (Kidd) (Lewis) (M) (S) NEC
  affecting management of pregnancy O36.11- ☑
   anti-A sensitization O36.11- ☑
   anti-B sensitization O36.19- ☑
  infusion or transfusion reaction T80.89 ☑
  newborn P55.8
 divorce or estrangement Z63.5
 Rh (blood group) (factor) Z31.82
  affecting management of pregnancy NEC O36.09- ☑
   anti-D antibody O36.01- ☑
  infusion or transfusion reaction — *see* Complication(s), transfusion, incompatibility reaction, Rh (factor)
  newborn P55.0
 rhesus — *see* Incompatibility, Rh
Incompetency, incompetent, incompetence
 annular
  aortic (valve) — *see* Insufficiency, aortic
  mitral (valve) I34.0
  pulmonary valve (heart) I37.1
 aortic (valve) — *see* Insufficiency, aortic
 cardiac valve — *see* Endocarditis
 cervix, cervical (os) N88.3
  in pregnancy O34.3- ☑
 chronotropic I45.89
  with
   autonomic dysfunction G90.8
   ischemic heart disease I25.89
   left ventricular dysfunction I51.89
   sinus node dysfunction I49.8
 esophagogastric (junction) (sphincter) K22.0
 mitral (valve) — *see* Insufficiency, mitral
 pelvic fundus N81.89
 pubocervical tissue N81.82
 pulmonary valve (heart) I37.1
  congenital Q22.3
 rectovaginal tissue N81.83
 tricuspid (annular) (valve) — *see* Insufficiency, tricuspid
 valvular — *see* Endocarditis
  congenital Q24.8
 vein, venous (saphenous) (varicose) — *see* Varix, leg
Incomplete (*see also* condition)
 bladder, emptying R33.9
 defecation R15.0
 expansion lungs (newborn) NEC — *see* Atelectasis
 rotation, intestine Q43.3
Inconclusive
 diagnostic imaging due to excess body fat of patient R93.9
 findings on diagnostic imaging of breast NEC R92.8
 mammogram (due to dense breasts) R92.2
Incontinence R32
 anal sphincter R15.9
 coital N39.491
 feces R15.9
  nonorganic origin F98.1
 insensible (urinary) N39.42
 overflow N39.490
 postural (urinary) N39.492
 psychogenic F45.8
 rectal R15.9
 reflex N39.498
 stress (female) (male) N39.3
  and urge N39.46
 urethral sphincter R32
 urge N39.41
  and stress (female) (male) N39.46
 urine (urinary) R32
  continuous N39.45
  due to cognitive impairment, or severe physical disability or immobility R39.81
  functional R39.81
  insensible N39.42
  mixed (stress and urge) N39.46
  nocturnal N39.44

Incontinence — *continued*
 urine — *continued*
  nonorganic origin F98.0
  overflow N39.490
  post dribbling N39.43
  postural N39.492
  reflex N39.498
  specified NEC N39.498
  stress (female) (male) N39.3
   and urge N39.46
  total N39.498
  unaware N39.42
  urge N39.41
   and stress (female) (male) N39.46
Incontinentia pigmenti Q82.3
Incoordinate, incoordination
 esophageal-pharyngeal (newborn) — *see* Dysphagia
 muscular R27.8
 uterus (action) (contractions) (complicating delivery) O62.4
Increase, increased
 abnormal, in development R63.8
 androgens (ovarian) E28.1
 anticoagulants (antithrombin) (anti-VIIIa) (anti-IXa) (anti-Xa) (anti-XIa) — *see* Circulating anticoagulants
 cold sense R20.8
 estrogen E28.0
 function
  adrenal
   cortex — *see* Cushing's, syndrome
   medulla E27.5
  pituitary (gland) (anterior) (lobe) E22.9
   posterior E22.2
 heat sense R20.8
 intracranial pressure (benign) G93.2
 permeability, capillaries I78.8
 pressure, intracranial G93.2
 secretion
  gastrin E16.4
  glucagon E16.3
  pancreas, endocrine E16.9
   growth hormone-releasing hormone E16.8
   pancreatic polypeptide E16.8
   somatostatin E16.8
   vasoactive-intestinal polypeptide E16.8
 sphericity, lens Q12.4
 splenic activity D73.1
 venous pressure I87.8
  portal K76.6
Increta placenta O43.22- ☑
Incrustation, cornea, foreign body (lead)(zinc) — *see* Foreign body, cornea
Incyclophoria H50.54
Incyclotropia — *see* Cyclotropia
Indeterminate sex Q56.4
India rubber skin Q82.8
Indigestion (acid) (bilious) (functional) K30
 catarrhal K31.89
 due to decomposed food NOS A05.9
 nervous F45.8
 psychogenic F45.8
Indirect — *see* condition
Induratio penis plastica N48.6
Induration, indurated
 brain G93.89
 breast (fibrous) N64.51
  puerperal, postpartum O92.29
 broad ligament N83.8
 chancre
  anus A51.1
   congenital A50.07
   extragenital NEC A51.2
 corpora cavernosa (penis) (plastic) N48.6
 liver (chronic) K76.89
 lung (black) (chronic) (fibroid) (*see also* Fibrosis, lung) J84.10
  essential brown J84.03
 penile (plastic) N48.6
 phlebitic — *see* Phlebitis
 skin R23.4
Inebriety (without dependence) — *see* Alcohol, intoxication
Inefficiency, kidney N28.9
Inelasticity, skin R23.4
Inequality, leg (length) (acquired) (*see also* Deformity, limb, unequal length)
 congenital — *see* Defect, reduction, lower limb

Inequality, leg — *continued*
 lower leg — *see* Deformity, limb, unequal length
Inertia
 bladder (neurogenic) N31.2
 stomach K31.89
  psychogenic F45.8
 uterus, uterine during labor O62.2
  during latent phase of labor O62.0
  primary O62.0
  secondary O62.1
 vesical (neurogenic) N31.2
Infancy, infantile, infantilism (*see also* condition)
 celiac K90.0
 genitalia, genitals (after puberty) E30.0
 Herter's (nontropical sprue) K90.0
 intestinal K90.0
 Lorain E23.0
 pancreatic K86.89
 pelvis M95.5
  with disproportion (fetopelvic) O33.1
   causing obstructed labor O65.1
 pituitary E23.0
 renal N25.0
 uterus — *see* Infantile, genitalia
Infant(s) (*see also* Infancy)
 excessive crying R68.11
 irritable child R68.12
 lack of care — *see* Neglect
 liveborn (singleton) Z38.2
  born in hospital Z38.00
   by cesarean Z38.01
  born outside hospital Z38.1
  multiple NEC Z38.8
   born in hospital Z38.68
    by cesarean Z38.69
   born outside hospital Z38.7
  quadruplet Z38.8
   born in hospital Z38.63
    by cesarean Z38.64
   born outside hospital Z38.7
  quintuplet Z38.8
   born in hospital Z38.65
    by cesarean Z38.66
   born outside hospital Z38.7
  triplet Z38.8
   born in hospital Z38.61
    by cesarean Z38.62
   born outside hospital Z38.7
  twin Z38.5
   born in hospital Z38.30
    by cesarean Z38.31
   born outside hospital Z38.4
  of diabetic mother (syndrome of) P70.1
   gestational diabetes P70.0
Infantile (*see also* condition)
 genitalia, genitals E30.0
 os, uterine E30.0
 penis E30.0
 testis E29.1
 uterus E30.0
Infantilism — *see* Infancy
Infarct, infarction
 adrenal (capsule) (gland) E27.49
 appendices epiploicae (*see also* Infarct, intestine) K55.069
 bowel (*see also* Infarct, intestine) K55.069
 brain (stem) — *see* Infarct, cerebral
 breast N64.89
 brewer's (kidney) N28.0
 cardiac — *see* Infarct, myocardium
 cerebellar — *see* Infarct, cerebral
 cerebral (*see also* Occlusion, artery cerebral or precerebral, with infarction) I63.9
  aborted I63.9
  cortical I63.9
  due to
   cerebral venous thrombosis, nonpyogenic I63.6
   embolism
    cerebral arteries I63.4- ☑
    precerebral arteries I63.1- ☑
   occlusion NEC
    cerebral arteries I63.5- ☑
    precerebral arteries I63.2- ☑
    small artery I63.81
   stenosis NEC
    cerebral arteries I63.5- ☑
    precerebral arteries I63.2- ☑
    small artery I63.81

Infarct, infarction — *continued*
cerebral (*see also* Occlusion, artery cerebral or precerebral, with infarction) — *continued*
  due to — *continued*
    thrombosis
      cerebral artery I63.3- ☑
      precerebral artery I63.0- ☑
    intraoperative
      during cardiac surgery I97.810
      during other surgery I97.811
    postprocedural
      following cardiac surgery I97.820
      following other surgery I97.821
    specified NEC I63.89
colon (acute) (agnogenic) (embolic) (hemorrhagic) (nonocclusive) (nonthrombotic) (occlusive) (segmental) (thrombotic) (with gangrene) (*see also* Infarct, intestine) K55.049
coronary artery — *see* Infarct, myocardium
embolic — *see* Embolism
fallopian tube N83.8
gallbladder K82.8
heart — *see* Infarct, myocardium
hepatic K76.3
hypophysis (anterior lobe) E23.6
impending (myocardium) I20.0
intestine (acute) (agnogenic) (embolic) (hemorrhagic) (nonocclusive) (nonthrombotic) (occlusive) (thrombotic) (with gangrene) K55.069
  diffuse K55.062
  focal K55.061
  large K55.049
    diffuse K55.042
    focal K55.041
  small K55.029
    diffuse K55.022
    focal K55.021
kidney N28.0
lacunar I63.81
liver K76.3
lung (embolic) (thrombotic) — *see* Embolism, pulmonary
lymph node I89.8
mesentery, mesenteric (embolic) (thrombotic) (with gangrene) (*see also* Infarct, intestine) K55.069
muscle (ischemic) M62.20
  ankle M62.27- ☑
  foot M62.27- ☑
  forearm M62.23- ☑
  hand M62.24- ☑
  lower leg M62.26- ☑
  pelvic region M62.25- ☑
  shoulder region M62.21- ☑
  specified site NEC M62.28
  thigh M62.25- ☑
  upper arm M62.22- ☑
myocardium, myocardial (acute) (with stated duration of 4 weeks or less) I21.9
  associated with revascularization procedure I21.A9
  diagnosed on ECG, but presenting no symptoms I25.2
  due to
    demand ischemia I21.A1
    ischemic imbalance I21.A1
  healed or old I25.2
  intraoperative (*see also* Infarct, myocardium, associated with revascularization procedure)
    during cardiac surgery I97.790
    during other surgery I97.791
  non-Q wave I21.4
  non-ST elevation (NSTEMI) I21.4
    subsequent I22.2
  nontransmural I21.4
  past (diagnosed on ECG or other investigation, but currently presenting no symptoms) I25.2
  postprocedural (*see also* Infarct, myocardium, associated with revascularization procedure)
    following cardiac surgery (*see also* Infarct, myocardium, type 4 or type 5) I97.190
    following other surgery I97.191
  Q wave (see also, Infarct, myocardium, by site) I21.3
  secondary to
    demand ischemia I21.A1
    ischemic imbalance I21.A1
  ST elevation (STEMI) I21.3
    anterior (anteroapical) (anterolateral) (anteroseptal) (Q wave) (wall) I21.09
      subsequent I22.0

Infarct, infarction — *continued*
myocardium, myocardial — *continued*
  ST elevation — *continued*
    inferior (diaphragmatic) (inferolateral) (inferoposterior) (wall) NEC I21.19
      subsequent I22.1
    inferoposterior transmural (Q wave) I21.11
    involving
      coronary artery of anterior wall NEC I21.09
      coronary artery of inferior wall NEC I21.19
      diagonal coronary artery I21.02
      left anterior descending coronary artery I21.02
      left circumflex coronary artery I21.21
      left main coronary artery I21.01
      oblique marginal coronary artery I21.21
      right coronary artery I21.11
    lateral (apical-lateral) (basal-lateral) (high) I21.29
      subsequent I22.8
    posterior (posterobasal) (posterolateral) (posteroseptal) (true) I21.29
      subsequent I22.8
    septal I21.29
      subsequent I22.8
    specified NEC I21.29
      subsequent I22.8
  subsequent (recurrent) (reinfarction) I22.9
    anterior (anteroapical) (anterolateral) (anteroseptal) (wall) I22.0
    diaphragmatic (wall) I22.1
    inferior (diaphragmatic) (inferolateral) (inferoposterior) (wall) I22.1
    lateral (apical-lateral) (basal-lateral) (high) I22.8
    non-ST elevation (NSTEMI) I22.2
    posterior (posterobasal) (posterolateral) (posteroseptal) (true) I22.8
    septal I22.8
    specified NEC I22.8
    ST elevation I22.9
      anterior (anteroapical) (anterolateral) (anteroseptal) (wall) I22.0
      inferior (diaphragmatic) (inferolateral) (inferoposterior) (wall) I22.1
      specified NEC I22.8
    subendocardial I22.2
    transmural I22.9
      anterior (anteroapical) (anterolateral) (anteroseptal) (wall) I22.0
      diaphragmatic (wall) I22.1
      inferior (diaphragmatic) (inferolateral) (inferoposterior) (wall) I22.1
      lateral (apical-lateral) (basal-lateral) (high) I22.8
      posterior (posterobasal) (posterolateral) (posteroseptal) (true) I22.8
      specified NEC I22.8
    type 1 (*see also* Infarction, myocardial, subsequent, by site, or by ST elevation or non-ST elevation) I22.9
    type 2 I21.A1
    type 3 I21.A9
    type 4 I21.A9
    type 5 I21.A9
  syphilitic A52.06
  transmural I21.9
    anterior (anteroapical) (anterolateral) (anteroseptal) (Q wave) (wall) NEC I21.09
    inferior (diaphragmatic) (inferolateral) (inferoposterior) (Q wave) (wall) NEC I21.19
    inferoposterior (Q wave) I21.11
    lateral (apical-lateral) (basal-lateral) (high) NEC I21.29
    posterior (posterobasal) (posterolateral) (posteroseptal) (true) NEC I21.29
    septal NEC I21.29
    specified NEC I21.29
  type 1 (*see also* Infarction, myocardial, by site, or by ST elevation or non-ST elevation) I21.9
  type 2 I21.A1
  type 3 I21.A9
  type 4 (a) (b) (c) I21.A9
  type 5 I21.A9
nontransmural I21.4
omentum (*see also* Infarct, intestine) K55.069
ovary N83.8
pancreas K86.89
papillary muscle — *see* Infarct, myocardium
parathyroid gland E21.4
pituitary (gland) E23.6

Infarct, infarction — *continued*
placenta O43.81- ☑
prostate N42.89
pulmonary (artery) (vein) (hemorrhagic) — *see* Embolism, pulmonary
renal (embolic) (thrombotic) N28.0
retina, retinal (artery) — *see* Occlusion, artery, retina
spinal (cord) (acute) (embolic) (nonembolic) G95.11
spleen D73.5
  embolic or thrombotic I74.8
subendocardial (acute) (nontransmural) I21.4
suprarenal (capsule) (gland) E27.49
testis N50.1
thrombotic (*see also* Thrombosis)
  artery, arterial — *see* Embolism
thyroid (gland) E07.89
ventricle (heart) — *see* Infarct, myocardium
Infecting — *see* condition
Infection, infected, infective (opportunistic) B99.9
with
  drug resistant organism — *see* Resistance (to), drug (*see also* specific organism)
  lymphangitis — *see* Lymphangitis
  organ dysfunction (acute) R65.20
    with septic shock R65.21
abscess (skin) — *code by* site under Abscess
Absidia — *see* Mucormycosis
Acanthamoeba — *see* Acanthamebiasis
Acanthocheilonema (perstans) (streptocerca) B74.4
accessory sinus (chronic) — *see* Sinusitis
achorion — *see* Dermatophytosis
Acremonium falciforme B47.0
acromioclavicular M00.9
Actinobacillus (actinomycetem-comitans) A28.8
  mallei A24.0
  muris A25.1
Actinomadura B47.1
Actinomyces (israelii) (*see also* Actinomycosis) A42.9
Actinomycetales — *see* Actinomycosis
actinomycotic NOS — *see* Actinomycosis
adenoid (and tonsil) J03.90
  chronic J35.02
adenovirus NEC
  as cause of disease classified elsewhere B97.0
  unspecified nature or site B34.0
aerogenes capsulatus A48.0
aertrycke — *see* Infection, salmonella
alimentary canal NOS — *see* Enteritis, infectious
Allescheria boydii B48.2
Alternaria B48.8
alveolus, alveolar (process) K04.7
Ameba, amebic (histolytica) — *see* Amebiasis
amniotic fluid, sac or cavity O41.10- ☑
  chorioamnionitis O41.12- ☑
  placentitis O41.14- ☑
amputation stump (surgical) — *see* Complication, amputation stump, infection
Ancylostoma (duodenalis) B76.0
Anisakis, Anisakis larvae B81.0
anthrax — *see* Anthrax
antrum (chronic) — *see* Sinusitis, maxillary
anus, anal (papillae) (sphincter) K62.89
arbovirus (arbor virus) A94
  specified type NEC A93.8
artificial insemination N98.0
Ascaris lumbricoides — *see* Ascariasis
Ascomycetes B47.0
Aspergillus (flavus) (fumigatus) (terreus) — *see* Aspergillosis
atypical
  acid-fast (bacilli) — *see* Mycobacterium, atypical
  mycobacteria — *see* Mycobacterium, atypical
  virus A81.9
    specified type NEC A81.89
auditory meatus (external) — *see* Otitis, externa, infective
auricle (ear) — *see* Otitis, externa, infective
axillary gland (lymph) L04.2
Bacillus A49.9
  abortus A23.1
  anthracis — *see* Anthrax
  Ducrey's (any location) A57
  Flexner's A03.1
  Friedländer's NEC A49.8
  gas (gangrene) A48.0
  mallei A24.0
  melitensis A23.0
  paratyphoid, paratyphosus A01.4

Infection, infected, infective — *continued*
    Bacillus — *continued*
        paratyphoid, paratyphosus — *continued*
            A A01.1
            B A01.2
            C A01.3
        Shiga (-Kruse) A03.0
        suipestifer — *see* Infection, salmonella
        swimming pool A31.1
        typhosa A01.00
        welchii — *see* Gangrene, gas
    bacterial NOS A49.9
        as cause of disease classified elsewhere B96.89
            Bacteroides fragilis [B. fragilis] B96.6
            Clostridium perfringens [C. perfringens] B96.7
            Enterobacter sakazakii B96.89
            Enterococcus B95.2
            Escherichia coli [E. coli] (*see also* Escherichia coli) B96.20
            Helicobacter pylori [H.pylori] B96.81
            Hemophilus influenzae [H. influenzae] B96.3
            Klebsiella pneumoniae [K. pneumoniae] B96.1
            Mycoplasma pneumoniae [M. pneumoniae] B96.0
            Proteus (mirabilis) (morganii) B96.4
            Pseudomonas (aeruginosa) (mallei) (pseudomallei) B96.5
            Staphylococcus B95.8
                aureus (methicillin susceptible) (MSSA) B95.61
                    methicillin resistant (MRSA) B95.62
                specified NEC B95.7
            Streptococcus B95.5
                group A B95.0
                group B B95.1
                pneumoniae B95.3
                specified NEC B95.4
            Vibrio vulnificus B96.82
            specified NEC A48.8
    Bacterium
        paratyphosum A01.4
            A A01.1
            B A01.2
            C A01.3
        typhosum A01.00
    Bacteroides NEC A49.8
        fragilis, as cause of disease classified elsewhere B96.6
    Balantidium coli A07.0
    Bartholin's gland N75.8
    Basidiobolus B46.8
    bile duct (common) (hepatic) — *see* Cholangitis
    bladder — *see* Cystitis
    Blastomyces, blastomycotic (*see also* Blastomycosis)
        brasiliensis — *see* Paracoccidioidomycosis
        dermatitidis — *see* Blastomycosis
        European — *see* Cryptococcosis
        Loboi B48.0
        North American B40.9
        South American — *see* Paracoccidioidomycosis
    bleb, postprocedure — *see* Blebitis
    bone — *see* Osteomyelitis
    Bordetella — *see* Whooping cough
    Borrelia bergdorfi A69.20
    brain (*see also* Encephalitis) G04.90
        membranes — *see* Meningitis
        septic G06.0
            meninges — *see* Meningitis, bacterial
    branchial cyst Q18.0
    breast — *see* Mastitis
    bronchus — *see* Bronchitis
    Brucella A23.9
        abortus A23.1
        canis A23.3
        melitensis A23.0
        mixed A23.8
        specified NEC A23.8
        suis A23.2
    Brugia (malayi) B74.1
        timori B74.2
    bursa — *see* Bursitis, infective
    buttocks (skin) L08.9
    Campylobacter, intestinal A04.5
        as cause of disease classified elsewhere B96.81
    Candida (albicans) (tropicalis) — *see* Candidiasis
    candiru B88.8
    Capillaria (intestinal) B81.1
        hepatica B83.8
        philippinensis B81.1

Infection, infected, infective — *continued*
    cartilage — *see* Disorder, cartilage, specified type NEC
    cat liver fluke B66.0
    catheter-related bloodstream (CRBSI) T80.211 ☑
    cellulitis — *code by* site under Cellulitis
    central line-associated T80.219 ☑
        bloodstream (CLABSI) T80.211 ☑
        specified NEC T80.218 ☑
    Cephalosporium falciforme B47.0
    cerebrospinal — *see* Meningitis
    cervical gland (lymph) L04.0
    cervix — *see* Cervicitis
    cesarean delivery wound (puerperal) O86.00
    cestodes — *see* Infestation, cestodes
    chest J22
    Chilomastix (intestinal) A07.8
    Chlamydia, chlamydial A74.9
        anus A56.3
        genitourinary tract A56.2
            lower A56.00
            specified NEC A56.19
        lymphogranuloma A55
        pharynx A56.4
        psittaci A70
        rectum A56.3
        sexually transmitted NEC A56.8
    cholera — *see* Cholera
    Cladosporium
        bantianum (brain abscess) B43.1
        carrionii B43.0
        castellanii B36.1
        trichoides (brain abscess) B43.1
        werneckii B36.1
    Clonorchis (sinensis) (liver) B66.1
    Clostridium NEC
        bifermentans A48.0
        botulinum (food poisoning) A05.1
            infant A48.51
            wound A48.52
        difficile
            as cause of disease classified elsewhere B96.89
            foodborne (disease)
                not specified as recurrent A04.72
                recurrent A04.71
            gas gangrene A48.0
            necrotizing enterocolitis
                not specified as recurrent A04.72
                recurrent A04.71
            sepsis A41.4
        gas-forming NEC A48.0
        histolyticum A48.0
        novyi, causing gas gangrene A48.0
        oedematiens A48.0
        perfringens
            as cause of disease classified elsewhere B96.7
            due to food A05.2
            foodborne (disease) A05.2
            gas gangrene A48.0
            sepsis A41.4
        septicum, causing gas gangrene A48.0
        sordellii, causing gas gangrene A48.0
        welchii
            as cause of disease classified elsewhere B96.7
            foodborne (disease) A05.2
            gas gangrene A48.0
            necrotizing enteritis A05.2
            sepsis A41.4
    Coccidioides (immitis) — *see* Coccidioidomycosis
    colon — *see* Enteritis, infectious
    colostomy K94.02
    common duct — *see* Cholangitis
    congenital P39.9
        Candida (albicans) P37.5
        cytomegalovirus P35.1
        hepatitis, viral P35.3
        herpes simplex P35.2
        infectious or parasitic disease P37.9
            specified NEC P37.8
        listeriosis (disseminated) P37.2
        malaria NEC P37.4
            falciparum P37.3
        Plasmodium falciparum P37.3
        poliomyelitis P35.8
        rubella P35.0
        skin P39.4
        toxoplasmosis (acute) (subacute) (chronic) P37.1
        tuberculosis P37.0
        urinary (tract) P39.3

Infection, infected, infective — *continued*
    congenital — *continued*
        vaccinia P35.8
        virus P35.9
            specified type NEC P35.8
    Conidiobolus B46.8
    coronavirus NEC B34.2
        as cause of disease classified elsewhere B97.29
        severe acute respiratory syndrome (SARS associated) B97.21
    corpus luteum — *see* Salpingo-oophoritis
    Corynebacterium diphtheriae — *see* Diphtheria
    cotia virus B08.8
    Coxiella burnetii A78
    coxsackie — *see* Coxsackie
    Cryptococcus neoformans — *see* Cryptococcosis
    Cryptosporidium A07.2
    Cunninghamella — *see* Mucormycosis
    cyst — *see* Cyst
    cystic duct (*see also* Cholecystitis) K81.9
    Cysticercus cellulosae — *see* Cysticercosis
    cytomegalovirus, cytomegaloviral B25.9
        congenital P35.1
        maternal, maternal care for (suspected) damage to fetus O35.3 ☑
        mononucleosis B27.10
            with
                complication NEC B27.19
                meningitis B27.12
                polyneuropathy B27.11
    delta-agent (acute), in hepatitis B carrier B17.0
    dental (pulpal origin) K04.7
    Deuteromycetes B47.0
    Dicrocoelium dendriticum B66.2
    Dipetalonema (perstans) (streptocerca) B74.4
    diphtherial — *see* Diphtheria
    Diphyllobothrium (adult) (latum) (pacificum) B70.0
        larval B70.1
    Diplogonoporus (grandis) B71.8
    Dipylidium caninum B67.4
    Dirofilaria B74.8
    Dracunculus medinensis B72
    Drechslera (hawaiiensis) B43.8
    Ducrey Haemophilus (any location) A57
    due to or resulting from
        artificial insemination N98.0
        central venous catheter T80.219 ☑
            bloodstream T80.211 ☑
            exit or insertion site T80.212 ☑
            localized T80.212 ☑
            port or reservoir T80.212 ☑
            specified NEC T80.218 ☑
            tunnel T80.212 ☑
        device, implant or graft (*see also* Complications, by site and type, infection or inflammation) T85.79 ☑
            arterial graft NEC T82.7 ☑
            breast (implant) T85.79 ☑
            catheter NEC T85.79 ☑
                dialysis (renal) T82.7 ☑
                    intraperitoneal T85.71 ☑
                infusion NEC T82.7 ☑
                    cranial T85.735 ☑
                    intrathecal T85.735 ☑
                    spinal (epidural) (subdural) T85.735 ☑
                    subarachnoid T85.735 ☑
                urinary T83.518 ☑
                    cystostomy T83.510 ☑
                    Hopkins T83.518 ☑
                    ileostomy T83.518 ☑
                    nephrostomy T83.512 ☑
                    specified NEC T83.518 ☑
                    urethral indwelling T83.511 ☑
                    urostomy T83.518 ☑
        electronic (electrode) (pulse generator) (stimulator)
            bone T84.7 ☑
            cardiac T82.7 ☑
            nervous system T85.738 ☑
                brain T85.731 ☑
                cranial nerve T85.732 ☑
                gastric nerve T85.732 ☑
                generator pocket T85.734 ☑
                neurostimulator generator T85.734 ☑
                peripheral nerve T85.732 ☑
                sacral nerve T85.732 ☑
                spinal cord T85.733 ☑

Infection, infected, infective — *continued*
  due to or resulting from — *continued*
    device, implant or graft (*see also* Complications, by
        site and type, infection or inflammation) —
        continued
      electronic — *continued*
        nervous system — *continued*
          vagal nerve T85.732 ☑
          urinary (indwelling) T83.51 ☑
        fixation, internal (orthopedic) NEC — *see* Compli-
          cation, fixation device, infection
        gastrointestinal (bile duct) (esophagus) T85.79 ☑
          neurostimulator electrode (lead) T85.732 ☑
        genital NEC T83.69 ☑
        heart NEC T82.7 ☑
          valve (prosthesis) T82.6 ☑
          graft T82.7 ☑
        joint prosthesis — *see* Complication, joint pros-
          thesis, infection
        ocular (corneal graft) (orbital implant) NEC
          T85.79 ☑
        orthopedic NEC T84.7 ☑
        penile (cylinder) (pump) (resevoir) T83.61 ☑
        specified NEC T85.79 ☑
        testicular T83.62 ☑
        urinary NEC T83.598 ☑
          ileal conduit stent T83.593 ☑
          implanted neurostimulation T83.590 ☑
          implanted sphincter T83.591 ☑
          indwelling ureteral stent T83.592 ☑
          nephroureteral stent T83.593 ☑
          specified stent NEC T83.593 ☑
        vascular NEC T82.7 ☑
        ventricular intracranial (communicating) shunt
          T85.730 ☑
    Hickman catheter T80.219 ☑
      bloodstream T80.211 ☑
      localized T80.212 ☑
      specified NEC T80.218 ☑
    immunization or vaccination T88.0 ☑
    infusion, injection or transfusion NEC T80.29 ☑
    injury NEC — *code by* site under Wound, open
    peripherally inserted central catheter (PICC)
      T80.219 ☑
      bloodstream T80.211 ☑
      localized T80.212 ☑
      specified NEC T80.218 ☑
    portacath (port-a-cath) T80.219 ☑
      bloodstream T80.211 ☑
      localized T80.212 ☑
      specified NEC T80.218 ☑
    pulmonary artery catheter — *see* Infection, due to
      or resulting from, central venous catheter
    surgery T81.40 ☑
    Swan Ganz catheter — *see* Infection, due to or re-
      sulting from, central venous catheter
    triple lumen catheter T80.219 ☑
      bloodstream T80.211 ☑
      localized T80.212 ☑
      specified NEC T80.218 ☑
    umbilical venous catheter T80.219 ☑
      bloodstream T80.211 ☑
      localized T80.212 ☑
      specified NEC T80.218 ☑
  during labor NEC O75.3
  ear (middle) (*see also* Otitis media)
    external — *see* Otitis, externa, infective
    inner — *see* subcategory H83.0 ☑
  Eberthella typhosa A01.00
  Echinococcus — *see* Echinococcus
  echovirus
    as cause of disease classified elsewhere B97.12
    unspecified nature or site B34.1
  endocardium I33.0
  endocervix — *see* Cervicitis
  Entamoeba — *see* Amebiasis
  enteric — *see* Enteritis, infectious
  Enterobacter sakazakii B96.89
  Enterobius vermicularis B80
  enterostomy K94.12
  enterovirus B34.1
    as cause of disease classified elsewhere B97.10
      coxsackievirus B97.11
      echovirus B97.12
      specified NEC B97.19
  Entomophthora B46.8

Infection, infected, infective — *continued*
  Epidermophyton — *see* Dermatophytosis
  epididymis — *see* Epididymitis
  episiotomy (puerperal) O86.09
  Erysipelothrix (insidiosa) (rhusiopathiae) — *see*
    Erysipeloid
  erythema infectiosum B08.3
  Escherichia (E.) coli NEC A49.8
    as cause of disease classified elsewhere (*see also*
      Escherichia coli) B96.20
    congenital P39.8
    sepsis P36.4
    generalized A41.51
    intestinal — *see* Enteritis, infectious, due to, Es-
      cherichia coli
  ethmoidal (chronic) (sinus) — *see* Sinusitis, ethmoidal
  eustachian tube (ear) — *see* Salpingitis, eustachian
  external auditory canal (meatus) NEC — *see* Otitis, ex-
    terna, infective
  eye (purulent) — *see* Endophthalmitis, purulent
  eyelid — *see* Inflammation, eyelid
  fallopian tube — *see* Salpingo-oophoritis
  Fasciola (gigantica) (hepatica) (indica) B66.3
  Fasciolopsis (buski) B66.5
  filarial — *see* Infestation, filarial
  finger (skin) L08.9
    nail L03.01- ☑
      fungus B35.1
  fish tapeworm B70.0
    larval B70.1
  flagellate, intestinal A07.9
  fluke — *see* Infestation, fluke
  focal
    teeth (pulpal origin) K04.7
    tonsils J35.01
  Fonsecaea (compactum) (pedrosoi) B43.0
  food — *see* Intoxication, foodborne
  foot (skin) L08.9
    dermatophytic fungus B35.3
  Francisella tularensis — *see* Tularemia
  frontal (sinus) (chronic) — *see* Sinusitis, frontal
  fungus NOS B49
    beard B35.0
    dermatophytic — *see* Dermatophytosis
    foot B35.3
    groin B35.6
    hand B35.2
    nail B35.1
    pathogenic to compromised host only B48.8
    perianal (area) B35.6
    scalp B35.0
    skin B36.9
      foot B35.3
      hand B35.2
      toenails B35.1
  Fusarium B48.8
  gallbladder — *see* Cholecystitis
  gas bacillus — *see* Gangrene, gas
  gastrointestinal — *see* Enteritis, infectious
  generalized NEC — *see* Sepsis
  generator pocket, implanted electronic neurostimulator
    T85.734 ☑
  genital organ or tract
    female — *see* Disease, pelvis, inflammatory
    male N49.9
      multiple sites N49.8
      specified NEC N49.8
  Ghon tubercle, primary A15.7
  Giardia lamblia A07.1
  gingiva (chronic) K05.10
    acute K05.00
      nonplaque induced K05.01
      plaque induced K05.00
    nonplaque induced K05.11
    plaque induced K05.10
  glanders A24.0
  glenosporopsis B48.0
  Gnathostoma (spinigerum) B83.1
  Gongylonema B83.8
  gonococcal — *see* Gonococcus
  gram-negative bacilli NOS A49.9
  guinea worm B72
  gum (chronic) K05.10
    acute K05.00
      nonplaque induced K05.01
      plaque induced K05.00
    nonplaque induced K05.11
    plaque induced K05.10

Infection, infected, infective — *continued*
  Haemophilus — *see* Infection, Hemophilus
  heart — *see* Carditis
  Helicobacter pylori A04.8
    as cause of disease classified elsewhere B96.81
  helminths B83.9
    intestinal B82.0
      mixed (types classifiable to more than one of the
        titles B65.0-B81.3 and B81.8) B81.4
      specified type NEC B81.8
    specified type NEC B83.8
  Hemophilus
    aegyptius, systemic A48.4
    ducrey (any location) A57
    generalized A41.3
    influenzae NEC A49.2
      as cause of disease classified elsewhere B96.3
  herpes (simplex) (*see also* Herpes)
    congenital P35.2
    disseminated B00.7
    zoster B02.9
  herpesvirus, herpesviral — *see* Herpes
  Heterophyes (heterophyes) B66.8
  hip (joint) NEC M00.9
    due to internal joint prosthesis
      left T84.52 ☑
      right T84.51 ☑
    skin NEC L08.9
  Histoplasma — *see* Histoplasmosis
    American B39.4
    capsulatum B39.4
  hookworm B76.9
  human
    papilloma virus A63.0
    T-cell lymphotropic virus type-1 (HTLV-1) B33.3
  hydrocele N43.0
  Hymenolepis B71.0
  hypopharynx — *see* Pharyngitis
  inguinal (lymph) glands L04.1
    due to soft chancre A57
  intervertebral disc, pyogenic M46.30
    cervical region M46.32
    cervicothoracic region M46.33
    lumbar region M46.36
    lumbosacral region M46.37
    multiple sites M46.39
    occipito-atlanto-axial region M46.31
    sacrococcygeal region M46.38
    thoracic region M46.34
    thoracolumbar region M46.35
  intestine, intestinal — *see* Enteritis, infectious
    specified NEC A08.8
  intra-amniotic affecting newborn NEC P39.2
  Isospora belli or hominis A07.3
  Japanese B encephalitis A83.0
  jaw (bone) (lower) (upper) M27.2
  joint NEC M00.9
    due to internal joint prosthesis T84.50 ☑
  kidney (cortex) (hematogenous) N15.9
    with calculus N20.0
      with hydronephrosis N13.6
    following ectopic gestation O08.83
    pelvis and ureter (cystic) N28.85
    puerperal (postpartum) O86.21
    specified NEC N15.8
  Klebsiella (K.) pneumoniae NEC A49.8
    as cause of disease classified elsewhere B96.1
  knee (joint) NEC M00.9
    joint M00.9
    due to internal joint prosthesis
      left T84.54 ☑
      right T84.53 ☑
    skin L08.9
  Koch's — *see* Tuberculosis
  labia (majora) (minora) (acute) — *see* Vulvitis
  lacrimal
    gland — *see* Dacryoadenitis
    passages (duct) (sac) — *see* Inflammation, lacrimal,
      passages
  lancet fluke B66.2
  larynx NEC J38.7
  leg (skin) NOS L08.9
  Legionella pneumophila A48.1
    nonpneumonic A48.2
  Leishmania (*see also* Leishmaniasis)
    aethiopica B55.1
    braziliensis B55.2
    chagasi B55.0

☑ **Additional Character Required** — Refer to the Tabular List for Character Selection ▽ **Subterms under main terms may continue to next column or page**

Infection, infected, infective — *continued*
  Leishmania (*see also* Leishmaniasis) — *continued*
    donovani B55.0
    infantum B55.0
    major B55.1
    mexicana B55.1
    tropica B55.1
  lentivirus, as cause of disease classified elsewhere B97.31
  Leptosphaeria senegalensis B47.0
  Leptospira interrogans A27.9
    autumnalis A27.89
    canicola A27.89
    hebdomadis A27.89
    icterohaemorrhagiae A27.0
    pomona A27.89
    specified type NEC A27.89
  leptospirochetal NEC — *see* Leptospirosis
  Listeria monocytogenes (*see also* Listeriosis)
    congenital P37.2
  Loa loa B74.3
    with conjunctival infestation B74.3
    eyelid B74.3
  Loboa loboi B48.0
  local, skin (staphylococcal) (streptococcal) L08.9
    abscess — *code by* site under Abscess
    cellulitis — *code by* site under Cellulitis
    specified NEC L08.89
    ulcer — *see* Ulcer, skin
  Loefflerella mallei A24.0
  lung (*see also* Pneumonia) J18.9
    atypical Mycobacterium A31.0
    spirochetal A69.8
    tuberculous — *see* Tuberculosis, pulmonary
    virus — *see* Pneumonia, viral
  lymph gland (*see also* Lymphadenitis, acute)
    mesenteric I88.0
  lymphoid tissue, base of tongue or posterior pharynx, NEC (chronic) J35.03
  Madurella (grisea) (mycetomii) B47.0
  major
    following ectopic or molar pregnancy O08.0
    puerperal, postpartum, childbirth O85
  Malassezia furfur B36.0
  Malleomyces
    mallei A24.0
    pseudomallei (whitmori) — *see* Melioidosis
  mammary gland N61.0
  Mansonella (ozzardi) (perstans) (streptocerca) B74.4
  mastoid — *see* Mastoiditis
  maxilla, maxillary M27.2
    sinus (chronic) — *see* Sinusitis, maxillary
  mediastinum J98.51
  Medina (worm) B72
  meibomian cyst or gland — *see* Hordeolum
  meninges — *see* Meningitis, bacterial
  meningococcal (*see also* condition) A39.9
    adrenals A39.1
    brain A39.81
    cerebrospinal A39.0
    conjunctiva A39.89
    endocardium A39.51
    heart A39.50
      endocardium A39.51
      myocardium A39.52
      pericardium A39.53
    joint A39.83
    meninges A39.0
    meningococcemia A39.4
      acute A39.2
      chronic A39.3
    myocardium A39.52
    pericardium A39.53
    retrobulbar neuritis A39.82
    specified site NEC A39.89
  mesenteric lymph nodes or glands NEC I88.0
  Metagonimus B66.8
  metatarsophalangeal M00.9
  methicillin
    resistant Staphylococcus aureus (MRSA) A49.02
    susceptible Staphylococcus aureus (MSSA) A49.01
  Microsporum, microsporic — *see* Dermatophytosis
  mixed flora (bacterial) NEC A49.8
  Monilia — *see* Candidiasis
  Monosporium apiospermum B48.2
  mouth, parasitic B37.0
  Mucor — *see* Mucormycosis
  muscle NEC — *see* Myositis, infective

Infection, infected, infective — *continued*
  mycelium NOS B49
  mycetoma B47.9
    actinomycotic NEC B47.1
    mycotic NEC B47.0
  Mycobacterium, mycobacterial — *see* Mycobacterium
  Mycoplasma NEC A49.3
    pneumoniae, as cause of disease classified elsewhere B96.0
  mycotic NOS B49
    pathogenic to compromised host only B48.8
    skin NOS B36.9
  myocardium NEC I40.0
  nail (chronic)
    with lymphangitis — *see* Lymphangitis, acute, digit
    finger L03.01- ☑
      fungus B35.1
    ingrowing L60.0
    toe L03.03- ☑
      fungus B35.1
  nasal sinus (chronic) — *see* Sinusitis
  nasopharynx — *see* Nasopharyngitis
  navel L08.82
  Necator americanus B76.1
  Neisseria — *see* Gonococcus
  Neotestudina rosatii B47.0
  newborn P39.9
    intra-amniotic NEC P39.2
    skin P39.4
    specified type NEC P39.8
  nipple N61.0
    associated with
      lactation O91.03
      pregnancy O91.01- ☑
      puerperium O91.02
  Nocardia — *see* Nocardiosis
  obstetrical surgical wound (puerperal) O86.00
    incisional site
      deep O86.02
      superficial O86.01
    organ and space site O86.03
    surgical site specified NEC O86.09
  Oesophagostomum (apiostomum) B81.8
  Oestrus ovis — *see* Myiasis
  Oidium albicans B37.9
  Onchocerca (volvulus) — *see* Onchocerciasis
  oncovirus, as cause of disease classified elsewhere B97.32
  operation wound T81.49 ☑
  Opisthorchis (felineus) (viverrini) B66.0
  orbit, orbital — *see* Inflammation, orbit
  orthopoxvirus NEC B08.09
  ovary — *see* Salpingo-oophoritis
  Oxyuris vermicularis B80
  pancreas (acute) — *see* Pancreatitis, acute
    abscess — *see* Pancreatitis, acute
    specified NEC (*see also* Pancreatitis, acute) K85.80
  papillomavirus, as cause of disease classified elsewhere B97.7
  papovavirus NEC B34.4
  Paracoccidioides brasiliensis — *see* Paracoccidioidomycosis
  Paragonimus (westermani) B66.4
  parainfluenza virus B34.8
  parameningococcus NOS A39.9
  parapoxvirus B08.60
    specified NEC B08.69
  parasitic B89
  Parastrongylus
    cantonensis B83.2
    costaricensis B81.3
    paratyphoid A01.4
      Type A A01.1
      Type B A01.2
      Type C A01.3
  paraurethral ducts N34.2
  parotid gland — *see* Sialoadenitis
  parvovirus NEC B34.3
    as cause of disease classified elsewhere B97.6
  Pasteurella NEC A28.0
    multocida A28.0
    pestis — *see* Plague
    pseudotuberculosis A28.0
    septica (cat bite) (dog bite) A28.0
    tularensis — *see* Tularemia
  pelvic, female — *see* Disease, pelvis, inflammatory
  Penicillium (marneffei) B48.4
  penis (glans) (retention) NEC N48.29

Infection, infected, infective — *continued*
  periapical K04.5
  peridental, periodontal K05.20
    generalized — *see* Peridontitis, aggressive, generalized
    localized — *see* Peridontitis, aggressive, localized
  perinatal period P39.9
    specified type NEC P39.8
  perineal repair (puerperal) O86.09
  periorbital — *see* Inflammation, orbit
  perirectal K62.89
  perirenal — *see* Infection, kidney
  peritoneal — *see* Peritonitis
  periureteral N28.89
  Petriellidium boydii B48.2
  pharynx (*see also* Pharyngitis)
    coxsackievirus B08.5
    posterior, lymphoid (chronic) J35.03
  Phialophora
    gougerotii (subcutaneous abscess or cyst) B43.2
    jeanselmei (subcutaneous abscess or cyst) B43.2
    verrucosa (skin) B43.0
  Piedraia hortae B36.3
  pinta A67.9
    intermediate A67.1
    late A67.2
    mixed A67.3
    primary A67.0
  pinworm B80
  pityrosporum furfur B36.0
  pleuro-pneumonia-like organism (PPLO) NEC A49.3
    as cause of disease classified elsewhere B96.0
  pneumococcus, pneumococcal NEC A49.1
    as cause of disease classified elsewhere B95.3
    generalized (purulent) A40.3
      with pneumonia J13
  Pneumocystis carinii (pneumonia) B59
  Pneumocystis jiroveci (pneumonia) B59
  port or reservoir T80.212 ☑
  postoperative T81.40 ☑
  postoperative wound T81.49 ☑
    surgical site
      deep incisional T81.42 ☑
      organ and space T81.43 ☑
      specified NEC T81.49 ☑
      superficial incisional T81.41 ☑
  postprocedural T81.40 ☑
  postvaccinal T88.0 ☑
  prepuce NEC N47.7
    with penile inflammation N47.6
  prion — *see* Disease, prion, central nervous system
  prostate (capsule) — *see* Prostatitis
  Proteus (mirabilis) (morganii) (vulgaris) NEC A49.8
    as cause of disease classified elsewhere B96.4
  protozoal NEC B64
    intestinal A07.9
      specified NEC A07.8
    specified NEC B60.8
  Pseudoallescheria boydii B48.2
  Pseudomonas NEC A49.8
    as cause of disease classified elsewhere B96.5
    mallei A24.0
    pneumonia J15.1
    pseudomallei — *see* Melioidosis
  puerperal O86.4
    genitourinary tract NEC O86.89
    major or generalized O85
    minor O86.4
    specified NEC O86.89
  pulmonary — *see* Infection, lung
  purulent — *see* Abscess
  Pyrenochaeta romeroi B47.0
  Q fever A78
  rectum (sphincter) K62.89
  renal (*see also* Infection, kidney)
    pelvis and ureter (cystic) N28.85
  reovirus, as cause of disease classified elsewhere B97.5
  respiratory (tract) NEC J98.8
    acute J22
    chronic J98.8
    influenzal (upper) (acute) — *see* Influenza, with, respiratory manifestations NEC
    lower (acute) J22
      chronic — *see* Bronchitis, chronic
    rhinovirus J00
    syncytial virus, as cause of disease classified elsewhere B97.4
    upper (acute) NOS J06.9

Infection, infected, infective — *continued*
respiratory — *continued*
  upper — *continued*
    chronic J39.8
    streptococcal J06.9
    viral NOS J06.9
  resulting from
    presence of internal prosthesis, implant, graft —
      see Complications, by site and type, infection
retortamoniasis A07.8
retroperitoneal NEC K68.9
retrovirus B33.3
  as cause of disease classified elsewhere B97.30
    human
      immunodeficiency, type 2 (HIV 2) B97.35
      T-cell lymphotropic
        type I (HTLV-I) B97.33
        type II (HTLV-II) B97.34
    lentivirus B97.31
    oncovirus B97.32
    specified NEC B97.39
Rhinosporidium (seeberi) B48.1
rhinovirus
  as cause of disease classified elsewhere B97.89
  unspecified nature or site B34.8
Rhizopus — *see* Mucormycosis
rickettsial NOS A79.9
roundworm (large) NEC B82.0
  Ascariasis (*see also* Ascariasis) B77.9
rubella — *see* Rubella
Saccharomyces — *see* Candidiasis
salivary duct or gland (any) — *see* Sialoadenitis
Salmonella (aertrycke) (arizonae) (callinarum) (cholerae-
  suis) (enteritidis) (suipestifer) (typhimurium)
  A02.9
  with
    (gastro)enteritis A02.0
    sepsis A02.1
    specified manifestation NEC A02.8
  due to food (poisoning) A02.9
  hirschfeldii A01.3
  localized A02.20
    arthritis A02.23
    meningitis A02.21
    osteomyelitis A02.24
    pneumonia A02.22
    pyelonephritis A02.25
    specified NEC A02.29
  paratyphi A01.4
    A A01.1
    B A01.2
    C A01.3
  schottmuelleri A01.2
  typhi, typhosa — *see* Typhoid
Sarcocystis A07.8
scabies B86
Schistosoma — *see* Infestation, Schistosoma
scrotum (acute) NEC N49.2
seminal vesicle — *see* Vesiculitis
septic
  localized, skin — *see* Abscess
sheep liver fluke B66.3
Shigella A03.9
  boydii A03.2
  dysenteriae A03.0
  flexneri A03.1
  group
    A A03.0
    B A03.1
    C A03.2
    D A03.3
  Schmitz (-Stutzer) A03.0
  schmitzii A03.0
  shigae A03.0
  sonnei A03.3
  specified NEC A03.8
shoulder (joint) NEC M00.9
  due to internal joint prosthesis T84.59 ☑
  skin NEC L08.9
sinus (accessory) (chronic) (nasal) (*see also* Sinusitis)
  pilonidal — *see* Sinus, pilonidal
  skin NEC L08.89
Skene's duct or gland — *see* Urethritis
skin (local) (staphylococcal) (streptococcal) L08.9
  abscess — *code by* site under Abscess
  cellulitis — *code by* site under Cellulitis
  due to fungus B36.9
    specified type NEC B36.8

Infection, infected, infective — *continued*
skin — *continued*
  mycotic B36.9
    specified type NEC B36.8
  newborn P39.4
  ulcer — *see* Ulcer, skin
slow virus A81.9
  specified NEC A81.89
Sparganum (mansoni) (proliferum) (baxteri) B70.1
specific (*see also* Syphilis)
  to perinatal period — *see* Infection, congenital
specified NEC B99.8
spermatic cord NEC N49.1
sphenoidal (sinus) — *see* Sinusitis, sphenoidal
spinal cord NOS (*see also* Myelitis) G04.91
  abscess G06.1
  meninges — *see* Meningitis
  streptococcal G04.89
Spirillum A25.0
spirochetal NOS A69.9
  lung A69.8
  specified NEC A69.8
Spirometra larvae B70.1
spleen D73.89
Sporotrichum, Sporothrix (schenckii) — *see* Sporotrichosis
staphylococcal, unspecified site
  as cause of disease classified elsewhere B95.8
    aureus (methicillin susceptible) (MSSA) B95.61
      methicillin resistant (MRSA) B95.62
    specified NEC B95.7
  aureus (methicillin susceptible) (MSSA) A49.01
    methicillin resistant (MRSA) A49.02
  food poisoning A05.0
  generalized (purulent) A41.2
  pneumonia — *see* Pneumonia, staphylococcal
Stellantchasmus falcatus B66.8
streptobacillus moniliformis A25.1
streptococcal NEC A49.1
  as cause of disease classified elsewhere B95.5
  B genitourinary complicating
    childbirth O98.82
    pregnancy O98.81- ☑
    puerperium O98.83
  congenital
    sepsis P36.10
      group B P36.0
      specified NEC P36.19
  generalized (purulent) A40.9
Streptomyces B47.1
Strongyloides (stercoralis) — *see* Strongyloidiasis
stump (amputation) (surgical) — *see* Complication,
  amputation stump, infection
subcutaneous tissue, local L08.9
suipestifer — *see* Infection, salmonella
swimming pool bacillus A31.1
Taenia — *see* Infestation, Taenia
Taeniarhynchus saginatus B68.1
tapeworm — *see* Infestation, tapeworm
tendon (sheath) — *see* Tenosynovitis, infective NEC
Ternidens diminutus B81.8
testis — *see* Orchitis
threadworm B80
throat — *see* Pharyngitis
thyroglossal duct K14.8
toe (skin) L08.9
  cellulitis L03.03- ☑
    fungus B35.1
  nail L03.03- ☑
    fungus B35.1
tongue NEC K14.0
  parasitic B37.0
tonsil (and adenoid) (faucial) (lingual) (pharyngeal) —
  see Tonsillitis
tooth, teeth K04.7
  periapical K04.7
  peridental, periodontal K05.20
    generalized — *see* Peridontitis, aggressive, gen-
      eralized
    localized — *see* Peridontitis, aggressive, localized
  pulp K04.01
    irreversible K04.02
    reversible K04.01
  socket M27.3
TORCH — *see* Infection, congenital
  without active infection P00.2
Torula histolytica — *see* Cryptococcosis
Toxocara (canis) (cati) (felis) B83.0

Infection, infected, infective — *continued*
Toxoplasma gondii — *see* Toxoplasma
trachea, chronic J42
trematode NEC — *see* Infestation, fluke
trench fever A79.0
Treponema pallidum — *see* Syphilis
Trichinella (spiralis) B75
Trichomonas A59.9
  cervix A59.09
  intestine A07.8
  prostate A59.02
  specified site NEC A59.8
  urethra A59.03
  urogenitalis A59.00
  vagina A59.01
  vulva A59.01
Trichophyton, trichophytic — *see* Dermatophytosis
Trichosporon (beigelii) cutaneum B36.2
Trichostrongylus B81.2
Trichuris (trichiura) B79
Trombicula (irritans) B88.0
Trypanosoma
  brucei
    gambiense B56.0
    rhodesiense B56.1
  cruzi — *see* Chagas' disease
  tubal — *see* Salpingo-oophoritis
tuberculous NEC — *see* Tuberculosis
tubo-ovarian — *see* Salpingo-oophoritis
tunica vaginalis N49.1
tunnel T80.212 ☑
tympanic membrane NEC — *see* Myringitis
typhoid (abortive) (ambulant) (bacillus) — *see* Typhoid
typhus A75.9
  flea-borne A75.2
  mite-borne A75.3
  recrudescent A75.1
  tick-borne A77.9
    African A77.1
    North Asian A77.2
umbilicus L08.82
ureter N28.86
urethra — *see* Urethritis
urinary (tract) N39.0
  bladder — *see* Cystitis
  complicating
    pregnancy O23.4- ☑
      specified type NEC O23.3- ☑
  kidney — *see* Infection, kidney
  newborn P39.3
  puerperal (postpartum) O86.20
  tuberculous A18.13
  urethra — *see* Urethritis
uterus, uterine — *see* Endometritis
vaccination T88.0 ☑
vaccinia not from vaccination B08.011
vagina (acute) — *see* Vaginitis
varicella B01.9
varicose veins — *see* Varix
vas deferens NEC N49.1
vesical — *see* Cystitis
Vibrio
  cholerae A00.0
    El Tor A00.1
  parahaemolyticus (food poisoning) A05.3
  vulnificus
    as cause of disease classified elsewhere B96.82
    foodborne intoxication A05.5
Vincent's (gum) (mouth) (tonsil) A69.1
virus, viral NOS B34.9
  adenovirus
    as cause of disease classified elsewhere B97.0
    unspecified nature or site B34.0
  arborvirus, arbovirus arthropod-borne A94
  as cause of disease classified elsewhere B97.89
    adenovirus B97.0
    coronavirus B97.29
      SARS-associated B97.21
    coxsackievirus B97.11
    echovirus B97.12
    enterovirus B97.10
      coxsackievirus B97.11
      echovirus B97.12
      specified NEC B97.19
    human
      immunodeficiency, type 2 (HIV 2) B97.35
      metapneumovirus B97.81

Infection, infected, infective — *continued*
  virus, viral — *continued*
    as cause of disease classified elsewhere — *continued*
      human — *continued*
        T-cell lymphotropic,
          type I (HTLV-I) B97.33
          type II (HTLV-II) B97.34
      papillomavirus B97.7
      parvovirus B97.6
      reovirus B97.5
      respiratory syncytial B97.4
      retrovirus B97.30
        human
          immunodeficiency, type 2 (HIV 2) B97.35
          T-cell lymphotropic,
            type I (HTLV-I) B97.33
            type II (HTLV-II) B97.34
        lentivirus B97.31
        oncovirus B97.32
        specified NEC B97.39
      specified NEC B97.89
    central nervous system A89
      atypical A81.9
        specified NEC A81.89
      enterovirus NEC A88.8
        meningitis A87.0
      slow virus A81.9
        specified NEC A81.89
      specified NEC A88.8
    chest J98.8
    cotia B08.8
    coxsackie (*see also* Infection, coxsackie) B34.1
      as cause of disease classified elsewhere B97.11
    ECHO
      as cause of disease classified elsewhere B97.12
      unspecified nature or site B34.1
    encephalitis, tick-borne A84.9
    enterovirus, as cause of disease classified elsewhere B97.10
      coxsackievirus B97.11
      echovirus B97.12
      specified NEC B97.19
    exanthem NOS B09
    human metapneumovirus as cause of disease classified elsewhere B97.81
    human papilloma as cause of disease classified elsewhere B97.7
    intestine — *see* Enteritis, viral
    respiratory syncytial
      as cause of disease classified elsewhere B97.4
      bronchopneumonia J12.1
      common cold syndrome J00
      nasopharyngitis (acute) J00
    rhinovirus
      as cause of disease classified elsewhere B97.89
      unspecified nature or site B34.8
    slow A81.9
      specified NEC A81.89
    specified type NEC B33.8
      as cause of disease classified elsewhere B97.89
      unspecified nature or site B34.8
    unspecified nature or site B34.9
    West Nile — *see* Virus, West Nile
  vulva (acute) — *see* Vulvitis
  West Nile — *see* Virus, West Nile
  whipworm B79
  worms B83.9
    specified type NEC B83.8
  Wuchereria (bancrofti) B74.0
    malayi B74.1
  yatapoxvirus B08.70
    specified NEC B08.79
  yeast (*see also* Candidiasis) B37.9
  yellow fever — *see* Fever, yellow
  Yersinia
    enterocolitica (intestinal) A04.6
    pestis — *see* Plague
    pseudotuberculosis A28.2
  Zeis' gland — *see* Hordeolum
  Zika virus A92.5
    congenital P35.4
  zoonotic bacterial NOS A28.9
  Zopfia senegalensis B47.0
Infective, infectious — *see* condition
Infertility
  female N97.9
    age-related N97.8

Infertility — *continued*
  female — *continued*
    associated with
      anovulation N97.0
      cervical (mucus) disease or anomaly N88.3
      congenital anomaly
        cervix N88.3
        fallopian tube N97.1
        uterus N97.2
        vagina N97.8
      dysmucorrhea N88.3
      fallopian tube disease or anomaly N97.1
      pituitary-hypothalamic origin E23.0
      specified origin NEC N97.8
      Stein-Leventhal syndrome E28.2
      uterine disease or anomaly N97.2
      vaginal disease or anomaly N97.8
    due to
      cervical anomaly N88.3
      fallopian tube anomaly N97.1
      ovarian failure E28.39
      Stein-Leventhal syndrome E28.2
      uterine anomaly N97.2
      vaginal anomaly N97.8
    nonimplantation N97.2
    origin
      cervical N88.3
      tubal (block) (occlusion) (stenosis) N97.1
      uterine N97.2
      vaginal N97.8
  male N46.9
    azoospermia N46.01
      extratesticular cause N46.029
        drug therapy N46.021
        efferent duct obstruction N46.023
        infection N46.022
        radiation N46.024
        specified cause NEC N46.029
        systemic disease N46.025
    oligospermia N46.11
      extratesticular cause N46.129
        drug therapy N46.121
        efferent duct obstruction N46.123
        infection N46.122
        radiation N46.124
        specified cause NEC N46.129
        systemic disease N46.125
    specified type NEC N46.8
Infestation B88.9
  Acanthocheilonema (perstans) (streptocerca) B74.4
  Acariasis B88.0
    demodex folliculorum B88.0
    sarcoptes scabiei B86
    trombiculae B88.0
  Agamofilaria streptocerca B74.4
  Ancylostoma, ankylostoma (braziliense) (caninum) (ceylanicum) (duodenale) B76.0
    americanum B76.1
    new world B76.1
  Anisakis larvae, anisakiasis B81.0
  arthropod NEC B88.2
  Ascaris lumbricoides — *see* Ascariasis
  Balantidium coli A07.0
  beef tapeworm B68.1
  Bothriocephalus (latus) B70.0
    larval B70.1
  broad tapeworm B70.0
    larval B70.1
  Brugia (malayi) B74.1
    timori B74.2
  candiru B88.8
  Capillaria
    hepatica B83.8
    philippinensis B81.1
  cat liver fluke B66.0
  cestodes B71.9
    diphyllobothrium — *see* Infestation, diphyllobothrium
    dipylidiasis B71.1
    hymenolepiasis B71.0
    specified type NEC B71.8
  chigger B88.0
  chigo, chigoe B88.1
  Clonorchis (sinensis) (liver) B66.1
  coccidial A07.3
  crab-lice B85.3
  Cysticercus cellulosae — *see* Cysticercosis
  Demodex (folliculorum) B88.0
  Dermanyssus gallinae B88.0

Infestation — *continued*
  Dermatobia (hominis) — *see* Myiasis
  Dibothriocephalus (latus) B70.0
    larval B70.1
  Dicrocoelium dendriticum B66.2
  Diphyllobothrium (adult) (latum) (intestinal) (pacificum) B70.0
    larval B70.1
  Diplogonoporus (grandis) B71.8
  Dipylidium caninum B67.4
  Distoma hepaticum B66.3
  dog tapeworm B67.4
  Dracunculus medinensis B72
  dragon worm B72
  dwarf tapeworm B71.0
  Echinococcus — *see* Echinococcus
  Echinostomum ilocanum B66.8
  Entamoeba (histolytica) — *see* Infection, Ameba
  Enterobius vermicularis B80
  eyelid
    in (due to)
      leishmaniasis B55.1
      loiasis B74.3
      onchocerciasis B73.09
      phthiriasis B85.3
      parasitic NOS B89
  eyeworm B74.3
  Fasciola (gigantica) (hepatica) (indica) B66.3
  Fasciolopsis (buski) (intestine) B66.5
  filarial B74.9
    bancroftian B74.0
    conjunctiva B74.9
    due to
      Acanthocheilonema (perstans) (streptocerca) B74.4
      Brugia (malayi) B74.1
        timori B74.2
      Dracunculus medinensis B72
      guinea worm B72
      loa loa B74.3
      Mansonella (ozzardi) (perstans) (streptocerca) B74.4
      Onchocerca volvulus B73.00
        eye B73.00
        eyelid B73.09
      Wuchereria (bancrofti) B74.0
    Malayan B74.1
    ozzardi B74.4
    specified type NEC B74.8
  fish tapeworm B70.0
    larval B70.1
  fluke B66.9
    blood NOS — *see* Schistosomiasis
    cat liver B66.0
    intestinal B66.5
    lancet B66.2
    liver (sheep) B66.3
      cat B66.0
      Chinese B66.1
      due to clonorchiasis B66.1
      oriental B66.1
    lung (oriental) B66.4
    sheep liver B66.3
    specified type NEC B66.8
  fly larvae — *see* Myiasis
  Gasterophilus (intestinalis) — *see* Myiasis
  Gastrodiscoides hominis B66.8
  Giardia lamblia A07.1
  Gnathostoma (spinigerum) B83.1
  Gongylonema B83.8
  guinea worm B72
  helminth B83.9
    angiostrongyliasis B83.2
      intestinal B81.3
    gnathostomiasis B83.1
    hirudiniasis, internal B83.4
    intestinal B82.0
      angiostrongyliasis B81.3
      anisakiasis B81.0
      ascariasis — *see* Ascariasis
      capillariasis B81.1
      cysticercosis — *see* Cysticercosis
      diphyllobothriasis — *see* Infestation, diphyllobothriasis
      dracunculiasis B72
      echinococcus — *see* Echinococcosis
      enterobiasis B80
      filariasis — *see* Infestation, filarial

Infestation — *continued*
  helminth — *continued*
    intestinal — *continued*
      fluke — *see* Infestation, fluke
      hookworm — *see* Infestation, hookworm
      mixed (types classifiable to more than one of the titles B65.Ø-B81.3 and B81.8) B81.4
      onchocerciasis — *see* Onchocerciasis
      schistosomiasis — *see* Infestation, schistosoma
      specified
        cestode NEC — *see* Infestation, cestode type NEC B81.8
      strongyloidiasis — *see* Strongyloidiasis
      taenia — *see* Infestation, taenia
      trichinellosis B75
      trichostrongyliasis B81.2
      trichuriasis B79
    specified type NEC B83.8
    syngamiasis B83.3
    visceral larva migrans B83.Ø
  Heterophyes (heterophyes) B66.8
  hookworm B76.9
    ancylostomiasis B76.Ø
    necatoriasis B76.1
    specified type NEC B76.8
  Hymenolepis (diminuta) (nana) B71.Ø
  intestinal NEC B82.9
  leeches (aquatic) (land) — *see* Hirudiniasis
  Leishmania — *see* Leishmaniasis
  lice, louse — *see* Infestation, Pediculus
  Linguatula B88.8
  Liponyssoides sanguineus B88.Ø
  Loa loa B74.3
    conjunctival B74.3
    eyelid B74.3
  louse — *see* Infestation, Pediculus
  maggots — *see* Myiasis
  Mansonella (ozzardi) (perstans) (streptocerca) B74.4
  Medina (worm) B72
  Metagonimus (yokogawai) B66.8
  microfilaria streptocerca — *see* Onchocerciasis
    eye B73.ØØ
    eyelid B73.Ø9
  mites B88.9
    scabic B86
  Monilia (albicans) — *see* Candidiasis
  mouth B37.Ø
  Necator americanus B76.1
  nematode NEC (intestinal) B82.Ø
    Ancylostoma B76.Ø
    conjunctiva NEC B83.9
    Enterobius vermicularis B8Ø
    Gnathostoma spinigerum B83.1
    physaloptera B8Ø
    specified NEC B81.8
    trichostrongylus B81.2
    trichuris (trichuria) B79
  Oesophagostomum (apiostomum) B81.8
  Oestrus ovis (*see also* Myiasis) B87.9
  Onchocerca (volvulus) — *see* Onchocerciasis
  Opisthorchis (felineus) (viverrini) B66.Ø
  orbit, parasitic NOS B89
  Oxyuris vermicularis B8Ø
  Paragonimus (westermani) B66.4
  parasite, parasitic B89
    eyelid B89
    intestinal NOS B82.9
    mouth B37.Ø
    skin B88.9
    tongue B37.Ø
  Parastrongylus
    cantonensis B83.2
    costaricensis B81.3
  Pediculus B85.2
    body B85.1
    capitis (humanus) (any site) B85.Ø
    corporis (humanus) (any site) B85.1
    head B85.Ø
    mixed (classifiable to more than one of the titles B85.Ø - B85.3) B85.4
    pubis (any site) B85.3
  Pentastoma B88.8
  Phthirus (pubis) (any site) B85.3
    with any infestation classifiable to B85.Ø - B85.2 B85.4
  pinworm B8Ø
  pork tapeworm (adult) B68.Ø
  protozoal NEC B64

Infestation — *continued*
  protozoal — *continued*
    intestinal AØ7.9
      specified NEC AØ7.8
    specified NEC B6Ø.8
  pubic, louse B85.3
  rat tapeworm B71.Ø
  red bug B88.Ø
  roundworm (large) NEC B82.Ø
    Ascariasis (*see also* Ascariasis) B77.9
  sandflea B88.1
  Sarcoptes scabiei B86
  scabies B86
  Schistosoma B65.9
    bovis B65.8
    cercariae B65.3
    haematobium B65.Ø
    intercalatum B65.8
    japonicum B65.2
    mansoni B65.1
    mattheei B65.8
    mekongi B65.8
    specified type NEC B65.8
    spindale B65.8
  screw worms — *see* Myiasis
  skin NOS B88.9
  Sparganum (mansoni) (proliferum) (baxteri) B7Ø.1
    larval B7Ø.1
  specified type NEC B88.8
  Spirometra larvae B7Ø.1
  Stellantchasmus falcatus B66.8
  Strongyloides stercoralis — *see* Strongyloidiasis
  Taenia B68.9
    diminuta B71.Ø
    echinococcus — *see* Echinococcus
    mediocanellata B68.1
    nana B71.Ø
    saginata B68.1
    solium (intestinal form) B68.Ø
      larval form — *see* Cysticercosis
  Taeniarhynchus saginatus B68.1
  tapeworm B71.9
    beef B68.1
    broad B7Ø.Ø
      larval B7Ø.1
    dog B67.4
    dwarf B71.Ø
    fish B7Ø.Ø
      larval B7Ø.1
    pork B68.Ø
    rat B71.Ø
  Ternidens diminutus B81.8
  Tetranychus molestissimus B88.Ø
  threadworm B8Ø
  tongue B37.Ø
  Toxocara (canis) (cati) (felis) B83.Ø
  trematode(s) NEC — *see* Infestation, fluke
  Trichinella (spiralis) B75
  Trichocephalus B79
  Trichomonas — *see* Trichomoniasis
  Trichostrongylus B81.2
  Trichuris (trichiura) B79
  Trombicula (irritans) B88.Ø
  Tunga penetrans B88.1
  Uncinaria americana B76.1
  Vandellia cirrhosa B88.8
  whipworm B79
  worms B83.9
    intestinal B82.Ø
  Wuchereria (bancrofti) B74.Ø

Infiltrate, infiltration
  amyloid (generalized) (localized) — *see* Amyloidosis
  calcareous NEC R89.7
    localized — *see* Degeneration, by site
  calcium salt R89.7
  cardiac
    fatty — *see* Degeneration, myocardial
    glycogenic E74.Ø2 [I43]
  corneal — *see* Edema, cornea
  eyelid — *see* Inflammation, eyelid
  glycogen, glycogenic — *see* Disease, glycogen storage
  heart, cardiac
    fatty — *see* Degeneration, myocardial
    glycogenic E74.Ø2 [I43]
  inflammatory in vitreous H43.89
  kidney N28.89
  leukemic — *see* Leukemia
  liver K76.89

Infiltrate, infiltration — *continued*
  liver — *continued*
    fatty — *see* Fatty, liver NEC
    glycogen (*see also* Disease, glycogen storage) E74.Ø3 [K77]
  lung R91.8
    eosinophilic J82
  lymphatic (*see also* Leukemia, lymphatic) C91.9- ☑
    gland I88.9
  muscle, fatty M62.89
  myocardium, myocardial
    fatty — *see* Degeneration, myocardial
    glycogenic E74.Ø2 [I43]
  on chest x-ray R91.8
  pulmonary R91.8
    with eosinophilia J82
  skin (lymphocytic) L98.6
  thymus (gland) (fatty) E32.8
  urine R39.Ø
  vesicant agent
    antineoplastic chemotherapy T8Ø.81Ø ☑
    other agent NEC T8Ø.818 ☑
  vitreous body H43.89
Infirmity R68.89
  senile R54
Inflammation, inflamed, inflammatory (with exudation)
  abducent (nerve) — *see* Strabismus, paralytic, sixth nerve
  accessory sinus (chronic) — *see* Sinusitis
  adrenal (gland) E27.8
  alveoli, teeth M27.3
    scorbutic E54
  anal canal, anus K62.89
  antrum (chronic) — *see* Sinusitis, maxillary
  appendix — *see* Appendicitis
  arachnoid — *see* Meningitis
  areola N61.Ø
    puerperal, postpartum or gestational — *see* Infection, nipple
  areolar tissue NOS LØ8.9
  artery — *see* Arteritis
  auditory meatus (external) — *see* Otitis, externa
  Bartholin's gland N75.8
  bile duct (common) (hepatic) or passage — *see* Cholangitis
  bladder — *see* Cystitis
  bone — *see* Osteomyelitis
  brain (*see also* Encephalitis)
    membrane — *see* Meningitis
  breast N61.Ø
    puerperal, postpartum, gestational — *see* Mastitis, obstetric
  broad ligament — *see* Disease, pelvis, inflammatory
  bronchi — *see* Bronchitis
  catarrhal JØØ
  cecum — *see* Appendicitis
  cerebral (*see also* Encephalitis)
    membrane — *see* Meningitis
  cerebrospinal
    meningococcal A39.Ø
  cervix (uteri) — *see* Cervicitis
  chest J98.8
  chorioretinal H3Ø.9- ☑
    cyclitis — *see* Cyclitis
    disseminated H3Ø.1Ø- ☑
      generalized H3Ø.13- ☑
      peripheral H3Ø.12- ☑
      posterior pole H3Ø.11- ☑
    epitheliopathy — *see* Epitheliopathy
    focal H3Ø.ØØ- ☑
      juxtapapillary H3Ø.Ø1- ☑
      macular H3Ø.Ø4- ☑
      paramacular — *see* Inflammation, chorioretinal, focal, macular
      peripheral H3Ø.Ø3- ☑
      posterior pole H3Ø.Ø2- ☑
    specified type NEC H3Ø.89- ☑
  choroid — *see* Inflammation, chorioretinal
  chronic, postmastoidectomy cavity — *see* Complications, postmastoidectomy, inflammation
  colon — *see* Enteritis
  connective tissue (diffuse) NEC — *see* Disorder, soft tissue, specified type NEC
  cornea — *see* Keratitis
  corpora cavernosa N48.29
  cranial nerve — *see* Disorder, nerve, cranial

Inflammation, inflamed, inflammatory —
continued
Douglas' cul-de-sac or pouch (chronic) N73.0
due to device, implant or graft (*see also* Complications, by site and type, infection or inflammation)
arterial graft T82.7 ☑
breast (implant) T85.79 ☑
catheter T85.79 ☑
dialysis (renal) T82.7 ☑
intraperitoneal T85.71 ☑
infusion T82.7 ☑
cranial T85.735 ☑
intrathecal T85.735 ☑
spinal (epidural) (subdural) T85.735 ☑
subarachnoid T85.735 ☑
urinary T83.518 ☑
cystostomy T83.510 ☑
Hopkins T83.518 ☑
ileostomy T83.518 ☑
nephrostomy T83.512 ☑
specified NEC T83.518 ☑
urethral indwelling T83.511 ☑
urostomy T83.518 ☑
electronic (electrode) (pulse generator) (stimulator)
bone T84.7 ☑
cardiac T82.7 ☑
nervous system T85.738 ☑
brain T85.731 ☑
cranial nerve T85.732 ☑
gastric nerve T85.732 ☑
neurostimulator generator T85.734 ☑
peripheral nerve T85.732 ☑
sacral nerve T85.732 ☑
spinal cord T85.733 ☑
vagal nerve T85.732 ☑
urinary T83.590 ☑
fixation, internal (orthopedic) NEC — *see* Complication, fixation device, infection
gastrointestinal (bile duct) (esophagus) T85.79 ☑
neurostimulator electrode (lead) T85.732 ☑
genital NEC T83.69 ☑
heart NEC T82.7 ☑
valve (prosthesis) T82.6 ☑
graft T82.7 ☑
joint prosthesis — *see* Complication, joint prosthesis, infection
ocular (corneal graft) (orbital implant) NEC T85.79 ☑
orthopedic NEC T84.7 ☑
penile (cylinder) (pump) (resevoir) T83.61 ☑
specified NEC T85.79 ☑
testicular T83.62 ☑
urinary NEC T83.598 ☑
ileal conduit stent T83.593 ☑
implanted neurostimulation T83.590 ☑
implanted sphincter T83.591 ☑
indwelling ureteral stent T83.592 ☑
nephroureteral stent T83.593 ☑
specified stent NEC T83.593 ☑
vascular NEC T82.7 ☑
ventricular intracranial (communicating) shunt T85.730 ☑
duodenum K29.80
with bleeding K29.81
dura mater — *see* Meningitis
ear (middle) (*see also* Otitis, media)
external — *see* Otitis, externa
inner — *see* subcategory H83.0 ☑
epididymis — *see* Epididymitis
esophagus K20.9
ethmoidal (sinus) (chronic) — *see* Sinusitis, ethmoidal
eustachian tube (catarrhal) — *see* Salpingitis, eustachian
eyelid H01.9
abscess — *see* Abscess, eyelid
blepharitis — *see* Blepharitis
chalazion — *see* Chalazion
dermatosis (noninfectious) — *see* Dermatosis, eyelid
hordeolum — *see* Hordeolum
specified NEC H01.8
fallopian tube — *see* Salpingo-oophoritis
fascia — *see* Myositis
follicular, pharynx J31.2
frontal (sinus) (chronic) — *see* Sinusitis, frontal
gallbladder — *see* Cholecystitis
gastric — *see* Gastritis
gastrointestinal — *see* Enteritis

Inflammation, inflamed, inflammatory —
continued
genital organ (internal) (diffuse)
female — *see* Disease, pelvis, inflammatory
male N49.9
multiple sites N49.8
specified NEC N49.8
gland (lymph) — *see* Lymphadenitis
glottis — *see* Laryngitis
granular, pharynx J31.2
gum K05.10
nonplaque induced K05.11
plaque induced K05.10
heart — *see* Carditis
hepatic duct — *see* Cholangitis
ileoanal (internal) pouch K91.850
ileum (*see also* Enteritis)
regional or terminal — *see* Enteritis, regional
intestinal pouch K91.850
intestine (any part) — *see* Enteritis
jaw (acute) (bone) (chronic) (lower) (suppurative) (upper) M27.2
joint NEC — *see* Arthritis
sacroiliac M46.1
kidney — *see* Nephritis
knee (joint) M13.169
tuberculous A18.02
labium (majus) (minus) — *see* Vulvitis
lacrimal
gland — *see* Dacryoadenitis
passages (duct) (sac) (*see also* Dacryocystitis)
canaliculitis — *see* Canaliculitis, lacrimal
larynx — *see* Laryngitis
leg NOS L08.9
lip K13.0
liver (capsule) (*see also* Hepatitis)
chronic K73.9
suppurative K75.0
lung (acute) (*see also* Pneumonia)
chronic J98.4
lymph gland or node — *see* Lymphadenitis
lymphatic vessel — *see* Lymphangitis
maxilla, maxillary M27.2
sinus (chronic) — *see* Sinusitis, maxillary
membranes of brain or spinal cord — *see* Meningitis
meninges — *see* Meningitis
mouth K12.1
muscle — *see* Myositis
myocardium — *see* Myocarditis
nasal sinus (chronic) — *see* Sinusitis
nasopharynx — *see* Nasopharyngitis
navel L08.82
nerve NEC — *see* Neuralgia
nipple N61.0
puerperal, postpartum or gestational — *see* Infection, nipple
nose — *see* Rhinitis
oculomotor (nerve) — *see* Strabismus, paralytic, third nerve
optic nerve — *see* Neuritis, optic
orbit (chronic) H05.10
acute H05.00
abscess — *see* Abscess, orbit
cellulitis — *see* Cellulitis, orbit
osteomyelitis — *see* Osteomyelitis, orbit
periostitis — *see* Periostitis, orbital
tenonitis — *see* Tenonitis, eye
granuloma — *see* Granuloma, orbit
myositis — *see* Myositis, orbital
ovary — *see* Salpingo-oophoritis
oviduct — *see* Salpingo-oophoritis
pancreas (acute) — *see* Pancreatitis
parametrium N73.0
parotid region L08.9
pelvis, female — *see* Disease, pelvis, inflammatory
penis (corpora cavernosa) N48.29
perianal K62.89
pericardium — *see* Pericarditis
perineum (female) (male) L08.9
periuterine — *see* Disease, pelvis, inflammatory
perivesical — *see* Cystitis
petrous bone (acute) (chronic) — *see* Petrositis
pharynx (acute) — *see* Pharyngitis
pia mater — *see* Meningitis
pleura — *see* Pleurisy

Inflammation, inflamed, inflammatory —
continued
polyp, colon (*see also* Polyp, colon, inflammatory) K51.40
prostate (*see also* Prostatitis)
specified type NEC N41.8
rectosigmoid — *see* Rectosigmoiditis
rectum (*see also* Proctitis) K62.89
respiratory, upper (*see also* Infection, respiratory, upper) J06.9
acute, due to radiation J70.0
chronic, due to external agent — *see* condition, respiratory, chronic, due to
due to
chemicals, gases, fumes or vapors (inhalation) J68.2
radiation J70.1
retina — *see* Chorioretinitis
retrocecal — *see* Appendicitis
retroperitoneal — *see* Peritonitis
salivary duct or gland (any) (suppurative) — *see* Sialoadenitis
scorbutic, alveoli, teeth E54
scrotum N49.2
seminal vesicle — *see* Vesiculitis
sigmoid — *see* Enteritis
sinus — *see* Sinusitis
Skene's duct or gland — *see* Urethritis
skin L08.9
spermatic cord N49.1
sphenoidal (sinus) — *see* Sinusitis, sphenoidal
spinal
cord — *see* Encephalitis
membrane — *see* Meningitis
nerve — *see* Disorder, nerve
spine — *see* Spondylopathy, inflammatory
spleen (capsule) D73.89
stomach — *see* Gastritis
subcutaneous tissue L08.9
suprarenal (gland) E27.8
synovial — *see* Tenosynovitis
tendon (sheath) NEC — *see* Tenosynovitis
testis — *see* Orchitis
throat (acute) — *see* Pharyngitis
thymus (gland) E32.8
thyroid (gland) — *see* Thyroiditis
tongue K14.0
tonsil — *see* Tonsillitis
trachea — *see* Tracheitis
trochlear (nerve) — *see* Strabismus, paralytic, fourth nerve
tubal — *see* Salpingo-oophoritis
tuberculous NEC — *see* Tuberculosis
tubo-ovarian — *see* Salpingo-oophoritis
tunica vaginalis N49.1
tympanic membrane — *see* Tympanitis
umbilicus, umbilical L08.82
uterine ligament — *see* Disease, pelvis, inflammatory
uterus (catarrhal) — *see* Endometritis
uveal tract (anterior) NOS (*see also* Iridocyclitis)
posterior — *see* Chorioretinitis
vagina — *see* Vaginitis
vas deferens N49.1
vein (*see also* Phlebitis)
intracranial or intraspinal (septic) G08
thrombotic I80.9
leg — *see* Phlebitis, leg
lower extremity — *see* Phlebitis, leg
vocal cord J38.3
vulva — *see* Vulvitis
Wharton's duct (suppurative) — *see* Sialoadenitis
Inflation, lung, imperfect (newborn) — *see* Atelectasis
Influenza (bronchial) (epidemic) (respiratory (upper)) (unidentified influenza virus) J11.1
with
digestive manifestations J11.2
encephalopathy J11.81
enteritis J11.2
gastroenteritis J11.2
gastrointestinal manifestations J11.2
laryngitis J11.1
myocarditis J11.82
otitis media J11.83
pharyngitis J11.1
pneumonia J11.00
specified type J11.08
respiratory manifestations NEC J11.1

Index

Influenza — *continued*
　with — *continued*
　　specified manifestation NEC J11.89
　A/H5N1 (*see also* Influenza, due to, identified novel influenza A virus) J09.X2
　avian (*see also* Influenza, due to, identified novel influenza A virus) J09.X2
　bird (*see also* Influenza, due to, identified novel influenza A virus) J09.X2
　novel (2009) H1N1 influenza (*see also* Influenza, due to, identified influenza NEC) J10.1
　novel influenza A/H1N1 (*see also* Influenza, due to, identified influenza virus NEC) J10.1
　due to
　　avian (*see also* Influenza, due to, identified novel influenza A virus) J09.X2
　　identified influenza virus NEC J10.1
　　　with
　　　　digestive manifestations J10.2
　　　　encephalopathy J10.81
　　　　enteritis J10.2
　　　　gastroenteritis J10.2
　　　　gastrointestinal manifestations J10.2
　　　　laryngitis J10.1
　　　　myocarditis J10.82
　　　　otitis media J10.83
　　　　pharyngitis J10.1
　　　　pneumonia (unspecified type) J10.00
　　　　　with same identified influenza virus J10.01
　　　　　specified type NEC J10.08
　　　　respiratory manifestations NEC J10.1
　　　　specified manifestation NEC J10.89
　　identified novel influenza A virus J09.X2
　　　with
　　　　digestive manifestations J09.X3
　　　　encephalopathy J09.X9
　　　　enteritis J09.X3
　　　　gastroenteritis J09.X3
　　　　gastrointestinal manifestations J09.X3
　　　　laryngitis J09.X2
　　　　myocarditis J09.X9
　　　　otitis media J09.X9
　　　　pharyngitis J09.X2
　　　　pneumonia J09.X1
　　　　respiratory manifestations NEC J09.X2
　　　　specified manifestation NEC J09.X9
　　　　upper respiratory symptoms J09.X2
　of other animal origin, not bird or swine (*see also* Influenza, due to, identified novel influenza A virus) J09.X2
　swine (viruses that normally cause infections in pigs) (*see also* Influenza, due to, identified novel influenza A virus) J09.X2
Influenzal — *see* Influenza
Influenza-like disease — *see* Influenza
Infraction, Freiberg's (metatarsal head) — *see* Osteochondrosis, juvenile, metatarsus
Infraeruption of tooth (teeth) M26.34
Infusion complication, misadventure, or reaction — *see* Complications, infusion
Ingestion
　chemical — *see* Table of Drugs and Chemicals, by substance, poisoning
　drug or medicament
　　correct substance properly administered — *see* Table of Drugs and Chemicals, by drug, adverse effect
　　overdose or wrong substance given or taken — *see* Table of Drugs and Chemicals, by drug, poisoning
　foreign body — *see* Foreign body, alimentary tract
　tularemia A21.3
Ingrowing
　hair (beard) L73.1
　nail (finger) (toe) L60.0
Inguinal (*see also* condition)
　testicle Q53.9
　　bilateral Q53.212
　　unilateral Q53.112
Inhalant-induced
　anxiety disorder F18.980
　depressive disorder F18.94
　major neurocognitive disorder F18.97
　mild neurocognitive disorder F18.988
　psychotic disorder F18.959
Inhalation
　anthrax A22.1

Inhalation — *continued*
　flame T27.3 ☑
　food or foreign body — *see* Foreign body, by site
　gases, fumes, or vapors NEC T59.9- ☑
　　specified agent — *see* Table of Drugs and Chemicals, by substance
　liquid or vomitus — *see* Asphyxia
　meconium (newborn) P24.00
　　with
　　　with respiratory symptoms P24.01
　　　pneumonia (pneumonitis) P24.01
　mucus — *see* Asphyxia, mucus
　oil or gasoline (causing suffocation) — *see* Foreign body, by site
　smoke J70.5
　　due to chemicals, gases, fumes and vapors J68.9
　steam — *see* Toxicity, vapors
　stomach contents or secretions — *see* Foreign body, by site
　　due to anesthesia (general) (local) or other sedation T88.59 ☑
　　in labor and delivery O74.0
　　in pregnancy O29.01- ☑
　　postpartum, puerperal O89.01
Inhibition, orgasm
　female F52.31
　male F52.32
Inhibitor, systemic lupus erythematosus (presence of) D68.62
Iniencephalus, iniencephaly Q00.2
Injection, traumatic jet (air) (industrial) (water) (paint or dye) T70.4 ☑
Injury (*see also* specified injury type) T14.90 ☑
　abdomen, abdominal S39.91 ☑
　　blood vessel — *see* Injury, blood vessel, abdomen
　　cavity — *see* Injury, intra-abdominal
　　contusion S30.1 ☑
　　internal — *see* Injury, intra-abdominal
　　intra-abdominal organ — *see* Injury, intra-abdominal
　　nerve — *see* Injury, nerve, abdomen
　　open — *see* Wound, open, abdomen
　　specified NEC S39.81 ☑
　　superficial — *see* Injury, superficial, abdomen
　Achilles tendon S86.00- ☑
　　laceration S86.02- ☑
　　specified type NEC S86.09- ☑
　　strain S86.01- ☑
　acoustic, resulting in deafness — *see* Injury, nerve, acoustic
　adrenal (gland) S37.819 ☑
　　contusion S37.812 ☑
　　laceration S37.813 ☑
　　specified type NEC S37.818 ☑
　alveolar (process) S09.93 ☑
　ankle S99.91- ☑
　　contusion — *see* Contusion, ankle
　　dislocation — *see* Dislocation, ankle
　　fracture — *see* Fracture, ankle
　　nerve — *see* Injury, nerve, ankle
　　open — *see* Wound, open, ankle
　　specified type NEC S99.81- ☑
　　sprain — *see* Sprain, ankle
　　superficial — *see* Injury, superficial, ankle
　anterior chamber, eye — *see* Injury, eye, specified site NEC
　anus — *see* Injury, abdomen
　aorta (thoracic) S25.00 ☑
　　abdominal S35.00 ☑
　　　laceration (minor) (superficial) S35.01 ☑
　　　　major S35.02 ☑
　　　specified type NEC S35.09 ☑
　　laceration (minor) (superficial) S25.01 ☑
　　　major S25.02 ☑
　　specified type NEC S25.09 ☑
　arm (upper) S49.9- ☑
　　blood vessel — *see* Injury, blood vessel, arm
　　contusion — *see* Contusion, arm, upper
　　fracture — *see* Fracture, humerus
　　lower — *see* Injury, forearm
　　muscle — *see* Injury, muscle, shoulder
　　nerve — *see* Injury, nerve, arm
　　open — *see* Wound, open, arm
　　specified type NEC S49.8- ☑
　　superficial — *see* Injury, superficial, arm

Injury — *continued*
　artery (complicating trauma) (*see also* Injury, blood vessel, by site)
　　cerebral or meningeal — *see* Injury, intracranial
　auditory canal (external) (meatus) S09.91 ☑
　auricle, auris, ear S09.91 ☑
　axilla — *see* Injury, shoulder
　back — *see* Injury, back, lower
　bile duct S36.13 ☑
　birth (*see also* Birth, injury) P15.9
　bladder (sphincter) S37.20 ☑
　　at delivery O71.5
　　contusion S37.22 ☑
　　laceration S37.23 ☑
　　obstetrical trauma O71.5
　　specified type NEC S37.29 ☑
　blast (air) (hydraulic) (immersion) (underwater) NEC T14.8 ☑
　　acoustic nerve trauma — *see* Injury, nerve, acoustic
　　bladder — *see* Injury, bladder
　　brain — *see* Concussion
　　colon — *see* Injury, intestine, large
　　ear (primary) S09.31- ☑
　　　secondary S09.39- ☑
　　generalized T70.8 ☑
　　lung — *see* Injury, intrathoracic, lung
　　multiple body organs T70.8 ☑
　　peritoneum S36.81 ☑
　　rectum S36.61 ☑
　　retroperitoneum S36.898 ☑
　　small intestine S36.419 ☑
　　　duodenum S36.410 ☑
　　　specified site NEC S36.418 ☑
　　specified
　　　intra-abdominal organ NEC S36.898 ☑
　　　pelvic organ NEC S37.899 ☑
　blood vessel NEC T14.8 ☑
　　abdomen S35.9 ☑
　　　aorta — *see* Injury, aorta, abdominal
　　　celiac artery — *see* Injury, blood vessel, celiac artery
　　　iliac vessel — *see* Injury, blood vessel, iliac
　　　laceration S35.91 ☑
　　　mesenteric vessel — *see* Injury, mesenteric
　　　portal vein — *see* Injury, blood vessel, portal vein
　　　renal vessel — *see* Injury, blood vessel, renal
　　　specified vessel NEC S35.8X- ☑
　　　splenic vessel — *see* Injury, blood vessel, splenic
　　　vena cava — *see* Injury, vena cava, inferior
　　ankle — *see* Injury, blood vessel, foot
　　aorta (abdominal) (thoracic) — *see* Injury, aorta
　　arm (upper) NEC S45.90- ☑
　　　forearm — *see* Injury, blood vessel, forearm
　　　laceration S45.91- ☑
　　　specified
　　　　site NEC S45.80- ☑
　　　　　laceration S45.81- ☑
　　　　　specified type NEC S45.89- ☑
　　　　type NEC S45.99- ☑
　　　superficial vein S45.30- ☑
　　　　laceration S45.31- ☑
　　　　specified type NEC S45.39- ☑
　　axillary
　　　artery S45.00- ☑
　　　　laceration S45.01- ☑
　　　　specified type NEC S45.09- ☑
　　　vein S45.20- ☑
　　　　laceration S45.21- ☑
　　　　specified type NEC S45.29- ☑
　　azygos vein — *see* Injury, blood vessel, thoracic, specified site NEC
　　brachial
　　　artery S45.10- ☑
　　　　laceration S45.11- ☑
　　　　specified type NEC S45.19- ☑
　　　vein S45.20- ☑
　　　　laceration S45.219 ☑
　　　　specified type NEC S45.29- ☑
　　carotid artery (common) (external) (internal, extracranial) S15.00- ☑
　　　internal, intracranial S06.8- ☑
　　　laceration (minor) (superficial) S15.01- ☑
　　　　major S15.02- ☑
　　　specified type NEC S15.09- ☑
　　celiac artery S35.219 ☑
　　　branch S35.299 ☑

Influenza — Injury

Injury — *continued*
  blood vessel — *continued*
    celiac artery — *continued*
      branch — *continued*
        laceration (minor) (superficial) S35.291 ☑
          major S35.292 ☑
        specified NEC S35.298 ☑
      laceration (minor) (superficial) S35.211 ☑
        major S35.212 ☑
      specified type NEC S35.218 ☑
    cerebral — *see* Injury, intracranial
    deep plantar — *see* Injury, blood vessel, plantar artery
    digital (hand) — *see* Injury, blood vessel, finger
    dorsal
      artery (foot) S95.00- ☑
        laceration S95.01- ☑
        specified type NEC S95.09- ☑
      vein (foot) S95.20- ☑
        laceration S95.21- ☑
        specified type NEC S95.29- ☑
    due to accidental laceration during procedure — *see* Laceration, accidental complicating surgery
    extremity — *see* Injury, blood vessel, limb
    femoral
      artery (common) (superficial) S75.00- ☑
        laceration (minor) (superficial) S75.01- ☑
          major S75.02- ☑
        specified type NEC S75.09- ☑
      vein (hip level) (thigh level) S75.10- ☑
        laceration (minor) (superficial) S75.11- ☑
          major S75.12- ☑
        specified type NEC S75.19- ☑
    finger S65.50- ☑
      index S65.50- ☑
        laceration S65.51- ☑
        specified type NEC S65.59- ☑
      laceration S65.51- ☑
      little S65.50- ☑
        laceration S65.51- ☑
        specified type NEC S65.59- ☑
      middle S65.50- ☑
        laceration S65.51- ☑
        specified type NEC S65.59- ☑
      specified type NEC S65.59- ☑
      thumb — *see* Injury, blood vessel, thumb
    foot S95.90- ☑
      dorsal
        artery — *see* Injury, blood vessel, dorsal, artery
        vein — *see* Injury, blood vessel, dorsal, vein
      laceration S95.91- ☑
      plantar artery — *see* Injury, blood vessel, plantar artery
      specified
        site NEC S95.80- ☑
          laceration S95.81- ☑
          specified type NEC S95.89- ☑
        specified type NEC S95.99- ☑
    forearm S55.90- ☑
      laceration S55.91- ☑
      radial artery — *see* Injury, blood vessel, radial artery
      specified
        site NEC S55.80- ☑
          laceration S55.81- ☑
          specified type NEC S55.89- ☑
        type NEC S55.99- ☑
      ulnar artery — *see* Injury, blood vessel, ulnar artery
      vein S55.20- ☑
        laceration S55.21- ☑
        specified type NEC S55.29- ☑
    gastric
      artery — *see* Injury, mesenteric, artery, branch
      vein — *see* Injury, blood vessel, abdomen
    gastroduodenal artery — *see* Injury, mesenteric, artery, branch
    greater saphenous vein (lower leg level) S85.30- ☑
      hip (and thigh) level S75.20- ☑
        laceration (minor) (superficial) S75.21- ☑
          major S75.22- ☑
        specified type NEC S75.29- ☑
      laceration S85.31- ☑
      specified type NEC S85.39- ☑

Injury — *continued*
  blood vessel — *continued*
    hand (level) S65.90- ☑
      finger — *see* Injury, blood vessel, finger
      laceration S65.91- ☑
      palmar arch — *see* Injury, blood vessel, palmar arch
      radial artery — *see* Injury, blood vessel, radial artery, hand
      specified
        site NEC S65.80- ☑
          laceration S65.81- ☑
          specified type NEC S65.89- ☑
        type NEC S65.99- ☑
      thumb — *see* Injury, blood vessel, thumb
      ulnar artery — *see* Injury, blood vessel, ulnar artery, hand
    head S09.0 ☑
      intracranial — *see* Injury, intracranial
      multiple S09.0 ☑
    hepatic
      artery — *see* Injury, mesenteric, artery
      vein — *see* Injury, vena cava, inferior
    hip S75.90- ☑
      femoral artery — *see* Injury, blood vessel, femoral, artery
      femoral vein — *see* Injury, blood vessel, femoral, vein
      greater saphenous vein — *see* Injury, blood vessel, greater saphenous, hip level
      laceration S75.91- ☑
      specified
        site NEC S75.80- ☑
          laceration S75.81- ☑
          specified type NEC S75.89- ☑
        type NEC S75.99- ☑
    hypogastric (artery) (vein) — *see* Injury, blood vessel, iliac
    iliac S35.5- ☑
      artery S35.51- ☑
      specified vessel NEC S35.5- ☑
      uterine vessel — *see* Injury, blood vessel, uterine
      vein S35.51- ☑
    innominate — *see* Injury, blood vessel, thoracic, innominate
    intercostal (artery) (vein) — *see* Injury, blood vessel, thoracic, intercostal
    jugular vein (external) S15.20- ☑
      internal S15.30- ☑
        laceration (minor) (superficial) S15.31- ☑
          major S15.32- ☑
        specified type NEC S15.39- ☑
      laceration (minor) (superficial) S15.21- ☑
        major S15.22- ☑
      specified type NEC S15.29- ☑
    leg (level) (lower) S85.90- ☑
      greater saphenous — *see* Injury, blood vessel, greater saphenous
      laceration S85.91- ☑
      lesser saphenous — *see* Injury, blood vessel, lesser saphenous
      peroneal artery — *see* Injury, blood vessel, peroneal artery
      popliteal
        artery — *see* Injury, blood vessel, popliteal, artery
        vein — *see* Injury, blood vessel, popliteal, vein
      specified
        site NEC S85.80- ☑
          laceration S85.81- ☑
          specified type NEC S85.89- ☑
        type NEC S85.99- ☑
      thigh — *see* Injury, blood vessel, hip
      tibial artery — *see* Injury, blood vessel, tibial artery
    lesser saphenous vein (lower leg level) S85.40- ☑
      laceration S85.41- ☑
      specified type NEC S85.49- ☑
    limb
      lower — *see* Injury, blood vessel, leg
      upper — *see* Injury, blood vessel, arm
    lower back — *see* Injury, blood vessel, abdomen
      specified NEC — *see* Injury, blood vessel, abdomen, specified, site NEC
    mammary (artery) (vein) — *see* Injury, blood vessel, thoracic, specified site NEC

Injury — *continued*
  blood vessel — *continued*
    mesenteric (inferior) (superior)
      artery — *see* Injury, mesenteric, artery
      vein — *see* Injury, blood vessel, mesenteric, vein
    neck S15.9
      specified site NEC S15.8 ☑
    ovarian (artery) (vein) — *see* subcategory S35.8
    palmar arch (superficial) S65.20- ☑
      deep S65.30- ☑
        laceration S65.31- ☑
        specified type NEC S65.39- ☑
      laceration S65.21- ☑
      specified type NEC S65.29- ☑
    pelvis — *see* Injury, blood vessel, abdomen
      specified NEC — *see* Injury, blood vessel, abdomen, specified, site NEC
    peroneal artery S85.20- ☑
      laceration S85.21- ☑
      specified type NEC S85.29- ☑
    plantar artery (deep) (foot) S95.10- ☑
      laceration S95.11- ☑
      specified type NEC S95.19- ☑
    popliteal
      artery S85.00- ☑
        laceration S85.01- ☑
        specified type NEC S85.09- ☑
      vein S85.50- ☑
        laceration S85.51- ☑
        specified type NEC S85.59- ☑
    portal vein S35.319 ☑
      laceration S35.311
      specified type NEC S35.318 ☑
    precerebral — *see* Injury, blood vessel, neck
    pulmonary (artery) (vein) — *see* Injury, blood vessel, thoracic, pulmonary
    radial artery (forearm level) S55.10- ☑
      hand and wrist (level) S65.10- ☑
        laceration S65.11- ☑
        specified type NEC S65.19- ☑
      laceration S55.11- ☑
      specified type NEC S55.19- ☑
    renal
      artery S35.40- ☑
        laceration S35.41- ☑
        specified NEC S35.49- ☑
      vein S35.40- ☑
        laceration S35.41- ☑
        specified NEC S35.49- ☑
    saphenous vein (greater) (lower leg level) — *see* Injury, blood vessel, greater saphenous
      hip and thigh level — *see* Injury, blood vessel, greater saphenous, hip level
      lesser — *see* Injury, blood vessel, lesser saphenous
    shoulder
      specified NEC — *see* Injury, blood vessel, arm, specified site NEC
      superficial vein — *see* Injury, blood vessel, arm, superficial vein
    specified NEC T14.8 ☑
    splenic
      artery — *see* Injury, blood vessel, celiac artery, branch
      vein S35.329 ☑
        laceration S35.321 ☑
        specified NEC S35.328 ☑
    subclavian — *see* Injury, blood vessel, thoracic, innominate
    thigh — *see* Injury, blood vessel, hip
    thoracic S25.90 ☑
      aorta S25.00 ☑
        laceration (minor) (superficial) S25.01 ☑
          major S25.02 ☑
        specified type NEC S25.09 ☑
      azygos vein — *see* Injury, blood vessel, thoracic, specified, site NEC
      innominate
        artery S25.10- ☑
          laceration (minor) (superficial) S25.11- ☑
            major S25.12- ☑
          specified type NEC S25.19- ☑
        vein S25.30- ☑
          laceration (minor) (superficial) S25.31- ☑
            major S25.32- ☑
          specified type NEC S25.39- ☑

Injury — *continued*
  blood vessel — *continued*
    thoracic — *continued*
      intercostal S25.50- ☑
        laceration S25.51- ☑
        specified type NEC S25.59- ☑
      laceration S25.91 ☑
      mammary vessel — *see* Injury, blood vessel, thoracic, specified, site NEC
      pulmonary S25.40- ☑
        laceration (minor) (superficial) S25.41- ☑
          major S25.42- ☑
        specified type NEC S25.49- ☑
      specified
        site NEC S25.80- ☑
          laceration S25.81 ☑
          specified type NEC S25.89 ☑
        type NEC S25.99 ☑
      subclavian — *see* Injury, blood vessel, thoracic, innominate
      vena cava (superior) S25.20 ☑
        laceration (minor) (superficial) S25.21 ☑
          major S25.22 ☑
        specified type NEC S25.29 ☑
    thumb S65.40- ☑
      laceration S65.41- ☑
      specified type NEC S65.49- ☑
    tibial artery S85.10- ☑
      anterior S85.13- ☑
        laceration S85.14- ☑
        specified injury NEC S85.15- ☑
      laceration S85.11- ☑
      posterior S85.16- ☑
        laceration S85.17- ☑
        specified injury NEC S85.18- ☑
      specified injury NEC S85.12- ☑
    ulnar artery (forearm level) S55.00- ☑
      hand and wrist (level) S65.00- ☑
        laceration S65.01- ☑
        specified type NEC S65.09- ☑
      laceration S55.01- ☑
      specified type NEC S55.09- ☑
    upper arm (level) — *see* Injury, blood vessel, arm
    superficial vein — *see* Injury, blood vessel, arm, superficial vein
  uterine S35.5- ☑
    artery S35.53- ☑
    vein S35.53- ☑
  vena cava — *see* Injury, vena cava
  vertebral artery S15.10- ☑
    laceration (minor) (superficial) S15.11- ☑
      major S15.12- ☑
    specified type NEC S15.19- ☑
  wrist (level) — *see* Injury, blood vessel, hand
brachial plexus S14.3 ☑
  newborn P14.3
brain (traumatic) S06.9- ☑
  diffuse (axonal) S06.2X- ☑
  focal S06.30- ☑
brainstem S06.38- ☑
breast NOS S29.9 ☑
broad ligament — *see* Injury, pelvic organ, specified site NEC
bronchus, bronchi — *see* Injury, intrathoracic, bronchus
brow S09.90 ☑
buttock S39.92 ☑
canthus, eye S05.90 ☑
cardiac plexus — *see* Injury, nerve, thorax, sympathetic
cauda equina S34.3 ☑
cavernous sinus — *see* Injury, intracranial
cecum — *see* Injury, colon
celiac ganglion or plexus — *see* Injury, nerve, lumbosacral, sympathetic
cerebellum — *see* Injury, intracranial
cerebral — *see* Injury, intracranial
cervix (uteri) — *see* Injury, uterus
cheek (wall) S09.93 ☑
chest — *see* Injury, thorax
childbirth (newborn) (*see also* Birth, injury)
  maternal NEC O71.9
chin S09.93 ☑
choroid (eye) — *see* Injury, eye, specified site NEC
clitoris S39.94 ☑
coccyx (*see also* Injury, back, lower)
  complicating delivery O71.6
colon — *see* Injury, intestine, large

Injury — *continued*
  common bile duct — *see* Injury, liver
  conjunctiva (superficial) — *see* Injury, eye, conjunctiva
  conus medullaris — *see* Injury, spinal, sacral
  cord
    spermatic (pelvic region) S37.898 ☑
      scrotal region S39.848 ☑
    spinal — *see* Injury, spinal cord, by region
  cornea — *see* Injury, eye, specified site NEC
    abrasion — *see* Injury, eye, cornea, abrasion
  cortex (cerebral) (*see also* Injury, intracranial)
    visual — *see* Injury, nerve, optic
  costal region NEC S29.9 ☑
  costochondral NEC S29.9 ☑
  cranial
    cavity — *see* Injury, intracranial
    nerve — *see* Injury, nerve, cranial
  crushing — *see* Crush
  cutaneous sensory nerve
  cystic duct — *see* Injury, liver
  deep tissue — *see* Contusion, by site
    meaning pressure ulcer — *see* Ulcer, pressure, unstageable, by site
  delivery (newborn) P15.9
    maternal NEC O71.9
  Descemet's membrane — *see* Injury, eyeball, penetrating
  diaphragm — *see* Injury, intrathoracic, diaphragm
  duodenum — *see* Injury, intestine, small, duodenum
  ear (auricle) (external) (canal) S09.91 ☑
    abrasion — *see* Abrasion, ear
    bite — *see* Bite, ear
    blister — *see* Blister, ear
    bruise — *see* Contusion, ear
    contusion — *see* Contusion, ear
    external constriction — *see* Constriction, external, ear
    hematoma — *see* Hematoma, ear
    inner — *see* Injury, ear, middle
    laceration — *see* Laceration, ear
    middle S09.30- ☑
      blast — *see* Injury, blast, ear
      specified NEC S09.39- ☑
    puncture — *see* Puncture, ear
    superficial — *see* Injury, superficial, ear
  eighth cranial nerve (acoustic or auditory) — *see* Injury, nerve, acoustic
  elbow S59.90- ☑
    contusion — *see* Contusion, elbow
    dislocation — *see* Dislocation, elbow
    fracture — *see* Fracture, ulna, upper end
    open — *see* Wound, open, elbow
    specified NEC S59.80- ☑
    sprain — *see* Sprain, elbow
    superficial — *see* Injury, superficial, elbow
  eleventh cranial nerve (accessory) — *see* Injury, nerve, accessory
  epididymis S39.94 ☑
  epigastric region S39.91 ☑
  epiglottis NEC S19.89 ☑
  esophageal plexus — *see* Injury, nerve, thorax, sympathetic
  esophagus (thoracic part) (*see also* Injury, intrathoracic, esophagus)
    cervical NEC S19.85 ☑
  eustachian tube S09.30 ☑
  eye S05.9- ☑
    avulsion S05.7- ☑
    ball — *see* Injury, eyeball
    conjunctiva S05.0- ☑
    cornea
      abrasion S05.0- ☑
      laceration S05.3- ☑
        with prolapse S05.2- ☑
    lacrimal apparatus S05.8X- ☑
    orbit penetration S05.4- ☑
    specified site NEC S05.8X- ☑
  eyeball S05.8X- ☑
    contusion S05.1- ☑
    penetrating S05.6- ☑
      with
        foreign body S05.5- ☑
        prolapse or loss of intraocular tissue S05.2- ☑
      without prolapse or loss of intraocular tissue S05.3- ☑
    specified type NEC S05.8- ☑

Injury — *continued*
  eyebrow S09.93 ☑
  eyelid S09.93 ☑
    abrasion — *see* Abrasion, eyelid
    contusion — *see* Contusion, eyelid
    open — *see* Wound, open, eyelid
  face S09.93 ☑
  fallopian tube S37.509 ☑
    bilateral S37.502 ☑
      blast injury S37.512 ☑
      contusion S37.522 ☑
      laceration S37.532 ☑
      specified type NEC S37.592 ☑
    blast injury (primary) S37.519 ☑
      bilateral S37.512 ☑
      secondary — *see* Injury, fallopian tube, specified type NEC
      unilateral S37.511 ☑
    contusion S37.529 ☑
      bilateral S37.522 ☑
      unilateral S37.521 ☑
    laceration S37.539 ☑
      bilateral S37.532 ☑
      unilateral S37.531 ☑
    specified type NEC S37.599 ☑
      bilateral S37.592 ☑
      unilateral S37.591 ☑
    unilateral S37.501 ☑
      blast injury S37.511 ☑
      contusion S37.521 ☑
      laceration S37.531 ☑
      specified type NEC S37.591 ☑
  fascia — *see* Injury, muscle
  fifth cranial nerve (trigeminal) — *see* Injury, nerve, trigeminal
  finger (nail) S69.9- ☑
    blood vessel — *see* Injury, blood vessel, finger
    contusion — *see* Contusion, finger
    dislocation — *see* Dislocation, finger
    fracture — *see* Fracture, finger
    muscle — *see* Injury, muscle, finger
    nerve — *see* Injury, nerve, digital, finger
    open — *see* Wound, open, finger
    specified NEC S69.8- ☑
    sprain — *see* Sprain, finger
    superficial — *see* Injury, superficial, finger
  first cranial nerve (olfactory) — *see* Injury, nerve, olfactory
  flank — *see* Injury, abdomen
  foot S99.92- ☑
    blood vessel — *see* Injury, blood vessel, foot
    contusion — *see* Contusion, foot
    dislocation — *see* Dislocation, foot
    fracture — *see* Fracture, foot
    muscle — *see* Injury, muscle, foot
    open — *see* Wound, open, foot
    specified type NEC S99.82- ☑
    sprain — *see* Sprain, foot
    superficial — *see* Injury, superficial, foot
  forceps NOS P15.9
  forearm S59.91- ☑
    blood vessel — *see* Injury, blood vessel, forearm
    contusion — *see* Contusion, forearm
    fracture — *see* Fracture, forearm
    muscle — *see* Injury, muscle, forearm
    nerve — *see* Injury, nerve, forearm
    open — *see* Wound, open, forearm
    specified NEC S59.81- ☑
    superficial — *see* Injury, superficial, forearm
  forehead S09.90 ☑
  fourth cranial nerve (trochlear) — *see* Injury, nerve, trochlear
  gallbladder S36.129 ☑
    contusion S36.122 ☑
    laceration S36.123 ☑
    specified NEC S36.128 ☑
  ganglion
    celiac, coeliac — *see* Injury, nerve, lumbosacral, sympathetic
    gasserian — *see* Injury, nerve, trigeminal
    stellate — *see* Injury, nerve, thorax, sympathetic
    thoracic sympathetic — *see* Injury, nerve, thorax, sympathetic
  gasserian ganglion — *see* Injury, nerve, trigeminal
  gastric artery — *see* Injury, blood vessel, celiac artery, branch

☑ **Additional Character Required** — Refer to the Tabular List for Character Selection   ▽ Subterms under main terms may continue to next column or page

Injury — *continued*
  gastroduodenal artery — *see* Injury, blood vessel, celiac artery, branch
  gastrointestinal tract — *see* Injury, intra-abdominal
    with open wound into abdominal cavity — *see* Wound, open, with penetration into peritoneal cavity
    colon — *see* Injury, intestine, large
    rectum — *see* Injury, intestine, large, rectum
      with open wound into abdominal cavity S36.61 ☑
    small intestine — *see* Injury, intestine, small
    specified site NEC — *see* Injury, intra-abdominal, specified, site NEC
    stomach — *see* Injury, stomach
  genital organ(s)
    external S39.94 ☑
      specified NEC S39.848 ☑
    internal S37.90 ☑
      fallopian tube — *see* Injury, fallopian tube
      ovary — *see* Injury, ovary
      prostate — *see* Injury, prostate
      seminal vesicle — *see* Injury, pelvis, organ, specified site NEC
      uterus — *see* Injury, uterus
      vas deferens — *see* Injury, pelvis, organ, specified site NEC
    obstetrical trauma O71.9
  gland
    lacrimal laceration — *see* Injury, eye, specified site NEC
    salivary S09.93 ☑
    thyroid NEC S19.84 ☑
  globe (eye) S05.90 ☑
    specified NEC S05.8X- ☑
  groin — *see* Injury, abdomen
  gum S09.90 ☑
  hand S69.9- ☑
    blood vessel — *see* Injury, blood vessel, hand
    contusion — *see* Contusion, hand
    fracture — *see* Fracture, hand
    muscle — *see* Injury, muscle, hand
    nerve — *see* Injury, nerve, hand
    open — *see* Wound, open, hand
    specified NEC S69.8- ☑
    sprain — *see* Sprain, hand
    superficial — *see* Injury, superficial, hand
  head S09.90 ☑
    with loss of consciousness S06.9- ☑
    specified NEC S09.8 ☑
  heart S26.90 ☑
    with hemopericardium S26.00 ☑
      contusion S26.01 ☑
      laceration (mild) S26.020 ☑
        major S26.022 ☑
        moderate S26.021 ☑
      specified type NEC S26.09 ☑
    contusion S26.91 ☑
    laceration S26.92 ☑
    specified type NEC S26.99 ☑
    without hemopericardium S26.10 ☑
      contusion S26.11 ☑
      laceration S26.12 ☑
      specified type NEC S26.19 ☑
  heel — *see* Injury, foot
  hepatic
    artery — *see* Injury, blood vessel, celiac artery, branch
    duct — *see* Injury, liver
    vein — *see* Injury, vena cava, inferior
  hip S79.91- ☑
    blood vessel — *see* Injury, blood vessel, hip
    contusion — *see* Contusion, hip
    dislocation — *see* Dislocation, hip
    fracture — *see* Fracture, femur, neck
    muscle — *see* Injury, muscle, hip
    nerve — *see* Injury, nerve, hip
    open — *see* Wound, open, hip
    specified NEC S79.81- ☑
    sprain — *see* Sprain, hip
    superficial — *see* Injury, superficial, hip
  hymen S39.94 ☑
  hypogastric
    blood vessel — *see* Injury, blood vessel, iliac
    plexus — *see* Injury, nerve, lumbosacral, sympathetic

Injury — *continued*
  ileum — *see* Injury, intestine, small
  iliac region S39.91 ☑
  instrumental (during surgery) — *see* Laceration, accidental complicating surgery
    birth injury — *see* Birth, injury
    nonsurgical — *see* Injury, by site
  obstetrical O71.9
    bladder O71.5
    cervix O71.3
    high vaginal O71.4
    perineal NOS O70.9
    urethra O71.5
    uterus O71.5
      with rupture or perforation O71.1
  internal T14.8 ☑
    aorta — *see* Injury, aorta
    bladder (sphincter) — *see* Injury, bladder
      with
        ectopic or molar pregnancy O08.6
        following ectopic or molar pregnancy O08.6
      obstetrical trauma O71.5
    bronchus, bronchi — *see* Injury, intrathoracic, bronchus
    cecum — *see* Injury, intestine, large
    cervix (uteri) (*see also* Injury, uterus)
      with ectopic or molar pregnancy O08.6
      following ectopic or molar pregnancy O08.6
      obstetrical trauma O71.3
    chest — *see* Injury, intrathoracic
    gastrointestinal tract — *see* Injury, intra-abdominal
    heart — *see* Injury, heart
    intestine NEC — *see* Injury, intestine
    intrauterine — *see* Injury, uterus
    mesentery — *see* Injury, intra-abdominal, specified, site NEC
    pelvis, pelvic (organ) S37.90 ☑
      following ectopic or molar pregnancy (subsequent episode) O08.6
      obstetrical trauma NEC O71.5
        rupture or perforation O71.1
      specified NEC S39.83 ☑
    rectum — *see* Injury, intestine, large, rectum
    stomach — *see* Injury, stomach
    ureter — *see* Injury, ureter
    urethra (sphincter) following ectopic or molar pregnancy O08.6
    uterus — *see* Injury, uterus
  interscapular area — *see* Injury, thorax
  intestine
    large S36.509 ☑
      ascending (right) S36.500 ☑
        blast injury (primary) S36.510 ☑
          secondary S36.590 ☑
        contusion S36.520 ☑
        laceration S36.530 ☑
        specified type NEC S36.590 ☑
      blast injury (primary) S36.519 ☑
        ascending (right) S36.510 ☑
        descending (left) S36.512 ☑
        rectum S36.61 ☑
        sigmoid S36.513 ☑
        specified site NEC S36.518 ☑
        transverse S36.511 ☑
      contusion S36.529 ☑
        ascending (right) S36.520 ☑
        descending (left) S36.522 ☑
        rectum S36.62 ☑
        sigmoid S36.523 ☑
        specified site NEC S36.528 ☑
        transverse S36.521 ☑
      descending (left) S36.502 ☑
        blast injury (primary) S36.512 ☑
          secondary S36.592 ☑
        contusion S36.522 ☑
        laceration S36.532 ☑
        specified type NEC S36.592 ☑
      laceration S36.539 ☑
        ascending (right) S36.530 ☑
        descending (left) S36.532 ☑
        rectum S36.63 ☑
        sigmoid S36.533 ☑
        specified site NEC S36.538 ☑
        transverse S36.531 ☑
      rectum S36.60 ☑
        blast injury (primary) S36.61 ☑
          secondary S36.69 ☑

Injury — *continued*
  intestine — *continued*
    large — *continued*
      rectum — *continued*
        contusion S36.62 ☑
        laceration S36.63 ☑
        specified type NEC S36.69 ☑
      sigmoid S36.503 ☑
        blast injury (primary) S36.513 ☑
          secondary S36.593 ☑
        contusion S36.523 ☑
        laceration S36.533 ☑
        specified type NEC S36.593 ☑
      specified
        site NEC S36.508 ☑
          blast injury (primary) S36.518 ☑
            secondary S36.598 ☑
          contusion S36.528 ☑
          laceration S36.538 ☑
          specified type NEC S36.598 ☑
        type NEC S36.599 ☑
          ascending (right) S36.590 ☑
          descending (left) S36.592 ☑
          rectum S36.69 ☑
          sigmoid S36.593 ☑
          specified site NEC S36.598 ☑
          transverse S36.591 ☑
      transverse S36.501 ☑
        blast injury (primary) S36.511 ☑
          secondary S36.591 ☑
        contusion S36.521 ☑
        laceration S36.531 ☑
        specified type NEC S36.591 ☑
    small S36.409 ☑
      blast injury (primary) S36.419 ☑
        duodenum S36.410 ☑
        secondary S36.499 ☑
          duodenum S36.490 ☑
          specified site NEC S36.498 ☑
        specified site NEC S36.418 ☑
      contusion S36.429 ☑
        duodenum S36.420 ☑
        specified site NEC S36.428 ☑
      duodenum S36.400 ☑
        blast injury (primary) S36.410 ☑
          secondary S36.490 ☑
        contusion S36.420 ☑
        laceration S36.430 ☑
        specified NEC S36.490 ☑
      laceration S36.439 ☑
        duodenum S36.430 ☑
        specified site NEC S36.438 ☑
      specified
        site NEC S36.408 ☑
        type NEC S36.499 ☑
          duodenum S36.490 ☑
          specified site NEC S36.498 ☑
  intra-abdominal S36.90 ☑
    adrenal gland — *see* Injury, adrenal gland
    bladder — *see* Injury, bladder
    colon — *see* Injury, intestine, large
    contusion S36.92 ☑
    fallopian tube — *see* Injury, fallopian tube
    gallbladder — *see* Injury, gallbladder
    intestine — *see* Injury, intestine
    kidney — *see* Injury, kidney
    laceration S36.93 ☑
    liver — *see* Injury, liver
    ovary — *see* Injury, ovary
    pancreas — *see* Injury, pancreas
    pelvic NOS S37.90 ☑
    peritoneum — *see* Injury, intra-abdominal, specified, site NEC
    prostate — *see* Injury, prostate
    rectum — *see* Injury, intestine, large, rectum
    retroperitoneum — *see* Injury, intra-abdominal, specified, site NEC
    seminal vesicle — *see* Injury, pelvis, organ, specified site NEC
    small intestine — *see* Injury, intestine, small
    specified
      pelvic S37.90 ☑
      specified
        site NEC S37.899 ☑
          specified type NEC S37.898 ☑
        type NEC S37.99 ☑

▽ **Subterms under main terms may continue to next column or page**   ☑ **Additional Character Required — Refer to the Tabular List for Character Selection**   193

Injury — Injury

Injury — *continued*
- intra-abdominal — *continued*
  - specified — *continued*
    - site NEC S36.899 ✓
      - contusion S36.892 ✓
      - laceration S36.893 ✓
      - specified type NEC S36.898 ✓
    - type NEC S36.99 ✓
  - spleen — *see* Injury, spleen
  - stomach — *see* Injury, stomach
  - ureter — *see* Injury, ureter
  - urethra — *see* Injury, urethra
  - uterus — *see* Injury, uterus
  - vas deferens — *see* Injury, pelvis, organ, specified site NEC
- intracranial (traumatic) S06.9- ✓
  - cerebellar hemorrhage, traumatic — *see* Injury, intracranial, focal
  - cerebral edema, traumatic S06.1X- ✓
    - diffuse S06.1X- ✓
    - focal S06.1X- ✓
  - diffuse (axonal) S06.2X- ✓
  - epidural hemorrhage (traumatic) S06.4X- ✓
  - focal brain injury S06.30- ✓
    - contusion — *see* Contusion, cerebral
    - laceration — *see* Laceration, cerebral
    - intracerebral hemorrhage, traumatic S06.36- ✓
      - left side S06.35- ✓
      - right side S06.34- ✓
    - subarachnoid hemorrhage, traumatic S06.6X- ✓
    - subdural hemorrhage, traumatic S06.5X- ✓
  - intraocular — *see* Injury, eyeball, penetrating
- intrathoracic S27.9 ✓
  - bronchus S27.409 ✓
    - bilateral S27.402 ✓
    - blast injury (primary) S27.419 ✓
      - bilateral S27.412 ✓
      - secondary — *see* Injury, intrathoracic, bronchus, specified type NEC
      - unilateral S27.411 ✓
    - contusion S27.429 ✓
      - bilateral S27.422 ✓
      - unilateral S27.421 ✓
    - laceration S27.439 ✓
      - bilateral S27.432 ✓
      - unilateral S27.431 ✓
    - specified type NEC S27.499 ✓
      - bilateral S27.492 ✓
      - unilateral S27.491 ✓
    - unilateral S27.401 ✓
  - diaphragm S27.809 ✓
    - contusion S27.802 ✓
    - laceration S27.803 ✓
    - specified type NEC S27.808 ✓
  - esophagus (thoracic) S27.819 ✓
    - contusion S27.812 ✓
    - laceration S27.813 ✓
    - specified type NEC S27.818 ✓
  - heart — *see* Injury, heart
  - hemopneumothorax S27.2 ✓
  - hemothorax S27.1 ✓
  - lung S27.309 ✓
    - aspiration J69.0
    - bilateral S27.302 ✓
    - blast injury (primary) S27.319 ✓
      - bilateral S27.312 ✓
      - secondary — *see* Injury, intrathoracic, lung, specified type NEC
      - unilateral S27.311 ✓
    - contusion S27.329 ✓
      - bilateral S27.322 ✓
      - unilateral S27.321 ✓
    - laceration S27.339 ✓
      - bilateral S27.332 ✓
      - unilateral S27.331 ✓
    - specified type NEC S27.399 ✓
      - bilateral S27.392 ✓
      - unilateral S27.391 ✓
    - unilateral S27.301 ✓
  - pleura S27.60 ✓
    - laceration S27.63 ✓
    - specified type NEC S27.69 ✓
  - pneumothorax S27.0 ✓
  - specified organ NEC S27.899 ✓
    - contusion S27.892 ✓
    - laceration S27.893 ✓

Injury — *continued*
- intrathoracic — *continued*
  - specified organ — *continued*
    - specified type NEC S27.898 ✓
  - thoracic duct — *see* Injury, intrathoracic, specified organ NEC
  - thymus gland — *see* Injury, intrathoracic, specified organ NEC
  - trachea, thoracic S27.50 ✓
    - blast (primary) S27.51 ✓
    - contusion S27.52 ✓
    - laceration S27.53 ✓
    - specified type NEC S27.59 ✓
- iris — *see* Injury, eye, specified site NEC
  - penetrating — *see* Injury, eyeball, penetrating
- jaw S09.93 ✓
- jejunum — *see* Injury, intestine, small
- joint NOS T14.8 ✓
  - old or residual — *see* Disorder, joint, specified type NEC
- kidney S37.00- ✓
  - acute (nontraumatic) N17.9
  - contusion — *see* Contusion, kidney
  - laceration — *see* Laceration, kidney
  - specified NEC S37.09- ✓
- knee S89.9- ✓
  - contusion — *see* Contusion, knee
  - dislocation — *see* Dislocation, knee
  - meniscus (lateral) (medial) — *see* Sprain, knee, specified site NEC
    - old injury or tear — *see* Derangement, knee, meniscus, due to old injury
  - open — *see* Wound, open, knee
  - specified NEC S89.8- ✓
  - sprain — *see* Sprain, knee
  - superficial — *see* Injury, superficial, knee
- labium (majus) (minus) S39.94 ✓
- labyrinth, ear S09.30- ✓
- lacrimal apparatus, duct, gland, or sac — *see* Injury, eye, specified site NEC
- larynx NEC S19.81 ✓
- leg (lower) S89.9- ✓
  - blood vessel — *see* Injury, blood vessel, leg
  - contusion — *see* Contusion, leg
  - fracture — *see* Fracture, leg
  - muscle — *see* Injury, muscle, leg
  - nerve — *see* Injury, nerve, leg
  - open — *see* Wound, open, leg
  - specified NEC S89.8- ✓
  - superficial — *see* Injury, superficial, leg
- lens, eye — *see* Injury, eye, specified site NEC
  - penetrating — *see* Injury, eyeball, penetrating
- limb NEC T14.8 ✓
- lip S09.93 ✓
- liver S36.119 ✓
  - contusion S36.112 ✓
  - laceration S36.113 ✓
    - major (stellate) S36.116 ✓
    - minor S36.114 ✓
    - moderate S36.115 ✓
  - specified NEC S36.118 ✓
- lower back S39.92 ✓
  - specified NEC S39.82 ✓
- lumbar, lumbosacral (region) S39.92 ✓
  - plexus — *see* Injury, lumbosacral plexus
- lumbosacral plexus S34.4 ✓
- lung (*see also* Injury, intrathoracic, lung)
  - aspiration J69.0
  - transfusion-related (TRALI) J95.84
- lymphatic thoracic duct — *see* Injury, intrathoracic, specified organ NEC
- malar region S09.93 ✓
- mastoid region S09.90 ✓
- maxilla S09.93 ✓
- mediastinum — *see* Injury, intrathoracic, specified organ NEC
- membrane, brain — *see* Injury, intracranial
- meningeal artery — *see* Injury, intracranial, subdural hemorrhage
- meninges (cerebral) — *see* Injury, intracranial
- mesenteric
  - artery
    - branch S35.299 ✓
      - laceration (minor) (superficial) S35.291 ✓
        - major S35.292 ✓
      - specified NEC S35.298 ✓

Injury — *continued*
- mesenteric — *continued*
  - artery — *continued*
    - inferior S35.239 ✓
      - laceration (minor) (superficial) S35.231 ✓
        - major S35.232 ✓
      - specified NEC S35.238 ✓
    - superior S35.229 ✓
      - laceration (minor) (superficial) S35.221 ✓
        - major S35.222 ✓
      - specified NEC S35.228 ✓
    - plexus (inferior) (superior) — *see* Injury, nerve, lumbosacral, sympathetic
  - vein
    - inferior S35.349 ✓
      - laceration S35.341 ✓
      - specified NEC S35.348 ✓
    - superior S35.339 ✓
      - laceration S35.331 ✓
      - specified NEC S35.338 ✓
- mesentery — *see* Injury, intra-abdominal, specified site NEC
- mesosalpinx — *see* Injury, pelvic organ, specified site NEC
- middle ear S09.30- ✓
- midthoracic region NOS S29.9 ✓
- mouth S09.93 ✓
- multiple NOS T07 ✓
- muscle (and fascia) (and tendon)
  - abdomen S39.001 ✓
    - laceration S39.021 ✓
    - specified type NEC S39.091 ✓
    - strain S39.011 ✓
  - abductor
    - thumb, forearm level — *see* Injury, muscle, thumb, abductor
  - adductor
    - thigh S76.20- ✓
      - laceration S76.22- ✓
      - specified type NEC S76.29- ✓
      - strain S76.21- ✓
  - ankle — *see* Injury, muscle, foot
  - anterior muscle group, at leg level (lower) S86.20- ✓
    - laceration S86.22- ✓
    - specified type NEC S86.29- ✓
    - strain S86.21- ✓
  - arm (upper) — *see* Injury, muscle, shoulder
  - biceps (parts NEC) S46.20- ✓
    - laceration S46.22- ✓
    - long head S46.10- ✓
      - laceration S46.12- ✓
      - specified type NEC S46.19- ✓
      - strain S46.11- ✓
    - specified type NEC S46.29- ✓
    - strain S46.21- ✓
  - extensor
    - finger(s) (other than thumb) — *see* Injury, muscle, finger by site, extensor
    - forearm level, specified NEC — *see* Injury, muscle, forearm, extensor
    - thumb — *see* Injury, muscle, thumb, extensor
    - toe (large) (ankle level) (foot level) — *see* Injury, muscle, toe, extensor
  - finger
    - extensor (forearm level) S56.40- ✓
      - hand level S66.309 ✓
        - laceration S66.329 ✓
        - specified type NEC S66.399 ✓
        - strain S66.319 ✓
      - laceration S56.429 ✓
      - specified type NEC S56.499 ✓
      - strain S56.419 ✓
    - flexor (forearm level) S56.10- ✓
      - hand level S66.109 ✓
        - laceration S66.129 ✓
        - specified type NEC S66.199 ✓
        - strain S66.119 ✓
      - laceration S56.129 ✓
      - specified type NEC S56.199 ✓
      - strain S56.119 ✓
    - index
      - extensor (forearm level)
        - hand level S66.308 ✓
          - laceration S66.32- ✓
          - specified type NEC S66.39- ✓
          - strain S66.31- ✓

☑ **Additional Character Required** — Refer to the Tabular List for Character Selection   ▽ **Subterms under main terms may continue to next column or page**

Injury — continued
  muscle — continued
    finger — continued
      index — continued
        extensor — continued
          specified type NEC S56.492- ☑
        flexor (forearm level)
          hand level S66.108 ☑
            laceration S66.12- ☑
            specified type NEC S66.19- ☑
            strain S66.11- ☑
          specified type NEC S56.19- ☑
          strain S56.11- ☑
        intrinsic S66.50- ☑
          laceration S66.52- ☑
          specified type NEC S66.59- ☑
          strain S66.51- ☑
      intrinsic S66.509 ☑
        laceration S66.529 ☑
        specified type NEC S66.599 ☑
        strain S66.519 ☑
      little
        extensor (forearm level)
          hand level S66.30- ☑
            laceration S66.32- ☑
            specified type NEC S66.39- ☑
            strain S66.31- ☑
          laceration S56.42- ☑
          specified type NEC S56.49- ☑
          strain S56.41- ☑
        flexor (forearm level)
          hand level S66.10- ☑
            laceration S66.12- ☑
            specified type NEC S66.19- ☑
            strain S66.11- ☑
          laceration S56.12- ☑
          specified type NEC S56.19- ☑
          strain S56.11- ☑
        intrinsic S66.50- ☑
          laceration S66.52- ☑
          specified type NEC S66.59- ☑
          strain S66.51- ☑
      middle
        extensor (forearm level)
          hand level S66.30- ☑
            laceration S66.32- ☑
            specified type NEC S66.39- ☑
            strain S66.31- ☑
          laceration S56.42- ☑
          specified type NEC S56.49- ☑
          strain S56.41- ☑
        flexor (forearm level)
          hand level S66.10- ☑
            laceration S66.12- ☑
            specified type NEC S66.19- ☑
            strain S66.11- ☑
          laceration S56.12- ☑
          specified type NEC S56.19- ☑
          strain S56.11- ☑
        intrinsic S66.50- ☑
          laceration S66.52- ☑
          specified type NEC S66.59- ☑
          strain S66.51- ☑
      ring
        extensor (forearm level)
          hand level S66.30- ☑
            laceration S66.32- ☑
            specified type NEC S66.39- ☑
            strain S66.31- ☑
          laceration S56.42- ☑
          specified type NEC S56.49- ☑
          strain S56.41- ☑
        flexor (forearm level)
          hand level S66.10- ☑
            laceration S66.12- ☑
            specified type NEC S66.19- ☑
            strain S66.11- ☑
          laceration S56.12- ☑
          specified type NEC S56.19- ☑
          strain S56.11- ☑
        intrinsic S66.50- ☑
          laceration S66.52- ☑
          specified type NEC S66.59- ☑
          strain S66.51- ☑

Injury — continued
  muscle — continued
    flexor
      finger(s) (other than thumb) — see Injury, muscle, finger
      forearm level, specified NEC — see Injury, muscle, forearm, flexor
      thumb — see Injury, muscle, thumb, flexor
      toe (long) (ankle level) (foot level) — see Injury, muscle, toe, flexor
    foot S96.90- ☑
      intrinsic S96.20- ☑
        laceration S96.22- ☑
        specified type NEC S96.29- ☑
        strain S96.21- ☑
      laceration S96.92- ☑
      long extensor, toe — see Injury, muscle, toe, extensor
      long flexor, toe — see Injury, muscle, toe, flexor
      specified
        site NEC S96.80- ☑
          laceration S96.82- ☑
          specified type NEC S96.89- ☑
          strain S96.81- ☑
        type S96.99- ☑
      strain S96.91- ☑
    forearm (level) S56.90- ☑
      extensor S56.50- ☑
        laceration S56.52- ☑
        specified type NEC S56.59- ☑
        strain S56.51- ☑
      flexor S56.20- ☑
        laceration S56.22- ☑
        specified type NEC S56.29- ☑
        strain S56.21- ☑
      laceration S56.92- ☑
      specified S56.99- ☑
        site NEC S56.80- ☑
          laceration S56.82- ☑
          strain S56.81- ☑
          type NEC S56.89- ☑
      strain S56.91- ☑
    hand (level) S66.90- ☑
      laceration S66.92- ☑
      specified
        site NEC S66.80- ☑
          laceration S66.82- ☑
          specified type NEC S66.89- ☑
          strain S66.81- ☑
          type NEC S66.99- ☑
      strain S66.91- ☑
    head S09.10 ☑
      laceration S09.12 ☑
      specified type NEC S09.19 ☑
      strain S09.11 ☑
    hip NEC S76.00- ☑
      laceration S76.02- ☑
      specified type NEC S76.09- ☑
      strain S76.01- ☑
    intrinsic
      ankle and foot level — see Injury, muscle, foot, intrinsic
      finger (other than thumb) — see Injury, muscle, finger by site, intrinsic
      foot (level) — see Injury, muscle, foot, intrinsic
      thumb — see Injury, muscle, thumb, intrinsic
    leg (level) (lower) S86.90- ☑
      Achilles tendon — see Injury, Achilles tendon
      anterior muscle group — see Injury, muscle, anterior muscle group
      laceration S86.92- ☑
      peroneal muscle group — see Injury, muscle, peroneal muscle group
      posterior muscle group — see Injury, muscle, posterior muscle group, leg level
      specified
        site NEC S86.80- ☑
          laceration S86.82- ☑
          specified type NEC S86.89- ☑
          strain S86.81- ☑
          type NEC S86.99- ☑
      strain S86.91- ☑
    long
      extensor toe, at ankle and foot level — see Injury, muscle, toe, extensor

Injury — continued
  muscle — continued
    long — continued
      flexor, toe, at ankle and foot level — see Injury, muscle, toe, flexor
      head, biceps — see Injury, muscle, biceps, long head
    lower back S39.002 ☑
      laceration S39.022 ☑
      specified type NEC S39.092 ☑
      strain S39.012 ☑
    neck (level) S16.9 ☑
      laceration S16.2 ☑
      specified type NEC S16.8 ☑
      strain S16.1 ☑
    pelvis S39.003 ☑
      laceration S39.023 ☑
      specified type NEC S39.093 ☑
      strain S39.013 ☑
    peroneal muscle group, at leg level (lower) S86.30- ☑
      laceration S86.32- ☑
      specified type NEC S86.39- ☑
      strain S86.31- ☑
    posterior muscle (group)
      leg level (lower) S86.10- ☑
        laceration S86.12- ☑
        specified type NEC S86.19- ☑
        strain S86.11- ☑
      thigh level S76.30- ☑
        laceration S76.32- ☑
        specified type NEC S76.39- ☑
        strain S76.31- ☑
    quadriceps (thigh) S76.10- ☑
      laceration S76.12- ☑
      specified type NEC S76.19- ☑
      strain S76.11- ☑
    shoulder S46.90- ☑
      laceration S46.92- ☑
      rotator cuff — see Injury, rotator cuff
      specified site NEC S46.80- ☑
        laceration S46.82- ☑
        specified type NEC S46.89- ☑
        strain S46.81- ☑
      specified type NEC S46.99- ☑
      strain S46.91- ☑
    thigh NEC (level) S76.90- ☑
      adductor — see Injury, muscle, adductor, thigh
      laceration S76.92- ☑
      posterior muscle (group) — see Injury, muscle, posterior muscle, thigh level
      quadriceps — see Injury, muscle, quadriceps
      specified
        site NEC S76.80- ☑
          laceration S76.82- ☑
          specified type NEC S76.89- ☑
          strain S76.81- ☑
        type NEC S76.99- ☑
      strain S76.91- ☑
    thorax (level) S29.009 ☑
      back wall S29.002 ☑
      front wall S29.001 ☑
      laceration S29.029 ☑
        back wall S29.022 ☑
        front wall S29.021 ☑
      specified type NEC S29.099 ☑
        back wall S29.092 ☑
        front wall S29.091 ☑
      strain S29.019 ☑
        back wall S29.012 ☑
        front wall S29.011 ☑
    thumb
      abductor (forearm level) S56.30- ☑
        laceration S56.32- ☑
        specified type NEC S56.39- ☑
        strain S56.31- ☑
      extensor (forearm level) S56.30- ☑
        hand level S66.20- ☑
          laceration S66.22- ☑
          specified type NEC S66.29- ☑
          strain S66.21- ☑
        laceration S56.32- ☑
        specified type NEC S56.39- ☑
        strain S56.31- ☑
      flexor (forearm level) S56.00- ☑
        hand level S66.00- ☑

Injury — *continued*
  muscle — *continued*
    thumb — *continued*
      flexor — *continued*
        hand level — *continued*
          laceration S66.02- ☑
          specified type NEC S66.09- ☑
          strain S66.01- ☑
        laceration S56.02- ☑
        specified type NEC S56.09- ☑
        strain S56.01- ☑
        wrist level — *see* Injury, muscle, thumb, flexor, hand level
      intrinsic S66.40- ☑
        laceration S66.42- ☑
        specified type NEC S66.49- ☑
        strain S66.41- ☑
    toe (*see also* Injury, muscle, foot)
      extensor, long S96.10- ☑
        laceration S96.12- ☑
        specified type NEC S96.19- ☑
        strain S96.11- ☑
      flexor, long S96.00- ☑
        laceration S96.02- ☑
        specified type NEC S96.09- ☑
        strain S96.01- ☑
    triceps S46.30- ☑
      laceration S46.32- ☑
      specified type NEC S46.39- ☑
      strain S46.31- ☑
    wrist (and hand) level — *see* Injury, muscle, hand
  musculocutaneous nerve — *see* Injury, nerve, musculocutaneous
  myocardium — *see* Injury, heart
  nape — *see* Injury, neck
  nasal (septum) (sinus) S09.92 ☑
  nasopharynx S09.92 ☑
  neck S19.9 ☑
    specified NEC S19.80 ☑
    specified site NEC S19.89 ☑
  nerve NEC T14.8 ☑
    abdomen S34.9 ☑
      peripheral S34.6 ☑
      specified site NEC S34.8 ☑
    abducens S04.4- ☑
      contusion S04.4- ☑
      laceration S04.4- ☑
      specified type NEC S04.4- ☑
    abducent — *see* Injury, nerve, abducens
    accessory S04.7- ☑
      contusion S04.7- ☑
      laceration S04.7- ☑
      specified type NEC S04.7- ☑
    acoustic S04.6- ☑
      contusion S04.6- ☑
      laceration S04.6- ☑
      specified type NEC S04.6- ☑
    ankle S94.9- ☑
      cutaneous sensory S94.3- ☑
      specified site NEC — *see* subcategory S94.8 ☑
    anterior crural, femoral — *see* Injury, nerve, femoral
    arm (upper) S44.9- ☑
      axillary — *see* Injury, nerve, axillary
      cutaneous — *see* Injury, nerve, cutaneous, arm
      median — *see* Injury, nerve, median, upper arm
      musculocutaneous — *see* Injury, nerve, musculocutaneous
      radial — *see* Injury, nerve, radial, upper arm
      specified site NEC — *see* subcategory S44.8 ☑
      ulnar — *see* Injury, nerve, ulnar, arm
    auditory — *see* Injury, nerve, acoustic
    axillary S44.3- ☑
    brachial plexus — *see* Injury, brachial plexus
    cervical sympathetic S14.5 ☑
    cranial S04.9 ☑
      contusion S04.9 ☑
      eighth (acoustic or auditory) — *see* Injury, nerve, acoustic
      eleventh (accessory) — *see* Injury, nerve, accessory
      fifth (trigeminal) — *see* Injury, nerve, trigeminal
      first (olfactory) — *see* Injury, nerve, olfactory
      fourth (trochlear) — *see* Injury, nerve, trochlear
      laceration S04.9 ☑
      ninth (glossopharyngeal) — *see* Injury, nerve, glossopharyngeal

Injury — *continued*
  nerve — *continued*
    cranial — *continued*
      second (optic) — *see* Injury, nerve, optic
      seventh (facial) — *see* Injury, nerve, facial
      sixth (abducent) — *see* Injury, nerve, abducens
      specified
        nerve NEC S04.89- ☑
          contusion S04.89- ☑
          laceration S04.89- ☑
          specified type NEC S04.89- ☑
        type NEC S04.9 ☑
      tenth (pneumogastric or vagus) — *see* Injury, nerve, vagus
      third (oculomotor) — *see* Injury, nerve, oculomotor
      twelfth (hypoglossal) — *see* Injury, nerve, hypoglossal
    cutaneous sensory
      ankle (level) S94.3- ☑
      arm (upper) (level) S44.5- ☑
      foot (level) — *see* Injury, nerve, cutaneous sensory, ankle
      forearm (level) S54.3- ☑
      hip (level) S74.2- ☑
      leg (lower level) S84.2- ☑
      shoulder (level) — *see* Injury, nerve, cutaneous sensory, arm
      thigh (level) — *see* Injury, nerve, cutaneous sensory, hip
    deep peroneal — *see* Injury, nerve, peroneal, foot
    digital
      finger S64.4- ☑
        index S64.49- ☑
        little S64.49- ☑
        middle S64.49- ☑
        ring S64.49- ☑
      thumb S64.3- ☑
      toe — *see* Injury, nerve, ankle, specified site NEC
    eighth cranial (acoustic or auditory) — *see* Injury, nerve, acoustic
    eleventh cranial (accessory) — *see* Injury, nerve, accessory
    facial S04.5- ☑
      contusion S04.5- ☑
      laceration S04.5- ☑
      newborn P11.3
      specified type NEC S04.5- ☑
    femoral (hip level) (thigh level) S74.1- ☑
    fifth cranial (trigeminal) — *see* Injury, nerve, trigeminal
    finger (digital) — *see* Injury, nerve, digital, finger
    first cranial (olfactory) — *see* Injury, nerve, olfactory
    foot S94.9- ☑
      cutaneous sensory S94.3- ☑
      deep peroneal S94.2- ☑
      lateral plantar S94.0- ☑
      medial plantar S94.1- ☑
      specified site NEC — *see* subcategory S94.8 ☑
    forearm (level) S54.9- ☑
      cutaneous sensory — *see* Injury, nerve, cutaneous sensory, forearm
      median — *see* Injury, nerve, median
      radial — *see* Injury, nerve, radial
      specified site NEC — *see* subcategory S54.8 ☑
      ulnar — *see* Injury, nerve, ulnar
    fourth cranial (trochlear) — *see* Injury, nerve, trochlear
    glossopharyngeal S04.89- ☑
      specified type NEC S04.89- ☑
    hand S64.9- ☑
      median — *see* Injury, nerve, median, hand
      radial — *see* Injury, nerve, radial, hand
      specified NEC — *see* subcategory S64.8 ☑
      ulnar — *see* Injury, nerve, ulnar, hand
    hip (level) S74.9- ☑
      cutaneous sensory — *see* Injury, nerve, cutaneous sensory, hip
      femoral — *see* Injury, nerve, femoral
      sciatic — *see* Injury, nerve, sciatic
      specified site NEC — *see* subcategory S74.8 ☑
    hypoglossal S04.89- ☑
      specified type NEC S04.89- ☑
    lateral plantar S94.0- ☑
    leg (lower) S84.9- ☑

Injury — *continued*
  nerve — *continued*
    leg — *continued*
      cutaneous sensory — *see* Injury, nerve, cutaneous sensory, leg
      peroneal — *see* Injury, nerve, peroneal
      specified site NEC — *see* subcategory S84.8 ☑
      tibial — *see* Injury, nerve, tibial
      upper — *see* Injury, nerve, thigh
    lower
      back — *see* Injury, nerve, abdomen, specified site NEC
      peripheral — *see* Injury, nerve, abdomen, peripheral
      limb — *see* Injury, nerve, leg
    lumbar plexus — *see* Injury, nerve, lumbosacral, sympathetic
    lumbar spinal — *see* Injury, nerve, spinal, lumbar
    lumbosacral
      plexus — *see* Injury, nerve, lumbosacral, sympathetic
      sympathetic S34.5 ☑
    medial plantar S94.1- ☑
    median (forearm level) S54.1- ☑
      hand (level) S64.1- ☑
      upper arm (level) S44.1- ☑
      wrist (level) — *see* Injury, nerve, median, hand
    musculocutaneous S44.4- ☑
    musculospiral (upper arm level) — *see* Injury, nerve, radial, upper arm
    neck S14.9 ☑
      peripheral S14.4 ☑
      specified site NEC S14.8 ☑
      sympathetic S14.5 ☑
    ninth cranial (glossopharyngeal) — *see* Injury, nerve, glossopharyngeal
    oculomotor S04.1- ☑
      contusion S04.1- ☑
      laceration S04.1- ☑
      specified type NEC S04.1- ☑
    olfactory S04.81- ☑
      specified type NEC S04.81- ☑
    optic S04.01- ☑
      contusion S04.01- ☑
      laceration S04.01- ☑
      specified type NEC S04.01- ☑
    pelvic girdle — *see* Injury, nerve, hip
    pelvis — *see* Injury, nerve, abdomen, specified site NEC
      peripheral — *see* Injury, nerve, abdomen, peripheral
    peripheral NEC T14.8 ☑
      abdomen — *see* Injury, nerve, abdomen, peripheral
      lower back — *see* Injury, nerve, abdomen, peripheral
      neck — *see* Injury, nerve, neck, peripheral
      pelvis — *see* Injury, nerve, abdomen, peripheral
      specified NEC T14.8 ☑
    peroneal (lower leg level) S84.1- ☑
      foot S94.2- ☑
    plexus
      brachial — *see* Injury, brachial plexus
      celiac, coeliac — *see* Injury, nerve, lumbosacral, sympathetic
      mesenteric, inferior — *see* Injury, nerve, lumbosacral, sympathetic
      sacral — *see* Injury, lumbosacral plexus
      spinal
        brachial — *see* Injury, brachial plexus
        lumbosacral — *see* Injury, lumbosacral plexus
    pneumogastric — *see* Injury, nerve, vagus
    radial (forearm level) S54.2- ☑
      hand (level) S64.2- ☑
      upper arm (level) S44.2- ☑
      wrist (level) — *see* Injury, nerve, radial, hand
    root — *see* Injury, nerve, spinal, root
    sacral plexus — *see* Injury, lumbosacral plexus
    sacral spinal — *see* Injury, nerve, spinal, sacral
    sciatic (hip level) (thigh level) S74.0- ☑
    second cranial (optic) — *see* Injury, nerve, optic
    seventh cranial (facial) — *see* Injury, nerve, facial
    shoulder — *see* Injury, nerve, arm
    sixth cranial (abducent) — *see* Injury, nerve, abducens

☑ Additional Character Required — Refer to the Tabular List for Character Selection   ▽ Subterms under main terms may continue to next column or page

Injury — *continued*
  nerve — *continued*
    spinal
      plexus — *see* Injury, nerve, plexus, spinal
      root
        cervical S14.2 ☑
        dorsal S24.2 ☑
        lumbar S34.21 ☑
        sacral S34.22 ☑
        thoracic — *see* Injury, nerve, spinal, root, dorsal
    splanchnic — *see* Injury, nerve, lumbosacral, sympathetic
    sympathetic NEC — *see* Injury, nerve, lumbosacral, sympathetic
      cervical — *see* Injury, nerve, cervical sympathetic
    tenth cranial (pneumogastric or vagus) — *see* Injury, nerve, vagus
    thigh (level) — *see* Injury, nerve, hip
      cutaneous sensory — *see* Injury, nerve, cutaneous sensory, hip
      femoral — *see* Injury, nerve, femoral
      sciatic — *see* Injury, nerve, sciatic
      specified NEC — *see* Injury, nerve, hip
    third cranial (oculomotor) — *see* Injury, nerve, oculomotor
    thorax S24.9 ☑
      peripheral S24.3 ☑
      specified site NEC S24.8 ☑
      sympathetic S24.4 ☑
    thumb, digital — *see* Injury, nerve, digital, thumb
    tibial (lower leg level) (posterior) S84.0- ☑
    toe — *see* Injury, nerve, ankle
    trigeminal S04.3- ☑
      contusion S04.3- ☑
      laceration S04.3- ☑
      specified type NEC S04.3- ☑
    trochlear S04.2- ☑
      contusion S04.2- ☑
      laceration S04.2- ☑
      specified type NEC S04.2- ☑
    twelfth cranial (hypoglossal) — *see* Injury, nerve, hypoglossal
    ulnar (forearm level) S54.0- ☑
      arm (upper) (level) S44.0- ☑
      hand (level) S64.0- ☑
      wrist (level) — *see* Injury, nerve, ulnar, hand
    vagus S04.89- ☑
      specified type NEC S04.89- ☑
    wrist (level) — *see* Injury, nerve, hand
    ninth cranial nerve (glossopharyngeal) — *see* Injury, nerve, glossopharyngeal
  nose (septum) S09.92 ☑
  obstetrical O71.9
    specified NEC O71.89
  occipital (region) (scalp) S09.90 ☑
    lobe — *see* Injury, intracranial
  optic chiasm S04.02 ☑
  optic radiation S04.03- ☑
  optic tract and pathways S04.03- ☑
  orbit, orbital (region) — *see* Injury, eye
    penetrating (with foreign body) — *see* Injury, eye, orbit, penetrating
    specified NEC — *see* Injury, eye, specified site NEC
  ovary, ovarian S37.409 ☑
    bilateral S37.402 ☑
      contusion S37.422 ☑
      laceration S37.432 ☑
      specified type NEC S37.492 ☑
    blood vessel — *see* Injury, blood vessel, ovarian
    contusion S37.429 ☑
      bilateral S37.422 ☑
      unilateral S37.421 ☑
    laceration S37.439 ☑
      bilateral S37.432 ☑
      unilateral S37.431 ☑
    specified type NEC S37.499 ☑
      bilateral S37.492 ☑
      unilateral S37.491 ☑
    unilateral S37.401 ☑
      contusion S37.421 ☑
      laceration S37.431 ☑
      specified type NEC S37.491 ☑
  palate (hard) (soft) S09.93 ☑
  pancreas S36.209 ☑
    body S36.201 ☑

Injury — *continued*
  pancreas — *continued*
    body — *continued*
      contusion S36.221 ☑
      laceration S36.231 ☑
        major S36.261 ☑
        minor S36.241 ☑
        moderate S36.251 ☑
        specified type NEC S36.291 ☑
    contusion S36.229 ☑
    head S36.200 ☑
      contusion S36.220 ☑
      laceration S36.230 ☑
        major S36.260 ☑
        minor S36.240 ☑
        moderate S36.250 ☑
        specified type NEC S36.290 ☑
    laceration S36.239 ☑
      major S36.269 ☑
      minor S36.249 ☑
      moderate S36.259 ☑
    specified type NEC S36.299 ☑
    tail S36.202 ☑
      contusion S36.222 ☑
      laceration S36.232 ☑
        major S36.262 ☑
        minor S36.242 ☑
        moderate S36.252 ☑
      specified type NEC S36.292 ☑
  parietal (region) (scalp) S09.90 ☑
    lobe — *see* Injury, intracranial
  patellar ligament (tendon) S76.10- ☑
    laceration S76.12- ☑
    specified NEC S76.19- ☑
    strain S76.11- ☑
  pelvis, pelvic (floor) S39.93 ☑
    complicating delivery O70.1
    joint or ligament, complicating delivery O71.6
    organ S37.90 ☑
      with ectopic or molar pregnancy O08.6
      complication of abortion — *see* Abortion
      contusion S37.92 ☑
      following ectopic or molar pregnancy O08.6
      laceration S37.93 ☑
      obstetrical trauma NEC O71.5
      specified
        site NEC S37.899 ☑
          contusion S37.892 ☑
          laceration S37.893 ☑
          specified type NEC S37.898 ☑
        type NEC S37.99 ☑
    specified NEC S39.83 ☑
  penis S39.94 ☑
  perineum S39.94 ☑
  peritoneum S36.81 ☑
    laceration S36.893 ☑
  periurethral tissue — *see* Injury, urethra
    complicating delivery O71.82
  phalanges
    foot — *see* Injury, foot
    hand — *see* Injury, hand
  pharynx NEC S19.85 ☑
  pleura — *see* Injury, intrathoracic, pleura
  plexus
    brachial — *see* Injury, brachial plexus
    cardiac — *see* Injury, nerve, thorax, sympathetic
    celiac, coeliac — *see* Injury, nerve, lumbosacral, sympathetic
    esophageal — *see* Injury, nerve, thorax, sympathetic
    hypogastric — *see* Injury, nerve, lumbosacral, sympathetic
    lumbar, lumbosacral — *see* Injury, lumbosacral plexus
    mesenteric — *see* Injury, nerve, lumbosacral, sympathetic
    pulmonary — *see* Injury, nerve, thorax, sympathetic
  postcardiac surgery (syndrome) I97.0
  prepuce S39.94 ☑
  prostate S37.829 ☑
    contusion S37.822 ☑
    laceration S37.823 ☑
    specified type NEC S37.828 ☑
  pubic region S39.94 ☑
  pudendum S39.94 ☑
  pulmonary plexus — *see* Injury, nerve, thorax, sympathetic

Injury — *continued*
  rectovaginal septum NEC S39.83 ☑
  rectum — *see* Injury, intestine, large, rectum
  retina — *see* Injury, eye, specified site NEC
    penetrating — *see* Injury, eyeball, penetrating
  retroperitoneal — *see* Injury, intra-abdominal, specified site NEC
  rotator cuff (muscle(s)) (tendon(s)) S46.00- ☑
    laceration S46.02- ☑
    specified type NEC S46.09- ☑
    strain S46.01- ☑
  round ligament — *see* Injury, pelvic organ, specified site NEC
  sacral plexus — *see* Injury, lumbosacral plexus
  salivary duct or gland S09.93 ☑
  scalp S09.90 ☑
    newborn (birth injury) P12.9
      due to monitoring (electrode) (sampling incision) P12.4
      specified NEC P12.89
        caput succedaneum P12.81
  scapular region — *see* Injury, shoulder
  sclera — *see* Injury, eye, specified site NEC
    penetrating — *see* Injury, eyeball, penetrating
  scrotum S39.94 ☑
  second cranial nerve (optic) — *see* Injury, nerve, optic
  seminal vesicle — *see* Injury, pelvic organ, specified site NEC
  seventh cranial nerve (facial) — *see* Injury, nerve, facial
  shoulder S49.9- ☑
    blood vessel — *see* Injury, blood vessel, arm
    contusion — *see* Contusion, shoulder
    dislocation — *see* Dislocation, shoulder
    fracture — *see* Fracture, shoulder
    muscle — *see* Injury, muscle, shoulder
    nerve — *see* Injury, nerve, shoulder
    open — *see* Wound, open, shoulder
    specified type NEC S49.8- ☑
    sprain — *see* Sprain, shoulder girdle
    superficial — *see* Injury, superficial, shoulder
  sinus
    cavernous — *see* Injury, intracranial
    nasal S09.92 ☑
  sixth cranial nerve (abducent) — *see* Injury, nerve, abducens
  skeleton, birth injury P13.9
    specified part NEC P13.8
  skin NEC T14.8 ☑
    surface intact — *see* Injury, superficial
  skull NEC S09.90 ☑
  specified NEC T14.8 ☑
  spermatic cord (pelvic region) S37.898 ☑
    scrotal region S39.848 ☑
  spinal (cord)
    cervical (neck) S14.109 ☑
      anterior cord syndrome S14.139 ☑
        C1 level S14.131 ☑
        C2 level S14.132 ☑
        C3 level S14.133 ☑
        C4 level S14.134 ☑
        C5 level S14.135 ☑
        C6 level S14.136 ☑
        C7 level S14.137 ☑
        C8 level S14.138 ☑
      Brown-Séquard syndrome S14.149 ☑
        C1 level S14.141 ☑
        C2 level S14.142 ☑
        C3 level S14.143 ☑
        C4 level S14.144 ☑
        C5 level S14.145 ☑
        C6 level S14.146 ☑
        C7 level S14.147 ☑
        C8 level S14.148 ☑
      C1 level S14.101 ☑
      C2 level S14.102 ☑
      C3 level S14.103 ☑
      C4 level S14.104 ☑
      C5 level S14.105 ☑
      C6 level S14.106 ☑
      C7 level S14.107 ☑
      C8 level S14.108 ☑
      central cord syndrome S14.129 ☑
        C1 level S14.121 ☑
        C2 level S14.122 ☑
        C3 level S14.123 ☑
        C4 level S14.124 ☑

☑ Subterms under main terms may continue to next column or page   ☑ Additional Character Required — Refer to the Tabular List for Character Selection   197

Injury — Injury

Injury — *continued*
  spinal — *continued*
    cervical — *continued*
      central cord syndrome — *continued*
        C5 level S14.125 ☑
        C6 level S14.126 ☑
        C7 level S14.127 ☑
        C8 level S14.128 ☑
      complete lesion S14.119 ☑
        C1 level S14.111 ☑
        C2 level S14.112 ☑
        C3 level S14.113 ☑
        C4 level S14.114 ☑
        C5 level S14.115 ☑
        C6 level S14.116 ☑
        C7 level S14.117 ☑
        C8 level S14.118 ☑
      concussion S14.0 ☑
      edema S14.0 ☑
      incomplete lesion specified NEC S14.159 ☑
        C1 level S14.151 ☑
        C2 level S14.152 ☑
        C3 level S14.153 ☑
        C4 level S14.154 ☑
        C5 level S14.155 ☑
        C6 level S14.156 ☑
        C7 level S14.157 ☑
        C8 level S14.158 ☑
      posterior cord syndrome S14.159 ☑
        C1 level S14.151 ☑
        C2 level S14.152 ☑
        C3 level S14.153 ☑
        C4 level S14.154 ☑
        C5 level S14.155 ☑
        C6 level S14.156 ☑
        C7 level S14.157 ☑
        C8 level S14.158 ☑
    dorsal — *see* Injury, spinal, thoracic
    lumbar S34.109 ☑
      complete lesion S34.119 ☑
        L1 level S34.111 ☑
        L2 level S34.112 ☑
        L3 level S34.113 ☑
        L4 level S34.114 ☑
        L5 level S34.115 ☑
      concussion S34.01 ☑
      edema S34.01 ☑
      incomplete lesion S34.129 ☑
        L1 level S34.121 ☑
        L2 level S34.122 ☑
        L3 level S34.123 ☑
        L4 level S34.124 ☑
        L5 level S34.125 ☑
      L1 level S34.101 ☑
      L2 level S34.102 ☑
      L3 level S34.103 ☑
      L4 level S34.104 ☑
      L5 level S34.105 ☑
    nerve root NEC
      cervical — *see* Injury, nerve, spinal, root, cervical
      dorsal — *see* Injury, nerve, spinal, root, dorsal
      lumbar S34.21 ☑
      sacral S34.22 ☑
      thoracic — *see* Injury, nerve, spinal, root, dorsal
    plexus
      brachial — *see* Injury, brachial plexus
      lumbosacral — *see* Injury, lumbosacral plexus
    sacral S34.139 ☑
      complete lesion S34.131 ☑
      incomplete lesion S34.132 ☑
    thoracic S24.109 ☑
      anterior cord syndrome S24.139 ☑
        T1 level S24.131 ☑
        T2-T6 level S24.132 ☑
        T7-T10 level S24.133 ☑
        T11-T12 level S24.134 ☑
      Brown-Séquard syndrome S24.149 ☑
        T1 level S24.141 ☑
        T2-T6 level S24.142 ☑
        T7-T10 level S24.143 ☑
        T11-T12 level S24.144 ☑
      complete lesion S24.119 ☑
        T1 level S24.111 ☑
        T2-T6 level S24.112 ☑
        T7-T10 level S24.113 ☑
        T11-T12 level S24.114 ☑

Injury — *continued*
  spinal — *continued*
    thoracic — *continued*
      concussion S24.0 ☑
      edema S24.0 ☑
      incomplete lesion specified NEC S24.159 ☑
        T1 level S24.151 ☑
        T2-T6 level S24.152 ☑
        T7-T10 level S24.153 ☑
        T11-T12 level S24.154 ☑
      posterior cord syndrome S24.159 ☑
        T1 level S24.151 ☑
        T2-T6 level S24.152 ☑
        T7-T10 level S24.153 ☑
        T11-T12 level S24.154 ☑
      T1 level S24.101 ☑
      T2-T6 level S24.102 ☑
      T7-T10 level S24.103 ☑
      T11-T12 level S24.104 ☑
  splanchnic nerve — *see* Injury, nerve, lumbosacral, sympathetic
  spleen S36.00 ☑
    contusion S36.029 ☑
      major S36.021 ☑
      minor S36.020 ☑
    laceration S36.039 ☑
      major (massive) (stellate) S36.032 ☑
      moderate S36.031 ☑
      superficial (capsular) (minor) S36.030 ☑
    specified type NEC S36.09 ☑
  splenic artery — *see* Injury, blood vessel, celiac artery, branch
  stellate ganglion — *see* Injury, nerve, thorax, sympathetic
  sternal region S29.9 ☑
  stomach S36.30 ☑
    contusion S36.32 ☑
    laceration S36.33 ☑
    specified type NEC S36.39 ☑
  subconjunctival — *see* Injury, eye, conjunctiva
  subcutaneous NEC T14.8 ☑
  submaxillary region S09.93 ☑
  submental region S09.93 ☑
  subungual
    fingers — *see* Injury, hand
    toes — *see* Injury, foot
  superficial NEC T14.8 ☑
    abdomen, abdominal (wall) S30.92 ☑
      abrasion S30.811 ☑
      bite S30.871 ☑
        insect S30.861 ☑
      contusion S30.1 ☑
      external constriction S30.841 ☑
      foreign body S30.851 ☑
    abrasion — *see* Abrasion, by site
    adnexa, eye NEC — *see* Injury, eye, specified site NEC
    alveolar process — *see* Injury, superficial, oral cavity
    ankle S90.91- ☑
      abrasion — *see* Abrasion, ankle
      bite — *see* Bite, ankle
      blister — *see* Blister, ankle
      contusion — *see* Contusion, ankle
      external constriction — *see* Constriction, external, ankle
      foreign body — *see* Foreign body, superficial, ankle
    anus S30.98 ☑
    arm (upper) S40.92- ☑
      abrasion — *see* Abrasion, arm
      bite — *see* Bite, superficial, arm
      blister — *see* Blister, arm (upper)
      contusion — *see* Contusion, arm
      external constriction — *see* Constriction, external, arm
      foreign body — *see* Foreign body, superficial, arm
    auditory canal (external) (meatus) — *see* Injury, superficial, ear
    auricle — *see* Injury, superficial, ear
    axilla — *see* Injury, superficial, arm
    back (*see also* Injury, superficial, thorax, back)
      lower S30.91 ☑
        abrasion S30.810 ☑
        contusion S30.0 ☑
        external constriction S30.840 ☑

Injury — *continued*
  superficial — *continued*
    back (*see also* Injury, superficial, thorax, back) — *continued*
      lower — *continued*
        superficial
          bite NEC S30.870 ☑
            insect S30.860 ☑
          foreign body S30.850 ☑
    bite NEC — *see* Bite, superficial NEC, by site
    blister — *see* Blister, by site
    breast S20.10- ☑
      abrasion — *see* Abrasion, breast
      bite — *see* Bite, superficial, breast
      contusion — *see* Contusion, breast
      external constriction — *see* Constriction, external, breast
      foreign body — *see* Foreign body, superficial, breast
    brow — *see* Injury, superficial, head, specified NEC
    buttock S30.91 ☑
    calf — *see* Injury, superficial, leg
    canthus, eye — *see* Injury, superficial, periocular area
    cheek (external) — *see* Injury, superficial, head, specified NEC
      internal — *see* Injury, superficial, oral cavity
    chest wall — *see* Injury, superficial, thorax
    chin — *see* Injury, superficial, head NEC
    clitoris S30.95 ☑
    conjunctiva — *see* Injury, eye, conjunctiva
      with foreign body (in conjunctival sac) — *see* Foreign body, conjunctival sac
    contusion — *see* Contusion, by site
    costal region — *see* Injury, superficial, thorax
    digit(s)
      hand — *see* Injury, superficial, finger
    ear (auricle) (canal) (external) S00.40- ☑
      abrasion — *see* Abrasion, ear
      bite — *see* Bite, superficial, ear
      contusion — *see* Contusion, ear
      external constriction — *see* Constriction, external, ear
      foreign body — *see* Foreign body, superficial, ear
    elbow S50.90- ☑
      abrasion — *see* Abrasion, elbow
      bite — *see* Bite, superficial, elbow
      blister — *see* Blister, elbow
      contusion — *see* Contusion, elbow
      external constriction — *see* Constriction, external, elbow
      foreign body — *see* Foreign body, superficial, elbow
    epididymis S30.94 ☑
    epigastric region S30.92 ☑
    epiglottis — *see* Injury, superficial, throat
    esophagus
      cervical — *see* Injury, superficial, throat
    external constriction — *see* Constriction, external, by site
    extremity NEC T14.8 ☑
    eyeball NEC — *see* Injury, eye, specified site NEC
    eyebrow — *see* Injury, superficial, periocular area
    eyelid S00.20- ☑
      abrasion — *see* Abrasion, eyelid
      bite — *see* Bite, superficial, eyelid
      contusion — *see* Contusion, eyelid
      external constriction — *see* Constriction, external, eyelid
      foreign body — *see* Foreign body, superficial, eyelid
    face NEC — *see* Injury, superficial, head, specified NEC
    finger(s) S60.949 ☑
      abrasion — *see* Abrasion, finger
      bite — *see* Bite, superficial, finger
      blister — *see* Blister, finger
      contusion — *see* Contusion, finger
      external constriction — *see* Constriction, external, finger
      foreign body — *see* Foreign body, superficial, finger
      index S60.94- ☑
      insect bite — *see* Bite, by site, superficial, insect
      little S60.94- ☑
      middle S60.94- ☑

☑ **Additional Character Required** — Refer to the Tabular List for Character Selection   ◀ **Subterms under main terms may continue to next column or page**

Injury — *continued*
  superficial — *continued*
    finger(s) — *continued*
      ring S60.94- ☑
    flank S30.92 ☑
    foot S90.92- ☑
      abrasion — *see* Abrasion, foot
      bite — *see* Bite, foot
      blister — *see* Blister, foot
      contusion — *see* Contusion, foot
      external constriction — *see* Constriction, external, foot
      foreign body — *see* Foreign body, superficial, foot
    forearm S50.91- ☑
      abrasion — *see* Abrasion, forearm
      bite — *see* Bite, forearm, superficial
      blister — *see* Blister, forearm
      contusion — *see* Contusion, forearm
      elbow only — *see* Injury, superficial, elbow
      external constriction — *see* Constriction, external, forearm
      foreign body — *see* Foreign body, superficial, forearm
    forehead — *see* Injury, superficial, head NEC
    foreign body — *see* Foreign body, superficial
    genital organs, external
      female S30.97 ☑
      male S30.96 ☑
    globe (eye) — *see* Injury, eye, specified site NEC
    groin S30.92 ☑
    gum — *see* Injury, superficial, oral cavity
    hand S60.92- ☑
      abrasion — *see* Abrasion, hand
      bite — *see* Bite, superficial, hand
      contusion — *see* Contusion, hand
      external constriction — *see* Constriction, external, hand
      foreign body — *see* Foreign body, superficial, hand
    head S00.90 ☑
      ear — *see* Injury, superficial, ear
      eyelid — *see* Injury, superficial, eyelid
      nose S00.30 ☑
      oral cavity S00.502 ☑
      scalp S00.00 ☑
      specified site NEC S00.80 ☑
    heel — *see* Injury, superficial, foot
    hip S70.91- ☑
      abrasion — *see* Abrasion, hip
      bite — *see* Bite, superficial, hip
      blister — *see* Blister, hip
      contusion — *see* Contusion, hip
      external constriction — *see* Constriction, external, hip
      foreign body — *see* Foreign body, superficial, hip
    iliac region — *see* Injury, superficial, abdomen
    inguinal region — *see* Injury, superficial, abdomen
    insect bite — *see* Bite, by site, superficial, insect
    interscapular region — *see* Injury, superficial, thorax, back
    jaw — *see* Injury, superficial, head, specified NEC
    knee S80.91- ☑
      abrasion — *see* Abrasion, knee
      bite — *see* Bite, superficial, knee
      blister — *see* Blister, knee
      contusion — *see* Contusion, knee
      external constriction — *see* Constriction, external, knee
      foreign body — *see* Foreign body, superficial, knee
    labium (majus) (minus) S30.95 ☑
    lacrimal (apparatus) (gland) (sac) — *see* Injury, eye, specified site NEC
    larynx — *see* Injury, superficial, throat
    leg (lower) S80.92- ☑
      abrasion — *see* Abrasion, leg
      bite — *see* Bite, superficial, leg
      contusion — *see* Contusion, leg
      external constriction — *see* Constriction, external, leg
      foreign body — *see* Foreign body, superficial, leg
      knee — *see* Injury, superficial, knee
    limb NEC T14.8 ☑

Injury — *continued*
  superficial — *continued*
    lip S00.501 ☑
    lower back S30.91 ☑
    lumbar region S30.91 ☑
    malar region — *see* Injury, superficial, head, specified NEC
    mammary — *see* Injury, superficial, breast
    mastoid region — *see* Injury, superficial, head, specified NEC
    mouth — *see* Injury, superficial, oral cavity
    muscle NEC T14.8 ☑
    nail NEC T14.8 ☑
      finger — *see* Injury, superficial, finger
      toe — *see* Injury, superficial, toe
    nasal (septum) — *see* Injury, superficial, nose
    neck S10.90 ☑
      specified site NEC S10.80 ☑
    nose (septum) S00.30 ☑
    occipital region — *see* Injury, superficial, scalp
    oral cavity S00.502 ☑
    orbital region — *see* Injury, superficial, periocular area
    palate — *see* Injury, superficial, oral cavity
    palm — *see* Injury, superficial, hand
    parietal region — *see* Injury, superficial, scalp
    pelvis S30.91 ☑
      girdle — *see* Injury, superficial, hip
    penis S30.93 ☑
    perineum
      female S30.95 ☑
      male S30.91 ☑
    periocular area S00.20- ☑
      abrasion — *see* Abrasion, eyelid
      bite — *see* Bite, superficial, eyelid
      contusion — *see* Contusion, eyelid
      external constriction — *see* Constriction, external, eyelid
      foreign body — *see* Foreign body, superficial, eyelid
    phalanges
      finger — *see* Injury, superficial, finger
      toe — *see* Injury, superficial, toe
    pharynx — *see* Injury, superficial, throat
    pinna — *see* Injury, superficial, ear
    popliteal space — *see* Injury, superficial, knee
    prepuce S30.93 ☑
    pubic region S30.91 ☑
    pudendum
      female S30.97 ☑
      male S30.96 ☑
    sacral region S30.91 ☑
    scalp S00.00 ☑
    scapular region — *see* Injury, superficial, shoulder
    sclera — *see* Injury, eye, specified site NEC
    scrotum S30.94 ☑
    shin — *see* Injury, superficial, leg
    shoulder S40.91- ☑
      abrasion — *see* Abrasion, shoulder
      bite — *see* Bite, superficial, shoulder
      blister — *see* Blister, shoulder
      contusion — *see* Contusion, shoulder
      external constriction — *see* Constriction, external, shoulder
      foreign body — *see* Foreign body, superficial, shoulder
    skin NEC T14.8 ☑
    sternal region — *see* Injury, superficial, thorax, front
    subconjunctival — *see* Injury, eye, specified site NEC
    subcutaneous NEC T14.8 ☑
    submaxillary region — *see* Injury, superficial, head, specified NEC
    submental region — *see* Injury, superficial, head, specified NEC
    subungual
      finger(s) — *see* Injury, superficial, finger
      toe(s) — *see* Injury, superficial, toe
    supraclavicular fossa — *see* Injury, superficial, neck
    supraorbital — *see* Injury, superficial, head, specified NEC
    temple — *see* Injury, superficial, head, specified NEC
    temporal region — *see* Injury, superficial, head, specified NEC
    testis S30.94 ☑
    thigh S70.92- ☑
      abrasion — *see* Abrasion, thigh

Injury — *continued*
  superficial — *continued*
    thigh — *continued*
      bite — *see* Bite, superficial, thigh
      blister — *see* Blister, thigh
      contusion — *see* Contusion, thigh
      external constriction — *see* Constriction, external, thigh
      foreign body — *see* Foreign body, superficial, thigh
    thorax, thoracic (wall) S20.90 ☑
      abrasion — *see* Abrasion, thorax
      back S20.40- ☑
      bite — *see* Bite, thorax, superficial
      blister — *see* Blister, thorax
      contusion — *see* Contusion, thorax
      external constriction — *see* Constriction, external, thorax
      foreign body — *see* Foreign body, superficial, thorax
      front S20.30- ☑
    throat S10.10 ☑
      abrasion S10.11 ☑
      bite S10.17 ☑
        insect S10.16 ☑
      blister S10.12 ☑
      contusion S10.0 ☑
      external constriction S10.14 ☑
      foreign body S10.15 ☑
    thumb S60.93- ☑
      abrasion — *see* Abrasion, thumb
      bite — *see* Bite, superficial, thumb
      blister — *see* Blister, thumb
      contusion — *see* Contusion, thumb
      external constriction — *see* Constriction, external, thumb
      foreign body — *see* Foreign body, superficial, thumb
      insect bite — *see* Bite, by site, superficial, insect
      specified type NEC S60.39 ☑
    toe(s) S90.93- ☑
      abrasion — *see* Abrasion, toe
      bite — *see* Bite, toe
      blister — *see* Blister, toe
      contusion — *see* Contusion, toe
      external constriction — *see* Constriction, external, toe
      foreign body — *see* Foreign body, superficial, toe
      great S90.93- ☑
    tongue — *see* Injury, superficial, oral cavity
    tooth, teeth — *see* Injury, superficial, oral cavity
    trachea S10.10 ☑
    tunica vaginalis S30.94 ☑
    tympanum, tympanic membrane — *see* Injury, superficial, ear
    uvula — *see* Injury, superficial, oral cavity
    vagina S30.95 ☑
    vocal cords — *see* Injury, superficial, throat
    vulva S30.95 ☑
    wrist S60.91- ☑
  supraclavicular region — *see* Injury, neck
  supraorbital S09.93 ☑
  suprarenal gland (multiple) — *see* Injury, adrenal
  surgical complication (external or internal site) — *see* Laceration, accidental complicating surgery
  temple S09.90 ☑
  temporal region S09.90 ☑
  tendon (*see also* Injury, muscle, by site)
    abdomen — *see* Injury, muscle, abdomen
    Achilles — *see* Injury, Achilles tendon
    lower back — *see* Injury, muscle, lower back
    pelvic organs — *see* Injury, muscle, pelvis
  tenth cranial nerve (pneumogastric or vagus) — *see* Injury, nerve, vagus
  testis S39.94 ☑
  thigh S79.92- ☑
    blood vessel — *see* Injury, blood vessel, hip
    contusion — *see* Contusion, thigh
    fracture — *see* Fracture, femur
    muscle — *see* Injury, muscle, thigh
    nerve — *see* Injury, nerve, thigh
    open — *see* Wound, open, thigh
    specified NEC S79.82- ☑
    superficial — *see* Injury, superficial, thigh

Injury — continued
- third cranial nerve (oculomotor) — see Injury, nerve, oculomotor
- thorax, thoracic S29.9 ☑
  - blood vessel — see Injury, blood vessel, thorax
  - cavity — see Injury, intrathoracic
  - dislocation — see Dislocation, thorax
  - external (wall) S29.9 ☑
    - contusion — see Contusion, thorax
    - nerve — see Injury, nerve, thorax
    - open — see Wound, open, thorax
    - specified NEC S29.8 ☑
    - sprain — see Sprain, thorax
    - superficial — see Injury, superficial, thorax
  - fracture — see Fracture, thorax
  - internal — see Injury, intrathoracic
  - intrathoracic organ — see Injury, intrathoracic
  - sympathetic ganglion — see Injury, nerve, thorax, sympathetic
- throat (see also Injury, neck) S19.9 ☑
- thumb S69.9- ☑
  - blood vessel — see Injury, blood vessel, thumb
  - contusion — see Contusion, thumb
  - dislocation — see Dislocation, thumb
  - fracture — see Fracture, thumb
  - muscle — see Injury, muscle, thumb
  - nerve — see Injury, nerve, digital, thumb
  - open — see Wound, open, thumb
  - specified NEC S69.8- ☑
  - sprain — see Sprain, thumb
  - superficial — see Injury, superficial, thumb
- thymus (gland) — see Injury, intrathoracic, specified organ NEC
- thyroid (gland) NEC S19.84 ☑
- toe S99.92- ☑
  - contusion — see Contusion, toe
  - dislocation — see Dislocation, toe
  - fracture — see Fracture, toe
  - muscle — see Injury, muscle, toe
  - open — see Wound, open, toe
  - specified type NEC S99.82- ☑
  - sprain — see Sprain, toe
  - superficial — see Injury, superficial, toe
- tongue S09.93 ☑
- tonsil S09.93 ☑
- tooth S09.93 ☑
- trachea (cervical) NEC S19.82 ☑
  - thoracic — see Injury, intrathoracic, trachea, thoracic
- transfusion-related acute lung (TRALI) J95.84
- tunica vaginalis S39.94 ☑
- twelfth cranial nerve (hypoglossal) — see Injury, nerve, hypoglossal
- ureter S37.10 ☑
  - contusion S37.12 ☑
  - laceration S37.13 ☑
  - specified type NEC S37.19 ☑
- urethra (sphincter) S37.30 ☑
  - at delivery O71.5
  - contusion S37.32 ☑
  - laceration S37.33 ☑
  - specified type NEC S37.39 ☑
- urinary organ S37.90 ☑
  - contusion S37.92 ☑
  - laceration S37.93 ☑
  - specified
    - site NEC S37.899 ☑
      - contusion S37.892 ☑
      - laceration S37.893 ☑
      - specified type NEC S37.898 ☑
    - type NEC S37.99 ☑
- uterus, uterine S37.60 ☑
  - with ectopic or molar pregnancy O08.6
  - blood vessel — see Injury, blood vessel, iliac
  - contusion S37.62 ☑
  - laceration S37.63 ☑
    - cervix at delivery O71.3
  - rupture associated with obstetrics — see Rupture, uterus
  - specified type NEC S37.69 ☑
- uvula S09.93 ☑
- vagina S39.93 ☑
  - abrasion S30.814 ☑
  - bite S31.45 ☑
    - insect S30.864 ☑
    - superficial NEC S30.874 ☑
  - contusion S30.23 ☑

Injury — continued
- vagina — continued
  - crush S38.03 ☑
  - during delivery — see Laceration, vagina, during delivery
  - external constriction S30.844 ☑
  - insect bite S30.864 ☑
  - laceration S31.41 ☑
    - with foreign body S31.42 ☑
  - open wound S31.40 ☑
  - puncture S31.43 ☑
    - with foreign body S31.44 ☑
  - superficial S30.95 ☑
    - foreign body S30.854 ☑
- vas deferens — see Injury, pelvic organ, specified site NEC
- vascular NEC T14.8 ☑
- vein — see Injury, blood vessel
- vena cava (superior) S25.20 ☑
  - inferior S35.10 ☑
    - laceration (minor) (superficial) S35.11 ☑
      - major S35.12 ☑
    - specified type NEC S35.19 ☑
  - laceration (minor) (superficial) S25.21 ☑
    - major S25.22 ☑
  - specified type NEC S25.29 ☑
- vesical (sphincter) — see Injury, bladder
- visual cortex S04.04- ☑
- vitreous (humor) S05.90 ☑
  - specified NEC S05.8X- ☑
- vocal cord NEC S19.83 ☑
- vulva S39.94 ☑
  - abrasion S30.814 ☑
  - bite S31.45 ☑
    - insect S30.864 ☑
    - superficial NEC S30.874 ☑
  - contusion S30.23 ☑
  - crush S38.03 ☑
  - during delivery — see Laceration, perineum, female, during delivery
  - external constriction S30.844 ☑
  - insect bite S30.864 ☑
  - laceration S31.41 ☑
    - with foreign body S31.42 ☑
  - open wound S31.40 ☑
  - puncture S31.43 ☑
    - with foreign body S31.44 ☑
  - superficial S30.95 ☑
    - foreign body S30.854 ☑
- whiplash (cervical spine) S13.4 ☑
- wrist S69.9- ☑
  - blood vessel — see Injury, blood vessel, hand
  - contusion — see Contusion, wrist
  - dislocation — see Dislocation, wrist
  - fracture — see Fracture, wrist
  - muscle — see Injury, muscle, hand
  - nerve — see Injury, nerve, hand
  - open — see Wound, open, wrist
  - specified NEC S69.8- ☑
  - sprain — see Sprain, wrist
  - superficial — see Injury, superficial, wrist

Inoculation (see also Vaccination)
- complication or reaction — see Complications, vaccination

Insanity, insane (see also Psychosis)
- adolescent — see Schizophrenia
- confusional F28
  - acute or subacute F05
- delusional F22
- senile F03 ☑

Insect
- bite — see Bite, by site, superficial, insect
- venomous, poisoning NEC (by) — see Venom, arthropod

Insensitivity
- adrenocorticotropin hormone (ACTH) E27.49
- androgen E34.50
  - complete E34.51
  - partial E34.52

Insertion
- cord (umbilical) lateral or velamentous O43.12- ☑
- intrauterine contraceptive device (encounter for) — see Intrauterine contraceptive device

Insolation (sunstroke) T67.0 ☑

Insomnia (organic) G47.00
- adjustment F51.02

Insomnia — continued
- adjustment disorder F51.02
- behavioral, of childhood Z73.819
  - combined type Z73.812
  - limit setting type Z73.811
  - sleep-onset association type Z73.810
- childhood Z73.819
- chronic F51.04
  - somatized tension F51.04
- conditioned F51.04
- due to
  - alcohol
    - abuse F10.182
    - dependence F10.282
    - use F10.982
  - amphetamines
    - abuse F15.182
    - dependence F15.282
    - use F15.982
  - anxiety disorder F51.05
  - caffeine
    - abuse F15.182
    - dependence F15.282
    - use F15.982
  - cocaine
    - abuse F14.182
    - dependence F14.282
    - use F14.982
  - depression F51.05
  - drug NEC
    - abuse F19.182
    - dependence F19.282
    - use F19.982
  - medical condition G47.01
  - mental disorder NEC F51.05
  - opioid
    - abuse F11.182
    - dependence F11.282
    - use F11.982
  - psychoactive substance NEC
    - abuse F19.182
    - dependence F19.182
    - use F19.982
  - sedative, hypnotic, or anxiolytic
    - abuse F13.182
    - dependence F13.282
    - use F13.982
  - stimulant NEC
    - abuse F15.182
    - dependence F15.282
    - use F15.982
- fatal familial (FFI) A81.83
- idiopathic F51.01
- learned F51.3
- nonorganic origin F51.01
- not due to a substance or known physiological condition F51.01
  - specified NEC F51.09
- paradoxical F51.03
- primary F51.01
- psychiatric F51.05
- psychophysiologic F51.04
- related to psychopathology F51.05
- short-term F51.02
- specified NEC G47.09
- stress-related F51.02
- transient F51.02
- without objective findings F51.02

Inspiration
- food or foreign body — see Foreign body, by site
- mucus — see Asphyxia, mucus

Inspissated bile syndrome (newborn) P59.1

Instability
- emotional (excessive) F60.3
- joint (post-traumatic) M25.30
  - ankle M25.37- ☑
  - due to old ligament injury — see Disorder, ligament
  - elbow M25.32- ☑
  - flail — see Flail, joint
  - foot M25.37- ☑
  - hand M25.34- ☑
  - hip M25.35- ☑
  - knee M25.36- ☑
  - lumbosacral — see subcategory M53.2 ☑
  - prosthesis — see Complications, joint prosthesis, mechanical, displacement, by site
  - sacroiliac — see subcategory M53.2 ☑

Instability — continued
  joint — continued
    secondary to
      old ligament injury — see Disorder, ligament
      removal of joint prosthesis M96.89
    shoulder (region) M25.31- ☑
    spine — see subcategory M53.2 ☑
    wrist M25.33- ☑
    knee (chronic) M23.5- ☑
    lumbosacral — see subcategory M53.2 ☑
  nervous F48.8
  personality (emotional) F60.3
  spine — see Instability, joint, spine
  vasomotor R55
Institutional syndrome (childhood) F94.2
Institutionalization, affecting child Z62.22
  disinhibited attachment F94.2
Insufficiency, insufficient
  accommodation, old age H52.4
  adrenal (gland) E27.40
    primary E27.1
  adrenocortical E27.40
    drug-induced E27.3
    iatrogenic E27.3
    primary E27.1
  anatomic crown height K08.89
  anterior (occlusal) guidance M26.54
  anus K62.89
  aortic (valve) I35.1
    with
      mitral (valve) disease I08.0
        with tricuspid (valve) disease I08.3
      stenosis I35.2
      tricuspid (valve) disease I08.2
        with mitral (valve) disease I08.3
    congenital Q23.1
    rheumatic I06.1
      with
        mitral (valve) disease I08.0
          with tricuspid (valve) disease I08.3
        stenosis I06.2
          with mitral (valve) disease I08.0
            with tricuspid (valve) disease I08.3
        tricuspid (valve) disease I08.2
          with mitral (valve) disease I08.3
    specified cause NEC I35.1
    syphilitic A52.03
  arterial I77.1
    basilar G45.0
    carotid (hemispheric) G45.1
    cerebral I67.81
    coronary (acute or subacute) I24.8
    mesenteric K55.1
    peripheral I73.9
    precerebral (multiple) (bilateral) G45.2
    vertebral G45.0
  arteriovenous I99.8
  biliary K83.8
  cardiac (see also Insufficiency, myocardial)
    due to presence of (cardiac) prosthesis I97.11- ☑
      postprocedural I97.11- ☑
  cardiorenal, hypertensive I13.2
  cardiovascular — see Disease, cardiovascular
  cerebrovascular (acute) I67.81
    with transient focal neurological signs and symp-
      toms G45.8
  circulatory NEC I99.8
    newborn P29.89
  clinical crown length K08.89
  convergence H51.11
  coronary (acute or subacute) I24.8
    chronic or with a stated duration of over 4 weeks
      I25.89
  corticoadrenal E27.40
    primary E27.1
  dietary E63.9
  divergence H51.8
  food T73.0 ☑
  gastroesophageal K22.8
  gonadal
    ovary E28.39
    testis E29.1
  heart (see also Insufficiency, myocardial)
    newborn P29.0
    valve — see Endocarditis
  hepatic — see Failure, hepatic
  idiopathic autonomic G90.09

Insufficiency, insufficient — continued
  interocclusal distance of fully erupted teeth (ridge)
    M26.36
  kidney N28.9
    acute N28.9
    chronic N18.9
  lacrimal (secretion) H04.12- ☑
    passages — see Stenosis, lacrimal
  liver — see Failure, hepatic
  lung — see Insufficiency, pulmonary
  mental (congenital) — see Disability, intellectual
  mesenteric K55.1
  mitral (valve) I34.0
    with
      aortic valve disease I08.0
        with tricuspid (valve) disease I08.3
      obstruction or stenosis I05.2
        with aortic valve disease I08.0
      tricuspid (valve) disease I08.1
        with aortic (valve) disease I08.3
    congenital Q23.3
    rheumatic I05.1
      with
        aortic valve disease I08.0
          with tricuspid (valve) disease I08.3
        obstruction or stenosis I05.2
          with aortic valve disease I08.0
            with tricuspid (valve) disease I08.3
        tricuspid (valve) disease I08.1
          with aortic (valve) disease I08.3
      active or acute I01.1
        with chorea, rheumatic (Sydenham's) I02.0
    specified cause, except rheumatic I34.0
  muscle (see also Disease, muscle)
    heart — see Insufficiency, myocardial
    ocular NEC H50.9
  myocardial, myocardium (with arteriosclerosis) (see
    also Failure, heart) I50.9
    with
      rheumatic fever (conditions in I00) I09.0
        active, acute or subacute I01.2
          with chorea I02.0
        inactive or quiescent (with chorea) I09.0
    congenital Q24.8
    hypertensive — see Hypertension, heart
    newborn P29.0
    rheumatic I09.0
      active, acute, or subacute I01.2
    syphilitic A52.06
  nourishment T73.0 ☑
  pancreatic K86.89
    exocrine K86.81
  parathyroid (gland) E20.9
  peripheral vascular (arterial) I73.9
  pituitary E23.0
  placental (mother) O36.51- ☑
  platelets D69.6
  prenatal care affecting management of pregnancy
    O09.3- ☑
  progressive pluriglandular E31.0
  pulmonary J98.4
    acute, following surgery (nonthoracic) J95.2
      thoracic J95.1
    chronic, following surgery J95.3
    following
      shock J98.4
      trauma J98.4
    newborn P28.5
    valve I37.1
      with stenosis I37.2
      congenital Q22.2
      rheumatic I09.89
        with aortic, mitral or tricuspid (valve) disease
          I08.8
  pyloric K31.89
  renal (acute) N28.9
    chronic N18.9
  respiratory R06.89
    newborn P28.5
  rotation — see Malrotation
  sleep syndrome F51.12
  social insurance Z59.7
  suprarenal E27.40
    primary E27.1
  tarso-orbital fascia, congenital Q10.3
  testis E29.1
  thyroid (gland) (acquired) E03.9
    congenital E03.1

Insufficiency, insufficient — continued
  tricuspid (valve) (rheumatic) I07.1
    with
      aortic (valve) disease I08.2
        with mitral (valve) disease I08.3
      mitral (valve) disease I08.1
        with aortic (valve) disease I08.3
      obstruction or stenosis I07.2
        with aortic (valve) disease I08.2
          with mitral (valve) disease I08.3
    congenital Q22.8
    nonrheumatic I36.1
      with stenosis I36.2
  urethral sphincter R32
  valve, valvular (heart) I38
    aortic — see Insufficiency, aortic (valve)
    congenital Q24.8
    mitral — see Insufficiency, mitral (valve)
    pulmonary — see Insufficiency, pulmonary, valve
    tricuspid — see Insufficiency, tricuspid (valve)
  vascular I99.8
    intestine K55.9
      acute (see also Ischemia, intestine, acute) K55.059
    mesenteric K55.1
    peripheral I73.9
    renal — see Hypertension, kidney
  velopharyngeal
    acquired K13.79
    congenital Q38.8
  venous (chronic) (peripheral) I87.2
  ventricular — see Insufficiency, myocardial
  welfare support Z59.7
Insufflation, fallopian Z31.41
Insular — see condition
Insulinoma
  pancreas
    benign D13.7
    malignant C25.4
    uncertain behavior D37.8
  specified site
    benign — see Neoplasm, by site, benign
    malignant — see Neoplasm, by site, malignant
    uncertain behavior — see Neoplasm, by site, uncer-
      tain behavior
  unspecified site
    benign D13.7
    malignant C25.4
    uncertain behavior D37.8
Insuloma — see Insulinoma
Interference
  balancing side M26.56
  non-working side M26.56
Intermenstrual — see condition
Intermittent — see condition
Internal — see condition
Interrogation
  cardiac defibrillator (automatic) (implantable) Z45.02
  cardiac pacemaker Z45.018
  cardiac (event) (loop) recorder Z45.09
  infusion pump (implanted) (intrathecal) Z45.1
  neurostimulator Z46.2
Interruption
  aortic arch Q25.21
  bundle of His I44.30
  phase-shift, sleep cycle — see Disorder, sleep, circadian
    rhythm
  sleep phase-shift, or 24 hour sleep-wake cycle — see
    Disorder, sleep, circadian rhythm
Interstitial — see condition
Intertrigo L30.4
  labialis K13.0
Intervertebral disc — see condition
Intestine, intestinal — see condition
Intolerance
  carbohydrate K90.49
  disaccharide, hereditary E73.0
  fat NEC K90.49
    pancreatic K90.3
  food K90.49
    dietary counseling and surveillance Z71.3
  fructose E74.10
    hereditary E74.12
  glucose (-galactose) E74.39
  gluten K90.41
  lactose E73.9
    specified NEC E73.8
  lysine E72.3
  milk NEC K90.49

Intolerance — *continued*
milk — *continued*
lactose E73.9
protein K90.49
starch NEC K90.49
sucrose (-isomaltose) E74.31
Intoxicated NEC (without dependence) — *see* Alcohol, intoxication
Intoxication
acid E87.2
alcoholic (acute) (without dependence) — *see* Alcohol, intoxication
alimentary canal K52.1
amphetamine (without dependence) — *see* Abuse, drug, stimulant, with intoxication
with dependence — *see* Dependence, drug, stimulant, with intoxication
anxiolytic (acute) (without dependence) — *see* Abuse, drug, sedative, with intoxication
with dependence — *see* Dependence, drug, sedative, with intoxication
caffeine F15.929
with dependence — *see* Dependence, drug, stimulant, with intoxication
cannabinoids (acute) (without dependence) — *see* Use, cannabis, with intoxication
with
abuse — *see* Abuse, drug, cannabis, with intoxication
dependence — *see* Dependence, drug, cannabis, with intoxication
chemical — *see* Table of Drugs and Chemicals
via placenta or breast milk — *see* - Absorption, chemical, through placenta
cocaine (acute) (without dependence) — *see* Abuse, drug, cocaine, with intoxication
with dependence — *see* Dependence, drug, cocaine, with intoxication
drug
acute (without dependence) — *see* Abuse, drug, by type with intoxication
with dependence — *see* Dependence, drug, by type with intoxication
addictive
via placenta or breast milk — *see* Absorption, drug, addictive, through placenta
newborn P93.8
gray baby syndrome P93.0
overdose or wrong substance given or taken — *see* Table of Drugs and Chemicals, by drug, poisoning
enteric K52.1
foodborne A05.9
bacterial A05.9
classical (Clostridium botulinum) A05.1
due to
Bacillus cereus A05.4
bacterium A05.9
specified NEC A05.8
Clostridium
botulinum A05.1
perfringens A05.2
welchii A05.2
Salmonella A02.9
with
(gastro)enteritis A02.0
localized infection(s) A02.20
arthritis A02.23
meningitis A02.21
osteomyelitis A02.24
pneumonia A02.22
pyelonephritis A02.25
specified NEC A02.29
sepsis A02.1
specified manifestation NEC A02.8
Staphylococcus A05.0
Vibrio
parahaemolyticus A05.3
vulnificus A05.5
enterotoxin, staphylococcal A05.0
noxious — *see* Poisoning, food, noxious
gastrointestinal K52.1
hallucinogenic (without dependence) — *see* Abuse, drug, hallucinogen, with intoxication
with dependence — *see* Dependence, drug, hallucinogen, with intoxication
hypnotic (acute) (without dependence) — *see* Abuse, drug, sedative, with intoxication

Intoxication — *continued*
hypnotic — *see* Abuse, drug, sedative, with intoxication — *continued*
with dependence — *see* Dependence, drug, sedative, with intoxication
inhalant (acute) (without dependence) — *see* Abuse, drug, inhalant, with intoxication
with dependence — *see* Dependence, drug, inhalant, with intoxication
meaning
inebriation — *see* category F10 ☑
poisoning — *see* Table of Drugs and Chemicals
methyl alcohol (acute) (without dependence) — *see* Alcohol, intoxication
opioid (acute) (without dependence) — *see* Abuse, drug, opioid, with intoxication
with dependence — *see* Dependence, drug, opioid, with intoxication
pathologic NEC (without dependence) — *see* Alcohol, intoxication
phencyclidine (without dependence) — *see* Abuse, drug, hallucinogen, with intoxication
with dependence — *see* Dependence, drug, hallucinogen, with intoxication
potassium (K) E87.5
psychoactive substance NEC (without dependence) — *see* Abuse, drug, psychoactive NEC, with intoxication
with dependence — *see* Dependence, drug, psychoactive NEC, with intoxication
sedative (acute) (without dependence) — *see* Abuse, drug, sedative, with intoxication
with dependence — *see* Dependence, drug, sedative, with intoxication
serum (*see also* Reaction, serum) T80.69 ☑
uremic — *see* Uremia
volatile solvents (acute) (without dependence) — *see* Abuse, drug, inhalant, with intoxication
with dependence — *see* Dependence, drug, inhalant, with intoxication
water E87.79
Intraabdominal testis, testes
bilateral Q53.211
unilateral Q53.111
Intracranial — *see* condition
Intrahepatic gallbladder Q44.1
Intraligamentous — *see* condition
Intrathoracic (*see also* condition)
kidney Q63.2
Intrauterine contraceptive device
checking Z30.431
in situ Z97.5
insertion Z30.430
immediately following removal Z30.433
management Z30.431
reinsertion Z30.433
removal Z30.432
replacement Z30.433
retention in pregnancy O26.3- ☑
Intraventricular — *see* condition
Intrinsic deformity — *see* Deformity
Intubation, difficult or failed T88.4 ☑
Intumescence, lens (eye) (cataract) — *see* Cataract
Intussusception (bowel) (colon) (enteric) (ileocecal) (ileocolic) (intestine) (rectum) K56.1
appendix K38.8
congenital Q43.8
ureter (with obstruction) N13.5
Invagination (bowel, colon, intestine or rectum) K56.1
Inversion
albumin-globulin (A-G) ratio E88.09
bladder N32.89
cecum — *see* Intussusception
cervix N88.8
chromosome in normal individual Q95.1
circadian rhythm — *see* Disorder, sleep, circadian rhythm
nipple N64.59
congenital Q83.8
gestational — *see* Retraction, nipple
puerperal, postpartum — *see* Retraction, nipple
nyctohemeral rhythm — *see* Disorder, sleep, circadian rhythm
optic papilla Q14.2
organ or site, congenital NEC — *see* Anomaly, by site
sleep rhythm — *see* Disorder, sleep, circadian rhythm
testis (congenital) Q55.29

Inversion — *continued*
uterus (chronic) (postinfectional) (postpartal, old) N85.5
postpartum O71.2
vagina (posthysterectomy) N99.3
ventricular Q20.5
Investigation (*see also* Examination) Z04.9
clinical research subject (control) (normal comparison) (participant) Z00.6
Involuntary movement, abnormal R25.9
Involution, involutional (*see also* condition)
breast, cystic — *see* Dysplasia, mammary, specified type NEC
depression (single episode) F32.89
recurrent episode F33.9
melancholia (single episode) F32.89
recurrent episode F33.8
ovary, senile — *see* Atrophy, ovary
thymus failure E32.8
I.Q.
20-34 F72
35-49 F71
50-69 F70
under 20 F73
IRDS (type I) P22.0
type II P22.1
Irideremia Q13.1
Iridis rubeosis — *see* Disorder, iris, vascular
Iridochoroiditis (panuveitis) — *see* Panuveitis
Iridocyclitis H20.9
acute H20.0- ☑
hypopyon H20.05- ☑
primary H20.01- ☑
recurrent H20.02- ☑
secondary (noninfectious) H20.04- ☑
infectious H20.03- ☑
chronic H20.1- ☑
due to allergy — *see* Iridocyclitis, acute, secondary
endogenous — *see* Iridocyclitis, acute, primary
Fuchs' — *see* Cyclitis, Fuchs' heterochromic
gonococcal A54.32
granulomatous — *see* Iridocyclitis, chronic
herpes, herpetic (simplex) B00.51
zoster B02.32
hypopyon — *see* Iridocyclitis, acute, hypopyon
in (due to)
ankylosing spondylitis M45.9
gonococcal infection A54.32
herpes (simplex) virus B00.51
zoster B02.32
infectious disease NOS B99 ☑
parasitic disease NOS B89 [H22]
sarcoidosis D86.83
syphilis A51.43
tuberculosis A18.54
zoster B02.32
lens-induced H20.2- ☑
nongranulomatous — *see* Iridocyclitis, acute
recurrent — *see* Iridocyclitis, acute, recurrent
rheumatic — *see* Iridocyclitis, chronic
subacute — *see* Iridocyclitis, acute
sympathetic — *see* Uveitis, sympathetic
syphilitic (secondary) A51.43
tuberculous (chronic) A18.54
Vogt-Koyanagi H20.82- ☑
Iridocyclochoroiditis (panuveitis) — *see* Panuveitis
Iridodialysis H21.53- ☑
Iridodonesis H21.89
Iridoplegia (complete) (partial) (reflex) H57.09
Iridoschisis H21.25- ☑
Iris (*see also* condition)
bombé — *see* Membrane, pupillary
Iritis (*see also* Iridocyclitis)
chronic — *see* Iridocyclitis, chronic
diabetic — *see* E08-E13 with .39
due to
herpes simplex B00.51
leprosy A30.9 [H22]
gonococcal A54.32
gouty (*see also* Gout, by type) M10.9 [H22]
granulomatous — *see* Iridocyclitis, chronic
lens induced — *see* Iridocyclitis, lens-induced
papulosa (syphilitic) A52.71
rheumatic — *see* Iridocyclitis, chronic
syphilitic (secondary) A51.43
congenital (early) A50.01
late A52.71
tuberculous A18.54

Iron — *see* condition
Iron-miner's lung J63.4
Irradiated enamel (tooth, teeth) K03.89
Irradiation effects, adverse T66 ☑
Irreducible, irreducibility — *see* condition
Irregular, irregularity
  action, heart I49.9
  alveolar process K08.89
  bleeding N92.6
  breathing R06.89
  contour of cornea (acquired) — *see* Deformity, cornea
    congenital Q13.4
  contour, reconstructed breast N65.0
  dentin (in pulp) K04.3
  eye movements H55.89
    nystagmus — *see* Nystagmus
    saccadic H55.81
  labor O62.2
  menstruation (cause unknown) N92.6
  periods N92.6
  prostate N42.9
  pupil — *see* Abnormality, pupillary
  reconstructed breast N65.0
  respiratory R06.89
  septum (nasal) J34.2
  shape, organ or site, congenital NEC — *see* Distortion
  sleep-wake pattern (rhythm) G47.23
Irritable, irritability R45.4
  bladder N32.89
  bowel (syndrome) K58.9
    with
      constipation K58.1
      diarrhea K58.0
    mixed K58.2
    psychogenic F45.8
    specified NEC K58.8
  bronchial — *see* Bronchitis
  cerebral, in newborn P91.3
  colon (see also Irritable, bowel) K58.9
    with diarrhea K58.0
    psychogenic F45.8
  duodenum K59.8
  heart (psychogenic) F45.8
  hip — *see* Derangement, joint, specified type NEC, hip
  ileum K59.8
  infant R68.12
  jejunum K59.8
  rectum K59.8
  stomach K31.89
    psychogenic F45.8
  sympathetic G90.8
  urethra N36.8
Irritation
  anus K62.89
  axillary nerve G54.0
  bladder N32.89
  brachial plexus G54.0
  bronchial — *see* Bronchitis
  cervical plexus G54.2
  cervix — *see* Cervicitis
  choroid, sympathetic — *see* Endophthalmitis
  cranial nerve — *see* Disorder, nerve, cranial
  gastric K31.89
    psychogenic F45.8
  globe, sympathetic — *see* Uveitis, sympathetic
  labyrinth — *see* subcategory H83.2 ☑
  lumbosacral plexus G54.1
  meninges (traumatic) — *see* Injury, intracranial
    nontraumatic — *see* Meningismus
  nerve — *see* Disorder, nerve
  nervous R45.0
  penis N48.89
  perineum NEC L29.3
  peripheral autonomic nervous system G90.8
  peritoneum — *see* Peritonitis
  pharynx J39.2
  plantar nerve — *see* Lesion, nerve, plantar
  spinal (cord) (traumatic) (see also Injury, spinal cord, by region)
    nerve G58.9
      root NEC — *see* Radiculopathy
    nontraumatic — *see* Myelopathy
  stomach K31.89
    psychogenic F45.8
  sympathetic nerve NEC G90.8
  ulnar nerve — *see* Lesion, nerve, ulnar
  vagina N89.8
Ischemia, ischemic I99.8

Ischemia, ischemic — *continued*
  bowel (transient)
    acute (see also Ischemia, intestine, acute) K55.059
    chronic K55.1
    due to mesenteric artery insufficiency K55.1
  brain — *see* Ischemia, cerebral
  cardiac (see Disease, heart, ischemic)
  cardiomyopathy I25.5
  cerebral (chronic) (generalized) I67.82
    arteriosclerotic I67.2
    intermittent G45.9
    newborn P91.0
    recurrent focal G45.8
    transient G45.9
  colon chronic (due to mesenteric artery insufficiency) K55.1
  coronary — *see* Disease, heart, ischemic
  demand (coronary) (see also Angina) I24.8
    with myocardial infarction I21.A1
    resulting in myocardial infarction I21.A1
  heart (chronic or with a stated duration of over 4 weeks) I25.9
    acute or with a stated duration of 4 weeks or less I24.9
    subacute I24.9
  infarction, muscle — *see* Infarct, muscle
  intestine (large) (small) (transient) K55.9
    acute K55.059
      diffuse K55.052
      focal K55.051
      large K55.039
        diffuse K55.032
        focal K55.031
      small K55.019
        diffuse K55.012
        focal K55.011
    chronic K55.1
    due to mesenteric artery insufficiency K55.1
  kidney N28.0
  mesenteric, acute (see also Ischemia, intestine, acute) K55.059
  muscle, traumatic T79.6 ☑
  myocardium, myocardial (chronic or with a stated duration of over 4 weeks) I25.9
    acute, without myocardial infarction I51.3
    silent (asymptomatic) I25.6
    transient of newborn P29.4
  renal N28.0
  retina, retinal — *see* Occlusion, artery, retina
  small bowel
    acute K55.019
      diffuse K55.012
      focal K55.011
    chronic K55.1
    due to mesenteric artery insufficiency K55.1
  spinal cord G95.11
  subendocardial — *see* Insufficiency, coronary
  supply (coronary) (see also Angina) I25.9
    due to vasospasm I20.1
Ischial spine — *see* condition
Ischialgia — *see* Sciatica
Ischiopagus Q89.4
Ischium, ischial — *see* condition
Ischuria R34
Iselin's disease or osteochondrosis — *see* Osteochondrosis, juvenile, metatarsus
Islands of
  parotid tissue in
    lymph nodes Q38.6
    neck structures Q38.6
  submaxillary glands in
    fascia Q38.6
    lymph nodes Q38.6
    neck muscles Q38.6
Islet cell tumor, pancreas D13.7
Isoimmunization NEC (see also Incompatibility)
  affecting management of pregnancy (ABO) (with hydrops fetalis) O36.11- ☑
    anti-A sensitization O36.11- ☑
    anti-B sensitization O36.19- ☑
    anti-c sensitization O36.09- ☑
    anti-C sensitization O36.09- ☑
    anti-e sensitization O36.09- ☑
    anti-E sensitization O36.09- ☑
    Rh NEC O36.09- ☑
      anti-D antibody O36.01- ☑
    specified NEC O36.19- ☑
  newborn P55.9

Isoimmunization — *continued*
  newborn — *continued*
    with
      hydrops fetalis P56.0
      kernicterus P57.0
    ABO (blood groups) P55.1
    Rhesus (Rh) factor P55.0
    specified type NEC P55.8
Isolation, isolated
  dwelling Z59.8
  family Z63.79
  social Z60.4
Isoleucinosis E71.19
Isomerism atrial appendages (with asplenia or polysplenia) Q20.6
Isosporiasis, isosporosis A07.3
Isovaleric acidemia E71.110
Issue of
  medical certificate Z02.79
    for disability determination Z02.71
  repeat prescription (appliance) (glasses) (medicinal substance, medicament, medicine) Z76.0
    contraception — *see* Contraception
Itch, itching (see also Pruritus)
  baker's L23.6
  barber's B35.0
  bricklayer's L24.5
  cheese B88.0
  clam digger's B65.3
  coolie B76.9
  copra B88.0
  dew B76.9
  dhobi B35.6
  filarial — *see* Infestation, filarial
  grain B88.0
  grocer's B88.0
  ground B76.9
  harvest B88.0
  jock B35.6
  Malabar B35.5
    beard B35.0
    foot B35.3
    scalp B35.0
  meaning scabies B86
  Norwegian B86
  perianal L29.0
  poultrymen's B88.0
  sarcoptic B86
  scabies B86
  scrub B88.0
  straw B88.0
  swimmer's B65.3
  water B76.9
  winter L29.8
Ivemark's syndrome (asplenia with congenital heart disease) Q89.01
Ivory bones Q78.2
Ixodiasis NEC B88.8

J

Jaccoud's syndrome — *see* Arthropathy, postrheumatic, chronic
Jackson's
  membrane Q43.3
  paralysis or syndrome G83.89
  veil Q43.3
Jacquet's dermatitis (diaper dermatitis) L22
Jadassohn-Pellizari's disease or anetoderma L90.2
Jadassohn's
  blue nevus — *see* Nevus
  intraepidermal epithelioma — *see* Neoplasm, skin, benign
Jaffe-Lichtenstein (-Uehlinger) **syndrome** — *see* Dysplasia, fibrous, bone NEC
Jakob-Creutzfeldt disease or syndrome — *see* Creutzfeldt-Jakob disease or syndrome
Jaksch-Luzet disease D64.89
Jamaican
  neuropathy G92
  paraplegic tropical ataxic-spastic syndrome G92
Janet's disease F48.8
Janiceps Q89.4
Jansky-Bielschowsky amaurotic idiocy E75.4
Japanese
  B-type encephalitis A83.0
  river fever A75.3
Jaundice (yellow) R17

▽ Subterms under main terms may continue to next column or page   ☑ Additional Character Required — Refer to the Tabular List for Character Selection   203

Iron — Jaundice

Keratoconjunctivitis — *continued*
- Acanthamoeba B6Ø.13
- adenoviral B3Ø.Ø
- epidemic B3Ø.Ø
- exposure H16.21- ☑
- herpes, herpetic (simplex) BØØ.52
  - zoster BØ2.33
- in exanthema (*see also* Exanthem) BØ9
- infectious B3Ø.Ø
- lagophthalmic — *see* Keratoconjunctivitis, specified type NEC
- neurotrophic H16.23- ☑
- phlyctenular H16.25- ☑
- postmeasles BØ5.81
- shipyard B3Ø.Ø
- sicca (Sjogren's) M35.Ø- ☑
  - not Sjogren's H16.22- ☑
- specified type NEC H16.29- ☑
- tuberculous (phlyctenular) A18.52
- vernal H16.26- ☑

Keratoconus H18.6Ø- ☑
- congenital Q13.4
- stable H18.61- ☑
- unstable H18.62- ☑

Keratocyst (dental) (odontogenic) — *see* Cyst, calcifying odontogenic

Keratoderma, keratodermia (congenital) (palmaris et plantaris) (symmetrical) Q82.8
- acquired L85.1
  - in diseases classified elsewhere L86
- climactericum L85.1
- gonococcal A54.89
- gonorrheal A54.89
- punctata L85.2
- Reiter's — *see* Reiter's disease

Keratodermatocele — *see* Descemetocele

Keratoglobus H18.79 ☑
- congenital Q15.8
  - with glaucoma Q15.Ø

Keratohemia — *see* Pigmentation, cornea, stromal

Keratoiritis (*see also* Iridocyclitis)
- syphilitic A5Ø.39
- tuberculous A18.54

Keratoma L57.Ø
- palmaris and plantaris hereditarium Q82.8
- senile L57.Ø

Keratomalacia H18.44- ☑
- vitamin A deficiency E5Ø.4

Keratomegaly Q13.4

Keratomycosis B49
- nigrans, nigricans (palmaris) B36.1

Keratopathy H18.9
- band H18.42- ☑
- bullous (aphakic), following cataract surgery H59.Ø1- ☑
- bullous H18.1- ☑

Keratoscleritis, tuberculous A18.52

Keratosis L57.Ø
- actinic L57.Ø
- arsenical L85.8
- congenital, specified NEC Q8Ø.8
- female genital NEC N94.89
- follicularis Q82.8
  - acquired L11.Ø
  - congenita Q82.8
  - et parafollicularis in cutem penetrans L87.Ø
  - spinulosa (decalvans) Q82.8
  - vitamin A deficiency E5Ø.8
- gonococcal A54.89
- male genital (external) N5Ø.89
- nigricans L83
- obturans, external ear (canal) — *see* Cholesteatoma, external ear
- palmaris et plantaris (inherited) (symmetrical) Q82.8
  - acquired L85.1
- penile N48.89
- pharynx J39.2
- pilaris, acquired L85.8
- punctata (palmaris et plantaris) L85.2
- scrotal N5Ø.89
- seborrheic L82.1
  - inflamed L82.Ø
- senile L57.Ø
- solar L57.Ø
- tonsillaris J35.8
- vagina N89.4
- vegetans Q82.8
- vitamin A deficiency E5Ø.8
- vocal cord J38.3

Kerato-uveitis — *see* Iridocyclitis

Kerion (celsi) B35.Ø

Kernicterus of newborn (not due to isoimmunization) P57.9
- due to isoimmunization (conditions in P55.Ø-P55.9) P57.Ø
- specified type NEC P57.8

Kerunoparalysis T75.Ø9 ☑

Keshan disease E59

Ketoacidosis E87.2
- diabetic — *see* Diabetes, by type, with ketoacidosis

Ketonuria R82.4

Ketosis NEC E88.89
- diabetic — *see* Diabetes, by type, with with ketoacidosis

Kew Garden fever A79.1

Kidney — *see* condition

Kienböck's disease (*see also* Osteochondrosis, juvenile, hand, carpal lunate)
- adult M93.1

Kimmelstiel (-Wilson) **disease** — *see* Diabetes, Kimmelstiel (-Wilson) disease

Kink, kinking
- artery I77.1
- hair (acquired) L67.8
- ileum or intestine — *see* Obstruction, intestine
- Lane's — *see* Obstruction, intestine
- organ or site, congenital NEC — *see* Anomaly, by site
- ureter (pelvic junction) N13.5
  - with
    - hydronephrosis N13.1
      - with infection N13.6
    - pyelonephritis (chronic) N11.1
  - congenital Q62.39
- vein(s) I87.8
  - caval I87.1
  - peripheral I87.1

Kinnier Wilson's disease (hepatolenticular degeneration) E83.Ø1

Kissing spine M48.2Ø
- cervical region M48.22
- cervicothoracic region M48.23
- lumbar region M48.26
- lumbosacral region M48.27
- occipito-atlanto-axial region M48.21
- thoracic region M48.24
- thoracolumbar region M48.25

Klatskin's tumor C22.1

Klauder's disease A26.8

Klebs' disease (*see also* Glomerulonephritis) NØ5- ☑

Klebsiella (K.) **pneumoniae, as cause of disease classified elsewhere** B96.1

Klein (e)-**Levin syndrome** G47.13

Kleptomania F63.2

Klinefelter's syndrome Q98.4
- karyotype 47,XXY Q98.Ø
- male with more than two X chromosomes Q98.1

Klippel-Feil deficiency, disease, or syndrome (brevicollis) Q76.1

Klippel's disease I67.2

Klippel-Trenaunay (-Weber) **syndrome** Q87.2

Klumpke (-Déjerine) **palsy, paralysis** (birth) (newborn) P14.1

Knee — *see* condition

Knock knee (acquired) M21.Ø6- ☑
- congenital Q74.1

Knot(s)
- intestinal, syndrome (volvulus) K56.2
- surfer S89.8- ☑
- umbilical cord (true) O69.2 ☑

Knotting (of)
- hair L67.8
- intestine K56.2

Knuckle pad (Garrod's) M72.1

Koch's
- infection — *see* Tuberculosis
- relapsing fever A68.9

Koch-Weeks' conjunctivitis — *see* Conjunctivitis, acute, mucopurulent

Köebner's syndrome Q81.8

Köenig's disease (osteochondritis dissecans) — *see* Osteochondritis, dissecans

Köhler-Pellegrini-Steida disease or syndrome (calcification, knee joint) — *see* Bursitis, tibial collateral

Köhler's disease
- patellar — *see* Osteochondrosis, juvenile, patella
- tarsal navicular — *see* Osteochondrosis, juvenile, tarsus

Koilonychia L6Ø.3
- congenital Q84.6

Kojevnikov's, epilepsy — *see* Kozhevnikof's epilepsy

Koplik's spots BØ5.9

Kopp's asthma E32.8

Korsakoff's (Wernicke) **disease, psychosis or syndrome** (alcoholic) F1Ø.96
- with dependence F1Ø.26
- drug-induced
  - due to drug abuse — *see* Abuse, drug, by type, with amnestic disorder
  - due to drug dependence — *see* Dependence, drug, by type, with amnestic disorder
- nonalcoholic FØ4

Korsakov's disease, psychosis or syndrome — *see* Korsakoff's disease

Korsakow's disease, psychosis or syndrome — *see* Korsakoff's disease

Kostmann's disease or syndrome (infantile genetic agranulocytosis) — *see* Agranulocytosis

Kozhevnikof's epilepsy G4Ø.1Ø9
- intractable G4Ø.119
  - with status epilepticus G4Ø.111
  - without status epilepticus G4Ø.119
- not intractable G4Ø.1Ø9
  - with status epilepticus G4Ø.1Ø1
  - without status epilepticus G4Ø.1Ø9

Krabbe's
- disease E75.23
- syndrome, congenital muscle hypoplasia Q79.8

Kraepelin-Morel disease — *see* Schizophrenia

Kraft-Weber-Dimitri disease Q85.8

Kraurosis
- ani K62.89
- penis N48.Ø
- vagina N89.8
- vulva N9Ø.4

Kreotoxism AØ5.9

Krukenberg's
- spindle — *see* Pigmentation, cornea, posterior
- tumor C79.6- ☑

Kufs' disease E75.4

Kugelberg-Welander disease G12.1

Kuhnt-Junius degeneration (*see also* Degeneration, macula) H35.32- ☑

Kümmell's disease or spondylitis — *see* Spondylopathy, traumatic

Kupffer cell sarcoma C22.3

Kuru A81.81

Kussmaul's
- disease M3Ø.Ø
- respiration E87.2
  - in diabetic acidosis — *see* Diabetes, by type, with ketoacidosis

Kwashiorkor E4Ø
- marasmic, marasmus type E42

Kyasanur Forest disease A98.2

Kyphoscoliosis, kyphoscoliotic (acquired) (*see also* Scoliosis) M41.9
- congenital Q67.5
- heart (disease) I27.1
- sequelae of rickets E64.3
- tuberculous A18.Ø1

Kyphosis, kyphotic (acquired) M4Ø.2Ø9
- cervical region M4Ø.2Ø2
- cervicothoracic region M4Ø.2Ø3
- congenital Q76.419
  - cervical region Q76.412
  - cervicothoracic region Q76.413
  - occipito-atlanto-axial region Q76.411
  - thoracic region Q76.414
  - thoracolumbar region Q76.415
- Morquio-Brailsford type (spinal) (*see also* subcategory M49.8) E76.219
- postlaminectomy M96.3
- postradiation therapy M96.2
- postural (adolescent) M4Ø.ØØ
  - cervicothoracic region M4Ø.Ø3
  - thoracic region M4Ø.Ø4
  - thoracolumbar region M4Ø.Ø5
- secondary NEC M4Ø.1Ø
  - cervical region M4Ø.12
  - cervicothoracic region M4Ø.13
  - thoracic region M4Ø.14
  - thoracolumbar region M4Ø.15
- sequelae of rickets E64.3
- specified type NEC M4Ø.299
  - cervical region M4Ø.292

Kyphosis, kyphotic — *continued*
  specified type — *continued*
    cervicothoracic region M40.293
    thoracic region M40.294
    thoracolumbar region M40.295
  syphilitic, congenital A50.56
  thoracic region M40.204
  thoracolumbar region M40.205
  tuberculous A18.01
Kyrle disease L87.0

L

Labia, labium — *see* condition
Labile
  blood pressure R09.89
  vasomotor system I73.9
Labioglossal paralysis G12.29
Labium leporinum — *see* Cleft, lip
Labor — *see* Delivery
Labored breathing — *see* Hyperventilation
Labyrinthitis (circumscribed) (destructive) (diffuse) (inner
  ear) (latent) (purulent) (suppurative) (*see also* subcategory) H83.0 ☑
  syphilitic A52.79
Laceration
  with abortion — *see* Abortion, by type, complicated
    by laceration of pelvic organs
  abdomen, abdominal
    wall S31.119 ☑
      with
        foreign body S31.129 ☑
        penetration into peritoneal cavity S31.619 ☑
          with foreign body S31.629 ☑
      epigastric region S31.112 ☑
        with
          foreign body S31.122 ☑
          penetration into peritoneal cavity
            S31.612 ☑
              with foreign body S31.622 ☑
      left
        lower quadrant S31.114 ☑
          with
            foreign body S31.124 ☑
            penetration into peritoneal cavity
              S31.614 ☑
                with foreign body S31.624 ☑
        upper quadrant S31.111 ☑
          with
            foreign body S31.121 ☑
            penetration into peritoneal cavity
              S31.611 ☑
                with foreign body S31.621 ☑
      periumbilic region S31.115 ☑
        with
          foreign body S31.125 ☑
          penetration into peritoneal cavity
            S31.615 ☑
              with foreign body S31.625 ☑
      right
        lower quadrant S31.113 ☑
          with
            foreign body S31.123 ☑
            penetration into peritoneal cavity
              S31.613 ☑
                with foreign body S31.623 ☑
        upper quadrant S31.110 ☑
          with
            foreign body S31.120 ☑
            penetration into peritoneal cavity
              S31.610 ☑
                with foreign body S31.620 ☑
  accidental, complicating surgery — *see* Complications,
    surgical, accidental puncture or laceration
  Achilles tendon S86.02- ☑
  adrenal gland S37.813 ☑
  alveolar (process) — *see* Laceration, oral cavity
  ankle S91.01- ☑
    with
      foreign body S91.02- ☑
  antecubital space — *see* Laceration, elbow
  anus (sphincter) S31.831 ☑
    with
      ectopic or molar pregnancy O08.6
      foreign body S31.832 ☑
    complicating delivery — *see* Delivery, complicated,
      by, laceration, anus (sphincter)

Laceration — *continued*
  anus — *continued*
    following ectopic or molar pregnancy O08.6
    nontraumatic, nonpuerperal — *see* Fissure, anus
  arm (upper) S41.11- ☑
    with foreign body S41.12- ☑
    lower — *see* Laceration, forearm
  auditory canal (external) (meatus) — *see* Laceration,
    ear
  auricle, ear — *see* Laceration, ear
  axilla — *see* Laceration, arm
  back (*see also* Laceration, thorax, back)
    lower S31.010 ☑
      with
        foreign body S31.020 ☑
          with penetration into retroperitoneal
            space S31.021 ☑
        penetration into retroperitoneal space
          S31.011 ☑
  bile duct S36.13 ☑
  bladder S37.23 ☑
    with ectopic or molar pregnancy O08.6
    following ectopic or molar pregnancy O08.6
    obstetrical trauma O71.5
  blood vessel — *see* Injury, blood vessel
  bowel (*see also* Laceration, intestine)
    with ectopic or molar pregnancy O08.6
    complicating abortion — *see* Abortion, by type,
      complicated by, specified condition NEC
    following ectopic or molar pregnancy O08.6
    obstetrical trauma O71.5
  brain (any part) (cortex) (diffuse) (membrane) (*see also*
    Injury, intracranial, diffuse)
    during birth P10.8
      with hemorrhage P10.1
    focal — *see* Injury, intracranial, focal brain injury
  brainstem S06.38- ☑
  breast S21.01- ☑
    with foreign body S21.02- ☑
  broad ligament S37.893 ☑
    with ectopic or molar pregnancy O08.6
    following ectopic or molar pregnancy O08.6
    laceration syndrome N83.8
    obstetrical trauma O71.6
    syndrome (laceration) N83.8
  buttock S31.801 ☑
    with foreign body S31.802 ☑
    left S31.821 ☑
      with foreign body S31.822 ☑
    right S31.811 ☑
      with foreign body S31.812 ☑
  calf — *see* Laceration, leg
  canaliculus lacrimalis — *see* Laceration, eyelid
  canthus, eye — *see* Laceration, eyelid
  capsule, joint — *see* Sprain
  causing eversion of cervix uteri (old) N86
  central (perineal), complicating delivery O70.9
  cerebellum, traumatic S06.37- ☑
  cerebral S06.33- ☑
    during birth P10.8
      with hemorrhage P10.1
    left side S06.32- ☑
    right side S06.31- ☑
  cervix (uteri)
    with ectopic or molar pregnancy O08.6
    following ectopic or molar pregnancy O08.6
    nonpuerperal, nontraumatic N88.1
    obstetrical trauma (current) O71.3
    old (postpartal) N88.1
    traumatic S37.63 ☑
  cheek (external) S01.41- ☑
    with foreign body S01.42- ☑
    internal — *see* Laceration, oral cavity
  chest wall — *see* Laceration, thorax
  chin — *see* Laceration, head, specified site NEC
  chordae tendinae NEC I51.1
    concurrent with acute myocardial infarction — *see*
      Infarct, myocardium
    following acute myocardial infarction (current
      complication) I23.4
  clitoris — *see* Laceration, vulva
  colon — *see* Laceration, intestine, large, colon
  common bile duct S36.13 ☑
  cortex (cerebral) — *see* Injury, intracranial, diffuse
  costal region — *see* Laceration, thorax
  cystic duct S36.13 ☑
  diaphragm S27.803 ☑

Laceration — *continued*
  digit(s)
    foot — *see* Laceration, toe
    hand — *see* Laceration, finger
  duodenum S36.430 ☑
  ear (canal) (external) S01.31- ☑
    with foreign body S01.32- ☑
    drum S09.2- ☑
  elbow S51.01- ☑
    with
      foreign body S51.02- ☑
  epididymis — *see* Laceration, testis
  epigastric region — *see* Laceration, abdomen, wall,
    epigastric region
  esophagus K22.8
    traumatic
      cervical S11.21 ☑
        with foreign body S11.22 ☑
      thoracic S27.813 ☑
  eye (ball) S05.3- ☑
    with prolapse or loss of intraocular tissue S05.2- ☑
    penetrating S05.6- ☑
  eyebrow — *see* Laceration, eyelid
  eyelid S01.11- ☑
    with foreign body S01.12- ☑
  face NEC — *see* Laceration, head, specified site NEC
  fallopian tube S37.539 ☑
    bilateral S37.532 ☑
    unilateral S37.531 ☑
  finger(s) S61.219 ☑
    with
      damage to nail S61.319 ☑
        with
          foreign body S61.329 ☑
      foreign body S61.229 ☑
    index S61.218 ☑
      with
        damage to nail S61.318 ☑
          with
            foreign body S61.328 ☑
        foreign body S61.228 ☑
      left S61.211 ☑
        with
          damage to nail S61.311 ☑
            with
              foreign body S61.321 ☑
          foreign body S61.221 ☑
      right S61.210 ☑
        with
          damage to nail S61.310 ☑
            with
              foreign body S61.320 ☑
          foreign body S61.220 ☑
    little S61.218 ☑
      with
        damage to nail S61.318 ☑
          with
            foreign body S61.328 ☑
        foreign body S61.228 ☑
      left S61.217 ☑
        with
          damage to nail S61.317 ☑
            with
              foreign body S61.327 ☑
          foreign body S61.227 ☑
      right S61.216 ☑
        with
          damage to nail S61.316 ☑
            with
              foreign body S61.326 ☑
          foreign body S61.226 ☑
    middle S61.218 ☑
      with
        damage to nail S61.318 ☑
          with
            foreign body S61.328 ☑
        foreign body S61.228 ☑
      left S61.213 ☑
        with
          damage to nail S61.313 ☑
            with
              foreign body S61.323 ☑
          foreign body S61.223 ☑
      right S61.212 ☑
        with
          damage to nail S61.312 ☑

Laceration — *continued*
  finger(s) — *continued*
    middle — *continued*
      right — *continued*
        with — *continued*
          damage to nail — *continued*
            with
              foreign body S61.322 ☑
          foreign body S61.222 ☑
    ring S61.218 ☑
      with
        damage to nail S61.318 ☑
          with
            foreign body S61.328 ☑
        foreign body S61.228 ☑
      left S61.215 ☑
        with
          damage to nail S61.315 ☑
            with
              foreign body S61.325 ☑
          foreign body S61.225 ☑
      right S61.214 ☑
        with
          damage to nail S61.314 ☑
            with
              foreign body S61.324 ☑
          foreign body S61.224 ☑
  flank S31.119 ☑
    with foreign body S31.129 ☑
  foot (except toe(s) alone) S91.319 ☑
    with foreign body S91.329 ☑
    left S91.312 ☑
      with foreign body S91.322 ☑
    right S91.311 ☑
      with foreign body S91.321 ☑
    toe — *see* Laceration, toe
  forearm S51.819 ☑
    with
      foreign body S51.829 ☑
    elbow only — *see* Laceration, elbow
    left S51.812 ☑
      with
        foreign body S51.822 ☑
    right S51.811 ☑
      with
        foreign body S51.821 ☑
  forehead S01.81 ☑
    with foreign body S01.82 ☑
  fourchette O70.0
    with ectopic or molar pregnancy O08.6
    complicating delivery O70.0
    following ectopic or molar pregnancy O08.6
  gallbladder S36.123 ☑
  genital organs, external
    female S31.512 ☑
      with foreign body S31.522 ☑
      vagina — *see* Laceration, vagina
      vulva — *see* Laceration, vulva
    male S31.511 ☑
      with foreign body S31.521 ☑
      penis — *see* Laceration, penis
      scrotum — *see* Laceration, scrotum
      testis — *see* Laceration, testis
  groin — *see* Laceration, abdomen, wall
  gum — *see* Laceration, oral cavity
  hand S61.419 ☑
    with
      foreign body S61.429 ☑
    finger — *see* Laceration, finger
    left S61.412 ☑
      with
        foreign body S61.422 ☑
    right S61.411 ☑
      with
        foreign body S61.421 ☑
    thumb — *see* Laceration, thumb
  head S01.91 ☑
    with foreign body S01.92 ☑
    cheek — *see* Laceration, cheek
    ear — *see* Laceration, ear
    eyelid — *see* Laceration, eyelid
    lip — *see* Laceration, lip
    nose — *see* Laceration, nose
    oral cavity — *see* Laceration, oral cavity
    scalp S01.01 ☑
      with foreign body S01.02 ☑

Laceration — *continued*
  head — *continued*
    specified site NEC S01.81 ☑
      with foreign body S01.82 ☑
    temporomandibular area — *see* Laceration, cheek
  heart — *see* Injury, heart, laceration
  heel — *see* Laceration, foot
  hepatic duct S36.13 ☑
  hip S71.019 ☑
    with foreign body S71.029 ☑
    left S71.012 ☑
      with foreign body S71.022 ☑
    right S71.011 ☑
      with foreign body S71.021 ☑
  hymen — *see* Laceration, vagina
  hypochondrium — *see* Laceration, abdomen, wall
  hypogastric region — *see* Laceration, abdomen, wall
  ileum S36.438 ☑
  inguinal region — *see* Laceration, abdomen, wall
  instep — *see* Laceration, foot
  internal organ — *see* Injury, by site
  interscapular region — *see* Laceration, thorax, back
  intestine
    large
      colon S36.539 ☑
        ascending S36.530 ☑
        descending S36.532 ☑
        sigmoid S36.533 ☑
        specified site NEC S36.538 ☑
      rectum S36.63 ☑
        transverse S36.531 ☑
    small S36.439 ☑
      duodenum S36.430 ☑
      specified site NEC S36.438 ☑
  intra-abdominal organ S36.93 ☑
    intestine — *see* Laceration, intestine
    liver — *see* Laceration, liver
    pancreas — *see* Laceration, pancreas
    peritoneum S36.81 ☑
    specified site NEC S36.893 ☑
    spleen — *see* Laceration, spleen
    stomach — *see* Laceration, stomach
  intracranial NEC (*see also* Injury, intracranial, diffuse)
    birth injury P10.9
  jaw — *see* Laceration, head, specified site NEC
  jejunum S36.438 ☑
  joint capsule — *see* Sprain, by site
  kidney S37.03- ☑
    major (greater than 3 cm) (massive) (stellate) S37.06- ☑
    minor (less than 1 cm) S37.04- ☑
    moderate (1 to 3 cm) S37.05- ☑
    multiple S37.06- ☑
  knee S81.01- ☑
    with foreign body S81.02- ☑
  labium (majus) (minus) — *see* Laceration, vulva
  lacrimal duct — *see* Laceration, eyelid
  large intestine — *see* Laceration, intestine, large
  larynx S11.011 ☑
    with foreign body S11.012 ☑
  leg (lower) S81.819 ☑
    with foreign body S81.829 ☑
    foot — *see* Laceration, foot
    knee — *see* Laceration, knee
    left S81.812 ☑
      with foreign body S81.822 ☑
    right S81.811 ☑
      with foreign body S81.821 ☑
    upper — *see* Laceration, thigh
  ligament — *see* Sprain
  lip S01.511 ☑
    with foreign body S01.521 ☑
  liver S36.113 ☑
    major (stellate) S36.116 ☑
    minor S36.114 ☑
    moderate S36.115 ☑
  loin — *see* Laceration, abdomen, wall
  lower back — *see* Laceration, back, lower
  lumbar region — *see* Laceration, back, lower
  lung S27.339 ☑
    bilateral S27.332 ☑
    unilateral S27.331 ☑
  malar region — *see* Laceration, head, specified site NEC
  mammary — *see* Laceration, breast
  mastoid region — *see* Laceration, head, specified site NEC

Laceration — *continued*
  meninges — *see* Injury, intracranial, diffuse
  meniscus — *see* Tear, meniscus
  mesentery S36.893 ☑
  mesosalpinx S37.893 ☑
  mouth — *see* Laceration, oral cavity
  muscle — *see* Injury, muscle, by site, laceration
  nail
    finger — *see* Laceration, finger, with damage to nail
    toe — *see* Laceration, toe, with damage to nail
  nasal (septum) (sinus) — *see* Laceration, nose
  nasopharynx — *see* Laceration, head, specified site NEC
  neck S11.91 ☑
    with foreign body S11.92 ☑
    involving
      cervical esophagus S11.21 ☑
        with foreign body S11.22 ☑
      larynx — *see* Laceration, larynx
      pharynx — *see* Laceration, pharynx
      thyroid gland — *see* Laceration, thyroid gland
      trachea — *see* Laceration, trachea
    specified site NEC S11.81 ☑
      with foreign body S11.82 ☑
  nerve — *see* Injury, nerve
  nose (septum) (sinus) S01.21 ☑
    with foreign body S01.22 ☑
  ocular NOS S05.3-
    adnexa NOS S01.11- ☑
  oral cavity S01.512 ☑
    with foreign body S01.522 ☑
  orbit (eye) — *see* Wound, open, ocular, orbit
  ovary S37.439 ☑
    bilateral S37.432 ☑
    unilateral S37.431 ☑
  palate — *see* Laceration, oral cavity
  palm — *see* Laceration, hand
  pancreas S36.239 ☑
  pelvic S31.010 ☑
    with
      foreign body S31.020 ☑
        penetration into retroperitoneal cavity S31.021 ☑
      penetration into retroperitoneal cavity S31.011 ☑
    floor (*see also* Laceration, back, lower)
      with ectopic or molar pregnancy O08.6
      complicating delivery O70.1
      following ectopic or molar pregnancy O08.6
      old (postpartal) N81.89
    organ S37.93 ☑
  penis S31.21 ☑
    with foreign body S31.22 ☑
  perineum
    female S31.41 ☑
      with
        ectopic or molar pregnancy O08.6
        foreign body S31.42 ☑
      during delivery O70.9
        first degree O70.0
        fourth degree O70.3
        second degree O70.1
        third degree (*see also* Delivery, complicated, by, laceration, perineum, third degree) O70.20
      old (postpartal) N81.89
      postpartal N81.89
      secondary (postpartal) O90.1
    male S31.119 ☑
      with foreign body S31.129 ☑
  periocular area (with or without lacrimal passages) — *see* Laceration, eyelid
  peritoneum S36.893 ☑
  periumbilic region — *see* Laceration, abdomen, wall, periumbilic
  periurethral tissue — *see* Laceration, urethra
  phalanges
    finger — *see* Laceration, finger
    toe — *see* Laceration, toe
  pharynx S11.21 ☑
    with foreign body S11.22 ☑
  pinna — *see* Laceration, ear
  popliteal space — *see* Laceration, knee
  prepuce — *see* Laceration, penis
  prostate S37.823 ☑
  pubic region S31.119 ☑
    with foreign body S31.129 ☑

▼ Subterms under main terms may continue to next column or page   ☑ Additional Character Required — Refer to the Tabular List for Character Selection   207

Laceration — Laceration

Laceration — *continued*
  pudendum — *see* Laceration, genital organs, external
  rectovaginal septum — *see* Laceration, vagina
  rectum S36.63
  retroperitoneum S36.893 ☑
  round ligament S37.893 ☑
  sacral region — *see* Laceration, back, lower
  sacroiliac region — *see* Laceration, back, lower
  salivary gland — *see* Laceration, oral cavity
  scalp S01.01 ☑
    with foreign body S01.02 ☑
  scapular region — *see* Laceration, shoulder
  scrotum S31.31 ☑
    with foreign body S31.32 ☑
  seminal vesicle S37.893 ☑
  shin — *see* Laceration, leg
  shoulder S41.019 ☑
    with foreign body S41.029 ☑
    left S41.012 ☑
      with foreign body S41.022 ☑
    right S41.011 ☑
      with foreign body S41.021 ☑
  small intestine — *see* Laceration, intestine, small
  spermatic cord — *see* Laceration, testis
  spinal cord (meninges) (*see also* Injury, spinal cord, by region)
    due to injury at birth P11.5
    newborn (birth injury) P11.5
  spleen S36.039 ☑
    major (massive) (stellate) S36.032 ☑
    moderate S36.031 ☑
    superficial (minor) S36.030 ☑
  sternal region — *see* Laceration, thorax, front
  stomach S36.33 ☑
  submaxillary region — *see* Laceration, head, specified site NEC
  submental region — *see* Laceration, head, specified site NEC
  subungual
    finger(s) — *see* Laceration, finger, with damage to nail
    toe(s) — *see* Laceration, toe, with damage to nail
  suprarenal gland — *see* Laceration, adrenal gland
  temple, temporal region — *see* Laceration, head, specified site NEC
  temporomandibular area — *see* Laceration, cheek
  tendon — *see* Injury, muscle, by site, laceration
    Achilles S86.02- ☑
  tentorium cerebelli — *see* Injury, intracranial, diffuse
  testis S31.31 ☑
    with foreign body S31.32 ☑
  thigh S71.11- ☑
    with foreign body S71.12- ☑
  thorax, thoracic (wall) S21.91 ☑
    with foreign body S21.92 ☑
      back S21.22-
        with penetration into thoracic cavity S21.42- ☑
      front S21.12- ☑
        with penetration into thoracic cavity S21.32- ☑
    back S21.21- ☑
      with
        foreign body S21.22-
          with penetration into thoracic cavity S21.42- ☑
        penetration into thoracic cavity S21.41- ☑
    breast — *see* Laceration, breast
    front S21.11- ☑
      with
        foreign body S21.12- ☑
          with penetration into thoracic cavity S21.32- ☑
        penetration into thoracic cavity S21.31- ☑
  thumb S61.019 ☑
    with
      damage to nail S61.119 ☑
        with
          foreign body S61.129 ☑
      foreign body S61.029 ☑
    left S61.012 ☑
      with
        damage to nail S61.112 ☑
          with
            foreign body S61.122 ☑
        foreign body S61.022 ☑

Laceration — *continued*
  thumb — *continued*
    right S61.011 ☑
      with
        damage to nail S61.111 ☑
          with
            foreign body S61.121 ☑
        foreign body S61.021 ☑
  thyroid gland S11.11 ☑
    with foreign body S11.12 ☑
  toe(s) S91.119 ☑
    with
      damage to nail S91.219 ☑
        with
          foreign body S91.229 ☑
      foreign body S91.129 ☑
    great S91.113 ☑
      with
        damage to nail S91.213 ☑
          with
            foreign body S91.223 ☑
        foreign body S91.123 ☑
      left S91.112 ☑
        with
          damage to nail S91.212 ☑
            with
              foreign body S91.222 ☑
          foreign body S91.122 ☑
      right S91.111 ☑
        with
          damage to nail S91.211 ☑
            with
              foreign body S91.221 ☑
          foreign body S91.121 ☑
    lesser S91.116 ☑
      with
        damage to nail S91.216 ☑
          with
            foreign body S91.226 ☑
        foreign body S91.126 ☑
      left S91.115 ☑
        with
          damage to nail S91.215 ☑
            with
              foreign body S91.225 ☑
          foreign body S91.125 ☑
      right S91.114 ☑
        with
          damage to nail S91.214 ☑
            with
              foreign body S91.224 ☑
          foreign body S91.124 ☑
  tongue — *see* Laceration, oral cavity
  trachea S11.021 ☑
    with foreign body S11.022 ☑
  tunica vaginalis — *see* Laceration, testis
  tympanum, tympanic membrane — *see* Laceration, ear, drum
  umbilical region S31.115 ☑
    with foreign body S31.125 ☑
  ureter S37.13 ☑
  urethra S37.33 ☑
    with or following ectopic or molar pregnancy O08.6
    obstetrical trauma O71.5
  urinary organ NEC S37.893 ☑
  uterus S37.63 ☑
    with ectopic or molar pregnancy O08.6
    following ectopic or molar pregnancy O08.6
    nonpuerperal, nontraumatic N85.8
    obstetrical trauma NEC O71.81
    old (postpartal) N85.8
  uvula — *see* Laceration, oral cavity
  vagina S31.41 ☑
    with
      ectopic or molar pregnancy O08.6
      foreign body S31.42 ☑
    during delivery O71.4
      with perineal laceration — *see* Laceration, perineum, female, during delivery
    following ectopic or molar pregnancy O08.6
    nonpuerperal, nontraumatic N89.8
    old (postpartal) N89.8
  vas deferens S37.893 ☑
  vesical — *see* Laceration, bladder
  vocal cords S11.031 ☑
    with foreign body S11.032 ☑
  vulva S31.41 ☑

Laceration — *continued*
  vulva — *continued*
    with
      ectopic or molar pregnancy O08.6
      foreign body S31.42 ☑
    complicating delivery O70.0
    following ectopic or molar pregnancy O08.6
    nonpuerperal, nontraumatic N90.89
    old (postpartal) N90.89
  wrist S61.519 ☑
    with
      foreign body S61.529 ☑
    left S61.512 ☑
      with
        foreign body S61.522 ☑
    right S61.511 ☑
      with
        foreign body S61.521 ☑

Lack of
  achievement in school Z55.3
  adequate
    food Z59.4
    intermaxillary vertical dimension of fully erupted teeth M26.36
    sleep Z72.820
  appetite (*see* Anorexia) R63.0
  awareness R41.9
  care
    in home Z74.2
    of infant (at or after birth) T76.02 ☑
      confirmed T74.02 ☑
  cognitive functions R41.9
  coordination R27.9
    ataxia R27.0
    specified type NEC R27.8
  development (physiological) R62.50
    failure to thrive (child over 28 days old) R62.51
      adult R62.7
      newborn P92.6
    short stature R62.52
    specified type NEC R62.59
  energy R53.83
  financial resources Z59.6
  food T73.0 ☑
  growth R62.52
  heating Z59.1
  housing (permanent) (temporary) Z59.0
    adequate Z59.1
  learning experiences in childhood Z62.898
  leisure time (affecting life-style) Z73.2
  material resources Z59.9
  memory (*see also* Amnesia)
    mild, following organic brain damage F06.8
  ovulation N97.0
  parental supervision or control of child Z62.0
  person able to render necessary care Z74.2
  physical exercise Z72.3
  play experience in childhood Z62.898
  posterior occlusal support M26.57
  relaxation (affecting life-style) Z73.2
  sexual
    desire F52.0
    enjoyment F52.1
  shelter Z59.0
  sleep (adequate) Z72.820
  supervision of child by parent Z62.0
  support, posterior occlusal M26.57
  water T73.1 ☑
Lacrimal — *see* condition
Lacrimation, abnormal — *see* Epiphora
Lacrimonasal duct — *see* condition
Lactation, lactating (breast) (puerperal, postpartum)
  associated
    cracked nipple O92.13
    retracted nipple O92.03
  defective O92.4
  disorder NEC O92.79
  excessive O92.6
  failed (complete) O92.3
    partial O92.4
  mastitis NEC — *see* Mastitis, obstetric
  mother (care and/or examination) Z39.1
  nonpuerperal N64.3
Lacticemia, excessive E87.2
Lacunar skull Q75.8
Laennec's cirrhosis K70.30
  with ascites K70.31
  nonalcoholic K74.69

☑ Additional Character Required — Refer to the Tabular List for Character Selection   Subterms under main terms may continue to next column or page

Lafora's disease — see Epilepsy, generalized, idiopathic
Lag, lid (nervous) — see Retraction, lid
Lagophthalmos (eyelid) (nervous) H02.209
  bilateral, upper and lower eyelids H02.20C
  cicatricial H02.219
    bilateral, upper and lower eyelids H02.21C
    left H02.216
      lower H02.215
      upper H02.214
      upper and lower eyelids H02.21B
    right H02.213
      lower H02.212
      upper H02.211
      upper and lower eyelids H02.21A
  keratoconjunctivitis — see Keratoconjunctivitis
  left H02.206
    lower H02.205
    upper H02.204
    upper and lower eyelids H02.20B
  mechanical H02.229
    bilateral, upper and lower eyelids H02.22C
    left H02.226
      lower H02.225
      upper H02.224
      upper and lower eyelids H02.22B
    right H02.223
      lower H02.222
      upper H02.221
      upper and lower eyelids H02.22A
  paralytic H02.239
    bilateral, upper and lower eyelids H02.23C
    left H02.236
      lower H02.235
      upper H02.234
      upper and lower eyelids H02.23B
    right H02.233
      lower H02.232
      upper H02.231
      upper and lower eyelids H02.23A
  right H02.203
    lower H02.202
    upper H02.201
    upper and lower eyelids H02.20A
Laki-Lorand factor deficiency — see Defect, coagulation, specified type NEC
Lalling F80.0
Lambert-Eaton syndrome — see Syndrome, Lambert-Eaton
Lambliasis, lambliosis A07.1
Landau-Kleffner syndrome — see Epilepsy, specified NEC
Landouzy-Déjérine dystrophy or facioscapulohumeral atrophy G71.02
Landouzy's disease (icterohemorrhagic leptospirosis) A27.0
Landry-Guillain-Barré, syndrome or paralysis G61.0
Landry's disease or paralysis G61.0
Lane's
  band Q43.3
  kink — see Obstruction, intestine
  syndrome K90.2
Langdon Down syndrome — see Trisomy, 21
Lapsed immunization schedule status Z28.3
Large
  baby (regardless of gestational age) (4000g to 4499g) P08.1
  ear, congenital Q17.1
  physiological cup Q14.2
  stature R68.89
Large-for-dates NEC (infant) (4000g to 4499g) P08.1
  affecting management of pregnancy O36.6- ☑
  exceptionally (4500g or more) P08.0
Larsen-Johansson disease or osteochondrosis — see Osteochondrosis, juvenile, patella
Larsen's syndrome (flattened facies and multiple congenital dislocations) Q74.8
Larva migrans
  cutaneous B76.9
    Ancylostoma B76.0
  visceral B83.0
Laryngeal — see condition
Laryngismus (stridulus) J38.5
  congenital P28.89
  diphtheritic A36.2
Laryngitis (acute) (edematous) (fibrinous) (infective) (infiltrative) (malignant) (membranous) (phlegmonous) (pneumococcal) (pseudomembranous) (septic) (subglottic) (suppurative) (ulcerative) J04.0

Laryngitis — continued
  with
    influenza, flu, or grippe — see Influenza, with, laryngitis
    tracheitis (acute) — see Laryngotracheitis
  atrophic J37.0
  catarrhal J37.0
  chronic J37.0
    with tracheitis (chronic) J37.1
  diphtheritic A36.2
  due to external agent — see Inflammation, respiratory, upper, due to
  H. influenzae J04.0
  Hemophilus influenzae J04.0
  hypertrophic J37.0
  influenzal — see Influenza, with, respiratory manifestations NEC
  obstructive J05.0
  sicca J37.0
  spasmodic J05.0
    acute J04.0
  streptococcal J04.0
  stridulous J05.0
  syphilitic (late) A52.73
    congenital A50.59 [J99]
      early A50.03 [J99]
  tuberculous A15.5
  Vincent's A69.1
Laryngocele (congenital) (ventricular) Q31.3
Laryngofissure J38.7
  congenital Q31.8
Laryngomalacia (congenital) Q31.5
Laryngopharyngitis (acute) J06.0
  chronic J37.0
  due to external agent — see Inflammation, respiratory, upper, due to
Laryngoplegia J38.00
  bilateral J38.02
  unilateral J38.01
Laryngoptosis J38.7
Laryngospasm J38.5
Laryngostenosis J38.6
Laryngotracheitis (acute) (Infectional) (infective) (viral) J04.2
  atrophic J37.1
  catarrhal J37.1
  chronic J37.1
  diphtheritic A36.2
  due to external agent — see Inflammation, respiratory, upper, due to
  Hemophilus influenzae J04.2
  hypertrophic J37.1
  influenzal — see Influenza, with, respiratory manifestations NEC
  pachydermic J38.7
  sicca J37.1
  spasmodic J38.5
    acute J05.0
  streptococcal J04.2
  stridulous J38.5
  syphilitic (late) A52.73
    congenital A50.59 [J99]
      early A50.03 [J99]
  tuberculous A15.5
  Vincent's A69.1
Laryngotracheobronchitis — see Bronchitis
Larynx, laryngeal — see condition
Lassa fever A96.2
Lassitude — see Weakness
Late
  talker R62.0
  walker R62.0
Late effect(s) — see Sequelae
Latent — see condition
Laterocession — see Lateroversion
Lateroflexion — see Lateroversion
Lateroversion
  cervix — see Lateroversion, uterus
  uterus, uterine (cervix) (postinfectional) (postpartal, old) N85.4
    congenital Q51.818
    in pregnancy or childbirth O34.59- ☑
Lathyrism — see Poisoning, food, noxious, plant
Launois' syndrome (pituitary gigantism) E22.0
Launois-Bensaude adenolipomatosis E88.89
Laurence-Moon (-Bardet)-**Biedl syndrome** Q87.89
Lax, laxity (see also Relaxation)
  ligament (ous) (see also Disorder, ligament)

Lax, laxity — continued
  ligament (see also Disorder, ligament) — continued
    familial M35.7
    knee — see Derangement, knee
  skin (acquired) L57.4
    congenital Q82.8
Laxative habit F55.2
Lazy leukocyte syndrome D70.8
Lead miner's lung J63.6
Leak, leakage
  air NEC J93.82
    postprocedural J95.812
  amniotic fluid — see Rupture, membranes, premature
  blood (microscopic), fetal, into maternal circulation affecting management of pregnancy — see Pregnancy, complicated by
  cerebrospinal fluid G96.0
    from spinal (lumbar) puncture G97.0
  device, implant or graft (see also Complications, by site and type, mechanical)
    arterial graft NEC — see Complication, cardiovascular device, mechanical, vascular
    breast (implant) T85.43 ☑
    catheter NEC T85.638 ☑
      dialysis (renal) T82.43 ☑
        intraperitoneal T85.631 ☑
      infusion NEC T82.534 ☑
        spinal (epidural) (subdural) T85.630 ☑
      urinary T83.038 ☑
        cystostomy T83.030 ☑
        Hopkins T83.038 ☑
        ileostomy T83.038 ☑
        indwelling T83.031 ☑
        nephrostomy T83.032 ☑
        specified T83.038 ☑
        urostomy T83.038 ☑
    gastrointestinal — see Complications, prosthetic device, mechanical, gastrointestinal device
    genital NEC T83.498 ☑
      penile prosthesis (cylinder) (implanted) (pump) (reservoir) T83.490 ☑
      testicular prosthesis T83.491 ☑
    heart NEC — see Complication, cardiovascular device, mechanical
    joint prosthesis — see Complications, joint prosthesis, mechanical, specified NEC, by site
    ocular NEC — see Complications, prosthetic device, mechanical, ocular device
    orthopedic NEC — see Complication, orthopedic, device, mechanical
    persistent air J93.82
    specified NEC T85.638 ☑
    urinary NEC (see also Complication, genitourinary, device, urinary, mechanical)
      graft T83.23 ☑
    vascular NEC — see Complication, cardiovascular device, mechanical
    ventricular intracranial shunt T85.03 ☑
  urine — see Incontinence
Leaky heart — see Endocarditis
Learning defect (specific) F81.9
Leather bottle stomach C16.9
Leber's
  congenital amaurosis H35.50
  optic atrophy (hereditary) H47.22
Lederer's anemia D59.1
Leeches (external) — see Hirudiniasis
Leg — see condition
Legg (-Calvé)-**Perthes disease, syndrome or osteochondrosis** M91.1- ☑
Legionellosis A48.1
  nonpneumonic A48.2
Legionnaires'
  disease A48.1
    nonpneumonic A48.2
  pneumonia A48.1
Leigh's disease G31.82
Leiner's disease L21.1
Leiofibromyoma — see Leiomyoma
Leiomyoblastoma — see Neoplasm, connective tissue, benign
Leiomyofibroma (see also Neoplasm, connective tissue, benign)
  uterus (cervix) (corpus) D25.9
Leiomyoma (see also Neoplasm, connective tissue, benign)

Leiomyoma — *continued*
  bizarre — *see* Neoplasm, connective tissue, benign
  cellular — *see* Neoplasm, connective tissue, benign
  epithelioid — *see* Neoplasm, connective tissue, benign
  uterus (cervix) (corpus) D25.9
    intramural D25.1
    submucous D25.0
    subserosal D25.2
  vascular — *see* Neoplasm, connective tissue, benign
Leiomyoma, leiomyomatosis (intravascular) — *see* Neoplasm, connective tissue, uncertain behavior
Leiomyosarcoma (*see also* Neoplasm, connective tissue, malignant)
  epithelioid — *see* Neoplasm, connective tissue, malignant
  myxoid — *see* Neoplasm, connective tissue, malignant
Leishmaniasis B55.9
  American (mucocutaneous) B55.2
    cutaneous B55.1
  Asian Desert B55.1
  Brazilian B55.2
  cutaneous (any type) B55.1
  dermal (*see also* Leishmaniasis, cutaneous)
    post-kala-azar B55.0
  eyelid B55.1
  infantile B55.0
  Mediterranean B55.0
  mucocutaneous (American) (New World) B55.2
  naso-oral B55.2
  nasopharyngeal B55.2
  old world B55.1
  tegumentaria diffusa B55.1
  visceral B55.0
Leishmanoid, dermal (*see also* Leishmaniasis, cutaneous)
  post-kala-azar B55.0
Lenegre's disease I44.2
Lengthening, leg — *see* Deformity, limb, unequal length
Lennert's lymphoma — *see* Lymphoma, Lennert's
Lennox-Gastaut syndrome G40.812
  intractable G40.814
    with status epilepticus G40.813
    without status epilepticus G40.814
  not intractable G40.812
    with status epilepticus G40.811
    without status epilepticus G40.812
Lens — *see* condition
Lenticonus (anterior) (posterior) (congenital) Q12.8
Lenticular degeneration, progressive E83.01
Lentiglobus (posterior) (congenital) Q12.8
Lentigo (congenital) L81.4
  maligna (*see also* Melanoma, in situ)
    melanoma — *see* Melanoma
Lentivirus, as cause of disease classified elsewhere B97.31
Leontiasis
  ossium M85.2
  syphilitic (late) A52.78
    congenital A50.59
Lepothrix A48.8
Lepra — *see* Leprosy
Leprechaunism E34.8
Leprosy A30.- ☑
  with muscle disorder A30.9 [M63.80]
    ankle A30.9 [M63.87-] ☑
    foot A30.9 [M63.87-] ☑
    forearm A30.9 [M63.83-] ☑
    hand A30.9 [M63.84-] ☑
    lower leg A30.9 [M63.86-] ☑
    multiple sites A30.9 [M63.89]
    pelvic region A30.9 [M63.85-] ☑
    shoulder region A30.9 [M63.81-] ☑
    specified site NEC A30.9 [M63.88]
    thigh A30.9 [M63.85-] ☑
    upper arm A30.9 [M63.82-] ☑
  anesthetic A30.9
  BB A30.3
  BL A30.4
  borderline (infiltrated) (neuritic) A30.3
    lepromatous A30.4
    tuberculoid A30.2
  BT A30.2
  dimorphous (infiltrated) (neuritic) A30.3
  I A30.0
  indeterminate (macular) (neuritic) A30.0
  lepromatous (diffuse) (infiltrated) (macular) (neuritic) (nodular) A30.5

Leprosy — *continued*
  LL A30.5
  macular (early) (neuritic) (simple) A30.9
  maculoanesthetic A30.9
  mixed A30.3
  neural A30.9
  nodular A30.5
  primary neuritic A30.3
  specified type NEC A30.8
  TT A30.1
  tuberculoid (major) (minor) A30.1
Leptocytosis, hereditary D56.9
Leptomeningitis (chronic) (circumscribed) (hemorrhagic) (nonsuppurative) — *see* Meningitis
Leptomeningopathy G96.19
Leptospiral — *see* condition
Leptospirochetal — *see* condition
Leptospirosis A27.9
  canicola A27.89
  due to Leptospira interrogans serovar icterohaemorrhagiae A27.0
  icterohemorrhagica A27.0
  pomona A27.89
  Weil's disease A27.0
Leptus dermatitis B88.0
Leriche's syndrome (aortic bifurcation occlusion) I74.09
Leri's pleonosteosis Q78.8
Leri-Weill syndrome Q77.8
Lermoyez' syndrome — *see* Vertigo, peripheral NEC
Lesch-Nyhan syndrome E79.1
Leser-Trélat disease L82.1
  inflamed L82.0
Lesion(s) (nontraumatic)
  abducens nerve — *see* Strabismus, paralytic, sixth nerve
  alveolar process K08.9
  angiocentric immunoproliferative D47.Z9 (*following* D47.4)
  anorectal K62.9
  aortic (valve) I35.9
  auditory nerve — *see* subcategory H93.3 ☑
  basal ganglion G25.9
  bile duct — *see* Disease, bile duct
  biomechanical M99.9
    specified type NEC M99.89
      abdomen M99.89
      acromioclavicular M99.87
      cervical region M99.81
      cervicothoracic M99.81
      costochondral M99.88
      costovertebral M99.88
      head region M99.80
      hip M99.85
      lower extremity M99.86
      lumbar region M99.83
      lumbosacral M99.83
      occipitocervical M99.80
      pelvic region M99.85
      pubic M99.85
      rib cage M99.88
      sacral region M99.84
      sacrococcygeal M99.84
      sacroiliac M99.84
      specified NEC M99.89
      sternochondral M99.88
      sternoclavicular M99.87
      thoracic region M99.82
      thoracolumbar M99.82
      upper extremity M99.87
  bladder N32.9
  bone — *see* Disorder, bone
  brachial plexus G54.0
  brain G93.9
    congenital Q04.9
    vascular I67.9
      degenerative I67.9
      hypertensive I67.4
  buccal cavity K13.79
  calcified — *see* Calcification
  canthus — *see* Disorder, eyelid
  carate — *see* Pinta, lesions
  cardia K31.9
  cardiac (*see also* Disease, heart) I51.9
    congenital Q24.9
    valvular — *see* Endocarditis
  cauda equina G83.4
  cecum K63.9
  cerebral — *see* Lesion, brain
  cerebrovascular I67.9

Lesion(s) — *continued*
  cerebrovascular — *continued*
    degenerative I67.9
    hypertensive I67.4
  cervical (nerve) root NEC G54.2
  chiasmal — *see* Disorder, optic, chiasm
  chorda tympani G51.8
  coin, lung R91.1
  colon K63.9
  combined periodontic - endodontic K05.5
  congenital — *see* Anomaly, by site
  conjunctiva H11.9
  conus medullaris — *see* Injury, conus medullaris
  coronary artery — *see* Ischemia, heart
  cranial nerve G52.9
    eighth — *see* Disorder, ear
    eleventh G52.9
    fifth G50.9
    first G52.0
    fourth — *see* Strabismus, paralytic, fourth nerve
    seventh G51.9
    sixth — *see* Strabismus, paralytic, sixth nerve
    tenth G52.2
    twelfth G52.3
  cystic — *see* Cyst
  degenerative — *see* Degeneration
  duodenum K31.9
  edentulous (alveolar) ridge, associated with trauma, due to traumatic occlusion K06.2
  en coup de sabre L94.1
  eyelid — *see* Disorder, eyelid
  gasserian ganglion G50.8
  gastric K31.9
  gastroduodenal K31.9
  gastrointestinal K63.9
  gingiva, associated with trauma K06.2
  glomerular
    focal and segmental (*see also* N00-N07 with fourth character .1) N05.1
    minimal change (*see also* N00-N07 with fourth character .0) N05.0
  heart (organic) — *see* Disease, heart
  hyperchromic, due to pinta (carate) A67.1
  hyperkeratotic — *see* Hyperkeratosis
  hypothalamic E23.7
  ileocecal K63.9
  ileum K63.9
  iliohypogastric nerve G57.8- ☑
  inflammatory — *see* Inflammation
  intestine K63.9
  intracerebral — *see* Lesion, brain
  intrachiasmal (optic) — *see* Disorder, optic, chiasm
  intracranial, space-occupying R90.0
  joint — *see* Disorder, joint
    sacroiliac (old) M53.3
  keratotic — *see* Keratosis
  kidney — *see* Disease, renal
  laryngeal nerve (recurrent) G52.2
  lip K13.0
  liver K76.9
  lumbosacral
    plexus G54.1
    root (nerve) NEC G54.4
  lung (coin) R91.1
  maxillary sinus J32.0
  mitral I05.9
  Morel-Lavallée — *see* Hematoma, by site
  motor cortex NEC G93.89
  mouth K13.79
  nerve G58.9
    femoral G57.2- ☑
    median G56.1- ☑
      carpal tunnel syndrome — *see* Syndrome, carpal tunnel
    plantar G57.6- ☑
    popliteal (lateral) G57.3- ☑
      medial G57.4- ☑
    radial G56.3- ☑
    sciatic G57.0- ☑
    spinal — *see* Injury, nerve, spinal
    ulnar G56.2- ☑
  nervous system, congenital Q07.9
  nonallopathic — *see* Lesion, biomechanical
  nose (internal) J34.89
  obstructive — *see* Obstruction
  obturator nerve G57.8- ☑
  oral mucosa K13.70

☑ **Additional Character Required** — Refer to the Tabular List for Character Selection   ▽ Subterms under main terms may continue to next column or page

Lesion(s) — *continued*
- organ or site NEC — *see* Disease, by site
- osteolytic — *see* Osteolysis
- peptic K27.9
- periodontal, due to traumatic occlusion K05.5
- pharynx J39.2
- pigment, pigmented (skin) L81.9
- pinta — *see* Pinta, lesions
- polypoid — *see* Polyp
- prechiasmal (optic) — *see* Disorder, optic, chiasm
- primary (*see also* Syphilis, primary) A51.0
  - carate A67.0
  - pinta A67.0
  - yaws A66.0
- pulmonary J98.4
  - valve I37.9
- pylorus K31.9
- rectosigmoid K63.9
- retina, retinal H35.9
- sacroiliac (joint) (old) M53.3
- salivary gland K11.9
  - benign lymphoepithelial K11.8
- saphenous nerve G57.8- ☑
- sciatic nerve G57.0- ☑
- secondary — *see* Syphilis, secondary
- shoulder (region) M75.9- ☑
  - specified NEC M75.8- ☑
- sigmoid K63.9
- sinus (accessory) (nasal) J34.89
- skin L98.9
  - suppurative L08.0
- SLAP S43.43- ☑
- spinal cord G95.9
  - congenital Q06.9
- spleen D73.89
- stomach K31.9
- superior glenoid labrum S43.43- ☑
- syphilitic — *see* Syphilis
- tertiary — *see* Syphilis, tertiary
- thoracic root (nerve) NEC G54.3
- tonsillar fossa J35.9
- tooth, teeth K08.9
  - white spot
    - chewing surface K02.51
    - pit and fissure surface K02.51
    - smooth surface K02.61
- traumatic — *see* specific type of injury by site
- tricuspid (valve) I07.9
  - nonrheumatic I36.9
- trigeminal nerve G50.9
- ulcerated or ulcerative — *see* Ulcer, skin
- uterus N85.9
- vagina N89.8
- vagus nerve G52.2
- valvular — *see* Endocarditis
- vascular I99.9
  - affecting central nervous system I67.9
  - following trauma NEC T14.8 ☑
  - umbilical cord, complicating delivery O69.5 ☑
- vulva N90.89
- warty — *see* Verruca
- white spot (tooth)
  - chewing surface K02.51
  - pit and fissure surface K02.51
  - smooth surface K02.61

Lethargic — *see* condition
Lethargy R53.83
Letterer-Siwe's disease C96.0
Leukemia, leukemic C95.9- ☑
- acute basophilic C94.8- ☑
- acute bilineal C95.0- ☑
- acute erythroid C94.0- ☑
- acute lymphoblastic C91.0- ☑
- acute megakaryoblastic C94.2- ☑
- acute megakaryocytic C94.2- ☑
- acute mixed lineage C95.0- ☑
- acute monoblastic (monoblastic/monocytic) C93.0- ☑
- acute monocytic (monoblastic/monocytic) C93.0- ☑
- acute myeloblastic (minimal differentiation) (with maturation) C92.0- ☑
- acute myeloid, NOS C92.0- ☑
  - with
    - 11q23-abnormality C92.6- ☑
    - dysplasia of remaining hematopoesis and/or myelodysplastic disease in its history C92.A- ☑ (*following* C92.6)

Leukemia, leukemic — *continued*
- acute myeloid, — *continued*
  - with — *continued*
    - multilineage dysplasia C92.A- ☑ (*following* C92.6)
    - variation of MLL-gene C92.6- ☑
  - M6 (a)(b) C94.0- ☑
  - M7 C94.2- ☑
- acute myelomonocytic C92.5- ☑
- acute promyelocytic C92.4- ☑
- adult T-cell (HTLV-1-associated) (acute variant) (chronic variant) (lymphomatoid variant) (smouldering variant) C91.5- ☑
- aggressive NK-cell C94.8- ☑
- AML (1/ETO) (M0) (M1) (M2) (without a FAB classification) C92.0- ☑
- AML M3 C92.4- ☑
- AML M4 (Eo with inv(16) or t(16;16)) C92.5- ☑
- AML M5 C93.0- ☑
- AML M5a C93.0- ☑
- AML M5b C93.0- ☑
- AML Me with t (15;17) and variants C92.4- ☑
- atypical chronic myeloid, BCR/ABL-negative C92.2- ☑
- biphenotypic acute C95.0- ☑
- blast cell C95.0- ☑
- Burkitt-type, mature B-cell C91.A- ☑ (*following* C91.6)
- chronic lymphocytic, of B-cell type C91.1- ☑
- chronic monocytic C93.1- ☑
- chronic myelogenous (Philadelphia chromosome (Ph1) positive) (t(9;22)) (q34;q11) (with crisis of blast cells) C92.1- ☑
- chronic myeloid, BCR/ABL-positive C92.1- ☑
  - atypical, BCR/ABL-negative C92.2- ☑
- chronic myelomonocytic C93.1- ☑
- chronic neutrophilic D47.1
- CMML (-1) (-2) (with eosinophilia) C93.1- ☑
- granulocytic (*see also* Category C92) C92.9- ☑
- hairy cell C91.4- ☑
- juvenile myelomonocytic C93.3- ☑
- lymphoid C91.9- ☑
  - specified NEC C91.Z- ☑ (*following* C91.6)
- mast cell C94.3- ☑
- mature B-cell, Burkitt-type C91.A- ☑ (*following* C91.6)
- monocytic (subacute) C93.9- ☑
  - specified NEC C93.Z- ☑ (*following* C93.3)
- myelogenous (*see also* Category C92) C92.9- ☑
- myeloid C92.9- ☑
  - specified NEC C92.Z- ☑ (*following* C92.6)
- plasma cell C90.1- ☑
- plasmacytic C90.1- ☑
- prolymphocytic
  - of B-cell type C91.3- ☑
  - of T-cell type C91.6- ☑
- specified NEC C94.8- ☑
- stem cell, of unclear lineage C95.0- ☑
- subacute lymphocytic C91.9- ☑
- T-cell large granular lymphocytic C91.Z- ☑ (*following* C91.6)
- unspecified cell type C95.9- ☑
  - acute C95.0- ☑
  - chronic C95.1- ☑

Leukemoid reaction (*see also* Reaction, leukemoid) D72.823
Leukoaraiosis (hypertensive) I67.81
Leukoariosis — *see* Leukoaraiosis
Leukocoria — *see* Disorder, globe, degenerated condition, leucocoria
Leukocytopenia D72.819
Leukocytosis D72.829
- eosinophilic D72.1
Leukoderma, leukodermia NEC L81.5
- syphilitic A51.39
  - late A52.79
Leukodystrophy E75.29
Leukoedema, oral epithelium K13.29
Leukoencephalitis G04.81
- acute (subacute) hemorrhagic G36.1
  - postimmunization or postvaccinal G04.02
- postinfectious G04.01
- subacute sclerosing A81.1
- van Bogaert's (sclerosing) A81.1
Leukoencephalopathy (*see also* Encephalopathy) G93.49
- Binswanger's I67.3
- heroin vapor G92
- metachromatic E75.25
- multifocal (progressive) A81.2

Leukoencephalopathy — *continued*
- postimmunization and postvaccinal G04.02
- progressive multifocal A81.2
- reversible, posterior G93.6
- van Bogaert's (sclerosing) A81.1
- vascular, progressive I67.3
Leukoerythroblastosis D75.9
Leukokeratosis (*see also* Leukoplakia)
- mouth K13.21
- nicotina palati K13.24
- oral mucosa K13.21
- tongue K13.21
- vocal cord J38.3
Leukokraurosis vulva (e) N90.4
Leukoma (cornea) (*see also* Opacity, cornea)
- adherent H17.0- ☑
- interfering with central vision — *see* Opacity, cornea, central
Leukomalacia, cerebral, newborn P91.2
- periventricular P91.2
Leukomelanopathy, hereditary D72.0
Leukonychia (punctata) (striata) L60.8
- congenital Q84.4
Leukopathia unguium L60.8
- congenital Q84.4
Leukopenia D72.819
- basophilic D72.818
- chemotherapy (cancer) induced D70.1
- congenital D70.0
- cyclic D70.0
- drug induced NEC D70.2
  - due to cytoreductive cancer chemotherapy D70.1
- eosinophilic D72.818
- familial D70.0
- infantile genetic D70.0
- malignant D70.9
- periodic D70.0
- transitory neonatal P61.5
Leukopenic — *see* condition
Leukoplakia
- anus K62.89
- bladder (postinfectional) N32.89
- buccal K13.21
- cervix (uteri) N88.0
- esophagus K22.8
- gingiva K13.21
- hairy (oral mucosa) (tongue) K13.3
- kidney (pelvis) N28.89
- larynx J38.7
- lip K13.21
- mouth K13.21
- oral epithelium, including tongue (mucosa) K13.21
- palate K13.21
- pelvis (kidney) N28.89
- penis (infectional) N48.0
- rectum K62.89
- syphilitic (late) A52.79
- tongue K13.21
- ureter (postinfectional) N28.89
- urethra (postinfectional) N36.8
- uterus N85.8
- vagina N89.4
- vocal cord J38.3
- vulva N90.4
Leukorrhea N89.8
- due to Trichomonas (vaginalis) A59.00
- trichomonal A59.00
Leukosarcoma C85.9- ☑
Levocardia (isolated) Q24.1
- with situs inversus Q89.3
Levotransposition Q20.5
Lev's disease or syndrome (acquired complete heart block) I44.2
Levulosuria — *see* Fructosuria
Levurid L30.2
Lewy body (ies) (dementia) (disease) G31.83
Leyden-Moebius dystrophy G71.09
Leydig cell
- carcinoma
  - specified site — *see* Neoplasm, malignant, by site
  - unspecified site
    - female C56.9
    - male C62.9- ☑
- tumor
  - benign
    - specified site — *see* Neoplasm, benign, by site
    - unspecified site
      - female D27.- ☑

Leydig cell — *continued*
　tumor — *continued*
　　benign — *continued*
　　　unspecified site — *continued*
　　　　male D29.2- ☑
　　　malignant
　　　　specified site — *see* Neoplasm, malignant, by
　　　　　site
　　　　unspecified site
　　　　　female C56.- ☑
　　　　　male C62.9- ☑
　　　specified site — *see* Neoplasm, uncertain behavior,
　　　　by site
　　　unspecified site
　　　　female D39.1- ☑
　　　　male D40.1- ☑
Leydig-Sertoli cell tumor
　specified site — *see* Neoplasm, benign, by site
　unspecified site
　　female D27.- ☑
　　male D29.2- ☑
LGSIL (Low grade squamous intraepithelial lesion on cy-
　tologic smear of)
　anus R85.612
　cervix R87.612
　vagina R87.622
Liar, pathologic F60.2
Libido
　decreased R68.82
Libman-Sacks disease M32.11
Lice (infestation) B85.2
　body (Pediculus corporis) B85.1
　crab B85.3
　head (Pediculus capitis) B85.0
　mixed (classifiable to more than one of the titles B85.0-
　　B85.3) B85.4
　pubic (Phthirus pubis) B85.3
Lichen L28.0
　albus L90.0
　　penis N48.0
　　vulva N90.4
　amyloidosis E85.4 [L99]
　atrophicus L90.0
　　penis N48.0
　　vulva N90.4
　congenital Q82.8
　myxedematosus L98.5
　nitidus L44.1
　pilaris Q82.8
　　acquired L85.8
　planopilaris L66.1
　planus (chronicus) L43.9
　　annularis L43.8
　　bullous L43.1
　　follicular L66.1
　　hypertrophic L43.0
　　moniliformis L44.3
　　of Wilson L43.9
　　specified NEC L43.8
　　subacute (active) L43.3
　　tropicus L43.3
　ruber
　　acuminatus L44.0
　　moniliformis L44.3
　　planus L43.9
　sclerosus (et atrophicus) L90.0
　　penis N48.0
　　vulva N90.4
　scrofulosus (primary) (tuberculous) A18.4
　simplex (chronicus) (circumscriptus) L28.0
　striatus L44.2
　urticatus L28.2
Lichenification L28.0
Lichenoides tuberculosis (primary) A18.4
Lichtheim's disease or syndrome — *see* Degeneration,
　combined
Lien migrans D73.89
Ligament — *see* condition
Light
　for gestational age — *see* Light for dates
　headedness R42
Light-for-dates (infant) P05.00
　with weight of
　　499 grams or less P05.01
　　500-749 grams P05.02
　　750-999 grams P05.03
　　1000-1249 grams P05.04
　　1250-1499 grams P05.05

Light-for-dates — *continued*
　with weight of — *continued*
　　1500-1749 grams P05.06
　　1750-1999 grams P05.07
　　2000-2499 grams P05.08
　　2500 grams and over P05.09
　affecting management of pregnancy O36.59- ☑
　and small-for-dates — *see* Small for dates
　specified NEC P05.09
Lightning (effects) (stroke) (struck by) T75.00 ☑
　burn — *see* Burn
　foot E53.8
　shock T75.01 ☑
　specified effect NEC T75.09 ☑
Lightwood-Albright syndrome N25.89
Lightwood's disease or syndrome (renal tubular acido-
　sis) N25.89
Lignac (-de Toni) (-Fanconi) (-Debré) **disease or syn-
　drome** E72.09
　with cystinosis E72.04
Ligneous thyroiditis E06.5
Likoff's syndrome I20.8
Limb — *see* condition
Limbic epilepsy personality syndrome F07.0
Limitation, limited
　activities due to disability Z73.6
　cardiac reserve — *see* Disease, heart
　eye muscle duction, traumatic — *see* Strabismus, me-
　　chanical
　mandibular range of motion M26.52
Lindau (-von Hippel) **disease** Q85.8
Line(s)
　Beau's L60.4
　Harris' — *see* Arrest, epiphyseal
　Hudson's (cornea) — *see* Pigmentation, cornea, anterior
　Stähli's (cornea) — *see* Pigmentation, cornea, anterior
Linea corneae senilis — *see* Change, cornea, senile
Lingua
　geographica K14.1
　nigra (villosa) K14.3
　plicata K14.5
　tylosis K13.29
Lingual — *see* condition
Linguatulosis B88.8
Linitis (gastric) **plastica** C16.9
Lip — *see* condition
Lipedema — *see* Edema
Lipemia (*see also* Hyperlipidemia)
　retina, retinalis E78.3
Lipidosis E75.6
　cerebral (infantile) (juvenile) (late) E75.4
　cerebroretinal E75.4
　cerebroside E75.22
　cholesterol (cerebral) E75.5
　glycolipid E75.21
　hepatosplenomegalic E78.3
　sphingomyelin — *see* Niemann-Pick disease or syn-
　　drome
　sulfatide E75.29
Lipoadenoma — *see* Neoplasm, benign, by site
Lipoblastoma — *see* Lipoma
Lipoblastomatosis — *see* Lipoma
Lipochondrodystrophy E76.01
Lipochrome histiocytosis (familial) D71
Lipodermatosclerosis — *see* Varix, leg, with, inflamma-
　tion
　ulcerated — *see* Varix, leg, with, ulcer, with inflamma-
　　tion by site
Lipodystrophia progressiva E88.1
Lipodystrophy (progressive) E88.1
　insulin E88.1
　intestinal K90.81
　mesenteric K65.4
Lipofibroma — *see* Lipoma
Lipofuscinosis, neuronal (with ceroidosis) E75.4
Lipogranuloma, sclerosing L92.8
Lipogranulomatosis E78.89
Lipoid (*see also* condition)
　histiocytosis D76.3
　　essential E75.29
　nephrosis N04.9
　proteinosis of Urbach E78.89
Lipoidemia — *see* Hyperlipidemia
Lipoidosis — *see* Lipidosis
Lipoma D17.9
　fetal D17.9
　　fat cell D17.9

Lipoma — *continued*
　infiltrating D17.9
　intramuscular D17.9
　pleomorphic D17.9
　site classification
　　arms (skin) (subcutaneous) D17.2- ☑
　　connective tissue D17.30
　　　intra-abdominal D17.5
　　　intrathoracic D17.4
　　　peritoneum D17.79
　　　retroperitoneum D17.79
　　　specified site NEC D17.39
　　　spermatic cord D17.6
　　face (skin) (subcutaneous) D17.0
　　genitourinary organ NEC D17.72
　　head (skin) (subcutaneous) D17.0
　　intra-abdominal D17.5
　　intrathoracic D17.4
　　kidney D17.71
　　legs (skin) (subcutaneous) D17.2- ☑
　　neck (skin) (subcutaneous) D17.0
　　peritoneum D17.79
　　retroperitoneum D17.79
　　skin D17.30
　　　specified site NEC D17.39
　　specified site NEC D17.79
　　spermatic cord D17.6
　　subcutaneous D17.30
　　　specified site NEC D17.39
　　trunk (skin) (subcutaneous) D17.1
　　unspecified D17.9
　spindle cell D17.9
Lipomatosis E88.2
　dolorosa (Dercum) E88.2
　fetal — *see* Lipoma
　Launois-Bensaude E88.89
Lipomyoma — *see* Lipoma
Lipomyxoma — *see* Lipoma
Lipomyxosarcoma — *see* Neoplasm, connective tissue,
　malignant
Lipoprotein metabolism disorder E78.9
Lipoproteinemia E78.5
　broad-beta E78.2
　floating-beta E78.2
　hyper-pre-beta E78.1
Liposarcoma (*see also* Neoplasm, connective tissue,
　malignant)
　dedifferentiated — *see* Neoplasm, connective tissue,
　　malignant
　differentiated type — *see* Neoplasm, connective tissue,
　　malignant
　embryonal — *see* Neoplasm, connective tissue, malig-
　　nant
　mixed type — *see* Neoplasm, connective tissue, malig-
　　nant
　myxoid — *see* Neoplasm, connective tissue, malignant
　pleomorphic — *see* Neoplasm, connective tissue, ma-
　　lignant
　round cell — *see* Neoplasm, connective tissue, malig-
　　nant
　well differentiated type — *see* Neoplasm, connective
　　tissue, malignant
Liposynovitis prepatellaris E88.89
Lipping, cervix N86
Lipschütz disease or ulcer N76.6
Lipuria R82.0
　schistosomiasis (bilharziasis) B65.0
Lisping F80.0
Lissauer's paralysis A52.17
Lissencephalia, lissencephaly Q04.3
Listeriosis, listerellosis A32.9
　congenital (disseminated) P37.2
　cutaneous A32.0
　neonatal, newborn (disseminated) P37.2
　oculoglandular A32.81
　specified NEC A32.89
Lithemia E79.0
Lithiasis — *see* Calculus
Lithosis J62.8
Lithuria R82.998
Litigation, anxiety concerning Z65.3
Little leaguer's elbow — *see* Epicondylitis, medial
Little's disease G80.9
Littre's
　gland — *see* condition
　hernia — *see* Hernia, abdomen
Littritis — *see* Urethritis

　☑ **Additional Character Required** — Refer to the Tabular List for Character Selection　　▽ **Subterms under main terms may continue to next column or page**

Index

Livedo (annularis) (racemosa) (reticularis) R23.1
Liver — *see* condition
Living alone (problems with) Z60.2
  with handicapped person Z74.2
Lloyd's syndrome — *see* Adenomatosis, endocrine
Loa loa, loaiasis, loasis B74.3
Lobar — *see* condition
Lobomycosis B48.0
Lobo's disease B48.0
Lobotomy syndrome F07.0
Lobstein (-Ekman) **disease or syndrome** Q78.0
Lobster-claw hand Q71.6- ☑
Lobulation (congenital) (*see also* Anomaly, by site)
  kidney, Q63.1
  liver, abnormal Q44.7
  spleen Q89.09
Lobule, lobular — *see* condition
Local, localized — *see* condition
Locked twins causing obstructed labor O66.1
Locked-in state G83.5
Locking
  joint — *see* Derangement, joint, specified type NEC
    knee — *see* Derangement, knee
Lockjaw — *see* Tetanus
Löffler's
  endocarditis I42.3
  eosinophilia J82
  pneumonia J82
  syndrome (eosinophilic pneumonitis) J82
Loiasis (with conjunctival infestation) (eyelid) B74.3
Lone Star fever A77.0
Long
  labor O63.9
    first stage O63.0
    second stage O63.1
  QT syndrome I45.81
Longitudinal stripes or grooves, nails L60.8
  congenital Q84.6
Long-term (current) (prophylactic) **drug therapy** (use of)
  agents affecting estrogen receptors and estrogen levels NEC Z79.818
  anastrozole (Arimidex) Z79.811
  antibiotics Z79.2
    short-term use — *omit code*
  anticoagulants Z79.01
  anti-inflammatory, non-steroidal (NSAID) Z79.1
  antiplatelet Z79.02
  antithrombotics Z79.02
  aromatase inhibitors Z79.811
  aspirin Z79.82
  birth control pill or patch Z79.3
  bisphosphonates Z79.83
  contraceptive, oral Z79.3
  drug, specified NEC Z79.899
  estrogen receptor downregulators Z79.818
  Evista Z79.810
  exemestane (Aromasin) Z79.811
  Fareston Z79.810
  fulvestrant (Faslodex) Z79.818
  gonadotropin-releasing hormone (GnRH) agonist Z79.818
  goserelin acetate (Zoladex) Z79.818
  hormone replacement Z79.890
  insulin Z79.4
  letrozole (Femara) Z79.811
  leuprolide acetate (leuprorelin) (Lupron) Z79.818
  megestrol acetate (Megace) Z79.818
  methadone for pain management Z79.891
  Nolvadex Z79.810
  non-steroidal anti-inflammatories (NSAID) Z79.1
  opiate analgesic Z79.891
  oral
    antidiabetic Z79.84
    contraceptive Z79.3
    hypoglycemic Z79.84
  raloxifene (Evista) Z79.810
  selective estrogen receptor modulators (SERMs) Z79.810
  steroids
    inhaled Z79.51
    systemic Z79.52
  tamoxifen (Nolvadex) Z79.810
  toremifene (Fareston) Z79.810
Loop
  intestine — *see* Volvulus
  vascular on papilla (optic) Q14.2
Loose (*see also* condition)

Loose — *continued*
  body
    joint M24.00
      ankle M24.07- ☑
      elbow M24.02- ☑
      hand M24.04- ☑
      hip M24.05- ☑
      knee M23.4- ☑
      shoulder (region) M24.01- ☑
      specified site NEC M24.08
      toe M24.07- ☑
      vertebra M24.08
      wrist M24.03- ☑
    knee M23.4- ☑
    sheath, tendon — *see* Disorder, tendon, specified type NEC
  cartilage — *see* Loose, body, joint
  skin and subcutaneous tissue (following bariatric surgery weight loss) (following dietary weight loss) L98.7
  tooth, teeth K08.89
Loosening
  aseptic
    joint prosthesis — *see* Complications, joint prosthesis, mechanical, loosening, by site
    epiphysis — *see* Osteochondropathy
  mechanical
    joint prosthesis — *see* Complications, joint prosthesis, mechanical, loosening, by site
Looser-Milkman (-Debray) **syndrome** M83.8
Lop ear (deformity) Q17.3
Lorain (-Levi) **short stature syndrome** E23.0
Lordosis M40.50
  acquired — *see* Lordosis, specified type NEC
  congenital Q76.429
    lumbar region Q76.426
    lumbosacral region Q76.427
    sacral region Q76.428
    sacrococcygeal region Q76.428
    thoracolumbar region Q76.425
  lumbar region M40.56
  lumbosacral region M40.57
  postsurgical M96.4
  postural — *see* Lordosis, specified type NEC
  rachitic (late effect) (sequelae) E64.3
  sequelae of rickets E64.3
  specified type NEC M40.40
    lumbar region M40.46
    lumbosacral region M40.47
    thoracolumbar region M40.45
  thoracolumbar region M40.55
  tuberculous A18.01
Loss (of)
  appetite (*see also* Anorexia) R63.0
    hysterical F50.89
    nonorganic origin F50.89
    psychogenic F50.89
  blood — *see* Hemorrhage
  bone —*see* Loss, substance of, bone
  consciousness, transient R55
    traumatic — *see* Injury, intracranial
  control, sphincter, rectum R15.9
    nonorganic origin F98.1
  elasticity, skin R23.4
  family (member) in childhood Z62.898
  fluid (acute) E86.9
  function of labyrinth — *see* subcategory H83.2 ☑
  hair, nonscarring — *see* Alopecia
  hearing (*see also* Deafness)
    central NOS H90.5
    conductive H90.2
      bilateral H90.0
      unilateral
        with
          restricted hearing on the contralateral side H90.A1- ☑
          unrestricted hearing on the contralateral side H90.1- ☑
    mixed conductive and sensorineural hearing loss H90.8
      bilateral H90.6
      unilateral
        with
          restricted hearing on the contralateral side H90.A3- ☑
          unrestricted hearing on the contralateral side H90.7- ☑
    neural NOS H90.5

Loss — *continued*
  hearing (*see also* Deafness) — *continued*
    perceptive NOS H90.5
    sensorineural NOS H90.5
      bilateral H90.3
      unilateral
        with
          restricted hearing onthe contralateral side H90.A2- ☑
          unrestricted hearing on the contralateral side H90.4- ☑
    sensory NOS H90.5
  height R29.890
  limb or member, traumatic, current — *see* Amputation, traumatic
  love relationship in childhood Z62.898
  memory (*see also* Amnesia)
    mild, following organic brain damage F06.8
  mind — *see* Psychosis
  occlusal vertical dimension of fully erupted teeth M26.37
  organ or part — *see* Absence, by site, acquired
  ossicles, ear (partial) H74.32- ☑
  parent in childhood Z63.4
  pregnancy, recurrent N96
    care in current pregnancy O26.2- ☑
    without current pregnancy N96
  recurrent pregnancy — *see* Loss, pregnancy, recurrent
  self-esteem, in childhood Z62.898
  sense of
    smell — *see* Disturbance, sensation, smell
    taste — *see* Disturbance, sensation, taste
    touch R20.8
  sensory R44.9
    dissociative F44.6
  sexual desire F52.0
  sight (acquired) (complete) (congenital) — *see* Blindness
  substance of
    bone — *see* Disorder, bone, density and structure, specified NEC
      horizontal alveolar K06.3
    cartilage — *see* Disorder, cartilage, specified type NEC
      auricle (ear) — *see* Disorder, pinna, specified type NEC
    vitreous (humor) H15.89
  tooth, teeth — *see* Absence, teeth, acquired
  vision, visual H54.7
    both eyes H54.3
    one eye H54.60
      left (normal vision on right) H54.62
      right (normal vision on left) H54.61
    specified as blindness — *see* Blindness
    subjective
      sudden H53.13- ☑
      transient H53.12- ☑
  vitreous — *see* Prolapse, vitreous
  voice — *see* Aphonia
  weight (abnormal) (cause unknown) R63.4
Louis-Bar syndrome (ataxia-telangiectasia) G11.3
Louping ill (encephalitis) A84.8
Louse, lousiness — *see* Lice
Low
  achiever, school Z55.3
  back syndrome M54.5
  basal metabolic rate R94.8
  birthweight (2499 grams or less) P07.10
    with weight of
      1000-1249 grams P07.14
      1250-1499 grams P07.15
      1500-1749 grams P07.16
      1750-1999 grams P07.17
      2000-2499 grams P07.18
    extreme (999 grams or less) P07.00
      with weight of
        499 grams or less P07.01
        500-749 grams P07.02
        750-999 grams P07.03
    for gestational age — *see* Light for dates
  blood pressure (*see also* Hypotension)
    reading (incidental) (isolated) (nonspecific) R03.1
  cardiac reserve — *see* Disease, heart
  function (*see also* Hypofunction)
    kidney N28.9
  hematocrit D64.9
  hemoglobin D64.9
  income Z59.6

Livedo — Low

Low — *continued*
  level of literacy Z55.Ø
  lying
    kidney N28.89
    organ or site, congenital — *see* Malposition, congenital
  output syndrome (cardiac) — *see* Failure, heart
  platelets (blood) — *see* Thrombocytopenia
  reserve, kidney N28.89
  salt syndrome E87.1
  self esteem R45.81
  set ears Q17.4
  vision H54.2X- ☑
    one eye (other eye normal) H54.5Ø
      left (normal vision on right) H54.52A- ☑
      other eye blind — *see* Blindness
      right (normal vision on left) H54.511- ☑
Low-density-lipoprotein-type (LDL) **hyperlipoproteinemia** E78.ØØ
Lowe's syndrome E72.Ø3
Lown-Ganong-Levine syndrome I45.6
LSD reaction (acute) (without dependence) F16.9Ø
  with dependence F16.2Ø
L-shaped kidney Q63.8
Ludwig's angina or disease K12.2
Lues (venerea), **luetic** — *see* Syphilis
Luetscher's syndrome (dehydration) E86.Ø
Lumbago, lumbalgia M54.5
  with sciatica M54.4- ☑
    due to intervertebral disc disorder M51.17
  due to displacement, intervertebral disc M51.27
    with sciatica M51.17
Lumbar — *see* condition
Lumbarization, vertebra, congenital Q76.49
Lumbermen's itch B88.Ø
Lump (*see also* Mass)
  breast N63.Ø
    axillary tail
      left N63.32
      right N63.31
    left
      lower inner quadrant N63.24
      lower outer quadrant N63.23
      unspecified quadrant N63.2Ø
      upper inner quadrant N63.22
      upper outer quadrant N63.21
    right
      lower inner quadrant N63.14
      lower outer quadrant N63.13
      unspecified quadrant N63.1Ø
      upper inner quadrant N63.12
      upper outer quadrant N63.11
    subareolar
      left N63.42
      right N63.41
Lunacy — *see* Psychosis
Lung — *see* condition
Lupoid (miliary) **of Boeck** D86.3
Lupus
  anticoagulant D68.62
    with
      hemorrhagic disorder D68.312
      hypercoagulable state D68.62
    finding without diagnosis R76.Ø
  discoid (local) L93.Ø
  erythematosus (discoid) (local) L93.Ø
    disseminated — *see* Lupus, erythematosus, systemic
    eyelid HØ1.129
      left HØ1.126
        lower HØ1.125
        upper HØ1.124
      right HØ1.123
        lower HØ1.122
        upper HØ1.121
    profundus L93.2
    specified NEC L93.2
    subacute cutaneous L93.1
    systemic M32.9
      with organ or system involvement M32.1Ø
        endocarditis M32.11
        lung M32.13
        pericarditis M32.12
        renal (glomerular) M32.14
          tubulo-interstitial M32.15
        specified organ or system NEC M32.19
      drug-induced M32.Ø
      inhibitor (presence of) D68.62

Lupus — *continued*
  erythematosus — *continued*
    systemic — *continued*
      inhibitor — *continued*
        with
          hemorrhagic disorder D68.312
          hypercoagulable state D68.62
        finding without diagnosis R76.Ø
      specified NEC M32.8
  exedens A18.4
  hydralazine M32.Ø
    correct substance properly administered — *see* Table of Drugs and Chemicals, by drug, adverse effect
    overdose or wrong substance given or taken — *see* Table of Drugs and Chemicals, by drug, poisoning
  nephritis (chronic) M32.14
  nontuberculous, not disseminated L93.Ø
  panniculitis L93.2
  pernio (Besnier) D86.3
  systemic — *see* Lupus, erythematosus, systemic
  tuberculous A18.4
    eyelid A18.4
  vulgaris A18.4
    eyelid A18.4
Luteinoma D27.- ☑
Lutembacher's disease or syndrome (atrial septal defect with mitral stenosis) Q21.1
Luteoma D27.- ☑
Lutz (-Splendore-de Almeida) **disease** — *see* Paracoccidioidomycosis
Luxation (*see also* Dislocation)
  eyeball (nontraumatic) — *see* Luxation, globe
    birth injury P15.3
  globe, nontraumatic H44.82- ☑
  lacrimal gland — *see* Dislocation, lacrimal gland
  lens (old) (partial) (spontaneous)
    congenital Q12.1
    syphilitic A5Ø.39
Lycanthropy F22
Lyell's syndrome L51.2
  due to drug L51.2
    correct substance properly administered — *see* Table of Drugs and Chemicals, by drug, adverse effect
    overdose or wrong substance given or taken — *see* Table of Drugs and Chemicals, by drug, poisoning
Lyme disease A69.2Ø
Lymph
  gland or node — *see* condition
  scrotum — *see* Infestation, filarial
Lymphadenitis I88.9
  with ectopic or molar pregnancy OØ8.Ø
  acute LØ4.9
    axilla LØ4.2
    face LØ4.Ø
    head LØ4.Ø
    hip LØ4.3
    limb
      lower LØ4.3
      upper LØ4.2
    neck LØ4.Ø
    shoulder LØ4.2
    specified site NEC LØ4.8
    trunk LØ4.1
  anthracosis (occupational) J6Ø
  any site, except mesenteric I88.9
    chronic I88.1
    subacute I88.1
  breast
    gestational — *see* Mastitis, obstetric
    puerperal, postpartum (nonpurulent) O91.22
  chancroidal (congenital) A57
  chronic I88.1
    mesenteric I88.Ø
  due to
    Brugia (malayi) B74.1
      timori B74.2
    chlamydial lymphogranuloma A55
    diphtheria (toxin) A36.89
    lymphogranuloma venereum A55
    Wuchereria bancrofti B74.Ø
  following ectopic or molar pregnancy OØ8.Ø
  gonorrheal A54.89
  infective — *see* Lymphadenitis, acute

Lymphadenitis — *continued*
  mesenteric (acute) (chronic) (nonspecific) (subacute) I88.Ø
    due to Salmonella typhi AØ1.Ø9
    tuberculous A18.39
  mycobacterial A31.8
  purulent — *see* Lymphadenitis, acute
  pyogenic — *see* Lymphadenitis, acute
  regional, nonbacterial I88.8
  septic — *see* Lymphadenitis, acute
  subacute, unspecified site I88.1
  suppurative — *see* Lymphadenitis, acute
  syphilitic (early) (secondary) A51.49
    late A52.79
  tuberculous — *see* Tuberculosis, lymph gland
  venereal (chlamydial) A55
Lymphadenoid goiter EØ6.3
Lymphadenopathy (generalized) R59.1
  angioimmunoblastic, with dysproteinemia (AILD) C86.5
  due to toxoplasmosis (acquired) B58.89
    congenital (acute) (subacute) (chronic) P37.1
  localized R59.Ø
  syphilitic (early) (secondary) A51.49
Lymphadenosis R59.1
Lymphangiectasis I89.Ø
  conjunctiva H11.89
  postinfectional I89.Ø
  scrotum I89.Ø
Lymphangiectatic elephantiasis, nonfilarial I89.Ø
Lymphangioendothelioma D18.1
  malignant — *see* Neoplasm, connective tissue, malignant
Lymphangioleiomyomatosis J84.81
Lymphangioma D18.1
  capillary D18.1
  cavernous D18.1
  cystic D18.1
  malignant — *see* Neoplasm, connective tissue, malignant
Lymphangiomyoma D18.1
Lymphangiomyomatosis J84.81
Lymphangiosarcoma — *see* Neoplasm, connective tissue, malignant
Lymphangitis I89.1
  with
    abscess — *code by* site under Abscess
    cellulitis — *code by* site under Cellulitis
    ectopic or molar pregnancy OØ8.Ø
  acute LØ3.91
    abdominal wall LØ3.321
    ankle — *see* Lymphangitis, acute, lower limb
    arm — *see* Lymphangitis, acute, upper limb
    auricle (ear) — *see* Lymphangitis, acute, ear
    axilla LØ3.12- ☑
    back (any part) LØ3.322
    buttock LØ3.327
    cervical (meaning neck) LØ3.222
    cheek (external) LØ3.212
    chest wall LØ3.323
    digit
      finger — *see* Lymphangitis, acute, finger
      toe — *see* Lymphangitis, acute, toe
    ear (external) H6Ø.1- ☑
    external auditory canal — *see* Lymphangitis, acute, ear
    eyelid — *see* Abscess, eyelid
    face NEC LØ3.212
    finger (intrathecal) (periosteal) (subcutaneous) (subcuticular) LØ3.Ø2- ☑
    foot — *see* Lymphangitis, acute, lower limb
    gluteal (region) LØ3.327
    groin LØ3.324
    hand — *see* Lymphangitis, acute, upper limb
    head NEC LØ3.891
      face (any part, except ear, eye and nose) LØ3.212
    heel — *see* Lymphangitis, acute, lower limb
    hip — *see* Lymphangitis, acute, lower limb
    jaw (region) LØ3.212
    knee — *see* Lymphangitis, acute, lower limb
    leg — *see* Lymphangitis, acute, lower limb
    lower limb LØ3.12- ☑
      toe — *see* Lymphangitis, acute, toe
    navel LØ3.326
    neck LØ3.222
    orbit, orbital — *see* Cellulitis, orbit
    pectoral (region) LØ3.323
    perineal, perineum LØ3.325

Lymphangitis — *continued*
  acute — *continued*
    scalp (any part) L03.891
    shoulder — *see* Lymphangitis, acute, upper limb
    specified site NEC L03.898
    thigh — *see* Lymphangitis, acute, lower limb
    thumb (intrathecal) (periosteal) (subcutaneous) (subcuticular) — *see* Lymphangitis, acute, finger
    toe (intrathecal) (periosteal) (subcutaneous) (subcuticular) L03.04- ☑
    trunk L03.329
      abdominal wall L03.321
      back (any part) L03.322
      buttock L03.327
      chest wall L03.323
      groin L03.324
      perineal, perineum L03.325
      umbilicus L03.326
    umbilicus L03.326
    upper limb L03.12- ☑
      axilla — *see* Lymphangitis, acute, axilla
      finger — *see* Lymphangitis, acute, finger
      thumb — *see* Lymphangitis, acute, finger
    wrist — *see* Lymphangitis, acute, upper limb
  breast
    gestational — *see* Mastitis, obstetric
  chancroidal A57
  chronic (any site) I89.1
  due to
    Brugia (malayi) B74.1
      timori B74.2
    Wuchereria bancrofti B74.0
  following ectopic or molar pregnancy O08.89
  penis
    acute N48.29
    gonococcal (acute) (chronic) A54.09
  puerperal, postpartum, childbirth O86.89
  strumous, tuberculous A18.2
  subacute (any site) I89.1
  tuberculous — *see* Tuberculosis, lymph gland
Lymphatic (vessel) — *see* condition
Lymphatism E32.8
Lymphectasia I89.0
Lymphedema (acquired) (*see also* Elephantiasis)
  congenital Q82.0
  hereditary (chronic) (idiopathic) Q82.0
  postmastectomy I97.2
  praecox I89.0
  secondary I89.0
  surgical NEC I97.89
    postmastectomy (syndrome) I97.2
Lymphoblastic — *see* condition
Lymphoblastoma (diffuse) — *see* Lymphoma, lymphoblastic (diffuse)
  giant follicular — *see* Lymphoma, lymphoblastic (diffuse)
  macrofollicular — *see* Lymphoma, lymphoblastic (diffuse)
Lymphocele I89.8
Lymphocytic
  chorioencephalitis (acute) (serous) A87.2
  choriomeningitis (acute) (serous) A87.2
  meningoencephalitis A87.2
Lymphocytoma, benign cutis L98.8
Lymphocytopenia D72.810
Lymphocytosis (symptomatic) D72.820
  infectious (acute) B33.8
Lymphoepithelioma — *see* Neoplasm, malignant, by site
Lymphogranuloma (malignant) (*see also* Lymphoma, Hodgkin)
  chlamydial A55
  inguinale A55
  venereum (any site) (chlamydial) (with stricture of rectum) A55
Lymphogranulomatosis (malignant) (*see also* Lymphoma, Hodgkin)
  benign (Boeck's sarcoid) (Schaumann's) D86.1
Lymphohistiocytosis, hemophagocytic (familial) D76.1
Lymphoid — *see* condition
Lymphoma (of) (malignant) C85.90
  adult T-cell (HTLV-1-associated) (acute variant) (chronic variant) (lymphomatoid variant) (smouldering variant) C91.5- ☑
  anaplastic large cell
    ALK-negative C84.7- ☑
    ALK-positive C84.6- ☑

Lymphoma — *continued*
  anaplastic large cell — *continued*
    CD30-positive C84.6- ☑
    primary cutaneous C86.6
  angioimmunoblastic T-cell C86.5
  BALT C88.4
  B-cell C85.1- ☑
  blastic NK-cell C86.4
  blastic plasmacytoid dendritic cell neoplasm (BPDCN) C86.4
  B-precursor C83.5- ☑
  bronchial-associated lymphoid tissue [BALT-lymphoma] C88.4
  Burkitt (atypical) C83.7- ☑
  Burkitt-like C83.7- ☑
  centrocytic C83.1- ☑
  cutaneous follicle center C82.6- ☑
  cutaneous T-cell C84.A- ☑ (*following* C84.7)
  diffuse follicle center C82.5- ☑
  diffuse large B-cell C83.3- ☑
    anaplastic C83.3- ☑
    B-cell C83.3- ☑
    CD30-positive C83.3- ☑
    centroblastic C83.3- ☑
    immunoblastic C83.3- ☑
    plasmablastic C83.3- ☑
    subtype not specified C83.3- ☑
    T-cell rich C83.3- ☑
  enteropathy-type (associated) (intestinal) T-cell C86.2
  extranodal marginal zone B-cell lymphoma of mucosa-associated lymphoid tissue [MALT-lymphoma] C88.4
  extranodal NK/T-cell, nasal type C86.0
  follicular C82.9- ☑
    grade
      I C82.0- ☑
      II C82.1- ☑
      III C82.2- ☑
      IIIa C82.3- ☑
      IIIb C82.4- ☑
    specified NEC C82.8- ☑
  hepatosplenic T-cell (alpha-beta) (gamma-delta) C86.1
  histiocytic C85.9- ☑
    true C96.A (*following* C96.6)
  Hodgkin C81.9 ☑
    lymphocyte depleted (classical) C81.3- ☑
    lymphocyte-rich (classical) C81.4- ☑
    mixed cellularity (classical) C81.2- ☑
    nodular
      lymphocyte predominant C81.0- ☑
      sclerosis (classical) C81.1- ☑
    nodular sclerosis (classical) C81.1- ☑
    specified NEC (classical) C81.7- ☑
  intravascular large B-cell C83.8- ☑
  Lennert's C84.4- ☑
  lymphoblastic (diffuse) C83.5- ☑
  lymphoblastic B-cell C83.5- ☑
  lymphoblastic T-cell C83.5- ☑
  lymphoepithelioid C84.4- ☑
  lymphoplasmacytic C83.0- ☑
    with IgM-production C88.0
  MALT C88.4
  mantle cell C83.1- ☑
  mature T-cell NEC C84.4- ☑
  mature T/NK-cell C84.9- ☑
    specified NEC C84.Z- ☑ (*following* C84.7)
  mediastinal (thymic) large B-cell C85.2- ☑
  Mediterranean C88.3
  mucosa-associated lymphoid tissue [MALT-lymphoma] C88.4
  NK/T cell C84.9- ☑
  nodal marginal zone C83.0- ☑
  non-follicular (diffuse) C83.9- ☑
    specified NEC C83.8- ☑
  non-Hodgkin (*see also* Lymphoma, by type) C85.9- ☑
    specified NEC C85.8- ☑
  non-leukemic variant of B-CLL C83.0- ☑
  peripheral T-cell, not classified C84.4- ☑
  primary cutaneous
    anaplastic large cell C86.6
    CD30-positive large T-cell C86.6
  primary effusion B-cell C83.8- ☑
  SALT C88.4
  skin-associated lymphoid tissue [SALT-lymphoma] C88.4
  small cell B-cell C83.0- ☑

Lymphoma — *continued*
  splenic marginal zone C83.0- ☑
  subcutaneous panniculitis-like T-cell C86.3
  T-precursor C83.5- ☑
  true histiocytic C96.A (*following* C96.6)
Lymphomatosis — *see* Lymphoma
Lymphopathia venereum, veneris A55
Lymphopenia D72.810
Lymphoplasmacytic leukemia — *see* Leukemia, chronic lymphocytic, B-cell type
Lymphoproliferation, X-linked disease D82.3
Lymphoreticulosis, benign (of inoculation) A28.1
Lymphorrhea I89.8
Lymphosarcoma (diffuse) (*see also* Lymphoma) C85.9- ☑
Lymphostasis I89.8
Lypemania — *see* Melancholia
Lysine and hydroxylysine metabolism disorder E72.3
Lyssa — *see* Rabies

M

Macacus ear Q17.3
Maceration, wet feet, tropical (syndrome) T69.02- ☑
MacLeod's syndrome J43.0
Macrocephalia, macrocephaly Q75.3
Macrocheilia, macrochilia (congenital) Q18.6
Macrocolon (*see also* Megacolon) Q43.1
Macrocornea Q15.8
  with glaucoma Q15.0
Macrocytic — *see* condition
Macrocytosis D75.89
Macrodactylia, macrodactylism (fingers) (thumbs) Q74.0
  toes Q74.2
Macrodontia K00.2
Macrogenia M26.05
Macrogenitosomia (adrenal) (male) (praecox) E25.9
  congenital E25.0
Macroglobulinemia (idiopathic) (primary) C88.0
  monoclonal (essential) D47.2
  Waldenström C88.0
Macroglossia (congenital) Q38.2
  acquired K14.8
Macrognathia, macrognathism (congenital) (mandibular) (maxillary) M26.09
Macrogyria (congenital) Q04.8
Macrohydrocephalus — *see* Hydrocephalus
Macromastia — *see* Hypertrophy, breast
Macrophthalmos Q11.3
  in congenital glaucoma Q15.0
Macropsia H53.15
Macrosigmoid K59.39
  congenital Q43.2
Macrospondylitis , acromegalic E22.0
Macrostomia (congenital) Q18.4
Macrotia (external ear) (congenital) Q17.1
Macula
  cornea, corneal — *see* Opacity, cornea
  degeneration (atrophic) (exudative) (senile) (*see also* Degeneration, macula)
  hereditary — *see* Dystrophy, retina
Maculae ceruleae B85.1
Maculopathy, toxic — *see* Degeneration, macula, toxic
Madarosis (eyelid) H02.729
  left H02.726
    lower H02.725
    upper H02.724
  right H02.723
    lower H02.722
    upper H02.721
Madelung's
  deformity (radius) Q74.0
  disease
    radial deformity Q74.0
    symmetrical lipomas, neck E88.89
Madness — *see* Psychosis
Madura
  foot B47.9
    actinomycotic B47.1
    mycotic B47.0
Maduromycosis B47.0
Maffucci's syndrome Q78.4
Magnesium metabolism disorder — *see* Disorder, metabolism, magnesium
Main en griffe (acquired) (*see also* Deformity, limb, clawhand)
  congenital Q74.0

Maintenance (encounter for)
 antineoplastic chemotherapy Z51.11
 antineoplastic radiation therapy Z51.0
 methadone F11.20
Majocchi's
 disease L81.7
 granuloma B35.8
Major — *see* condition
Mal de los pintos — *see* Pinta
Mal de mer T75.3 ☑
Malabar itch (any site) B35.5
Malabsorption K90.9
 calcium K90.89
 carbohydrate K90.49
 disaccharide E73.9
 fat K90.49
 galactose E74.20
 glucose (-galactose) E74.39
 intestinal K90.9
  specified NEC K90.89
 isomaltose E74.31
 lactose E73.9
 methionine E72.19
 monosaccharide E74.39
 postgastrectomy K91.2
 postsurgical K91.2
 protein K90.49
 starch K90.49
 sucrose E74.39
 syndrome K90.9
  postsurgical K91.2
Malacia, bone (adult) M83.9
 juvenile — *see* Rickets
Malacoplakia
 bladder N32.89
 pelvis (kidney) N28.89
 ureter N28.89
 urethra N36.8
Malacosteon, juvenile — *see* Rickets
Maladaptation — *see* Maladjustment
Maladie de Roger Q21.0
Maladjustment
 conjugal Z63.0
  involving divorce or estrangement Z63.5
 educational Z55.4
 family Z63.9
 marital Z63.0
  involving divorce or estrangement Z63.5
 occupational NEC Z56.89
 simple, adult — *see* Disorder, adjustment
 situational — *see* Disorder, adjustment
 social Z60.9
  due to
   acculturation difficulty Z60.3
   discrimination and persecution (perceived) Z60.5
   exclusion and isolation Z60.4
   life-cycle (phase of life) transition Z60.0
   rejection Z60.4
   specified reason NEC Z60.8
Malaise R53.81
Malakoplakia — *see* Malacoplakia
Malaria, malarial (fever) B54
 with
  blackwater fever B50.8
   hemoglobinuric (bilious) B50.8
  hemoglobinuria B50.8
 accidentally induced (therapeutically) — *code by* type
  under Malaria
 algid B50.9
 cerebral B50.0 [G94]
 clinically diagnosed (without parasitological confirmation) B54
 congenital NEC P37.4
  falciparum P37.3
 congestion, congestive B54
 continued (fever) B50.9
 estivo-autumnal B50.9
 falciparum B50.9
  with complications NEC B50.8
   cerebral B50.0 [G94]
  severe B50.8
 hemorrhagic B54
 malariae B52.9
  with
   complications NEC B52.8
   glomerular disorder B52.0
 malignant (tertian) — *see* Malaria, falciparum

Malaria, malarial — *continued*
 mixed infections — *code to* first listed type in B50-B53
 ovale B53.0
 parasitologically confirmed NEC B53.8
 pernicious, acute — *see* Malaria, falciparum
 Plasmodium (P.)
  falciparum NEC — *see* Malaria, falciparum
  malariae NEC B52.9
   with Plasmodium
    falciparum (and or vivax) — *see* Malaria, falciparum
    vivax (*see also* Malaria, vivax)
     and falciparum — *see* Malaria, falciparum
  ovale B53.0
   with Plasmodium malariae (*see also* Malaria, malariae)
    and vivax (*see also* Malaria, vivax)
     and falciparum — *see* Malaria, falciparum
  simian B53.1
   with Plasmodium malariae (*see also* Malaria, malariae)
    and vivax (*see also* Malaria, vivax)
     and falciparum — *see* Malaria, falciparum
  vivax NEC B51.9
   with Plasmodium falciparum — *see* Malaria, falciparum
 quartan — *see* Malaria, malariae
 quotidian — *see* Malaria, falciparum
 recurrent B54
 remittent B54
 specified type NEC (parasitologically confirmed) B53.8
 spleen B54
 subtertian (fever) — *see* Malaria, falciparum
 tertian (benign) (*see also* Malaria, vivax)
  malignant B50.9
 tropical B50.9
 typhoid B54
 vivax B51.9
  with
   complications NEC B51.8
   ruptured spleen B51.0
Malassez's disease (cystic) N50.89
Malassimilation K90.9
Maldescent, testis Q53.9
 bilateral Q53.20
  abdominal Q53.211
  perineal Q53.22
 unilateral Q53.10
  abdominal Q53.111
  perineal Q53.12
Maldevelopment (*see also* Anomaly)
 brain Q07.9
 colon Q43.9
 hip Q74.2
  congenital dislocation Q65.2
   bilateral Q65.1
   unilateral Q65.0- ☑
 mastoid process Q75.8
 middle ear Q16.4
  except ossicles Q16.4
  ossicles Q16.3
 ossicles Q16.3
 spine Q76.49
 toe Q74.2
Male type pelvis Q74.2
 with disproportion (fetopelvic) O33.3 ☑
  causing obstructed labor O65.3
Malformation (congenital) (*see also* Anomaly)
 adrenal gland Q89.1
 affecting multiple systems with skeletal changes NEC Q87.5
 alimentary tract Q45.9
  specified type NEC Q45.8
  upper Q40.9
   specified type NEC Q40.8
 aorta Q25.40
  absence Q25.41
  aneurysm, congenital Q25.43
  aplasia Q25.41
  atresia Q25.29
   aortic arch Q25.21
  coarctation (preductal) (postductal) Q25.1
  dilatation, congenital Q25.44
  hypoplasia Q25.42
  patent ductus arteriosus Q25.0
  specified type NEC Q25.49
  stenosis Q25.1
   supravalvular Q25.3

Malformation — *continued*
 aortic valve Q23.9
  specified NEC Q23.8
 arteriovenous, aneurysmatic (congenital) Q27.30
  brain Q28.2
  cerebral Q28.2
  peripheral Q27.30
   digestive system Q27.33
   lower limb Q27.32
   other specified site Q27.39
   renal vessel Q27.34
   upper limb Q27.31
  precerebral vessels (nonruptured) Q28.0
 auricle
  ear (congenital) Q17.3
   acquired H61.119
    left H61.112
     with right H61.113
    right H61.111
     with left H61.113
 bile duct Q44.5
 bladder Q64.79
  aplasia Q64.5
  diverticulum Q64.6
  exstrophy — *see* Exstrophy, bladder
  neck obstruction Q64.31
 bone Q79.9
  face Q75.9
   specified type NEC Q75.8
  skull Q75.9
   specified type NEC Q75.8
 brain (multiple) Q04.9
  arteriovenous Q28.2
  specified type NEC Q04.8
 branchial cleft Q18.2
 breast Q83.9
  specified type NEC Q83.8
 broad ligament Q50.6
 bronchus Q32.4
 bursa Q79.9
 cardiac
  chambers Q20.9
   specified type NEC Q20.8
  septum Q21.9
   specified type NEC Q21.8
 cerebral Q04.9
  vessels Q28.3
 cervix uteri Q51.9
  specified type NEC Q51.828
 Chiari
  Type I G93.5
  Type II Q07.01
 choroid (congenital) Q14.3
  plexus Q07.8
 circulatory system Q28.9
 cochlea Q16.5
 cornea Q13.4
 coronary vessels Q24.5
 corpus callosum (congenital) Q04.0
 diaphragm Q79.1
 digestive system NEC, specified type NEC Q45.8
 dura Q07.9
  brain Q04.9
  spinal Q06.9
 ear Q17.9
  causing impairment of hearing Q16.9
  external Q17.9
   accessory auricle Q17.0
   causing impairment of hearing Q16.9
    absence of
     auditory canal Q16.1
     auricle Q16.0
   macrotia Q17.1
   microtia Q17.2
   misplacement Q17.4
   misshapen NEC Q17.3
   prominence Q17.5
   specified type NEC Q17.8
  inner Q16.5
  middle Q16.4
   absence of eustachian tube Q16.2
   ossicles (fusion) Q16.3
  ossicles Q16.3
  specified type NEC Q17.8
 epididymis Q55.4
 esophagus Q39.9
  specified type NEC Q39.8
 eye Q15.9
  lid Q10.3

Malformation — continued
eye — continued
  specified NEC Q15.8
fallopian tube Q50.6
genital organ — see Anomaly, genitalia
great
  artery Q25.9
    aorta — see Malformation, aorta
    pulmonary artery — see Malformation, pulmonary, artery
    specified type NEC Q25.8
  vein Q26.9
    anomalous
      portal venous connection Q26.5
      pulmonary venous connection Q26.4
        partial Q26.3
        total Q26.2
    persistent left superior vena cava Q26.1
    portal vein-hepatic artery fistula Q26.6
    specified type NEC Q26.8
    vena cava stenosis, congenital Q26.0
gum Q38.6
hair Q84.2
heart Q24.9
  specified type NEC Q24.8
integument Q84.9
  specified type NEC Q84.8
internal ear Q16.5
intestine Q43.9
  specified type NEC Q43.8
iris Q13.2
joint Q74.9
  ankle Q74.2
  lumbosacral Q76.49
  sacroiliac Q74.2
  specified type NEC Q74.8
kidney Q63.9
  accessory Q63.0
  giant Q63.3
  horseshoe Q63.1
  hydronephrosis Q62.0
  malposition Q63.2
  specified type NEC Q63.8
lacrimal apparatus Q10.6
lingual Q38.3
lip Q38.0
liver Q44.7
lung Q33.9
meninges or membrane (congenital) Q07.9
  cerebral Q04.8
  spinal (cord) Q06.9
middle ear Q16.4
  ossicles Q16.3
mitral valve Q23.9
  specified NEC Q23.8
Mondini's (congenital) (malformation, cochlea) Q16.5
mouth (congenital) Q38.6
multiple types NEC Q89.7
musculoskeletal system Q79.9
myocardium Q24.8
nail Q84.6
nervous system (central) Q07.9
nose Q30.9
  specified type NEC Q30.8
optic disc Q14.2
orbit Q10.7
ovary Q50.39
palate Q38.5
parathyroid gland Q89.2
pelvic organs or tissues NEC
  in pregnancy or childbirth O34.8- ☑
    causing obstructed labor O65.5
penis Q55.69
  aplasia Q55.5
  curvature (lateral) Q55.61
  hypoplasia Q55.62
pericardium Q24.8
peripheral vascular system Q27.9
  specified type NEC Q27.8
pharynx Q38.8
precerebral vessels Q28.1
prostate Q55.4
pulmonary
  arteriovenous Q25.72
  artery Q25.9
    atresia Q25.5
    specified type NEC Q25.79
    stenosis Q25.6
  valve Q22.3

Malformation — continued
renal artery Q27.2
respiratory system Q34.9
retina Q14.1
scrotum — see Malformation, testis and scrotum
seminal vesicles Q55.4
sense organs NEC Q07.9
skin Q82.9
specified NEC Q89.8
spinal
  cord Q06.9
  nerve root Q07.8
spine Q76.49
  kyphosis — see Kyphosis, congenital
  lordosis — see Lordosis, congenital
spleen Q89.09
stomach Q40.3
  specified type NEC Q40.2
teeth, tooth K00.9
tendon Q79.9
testis and scrotum Q55.20
  aplasia Q55.0
  hypoplasia Q55.1
  polyorchism Q55.21
  retractile testis Q55.22
  scrotal transposition Q55.23
  specified type NEC Q55.29
thorax, bony Q76.9
throat Q38.8
thyroid gland Q89.2
tongue (congenital) Q38.3
  hypertrophy Q38.2
  tie Q38.1
trachea Q32.1
tricuspid valve Q22.9
  specified type NEC Q22.8
umbilical cord NEC (complicating delivery) O69.89 ☑
umbilicus Q89.9
ureter Q62.8
  agenesis Q62.4
  duplication Q62.5
  malposition — see Malposition, congenital, ureter
  obstructive defect — see Defect, obstructive, ureter
  vesico-uretero-renal reflux Q62.7
urethra Q64.79
  aplasia Q64.5
  duplication Q64.74
  posterior valves Q64.2
  prolapse Q64.71
  stricture Q64.32
urinary system Q64.9
uterus Q51.9
  specified type NEC Q51.818
vagina Q52.4
vas deferens Q55.4
  atresia Q55.3
vascular system, peripheral Q27.9
venous — see Anomaly, vein(s)
vulva Q52.70

Malfunction (see also Dysfunction)
cardiac electronic device T82.119 ☑
  electrode T82.110 ☑
  pulse generator T82.111 ☑
  specified type NEC T82.118 ☑
catheter device NEC T85.618 ☑
  cystostomy T83.010 ☑
  dialysis (renal) (vascular) T82.41 ☑
    intraperitoneal T85.611 ☑
  infusion NEC T82.514 ☑
    cranial T85.610 ☑
    epidural T85.610 ☑
    intrathecal T85.610 ☑
    spinal T85.610 ☑
    subarachnoid T85.610 ☑
    subdural T85.610 ☑
  urinary (see also Breakdown, device, catheter) T83.018 ☑
colostomy K94.03
  valve K94.03
cystostomy (stoma) N99.512
  catheter T83.010 ☑
enteric stoma K94.13
enterostomy K94.13
esophagostomy K94.33
gastroenteric K31.89
gastrostomy K94.23
ileostomy K94.13
  valve K94.13

Malfunction — continued
intrathecal infusion pump T85.615 ☑
jejunostomy K94.13
nervous system device, implant or graft, specified NEC T85.615 ☑
pacemaker — see Malfunction, cardiac electronic device
prosthetic device, internal — see Complications, prosthetic device, by site, mechanical
tracheostomy J95.03
urinary device NEC — see Complication, genitourinary, device, urinary, mechanical
valve
  colostomy K94.03
  heart T82.09 ☑
  ileostomy K94.13
vascular graft or shunt NEC — see Complication, cardiovascular device, mechanical, vascular
ventricular (communicating shunt) T85.01 ☑
Malherbe's tumor — see Neoplasm, skin, benign
Malibu disease L98.8
Malignancy (see also Neoplasm, malignant, by site)
unspecified site (primary) C80.1
Malignant — see condition
Malingerer, malingering Z76.5
Mallet finger (acquired) — see Deformity, finger, mallet finger
congenital Q74.0
sequelae of rickets E64.3
Malleus A24.0
Mallory's bodies R89.7
Mallory-Weiss syndrome K22.6
Malnutrition E46
degree
  first E44.1
    mild (protein) E44.1
    moderate (protein) E44.0
  second E44.0
  severe (protein-energy) E43
    intermediate form E42
      with
        kwashiorkor (and marasmus) E42
        marasmus E41
  third E43
following gastrointestinal surgery K91.2
intrauterine
  light-for-dates — see Light for dates
  small-for-dates — see Small for dates
lack of care, or neglect (child) (infant) T76.02 ☑
  confirmed T74.02 ☑
malignant E40
protein E46
  calorie E46
    mild E44.1
    moderate E44.0
    severe E43
      intermediate form E42
        with
          kwashiorkor (and marasmus) E42
          marasmus E41
  energy E46
    mild E44.1
    moderate E44.0
    severe E43
      intermediate form E42
        with
          kwashiorkor (and marasmus) E42
          marasmus E41
severe (protein-energy) E43
  with
    kwashiorkor (and marasmus) E42
    marasmus E41
Malocclusion (teeth) M26.4
Angle's M26.219
  class I M26.211
  class II M26.212
  class III M26.213
due to
  abnormal swallowing M26.59
  mouth breathing M26.59
  tongue, lip or finger habits M26.59
  temporomandibular (joint) M26.69
Malposition
cervix — see Malposition, uterus
congenital
  adrenal (gland) Q89.1
  alimentary tract Q45.8
    lower Q43.8

Malposition — *continued*
  congenital — *continued*
    alimentary tract — *continued*
      upper Q40.8
    aorta Q25.49
    appendix Q43.8
    arterial trunk Q20.0
    artery (peripheral) Q27.8
      coronary Q24.5
      digestive system Q27.8
      lower limb Q27.8
      pulmonary Q25.79
      specified site NEC Q27.8
      upper limb Q27.8
    auditory canal Q17.8
      causing impairment of hearing Q16.9
    auricle (ear) Q17.4
      causing impairment of hearing Q16.9
      cervical Q18.2
    biliary duct or passage Q44.5
    bladder (mucosa) — *see* Exstrophy, bladder
    brachial plexus Q07.8
    brain tissue Q04.8
    breast Q83.8
    bronchus Q32.4
    cecum Q43.8
    clavicle Q74.0
    colon Q43.8
    digestive organ or tract NEC Q45.8
      lower Q43.8
      upper Q40.8
    ear (auricle) (external) Q17.4
      ossicles Q16.3
    endocrine (gland) NEC Q89.2
    epiglottis Q31.8
    eustachian tube Q17.8
    eye Q15.8
    facial features Q18.8
    fallopian tube Q50.6
    finger(s) Q68.1
      supernumerary Q69.0
    foot Q66.9
    gallbladder Q44.1
    gastrointestinal tract Q45.8
    genitalia, genital organ(s) or tract
      female Q52.8
        external Q52.79
        internal NEC Q52.8
      male Q55.8
    glottis Q31.8
    hand Q68.1
    heart Q24.8
      dextrocardia Q24.0
        with complete transposition of viscera Q89.3
    hepatic duct Q44.5
    hip (joint) Q65.89
    intestine (large) (small) Q43.8
      with anomalous adhesions, fixation or malrotation Q43.3
    joint NEC Q68.8
    kidney Q63.2
    larynx Q31.8
    limb Q68.8
      lower Q68.8
      upper Q68.8
    liver Q44.7
    lung (lobe) Q33.8
    nail(s) Q84.6
    nerve Q07.8
    nervous system NEC Q07.8
    nose, nasal (septum) Q30.8
    organ or site not listed — *see* Anomaly, by site
    ovary Q50.39
    pancreas Q45.3
    parathyroid (gland) Q89.2
    patella Q74.1
    peripheral vascular system Q27.8
    pituitary (gland) Q89.2
    respiratory organ or system NEC Q34.8
    rib (cage) Q76.6
      supernumerary in cervical region Q76.5
    scapula Q74.0
    shoulder Q74.0
    spinal cord Q06.8
    spleen Q89.09
    sternum NEC Q76.7
    stomach Q40.2
    symphysis pubis Q74.2
    thymus (gland) Q89.2

Malposition — *continued*
  congenital — *continued*
    thyroid (gland) (tissue) Q89.2
      cartilage Q31.8
    toe(s) Q66.9
      supernumerary Q69.2
    tongue Q38.3
    trachea Q32.1
    ureter Q62.60
      deviation Q62.61
      displacement Q62.62
      ectopia Q62.63
      specified type NEC Q62.69
    uterus Q51.818
    vein(s) (peripheral) Q27.8
      great Q26.8
    vena cava (inferior) (superior) Q26.8
  device, implant or graft (*see also* Complications, by site and type, mechanical) T85.628 ☑
    arterial graft NEC — *see* Complication, cardiovascular device, mechanical, vascular
    breast (implant) T85.42 ☑
    catheter NEC T85.628 ☑
      cystostomy T83.020 ☑
      dialysis (renal) T82.42 ☑
        intraperitoneal T85.621 ☑
      infusion NEC T82.524 ☑
        spinal (epidural) (subdural) T85.620 ☑
      urinary (*see also* Displacement, device, catheter, urinary) T83.028 ☑
    electronic (electrode) (pulse generator) (stimulator)
      bone T84.320 ☑
      cardiac T82.129 ☑
        electrode T82.120 ☑
        pulse generator T82.121 ☑
        specified type NEC T82.128 ☑
      nervous system — *see* Complication, prosthetic device, mechanical, electronic nervous system stimulator
      urinary — *see* Complication, genitourinary, device, urinary, mechanical
    fixation, internal (orthopedic) NEC — *see* Complication, fixation device, mechanical
    gastrointestinal — *see* Complications, prosthetic device, mechanical, gastrointestinal device
    genital NEC T83.428 ☑
      intrauterine contraceptive device (string) T83.32 ☑
      penile prosthesis (cylinder) (implanted) (pump) (reservoir) T83.420 ☑
      testicular prosthesis T83.421 ☑
    heart NEC — *see* Complication, cardiovascular device, mechanical
    joint prosthesis — *see* Complication, joint prosthesis, mechanical
    ocular NEC — *see* Complications, prosthetic device, mechanical, ocular device
    orthopedic NEC — *see* Complication, orthopedic, device, mechanical
    specified NEC T85.628 ☑
    urinary NEC (*see also* Complication, genitourinary, device, urinary, mechanical)
      graft T83.22 ☑
    vascular NEC — *see* Complication, cardiovascular device, mechanical
    ventricular intracranial shunt T85.02 ☑
  fetus — *see* Pregnancy, complicated by (management affected by), presentation, fetal
  gallbladder K82.8
  gastrointestinal tract, congenital Q45.8
  heart, congenital NEC Q24.8
  joint prosthesis — *see* Complications, joint prosthesis, mechanical, displacement, by site
  stomach K31.89
    congenital Q40.2
  tooth, teeth, fully erupted M26.30
  uterus (acute) (acquired) (adherent) (asymptomatic) (postinfectional) (postpartal, old) N85.4
    anteflexion or anteversion N85.4
      congenital Q51.818
    flexion N85.4
      lateral — *see* Lateroversion, uterus
    inversion N85.5
    lateral (flexion) (version) — *see* Lateroversion, uterus
      in pregnancy or childbirth — *see* subcategory O34.5 ☑

Malposition — *continued*
  uterus — *continued*
    retroflexion or retroversion — *see* Retroversion, uterus
Malposture R29.3
Malrotation
  cecum Q43.3
  colon Q43.3
  intestine Q43.3
  kidney Q63.2
Malta fever — *see* Brucellosis
Maltreatment
  adult
    abandonment
      confirmed T74.01 ☑
      suspected T76.01 ☑
    bullying
      confirmed T74.31 ☑
      suspected T76.31 ☑
    confirmed T74.91 ☑
    history of Z91.419
    intimidation (through social media)
      confirmed T74.31 ☑
      suspected T76.31 ☑
    neglect
      confirmed T74.01 ☑
      suspected T76.01 ☑
    physical abuse
      confirmed T74.11 ☑
      suspected T76.11 ☑
    psychological abuse
      confirmed T74.31 ☑
      history of Z91.411
      suspected T76.31 ☑
    sexual abuse
      confirmed T74.21 ☑
      suspected T76.21 ☑
    suspected T76.91 ☑
  child
    abandonment
      confirmed T74.02 ☑
      suspected T76.02 ☑
    bullying
      confirmed T74.32 ☑
      suspected T76.32 ☑
    confirmed T74.92 ☑
    history of — *see* History, personal (of), abuse
    intimidation (through social media)
      confirmed T74.32 ☑
      suspected T76.32 ☑
    neglect
      confirmed T74.02 ☑
      history of — *see* History, personal (of), abuse
      suspected T76.02 ☑
    physical abuse
      confirmed T74.12 ☑
      history of — *see* History, personal (of), abuse
      suspected T76.12 ☑
    psychological abuse
      confirmed T74.32 ☑
      history of — *see* History, personal (of), abuse
      suspected T76.32 ☑
    sexual abuse
      confirmed T74.22 ☑
      history of — *see* History, personal (of), abuse
      suspected T76.22 ☑
    suspected T76.92 ☑
  personal history of Z91.89
Maltworker's lung J67.4
Malunion, fracture — *see* Fracture, by site
Mammillitis N61.0
  puerperal, postpartum O91.02
Mammitis — *see* Mastitis
Mammogram (examination) Z12.39
  routine Z12.31
Mammoplasia N62
Management (of)
  bone conduction hearing device (implanted) Z45.320
  cardiac pacemaker NEC Z45.018
  cerebrospinal fluid drainage device Z45.41
  cochlear device (implanted) Z45.321
  contraceptive Z30.9
    specified NEC Z30.8
  implanted device Z45.9
    specified NEC Z45.89
  infusion pump Z45.1
  procreative Z31.9

Management — *continued*
  procreative — *continued*
    male factor infertility in female Z31.81
    specified NEC Z31.89
  prosthesis (external) (*see also* Fitting) Z44.9
    implanted Z45.9
      specified NEC Z45.89
  renal dialysis catheter Z49.01
  vascular access device Z45.2
Mangled — *see* specified injury by site
Mania (monopolar) (*see also* Disorder, mood, manic
    episode)
  with psychotic symptoms F30.2
  without psychotic symptoms F30.10
    mild F30.11
    moderate F30.12
    severe F30.13
  Bell's F30.8
  chronic (recurrent) F31.89
  hysterical F44.89
  puerperal F30.8
  recurrent F31.89
Manic depression F31.9
Manic-depressive insanity, psychosis, or syndrome
    — *see* Disorder, bipolar
Mannosidosis E77.1
Mansonelliasis, mansonellosis B74.4
Manson's
  disease B65.1
  schistosomiasis B65.1
Manual — *see* condition
Maple-bark-stripper's lung (disease) J67.6
Maple-syrup-urine disease E71.0
Marable's syndrome (celiac artery compression) I77.4
Marasmus E41
  due to malnutrition E41
  intestinal E41
  nutritional E41
  senile R54
  tuberculous NEC — *see* Tuberculosis
Marble
  bones Q78.2
  skin R23.8
Marburg virus disease A98.3
March
  fracture — *see* Fracture, traumatic, stress, by site
  hemoglobinuria D59.6
Marchesani (-Weill) **syndrome** Q87.0
Marchiafava (-Bignami) **syndrome or disease** G37.1
Marchiafava-Micheli syndrome D59.5
Marcus Gunn's syndrome Q07.8
Marfan's syndrome — *see* Syndrome, Marfan's
Marie-Bamberger disease — *see* Osteoarthropathy,
  hypertrophic, specified NEC
Marie-Charcot-Tooth neuropathic muscular atrophy
  G60.0
Marie's
  cerebellar ataxia (late-onset) G11.2
  disease or syndrome (acromegaly) E22.0
Marie-Strümpell arthritis, disease or spondylitis —
  see Spondylitis, ankylosing
Marion's disease (bladder neck obstruction) N32.0
Marital conflict Z63.0
Mark
  port wine Q82.5
  raspberry Q82.5
  strawberry Q82.5
  stretch L90.6
  tattoo L81.8
Marker heterochromatin — *see* Extra, marker chromo-
  somes
Maroteaux-Lamy syndrome (mild) (severe) E76.29
Marrow (bone)
  arrest D61.9
  poor function D75.89
Marseilles fever A77.1
Marsh fever — *see* Malaria
Marshall's (hidrotic) **ectodermal dysplasia** Q82.4
Marsh's disease (exophthalmic goiter) E05.00
  with storm E05.01
Masculinization (female) **with adrenal hyperplasia**
  E25.9
  congenital E25.0
Masculinovoblastoma D27.- ☑
Masochism (sexual) F65.51
Mason's lung J62.8

Mass
  abdominal R19.00
    epigastric R19.06
    generalized R19.07
    left lower quadrant R19.04
    left upper quadrant R19.02
    periumbilic R19.05
    right lower quadrant R19.03
    right upper quadrant R19.01
    specified site NEC R19.09
  breast (*see also* Lump, breast) N63.0
  chest R22.2
  cystic — *see* Cyst
  ear H93.8- ☑
  head R22.0
  intra-abdominal (diffuse) (generalized) — *see* Mass,
    abdominal
  kidney N28.89
  liver R16.0
  localized (skin) R22.9
    chest R22.2
    head R22.0
    limb
      lower R22.4- ☑
      upper R22.3- ☑
    neck R22.1
    trunk R22.2
  lung R91.8
  malignant — *see* Neoplasm, malignant, by site
  neck R22.1
  pelvic (diffuse) (generalized) — *see* Mass, abdominal
  specified organ NEC — *see* Disease, by site
  splenic R16.1
  substernal thyroid — *see* Goiter
  superficial (localized) R22.9
  umbilical (diffuse) (generalized) R19.09
Massive — *see* condition
Mast cell
  disease, systemic tissue D47.02
  leukemia C94.3- ☑
  neoplasm
    malignant C96.20
      specified type NEC C96.29
    of uncertain behavior NEC D47.09
  sarcoma C96.22
  tumor D47.09
Mastalgia N64.4
Masters-Allen syndrome N83.8
Mastitis (acute) (diffuse) (nonpuerperal) (subacute) N61.0
  with abscess N61.1
  chronic (cystic) — *see* Mastopathy, cystic
  cystic (Schimmelbusch's type) — *see* Mastopathy, cystic
  fibrocystic — *see* Mastopathy, cystic
  infective N61.0
    newborn P39.0
  interstitial, gestational or puerperal — *see* Mastitis,
    obstetric
  neonatal (noninfective) P83.4
    infective P39.0
  obstetric (interstitial) (nonpurulent)
    associated with
      lactation O91.23
      pregnancy O91.21- ☑
      puerperium O91.22
    purulent
      associated with
        lactation O91.13
        pregnancy O91.11- ☑
        puerperium O91.12
  periductal — *see* Ectasia, mammary duct
  phlegmonous — *see* Mastopathy, cystic
  plasma cell — *see* Ectasia, mammary duct
  without abscess N61.0
Mastocytoma (extracutaneous) D47.09
  malignant C96.29
  solitary D47.01
Mastocytosis D47.09
  aggressive systemic C96.21
  cutaneous (diffuse) (maculopapular) D47.01
    congenital Q82.2
    of neonatal onset Q82.2
    of newborn onset Q82.2
  indolent systemic D47.02
  isolated bone marrow D47.02
  malignant C96.29
  systemic (indolent) (smoldering)
    with an associated hematological non-mast cell
      lineage disease (SM-AHNMD) D47.02

Mastodynia N64.4
Mastoid — *see* condition
Mastoidalgia — *see* subcategory H92.0 ☑
Mastoiditis (coalescent) (hemorrhagic) (suppurative)
  H70.9-
  acute, subacute H70.00- ☑
    complicated NEC H70.09- ☑
    subperiosteal H70.01- ☑
  chronic (necrotic) (recurrent) H70.1- ☑
  in (due to)
    infectious disease NEC B99 [H75.0-] ☑
    parasitic disease NEC B89 [H75.0-] ☑
    tuberculosis A18.03
  petrositis — *see* Petrositis
  postauricular fistula — *see* Fistula, postauricular
  specified NEC H70.89- ☑
  tuberculous A18.03
Mastopathy, mastopathia N64.9
  chronica cystica — *see* Mastopathy, cystic
  cystic (chronic) (diffuse) N60.1- ☑
    with epithelial proliferation N60.3- ☑
  diffuse cystic — *see* Mastopathy, cystic
  estrogenic, oestrogenica N64.89
  ovarian origin N64.89
Mastoplasia, mastoplastia N62
Masturbation (excessive) F98.8
Maternal care (for) — *see* Pregnancy (complicated by)
  (management affected by)
Matheiu's disease (leptospiral jaundice) A27.0
Mauclaire's disease or osteochondrosis — *see* Osteo-
  chondrosis, juvenile, hand, metacarpal
Maxcy's disease A75.2
Maxilla, maxillary — *see* condition
May (-Hegglin) **anomaly or syndrome** D72.0
McArdle (-Schmid)(-Pearson) **disease** (glycogen storage)
  E74.04
McCune-Albright syndrome Q78.1
McQuarrie's syndrome (idiopathic familial hypo-
  glycemia) E16.2
Meadow's syndrome Q86.1
Measles (black) (hemorrhagic) (suppressed) B05.9
  with
    complications NEC B05.89
    encephalitis B05.0
    intestinal complications B05.4
    keratitis (keratoconjunctivitis) B05.81
    meningitis B05.1
    otitis media B05.3
    pneumonia B05.2
  French — *see* Rubella
  German — *see* Rubella
  Liberty — *see* Rubella
Meatitis, urethral — *see* Urethritis
Meatus, meatal — *see* condition
Meat-wrappers' asthma J68.9
Meckel-Gruber syndrome Q61.9
Meckel's diverticulitis, diverticulum (displaced) (hypertrophic) Q43.0
  malignant — *see* Table of Neoplasms, small intestine,
    malignant
Meconium
  ileus, newborn P76.0
    in cystic fibrosis E84.11
    meaning meconium plug (without cystic fibrosis)
      P76.0
  obstruction, newborn P76.0
    due to fecaliths P76.0
    in mucoviscidosis E84.11
  peritonitis P78.0
  plug syndrome (newborn) NEC P76.0
Median (*see also* condition)
  arcuate ligament syndrome I77.4
  bar (prostate) (vesical orifice) — *see* Hyperplasia,
    prostate
  rhomboid glossitis K14.2
Mediastinal shift R93.89
Mediastinitis (acute) (chronic) J98.51
  syphilitic A52.73
  tuberculous A15.8
Mediastinopericarditis (*see also* Pericarditis)
  acute I30.9
  adhesive I31.0
  chronic I31.8
    rheumatic I09.2
Mediastinum, mediastinal — *see* condition
Medicine poisoning — *see* Table of Drugs and Chemicals, by drug, poisoning

Mediterranean
fever — *see* Brucellosis
familial M04.1
tick A77.1
kala-azar B55.0
leishmaniasis B55.0
tick fever A77.1
Medulla — *see* condition
Medullary cystic kidney Q61.5
Medullated fibers
optic (nerve) Q14.8
retina Q14.1
Medulloblastoma
desmoplastic C71.6
specified site — *see* Neoplasm, malignant, by site
unspecified site C71.6
Medulloepithelioma (*see also* Neoplasm, malignant, by site)
teratoid — *see* Neoplasm, malignant, by site
Medullomyoblastoma
specified site — *see* Neoplasm, malignant, by site
unspecified site C71.6
Meekeren-Ehlers-Danlos syndrome Q79.6
Megacolon (acquired) (functional) (not Hirschsprung's disease) (in) K59.39
Chagas' disease B57.32
congenital, congenitum (aganglionic) Q43.1
Hirschsprung's (disease) Q43.1
toxic NEC K59.31
due to Clostridium difficile
not specified as recurrent A04.72
recurrent A04.71
Megaesophagus (functional) K22.0
congenital Q39.5
in (due to) Chagas' disease B57.31
Megalencephaly Q04.5
Megalerythema (epidemic) B08.3
Megaloappendix Q43.8
Megalocephalus, megalocephaly NEC Q75.3
Megalocornea Q15.8
with glaucoma Q15.0
Megalocytic anemia D53.1
Megalodactylia (fingers) (thumbs) (congenital) Q74.0
toes Q74.2
Megaloduodenum Q43.8
Megaloesophagus (functional) K22.0
congenital Q39.5
Megalogastria (acquired) K31.89
congenital Q40.2
Megalophthalmos Q11.3
Megalopsia H53.15
Megalosplenia — *see* Splenomegaly
Megaloureter N28.82
congenital Q62.2
Megarectum K62.89
Megasigmoid K59.39
congenital Q43.2
Megaureter N28.82
congenital Q62.2
Megavitamin-B6 syndrome E67.2
Megrim — *see* Migraine
Meibomian
cyst, infected — *see* Hordeolum
gland — *see* condition
sty, stye — *see* Hordeolum
Meibomitis — *see* Hordeolum
Meige-Milroy disease (chronic hereditary edema) Q82.0
Meige's syndrome Q82.0
Melalgia, nutritional E53.8
Melancholia F32.9
climacteric (single episode) F32.89
recurrent episode F33.8
hypochondriac F45.29
intermittent (single episode) F32.89
recurrent episode F33.8
involutional (single episode) F32.89
recurrent episode F33.8
menopausal (single episode) F32.89
recurrent episode F33.8
puerperal F32.89
reactive (emotional stress or trauma) F32.3
recurrent F33.9
senile F03 ☑
stuporous (single episode) F32.89
recurrent episode F33.8
Melanemia R79.89
Melanoameloblastoma — *see* Neoplasm, bone, benign

Melanoblastoma — *see* Melanoma
Melanocarcinoma — *see* Melanoma
Melanocytoma, eyeball D31.9- ☑
Melanocytosis, neurocutaneous Q82.8
Melanoderma, melanodermia L81.4
Melanodontia, infantile K03.89
Melanodontoclasia K03.89
Melanoepithelioma — *see* Melanoma
Melanoma (malignant) C43.9
acral lentiginous, malignant — *see* Melanoma, skin, by site
amelanotic — *see* Melanoma, skin, by site
balloon cell — *see* Melanoma, skin, by site
benign — *see* Nevus
desmoplastic, malignant — *see* Melanoma, skin, by site
epithelioid cell — *see* Melanoma, skin, by site
with spindle cell, mixed — *see* Melanoma, skin, by site
in
giant pigmented nevus — *see* Melanoma, skin, by site
Hutchinson's melanotic freckle — *see* Melanoma, skin, by site
junctional nevus — *see* Melanoma, skin, by site
precancerous melanosis — *see* Melanoma, skin, by site
in situ D03.9
abdominal wall D03.59
ala nasi D03.39
ankle D03.7- ☑
anus, anal (margin) (skin) D03.51
arm D03.6- ☑
auditory canal D03.2- ☑
auricle (ear) D03.2- ☑
auricular canal (external) D03.2- ☑
axilla, axillary fold D03.59
back D03.59
breast D03.52
brow D03.39
buttock D03.59
canthus (eye) D03.1- ☑
cheek (external) D03.39
chest wall D03.59
chin D03.39
choroid D03.8
conjunctiva D03.8
ear (external) D03.2- ☑
external meatus (ear) D03.2- ☑
eye D03.8
eyebrow D03.39
eyelid (lower) (upper) D03.1- ☑
face D03.30
specified NEC D03.39
female genital organ (external) NEC D03.8
finger D03.6- ☑
flank D03.59
foot D03.7- ☑
forearm D03.6- ☑
forehead D03.39
foreskin D03.8
gluteal region D03.59
groin D03.59
hand D03.6- ☑
heel D03.7- ☑
helix D03.2- ☑
hip D03.7- ☑
interscapular region D03.59
iris D03.8
jaw D03.39
knee D03.7- ☑
labium (majus) (minus) D03.8
lacrimal gland D03.8
leg D03.7- ☑
lip (lower) (upper) D03.0
lower limb NEC D03.7- ☑
male genital organ (external) NEC D03.8
nail D03.9
finger D03.6- ☑
toe D03.7- ☑
neck D03.4
nose (external) D03.39
orbit D03.8
penis D03.8
perianal skin D03.51
perineum D03.51
pinna D03.2- ☑

Melanoma — *continued*
in situ — *continued*
popliteal fossa or space D03.7- ☑
prepuce D03.8
pudendum D03.8
retina D03.8
retrobulbar D03.8
scalp D03.4
scrotum D03.8
shoulder D03.6- ☑
specified site NEC D03.8
submammary fold D03.52
temple D03.39
thigh D03.7- ☑
toe D03.7- ☑
trunk NEC D03.59
umbilicus D03.59
upper limb NEC D03.6- ☑
vulva D03.8
juvenile — *see* Nevus
malignant, of soft parts except skin — *see* Neoplasm, connective tissue, malignant
metastatic
breast C79.81
genital organ C79.82
specified site NEC C79.89
neurotropic, malignant — *see* Melanoma, skin, by site
nodular — *see* Melanoma, skin, by site
regressing, malignant — *see* Melanoma, skin, by site
skin C43.9
abdominal wall C43.59
ala nasi C43.31
ankle C43.7- ☑
anus, anal (skin) C43.51
arm C43.6- ☑
auditory canal (external) C43.2- ☑
auricle (ear) C43.2- ☑
auricular canal (external) C43.2- ☑
axilla, axillary fold C43.59
back C43.59
breast (female) (male) C43.52
brow C43.39
buttock C43.59
canthus (eye) C43.1- ☑
cheek (external) C43.39
chest wall C43.59
chin C43.39
ear (external) C43.2- ☑
elbow C43.6- ☑
external meatus (ear) C43.2- ☑
eyebrow C43.39
eyelid (lower) (upper) C43.1- ☑
face C43.30
specified NEC C43.39
female genital organ (external) NEC C51.9
finger C43.6- ☑
flank C43.59
foot C43.7- ☑
forearm C43.6- ☑
forehead C43.39
foreskin C60.0
glabella C43.39
gluteal region C43.59
groin C43.59
hand C43.6- ☑
heel C43.7- ☑
helix C43.2- ☑
hip C43.7- ☑
interscapular region C43.59
jaw (external) C43.39
knee C43.7- ☑
labium C51.9
majus C51.0
minus C51.1
leg C43.7- ☑
lip (lower) (upper) C43.0
lower limb NEC C43.7- ☑
male genital organ (external) NEC C63.9
nail
finger C43.6- ☑
toe C43.7- ☑
nasolabial groove C43.39
nates C43.59
neck C43.4
nose (external) C43.31
overlapping site C43.8
palpebra C43.1- ☑

☑ Additional Character Required — Refer to the Tabular List for Character Selection   Subterms under main terms may continue to next column or page

Melanoma — *continued*
  skin — *continued*
    penis C60.9
    perianal skin C43.51
    perineum C43.51
    pinna C43.2- ☑
    popliteal fossa or space C43.7- ☑
    prepuce C60.0
    pudendum C51.9
    scalp C43.4
    scrotum C63.2
    shoulder C43.6- ☑
    skin NEC C43.9
    submammary fold C43.52
    temple C43.39
    thigh C43.7- ☑
    toe C43.7- ☑
    trunk NEC C43.59
    umbilicus C43.59
    upper limb NEC C43.6- ☑
    vulva C51.9
      overlapping sites C51.8
  spindle cell
    with epithelioid, mixed — *see* Melanoma, skin, by site
    type A C69.4- ☑
    type B C69.4- ☑
  superficial spreading — *see* Melanoma, skin, by site
Melanosarcoma (*see also* Melanoma)
  epithelioid cell — *see* Melanoma
Melanosis L81.4
  addisonian E27.1
    tuberculous A18.7
  adrenal E27.1
  colon K63.89
  conjunctiva — *see* Pigmentation, conjunctiva
    congenital Q13.89
  cornea (presenile) (senile) (*see also* Pigmentation, cornea)
    congenital Q13.4
  eye NEC H57.89
    congenital Q15.8
  lenticularis progressiva Q82.1
  liver K76.89
  precancerous (*see also* Melanoma, in situ)
    malignant melanoma in — *see* Melanoma
  Riehl's L81.4
  sclera H15.89
    congenital Q13.89
  suprarenal E27.1
  tar L81.4
  toxic L81.4
Melanuria R82.998
MELAS syndrome E88.41
Melasma L81.1
  adrenal (gland) E27.1
  suprarenal (gland) E27.1
Melena K92.1
  with ulcer — *code by* site under Ulcer, with hemorrhage K27.4
  due to swallowed maternal blood P78.2
  newborn, neonatal P54.1
    due to swallowed maternal blood P78.2
Meleney's
  gangrene (cutaneous) — *see* Ulcer, skin
  ulcer (chronic undermining) — *see* Ulcer, skin
Melioidosis A24.9
  acute A24.1
  chronic A24.2
  fulminating A24.1
  pneumonia A24.1
  pulmonary (chronic) A24.2
    acute A24.1
    subacute A24.2
  sepsis A24.1
  specified NEC A24.3
  subacute A24.2
Melitensis, febris A23.0
Melkersson (-Rosenthal) **syndrome** G51.2
Mellitus, diabetes — *see* Diabetes
Melorheostosis (bone) — *see* Disorder, bone, density and structure, specified NEC
Meloschisis Q18.4
Melotia Q17.4
Membrana
  capsularis lentis posterior Q13.89
  epipapillaris Q14.2
Membranacea placenta O43.19- ☑

Membranaceous uterus N85.8
Membrane(s), membranous (*see also* condition)
  cyclitic — *see* Membrane, pupillary
  folds, congenital — *see* Web
  Jackson's Q43.3
  over face of newborn P28.9
  premature rupture — *see* Rupture, membranes, premature
  pupillary H21.4- ☑
    persistent Q13.89
  retained (with hemorrhage) (complicating delivery) O72.2
    without hemorrhage O73.1
  secondary cataract — *see* Cataract, secondary
  unruptured (causing asphyxia) — *see* Asphyxia, newborn
  vitreous — *see* Opacity, vitreous, membranes and strands
Membranitis — *see* Chorioamnionitis
Memory disturbance, lack or loss (*see also* Amnesia)
  mild, following organic brain damage F06.8
Menadione deficiency E56.1
Menarche
  delayed E30.0
  precocious E30.1
Mendacity, pathologic F60.2
Mendelson's syndrome (due to anesthesia) J95.4
  in labor and delivery O74.0
  in pregnancy O29.01- ☑
  obstetric O74.0
  postpartum, puerperal O89.01
Ménétrier's disease or syndrome K29.60
  with bleeding K29.61
Ménière's disease, syndrome or vertigo H81.0- ☑
Meninges, meningeal — *see* condition
Meningioma (*see also* Neoplasm, meninges, benign)
  angioblastic — *see* Neoplasm, meninges, benign
  angiomatous — *see* Neoplasm, meninges, benign
  endotheliomatous — *see* Neoplasm, meninges, benign
  fibroblastic — *see* Neoplasm, meninges, benign
  fibrous — *see* Neoplasm, meninges, benign
  hemangioblastic — *see* Neoplasm, meninges, benign
  hemangiopericytic — *see* Neoplasm, meninges, benign
  malignant — *see* Neoplasm, meninges, malignant
  meningiothelial — *see* Neoplasm, meninges, benign
  meningotheliomatous — *see* Neoplasm, meninges, benign
  mixed — *see* Neoplasm, meninges, benign
  multiple — *see* Neoplasm, meninges, uncertain behavior
  papillary — *see* Neoplasm, meninges, uncertain behavior
  psammomatous — *see* Neoplasm, meninges, benign
  syncytial — *see* Neoplasm, meninges, benign
  transitional — *see* Neoplasm, meninges, benign
Meningiomatosis (diffuse) — *see* Neoplasm, meninges, uncertain behavior
Meningism — *see* Meningismus
Meningismus (infectional) (pneumococcal) R29.1
  due to serum or vaccine R29.1
  influenzal — *see* Influenza, with, manifestations NEC
Meningitis (basal) (basic) (brain) (cerebral) (cervical) (congestive) (diffuse) (hemorrhagic) (infantile) (membranous) (metastatic) (nonspecific) (pontine) (progressive) (simple) (spinal) (subacute) (sympathetic) (toxic) G03.9
  abacterial G03.0
  actinomycotic A42.81
  adenoviral A87.1
  arbovirus A87.8
  aseptic (acute) G03.0
  bacterial G00.9
    Escherichia coli (E. coli) G00.8
    Friedländer (bacillus) G00.8
    gram-negative G00.9
    H. influenzae G00.0
    Klebsiella G00.8
    pneumococcal G00.1
    specified organism NEC G00.8
    staphylococcal G00.3
    streptococcal (acute) G00.2
  benign recurrent (Mollaret) G03.2
  candidal B37.5
  caseous (tuberculous) A17.0
  cerebrospinal A39.0
  chronic NEC G03.1
  clear cerebrospinal fluid NEC G03.0

Meningitis — *continued*
  coxsackievirus A87.0
  cryptococcal B45.1
  diplococcal (gram positive) A39.0
  echovirus A87.0
  enteroviral A87.0
  eosinophilic B83.2
  epidemic NEC A39.0
  Escherichia coli (E. coli) G00.8
  fibrinopurulent G00.9
    specified organism NEC G00.8
  Friedländer (bacillus) G00.8
  gonococcal A54.81
  gram-negative cocci G00.9
  gram-positive cocci G00.9
  H. influenzae G00.0
  Haemophilus (influenzae) G00.0
  in (due to)
    adenovirus A87.1
    African trypanosomiasis B56.9 [G02]
    anthrax A22.8
    bacterial disease NEC A48.8 [G01]
    Chagas' disease (chronic) B57.41
    chickenpox B01.0
    coccidioidomycosis B38.4
    Diplococcus pneumoniae G00.1
    enterovirus A87.0
    herpes (simplex) virus B00.3
      zoster B02.1
    infectious mononucleosis B27.92
    leptospirosis A27.81
    Listeria monocytogenes A32.11
    Lyme disease A69.21
    measles B05.1
    mumps (virus) B26.1
    neurosyphilis (late) A52.13
    parasitic disease NEC B89 [G02]
    poliovirus A80.9 [G02]
    preventive immunization, inoculation or vaccination G03.8
    rubella B06.02
    Salmonella infection A02.21
    specified cause NEC G03.8
    Streptococcal pneumoniae G00.1
    typhoid fever A01.01
    varicella B01.0
    viral disease NEC A87.8
    whooping cough A37.90
    zoster B02.1
  infectious G00.9
  influenzal (H. influenzae) G00.0
  Klebsiella G00.8
  leptospiral (aseptic) A27.81
  lymphocytic (acute) (benign) (serous) A87.2
  meningococcal A39.0
  Mima polymorpha G00.8
  Mollaret (benign recurrent) G03.2
  monilial B37.5
  mycotic NEC B49 [G02]
  Neisseria A39.0
  nonbacterial G03.0
  nonpyogenic NEC G03.0
  ossificans G96.19
  pneumococcal streptococcus pneumoniae G00.1
  poliovirus A80.9 [G02]
  postmeasles B05.1
  purulent G00.9
    specified organism NEC G00.8
  pyogenic G00.9
    specified organism NEC G00.8
  Salmonella (arizonae) (Cholerae-Suis) (enteritidis) (typhimurium) A02.21
  septic G00.9
    specified organism NEC G00.8
  serosa circumscripta NEC G03.0
  serous NEC G93.2
  specified organism NEC G00.8
  sporotrichosis B42.81
  staphylococcal G00.3
  sterile G03.0
  Streptococcal (acute) G00.2
    pneumoniae G00.1
  suppurative G00.9
    specified organism NEC G00.8
  syphilitic (late) (tertiary) A52.13
    acute A51.41
    congenital A50.41
    secondary A51.41
  Torula histolytica (cryptococcal) B45.1

Meningitis — *continued*
  traumatic (complication of injury) T79.8 ☑
  tuberculous A17.0
  typhoid A01.01
  viral NEC A87.9
  Yersinia pestis A20.3
Meningocele (spinal) (*see also* Spina bifida)
  with hydrocephalus — *see* Spina bifida, by site, with
    hydrocephalus
  acquired (traumatic) G96.19
  cerebral — *see* Encephalocele
Meningocerebritis — *see* Meningoencephalitis
Meningococcemia A39.4
  acute A39.2
  chronic A39.3
Meningococcus, meningococcal (*see also* condition)
    A39.9
  adrenalitis, hemorrhagic A39.1
  carrier (suspected) of Z22.31
  meningitis (cerebrospinal) A39.0
Meningoencephalitis (*see also* Encephalitis) G04.90
  acute NEC (*see also* Encephalitis, viral) A86
  bacterial NEC G04.2
  California A83.5
  diphasic A84.1
  eosinophilic B83.2
  epidemic A39.81
  herpesviral, herpetic B00.4
    due to herpesvirus 6 B10.01
    due to herpesvirus 7 B10.09
    specified NEC B10.09
  in (due to)
    blastomycosis NEC B40.81
    diseases classified elsewhere G05.3
    free-living amebae B60.2
    H. influenzae G00.0
    Hemophilus influenzae (H .influenzae) G00.0
    herpes B00.4
      due to herpesvirus 6 B10.01
      due to herpesvirus 7 B10.09
      specified NEC B10.09
    Lyme disease A69.22
    mercury — *see* subcategory T56.1 ☑
    mumps B26.2
    Naegleria (amebae) (organisms) (fowleri) B60.2
    Parastrongylus cantonensis B83.2
    toxoplasmosis (acquired) B58.2
      congenital P37.1
  infectious (acute) (viral) A86
  influenzal (H. influenzae) G00.0
  Listeria monocytogenes A32.12
  lymphocytic (serous) A87.2
  mumps B26.2
  parasitic NEC B89 [G05.3]
  pneumococcal G04.2
  primary amebic B60.2
  specific (syphilitic) A52.14
  specified organism NEC G04.81
  staphylococcal G04.2
  streptococcal G04.2
  syphilitic A52.14
  toxic NEC G92
    due to mercury — *see* subcategory T56.1 ☑
  tuberculous A17.82
  virus NEC A86
Meningoencephalocele (*see also* Encephalocele)
  syphilitic A52.19
    congenital A50.49
Meningoencephalomyelitis (*see also* Meningoencephali-
    tis)
  acute NEC (viral) A86
    disseminated G04.00
      postimmunization or postvaccination G04.02
      postinfectious G04.01
    due to
      actinomycosis A42.82
      Torula B45.1
      Toxoplasma or toxoplasmosis (acquired) B58.2
        congenital P37.1
    postimmunization or postvaccination G04.02
Meningoencephalomyelopathy G96.9
Meningoencephalopathy G96.9
Meningomyelitis (*see also* Meningoencephalitis)
  bacterial NEC G04.2
  blastomycotic NEC B40.81
  cryptococcal B45.1
  in diseases classified elsewhere G05.4
  meningococcal A39.81

Meningomyelitis — *continued*
  syphilitic A52.14
  tuberculous A17.82
Meningomyelocele (*see also* Spina bifida)
  syphilitic A52.19
Meningomyeloneuritis — *see* Meningoencephalitis
Meningoradiculitis — *see* Meningitis
Meningovascular — *see* condition
Menkes' disease or syndrome E83.09
  meaning maple-syrup-urine disease E71.0
Menometrorrhagia N92.1
Menopause, menopausal (asymptomatic) (state) Z78.0
  arthritis (any site) NEC — *see* Arthritis, specified form
    NEC
  bleeding N92.4
  depression (single episode) F32.89
    agitated (single episode) F32.2
      recurrent episode F33.9
    psychotic (single episode) F32.89
      recurrent episode F33.9
    recurrent episode F33.8
  melancholia (single episode) F32.89
    recurrent episode F33.8
  paranoid state F22
  premature E28.319
    asymptomatic E28.319
      postirradiation E89.40
      postsurgical E89.40
    symptomatic E28.310
      postirradiation E89.41
      postsurgical E89.41
  psychosis NEC F28
  symptomatic N95.1
  toxic polyarthritis NEC — *see* Arthritis, specified form
    NEC
Menorrhagia (primary) N92.0
  climacteric N92.4
    menopausal N92.4
  menopausal N92.4
  postclimacteric N95.0
  postmenopausal N95.0
  preclimacteric or premenopausal N92.4
  pubertal (menses retained) N92.2
Menostaxis N92.0
Menses, retention N94.89
Menstrual — *see* Menstruation
Menstruation
  absent — *see* Amenorrhea
  anovulatory N97.0
  cycle, irregular N92.6
  delayed N91.0
  disorder N93.9
    psychogenic F45.8
  during pregnancy O20.8
  excessive (with regular cycle) N92.0
    with irregular cycle N92.1
    at puberty N92.2
  frequent N92.0
  infrequent — *see* Oligomenorrhea
  irregular N92.6
    specified NEC N92.5
  latent N92.5
  membranous N92.5
  painful (*see also* Dysmenorrhea) N94.6
    primary N94.4
    psychogenic F45.8
    secondary N94.5
  passage of clots N92.0
  precocious E30.1
  protracted N92.5
  rare — *see* Oligomenorrhea
  retained N94.89
  retrograde N92.5
  scanty — *see* Oligomenorrhea
  suppression N94.89
  vicarious (nasal) N94.89
Mental (*see also* condition)
  deficiency — *see* Disability, intellectual
  deterioration — *see* Psychosis
  disorder — *see* Disorder, mental
  exhaustion F48.8
  insufficiency (congenital) — *see* Disability, intellectual
  observation without need for further medical care
    Z03.89
  retardation — *see* Disability, intellectual
  subnormality — *see* Disability, intellectuall
  upset — *see* Disorder, mental
Meralgia paresthetica G57.1- ☑

Mercurial — *see* condition
Mercurialism — *see* subcategory T56.1 ☑
Merkel cell tumor — *see* Carcinoma, Merkel cell
Merocele — *see* Hernia, femoral
Meromelia
  lower limb — *see* Defect, reduction, lower limb
    intercalary
      femur — *see* Defect, reduction, lower limb,
        specified type NEC
        tibiofibular (complete) (incomplete) — *see*
          Defect, reduction, lower limb
  upper limb — *see* Defect, reduction, upper limb
    intercalary, humeral, radioulnar — *see* Agenesis,
      arm, with hand present
MERRF syndrome (myoclonic epilepsy associated with
    ragged-red fiber) E88.42
Merzbacher-Pelizaeus disease E75.29
Mesaortitis — *see* Aortitis
Mesarteritis — *see* Arteritis
Mesencephalitis — *see* Encephalitis
Mesenchymoma (*see also* Neoplasm, connective tissue,
    uncertain behavior)
  benign — *see* Neoplasm, connective tissue, benign
  malignant — *see* Neoplasm, connective tissue, malig-
    nant
Mesenteritis
  retractile K65.4
  sclerosing K65.4
Mesentery, mesenteric — *see* condition
Mesiodens, mesiodentes K00.1
Mesio-occlusion M26.213
Mesocolon — *see* condition
Mesonephroma (malignant) — *see* Neoplasm, malig-
    nant, by site
  benign — *see* Neoplasm, benign, by site
Mesophlebitis — *see* Phlebitis
Mesostromal dysgenesia Q13.89
Mesothelioma (malignant) C45.9
  benign
    mesentery D19.1
    mesocolon D19.1
    omentum D19.1
    peritoneum D19.1
    pleura D19.0
    specified site NEC D19.7
    unspecified site D19.9
  biphasic C45.9
    benign
      mesentery D19.1
      mesocolon D19.1
      omentum D19.1
      peritoneum D19.1
      pleura D19.0
      specified site NEC D19.7
      unspecified site D19.9
  cystic D48.4
  epithelioid C45.9
    benign
      mesentery D19.1
      mesocolon D19.1
      omentum D19.1
      peritoneum D19.1
      pleura D19.0
      specified site NEC D19.7
      unspecified site D19.9
  fibrous C45.9
    benign
      mesentery D19.1
      mesocolon D19.1
      omentum D19.1
      peritoneum D19.1
      pleura D19.0
      specified site NEC D19.7
      unspecified site D19.9
  site classification
    liver C45.7
    lung C45.7
    mediastinum C45.7
    mesentery C45.1
    mesocolon C45.1
    omentum C45.1
    pericardium C45.2
    peritoneum C45.1
    pleura C45.0
      parietal C45.0
    retroperitoneum C45.7
    specified site NEC C45.7
    unspecified C45.9

Metabolic syndrome E88.81
Metagonimiasis B66.8
Metagonimus infestation (intestine) B66.8
Metal
  pigmentation L81.8
  polisher's disease J62.8
Metamorphopsia H53.15
Metaplasia
  apocrine (breast) — *see* Dysplasia, mammary, specified type NEC
  cervix (squamous) — *see* Dysplasia, cervix
  endometrium (squamous) (uterus) N85.8
  esophagus K22.7- ☑
  kidney (pelvis) (squamous) N28.89
  myelogenous D73.1
  myeloid (agnogenic) (megakaryocytic) D73.1
  spleen D73.1
  squamous cell, bladder N32.89
Metastasis, metastatic
  abscess — *see* Abscess
  calcification E83.59
  cancer
    from specified site — *see* Neoplasm, malignant, by site
    to specified site — *see* Neoplasm, secondary, by site
  deposits (in) — *see* Neoplasm, secondary, by site
  disease (*see also* Neoplasm, secondary, by site) C79.9
  spread (to) — *see* Neoplasm, secondary, by site
Metastrongyliasis B83.8
Metatarsalgia M77.4- ☑
  anterior G57.6- ☑
  Morton's G57.6- ☑
Metatarsus, metatarsal (*see also* condition)
  adductus, congenital Q66.22
  valgus (abductus), congenital Q66.6
  varus (congenital) Q66.22
    primus Q66.21
Methadone use — *see* Use, opioid
Methemoglobinemia D74.9
  acquired (with sulfhemoglobinemia) D74.8
  congenital D74.0
  enzymatic (congenital) D74.0
  Hb M disease D74.0
  hereditary D74.0
  toxic D74.8
Methemoglobinuria — *see* Hemoglobinuria
Methioninemia E72.19
Methylmalonic acidemia E71.120
Metritis (catarrhal) (hemorrhagic) (septic) (suppurative) (*see also* Endometritis)
  cervical — *see* Cervicitis
Metropathia hemorrhagica N93.8
Metroperitonitis — *see* Peritonitis, pelvic, female
Metrorrhagia N92.1
  climacteric N92.4
  menopausal N92.4
  postpartum NEC (atonic) (following delivery of placenta) O72.1
    delayed or secondary O72.2
  preclimacteric or premenopausal N92.4
  psychogenic F45.8
Metrorrhexis — *see* Rupture, uterus
Metrosalpingitis N70.91
Metrostaxis N93.8
Metrovaginitis — *see* Endometritis
Meyer-Schwickerath and Weyers syndrome Q87.0
Meynert's amentia (nonalcoholic) F04
  alcoholic F10.96
    with dependence F10.26
Mibelli's disease (porokeratosis) Q82.8
Mice, joint — *see* Loose, body, joint
  knee M23.4- ☑
Micrencephalon, micrencephaly Q02
Microalbuminuria R80.9
Microaneurysm, retinal (*see also* Disorder, retina, microaneurysms)
  diabetic — *see* E08-E13 with .31
Microangiopathy (peripheral) I73.9
  thrombotic M31.1
Microcalcifications, breast R92.0
Microcephalus, microcephalic, microcephaly Q02
  due to toxoplasmosis (congenital) P37.1
Microcheilia Q18.7
Microcolon (congenital) Q43.8
Microcornea (congenital) Q13.4
Microcytic — *see* condition
Microdeletions NEC Q93.88

Microdontia K00.2
Microdrepanocytosis D57.40
  with crisis (vasoocclusive pain) D57.419
    with
      acute chest syndrome D57.411
      splenic sequestration D57.412
Microembolism
  atherothrombotic — *see* Atheroembolism
  retinal — *see* Occlusion, artery, retina
Microencephalon Q02
Microfilaria streptocerca infestation — *see* Onchocerciasis
Microgastria (congenital) Q40.2
Microgenia M26.06
Microgenitalia, congenital
  female Q52.8
  male Q55.8
Microglioma — *see* Lymphoma, non-Hodgkin, specified NEC
Microglossia (congenital) Q38.3
Micrognathia, micrognathism (congenital) (mandibular) (maxillary) M26.09
Microgyria (congenital) Q04.3
Microinfarct of heart — *see* Insufficiency, coronary
Microlentia (congenital) Q12.8
Microlithiasis, alveolar, pulmonary J84.02
Micromastia N64.82
Micromyelia (congenital) Q06.8
Micropenis Q55.62
Microphakia (congenital) Q12.8
Microphthalmos, microphthalmia (congenital) Q11.2
  due to toxoplasmosis P37.1
Micropsia H53.15
Microscopic polyangiitis (polyarteritis) M31.7
Microsporidiosis B60.8
  intestinal A07.8
Microsporon furfur infestation B36.0
Microsporosis (*see also* Dermatophytosis)
  nigra B36.1
Microstomia (congenital) Q18.5
Microtia (congenital) (external ear) Q17.2
Microtropia H50.40
Microvillus inclusion disease (MVD) (MVID) Q43.8
Micturition
  disorder NEC (*see also* Difficulty, micturition) R39.198
    psychogenic F45.8
  frequency R35.0
    psychogenic F45.8
  hesitancy R39.11
  incomplete emptying R39.14
  nocturnal R35.1
  painful R30.9
    dysuria R30.0
    psychogenic F45.8
    tenesmus R30.1
  poor stream R39.12
  position dependent R39.192
  split stream R39.13
  straining R39.16
  urgency R39.15
Mid plane — *see* condition
Middle
  ear — *see* condition
  lobe (right) syndrome J98.19
Miescher's elastoma L87.2
Mietens' syndrome Q87.2
Migraine (idiopathic) G43.909
  with refractory migraine G43.919
    with status migrainosus G43.911
    without status migrainosus G43.919
  with aura (acute-onset) (prolonged) (typical) (without headache) G43.109
    with refractory migraine G43.119
      with status migrainosus G43.111
      without status migrainosus G43.119
    intractable G43.119
      with status migrainosus G43.111
      without status migrainosus G43.119
    not intractable G43.109
      with status migrainosus G43.101
      without status migrainosus G43.109
    persistent G43.509
      with cerebral infarction G43.609
        with refractory migraine G43.619
          with status migrainosus G43.611
          without status migrainosus G43.619
        intractable G43.619
          with status migrainosus G43.611

Migraine — *continued*
  with aura — *continued*
    persistent — *continued*
      with cerebral infarction — *continued*
        intractable — *continued*
          without status migrainosus G43.619
          not intractable G43.609
            with status migrainosus G43.601
            without status migrainosus G43.609
          without refractory migraine G43.609
            with status migrainosus G43.601
            without status migrainosus G43.609
        without cerebral infarction G43.509
          with refractory migraine G43.519
            with status migrainosus G43.511
            without status migrainosus G43.519
          intractable G43.519
            with status migrainosus G43.511
            without status migrainosus G43.519
          not intractable G43.509
            with status migrainosus G43.501
            without status migrainosus G43.509
          without refractory migraine G43.509
            with status migrainosus G43.501
            without status migrainosus G43.509
      without mention of refractory migraine G43.109
        with status migrainosus G43.101
        without status migrainosus G43.109
  abdominal G43.D0 (following G43.7)
    with refractory migraine G43.D1 (*following* G43.7)
    intractable G43.D1 (*following* G43.7)
    not intractable G43.D0 (*following* G43.7)
    without refractory migraine G43.D0 (*following* G43.7)
  basilar — *see* Migraine, with aura
  classical — *see* Migraine, with aura
  common — *see* Migraine, without aura
  complicated G43.109
  equivalents — *see* Migraine, with aura
  familiar — *see* Migraine, hemiplegic
  hemiplegic G43.409
    with refractory migraine G43.419
      with status migrainosus G43.411
      without status migrainosus G43.419
    intractable G43.419
      with status migrainosus G43.411
      without status migrainosus G43.419
    not intractable G43.409
      with status migrainosus G43.401
      without status migrainosus G43.409
    without refractory migraine G43.409
      with status migrainosus G43.401
      without status migrainosus G43.409
  intractable G43.919
    with status migrainosus G43.911
    without status migrainosus G43.919
  menstrual G43.829
    with refractory migraine G43.839
      with status migrainosus G43.831
      without status migrainosus G43.839
    intractable G43.839
      with status migrainosus G43.831
      without status migrainosus G43.839
    not intractable 4G43.829
      with status migrainosus G43.821
      without status migrainosus G43.829
    without refractory migraine G43.829
      with status migrainosus G43.821
      without status migrainosus G43.829
  menstrually related — *see* Migraine, menstrual
  not intractable G43.909
    with status migrainosus G43.901
    without status migrainosus G43.919
  ophthalmoplegic G43.B0 (following G43.7)
    with refractory migraine G43.B1 (*following* G43.7)
    intractable G43.B1 (*following* G43.7)
    not intractable G43.B0 (*following* G43.7)
    without refractory migraine G43.B0 (*following* G43.7)
  persistent aura (with, without) cerebral infarction — *see* Migraine, with aura, persistent
  preceded or accompanied by transient focal neurological phenomena — *see* Migraine, with aura
  pre-menstrual — *see* Migraine, menstrual
  pure menstrual — *see* Migraine, menstrual
  retinal — *see* Migraine, with aura
  specified NEC G43.809
    intractable G43.819
      with status migrainosus G43.811
      without status migrainosus G43.819

Migraine — *continued*
  specified — *continued*
    not intractable G43.809
      with status migrainosus G43.801
      without status migrainosus G43.809
  sporadic — *see* Migraine, hemiplegic
  transformed — *see* Migraine, without aura, chronic
  triggered seizures — *see* Migraine, with aura
  without aura G43.009
    with refractory migraine G43.019
      with status migrainosus G43.011
      without status migrainosus G43.019
    chronic G43.709
      with refractory migraine G43.719
        with status migrainosus G43.711
        without status migrainosus G43.719
      intractable
        with status migrainosus G43.711
        without status migrainosus G43.719
      not intractable
        with status migrainosus G43.701
        without status migrainosus G43.709
      without refractory migraine G43.709
        with status migrainosus G43.701
        without status migrainosus G43.709
    intractable
      with status migrainosus G43.011
      without status migrainosus G43.019
    not intractable
      with status migrainosus G43.001
      without status migrainosus G43.009
    without mention of refractory migraine G43.009
      with status migrainosus G43.001
      without status migrainosus G43.009
  without refractory migraine G43.909
    with status migrainosus G43.901
    without status migrainosus G43.919
Migrant, social Z59.0
Migration, anxiety concerning Z60.3
Migratory, migrating (*see also* condition)
  person Z59.0
  testis Q55.29
Mikity-Wilson disease or syndrome P27.0
Mikulicz' disease or syndrome K11.8
Miliaria L74.3
  alba L74.1
  apocrine L75.2
  crystallina L74.1
  profunda L74.2
  rubra L74.0
  tropicalis L74.2
Miliary — *see* condition
Milium L72.0
  colloid L57.8
Milk
  crust L21.0
  excessive secretion O92.6
  poisoning — *see* Poisoning, food, noxious
  retention O92.79
  sickness — *see* Poisoning, food, noxious
  spots I31.0
Milk-alkali disease or syndrome E83.52
Milk-leg (deep vessels) (nonpuerperal) — *see* Embolism, vein, lower extremity
  complicating pregnancy O22.3- ☑
  puerperal, postpartum, childbirth O87.1
Milkman's disease or syndrome M83.8
Milky urine — *see* Chyluria
Millard-Gubler (-Foville) **paralysis or syndrome** G46.3
Millar's asthma J38.5
Miller Fisher syndrome G61.0
Mills' disease — *see* Hemiplegia
Millstone maker's pneumoconiosis J62.8
Milroy's disease (chronic hereditary edema) Q82.0
Minamata disease T56.1 ☑
Miners' asthma or lung J60
Minkowski-Chauffard syndrome — *see* Spherocytosis
Minor — *see* condition
Minor's disease (hematomyelia) G95.19
Minot's disease (hemorrhagic disease), newborn P53
Minot-von Willebrand-Jurgens disease or syndrome (angiohemophilia) D68.0
Minus (and plus) **hand** (intrinsic) — *see* Deformity, limb, specified type NEC, forearm
Miosis (pupil) H57.03
Mirizzi's syndrome (hepatic duct stenosis) K83.1
Mirror writing F81.0

Misadventure (of) (prophylactic) (therapeutic) (*see also* Complications) T88.9 ☑
  administration of insulin (by accident) — *see* subcategory T38.3
  infusion — *see* Complications, infusion
  local applications (of fomentations, plasters, etc.) T88.9 ☑
    burn or scald — *see* Burn
    specified NEC T88.8 ☑
  medical care (early) (late) T88.9 ☑
    adverse effect of drugs or chemicals — *see* Table of Drugs and Chemicals
    burn or scald — *see* Burn
    specified NEC T88.8 ☑
  specified NEC T88.8 ☑
  surgical procedure (early) (late) — *see* Complications, surgical procedure
  transfusion — *see* Complications, transfusion
  vaccination or other immunological procedure — *see* Complications, vaccination
Miscarriage O03.9
Misdirection, aqueous H40.83- ☑
Misperception, sleep state F51.02
Misplaced, misplacement
  ear Q17.4
  kidney (acquired) N28.89
    congenital Q63.2
  organ or site, congenital NEC — *see* Malposition, congenital
Missed
  abortion O02.1
  delivery O36.4 ☑
Missing (*see also* Absence)
  string of intrauterine contraceptive device T83.32- ☑
Misuse of drugs F19.99
Mitchell's disease (erythromelalgia) I73.81
Mite(s) (infestation) B88.9
  diarrhea B88.0
  grain (itch) B88.0
  hair follicle (itch) B88.0
  in sputum B88.0
Mitral — *see* condition
Mittelschmerz N94.0
Mixed — *see* condition
MMN (multifocal motor neuropathy) G61.82
MNGIE (Mitochondrial Neurogastrointestinal Encephalopathy) **syndrome** E88.49
Mobile, mobility
  cecum Q43.3
  excessive — *see* Hypermobility
  gallbladder, congenital Q44.1
  kidney N28.89
  organ or site, congenital NEC — *see* Malposition, congenital
Mobitz heart block (atrioventricular) I44.1
Moebius, Möbius
  disease (ophthalmoplegic migraine) — *see* Migraine, ophthalmoplegic
  syndrome Q87.0
    congenital oculofacial paralysis (with other anomalies) Q87.0
    ophthalmoplegic migraine — *see* Migraine, ophthalmoplegic
Moeller's glossitis K14.0
Mohr's syndrome (Types I and II) Q87.0
Mola destruens D39.2
Molar pregnancy O02.0
Molarization of premolars K00.2
Molding, head (during birth) — *omit code*
Mole (pigmented) (*see also* Nevus)
  blood O02.0
  Breus' O02.0
  cancerous — *see* Melanoma
  carneous O02.0
  destructive D39.2
  fleshy O02.0
  hydatid, hydatidiform (benign) (complicating pregnancy) (delivered) (undelivered) O01.9
    classical O01.0
    complete O01.0
    incomplete O01.1
    invasive D39.2
    malignant D39.2
    partial O01.1
  intrauterine O02.0
  invasive (hydatidiform) D39.2

Mole — *continued*
  malignant
    meaning
      malignant hydatidiform mole D39.2
      melanoma — *see* Melanoma
  nonhydatidiform O02.0
  nonpigmented — *see* Nevus
  pregnancy NEC O02.0
  skin — *see* Nevus
  tubal O00.10- ☑
    with intrauterine pregnancy O00.11- ☑
  vesicular — *see* Mole, hydatidiform
Molimen, molimina (menstrual) N94.3
Molluscum contagiosum (epitheliale) B08.1
Mönckeberg's arteriosclerosis, disease, or sclerosis — *see* Arteriosclerosis, extremities
Mondini's malformation (cochlea) Q16.5
Mondor's disease I80.8
Monge's disease T70.29 ☑
Monilethrix (congenital) Q84.1
Moniliasis (*see also* Candidiasis) B37.9
  neonatal P37.5
Monitoring (encounter for)
  therapeutic drug level Z51.81
Monkey malaria B53.1
Monkeypox B04
Monoarthritis M13.10
  ankle M13.17- ☑
  elbow M13.12- ☑
  foot joint M13.17- ☑
  hand joint M13.14- ☑
  hip M13.15- ☑
  knee M13.16- ☑
  shoulder M13.11- ☑
  wrist M13.13- ☑
Monoblastic — *see* condition
Monochromat (ism), monochromatopsia (acquired) (congenital) H53.51
Monocytic — *see* condition
Monocytopenia D72.818
Monocytosis (symptomatic) D72.821
Monomania — *see* Psychosis
Mononeuritis G58.9
  cranial nerve — *see* Disorder, nerve, cranial
  femoral nerve G57.2- ☑
  lateral
    cutaneous nerve of thigh G57.1- ☑
    popliteal nerve G57.3- ☑
  lower limb G57.9-
    specified nerve NEC G57.8- ☑
  medial popliteal nerve G57.4- ☑
  median nerve G56.1- ☑
  multiplex G58.7
  plantar nerve G57.6- ☑
  posterior tibial nerve G57.5- ☑
  radial nerve G56.3- ☑
  sciatic nerve G57.0- ☑
  specified NEC G58.8
  tibial nerve G57.4- ☑
  ulnar nerve G56.2- ☑
  upper limb G56.9-
    specified nerve NEC G56.8- ☑
  vestibular — *see* subcategory H93.3 ☑
Mononeuropathy G58.9
  carpal tunnel syndrome — *see* Syndrome, carpal tunnel
  diabetic NEC — *see* E08-E13 with .41
  femoral nerve — *see* Lesion, nerve, femoral
  ilioinguinal nerve G57.8- ☑
  in diseases classified elsewhere — *see* category G59
  intercostal G58.0
  lower limb G57.9-
    causalgia — *see* Causalgia, lower limb
    femoral nerve — *see* Lesion, nerve, femoral
    meralgia paresthetica G57.1- ☑
    plantar nerve — *see* Lesion, nerve, plantar
    popliteal nerve — *see* Lesion, nerve, popliteal
    sciatic nerve — *see* Lesion, nerve, sciatic
    specified NEC G57.8- ☑
    tarsal tunnel syndrome — *see* Syndrome, tarsal tunnel
  median nerve — *see* Lesion, nerve, median
  multiplex G58.7
  obturator nerve G57.8- ☑
  popliteal nerve — *see* Lesion, nerve, popliteal
  radial nerve — *see* Lesion, nerve, radial
  saphenous nerve G57.8- ☑

Mononeuropathy — *continued*
  specified NEC G58.8
  tarsal tunnel syndrome — *see* Syndrome, tarsal tunnel
  tuberculous A17.83
  ulnar nerve — *see* Lesion, nerve, ulnar
  upper limb G56.9- ☑
    carpal tunnel syndrome — *see* Syndrome, carpal
      tunnel
    causalgia — *see* Causalgia
    median nerve — *see* Lesion, nerve, median
    radial nerve — *see* Lesion, nerve, radial
    specified site NEC G56.8- ☑
    ulnar nerve — *see* Lesion, nerve, ulnar
Mononucleosis, infectious B27.90
  with
    complication NEC B27.99
    meningitis B27.92
    polyneuropathy B27.91
  cytomegaloviral B27.10
    with
      complication NEC B27.19
      meningitis B27.12
      polyneuropathy B27.11
  Epstein-Barr (virus) B27.00
    with
      complication NEC B27.09
      meningitis B27.02
      polyneuropathy B27.01
  gammaherpesviral B27.00
    with
      complication NEC B27.09
      meningitis B27.02
      polyneuropathy B27.01
  specified NEC B27.80
    with
      complication NEC B27.89
      meningitis B27.82
      polyneuropathy B27.81
Monoplegia G83.3- ☑
  congenital (cerebral) G80.8
    spastic G80.1
  embolic (current episode) I63.4- ☑
  following
    cerebrovascular disease
      cerebral infarction
        lower limb I69.34- ☑
        upper limb I69.33- ☑
      intracerebral hemorrhage
        lower limb I69.14- ☑
        upper limb I69.13- ☑
      lower limb I69.94- ☑
      nontraumatic intracranial hemorrhage NEC
        lower limb I69.24- ☑
        upper limb I69.23- ☑
      specified disease NEC
        lower limb I69.84- ☑
        upper limb I69.83- ☑
      stroke NOS
        lower limb I69.34- ☑
        upper limb I69.33- ☑
      subarachnoid hemorrhage
        lower limb I69.04- ☑
        upper limb I69.03- ☑
      upper limb I69.93- ☑
  hysterical (transient) F44.4
  lower limb G83.1- ☑
  psychogenic (conversion reaction) F44.4
  thrombotic (current episode) I63.3- ☑
  transient R29.818
  upper limb G83.2- ☑
Monorchism, monorchidism Q55.0
Monosomy (*see also* Deletion, chromosome) Q93.9
  specified NEC Q93.89
  whole chromosome
    meiotic nondisjunction Q93.0
    mitotic nondisjunction Q93.1
    mosaicism Q93.1
  X Q96.9
Monster, monstrosity (single) Q89.7
  acephalic Q00.0
  twin Q89.4
Monteggia's fracture (-dislocation) S52.27- ☑
Mooren's ulcer (cornea) — *see* Ulcer, cornea, Mooren's
Moore's syndrome — *see* Epilepsy, specified NEC
Mooser-Neill reaction A75.2
Mooser's bodies A75.2
Morbidity not stated or unknown R69

Morbilli — *see* Measles
Morbus (*see also* Disease)
  angelicus, anglorum E55.0
  Beigel B36.2
  caducus — *see* Epilepsy
  celiacus K90.0
  comitialis — *see* Epilepsy
  cordis (*see also* Disease, heart) I51.9
    valvulorum — *see* Endocarditis
  coxae senilis M16.9
    tuberculous A18.02
  hemorrhagicus neonatorum P53
  maculosus neonatorum P54.5
Morel (-Stewart)(-Morgagni) **syndrome** M85.2
Morel-Kraepelin disease — *see* Schizophrenia
Morel-Moore syndrome M85.2
Morgagni's
  cyst, organ, hydatid, or appendage
    female Q50.5
    male (epididymal) Q55.4
      testicular Q55.29
  syndrome M85.2
Morgagni-Stewart-Morel syndrome M85.2
Morgagni-Stokes-Adams syndrome I45.9
Morgagni-Turner (-Albright) **syndrome** Q96.9
Moria F07.0
Moron (I.Q. 50-69) F70
Morphea L94.0
Morphinism (without remission) F11.20
  with remission F11.21
Morphinomania (without remission) F11.20
  with remission F11.21
Morquio (-Ullrich)(-Brailsford) **disease or syndrome** —
  see Mucopolysaccharidosis
Mortification (dry) (moist) — *see* Gangrene
Morton's metatarsalgia (neuralgia)(neuroma) (syn-
  drome) G57.6- ☑
Morvan's disease or syndrome G60.8
Mosaicism, mosaic (autosomal) (chromosomal)
  45,X/46,XX Q96.3
  45,X/other cell lines NEC with abnormal sex chromo-
    some Q96.4
  sex chromosome
    female Q97.8
    lines with various numbers of X chromosomes Q97.2
    male Q98.7
  XY Q96.3
Moschowitz' disease M31.1
Mother yaw A66.0
Motion sickness (from travel, any vehicle) (from round-
  abouts or swings) T75.3 ☑
Mottled, mottling, teeth (enamel) (endemic) (nonen-
  demic) K00.3
Mounier-Kuhn syndrome Q32.4
  with bronchiectasis J47.9
    exacerbation (acute) J47.1
    lower respiratory infection J47.0
  acquired J98.09
    with bronchiectasis J47.9
      with
        exacerbation (acute) J47.1
        lower respiratory infection J47.0
Mountain
  sickness T70.29 ☑
    with polycythemia , acquired (acute) D75.1
  tick fever A93.2
Mouse, joint — *see* Loose, body, joint
  knee M23.4- ☑
Mouth — *see* condition
Movable
  coccyx — *see* subcategory M53.2 ☑
  kidney N28.89
    congenital Q63.8
  spleen D73.89
Movements, dystonic R25.8
Moyamoya disease I67.5
MRSA (Methicillin resistant Staphylococcus aureus)
  infection A49.02
    as the cause of diseases classified elsewhere B95.62
  sepsis A41.02
MSD (multiple sulfatase deficiency) E75.26
MSSA (Methicillin susceptible Staphylococcus aureus)
  infection A49.01
    as the cause of diseases classified elsewhere B95.61
  sepsis A41.01
Mucha-Habermann disease L41.0
Mucinosis (cutaneous) (focal) (papular) (skin) L98.5

Mucinosis — *continued*
  oral K13.79
Mucocele
  appendix K38.8
  buccal cavity K13.79
  gallbladder K82.1
  lacrimal sac, chronic H04.43- ☑
  nasal sinus J34.1
  nose J34.1
  salivary gland (any) K11.6
  sinus (accessory) (nasal) J34.1
  turbinate (bone) (middle) (nasal) J34.1
  uterus N85.8
Mucolipidosis
  I E77.1
  II, III E77.0
  IV E75.11
Mucopolysaccharidosis E76.3
  beta-gluduronidase deficiency E76.29
  cardiopathy E76.3 [I52]
  Hunter's syndrome E76.1
  Hurler's syndrome E76.01
  Hurler-Scheie syndrome E76.02
  Maroteaux-Lamy syndrome E76.29
  Morquio syndrome E76.219
    A E76.210
    B E76.211
    classic E76.210
  Sanfilippo syndrome E76.22
  Scheie's syndrome E76.03
  specified NEC E76.29
  type
    I
      Hurler's syndrome E76.01
      Hurler-Scheie syndrome E76.02
      Scheie's syndrome E76.03
    II E76.1
    III E76.22
    IV E76.219
    IVA E76.210
    IVB E76.211
    VI E76.29
    VII E76.29
Mucormycosis B46.5
  cutaneous B46.3
  disseminated B46.4
  gastrointestinal B46.2
  generalized B46.4
  pulmonary B46.0
  rhinocerebral B46.1
  skin B46.3
  subcutaneous B46.3
Mucositis (ulcerative) K12.30
  due to drugs NEC K12.32
  gastrointestinal K92.81
  mouth (oral) (oropharyngeal) K12.30
    due to antineoplastic therapy K12.31
    due to drugs NEC K12.32
    due to radiation K12.33
    specified NEC K12.39
    viral K12.39
  nasal J34.81
  oral cavity — *see* Mucositis, mouth
  oral soft tissues — *see* Mucositis, mouth
  vagina and vulva N76.81
Mucositis necroticans agranulocytica — *see* Agranulocytosis
Mucous (*see also* condition)
  patches (syphilitic) A51.39
    congenital A50.07
Mucoviscidosis E84.9
  with meconium obstruction E84.11
Mucus
  asphyxia or suffocation — *see* Asphyxia, mucus
  in stool R19.5
  plug — *see* Asphyxia, mucus
Muguet B37.0
Mulberry molars (congenital syphilis) A50.52
Müllerian mixed tumor
  specified site — *see* Neoplasm, malignant, by site
  unspecified site C54.9
Multicystic kidney (development) Q61.4
Multiparity (grand) Z64.1
  affecting management of pregnancy, labor and delivery
    (supervision only) O09.4- ☑
  requiring contraceptive management — *see* Contra-
    ception
Multipartita placenta O43.19- ☑

Multiple, multiplex (see also condition)
- digits (congenital) Q69.9
- endocrine neoplasia — see Neoplasia, endocrine, multiple (MEN)
- personality F44.81

Mumps B26.9
- arthritis B26.85
- complication NEC B26.89
- encephalitis B26.2
- hepatitis B26.81
- meningitis (aseptic) B26.1
- meningoencephalitis B26.2
- myocarditis B26.82
- oophoritis B26.89
- orchitis B26.0
- pancreatitis B26.3
- polyneuropathy B26.84

Mumu (see also Infestation, filarial) B74.9 [N51]
Münchhausen's syndrome — see Disorder, factitious
Münchmeyer's syndrome — see Myositis, ossificans, progressiva
Mural — see condition
Murmur (cardiac) (heart) (organic) R01.1
- abdominal R19.15
- aortic (valve) — see Endocarditis, aortic
- benign R01.0
- diastolic — see Endocarditis
- Flint I35.1
- functional R01.0
- Graham Steell I37.1
- innocent R01.0
- mitral (valve) — see Insufficiency, mitral
- nonorganic R01.0
- presystolic, mitral — see Insufficiency, mitral
- pulmonic (valve) I37.8
- systolic R01.1
- tricuspid (valve) I07.9
- valvular — see Endocarditis

Murri's disease (intermittent hemoglobinuria) D59.6
Muscle, muscular (see also condition)
- carnitine (palmityltransferase) deficiency E71.314

Musculoneuralgia — see Neuralgia
Mushrooming hip — see Derangement, joint, specified NEC, hip
Mushroom-workers' (pickers') disease or lung J67.5
Mutation(s)
- factor V Leiden D68.51
- prothrombin gene D68.52
- surfactant, of lung J84.83

Mutism (see also Aphasia)
- deaf (acquired) (congenital) NEC H91.3
- elective (adjustment reaction) (childhood) F94.0
- hysterical F44.4
- selective (childhood) F94.0

MVD (microvillus inclusion disease) Q43.8
MVID (microvillus inclusion disease) Q43.8
Myalgia M79.10
- auxiliary muscles, head and neck M79.12
- epidemic (cervical) B33.0
- mastication muscle M79.11
- site specified NEC M79.18
- traumatic NEC T14.8 ☑

Myasthenia G70.9
- congenital G70.2
- cordis — see Failure, heart
- developmental G70.2
- gravis G70.00
  - with exacerbation (acute) G70.01
  - in crisis G70.01
  - neonatal, transient P94.0
  - pseudoparalytica G70.00
    - with exacerbation (acute) G70.01
    - in crisis G70.01
- stomach, psychogenic F45.8
- syndrome
  - in
    - diabetes mellitus — see E08-E13 with .44
    - neoplastic disease (see also Neoplasm) D49.9 [G73.3]
    - pernicious anemia D51.0 [G73.3]
    - thyrotoxicosis E05.90 [G73.3]
      - with thyroid storm E05.91 [G73.3]

Myasthenic M62.81
Mycelium infection B49
Mycetismus — see Poisoning, food, noxious, mushroom
Mycetoma B47.9
- actinomycotic B47.1
- bone (mycotic) B47.9 [M90.80]

Mycetoma — continued
- eumycotic B47.0
- foot B47.9
  - actinomycotic B47.1
  - mycotic B47.0
- madurae NEC B47.9
  - mycotic B47.0
- maduromycotic B47.0
- mycotic B47.0
- nocardial B47.1

Mycobacteriosis — see Mycobacterium
Mycobacterium, mycobacterial (infection) A31.9
- anonymous A31.9
- atypical A31.9
  - cutaneous A31.1
  - pulmonary A31.0
    - tuberculous — see Tuberculosis, pulmonary
  - specified site NEC A31.8
- avium (intracellulare complex) A31.0
- balnei A31.1
- Battey A31.0
- chelonei A31.8
- cutaneous A31.1
- extrapulmonary systemic A31.8
- fortuitum A31.8
- intracellulare (Battey bacillus) A31.0
- kakaferifu A31.8
- kansasii (yellow bacillus) A31.0
- kasongo A31.8
- leprae (see also Leprosy) A30.9
- luciflavum A31.1
- marinum (M. balnei) A31.1
- nonspecific — see Mycobacterium, atypical
- pulmonary (atypical) A31.0
  - tuberculous — see Tuberculosis, pulmonary
- scrofulaceum A31.8
- simiae A31.8
- systemic, extrapulmonary A31.8
- szulgai A31.8
- terrae A31.8
- triviale A31.8
- tuberculosis (human, bovine) — see Tuberculosis
- ulcerans A31.1
- xenopi A31.8

Mycoplasma (M.) **pneumoniae, as cause of disease classified elsewhere** B96.0
Mycosis, mycotic B49
- cutaneous NEC B36.9
- ear B36.9
  - in
    - aspergillosis B44.89
    - candidiasis B37.84
    - moniliasis B37.84
- fungoides (extranodal) (solid organ) C84.0- ☑
- mouth B37.0
- nails B35.1
- opportunistic B48.8
- skin NEC B36.9
- specified NEC B48.8
- stomatitis B37.0
- vagina, vaginitis (candidal) B37.3

Mydriasis (pupil) H57.04
Myelatelia Q06.1
Myelinolysis, pontine, central G37.2
Myelitis (acute) (ascending) (childhood) (chronic) (descending) (diffuse) (disseminated) (idiopathic) (pressure) (progressive) (spinal cord) (subacute) (see also Encephalitis) G04.91
- herpes simplex B00.82
- herpes zoster B02.24
- in diseases classified elsewhere G05.4
- necrotizing, subacute G37.4
- optic neuritis in G36.0
- postchickenpox B01.12
- postherpetic B02.24
- postimmunization G04.02
- postinfectious NEC G04.89
- postvaccinal G04.02
- specified NEC G04.89
- syphilitic (transverse) A52.14
- toxic G92
- transverse (in demyelinating diseases of central nervous system) G37.3
- tuberculous A17.82
- varicella B01.12

Myeloblastic — see condition
Myeloblastoma
- granular cell (see also Neoplasm, connective tissue)

Myeloblastoma — continued
- granular cell (see also Neoplasm, connective tissue) — continued
  - malignant — see Neoplasm, connective tissue, malignant
  - tongue D10.1

Myelocele — see Spina bifida
Myelocystocele — see Spina bifida
Myelocytic — see condition
Myelodysplasia D46.9
- specified NEC D46.Z (following D46.4)
- spinal cord (congenital) Q06.1

Myelodysplastic syndrome D46.9
- with
  - 5q deletion D46.C (following D46.2)
  - isolated del (5q) chromosomal abnormality D46.C (following D46.2)
- specified NEC D46.Z (following D46.4)

Myeloencephalitis — see Encephalitis
Myelofibrosis D75.81
- with myeloid metaplasia D47.4
- acute C94.4- ☑
- idiopathic (chronic) D47.4
- primary D47.1
- secondary D75.81
  - in myeloproliferative disease D47.4

Myelogenous — see condition
Myeloid — see condition
Myelokathexis D70.9
Myeloleukodystrophy E75.29
Myelolipoma — see Lipoma
Myeloma (multiple) C90.0- ☑
- monostotic C90.3 ☑
  - plasma cell C90.0- ☑
- plasma cell C90.0- ☑
- solitary (see also Plasmacytoma, solitary) C90.3- ☑

Myelomalacia G95.89
Myelomatosis C90.0- ☑
Myelomeningitis — see Meningoencephalitis
Myelomeningocele (spinal cord) — see Spina bifida
Myelo-osteo-musculodysplasia hereditaria Q79.8
Myelopathic
- anemia D64.89
- muscle atrophy — see Atrophy, muscle, spinal
- pain syndrome G89.0

Myelopathy (spinal cord) G95.9
- drug-induced G95.89
- in (due to)
  - degeneration or displacement, intervertebral disc NEC — see Disorder, disc, with, myelopathy
  - infection — see Encephalitis
  - intervertebral disc disorder (see also Disorder, disc, with, myelopathy)
  - mercury — see subcategory T56.1 ☑
  - neoplastic disease (see also Neoplasm) D49.9 [G99.2]
  - pernicious anemia D51.0 [G99.2]
  - spondylosis — see Spondylosis, with myelopathy NEC
- necrotic (subacute) (vascular) G95.19
- radiation-induced G95.89
- spondylogenic NEC — see Spondylosis, with myelopathy NEC
- toxic G95.89
- transverse, acute G37.3
- vascular G95.19
- vitamin B12 E53.8 [G32.0]

Myelophthisis D61.82
Myeloradiculitis G04.91
Myeloradiculodysplasia (spinal) Q06.1
Myelosarcoma C92.3- ☑
Myelosclerosis D75.89
- with myeloid metaplasia D47.4
- disseminated, of nervous system G35
- megakaryocytic D47.4
  - with myeloid metaplasia D47.4

Myelosis
- acute C92.0- ☑
- aleukemic C92.9- ☑
- chronic D47.1
- erythremic (acute) C94.0- ☑
- megakaryocytic C94.2- ☑
- nonleukemic D72.828
- subacute C92.9- ☑

Myiasis (cavernous) B87.9
- aural B87.4
- creeping B87.0
- cutaneous B87.0

Myiasis — *continued*
  dermal B87.0
  ear (external) (middle) B87.4
  eye B87.2
  genitourinary B87.81
  intestinal B87.82
  laryngeal B87.3
  nasopharyngeal B87.3
  ocular B87.2
  orbit B87.2
  skin B87.0
  specified site NEC B87.89
  traumatic B87.1
  wound B87.1
Myoadenoma, prostate — *see* Hyperplasia, prostate
Myoblastoma
  granular cell (*see also* Neoplasm, connective tissue, benign)
    malignant — *see* Neoplasm, connective tissue, malignant
  tongue D10.1
Myocardial — *see* condition
Myocardiopathy (congestive) (constrictive) (familial) (hypertrophic nonobstructive) (idiopathic) (infiltrative) (obstructive) (primary) (restrictive) (sporadic) (*see also* Cardiomyopathy) I42.9
  alcoholic I42.6
  cobalt-beer I42.6
  glycogen storage E74.02 [I43]
  hypertrophic obstructive I42.1
  in (due to)
    beriberi E51.12
    cardiac glycogenosis E74.02 [I43]
    Friedreich's ataxia G11.1 [I43]
    myotonia atrophica G71.11 [I43]
    progressive muscular dystrophy G71.09 [I43]
  obscure (African) I42.8
  secondary I42.9
  thyrotoxic E05.90 [I43]
    with storm E05.91 [I43]
  toxic NEC I42.7
Myocarditis (with arteriosclerosis)(chronic)(fibroid) (interstitial) (old) (progressive) (senile) I51.4
  with
    rheumatic fever (conditions in I00) I09.0
      active — *see* Myocarditis, acute, rheumatic
      inactive or quiescent (with chorea) I09.0
  active I40.9
    rheumatic I01.2
      with chorea (acute) (rheumatic) (Sydenham's) I02.0
  acute or subacute (interstitial) I40.9
    due to
      streptococcus (beta-hemolytic) I01.2
    idiopathic I40.1
    rheumatic I01.2
      with chorea (acute) (rheumatic) (Sydenham's) I02.0
    specified NEC I40.8
  aseptic of newborn B33.22
  bacterial (acute) I40.0
  Coxsackie (virus) B33.22
  diphtheritic A36.81
  eosinophilic I40.1
  epidemic of newborn (Coxsackie) B33.22
  Fiedler's (acute) (isolated) I40.1
  giant cell (acute) (subacute) I40.1
  gonococcal A54.83
  granulomatous (idiopathic) (isolated) (nonspecific) I40.1
  hypertensive — *see* Hypertension, heart
  idiopathic (granulomatous) I40.1
  in (due to)
    diphtheria A36.81
    epidemic louse-borne typhus A75.0 [I41]
    Lyme disease A69.29
    sarcoidosis D86.85
    scarlet fever A38.1
    toxoplasmosis (acquired) B58.81
    typhoid A01.02
    typhus NEC A75.9 [I41]
  infective I40.0
  influenzal — *see* Influenza, with, myocarditis
  isolated (acute) I40.1
  meningococcal A39.52
  mumps B26.82
  nonrheumatic, active I40.9
  parenchymatous I40.9
  pneumococcal I40.0

Myocarditis — *continued*
  rheumatic (chronic) (inactive) (with chorea) I09.0
    active or acute I01.2
      with chorea (acute) (rheumatic) (Sydenham's) I02.0
  rheumatoid — *see* Rheumatoid, carditis
  septic I40.0
  staphylococcal I40.0
  suppurative I40.0
  syphilitic (chronic) A52.06
  toxic I40.8
    rheumatic — *see* Myocarditis, acute, rheumatic
  tuberculous A18.84
  typhoid A01.02
  valvular — *see* Endocarditis
  virus, viral I40.0
    of newborn (Coxsackie) B33.22
Myocardium, myocardial — *see* condition
Myocardosis — *see* Cardiomyopathy
Myoclonus, myoclonic, myoclonia (familial) (essential) (multifocal) (simplex) G25.3
  drug-induced G25.3
  epilepsy (*see also* Epilepsy, generalized, specified NEC) G40.4- ☑
    familial (progressive) G25.3
  epileptica G40.409
    with status epilepticus G40.401
  facial G51.3- ☑
  familial progressive G25.3
  Friedreich's G25.3
  jerks G25.3
  massive G25.3
  palatal G25.3
  pharyngeal G25.3
Myocytolysis I51.5
Myodiastasis — *see* Diastasis, muscle
Myoendocarditis — *see* Endocarditis
Myoepithelioma — *see* Neoplasm, benign, by site
Myofasciitis (acute) — *see* Myositis
Myofibroma (*see also* Neoplasm, connective tissue, benign)
  uterus (cervix) (corpus) — *see* Leiomyoma
Myofibromatosis D48.1
  infantile Q89.8
Myofibrosis M62.89
  heart — *see* Myocarditis
  scapulohumeral — *see* Lesion, shoulder, specified NEC
Myofibrositis M79.7
  scapulohumeral — *see* Lesion, shoulder, specified NEC
Myoglobulinuria, myoglobinuria (primary) R82.1
Myokymia, facial G51.4
Myolipoma — *see* Lipoma
Myoma (*see also* Neoplasm, connective tissue, benign)
  malignant — *see* Neoplasm, connective tissue, malignant
  prostate D29.1
  uterus (cervix) (corpus) — *see* Leiomyoma
Myomalacia M62.89
Myometritis — *see* Endometritis
Myometrium — *see* condition
Myonecrosis, clostridial A48.0
Myopathy G72.9
  acute
    necrotizing G72.81
    quadriplegic G72.81
  alcoholic G72.1
  benign congenital G71.2
  central core G71.2
  centronuclear G71.2
  congenital (benign) G71.2
  critical illness G72.81
  distal G71.09
  drug-induced G72.0
  endocrine NEC E34.9 [G73.7]
  extraocular muscles H05.82- ☑
  facioscapulohumeral G71.02
  hereditary G71.9
    specified NEC G71.8
  immune NEC G72.49
  in (due to)
    Addison's disease E27.1 [G73.7]
    alcohol G72.1
    amyloidosis E85.0 [G73.7]
    cretinism E00.9 [G73.7]
    Cushing's syndrome E24.9 [G73.7]
    drugs G72.0
    endocrine disease NEC E34.9 [G73.7]
    giant cell arteritis M31.6 [G73.7]

Myopathy — *continued*
  in — *continued*
    glycogen storage disease E74.00 [G73.7]
    hyperadrenocorticism E24.9 [G73.7]
    hyperparathyroidism NEC E21.3 [G73.7]
    hypoparathyroidism E20.9 [G73.7]
    hypopituitarism E23.0 [G73.7]
    hypothyroidism E03.9 [G73.7]
    infectious disease NEC B99 ☑ [G73.7]
    lipid storage disease E75.6 [G73.7]
    metabolic disease NEC E88.9 [G73.7]
    myxedema E03.9 [G73.7]
    parasitic disease NEC B89 [G73.7]
    polyarteritis nodosa M30.0 [G73.7]
    rheumatoid arthritis — *see* Rheumatoid, myopathy
    sarcoidosis D86.87
    scleroderma M34.82
    sicca syndrome M35.03
    Sjögren's syndrome M35.03
    systemic lupus erythematosus M32.19
    thyrotoxicosis (hyperthyroidism) E05.90 [G73.7]
      with thyroid storm E05.91 [G73.7]
    toxic agent NEC G72.2
  inflammatory NEC G72.49
  intensive care (ICU) G72.81
  limb-girdle G71.09
  mitochondrial NEC G71.3
  myotubular G71.2
  mytonic, proximal (PROMM) G71.11
  nemaline G71.2
  ocular G71.09
  oculopharyngeal G71.09
  of critical illness G72.81
  primary G71.9
    specified NEC G71.8
  progressive NEC G72.89
  proximal myotonic (PROMM) G71.11
  rod G71.2
  scapulohumeral G71.02
  specified NEC G72.89
  toxic G72.2
Myopericarditis (*see also* Pericarditis)
  chronic rheumatic I09.2
Myopia (axial) (congenital) H52.1- ☑
  degenerative (malignant) H44.20
    with
      choroidal neovascularization H44.2A- ☑
      foveoschisis H44.2D- ☑
      macular hole H44.2B- ☑
      retinal detachment H44.2C- ☑
      specified maculopathy NEC H44.2E- ☑
    bilateral H44.23
    left eye H44.22
    right eye H44.21
  malignant (*see also* Myopia, degenerative) H44.2- ☑
  pernicious (*see also* Myopia, degenerative) H44.2- ☑
  progressive high (degenerative) (*see also* Myopia, degenerative) H44.2- ☑
Myosarcoma — *see* Neoplasm, connective tissue, malignant
Myosis (pupil) H57.03
  stromal (endolymphatic) D39.0
Myositis M60.9
  clostridial A48.0
  due to posture — *see* Myositis, specified type NEC
  epidemic B33.0
  fibrosa or fibrous (chronic), Volkmann's T79.6 ☑
  foreign body granuloma — *see* Granuloma, foreign body
  in (due to)
    bilharziasis B65.9 [M63.8-] ☑
    cysticercosis B69.81
    leprosy A30.9 [M63.8-] ☑
    mycosis B49 [M63.8-] ☑
    sarcoidosis D86.87
    schistosomiasis B65.9 [M63.8-] ☑
    syphilis
      late A52.78
      secondary A51.49
    toxoplasmosis (acquired) B58.82
    trichinellosis B75 [M63.8-] ☑
    tuberculosis A18.09
  inclusion body [IBM] G72.41
  infective M60.009
    arm M60.002
      left M60.001
      right M60.000
    leg M60.005

▽ Subterms under main terms may continue to next column or page   ☑ Additional Character Required — Refer to the Tabular List for Character Selection   **227**

Myiasis — Myositis

Myositis — *continued*
  infective — *continued*
    leg — *continued*
      left M60.004
      right M60.003
      lower limb M60.005
        ankle M60.07- ☑
        foot M60.07- ☑
        lower leg M60.06- ☑
        thigh M60.05- ☑
        toe M60.07- ☑
      multiple sites M60.09
      specified site NEC M60.08
      upper limb M60.002
        finger M60.04- ☑
        forearm M60.03- ☑
        hand M60.04- ☑
        shoulder region M60.01- ☑
        upper arm M60.02- ☑
  interstitial M60.10
    ankle M60.17- ☑
    foot M60.17- ☑
    forearm M60.13- ☑
    hand M60.14- ☑
    lower leg M60.16- ☑
    multiple sites M60.19
    shoulder region M60.11- ☑
    specified site NEC M60.18
    thigh M60.15- ☑
    upper arm M60.12- ☑
  mycotic B49 [M63.8-] ☑
  orbital, chronic H05.12- ☑
  ossificans or ossifying (circumscripta) (*see also* Ossification, muscle, specified NEC)
    in (due to)
      burns M61.30
        ankle M61.37- ☑
        foot M61.37- ☑
        forearm M61.33- ☑
        hand M61.34- ☑
        lower leg M61.36- ☑
        multiple sites M61.39
        pelvic region M61.35- ☑
        shoulder region M61.31- ☑
        specified site NEC M61.38
        thigh M61.35- ☑
        upper arm M61.32- ☑
      quadriplegia or paraplegia M61.20
        ankle M61.27- ☑
        foot M61.27- ☑
        forearm M61.23- ☑
        hand M61.24- ☑

Myositis — *continued*
  ossificans or ossifying (*see also* Ossification, muscle, specified) — *continued*
    in — *continued*
      quadriplegia or paraplegia — *continued*
        lower leg M61.26- ☑
        multiple sites M61.29
        pelvic region M61.25- ☑
        shoulder region M61.21- ☑
        specified site NEC M61.28
        thigh M61.25- ☑
        upper arm M61.22- ☑
    progressiva M61.10
      ankle M61.17- ☑
      finger M61.14- ☑
      foot M61.17- ☑
      forearm M61.13- ☑
      hand M61.14- ☑
      lower leg M61.16- ☑
      multiple sites M61.19
      pelvic region M61.15- ☑
      shoulder region M61.11- ☑
      specified site NEC M61.18
      thigh M61.15- ☑
      toe M61.17- ☑
      upper arm M61.12- ☑
    traumatica M61.00
      ankle M61.07- ☑
      foot M61.07- ☑
      forearm M61.03- ☑
      hand M61.04- ☑
      lower leg M61.06- ☑
      multiple sites M61.09
      pelvic region M61.05- ☑
      shoulder region M61.01- ☑
      specified site NEC M61.08
      thigh M61.05- ☑
      upper arm M61.02- ☑
  purulent — *see* Myositis, infective
  specified type NEC M60.80
    ankle M60.87- ☑
    foot M60.87- ☑
    forearm M60.83- ☑
    hand M60.84- ☑
    lower leg M60.86- ☑
    multiple sites M60.89
    pelvic region M60.85- ☑
    shoulder region M60.81- ☑
    specified site NEC M60.88
    thigh M60.85- ☑
    upper arm M60.82- ☑
  suppurative — *see* Myositis, infective

Myositis — *continued*
  traumatic (old) — *see* Myositis, specified type NEC
Myospasia impulsiva F95.2
Myotonia (acquisita) (intermittens) M62.89
  atrophica G71.11
  chondrodystrophic G71.13
  congenita (acetazolamide responsive) (dominant) (recessive) G71.12
  drug-induced G71.14
  dystrophica G71.11
  fluctuans G71.19
  levior G71.12
  permanens G71.19
  symptomatic G71.19
Myotonic pupil — *see* Anomaly, pupil, function, tonic pupil
Myriapodiasis B88.2
Myringitis H73.2- ☑
  with otitis media — *see* Otitis, media
  acute H73.00- ☑
    bullous H73.01- ☑
    specified NEC H73.09- ☑
  bullous — *see* Myringitis, acute, bullous
  chronic H73.1- ☑
Mysophobia F40.228
Mytilotoxism — *see* Poisoning, fish
Myxadenitis labialis K13.0
Myxedema (adult) (idiocy) (infantile) (juvenile) (*see also* Hypothyroidism) E03.9
  circumscribed E05.90
    with storm E05.91
  coma E03.5
  congenital E00.1
  cutis L98.5
  localized (pretibial) E05.90
    with storm E05.91
  papular L98.5
Myxochondrosarcoma — *see* Neoplasm, cartilage, malignant
Myxofibroma — *see* Neoplasm, connective tissue, benign
  odontogenic — *see* Cyst, calcifying odontogenic
Myxofibrosarcoma — *see* Neoplasm, connective tissue, malignant
Myxolipoma D17.9
Myxoliposarcoma — *see* Neoplasm, connective tissue, malignant
Myxoma (*see also* Neoplasm, connective tissue, benign)
  nerve sheath — *see* Neoplasm, nerve, benign
  odontogenic — *see* Cyst, calcifying odontogenic
Myxosarcoma — *see* Neoplasm, connective tissue, malignant

☑ **Additional Character Required** — **Refer to the Tabular List for Character Selection**   🔻 **Subterms under main terms may continue to next column or page**

N

Naegeli's
  disease Q82.8
  leukemia, monocytic C93.1- ☑
Naegleriasis (with meningoencephalitis) B60.2
Naffziger's syndrome G54.0
Naga sore — *see* Ulcer, skin
Nägele's pelvis M95.5
  with disproportion (fetopelvic) O33.0
    causing obstructed labor O65.0
Nail (*see also* condition)
  biting F98.8
  patella syndrome Q87.2
Nanism, nanosomia — *see* Dwarfism
Nanophyetiasis B66.8
Nanukayami A27.89
Napkin rash L22
Narcolepsy G47.419
  with cataplexy G47.411
  in conditions classified elsewhere G47.429
    with cataplexy G47.421
Narcosis R06.89
Narcotism — *see* Dependence
NARP (Neuropathy, Ataxia and Retinitis pigmentosa)
    syndrome E88.49
Narrow
  anterior chamber angle H40.03- ☑
  gingival width (of periodontal soft tissue) K05.5
  pelvis — *see* Contraction, pelvis
Narrowing (*see also* Stenosis)
  artery I77.1
    auditory, internal I65.8
    basilar — *see* Occlusion, artery, basilar
    carotid — *see* Occlusion, artery, carotid
    cerebellar — *see* Occlusion, artery, cerebellar
    cerebral — *see* Occlusion artery, cerebral
    choroidal — *see* Occlusion, artery, cerebral, specified
      NEC
    communicating posterior — *see* Occlusion, artery,
      cerebral, specified NEC
    coronary (*see also* Disease, heart, ischemic,
      atherosclerotic)
      congenital Q24.5
        syphilitic A50.54 [I52]
      due to syphilis NEC A52.06
    hypophyseal — *see* Occlusion, artery, cerebral,
      specified NEC
    pontine — *see* Occlusion, artery, cerebral, specified
      NEC
    precerebral — *see* Occlusion, artery, precerebral
    vertebral — *see* Occlusion, artery, vertebral
  auditory canal (external) — *see* Stenosis, external ear
    canal
  eustachian tube — *see* Obstruction, eustachian tube
  eyelid — *see* Disorder, eyelid function
  larynx J38.6
  mesenteric artery (*see also* Ischemia, intestine, acute)
    K55.059
  palate M26.89
  palpebral fissure — *see* Disorder, eyelid function
  ureter N13.5
    with infection N13.6
  urethra — *see* Stricture, urethra
Narrowness, abnormal, eyelid Q10.3
Nasal — *see* condition
Nasolachrymal, nasolacrimal — *see* condition
Nasopharyngeal (*see also* condition)
  pituitary gland Q89.2
  torticollis M43.6
Nasopharyngitis (acute) (infective) (streptococcal)
    (subacute) J00
  chronic (suppurative) (ulcerative) J31.1
Nasopharynx, nasopharyngeal — *see* condition
Natal tooth, teeth K00.6
Nausea (without vomiting) R11.0
  with vomiting R11.2
  gravidarum — *see* Hyperemesis, gravidarum
  marina T75.3 ☑
  navalis T75.3 ☑
Navel — *see* condition
Neapolitan fever — *see* Brucellosis
Near drowning T75.1 ☑
Nearsightedness — *see* Myopia
Near-syncope R55
Nebula, cornea — *see* Opacity, cornea

Necator americanus infestation B76.1
Necatoriasis B76.1
Neck — *see* condition
Necrobiosis R68.89
  lipoidica NEC L92.1
    with diabetes — *see* E08-E13 with .620
Necrolysis, toxic epidermal L51.2
  due to drug
    correct substance properly administered — *see* Ta-
      ble of Drugs and Chemicals, by drug, adverse
      effect
    overdose or wrong substance given or taken — *see*
      Table of Drugs and Chemicals, by drug, poi-
      soning
Necrophilia F65.89
Necrosis, necrotic (ischemic) (*see also* Gangrene)
  adrenal (capsule) (gland) E27.49
  amputation stump (surgical) (late) T87.50
    arm T87.5- ☑
    leg T87.5- ☑
  antrum J32.0
  aorta (hyaline) (*see also* Aneurysm, aorta)
    cystic medial — *see* Dissection, aorta
  artery I77.5
  bladder (aseptic) (sphincter) N32.89
  bone (*see also* Osteonecrosis) M87.9
    aseptic or avascular — *see* Osteonecrosis
      idiopathic M87.00
    ethmoid J32.2
    jaw M27.2
    tuberculous — *see* Tuberculosis, bone
  brain I67.89
  breast (aseptic) (fat) (segmental) N64.1
  bronchus J98.09
  central nervous system NEC I67.89
  cerebellar I67.89
  cerebral I67.89
  colon (*see also* Infarct, intestine) K55.049
  cornea H18.89- ☑
  cortical (acute) (renal) N17.1
  cystic medial (aorta) — *see* Dissection, aorta
  dental pulp K04.1
  esophagus K22.8
  ethmoid (bone) J32.2
  eyelid — *see* Disorder, eyelid, degenerative
  fat, fatty (generalized) (*see also* Disorder, soft tissue,
      specified type NEC)
    abdominal wall K65.4
    breast (aseptic) (segmental) N64.1
    localized — *see* Degeneration, by site, fatty
    mesentery K65.4
    omentum K65.4
    pancreas K86.89
    peritoneum K65.4
    skin (subcutaneous), newborn P83.0
    subcutaneous, due to birth injury P15.6
  gallbladder — *see* Cholecystitis, acute
  heart — *see* Infarct, myocardium
  hip, aseptic or avascular — *see* Osteonecrosis, by type,
    femur
  intestine (acute) (hemorrhagic) (massive) (*see also* In-
    farct, intestine) K55.069
  jaw M27.2
  kidney (bilateral) N28.0
    acute N17.9
    cortical (acute) (bilateral) N17.1
      with ectopic or molar pregnancy O08.4
    medullary (bilateral) (in acute renal failure) (papil-
      lary) N17.2
    papillary (bilateral) (in acute renal failure) N17.2
    tubular N17.0
      with ectopic or molar pregnancy O08.4
      complicating
        abortion — *see* Abortion, by type, complicat-
          ed by, tubular necrosis
        ectopic or molar pregnancy O08.4
        pregnancy — *see* Pregnancy, complicated by,
          diseases of, specified type or system
          NEC
      following ectopic or molar pregnancy O08.4
      traumatic T79.5 ☑
  larynx J38.7
  liver (with hepatic failure) (cell) — *see* Failure, hepatic
    hemorrhagic, central K76.2
  lung J85.0
  lymphatic gland — *see* Lymphadenitis, acute
  mammary gland (fat) (segmental) N64.1
  mastoid (chronic) — *see* Mastoiditis, chronic

Necrosis, necrotic — *continued*
  medullary (acute) (renal) N17.2
  mesentery (*see also* Infarct, intestine) K55.069
    fat K65.4
  mitral valve — *see* Insufficiency, mitral
  myocardium, myocardial — *see* Infarct, myocardium
  nose J34.0
  omentum (with mesenteric infarction) (*see also* Infarct,
      intestine) K55.069
    fat K65.4
  orbit, orbital — *see* Osteomyelitis, orbit
  ossicles, ear — *see* Abnormal, ear ossicles
  ovary N70.92
  pancreas (aseptic) (duct) (fat) K86.89
    acute (infective) — *see* Pancreatitis, acute
    infective — *see* Pancreatitis, acute
  papillary (acute) (renal) N17.2
  perineum N90.89
  peritoneum (with mesenteric infarction) (*see also* In-
    farct, intestine) K55.069
    fat K65.4
  pharynx J02.9
    in granulocytopenia — *see* Neutropenia
    Vincent's A69.1
  phosphorus — *see* subcategory T54.2 ☑
  pituitary (gland) E23.0
    postpartum O99.285
    Sheehan O99.285
  pressure — *see* Ulcer, pressure, by site
  pulmonary J85.0
  pulp (dental) K04.1
  radiation — *see* Necrosis, by site
  radium — *see* Necrosis, by site
  renal — *see* Necrosis, kidney
  sclera H15.89
  scrotum N50.89
  skin or subcutaneous tissue NEC I96
  spine, spinal (column) (*see also* Osteonecrosis, by type,
      vertebra)
    cord G95.19
  spleen D73.5
  stomach K31.89
  stomatitis (ulcerative) A69.0
  subcutaneous fat, newborn P83.88
  subendocardial (acute) I21.4
    chronic I25.89
  suprarenal (capsule) (gland) E27.49
  testis N50.89
  thymus (gland) E32.8
  tonsil J35.8
  trachea J39.8
  tuberculous NEC — *see* Tuberculosis
  tubular (acute) (anoxic) (renal) (toxic) N17.0
    postprocedural N99.0
  vagina N89.8
  vertebra (*see also* Osteonecrosis, by type, vertebra)
    tuberculous A18.01
  vulva N90.89
  X-ray — *see* Necrosis, by site
Necrospermia — *see* Infertility, male
Need (for)
  care provider because (of)
    assistance with personal care Z74.1
    continuous supervision required Z74.3
    impaired mobility Z74.09
    no other household member able to render care
      Z74.2
    specified reason NEC Z74.8
  immunization — *see* Vaccination
  vaccination — *see* Vaccination
Neglect
  adult
    confirmed T74.01 ☑
    history of Z91.412
    suspected T76.01 ☑
  child (childhood)
    confirmed T74.02 ☑
    history of Z62.812
    suspected T76.02 ☑
  emotional, in childhood Z62.898
  hemispatial R41.4
  left-sided R41.4
  sensory R41.4
  visuospatial R41.4
Neisserian infection NEC — *see* Gonococcus
Nelaton's syndrome G60.8
Nelson's syndrome E24.1
Nematodiasis (intestinal) B82.0

Nematodiasis — *continued*
  Ancylostoma B76.0
Neonatal (*see also* Newborn)
  acne L70.4
  bradycardia P29.12
  screening, abnormal findings on P09
  tachycardia P29.11
  tooth, teeth K00.6
Neonatorum — *see* condition
Neoplasia
  endocrine, multiple (MEN) E31.20
    type I E31.21
    type IIA E31.22
    type IIB E31.23
  intraepithelial (histologically confirmed)
    anal (AIN) (histologically confirmed) K62.82
      grade I K62.82
      grade II K62.82
      severe D01.3
    cervical glandular (histologically confirmed) D06.9
    cervix (uteri) (CIN) (histologically confirmed) N87.9
      glandular D06.9
      grade I N87.0
      grade II N87.1
      grade III (severe dysplasia) (*see also* Carcinoma, cervix uteri, in situ) D06.9
    prostate (histologically confirmed) (PIN) N42.31
      grade I N42.31
      grade II N42.31
      grade III (severe dysplasia) D07.5
    vagina (histologically confirmed) (VAIN) N89.3
      grade I N89.0
      grade II N89.1
      grade III (severe dysplasia) D07.2
    vulva (histologically confirmed) (VIN) N90.3
      grade I N90.0
      grade II N90.1
      grade III (severe dysplasia) D07.1
Neoplasm, neoplastic (*see also* Table of Neoplasms)
  lipomatous, benign — *see* Lipoma
  malignant mast cell C96.20
    specified type NEC C96.29
  mast cell, of uncertain behavior NEC D47.09
Neovascularization
  ciliary body — *see* Disorder, iris, vascular
  cornea H16.40- ☑
    deep H16.44- ☑
    ghost vessels — *see* Ghost, vessels
    localized H16.43- ☑
    pannus — *see* Pannus
  iris — *see* Disorder, iris, vascular
  retina H35.05- ☑
Nephralgia N23
Nephritis, nephritic (albuminuric) (azotemic) (congenital) (disseminated) (epithelial) (familial) (focal) (granulomatous) (hemorrhagic) (infantile) (nonsuppurative, excretory) (uremic) N05.9
  with
    dense deposit disease N05.6
    diffuse
      crescentic glomerulonephritis N05.7
      endocapillary proliferative glomerulonephritis N05.4
      membranous glomerulonephritis N05.2
      mesangial proliferative glomerulonephritis N05.3
      mesangiocapillary glomerulonephritis N05.5
    edema — *see* Nephrosis
    focal and segmental glomerular lesions N05.1
    foot process disease N04.9
    glomerular lesion
      diffuse sclerosing N05.8
      hypocomplementemic — *see* Nephritis, membranoproliferative
      IgA — *see* Nephropathy, IgA
      lobular, lobulonodular — *see* Nephritis, membranoproliferative
      nodular — *see* Nephritis, membranoproliferative
    lesion of
      glomerulonephritis, proliferative N05.8
      renal necrosis N05.9
    minor glomerular abnormality N05.0
    specified morphological changes NEC N05.8
  acute N00.9
    with
      dense deposit disease N00.6
      diffuse
        crescentic glomerulonephritis N00.7

Nephritis, nephritic — *continued*
  acute — *continued*
    with — *continued*
      diffuse — *continued*
        endocapillary proliferative glomerulonephritis N00.4
        membranous glomerulonephritis N00.2
        mesangial proliferative glomerulonephritis N00.3
        mesangiocapillary glomerulonephritis N00.5
      focal and segmental glomerular lesions N00.1
      minor glomerular abnormality N00.0
      specified morphological changes NEC N00.8
  amyloid E85.4 [N08]
  antiglomerular basement membrane (anti-GBM) antibody NEC
    in Goodpasture's syndrome M31.0
  antitubular basement membrane (tubulo-interstitial) NEC N12
    toxic — *see* Nephropathy, toxic
  arteriolar — *see* Hypertension, kidney
  arteriosclerotic — *see* Hypertension, kidney
  ascending — *see* Nephritis, tubulo-interstitial
  atrophic N03.9
  Balkan (endemic) N15.0
  calculous, calculus — *see* Calculus, kidney
  cardiac — *see* Hypertension, kidney
  cardiovascular — *see* Hypertension, kidney
  chronic N03.9
    with
      dense deposit disease N03.6
      diffuse
        crescentic glomerulonephritis N03.7
        endocapillary proliferative glomerulonephritis N03.4
        membranous glomerulonephritis N03.2
        mesangial proliferative glomerulonephritis N03.3
        mesangiocapillary glomerulonephritis N03.5
      focal and segmental glomerular lesions N03.1
      minor glomerular abnormality N03.0
      specified morphological changes NEC N03.8
    arteriosclerotic — *see* Hypertension, kidney
  cirrhotic N26.9
  complicating pregnancy O26.83- ☑
  croupous N00.9
  degenerative — *see* Nephrosis
  diffuse sclerosing N05.8
  due to
    diabetes mellitus — *see* E08-E13 with .21
    subacute bacterial endocarditis I33.0
    systemic lupus erythematosus (chronic) M32.14
    typhoid fever A01.09
  gonococcal (acute) (chronic) A54.21
  hypocomplementemic — *see* Nephritis, membranoproliferative
  IgA — *see* Nephropathy, IgA
  immune complex (circulating) NEC N05.8
  infective — *see* Nephritis, tubulo-interstitial
  interstitial — *see* Nephritis, tubulo-interstitial
  lead N14.3
  membranoproliferative (diffuse) (type 1 or 3) (*see also* N00-N07 with fourth character .5) N05.5
    type 2 (*see also* N00-N07 with fourth character .6) N05.6
  minimal change N05.0
  necrotic, necrotizing NEC (*see also* N00-N07 with fourth character .8) N05.8
  nephrotic — *see* Nephrosis
  nodular — *see* Nephritis, membranoproliferative
  polycystic Q61.3
    adult type Q61.2
    autosomal
      dominant Q61.2
      recessive NEC Q61.19
    childhood type NEC Q61.19
    infantile type NEC Q61.19
  poststreptococcal N05.9
    acute N00.9
    chronic N03.9
    rapidly progressive N01.9
  proliferative NEC (*see also* N00-N07 with fourth character .8) N05.8
  purulent — *see* Nephritis, tubulo-interstitial
  rapidly progressive N01.9
    with
      dense deposit disease N01.6
      diffuse

Nephritis, nephritic — *continued*
  rapidly progressive — *continued*
    with — *continued*
      diffuse — *continued*
        crescentic glomerulonephritis N01.7
        endocapillary proliferative glomerulonephritis N01.4
        membranous glomerulonephritis N01.2
        mesangial proliferative glomerulonephritis N01.3
        mesangiocapillary glomerulonephritis N01.5
      focal and segmental glomerular lesions N01.1
      minor glomerular abnormality N01.0
      specified morphological changes NEC N01.8
  salt losing or wasting NEC N28.89
  saturnine N14.3
  sclerosing, diffuse N05.8
  septic — *see* Nephritis, tubulo-interstitial
  specified pathology NEC (*see also* N00-N07 with fourth character .8) N05.8
  subacute N01.9
  suppurative — *see* Nephritis, tubulo-interstitial
  syphilitic (late) A52.75
    congenital A50.59 [N08]
    early (secondary) A51.44
  toxic — *see* Nephropathy, toxic
  tubal, tubular — *see* Nephritis, tubulo-interstitial
  tuberculous A18.11
  tubulo-interstitial (in) N12
    acute (infectious) N10
    chronic (infectious) N11.9
      nonobstructive N11.8
        reflux-associated N11.0
      obstructive N11.1
      specified NEC N11.8
    due to
      brucellosis A23.9 [N16]
      cryoglobulinemia D89.1 [N16]
      glycogen storage disease E74.00 [N16]
      Sjögren's syndrome M35.04
  vascular — *see* Hypertension, kidney
  war N00.9
Nephroblastoma (epithelial) (mesenchymal) C64- ☑
Nephrocalcinosis E83.59 [N29]
Nephrocystitis, pustular — *see* Nephritis, tubulo-interstitial
Nephrolithiasis (congenital) (pelvis) (recurrent) (*see also* Calculus, kidney)
Nephroma C64- ☑
  mesoblastic D41.0- ☑
Nephronephritis — *see* Nephrosis
Nephronophthisis Q61.5
Nephropathia epidemica A98.5
Nephropathy (*see also* Nephritis) N28.9
  with
    edema — *see* Nephrosis
    glomerular lesion — *see* Glomerulonephritis
  amyloid, hereditary E85.0
  analgesic N14.0
    with medullary necrosis, acute N17.2
  Balkan (endemic) N15.0
  chemical — *see* Nephropathy, toxic
  diabetic — *see* E08-E13 with .21
  drug-induced N14.2
    specified NEC N14.1
  focal and segmental hyalinosis or sclerosis N02.1
  heavy metal-induced N14.3
  hereditary NEC N07.9
    with
      dense deposit disease N07.6
      diffuse
        crescentic glomerulonephritis N07.7
        endocapillary proliferative glomerulonephritis N07.4
        membranous glomerulonephritis N07.2
        mesangial proliferative glomerulonephritis N07.3
        mesangiocapillary glomerulonephritis N07.5
      focal and segmental glomerular lesions N07.1
      minor glomerular abnormality N07.0
      specified morphological changes NEC N07.8
  hypercalcemic N25.89
  hypertensive — *see* Hypertension, kidney
  hypokalemic (vacuolar) N25.89
  IgA N02.8
    with glomerular lesion N02.9
      focal and segmental hyalinosis or sclerosis N02.1
      membranoproliferative (diffuse) N02.5

Nephropathy — *continued*
  IgA — *continued*
    with glomerular lesion — *continued*
      membranous (diffuse) N02.2
      mesangial proliferative (diffuse) N02.3
      mesangiocapillary (diffuse) N02.5
      proliferative NEC N02.8
      specified pathology NEC N02.8
  lead N14.3
  membranoproliferative (diffuse) N02.5
  membranous (diffuse) N02.2
  mesangial (IgA/IgG) — *see* Nephropathy, IgA
    proliferative (diffuse) N02.3
  mesangiocapillary (diffuse) N02.5
  obstructive N13.8
  phenacetin N17.2
  phosphate-losing N25.0
  potassium depletion N25.89
  pregnancy-related O26.83- ☑
  proliferative NEC (*see also* N00-N07 with fourth character .8) N05.8
  protein-losing N25.89
  saturnine N14.3
  sickle-cell D57.- ☑ [N08]
  toxic NEC N14.4
    due to
      drugs N14.2
        analgesic N14.0
        specified NEC N14.1
      heavy metals N14.3
  vasomotor N17.0
  water-losing N25.89
Nephroptosis N28.83
Nephropyosis — *see* Abscess, kidney
Nephrorrhagia N28.89
Nephrosclerosis (arteriolar)(arteriosclerotic) (chronic) (hyaline) (*see also* Hypertension, kidney)
  hyperplastic — *see* Hypertension, kidney
  senile N26.9
Nephrosis, nephrotic (Epstein's) (syndrome) (congenital) N04.9
  with
    foot process disease N04.9
    glomerular lesion N04.1
    hypocomplementemic N04.5
  acute N04.9
  anoxic — *see* Nephrosis, tubular
  chemical — *see* Nephrosis, tubular
  cholemic K76.7
  diabetic — *see* E08-E13 with .21
  Finnish type (congenital) Q89.8
  hemoglobin N10
  hemoglobinuric — *see* Nephrosis, tubular
  in
    amyloidosis E85.4 [N08]
    diabetes mellitus — *see* E08-E13 with .21
    epidemic hemorrhagic fever A98.5
    malaria (malariae) B52.0
  ischemic — *see* Nephrosis, tubular
  lipoid N04.9
  lower nephron — *see* Nephrosis, tubular
  malarial (malariae) B52.0
  minimal change N04.0
  myoglobin N10
  necrotizing — *see* Nephrosis, tubular
  osmotic (sucrose) N25.89
  radiation N04.9
  syphilitic (late) A52.75
  toxic — *see* Nephrosis, tubular
  tubular (acute) N17.0
    postprocedural N99.0
    radiation N04.9
Nephrosonephritis, hemorrhagic (endemic) A98.5
Nephrostomy
  attention to Z43.6
  status Z93.6
Nerve (*see also* condition)
  injury — *see* Injury, nerve, by body site
Nerves R45.0
Nervous (*see also* condition) R45.0
  heart F45.8
  stomach F45.8
  tension R45.0
Nervousness R45.0
Nesidioblastoma
  pancreas D13.7
  specified site NEC — *see* Neoplasm, benign, by site
  unspecified site D13.7

Nettleship's syndrome — *see* Urticaria pigmentosa
Neumann's disease or syndrome L10.1
Neuralgia, neuralgic (acute) M79.2
  accessory (nerve) G52.8
  acoustic (nerve) — *see* subcategory H93.3 ☑
  auditory (nerve) — *see* subcategory H93.3 ☑
  ciliary G44.009
    intractable G44.001
    not intractable G44.009
  cranial
    nerve (*see also* Disorder, nerve, cranial)
      fifth or trigeminal — *see* Neuralgia, trigeminal
      postherpetic, postzoster B02.29
  ear — *see* subcategory H92.0 ☑
  facialis vera G51.1
  Fothergill's — *see* Neuralgia, trigeminal
  glossopharyngeal (nerve) G52.1
  Horton's G44.009
    intractable G44.091
    not intractable G44.099
  Hunt's B02.21
  hypoglossal (nerve) G52.3
  infraorbital — *see* Neuralgia, trigeminal
  malarial — *see* Malaria
  migrainous G44.009
    intractable G44.001
    not intractable G44.009
  Morton's G57.6- ☑
  nerve, cranial — *see* Disorder, nerve, cranial
  nose G52.0
  occipital M54.81
  olfactory G52.0
  penis N48.9
  perineum R10.2
  postherpetic NEC B02.29
    trigeminal B02.22
  pubic region R10.2
  scrotum R10.2
  Sluder's G44.89
  specified nerve NEC G58.8
  spermatic cord R10.2
  sphenopalatine (ganglion) G90.09
  trifacial — *see* Neuralgia, trigeminal
  trigeminal G50.0
    postherpetic, postzoster B02.22
  vagus (nerve) G52.2
  writer's F48.8
    organic G25.89
Neurapraxia — *see* Injury, nerve
Neurasthenia F48.8
  cardiac F45.8
  gastric F45.8
  heart F45.8
Neurilemmoma (*see also* Neoplasm, nerve, benign)
  acoustic (nerve) D33.3
  malignant (*see also* Neoplasm, nerve, malignant)
    acoustic (nerve) C72.4- ☑
Neurilemmosarcoma — *see* Neoplasm, nerve, malignant
Neurinoma — *see* Neoplasm, nerve, benign
Neurinomatosis — *see* Neoplasm, nerve, uncertain behavior
Neuritis (rheumatoid) M79.2
  abducens (nerve) — *see* Strabismus, paralytic, sixth nerve
  accessory (nerve) G52.8
  acoustic (nerve) (*see also* subcategory) H93.3 ☑
    in (due to)
      infectious disease NEC B99 ☑ [H94.0-] ☑
      parasitic disease NEC B89 [H94.0-] ☑
      syphilitic A52.15
  alcoholic G62.1
    with psychosis — *see* Psychosis, alcoholic
  amyloid, any site E85.4 [G63]
  auditory (nerve) — *see* subcategory H93.3 ☑
  brachial — *see* Radiculopathy
    due to displacement, intervertebral disc — *see* Disorder, disc, cervical, with neuritis
  cranial nerve
    due to Lyme disease A69.22
    eighth or acoustic or auditory — *see* subcategory H93.3 ☑
    eleventh or accessory G52.8
    fifth or trigeminal G51.0
    first or olfactory G52.0
    fourth or trochlear — *see* Strabismus, paralytic, fourth nerve
    second or optic — *see* Neuritis, optic
    seventh or facial G51.8

Neuritis — *continued*
  cranial nerve — *continued*
    seventh or facial — *continued*
      newborn (birth injury) P11.3
    sixth or abducent — *see* Strabismus, paralytic, sixth nerve
    tenth or vagus G52.2
    third or oculomotor — *see* Strabismus, paralytic, third nerve
    twelfth or hypoglossal G52.3
  Déjérine-Sottas G60.0
  diabetic (mononeuropathy) — *see* E08-E13 with .41
    polyneuropathy — *see* E08-E13 with .42
  due to
    beriberi E51.11
    displacement, prolapse or rupture, intervertebral disc — *see* Disorder, disc, with, radiculopathy
    herniation, nucleus pulposus M51.9 [G55]
  endemic E51.11
  facial G51.8
    newborn (birth injury) P11.3
  general — *see* Polyneuropathy
  geniculate ganglion G51.1
    due to herpes (zoster) B02.21
  gouty (*see also* Gout, by type) M10.9 [G63]
  hypoglossal (nerve) G52.3
  ilioinguinal (nerve) G57.9- ☑
  infectious (multiple) NEC G61.0
  interstitial hypertrophic progressive G60.0
  lumbar M54.16
  lumbosacral M54.17
  multiple (*see also* Polyneuropathy)
    endemic E51.11
    infective, acute G61.0
  multiplex endemica E51.11
  nerve root — *see* Radiculopathy
  oculomotor (nerve) — *see* Strabismus, paralytic, third nerve
  olfactory nerve G52.0
  optic (nerve) (hereditary) (sympathetic) H46.9
    with demyelination G36.0
    in myelitis G36.0
    nutritional H46.2
    papillitis — *see* Papillitis, optic
    retrobulbar H46.1- ☑
    specified type NEC H46.8
    toxic H46.3
  peripheral (nerve) G62.9
    multiple — *see* Polyneuropathy
    single — *see* Mononeuritis
  pneumogastric (nerve) G52.2
  postherpetic, postzoster B02.29
  progressive hypertrophic interstitial G60.0
  retrobulbar (*see also* Neuritis, optic, retrobulbar)
    in (due to)
      late syphilis A52.15
      meningococcal infection A39.82
    meningococcal A39.82
    syphilitic A52.15
  sciatic (nerve) (*see also* Sciatica)
    due to displacement of intervertebral disc — *see* Disorder, disc, with, radiculopathy
  serum (*see also* Reaction, serum) T80.69 ☑
  shoulder-girdle G54.5
  specified nerve NEC G58.8
  spinal (nerve) root — *see* Radiculopathy
  syphilitic A52.15
  thenar (median) G56.1- ☑
  thoracic M54.14
  toxic NEC G62.2
  trochlear (nerve) — *see* Strabismus, paralytic, fourth nerve
  vagus (nerve) G52.2
Neuroastrocytoma — *see* Neoplasm, uncertain behavior, by site
Neuroavitaminosis E56.9 [G99.8]
Neuroblastoma
  olfactory C30.0
  specified site — *see* Neoplasm, malignant, by site
  unspecified site C74.90
Neurochorioretinitis — *see* Chorioretinitis
Neurocirculatory asthenia F45.8
Neurocysticercosis B69.0
Neurocytoma — *see* Neoplasm, benign, by site
Neurodermatitis (circumscribed) (circumscripta) (local) L28.0
  atopic L20.81
  diffuse (Brocq) L20.81

Neurodermatitis — *continued*
  disseminated L20.81
Neuroencephalomyelopathy, optic G36.0
Neuroepithelioma (*see also* Neoplasm, malignant, by site)
  olfactory C30.0
Neurofibroma (*see also* Neoplasm, nerve, benign)
  melanotic — *see* Neoplasm, nerve, benign
  multiple — *see* Neurofibromatosis
  plexiform — *see* Neoplasm, nerve, benign
Neurofibromatosis (multiple) (nonmalignant) Q85.00
  acoustic Q85.02
  malignant — *see* Neoplasm, nerve, malignant
  specified NEC Q85.09
  type 1 (von Recklinghausen) Q85.01
  type 2 Q85.02
Neurofibrosarcoma — *see* Neoplasm, nerve, malignant
Neurogenic (*see also* condition)
  bladder (*see also* Dysfunction, bladder, neuromuscular) N31.9
    cauda equina syndrome G83.4
  bowel NEC K59.2
  heart F45.8
Neuroglioma — *see* Neoplasm, uncertain behavior, by site
Neurolabyrinthitis (of Dix and Hallpike) — *see* Neuronitis, vestibular
Neurolathyrism — *see* Poisoning, food, noxious, plant
Neuroleprosy A30.9
Neuroma (*see also* Neoplasm, nerve, benign)
  acoustic (nerve) D33.3
  amputation (stump) (traumatic) (surgical complication) (late) T87.3- ☑
    arm T87.3- ☑
    leg T87.3- ☑
  digital (toe) G57.6- ☑
  interdigital G58.8
    lower limb (toe) G57.8- ☑
    upper limb G56.8- ☑
  intermetatarsal G57.8- ☑
  Morton's G57.6- ☑
  nonneoplastic
    arm G56.9- ☑
    leg G57.9- ☑
    lower extremity G57.9- ☑
    upper extremity G56.9- ☑
  optic (nerve) D33.3
  plantar G57.6- ☑
  plexiform — *see* Neoplasm, nerve, benign
  surgical (nonneoplastic)
    arm G56.9- ☑
    leg G57.9- ☑
    lower extremity G57.9- ☑
    upper extremity G56.9- ☑
Neuromyalgia — *see* Neuralgia
Neuromyasthenia (epidemic) (postinfectious) G93.3
Neuromyelitis G36.9
  ascending G61.0
  optica G36.0
Neuromyopathy G70.9
  paraneoplastic D49.9 [G13.0]
Neuromyotonia (Isaacs) G71.19
Neuronevus — *see* Nevus
Neuronitis G58.9
  ascending (acute) G57.2- ☑
  vestibular H81.2- ☑
Neuroparalytic — *see* condition
Neuropathy, neuropathic G62.9
  acute motor G62.81
  alcoholic G62.1
    with psychosis — *see* Psychosis, alcoholic
  arm G56.9- ☑
  autonomic, peripheral — *see* Neuropathy, peripheral, autonomic
  axillary G56.9- ☑
  bladder N31.9
    atonic (motor) (sensory) N31.2
    autonomous N31.2
    flaccid N31.2
    nonreflex N31.2
    reflex N31.1
    uninhibited N31.0
  brachial plexus G54.0
  cervical plexus G54.2
  chronic
    progressive segmentally demyelinating G62.89
    relapsing demyelinating G62.89

Neuropathy, neuropathic — *continued*
  Déjérine-Sottas G60.0
  diabetic — *see* E08-E13 with .40
    mononeuropathy — *see* E08-E13 with .41
    polyneuropathy — *see* E08-E13 with .42
  entrapment G58.9
    iliohypogastric nerve G57.8- ☑
    ilioinguinal nerve G57.8- ☑
    lateral cutaneous nerve of thigh G57.1- ☑
    median nerve G56.0- ☑
    obturator nerve G57.8- ☑
    peroneal nerve G57.3- ☑
    posterior tibial nerve G57.5- ☑
    saphenous nerve G57.8- ☑
    ulnar nerve G56.2- ☑
  facial nerve G51.9
  hereditary G60.9
    motor and sensory (types I-IV) G60.0
    sensory G60.8
    specified NEC G60.8
  hypertrophic G60.0
    Charcot-Marie-Tooth G60.0
    Déjérine-Sottas G60.0
    interstitial progressive G60.0
    of infancy G60.0
    Refsum G60.1
  idiopathic G60.9
    progressive G60.3
    specified NEC G60.8
  in association with hereditary ataxia G60.2
  intercostal G58.0
  ischemic — *see* Disorder, nerve
  Jamaica (ginger) G62.2
  leg NEC G57.9- ☑
  lower extremity G57.9- ☑
  lumbar plexus G54.1
  median nerve G56.1- ☑
  motor and sensory (*see also* Polyneuropathy)
    hereditary (types I-IV) G60.0
    multifocal motor (MMN) G61.82
  multiple (acute) (chronic) — *see* Polyneuropathy
  optic (nerve) (*see also* Neuritis, optic)
    ischemic H47.01- ☑
  paraneoplastic (sensorial) (Denny Brown) D49.9 [G13.0]
  peripheral (nerve) (*see also* Polyneuropathy) G62.9
    autonomic G90.9
      idiopathic G90.09
      in (due to)
        amyloidosis E85.4 [G99.0]
        diabetes mellitus — *see* E08-E13 with .43
        endocrine disease NEC E34.9 [G99.0]
        gout M10.00 [G99.0]
        hyperthyroidism E05.90 [G99.0]
          with thyroid storm E05.91 [G99.0]
        metabolic disease NEC E88.9 [G99.0]
    idiopathic G60.9
      progressive G60.3
    in (due to)
      antitetanus serum G62.0
      arsenic G62.2
      drugs NEC G62.0
      lead G62.2
      organophosphate compounds G62.2
      toxic agent NEC G62.2
  plantar nerves G57.6- ☑
  progressive
    hypertrophic interstitial G60.0
    inflammatory G62.81
  radicular NEC — *see* Radiculopathy
  sacral plexus G54.1
  sciatic G57.0- ☑
  serum G61.1
  toxic NEC G62.2
  trigeminal sensory G50.8
  ulnar nerve G56.2- ☑
  uremic N18.9 [G63]
  vitamin B12 E53.8 [G63]
    with anemia (pernicious) D51.0 [G63]
      due to dietary deficiency D51.3 [G63]
Neurophthisis (*see also* Disorder, nerve)
  peripheral, diabetic — *see* E08-E13 with .42
Neuroretinitis — *see* Chorioretinitis
Neuroretinopathy, hereditary optic H47.22
Neurosarcoma — *see* Neoplasm, nerve, malignant
Neurosclerosis — *see* Disorder, nerve
Neurosis, neurotic F48.9
  anankastic F42.8
  anxiety (state) F41.1

Neurosis, neurotic — *continued*
  anxiety — *continued*
    panic type F41.0
  asthenic F48.8
  bladder F45.8
  cardiac (reflex) F45.8
  cardiovascular F45.8
  character F60.9
  colon F45.8
  compensation F68.10
  compulsive, compulsion F42.8
  conversion F44.9
  craft F48.8
  cutaneous F45.8
  depersonalization F48.1
  depressive (reaction) (type) F34.1
  environmental F48.8
  excoriation L98.1
  fatigue F48.8
  functional — *see* Disorder, somatoform
  gastric F45.8
  gastrointestinal F45.8
  heart F45.8
  hypochondriacal F45.21
  hysterical F44.9
  incoordination F45.8
    larynx F45.8
    vocal cord F45.8
  intestine F45.8
  larynx (sensory) F45.8
    hysterical F44.4
  mixed NEC F48.8
  musculoskeletal F45.8
  obsessional F42.8
  obsessive-compulsive F42.8
  occupational F48.8
  ocular NEC F45.8
  organ — *see* Disorder, somatoform
  pharynx F45.8
  phobic F40.9
  posttraumatic (situational) F43.10
    acute F43.11
    chronic F43.12
  psychasthenic (type) F48.8
  railroad F48.8
  rectum F45.8
  respiratory F45.8
  rumination F45.8
  sexual F65.9
  situational F48.8
  social F40.10
    generalized F40.11
  specified type NEC F48.8
  state F48.9
    with depersonalization episode F48.1
  stomach F45.8
  traumatic F43.10
    acute F43.11
    chronic F43.12
  vasomotor F45.8
  visceral F45.8
  war F48.8
Neurospongioblastosis diffusa Q85.1
Neurosyphilis (arrested) (early) (gumma) (late) (latent) (recurrent) (relapse) A52.3
  with ataxia (cerebellar) (locomotor) (spastic) (spinal) A52.19
  aneurysm (cerebral) A52.05
  arachnoid (adhesive) A52.13
  arteritis (any artery) (cerebral) A52.04
  asymptomatic A52.2
  congenital A50.40
  dura (mater) A52.13
  general paresis A52.17
  hemorrhagic A52.05
  juvenile (asymptomatic) (meningeal) A50.40
  leptomeninges (aseptic) A52.13
  meningeal, meninges (adhesive) A52.13
  meningitis A52.13
  meningovascular (diffuse) A52.13
  optic atrophy A52.15
  parenchymatous (degenerative) A52.19
  paresis, paretic A52.17
    juvenile A50.45
  remission in (sustained) A52.3
  serological (without symptoms) A52.2
  specified nature or site NEC A52.19
  tabes, tabetic (dorsalis) A52.11
    juvenile A50.45

☑ **Additional Character Required** — Refer to the Tabular List for Character Selection   ▽ **Subterms under main terms may continue to next column or page**

Neurosyphilis — continued
　taboparesis A52.17
　　juvenile A50.45
　thrombosis (cerebral) A52.05
　vascular (cerebral) NEC A52.05
Neurothekeoma — see Neoplasm, nerve, benign
Neurotic — see Neurosis
Neurotoxemia — see Toxemia
Neutroclusion M26.211
Neutropenia, neutropenic (chronic) (genetic) (idiopathic) (immune) (infantile) (malignant) (pernicious) (splenic) D70.9
　congenital (primary) D70.0
　cyclic D70.4
　cytoreductive cancer chemotherapy sequela D70.1
　drug-induced D70.2
　　due to cytoreductive cancer chemotherapy D70.1
　due to infection D70.3
　fever D70.9
　neonatal, transitory (isoimmune) (maternal transfer) P61.5
　periodic D70.4
　secondary (cyclic) (periodic) (splenic) D70.4
　　drug-induced D70.2
　　　due to cytoreductive cancer chemotherapy D70.1
　toxic D70.8
Neutrophilia, hereditary giant D72.0
Nevocarcinoma — see Melanoma
Nevus D22.9
　achromic — see Neoplasm, skin, benign
　amelanotic — see Neoplasm, skin, benign
　angiomatous D18.00
　　intra-abdominal D18.03
　　intracranial D18.02
　　skin D18.01
　　specified site NEC D18.09
　araneus I78.1
　balloon cell — see Neoplasm, skin, benign
　bathing trunk D48.5
　blue — see Neoplasm, skin, benign
　　cellular — see Neoplasm, skin, benign
　　giant — see Neoplasm, skin, benign
　　Jadassohn's — see Neoplasm, skin, benign
　　malignant — see Melanoma
　capillary D18.00
　　intra-abdominal D18.03
　　intracranial D18.02
　　skin D18.01
　　specified site NEC D18.09
　cavernous D18.00
　　intra-abdominal D18.03
　　intracranial D18.02
　　skin D18.01
　　specified site NEC D18.09
　cellular — see Neoplasm, skin, benign
　　blue — see Neoplasm, skin, benign
　choroid D31.3- ☑
　comedonicus Q82.5
　conjunctiva D31.0- ☑
　dermal — see Neoplasm, skin, benign
　　with epidermal nevus — see Neoplasm, skin, benign
　dysplastic — see Neoplasm, skin, benign
　eye D31.9- ☑
　flammeus Q82.5
　hemangiomatous D18.00
　　intra-abdominal D18.03
　　intracranial D18.02
　　skin D18.01
　　specified site NEC D18.09
　iris D31.4- ☑
　lacrimal gland D31.5- ☑
　lymphatic D18.1
　magnocellular
　　specified site — see Neoplasm, benign, by site
　　unspecified site D31.40
　malignant — see Melanoma
　meaning hemangioma D18.00
　　intra-abdominal D18.03
　　intracranial D18.02
　　skin D18.01
　　specified site NEC D18.09
　mouth (mucosa) D10.30
　　specified site NEC D10.39
　　white sponge Q38.6
　multiplex Q85.1
　non-neoplastic I78.1
　oral mucosa D10.30
　　specified site NEC D10.39

Nevus — continued
　oral mucosa — continued
　　white sponge Q38.6
　orbit D31.6- ☑
　pigmented
　　giant (see also Neoplasm, skin, uncertain behavior) D48.5
　　malignant melanoma in — see Melanoma
　portwine Q82.5
　retina D31.2- ☑
　retrobulbar D31.6- ☑
　sanguineous Q82.5
　senile I78.1
　skin D22.9
　　abdominal wall D22.5
　　ala nasi D22.39
　　ankle D22.7- ☑
　　anus, anal D22.5
　　arm D22.6- ☑
　　auditory canal (external) D22.2- ☑
　　auricle (ear) D22.2- ☑
　　auricular canal (external) D22.2- ☑
　　axilla, axillary fold D22.5
　　back D22.5
　　breast D22.5
　　brow D22.39
　　buttock D22.5
　　canthus (eye) D22.1- ☑
　　cheek (external) D22.39
　　chest wall D22.5
　　chin D22.39
　　ear (external) D22.2- ☑
　　external meatus (ear) D22.2- ☑
　　eyebrow D22.39
　　eyelid (lower) (upper) D22.1- ☑
　　face D22.30
　　　specified NEC D22.39
　　female genital organ (external) NEC D28.0
　　finger D22.6- ☑
　　flank D22.5
　　foot D22.7- ☑
　　forearm D22.6- ☑
　　forehead D22.39
　　foreskin D29.0
　　genital organ (external) NEC
　　　female D28.0
　　　male D29.9
　　gluteal region D22.5
　　groin D22.5
　　hand D22.6- ☑
　　heel D22.7- ☑
　　helix D22.2- ☑
　　hip D22.7- ☑
　　interscapular region D22.5
　　jaw D22.39
　　knee D22.7- ☑
　　labium (majus) (minus) D28.0
　　leg D22.7- ☑
　　lip (lower) (upper) D22.0
　　lower limb D22.7- ☑
　　male genital organ (external) D29.9
　　nail D22.9
　　　finger D22.6- ☑
　　　toe D22.7- ☑
　　nasolabial groove D22.39
　　nates D22.5
　　neck D22.4
　　nose (external) D22.39
　　palpebra D22.1- ☑
　　penis D29.0
　　perianal skin D22.5
　　perineum D22.5
　　pinna D22.2- ☑
　　popliteal fossa or space D22.7- ☑
　　prepuce D29.0
　　pudendum D28.0
　　scalp D22.4
　　scrotum D29.4
　　shoulder D22.6- ☑
　　submammary fold D22.5
　　temple D22.39
　　thigh D22.7- ☑
　　toe D22.7- ☑
　　trunk NEC D22.5
　　umbilicus D22.5
　　upper limb D22.6- ☑
　　vulva D28.0

Nevus — continued
　specified site NEC — see Neoplasm, by site, benign
　spider I78.1
　stellar I78.1
　strawberry Q82.5
　Sutton's benign D22.9
　unius lateris Q82.5
　Unna's Q82.5
　vascular Q82.5
　verrucous Q82.5
Newborn (infant) (liveborn) (singleton) Z38.2
　abstinence syndrome P96.1
　acne L70.4
　affected by
　　abnormalities of membranes P02.9
　　　specified NEC P02.8
　　abruptio placenta P02.1
　　amino-acid metabolic disorder, transitory P74.8
　　amniocentesis (while in utero) P00.6
　　amnionitis P02.78
　　apparent life threatening event (ALTE) R68.13
　　bleeding (into)
　　　cerebral cortex P52.22
　　　germinal matrix P52.0
　　　ventricles P52.1
　　breech delivery P03.0
　　cardiac arrest P29.81
　　cardiomyopathy I42.8
　　　congenital I42.4
　　cerebral ischemia P91.0
　　Cesarean delivery P03.4
　　chemotherapy agents P04.11
　　chorioamnionitis P02.78
　　cocaine (crack) P04.41
　　complications of labor and delivery P03.9
　　　specified NEC P03.89
　　compression of umbilical cord NEC P02.5
　　contracted pelvis P03.1
　　delivery P03.9
　　　Cesarean P03.4
　　　forceps P03.2
　　　vacuum extractor P03.3
　　drugs of addiction P04.40
　　　cocaine P04.41
　　　hallucinogens P04.42
　　　specified drug NEC P04.49
　　entanglement (knot) in umbilical cord P02.5
　　environmental chemicals P04.6
　　fetal (intrauterine)
　　　growth retardation P05.9
　　　inflammatory response syndrome (FIRS) P02.70
　　　malnutrition not light or small for gestational age P05.2
　　FIRS (fetal inflammatory response syndrome) P02.70
　　forceps delivery P03.2
　　heart rate abnormalities
　　　bradycardia P29.12
　　　intrauterine P03.819
　　　　before onset of labor P03.810
　　　　during labor P03.811
　　　tachycardia P29.11
　　hemorrhage (antepartum) P02.1
　　　cerebellar (nontraumatic) P52.6
　　　intracerebral (nontraumatic) P52.4
　　　intracranial (nontraumatic) P52.9
　　　　specified NEC P52.8
　　　intraventricular (nontraumatic) P52.3
　　　　grade 1 P52.0
　　　　grade 2 P52.1
　　　　grade 3 P52.21
　　　　grade 4 P52.22
　　　posterior fossa (nontraumatic) P52.6
　　　subarachnoid (nontraumatic) P52.5
　　　subependymal P52.0
　　　　with intracerebral extension P52.22
　　　　with intraventricular extension P52.1
　　　　　with enlargement of ventricles P52.21
　　　　without intraventricular extension P52.0
　　hypoxic ischemic encephalopathy [HIE] P91.60
　　　mild P91.61
　　　moderate P91.62
　　　severe P91.63
　　induction of labor P03.89
　　intestinal perforation P78.0
　　intrauterine (fetal) blood loss P50.9
　　　due to (from)
　　　　cut end of co-twin cord P50.5
　　　　hemorrhage into
　　　　　co-twin P50.3

Newborn — *continued*
  affected by — *continued*
    intrauterine blood loss — *continued*
      due to — *continued*
        hemorrhage into — *continued*
          maternal circulation P50.4
        placenta P50.2
        ruptured cord blood P50.1
        vasa previa P50.0
      specified NEC P50.8
    intrauterine (fetal) hemorrhage P50.9
    intrauterine (in utero) procedure P96.5
    malpresentation (malposition) NEC P03.1
    maternal (complication of) (use of)
      alcohol P04.3
      amphetamines P04.16
      analgesia (maternal) P04.0
      anesthesia (maternal) P04.0
      anticonvulsants P04.13
      antidepressants P04.15
      antineoplastic chemotherapy P04.11
      anxiolytics P04.1A
      blood loss P02.1
      cannabis P04.81
      circulatory disease P00.3
      condition P00.9
        specified NEC P00.89
      cytotoxic drugs P04.12
      delivery P03.9
        Cesarean P03.4
        forceps P03.2
        vacuum extractor P03.3
      diabetes mellitus (pre-existing) P70.1
      disorder P00.9
        specified NEC P00.89
      drugs (addictive) (illegal) NEC P04.49
      ectopic pregnancy P01.4
      gestational diabetes P70.0
      hemorrhage P02.1
      hypertensive disorder P00.0
      incompetent cervix P01.0
      infectious disease P00.2
      injury P00.5
      labor and delivery P03.9
      malpresentation before labor P01.7
      maternal death P01.6
      medical procedure P00.7
      medication P04.19
        specified type NEC P04.18
      multiple pregnancy P01.5
      nutritional disorder P00.4
      oligohydramnios P01.2
      opiates P04.14
        administered for procedures during pregnancy or labor and delivery P04.0
      parasitic disease P00.2
      periodontal disease P00.81
      placenta previa P02.0
      polyhydramnios P01.3
      precipitate delivery P03.5
      pregnancy P01.9
        specified P01.8
      premature rupture of membranes P01.1
      renal disease P00.1
      respiratory disease P00.3
      sedative-hypnotics P04.17
      surgical procedure P00.6
      tranquilizers administered for procedures during pregnancy or labor and delivery P04.0
      urinary tract disease P00.1
      uterine contraction (abnormal) P03.6
    meconium peritonitis P78.0
    medication (legal) (maternal use) (prescribed) P04.19
    membrane abnormalities P02.9
      specified NEC P02.8
    membranitis P02.78
    methamphetamine(s) P04.49
    mixed metabolic and respiratory acidosis P84
    neonatal abstinence syndrome P96.1
    noxious substances transmitted via placenta or breast milk P04.9
      cannabis P04.81
      specified NEC P04.89
    nutritional supplements P04.5
    placenta previa P02.0
    placental
      abnormality (functional) (morphological) P02.20
        specified NEC P02.29

Newborn — *continued*
  affected by — *continued*
    placental — *continued*
      dysfunction P02.29
      infarction P02.29
      insufficiency P02.29
      separation NEC P02.1
      transfusion syndromes P02.3
    placentitis P02.78
    precipitate delivery P03.5
    prolapsed cord P02.4
    respiratory arrest P28.81
    slow intrauterine growth P05.9
    tobacco P04.2
    twin to twin transplacental transfusion P02.3
    umbilical cord (tightly) around neck P02.5
    umbilical cord condition P02.60
      short cord P02.69
      specified NEC P02.69
    uterine contractions (abnormal) P03.6
    vasa previa P02.69
      from intrauterine blood loss P50.0
  apnea P28.4
    obstructive P28.4
    primary P28.3
    sleep (central) (obstructive) (primary) P28.3
  born in hospital Z38.00
    by cesarean Z38.01
  born outside hospital Z38.1
  breast buds P96.89
  breast engorgement P83.4
  check-up — *see* Newborn, examination
  convulsion P90
  dehydration P74.1
  examination
    8 to 28 days old Z00.111
    under 8 days old Z00.110
  fever P81.9
    environmentally-induced P81.0
  hyperbilirubinemia P59.9
    of prematurity P59.0
  hypernatremia P74.21
  hyponatremia P74.22
  infection P39.9
    candidal P37.5
    specified NEC P39.8
    urinary tract P39.3
  jaundice P59.9
    due to
      breast milk inhibitor P59.3
      hepatocellular damage P59.20
        specified NEC P59.29
      preterm delivery P59.0
    of prematurity P59.0
    specified NEC P59.8
  late metabolic acidosis P74.0
  mastitis P39.0
    infective P39.0
    noninfective P83.4
  multiple born NEC Z38.8
    born in hospital Z38.68
      by cesarean Z38.69
    born outside hospital Z38.7
  omphalitis P38.9
    with mild hemorrhage P38.1
    without hemorrhage P38.9
  post-term P08.21
  prolonged gestation (over 42 completed weeks) P08.22
  quadruplet Z38.8
    born in hospital Z38.63
      by cesarean Z38.64
    born outside hospital Z38.7
  quintuplet Z38.8
    born in hospital Z38.65
      by cesarean Z38.66
    born outside hospital Z38.7
  seizure P90
  sepsis (congenital) P36.9
    due to
      anaerobes NEC P36.5
      Escherichia coli P36.4
      Staphylococcus P36.30
        aureus P36.2
        specified NEC P36.39
      Streptococcus P36.10
        group B P36.0
        specified NEC P36.19
    specified NEC P36.8
  triplet Z38.8

Newborn — *continued*
  triplet — *continued*
    born in hospital Z38.61
      by cesarean Z38.62
    born outside hospital Z38.7
  twin Z38.5
    born in hospital Z38.30
      by cesarean Z38.31
    born outside hospital Z38.4
  vomiting P92.09
    bilious P92.01
  weight check Z00.111
Newcastle conjunctivitis or disease B30.8
Nezelof's syndrome (pure alymphocytosis) D81.4
Niacin (amide) **deficiency** E52
Nicolas (-Durand)-**Favre disease** A55
Nicotine — *see* Tobacco
Nicotinic acid deficiency E52
Niemann-Pick disease or syndrome E75.249
  specified NEC E75.248
  type
    A E75.240
    B E75.241
    C E75.242
    D E75.243
Night
  blindness — *see* Blindness, night
  sweats R61
  terrors (child) F51.4
Nightmares (REM sleep type) F51.5
NIHSS (National Institutes of Health Stroke Scale) **score** R29.7- ☑
Nipple — *see* condition
Nisbet's chancre A57
Nishimoto (-Takeuchi) **disease** I67.5
Nitritoid crisis or reaction — *see* Crisis, nitritoid
Nitrosohemoglobinemia D74.8
Njovera A65
Nocardiosis, nocardiasis A43.9
  cutaneous A43.1
  lung A43.0
  pneumonia A43.0
  pulmonary A43.0
  specified site NEC A43.8
Nocturia R35.1
  psychogenic F45.8
Nocturnal — *see* condition
Nodal rhythm I49.8
Node(s) (*see also* Nodule)
  Bouchard's (with arthropathy) M15.2
  Haygarth's M15.8
  Heberden's (with arthropathy) M15.1
  larynx J38.7
  lymph — *see* condition
  milker's B08.03
  Osler's I33.0
  Schmorl's — *see* Schmorl's disease
  singer's J38.2
  teacher's J38.2
  tuberculous — *see* Tuberculosis, lymph gland
  vocal cord J38.2
Nodule(s), **nodular**
  actinomycotic — *see* Actinomycosis
  breast NEC (*see also* Lump, breast) N63.0
  colloid (cystic), thyroid E04.1
  cutaneous — *see* Swelling, localized
  endometrial (stromal) D26.1
  Haygarth's M15.8
  inflammatory — *see* Inflammation
  juxta-articular
    syphilitic A52.77
    yaws A66.7
  larynx J38.7
  lung, solitary (subsegmental branch of the bronchial tree) R91.1
    multiple R91.8
  milker's B08.03
  prostate N40.2
    with lower urinary tract symptoms (LUTS) N40.3
    without lower urinary tract symtpoms (LUTS) N40.2
  pulmonary, solitary (subsegmental branch of the bronchial tree) R91.1
  retrocardiac R09.89
  rheumatoid M06.30
    ankle M06.37- ☑
    elbow M06.32- ☑
    foot joint M06.37- ☑
    hand joint M06.34- ☑

☑ **Additional Character Required** — Refer to the Tabular List for Character Selection   ▽ **Subterms under main terms may continue to next column or page**

Nodule(s), **nodular** — *continued*
  rheumatoid — *continued*
    hip M06.35- ☑
    knee M06.36- ☑
    multiple site M06.39
    shoulder M06.31- ☑
    vertebra M06.38
    wrist M06.33- ☑
  scrotum (inflammatory) N49.2
  singer's J38.2
  solitary, lung (subsegmental branch of the bronchial tree) R91.1
    multiple R91.8
  subcutaneous — *see* Swelling, localized
  teacher's J38.2
  thyroid (cold) (gland) (nontoxic) E04.1
    with thyrotoxicosis E05.20
      with thyroid storm E05.21
    toxic or with hyperthyroidism E05.20
      with thyroid storm E05.21
  vocal cord J38.2
Noma (gangrenous) (hospital) (infective) A69.0
  auricle I96
  mouth A69.0
  pudendi N76.89
  vulvae N76.89
Nomad, nomadism Z59.0
NOMID (neonatal onset multisystemic inflammatory disorder) M04.2
Nonadherence to medical treatment Z91.19
Nonautoimmune hemolytic anemia D59.4
  drug-induced D59.2
Nonclosure (*see also* Imperfect, closure)
  ductus arteriosus (Botallo's) Q25.0
  foramen
    botalli Q21.1
    ovale Q21.1
Noncompliance Z91.19
  with
    dialysis Z91.15
    dietary regimen Z91.11
    medical treatment Z91.19
    medication regimen NEC Z91.14
      underdosing (*see also* Table of Drugs and Chemicals, categories T36-T50, with final character 6) Z91.14
        intentional NEC Z91.128
          due to financial hardship of patient Z91.120
        unintentional NEC Z91.138
          due to patient's age related debility Z91.130
    renal dialysis Z91.15
Nondescent (congenital) (*see also* Malposition, congenital)
  cecum Q43.3
  colon Q43.3
  testicle Q53.9
    bilateral Q53.20
      abdominal Q53.211
      perineal Q53.22
    unilateral Q53.10
      abdominal Q53.111
      perineal Q53.12
Nondevelopment
  brain Q02
    part of Q04.3
  heart Q24.8
  organ or site, congenital NEC — *see* Hypoplasia
Nonengagement
  head NEC O32.4 ☑
    in labor, causing obstructed labor O64.8 ☑
Nonexanthematous tick fever A93.2
Nonexpansion, lung (newborn) P28.0
Nonfunctioning
  cystic duct (*see also* Disease, gallbladder) K82.8
  gallbladder (*see also* Disease, gallbladder) K82.8
  kidney N28.9
  labyrinth — *see* subcategory H83.2 ☑
Non-Hodgkin lymphoma NEC — *see* Lymphoma, non-Hodgkin
Nonimplantation, ovum N97.2
Noninsufflation, fallopian tube N97.1
Non-ketotic hyperglycinemia E72.51
Nonne-Milroy syndrome Q82.0
Nonovulation N97.0
Non-palpable testicle(s)
  bilateral R39.84

Non-palpable testicle(s) — *continued*
  unilateral R39.83
Nonpatent fallopian tube N97.1
Nonpneumatization, lung NEC P28.0
Nonrotation — *see* Malrotation
Nonsecretion, urine — *see* Anuria
Nonunion
  fracture — *see* Fracture, by site
  joint, following fusion or arthrodesis M96.0
  organ or site, congenital NEC — *see* Imperfect, closure
  symphysis pubis, congenital Q74.2
Nonvisualization, gallbladder R93.2
Nonvital, nonvitalized tooth K04.99
Non-working side interference M26.56
Noonan's syndrome Q87.1
Normocytic anemia (infectional) due to blood loss (chronic) D50.0
  acute D62
Norrie's disease (congenital) Q15.8
North American blastomycosis B40.9
Norwegian itch B86
Nose, nasal — *see* condition
Nosebleed R04.0
Nose-picking F98.8
Nosomania F45.21
Nosophobia F45.22
Nostalgia F43.20
Notch of iris Q13.2
Notching nose, congenital (tip) Q30.2
Nothnagel's
  syndrome — *see* Strabismus, paralytic, third nerve
  vasomotor acroparesthesia I73.89
Novy's relapsing fever A68.9
  louse-borne A68.0
  tick-borne A68.1
Noxious
  foodstuffs, poisoning by — *see* Poisoning, food, noxious, plant
  substances transmitted through placenta or breast milk P04.9
Nucleus pulposus — *see* condition
Numbness R20.0
Nuns' knee — *see* Bursitis, prepatellar
Nursemaid's elbow S53.03- ☑
Nutcracker esophagus K22.4
Nutmeg liver K76.1
Nutrient element deficiency E61.9
  specified NEC E61.8
Nutrition deficient or insufficient (*see also* Malnutrition) E46
  due to
    insufficient food T73.0 ☑
    lack of
      care (child) T76.02 ☑
        adult T76.01 ☑
      food T73.0 ☑
Nutritional stunting E45
Nyctalopia (night blindness) — *see* Blindness, night
Nycturia R35.1
  psychogenic F45.8
Nymphomania F52.8
Nystagmus H55.00
  benign paroxysmal — *see* Vertigo, benign paroxysmal
  central positional H81.4- ☑
  congenital H55.01
  dissociated H55.04
  latent H55.02
  miners' H55.09
  positional
    benign paroxysmal H81.4- ☑
    central H81.4- ☑
  specified form NEC H55.09
  visual deprivation H55.03

O

Obermeyer's relapsing fever (European) A68.0
Obesity E66.9
  with alveolar hypoventilation E66.2
  adrenal E27.8
  complicating
    childbirth O99.214
    pregnancy O99.21- ☑
    puerperium O99.215
  constitutional E66.8
  dietary counseling and surveillance Z71.3
  drug-induced E66.1

Obesity — *continued*
  due to
    drug E66.1
    excess calories E66.09
      morbid E66.01
      severe E66.01
  endocrine E66.8
  endogenous E66.8
  exogenous E66.09
  familial E66.8
  glandular E66.8
  hypothyroid — *see* Hypothyroidism
  hypoventilation syndrome (OHS) E66.2
  morbid E66.01
    with
      alveolar hypoventilation E66.2
      obesity hypoventilation syndrome (OHS) E66.2
    due to excess calories E66.01
  nutritional E66.09
  pituitary E23.6
  severe E66.01
  specified type NEC E66.8
Oblique — *see* condition
Obliteration
  appendix (lumen) K38.8
  artery I77.1
  bile duct (noncalculous) K83.1
  common duct (noncalculous) K83.1
  cystic duct — *see* Obstruction, gallbladder
  disease, arteriolar I77.1
  endometrium N85.8
  eye, anterior chamber — *see* Disorder, globe, hypotony
  fallopian tube N97.1
  lymphatic vessel I89.0
    due to mastectomy I97.2
  organ or site, congenital NEC — *see* Atresia, by site
  ureter N13.5
    with infection N13.6
  urethra — *see* Stricture, urethra
  vein I87.8
  vestibule (oral) K08.89
Observation (following) (for) (without need for further medical care) Z04.9
  accident NEC Z04.3
    at work Z04.2
    transport Z04.1
  adverse effect of drug Z03.6
  alleged rape or sexual assault (victim), ruled out
    adult Z04.41
    child Z04.42
  criminal assault Z04.89
  development state
    adolescent Z00.3
    period of rapid growth in childhood Z00.2
    puberty Z00.3
  disease, specified NEC Z03.89
  following work accident Z04.2
  forced sexual exploitation Z04.81
  forced labor exploitation Z04.82
  growth and development state — *see* Observation, development state
  injuries (accidental) NEC (*see also* Observation, accident)
  newborn (for)
    suspected condition, related to exposure from the mother or birth process — *see* Newborn, affected by, maternal
      ruled out Z05.9
        cardiac Z05.0
        connective tissue Z05.73
        gastrointestinal Z05.5
        genetic Z05.41
        genitourinary Z05.6
        immunologic Z05.43
        infectious Z05.1
        metabolic Z05.42
        musculoskeletal Z05.72
        neurological Z05.2
        respiratory Z05.3
        skin and subcutaneous tissue Z05.71
        specified condition NEC Z05.8
  postpartum
    immediately after delivery Z39.0
    routine follow-up Z39.2
  pregnancy (normal) (without complication) Z34.9- ☑
    high risk O09.9- ☑
  suicide attempt, alleged NEC Z03.89
    self-poisoning Z03.6

Observation — *continued*
  suspected, ruled out (*see also* Suspected condition, ruled out)
    abuse, physical
      adult Z04.71
      child Z04.72
    accident at work Z04.2
    adult battering victim Z04.71
    child battering victim Z04.72
    condition NEC Z03.89
      newborn (*see also* Observation, newborn (for), suspected condition, ruled out) Z05.9
    drug poisoning or adverse effect Z03.6
    exposure (to)
      anthrax Z03.810
      biological agent NEC Z03.818
    inflicted injury NEC Z04.89
    suicide attempt, alleged Z03.89
      self-poisoning Z03.6
    toxic effects from ingested substance (drug) (poison) Z03.6
  toxic effects from ingested substance (drug) (poison) Z03.6
Obsession, obsessional state F42.8
  mixed thoughts and acts F42.2
Obsessive-compulsive neurosis or reaction F42.8
Obstetric embolism, septic — *see* Embolism, obstetric, septic
Obstetrical trauma (complicating delivery) O71.9
  with or following ectopic or molar pregnancy O08.6
  specified type NEC O71.89
Obstipation — *see* Constipation
Obstruction, obstructed, obstructive
  airway J98.8
    with
      allergic alveolitis J67.9
      asthma J45.909
        with
          exacerbation (acute) J45.901
          status asthmaticus J45.902
      bronchiectasis J47.9
        with
          exacerbation (acute) J47.1
          lower respiratory infection J47.0
      bronchitis (chronic) J44.9
      emphysema J43.9
    chronic J44.9
      with
        allergic alveolitis — *see* Pneumonitis, hypersensitivity
        bronchiectasis J47.9
          with
            exacerbation (acute) J47.1
            lower respiratory infection J47.0
    due to
      foreign body — *see* Foreign body, by site, causing asphyxia
      inhalation of fumes or vapors J68.9
      laryngospasm J38.5
  ampulla of Vater K83.1
  aortic (heart) (valve) — *see* Stenosis, aortic
  aortoiliac I74.09
  aqueduct of Sylvius G91.1
    congenital Q03.0
      with spina bifida — *see* Spina bifida, by site, with hydrocephalus
  Arnold-Chiari — *see* Arnold-Chiari disease
  artery (*see also* Atherosclerosis, artery) I70.9 ☑
    basilar (complete) (partial) — *see* Occlusion, artery, basilar
    carotid (complete) (partial) — *see* Occlusion, artery, carotid
    cerebellar — *see* Occlusion, artery, cerebellar
    cerebral (anterior) (middle) (posterior) — *see* Occlusion, artery, cerebral
    precerebral — *see* Occlusion, artery, precerebral
    renal N28.0
    retinal NEC — *see* Occlusion, artery, retina
    stent — *see* Restenosis, stent
    vertebral (complete) (partial) — *see* Occlusion, artery, vertebral
  band (intestinal) (*see also* Obstruction, intestine, specified NEC) K56.699
  bile duct or passage (common) (hepatic) (noncalculous) K83.1
    with calculus K80.51
    congenital (causing jaundice) Q44.3
  biliary (duct) (tract) K83.1

Obstruction, obstructed, obstructive — *continued*
  biliary — *continued*
    gallbladder K82.0
  bladder-neck (acquired) N32.0
    congenital Q64.31
    due to hyperplasia (hypertrophy) of prostate — *see* Hyperplasia, prostate
  bowel — *see* Obstruction, intestine
  bronchus J98.09
  canal, ear — *see* Stenosis, external ear canal
  cardia K22.2
  caval veins (inferior) (superior) I87.1
  cecum — *see* Obstruction, intestine
  circulatory I99.8
  colon — *see* Obstruction, intestine
  common duct (noncalculous) K83.1
  coronary (artery) — *see* Occlusion, coronary
  cystic duct (*see also* Obstruction, gallbladder)
    with calculus K80.21
  device, implant or graft (*see also* Complications, by site and type, mechanical) T85.698 ☑
    arterial graft NEC — *see* Complication, cardiovascular device, mechanical, vascular
    catheter NEC T85.628 ☑
      cystostomy T83.090 ☑
      dialysis (renal) T82.49 ☑
        intraperitoneal T85.691 ☑
      Hopkins T83.098 ☑
      ileostomy T83.098 ☑
      infusion NEC T82.594 ☑
        spinal (epidural) (subdural) T85.690 ☑
      nephrostomy T83.092 ☑
      urethral indwelling T83.091 ☑
      urinary T83.098 ☑
      urostomy T83.098 ☑
    due to infection T85.79 ☑
    gastrointestinal — *see* Complications, prosthetic device, mechanical, gastrointestinal device
    genital NEC T83.498 ☑
      intrauterine contraceptive device T83.39 ☑
      penile prosthesis (cylinder) (implanted) (pump) (resevoir) T83.490 ☑
      testicular prosthesis T83.491 ☑
    heart NEC — *see* Complication, cardiovascular device, mechanical
    joint prosthesis — *see* Complications, joint prosthesis, mechanical, specified NEC, by site
    orthopedic NEC — *see* Complication, orthopedic, device, mechanical
    specified NEC T85.628 ☑
    urinary NEC (*see also* Complication, genitourinary, device, urinary, mechanical)
      graft T83.29 ☑
    vascular NEC — *see* Complication, cardiovascular device, mechanical
    ventricular intracranial shunt T85.09 ☑
  due to foreign body accidentally left in operative wound T81.529 ☑
  duodenum K31.5
  ejaculatory duct N50.89
  esophagus K22.2
  eustachian tube (complete) (partial) H68.10- ☑
    cartilagenous (extrinsic) H68.13- ☑
    intrinsic H68.12- ☑
    osseous H68.11- ☑
  fallopian tube (bilateral) N97.1
  fecal K56.41
    with hernia — *see* Hernia, by site, with obstruction
  foramen of Monro (congenital) Q03.8
    with spina bifida — *see* Spina bifida, by site, with hydrocephalus
  foreign body — *see* Foreign body
  gallbladder K82.0
    with calculus, stones K80.21
    congenital Q44.1
  gastric outlet K31.1
  gastrointestinal — *see* Obstruction, intestine
  hepatic K76.89
    duct (noncalculous) K83.1
  ileum — *see* Obstruction, intestine
  iliofemoral (artery) I74.5
  intestine K56.609
    with
      adhesions (intestinal) (peritoneal) K56.50
        complete K56.52
        incomplete K56.51
        partial K56.51

Obstruction, obstructed, obstructive — *continued*
  intestine — *continued*
    adynamic K56.0
    by gallstone K56.3
    complete K56.601
    congenital (small) Q41.9
      large Q42.9
        specified part NEC Q42.8
    incomplete K56.600
    neurogenic K56.0
      Hirschsprung's disease or megacolon Q43.1
    newborn P76.9
      due to
        fecaliths P76.8
        inspissated milk P76.2
        meconium (plug) P76.0
          in mucoviscidosis E84.11
      specified NEC P76.8
    partial K56.600
    postoperative K91.30
      complete K91.32
      incomplete K91.31
      partial K91.31
    reflex K56.0
    specified NEC K56.699
      complete K56.691
      incomplete K56.690
      partial K56.690
    volvulus K56.2
  intracardiac ball valve prosthesis T82.09 ☑
  jejunum — *see* Obstruction, intestine
  joint prosthesis — *see* Complications, joint prosthesis, mechanical, specified NEC, by site
  kidney (calices) N28.89
  labor — *see* Delivery
  lacrimal (passages) (duct)
    by
      dacryolith — *see* Dacryolith
      stenosis — *see* Stenosis, lacrimal
    congenital Q10.5
    neonatal H04.53- ☑
  lacrimonasal duct — *see* Obstruction, lacrimal
  lacteal, with steatorrhea K90.2
  laryngitis — *see* Laryngitis
  larynx NEC J38.6
    congenital Q31.8
  lung J98.4
    disease, chronic J44.9
  lymphatic I89.0
  meconium (plug)
    newborn P76.0
      due to fecaliths P76.0
      in mucoviscidosis E84.11
  mitral — *see* Stenosis, mitral
  nasal J34.89
  nasolacrimal duct (*see also* Obstruction, lacrimal)
    congenital Q10.5
  nasopharynx J39.2
  nose J34.89
  organ or site, congenital NEC — *see* Atresia, by site
  pancreatic duct K86.89
  parotid duct or gland K11.8
  pelviureteral junction N13.5
    with hydronephrosis N13.0
    congenital Q62.39
  pharynx J39.2
  portal (circulation) (vein) I81
  prostate (*see also* Hyperplasia, prostate)
    valve (urinary) N32.0
  pulmonary valve (heart) I37.0
  pyelonephritis (chronic) N11.1
  pylorus
    adult K31.1
    congenital or infantile Q40.0
  rectosigmoid — *see* Obstruction, intestine
  rectum K62.4
  renal N28.89
    outflow N13.8
    pelvis, congenital Q62.39
  respiratory J98.8
    chronic J44.9
  retinal (vessels) H34.9
  salivary duct (any) K11.8
    with calculus K11.5
  sigmoid — *see* Obstruction, intestine
  sinus (accessory) (nasal) J34.89
  Stensen's duct K11.8
  stomach NEC K31.89

☑ **Additional Character Required** — Refer to the Tabular List for Character Selection   ▽ **Subterms under main terms may continue to next column or page**

Obstruction, obstructed, obstructive — continued
- stomach — continued
  - acute K31.0
  - congenital Q40.2
  - due to pylorospasm K31.3
- submandibular duct K11.8
- submaxillary gland K11.8
  - with calculus K11.5
- thoracic duct I89.0
- thrombotic — see Thrombosis
- trachea J39.8
- tracheostomy airway J95.03
- tricuspid (valve) — see Stenosis, tricuspid
- upper respiratory, congenital Q34.8
- ureter (functional) (pelvic junction) NEC N13.5
  - with
    - hydronephrosis N13.1
      - with infection N13.6
    - pyelonephritis (chronic) N11.1
  - congenital Q62.39
  - due to calculus — see Calculus, ureter
- urethra NEC N36.8
  - congenital Q64.39
- urinary (moderate) N13.9
  - due to hyperplasia (hypertrophy) of prostate — see Hyperplasia, prostate
  - organ or tract (lower) N13.9
  - prostatic valve N32.0
  - specified NEC N13.8
- uropathy N13.9
- uterus N85.8
- vagina N89.5
- valvular — see Endocarditis
- vein, venous I87.1
  - caval (inferior) (superior) I87.1
  - thrombotic — see Thrombosis
- vena cava (inferior) (superior) I87.1
- vesical NEC N32.0
- vesicourethral orifice N32.0
  - congenital Q64.31
- vessel NEC I99.8
  - stent — see Restenosis, stent

Obturator — see condition
Occlusal wear, teeth K03.0
Occlusio pupillae — see Membrane, pupillary
Occlusion, occluded
- anus K62.4
  - congenital Q42.3
    - with fistula Q42.2
- aortoiliac (chronic) I74.09
- aqueduct of Sylvius G91.1
  - congenital Q03.0
    - with spina bifida — see Spina bifida, by site, with hydrocephalus
- artery (see also Atherosclerosis, artery) I70.9 ☑
  - auditory, internal I65.8
  - basilar I65.1
    - with
      - infarction I63.22
        - due to
          - embolism I63.12
          - thrombosis I63.02
  - brain or cerebral I66.9
    - with infarction (due to) I63.5- ☑
      - embolism I63.4- ☑
      - thrombosis I63.3- ☑
  - carotid I65.2- ☑
    - with
      - infarction I63.23- ☑
        - due to
          - embolism I63.13- ☑
          - thrombosis I63.03- ☑
  - cerebellar (anterior inferior) (posterior inferior) (superior) I66.3
    - with infarction I63.54- ☑
      - due to
        - embolism I63.44- ☑
        - thrombosis I63.34- ☑
  - cerebral I66.9
    - with infarction I63.50
      - due to
        - embolism I63.40
          - specified NEC I63.49
        - thrombosis I63.30
          - specified NEC I63.39
    - anterior I66.1- ☑
      - with infarction I63.52- ☑

- artery (see also Atherosclerosis, artery) — continued
  - cerebral — continued
    - anterior
      - with infarction — continued
        - due to
          - embolism I63.42- ☑
          - thrombosis I63.32- ☑
    - middle I66.0- ☑
      - with infarction I63.51- ☑
        - due to
          - embolism I63.41- ☑
          - thrombosis I63.31- ☑
    - posterior I66.2- ☑
      - with infarction I63.53- ☑
        - due to
          - embolism I63.43- ☑
          - thrombosis I63.33- ☑
    - specified NEC I66.8
      - with infarction I63.59
        - due to
          - embolism I63.4- ☑
          - thrombosis I63.3- ☑
  - choroidal (anterior) — see Occlusion, artery, precerebral, specified NEC
  - communicating posterior — see Occlusion, artery, precerebral, specified NEC
  - complete
    - coronary I25.82
    - extremities I70.92
  - coronary (acute) (thrombotic) (without myocardial infarction) I24.0
    - with myocardial infarction — see Infarction, myocardium
    - chronic total I25.82
    - complete I25.82
    - healed or old I25.2
    - total (chronic) I25.82
  - hypophyseal — see Occlusion, artery, precerebral, specified NEC
  - iliac I74.5
  - lower extremities due to stenosis or stricture I77.1
  - mesenteric (embolic) (thrombotic) (see also Infarct, intestine) K55.069
  - perforating — see Occlusion, artery, cerebral, specified NEC
  - peripheral I77.9
    - thrombotic or embolic I74.4
  - pontine — see Occlusion, artery, precerebral, specified NEC
  - precerebral I65.9
    - with infarction I63.20
      - specified NEC I63.29
      - due to
        - embolism I63.10
          - specified NEC I63.19
        - thrombosis I63.00
          - specified NEC I63.09
    - basilar — see Occlusion, artery, basilar
    - carotid — see Occlusion, artery, carotid
    - puerperal O88.23
    - specified NEC I65.8
      - with infarction I63.29
        - due to
          - embolism I63.19
          - thrombosis I63.09
    - vertebral — see Occlusion, artery, vertebral
  - renal N28.0
  - retinal
    - branch H34.23- ☑
    - central H34.1- ☑
    - partial H34.21- ☑
    - transient H34.0- ☑
  - spinal — see Occlusion, artery, precerebral, vertebral
  - total (chronic)
    - coronary I25.82
    - extremities I70.92
  - vertebral I65.0- ☑
    - with
      - infarction I63.21- ☑
        - due to
          - embolism I63.11- ☑
          - thrombosis I63.01- ☑
  - basilar artery — see Occlusion, artery, basilar
  - bile duct (common) (hepatic) (noncalculous) K83.1
  - bowel — see Obstruction, intestine

- carotid (artery) (common) (internal) — see Occlusion, artery, carotid
- centric (of teeth) M26.59
  - maximum intercuspation discrepancy M26.55
- cerebellar (artery) — see Occlusion, artery, cerebellar
- cerebral (artery) — see Occlusion, artery, cerebral
- cerebrovascular (see also Occlusion, artery, cerebral)
  - with infarction I63.5- ☑
- cervical canal — see Stricture, cervix
- cervix (uteri) — see Stricture, cervix
- choanal Q30.0
- choroidal (artery) — see Occlusion, artery, precerebral, specified NEC
- colon — see Obstruction, intestine
- communicating posterior artery — see Occlusion, artery, precerebral, specified NEC
- coronary (artery) (vein) (thrombotic) (see also Infarct, myocardium)
  - chronic total I25.82
  - healed or old I25.2
  - not resulting in infarction I24.0
  - total (chronic) I25.82
- cystic duct — see Obstruction, gallbladder
- embolic — see Embolism
- fallopian tube N97.1
  - congenital Q50.6
- gallbladder (see also Obstruction, gallbladder)
  - congenital (causing jaundice) Q44.1
- gingiva, traumatic K06.2
- hymen N89.6
  - congenital Q52.3
- hypophyseal (artery) — see Occlusion, artery, precerebral, specified NEC
- iliac artery I74.5
- intestine — see Obstruction, intestine
- lacrimal passages — see Obstruction, lacrimal
- lung J98.4
- lymph or lymphatic channel I89.0
- mammary duct N64.89
- mesenteric artery (embolic) (thrombotic) (see also Infarct, intestine) K55.069
- nose J34.89
  - congenital Q30.0
- organ or site, congenital NEC — see Atresia, by site
- oviduct N97.1
  - congenital Q50.6
- peripheral arteries
  - due to stricture or stenosis I77.1
  - upper extremity I74.2
- pontine (artery) — see Occlusion, artery, precerebral, specified NEC
- posterior lingual, of mandibular teeth M26.29
- precerebral artery — see Occlusion, artery, precerebral
- punctum lacrimale — see Obstruction, lacrimal
- pupil — see Membrane, pupillary
- pylorus, adult (see also Stricture, pylorus) K31.1
- renal artery N28.0
- retina, retinal
  - artery — see Occlusion, artery, retinal
  - vein (central) H34.81- ☑
    - engorgement H34.82- ☑
    - tributary H34.83- ☑
  - vessels H34.9
- spinal artery — see Occlusion, artery, precerebral, vertebral
- teeth (mandibular) (posterior lingual) M26.29
- thoracic duct I89.0
- thrombotic — see Thrombosis, artery
- traumatic
  - edentulous (alveolar) ridge K06.2
  - gingiva K06.2
  - periodontal K05.5
- tubal N97.1
- ureter (complete) (partial) N13.5
  - congenital Q62.10
- ureteropelvic junction N13.5
  - congenital Q62.11
- ureterovesical orifice N13.5
  - congenital Q62.12
- urethra — see Stricture, urethra
- uterus N85.8
- vagina N89.5
- vascular NEC I99.8
- vein — see Thrombosis
  - retinal — see Occlusion, retinal, vein
- vena cava (inferior) (superior) — see Embolism, vena cava

Occlusion, occluded — continued
  ventricle (brain) NEC G91.1
  vertebral (artery) — see Occlusion, artery, vertebral
  vessel (blood) I99.8
  vulva N90.5
Occult
  blood in feces (stools) R19.5
Occupational
  problems NEC Z56.89
Ochlophobia — see Agoraphobia
Ochronosis (endogenous) E70.29
Ocular muscle — see condition
Oculogyric crisis or disturbance H51.8
  psychogenic F45.8
Oculomotor syndrome H51.9
Oculopathy
  syphilitic NEC A52.71
    congenital
      early A50.01
      late A50.30
    early (secondary) A51.43
    late A52.71
Oddi's sphincter spasm K83.4
Odontalgia K08.89
Odontoameloblastoma — see Cyst, calcifying odontogenic
Odontoclasia K03.89
Odontodysplasia, regional K00.4
Odontogenesis imperfecta K00.5
Odontoma (ameloblastic) (complex) (compound) (fibroameloblastic) — see Cyst, calcifying odontogenic
Odontomyelitis (closed) (open) K04.01
  irreversible K04.02
  reversible K04.01
Odontorrhagia K08.89
Odontosarcoma, ameloblastic C41.1
  upper jaw (bone) C41.0
Oestriasis — see Myiasis
Oguchi's disease H53.63
Ohara's disease — see Tularemia
OHS (obesity hypoventilation syndrome) E66.2
Oidiomycosis — see Candidiasis
Oidium albicans infection — see Candidiasis
Old age (without mention of debility) R54
  dementia F03 ☑
Old (previous) **myocardial infarction** I25.2
Olfactory — see condition
Oligemia — see Anemia
Oligoastrocytoma
  specified site — see Neoplasm, malignant, by site
  unspecified site C71.9
Oligocythemia D64.9
Oligodendroblastoma
  specified site — see Neoplasm, malignant
  unspecified site C71.9
Oligodendroglioma
  anaplastic type
    specified site — see Neoplasm, malignant, by site
    unspecified site C71.9
  specified site — see Neoplasm, malignant, by site
  unspecified site C71.9
Oligodontia — see Anodontia
Oligoencephalon Q02
Oligohidrosis L74.4
Oligohydramnios O41.0- ☑
Oligohydrosis L74.4
Oligomenorrhea N91.5
  primary N91.3
  secondary N91.4
Oligophrenia (see also Disability, intellectual)
  phenylpyruvic E70.0
Oligospermia N46.11
  due to
    drug therapy N46.121
    efferent duct obstruction N46.123
    infection N46.122
    radiation N46.124
    specified cause NEC N46.129
    systemic disease N46.125
Oligotrichia — see Alopecia
Oliguria R34
  with, complicating or following ectopic or molar pregnancy O08.4
  postprocedural N99.0
Ollier's disease Q78.4
Omenotocele — see Hernia, abdomen, specified site NEC
Omentitis — see Peritonitis

Omentum, omental — see condition
Omphalitis (congenital) (newborn) P38.9
  with mild hemorrhage P38.1
  without hemorrhage P38.9
  not of newborn L08.82
  tetanus A33
Omphalocele Q79.2
Omphalomesenteric duct, persistent Q43.0
Omphalorrhagia, newborn P51.9
Omsk hemorrhagic fever A98.1
Onanism (excessive) F98.8
Onchocerciasis, onchocercosis B73.1
  with
    eye disease B73.00
      endophthalmitis B73.01
      eyelid B73.09
      glaucoma B73.02
      specified NEC B73.09
    eyelid B73.09
    eye NEC B73.00
Oncocytoma — see Neoplasm, benign, by site
Oncovirus, as cause of disease classified elsewhere B97.32
Ondine's curse — see Apnea, sleep
Oneirophrenia F23
Onychauxis L60.2
  congenital Q84.5
Onychia (see also Cellulitis, digit)
  with lymphangitis — see Lymphangitis, acute, digit
  candidal B37.2
  dermatophytic B35.1
Onychitis (see also Cellulitis, digit)
  with lymphangitis — see Lymphangitis, acute, digit
Onychocryptosis L60.0
Onychodystrophy L60.3
  congenital Q84.6
Onychogryphosis, onychogryposis L60.2
Onycholysis L60.1
Onychomadesis L60.8
Onychomalacia L60.3
Onychomycosis (finger) (toe) B35.1
Onycho-osteodysplasia Q87.2
Onychophagia F98.8
Onychophosis L60.8
Onychoptosis L60.8
Onychorrhexis L60.3
  congenital Q84.6
Onychoschizia L60.3
Onyxis (finger) (toe) L60.0
Onyxitis (see also Cellulitis, digit)
  with lymphangitis — see Lymphangitis, acute, digit
Oophoritis (cystic) (infectional) (interstitial) N70.92
  with salpingitis N70.93
  acute N70.02
    with salpingitis N70.03
  chronic N70.12
    with salpingitis N70.13
  complicating abortion — see Abortion, by type, complicated by, oophoritis
Oophorocele N83.4- ☑
Opacity, opacities
  cornea H17.- ☑
    central H17.1- ☑
    congenital Q13.3
    degenerative — see Degeneration, cornea
    hereditary — see Dystrophy, cornea
    inflammatory — see Keratitis
    minor H17.81- ☑
    peripheral H17.82- ☑
    sequelae of trachoma (healed) B94.0
    specified NEC H17.89
  enamel (teeth) (fluoride) (nonfluoride) K00.3
  lens — see Cataract
  snowball — see Deposit, crystalline
  vitreous (humor) NEC H43.39- ☑
    congenital Q14.0
    membranes and strands H43.31- ☑
Opalescent dentin (hereditary) K00.5
Open, opening
  abnormal, organ or site, congenital — see Imperfect, closure
  angle with
    borderline
      findings
        high risk H40.02- ☑
        low risk H40.01- ☑
      intraocular pressure H40.00- ☑

Open, opening — continued
  angle with — continued
    cupping of discs H40.01- ☑
    glaucoma (primary) — see Glaucoma, open angle
  bite
    anterior M26.220
    posterior M26.221
  false — see Imperfect, closure
  margin on tooth restoration K08.51
  restoration margins of tooth K08.51
  wound — see Wound, open
Operational fatigue F48.8
Operative — see condition
Operculitis — see Periodontitis
Operculum — see Break, retina
Ophiasis L63.2
Ophthalmia (see also Conjunctivitis) H10.9
  actinic rays — see Photokeratitis
  allergic (acute) — see Conjunctivitis, acute, atopic
  blennorrhagic (gonococcal) (neonatorum) A54.31
  diphtheritic A36.86
  Egyptian A71.1
  electrica — see Photokeratitis
  gonococcal (neonatorum) A54.31
  metastatic — see Endophthalmitis, purulent
  migraine — see Migraine, ophthalmoplegic
  neonatorum, newborn P39.1
    gonococcal A54.31
  nodosa H16.24- ☑
  purulent — see Conjunctivitis, acute, mucopurulent
  spring — see Conjunctivitis, acute, atopic
  sympathetic — see Uveitis, sympathetic
Ophthalmitis — see Ophthalmia
Ophthalmocele (congenital) Q15.8
Ophthalmoneuromyelitis G36.0
Ophthalmoplegia (see also Strabismus, paralytic)
  anterior internuclear — see Ophthalmoplegia, internuclear
  ataxia-areflexia G61.0
  diabetic — see E08-E13 with .39
  exophthalmic E05.00
    with thyroid storm E05.01
  external H49.88- ☑
    progressive H49.4- ☑
      with pigmentary retinopathy — see Kearns-Sayre syndrome
    total H49.3- ☑
  internal (complete) (total) H52.51- ☑
  internuclear H51.2- ☑
  migraine — see Migraine, ophthalmoplegic
  Parinaud's H49.88- ☑
  progressive external — see Ophthalmoplegia, external, progressive
  supranuclear, progressive G23.1
  total (external) — see Ophthalmoplegia, external, total
Opioid(s)
  abuse — see Abuse, drug, opioids
  dependence — see Dependence, drug, opioids
  induced, without use disorder
    anxiety disorder F11.988
    delirium F11.921
    depressive disorder F11.94
    sexual dysfunction F11.981
    sleep disorder F11.982
Opisthognathism M26.09
Opisthorchiasis (felineus) (viverrini) B66.0
Opitz' disease D73.2
Opiumism — see Dependence, drug, opioid
Oppenheim's disease G70.2
Oppenheim-Urbach disease (necrobiosis lipoidica diabeticorum) — see E08-E13 with .620
Optic nerve — see condition
Orbit — see condition
Orchioblastoma C62.9- ☑
Orchitis (gangrenous) (nonspecific) (septic) (suppurative) N45.2
  blennorrhagic (gonococcal) (acute) (chronic) A54.23
  chlamydial A56.19
  filarial (see also Infestation, filarial) B74.9 [N51]
  gonococcal (acute) (chronic) A54.23
  mumps B26.0
  syphilitic A52.76
  tuberculous A18.15
Orf (virus disease) B08.02
Organic (see also condition)
  brain syndrome F09
  heart — see Disease, heart

☑ **Additional Character Required** — Refer to the Tabular List for Character Selection

Subterms under main terms may continue to next column or page

Organic — *continued*
  mental disorder F09
  psychosis F09
Orgasm
  anejaculatory N53.13
Oriental
  bilharziasis B65.2
  schistosomiasis B65.2
Orifice — *see* condition
Origin of both great vessels from right ventricle
  Q20.1
Ormond's disease (with ureteral obstruction) N13.5
  with infection N13.6
Ornithine metabolism disorder E72.4
Ornithinemia (Type I) (Type II) E72.4
Ornithosis A70
Orotaciduria, oroticaciduria (congenital) (hereditary)
  (pyrimidine deficiency) E79.8
  anemia D53.0
Orthodontics
  adjustment Z46.4
  fitting Z46.4
Orthopnea R06.01
Orthopoxvirus B08.09
  specified NEC B08.09
Os, uterus — *see* condition
Osgood-Schlatter disease or osteochondrosis — *see*
  Osteochondrosis, juvenile, tibia
Osler (-Weber)-**Rendu disease** I78.0
Osler's nodes I33.0
Osmidrosis L75.0
Osseous — *see* condition
Ossification
  artery — *see* Arteriosclerosis
  auricle (ear) — *see* Disorder, pinna, specified type NEC
  bronchial J98.09
  cardiac — *see* Degeneration, myocardial
  cartilage (senile) — *see* Disorder, cartilage, specified
    type NEC
  coronary (artery) — *see* Disease, heart, ischemic,
    atherosclerotic
  diaphragm J98.6
  ear, middle — *see* Otosclerosis
  falx cerebri G96.19
  fontanel, premature Q75.0
  heart (see also Degeneration, myocardial)
    valve — *see* Endocarditis
  larynx J38.7
  ligament — *see* Disorder, tendon, specified type NEC
    posterior longitudinal — *see* Spondylopathy, spec-
      ified NEC
  meninges (cerebral) (spinal) G96.19
  multiple, eccentric centers — *see* Disorder, bone, de-
    velopment or growth
  muscle (see also Calcification, muscle)
    due to burns — *see* Myositis, ossificans, in, burns
    paralytic — *see* Myositis, ossificans, in, quadriplegia
    progressive — *see* Myositis, ossificans, progressiva
    specified NEC M61.50
      ankle M61.57- ☑
      foot M61.57- ☑
      forearm M61.53- ☑
      hand M61.54- ☑
      lower leg M61.56- ☑
      multiple sites M61.59
      pelvic region M61.55- ☑
      shoulder region M61.51- ☑
      specified site NEC M61.58
      thigh M61.55- ☑
      upper arm M61.52- ☑
    traumatic — *see* Myositis, ossificans, traumatica
  myocardium, myocardial — *see* Degeneration, myocar-
    dial
  penis N48.89
  periarticular — *see* Disorder, joint, specified type NEC
  pinna — *see* Disorder, pinna, specified type NEC
  rider's bone — *see* Ossification, muscle, specified NEC
  sclera H15.89
  subperiosteal, post-traumatic M89.8X- ☑
  tendon — *see* Disorder, tendon, specified type NEC
  trachea J39.8
  tympanic membrane — *see* Disorder, tympanic mem-
    brane, specified NEC
  vitreous (humor) — *see* Deposit, crystalline
Osteitis (*see also* Osteomyelitis)
  alveolar M27.3
  condensans M85.30

Osteitis — *continued*
  condensans — *continued*
    ankle M85.37- ☑
    foot M85.37- ☑
    forearm M85.33- ☑
    hand M85.34- ☑
    lower leg M85.36- ☑
    multiple site M85.39
    neck M85.38
    rib M85.38
    shoulder M85.31- ☑
    skull M85.38
    specified site NEC M85.38
    thigh M85.35- ☑
    toe M85.37- ☑
    upper arm M85.32- ☑
    vertebra M85.38
  deformans M88.9
    in (due to)
      malignant neoplasm of bone C41.9 [M90.60]
      neoplastic disease (*see also* Neoplasm)
        D49.9 [M90.60]
        carpus D49.9 [M90.64-] ☑
        clavicle D49.9 [M90.61-] ☑
        femur D49.9 [M90.65-] ☑
        fibula D49.9 [M90.66-] ☑
        finger D49.9 [M90.64-] ☑
        humerus D49.9 [M90.62-] ☑
        ilium D49.9 [M90.65-] ☑
        ischium D49.9 [M90.65-] ☑
        metacarpus D49.9 [M90.64-] ☑
        metatarsus D49.9 [M90.67-] ☑
        multiple sites D49.9 [M90.69]
        neck D49.9 [M90.68]
        radius D49.9 [M90.63-] ☑
        rib D49.9 [M90.68]
        scapula D49.9 [M90.61-] ☑
        skull D49.9 [M90.68]
        tarsus D49.9 [M90.67-] ☑
        tibia D49.9 [M90.66-] ☑
        toe D49.9 [M90.67-] ☑
        ulna D49.9 [M90.63-] ☑
        vertebra D49.9 [M90.68]
    skull M88.0
    specified NEC — *see* Paget's disease, bone, by site
    vertebra M88.1
  due to yaws A66.6
  fibrosa NEC — *see* Cyst, bone, by site
    circumscripta — *see* Dysplasia, fibrous, bone NEC
    cystica (generalisata) E21.0
    disseminata Q78.1
    osteoplastica E21.0
  fragilitans Q78.0
  Garr's (sclerosing) — *see* Osteomyelitis, specified type
    NEC
  jaw (acute) (chronic) (lower) (suppurative) (upper)
    M27.2
  parathyroid E21.0
  petrous bone (acute) (chronic) — *see* Petrositis
  sclerotic, nonsuppurative — *see* Osteomyelitis, speci-
    fied type NEC
  tuberculosa A18.09
    cystica D86.89
    multiplex cystoides D86.89
Osteoarthritis M19.90
  ankle M19.07- ☑
  elbow M19.02- ☑
  foot joint M19.07- ☑
  generalized M15.9
    erosive M15.4
    primary M15.0
    specified NEC M15.8
  hand joint M19.04- ☑
    first carpometacarpal joint M18.9
  hip M16.1- ☑
    bilateral M16.0
    due to hip dysplasia (unilateral) M16.3- ☑
      bilateral M16.2
  interphalangeal
    distal (Heberden) M15.1
    proximal (Bouchard) M15.2
  knee M17.1- ☑
    bilateral M17.0
  post-traumatic NEC M19.92
    ankle M19.17- ☑
    elbow M19.12- ☑
    foot joint M19.17- ☑

Osteoarthritis — *continued*
  post-traumatic — *continued*
    hand joint M19.14- ☑
      first carpometacarpal joint M18.3- ☑
        bilateral M18.2
    hip M16.5- ☑
      bilateral M16.4
    knee M17.3- ☑
      bilateral M17.2
    shoulder M19.11- ☑
    wrist M19.13- ☑
  primary M19.91
    ankle M19.07- ☑
    elbow M19.02- ☑
    foot joint M19.07- ☑
    hand joint M19.04- ☑
      first carpometacarpal joint M18.1- ☑
        bilateral M18.0
    hip M16.1- ☑
      bilateral M16.0
    knee M17.1- ☑
      bilateral M17.0
    shoulder M19.01- ☑
    spine — *see* Spondylosis
    wrist M19.03- ☑
  secondary M19.93
    ankle M19.27- ☑
    elbow M19.22- ☑
    foot joint M19.27- ☑
    hand joint M19.24- ☑
      first carpometacarpal joint M18.5- ☑
        bilateral M18.4
    hip M16.7
      bilateral M16.6
    knee M17.5
      bilateral M17.4
    multiple M15.3
    shoulder M19.21- ☑
    spine — *see* Spondylosis
    wrist M19.23- ☑
  shoulder M19.01- ☑
  spine — *see* Spondylosis
  wrist M19.03- ☑
Osteoarthropathy (hypertrophic) M19.90
  ankle — *see* Osteoarthritis, primary, ankle
  elbow — *see* Osteoarthritis, primary, elbow
  foot joint — *see* Osteoarthritis, primary, foot
  hand joint — *see* Osteoarthritis, primary, hand joint
  knee joint — *see* Osteoarthritis, primary, knee
  multiple site — *see* Osteoarthritis, primary, multiple
    joint
  pulmonary (*see also* Osteoarthropathy, specified type
    NEC)
    hypertrophic — *see* Osteoarthropathy, hypertrophic,
      specified type NEC
  secondary — *see* Osteoarthropathy, specified type NEC
  secondary hypertrophic — *see* Osteoarthropathy,
    specified type NEC
  shoulder — *see* Osteoarthritis, primary, shoulder
  specified joint NEC — *see* Osteoarthritis, primary,
    specified joint NEC
  specified type NEC M89.40
    carpus M89.44- ☑
    clavicle M89.41- ☑
    femur M89.45- ☑
    fibula M89.46- ☑
    finger M89.44- ☑
    humerus M89.42- ☑
    ilium M89.459
    ischium M89.459
    metacarpus M89.44- ☑
    metatarsus M89.47- ☑
    multiple sites M89.49
    neck M89.48
    radius M89.43- ☑
    rib M89.48
    scapula M89.41- ☑
    skull M89.48
    tarsus M89.47- ☑
    tibia M89.46- ☑
    toe M89.47- ☑
    ulna M89.43- ☑
    vertebra M89.48
  spine — *see* Spondylosis
  wrist — *see* Osteoarthritis, primary, wrist
Osteoarthrosis (degenerative) (hypertrophic) (joint) (*see*
  also Osteoarthritis)

Osteoarthrosis — continued
  deformans alkaptonurica E70.29 [M36.8]
  erosive M15.4
  generalized M15.9
    primary M15.0
  polyarticular M15.9
  spine — see Spondylosis
Osteoblastoma — see Neoplasm, bone, benign
  aggressive — see Neoplasm, bone, uncertain behavior
Osteochondritis (see also Osteochondropathy, by site)
  Brailsford's — see Osteochondrosis, juvenile, radius
  dissecans M93.20
    ankle M93.27- ☑
    elbow M93.22- ☑
    foot M93.27- ☑
    hand M93.24- ☑
    hip M93.25- ☑
    knee M93.26- ☑
    multiple sites M93.29
    shoulder joint M93.21- ☑
    specified site NEC M93.28
    wrist M93.23- ☑
  juvenile M92.9
    patellar — see Osteochondrosis, juvenile, patella
  syphilitic (congenital) (early) A50.02 [M90.80]
    ankle A50.02 [M90.87-] ☑
    elbow A50.02 [M90.82-] ☑
    foot A50.02 [M90.87-] ☑
    forearm A50.02 [M90.83-] ☑
    hand A50.02 [M90.84-] ☑
    hip A50.02 [M90.85-] ☑
    knee A50.02 [M90.86-] ☑
    multiple sites A50.02 [M90.89]
    shoulder joint A50.02 [M90.81-] ☑
    specified site NEC A50.02 [M90.88]
Osteochondroarthrosis deformans endemica — see
  Disease, Kaschin-Beck
Osteochondrodysplasia Q78.9
  with defects of growth of tubular bones and spine
    Q77.9
    specified NEC Q77.8
  specified NEC Q78.8
Osteochondrodystrophy E78.9
Osteochondrolysis — see Osteochondritis, dissecans
Osteochondroma — see Neoplasm, bone, benign
Osteochondromatosis D48.0
  syndrome Q78.4
Osteochondromyxosarcoma — see Neoplasm, bone,
  malignant
Osteochondropathy M93.90
  ankle M93.97- ☑
  elbow M93.92- ☑
  foot M93.97- ☑
  hand M93.94- ☑
  hip M93.95- ☑
  Kienböck's disease of adults M93.1
  knee M93.96- ☑
  multiple joints M93.99
  osteochondritis dissecans — see Osteochondritis, dis-
    secans
  osteochondrosis — see Osteochondrosis
  shoulder region M93.91- ☑
  slipped upper femoral epiphysis — see Slipped, epiph-
    ysis, upper femoral
  specified joint NEC M93.98
  specified type NEC M93.80
    ankle M93.87- ☑
    elbow M93.82- ☑
    foot M93.87- ☑
    hand M93.84- ☑
    hip M93.85- ☑
    knee M93.86- ☑
    multiple joints M93.89
    shoulder region M93.81- ☑
    specified joint NEC M93.88
    wrist M93.83- ☑
  syphilitic, congenital
    early A50.02 [M90.80]
    late A50.56 [M90.80]
  wrist M93.93- ☑
Osteochondrosarcoma — see Neoplasm, bone, malignant
Osteochondrosis (see also Osteochondropathy, by site)
  acetabulum (juvenile) M91.0
  adult — see Osteochondropathy, specified type NEC,
    by site

Osteochondrosis — continued
  astragalus (juvenile) — see Osteochondrosis, juvenile,
    tarsus
  Blount's — see Osteochondrosis, juvenile, tibia
  Buchanan's M91.0
  Burns' — see Osteochondrosis, juvenile, ulna
  calcaneus (juvenile) — see Osteochondrosis, juvenile,
    tarsus
  capitular epiphysis (femur) (juvenile) — see Legg-Calvé-
    Perthes disease
  carpal (juvenile) (lunate) (scaphoid) — see Osteochon-
    drosis, juvenile, hand, carpal lunate
    adult M93.1
  coxae juvenilis — see Legg-Calvé-Perthes disease
  deformans juvenilis, coxae — see Legg-Calvé-Perthes
    disease
  Diaz's — see Osteochondrosis, juvenile, tarsus
  dissecans (knee) (shoulder) — see Osteochondritis,
    dissecans
  femoral capital epiphysis (juvenile) — see Legg-Calvé-
    Perthes disease
  femur (head), juvenile — see Legg-Calvé-Perthes dis-
    ease
  fibula (juvenile) — see Osteochondrosis, juvenile,
    fibula
  foot NEC (juvenile) M92.8
  Freiberg's — see Osteochondrosis, juvenile, metatarsus
  Haas' — see Osteochondrosis, juvenile,
    humerus
  Haglund's — see Osteochondrosis, juvenile, tarsus
  hip (juvenile) — see Legg-Calvé-Perthes disease
  humerus (capitulum) (head) (juvenile) — see Osteo-
    chondrosis, juvenile, humerus
  ilium, iliac crest (juvenile) M91.0
  ischiopubic synchondrosis M91.0
  Iselin's — see Osteochondrosis, juvenile, metatarsus
  juvenile, juvenilis M92.9
    after congenital dislocation of hip reduction — see
      Osteochondrosis, juvenile, hip, specified NEC
    arm — see Osteochondrosis, juvenile, upper limb
      NEC
    capitular epiphysis (femur) — see Legg-Calvé-
      Perthes disease
    clavicle, sternal epiphysis — see Osteochondrosis,
      juvenile, upper limb NEC
    coxae — see Legg-Calvé-Perthes disease
    deformans M92.9
    fibula M92.5- ☑
    foot NEC M92.8
    hand M92.20- ☑
      carpal lunate M92.21- ☑
      metacarpal head M92.22- ☑
      specified site NEC M92.29- ☑
    head of femur — see Legg-Calvé-Perthes disease
    hip and pelvis M91.9- ☑
      coxa plana — see Coxa, plana
      femoral head — see Legg-Calvé-Perthes disease
      pelvis M91.0
      pseudocoxalgia — see Pseudocoxalgia
      specified NEC M91.8- ☑
    humerus M92.0- ☑
    limb
      lower NEC M92.8
      upper NEC — see Osteochondrosis, juvenile,
        upper limb NEC
    medial cuneiform bone — see Osteochondrosis,
      juvenile, tarsus
    metatarsus M92.7- ☑
    patella M92.4- ☑
    radius M92.1- ☑
    specified site NEC M92.8
    spine M42.00
      cervical region M42.02
      cervicothoracic region M42.03
      lumbar region M42.06
      lumbosacral region M42.07
      multiple sites M42.09
      occipito-atlanto-axial region M42.01
      sacrococcygeal region M42.08
      thoracic region M42.04
      thoracolumbar region M42.05
    tarsus M92.6- ☑
    tibia M92.5- ☑
    ulna M92.1- ☑
    upper limb NEC M92.3- ☑

Osteochondrosis — continued
  juvenile, juvenilis — continued
    vertebra (body) (epiphyseal plates) (Calvé's)
      (Scheuermann's) — see Osteochondrosis, ju-
      venile, spine
  Kienböck's — see Osteochondrosis, juvenile, hand,
    carpal lunate
    adult M93.1
  Köhler's
    patellar — see Osteochondrosis, juvenile, patella
    tarsal navicular — see Osteochondrosis, juvenile,
      tarsus
  Legg-Perthes (-Calvé)(-Waldenström) — see Legg-
    Calvé-Perthes disease
  limb
    lower NEC (juvenile) M92.8
    upper NEC (juvenile) — see Osteochondrosis, juve-
      nile, upper limb NEC
  lunate bone (carpal) (juvenile) (see also Osteochondro-
    sis, juvenile, hand, carpal lunate)
    adult M93.1
  Mauclaire's — see Osteochondrosis, juvenile, hand,
    metacarpal
  metacarpal (head) (juvenile) — see Osteochondrosis,
    juvenile, hand, metacarpal
  metatarsus (fifth) (head) (juvenile) (second) — see Os-
    teochondrosis, juvenile, metatarsus
  navicular (juvenile) — see Osteochondrosis, juvenile,
    tarsus
  os
    calcis (juvenile) — see Osteochondrosis, juvenile,
      tarsus
    tibiale externum (juvenile) — see Osteochondrosis,
      juvenile, tarsus
  Osgood-Schlatter — see Osteochondrosis, juvenile,
    tibia
  Panner's — see Osteochondrosis, juvenile, humerus
  patellar center (juvenile) (primary) (secondary) — see
    Osteochondrosis, juvenile, patella
  pelvis (juvenile) M91.0
  Pierson's M91.0
  radius (head) (juvenile) — see Osteochondrosis, juve-
    nile, radius
  Scheuermann's — see Osteochondrosis, juvenile, spine
  Sever's — see Osteochondrosis, juvenile, tarsus
  Sinding-Larsen — see Osteochondrosis, juvenile,
    patella
  spine M42.9
    adult M42.10
      cervical region M42.12
      cervicothoracic region M42.13
      lumbar region M42.16
      lumbosacral region M42.17
      multiple sites M42.19
      occipito-atlanto-axial region M42.11
      sacrococcygeal region M42.18
      thoracic region M42.14
      thoracolumbar region M42.15
    juvenile — see Osteochondrosis, juvenile, spine
  symphysis pubis (juvenile) M91.0
  syphilitic (congenital) A50.02
  talus (juvenile) — see Osteochondrosis, juvenile, tarsus
  tarsus (navicular) (juvenile) — see Osteochondrosis,
    juvenile, tarsus
  tibia (proximal) (tubercle) (juvenile) — see Osteochon-
    drosis, juvenile, tibia
  tuberculous — see Tuberculosis, bone
  ulna (lower) (juvenile) — see Osteochondrosis, juvenile,
    ulna
  van Neck's M91.0
  vertebral — see Osteochondrosis, spine
Osteoclastoma D48.0
  malignant — see Neoplasm, bone, malignant
Osteodynia — see Disorder, bone, specified type NEC
Osteodystrophy Q78.9
  azotemic N25.0
  congenital Q78.9
  parathyroid, secondary E21.1
  renal N25.0
Osteofibroma — see Neoplasm, bone, benign
Osteofibrosarcoma — see Neoplasm, bone, malignant
Osteogenesis imperfecta Q78.0
Osteogenic — see condition
Osteolysis M89.50
  carpus M89.54- ☑
  clavicle M89.51- ☑
  femur M89.55- ☑

Osteolysis — *continued*
  fibula M89.56- ☑
  finger M89.54- ☑
  humerus M89.52- ☑
  ilium M89.559
  ischium M89.559
  joint prosthesis (periprosthetic) — *see* Complications, joint prosthesis, mechanical, periprosthetic, osteolysis, by site
  metacarpus M89.54- ☑
  metatarsus M89.57- ☑
  multiple sites M89.59
  neck M89.58
  periprosthetic — *see* Complications, joint prosthesis, mechanical, periprosthetic, osteolysis, by site
  radius M89.53- ☑
  rib M89.58
  scapula M89.51- ☑
  skull M89.58
  tarsus M89.57- ☑
  tibia M89.56- ☑
  toe M89.57- ☑
  ulna M89.53- ☑
  vertebra M89.58

Osteoma (*see also* Neoplasm, bone, benign)
  osteoid (*see also* Neoplasm, bone, benign)
    giant — *see* Neoplasm, bone, benign
Osteomalacia M83.9
  adult M83.9
    drug-induced NEC M83.5
    due to
      malabsorption (postsurgical) M83.2
      malnutrition M83.3
    specified NEC M83.8
  aluminium-induced M83.4
  infantile — *see* Rickets
  juvenile — *see* Rickets
  oncogenic E83.89
  pelvis M83.8
  puerperal M83.0
  senile M83.1
  vitamin-D-resistant in adults E83.31 [M90.8-] ☑
    carpus E83.31 [M90.84-] ☑
    clavicle E83.31 [M90.81-] ☑
    femur E83.31 [M90.85-] ☑
    fibula E83.31 [M90.86-] ☑
    finger E83.31 [M90.84-] ☑
    humerus E83.31 [M90.82-] ☑
    ilium E83.31 [M90.859]
    ischium E83.31 [M90.859]
    metacarpus E83.31 [M90.84-] ☑
    metatarsus E83.31 [M90.87-] ☑
    multiple sites E83.31 [M90.89]
    neck E83.31 [M90.88]
    radius E83.31 [M90.83-] ☑
    rib E83.31 [M90.88]
    scapula E83.31 [M90.819]
    skull E83.31 [M90.88]
    tarsus E83.31 [M90.879]
    tibia E83.31 [M90.869]
    toe E83.31 [M90.879]
    ulna E83.31 [M90.839]
    vertebra E83.31 [M90.88]

Osteomyelitis (general) (infective) (localized) (neonatal) (purulent) (septic) (staphylococcal) (streptococcal) (suppurative) (with periostitis) M86.9
  acute M86.10
    carpus M86.14- ☑
    clavicle M86.11- ☑
    femur M86.15- ☑
    fibula M86.16- ☑
    finger M86.14- ☑
    hematogenous M86.00
      carpus M86.04- ☑
      clavicle M86.01- ☑
      femur M86.05- ☑
      fibula M86.06- ☑
      finger M86.04- ☑
      humerus M86.02- ☑
      ilium M86.059
      ischium M86.059
      mandible M27.2
      metacarpus M86.04- ☑
      metatarsus M86.07- ☑
      multiple sites M86.09
      neck M86.08
      orbit H05.02- ☑

Osteomyelitis — *continued*
  acute — *continued*
    hematogenous — *continued*
      petrous bone — *see* Petrositis
      radius M86.03- ☑
      rib M86.08
      scapula M86.01- ☑
      skull M86.08
      tarsus M86.07- ☑
      tibia M86.06- ☑
      toe M86.07- ☑
      ulna M86.03- ☑
      vertebra — *see* Osteomyelitis, vertebra
    humerus M86.12- ☑
    ilium M86.159
    ischium M86.159
    mandible M27.2
    metacarpus M86.14- ☑
    metatarsus M86.17- ☑
    multiple sites M86.19
    neck M86.18
    orbit H05.02- ☑
    petrous bone — *see* Petrositis
    radius M86.13- ☑
    rib M86.18
    scapula M86.11- ☑
    skull M86.18
    tarsus M86.17- ☑
    tibia M86.16- ☑
    toe M86.17- ☑
    ulna M86.13- ☑
    vertebra — *see* Osteomyelitis, vertebra
  chronic (or old) M86.60
    with draining sinus M86.40
      carpus M86.44- ☑
      clavicle M86.41- ☑
      femur M86.45- ☑
      fibula M86.46- ☑
      finger M86.44- ☑
      humerus M86.42- ☑
      ilium M86.459
      ischium M86.459
      mandible M27.2
      metacarpus M86.44- ☑
      metatarsus M86.47- ☑
      multiple sites M86.49
      neck M86.48
      orbit H05.02- ☑
      petrous bone — *see* Petrositis
      radius M86.43- ☑
      rib M86.48
      scapula M86.41- ☑
      skull M86.48
      tarsus M86.47- ☑
      tibia M86.46- ☑
      toe M86.47- ☑
      ulna M86.43- ☑
      vertebra — *see* Osteomyelitis, vertebra
    carpus M86.64- ☑
    clavicle M86.61- ☑
    femur M86.65- ☑
    fibula M86.66- ☑
    finger M86.64- ☑
    hematogenous NEC M86.50
      carpus M86.54- ☑
      clavicle M86.51- ☑
      femur M86.55- ☑
      fibula M86.56- ☑
      finger M86.54- ☑
      humerus M86.52- ☑
      ilium M86.559
      ischium M86.559
      mandible M27.2
      metacarpus M86.54- ☑
      metatarsus M86.57- ☑
      multifocal M86.30
        carpus M86.34- ☑
        clavicle M86.31- ☑
        femur M86.35- ☑
        fibula M86.36- ☑
        finger M86.34- ☑
        humerus M86.32- ☑
        ilium M86.359
        ischium M86.359
        metacarpus M86.34- ☑
        metatarsus M86.37- ☑

Osteomyelitis — *continued*
  chronic — *continued*
    hematogenous — *continued*
      multifocal — *continued*
        multiple sites M86.39
        neck M86.38
        radius M86.33- ☑
        rib M86.38
        scapula M86.31- ☑
        skull M86.38
        tarsus M86.37- ☑
        tibia M86.36- ☑
        toe M86.37- ☑
        ulna M86.33- ☑
        vertebra — *see* Osteomyelitis, vertebra
      multiple sites M86.59
      neck M86.58
      orbit H05.02- ☑
      petrous bone — *see* Petrositis
      radius M86.53- ☑
      rib M86.58
      scapula M86.51- ☑
      skull M86.58
      tarsus M86.57- ☑
      tibia M86.56- ☑
      toe M86.57- ☑
      ulna M86.53- ☑
      vertebra — *see* Osteomyelitis, vertebra
    humerus M86.62- ☑
    ilium M86.659
    ischium M86.659
    mandible M27.2
    metacarpus M86.64- ☑
    metatarsus M86.67- ☑
    multifocal — *see* Osteomyelitis, chronic, hematogenous, multifocal
    multiple sites M86.69
    neck M86.68
    orbit H05.02- ☑
    petrous bone — *see* Petrositis
    radius M86.63- ☑
    rib M86.68
    scapula M86.61- ☑
    skull M86.68
    tarsus M86.67- ☑
    tibia M86.66- ☑
    toe M86.67- ☑
    ulna M86.63- ☑
    vertebra — *see* Osteomyelitis, vertebra
  echinococcal B67.2
  Garr's — *see* Osteomyelitis, specified type NEC
  in diabetes mellitus — *see* E08-E13 with .69
  jaw (acute) (chronic) (lower) (neonatal) (suppurative) (upper) M27.2
  nonsuppurating — *see* Osteomyelitis, specified type NEC
  orbit H05.02- ☑
  petrous bone — *see* Petrositis
  Salmonella (arizonae) (cholerae-suis) (enteritidis) (typhimurium) A02.24
  sclerosing, nonsuppurative — *see* Osteomyelitis, specified type NEC
  specified type NEC (*see also* subcategory) M86.8X- ☑
    mandible M27.2
    orbit H05.02- ☑
    petrous bone — *see* Petrositis
    vertebra — *see* Osteomyelitis, vertebra
  subacute M86.20
    carpus M86.24- ☑
    clavicle M86.21- ☑
    femur M86.25- ☑
    fibula M86.26- ☑
    finger M86.24- ☑
    humerus M86.22- ☑
    mandible M27.2
    metacarpus M86.24- ☑
    metatarsus M86.27- ☑
    multiple sites M86.29
    neck M86.28
    orbit H05.02- ☑
    petrous bone — *see* Petrositis
    radius M86.23- ☑
    rib M86.28
    scapula M86.21- ☑
    skull M86.28
    tarsus M86.27- ☑
    tibia M86.26- ☑

Index

Osteolysis — Osteomyelitis

Osteomyelitis — *continued*
  subacute — *continued*
    toe M86.27- ☑
    ulna M86.23- ☑
    vertebra — *see* Osteomyelitis, vertebra
  syphilitic A52.77
    congenital (early) A50.02 [M90.80]
  tuberculous — *see* Tuberculosis, bone
  typhoid A01.05
  vertebra M46.20
    cervical region M46.22
    cervicothoracic region M46.23
    lumbar region M46.26
    lumbosacral region M46.27
    occipito-atlanto-axial region M46.21
    sacrococcygeal region M46.28
    thoracic region M46.24
    thoracolumbar region M46.25
Osteomyelofibrosis D47.4
Osteomyelosclerosis D75.89
Osteonecrosis M87.9
  due to
    drugs — *see* Osteonecrosis, secondary, due to, drugs
    trauma — *see* Osteonecrosis, secondary, due to, trauma
  idiopathic aseptic M87.00
    ankle M87.07- ☑
    carpus M87.03- ☑
    clavicle M87.01- ☑
    femur M87.05- ☑
    fibula M87.06- ☑
    finger M87.04- ☑
    humerus M87.02- ☑
    ilium M87.050
    ischium M87.050
    metacarpus M87.04- ☑
    metatarsus M87.07- ☑
    multiple sites M87.09
    neck M87.08
    pelvis M87.050
    radius M87.03- ☑
    rib M87.08
    scapula M87.01- ☑
    skull M87.08
    tarsus M87.07- ☑
    tibia M87.06- ☑
    toe M87.07- ☑
    ulna M87.03- ☑
    vertebra M87.08
  secondary NEC M87.30
    carpus M87.33- ☑
    clavicle M87.31- ☑
    due to
      drugs M87.10
        carpus M87.13- ☑
        clavicle M87.11- ☑
        femur M87.15- ☑
        fibula M87.16- ☑
        finger M87.14- ☑
        humerus M87.12- ☑
        ilium M87.159
        ischium M87.159
        jaw M87.180
        metacarpus M87.14- ☑
        metatarsus M87.17- ☑
        multiple sites M87.19
        neck M87.18 ☑
        radius M87.13- ☑
        rib M87.18
        scapula M87.11- ☑
        skull M87.18 ☑
        tarsus M87.17- ☑
        tibia M87.16- ☑
        toe M87.17- ☑
        ulna M87.13- ☑
        vertebra M87.18 ☑
      hemoglobinopathy NEC D58.2 [M90.50]
        carpus D58.2 [M90.54-] ☑
        clavicle D58.2 [M90.51-] ☑
        femur D58.2 [M90.55-] ☑
        fibula D58.2 [M90.56-] ☑
        finger D58.2 [M90.54-] ☑
        humerus D58.2 [M90.52-] ☑
        ilium D58.2 [M90.55-] ☑
        ischium D58.2 [M90.55-] ☑
        metacarpus D58.2 [M90.54-] ☑
        metatarsus D58.2 [M90.57-] ☑

Osteonecrosis — *continued*
  secondary — *continued*
    due to — *continued*
      hemoglobinopathy — *continued*
        multiple sites D58.2 [M90.58]
        neck D58.2 [M90.58]
        radius D58.2 [M90.53-] ☑
        rib D58.2 [M90.58]
        scapula D58.2 [M90.51-] ☑
        skull D58.2 [M90.58]
        tarsus D58.2 [M90.57-] ☑
        tibia D58.2 [M90.56-] ☑
        toe D58.2 [M90.57-] ☑
        ulna D58.2 [M90.53-] ☑
        vertebra D58.2 [M90.58]
      trauma (previous) M87.20
        carpus M87.23- ☑
        clavicle M87.21- ☑
        femur M87.25- ☑
        fibula M87.26- ☑
        finger M87.24- ☑
        humerus M87.22- ☑
        ilium M87.25- ☑
        ischium M87.25- ☑
        metacarpus M87.24- ☑
        metatarsus M87.27- ☑
        multiple sites M87.29
        neck M87.28
        radius M87.23- ☑
        rib M87.28
        scapula M87.21- ☑
        skull M87.28
        tarsus M87.27- ☑
        tibia M87.26- ☑
        toe M87.27- ☑
        ulna M87.23- ☑
        vertebra M87.28
    femur M87.35- ☑
    fibula M87.36- ☑
    finger M87.34- ☑
    humerus M87.32- ☑
    ilium M87.350
    in
      caisson disease T70.3 ☑ [M90.50]
        carpus T70.3 [M90.54-] ☑
        clavicle T70.3 [M90.51-] ☑
        femur T70.3 [M90.55-] ☑
        fibula T70.3 [M90.56-] ☑
        finger T70.3 [M90.54-] ☑
        humerus T70.3 ☑ [M90.52-] ☑
        ilium T70.3 ☑ [M90.55-]
        ischium T70.3 ☑ [M90.55-] ☑
        metacarpus T70.3 ☑ [M90.54-] ☑
        metatarsus T70.3 [M90.57-] ☑
        multiple sites T70.3 ☑ [M90.59]
        neck T70.3 ☑ [M90.58]
        radius T70.3 [M90.53-] ☑
        rib T70.3 ☑ [M90.58]
        scapula T70.3 [M90.51-] ☑
        skull T70.3 ☑ [M90.58]
        tarsus T70.3 [M90.57-] ☑
        tibia T70.3 [M90.56-] ☑
        toe T70.3 ☑ [M90.57-] ☑
        ulna T70.3 [M90.53-] ☑
        vertebra T70.3 ☑ [M90.58]
    ischium M87.350
    metacarpus M87.34- ☑
    metatarsus M87.37- ☑
    multiple site M87.39
    neck M87.38
    radius M87.33- ☑
    rib M87.38
    scapula M87.319
    skull M87.38
    tarsus M87.379
    tibia M87.366
    toe M87.379
    ulna M87.33- ☑
    vertebra M87.38
  specified type NEC M87.80
    carpus M87.83- ☑
    clavicle M87.81- ☑
    femur M87.85- ☑
    fibula M87.86- ☑
    finger M87.84- ☑
    humerus M87.82- ☑

Osteonecrosis — *continued*
  specified type — *continued*
    ilium M87.85- ☑
    ischium M87.85- ☑
    metacarpus M87.84- ☑
    metatarsus M87.87- ☑
    multiple sites M87.89
    neck M87.88
    radius M87.83- ☑
    rib M87.88
    scapula M87.81- ☑
    skull M87.88
    tarsus M87.87- ☑
    tibia M87.86- ☑
    toe M87.87- ☑
    ulna M87.83- ☑
    vertebra M87.88
Osteo-onycho-arthro-dysplasia Q87.2
Osteo-onychodysplasia, hereditary Q87.2
Osteopathia condensans disseminata Q78.8
Osteopathy (*see also* Osteomyelitis, Osteonecrosis, Osteoporosis)
  after poliomyelitis M89.60
    carpus M89.64- ☑
    clavicle M89.61- ☑
    femur M89.65- ☑
    fibula M89.66- ☑
    finger M89.64- ☑
    humerus M89.62- ☑
    ilium M89.659
    ischium M89.659
    metacarpus M89.64- ☑
    metatarsus M89.67- ☑
    multiple sites M89.69
    neck M89.68
    radius M89.63- ☑
    rib M89.68
    scapula M89.61- ☑
    skull M89.68
    tarsus M89.67- ☑
    tibia M89.66- ☑
    toe M89.67- ☑
    ulna M89.63- ☑
    vertebra M89.68
  in (due to)
    renal osteodystrophy N25.0
    specified diseases classified elsewhere — *see* subcategory M90.8 ☑
Osteopenia M85.8- ☑
  borderline M85.8- ☑
Osteoperiostitis — *see* Osteomyelitis, specified type NEC
Osteopetrosis (familial) Q78.2
Osteophyte M25.70
  ankle M25.77- ☑
  elbow M25.72- ☑
  foot joint M25.77- ☑
  hand joint M25.74- ☑
  hip M25.75- ☑
  knee M25.76- ☑
  shoulder M25.71- ☑
  spine M25.78
  vertebrae M25.78
  wrist M25.73- ☑
Osteopoikilosis Q78.8
Osteoporosis (female) (male) M81.0
  with current pathological fracture M80.00 ☑
  age-related M81.0
    with current pathologic fracture M80.00 ☑
      carpus M80.04- ☑
      clavicle M80.01- ☑
      fibula M80.06- ☑
      finger M80.04- ☑
      humerus M80.02- ☑
      ilium M80.05- ☑
      ischium M80.05- ☑
      metacarpus M80.04- ☑
      metatarsus M80.07- ☑
      pelvis M80.05- ☑
      radius M80.03- ☑
      scapula M80.01- ☑
      tarsus M80.07- ☑
      tibia M80.06- ☑
      toe M80.07- ☑
      ulna M80.03- ☑
      vertebra M80.08 ☑

☑ **Additional Character Required** — Refer to the Tabular List for Character Selection   ▽ **Subterms under main terms may continue to next column or page**

Osteoporosis — *continued*
  disuse M81.8
    with current pathological fracture M80.80 ☑
      carpus M80.84- ☑
      clavicle M80.81- ☑
      fibula M80.86- ☑
      finger M80.84- ☑
      humerus M80.82- ☑
      ilium M80.85- ☑
      ischium M80.85- ☑
      metacarpus M80.84- ☑
      metatarsus M80.87- ☑
      pelvis M80.85- ☑
      radius M80.83- ☑
      scapula M80.81- ☑
      tarsus M80.87- ☑
      tibia M80.86- ☑
      toe M80.87- ☑
      ulna M80.83- ☑
      vertebra M80.88 ☑
  drug-induced — *see* Osteoporosis, specified type NEC
  idiopathic — *see* Osteoporosis, specified type NEC
  involutional — *see* Osteoporosis, age-related
  Lequesne M81.6
  localized M81.6
  postmenopausal M81.0
    with pathological fracture M80.00 ☑
      carpus M80.04- ☑
      clavicle M80.01- ☑
      fibula M80.06- ☑
      finger M80.04- ☑
      humerus M80.02- ☑
      ilium M80.05- ☑
      ischium M80.05- ☑
      metacarpus M80.04- ☑
      metatarsus M80.07- ☑
      pelvis M80.05- ☑
      radius M80.03- ☑
      scapula M80.01- ☑
      tarsus M80.07- ☑
      tibia M80.06- ☑
      toe M80.07- ☑
      ulna M80.03- ☑
      vertebra M80.08 ☑
  postoophorectomy — *see* Osteoporosis, specified type NEC
  postsurgical malabsorption — *see* Osteoporosis, specified type NEC
  post-traumatic — *see* Osteoporosis, specified type NEC
  senile — *see* Osteoporosis, age-related
  specified type NEC M81.8
    with pathological fracture M80.80 ☑
      carpus M80.84- ☑
      clavicle M80.81- ☑
      fibula M80.86- ☑
      finger M80.84- ☑
      humerus M80.82- ☑
      ilium M80.85- ☑
      ischium M80.85- ☑
      metacarpus M80.84- ☑
      metatarsus M80.87- ☑
      pelvis M80.85- ☑
      radius M80.83- ☑
      scapula M80.81- ☑
      tarsus M80.87- ☑
      tibia M80.86- ☑
      toe M80.87- ☑
      ulna M80.83- ☑
      vertebra M80.88 ☑
Osteopsathyrosis (idiopathica) Q78.0
Osteoradionecrosis, jaw (acute) (chronic) (lower) (suppurative) (upper) M27.2
Osteosarcoma (any form) — *see* Neoplasm, bone, malignant
Osteosclerosis Q78.2
  acquired M85.8- ☑
  congenita Q77.4
  fragilitas (generalisata) Q78.2
  myelofibrosis D75.81
Osteosclerotic anemia D64.89
Osteosis
  cutis L94.2
  renal fibrocystic N25.0
Österreicher-Turner syndrome Q87.2
Ostium
  atrioventriculare commune Q21.2

Ostium — *continued*
  primum (arteriosum) (defect) (persistent) Q21.2
  secundum (arteriosum) (defect) (patent) (persistent) Q21.1
Ostrum-Furst syndrome Q75.8
Otalgia H92.0 ☑
Otitis (acute) H66.90
  with effusion (*see also* Otitis, media, nonsuppurative)
    purulent — *see* Otitis, media, suppurative
  adhesive — *see* subcategory H74.1 ☑
  chronic (*see also* Otitis, media, chronic)
    with effusion (*see also* Otitis, media, nonsuppurative, chronic)
  externa H60.9- ☑
    abscess — *see* Abscess, ear, external
    acute (noninfective) H60.50- ☑
      actinic H60.51- ☑
      chemical H60.52- ☑
      contact H60.53- ☑
      eczematoid H60.54- ☑
      infective — *see* Otitis, externa, infective
      reactive H60.55- ☑
      specified NEC H60.59- ☑
    cellulitis — *see* Cellulitis, ear
    chronic H60.6- ☑
    diffuse — *see* Otitis, externa, infective, diffuse
    hemorrhagic — *see* Otitis, externa, infective, hemorrhagic
    in (due to)
      aspergillosis B44.89
      candidiasis B37.84
      erysipelas A46 [H62.40]
      herpes (simplex) virus infection B00.1
        zoster B02.8
      impetigo L01.00 [H62.40]
      infectious disease NEC B99 ☑ [H62.4-] ☑
      mycosis NEC B36.9 [H62.40]
      parasitic disease NEC B89 [H62.40]
      viral disease NEC B34.9 [H62.40]
      zoster B02.8
    infective NEC H60.39- ☑
      abscess — *see* Abscess, ear, external
      cellulitis — *see* Cellulitis, ear
      diffuse H60.31- ☑
      hemorrhagic H60.32- ☑
      swimmer's ear — *see* Swimmer's, ear
    malignant H60.2- ☑
    mycotic NEC B36.9 [H62.40]
      in
        aspergillosis B44.89
        candidiasis B37.84
        moniliasis B37.84
    necrotizing — *see* Otitis, externa, malignant
    Pseudomonas aeruginosa — *see* Otitis, externa, malignant
    reactive — *see* Otitis, externa, acute, reactive
    specified NEC — *see* subcategory H60.8 ☑
    tropical NEC B36.9 [H62.40]
      aspergillosis B44.89
      candidiasis B37.84
      moniliasis B37.84
  insidiosa — *see* Otosclerosis
  interna H83.0 ☑
  media (hemorrhagic) (staphylococcal) (streptococcal) H66.9- ☑
    with effusion (nonpurulent) — *see* Otitis, media, nonsuppurative
    acute, subacute H66.90
      allergic — *see* Otitis, media, nonsuppurative, acute, allergic
      exudative — *see* Otitis, media, suppurative, acute
      mucoid — *see* Otitis, media, nonsuppurative, acute
      necrotizing (*see also* Otitis, media, suppurative, acute)
        in
          measles B05.3
          scarlet fever A38.0
      nonsuppurative NEC — *see* Otitis, media, nonsuppurative, acute
      purulent — *see* Otitis, media, suppurative, acute
      sanguinous — *see* Otitis, media, nonsuppurative, acute
      secretory — *see* Otitis, media, nonsuppurative, acute, serous
      seromucinous — *see* Otitis, media, nonsuppurative, acute

Otitis — *continued*
  media — *continued*
    acute, subacute — *continued*
      serous — *see* Otitis, media, nonsuppurative, acute, serous
      suppurative — *see* Otitis, media, suppurative, acute
    allergic — *see* Otitis, media, nonsuppurative
    catarrhal — *see* Otitis, media, nonsuppurative
    chronic H66.90
      with effusion (nonpurulent) — *see* Otitis, media, nonsuppurative, chronic
      allergic — *see* Otitis, media, nonsuppurative, chronic, allergic
      benign suppurative — *see* Otitis, media, suppurative, chronic, tubotympanic
      catarrhal — *see* Otitis, media, nonsuppurative, chronic, serous
      exudative — *see* Otitis, media, nonsuppurative, chronic
      mucinous — *see* Otitis, media, nonsuppurative, chronic, mucoid
      mucoid — *see* Otitis, media, nonsuppurative, chronic, mucoid
      nonsuppurative NEC — *see* Otitis, media, nonsuppurative, chronic
      purulent — *see* Otitis, media, suppurative, chronic
      secretory — *see* Otitis, media, nonsuppurative, chronic, mucoid
      seromucinous — *see* Otitis, media, nonsuppurative, chronic
      serous — *see* Otitis, media, nonsuppurative, chronic, serous
      suppurative — *see* Otitis, media, suppurative, chronic
      transudative — *see* Otitis, media, nonsuppurative, chronic, mucoid
    exudative — *see* Otitis, media, suppurative
    in (due to) (with)
      influenza — *see* Influenza, with, otitis media
      measles B05.3
      scarlet fever A38.0
      tuberculosis A18.6
      viral disease NEC B34.- ☑ [H67.-] ☑
    mucoid — *see* Otitis, media, nonsuppurative
    nonsuppurative H65.9- ☑
      acute or subacute NEC H65.19- ☑
        allergic H65.11- ☑
          recurrent H65.11- ☑
        recurrent H65.19- ☑
        secretory — *see* Otitis, media, nonsuppurative, serous
        serous H65.0- ☑
          recurrent H65.0- ☑
      chronic H65.49- ☑
        allergic H65.41- ☑
        mucoid H65.3- ☑
        serous H65.2- ☑
    postmeasles B05.3
    purulent — *see* Otitis, media, suppurative
    secretory — *see* Otitis, media, nonsuppurative
    seromucinous — *see* Otitis, media, nonsuppurative
    serous — *see* Otitis, media, nonsuppurative
    suppurative H66.4- ☑
      acute H66.00- ☑
        with rupture of ear drum H66.01- ☑
        recurrent H66.00- ☑
          with rupture of ear drum H66.01- ☑
      chronic (*see also* subcategory) H66.3 ☑
        atticoantral H66.2- ☑
        benign — *see* Otitis, media, suppurative, chronic, tubotympanic
        tubotympanic H66.1- ☑
    transudative — *see* Otitis, media, nonsuppurative
    tuberculous A18.6
Otocephaly Q18.2
Otolith syndrome — *see* subcategory H81.8 ☑
Otomycosis (diffuse) **NEC** B36.9 [H62.40]
  in
    aspergillosis B44.89
    candidiasis B37.84
    moniliasis B37.84
Otoporosis — *see* Otosclerosis
Otorrhagia (nontraumatic) H92.2- ☑
  traumatic — *code by* Type of injury
Otorrhea H92.1- ☑

Index

Otorrhea — *continued*
  cerebrospinal G96.0
Otosclerosis (general) H80.9- ☑
  cochlear (endosteal) H80.2- ☑
  involving
    otic capsule — *see* Otosclerosis, cochlear
    oval window
      nonobliterative H80.0- ☑
      obliterative H80.1- ☑
    round window — *see* Otosclerosis, cochlear
  nonobliterative — *see* Otosclerosis, involving, oval
      window, nonobliterative
  obliterative — *see* Otosclerosis, involving, oval window,
      obliterative
  specified NEC H80.8- ☑
Otospongiosis — *see* Otosclerosis
Otto's disease or pelvis M24.7
Outcome of delivery Z37.9
  multiple births Z37.9
    all liveborn Z37.50
      quadruplets Z37.52
      quintuplets Z37.53
      sextuplets Z37.54
      specified number NEC Z37.59
      triplets Z37.51
    all stillborn Z37.7
    some liveborn Z37.60
      quadruplets Z37.62
      quintuplets Z37.63
      sextuplets Z37.64
      specified number NEC Z37.69
      triplets Z37.61
    single NEC Z37.9
      liveborn Z37.0
      stillborn Z37.1
    twins NEC Z37.9
      both liveborn Z37.2
      both stillborn Z37.4
      one liveborn, one stillborn Z37.3
Outlet — *see* condition
Ovalocytosis (congenital) (hereditary) — *see* Elliptocyto-
      sis
Ovarian — *see* Condition
Ovariocele N83.4- ☑
Ovaritis (cystic) — *see* Oophoritis
Ovary, ovarian (*see also* condition)
  resistant syndrome E28.39
  vein syndrome N13.8
Overactive (*see also* Hyperfunction)
  adrenal cortex NEC E27.0
  bladder N32.81
  hypothalamus E23.3
  thyroid — *see* Hyperthyroidism
Overactivity R46.3
  child — *see* Disorder, attention-deficit hyperactivity
Overbite (deep) (excessive) (horizontal) (vertical) M26.29
Overbreathing — *see* Hyperventilation
Overconscientious personality F60.5
Overdevelopment — *see* Hypertrophy
Overdistension — *see* Distension
Overdose, overdosage (drug) — *see* Table of Drugs and
      Chemicals, by drug, poisoning
Overeating R63.2
  nonorganic origin F50.89
  psychogenic F50.89
Overexertion (effects) (exhaustion) T73.3 ☑
Overexposure (effects) T73.9 ☑
  exhaustion T73.2 ☑
Overfeeding — *see* Overeating
  newborn P92.4
Overfill, endodontic M27.52
Overgrowth, bone — *see* Hypertrophy, bone
Overhanging of dental restorative material (unre-
      pairable) K08.52
Overheated (places) (effects) — *see* Heat
Overjet (excessive horizontal) M26.23
Overlaid, overlying (suffocation) — *see* Asphyxia, trau-
      matic, due to mechanical threat
Overlap, excessive horizontal (teeth) M26.23
Overlapping toe (acquired) (*see also* Deformity, toe,
      specified NEC)
  congenital (fifth toe) Q66.89
Overload
  circulatory, due to transfusion (blood) (blood compo-
      nents) (TACO) E87.71
  fluid E87.70

Overload — *continued*
  fluid — *continued*
    due to transfusion (blood) (blood components)
        E87.71
    specified NEC E87.79
  iron, due to repeated red blood cell transfusions
      E83.111
  potassium (K) E87.5
  sodium (Na) E87.0
Overnutrition — *see* Hyperalimentation
Overproduction (*see also* Hypersecretion)
  ACTH E27.0
  catecholamine E27.5
  growth hormone E22.0
Overprotection, child by parent Z62.1
Overriding
  aorta Q25.49
  finger (acquired) — *see* Deformity, finger
    congenital Q68.1
  toe (acquired) (*see also* Deformity, toe, specified NEC)
    congenital Q66.89
Overstrained R53.83
  heart — *see* Hypertrophy, cardiac
Overuse, muscle NEC M70.8- ☑
Overweight E66.3
Overworked R53.83
Oviduct — *see* condition
Ovotestis Q56.0
Ovulation (cycle)
  failure or lack of N97.0
  pain N94.0
Ovum — *see* condition
Owren's disease or syndrome (parahemophilia) D68.2
Ox heart — *see* Hypertrophy, cardiac
Oxalosis E72.53
Oxaluria E72.53
Oxycephaly, oxycephalic Q75.0
  syphilitic, congenital A50.02
Oxyuriasis B80
Oxyuris vermicularis (infestation) B80
Ozena J31.0

P

Pachyderma, pachydermia L85.9
  larynx (verrucosa) J38.7
Pachydermatocele (congenital) Q82.8
Pachydermoperiostosis (*see also* Osteoarthropathy,
      hypertrophic, specified type NEC)
  clubbed nail M89.40 [L62]
Pachygyria Q04.3
Pachymeningitis (adhesive) (basal) (brain) (cervical)
      (chronic)(circumscribed) (external) (fibrous) (hemor-
      rhagic) (hypertrophic) (internal) (purulent) (spinal)
      (suppurative) — *see* Meningitis
Pachyonychia (congenital) Q84.5
Pacinian tumor — *see* Neoplasm, skin, benign
Pad, knuckle or Garrod's M72.1
Paget's disease
  with infiltrating duct carcinoma — *see* Neoplasm,
      breast, malignant
  bone M88.9
    carpus M88.84- ☑
    clavicle M88.81- ☑
    femur M88.85- ☑
    fibula M88.86- ☑
    finger M88.84- ☑
    humerus M88.82- ☑
    ilium M88.85- ☑
    in neoplastic disease — *see* Osteitis, deformans, in
        neoplastic disease
    ischium M88.85- ☑
    metacarpus M88.84- ☑
    metatarsus M88.87- ☑
    multiple sites M88.89
    neck M88.88
    radius M88.83- ☑
    rib M88.88
    scapula M88.81- ☑
    skull M88.0
    tarsus M88.87- ☑
    tibia M88.86- ☑
    toe M88.87- ☑
    ulna M88.83- ☑
    vertebra M88.88
  breast (female) C50.01- ☑

Paget's disease — *continued*
  breast — *continued*
    male C50.02- ☑
  extramammary (*see also* Neoplasm, skin, malignant)
    anus C21.0
      margin C44.590
      skin C44.590
    intraductal carcinoma — *see* Neoplasm, breast, malig-
        nant
    malignant — *see* Neoplasm, skin, malignant
      breast (female) C50.01- ☑
        male C50.02- ☑
      unspecified site (female) C50.01- ☑
        male C50.02- ☑
  mammary — *see* Paget's disease, breast
  nipple — *see* Paget's disease, breast
  osteitis deformans — *see* Paget's disease, bone
Paget-Schroetter syndrome I82.890
Pain(s) (*see also* Painful) R52
  abdominal R10.9
    colic R10.83
    generalized R10.84
      with acute abdomen R10.0
    lower R10.30
      left quadrant R10.32
      pelvic or perineal R10.2
      periumbilical R10.33
      right quadrant R10.31
    rebound — *see* Tenderness, abdominal, rebound
    severe with abdominal rigidity R10.0
    tenderness — *see* Tenderness, abdominal
    upper R10.10
      epigastric R10.13
      left quadrant R10.12
      right quadrant R10.11
  acute R52
    due to trauma G89.11
    neoplasm related G89.3
    postprocedural NEC G89.18
    post-thoracotomy G89.12
    specified by site — *code to* Pain, by site
  adnexa (uteri) R10.2
  anginoid — *see* Pain, precordial
  anus K62.89
  arm — *see* Pain, limb, upper
  axillary (axilla) M79.62- ☑
  back (postural) M54.9
  bladder R39.89
    associated with micturition — *see* Micturition,
        painful
    chronic R39.82
  bone — *see* Disorder, bone, specified type NEC
  breast N64.4
  broad ligament R10.2
  cancer associated (acute) (chronic) G89.3
  cecum — *see* Pain, abdominal
  cervicobrachial M53.1
  chest (central) R07.9
    anterior wall R07.89
    atypical I07.89
    ischemic I20.9
    musculoskeletal R07.89
    non-cardiac R07.89
    on breathing R07.1
    pleurodynia R07.81
    precordial R07.2
    wall (anterior) R07.89
  chronic G89.29
    associated with significant psychosocial dysfunction
        G89.4
    due to trauma G89.21
    neoplasm related G89.3
    postoperative NEC G89.28
    postprocedural NEC G89.28
    post-thoracotomy G89.22
    specified NEC G89.29
  coccyx M53.3
  colon — *see* Pain, abdominal
  coronary — *see* Angina
  costochondral R07.1
  diaphragm R07.1
  due to cancer G89.3
  due to device, implant or graft (*see also* Complications,
      by site and type, specified NEC) T85.848 ☑
    arterial graft NEC T82.848 ☑
    breast (implant) T85.848 ☑
    catheter NEC T85.848 ☑
      dialysis (renal) T82.848 ☑

☑ **Additional Character Required** — Refer to the Tabular List for Character Selection   ◥ **Subterms under main terms may continue to next column or page**

Pain(s) — continued
   due to device, implant or graft (see also Complications, by site and type, specified) — continued
     catheter — continued
      dialysis — continued
       intraperitoneal T85.848 ☑
      infusion NEC T82.848 ☑
       spinal (epidural) (subdural) T85.840 ☑
      urinary (indwelling) T83.84 ☑
     electronic (electrode) (pulse generator) (stimulator)
      bone T85.840 ☑
      cardiac T82.847 ☑
      nervous system (brain) (peripheral nerve) (spinal) T85.84 ☑
      urinary T83.84 ☑
     fixation, internal (orthopedic) NEC T84.84 ☑
     gastrointestinal (bile duct) (esophagus) T85.848 ☑
     genital NEC T83.84 ☑
     heart NEC T82.847 ☑
     infusion NEC T85.848 ☑
     joint prosthesis T84.84 ☑
     ocular (corneal graft) (orbital implant) NEC T85.848 ☑
     orthopedic NEC T84.84 ☑
     specified NEC T85.848 ☑
     urinary NEC T83.84 ☑
     vascular NEC T82.848 ☑
     ventricular intracranial shunt T85.840 ☑
   due to malignancy (primary) (secondary) G89.3
   ear — see subcategory H92.0 ☑
   epigastric, epigastrium R10.13
   eye — see Pain, ocular
   face, facial R51
     atypical G50.1
   female genital organs NEC N94.89
   finger — see Pain, limb, upper
   flank — see Pain, abdominal
   foot — see Pain, limb, lower
   gallbladder K82.9
   gas (intestinal) R14.1
   gastric — see Pain, abdominal
   generalized NOS R52
   genital organ
     female N94.89
     male N50.89
   groin — see Pain, abdominal, lower
   hand — see Pain, limb, upper
   head — see Headache
   heart — see Pain, precordial
   infra-orbital — see Neuralgia, trigeminal
   intercostal R07.82
   intermenstrual N94.0
   jaw R68.84
   joint M25.50
     ankle M25.57- ☑
     elbow M25.52- ☑
     finger M25.54- ☑
     foot M25.57- ☑
     hand M25.54- ☑
     hip M25.55- ☑
     knee M25.56- ☑
     shoulder M25.51- ☑
     toe M25.57- ☑
     wrist M25.53- ☑
   kidney N23
   laryngeal R07.0
   leg — see Pain, limb, lower
   limb M79.609
     lower M79.60- ☑
      foot M79.67- ☑
      lower leg M79.66- ☑
      thigh M79.65- ☑
      toe M79.67- ☑
     upper M79.60- ☑
      axilla M79.62- ☑
      finger M79.64- ☑
      forearm M79.63- ☑
      hand M79.64- ☑
      upper arm M79.62- ☑
   loin M54.5
   low back M54.5
   lumbar region M54.5
   mandibular R68.84
   mastoid — see subcategory H92.0 ☑
   maxilla R68.84
   menstrual (see also Dysmenorrhea) N94.6
   metacarpophalangeal (joint) — see Pain, joint, hand

Pain(s) — continued
   metatarsophalangeal (joint) — see Pain, joint, foot
   mouth K13.79
   muscle — see Myalgia
   musculoskeletal (see also Pain, by site) M79.18
   myofascial M79.18
   nasal J34.89
   nasopharynx J39.2
   neck NEC M54.2
   nerve NEC — see Neuralgia
   neuromuscular — see Neuralgia
   nose J34.89
   ocular H57.1- ☑
   ophthalmic — see Pain, ocular
   orbital region — see Pain, ocular
   ovary N94.89
   over heart — see Pain, precordial
   ovulation N94.0
   pelvic (female) R10.2
   penis N48.89
   pericardial — see Pain, precordial
   perineal, perineum R10.2
   pharynx J39.2
   pleura, pleural, pleuritic R07.81
   postoperative NOS G89.18
   postprocedural NOS G89.18
   post-thoracotomy G89.12
   precordial (region) R07.2
   premenstrual N94.3
   psychogenic (persistent) (any site) F45.41
   radicular (spinal) — see Radiculopathy
   rectum K62.89
   respiration R07.1
   retrosternal R07.2
   rheumatoid, muscular — see Myalgia
   rib R07.81
   root (spinal) — see Radiculopathy
   round ligament (stretch) R10.2
   sacroiliac M53.3
   sciatic — see Sciatica
   scrotum N50.82
   seminal vesicle N50.89
   shoulder M25.51- ☑
   spermatic cord N50.89
   spinal root — see Radiculopathy
   spine M54.9
     cervical M54.2
     low back M54.5
      with sciatica M54.4- ☑
     thoracic M54.6
   stomach — see Pain, abdominal
   substernal R07.2
   temporomandibular (joint) M26.62- ☑
   testis N50.81- ☑
   thoracic spine M54.6
     with radicular and visceral pain M54.14
   throat R07.0
   tibia — see Pain, limb, lower
   toe — see Pain, limb, lower
   tongue K14.6
   tooth K08.89
   trigeminal — see Neuralgia, trigeminal
   tumor associated G89.3
   ureter N23
   urinary (organ) (system) N23
   uterus NEC N94.89
   vagina R10.2
   vertebrogenic (syndrome) M54.89
   vesical R39.89
     associated with micturition — see Micturition, painful
   vulva R10.2
Painful (see also Pain)
   coitus
     female N94.10
     male N53.12
     psychogenic F52.6
   ejaculation (semen) N53.12
     psychogenic F52.6
   erection — see Priapism
   feet syndrome E53.8
   joint replacement (hip) (knee) T84.84 ☑
   menstruation — see Dysmenorrhea
     psychogenic F45.8
   micturition — see Micturition, painful
   respiration R07.1
   scar NEC L90.5
   wire sutures T81.89 ☑

Painter's colic — see subcategory T56.0 ☑
Palate — see condition
Palatoplegia K13.79
Palatoschisis — see Cleft, palate
Palilalia R48.8
Palliative care Z51.5
Pallor R23.1
   optic disc, temporal — see Atrophy, optic
Palmar (see also condition)
   fascia — see condition
Palpable
   cecum K63.89
   kidney N28.89
   ovary N83.8
   prostate N42.9
   spleen — see Splenomegaly
Palpitations (heart) R00.2
   psychogenic F45.8
Palsy (see also Paralysis) G83.9
   atrophic diffuse (progressive) G12.22
   Bell's (see also Palsy, facial)
     newborn P11.3
   brachial plexus NEC G54.0
     newborn (birth injury) P14.3
   brain — see Palsy, cerebral
   bulbar (progressive) (chronic) G12.22
     of childhood (Fazio-Londe) G12.1
     pseudo NEC G12.29
     supranuclear (progressive) G23.1
   cerebral (congenital) G80.9
     ataxic G80.4
     athetoid G80.3
     choreathetoid G80.3
     diplegic G80.8
      spastic G80.1
     dyskinetic G80.3
      athetoid G80.3
      choreathetoid G80.3
      distonic G80.3
     dystonic G80.3
     hemiplegic G80.8
      spastic G80.2
     mixed G80.8
     monoplegic G80.8
      spastic G80.1
     paraplegic G80.8
      spastic G80.1
     quadriplegic G80.8
      spastic G80.0
     spastic G80.1
      diplegic G80.1
      hemiplegic G80.2
      monoplegic G80.1
      quadriplegic G80.0
      specified NEC G80.1
      tetrapelgic G80.0
     specified NEC G80.8
     syphilitic A52.12
      congenital A50.49
     tetraplegic G80.8
      spastic G80.0
   cranial nerve (see also Disorder, nerve, cranial)
     multiple G52.7
      in
       infectious disease B99 ☑ [G53]
       neoplastic disease (see also Neoplasm) D49.9 [G53]
       parasitic disease B89 [G53]
       sarcoidosis D86.82
   creeping G12.22
   diver's T70.3 ☑
   Erb's P14.0
   facial G51.0
     newborn (birth injury) P11.3
   glossopharyngeal G52.1
   Klumpke (-Déjérine) P14.1
   lead — see subcategory T56.0 ☑
   median nerve (tardy) G56.1- ☑
   nerve G58.9
     specified NEC G58.8
   peroneal nerve (acute) (tardy) G57.3- ☑
   progressive supranuclear G23.1
   pseudobulbar NEC G12.29
   radial nerve (acute) G56.3- ☑
   seventh nerve (see also Palsy, facial)
     newborn P11.3
   shaking — see Parkinsonism
   spastic (cerebral) (spinal) G80.1

✎ Subterms under main terms may continue to next column or page   ☑ Additional Character Required — Refer to the Tabular List for Character Selection

Palsy — *continued*
  ulnar nerve (tardy) G56.2- ☑
  wasting G12.29
Paludism — *see* Malaria
Panangiitis M30.0
Panaris, panaritium (*see also* Cellulitis, digit)
  with lymphangitis — *see* Lymphangitis, acute, digit
Panarteritis nodosa M30.0
  brain or cerebral I67.7
Pancake heart R93.1
  with cor pulmonale (chronic) I27.81
Pancarditis (acute) (chronic) I51.89
  rheumatic I09.89
    active or acute I01.8
Pancoast's syndrome or tumor C34.1- ☑
Pancolitis, ulcerative (chronic) K51.00
  with
    abscess K51.014
    complication K51.019
    fistula K51.013
    obstruction K51.012
    rectal bleeding K51.011
    specified complication NEC K51.018
Pancreas, pancreatic — *see* condition
Pancreatitis (annular) (apoplectic) (calcareous) (edematous) (hemorrhagic) (malignant) (recurrent) (subacute) (suppurative) K85.90
  with necrosis (uninfected) K85.91
    infected K85.92
  acute (without necrosis or infection) K85.90
    with necrosis (uninfected) K85.91
      infected K85.92
    alcohol induced (without necrosis or infection) K85.20
      with necrosis (uninfected) K85.21
        infected K85.22
    biliary (without necrosis or infection) K85.10
      with necrosis (uninfected) K85.11
        infected K85.12
    drug induced (without necrosis or infection) K85.30
      with necrosis (uninfected) K85.31
        infected K85.32
    gallstone (without necrosis or infection) K85.10
      with necrosis (uninfected) K85.11
        infected K85.12
    idiopathic (without necrosis or infection) K85.00
      with necrosis (uninfected) K85.01
        infected K85.02
    specified NEC (without necrosis or infection) K85.80
      with necrosis (uninfected) K85.81
        infected K85.82
  chronic (infectious) K86.1
    alcohol-induced K86.0
    recurrent K86.1
    relapsing K86.1
  cystic (chronic) K86.1
  cytomegaloviral B25.2
  fibrous (chronic) K86.1
  gallstone (without necrosis or infection) K85.10
    with necrosis (uninfected) K85.11
      infected K85.12
  gangrenous — *see* Pancreatitis, acute
  interstitial (chronic) K86.1
    acute (*see also* Pancreatitis, acute) K85.80
  mumps B26.3
  recurrent (chronic) K86.1
  relapsing, chronic K86.1
  syphilitic A52.74
Pancreatoblastoma — *see* Neoplasm, pancreas, malignant
Pancreolithiasis K86.89
Pancytolysis D75.89
Pancytopenia (acquired) D61.818
  with
    malformations D61.09
    myelodysplastic syndrome — *see* Syndrome, myelodysplastic
  antineoplastic chemotherapy induced D61.810
  congenital D61.09
  drug-induced NEC D61.811
PANDAS (pediatric autoimmune neuropsychiatric disorders associated with streptococcal infections syndrome) D89.89
Panencephalitis, subacute, sclerosing A81.1
Panhematopenia D61.9
  congenital D61.09
  constitutional D61.09
  splenic, primary D73.1

Panhemocytopenia D61.9
  congenital D61.09
  constitutional D61.09
Panhypogonadism E29.1
Panhypopituitarism E23.0
  prepubertal E23.0
Panic (attack) (state) F41.0
  reaction to exceptional stress (transient) F43.0
Panmyelopathy, familial, constitutional D61.09
Panmyelophthisis D61.82
  congenital D61.09
Panmyelosis (acute) (with myelofibrosis) C94.4- ☑
Panner's disease — *see* Osteochondrosis, juvenile, humerus
Panneuritis endemica E51.11
Panniculitis (nodular) (nonsuppurative) M79.3
  back M54.00
    cervical region M54.02
    cervicothoracic region M54.03
    lumbar region M54.06
    lumbosacral region M54.07
    multiple sites M54.09
    occipito-atlanto-axial region M54.01
    sacrococcygeal region M54.08
    thoracic region M54.04
    thoracolumbar region M54.05
  lupus L93.2
  mesenteric K65.4
  neck M54.02
    cervicothoracic region M54.03
    occipito-atlanto-axial region M54.01
  relapsing M35.6
Panniculus adiposus (abdominal) E65
Pannus (allergic) (cornea) (degenerativus) (keratic) H16.42- ☑
  abdominal (symptomatic) E65
  trachomatosus, trachomatous (active) A71.1
Panophthalmitis H44.01- ☑
Pansinusitis (chronic) (hyperplastic) (nonpurulent) (purulent) J32.4
  acute J01.40
    recurrent J01.41
  tuberculous A15.8
Panuveitis (sympathetic) H44.11- ☑
Panvalvular disease I08.9
  specified NEC I08.8
PAPA (pyogenic arthritis, pyoderma gangrenosum, and acne syndrome) M04.8
Papanicolaou smear, cervix Z12.4
  as part of routine gynecological examination Z01.419
    with abnormal findings Z01.411
  for suspected neoplasm Z12.4
  nonspecific abnormal finding R87.619
  routine Z01.419
    with abnormal findings Z01.411
Papilledema (choked disc) H47.10
  associated with
    decreased ocular pressure H47.12
    increased intracranial pressure H47.11
    retinal disorder H47.13
  Foster-Kennedy syndrome H47.14- ☑
Papillitis H46.00
  anus K62.89
  chronic lingual K14.4
  necrotizing, kidney N17.2
  optic H46.0- ☑
  rectum K62.89
  renal, necrotizing N17.2
  tongue K14.0
Papilloma (*see also* Neoplasm, benign, by site)
  acuminatum (female) (male) (anogenital) A63.0
  basal cell L82.1
    inflamed L82.0
  benign pinta (primary) A67.0
  bladder (urinary) (transitional cell) D41.4
  choroid plexus (lateral ventricle) (third ventricle) D33.0
    anaplastic C71.5
    fourth ventricle D33.1
    malignant C71.5
  renal pelvis (transitional cell) D41.1- ☑
    benign D30.1- ☑
  Schneiderian
    specified site — *see* Neoplasm, benign, by site
    unspecified site D14.0
  serous surface
    borderline malignancy
      specified site — *see* Neoplasm, uncertain behavior, by site

Papilloma — *continued*
  serous surface — *continued*
    borderline malignancy — *continued*
      unspecified site D39.10
    specified site — *see* Neoplasm, benign, by site
    unspecified site D27.9
  transitional (cell)
    bladder (urinary) D41.4
    inverted type — *see* Neoplasm, uncertain behavior, by site
    renal pelvis D41.1- ☑
    ureter D41.2- ☑
  ureter (transitional cell) D41.2- ☑
    benign D30.2- ☑
  urothelial — *see* Neoplasm, uncertain behavior, by site
  villous — *see* Neoplasm, uncertain behavior, by site
    adenocarcinoma in — *see* Neoplasm, malignant, by site
    in situ — *see* Neoplasm, in situ
  yaws, plantar or palmar A66.1
Papillomata, multiple, of yaws A66.1
Papillomatosis (*see also* Neoplasm, benign, by site)
  confluent and reticulated L83
  cystic, breast — *see* Mastopathy, cystic
  ductal, breast — *see* Mastopathy, cystic
  intraductal (diffuse) — *see* Neoplasm, benign, by site
  subareolar duct D24- ☑
Papillomavirus, as cause of disease classified elsewhere B97.7
Papillon-Léage and Psaume syndrome Q87.0
Papule(s) R23.8
  carate (primary) A67.0
  fibrous, of nose D22.39
  Gottron's L94.4
  pinta (primary) A67.0
Papulosis
  lymphomatoid C86.6
  malignant I77.89
Papyraceous fetus O31.0- ☑
Para-albuminemia E88.09
Paracephalus Q89.7
Parachute mitral valve Q23.2
Paracoccidioidomycosis B41.9
  disseminated B41.7
  generalized B41.7
  mucocutaneous-lymphangitic B41.8
  pulmonary B41.0
  specified NEC B41.8
  visceral B41.8
Paradentosis K05.4
Paraffinoma T88.8 ☑
Paraganglioma D44.7
  adrenal D35.0- ☑
    malignant C74.1- ☑
  aortic body D44.7
    malignant C75.5
  carotid body D44.6
    malignant C75.4
  chromaffin (*see also* Neoplasm, benign, by site)
    malignant — *see* Neoplasm, malignant, by site
  extra-adrenal D44.7
    malignant C75.5
      specified site — *see* Neoplasm, malignant, by site
      unspecified site C75.5
    specified site — *see* Neoplasm, uncertain behavior, by site
    unspecified site D44.7
  gangliocytic D13.2
    specified site — *see* Neoplasm, benign, by site
    unspecified site D13.2
  glomus jugulare D44.7
    malignant C75.5
  jugular D44.7
  malignant C75.5
    specified site — *see* Neoplasm, malignant, by site
    unspecified site C75.5
  nonchromaffin D44.7
    malignant C75.5
      specified site — *see* Neoplasm, malignant, by site
      unspecified site C75.5
    specified site — *see* Neoplasm, uncertain behavior, by site
    unspecified site D44.7
  parasympathetic D44.7

☑ **Additional Character Required** — Refer to the Tabular List for Character Selection   ▽ **Subterms under main terms may continue to next column or page**

Paraganglioma — continued
  parasympathetic — continued
    specified site — see Neoplasm, uncertain behavior, by site
    unspecified site D44.7
  specified site — see Neoplasm, uncertain behavior, by site
  sympathetic D44.7
    specified site — see Neoplasm, uncertain behavior, by site
    unspecified site D44.7
  unspecified site D44.7
Parageusia R43.2
  psychogenic F45.8
Paragonimiasis B66.4
Paragranuloma, Hodgkin — see Lymphoma, Hodgkin, specified NEC
Parahemophilia (see also Defect, coagulation) D68.2
Parakeratosis R23.4
  variegata L41.0
Paralysis, paralytic (complete) (incomplete) G83.9
  with
    syphilis A52.17
  abducens, abducent (nerve) — see Strabismus, paralytic, sixth nerve
  abductor, lower extremity G57.9- ☑
  accessory nerve G52.8
  accommodation (see also Paresis, of accommodation)
    hysterical F44.89
  acoustic nerve (except Deafness) H93.3 ☑
  agitans (see also Parkinsonism) G20
    arteriosclerotic G21.4
  alternating (oculomotor) G83.89
  amyotrophic G12.21
  ankle G57.9- ☑
  anus (sphincter) K62.89
  arm — see Monoplegia, upper limb
  ascending (spinal), acute G61.0
  association G12.29
  asthenic bulbar G70.00
    with exacerbation (acute) G70.01
    in crisis G70.01
  ataxic (hereditary) G11.9
    general (syphilitic) A52.17
  atrophic G58.9
    infantile, acute — see Poliomyelitis, paralytic
    progressive G12.22
    spinal (acute) — see Poliomyelitis, paralytic
  axillary G54.0
  Babinski-Nageotte's G83.89
  Bell's G51.0
    newborn P11.3
  Benedikt's G46.3
  birth injury P14.9
    spinal cord P11.5
  bladder (neurogenic) (sphincter) N31.2
  bowel, colon or intestine K56.0
  brachial plexus G54.0
    birth injury P14.3
    newborn (birth injury) P14.3
  brain G83.9
    diplegia G83.0
    triplegia G83.89
  bronchial J98.09
  Brown-Séquard G83.81
  bulbar (chronic) (progressive) G12.22
    infantile — see Poliomyelitis, paralytic
    poliomyelitic — see Poliomyelitis, paralytic
    pseudo G12.29
  bulbospinal G70.00
    with exacerbation (acute) G70.01
    in crisis G70.01
  cardiac (see also Failure, heart) I50.9
  cerebrocerebellar, diplegic G80.1
  cervical
    plexus G54.2
    sympathetic G90.09
  Céstan-Chenais G46.3
  Charcot-Marie-Tooth type G60.0
  Clark's G80.9
  colon K56.0
  compressed air T70.3 ☑
  compression
    arm G56.9- ☑
    leg G57.9- ☑
    lower extremity G57.9- ☑
    upper extremity G56.9- ☑
  congenital (cerebral) — see Palsy, cerebral

Paralysis, paralytic — continued
  conjugate movement (gaze) (of eye) H51.0
    cortical (nuclear) (supranuclear) H51.0
  cordis — see Failure, heart
  cranial or cerebral nerve G52.9
  creeping G12.22
  crossed leg G83.89
  crutch — see Injury, brachial plexus
  deglutition R13.0
    hysterical F44.4
  dementia A52.17
  descending (spinal) NEC G12.29
  diaphragm (flaccid) J98.6
    due to accidental dissection of phrenic nerve during procedure — see Puncture, accidental complicating surgery
  digestive organs NEC K59.8
  diplegic — see Diplegia
  divergence (nuclear) H51.8
  diver's T70.3 ☑
  Duchenne's
    birth injury P14.0
    due to or associated with
      motor neuron disease G12.22
      muscular dystrophy G71.01
  due to intracranial or spinal birth injury — see Palsy, cerebral
  embolic (current episode) I63.4- ☑
  Erb (-Duchenne) (birth) (newborn) P14.0
  Erb's syphilitic spastic spinal A52.17
  esophagus K22.8
  eye muscle (extrinsic) H49.9
    intrinsic (see also Paresis, of accommodation)
  facial (nerve) G51.0
    birth injury P11.3
    congenital P11.3
    following operation NEC — see Puncture, accidental complicating surgery
    newborn (birth injury) P11.3
  familial (recurrent) (periodic) G72.3
    spastic G11.4
  fauces J39.2
  finger G56.9- ☑
  gait R26.1
  gastric nerve (nondiabetic) G52.2
  gaze, conjugate H51.0
  general (progressive) (syphilitic) A52.17
    juvenile A50.45
  glottis J38.00
    bilateral J38.02
    unilateral J38.01
  gluteal G54.1
  Gubler (-Millard) G46.3
  hand — see Monoplegia, upper limb
  heart — see Arrest, cardiac
  hemiplegic — see Hemiplegia
  hyperkalemic periodic (familial) G72.3
  hypoglossal (nerve) G52.3
  hypokalemic periodic G72.3
  hysterical F44.4
  ileus K56.0
  infantile (see also Poliomyelitis, paralytic) A80.30
    bulbar — see Poliomyelitis, paralytic
    cerebral — see Palsy, cerebral
    spastic — see Palsy, cerebral, spastic
  infective — see Poliomyelitis, paralytic
  inferior nuclear G83.9
  internuclear — see Ophthalmoplegia, internuclear
  intestine K56.0
  iris H57.09
    due to diphtheria (toxin) A36.89
  ischemic, Volkmann's (complicating trauma) T79.6 ☑
  Jackson's G83.89
  jake — see Poisoning, food, noxious, plant
  Jamaica ginger (jake) G62.2
  juvenile general A50.45
  Klumpke (-Déjérine) (birth) (newborn) P14.1
  labioglossal (laryngeal) (pharyngeal) G12.29
  Landry's G61.0
  laryngeal nerve (recurrent) (superior) (unilateral) J38.00
    bilateral J38.02
    unilateral J38.01
  larynx J38.00
    bilateral J38.02
    due to diphtheria (toxin) A36.2
    unilateral J38.01
  lateral G12.23
  lead T56.0 ☑

Paralysis, paralytic — continued
  left side — see Hemiplegia
  leg G83.1- ☑
    both — see Paraplegia
    crossed G83.89
    hysterical F44.4
    psychogenic F44.4
    transient or transitory R29.818
      traumatic NEC — see Injury, nerve, leg
  levator palpebrae superioris — see Blepharoptosis, paralytic
  limb — see Monoplegia
  lip K13.0
  Lissauer's A52.17
  lower limb — see Monoplegia, lower limb
    both — see Paraplegia
  lung J98.4
  median nerve G56.1- ☑
  medullary (tegmental) G83.89
  mesencephalic NEC G83.89
    tegmental G83.89
  middle alternating G83.89
  Millard-Gubler-Foville G46.3
  monoplegic — see Monoplegia
  motor G83.9
  muscle, muscular NEC G72.89
    due to nerve lesion G58.9
    eye (extrinsic) H49.9
      intrinsic — see Paresis, of accommodation
      oblique — see Strabismus, paralytic, fourth nerve
    iris sphincter H21.9
    ischemic (Volkmann's) (complicating trauma) T79.6 ☑
    progressive G12.21
    pseudohypertrophic G71.02
  musculocutaneous nerve G56.9- ☑
  musculospiral G56.9- ☑
  nerve (see also Disorder, nerve)
    abducent — see Strabismus, paralytic, sixth nerve
    accessory G52.8
    auditory (except Deafness) H93.3 ☑
    birth injury P14.9
    cranial or cerebral G52.9
    facial G51.0
      birth injury P11.3
      congenital P11.3
      newborn (birth injury) P11.3
    fourth or trochlear — see Strabismus, paralytic, fourth nerve
    newborn (birth injury) P14.9
    oculomotor — see Strabismus, paralytic, third nerve
    phrenic (birth injury) P14.2
    radial G56.3- ☑
    seventh or facial G51.0
      newborn (birth injury) P11.3
    sixth or abducent — see Strabismus, paralytic, sixth nerve
    syphilitic A52.15
    third or oculomotor — see Strabismus, paralytic, third nerve
    trigeminal G50.9
    trochlear — see Strabismus, paralytic, fourth nerve
    ulnar G56.2- ☑
  normokalemic periodic G72.3
  ocular H49.9
    alternating G83.89
  oculofacial, congenital (Moebius) Q87.0
  oculomotor (external bilateral) (nerve) — see Strabismus, paralytic, third nerve
  palate (soft) K13.79
  paratrigeminal G50.9
  periodic (familial) (hyperkalemic) (hypokalemic) (myotonic) (normokalemic) (potassium sensitive) (secondary) G72.3
  peripheral autonomic nervous system — see Neuropathy, peripheral, autonomic
  peroneal (nerve) G57.3- ☑
  pharynx J39.2
  phrenic nerve G56.8- ☑
  plantar nerve(s) G57.6- ☑
  pneumogastric nerve G52.2
  poliomyelitis (current) — see Poliomyelitis, paralytic
  popliteal nerve G57.3- ☑
  postepileptic transitory G83.84
  progressive (atrophic) (bulbar) (spinal) G12.22
    general A52.17
    infantile acute — see Poliomyelitis, paralytic
    supranuclear G23.1

Paralysis, paralytic — *continued*
  pseudobulbar G12.29
  pseudohypertrophic (muscle) G71.09
  psychogenic F44.4
  quadriceps G57.9- ☑
  quadriplegic — *see* Tetraplegia
  radial nerve G56.3- ☑
  rectus muscle (eye) H49.9
  recurrent isolated sleep G47.53
  respiratory (muscle) (system) (tract) R06.81
    center NEC G93.89
    congenital P28.89
    newborn P28.89
  right side — *see* Hemiplegia
  saturnine T56.0 ☑
  sciatic nerve G57.0- ☑
  senile G83.9
  shaking — *see* Parkinsonism
  shoulder G56.9- ☑
  sleep, recurrent isolated G47.53
  spastic G83.9
    cerebral — *see* Palsy, cerebral, spastic
    congenital (cerebral) — *see* Palsy, cerebral, spastic
    familial G11.4
    hereditary G11.4
    quadriplegic G80.0
    syphilitic (spinal) A52.17
  sphincter, bladder — *see* Paralysis, bladder
  spinal (cord) G83.9
    accessory nerve G52.8
    acute — *see* Poliomyelitis, paralytic
    ascending acute G61.0
    atrophic (acute) (*see also* Poliomyelitis, paralytic)
      spastic, syphilitic A52.17
    congenital NEC — *see* Palsy, cerebral
    hereditary G95.89
    infantile — *see* Poliomyelitis, paralytic
    progressive G12.21
    sequelae NEC G83.89
  sternomastoid G52.8
  stomach K31.84
    diabetic — *see* Diabetes, by type, with gastroparesis
    nerve G52.2
      diabetic — *see* Diabetes, by type, with gastro-paresis
  stroke — *see* Infarct, brain
  subcapsularis G56.8- ☑
  supranuclear (progressive) G23.1
  sympathetic G90.8
    cervical G90.09
    nervous system — *see* Neuropathy, peripheral, autonomic
  syndrome G83.9
    specified NEC G83.89
  syphilitic spastic spinal (Erb's) A52.17
  thigh G57.9- ☑
  throat J39.2
    diphtheritic A36.0
    muscle J39.2
  thrombotic (current episode) I63.3- ☑
  thumb G56.9- ☑
  tick — *see* Toxicity, venom, arthropod, specified NEC
  Todd's (postepileptic transitory paralysis) G83.84
  toe G57.6- ☑
  tongue K14.8
  transient R29.5
    arm or leg NEC R29.818
    traumatic NEC — *see* Injury, nerve
  trapezius G52.8
  traumatic, transient NEC — *see* Injury, nerve
  trembling — *see* Parkinsonism
  triceps brachii G56.9- ☑
  trigeminal nerve G50.9
  trochlear (nerve) — *see* Strabismus, paralytic, fourth nerve
  ulnar nerve G56.2- ☑
  upper limb — *see* Monoplegia, upper limb
  uremic N18.9 [G99.8]
  uveoparotitic D86.89
  uvula K13.79
    postdiphtheritic A36.0
  vagus nerve G52.2
  vasomotor NEC G90.8
  velum palati K13.79
  vesical — *see* Paralysis, bladder
  vestibular nerve (except Vertigo) H93.3 ☑
  vocal cords J38.00
    bilateral J38.02

Paralysis, paralytic — *continued*
  vocal cords — *continued*
    unilateral J38.01
  Volkmann's (complicating trauma) T79.6 ☑
  wasting G12.29
  Weber's G46.3
  wrist G56.9- ☑
Paramedial urethrovesical orifice Q64.79
Paramenia N92.6
Parametritis (*see also* Disease, pelvis, inflammatory) N73.2
  acute N73.0
  complicating abortion — *see* Abortion, by type, complicated by, parametritis
Parametrium, parametric — *see* condition
Paramnesia — *see* Amnesia
Paramolar K00.1
Paramyloidosis E85.89
Paramyoclonus multiplex G25.3
Paramyotonia (congenita) G71.19
Parangi — *see* Yaws
Paranoia (querulans) F22
  senile F03 ☑
Paranoid
  dementia (senile) F03 ☑
    praecox — *see* Schizophrenia
  personality F60.0
  psychosis (climacteric) (involutional) (menopausal) F22
    psychogenic (acute) F23
    senile F03 ☑
  reaction (acute) F23
    chronic F22
  schizophrenia F20.0
  state (climacteric) (involutional) (menopausal) (simple) F22
    senile F03 ☑
  tendencies F60.0
  traits F60.0
  trends F60.0
  type, psychopathic personality F60.0
Paraparesis — *see* Paraplegia
Paraphasia R47.02
Paraphilia F65.9
Paraphimosis (congenital) N47.2
  chancroidal A57
Paraphrenia, paraphrenic (late) F22
  schizophrenia F20.0
Paraplegia (lower) G82.20
  ataxic — *see* Degeneration, combined, spinal cord
  complete G82.21
  congenital (cerebral) G80.8
    spastic G80.1
  familial spastic G11.4
  functional (hysterical) F44.4
  hereditary, spastic G11.4
  hysterical F44.4
  incomplete G82.22
  Pott's A18.01
  psychogenic F44.4
  spastic
    Erb's spinal, syphilitic A52.17
    hereditary G11.4
    tropical G04.1
  syphilitic (spastic) A52.17
  traumatic
    current injury — code to injury with seventh character A
    sequela of previous injury — code to injury with seventh character S
  tropical spastic G04.1
Parapoxvirus B08.60
  specified NEC B08.69
Paraproteinemia D89.2
  benign (familial) D89.2
  monoclonal D47.2
  secondary to malignant disease D47.2
Parapsoriasis L41.9
  en plaques L41.4
  guttata L41.1
  large plaque L41.4
  retiform, retiformis L41.5
  small plaque L41.3
  specified NEC L41.8
  varioliformis (acuta) L41.0
Parasitic (*see also* condition)
  disease NEC B89
  stomatitis B37.0
  sycosis (beard) (scalp) B35.0

Parasitic — *continued*
  twin Q89.4
Parasitism B89
  intestinal B82.9
  skin B88.9
  specified — *see* Infestation
Parasitophobia F40.218
Parasomnia G47.50
  due to
    alcohol
      abuse F10.182
      dependence F10.282
      use F10.982
    amphetamines
      abuse F15.182
      dependence F15.282
      use F15.982
    caffeine
      abuse F15.182
      dependence F15.282
      use F15.982
    cocaine
      abuse F14.182
      dependence F14.282
      use F14.982
    drug NEC
      abuse F19.182
      dependence F19.282
      use F19.982
    opioid
      abuse F11.182
      dependence F11.282
      use F11.982
    psychoactive substance NEC
      abuse F19.182
      dependence F19.282
      use F19.982
    sedative, hypnotic, or anxiolytic
      abuse F13.182
      dependence F13.282
      use F13.982
    stimulant NEC
      abuse F15.182
      dependence F15.282
      use F15.982
  in conditions classified elsewhere G47.54
  nonorganic origin F51.8
  organic G47.50
  specified NEC G47.59
Paraspadias Q54.9
Paraspasmus facialis G51.8
Parasuicide (attempt)
  history of (personal) Z91.5
    in family Z81.8
Parathyroid gland — *see* condition
Parathyroid tetany E20.9
Paratrachoma A74.0
Paratyphilitis — *see* Appendicitis
Paratyphoid (fever) — *see* Fever, paratyphoid
Paratyphus — *see* Fever, paratyphoid
Paraurethral duct Q64.79
  nonorganic origin F51.5
Paraurethritis (*see also* Urethritis)
  gonococcal (acute) (chronic) (with abscess) A54.1
Paravaccinia NEC B08.04
Paravaginitis — *see* Vaginitis
Parencephalitis (*see also* Encephalitis)
  sequelae G09
Parent-child conflict — *see* Conflict, parent-child
  estrangement NEC Z62.890
Paresis (*see also* Paralysis)
  accommodation — *see* Paresis, of accommodation
  Bernhardt's G57.1- ☑
  bladder (sphincter) (*see also* Paralysis, bladder)
    tabetic A52.17
  bowel, colon or intestine K56.0
  extrinsic muscle, eye H49.9
  general (progressive) (syphilitic) A52.17
    juvenile A50.45
  heart — *see* Failure, heart
  insane (syphilitic) A52.17
  juvenile (general) A50.45
  of accommodation H52.52- ☑
  peripheral progressive (idiopathic) G60.3
  pseudohypertrophic G71.09
  senile G83.9
  syphilitic (general) A52.17
    congenital A50.45

☑ **Additional Character Required** — Refer to the Tabular List for Character Selection ⑦ **Subterms under main terms may continue to next column or page**

Paresis — *continued*
vesical NEC N31.2
Paresthesia (*see also* Disturbance, sensation, skin) R20.2
Bernhardt G57.1- ☑
Paretic — *see* condition
Parinaud's
conjunctivitis H10.89
oculoglandular syndrome H10.89
ophthalmoplegia H49.88- ☑
Parkinsonism (idiopathic) (primary) G20
with neurogenic orthostatic hypotension (symptomatic) G90.3
arteriosclerotic G21.4
dementia G31.83 [F02.80]
with behavioral disturbance G31.83 [F02.81]
due to
drugs NEC G21.19
neuroleptic G21.11
medication-induced NEC G21.19
neuroleptic induced G21.11
postencephalitic G21.3
secondary G21.9
due to
arteriosclerosis G21.4
drugs NEC G21.19
neuroleptic G21.11
encephalitis G21.3
external agents NEC G21.2
syphilis A52.19
specified NEC G21.8
syphilitic A52.19
treatment-induced NEC G21.19
vascular G21.4
Parkinson's disease, syndrome or tremor — *see* Parkinsonism
Parodontitis — *see* Periodontitis
Parodontosis K05.4
Paronychia (*see also* Cellulitis, digit)
with lymphangitis — *see* Lymphangitis, acute, digit
candidal (chronic) B37.2
tuberculous (primary) A18.4
Parorexia (psychogenic) F50.89
Parosmia R43.1
psychogenic F45.8
Parotid gland — *see* condition
Parotitis, parotiditis (allergic)(nonspecific toxic) (purulent) (septic) (suppurative) (*see also* Sialoadenitis)
epidemic — *see* Mumps
infectious — *see* Mumps
postoperative K91.89
surgical K91.89
Parrot fever A70
Parrot's disease (early congenital syphilitic pseudoparalysis) A50.02
Parry-Romberg syndrome G51.8
Parry's disease or syndrome E05.00
with thyroid storm E05.01
Pars planitis — *see* Cyclitis
Parsonage (-Aldren)-**Turner syndrome** G54.5
Parson's disease (exophthalmic goiter) E05.00
with thyroid storm E05.01
Particolored infant Q82.8
Parturition — *see* Delivery
Parulis K04.7
with sinus K04.6
Parvovirus, as cause of disease classified elsewhere B97.6
Pasini and Pierini's atrophoderma L90.3
Passage
false, urethra N36.5
meconium (newborn) during delivery P03.82
of sounds or bougies — *see* Attention to, artificial, opening
Passive — *see* condition
smoking Z77.22
Pasteurella septica A28.0
Pasteurellosis — *see* Infection, Pasteurella
PAT (paroxysmal atrial tachycardia) I47.1
Patau's syndrome — *see* Trisomy, 13
Patches
mucous (syphilitic) A51.39
congenital A50.07
smokers' (mouth) K13.24
Patellar — *see* condition
Patent (*see also* Imperfect, closure)
canal of Nuck Q52.4
cervix N88.3

Patent — *continued*
ductus arteriosus or Botallo's Q25.0
foramen
botalli Q21.1
ovale Q21.1
interauricular septum Q21.1
interventricular septum Q21.0
omphalomesenteric duct Q43.0
os (uteri) — *see* Patent, cervix
ostium secundum Q21.1
urachus Q64.4
vitelline duct Q43.0
Paterson (-Brown)(-Kelly) **syndrome or web** D50.1
Pathologic, pathological (*see also* condition)
asphyxia R09.01
fire-setting F63.1
gambling F63.0
ovum O02.0
resorption, tooth K03.3
stealing F63.2
Pathology (of) — *see* Disease
periradicular, associated with previous endodontic treatment NEC M27.59
Pattern, sleep-wake, irregular G47.23
Patulous (*see also* Imperfect, closure (congenital))
alimentary tract Q45.8
lower Q43.8
upper Q40.8
eustachian tube H69.0- ☑
Pause, sinoatrial I49.5
Paxton's disease B36.2
Pearl(s)
enamel K00.2
Epstein's K09.8
Pearl-worker's disease — *see* Osteomyelitis, specified type NEC
Pectenosis K62.4
Pectoral — *see* condition
Pectus
carinatum (congenital) Q67.7
acquired M95.4
rachitic sequelae (late effect) E64.3
excavatum (congenital) Q67.6
acquired M95.4
rachitic sequelae (late effect) E64.3
recurvatum (congenital) Q67.6
Pedatrophia E41
Pederosis F65.4
Pediculosis (infestation) B85.2
capitis (head-louse) (any site) B85.0
corporis (body-louse) (any site) B85.1
eyelid B85.0
mixed (classifiable to more than one of the titles B85.0-B85.3) B85.4
pubis (pubic louse) (any site) B85.3
vestimenti B85.1
vulvae B85.3
Pediculus (infestation) — *see* Pediculosis
Pedophilia F65.4
Peg-shaped teeth K00.2
Pelade — *see* Alopecia, areata
Pelger-Huët anomaly or syndrome D72.0
Peliosis (rheumatica) D69.0
hepatis K76.4
with toxic liver disease K71.8
Pelizaeus-Merzbacher disease E75.29
Pellagra (alcoholic) (with polyneuropathy) E52
Pellagra-cerebellar-ataxia-renal aminoaciduria syndrome E72.02
Pellegrini (-Stieda) **disease or syndrome** — *see* Bursitis, tibial collateral
Pellizzi's syndrome E34.8
Pel's crisis A52.11
Pelvic (*see also* condition)
examination (periodic) (routine) Z01.419
with abnormal findings Z01.411
kidney, congenital Q63.2
Pelviolithiasis — *see* Calculus, kidney
Pelviperitonitis (*see also* Peritonitis, pelvic)
gonococcal A54.24
puerperal O85
Pelvis — *see* condition or type
Pemphigoid L12.9
benign, mucous membrane L12.1
bullous L12.0
cicatricial L12.1
juvenile L12.2
ocular L12.1

Pemphigoid — *continued*
specified NEC L12.8
Pemphigus L10.9
benign familial (chronic) Q82.8
Brazilian L10.3
circinatus L13.0
conjunctiva L12.1
drug-induced L10.5
erythematosus L10.4
foliaceous L10.2
gangrenous — *see* Gangrene
neonatorum L01.03
ocular L12.1
paraneoplastic L10.81
specified NEC L10.89
syphilitic (congenital) A50.06
vegetans L10.1
vulgaris L10.0
wildfire L10.3
Pendred's syndrome E07.1
Pendulous
abdomen, in pregnancy — *see* Pregnancy, complicated by, abnormal, pelvic organs or tissues NEC
breast N64.89
Penetrating wound (*see also* Puncture)
with internal injury — *see* Injury, by site
eyeball — *see* Puncture, eyeball
orbit (with or without foreign body) — *see* Puncture, orbit
uterus by instrument with or following ectopic or molar pregnancy O08.6
Penicillosis B48.4
Penis — *see* condition
Penitis N48.29
Pentalogy of Fallot Q21.8
Pentasomy X syndrome Q97.1
Pentosuria (essential) E74.8
Percreta placenta - O43.23 ☑
Peregrinating patient — *see* Disorder, factitious
Perforation, perforated (nontraumatic) (of)
accidental during procedure (blood vessel) (nerve) (organ) — *see* Complication, accidental puncture or laceration
antrum — *see* Sinusitis, maxillary
appendix K35.32
with localized peritonitis K35.32
atrial septum, multiple Q21.1
attic, ear — *see* Perforation, tympanum, attic
bile duct (common) (hepatic) K83.2
cystic K82.2
bladder (urinary)
with or following ectopic or molar pregnancy O08.6
obstetrical trauma O71.5
traumatic S37.29 ☑
at delivery O71.5
bowel K63.1
with or following ectopic or molar pregnancy O08.6
newborn P78.0
obstetrical trauma O71.5
traumatic — *see* Laceration, intestine
broad ligament N83.8
with or following ectopic or molar pregnancy O08.6
obstetrical trauma O71.6
by
device, implant or graft (*see also* Complications, by site and type, mechanical) T85.628 ☑
arterial graft NEC — *see* Complication, cardiovascular device, mechanical, vascular
breast (implant) T85.49 ☑
catheter NEC T85.698 ☑
cystostomy T83.090 ☑
dialysis (renal) T82.49 ☑
intraperitoneal T85.691 ☑
infusion NEC T82.594 ☑
spinal (epidural) (subdural) T85.690 ☑
urinary (*see also* Complications, catheter, urinary T83.098 ☑
electronic (electrode) (pulse generator) (stimulator)
bone T84.390 ☑
cardiac T82.199 ☑
electrode T82.190 ☑
pulse generator T82.191 ☑
specified type NEC T82.198 ☑
nervous system — *see* Complication, prosthetic device, mechanical, electronic nervous system stimulator

Perforation, perforated — *continued*
- by — *continued*
  - device, implant or graft (*see also* Complications, by site and type, mechanical) — *continued*
    - electronic — *continued*
      - urinary — *see* Complication, genitourinary, device, urinary, mechanical
    - fixation, internal (orthopedic) NEC — *see* Complication, fixation device, mechanical
    - gastrointestinal — *see* Complications, prosthetic device, mechanical, gastrointestinal device
    - genital NEC T83.498 ☑
      - intrauterine contraceptive device T83.39 ☑
      - penile prosthesis T83.490 ☑
    - heart NEC — *see* Complication, cardiovascular device, mechanical
    - joint prosthesis — *see* Complications, joint prosthesis, mechanical, specified NEC, by site
    - ocular NEC — *see* Complications, prosthetic device, mechanical, ocular device
    - orthopedic NEC — *see* Complication, orthopedic, device, mechanical
    - specified NEC T85.628 ☑
    - urinary NEC (*see also* Complication, genitourinary, device, urinary, mechanical)
      - graft T83.29 ☑
    - vascular NEC — *see* Complication, cardiovascular device, mechanical
    - ventricular intracranial shunt T85.09 ☑
  - foreign body left accidentally in operative wound T81.539 ☑
  - instrument (any) during a procedure, accidental — *see* Puncture, accidental complicating surgery
- cecum K35.32
  - with localized peritonitis K35.32
- cervix (uteri) N88.8
  - with or following ectopic or molar pregnancy O08.6
  - obstetrical trauma O71.3
- colon K63.1
  - newborn P78.0
  - obstetrical trauma O71.5
  - traumatic — *see* Laceration, intestine, large
- common duct (bile) K83.2
- cornea (due to ulceration) — *see* Ulcer, cornea, perforated
- cystic duct K82.2
- diverticulum (intestine) K57.80
  - with bleeding K57.81
  - large intestine K57.20
    - with
      - bleeding K57.21
      - small intestine K57.40
        - with bleeding K57.41
  - small intestine K57.00
    - with
      - bleeding K57.01
      - large intestine K57.40
        - with bleeding K57.41
- ear drum — *see* Perforation, tympanum
- esophagus K22.3
- ethmoidal sinus — *see* Sinusitis, ethmoidal
- frontal sinus — *see* Sinusitis, frontal
- gallbladder K82.2
- heart valve — *see* Endocarditis
- ileum K63.1
  - newborn P78.0
  - obstetrical trauma O71.5
  - traumatic — *see* Laceration, intestine, small
- instrumental, surgical (accidental) (blood vessel) (nerve) (organ) — *see* Puncture, accidental complicating surgery
- intestine NEC K63.1
  - with ectopic or molar pregnancy O08.6
  - newborn P78.0
  - obstetrical trauma O71.5
  - traumatic — *see* Laceration, intestine
  - ulcerative NEC K63.1
    - newborn P78.0
- jejunum, jejunal K63.1
  - obstetrical trauma O71.5
  - traumatic — *see* Laceration, intestine, small
  - ulcer — *see* Ulcer, gastrojejunal, with perforation
- joint prosthesis — *see* Complications, joint prosthesis, mechanical, specified NEC, by site
- mastoid (antrum) (cell) — *see* Disorder, mastoid, specified NEC
- maxillary sinus — *see* Sinusitis, maxillary

Perforation, perforated — *continued*
- membrana tympani — *see* Perforation, tympanum
- nasal
  - septum J34.89
    - congenital Q30.3
    - syphilitic A52.73
  - sinus J34.89
    - congenital Q30.8
    - due to sinusitis — *see* Sinusitis
- palate (*see also* Cleft, palate) Q35.9
  - syphilitic A52.79
- palatine vault (*see also* Cleft, palate, hard) Q35.1
  - syphilitic A52.79
  - congenital A50.59
- pars flaccida (ear drum) — *see* Perforation, tympanum, attic
- pelvic
  - floor S31.030 ☑
    - with
      - ectopic or molar pregnancy O08.6
      - penetration into retroperitoneal space S31.031 ☑
      - retained foreign body S31.040 ☑
        - with penetration into retroperitoneal space S31.041 ☑
    - following ectopic or molar pregnancy O08.6
    - obstetrical trauma O70.1
  - organ S37.99 ☑
    - adrenal gland S37.818 ☑
    - bladder — *see* Perforation, bladder
    - fallopian tube S37.599 ☑
      - bilateral S37.592 ☑
      - unilateral S37.591 ☑
    - kidney S37.09- ☑
      - obstetrical trauma O71.5
    - ovary S37.499 ☑
      - bilateral S37.492 ☑
      - unilateral S37.491 ☑
    - prostate S37.828 ☑
    - specified organ NEC S37.898 ☑
    - ureter — *see* Perforation, ureter
    - urethra — *see* Perforation, urethra
    - uterus — *see* Perforation, uterus
- perineum — *see* Laceration, perineum
- pharynx J39.2
- rectum K63.1
  - newborn P78.0
  - obstetrical trauma O71.5
  - traumatic S36.63 ☑
- root canal space due to endodontic treatment M27.51
- sigmoid K63.1
  - newborn P78.0
  - obstetrical trauma O71.5
  - traumatic S36.533 ☑
- sinus (accessory) (chronic) (nasal) J34.89
- sphenoidal sinus — *see* Sinusitis, sphenoidal
- surgical (accidental) (by instrument) (blood vessel) (nerve) (organ) — *see* Puncture, accidental complicating surgery
- traumatic
  - external — *see* Puncture
  - eye — *see* Puncture, eyeball
  - internal organ — *see* Injury, by site
- tympanum, tympanic (membrane) (persistent post-traumatic) (postinflammatory) H72.9- ☑
  - attic H72.1- ☑
    - multiple — *see* Perforation, tympanum, multiple
    - total — *see* Perforation, tympanum, total
  - central H72.0- ☑
    - multiple — *see* Perforation, tympanum, multiple
    - total — *see* Perforation, tympanum, total
  - marginal NEC — *see* subcategory H72.2
  - multiple H72.81- ☑
  - pars flaccida — *see* Perforation, tympanum, attic
  - total H72.82- ☑
  - traumatic, current episode S09.2- ☑
- typhoid, gastrointestinal — *see* Typhoid
- ulcer — *see* Ulcer, by site, with perforation
- ureter N28.89
  - traumatic S37.19 ☑
- urethra N36.8
  - with ectopic or molar pregnancy O08.6
  - following ectopic or molar pregnancy O08.6
  - obstetrical trauma O71.5
  - traumatic S37.39 ☑
    - at delivery O71.5

Perforation, perforated — *continued*
- uterus
  - with ectopic or molar pregnancy O08.6
  - by intrauterine contraceptive device T83.39 ☑
  - following ectopic or molar pregnancy O08.6
  - obstetrical trauma O71.1
  - traumatic S37.69 ☑
    - obstetric O71.1
- uvula K13.79
  - syphilitic A52.79
- vagina O71.4
  - obstetrical trauma O71.4
  - other trauma — *see* Puncture, vagina

Periadenitis mucosa necrotica recurrens K12.0
Periappendicitis (acute) — *see* Appendicitis
Periarteritis nodosa (disseminated) (infectious) (necrotizing) M30.0
Periarthritis (joint) (*see also* Enthesopathy)
- Duplay's M75.0- ☑
- gonococcal A54.42
- humeroscapularis — *see* Capsulitis, adhesive
- scapulohumeral — *see* Capsulitis, adhesive
- shoulder — *see* Capsulitis, adhesive
- wrist M77.2- ☑

Periarthrosis (angioneural) — *see* Enthesopathy
Pericapsulitis, adhesive (shoulder) — *see* Capsulitis, adhesive
Pericarditis (with decompensation) (with effusion) I31.9
- with rheumatic fever (conditions in I00)
  - active — *see* Pericarditis, rheumatic
  - inactive or quiescent I09.2
- acute (hemorrhagic) (nonrheumatic) (Sicca) I30.9
  - with chorea (acute) (rheumatic) (Sydenham's) I02.0
  - benign I30.8
  - nonspecific I30.0
  - rheumatic I01.0
    - with chorea (acute) (Sydenham's) I02.0
- adhesive or adherent (chronic) (external) (internal) I31.0
  - acute — *see* Pericarditis, acute
  - rheumatic I09.2
- bacterial (acute) (subacute) (with serous or seropurulent effusion) I30.1
- calcareous I31.1
- cholesterol (chronic) I31.8
  - acute I30.9
- chronic (nonrheumatic) I31.9
  - rheumatic I09.2
- constrictive (chronic) I31.1
- coxsackie B33.23
- fibrinocaseous (tuberculous) A18.84
- fibrinopurulent I30.1
- fibrinous I30.8
- fibrous I31.0
- gonococcal A54.83
- idiopathic I30.0
- in systemic lupus erythematosus M32.12
- infective I30.1
- meningococcal A39.53
- neoplastic (chronic) I31.8
  - acute I30.9
- obliterans, obliterating I31.0
- plastic I31.0
- pneumococcal I30.1
- postinfarction I24.1
- purulent I30.1
- rheumatic (active) (acute) (with effusion) (with pneumonia) I01.0
  - with chorea (acute) (rheumatic) (Sydenham's) I02.0
  - chronic or inactive (with chorea) I09.2
- rheumatoid — *see* Rheumatoid, carditis
- septic I30.1
- serofibrinous I30.8
- staphylococcal I30.1
- streptococcal I30.1
- suppurative I30.1
- syphilitic A52.06
- tuberculous A18.84
- uremic N18.9 [I32]
- viral I30.1

Pericardium, pericardial — *see* condition
Pericellulitis — *see* Cellulitis
Pericementitis (chronic) (suppurative) (*see also* Periodontitis)
- acute K05.20
  - generalized — *see* Peridontitis, aggressive, generalized
  - localized — *see* Peridontitis, aggressive, localized

Perichondritis
auricle — *see* Perichondritis, ear
bronchus J98.09
ear (external) H61.00- ✓
    acute H61.01- ✓
    chronic H61.02- ✓
external auditory canal — *see* Perichondritis, ear
larynx J38.7
    syphilitic A52.73
    typhoid A01.09
nose J34.89
pinna — *see* Perichondritis, ear
trachea J39.8
Periclasia K05.4
Pericoronitis — *see* Periodontitis
Pericystitis N30.90
with hematuria N30.91
Peridiverticulitis (intestine) K57.92
cecum — *see* Diverticulitis, intestine, large
colon — *see* Diverticulitis, intestine, large
duodenum — *see* Diverticulitis, intestine, small
intestine — *see* Diverticulitis, intestine
jejunum — *see* Diverticulitis, intestine, small
rectosigmoid — *see* Diverticulitis, intestine, large
rectum — *see* Diverticulitis, intestine, large
sigmoid — *see* Diverticulitis, intestine, large
Periendocarditis — *see* Endocarditis
Periepididymitis N45.1
Perifolliculitis L01.02
abscedens, caput, scalp L66.3
capitis, abscedens (et suffodiens) L66.3
superficial pustular L01.02
Perihepatitis K65.8
Perilabyrinthitis (acute) — *see* subcategory H83.0 ✓
Perimeningitis — *see* Meningitis
Perimetritis — *see* Endometritis
Perimetrosalpingitis — *see* Salpingo-oophoritis
Perineocele N81.81
Perinephric, perinephritic — *see* condition
Perinephritis (*see also* Infection, kidney)
purulent — *see* Abscess, kidney
Perineum, perineal — *see* condition
Perineuritis NEC — *see* Neuralgia
Periodic — *see* condition
Periodontitis (chronic) (complex) (compound) (local)
    (simplex) K05.30
acute K05.20
    generalized K05.229
        moderate K05.222
        severe K05.223
        slight K05.221
    localized K05.219
        moderate K05.212
        severe K05.213
        slight K05.211
apical K04.5
    acute (pulpal origin) K04.4
generalized K05.329
    moderate K05.322
    severe K05.323
    slight K05.321
localized K05.319
    moderate K05.312
    severe K05.313
    slight K05.311
Periodontoclasia K05.4
Periodontosis (juvenile) K05.4
Periods (*see also* Menstruation)
heavy N92.0
irregular N92.6
shortened intervals (irregular) N92.1
Perionychia (*see also* Cellulitis, digit)
with lymphangitis — *see* Lymphangitis, acute, digit
Perioophoritis — *see* Salpingo-oophoritis
Periorchitis N45.2
Periosteum, periosteal — *see* condition
Periostitis (albuminosa) (circumscribed) (diffuse) (infective) (monomelic) (*see also* Osteomyelitis)
alveolar M27.3
alveolodental M27.3
dental M27.3
gonorrheal A54.43
jaw (lower) (upper) M27.2
orbit H05.03- ✓
syphilitic A52.77
    congenital (early) A50.02 [M90.80]
    secondary A51.46

Periostitis — *continued*
tuberculous — *see* Tuberculosis, bone
yaws (hypertrophic) (early) (late) A66.6 [M90.80]
Periostosis (hyperplastic) (*see also* Disorder, bone, spec-
ified type NEC)
with osteomyelitis — *see* Osteomyelitis, specified type
NEC
Peripartum
cardiomyopathy O90.3
Periphlebitis — *see* Phlebitis
Periproctitis K62.89
Periprostatitis — *see* Prostatitis
Perirectal — *see* condition
Perirenal — *see* condition
Perisalpingitis — *see* Salpingo-oophoritis
Perisplenitis (infectional) D73.89
Peristalsis, visible or reversed R19.2
Peritendinitis — *see* Enthesopathy
Peritoneum, peritoneal — *see* condition
Peritonitis (adhesive) (bacterial) (fibrinous) (hemorrhagic)
    (idiopathic) (localized) (perforative) (primary) (with
    adhesions) (with effusion) K65.9
with or following
    abscess K65.1
    appendicitis
        with perforation or rupture K35.32
        generalized (*see also* Appendicitis) K35.20
        localized (*see also* Appendicitis) K35.30
    diverticular disease (intestine) K57.80
        with bleeding K57.81
        ectopic or molar pregnancy O08.0
        large intestine K57.20
            with
                bleeding K57.21
                small intestine K57.40
                    with bleeding K57.41
        small intestine K57.00
            with
                bleeding K57.01
                large intestine K57.40
                    with bleeding K57.41
acute (generalized) K65.0
aseptic T81.61 ✓
bile, biliary K65.3
chemical T81.61 ✓
chlamydial A74.81
chronic proliferative K65.8
complicating abortion — *see* Abortion, by type, complicated by, pelvic peritonitis
congenital P78.1
diaphragmatic K65.0
diffuse K65.0
diphtheritic A36.89
disseminated K65.0
due to
    bile K65.3
    foreign
        body or object accidentally left during a proce-
            dure (instrument) (sponge) (swab)
            T81.599 ✓
        substance accidentally left during a procedure
            (chemical) (powder) (talc) T81.61 ✓
    talc T81.61 ✓
    urine K65.8
eosinophilic K65.8
    acute K65.0
fibrocaseous (tuberculous) A18.31
fibropurulent K65.0
following ectopic or molar pregnancy O08.0
general (ized) K65.0
gonococcal A54.85
meconium (newborn) P78.0
neonatal P78.1
    meconium P78.0
pancreatic K65.0
paroxysmal, familial E85.0
    benign E85.0
pelvic
    female N73.5
        acute N73.3
        chronic N73.4
            with adhesions N73.6
    male K65.0
periodic, familial E85.0
proliferative, chronic K65.8
puerperal, postpartum, childbirth O85
purulent K65.0
septic K65.0

Peritonitis — *continued*
specified NEC K65.8
spontaneous bacterial K65.2
subdiaphragmatic K65.0
subphrenic K65.0
suppurative K65.0
syphilitic A52.74
    congenital (early) A50.08 [K67]
talc T81.61 ✓
tuberculous A18.31
urine K65.8
Peritonsillar — *see* condition
Peritonsillitis J36
Perityphlitis K37
Periureteritis N28.89
Periurethral — *see* condition
Periurethritis (gangrenous) — *see* Urethritis
Periuterine — *see* condition
Perivaginitis — *see* Vaginitis
Perivasculitis, retinal H35.06- ✓
Perivasitis (chronic) N49.1
Perivesiculitis (seminal) — *see* Vesiculitis
Perlèche NEC K13.0
due to
    candidiasis B37.83
    moniliasis B37.83
    riboflavin deficiency E53.0
    vitamin B2 (riboflavin) deficiency E53.0
Pernicious — *see* condition
Pernio, perniosis T69.1 ✓
Perpetrator (of abuse) — *see* Index to External Causes
of Injury, Perpetrator
Persecution
delusion F22
social Z60.5
Perseveration (tonic) R48.8
Persistence, persistent (congenital)
anal membrane Q42.3
    with fistula Q42.2
arteria stapedia Q16.3
atrioventricular canal Q21.2
branchial cleft NOS Q18.2
    cyst Q18.0
    fistula Q18.0
    sinus Q18.0
bulbus cordis in left ventricle Q21.8
canal of Cloquet Q14.0
capsule (opaque) Q12.8
cilioretinal artery or vein Q14.8
cloaca Q43.7
communication — *see* Fistula, congenital
convolutions
    aortic arch Q25.46
    fallopian tube Q50.6
    oviduct Q50.6
    uterine tube Q50.6
double aortic arch Q25.45
ductus arteriosus (Botalli) Q25.0
fetal
    circulation P29.38
    form of cervix (uteri) Q51.828
    hemoglobin, hereditary (HPFH) D56.4
foramen
    Botalli Q21.1
    ovale Q21.1
Gartner's duct Q52.4
hemoglobin, fetal (hereditary) (HPFH) D56.4
hyaloid
    artery (generally incomplete) Q14.0
    system Q14.8
hymen, in pregnancy or childbirth — *see* Pregnancy,
    complicated by, abnormal, vulva
lanugo Q84.2
left
    posterior cardinal vein Q26.8
    root with right arch of aorta Q25.49
    superior vena cava Q26.1
Meckel's diverticulum Q43.0
    malignant — *see* Table of Neoplasms, small intes-
        tine, malignant
mucosal disease (middle ear) — *see* Otitis, media,
    suppurative, chronic, tubotympanic
nail(s), anomalous Q84.6
omphalomesenteric duct Q43.0
organ or site not listed — *see* Anomaly, by site
ostium
    atrioventriculare commune Q21.2
    primum Q21.2

▽ **Subterms under main terms may continue to next column or page**   ✓ **Additional Character Required — Refer to the Tabular List for Character Selection**

Persistence, persistent — *continued*
- ostium — *continued*
  - secundum Q21.1
- ovarian rests in fallopian tube Q50.6
- pancreatic tissue in intestinal tract Q43.8
- primary (deciduous)
  - teeth K00.6
  - vitreous hyperplasia Q14.0
- pupillary membrane Q13.89
- rhesus (Rh) titer — *see* Complication(s), transfusion, incompatibility reaction, Rh (factor)
- right aortic arch Q25.47
- sinus
  - urogenitalis
    - female Q52.8
    - male Q55.8
  - venosus with imperfect incorporation in right auricle Q26.8
- thymus (gland) (hyperplasia) E32.0
- thyroglossal duct Q89.2
- thyrolingual duct Q89.2
- truncus arteriosus or communis Q20.0
- tunica vasculosa lentis Q12.2
- umbilical sinus Q64.4
- urachus Q64.4
- vitelline duct Q43.0
Person (with)
- admitted for clinical research, as a control subject (normal comparison) (participant) Z00.6
- awaiting admission to adequate facility elsewhere Z75.1
- concern (normal) about sick person in family Z63.6
- consulting on behalf of another Z71.0
- feigning illness Z76.5
- living (in)
  - alone Z60.2
  - boarding school Z59.3
  - residential institution Z59.3
  - without
    - adequate housing (heating) (space) Z59.1
    - housing (permanent) (temporary) Z59.0
    - person able to render necessary care Z74.2
    - shelter Z59.0
- on waiting list Z75.1
- sick or handicapped in family Z63.6
Personality (disorder) F60.9
- accentuation of traits (type A pattern) Z73.1
- affective F34.0
- aggressive F60.3
- amoral F60.2
- anacastic, anankastic F60.5
- antisocial F60.2
- anxious F60.6
- asocial F60.2
- asthenic F60.7
- avoidant F60.6
- borderline F60.3
- change due to organic condition (enduring) F07.0
- compulsive F60.5
- cycloid F34.0
- cyclothymic F34.0
- dependent F60.7
- depressive F34.1
- dissocial F60.2
- dual F44.81
- eccentric F60.89
- emotionally unstable F60.3
- expansive paranoid F60.0
- explosive F60.3
- fanatic F60.0
- haltose type F60.89
- histrionic F60.4
- hyperthymic F34.0
- hypothymic F34.1
- hysterical F60.4
- immature F60.89
- inadequate F60.7
- labile (emotional) F60.3
- mixed (nonspecific) F60.89
- morally defective F60.2
- multiple F44.81
- narcissistic F60.81
- obsessional F60.5
- obsessive (-compulsive) F60.5
- organic F07.0
- overconscientious F60.5
- paranoid F60.0
- passive (-dependent) F60.7
- passive-aggressive F60.89

Personality — *continued*
- pathologic F60.9
- pattern defect or disturbance F60.9
- pseudopsychopathic (organic) F07.0
- pseudoretarded (organic) F07.0
- psychoinfantile F60.4
- psychoneurotic NEC F60.89
- psychopathic F60.2
- querulant F60.0
- sadistic F60.89
- schizoid F60.1
- self-defeating F60.7
- sensitive paranoid F60.0
- sociopathic (amoral) (antisocial) (asocial) (dissocial) F60.2
- specified NEC F60.89
- type A Z73.1
- unstable (emotional) F60.3
Perthes' disease — *see* Legg-Calvé-Perthes disease
Pertussis (*see also* Whooping cough) A37.90
Perversion, perverted
- appetite F50.89
  - psychogenic F50.89
- function
  - pituitary gland E23.2
    - posterior lobe E22.2
- sense of smell and taste R43.8
  - psychogenic F45.8
- sexual — *see* Deviation, sexual
Pervious, congenital (*see also* Imperfect, closure)
- ductus arteriosus Q25.0
Pes (congenital) (*see also* Talipes)
- acquired (*see also* Deformity, limb, foot, specified NEC)
  - planus — *see* Deformity, limb, flat foot
- adductus Q66.89
- cavus Q66.7
- deformity NEC, acquired — *see* Deformity, limb, foot, specified NEC
- planus (acquired) (any degree) (*see also* Deformity, limb, flat foot)
  - rachitic sequelae (late effect) E64.3
- valgus Q66.6
Pest, pestis — *see* Plague
Petechia, petechiae R23.3
- newborn P54.5
Petechial typhus A75.9
Peter's anomaly Q13.4
Petit mal seizure — *see* Epilepsy, generalized, specified NEC
Petit's hernia — *see* Hernia, abdomen, specified site NEC
Petrellidosis B48.2
Petrositis H70.20- ☑
- acute H70.21- ☑
- chronic H70.22- ☑
Peutz-Jeghers disease or syndrome Q85.8
Peyronie's disease N48.6
PFAPA (periodic fever, aphthous stomatitis, pharyngitis, and adenopathy syndrome) M04.8
Pfeiffer's disease — *see* Mononucleosis, infectious
Phagedena (dry) (moist) (sloughing) (*see also* Gangrene)
- geometric L88
- penis N48.29
- tropical — *see* Ulcer, skin
- vulva N76.6
Phagedenic — *see* condition
Phakoma H35.89
Phakomatosis (*see also* specific eponymous syndromes) Q85.9
- Bourneville's Q85.1
- specified NEC Q85.8
Phantom limb syndrome (without pain) G54.7
- with pain G54.6
Pharyngeal pouch syndrome D82.1
Pharyngitis (acute) (catarrhal)(gangrenous) (infective) (malignant) (membranous) (phlegmonous) (pseudomembranous) (simple) (subacute) (suppurative) (ulcerative) (viral) J02.9
- with influenza, flu, or grippe — *see* Influenza, with, pharyngitis
- aphthous B08.5
- atrophic J31.2
- chlamydial A56.4
- chronic (atrophic) (granular) (hypertrophic) J31.2
- coxsackievirus B08.5
- diphtheritic A36.0
- enteroviral vesicular B08.5
- follicular (chronic) J31.2
- fusospirochetal A69.1

Pharyngitis — *continued*
- gonococcal A54.5
- granular (chronic) J31.2
- herpesviral B00.2
- hypertrophic J31.2
- infectional, chronic J31.2
- influenzal — *see* Influenza, with, respiratory manifestations NEC
- lymphonodular, acute (enteroviral) B08.8
- pneumococcal J02.8
- purulent J02.9
- putrid J02.9
- septic J02.0
- sicca J31.2
- specified organism NEC J02.8
- staphylococcal J02.8
- streptococcal J02.0
- syphilitic, congenital (early) A50.03
- tuberculous A15.8
- vesicular, enteroviral B08.5
- viral NEC J02.8
Pharyngoconjunctivitis, viral B30.2
Pharyngolaryngitis (acute) J06.0
- chronic J37.0
Pharyngoplegia J39.2
Pharyngotonsillitis, herpesviral B00.2
Pharyngotracheitis, chronic J42
Pharynx, pharyngeal — *see* condition
Phencyclidine-induced
- anxiety disorder F16.980
- bipolar and related disorder F16.94
- depressive disorder F16.94
- psychotic disorder F16.959
Phenomenon
- Arthus' — *see* Arthus' phenomenon
- jaw-winking Q07.8
- lupus erythematosus (LE) cell M32.9
- Raynaud's (secondary) I73.00
  - with gangrene I73.01
- vasomotor R55
- vasospastic I73.9
- vasovagal R55
- Wenckebach's I44.1
Phenylketonuria E70.1
- classical E70.0
- maternal E70.1
Pheochromoblastoma
- specified site — *see* Neoplasm, malignant, by site
- unspecified site C74.10
Pheochromocytoma
- malignant
  - specified site — *see* Neoplasm, malignant, by site
  - unspecified site C74.10
- specified site — *see* Neoplasm, benign, by site
- unspecified site D35.00
Pheohyphomycosis — *see* Chromomycosis
Pheomycosis — *see* Chromomycosis
Phimosis (congenital) (due to infection) N47.1
- chancroidal A57
Phlebectasia (*see also* Varix)
- congenital Q27.4
Phlebitis (infective) (pyemic) (septic) (suppurative) I80.9
- antepartum — *see* Thrombophlebitis, antepartum
- blue — *see* Phlebitis, leg, deep
- breast, superficial I80.8
- cavernous (venous) sinus — *see* Phlebitis, intracranial (venous) sinus
- cerebral (venous) sinus — *see* Phlebitis, intracranial (venous) sinus
- chest wall, superficial I80.8
- cranial (venous) sinus — *see* Phlebitis, intracranial (venous) sinus
- deep (vessels) — *see* Phlebitis, leg, deep
- due to implanted device — *see* Complications, by site and type, specified NEC
- during or resulting from a procedure T81.72 ☑
- femoral vein (superficial) I80.1- ☑
- femoropopliteal vein I80.0- ☑
- gestational — *see* Phlebopathy, gestational
- hepatic veins I80.8
- iliofemoral — *see* Phlebitis, femoral vein
- intracranial (venous) sinus (any) G08
  - nonpyogenic I67.6
- intraspinal venous sinuses and veins G08
  - nonpyogenic G95.19
- lateral (venous) sinus — *see* Phlebitis, intracranial (venous) sinus
- leg I80.3

☑ **Additional Character Required** — Refer to the Tabular List for Character Selection   ⬇ **Subterms under main terms may continue to next column or page**

Phlebitis — continued
- leg — continued
  - antepartum — see Thrombophlebitis, antepartum
  - deep (vessels) NEC I80.20- ☑
    - iliac I80.21- ☑
    - popliteal vein I80.22- ☑
    - specified vessel NEC I80.29- ☑
    - tibial vein I80.23- ☑
  - femoral vein (superficial) I80.1- ☑
  - superficial (vessels) I80.0- ☑
- longitudinal sinus — see Phlebitis, intracranial (venous) sinus
- lower limb — see Phlebitis, leg
- migrans, migrating (superficial) I82.1
- pelvic
  - with ectopic or molar pregnancy O08.0
  - following ectopic or molar pregnancy O08.0
  - puerperal, postpartum O87.1
- popliteal vein — see Phlebitis, leg, deep, popliteal
- portal (vein) K75.1
- postoperative T81.72 ☑
- pregnancy — see Thrombophlebitis, antepartum
- puerperal, postpartum, childbirth O87.0
  - deep O87.1
  - pelvic O87.1
  - superficial O87.0
- retina — see Vasculitis, retina
- saphenous (accessory) (great) (long) (small) — see Phlebitis, leg, superficial
- sinus (meninges) — see Phlebitis, intracranial (venous) sinus
- specified site NEC I80.8
- syphilitic A52.09
- tibial vein — see Phlebitis, leg, deep, tibial
- ulcerative I80.9
  - leg — see Phlebitis, leg
- umbilicus I80.8
- uterus (septic) — see Endometritis
- varicose (leg) (lower limb) — see Varix, leg, with, inflammation

Phlebofibrosis I87.8
Phleboliths I87.8
Phlebopathy,
- gestational O22.9- ☑
- puerperal O87.9
Phlebosclerosis I87.8
Phlebothrombosis (see also Thrombosis)
- antepartum — see Thrombophlebitis, antepartum
- pregnancy — see Thrombophlebitis, antepartum
- puerperal — see Thrombophlebitis, puerperal
Phlebotomus fever A93.1
Phlegmasia
- alba dolens O87.1
  - nonpuerperal — see Phlebitis, femoral vein
- cerulea dolens — see Phlebitis, leg, deep
Phlegmon — see Abscess
Phlegmonous — see condition
Phlyctenulosis (allergic) (keratoconjunctivitis) (nontuberculous) (see also Keratoconjunctivitis)
- cornea — see Keratoconjunctivitis
- tuberculous A18.52
Phobia, phobic F40.9
- animal F40.218
  - spiders F40.210
- examination F40.298
- reaction F40.9
- simple F40.298
- social F40.10
  - generalized F40.11
- specific (isolated) F40.298
  - animal F40.218
    - spiders F40.210
  - blood F40.230
  - injection F40.231
  - injury F40.233
  - men F40.290
  - natural environment F40.228
    - thunderstorms F40.220
  - situational F40.248
    - bridges F40.242
    - closed in spaces F40.240
    - flying F40.243
    - heights F40.241
  - specified focus NEC F40.298
  - transfusion F40.231
  - women F40.291
- specified NEC F40.8

Phobia, phobic — continued
- specified — continued
  - medical care NEC F40.232
- state F40.9
Phocas' disease — see Mastopathy, cystic
Phocomelia Q73.1
- lower limb — see Agenesis, leg, with foot present
- upper limb — see Agenesis, arm, with hand present
Phoria H50.50
Phosphate-losing tubular disorder N25.0
Phosphatemia E83.39
Phosphaturia E83.39
Photodermatitis (sun) L56.8
- chronic L57.8
- due to drug L56.8
- light other than sun L59.8
Photokeratitis H16.13- ☑
Photophobia H53.14- ☑
Photophthalmia — see Photokeratitis
Photopsia H53.19
Photoretinitis — see Retinopathy, solar
Photosensitivity, photosensitization (sun) skin L56.8
- light other than sun L59.8
Phrenitis — see Encephalitis
Phrynoderma (vitamin A deficiency) E50.8
Phthiriasis (pubis) B85.3
- with any infestation classifiable to B85.0-B85.2 B85.4
Phthirus infestation — see Phthiriasis
Phthisis (see also Tuberculosis)
- bulbi (infectional) — see Disorder, globe, degenerated condition, atrophy
- eyeball (due to infection) — see Disorder, globe, degenerated condition, atrophy
Phycomycosis — see Zygomycosis
Physalopteriasis B81.8
Physical restraint status Z78.1
Phytobezoar T18.9 ☑
- intestine T18.3 ☑
- stomach T18.2 ☑
Pian — see Yaws
Pianoma A66.1
Pica F50.89
- in adults F50.89
- infant or child F98.3
Picking, nose F98.8
Pick-Niemann disease — see Niemann-Pick disease or syndrome
Pick's
- cerebral atrophy G31.01 [F02.80]
  - with behavioral disturbance G31.01 [F02.81]
- disease or syndrome (brain) G31.01 [F02.80]
  - with behavioral disturbance G31.01 [F02.81]
  - brain G31.01 [F02.80]
    - with behavioral disturbance G31.01 [F02.81]
  - pericardium (pericardial pseudocirrhosis of liver) I31.1
- syndrome
  - brain G31.01 [F02.80]
    - with behavioral disturbance G31.01 [F02.81]
  - of heart (pericardial pseudocirrhosis of liver) I31.1
Pickwickian syndrome E66.2
Piebaldism E70.39
Piedra (beard) (scalp) B36.8
- black B36.3
- white B36.2
Pierre Robin deformity or syndrome Q87.0
Pierson's disease or osteochondrosis M91.0
Pig-bel A05.2
Pigeon
- breast or chest (acquired) M95.4
  - congenital Q67.7
  - rachitic sequelae (late effect) E64.3
- breeder's disease or lung J67.2
- fancier's disease or lung J67.2
- toe — see Deformity, toe, specified NEC
Pigmentation (abnormal) (anomaly) L81.9
- conjunctiva H11.13- ☑
- cornea (anterior) H18.01- ☑
  - posterior H18.05- ☑
  - stromal H18.06- ☑
- diminished melanin formation NEC L81.6
- iron L81.8
- lids, congenital Q82.8
- limbus corneae — see Pigmentation, cornea
- metals L81.8
- optic papilla, congenital Q14.2
- retina, congenital (grouped) (nevoid) Q14.1

Pigmentation — continued
- scrotum, congenital Q82.8
- tattoo L81.8
Piles (see also Hemorrhoids) K64.9
Pili
- annulati or torti (congenital) Q84.1
- incarnati L73.1
Pill roller hand (intrinsic) — see Parkinsonism
Pilomatrixoma — see Neoplasm, skin, benign
- malignant — see Neoplasm, skin, malignant
Pilonidal — see condition
Pimple R23.8
PIN — see Neoplasia, intraepithelial, prostate
Pinched nerve — see Neuropathy, entrapment
Pindborg tumor — see Cyst, calcifying odontogenic
Pineal body or gland — see condition
Pinealoblastoma C75.3
Pinealoma D44.5
- malignant C75.3
Pineoblastoma C75.3
Pineocytoma D44.5
Pinguecula H11.15- ☑
Pingueculitis H10.81- ☑
Pinhole meatus (see also Stricture, urethra) N35.919
Pink
- disease — see subcategory T56.1 ☑
- eye — see Conjunctivitis, acute, mucopurulent
Pinkus' disease (lichen nitidus) L44.1
Pinpoint
- meatus — see Stricture, urethra
- os (uteri) — see Stricture, cervix
Pins and needles R20.2
Pinta A67.9
- cardiovascular lesions A67.2
- chancre (primary) A67.0
- erythematous plaques A67.1
- hyperchromic lesions A67.1
- hyperkeratosis A67.1
- lesions A67.9
  - cardiovascular A67.2
  - hyperchromic A67.1
  - intermediate A67.1
  - late A67.2
  - mixed A67.3
  - primary A67.0
  - skin (achromic) (cicatricial) (dyschromic) A67.2
    - hyperchromic A67.1
    - mixed (achromic and hyperchromic) A67.3
- papule (primary) A67.0
- skin lesions (achromic) (cicatricial) (dyschromic) A67.2
  - hyperchromic A67.1
  - mixed (achromic and hyperchromic) A67.3
- vitiligo A67.2
Pintids A67.1
Pinworm (disease) (infection) (infestation) B80
Piroplasmosis B60.0
Pistol wound — see Gunshot wound
Pitchers' elbow — see Derangement, joint, specified type NEC, elbow
Pithecoid pelvis Q74.2
- with disproportion (fetopelvic) O33.0
  - causing obstructed labor O65.0
Pithiatism F48.8
Pitted — see Pitting
Pitting (see also Edema) R60.9
- lip R60.0
- nail L60.8
- teeth K00.4
Pituitary gland — see condition
Pituitary-snuff-taker's disease J67.8
Pityriasis (capitis) L21.0
- alba L30.5
- circinata (et maculata) L42
- furfuracea L21.0
- Hebra's L26
- lichenoides L41.0
  - chronica L41.1
  - et varioliformis (acuta) L41.0
- maculata (et circinata) L30.5
- nigra B36.1
- pilaris, Hebra's L44.0
- rosea L42
- rotunda L44.8
- rubra (Hebra) pilaris L44.0
- simplex L30.5
- specified type NEC L30.5
- streptogenes L30.5

Pityriasis — continued
  versicolor (scrotal) B36.0
Placenta, placental — see Pregnancy, complicated by (care of) (management affected by), specified condition
Placentitis O41.14- ☑
Plagiocephaly Q67.3
Plague A20.9
  abortive A20.8
  ambulatory A20.8
  asymptomatic A20.8
  bubonic A20.0
  cellulocutaneous A20.1
  cutaneobubonic A20.1
  lymphatic gland A20.0
  meningitis A20.3
  pharyngeal A20.8
  pneumonic (primary) (secondary) A20.2
  pulmonary, pulmonic A20.2
  septicemic A20.7
  tonsillar A20.8
    septicemic A20.7
Planning, family
  contraception Z30.9
  procreation Z31.69
Plaque(s)
  artery, arterial — see Arteriosclerosis
  calcareous — see Calcification
  coronary, lipid rich I25.83
  epicardial I31.8
  erythematous, of pinta A67.1
  Hollenhorst's — see Occlusion, artery, retina
  lipid rich, coronary I25.83
  pleural (without asbestos) J92.9
    with asbestos J92.0
  tongue K13.29
Plasmacytoma C90.3- ☑
  extramedullary C90.2- ☑
  medullary C90.0- ☑
  solitary C90.3- ☑
Plasmacytopenia D72.818
Plasmacytosis D72.822
Plaster ulcer — see Ulcer, pressure, by site
Plateau iris syndrome (post-iridectomy) (postprocedural) (without glaucoma) H21.82
  with glaucoma H40.22- ☑
Platybasia Q75.8
Platyonychia (congenital) Q84.6
  acquired L60.8
Platypelloid pelvis M95.5
  with disproportion (fetopelvic) O33.0
    causing obstructed labor O65.0
  congenital Q74.2
Platyspondylisis Q76.49
Plaut (-Vincent) **disease** (see also Vincent's) A69.1
Plethora R23.2
  newborn P61.1
Pleura, pleural — see condition
Pleuralgia R07.81
Pleurisy (acute) (adhesive) (chronic) (costal) (diaphragmatic) (double) (dry) (fibrinous) (fibrous) (interlobar) (latent) (plastic) (primary) (residual) (sicca) (sterile) (subacute) (unresolved) R09.1
  with
    adherent pleura J86.0
    effusion J90
      chylous, chyliform J94.0
      tuberculous (non primary) A15.6
        primary (progressive) A15.7
    tuberculosis — see Pleurisy, tuberculous (non primary)
  encysted — see Pleurisy, with effusion
  exudative — see Pleurisy, with effusion
  fibrinopurulent, fibropurulent — see Pyothorax
  hemorrhagic — see Hemothorax
  pneumococcal J90
  purulent — see Pyothorax
  septic — see Pyothorax
  serofibrinous — see Pleurisy, with effusion
  seropurulent — see Pyothorax
  serous — see Pleurisy, with effusion
  staphylococcal J86.9
  streptococcal J90
  suppurative — see Pyothorax
  traumatic (post) (current) — see Injury, intrathoracic, pleura
  tuberculous (with effusion) (non primary) A15.6

Pleurisy — continued
  tuberculous — continued
    primary (progressive) A15.7
Pleuritis sicca — see Pleurisy
Pleurobronchopneumonia — see Pneumonia, broncho-
Pleurodynia R07.81
  epidemic B33.0
  viral B33.0
Pleuropericarditis (see also Pericarditis)
  acute I30.9
Pleuropneumonia (acute) (bilateral) (double) (septic) (see also Pneumonia) J18.8
  chronic — see Fibrosis, lung
Pleuro-pneumonia-like-organism (PPLO), as cause of disease classified elsewhere B96.0
Pleurorrhea — see Pleurisy, with effusion
Plexitis, brachial G54.0
Plica
  polonica B85.0
  syndrome, knee M67.5- ☑
  tonsil J35.8
Plicated tongue K14.5
Plug
  bronchus NEC J98.09
  meconium (newborn) NEC syndrome P76.0
  mucus — see Asphyxia, mucus
Plumbism — see subcategory T56.0 ☑
Plummer's disease E05.20
  with thyroid storm E05.21
Plummer-Vinson syndrome D50.1
Pluricarential syndrome of infancy E40
Plus (and minus) **hand** (intrinsic) — see Deformity, limb, specified type NEC, forearm
Pneumathemia — see Air, embolism
Pneumatic hammer (drill) syndrome T75.21 ☑
Pneumatocele (lung) J98.4
  intracranial G93.89
  tension J44.9
Pneumatosis
  cystoides intestinalis K63.89
  intestinalis K63.89
  peritonei K66.8
Pneumaturia R39.89
Pneumoblastoma — see Neoplasm, lung, malignant
Pneumocephalus G93.89
Pneumococcemia A40.3
Pneumococcus, pneumococcal — see condition
Pneumoconiosis (due to) (inhalation of) J64
  with tuberculosis (any type in A15) J65
  aluminum J63.0
  asbestos J61
  bagasse, bagassosis J67.1
  bauxite J63.1
  beryllium J63.2
  coal miners' (simple) J60
  coalworkers' (simple) J60
  collier's J60
  cotton dust J66.0
  diatomite (diatomaceous earth) J62.8
  dust
    inorganic NEC J63.6
    lime J62.8
    marble J62.8
    organic NEC J66.8
  fumes or vapors (from silo) J68.9
  graphite J63.3
  grinder's J62.8
  kaolin J62.8
  mica J62.8
  millstone maker's J62.8
  mineral fibers NEC J61
  miner's J60
  moldy hay J67.0
  potter's J62.8
  rheumatoid — see Rheumatoid, lung
  sandblaster's J62.8
  silica, silicate NEC J62.8
    with carbon J60
  stonemason's J62.8
  talc (dust) J62.0
Pneumocystis carinii pneumonia B59
Pneumocystis jiroveci (pneumonia) B59
Pneumocystosis (with pneumonia) B59
Pneumohemopericardium I31.2
Pneumohemothorax J94.2
  traumatic S27.2 ☑
Pneumohydropericardium — see Pericarditis

Pneumohydrothorax — see Hydrothorax
Pneumomediastinum J98.2
  congenital or perinatal P25.2
Pneumomycosis B49 [J99]
Pneumonia (acute) (double) (migratory) (purulent) (septic) (unresolved) J18.9
  with
    influenza — see Influenza, with, pneumonia
    lung abscess J85.1
      due to specified organism — see Pneumonia, in (due to)
  adenoviral J12.0
  adynamic J18.2
  alba A50.04
  allergic (eosinophilic) J82
  alveolar — see Pneumonia, lobar
  anaerobes J15.8
  anthrax A22.1
  apex, apical — see Pneumonia, lobar
  Ascaris B77.81
  aspiration J69.0
    due to
      aspiration of microorganisms
        bacterial J15.9
        viral J12.9
      food (regurgitated) J69.0
      gastric secretions J69.0
      milk (regurgitated) J69.0
      oils, essences J69.1
      solids, liquids NEC J69.8
      vomitus J69.0
    newborn P24.81
      amniotic fluid (clear) P24.11
      blood P24.21
      food (regurgitated) P24.31
      liquor (amnii) P24.11
      meconium P24.01
      milk P24.31
      mucus P24.11
      specified NEC P24.81
      stomach contents P24.31
    postprocedural J95.4
  atypical NEC J18.9
  bacillus J15.9
    specified NEC J15.8
  bacterial J15.9
    specified NEC J15.8
  Bacteroides (fragilis) (oralis) (melaninogenicus) J15.8
  basal, basic, basilar — see Pneumonia, by type
  bronchiolitis obliterans organized (BOOP) J84.89
  broncho-, bronchial (confluent) (croupous) (diffuse) (disseminated) (hemorrhagic) (involving lobes) (lobar) (terminal) J18.0
    allergic (eosinophilic) J82
    aspiration — see Pneumonia, aspiration
    bacterial J15.9
      specified NEC J15.8
    chronic — see Fibrosis, lung
    diplococcal J13
    Eaton's agent J15.7
    Escherichia coli (E. coli) J15.5
    Friedländer's bacillus J15.0
    Hemophilus influenzae J14
    hypostatic J18.2
    inhalation (see also Pneumonia, aspiration)
      due to fumes or vapors (chemical) J68.0
      of oils or essences J69.1
    Klebsiella (pneumoniae) J15.0
    lipid, lipoid J69.1
      endogenous J84.89
    Mycoplasma (pneumoniae) J15.7
    pleuro-pneumonia-like-organisms (PPLO) J15.7
    pneumococcal J13
    Proteus J15.6
    Pseudomonas J15.1
    Serratia marcescens J15.6
    specified organism NEC J16.8
    staphylococcal — see Pneumonia, staphylococcal
    streptococcal NEC J15.4
      group B J15.3
      pneumoniae J13
    viral, virus — see Pneumonia, viral
  Butyrivibrio (fibriosolvens) J15.8
  Candida B37.1
  caseous — see Tuberculosis, pulmonary
  catarrhal — see Pneumonia, broncho
  chlamydial J16.0
    congenital P23.1

Pneumonia — *continued*
  cholesterol J84.89
  cirrhotic (chronic) — *see* Fibrosis, lung
  Clostridium (haemolyticum) (novyi) J15.8
  confluent — *see* Pneumonia, broncho
  congenital (infective) P23.9
    due to
      bacterium NEC P23.6
      Chlamydia P23.1
      Escherichia coli P23.4
      Haemophilus influenzae P23.6
      infective organism NEC P23.8
      Klebsiella pneumoniae P23.6
      Mycoplasma P23.6
      Pseudomonas P23.5
      Staphylococcus P23.2
      Streptococcus (except group B) P23.6
        group B P23.3
      viral agent P23.0
    specified NEC P23.8
  croupous — *see* Pneumonia, lobar
  cryptogenic organizing J84.116
  cytomegalic inclusion B25.0
  cytomegaloviral B25.0
  deglutition — *see* Pneumonia, aspiration
  desquamative interstitial J84.117
  diffuse — *see* Pneumonia, broncho
  diplococcal, diplococcus (broncho-) (lobar) J13
  disseminated (focal) — *see* Pneumonia, broncho
  Eaton's agent J15.7
  embolic, embolism — *see* Embolism, pulmonary
  Enterobacter J15.6
  eosinophilic J82
  Escherichia coli (E. coli) J15.5
  Eubacterium J15.8
  fibrinous — *see* Pneumonia, lobar
  fibroid, fibrous (chronic) — *see* Fibrosis, lung
  Friedländer's bacillus J15.0
  Fusobacterium (nucleatum) J15.8
  gangrenous J85.0
  giant cell (measles) B05.2
  gonococcal A54.84
  gram-negative bacteria NEC J15.6
    anaerobic J15.8
  Hemophilus influenzae (broncho) (lobar) J14
  human metapneumovirus J12.3
  hypostatic (broncho) (lobar) J18.2
  in (due to)
    actinomycosis A42.0
    adenovirus J12.0
    anthrax A22.1
    ascariasis B77.81
    aspergillosis B44.9
    Bacillus anthracis A22.1
    Bacterium anitratum J15.6
    candidiasis B37.1
    chickenpox B01.2
    Chlamydia J16.0
      neonatal P23.1
    coccidioidomycosis B38.2
      acute B38.0
      chronic B38.1
    cytomegalovirus disease B25.0
    Diplococcus (pneumoniae) J13
    Eaton's agent J15.7
    Enterobacter J15.6
    Escherichia coli (E. coli) J15.5
    Friedländer's bacillus J15.0
    fumes and vapors (chemical) (inhalation) J68.0
    gonorrhea A54.84
    Hemophilus influenzae (H. influenzae) J14
    Herellea J15.6
    histoplasmosis B39.2
      acute B39.0
      chronic B39.1
    human metapneumovirus J12.3
    Klebsiella (pneumoniae) J15.0
    measles B05.2
    Mycoplasma (pneumoniae) J15.7
    nocardiosis, nocardiasis A43.0
    ornithosis A70
    parainfluenza virus J12.2
    pleuro-pneumonia-like-organism (PPLO) J15.7
    pneumococcus J13
    pneumocystosis (Pneumocystis carinii) (Pneumocystis jiroveci) B59
    Proteus J15.6
    Pseudomonas NEC J15.1

Pneumonia — *continued*
  in — *continued*
    Pseudomonas — *continued*
      pseudomallei A24.1
    psittacosis A70
    Q fever A78
    respiratory syncytial virus J12.1
    rheumatic fever I00 [J17]
    rubella B06.81
    Salmonella (infection) A02.22
      typhi A01.03
    schistosomiasis B65.9 [J17]
    Serratia marcescens J15.6
    specified
      bacterium NEC J15.8
      organism NEC J16.8
    spirochetal NEC A69.8
    Staphylococcus J15.20
      aureus (methicillin susceptible) (MSSA) J15.211
        methicillin resistant (MRSA) J15.212
      specified NEC J15.29
    Streptococcus J15.4
      group B J15.3
      pneumoniae J13
      specified NEC J15.4
    toxoplasmosis B58.3
    tularemia A21.2
    typhoid (fever) A01.03
    varicella B01.2
    virus — *see* Pneumonia, viral
    whooping cough A37.91
      due to
        Bordetella parapertussis A37.11
        Bordetella pertussis A37.01
        specified NEC A37.81
    Yersinia pestis A20.2
  inhalation of food or vomit — *see* Pneumonia, aspiration
  interstitial J84.9
    chronic J84.111
    desquamative J84.117
    due to
      collagen vascular disease J84.17
      known underlying cause J84.17
    idiopathic NOS J84.111
    in disease classified elsewhere J84.17
    lymphocytic (due to collagen vascular disease) (in diseases classified elsewhere) J84.17
    lymphoid J84.2
    non-specific J84.89
      due to
        collagen vascular disease J84.17
        known underlying cause J84.17
      idiopathic J84.113
      in diseases classified elsewhere J84.17
    plasma cell B59
    pseudomonas J15.1
    usual J84.112
      due to collagen vascular disease J84.17
      idiopathic J84.112
      in diseases classified elsewhere J84.17
  Klebsiella (pneumoniae) J15.0
  lipid, lipoid (exogenous) J69.1
    endogenous J84.89
  lobar (disseminated) (double) (interstitial) J18.1
    bacterial J15.9
      specified NEC J15.8
    chronic — *see* Fibrosis, lung
    Escherichia coli (E. coli) J15.5
    Friedländer's bacillus J15.0
    Hemophilus influenzae J14
    hypostatic J18.2
    Klebsiella (pneumoniae) J15.0
    pneumococcal J13
    Proteus J15.6
    Pseudomonas J15.1
    specified organism NEC J16.8
    staphylococcal — *see* Pneumonia, staphylococcal
    streptococcal NEC J15.4
    Streptococcus pneumoniae J13
    viral, virus — *see* Pneumonia, viral
  lobular — *see* Pneumonia, broncho
  Löffler's J82
  lymphoid interstitial J84.2
  massive — *see* Pneumonia, lobar
  meconium P24.01
  MRSA (methicillin resistant Staphylococcus aureus) J15.212

Pneumonia — *continued*
  MSSA (methicillin susceptible Staphylococcus aureus) J15.211
  multilobar — *see* Pneumonia, by type
  Mycoplasma (pneumoniae) J15.7
  necrotic J85.0
  neonatal P23.9
    aspiration — *see* Aspiration, by substance, with pneumonia
  nitrogen dioxide J68.0
  organizing J84.89
    due to
      collagen vascular disease J84.17
      known underlying cause J84.17
    in diseases classified elsewhere J84.17
  orthostatic J18.2
  parainfluenza virus J12.2
  parenchymatous — *see* Fibrosis, lung
  passive J18.2
  patchy — *see* Pneumonia, broncho
  Peptococcus J15.8
  Peptostreptococcus J15.8
  plasma cell (of infants) B59
  pleurolobar — *see* Pneumonia, lobar
  pleuro-pneumonia-like organism (PPLO) J15.7
  pneumococcal (broncho) (lobar) J13
  Pneumocystis (carinii) (jiroveci) B59
  postinfectional NEC B99 ☑ [J17]
  postmeasles B05.2
  Proteus J15.6
  Pseudomonas J15.1
  psittacosis A70
  radiation J70.0
  respiratory syncytial virus J12.1
  resulting from a procedure J95.89
  rheumatic I00 [J17]
  Salmonella (arizonae) (cholerae-suis) (enteritidis) (typhimurium) A02.22
    typhi A01.03
    typhoid fever A01.03
  SARS-associated coronavirus J12.81
  segmented, segmental — *see* Pneumonia, broncho-
  Serratia marcescens J15.6
  specified NEC J18.8
    bacterium NEC J15.8
    organism NEC J16.8
    virus NEC J12.89
  spirochetal NEC A69.8
  staphylococcal (broncho) (lobar) J15.20
    aureus (methicillin susceptible) (MSSA) J15.211
      methicillin resistant (MRSA) J15.212
    specified NEC J15.29
  static, stasis J18.2
  streptococcal NEC (broncho) (lobar) J15.4
    group
      A J15.4
      B J15.3
      specified NEC J15.4
  Streptococcus pneumoniae J13
  syphilitic, congenital (early) A50.04
  traumatic (complication) (early) (secondary) T79.8 ☑
  tuberculous (any) — *see* Tuberculosis, pulmonary
  tularemic A21.2
  varicella B01.2
  Veillonella J15.8
  ventilator associated J95.851
  viral, virus (broncho) (interstitial) (lobar) J12.9
    adenoviral J12.0
    congenital P23.0
    human metapneumovirus J12.3
    parainfluenza J12.2
    respiratory syncytial J12.1
    SARS-associated coronavirus J12.81
    specified NEC J12.89
  white (congenital) A50.04
Pneumonic — *see* condition
Pneumonitis (acute) (primary) (*see also* Pneumonia)
  air-conditioner J67.7
  allergic (due to) J67.9
    organic dust NEC J67.8
    red cedar dust J67.8
    sequoiosis J67.8
    wood dust J67.8
  aspiration J69.0
    due to
      anesthesia J95.4
        during
          labor and delivery O74.0

Pneumonitis — *continued*
  aspiration — *continued*
    due to — *continued*
      anesthesia — *continued*
        during — *continued*
          pregnancy O29.01- ☑
          puerperium O89.01
      fumes or gases J68.0
    obstetric O74.0
  chemical (due to gases, fumes or vapors) (inhalation) J68.0
    due to anesthesia J95.4
  cholesterol J84.89
  chronic — *see* Fibrosis, lung
  congenital rubella P35.0
  crack (cocaine) J68.0
  due to
    beryllium J68.0
    cadmium J68.0
    crack (cocaine) J68.0
    detergent J69.8
    fluorocarbon-polymer J68.0
    food, vomit (aspiration) J69.0
    fumes or vapors J68.0
    gases, fumes or vapors (inhalation) J68.0
    inhalation
      blood J69.8
      essences J69.1
      food (regurgitated), milk, vomit J69.0
      oils, essences J69.1
      saliva J69.0
      solids, liquids NEC J69.8
    manganese J68.0
    nitrogen dioxide J68.0
    oils, essences J69.1
    solids, liquids NEC J69.8
    toxoplasmosis (acquired) B58.3
      congenital P37.1
    vanadium J68.0
    ventilator J95.851
  eosinophilic J82
  hypersensitivity J67.9
    air conditioner lung J67.7
    bagassosis J67.1
    bird fancier's lung J67.2
    farmer's lung J67.0
    maltworker's lung J67.4
    maple bark-stripper's lung J67.6
    mushroom worker's lung J67.5
    specified organic dust NEC J67.8
    suberosis J67.3
  interstitial (chronic) J84.89
    acute J84.114
    lymphoid J84.2
    non-specific J84.89
      idiopathic J84.113
  lymphoid, interstitial J84.2
  meconium P24.01
  postanesthetic J95.4
    correct substance properly administered — *see* Table of Drugs and Chemicals, by drug, adverse effect
    in labor and delivery O74.0
    in pregnancy O29.01- ☑
    obstetric O74.0
    overdose or wrong substance given or taken (by accident) — *see* Table of Drugs and Chemicals, by drug, poisoning
    postpartum, puerperal O89.01
  postoperative J95.4
    obstetric O74.0
  radiation J70.0
  rubella, congenital P35.0
  ventilation (air-conditioning) J67.7
  ventilator associated J95.851
  wood-dust J67.8
Pneumonoconiosis — *see* Pneumoconiosis
Pneumoparotid K11.8
Pneumopathy NEC J98.4
  alveolar J84.09
  due to organic dust NEC J66.8
  parietoalveolar J84.09
Pneumopericarditis (*see also* Pericarditis)
  acute I30.9
Pneumopericardium (*see also* Pericarditis)
  congenital P25.3
  newborn P25.3
  traumatic (post) — *see* Injury, heart

Pneumophagia (psychogenic) F45.8
Pneumopleurisy, pneumopleuritis (*see also* Pneumonia) J18.8
Pneumopyopericardium I30.1
Pneumopyothorax — *see* Pyopneumothorax
  with fistula J86.0
Pneumorrhagia (*see also* Hemorrhage, lung)
  tuberculous — *see* Tuberculosis, pulmonary
Pneumothorax NOS J93.9
  acute J93.83
  chronic J93.81
  congenital P25.1
  perinatal period P25.1
  postprocedural J95.811
  specified NEC J93.83
  spontaneous NOS J93.83
    newborn P25.1
    primary J93.11
    secondary J93.12
    tension J93.0
  tense valvular, infectional J93.0
  tension (spontaneous) J93.0
  traumatic S27.0 ☑
    with hemothorax S27.2 ☑
  tuberculous — *see* Tuberculosis, pulmonary
Podagra (*see also* Gout) M10.9
Podencephalus Q01.9
Poikilocytosis R71.8
Poikiloderma L81.6
  Civatte's L57.3
  congenital Q82.8
  vasculare atrophicans L94.5
Poikilodermatomyositis M33.10
  with
    myopathy M33.12
    respiratory involvement M33.11
    specified organ involvement NEC M33.19
Pointed ear (congenital) Q17.3
Poison ivy, oak, sumac or other plant dermatitis (allergic) (contact) L23.7
Poisoning (acute) (*see also* Table of Drugs and Chemicals)
  algae and toxins T65.82- ☑
  Bacillus B (aertrycke) (cholerae (suis)) (paratyphosus) (suipestifer) A02.9
    botulinus A05.1
  bacterial toxins A05.9
  berries, noxious — *see* Poisoning, food, noxious, berries
  botulism A05.1
  ciguatera fish T61.0- ☑
  Clostridium botulinum A05.1
  death-cap (Amanita phalloides) (Amanita verna) — *see* Poisoning, food, noxious, mushrooms
  drug — *see* Table of Drugs and Chemicals, by drug, poisoning
  epidemic, fish (noxious) — *see* Poisoning, seafood
    bacterial A05.9
  fava bean D55.0
  fish (noxious) T61.9- ☑
    bacterial — *see* Intoxication, foodborne, by agent
    ciguatera fish — *see* Poisoning, ciguatera fish
    scombroid fish — *see* Poisoning, scombroid fish
    specified type NEC T61.77- ☑
  food (acute) (diseased) (infected) (noxious) NEC T62.9- ☑
    bacterial — *see* Intoxication, foodborne, by agent
    due to
      Bacillus (aertrycke) (choleraesuis) (paratyphosus) (suipestifer) A02.9
        botulinus A05.1
      Clostridium (perfringens) (Welchii) A05.2
      salmonella (aertrycke) (callinarum) (choleraesuis) (enteritidis) (paratyphi) (suipestifer) A02.9
        with
          gastroenteritis A02.0
          sepsis A02.1
      staphylococcus A05.0
      Vibrio
        parahaemolyticus A05.3
        vulnificus A05.5
    noxious or naturally toxic T62.9- ☑
      berries — *see* subcategory T62.1 ☑
      fish — *see* Poisoning, seafood
      mushrooms — *see* subcategory T62.0X ☑
      plants NEC — *see* subcategory T62.2X ☑
      seafood — *see* Poisoning, seafood
      specified NEC — *see* subcategory T62.8X ☑
  ichthyotoxism — *see* Poisoning, seafood

Poisoning — *continued*
  kreotoxism, food A05.9
  latex T65.81- ☑
  lead T56.0- ☑
  mushroom — *see* Poisoning, food, noxious, mushroom
  mussels (*see also* Poisoning, shellfish)
    bacterial — *see* Intoxication, foodborne, by agent
  nicotine (tobacco) T65.2- ☑
  noxious foodstuffs — *see* Poisoning, food, noxious
  plants, noxious — *see* Poisoning, food, noxious, plants NEC
  ptomaine — *see* Poisoning, food
  radiation J70.0
  Salmonella (arizonae) (cholerae-suis) (enteritidis) (typhimurium) A02.9
  scombroid fish T61.1- ☑
  seafood (noxious) T61.9- ☑
    bacterial — *see* Intoxication, foodborne, by agent
    fish — *see* Poisoning, fish
    shellfish — *see* Poisoning, shellfish
    specified NEC — *see* subcategory T61.8X ☑
  shellfish (amnesic) (azaspiracid) (diarrheic) (neurotoxic) (noxious) (paralytic) T61.78- ☑
    bacterial — *see* Intoxication, foodborne, by agent
    ciguatera mollusk — *see* Poisoning, ciguatera fish
  specified substance NEC T65.891 ☑
  Staphylococcus, food A05.0
  tobacco (nicotine) T65.2- ☑
  water E87.79
Poker spine — *see* Spondylitis, ankylosing
Poland syndrome Q79.8
Polioencephalitis (acute) (bulbar) A80.9
  inferior G12.22
  influenzal — *see* Influenza, with, encephalopathy
  superior hemorrhagic (acute) (Wernicke's) E51.2
  Wernicke's E51.2
Polioencephalomyelitis (acute) (anterior) A80.9
  with beriberi E51.2
Polioencephalopathy, superior hemorrhagic E51.2
  with
    beriberi E51.11
    pellagra E52
Poliomeningoencephalitis — *see* Meningoencephalitis
Poliomyelitis (acute) (anterior) (epidemic) A80.9
  with paralysis (bulbar) — *see* Poliomyelitis, paralytic
  abortive A80.4
  ascending (progressive) — *see* Poliomyelitis, paralytic
  bulbar (paralytic) — *see* Poliomyelitis, paralytic
  congenital P35.8
  nonepidemic A80.9
  nonparalytic A80.4
  paralytic A80.30
    specified NEC A80.39
    vaccine-associated A80.0
    wild virus
      imported A80.1
      indigenous A80.2
  spinal, acute A80.9
Poliosis (eyebrow) (eyelashes) L67.1
  circumscripta, acquired L67.1
Pollakiuria R35.0
  psychogenic F45.8
Pollinosis J30.1
Pollitzer's disease L73.2
Polyadenitis (*see also* Lymphadenitis)
  malignant A20.0
Polyalgia M79.89
Polyangiitis M30.0
  microscopic M31.7
  overlap syndrome M30.8
Polyarteritis
  microscopic M31.7
  nodosa M30.0
    with lung involvement M30.1
    juvenile M30.2
    related condition NEC M30.8
Polyarthralgia — *see* Pain, joint
Polyarthritis, polyarthropathy (*see also* Arthritis) M13.0
  due to or associated with other specified conditions — *see* Arthritis
  epidemic (Australian) (with exanthema) B33.1
  infective — *see* Arthritis, pyogenic or pyemic
  inflammatory M06.4
  juvenile (chronic) (seronegative) M08.3
  migratory — *see* Fever, rheumatic
  rheumatic, acute — *see* Fever, rheumatic
Polyarthrosis M15.9

Polyarthrosis — *continued*
 post-traumatic M15.3
 primary M15.0
 specified NEC M15.8
Polycarential syndrome of infancy E40
Polychondritis (atrophic) (chronic) (*see also* Disorder,
 cartilage, specified type NEC)
 relapsing M94.1
Polycoria Q13.2
Polycystic (disease)
 degeneration, kidney Q61.3
  autosomal dominant (adult type) Q61.2
  autosomal recessive (infantile type) NEC Q61.19
 kidney Q61.3
  autosomal
   dominant Q61.2
   recessive NEC Q61.19
  autosomal dominant (adult type) Q61.2
  autosomal recessive (childhood type) NEC Q61.19
  infantile type NEC Q61.19
 liver Q44.6
 lung J98.4
  congenital Q33.0
 ovary, ovaries E28.2
 spleen Q89.09
Polycythemia (secondary) D75.1
 acquired D75.1
 benign (familial) D75.0
 due to
  donor twin P61.1
  erythropoietin D75.1
  fall in plasma volume D75.1
  high altitude D75.1
  maternal-fetal transfusion P61.1
  stress D75.1
 emotional D75.1
 erythropoietin D75.1
 familial (benign) D75.0
 Gaisböck's (hypertonica) D75.1
 high altitude D75.1
 hypertonica D75.1
 hypoxemic D75.1
 neonatorum P61.1
 nephrogenous D75.1
 relative D75.1
 secondary D75.1
 spurious D75.1
 stress D75.1
 vera D45
Polycytosis cryptogenica D75.1
Polydactylism, polydactyly Q69.9
 toes Q69.2
Polydipsia R63.1
Polydystrophy, pseudo-Hurler E77.0
Polyembryoma — *see* Neoplasm, malignant, by site
Polyglandular
 deficiency E31.0
 dyscrasia E31.9
 dysfunction E31.9
 syndrome E31.8
Polyhydramnios O40.- ☑
Polymastia Q83.1
Polymenorrhea N92.0
Polymyalgia M35.3
 arteritica, giant cell M31.5
 rheumatica M35.3
  with giant cell arteritis M31.5
Polymyositis (acute) (chronic) (hemorrhagic) M33.20
 with
  myopathy M33.22
  respiratory involvement M33.21
  skin involvement — *see* Dermatopolymyositis
  specified organ involvement NEC M33.29
 ossificans (generalisata) (progressiva) — *see* Myositis,
  ossificans, progressiva
Polyneuritis, polyneuritic (*see also* Polyneuropathy)
 acute (post-)infective G61.0
 alcoholic G62.1
 cranialis G52.7
 demyelinating, chronic inflammatory (CIDP) G61.81
 diabetic — *see* Diabetes, polyneuropathy
 diphtheritic A36.83
 due to lack of vitamin NEC E56.9 [G63]
 endemic E51.11
 erythredema — *see* subcategory T56.1 ☑
 febrile, acute G61.0
 hereditary ataxic G60.1
 idiopathic, acute G61.0

Polyneuritis, polyneuritic — *continued*
 infective (acute) G61.0
 inflammatory, chronic demyelinating (CIDP) G61.81
 nutritional E63.9 [G63]
 postinfective (acute) G61.0
 specified NEC G62.89
Polyneuropathy (peripheral) G62.9
 alcoholic G62.1
 amyloid (Portuguese) E85.1 [G63]
  transthyretin-related (ATTR) familial E85.1
 arsenical G62.2
 critical illness G62.81
 demyelinating, chronic inflammatory (CIDP) G61.81
 diabetic — *see* Diabetes, polyneuropathy
 drug-induced G62.0
 hereditary G60.9
  specified NEC G60.8
 idiopathic G60.9
  progressive G60.3
 in (due to)
  alcohol G62.1
   sequelae G65.2
  amyloidosis, familial (Portuguese) E85.1 [G63]
  antitetanus serum G61.1
  arsenic G62.2
   sequelae G65.2
  avitaminosis NEC E56.9 [G63]
  beriberi E51.11
  collagen vascular disease NEC M35.9 [G63]
  deficiency (of)
   B (-complex) vitamins E53.9 [G63]
   vitamin B6 E53.1 [G63]
  diabetes — *see* Diabetes, polyneuropathy
  diphtheria A36.83
  drug or medicament G62.0
   correct substance properly administered — *see*
    Table of Drugs and Chemicals, by drug,
    adverse effect
   overdose or wrong substance given or taken —
    see Table of Drugs and Chemicals, by drug,
    poisoning
  endocrine disease NEC E34.9 [G63]
  herpes zoster B02.23
  hypoglycemia E16.2 [G63]
  infectious
   disease NEC B99 ☑ [G63]
   mononucleosis B27.91
  lack of vitamin NEC E56.9 [G63]
  lead G62.2
   sequelae G65.2
  leprosy A30.9 [G63]
  Lyme disease A69.22
  metabolic disease NEC E88.9 [G63]
  microscopic polyangiitis M31.7 [G63]
  mumps B26.84
  neoplastic disease (*see also* Neoplasm) D49.9 [G63]
  nutritional deficiency NEC E63.9 [G63]
  organophosphate compounds G62.2
   sequelae G65.2
  parasitic disease NEC B89 [G63]
  pellagra E52 [G63]
  polyarteritis nodosa M30.0
  porphyria E80.20 [G63]
  radiation G62.82
  rheumatoid arthritis — *see* Rheumatoid, polyneuropathy
  sarcoidosis D86.89
  serum G61.1
  syphilis (late) A52.15
   congenital A50.43
  systemic
   connective tissue disorder M35.9 [G63]
   lupus erythematosus M32.19
  toxic agent NEC G62.2
   sequelae G65.2
 inflammatory G61.9
  chronic demyelinating (CIDP) G61.81
  sequelae G65.1
  specified NEC G61.89
 lead G62.2
  sequelae G65.2
 nutritional NEC E63.9 [G63]
 postherpetic (zoster) B02.23
 progressive G60.3
 radiation-induced G62.82
 sensory (hereditary) (idiopathic) G60.8
 specified NEC G62.89
 syphilitic (late) A52.15

Polyneuropathy — *continued*
 syphilitic — *continued*
  congenital A50.43
 transthyretin-related (ATTR) familial amyloid E85.1
  triorthocresyl phosphate G62.2
   sequelae G65.2
  tuberculosis A17.89
  uremia N18.9 [G63]
  vitamin B12 deficiency E53.8 [G63]
   with anemia (pernicious) D51.0 [G63]
    due to dietary deficiency D51.3 [G63]
  zoster B02.23
Polyopia H53.8
Polyorchism, polyorchidism Q55.21
Polyosteoarthritis (*see also* Osteoarthritis, generalized)
 M15.9
 post-traumatic M15.3
 specified NEC M15.8
Polyostotic fibrous dysplasia Q78.1
Polyotia Q17.0
Polyp, polypus
 accessory sinus J33.8
 adenocarcinoma in — *see* Neoplasm, malignant, by
  site
 adenocarcinoma in situ in — *see* Neoplasm, in situ, by
  site
 adenoid tissue J33.0
 adenomatous (*see also* Neoplasm, benign, by site)
  adenocarcinoma in — *see* Neoplasm, malignant, by
   site
  adenocarcinoma in situ in — *see* Neoplasm, in situ,
   by site
  carcinoma in — *see* Neoplasm, malignant, by site
  carcinoma in situ in — *see* Neoplasm, in situ, by site
  multiple — *see* Neoplasm, benign
   adenocarcinoma in — *see* Neoplasm, malignant,
    by site
   adenocarcinoma in situ in — *see* Neoplasm, in
    situ, by site
 antrum J33.8
 anus, anal (canal) K62.0
 Bartholin's gland N84.3
 bladder D41.4
 carcinoma in — *see* Neoplasm, malignant, by site
 carcinoma in situ in — *see* Neoplasm, in situ, by site
 cecum D12.0
 cervix (uteri) N84.1
  in pregnancy or childbirth — *see* Pregnancy, complicated by, abnormal, cervix
  mucous N84.1
  nonneoplastic N84.1
 choanal J33.0
 cholesterol K82.4
 clitoris N84.3
 colon K63.5
  adenomatous D12.6
  ascending D12.2
  cecum D12.0
  descending D12.4
  inflammatory K51.40
   with
    abscess K51.414
    complication K51.419
     specified NEC K51.418
    fistula K51.413
    intestinal obstruction K51.412
    rectal bleeding K51.411
  sigmoid D12.5
  transverse D12.3
 corpus uteri N84.0
 dental K04.01
  irreversible K04.02
  reversible K04.01
 duodenum K31.7
 ear (middle) H74.4- ☑
 endometrium N84.0
 ethmoidal (sinus) J33.8
 fallopian tube N84.8
 female genital tract N84.9
  specified NEC N84.8
 frontal (sinus) J33.8
 gallbladder K82.4
 gingiva, gum K06.8
 labia, labium (majus) (minus) N84.3
 larynx (mucous) J38.1
  adenomatous D14.1
 malignant — *see* Neoplasm, malignant, by site
 maxillary (sinus) J33.8

Polyp, polypus — *continued*
  middle ear — *see* Polyp, ear (middle)
  myometrium N84.0
  nares
    anterior J33.9
    posterior J33.0
  nasal (mucous) J33.9
    cavity J33.0
    septum J33.0
  nasopharyngeal J33.0
  nose (mucous) J33.9
  oviduct N84.8
  pharynx J39.2
  placenta O90.89
  prostate — *see* Enlargement, enlarged, prostate
  pudenda, pudendum N84.3
  pulpal (dental) K04.01
    irreversible K04.02
    reversible K04.01
  rectum (nonadenomatous) K62.1
    adenomatous — *see* Polyp, adenomatous
  septum (nasal) J33.0
  sinus (accessory) (ethmoidal) (frontal) (maxillary)
    (sphenoidal) J33.8
  sphenoidal (sinus) J33.8
  stomach K31.7
    adenomatous D13.1
  tube, fallopian N84.8
  turbinate, mucous membrane J33.8
  umbilical, newborn P83.6
  ureter N28.89
  urethra N36.2
  uterus (body) (corpus) (mucous) N84.0
    cervix N84.1
    in pregnancy or childbirth — *see* Pregnancy, complicated by, tumor, uterus
  vagina N84.2
  vocal cord (mucous) J38.1
  vulva N84.3
Polyphagia R63.2
Polyploidy Q92.7
Polypoid — *see* condition
Polyposis (*see also* Polyp)
  coli (adenomatous) D12.6
    adenocarcinoma in C18.9
    adenocarcinoma in situ in — *see* Neoplasm, in situ, by site
    carcinoma in C18.9
  colon (adenomatous) D12.6
  familial D12.6
    adenocarcinoma in situ in — *see* Neoplasm, in situ, by site
  intestinal (adenomatous) D12.6
  malignant lymphomatous C83.1- ☑
  multiple, adenomatous (*see also* Neoplasm, benign) D36.9
Polyradiculitis — *see* Polyneuropathy
Polyradiculoneuropathy (acute) (postinfective) (segmentally demyelinating) G61.0
Polyserositis
  due to pericarditis I31.1
  pericardial I31.1
  periodic, familial E85.0
  tuberculous A19.9
    acute A19.1
    chronic A19.8
Polysplenia syndrome Q89.09
Polysyndactyly (*see also* Syndactylism, syndactyly) Q70.4
Polytrichia L68.3
Polyunguia Q84.6
Polyuria R35.8
  nocturnal R35.1
  psychogenic F45.8
Pompe's disease (glycogen storage) E74.02
Pompholyx L30.1
Poncet's disease (tuberculous rheumatism) A18.09
Pond fracture — *see* Fracture, skull
Ponos B55.0
Pons, pontine — *see* condition
Poor
  aesthetic of existing restoration of tooth K08.56
  contractions, labor O62.2
  gingival margin to tooth restoration K08.51
  personal hygiene R46.0
  prenatal care, affecting management of pregnancy — *see* Pregnancy, complicated by, insufficient, prenatal care
  sucking reflex (newborn) R29.2

Poor — *continued*
  urinary stream R39.12
  vision NEC H54.7
Poradenitis, nostras inguinalis or venerea A55
Porencephaly (congenital) (developmental) (true) Q04.6
  acquired G93.0
  nondevelopmental G93.0
  traumatic (post) F07.89
Porocephaliasis B88.8
Porokeratosis Q82.8
Poroma, eccrine — *see* Neoplasm, skin, benign
Porphyria (South African) E80.20
  acquired E80.20
  acute intermittent (hepatic) (Swedish) E80.21
  cutanea tarda (hereditary) (symptomatic) E80.1
  due to drugs E80.20
    correct substance properly administered — *see* Table of Drugs and Chemicals, by drug, adverse effect
    overdose or wrong substance given or taken — *see* Table of Drugs and Chemicals, by drug, poisoning
  erythropoietic (congenital) (hereditary) E80.0
  hepatocutaneous type E80.1
  secondary E80.20
  toxic NEC E80.20
  variegata E80.20
Porphyrinuria — *see* Porphyria
Porphyruria — *see* Porphyria
Port wine nevus, mark, or stain Q82.5
Portal — *see* condition
Posadas-Wernicke disease B38.9
Positive
  culture (nonspecific)
    blood R78.81
    bronchial washings R84.5
    cerebrospinal fluid R83.5
    cervix uteri R87.5
    nasal secretions R84.5
    nipple discharge R89.5
    nose R84.5
      staphylococcus (Methicillin susceptible) Z22.321
        Methicillin resistant Z22.322
    peritoneal fluid R85.5
    pleural fluid R84.5
    prostatic secretions R86.5
    saliva R85.5
    seminal fluid R86.5
    sputum R84.5
    synovial fluid R89.5
    throat scrapings R84.5
    urine R82.79
    vagina R87.5
    vulva R87.5
    wound secretions R89.5
  PPD (skin test) R76.11
  serology for syphilis A53.0
    false R76.8
    with signs or symptoms — *code as* Syphilis, by site and stage
  skin test, tuberculin (without active tuberculosis) R76.11
  test, human immunodeficiency virus (HIV) R75
  VDRL A53.0
    with signs or symptoms — *code by* site and stage under Syphilis A53.9
  Wassermann reaction A53.0
Postcardiotomy syndrome I97.0
Postcaval ureter Q62.62
Postcholecystectomy syndrome K91.5
Postclimacteric bleeding N95.0
Postcommissurotomy syndrome I97.0
Postconcussional syndrome F07.81
Postcontusional syndrome F07.81
Postcricoid region — *see* condition
Post-dates (40-42 weeks) (pregnancy) (mother) O48.0
  more than 42 weeks gestation O48.1
Postencephalitic syndrome F07.89
Posterior — *see* condition
Posterolateral sclerosis (spinal cord) — *see* Degeneration, combined
Postexanthematous — *see* condition
Postfebrile — *see* condition
Postgastrectomy dumping syndrome K91.1
Posthemiplegic chorea — *see* Monoplegia
Posthemorrhagic anemia (chronic) D50.0
  acute D62
  newborn P61.3
Postherpetic neuralgia (zoster) B02.29

Postherpetic neuralgia — *continued*
  trigeminal B02.22
Posthitis N47.7
Postimmunization complication or reaction — *see* Complications, vaccination
Postinfectious — *see* condition
Postlaminectomy syndrome NEC M96.1
Postleukotomy syndrome F07.0
Postmastectomy lymphedema (syndrome) I97.2
Postmaturity, postmature (over 42 weeks)
  maternal (over 42 weeks gestation) O48.1
  newborn P08.22
Postmeasles complication NEC (*see also* condition) B05.89
Postmenopausal
  endometrium (atrophic) N95.8
    suppurative (*see also* Endometritis) N71.9
  osteoporosis — *see* Osteoporosis, postmenopausal
Postnasal drip R09.82
  due to
    allergic rhinitis — *see* Rhinitis, allergic
    common cold J00
    gastroesophageal reflux — *see* Reflux, gastroesophageal
    nasopharyngitis — *see* Nasopharyngitis
    other known condition — *code to* condition
    sinusitis — *see* Sinusitis
Postnatal — *see* condition
Postoperative (postprocedural) — *see* Complication, postoperative
  pneumothorax, therapeutic Z98.3
  state NEC Z98.890
Postpancreatectomy hyperglycemia E89.1
Postpartum — *see* Puerperal
Postphlebitic syndrome — *see* Syndrome, postthrombotic
Postpolio (myelitic) **syndrome** G14
Postpoliomyelitic (*see also* condition)
  osteopathy — *see* Osteopathy, after poliomyelitis
Postprocedural (*see also* Postoperative)
  hypoinsulinemia E89.1
Postschizophrenic depression F32.89
Postsurgery status (*see also* Status (post))
  pneumothorax, therapeutic Z98.3
Post-term (40-42 weeks) (pregnancy) (mother) O48.0
  infant P08.21
  more than 42 weeks gestation (mother) O48.1
Post-traumatic brain syndrome, nonpsychotic F07.81
Post-typhoid abscess A01.09
Postures, hysterical F44.2
Postvaccinal reaction or complication — *see* Complications, vaccination
Postvalvulotomy syndrome I97.0
Potain's
  disease (pulmonary edema) — *see* Edema, lung
  syndrome (gastrectasis with dyspepsia) K31.0
Potter's
  asthma J62.8
  facies Q60.6
  lung J62.8
  syndrome (with renal agenesis) Q60.6
Pott's
  curvature (spinal) A18.01
  disease or paraplegia A18.01
  spinal curvature A18.01
  tumor, puffy — *see* Osteomyelitis, specified type NEC
Pouch
  bronchus Q32.4
  Douglas' — *see* condition
  esophagus, esophageal, congenital Q39.6
    acquired K22.5
  gastric K31.4
  Hartmann's K82.8
  pharynx, pharyngeal (congenital) Q38.7
Pouchitis K91.850
Poultrymen's itch B88.0
Poverty NEC Z59.6
  extreme Z59.5
Poxvirus NEC B08.8
Prader-Willi syndrome Q87.1
Preauricular appendage or tag Q17.0
Prebetalipoproteinemia (acquired) (essential) (familial) (hereditary) (primary) (secondary) E78.1
  with chylomicronemia E78.3
Precipitate labor or delivery O62.3
Preclimacteric bleeding (menorrhagia) N92.4

☑ **Additional Character Required** — **Refer to the Tabular List for Character Selection**

▽ **Subterms under main terms may continue to next column or page**

Precocious
adrenarche E30.1
menarche E30.1
menstruation E30.1
pubarche E30.1
puberty E30.1
central E22.8
sexual development NEC E30.1
thelarche E30.8
Precocity, sexual (constitutional) (cryptogenic) (female) (idiopathic) (male) E30.1
with adrenal hyperplasia E25.9
congenital E25.0
Precordial pain R07.2
Predeciduous teeth K00.2
Prediabetes, prediabetic R73.03
complicating
pregnancy — *see* Pregnancy, complicated by, diseases of, specified type or system NEC
puerperium O99.89
Predislocation status of hip at birth Q65.6
Pre-eclampsia O14.9- ☑
with pre-existing hypertension — *see* Hypertension, complicating pregnancy, pre-existing, with, pre-eclampsia
complicating
childbirth O14.94
puerperium O14.95
mild O14.0- ☑
complicating
childbirth O14.04
puerperium O14.05
moderate O14.0- ☑
complicating
childbirth O14.04
puerperium O14.05
severe O14.1- ☑
with hemolysis, elevated liver enzymes and low platelet count (HELLP) O14.2- ☑
complicating
childbirth O14.24
puerperium O14.25
complicating
childbirth O14.14
puerperium O14.15
Pre-eruptive color change, teeth, tooth K00.8
Pre-excitation atrioventricular conduction I45.6
Preglaucoma H40.00- ☑
Pregnancy (single) (uterine) (*see also* Delivery and Puerperal)

Note: The Tabular must be reviewed for assignment of appropriate seventh character for multiple gestation codes in Chapter 15

Note: The Tabular must be reviewed for assignment of the appropriate character indicating the trimester of the pregnancy

abdominal (ectopic) O00.00
with intrauterine pregnancy O00.01
with viable fetus O36.7- ☑
ampullar O00.10- ☑
with intrauterine pregnancy O00.11- ☑
biochemical O02.81
broad ligament O00.80
with intrauterine pregnancy O00.81
cervical O00.8
with intrauterine pregnancy O00.81
chemical O02.81
complicated by (care of) (management affected by)
abnormal, abnormality
cervix O34.4- ☑
causing obstructed labor O65.5
cord (umbilical) O69.9 ☑
fetal heart rate or rhythm O36.83- ☑
findings on antenatal screening of mother O28.9
biochemical O28.1
chromosomal O28.5
cytological O28.2
genetic O28.5
hematological O28.0
radiological O28.4
specified NEC O28.8
ultrasonic O28.3
glucose (tolerance) NEC O99.810
pelvic organs O34.9- ☑
specified NEC O34.8- ☑
causing obstructed labor O65.5

Pregnancy — *continued*
complicated by — *continued*
abnormal, abnormality — *continued*
pelvis (bony) (major) NEC O33.0
perineum O34.7- ☑
position
placenta O44.0- ☑
with hemorrhage O44.1- ☑
uterus O34.59- ☑
uterus O34.59- ☑
causing obstructed labor O65.5
congenital O34.0- ☑
vagina O34.6- ☑
causing obstructed labor O65.5
vulva O34.7- ☑
causing obstructed labor O65.5
abruptio placentae — *see* Abruptio placentae
abscess or cellulitis
bladder O23.1- ☑
breast O91.11- ☑
genital organ or tract O23.9- ☑
abuse
physical O9A.31 ☑ (*following* O99)
psychological O9A.51 ☑ (*following* O99)
sexual O9A.41 ☑ (*following* O99)
adverse effect anesthesia O29.9- ☑
aspiration pneumonitis O29.01- ☑
cardiac arrest O29.11- ☑
cardiac complication NEC O29.19- ☑
cardiac failure O29.12- ☑
central nervous system complication NEC O29.29- ☑
cerebral anoxia O29.21- ☑
failed or difficult intubation O29.6- ☑
inhalation of stomach contents or secretions NOS O29.01- ☑
local, toxic reaction O29.3X
Mendelson's syndrome O29.01- ☑
pressure collapse of lung O29.02- ☑
pulmonary complications NEC O29.09- ☑
specified NEC O29.8X- ☑
spinal and epidural type NEC O29.5X ☑
induced headache O29.4- ☑
albuminuria (*see also* Proteinuria, gestational) O12.1- ☑
alcohol use O99.31- ☑
amnionitis O41.12- ☑
anaphylactoid syndrome of pregnancy O88.01- ☑
anemia (conditions in D50-D64) (pre-existing) O99.01- ☑
complicating the puerperium O99.03
antepartum hemorrhage O46.9- ☑
with coagulation defect — *see* Hemorrhage, antepartum, with coagulation defect
specified NEC O46.8X- ☑
appendicitis O99.61- ☑
atrophy (yellow) (acute) liver (subacute) O26.61- ☑
bariatric surgery status O99.84- ☑
bicornis or bicornuate uterus O34.0- ☑
biliary tract problems O26.61- ☑
breech presentation O32.1 ☑
cardiovascular diseases (conditions in I00-I09, I20-I52, I70-I99) O99.41- ☑
cerebrovascular disorders (conditions in I60-I69) O99.41- ☑
cervical shortening O26.87- ☑
cervicitis O23.51- ☑
chloasma (gravidarum) O26.89- ☑
cholecystitis O99.61- ☑
cholestasis (intrahepatic) O26.61- ☑
chorioamnionitis O41.12- ☑
circulatory system disorder (conditions in I00-I09, I20-I99, O99.41-)
compound presentation O32.6 ☑
conjoined twins O30.02- ☑
connective system disorders (conditions in M00-M99) O99.89
contracted pelvis (general) O33.1
inlet O33.2
outlet O33.3 ☑
convulsions (eclamptic) (uremic) (*see also* Eclampsia) O15.9
cracked nipple O92.11- ☑
cystitis O23.1- ☑
cystocele O34.8- ☑
death of fetus (near term) O36.4 ☑

Pregnancy — *continued*
complicated by — *continued*
death of fetus — *continued*
early pregnancy O02.1
of one fetus or more in multiple gestation O31.2- ☑
deciduitis O41.14- ☑
decreased fetal movement O36.81- ☑
dental problems O99.61- ☑
diabetes (mellitus) O24.91- ☑
gestational (pregnancy induced) — *see* Diabetes, gestational
pre-existing O24.31- ☑
specified NEC O24.81- ☑
type 1 O24.01- ☑
type 2 O24.11- ☑
digestive system disorders (conditions in K00-K93) O99.61- ☑
diseases of — *see* Pregnancy, complicated by, specified body system disease
biliary tract O26.61- ☑
blood NEC (conditions in D65-D77) O99.11- ☑
liver O26.61- ☑
specified NEC O99.89
disorders of — *see* Pregnancy, complicated by, specified body system disorder
amniotic fluid and membranes O41.9- ☑
specified NEC O41.8X- ☑
biliary tract O26.61- ☑
ear and mastoid process (conditions in H60-H95) O99.89
eye and adnexa (conditions in H00-H59) O99.89
liver O26.61- ☑
skin (conditions in L00-L99) O99.71- ☑
specified NEC O99.89
displacement, uterus NEC O34.59- ☑
causing obstructed labor O65.5
disproportion (due to) O33.9
fetal (ascites) (hydrops) (meningomyelocele) (sacral teratoma) (tumor) deformities NEC O33.7 ☑
generally contracted pelvis O33.1
hydrocephalic fetus O33.6 ☑
inlet contraction of pelvis O33.2
mixed maternal and fetal origin O33.4 ☑
specified NEC O33.8
double uterus O34.0- ☑
causing obstructed labor O65.5
drug use (conditions in F11-F19) O99.32- ☑
eclampsia, eclamptic (coma) (convulsions) (delirium) (nephritis) (uremia) (*see also* Eclampsia) O15.- ☑
ectopic pregnancy — *see* Pregnancy, ectopic
edema O12.0- ☑
with
gestational hypertension, mild (*see also* Pre-eclampsia) O14.0- ☑
proteinuria O12.2- ☑
effusion, amniotic fluid — *see* Pregnancy, complicated by, premature rupture of membranes
elderly
multigravida O09.52- ☑
primigravida O09.51- ☑
embolism (*see also* Embolism, obstetric, pregnancy) O88.- ☑
endocrine diseases NEC O99.28- ☑
endometritis O86.12
excessive weight gain O26.0- ☑
exhaustion O26.81- ☑
during labor and delivery O75.81
face presentation O32.3 ☑
failed induction of labor O61.9
instrumental O61.1
mechanical O61.1
medical O61.0
specified NEC O61.8
surgical O61.1
failed or difficult intubation for anesthesia O29.6- ☑
false labor (pains) O47.9
at or after 37 completed weeks of pregnancy O47.1
before 37 completed weeks of pregnancy O47.0- ☑
fatigue O26.81- ☑
during labor and delivery O75.81
fatty metamorphosis of liver O26.61- ☑
female genital mutilation O34.8- ☑ [N90.81-] ☑

Pregnancy — *continued*
  complicated by — *continued*
    fetal (maternal care for)
      abnormality or damage O35.9 ☑
        acid-base balance O68
        specified type NEC O35.8 ☑
      acidemia O68
      acidosis O68
      alkalosis O68
      anemia and thrombocytopenia O36.82- ☑
      anencephaly O35.0 ☑
      chromosomal abnormality (conditions in Q90-Q99) O35.1 ☑
      conjoined twins O30.02- ☑
      damage from
        amniocentesis O35.7 ☑
        biopsy procedures O35.7 ☑
        drug addiction O35.5 ☑
        hematological investigation O35.7 ☑
        intrauterine contraceptive device O35.7 ☑
        maternal
          alcohol addiction O35.4 ☑
          cytomegalovirus infection O35.3 ☑
          disease NEC O35.8 ☑
          drug addiction O35.5 ☑
          listeriosis O35.8 ☑
          rubella O35.3 ☑
          toxoplasmosis O35.8 ☑
          viral infection O35.3 ☑
        medical procedure NEC O35.7 ☑
        radiation O35.6 ☑
      death (near term) O36.4 ☑
        early pregnancy O02.1
      decreased movement O36.81- ☑
      disproportion due to deformity (fetal) O33.7 ☑
      excessive growth (large for dates) O36.6- ☑
      growth retardation O36.59- ☑
        light for dates O36.59- ☑
        small for dates O36.59- ☑
      heart rate irregularity (bradycardia) (decelerations) (tachycardia) O76
      hereditary disease O35.2 ☑
      hydrocephalus O35.0 ☑
      intrauterine death O36.4 ☑
      poor growth O36.59- ☑
        light for dates O36.59- ☑
        small for dates O36.59- ☑
      problem O36.9- ☑
        specified NEC O36.89- ☑
      reduction (elective) O31.3- ☑
      selective termination O31.3- ☑
      spina bifida O35.0 ☑
      thrombocytopenia O36.82- ☑
    fibroid (tumor) (uterus) O34.1- ☑
    fissure of nipple O92.11- ☑
    gallstones O99.61- ☑
    gastric banding status O99.84- ☑
    gastric bypass status O99.84- ☑
    genital herpes (asymptomatic) (history of) (inactive) O98.3- ☑
    genital tract infection O23.9- ☑
    glomerular diseases (conditions in N00-N07) O26.83- ☑
      with hypertension, pre-existing — *see* Hypertension, complicating, pregnancy, pre-existing, with, renal disease
    gonorrhea O98.21- ☑
    grand multiparity O09.4 ☑
    habitual aborter — *see* Pregnancy, complicated by, recurrent pregnancy loss
    HELLP syndrome (hemolysis, elevated liver enzymes and low platelet count) O14.2- ☑
    hemorrhage
      antepartum — *see* Hemorrhage, antepartum
      before 20 completed weeks gestation O20.9
        specified NEC O20.8
      due to premature separation, placenta (*see also* Abruptio placentae) O45.9- ☑
      early O20.9
        specified NEC O20.8
      threatened abortion O20.0
    hemorrhoids O22.4- ☑
    hepatitis (viral) O98.41- ☑
    herniation of uterus O34.59- ☑
    high
      head at term O32.4 ☑

Pregnancy — *continued*
  complicated by — *continued*
    high — *continued*
      risk — *see* Supervision (of) (for), high-risk
    history of in utero procedure during previous pregnancy O09.82- ☑
    HIV O98.71- ☑
    human immunodeficiency virus (HIV) disease O98.71- ☑
    hydatidiform mole (*see also* Mole, hydatidiform) O01.9
    hydramnios O40.- ☑
    hydrocephalic fetus (disproportion) O33.6 ☑
    hydrops
      amnii O40.- ☑
      fetalis O36.2- ☑
        associated with isoimmunization (*see also* Pregnancy, complicated by, isoimmunization) O36.11- ☑
    hydrorrhea O42.90
    hyperemesis (gravidarum) (mild) (*see also* Hyperemesis, gravidarum) O21.0
    hypertension — *see* Hypertension, complicating pregnancy
    hypertensive
      heart and renal disease, pre-existing — *see* Hypertension, complicating, pregnancy, pre-existing, with, heart disease, with renal disease
      heart disease, pre-existing — *see* Hypertension, complicating, pregnancy, pre-existing, with, heart disease
      renal disease, pre-existing — *see* Hypertension, complicating, pregnancy, pre-existing, with, renal disease
    hypotension O26.5- ☑
    immune disorders NEC (conditions in D80-D89) O99.11- ☑
    incarceration, uterus O34.51- ☑
    incompetent cervix O34.3- ☑
    inconclusive fetal viability O36.80 ☑
    infection(s) O98.91- ☑
      amniotic fluid or sac O41.10- ☑
      bladder O23.1- ☑
      carrier state NEC O99.830
        streptococcus B O99.820
      genital organ or tract O23.9- ☑
        specified NEC O23.59- ☑
      genitourinary tract O23.9- ☑
      gonorrhea O98.21- ☑
      hepatitis (viral) O98.41- ☑
      HIV O98.71- ☑
      human immunodeficiency virus (HIV) O98.71- ☑
      kidney O23.0- ☑
      nipple O91.01- ☑
      parasitic disease O98.91- ☑
        specified NEC O98.81- ☑
      protozoal disease O98.61- ☑
      sexually transmitted NEC O98.31- ☑
      specified type NEC O98.81- ☑
      syphilis O98.11- ☑
      tuberculosis O98.01- ☑
      urethra O23.2- ☑
      urinary (tract) O23.4- ☑
        specified NEC O23.3- ☑
      viral disease O98.51- ☑
    injury or poisoning (conditions in S00-T88) O9A.21- ☑ (*following* O99)
      due to abuse
        physical O9A.31- ☑ (*following* O99)
        psychological O9A.51- ☑ (*following* O99)
        sexual O9A.41- ☑ (*following* O99)
    insufficient
      prenatal care O09.3- ☑
      weight gain O26.1- ☑
    insulin resistance O26.89 ☑
    intrauterine fetal death (near term) O36.4 ☑
      early pregnancy O02.1
      multiple gestation (one fetus or more) O31.2- ☑
    isoimmunization O36.11- ☑
      anti-A sensitization O36.11- ☑
      anti-B sensitization O36.19- ☑
      Rh O36.09- ☑
        anti-D antibody O36.01- ☑
      specified NEC O36.19- ☑
    laceration of uterus NEC O71.81

Pregnancy — *continued*
  complicated by — *continued*
    malformation
      placenta, placental (vessel) O43.10- ☑
        specified NEC O43.19- ☑
      uterus (congenital) O34.0- ☑
    malnutrition (conditions in E40-E46) O25.1- ☑
    maternal hypotension syndrome O26.5- ☑
    mental disorders (conditions in F01-F09, F20-F99) O99.34- ☑
      alcohol use O99.31- ☑
      drug use O99.32- ☑
      smoking O99.33- ☑
    mentum presentation O32.3 ☑
    metabolic disorders O99.28- ☑
    missed
      abortion O02.1
      delivery O36.4 ☑
    multiple gestations O30.9- ☑
      conjoined twins O30.02- ☑
      quadruplet — *see* Pregnancy, quadruplet
      specified complication NEC O31.8X- ☑
      specified number of multiples NEC — *see* Pregnancy, multiple (gestation), specified NEC
      triplet — *see* Pregnancy, triplet
      twin — *see* Pregnancy, twin
    musculoskeletal condition (conditions is M00-M99) O99.89
    necrosis, liver (conditions in K72) O26.61- ☑
    neoplasm
      benign
        cervix O34.4- ☑
        corpus uteri O34.1- ☑
        uterus O34.1- ☑
      malignant O9A.11- ☑ (*following* O99)
    nephropathy NEC O26.83- ☑
    nervous system condition (conditions in G00-G99) O99.35- ☑
    nutritional diseases NEC O99.28- ☑
    obesity (pre-existing) O99.21- ☑
    obesity surgery status O99.84- ☑
    oblique lie or presentation O32.2 ☑
    older mother — *see* Pregnancy, complicated by, elderly
    oligohydramnios O41.0- ☑
      with premature rupture of membranes (*see also* Pregnancy, complicated by, premature rupture of membranes) O42.- ☑
    onset (spontaneous) of labor after 37 completed weeks of gestation but before 39 completed weeks gestation, with delivery by (planned) cesarean section O75.82
    oophoritis O23.52- ☑
    overdose, drug (*see also* Table of Drugs and Chemicals, by drug, poisoning) O9A.21- ☑ (*following* O99)
    oversize fetus O33.5 ☑
    papyraceous fetus O31.0- ☑
    pelvic inflammatory disease O99.89
    periodontal disease O99.61- ☑
    peripheral neuritis O26.82- ☑
    peritoneal (pelvic) adhesions O99.89
    phlebitis O22.9- ☑
    phlebopathy O22.9- ☑
    phlebothrombosis (superficial) O22.2- ☑
      deep O22.3- ☑
    placenta accreta O43.21- ☑
    placenta increta O43.22- ☑
    placenta percreta O43.23- ☑
    placenta previa O44.0- ☑
      complete O44.0- ☑
        with hemorrhage O44.1- ☑
      marginal O44.2- ☑
        with hemorrhage O44.3- ☑
      partial O44.2- ☑
        with hemorrhage O44.3- ☑
    placental disorder O43.9- ☑
      specified NEC O43.89- ☑
    placental dysfunction O43.89- ☑
    placental infarction O43.81- ☑
    placental insufficiency O36.51- ☑
    placental transfusion syndromes
      fetomaternal O43.01- ☑
      fetus to fetus O43.02- ☑
      maternofetal O43.01- ☑
    placentitis O41.14- ☑

☑ Additional Character Required — Refer to the Tabular List for Character Selection   ▽ Subterms under main terms may continue to next column or page

Pregnancy — *continued*
  complicated by — *continued*
    pneumonia O99.51-
    poisoning (*see also* Table of Drugs and Chemicals)
      O9A.21 ☑ (*following* O99)
    polyhydramnios O40- ☑
    polymorphic eruption of pregnancy O26.86
    poor obstetric history NEC O09.29-
    postmaturity (post-term) (40 to 42 weeks) O48.0
      more than 42 completed weeks gestation (prolonged) O48.1
    pre-eclampsia O14.9- ☑
      mild O14.0- ☑
      moderate O14.0- ☑
      severe O14.1- ☑
        with hemolysis, elevated liver enzymes and low platelet count (HELLP) O14.2- ☑
    premature labor — *see* Pregnancy, complicated by, preterm labor
    premature rupture of membranes O42.90
      with onset of labor
        within 24 hours O42.00
          at or after 37 weeks gestation, onset of labor within 24 hours of rupture O42.02
          pre-term (before 37 completed weeks of gestation) O42.01- ☑
        after 24 hours O42.10
          at or after 37 weeks gestation, onset of labor more than 24 hours following rupture O42.12
          pre-term (before 37 completed weeks of gestation) O42.11- ☑
      at or after 37 weeks gestation, unspecified as to length of time between rupture and onset of labor O42.92
      full-term, unspecified as to length of time between rupture and onset of labor O42.92
      pre-term (before 37 completed weeks of gestation) O42.91- ☑
    premature separation of placenta (*see also* Abruptio placentae) O45.9- ☑
    presentation, fetal — *see* Delivery, complicated by, malposition
    preterm delivery O60.10 ☑
    preterm labor
      with delivery O60.10 ☑
        preterm O60.10 ☑
        term O60.20 ☑
      second trimester
        with term delivery O60.22 ☑
        without delivery O60.02 ☑
        with preterm delivery
          second trimester O60.12 ☑
          third trimester O60.13 ☑
      third trimester
        with term delivery O60.23 ☑
        without delivery O60.03 ☑
        with third trimester preterm delivery O60.14 ☑
      without delivery O60.00
        second trimester O60.02
        third trimester O60.03
    previous history of — *see* Pregnancy, supervision of, high-risk
    prolapse, uterus O34.52- ☑
    proteinuria (gestational) (*see also* Proteinuria, gestational) O12.1- ☑
      with edema O12.2- ☑
    pruritic urticarial papules and plaques of pregnancy (PUPPP) O26.86
    pruritus (neurogenic) O26.89-
    psychosis or psychoneurosis (puerperal) F53.1
    ptyalism O26.89- ☑
    PUPPP (pruritic urticarial papules and plaques of pregnancy) O26.86
    pyelitis O23.0- ☑
    recurrent pregnancy loss O26.2- ☑
    renal disease or failure NEC O26.83- ☑
      with secondary hypertension, pre-existing — *see* Hypertension, complicating, pregnancy, pre-existing, secondary
      hypertensive, pre-existing — *see* Hypertension, complicating, pregnancy, pre-existing, with, renal disease
    respiratory condition (conditions in J00-J99) O99.51- ☑

Pregnancy — *continued*
  complicated by — *continued*
    retained, retention
      dead ovum O02.0
      intrauterine contraceptive device O26.3- ☑
    retroversion, uterus O34.53- ☑
    Rh immunization, incompatibility or sensitization NEC O36.09- ☑
      anti-D antibody O36.01- ☑
    rupture
      amnion (premature) (*see also* Pregnancy, complicated by, premature rupture of membranes) O42- ☑
      membranes (premature) (*see also* Pregnancy, complicated by, premature rupture of membranes) O42- ☑
      uterus (during labor) O71.1
        before onset of labor O71.0- ☑
    salivation (excessive) O26.89- ☑
    salpingitis O23.52- ☑
    salpingo-oophoritis O23.52- ☑
    sepsis (conditions in A40, A41) O98.81- ☑
    size date discrepancy (uterine) O26.84- ☑
    skin condition (conditions in L00-L99) O99.71- ☑
    smoking (tobacco) O99.33- ☑
    social problem O09.7- ☑
    specified condition NEC O26.89- ☑
    spotting O26.85- ☑
    streptococcus group B (GBS) carrier state O99.820
    subluxation of symphysis (pubis) O26.71- ☑
    syphilis (conditions in A50-A53) O98.11- ☑
    threatened
      abortion O20.0
      labor O47.9
        at or after 37 completed weeks of gestation O47.1
        before 37 completed weeks of gestation O47.0- ☑
    thrombophlebitis (superficial) O22.2- ☑
    thrombosis O22.9- ☑
      cerebral venous O22.5- ☑
      cerebrovenous sinus O22.5- ☑
      deep O22.3- ☑
    tobacco use disorder (smoking) O99.33- ☑
    torsion of uterus O34.59- ☑
    toxemia O14.9- ☑
    transverse lie or presentation O32.2 ☑
    tuberculosis (conditions in A15-A19) O98.01- ☑
    tumor (benign)
      cervix O34.4- ☑
      malignant O9A.11- ☑ (*following* O99)
      uterus O34.1- ☑
    unstable lie O32.0 ☑
    upper respiratory infection O99.51- ☑
    urethritis O23.2- ☑
    uterine size date discrepancy O26.84- ☑
    vaginitis or vulvitis O23.59- ☑
    varicose veins (lower extremities) O22.0- ☑
      genitals O22.1- ☑
      legs O22.0- ☑
      perineal O22.1- ☑
      vaginal or vulval O22.1- ☑
    venereal disease NEC (conditions in A63.8) O98.31- ☑
    venous disorders O22.9- ☑
      specified NEC O22.8X- ☑
    very young mother — *see* Pregnancy, complicated by, young mother
    viral diseases (conditions in A80-B09, B25-B34) O98.51- ☑
    vomiting O21.9
      due to diseases classified elsewhere O21.8
      hyperemesis gravidarum (mild) (*see also* Hyperemesis, gravidarum) O21.0
      late (occurring after 20 weeks of gestation) O21.2
    young mother
      multigravida O09.62- ☑
      primigravida O09.61- ☑
  complicated NOS O26.9- ☑
  concealed O09.3- ☑
  continuing following
    elective fetal reduction of one or more fetus O31.3- ☑
    intrauterine death of one or more fetus O31.2- ☑
    spontaneous abortion of one or more fetus O31.1- ☑
  cornual O00.80

Pregnancy — *continued*
  cornual — *continued*
    with intrauterine pregnancy O00.81
  ectopic (ruptured) O00.90
    with intrauterine pregnancy O00.91
    abdominal O00.00
      with
        intrauterine pregnancy O00.01
        viable fetus O36.7- ☑
    cervical O00.80
      with intrauterine pregnancy O00.81
    complicated (by) O08.9
      afibrinogenemia O08.1
      cardiac arrest O08.81
      chemical damage of pelvic organ(s) O08.6
      circulatory collapse O08.3
      defibrination syndrome O08.1
      electrolyte imbalance O08.5
      embolism (amniotic fluid) (blood clot) (pulmonary) (septic) O08.2
      endometritis O08.0
      genital tract and pelvic infection O08.0
      hemorrhage (delayed) (excessive) O08.1
      infection
        genital tract or pelvic O08.0
        kidney O08.83
        urinary tract O08.3
      intravascular coagulation O08.1
      laceration of pelvic organ(s) O08.6
      metabolic disorder O08.5
      oliguria O08.4
      oophoritis O08.0
      parametritis O08.0
      pelvic peritonitis O08.0
      perforation of pelvic organ(s) O08.6
      renal failure or shutdown O08.4
      salpingitis or salpingo-oophoritis O08.0
      sepsis O08.82
      shock O08.83
        septic O08.82
      specified condition NEC O08.89
      tubular necrosis (renal) O08.4
      uremia O08.4
      urinary infection O08.83
      venous complication NEC O08.7
        embolism O08.2
    cornual O00.80
      with intrauterine pregnancy O00.81
    intraligamentous O00.80
      with intrauterine pregnancy O00.81
    mural O00.80
      with intrauterine pregnancy O00.81
    ovarian O00.20- ☑
      with intrauterine pregnancy O00.21- ☑
    specified site NEC O00.80
      with intrauterine pregnancy O00.81
    tubal (ruptured) O00.10- ☑
      with intrauterine pregnancy O00.11- ☑
  examination (normal) Z34.9- ☑
    first Z34.0- ☑
    high-risk — *see* Pregnancy, supervision of, high-risk
    specified Z34.8- ☑
  extrauterine — *see* Pregnancy, ectopic
  fallopian O00.10- ☑
    with intrauterine pregnancy O00.11- ☑
  false F45.8
  gestational carrier Z33.3
  heptachorionic, hepta-amniotic (septuplets) O30.83- ☑
  hexachorionic, hexa-amniotic (sextuplets) O30.83- ☑
  hidden O09.3- ☑
  high-risk — *see* Pregnancy, supervision of, high-risk
  incidental finding Z33.1
  interstitial O00.80
    with intrauterine pregnancy O00.81
  intraligamentous O00.80
    with intrauterine pregnancy O00.81
  intramural O00.80
    with intrauterine pregnancy O00.81
  intraperitoneal O00.00
    with intrauterine pregnancy O00.01
  isthmian O00.10- ☑
    with intrauterine pregnancy O00.11- ☑
  mesometric (mural) O00.80
    with intrauterine pregnancy O00.81
  molar NEC O02.0
    complicated (by) O08.9
      afibrinogenemia O08.1
      cardiac arrest O08.81

▽ Subterms under main terms may continue to next column or page   ☑ Additional Character Required — Refer to the Tabular List for Character Selection   **261**

Pregnancy — Pregnancy

Pregnancy — *continued*
  molar — *continued*
    complicated — *continued*
      chemical damage of pelvic organ(s) O08.6
      circulatory collapse O08.3
      defibrination syndrome O08.1
      electrolyte imbalance O08.5
      embolism (amniotic fluid) (blood clot) (pulmonary) (septic) O08.2
      endometritis O08.0
      genital tract and pelvic infection O08.0
      hemorrhage (delayed) (excessive) O08.1
      infection
        genital tract or pelvic O08.0
        kidney O08.83
        urinary tract O08.83
      intravascular coagulation O08.1
      laceration of pelvic organ(s) O08.6
      metabolic disorder O08.5
      oliguria O08.4
      oophoritis O08.0
      parametritis O08.0
      pelvic peritonitis O08.0
      perforation of pelvic organ(s) O08.6
      renal failure or shutdown O08.4
      salpingitis or salpingo-oophoritis O08.0
      sepsis O08.82
      shock O08.3
        septic O08.82
      specified condition NEC O08.89
      tubular necrosis (renal) O08.4
      uremia O08.4
      urinary infection O08.83
      venous complication NEC O08.7
        embolism O08.2
  hydatidiform (*see also* Mole, hydatidiform) O01.9
  multiple (gestation) O30.9- ☑
    greater than quadruplets — *see* Pregnancy, multiple (gestation), specified NEC
    specified NEC O30.80- ☑
      with
        two or more monoamniotic fetuses O30.82- ☑
        two or more monochorionic fetuses O30.81- ☑
      number of chorions and amnions are both equal to the number of fetuses O30.83- ☑
      two or more monoamniotic fetuses O30.82- ☑
      two or more monochorionic fetuses O30.81- ☑
      unable to determine number of placenta and number of amniotic sacs O30.89- ☑
      unspecified number of placenta and unspecified number of amniotic sacs O30.80- ☑
  mural O00.80
    with intrauterine pregnancy O00.81
  normal (supervision of) Z34.9- ☑
    first Z34.0- ☑
    high-risk — *see* Pregnancy, supervision of, high-risk
    specified Z34.8- ☑
  ovarian O00.20- ☑
    with intrauterine pregnancy O00.21- ☑
  pentachorionic, penta-amniotic (quintuplets) O30.83- ☑
  postmature (40 to 42 weeks) O48.0
    more than 42 weeks gestation O48.1
  post-term (40 to 42 weeks) O48.0
  prenatal care only Z34.9- ☑
    first Z34.0- ☑
    high-risk — *see* Pregnancy, supervision of, high-risk
    specified Z34.8- ☑
  prolonged (more than 42 weeks gestation) O48.1
  quadruplet O30.20- ☑
    with
      two or more monoamniotic fetuses O30.22- ☑
      two or more monochorionic fetuses O30.21- ☑
      quadrachorionic/quadra-amniotic O30.23- ☑
      two or more monoamniotic fetuses O30.22- ☑
      two or more monochorionic fetuses O30.21- ☑
      unable to determine number of placenta and number of amniotic sacs O30.29- ☑
      unspecified number of placenta and unspecified number of amniotic sacs O30.20- ☑
  quintuplet — *see* Pregnancy, multiple (gestation), specified NEC
  sextuplet — *see* Pregnancy, multiple (gestation), specified NEC

Pregnancy — *continued*
  supervision of
    concealed pregnancy O09.3- ☑
    elderly mother
      multigravida O09.52- ☑
      primigravida O09.51- ☑
    hidden pregnancy O09.3- ☑
    high-risk O09.9- ☑
      due to (history of)
        ectopic pregnancy O09.1- ☑
        elderly — *see* Pregnancy, supervision, elderly mother
        grand multiparity O09.4 ☑
        in utero procedure during previous pregnancy O09.82- ☑
        in vitro fertilization O09.81- ☑
        infertility O09.0- ☑
        insufficient prenatal care O09.3- ☑
        molar pregnancy O09.A- ☑
        multiple previous pregnancies O09.4- ☑
        older mother — *see* Pregnancy, supervision of, elderly mother
        poor reproductive or obstetric history NEC O09.29- ☑
        pre-term labor O09.21- ☑
        previous
          neonatal death O09.29- ☑
        social problems O09.7- ☑
        specified NEC O09.89- ☑
        very young mother — *see* Pregnancy, supervision, young mother
      resulting from in vitro fertilization O09.81- ☑
    normal Z34.9- ☑
      first Z34.0- ☑
      specified NEC Z34.8- ☑
    young mother
      multigravida O09.62- ☑
      primigravida O09.61- ☑
  triplet O30.10- ☑
    with
      two or more monoamniotic fetuses O30.12- ☑
      two or more monochorionic fetuses O30.11- ☑
      trichorionic/triamniotic O30.13- ☑
      two or more monoamniotic fetuses O30.12- ☑
      two or more monochorionic fetuses O30.11- ☑
      unable to determine number of placenta and number of amniotic sacs O30.19- ☑
      unspecified number of placenta and unspecified number of amniotic sacs O30.10- ☑
  tubal (with abortion) (with rupture) O00.10- ☑
    with intrauterine pregnancy O00.11- ☑
  twin O30.00- ☑
    conjoined O30.02- ☑
    dichorionic/diamniotic (two placenta, two amniotic sacs) O30.04- ☑
    monochorionic/diamniotic (one placenta, two amniotic sacs) O30.03- ☑
    monochorionic/monoamniotic (one placenta, one amniotic sac) O30.01- ☑
    unable to determine number of placenta and number of amniotic sacs O30.09- ☑
    unspecified number of placenta and unspecified number of amniotic sacs O30.00- ☑
  unwanted Z64.0
  weeks of gestation
    8 weeks Z3A.08 (*following* Z36)
    9 weeks Z3A.09 (*following* Z36)
    10 weeks Z3A.10 (*following* Z36)
    11 weeks Z3A.11 (*following* Z36)
    12 weeks Z3A.12 (*following* Z36)
    13 weeks Z3A.13 (*following* Z36)
    14 weeks Z3A.14 (*following* Z36)
    15 weeks Z3A.15 (*following* Z36)
    16 weeks Z3A.16 (*following* Z36)
    17 weeks Z3A.17 (*following* Z36)
    18 weeks Z3A.18 (*following* Z36)
    19 weeks Z3A.19 (*following* Z36)
    20 weeks Z3A.20 (*following* Z36)
    21 weeks Z3A.21 (*following* Z36)
    22 weeks Z3A.22 (*following* Z36)
    23 weeks Z3A.23 (*following* Z36)
    24 weeks Z3A.24 (*following* Z36)
    25 weeks Z3A.25 (*following* Z36)
    26 weeks Z3A.26 (*following* Z36)
    27 weeks Z3A.27 (*following* Z36)
    28 weeks Z3A.28 (*following* Z36)
    29 weeks Z3A.29 (*following* Z36)

Pregnancy — *continued*
  weeks of gestation — *continued*
    30 weeks Z3A.30 (*following* Z36)
    31 weeks Z3A.31 (*following* Z36)
    32 weeks Z3A.32 (*following* Z36)
    33 weeks Z3A.33 (*following* Z36)
    34 weeks Z3A.34 (*following* Z36)
    35 weeks Z3A.35 (*following* Z36)
    36 weeks Z3A.36 (*following* Z36)
    37 weeks Z3A.37 (*following* Z36)
    38 weeks Z3A.38 (*following* Z36)
    39 weeks Z3A.39 (*following* Z36)
    40 weeks Z3A.40 (*following* Z36)
    41 weeks Z3A.41 (*following* Z36)
    42 weeks Z3A.42 (*following* Z36)
    greater than 42 weeks Z3A.49 (*following* Z36)
    less than 8 weeks Z3A.01 (*following* Z36)
    not specified Z3A.00 (*following* Z36)
Preiser's disease — *see* Osteonecrosis, secondary, due to, trauma, metacarpus
Pre-kwashiorkor — *see* Malnutrition, severe
Preleukemia (syndrome) D46.9
Preluxation, hip, congenital Q65.6
Premature (*see also* condition)
  adrenarche E27.0
  aging E34.8
  beats I49.40
    atrial I49.1
    auricular I49.1
    supraventricular I49.1
  birth NEC — *see* Preterm, newborn
  closure, foramen ovale Q21.8
  contraction
    atrial I49.1
    atrioventricular I49.2
    auricular I49.1
    auriculoventricular I49.49
    heart (extrasystole) I49.49
    junctional I49.2
    ventricular I49.3
  delivery (*see also* Pregnancy, complicated by, preterm labor) O60.10 ☑
  ejaculation F52.4
  infant NEC — *see* Preterm, newborn
    light-for-dates — *see* Light for dates
  labor — *see* Pregnancy, complicated by, preterm labor
  lungs P28.0
  menopause E28.319
    asymptomatic E28.319
    symptomatic E28.310
  newborn
    extreme (less than 28 completed weeks) — *see* Immaturity, extreme
    less than 37 completed weeks — *see* Preterm, newborn
  puberty E30.1
  rupture membranes or amnion — *see* Pregnancy, complicated by, premature rupture of membranes
  senility E34.8
  thelarche E30.8
  ventricular systole I49.3
Prematurity NEC (less than 37 completed weeks) — *see* Preterm, newborn
  extreme (less than 28 completed weeks) — *see* Immaturity, extreme
Premenstrual
  dysphoric disorder (PMDD) F32.81
  tension (syndrome) N94.3
Premolarization, cuspids K00.2
Prenatal
  care, normal pregnancy — *see* Pregnancy, normal
  screening of mother (*see also* Encounter, antenatal screening) Z36.9
  teeth K00.6
Preparatory care for subsequent treatment NEC
  for dialysis Z49.01
    peritoneal Z49.02
Prepartum — *see* condition
Preponderance, left or right ventricular I51.7
Prepuce — *see* condition
PRES (posterior reversible encephalopathy syndrome) I67.83
Presbycardia R54
Presbycusis, presbyacusia H91.1- ☑
Presbyesophagus K22.8
Presbyophrenia F03 ☑
Presbyopia H52.4

☑ **Additional Character Required** — Refer to the Tabular List for Character Selection   ▽ Subterms under main terms may continue to next column or page

Prescription of contraceptives (initial) Z30.019
  barrier Z30.018
  diaphragm Z30.018
  emergency (postcoital) Z30.012
  implantable subdermal Z30.017
  injectable Z30.013
  intrauterine contraceptive device Z30.014
  pills Z30.011
  postcoital (emergency) Z30.012
  repeat Z30.40
    barrier Z30.49
    diaphragm Z30.49
    implantable subdermal Z30.46
    injectable Z30.42
    pills Z30.41
    specified type NEC Z30.49
    transdermal patch hormonal Z30.45
    vaginal ring hormonal Z30.44
  specified type NEC Z30.018
    transdermal patch hormonal Z30.016
    vaginal ring hormonal Z30.015
Presence (of)
  ankle-joint implant (functional) (prosthesis) Z96.66- ☑
  aortocoronary (bypass) graft Z95.1
  arterial-venous shunt (dialysis) Z99.2
  artificial
    eye (globe) Z97.0
    heart (fully implantable) (mechanical) Z95.812
      valve Z95.2
    larynx Z96.3
    lens (intraocular) Z96.1
    limb (complete) (partial) Z97.1- ☑
      arm Z97.1- ☑
        bilateral Z97.15
      leg Z97.1- ☑
        bilateral Z97.16
  audiological implant (functional) Z96.29
  bladder implant (functional) Z96.0
  bone
    conduction hearing device Z96.29
    implant (functional) NEC Z96.7
    joint (prosthesis) — *see* Presence, joint implant
  cardiac
    defibrillator (functional) (with synchronous cardiac
      pacemaker) Z95.810
    implant or graft Z95.9
      specified type NEC Z95.818
    pacemaker Z95.0
    resynchronization therapy
      defibrillator Z95.810
      pacemaker Z95.0
  cardioverter-defibrillator (ICD) Z95.810
  cerebrospinal fluid drainage device Z98.2
  cochlear implant (functional) Z96.21
  contact lens (es) Z97.3
  coronary artery graft or prosthesis Z95.5
  CRT-D (cardiac resynchronization therapy defibrillator)
    Z95.810
  CRT-P (cardiac resynchronization therapy pacemaker)
    Z95.0
  CSF shunt Z98.2
  dental prosthesis device Z97.2
  dentures Z97.2
  device (external) NEC Z97.8
    cardiac NEC Z95.818
    heart assist Z95.811
    implanted (functional) Z96.9
      specified NEC Z96.89
    prosthetic Z97.8
  ear implant Z96.20
    cochlear implant Z96.21
    myringotomy tube Z96.22
    specified type NEC Z96.29
  elbow-joint implant (functional) (prosthesis) Z96.62- ☑
  endocrine implant (functional) NEC Z96.49
  eustachian tube stent or device (functional) Z96.29
  external hearing-aid or device Z97.4
  finger-joint implant (functional) (prosthetic) Z96.69- ☑
  functional implant Z96.9
    specified NEC Z96.89
  graft
    cardiac NEC Z95.818
    vascular NEC Z95.828
  hearing-aid or device (external) Z97.4
    implant (bone) (cochlear) (functional) Z96.21
  heart assist device Z95.811
  heart valve implant (functional) Z95.2
    prosthetic Z95.2

Presence — *continued*
  heart valve implant — *continued*
    specified type NEC Z95.4
    xenogenic Z95.3
  hip-joint implant (functional) (prosthesis) Z96.64- ☑
  ICD (cardioverter-defibrillator) Z95.810
  implanted device (artificial) (functional) (prosthetic)
    Z96.9
    automatic cardiac defibrillator (with synchronous
      cardiac pacemaker) Z95.810
    cardiac pacemaker Z95.0
    cochlear Z96.21
    dental Z96.5
    heart Z95.812
    heart valve Z95.2
      prosthetic Z95.2
      specified NEC Z95.4
      xenogenic Z95.3
    insulin pump Z96.41
    intraocular lens Z96.1
    joint Z96.60
      ankle Z96.66- ☑
      elbow Z96.62- ☑
      finger Z96.69- ☑
      hip Z96.64- ☑
      knee Z96.65- ☑
      shoulder Z96.61- ☑
      specified NEC Z96.698
      wrist Z96.63- ☑
    larynx Z96.3
    myringotomy tube Z96.22
    otological Z96.20
      cochlear Z96.21
      eustachian stent Z96.29
      myringotomy Z96.22
      specified NEC Z96.29
      stapes Z96.29
    skin Z96.81
    skull plate Z96.7
    specified NEC Z96.89
    urogenital Z96.0
  insulin pump (functional) Z96.41
  intestinal bypass or anastomosis Z98.0
  intraocular lens (functional) Z96.1
  intrauterine contraceptive device (IUD) Z97.5
  intravascular implant (functional) (prosthetic) NEC
    Z95.9
    coronary artery Z95.5
    defibrillator (with synchronous cardiac pacemaker)
      Z95.810
    peripheral vessel (with angioplasty) Z95.820
  joint implant (prosthetic) (any) Z96.60
    ankle — *see* Presence, ankle joint implant
    elbow — *see* Presence, elbow joint implant
    finger — *see* Presence, finger joint implant
    hip — *see* Presence, hip joint implant
    knee — *see* Presence, knee joint implant
    shoulder — *see* Presence, shoulder joint implant
    specified joint NEC Z96.698
    wrist — *see* Presence, wrist joint implant
  knee-joint implant (functional) (prosthesis) Z96.65- ☑
  laryngeal implant (functional) Z96.3
  mandibular implant (dental) Z96.5
  myringotomy tube(s) Z96.22
  orthopedic-joint implant (prosthetic) (any) — *see*
    Presence, joint implant
  otological implant (functional) Z96.29
  shoulder-joint implant (functional) (prosthesis)
    Z96.61- ☑
  skull-plate implant Z96.7
  spectacles Z97.3
  stapes implant (functional) Z96.29
  systemic lupus erythematosus [SLE] inhibitor D68.62
  tendon implant (functional) (graft) Z96.7
  tooth root(s) implant Z96.5
  ureteral stent Z96.0
  urethral stent Z96.0
  urogenital implant (functional) Z96.0
  vascular implant or device Z95.9
    access port device Z95.828
    specified type NEC Z95.828
  wrist-joint implant (functional) (prosthesis) Z96.63- ☑
Presenile (*see also* condition)
  dementia F03
  premature aging E34.8
Presentation, fetal — *see* Delivery, complicated by,
  malposition
Prespondylolisthesis (congenital) Q76.2

Pressure
  area, skin — *see* Ulcer, pressure, by site
  brachial plexus G54.0
  brain G93.5
    injury at birth NEC P11.1
  cerebral — *see* Pressure, brain
  chest R07.89
  cone, tentorial G93.5
  hyposystolic (*see also* Hypotension)
    incidental reading, without diagnosis of hypoten-
      sion R03.1
  increased
    intracranial (benign) G93.2
      injury at birth P11.0
    intraocular H40.05- ☑
  lumbosacral plexus G54.1
  mediastinum J98.59
  necrosis (chronic) — *see* Ulcer, pressure, by site
  parental, inappropriate (excessive) Z62.6
  sore (chronic) — *see* Ulcer, pressure, by site
  spinal cord G95.20
  ulcer (chronic) — *see* Ulcer, pressure, by site
  venous, increased I87.8
Pre-syncope R55
Preterm
  delivery (*see also* Pregnancy, complicated by, preterm
    labor) O60.10- ☑
  labor — *see* Pregnancy, complicated by, preterm labor
  newborn (infant) P07.30
    gestational age
      28 completed weeks (28 weeks, 0 days through
        28 weeks, 6 days) P07.31
      29 completed weeks (29 weeks, 0 days through
        29 weeks, 6 days) P07.32
      30 completed weeks (30 weeks, 0 days through
        30 weeks, 6 days) P07.33
      31 completed weeks (31 weeks, 0 days through
        31 weeks, 6 days) P07.34
      32 completed weeks (32 weeks, 0 days through
        32 weeks, 6 days) P07.35
      33 completed weeks (33 weeks, 0 days through
        33 weeks, 6 days) P07.36
      34 completed weeks (34 weeks, 0 days through
        34 weeks, 6 days) P07.37
      35 completed weeks (35 weeks, 0 days through
        35 weeks, 6 days) P07.38
      36 completed weeks (36 weeks, 0 days through
        36 weeks, 6 days) P07.39
Previa
  placenta (total) (without hemorrhage) O44.0- ☑
    with hemorrhage O44.1- ☑
    complete O44.0- ☑
      with hemorrhage O44.1- ☑
    low (*see also* Delivery, complicated, by, placenta,
      low) O44.4- ☑
      with hemorrhage O44.5- ☑
    marginal O44.2- ☑
      with hemorrhage O44.3- ☑
    partial O44.2- ☑
      with hemorrhage O44.3- ☑
  vasa O69.4 ☑
Priapism N48.30
  due to
    disease classified elsewhere N48.32
    drug N48.33
    specified cause NEC N48.39
    trauma N48.31
Prickling sensation (skin) R20.2
Prickly heat L74.0
Primary — *see* condition
Primigravida
  elderly, affecting management of pregnancy, labor and
    delivery (supervision only) — *see* Pregnancy,
    complicated by, elderly, primigravida
  older, affecting management of pregnancy, labor and
    delivery (supervision only) — *see* Pregnancy,
    complicated by, elderly, primigravida
  very young, affecting management of pregnancy, labor
    and delivery (supervision only) — *see* Pregnancy,
    complicated by, young mother, primigravida
Primipara
  elderly, affecting management of pregnancy, labor and
    delivery (supervision only) — *see* Pregnancy,
    complicated by, elderly, primigravida
  older, affecting management of pregnancy, labor and
    delivery (supervision only) — *see* Pregnancy,
    complicated by, elderly, primigravida

Primipara — *continued*
very young, affecting management of pregnancy, labor and delivery (supervision only) — *see* Pregnancy, complicated by, young mother, primigravida
Primus varus (bilateral) Q66.2 ✓
PRIND (Prolonged reversible ischemic neurologic deficit) I63.9
Pringle's disease (tuberous sclerosis) Q85.1
Prinzmetal angina I20.1
Prizefighter ear — *see* Cauliflower ear
Problem (with) (related to)
academic Z55.8
acculturation Z60.3
adjustment (to)
change of job Z56.1
life-cycle transition Z60.0
pension Z60.0
retirement Z60.0
adopted child Z62.821
alcoholism in family Z63.72
atypical parenting situation Z62.9
bankruptcy Z59.8
behavioral (adult) F69
drug seeking Z76.5
birth of sibling affecting child Z62.898
care (of)
provider dependency Z74.9
specified NEC Z74.8
sick or handicapped person in family or household Z63.6
child
abuse (affecting the child) — *see* Maltreatment, child
custody or support proceedings Z65.3
in care of non-parental family member Z62.21
in foster care Z62.21
in welfare custody Z62.21
living in orphanage or group home Z62.22
child-rearing Z62.9
specified NEC Z62.898
communication (developmental) F80.9
conflict or discord (with)
boss Z56.4
classmates Z55.4
counselor Z64.4
employer Z56.4
family Z63.9
specified NEC Z63.8
probation officer Z64.4
social worker Z64.4
teachers Z55.4
workmates Z56.4
conviction in legal proceedings Z65.0
with imprisonment Z65.1
counselor Z64.4
creditors Z59.8
digestive K92.9
drug addict in family Z63.72
ear — *see* Disorder, ear
economic Z59.9
affecting care Z59.9
specified NEC Z59.8
education Z55.9
specified NEC Z55.8
employment Z56.9
change of job Z56.1
discord Z56.4
environment Z56.5
sexual harassment Z56.81
specified NEC Z56.89
stressful schedule Z56.3
stress NEC Z56.6
threat of job loss Z56.2
unemployment Z56.0
enuresis, child F98.0
eye H57.9
failed examinations (school) Z55.2
falling Z91.81
family (*see also* Disruption, family) Z63.9
specified NEC Z63.8
feeding (elderly) (infant) R63.3
newborn P92.9
breast P92.5
overfeeding P92.4
slow P92.2
specified NEC P92.8
underfeeding P92.3
nonorganic F50.89

Problem — *continued*
finance Z59.9
specified NEC Z59.8
foreclosure on loan Z59.8
foster child Z62.822
frightening experience(s) in childhood Z62.898
genital NEC
female N94.9
male N50.9
health care Z75.9
specified NEC Z75.8
hearing — *see* Deafness
homelessness Z59.0
housing Z59.9
inadequate Z59.1
isolated Z59.8
specified NEC Z59.8
identity (of childhood) F93.8
illegitimate pregnancy (unwanted) Z64.0
illiteracy Z55.0
impaired mobility Z74.09
imprisonment or incarceration Z65.1
inadequate teaching affecting education Z55.8
inappropriate (excessive) parental pressure Z62.6
influencing health status NEC Z78.9
in-law Z63.1
institutionalization, affecting child Z62.22
intrafamilial communication Z63.8
jealousy, child F93.8
landlord Z59.2
language (developmental) F80.9
learning (developmental) F81.9
legal Z65.3
conviction without imprisonment Z65.0
imprisonment Z65.1
release from prison Z65.2
life-management Z73.9
specified NEC Z73.89
life-style Z72.9
gambling Z72.6
high-risk sexual behavior (heterosexual) Z72.51
bisexual Z72.53
homosexual Z72.52
inappropriate eating habits Z72.4
self-damaging behavior NEC Z72.89
specified NEC Z72.89
tobacco use Z72.0
literacy Z55.9
low level Z55.0
specified NEC Z55.8
living alone Z60.2
lodgers Z59.2
loss of love relationship in childhood Z62.898
marital Z63.0
involving
divorce Z63.5
estrangement Z63.5
gender identity F66
mastication K08.89
medical
care, within family Z63.6
facilities Z75.9
specified NEC Z75.8
mental F48.9
multiparity Z64.1
negative life events in childhood Z62.9
altered pattern of family relationships Z62.898
frightening experience Z62.898
loss of
love relationship Z62.898
self-esteem Z62.898
physical abuse (alleged) — *see* Maltreatment, child
removal from home Z62.29
specified event NEC Z62.898
neighbor Z59.2
neurological NEC R29.818
new step-parent affecting child Z62.898
none (feared complaint unfounded) Z71.1
occupational NEC Z56.89
parent-child — *see* Conflict, parent-child
personal hygiene Z91.89
personality F69
phase-of-life transition, adjustment Z60.0
presence of sick or disabled person in family or household Z63.79
needing care Z63.6
primary support group (family) Z63.9
specified NEC Z63.8
probation officer Z64.4

Problem — *continued*
psychiatric F99
psychosexual (development) F66
psychosocial Z65.9
religious or spiritual Z65.8
specified NEC Z65.8
relationship Z63.9
childhood F93.8
release from prison Z65.2
religious or spiritual Z65.8
removal from home affecting child Z62.29
seeking and accepting known hazardous and harmful behavioral or psychological interventions Z65.8
chemical, nutritional or physical interventions Z65.8
sexual function (nonorganic) F52.9
sight H54.7
sleep disorder, child F51.9
smell — *see* Disturbance, sensation, smell
social
environment Z60.9
specified NEC Z60.8
exclusion and rejection Z60.4
worker Z64.4
speech R47.9
developmental F80.9
specified NEC R47.89
swallowing — *see* Dysphagia
taste — *see* Disturbance, sensation, taste
tic, child F95.0
underachievement in school Z55.3
unemployment Z56.0
threatened Z56.2
unwanted pregnancy Z64.0
upbringing Z62.9
specified NEC Z62.898
urinary N39.9
voice production R47.89
work schedule (stressful) Z56.3
Procedure (surgical)
converted
arthroscopic to open Z53.33
laparoscopic to open Z53.31
specified procedure NEC to open Z53.39
thoracoscopic to open Z53.32
for purpose other than remedying health state Z41.9
specified NEC Z41.8
not done Z53.9
because of
administrative reasons Z53.8
contraindication Z53.09
smoking Z53.01
patient's decision Z53.20
for reasons of belief or group pressure Z53.1
left against medical advice (AMA) Z53.21
specified reason NEC Z53.29
specified reason NEC Z53.8
Procidentia (uteri) N81.3
Proctalgia K62.89
fugax K59.4
spasmodic K59.4
Proctitis K62.89
amebic (acute) A06.0
chlamydial A56.3
gonococcal A54.6
granulomatous — *see* Enteritis, regional, large intestine
herpetic A60.1
radiation K62.7
tuberculous A18.32
ulcerative (chronic) K51.20
with
complication K51.219
abscess K51.214
fistula K51.213
obstruction K51.212
rectal bleeding K51.211
specified NEC K51.218
Proctocele
female (without uterine prolapse) N81.6
with uterine prolapse N81.2
complete N81.3
male K62.3
Proctocolitis
food protein-induced K52.82
food-induced eosinophilic K52.82
milk protein-induced K52.82
mucosal — *see* Rectosigmoiditis, ulcerative
Proctoptosis K62.3
Proctorrhagia K62.5

Proctosigmoiditis K63.89
   ulcerative (chronic) — *see* Rectosigmoiditis, ulcerative
Proctospasm K59.4
   psychogenic F45.8
Profichet's disease — *see* Disorder, soft tissue, specified
      type NEC
Progeria E34.8
Prognathism (mandibular) (maxillary) M26.19
Progonoma (melanotic) — *see* Neoplasm, benign, by
   site
Progressive — *see* condition
Prolactinoma
   specified site — *see* Neoplasm, benign, by site
   unspecified site D35.2
Prolapse, prolapsed
   anus, anal (canal) (sphincter) K62.2
   arm or hand O32.2 ☑
      causing obstructed labor O64.4 ☑
   bladder (mucosa) (sphincter) (acquired)
      congenital Q79.4
      female — *see* Cystocele
      male N32.89
   breast implant (prosthetic) T85.49 ☑
   cecostomy K94.09
   cecum K63.4
   cervix, cervical (hypertrophied) N81.2
      anterior lip, obstructing labor O65.5
      congenital Q51.828
      postpartal, old N81.2
      stump N81.85
   ciliary body (traumatic) — *see* Laceration, eye(ball),
      with prolapse or loss of interocular tissue
   colon (pedunculated) K63.4
   colostomy K94.09
   disc (intervertebral) — *see* Displacement, intervertebral
      disc
   eye implant (orbital) T85.398 ☑
      lens (ocular) — *see* Complications, intraocular lens
   fallopian tube N83.4- ☑
   gastric (mucosa) K31.89
   genital, female N81.9
      specified NEC N81.89
   globe, nontraumatic — *see* Luxation, globe
   ileostomy bud K94.19
   intervertebral disc — *see* Displacement, intervertebral
      disc
   intestine (small) K63.4
   iris (traumatic) — *see* Laceration, eye(ball), with pro-
      lapse or loss of interocular tissue
      nontraumatic H21.89
   kidney N28.83
      congenital Q63.2
   laryngeal muscles or ventricle J38.7
   liver K76.89
   meatus urinarius N36.8
   mitral (valve) I34.1
   ocular lens implant — *see* Complications, intraocular
      lens
   organ or site, congenital NEC — *see* Malposition, con-
      genital
   ovary N83.4- ☑
   pelvic floor, female N81.89
   perineum, female N81.89
   rectum (mucosa) (sphincter) K62.3
      due to trichuris trichuria B79
   spleen D73.89
   stomach K31.89
   umbilical cord
      complicating delivery O69.0 ☑
   urachus, congenital Q64.4
   ureter N28.89
      with obstruction N13.5
         with infection N13.6
   ureterovesical orifice N28.89
   urethra (acquired) (infected) (mucosa) N36.8
      congenital Q64.71
   urinary meatus N36.8
      congenital Q64.72
   uterovaginal N81.4
      complete N81.3
      incomplete N81.2
   uterus (with prolapse of vagina) N81.4
      complete N81.3
      congenital Q51.818
      first degree N81.2
      in pregnancy or childbirth — *see* Pregnancy, com-
         plicated by, abnormal, uterus
      incomplete N81.2

Prolapse, prolapsed — *continued*
   uterus — *continued*
      postpartal (old) N81.4
      second degree N81.2
      third degree N81.3
   uveal (traumatic) — *see* Laceration, eye(ball), with
      prolapse or loss of interocular tissue
   vagina (anterior) (wall) — *see* Cystocele
      with prolapse of uterus N81.4
         complete N81.3
         incomplete N81.2
      posterior wall N81.6
      posthysterectomy N99.3
   vitreous (humor) H43.0- ☑
      in wound — *see* Laceration, eye(ball), with prolapse
         or loss of interocular tissue
   womb — *see* Prolapse, uterus
Prolapsus, female N81.9
   specified NEC N81.89
Proliferation(s)
   primary cutaneous CD30-positive large T-cell C86.6
   prostate, atypical small acinar N42.32
Proliferative — *see* condition
Prolonged, prolongation (of)
   bleeding (time) (idiopathic) R79.1
   coagulation (time) R79.1
   gestation (over 42 completed weeks)
      mother O48.1
      newborn P08.22
   interval I44.0
   labor O63.9
      first stage O63.0
      second stage O63.1
   partial thromboplastin time (PTT) R79.1
   pregnancy (more than 42 weeks gestation) O48.1
   prothrombin time R79.1
   QT interval I45.81
   uterine contractions in labor O62.4
Prominence, prominent
   auricle (congenital) (ear) Q17.5
   ischial spine or sacral promontory with disproportion
      (fetopelvic)
      with disproportion (fetopelvic) O33.0
         causing obstructed labor O65.0-
   nose (congenital) acquired M95.0
Promiscuity — *see* High, risk, sexual behavior
Pronation
   ankle — *see* Deformity, limb, foot, specified NEC
   foot (*see also* Deformity, limb, foot, specified NEC)
      congenital Q74.2
Prophylactic
   administration of
      antibiotics, long-term Z79.2
         short-term use — *omit code*
      drug (*see also* Long-term (current) drug therapy
         (use of)) Z79.899
   medication Z79.899
   organ removal (for neoplasia management) Z40.00
      breast Z40.01
      fallopian tube(s) Z40.03
         with ovary(s) Z40.02
      ovary(s) Z40.02
      specified site NEC Z40.09
   surgery Z40.9
      for risk factors related to malignant neoplasm —
         see Prophylactic, organ removal
      specified NEC Z40.8
   vaccination Z23
Propionic acidemia E71.121
Proptosis (ocular) (*see also* Exophthalmos)
   thyroid — *see* Hyperthyroidism, with goiter
Prosecution, anxiety concerning Z65.3
Prosopagnosia R48.3
Prostadynia N42.81
Prostate, prostatic — *see* condition
Prostatism — *see* Hyperplasia, prostate
Prostatitis (congestive) (suppurative) (with cystitis) N41.9
   acute N41.0
   cavitary N41.8
   chronic N41.1
   diverticular N41.8
   due to Trichomonas (vaginalis) A59.02
   fibrous N41.1
   gonococcal (acute) (chronic) A54.22
   granulomatous N41.4
   hypertrophic N41.1
   subacute N41.1
   trichomonal A59.02

Prostatitis — *continued*
   tuberculous A18.14
Prostatocystitis N41.3
Prostatorrhea N42.89
Prostatosis N42.82
Prostration R53.83
   heat (*see also* Heat, exhaustion)
      anhydrotic T67.3 ☑
      due to
         salt (and water) depletion T67.4 ☑
         water depletion T67.3 ☑
   nervous F48.8
   senile R54
Protanomaly (anomalous trichromat) H53.54
Protanopia (complete) (incomplete) H53.54
Protection (against) (from) — *see* Prophylactic
Protein
   deficiency NEC — *see* Malnutrition
   malnutrition — *see* Malnutrition
   sickness (*see also* Reaction, serum) T80.69 ☑
Proteinemia R77.9
Proteinosis
   alveolar (pulmonary) J84.01
   lipid or lipoid (of Urbach) E78.89
Proteinuria R80.9
   Bence Jones R80.3
   complicating pregnancy — *see* Proteinuria, gestational
   gestational
      complicating
         childbirth O12.14
         pregnancy O12.1- ☑
            with edema O12.2- ☑
         puerperium O12.15
   idiopathic R80.0
   isolated R80.0
      with glomerular lesion N06.9
         dense deposit disease N06.6
         diffuse
            crescentic glomerulonephritis N06.7
            endocapillary proliferative glomerulonephritis
               N06.4
            mesangiocapillary glomerulonephritis N06.5
         focal and segmental hyalinosis or sclerosis N06.1
         membranous (diffuse) N06.2
         mesangial proliferative (diffuse) N06.3
         minimal change N06.0
         specified pathology NEC N06.8
   orthostatic R80.2
      with glomerular lesion — *see* Proteinuria, isolated,
         with glomerular lesion
   persistent R80.1
      with glomerular lesion — *see* Proteinuria, isolated,
         with glomerular lesion
   postural R80.2
      with glomerular lesion — *see* Proteinuria, isolated,
         with glomerular lesion
   pre-eclamptic — *see* Pre-eclampsia
   puerperal O12.15
   specified type NEC R80.8
Proteolysis, pathologic D65
Proteus (mirabilis) (morganii), **as cause of disease**
      classified elsewhere B96.4
Prothrombin gene mutation D68.52
Protoporphyria, erythropoietic E80.0
Protozoal (*see also* condition)
   disease B64
      specified NEC B60.8
Protrusion, protrusio
   acetabuli M24.7
   acetabulum (into pelvis) M24.7
   device, implant or graft (*see also* Complications, by site
         and type, mechanical) T85.698 ☑
      arterial graft NEC — *see* Complication, cardiovascu-
         lar device, mechanical, vascular
      breast (implant) T85.49 ☑
      catheter NEC T85.698 ☑
         cystostomy T83.090 ☑
         dialysis (renal) T82.49 ☑
            intraperitoneal T85.691 ☑
         infusion NEC T82.594 ☑
            spinal (epidural) (subdural) T85.690 ☑
         urinary (*see also* Complications, catheter, urinary)
            T83.098 ☑
      electronic (electrode) (pulse generator) (stimulator)
         bone T84.390 ☑

Protrusion, protrusio — continued
  device, implant or graft (see also Complications, by site and type, mechanical) — continued
    electronic — continued
      nervous system — see Complication, prosthetic device, mechanical, electronic nervous system stimulator
    fixation, internal (orthopedic) NEC — see Complication, fixation device, mechanical
    gastrointestinal — see Complications, prosthetic device, mechanical, gastrointestinal device
    genital NEC T83.498 ☑
      intrauterine contraceptive device T83.39 ☑
      penile prosthesis (cylinder) (implanted) (pump) (resevoir) T83.490 ☑
      testicular prosthesis T83.491 ☑
    heart NEC — see Complication, cardiovascular device, mechanical
    joint prosthesis — see Complications, joint prosthesis, mechanical, specified NEC, by site
    ocular NEC — see Complications, prosthetic device, mechanical, ocular device
    orthopedic NEC — see Complication, orthopedic, device, mechanical
    specified NEC T85.628 ☑
    urinary NEC (see also Complication, genitourinary, device, urinary, mechanical)
      graft T83.29 ☑
    vascular NEC — see Complication, cardiovascular device, mechanical
    ventricular intracranial shunt T85.09 ☑
  intervertebral disc — see Displacement, intervertebral disc
  joint prosthesis — see Complications, joint prosthesis, mechanical, specified NEC, by site
  nucleus pulposus — see Displacement, intervertebral disc
Prune belly (syndrome) Q79.4
Prurigo (ferox) (gravis) (Hebrae) (Hebra's) (mitis) (simplex) L28.2
  Besnier's L20.0
  estivalis L56.4
  nodularis L28.1
  psychogenic F45.8
Pruritus, pruritic (essential) L29.9
  ani, anus L29.0
    psychogenic F45.8
  anogenital L29.3
    psychogenic F45.8
  due to onchocerca volvulus B73.1
  gravidarum — see Pregnancy, complicated by, specified pregnancy-related condition NEC
  hiemalis L29.8
  neurogenic (any site) F45.8
  perianal L29.0
  psychogenic (any site) F45.8
  scroti, scrotum L29.1
    psychogenic F45.8
  senile, senilis L29.8
  specified NEC L29.8
    psychogenic F45.8
  Trichomonas A59.9
  vulva, vulvae L29.2
    psychogenic F45.8
Pseudarthrosis, pseudoarthrosis (bone) — see Nonunion, fracture
  clavicle, congenital Q74.0
  joint, following fusion or arthrodesis M96.0
Pseudoaneurysm — see Aneurysm
Pseudoangina (pectoris) — see Angina
Pseudoangioma I81
Pseudoarteriosus Q28.8
Pseudoarthrosis — see Pseudarthrosis
Pseudobulbar affect (PBA) F48.2
Pseudochromhidrosis L67.8
Pseudocirrhosis, liver, pericardial I31.1
Pseudocowpox B08.03
Pseudocoxalgia M91.3- ☑
Pseudocroup J38.5
Pseudo-Cushing's syndrome, alcohol-induced E24.4
Pseudocyesis F45.8
Pseudocyst
  lung J98.4
  pancreas K86.3
  retina — see Cyst, retina
Pseudoelephantiasis neuroarthritica Q82.0

Pseudoexfoliation, capsule (lens) — see Cataract, specified NEC
Pseudofolliculitis barbae L73.1
Pseudoglioma H44.89
Pseudohemophilia (Bernuth's) (hereditary) (type B) D68.0
  Type A D69.8
  vascular D69.8
Pseudohermaphroditism Q56.3
  adrenal E25.8
  female Q56.2
    with adrenocortical disorder E25.8
    without adrenocortical disorder Q56.2
    adrenal (congenital) E25.0
    unspecified E25.9
  male Q56.1
    with
      5-alpha-reductase deficiency E29.1
      adrenocortical disorder E25.8
      androgen resistance E34.51
      cleft scrotum Q56.1
      feminizing testis E34.51
    without gonadal disorder Q56.1
    adrenal E25.8
    unspecified E25.9
Pseudo-Hurler's polydystrophy E77.0
Pseudohydrocephalus G93.2
Pseudohypertrophic muscular dystrophy (Erb's) G71.02
Pseudohypertrophy, muscle G71.09
Pseudohypoparathyroidism E20.1
Pseudoinsomnia F51.03
Pseudoleukemia, infantile D64.89
Pseudomembranous — see condition
Pseudomeningocele (cerebral) (infective) (post-traumatic) G96.19
  postprocedural (spinal) G97.82
Pseudomenses (newborn) P54.6
Pseudomenstruation (newborn) P54.6
Pseudomonas
  aeruginosa, as cause of disease classified elsewhere B96.5
  mallei infection A24.0
    as cause of disease classified elsewhere B96.5
  pseudomallei, as cause of disease classified elsewhere B96.5
Pseudomyotonia G71.19
Pseudomyxoma peritonei C78.6
Pseudoneuritis, optic (nerve) (disc) (papilla), **congenital** Q14.2
Pseudo-obstruction intestine (acute) (chronic) (idiopathic) (intermittent secondary) (primary) K59.8
Pseudopapilledema H47.33- ☑
  congenital Q14.2
Pseudoparalysis
  arm or leg R29.818
  atonic, congenital P94.2
Pseudopelade L66.0
Pseudophakia Z96.1
Pseudopolyarthritis, rhizomelic M35.3
Pseudopolycythemia D75.1
Pseudopseudohypoparathyroidism E20.1
Pseudopterygium H11.81- ☑
Pseudoptosis (eyelid) — see Blepharochalasis
Pseudopuberty, precocious
  female heterosexual E25.8
  male isosexual E25.8
Pseudorickets (renal) N25.0
Pseudorubella B08.20
Pseudosclerema, newborn P83.88
Pseudosclerosis (brain)
  Jakob's — see Creutzfeldt-Jakob disease or syndrome of Westphal (Strümpell) E83.01
  spastic — see Creutzfeldt-Jakob disease or syndrome
Pseudotetanus — see Convulsions
Pseudotetany R29.0
  hysterical F44.5
Pseudotruncus arteriosus Q25.49
Pseudotuberculosis A28.2
  enterocolitis A04.8
  pasteurella (infection) A28.0
Pseudotumor
  cerebri G93.2
  orbital H05.11 ☑
Pseudoxanthoma elasticum Q82.8
Psilosis (sprue) (tropical) K90.1
  nontropical K90.0

Psittacosis A70
Psoitis M60.88
Psoriasis L40.9
  arthropathic L40.50
    arthritis mutilans L40.52
    distal interphalangeal L40.51
    juvenile L40.54
    other specified L40.59
    spondylitis L40.53
  buccal K13.29
  flexural L40.8
  guttate L40.4
  mouth K13.29
  nummular L40.0
  plaque L40.0
  psychogenic F54
  pustular (generalized) L40.1
    palmaris et plantaris L40.3
  specified NEC L40.8
  vulgaris L40.0
Psychasthenia F48.8
Psychiatric disorder or problem F99
Psychogenic (see also condition)
  factors associated with physical conditions F54
Psychological and behavioral factors affecting medical condition F59
Psychoneurosis, psychoneurotic (see also Neurosis)
  anxiety (state) F41.1
  depersonalization F48.1
  hypochondriacal F45.21
  hysteria F44.9
  neurasthenic F48.8
  personality NEC F60.89
Psychopathy, psychopathic
  affectionless F94.2
  autistic F84.5
  constitution, post-traumatic F07.81
  personality — see Disorder, personality
  sexual — see Deviation, sexual
  state F60.2
Psychosexual identity disorder of childhood F64.2
Psychosis, psychotic F29
  acute (transient) F23
    hysterical F44.9
  affective — see Disorder, mood
  alcoholic F10.959
    with
      abuse F10.159
      anxiety disorder F10.980
        with
          abuse F10.180
          dependence F10.280
      delirium tremens F10.231
      delusions F10.950
        with
          abuse F10.150
          dependence F10.250
      dementia F10.97
        with dependence F10.27
      dependence F10.259
      hallucinosis F10.951
        with
          abuse F10.151
          dependence F10.251
      mood disorder F10.94
        with
          abuse F10.14
          dependence F10.24
      paranoia F10.950
        with
          abuse F10.150
          dependence F10.250
      persisting amnesia F10.96
        with dependence F10.26
    amnestic confabulatory F10.96
      with dependence F10.26
    delirium tremens F10.231
    Korsakoff's, Korsakov's, Korsakow's F10.26
    paranoid type F10.950
      with
        abuse F10.150
        dependence F10.250
  anergastic — see Psychosis, organic
  arteriosclerotic (simple type) (uncomplicated) F01.50
    with behavioral disturbance F01.51
  childhood F84.0
    atypical F84.8
  climacteric — see Psychosis, involutional

Psychosis, psychotic — continued
  confusional F29
    acute or subacute F05
    reactive F23
  cycloid F23
  depressive — see Disorder, depressive
  disintegrative (childhood) F84.3
  drug-induced — see F11-F19 with .X59
    paranoid and hallucinatory states — see F11-F19
        with .X50 or .X51
  due to or associated with
    addiction, drug — see F11-F19 with .X59
    dependence
      alcohol F10.259
      drug — see F11-F19 with .X59
    epilepsy F06.8
    Huntington's chorea F06.8
    ischemia, cerebrovascular (generalized) F06.8
    multiple sclerosis F06.8
    physical disease F06.8
    presenile dementia F03 ☑
    senile dementia F03 ☑
    vascular disease (arteriosclerotic) (cerebral) F01.50
      with behavioral disturbance F01.51
  epileptic F06.8
  episode F23
    due to or associated with physical condition F06.8
  exhaustive F43.0
  hallucinatory, chronic F28
  hypomanic F30.8
  hysterical (acute) F44.9
  induced F24
  infantile F84.0
    atypical F84.8
  infective (acute) (subacute) F05
  involutional F28
    depressive — see Disorder, depressive
    melancholic — see Disorder, depressive
    paranoid (state) F22
  Korsakoff's, Korsakov's, Korsakow's (nonalcoholic) F04
    alcoholic F10.96
      in dependence F10.26
    induced by other psychoactive substance — see
        categories F11-F19 with .X5X
  mania, manic (single episode) F30.2
    recurrent type F31.89
  manic-depressive — see Disorder, bipolar
  menopausal — see Psychosis, involutional
  mixed schizophrenic and affective F25.8
  multi-infarct (cerebrovascular) F01.50
    with behavioral disturbance F01.51
  nonorganic F29
    specified NEC F28
  organic F09
    due to or associated with
      arteriosclerosis (cerebral) — see Psychosis, arte-
          riosclerotic
      cerebrovascular disease, arteriosclerotic — see
          Psychosis, arteriosclerotic
      childbirth — see Psychosis, puerperal
      Creutzfeldt-Jakob disease or syndrome — see
          Creutzfeldt-Jakob disease or syndrome
      dependence, alcohol F10.259
      disease
        alcoholic liver F10.259
        brain, arteriosclerotic — see Psychosis, arte-
            riosclerotic
        cerebrovascular F01.50
          with behavioral disturbance F01.51
        Creutzfeldt-Jakob — see Creutzfeldt-Jakob
            disease or syndrome
        endocrine or metabolic F06.8
          acute or subacute F05
        liver, alcoholic F10.259
      epilepsy transient (acute) F05
      infection
        brain (intracranial) F06.8
          acute or subacute F05
      intoxication
        alcoholic (acute) F10.259
        drug F11-F19 with .x59
      ischemia, cerebrovascular (generalized) — see
          Psychosis, arteriosclerotic
      puerperium — see Psychosis, puerperal
      trauma, brain (birth) (from electric current) (sur-
          gical) F06.8
        acute or subacute F05
    infective F06.8

Psychosis, psychotic — continued
  organic — continued
    infective — continued
      acute or subacute F05
      post-traumatic F06.8
        acute or subacute F05
    paranoiac F22
    paranoid (climacteric) (involutional) (menopausal) F22
      psychogenic (acute) F23
      schizophrenic F20.0
      senile F03 ☑
    postpartum (NOS) F53.1
    presbyophrenic (type) F03 ☑
    presenile F03 ☑
    psychogenic (paranoid) F23
      depressive F32.3
    puerperal (NOS) F53.1
      specified type — see Psychosis, by type
    reactive (brief) (transient) (emotional stress) (psycho-
        logical trauma) F23
      depressive F32.3
        recurrent F33.3
      excitative type F30.8
    schizoaffective F25.9
      depressive type F25.1
      manic type F25.0
    schizophrenia, schizophrenic — see Schizophrenia
    schizophrenia-like, in epilepsy F06.2
    schizophreniform F20.81
      affective type F25.9
      brief F23
      confusional type F23
      mixed type F25.0
    senile NEC F03 ☑
      depressed or paranoid type F03 ☑
      simple deterioration F03 ☑
      specified type — code to condition
    shared F24
    situational (reactive) F23
    symbiotic (childhood) F84.3
    symptomatic F09
Psychosomatic — see Disorder, psychosomatic
Psychosyndrome, organic F07.9
**Psychotic episode due to or associated with physical
    condition** F06.8
Pterygium (eye) H11.00- ☑
  amyloid H11.01- ☑
  central H11.02- ☑
  colli Q18.3
  double H11.03- ☑
  peripheral
    progressive H11.05- ☑
    stationary H11.04- ☑
  recurrent H11.06- ☑
Ptilosis (eyelid) — see Madarosis
Ptomaine (poisoning) — see Poisoning, food
Ptosis (see also Blepharoptosis)
  adiposa (false) — see Blepharoptosis
  breast N64.81-
  brow H57.81- ☑
  cecum K63.4
  colon K63.4
  congenital (eyelid) Q10.0
    specified site NEC — see Anomaly, by site
  eyebrow H57.81- ☑
  eyelid — see Blepharoptosis
    congenital Q10.0
  gastric K31.89
  intestine K63.4
  kidney N28.83
  liver K76.89
  renal N28.83
  splanchnic K63.4
  spleen D73.89
  stomach K31.89
  viscera K63.4
PTP D69.51
Ptyalism (periodic) K11.7
  hysterical F45.8
  pregnancy — see Pregnancy, complicated by, specified
      pregnancy-related condition NEC
  psychogenic F45.8
Ptyalolithiasis K11.5
Pubarche, precocious E30.1
Pubertas praecox E30.1
Puberty (development state) Z00.3
  bleeding (excessive) N92.2

Puberty — continued
  delayed E30.0
  precocious (constitutional) (cryptogenic) (idiopathic)
      E30.1
    central E22.8
    due to
      ovarian hyperfunction E28.1
        estrogen E28.0
      testicular hyperfunction E29.0
  premature E30.1
    due to
      adrenal cortical hyperfunction E25.8
      pineal tumor E34.8
      pituitary (anterior) hyperfunction E22.8
Puckering, macula — see Degeneration, macula, puck-
    ering
Pudenda, pudendum — see condition
Puente's disease (simple glandular cheilitis) K13.0
Puerperal, puerperium (complicated by, complications)
  abnormal glucose (tolerance test) O99.815
  abscess
    areola O91.02
      associated with lactation O91.03
    Bartholin's gland O86.19
    breast O91.12
      associated with lactation O91.13
    cervix (uteri) O86.11
    genital organ NEC O86.19
    kidney O86.21
    mammary O91.12
      associated with lactation O91.13
    nipple O91.02
      associated with lactation O91.03
    peritoneum O85
    subareolar O91.12
      associated with lactation O91.13
    urinary tract — see Puerperal, infection, urinary
    uterus O86.12
    vagina (wall) O86.13
    vaginorectal O86.13
    vulvovaginal gland O86.13
  adnexitis O86.19
  afibrinogenemia, or other coagulation defect O72.3
  albuminuria (acute) (subacute) — see Proteinuria,
      gestational
  alcohol use O99.315
  anemia O90.81
    pre-existing (pre-pregnancy) O99.03
  anesthetic death O89.8
  apoplexy O99.43
  bariatric surgery status O99.845
  blood disorder NEC O99.13
  blood dyscrasia O72.3
  cardiomyopathy O90.3
  cerebrovascular disorder (conditions in I60-I69) O99.43
  cervicitis O86.11
  circulatory system disorder O99.43
  coagulopathy (any) O99.13
    with hemorrhage O72.3
  complications O90.9
    specified NEC O90.89
  convulsions — see Eclampsia
  cystitis O86.22
  cystopyelitis O86.29
  delirium NEC F05
  diabetes O24.93
    gestational — see Puerperal, gestational diabetes
    pre-existing O24.33
      specified NEC O24.83
      type 1 O24.03
      type 2 O24.13
  digestive system disorder O99.63
  disease O90.9
    breast NEC O92.29
    cerebrovascular (acute) O99.43
    nonobstetric NEC O99.89
    tubo-ovarian O86.19
    Valsuani's O99.03
  disorder O90.9
    biliary tract O26.63
    lactation O92.70
    liver O26.63
    nonobstetric NEC O99.89
  disruption
    cesarean wound O90.0
    episiotomy wound O90.1
    perineal laceration wound O90.1
  drug use O99.325

Puerperal, puerperium — *continued*
eclampsia (with pre-existing hypertension) O15.2
embolism (pulmonary) (blood clot) — *see* Embolism, obstetric, puerperal
endocrine, nutritional or metabolic disease NEC O99.285
endophlebitis — *see* Puerperal, phlebitis
endotrachelitis O86.11
failure
  lactation (complete) O92.3
    partial O92.4
  renal, acute O90.4
fever (of unknown origin) O86.4
  septic O85
fissure, nipple O92.12
  associated with lactation O92.13
fistula
  breast (due to mastitis) O91.12
    associated with lactation O91.13
  nipple O91.02
    associated with lactation O91.03
galactophoritis O91.22
  associated with lactation O91.23
galactorrhea O92.6
gastric banding status O99.845
gastric bypass status O99.845
gastrointestinal disease NEC O99.63
gestational
  diabetes O24.439
    diet controlled O24.430
    insulin (and diet) controlled O24.434
    oral drug controlled (antidiabetic) (hypo-glycemic) O24.435
  edema O12.05
    with proteinuria O12.25
  proteinuria O12.15
gonorrhea O98.23
hematoma, subdural O99.43
hemiplegia, cerebral O99.355
  due to cerbrovascular disorder O99.43
hemorrhage O72.1
  brain O99.43
  bulbar O99.43
  cerebellar O99.43
  cerebral O99.43
  cortical O99.43
  delayed or secondary O72.2
  extradural O99.43
  internal capsule O99.43
  intracranial O99.43
  intrapontine O99.43
  meningeal O99.43
  pontine O99.43
  retained placenta O72.0
  subarachnoid O99.43
  subcortical O99.43
  subdural O99.43
  third stage O72.0
  uterine, delayed O72.2
  ventricular O99.43
hemorrhoids O87.2
hepatorenal syndrome O90.4
hypertension — *see* Hypertension, complicating, puerperium
hypertrophy, breast O92.29
induration breast (fibrous) O92.29
infection O86.4
  cervix O86.11
  generalized O85
  genital tract NEC O86.19
    obstetric surgical wound O86.09
  kidney (bacillus coli) O86.21
  maternal O98.93
    carrier state NEC O99.835
    gonorrhea O98.23
    human immunodeficiency virus (HIV) O98.73
    protozoal O98.63
    sexually transmitted NEC O98.33
    specified NEC O98.83
    streptococcus group B (GBS) carrier state O99.825
    syphilis O98.13
    tuberculosis O98.03
    viral hepatitis O98.43
    viral NEC O98.53
  nipple O91.02
    associated with lactation O91.03
  peritoneum O85
  renal O86.21
  specified NEC O86.89

Puerperal, puerperium — *continued*
infection — *continued*
  urinary (asymptomatic) (tract) NEC O86.20
    bladder O86.22
    kidney O86.21
    specified site NEC O86.29
    urethra O86.22
  vagina O86.13
  vein — *see* Puerperal, phlebitis
ischemia, cerebral O99.43
lymphangitis O86.89
  breast O91.22
    associated with lactation O91.23
malignancy O9A.13 (*following* O99)
malnutrition O25.3
mammillitis O91.02
  associated with lactation O91.03
mammitis O91.22
  associated with lactation O91.23
mania F30.8
mastitis O91.22
  associated with lactation O91.23
  purulent O91.12
    associated with lactation O91.13
melancholia — *see* Disorder, depressive
mental disorder NEC O99.345
metroperitonitis O85
metrorrhagia — *see* Hemorrhage, postpartum
metrosalpingitis O86.19
metrovaginitis O86.13
milk leg O87.1
monoplegia, cerebral O99.43
mood disturbance O90.6
necrosis, liver (acute) (subacute) (conditions in subcat-egory K72.0) O26.63
  with renal failure O90.4
nervous system disorder O99.355
obesity (pre-existing prior to pregnancy) O99.215
obesity surgery status O99.845
occlusion, precerebral artery O99.43
paralysis
  bladder (sphincter) O90.89
  cerebral O99.43
paralytic stroke O99.43
parametritis O85
paravaginitis O86.13
pelviperitonitis O85
perimetritis O86.12
perimetrosalpingitis O86.19
perinephritis O86.21
periphlebitis — *see* Puerperal phlebitis
peritoneal infection O85
peritonitis (pelvic) O85
perivaginitis O86.13
phlebitis O87.0
  deep O87.1
  pelvic O87.1
  superficial O87.0
phlebothrombosis, deep O87.1
phlegmasia alba dolens O87.1
placental polyp O90.89
pneumonia, embolic — *see* Embolism, obstetric, puerperal
pre-eclampsia — *see* Pre-eclampsia
psychosis (NOS) F53.1
pyelitis O86.21
pyelocystitis O86.29
pyelonephritis O86.21
pyelonephrosis O86.21
pyemia O85
pyocystitis O86.29
pyohemia O85
pyometra O86.12
pyonephritis O86.21
pyosalpingitis O86.19
pyrexia (of unknown origin) O86.4
renal
  disease NEC O90.89
  failure O90.4
respiratory disease NEC O99.53
retention
  decidua — *see* Retention, decidua
  placenta O72.0
  secundines — *see* Retention, secundines
retrated nipple O92.02
salpingo-ovaritis O86.19
salpingoperitonitis O85
secondary perineal tear O90.1

Puerperal, puerperium — *continued*
sepsis (pelvic) O85
sepsis O85
septic thrombophlebitis O86.81
skin disorder NEC O99.73
specified condition NEC O99.89
stroke O99.43
subinvolution (uterus) O90.89
subluxation of symphysis (pubis) O26.73
suppuration — *see* Puerperal, abscess
tetanus A34
thelitis O91.02
  associated with lactation O91.03
thrombocytopenia O72.3
thrombophlebitis (superficial) O87.0
  deep O87.1
  pelvic O87.1
  septic O86.81
thrombosis (venous) — *see* Thrombosis, puerperal
thyroiditis O90.5
toxemia (eclamptic) (pre-eclamptic) (with convulsions) O15.2
trauma, non-obstetric O9A.23 (*following* O99)
  caused by abuse (physical) (suspected) O9A.33 (*following* O99)
    confirmed O9A.33 (*following* O99)
    psychological (suspected) O9A.53 (*following* O99)
      confirmed O9A.53 (*following* O99)
    sexual (suspected) O9A.43 (*following* O99)
      confirmed O9A.43 (*following* O99)
uremia (due to renal failure) O90.4
urethritis O86.22
vaginitis O86.13
varicose veins (legs) O87.4
  vulva or perineum O87.8
venous O87.9
vulvitis O86.19
vulvovaginitis O86.13
white leg O87.1
Puerperium — *see* Puerperal
Pulmolithiasis J98.4
Pulmonary — *see* condition
Pulpitis (acute) (anachoretic) (chronic) (hyperplastic) (putrescent) (suppurative) (ulcerative) K04.01
  irreversible K04.02
  reversible K04.01
Pulpless tooth K04.99
Pulse
  alternating R00.8
  bigeminal R00.8
  fast R00.0
  feeble, rapid due to shock following injury T79.4 ☑
  rapid R00.0
  weak R09.89
Pulsus alternans or trigeminus R00.8
Punch drunk F07.81
Punctum lacrimale occlusion — *see* Obstruction, lacrimal
Puncture
abdomen, abdominal
  wall S31.139 ☑
    with
      foreign body S31.149 ☑
      penetration into peritoneal cavity S31.639 ☑
        with foreign body S31.649 ☑
    epigastric region S31.132 ☑
      with
        foreign body S31.142 ☑
        penetration into peritoneal cavity S31.632 ☑
          with foreign body S31.642 ☑
    left
      lower quadrant S31.134 ☑
        with
          foreign body S31.144 ☑
          penetration into peritoneal cavity S31.634 ☑
            with foreign body S31.644 ☑
      upper quadrant S31.131 ☑
        with
          foreign body S31.141 ☑
          penetration into peritoneal cavity S31.631 ☑
            with foreign body S31.641 ☑
    periumbilic region S31.135 ☑
      with
        foreign body S31.145 ☑

☑ **Additional Character Required** — Refer to the Tabular List for Character Selection   ⬆ **Subterms under main terms may continue to next column or page**

Puncture — *continued*
  abdomen, abdominal — *continued*
    wall — *continued*
      periumbilic region — *continued*
        with — *continued*
          penetration into peritoneal cavity S31.635 ☑
            with foreign body S31.645 ☑
      right
        lower quadrant S31.133 ☑
          with
            foreign body S31.143 ☑
            penetration into peritoneal cavity S31.633 ☑
              with foreign body S31.643 ☑
        upper quadrant S31.130 ☑
          with
            foreign body S31.140 ☑
            penetration into peritoneal cavity S31.630 ☑
              with foreign body S31.640 ☑
  accidental, complicating surgery — *see* Complication, accidental puncture or laceration
  alveolar (process) — *see* Puncture, oral cavity
  ankle S91.039 ☑
    with
      foreign body S91.049 ☑
    left S91.032 ☑
      with
        foreign body S91.042 ☑
    right S91.031 ☑
      with
        foreign body S91.041 ☑
  anus S31.833 ☑
    with foreign body S31.834 ☑
  arm (upper) S41.139 ☑
    with foreign body S41.149 ☑
    left S41.132 ☑
      with foreign body S41.142 ☑
    lower — *see* Puncture, forearm
    right S41.131 ☑
      with foreign body S41.141 ☑
  auditory canal (external) (meatus) — *see* Puncture, ear
  auricle, ear — *see* Puncture, ear
  axilla — *see* Puncture, arm
  back (*see also* Puncture, thorax, back)
    lower S31.030 ☑
      with
        foreign body S31.040 ☑
          with penetration into retroperitoneal space S31.041 ☑
        penetration into retroperitoneal space S31.031 ☑
  bladder (traumatic) S37.29 ☑
    nontraumatic N32.89
  breast S21.039 ☑
    with foreign body S21.049 ☑
    left S21.032 ☑
      with foreign body S21.042 ☑
    right S21.031 ☑
      with foreign body S21.041 ☑
  buttock S31.803 ☑
    with foreign body S31.804 ☑
    left S31.823 ☑
      with foreign body S31.824 ☑
    right S31.813 ☑
      with foreign body S31.814 ☑
  by
    device, implant or graft — *see* Complications, by site and type, mechanical
    foreign body left accidentally in operative wound T81.539 ☑
    instrument (any) during a procedure, accidental — *see* Puncture, accidental complicating surgery
  calf — *see* Puncture, leg
  canaliculus lacrimalis — *see* Puncture, eyelid
  canthus, eye — *see* Puncture, eyelid
  cervical esophagus S11.23 ☑
    with foreign body S11.24 ☑
  cheek (external) S01.439 ☑
    with foreign body S01.449 ☑
    internal — *see* Puncture, oral cavity
    left S01.432 ☑
      with foreign body S01.442 ☑
    right S01.431 ☑
      with foreign body S01.441 ☑

Puncture — *continued*
  chest wall — *see* Puncture, thorax
  chin — *see* Puncture, head, specified site NEC
  clitoris — *see* Puncture, vulva
  costal region — *see* Puncture, thorax
  digit(s)
    foot — *see* Puncture, toe
    hand — *see* Puncture, finger
  ear (canal) (external) S01.339 ☑
    with foreign body S01.349 ☑
    drum S09.2- ☑
    left S01.332 ☑
      with foreign body S01.342 ☑
    right S01.331 ☑
      with foreign body S01.341 ☑
  elbow S51.039 ☑
    with
      foreign body S51.049 ☑
    left S51.032 ☑
      with
        foreign body S51.042 ☑
    right S51.031 ☑
      with
        foreign body S51.041 ☑
  epididymis — *see* Puncture, testis
  epigastric region — *see* Puncture, abdomen, wall, epigastric
  epiglottis S11.83 ☑
    with foreign body S11.84 ☑
  esophagus
    cervical S11.23 ☑
      with foreign body S11.24 ☑
    thoracic S27.818 ☑
  eyeball S05.6- ☑
    with foreign body S05.5- ☑
  eyebrow — *see* Puncture, eyelid
  eyelid S01.13- ☑
    with foreign body S01.14- ☑
    left S01.132 ☑
      with foreign body S01.142 ☑
    right S01.131 ☑
      with foreign body S01.141 ☑
  face NEC — *see* Puncture, head, specified site NEC
  finger(s) S61.239 ☑
    with
      damage to nail S61.339 ☑
        with
          foreign body S61.349 ☑
      foreign body S61.249 ☑
    index S61.238 ☑
      with
        damage to nail S61.338 ☑
          with
            foreign body S61.348 ☑
        foreign body S61.248 ☑
      left S61.231 ☑
        with
          damage to nail S61.331 ☑
            with
              foreign body S61.341 ☑
          foreign body S61.241 ☑
      right S61.230 ☑
        with
          damage to nail S61.330 ☑
            with
              foreign body S61.340 ☑
          foreign body S61.240 ☑
    little S61.238 ☑
      with
        damage to nail S61.338 ☑
          with
            foreign body S61.348 ☑
        foreign body S61.248 ☑
      left S61.237 ☑
        with
          damage to nail S61.337 ☑
            with
              foreign body S61.347 ☑
          foreign body S61.247 ☑
      right S61.236 ☑
        with
          damage to nail S61.336 ☑
            with
              foreign body S61.346 ☑
          foreign body S61.246 ☑
    middle S61.238 ☑

Puncture — *continued*
  finger(s) — *continued*
    middle — *continued*
      with
        damage to nail S61.338 ☑
          with
            foreign body S61.348 ☑
        foreign body S61.248 ☑
      left S61.233 ☑
        with
          damage to nail S61.333 ☑
            with
              foreign body S61.343 ☑
          foreign body S61.243 ☑
      right S61.232 ☑
        with
          damage to nail S61.332 ☑
            with
              foreign body S61.342 ☑
          foreign body S61.242 ☑
    ring S61.238 ☑
      with
        damage to nail S61.338 ☑
          with
            foreign body S61.348 ☑
        foreign body S61.248 ☑
      left S61.235 ☑
        with
          damage to nail S61.335 ☑
            with
              foreign body S61.345 ☑
          foreign body S61.245 ☑
      right S61.234 ☑
        with
          damage to nail S61.334 ☑
            with
              foreign body S61.344 ☑
          foreign body S61.244 ☑
  flank S31.139 ☑
    with foreign body S31.149 ☑
  foot (except toe(s) alone) S91.339 ☑
    with foreign body S91.349 ☑
    left S91.332 ☑
      with foreign body S91.342 ☑
    right S91.331 ☑
      with foreign body S91.341 ☑
    toe — *see* Puncture, toe
  forearm S51.839 ☑
    with
      foreign body S51.849 ☑
    elbow only — *see* Puncture, elbow
    left S51.832 ☑
      with
        foreign body S51.842 ☑
    right S51.831 ☑
      with
        foreign body S51.841 ☑
  forehead — *see* Puncture, head, specified site NEC
  genital organs, external
    female S31.532 ☑
      with foreign body S31.542 ☑
      vagina — *see* Puncture, vagina
      vulva — *see* Puncture, vulva
    male S31.531 ☑
      with foreign body S31.541 ☑
      penis — *see* Puncture, penis
      scrotum — *see* Puncture, scrotum
      testis — *see* Puncture, testis
  groin — *see* Puncture, abdomen, wall
  gum — *see* Puncture, oral cavity
  hand S61.439 ☑
    with
      foreign body S61.449 ☑
    finger — *see* Puncture, finger
    left S61.432 ☑
      with
        foreign body S61.442 ☑
    right S61.431 ☑
      with
        foreign body S61.441 ☑
    thumb — *see* Puncture, thumb
  head S01.93 ☑
    with foreign body S01.94 ☑
    cheek — *see* Puncture, cheek
    ear — *see* Puncture, ear
    eyelid — *see* Puncture, eyelid

☑ Subterms under main terms may continue to next column or page   ☑ Additional Character Required — Refer to the Tabular List for Character Selection   269

Puncture—Puncture

Puncture — *continued*
  head — *continued*
    lip — *see* Puncture, oral cavity
    nose — *see* Puncture, nose
    oral cavity — *see* Puncture, oral cavity
    scalp S01.03 ☑
      with foreign body S01.04 ☑
    specified site NEC S01.83 ☑
      with foreign body S01.84 ☑
    temporomandibular area — *see* Puncture, cheek
  heart S26.99 ☑
    with hemopericardium S26.09 ☑
    without hemopericardium S26.19 ☑
  heel — *see* Puncture, foot
  hip S71.039 ☑
    with foreign body S71.049 ☑
    left S71.032 ☑
      with foreign body S71.042 ☑
    right S71.031 ☑
      with foreign body S71.041 ☑
  hymen — *see* Puncture, vagina
  hypochondrium — *see* Puncture, abdomen, wall
  hypogastric region — *see* Puncture, abdomen, wall
  inguinal region — *see* Puncture, abdomen, wall
  instep — *see* Puncture, foot
  internal organs — *see* Injury, by site
  interscapular region — *see* Puncture, thorax, back
  intestine
    large
      colon S36.599 ☑
        ascending S36.590 ☑
        descending S36.592 ☑
        sigmoid S36.593 ☑
        specified site NEC S36.598 ☑
        transverse S36.591 ☑
      rectum S36.69 ☑
    small S36.499 ☑
      duodenum S36.490 ☑
      specified site NEC S36.498 ☑
  intra-abdominal organ S36.99 ☑
    gallbladder S36.128 ☑
    intestine — *see* Puncture, intestine
    liver S36.118 ☑
    pancreas — *see* Puncture, pancreas
    peritoneum S36.81 ☑
    specified site NEC S36.898 ☑
    spleen S36.09 ☑
    stomach S36.39 ☑
  jaw — *see* Puncture, head, specified site NEC
  knee S81.039 ☑
    with foreign body S81.049 ☑
    left S81.032 ☑
      with foreign body S81.042 ☑
    right S81.031 ☑
      with foreign body S81.041 ☑
  labium (majus) (minus) — *see* Puncture, vulva
  lacrimal duct — *see* Puncture, eyelid
  larynx S11.013 ☑
    with foreign body S11.014 ☑
  leg (lower) S81.839 ☑
    with foreign body S81.849 ☑
    foot — *see* Puncture, foot
    knee — *see* Puncture, knee
    left S81.832 ☑
      with foreign body S81.842 ☑
    right S81.831 ☑
      with foreign body S81.841 ☑
    upper — *see* Puncture, thigh
  lip S01.531 ☑
    with foreign body S01.541 ☑
  loin — *see* Puncture, abdomen, wall
  lower back — *see* Puncture, back, lower
  lumbar region — *see* Puncture, back, lower
  malar region — *see* Puncture, head, specified site NEC
  mammary — *see* Puncture, breast
  mastoid region — *see* Puncture, head, specified site NEC
  mouth — *see* Puncture, oral cavity
  nail
    finger — *see* Puncture, finger, with damage to nail
    toe — *see* Puncture, toe, with damage to nail
  nasal (septum) (sinus) — *see* Puncture, nose
  nasopharynx — *see* Puncture, head, specified site NEC
  neck S11.93 ☑
    with foreign body S11.94 ☑

Puncture — *continued*
  neck — *continued*
    involving
      cervical esophagus — *see* Puncture, cervical esophagus
      larynx — *see* Puncture, larynx
      pharynx — *see* Puncture, pharynx
      thyroid gland — *see* Puncture, thyroid gland
      trachea — *see* Puncture, trachea
    specified site NEC S11.83 ☑
      with foreign body S11.84 ☑
  nose (septum) (sinus) S01.23 ☑
    with foreign body S01.24 ☑
  ocular — *see* Puncture, eyeball
  oral cavity S01.532 ☑
    with foreign body S01.542 ☑
  orbit S05.4- ☑
  palate — *see* Puncture, oral cavity
  palm — *see* Puncture, hand
  pancreas S36.299 ☑
    body S36.291 ☑
    head S36.290 ☑
    tail S36.292 ☑
  pelvis — *see* Puncture, back, lower
  penis S31.23 ☑
    with foreign body S31.24 ☑
  perineum
    female S31.43 ☑
      with foreign body S31.44 ☑
    male S31.139 ☑
      with foreign body S31.149 ☑
  periocular area (with or without lacrimal passages) — *see* Puncture, eyelid
  phalanges
    finger — *see* Puncture, finger
    toe — *see* Puncture, toe
  pharynx S11.23 ☑
    with foreign body S11.24 ☑
  pinna — *see* Puncture, ear
  popliteal space — *see* Puncture, knee
  prepuce — *see* Puncture, penis
  pubic region S31.139 ☑
    with foreign body S31.149 ☑
  pudendum — *see* Puncture, genital organs, external
  rectovaginal septum — *see* Puncture, vagina
  sacral region — *see* Puncture, back, lower
  sacroiliac region — *see* Puncture, back, lower
  salivary gland — *see* Puncture, oral cavity
  scalp S01.03 ☑
    with foreign body S01.04 ☑
  scapular region — *see* Puncture, shoulder
  scrotum S31.33 ☑
    with foreign body S31.34 ☑
  shin — *see* Puncture, leg
  shoulder S41.039 ☑
    with foreign body S41.049 ☑
    left S41.032 ☑
      with foreign body S41.042 ☑
    right S41.031 ☑
      with foreign body S41.041 ☑
  spermatic cord — *see* Puncture, testis
  sternal region — *see* Puncture, thorax, front
  submaxillary region — *see* Puncture, head, specified site NEC
  submental region — *see* Puncture, head, specified site NEC
  subungual
    finger(s) — *see* Puncture, finger, with damage to nail
    toe — *see* Puncture, toe, with damage to nail
  supraclavicular fossa — *see* Puncture, neck, specified site NEC
  temple, temporal region — *see* Puncture, head, specified site NEC
  temporomandibular area — *see* Puncture, cheek
  testis S31.33 ☑
    with foreign body S31.34 ☑
  thigh S71.139 ☑
    with foreign body S71.149 ☑
    left S71.132 ☑
      with foreign body S71.142 ☑
    right S71.131 ☑
      with foreign body S71.141 ☑
  thorax, thoracic (wall) S21.93 ☑
    with foreign body S21.94 ☑
    back S21.23- ☑

Puncture — *continued*
  thorax, thoracic — *continued*
    back — *continued*
      with
        foreign body S21.24- ☑
          with penetration S21.44 ☑
        penetration S21.43 ☑
    breast — *see* Puncture, breast
    front S21.13- ☑
      with
        foreign body S21.14- ☑
          with penetration S21.34 ☑
        penetration S21.33 ☑
    throat — *see* Puncture, neck
  thumb S61.039 ☑
    with
      damage to nail S61.139 ☑
        with
          foreign body S61.149 ☑
      foreign body S61.049 ☑
    left S61.032 ☑
      with
        damage to nail S61.132 ☑
          with
            foreign body S61.142 ☑
        foreign body S61.042 ☑
    right S61.031 ☑
      with
        damage to nail S61.131 ☑
          with
            foreign body S61.141 ☑
        foreign body S61.041 ☑
  thyroid gland S11.13 ☑
    with foreign body S11.14 ☑
  toe(s) S91.139 ☑
    with
      damage to nail S91.239 ☑
        with
          foreign body S91.249 ☑
      foreign body S91.149 ☑
    great S91.133 ☑
      with
        damage to nail S91.233 ☑
          with
            foreign body S91.243 ☑
        foreign body S91.143 ☑
      left S91.132 ☑
        with
          damage to nail S91.232 ☑
            with
              foreign body S91.242 ☑
          foreign body S91.142 ☑
      right S91.131 ☑
        with
          damage to nail S91.231 ☑
            with
              foreign body S91.241 ☑
          foreign body S91.141 ☑
    lesser S91.136 ☑
      with
        damage to nail S91.236 ☑
          with
            foreign body S91.246 ☑
        foreign body S91.146 ☑
      left S91.135 ☑
        with
          damage to nail S91.235 ☑
            with
              foreign body S91.245 ☑
          foreign body S91.145 ☑
      right S91.134 ☑
        with
          damage to nail S91.234 ☑
            with
              foreign body S91.244 ☑
          foreign body S91.144 ☑
  tongue — *see* Puncture, oral cavity
  trachea S11.023 ☑
    with foreign body S11.024 ☑
  tunica vaginalis — *see* Puncture, testis
  tympanum, tympanic membrane S09.2- ☑
  umbilical region S31.135 ☑
    with foreign body S31.145 ☑
  uvula — *see* Puncture, oral cavity
  vagina S31.43 ☑
    with foreign body S31.44 ☑

☑ **Additional Character Required** — Refer to the Tabular List for Character Selection   ⬙ **Subterms under main terms may continue to next column or page**

Puncture — *continued*
  vocal cords S11.033 ☑
    with foreign body S11.034 ☑
  vulva S31.43 ☑
    with foreign body S31.44 ☑
  wrist S61.539 ☑
    with
      foreign body S61.549 ☑
    left S61.532 ☑
      with
        foreign body S61.542 ☑
    right S61.531 ☑
      with
        foreign body S61.541 ☑
PUO (pyrexia of unknown origin) R50.9
Pupillary membrane (persistent) Q13.89
Pupillotonia — *see* Anomaly, pupil, function, tonic pupil
Purpura D69.2
  abdominal D69.0
  allergic D69.0
  anaphylactoid D69.0
  annularis telangiectodes L81.7
  arthritic D69.0
  autoerythrocyte sensitization D69.2
  autoimmune D69.0
  bacterial D69.0
  Bateman's (senile) D69.2
  capillary fragility (hereditary) (idiopathic) D69.8
  cryoglobulinemic D89.1
  Devil's pinches D69.2
  fibrinolytic — *see* Fibrinolysis
  fulminans, fulminous D65
  gangrenous D65
  hemorrhagic, hemorrhagica D69.3
    not due to thrombocytopenia D69.0
  Henoch (-Schönlein) (allergic) D69.0
  hypergammaglobulinemic (benign) (Waldenström)
    D89.0
  idiopathic (thrombocytopenic) D69.3
    nonthrombocytopenic D69.0
  immune thrombocytopenic D69.3
  infectious D69.0
  malignant D69.0
  neonatorum P54.5
  nervosa D69.0
  newborn P54.5
  nonthrombocytopenic D69.2
    hemorrhagic D69.0
    idiopathic D69.0
  nonthrombopenic D69.2
  peliosis rheumatica D69.0
  posttransfusion (post-transfusion) (from (fresh) whole
    blood or blood products) D69.51
  primary D69.49
  red cell membrane sensitivity D69.2
  rheumatica D69.0
  Schönlein (-Henoch) (allergic) D69.0
  scorbutic E54 [D77]
  senile D69.2
  simplex D69.2
  symptomatica D69.0
  telangiectasia annularis L81.7
  thrombocytopenic D69.49
    congenital D69.42
    hemorrhagic D69.3
    hereditary D69.42
    idiopathic D69.3
    immune D69.3
    neonatal, transitory P61.0
    thrombotic M31.1
  thrombohemolytic — *see* Fibrinolysis
  thrombolytic — *see* Fibrinolysis
  thrombopenic D69.49
  thrombotic, thrombocytopenic M31.1
  toxic D69.0
  vascular D69.0
  visceral symptoms D69.0
Purpuric spots R23.3
Purulent — *see* condition
Pus
  in
    stool R19.5
    urine N39.0
  tube (rupture) — *see* Salpingo-oophoritis
Pustular rash L08.0
Pustule (nonmalignant) L08.9
  malignant A22.0
Pustulosis palmaris et plantaris L40.3

Putnam (-Dana) **disease or syndrome** — *see* Degeneration, combined
Putrescent pulp (dental) K04.1
Pyarthritis, pyarthrosis — *see* Arthritis, pyogenic or pyemic
  tuberculous — *see* Tuberculosis, joint
Pyelectasis — *see* Hydronephrosis
Pyelitis (congenital) (uremic) (*see also* Pyelonephritis)
  with
    calculus — *see* category N20 ☑
      with hydronephrosis N13.2
    contracted kidney N11.9
  acute N10
  chronic N11.9
    with calculus — *see* category N20 ☑
      with hydronephrosis N13.2
  cystica N28.84
  puerperal (postpartum) O86.21
  tuberculous A18.11
Pyelocystitis — *see* Pyelonephritis
Pyelonephritis (*see also* Nephritis, tubulo-interstitial)
  with
    calculus — *see* category N20 ☑
      with hydronephrosis N13.2
    contracted kidney N11.9
  acute N10
  calculous — *see* category N20 ☑
    with hydronephrosis N13.2
  chronic N11.9
    with calculus — *see* category N20 ☑
      with hydronephrosis N13.2
    associated with ureteral obstruction or stricture
      N11.1
    nonobstructive N11.8
      with reflux (vesicoureteral) N11.0
    obstructive N11.1
    specified NEC N11.8
  in (due to)
    brucellosis A23.9 [N16]
    cryoglobulinemia (mixed) D89.1 [N16]
    cystinosis E72.04
    diphtheria A36.84
    glycogen storage disease E74.09 [N16]
    leukemia NEC C95.9- ☑ [N16]
    lymphoma NEC C85.90 [N16]
    multiple myeloma C90.0- ☑ [N16]
    obstruction N11.1
    Salmonella infection A02.25
    sarcoidosis D86.84
    sepsis A41.9 [N16]
    Sjögren's disease M35.04
    toxoplasmosis B58.83
    transplant rejection T86.91 [N16]
    Wilson's disease E83.01 [N16]
  nonobstructive N12
    with reflux (vesicoureteral) N11.0
    chronic N11.8
  syphilitic A52.75
Pyelonephrosis (obstructive) N11.1
  chronic N11.9
Pyelophlebitis I80.8
Pyeloureteritis cystica N28.85
Pyemia, pyemic (fever) (infection) (purulent) (*see also* Sepsis)
  joint — *see* Arthritis, pyogenic or pyemic
  liver K75.1
  pneumococcal A40.3
  portal K75.1
  postvaccinal T88.0 ☑
  puerperal, postpartum, childbirth O85
  specified organism NEC A41.89
  tuberculous — *see* Tuberculosis, miliary
Pygopagus Q89.4
Pyknoepilepsy (idiopathic) — *see* Pyknolepsy
Pyknolepsy G40.A09 (*following* G40.3)
  intractable G40.A19 (*following* G40.3)
    with status epilepticus G40.A11 (*following* G40.3)
    without status epilepticus G40.A19 (*following* G40.3)
  not intractable G40.A09 (*following* G40.3)
    with status epilepticus G40.A01 (*following* G40.3)
    without status epilepticus G40.A09 (*following* G40.3)
Pylephlebitis K75.1
Pyle's syndrome Q78.5
Pylethrombophlebitis K75.1
Pylethrombosis K75.1
Pyloritis K29.90
  with bleeding K29.91
Pylorospasm (reflex) **NEC** K31.3

Pylorospasm (reflex) **NEC** — *continued*
  congenital or infantile Q40.0
  neurotic F45.8
  newborn Q40.0
  psychogenic F45.8
Pylorus, pyloric — *see* condition
Pyoarthrosis — *see* Arthritis, pyogenic or pyemic
Pyocele
  mastoid — *see* Mastoiditis, acute
  sinus (accessory) — *see* Sinusitis
  turbinate (bone) J32.9
  urethra (*see also* Urethritis) N34.0
Pyocolpos — *see* Vaginitis
Pyocystitis N30.80
  with hematuria N30.81
Pyoderma, pyodermia L08.0
  gangrenosum L88
  newborn P39.4
  phagedenic L88
  vegetans L08.81
Pyodermatitis L08.0
  vegetans L08.81
Pyogenic — *see* condition
Pyohydronephrosis N13.6
Pyometra, pyometrium, pyometritis — *see* Endometritis
Pyomyositis (tropical) — *see* Myositis, infective
Pyonephritis N12
Pyonephrosis N13.6
  tuberculous A18.11
Pyo-oophoritis — *see* Salpingo-oophoritis
Pyo-ovarium — *see* Salpingo-oophoritis
Pyopericarditis, pyopericardium I30.1
Pyophlebitis — *see* Phlebitis
Pyopneumopericardium I30.1
Pyopneumothorax (infective) J86.9
  with fistula J86.0
  tuberculous NEC A15.6
Pyosalpinx, pyosalpingitis (*see also* Salpingo-oophoritis)
Pyothorax J86.9
  with fistula J86.0
  tuberculous NEC A15.6
Pyoureter N28.89
  tuberculous A18.11
Pyramidopallidonigral syndrome G20
Pyrexia (of unknown origin) R50.9
  atmospheric T67.0 ☑
  during labor NEC O75.2
  heat T67.0 ☑
  newborn P81.9
    environmentally-induced P81.0
  persistent R50.9
  puerperal O86.4
Pyroglobulinemia NEC E88.09
Pyromania F63.1
Pyrosis R12
Pyuria (bacterial) N39.0

Q

Q fever A78
  with pneumonia A78
Quadricuspid aortic valve Q23.8
Quadrilateral fever A78
Quadriparesis — *see* Quadriplegia
  meaning muscle weakness M62.81
Quadriplegia G82.50
  complete
    C1-C4 level G82.51
    C5-C7 level G82.53
  congenital (cerebral) (spinal) G80.8
    spastic G80.0
  embolic (current episode) I63.4- ☑
  functional R53.2
  incomplete
    C1-C4 level G82.52
    C5-C7 level G82.54
  thrombotic (current episode) I63.3- ☑
  traumatic — *code to* injury with seventh character S
    current episode — *see* Injury, spinal (cord), cervical
Quadruplet, pregnancy — *see* Pregnancy, quadruplet
Quarrelsomeness F60.3
Queensland fever A77.3
Quervain's disease M65.4
  thyroid E06.1
Queyrat's erythroplasia D07.4

Queyrat's erythroplasia — *continued*
  penis D07.4
  specified site — *see* Neoplasm, skin, in situ
  unspecified site D07.4
Quincke's disease or edema T78.3 ☑
  hereditary D84.1
Quinsy (gangrenous) J36
Quintan fever A79.0
Quintuplet, pregnancy — *see* Pregnancy, quintuplet

R

Rabbit fever — *see* Tularemia
Rabies A82.9
  contact Z20.3
  exposure to Z20.3
  inoculation reaction — *see* Complications, vaccination
  sylvatic A82.0
  urban A82.1
Rachischisis — *see* Spina bifida
Rachitic (*see also* condition)
  deformities of spine (late effect) (sequelae) E64.3
  pelvis (late effect) (sequelae) E64.3
    with disproportion (fetopelvic) O33.0
      causing obstructed labor O65.0
Rachitis, rachitism (acute) (tarda) (*see also* Rickets)
  renalis N25.0
  sequelae E64.3
Radial nerve — *see* condition
Radiation
  burn — *see* Burn
  effects NOS T66 ☑
  sickness NOS T66 ☑
  therapy, encounter for Z51.0
Radiculitis (pressure) (vertebrogenic) — *see* Radiculopathy
Radiculomyelitis (*see also* Encephalitis)
  toxic, due to
    Clostridium tetani A35
    Corynebacterium diphtheriae A36.82
Radiculopathy M54.10
  cervical region M54.12
  cervicothoracic region M54.13
  due to
    disc disorder
      C3 M50.11
      C4 M50.11
      C5 M50.121
      C6 M50.122
      C7 M50.123
    displacement of intervertebral disc — *see* Disorder, disc, with, radiculopathy
  leg M54.1- ☑
  lumbar region M54.16
  lumbosacral region M54.17
  occipito-atlanto-axial region M54.11
  postherpetic B02.29
  sacrococcygeal region M54.18
  syphilitic A52.11
  thoracic region (with visceral pain) M54.14
  thoracolumbar region M54.15
Radiodermal burns (acute, chronic, or occupational) — *see* Burn
Radiodermatitis L58.9
  acute L58.0
  chronic L58.1
Radiotherapy session Z51.0
RAEB (refractory anemia with excess blasts) D46.2- ☑
Rage, meaning rabies — *see* Rabies
Ragpicker's disease A22.1
Ragsorter's disease A22.1
Raillietiniasis B71.8
Railroad neurosis F48.8
Railway spine F48.8
Raised (*see also* Elevated)
  antibody titer R76.0
Rake teeth, tooth M26.39
Rales R09.89
Ramifying renal pelvis Q63.8
Ramsay-Hunt disease or syndrome (*see also* Hunt's disease) B02.21
  meaning dyssynergia cerebellaris myoclonica G11.1
Ranula K11.6
  congenital Q38.4
Rape
  adult
    confirmed T74.21 ☑

Rape — *continued*
  adult — *continued*
    suspected T76.21 ☑
    alleged, observation or examination, ruled out
      adult Z04.41
      child Z04.42
    child
      confirmed T74.22 ☑
      suspected T76.22 ☑
Rapid
  feeble pulse, due to shock, following injury T79.4 ☑
  heart (beat) R00.0
    psychogenic F45.8
  second stage (delivery) O62.3
  time-zone change syndrome G47.25
Rarefaction, bone — *see* Disorder, bone, density and structure, specified NEC
Rash (toxic) R21
  canker A38.9
  diaper L22
  drug (internal use) L27.0
    contact (*see also* Dermatitis, due to, drugs, external) L25.1
  following immunization T88.1 ☑
  food — *see* Dermatitis, due to, food
  heat L74.0
  napkin (psoriasiform) L22
  nettle — *see* Urticaria
  pustular L08.0
  rose R21
    epidemic B06.9
  scarlet A38.9
  serum (*see also* Reaction, serum) T80.69 ☑
  wandering tongue K14.1
Rasmussen aneurysm — *see* Tuberculosis, pulmonary
Rasmussen encephalitis G04.81
Rat-bite fever A25.9
  due to Streptobacillus moniliformis A25.1
  spirochetal (morsus muris) A25.0
Rathke's pouch tumor D44.3
Raymond (-Céstan) **syndrome** I65.8
Raynaud's disease, phenomenon or syndrome (secondary) I73.00
  with gangrene (symmetric) I73.01
RDS (newborn) (type I) P22.0
  type II P22.1
Reaction (*see also* Disorder)
  withdrawing, child or adolescent F93.8
  adaptation — *see* Disorder, adjustment
  adjustment (anxiety) (conduct disorder) (depressiveness) (distress) — *see* Disorder, adjustment
    with
      mutism, elective (child) (adolescent) F94.0
  adverse
    food (any) (ingested) NEC T78.1 ☑
      anaphylactic — *see* Shock, anaphylactic, due to food
  affective — *see* Disorder, mood
  allergic — *see* Allergy
  anaphylactic — *see* Shock, anaphylactic
  anaphylactoid — *see* Shock, anaphylactic
  anesthesia — *see* Anesthesia, complication
  antitoxin (prophylactic) (therapeutic) — *see* Complications, vaccination
  anxiety F41.1
  Arthus — *see* Arthus' phenomenon
  asthenic F48.8
  combat and operational stress F43.0
  compulsive F42.8
  conversion F44.9
  crisis, acute F43.0
  deoxyribonuclease (DNA) (DNase) hypersensitivity D69.2
  depressive (single episode) F32.9
    affective (single episode) F31.4
      recurrent episode F33.9
    neurotic F34.1
    psychoneurotic F34.1
    psychotic F32.3
    recurrent — *see* Disorder, depressive, recurrent
  dissociative F44.9
  drug NEC T88.7 ☑
    addictive — *see* Dependence, drug
      transmitted via placenta or breast milk — *see* Absorption, drug, addictive, through placenta
    allergic — *see* Allergy, drug
    lichenoid L43.2

Reaction — *continued*
  drug — *continued*
    newborn P93.8
      gray baby syndrome P93.0
    overdose or poisoning (by accident) — *see* Table of Drugs and Chemicals, by drug, poisoning
    photoallergic L56.1
    phototoxic L56.0
    withdrawal — *see* Dependence, by drug, with, withdrawal
      infant of dependent mother P96.1
      newborn P96.1
    wrong substance given or taken (by accident) — *see* Table of Drugs and Chemicals, by drug, poisoning
  fear F40.9
    child (abnormal) F93.8
  febrile nonhemolytic transfusion (FNHTR) R50.84
  fluid loss, cerebrospinal G97.1
  foreign
    body NEC — *see* Granuloma, foreign body
      in operative wound (inadvertently left) — *see* Foreign body, accidentally left during a procedure
    substance accidentally left during a procedure (chemical) (powder) (talc) T81.60 ☑
      aseptic peritonitis T81.61 ☑
      body or object (instrument) (sponge) (swab) — *see* Foreign body, accidentally left during a procedure
      specified reaction NEC T81.69 ☑
  grief — *see* Disorder, adjustment
  Herxheimer's R68.89
  hyperkinetic — *see* Hyperkinesia
  hypochondriacal F45.20
  hypoglycemic, due to insulin E16.0
    with coma (diabetic) — *see* Diabetes, coma
    nondiabetic E15
    therapeutic misadventure — *see* subcategory T38.3 ☑
  hypomanic F30.8
  hysterical F44.9
  immunization — *see* Complications, vaccination
  incompatibility
    ABO blood group (infusion) (transfusion) — *see* Complication(s), transfusion, incompatibility reaction, ABO
    delayed serologic T80.39 ☑
    minor blood group (Duffy) (E) (K) (Kell) (Kidd) (Lewis) (M) (N) (P) (S) T80.89 ☑
    Rh (factor) (infusion) (transfusion) — *see* Complication(s), transfusion, incompatibility reaction, Rh (factor)
  inflammatory — *see* Infection
  infusion — *see* Complications, infusion
  inoculation (immune serum) — *see* Complications, vaccination
  insulin T38.3- ☑
  involutional psychotic — *see* Disorder, depressive
  leukemoid D72.823
    basophilic D72.823
    lymphocytic D72.823
    monocytic D72.823
    myelocytic D72.823
    neutrophilic D72.823
  LSD (acute)
    due to drug abuse — *see* Abuse, drug, hallucinogen
    due to drug dependence — *see* Dependence, drug, hallucinogen
  lumbar puncture G97.1
  manic-depressive — *see* Disorder, bipolar
  neurasthenic F48.8
  neurogenic — *see* Neurosis
  neurotic F48.9
  neurotic-depressive F34.1
  nitritoid — *see* Crisis, nitritoid
  nonspecific
    to
      cell mediated immunity measurement of gamma interferon antigen response without active tuberculosis R76.12
      QuantiFERON-TB test (QFT) without active tuberculosis R76.12
      tuberculin test (*see also* Reaction, tuberculin skin test) R76.11
  obsessive-compulsive F42.8
  organic, acute or subacute — *see* Delirium
  paranoid (acute) F23

☑ **Additional Character Required — Refer to the Tabular List for Character Selection**   ☑ Subterms under main terms may continue to next column or page

Reaction — *continued*
  paranoid — *continued*
    chronic F22
    senile F03 ☑
  passive dependency F60.7
  phobic F40.9
  post-traumatic stress, uncomplicated Z73.3
  psychogenic F99
  psychoneurotic (*see also* Neurosis)
    compulsive F42.8
    depersonalization F48.1
    depressive F34.1
    hypochondriacal F45.20
    neurasthenic F48.8
    obsessive F42.8
  psychophysiologic — *see* Disorder, somatoform
  psychosomatic — *see* Disorder, somatoform
  psychotic — *see* Psychosis
  scarlet fever toxin — *see* Complications, vaccination
  schizophrenic F23
    acute (brief) (undifferentiated) F23
    latent F21
    undifferentiated (acute) (brief) F23
  serological for syphilis — *see* Serology for syphilis
  serum T80.69 ☑
    anaphylactic (immediate) (*see also* Shock, anaphylactic) T80.59 ☑
    specified reaction NEC
      due to
        administration of blood and blood products T80.61 ☑
        immunization T80.62 ☑
        serum specified NEC T80.69 ☑
        vaccination T80.62 ☑
  situational — *see* Disorder, adjustment
  somatization — *see* Disorder, somatoform
  spinal puncture G97.1
  stress (severe) F43.9
    acute (agitation) ("daze") (disorientation) (disturbance of consciousness) (flight reaction) (fugue) F43.0
    specified NEC F43.8
  surgical procedure — *see* Complications, surgical procedure
  tetanus antitoxin — *see* Complications, vaccination
  toxic, to local anesthesia T88.59 ☑
    in labor and delivery O74.4
    in pregnancy O29.3X- ☑
    postpartum, puerperal O89.3
  toxin-antitoxin — *see* Complications, vaccination
  transfusion (blood) (bone marrow) (lymphocytes) (allergic) — *see* Complications, transfusion
  tuberculin skin test, abnormal R76.11
  vaccination (any) — *see* Complications, vaccination
Reactive airway disease — *see* Asthma
Reactive depression — *see* Reaction, depressive
Rearrangement
  chromosomal
    balanced (in) Q95.9
      abnormal individual (autosomal) Q95.2
        non-sex (autosomal) chromosomes Q95.2
        sex/non-sex chromosomes Q95.3
      specified NEC Q95.8
Recalcitrant patient — *see* Noncompliance
Recanalization, thrombus — *see* Thrombosis
Recession, receding
  chamber angle (eye) H21.55- ☑
  chin M26.09
  gingival (postinfective) (postoperative)
    generalized K06.020
      minimal K06.021
      moderate K06.022
      severe K06.023
    localized K06.010
      minimal K06.011
      moderate K06.012
      severe K06.013
Recklinghausen disease Q85.01
  bones E21.0
Reclus' disease (cystic) — *see* Mastopathy, cystic
Recrudescent typhus (fever) A75.1
Recruitment, auditory H93.21- ☑
Rectalgia K62.89
Rectitis K62.89
Rectocele
  female (without uterine prolapse) N81.6
    with uterine prolapse N81.4

Rectocele — *continued*
  female — *continued*
    with uterine prolapse — *continued*
      incomplete N81.2
  in pregnancy — *see* Pregnancy, complicated by, abnormal, pelvic organs or tissues NEC
  male K62.3
Rectosigmoid junction — *see* condition
Rectosigmoiditis K63.89
  ulcerative (chronic) K51.30
    with
      complication K51.319
        abscess K51.314
        fistula K51.313
        obstruction K51.312
        rectal bleeding K51.311
        specified NEC K51.318
Rectourethral — *see* condition
Rectovaginal — *see* condition
Rectovesical — *see* condition
Rectum, rectal — *see* condition
Recurrent — *see* condition
  pregnancy loss — *see* Loss (of), pregnancy, recurrent
Red bugs B88.0
Red tide (*see also* Table of Drugs and Chemicals) T65.82- ☑
Red-cedar lung or pneumonitis J67.8
Reduced
  mobility Z74.09
  ventilatory or vital capacity R94.2
Redundant, redundancy
  anus (congenital) Q43.8
  clitoris N90.89
  colon (congenital) Q43.8
  foreskin (congenital) N47.8
  intestine (congenital) Q43.8
  labia N90.69
  organ or site, congenital NEC — *see* Accessory
  panniculus (abdominal) E65
  prepuce (congenital) N47.8
  pylorus K31.89
  rectum (congenital) Q43.8
  scrotum N50.89
  sigmoid (congenital) Q43.8
  skin L98.7
    and subcutaneous tissue L98.7
    of face L57.4
      eyelids — *see* Blepharochalasis
  stomach K31.89
Reduplication — *see* Duplication
Reflex R29.2
  hyperactive gag J39.2
  pupillary, abnormal — *see* Anomaly, pupil, function
  vasoconstriction I73.9
  vasovagal R55
Reflux K21.9
  acid K21.9
  esophageal K21.9
    with esophagitis K21.0
    newborn P78.83
  gastroesophageal K21.9
    with esophagitis K21.0
  mitral — *see* Insufficiency, mitral
  ureteral — *see* Reflux, vesicoureteral
  vesicoureteral (with scarring) N13.70
    with
      nephropathy N13.729
        with hydroureter N13.739
          bilateral N13.732
          unilateral N13.731
        bilateral N13.722
        unilateral N13.721
        without hydroureter N13.729
          bilateral N13.722
          unilateral N13.721
      pyelonephritis (chronic) N11.0
    congenital Q62.7
    without nephropathy N13.71
Reforming, artificial openings — *see* Attention to, artificial, opening
Refractive error — *see* Disorder, refraction
Refsum's disease or syndrome G60.1
Refusal of
  food, psychogenic F50.89
  treatment (because of) Z53.20
    left against medical advice (AMA) Z53.21
    patient's decision NEC Z53.29
    reasons of belief or group pressure Z53.1

Regional — *see* condition
Regurgitation R11.10
  aortic (valve) — *see* Insufficiency, aortic
  food (*see also* Vomiting)
    with reswallowing — *see* Rumination
    newborn P92.1
  gastric contents — *see* Vomiting
  heart — *see* Endocarditis
  mitral (valve) — *see* Insufficiency, mitral
    congenital Q23.3
  myocardial — *see* Endocarditis
  pulmonary (valve) (heart) I37.1
    congenital Q22.2
    syphilitic A52.03
  tricuspid — *see* Insufficiency, tricuspid
  valve, valvular — *see* Endocarditis
    congenital Q24.8
  vesicoureteral — *see* Reflux, vesicoureteral
Reichmann's disease or syndrome K31.89
Reifenstein syndrome E34.52
Reinsertion
  implantable subdermal contraceptive Z30.46
  intrauterine contraceptive device Z30.433
Reiter's disease, syndrome, or urethritis M02.30
  ankle M02.37- ☑
  elbow M02.32- ☑
  foot joint M02.37- ☑
  hand joint M02.34- ☑
  hip M02.35- ☑
  knee M02.36- ☑
  multiple site M02.39
  shoulder M02.31- ☑
  vertebra M02.38
  wrist M02.33- ☑
Rejection
  food, psychogenic F50.89
  transplant T86.91
    bone T86.830
      marrow T86.01
    cornea T86.840
    heart T86.21
      with lung(s) T86.31
    intestine T86.850
    kidney T86.11
    liver T86.41
    lung(s) T86.810
      with heart T86.31
    organ (immune or nonimmune cause) T86.91
    pancreas T86.890
    skin (allograft) (autograft) T86.820
    specified NEC T86.890
    stem cell (peripheral blood) (umbilical cord) T86.5
Relapsing fever A68.9
  Carter's (Asiatic) A68.1
  Dutton's (West African) A68.1
  Koch's A68.9
  louse-borne (epidemic) A68.0
  Novy's (American) A68.1
  Obermeyers's (European) A68.0
  Spirillum A68.9
  tick-borne (endemic) A68.1
Relationship
  occlusal
    open anterior M26.220
    open posterior M26.221
Relaxation
  anus (sphincter) K62.89
    psychogenic F45.8
  arch (foot) (*see also* Deformity, limb, flat foot)
  back ligaments — *see* Instability, joint, spine
  bladder (sphincter) N31.2
  cardioesophageal K21.9
  cervix — *see* Incompetency, cervix
  diaphragm J98.6
  joint (capsule) (ligament) (paralytic) — *see* Flail, joint
    congenital NEC Q74.8
  lumbosacral (joint) — *see* subcategory M53.2 ☑
  pelvic floor N81.89
  perineum N81.89
  posture R29.3
  rectum (sphincter) K62.89
  sacroiliac (joint) — *see* subcategory M53.2 ☑
  scrotum N50.89
  urethra (sphincter) N36.44
  vesical N31.2
Release from prison, anxiety concerning Z65.2
Remains
  canal of Cloquet Q14.0

Remains — continued
  capsule (opaque) Q14.8
Remittent fever (malarial) B54
Remnant
  canal of Cloquet Q14.0
  capsule (opaque) Q14.8
  cervix, cervical stump (acquired) (postoperative) N88.8
  cystic duct, postcholecystectomy K91.5
  fingernail L60.8
    congenital Q84.6
  meniscus, knee — see Derangement, knee, meniscus, specified NEC
  thyroglossal duct Q89.2
  tonsil J35.8
    infected (chronic) J35.01
  urachus Q64.4
Removal (from) (of)
  artificial
    arm Z44.00- ☑
      complete Z44.01- ☑
      partial Z44.02- ☑
    eye Z44.2- ☑
    leg Z44.10- ☑
      complete Z44.11- ☑
      partial Z44.12- ☑
  breast implant Z45.81 ☑
  cardiac pulse generator (battery) (end-of-life) Z45.010
  catheter (urinary) (indwelling) Z46.6
    from artificial opening — see Attention to, artificial, opening
    non-vascular Z46.82
    vascular NEC Z45.2
  device Z46.9
    contraceptive Z30.432
      implantable subdermal Z30.46
    implanted NEC Z45.89
    specified NEC Z46.89
  drains Z48.03
  dressing (nonsurgical) Z48.00
    surgical Z48.01
  external
    fixation device — code to fracture with seventh character D
    prosthesis, prosthetic device Z44.9
      breast Z44.3- ☑
      specified NEC Z44.8
  home in childhood (to foster home or institution) Z62.29
  ileostomy Z43.2
  insulin pump Z46.81
  myringotomy device (stent) (tube) Z45.82
  nervous system device NEC Z46.2
    brain neuropacemaker Z46.2
    visual substitution device Z46.2
      implanted Z45.31
  non-vascular catheter Z46.82
  organ, prophylactic (for neoplasia management) — see Prophylactic, organ removal
  orthodontic device Z46.4
  staples Z48.02
  stent
    ureteral Z46.6
  suture Z48.02
  urinary device Z46.6
  vascular access device or catheter Z45.2
Ren
  arcuatus Q63.1
  mobile, mobilis N28.89
    congenital Q63.8
  unguliformis Q63.1
Renal — see condition
Rendu-Osler-Weber disease or syndrome I78.0
Reninoma D41.0- ☑
Renon-Delille syndrome E23.3
Reovirus, as cause of disease classified elsewhere B97.5
Repeated falls NEC R29.6
Replaced chromosome by dicentric ring Q93.2
Replacement by artificial or mechanical device or prosthesis of
  bladder Z96.0
  blood vessel NEC Z95.828
  bone NEC Z96.7
  cochlea Z96.21
  coronary artery Z95.5
  eustachian tube Z96.29
  eye globe Z97.0
  heart Z95.812

Replacement by artificial or mechanical device or prosthesis of — continued
  heart — continued
    valve Z95.2
      prosthetic Z95.2
      specified NEC Z95.4
      xenogenic Z95.3
  intestine Z96.89
  joint Z96.60
    hip — see Presence, hip joint implant
    knee — see Presence, knee joint implant
    specified site NEC Z96.698
  larynx Z96.3
  lens Z96.1
  limb(s) — see Presence, artificial, limb
  mandible NEC (for tooth root implant(s)) Z96.5
  organ NEC Z96.89
  peripheral vessel NEC Z95.828
  stapes Z96.29
  teeth Z97.2
  tendon Z96.7
  tissue NEC Z96.89
  tooth root(s) Z96.5
  vessel NEC Z95.828
    coronary (artery) Z95.5
Request for expert evidence Z04.89
Reserve, decreased or low
  cardiac — see Disease, heart
  kidney N28.89
Residual (see also condition)
  ovary syndrome N99.83
  state, schizophrenic F20.5
  urine R39.198
Resistance, resistant (to)
  activated protein C D68.51
  complicating pregnancy O26.89 ☑
  insulin E88.81
  organism(s)
    to
      drug Z16.30
        aminoglycosides Z16.29
        amoxicillin Z16.11
        ampicillin Z16.11
        antibiotic(s) Z16.20
          multiple Z16.24
          specified NEC Z16.29
        antifungal Z16.32
        antimicrobial (single) Z16.30
          multiple Z16.35
          specified NEC Z16.39
        antimycobacterial (single) Z16.341
          multiple Z16.342
        antiparasitic Z16.31
        antiviral Z16.33
        beta lactam antibiotics Z16.10
          specified NEC Z16.19
        cephalosporins Z16.19
        extended beta lactamase (ESBL) Z16.12
        fluoroquinolones Z16.23
        macrolides Z16.29
        methicillin — see MRSA
        multiple drugs (MDRO)
          antibiotics Z16.24
          antimicrobial Z16.35
          antimycobacterials Z16.342
        penicillins Z16.11
        quinine (and related compounds) Z16.31
        quinolones Z16.23
        sulfonamides Z16.29
        tetracyclines Z16.29
        tuberculostatics (single) Z16.341
          multiple Z16.342
        vancomycin Z16.21
          related antibiotics Z16.22
  thyroid hormone E07.89
Resorption
  dental (roots) K03.3
    alveoli M26.79
  teeth (external) (internal) (pathological) (roots) K03.3
Respiration
  Cheyne-Stokes R06.3
  decreased due to shock, following injury T79.4 ☑
  disorder of, psychogenic F45.8
  insufficient, or poor R06.89
    newborn P28.5
  painful R07.1
  sighing, psychogenic F45.8
Respiratory (see also condition)

Respiratory — continued
  distress syndrome (newborn) (type I) P22.0
    type II P22.1
  syncytial virus, as cause of disease classified elsewhere B97.4
Respite care Z75.5
Response (drug)
  photoallergic L56.1
  phototoxic L56.0
Restenosis
  stent
    vascular
      end stent
        adjacent to stent — see Arteriosclerosis
        within the stent
          coronary T82.855 ☑
          peripheral T82.856 ☑
      in stent
        coronary vessel T82.855 ☑
        peripheral vessel T82.856 ☑
Restless legs (syndrome) G25.81
Restlessness R45.1
Restoration (of)
  dental
    aesthetically inadequate or displeasing K08.56
    defective K08.50
      specified NEC K08.59
    failure of marginal integrity K08.51
    failure of periodontal anatomical intergrity K08.54
    organ continuity from previous sterilization (tuboplasty) (vasoplasty) Z31.0
      aftercare Z31.42
    tooth (existing)
      contours biologically incompatible with oral health K08.54
      open margins K08.51
      overhanging K08.52
      poor aesthetic K08.56
      poor gingival margins K08.51
    unsatisfactory, of tooth K08.50
      specified NEC K08.59
Restorative material (dental)
  allergy to K08.55
  fractured K08.539
    with loss of material K08.531
    without loss of material K08.530
  unrepairable overhanging of K08.52
Restriction of housing space Z59.1
Rests, ovarian, in fallopian tube Q50.6
Restzustand (schizophrenic) F20.5
Retained (see also Retention)
  cholelithiasis following cholecystectomy K91.86
  foreign body fragments (type of) Z18.9
    acrylics Z18.2
    animal quill(s) or spines Z18.31
    cement Z18.83
    concrete Z18.83
    crystalline Z18.83
    depleted isotope Z18.09
    depleted uranium Z18.01
    diethylhexyl phthalates Z18.2
    glass Z18.81
    isocyanate Z18.2
    magnetic metal Z18.11
    metal Z18.10
    nonmagnectic metal Z18.12
    nontherapeutic radioactive Z18.09
    organic NEC Z18.39
    plastic Z18.2
    quill(s) (animal) Z18.31
    radioactive (nontherapeutic) NEC Z18.09
    specified NEC Z18.89
    spine(s) (animal) Z18.31
    stone Z18.83
    tooth (teeth) Z18.32
    wood Z18.33
  fragments (type of) Z18.9
    acrylics Z18.2
    animal quill(s) or spines Z18.31
    cement Z18.83
    concrete Z18.83
    crystalline Z18.83
    depleted isotope Z18.09
    depleted uranium Z18.01
    diethylhexyl phthalates Z18.2
    glass Z18.81
    isocyanate Z18.2
    magnetic metal Z18.11

☑ **Additional Character Required** — Refer to the Tabular List for Character Selection   ⑯ **Subterms under main terms may continue to next column or page**

Retained — *continued*
  fragments — *continued*
    metal Z18.10
    nonmagnectic metal Z18.12
    nontherapeutic radioactive Z18.09
    organic NEC Z18.39
    plastic Z18.2
    quill(s) (animal) Z18.31
    radioactive (nontherapeutic) NEC Z18.09
    specified NEC Z18.89
    spine(s) (animal) Z18.31
    stone Z18.83
    tooth (teeth) Z18.32
    wood Z18.33
  gallstones, following cholecystectomy K91.86
Retardation
  development, developmental, specific — *see* Disorder, developmental
  endochondral bone growth — *see* Disorder, bone, development or growth
  growth R62.50
    due to malnutrition E45
  mental — *see* Disability, intellectual
  motor function, specific F82
  physical (child) R62.52
    due to malnutrition E45
  reading (specific) F81.0
  spelling (specific) (without reading disorder) F81.81
Retching — *see* Vomiting
Retention (*see also* Retained)
  bladder — *see* Retention, urine
  carbon dioxide E87.2
  cholelithiasis following cholecystectomy K91.86
  cyst — *see* Cyst
  dead
    fetus (at or near term) (mother) O36.4 ☑
      early fetal death O02.1
      ovum O02.0
  decidua (fragments) (following delivery) (with hemorrhage) O72.2
    without hemorrhage O73.1
  deciduous tooth K00.6
  dental root K08.3
  fecal — *see* Constipation
  fetus
    dead O36.4 ☑
      early O02.1
  fluid R60.9
  foreign body (*see also* Foreign body, retained)
    current trauma — *code as* Foreign body, by site or type
  gallstones, following cholecystectomy K91.86
  gastric K31.89
  intrauterine contraceptive device, in pregnancy — *see* Pregnancy, complicated by, retention, intrauterine device
  membranes (complicating delivery) (with hemorrhage) O72.2
    with abortion — *see* Abortion, by type
    without hemorrhage O73.1
  meniscus — *see* Derangement, meniscus
  menses N94.89
  milk (puerperal, postpartum) O92.79
  nitrogen, extrarenal R39.2
  ovary syndrome N99.83
  placenta (total) (with hemorrhage) O72.0
    without hemorrhage O73.0
    portions or fragments (with hemorrhage) O72.2
      without hemorrhage O73.1
  products of conception
    early pregnancy (dead fetus) O02.1
    following
      delivery (with hemorrhage) O72.2
        without hemorrhage O73.1
  secundines (following delivery) (with hemorrhage) O72.2
    without hemorrhage O73.0
    complicating puerperium (delayed hemorrhage) O72.2
    partial O72.2
      without hemorrhage O73.1
  smegma, clitoris N90.89
  urine R33.9
    due to hyperplasia (hypertrophy) of prostate — *see* Hyperplasia, prostate
    drug-induced R33.0
    organic R33.8
      drug-induced R33.0

Retention — *continued*
  urine — *continued*
    psychogenic F45.8
    specified NEC R33.8
  water (in tissues) — *see* Edema
Reticulation, dust — *see* Pneumoconiosis
Reticulocytosis R70.1
Reticuloendotheliosis
  acute infantile C96.0
  leukemic C91.4- ☑
  nonlipid C96.0
Reticulohistiocytoma (giant-cell) D76.3
Reticuloid, actinic L57.1
Reticulosis (skin)
  acute of infancy C96.0
  hemophagocytic, familial D76.1
  histiocytic medullary C96.A (*following* C96.6)
  lipomelanotic I89.8
  malignant (midline) C86.0
  polymorphic C83.8- ☑
  Sézary — *see* Sézary disease
Retina, retinal (*see also* condition)
  dark area D49.81
Retinitis (*see also* Inflammation, chorioretinal)
  albuminurica N18.9 [H32]
  diabetic — *see* Diabetes, retinitis
  disciformis — *see* Degeneration, macula
  focal — *see* Inflammation, chorioretinal, focal
  gravidarum — *see* Pregnancy, complicated by, specified pregnancy-related condition NEC
  juxtapapillaris — *see* Inflammation, chorioretinal, focal, juxtapapillary
  luetic — *see* Retinitis, syphilitic
  pigmentosa H35.52
  proliferans — *see* Disorder, globe, degenerative, specified type NEC
  proliferating — *see* Disorder, globe, degenerative, specified type NEC
  renal N18.9 [H32]
  syphilitic (early) (secondary) A51.43
    central, recurrent A52.71
    congenital (early) A50.01 [H32]
    late A52.71
  tuberculous A18.53
Retinoblastoma C69.2- ☑
  differentiated C69.2- ☑
  undifferentiated C69.2- ☑
Retinochoroiditis (*see also* Inflammation, chorioretinal)
  disseminated — *see* Inflammation, chorioretinal, disseminated
    syphilitic A52.71
  focal — *see* Inflammation, chorioretinal
  juxtapapillaris — *see* Inflammation, chorioretinal, focal, juxtapapillary
Retinopathy (background) H35.00
  arteriosclerotic I70.8 [H35.0-] ☑
  atherosclerotic I70.8 [H35.0-] ☑
  central serous — *see* Chorioretinopathy, central serous
  Coats H35.02- ☑
  diabetic — *see* Diabetes, retinopathy
  exudative H35.02- ☑
  hypertensive H35.03- ☑
  in (due to)
    diabetes — *see* Diabetes, retinopathy
    sickle-cell disorders D57.- ☑ [H36]
  of prematurity H35.10- ☑
    stage 0 H35.11- ☑
    stage 1 H35.12- ☑
    stage 2 H35.13- ☑
    stage 3 H35.14- ☑
    stage 4 H35.15- ☑
    stage 5 H35.16- ☑
  pigmentary, congenital — *see* Dystrophy, retina
  proliferative NEC H35.2- ☑
    diabetic — *see* Diabetes, retinopathy, proliferative
    sickle-cell D57.- ☑ [H36]
  solar H31.02- ☑
Retinoschisis H33.10- ☑
  congenital Q14.1
  specified type NEC H33.19- ☑
Retortamoniasis A07.8
Retractile testis Q55.22
Retraction
  cervix — *see* Retroversion, uterus
  drum (membrane) — *see* Disorder, tympanic membrane, specified NEC
  finger — *see* Deformity, finger

Retraction — *continued*
  lid H02.539
    left H02.536
      lower H02.535
      upper H02.534
    right H02.533
      lower H02.532
      upper H02.531
  lung J98.4
  mediastinum J98.59
  nipple N64.53
    associated with
      lactation O92.03
      pregnancy O92.01- ☑
      puerperium O92.02
    congenital Q83.8
  palmar fascia M72.0
  pleura — *see* Pleurisy
  ring, uterus (Bandl's) (pathological) O62.4
  sternum (congenital) Q76.7
    acquired M95.4
  uterus — *see* Retroversion, uterus
  valve (heart) — *see* Endocarditis
Retrobulbar — *see* condition
Retrocecal — *see* condition
Retrocession — *see* Retroversion
Retrodisplacement — *see* Retroversion
Retroflection, retroflexion — *see* Retroversion
Retrognathia, retrognathism (mandibular) (maxillary) M26.19
Retrograde menstruation N92.5
Retroperineal — *see* condition
Retroperitoneal — *see* condition
Retroperitonitis K68.9
Retropharyngeal — *see* condition
Retroplacental — *see* condition
Retroposition — *see* Retroversion
Retroprosthetic membrane T85.398 ☑
Retrosternal thyroid (congenital) Q89.2
Retroversion, retroverted
  cervix — *see* Retroversion, uterus
  female NEC — *see* Retroversion, uterus
  iris H21.89
  testis (congenital) Q55.29
  uterus (acquired) (acute) (any degree) (asymptomatic) (cervix) (postinfectional) (postpartal, old) N85.4
    congenital Q51.818
    in pregnancy O34.53- ☑
Retrovirus, as cause of disease classified elsewhere B97.30
  human
    immunodeficiency, type 2 (HIV 2) B97.35
    T-cell lymphotropic
      type I (HTLV-I) B97.33
      type II (HTLV-II) B97.34
  lentivirus B97.31
  oncovirus B97.32
  specified NEC B97.39
Retrusion, premaxilla (developmental) M26.09
Rett's disease or syndrome F84.2
Reverse peristalsis R19.2
Reye's syndrome G93.7
Rh (factor)
  hemolytic disease (newborn) P55.0
  incompatibility, immunization or sensitization
    affecting management of pregnancy NEC O36.09- ☑
      anti-D antibody O36.01- ☑
    newborn P55.0
    transfusion reaction — *see* Complication(s), transfusion, incompatibility reaction, Rh (factor)
  negative mother affecting newborn P55.0
  titer elevated — *see* Complication(s), transfusion, incompatibility reaction, Rh (factor)
  transfusion reaction — *see* Complication(s), transfusion, incompatibility reaction, Rh (factor)
Rhabdomyolysis (idiopathic) NEC M62.82
  traumatic T79.6 ☑
Rhabdomyoma (*see also* Neoplasm, connective tissue, benign)
  adult — *see* Neoplasm, connective tissue, benign
  fetal — *see* Neoplasm, connective tissue, benign
  glycogenic — *see* Neoplasm, connective tissue, benign
Rhabdomyosarcoma (any type) — *see* Neoplasm, connective tissue, malignant
Rhabdosarcoma — *see* Rhabdomyosarcoma
Rhesus (factor) **incompatibility** — *see* Rh, incompatibility

Rheumatic (acute) (subacute) (chronic)
  adherent pericarditis I09.2
  coronary arteritis I01.9
  degeneration, myocardium I09.0
  fever (acute) — see Fever, rheumatic
  heart — see Disease, heart, rheumatic
  myocardial degeneration — see Degeneration, myocardium
  myocarditis (chronic) (inactive) (with chorea) I09.0
    active or acute I01.2
      with chorea (acute) (rheumatic) (Sydenham's) I02.0
  pancarditis, acute I01.8
    with chorea (acute) (rheumatic) Sydenham's) I02.0
  pericarditis (active) (acute) (with effusion) (with pneumonia) I01.0
    with chorea (acute) (rheumatic) (Sydenham's) I02.0
    chronic or inactive I09.2
  pneumonia I00 [J17]
  torticollis M43.6
  typhoid fever A01.09
Rheumatism (articular) (neuralgic) (nonarticular) M79.0
  gout — see Arthritis, rheumatoid
  intercostal, meaning Tietze's disease M94.0
  palindromic (any site) M12.30
    ankle M12.37- ☑
    elbow M12.32- ☑
    foot joint M12.37- ☑
    hand joint M12.34- ☑
    hip M12.35- ☑
    knee M12.36- ☑
    multiple site M12.39
    shoulder M12.31- ☑
    specified joint NEC M12.38
    vertebrae M12.38
    wrist M12.33- ☑
  sciatic M54.4- ☑
Rheumatoid (see also condition)
  arthritis (see also Arthritis, rheumatoid)
    with involvement of organs NEC M05.60
      ankle M05.67- ☑
      elbow M05.62- ☑
      foot joint M05.67- ☑
      hand joint M05.64- ☑
      hip M05.65- ☑
      knee M05.66- ☑
      multiple site M05.69
      shoulder M05.61- ☑
      vertebra — see Spondylitis, ankylosing
      wrist M05.63- ☑
    seronegative — see Arthritis, rheumatoid, seronegative
    seropositive — see Arthritis, rheumatoid, seropositive
  carditis M05.30
    ankle M05.37- ☑
    elbow M05.32- ☑
    foot joint M05.37- ☑
    hand joint M05.34- ☑
    hip M05.35- ☑
    knee M05.36- ☑
    multiple site M05.39
    shoulder M05.31- ☑
    vertebra — see Spondylitis, ankylosing
    wrist M05.33- ☑
  endocarditis — see Rheumatoid, carditis
  lung (disease) M05.10
    ankle M05.17- ☑
    elbow M05.12- ☑
    foot joint M05.17- ☑
    hand joint M05.14- ☑
    hip M05.15- ☑
    knee M05.16- ☑
    multiple site M05.19
    shoulder M05.11- ☑
    vertebra — see Spondylitis, ankylosing
    wrist M05.13- ☑
  myocarditis — see Rheumatoid, carditis
  myopathy M05.40
    ankle M05.47- ☑
    elbow M05.42- ☑
    foot joint M05.47- ☑
    hand joint M05.44- ☑
    hip M05.45- ☑
    knee M05.46- ☑
    multiple site M05.49
    shoulder M05.41- ☑
    vertebra — see Spondylitis, ankylosing

Rheumatoid — continued
  myopathy — continued
    wrist M05.43- ☑
  pericarditis — see Rheumatoid, carditis
  polyarthritis — see Arthritis, rheumatoid
  polyneuropathy M05.50
    ankle M05.57- ☑
    elbow M05.52- ☑
    foot joint M05.57- ☑
    hand joint M05.54- ☑
    hip M05.55- ☑
    knee M05.56- ☑
    multiple site M05.59
    shoulder M05.51- ☑
    vertebra — see Spondylitis, ankylosing
    wrist M05.53- ☑
  vasculitis M05.20
    ankle M05.27- ☑
    elbow M05.22- ☑
    foot joint M05.27- ☑
    hand joint M05.24- ☑
    hip M05.25- ☑
    knee M05.26- ☑
    multiple site M05.29
    shoulder M05.21- ☑
    vertebra — see Spondylitis, ankylosing
    wrist M05.23- ☑
Rhinitis (atrophic) (catarrhal) (chronic) (croupous) (fibrinous) (granulomatous) (hyperplastic) (hypertrophic) (membranous) (obstructive) (purulent) (suppurative) (ulcerative) J31.0
  with
    sore throat — see Nasopharyngitis
  acute J00
  allergic J30.9
    with asthma J45.909
      with
        exacerbation (acute) J45.901
        status asthmaticus J45.902
    due to
      food J30.5
      pollen J30.1
    nonseasonal J30.89
    perennial J30.89
    seasonal NEC J30.2
    specified NEC J30.89
  infective J00
  pneumococcal J00
  syphilitic A52.73
    congenital A50.05 [J99]
  tuberculous A15.8
  vasomotor J30.0
Rhinoantritis (chronic) — see Sinusitis, maxillary
Rhinodacryolith — see Dacryolith
Rhinolith (nasal sinus) J34.89
Rhinomegaly J34.89
Rhinopharyngitis (acute) (subacute) (see also Nasopharyngitis)
  chronic J31.1
  destructive ulcerating A66.5
  mutilans A66.5
Rhinophyma L71.1
Rhinorrhea J34.89
  cerebrospinal (fluid) G96.0
  paroxysmal — see Rhinitis, allergic
  spasmodic — see Rhinitis, allergic
Rhinosalpingitis — see Salpingitis, eustachian
Rhinoscleroma A48.8
Rhinosporidiosis B48.1
Rhinovirus infection NEC B34.8
Rhizomelic chondrodysplasia punctata E71.540
Rhythm
  atrioventricular nodal I49.8
  disorder I49.9
    coronary sinus I49.8
    ectopic I49.8
    nodal I49.8
  escape I49.9
  heart, abnormal I49.9
  idioventricular I44.2
  nodal I49.8
  sleep, inversion G47.2- ☑
    nonorganic origin — see Disorder, sleep, circadian rhythm, psychogenic
Rhytidosis facialis L98.8
Rib (see also condition)
  cervical Q76.5

Riboflavin deficiency E53.0
Rice bodies (see also Loose, body, joint)
  knee M23.4- ☑
Richter syndrome — see Leukemia, chronic lymphocytic, B-cell type
Richter's hernia — see Hernia, abdomen, with obstruction
Ricinism — see Poisoning, food, noxious, plant
Rickets (active) (acute) (adolescent) (chest wall) (congenital) (current) (infantile) (intestinal) E55.0
  adult — see Osteomalacia
  celiac K90.0
  hypophosphatemic with nephrotic-glycosuric dwarfism E72.09
  inactive E64.3
  kidney N25.0
  renal N25.0
  sequelae, any E64.3
  vitamin-D-resistant E83.31 [M90.80]
Rickettsial disease A79.9
  specified type NEC A79.89
Rickettsialpox (Rickettsia akari) A79.1
Rickettsiosis A79.9
  due to
    Ehrlichia sennetsu A79.81
    Rickettsia akari (rickettsialpox) A79.1
  specified type NEC A79.89
  tick-borne A77.9
  vesicular A79.1
Rider's bone — see Ossification, muscle, specified NEC
Ridge, alveolus (see also condition)
  flabby K06.8
Ridged ear, congenital Q17.3
Riedel's
  lobe, liver Q44.7
  struma, thyroiditis or disease E06.5
Rieger's anomaly or syndrome Q13.81
Riehl's melanosis L81.4
Rietti-Greppi-Micheli anemia D56.9
Rieux's hernia — see Hernia, abdomen, specified site NEC
Riga (-Fede) **disease** K14.0
Riggs' disease — see Periodontitis
Right aortic arch Q25.47
Right middle lobe syndrome J98.11
Rigid, rigidity (see also condition)
  abdominal R19.30
    with severe abdominal pain R10.0
    epigastric R19.36
    generalized R19.37
    left lower quadrant R19.34
    left upper quadrant R19.32
    periumbilic R19.35
    right lower quadrant R19.33
    right upper quadrant R19.31
  articular, multiple, congenital Q68.8
  cervix (uteri) in pregnancy — see Pregnancy, complicated by, abnormal, cervix
  hymen (acquired) (congenital) N89.6
  nuchal R29.1
  pelvic floor in pregnancy — see Pregnancy, complicated by, abnormal, pelvic organs or tissues NEC
  perineum or vulva in pregnancy — see Pregnancy, complicated by, abnormal, vulva
  spine — see Dorsopathy, specified NEC
  vagina in pregnancy — see Pregnancy, complicated by, abnormal, vagina
Rigors R68.89
  with fever R50.9
Riley-Day syndrome G90.1
RIND (reversible ischemic neurologic deficit) I63.9
Ring(s)
  aorta (vascular) Q25.45
  Bandl's O62.4
  contraction, complicating delivery O62.4
  esophageal, lower (muscular) K22.2
  Fleischer's (cornea) H18.04- ☑
  hymenal, tight (acquired) (congenital) N89.6
  Kayser-Fleischer (cornea) H18.04- ☑
  retraction, uterus, pathological O62.4
  Schatzki's (esophagus) (lower) K22.2
    congenital Q39.3
  Soemmerring's — see Cataract, secondary
  vascular (congenital) Q25.8
    aorta Q25.45
Ringed hair (congenital) Q84.1
Ringworm B35.9
  beard B35.0

☑ **Additional Character Required** — Refer to the Tabular List for Character Selection   Subterms under main terms may continue to next column or page

Ringworm — *continued*
  black dot B35.0
  body B35.4
  Burmese B35.5
  corporeal B35.4
  foot B35.3
  groin B35.6
  hand B35.2
  honeycomb B35.0
  nails B35.1
  perianal (area) B35.6
  scalp B35.0
  specified NEC B35.8
  Tokelau B35.5
Rise, venous pressure I87.8
Rising, PSA following treatment for malignant neoplasm of prostate R97.21
Risk
  for
    dental caries Z91.849
      high Z91.843
      low Z91.841
      moderate Z91.842
  suicidal
    meaning personal history of attempted suicide Z91.5
    meaning suicidal ideation — *see* Ideation, suicidal
Ritter's disease L00
Rivalry, sibling Z62.891
Rivalta's disease A42.2
River blindness B73.01
Robert's pelvis Q74.2
  with disproportion (fetopelvic) O33.0
    causing obstructed labor O65.0
Robin (-Pierre) **syndrome** Q87.0
Robinow-Silvermann-Smith syndrome Q87.1
Robinson's (hidrotic) **ectodermal dysplasia or syndrome** Q82.4
Robles' disease B73.01
Rocky Mountain (spotted) **fever** A77.0
Roetheln — *see* Rubella
Roger's disease Q21.0
Rokitansky-Aschoff sinuses (gallbladder) K82.8
Rolando's fracture (displaced) S62.22- ☑
  nondisplaced S62.22- ☑
Romano-Ward (prolonged QT interval) **syndrome** I45.81
Romberg's disease or syndrome G51.8
Roof, mouth — *see* condition
Rosacea L71.9
  acne L71.9
  keratitis L71.8
  specified NEC L71.8
Rosary, rachitic E55.0
Rose
  cold J30.1
  fever J30.1
  rash R21
    epidemic B06.9
Rosenbach's erysipeloid A26.0
Rosenthal's disease or syndrome D68.1
Roseola B09
  infantum B08.20
    due to human herpesvirus 6 B08.21
    due to human herpesvirus 7 B08.22
Ross River disease or fever B33.1
Rossbach's disease K31.89
  psychogenic F45.8
Rostan's asthma (cardiac) — *see* Failure, ventricular, left
Rotation
  anomalous, incomplete or insufficient, intestine Q43.3
  cecum (congenital) Q43.3
  colon (congenital) Q43.3
  spine, incomplete or insufficient — *see* Dorsopathy, deforming, specified NEC
  tooth, teeth, fully erupted M26.35
  vertebra, incomplete or insufficient — *see* Dorsopathy, deforming, specified NEC
Rotes Quérol disease or syndrome — *see* Hyperostosis, ankylosing
Roth (-Bernhardt) **disease or syndrome** — *see* Meralgia paraesthetica
Rothmund (-Thomson) **syndrome** Q82.8
Rotor's disease or syndrome E80.6
Round
  back (with wedging of vertebrae) — *see* Kyphosis
    sequelae (late effect) of rickets E64.3
  worms (large) (infestation) NEC B82.0
    Ascariasis (*see also* Ascariasis) B77.9

Roussy-Lévy syndrome G60.0
Rubella (German measles) B06.9
  complication NEC B06.09
    neurological B06.00
  congenital P35.0
  contact Z20.4
  exposure to Z20.4
  maternal
    care for (suspected) damage to fetus O35.3 ☑
    manifest rubella in infant P35.0
    suspected damage to fetus affecting management of pregnancy O35.3 ☑
  specified complications NEC B06.89
Rubeola (meaning measles) — *see* Measles
  meaning rubella — *see* Rubella
Rubeosis, iris — *see* Disorder, iris, vascular
Rubinstein-Taybi syndrome Q87.2
Rudimentary (congenital) (*see also* Agenesis)
  arm — *see* Defect, reduction, upper limb
  bone Q79.9
  cervix uteri Q51.828
  eye Q11.2
  lobule of ear Q17.3
  patella Q74.1
  respiratory organs in thoracopagus Q89.4
  tracheal bronchus Q32.4
  uterus Q51.818
    in male Q56.1
  vagina Q52.0
Ruled out condition — *see* Observation, suspected
Rumination R11.10
  with nausea R11.2
  disorder of infancy F98.21
  neurotic F42.8
  newborn P92.1
  obsessional F42.8
  psychogenic F42.8
Runeberg's disease D51.0
Runny nose R09.89
Rupia (syphilitic) A51.39
  congenital A50.06
  tertiary A52.79
Rupture, ruptured
  abscess (spontaneous) — *code by* site under Abscess
  aneurysm — *see* Aneurysm
  anus (sphincter) — *see* Laceration, anus
  aorta, aortic I71.8
    abdominal I71.3
    arch I71.1
    ascending I71.1
    descending I71.8
      abdominal I71.3
      thoracic I71.1
    syphilitic A52.01
    thoracoabdominal I71.5
    thorax, thoracic I71.1
    transverse I71.1
    traumatic — *see* Injury, aorta, laceration, major
    valve or cusp (*see also* Endocarditis, aortic) I35.8
  appendix (with peritonitis) (*see also* Appendicitis) K35.32
    with localized peritonitis (*see also* Appendicitis) K35.32
  arteriovenous fistula, brain I60.8
  artery I77.2
    brain — *see* Hemorrhage, intracranial, intracerebral
    coronary — *see* Infarct, myocardium
    heart — *see* Infarct, myocardium
    pulmonary I28.8
    traumatic (complication) — *see* Injury, blood vessel
  bile duct (common) (hepatic) K83.2
    cystic K82.2
  bladder (sphincter) (nontraumatic) (spontaneous) N32.89
    following ectopic or molar pregnancy O08.6
    obstetrical trauma O71.5
    traumatic S37.29 ☑
  blood vessel (*see also* Hemorrhage)
    brain — *see* Hemorrhage, intracranial, intracerebral
    heart — *see* Infarct, myocardium
    traumatic (complication) — *see* Injury, blood vessel, laceration, major, by site
  bone — *see* Fracture
  bowel (nontraumatic) K63.1
  brain
    aneurysm (congenital) (*see also* Hemorrhage, intracranial, subarachnoid)
      syphilitic A52.05

Rupture, ruptured — *continued*
  brain — *continued*
    hemorrhagic — *see* Hemorrhage, intracranial, intracerebral
  capillaries I78.8
  cardiac (auricle) (ventricle) (wall) I23.3
    with hemopericardium I23.0
    infectional I40.9
    traumatic — *see* Injury, heart
  cartilage (articular) (current) (*see also* Sprain)
    knee S83.3-
    semilunar — *see* Tear, meniscus
  cecum (with peritonitis) K65.0
    with peritoneal abscess K35.33
    traumatic S36.598 ☑
  celiac artery, traumatic — *see* Injury, blood vessel, celiac artery, laceration, major
  cerebral aneurysm (congenital) (see Hemorrhage, intracranial, subarachnoid)
  cervix (uteri)
    with ectopic or molar pregnancy O08.6
    following ectopic or molar pregnancy O08.6
    obstetrical trauma O71.3
    traumatic S37.69 ☑
  chordae tendineae NEC I51.1
    concurrent with acute myocardial infarction — *see* Infarct, myocardium
    following acute myocardial infarction (current complication) I23.4
  choroid (direct) (indirect) (traumatic) H31.32- ☑
  circle of Willis I60.6
  colon (nontraumatic) K63.1
    traumatic — *see* Injury, intestine, large
  cornea (traumatic) — *see* Injury, eye, laceration
  coronary (artery) (thrombotic) — *see* Infarct, myocardium
  corpus luteum (infected) (ovary) N83.1- ☑
  cyst — *see* Cyst
  cystic duct K82.2
  Descemet's membrane — *see* Change, corneal membrane, Descemet's, rupture
    traumatic — *see* Injury, eye, laceration
  diaphragm, traumatic — *see* Injury, intrathoracic, diaphragm
  disc — *see* Rupture, intervertebral disc
  diverticulum (intestine) K57.80
    with bleeding K57.81
    bladder N32.3
    large intestine K57.20
      with
        bleeding K57.21
        small intestine K57.40
          with bleeding K57.41
    small intestine K57.00
      with
        bleeding K57.01
        large intestine K57.40
          with bleeding K57.41
  duodenal stump K31.89
  ear drum (nontraumatic) (*see also* Perforation, tympanum)
    traumatic S09.2- ☑
    due to blast injury — *see* Injury, blast, ear
  esophagus K22.3
  eye (without prolapse or loss of intraocular tissue) — *see* Injury, eye, laceration
  fallopian tube NEC (nonobstetric) (nontraumatic) N83.8
    due to pregnancy O00.10- ☑
    with intrauterine pregnancy O00.11- ☑
  fontanel P13.1
  gallbladder K82.2
    traumatic S36.128 ☑
  gastric (*see also* Rupture, stomach)
    vessel K92.2
  globe (eye) (traumatic) — *see* Injury, eye, laceration
  graafian follicle (hematoma) N83.0- ☑
  heart — *see* Rupture, cardiac
  hymen (nontraumatic) (nonintentional) N89.8
  internal organ, traumatic — *see* Injury, by site
  intervertebral disc — *see* Displacement, intervertebral disc
    traumatic — *see* Rupture, traumatic, intervertebral disc
  intestine NEC (nontraumatic) K63.1
    traumatic — *see* Injury, intestine
  iris (*see also* Abnormality, pupillary)
    traumatic — *see* Injury, eye, laceration

⏷ Subterms under main terms may continue to next column or page
☑ Additional Character Required — Refer to the Tabular List for Character Selection
277

Rupture, ruptured — *continued*
- joint capsule, traumatic — *see* Sprain
- kidney (traumatic) S37.06- ☑
  - birth injury P15.8
  - nontraumatic N28.89
- lacrimal duct (traumatic) — *see* Injury, eye, specified site NEC
- lens (cataract) (traumatic) — *see* Cataract, traumatic
- ligament, traumatic — *see* Rupture, traumatic, ligament, by site
- liver S36.116 ☑
  - birth injury P15.0
- lymphatic vessel I89.8
- marginal sinus (placental) (with hemorrhage) — *see* Hemorrhage, antepartum, specified cause NEC
- membrana tympani (nontraumatic) — *see* Perforation, tympanum
- membranes (spontaneous)
  - artificial
    - delayed delivery following O75.5
  - delayed delivery following — *see* Pregnancy, complicated by, premature rupture of membranes
- meningeal artery I60.8
- meniscus (knee) (*see also* Tear, meniscus)
  - old — *see* Derangement, meniscus
  - site other than knee — *code as* Sprain
- mesenteric artery, traumatic — *see* Injury, mesenteric, artery, laceration, major
- mesentery (nontraumatic) K66.8
  - traumatic — *see* Injury, intra-abdominal, specified, site NEC
- mitral (valve) I34.8
- muscle (traumatic) (*see also* Strain)
  - diastasis — *see* Diastasis, muscle
  - nontraumatic M62.10
    - ankle M62.17- ☑
    - foot M62.17- ☑
    - forearm M62.13- ☑
    - hand M62.14- ☑
    - lower leg M62.16- ☑
    - pelvic region M62.15- ☑
    - shoulder region M62.11- ☑
    - specified site NEC M62.18
    - thigh M62.15- ☑
    - upper arm M62.12- ☑
  - traumatic — *see* Strain, by site
- musculotendinous junction NEC, nontraumatic — *see* Rupture, tendon, spontaneous
- mycotic aneurysm causing cerebral hemorrhage — *see* Hemorrhage, intracranial, subarachnoid
- myocardium, myocardial — *see* Rupture, cardiac
  - traumatic — *see* Injury, heart
- nontraumatic, meaning hernia — *see* Hernia
- obstructed — *see* Hernia, by site, obstructed
- operation wound — *see* Disruption, wound, operation
- ovary, ovarian N83.8
  - corpus luteum cyst N83.1- ☑
  - follicle (graafian) N83.0- ☑
- oviduct (nonobstetric) (nontraumatic) N83.8
  - due to pregnancy O00.10- ☑
    - with intrauterine pregnancy O00.11- ☑
- pancreas (nontraumatic) K86.89
  - traumatic S36.299 ☑
- papillary muscle NEC I51.2
  - following acute myocardial infarction (current complication) I23.5
- pelvic
  - floor, complicating delivery O70.1
  - organ NEC, obstetrical trauma O71.5
- perineum (nonobstetric) (nontraumatic) N90.89
  - complicating delivery — *see* Delivery, complicated, by, laceration, anus (sphincter)
- postoperative wound — *see* Disruption, wound, operation
- prostate (traumatic) S37.828 ☑
- pulmonary
  - artery I28.8
  - valve (heart) I37.8
  - vein I28.8
  - vessel I28.8
- pus tube — *see* Salpingitis
- pyosalpinx — *see* Salpingitis
- rectum (nontraumatic) K63.1
  - traumatic S36.69 ☑
- retina, retinal (traumatic) (without detachment) (*see also* Break, retina)

Rupture, ruptured — *continued*
- retina, retinal (*see also* Break, retina) — *continued*
  - with detachment — *see* Detachment, retina, with retinal, break
- rotator cuff (nontraumatic) M75.10- ☑
  - complete M75.12- ☑
  - incomplete M75.11- ☑
- sclera — *see* Injury, eye, laceration
- sigmoid (nontraumatic) K63.1
  - traumatic S36.593 ☑
- spinal cord (*see also* Injury, spinal cord, by region)
  - due to injury at birth P11.5
  - newborn (birth injury) P11.5
- spleen (traumatic) S36.09 ☑
  - birth injury P15.1
  - congenital (birth injury) P15.1
  - due to P. vivax malaria B51.0
  - nontraumatic D73.5
  - spontaneous D73.5
- splenic vein R58
  - traumatic — *see* Injury, blood vessel, splenic vein
- stomach (nontraumatic) (spontaneous) K31.89
  - traumatic S36.39 ☑
- supraspinatus (complete) (incomplete) (nontraumatic) — *see* Tear, rotator cuff
- symphysis pubis
  - obstetric O71.6
  - traumatic S33.4 ☑
- synovium (cyst) M66.10
  - ankle M66.17- ☑
  - elbow M66.12- ☑
  - finger M66.14- ☑
  - foot M66.17- ☑
  - forearm M66.13- ☑
  - hand M66.14- ☑
  - pelvic region M66.15- ☑
  - shoulder region M66.11- ☑
  - specified site NEC M66.18
  - thigh M66.15- ☑
  - toe M66.17- ☑
  - upper arm M66.12- ☑
  - wrist M66.13- ☑
- tendon (traumatic) — *see* Strain
  - nontraumatic (spontaneous) M66.9
    - ankle M66.87- ☑
    - extensor M66.20
      - ankle M66.27- ☑
      - foot M66.27- ☑
      - forearm M66.23- ☑
      - hand M66.24- ☑
      - lower leg M66.26- ☑
      - multiple sites M66.29
      - pelvic region M66.25- ☑
      - shoulder region M66.21- ☑
      - specified site NEC M66.28
      - thigh M66.25- ☑
      - upper arm M66.22- ☑
    - flexor M66.30
      - ankle M66.37- ☑
      - foot M66.37- ☑
      - forearm M66.33- ☑
      - hand M66.34- ☑
      - lower leg M66.36- ☑
      - multiple sites M66.39
      - pelvic region M66.35- ☑
      - shoulder region M66.31- ☑
      - specified site NEC M66.38
      - thigh M66.35- ☑
      - upper arm M66.32- ☑
    - foot M66.87- ☑
    - forearm M66.83- ☑
    - hand M66.84- ☑
    - lower leg M66.86- ☑
    - multiple sites M66.89
    - pelvic region M66.85- ☑
    - shoulder region M66.81- ☑
    - specified
      - site NEC M66.88
      - tendon M66.80
    - thigh M66.85- ☑
    - upper arm M66.82- ☑
- thoracic duct I89.8
- tonsil J35.8
- traumatic
  - aorta — *see* Injury, aorta, laceration, major
  - diaphragm — *see* Injury, intrathoracic, diaphragm
  - external site — *see* Wound, open, by site

Rupture, ruptured — *continued*
- traumatic — *continued*
  - eye — *see* Injury, eye, laceration
  - internal organ — *see* Injury, by site
  - intervertebral disc
    - cervical S13.0 ☑
    - lumbar S33.0 ☑
    - thoracic S23.0 ☑
  - kidney S37.06- ☑
  - ligament (*see also* Sprain)
    - ankle — *see* Sprain, ankle
    - carpus — *see* Rupture, traumatic, ligament, wrist
    - collateral (hand) — *see* Rupture, traumatic, ligament, finger, collateral
    - finger (metacarpophalangeal) (interphalangeal) S63.40- ☑
      - collateral S63.41- ☑
        - index S63.41- ☑
        - little S63.41- ☑
        - middle S63.41- ☑
        - ring S63.41- ☑
      - index S63.40- ☑
      - little S63.40- ☑
      - middle S63.40- ☑
      - palmar S63.42- ☑
        - index S63.42- ☑
        - little S63.42- ☑
        - middle S63.42- ☑
        - ring S63.42- ☑
      - ring S63.40- ☑
      - specified site NEC S63.499 ☑
        - index S63.49- ☑
        - little S63.49- ☑
        - middle S63.49- ☑
        - ring S63.49- ☑
      - volar plate S63.43- ☑
        - index S63.43- ☑
        - little S63.43- ☑
        - middle S63.43- ☑
        - ring S63.43- ☑
    - foot — *see* Sprain, foot
    - radial collateral S53.2- ☑
    - radiocarpal — *see* Rupture, traumatic, ligament, wrist, radiocarpal
    - ulnar collateral S53.3- ☑
    - ulnocarpal — *see* Rupture, traumatic, ligament, wrist, ulnocarpal
    - wrist S63.30- ☑
      - collateral S63.31- ☑
      - radiocarpal S63.32- ☑
      - specified site NEC S63.39- ☑
      - ulnocarpal (palmar) S63.33- ☑
  - liver S36.116 ☑
  - membrana tympani — *see* Rupture, ear drum, traumatic
  - muscle or tendon — *see* Strain
  - myocardium — *see* Injury, heart
  - pancreas S36.299 ☑
  - rectum S36.69 ☑
  - sigmoid S36.593 ☑
  - spleen S36.09 ☑
  - stomach S36.39 ☑
  - symphysis pubis S33.4 ☑
  - tympanum, tympanic (membrane) — *see* Rupture, ear drum, traumatic
  - ureter S37.19 ☑
  - uterus S37.69 ☑
  - vagina — *see* Injury, vagina
  - vena cava — *see* Injury, vena cava, laceration, major
- tricuspid (heart) (valve) I07.8
- tube, tubal (nonobstetric) (nontraumatic) N83.8
  - abscess — *see* Salpingitis
  - due to pregnancy O00.10- ☑
    - with intrauterine pregnancy O00.11- ☑
- tympanum, tympanic (membrane) (nontraumatic) (*see also* Perforation, tympanic membrane) H72.9- ☑
  - traumatic — *see* Rupture, ear drum, traumatic
- umbilical cord, complicating delivery O69.89 ☑
- ureter (traumatic) S37.19 ☑
  - nontraumatic N28.89
- urethra (nontraumatic) N36.8
  - with ectopic or molar pregnancy O08.6
  - following ectopic or molar pregnancy O08.6
  - obstetrical trauma O71.5
  - traumatic S37.39 ☑

☑ **Additional Character Required** — Refer to the Tabular List for Character Selection   ▽ **Subterms under main terms may continue to next column or page**

Rupture, ruptured — *continued*
   uterosacral ligament (nonobstetric) (nontraumatic)
      N83.8
   uterus (traumatic) S37.69 ☑
      before labor O71.0- ☑
      during or after labor O71.1
      nonpuerperal, nontraumatic N85.8
      pregnant (during labor) O71.1
         before labor O71.0- ☑
   vagina — *see* Injury, vagina
   valve, valvular (heart) — *see* Endocarditis
   varicose vein — *see* Varix
   varix — *see* Varix
   vena cava R58
      traumatic — *see* Injury, vena cava, laceration, major
   vesical (urinary) N32.89
   vessel (blood) R58
      pulmonary I28.8
      traumatic — *see* Injury, blood vessel
   viscus R19.8
   vulva complicating delivery O70.0
Russell-Silver syndrome Q87.1
Russian spring-summer type encephalitis A84.0
Rust's disease (tuberculous cervical spondylitis) A18.01
Ruvalcaba-Myhre-Smith syndrome E71.440
Rytand-Lipsitch syndrome I44.2

S

Saber, sabre shin or tibia (syphilitic) A50.56 [M90.8-] ☑
Sac lacrimal — *see* condition
Saccharomyces infection B37.9
Saccharopinuria E72.3
Saccular — *see* condition
Sacculation
   aorta (nonsyphilitic) — *see* Aneurysm, aorta
   bladder N32.3
   intralaryngeal (congenital) (ventricular) Q31.3
   larynx (congenital) (ventricular) Q31.3
   organ or site, congenital — *see* Distortion
   pregnant uterus — *see* Pregnancy, complicated by, abnormal, uterus
   ureter N28.89
   urethra N36.1
   vesical N32.3
Sachs' amaurotic familial idiocy or disease E75.02
Sachs-Tay disease E75.02
Sacks-Libman disease M32.11
Sacralgia M53.3
Sacralization Q76.49
Sacrodynia M53.3
Sacroiliac joint — *see* condition
Sacroiliitis NEC M46.1
Sacrum — *see* condition
Saddle
   back — *see* Lordosis
   embolus
      abdominal aorta I74.01
      pulmonary artery I26.92
         with acute cor pulmonale I26.02
   injury — *code to* condition
   nose M95.0
      due to syphilis A50.57
Sadism (sexual) F65.52
Sadness, postpartal O90.6
Sadomasochism F65.50
Saemisch's ulcer (cornea) — *see* Ulcer, cornea, central
Sagging
   skin and subcutaneous tissue (following bariatric surgery weight loss) (following dietary weight loss) L98.7
Sahib disease B55.0
Sailors' skin L57.8
Saint
   Anthony's fire — *see* Erysipelas
   triad — *see* Hernia, diaphragm
   Vitus' dance — *see* Chorea, Sydenham's
Salaam
   attack(s) — *see* Epilepsy, spasms
   tic R25.8
Salicylism
   abuse F55.8
   overdose or wrong substance given — *see* Table of Drugs and Chemicals, by drug, poisoning
Salivary duct or gland — *see* condition
Salivation, excessive K11.7
Salmonella — *see* Infection, Salmonella

Salmonellosis A02.0
Salpingitis (catarrhal) (fallopian tube) (nodular) (pseud-ofollicular) (purulent) (septic) N70.91
   with oophoritis N70.93
   acute N70.01
      with oophoritis N70.03
   chlamydial A56.11
   chronic N70.11
      with oophoritis N70.13
   complicating abortion — *see* Abortion, by type, complicated by, salpingitis
   ear — *see* Salpingitis, eustachian
   eustachian (tube) H68.00- ☑
      acute H68.01- ☑
      chronic H68.02- ☑
   follicularis N70.11
      with oophoritis N70.13
   gonococcal (acute) (chronic) A54.24
   interstitial, chronic N70.11
      with oophoritis N70.13
   isthmica nodosa N70.11
      with oophoritis N70.13
   specific (gonococcal) (acute) (chronic) A54.24
   tuberculous (acute) (chronic) A18.17
   venereal (gonococcal) (acute) (chronic) A54.24
Salpingocele N83.4- ☑
Salpingo-oophoritis (catarrhal) (purulent) (ruptured) (septic) (suppurative) N70.93
   acute N70.03
      with ectopic or molar pregnancy O08.0
      following ectopic or molar pregnancy O08.0
      gonococcal A54.24
   chronic N70.13
   following ectopic or molar pregnancy O08.0
   gonococcal (acute) (chronic) A54.24
   puerperal O86.19
   specific (gonococcal) (acute) (chronic) A54.24
   subacute N70.03
   tuberculous (acute) (chronic) A18.17
   venereal (gonococcal) (acute) (chronic) A54.24
Salpingo-ovaritis — *see* Salpingo-oophoritis
Salpingoperitonitis — *see* Salpingo-oophoritis
Salzmann's nodular dystrophy — *see* Degeneration, cornea, nodular
Sampson's cyst or tumor N80.1
San Joaquin (Valley) **fever** B38.0
Sandblaster's asthma, lung or pneumoconiosis J62.8
Sander's disease (paranoia) F22
Sandfly fever A93.1
Sandhoff's disease E75.01
Sanfilippo (Type B) (Type C) (Type D) **syndrome** E76.22
Sanger-Brown ataxia G11.2
Sao Paulo fever or typhus A77.0
Saponification, mesenteric K65.8
Sarcocele (benign)
   syphilitic A52.76
      congenital A50.59
Sarcocystosis A07.8
Sarcoepiplocele — *see* Hernia
Sarcoepiplomphalocele Q79.2
Sarcoid (*see also* Sarcoidosis)
   arthropathy D86.86
   Boeck's D86.9
   Darier-Roussy D86.3
   iridocyclitis D86.83
   meningitis D86.81
   myocarditis D86.85
   myositis D86.87
   pyelonephritis D86.84
   Spiegler-Fendt L08.89
Sarcoidosis D86.9
   with
      cranial nerve palsies D86.82
      hepatic granuloma D86.89
      polyarthritis D86.86
      tubulo-interstitial nephropathy D86.84
   combined sites NEC D86.89
   lung D86.0
      and lymph nodes D86.2
   lymph nodes D86.1
      and lung D86.2
   meninges D86.81
   skin D86.3
   specified type NEC D86.89
Sarcoma (of) (*see also* Neoplasm, connective tissue, malignant)
   alveolar soft part — *see* Neoplasm, connective tissue, malignant

Sarcoma — *continued*
   ameloblastic C41.1
      upper jaw (bone) C41.0
   botryoid — *see* Neoplasm, connective tissue, malignant
   botryoides — *see* Neoplasm, connective tissue, malignant
   cerebellar C71.6
      circumscribed (arachnoidal) C71.6
   circumscribed (arachnoidal) cerebellar C71.6
   clear cell (*see also* Neoplasm, connective tissue, malignant)
      kidney C64.- ☑
   dendritic cells (accessory cells) C96.4
   embryonal — *see* Neoplasm, connective tissue, malignant
   endometrial (stromal) C54.1
      isthmus C54.0
   epithelioid (cell) — *see* Neoplasm, connective tissue, malignant
   Ewing's — *see* Neoplasm, bone, malignant
   follicular dendritic cell C96.4
   germinoblastic (diffuse) — *see* Lymphoma, diffuse large cell
      follicular — *see* Lymphoma, follicular, specified NEC
   giant cell (except of bone) (*see also* Neoplasm, connective tissue, malignant)
      bone — *see* Neoplasm, bone, malignant
   glomoid — *see* Neoplasm, connective tissue, malignant
   granulocytic C92.3- ☑
   hemangioendothelial — *see* Neoplasm, connective tissue, malignant
   hemorrhagic, multiple — *see* Sarcoma, Kaposi's
   histiocytic C96.A (*following* C96.6)
   Hodgkin — *see* Lymphoma, Hodgkin
   immunoblastic (diffuse) — *see* Lymphoma, diffuse large cell
   interdigitating dendritic cell C96.4
   Kaposi's
      colon C46.4
      connective tissue C46.1
      gastrointestinal organ C46.4
      lung C46.5- ☑
      lymph node(s) C46.3
      palate (hard) (soft) C46.2
      rectum C46.4
      skin C46.0
      specified site NEC C46.7
      stomach C46.4
      unspecified site C46.9
   Kupffer cell C22.3
   Langerhans cell C96.4
   leptomeningeal — *see* Neoplasm, meninges, malignant
   liver NEC C22.4
   lymphangioendothelial — *see* Neoplasm, connective tissue, malignant
   lymphoblastic — *see* Lymphoma, lymphoblastic (diffuse)
   lymphocytic — *see* Lymphoma, small cell B-cell
   mast cell C96.22
   melanotic — *see* Melanoma
   meningeal — *see* Neoplasm, meninges, malignant
   meningothelial — *see* Neoplasm, meninges, malignant
   mesenchymal (*see also* Neoplasm, connective tissue, malignant)
      mixed — *see* Neoplasm, connective tissue, malignant
   mesothelial — *see* Mesothelioma
   monstrocellular
      specified site — *see* Neoplasm, malignant, by site
      unspecified site C71.9
   myeloid C92.3- ☑
   neurogenic — *see* Neoplasm, nerve, malignant
   odontogenic C41.1
      upper jaw (bone) C41.0
   osteoblastic — *see* Neoplasm, bone, malignant
   osteogenic (*see also* Neoplasm, bone, malignant)
      juxtacortical — *see* Neoplasm, bone, malignant
      periosteal — *see* Neoplasm, bone, malignant
   periosteal (*see also* Neoplasm, bone, malignant)
      osteogenic — *see* Neoplasm, bone, malignant
   pleomorphic cell — *see* Neoplasm, connective tissue, malignant
   reticulum cell (diffuse) — *see* Lymphoma, diffuse large cell
      nodular — *see* Lymphoma, follicular
      pleomorphic cell type — *see* Lymphoma, diffuse large cell

---

Sarcoma — *continued*
 rhabdoid — *see* Neoplasm, malignant, by site
 round cell — *see* Neoplasm, connective tissue, malignant
 small cell — *see* Neoplasm, connective tissue, malignant
 soft tissue — *see* Neoplasm, connective tissue, malignant
 spindle cell — *see* Neoplasm, connective tissue, malignant
 stromal (endometrial) C54.1
  isthmus C54.0
 synovial (*see also* Neoplasm, connective tissue, malignant)
  biphasic — *see* Neoplasm, connective tissue, malignant
  epithelioid cell — *see* Neoplasm, connective tissue, malignant
  spindle cell — *see* Neoplasm, connective tissue, malignant
Sarcomatosis
 meningeal — *see* Neoplasm, meninges, malignant
 specified site NEC — *see* Neoplasm, connective tissue, malignant
 unspecified site C80.1
Sarcopenia (age-related) M62.84
Sarcosinemia E72.59
Sarcosporidiosis (intestinal) A07.8
Satiety, early R68.81
Saturnine — *see* condition
Saturnism
 overdose or wrong substance given or taken — *see* Table of Drugs and Chemicals, by drug, poisoning
Satyriasis F52.8
Sauriasis — *see* Ichthyosis
SBE (subacute bacterial endocarditis) I33.0
Scabies (any site) B86
Scabs R23.4
Scaglietti-Dagnini syndrome E22.0
Scald — *see* Burn
Scalenus anticus (anterior) **syndrome** G54.0
Scales R23.4
Scaling, skin R23.4
Scalp — *see* condition
Scapegoating affecting child Z62.3
Scaphocephaly Q75.0
Scapulalgia M89.8X1
Scapulohumeral myopathy G71.02
Scar, scarring (*see also* Cicatrix) L90.5
 adherent L90.5
 atrophic L90.5
 cervix
  in pregnancy or childbirth — *see* Pregnancy, complicated by, abnormal cervix
 cheloid L91.0
 chorioretinal H31.00- ☑
  posterior pole macula H31.01- ☑
  postsurgical H59.81- ☑
  solar retinopathy H31.02- ☑
  specified type NEC H31.09- ☑
 choroid — *see* Scar, chorioretinal
 conjunctiva H11.24- ☑
 cornea H17.9
  xerophthalmic (*see also* Opacity, cornea)
   vitamin A deficiency E50.6
 duodenum, obstructive K31.5
 hypertrophic L91.0
 keloid L91.0
 labia N90.89
 lung (base) J98.4
 macula — *see* Scar, chorioretinal, posterior pole
 muscle M62.89
 myocardium, myocardial I25.2
 painful L90.5
 posterior pole (eye) — *see* Scar, chorioretinal, posterior pole
 retina — *see* Scar, chorioretinal
 trachea J39.8
 transmural uterine, in pregnancy O34.29
 uterus N85.8
  in pregnancy O34.29
 vagina N89.8
  postoperative N99.2
 vulva N90.89
Scarabiasis B88.2
Scarlatina (anginosa) (maligna) A38.9
 myocarditis (acute) A38.1

Scarlatina — *continued*
 myocarditis — *continued*
  old — *see* Myocarditis
 otitis media A38.0
 ulcerosa A38.8
Scarlet fever (albuminuria) (angina) A38.9
Schamberg's disease (progressive pigmentary dermatosis) L81.7
Schatzki's ring (acquired) (esophagus) (lower) K22.2
 congenital Q39.3
Schaufenster krankheit I20.8
Schaumann's
 benign lymphogranulomatosis D86.1
 disease or syndrome — *see* Sarcoidosis
Scheie's syndrome E76.03
Schenck's disease B42.1
Scheuermann's disease or osteochondrosis — *see* Osteochondrosis, juvenile, spine
Schilder (-Flatau) **disease** G37.0
Schilling-type monocytic leukemia C93.0- ☑
Schimmelbusch's disease, cystic mastitis, or hyperplasia — *see* Mastopathy, cystic
Schistosoma infestation — *see* Infestation, Schistosoma
Schistosomiasis B65.9
 with muscle disorder B65.9 [M63.80]
  ankle B65.9 [M63.87-] ☑
  foot B65.9 [M63.87-] ☑
  forearm B65.9 [M63.83-] ☑
  hand B65.9 [M63.84-] ☑
  lower leg B65.9 [M63.86-] ☑
  multiple sites B65.9 [M63.89]
  pelvic region B65.9 [M63.85-] ☑
  shoulder region B65.9 [M63.81-] ☑
  specified site NEC B65.9 [M63.88]
  thigh B65.9 [M63.85-] ☑
  upper arm B65.9 [M63.82-] ☑
 Asiatic B65.2
 bladder B65.0
 chestermani B65.8
 colon B65.1
 cutaneous B65.3
 due to
  S. haematobium B65.0
  S. japonicum B65.2
  S. mansoni B65.1
  S. mattheii B65.8
 Eastern B65.2
 genitourinary tract B65.0
 intestinal B65.1
 lung NEC B65.9 [J99]
  pneumonia B65.9 [J17]
 Manson's (intestinal) B65.1
 oriental B65.2
 pulmonary NEC B65.9 [J99]
  pneumonia B65.9
 Schistosoma
  haematobium B65.0
  japonicum B65.2
  mansoni B65.1
 specified type NEC B65.8
 urinary B65.0
 vesical B65.0
Schizencephaly Q04.6
Schizoaffective psychosis F25.9
Schizodontia K00.2
Schizoid personality F60.1
Schizophrenia, schizophrenic F20.9
 acute (brief) (undifferentiated) F23
 atypical (form) F20.3
 borderline F21
 catalepsy F20.2
 catatonic (type) (excited) (withdrawn) F20.2
 cenesthopathic, cenesthesiopathic F20.89
 childhood type F84.5
 chronic undifferentiated F20.5
 cyclic F25.0
 disorganized (type) F20.1
 flexibilitas cerea F20.2
 hebephrenic (type) F20.1
 incipient F21
 latent F21
 negative type F20.5
 paranoid (type) F20.0
 paraphrenic F20.0
 post-psychotic depression F32.89
 prepsychotic F21
 prodromal F21
 pseudoneurotic F21

Schizophrenia, schizophrenic — *continued*
 pseudopsychopathic F21
 reaction F23
 residual (state) (type) F20.5
 restzustand F20.5
 schizoaffective (type) — *see* Psychosis, schizoaffective
 simple (type) F20.89
 simplex F20.89
 specified type NEC F20.89
 spectrum and other psychotic disorder F29
  specified NEC F28
 stupor F20.2
 syndrome of childhood F84.5
 undifferentiated (type) F20.3
  chronic F20.5
Schizothymia (persistent) F60.1
Schlatter-Osgood disease or osteochondrosis — *see* Osteochondrosis, juvenile, tibia
Schlatter's tibia — *see* Osteochondrosis, juvenile, tibia
Schmidt's syndrome (polyglandular, autoimmune) E31.0
Schmincke's carcinoma or tumor — *see* Neoplasm, nasopharynx, malignant
Schmitz (-Stutzer) **dysentery** A03.0
Schmorl's disease or nodes
 lumbar region M51.46
 lumbosacral region M51.47
 sacrococcygeal region M53.3
 thoracic region M51.44
 thoracolumbar region M51.45
Schneiderian
 papilloma — *see* Neoplasm, nasopharynx, benign
  specified site — *see* Neoplasm, benign, by site
  unspecified site D14.0
  specified site — *see* Neoplasm, malignant, by site
   unspecified site C30.0
Scholte's syndrome (malignant carcinoid) E34.0
Scholz (-Bielchowsky-Henneberg) **disease or syndrome** E75.25
Schönlein (-Henoch) disease or purpura (primary) (rheumatic) D69.0
Schottmuller's disease A01.4
Schroeder's syndrome (endocrine hypertensive) E27.0
Schüller-Christian disease or syndrome C96.5
Schultze's type acroparesthesia, simple I73.89
Schultz's disease or syndrome — *see* Agranulocytosis
Schwalbe-Ziehen-Oppenheim disease G24.1
Schwannoma (*see also* Neoplasm, nerve, benign)
 malignant (*see also* Neoplasm, nerve, malignant)
  with rhabdomyoblastic differentiation — *see* Neoplasm, nerve, malignant
 melanocytic — *see* Neoplasm, nerve, benign
 pigmented — *see* Neoplasm, nerve, benign
Schwannomatosis Q85.03
Schwartz (-Jampel) **syndrome** G71.13
Schwartz-Bartter syndrome E22.2
Schweniger-Buzzi anetoderma L90.1
Sciatic — *see* condition
Sciatica (infective)
 with lumbago M54.4- ☑
  due to intervertebral disc disorder — *see* Disorder, disc, with, radiculopathy
 due to displacement of intervertebral disc (with lumbago) — *see* Disorder, disc, with, radiculopathy
 wallet M54.3- ☑
Scimitar syndrome Q26.8
Sclera — *see* condition
Sclerectasia H15.84- ☑
Scleredema
 adultorum — *see* Sclerosis, systemic
 Buschke's — *see* Sclerosis, systemic
 newborn P83.0
Sclerema (adiposum) (edematosum) (neonatorum) (newborn) P83.0
 adultorum — *see* Sclerosis, systemic
Scleriasis — *see* Scleroderma
Scleritis H15.00- ☑
 with corneal involvement H15.04- ☑
 anterior H15.01- ☑
 brawny H15.02- ☑
 in (due to) zoster B02.34
 posterior H15.03- ☑
 specified type NEC H15.09- ☑
 syphilitic A52.71
 tuberculous (nodular) A18.51
Sclerochoroiditis H31.8
Scleroconjunctivitis — *see* Scleritis
Sclerocystic ovary syndrome E28.2

Sclerodactyly, sclerodactylia L94.3
Scleroderma, sclerodermia (acrosclerotic) (diffuse) (generalized) (progressive) (pulmonary) (*see also* Sclerosis, systemic) M34.9
  circumscribed L94.0
  linear L94.1
  localized L94.0
  newborn P83.88
  systemic M34.9
Sclerokeratitis H16.8
  tuberculous A18.52
Scleroma nasi A48.8
Scleromalacia (perforans) H15.05- ☑
Scleromyxedema L98.5
Sclérose en plaques G35
Sclerosis, sclerotic
  adrenal (gland) E27.8
  Alzheimer's — *see* Disease, Alzheimer's
  amyotrophic (lateral) G12.21
  aorta, aortic I70.0
    valve — *see* Endocarditis, aortic
  artery, arterial, arteriolar, arteriovascular — *see* Arteriosclerosis
  ascending multiple G35
  brain (generalized) (lobular) G37.9
    artery, arterial I67.2
    diffuse G37.0
    disseminated G35
    insular G35
    Krabbe's E75.23
    miliary G35
    multiple G35
    presenile (Alzheimer's) — *see* Disease, Alzheimer's, early onset
    senile (arteriosclerotic) I67.2
    stem, multiple G35
    tuberous Q85.1
  bulbar, multiple G35
  bundle of His I44.39
  cardiac — *see* Disease, heart, ischemic, atherosclerotic
  cardiorenal — *see* Hypertension, cardiorenal
  cardiovascular (*see also* Disease, cardiovascular)
    renal — *see* Hypertension, cardiorenal
  cerebellar — *see* Sclerosis, brain
  cerebral — *see* Sclerosis, brain
  cerebrospinal (disseminated) (multiple) G35
  cerebrovascular I67.2
  choroid — *see* Degeneration, choroid
  combined (spinal cord) (*see also* Degeneration, combined)
    multiple G35
  concentric (Balo) G37.5
  cornea — *see* Opacity, cornea
  coronary (artery) I25.10
    with angina pectoris — *see* Arteriosclerosis, coronary (artery),
  corpus cavernosum
    female N90.89
    male N48.6
  diffuse (brain) (spinal cord) G37.0
  disseminated G35
  dorsal G35
  dorsolateral (spinal cord) — *see* Degeneration, combined
  endometrium N85.5
  extrapyramidal G25.9
  eye, nuclear (senile) — *see* Cataract, senile, nuclear
  focal and segmental (glomerular) (*see also* N00-N07 with fourth character .1) N05.1
  Friedreich's (spinal cord) G11.1
  funicular (spermatic cord) N50.89
  general (vascular) — *see* Arteriosclerosis
  gland (lymphatic) I89.8
  hepatic K74.1
    alcoholic K70.2
  hereditary
    cerebellar G11.9
    spinal (Friedreich's ataxia) G11.1
  hippocampal G93.81
  insular G35
  kidney — *see* Sclerosis, renal
  larynx J38.7
  lateral (amyotrophic) (descending) (spinal) G12.21
    primary G12.23
  lens, senile nuclear — *see* Cataract, senile, nuclear
  liver K74.1
    with fibrosis K74.2
      alcoholic K70.2

Sclerosis, sclerotic — *continued*
  liver — *continued*
    alcoholic K70.2
    cardiac K76.1
  lung — *see* Fibrosis, lung
  mastoid — *see* Mastoiditis, chronic
  mesial temporal G93.81
  mitral I05.8
  Mönckeberg's (medial) — *see* Arteriosclerosis, extremities
  multiple (brain stem) (cerebral) (generalized) (spinal cord) G35
  myocardium, myocardial — *see* Disease, heart, ischemic, atherosclerotic
  nuclear (senile), eye — *see* Cataract, senile, nuclear
  ovary N83.8
  pancreas K86.89
  penis N48.6
  peripheral arteries — *see* Arteriosclerosis, extremities
  plaques G35
  pluriglandular E31.8
  polyglandular E31.8
  posterolateral (spinal cord) — *see* Degeneration, combined
  presenile (Alzheimer's) — *see* Disease, Alzheimer's, early onset
  primary, lateral G12.23
  progressive, systemic M34.0
  pulmonary — *see* Fibrosis, lung
    artery I27.0
    valve (heart) — *see* Endocarditis, pulmonary
  renal N26.9
    with
      cystine storage disease E72.09
      hypertensive heart disease (conditions in I11) — *see* Hypertension, cardiorenal
    arteriolar (hyaline) (hyperplastic) — *see* Hypertension, kidney
  retina (senile) (vascular) H35.00
  senile (vascular) — *see* Arteriosclerosis
  spinal (cord) (progressive) G95.89
    ascending G61.0
    combined (*see also* Degeneration, combined)
      multiple G35
      syphilitic A52.11
    disseminated G35
    dorsolateral — *see* Degeneration, combined
    hereditary (Friedreich's) (mixed form) G11.1
    lateral (amyotrophic) G12.23
    multiple G35
    posterior (syphilitic) A52.11
  stomach K31.89
  subendocardial, congenital I42.4
  systemic M34.9
    with
      lung involvement M34.81
      myopathy M34.82
      polyneuropathy M34.83
    drug-induced M34.2
    due to chemicals NEC M34.2
    progressive M34.0
    specified NEC M34.89
  temporal (mesial) G93.81
  tricuspid (heart) (valve) I07.8
  tuberous (brain) Q85.1
  tympanic membrane — *see* Disorder, tympanic membrane, specified NEC
  valve, valvular (heart) — *see* Endocarditis
  vascular — *see* Arteriosclerosis
  vein I87.8
Scoliosis (acquired) (postural) M41.9
  adolescent (idiopathic) — *see* Scoliosis, idiopathic, adolescent
  congenital Q67.5
    due to bony malformation Q76.3
    failure of segmentation (hemivertebra) Q76.3
    hemivertebra fusion Q76.3
    postural Q67.5
  idiopathic M41.20
    adolescent M41.129
      cervical region M41.122
      cervicothoracic region M41.123
      lumbar region M41.126
      lumbosacral region M41.127
      thoracic region M41.124
      thoracolumbar region M41.125
    cervical region M41.22
    cervicothoracic region M41.23

Scoliosis — *continued*
  idiopathic — *continued*
    infantile M41.00
      cervical region M41.02
      cervicothoracic region M41.03
      lumbar region M41.06
      lumbosacral region M41.07
      sacrococcygeal region M41.08
      thoracic region M41.04
      thoracolumbar region M41.05
    juvenile M41.119
      cervical region M41.112
      cervicothoracic region M41.113
      lumbar region M41.116
      lumbosacral region M41.117
      thoracic region M41.114
      thoracolumbar region M41.115
    lumbar region M41.26
    lumbosacral region M41.27
    thoracic region M41.24
    thoracolumbar region M41.25
  infantile — *see* Scoliosis, idiopathic, infantile
  neuromuscular M41.40
    cervical region M41.42
    cervicothoracic region M41.43
    lumbar region M41.46
    lumbosacral region M41.47
    occipito-atlanto-axial region M41.41
    thoracic region M41.44
    thoracolumbar region M41.45
  paralytic — *see* Scoliosis, neuromuscular
  postradiation therapy M96.5
  rachitic (late effect or sequelae) E64.3 [M49.80]
    cervical region E64.3 [M49.82]
    cervicothoracic region E64.3 [M49.83]
    lumbar region E64.3 [M49.86]
    lumbosacral region E64.3 [M49.87]
    multiple sites E64.3 [M49.89]
    occipito-atlanto-axial region E64.3 [M49.81]
    sacrococcygeal region E64.3 [M49.88]
    thoracic region E64.3 [M49.84]
    thoracolumbar region E64.3 [M49.85]
  sciatic M54.4- ☑
  secondary (to) NEC M41.50
    cerebral palsy, Friedreich's ataxia, poliomyelitis, neuromuscular disorders — *see* Scoliosis, neuromuscular
    cervical region M41.52
    cervicothoracic region M41.53
    lumbar region M41.56
    lumbosacral region M41.57
    thoracic region M41.54
    thoracolumbar region M41.55
  specified form NEC M41.80
    cervical region M41.82
    cervicothoracic region M41.83
    lumbar region M41.86
    lumbosacral region M41.87
    thoracic region M41.84
    thoracolumbar region M41.85
  thoracogenic M41.30
    thoracic region M41.34
    thoracolumbar region M41.35
  tuberculous A18.01
Scoliotic pelvis
  with disproportion (fetopelvic) O33.0
    causing obstructed labor O65.0
Scorbutus, scorbutic (*see also* Scurvy)
  anemia D53.2
Score, NIHSS (National Institutes of Health Stroke Scale) R29.7- ☑
Scotoma (arcuate) (Bjerrum) (central) (ring) (*see also* Defect, visual field, localized, scotoma)
  scintillating H53.19
Scratch — *see* Abrasion
Scratchy throat R09.89
Screening (for) Z13.9
  alcoholism Z13.39
  anemia Z13.0
  anomaly, congenital Z13.89
  antenatal, of mother (*see also* Encounter, antenatal screening) Z36.9
  arterial hypertension Z13.6
  arthropod-borne viral disease NEC Z11.59
  autism Z13.41
  bacteriuria, asymptomatic Z13.89
  behavioral disorder Z13.30
    specified NEC Z13.39

Screening — *continued*
  brain injury, traumatic Z13.85Ø
  bronchitis, chronic Z13.83
  brucellosis Z11.2
  cardiovascular disorder Z13.6
  cataract Z13.5
  chlamydial diseases Z11.8
  cholera Z11.Ø
  chromosomal abnormalities (nonprocreative) NEC
    Z13.79
  colonoscopy Z12.11
  congenital
    dislocation of hip Z13.89
    eye disorder Z13.5
    malformation or deformation Z13.89
  contamination NEC Z13.88
  cystic fibrosis Z13.228
  dengue fever Z11.59
  dental disorder Z13.84
  depression (adult) (adolescent) (child) Z13.31
    maternal Z13.32
    perinatal Z13.32
  developmental
    delays Z13.4Ø
      global (milestones) Z13.42
      specified NEC Z13.49
    handicap Z13.42
      in early childhood Z13.42
  diabetes mellitus Z13.1
  diphtheria Z11.2
  disability, intellectual Z13.39
  disease or disorder Z13.9
    bacterial NEC Z11.2
      intestinal infectious Z11.Ø
      respiratory tuberculosis Z11.1
    behavioral Z13.3Ø
      specified NEC Z13.39
    blood or blood-forming organ Z13.Ø
    cardiovascular Z13.6
    Chagas' Z11.6
    chlamydial Z11.8
    dental Z13.89
    developmental delays Z13.4Ø
      global (milestones) Z13.42
      specified NEC Z13.49
    digestive tract NEC Z13.818
      lower GI Z13.811
      upper GI Z13.81Ø
    ear Z13.5
    endocrine Z13.29
    eye Z13.5
    genitourinary Z13.89
    heart Z13.6
    human immunodeficiency virus (HIV) infection Z11.4
    immunity Z13.Ø
    infection
      intestinal Z11.Ø
        specified NEC Z11.6
    infectious Z11.9
    mental health and behavioral Z13.3Ø
      specified NEC Z13.39
    metabolic Z13.228
    neurological Z13.89
    nutritional Z13.21
      metabolic Z13.228
      lipoid disorders Z13.22Ø
    protozoal Z11.6
      intestinal Z11.Ø
    respiratory Z13.83
    rheumatic Z13.828
    rickettsial Z11.8
    sexually-transmitted NEC Z11.3
      human immunodeficiency virus (HIV) Z11.4
    sickle-cell (trait) Z13.Ø
    skin Z13.89
    specified NEC Z13.89
    spirochetal Z11.8
    thyroid Z13.29
    vascular Z13.6
    venereal Z11.3
    viral NEC Z11.59
      human immunodeficiency virus (HIV) Z11.4
      intestinal Z11.Ø
  elevated titer Z13.89
  emphysema Z13.83
  encephalitis, viral (mosquito- or tick-borne) Z11.59
  exposure to contaminants (toxic) Z13.88
  fever
    dengue Z11.59

Screening — *continued*
  fever — *continued*
    hemorrhagic Z11.59
    yellow Z11.59
  filariasis Z11.6
  galactosemia Z13.228
  gastrointestinal condition Z13.818
  genetic (nonprocreative) - for procreative management
    — *see* Testing, genetic, for procreative manage-
    ment
    disease carrier status (nonprocreative) Z13.71
    specified NEC (nonprocreative) Z13.79
  genitourinary condition Z13.89
  glaucoma Z13.5
  gonorrhea Z11.3
  gout Z13.89
  helminthiasis (intestinal) Z11.6
  hematopoietic malignancy Z12.89
  hemoglobinopathies NEC Z13.Ø
  hemorrhagic fever Z11.59
  Hodgkin disease Z12.89
  human immunodeficiency virus (HIV) Z11.4
  human papillomavirus Z11.51
  hypertension Z13.6
  immunity disorders Z13.Ø
  infant or child (over 28 days old) ZØØ.129
    with abnormal findings ZØØ.121
  infection
    mycotic Z11.8
    parasitic Z11.8
  ingestion of radioactive substance Z13.88
  intellectual disability Z13.39
  intestinal
    helminthiasis Z11.6
    infectious disease Z11.Ø
  leishmaniasis Z11.6
  leprosy Z11.2
  leptospirosis Z11.8
  leukemia Z12.89
  lymphoma Z12.89
  malaria Z11.6
  malnutrition Z13.29
    metabolic Z13.228
    nutritional Z13.21
  measles Z11.59
  mental health disorder Z13.3Ø
    specified NEC Z13.39
  metabolic errors, inborn Z13.228
  multiphasic Z13.89
  musculoskeletal disorder Z13.828
    osteoporosis Z13.82Ø
  mycoses Z11.8
  myocardial infarction (acute) Z13.6
  neoplasm (malignant) (of) Z12.9
    bladder Z12.6
    blood Z12.89
    breast Z12.39
      routine mammogram Z12.31
    cervix Z12.4
    colon Z12.11
    genitourinary organs NEC Z12.79
      bladder Z12.6
      cervix Z12.4
      ovary Z12.73
      prostate Z12.5
      testis Z12.71
      vagina Z12.72
    hematopoietic system Z12.89
    intestinal tract Z12.1Ø
      colon Z12.11
      rectum Z12.12
      small intestine Z12.13
    lung Z12.2
    lymph (glands) Z12.89
    nervous system Z12.82
    oral cavity Z12.81
    prostate Z12.5
    rectum Z12.12
    respiratory organs Z12.2
    skin Z12.83
    small intestine Z12.13
    specified site NEC Z12.89
    stomach Z12.Ø
  nephropathy Z13.89
  nervous system disorders NEC Z13.858
  neurological condition Z13.89
  osteoporosis Z13.82Ø
  parasitic infestation Z11.9
    specified NEC Z11.8

Screening — *continued*
  phenylketonuria Z13.228
  plague Z11.2
  poisoning (chemical) (heavy metal) Z13.88
  poliomyelitis Z11.59
  postnatal, chromosomal abnormalities Z13.89
  prenatal, of mother (*see also* Encounter, antenatal
    screening) Z36.9
  protozoal disease Z11.6
    intestinal Z11.Ø
  pulmonary tuberculosis Z11.1
  radiation exposure Z13.88
  respiratory condition Z13.83
  respiratory tuberculosis Z11.1
  rheumatoid arthritis Z13.828
  rubella Z11.59
  schistosomiasis Z11.6
  sexually-transmitted disease NEC Z11.3
    human immunodeficiency virus (HIV) Z11.4
  sickle-cell disease or trait Z13.Ø
  skin condition Z13.89
  sleeping sickness Z11.6
  special Z13.9
    specified NEC Z13.89
  syphilis Z11.3
  tetanus Z11.2
  trachoma Z11.8
  traumatic brain injury Z13.85Ø
  trypanosomiasis Z11.6
  tuberculosis, respiratory Z11.1
  venereal disease Z11.3
  viral encephalitis (mosquito- or tick-borne) Z11.59
  whooping cough Z11.2
  worms, intestinal Z11.6
  yaws Z11.8
  yellow fever Z11.59
Scrofula, scrofulosis (tuberculosis of cervical lymph
    glands) A18.2
Scrofulide (primary) (tuberculous) A18.4
Scrofuloderma, scrofulodermia (any site) (primary)
    A18.4
Scrofulosus lichen (primary) (tuberculous) A18.4
Scrofulous — *see* condition
Scrotal tongue K14.5
Scrotum — *see* condition
Scurvy, scorbutic E54
  anemia D53.2
  gum E54
  infantile E54
  rickets E55.Ø [M9Ø.8Ø]
Sealpox BØ8.62
Seasickness T75.3 ☑
Seatworm (infection) (infestation) B8Ø
Sebaceous (*see also* condition)
  cyst — *see* Cyst, sebaceous
Seborrhea, seborrheic L21.9
  capillitii R23.8
  capitis L21.Ø
  dermatitis L21.9
    infantile L21.1
  eczema L21.9
    infantile L21.1
  sicca L21.Ø
Seckel's syndrome Q87.1
Seclusion, pupil — *see* Membrane, pupillary
Second hand tobacco smoke exposure (acute)
    (chronic) Z77.22
  in the perinatal period P96.81
Secondary
  dentin (in pulp) KØ4.3
  neoplasm, secondaries — *see* Table of Neoplasms,
    secondary
Secretion
  antidiuretic hormone, inappropriate E22.2
  catecholamine, by pheochromocytoma E27.5
  hormone
    antidiuretic, inappropriate (syndrome) E22.2
    by
      carcinoid tumor E34.Ø
      pheochromocytoma E27.5
    ectopic NEC E34.2
  urinary
    excessive R35.8
    suppression R34
Section
  nerve, traumatic — *see* Injury, nerve
Sedative, hypnotic, or anxiolytic-induced
  anxiety disorder F13.98Ø

☑ **Additional Character Required** — Refer to the Tabular List for Character Selection   ⁿᵉʷ **Subterms under main terms may continue to next column or page**

Sedative, hypnotic, or anxiolytic-induced — *continued*
  bipolar and related disorder F13.94
  delirium F13.921
  depressive disorder F13.94
  major neurocognitive disorder F13.97
  mild neurocognitive disorder F13.988
  psychotic disorder F13.959
  sexual dysfunction F13.981
  sleep disorder F13.982
Segmentation, incomplete (congenital) (*see also* Fusion)
  bone NEC Q78.8
  lumbosacral (joint) (vertebra) Q76.49
Seitelberger's syndrome (infantile neuraxonal dystrophy) G31.89
Seizure(s) (*see also* Convulsions) R56.9
  akinetic — *see* Epilepsy, generalized, specified NEC
  atonic — *see* Epilepsy, generalized, specified NEC
  autonomic (hysterical) F44.5
  convulsive — *see* Convulsions
  cortical (focal) (motor) — *see* Epilepsy, localization-related, symptomatic, with simple partial seizures
  disorder (*see also* Epilepsy) G40.909
  due to stroke — *see* Sequelae (of), disease, cerebrovascular, by type, specified NEC
  epileptic — *see* Epilepsy
  febrile (simple) R56.00
    with status epilepticus G40.901
    complex (atypical) (complicated) R56.01
      with status epilepticus G40.901
  grand mal G40.409
    intractable G40.419
      with status epilepticus G40.411
      without status epilepticus G40.419
    not intractable G40.409
      with status epilepticus G40.401
      without status epilepticus G40.409
  heart — *see* Disease, heart
  hysterical F44.5
  intractable G40.919
    with status epilepticus G40.911
  Jacksonian (focal) (motor type) (sensory type) — *see* Epilepsy, localization-related, symptomatic, with simple partial seizures
  newborn P90
  nonspecific epileptic
    atonic — *see* Epilepsy, generalized, specified NEC
    clonic — *see* Epilepsy, generalized, specified NEC
    myoclonic — *see* Epilepsy, generalized, specified NEC
    tonic — *see* Epilepsy, generalized, specified NEC
    tonic-clonic — *see* Epilepsy, generalized, specified NEC
  partial, developing into secondarily generalized seizures
    complex — *see* Epilepsy, localization-related, symptomatic, with complex partial seizures
    simple — *see* Epilepsy, localization-related, symptomatic, with simple partial seizures
  petit mal G40.409
    intractable G40.419
      with status epilepticus G40.411
      without status epilepticus G40.419
    not intractable G40.409
      with status epilepticus G40.401
      without status epilepticus G40.409
  post traumatic R56.1
  recurrent G40.909
  specified NEC G40.89
  uncinate — *see* Epilepsy, localization-related, symptomatic, with complex partial seizures
Selenium deficiency, dietary E59
Self-damaging behavior (life-style) Z72.89
Self-harm (attempted)
  history (personal) Z91.5
    in family Z81.8
Self-mutilation (attempted)
  history (personal) Z91.5
    in family Z81.8
Self-poisoning
  history (personal) Z91.5
    in family Z81.8
  observation following (alleged) attempt Z03.6
Semicoma R40.1
Seminal vesiculitis N49.0
Seminoma C62.9- ☑
  specified site — *see* Neoplasm, malignant, by site

Senear-Usher disease or syndrome L10.4
Senectus R54
Senescence (without mention of psychosis) R54
Senile, senility (*see also* condition) R41.81
  with
    acute confusional state F05
    mental changes NOS F03 ☑
    psychosis NEC — *see* Psychosis, senile
  asthenia R54
  cervix (atrophic) N88.8
  debility R54
  endometrium (atrophic) N85.8
  fallopian tube (atrophic) — *see* Atrophy, fallopian tube
  heart (failure) R54
  ovary (atrophic) — *see* Atrophy, ovary
  premature E34.8
  vagina, vaginitis (atrophic) N95.2
  wart L82.1
Sensation
  burning (skin) R20.8
    tongue K14.6
  loss of R20.8
  prickling (skin) R20.2
  tingling (skin) R20.2
Sense loss
  smell — *see* Disturbance, sensation, smell
  taste — *see* Disturbance, sensation, taste
  touch R20.8
Sensibility disturbance (cortical) (deep) (vibratory) R20.9
Sensitive, sensitivity (*see also* Allergy)
  carotid sinus G90.01
  child (excessive) F93.8
  cold, autoimmune D59.1
  dentin K03.89
  gluten (non-celiac) K90.41
  latex Z91.040
  methemoglobin D74.8
  tuberculin, without clinical or radiological symptoms R76.11
  visual
    glare H53.71
    impaired contrast H53.72
Sensitiver Beziehungswahn F22
Sensitization, auto-erythrocytic D69.2
Separation
  anxiety, abnormal (of childhood) F93.0
  apophysis, traumatic — *code as* Fracture, by site
  choroid — *see* Detachment, choroid
  epiphysis, epiphyseal
    nontraumatic (*see also* Osteochondropathy, specified type NEC)
      upper femoral — *see* Slipped, epiphysis, upper femoral
    traumatic — *code as* Fracture, by site
  fracture — *see* Fracture
  infundibulum cardiac from right ventricle by a partition Q24.3
  joint (traumatic) (current) — *code by* site under Dislocation
  pubic bone, obstetrical trauma O71.6
  retina, retinal — *see* Detachment, retina
  symphysis pubis, obstetrical trauma O71.6
  tracheal ring, incomplete, congenital Q32.1
Sepsis (generalized) (unspecified organism) A41.9
  with
    organ dysfunction (acute) (multiple) R65.20
      with septic shock R65.21
  actinomycotic A42.7
  adrenal hemorrhage syndrome (meningococcal) A39.1
  anaerobic A41.4
  Bacillus anthracis A22.7
  Brucella (*see also* Brucellosis) A23.9
  candidal B37.7
  cryptogenic A41.9
  due to device, implant or graft T85.79 ☑
    arterial graft NEC T82.7 ☑
    breast (implant) T85.79 ☑
    catheter NEC T85.79 ☑
      dialysis (renal) T82.7 ☑
        intraperitoneal T85.71 ☑
      infusion NEC T82.7 ☑
        spinal (cranial) (epidural) (intrathecal) (spinal) (subarachnoid) (subdural) T85.735 ☑
      urethral indwelling T83.511 ☑
      urinary T83.518 ☑
    ectopic or molar pregnancy O08.82

Sepsis — *continued*
  due to device, implant or graft — *continued*
    electronic (electrode) (pulse generator) (stimulator)
      bone T84.7 ☑
      cardiac T82.7 ☑
      nervous system T85.738 ☑
        brain T85.731 ☑
        neurostimulator generator T85.734 ☑
        peripheral nerve T85.732 ☑
        spinal cord T85.733 ☑
      urinary T83.590 ☑
    fixation, internal (orthopedic) — *see* Complication, fixation device, infection
    gastrointestinal (bile duct) (esophagus) T85.79 ☑
      neurostimulator electrode (lead) T85.732 ☑
    genital T83.69 ☑
    heart NEC T82.7 ☑
      valve (prosthesis) T82.6 ☑
        graft T82.7 ☑
    joint prosthesis — *see* Complication, joint prosthesis, infection
    ocular (corneal graft) (orbital implant) T85.79 ☑
    orthopedic NEC T84.7 ☑
      fixation device, internal — *see* Complication, fixation device, infection
    specified NEC T85.79 ☑
    vascular T82.7 ☑
    ventricular intracranial (communicating) shunt T85.730 ☑
  during labor O75.3
  Enterococcus A41.81
  Erysipelothrix (rhusiopathiae) (erysipeloid) A26.7
  Escherichia coli (E. coli) A41.5 ☑
  extraintestinal yersiniosis A28.2
  following
    abortion (subsequent episode) O08.0
      current episode — *see* Abortion
    ectopic or molar pregnancy O08.82
    immunization T88.0 ☑
    infusion, therapeutic injection or transfusion NEC T80.29 ☑
    obstetrical procedure O86.04
  gangrenous A41.9
  gonococcal A54.86
  Gram-negative (organism) A41.5 ☑
    anaerobic A41.4
  Haemophilus influenzae A41.3
  herpesviral B00.7
  intra-abdominal K65.1
  intraocular — *see* Endophthalmitis, purulent
  Listeria monocytogenes A32.7
  localized — *code to* specific localized infection
    in operation wound T81.49 ☑
    skin — *see* Abscess
  malleus A24.0
  melioidosis A24.1
  meningeal — *see* Meningitis
  meningococcal A39.4
    acute A39.2
    chronic A39.3
  MSSA (Methicillin susceptible Staphylococcus aureus) A41.01
  newborn P36.9
    due to
      anaerobes NEC P36.5
      Escherichia coli P36.4
      Staphylococcus P36.30
        aureus P36.2
        specified NEC P36.39
      Streptococcus P36.10
        group B P36.0
        specified NEC P36.19
    specified NEC P36.8
  Pasteurella multocida A28.0
  pelvic, puerperal, postpartum, childbirth O85
  pneumococcal A40.3
  postprocedural T81.44 ☑
  puerperal, postpartum, childbirth (pelvic) O85
  Salmonella (arizonae) (cholerae-suis) (enteritidis) (typhimurium) A02.1
  severe R65.20
    with septic shock R65.21
  Shigella (*see also* Dysentery, bacillary) A03.9
  skin, localized — *see* Abscess
  specified organism NEC A41.89
  Staphylococcus, staphylococcal A41.2
    aureus (methicillin susceptible) (MSSA) A41.01

Sepsis — *continued*
  Staphylococcus, staphylococcal — *continued*
    aureus — *continued*
      methicillin resistant (MRSA) A41.02
    coagulase-negative A41.1
    specified NEC A41.1
  Streptococcus, streptococcal A40.9
    agalactiae A40.1
    group
      A A40.0
      B A40.1
      D A41.81
    neonatal P36.10
      group B P36.0
      specified NEC P36.19
    pneumoniae A40.3
    pyogenes A40.0
    specified NEC A40.8
  tracheostomy stoma J95.02
  tularemic A21.7
  umbilical, umbilical cord (newborn) — *see* Sepsis, newborn
  Yersinia pestis A20.7
Septate — *see* Septum
Septic — *see* condition
  arm — *see* Cellulitis, upper limb
    with lymphangitis — *see* Lymphangitis, acute, upper limb
  embolus — *see* Embolism
  finger — *see* Cellulitis, digit
    with lymphangitis — *see* Lymphangitis, acute, digit
  foot — *see* Cellulitis, lower limb
    with lymphangitis — *see* Lymphangitis, acute, lower limb
  gallbladder (acute) K81.0
  hand — *see* Cellulitis, upper limb
    with lymphangitis — *see* Lymphangitis, acute, upper limb
  joint — *see* Arthritis, pyogenic or pyemic
  leg — *see* Cellulitis, lower limb
    with lymphangitis — *see* Lymphangitis, acute, lower limb
  nail (*see also* Cellulitis, digit)
    with lymphangitis — *see* Lymphangitis, acute, digit
  sore (*see also* Abscess)
    throat J02.0
      streptococcal J02.0
  spleen (acute) D73.89
  teeth, tooth (pulpal origin) K04.4
  throat — *see* Pharyngitis
  thrombus — *see* Thrombosis
  toe — *see* Cellulitis, digit
    with lymphangitis — *see* Lymphangitis, acute, digit
  tonsils, chronic J35.01
    with adenoiditis J35.03
  uterus — *see* Endometritis
Septicemia A41.9
  meaning sepsis — *see* Sepsis
Septum, septate (congenital) (*see also* Anomaly, by site)
  anal Q42.3
    with fistula Q42.2
  aqueduct of Sylvius Q03.0
    with spina bifida — *see* Spina bifida, by site, with hydrocephalus
  uterus Q51.20
    complete Q51.21
    partial Q51.22
    specified NEC Q51.28
  vagina Q52.10
    in pregnancy — *see* Pregnancy, complicated by, abnormal vagina
      causing obstructed labor O65.5
    longitudinal Q52.129
      microperforate
        left side Q52.124
        right side Q52.123
      nonobstruction Q52.120
      obstructing Q52.129
        left side Q52.122
        right side Q52.121
    transverse Q52.11
Sequelae (of) (*see also* condition)
  abscess, intracranial or intraspinal (conditions in G06) G09

Sequelae — *continued*
  amputation — *code to* injury with seventh character S
  burn and corrosion — *code to* injury with seventh character S
  calcium deficiency E64.8
  cerebrovascular disease — *see* Sequelae, disease, cerebrovascular
  childbirth O94
  contusion — *code to* injury with seventh character S
  corrosion — *see* Sequelae, burn and corrosion
  crushing injury — *code to* injury with seventh character S
  disease
    cerebrovascular I69.90
      alteration of sensation I69.998
      aphasia I69.920
      apraxia I69.990
      ataxia I69.993
      cognitive deficits I69.91 ☑
      disturbance of vision I69.998
      dysarthria I69.922
      dysphagia I69.991
      dysphasia I69.921
      facial droop I69.992
      facial weakness I69.992
      fluency disorder I69.923
      hemiplegia I69.95- ☑
      hemorrhage
        intracerebral — *see* Sequelae, hemorrhage, intracerebral
        intracranial, nontraumatic NEC — *see* Sequelae, hemorrhage, intracranial, nontraumatic
        subarachnoid — *see* Sequelae, hemorrhage, subarachnoid
      language deficit I69.928
      monoplegia
        lower limb I69.94- ☑
        upper limb I69.93- ☑
      paralytic syndrome I69.96- ☑
      specified effect NEC I69.998
      specified type NEC I69.80
        alteration of sensation I69.898
        aphasia I69.820
        apraxia I69.890
        ataxia I69.893
        cognitive deficits I69.81 ☑
        disturbance of vision I69.898
        dysarthria I69.822
        dysphagia I69.891
        dysphasia I69.821
        facial droop I69.892
        facial weakness I69.892
        fluency disorder I69.823
        hemiplegia I69.85- ☑
        language deficit I69.828
        monoplegia
          lower limb I69.84- ☑
          upper limb I69.83- ☑
        paralytic syndrome I69.86- ☑
        specified effect NEC I69.898
      speech deficit I69.928
        speech deficit I69.828
      stroke NOS — *see* Sequelae, stroke NOS
  dislocation — *code to* injury with seventh character S
  encephalitis or encephalomyelitis (conditions in G04) G09
    in infectious disease NEC B94.8
    viral B94.1
  external cause — *code to* injury with seventh character S
  foreign body entering natural orifice — *code to* injury with seventh character S
  fracture — *code to* injury with seventh character S
  frostbite — *code to* injury with seventh character S
  Hansen's disease B92
  hemorrhage
    intracerebral I69.10
      alteration of sensation I69.198
      aphasia I69.120
      apraxia I69.190
      ataxia I69.193
      cognitive deficits I69.11 ☑
      disturbance of vision I69.198
      dysarthria I69.122
      dysphagia I69.191
      dysphasia I69.121

Sequelae — *continued*
  hemorrhage — *continued*
    intracerebral — *continued*
      facial droop I69.192
      facial weakness I69.192
      fluency disorder I69.123
      hemiplegia I69.15- ☑
      language deficit NEC I69.128
      monoplegia
        lower limb I69.14- ☑
        upper limb I69.13- ☑
      paralytic syndrome I69.16- ☑
      specified effect NEC I69.198
      speech deficit NEC I69.128
    intracranial, nontraumatic NEC I69.20
      alteration of sensation I69.298
      aphasia I69.220
      apraxia I69.290
      ataxia I69.293
      cognitive deficits I69.21 ☑
      disturbance of vision I69.298
      dysarthria I69.222
      dysphagia I69.291
      dysphasia I69.221
      facial droop I69.292
      facial weakness I69.292
      fluency disorder I69.223
      hemiplegia I69.25- ☑
      language deficit NEC I69.228
      monoplegia
        lower limb I69.24- ☑
        upper limb I69.23- ☑
      paralytic syndrome I69.26- ☑
      specified effect NEC I69.298
      speech deficit NEC I69.228
    subarachnoid I69.00
      alteration of sensation I69.098
      aphasia I69.020
      apraxia I69.090
      ataxia I69.093
      cognitive deficits — *see* subcategory I69.01- ☑
      disturbance of vision I69.098
      dysarthria I69.022
      dysphagia I69.091
      dysphasia I69.021
      facial droop I69.092
      facial weakness I69.092
      fluency disorder I69.023
      hemiplegia I69.05- ☑
      language deficit NEC I69.028
      monoplegia
        lower limb I69.04- ☑
        upper limb I69.03- ☑
      paralytic syndrome I69.06- ☑
      specified effect NEC I69.098
      speech deficit NEC I69.028
  hepatitis, viral B94.2
  hyperalimentation E68
  infarction
    cerebral I69.30
      alteration of sensation I69.398
      aphasia I69.320
      apraxia I69.390
      ataxia I69.393
      cognitive deficits I69.31 ☑
      disturbance of vision I69.398
      dysarthria I69.322
      dysphagia I69.391
      dysphasia I69.321
      facial droop I69.392
      facial weakness I69.392
      fluency disorder I69.323
      hemiplegia I69.35- ☑
      language deficit NEC I69.328
      monoplegia
        lower limb I69.34- ☑
        upper limb I69.33- ☑
      paralytic syndrome I69.36- ☑
      specified effect NEC I69.398
      speech deficit NEC I69.328
  infection, pyogenic, intracranial or intraspinal G09
  infectious disease B94.9
    specified NEC B94.8
  injury — *code to* injury with seventh character S
  leprosy B92
  meningitis
    bacterial (conditions in G00) G09
    other or unspecified cause (conditions in G03) G09

Sequelae — *continued*
- muscle (and tendon) injury — *code to* injury with seventh character S
- myelitis — *see* Sequelae, encephalitis
- niacin deficiency E64.8
- nutritional deficiency E64.9
  - specified NEC E64.8
- obstetrical condition O94
- parasitic disease B94.9
- phlebitis or thrombophlebitis of intracranial or intraspinal venous sinuses and veins (conditions in G08) G09
- poisoning — *code to* poisoning with seventh character S
  - nonmedicinal substance — *see* Sequelae, toxic effect, nonmedicinal substance
- poliomyelitis (acute) B91
- pregnancy O94
- protein-energy malnutrition E64.0
- puerperium O94
- rickets E64.3
- selenium deficiency E64.8
- sprain and strain — *code to* injury with seventh character S
- stroke NOS I69.30
  - alteration in sensation I69.398
  - aphasia I69.320
  - apraxia I69.390
  - ataxia I69.393
  - cognitive deficits I69.31 ☑
  - disturbance of vision I69.398
  - dysarthria I69.322
  - dysphagia I69.391
  - dysphasia I69.321
  - facial droop I69.392
  - facial weakness I69.392
  - hemiplegia I69.35- ☑
  - language deficit NEC I69.328
  - monoplegia
    - lower limb I69.34- ☑
    - upper limb I69.33- ☑
  - paralytic syndrome I69.36- ☑
  - specified effect NEC I69.398
  - speech deficit NEC I69.328
- tendon and muscle injury — *code to* injury with seventh character S
- thiamine deficiency E64.8
- trachoma B94.0
- tuberculosis B90.9
  - bones and joints B90.2
  - central nervous system B90.0
  - genitourinary B90.1
  - pulmonary (respiratory) B90.9
  - specified organs NEC B90.8
- viral
  - encephalitis B94.1
  - hepatitis B94.2
- vitamin deficiency NEC E64.8
  - A E64.1
  - B E64.8
  - C E64.2
- wound, open — *code to* injury with seventh character S

Sequestration (*see also* Sequestrum)
- disk — *see* Displacement, intervertebral disk
- lung, congenital Q33.2

Sequestrum
- bone — *see* Osteomyelitis, chronic
- dental M27.2
- jaw bone M27.2
- orbit — *see* Osteomyelitis, orbit
- sinus (accessory) (nasal) — *see* Sinusitis

Sequoiosis lung or pneumonitis J67.8
Serology for syphilis
- doubtful
  - with signs or symptoms — *code by* site and stage under Syphilis
  - follow-up of latent syphilis — *see* Syphilis, latent
  - negative, with signs or symptoms — *code by* site and stage under Syphilis
- positive A53.0
  - with signs or symptoms — *code by* site and stage under Syphilis
- reactivated A53.0

Seroma (*see also* Hematoma)
- postprocedural — *see* Complication, postprocedural, seroma
- traumatic, secondary and recurrent T79.2 ☑

Seropurulent — *see* condition
Serositis, multiple K65.8
- pericardial I31.1
- peritoneal K65.8
Serous — *see* condition
Sertoli cell
- adenoma
  - specified site — *see* Neoplasm, benign, by site
  - unspecified site
    - female D27.9
    - male D29.20
- carcinoma
  - specified site — *see* Neoplasm, malignant, by site
  - unspecified site (male) C62.9- ☑
    - female C56.9
- tumor
  - with lipid storage
    - specified site — *see* Neoplasm, benign, by site
    - unspecified site
      - female D27.9
      - male D29.20
  - specified site — *see* Neoplasm, benign, by site
  - unspecified site
    - female D27.9
    - male D29.20
Sertoli-Leydig cell tumor — *see* Neoplasm, benign, by site
- specified site — *see* Neoplasm, benign, by site
- unspecified site
  - female D27.9
  - male D29.20
Serum
- allergy, allergic reaction (*see also* Reaction, serum) T80.69 ☑
  - shock (*see also* Shock, anaphylactic) T80.59 ☑
- arthritis (*see also* Reaction, serum) T80.69 ☑
- complication or reaction NEC (*see also* Reaction, serum) T80.69 ☑
- disease NEC (*see also* Reaction, serum) T80.69 ☑
- hepatitis (*see also* Hepatitis, viral, type B)
  - carrier (suspected) of B18.1
- intoxication (*see also* Reaction, serum) T80.69 ☑
- neuritis (*see also* Reaction, serum) T80.69 ☑
- neuropathy G61.1
- poisoning NEC (*see also* Reaction, serum) T80.69 ☑
- rash NEC (*see also* Reaction, serum) T80.69 ☑
- reaction NEC (*see also* Reaction, serum) T80.69 ☑
- sickness NEC (*see also* Reaction, serum) T80.69 ☑
- urticaria (*see also* Reaction, serum) T80.69 ☑
Sesamoiditis M25.8- ☑
Severe sepsis R65.20
- with septic shock R65.21
Sever's disease or osteochondrosis — *see* Osteochondrosis, juvenile, tarsus
Sex
- chromosome mosaics Q97.8
  - lines with various numbers of X chromosomes Q97.2
- education Z70.8
- reassignment surgery status Z87.890
Sextuplet pregnancy — *see* Pregnancy, sextuplet
Sexual
- function, disorder of (psychogenic) F52.9
- immaturity (female) (male) E30.0
- impotence (psychogenic) organic origin NEC — *see* Dysfunction, sexual, male
- precocity (constitutional) (cryptogenic) (female) (idiopathic) (male) E30.1
Sexuality, pathologic — *see* Deviation, sexual
Sézary disease C84.1- ☑
Shadow, lung R91.8
Shaking palsy or paralysis — *see* Parkinsonism
Shallowness, acetabulum — *see* Derangement, joint, specified type NEC, hip
Shaver's disease J63.1
Sheath (tendon) — *see* condition
Sheathing, retinal vessels H35.01- ☑
Shedding
- nail L60.8
- premature, primary (deciduous) teeth K00.6
Sheehan's disease or syndrome E23.0
Shelf, rectal K62.89
Shell teeth K00.5
Shellshock (current) F43.0
- lasting state — *see* Disorder, post-traumatic stress
Shield kidney Q63.1
Shift
- auditory threshold (temporary) H93.24- ☑

Shift — *continued*
- mediastinal R93.89
Shifting sleep-work schedule (affecting sleep) G47.26
Shiga (-Kruse) **dysentery** A03.0
Shiga's bacillus A03.0
Shigella (dysentery) — *see* Dysentery, bacillary
Shigellosis A03.9
- Group A A03.0
- Group B A03.1
- Group C A03.2
- Group D A03.3
Shin splints S86.89- ☑
Shingles — *see* Herpes, zoster
Shipyard disease or eye B30.0
Shirodkar suture, in pregnancy — *see* Pregnancy, complicated by, incompetent cervix
Shock R57.9
- with ectopic or molar pregnancy O08.3
- adrenal (cortical) (Addisonian) E27.2
- adverse food reaction (anaphylactic) — *see* Shock, anaphylactic, due to food
- allergic — *see* Shock, anaphylactic
- anaphylactic T78.2 ☑
  - chemical — *see* Table of Drugs and Chemicals
  - due to drug or medicinal substance
    - correct substance properly administered T88.6 ☑
    - overdose or wrong substance given or taken (by accident) — *see* Table of Drugs and Chemicals, by drug, poisoning
  - due to food (nonpoisonous) T78.00 ☑
    - additives T78.06 ☑
    - dairy products T78.07 ☑
    - eggs T78.08 ☑
    - fish T78.03 ☑
      - shellfish T78.02 ☑
    - fruit T78.04 ☑
    - milk T78.07 ☑
    - nuts T78.05 ☑
      - multiple types T78.05 ☑
      - peanuts T78.01 ☑
    - peanuts T78.01 ☑
    - seeds T78.05 ☑
    - specified type NEC T78.09 ☑
    - vegetable T78.04 ☑
  - following sting(s) — *see* Venom
  - immunization T80.52 ☑
  - serum T80.59 ☑
    - blood and blood products T80.51 ☑
    - immunization T80.52 ☑
    - specified NEC T80.59 ☑
    - vaccination T80.52 ☑
- anaphylactoid — *see* Shock, anaphylactic
- anesthetic
  - correct substance properly administered T88.2 ☑
  - overdose or wrong substance given or taken — *see* Table of Drugs and Chemicals, by drug, poisoning
  - specified anesthetic — *see* Table of Drugs and Chemicals, by drug, poisoning
- cardiogenic R57.0
- chemical substance — *see* Table of Drugs and Chemicals
- complicating ectopic or molar pregnancy O08.3
- culture — *see* Disorder, adjustment
- drug
  - due to correct substance properly administered T88.6 ☑
  - overdose or wrong substance given or taken (by accident) — *see* Table of Drugs and Chemicals, by drug, poisoning
- during or after labor and delivery O75.1
- electric T75.4 ☑
  - (taser) T75.4 ☑
- endotoxic R65.21
  - postprocedural (resulting from a procedure, not elsewhere classified) T81.12 ☑
- following
  - ectopic or molar pregnancy O08.3
  - injury (immediate) (delayed) T79.4 ☑
  - labor and delivery O75.1
- food (anaphylactic) — *see* Shock, anaphylactic, due to food
- from electroshock gun (taser) T75.4 ☑
- gram-negative R65.21
  - postprocedural (resulting from a procedure, not elsewhere classified) T81.12 ☑
- hematologic R57.8

Shock — *continued*
hemorrhagic R57.8
surgery (intraoperative) (postoperative) T81.19 ☑
trauma T79.4 ☑
hypovolemic R57.1
surgical T81.19 ☑
traumatic T79.4 ☑
insulin E15
therapeutic misadventure — *see* subcategory
T38.3 ☑
kidney N17.0
traumatic (following crushing) T79.5 ☑
lightning T75.01 ☑
liver K72.00
lung J80
obstetric O75.1
with ectopic or molar pregnancy O08.3
following ectopic or molar pregnancy O08.3
pleural (surgical) T81.19 ☑
due to trauma T79.4 ☑
postprocedural (postoperative) T81.10 ☑
with ectopic or molar pregnancy O08.3
cardiogenic T81.11 ☑
endotoxic T81.12 ☑
following ectopic or molar pregnancy O08.3
gram-negative T81.12 ☑
hypovolemic T81.19 ☑
septic T81.12 ☑
specified type NEC T81.19 ☑
psychic F43.0
septic (due to severe sepsis) R65.21
specified NEC R57.8
surgical T81.10 ☑
taser gun (taser) T75.4 ☑
therapeutic misadventure NEC T81.10 ☑
thyroxin
overdose or wrong substance given or taken — *see*
Table of Drugs and Chemicals, by drug, poisoning
toxic, syndrome A48.3
transfusion — *see* Complications, transfusion
traumatic (immediate) (delayed) T79.4 ☑
Shoemaker's chest M95.4
Short, shortening, shortness
arm (acquired) (*see also* Deformity, limb, unequal
length)
congenital Q71.81-
forearm — *see* Deformity, limb, unequal length
bowel syndrome K91.2
breath R06.02
cervical (complicating pregnancy) O26.87- ☑
non-gravid uterus N88.3
common bile duct, congenital Q44.5
cord (umbilical), complicating delivery O69.3 ☑
cystic duct, congenital Q44.5
esophagus (congenital) Q39.8
femur (acquired) — *see* Deformity, limb, unequal
length, femur
congenital — *see* Defect, reduction, lower limb,
longitudinal, femur
frenum, frenulum, linguae (congenital) Q38.1
hip (acquired) (*see also* Deformity, limb, unequal
length)
congenital Q65.89
leg (acquired) (*see also* Deformity, limb, unequal
length)
congenital Q72.81- ☑
lower leg (*see also* Deformity, limb, unequal length)
limbed stature, with immunodeficiency D82.2
lower limb (acquired) (*see also* Deformity, limb, unequal
length)
congenital Q72.81- ☑
organ or site, congenital NEC — *see* Distortion
palate, congenital Q38.5
radius (acquired) (*see also* Deformity, limb, unequal
length)
congenital — *see* Defect, reduction, upper limb,
longitudinal, radius
rib syndrome Q77.2
stature (child) (hereditary) (idiopathic) NEC R62.52
constitutional E34.3
due to endocrine disorder E34.3
Laron-type E34.3
tendon (*see also* Contraction, tendon)
with contracture of joint — *see* Contraction, joint
Achilles (acquired) M67.0- ☑
congenital Q66.89

Short, shortening, shortness — *continued*
tendon (*see also* Contraction, tendon) — *continued*
congenital Q79.8
thigh (acquired) (*see also* Deformity, limb, unequal
length, femur)
congenital — *see* Defect, reduction, lower limb,
longitudinal, femur
tibialis anterior (tendon) — *see* Contraction, tendon
umbilical cord
complicating delivery O69.3 ☑
upper limb, congenital — *see* Defect, reduction, upper
limb, specified type NEC
urethra N36.8
uvula, congenital Q38.5
vagina (congenital) Q52.4
Shortsightedness — *see* Myopia
Shoshin (acute fulminating beriberi) E51.11
Shoulder — *see* condition
Shovel-shaped incisors K00.2
Shower, thromboembolic — *see* Embolism
Shunt
arterial-venous (dialysis) Z99.2
arteriovenous, pulmonary (acquired) I28.0
congenital Q25.72
cerebral ventricle (communicating) in situ Z98.2
surgical, prosthetic, with complications — *see* Compli-
cations, cardiovascular, device or implant
Shutdown, renal N28.9
Shy-Drager syndrome G90.3
Sialadenitis, sialadenosis (any gland) (chronic) (period-
ic) (suppurative) — *see* Sialoadenitis
Sialectasia K11.8
Sialidosis E77.1
Sialitis, silitis (any gland) (chronic) (suppurative) — *see*
Sialoadenitis
Sialoadenitis (any gland) (periodic) (suppurative) K11.20
acute K11.21
recurrent K11.22
chronic K11.23
Sialoadenopathy K11.9
Sialoangitis — *see* Sialoadenitis
Sialodochitis (fibrinosa) — *see* Sialoadenitis
Sialodocholithiasis K11.5
Sialolithiasis K11.5
Sialometaplasia, necrotizing K11.8
Sialorrhea (*see also* Ptyalism)
periodic — *see* Sialoadenitis
Sialosis K11.7
Siamese twin Q89.4
Sibling rivalry Z62.891
Sicard's syndrome G52.7
Sicca syndrome M35.00
with
keratoconjunctivitis M35.01
lung involvement M35.02
myopathy M35.03
renal tubulo-interstitial disorders M35.04
specified organ involvement NEC M35.09
Sick R69
or handicapped person in family Z63.79
needing care at home Z63.6
sinus (syndrome) I49.5
Sick-euthyroid syndrome E07.81
Sickle-cell
anemia — *see* Disease, sickle-cell
trait D57.3
Sicklemia (*see also* Disease, sickle-cell)
trait D57.3
Sickness
air (travel) T75.3 ☑
airplane T75.3 ☑
alpine T70.29 ☑
altitude T70.20 ☑
Andes T70.29 ☑
aviator's T70.29 ☑
balloon T70.29 ☑
car T75.3 ☑
compressed air T70.3 ☑
decompression T70.3 ☑
green D50.8
milk — *see* Poisoning, food, noxious
motion T75.3 ☑
mountain T70.29 ☑
acute D75.1
protein (*see also* Reaction, serum) T80.69 ☑
radiation T66 ☑
roundabout (motion) T75.3 ☑

Sickness — *continued*
sea T75.3 ☑
serum NEC (*see also* Reaction, serum) T80.69 ☑
sleeping (African) B56.9
by Trypanosoma B56.9
brucei
gambiense B56.0
rhodesiense B56.1
East African B56.1
Gambian B56.0
Rhodesian B56.1
West African B56.0
swing (motion) T75.3 ☑
train (railway) (travel) T75.3 ☑
travel (any vehicle) T75.3 ☑
Sideropenia — *see* Anemia, iron deficiency
Siderosilicosis J62.8
Siderosis (lung) J63.4
eye (globe) — *see* Disorder, globe, degenerative,
siderosis
Siemens' syndrome (ectodermal dysplasia) Q82.8
Sighing R06.89
psychogenic F45.8
Sigmoid (*see also* condition)
flexure — *see* condition
kidney Q63.1
Sigmoiditis (*see also* Enteritis) K52.9
infectious A09
noninfectious K52.9
Silfversköld's syndrome Q78.9
Silicosiderosis J62.8
Silicosis, silicotic (simple) (complicated) J62.8
with tuberculosis J65
Silicotuberculosis J65
Silo-fillers' disease J68.8
bronchitis J68.0
pneumonitis J68.0
pulmonary edema J68.1
Silver's syndrome Q87.1
Simian malaria B53.1
Simmonds' cachexia or disease E23.0
Simons' disease or syndrome (progressive lipodystro-
phy) E88.1
Simple, simplex — *see* condition
Simulation, conscious (of illness) Z76.5
Simultanagnosia (asimultagnosia) R48.3
Sin Nombre virus disease (Hantavirus) (cardio)-pul-
monary syndrome) B33.4
Sinding-Larsen disease or osteochondrosis — *see*
Osteochondrosis, juvenile, patella
Singapore hemorrhagic fever A91
Singer's node or nodule J38.2
Single
atrium Q21.2
coronary artery Q24.5
umbilical artery Q27.0
ventricle Q20.4
Singultus R06.6
epidemicus B33.0
Sinus (*see also* Fistula)
abdominal K63.89
arrest I45.5
arrhythmia I49.8
bradycardia R00.1
branchial cleft (internal) (external) Q18.0
coccygeal — *see* Sinus, pilonidal
dental K04.6
dermal (congenital) Q06.8
with abscess Q06.8
coccygeal, pilonidal — *see* Sinus, coccygeal
infected, skin NEC L08.89
marginal, ruptured or bleeding — *see* Hemorrhage,
antepartum, specified cause NEC
medial, face and neck Q18.8
pause I45.5
pericranii Q01.9
pilonidal (infected) (rectum) L05.92
with abscess L05.02
preauricular Q18.1
rectovaginal N82.3
Rokitansky-Aschoff (gallbladder) K82.8
sacrococcygeal (dermoid) (infected) — *see* Sinus, pilonidal
tachycardia R00.0
paroxysmal I47.1
tarsi syndrome M25.57- ☑
testis N50.89

☑ **Additional Character Required** — Refer to the Tabular List for Character Selection
▽ **Subterms under main terms may continue to next column or page**

Sinus — *continued*
  tract (postinfective) — *see* Fistula
  urachus Q64.4
Sinusitis (accessory) (chronic) (hyperplastic) (nasal)
  (nonpurulent) (purulent) J32.9
  acute J01.90
    ethmoidal J01.20
      recurrent J01.21
    frontal J01.10
      recurrent J01.11
    involving more than one sinus, other than pansinusi-
      tis J01.80
      recurrent J01.81
    maxillary J01.00
      recurrent J01.01
    pansinusitis J01.40
      recurrent J01.41
    recurrent J01.91
    specified NEC J01.80
      recurrent J01.81
    sphenoidal J01.30
      recurrent J01.31
  allergic — *see* Rhinitis, allergic
  due to high altitude T70.1 ☑
  ethmoidal J32.2
    acute J01.20
      recurrent J01.21
  frontal J32.1
    acute J01.10
      recurrent J01.11
  influenzal — *see* Influenza, with, respiratory manifesta-
    tions NEC
  involving more than one sinus but not pansinusitis
    J32.8
    acute J01.80
      recurrent J01.81
  maxillary J32.0
    acute J01.00
      recurrent J01.01
  sphenoidal J32.3
    acute J01.30
      recurrent J01.31
  tuberculous, any sinus A15.8
Sinusitis-bronchiectasis-situs inversus (syndrome)
  (triad) Q89.3
Sipple's syndrome E31.22
Sirenomelia (syndrome) Q87.2
Siriasis T67.0 ☑
Sirkari's disease B55.0
Siti A65
Situation, psychiatric F99
Situational
  disturbance (transient) — *see* Disorder, adjustment
    acute F43.0
  maladjustment — *see* Disorder, adjustment
  reaction — *see* Disorder, adjustment
    acute F43.0
Situs inversus or transversus (abdominalis) (thoracis)
  Q89.3
Sixth disease B08.20
  due to human herpesvirus 6 B08.21
  due to human herpesvirus 7 B08.22
Sjögren-Larsson syndrome Q87.1
Sjögren's syndrome or disease — *see* Sicca syndrome
Skeletal — *see* condition
Skene's gland — *see* condition
Skenitis — *see* Urethritis
Skerljevo A65
Skevas-Zerfus disease — *see* Toxicity, venom, marine
  animal, sea anemone
Skin (*see also* condition)
  clammy R23.1
  donor — *see* Donor, skin
  hidebound M35.9
Slate-dressers' or slate-miners' lung J62.8
Sleep
  apnea — *see* Apnea, sleep
  deprivation Z72.820
  disorder or disturbance G47.9
    child F51.9
      nonorganic origin F51.9
      specified NEC G47.8
  disturbance G47.9
    nonorganic origin F51.9
  drunkenness F51.9
  rhythm inversion G47.2- ☑
  terrors F51.4
  walking F51.3

Sleep — *continued*
  walking — *continued*
    hysterical F44.89
Sleep hygiene
  abuse Z72.821
  inadequate Z72.821
  poor Z72.821
Sleeping sickness — *see* Sickness, sleeping
Sleeplessness — *see* Insomnia
  menopausal N95.1
Sleep-wake schedule disorder G47.20
Slim disease (in HIV infection) B20
Slipped, slipping
  epiphysis (traumatic) (*see also* Osteochondropathy,
    specified type NEC)
    capital femoral (traumatic)
      acute (on chronic) S79.01- ☑
    current traumatic — *code as* Fracture, by site
    upper femoral (nontraumatic) M93.00- ☑
      acute M93.01- ☑
        on chronic M93.03- ☑
      chronic M93.02- ☑
  intervertebral disc — *see* Displacement, intervertebral
    disc
  ligature, umbilical P51.8
  patella — *see* Disorder, patella, derangement NEC
  rib M89.8X8
  sacroiliac joint — *see* subcategory M53.2 ☑
  tendon — *see* Disorder, tendon
  ulnar nerve, nontraumatic — *see* Lesion, nerve, ulnar
  vertebra NEC — *see* Spondylolisthesis
Slocumb's syndrome E27.0
Sloughing (multiple) (phagedena) (skin) (*see also* Gangrene)
  abscess — *see* Abscess
  appendix K38.8
  fascia — *see* Disorder, soft tissue, specified type NEC
  scrotum N50.89
  tendon — *see* Disorder, tendon
  transplanted organ — *see* Rejection, transplant
  ulcer — *see* Ulcer, skin
Slow
  feeding, newborn P92.2
  flow syndrome, coronary I20.8
  heart (beat) R00.1
Slowing, urinary stream R39.198
Sluder's neuralgia (syndrome) G44.89
Slurred, slurring speech R47.81
Small (ness)
  for gestational age — *see* Small for dates
  introitus, vagina N89.6
  kidney (unknown cause) N27.9
    bilateral N27.1
    unilateral N27.0
  ovary (congenital) Q50.39
  pelvis
    with disproportion (fetopelvic) O33.1
      causing obstructed labor O65.1
  uterus N85.8
  white kidney N03.9
Small-and-light-for-dates — *see* Small for dates
Small-for-dates (infant) P05.10
  with weight of
    499 grams or less P05.11
    500-749 grams P05.12
    750-999 grams P05.13
    1000-1249 grams P05.14
    1250-1499 grams P05.15
    1500-1749 grams P05.16
    1750-1999 grams P05.17
    2000-2499 grams P05.18
    2500 grams and over P05.19
  specified NEC P05.19
Smallpox B03
Smearing, fecal R15.1
Smith-Lemli-Opitz syndrome E78.72
Smith's fracture S52.54- ☑
Smoker — *see* Dependence, drug, nicotine
Smoker's
  bronchitis J41.0
  cough J41.0
  palate K13.24
  throat J31.2
  tongue K13.24
Smoking
  passive Z77.22
Smothering spells R06.81

Snaggle teeth, tooth M26.39
Snapping
  finger — *see* Trigger finger
  hip — *see* Derangement, joint, specified type NEC, hip
    involving the iliotibial band M76.3- ☑
  knee — *see* Derangement, knee
    involving the iliotibial band M76.3- ☑
Sneddon-Wilkinson disease or syndrome (sub-corneal
  pustular dermatosis) L13.1
Sneezing (intractable) R06.7
Sniffing
  cocaine
    abuse — *see* Abuse, drug, cocaine
    dependence — *see* Dependence, drug, cocaine
  gasoline
    abuse — *see* Abuse, drug, inhalant
    dependence — *see* Dependence, drug, inhalant
  glue (airplane)
    abuse — *see* Abuse, drug, inhalant
    drug dependence — *see* Dependence, drug, in-
      halant
Sniffles
  newborn P28.89
Snoring R06.83
Snow blindness — *see* Photokeratitis
Snuffles (non-syphilitic) R06.5
  newborn P28.89
  syphilitic (infant) A50.05 [J99]
Social
  exclusion Z60.4
    due to discrimination or persecution (perceived)
      Z60.5
  migrant Z59.0
    acculturation difficulty Z60.3
  rejection Z60.4
    due to discrimination or persecution Z60.5
  role conflict NEC Z73.5
  skills inadequacy NEC Z73.4
  transplantation Z60.3
Sodoku A25.0
Soemmerring's ring — *see* Cataract, secondary
Soft (*see also* condition)
  nails L60.3
Softening
  bone — *see* Osteomalacia
  brain (necrotic) (progressive) G93.89
    congenital Q04.8
    embolic I63.4- ☑
    hemorrhagic — *see* Hemorrhage, intracranial, intrac-
      erebral
    occlusive I63.5- ☑
    thrombotic I63.3- ☑
  cartilage M94.2- ☑
    patella M22.4- ☑
  cerebellar — *see* Softening, brain
  cerebral — *see* Softening, brain
  cerebrospinal — *see* Softening, brain
  myocardial, heart — *see* Degeneration, myocardial
  spinal cord G95.89
  stomach K31.89
Soldier's
  heart F45.8
  patches I31.0
Solitary
  cyst, kidney N28.1
  kidney, congenital Q60.0
Solvent abuse — *see* Abuse, drug, inhalant
  dependence — *see* Dependence, drug, inhalant
Somatization reaction, somatic reaction — *see* Disorder, somatoform
Somnambulism F51.3
  hysterical F44.89
Somnolence R40.0
  nonorganic origin F51.11
Sonne dysentery A03.3
Soor B37.0
Sore
  bed — *see* Ulcer, pressure, by site
  chiclero B55.1
  Delhi B55.1
  desert — *see* Ulcer, skin
  eye H57.1- ☑
  Lahore B55.1
  mouth K13.79
    canker K12.0
  muscle M79.10
  Naga — *see* Ulcer, skin

Sore — *continued*
of skin — *see* Ulcer, skin
oriental B55.1
pressure — *see* Ulcer, pressure, by site
skin L98.9
soft A57
throat (acute) (*see also* Pharyngitis)
　with influenza, flu, or grippe — *see* Influenza, with, respiratory manifestations NEC
　chronic J31.2
　coxsackie (virus) B08.5
　diphtheritic A36.0
　herpesviral B00.2
　influenzal — *see* Influenza, with, respiratory manifestations NEC
　septic J02.0
　streptococcal (ulcerative) J02.0
　viral NEC J02.8
　　coxsackie B08.5
tropical — *see* Ulcer, skin
veldt — *see* Ulcer, skin
Soto's syndrome (cerebral gigantism) Q87.3
South African cardiomyopathy syndrome I42.8
Southeast Asian hemorrhagic fever A91
Spacing
abnormal, tooth, teeth, fully erupted M26.30
excessive, tooth, fully erupted M26.32
Spade-like hand (congenital) Q68.1
Spading nail L60.8
congenital Q84.6
Spanish collar N47.1
Sparganosis B70.1
Spasm(s), **spastic, spasticity** (*see also* condition) R25.2
accommodation — *see* Spasm, of accommodation
ampulla of Vater K83.4
anus, ani (sphincter) (reflex) K59.4
　psychogenic F45.8
artery I73.9
　cerebral G45.9
Bell's G51.3- ☑
bladder (sphincter, external or internal) N32.89
　psychogenic F45.8
bronchus, bronchiole J98.01
cardia K22.0
cardiac I20.1
carpopedal — *see* Tetany
cerebral (arteries) (vascular) G45.9
cervix, complicating delivery O62.4
ciliary body (of accommodation) — *see* Spasm, of accommodation
colon (*see also* Irritable, bowel) K58.9
　with diarrhea K58.0
　psychogenic F45.8
common duct K83.8
compulsive — *see* Tic
conjugate H51.8
coronary (artery) I20.1
diaphragm (reflex) R06.6
　epidemic B33.0
　psychogenic F45.8
duodenum K59.8
epidemic diaphragmatic (transient) B33.0
esophagus (diffuse) K22.4
　psychogenic F45.8
facial G51.3- ☑
fallopian tube N83.8
gastrointestinal (tract) K31.89
　psychogenic F45.8
glottis J38.5
　hysterical F44.4
　psychogenic F45.8
　　conversion reaction F44.4
　reflex through recurrent laryngeal nerve J38.5
habit — *see* Tic
heart I20.1
hemifacial (clonic) G51.3- ☑
hourglass — *see* Contraction, hourglass
hysterical F44.4
infantile — *see* Epilepsy, spasms
inferior oblique, eye H51.8
intestinal (*see also* Syndrome, irritable bowel) K58.9
　psychogenic F45.8
larynx, laryngeal J38.5
　hysterical F44.4
　psychogenic F45.8
　　conversion reaction F44.4
levator palpebrae superioris — *see* Disorder, eyelid function

Spasm(s), **spastic, spasticity** — *continued*
muscle NEC M62.838
　back M62.830
nerve, trigeminal G51.0
nervous F45.8
nodding F98.4
occupational F48.8
oculogyric H51.8
　psychogenic F45.8
of accommodation H52.53- ☑
ophthalmic artery — *see* Occlusion, artery, retina
perineal, female N94.89
peroneo-extensor (*see also* Deformity, limb, flat foot)
pharynx (reflex) J39.2
　hysterical F45.8
　psychogenic F45.8
psychogenic F45.8
pylorus NEC K31.3
　adult hypertrophic K31.89
　congenital or infantile Q40.0
　psychogenic F45.8
rectum (sphincter) K59.4
　psychogenic F45.8
retinal (artery) — *see* Occlusion, artery, retina
sigmoid (*see also* Syndrome, irritable bowel) K58.9
　psychogenic F45.8
sphincter of Oddi K83.4
stomach K31.89
　neurotic F45.8
throat J39.2
　hysterical F45.8
　psychogenic F45.8
tic F95.9
　chronic F95.1
　transient of childhood F95.0
tongue K14.8
torsion (progressive) G24.1
trigeminal nerve — *see* Neuralgia, trigeminal
ureter N13.5
urethra (sphincter) N35.919
uterus N85.8
　complicating labor O62.4
vagina N94.2
　psychogenic F52.5
vascular I73.9
vasomotor I73.9
vein NEC I87.8
viscera — *see* Pain, abdominal
Spasmodic — *see* condition
Spasmophilia — *see* Tetany
Spasmus nutans F98.4
Spastic, spasticity (*see also* Spasm)
child (cerebral) (congenital) (paralysis) G80.1
Speaker's throat R49.8
Specific, specified — *see* condition
Speech
defect, disorder, disturbance, impediment R47.9
　psychogenic, in childhood and adolescence F98.8
　slurring R47.81
　specified NEC R47.89
Spencer's disease A08.19
Spens' syndrome (syncope with heart block) I45.9
Sperm counts (fertility testing) Z31.41
postvasectomy Z30.8
reversal Z31.42
Spermatic cord — *see* condition
Spermatocele N43.40
congenital Q55.4
multiple N43.42
single N43.41
Spermatocystitis N49.0
Spermatocytoma C62.9- ☑
specified site — *see* Neoplasm, malignant, by site
Spermatorrhea N50.89
Sphacelus — *see* Gangrene
Sphenoidal — *see* condition
Sphenoiditis (chronic) — *see* Sinusitis, sphenoidal
Sphenopalatine ganglion neuralgia G90.09
Sphericity, increased, lens (congenital) Q12.4
Spherocytosis (congenital) (familial) (hereditary) D58.0
hemoglobin disease D58.0
sickle-cell (disease) D57.8- ☑
Spherophakia Q12.4
Sphincter — *see* condition
Sphincteritis, sphincter of Oddi — *see* Cholangitis
Sphingolipidosis E75.3
specified NEC E75.29
Sphingomyelinosis E75.3

Spicule tooth K00.2
Spider
bite — *see* Toxicity, venom, spider
fingers — *see* Syndrome, Marfan's
nevus I78.1
toes — *see* Syndrome, Marfan's
vascular I78.1
Spiegler-Fendt
benign lymphocytoma L98.8
sarcoid L08.89
Spielmeyer-Vogt disease E75.4
Spina bifida (aperta) Q05.9
with hydrocephalus NEC Q05.4
cervical Q05.5
　with hydrocephalus Q05.0
dorsal Q05.6
　with hydrocephalus Q05.1
lumbar Q05.7
　with hydrocephalus Q05.2
lumbosacral Q05.7
　with hydrocephalus Q05.2
occulta Q76.0
sacral Q05.8
　with hydrocephalus Q05.3
thoracic Q05.6
　with hydrocephalus Q05.1
thoracolumbar Q05.6
　with hydrocephalus Q05.1
Spindle, Krukenberg's — *see* Pigmentation, cornea, posterior
Spine, spinal — *see* condition
Spiradenoma (eccrine) — *see* Neoplasm, skin, benign
Spirillosis A25.0
Spirillum
minus A25.0
obermeieri infection A68.0
Spirochetal — *see* condition
Spirochetosis A69.9
arthritic, arthritica A69.9
bronchopulmonary A69.8
icterohemorrhagic A27.0
lung A69.8
Spirometrosis B70.1
Spitting blood — *see* Hemoptysis
Splanchnoptosis K63.4
Spleen, splenic — *see* condition
Splenectasis — *see* Splenomegaly
Splenitis (interstitial) (malignant) (nonspecific) D73.89
malarial (*see also* Malaria) B54 [D77]
tuberculous A18.85
Splenocele D73.89
Splenomegaly, splenomegalia (Bengal) (cryptogenic) (idiopathic) (tropical) R16.1
with hepatomegaly R16.2
cirrhotic D73.2
congenital Q89.09
congestive, chronic D73.2
Egyptian B65.1
Gaucher's E75.22
malarial (*see also* Malaria) B54 [D77]
neutropenic D73.81
Niemann-Pick — *see* Niemann-Pick disease or syndrome
siderotic D73.2
syphilitic A52.79
　congenital (early) A50.08 [D77]
Splenopathy D73.9
Splenoptosis D73.89
Splenosis D73.89
Splinter — *see* Foreign body, superficial, by site
Split, splitting
foot Q72.7- ☑
hand Q71.6- ☑
heart sounds R01.2
lip, congenital — *see* Cleft, lip
nails L60.3
urinary stream R39.13
Spondylarthrosis — *see* Spondylosis
Spondylitis (chronic) (*see also* Spondylopathy, inflammatory)
ankylopoietica — *see* Spondylitis, ankylosing
ankylosing (chronic) M45.9
　with lung involvement M45.9 [J99]
　cervical region M45.2
　cervicothoracic region M45.3
　juvenile M08.1
　lumbar region M45.6
　lumbosacral region M45.7

☑ Additional Character Required — Refer to the Tabular List for Character Selection　　　 Subterms under main terms may continue to next column or page

Spondylitis — *continued*
  ankylosing — *continued*
    multiple sites M45.0
    occipito-atlanto-axial region M45.1
    sacrococcygeal region M45.8
    thoracic region M45.4
    thoracolumbar region M45.5
  atrophic (ligamentous) — *see* Spondylitis, ankylosing
  deformans (chronic) — *see* Spondylosis
  gonococcal A54.41
  gouty (*see also* Gout, by type, vertebrae) M10.08
  in (due to)
    brucellosis A23.9 [M49.80]
      cervical region A23.9 [M49.82]
      cervicothoracic region A23.9 [M49.83]
      lumbar region A23.9 [M49.86]
      lumbosacral region A23.9 [M49.87]
      multiple sites A23.9 [M49.89]
      occipito-atlanto-axial region A23.9 [M49.81]
      sacrococcygeal region A23.9 [M49.88]
      thoracic region A23.9 [M49.84]
      thoracolumbar region A23.9 [M49.85]
    enterobacteria (*see also* subcategory M49.8) A04.9
    tuberculosis A18.01
  infectious NEC — *see* Spondylopathy, infective
  juvenile ankylosing (chronic) M08.1
  Kümmell's — *see* Spondylopathy, traumatic
  Marie-Strümpell — *see* Spondylitis, ankylosing
  muscularis — *see* Spondylopathy, specified NEC
  psoriatic L40.53
  rheumatoid — *see* Spondylitis, ankylosing
  rhizomelica — *see* Spondylitis, ankylosing
  sacroiliac NEC M46.1
  senescent, senile — *see* Spondylosis
  traumatic (chronic) or post-traumatic — *see* Spondylopathy, traumatic
  tuberculous A18.01
  typhosa A01.05
Spondylolisthesis (acquired) (degenerative) M43.10
  with disproportion (fetopelvic) O33.0
    causing obstructed labor O65.0
  cervical region M43.12
  cervicothoracic region M43.13
  congenital Q76.2
  lumbar region M43.16
  lumbosacral region M43.17
  multiple sites M43.19
  occipito-atlanto-axial region M43.11
  sacrococcygeal region M43.18
  thoracic region M43.14
  thoracolumbar region M43.15
  traumatic (old) M43.10
    acute
      fifth cervical (displaced) S12.430 ☑
        nondisplaced S12.431 ☑
        specified type NEC (displaced) S12.450 ☑
          nondisplaced S12.451 ☑
        type III S12.44 ☑
      fourth cervical (displaced) S12.330 ☑
        nondisplaced S12.331 ☑
        specified type NEC (displaced) S12.350 ☑
          nondisplaced S12.351 ☑
        type III S12.34 ☑
      second cervical (displaced) S12.130 ☑
        nondisplaced S12.131 ☑
        specified type NEC (displaced) S12.150 ☑
          nondisplaced S12.151 ☑
        type III S12.14 ☑
      seventh cervical (displaced) S12.630 ☑
        nondisplaced S12.631 ☑
        specified type NEC (displaced) S12.650 ☑
          nondisplaced S12.651 ☑
        type III S12.64 ☑
      sixth cervical (displaced) S12.530 ☑
        nondisplaced S12.531 ☑
        specified type NEC (displaced) S12.550 ☑
          nondisplaced S12.551 ☑
        type III S12.54 ☑
      third cervical (displaced) S12.230 ☑
        nondisplaced S12.231 ☑
        specified type NEC (displaced) S12.250 ☑
          nondisplaced S12.251 ☑
        type III S12.24 ☑
Spondylolysis (acquired) M43.00
  cervical region M43.02
  cervicothoracic region M43.03
  congenital Q76.2

Spondylolysis — *continued*
  lumbar region M43.06
  lumbosacral region M43.07
    with disproportion (fetopelvic) O33.0
      causing obstructed labor O65.8
  multiple sites M43.09
  occipito-atlanto-axial region M43.01
  sacrococcygeal region M43.08
  thoracic region M43.04
  thoracolumbar region M43.05
Spondylopathy M48.9
  infective NEC M46.50
    cervical region M46.52
    cervicothoracic region M46.53
    lumbar region M46.56
    lumbosacral region M46.57
    multiple sites M46.59
    occipito-atlanto-axial region M46.51
    sacrococcygeal region M46.58
    thoracic region M46.54
    thoracolumbar region M46.55
  inflammatory M46.90
    cervical region M46.92
    cervicothoracic region M46.93
    lumbar region M46.96
    lumbosacral region M46.97
    multiple sites M46.99
    occipito-atlanto-axial region M46.91
    sacrococcygeal region M46.98
    specified type NEC M46.80
      cervical region M46.82
      cervicothoracic region M46.83
      lumbar region M46.86
      lumbosacral region M46.87
      multiple sites M46.89
      occipito-atlanto-axial region M46.81
      sacrococcygeal region M46.88
      thoracic region M46.84
      thoracolumbar region M46.85
    thoracic region M46.94
    thoracolumbar region M46.95
  neuropathic, in
    syringomyelia and syringobulbia G95.0
    tabes dorsalis A52.11
  specified NEC — *see* subcategory M48.8 ☑
  traumatic M48.30
    cervical region M48.32
    cervicothoracic region M48.33
    lumbar region M48.36
    lumbosacral region M48.37
    occipito-atlanto-axial region M48.31
    sacrococcygeal region M48.38
    thoracic region M48.34
    thoracolumbar region M48.35
Spondylosis M47.9
  with
    disproportion (fetopelvic) O33.0
      causing obstructed labor O65.0
    myelopathy NEC M47.10
      cervical region M47.12
      cervicothoracic region M47.13
      lumbar region M47.16
      occipito-atlanto-axial region M47.11
      thoracic region M47.14
      thoracolumbar region M47.15
    radiculopathy M47.20
      cervical region M47.22
      cervicothoracic region M47.23
      lumbar region M47.26
      lumbosacral region M47.27
      occipito-atlanto-axial region M47.21
      sacrococcygeal region M47.28
      thoracic region M47.24
      thoracolumbar region M47.25
  specified NEC M47.899
    cervical region M47.892
    cervicothoracic region M47.893
    lumbar region M47.896
    lumbosacral region M47.897
    occipito-atlanto-axial region M47.891
    sacrococcygeal region M47.898
    thoracic region M47.894
    thoracolumbar region M47.895
  traumatic — *see* Spondylopathy, traumatic
  without myelopathy or radiculopathy M47.819
    cervical region M47.812
    cervicothoracic region M47.813
    lumbar region M47.816
    lumbosacral region M47.817

Spondylosis — *continued*
  without myelopathy or radiculopathy — *continued*
    occipito-atlanto-axial region M47.811
    sacrococcygeal region M47.818
    thoracic region M47.814
    thoracolumbar region M47.815
Sponge
  inadvertently left in operation wound — *see* Foreign body, accidentally left during a procedure
  kidney (medullary) Q61.5
Sponge-diver's disease — *see* Toxicity, venom, marine animal, sea anemone
Spongioblastoma (any type) — *see* Neoplasm, malignant, by site
  specified site — *see* Neoplasm, malignant, by site
  unspecified site C71.9
Spongioneuroblastoma — *see* Neoplasm, malignant, by site
Spontaneous (*see also* condition)
  fracture (cause unknown) — *see* Fracture, pathological
Spoon nail L60.3
  congenital Q84.6
Sporadic — *see* condition
Sporothrix schenckii infection — *see* Sporotrichosis
Sporotrichosis B42.9
  arthritis B42.82
  disseminated B42.7
  generalized B42.7
  lymphocutaneous (fixed) (progressive) B42.1
  pulmonary B42.0
  specified NEC B42.89
Spots, spotting (in) (of)
  Bitot's (*see also* Pigmentation, conjunctiva)
    in the young child E50.1
    vitamin A deficiency E50.1
  café, au lait L81.3
  Cayenne pepper I78.1
  cotton wool, retina — *see* Occlusion, artery, retina
  de Morgan's (senile angiomas) I78.1
  Fuchs' black (myopic) (*see also* Myopia, degenerative) H44.2- ☑
  intermenstrual (regular) N92.0
    irregular N92.1
  Koplik's B05.9
  liver L81.4
  pregnancy O26.85- ☑
  purpuric R23.3
  ruby I78.1
Spotted fever — *see* Fever, spotted N92.3
Sprain (joint) (ligament)
  acromioclavicular joint or ligament S43.5- ☑
  ankle S93.40- ☑
    calcaneofibular ligament S93.41- ☑
    deltoid ligament S93.42- ☑
    internal collateral ligament — *see* Sprain, ankle, specified ligament NEC
    specified ligament NEC S93.49- ☑
    talofibular ligament — *see* Sprain, ankle, specified ligament NEC
    tibiofibular ligament S93.43- ☑
  anterior longitudinal, cervical S13.4 ☑
  atlas, atlanto-axial, atlanto-occipital S13.4 ☑
  breast bone — *see* Sprain, sternum
  calcaneofibular — *see* Sprain, ankle
  carpal — *see* Sprain, wrist
  carpometacarpal — *see* Sprain, hand, specified site NEC
  cartilage
    costal S23.41 ☑
    semilunar (knee) — *see* Sprain, knee, specified site NEC
      with current tear — *see* Tear, meniscus
    thyroid region S13.5 ☑
    xiphoid — *see* Sprain, sternum
  cervical, cervicodorsal, cervicothoracic S13.4 ☑
  chondrosternal S23.421 ☑
  coracoclavicular S43.8- ☑
  coracohumeral S43.41- ☑
  coronary, knee — *see* Sprain, knee, specified site NEC
  costal cartilage S23.41 ☑
  cricoarytenoid articulation or ligament S13.5 ☑
  cricothyroid articulation S13.5 ☑
  cruciate, knee — *see* Sprain, knee, cruciate
  deltoid, ankle — *see* Sprain, ankle
  dorsal (spine) S23.3 ☑
  elbow S53.40- ☑

▽ Subterms under main terms may continue to next column or page   ☑ Additional Character Required — Refer to the Tabular List for Character Selection   289

Spondylitis — Sprain

Index

Sprain — Stanton's disease

Sprain — *continued*
  elbow — *continued*
    radial collateral ligament S53.43- ☑
    radiohumeral S53.41- ☑
    rupture
      radial collateral ligament — *see* Rupture, traumatic, ligament, radial collateral
      ulnar collateral ligament — *see* Rupture, traumatic, ligament, ulnar collateral
    specified type NEC S53.49- ☑
    ulnar collateral ligament S53.44- ☑
    ulnohumeral S53.42- ☑
  femur, head — *see* Sprain, hip
  fibular collateral, knee — *see* Sprain, knee, collateral
  fibulocalcaneal — *see* Sprain, ankle
  finger(s) S63.61- ☑
    index S63.61- ☑
    interphalangeal (joint) S63.63- ☑
      index S63.63- ☑
      little S63.63- ☑
      middle S63.63- ☑
      ring S63.63- ☑
    little S63.61- ☑
    metacarpophalangeal (joint) S63.65- ☑
    middle S63.61- ☑
    ring S63.61- ☑
    specified site NEC S63.69- ☑
      index S63.69- ☑
      little S63.69- ☑
      middle S63.69- ☑
      ring S63.69- ☑
  foot S93.60- ☑
    specified ligament NEC S93.69- ☑
    tarsal ligament S93.61- ☑
    tarsometatarsal ligament S93.62- ☑
    toe — *see* Sprain, toe
  hand S63.9- ☑
    finger — *see* Sprain, finger
    specified site NEC — *see* subcategory S63.8 ☑
    thumb — *see* Sprain, thumb
  head S03.9 ☑
  hip S73.10- ☑
    iliofemoral ligament S73.11- ☑
    ischiocapsular (ligament) S73.12- ☑
    specified NEC S73.19- ☑
  iliofemoral — *see* Sprain, hip
  innominate
    acetabulum — *see* Sprain, hip
    sacral junction S33.6 ☑
  internal
    collateral, ankle — *see* Sprain, ankle
    semilunar cartilage — *see* Sprain, knee, specified site NEC
  interphalangeal
    finger — *see* Sprain, finger, interphalangeal (joint)
    toe — *see* Sprain, toe, interphalangeal joint
  ischiocapsular — *see* Sprain, hip
  ischiofemoral — *see* Sprain, hip
  jaw (articular disc) (cartilage) (meniscus) S03.4- ☑
    old M26.69
  knee S83.9- ☑
    collateral ligament S83.40- ☑
      lateral (fibular) S83.42- ☑
      medial (tibial) S83.41- ☑
    cruciate ligament S83.50- ☑
      anterior S83.51- ☑
      posterior S83.52- ☑
    lateral (fibular) collateral ligament S83.42- ☑
    medial (tibial) collateral ligament S83.41- ☑
    patellar ligament S76.11- ☑
    specified site NEC S83.8X- ☑
    superior tibiofibular joint (ligament) S83.6- ☑
  lateral collateral, knee — *see* Sprain, knee, collateral
  lumbar (spine) S33.5 ☑
  lumbosacral S33.9 ☑
  mandible (articular disc) S03.4- ☑
    old M26.69
  medial collateral, knee — *see* Sprain, knee, collateral
  meniscus
    jaw S03.4- ☑
      old M26.69
    knee — *see* Sprain, knee, specified site NEC
      with current tear — *see* Tear, meniscus
        old — *see* Derangement, knee, meniscus, due to old tear
    mandible S03.4- ☑

Sprain — *continued*
  meniscus — *continued*
    mandible — *continued*
      old M26.69
  metacarpal (distal) (proximal) — *see* Sprain, hand, specified site NEC
  metacarpophalangeal — *see* Sprain, finger, metacarpophalangeal (joint)
  metatarsophalangeal — *see* Sprain, toe, metatarsophalangeal joint
  midcarpal — *see* Sprain, hand, specified site NEC
  midtarsal — *see* Sprain, foot, specified site NEC
  neck S13.9 ☑
    anterior longitudinal cervical ligament S13.4 ☑
    atlanto-axial joint S13.4 ☑
    atlanto-occipital joint S13.4 ☑
    cervical spine S13.4 ☑
    cricoarytenoid ligament S13.5 ☑
    cricothyroid ligament S13.5 ☑
    specified site NEC S13.8 ☑
    thyroid region (cartilage) S13.5 ☑
  nose S03.8 ☑
  orbicular, hip — *see* Sprain, hip
  patella — *see* Sprain, knee, specified site NEC
  patellar ligament S76.11- ☑
  pelvis NEC S33.8 ☑
  phalanx
    finger — *see* Sprain, finger
    toe — *see* Sprain, toe
  pubofemoral — *see* Sprain, hip
  radiocarpal — *see* Sprain, wrist
  radiohumeral — *see* Sprain, elbow
  radius, collateral — *see* Rupture, traumatic, ligament, radial collateral
  rib (cage) S23.41 ☑
  rotator cuff (capsule) S43.42- ☑
  sacroiliac (region)
    chronic or old — *see* subcategory M53.2 ☑
    joint S33.6 ☑
  scaphoid (hand) — *see* Sprain, hand, specified site NEC
  scapula (r) — *see* Sprain, shoulder girdle, specified site NEC
  semilunar cartilage (knee) — *see* Sprain, knee, specified site NEC
    with current tear — *see* Tear, meniscus
      old — *see* Derangement, knee, meniscus, due to old tear
  shoulder joint S43.40- ☑
    acromioclavicular joint (ligament) — *see* Sprain, acromioclavicular joint
    blade — *see* Sprain, shoulder, girdle, specified site NEC
    coracoclavicular joint (ligament) — *see* Sprain, coracoclavicular joint
    coracohumeral ligament — *see* Sprain, coracohumeral joint
    girdle S43.9- ☑
      specified site NEC S43.8- ☑
    rotator cuff — *see* Sprain, rotator cuff
    specified site NEC S43.49- ☑
    sternoclavicular joint (ligament) — *see* Sprain, sternoclavicular joint
  spine
    cervical S13.4 ☑
    lumbar S33.5 ☑
    thoracic S23.3 ☑
  sternoclavicular joint S43.6- ☑
  sternum S23.429 ☑
    chondrosternal joint S23.421 ☑
    specified site NEC S23.428 ☑
    sternoclavicular (joint) (ligament) S23.420 ☑
  symphysis
    jaw S03.4- ☑
      old M26.69
    mandibular S03.4- ☑
      old M26.69
  talofibular — *see* Sprain, ankle
  tarsal — *see* Sprain, foot, specified site NEC
  tarsometatarsal — *see* Sprain, foot, specified site NEC
  temporomandibular S03.4- ☑
    old M26.69
  thorax S23.9 ☑
    ribs S23.41 ☑
    specified site NEC S23.8 ☑
    spine S23.3 ☑
    sternum — *see* Sprain, sternum

Sprain — *continued*
  thumb S63.60- ☑
    interphalangeal (joint) S63.62- ☑
    metacarpophalangeal (joint) S63.64- ☑
    specified site NEC S63.68- ☑
  thyroid cartilage or region S13.5 ☑
  tibia (proximal end) — *see* Sprain, knee, specified site NEC
  tibial collateral, knee — *see* Sprain, knee, collateral
  tibiofibular
    distal — *see* Sprain, ankle
    superior — *see* Sprain, knee, specified site NEC
  toe(s) S93.50- ☑
    great S93.50- ☑
    interphalangeal joint S93.51- ☑
      great S93.51- ☑
      lesser S93.51- ☑
    lesser S93.50- ☑
    metatarsophalangeal joint S93.52- ☑
      great S93.52- ☑
      lesser S93.52- ☑
  ulna, collateral — *see* Rupture, traumatic, ligament, ulnar collateral
  ulnohumeral — *see* Sprain, elbow
  wrist S63.50- ☑
    carpal S63.51- ☑
    radiocarpal S63.52- ☑
    specified site NEC S63.59- ☑
  xiphoid cartilage — *see* Sprain, sternum
Sprengel's deformity (congenital) Q74.0
Sprue (tropical) K90.1
  celiac K90.0
  idiopathic K90.49
  meaning thrush B37.0
  nontropical K90.0
Spur, bone (*see also* Enthesopathy)
  calcaneal M77.3-
  iliac crest M76.2-
  nose (septum) J34.89
Spurway's syndrome Q78.0
Sputum
  abnormal (amount) (color) (odor) (purulent) R09.3
  blood-stained R04.2
  excessive (cause unknown) R09.3
Squamous (*see also* condition)
  epithelium in
    cervical canal (congenital) Q51.828
    uterine mucosa (congenital) Q51.818
Squashed nose M95.0
  congenital Q67.4
Squeeze, diver's T70.3 ☑
Squint (*see also* Strabismus)
  accommodative — *see* Strabismus, convergent concomitant
SSADHD (succinic semialdehyde dehydrogenase deficiency) E72.81
St. Hubert's disease A82.9
Stab (*see also* Laceration)
  internal organs — *see* Injury, by site
Stafne's cyst or cavity M27.0
Staggering gait R26.0
  hysterical F44.4
Staghorn calculus — *see* Calculus, kidney
Stähli's line (cornea) (pigment) — *see* Pigmentation, cornea, anterior
Stain, staining
  meconium (newborn) P96.83
  port wine Q82.5
  tooth, teeth (hard tissues) (extrinsic) K03.6
    due to
      accretions K03.6
      deposits (betel) (black) (green) (materia alba) (orange) (soft) (tobacco) K03.6
      metals (copper) (silver) K03.7
      nicotine K03.6
      pulpal bleeding K03.7
      tobacco K03.6
    intrinsic K00.8
Stammering (*see also* Disorder, fluency) F80.81
Standstill
  auricular I45.5
  cardiac — *see* Arrest, cardiac
  sinoatrial I45.5
  ventricular — *see* Arrest, cardiac
Stannosis J63.5
Stanton's disease — *see* Melioidosis

☑ Additional Character Required — Refer to the Tabular List for Character Selection   ☑ Subterms under main terms may continue to next column or page

Staphylitis (acute) (catarrhal) (chronic) (gangrenous) (membranous) (suppurative) (ulcerative) K12.2
Staphylococcal scalded skin syndrome L00
Staphylococcemia A41.2
Staphylococcus, staphylococcal (see also condition)
  as cause of disease classified elsewhere B95.8
    aureus (methicillin susceptible) (MSSA) B95.61
      methicillin resistant (MRSA) B95.62
    specified NEC, as cause of disease classified elsewhere B95.7
Staphyloma (sclera)
  cornea H18.72- ☑
  equatorial H15.81- ☑
  localized (anterior) H15.82- ☑
  posticum H15.83- ☑
  ring H15.85- ☑
Stargardt's disease — see Dystrophy, retina
Starvation (inanition) (due to lack of food) T73.0 ☑
  edema — see Malnutrition, severe
Stasis
  bile (noncalculous) K83.1
  bronchus J98.09
    with infection — see Bronchitis
  cardiac — see Failure, heart, congestive
  cecum K59.8
  colon K59.8
  dermatitis I87.2
    with
      varicose ulcer — see Varix, leg, with ulcer, with inflammation
      varicose veins — see Varix, leg, with, inflammation
      due to postthrombotic syndrome — see Syndrome, postthrombotic
  duodenal K31.5
  eczema — see Varix, leg, with, inflammation
  edema — see Hypertension, venous (chronic), idiopathic
  foot T69.0- ☑
  ileocecal coil K59.8
  ileum K59.8
  intestinal K59.8
  jejunum K59.8
  kidney N19
  liver (cirrhotic) K76.1
  lymphatic I89.8
  pneumonia J18.2
  pulmonary — see Edema, lung
  rectal K59.8
  renal N19
    tubular N17.0
  ulcer — see Varix, leg, with, ulcer
    without varicose veins I87.2
  urine — see Retention, urine
  venous I87.8
State (of)
  affective and paranoid, mixed, organic psychotic F06.8
  agitated R45.1
    acute reaction to stress F43.0
  anxiety (neurotic) F41.1
  apprehension F41.1
  burn-out Z73.0
  climacteric, female Z78.0
    symptomatic N95.1
  compulsive F42.8
    mixed with obsessional thoughts F42.2
  confusional (psychogenic) F44.89
    acute (see also Delirium)
      with
        arteriosclerotic dementia F01.50
          with behavioral disturbance F01.51
        senility or dementia F05
      alcoholic F10.231
      epileptic F05
      reactive (from emotional stress, psychological trauma) F44.89
      subacute — see Delirium
  convulsive — see Convulsions
  crisis F43.0
  depressive F32.9
    neurotic F34.1
  dissociative F44.9
  emotional shock (stress) R45.7
  hypercoagulation — see Hypercoagulable
  locked-in G83.5
  menopausal Z78.0
    symptomatic N95.1
  neurotic F48.9

State — continued
  neurotic — continued
    with depersonalization F48.1
  obsessional F42.8
  oneiroid (schizophrenia-like) F23
  organic
    hallucinatory (nonalcoholic) F06.0
    paranoid (-hallucinatory) F06.2
  panic F41.0
  paranoid F22
    climacteric F22
    involutional F22
    menopausal F22
    organic F06.2
    senile F03 ☑
    simple F22
  persistent vegetative R40.3
  phobic F40.9
  postleukotomy F07.0
  pregnant
    gestational carrier Z33.3
    incidental Z33.1
  psychogenic, twilight F44.89
  psychopathic (constitutional) F60.2
  psychotic, organic (see also Psychosis, organic)
    mixed paranoid and affective F06.8
    senile or presenile F03 ☑
    transient NEC F06.8
      with
        depression F06.31
        hallucinations F06.0
  residual schizophrenic F20.5
  restlessness R45.1
  stress (emotional) R45.7
  tension (mental) F48.9
    specified NEC F48.8
  transient organic psychotic NEC F06.8
    depressive type F06.31
    hallucinatory type F06.0
  twilight
    epileptic F05
    psychogenic F44.89
  vegetative, persistent R40.3
  vital exhaustion Z73.0
  withdrawal, — see Withdrawal, state
Status (post) (see also Presence (of))
  absence, epileptic — see Epilepsy, by type, with status epilepticus
  administration of tPA (rtPA) in a different facility within the last 24 hours prior to admission to current facility Z92.82
  adrenalectomy (unilateral) (bilateral) E89.6
  anastomosis Z98.0
  anginosus I20.9
  angioplasty (peripheral) Z98.62
    with implant Z95.820
    coronary artery Z98.61
      with implant Z95.5
  aortocoronary bypass Z95.1
  arthrodesis Z98.1
  artificial opening (of) Z93.9
    gastrointestinal tract Z93.4
    specified NEC Z93.8
    urinary tract Z93.6
    vagina Z93.8
  asthmaticus — see Asthma, by type, with status asthmaticus
  awaiting organ transplant Z76.82
  bariatric surgery Z98.84
  bed confinement Z74.01
  bleb, filtering (vitreous), after glaucoma surgery Z98.83
  breast implant Z98.82
    removal Z98.86
  cataract extraction Z98.4- ☑
  cholecystectomy Z90.49
  clitorectomy N90.811
    with excision of labia minora N90.812
  colectomy (complete) (partial) Z90.49
  colonization — see Carrier (suspected) of
  colostomy Z93.3
  convulsivus idiopathicus — see Epilepsy, by type, with status epilepticus
  coronary artery angioplasty — see Status, angioplasty, coronary artery
  coronary artery bypass graft Z95.1
  cystectomy (urinary bladder) Z90.6
  cystostomy Z93.50
    appendico-vesicostomy Z93.52

Status — continued
  cystostomy — continued
    cutaneous Z93.51
    specified NEC Z93.59
  delinquent immunization Z28.3
  dental Z98.818
    crown Z98.811
    fillings Z98.811
    restoration Z98.811
    sealant Z98.810
    specified NEC Z98.818
  deployment (current) (military) Z56.82
  dialysis (hemodialysis) (peritoneal) Z99.2
  do not resuscitate (DNR) Z66
  donor — see Donor
  embedded fragments — see Retained, foreign body fragments (type of)
  embedded splinter — see Retained, foreign body fragments (type of)
  enterostomy Z93.4
  epileptic, epilepticus (see also Epilepsy, by type, with status epilepticus) G40.901
  estrogen receptor
    negative Z17.1
    positive Z17.0
  female genital cutting — see Female genital mutilation status
  female genital mutilation — see Female genital mutilation status
  filtering (vitreous) bleb after glaucoma surgery Z98.83
  gastrectomy (complete) (partial) Z90.3
  gastric banding Z98.84
  gastric bypass for obesity Z98.84
  gastrostomy Z93.1
  human immunodeficiency virus (HIV) infection, asymptomatic Z21
  hysterectomy (complete) (total) Z90.710
    partial (with remaining cervial stump) Z90.711
  ileostomy Z93.2
  implant
    breast Z98.82
  infibulation N90.813
  intestinal bypass Z98.0
  jejunostomy Z93.4
  lapsed immunization schedule Z28.3
  laryngectomy Z90.02
  lymphaticus E32.8
  malignancy
    castrate resistant prostate Z19.2
    hormone resistant Z19.2
    hormone sensitive Z19.1
  marmoratus G80.3
  mastectomy (unilateral) (bilateral) Z90.1- ☑
  military deployment status (current) Z56.82
    in theater or in support of military war, peacekeeping and humanitarian operations Z56.82
  nephrectomy (unilateral) (bilateral) Z90.5
  nephrostomy Z93.6
  obesity surgery Z98.84
  oophorectomy
    bilateral Z90.722
    unilateral Z90.721
  organ replacement
    by artificial or mechanical device or prosthesis of
      artery Z95.828
      bladder Z96.0
      blood vessel Z95.828
      breast Z97.8
      eye globe Z97.0
      heart Z95.812
        valve Z95.2
      intestine Z97.8
      joint Z96.60
        hip — see Presence, hip joint implant
        knee — see Presence, knee joint implant
        specified site NEC Z96.698
      kidney Z97.8
      larynx Z96.3
      lens Z96.1
      limbs — see Presence, artificial, limb
      liver Z97.8
      lung Z97.8
      pancreas Z97.8
    by organ transplant (heterologous)(homologous) — see Transplant
  pacemaker
    brain Z96.89
    cardiac Z95.0

Status — *continued*
  pacemaker — *continued*
    specified NEC Z96.89
  pancreatectomy Z90.410
    complete Z90.410
    partial Z90.411
    total Z90.410
  physical restraint Z78.1
  pneumonectomy (complete) (partial) Z90.2
  pneumothorax, therapeutic Z98.3
  postcommotio cerebri F07.81
  postoperative (postprocedural) NEC Z98.890
    breast implant Z98.82
    dental Z98.818
      crown Z98.811
      fillings Z98.811
      restoration Z98.811
      sealant Z98.810
      specified NEC Z98.818
    pneumothorax, therapeutic Z98.3
    uterine scar Z98.891
  postpartum (routine follow-up) Z39.2
    care immediately after delivery Z39.0
  postsurgical (postprocedural) NEC Z98.890
    pneumothorax, therapeutic Z98.3
  pregnancy, incidental Z33.1
  prosthesis coronary angioplasty Z95.5
  pseudophakia Z96.1
  renal dialysis (hemodialysis) (peritoneal) Z99.2
  retained foreign body — *see* Retained, foreign body
      fragments (type of)
  reversed jejunal transposition (for bypass) Z98.0
  salpingo-oophorectomy
    bilateral Z90.722
    unilateral Z90.721
  sex reassignment surgery status Z87.890
  shunt
    arteriovenous (for dialysis) Z99.2
    cerebrospinal fluid Z98.2
    ventricular (communicating) (for drainage) Z98.2
  splenectomy Z90.81
  thymicolymphaticus E32.8
  thymicus E32.8
  thymolymphaticus E32.8
  thyroidectomy (hypothyroidism) E89.0
  tooth (teeth) extraction (*see also* Absence, teeth, ac-
      quired) K08.409
  tPA (rtPA) administration in a different facility within
      the last 24 hours prior to admission to current
      facility Z92.82
  tracheostomy Z93.0
  transplant — *see* Transplant
    organ removed Z98.85
  tubal ligation Z98.51
  underimmunization Z28.3
  ureterostomy Z93.6
  urethrostomy Z93.6
  vagina, artificial Z93.8
  vasectomy Z98.52
  wheelchair confinement Z99.3
Stealing
  child problem F91.8
    in company with others Z72.810
  pathological (compulsive) F63.2
Steam burn — *see* Burn
Steatocystoma multiplex L72.2
Steatohepatitis (nonalcoholic) (NASH) K75.81
Steatoma L72.3
  eyelid (cystic) — *see* Dermatosis, eyelid
    infected — *see* Hordeolum
Steatorrhea (chronic) K90.9
  with lacteal obstruction K90.2
  idiopathic (adult) (infantile) K90.9
  pancreatic K90.3
  primary K90.0
  tropical K90.1
Steatosis E88.89
  heart — *see* Degeneration, myocardial
  kidney N28.89
  liver NEC K76.0
Steele-Richardson-Olszewski disease or syndrome
    G23.1
Steinbrocker's syndrome G90.8
Steinert's disease G71.11
Stein-Leventhal syndrome E28.2
Stein's syndrome E28.2
STEMI (*see also* Infarct, myocardium, ST elevation) I21.3
Stenocardia I20.8

Stenocephaly Q75.8
Stenosis, stenotic (cicatricial) (*see also* Stricture)
  ampulla of Vater K83.1
  anus, anal (canal) (sphincter) K62.4
    and rectum K62.4
    congenital Q42.3
      with fistula Q42.2
  aorta (ascending) (supraventricular) (congenital) Q25.1
    arteriosclerotic I70.0
    calcified I70.0
    supravalvular Q25.3
  aortic (valve) I35.0
    with insufficiency I35.2
    congenital Q23.0
    rheumatic I06.0
      with
        incompetency, insufficiency or regurgitation
            I06.2
          with mitral (valve) disease I08.0
            with tricuspid (valve) disease I08.3
        mitral (valve) disease I08.0
          with tricuspid (valve) disease I08.3
        tricuspid (valve) disease I08.2
          with mitral (valve) disease I08.3
    specified cause NEC I35.0
    syphilitic A52.03
  aqueduct of Sylvius (congenital) Q03.0
    with spina bifida — *see* Spina bifida, by site, with
        hydrocephalus
    acquired G91.1
  artery NEC (*see also* Arteriosclerosis) I77.1
    celiac I77.4
    cerebral — *see* Occlusion, artery, cerebral
    extremities — *see* Arteriosclerosis, extremities
    precerebral — *see* Occlusion, artery, precerebral
    pulmonary (congenital) Q25.6
      acquired I28.8
    renal I70.1
    stent
      coronary T82.855 ☑
      peripheral T82.856 ☑
  bile duct (common) (hepatic) K83.1
    congenital Q44.3
  bladder-neck (acquired) N32.0
    congenital Q64.31
  brain G93.89
  bronchus J98.09
    congenital Q32.3
    syphilitic A52.72
  cardia (stomach) K22.2
    congenital Q39.3
  cardiovascular — *see* Disease, cardiovascular
  caudal M48.08
  cervix, cervical (canal) N88.2
    congenital Q51.828
    in pregnancy or childbirth — *see* Pregnancy, com-
        plicated by, abnormal cervix
  colon (*see also* Obstruction, intestine)
    congenital Q42.9
      specified NEC Q42.8
  colostomy K94.03
  common (bile) duct K83.1
    congenital Q44.3
  coronary (artery) — *see* Disease, heart, ischemic,
      atherosclerotic
  cystic duct — *see* Obstruction, gallbladder
  due to presence of device, implant or graft (*see also*
      Complications, by site and type, specified NEC)
      T85.858 ☑
    arterial graft NEC T82.858 ☑
    breast (implant) T85.858 ☑
    catheter T85.858 ☑
      dialysis (renal) T82.858 ☑
        intraperitoneal T85.858 ☑
      infusion NEC T82.858 ☑
        spinal (epidural) (subdural) T85.850 ☑
      urinary (indwelling) T83.85 ☑
    fixation, internal (orthopedic) NEC T84.85 ☑
    gastrointestinal (bile duct) (esophagus) T85.858 ☑
    genital NEC T83.85 ☑
    heart NEC T82.857 ☑
    joint prosthesis T84.85 ☑
    ocular (corneal graft) (orbital implant) NEC
        T85.858 ☑
    orthopedic NEC T84.85 ☑
    specified NEC T85.858 ☑
    urinary NEC T83.85 ☑
    vascular NEC T82.858 ☑

Stenosis, stenotic — *continued*
  due to presence of device, implant or graft (*see also*
      Complications, by site and type, specified) —
      continued
    ventricular intracranial shunt T85.850 ☑
  duodenum K31.5
    congenital Q41.0
  ejaculatory duct NEC N50.89
    stent
      vascular
        end stent
          adjacent to stent — *see* Arteriosclerosis
          within the stent
            coronary T82.855 ☑
            peripheral T82.856 ☑
        in stent
          coronary vessel T82.855 ☑
          peripheral vessel T82.856 ☑
  endocervical os — *see* Stenosis, cervix
  enterostomy K94.13
  esophagus K22.2
    congenital Q39.3
    syphilitic A52.79
      congenital A50.59 [K23]
  eustachian tube — *see* Obstruction, eustachian tube
  external ear canal (acquired) H61.30- ☑
    congenital Q16.1
    due to
      inflammation H61.32- ☑
      trauma H61.31- ☑
    postprocedural H95.81- ☑
    specified cause NEC H61.39- ☑
  gallbladder — *see* Obstruction, gallbladder
  glottis J38.6
  heart valve (congenital) Q24.8
    aortic Q23.0
    mitral Q23.2
    pulmonary Q22.1
    tricuspid Q22.4
  hepatic duct K83.1
  hymen N89.6
  hypertrophic subaortic (idiopathic) I42.1
  ileum (*see also* Obstruction, intestine, specified NEC)
      K56.699
    congenital Q41.2
  infundibulum cardia Q24.3
  intervertebral foramina (*see also* Lesion, biomechanical,
      specified NEC)
    connective tissue M99.79
      abdomen M99.79
      cervical region M99.71
      cervicothoracic M99.71
      head region M99.70
      lumbar region M99.73
      lumbosacral M99.73
      occipitocervical M99.70
      sacral region M99.74
      sacrococcygeal M99.74
      sacroiliac M99.74
      specified NEC M99.79
      thoracic region M99.72
      thoracolumbar M99.72
    disc M99.79
      abdomen M99.79
      cervical region M99.71
      cervicothoracic M99.71
      head region M99.70
      lower extremity M99.76
      lumbar region M99.73
      lumbosacral M99.73
      occipitocervical M99.70
      pelvic M99.75
      rib cage M99.78
      sacral region M99.74
      sacrococcygeal M99.74
      sacroiliac M99.74
      specified NEC M99.79
      thoracic region M99.72
      thoracolumbar M99.72
      upper extremity M99.77
    osseous M99.69
      abdomen M99.69
      cervical region M99.61
      cervicothoracic M99.61
      head region M99.60
      lower extremity M99.66
      lumbar region M99.63
      lumbosacral M99.63

Stenosis, stenotic — *continued*
  intervertebral foramina (*see also* Lesion, biomechanical, specified) — *continued*
    osseous — *continued*
      occipitocervical M99.60
      pelvic M99.65
      rib cage M99.68
      sacral region M99.64
      sacrococcygeal M99.64
      sacroiliac M99.64
      specified NEC M99.69
      thoracic region M99.62
      thoracolumbar M99.62
      upper extremity M99.67
    subluxation — *see* Stenosis, intervertebral foramina, osseous
  intestine (*see also* Obstruction, intestine)
    congenital (small) Q41.9
      large Q42.9
        specified NEC Q42.8
      specified NEC Q41.8
  jejunum (*see also* Obstruction, intestine, specified NEC) K56.699
    congenital Q41.1
  lacrimal (passage)
    canaliculi H04.54- ☑
    congenital Q10.5
    duct H04.55- ☑
    punctum H04.56- ☑
    sac H04.57- ☑
  lacrimonasal duct — *see* Stenosis, lacrimal, duct
    congenital Q10.5
  larynx J38.6
    congenital NEC Q31.8
      subglottic Q31.1
    syphilitic A52.73
      congenital A50.59 [J99]
  mitral (chronic) (inactive) (valve) I05.0
    with
      aortic valve disease I08.0
      incompetency, insufficiency or regurgitation I05.2
    active or acute I01.1
      with rheumatic or Sydenham's chorea I02.0
    congenital Q23.2
    specified cause, except rheumatic I34.2
    syphilitic A52.03
  myocardium, myocardial (*see also* Degeneration, myocardial)
    hypertrophic subaortic (idiopathic) I42.1
  nares (anterior) (posterior) J34.89
    congenital Q30.0
  nasal duct (*see also* Stenosis, lacrimal, duct)
    congenital Q10.5
  nasolacrimal duct (*see also* Stenosis, lacrimal, duct)
    congenital Q10.5
  neural canal (*see also* Lesion, biomechanical, specified NEC)
    connective tissue M99.49
      abdomen M99.49
      cervical region M99.41
      cervicothoracic M99.41
      head region M99.40
      lower extremity M99.46
      lumbar region M99.43
      lumbosacral M99.43
      occipitocervical M99.40
      pelvic M99.45
      rib cage M99.48
      sacral region M99.44
      sacrococcygeal M99.44
      sacroiliac M99.44
      specified NEC M99.49
      thoracic region M99.42
      thoracolumbar M99.42
      upper extremity M99.47
    intervertebral disc M99.59
      abdomen M99.59
      cervical region M99.51
      cervicothoracic M99.51
      head region M99.50
      lower extremity M99.56
      lumbar region M99.53
      lumbosacral M99.53
      occipitocervical M99.50
      pelvic M99.55
      rib cage M99.58
      sacral region M99.54

Stenosis, stenotic — *continued*
  neural canal (*see also* Lesion, biomechanical, specified) — *continued*
    intervertebral disc — *continued*
      sacrococcygeal M99.54
      sacroiliac M99.54
      specified NEC M99.59
      thoracic region M99.52
      thoracolumbar M99.52
      upper extremity M99.57
    osseous M99.39
      abdomen M99.39
      cervical region M99.31
      cervicothoracic M99.31
      head region M99.30
      lower extremity M99.36
      lumbar region M99.33
      lumbosacral M99.33
      occipitocervical M99.30
      pelvic M99.35
      rib cage M99.38
      sacral region M99.34
      sacrococcygeal M99.34
      sacroiliac M99.34
      specified NEC M99.39
      thoracic region M99.32
      thoracolumbar M99.32
      upper extremity M99.37
    subluxation M99.29
      cervical region M99.21
      cervicothoracic M99.21
      head region M99.20
      lower extremity M99.26
      lumbar region M99.23
      lumbosacral M99.23
      occipitocervical M99.20
      pelvic M99.25
      rib cage M99.28
      sacral region M99.24
      sacrococcygeal M99.24
      sacroiliac M99.24
      specified NEC M99.29
      thoracic region M99.22
      thoracolumbar M99.22
      upper extremity M99.27
  organ or site, congenital NEC — *see* Atresia, by site
  papilla of Vater K83.1
  pulmonary (artery) (congenital) Q25.6
    with ventricular septal defect, transposition of aorta, and hypertrophy of right ventricle Q21.3
    acquired I28.8
    in tetralogy of Fallot Q21.3
    infundibular Q24.3
    subvalvular Q24.3
    supravalvular Q25.6
    valve I37.0
      with insufficiency I37.2
      congenital Q22.1
      rheumatic I09.89
        with aortic, mitral or tricuspid (valve) disease I08.8
    vein, acquired I28.8
    vessel NEC I28.8
  pulmonic (congenital) Q22.1
    infundibular Q24.3
    subvalvular Q24.3
  pylorus (hypertrophic) (acquired) K31.1
    adult K31.1
    congenital Q40.0
    infantile Q40.0
  rectum (sphincter) — *see* Stricture, rectum
  renal artery I70.1
    congenital Q27.1
  salivary duct (any) K11.8
  sphincter of Oddi K83.1
  spinal M48.00
    cervical region M48.02
    cervicothoracic region M48.03
    lumbar region (NOS) (without neurogenic claudication) M48.061
      with neurogenic claudication M48.062
    lumbosacral region M48.07
    occipito-atlanto-axial region M48.01
    sacrococcygeal region M48.08
    thoracic region M48.04
    thoracolumbar region M48.05
  stomach, hourglass K31.2
  subaortic (congenital) Q24.4
    hypertrophic (idiopathic) I42.1

Stenosis, stenotic — *continued*
  subglottic J38.6
    congenital Q31.1
    postprocedural J95.5
  trachea J39.8
    congenital Q32.1
    syphilitic A52.73
    tuberculous NEC A15.5
  tracheostomy J95.03
  tricuspid (valve) I07.0
    with
      aortic (valve) disease I08.2
      incompetency, insufficiency or regurgitation I07.2
        with aortic (valve) disease I08.2
          with mitral (valve) disease I08.3
        mitral (valve) disease I08.1
          with aortic (valve) disease I08.3
    congenital Q22.4
    nonrheumatic I36.0
      with insufficiency I36.2
  tubal N97.1
  ureter — *see* Atresia, ureter
  ureteropelvic junction, congenital Q62.11
  ureterovesical orifice, congenital Q62.12
  urethra (valve) (*see also* Stricture, urethra)
    congenital Q64.32
  urinary meatus, congenital Q64.33
  vagina N89.5
    congenital Q52.4
    in pregnancy — *see* Pregnancy, complicated by, abnormal vagina
    causing obstructed labor O65.5
  valve (cardiac) (heart) (*see also* Endocarditis) I38
    congenital Q24.8
      aortic Q23.0
      mitral Q23.2
      pulmonary Q22.1
      tricuspid Q22.4
  vena cava (inferior) (superior) I87.1
    congenital Q26.0
  vesicourethral orifice Q64.31
  vulva N90.5
Stent jail T82.897 ☑
Stercolith (impaction) K56.41
  appendix K38.1
Stercoraceous, stercoral ulcer K63.3
  anus or rectum K62.6
Stereotypies NEC F98.4
Sterility — *see* Infertility
Sterilization — *see* Encounter (for), sterilization
Sternalgia — *see* Angina
Sternopagus Q89.4
Sternum bifidum Q76.7
Steroid
  effects (adverse) (adrenocortical) (iatrogenic)
    cushingoid E24.2
      correct substance properly administered — *see* Table of Drugs and Chemicals, by drug, adverse effect
      overdose or wrong substance given or taken — *see* Table of Drugs and Chemicals, by drug, poisoning
    diabetes — *see* subcategory E09 ☑
      correct substance properly administered — *see* Table of Drugs and Chemicals, by drug, adverse effect
      overdose or wrong substance given or taken — *see* Table of Drugs and Chemicals, by drug, poisoning
    fever R50.2
    insufficiency E27.3
      correct substance properly administered — *see* Table of Drugs and Chemicals, by drug, adverse effect
      overdose or wrong substance given or taken — *see* Table of Drugs and Chemicals, by drug, poisoning
  responder H40.04- ☑
Stevens-Johnson disease or syndrome L51.1
  toxic epidermal necrolysis overlap L51.3
Stewart-Morel syndrome M85.2
Sticker's disease B08.3
Sticky eye — *see* Conjunctivitis, acute, mucopurulent
Stieda's disease — *see* Bursitis, tibial collateral
Stiff neck — *see* Torticollis
Stiff-man syndrome G25.82
Stiffness, joint NEC M25.60

Stiffness, joint — continued
  ankle M25.67- ☑
  ankylosis — see Ankylosis, joint
  contracture — see Contraction, joint
  elbow M25.62- ☑
  foot M25.67- ☑
  hand M25.64- ☑
  hip M25.65- ☑
  knee M25.66- ☑
  shoulder M25.61- ☑
  wrist M25.63- ☑
Stigmata congenital syphilis A50.59
Stillbirth P95
Still-Felty syndrome — see Felty's syndrome
Still's disease or syndrome (juvenile) M08.20
  adult-onset M06.1
  ankle M08.27- ☑
  elbow M08.22- ☑
  foot joint M08.27- ☑
  hand joint M08.24- ☑
  hip M08.25- ☑
  knee M08.26- ☑
  multiple site M08.29
  shoulder M08.21- ☑
  vertebra M08.28
  wrist M08.23- ☑
Stimulation, ovary E28.1
Sting (venomous) (with allergic or anaphylactic shock)
    — see Table of Drugs and Chemicals, by animal or
    substance, poisoning
Stippled epiphyses Q78.8
Stitch
  abscess T81.41 ☑
  burst (in operation wound) — see Disruption, wound,
    operation
Stokes' disease E05.00
  with thyroid storm E05.01
Stokes-Adams disease or syndrome I45.9
Stokvis (-Talma) **disease** D74.8
Stoma malfunction
  colostomy K94.03
  enterostomy K94.13
  gastrostomy K94.23
  ileostomy K94.13
  tracheostomy J95.03
Stomach — see condition
Stomatitis (denture) (ulcerative) K12.1
  angular K13.0
    due to dietary or vitamin deficiency E53.0
  aphthous K12.0
  bovine B08.61
  candidal B37.0
  catarrhal K12.1
  diphtheritic A36.89
  due to
    dietary deficiency E53.0
    thrush B37.0
    vitamin deficiency
      B group NEC E53.9
      B2 (riboflavin) E53.0
  epidemic B08.8
  epizootic B08.8
  follicular K12.1
  gangrenous A69.0
  Geotrichum B48.3
  herpesviral, herpetic B00.2
  herpetiformis K12.0
  malignant K12.1
  membranous acute K12.1
  monilial B37.0
  mycotic B37.0
  necrotizing ulcerative A69.0
  parasitic B37.0
  septic K12.1
  spirochetal A69.1
  suppurative (acute) K12.2
  ulceromembranous A69.1
  vesicular K12.1
    with exanthem (enteroviral) B08.4
    virus disease A93.8
  Vincent's A69.1
Stomatocytosis D58.8
Stomatomycosis B37.0
Stomatorrhagia K13.79
Stone(s) (see also Calculus)
  bladder (diverticulum) N21.0
  cystine E72.09

Stone(s) — continued
  heart syndrome I50.1
  kidney N20.0
  prostate N42.0
  pulpal (dental) K04.2
  renal N20.0
  salivary gland or duct (any) K11.5
  urethra (impacted) N21.1
  urinary (duct) (impacted) (passage) N20.9
    bladder (diverticulum) N21.0
    lower tract N21.9
    specified NEC N21.8
  xanthine E79.8 [N22]
Stonecutter's lung J62.8
**Stonemason's asthma, disease, lung or pneumoco-
    niosis** J62.8
Stoppage
  heart — see Arrest, cardiac
  urine — see Retention, urine
Storm, thyroid — see Thyrotoxicosis
Strabismus (congenital) (nonparalytic) H50.9
  concomitant H50.40
    convergent — see Strabismus, convergent concomi-
      tant
    divergent — see Strabismus, divergent concomitant
  convergent concomitant H50.00
    accommodative component H50.43
    alternating H50.05
      with
        A pattern H50.06
        specified nonconcomitances NEC H50.08
        V pattern H50.07
    monocular H50.01- ☑
      with
        A pattern H50.02- ☑
        specified nonconcomitances NEC H50.04- ☑
        V pattern H50.03- ☑
      intermittent H50.31- ☑
        alternating H50.32
  cyclotropia H50.41 ☑
  divergent concomitant H50.10
    alternating H50.15
      with
        A pattern H50.16
        specified noncomitances NEC H50.18
        V pattern H50.17
    monocular H50.11- ☑
      with
        A pattern H50.12- ☑
        specified noncomitances NEC H50.14- ☑
        V pattern H50.13- ☑
      intermittent H50.33 ☑
        alternating H50.34
  Duane's syndrome H50.81- ☑
  due to adhesions, scars H50.69
  heterophoria H50.50
    alternating H50.55
    cyclophoria H50.54
    esophoria H50.51
    exophoria H50.52
    vertical H50.53
  heterotropia H50.40
    intermittent H50.30
  hypertropia H50.2- ☑
  hypotropia — see Hypertropia
  latent H50.50
  mechanical H50.60
    Brown's sheath syndrome H50.61- ☑
    specified type NEC H50.69
  monofixation syndrome H50.42
  paralytic H49.9
    abducens nerve H49.2- ☑
    fourth nerve H49.1- ☑
    Kearns-Sayre syndrome H49.81- ☑
    ophthalmoplegia (external)
      progressive H49.4- ☑
        with pigmentary retinopathy H49.81- ☑
      total H49.3- ☑
    sixth nerve H49.2- ☑
    specified type NEC H49.88- ☑
    third nerve H49.0- ☑
    trochlear nerve H49.1- ☑
  specified type NEC H50.89
  vertical H50.2- ☑
Strain
  back S39.012 ☑
  cervical S16.1 ☑

Strain — continued
  eye NEC — see Disturbance, vision, subjective
  heart — see Disease, heart
  low back S39.012 ☑
  mental NOS Z73.3
    work-related Z56.6
  muscle (tendon) — see Injury, muscle, by site, strain
  neck S16.1 ☑
  physical NOS Z73.3
    work-related Z56.6
  postural (see also Disorder, soft tissue, due to use)
  psychological NEC Z73.3
  tendon — see Injury, muscle, by site, strain
Straining, on urination R39.16
Strand, vitreous — see Opacity, vitreous, membranes
    and strands
Strangulation, strangulated (see also Asphyxia, trau-
    matic)
  appendix K38.8
  bladder-neck N32.0
  bowel or colon K56.2
  food or foreign body — see Foreign body, by site
  hemorrhoids — see Hemorrhoids, with complication
  hernia (see also Hernia, by site, with obstruction)
    with gangrene — see Hernia, by site, with gangrene
  intestine (large) (small) K56.2
    with hernia (see also Hernia, by site, with obstruc-
      tion)
      with gangrene — see Hernia, by site, with gan-
        grene
  mesentery K56.2
  mucus — see Asphyxia, mucus
  omentum K56.2
  organ or site, congenital NEC — see Atresia, by site
  ovary — see Torsion, ovary
  penis N48.89
    foreign body T19.4 ☑
  rupture — see Hernia, by site, with obstruction
  stomach due to hernia (see also Hernia, by site, with
    obstruction)
    with gangrene — see Hernia, by site, with gangrene
  vesicourethral orifice N32.0
Strangury R30.0
Straw itch B88.0
Strawberry
  gallbladder K82.4
  mark Q82.5
  tongue (red) (white) K14.3
Streak(s)
  macula, angioid H35.33
  ovarian Q50.32
Strephosymbolia F81.0
  secondary to organic lesion R48.8
Streptobacillary fever A25.1
Streptobacillosis A25.1
Streptobacillus moniliformis A25.1
Streptococcus, streptococcal (see also condition)
  as cause of disease classified elsewhere B95.5
  group
    A, as cause of disease classified elsewhere B95.0
    B, as cause of disease classified elsewhere B95.1
    D, as cause of disease classified elsewhere B95.2
  pneumoniae, as cause of disease classified elsewhere
    B95.3
  specified NEC, as cause of disease classified elsewhere
    B95.4
Streptomycosis B47.1
Streptotrichosis A48.8
Stress F43.9
  family — see Disruption, family
  fetal P84
    complicating pregnancy O77.9
      due to drug administration O77.1
  mental NEC Z73.3
    work-related Z56.6
  physical NEC Z73.3
    work-related Z56.6
  polycythemia D75.1
  reaction (see also Reaction, stress) F43.9
  work schedule Z56.3
Stretching, nerve — see Injury, nerve
Striae albicantes, atrophicae or distensae (cutis) L90.6
Stricture (see also Stenosis)
  ampulla of Vater K83.1
  anus (sphincter) K62.4
    congenital Q42.3
      with fistula Q42.2

☑ **Additional Character Required** — Refer to the Tabular List for Character Selection   ▽ **Subterms under main terms may continue to next column or page**

Stricture — *continued*
- anus — *continued*
  - infantile Q42.3
    - with fistula Q42.2
- aorta (ascending) (congenital) Q25.1
  - arteriosclerotic I70.0
  - calcified I70.0
  - supravalvular, congenital Q25.3
- aortic (valve) — *see* Stenosis, aortic
- aqueduct of Sylvius (congenital) Q03.0
  - with spina bifida — *see* Spina bifida, by site, with hydrocephalus
  - acquired G91.1
- artery I77.1
  - basilar — *see* Occlusion, artery, basilar
  - carotid — *see* Occlusion, artery, carotid
  - celiac I77.4
  - congenital (peripheral) Q27.8
    - cerebral Q28.3
    - coronary Q24.5
    - digestive system Q27.8
    - lower limb Q27.8
    - retinal Q14.1
    - specified site NEC Q27.8
    - umbilical Q27.0
    - upper limb Q27.8
  - coronary — *see* Disease, heart, ischemic, atherosclerotic
    - congenital Q24.5
  - precerebral — *see* Occlusion, artery, precerebral
  - pulmonary (congenital) Q25.6
    - acquired I28.8
  - renal I70.1
  - vertebral — *see* Occlusion, artery, vertebral
- auditory canal (external) (congenital)
  - acquired — *see* Stenosis, external ear canal
- bile duct (common) (hepatic) K83.1
  - congenital Q44.3
  - postoperative K91.89
- bladder N32.89
  - neck N32.0
- bowel — *see* Obstruction, intestine
- brain G93.89
- bronchus J98.09
  - congenital Q32.3
  - syphilitic A52.72
- cardia (stomach) K22.2
  - congenital Q39.3
- cardiac (*see also* Disease, heart)
  - orifice (stomach) K22.2
- cecum — *see* Obstruction, intestine
- cervix, cervical (canal) N88.2
  - congenital Q51.828
  - in pregnancy — *see* Pregnancy, complicated by, abnormal cervix
    - causing obstructed labor O65.5
- colon (*see also* Obstruction, intestine)
  - congenital Q42.9
    - specified NEC Q42.8
- colostomy K94.03
- common (bile) duct K83.1
- coronary (artery) — *see* Disease, heart, ischemic, atherosclerotic
- cystic duct — *see* Obstruction, gallbladder
- digestive organs NEC, congenital Q45.8
- duodenum K31.5
  - congenital Q41.0
- ear canal (external) (congenital) Q16.1
  - acquired — *see* Stricture, auditory canal, acquired
- ejaculatory duct N50.89
- enterostomy K94.13
- esophagus K22.2
  - congenital Q39.3
  - syphilitic A52.79
    - congenital A50.59 [K23]
- eustachian tube (*see also* Obstruction, eustachian tube)
  - congenital Q17.8
- fallopian tube N97.1
  - gonococcal A54.24
  - tuberculous A18.17
- gallbladder — *see* Obstruction, gallbladder
- glottis J38.6
- heart (*see also* Disease, heart)
  - valve (*see also* Endocarditis) I38
    - aortic Q23.0
    - mitral Q23.2
    - pulmonary Q22.1
    - tricuspid Q22.4

Stricture — *continued*
- hepatic duct K83.1
- hourglass, of stomach K31.2
- hymen N89.6
- hypopharynx J39.2
- ileum (*see also* Obstruction, intestine, specified NEC) K56.699
  - congenital Q41.2
- intestine (*see also* Obstruction, intestine)
  - congenital (small) Q41.9
    - large Q42.9
      - specified NEC Q42.8
    - specified NEC Q41.8
  - ischemic K55.1
- jejunum (*see also* Obstruction, intestine, specified NEC) K56.699
  - congenital Q41.1
- lacrimal passages (*see also* Stenosis, lacrimal)
  - congenital Q10.5
- larynx J38.6
  - congenital NEC Q31.8
    - subglottic Q31.1
  - syphilitic A52.73
    - congenital A50.59 [J99]
- meatus
  - ear (congenital) Q16.1
    - acquired — *see* Stricture, auditory canal, acquired
  - osseous (ear) (congenital) Q16.1
    - acquired — *see* Stricture, auditory canal, acquired
  - urinarius (*see also* Stricture, urethra)
    - congenital Q64.33
- mitral (valve) — *see* Stenosis, mitral
- myocardium, myocardial I51.5
  - hypertrophic subaortic (idiopathic) I42.1
- nares (anterior) (posterior) J34.89
  - congenital Q30.0
- nasal duct (*see also* Stenosis, lacrimal, duct)
  - congenital Q10.5
- nasolacrimal duct (*see also* Stenosis, lacrimal, duct)
  - congenital Q10.5
- nasopharynx J39.2
  - syphilitic A52.73
- nose J34.89
  - congenital Q30.0
- nostril (anterior) (posterior) J34.89
  - congenital Q30.0
  - syphilitic A52.73
    - congenital A50.59 [J99]
- organ or site, congenital NEC — *see* Atresia, by site
- os uteri — *see* Stricture, cervix
- osseous meatus (ear) (congenital) Q16.1
  - acquired — *see* Stricture, auditory canal, acquired
- oviduct — *see* Stricture, fallopian tube
- pelviureteric junction (congenital) Q62.11
  - acquired, with hydronephrosis N13.0
- penis, by foreign body T19.4 ☑
- pharynx J39.2
- prostate N42.89
- pulmonary, pulmonic
  - artery (congenital) Q25.6
    - acquired I28.8
    - noncongenital I28.8
  - infundibulum (congenital) Q24.3
  - valve I37.0
    - congenital Q22.1
  - vein, acquired I28.8
  - vessel NEC I28.8
- punctum lacrimale (*see also* Stenosis, lacrimal, punctum)
  - congenital Q10.5
- pylorus (hypertrophic) K31.1
  - adult K31.1
  - congenital Q40.0
  - infantile Q40.0
- rectosigmoid (*see also* Obstruction, intestine, specified NEC) K56.699
- rectum (sphincter) K62.4
  - congenital Q42.1
    - with fistula Q42.0
  - due to
    - chlamydial lymphogranuloma A55
    - irradiation K91.89
    - lymphogranuloma venereum A55
  - gonococcal A54.6
  - inflammatory (chlamydial) A55
  - syphilitic A52.74

Stricture — *continued*
- rectum — *continued*
  - tuberculous A18.32
- renal artery I70.1
  - congenital Q27.1
- salivary duct or gland (any) K11.8
- sigmoid (flexure) — *see* Obstruction, intestine
- spermatic cord N50.89
- stoma (following) (of)
  - colostomy K94.03
  - enterostomy K94.13
  - gastrostomy K94.23
  - ileostomy K94.13
  - tracheostomy J95.03
- stomach K31.89
  - congenital Q40.2
  - hourglass K31.2
- subaortic Q24.4
  - hypertrophic (acquired) (idiopathic) I42.1
- subglottic J38.6
- syphilitic NEC A52.79
- trachea J39.8
  - congenital Q32.1
  - syphilitic A52.73
  - tuberculous NEC A15.5
- tracheostomy J95.03
- tricuspid (valve) — *see* Stenosis, tricuspid
- tunica vaginalis N50.89
- ureter (postoperative) N13.5
  - with
    - hydronephrosis N13.1
      - with infection N13.6
    - pyelonephritis (chronic) N11.1
  - congenital — *see* Atresia, ureter
  - tuberculous A18.11
- ureteropelvic junction (congenital) Q62.11
  - acquired, with hydronephrosis N13.0
- ureterovesical orifice N13.5
  - with infection N13.6
- urethra (organic) (spasmodic) (*see also* Stricture, urethra, male) N35.919
  - associated with schistosomiasis B65.0 [N37]
  - congenital Q64.39
    - valvular (posterior) Q64.2
  - due to
    - infection — *see* Stricture, urethra, postinfective
    - trauma — *see* Stricture, urethra, post-traumatic
  - female N35.92
  - gonococcal, gonorrheal A54.01
  - infective NEC — *see* Stricture, urethra, postinfective
  - late effect (sequelae) of injury — *see* Stricture, urethra, post-traumatic
  - male N35.919
    - anterior urethra N35.914
    - bulbous urethra N35.912
    - meatal N35.911
    - membranous urethra N35.913
    - overlapping sites N35.916
  - postcatheterization — *see* Stricture, urethra, post-procedural
  - postinfective NEC
    - female N35.12
    - male N35.119
      - anterior urethra N35.114
      - bulbous urethra N35.112
      - meatal N35.111
      - membranous urethra N35.113
      - overlapping sites N35.116
  - postobstetric N35.021
  - postoperative — *see* Stricture, urethra, postprocedural
  - postprocedural
    - female N99.12
    - male N99.114
      - anterior bulbous urethra N99.113
      - bulbous urethra N99.111
      - fossa navicularis N99.115
      - meatal N99.110
      - membranous urethra N99.112
      - overlapping sites N99.116
  - post-traumatic
    - female N35.028
      - due to childbirth N35.021
    - male N35.014
      - anterior urethra N35.013
      - bulbous urethra N35.011
      - meatal N35.010
      - membranous urethra N35.012

Stricture — *continued*
  urethra (*see also* Stricture, urethra, male) —
      continued
    post-traumatic — *continued*
      male — *continued*
        overlapping sites N35.016
    sequela (late effect) of
      childbirth N35.021
      injury — *see* Stricture, urethra, post-traumatic
    specified cause NEC
      female N35.82
      male N35.819
        anterior urethra N35.814
        bulbous urethra N35.812
        meatal N35.811
        membranous urethra N35.813
        overlapping sites N35.816
    syphilitic A52.76
    traumatic — *see* Stricture, urethra, post-traumatic
    valvular (posterior), congenital Q64.2
  urinary meatus — *see* Stricture, urethra
  uterus, uterine (synechiae) N85.6
    os (external) (internal) — *see* Stricture, cervix
  vagina (outlet) — *see* Stenosis, vagina
  valve (cardiac) (heart) (*see also* Endocarditis)
    congenital
      aortic Q23.0
      mitral Q23.2
      pulmonary Q22.1
      tricuspid Q22.4
  vas deferens N50.89
    congenital Q55.4
  vein I87.1
  vena cava (inferior) (superior) NEC I87.1
    congenital Q26.0
  vesicourethral orifice N32.0
    congenital Q64.31
  vulva (acquired) N90.5
Stridor R06.1
  congenital (larynx) P28.89
Stridulous — *see* condition
Stroke (apoplectic) (brain) (embolic) (ischemic) (paralytic)
    (thrombotic) I63.9
  cryptogenic (*see also* infarction, cerebral) I63.9
  epileptic — *see* Epilepsy
  heat T67.0 ☑
  in evolution I63.9
  intraoperative
    during cardiac surgery I97.810
    during other surgery I97.811
  lightning — *see* Lightning
  meaning
    cerebral hemorrhage — *code to* Hemorrhage, in-
        tracranial
    cerebral infarction — *code to* Infarction, cerebral
  postprocedural
    following cardiac surgery I97.820
    following other surgery I97.821
  unspecified (NOS) I63.9
Stromatosis, endometrial D39.0
Strongyloidiasis, strongyloidosis B78.9
  cutaneous B78.1
  disseminated B78.7
  intestinal B78.0
Strophulus pruriginosus L28.2
Struck by lightning — *see* Lightning
Struma (*see also* Goiter)
  Hashimoto E06.3
  lymphomatosa E06.3
  nodosa (simplex) E04.9
    endemic E01.2
      multinodular E01.1
    multinodular E04.2
      iodine-deficiency related E01.1
    toxic or with hyperthyroidism E05.20
      with thyroid storm E05.21
      multinodular E05.20
        with thyroid storm E05.21
      uninodular E05.10
        with thyroid storm E05.11
    toxicosa E05.20
      with thyroid storm E05.21
      multinodular E05.20
        with thyroid storm E05.21
      uninodular E05.10
        with thyroid storm E05.11
    uninodular E04.1
  ovarii D27.- ☑

Struma — *continued*
  Riedel's E06.5
Strumipriva cachexia E03.4
Strümpell-Marie spine — *see* Spondylitis, ankylosing
Strümpell-Westphal pseudosclerosis E83.01
Stuart deficiency disease (factor X) D68.2
Stuart-Prower factor deficiency (factor X) D68.2
Student's elbow — *see* Bursitis, elbow, olecranon
Stump — *see* Amputation
Stunting, nutritional E45
Stupor (catatonic) R40.1
  depressive (single episode) F32.89
    recurrent episode F33.8
  dissociative F44.2
  manic F30.2
  manic-depressive F31.89
  psychogenic (anergic) F44.2
  reaction to exceptional stress (transient) F43.0
Sturge (-Weber) (-Dimitri) (-Kalischer) **disease or syn-
    drome** Q85.8
Stuttering F80.81
  adult onset F98.5
  childhood onset F80.81
  following cerebrovascular disease — *see* Disorder, flu-
      ency. following cerebrovascular disease
  in conditions classified elsewhere R47.82
Sty, stye (external) (internal) (meibomian) (zeisian) —
    see Hordeolum
Subacidity, gastric K31.89
  psychogenic F45.8
Subacute — *see* condition
Subarachnoid — *see* condition
Subcortical — *see* condition
Subcostal syndrome, nerve compression — *see*
    Mononeuropathy, upper limb, specified site NEC
Subcutaneous, subcuticular — *see* condition
Subdural — *see* condition
Subendocardium — *see* condition
Subependymoma
  specified site — *see* Neoplasm, uncertain behavior, by
      site
  unspecified site D43.2
Suberosis J67.3
Subglossitis — *see* Glossitis
Subhemophilia D66
Subinvolution
  breast (postlactational) (postpuerperal) N64.89
  puerperal O90.89
  uterus (chronic) (nonpuerperal) N85.3
    puerperal O90.89
Sublingual — *see* condition
Sublinguitis — *see* Sialoadenitis
Subluxatable hip Q65.6
Subluxation (*see also* Dislocation)
  acromioclavicular S43.11- ☑
  ankle S93.0- ☑
  atlantoaxial, recurrent M43.4
    with myelopathy M43.3
  carpometacarpal (joint) NEC S63.05- ☑
    thumb S63.04- ☑
  complex, vertebral — *see* Complex, subluxation
  congenital (*see also* Malposition, congenital)
    hip — *see* Dislocation, hip, congenital, partial
    joint (excluding hip)
      lower limb Q68.8
      shoulder Q68.8
      upper limb Q68.8
  elbow (traumatic) S53.10- ☑
    anterior S53.11- ☑
    lateral S53.14- ☑
    medial S53.13- ☑
    posterior S53.12- ☑
    specified type NEC S53.19- ☑
  finger S63.20- ☑
    index S63.20- ☑
    interphalangeal S63.22- ☑
      distal S63.24- ☑
        index S63.24- ☑
        little S63.24- ☑
        middle S63.24- ☑
        ring S63.24- ☑
      index S63.22- ☑
      little S63.22- ☑
      middle S63.22- ☑
      proximal S63.23- ☑
        index S63.23- ☑
        little S63.23- ☑

Subluxation — *continued*
  finger — *continued*
    interphalangeal — *continued*
      proximal — *continued*
        middle S63.23- ☑
        ring S63.23- ☑
      ring S63.22- ☑
    little S63.20- ☑
    metacarpophalangeal S63.21- ☑
      index S63.21- ☑
      little S63.21- ☑
      middle S63.21- ☑
      ring S63.21- ☑
    middle S63.20- ☑
    ring S63.20- ☑
  foot S93.30- ☑
    specified site NEC S93.33- ☑
    tarsal joint S93.31- ☑
    tarsometatarsal joint S93.32- ☑
    toe — *see* Subluxation, toe
  hip S73.00- ☑
    anterior S73.03- ☑
      obturator S73.02- ☑
    central S73.04- ☑
    posterior S73.01- ☑
  interphalangeal (joint)
    finger S63.22- ☑
      distal joint S63.24- ☑
        index S63.24- ☑
        little S63.24- ☑
        middle S63.24- ☑
        ring S63.24- ☑
      index S63.22- ☑
      little S63.22- ☑
      middle S63.22- ☑
      proximal joint S63.23- ☑
        index S63.23- ☑
        little S63.23- ☑
        middle S63.23- ☑
        ring S63.23- ☑
      ring S63.22- ☑
      thumb S63.12- ☑
    toe S93.13- ☑
      great S93.13- ☑
      lesser S93.13- ☑
  joint prosthesis — *see* Complications, joint prosthesis,
      mechanical, displacement, by site
  knee S83.10- ☑
    cap — *see* Subluxation, patella
    patella — *see* Subluxation, patella
    proximal tibia
      anteriorly S83.11- ☑
      laterally S83.14- ☑
      medially S83.13- ☑
      posteriorly S83.12- ☑
    specified type NEC S83.19- ☑
  lens — *see* Dislocation, lens, partial
  ligament, traumatic — *see* Sprain, by site
  metacarpal (bone)
    proximal end S63.06- ☑
  metacarpophalangeal (joint)
    finger S63.21- ☑
      index S63.21- ☑
      little S63.21- ☑
      middle S63.21- ☑
      ring S63.21- ☑
    thumb S63.11- ☑
  metatarsophalangeal joint S93.14- ☑
    great toe S93.14- ☑
    lesser toe S93.14- ☑
  midcarpal (joint) S63.03- ☑
  patella S83.00- ☑
    lateral S83.01- ☑
    recurrent (nontraumatic) — *see* Dislocation, patella,
        recurrent, incomplete
    specified type NEC S83.09- ☑
  pathological — *see* Dislocation, pathological
  radial head S53.00- ☑
    anterior S53.01- ☑
    nursemaid's elbow S53.03- ☑
    posterior S53.02- ☑
    specified type NEC S53.09- ☑
  radiocarpal (joint) S63.02- ☑
  radioulnar (joint)
    distal S63.01- ☑
    proximal — *see* Subluxation, elbow

☑ **Additional Character Required** — Refer to the Tabular List for Character Selection   ▽ **Subterms under main terms may continue to next column or page**

Subluxation — *continued*
  shoulder
    congenital Q68.8
    girdle S43.3Ø- ☑
      scapula S43.31- ☑
      specified site NEC S43.39- ☑
    traumatic S43.ØØ- ☑
      anterior S43.Ø1- ☑
      inferior S43.Ø3- ☑
      posterior S43.Ø2- ☑
      specified type NEC S43.Ø8- ☑
  sternoclavicular (joint) S43.2Ø- ☑
    anterior S43.21- ☑
    posterior S43.22- ☑
  symphysis (pubis)
  thumb S63.1Ø3 ☑
    interphalangeal joint — *see* Subluxation, interpha-
        langeal (joint), thumb
    metacarpophalangeal joint — *see* Subluxation,
        metacarpophalangeal (joint), thumb
  toe(s) S93.1Ø- ☑
    great S93.1Ø- ☑
      interphalangeal joint S93.13- ☑
      metatarsophalangeal joint S93.14- ☑
    interphalangeal joint S93.13- ☑
    lesser S93.1Ø- ☑
      interphalangeal joint S93.13- ☑
      metatarsophalangeal joint S93.14- ☑
    metatarsophalangeal joint S93.149 ☑
  ulna
    distal end S63.Ø7- ☑
    proximal end — *see* Subluxation, elbow
  ulnohumeral joint — *see* Subluxation, elbow
  vertebral
    recurrent NEC — *see* subcategory M43.5 ☑
    traumatic
      cervical S13.1ØØ ☑
        atlantoaxial joint S13.12Ø ☑
        atlantooccipital joint S13.11Ø ☑
        atloidooccipital joint S13.11Ø ☑
        joint between
          CØ and C1 S13.11Ø ☑
          C1 and C2 S13.12Ø ☑
          C2 and C3 S13.13Ø ☑
          C3 and C4 S13.14Ø ☑
          C4 and C5 S13.15Ø ☑
          C5 and C6 S13.16Ø ☑
          C6 and C7 S13.17Ø ☑
          C7 and T1 S13.18Ø ☑
        occipitoatloid joint S13.11Ø ☑
      lumbar S33.1ØØ ☑
        joint between
          L1 and L2 S33.11Ø ☑
          L2 and L3 S33.12Ø ☑
          L3 and L4 S33.13Ø ☑
          L4 and L5 S33.14Ø ☑
      thoracic S23.1ØØ ☑
        joint between
          T1 and T2 S23.11Ø ☑
          T2 and T3 S23.12Ø ☑
          T3 and T4 S23.122 ☑
          T4 and T5 S23.13Ø ☑
          T5 and T6 S23.132 ☑
          T6 and T7 S23.14Ø ☑
          T7 and T8 S23.142 ☑
          T8 and T9 S23.15Ø ☑
          T9 and T1Ø S23.152 ☑
          T1Ø and T11 S23.16Ø ☑
          T11 and T12 S23.162 ☑
          T12 and L1 S23.17Ø ☑
  wrist (carpal bone) S63.ØØ- ☑
    carpometacarpal joint — *see* Subluxation, car-
        pometacarpal (joint)
    distal radioulnar joint — *see* Subluxation, radioulnar
        (joint), distal
    metacarpal bone, proximal — *see* Subluxation,
        metacarpal (bone), proximal end
    midcarpal — *see* Subluxation, midcarpal (joint)
    radiocarpal joint — *see* Subluxation, radiocarpal
        (joint)
    recurrent — *see* Dislocation, recurrent, wrist
    specified site NEC S63.Ø9- ☑
    ulna — *see* Subluxation, ulna, distal end
Submaxillary — *see* condition
Submersion (fatal) (nonfatal) T75.1 ☑
Submucous — *see* condition

Subnormal, subnormality
  accommodation (old age) H52.4
  mental — *see* Disability, intellectual
  temperature (accidental) T68 ☑
Subphrenic — *see* condition
Subscapular nerve — *see* condition
Subseptus uterus Q51.28
Subsiding appendicitis K36
Substance (other psychoactive) **-induced**
  anxiety disorder F19.98Ø
  bipolar and related disorder F19.94
  delirium F19.921
  depressive disorder F19.94
  major neurocognitive disorder F19.97
  mild neurocognitive disorder F19.988
  obsessive-compulsive and related disorder F19.988
  psychotic disorder F19.959
  sexual dysfunction F19.981
  sleep disorder F19.982
Substernal thyroid EØ4.9
  congenital Q89.2
Substitution disorder F44.9
Subtentorial — *see* condition
Subthyroidism (acquired) (*see also* Hypothyroidism)
  congenital EØ3.1
Succenturiate placenta O43.19- ☑
Sucking thumb, child (excessive) F98.8
Sudamen, sudamina L74.1
Sudanese kala-azar B55.Ø
Sudden
  hearing loss — *see* Deafness, sudden
  heart failure — *see* Failure, heart
Sudeck's atrophy, disease, or syndrome — *see* Algo-
    neurodystrophy
Suffocation — *see* Asphyxia, traumatic
Sugar
  blood
    high (transient) R73.9
    low (transient) E16.2
  in urine R81
Suicide, suicidal (attempted) T14.91 ☑
  by poisoning — *see* Table of Drugs and Chemicals
  history of (personal) Z91.5
    in family Z81.8
  ideation — *see* Ideation, suicidal
  risk
    meaning personal history of attempted suicide Z91.5
    meaning suicidal ideation — *see* Ideation, suicidal
  tendencies
    meaning personal history of attempted suicide Z91.5
    meaning suicidal ideation — *see* Ideation, suicidal
  trauma — *see* nature of injury by site
Suipestifer infection — *see* Infection, salmonella
Sulfhemoglobinemia, sulphemoglobinemia (ac-
    quired) (with methemoglobinemia) D74.8
Sumatran mite fever A75.3
Summer — *see* condition
Sunburn L55.9
  due to
    tanning bed (acute) L56.8
      chronic L57.8
    ultraviolet radiation (acute) L56.8
      chronic L57.8
  first degree L55.Ø
  second degree L55.1
  third degree L55.2
SUNCT (short lasting unilateral neuralgiform headache
    with conjunctival injection and tearing) G44.Ø59
  intractable G44.Ø51
  not intractable G44.Ø59
Sundowning FØ5
Sunken acetabulum — *see* Derangement, joint, speci-
    fied type NEC, hip
Sunstroke T67.Ø ☑
Superfecundation — *see* Pregnancy, multiple
Superfetation — *see* Pregnancy, multiple
Superinvolution (uterus) N85.8
Supernumerary (congenital)
  aortic cusps Q23.8
  auditory ossicles Q16.3
  bone Q79.8
  breast Q83.1
  carpal bones Q74.Ø
  cusps, heart valve NEC Q24.8
    aortic Q23.8
    mitral Q23.2
    pulmonary Q22.3

Supernumerary — *continued*
  digit(s) Q69.9
  ear (lobule) Q17.Ø
  fallopian tube Q5Ø.6
  finger Q69.Ø
  hymen Q52.4
  kidney Q63.Ø
  lacrimonasal duct Q1Ø.6
  lobule (ear) Q17.Ø
  mitral cusps Q23.2
  muscle Q79.8
  nipple(s) Q83.3
  organ or site not listed — *see* Accessory
  ossicles, auditory Q16.3
  ovary Q5Ø.31
  oviduct Q5Ø.6
  pulmonary, pulmonic cusps Q22.3
  rib Q76.6
    cervical or first (syndrome) Q76.5
  roots (of teeth) KØØ.2
  spleen Q89.Ø9
  tarsal bones Q74.2
  teeth KØØ.1
  testis Q55.29
  thumb Q69.1
  toe Q69.2
  uterus Q51.28
  vagina Q52.1
  vertebra Q76.49
Supervision (of)
  contraceptive — *see* Prescription, contraceptives
  dietary (for) Z71.3
    allergy (food) Z71.3
    colitis Z71.3
    diabetes mellitus Z71.3
    food allergy or intolerance Z71.3
    gastritis Z71.3
    hypercholesterolemia Z71.3
    hypoglycemia Z71.3
    intolerance (food) Z71.3
    obesity Z71.3
    specified NEC Z71.3
  healthy infant or child Z76.2
    foundling Z76.1
  high-risk pregnancy — *see* Pregnancy, complicated
      by, high, risk
  lactation Z39.1
  pregnancy — *see* Pregnancy, supervision of
Supplemental teeth KØØ.1
Suppression
  binocular vision H53.34
  lactation O92.5
  menstruation N94.89
  ovarian secretion E28.39
  renal N28.9
  urine, urinary secretion R34
Suppuration, suppurative (*see also* condition)
  accessory sinus (chronic) — *see* Sinusitis
  adrenal gland
  antrum (chronic) — *see* Sinusitis, maxillary
  bladder — *see* Cystitis
  brain GØ6.Ø
    sequelae GØ9
  breast N61.1
    puerperal, postpartum or gestational — *see* Mastitis,
        obstetric, purulent
  dental periosteum M27.3
  ear (middle) (*see also* Otitis, media)
    external NEC — *see* Otitis, externa, infective
    internal — *see* subcategory H83.Ø ☑
  ethmoidal (chronic) (sinus) — *see* Sinusitis, ethmoidal
  fallopian tube — *see* Salpingo-oophoritis
  frontal (chronic) (sinus) — *see* Sinusitis, frontal
  gallbladder (acute) K81.Ø
  gum KØ5.2Ø
    generalized — *see* Peridontitis, aggressive, general-
        ized
    localized — *see* Peridontitis, aggressive, localized
  intracranial GØ6.Ø
  joint — *see* Arthritis, pyogenic or pyemic
  labyrinthine — *see* subcategory H83.Ø ☑
  lung — *see* Abscess, lung
  mammary gland N61.1
    puerperal, postpartum O91.12
      associated with lactation O91.13
  maxilla, maxillary M27.2
    sinus (chronic) — *see* Sinusitis, maxillary
  muscle — *see* Myositis, infective

Suppuration, suppurative — *continued*
  nasal sinus (chronic) — *see* Sinusitis
  pancreas, acute (*see also* Pancreatitis, acute) K85.80
  parotid gland — *see* Sialoadenitis
  pelvis, pelvic
    female — *see* Disease, pelvis, inflammatory
    male K65.0
  pericranial — *see* Osteomyelitis
  salivary duct or gland (any) — *see* Sialoadenitis
  sinus (accessory) (chronic) (nasal) — *see* Sinusitis
  sphenoidal sinus (chronic) — *see* Sinusitis, sphenoidal
  thymus (gland) E32.1
  thyroid (gland) E06.0
  tonsil — *see* Tonsillitis
  uterus — *see* Endometritis
Supraeruption of tooth (teeth) M26.34
Supraglottitis J04.30
  with obstruction J04.31
Suprarenal (gland) — *see* condition
Suprascapular nerve — *see* condition
Suprasellar — *see* condition
Surfer's knots or nodules S89.8- ☑
Surgical
  emphysema T81.82 ☑
  procedures, complication or misadventure — *see*
    Complications, surgical procedures
  shock T81.10 ☑
Surveillance (of) (for) (*see also* Observation)
  alcohol abuse Z71.41
  contraceptive — *see* Prescription, contraceptives
  dietary Z71.3
  drug abuse Z71.51
Susceptibility to disease, genetic Z15.89
  malignant neoplasm Z15.09
    breast Z15.01
    endometrium Z15.04
    ovary Z15.02
    prostate Z15.03
    specified NEC Z15.09
  multiple endocrine neoplasia Z15.81
Suspected condition, ruled out (*see also* Observation, suspected)
  amniotic cavity and membrane Z03.71
  cervical shortening Z03.75
  fetal anomaly Z03.73
  fetal growth Z03.74
  maternal and fetal conditions NEC Z03.79
  newborn (*see also* Observation, newborn, suspected condition ruled out) Z05.9
  oligohydramnios Z03.71
  placental problem Z03.72
  polyhydramnios Z03.71
Suspended uterus
  in pregnancy or childbirth — *see* Pregnancy, complicated by, abnormal uterus
Sutton's nevus D22.9
Suture
  burst (in operation wound) T81.31 ☑
    external operation wound T81.31 ☑
    internal operation wound T81.32 ☑
  inadvertently left in operation wound — *see* Foreign body, accidentally left during a procedure
  removal Z48.02
Swab inadvertently left in operation wound — *see* Foreign body, accidentally left during a procedure
Swallowed, swallowing
  difficulty — *see* Dysphagia
  foreign body — *see* Foreign body, alimentary tract
Swan-neck deformity (finger) — *see* Deformity, finger, swan-neck
Swearing, compulsive F42.8
  in Gilles de la Tourette's syndrome F95.2
Sweat, sweats
  fetid L75.0
  night R61
Sweating, excessive R61
Sweeley-Klionsky disease E75.21
Sweet's disease or dermatosis L98.2
Swelling (of) R60.9
  abdomen, abdominal (not referable to any particular organ) — *see* Mass, abdominal
  ankle — *see* Effusion, joint, ankle
  arm M79.89
    forearm M79.89
  breast (*see also* Lump, breast) N63.0
  Calabar B74.3
  cervical gland R59.0

Swelling — *continued*
  chest, localized R22.2
  ear H93.8- ☑
  extremity (lower) (upper) — *see* Disorder, soft tissue, specified type NEC
  finger M79.89
  foot M79.89
  glands R59.9
    generalized R59.1
    localized R59.0
  hand M79.89
  head (localized) R22.0
  inflammatory — *see* Inflammation
  intra-abdominal — *see* Mass, abdominal
  joint — *see* Effusion, joint
  leg M79.89
    lower M79.89
  limb — *see* Disorder, soft tissue, specified type NEC
  localized (skin) R22.9
    chest R22.2
    head R22.0
    limb
      lower — *see* Mass, localized, limb, lower
      upper — *see* Mass, localized, limb, upper
    neck R22.1
    trunk R22.2
  neck (localized) R22.1
  pelvic — *see* Mass, abdominal
  scrotum N50.89
  splenic — *see* Splenomegaly
  testis N50.89
  toe M79.89
  umbilical R19.09
  wandering, due to Gnathostoma (spinigerum) B83.1
  white — *see* Tuberculosis, arthritis
Swift (-Feer) **disease**
  overdose or wrong substance given or taken — *see* Table of Drugs and Chemicals, by drug, poisoning
Swimmer's
  cramp T75.1 ☑
  ear H60.33- ☑
  itch B65.3
Swimming in the head R42
Swollen — *see* Swelling
Swyer syndrome Q99.1
Sycosis L73.8
  barbae (not parasitic) L73.8
  contagiosa (mycotic) B35.0
  lupoides L73.8
  mycotic B35.0
  parasitic B35.0
  vulgaris L73.8
Sydenham's chorea — *see* Chorea, Sydenham's
Sylvatic yellow fever A95.0
Sylvest's disease B33.0
Symblepharon H11.23- ☑
  congenital Q10.3
Symond's syndrome G93.2
Sympathetic — *see* condition
Sympatheticotonia G90.8
Sympathicoblastoma
  specified site — *see* Neoplasm, malignant, by site
  unspecified site C74.90
Sympathogonioma — *see* Sympathicoblastoma
Symphalangy (fingers) (toes) Q70.9
Symptoms NEC R68.89
  breast NEC N64.59
  cold J00
  development NEC R63.8
  factitious, self-induced — *see* Disorder, factitious
  genital organs, female R10.2
  involving
    abdomen NEC R19.8
    appearance NEC R46.89
    awareness R41.9
      altered mental status R41.82
      amnesia — *see* Amnesia
      borderline intellectual functioning R41.83
      coma — *see* Coma
      disorientation R41.0
      neurologic neglect syndrome R41.4
      senile cognitive decline R41.81
      specified symptom NEC R41.89
    behavior NEC R46.89
    cardiovascular system NEC R09.89
    chest NEC R09.89
    circulatory system NEC R09.89
    cognitive functions R41.9

Symptoms — *continued*
  involving — *continued*
    cognitive functions — *continued*
      altered mental status R41.82
      amnesia — *see* Amnesia
      borderline intellectual functioning R41.83
      coma — *see* Coma
      disorientation R41.0
      neurologic neglect syndrome R41.4
      senile cognitive decline R41.81
      specified symptom NEC R41.89
    development NEC R62.50
    digestive system NEC R19.8
    emotional state NEC R45.89
      emotional lability R45.86
    food and fluid intake R63.8
    general perceptions and sensations R44.9
      specified NEC R44.8
    musculoskeletal system R29.91
      specified NEC R29.898
    nervous system R29.90
      specified NEC R29.818
    pelvis NEC R19.8
    respiratory system NEC R09.89
    skin and integument R23.9
    urinary system R39.9
  menopausal N95.1
  metabolism NEC R63.8
  neurotic F48.8
  of infancy R68.19
  pelvis NEC, female R10.2
  skin and integument NEC R23.9
  subcutaneous tissue NEC R23.9
  viral cold J00
Sympus Q74.2
Syncephalus Q89.4
Synchondrosis
  abnormal (congenital) Q78.8
  ischiopubic M91.0
Synchysis (scintillans) (senile) (vitreous body) H43.89
Syncope (near) (pre-) R55
  anginosa I20.8
  bradycardia R00.1
  cardiac R55
  carotid sinus G90.01
  due to spinal (lumbar) puncture G97.1
  heart R55
  heat T67.1 ☑
  laryngeal R05
  psychogenic F48.8
  tussive R05
  vasoconstriction R55
  vasodepressor R55
  vasomotor R55
  vasovagal R55
Syndactylism, syndactyly Q70.9
  complex (with synostosis)
    fingers Q70.0- ☑
    toes Q70.2- ☑
  simple (without synostosis)
    fingers Q70.1- ☑
    toes Q70.3- ☑
Syndrome (*see also* Disease)
  5q minus NOS D46.C (*following* D46.2)
  48,XXXX Q97.1
  49,XXXXX Q97.1
  abdominal
    acute R10.0
    muscle deficiency Q79.4
  abnormal innervation H02.519
    left H02.516
      lower H02.515
      upper H02.514
    right H02.513
      lower H02.512
      upper H02.511
  abstinence, neonatal P96.1
  acid pulmonary aspiration, obstetric O74.0
  acquired immunodeficiency — *see* Human, immunodeficiency virus (HIV) disease
  acute abdominal R10.0
  acute respiratory distress (adult) (child) J80
    idiopathic J84.114
  Adair-Dighton Q78.0
  Adams-Stokes (-Morgagni) I45.9
  adiposogenital E23.6
  adrenal
    hemorrhage (meningococcal) A39.1

☑ Additional Character Required — Refer to the Tabular List for Character Selection   ᴺᴱ Subterms under main terms may continue to next column or page

Syndrome — *continued*
- adrenal — *continued*
  - meningococcic A39.1
- adrenocortical — *see* Cushing's, syndrome
- adrenogenital E25.9
  - congenital, associated with enzyme deficiency E25.0
- afferent loop NEC K91.89
- Alagille's Q44.7
- alcohol withdrawal (without convulsions) — *see* Dependence, alcohol, with, withdrawal
- Alder's D72.0
- Aldrich (-Wiskott) D82.0
- alien hand R41.4
- Alport Q87.81
- alveolar hypoventilation E66.2
- alveolocapillary block J84.10
- amnesic, amnestic (confabulatory) (due to) — *see* Disorder, amnesic
- amyostatic (Wilson's disease) E83.01
- androgen insensitivity E34.50
  - complete E34.51
  - partial E34.52
- androgen resistance (*see also* Syndrome, androgen insensitivity) E34.50
- Angelman Q93.51
- anginal — *see* Angina
- ankyloglossia superior Q38.1
- anterior
  - chest wall R07.89
  - cord G83.82
  - spinal artery G95.19
    - compression M47.019
      - cervical region M47.012
      - cervicothoracic region M47.013
      - lumbar region M47.016
      - occipito-atlanto-axial region M47.011
      - thoracic region M47.014
      - thoracolumbar region M47.015
  - tibial M76.81- ☑
- antibody deficiency D80.9
  - agammaglobulinemic D80.1
    - hereditary D80.0
  - congenital D80.0
  - hypogammaglobulinemic D80.1
    - hereditary D80.0
- anticardiolipin (-antibody) D68.61
- antidepressant discontinuation T43.205 ☑
- antiphospholipid (-antibody) D68.61
- aortic
  - arch M31.4
  - bifurcation I74.09
- aortomesenteric duodenum occlusion K31.5
- apical ballooning (transient left ventricular) I51.81
- arcuate ligament I77.4
- argentaffin, argintaffinoma E34.0
- Arnold-Chiari — *see* Arnold-Chiari disease
- Arrillaga-Ayerza I27.0
- arterial tortuosity Q87.82
- arteriovenous steal T82.898- ☑
- Asherman's N85.6
- aspiration, of newborn — *see* Aspiration, by substance, with pneumonia
  - meconium P24.01
- ataxia-telangiectasia G11.3
- auriculotemporal G50.8
- autoerythrocyte sensitization (Gardner-Diamond) D69.2
- autoimmune lymphoproliferative [ALPS] D89.82
- autoimmune polyglandular E31.0
- autoinflammatory M04.9
  - specified type NEC M04.8
- autosomal — *see* Abnormal, autosomes
- Avellis' G46.8
- Babinski-Nageotte G83.89
- Bakwin-Krida Q78.5
- bare lymphocyte D81.6
- Barré-Guillain G61.0
- Barré-Liéou M53.0
- Barrett's — *see* Barrett's, esophagus
- Barsony-Polgar K22.4
- Bársony-Teschendorf K22.4
- Barth E78.71
- Bartter's E26.81
- basal cell nevus Q87.89
- Basedow's E05.00
  - with thyroid storm E05.01
- basilar artery G45.0
- Batten-Steinert G71.11

Syndrome — *continued*
- battered
  - baby or child — *see* Maltreatment, child, physical abuse
  - spouse — *see* Maltreatment, adult, physical abuse
- Beals Q87.40
- Beau's I51.5
- Beck's I65.8
- Benedikt's G46.3
- Béquez César (-Steinbrinck-Chédiak-Higashi) E70.330
- Bernhardt-Roth — *see* Meralgia paresthetica
- Bernheim's — *see* Failure, heart, right
- big spleen D73.1
- Bing-Horton's — *see* Horton's headache
- Birt-Hogg-Dube syndrome Q87.89
- Björck (-Thorsen) E34.0
- black
  - lung J60
  - widow spider bite — *see* Toxicity, venom, spider, black widow
- Blackfan-Diamond D61.01
- Blau M04.8
- blind loop K90.2
  - congenital Q43.8
  - postsurgical K91.2
- blue sclera Q78.0
- blue toe I75.02- ☑
- Boder-Sedgewick G11.3
- Boerhaave's K22.3
- Borjeson Forssman Lehmann Q89.8
- Bouillaud's I01.9
- Bourneville (-Pringle) Q85.1
- Bouveret (-Hoffman) I47.9
- brachial plexus G54.0
- bradycardia-tachycardia I49.5
- brain (nonpsychotic) F09
  - with psychosis, psychotic reaction F09
    - acute or subacute — *see* Delirium
  - congenital — *see* Disability, intellectual
  - organic F09
    - post-traumatic (nonpsychotic) F07.81
      - psychotic F09
    - personality change F07.0
  - postcontusional F07.81
  - post-traumatic, nonpsychotic F07.81
  - psycho-organic F09
  - psychotic F06.8
- brain stem stroke G46.3
- Brandt's (acrodermatitis enteropathica) E83.2
- broad ligament laceration N83.8
- Brock's J98.11
- bronze baby P83.88
- Brown-Sequard G83.81
- Brugada I49.8
- bubbly lung P27.0
- Buchem's M85.2
- Budd-Chiari I82.0
- bulbar (progressive) G12.22
- Bürger-Grütz E78.3
- Burke's K86.89
- Burnett's (milk-alkali) E83.52
- burning feet E53.9
- Bywaters' T79.5 ☑
- Call-Fleming I67.841
- carbohydrate-deficient glycoprotein (CDGS) E77.8
- carcinogenic thrombophlebitis I82.1
- carcinoid E34.0
- cardiac asthma I50.1
- cardiacos negros I27.0
- cardiofaciocutaneous Q87.89
- cardiopulmonary-obesity E66.2
- cardiorenal — *see* Hypertension, cardiorenal
- cardiorespiratory distress (idiopathic), newborn P22.0
- cardiovascular renal — *see* Hypertension, cardiorenal
- carotid
  - artery (hemispheric) (internal) G45.1
  - body G90.01
  - sinus G90.01
- carpal tunnel G56.0- ☑
- Cassidy (-Scholte) E34.0
- cat cry Q93.4
- cat eye Q92.8
- cauda equina G83.4
- causalgia — *see* Causalgia
- celiac K90.0
  - artery compression I77.4
  - axis I77.4

Syndrome — *continued*
- central pain G89.0
- cerebellar
  - hereditary G11.9
  - stroke G46.4
- cerebellomedullary malformation — *see* Spina bifida
- cerebral
  - artery
    - anterior G46.1
    - middle G46.0
    - posterior G46.2
  - gigantism E22.0
- cervical (root) M53.1
  - disc — *see* Disorder, disc, cervical, with neuritis
  - fusion Q76.1
  - posterior, sympathicus M53.0
  - rib Q76.5
  - sympathetic paralysis G90.2
- cervicobrachial (diffuse) M53.1
- cervicocranial M53.0
- cervicodorsal outlet G54.2
- cervicothoracic outlet G54.0
- Céstan (-Raymond) I65.8
- Charcot's (angina cruris) (intermittent claudication) I73.9
- Charcot-Weiss-Baker G90.09
- CHARGE Q89.8
- Chédiak-Higashi (-Steinbrinck) E70.330
- chest wall R07.1
- Chiari's (hepatic vein thrombosis) I82.0
- Chilaiditi's Q43.3
- child maltreatment — *see* Maltreatment, child
- chondrocostal junction M94.0
- chondroectodermal dysplasia Q77.6
- chromosome 4 short arm deletion Q93.3
- chromosome 5 short arm deletion Q93.4
- chronic
  - infantile neurological, cutaneous and articular (CINCA) M04.2
  - pain G89.4
    - personality F68.8
- Clarke-Hadfield K86.89
- Clerambault's automatism G93.89
- Clouston's (hidrotic ectodermal dysplasia) Q82.4
- clumsiness, clumsy child F82
- cluster headache G44.009
  - intractable G44.001
  - not intractable G44.009
- Coffin-Lowry Q89.8
- cold injury (newborn) P80.0
- combined immunity deficiency D81.9
- compartment (deep) (posterior) (traumatic) T79.A0 ☑ (*following* T79.7)
  - abdomen T79.A3 ☑ (*following* T79.7)
  - lower extremity (hip, buttock, thigh, leg, foot, toes) T79.A2 ☑ (*following* T79.7)
  - nontraumatic
    - abdomen M79.A3 (*following* M79.7)
    - lower extremity (hip, buttock, thigh, leg, foot, toes) M79.A2- ☑ (*following* M79.7)
    - specified site NEC M79.A9 (*following* M79.7)
    - upper extremity (shoulder, arm, forearm, wrist, hand, fingers) M79.A1- ☑ (*following* M79.7)
  - postprocedural — *see* Syndrome, compartment, nontraumatic
  - specified site NEC T79.A9 ☑ (*following* T79.7)
  - upper extremity (shoulder, arm, forearm, wrist, hand, fingers) T79.A1 ☑ (*following* T79.7)
- complex regional pain — *see* Syndrome, pain, complex regional
- compression T79.5 ☑
  - anterior spinal — *see* Syndrome, anterior, spinal artery, compression
  - cauda equina G83.4
  - celiac artery I77.4
  - vertebral artery M47.029
    - cervical region M47.022
    - occipito-atlanto-axial region M47.021
- concussion F07.81
- congenital
  - affecting multiple systems NEC Q87.89
  - central alveolar hypoventilation G47.35
  - facial diplegia Q87.0
  - muscular hypertrophy-cerebral Q87.89
  - oculo-auriculovertebral Q87.0
  - oculofacial diplegia (Moebius) Q87.0
  - rubella (manifest) P35.0

Syndrome — *continued*

congestion-fibrosis (pelvic), female N94.89
congestive dysmenorrhea N94.6
connective tissue M35.9
    overlap NEC M35.1
Conn's E26.01
conus medullaris G95.81
cord
    anterior G83.82
    posterior G83.83
coronary
    acute NEC I24.9
    insufficiency or intermediate I20.0
    slow flow I20.8
Costen's (complex) M26.69
costochondral junction M94.0
costoclavicular G54.0
costovertebral E22.0
Cowden Q85.8
craniovertebral M53.0
Creutzfeldt-Jakob — *see* Creutzfeldt-Jakob disease or
    syndrome
crib death R99
cricopharyngeal — *see* Dysphagia
cri-du-chat Q93.4
croup J05.0
CRPS I — *see* Syndrome, pain, complex regional I
crush T79.5 ☑
cryopyrin-associated perodic M04.2
cryptophthalmos Q87.0
cubital tunnel — *see* Lesion, nerve, ulnar
Curschmann (-Batten) (-Steinert) G71.11
Cushing's E24.9
    alcohol-induced E24.4
    due to
        alcohol
        drugs E24.2
        ectopic ACTH E24.3
        overproduction of pituitary ACTH E24.0
    drug-induced E24.2
    overdose or wrong substance given or taken — *see*
        Table of Drugs and Chemicals, by drug, poi-
        soning
    pituitary-dependent E24.0
    specified type NEC E24.8
cystic duct stump K91.5
Dana-Putnam D51.0
Danbolt (-Cross) (acrodermatitis enteropathica) E83.2
Dandy-Walker Q03.1
    with spina bifida Q07.01
Danlos' Q79.6
De Quervain E34.51
de Toni-Fanconi (-Debré) E72.09
    with cystinosis E72.04
defibrination (*see also* Fibrinolysis)
    with
        antepartum hemorrhage — *see* Hemorrhage,
            antepartum, with coagulation defect
        intrapartum hemorrhage — *see* Hemorrhage,
            complicating, delivery
    newborn P60
    postpartum O72.3
Degos' I77.89
Déjérine-Roussy G89.0
delayed sleep phase G47.21
demyelinating G37.9
dependence — *see* F10-F19 with fourth character .2
depersonalization (-derealization) F48.1
di George's D82.1
diabetes mellitus in newborn infant P70.2
diabetes mellitus-hypertension-nephrosis — *see* Dia-
    betes, nephrosis
diabetes-nephrosis — *see* Diabetes, nephrosis
diabetic amyotrophy — *see* Diabetes, amyotrophy
dialysis associated steal T82.898- ☑
Diamond-Blackfan D61.01
Diamond-Gardener D69.2
DIC (diffuse or disseminated intravascular coagulopa-
    thy) D65
Dighton's Q78.0
disequilibrium E87.8
Döhle body-panmyelopathic D72.0
dorsolateral medullary G46.4
double athetosis G80.3
Down (*see also* Down syndrome) Q90.9
Dresbach's (elliptocytosis) D58.1
Dressler's (postmyocardial infarction) I24.1
    postcardiotomy I97.0

Syndrome — *continued*

drug withdrawal, infant of dependent mother P96.1
dry eye H04.12- ☑
due to abnormality
    chromosomal Q99.9
        sex
            female phenotype Q97.9
            male phenotype Q98.9
        specified NEC Q99.8
dumping (postgastrectomy) K91.1
    nonsurgical K31.89
Dupré's (meningism) R29.1
dysmetabolic X E88.81
dyspraxia, developmental F82
Eagle-Barrett Q79.4
Eaton-Lambert — *see* Syndrome, Lambert-Eaton
Ebstein's Q22.5
ectopic ACTH E24.3
eczema-thrombocytopenia D82.0
Eddowes' Q78.0
effort (psychogenic) F45.8
Ehlers-Danlos Q79.6
Eisenmenger's I27.83
Ekman's Q78.0
electric feet E53.8
Ellis-van Creveld Q77.6
empty nest Z60.0
endocrine-hypertensive E27.0
entrapment — *see* Neuropathy, entrapment
eosinophilia-myalgia M35.8
epileptic (*see also* Epilepsy, by type)
    absence G40.A09 (*following* G40.3)
        intractable G40.A19 (*following* G40.3)
            with status epilepticus G40.A11 (*following*
                G40.3)
            without status epilepticus G40.A19 (*following*
                G40.3)
        not intractable G40.A09 (*following* G40.3)
            with status epilepticus G40.A01 (*following*
                G40.3)
            without status epilepticus G40.A09 (*following*
                G40.3)
Erdheim-Chester (ECD) E88.89
Erdheim's E22.0
erythrocyte fragmentation D59.4
Evans D69.41
exhaustion F48.8
extrapyramidal G25.9
    specified NEC G25.89
eye retraction — *see* Strabismus
eyelid-malar-mandible Q87.0
Faber's D50.9
facial pain, paroxysmal G50.0
Fallot's Q21.3
familial cold autoinflammatory M04.2
familial eczema-thrombocytopenia (Wiskott-Aldrich)
    D82.0
Fanconi (-de Toni) (-Debré) E72.09
    with cystinosis E72.04
Fanconi's (anemia) (congenital pancytopenia) D61.09
fatigue
    chronic R53.82
    psychogenic F48.8
faulty bowel habit K59.39
Feil-Klippel (brevicollis) Q76.1
Felty's — *see* Felty's syndrome
fertile eunuch E23.0
fetal
    alcohol (dysmorphic) Q86.0
    hydantoin Q86.1
Fiedler's I40.1
first arch Q87.0
fish odor E72.89
Fisher's G61.0
Fitzhugh-Curtis
    due to
        Chlamydia trachomatis A74.81
        Neisseria gonorrhorea (gonococcal peritonitis)
            A54.85
Fitz's (*see also* Pancreatitis, acute) K85.80
Flajani (-Basedow) E05.00
    with thyroid storm E05.01
flatback — *see* Flatback syndrome
floppy
    baby P94.2
    iris (intraoeprative) (IFIS) H21.81
    mitral valve I34.1
flush E34.0

Syndrome — *continued*

Foix-Alajouanine G95.19
Fong's Q87.2
food protein-induced enterocolitis (FPIES) K52.21
foramen magnum G93.5
Foster-Kennedy H47.14- ☑
Foville's (peduncular) G46.3
fragile X Q99.2
Franceschetti Q75.4
Frey's
    auriculotemporal G50.8
    hyperhidrosis L74.52
Friderichsen-Waterhouse A39.1
Froin's G95.89
frontal lobe F07.0
Fukuhara E88.49
functional
    bowel K59.9
    prepubertal castrate E29.1
Gaisböck's D75.1
ganglion (basal ganglia brain) G25.9
    geniculi G51.1
Gardner-Diamond D69.2
gastroesophageal
    junction K22.0
    laceration-hemorrhage K22.6
gastrojejunal loop obstruction K91.89
Gee-Herter-Heubner K90.0
Gelineau's G47.419
    with cataplexy G47.411
genito-anorectal A55
Gerstmann-Sträussler-Scheinker (GSS) A81.82
Gianotti-Crosti L44.4
giant platelet (Bernard-Soulier) D69.1
Gilles de la Tourette's F95.2
goiter-deafness E07.1
Goldberg Q89.8
Goldberg-Maxwell E34.51
Good's D83.8
Gopalan' (burning feet) E53.8
Gorlin's Q87.89
Gougerot-Blum L81.7
Gouley's I31.1
Gower's R55
gray or grey (newborn) P93.0
    platelet D69.1
Gubler-Millard G46.3
Guillain-Barré (-Strohl) G61.0
gustatory sweating G50.8
Hadfield-Clarke K86.89
hair tourniquet — *see* Constriction, external, by site
Hamman's J98.19
hand-foot L27.1
hand-shoulder G90.8
hantavirus (cardio)-pulmonary (HPS) (HCPS) B33.4
happy puppet Q93.51
Harada's H30.81- ☑
Hayem-Faber D50.9
Hegglin's D72.0
HELLP (hemolysis, elevated liver enzymes and low
    platelet count) O14.2- ☑
    complicating
        childbirth O14.24
        puerperium O14.25
hemolytic-uremic D59.3
hemophagocytic, infection-associated D76.2
Henoch-Schönlein D69.0
hepatic flexure K59.8
hepatopulmonary K76.81
hepatorenal K76.7
    following delivery O90.4
    postoperative or postprocedural K91.83
    postpartum, puerperal O90.4
hepatourologic K76.7
Herter (-Gee) (nontropical sprue) K90.0
Heubner-Herter K90.0
Heyd's K76.7
Hilger's G90.09
histamine-like (fish poisoning) — *see* Poisoning, fish
histiocytic D76.3
histiocytosis NEC D76.3
HIV infection, acute B20
Hoffmann-Werdnig G12.0
Hollander-Simons E88.1
Hoppe-Goldflam G70.00

300   ☑ **Additional Character Required** — Refer to the Tabular List for Character Selection   ▽ **Subterms under main terms may continue to next column or page**

Syndrome — Syndrome

Syndrome — *continued*
  Hoppe-Goldflam — *continued*
    with exacerbation (acute) G70.01
      in crisis G70.01
  Horner's G90.2
  hungry bone E83.81
  hunterian glossitis D51.0
  Hutchinson's triad A50.53
  hyperabduction G54.0
  hyperammonemia-hyperornithinemia-homocitrulline-
    mia E72.4
  hypereosinophilic (idiopathic) D72.1
  hyperimmunoglobulin D M04.1
  hyperimmunoglobulin E (IgE) D82.4
  hyperkalemic E87.5
  hyperkinetic — *see* Hyperkinesia
  hypermobility M35.7
  hypernatremia E87.0
  hyperosmolarity E87.0
  hyperperfusion G97.82
  hypersplenic D73.1
  hypertransfusion, newborn P61.1
  hyperventilation F45.8
  hyperviscosity (of serum)
    polycythemic D75.1
    sclerothymic D58.8
  hypoglycemic (familial) (neonatal) E16.2
  hypokalemic E87.6
  hyponatremic E87.1
  hypopituitarism E23.0
  hypoplastic left-heart Q23.4
  hypopotassemia E87.6
  hyposmolality E87.1
  hypotension, maternal O26.5- ☑
  hypothenar hammer I73.89
  hypoventilation, obesity (OHS) E66.2
  ICF (intravascular coagulation-fibrinolysis) D65
  idiopathic
    cardiorespiratory distress, newborn P22.0
    nephrotic (infantile) N04.9
  iliotibial band M76.3- ☑
  immobility, immobilization (paraplegic) M62.3
  immune reconstitution D89.3
  immune reconstitution inflammatory [IRIS] D89.3
  immunity deficiency, combined D81.9
  immunodeficiency
    acquired — *see* Human, immunodeficiency virus
      (HIV) disease
    combined D81.9
  impending coronary I20.0
  impingement, shoulder M75.4- ☑
  inappropriate secretion of antidiuretic hormone E22.2
  infant
    gestational diabetes P70.0
    of diabetic mother P70.1
  infantilism (pituitary) E23.0
  inferior vena cava I87.1
  inspissated bile (newborn) P59.1
  institutional (childhood) F94.2
  insufficient sleep F51.12
  intermediate coronary (artery) I20.0
  interspinous ligament — *see* Spondylopathy, specified
    NEC
  intestinal
    carcinoid E34.0
    knot K56.2
  intravascular coagulation-fibrinolysis (ICF) D65
  iodine-deficiency, congenital E00.9
    type
      mixed E00.2
      myxedematous E00.1
      neurological E00.0
  IRDS (idiopathic respiratory distress, newborn) P22.0
  irritable
    bowel K58.9
      with
        constipation K58.1
        diarrhea K58.0
      mixed K58.2
      psychogenic F45.8
      specified NEC K58.8
    heart (psychogenic) F45.8
    weakness F48.8
  ischemic
    bowel (transient) K55.9
      chronic K55.1
      due to mesenteric artery insufficiency K55.1
    steal T82.898 ☑

Syndrome — *continued*
  IVC (intravascular coagulopathy) D65
  Ivemark's Q89.01
  Jaccoud's — *see* Arthropathy, postrheumatic, chronic
  Jackson's G83.89
  Jakob-Creutzfeldt — *see* Creutzfeldt-Jakob disease or
    syndrome
  jaw-winking Q07.8
  Jervell-Lange-Nielsen I45.81
  jet lag G47.25
  Job's D71
  Joseph-Diamond-Blackfan D61.01
  jugular foramen G52.7
  Kabuki Q89.8
  Kanner's (autism) F84.0
  Kartagener's Q89.3
  Kelly's D50.1
  Kimmelsteil-Wilson — *see* Diabetes, specified type,
    with Kimmelsteil-Wilson disease
  Klein (e)-Levine G47.13
  Klippel-Feil (brevicollis) Q76.1
  Köhler-Pellegrini-Steida — *see* Bursitis, tibial collateral
  König's K59.8
  Korsakoff (-Wernicke) (nonalcoholic) F04
    alcoholic F10.26
  Kostmann's D70.0
  Krabbe's congenital muscle hypoplasia Q79.8
  labyrinthine — *see* subcategory H83.2 ☑
  lacunar NEC G46.7
  Lambert-Eaton G70.80
    in
      neoplastic disease G73.1
      specified disease NEC G70.81
  Landau-Kleffner — *see* Epilepsy, specified NEC
  Larsen's Q74.8
  lateral
    cutaneous nerve of thigh G57.1- ☑
    medullary G46.4
  Launois' E22.0
  lazy
    leukocyte D70.8
    posture M62.3
  Lemiere I80.8
  Lennox-Gastaut G40.812
    intractable G40.814
      with status epilepticus G40.813
      without status epilepticus G40.814
    not intractable G40.812
      with status epilepticus G40.811
      without status epilepticus G40.812
  lenticular, progressive E83.01
  Leopold-Levi's E05.90
  Lev's I44.2
  Lichtheim's D51.0
  Li-Fraumeni Z15.01
  Lightwood's N25.89
  Lignac (de Toni) (-Fanconi) (-Debré) E72.09
    with cystinosis E72.04
  Likoff's I20.8
  limbic epilepsy personality F07.0
  liver-kidney K76.7
  lobotomy F07.0
  Loffler's J82
  long arm 18 or 21 deletion Q93.89
  long QT I45.81
  Louis-Barré G11.3
  low
    atmospheric pressure T70.29 ☑
    back M54.5
    output (cardiac) I50.9
  lower radicular, newborn (birth injury) P14.8
  Luetscher's (dehydration) E86.0
  Lupus anticoagulant D68.62
  Lutembacher's Q21.1
  macrophage activation D76.1
    due to infection D76.2
  magnesium-deficiency R29.0
  Majeed M04.8
  Mal de Debarquement R42
  malabsorption K90.9
    postsurgical K91.2
  malformation, congenital, due to
    alcohol Q86.0
    exogenous cause NEC Q86.8
    hydantoin Q86.1
    warfarin Q86.2
  malignant
    carcinoid E34.0

Syndrome — *continued*
  malignant — *continued*
    neuroleptic G21.0
  Mallory-Weiss K22.6
  mandibulofacial dysostosis Q75.4
  manic-depressive — *see* Disorder, bipolar
  maple-syrup-urine E71.0
  Marable's I77.4
  Marfan's Q87.40
    with
      cardiovascular manifestations Q87.418
        aortic dilation Q87.410
      ocular manifestations Q87.42
      skeletal manifestations Q87.43
  Marie's (acromegaly) E22.0
  mast cell activation — *see* Activation, mast cell
  maternal hypotension — *see* Syndrome, hypotension,
    maternal
  May (-Hegglin) D72.0
  McArdle (-Schmidt) (-Pearson) E74.04
  McQuarrie's E16.2
  meconium plug (newborn) P76.0
  median arcuate ligament I77.4
  Meekeren-Ehlers-Danlos Q79.6
  megavitamin-B6 E67.2
  Meige G24.4
  MELAS E88.41
  Mendelson's O74.0
  MERRF (myoclonic epilepsy associated with ragged-
    red fibers) E88.42
  mesenteric
    artery (superior) K55.1
    vascular insufficiency K55.1
  metabolic E88.81
  metastatic carcinoid E34.0
  micrognathia-glossoptosis Q87.0
  midbrain NEC G93.89
  middle lobe (lung) J98.19
  middle radicular G54.0
  migraine (*see also* Migraine) G43.909
  Mikulicz' K11.8
  milk-alkali E83.52
  Millard-Gubler G46.3
  Miller-Dieker Q93.88
  Miller-Fisher G61.0
  Minkowski-Chauffard D58.0
  Mirizzi's K83.1
  MNGIE (Mitochondrial Neurogastrointestinal En-
    cephalopathy) E88.49
  Möbius, ophthalmoplegic migraine — *see* Migraine,
    ophthalmoplegic
  monofixation H50.42
  Morel-Moore M85.2
  Morel-Morgagni M85.2
  Morgagni (-Morel) (-Stewart) M85.2
  Morgagni-Adams-Stokes I45.9
  Mounier-Kuhn Q32.4
    with bronchiectasis J47.9
      with
        exacerbation (acute) J47.1
        lower respiratory infection J47.0
    acquired J98.09
      with bronchiectasis J47.9
        with
          exacerbation (acute) J47.1
          lower respiratory infection J47.0
  Muckle-Wells M04.2
  mucocutaneous lymph node (acute febrile) (MCLS)
    M30.3
  multiple endocrine neoplasia (MEN) — *see* Neoplasia,
    endocrine, multiple (MEN)
  multiple operations — *see* Disorder, factitious
  myasthenic G70.9
    in
      diabetes mellitus — *see* Diabetes, amyotrophy
      endocrine disease NEC E34.9 [G73.3]
      neoplastic disease (*see also* Neoplasm)
        D49.9 [G73.3]
      thyrotoxicosis (hyperthyroidism) E05.90 [G73.3]
        with thyroid storm E05.91 [G73.3]
  myelodysplastic D46.9
    with
      5q deletion D46.C (*following* D46.2)
      isolated del (5q) chromosomal abnormality D46.C
        (*following* D46.2)
    lesions, low grade D46.20
    specified NEC D46.Z (*following* D46.4)
  myelopathic pain G89.0

Syndrome — *continued*

myeloproliferative (chronic) D47.1
myofascial pain M79.18
Naffziger's G54.0
nail patella Q87.2
NARP (Neuropathy, Ataxia and Retinitis pigmentosa) E88.49
neonatal abstinence P96.1
nephritic (*see also* Nephritis)
  with edema — *see* Nephrosis
  acute N00.9
  chronic N03.9
  rapidly progressive N01.9
nephrotic (congenital) (*see also* Nephrosis) N04.9
  with
    dense deposit disease N04.6
    diffuse
      crescentic glomerulonephritis N04.7
      endocapillary proliferative glomerulonephritis N04.4
      membranous glomerulonephritis N04.2
      mesangial proliferative glomerulonephritis N04.3
      mesangiocapillary glomerulonephritis N04.5
    focal and segmental glomerular lesions N04.1
    minor glomerular abnormality N04.0
    specified morphological changes NEC N04.8
  diabetic — *see* Diabetes, nephrosis
neurologic neglect R41.4
Nezelof's D81.4
Nonne-Milroy-Meige Q82.0
Nothnagel's vasomotor acroparesthesia I73.89
obesity hypoventilation (OHS) E66.2
oculomotor H51.9
ophthalmoplegia-cerebellar ataxia — *see* Strabismus, paralytic, third nerve
oral allergy T78.1 ☑
oral-facial-digital Q87.0
organic
  affective F06.30
  amnesic (not alcohol- or drug-induced) F04
  brain F09
  depressive F06.31
  hallucinosis F06.0
  personality F07.0
Ormond's N13.5
oro-facial-digital Q87.0
os trigonum Q68.8
Osler-Weber-Rendu I78.0
osteoporosis-osteomalacia M83.8
Osterreicher-Turner Q87.2
otolith — *see* subcategory H81.8 ☑
oto-palatal-digital Q87.0
outlet (thoracic) G54.0
ovary
  polycystic E28.2
  resistant E28.39
  sclerocystic E28.2
Owren's D68.2
Paget-Schroetter I82.890
pain (*see also* Pain)
  complex regional I G90.50
    lower limb G90.52- ☑
    specified site NEC G90.59
    upper limb G90.51- ☑
  complex regional II — *see* Causalgia
painful
  bruising D69.2
  feet E53.8
  prostate N42.81
paralysis agitans — *see* Parkinsonism
paralytic G83.9
  specified NEC G83.89
Parinaud's H51.0
parkinsonian — *see* Parkinsonism
Parkinson's — *see* Parkinsonism
paroxysmal facial pain G50.0
Parry's E05.00
  with thyroid storm E05.01
Parsonage (-Aldren)-Turner G54.5
patella clunk M25.86- ☑
Paterson (-Brown) (-Kelly) D50.1
pectoral girdle I77.89
pectoralis minor I77.89
pediatric autoimmune neuropsychiatric disorders associated with streptococcal infections (PANDAS) D89.89
Pelger-Huet D72.0

Syndrome — *continued*

pellagra-cerebellar ataxia-renal aminoaciduria E72.02
pellagroid E52
Pellegrini-Stieda — *see* Bursitis, tibial collateral
pelvic congestion-fibrosis, female N94.89
penta X Q97.1
peptic ulcer — *see* Ulcer, peptic
perabduction I77.89
periodic fever M04.1
periodic fever, aphthous stomatitis, pharyngitis, and adenopathy [PFAPA] M04.8
periodic headache, in adults and children — *see* Headache, periodic syndromes in adults and children
periurethral fibrosis N13.5
phantom limb (without pain) G54.7
  with pain G54.6
pharyngeal pouch D82.1
Pick's — *see* Disease, Pick's
Pickwickian E66.2
PIE (pulmonary infiltration with eosinophilia) J82
pigmentary pallidal degeneration (progressive) G23.0
pineal E34.8
pituitary E22.0
placental transfusion — *see* Pregnancy, complicated by, placental transfusion syndromes
plantar fascia M72.2
plateau iris (post-iridectomy) (postprocedural) H21.82
Plummer-Vinson D50.1
pluricarential of infancy E40
plurideficiency E40
pluriglandular (compensatory) E31.8
  autoimmune E31.0
pneumatic hammer T75.21 ☑
polyangiitis overlap M30.8
polycarential of infancy E40
polyglandular E31.8
  autoimmune E31.0
polysplenia Q89.09
pontine NEC G93.89
popliteal
  artery entrapment I77.89
  web Q87.89
post chemoembolization — *code to* associated conditions
postcardiac injury
  postcardiotomy I97.0
  postmyocardial infarction I24.1
postcardiotomy I97.0
postcholecystectomy K91.5
postcommissurotomy I97.0
postconcussional F07.81
postcontusional F07.81
postencephalitic F07.89
posterior
  cervical sympathetic M53.0
  cord G83.83
  fossa compression G93.5
  reversible encephalopathy (PRES) I67.83
postgastrectomy (dumping) K91.1
postgastric surgery K91.1
postinfarction I24.1
postlaminectomy NEC M96.1
postleukotomy F07.0
postmastectomy lymphedema I97.2
postmyocardial infarction I24.1
postoperative NEC T81.9 ☑
  blind loop K90.2
postpartum panhypopituitary (Sheehan) E23.0
postpolio (myelitic) G14
postthrombotic I87.009
  with
    inflammation I87.02- ☑
      with ulcer I87.03- ☑
    specified complication NEC I87.09- ☑
    ulcer I87.01- ☑
      with inflammation I87.03- ☑
  asymptomatic I87.00- ☑
postvagotomy K91.1
postvalvulotomy I97.0
postviral NEC G93.3
  fatigue G93.3
Potain's K31.0
potassium intoxication E87.5
precerebral artery (multiple) (bilateral) G45.2
preinfarction I20.0
preleukemic D46.9
premature senility E34.8

Syndrome — *continued*

premenstrual dysphoric F32.89
premenstrual tension N94.3
Prinzmetal-Massumi R07.1
prune belly Q79.4
pseudo -Turner's Q87.1
pseudocarpal tunnel (sublimis) — *see* Syndrome, carpal tunnel
pseudoparalytica G70.00
  with exacerbation (acute) G70.01
  in crisis G70.01
psycho-organic (nonpsychotic severity) F07.9
  acute or subacute F05
  depressive type F06.31
  hallucinatory type F06.0
  nonpsychotic severity F07.0
  specified NEC F07.89
pulmonary
  arteriosclerosis I27.0
  dysmaturity (Wilson-Mikity) P27.0
  hypoperfusion (idiopathic) P22.0
  renal (hemorrhagic) (Goodpasture's) M31.0
pure
  motor lacunar G46.5
  sensory lacunar G46.6
Putnam-Dana D51.0
pyogenic arthritis, pyoderma gangrenosum, and acne [PAPA] M04.8
pyramidopallidonigral G20
pyriformis — *see* Lesion, nerve, sciatic
QT interval prolongation I45.81
radicular NEC — *see* Radiculopathy
  upper limbs, newborn (birth injury) P14.3
rapid time-zone change G47.25
Rasmussen G04.81
Raymond (-Céstan) I65.8
Raynaud's I73.00
  with gangrene I73.01
RDS (respiratory distress syndrome, newborn) P22.0
reactive airways dysfunction J68.3
Refsum's G60.1
Reifenstein E34.52
renal glomerulohyalinosis-diabetic — *see* Diabetes, nephrosis
Rendu-Osler-Weber I78.0
residual ovary N99.83
resistant ovary E28.39
respiratory
  distress
    acute J80
      adult J80
      child J80
      idiopathic J84.114
    newborn (idiopathic) (type I) P22.0
      type II P22.1
restless legs G25.81
retinoblastoma (familial) C69.2 ☑
retroperitoneal fibrosis N13.5
retroviral seroconversion (acute) Z21
Reye's G93.7
Richter — *see* Leukemia, chronic lymphocytic, B-cell type
Ridley's I50.1
right
  heart, hypoplastic Q22.6
  ventricular obstruction — *see* Failure, heart, congestive
Romano-Ward (prolonged QT interval) I45.81
rotator cuff, shoulder (*see also* Tear, rotator cuff) M75.10- ☑
Rotes Quérol — *see* Hyperostosis, ankylosing
Roth — *see* Meralgia paresthetica
rubella (congenital) P35.0
Ruvalcaba-Myhre-Smith E71.440
Rytand-Lipsitch I44.2
salt
  depletion E87.1
    due to heat NEC T67.8 ☑
      causing heat exhaustion or prostration T67.4 ☑
  low E87.1
salt-losing N28.89
Scaglietti-Dagnini E22.0
scalenus anticus (anterior) G54.0
scapulocostal — *see* Mononeuropathy, upper limb, specified site NEC
scapuloperoneal G71.09
schizophrenic, of childhood NEC F84.5

☑ **Additional Character Required** — Refer to the Tabular List for Character Selection   Subterms under main terms may continue to next column or page

Syndrome — *continued*

Schnitzler D47.2
Scholte's E34.0
Schroeder's E27.0
Schüller-Christian C96.5
Schwachman's — *see* Syndrome, Shwachman's
Schwartz (-Jampel) G71.13
Schwartz-Bartter E22.2
scimitar Q26.8
sclerocystic ovary E28.2
Seitelberger's G31.89
septicemic adrenal hemorrhage A39.1
seroconversion, retroviral (acute) Z21
serous meningitis G93.2
severe acute respiratory (SARS) J12.81
shaken infant T74.4 ☑
shock (traumatic) T79.4 ☑
    kidney N17.0
       following crush injury T79.5 ☑
    toxic A48.3
shock-lung J80
Shone's — *code to* specific anomalies
short
    bowel K91.2
    rib Q77.2
shoulder-hand — *see* Algoneurodystrophy
Shwachman's D70.4
sicca — *see* Sicca syndrome
sick
    cell E87.1
    sinus I49.5
sick-euthyroid E07.81
sideropenic D50.1
Siemens' ectodermal dysplasia Q82.4
Silfversköld's Q78.9
Simons' E88.1
sinus tarsi M25.57- ☑
sinusitis-bronchiectasis-situs inversus Q89.3
Sipple's E31.22
sirenomelia Q87.2
Slocumb's E27.0
slow flow, coronary I20.8
Sluder's G44.89
Smith-Magenis Q93.88
Sneddon-Wilkinson L13.1
Sotos' Q87.3
South African cardiomyopathy I42.8
spasmodic
    upward movement, eyes H51.8
    winking F95.8
Spen's I45.9
splenic
    agenesis Q89.01
    flexure K59.8
    neutropenia D73.81
Spurway's Q78.0
staphylococcal scalded skin L00
steal
    arteriovenous T82.898- ☑
    ischemic T82.898- ☑
    subclavian G45.8
Stein-Leventhal E28.2
Stein's E28.2
Stevens-Johnson syndrome L51.1
    toxic epidermal necrolysis overlap L51.3
Stewart-Morel M85.2
Stickler Q89.8
stiff baby Q89.8
stiff man G25.82
Still-Felty — *see* Felty's syndrome
Stokes (-Adams) I45.9
stone heart I50.1
straight back, congenital Q76.49
subclavian steal G45.8
subcoracoid-pectoralis minor G54.0
subcostal nerve compression I77.89
subphrenic interposition Q43.3
superior
    cerebellar artery I63.89
    mesenteric artery K55.1
    semi-circular canal dehiscence H83.8X- ☑
    vena cava I87.1
supine hypotensive (maternal) — *see* Syndrome, hypotension, maternal
suprarenal cortical E27.0
supraspinatus (*see also* Tear, rotator cuff) M75.10- ☑
Susac G93.49
swallowed blood P78.2

Syndrome — *continued*

sweat retention L74.0
Swyer Q99.1
Symond's G93.2
sympathetic
    cervical paralysis G90.2
    pelvic, female N94.89
systemic inflammatory response (SIRS), of non-infectious origin (without organ dysfunction) R65.10
    with acute organ dysfunction R65.11
tachycardia-bradycardia I49.5
takotsubo I51.81
TAR (thrombocytopenia with absent radius) Q87.2
tarsal tunnel G57.5- ☑
teething K00.7
tegmental G93.89
telangiectasic-pigmentation-cataract Q82.8
temporal pyramidal apex — *see* Otitis, media, suppurative, acute
temporomandibular joint-pain-dysfunction M26.62- ☑
Terry's (*see also* Myopia, degenerative) H44.2- ☑
testicular feminization (*see also* Syndrome, androgen insensitivity) E34.51
thalamic pain (hyperesthetic) G89.0
thoracic outlet (compression) G54.0
Thorson-Björck E34.0
thrombocytopenia with absent radius (TAR) Q87.2
thyroid-adrenocortical insufficiency E31.0
tibial
    anterior M76.81- ☑
    posterior M76.82- ☑
Tietze's M94.0
time-zone (rapid) G47.25
Toni-Fanconi E72.09
    with cystinosis E72.04
Touraine's Q79.8
tourniquet — *see* Constriction, external, by site
toxic shock A48.3
transient left ventricular apical ballooning I51.81
traumatic vasospastic T75.22 ☑
Treacher Collins Q75.4
triple X, female Q97.0
trisomy Q92.9
    13 Q91.7
       meiotic nondisjunction Q91.4
       mitotic nondisjunction Q91.5
       mosaicism Q91.5
       translocation Q91.6
    18 Q91.3
       meiotic nondisjunction Q91.0
       mitotic nondisjunction Q91.1
       mosaicism Q91.1
       translocation Q91.2
    20 (q)(p) Q92.8
    21 Q90.9
       meiotic nondisjunction Q90.0
       mitotic nondisjunction Q90.1
       mosaicism Q90.1
       translocation Q90.2
    22 Q92.8
tropical wet feet T69.0- ☑
Trousseau's I82.1
tumor lysis (following antineoplastic chemotherapy) (spontaneous) NEC E88.3
tumor necrosis factor receptor associated periodic (TRAPS) M04.1
Twiddler's (due to)
    automatic implantable defibrillator T82.198 ☑
    cardiac pacemaker T82.198 ☑
Unverricht (-Lundborg) — *see* Epilepsy, generalized, idiopathic
upward gaze H51.8
uremia, chronic (*see also* Disease, kidney, chronic) N18.9
urethral N34.3
urethro-oculo-articular — *see* Reiter's disease
urohepatic K76.7
vago-hypoglossal G52.7
van Buchem's M85.2
van der Hoeve's Q78.0
vascular NEC in cerebrovascular disease G46.8
vasoconstriction, reversible cerebrovascular I67.841
vasomotor I73.9
vasospastic (traumatic) T75.22 ☑
vasovagal R55
VATER Q87.2
velo-cardio-facial Q93.81
vena cava (inferior) (superior) (obstruction) I87.1

Syndrome — *continued*

vertebral
    artery G45.0
       compression — *see* Syndrome, anterior, spinal artery, compression
    steal G45.0
vertebro-basilar artery G45.0
vertebrogenic (pain) M54.89
vertiginous — *see* Disorder, vestibular function
Vinson-Plummer D50.1
virus B34.9
visceral larva migrans B83.0
visual disorientation H53.8
vitamin B6 deficiency E53.1
vitreal corneal H59.01- ☑
vitreous (touch) H59.01- ☑
Vogt-Koyanagi H20.82- ☑
Volkmann's T79.6 ☑
von Schroetter's I82.890
von Willebrand (-Jürgen) D68.0
Waldenström-Kjellberg D50.1
Wallenberg's G46.3
water retention E87.79
Waterhouse (-Friderichsen) A39.1
Weber-Gubler G46.3
Weber-Leyden G46.3
Weber's G46.3
Wegener's M31.30
    with
       kidney involvement M31.31
       lung involvement M31.30
        with kidney involvement M31.31
Weingarten's (tropical eosinophilia) J82
Weiss-Baker G90.09
Werdnig-Hoffman G12.0
Wermer's E31.21
Werner's E34.8
Wernicke-Korsakoff (nonalcoholic) F04
    alcoholic F10.26
Westphal-Strümpell E83.01
West's — *see* Epilepsy, spasms
wet
    feet (maceration) (tropical) T69.0- ☑
    lung, newborn P22.1
whiplash S13.4 ☑
whistling face Q87.0
Wilkie's K55.1
Wilkinson-Sneddon L13.1
Willebrand (-Jürgens) D68.0
Williams Q93.82
Wilson's (hepatolenticular degeneration) E83.01
Wiskott-Aldrich D82.0
withdrawal — *see* Withdrawal, state
    drug
       infant of dependent mother P96.1
       therapeutic use, newborn P96.2
Woakes' (ethmoiditis) J33.1
Wright's (hyperabduction) G54.0
X I20.9
XXXX Q97.1
XXXXX Q97.1
XXXXY Q98.1
XXY Q98.0
Yao M04.8
yellow nail L60.5
Zahorsky's B08.5
Zellweger syndrome E71.510
Zellweger-like syndrome E71.541

Synechia (anterior) (iris) (posterior) (pupil) (*see also* Adhesions, iris)
    intra-uterine (traumatic) N85.6
Synesthesia R20.8
Syngamiasis, syngamosis B83.3
Synodontia K00.2
Synorchidism, synorchism Q55.1
Synostosis (congenital) Q78.8
    astragalo-scaphoid Q74.2
    radioulnar Q74.0
Synovial sarcoma — *see* Neoplasm, connective tissue, malignant
Synovioma (malignant) (*see also* Neoplasm, connective tissue, malignant)
    benign — *see* Neoplasm, connective tissue, benign
Synoviosarcoma — *see* Neoplasm, connective tissue, malignant
Synovitis (*see also* Tenosynovitis) M65.9
    crepitant
       hand M70.0- ☑

Synovitis — *continued*
  crepitant — *continued*
    wrist M70.03- ☑
  gonococcal A54.49
  gouty — *see* Gout
  in (due to)
    crystals M65.8- ☑
    gonorrhea A54.49
    syphilis (late) A52.78
    use, overuse, pressure — *see* Disorder, soft tissue, due to use
  infective NEC — *see* Tenosynovitis, infective NEC
  specified NEC — *see* Tenosynovitis, specified type NEC
  syphilitic A52.78
    congenital (early) A50.02
  toxic — *see* Synovitis, transient
  transient M67.3- ☑
    ankle M67.37- ☑
    elbow M67.32- ☑
    foot joint M67.37- ☑
    hand joint M67.34- ☑
    hip M67.35- ☑
    knee M67.36- ☑
    multiple site M67.39
    pelvic region M67.35- ☑
    shoulder M67.31- ☑
    specified joint NEC M67.38
    wrist M67.33- ☑
  traumatic, current — *see* Sprain
  tuberculous — *see* Tuberculosis, synovitis
  villonodular (pigmented) M12.2- ☑
    ankle M12.27- ☑
    elbow M12.22- ☑
    foot joint M12.27- ☑
    hand joint M12.24- ☑
    hip M12.25- ☑
    knee M12.26- ☑
    multiple site M12.29
    pelvic region M12.25- ☑
    shoulder M12.21- ☑
    specified joint NEC M12.28
    vertebrae M12.28
    wrist M12.23- ☑
Syphilid A51.39
  congenital A50.06
  newborn A50.06
  tubercular (late) A52.79
Syphilis, syphilitic (acquired) A53.9
  abdomen (late) A52.79
  acoustic nerve A52.15
  adenopathy (secondary) A51.49
  adrenal (gland) (with cortical hypofunction) A52.79
  age under 2 years NOS (*see also* Syphilis, congenital, early)
    acquired A51.9
  alopecia (secondary) A51.32
  anemia (late) A52.79 [D63.8]
  aneurysm (aorta) (ruptured) A52.01
    central nervous system A52.05
    congenital A50.54 [I79.0]
  anus (late) A52.74
    primary A51.1
    secondary A51.39
  aorta (arch) (abdominal) (thoracic) A52.02
    aneurysm A52.01
  aortic (insufficiency) (regurgitation) (stenosis) A52.03
    aneurysm A52.01
  arachnoid (adhesive) (cerebral) (spinal) A52.13
  asymptomatic — *see* Syphilis, latent
  ataxia (locomotor) A52.11
  atrophoderma maculatum A51.39
  auricular fibrillation A52.06
  bladder (late) A52.76
  bone A52.77
    secondary A51.46
  brain A52.17
  breast (late) A52.79
  bronchus (late) A52.72
  bubo (primary) A51.0
  bulbar palsy A52.19
  bursa (late) A52.78
  cardiac decompensation A52.06
  cardiovascular A52.00
  central nervous system (late) (recurrent) (relapse) (tertiary) A52.3
    with
      ataxia A52.11
      general paralysis A52.17

Syphilis, syphilitic — *continued*
  central nervous system — *continued*
    with — *continued*
      general paralysis — *continued*
        juvenile A50.45
      paresis (general) A52.17
        juvenile A50.45
      tabes (dorsalis) A52.11
        juvenile A50.45
      taboparesis A52.17
        juvenile A50.45
    aneurysm A52.05
    congenital A50.40
    juvenile A50.40
    remission in (sustained) A52.3
    serology doubtful, negative, or positive A52.3
    specified nature or site NEC A52.19
    vascular A52.05
  cerebral A52.17
    meningovascular A52.13
    nerves (multiple palsies) A52.15
    sclerosis A52.17
    thrombosis A52.05
  cerebrospinal (tabetic type) A52.12
  cerebrovascular A52.05
  cervix (late) A52.76
  chancre (multiple) A51.0
    extragenital A51.2
    Rollet's A51.0
  Charcot's joint A52.16
  chorioretinitis A51.43
    congenital A50.01
    late A52.71
    prenatal A50.01
  choroiditis — *see* Syphilitic chorioretinitis
  choroidoretinitis — *see* Syphilitic chorioretinitis
  ciliary body (secondary) A51.43
    late A52.71
  colon (late) A52.74
  combined spinal sclerosis A52.11
  condyloma (latum) A51.31
  congenital A50.9
    with
      paresis (general) A50.45
      tabes (dorsalis) A50.45
      taboparesis A50.45
    chorioretinitis, choroiditis A50.01 [H32]
    early, or less than 2 years after birth NEC A50.2
      with manifestations — *see* Syphilis, congenital, early, symptomatic
      latent (without manifestations) A50.1
        negative spinal fluid test A50.1
        serology positive A50.1
      symptomatic A50.09
        cutaneous A50.06
        mucocutaneous A50.07
        oculopathy A50.01
        osteochondropathy A50.02
        pharyngitis A50.03
        pneumonia A50.04
        rhinitis A50.05
        visceral A50.08
    interstitial keratitis A50.31
    juvenile neurosyphilis A50.45
    late, or 2 years or more after birth NEC A50.7
      chorioretinitis, choroiditis A50.32
      interstitial keratitis A50.31
      juvenile neurosyphilis A50.45
      latent (without manifestations) A50.6
        negative spinal fluid test A50.6
        serology positive A50.6
      symptomatic or with manifestations NEC A50.59
        arthropathy A50.55
        cardiovascular A50.54
        Clutton's joints A50.51
        Hutchinson's teeth A50.52
        Hutchinson's triad A50.53
        osteochondropathy A50.56
        saddle nose A50.57
  conjugal A53.9
    tabes A52.11
  conjunctiva (late) A52.71
  contact Z20.2
  cord bladder A52.19
  cornea, late A52.71
  coronary (artery) (sclerosis) A52.06
  coryza, congenital A50.05
  cranial nerve A52.15
    multiple palsies A52.15

Syphilis, syphilitic — *continued*
  cutaneous — *see* Syphilis, skin
  dacryocystitis (late) A52.71
  degeneration, spinal cord A52.12
  dementia paralytica A52.17
    juvenilis A50.45
  destruction of bone A52.77
  dilatation, aorta A52.01
  due to blood transfusion A53.9
  dura mater A52.13
  ear A52.79
    inner A52.79
      nerve (eighth) A52.15
      neurorecurrence A52.15
  early A51.9
    cardiovascular A52.00
    central nervous system A52.3
    latent (without manifestations) (less than 2 years after infection) A51.5
      negative spinal fluid test A51.5
      serological relapse after treatment A51.5
      serology positive A51.5
    relapse (treated, untreated) A51.9
    skin A51.39
    symptomatic A51.9
      extragenital chancre A51.2
      primary, except extragenital chancre A51.0
      secondary (*see also* Syphilis, secondary) A51.39
        relapse (treated, untreated) A51.49
    ulcer A51.39
  eighth nerve (neuritis) A52.15
  endemic A65
  endocarditis A52.03
    aortic A52.03
    pulmonary A52.03
  epididymis (late) A52.76
  epiglottis (late) A52.73
  epiphysitis (congenital) (early) A50.02
  episcleritis (late) A52.71
  esophagus A52.79
  eustachian tube A52.73
  exposure to Z20.2
  eye A52.71
  eyelid (late) (with gumma) A52.71
  fallopian tube (late) A52.76
  fracture A52.77
  gallbladder (late) A52.74
  gastric (polyposis) (late) A52.74
  general A53.9
    paralysis A52.17
      juvenile A50.45
  genital (primary) A51.0
  glaucoma A52.71
  gumma NEC A52.79
    cardiovascular system A52.00
    central nervous system A52.3
    congenital A50.59
  heart (block) (decompensation) (disease) (failure) A52.06 [I52]
    valve NEC A52.03
  hemianesthesia A52.19
  hemianopsia A52.71
  hemiparesis A52.17
  hemiplegia A52.17
  hepatic artery A52.09
  hepatis A52.74
  hepatomegaly, congenital A50.08
  hereditaria tarda — *see* Syphilis, congenital, late
  hereditary — *see* Syphilis, congenital
  Hutchinson's teeth A50.52
  hyalitis A52.71
  inactive — *see* Syphilis, latent
  infantum — *see* Syphilis, congenital
  inherited — *see* Syphilis, congenital
  internal ear A52.79
  intestine (late) A52.74
  iris, iritis (secondary) A51.43
    late A52.71
  joint (late) A52.77
  keratitis (congenital) (interstitial) (late) A50.31
  kidney (late) A52.75
  lacrimal passages (late) A52.71
  larynx (late) A52.73
  late A52.9
    cardiovascular A52.00
    central nervous system A52.3
    kidney A52.75

☑ Additional Character Required — Refer to the Tabular List for Character Selection   ▽ Subterms under main terms may continue to next column or page

Syphilis, syphilitic — continued
  late — continued
    latent or 2 years or more after infection (without
      manifestations) A52.8
      negative spinal fluid test A52.8
      serology positive A52.8
    paresis A52.17
    specified site NEC A52.79
    symptomatic or with manifestations A52.79
    tabes A52.11
  latent A53.0
    with signs or symptoms — code by site and stage
      under Syphilis
    central nervous system A52.2
    date of infection unspecified A53.0
    early, or less than 2 years after infection A51.5
    follow-up of latent syphilis A53.0
      date of infection unspecified A53.0
      late, or 2 years or more after infection A52.8
    late, or 2 years or more after infection A52.8
    positive serology (only finding) A53.0
      date of infection unspecified A53.0
      early, or less than 2 years after infection A51.5
      late, or 2 years or more after infection A52.8
  lens (late) A52.71
  leukoderma A51.39
    late A52.79
  lienitis A52.79
  lip A51.39
    chancre (primary) A51.2
    late A52.79
  Lissauer's paralysis A52.17
  liver A52.74
  locomotor ataxia A52.11
  lung A52.72
  lymph gland (early) (secondary) A51.49
    late A52.79
  lymphadenitis (secondary) A51.49
  macular atrophy of skin A51.39
    striated A52.79
  mediastinum (late) A52.73
  meninges (adhesive) (brain) (spinal cord) A52.13
  meningitis A52.13
    acute (secondary) A51.41
    congenital A50.41
  meningoencephalitis A52.14
  meningovascular A52.13
    congenital A50.41
  mesarteritis A52.09
    brain A52.04
  middle ear A52.77
  mitral stenosis A52.03
  monoplegia A52.17
  mouth (secondary) A51.39
    late A52.79
  mucocutaneous (secondary) A51.39
    late A52.79
  mucous
    membrane (secondary) A51.39
      late A52.79
    patches A51.39
      congenital A50.07
  mulberry molars A50.52
  muscle A52.78
  myocardium A52.06
  nasal sinus (late) A52.73
  neonatorum — see Syphilis, congenital
  nephrotic syndrome (secondary) A51.44
  nerve palsy (any cranial nerve) A52.15
    multiple A52.15
  nervous system, central A52.3
  neuritis A52.15
    acoustic A52.15
  neurorecidive of retina A52.19
  neuroretinitis A52.19
  newborn — see Syphilis, congenital
  nodular superficial (late) A52.79
  nonvenereal A65
  nose (late) A52.73
    saddle back deformity A50.57
  occlusive arterial disease A52.09
  oculopathy A52.71
  ophthalmic (late) A52.71
  optic nerve (atrophy) (neuritis) (papilla) A52.15
  orbit (late) A52.71

Syphilis, syphilitic — continued
  organic A53.9
  osseous (late) A52.77
  osteochondritis (congenital) (early) A50.02 [M90.80]
  osteoporosis A52.77
  ovary (late) A52.76
  oviduct (late) A52.76
  palate (late) A52.79
  pancreas (late) A52.74
  paralysis A52.17
    general A52.17
      juvenile A50.45
  paresis (general) A52.17
    juvenile A50.45
  paresthesia A52.19
  Parkinson's disease or syndrome A52.19
  paroxysmal tachycardia A52.06
  pemphigus (congenital) A50.06
  penis (chancre) A51.0
    late A52.76
  pericardium A52.06
  perichondritis, larynx (late) A52.73
  periosteum (late) A52.77
    congenital (early) A50.02 [M90.80]
    early (secondary) A51.46
  peripheral nerve A52.79
  petrous bone (late) A52.77
  pharynx (late) A52.73
    secondary A51.39
  pituitary (gland) A52.79
  pleura (late) A52.73
  pneumonia, white A50.04
  pontine lesion A52.17
  portal vein A52.09
  primary A51.0
    anal A51.1
    and secondary — see Syphilis, secondary
    central nervous system A52.3
    extragenital chancre NEC A51.2
    fingers A51.2
    genital A51.0
    lip A51.2
    specified site NEC A51.2
    tonsils A51.2
  prostate (late) A52.76
  ptosis (eyelid) A52.71
  pulmonary (late) A52.72
    artery A52.09
  pyelonephritis (late) A52.75
  recently acquired, symptomatic A51.9
  rectum (late) A52.74
  respiratory tract (late) A52.73
  retina, late A52.71
  retrobulbar neuritis A52.15
  salpingitis A52.76
  sclera (late) A52.71
  sclerosis
    cerebral A52.17
    coronary A52.06
    multiple A52.11
  scotoma (central) A52.71
  scrotum (late) A52.76
  secondary (and primary) A51.49
    adenopathy A51.49
    anus A51.39
    bone A51.46
    chorioretinitis, choroiditis A51.43
    hepatitis A51.45
    liver A51.45
    lymphadenitis A51.49
    meningitis (acute) A51.41
    mouth A51.39
    mucous membranes A51.39
    periosteum, periostitis A51.46
    pharynx A51.39
    relapse (treated, untreated) A51.49
    skin A51.39
    specified form NEC A51.49
    tonsil A51.39
    ulcer A51.39
    viscera NEC A51.49
    vulva A51.39
  seminal vesicle (late) A52.76
  seronegative with signs or symptoms — code by site
    and stage under Syphilis

Syphilis, syphilitic — continued
  seropositive
    with signs or symptoms — code by site and stage
      under Syphilis
    follow-up of latent syphilis — see Syphilis, latent
    only finding — see Syphilis, latent
  seventh nerve (paralysis) A52.15
  sinus, sinusitis (late) A52.73
  skeletal system A52.77
  skin (with ulceration) (early) (secondary) A51.39
    late or tertiary A52.79
  small intestine A52.74
  spastic spinal paralysis A52.17
  spermatic cord (late) A52.76
  spinal (cord) A52.12
  spleen A52.79
  splenomegaly A52.79
  spondylitis A52.77
  staphyloma A52.71
  stigmata (congenital) A50.59
  stomach A52.74
  synovium A52.78
  tabes dorsalis (late) A52.11
    juvenile A50.45
  tabetic type A52.11
    juvenile A50.45
  taboparesis A52.17
    juvenile A50.45
  tachycardia A52.06
  tendon (late) A52.78
  tertiary A52.9
    with symptoms NEC A52.79
    cardiovascular A52.00
    central nervous system A52.3
    multiple NEC A52.79
    specified site NEC A52.79
  testis A52.76
  thorax A52.73
  throat A52.73
  thymus (gland) (late) A52.79
  thyroid (late) A52.79
  tongue (late) A52.79
  tonsil (lingual) (late) A52.73
    primary A51.2
    secondary A51.39
  trachea (late) A52.73
  tunica vaginalis (late) A52.76
  ulcer (any site) (early) (secondary) A51.39
    late A52.79
    perforating A52.79
      foot A52.11
  urethra (late) A52.76
  urogenital (late) A52.76
  uterus (late) A52.76
  uveal tract (secondary) A51.43
    late A52.71
  uveitis (secondary) A51.43
    late A52.71
  uvula (late) (perforated) A52.79
  vagina A51.0
    late A52.76
  valvulitis NEC A52.03
  vascular A52.00
    brain (cerebral) A52.05
  ventriculi A52.74
  vesicae urinariae (late) A52.76
  viscera (abdominal) (late) A52.74
    secondary A51.49
  vitreous (opacities) (late) A52.71
    hemorrhage A52.71
  vulva A51.0
    late A52.76
    secondary A51.39
Syphiloma A52.79
  cardiovascular system A52.00
  central nervous system A52.3
  circulatory system A52.00
  congenital A50.59
Syphilophobia F45.29
Syringadenoma (see also Neoplasm, skin, benign)
  papillary — see Neoplasm, skin, benign
Syringobulbia G95.0

Index

Syringocystadenoma — *see* Neoplasm, skin, benign
   papillary — *see* Neoplasm, skin, benign
Syringoma (*see also* Neoplasm, skin, benign)
   chondroid — *see* Neoplasm, skin, benign

Syringomyelia G95.0
Syringomyelitis — *see* Encephalitis
Syringomyelocele — *see* Spina bifida
Syringopontia G95.0

System, systemic (*see also* condition)
   disease, combined — *see* Degeneration, combined
   inflammatory response syndrome (SIRS) of non-infec-
     tious origin (without organ dysfunction) R65.10
   lupus erythematosus M32.9
     with acute organ dysfunction R65.11
     inhibitor present D68.62

☑ **Additional Character Required** — **Refer to the Tabular List for Character Selection**

▽ **Subterms under main terms may continue to next column or page**

Syringocystadenoma — System, systemic

T

Tabacism, tabacosis, tabagism (*see also* Poisoning, tobacco)
  meaning dependence (without remission) F17.200
    with
      disorder F17.299
        in remission F17.211
          specified disorder NEC F17.298
        withdrawal F17.203
Tabardillo A75.9
  flea-borne A75.2
  louse-borne A75.0
Tabes, tabetic A52.10
  with
    central nervous system syphilis A52.10
    Charcot's joint A52.16
    cord bladder A52.19
    crisis, viscera (any) A52.19
    paralysis, general A52.17
    paresis (general) A52.17
    perforating ulcer (foot) A52.19
  arthropathy (Charcot) A52.16
  bladder A52.19
  bone A52.11
  cerebrospinal A52.12
  congenital A50.45
  conjugal A52.10
  dorsalis A52.11
    juvenile A50.49
  juvenile A50.49
  latent A52.19
  mesenterica A18.39
  paralysis, insane, general A52.17
  spasmodic A52.17
  syphilis (cerebrospinal) A52.12
Taboparalysis A52.17
Taboparesis (remission) A52.17
  juvenile A50.45
TAC (trigeminal autonomic cephalgia) **NEC** G44.099
  intractable G44.091
  not intractable G44.099
Tache noir S60.22- ☑
Tachyalimentation K91.2
Tachyarrhythmia, tachyrhythmia — *see* Tachycardia
Tachycardia R00.0
  atrial (paroxysmal) I47.1
  auricular I47.1
  AV nodal re-entry (re-entrant) I47.1
  junctional (paroxysmal) I47.1
  newborn P29.11
  nodal (paroxysmal) I47.1
  non-paroxysmal AV nodal I45.89
  paroxysmal (sustained) (nonsustained) I47.9
    with sinus bradycardia I49.5
    atrial (PAT) I47.1
    atrioventricular (AV) (re-entrant) I47.1
      psychogenic F54
    junctional I47.1
      ectopic I47.1
    nodal I47.1
    psychogenic (atrial) (supraventricular) (ventricular) F54
    supraventricular (sustained) I47.1
      psychogenic F54
    ventricular I47.2
      psychogenic F54
  psychogenic F45.8
  sick sinus I49.5
  sinoauricular NOS R00.0
    paroxysmal I47.1
  sinus [sinusal] NOS R00.0
    paroxysmal I47.1
  supraventricular I47.1
  ventricular (paroxysmal) (sustained) I47.2
    psychogenic F54
Tachygastria K31.89
Tachypnea R06.82
  hysterical F45.8
  newborn (idiopathic) (transitory) P22.1
  psychogenic F45.8
  transitory, of newborn P22.1
TACO (transfusion associated circulatory overload) E87.71
Taenia (infection) (infestation) B68.9
  diminuta B71.0
  echinococcal infestation B67.90
  mediocanellata B68.1

Taenia — *continued*
  nana B71.0
  saginata B68.1
  solium (intestinal form) B68.0
    larval form — *see* Cysticercosis
Taeniasis (intestine) — *see* Taenia
Tag (hypertrophied skin) (infected) L91.8
  adenoid J35.8
  anus K64.4
  hemorrhoidal K64.4
  hymen N89.8
  perineal N90.89
  preauricular Q17.0
  sentinel K64.4
  skin L91.8
    accessory (congenital) Q82.8
    anus K64.4
    congenital Q82.8
    preauricular Q17.0
  tonsil J35.8
  urethra, urethral N36.8
  vulva N90.89
Tahyna fever B33.8
Takahara's disease E80.3
Takayasu's disease or syndrome M31.4
Talcosis (pulmonary) J62.0
Talipes (congenital) Q66.89
  acquired, planus — *see* Deformity, limb, flat foot
  asymmetric Q66.89
  calcaneovalgus Q66.4
  calcaneovarus Q66.1
  calcaneus Q66.89
  cavus Q66.7
  equinovalgus Q66.6
  equinovarus Q66.0
  equinus Q66.89
  percavus Q66.7
  planovalgus Q66.6
  planus (acquired) (any degree) (*see also* Deformity, limb, flat foot)
    congenital Q66.5- ☑
    due to rickets (sequelae) E64.3
  valgus Q66.6
  varus Q66.3
Tall stature, constitutional E34.4
Talma's disease M62.89
Talon noir S90.3- ☑
  hand S60.22- ☑
  heel S90.3- ☑
  toe S90.1- ☑
Tamponade, heart I31.4
Tanapox (virus disease) B08.71
Tangier disease E78.6
Tantrum, child problem F91.8
Tapeworm (infection) (infestation) — *see* Infestation, tapeworm
Tapia's syndrome G52.7
TAR (thrombocytopenia with absent radius) **syndrome** Q87.2
Tarral-Besnier disease L44.0
Tarsal tunnel syndrome — *see* Syndrome, tarsal tunnel
Tarsalgia — *see* Pain, limb, lower
Tarsitis (eyelid) H01.8
  syphilitic A52.71
  tuberculous A18.4
Tartar (teeth) (dental calculus) K03.6
Tattoo (mark) L81.8
Tauri's disease E74.09
Taurodontism K00.2
Taussig-Bing syndrome Q20.1
Taybi's syndrome Q87.2
Tay-Sachs amaurotic familial idiocy or disease E75.02
TBI (traumatic brain injury) S06.9 ☑
Teacher's node or nodule J38.2
Tear, torn (traumatic) (*see also* Laceration)
  with abortion — *see* Abortion
  annular fibrosis M51.35
  anus, anal (sphincter) S31.831 ☑
    complicating delivery
      with third degree perineal laceration (*see also* Delivery, complicated, by, laceration, perineum, third degree) O70.20
        with mucosa O70.3
      without third degree perineal laceration O70.4
    nontraumatic (healed) (old) K62.81
  articular cartilage, old — *see* Derangement, joint, articular cartilage, by site

Tear, torn — *continued*
  bladder
    with ectopic or molar pregnancy O08.6
    following ectopic or molar pregnancy O08.6
    obstetrical O71.5
    traumatic — *see* Injury, bladder
  bowel
    with ectopic or molar pregnancy O08.6
    following ectopic or molar pregnancy O08.6
    obstetrical trauma O71.5
  broad ligament
    with ectopic or molar pregnancy O08.6
    following ectopic or molar pregnancy O08.6
    obstetrical trauma O71.6
  bucket handle (knee) (meniscus) — *see* Tear, meniscus
  capsule, joint — *see* Sprain
  cartilage (*see also* Sprain)
    articular, old — *see* Derangement, joint, articular cartilage, by site
  cervix
    with ectopic or molar pregnancy O08.6
    following ectopic or molar pregnancy O08.6
    obstetrical trauma (current) O71.3
    old N88.1
    traumatic — *see* Injury, uterus
  dural G97.41
    nontraumatic G96.11
  internal organ — *see* Injury, by site
  knee cartilage
    articular (current) S83.3- ☑
    old — *see* Derangement, knee, meniscus, due to old tear
  ligament — *see* Sprain
  meniscus (knee) (current injury) S83.209 ☑
    bucket-handle S83.20- ☑
    lateral
      bucket-handle S83.25- ☑
      complex S83.27- ☑
      peripheral S83.26- ☑
      specified type NEC S83.28- ☑
    medial
      bucket-handle S83.21- ☑
      complex S83.23- ☑
      peripheral S83.22- ☑
      specified type NEC S83.24- ☑
    old — *see* Derangement, knee, meniscus, due to old tear
    site other than knee — *code as* Sprain
    specified type NEC S83.20- ☑
  muscle — *see* Strain
  pelvic
    floor, complicating delivery O70.1
    organ NEC, obstetrical trauma O71.5
      with ectopic or molar pregnancy O08.6
      following ectopic or molar pregnancy O08.6
  perineal, secondary O90.1
  periurethral tissue, obstetrical trauma O71.82
    with ectopic or molar pregnancy O08.6
    following ectopic or molar pregnancy O08.6
  rectovaginal septum — *see* Laceration, vagina
  retina, retinal (without detachment) (horseshoe) (*see also* Break, retina, horseshoe)
    with detachment — *see* Detachment, retina, with retinal, break
  rotator cuff (nontraumatic) M75.10- ☑
    complete M75.12- ☑
    incomplete M75.11- ☑
    traumatic S46.01- ☑
      capsule S43.42- ☑
  semilunar cartilage, knee — *see* Tear, meniscus
  supraspinatus (complete) (incomplete) (nontraumatic) (*see also* Tear, rotator cuff) M75.10- ☑
  tendon — *see* Strain
  tentorial, at birth P10.4
  umbilical cord
    complicating delivery O69.89 ☑
  urethra
    with ectopic or molar pregnancy O08.6
    following ectopic or molar pregnancy O08.6
    obstetrical trauma O71.5
  uterus — *see* Injury, uterus
  vagina — *see* Laceration, vagina
  vessel, from catheter — *see* Puncture, accidental complicating surgery
  vulva, complicating delivery O70.0
Tear-stone — *see* Dacryolith
Teeth (*see also* condition)

Teeth — *continued*
  grinding
    psychogenic F45.8
    sleep related G47.63
Teething (syndrome) K00.7
Telangiectasia, telangiectasis (verrucous) I78.1
  ataxic (cerebellar) (Louis-Bar) G11.3
  familial I78.0
  hemorrhagic, hereditary (congenital) (senile) I78.0
  hereditary, hemorrhagic (congenital) (senile) I78.0
  juxtafoveal H35.07- ☑
  macular H35.07- ☑
  macularis eruptiva perstans D47.01
  parafoveal H35.07- ☑
  retinal (idiopathic) (juxtafoveal) (macular) (parafoveal) H35.07- ☑
  spider I78.1
Telephone scatologia F65.89
Telescoped bowel or intestine K56.1
  congenital Q43.8
Temperature
  body, high (of unknown origin) R50.9
  cold, trauma from T69.9 ☑
    newborn P80.0
    specified effect NEC T69.8 ☑
Temple — *see* condition
Temporal — *see* condition
Temporomandibular joint pain-dysfunction syndrome M26.62- ☑
Temporosphenoidal — *see* condition
Tendency
  bleeding — *see* Defect, coagulation
  suicide
    meaning personal history of attempted suicide Z91.5
    meaning suicidal ideation — *see* Ideation, suicidal
  to fall R29.6
Tenderness, abdominal R10.819
  epigastric R10.816
  generalized R10.817
  left lower quadrant R10.814
  left upper quadrant R10.812
  periumbilic R10.815
  rebound R10.829
    epigastric R10.826
    generalized R10.827
    left lower quadrant R10.824
    left upper quadrant R10.822
    periumbilic R10.825
    right lower quadrant R10.823
    right upper quadrant R10.821
  right lower quadrant R10.813
  right upper quadrant R10.811
Tendinitis, tendonitis (*see also* Enthesopathy)
  Achilles M76.6- ☑
  adhesive — *see* Tenosynovitis, specified type NEC
    shoulder — *see* Capsulitis, adhesive
  bicipital M75.2- ☑
  calcific M65.2- ☑
    ankle M65.27- ☑
    foot M65.27- ☑
    forearm M65.23- ☑
    hand M65.24- ☑
    lower leg M65.26- ☑
    multiple sites M65.29
    pelvic region M65.25- ☑
    shoulder M75.3- ☑
    specified site NEC M65.28
    thigh M65.25- ☑
    upper arm M65.22- ☑
  due to use, overuse, pressure (*see also* Disorder, soft tissue, due to use)
    specified NEC — *see* Disorder, soft tissue, due to use, specified NEC
  gluteal M76.0- ☑
  patellar M76.5- ☑
  peroneal M76.7- ☑
  psoas M76.1- ☑
  tibial (posterior) M76.82- ☑
    anterior M76.81- ☑
  trochanteric — *see* Bursitis, hip, trochanteric
Tendon — *see* condition
Tendosynovitis — *see* Tenosynovitis
Tenesmus (rectal) R19.8
  vesical R30.1
Tennis elbow — *see* Epicondylitis, lateral
Tenonitis (*see also* Tenosynovitis)
  eye (capsule) H05.04- ☑

Tenontosynovitis — *see* Tenosynovitis
Tenontothecitis — *see* Tenosynovitis
Tenophyte — *see* Disorder, synovium, specified type NEC
Tenosynovitis (*see also* Synovitis) M65.9
  adhesive — *see* Tenosynovitis, specified type NEC
    shoulder — *see* Capsulitis, adhesive
  bicipital (calcifying) — *see* Tendinitis, bicipital
  gonococcal A54.49
  in (due to)
    crystals M65.8- ☑
    gonorrhea A54.49
    syphilis (late) A52.78
    use, overuse, pressure (*see also* Disorder, soft tissue, due to use)
      specified NEC — *see* Disorder, soft tissue, due to use, specified NEC
  infective NEC M65.1- ☑
    ankle M65.17- ☑
    foot M65.17- ☑
    forearm M65.13- ☑
    hand M65.14- ☑
    lower leg M65.16- ☑
    multiple sites M65.19
    pelvic region M65.15- ☑
    shoulder region M65.11- ☑
    specified site NEC M65.18
    thigh M65.15- ☑
    upper arm M65.12- ☑
  radial styloid M65.4
  shoulder region M65.81- ☑
    adhesive — *see* Capsulitis, adhesive
  specified type NEC M65.88
    ankle M65.87- ☑
    foot M65.87- ☑
    forearm M65.83- ☑
    hand M65.84- ☑
    lower leg M65.86- ☑
    multiple sites M65.89
    pelvic region M65.85- ☑
    shoulder region M65.81- ☑
    specified site NEC M65.88
    thigh M65.85- ☑
    upper arm M65.82- ☑
  tuberculous — *see* Tuberculosis, tenosynovitis
Tenovaginitis — *see* Tenosynovitis
Tension
  arterial, high (*see also* Hypertension)
    without diagnosis of hypertension R03.0
  headache G44.209
    intractable G44.201
    not intractable G44.209
  nervous R45.0
  pneumothorax J93.0
  premenstrual N94.3
  state (mental) F48.9
Tentorium — *see* condition
Teratencephalus Q89.8
Teratism Q89.7
Teratoblastoma (malignant) — *see* Neoplasm, malignant, by site
Teratocarcinoma (*see also* Neoplasm, malignant, by site)
  liver C22.7
Teratoma (solid) (*see also* Neoplasm, uncertain behavior, by site)
  with embryonal carcinoma, mixed — *see* Neoplasm, malignant, by site
  with malignant transformation — *see* Neoplasm, malignant, by site
  adult (cystic) — *see* Neoplasm, benign, by site
  benign — *see* Neoplasm, benign, by site
  combined with choriocarcinoma — *see* Neoplasm, malignant, by site
  cystic (adult) — *see* Neoplasm, benign, by site
  differentiated — *see* Neoplasm, benign, by site
  embryonal (*see also* Neoplasm, malignant, by site)
    liver C22.7
  immature — *see* Neoplasm, malignant, by site
  liver C22.7
    adult, benign, cystic, differentiated type or mature D13.4
  malignant (*see also* Neoplasm, malignant, by site)
    anaplastic — *see* Neoplasm, malignant, by site
    intermediate — *see* Neoplasm, malignant, by site
      specified site — *see* Neoplasm, malignant, by site
    unspecified site C62.90

Teratoma — *continued*
  malignant (*see also* Neoplasm, malignant, by site) — *continued*
    undifferentiated — *see* Neoplasm, malignant, by site
  mature — *see* Neoplasm, uncertain behavior, by site
    malignant — *see* Neoplasm, by site, malignant, by site
  ovary D27.- ☑
    embryonal, immature or malignant C56- ☑
  solid — *see* Neoplasm, uncertain behavior, by site
  testis C62.9- ☑
    adult, benign, cystic, differentiated type or mature D29.2- ☑
    scrotal C62.1- ☑
    undescended C62.0- ☑
Termination
  anomalous (*see also* Malposition, congenital)
    right pulmonary vein Q26.3
  pregnancy, elective Z33.2
Ternidens diminutus infestation B81.8
Ternidensiasis B81.8
Terror(s) night (child) F51.4
Terrorism, victim of Z65.4
Terry's syndrome (*see also* Myopia, degenerative) H44.2- ☑
Tertiary — *see* condition
Test, tests, testing (for)
  adequacy (for dialysis)
    hemodialysis Z49.31
    peritoneal Z49.32
  blood pressure Z01.30
    abnormal reading — *see* Blood, pressure
  blood typing Z01.83
    Rh typing Z01.83
  blood-alcohol Z04.89
    positive — *see* Findings, abnormal, in blood
  blood-drug Z04.89
    positive — *see* Findings, abnormal, in blood
  cardiac pulse generator (battery) Z45.010
  fertility Z31.41
  genetic
    disease carrier status for procreative management
      female Z31.430
      male Z31.440
    male partner of patient with recurrent pregnancy loss Z31.441
    procreative management NEC
      female Z31.438
      male Z31.448
  hearing Z01.10
    with abnormal findings NEC Z01.118
    infant or child (over 28 days old) Z00.129
      with abnormal findings Z00.121
  HIV (human immunodeficiency virus)
    nonconclusive (in infants) R75
    positive Z21
    seropositive Z21
  immunity status Z01.84
  intelligence NEC Z01.89
  laboratory (as part of a general medical examination) Z00.00
    with abnormal finding Z00.01
    for medicolegal reason NEC Z04.89
  male partner of patient with recurrent pregnancy loss Z31.441
  Mantoux (for tuberculosis) Z11.1
    abnormal result R76.11
  pregnancy, positive first pregnancy — *see* Pregnancy, normal, first
  procreative Z31.49
    fertility Z31.41
  skin, diagnostic
    allergy Z01.82
      special screening examination — *see* Screening, by name of disease
    Mantoux Z11.1
    tuberculin Z11.1
  specified NEC Z01.89
  tuberculin Z11.1
    abnormal result R76.11
  vision Z01.00
    with abnormal findings Z01.01
    infant or child (over 28 days old) Z00.129
      with abnormal findings Z00.121
  Wassermann Z11.3
    positive — *see* Serology for syphilis, positive
Testicle, testicular, testis (*see also* condition)

☑ Additional Character Required — Refer to the Tabular List for Character Selection   ▽ Subterms under main terms may continue to next column or page

Testicle, testicular, testis — *continued*
feminization syndrome (*see also* Syndrome, androgen insensitivity) E34.51
migrans Q55.29
Tetanus, tetanic (cephalic) (convulsions) A35
with
abortion A34
ectopic or molar pregnancy O08.0
following ectopic or molar pregnancy O08.0
inoculation reaction (due to serum) — *see* Complications, vaccination
neonatorum A33
obstetrical A34
puerperal, postpartum, childbirth A34
Tetany (due to) R29.0
alkalosis E87.3
associated with rickets E55.0
convulsions R29.0
hysterical F44.5
functional (hysterical) F44.5
hyperkinetic R29.0
hysterical F44.5
hyperpnea R06.4
hysterical F44.5
psychogenic F45.8
hyperventilation (*see also* Hyperventilation) R06.4
hysterical F44.5
neonatal (without calcium or magnesium deficiency) P71.3
parathyroid (gland) E20.9
parathyroprival E89.2
post- (para)thyroidectomy E89.2
postoperative E89.2
pseudotetany R29.0
psychogenic (conversion reaction) F44.5
Tetralogy of Fallot Q21.3
Tetraplegia (chronic) (*see also* Quadriplegia) G82.50
Thailand hemorrhagic fever A91
Thalassanemia — *see* Thalassemia
Thalassemia (anemia) (disease) D56.9
with other hemoglobinopathy D56.8
alpha (major) (severe) (triple gene defect) D56.0
minor D56.3
silent carrier D56.3
trait D56.3
beta (severe) D56.1
homozygous D56.1
major D56.1
minor D56.3
trait D56.3
delta-beta (homozygous) D56.2
minor D56.3
trait D56.3
dominant D56.8
hemoglobin
C D56.8
E-beta D56.5
intermedia D56.1
major D56.1
minor D56.3
mixed D56.8
sickle-cell — *see* Disease, sickle-cell, thalassemia
specified type NEC D56.8
trait D56.3
variants D56.8
Thanatophoric dwarfism or short stature Q77.1
Thaysen-Gee disease (nontropical sprue) K90.0
Thaysen's disease K90.0
Thecoma D27- ☑
luteinized D27- ☑
malignant C56- ☑
Thelarche, premature E30.8
Thelaziasis B83.8
Thelitis N61.0
puerperal, postpartum or gestational — *see* Infection, nipple
Therapeutic — *see* condition
Therapy
drug, long-term (current) (prophylactic)
agents affecting estrogen receptors and estrogen levels NEC Z79.818
anastrozole (Arimidex) Z79.811
antibiotics Z79.2
short-term use — *omit code*
anticoagulants Z79.01
anti-inflammatory Z79.1
antiplatelet Z79.02
antithrombotics Z79.02

Therapy — *continued*
drug, long-term — *continued*
aromatase inhibitors Z79.811
aspirin Z79.82
birth control pill or patch Z79.3
bisphosphonates Z79.83
contraceptive, oral Z79.3
drug, specified NEC Z79.899
estrogen receptor downregulators Z79.818
Evista Z79.810
exemestane (Aromasin) Z79.811
Fareston Z79.810
fulvestrant (Faslodex) Z79.818
gonadotropin-releasing hormone (GnRH) agonist Z79.818
goserelin acetate (Zoladex) Z79.818
hormone replacement Z79.890
insulin Z79.4
letrozole (Femara) Z79.811
leuprolide acetate (leuprorelin) (Lupron) Z79.818
megestrol acetate (Megace) Z79.818
methadone
for pain management Z79.891
maintenance therapy F11.20
Nolvadex Z79.810
opiate analgesic Z79.891
oral contraceptive Z79.3
raloxifene (Evista) Z79.810
selective estrogen receptor modulators (SERMs) Z79.810
short term — *omit code*
steroids
inhaled Z79.51
systemic Z79.52
tamoxifen (Nolvadex) Z79.810
toremifene (Fareston) Z79.810
Thermic — *see* condition
Thermography (abnormal) (*see also* Abnormal, diagnostic imaging) R93.89
breast R92.8
Thermoplegia T67.0 ☑
Thesaurismosis, glycogen — *see* Disease, glycogen storage
Thiamin deficiency E51.9
specified NEC E51.8
Thiaminic deficiency with beriberi E51.11
Thibierge-Weissenbach syndrome — *see* Sclerosis, systemic
Thickening
bone — *see* Hypertrophy, bone
breast N64.59
endometrium R93.89
epidermal L85.9
specified NEC L85.8
hymen N89.6
larynx J38.7
nail L60.2
congenital Q84.5
periosteal — *see* Hypertrophy, bone
pleura J92.9
with asbestos J92.0
skin R23.4
subepiglottic J38.7
tongue K14.8
valve, heart — *see* Endocarditis
Thigh — *see* condition
Thinning vertebra — *see* Spondylopathy, specified NEC
Thirst, excessive R63.1
due to deprivation of water T73.1 ☑
Thomsen disease G71.12
Thoracic (*see also* condition)
kidney Q63.2
outlet syndrome G54.0
Thoracogastroschisis (congenital) Q79.8
Thoracopagus Q89.4
Thorax — *see* condition
Thorn's syndrome N28.89
Thorson-Björck syndrome E34.0
Threadworm (infection) (infestation) B80
Threatened
abortion O20.0
with subsequent abortion O03.9
job loss, anxiety concerning Z56.2
labor (without delivery) O47.9
at or after 37 completed weeks of gestation O47.1
before 37 completed weeks of gestation O47.0- ☑
loss of job, anxiety concerning Z56.2
miscarriage O20.0

Threatened — *continued*
unemployment, anxiety concerning Z56.2
Three-day fever A93.1
Threshers' lung J67.0
Thrix annulata (congenital) Q84.1
Throat — *see* condition
Thrombasthenia (Glanzmann) (hemorrhagic) (hereditary) D69.1
Thromboangiitis I73.1
obliterans (general) I73.1
cerebral I67.89
vessels
brain I67.89
spinal cord I67.89
Thromboarteritis — *see* Arteritis
Thromboasthenia (Glanzmann) (hemorrhagic) (hereditary) D69.1
Thrombocytasthenia (Glanzmann) D69.1
Thrombocythemia (essential) (hemorrhagic) (idiopathic) (primary) D47.3
Thrombocytopathy (dystrophic) (granulopenic) D69.1
Thrombocytopenia, thrombocytopenic D69.6
with absent radius (TAR) Q87.2
congenital D69.42
dilutional D69.59
due to
(massive) blood transfusion D69.59
drugs D69.59
extracorporeal circulation of blood D69.59
platelet alloimmunization D69.59
essential D69.3
heparin induced (HIT) D75.82
hereditary D69.42
idiopathic D69.3
neonatal, transitory P61.0
due to
exchange transfusion P61.0
idiopathic maternal thrombocytopenia P61.0
isoimmunization P61.0
primary NEC D69.49
idiopathic D69.3
puerperal, postpartum O72.3
secondary D69.59
transient neonatal P61.0
Thrombocytosis, essential D47.3
primary D47.3
Thromboembolism — *see* Embolism
Thrombopathy (Bernard-Soulier) D69.1
constitutional D68.0
Willebrand-Jurgens D68.0
Thrombopenia — *see* Thrombocytopenia
Thrombophilia D68.59
primary NEC D68.59
secondary NEC D68.69
specified NEC D68.69
Thrombophlebitis I80.9
antepartum O22.2- ☑
deep O22.3- ☑
superficial O22.2- ☑
cavernous (venous) sinus G08
complicating pregnancy O22.5- ☑
nonpyogenic I67.6
cerebral (sinus) (vein) G08
nonpyogenic I67.6
sequelae G09
due to implanted device — *see* Complications, by site and type, specified NEC
during or resulting from a procedure NEC T81.72 ☑
femoral vein (superficial) I80.1- ☑
femoropopliteal vein I80.0- ☑
hepatic (vein) I80.8
idiopathic, recurrent I82.1
iliofemoral I80.1- ☑
intracranial venous sinus (any) G08
nonpyogenic I67.6
sequelae G09
intraspinal venous sinuses and veins G08
nonpyogenic G95.19
lateral (venous) sinus G08
nonpyogenic I67.6
leg I80.3
superficial I80.0- ☑
longitudinal (venous) sinus G08
nonpyogenic I67.6
lower extremity I80.299
migrans, migrating I82.1
pelvic
with ectopic or molar pregnancy O08.0

Thrombophlebitis — *continued*
pelvic — *continued*
following ectopic or molar pregnancy O08.0
puerperal O87.1
popliteal vein — *see* Phlebitis, leg, deep, popliteal
portal (vein) K75.1
postoperative T81.72 ☑
pregnancy — *see* Thrombophlebitis, antepartum
puerperal, postpartum, childbirth O87.0
deep O87.1
pelvic O87.1
septic O86.81
superficial O87.0
saphenous (greater) (lesser) I80.0- ☑
sinus (intracranial) G08
nonpyogenic I67.6
specified site NEC I80.8
tibial vein I80.23- ☑

Thrombosis, thrombotic (bland) (multiple) (progressive) (silent) (vessel) I82.90
anal K64.5
antepartum — *see* Thrombophlebitis, antepartum
aorta, aortic I74.10
abdominal I74.09
saddle I74.01
bifurcation I74.09
saddle I74.01
specified site NEC I74.19
terminal I74.09
thoracic I74.11
valve — *see* Endocarditis, aortic
apoplexy I63.3- ☑
artery, arteries (postinfectional) I74.9
auditory, internal — *see* Occlusion, artery, precerebral, specified NEC
basilar — *see* Occlusion, artery, basilar
carotid (common) (internal) — *see* Occlusion, artery, carotid
cerebellar (anterior inferior) (posterior inferior) (superior) — *see* Occlusion, artery, cerebellar
cerebral — *see* Occlusion, artery, cerebral
choroidal (anterior) — *see* Occlusion, artery, precerebral, specified NEC
communicating, posterior — *see* Occlusion, artery, precerebral, specified NEC
coronary (*see also* Infarct, myocardium)
not resulting in infarction I24.0
hepatic I74.8
hypophyseal — *see* Occlusion, artery, precerebral, specified NEC
iliac I74.5
limb I74.4
lower I74.3
upper I74.2
meningeal, anterior or posterior — *see* Occlusion, artery, cerebral, specified NEC
mesenteric (with gangrene) (*see also* Infarct, intestine) K55.069
ophthalmic — *see* Occlusion, artery, retina
pontine — *see* Occlusion, artery, precerebral, specified NEC
precerebral — *see* Occlusion, artery, precerebral
pulmonary (iatrogenic) — *see* Embolism, pulmonary
renal N28.0
retinal — *see* Occlusion, artery, retina
spinal, anterior or posterior G95.11
traumatic NEC T14.8 ☑
vertebral — *see* Occlusion, artery, vertebral
atrium, auricular (*see also* Infarct, myocardium)
following acute myocardial infarction (current complication) I23.6
not resulting in infarction I51.3
old I51.3
basilar (artery) — *see* Occlusion, artery, basilar
brain (artery) (stem) (*see also* Occlusion, artery, cerebral)
due to syphilis A52.05
puerperal O99.43
sinus — *see* Thrombosis, intracranial venous sinus
capillary I78.8
cardiac (*see also* Infarct, myocardium)
not resulting in infarction I51.3
old I51.3
valve — *see* Endocarditis
carotid (artery) (common) (internal) — *see* Occlusion, artery, carotid
cavernous (venous) sinus — *see* Thrombosis, intracranial venous sinus

Thrombosis, thrombotic — *continued*
cerebellar artery (anterior inferior) (posterior inferior) (superior) I66.3
cerebral (artery) — *see* Occlusion, artery, cerebral
cerebrovenous sinus (*see also* Thrombosis, intracranial venous sinus)
puerperium O87.3
chronic I82.91
coronary (artery) (vein) (*see also* Infarct, myocardium)
not resulting in infarction I24.0
corpus cavernosum N48.89
cortical I66.9
deep — *see* Embolism, vein, lower extremity
due to device, implant or graft (*see also* Complications, by site and type, specified NEC) T85.868 ☑
arterial graft NEC T82.868 ☑
breast (implant) T85.868 ☑
catheter NEC T85.868 ☑
dialysis (renal) T82.868 ☑
intraperitoneal T85.868 ☑
infusion NEC T82.868 ☑
spinal (epidural) (subdural) T85.860 ☑
urinary (indwelling) T83.86 ☑
electronic (electrode) (pulse generator) (stimulator)
bone T84.86 ☑
cardiac T82.867 ☑
nervous system (brain) (peripheral nerve) (spinal) T85.860 ☑
urinary T83.86 ☑
fixation, internal (orthopedic) NEC T84.86 ☑
gastrointestinal (bile duct) (esophagus) T85.868 ☑
genital NEC T83.86 ☑
heart T82.867 ☑
joint prosthesis T84.86 ☑
ocular (corneal graft) (orbital implant) NEC T85.868 ☑
orthopedic NEC T84.86 ☑
specified NEC T85.868 ☑
urinary NEC T83.86 ☑
vascular NEC T82.868 ☑
ventricular intracranial shunt T85.860 ☑
during the puerperium — *see* Thrombosis, puerperal
endocardial (*see also* Infarct, myocardium)
not resulting in infarction I51.3
eye — *see* Occlusion, retina
genital organ
female NEC N94.89
pregnancy — *see* Thrombophlebitis, antepartum
male N50.1
gestational — *see* Phlebopathy, gestational
heart (chamber) (*see also* Infarct, myocardium)
not resulting in infarction I51.3
old I51.3
hepatic (vein) I82.0
artery I74.8
history (of) Z86.718
intestine (with gangrene) (*see also* Infarct, intestine) K55.069
intracardiac NEC (apical) (atrial) (auricular) (ventricular) (old) I51.3
intracranial (arterial) I66.9
venous sinus (any) G08
nonpyogenic origin I67.6
puerperium O87.3
intramural (*see also* Infarct, myocardium)
not resulting in infarction I51.3
old I51.3
intraspinal venous sinuses and veins G08
nonpyogenic G95.19
kidney (artery) N28.0
lateral (venous) sinus — *see* Thrombosis, intracranial venous sinus
leg — *see* Thrombosis, vein, lower extremity
arterial I74.3
liver (venous) I82.0
artery I74.8
portal vein I81
longitudinal (venous) sinus — *see* Thrombosis, intracranial venous sinus
lower limb — *see* Thrombosis, vein, lower extremity
lung (iatrogenic) (postoperative) — *see* Embolism, pulmonary
meninges (brain) (arterial) I66.8
mesenteric (artery) (with gangrene) (*see also* Infarct, intestine) K55.069
vein (inferior) (superior) I81
mitral I34.8

Thrombosis, thrombotic — *continued*
mural (*see also* Infarct, myocardium)
due to syphilis A52.06
not resulting in infarction I51.3
old I51.3
omentum (with gangrene) (*see also* Infarct, intestine) K55.069
ophthalmic — *see* Occlusion, retina
pampiniform plexus (male) N50.1
parietal (*see also* Infarct, myocardium)
not resulting in infarction I24.0
penis, superficial vein N48.81
perianal venous K64.5
peripheral arteries I74.4
upper I74.2
personal history (of) Z86.718
portal I81
due to syphilis A52.09
precerebral artery — *see* Occlusion, artery, precerebral
puerperal, postpartum O87.0
brain (artery) O99.43
venous (sinus) O87.3
cardiac O99.43
cerebral (artery) O99.43
venous (sinus) O87.3
superficial O87.0
pulmonary (artery) (iatrogenic) (postoperative) (vein) — *see* Embolism, pulmonary
renal (artery) N28.0
vein I82.3
resulting from presence of device, implant or graft — *see* Complications, by site and type, specified NEC
retina, retinal — *see* Occlusion, retina
scrotum N50.1
seminal vesicle N50.1
sigmoid (venous) sinus — *see* Thrombosis, intracranial venous sinus
sinus, intracranial (any) — *see* Thrombosis, intracranial venous sinus
specified site NEC I82.890
chronic I82.891
spermatic cord N50.1
spinal cord (arterial) G95.11
due to syphilis A52.09
pyogenic origin G06.1
spleen, splenic D73.5
artery I74.8
testis N50.1
traumatic NEC T14.8 ☑
tricuspid I07.8
tumor — *see* Neoplasm, unspecified behavior, by site
tunica vaginalis N50.1
umbilical cord (vessels), complicating delivery O69.5 ☑
vas deferens N50.1
vein (acute) I82.90
antecubital I82.61- ☑
chronic I82.71- ☑
axillary I82.A1- ☑ (*following* I82.7)
chronic I82.A2- ☑ (*following* I82.7)
basilic I82.61- ☑
chronic I82.71- ☑
brachial I82.62- ☑
chronic I82.72- ☑
brachiocephalic (innominate) I82.290
chronic I82.291
cephalic I82.61- ☑
chronic I82.71- ☑
cerebral, nonpyogenic I67.6
chronic I82.91
deep (DVT) I82.40- ☑
calf I82.4Z- ☑
chronic I82.5Z- ☑
lower leg I82.4Z- ☑
chronic I82.5Z- ☑
thigh I82.4Y- ☑
chronic I82.5Y- ☑
upper leg I82.4Y ☑
chronic I82.5Y- ☑
femoral I82.41- ☑
chronic I82.51- ☑
iliac (iliofemoral) I82.42- ☑
chronic I82.52- ☑
innominate I82.290
chronic I82.291
internal jugular I82.C1- ☑ (*following* I82.7)
chronic I82.C2- ☑ (*following* I82.7)

Thrombosis, thrombotic — continued
  vein — continued
    lower extremity
      deep I82.40- ☑
        chronic I82.50- ☑
        specified NEC I82.49- ☑
          chronic NEC I82.59- ☑
      distal
        deep I82.4Z- ☑
      proximal
        deep I82.4Y- ☑
          chronic I82.5Y- ☑
      superficial I82.81- ☑
    perianal K64.5
    popliteal I82.43- ☑
      chronic I82.53- ☑
    radial I82.62- ☑
      chronic I82.72- ☑
    renal I82.3
    saphenous (greater) (lesser) I82.81- ☑
    specified NEC I82.890
      chronic NEC I82.891
    subclavian I82.B1- ☑ (following I82.7)
      chronic I82.B2- ☑ (following I82.7)
    thoracic NEC I82.290
      chronic I82.291
    tibial I82.44- ☑
      chronic I82.54- ☑
    ulnar I82.62- ☑
      chronic I82.72- ☑
    upper extremity I82.60- ☑
      chronic I82.70- ☑
      deep I82.62- ☑
        chronic I82.72- ☑
      superficial I82.61- ☑
        chronic I82.71- ☑
  vena cava
    inferior I82.220
      chronic I82.221
    superior I82.210
      chronic I82.211
  venous, perianal K64.5
  ventricle (see also Infarct, myocardium)
    following acute myocardial infarction (current
      complication) I23.6
    not resulting in infarction I24.0
    old I51.3
Thrombus — see Thrombosis
Thrush (see also Candidiasis)
  newborn P37.5
  oral B37.0
  vaginal B37.3
Thumb (see also condition)
  sucking (child problem) F98.8
Thymitis E32.8
Thymoma (benign) D15.0
  malignant C37
Thymus, thymic (gland) — see condition
Thyrocele — see Goiter
Thyroglossal (see also condition)
  cyst Q89.2
  duct, persistent Q89.2
Thyroid (gland) (body) (see also condition)
  hormone resistance E07.89
  lingual Q89.2
  nodule (cystic) (nontoxic) (single) E04.1
Thyroiditis E06.9
  acute (nonsuppurative) (pyogenic) (suppurative) E06.0
  autoimmune E06.3
  chronic (nonspecific) (sclerosing) E06.5
    with thyrotoxicosis, transient E06.2
    fibrous E06.5
    lymphadenoid E06.3
    lymphocytic E06.3
    lymphoid E06.3
  de Quervain's E06.1
  drug-induced E06.4
  fibrous (chronic) E06.5
  giant-cell (follicular) E06.1
  granulomatous (de Quervain) (subacute) E06.1
  Hashimoto's (struma lymphomatosa) E06.3
  iatrogenic E06.4
  ligneous E06.5
  lymphocytic (chronic) E06.3
  lymphoid E06.3
  lymphomatous E06.3
  nonsuppurative E06.1

Thyroiditis — continued
  postpartum, puerperal O90.5
  pseudotuberculous E06.1
  pyogenic E06.0
  radiation E06.4
  Riedel's E06.5
  subacute (granulomatous) E06.1
  suppurative E06.0
  tuberculous A18.81
  viral E06.1
  woody E06.5
Thyrolingual duct, persistent Q89.2
Thyromegaly E01.0
Thyrotoxic
  crisis — see Thyrotoxicosis
  heart disease or failure (see also Thyrotoxicosis)
    E05.90 [I43]
    with thyroid storm E05.91 [I43]
  storm — see Thyrotoxicosis
Thyrotoxicosis (recurrent) E05.90
  with
    goiter (diffuse) E05.00
      with thyroid storm E05.01
      adenomatous uninodular E05.10
        with thyroid storm E05.11
      multinodular E05.20
        with thyroid storm E05.21
      nodular E05.20
        with thyroid storm E05.21
      uninodular E05.10
        with thyroid storm E05.11
    infiltrative
      dermopathy E05.00
        with thyroid storm E05.01
      ophthalmopathy E05.00
        with thyroid storm E05.01
    single thyroid nodule E05.10
      with thyroid storm E05.11
    thyroid storm E05.91
  due to
    ectopic thyroid nodule or tissue E05.30
      with thyroid storm E05.31
    ingestion of (excessive) thyroid material E05.40
      with thyroid storm E05.41
    overproduction of thyroid-stimulating hormone
      E05.80
      with thyroid storm E05.81
    specified cause NEC E05.80
      with thyroid storm E05.81
  factitia E05.40
    with thyroid storm E05.41
  heart (see also Failure, heart, high-output) E05.90 [I43]
    with thyroid storm (see also Failure, heart, high-
      output) E05.91 [I43]
    failure (see also Failure, heart, high-output)
      E05.90 [I43]
  neonatal (transient) P72.1
  transient with chronic thyroiditis E06.2
Tibia vara — see Osteochondrosis, juvenile, tibia
Tic (disorder) F95.9
  breathing F95.8
  child problem F95.0
  compulsive F95.1
  de la Tourette F95.2
  degenerative (generalized) (localized) G25.69
    facial G25.69
  disorder
    chronic
      motor F95.1
      vocal F95.1
    combined vocal and multiple motor F95.2
    transient F95.0
  douloureux G50.0
    atypical G50.1
    postherpetic, postzoster B02.22
  drug-induced G25.61
  eyelid F95.8
  habit F95.9
    chronic F95.1
    transient of childhood F95.0
  lid, transient of childhood F95.0
  motor-verbal F95.2
  occupational F48.8
  orbicularis F95.8
    transient of childhood F95.0
  organic origin G25.69
  postchoreic G25.69
  provisional F95.0

Tic — continued
  psychogenic, compulsive F95.1
  salaam R25.8
  spasm (motor or vocal) F95.9
    chronic F95.1
    transient of childhood F95.0
  specified NEC F95.8
Tick-borne — see condition
Tietze's disease or syndrome M94.0
Tight, tightness
  anus K62.89
  chest R07.89
  fascia (lata) M62.89
  foreskin (congenital) N47.1
  hymen, hymenal ring N89.6
  introitus (acquired) (congenital) N89.6
  rectal sphincter K62.89
  tendon — see Short, tendon
  urethral sphincter N35.919
Tilting vertebra — see Dorsopathy, deforming, specified
  NEC
Timidity, child F93.8
Tinea (intersecta) (tarsi) B35.9
  amiantacea L44.8
  asbestina B35.0
  barbae B35.0
  beard B35.0
  black dot B35.0
  blanca B36.2
  capitis B35.0
  corporis B35.4
  cruris B35.6
  flava B36.0
  foot B35.3
  furfuracea B36.0
  imbricata (Tokelau) B35.5
  kerion B35.0
  manuum B35.2
  microsporic — see Dermatophytosis
  nigra B36.1
  nodosa — see Piedra
  pedis B35.3
  scalp B35.0
  specified NEC B35.8
  sycosis B35.0
  tonsurans B35.0
  trichophytic — see Dermatophytosis
  unguium B35.1
  versicolor B36.0
Tingling sensation (skin) R20.2
Tin-miner's lung J63.5
Tinnitus NOS H93.1- ☑
  audible H93.1- ☑
  aurium H93.1- ☑
  pulsatile H93.A- ☑
  subjective H93.1- ☑
Tipped tooth (teeth) M26.33
Tipping
  pelvis M95.5
    with disproportion (fetopelvic) O33.0
      causing obstructed labor O65.0
  tooth (teeth), fully erupted M26.33
Tiredness R53.83
Tissue — see condition
Tobacco (nicotine)
  abuse — see Tobacco, use
  dependence — see Dependence, drug, nicotine
  harmful use Z72.0
  heart — see Tobacco, toxic effect
  maternal use, affecting newborn P04.2
  toxic effect — see Table of Drugs and Chemicals, by
    substance, poisoning
    chewing tobacco — see Table of Drugs and Chemi-
      cals, by substance, poisoning
    cigarettes — see Table of Drugs and Chemicals, by
      substance, poisoning
  use Z72.0
    complicating
      childbirth O99.334
      pregnancy O99.33- ☑
      puerperium O99.335
    counseling and surveillance Z71.6
    history Z87.891
    withdrawal state (see also Dependence, drug, nicotine)
      F17.203
Tocopherol deficiency E56.0
Todd's
  cirrhosis K74.3

Todd's — *continued*
  paralysis (postepileptic) (transitory) G83.84
Toe — *see* condition
Toilet, artificial opening — *see* Attention to, artificial, opening
Tokelau (ringworm) B35.5
Tollwut — *see* Rabies
Tommaselli's disease R31.9
  correct substance properly administered — *see* Table of Drugs and Chemicals, by drug, adverse effect
  overdose or wrong substance given or taken — *see* Table of Drugs and Chemicals, by drug, poisoning
Tongue (*see also* condition)
  tie Q38.1
Tonic pupil — *see* Anomaly, pupil, function, tonic pupil
Toni-Fanconi syndrome (cystinosis) E72.09
  with cystinosis E72.04
Tonsil — *see* condition
Tonsillitis (acute) (catarrhal) (croupous) (follicular) (gangrenous) (infective) (lacunar) (lingual) (malignant) (membranous) (parenchymatous) (phlegmonous) (pseudomembranous) (purulent) (septic) (subacute) (suppurative) (toxic) (ulcerative) (vesicular) (viral) J03.90
  chronic J35.01
    with adenoiditis J35.03
  diphtheritic A36.0
  hypertrophic J35.01
    with adenoiditis J35.03
  recurrent J03.91
  specified organism NEC J03.80
    recurrent J03.81
  staphylococcal J03.80
    recurrent J03.81
  streptococcal J03.00
    recurrent J03.01
  tuberculous A15.8
  Vincent's A69.1
Tooth, teeth — *see* condition
Toothache K08.89
Topagnosis R20.8
Tophi — *see* Gout, chronic
TORCH infection — *see* Infection, congenital
  without active infection P00.2
Torn — *see* Tear
Tornwaldt's cyst or disease J39.2
Torsion
  accessory tube — *see* Torsion, fallopian tube
  adnexa (female) — *see* Torsion, fallopian tube
  aorta, acquired I77.1
  appendix epididymis N44.04
  appendix testis N44.03
  bile duct (common) (hepatic) K83.8
    congenital Q44.5
  bowel, colon or intestine K56.2
  cervix — *see* Malposition, uterus
  cystic duct K82.8
  dystonia — *see* Dystonia, torsion
  epididymis (appendix) N44.04
  fallopian tube N83.52- ☑
    with ovary N83.53
  gallbladder K82.8
    congenital Q44.1
  hydatid of Morgagni
    female N83.52- ☑
    male N44.03
  kidney (pedicle) (leading to infarction) N28.0
  Meckel's diverticulum (congenital) Q43.0
    malignant — *see* Table of Neoplasms, small intestine, malignant
  mesentery K56.2
  omentum K56.2
  organ or site, congenital NEC — *see* Anomaly, by site
  ovary (pedicle) N83.51- ☑
    with fallopian tube N83.53
    congenital Q50.2
  oviduct — *see* Torsion, fallopian tube
  penis (acquired) N48.82
    congenital Q55.63
  spasm — *see* Dystonia, torsion
  spermatic cord N44.02
    extravaginal N44.01
    intravaginal N44.02
  spleen D73.5
  testis, testicle N44.00
    appendix N44.03
  tibia — *see* Deformity, limb, specified type NEC, lower leg

Torsion — *continued*
  uterus — *see* Malposition, uterus
Torticollis (intermittent) (spastic) M43.6
  congenital (sternomastoid) Q68.0
  due to birth injury P15.8
  hysterical F44.4
  ocular R29.891
  psychogenic F45.8
    conversion reaction F44.4
  rheumatic M43.6
  rheumatoid M06.88
  spasmodic G24.3
  traumatic, current S13.4 ☑
Tortipelvis G24.1
Tortuous
  aortic arch Q25.46
  artery I77.1
  organ or site, congenital NEC — *see* Distortion
  retinal vessel, congenital Q14.1
  ureter N13.8
  urethra N36.8
  vein — *see* Varix
Torture, victim of Z65.4
Torula, torular (histolytica) (infection) — *see* Cryptococcosis
Torulosis — *see* Cryptococcosis
Torus (mandibularis) (palatinus) M27.0
  fracture — *see* Fracture, by site, torus
Touraine's syndrome Q79.8
Tourette's syndrome F95.2
Tourniquet syndrome — *see* Constriction, external, by site
Tower skull Q75.0
  with exophthalmos Q87.0
Toxemia R68.89
  bacterial — *see* Sepsis
  burn — *see* Burn
  eclamptic (with pre-existing hypertension) — *see* Eclampsia
  erysipelatous — *see* Erysipelas
  fatigue R68.89
  food — *see* Poisoning, food
  gastrointestinal K52.1
  intestinal K52.1
  kidney — *see* Uremia
  malarial — *see* Malaria
  myocardial — *see* Myocarditis, toxic
  of pregnancy — *see* Pre-eclampsia
  pre-eclamptic — *see* Pre-eclampsia
  small intestine K52.1
  staphylococcal, due to food A05.0
  stasis R68.89
  uremic — *see* Uremia
  urinary — *see* Uremia
Toxemica cerebropathia psychica (nonalcoholic) F04
  alcoholic — *see* Alcohol, amnestic disorder
Toxic (poisoning) (*see also* condition) T65.91 ☑
  effect — *see* Table of Drugs and Chemicals, by substance, poisoning
  shock syndrome A48.3
  thyroid (gland) — *see* Thyrotoxicosis
Toxicemia — *see* Toxemia
Toxicity — *see* Table of Drugs and Chemicals, by substance, poisoning
  fava bean D55.0
  food, noxious — *see* Poisoning, food
  from drug or nonmedicinal substance — *see* Table of Drugs and Chemicals, by drug
Toxicosis (*see also* Toxemia)
  capillary, hemorrhagic D69.0
Toxinfection, gastrointestinal K52.1
Toxocariasis B83.0
Toxoplasma, toxoplasmosis (acquired) B58.9
  with
    hepatitis B58.1
    meningoencephalitis B58.2
    ocular involvement B58.00
    other organ involvement B58.89
    pneumonia, pneumonitis B58.3
  congenital (acute) (subacute) (chronic) P37.1
  maternal, manifest toxoplasmosis in infant (acute) (subacute) (chronic) P37.1
tPA (rtPA) **administration in a different facility within the last 24 hours prior to admission to current facility** Z92.82
Trabeculation, bladder N32.89
Trachea — *see* condition

Tracheitis (catarrhal) (infantile) (membranous) (plastic) (septal) (suppurative) (viral) J04.10
  with
    bronchitis (15 years of age and above) J40
      acute or subacute — *see* Bronchitis, acute
      chronic J42
      tuberculous NEC A15.5
      under 15 years of age J20.9
    laryngitis (acute) J04.2
      chronic J37.1
      tuberculous NEC A15.5
  acute J04.10
    with obstruction J04.11
  chronic J42
    with
      bronchitis (chronic) J42
      laryngitis (chronic) J37.1
  diphtheritic (membranous) A36.89
  due to external agent — *see* Inflammation, respiratory, upper, due to
  syphilitic A52.73
  tuberculous A15.5
Trachelitis (nonvenereal) — *see* Cervicitis
Tracheobronchial — *see* condition
Tracheobronchitis (15 years of age and above) (*see also* Bronchitis)
  due to
    Bordetella bronchiseptica A37.80
      with pneumonia A37.81
    Francisella tularensis A21.8
Tracheobronchomegaly Q32.4
  with bronchiectasis J47.9
    with
      exacerbation (acute) J47.1
      lower respiratory infection J47.0
  acquired J98.09
    with bronchiectasis J47.9
      with
        exacerbation (acute) J47.1
        lower respiratory infection J47.0
Tracheobronchopneumonitis — *see* Pneumonia, broncho-
Tracheocele (external) (internal) J39.8
  congenital Q32.1
Tracheomalacia J39.8
  congenital Q32.0
Tracheopharyngitis (acute) J06.9
  chronic J42
  due to external agent — *see* Inflammation, respiratory, upper, due to
Tracheostenosis J39.8
Tracheostomy
  complication — *see* Complication, tracheostomy
  status Z93.0
    attention to Z43.0
    malfunctioning J95.03
Trachoma, trachomatous A71.9
  active (stage) A71.1
  contraction of conjunctiva A71.1
  dubium A71.0
  healed or sequelae B94.0
  initial (stage) A71.0
  pannus A71.1
  Türck's J37.0
Traction, vitreomacular H43.82- ☑
Train sickness T75.3 ☑
Trait(s)
  Hb-S D57.3
  hemoglobin
    abnormal NEC D58.2
      with thalassemia D56.3
    C — *see* Disease, hemoglobin C
    S (Hb-S) D57.3
  Lepore D56.3
  personality, accentuated Z73.1
  sickle-cell D57.3
    with elliptocytosis or spherocytosis D57.3
  type A personality Z73.1
Tramp Z59.0
Trance R41.89
  hysterical F44.89
Transaminasemia R74.0
Transection
  abdomen (partial) S38.3 ☑
  aorta (incomplete) (*see also* Injury, aorta)
    complete — *see* Injury, aorta, laceration, major
  carotid artery (incomplete) (*see also* Injury, blood vessel, carotid, laceration)

Transection — *continued*
  carotid artery (*see also* Injury, blood vessel, carotid, laceration) — *continued*
    complete — *see* Injury, blood vessel, carotid, laceration, major
  celiac artery (incomplete) S35.211 ☑
    branch (incomplete) S35.291 ☑
      complete S35.292 ☑
    complete S35.212 ☑
  innominate
    artery (incomplete) (*see also* Injury, blood vessel, thoracic, innominate, artery, laceration)
      complete — *see* Injury, blood vessel, thoracic, innominate, artery, laceration, major
    vein (incomplete) (*see also* Injury, blood vessel, thoracic, innominate, vein, laceration)
      complete — *see* Injury, blood vessel, thoracic, innominate, vein, laceration, major
  jugular vein (external) (incomplete) (*see also* Injury, blood vessel, jugular vein, laceration)
    complete — *see* Injury, blood vessel, jugular vein, laceration, major
    internal (incomplete) (*see also* Injury, blood vessel, jugular vein, internal, laceration)
      complete — *see* Injury, blood vessel, jugular vein, internal, laceration, major
  mesenteric artery (incomplete) (*see also* Injury, mesenteric, artery, laceration)
    complete — *see* Injury, mesenteric artery, laceration, major
  pulmonary vessel (incomplete) (*see also* Injury, blood vessel, thoracic, pulmonary, laceration)
    complete — *see* Injury, blood vessel, thoracic, pulmonary, laceration, major
  subclavian — *see* Transection, innominate
  vena cava (incomplete) (*see also* Injury, vena cava)
    complete — *see* Injury, vena cava, laceration, major
  vertebral artery (incomplete) (*see also* Injury, blood vessel, vertebral, laceration)
    complete — *see* Injury, blood vessel, vertebral, laceration, major
Transfusion
  associated (red blood cell) hemochromatosis E83.111
  blood
    ABO incompatible — *see* Complication(s), transfusion, incompatibility reaction, ABO
    minor blood group (Duffy) (E) (K) (Kell) (Kidd) (Lewis) (M) (N) (P) (S) T80.89 ☑
    reaction or complication — *see* Complications, transfusion
  fetomaternal (mother) — *see* Pregnancy, complicated by, placenta, transfusion syndrome
  maternofetal (mother) — *see* Pregnancy, complicated by, placenta, transfusion syndrome
  placental (syndrome) (mother) — *see* Pregnancy, complicated by, placenta, transfusion syndrome
  reaction (adverse) — *see* Complications, transfusion
  related acute lung injury (TRALI) J95.84
  twin-to-twin — *see* Pregnancy, complicated by, placenta, transfusion syndrome, fetus to fetus
Transient (meaning homeless) (*see also* condition) Z59.0
Translocation
  balanced autosomal Q95.9
    in normal individual Q95.0
  chromosomes NEC Q99.8
    balanced and insertion in normal individual Q95.0
  Down syndrome Q90.2
  trisomy
    13 Q91.6
    18 Q91.2
    21 Q90.2
Translucency, iris — *see* Degeneration, iris
Transmission of chemical substances through the placenta — *see* Absorption, chemical, through placenta
Transparency, lung, unilateral J43.0
Transplant (ed) (status) Z94.9
  awaiting organ Z76.82
  bone Z94.6
    marrow Z94.81
  candidate Z76.82
  complication — *see* Complication, transplant
  cornea Z94.7
  heart Z94.1
    and lung(s) Z94.3
    valve Z95.2
      prosthetic Z95.2

Transplant — *continued*
  heart — *continued*
    valve — *continued*
      specified NEC Z95.4
      xenogenic Z95.3
  intestine Z94.82
  kidney Z94.0
  liver Z94.4
  lung(s) Z94.2
    and heart Z94.3
  organ (failure) (infection) (rejection) Z94.9
    removal status Z98.85
  pancreas Z94.83
  skin Z94.5
  social Z60.3
  specified organ or tissue NEC Z94.89
  stem cells Z94.84
  tissue Z94.9
Transplants, ovarian, endometrial N80.1
Transposed — *see* Transposition
Transposition (congenital) (*see also* Malposition, congenital)
  abdominal viscera Q89.3
  aorta (dextra) Q20.3
  appendix Q43.8
  colon Q43.8
  corrected Q20.5
  great vessels (complete) (partial) Q20.3
  heart Q24.0
    with complete transposition of viscera Q89.3
  intestine (large) (small) Q43.8
  reversed jejunal (for bypass) (status) Z98.0
  scrotum Q55.23
  stomach Q40.2
    with general transposition of viscera Q89.3
  tooth, teeth, fully erupted M26.30
  vessels, great (complete) (partial) Q20.3
  viscera (abdominal) (thoracic) Q89.3
Transsexualism F64.0
Transverse (*see also* condition)
  arrest (deep), in labor O64.0 ☑
  lie (mother) O32.2 ☑
    causing obstructed labor O64.8 ☑
Transvestism, transvestitism (dual-role) F64.1
  fetishistic F65.1
Trapped placenta (with hemorrhage) O72.0
  without hemorrhage O73.0
TRAPS (tumor necrosis factor receptor associated periodic syndrome) M04.1
Trauma, traumatism (*see also* Injury)
  acoustic — *see* subcategory H83.3 ☑
  birth — *see* Birth, injury
  complicating ectopic or molar pregnancy O08.6
  during delivery O71.9
  following ectopic or molar pregnancy O08.6
  obstetric O71.9
    specified NEC O71.89
  occusal
    primary K08.81
    secondary K08.82
Traumatic (*see also* condition)
  brain injury S06.9 ☑
Treacher Collins syndrome Q75.4
Treitz's hernia — *see* Hernia, abdomen, specified site NEC
Trematode infestation — *see* Infestation, fluke
Trematodiasis — *see* Infestation, fluke
Trembling paralysis — *see* Parkinsonism
Tremor(s) R25.1
  drug induced G25.1
  essential (benign) G25.0
  familial G25.0
  hereditary G25.0
  hysterical F44.4
  intention G25.2
  medication induced postural G25.1
  mercurial — *see* subcategory T56.1 ☑
  Parkinson's — *see* Parkinsonism
  psychogenic (conversion reaction) F44.4
  senilis R54
  specified type NEC G25.2
Trench
  fever A79.0
  foot — *see* Immersion, foot
  mouth A69.1
Treponema pallidum infection — *see* Syphilis

Treponematosis
  due to
    T. pallidum — *see* Syphilis
    T. pertenue — *see* Yaws
Triad
  Hutchinson's (congenital syphilis) A50.53
  Kartagener's Q89.3
  Saint's — *see* Hernia, diaphragm
Trichiasis (eyelid) H02.059
  with entropion — *see* Entropion
  left H02.056
    lower H02.055
    upper H02.054
  right H02.053
    lower H02.052
    upper H02.051
Trichinella spiralis (infection) (infestation) B75
Trichinellosis, trichiniasis, trichinelliasis, trichinosis B75
  with muscle disorder B75 [M63.80]
    ankle B75 [M63.87-] ☑
    foot B75 [M63.87-] ☑
    forearm B75 [M63.83-] ☑
    hand B75 [M63.84-] ☑
    lower leg B75 [M63.86-] ☑
    multiple sites B75 [M63.89]
    pelvic region B75 [M63.85-] ☑
    shoulder region B75 [M63.81-] ☑
    specified site NEC B75 [M63.88]
    thigh B75 [M63.85-] ☑
    upper arm B75 [M63.82-] ☑
Trichobezoar T18.9 ☑
  intestine T18.3 ☑
  stomach T18.2 ☑
Trichocephaliasis, trichocephalosis B79
Trichocephalus infestation B79
Trichoclasis L67.8
Trichoepithelioma (*see also* Neoplasm, skin, benign)
  malignant — *see* Neoplasm, skin, malignant
Trichofolliculoma — *see* Neoplasm, skin, benign
Tricholemmoma — *see* Neoplasm, skin, benign
Trichomoniasis A59.9
  bladder A59.03
  cervix A59.09
  intestinal A07.8
  prostate A59.02
  seminal vesicles A59.09
  specified site NEC A59.8
  urethra A59.03
  urogenitalis A59.00
  vagina A59.01
  vulva A59.01
Trichomycosis
  axillaris A48.8
  nodosa, nodularis B36.8
Trichonodosis L67.8
Trichophytid, trichophyton infection — *see* Dermatophytosis
Trichophytobezoar T18.9 ☑
  intestine T18.3 ☑
  stomach T18.2 ☑
Trichophytosis — *see* Dermatophytosis
Trichoptilosis L67.8
Trichorrhexis (nodosa) (invaginata) L67.0
Trichosis axillaris A48.8
Trichosporosis nodosa B36.2
Trichostasis spinulosa (congenital) Q84.1
Trichostrongyliasis, trichostrongylosis (small intestine) B81.2
Trichostrongylus infection B81.2
Trichotillomania F63.3
Trichromat, trichromatopsia, anomalous (congenital) H53.55
Trichuriasis B79
Trichuris trichiura (infection) (infestation) (any site) B79
Tricuspid (valve) — *see* condition
Trifid (*see also* Accessory)
  kidney (pelvis) Q63.8
  tongue Q38.3
Trigeminal neuralgia — *see* Neuralgia, trigeminal
Trigeminy R00.8
Trigger finger (acquired) M65.30
  congenital Q74.0
  index finger M65.32- ☑
  little finger M65.35- ☑
  middle finger M65.33- ☑
  ring finger M65.34- ☑

Trigger finger — *continued*
  thumb M65.31- ☑
Trigonitis (bladder) (chronic) (pseudomembranous) N30.30
  with hematuria N30.31
Trigonocephaly Q75.0
Trilocular heart — *see* Cor triloculare
Trimethylaminuria E72.52
Tripartite placenta O43.19- ☑
Triphalangeal thumb Q74.0
Triple (*see also* Accessory)
  kidneys Q63.0
  uteri Q51.818
  X, female Q97.0
Triplegia G83.89
  congenital G80.8
Triplet (newborn) (*see also* Newborn, triplet)
  complicating pregnancy — *see* Pregnancy, triplet
Triplication — *see* Accessory
Triploidy Q92.7
Trismus R25.2
  neonatorum A33
  newborn A33
Trisomy (syndrome) Q92.9
  13 (partial) Q91.7
    meiotic nondisjunction Q91.4
    mitotic nondisjunction Q91.5
    mosaicism Q91.5
    translocation Q91.6
  18 (partial) Q91.3
    meiotic nondisjunction Q91.0
    mitotic nondisjunction Q91.1
    mosaicism Q91.1
    translocation Q91.2
  20 Q92.8
  21 (partial) Q90.9
    meiotic nondisjunction Q90.0
    mitotic nondisjunction Q90.1
    mosaicism Q90.1
    translocation Q90.2
  22 Q92.8
  autosomes Q92.9
  chromosome specified NEC Q92.8
    partial Q92.2
      due to unbalanced translocation Q92.5
    specified NEC Q92.8
    whole (nonsex chromosome)
      meiotic nondisjunction Q92.0
      mitotic nondisjunction Q92.1
      mosaicism Q92.1
  due to
    dicentrics — *see* Extra, marker chromosomes
    extra rings — *see* Extra, marker chromosomes
    isochromosomes — *see* Extra, marker chromosomes
  specified NEC Q92.8
  whole chromosome Q92.9
    meiotic nondisjunction Q92.0
    mitotic nondisjunction Q92.1
    mosaicism Q92.1
    partial Q92.9
    specified NEC Q92.8
Tritanomaly, tritanopia H53.55
Trombiculosis, trombiculiasis, trombidiosis B88.0
Trophedema (congenital) (hereditary) Q82.0
Trophoblastic disease (*see also* Mole, hydatidiform) O01.9
Tropholymphedema Q82.0
Trophoneurosis NEC G96.8
  disseminated M34.9
Tropical — *see* condition
Trouble (*see also* Disease)
  heart — *see* Disease, heart
  kidney — *see* Disease, renal
  nervous R45.0
  sinus — *see* Sinusitis
Trousseau's syndrome (thrombophlebitis migrans) I82.1
Truancy, childhood
  from school Z72.810
Truncus
  arteriosus (persistent) Q20.0
  communis Q20.0
Trunk — *see* condition
Trypanosomiasis
  African B56.9
    by Trypanosoma brucei
      gambiense B56.0
      rhodesiense B56.1
  American — *see* Chagas' disease

Trypanosomiasis — *continued*
  Brazilian — *see* Chagas' disease
  by Trypanosoma
    brucei gambiense B56.0
    brucei rhodesiense B56.1
    cruzi — *see* Chagas' disease
    gambiensis, Gambian B56.0
    rhodesiensis, Rhodesian B56.1
  South American — *see* Chagas' disease
  where
    African trypanosomiasis is prevalent B56.9
    Chagas' disease is prevalent B57.2
T-shaped incisors K00.2
Tsutsugamushi (disease) (fever) A75.3
Tube, tubal, tubular — *see* condition
Tubercle (*see also* Tuberculosis)
  brain, solitary A17.81
  Darwin's Q17.8
  Ghon, primary infection A15.7
Tuberculid, tuberculide (indurating, subcutaneous) (lichenoid) (miliary) (papulonecrotic) (primary) (skin) A18.4
Tuberculoma (*see also* Tuberculosis)
  brain A17.81
  meninges (cerebral) (spinal) A17.1
  spinal cord A17.81
Tuberculosis, tubercular, tuberculous (calcification) (calcified) (caseous) (chromogenic acid-fast bacilli) (degeneration) (fibrocaseous) (fistula) (interstitial) (isolated circumscribed lesions) (necrosis) (parenchymatous) (ulcerative) A15.9
  with pneumoconiosis (any condition in J60-J64) J65
  abdomen (lymph gland) A18.39
  abscess (respiratory) A15.9
    bone A18.03
      hip A18.02
      knee A18.02
      sacrum A18.01
      specified site NEC A18.03
      spinal A18.01
      vertebra A18.01
    brain A17.81
    breast A18.89
    Cowper's gland A18.15
    dura (mater) (cerebral) (spinal) A17.81
    epidural (cerebral) (spinal) A17.81
    female pelvis A18.17
    frontal sinus A15.8
    genital organs NEC A18.10
    genitourinary A18.10
    gland (lymphatic) — *see* Tuberculosis, lymph gland
    hip A18.02
    intestine A18.32
    ischiorectal A18.32
    joint NEC A18.02
      hip A18.02
      knee A18.02
      specified NEC A18.02
      vertebral A18.01
    kidney A18.11
    knee A18.02
    latent R76.11
    lumbar (spine) A18.01
    lung — *see* Tuberculosis, pulmonary
    meninges (cerebral) (spinal) A17.0
    muscle A18.09
    perianal (fistula) A18.32
    perinephric A18.11
    perirectal A18.32
    rectum A18.32
    retropharyngeal A15.8
    sacrum A18.01
    scrofulous A18.2
    scrotum A18.15
    skin (primary) A18.4
    spinal cord A17.81
    spine or vertebra (column) A18.01
    subdiaphragmatic A18.31
    testis A18.15
    urinary A18.13
    uterus A18.17
  accessory sinus — *see* Tuberculosis, sinus
  Addison's disease A18.7
  adenitis — *see* Tuberculosis, lymph gland
  adenoids A15.8
  adenopathy — *see* Tuberculosis, lymph gland
  adherent pericardium A18.84
  adnexa (uteri) A18.17

Tuberculosis, tubercular, tuberculous — *continued*
  adrenal (capsule) (gland) A18.7
  alimentary canal A18.32
  anemia A18.89
  ankle (joint) (bone) A18.02
  anus A18.32
  apex, apical — *see* Tuberculosis, pulmonary
  appendicitis, appendix A18.32
  arachnoid A17.0
  artery, arteritis A18.89
    cerebral A18.89
  arthritis (chronic) (synovial) A18.02
    spine or vertebra (column) A18.01
  articular — *see* Tuberculosis, joint
  ascites A18.31
  asthma — *see* Tuberculosis, pulmonary
  axilla, axillary (gland) A18.2
  bladder A18.12
  bone A18.03
    hip A18.02
    knee A18.02
    limb NEC A18.03
    sacrum A18.01
    spine or vertebral column A18.01
  bowel (miliary) A18.32
  brain A17.81
  breast A18.89
  broad ligament A18.17
  bronchi, bronchial, bronchus A15.5
    ectasia, ectasis (bronchiectasis) — *see* Tuberculosis, pulmonary
    fistula A15.5
      primary (progressive) A15.7
    gland or node A15.4
      primary (progressive) A15.7
    lymph gland or node A15.4
      primary (progressive) A15.7
  bronchiectasis — *see* Tuberculosis, pulmonary
  bronchitis A15.5
  bronchopleural A15.6
  bronchopneumonia, bronchopneumonic — *see* Tuberculosis, pulmonary
  bronchorrhagia A15.5
  bronchotracheal A15.5
  bronze disease A18.7
  buccal cavity A18.83
  bulbourethral gland A18.15
  bursa A18.09
  cachexia A15.9
  cardiomyopathy A18.84
  caries — *see* Tuberculosis, bone
  cartilage A18.02
    intervertebral A18.01
  catarrhal — *see* Tuberculosis, respiratory
  cecum A18.32
  cellulitis (primary) A18.4
  cerebellum A17.81
  cerebral, cerebrum A17.81
  cerebrospinal A17.81
    meninges A17.0
  cervical (lymph gland or node) A18.2
  cervicitis, cervix (uteri) A18.16
  chest — *see* Tuberculosis, respiratory
  chorioretinitis A18.53
  choroid, choroiditis A18.53
  ciliary body A18.54
  colitis A18.32
  collier's J65
  colliquativa (primary) A18.4
  colon A18.32
  complex, primary A15.7
  congenital P37.0
  conjunctiva A18.59
  connective tissue (systemic) A18.89
  contact Z20.1
  cornea (ulcer) A18.52
  Cowper's gland A18.15
  coxae A18.02
  coxalgia A18.02
  cul-de-sac of Douglas A18.17
  curvature, spine A18.01
  cutis (colliquativa) (primary) A18.4
  cyst, ovary A18.18
  cystitis A18.12
  dactylitis A18.03
  diarrhea A18.32
  diffuse — *see* Tuberculosis, miliary
  digestive tract A18.32

☑ **Additional Character Required** — Refer to the Tabular List for Character Selection   ▽ **Subterms under main terms may continue to next column or page**

Tuberculosis, tubercular, tuberculous — *continued*

disseminated — *see* Tuberculosis, miliary
duodenum A18.32
dura (mater) (cerebral) (spinal) A17.0
   abscess (cerebral) (spinal) A17.81
dysentery A18.32
ear (inner) (middle) A18.6
   bone A18.03
   external (primary) A18.4
   skin (primary) A18.4
elbow A18.02
emphysema — *see* Tuberculosis, pulmonary
empyema A15.6
encephalitis A17.82
endarteritis A18.89
endocarditis A18.84
   aortic A18.84
   mitral A18.84
   pulmonary A18.84
   tricuspid A18.84
endocrine glands NEC A18.82
endometrium A18.17
enteric, enterica, enteritis A18.32
enterocolitis A18.32
epididymis, epididymitis A18.15
epidural abscess (cerebral) (spinal) A17.81
epiglottis A15.5
episcleritis A18.51
erythema (induratum) (nodosum) (primary) A18.4
esophagus A18.83
eustachian tube A18.6
exposure (to) Z20.1
exudative — *see* Tuberculosis, pulmonary
eye A18.50
eyelid (primary) (lupus) A18.4
fallopian tube (acute) (chronic) A18.17
fascia A18.09
fauces A15.8
female pelvic inflammatory disease A18.17
finger A18.03
first infection A15.7
gallbladder A18.83
ganglion A18.09
gastritis A18.83
gastrocolic fistula A18.32
gastroenteritis A18.32
gastrointestinal tract A18.32
general, generalized — *see* Tuberculosis, miliary
genital organs A18.10
genitourinary A18.10
genu A18.02
glandula suprarenalis A18.7
glandular, general A18.2
glottis A15.5
grinder's J65
gum A18.83
hand A18.03
heart A18.84
hematogenous — *see* Tuberculosis, miliary
hemoptysis — *see* Tuberculosis, pulmonary
hemorrhage NEC — *see* Tuberculosis, pulmonary
hemothorax A15.6
hepatitis A18.83
hilar lymph nodes A15.4
   primary (progressive) A15.7
hip (joint) (disease) (bone) A18.02
hydropneumothorax A15.6
hydrothorax A15.6
hypoadrenalism A18.7
hypopharynx A15.8
ileocecal (hyperplastic) A18.32
ileocolitis A18.32
ileum A18.32
iliac spine (superior) A18.03
immunological findings only A15.7
indurativa (primary) A18.4
infantile A15.7
infection A15.9
   without clinical manifestations A15.7
infraclavicular gland A18.2
inguinal gland A18.2
inguinalis A18.2
intestine (any part) A18.32
iridocyclitis A18.54
iris, iritis A18.54
ischiorectal A18.32
jaw A18.03
jejunum A18.32

Tuberculosis, tubercular, tuberculous — *continued*

joint A18.02
   vertebral A18.01
keratitis (interstitial) A18.52
keratoconjunctivitis A18.52
kidney A18.11
knee (joint) A18.02
kyphosis, kyphoscoliosis A18.01
laryngitis A15.5
larynx A15.5
latent R76.11
leptomeninges, leptomeningitis (cerebral) (spinal) A17.0
lichenoides (primary) A18.4
linguae A18.83
lip A18.83
liver A18.83
lordosis A18.01
lung — *see* Tuberculosis, pulmonary
lupus vulgaris A18.4
lymph gland or node (peripheral) A18.2
   abdomen A18.39
   bronchial A15.4
      primary (progressive) A15.7
   cervical A18.2
   hilar A15.4
      primary (progressive) A15.7
   intrathoracic A15.4
      primary (progressive) A15.7
   mediastinal A15.4
      primary (progressive) A15.7
   mesenteric A18.39
   retroperitoneal A18.39
   tracheobronchial A15.4
      primary (progressive) A15.7
lymphadenitis — *see* Tuberculosis, lymph gland
lymphangitis — *see* Tuberculosis, lymph gland
lymphatic (gland) (vessel) — *see* Tuberculosis, lymph gland
mammary gland A18.89
marasmus A15.7
mastoiditis A18.03
mediastinal lymph gland or node A15.4
   primary (progressive) A15.7
mediastinitis A15.8
   primary (progressive) A15.7
mediastinum A15.8
   primary (progressive) A15.7
medulla A17.81
melanosis, Addisonian A18.7
meninges, meningitis (basilar) (cerebral) (cerebrospinal) (spinal) A17.0
meningoencephalitis A17.82
mesentery, mesenteric (gland or node) A18.39
miliary A19.9
   acute A19.2
      multiple sites A19.1
      single specified site A19.0
   chronic A19.8
   specified NEC A19.8
millstone makers' J65
miner's J65
molder's J65
mouth A18.83
multiple A19.9
   acute A19.1
   chronic A19.8
muscle A18.09
myelitis A17.82
myocardium, myocarditis A18.84
nasal (passage) (sinus) A15.8
nasopharynx A15.8
neck gland A18.2
nephritis A18.11
nerve (mononeuropathy) A17.83
nervous system A17.9
nose (septum) A15.8
ocular A18.50
omentum A18.31
oophoritis (acute) (chronic) A18.17
optic (nerve trunk) (papilla) A18.59
orbit A18.59
orchitis A18.15
organ, specified NEC A18.89
osseous — *see* Tuberculosis, bone
osteitis — *see* Tuberculosis, bone
osteomyelitis — *see* Tuberculosis, bone
otitis media A18.6

Tuberculosis, tubercular, tuberculous — *continued*

ovary, ovaritis (acute) (chronic) A18.17
oviduct (acute) (chronic) A18.17
pachymeningitis A17.0
palate (soft) A18.83
pancreas A18.83
papulonecrotic (a) (primary) A18.4
parathyroid glands A18.82
paronychia (primary) A18.4
parotid gland or region A18.83
pelvis (bony) A18.03
penis A18.15
peribronchitis A15.5
pericardium, pericarditis A18.84
perichondritis, larynx A15.5
periostitis — *see* Tuberculosis, bone
perirectal fistula A18.32
peritoneum NEC A18.31
peritonitis A18.31
pharynx, pharyngitis A15.8
phlyctenulosis (keratoconjunctivitis) A18.52
phthisis NEC — *see* Tuberculosis, pulmonary
pituitary gland A18.82
pleura, pleural, pleurisy, pleuritis (fibrinous) (obliterative) (purulent) (simple plastic) (with effusion) A15.6
   primary (progressive) A15.7
pneumonia, pneumonic — *see* Tuberculosis, pulmonary
pneumothorax (spontaneous) (tense valvular) — *see* Tuberculosis, pulmonary
polyneuropathy A17.89
polyserositis A19.9
   acute A19.1
   chronic A19.8
potter's J65
prepuce A18.15
primary (complex) A15.7
proctitis A18.32
prostate, prostatitis A18.14
pulmonalis — *see* Tuberculosis, pulmonary
pulmonary (cavitated) (fibrotic) (infiltrative) (nodular) A15.0
   childhood type or first infection A15.7
      primary (complex) A15.7
pyelitis A18.11
pyelonephritis A18.11
pyemia — *see* Tuberculosis, miliary
pyonephrosis A18.11
pyopneumothorax A15.6
pyothorax A15.6
rectum (fistula) (with abscess) A18.32
reinfection stage — *see* Tuberculosis, pulmonary
renal A18.11
renis A18.11
respiratory A15.9
   primary A15.7
   specified site NEC A15.8
retina, retinitis A18.53
retroperitoneal (lymph gland or node) A18.39
rheumatism NEC A18.09
rhinitis A15.8
sacroiliac (joint) A18.01
sacrum A18.01
salivary gland A18.83
salpingitis (acute) (chronic) A18.17
sandblaster's J65
sclera A18.51
scoliosis A18.01
scrofulous A18.2
scrotum A18.15
seminal tract or vesicle A18.15
senile A15.9
septic — *see* Tuberculosis, miliary
shoulder (joint) A18.02
   blade A18.03
sigmoid A18.32
sinus (any nasal) A15.8
   bone A18.03
   epididymis A18.15
skeletal NEC A18.03
skin (any site) (primary) A18.4
small intestine A18.32
soft palate A18.83
spermatic cord A18.15
spine, spinal (column) A18.01
   cord A17.81
   medulla A17.81

Tuberculosis, tubercular, tuberculous — *continued*
spine, spinal — *continued*
membrane A17.0
meninges A17.0
spleen, splenitis A18.85
spondylitis A18.01
sternoclavicular joint A18.02
stomach A18.83
stonemason's J65
subcutaneous tissue (cellular) (primary) A18.4
subcutis (primary) A18.4
subdeltoid bursa A18.83
submaxillary (region) A18.83
supraclavicular gland A18.2
suprarenal (capsule) (gland) A18.7
swelling, joint (*see also* category M01) (*see also* Tuberculosis, joint) A18.02
symphysis pubis A18.02
synovitis A18.09
articular A18.02
spine or vertebra A18.01
systemic — *see* Tuberculosis, miliary
tarsitis A18.4
tendon (sheath) — *see* Tuberculosis, tenosynovitis
tenosynovitis A18.09
spine or vertebra A18.01
testis A18.15
throat A15.8
thymus gland A18.82
thyroid gland A18.81
tongue A18.83
tonsil, tonsillitis A15.8
trachea, tracheal A15.5
lymph gland or node A15.4
primary (progressive) A15.7
tracheobronchial A15.5
lymph gland or node A15.4
primary (progressive) A15.7
tubal (acute) (chronic) A18.17
tunica vaginalis A18.15
ulcer (skin) (primary) A18.4
bowel or intestine A18.32
specified NEC — *see* Tuberculosis, by site
unspecified site A15.9
ureter A18.11
urethra, urethral (gland) A18.13
urinary organ or tract A18.13
uterus A18.17
uveal tract A18.54
uvula A18.83
vagina A18.18
vas deferens A18.15
verruca, verrucosa (cutis) (primary) A18.4
vertebra (column) A18.01
vesiculitis A18.15
vulva A18.18
wrist (joint) A18.02
Tuberculum
Carabelli — *see* Excludes Note at K00.2
occlusal — *see* Excludes Note at K00.2
paramolare K00.2
Tuberosity, enitre maxillary M26.07
Tuberous sclerosis (brain) Q85.1
Tubo-ovarian — *see* condition
Tuboplasty, after previous sterilization Z31.0
aftercare Z31.42
Tubotympanitis, catarrhal (chronic) — *see* Otitis, media, nonsuppurative, chronic, serous
Tularemia A21.9
with
conjunctivitis A21.1
pneumonia A21.2
abdominal A21.3
bronchopneumonic A21.2
conjunctivitis A21.1
cryptogenic A21.3
enteric A21.3
gastrointestinal A21.3
generalized A21.7
ingestion A21.3
intestinal A21.3
oculoglandular A21.1
ophthalmic A21.1
pneumonia (any), pneumonic A21.2
pulmonary A21.2
sepsis A21.7
specified NEC A21.8
typhoidal A21.7

Tularemia — *continued*
ulceroglandular A21.0
Tularensis conjunctivitis A21.1
Tumefaction (*see also* Swelling)
liver — *see* Hypertrophy, liver
Tumor (*see also* Neoplasm, unspecified behavior, by site)
acinar cell — *see* Neoplasm, uncertain behavior, by site
acinic cell — *see* Neoplasm, uncertain behavior, by site
adenocarcinoid — *see* Neoplasm, malignant, by site
adenomatoid (*see also* Neoplasm, benign, by site)
odontogenic — *see* Cyst, calcifying odontogenic
adnexal (skin) — *see* Neoplasm, skin, benign, by site
adrenal
cortical (benign) D35.0- ☑
malignant C74.0- ☑
rest — *see* Neoplasm, benign, by site
alpha-cell
malignant
pancreas C25.4
specified site NEC — *see* Neoplasm, malignant, by site
unspecified site C25.4
pancreas D13.7
specified site NEC — *see* Neoplasm, benign, by site
unspecified site D13.7
aneurysmal — *see* Aneurysm
aortic body D44.7
malignant C75.5
Askin's — *see* Neoplasm, connective tissue, malignant
basal cell (*see also* Neoplasm, skin, uncertain behavior) D48.5
Bednar — *see* Neoplasm, skin, malignant
benign (unclassified) — *see* Neoplasm, benign, by site
beta-cell
malignant
pancreas C25.4
specified site NEC — *see* Neoplasm, malignant, by site
unspecified site C25.4
pancreas D13.7
specified site NEC — *see* Neoplasm, benign, by site
unspecified site D13.7
Brenner D27.9
borderline malignancy D39.1- ☑
malignant C56- ☑
proliferating D39.1- ☑
bronchial alveolar, intravascular D38.1
Brooke's — *see* Neoplasm, skin, benign
brown fat — *see* Lipoma
Burkitt — *see* Lymphoma, Burkitt
calcifying epithelial odontogenic — *see* Cyst, calcifying odontogenic
carcinoid
benign D3A.00 (*following* D36)
appendix D3A.020 (*following* D36)
ascending colon D3A.022 (*following* D36)
bronchus (lung) D3A.090 (*following* D36)
cecum D3A.021 (*following* D36)
colon D3A.029 (*following* D36)
descending colon D3A.024 (*following* D36)
duodenum D3A.010 (*following* D36)
foregut NOS D3A.094 (*following* D36)
hindgut NOS D3A.096 (*following* D36)
ileum D3A.012 (*following* D36)
jejunum D3A.011 (*following* D36)
kidney D3A.093 (*following* D36)
large intestine D3A.029 (*following* D36)
lung (bronchus) D3A.090 (*following* D36)
midgut NOS D3A.095 (*following* D36)
rectum D3A.026 (*following* D36)
sigmoid colon D3A.025 (*following* D36)
small intestine D3A.019 (*following* D36)
specified NEC D3A.098 (*following* D36)
stomach D3A.092 (*following* D36)
thymus D3A.091 (*following* D36)
transverse colon D3A.023 (*following* D36)
malignant C7A.00 (*following* C75)
appendix C7A.020 (*following* C75)
ascending colon C7A.022 (*following* C75)
bronchus (lung) C7A.090 (*following* C75)
cecum C7A.021 (*following* C75)
colon C7A.029 (*following* C75)
descending colon C7A.024 (*following* C75)
duodenum C7A.010 (*following* C75)
foregut NOS C7A.094 (*following* C75)
hindgut NOS C7A.096 (*following* C75)
ileum C7A.012 (*following* C75)
jejunum C7A.011 (*following* C75)

Tumor — *continued*
carcinoid — *continued*
malignant — *continued*
kidney C7A.093 (*following* C75)
large intestine C7A.029 (*following* C75)
lung (bronchus) C7A.090 (*following* C75)
midgut NOS C7A.095 (*following* C75)
rectum C7A.026 (*following* C75)
sigmoid colon C7A.025 (*following* C75)
small intestine C7A.019 (*following* C75)
specified NEC C7A.098 (*following* C75)
stomach C7A.092 (*following* C75)
thymus C7A.091 (*following* C75)
transverse colon C7A.023 (*following* C75)
mesentery metastasis C7B.04 (*following* C75)
secondary C7B.00 (*following* C75)
bone C7B.03 (*following* C75)
distant lymph nodes C7B.01 (*following* C75)
liver C7B.02 (*following* C75)
peritoneum C7B.04 (*following* C75)
specified NEC C7B.09 (*following* C75)
carotid body D44.6
malignant C75.4
cells (*see also* Neoplasm, unspecified behavior, by site)
benign — *see* Neoplasm, benign, by site
malignant — *see* Neoplasm, malignant, by site
uncertain whether benign or malignant — *see* Neoplasm, uncertain behavior, by site
cervix, in pregnancy or childbirth — *see* Pregnancy, complicated by, tumor, cervix
chondromatous giant cell — *see* Neoplasm, bone, benign
chromaffin (*see also* Neoplasm, benign, by site)
malignant — *see* Neoplasm, malignant, by site
Cock's peculiar L72.3
Codman's — *see* Neoplasm, bone, benign
dentigerous, mixed — *see* Cyst, calcifying odontogenic
dermoid — *see* Neoplasm, benign, by site
with malignant transformation C56- ☑
desmoid (extra-abdominal) (*see also* Neoplasm, connective tissue, uncertain behavior)
abdominal — *see* Neoplasm, connective tissue, uncertain behavior
embolus — *see* Neoplasm, secondary, by site
embryonal (mixed) (*see also* Neoplasm, uncertain behavior, by site)
liver C22.7
endodermal sinus
specified site — *see* Neoplasm, malignant, by site
unspecified site
female C56.- ☑
male C62.90
epithelial
benign — *see* Neoplasm, benign, by site
malignant — *see* Neoplasm, malignant, by site
Ewing's — *see* Neoplasm, bone, malignant, by site
fatty — *see* Lipoma
fibroid — *see* Leiomyoma
G cell
malignant
pancreas C25.4
specified site NEC — *see* Neoplasm, malignant, by site
unspecified site C25.4
specified site — *see* Neoplasm, uncertain behavior, by site
unspecified site D37.8
germ cell (*see also* Neoplasm, malignant, by site)
mixed — *see* Neoplasm, malignant, by site
ghost cell, odontogenic — *see* Cyst, calcifying odontogenic
giant cell (*see also* Neoplasm, uncertain behavior, by site)
bone D48.0
malignant — *see* Neoplasm, bone, malignant
chondromatous — *see* Neoplasm, bone, benign
malignant — *see* Neoplasm, malignant, by site
soft parts — *see* Neoplasm, connective tissue, uncertain behavior
malignant — *see* Neoplasm, connective tissue, malignant
glomus D18.00
intra-abdominal D18.03
intracranial D18.02
jugulare D44.7
malignant C75.5
skin D18.01
specified site NEC D18.09

☑ **Additional Character Required** — **Refer to the Tabular List for Character Selection**   ▦ **Subterms under main terms may continue to next column or page**

Tumor — *continued*
  gonadal stromal — *see* Neoplasm, uncertain behavior,
    by site
  granular cell (*see also* Neoplasm, connective tissue,
    benign)
    malignant — *see* Neoplasm, connective tissue, ma-
      lignant
  granulosa cell D39.1- ☑
    juvenile D39.1- ☑
    malignant C56- ☑
  granulosa cell-theca cell D39.1- ☑
    malignant C56- ☑
  Grawitz's C64- ☑
  hemorrhoidal — *see* Hemorrhoids
  hilar cell D27- ☑
  hilus cell D27- ☑
  Hurthle cell (benign) D34
    malignant C73
  hydatid — *see* Echinococcus
  hypernephroid (*see also* Neoplasm, uncertain behavior,
    by site)
  interstitial cell (*see also* Neoplasm, uncertain behavior,
    by site)
    benign — *see* Neoplasm, benign, by site
    malignant — *see* Neoplasm, malignant, by site
  intravascular bronchial alveolar D38.1
  islet cell — *see* Neoplasm, benign, by site
    malignant — *see* Neoplasm, malignant, by site
      pancreas C25.4
      specified site NEC — *see* Neoplasm, malignant,
        by site
      unspecified site C25.4
    pancreas D13.7
    specified site NEC — *see* Neoplasm, benign, by site
    unspecified site D13.7
  juxtaglomerular D41.0- ☑
  Klatskin's C22.1
  Krukenberg's C79.6- ☑
  Leydig cell — *see* Neoplasm, uncertain behavior, by
    site
    benign — *see* Neoplasm, benign, by site
      specified site — *see* Neoplasm, benign, by site
      unspecified site
        female D27.9
        male D29.20
    malignant — *see* Neoplasm, malignant, by site
      specified site — *see* Neoplasm, malignant, by
        site
      unspecified site
        female C56.9
        male C62.90
    specified site — *see* Neoplasm, uncertain behavior,
      by site
    unspecified site
      female D39.10
      male D40.10
  lipid cell, ovary D27- ☑
  lipoid cell, ovary D27- ☑
  malignant (*see also* Neoplasm, malignant, by site) C80.1
    fusiform cell (type) C80.1
    giant cell (type) C80.1
    localized, plasma cell — *see* Plasmacytoma, solitary
    mixed NEC C80.1
    small cell (type) C80.1
    spindle cell (type) C80.1
    unclassified C80.1
  mast cell D47.09
  melanotic, neuroectodermal — *see* Neoplasm, benign,
    by site
  Merkel cell — *see* Carcinoma, Merkel cell
  mesenchymal
    malignant — *see* Neoplasm, connective tissue, ma-
      lignant
    mixed — *see* Neoplasm, connective tissue, uncertain
      behavior
  mesodermal, mixed (*see also* Neoplasm, malignant, by
    site)
    liver C22.4
  mesonephric (*see also* Neoplasm, uncertain behavior,
    by site)
    malignant — *see* Neoplasm, malignant, by site
  metastatic
    from specified site — *see* Neoplasm, malignant, by
      site
    of specified site — *see* Neoplasm, malignant, by site
    to specified site — *see* Neoplasm, secondary, by site
  mixed NEC (*see also* Neoplasm, benign, by site)

Tumor — *continued*
  mixed (*see also* Neoplasm, benign, by site) — *contin-*
    ued
    malignant — *see* Neoplasm, malignant, by site
  mucinous of low malignant potential
    specified site — *see* Neoplasm, malignant, by site
    unspecified site C56.9
  mucocarcinoid
    specified site — *see* Neoplasm, malignant, by site
    unspecified site C18.1
  mucoepidermoid — *see* Neoplasm, uncertain behavior,
    by site
  Müllerian, mixed
    specified site — *see* Neoplasm, malignant, by site
    unspecified site C54.9
  myoepithelial — *see* Neoplasm, benign, by site
  neuroectodermal (peripheral) — *see* Neoplasm, malig-
    nant, by site
    primitive
      specified site — *see* Neoplasm, malignant, by
        site
      unspecified site C71.9
  neuroendocrine D3A.8 (*following* D36)
    malignant poorly differentiated C7A.1 (*following*
      C75)
    secondary NEC C7B.8 (*following* C75)
    specified NEC C7A.8 (*following* C75)
  neurogenic olfactory C30.0
  nonencapsulated sclerosing C73
  odontogenic (adenomatoid) (benign) (calcifying epithe-
    lial) (keratocystic) (squamous) — *see* Cyst, calci-
    fying odontogenic
    malignant C41.1
      upper jaw (bone) C41.0
  ovarian stromal D39.1- ☑
  ovary, in pregnancy — *see* Pregnancy, complicated by
  pacinian — *see* Neoplasm, skin, benign
  Pancoast's — *see* Pancoast's syndrome
  papillary (*see also* Papilloma)
    cystic D37.9
    mucinous of low malignant potential C56- ☑
      specified site — *see* Neoplasm, malignant, by
        site
      unspecified site C56.9
    serous of low malignant potential
      specified site — *see* Neoplasm, malignant, by
        site
      unspecified site C56.9
  pelvic, in pregnancy or childbirth — *see* Pregnancy,
    complicated by
  phantom F45.8
  phyllodes D48.6- ☑
    benign D24- ☑
    malignant — *see* Neoplasm, breast, malignant
  Pindborg — *see* Cyst, calcifying odontogenic
  placental site trophoblastic D39.2
  plasma cell (malignant) (localized) — *see* Plasmacy-
    toma, solitary
  polyvesicular vitelline
    specified site — *see* Neoplasm, malignant, by site
    unspecified site
      female C56.9
      male C62.90
  Pott's puffy — *see* Osteomyelitis, specified NEC
  Rathke's pouch D44.3
  retinal anlage — *see* Neoplasm, benign, by site
  salivary gland type, mixed — *see* Neoplasm, salivary
    gland, benign
    malignant — *see* Neoplasm, salivary gland, malig-
      nant
  Sampson's N80.1
  Schmincke's — *see* Neoplasm, nasopharynx, malignant
  sclerosing stromal D27- ☑
  sebaceous — *see* Cyst, sebaceous
  secondary — *see* Neoplasm, secondary, by site
    carcinoid C7B.00 (*following* C75)
      bone C7B.03 (*following* C75)
      distant lymph nodes C7B.01 (*following* C75)
      liver C7B.02 (*following* C75)
      peritoneum C7B.04 (*following* C75)
      specified NEC C7B.09 (*following* C75)
    neuroendocrine NEC C7B.8 (*following* C75)
  serous of low malignant potential
    specified site — *see* Neoplasm, malignant, by site
    unspecified site C56.9
  Sertoli cell — *see* Neoplasm, benign, by site
    with lipid storage
      specified site — *see* Neoplasm, benign, by site

Tumor — *continued*
  Sertoli cell — *see* Neoplasm, benign, by site —
    continued
    with lipid storage — *continued*
      unspecified site
        female D27.9
        male D29.20
    specified site — *see* Neoplasm, benign, by site
    unspecified site
      female D27.9
      male D29.20
  Sertoli-Leydig cell — *see* Neoplasm, benign, by site
    specified site — *see* Neoplasm, benign, by site
    unspecified site
      female D27.9
      male D29.20
  sex cord (-stromal) — *see* Neoplasm, uncertain behav-
    ior, by site
    with annular tubules D39.1- ☑
  skin appendage — *see* Neoplasm, skin, benign
  smooth muscle — *see* Neoplasm, connective tissue,
    uncertain behavior
  soft tissue
    benign — *see* Neoplasm, connective tissue, benign
    malignant — *see* Neoplasm, connective tissue, ma-
      lignant
  sternomastoid (congenital) Q68.0
  stromal
    endometrial D39.0
    gastric D48.1
      benign D21.4
      malignant C16.9
      uncertain behavior D48.1
    gastrointestinal C49.A- ☑
      benign D21.4
      esophagus C49.A1
      malignant C49.A0
        colon C49.A4
        duodenum C49.A3
        esophagus C49.A1
        ileum C49.A3
        jejunum C49.A3
        large intestine C49.A4
        Meckel diverticulum C49.A3
        omentum C49.A9
        peritoneum C49.A9
        rectum C49.A5
        small intestine C49.A3
        specified site NEC C49.A9
        stomach C49.A2
      rectum C49.A5
      small intestine C49.A3
      specified site NEC C49.A9
      stomach C49.A2
      uncertain behavior D48.1
    intestine
      benign D21.4
      malignant
        large C49.A4
        small C49.A3
      uncertain behavior D48.1
    ovarian D39.1- ☑
    stomach C49.A2
      benign D21.4
      malignant C49.A2
      uncertain behavior D48.1
  sweat gland (*see also* Neoplasm, skin, uncertain behav-
    ior)
    benign — *see* Neoplasm, skin, benign
    malignant — *see* Neoplasm, skin, malignant
  syphilitic, brain A52.17
  testicular D40.10
  testicular stromal D40.1- ☑
  theca cell D27.- ☑
  theca cell-granulosa cell D39.1- ☑
  Triton, malignant — *see* Neoplasm, nerve, malignant
  trophoblastic, placental site D39.2
  turban D23.4
  uterus (body), in pregnancy or childbirth — *see* Preg-
    nancy, complicated by, tumor, uterus
  vagina, in pregnancy or childbirth — *see* Pregnancy,
    complicated by
  varicose — *see* Varix
  von Recklinghausen's — *see* Neurofibromatosis
  vulva or perineum, in pregnancy or childbirth — *see*
    Pregnancy, complicated by
    causing obstructed labor O65.5
  Warthin's — *see* Neoplasm, salivary gland, benign

Tumor — continued
  Wilms' C64- ☑
  yolk sac — see Neoplasm, malignant, by site
    specified site — see Neoplasm, malignant, by site
    unspecified site
      female C56.9
      male C62.90
Tumor lysis syndrome (following antineoplastic chemotherapy) (spontaneous) NEC E88.3
Tumorlet — see Neoplasm, uncertain behavior, by site
Tungiasis B88.1
Tunica vasculosa lentis Q12.2
Turban tumor D23.4
Türck's trachoma J37.0
Turner-Kieser syndrome Q87.2
Turner-like syndrome Q87.1
Turner's
  hypoplasia (tooth) K00.4
  syndrome Q96.9
    specified NEC Q96.8
  tooth K00.4
Turner-Ullrich syndrome Q96.9
Tussis convulsiva — see Whooping cough
Twiddler's syndrome (due to)
  automatic implantable defibrillatorT82.198
  cardiac pacemaker T82.198 ☑
Twilight state
  epileptic F05
  psychogenic F44.89
Twin (newborn) (see also Newborn, twin)
  conjoined Q89.4
  pregnancy — see Pregnancy, twin
Twinning, teeth K00.2
Twist, twisted
  bowel, colon or intestine K56.2
  hair (congenital) Q84.1
  mesentery K56.2
  omentum K56.2
  organ or site, congenital NEC — see Anomaly, by site
  ovarian pedicle — see Torsion, ovary
Twitching R25.3
Tylosis (acquired) L84
  buccalis K13.29
  linguae K13.29
  palmaris et plantaris (congenital) (inherited) Q82.8
    acquired L85.1
Tympanism R14.0
Tympanites (abdominal) (intestinal) R14.0
Tympanitis — see Myringitis
Tympanosclerosis H74.0 ☑
Tympanum — see condition
Tympany
  abdomen R14.0
  chest R09.89
Type A behavior pattern Z73.1
Typhlitis — see Appendicitis
Typhoenteritis — see Typhoid
Typhoid (abortive) (ambulant) (any site) (clinical) (fever) (hemorrhagic) (infection) (intermittent) (malignant) (rheumatic) (Widal negative) A01.00
  with pneumonia A01.03
  abdominal A01.09
  arthritis A01.04
  carrier (suspected) of Z22.0
  cholecystitis (current) A01.09
  endocarditis A01.02
  heart involvement A01.02
  inoculation reaction — see Complications, vaccination
  meningitis A01.01
  mesenteric lymph nodes A01.09
  myocarditis A01.02
  osteomyelitis A01.05
  perichondritis, larynx A01.09
  pneumonia A01.03
  specified NEC A01.09
  spine A01.05
  ulcer (perforating) A01.09
Typhomalaria (fever) — see Malaria
Typhomania A01.00
Typhoperitonitis A01.09
Typhus (fever) A75.9
  abdominal, abdominalis — see Typhoid
  African tick A77.1
  amarillic A95.9
  brain A75.9 [G94]
  cerebral A75.9 [G94]
  classical A75.0

Typhus — continued
  due to Rickettsia
    prowazekii A75.0
      recrudescent A75.1
    tsutsugamushi A75.3
    typhi A75.2
  endemic (flea-borne) A75.2
  epidemic (louse-borne) A75.0
  exanthematicus SAI A75.0
    brillii SAI A75.1
    mexicanus SAI A75.2
    typhus murinus A75.2
  exanthematic NEC A75.0
  flea-borne A75.2
  India tick A77.1
  Kenya (tick) A77.1
  louse-borne A75.0
  Mexican A75.2
  mite-borne A75.3
  murine A75.2
  North Asian tick-borne A77.2
  petechial A75.9
  Queensland tick A77.3
  rat A75.2
  recrudescent A75.1
  recurrens — see Fever, relapsing
  Sao Paulo A77.0
  scrub (China) (India) (Malaysia) (New Guinea) A75.3
  shop (of Malaysia) A75.2
  Siberian tick A77.2
  tick-borne A77.9
  tropical (mite-borne) A75.3
Tyrosinemia E70.21
  newborn, transitory P74.5
Tyrosinosis E70.21
Tyrosinuria E70.29

U

Uhl's anomaly or disease Q24.8
Ulcer, ulcerated, ulcerating, ulceration, ulcerative
  alveolar process M27.3
  amebic (intestine) A06.1
    skin A06.7
  anastomotic — see Ulcer, gastrojejunal
  anorectal K62.6
  antral — see Ulcer, stomach
  anus (sphincter) (solitary) K62.6
  aorta — see Aneurysm
  aphthous (oral) (recurrent) K12.0
    genital organ(s)
      female N76.6
      male N50.89
  artery I77.2
  atrophic — see Ulcer, skin
    decubitus — see Ulcer, pressure, by site
  back L98.429
    with
      bone involvement without evidence of necrosis L98.426
      bone necrosis L98.424
      exposed fat layer L98.422
      muscle involvement without evidence of necrosis L98.425
      muscle necrosis L98.423
      skin breakdown only L98.421
      specified severity NEC L98.428
  Barrett's (esophagus) K22.10
    with bleeding K22.11
  bile duct (common) (hepatic) K83.8
  bladder (solitary) (sphincter) NEC N32.89
    bilharzial B65.9 [N33]
    in schistosomiasis (bilharzial) B65.9 [N33]
    submucosal — see Cystitis, interstitial
    tuberculous A18.12
  bleeding K27.4
  bone — see Osteomyelitis, specified type NEC
  bowel — see Ulcer, intestine
  breast N61.1
  bronchus J98.09
  buccal (cavity) (traumatic) K12.1
  Buruli A31.1
  buttock L98.419
    with
      bone involvement without evidence of necrosis L98.416
      bone necrosis L98.414
      exposed fat layer L98.412

Ulcer, ulcerated, ulcerating, ulceration, ulcerative
— continued
  buttock — continued
    with — continued
      muscle involvement without evidence of necrosis L98.415
      muscle necrosis L98.413
      skin breakdown only L98.411
      specified severity NEC L98.418
  cancerous — see Neoplasm, malignant, by site
  cardia K22.10
    with bleeding K22.11
  cardioesophageal (peptic) K22.10
    with bleeding K22.11
  cecum — see Ulcer, intestine
  cervix (uteri) (decubitus) (trophic) N86
    with cervicitis N72
  chancroidal A57
  chiclero B55.1
  chronic (cause unknown) — see Ulcer, skin
  Cochin-China B55.1
  colon — see Ulcer, intestine
  conjunctiva H10.89
  cornea H16.00- ☑
    with hypopyon H16.03- ☑
    central H16.01- ☑
    dendritic (herpes simplex) B00.52
    marginal H16.04- ☑
    Mooren's H16.05- ☑
    mycotic H16.06- ☑
    perforated H16.07- ☑
    ring H16.02- ☑
    tuberculous (phlyctenular) A18.52
  corpus cavernosum (chronic) N48.5
  crural — see Ulcer, lower limb
  Curling's — see Ulcer, peptic, acute
  Cushing's — see Ulcer, peptic, acute
  cystic duct K82.8
  cystitis (interstitial) — see Cystitis, interstitial
  decubitus — see Ulcer, pressure, by site
  dendritic, cornea (herpes simplex) B00.52
  diabetes, diabetic — see Diabetes, ulcer
  Dieulafoy's K25.0
  due to
    infection NEC — see Ulcer, skin
    radiation NEC L59.8
    trophic disturbance (any region) — see Ulcer, skin
    X-ray L58.1
  duodenum, duodenal (eroded) (peptic) K26.9
    with
      hemorrhage K26.4
        and perforation K26.6
      perforation K26.5
    acute K26.3
      with
        hemorrhage K26.0
          and perforation K26.2
        perforation K26.1
    chronic K26.7
      with
        hemorrhage K26.4
          and perforation K26.6
        perforation K26.5
  dysenteric A09
  elusive — see Cystitis, interstitial
  endocarditis (acute) (chronic) (subacute) I28.8
  epiglottis J38.7
  esophagus (peptic) K22.10
    with bleeding K22.11
    due to
      aspirin K22.10
        with bleeding K22.11
      gastrointestinal reflux disease K21.0
      ingestion of chemical or medicament K22.10
        with bleeding K22.11
    fungal K22.10
      with bleeding K22.11
    infective K22.10
      with bleeding K22.11
    varicose — see Varix, esophagus
  eyelid (region) H01.8
  fauces J39.2
  Fenwick (-Hunner) (solitary) — see Cystitis, interstitial
  fistulous — see Ulcer, skin
  foot (indolent) (trophic) — see Ulcer, lower limb
  frambesial, initial A66.0
  frenum (tongue) K14.0
  gallbladder or duct K82.8

☑ Additional Character Required — Refer to the Tabular List for Character Selection   ▼ Subterms under main terms may continue to next column or page

Ulcer, ulcerated, ulcerating, ulceration, ulcerative — *continued*
gangrenous — *see* Gangrene
gastric — *see* Ulcer, stomach
gastrocolic — *see* Ulcer, gastrojejunal
gastroduodenal — *see* Ulcer, peptic
gastroesophageal — *see* Ulcer, stomach
gastrointestinal — *see* Ulcer, gastrojejunal
gastrojejunal (peptic) K28.9
  with
    hemorrhage K28.4
      and perforation K28.6
    perforation K28.5
  acute K28.3
    with
      hemorrhage K28.0
        and perforation K28.2
      perforation K28.1
  chronic K28.7
    with
      hemorrhage K28.4
        and perforation K28.6
      perforation K28.5
gastrojejunocolic — *see* Ulcer, gastrojejunal
gingiva K06.8
gingivitis K05.10
  nonplaque induced K05.11
  plaque induced K05.10
glottis J38.7
granuloma of pudenda A58
gum K06.8
gumma, due to yaws A66.4
heel — *see* Ulcer, lower limb
hemorrhoid (*see also* Hemorrhoids, by degree) K64.8
Hunner's — *see* Cystitis, interstitial
hypopharynx J39.2
hypopyon (chronic) (subacute) — *see* Ulcer, cornea, with hypopyon
hypostaticum — *see* Ulcer, varicose
ileum — *see* Ulcer, intestine
intestine, intestinal K63.3
  with perforation K63.1
  amebic A06.1
  duodenal — *see* Ulcer, duodenum
  granulocytopenic (with hemorrhage) — *see* Neutropenia
  marginal — *see* Ulcer, gastrojejunal
  perforating K63.1
    newborn P78.0
  primary, small intestine K63.3
  rectum K62.6
  stercoraceous, stercoral K63.3
  tuberculous A18.32
  typhoid (fever) — *see* Typhoid
  varicose I86.8
jejunum, jejunal — *see* Ulcer, gastrojejunal
keratitis — *see* Ulcer, cornea
knee — *see* Ulcer, lower limb
labium (majus) (minus) N76.6
laryngitis — *see* Laryngitis
larynx (aphthous) (contact) J38.7
  diphtheritic A36.2
leg — *see* Ulcer, lower limb
lip K13.0
Lipschütz's N76.6
lower limb (atrophic) (chronic) (neurogenic) (perforating) (pyogenic) (trophic) (tropical) L97.909
  with
    bone involvement without evidence of necrosis L97.906
    bone necrosis L97.904
    exposed fat layer L97.902
    muscle involvement without evidence of necrosis L97.905
    muscle necrosis L97.903
    skin breakdown only L97.901
    specified severity NEC L97.908
  ankle L97.309
    with
      bone involvement without evidence of necrosis L97.306
      bone necrosis L97.304
      exposed fat layer L97.302
      muscle involvement without evidence of necrosis L97.305
      muscle necrosis L97.303
      skin breakdown only L97.301
      specified severity NEC L97.308

Ulcer, ulcerated, ulcerating, ulceration, ulcerative — *continued*
lower limb — *continued*
  ankle — *continued*
    left L97.329
      with
        bone involvement without evidence of necrosis L97.326
        bone necrosis L97.324
        exposed fat layer L97.322
        muscle involvement without evidence of necrosis L97.325
        muscle necrosis L97.323
        skin breakdown only L97.321
        specified severity NEC L97.328
    right L97.319
      with
        bone involvement without evidence of necrosis L97.316
        bone necrosis L97.314
        exposed fat layer L97.312
        muscle involvement without evidence of necrosis L97.315
        muscle necrosis L97.313
        skin breakdown only L97.311
        specified severity NEC L97.318
  calf L97.209
    with
      bone involvement without evidence of necrosis L97.206
      bone necrosis L97.204
      exposed fat layer L97.202
      muscle involvement without evidence of necrosis L97.205
      muscle necrosis L97.203
      skin breakdown only L97.201
      specified severity NEC L97.208
    left L97.229
      with
        bone involvement without evidence of necrosis L97.226
        bone necrosis L97.224
        exposed fat layer L97.222
        muscle involvement without evidence of necrosis L97.225
        muscle necrosis L97.223
        skin breakdown only L97.221
        specified severity NEC L97.228
    right L97.219
      with
        bone involvement without evidence of necrosis L97.216
        bone necrosis L97.214
        exposed fat layer L97.212
        muscle involvement without evidence of necrosis L97.215
        muscle necrosis L97.213
        skin breakdown only L97.211
        specified severity NEC L97.218
  decubitus — *see* Ulcer, pressure, by site
  foot specified NEC L97.509
    with
      bone involvement without evidence of necrosis L97.506
      bone necrosis L97.504
      exposed fat layer L97.502
      muscle involvement without evidence of necrosis L97.505
      muscle necrosis L97.503
      skin breakdown only L97.501
      specified severity NEC L97.508
    left L97.529
      with
        bone involvement without evidence of necrosis L97.526
        bone necrosis L97.524
        exposed fat layer L97.522
        muscle involvement without evidence of necrosis L97.525
        muscle necrosis L97.523
        skin breakdown only L97.521
        specified severity NEC L97.528
    right L97.519
      with
        bone involvement without evidence of necrosis L97.516
        bone necrosis L97.514
        exposed fat layer L97.512

Ulcer, ulcerated, ulcerating, ulceration, ulcerative — *continued*
lower limb — *continued*
  foot specified — *continued*
    right — *continued*
      with — *continued*
        muscle involvement without evidence of necrosis L97.515
        muscle necrosis L97.513
        skin breakdown only L97.511
        specified severity NEC L97.518
  heel L97.409
    with
      bone involvement without evidence of necrosis L97.406
      bone necrosis L97.404
      exposed fat layer L97.402
      muscle involvement without evidence of necrosis L97.405
      muscle necrosis L97.403
      skin breakdown only L97.401
      specified severity NEC L97.408
    left L97.429
      with
        bone involvement without evidence of necrosis L97.426
        bone necrosis L97.424
        exposed fat layer L97.422
        muscle involvement without evidence of necrosis L97.425
        muscle necrosis L97.423
        skin breakdown only L97.421
        specified severity NEC L97.428
    right L97.419
      with
        bone involvement without evidence of necrosis L97.416
        bone necrosis L97.414
        exposed fat layer L97.412
        muscle involvement without evidence of necrosis L97.415
        muscle necrosis L97.413
        skin breakdown only L97.411
        specified severity NEC L97.418
  left L97.929
    with
      bone involvement without evidence of necrosis L97.926
      bone necrosis L97.924
      exposed fat layer L97.922
      muscle involvement without evidence of necrosis L97.925
      muscle necrosis L97.923
      skin breakdown only L97.921
      specified severity NEC L97.928
  leprous A30.1
  lower leg NOS L97.909
    with
      bone involvement without evidence of necrosis L97.906
      bone necrosis L97.904
      exposed fat layer L97.902
      muscle involvement without evidence of necrosis L97.905
      muscle necrosis L97.903
      skin breakdown only L97.901
      specified severity NEC L97.908
    left L97.929
      with
        bone involvement without evidence of necrosis L97.926
        bone necrosis L97.924
        exposed fat layer L97.922
        muscle involvement without evidence of necrosis L97.925
        muscle necrosis L97.923
        skin breakdown only L97.921
        specified severity NEC L97.928
    right L97.919
      with
        bone involvement without evidence of necrosis L97.916
        bone necrosis L97.914
        exposed fat layer L97.912
        muscle involvement without evidence of necrosis L97.915
        muscle necrosis L97.913
        skin breakdown only L97.911
        specified severity NEC L97.918

Ulcer, ulcerated, ulcerating, ulceration, ulcerative
— *continued*
lower limb — *continued*
  lower leg — *continued*
    specified site NEC L97.809
      with
        bone involvement without evidence of
          necrosis L97.806
        bone necrosis L97.804
        exposed fat layer L97.802
        muscle involvement without evidence of
          necrosis L97.805
        muscle necrosis L97.803
        skin breakdown only L97.801
        specified severity NEC L97.808
    left L97.829
      with
        bone involvement without evidence
          of necrosis L97.826
        bone necrosis L97.824
        exposed fat layer L97.822
        muscle involvement without evidence
          of necrosis L97.825
        muscle necrosis L97.823
        skin breakdown only L97.821
        specified severity NEC L97.828
    right L97.819
      with
        bone involvement without evidence
          of necrosis L97.816
        bone necrosis L97.814
        exposed fat layer L97.812
        muscle involvement without evidence
          of necrosis L97.815
        muscle necrosis L97.813
        skin breakdown only L97.811
        specified severity NEC L97.818
  midfoot L97.409
    with
      bone involvement without evidence of
        necrosis L97.406
      bone necrosis L97.404
      exposed fat layer L97.402
      muscle involvement without evidence of
        necrosis L97.405
      muscle necrosis L97.403
      skin breakdown only L97.401
      specified severity NEC L97.408
    left L97.429
      with
        bone involvement without evidence of
          necrosis L97.426
        bone necrosis L97.424
        exposed fat layer L97.422
        muscle involvement without evidence of
          necrosis L97.425
        muscle necrosis L97.423
        skin breakdown only L97.421
        specified severity NEC L97.428
    right L97.419
      with
        bone involvement without evidence of
          necrosis L97.416
        bone necrosis L97.414
        exposed fat layer L97.412
        muscle involvement without evidence of
          necrosis L97.415
        muscle necrosis L97.413
        skin breakdown only L97.411
        specified severity NEC L97.418
  right L97.919
    with
      bone involvement without evidence of
        necrosis L97.916
      bone necrosis L97.914
      exposed fat layer L97.912
      muscle involvement without evidence of
        necrosis L97.915
      muscle necrosis L97.913
      skin breakdown only L97.911
      specified severity NEC L97.918
  syphilitic A52.19
  thigh L97.109
    with
      bone involvement without evidence of
        necrosis L97.106
      bone necrosis L97.104
      exposed fat layer L97.102

Ulcer, ulcerated, ulcerating, ulceration, ulcerative
— *continued*
lower limb — *continued*
  thigh — *continued*
    with — *continued*
      muscle involvement without evidence of
        necrosis L97.105
      muscle necrosis L97.103
      skin breakdown only L97.101
      specified severity NEC L97.108
    left L97.129
      with
        bone involvement without evidence of
          necrosis L97.126
        bone necrosis L97.124
        exposed fat layer L97.122
        muscle involvement without evidence of
          necrosis L97.125
        muscle necrosis L97.123
        skin breakdown only L97.121
        specified severity NEC L97.128
    right L97.119
      with
        bone involvement without evidence of
          necrosis L97.116
        bone necrosis L97.114
        exposed fat layer L97.112
        muscle involvement without evidence of
          necrosis L97.115
        muscle necrosis L97.113
        skin breakdown only L97.111
        specified severity NEC L97.118
  toe L97.509
    with
      bone involvement without evidence of
        necrosis L97.506
      bone necrosis L97.504
      exposed fat layer L97.502
      muscle involvement without evidence of
        necrosis L97.505
      muscle necrosis L97.503
      skin breakdown only L97.501
      specified severity NEC L97.508
    left L97.529
      with
        bone involvement without evidence of
          necrosis L97.526
        bone necrosis L97.524
        exposed fat layer L97.522
        muscle involvement without evidence of
          necrosis L97.525
        muscle necrosis L97.523
        skin breakdown only L97.521
        specified severity NEC L97.528
    right L97.519
      with
        bone involvement without evidence of
          necrosis L97.516
        bone necrosis L97.514
        exposed fat layer L97.512
        muscle involvement without evidence of
          necrosis L97.515
        muscle necrosis L97.513
        skin breakdown only L97.511
        specified severity NEC L97.518
  varicose — *see* Varix, leg, with, ulcer
luetic — *see* Ulcer, syphilitic
lung J98.4
  tuberculous — *see* Tuberculosis, pulmonary
malignant — *see* Neoplasm, malignant, by site
marginal NEC — *see* Ulcer, gastrojejunal
meatus (urinarius) N34.2
Meckel's diverticulum Q43.0
  malignant — *see* Table of Neoplasms, small intes-
    tine, malignant
Meleney's (chronic undermining) — *see* Ulcer, skin
Mooren's (cornea) — *see* Ulcer, cornea, Mooren's
mycobacterial (skin) A31.1
nasopharynx J39.2
neck, uterus N86
neurogenic NEC — *see* Ulcer, skin
nose, nasal (passage) (infective) (septum) J34.0
  skin — *see* Ulcer, skin
  spirochetal A69.8
  varicose (bleeding) I86.8
oral mucosa (traumatic) K12.1
palate (soft) K12.1
penis (chronic) N48.5

Ulcer, ulcerated, ulcerating, ulceration, ulcerative
— *continued*
peptic (site unspecified) K27.9
  with
    hemorrhage K27.4
      and perforation K27.6
    perforation K27.5
  acute K27.3
    with
      hemorrhage K27.0
        and perforation K27.2
      perforation K27.1
  chronic K27.7
    with
      hemorrhage K27.4
        and perforation K27.6
      perforation K27.5
  esophagus K22.10
    with bleeding K22.11
  newborn P78.82
perforating K27.5
  skin — *see* Ulcer, skin
peritonsillar J35.8
phagedenic (tropical) — *see* Ulcer, skin
pharynx J39.2
phlebitis — *see* Phlebitis
plaster — *see* Ulcer, pressure, by site
popliteal space — *see* Ulcer, lower limb
postpyloric — *see* Ulcer, duodenum
prepuce N47.7
prepyloric — *see* Ulcer, stomach
pressure (pressure area) L89.9- ☑
  ankle L89.5- ☑
  back L89.1- ☑
  buttock L89.3- ☑
  coccyx L89.15- ☑
  contiguous site of back, buttock, hip L89.4- ☑
  elbow L89.0- ☑
  face L89.81- ☑
  head L89.81- ☑
  heel L89.6- ☑
  hip L89.2- ☑
  sacral region (tailbone) L89.15- ☑
  specified site NEC L89.89- ☑
  stage 1 (healing) (pre-ulcer skin changes limited to
      persistent focal edema)
    ankle L89.5- ☑
    back L89.1- ☑
    buttock L89.3- ☑
    coccyx L89.15- ☑
    contiguous site of back, buttock, hip L89.4- ☑
    elbow L89.0- ☑
    face L89.81- ☑
    head L89.81- ☑
    heel L89.6- ☑
    hip L89.2- ☑
    sacral region (tailbone) L89.15- ☑
    specified site NEC L89.89- ☑
  stage 2 (healing) (abrasion, blister, partial thickness
      skin loss involving epidermis and/or dermis)
    ankle L89.5- ☑
    back L89.1- ☑
    buttock L89.3- ☑
    coccyx L89.15- ☑
    contiguous site of back, buttock, hip L89.4- ☑
    elbow L89.0- ☑
    face L89.81- ☑
    head L89.81- ☑
    heel L89.6- ☑
    hip L89.2- ☑
    sacral region (tailbone) L89.15- ☑
    specified site NEC L89.89- ☑
  stage 3 (healing) (full thickness skin loss involving
      damage or necrosis of subcutaneous tissue)
    ankle L89.5- ☑
    back L89.1- ☑
    buttock L89.3- ☑
    coccyx L89.15- ☑
    contiguous site of back, buttock, hip L89.4- ☑
    elbow L89.0- ☑
    face L89.81- ☑
    head L89.81- ☑
    heel L89.6- ☑
    hip L89.2- ☑
    sacral region (tailbone) L89.15- ☑
    specified site NEC L89.89- ☑

☑ Additional Character Required — Refer to the Tabular List for Character Selection   ▽ Subterms under main terms may continue to next column or page

Ulcer, ulcerated, ulcerating, ulceration, ulcerative
— *continued*
  pressure — *continued*
    stage 4 (healing) (necrosis of soft tissues through to underlying muscle, tendon, or bone)
      ankle L89.5- ☑
      back L89.1- ☑
      buttock L89.3- ☑
      coccyx L89.15- ☑
      contiguous site of back, buttock, hip L89.4- ☑
      elbow L89.0- ☑
      face L89.81- ☑
      head L89.81- ☑
      heel L89.6- ☑
      hip L89.2- ☑
      sacral region (tailbone) L89.15- ☑
      specified site NEC L89.89- ☑
    unspecified stage
      ankle L89.5- ☑
      back L89.1- ☑
      buttock L89.3- ☑
      coccyx L89.15- ☑
      contiguous site of back, buttock, hip L89.4- ☑
      elbow L89.0- ☑
      face L89.81- ☑
      head L89.81- ☑
      heel L89.6- ☑
      hip L89.2- ☑
      sacral region (tailbone) L89.15- ☑
      specified site NEC L89.89- ☑
    unstageable
      ankle L89.5- ☑
      back L89.1- ☑
      buttock L89.3- ☑
      coccyx L89.15- ☑
      contiguous site of back, buttock, hip L89.4- ☑
      elbow L89.0- ☑
      face L89.81- ☑
      head L89.81- ☑
      heel L89.6- ☑
      hip L89.2- ☑
      sacral region (tailbone) L89.15- ☑
      specified site NEC L89.89- ☑
  primary of intestine K63.3
    with perforation K63.1
  prostate N41.9
  pyloric — *see* Ulcer, stomach
  rectosigmoid K63.3
    with perforation K63.1
  rectum (sphincter) (solitary) K62.6
    stercoraceous, stercoral K62.6
  retina — *see* Inflammation, chorioretinal
  rodent (*see also* Neoplasm, skin, malignant)
  sclera — *see* Scleritis
  scrofulous (tuberculous) A18.2
  scrotum N50.89
    tuberculous A18.15
    varicose I86.1
  seminal vesicle N50.89
  sigmoid — *see* Ulcer, intestine
  skin (atrophic) (chronic) (neurogenic) (non-healing) (perforating) (pyogenic) (trophic) (tropical) L98.499
    with gangrene — *see* Gangrene
    amebic A06.7
    back — *see* Ulcer, back
    buttock — *see* Ulcer, buttock
    decubitus — *see* Ulcer, pressure
    lower limb — *see* Ulcer, lower limb
    mycobacterial A31.1
    specified site NEC L98.499
      with
        bone involvement without evidence of necrosis L98.496
        bone necrosis L98.494
        exposed fat layer L98.492
        muscle involvement without evidence of necrosis L98.495
        muscle necrosis L98.493
        skin breakdown only L98.491
        specified severity NEC L98.498
    tuberculous (primary) A18.4
    varicose — *see* Ulcer, varicose
  sloughing — *see* Ulcer, skin
  solitary, anus or rectum (sphincter) K62.6
  sore throat J02.9
    streptococcal J02.0

Ulcer, ulcerated, ulcerating, ulceration, ulcerative
— *continued*
  spermatic cord N50.89
  spine (tuberculous) A18.01
  stasis (venous) — *see* Varix, leg, with, ulcer
    without varicose veins I87.2
  stercoraceous, stercoral K63.3
    with perforation K63.1
    anus or rectum K62.6
  stoma, stomal — *see* Ulcer, gastrojejunal
  stomach (eroded) (peptic) (round) K25.9
    with
      hemorrhage K25.4
        and perforation K25.6
      perforation K25.5
    acute K25.3
      with
        hemorrhage K25.0
          and perforation K25.2
        perforation K25.1
    chronic K25.7
      with
        hemorrhage K25.4
          and perforation K25.6
        perforation K25.5
  stomal — *see* Ulcer, gastrojejunal
  stomatitis K12.1
  stress — *see* Ulcer, peptic
  strumous (tuberculous) A18.2
  submucosal, bladder — *see* Cystitis, interstitial
  syphilitic (any site) (early) (secondary) A51.39
    late A52.79
      perforating A52.79
        foot A52.11
  testis N50.89
  thigh — *see* Ulcer, lower limb
  throat J39.2
    diphtheritic A36.0
  toe — *see* Ulcer, lower limb
  tongue (traumatic) K14.0
  tonsil J35.8
    diphtheritic A36.0
  trachea J39.8
  trophic — *see* Ulcer, skin
  tropical — *see* Ulcer, skin
  tuberculous — *see* Tuberculosis, ulcer
  tunica vaginalis N50.89
  turbinate J34.89
  typhoid (perforating) — *see* Typhoid
  unspecified site — *see* Ulcer, skin
  urethra (meatus) — *see* Urethritis
  uterus N85.8
    cervix N86
      with cervicitis N72
    neck N86
      with cervicitis N72
  vagina N76.5
    in Behçet's disease M35.2 [N77.0]
    pessary N89.8
  valve, heart I33.0
  varicose (lower limb, any part) (*see also* Varix, leg, with, ulcer)
    broad ligament I86.2
    esophagus — *see* Varix, esophagus
    inflamed or infected — *see* Varix, leg, with ulcer, with inflammation
    nasal septum I86.8
    perineum I86.3
    scrotum I86.1
    specified site NEC I86.8
    sublingual I86.0
    vulva I86.3
  vas deferens N50.89
  vulva (acute) (infectional) N76.6
    in (due to)
      Behçet's disease M35.2 [N77.0]
      herpesviral (herpes simplex) infection A60.04
      tuberculosis A18.18
  vulvobuccal, recurring N76.6
  X-ray L58.1
  yaws A66.4

Ulcerosa scarlatina A38.8
Ulcus (*see also* Ulcer)
  cutis tuberculosum A18.4
  duodeni — *see* Ulcer, duodenum
  durum (syphilitic) A51.0
    extragenital A51.2
  gastrojejunale — *see* Ulcer, gastrojejunal

Ulcus — *continued*
  hypostaticum — *see* Ulcer, varicose
  molle (cutis) (skin) A57
  serpens corneae — *see* Ulcer, cornea, central
  ventriculi — *see* Ulcer, stomach
Ulegyria Q04.8
Ulerythema
  ophryogenes, congenital Q84.2
  sycosiforme L73.8
Ullrich (-Bonnevie)(-Turner) **syndrome** (*see also* Turner's syndrome) Q87.1
Ullrich-Feichtiger syndrome Q87.0
Ulnar — *see* condition
Ulorrhagia, ulorrhea K06.8
Umbilicus, umbilical — *see* condition
Unacceptable
  contours of tooth K08.54
  morphology of tooth K08.54
Unavailability (of)
  bed at medical facility Z75.1
  health service-related agencies Z75.4
  medical facilities (at) Z75.3
    due to
      investigation by social service agency Z75.2
      lack of services at home Z75.0
      remoteness from facility Z75.3
      waiting list Z75.1
    home Z75.0
    outpatient clinic Z75.3
  schooling Z55.1
  social service agencies Z75.4
Uncinaria americana infestation B76.1
Uncinariasis B76.9
Uncongenial work Z56.5
Unconscious (ness) — *see* Coma
Under observation — *see* Observation
Underachievement in school Z55.3
Underdevelopment (*see also* Undeveloped)
  nose Q30.1
  sexual E30.0
Underdosing (*see also* Table of Drugs and Chemicals, categories T36-T50, with final character 6) Z91.14
  intentional NEC Z91.128
    due to financial hardship of patient Z91.120
  unintentional NEC Z91.138
    due to patient's age related debility Z91.130
Underfeeding, newborn P92.3
Underfill, endodontic M27.53
Underimmunization status Z28.3
Undernourishment — *see* Malnutrition
Undernutrition — *see* Malnutrition
Underweight R63.6
  for gestational age — *see* Light for dates
Underwood's disease P83.0
Undescended (*see also* Malposition, congenital)
  cecum Q43.3
  colon Q43.3
  testicle — *see* Cryptorchid
Undeveloped, undevelopment (*see also* Hypoplasia)
  brain (congenital) Q02
  cerebral (congenital) Q02
  heart Q24.8
  lung Q33.6
  testis E29.1
  uterus E30.0
Undiagnosed (disease) R69
Undulant fever — *see* Brucellosis
Unemployment, anxiety concerning Z56.0
  threatened Z56.2
Unequal length (acquired) (limb) (*see also* Deformity, limb, unequal length)
  leg (*see also* Deformity, limb, unequal length)
    congenital Q72.9- ☑
Unextracted dental root K08.3
Unguis incarnatus L60.0
Unhappiness R45.2
Unicornate uterus Q51.4
  in pregnancy or childbirth O34.00
Unilateral (*see also* condition)
  development, breast N64.89
  organ or site, congenital NEC — *see* Agenesis, by site
Unilocular heart Q20.8
Union, abnormal (*see also* Fusion)
  larynx and trachea Q34.8
Universal mesentery Q43.3
Unrepairable overhanging of dental restorative materials K08.52

Unsatisfactory
restoration of tooth K08.50
specified NEC K08.59
sample of cytologic smear
anus R85.615
cervix R87.615
vagina R87.625
surroundings Z59.1
work Z56.5
Unsoundness of mind — *see* Psychosis
Unstable
back NEC — *see* Instability, joint, spine
hip (congenital) Q65.6
acquired — *see* Derangement, joint, specified type NEC, hip
joint — *see* Instability, joint
secondary to removal of joint prosthesis M96.89
lie (mother) O32.0 ☑
lumbosacral joint (congenital)
acquired — *see* subcategory M53.2 ☑
sacroiliac — *see* subcategory M53.2 ☑
spine NEC — *see* Instability, joint, spine
Unsteadiness on feet R26.81
Untruthfulness, child problem F91.8
Unverricht (-Lundborg) **disease or epilepsy** — *see* Epilepsy, generalized, idiopathic
Unwanted pregnancy Z64.0
Upbringing, institutional Z62.22
away from parents NEC Z62.29
in care of non-parental family member Z62.21
in foster care Z62.21
in orphanage or group home Z62.22
in welfare custody Z62.21
Upper respiratory — *see* condition
Upset
gastric K30
gastrointestinal K30
psychogenic F45.8
intestinal (large) (small) K59.9
psychogenic F45.8
menstruation N93.9
mental F48.9
stomach K30
psychogenic F45.8
Urachus (*see also* condition)
patent or persistent Q64.4
Urbach-Oppenheim disease (necrobiosis lipoidica diabeticorum) — *see* E08-E13 with .620
Urbach's lipoid proteinosis E78.89
Urbach-Wiethe disease E78.89
Urban yellow fever A95.1
Urea
blood, high — *see* Uremia
cycle metabolism disorder — *see* Disorder, urea cycle metabolism
Uremia, uremic N19
with
ectopic or molar pregnancy O08.4
polyneuropathy N18.9 [G63]
chronic NOS (*see also* Disease, kidney, chronic) N18.9
due to hypertension — *see* Hypertensive, kidney
complicating
ectopic or molar pregnancy O08.4
congenital P96.0
extrarenal R39.2
following ectopic or molar pregnancy O08.4
newborn P96.0
prerenal R39.2
Ureter, ureteral — *see* condition
Ureteralgia N23
Ureterectasis — *see* Hydroureter
Ureteritis N28.89
cystica N28.86
due to calculus N20.1
with calculus, kidney N20.2
with hydronephrosis N13.2
gonococcal (acute) (chronic) A54.21
nonspecific N28.89
Ureterocele N28.89
congenital (orthotopic) Q62.31
ectopic Q62.32
Ureterolith, ureterolithiasis — *see* Calculus, ureter
Ureterostomy
attention to Z43.6
status Z93.6
Urethra, urethral — *see* condition
Urethralgia R39.89

Urethritis (anterior) (posterior) N34.2
calculous N21.1
candidal B37.41
chlamydial A56.01
diplococcal (gonococcal) A54.01
with abscess (accessory gland) (periurethral) A54.1
gonococcal A54.01
with abscess (accessory gland) (periurethral) A54.1
nongonococcal N34.1
Reiter's — *see* Reiter's disease
nonspecific N34.1
nonvenereal N34.1
postmenopausal N34.2
puerperal O86.22
Reiter's — *see* Reiter's disease
specified NEC N34.2
trichomonal or due to Trichomonas (vaginalis) A59.03
Urethrocele N81.0
with
cystocele — *see* Cystocele
prolapse of uterus — *see* Prolapse, uterus
Urethrolithiasis (with colic or infection) N21.1
Urethrorectal — *see* condition
Urethrorrhagia N36.8
Urethrorrhea R36.9
Urethrostomy
attention to Z43.6
status Z93.6
Urethrotrigonitis — *see* Trigonitis
Urethrovaginal — *see* condition
Urgency
fecal R15.2
hypertensive — *see* Hypertension
urinary R39.15
Urhidrosis, uridrosis L74.8
Uric acid in blood (increased) E79.0
Uricacidemia (asymptomatic) E79.0
Uricemia (asymptomatic) E79.0
Uricosuria R82.998
Urinary — *see* condition
Urination
frequent R35.0
painful R30.9
Urine
blood in — *see* Hematuria
discharge, excessive R35.8
enuresis, nonorganic origin F98.0
extravasation R39.0
frequency R35.0
incontinence R32
nonorganic origin F98.0
intermittent stream R39.198
pus in N39.0
retention or stasis R33.9
organic R33.8
drug-induced R33.0
psychogenic F45.8
secretion
deficient R34
excessive R35.8
frequency R35.0
stream
intermittent R39.198
slowing R39.198
splitting R39.13
weak R39.12
Urinemia — *see* Uremia
Urinoma, urethra N36.8
Uroarthritis, infectious (Reiter's) — *see* Reiter's disease
Urodialysis R34
Urolithiasis — *see* Calculus, urinary
Uronephrosis — *see* Hydronephrosis
Uropathy N39.9
obstructive N13.9
specified NEC N13.8
reflux N13.9
specified NEC N13.8
vesicoureteral reflux-associated — *see* Reflux, vesicoureteral
Urosepsis — *code to* condition
Urticaria L50.9
with angioneurotic edema T78.3 ☑
hereditary D84.1
allergic L50.0
cholinergic L50.5
chronic L50.8
cold, familial L50.2
contact L50.6

Urticaria — *continued*
dermatographic L50.3
due to
cold or heat L50.2
drugs L50.0
food L50.0
inhalants L50.0
plants L50.6
serum (*see also* Reaction, serum) T80.69 ☑
factitial L50.3
familial cold M04.2
giant T78.3 ☑
hereditary D84.1
gigantea T78.3 ☑
idiopathic L50.1
larynx T78.3 ☑
hereditary D84.1
neonatorum P83.88
nonallergic L50.1
papulosa (Hebra) L28.2
pigmentosa D47.01
congenital Q82.2
of neonatal onset Q82.2
of newborn onset Q82.2
recurrent periodic L50.8
serum (*see also* Reaction, serum) T80.69 ☑
solar L56.3
specified type NEC L50.8
thermal (cold) (heat) L50.2
vibratory L50.4
xanthelasmoidea — *see* Urticaria pigmentosa
Use (of)
alcohol Z72.89
with
intoxication F10.929
sleep disorder F10.982
harmful — *see* Abuse, alcohol
amphetamines — *see* Use, stimulant NEC
caffeine — *see* Use, stimulant NEC
cannabis F12.90
with
anxiety disorder F12.980
intoxication F12.929
with
delirium F12.921
perceptual disturbance F12.922
uncomplicated F12.920
other specified disorder F12.988
psychosis F12.959
delusions F12.950
hallucinations F12.951
unspecified disorder F12.99
withdrawal F12.93
cocaine F14.90
with
anxiety disorder F14.980
intoxication F14.929
with
delirium F14.921
perceptual disturbance F14.922
uncomplicated F14.920
other specified disorder F14.988
psychosis F14.959
delusions F14.950
hallucinations F14.951
sexual dysfunction F14.981
sleep disorder F14.982
unspecified disorder F14.99
harmful — *see* Abuse, drug, cocaine
drug(s) NEC F19.90
with sleep disorder F19.982
harmful — *see* Abuse, drug, by type
hallucinogen NEC F16.90
with
anxiety disorder F16.980
intoxication F16.929
with
delirium F16.921
uncomplicated F16.920
mood disorder F16.94
other specified disorder F16.988
perception disorder (flashbacks) F16.983
psychosis F16.959
delusions F16.950
hallucinations F16.951
unspecified disorder F16.99
harmful — *see* Abuse, drug, hallucinogen NEC
inhalants F18.90

☑ **Additional Character Required** — Refer to the Tabular List for Character Selection   ▽ **Subterms under main terms may continue to next column or page**

Unsatisfactory — Use

Use — *continued*
  inhalants — *continued*
    with
      anxiety disorder F18.980
      intoxication F18.929
        with delirium F18.921
        uncomplicated F18.920
      mood disorder F18.94
      other specified disorder F18.988
      persisting dementia F18.97
      psychosis F18.959
        delusions F18.950
        hallucinations F18.951
      unspecified disorder F18.99
    harmful — *see* Abuse, drug, inhalant
  methadone — *see* Use, opioid
  nonprescribed drugs F19.90
    harmful — *see* Abuse, non-psychoactive substance
  opioid F11.90
    with
      disorder F11.99
        mood F11.94
        sleep F11.982
        specified type NEC F11.988
      intoxication F11.929
        with
          delirium F11.921
          perceptual disturbance F11.922
        uncomplicated F11.920
      withdrawal F11.93
    harmful — *see* Abuse, drug, opioid
  patent medicines F19.90
    harmful — *see* Abuse, non-psychoactive substance
  psychoactive drug NEC F19.90
    with
      anxiety disorder F19.980
      intoxication F19.929
        with
          delirium F19.921
          perceptual disturbance F19.922
        uncomplicated F19.920
      mood disorder F19.94
      other specified disorder F19.988
      persisting
        amnestic disorder F19.96
        dementia F19.97
      psychosis F19.959
        delusions F19.950
        hallucinations F19.951
      sexual dysfunction F19.981
      sleep disorder F19.982
      unspecified disorder F19.99
      withdrawal F19.939
        with
          delirium F19.931
          perceptual disturbance F19.932
        uncomplicated F19.930
    harmful — *see* Abuse, drug NEC, psychoactive NEC
  sedative, hypnotic, or anxiolytic F13.90
    with
      anxiety disorder F13.980
      intoxication F13.929
        with
          delirium F13.921
        uncomplicated F13.920
      other specified disorder F13.988
      persisting
        amnestic disorder F13.96
        dementia F13.97
      psychosis F13.959
        delusions F13.950
        hallucinations F13.951
      sexual dysfunction F13.981
      sleep disorder F13.982
      unspecified disorder F13.99
    harmful — *see* Abuse, drug, sedative, hypnotic, or anxiolytic
  stimulant NEC F15.90
    with
      anxiety disorder F15.980
      intoxication F15.929
        with
          delirium F15.921
          perceptual disturbance F15.922
        uncomplicated F15.920
      mood disorder F15.94
      other specified disorder F15.988
      psychosis F15.959

Use — *continued*
  stimulant — *continued*
    with — *continued*
      psychosis — *continued*
        delusions F15.950
        hallucinations F15.951
      sexual dysfunction F15.981
      sleep disorder F15.982
      unspecified disorder F15.99
      withdrawal F15.93
    harmful — *see* Abuse, drug, stimulant NEC
  tobacco Z72.0
    with dependence — *see* Dependence, drug, nicotine
  volatile solvents (*see also* Use, inhalant) F18.90
    harmful — *see* Abuse, drug, inhalant
Usher-Senear disease or syndrome L10.4
Uta B55.1
Uteromegaly N85.2
Uterovaginal — *see* condition
Uterovesical — *see* condition
Uveal — *see* condition
Uveitis (anterior) (*see also* Iridocyclitis)
  acute — *see* Iridocyclitis, acute
  chronic — *see* Iridocyclitis, chronic
  due to toxoplasmosis (acquired) B58.09
    congenital P37.1
  granulomatous — *see* Iridocyclitis, chronic
  heterochromic — *see* Cyclitis, Fuchs' heterochromic
  lens-induced — *see* Iridocyclitis, lens-induced
  posterior — *see* Chorioretinitis
  sympathetic H44.13-☑
  syphilitic (secondary) A51.43
    congenital (early) A50.01
    late A52.71
  tuberculous A18.54
Uveoencephalitis — *see* Inflammation, chorioretinal
Uveokeratitis — *see* Iridocyclitis
Uveoparotitis D86.89
Uvula — *see* condition
Uvulitis (acute) (catarrhal) (chronic) (membranous) (suppurative) (ulcerative) K12.2

V

Vaccination (prophylactic)
  complication or reaction — *see* Complications, vaccination
  delayed Z28.9
  encounter for Z23
  not done — *see* Immunization, not done, because (of)
Vaccinia (generalized) (localized) T88.1 ☑
  congenital P35.8
  without vaccination B08.011
Vacuum, in sinus (accessory) (nasal) J34.89
Vagabond, vagabondage Z59.0
Vagabond's disease B85.1
Vagina, vaginal — *see* condition
Vaginalitis (tunica) (testis) N49.1
Vaginismus (reflex) N94.2
  functional F52.5
  nonorganic F52.5
  psychogenic F52.5
  secondary N94.2
Vaginitis (acute) (circumscribed) (diffuse) (emphysematous) (nonvenereal) (ulcerative) N76.0
  with ectopic or molar pregnancy O08.0
  amebic A06.82
  atrophic, postmenopausal N95.2
  bacterial N76.0
  blennorrhagic (gonococcal) A54.02
  candidal B37.3
  chlamydial A56.02
  chronic N76.1
  due to Trichomonas (vaginalis) A59.01
  following ectopic or molar pregnancy O08.0
  gonococcal A54.02
    with abscess (accessory gland) (periurethral) A54.1
  granuloma A58
  in (due to)
    candidiasis B37.3
    herpesviral (herpes simplex) infection A60.04
    pinworm infection B80 [N77.1]
  monilial B37.3
  mycotic (candidal) B37.3
  postmenopausal atrophic N95.2
  puerperal (postpartum) O86.13
  senile (atrophic) N95.2

Vaginitis — *continued*
  subacute or chronic N76.1
  syphilitic (early) A51.0
    late A52.76
  trichomonal A59.01
  tuberculous A18.18
Vaginosis — *see* Vaginitis
Vagotonia G52.2
Vagrancy Z59.0
VAIN — *see* Neoplasia, intraepithelial, vagina
Vallecula — *see* condition
Valley fever B38.0
Valsuani's disease — *see* Anemia, obstetric
Valve, valvular (formation) (*see also* condition)
  cerebral ventricle (communicating) in situ Z98.2
  cervix, internal os Q51.828
  congenital NEC — *see* Atresia, by site
  ureter (pelvic junction) (vesical orifice) Q62.39
  urethra (congenital) (posterior) Q64.2
Valvulitis (chronic) — *see* Endocarditis
Valvulopathy — *see* Endocarditis
Van Bogaert's leukoencephalopathy (sclerosing) (subacute) A81.1
Van Bogaert-Scherer-Epstein disease or syndrome E75.5
Van Buchem's syndrome M85.2
Van Creveld-von Gierke disease E74.01
Van der Hoeve (-de Kleyn) **syndrome** Q78.0
Van der Woude's syndrome Q38.0
Van Neck's disease or osteochondrosis M91.0
Vanishing lung J44.9
Vapor asphyxia or suffocation T59.9 ☑
  specified agent — *see* Table of Drugs and Chemicals
Variance, lethal ball, prosthetic heart valve T82.09 ☑
Variants, thalassemic D56.8
Variations in hair color L67.1
Varicella B01.9
  with
    complications NEC B01.89
    encephalitis B01.11
    encephalomyelitis B01.11
    meningitis B01.0
    myelitis B01.12
    pneumonia B01.2
  congenital P35.8
Varices — *see* Varix
Varicocele (scrotum) (thrombosed) I86.1
  ovary I86.2
  perineum I86.3
  spermatic cord (ulcerated) I86.1
Varicose
  aneurysm (ruptured) I77.0
  dermatitis — *see* Varix, leg, with, inflammation
  eczema — *see* Varix, leg, with, inflammation
  phlebitis — *see* Varix, with, inflammation
  tumor — *see* Varix
  ulcer (lower limb, any part) (*see also* Varix, leg, with, ulcer)
    anus (*see also* Hemorrhoids) K64.8
    esophagus — *see* Varix, esophagus
    inflamed or infected — *see* Varix, leg, with ulcer, with inflammation
    nasal septum I86.8
    perineum I86.3
    scrotum I86.1
    specified site NEC I86.8
  vein — *see* Varix
  vessel — *see* Varix, leg
Varicosis, varicosities, varicosity — *see* Varix
Variola (major) (minor) B03
Varioloid B03
Varix (lower limb) (ruptured) I83.90
  with
    edema I83.899
    inflammation I83.10
      with ulcer (venous) I83.209
    pain I83.819
    specified complication NEC I83.899
    stasis dermatitis I83.10
      with ulcer (venous) I83.209
    swelling I83.899
    ulcer I83.009
      with inflammation I83.209
  aneurysmal I77.0
  asymptomatic I83.9- ☑
  bladder I86.2
  broad ligament I86.2

Index

Varix — *continued*
  complicating
    childbirth (lower extremity) O87.4
      anus or rectum O87.2
      genital (vagina, vulva or perineum) O87.8
    pregnancy (lower extremity) O22.0- ☑
      anus or rectum O22.4- ☑
      genital (vagina, vulva or perineum) O22.1- ☑
    puerperium (lower extremity) O87.4
      anus or rectum O87.2
      genital (vagina, vulva, perineum) O87.8
  congenital (any site) Q27.8
  esophagus (idiopathic) (primary) (ulcerated) I85.00
    bleeding I85.01
    congenital Q27.8
    in (due to)
      alcoholic liver disease I85.10
        bleeding I85.11
      cirrhosis of liver I85.10
        bleeding I85.11
      portal hypertension I85.10
        bleeding I85.11
      schistosomiasis I85.10
        bleeding I85.11
      toxic liver disease I85.10
        bleeding I85.11
    secondary I85.10
      bleeding I85.11
  gastric I86.4
  inflamed or infected I83.10
    ulcerated I83.209
  labia (majora) I86.3
  leg (asymptomatic) I83.90
    with
      edema I83.899
      inflammation I83.10
        with ulcer — *see* Varix, leg, with, ulcer, with
          inflammation by site
      pain I83.819
      specified complication NEC I83.899
      swelling I83.899
      ulcer I83.009
        with inflammation I83.209
        ankle I83.003
          with inflammation I83.203
        calf I83.002
          with inflammation I83.202
        foot NEC I83.005
          with inflammation I83.205
        heel I83.004
          with inflammation I83.204
        lower leg NEC I83.008
          with inflammation I83.208
        midfoot I83.004
          with inflammation I83.204
        thigh I83.001
          with inflammation I83.201
    bilateral (asymptomatic) I83.93
      with
        edema I83.893
        pain I83.813
        specified complication NEC I83.893
        swelling I83.893
        ulcer I83.0- ☑
          with inflammation I83.209
    left (asymptomatic) I83.92
      with
        edema I83.892
        inflammation I83.12
          with ulcer — *see* Varix, leg, with, ulcer,
            with inflammation by site
        pain I83.812
        specified complication NEC I83.892
        swelling I83.892
        ulcer I83.029
          with inflammation I83.229
          ankle I83.023
            with inflammation I83.223
          calf I83.022
            with inflammation I83.222
          foot NEC I83.025
            with inflammation I83.225
          heel I83.024
            with inflammation I83.224
          lower leg NEC I83.028
            with inflammation I83.228
          midfoot I83.024
            with inflammation I83.224

Varix — *continued*
  leg — *continued*
    left — *continued*
      with — *continued*
        ulcer — *continued*
          thigh I83.021
            with inflammation I83.221
    right (asymptomatic) I83.91
      with
        edema I83.891
        inflammation I83.11
          with ulcer — *see* Varix, leg, with, ulcer,
            with inflammation by site
        pain I83.811
        specified complication NEC I83.891
        swelling I83.891
        ulcer I83.019
          with inflammation I83.219
          ankle I83.013
            with inflammation I83.213
          calf I83.012
            with inflammation I83.212
          foot NEC I83.015
            with inflammation I83.215
          heel I83.014
            with inflammation I83.214
          lower leg NEC I83.018
            with inflammation I83.218
          midfoot I83.014
            with inflammation I83.214
          thigh I83.011
            with inflammation I83.211
  nasal septum I86.8
  orbit I86.8
    congenital Q27.8
  ovary I86.2
  papillary I78.1
  pelvis I86.2
  perineum I86.3
  pharynx I86.8
  placenta O43.89- ☑
  renal papilla I86.8
  retina H35.09
  scrotum (ulcerated) I86.1
  sigmoid colon I86.8
  specified site NEC I86.8
  spinal (cord) (vessels) I86.8
  spleen, splenic (vein) (with phlebolith) I86.8
  stomach I86.4
  sublingual I86.0
  ulcerated I83.009
    inflamed or infected I83.209
  uterine ligament I86.2
  vagina I86.8
  vocal cord I86.8
  vulva I86.3
Vas deferens — *see* condition
Vas deferentitis N49.1
Vasa previa O69.4 ☑
  hemorrhage from, affecting newborn P50.0
Vascular (*see also* condition)
  loop on optic papilla Q14.2
  spasm I73.9
  spider I78.1
Vascularization, cornea — *see* Neovascularization,
  cornea
Vasculitis I77.6
  allergic D69.0
  cryoglobulinemic D89.1
  disseminated I77.6
  hypocomplementemic M31.8
  kidney I77.89
  livedoid L95.0
  nodular L95.8
  retina H35.06- ☑
  rheumatic — *see* Fever, rheumatic
  rheumatoid — *see* Rheumatoid, vasculitis
  skin (limited to) L95.9
    specified NEC L95.8
  systemic M31.8
Vasculopathy, necrotizing M31.9
  cardiac allograft T86.290
  specified NEC M31.8
Vasitis (nodosa) N49.1
  tuberculous A18.15
Vasodilation I73.9
Vasomotor — *see* condition
Vasoplasty, after previous sterilization Z31.0

Vasoplasty, after previous sterilization —
  continued
  aftercare Z31.42
Vasospasm (vasoconstriction) I73.9
  cerebral (cerebrovascular) (artery) I67.848
    reversible I67.841
  coronary I20.1
  nerve
    arm — *see* Mononeuropathy, upper limb
    brachial plexus G54.0
    cervical plexus G54.2
    leg — *see* Mononeuropathy, lower limb
  peripheral NOS I73.9
  retina (artery) — *see* Occlusion, artery, retina
Vasospastic — *see* condition
Vasovagal attack (paroxysmal) R55
  psychogenic F45.8
VATER syndrome Q87.2
Vater's ampulla — *see* condition
Vegetation, vegetative
  adenoid (nasal fossa) J35.8
  endocarditis (acute) (any valve) (subacute) I33.0
  heart (mycotic) (valve) I33.0
Veil
  Jackson's Q43.3
Vein, venous — *see* condition
Veldt sore — *see* Ulcer, skin
Velpeau's hernia — *see* Hernia, femoral
Venereal
  bubo A55
  disease A64
  granuloma inguinale A58
  lymphogranuloma (Durand-Nicolas-Favre) A55
Venofibrosis I87.8
Venom, venomous — *see* Table of Drugs and Chemicals,
  by animal or substance, poisoning
Venous — *see* condition
Ventilator lung, newborn P27.8
Ventral — *see* condition
Ventricle, ventricular (*see also* condition)
  escape I49.3
  inversion Q20.5
Ventriculitis (cerebral) (*see also* Encephalitis) G04.90
Ventriculostomy status Z98.2
Vernet's syndrome G52.7
Verneuil's disease (syphilitic bursitis) A52.78
Verruca (due to HPV) (filiformis) (simplex) (viral) (vulgaris)
  B07.9
  acuminata A63.0
  necrogenica (primary) (tuberculosa) A18.4
  plana B07.8
  plantaris B07.0
  seborrheica L82.1
    inflamed L82.0
  senile (seborrheic) L82.1
    inflamed L82.0
  tuberculosa (primary) A18.4
  venereal A63.0
Verrucosities — *see* Verruca
Verruga peruana, peruviana A44.1
Version
  with extraction
  cervix — *see* Malposition, uterus
  uterus (postinfectional) (postpartal, old) — *see* Malpo-
    sition, uterus
Vertebra, vertebral — *see* condition
Vertical talus (congenital) Q66.80
  left foot Q66.82
  right foot Q66.81
Vertigo R42
  auditory — *see* Vertigo, aural
  aural H81.31- ☑
  benign paroxysmal (positional) H81.1- ☑
  central (origin) H81.4- ☑
  cerebral H81.4- ☑
  Dix and Hallpike (epidemic) — *see* Neuronitis,
    vestibular
  due to infrasound T75.23 ☑
  epidemic A88.1
    Dix and Hallpike — *see* Neuronitis, vestibular
    Pedersen's — *see* Neuronitis, vestibular
    vestibular neuronitis — *see* Neuronitis, vestibular
  hysterical F44.89
  infrasound T75.23 ☑
  labyrinthine — *see* subcategory H81.0 ☑
  laryngeal R05
  malignant positional H81.4- ☑

Varix — Vertigo

324   ☑ **Additional Character Required** — Refer to the Tabular List for Character Selection   ▽ᵇ **Subterms under main terms may continue to next column or page**

Vertigo — *continued*
  Ménière's — *see* subcategory H81.0 ☑
  menopausal N95.1
  otogenic — *see* Vertigo, aural
  paroxysmal positional, benign — *see* Vertigo, benign
    paroxysmal
  Pedersen's (epidemic) — *see* Neuronitis, vestibular
  peripheral NEC H81.39- ☑
  positional
    benign paroxysmal — *see* Vertigo, benign paroxys-
      mal
    malignant H81.4- ☑
Very-low-density-lipoprotein-type (VLDL) **hyper-**
  lipoproteinemia E78.1
Vesania — *see* Psychosis
Vesical — *see* condition
Vesicle
  cutaneous R23.8
  seminal — *see* condition
  skin R23.8
Vesicocolic — *see* condition
Vesicoperineal — *see* condition
Vesicorectal — *see* condition
Vesicourethrorectal — *see* condition
Vesicovaginal — *see* condition
Vesicular — *see* condition
Vesiculitis (seminal) N49.0
  amebic A06.82
  gonorrheal (acute) (chronic) A54.23
  trichomonal A59.09
  tuberculous A18.15
Vestibulitis (ear) (*see also* subcategory H83.0 ☑
  nose (external) J34.89
  vulvar N94.810
Vestibulopathy , acute peripheral (recurrent) — *see*
  Neuronitis, vestibular
Vestige, vestigial (*see also* Persistence)
  branchial Q18.0
  structures in vitreous Q14.0
Vibration
  adverse effects T75.20 ☑
    pneumatic hammer syndrome T75.21 ☑
    specified effect NEC T75.29 ☑
    vasospastic syndrome T75.22 ☑
    vertigo from infrasound T75.23 ☑
  exposure (occupational) Z57.7
  vertigo T75.23 ☑
Vibriosis A28.9
Victim (of)
  crime Z65.4
  disaster Z65.5
  terrorism Z65.4
  torture Z65.4
  war Z65.5
Vidal's disease L28.0
Villaret's syndrome G52.7
Villous — *see* condition
VIN — *see* Neoplasia, intraepithelial, vulva
Vincent's infection (angina) (gingivitis) A69.1
  stomatitis NEC A69.1
Vinson-Plummer syndrome D50.1
Violence, physical R45.6
Viosterol deficiency — *see* Deficiency, calciferol
Vipoma — *see* Neoplasm, malignant, by site
Viremia B34.9
Virilism (adrenal) E25.9
  congenital E25.0
Virilization (female) (suprarenal) E25.9
  congenital E25.0
  isosexual E28.2
Virulent bubo A57
Virus, viral (*see also* condition)
  as cause of disease classified elsewhere B97.89
  cytomegalovirus B25.9
  human immunodeficiency (HIV) — *see* Human, immun-
    odeficiency virus (HIV) disease
  infection — *see* Infection, virus
  specified NEC B34.8
  swine influenza (viruses that normally cause infections
    in pigs) (*see also* Influenza, due to, identified
    novel influenza A virus) J09.X2
  West Nile (fever) A92.30
    with
      complications NEC A92.39
      cranial nerve disorders A92.32
      encephalitis A92.31
      encephalomyelitis A92.31

Virus, viral — *continued*
  West Nile — *continued*
    with — *continued*
      neurologic manifestation NEC A92.32
      optic neuritis A92.32
      polyradiculitis A92.32
Viscera, visceral — *see* condition
Visceroptosis K63.4
Visible peristalsis R19.2
Vision, visual
  binocular, suppression H53.34
  blurred, blurring H53.8
    hysterical F44.6
  defect, defective NEC H54.7
  disorientation (syndrome) H53.8
  disturbance H53.9
    hysterical F44.6
  double H53.2
  examination Z01.00
    with abnormal findings Z01.01
  field, limitation (defect) — *see* Defect, visual field
  hallucinations R44.1
  halos H53.19
  loss — *see* Loss, vision
    sudden — *see* Disturbance, vision, subjective, loss,
      sudden
  low (both eyes) — *see* Low, vision
  perception, simultaneous without fusion H53.33
Vitality, lack or want of R53.83
  newborn P96.89
Vitamin deficiency — *see* Deficiency, vitamin
Vitelline duct, persistent Q43.0
Vitiligo L80
  eyelid H02.739
    left H02.736
      lower H02.735
      upper H02.734
    right H02.733
      lower H02.732
      upper H02.731
  pinta A67.2
  vulva N90.89
Vitreal corneal syndrome H59.01- ☑
Vitreoretinopathy, proliferative (*see also* Retinopathy,
  proliferative)
  with retinal detachment — *see* Detachment, retina,
    traction
Vitreous (*see also* condition)
  touch syndrome — *see* Complication, postprocedural,
    following cataract surgery
Vocal cord — *see* condition
Vogt-Koyanagi syndrome H20.82- ☑
Vogt's disease or syndrome G80.3
Vogt-Spielmeyer amaurotic idiocy or disease E75.4
Voice
  change R49.9
    specified NEC R49.8
  loss — *see* Aphonia
Volhynian fever A79.0
Volkmann's ischemic contracture or paralysis (complicating trauma) T79.6 ☑
Volvulus (bowel) (colon) (intestine) K56.2
  with perforation K56.2
  congenital Q43.8
  duodenum K31.5
  fallopian tube — *see* Torsion, fallopian tube
  oviduct — *see* Torsion, fallopian tube
  stomach (due to absence of gastrocolic ligament)
    K31.89
Vomiting R11.10
  with nausea R11.2
  asphyxia — *see* Foreign body, by site, causing asphyxia,
    gastric contents
  bilious (cause unknown) R11.14
    following gastro-intestinal surgery K91.0
    in newborn P92.01
  blood — *see* Hematemesis
  causing asphyxia, choking, or suffocation — *see* For-
    eign body, by site
  cyclical G43.A0 (*following* G43.7)
    with refractory migraine G43.A1 (*following* G43.7)
    intractable G43.A1 (*following* G43.7)
    not intractable G43.A0 (*following* G43.7)
    psychogenic F50.89
    without refractory migraine G43.A0 (*following* G43.7)
  fecal mater R11.13
  following gastrointestinal surgery K91.0
    psychogenic F50.89

Vomiting — *continued*
  functional K31.89
  hysterical F50.89
  nervous F50.89
  neurotic F50.89
  newborn NEC P92.09
    bilious P92.01
  periodic R11.10
    psychogenic F50.89
  projectile R11.12
  psychogenic F50.89
  uremic — *see* Uremia
  without nausea R11.11
Vomito negro — *see* Fever, yellow
Von Bezold's abscess — *see* Mastoiditis, acute
Von Economo-Cruchet disease A85.8
Von Eulenburg's disease G71.19
Von Gierke's disease E74.01
Von Hippel (-Lindau) **disease or syndrome** Q85.8
Von Jaksch's anemia or disease D64.89
Von Recklinghausen
  disease (neurofibromatosis) Q85.01
    bones E21.0
Von Schroetter's syndrome I82.890
Von Willebrand (-Jurgens)(-Minot) **disease or syn-**
  drome D68.0
Von Zumbusch's disease L40.1
Voyeurism F65.3
Vrolik's disease Q78.0
Vulva — *see* condition
Vulvismus N94.2
Vulvitis (acute) (allergic) (atrophic) (hypertrophic) (intertriginous) (senile) N76.2
  with ectopic or molar pregnancy O08.0
  adhesive, congenital Q52.79
  blennorrhagic (gonococcal) A54.02
  candidal B37.3
  chlamydial A56.02
  due to Haemophilus ducreyi A57
  following ectopic or molar pregnancy O08.0
  gonococcal A54.02
    with abscess (accessory gland) (periurethral) A54.1
  herpesviral A60.04
  leukoplakic N90.4
  monilial B37.3
  puerperal (postpartum) O86.19
  subacute or chronic N76.3
  syphilitic (early) A51.0
    late A52.76
  trichomonal A59.01
  tuberculous A18.18
Vulvodynia N94.819
  specified NEC N94.818
Vulvorectal — *see* condition
Vulvovaginitis (acute) — *see* Vaginitis

W

Waiting list, person on Z75.1
  for organ transplant Z76.82
  undergoing social agency investigation Z75.2
Waldenström
  hypergammaglobulinemia D89.0
  syndrome or macroglobulinemia C88.0
Waldenström-Kjellberg syndrome D50.1
Walking
  difficulty R26.2
    psychogenic F44.4
  sleep F51.3
    hysterical F44.89
Wall, abdominal — *see* condition
Wallenberg's disease or syndrome G46.3
Wallgren's disease I87.8
Wandering
  gallbladder, congenital Q44.1
  in diseases classified elsewhere Z91.83
  kidney, congenital Q63.8
  organ or site, congenital NEC — *see* Malposition, con-
    genital, by site
  pacemaker (heart) I49.8
  spleen D73.89
War neurosis F48.8
Wart (due to HPV) (filiform) (infectious) (viral) B07.9
  anogenital region (venereal) A63.0
  common B07.8
  external genital organs (venereal) A63.0
  flat B07.8
  Hassal-Henle's (of cornea) H18.49

▽ **Subterms under main terms may continue to next column or page**   ☑ **Additional Character Required — Refer to the Tabular List for Character Selection**   **325**

Vertigo — Wart

Wart — *continued*
  Peruvian A44.1
  plantar B07.0
  prosector (tuberculous) A18.4
  seborrheic L82.1
    inflamed L82.0
  senile (seborrheic) L82.1
    inflamed L82.0
  tuberculous A18.4
  venereal A63.0
Warthin's tumor — *see* Neoplasm, salivary gland, benign
Wassilieff's disease A27.0
Wasting
  disease R64
    due to malnutrition E41
  extreme (due to malnutrition) E41
  muscle NEC — *see* Atrophy, muscle
Water
  clefts (senile cataract) — *see* Cataract, senile, incipient
  deprivation of T73.1 ☑
  intoxication E87.79
  itch B76.9
  lack of T73.1 ☑
  loading E87.70
  on
    brain — *see* Hydrocephalus
    chest J94.8
  poisoning E87.79
Waterbrash R12
Waterhouse (-Friderichsen) **syndrome or disease**
  (meningococcal) A39.1
Water-losing nephritis N25.89
Watermelon stomach K31.819
  with hemorrhage K31.811
  without hemorrhage K31.819
Watsoniasis B66.8
Wax in ear — *see* Impaction, cerumen
Weak, weakening, weakness (generalized) R53.1
  arches (acquired) (*see also* Deformity, limb, flat foot)
  bladder (sphincter) R32
  facial R29.810
    following
      cerebrovascular disease I69.992
        cerebral infarction I69.392
        intracerebral hemorrhage I69.192
        nontraumatic intracranial hemorrhage NEC
          I69.292
        specified disease NEC I69.892
        stroke I69.392
        subarachnoid hemorrhage I69.092
  foot (double) — *see* Weak, arches
  heart, cardiac — *see* Failure, heart
  mind F70
  muscle M62.81
  myocardium — *see* Failure, heart
  newborn P96.89
  pelvic fundus N81.89
  pubocervical tissue N81.82
  rectovaginal tissue N81.83
  senile R54
  urinary stream R39.12
  valvular — *see* Endocarditis
Wear, worn (with normal or routine use)
  articular bearing surface of internal joint prosthesis —
    see Complications, joint prosthesis, mechanical,
    wear of articular bearing surfaces, by site
  device, implant or graft — *see* Complications, by site,
    mechanical complication
  tooth, teeth (approximal) (hard tissues) (interproximal)
    (occlusal) K03.0
Weather, weathered
  effects of
    cold T69.9 ☑
      specified effect NEC T69.8 ☑
    hot — *see* Heat
  skin L57.8
Weaver's syndrome Q87.3
Web, webbed (congenital)
  duodenal Q43.8
  esophagus Q39.4
  fingers Q70.1- ☑
  larynx (glottic) (subglottic) Q31.0
  neck (pterygium colli) Q18.3
  Paterson-Kelly D50.1
  popliteal syndrome Q87.89
  toes Q70.3- ☑
Weber-Christian disease M35.6

Weber-Cockayne syndrome (epidermolysis bullosa)
  Q81.8
Weber-Gubler syndrome G46.3
Weber-Leyden syndrome G46.3
Weber-Osler syndrome I78.0
Weber's paralysis or syndrome G46.3
Wedge-shaped or wedging vertebra — *see* Collapse,
  vertebra NEC
Wegener's granulomatosis or syndrome M31.30
  with
    kidney involvement M31.31
    lung involvement M31.30
      with kidney involvement M31.31
Wegner's disease A50.02
Weight
  1000-2499 grams at birth (low) — *see* Low, birthweight
  999 grams or less at birth (extremely low) — *see* Low,
    birthweight, extreme
  and length below 10th percentile for gestational age
    P05.1- ☑
    below but length above 10th percentile for gestational
      age P05.0- ☑
  gain (abnormal) (excessive) R63.5
    in pregnancy — *see* Pregnancy, complicated by,
      excessive weight gain
    low — *see* Pregnancy, complicated by, insuffi-
      cient, weight gain
  loss (abnormal) (cause unknown) R63.4
Weightlessness (effect of) T75.82 ☑
Weil (I)-**Marchesani syndrome** Q87.1
Weil's disease A27.0
Weingarten's syndrome J82
Weir Mitchell's disease I73.81
Weiss-Baker syndrome G90.09
Wells' disease L98.3
Wen — *see* Cyst, sebaceous
Wenckebach's block or phenomenon I44.1
Werdnig-Hoffmann syndrome (muscular atrophy)
  G12.0
Werlhof's disease D69.3
Wermer's disease or syndrome E31.21
Werner-His disease A79.0
Werner's disease or syndrome E34.8
Wernicke-Korsakoff's syndrome or psychosis (alco-
  holic) F10.96
  with dependence F10.26
  drug-induced
    due to drug abuse — *see* Abuse, drug, by type, with
      amnestic disorder
    due to drug dependence — *see* Dependence, drug,
      by type, with amnestic disorder
  nonalcoholic F04
Wernicke-Posadas disease B38.9
Wernicke's
  developmental aphasia F80.2
  disease or syndrome E51.2
  encephalopathy E51.2
  polioencephalitis, superior E51.2
West African fever B50.8
Westphal-Strümpell syndrome E83.01
West's syndrome — *see* Epilepsy, spasms
Wet
  feet, tropical (maceration) (syndrome) — *see* Immer-
    sion, foot
  lung (syndrome), newborn P22.1
Wharton's duct — *see* condition
Wheal — *see* Urticaria
Wheezing R06.2
Whiplash injury S13.4 ☑
Whipple's disease (*see also* subcategory M14.8-) K90.81
Whipworm (disease) (infection) (infestation) B79
Whistling face Q87.0
White (*see also* condition)
  kidney, small N03.9
  leg, puerperal, postpartum, childbirth O87.1
  mouth B37.0
  patches of mouth K13.29
  spot lesions, teeth
    chewing surface K02.51
    pit and fissure surface K02.51
    smooth surface K02.61
Whitehead L70.0
Whitlow (*see also* Cellulitis, digit)
  with lymphangitis — *see* Lymphangitis, acute, digit
  herpesviral B00.89
Whitmore's disease or fever — *see* Melioidosis
Whooping cough A37.90

Whooping cough — *continued*
  with pneumonia A37.91
    due to Bordetella
      bronchiseptica A37.81
      parapertussis A37.11
      pertussis A37.01
    specified organism NEC A37.81
  due to
    Bordetella
      bronchiseptica A37.80
        with pneumonia A37.81
      parapertussis A37.10
        with pneumonia A37.11
      pertussis A37.00
        with pneumonia A37.01
    specified NEC A37.80
      with pneumonia A37.81
Wichman's asthma J38.5
Wide cranial sutures, newborn P96.3
Widening aorta — *see* Ectasia, aorta
  with aneurysm — *see* Aneurysm, aorta
Wilkie's disease or syndrome K55.1
Wilkinson-Sneddon disease or syndrome L13.1
Willebrand (-Jürgens) **thrombopathy** D68.0
Williams syndrome Q93.82
Willige-Hunt disease or syndrome G23.1
Wilms' tumor C64- ☑
Wilson-Mikity syndrome P27.0
Wilson's
  disease or syndrome E83.01
  hepatolenticular degeneration E83.01
  lichen ruber L43.9
Window (*see also* Imperfect, closure)
  aorticopulmonary Q21.4
Winter — *see* condition
Wiskott-Aldrich syndrome D82.0
Withdrawal state (*see also* Dependence, drug by type,
  with withdrawal)
  alcohol
    with perceptual disturbances F10.232
    without perceptual disturbances F10.239
  caffeine F15.93
  cannabis F12.23
  newborn
    correct therapeutic substance properly administered
      P96.2
    infant of dependent mother P96.1
  therapeutic substance, neonatal P96.2
Witts' anemia D50.8
Witzelsucht F07.0
Woakes' ethmoiditis or syndrome J33.1
Wolff-Hirschorn syndrome Q93.3
Wolff-Parkinson-White syndrome I45.6
Wolhynian fever A79.0
Wolman's disease E75.5
Wood lung or pneumonitis J67.8
Woolly, wooly hair (congenital) (nevus) Q84.1
Woolsorter's disease A22.1
Word
  blindness (congenital) (developmental) F81.0
  deafness (congenital) (developmental) H93.25
Worm(s) (infection) (infestation) (*see also* Infestation,
  helminth)
  guinea B72
  in intestine NEC B82.0
Worm-eaten soles A66.3
Worn out — *see* Exhaustion
  cardiac
    defibrillator (with synchronous cardiace pacemaker)
      Z45.02
    pacemaker
      battery Z45.010
      lead Z45.018
  device, implant or graft — *see* Complications, by site,
    mechanical
Worried well Z71.1
Worries R45.82
Wound check Z48.0- ☑
  due to injury — *code* to Injury, by site, using appropri-
    ate seventh character for subsequent encounter
Wound, open T14.8- ☑
  abdomen, abdominal
    wall S31.109 ☑
      with penetration into peritoneal cavity
        S31.609 ☑
      bite — *see* Bite, abdomen, wall
      epigastric region S31.102 ☑

☑ **Additional Character Required** — **Refer to the Tabular List for Character Selection**   ▽ **Subterms under main terms may continue to next column or page**

Wound, open — *continued*
  abdomen, abdominal — *continued*
    wall — *continued*
      epigastric region — *continued*
        with penetration into peritoneal cavity S31.602 ☑
          bite — *see* Bite, abdomen, wall, epigastric region
          laceration — *see* Laceration, abdomen, wall, epigastric region
          puncture — *see* Puncture, abdomen, wall, epigastric region
      laceration — *see* Laceration, abdomen, wall
      left
        lower quadrant S31.104 ☑
          with penetration into peritoneal cavity S31.604 ☑
            bite — *see* Bite, abdomen, wall, left, lower quadrant
            laceration — *see* Laceration, abdomen, wall, left, lower quadrant
            puncture — *see* Puncture, abdomen, wall, left, lower quadrant
        upper quadrant S31.101 ☑
          with penetration into peritoneal cavity S31.601 ☑
            bite — *see* Bite, abdomen, wall, left, upper quadrant
            laceration — *see* Laceration, abdomen, wall, left, upper quadrant
            puncture — *see* Puncture, abdomen, wall, left, upper quadrant
      periumbilic region S31.105 ☑
        with penetration into peritoneal cavity S31.605 ☑
          bite — *see* Bite, abdomen, wall, periumbilic region
          laceration — *see* Laceration, abdomen, wall, periumbilic region
          puncture — *see* Puncture, abdomen, wall, periumbilic region
      puncture — *see* Puncture, abdomen, wall
      right
        lower quadrant S31.103 ☑
          with penetration into peritoneal cavity S31.603 ☑
            bite — *see* Bite, abdomen, wall, right, lower quadrant
            laceration — *see* Laceration, abdomen, wall, right, lower quadrant
            puncture — *see* Puncture, abdomen, wall, right, lower quadrant
        upper quadrant S31.100 ☑
          with penetration into peritoneal cavity S31.600 ☑
            bite — *see* Bite, abdomen, wall, right, upper quadrant
            laceration — *see* Laceration, abdomen, wall, right, upper quadrant
            puncture — *see* Puncture, abdomen, wall, right, upper quadrant
  alveolar (process) — *see* Wound, open, oral cavity
  ankle S91.00- ☑
    bite — *see* Bite, ankle
    laceration — *see* Laceration, ankle
    puncture — *see* Puncture, ankle
  antecubital space — *see* Wound, open, elbow
  anterior chamber, eye — *see* Wound, open, ocular
  anus S31.839 ☑
    bite S31.835 ☑
    laceration — *see* Laceration, anus
    puncture — *see* Puncture, anus
  arm (upper) S41.10- ☑
    with amputation — *see* Amputation, traumatic, arm
    bite — *see* Bite, arm
    forearm — *see* Wound, open, forearm
    laceration — *see* Laceration, arm
    puncture — *see* Puncture, arm
  auditory canal (external) (meatus) — *see* Wound, open, ear
  auricle, ear — *see* Wound, open, ear
  axilla — *see* Wound, open, arm
  back (*see also* Wound, open, thorax, back)
    lower S31.000 ☑
      with penetration into retroperitoneal space S31.001 ☑
        bite — *see* Bite, back, lower

Wound, open — *continued*
  back (*see also* Wound, open, thorax, back) — *continued*
    lower — *continued*
      laceration — *see* Laceration, back, lower
      puncture — *see* Puncture, back, lower
  bite — *see* Bite
  blood vessel — *see* Injury, blood vessel
  breast S21.00- ☑
    with amputation — *see* Amputation, traumatic, breast
    bite — *see* Bite, breast
    laceration — *see* Laceration, breast
    puncture — *see* Puncture, breast
  buttock S31.809 ☑
    bite — *see* Bite, buttock
    laceration — *see* Laceration, buttock
    left S31.829 ☑
    puncture — *see* Puncture, buttock
    right S31.819 ☑
  calf — *see* Wound, open, leg
  canaliculus lacrimalis — *see* Wound, open, eyelid
  canthus, eye — *see* Wound, open, eyelid
  cervical esophagus S11.20 ☑
    bite S11.25 ☑
    laceration — *see* Laceration, esophagus, traumatic, cervical
    puncture — *see* Puncture, cervical esophagus
  cheek (external) S01.40- ☑
    bite — *see* Bite, cheek
    internal — *see* Wound, open, oral cavity
    laceration — *see* Laceration, cheek
    puncture — *see* Puncture, cheek
  chest wall — *see* Wound, open, thorax
  chin — *see* Wound, open, head, specified site NEC
  choroid — *see* Wound, open, ocular
  ciliary body (eye) — *see* Wound, open, ocular
  clitoris S31.40 ☑
    with amputation — *see* Amputation, traumatic, clitoris
    bite S31.45 ☑
    laceration — *see* Laceration, vulva
    puncture — *see* Puncture, vulva
  conjunctiva — *see* Wound, open, ocular
  cornea — *see* Wound, open, ocular
  costal region — *see* Wound, open, thorax
  Descemet's membrane — *see* Wound, open, ocular
  digit(s)
    foot — *see* Wound, open, toe
    hand — *see* Wound, open, finger
  ear (canal) (external) S01.30- ☑
    with amputation — *see* Amputation, traumatic, ear
    bite — *see* Bite, ear
    drum S09.2- ☑
    laceration — *see* Laceration, ear
    puncture — *see* Puncture, ear
  elbow S51.00- ☑
    bite — *see* Bite, elbow
    laceration — *see* Laceration, elbow
    puncture — *see* Puncture, elbow
  epididymis — *see* Wound, open, testis
  epigastric region S31.102 ☑
    with penetration into peritoneal cavity S31.602 ☑
    bite — *see* Bite, abdomen, wall, epigastric region
    laceration — *see* Laceration, abdomen, wall, epigastric region
    puncture — *see* Puncture, abdomen, wall, epigastric region
  epiglottis — *see* Wound, open, neck, specified site NEC
  esophagus (thoracic) S27.819 ☑
    cervical — *see* Wound, open, cervical esophagus
    laceration S27.813 ☑
    specified type NEC S27.818 ☑
  eye — *see* Wound, open, ocular
  eyeball — *see* Wound, open, ocular
  eyebrow — *see* Wound, open, eyelid
  eyelid S01.10- ☑
    bite — *see* Bite, eyelid
    laceration — *see* Laceration, eyelid
    puncture — *see* Puncture, eyelid
  face NEC — *see* Wound, open, head, specified site NEC
  finger(s) S61.209 ☑
    with
      amputation — *see* Amputation, traumatic, finger
      damage to nail S61.309 ☑
    bite — *see* Bite, finger

Wound, open — *continued*
  finger(s) — *continued*
    index S61.208 ☑
      with
        damage to nail S61.308 ☑
      left S61.201 ☑
        with
          damage to nail S61.301 ☑
      right S61.200 ☑
        with
          damage to nail S61.300 ☑
    laceration — *see* Laceration, finger
    little S61.208 ☑
      with
        damage to nail S61.308 ☑
      left S61.207 ☑
        with damage to nail S61.307 ☑
      right S61.206 ☑
        with damage to nail S61.306 ☑
    middle S61.208 ☑
      with
        damage to nail S61.308 ☑
      left S61.203 ☑
        with damage to nail S61.303 ☑
      right S61.202 ☑
        with damage to nail S61.302 ☑
    puncture — *see* Puncture, finger
    ring S61.208 ☑
      with
        damage to nail S61.308 ☑
      left S61.205 ☑
        with damage to nail S61.305 ☑
      right S61.204 ☑
        with damage to nail S61.304 ☑
  flank — *see* Wound, open, abdomen, wall
  foot (except toe(s) alone) S91.30- ☑
    with amputation — *see* Amputation, traumatic, foot
    bite — *see* Bite, foot
    laceration — *see* Laceration, foot
    puncture — *see* Puncture, foot
    toe — *see* Wound, open, toe
  forearm S51.80- ☑
    with
      amputation — *see* Amputation, traumatic, forearm
    bite — *see* Bite, forearm
    elbow only — *see* Wound, open, elbow
    laceration — *see* Laceration, forearm
    puncture — *see* Puncture, forearm
  forehead — *see* Wound, open, head, specified site NEC
  genital organs, external
    with amputation — *see* Amputation, traumatic, genital organs
    bite — *see* Bite, genital organ
    female S31.502 ☑
      vagina S31.40 ☑
      vulva S31.40 ☑
    laceration — *see* Laceration, genital organ
    male S31.501 ☑
      penis S31.20 ☑
      scrotum S31.30 ☑
      testes S31.30 ☑
    puncture — *see* Puncture, genital organ
  globe (eye) — *see* Wound, open, ocular
  groin — *see* Wound, open, abdomen, wall
  gum — *see* Wound, open, oral cavity
  hand S61.40- ☑
    with
      amputation — *see* Amputation, traumatic, hand
    bite — *see* Bite, hand
    finger(s) — *see* Wound, open, finger
    laceration — *see* Laceration, hand
    puncture — *see* Puncture, hand
    thumb — *see* Wound, open, thumb
  head S01.90 ☑
    bite — *see* Bite, head
    cheek — *see* Wound, open, cheek
    ear — *see* Wound, open, ear
    eyelid — *see* Wound, open, eyelid
    laceration — *see* Laceration, head
    lip — *see* Wound, open, lip
    nose S01.20 ☑
    oral cavity — *see* Wound, open, oral cavity
    puncture — *see* Puncture, head
    scalp — *see* Wound, open, scalp
    specified site NEC S01.80 ☑

Wound, open — *continued*
head — *continued*
temporomandibular area — *see* Wound, open,
cheek
heel — *see* Wound, open, foot
hip S71.00- ☑
with amputation — *see* Amputation, traumatic, hip
bite — *see* Bite, hip
laceration — *see* Laceration, hip
puncture — *see* Puncture, hip
hymen S31.40 ☑
bite — *see* Bite, vulva
laceration — *see* Laceration, vagina
puncture — *see* Puncture, vagina
hypochondrium S31.109 ☑
bite — *see* Bite, hypochondrium
laceration — *see* Laceration, hypochondrium
puncture — *see* Puncture, hypochondrium
hypogastric region S31.109 ☑
bite — *see* Bite, hypogastric region
laceration — *see* Laceration, hypogastric region
puncture — *see* Puncture, hypogastric region
iliac (region) — *see* Wound, open, inguinal region
inguinal region S31.109 ☑
bite — *see* Bite, abdomen, wall, lower quadrant
laceration — *see* Laceration, inguinal region
puncture — *see* Puncture, inguinal region
instep — *see* Wound, open, foot
interscapular region — *see* Wound, open, thorax, back
intraocular — *see* Wound, open, ocular
iris — *see* Wound, open, ocular
jaw — *see* Wound, open, head, specified site NEC
knee S81.00- ☑
bite — *see* Bite, knee
laceration — *see* Laceration, knee
puncture — *see* Puncture, knee
labium (majus) (minus) — *see* Wound, open, vulva
laceration — *see* Laceration, by site
lacrimal duct — *see* Wound, open, eyelid
larynx S11.019 ☑
bite — *see* Bite, larynx
laceration — *see* Laceration, larynx
puncture — *see* Puncture, larynx
left
lower quadrant S31.104 ☑
with penetration into peritoneal cavity
S31.604 ☑
bite — *see* Bite, abdomen, wall, lower
quadrant
laceration — *see* Laceration, abdomen, wall, left,
lower quadrant
puncture — *see* Puncture, abdomen, wall, left,
lower quadrant
upper quadrant S31.101 ☑
with penetration into peritoneal cavity
S31.601 ☑
bite — *see* Bite, abdomen, wall, left, upper
quadrant
laceration — *see* Laceration, abdomen, wall, left,
upper quadrant
puncture — *see* Puncture, abdomen, wall, left,
upper quadrant
leg (lower) S81.80- ☑
with amputation — *see* Amputation, traumatic, leg
ankle — *see* Wound, open, ankle
bite — *see* Bite, leg
foot — *see* Wound, open, foot
knee — *see* Wound, open, knee
laceration — *see* Laceration, leg
puncture — *see* Puncture, leg
toe — *see* Wound, open, toe
upper — *see* Wound, open, thigh
lip S01.501 ☑
bite — *see* Bite, lip
laceration — *see* Laceration, lip
puncture — *see* Puncture, lip
loin S31.109 ☑
bite — *see* Bite, abdomen, wall
laceration — *see* Laceration, loin
puncture — *see* Puncture, loin
lower back — *see* Wound, open, back, lower
lumbar region — *see* Wound, open, back, lower
malar region — *see* Wound, open, head, specified site
NEC
mammary — *see* Wound, open, breast

Wound, open — *continued*
mastoid region — *see* Wound, open, head, specified
site NEC
mouth — *see* Wound, open, oral cavity
nail
finger — *see* Wound, open, finger, with damage to
nail
toe — *see* Wound, open, toe, with damage to nail
nape (neck) — *see* Wound, open, neck
nasal (septum) (sinus) — *see* Wound, open, nose
nasopharynx — *see* Wound, open, head, specified site
NEC
neck S11.90 ☑
bite — *see* Bite, neck
involving
cervical esophagus S11.20 ☑
larynx — *see* Wound, open, larynx
pharynx S11.20 ☑
thyroid S11.10 ☑
trachea (cervical) S11.029 ☑
bite — *see* Bite, trachea
laceration S11.021 ☑
with foreign body S11.022 ☑
puncture S11.023 ☑
with foreign body S11.024 ☑
laceration — *see* Laceration, neck
puncture — *see* Puncture, neck
specified site NEC S11.80 ☑
specified type NEC S11.89 ☑
nose (septum) (sinus) S01.20 ☑
with amputation — *see* Amputation, traumatic,
nose
bite — *see* Bite, nose
laceration — *see* Laceration, nose
puncture — *see* Puncture, nose
ocular S05.90 ☑
avulsion (traumatic enucleation) S05.7- ☑
eyeball S05.6- ☑
with foreign body S05.5- ☑
eyelid — *see* Wound, open, eyelid
laceration and rupture S05.3- ☑
with prolapse or loss of intraocular tissue
S05.2- ☑
orbit (penetrating) (with or without foreign body)
S05.4- ☑
periocular area — *see* Wound, open, eyelid
specified NEC S05.8X- ☑
oral cavity S01.502 ☑
bite S01.552 ☑
laceration — *see* Laceration, oral cavity
puncture — *see* Puncture, oral cavity
orbit — *see* Wound, open, ocular, orbit
palate — *see* Wound, open, oral cavity
palm — *see* Wound, open, hand
pelvis, pelvic (*see also* Wound, open, back, lower)
girdle — *see* Wound, open, hip
penetrating — *see* Puncture, by site
penis S31.20 ☑
with amputation — *see* Amputation, traumatic,
penis
bite S31.25 ☑
laceration — *see* Laceration, penis
puncture — *see* Puncture, penis
perineum
bite — *see* Bite, perineum
female S31.502 ☑
laceration — *see* Laceration, perineum
male S31.501 ☑
puncture — *see* Puncture, perineum
periocular area (with or without lacrimal passages) —
see Wound, open, eyelid
periumbilic region S31.105 ☑
with penetration into peritoneal cavity S31.605 ☑
bite — *see* Bite, abdomen, wall, periumbilic region
laceration — *see* Laceration, abdomen, wall, periumbilic region
puncture — *see* Puncture, abdomen, wall, periumbilic region
phalanges
finger — *see* Wound, open, finger
toe — *see* Wound, open, toe
pharynx S11.20 ☑
pinna — *see* Wound, open, ear
popliteal space — *see* Wound, open, knee
prepuce — *see* Wound, open, penis
pubic region — *see* Wound, open, back, lower

Wound, open — *continued*
pudendum — *see* Wound, open, genital organs, external
puncture wound — *see* Puncture
rectovaginal septum — *see* Wound, open, vagina
right
lower quadrant S31.103 ☑
with penetration into peritoneal cavity
S31.603 ☑
bite — *see* Bite, abdomen, wall, right, lower
quadrant
laceration — *see* Laceration, abdomen, wall,
right, lower quadrant
puncture — *see* Puncture, abdomen, wall, right,
lower quadrant
upper quadrant S31.100 ☑
with penetration into peritoneal cavity
S31.600 ☑
bite — *see* Bite, abdomen, wall, right, upper
quadrant
laceration — *see* Laceration, abdomen, wall,
right, upper quadrant
puncture — *see* Puncture, abdomen, wall, right,
upper quadrant
sacral region — *see* Wound, open, back, lower
sacroiliac region — *see* Wound, open, back, lower
salivary gland — *see* Wound, open, oral cavity
scalp S01.00 ☑
bite S01.05 ☑
laceration — *see* Laceration, scalp
puncture — *see* Puncture, scalp
scalpel, newborn (birth injury) P15.8
scapular region — *see* Wound, open, shoulder
sclera — *see* Wound, open, ocular
scrotum S31.30 ☑
with amputation — *see* Amputation, traumatic,
scrotum
bite S31.35 ☑
laceration — *see* Laceration, scrotum
puncture — *see* Puncture, scrotum
shin — *see* Wound, open, leg
shoulder S41.00- ☑
with amputation — *see* Amputation, traumatic, arm
bite — *see* Bite, shoulder
laceration — *see* Laceration, shoulder
puncture — *see* Puncture, shoulder
skin NOS T14.8 ☑
spermatic cord — *see* Wound, open, testis
sternal region — *see* Wound, open, thorax, front wall
submaxillary region — *see* Wound, open, head, specified site NEC
submental region — *see* Wound, open, head, specified
site NEC
subungual
finger(s) — *see* Wound, open, finger
toe(s) — *see* Wound, open, toe
supraclavicular region — *see* Wound, open, neck,
specified site NEC
temple, temporal region — *see* Wound, open, head,
specified site NEC
temporomandibular area — *see* Wound, open, cheek
testis S31.30 ☑
with amputation — *see* Amputation, traumatic,
testes
bite S31.35 ☑
laceration — *see* Laceration, testis
puncture — *see* Puncture, testis
thigh S71.10- ☑
with amputation — *see* Amputation, traumatic, hip
bite — *see* Bite, thigh
laceration — *see* Laceration, thigh
puncture — *see* Puncture, thigh
thorax, thoracic (wall) S21.90 ☑
back S21.20- ☑
with penetration S21.40 ☑
bite — *see* Bite, thorax
breast — *see* Wound, open, breast
front S21.10- ☑
with penetration S21.30 ☑
laceration — *see* Laceration, thorax
puncture — *see* Puncture, thorax
throat — *see* Wound, open, neck
thumb S61.009 ☑
with
amputation — *see* Amputation, traumatic,
thumb

☑ **Additional Character Required** — Refer to the Tabular List for Character Selection   ▽ **Subterms under main terms may continue to next column or page**

Wound, open — *continued*
  thumb — *continued*
    with — *continued*
      damage to nail S61.109 ☑
    bite — *see* Bite, thumb
    laceration — *see* Laceration, thumb
    left S61.002 ☑
      with
        damage to nail S61.102 ☑
      puncture — *see* Puncture, thumb
    right S61.001 ☑
      with
        damage to nail S61.101 ☑
  thyroid (gland) — *see* Wound, open, neck, thyroid
  toe(s) S91.109 ☑
    with
      amputation — *see* Amputation, traumatic, toe
      damage to nail S91.209 ☑
    bite — *see* Bite, toe
    great S91.103 ☑
      with
        damage to nail S91.203 ☑
      left S91.102 ☑
        with
          damage to nail S91.202 ☑
      right S91.101 ☑
        with
          damage to nail S91.201 ☑
    laceration — *see* Laceration, toe
    lesser S91.106 ☑
      with
        damage to nail S91.206 ☑
      left S91.105 ☑
        with
          damage to nail S91.205 ☑
      right S91.104 ☑
        with
          damage to nail S91.204 ☑
    puncture — *see* Puncture, toe
  tongue — *see* Wound, open, oral cavity
  trachea (cervical region) — *see* Wound, open, neck, trachea
  tunica vaginalis — *see* Wound, open, testis
  tympanum, tympanic membrane S09.2- ☑
    laceration — *see* Laceration, ear, drum
    puncture — *see* Puncture, tympanum
  umbilical region — *see* Wound, open, abdomen, wall, periumbilic region
  uvula — *see* Wound, open, oral cavity
  vagina S31.40 ☑
    bite S31.45 ☑
    laceration — *see* Laceration, vagina
    puncture — *see* Puncture, vagina
  vitreous (humor) — *see* Wound, open, ocular
  vocal cord S11.039 ☑
    bite — *see* Bite, vocal cord
    laceration S11.031 ☑
      with foreign body S11.032 ☑
    puncture S11.033 ☑
      with foreign body S11.034 ☑
  vulva S31.40 ☑
    with amputation — *see* Amputation, traumatic, vulva
    bite S31.45 ☑
    laceration — *see* Laceration, vulva
    puncture — *see* Puncture, vulva
  wrist S61.50- ☑
    bite — *see* Bite, wrist
    laceration — *see* Laceration, wrist
    puncture — *see* Puncture, wrist
Wound, superficial — *see* Injury (*see also* specified injury type)
Wright's syndrome G54.0
Wrist — *see* condition
Wrong drug (by accident) (given in error) — *see* Table of Drugs and Chemicals, by drug, poisoning
Wry neck — *see* Torticollis
Wuchereria (bancrofti) **infestation** B74.0
Wuchereriasis B74.0

Wuchernde Struma Langhans C73

X

Xanthelasma (eyelid) (palpebrarum) H02.60
  left H02.66
    lower H02.65
    upper H02.64
  right H02.63
    lower H02.62
    upper H02.61
Xanthelasmatosis (essential) E78.2
Xanthinuria, hereditary E79.8
Xanthoastrocytoma
  specified site — *see* Neoplasm, malignant, by site
  unspecified site C71.9
Xanthofibroma — *see* Neoplasm, connective tissue, benign
Xanthogranuloma D76.3
Xanthoma(s), xanthomatosis (primary) (familial) (hereditary) E75.5
  with
    hyperlipoproteinemia
      Type I E78.3
      Type III E78.2
      Type IV E78.1
      Type V E78.3
  bone (generalisata) C96.5
  cerebrotendinous E75.5
  cutaneotendinous E75.5
  disseminatum (skin) E78.2
  eruptive E78.2
  hypercholesterinemic E78.00
  hypercholesterolemic E78.00
  hyperlipidemic E78.5
  joint E75.5
  multiple (skin) E78.2
  tendon (sheath) E75.5
  tuberosum E78.2
  tuberous E78.2
  tubo-eruptive E78.2
  verrucous, oral mucosa K13.4
Xanthosis R23.8
Xenophobia F40.10
Xeroderma (*see also* Ichthyosis)
  acquired L85.0
  eyelid H01.149
    left H01.146
      lower H01.145
      upper H01.144
    right H01.143
      lower H01.142
      upper H01.141
  pigmentosum Q82.1
  vitamin A deficiency E50.8
Xerophthalmia (vitamin A deficiency) E50.7
  unrelated to vitamin A deficiency — *see* Keratoconjunctivitis
Xerosis
  conjunctiva H11.14- ☑
    with Bitot's spots (*see also* Pigmentation, conjunctiva)
    vitamin A deficiency E50.1
    vitamin A deficiency E50.0
  cornea H18.89- ☑
    with ulceration — *see* Ulcer, cornea
    vitamin A deficiency E50.3
    vitamin A deficiency E50.2
  cutis L85.3
  skin L85.3
Xerostomia K11.7
Xiphopagus Q89.4
XO syndrome Q96.9
X-ray (of)
  abnormal findings — *see* Abnormal, diagnostic imaging
  breast (mammogram) (routine) Z12.31
  chest
    routine (as part of a general medical examination) Z00.00
      with abnormal findings Z00.01

X-ray — *continued*
  routine (as part of a general medical examination) Z00.00
    with abnormal findings Z00.01
XXXXY syndrome Q98.1
XXY syndrome Q98.0

Y

Yaba pox (virus disease) B08.72
Yatapoxvirus B08.70
  specified NEC B08.79
Yawning R06.89
  psychogenic F45.8
Yaws A66.9
  bone lesions A66.6
  butter A66.1
  chancre A66.0
  cutaneous, less than five years after infection A66.2
  early (cutaneous) (macular) (maculopapular) (micropapular) (papular) A66.2
    frambeside A66.2
    skin lesions NEC A66.2
  eyelid A66.2
  ganglion A66.6
  gangosis, gangosa A66.5
  gumma, gummata A66.4
    bone A66.6
  gummatous
    frambeside A66.4
    osteitis A66.6
    periostitis A66.6
  hydrarthrosis (*see also* subcategory M14.8-) A66.6
  hyperkeratosis (early) (late) A66.3
  initial lesions A66.0
  joint lesions (*see also* subcategory M14.8-) A66.6
  juxta-articular nodules A66.7
  late nodular (ulcerated) A66.4
  latent (without clinical manifestations) (with positive serology) A66.8
  mother A66.0
  mucosal A66.7
  multiple papillomata A66.1
  nodular, late (ulcerated) A66.4
  osteitis A66.6
  papilloma, plantar or palmar A66.1
  periostitis (hypertrophic) A66.6
  specified NEC A66.7
  ulcers A66.4
  wet crab A66.1
Yeast infection (*see also* Candidiasis) B37.9
Yellow
  atrophy (liver) — *see* Failure, hepatic
  fever — *see* Fever, yellow
  jack — *see* Fever, yellow
  jaundice — *see* Jaundice
  nail syndrome L60.5
Yersiniosis (*see also* Infection, Yersinia)
  extraintestinal A28.2
  intestinal A04.6

Z

Zahorsky's syndrome (herpangina) B08.5
Zellweger's syndrome Q87.89
Zenker's diverticulum (esophagus) K22.5
Ziehen-Oppenheim disease G24.1
Zieve's syndrome K70.0
Zika NOS A92.5
  congenital P35.4
Zinc
  deficiency, dietary E60
  metabolism disorder E83.2
Zollinger-Ellison syndrome E16.4
Zona — *see* Herpes, zoster
Zoophobia F40.218
Zoster (herpes) — *see* Herpes, zoster
Zygomycosis B46.9
  specified NEC B46.8
Zymotic — *see* condition

Note: The list below gives the code number for neoplasms by anatomical site. For each site there are six possible code numbers according to whether the neoplasm in question is malignant, benign, in situ, of uncertain behavior, or of unspecified nature. The description of the neoplasm will often indicate which of the six columns is appropriate; e.g., malignant melanoma of skin, benign fibroadenoma of breast, carcinoma in situ of cervix uteri. Where such descriptors are not present, the remainder of the Index should be consulted where guidance is given to the appropriate column for each morphological (histological) variety listed; e.g., Mesonephroma – see Neoplasm, malignant; Embryoma (see also Neoplasm, uncertain behavior); Disease, Bowen's – see Neoplasm, skin, in situ. However, the guidance in the Index can be overridden if one of the descriptors mentioned above is present; e.g., malignant adenoma of colon is coded to C18.9 and not to D12.6 as the adjective "malignant" overrides the Index entry "Adenoma (see also Neoplasm, benign, by site)." Codes listed with a dash -, following the code have a required additional character for laterality. The tabular list must be reviewed for the complete code.

	Malignant Primary	Malignant Secondary	Ca in situ	Benign	Uncertain	Unspecified Behavior
Neoplasm, neoplastic	C80.1	C79.9	D09.9	D36.9	D48.9	D49.9
abdomen,						
abdominal	C76.2	C79.8-✓	D09.8	D36.7	D48.7	D49.89
cavity	C76.2	C79.8-✓	D09.8	D36.7	D48.7	D49.89
organ	C76.2	C79.8-✓	D09.8	D36.7	D48.7	D49.89
viscera	C76.2	C79.8-✓	D09.8	D36.7	D48.7	D49.89
wall — *see also* Neoplasm, abdomen, wall,						
skin	C44.509	C79.2	D04.5	D23.5	D48.5	D49.2
connective tissue	C49.4	C79.8-✓	—	D21.4	D48.1	D49.2
skin	C44.509	—	—	—	—	—
basal cell carcinoma	C44.519	—	—	—	—	—
specified type NEC	C44.599	—	—	—	—	—
squamous cell carcinoma	C44.529	—	—	—	—	—
abdominopelvic	C76.8	C79.8-✓	—	D36.7	D48.7	D49.89
accessory sinus — *see* Neoplasm, sinus						
acoustic nerve	C72.4-✓	C79.49	—	D33.3	D43.3	D49.7
adenoid (pharynx) (tissue)	C11.1	C79.89	D00.08	D10.6	D37.05	D49.0
adipose tissue — *see also* Neoplasm, connective tissue	C49.4	C79.89		D21.9	D48.1	D49.2
adnexa (uterine)	C57.4	C79.89	D07.39	D28.7	D39.8	D49.59
adrenal	C74.9-✓	C79.7-✓	D09.3	D35.0-✓	D44.1-✓	D49.7
capsule	C74.9-✓	C79.7-✓	D09.3	D35.0-✓	D44.1-✓	D49.7
cortex	C74.0-✓	C79.7-✓	D09.3	D35.0-✓	D44.1-✓	D49.7
gland	C74.9-✓	C79.7-✓	D09.3	D35.0-✓	D44.1-✓	D49.7
medulla	C74.1-✓	C79.7-✓	D09.3	D35.0-✓	D44.1-✓	D49.7
ala nasi (external) — *see also* Neoplasm, skin, nose	C44.301	C79.2	D04.39	D23.39	D48.5	D49.2
alimentary canal or tract NEC	C26.9	C78.80	D01.9	D13.9	D37.9	D49.0
alveolar	C03.9	C79.89	D00.03	D10.39	D37.09	D49.0
mucosa	C03.9	C79.89	D00.03	D10.39	D37.09	D49.0
lower	C03.1	C79.89	D00.03	D10.39	D37.09	D49.0
upper	C03.0	C79.89	D00.03	D10.39	D37.09	D49.0
ridge or process	C41.1	C79.51	—	D16.5	D48.0	D49.2
carcinoma	C03.9	C79.8-✓	—	—	—	—
lower	C03.1	C79.8-✓	—	—	—	—
upper	C03.0	C79.8-✓	—	—	—	—
lower	C41.1	C79.51	—	D16.5	D48.0	D49.2
mucosa	C03.9	C79.89	D00.03	D10.39	D37.09	D49.0
lower	C03.1	C79.89	D00.03	D10.39	D37.09	D49.0
upper	C03.0	C79.89	D00.03	D10.39	D37.09	D49.0
upper	C41.0	C79.51	—	D16.4	D48.0	D49.2
sulcus	C06.1	C79.89	D00.02	D10.39	D37.09	D49.0
alveolus	C03.9	C79.89	D00.03	D10.39	D37.09	D49.0
lower	C03.1	C79.89	D00.03	D10.39	D37.09	D49.0
upper	C03.0	C79.89	D00.03	D10.39	D37.09	D49.0
ampulla of Vater	C24.1	C78.89	D01.5	D13.5	D37.6	D49.0
ankle NEC	C76.5-✓	C79.89	D04.7-✓	D36.7	D48.7	D49.89
anorectum, anorectal (junction)	C21.8	C78.5	D01.3	D12.9	D37.8	D49.0
antecubital fossa or space	C76.4-✓	C79.89	D04.6-✓	D36.7	D48.7	D49.89

Neoplasm, neoplastic — *continued*	Malignant Primary	Malignant Secondary	Ca in situ	Benign	Uncertain	Unspecified Behavior
antrum (Highmore) (maxillary)	C31.0	C78.39	D02.3	D14.0	D38.5	D49.1
pyloric	C16.3	C78.89	D00.2	D13.1	D37.1	D49.0
tympanicum	C30.1	C78.39	D02.3	D14.0	D38.5	D49.1
anus, anal	C21.0	C78.5	D01.3	D12.9	D37.8	D49.0
canal	C21.1	C78.5	D01.3	D12.9	D37.8	D49.0
cloacogenic zone	C21.2	C78.5	D01.3	D12.9	D37.8	D49.0
margin — *see also* Neoplasm, anus, skin	C44.500	C79.2	D04.5	D23.5	D48.5	D49.2
overlapping lesion with rectosigmoid junction or rectum	C21.8	—	—	—	—	—
skin	C44.500	C79.2	D04.5	D23.5	D48.5	D49.2
basal cell carcinoma	C44.510	—	—	—	—	—
specified type NEC	C44.590	—	—	—	—	—
squamous cell carcinoma	C44.520	—	—	—	—	—
sphincter	C21.1	C78.5	D01.3	D12.9	D37.8	D49.0
aorta (thoracic)	C49.3	C79.89	—	D21.3	D48.1	D49.2
abdominal	C49.4	C79.89	—	D21.4	D48.1	D49.2
aortic body	C75.5	C79.89	—	D35.6	D44.7	D49.7
aponeurosis	C49.9	C79.89	—	D21.9	D48.1	D49.2
palmar	C49.1-✓	C79.89	—	D21.1-✓	D48.1	D49.2
plantar	C49.2-✓	C79.89	—	D21.2-✓	D48.1	D49.2
appendix	C18.1	C78.5	D01.0	D12.1	D37.3	D49.0
arachnoid	C70.9	C79.49	—	D32.9	D42.9	D49.7
cerebral	C70.0	C79.32	—	D32.0	D42.0	D49.7
spinal	C70.1	C79.49	—	D32.1	D42.1	D49.7
areola	C50.0-✓	C79.81	D05-✓	D24-✓	D48.6-✓	D49.3
arm NEC	C76.4-✓	C79.89	D04.6-✓	D36.7	D48.7	D49.89
artery — *see* Neoplasm, connective tissue						
aryepiglottic fold	C13.1	C79.89	D00.08	D10.7	D37.05	D49.0
hypopharyngeal aspect	C13.1	C79.89	D00.08	D10.7	D37.05	D49.0
laryngeal aspect	C32.1	C78.39	D02.0	D14.1	D38.0	D49.1
marginal zone	C13.1	C79.89	D00.08	D10.7	D37.05	D49.0
arytenoid (cartilage)	C32.3	C78.39	D02.0	D14.1	D38.0	D49.1
fold — *see* Neoplasm, aryepiglottic						
associated with transplanted organ	C80.2	—	—	—	—	—
atlas	C41.2	C79.51	—	D16.6	D48.0	D49.2
atrium, cardiac	C38.0	C79.89	—	D15.1	D48.7	D49.89
auditory						
canal (external) (skin)	C44.20-✓	C79.2	D04.2-✓	D23.2-✓	D48.5	D49.2
internal	C30.1	C78.39	D02.3	D14.0	D38.5	D49.1
nerve	C72.4-✓	C79.49	—	D33.3	D43.3	D49.7
tube	C30.1	C78.39	D02.3	D14.0	D38.5	D49.1
opening	C11.2	C79.89	D00.08	D10.6	D37.05	D49.0
auricle, ear — *see also* Neoplasm, skin, ear	C44.20-✓	C79.2	D04.2-✓	D23.2-✓	D48.5	D49.2
auricular canal (external) — *see also* Neoplasm, skin, ear	C44.20-✓	C79.2	D04.2-✓	D23.2-✓	D48.5	D49.2
internal	C30.1	C78.39	D02.3	D14.0	D38.5	D49.2
autonomic nerve or nervous system NEC (see Neoplasm, nerve, peripheral)						
axilla, axillary	C76.1	C79.89	D09.8	D36.7	D48.7	D49.89
fold — *see also* Neoplasm, skin, trunk	C44.509	C79.2	D04.5	D23.5	D48.5	D49.2
back NEC	C76.8	C79.89	D04.5	D36.7	D48.7	D49.89
Bartholin's gland	C51.0	C79.82	D07.1	D28.0	D39.8	D49.59
basal ganglia	C71.0	C79.31	—	D33.0	D43.0	D49.6
basis pedunculi	C71.7	C79.31	—	D33.1	D43.1	D49.6
bile or biliary (tract)	C24.9	C78.89	D01.5	D13.5	D37.6	D49.0

Neoplasm Table

Neoplasm, bile or biliary — Neoplasm, brain NEC

Neoplasm, neoplastic — continued / bile or biliary — continued

	Malignant Primary	Malignant Secondary	Ca in situ	Benign	Uncertain	Unspecified Behavior
canaliculi (biliferi) (intrahepatic)	C22.1	C78.7	D01.5	D13.4	D37.6	D49.0
canals, interlobular	C22.1	C78.89	D01.5	D13.4	D37.6	D49.0
duct or passage (common) (cystic) (extrahepatic)	C24.0	C78.89	D01.5	D13.5	D37.6	D49.0
interlobular	C22.1	C78.89	D01.5	D13.4	D37.6	D49.0
intrahepatic	C22.1	C78.7	D01.5	D13.4	D37.6	D49.0
and extrahepatic	C24.8	C78.89	D01.5	D13.5	D37.6	D49.0
bladder (urinary)	C67.9	C79.11	D09.0	D30.3	D41.4	D49.4
dome	C67.1	C79.11	D09.0	D30.3	D41.4	D49.4
neck	C67.5	C79.11	D09.0	D30.3	D41.4	D49.4
orifice	C67.9	C79.11	D09.0	D30.3	D41.4	D49.4
ureteric	C67.6	C79.11	D09.0	D30.3	D41.4	D49.4
urethral	C67.5	C79.11	D09.0	D30.3	D41.4	D49.4
overlapping lesion	C67.8	—	—	—	—	—
sphincter	C67.8	C79.11	D09.0	D30.3	D41.4	D49.4
trigone	C67.0	C79.11	D09.0	D30.3	D41.4	D49.4
urachus	C67.7	C79.11	D09.0	D30.3	D41.4	D49.4
wall	C67.9	C79.11	D09.0	D30.3	D41.4	D49.4
anterior	C67.3	C79.11	D09.0	D30.3	D41.4	D49.4
lateral	C67.2	C79.11	D09.0	D30.3	D41.4	D49.4
posterior	C67.4	C79.11	D09.0	D30.3	D41.4	D49.4
blood vessel — see Neoplasm, connective tissue						
bone (periosteum)	C41.9	C79.51	—	D16.9	D48.0	D49.2
acetabulum	C41.4	C79.51	—	D16.8	D48.0	D49.2
ankle	C40.3-☑	C79.51	—	D16.3-☑	—	—
arm NEC	C40.0-☑	C79.51	—	D16.0-☑	—	—
astragalus	C40.3-☑	C79.51	—	D16.3-☑	—	—
atlas	C41.2	C79.51	—	D16.6	D48.0	D49.2
axis	C41.2	C79.51	—	D16.6	D48.0	D49.2
back NEC	C41.2	C79.51	—	D16.6	D48.0	D49.2
calcaneus	C40.3-☑	C79.51	—	D16.3-☑	—	—
calvarium	C41.0	C79.51	—	D16.4	D48.0	D49.2
carpus (any)	C40.1-☑	C79.51	—	D16.1-☑	—	—
cartilage NEC	C41.9	C79.51	—	D16.9	D48.0	D49.2
clavicle	C41.3	C79.51	—	D16.7	D48.0	D49.2
clivus	C41.0	C79.51	—	D16.4	D48.0	D49.2
coccygeal vertebra	C41.4	C79.51	—	D16.8	D48.0	D49.2
coccyx	C41.4	C79.51	—	D16.8	D48.0	D49.2
costal cartilage	C41.3	C79.51	—	D16.7	D48.0	D49.2
costovertebral joint	C41.3	C79.51	—	D16.7	D48.0	D49.2
cranial	C41.0	C79.51	—	D16.4	D48.0	D49.2
cuboid	C40.3-☑	C79.51	—	D16.3-☑	—	—
cuneiform	C41.9	C79.51	—	D16.9	D48.0	D49.2
elbow	C40.0-☑	C79.51	—	D16.0-☑	—	—
ethmoid (labyrinth)	C41.0	C79.51	—	D16.4	D48.0	D49.2
face	C41.0	C79.51	—	D16.4	D48.0	D49.2
femur (any part)	C40.2-☑	C79.51	—	D16.2-☑	—	—
fibula (any part)	C40.2-☑	C79.51	—	D16.2-☑	—	—
finger (any)	C40.1-☑	C79.51	—	D16.1-☑	—	—
foot	C40.3-☑	C79.51	—	D16.3-☑	—	—
forearm	C40.0-☑	C79.51	—	D16.0-☑	—	—
frontal	C41.0	C79.51	—	D16.4	D48.0	D49.2
hand	C40.1-☑	C79.51	—	D16.1-☑	—	—
heel	C40.3-☑	C79.51	—	D16.3-☑	—	—
hip	C41.4	C79.51	—	D16.8	D48.0	D49.2
humerus (any part)	C40.0-☑	C79.51	—	D16.0-☑	—	—
hyoid	C41.0	C79.51	—	D16.4	D48.0	D49.2
ilium	C41.4	C79.51	—	D16.8	D48.0	D49.2
innominate	C41.4	C79.51	—	D16.8	D48.0	D49.2
intervertebral cartilage or disc	C41.2	C79.51	—	D16.6	D48.0	D49.2
ischium	C41.4	C79.51	—	D16.8	D48.0	D49.2
jaw (lower)	C41.1	C79.51	—	D16.5	D48.0	D49.2
knee	C40.2-☑	C79.51	—	D16.2-☑	—	—
leg NEC	C40.2-☑	C79.51	—	D16.2-☑	—	—
limb NEC	C40.9-☑	C79.51	—	D16.9	—	—

Neoplasm, neoplastic — continued / bone — continued / limb — continued

	Malignant Primary	Malignant Secondary	Ca in situ	Benign	Uncertain	Unspecified Behavior
lower (long bones)	C40.2-☑	C79.51	—	D16.2-☑	—	—
short bones	C40.3-☑	C79.51	—	D16.3-☑	—	—
upper (long bones)	C40.0-☑	C79.51	—	D16.0-☑	—	—
short bones	C40.1-☑	C79.51	—	D16.1-☑	—	—
malar	C41.0	C79.51	—	D16.4	D48.0	D49.2
mandible	C41.1	C79.51	—	D16.5	D48.0	D49.2
marrow NEC (any bone)	C96.9	C79.52	—	—	D47.9	D49.89
mastoid	C41.0	C79.51	—	D16.4	D48.0	D49.2
maxilla, maxillary (superior)	C41.0	C79.51	—	D16.4	D48.0	D49.2
inferior	C41.1	C79.51	—	D16.5	D48.0	D49.2
metacarpus (any)	C40.1-☑	C79.51	—	D16.1-☑	—	—
metatarsus (any)	C40.3-☑	C79.51	—	D16.3-☑	—	—
navicular ankle	C40.3-☑	C79.51	—	—	—	—
hand	C40.1-☑	C79.51	—	—	—	—
nose, nasal	C41.0	C79.51	—	D16.4	D48.0	D49.2
occipital	C41.0	C79.51	—	D16.4	D48.0	D49.2
orbit	C41.0	C79.51	—	D16.4	D48.0	D49.2
overlapping sites	C40.8-☑	—	—	—	—	—
parietal	C41.0	C79.51	—	D16.4	D48.0	D49.2
patella	C40.2-☑	C79.51	—	—	—	—
pelvic	C41.4	C79.51	—	D16.8	D48.0	D49.2
phalanges foot	C40.3-☑	C79.51	—	—	—	—
hand	C40.1-☑	C79.51	—	—	—	—
pubic	C41.4	C79.51	—	D16.8	D48.0	D49.2
radius (any part)	C40.0-☑	C79.51	—	D16.0-☑	—	—
rib	C41.3	C79.51	—	D16.7	D48.0	D49.2
sacral vertebra	C41.4	C79.51	—	D16.8	D48.0	D49.2
sacrum	C41.4	C79.51	—	D16.8	D48.0	D49.2
scaphoid of ankle	C40.3-☑	C79.51	—	—	—	—
of hand	C40.1-☑	C79.51	—	—	—	—
scapula (any part)	C40.0-☑	C79.51	—	D16.0-☑	—	—
sella turcica	C41.0	C79.51	—	D16.4	D48.0	D49.2
shoulder	C40.0-☑	C79.51	—	D16.0-☑	—	—
skull	C41.0	C79.51	—	D16.4	D48.0	D49.2
sphenoid	C41.0	C79.51	—	D16.4	D48.0	D49.2
spine, spinal (column)	C41.2	C79.51	—	D16.6	D48.0	D49.2
coccyx	C41.4	C79.51	—	D16.8	D48.0	D49.2
sacrum	C41.4	C79.51	—	D16.8	D48.0	D49.2
sternum	C41.3	C79.51	—	D16.7	D48.0	D49.2
tarsus (any)	C40.3-☑	C79.51	—	—	—	—
temporal	C41.0	C79.51	—	D16.4	D48.0	D49.2
thumb	C40.1-☑	C79.51	—	—	—	—
tibia (any part)	C40.2-☑	C79.51	—	—	—	—
toe (any)	C40.3-☑	C79.51	—	—	—	—
trapezium	C40.1-☑	C79.51	—	—	—	—
trapezoid	C40.1-☑	C79.51	—	—	—	—
turbinate	C41.0	C79.51	—	D16.4	D48.0	D49.2
ulna (any part)	C40.0-☑	C79.51	—	D16.0-☑	—	—
unciform	C40.1-☑	C79.51	—	—	—	—
vertebra (column)	C41.2	C79.51	—	D16.6	D48.0	D49.2
coccyx	C41.4	C79.51	—	D16.8	D48.0	D49.2
sacrum	C41.4	C79.51	—	D16.8	D48.0	D49.2
vomer	C41.0	C79.51	—	D16.4	D48.0	D49.2
wrist	C40.1-☑	C79.51	—	—	—	—
xiphoid process	C41.3	C79.51	—	D16.7	D48.0	D49.2
zygomatic	C41.0	C79.51	—	D16.4	D48.0	D49.2
book-leaf (mouth) — ventral surface of tongue and floor of mouth	C06.89	C79.89	D00.00	D10.39	D37.09	D49.0
bowel — see Neoplasm, intestine						
brachial plexus	C47.1-☑	C79.89	—	D36.12	D48.2	D49.2
brain NEC	C71.9	C79.31	—	D33.2	D43.2	D49.6

☑ Additional Character Required — Refer to the Tabular List for Character Selection   Subterms under main terms may continue to next column or page

	Malignant Primary	Malignant Secondary	Ca in situ	Benign	Uncertain	Unspecified Behavior
Neoplasm, neoplastic						
— continued						
brain — continued						
basal ganglia	C71.0	C79.31	—	D33.0	D43.0	D49.6
cerebellopontine angle	C71.6	C79.31	—	D33.1	D43.1	D49.6
cerebellum NOS	C71.6	C79.31	—	D33.1	D43.1	D49.6
cerebrum	C71.0	C79.31	—	D33.0	D43.0	D49.6
choroid plexus	C71.7	C79.31	—	D33.1	D43.1	D49.6
corpus callosum	C71.8	C79.31	—	D33.2	D43.2	D49.6
corpus striatum	C71.0	C79.31	—	D33.0	D43.0	D49.6
cortex (cerebral)	C71.0	C79.31	—	D33.0	D43.0	D49.6
frontal lobe	C71.1	C79.31	—	D33.0	D43.0	D49.6
globus pallidus	C71.0	C79.31	—	D33.0	D43.0	D49.6
hippocampus	C71.2	C79.31	—	D33.0	D43.0	D49.6
hypothalamus	C71.0	C79.31	—	D33.0	D43.0	D49.6
internal capsule	C71.0	C79.31	—	D33.0	D43.0	D49.6
medulla oblongata	C71.7	C79.31	—	D33.1	D43.1	D49.6
meninges	C70.0	C79.32	—	D32.0	D42.0	D49.7
midbrain	C71.7	C79.31	—	D33.1	D43.1	D49.6
occipital lobe	C71.4	C79.31	—	D33.0	D43.0	D49.6
overlapping lesion	C71.8	C79.31	—	—	—	—
parietal lobe	C71.3	C79.31	—	D33.0	D43.0	D49.6
peduncle	C71.7	C79.31	—	D33.1	D43.1	D49.6
pons	C71.7	C79.31	—	D33.1	D43.1	D49.6
stem	C71.7	C79.31	—	D33.1	D43.1	D49.6
tapetum	C71.8	C79.31	—	D33.2	D43.2	D49.6
temporal lobe	C71.2	C79.31	—	D33.0	D43.0	D49.6
thalamus	C71.0	C79.31	—	D33.0	D43.0	D49.6
uncus	C71.2	C79.31	—	D33.0	D43.0	D49.6
ventricle (floor)	C71.5	C79.31	—	D33.0	D43.0	D49.6
fourth	C71.7	C79.31	—	D33.1	D43.1	D49.6
branchial (cleft) (cyst) (vestiges)	C10.4	C79.89	D00.08	D10.5	D37.05	D49.0
breast (connective tissue) (glandular tissue) (soft parts)	C50.9-✓	C79.81	D05.-✓	D24.-✓	D48.6-✓	D49.3
areola	C50.0-✓	C79.81	D05.-✓	D24.-✓	D48.6-✓	D49.3
axillary tail	C50.6-✓	C79.81	D05.-✓	D24.-✓	D48.6-✓	D49.3
central portion	C50.1-✓	C79.81	D05.-✓	D24.-✓	D48.6-✓	D49.3
inner	C50.8-✓	C79.81	D05.-✓	D24.-✓	D48.6-✓	D49.3
lower	C50.8-✓	C79.81	D05.-✓	D24.-✓	D48.6-✓	D49.3
lower-inner quadrant	C50.3-✓	C79.81	D05.-✓	D24.-✓	D48.6-✓	D49.3
lower-outer quadrant	C50.5-✓	C79.81	D05.-✓	D24.-✓	D48.6-✓	D49.3
mastectomy site (skin) — see also Neoplasm, breast, skin	C44.501	C79.2	—	—	—	—
specified as breast tissue	C50.8-✓	C79.81	—	—	—	—
midline	C50.8-✓	C79.81	D05.-✓	D24.-✓	D48.6-✓	D49.3
nipple	C50.0-✓	C79.81	D05.-✓	D24.-✓	D48.6-✓	D49.3
outer	C50.8-✓	C79.81	D05.-✓	D24.-✓	D48.6-✓	D49.3
overlapping lesion	C50.8-✓	—	—	—	—	—
skin	C44.501	C79.2	D04.5	D23.5	D48.5	D49.2
basal cell carcinoma	C44.511	—	—	—	—	—
specified type NEC	C44.591	—	—	—	—	—
squamous cell carcinoma	C44.521	—	—	—	—	—
tail (axillary)	C50.6-✓	C79.81	D05.-✓	D24.-✓	D48.6-✓	D49.3
upper	C50.8-✓	C79.81	D05.-✓	D24.-✓	D48.6-✓	D49.3
upper-inner quadrant	C50.2-✓	C79.81	D05.-✓	D24.-✓	D48.6-✓	D49.3
upper-outer quadrant	C50.4-✓	C79.81	D05.-✓	D24.-✓	D48.6-✓	D49.3
broad ligament	C57.1-✓	C79.82	D07.39	D28.2	D39.8	D49.59
bronchiogenic, bronchogenic (lung)	C34.9-✓	C78.0-✓	D02.2-✓	D14.3-✓	D38.1	D49.1
bronchiole	C34.9-✓	C78.0-✓	D02.2-✓	D14.3-✓	D38.1	D49.1
bronchus	C34.9-✓	C78.0-✓	D02.2-✓	D14.3-✓	D38.1	D49.1
carina	C34.0-✓	C78.0-✓	D02.2-✓	D14.3-✓	D38.1	D49.1
lower lobe of lung	C34.3-✓	C78.0-✓	D02.2-✓	D14.3-✓	D38.1	D49.1
Neoplasm, neoplastic						
— continued						
bronchus — continued						
main	C34.0-✓	C78.0-✓	D02.2-✓	D14.3-✓	D38.1	D49.1
middle lobe of lung	C34.2	C78.0-✓	D02.21	D14.31	D38.1	D49.1
overlapping lesion	C34.8-✓	—	—	—	—	—
upper lobe of lung	C34.1-✓	C78.0-✓	D02.2-✓	D14.3-✓	D38.1	D49.1
brow	C44.309	C79.2	D04.39	D23.39	D48.5	D49.2
basal cell carcinoma	C44.319	—	—	—	—	—
specified type NEC	C44.399	—	—	—	—	—
squamous cell carcinoma	C44.329	—	—	—	—	—
buccal (cavity)	C06.9	C79.89	D00.00	D10.39	D37.09	D49.0
commissure	C06.0	C79.89	D00.02	D10.39	D37.09	D49.0
groove (lower) (upper)	C06.1	C79.89	D00.02	D10.39	D37.09	D49.0
mucosa	C06.0	C79.89	D00.02	D10.39	D37.09	D49.0
sulcus (lower) (upper)	C06.1	C79.89	D00.02	D10.39	D37.09	D49.0
bulbourethral gland	C68.0	C79.19	D09.19	D30.4	D41.3	D49.59
bursa — see Neoplasm, connective tissue						
buttock NEC	C76.3	C79.89	D04.5	D36.7	D48.7	D49.89
calf	C76.5-✓	C79.89	D04.7-✓	D36.7	D48.7	D49.89
calvarium	C41.0	C79.51	—	D16.4	D48.0	D49.2
calyx, renal	C65.-✓	C79.0-✓	D09.19	D30.1-✓	D41.1-✓	D49.51-✓
canal						
anal	C21.1	C78.5	D01.3	D12.9	D37.8	D49.0
auditory (external) — see also Neoplasm, skin, ear	C44.20-✓	C79.2	D04.2-✓	D23.2-✓	D48.5	D49.2
auricular (external) — see also Neoplasm, skin, ear	C44.20-✓	C79.2	D04.2-✓	D23.2-✓	D48.5	D49.2
canaliculi, biliary (biliferi) (intrahepatic)	C22.1	C78.7	D01.5	D13.4	D37.6	D49.0
canthus (eye) (inner) (outer)	C44.10-✓	C79.2	D04.1-✓	D23.1-✓	D48.5	D49.2
basal cell carcinoma	C44.11-✓	—	—	—	—	—
sebaceous cell	C44.13-✓	—	—	—	—	—
specified type NEC	C44.19-✓	—	—	—	—	—
squamous cell carcinoma	C44.12-✓	—	—	—	—	—
capillary — see Neoplasm, connective tissue						
caput coli	C18.0	C78.5	D01.0	D12.0	D37.4	D49.0
carcinoid — see Tumor, carcinoid						
cardia (gastric)	C16.0	C78.89	D00.2	D13.1	D37.1	D49.0
cardiac orifice (stomach)	C16.0	C78.89	D00.2	D13.1	D37.1	D49.0
cardio-esophageal junction	C16.0	C78.89	D00.2	D13.1	D37.1	D49.0
cardio-esophagus	C16.0	C78.89	D00.2	D13.1	D37.1	D49.0
carina (bronchus)	C34.0-✓	C78.0-✓	D02.2-✓	D14.3-✓	D38.1	D49.1
carotid (artery)	C49.0	C79.89	—	D21.0	D48.1	D49.2
body	C75.4	C79.89	—	D35.5	D44.6	D49.7
carpus (any bone)	C40.1-✓	C79.51	—	D16.1-✓	—	—
cartilage (articular) (joint) NEC — see also Neoplasm, bone	C41.9	C79.51	—	D16.9	D48.0	D49.2
arytenoid	C32.3	C78.39	D02.0	D14.1	D38.0	D49.1
auricular	C49.0	C79.89	—	D21.0	D48.1	D49.2
bronchi	C34.0-✓	C78.39	—	D14.3-✓	D38.1	D49.1
costal	C41.3	C79.51	—	D16.7	D48.0	D49.2
cricoid	C32.3	C78.39	D02.0	D14.1	D38.0	D49.1
cuneiform	C32.3	C78.39	D02.0	D14.1	D38.0	D49.1
ear (external)	C49.0	C79.89	—	D21.0	D48.1	D49.2
ensiform	C41.3	C79.51	—	D16.7	D48.0	D49.2
epiglottis	C32.1	C78.39	D02.0	D14.1	D38.0	D49.1

Neoplasm, neoplastic
— *continued*

	Malignant Primary	Malignant Secondary	Ca in situ	Benign	Uncertain	Unspecified Behavior
cartilage — *see also* Neoplasm, bone — *continued*						
epiglottis — *continued*						
anterior						
surface	C10.1	C79.89	D00.08	D10.5	D37.05	D49.0
eyelid	C49.0	C79.89	—	D21.0	D48.1	D49.2
intervertebral	C41.2	C79.51	—	D16.6	D48.0	D49.2
larynx, laryngeal	C32.3	C78.39	D02.0	D14.1	D38.0	D49.1
nose, nasal	C30.0	C78.39	D02.3	D14.0	D38.5	D49.1
pinna	C49.0	C79.89	—	D21.0	D48.1	D49.2
rib	C41.3	C79.51	—	D16.7	D48.0	D49.2
semilunar (knee)	C40.2-☑	C79.51	—	D16.2-☑	D48.0	D49.2
thyroid	C32.3	C78.39	D02.0	D14.1	D38.0	D49.1
trachea	C33	C78.39	D02.1	D14.2	D38.1	D49.1
cauda equina	C72.1	C79.49	—	D33.4	D43.4	D49.7
cavity						
buccal	C06.9	C79.89	D00.00	D10.30	D37.09	D49.0
nasal	C30.0	C78.39	D02.3	D14.0	D38.5	D49.1
oral	C06.9	C79.89	D00.00	D10.30	D37.09	D49.0
peritoneal	C48.2	C78.6	—	D20.1	D48.4	D49.0
tympanic	C30.1	C78.39	D02.3	D14.0	D38.5	D49.1
cecum	C18.0	C78.5	D01.0	D12.0	D37.4	D49.0
central nervous system	C72.9	C79.40	—	—	—	—
cerebellopontine (angle)	C71.6	C79.31		D33.1	D43.1	D49.6
cerebellum, cerebellar	C71.6	C79.31		D33.1	D43.1	D49.6
cerebrum, cerebral (cortex) (hemisphere) (white matter)	C71.0	C79.31		D33.0	D43.0	D49.6
meninges	C70.0	C79.32		D32.0	D42.0	D49.7
peduncle	C71.7	C79.31	—	D33.1	D43.1	D49.6
ventricle	C71.5	C79.31	—	D33.0	D43.0	D49.6
fourth	C71.7	C79.31	—	D33.1	D43.1	D49.6
cervical region	C76.0	C79.89	D09.8	D36.7	D48.7	D49.89
cervix (cervical) (uteri) (uterus)	C53.9	C79.82	D06.9	D26.0	D39.0	D49.59
canal	C53.0	C79.82	D06.0	D26.0	D39.0	D49.59
endocervix (canal) (gland)	C53.0	C79.82	D06.0	D26.0	D39.0	D49.59
exocervix	C53.1	C79.82	D06.1	D26.0	D39.0	D49.59
external os	C53.1	C79.82	D06.1	D26.0	D39.0	D49.59
internal os	C53.0	C79.82	D06.0	D26.0	D39.0	D49.59
nabothian gland	C53.0	C79.82	D06.0	D26.0	D39.0	D49.59
overlapping lesion	C53.8	—	—	—	—	—
squamocolumnar junction	C53.8	C79.82	D06.7	D26.0	D39.0	D49.59
stump	C53.8	C79.82	D06.7	D26.0	D39.0	D49.59
cheek	C76.0	C79.89	D09.8	D36.7	D48.7	D49.89
external	C44.309	C79.2	D04.39	D23.39	D48.5	D49.2
basal cell carcinoma	C44.319	—	—	—	—	—
specified type NEC	C44.399	—	—	—	—	—
squamous cell carcinoma	C44.329	—	—	—	—	—
inner aspect	C06.0	C79.89	D00.02	D10.39	D37.09	D49.0
internal	C06.0	C79.89	D00.02	D10.39	D37.09	D49.0
mucosa	C06.0	C79.89	D00.02	D10.39	D37.09	D49.0
chest (wall) NEC	C76.1	C79.89	D09.8	D36.7	D48.7	D49.89
chiasma opticum	C72.3-☑	C79.49		D33.3	D43.3	D49.7
chin	C44.309	C79.2	D04.39	D23.39	D48.5	D49.2
basal cell carcinoma	C44.319	—	—	—	—	—
specified type NEC	C44.399	—	—	—	—	—
squamous cell carcinoma	C44.329	—	—	—	—	—
choana	C11.3	C79.89	D00.08	D10.6	D37.05	D49.0
cholangiole	C22.1	C78.89	D01.5	D13.4	D37.6	D49.0
choledochal duct	C24.0	C78.89	D01.5	D13.5	D37.6	D49.0
choroid	C69.3-☑	C79.49	D09.2-☑	D31.3-☑	D48.7	D49.81
plexus	C71.5	C79.31		D33.0	D43.0	D49.6
ciliary body	C69.4-☑	C79.49	D09.2-☑	D31.4-☑	D48.7	D49.89
clavicle	C41.3	C79.51		D16.7	D48.0	D49.2

Neoplasm, neoplastic
— *continued*

	Malignant Primary	Malignant Secondary	Ca in situ	Benign	Uncertain	Unspecified Behavior
clitoris	C51.2	C79.82	D07.1	D28.0	D39.8	D49.59
clivus	C41.0	C79.51	—	D16.4	D48.0	D49.2
cloacogenic zone	C21.2	C78.5	D01.3	D12.9	D37.8	D49.0
coccygeal						
body or glomus	C49.5	C79.89	—	D21.5	D48.1	D49.2
vertebra	C41.4	C79.51	—	D16.8	D48.0	D49.2
coccyx	C41.4	C79.51	—	D16.8	D48.0	D49.2
colon — *see also* Neoplasm, intestine, large	C18.9	C78.5		—	—	—
with rectum	C19	C78.5	D01.1	D12.7	D37.5	D49.0
columnella — *see also* Neoplasm, skin, face	C44.390	C79.2	D04.39	D23.39	D48.5	D49.2
column, spinal — *see* Neoplasm, spine						
commissure						
labial, lip	C00.6	C79.89	D00.01	D10.39	D37.01	D49.0
laryngeal	C32.0	C78.39	D02.0	D14.1	D38.0	D49.1
common (bile) duct	C24.0	C78.89	D01.5	D13.5	D37.6	D49.0
concha — *see also* Neoplasm, skin, ear	C44.20-☑	C79.2	D04.2-☑	D23.2-☑	D48.5	D49.2
nose	C30.0	C78.39	D02.3	D14.0	D38.5	D49.1
conjunctiva	C69.0-☑	C79.49	D09.2-☑	D31.0-☑	D48.7	D49.89
connective tissue NEC	C49.9	C79.89	—	D21.9	D48.1	D49.2

> **Note:** For neoplasms of connective tissue (blood vessel, bursa, fascia, ligament, muscle, peripheral nerves, sympathetic and parasympathetic nerves and ganglia, synovia, tendon, etc.) or of morphological types that indicate connective tissue, code according to the list under "Neoplasm, connective tissue". For sites that do not appear in this list, code to neoplasm of that site; e.g., fibrosarcoma, pancreas (C25.9)

> **Note:** Morphological types that indicate connective tissue appear in their proper place in the alphabetic index with the instruction "see Neoplasm, connective tissue ...."

	Malignant Primary	Malignant Secondary	Ca in situ	Benign	Uncertain	Unspecified Behavior
abdomen	C49.4	C79.89	—	D21.4	D48.1	D49.2
abdominal wall	C49.4	C79.89	—	D21.4	D48.1	D49.2
ankle	C49.2-☑	C79.89	—	D21.2-☑	D48.1	D49.2
antecubital fossa or space	C49.1-☑	C79.89	—	D21.1-☑	D48.1	D49.2
arm	C49.1-☑	C79.89	—	D21.1-☑	D48.1	D49.2
auricle (ear)	C49.0	C79.89	—	D21.0	D48.1	D49.2
axilla	C49.3	C79.89	—	D21.3	D48.1	D49.2
back	C49.6	C79.89	—	D21.6	D48.1	D49.2
breast — *see* Neoplasm, breast						
buttock	C49.5	C79.89	—	D21.5	D48.1	D49.2
calf	C49.2-☑	C79.89	—	D21.2-☑	D48.1	D49.2
cervical region	C49.0	C79.89	—	D21.0	D48.1	D49.2
cheek	C49.0	C79.89	—	D21.0	D48.1	D49.2
chest (wall)	C49.3	C79.89	—	D21.3	D48.1	D49.2
chin	C49.0	C79.89	—	D21.0	D48.1	D49.2
diaphragm	C49.3	C79.89	—	D21.3	D48.1	D49.2
ear (external)	C49.0	C79.89	—	D21.0	D48.1	D49.2
elbow	C49.1-☑	C79.89	—	D21.1-☑	D48.1	D49.2
extrarectal	C49.5	C79.89	—	D21.5	D48.1	D49.2
extremity	C49.9	C79.89	—	D21.9	D48.1	D49.2
lower	C49.2-☑	C79.89	—	D21.2-☑	D48.1	D49.2
upper	C49.1-☑	C79.89	—	D21.1-☑	D48.1	D49.2
eyelid	C49.0	C79.89	—	D21.0	D48.1	D49.2
face	C49.0	C79.89	—	D21.0	D48.1	D49.2
finger	C49.1-☑	C79.89	—	D21.1-☑	D48.1	D49.2
flank	C49.6	C79.89	—	D21.6	D48.1	D49.2
foot	C49.2-☑	C79.89	—	D21.2-☑	D48.1	D49.2
forearm	C49.1-☑	C79.89	—	D21.1-☑	D48.1	D49.2
forehead	C49.0	C79.89	—	D21.0	D48.1	D49.2
gastric	C49.4	C79.89	—	D21.4	D48.1	D49.2
gastrointestinal	C49.4	C79.89	—	D21.4	D48.1	D49.2
gluteal region	C49.5	C79.89	—	D21.5	D48.1	D49.2
great vessels NEC	C49.3	C79.89	—	D21.3	D48.1	D49.2
groin	C49.5	C79.89	—	D21.5	D48.1	D49.2
hand	C49.1-☑	C79.89	—	D21.1-☑	D48.1	D49.2
head	C49.0	C79.89	—	D21.0	D48.1	D49.2

☑ **Additional Character Required** — Refer to the Tabular List for Character Selection   ⬁ **Subterms under main terms may continue to next column or page**

Neoplasm, neoplastic — continued

	Malignant Primary	Malignant Secondary	Ca in situ	Benign	Uncertain	Unspecified Behavior
Neoplasm, neoplastic — *continued*						
connective tissue — *continued*						
heel	C49.2-☑	C79.89	—	D21.2-☑	D48.1	D49.2
hip	C49.2-☑	C79.89	—	D21.2-☑	D48.1	D49.2
hypochondrium	C49.4	C79.89	—	D21.4	D48.1	D49.2
iliopsoas muscle	C49.5	C79.89	—	D21.5	D48.1	D49.2
infraclavicular region	C49.3	C79.89	—	D21.3	D48.1	D49.2
inguinal (canal) (region)	C49.5	C79.89	—	D21.5	D48.1	D49.2
intestinal	C49.4	C79.89	—	D21.4	D48.1	D49.2
intrathoracic	C49.3	C79.89	—	D21.3	D48.1	D49.2
ischiorectal fossa	C49.5	C79.89	—	D21.5	D48.1	D49.2
jaw	C03.9	C79.89	D00.03	D10.39	D48.1	D49.0
knee	C49.2-☑	C79.89	—	D21.2-☑	D48.1	D49.2
leg	C49.2-☑	C79.89	—	D21.2-☑	D48.1	D49.2
limb NEC	C49.9	C79.89	—	D21.9	D48.1	D49.2
lower	C49.2-☑	C79.89	—	D21.2-☑	D48.1	D49.2
upper	C49.1-☑	C79.89	—	D21.1-☑	D48.1	D49.2
nates	C49.5	C79.89	—	D21.5	D48.1	D49.2
neck	C49.0	C79.89	—	D21.0	D48.1	D49.2
orbit	C69.6-☑	C79.49	D09.2-☑	D31.6-☑	D48.1	D49.89
overlapping lesion	C49.8	—	—	—	—	—
pararectal	C49.5	C79.89	—	D21.5	D48.1	D49.2
para-urethral	C49.5	C79.89	—	D21.5	D48.1	D49.2
paravaginal	C49.5	C79.89	—	D21.5	D48.1	D49.2
pelvis (floor)	C49.5	C79.89	—	D21.5	D48.1	D49.2
pelvo-abdominal	C49.8	C79.89	—	D21.6	D48.1	D49.2
perineum	C49.5	C79.89	—	D21.5	D48.1	D49.2
perirectal (tissue)	C49.5	C79.89	—	D21.5	D48.1	D49.2
periurethral (tissue)	C49.5	C79.89	—	D21.5	D48.1	D49.2
popliteal fossa or space	C49.2-☑	C79.89	—	D21.2-☑	D48.1	D49.2
presacral	C49.5	C79.89	—	D21.5	D48.1	D49.2
psoas muscle	C49.4	C79.89	—	D21.4	D48.1	D49.2
pterygoid fossa	C49.0	C79.89	—	D21.0	D48.1	D49.2
rectovaginal septum or wall	C49.5	C79.89	—	D21.5	D48.1	D49.2
rectovesical	C49.5	C79.89	—	D21.5	D48.1	D49.2
retroperitoneum	C48.0	C78.6	—	D20.0	D48.3	D49.0
sacrococcygeal region	C49.5	C79.89	—	D21.5	D48.1	D49.2
scalp	C49.0	C79.89	—	D21.0	D48.1	D49.2
scapular region	C49.3	C79.89	—	D21.3	D48.1	D49.2
shoulder	C49.1-☑	C79.89	—	D21.1-☑	D48.1	D49.2
skin (dermis) NEC — *see also* Neoplasm, skin, by site	C44.90	C79.2	D04.9	D23.9	D48.5	D49.2
stomach	C49.4	C79.89	—	D21.4	D48.1	D49.2
submental	C49.0	C79.89	—	D21.0	D48.1	D49.2
supraclavicular region	C49.0	C79.89	—	D21.0	D48.1	D49.2
temple	C49.0	C79.89	—	D21.0	D48.1	D49.2
temporal region	C49.0	C79.89	—	D21.0	D48.1	D49.2
thigh	C49.2-☑	C79.89	—	D21.2-☑	D48.1	D49.2
thoracic (duct) (wall)	C49.3	C79.89	—	D21.3	D48.1	D49.2
thorax	C49.3	C79.89	—	D21.3	D48.1	D49.2
thumb	C49.1-☑	C79.89	—	D21.1-☑	D48.1	D49.2
toe	C49.2-☑	C79.89	—	D21.2-☑	D48.1	D49.2
trunk	C49.6	C79.89	—	D21.6	D48.1	D49.2
umbilicus	C49.4	C79.89	—	D21.4	D48.1	D49.2
vesicorectal	C49.5	C79.89	—	D21.5	D48.1	D49.2
wrist	C49.1-☑	C79.89	—	D21.1-☑	D48.1	D49.2
conus medullaris	C72.0	C79.49	—	D33.4	D43.4	D49.7
cord (true) (vocal)	C32.0	C78.39	D02.0	D14.1	D38.0	D49.1
false	C32.1	C78.39	D02.0	D14.1	D38.0	D49.1
spermatic	C63.1-☑	C79.82	D07.69	D29.8	D40.8	D49.59
spinal (cervical) (lumbar) (thoracic)	C72.0	C79.49	—	D33.4	D43.4	D49.7
cornea (limbus)	C69.1-☑	C79.49	D09.2-☑	D31.1-☑	D48.7	D49.89
corpus						
albicans	C56.-☑	C79.6-☑	D07.39	D27.-☑	D39.1-☑	D49.59
callosum, brain	C71.0	C79.31	—	D33.2	D43.2	D49.6

Neoplasm, neoplastic — continued

	Malignant Primary	Malignant Secondary	Ca in situ	Benign	Uncertain	Unspecified Behavior
Neoplasm, neoplastic — *continued*						
corpus — *continued*						
cavernosum	C60.2	C79.82	D07.4	D29.0	D40.8	D49.59
gastric	C16.2	C78.89	D00.2	D13.1	D37.1	D49.0
overlapping sites	C54.8	—	—	—	—	—
penis	C60.2	C79.82	D07.4	D29.0	D40.8	D49.59
striatum, cerebrum	C71.0	C79.31	—	D33.0	D43.0	D49.6
uteri	C54.9	C79.82	D07.0	D26.1	D39.0	D49.59
isthmus	C54.0	C79.82	D07.0	D26.1	D39.0	D49.59
cortex						
adrenal	C74.0-☑	C79.7-☑	D09.3	D35.0-☑	D44.1-☑	D49.7
cerebral	C71.0	C79.31	—	D33.0	D43.0	D49.6
costal cartilage	C41.3	C79.51	—	D16.7	D48.0	D49.2
costovertebral joint	C41.3	C79.51	—	D16.7	D48.0	D49.2
Cowper's gland	C68.0	C79.19	D09.19	D30.4	D41.3	D49.59
cranial (fossa, any)	C71.9	C79.31	—	D33.2	D43.2	D49.6
meninges	C70.0	C79.32	—	D32.0	D42.0	D49.7
nerve	C72.50	C79.49	—	D33.3	D43.3	D49.7
specified NEC	C72.59	C79.49	—	D33.3	D43.3	D49.7
craniobuccal pouch	C75.2	C79.89	D09.3	D35.2	D44.3	D49.7
craniopharyngeal (duct) (pouch)	C75.2	C79.89	D09.3	D35.3	D44.4	D49.7
cricoid	C13.0	C79.89	D00.08	D10.7	D37.05	D49.0
cartilage	C32.3	C78.39	D02.0	D14.1	D38.0	D49.1
cricopharynx	C13.0	C79.89	D00.08	D10.7	D37.05	D49.0
crypt of Morgagni	C21.8	C78.5	D01.3	D12.9	D37.8	D49.0
crystalline lens	C69.4-☑	C79.49	D09.2-☑	D31.4-☑	D48.7	D49.89
cul-de-sac (Douglas')	C48.1	C78.6	—	D20.1	D48.4	D49.0
cuneiform cartilage	C32.3	C78.39	D02.0	D14.1	D38.0	D49.1
cutaneous — *see* Neoplasm, skin						
cutis — *see* Neoplasm, skin						
cystic (bile) duct (common)	C24.0	C78.89	D01.5	D13.5	D37.6	D49.0
dermis — *see* Neoplasm, skin						
diaphragm	C49.3	C79.89	—	D21.3	D48.1	D49.2
digestive organs, system, tube, or tract NEC	C26.9	C78.89	D01.9	D13.9	D37.9	D49.0
disc, intervertebral	C41.2	C79.51	—	D16.6	D48.0	D49.2
disease, generalized	C80.0	—	—	—	—	—
disseminated	C80.0	—	—	—	—	—
Douglas' cul-de-sac or pouch	C48.1	C78.6	—	D20.1	D48.4	D49.0
duodenojejunal junction	C17.8	C78.4	D01.49	D13.39	D37.2	D49.0
duodenum	C17.0	C78.4	D01.49	D13.2	D37.2	D49.0
dura (cranial) (mater)	C70.9	C79.49	—	D32.9	D42.9	D49.7
cerebral	C70.0	C79.32	—	D32.0	D42.0	D49.7
spinal	C70.1	C79.49	—	D32.1	D42.1	D49.7
ear (external) — *see also* Neoplasm, skin, ear	C44.20-☑	C79.2	D04.2-☑	D23.2-☑	D48.5	D49.2
auricle or auris — *see also* Neoplasm, skin, ear	C44.20-☑	C79.2	D04.2-☑	D23.2-☑	D48.5	D49.2
canal, external — *see also* Neoplasm, skin, ear	C44.20-☑	C79.2	D04.2-☑	D23.2-☑	D48.5	D49.2
cartilage	C49.0	C79.89	—	D21.0	D48.1	D49.2
external meatus — *see also* Neoplasm, skin, ear	C44.20-☑	C79.2	D04.2-☑	D23.2-☑	D48.5	D49.2
inner	C30.1	C78.39	D02.3	D14.0	D38.5	D49.1
lobule — *see also* Neoplasm, skin, ear	C44.20-☑	C79.2	D04.2-☑	D23.2-☑	D48.5	D49.2
middle	C30.1	C78.39	D02.3	D14.0	D38.5	D49.1
overlapping lesion with accessory sinuses	C31.8	—	—	—	—	—

Neoplasm Table

Neoplasm, ear — Neoplasm, frenulum

Neoplasm, neoplastic	Malignant Primary	Malignant Secondary	Ca in situ	Benign	Uncertain	Unspecified Behavior
— continued						
ear — see also						
Neoplasm, skin, ear						
— continued						
skin	C44.20-☑	C79.2	D04.2-☑	D23.2-☑	D48.5	D49.2
basal cell						
carcinoma	C44.21-☑	—	—	—	—	—
specified type NEC	C44.29-☑	—	—	—	—	—
squamous cell carcinoma	C44.22-☑	—	—	—	—	—
earlobe	C44.20-☑	C79.2	D04.2-☑	D23.2-☑	D48.5	D49.2
basal cell						
carcinoma	C44.21-☑	—	—	—	—	—
specified type NEC	C44.29-☑	—	—	—	—	—
squamous cell carcinoma	C44.22-☑	—	—	—	—	—
ejaculatory duct	C63.7	C79.82	D07.69	D29.8	D40.8	D49.59
elbow NEC	C76.4-☑	C79.89	D04.6-☑	D36.7	D48.7	D49.89
endocardium	C38.0	C79.89	—	D15.1	D48.7	D49.89
endocervix (canal) (gland)	C53.0	C79.82	D06.0	D26.0	D39.0	D49.59
endocrine gland NEC	C75.9	C79.89	D09.3	D35.9	D44.9	D49.7
pluriglandular	C75.8	C79.89	D09.3	D35.7	D44.9	D49.7
endometrium (gland) (stroma)	C54.1	C79.82	D07.0	D26.1	D39.0	D49.59
ensiform cartilage	C41.3	C79.51	—	D16.7	D48.0	D49.2
enteric — see Neoplasm, intestine						
ependyma (brain)	C71.5	C79.31	—	D33.0	D43.0	D49.6
fourth ventricle	C71.7	C79.31	—	D33.1	D43.1	D49.6
epicardium	C38.0	C79.89	—	D15.1	D48.7	D49.89
epididymis	C63.0-☑	C79.82	D07.69	D29.3-☑	D40.8	D49.59
epidural	C72.9	C79.49	—	D33.9	D43.9	D49.7
epiglottis	C32.1	C78.39	D02.0	D14.1	D38.0	D49.1
anterior aspect or surface	C10.1	C79.89	D00.08	D10.5	D37.05	D49.0
cartilage	C32.3	C78.39	D02.0	D14.1	D38.0	D49.1
free border (margin)	C10.1	C79.89	D00.08	D10.5	D37.05	D49.0
junctional region	C10.8	C79.89	D00.08	D10.5	D37.05	D49.0
posterior (laryngeal) surface	C32.1	C78.39	D02.0	D14.1	D38.0	D49.1
suprahyoid portion	C32.1	C78.39	D02.0	D14.1	D38.0	D49.1
esophagogastric junction	C16.0	C78.89	D00.2	D13.1	D37.1	D49.0
esophagus	C15.9	C78.89	D00.1	D13.0	D37.8	D49.0
abdominal	C15.5	C78.89	D00.1	D13.0	D37.8	D49.0
cervical	C15.3	C78.89	D00.1	D13.0	D37.8	D49.0
distal (third)	C15.5	C78.89	D00.1	D13.0	D37.8	D49.0
lower (third)	C15.5	C78.89	D00.1	D13.0	D37.8	D49.0
middle (third)	C15.4	C78.89	D00.1	D13.0	D37.8	D49.0
overlapping lesion	C15.8	—	—	—	—	—
proximal (third)	C15.3	C78.89	D00.1	D13.0	D37.8	D49.0
thoracic	C15.4	C78.89	D00.1	D13.0	D37.8	D49.0
upper (third)	C15.3	C78.89	D00.1	D13.0	D37.8	D49.0
ethmoid (sinus)	C31.1	C78.39	D02.3	D14.0	D38.5	D49.1
bone or labyrinth	C41.0	C79.51	—	D16.4	D48.0	D49.2
eustachian tube	C30.1	C78.39	D02.3	D14.0	D38.5	D49.1
exocervix	C53.1	C79.82	D06.1	D26.0	D39.0	D49.59
external						
meatus (ear) — see also Neoplasm, skin, ear	C44.20-☑	C79.2	D04.2-☑	D23.2-☑	D48.5	D49.2
os, cervix uteri	C53.1	C79.82	D06.1	D26.0	D39.0	D49.59
extradural	C72.9	C79.49	—	D33.9	D43.9	D49.7
extrahepatic (bile) duct	C24.0	C78.89	D01.5	D13.5	D37.6	D49.0
overlapping lesion with gallbladder	C24.8	—	—	—	—	—
extraocular muscle	C69.6-☑	C79.49	D09.2-☑	D31.6-☑	D48.7	D49.89
extrarectal	C76.3	C79.89	D09.8	D36.7	D48.7	D49.89
extremity	C76.8	C79.89	D04.8	D36.7	D48.7	D49.89

Neoplasm, neoplastic	Malignant Primary	Malignant Secondary	Ca in situ	Benign	Uncertain	Unspecified Behavior
— continued						
extremity — continued						
lower	C76.5-☑	C79.89	D04.7-☑	D36.7	D48.7	D49.89
upper	C76.4-☑	C79.89	D04.6-☑	D36.7	D48.7	D49.89
eyeball	C69.9-☑	C79.49	D09.2-☑	D31.9-☑	D48.7	D49.89
eyebrow	C44.309	C79.2	D04.39	D23.39	D48.5	D49.2
basal cell carcinoma	C44.319	—	—	—	—	—
specified type NEC	C44.399	—	—	—	—	—
squamous cell carcinoma	C44.329	—	—	—	—	—
eyelid (lower) (skin) (upper)	C44.10-☑					
basal cell carcinoma	C44.11-☑					
cartilage	C49.0	C79.89		D21.0	D48.1	D49.2
sebaceous cell	C44.13-☑					
specified type NEC	C44.19-☑					
squamous cell carcinoma	C44.12-☑					
eye NEC	C69.9-☑	C79.49	D09.2-☑	D31.9-☑	D48.7	D49.89
overlapping sites	C69.8-☑					
face NEC	C76.0	C79.89	D04.39	D36.7	D48.7	D49.89
fallopian tube (accessory)	C57.0-☑	C79.82	D07.39	D28.2	D39.8	D49.59
falx (cerebella) (cerebri)	C70.0	C79.32		D32.0	D42.0	D49.7
fascia — see also Neoplasm, connective tissue						
palmar	C49.1-☑	C79.89		D21.1-☑	D48.1	D49.2
plantar	C49.2-☑	C79.89		D21.2-☑	D48.1	D49.2
fatty tissue — see Neoplasm, connective tissue						
fauces, faucial NEC	C10.9	C79.89	D00.08	D10.5	D37.05	D49.0
pillars	C09.1	C79.89	D00.08	D10.5	D37.05	D49.0
tonsil	C09.9	C79.89	D00.08	D10.4	D37.05	D49.0
femur (any part)	C40.2-☑	C79.51	—	D16.2-☑	—	—
fetal membrane	C58	C79.82	D07.0	D26.7	D39.2	D49.59
fibrous tissue — see Neoplasm, connective tissue						
fibula (any part)	C40.2-☑	C79.51	—	D16.2-☑	—	—
filum terminale	C72.0	C79.49		D33.4	D43.4	D49.7
finger NEC	C76.4-☑	C79.89	D04.6-☑	D36.7	D48.7	D49.89
flank NEC	C76.8	C79.89	D04.5	D36.7	D48.7	D49.89
follicle, nabothian	C53.0	C79.82	D06.0	D26.0	D39.0	D49.59
foot NEC	C76.5-☑	C79.89	D04.7-☑	D36.7	D48.7	D49.89
forearm NEC	C76.4-☑	C79.89	D04.6-☑	D36.7	D48.7	D49.89
forehead (skin)	C44.309	C79.2	D04.39	D23.39	D48.5	D49.2
basal cell carcinoma	C44.319	—	—	—	—	—
specified type NEC	C44.399	—	—	—	—	—
squamous cell carcinoma	C44.329					
foreskin	C60.0	C79.82	D07.4	D29.0	D40.8	D49.59
fornix						
pharyngeal	C11.3	C79.89	D00.08	D10.6	D37.05	D49.0
vagina	C52	C79.82	D07.2	D28.1	D39.8	D49.59
fossa (of)						
anterior (cranial)	C71.9	C79.31	—	D33.2	D43.2	D49.6
cranial	C71.9	C79.31	—	D33.2	D43.2	D49.6
ischiorectal	C76.3	C79.89	D09.8	D36.7	D48.7	D49.89
middle (cranial)	C71.9	C79.31	—	D33.2	D43.2	D49.6
piriform	C12	C79.89	D00.08	D10.7	D37.05	D49.0
pituitary	C75.1	C79.89	D09.3	D35.2	D44.3	D49.7
posterior (cranial)	C71.9	C79.31	—	D33.2	D43.2	D49.6
pterygoid	C49.0	C79.89	—	D21.0	D48.1	D49.2
pyriform	C12	C79.89	D00.08	D10.7	D37.05	D49.0
Rosenmuller	C11.2	C79.89	D00.08	D10.6	D37.05	D49.0
tonsillar	C09.0	C79.89	D00.08	D10.5	D37.05	D49.0
fourchette	C51.9	C79.82	D07.1	D28.0	D39.8	D49.59
frenulum						
labii — see Neoplasm, lip, internal						

☑ Additional Character Required — Refer to the Tabular List for Character Selection ▽ Subterms under main terms may continue to next column or page

Neoplasm, neoplastic	Malignant Primary	Malignant Secondary	Ca in situ	Benign	Uncertain	Unspecified Behavior
— continued						
frenulum — continued						
linguae	C02.2	C79.89	D00.07	D10.1	D37.02	D49.0
frontal						
bone	C41.0	C79.51	—	D16.4	D48.0	D49.2
lobe, brain	C71.1	C79.31	—	D33.0	D43.0	D49.6
pole	C71.1	C79.31	—	D33.0	D43.0	D49.6
sinus	C31.2	C78.39	D02.3	D14.0	D38.5	D49.1
fundus						
stomach	C16.1	C78.89	D00.2	D13.1	D37.1	D49.0
uterus	C54.3	C79.82	D07.0	D26.1	D39.0	D49.59
gallbladder	C23	C78.89	D01.5	D13.5	D37.6	D49.0
overlapping lesion with extrahepatic bile ducts	C24.8	—	—	—	—	—
gall duct (extrahepatic)	C24.0	C78.89	D01.5	D13.5	D37.6	D49.0
intrahepatic	C22.1	C78.7	D01.5	D13.4	D37.6	D49.0
ganglia — see also Neoplasm, nerve, peripheral	C47.9	C79.89	—	D36.10	D48.2	D49.2
basal	C71.0	C79.31	—	D33.0	D43.0	D49.6
cranial nerve	C72.50	C79.49	—	D33.3	D43.3	D49.7
Gartner's duct	C52	C79.82	D07.2	D28.1	D39.8	D49.59
gastric — see Neoplasm, stomach						
gastrocolic	C26.9	C78.89	D01.9	D13.9	D37.9	D49.0
gastroesophageal junction	C16.0	C78.89	D00.2	D13.1	D37.1	D49.0
gastrointestinal (tract) NEC	C26.9	C78.89	D01.9	D13.9	D37.9	D49.0
generalized	C80.0	—	—	—	—	—
genital organ or tract						
female NEC	C57.9	C79.82	D07.30	D28.9	D39.9	D49.59
overlapping lesion	C57.8	—	—	—	—	—
specified site NEC	C57.7	C79.82	D07.39	D28.7	D39.8	D49.59
male NEC	C63.9	C79.82	D07.60	D29.9	D40.9	D49.59
overlapping lesion	C63.8	—	—	—	—	—
specified site NEC	C63.7	C79.82	D07.69	D29.8	D40.8	D49.59
genitourinary tract						
female	C57.9	C79.82	D07.30	D28.9	D39.9	D49.59
male	C63.9	C79.82	D07.60	D29.9	D40.9	D49.59
gingiva (alveolar) (marginal)	C03.9	C79.89	D00.03	D10.39	D37.09	D49.0
lower	C03.1	C79.89	D00.03	D10.39	D37.09	D49.0
mandibular	C03.1	C79.89	D00.03	D10.39	D37.09	D49.0
maxillary	C03.0	C79.89	D00.03	D10.39	D37.09	D49.0
upper	C03.0	C79.89	D00.03	D10.39	D37.09	D49.0
gland, glandular (lymphatic) (system) — see also Neoplasm, lymph gland						
endocrine NEC	C75.9	C79.89	D09.3	D35.9	D44.9	D49.7
salivary — see Neoplasm, salivary gland						
glans penis	C60.1	C79.82	D07.4	D29.0	D40.8	D49.59
globus pallidus	C71.0	C79.31	—	D33.0	D43.0	D49.6
glomus						
coccygeal	C49.5	C79.89	—	D21.5	D48.1	D49.2
jugularis	C75.5	C79.89	—	D35.6	D44.7	D49.7
glosso-epiglottic fold(s)	C10.1	C79.89	D00.08	D10.5	D37.05	D49.0
glossopalatine fold	C09.1	C79.89	D00.08	D10.5	D37.05	D49.0
glossopharyngeal sulcus	C09.0	C79.89	D00.08	D10.5	D37.05	D49.0
glottis	C32.0	C78.39	D02.0	D14.1	D38.0	D49.1
gluteal region	C76.3	C79.89	D04.5	D36.7	D48.7	D49.89
great vessels NEC	C49.3	C79.89	—	D21.3	D48.1	D49.2
groin NEC	C76.3	C79.89	D04.5	D36.7	D48.7	D49.89
gum	C03.9	C79.89	D00.03	D10.39	D37.09	D49.0
lower	C03.1	C79.89	D00.03	D10.39	D37.09	D49.0
upper	C03.0	C79.89	D00.03	D10.39	D37.09	D49.0
hand NEC	C76.4-☑	C79.89	D04.6-☑	D36.7	D48.7	D49.89
head NEC	C76.0	C79.89	D04.4	D36.7	D48.7	D49.89
heart	C38.0	C79.89	—	D15.1	D48.7	D49.89

Neoplasm, neoplastic	Malignant Primary	Malignant Secondary	Ca in situ	Benign	Uncertain	Unspecified Behavior
— continued						
heel NEC	C76.5-☑	C79.89	D04.7-☑	D36.7	D48.7	D49.89
helix — see also Neoplasm, skin, ear	C44.20-☑	C79.2	D04.2-☑	D23.2-☑	D48.5	D49.2
hematopoietic, hemopoietic tissue NEC	C96.9	—	—	—	—	—
specified NEC	C96.Z	—	—	—	—	—
hemisphere, cerebral	C71.0	C79.31	—	D33.0	D43.0	D49.6
hemorrhoidal zone	C21.1	C78.5	D01.3	D12.9	D37.8	D49.0
hepatic — see also Index to disease, by histology	C22.9	C78.7	D01.5	D13.4	D37.6	D49.0
duct (bile)	C24.0	C78.89	D01.5	D13.5	D37.6	D49.0
flexure (colon)	C18.3	C78.5	D01.0	D12.3	D37.4	D49.0
primary	C22.8	C78.7	D01.5	D13.4	D37.6	D49.0
hepatobiliary	C24.9	C78.89	D01.5	D13.5	D37.6	D49.0
hepatoblastoma	C22.2	C78.7	D01.5	D13.4	D37.6	D49.0
hepatoma	C22.0	C78.7	D01.5	D13.4	D37.6	D49.0
hilus of lung	C34.0-☑	C78.0-☑	D02.2-☑	D14.3-☑	D38.1	D49.1
hippocampus, brain	C71.2	C79.31	—	D33.0	D43.0	D49.6
hip NEC	C76.5-☑	C79.89	D04.7-☑	D36.7	D48.7	D49.89
humerus (any part)	C40.0-☑	C79.51	—	D16.0-☑	—	—
hymen	C52	C79.82	D07.2	D28.1	D39.8	D49.59
hypopharynx, hypopharyngeal NEC	C13.9	C79.89	D00.08	D10.7	D37.05	D49.0
overlapping lesion	C13.8	—	—	—	—	—
postcricoid region	C13.0	C79.89	D00.08	D10.7	D37.05	D49.0
posterior wall	C13.2	C79.89	D00.08	D10.7	D37.05	D49.0
pyriform fossa (sinus)	C12	C79.89	D00.08	D10.7	D37.05	D49.0
hypophysis	C75.1	C79.89	D09.3	D35.2	D44.3	D49.7
hypothalamus	C71.0	C79.31	—	D33.0	D43.0	D49.6
ileocecum, ileocecal (coil) (junction) (valve)	C18.0	C78.5	D01.0	D12.0	D37.4	D49.0
ileum	C17.2	C78.4	D01.49	D13.39	D37.2	D49.0
ilium	C41.4	C79.51	—	D16.8	D48.0	D49.2
immunoproliferative NEC	C88.9	—	—	—	—	—
infraclavicular (region)	C76.1	C79.89	D04.5	D36.7	D48.7	D49.89
inguinal (region)	C76.3	C79.89	D04.5	D36.7	D48.7	D49.89
insula	C71.0	C79.31	—	D33.0	D43.0	D49.6
insular tissue (pancreas)	C25.4	C78.89	D01.7	D13.7	D37.8	D49.0
brain	C71.0	C79.31	—	D33.0	D43.0	D49.6
interarytenoid fold	C13.1	C78.39	D00.08	D10.7	D37.05	D49.0
hypopharyngeal aspect	C13.1	C79.89	D00.08	D10.7	D37.05	D49.0
laryngeal aspect	C32.1	C78.39	D02.0	D14.1	D38.0	D49.1
marginal zone	C13.1	C79.89	D00.08	D10.7	D37.05	D49.0
interdental						
papillae	C03.9	C79.89	D00.03	D10.39	D37.09	D49.0
lower	C03.1	C79.89	D00.03	D10.39	D37.09	D49.0
upper	C03.0	C79.89	D00.03	D10.39	D37.09	D49.0
internal						
capsule	C71.0	C79.31	—	D33.0	D43.0	D49.6
os (cervix)	C53.0	C79.82	D06.0	D26.0	D39.0	D49.59
intervertebral cartilage or disc	C41.2	C79.51	—	D16.6	D48.0	D49.2
intestine, intestinal	C26.0	C78.80	D01.40	D13.9	D37.8	D49.0
large	C18.9	C78.5	D01.0	D12.6	D37.4	D49.0
appendix	C18.1	C78.5	D01.0	D12.1	D37.3	D49.0
caput coli	C18.0	C78.5	D01.0	D12.0	D37.4	D49.0
cecum	C18.0	C78.5	D01.0	D12.0	D37.4	D49.0
colon	C18.9	C78.5	D01.0	D12.6	D37.4	D49.0
and rectum	C19	C78.5	D01.1	D12.7	D37.5	D49.0
ascending	C18.2	C78.5	D01.0	D12.2	D37.4	D49.0
caput	C18.0	C78.5	D01.0	D12.0	D37.4	D49.0
descending	C18.6	C78.5	D01.0	D12.4	D37.4	D49.0
distal	C18.6	C78.5	D01.0	D12.4	D37.4	D49.0

Neoplasm, neoplastic — continued

	Malignant Primary	Malignant Secondary	Ca in situ	Benign	Uncertain	Unspecified Behavior
intestine, intestinal — continued						
large — continued						
colon — continued						
left	C18.6	C78.5	D01.0	D12.4	D37.4	D49.0
overlapping lesion	C18.8	—	—	—	—	—
pelvic	C18.7	C78.5	D01.0	D12.5	D37.4	D49.0
right	C18.2	C78.5	D01.0	D12.2	D37.4	D49.0
sigmoid (flexure)	C18.7	C78.5	D01.0	D12.5	D37.4	D49.0
transverse	C18.4	C78.5	D01.0	D12.3	D37.4	D49.0
hepatic flexure	C18.3	C78.5	D01.0	D12.3	D37.4	D49.0
ileocecum, ileocecal (coil) (valve)	C18.0	C78.5	D01.0	D12.0	D37.4	D49.0
overlapping lesion	C18.8	—	—	—	—	—
sigmoid flexure (lower) (upper)	C18.7	C78.5	D01.0	D12.5	D37.4	D49.0
splenic flexure	C18.5	C78.5	D01.0	D12.3	D37.4	D49.0
small	C17.9	C78.4	D01.40	D13.30	D37.2	D49.0
duodenum	C17.0	C78.4	D01.49	D13.2	D37.2	D49.0
ileum	C17.2	C78.4	D01.49	D13.39	D37.2	D49.0
jejunum	C17.1	C78.4	D01.49	D13.39	D37.2	D49.0
overlapping lesion	C17.8	—	—	—	—	—
tract NEC	C26.0	C78.89	D01.40	D13.9	D37.8	D49.0
intra-abdominal	C76.2	C79.89	D09.8	D36.7	D48.7	D49.89
intracranial NEC	C71.9	C79.31	—	D33.2	D43.2	D49.6
intrahepatic (bile) duct	C22.1	C78.7	D01.5	D13.4	D37.6	D49.0
intraocular	C69.9-☑	C79.49	D09.2-☑	D31.9-☑	D48.7	D49.89
intraorbital	C69.6-☑	C79.49	D09.2-☑	D31.6-☑	D48.7	D49.89
intrasellar	C75.1	C79.89	D09.3	D35.2	D44.3	D49.7
intrathoracic (cavity) (organs)	C76.1	C79.89	D09.8	D15.9	D48.7	D49.89
specified NEC	C76.1	C79.89	D09.8	D15.7	—	—
iris	C69.4-☑	C79.49	D09.2-☑	D31.4-☑	D48.7	D49.89
ischiorectal (fossa)	C76.3	C79.89	D09.8	D36.7	D48.7	D49.89
ischium	C41.4	C79.51	—	D16.8	D48.0	D49.2
island of Reil	C71.0	C79.31	—	D33.0	D43.0	D49.6
islands or islets of Langerhans	C25.4	C78.89	D01.7	D13.7	D37.8	D49.0
isthmus uteri	C54.0	C79.82	D07.0	D26.1	D39.0	D49.59
jaw	C76.0	C79.89	D09.8	D36.7	D48.7	D49.89
bone	C41.1	C79.51	—	D16.5	D48.0	D49.2
lower	C41.1	C79.51	—	D16.5	—	—
upper	C41.0	C79.51	—	D16.4	—	—
carcinoma (any type) (lower) (upper)	C76.0	C79.89				
skin — see also Neoplasm, skin, face	C44.309	C79.2	D04.39	D23.39	D48.5	D49.2
soft tissues	C03.9	C79.89	D00.03	D10.39	D37.09	D49.0
lower	C03.1	C79.89	D00.03	D10.39	D37.09	D49.0
upper	C03.0	C79.89	D00.03	D10.39	D37.09	D49.0
jejunum	C17.1	C78.4	D01.49	D13.39	D37.2	D49.0
joint NEC — see also Neoplasm, bone	C41.9	C79.51	—	D16.9	D48.0	D49.2
acromioclavicular	C40.0-☑	C79.51	—	D16.0-☑	—	—
bursa or synovial membrane — see Neoplasm, connective tissue						
costovertebral	C41.3	C79.51	—	D16.7	D48.0	D49.2
sternocostal	C41.3	C79.51	—	D16.7	D48.0	D49.2
temporomandibular	C41.1	C79.51	—	D16.5	D48.0	D49.2
junction						
anorectal	C21.8	C78.5	D01.3	D12.9	D37.8	D49.0
cardioesophageal	C16.0	C78.89	D00.2	D13.1	D37.1	D49.0
esophagogastric	C16.0	C78.89	D00.2	D13.1	D37.1	D49.0
gastroesophageal	C16.0	C78.89	D00.2	D13.1	D37.1	D49.0
hard and soft palate	C05.9	C79.89	D00.00	D10.39	D37.09	D49.0
ileocecal	C18.0	C78.5	D01.0	D12.0	D37.4	D49.0

Neoplasm, neoplastic — continued

	Malignant Primary	Malignant Secondary	Ca in situ	Benign	Uncertain	Unspecified Behavior
junction — continued						
pelvirectal	C19	C78.5	D01.1	D12.7	D37.5	D49.0
pelviureteric	C65.-☑	C79.0-☑	D09.19	D30.1-☑	D41.1-☑	D49.59
rectosigmoid	C19	C78.5	D01.1	D12.7	D37.5	D49.0
squamocolumnar, of cervix	C53.8	C79.82	D06.7	D26.0	D39.0	D49.59
Kaposi's sarcoma — see Kaposi's, sarcoma						
kidney (parenchymal)	C64.-☑	C79.0-☑	D09.19	D30.0-☑	D41.0-☑	D49.51-☑
calyx	C65.-☑	C79.0-☑	D09.19	D30.1-☑	D41.1-☑	D49.51-☑
hilus	C65.-☑	C79.0-☑	D09.19	D30.1-☑	D41.1-☑	D49.51-☑
pelvis	C65.-☑	C79.0-☑	D09.19	D30.1-☑	D41.1-☑	D49.51-☑
knee NEC	C76.5-☑	C79.89	D04.7-☑	D36.7	D48.7	D49.89
labia (skin)	C51.9	C79.82	D07.1	D28.0	D39.8	D49.59
majora	C51.0	C79.82	D07.1	D28.0	D39.8	D49.59
minora	C51.1	C79.82	D07.1	D28.0	D39.8	D49.59
labial — see also Neoplasm, lip sulcus (lower)	C00.9	C79.89	D00.01	D10.0	D37.01	D49.0
(upper)	C06.1	C79.89	D00.02	D10.39	D37.09	D49.0
labium (skin)	C51.9	C79.82	D07.1	D28.0	D39.8	D49.59
majus	C51.0	C79.82	D07.1	D28.0	D39.8	D49.59
minus	C51.1	C79.82	D07.1	D28.0	D39.8	D49.59
lacrimal						
canaliculi	C69.5-☑	C79.49	D09.2-☑	D31.5-☑	D48.7	D49.89
duct (nasal)	C69.5-☑	C79.49	D09.2-☑	D31.5-☑	D48.7	D49.89
gland	C69.5-☑	C79.49	D09.2-☑	D31.5-☑	D48.7	D49.89
punctum	C69.5-☑	C79.49	D09.2-☑	D31.5-☑	D48.7	D49.89
sac	C69.5-☑	C79.49	D09.2-☑	D31.5-☑	D48.7	D49.89
Langerhans, islands or islets	C25.4	C78.89	D01.7	D13.7	D37.8	D49.0
laryngopharynx	C13.9	C79.89	D00.08	D10.7	D37.05	D49.0
larynx, laryngeal NEC	C32.9	C78.39	D02.0	D14.1	D38.0	D49.1
aryepiglottic fold	C32.1	C78.39	D02.0	D14.1	D38.0	D49.1
cartilage (arytenoid) (cricoid) (cuneiform) (thyroid)	C32.3	C78.39	D02.0	D14.1	D38.0	D49.1
commissure (anterior) (posterior)	C32.0	C78.39	D02.0	D14.1	D38.0	D49.1
extrinsic NEC	C32.1	C78.39	D02.0	D14.1	D38.0	D49.1
meaning hypopharynx	C13.9	C79.89	D00.08	D10.7	D37.05	D49.0
interarytenoid fold	C32.1	C78.39	D02.0	D14.1	D38.0	D49.1
intrinsic	C32.0	C78.39	D02.0	D14.1	D38.0	D49.1
overlapping lesion	C32.8	—	—	—	—	—
ventricular band	C32.1	C78.39	D02.0	D14.1	D38.0	D49.1
leg NEC	C76.5-☑	C79.89	D04.7-☑	D36.7	D48.7	D49.89
lens, crystalline	C69.4-☑	C79.49	D09.2-☑	D31.4-☑	D48.7	D49.89
lid (lower) (upper)	C44.10-☑	C79.2	D04.1-☑	D23.1-☑	D48.5	D49.2
basal cell carcinoma	C44.11-☑	—	—	—	—	—
sebaceous cell	C44.13-☑	—	—	—	—	—
specified type NEC	C44.19-☑	—	—	—	—	—
squamous cell carcinoma	C44.12-☑	—	—	—	—	—
ligament — see also Neoplasm, connective tissue						
broad	C57.1-☑	C79.82	D07.39	D28.2	D39.8	D49.59
Mackenrodt's	C57.7	C79.82	D07.39	D28.7	D39.8	D49.59
non-uterine — see Neoplasm, connective tissue						
round	C57.2-☑	C79.82	—	D28.2	D39.8	D49.59
sacro-uterine	C57.3	C79.82	—	D28.2	D39.8	D49.59
uterine	C57.3	C79.82	—	D28.2	D39.8	D49.59
utero-ovarian	C57.7	C79.82	D07.39	D28.2	D39.8	D49.59
uterosacral	C57.3	C79.82	—	D28.2	D39.8	D49.59
limb	C76.8	C79.89	D04.8	D36.7	D48.7	D49.89
lower	C76.5-☑	C79.89	D04.7-☑	D36.7	D48.7	D49.89
upper	C76.4-☑	C79.89	D04.6-☑	D36.7	D48.7	D49.89
limbus of cornea	C69.1-☑	C79.49	D09.2-☑	D31.1-☑	D48.7	D49.89

Neoplasm, neoplastic — continued

	Malignant Primary	Malignant Secondary	Ca in situ	Benign	Uncertain	Unspecified Behavior
lingual NEC — see also Neoplasm, tongue	C02.9	C79.89	D00.07	D10.1	D37.02	D49.0
lingula, lung	C34.1-✓	C78.0-✓	D02.2-✓	D14.3-✓	D38.1	D49.1
lip	C00.9	C79.89	D00.01	D10.0	D37.01	D49.0
buccal aspect — see Neoplasm, lip, internal						
commissure	C00.6	C79.89	D00.01	D10.0	D37.01	D49.0
external	C00.2	C79.89	D00.01	D10.0	D37.01	D49.0
lower	C00.1	C79.89	D00.01	D10.0	D37.01	D49.0
upper	C00.0	C79.89	D00.01	D10.0	D37.01	D49.0
frenulum — see Neoplasm, lip, internal						
inner aspect — see Neoplasm, lip, internal						
internal	C00.5	C79.89	D00.01	D10.0	D37.01	D49.0
lower	C00.4	C79.89	D00.01	D10.0	D37.01	D49.0
upper	C00.3	C79.89	D00.01	D10.0	D37.01	D49.0
lipstick area	C00.2	C79.89	D00.01	D10.0	D37.01	D49.0
lower	C00.1	C79.89	D00.01	D10.0	D37.01	D49.0
upper	C00.0	C79.89	D00.01	D10.0	D37.01	D49.0
lower	C00.1	C79.89	D00.01	D10.0	D37.01	D49.0
internal	C00.4	C79.89	D00.01	D10.0	D37.01	D49.0
mucosa — see Neoplasm, lip, internal						
oral aspect — see Neoplasm, lip, internal						
overlapping lesion	C00.8	—	—	—	—	—
with oral cavity or pharynx	C14.8	—	—	—	—	—
skin (commissure) (lower) (upper)	C44.00	C79.2	D04.0	D23.0	D48.5	D49.2
basal cell carcinoma	C44.01	—	—	—	—	—
specified type NEC	C44.09	—	—	—	—	—
squamous cell carcinoma	C44.02	—	—	—	—	—
upper	C00.0	C79.89	D00.01	D10.0	D37.01	D49.0
internal	C00.3	C79.89	D00.01	D10.0	D37.01	D49.0
vermilion border	C00.2	C79.89	D00.01	D10.0	D37.01	D49.0
lower	C00.1	C79.89	D00.01	D10.0	D37.01	D49.0
upper	C00.0	C79.89	D00.01	D10.0	D37.01	D49.0
lipomatous — see Lipoma, by site						
liver — see also Index to disease, by histology	C22.9	C78.7	D01.5	D13.4	D37.6	D49.0
primary	C22.8	C78.7	D01.5	D13.4	D37.6	D49.0
lumbosacral plexus	C47.5	C79.89	—	D36.16	D48.2	D49.2
lung	C34.9-✓	C78.0-✓	D02.2-✓	D14.3-✓	D38.1	D49.1
azygos lobe	C34.1-✓	C78.0-✓	D02.2-✓	D14.3-✓	D38.1	D49.1
carina	C34.0-✓	C78.0-✓	D02.2-✓	D14.3-✓	D38.1	D49.1
hilus	C34.0-✓	C78.0-✓	D02.2-✓	D14.3-✓	D38.1	D49.1
lingula	C34.1-✓	C78.0-✓	D02.2-✓	D14.3-✓	D38.1	D49.1
lobe NEC	C34.9-✓	C78.0-✓	D02.2-✓	D14.3-✓	D38.1	D49.1
lower lobe	C34.3-✓	C78.0-✓	D02.2-✓	D14.3-✓	D38.1	D49.1
main bronchus	C34.0-✓	C78.0-✓	D02.2-✓	D14.3-✓	D38.1	D49.1
mesothelioma — see Mesothelioma						
middle lobe	C34.2	C78.0-✓	D02.21	D14.31	D38.1	D49.1
overlapping lesion	C34.8-✓	—	—	—	—	—
upper lobe	C34.1-✓	C78.0-✓	D02.2-✓	D14.3-✓	D38.1	D49.1
lymph, lymphatic channel NEC	C49.9	C79.89	—	D21.9	D48.1	D49.2
gland (secondary)	—	C77.9	—	D36.0	D48.7	D49.89
abdominal	—	C77.2	—	D36.0	D48.7	D49.89
aortic	—	C77.2	—	D36.0	D48.7	D49.89
arm	—	C77.3	—	D36.0	D48.7	D49.89

Neoplasm, neoplastic — continued
lymph, lymphatic channel — continued
gland — continued

	Malignant Primary	Malignant Secondary	Ca in situ	Benign	Uncertain	Unspecified Behavior
auricular (anterior) (posterior)	—	C77.0	—	D36.0	D48.7	D49.89
axilla, axillary	—	C77.3	—	D36.0	D48.7	D49.89
brachial	—	C77.3	—	D36.0	D48.7	D49.89
bronchial	—	C77.1	—	D36.0	D48.7	D49.89
bronchopulmonary	—	C77.1	—	D36.0	D48.7	D49.89
celiac	—	C77.2	—	D36.0	D48.7	D49.89
cervical	—	C77.0	—	D36.0	D48.7	D49.89
cervicofacial	—	C77.0	—	D36.0	D48.7	D49.89
Cloquet	—	C77.4	—	D36.0	D48.7	D49.89
colic	—	C77.2	—	D36.0	D48.7	D49.89
common duct	—	C77.2	—	D36.0	D48.7	D49.89
cubital	—	C77.3	—	D36.0	D48.7	D49.89
diaphragmatic	—	C77.1	—	D36.0	D48.7	D49.89
epigastric, inferior	—	C77.1	—	D36.0	D48.7	D49.89
epitrochlear	—	C77.3	—	D36.0	D48.7	D49.89
esophageal	—	C77.1	—	D36.0	D48.7	D49.89
face	—	C77.0	—	D36.0	D48.7	D49.89
femoral	—	C77.4	—	D36.0	D48.7	D49.89
gastric	—	C77.2	—	D36.0	D48.7	D49.89
groin	—	C77.4	—	D36.0	D48.7	D49.89
head	—	C77.0	—	D36.0	D48.7	D49.89
hepatic	—	C77.2	—	D36.0	D48.7	D49.89
hilar (pulmonary)	—	C77.1	—	D36.0	D48.7	D49.89
splenic	—	C77.2	—	D36.0	D48.7	D49.89
hypogastric	—	C77.5	—	D36.0	D48.7	D49.89
ileocolic	—	C77.2	—	D36.0	D48.7	D49.89
iliac	—	C77.5	—	D36.0	D48.7	D49.89
infraclavicular	—	C77.3	—	D36.0	D48.7	D49.89
inguina, inguinal	—	C77.4	—	D36.0	D48.7	D49.89
innominate	—	C77.1	—	D36.0	D48.7	D49.89
intercostal	—	C77.1	—	D36.0	D48.7	D49.89
intestinal	—	C77.2	—	D36.0	D48.7	D49.89
intrabdominal	—	C77.2	—	D36.0	D48.7	D49.89
intrapelvic	—	C77.5	—	D36.0	D48.7	D49.89
intrathoracic	—	C77.1	—	D36.0	D48.7	D49.89
jugular	—	C77.0	—	D36.0	D48.7	D49.89
leg	—	C77.4	—	D36.0	D48.7	D49.89
limb lower	—	C77.4	—	D36.0	D48.7	D49.89
upper	—	C77.3	—	D36.0	D48.7	D49.89
lower limb	—	C77.4	—	D36.0	D48.7	D49.89
lumbar	—	C77.2	—	D36.0	D48.7	D49.89
mandibular	—	C77.0	—	D36.0	D48.7	D49.89
mediastinal	—	C77.1	—	D36.0	D48.7	D49.89
mesenteric (inferior) (superior)	—	C77.2	—	D36.0	D48.7	D49.89
midcolic	—	C77.2	—	D36.0	D48.7	D49.89
multiple sites in categories C77.0 - C77.5	—	C77.8	—	D36.0	D48.7	D49.89
neck	—	C77.0	—	D36.0	D48.7	D49.89
obturator	—	C77.5	—	D36.0	D48.7	D49.89
occipital	—	C77.0	—	D36.0	D48.7	D49.89
pancreatic	—	C77.2	—	D36.0	D48.7	D49.89
para-aortic	—	C77.2	—	D36.0	D48.7	D49.89
paracervical	—	C77.5	—	D36.0	D48.7	D49.89
parametrial	—	C77.5	—	D36.0	D48.7	D49.89
parasternal	—	C77.1	—	D36.0	D48.7	D49.89
parotid	—	C77.0	—	D36.0	D48.7	D49.89
pectoral	—	C77.3	—	D36.0	D48.7	D49.89
pelvic	—	C77.5	—	D36.0	D48.7	D49.89
peri-aortic	—	C77.2	—	D36.0	D48.7	D49.89
peripancreatic	—	C77.2	—	D36.0	D48.7	D49.89
popliteal	—	C77.4	—	D36.0	D48.7	D49.89
porta hepatis	—	C77.2	—	D36.0	D48.7	D49.89
portal	—	C77.2	—	D36.0	D48.7	D49.89
preauricular	—	C77.0	—	D36.0	D48.7	D49.89
prelaryngeal	—	C77.0	—	D36.0	D48.7	D49.89
presymphysial	—	C77.5	—	D36.0	D48.7	D49.89
pretracheal	—	C77.0	—	D36.0	D48.7	D49.89
primary (any site) NEC	C96.9	—	—	—	—	—

Neoplasm, neoplastic	Malignant Primary	Malignant Secondary	Ca in situ	Benign	Uncertain	Unspecified Behavior
— continued						
lymph, lymphatic channel — continued						
gland — continued						
pulmonary (hiler)	—	C77.1	—	D36.0	D48.7	D49.89
pyloric	—	C77.2	—	D36.0	D48.7	D49.89
retroperitoneal	—	C77.2	—	D36.0	D48.7	D49.89
retropharyngeal	—	C77.0	—	D36.0	D48.7	D49.89
Rosenmuller's	—	C77.4	—	D36.0	D48.7	D49.89
sacral	—	C77.5	—	D36.0	D48.7	D49.89
scalene	—	C77.0	—	D36.0	D48.7	D49.89
site NEC	—	C77.9	—	D36.0	D48.7	D49.89
splenic (hilar)	—	C77.2	—	D36.0	D48.7	D49.89
subclavicular	—	C77.3	—	D36.0	D48.7	D49.89
subinguinal	—	C77.4	—	D36.0	D48.7	D49.89
sublingual	—	C77.0	—	D36.0	D48.7	D49.89
submandibular	—	C77.0	—	D36.0	D48.7	D49.89
submaxillary	—	C77.0	—	D36.0	D48.7	D49.89
submental	—	C77.0	—	D36.0	D48.7	D49.89
subscapular	—	C77.3	—	D36.0	D48.7	D49.89
supraclavicular	—	C77.0	—	D36.0	D48.7	D49.89
thoracic	—	C77.1	—	D36.0	D48.7	D49.89
tibial	—	C77.4	—	D36.0	D48.7	D49.89
tracheal	—	C77.1	—	D36.0	D48.7	D49.89
tracheobronchial	—	C77.1	—	D36.0	D48.7	D49.89
upper limb	—	C77.3	—	D36.0	D48.7	D49.89
Virchow's	—	C77.0	—	D36.0	D48.7	D49.89
node — see also Neoplasm, lymph gland						
primary NEC	C96.9	—	—	—	—	—
vessel — see also Neoplasm, connective tissue	C49.9	C79.89	—	D21.9	D48.1	D49.2
Mackenrodt's ligament	C57.7	C79.82	D07.39	D28.7	D39.8	D49.59
malar	C41.0	C79.51		D16.4	D48.0	D49.2
region — see Neoplasm, cheek						
mammary gland — see Neoplasm, breast						
mandible	C41.1	C79.51	—	D16.5	D48.0	D49.2
alveolar						
mucosa (carcinoma)	C03.1	C79.89	D00.03	D10.39	D37.09	D49.0
ridge or process	C41.1	C79.51	—	D16.5	D48.0	D49.2
marrow (bone) NEC	C96.9	C79.52	—	—	D47.9	D49.89
mastectomy site (skin) — see also Neoplasm, breast, skin	C44.501	C79.2	—	—	—	—
specified as breast tissue	C50.8-☑	C79.81	—	—	—	—
mastoid (air cells) (antrum) (cavity)	C30.1	C78.39	D02.3	D14.0	D38.5	D49.1
bone or process	C41.0	C79.51	—	D16.4	D48.0	D49.2
maxilla, maxillary (superior)	C41.0	C79.51	—	D16.4	D48.0	D49.2
alveolar						
mucosa	C03.0	C79.89	D00.03	D10.39	D37.09	D49.0
ridge or process (carcinoma)	C41.0	C79.51	—	D16.4	D48.0	D49.2
antrum	C31.0	C78.39	D02.3	D14.0	D38.5	D49.1
carcinoma	C03.0	C79.51	—	—	—	—
inferior — see Neoplasm, mandible						
sinus	C31.0	C78.39	D02.3	D14.0	D38.5	D49.1
meatus external (ear) — see also Neoplasm, skin, ear	C44.20-☑	C79.2	D04.2-☑	D23.2-☑	D48.5	D49.2
Meckel diverticulum, malignant	C17.3	C78.4	D01.49	D13.39	D37.2	D49.0
mediastinum, mediastinal	C38.3	C78.1		D15.2	D38.3	D49.89
anterior	C38.1	C78.1		D15.2	D38.3	D49.89

Neoplasm, neoplastic	Malignant Primary	Malignant Secondary	Ca in situ	Benign	Uncertain	Unspecified Behavior
— continued						
mediastinum, mediastinal — continued						
posterior	C38.2	C78.1		D15.2	D38.3	D49.89
medulla						
adrenal	C74.1-☑	C79.7-☑	D09.3	D35.0-☑	D44.1-☑	D49.7
oblongata	C71.7	C79.31		D33.1	D43.1	D49.6
meibomian gland	C44.10-☑	C79.2	D04.1-☑	D23.1-☑	D48.5	D49.2
basal cell carcinoma	C44.11-☑	—	—	—	—	—
sebaceous cell	C44.13-☑	—	—	—	—	—
specified type NEC	C44.19-☑	—	—	—	—	—
squamous cell carcinoma	C44.12-☑	—	—	—	—	—
melanoma — see Melanoma						
meninges	C70.9	C79.49	—	D32.9	D42.9	D49.7
brain	C70.0	C79.32	—	D32.0	D42.0	D49.7
cerebral	C70.0	C79.32	—	D32.0	D42.0	D49.7
crainial	C70.0	C79.32	—	D32.0	D42.0	D49.7
intracranial	C70.0	C79.32	—	D32.0	D42.0	D49.7
spinal (cord)	C70.1	C79.49	—	D32.1	D42.1	D49.7
meniscus, knee joint (lateral) (medial)	C40.2-☑	C79.51	—	D16.2-☑	D48.0	D49.2
Merkel cell — see Carcinoma, Merkel cell						
mesentery, mesenteric	C48.1	C78.6	—	D20.1	D48.4	D49.0
mesoappendix	C48.1	C78.6	—	D20.1	D48.4	D49.0
mesocolon	C48.1	C78.6	—	D20.1	D48.4	D49.0
mesopharynx — see Neoplasm, oropharynx						
mesosalpinx	C57.1-☑	C79.82	D07.39	D28.2	D39.8	D49.59
mesothelial tissue — see Mesothelioma						
mesothelioma — see Mesothelioma						
mesovarium	C57.1-☑	C79.82	D07.39	D28.2	D39.8	D49.59
metacarpus (any bone)	C40.1-☑	C79.51	—	D16.1-☑	—	—
metastatic NEC — see also Neoplasm, by site, secondary	—	C79.9	—	—	—	—
metatarsus (any bone)	C40.3-☑	C79.51	—	D16.3-☑	—	—
midbrain	C71.7	C79.31	—	D33.1	D43.1	D49.6
milk duct — see Neoplasm, breast						
mons						
pubis	C51.9	C79.82	D07.1	D28.0	D39.8	D49.59
veneris	C51.9	C79.82	D07.1	D28.0	D39.8	D49.59
motor tract	C72.9	C79.49	—	D33.9	D43.9	D49.7
brain	C71.9	C79.31	—	D33.2	D43.2	D49.6
cauda equina	C72.1	C79.49	—	D33.4	D43.4	D49.7
spinal	C72.0	C79.49	—	D33.4	D43.4	D49.7
mouth	C06.9	C79.89	D00.00	D10.30	D37.09	D49.0
book-leaf	C06.89	C79.89	—	—	—	—
floor	C04.9	C79.89	D00.06	D10.2	D37.09	D49.0
anterior portion	C04.0	C79.89	D00.06	D10.2	D37.09	D49.0
lateral portion	C04.1	C79.89	D00.06	D10.2	D37.09	D49.0
overlapping lesion	C04.8	—	—	—	—	—
overlapping NEC	C06.80	—	—	—	—	—
roof	C05.9	C79.89	D00.00	D10.39	D37.09	D49.0
specified part NEC	C06.89	C79.89	D00.00	D10.39	D37.09	D49.0
vestibule	C06.1	C79.89	D00.00	D10.39	D37.09	D49.0
mucosa						
alveolar (ridge or process)	C03.9	C79.89	D00.03	D10.39	D37.09	D49.0
lower	C03.1	C79.89	D00.03	D10.39	D37.09	D49.0
upper	C03.0	C79.89	D00.03	D10.39	D37.09	D49.0
buccal	C06.0	C79.89	D00.02	D10.39	D37.09	D49.0
cheek	C06.0	C79.89	D00.02	D10.39	D37.09	D49.0

☑ Additional Character Required — Refer to the Tabular List for Character Selection   Subterms under main terms may continue to next column or page

Neoplasm, neoplastic	Malignant Primary	Malignant Secondary	Ca in situ	Benign	Uncertain	Unspecified Behavior
— continued						
mucosa — continued						
lip — see Neoplasm, lip, internal						
nasal	C30.0	C78.39	D02.3	D14.0	D38.5	D49.1
oral	C06.0	C79.89	D00.02	D10.39	D37.09	D49.0
Mullerian duct						
female	C57.7	C79.82	D07.39	D28.7	D39.8	D49.59
male	C63.7	C79.82	D07.69	D29.8	D40.8	D49.59
muscle — see also Neoplasm, connective tissue						
extraocular	C69.6-☑	C79.49	D09.2-☑	D31.6-☑	D48.7	D49.89
myocardium	C38.0	C79.89	—	D15.1	D48.7	D49.89
myometrium	C54.2	C79.82	D07.0	D26.1	D39.0	D49.59
myopericardium	C38.0	C79.89	—	D15.1	D48.7	D49.89
nabothian gland (follicle)	C53.0	C79.82	D06.0	D26.0	D39.0	D49.59
nail — see also Neoplasm, skin, limb	C44.90	C79.2	D04.9	D23.9	D48.5	D49.2
finger — see also Neoplasm, skin, limb, upper	C44.60-☑	C79.2	D04.6-☑	D23.6-☑	D48.5	D49.2
toe — see also Neoplasm, skin, limb, lower	C44.70-☑	C79.2	D04.7-☑	D23.7-☑	D48.5	D49.2
nares, naris (anterior) (posterior)	C30.0	C78.39	D02.3	D14.0	D38.5	D49.1
nasal — see Neoplasm, nose						
nasolabial groove — see also Neoplasm, skin, face	C44.309	C79.2	D04.39	D23.39	D48.5	D49.2
nasolacrimal duct	C69.5-☑	C79.49	D09.2-☑	D31.5-☑	D48.7	D49.89
nasopharynx, nasopharyngeal	C11.9	C79.89	D00.08	D10.6	D37.05	D49.0
floor	C11.3	C79.89	D00.08	D10.6	D37.05	D49.0
overlapping lesion	C11.8	—	—	—	—	—
roof	C11.0	C79.89	D00.08	D10.6	D37.05	D49.0
wall	C11.9	C79.89	D00.08	D10.6	D37.05	D49.0
anterior	C11.3	C79.89	D00.08	D10.6	D37.05	D49.0
lateral	C11.2	C79.89	D00.08	D10.6	D37.05	D49.0
posterior	C11.1	C79.89	D00.08	D10.6	D37.05	D49.0
superior	C11.0	C79.89	D00.08	D10.6	D37.05	D49.0
nates — see also Neoplasm, skin, trunk	C44.509	C79.2	D04.5	D23.5	D48.5	D49.2
neck NEC	C76.0	C79.89	D09.8	D36.7	D48.7	D49.89
skin	C44.40	—	—	—	—	—
basal cell carcinoma	C44.41	—	—	—	—	—
specified type NEC	C44.49	—	—	—	—	—
squamous cell carcinoma	C44.42	—	—	—	—	—
nerve (ganglion)	C47.9	C79.89	—	D36.10	D48.2	D49.2
abducens	C72.59	C79.49	—	D33.3	D43.3	D49.7
accessory (spinal)	C72.59	C79.49	—	D33.3	D43.3	D49.7
acoustic	C72.4-☑	C79.49	—	D33.3	D43.3	D49.7
auditory	C72.4-☑	C79.49	—	D33.3	D43.3	D49.7
autonomic NEC — see also Neoplasm, nerve, peripheral	C47.9	C79.89	—	D36.10	D48.2	D49.2
brachial	C47.1-☑	C79.89	—	D36.12	D48.2	D49.2
cranial	C72.50	C79.49	—	D33.3	D43.3	D49.7
specified NEC	C72.59	C79.49	—	D33.3	D43.3	D49.7
facial	C72.59	C79.49	—	D33.3	D43.3	D49.7
femoral	C47.2-☑	C79.89	—	D36.13	D48.2	D49.2
ganglion NEC — see also Neoplasm, nerve, peripheral	C47.9	C79.89	—	D36.10	D48.2	D49.2
glossopharyngeal	C72.59	C79.49	—	D33.3	D43.3	D49.7
hypoglossal	C72.59	C79.49	—	D33.3	D43.3	D49.7
intercostal	C47.3	C79.89	—	D36.14	D48.2	D49.2
lumbar	C47.6	C79.89	—	D36.17	D48.2	D49.2
median	C47.1-☑	C79.89	—	D36.12	D48.2	D49.2
obturator	C47.2-☑	C79.89	—	D36.13	D48.2	D49.2

Neoplasm, neoplastic	Malignant Primary	Malignant Secondary	Ca in situ	Benign	Uncertain	Unspecified Behavior
— continued						
nerve — continued						
oculomotor	C72.59	C79.49	—	D33.3	D43.3	D49.7
olfactory	C47.2-☑	C79.49	—	D33.3	D43.3	D49.7
optic	C72.3-☑	C79.49	—	D33.3	D43.3	D49.7
parasympathetic NEC	C47.9	C79.89	—	D36.10	D48.2	D49.2
peripheral NEC	C47.9	C79.89	—	D36.10	D48.2	D49.2
abdomen	C47.4	C79.89	—	D36.15	D48.2	D49.2
abdominal wall	C47.4	C79.89	—	D36.15	D48.2	D49.2
ankle	C47.2-☑	C79.89	—	D36.13	D48.2	D49.2
antecubital fossa or space	C47.1-☑	C79.89	—	D36.12	D48.2	D49.2
arm	C47.1-☑	C79.89	—	D36.12	D48.2	D49.2
auricle (ear)	C47.0	C79.89	—	D36.11	D48.2	D49.2
axilla	C47.3	C79.89	—	D36.12	D48.2	D49.2
back	C47.6	C79.89	—	D36.17	D48.2	D49.2
buttock	C47.5	C79.89	—	D36.16	D48.2	D49.2
calf	C47.2-☑	C79.89	—	D36.13	D48.2	D49.2
cervical region	C47.0	C79.89	—	D36.11	D48.2	D49.2
cheek	C47.0	C79.89	—	D36.11	D48.2	D49.2
chest (wall)	C47.3	C79.89	—	D36.14	D48.2	D49.2
chin	C47.0	C79.89	—	D36.11	D48.2	D49.2
ear (external)	C47.0	C79.89	—	D36.11	D48.2	D49.2
elbow	C47.1-☑	C79.89	—	D36.12	D48.2	D49.2
extrarectal	C47.5	C79.89	—	D36.16	D48.2	D49.2
extremity	C47.9	C79.89	—	D36.10	D48.2	D49.2
lower	C47.2-☑	C79.89	—	D36.13	D48.2	D49.2
upper	C47.1-☑	C79.89	—	D36.12	D48.2	D49.2
eyelid	C47.0	C79.89	—	D36.11	D48.2	D49.2
face	C47.0	C79.89	—	D36.11	D48.2	D49.2
finger	C47.1-☑	C79.89	—	D36.12	D48.2	D49.2
flank	C47.6	C79.89	—	D36.17	D48.2	D49.2
foot	C47.2-☑	C79.89	—	D36.13	D48.2	D49.2
forearm	C47.1-☑	C79.89	—	D36.12	D48.2	D49.2
forehead	C47.0	C79.89	—	D36.11	D48.2	D49.2
gluteal region	C47.5	C79.89	—	D36.16	D48.2	D49.2
groin	C47.5	C79.89	—	D36.16	D48.2	D49.2
hand	C47.1-☑	C79.89	—	D36.12	D48.2	D49.2
head	C47.0	C79.89	—	D36.11	D48.2	D49.2
heel	C47.2-☑	C79.89	—	D36.13	D48.2	D49.2
hip	C47.2-☑	C79.89	—	D36.13	D48.2	D49.2
infraclavicular region	C47.3	C79.89	—	D36.14	D48.2	D49.2
inguinal (canal) (region)	C47.5	C79.89	—	D36.16	D48.2	D49.2
intrathoracic	C47.3	C79.89	—	D36.14	D48.2	D49.2
ischiorectal fossa	C47.5	C79.89	—	D36.16	D48.2	D49.2
knee	C47.2-☑	C79.89	—	D36.13	D48.2	D49.2
leg	C47.2-☑	C79.89	—	D36.13	D48.2	D49.2
limb NEC	C47.9	C79.89	—	D36.10	D48.2	D49.2
lower	C47.2-☑	C79.89	—	D36.13	D48.2	D49.2
upper	C47.1-☑	C79.89	—	D36.12	D48.2	D49.2
nates	C47.5	C79.89	—	D36.16	D48.2	D49.2
neck	C47.0	C79.89	—	D36.11	D48.2	D49.2
orbit	C69.6-☑	C79.49	—	D31.6-☑	D48.7	D49.2
pararectal	C47.5	C79.89	—	D36.16	D48.2	D49.2
paraurethral	C47.5	C79.89	—	D36.16	D48.2	D49.2
paravaginal	C47.5	C79.89	—	D36.16	D48.2	D49.2
pelvis (floor)	C47.5	C79.89	—	D36.16	D48.2	D49.2
pelvoabdominal	C47.8	C79.89	—	D36.17	D48.2	D49.2
perineum	C47.5	C79.89	—	D36.16	D48.2	D49.2
perirectal (tissue)	C47.5	C79.89	—	D36.16	D48.2	D49.2
periurethral (tissue)	C47.5	C79.89	—	D36.16	D48.2	D49.2
popliteal fossa or space	C47.2-☑	C79.89	—	D36.13	D48.2	D49.2
presacral	C47.5	C79.89	—	D36.16	D48.2	D49.2
pterygoid fossa	C47.0	C79.89	—	D36.11	D48.2	D49.2
rectovaginal septum or wall	C47.5	C79.89	—	D36.16	D48.2	D49.2
rectovesical	C47.5	C79.89	—	D36.16	D48.2	D49.2
sacrococcygeal region	C47.5	C79.89	—	D36.16	D48.2	D49.2
scalp	C47.0	C79.89	—	D36.11	D48.2	D49.2

Neoplasm, neoplastic	Malignant Primary	Malignant Secondary	Ca in situ	Benign	Uncertain	Unspecified Behavior
— continued						
nerve — continued						
peripheral — continued						
scapular						
region	C47.3	C79.89	—	D36.14	D48.2	D49.2
shoulder	C47.1-☑	C79.89	—	D36.12	D48.2	D49.2
submental	C47.0	C79.89	—	D36.11	D48.2	D49.2
supraclavicular						
region	C47.0	C79.89	—	D36.11	D48.2	D49.2
temple	C47.0	C79.89	—	D36.11	D48.2	D49.2
temporal						
region	C47.0	C79.89	—	D36.11	D48.2	D49.2
thigh	C47.2-☑	C79.89	—	D36.13	D48.2	D49.2
thoracic (duct)						
(wall)	C47.3	C79.89	—	D36.14	D48.2	D49.2
thorax	C47.3	C79.89	—	D36.14	D48.2	D49.2
thumb	C47.1-☑	C79.89	—	D36.12	D48.2	D49.2
toe	C47.2-☑	C79.89	—	D36.13	D48.2	D49.2
trunk	C47.6	C79.89	—	D36.17	D48.2	D49.2
umbilicus	C47.4	C79.89	—	D36.15	D48.2	D49.2
vesicorectal	C47.5	C79.89	—	D36.16	D48.2	D49.2
wrist	C47.1-☑	C79.89	—	D36.12	D48.2	D49.2
radial	C47.1-☑	C79.89	—	D36.12	D48.2	D49.2
sacral	C47.5	C79.89	—	D36.16	D48.2	D49.2
sciatic	C47.2-☑	C79.89	—	D36.13	D48.2	D49.2
spinal NEC	C47.9	C79.89	—	D36.10	D48.2	D49.2
accessory	C72.59	C79.49		D33.3	D43.3	D49.7
sympathetic NEC — see also						
Neoplasm, nerve, peripheral	C47.9	C79.89	—	D36.10	D48.2	D49.2
trigeminal	C72.59	C79.49		D33.3	D43.3	D49.7
trochlear	C72.59	C79.49		D33.3	D43.3	D49.7
ulnar	C47.1-☑	C79.89	—	D36.12	D48.2	D49.2
vagus	C72.59	C79.49		D33.3	D43.3	D49.7
nervous system						
(central)	C72.9	C79.40		D33.9	D43.9	D49.7
autonomic — see Neoplasm, nerve, peripheral						
parasympathetic — see Neoplasm, nerve, peripheral						
specified site NEC	—	C79.49	—	D33.7	D43.8	—
sympathetic — see Neoplasm, nerve, peripheral						
nevus — see Nevus						
nipple	C50.0-☑	C79.81	D05.-☑	D24.-☑	—	—
nose, nasal	C76.0	C79.89	D09.8	D36.7	D48.7	D49.89
ala (external) (nasi) — see also Neoplasm, nose, skin	C44.301	C79.2	D04.39	D23.39	D48.5	D49.2
bone	C41.0	C79.51	—	D16.4	D48.0	D49.2
cartilage	C30.0	C78.39	D02.3	D14.0	D38.5	D49.1
cavity	C30.0	C78.39	D02.3	D14.0	D38.5	D49.1
choana	C11.3	C79.89	D00.08	D10.6	D37.05	D49.0
external (skin) — see also Neoplasm, nose, skin	C44.301	C79.2	D04.39	D23.39	D48.5	D49.2
fossa	C30.0	C78.39	D02.3	D14.0	D38.5	D49.1
internal	C30.0	C78.39	D02.3	D14.0	D38.5	D49.1
mucosa	C30.0	C78.39	D02.3	D14.0	D38.5	D49.1
septum	C30.0	C78.39	D02.3	D14.0	D38.5	D49.1
posterior margin	C11.3	C79.89	D00.08	D10.6	D37.05	D49.0
sinus — see Neoplasm, sinus						
skin	C44.301	C79.2	D04.39	D23.39	D48.5	D49.2
basal cell carcinoma	C44.311	—	—	—	—	—
specified type NEC	C44.391	—	—	—	—	—
squamous cell carcinoma	C44.321	—	—	—	—	—
turbinate (mucosa)	C30.0	C78.39	D02.3	D14.0	D38.5	D49.1
bone	C41.0	C79.51	—	D16.4	D48.0	D49.2
vestibule	C30.0	C78.39	D02.3	D14.0	D38.5	D49.1

Neoplasm, neoplastic	Malignant Primary	Malignant Secondary	Ca in situ	Benign	Uncertain	Unspecified Behavior
— continued						
nostril	C30.0	C78.39	D02.3	D14.0	D38.5	D49.1
nucleus pulposus	C41.2	C79.51	—	D16.6	D48.0	D49.2
occipital						
bone	C41.0	C79.51	—	D16.4	D48.0	D49.2
lobe or pole, brain	C71.4	C79.31		D33.0	D43.0	D49.6
odontogenic — see Neoplasm, jaw bone						
olfactory nerve or bulb	C72.2-☑	C79.49	—	D33.3	D43.3	D49.7
olive (brain)	C71.7	C79.31	—	D33.1	D43.1	D49.6
omentum	C48.1	C78.6		D20.1	D48.4	D49.0
operculum (brain)	C71.0	C79.31	—	D33.0	D43.0	D49.6
optic nerve, chiasm, or tract	C72.3-☑	C79.49	—	D33.3	D43.3	D49.7
oral (cavity)	C06.9	C79.89	D00.00	D10.30	D37.09	D49.0
ill-defined	C14.8	C79.89	D00.00	D10.30	D37.09	D49.0
mucosa	C06.0	C79.89	D00.02	D10.39	D37.09	D49.0
orbit	C69.6-☑	C79.49	D09.2-☑	D31.6-☑	D48.7	D49.89
autonomic nerve	C69.6-☑	C79.49		D31.6-☑	D48.7	D49.2
bone	C41.0	C79.51	—	D16.4	D48.0	D49.2
eye	C69.6-☑	C79.49	D09.2-☑	D31.6-☑	D48.7	D49.89
peripheral nerves	C69.6-☑	C79.49		D31.6-☑	D48.7	D49.2
soft parts	C69.6-☑	C79.49	D09.2-☑	D31.6-☑	D48.7	D49.89
organ of Zuckerkandl	C75.5	C79.89	—	D35.6	D44.7	D49.7
oropharynx	C10.9	C79.89	D00.08	D10.5	D37.05	D49.0
branchial cleft (vestige)	C10.4	C79.89	D00.08	D10.5	D37.05	D49.0
junctional region	C10.8	C79.89	D00.08	D10.5	D37.05	D49.0
lateral wall	C10.2	C79.89	D00.08	D10.5	D37.05	D49.0
overlapping lesion	C10.8	—	—	—	—	—
pillars or fauces	C09.1	C79.89	D00.08	D10.5	D37.05	D49.0
posterior wall	C10.3	C79.89	D00.08	D10.5	D37.05	D49.0
vallecula	C10.0	C79.89	D00.08	D10.5	D37.05	D49.0
os						
external	C53.1	C79.82	D06.1	D26.0	D39.0	D49.59
internal	C53.0	C79.82	D06.0	D26.0	D39.0	D49.59
ovary	C56.-☑	C79.6-☑	D07.39	D27.-☑	D39.1-☑	D49.59
oviduct	C57.0-☑	C79.82	D07.39	D28.2	D39.8	D49.59
palate	C05.9	C79.89	D00.00	D10.39	D37.09	D49.0
hard	C05.0	C79.89	D00.05	D10.39	D37.09	D49.0
junction of hard and soft palate	C05.9	C79.89	D00.00	D10.39	D37.09	D49.0
overlapping lesions	C05.8	—	—	—	—	—
soft	C05.1	C79.89	D00.04	D10.39	D37.09	D49.0
nasopharyngeal surface	C11.3	C79.89	D00.08	D10.6	D37.05	D49.0
posterior surface	C11.3	C79.89	D00.08	D10.6	D37.05	D49.0
superior surface	C11.3	C79.89	D00.08	D10.6	D37.05	D49.0
palatoglossal arch	C09.1	C79.89	D00.00	D10.5	D37.09	D49.0
palatopharyngeal arch	C09.1	C79.89	D00.00	D10.5	D37.09	D49.0
pallium	C71.0	C79.31	—	D33.0	D43.0	D49.6
palpebra	C44.10-☑	C79.2	D04.1-☑	D23.1-☑	D48.5	D49.2
basal cell carcinoma	C44.11-☑	—	—	—	—	—
sebaceous cell	C44.13-☑	—				
specified type NEC	C44.19-☑	—				
squamous cell carcinoma	C44.12-☑	—	—	—	—	—
pancreas	C25.9	C78.89	D01.7	D13.6	D37.8	D49.0
body	C25.1	C78.89	D01.7	D13.6	D37.8	D49.0
duct (of Santorini) (of Wirsung)	C25.3	C78.89	D01.7	D13.6	D37.8	D49.0
ectopic tissue	C25.7	C78.89	—	D13.6	D37.8	D49.0
head	C25.0	C78.89	D01.7	D13.6	D37.8	D49.0
islet cells	C25.4	C78.89	D01.7	D13.7	D37.8	D49.0
neck	C25.7	C78.89	D01.7	D13.6	D37.8	D49.0
overlapping lesion	C25.8	—	—	—	—	—
tail	C25.2	C78.89	D01.7	D13.6	D37.8	D49.0

☑ Additional Character Required — Refer to the Tabular List for Character Selection   ▽ Subterms under main terms may continue to next column or page

Neoplasm, neoplastic — continued

	Malignant Primary	Malignant Secondary	Ca in situ	Benign	Uncertain	Unspecified Behavior
para-aortic body	C75.5	C79.89	—	D35.6	D44.7	D49.7
paraganglion NEC	C75.5	C79.89	—	D35.6	D44.7	D49.7
parametrium	C57.3	C79.82	—	D28.2	D39.8	D49.59
paranephric	C48.0	C78.6	—	D20.0	D48.3	D49.0
pararectal	C76.3	C79.89	—	D36.7	D48.7	D49.89
parasagittal (region)	C76.0	C79.89	D09.8	D36.7	D48.7	D49.89
parasellar	C72.9	C79.49	—	D33.9	D43.8	D49.7
parathyroid (gland)	C75.0	C79.89	D09.3	D35.1	D44.2	D49.7
paraurethral	C76.3	C79.89	—	D36.7	D48.7	D49.89
gland	C68.1	C79.19	D09.19	D30.8	D41.8	D49.59
paravaginal	C76.3	C79.89	—	D36.7	D48.7	D49.89
parenchyma, kidney	C64.-☑	C79.0-☑	D09.19	D30.0-☑	D41.0-☑	D49.51-☑
parietal						
bone	C41.0	C79.51	—	D16.4	D48.0	D49.2
lobe, brain	C71.3	C79.31	—	D33.0	D43.0	D49.6
paroophoron	C57.1-☑	C79.82	D07.39	D28.2	D39.8	D49.59
parotid (duct) (gland)	C07	C79.89	D00.00	D11.0	D37.030	D49.0
parovarium	C57.1-☑	C79.82	D07.39	D28.2	D39.8	D49.59
patella	C40.20	C79.51	—	—	—	—
peduncle, cerebral	C71.7	C79.31	—	D33.1	D43.1	D49.6
pelvirectal junction	C19	C78.5	D01.1	D12.7	D37.5	D49.0
pelvis, pelvic	C76.3	C79.89	D09.8	D36.7	D48.7	D49.89
bone	C41.4	C79.51	—	D16.8	D48.0	D49.2
floor	C76.3	C79.89	D09.8	D36.7	D48.7	D49.89
renal	C65.-☑	C79.0-☑	D09.19	D30.1-☑	D41.1-☑	D49.51-☑
viscera	C76.3	C79.89	D09.8	D36.7	D48.7	D49.89
wall	C76.3	C79.89	D09.8	D36.7	D48.7	D49.89
pelvo-abdominal	C76.8	C79.89	D09.8	D36.7	D48.7	D49.89
penis	C60.9	C79.82	D07.4	D29.0	D40.8	D49.59
body	C60.2	C79.82	D07.4	D29.0	D40.8	D49.59
corpus (cavernosum)	C60.2	C79.82	D07.4	D29.0	D40.8	D49.59
glans	C60.1	C79.82	D07.4	D29.0	D40.8	D49.59
overlapping sites	C60.8	—	—	—	—	—
skin NEC	C60.9	C79.82	D07.4	D29.0	D40.8	D49.59
periadrenal (tissue)	C48.0	C78.6	—	D20.0	D48.3	D49.0
perianal (skin) — see also Neoplasm, anus, skin	C44.500	C79.2	D04.5	D23.5	D48.5	D49.2
pericardium	C38.0	C79.89	—	D15.1	D48.7	D49.89
perinephric	C48.0	C78.6	—	D20.0	D48.3	D49.0
perineum	C76.3	C79.89	D09.8	D36.7	D48.7	D49.89
periodontal tissue NEC	C03.9	C79.89	D00.03	D10.39	D37.09	D49.0
periosteum — see Neoplasm, bone						
peripancreatic	C48.0	C78.6	—	D20.0	D48.3	D49.0
peripheral nerve NEC	C47.9	C79.89	—	D36.10	D48.2	D49.2
perirectal (tissue)	C76.3	C79.89	—	D36.7	D48.7	D49.89
perirenal (tissue)	C48.0	C78.6	—	D20.0	D48.3	D49.0
peritoneum, peritoneal (cavity)	C48.2	C78.6	—	D20.1	D48.4	D49.0
benign mesothelial tissue — see Mesothelioma, benign						
overlapping lesion	C48.8	—	—	—	—	—
with digestive organs	C26.9	—	—	—	—	—
parietal	C48.1	C78.6	—	D20.1	D48.4	D49.0
pelvic	C48.1	C78.6	—	D20.1	D48.4	D49.0
specified part NEC	C48.1	C78.6	—	D20.1	D48.4	D49.0
peritonsillar (tissue)	C76.0	C79.89	D09.8	D36.7	D48.7	D49.89
periurethral tissue	C76.3	C79.89	—	D36.7	D48.7	D49.89
phalanges						
foot	C40.3-☑	C79.51	—	D16.3-☑	—	—
hand	C40.1-☑	C79.51	—	D16.1-☑	—	—
pharynx, pharyngeal	C14.0	C79.89	D00.08	D10.9	D37.05	D49.0
bursa	C11.1	C79.89	D00.08	D10.6	D37.05	D49.0

Neoplasm, neoplastic — continued

	Malignant Primary	Malignant Secondary	Ca in situ	Benign	Uncertain	Unspecified Behavior
pharynx, pharyngeal — continued						
fornix	C11.3	C79.89	D00.08	D10.6	D37.05	D49.0
recess	C11.2	C79.89	D00.08	D10.6	D37.05	D49.0
region	C14.0	C79.89	D00.08	D10.9	D37.05	D49.0
tonsil	C11.1	C79.89	D00.08	D10.6	D37.05	D49.0
wall (lateral) (posterior)	C14.0	C79.89	D00.08	D10.9	D37.05	D49.0
pia mater	C70.9	C79.40	—	D32.9	D42.9	D49.7
cerebral	C70.0	C79.32	—	D32.0	D42.0	D49.7
cranial	C70.0	C79.32	—	D32.0	D42.0	D49.7
spinal	C70.1	C79.49	—	D32.1	D42.1	D49.7
pillars of fauces	C09.1	C79.89	D00.08	D10.5	D37.05	D49.0
pineal (body) (gland)	C75.3	C79.89	D09.3	D35.4	D44.5	D49.7
pinna (ear) NEC — see also Neoplasm, skin, ear	C44.20-☑	C79.2	D04.2-☑	D23.2-☑	D48.5	D49.2
piriform fossa or sinus	C12	C79.89	D00.08	D10.7	D37.05	D49.0
pituitary (body) (fossa) (gland) (lobe)	C75.1	C79.89	D09.3	D35.2	D44.3	D49.7
placenta	C58	C79.82	D07.0	D26.7	D39.2	D49.59
pleura, pleural (cavity)	C38.4	C78.2	—	D19.0	D38.2	D49.1
overlapping lesion with heart or mediastinum	C38.8	—	—	—	—	—
parietal	C38.4	C78.2	—	D19.0	D38.2	D49.1
visceral	C38.4	C78.2	—	D19.0	D38.2	D49.1
plexus						
brachial	C47.1-☑	C79.89	—	D36.12	D48.2	D49.2
cervical	C47.0	C79.89	—	D36.11	D48.2	D49.2
choroid	C71.5	C79.31	—	D33.0	D43.0	D49.6
lumbosacral	C47.5	C79.89	—	D36.16	D48.2	D49.2
sacral	C47.5	C79.89	—	D36.16	D48.2	D49.2
pluriendocrine	C75.8	C79.89	D09.3	D35.7	D44.9	D49.7
pole						
frontal	C71.1	C79.31	—	D33.0	D43.0	D49.6
occipital	C71.4	C79.31	—	D33.0	D43.0	D49.6
pons (varolii)	C71.7	C79.31	—	D33.1	D43.1	D49.6
popliteal fossa or space	C76.5-☑	C79.89	D04.7-☑	D36.7	D48.7	D49.89
postcricoid (region)	C13.0	C79.89	D00.08	D10.7	D37.05	D49.0
posterior fossa (cranial)	C71.9	C79.31	—	D33.2	D43.2	D49.6
postnasal space	C11.9	C79.89	D00.08	D10.6	D37.05	D49.0
prepuce	C60.0	C79.82	D07.4	D29.0	D40.8	D49.59
prepylorus	C16.4	C78.89	D00.2	D13.1	D37.1	D49.0
presacral (region)	C76.3	C79.89	—	D36.7	D48.7	D49.89
prostate (gland)	C61	C79.82	D07.5	D29.1	D40.0	D49.59
utricle	C68.0	C79.19	D09.19	D30.4	D41.3	D49.59
pterygoid fossa	C49.0	C79.89	—	D21.0	D48.1	D49.2
pubic bone	C41.4	C79.51	—	D16.8	D48.0	D49.2
pudenda, pudendum (femaie)	C51.9	C79.82	D07.1	D28.0	D39.8	D49.59
pulmonary — see also Neoplasm, lung	C34.9-☑	C78.0-☑	D02.2-☑	D14.3-☑	D38.1	D49.1
putamen	C71.0	C79.31	—	D33.0	D43.0	D49.6
pyloric						
antrum	C16.3	C78.89	D00.2	D13.1	D37.1	D49.0
canal	C16.4	C78.89	D00.2	D13.1	D37.1	D49.0
pylorus	C16.4	C78.89	D00.2	D13.1	D37.1	D49.0
pyramid (brain)	C71.7	C79.31	—	D33.1	D43.1	D49.6
pyriform fossa or sinus	C12	C79.89	D00.08	D10.7	D37.05	D49.0
radius (any part)	C40.0-☑	C79.51	—	D16.0-☑	—	—
Rathke's pouch	C75.1	C79.89	D09.3	D35.2	D44.3	D49.7
rectosigmoid (junction)	C19	C78.5	D01.1	D12.7	D37.5	D49.0
overlapping lesion with anus or rectum	C21.8	—	—	—	—	—
rectouterine pouch	C48.1	C78.6	—	D20.1	D48.4	D49.0
rectovaginal septum or wall	C76.3	C79.89	D09.8	D36.7	D48.7	D49.89
rectovesical septum	C76.3	C79.89	D09.8	D36.7	D48.7	D49.89
rectum (ampulla)	C20	C78.5	D01.2	D12.8	D37.5	D49.0

Neoplasm, neoplastic — continued

	Malignant Primary	Malignant Secondary	Ca in situ	Benign	Uncertain	Unspecified Behavior
rectum — *continued*						
and colon	C19	C78.5	D01.1	D12.7	D37.5	D49.0
overlapping lesion with anus or rectosigmoid junction	C21.8	—	—	—	—	—
renal	C64.-☑	C79.0-☑	D09.19	D30.0-☑	D41.0-☑	D49.51-☑
calyx	C65.-☑	C79.0-☑	D09.19	D30.1-☑	D41.1-☑	D49.51-☑
hilus	C65.-☑	C79.0-☑	D09.19	D30.1-☑	D41.1-☑	D49.51-☑
parenchyma	C64.-☑	C79.0-☑	D09.19	D30.0-☑	D41.0-☑	D49.51-☑
pelvis	C65.-☑	C79.0-☑	D09.19	D30.1-☑	D41.1-☑	D49.51-☑
respiratory						
organs or system NEC	C39.9	C78.30	D02.4	D14.4	D38.6	D49.1
tract NEC	C39.9	C78.30	D02.4	D14.4	D38.5	D49.1
upper	C39.0	C78.30	D02.4	D14.4	D38.5	D49.1
retina	C69.2-☑	C79.49	D09.2-☑	D31.2-☑	D48.7	D49.81
retrobulbar	C69.6-☑	C79.49	—	D31.6-☑	D48.7	D49.89
retrocecal	C48.0	C78.6	—	D20.0	D48.3	D49.0
retromolar (area) (triangle) (trigone)	C06.2	C79.89	D00.00	D10.39	D37.09	D49.0
retro-orbital	C76.0	C79.89	D09.8	D36.7	D48.7	D49.89
retroperitoneal (space) (tissue)	C48.0	C78.6	—	D20.0	D48.3	D49.0
retroperitoneum	C48.0	C78.6	—	D20.0	D48.3	D49.0
retropharyngeal	C14.0	C79.89	D00.08	D10.9	D37.05	D49.0
retrovesical (septum)	C76.3	C79.89	D09.8	D36.7	D48.7	D49.89
rhinencephalon	C71.0	C79.31	—	D33.0	D43.0	D49.6
rib	C41.3	C79.51	—	D16.7	D48.0	D49.2
Rosenmuller's fossa	C11.2	C79.89	D00.08	D10.6	D37.05	D49.0
round ligament	C57.2-☑	C79.82	—	D28.2	D39.8	D49.59
sacrococcyx, sacrococcygeal	C41.4	C79.51	—	D16.8	D48.0	D49.2
region	C76.3	C79.89	D09.8	D36.7	D48.7	D49.89
sacrouterine ligament	C57.3	C79.82	—	D28.2	D39.8	D49.59
sacrum, sacral (vertebra)	C41.4	C79.51	—	D16.8	D48.0	D49.2
salivary gland or duct (major)	C08.9	C79.89	D00.00	D11.9	D37.039	D49.0
minor NEC	C06.9	C79.89	D00.00	D10.39	D37.04	D49.0
overlapping lesion	C08.9	—	—	—	—	—
parotid	C07	C79.89	D00.00	D11.0	D37.030	D49.0
pluriglandular	C08.9	C79.89	D00.00	D11.9	D37.039	D49.0
sublingual	C08.1	C79.89	D00.00	D11.7	D37.031	D49.0
submandibular	C08.0	C79.89	D00.00	D11.7	D37.032	D49.0
submaxillary	C08.0	C79.89	D00.00	D11.7	D37.032	D49.0
salpinx (uterine)	C57.0-☑	C79.82	D07.39	D28.2	D39.8	D49.59
Santorini's duct	C25.3	C78.89	D01.7	D13.6	D37.8	D49.0
scalp	C44.40	C79.2	D04.4	D23.4	D48.5	D49.2
basal cell carcinoma	C44.41	—	—	—	—	—
specified type NEC	C44.49	—	—	—	—	—
squamous cell carcinoma	C44.42	—	—	—	—	—
scapula (any part)	C40.0-☑	C79.51	—	D16.0-☑	—	—
scapular region	C76.1	C79.89	D09.8	D36.7	D48.7	D49.89
scar NEC — *see also* Neoplasm, skin, by site	C44.90	C79.2	D04.9	D23.9	D48.5	D49.2
sciatic nerve	C47.2-☑	C79.89	—	D36.13	D48.2	D49.2
sclera	C69.4-☑	C79.49	D09.2-☑	D31.4-☑	D48.7	D49.89
scrotum (skin)	C63.2	C79.82	D07.61	D29.4	D40.8	D49.59
sebaceous gland — *see* Neoplasm, skin						
sella turcica	C75.1	C79.89	D09.3	D35.2	D44.3	D49.7
bone	C41.0	C79.51	—	D16.4	D48.0	D49.2
semilunar cartilage (knee)	C40.2-☑	C79.51	—	D16.2-☑	D48.0	D49.2
seminal vesicle	C63.7	C79.82	D07.69	D29.8	D40.8	D49.59
septum						
nasal	C30.0	C78.39	D02.3	D14.0	D38.5	D49.1
posterior margin	C11.3	C79.89	D00.08	D10.6	D37.05	D49.0
rectovaginal	C76.3	C79.89	D09.8	D36.7	D48.7	D49.89
rectovesical	C76.3	C79.89	D09.8	D36.7	D48.7	D49.89
septum — *continued*						
urethrovaginal	C57.9	C79.82	D07.30	D28.9	D39.9	D49.59
vesicovaginal	C57.9	C79.82	D07.30	D28.9	D39.9	D49.59
shoulder NEC	C76.4-☑	C79.89	D04.6-☑	D36.7	D48.7	D49.89
sigmoid flexure (lower) (upper)	C18.7	C78.5	D01.0	D12.5	D37.4	D49.0
sinus (accessory)	C31.9	C78.39	D02.3	D14.0	D38.5	D49.1
bone (any)	C41.0	C79.51	—	D16.4	D48.0	D49.2
ethmoidal	C31.1	C78.39	D02.3	D14.0	D38.5	D49.1
frontal	C31.2	C78.39	D02.3	D14.0	D38.5	D49.1
maxillary	C31.0	C78.39	D02.3	D14.0	D38.5	D49.1
nasal, paranasal NEC	C31.9	C78.39	D02.3	D14.0	D38.5	D49.1
overlapping lesion	C31.8	—	—	—	—	—
pyriform	C12	C79.89	D00.08	D10.7	D37.05	D49.0
sphenoid	C31.3	C78.39	D02.3	D14.0	D38.5	D49.1
skeleton, skeletal NEC	C41.9	C79.51	—	D16.9	D48.0	D49.2
Skene's gland	C68.1	C79.19	D09.19	D30.8	D41.8	D49.59
skin NOS	C44.90	C79.2	D04.9	D23.9	D48.5	D49.2
abdominal wall	C44.509	C79.2	D04.5	D23.5	D48.5	D49.2
basal cell carcinoma	C44.519	—	—	—	—	—
specified type NEC	C44.599	—	—	—	—	—
squamous cell carcinoma	C44.529	—	—	—	—	—
ala nasi — *see also* Neoplasm, nose, skin	C44.301	C79.2	D04.39	D23.39	D48.5	D49.2
ankle — *see also* Neoplasm, skin, limb, lower	C44.70-☑	C79.2	D04.7-☑	D23.7-☑	D48.5	D49.2
antecubital space — *see also* Neoplasm, skin, limb, upper	C44.60-☑	C79.2	D04.6-☑	D23.6-☑	D48.5	D49.2
anus	C44.500	C79.2	D04.5	D23.5	D48.5	D49.2
basal cell carcinoma	C44.510	—	—	—	—	—
specified type NEC	C44.590	—	—	—	—	—
squamous cell carcinoma	C44.520	—	—	—	—	—
arm — *see also* Neoplasm, skin, limb, upper	C44.60-☑	C79.2	D04.6-☑	D23.6-☑	D48.5	D49.2
auditory canal (external) — *see also* Neoplasm, skin, ear	C44.20-☑	C79.2	D04.2-☑	D23.2-☑	D48.5	D49.2
auricle (ear) — *see also* Neoplasm, skin, ear	C44.20-☑	C79.2	D04.2-☑	D23.2-☑	D48.5	D49.2
auricular canal (external) — *see also* Neoplasm, skin, ear	C44.20-☑	C79.2	D04.2-☑	D23.2-☑	D48.5	D49.2
axilla, axillary fold — *see also* Neoplasm, skin, trunk	C44.509	C79.2	D04.5	D23.5	D48.5	D49.2
back — *see also* Neoplasm, skin, trunk	C44.509	C79.2	D04.5	D23.5	D48.5	D49.2
basal cell carcinoma	C44.91	—	—	—	—	—
breast	C44.501	C79.2	D04.5	D23.5	D48.5	D49.2
basal cell carcinoma	C44.511	—	—	—	—	—
specified type NEC	C44.591	—	—	—	—	—
squamous cell carcinoma	C44.521	—	—	—	—	—
brow — *see also* Neoplasm, skin, face	C44.309	C79.2	D04.39	D23.39	D48.5	D49.2
buttock — *see also* Neoplasm, skin, trunk	C44.509	C79.2	D04.5	D23.5	D48.5	D49.2

Neoplasm, neoplastic — continued / skin — continued (left)

	Malignant Primary	Malignant Secondary	Ca in situ	Benign	Uncertain	Unspecified Behavior
calf — see also Neoplasm, skin, limb, lower	C44.70-☑	C79.2	D04.7-☑	D23.7-☑	D48.5	D49.2
canthus (eye) (inner) (outer)	C44.10-☑	C79.2	D04.1-☑	D23.1-☑	D48.5	D49.2
basal cell carcinoma	C44.11-☑	—	—	—	—	—
sebaceous cell	C44.13-☑	—	—	—	—	—
specified type NEC	C44.19-☑	—	—	—	—	—
squamous cell carcinoma	C44.12-☑	—	—	—	—	—
cervical region — see also Neoplasm, skin, neck	C44.40	C79.2	D04.4	D23.4	D48.5	D49.2
cheek (external) — see also Neoplasm, skin, face	C44.309	C79.2	D04.39	D23.39	D48.5	D49.2
chest (wall) — see also Neoplasm, skin, trunk	C44.509	C79.2	D04.5	D23.5	D48.5	D49.2
chin — see also Neoplasm, skin, face	C44.309	C79.2	D04.39	D23.39	D48.5	D49.2
clavicular area — see also Neoplasm, skin, trunk	C44.509	C79.2	D04.5	D23.5	D48.5	D49.2
clitoris	C51.2	C79.82	D07.1	D28.0	D39.8	D49.59
columnella — see also Neoplasm, skin, face	C44.309	C79.2	D04.39	D23.39	D48.5	D49.2
concha — see also Neoplasm, skin, ear	C44.20-☑	C79.2	D04.2-☑	D23.2-☑	D48.5	D49.2
ear (external)	C44.20-☑	C79.2	D04.2-☑	D23.2-☑	D48.5	D49.2
basal cell carcinoma	C44.21-☑	—	—	—	—	—
specified type NEC	C44.29-☑	—	—	—	—	—
squamous cell carcinoma	C44.22-☑	—	—	—	—	—
elbow — see also Neoplasm, skin, limb, upper	C44.60-☑	C79.2	D04.6-☑	D23.6-☑	D48.5	D49.2
eyebrow — see also Neoplasm, skin, face	C44.309	C79.2	D04.39	D23.39	D48.5	D49.2
eyelid	C44.10-☑	C79.2	D04.1-☑	D23.1-☑	D48.5	D49.2
basal cell carcinoma	C44.11-☑	—	—	—	—	—
sebaceous cell	C44.13-☑	—	—	—	—	—
specified type NEC	C44.19-☑	—	—	—	—	—
squamous cell carcinoma	C44.12-☑	—	—	—	—	—
face NOS	C44.300	C79.2	D04.30	D23.30	D48.5	D49.2
basal cell carcinoma	C44.310	—	—	—	—	—
specified type NEC	C44.390	—	—	—	—	—
squamous cell carcinoma	C44.320	—	—	—	—	—
female genital organs (external)	C51.9	C79.82	D07.1	D28.0	D39.8	D49.59
clitoris	C51.2	C79.82	D07.1	D28.0	D39.8	D49.59
labium NEC	C51.9	C79.82	D07.1	D28.0	D39.8	D49.59
majus	C51.0	C79.82	D07.1	D28.0	D39.8	D49.59
minus	C51.1	C79.82	D07.1	D28.0	D39.8	D49.59
pudendum	C51.9	C79.82	D07.1	D28.0	D39.8	D49.59
vulva	C51.9	C79.82	D07.1	D28.0	D39.8	D49.59
finger — see also Neoplasm, skin, limb, upper	C44.60-☑	C79.2	D04.6-☑	D23.6-☑	D48.5	D49.2
flank — see also Neoplasm, skin, trunk	C44.509	C79.2	D04.5	D23.5	D48.5	D49.2
foot — see also Neoplasm, skin, limb, lower	C44.70-☑	C79.2	D04.7-☑	D23.7-☑	D48.5	D49.2

Neoplasm, neoplastic — continued / skin — continued (right)

	Malignant Primary	Malignant Secondary	Ca in situ	Benign	Uncertain	Unspecified Behavior
forearm — see also Neoplasm, skin, limb, upper	C44.60-☑	C79.2	D04.6-☑	D23.6-☑	D48.5	D49.2
forehead — see also Neoplasm, skin, face	C44.309	C79.2	D04.39	D23.39	D48.5	D49.2
glabella — see also Neoplasm, skin, face	C44.309	C79.2	D04.39	D23.39	D48.5	D49.2
gluteal region — see also Neoplasm, skin, trunk	C44.509	C79.2	D04.5	D23.5	D48.5	D49.2
groin — see also Neoplasm, skin, trunk	C44.509	C79.2	D04.5	D23.5	D48.5	D49.2
hand — see also Neoplasm, skin, limb, upper	C44.60-☑	C79.2	D04.6-☑	D23.6-☑	D48.5	D49.2
head NEC — see also Neoplasm, skin, scalp	C44.40	C79.2	D04.4	D23.4	D48.5	D49.2
heel — see also Neoplasm, skin, limb, lower	C44.70-☑	C79.2	D04.7-☑	D23.7-☑	D48.5	D49.2
helix — see also Neoplasm, skin, ear	C44.20-☑	C79.2	D04.2-☑	D23.2-☑	D48.5	D49.2
hip — see also Neoplasm, skin, limb, lower	C44.70-☑	C79.2	D04.7-☑	D23.7-☑	D48.5	D49.2
infraclavicular region — see also Neoplasm, skin, trunk	C44.509	C79.2	D04.5	D23.5	D48.5	D49.2
inguinal region — see also Neoplasm, skin, trunk	C44.509	C79.2	D04.5	D23.5	D48.5	D49.2
jaw — see also Neoplasm, skin, face	C44.309	C79.2	D04.39	D23.39	D48.5	D49.2
Kaposi's sarcoma — see Kaposi's, sarcoma, skin						
knee — see also Neoplasm, skin, limb, lower	C44.70-☑	C79.2	D04.7-☑	D23.7-☑	D48.5	D49.2
labia majora	C51.0	C79.82	D07.1	D28.0	D39.8	D49.59
minora	C51.1	C79.82	D07.1	D28.0	D39.8	D49.59
leg — see also Neoplasm, skin, limb, lower	C44.70-☑	C79.2	D04.7-☑	D23.7-☑	D48.5	D49.2
lid (lower) (upper)	C44.10-☑	C79.2	D04.1-☑	D23.1-☑	D48.5	D49.2
basal cell carcinoma	C44.11-☑	—	—	—	—	—
sebaceous cell	C44.13-☑	—	—	—	—	—
specified type NEC	C44.19-☑	—	—	—	—	—
squamous cell carcinoma	C44.12-☑	—	—	—	—	—
limb NEC	C44.90	C79.2	D04.9	D23.9	D48.5	D49.2
basal cell carcinoma	C44.91	—	—	—	—	—
lower	C44.70-☑	C79.2	D04.7-☑	D23.7-☑	D48.5	D49.2
basal cell carcinoma	C44.71-☑	—	—	—	—	—
specified type NEC	C44.79-☑	—	—	—	—	—
squamous cell carcinoma	C44.72-☑	—	—	—	—	—
upper	C44.60-☑	C79.2	D04.6-☑	D23.6-☑	D48.5	D49.2
basal cell carcinoma	C44.61-☑	—	—	—	—	—
specified type NEC	C44.69-☑	—	—	—	—	—
squamous cell carcinoma	C44.62-☑	—	—	—	—	—
lip (lower) (upper)	C44.00	C79.2	D04.0	D23.0	D48.5	D49.2

Neoplasm, neoplastic — continued / skin — continued / lip — continued

	Malignant Primary	Malignant Secondary	Ca in situ	Benign	Uncertain	Unspecified Behavior
basal cell carcinoma	C44.01	—	—	—	—	—
specified type NEC	C44.09	—	—	—	—	—
squamous cell carcinoma	C44.02	—	—	—	—	—
male genital organs	C63.9	C79.82	D07.60	D29.9	D40.8	D49.59
penis	C60.9	C79.82	D07.4	D29.0	D40.8	D49.59
prepuce	C60.0	C79.82	D07.4	D29.0	D40.8	D49.59
scrotum	C63.2	C79.82	D07.61	D29.4	D40.8	D49.59
mastectomy site (skin) — see also Neoplasm, skin, breast	C44.501	C79.2	—	—	—	—
specified as breast tissue	C50.8-☑	C79.81	—	—	—	—
meatus, acoustic (external) — see also Neoplasm, skin, ear	C44.20-☑	C79.2	D04.2-☑	D23.2-☑	D48.5	D49.2
melanotic — see Melanoma						
Merkel cell — see Carcinoma, Merkel cell						
nates — see also Neoplasm, skin, trunk	C44.509	C79.2	D04.5	D23.5	D48.5	D49.2
neck	C44.40	C79.2	D04.4	D23.4	D48.5	D49.2
basal cell carcinoma	C44.41	—	—	—	—	—
specified type NEC	C44.49	—	—	—	—	—
squamous cell carcinoma	C44.42	—	—	—	—	—
nevus — see Nevus, skin						
nose (external) — see also Neoplasm, nose, skin	C44.301	C79.2	D04.39	D23.39	D48.5	D49.2
overlapping lesion	C44.80	—	—	—	—	—
basal cell carcinoma	C44.81	—	—	—	—	—
specified type NEC	C44.89	—	—	—	—	—
squamous cell carcinoma	C44.82	—	—	—	—	—
palm — see also Neoplasm, skin, limb, upper	C44.60-☑	C79.2	D04.6-☑	D23.6-☑	D48.5	D49.2
palpebra	C44.10-☑	C79.2	D04.1-☑	D23.1-☑	D48.5	D49.2
basal cell carcinoma	C44.11-☑	—	—	—	—	—
sebaceous cell	C44.13-☑	—	—	—	—	—
specified type NEC	C44.19-☑	—	—	—	—	—
squamous cell carcinoma	C44.12-☑	—	—	—	—	—
penis NEC	C60.9	C79.82	D07.4	D29.0	D40.8	D49.59
perianal — see also Neoplasm, skin, anus	C44.500	C79.2	D04.5	D23.5	D48.5	D49.2
perineum — see also Neoplasm, skin, anus	C44.500	C79.2	D04.5	D23.5	D48.5	D49.2
pinna — see also Neoplasm, skin, ear	C44.20-☑	C79.2	D04.2-☑	D23.2-☑	D48.5	D49.2
plantar — see also Neoplasm, skin, limb, lower	C44.70-☑	C79.2	D04.7-☑	D23.7-☑	D48.5	D49.2
popliteal fossa or space — see also Neoplasm, skin, limb, lower	C44.70-☑	C79.2	D04.7-☑	D23.7-☑	D48.5	D49.2
prepuce	C60.0	C79.82	D07.4	D29.0	D40.8	D49.59

Neoplasm, neoplastic — continued / skin — continued

	Malignant Primary	Malignant Secondary	Ca in situ	Benign	Uncertain	Unspecified Behavior
pubes — see also Neoplasm, skin, trunk	C44.509	C79.2	D04.5	D23.5	D48.5	D49.2
sacrococcygeal region — see also Neoplasm, skin, trunk	C44.509	C79.2	D04.5	D23.5	D48.5	D49.2
scalp	C44.40	C79.2	D04.4	D23.4	D48.5	D49.2
basal cell carcinoma	C44.41	—	—	—	—	—
specified type NEC	C44.49	—	—	—	—	—
squamous cell carcinoma	C44.42	—	—	—	—	—
scapular region — see also Neoplasm, skin, trunk	C44.509	C79.2	D04.5	D23.5	D48.5	D49.2
scrotum	C63.2	C79.82	D07.61	D29.4	D40.8	D49.59
shoulder — see also Neoplasm, skin, limb, upper	C44.60-☑	C79.2	D04.6-☑	D23.6-☑	D48.5	D49.2
sole (foot) — see also Neoplasm, skin, limb, lower	C44.70-☑	C79.2	D04.7-☑	D23.7-☑	D48.5	D49.2
specified sites NEC	C44.80	C79.2	D04.8	D23.9	D48.5	D49.2
basal cell carcinoma	C44.81	—	—	—	—	—
specified type NEC	C44.89	—	—	—	—	—
squamous cell carcinoma	C44.82	—	—	—	—	—
specified type NEC	C44.99	—	—	—	—	—
squamous cell carcinoma	C44.92	—	—	—	—	—
submammary fold — see also Neoplasm, skin, trunk	C44.509	C79.2	D04.5	D23.5	D48.5	D49.2
supraclavicular region — see also Neoplasm, skin, neck	C44.40	C79.2	D04.4	D23.4	D48.5	D49.2
temple — see also Neoplasm, skin, face	C44.309	C79.2	D04.39	D23.39	D48.5	D49.2
thigh — see also Neoplasm, skin, limb, lower	C44.70-☑	C79.2	D04.7-☑	D23.7-☑	D48.5	D49.2
thoracic wall — see also Neoplasm, skin, trunk	C44.509	C79.2	D04.5	D23.5	D48.5	D49.2
thumb — see also Neoplasm, skin, limb, upper	C44.60-☑	C79.2	D04.6-☑	D23.6-☑	D48.5	D49.2
toe — see also Neoplasm, skin, limb, lower	C44.70-☑	C79.2	D04.7-☑	D23.7-☑	D48.5	D49.2
tragus — see also Neoplasm, skin, ear	C44.20-☑	C79.2	D04.2-☑	D23.2-☑	D48.5	D49.2
trunk	C44.509	C79.2	D04.5	D23.5	D48.5	D49.2
basal cell carcinoma	C44.519	—	—	—	—	—
specified type NEC	C44.599	—	—	—	—	—
squamous cell carcinoma	C44.529	—	—	—	—	—
umbilicus — see also Neoplasm, skin, trunk	C44.509	C79.2	D04.5	D23.5	D48.5	D49.2
vulva	C51.9	C79.82	D07.1	D28.0	D39.8	D49.59
overlapping lesion	C51.8	—	—	—	—	—
wrist — see also Neoplasm, skin, limb, upper	C44.60-☑	C79.2	D04.6-☑	D23.6-☑	D48.5	D49.2
skull	C41.0	C79.51	—	D16.4	D48.0	D49.2

☑ Additional Character Required — Refer to the Tabular List for Character Selection   ⏷ Subterms under main terms may continue to next column or page

Neoplasm, neoplastic	Malignant Primary	Malignant Secondary	Ca in situ	Benign	Uncertain	Unspecified Behavior
— continued						
soft parts or tissues —						
see Neoplasm,						
connective tissue						
specified site NEC	C76.8	C79.89	D09.8	D36.7	D48.7	D49.89
spermatic cord	C63.1-☑	C79.82	D07.69	D29.8	D40.8	D49.59
sphenoid	C31.3	C78.39	D02.3	D14.0	D38.5	D49.1
bone	C41.0	C79.51	—	D16.4	D48.0	D49.2
sinus	C31.3	C78.39	D02.3	D14.0	D38.5	D49.1
sphincter						
anal	C21.1	C78.5	D01.3	D12.9	D37.8	D49.0
of Oddi	C24.0	C78.89	D01.5	D13.5	D37.6	D49.0
spine, spinal						
(column)	C41.2	C79.51	—	D16.6	D48.0	D49.2
bulb	C71.7	C79.31	—	D33.1	D43.1	D49.6
coccyx	C41.4	C79.51	—	D16.8	D48.0	D49.2
cord (cervical)						
(lumbar) (sacral)						
(thoracic)	C72.0	C79.49	—	D33.4	D43.4	D49.7
dura mater	C70.1	C79.49	—	D32.1	D42.1	D49.7
lumbosacral	C41.2	C79.51	—	D16.6	D48.0	D49.2
marrow NEC	C96.9	C79.52	—	—	D47.9	D49.89
membrane	C70.1	C79.49	—	D32.1	D42.1	D49.7
meninges	C70.1	C79.49	—	D32.1	D42.1	D49.7
nerve (root)	C47.9	C79.89	—	D36.10	D48.2	D49.2
pia mater	C70.1	C79.49	—	D32.1	D42.1	D49.7
root	C47.9	C79.89	—	D36.10	D48.2	D49.2
sacrum	C41.4	C79.51	—	D16.8	D48.0	D49.2
spleen, splenic						
NEC	C26.1	C78.89	D01.7	D13.9	D37.8	D49.0
flexure (colon)	C18.5	C78.5	D01.0	D12.3	D37.4	D49.0
stem, brain	C71.7	C79.31	—	D33.1	D43.1	D49.6
Stensen's duct	C07	C79.89	D00.00	D11.0	D37.030	D49.0
sternum	C41.3	C79.51	—	D16.7	D48.0	D49.2
stomach	C16.9	C78.89	D00.2	D13.1	D37.1	D49.0
antrum (pyloric)	C16.3	C78.89	D00.2	D13.1	D37.1	D49.0
body	C16.2	C78.89	D00.2	D13.1	D37.1	D49.0
cardia	C16.0	C78.89	D00.2	D13.1	D37.1	D49.0
cardiac orifice	C16.0	C78.89	D00.2	D13.1	D37.1	D49.0
corpus	C16.2	C78.89	D00.2	D13.1	D37.1	D49.0
fundus	C16.1	C78.89	D00.2	D13.1	D37.1	D49.0
greater curvature						
NEC	C16.6	C78.89	D00.2	D13.1	D37.1	D49.0
lesser curvature						
NEC	C16.5	C78.89	D00.2	D13.1	D37.1	D49.0
overlapping						
lesion	C16.8	—	—	—	—	—
prepylorus	C16.4	C78.89	D00.2	D13.1	D37.1	D49.0
pylorus	C16.4	C78.89	D00.2	D13.1	D37.1	D49.0
wall NEC	C16.9	C78.89	D00.2	D13.1	D37.1	D49.0
anterior NEC	C16.8	C78.89	D00.2	D13.1	D37.1	D49.0
posterior NEC	C16.8	C78.89	D00.2	D13.1	D37.1	D49.0
stroma,						
endometrial	C54.1	C79.82	D07.0	D26.1	D39.0	D49.59
stump, cervical	C53.8	C79.82	D06.7	D26.0	D39.0	D49.59
subcutaneous (nodule)						
(tissue) NEC — see						
Neoplasm,						
connective tissue						
subdural	C70.9	C79.32	—	D32.9	D42.9	D49.7
subglottis,						
subglottic	C32.2	C78.39	D02.0	D14.1	D38.0	D49.1
sublingual	C04.9	C79.89	D00.06	D10.2	D37.09	D49.0
gland or duct	C08.1	C79.89	D00.00	D11.7	D37.031	D49.0
submandibular						
gland	C08.0	C79.89	D00.00	D11.7	D37.032	D49.0
submaxillary gland or						
duct	C08.0	C79.89	D00.00	D11.7	D37.032	D49.0
submental	C76.0	C79.89	D09.8	D36.7	D48.7	D49.89
subpleural	C34.9-☑	C78.0-☑	D02.2-☑	D14.3-☑	D38.1	D49.1
substernal	C38.1	C78.1	—	D15.2	D38.3	D49.89
sudoriferous,						
sudoriparous gland,						
site						
unspecified	C44.90	C79.2	D04.9	D23.9	D48.5	D49.2
specified site — see						
Neoplasm, skin						
supraclavicular						
region	C76.0	C79.89	D09.8	D36.7	D48.7	D49.89
supraglottis	C32.1	C78.39	D02.0	D14.1	D38.0	D49.1
suprarenal	C74.9-☑	C79.7-☑	D09.3	D35.0-☑	D44.1-☑	D49.7
capsule	C74.9-☑	C79.7-☑	D09.3	D35.0-☑	D44.1-☑	D49.7

Neoplasm, neoplastic	Malignant Primary	Malignant Secondary	Ca in situ	Benign	Uncertain	Unspecified Behavior
— continued						
suprarenal —						
continued						
cortex	C74.0-☑	C79.7-☑	D09.3	D35.0-☑	D44.1-☑	D49.7
gland	C74.9-☑	C79.7-☑	D09.3	D35.0-☑	D44.1-☑	D49.7
medulla	C74.1-☑	C79.7-☑	D09.3	D35.0-☑	D44.1-☑	D49.7
suprasellar						
(region)	C71.9	C79.31	—	D33.2	D43.2	D49.6
supratentorial (brain)						
NEC	C71.0	C79.31	—	D33.0	D43.0	D49.6
sweat gland (apocrine)						
(eccrine), site						
unspecified	C44.90	C79.2	D04.9	D23.9	D48.5	D49.2
specified site — see						
Neoplasm, skin						
sympathetic nerve or						
nervous system						
NEC	C47.9	C79.89	—	D36.10	D48.2	D49.2
symphysis pubis	C41.4	C79.51	—	D16.8	D48.0	D49.2
synovial membrane —						
see Neoplasm,						
connective tissue						
tapetum, brain	C71.8	C79.31	—	D33.2	D43.2	D49.6
tarsus (any bone)	C40.3-☑	C79.51	—	D16.3-☑	—	—
temple (skin) — see						
also Neoplasm, skin,						
face	C44.309	C79.2	D04.39	D23.39	D48.5	D49.2
temporal						
bone	C41.0	C79.51	—	D16.4	D48.0	D49.2
lobe or pole	C71.2	C79.31	—	D33.0	D43.0	D49.6
region	C76.0	C79.89	D09.8	D36.7	D48.7	D49.89
skin — see also						
Neoplasm, skin,						
face	C44.309	C79.2	D04.39	D23.39	D48.5	D49.2
tendon (sheath) — see						
Neoplasm,						
connective tissue						
tentorium						
(cerebelli)	C70.0	C79.32	—	D32.0	D42.0	D49.7
testis, testes	C62.9-☑	C79.82	D29.2-☑	D40.1-☑	D49.59	
descended	C62.1-☑	C79.82	D07.69	D29.2-☑	D40.1-☑	D49.59
ectopic	C62.0-☑	C79.82	D07.69	D29.2-☑	D40.1-☑	D49.59
retained	C62.0-☑	C79.82	D07.69	D29.2-☑	D40.1-☑	D49.59
scrotal	C62.1-☑	C79.82	D07.69	D29.2-☑	D40.1-☑	D49.59
undescended	C62.0-☑	C79.82	D07.69	D29.2-☑	D40.1-☑	D49.59
unspecified whether						
descended or						
undescended	C62.9-☑	C79.82	D07.69	D29.2-☑	D40.1-☑	D49.59
thalamus	C71.0	C79.31	—	D33.0	D43.0	D49.6
thigh NEC	C76.5-☑	C79.89	D04.7-☑	D36.7	D48.7	D49.89
thorax, thoracic (cavity)						
(organs NEC)	C76.1	C79.89	D09.8	D36.7	D48.7	D49.89
duct	C49.3	C79.89	—	D21.3	D48.1	D49.2
wall NEC	C76.1	C79.89	D09.8	D36.7	D48.7	D49.89
throat	C14.0	C79.89	D00.08	D10.9	D37.05	D49.0
thumb NEC	C76.4-☑	C79.89	D04.6-☑	D36.7	D48.7	D49.89
thymus (gland)	C37	C79.89	D09.3	D15.0	D38.4	D49.89
thyroglossal duct	C73	C79.89	D09.3	D34	D44.0	D49.7
thyroid (gland)	C73	C79.89	D09.3	D34	D44.0	D49.7
cartilage	C32.3	C78.39	D02.0	D14.1	D38.0	D49.1
tibia (any part)	C40.2-☑	C79.51	—	D16.2-☑	—	—
toe NEC	C76.5-☑	C79.89	D04.7-☑	D36.7	D48.7	D49.89
tongue	C02.9	C79.89	D00.07	D10.1	D37.02	D49.0
anterior (two-thirds)						
NEC	C02.3	C79.89	D00.07	D10.1	D37.02	D49.0
dorsal surface	C02.0	C79.89	D00.07	D10.1	D37.02	D49.0
ventral surface	C02.2	C79.89	D00.07	D10.1	D37.02	D49.0
base (dorsal						
surface)	C01	C79.89	D00.07	D10.1	D37.02	D49.0
border (lateral)	C02.1	C79.89	D00.07	D10.1	D37.02	D49.0
dorsal surface						
NEC	C02.0	C79.89	D00.07	D10.1	D37.02	D49.0
fixed part NEC	C01	C79.89	D00.07	D10.1	D37.02	D49.0
foreamen						
cecum	C02.0	C79.89	D00.07	D10.1	D37.02	D49.0
frenulum						
linguae	C02.2	C79.89	D00.07	D10.1	D37.02	D49.0
junctional zone	C02.8	C79.89	D00.07	D10.1	D37.02	D49.0
margin (lateral)	C02.1	C79.89	D00.07	D10.1	D37.02	D49.0
midline NEC	C02.0	C79.89	D00.07	D10.1	D37.02	D49.0
mobile part NEC	C02.3	C79.89	D00.07	D10.1	D37.02	D49.0

Neoplasm, neoplastic — continued	Malignant Primary	Malignant Secondary	Ca in situ	Benign	Uncertain	Unspecified Behavior
tongue — continued						
overlapping lesion	C02.8	—	—	—	—	—
posterior (third)	C01	C79.89	D00.07	D10.1	D37.02	D49.0
root	C01	C79.89	D00.07	D10.1	D37.02	D49.0
surface (dorsal)	C02.0	C79.89	D00.07	D10.1	D37.02	D49.0
base	C01	C79.89	D00.07	D10.1	D37.02	D49.0
ventral	C02.2	C79.89	D00.07	D10.1	D37.02	D49.0
tip	C02.1	C79.89	D00.07	D10.1	D37.02	D49.0
tonsil	C02.4	C79.89	D00.07	D10.1	D37.02	D49.0
tonsil	C09.9	C79.89	D00.08	D10.4	D37.05	D49.0
fauces, faucial	C09.9	C79.89	D00.08	D10.4	D37.05	D49.0
lingual	C02.4	C79.89	D00.07	D10.1	D37.02	D49.0
overlapping sites	C09.8	—	—	—	—	—
palatine	C09.9	C79.89	D00.08	D10.4	D37.05	D49.0
pharyngeal	C11.1	C79.89	D00.08	D10.6	D37.05	D49.0
pillar (anterior) (posterior)	C09.1	C79.89	D00.08	D10.5	D37.05	D49.0
tonsillar fossa	C09.0	C79.89	D00.08	D10.5	D37.05	D49.0
tooth socket NEC	C03.9	C79.89	D00.03	D10.39	D37.09	D49.0
trachea (cartilage) (mucosa)	C33	C78.39	D02.1	D14.2	D38.1	D49.1
overlapping lesion with bronchus or lung	C34.8-☑	—	—	—	—	—
tracheobronchial	C34.8-☑	C78.39	D02.1	D14.2	D38.1	D49.1
overlapping lesion with lung	C34.8-☑	—				
tragus — see also Neoplasm, skin, ear	C44.20-☑	C79.2	D04.2-☑	D23.2-☑	D48.5	D49.2
trunk NEC	C76.8	C79.89	D04.5	D36.7	D48.7	D49.89
tubo-ovarian	C57.8	C79.82	D07.39	D28.7	D39.8	D49.59
tunica vaginalis	C63.7	C79.82	D07.69	D29.8	D40.8	D49.59
turbinate (bone)	C41.0	C79.51	—	D16.4	D48.0	D49.2
nasal	C30.0	C78.39	D02.3	D14.0	D38.5	D49.1
tympanic cavity	C30.1	C78.39	D02.3	D14.0	D38.5	D49.1
ulna (any part)	C40.0-☑	C79.51	—	D16.0-☑	D48.0	D49.2
umbilicus, umbilical — see also Neoplasm, skin, trunk	C44.509	C79.2	D04.5	D23.5	D48.5	D49.2
uncus, brain	C71.2	C79.31	—	D33.0	D43.0	D49.6
unknown site or unspecified	C80.1	C79.9	D09.9	D36.9	D48.9	D49.9
urachus	C67.7	C79.11	D09.0	D30.3	D41.4	D49.4
ureter-bladder (junction)	C67.6	C79.11	D09.0	D30.3	D41.4	D49.4
ureter, ureteral	C66.-☑	C79.19	D09.19	D30.2-☑	D41.2-☑	D49.59
orifice (bladder)	C67.6	C79.11	D09.0	D30.3	D41.4	D49.4
urethra, urethral (gland)	C68.0	C79.19	D09.19	D30.4	D41.3	D49.59
orifice, internal	C67.5	C79.11	D09.0	D30.3	D41.4	D49.4
urethrovaginal (septum)	C57.9	C79.82	D07.30	D28.9	D39.8	D49.59
urinary organ or system	C68.9	C79.10	D09.10	D30.9	D41.9	D49.59
bladder — see Neoplasm, bladder						
overlapping lesion	C68.8	—	—	—	—	—
specified sites NEC	C68.8	C79.19	D09.19	D30.8	D41.8	D49.59
utero-ovarian	C57.8	C79.82	D07.39	D28.7	D39.8	D49.59
ligament	C57.1-☑	C79.82	D07.39	D28.2	D39.8	D49.59
uterosacral ligament	C57.3	C79.82	—	D28.2	D39.8	D49.59
uterus, uteri, uterine	C55	C79.82	D07.0	D26.9	D39.0	D49.59
adnexa NEC	C57.4	C79.82	D07.39	D28.7	D39.8	D49.59
body	C54.9	C79.82	D07.0	D26.1	D39.0	D49.59
cervix	C53.9	C79.82	D06.9	D26.0	D39.0	D49.59
cornu	C54.9	C79.82	D07.0	D26.1	D39.0	D49.59
corpus	C54.9	C79.82	D07.0	D26.1	D39.0	D49.59
endocervix (canal) (gland)	C53.0	C79.82	D06.0	D26.0	D39.0	D49.59
endometrium	C54.1	C79.82	D07.0	D26.1	D39.0	D49.59
exocervix	C53.1	C79.82	D06.1	D26.0	D39.0	D49.59
external os	C53.1	C79.82	D06.1	D26.0	D39.0	D49.59
fundus	C54.3	C79.82	D07.0	D26.1	D39.0	D49.59

Neoplasm, neoplastic — continued	Malignant Primary	Malignant Secondary	Ca in situ	Benign	Uncertain	Unspecified Behavior
uterus, uteri, uterine — continued						
internal os	C53.0	C79.82	D06.0	D26.0	D39.0	D49.59
isthmus	C54.0	C79.82	D07.0	D26.1	D39.0	D49.59
ligament	C57.3	C79.82	—	D28.2	D39.8	D49.59
broad	C57.1-☑	C79.82	D07.39	D28.2	D39.8	D49.59
round	C57.2-☑	C79.82	—	D28.2	D39.8	D49.59
lower segment	C54.0	C79.82	D07.0	D26.1	D39.0	D49.59
myometrium	C54.2	C79.82	D07.0	D26.1	D39.0	D49.59
overlapping sites	C54.8	—	—	—	—	—
squamocolumnar junction	C53.8	C79.82	D06.7	D26.0	D39.0	D49.59
tube	C57.0-☑	C79.82	D07.39	D28.2	D39.8	D49.59
utricle, prostatic	C68.0	C79.19	D09.19	D30.4	D41.3	D49.59
uveal tract	C69.4-☑	C79.49	D09.2-☑	D31.4-☑	D48.7	D49.89
uvula	C05.2	C79.89	D00.04	D10.39	D37.09	D49.0
vagina, vaginal (fornix) (vault) (wall)	C52	C79.82	D07.2	D28.1	D39.8	D49.59
vaginovesical	C57.9	C79.82	D07.30	D28.9	D39.9	D49.59
septum	C57.9	C79.82	D07.30	D28.9	D39.9	D49.59
vallecula (epigiottis)	C10.0	C79.89	D00.08	D10.5	D37.05	D49.0
vascular — see Neoplasm, connective tissue						
vas deferens	C63.1-☑	C79.82	D07.69	D29.8	D40.8	D49.59
Vater's ampulla	C24.1	C78.89	D01.5	D13.5	D37.6	D49.0
vein, venous — see Neoplasm, connective tissue						
vena cava (abdominal) (inferior)	C49.4	C79.89	—	D21.4	D48.1	D49.2
superior	C49.3	C79.89	—	D21.3	D48.1	D49.2
ventricle (cerebral) (floor) (lateral) (third)	C71.5	C79.31	—	D33.0	D43.0	D49.6
cardiac (left) (right)	C38.0	C79.89	—	D15.1	D48.7	D49.89
fourth	C71.7	C79.31	—	D33.1	D43.1	D49.6
ventricular band of larynx	C32.1	C78.39	D02.0	D14.1	D38.0	D49.1
ventriculus — see Neoplasm, stomach						
vermillion border — see Neoplasm, lip						
vermis, cerebellum	C71.6	C79.31	—	D33.1	D43.1	D49.6
vertebra (column)	C41.2	C79.51	—	D16.6	D48.0	D49.2
coccyx	C41.4	C79.51	—	D16.8	D48.0	D49.2
marrow NEC	C96.9	C79.52	—	—	D47.9	D49.89
sacrum	C41.4	C79.51	—	D16.8	D48.0	D49.2
vesical — see Neoplasm, bladder						
vesicle, seminal	C63.7	C79.82	D07.69	D29.8	D40.8	D49.59
vesicocervical tissue	C57.9	C79.82	D07.30	D28.9	D39.9	D49.59
vesicorectal	C76.3	C79.82	D09.8	D36.7	D48.7	D49.89
vesicovaginal	C57.9	C79.82	D07.30	D28.9	D39.9	D49.59
septum	C57.9	C79.82	D07.30	D28.9	D39.8	D49.59
vessel (blood) — see Neoplasm, connective tissue						
vestibular gland, greater	C51.0	C79.82	D07.1	D28.0	D39.8	D49.59
vestibule						
mouth	C06.1	C79.89	D00.00	D10.39	D37.09	D49.0
nose	C30.0	C78.39	D02.3	D14.0	D38.5	D49.1
Virchow's gland	C77.0	C77.0	—	D36.0	D48.7	D49.89
viscera NEC	C76.8	C79.89	D09.8	D36.7	D48.7	D49.89
vocal cords (true)	C32.0	C78.39	D02.0	D14.1	D38.0	D49.1
false	C32.1	C78.39	D02.0	D14.1	D38.0	D49.1
vomer	C41.0	C79.51	—	D16.4	D48.0	D49.2
vulva	C51.9	C79.82	D07.1	D28.0	D39.8	D49.59
vulvovaginal gland	C51.9	C79.82	D07.1	D28.0	D39.8	D49.59
Waldeyer's ring	C14.2	C79.89	D00.08	D10.9	D37.05	D49.0
Wharton's duct	C08.0	C79.89	D00.00	D11.7	D37.032	D49.0
white matter (central) (cerebral)	C71.0	C79.31	—	D33.0	D43.0	D49.6

☑ Additional Character Required — Refer to the Tabular List for Character Selection   ▽ Subterms under main terms may continue to next column or page

	Malignant Primary	Malignant Secondary	Ca in situ	Benign	Uncertain	Unspecified Behavior
Neoplasm, neoplastic						
— *continued*						
windpipe	C33	C78.39	D02.1	D14.2	D38.1	D49.1
Wirsung's duct	C25.3	C78.89	D01.7	D13.6	D37.8	D49.0
wolffian (body) (duct)						
female	C57.7	C79.82	D07.39	D28.7	D39.8	D49.59
male	C63.7	C79.82	D07.69	D29.8	D40.8	D49.59
womb — *see*						
Neoplasm, uterus						
wrist NEC	C76.4-☑	C79.89	D04.6-☑	D36.7	D48.7	D49.89
xiphoid process	C41.3	C79.51	—	D16.7	D48.0	D49.2
Zuckerkandl						
organ	C75.5	C79.89	—	D35.6	D44.7	D49.7

Substance	Poisoning, Accidental (unintentional)	Poisoning, Intentional Self-harm	Poisoning, Assault	Poisoning, Undetermined	Adverse Effect	Under-dosing
14-Hydroxydihydromorphinone	T40.2X1	T40.2X2	T40.2X3	T40.2X4	T40.2X5	T40.2X6
1-Propanol	T51.3X1	T51.3X2	T51.3X3	T51.3X4	—	—
2,3,7,8-Tetrachlorodibenzo-p-dioxin	T53.7X1	T53.7X2	T53.7X3	T53.7X4	—	—
2,4,5-T (trichlorophenoxyacetic acid)	T60.1X1	T60.1X2	T60.1X3	T60.1X4	—	—
2,4,5-Trichlorophenoxyacetic acid	T60.3X1	T60.3X2	T60.3X3	T60.3X4	—	—
2,4-D (dichlorophenoxyacetic acid)	T60.3X1	T60.3X2	T60.3X3	T60.3X4	—	—
2,4-Toluene diisocyanate	T65.0X1	T65.0X2	T65.0X3	T65.0X4	—	—
2-Deoxy-5-fluorouridine	T45.1X1	T45.1X2	T45.1X3	T45.1X4	T45.1X5	T45.1X6
2-Ethoxyethanol	T52.3X1	T52.3X2	T52.3X3	T52.3X4	—	—
2-Methoxyethanol	T52.3X1	T52.3X2	T52.3X3	T52.3X4	—	—
2-Propanol	T51.2X1	T51.2X2	T51.2X3	T51.2X4	—	—
3,4-methylenedioxymeth-amphetamine	T43.641	T43.642	T43.643	T43.644	—	—
4-Aminobutyric acid	T43.8X1	T43.8X2	T43.8X3	T43.8X4	T43.8X5	T43.8X6
4-Aminophenol derivatives	T39.1X1	T39.1X2	T39.1X3	T39.1X4	T39.1X5	T39.1X6
5-Deoxy-5-fluorouridine	T45.1X1	T45.1X2	T45.1X3	T45.1X4	T45.1X5	T45.1X6
5-Methoxypsoralen (5-MOP)	T50.991	T50.992	T50.993	T50.994	T50.995	T50.996
8-Aminoquinoline drugs	T37.2X1	T37.2X2	T37.2X3	T37.2X4	T37.2X5	T37.2X6
8-Methoxypsoralen (8-MOP)	T50.991	T50.992	T50.993	T50.994	T50.995	T50.996
ABOB	T37.5X1	T37.5X2	T37.5X3	T37.5X4	T37.5X5	T37.5X6
Abrine	T62.2X1	T62.2X2	T62.2X3	T62.2X4	—	—
Abrus (seed)	T62.2X1	T62.2X2	T62.2X3	T62.2X4	—	—
Absinthe	T51.0X1	T51.0X2	T51.0X3	T51.0X4	—	—
beverage	T51.0X1	T51.0X2	T51.0X3	T51.0X4	—	—
Acaricide	T60.8X1	T60.8X2	T60.8X3	T60.8X4	—	—
Acebutolol	T44.7X1	T44.7X2	T44.7X3	T44.7X4	T44.7X5	T44.7X6
Acecarbromal	T42.6X1	T42.6X2	T42.6X3	T42.6X4	T42.6X5	T42.6X6
Aceclidine	T44.1X1	T44.1X2	T44.1X3	T44.1X4	T44.1X5	T44.1X6
Acedapsone	T37.0X1	T37.0X2	T37.0X3	T37.0X4	T37.0X5	T37.0X6
Acefylline piperazine	T48.6X1	T48.6X2	T48.6X3	T48.6X4	T48.6X5	T48.6X6
Acemorphan	T40.2X1	T40.2X2	T40.2X3	T40.2X4	T40.2X5	T40.2X6
Acenocoumarin	T45.511	T45.512	T45.513	T45.514	T45.515	T45.516
Acenocoumarol	T45.511	T45.512	T45.513	T45.514	T45.515	T45.516
Acepifylline	T48.6X1	T48.6X2	T48.6X3	T48.6X4	T48.6X5	T48.6X6
Acepromazine	T43.3X1	T43.3X2	T43.3X3	T43.3X4	T43.3X5	T43.3X6
Acesulfamethoxypyridazine	T37.0X1	T37.0X2	T37.0X3	T37.0X4	T37.0X5	T37.0X6
Acetal	T52.8X1	T52.8X2	T52.8X3	T52.8X4	—	—
Acetaldehyde (vapor)	T52.8X1	T52.8X2	T52.8X3	T52.8X4	—	—
liquid	T65.891	T65.892	T65.893	T65.894	—	—
Acetaminophen	T39.1X1	T39.1X2	T39.1X3	T39.1X4	T39.1X5	T39.1X6
Acetaminosalol	T39.1X1	T39.1X2	T39.1X3	T39.1X4	T39.1X5	T39.1X6
Acetanilide	T39.1X1	T39.1X2	T39.1X3	T39.1X4	T39.1X5	T39.1X6
Acetarsol	T37.3X1	T37.3X2	T37.3X3	T37.3X4	T37.3X5	T37.3X6
Acetazolamide	T50.2X1	T50.2X2	T50.2X3	T50.2X4	T50.2X5	T50.2X6
Acetiamine	T45.2X1	T45.2X2	T45.2X3	T45.2X4	T45.2X5	T45.2X6
Acetic						
acid	T54.2X1	T54.2X2	T54.2X3	T54.2X4	—	—
with sodium acetate (ointment)	T49.3X1	T49.3X2	T49.3X3	T49.3X4	T49.3X5	T49.3X6
ester (solvent)(vapor)	T52.8X1	T52.8X2	T52.8X3	T52.8X4	—	—
irrigating solution	T50.3X1	T50.3X2	T50.3X3	T50.3X4	T50.3X5	T50.3X6
medicinal (lotion)	T49.2X1	T49.2X2	T49.2X3	T49.2X4	T49.2X5	T49.2X6
anhydride	T65.891	T65.892	T65.893	T65.894	—	—
ether (vapor)	T52.8X1	T52.8X2	T52.8X3	T52.8X4	—	—
Acetohexamide	T38.3X1	T38.3X2	T38.3X3	T38.3X4	T38.3X5	T38.3X6
Acetohydroxamic acid	T50.991	T50.992	T50.993	T50.994	T50.995	T50.996
Acetomenaphthone	T45.7X1	T45.7X2	T45.7X3	T45.7X4	T45.7X5	T45.7X6
Acetomorphine	T40.1X1	T40.1X2	T40.1X3	T40.1X4	—	—
Acetone (oils)	T52.4X1	T52.4X2	T52.4X3	T52.4X4	—	—
chlorinated	T52.4X1	T52.4X2	T52.4X3	T52.4X4	—	—
vapor	T52.4X1	T52.4X2	T52.4X3	T52.4X4	—	—
Acetonitrile	T52.8X1	T52.8X2	T52.8X3	T52.8X4	—	—
Acetophenazine	T43.3X1	T43.3X2	T43.3X3	T43.3X4	T43.3X5	T43.3X6
Acetophenetedin	T39.1X1	T39.1X2	T39.1X3	T39.1X4	T39.1X5	T39.1X6
Acetophenone	T52.4X1	T52.4X2	T52.4X3	T52.4X4	—	—
Acetorphine	T40.2X1	T40.2X2	T40.2X3	T40.2X4	—	—
Acetosulfone (sodium)	T37.1X1	T37.1X2	T37.1X3	T37.1X4	T37.1X5	T37.1X6
Acetrizoate (sodium)	T50.8X1	T50.8X2	T50.8X3	T50.8X4	T50.8X5	T50.8X6
Acetrizoic acid	T50.8X1	T50.8X2	T50.8X3	T50.8X4	T50.8X5	T50.8X6
Acetyl						
bromide	T53.6X1	T53.6X2	T53.6X3	T53.6X4	—	—
Acetyl — continued						
chloride	T53.6X1	T53.6X2	T53.6X3	T53.6X4	—	—
Acetylcarbromal	T42.6X1	T42.6X2	T42.6X3	T42.6X4	T42.6X5	T42.6X6
Acetylcholine						
chloride	T44.1X1	T44.1X2	T44.1X3	T44.1X4	T44.1X5	T44.1X6
derivative	T44.1X1	T44.1X2	T44.1X3	T44.1X4	T44.1X5	T44.1X6
Acetylcysteine	T48.4X1	T48.4X2	T48.4X3	T48.4X4	T48.4X5	T48.4X6
Acetyldigitoxin	T46.0X1	T46.0X2	T46.0X3	T46.0X4	T46.0X5	T46.0X6
Acetyldigoxin	T46.0X1	T46.0X2	T46.0X3	T46.0X4	T46.0X5	T46.0X6
Acetyldihydrocodeine	T40.2X1	T40.2X2	T40.2X3	T40.2X4	—	—
Acetyldihydrocodeinone	T40.2X1	T40.2X2	T40.2X3	T40.2X4	—	—
Acetylene (gas)	T59.891	T59.892	T59.893	T59.894	—	—
dichloride	T53.6X1	T53.6X2	T53.6X3	T53.6X4	—	—
incomplete combustion of	T58.11	T58.12	T58.13	T58.14	—	—
industrial	T59.891	T59.892	T59.893	T59.894	—	—
tetrachloride	T53.6X1	T53.6X2	T53.6X3	T53.6X4	—	—
vapor	T53.6X1	T53.6X2	T53.6X3	T53.6X4	—	—
Acetylpheneturide	T42.6X1	T42.6X2	T42.6X3	T42.6X4	T42.6X5	T42.6X6
Acetylphenylhydrazine	T39.8X1	T39.8X2	T39.8X3	T39.8X4	T39.8X5	T39.8X6
Acetylsalicylic acid (salts)	T39.011	T39.012	T39.013	T39.014	T39.015	T39.016
enteric coated	T39.011	T39.012	T39.013	T39.014	T39.015	T39.016
Acetylsulfamethoxypyridazine	T37.0X1	T37.0X2	T37.0X3	T37.0X4	T37.0X5	T37.0X6
Achromycin	T36.4X1	T36.4X2	T36.4X3	T36.4X4	T36.4X5	T36.4X6
ophthalmic preparation	T49.5X1	T49.5X2	T49.5X3	T49.5X4	T49.5X5	T49.5X6
topical NEC	T49.0X1	T49.0X2	T49.0X3	T49.0X4	T49.0X5	T49.0X6
Aciclovir	T37.5X1	T37.5X2	T37.5X3	T37.5X4	T37.5X5	T37.5X6
Acidifying agent NEC	T50.901	T50.902	T50.903	T50.904	T50.905	T50.906
Acid (corrosive) NEC	T54.2X1	T54.2X2	T54.2X3	T54.2X4	—	—
Acipimox	T46.6X1	T46.6X2	T46.6X3	T46.6X4	T46.6X5	T46.6X6
Acitretin	T50.991	T50.992	T50.993	T50.994	T50.995	T50.996
Aclarubicin	T45.1X1	T45.1X2	T45.1X3	T45.1X4	T45.1X5	T45.1X6
Aclatonium napadisilate	T48.1X1	T48.1X2	T48.1X3	T48.1X4	T48.1X5	T48.1X6
Aconite (wild)	T46.991	T46.992	T46.993	T46.994	T46.995	T46.996
Aconitine	T46.991	T46.992	T46.993	T46.994	T46.995	T46.996
Aconitum ferox	T46.991	T46.992	T46.993	T46.994	T46.995	T46.996
Acridine	T65.6X1	T65.6X2	T65.6X3	T65.6X4	—	—
vapor	T59.891	T59.892	T59.893	T59.894	—	—
Acriflavine	T37.91	T37.92	T37.93	T37.94	T37.95	T37.96
Acriflavinium chloride	T49.0X1	T49.0X2	T49.0X3	T49.0X4	T49.0X5	T49.0X6
Acrinol	T49.0X1	T49.0X2	T49.0X3	T49.0X4	T49.0X5	T49.0X6
Acrisorcin	T49.0X1	T49.0X2	T49.0X3	T49.0X4	T49.0X5	T49.0X6
Acrivastine	T45.0X1	T45.0X2	T45.0X3	T45.0X4	T45.0X5	T45.0X6
Acrolein (gas)	T59.891	T59.892	T59.893	T59.894	—	—
liquid	T54.1X1	T54.1X2	T54.1X3	T54.1X4	—	—
Acrylamide	T65.891	T65.892	T65.893	T65.894	—	—
Acrylic resin	T49.3X1	T49.3X2	T49.3X3	T49.3X4	T49.3X5	T49.3X6
Acrylonitrile	T65.891	T65.892	T65.893	T65.894	—	—
Actaea spicata	T62.2X1	T62.2X2	T62.2X3	T62.2X4	—	—
berry	T62.1X1	T62.1X2	T62.1X3	T62.1X4	—	—
Acterol	T37.3X1	T37.3X2	T37.3X3	T37.3X4	T37.3X5	T37.3X6
ACTH	T38.811	T38.812	T38.813	T38.814	T38.815	T38.816
Actinomycin C	T45.1X1	T45.1X2	T45.1X3	T45.1X4	T45.1X5	T45.1X6
Actinomycin D	T45.1X1	T45.1X2	T45.1X3	T45.1X4	T45.1X5	T45.1X6
Activated charcoal — see also Charcoal, medicinal	T47.6X1	T47.6X2	T47.6X3	T47.6X4	T47.6X5	T47.6X6
Acyclovir	T37.5X1	T37.5X2	T37.5X3	T37.5X4	T37.5X5	T37.5X6
Adenine	T45.2X1	T45.2X2	T45.2X3	T45.2X4	T45.2X5	T45.2X6
arabinoside	T37.5X1	T37.5X2	T37.5X3	T37.5X4	T37.5X5	T37.5X6
Adenosine (phosphate)	T46.2X1	T46.2X2	T46.2X3	T46.2X4	T46.2X5	T46.2X6
ADH	T38.891	T38.892	T38.893	T38.894	T38.895	T38.896
Adhesive NEC	T65.891	T65.892	T65.893	T65.894	—	—
Adicillin	T36.0X1	T36.0X2	T36.0X3	T36.0X4	T36.0X5	T36.0X6
Adiphenine	T44.3X1	T44.3X2	T44.3X3	T44.3X4	T44.3X5	T44.3X6
Adipiodone	T50.8X1	T50.8X2	T50.8X3	T50.8X4	T50.8X5	T50.8X6
Adjunct, pharmaceutical	T50.901	T50.902	T50.903	T50.904	T50.905	T50.906
Adrenal (extract, cortex or medulla) (glucocorticoids) (hormones) (mineralocorticoids)	T38.0X1	T38.0X2	T38.0X3	T38.0X4	T38.0X5	T38.0X6
ENT agent	T49.6X1	T49.6X2	T49.6X3	T49.6X4	T49.6X5	T49.6X6
ophthalmic preparation	T49.5X1	T49.5X2	T49.5X3	T49.5X4	T49.5X5	T49.5X6
topical NEC	T49.0X1	T49.0X2	T49.0X3	T49.0X4	T49.0X5	T49.0X6
Adrenalin — see Adrenaline						
Adrenaline	T44.5X1	T44.5X2	T44.5X3	T44.5X4	T44.5X5	T44.5X6
Adrenergic NEC	T44.901	T44.902	T44.903	T44.904	T44.905	T44.906
blocking agent NEC	T44.8X1	T44.8X2	T44.8X3	T44.8X4	T44.8X5	T44.8X6
beta, heart	T44.7X1	T44.7X2	T44.7X3	T44.7X4	T44.7X5	T44.7X6
specified NEC	T44.991	T44.992	T44.993	T44.994	T44.995	T44.996

Table of Drugs and Chemicals

Substance	Poisoning, Accidental (unintentional)	Poisoning, Intentional Self-harm	Poisoning, Assault	Poisoning, Undetermined	Adverse Effect	Under-dosing
Adrenochrome						
derivative	T46.991	T46.992	T46.993	T46.994	T46.995	T46.996
(mono) semicarbazone	T46.991	T46.992	T46.993	T46.994	T46.995	T46.996
Adrenocorticotrophic hormone	T38.811	T38.812	T38.813	T38.814	T38.815	T38.816
Adrenocorticotrophin	T38.811	T38.812	T38.813	T38.814	T38.815	T38.816
Adriamycin	T45.1X1	T45.1X2	T45.1X3	T45.1X4	T45.1X5	T45.1X6
Aerosol spray NEC	T65.91	T65.92	T65.93	T65.94		
Aerosporin	T36.8X1	T36.8X2	T36.8X3	T36.8X4	T36.8X5	T36.8X6
ENT agent	T49.6X1	T49.6X2	T49.6X3	T49.6X4	T49.6X5	T49.6X6
ophthalmic preparation	T49.5X1	T49.5X2	T49.5X3	T49.5X4	T49.5X5	T49.5X6
topical NEC	T49.0X1	T49.0X2	T49.0X3	T49.0X4	T49.0X5	T49.0X6
Aethusa cynapium	T62.2X1	T62.2X2	T62.2X3	T62.2X4		
Afghanistan black	T40.7X1	T40.7X2	T40.7X3	T40.7X4	T40.7X5	T40.7X6
Aflatoxin	T64.01	T64.02	T64.03	T64.04		
Afloqualone	T42.8X1	T42.8X2	T42.8X3	T42.8X4	T42.8X5	T42.8X6
African boxwood	T62.2X1	T62.2X2	T62.2X3	T62.2X4		
Agar	T47.4X1	T47.4X2	T47.4X3	T47.4X4	T47.4X5	T47.4X6
Agonist						
predominantly						
alpha-adrenoreceptor	T44.4X1	T44.4X2	T44.4X3	T44.4X4	T44.4X5	T44.4X6
beta-adrenoreceptor	T44.5X1	T44.5X2	T44.5X3	T44.5X4	T44.5X5	T44.5X6
Agricultural agent NEC	T65.91	T65.92	T65.93	T65.94		
Agrypnal	T42.3X1	T42.3X2	T42.3X3	T42.3X4	T42.3X5	T42.3X6
AHLG	T50.Z11	T50.Z12	T50.Z13	T50.Z14	T50.Z15	T50.Z16
Air contaminant(s), **source/type NOS**	T65.91	T65.92	T65.93	T65.94		
Ajmaline	T46.2X1	T46.2X2	T46.2X3	T46.2X4	T46.2X5	T46.2X6
Akee	T62.1X1	T62.1X2	T62.1X3	T62.1X4		
Akrinol	T49.0X1	T49.0X2	T49.0X3	T49.0X4	T49.0X5	T49.0X6
Akritoin	T37.8X1	T37.8X2	T37.8X3	T37.8X4	T37.8X5	T37.8X6
Alacepril	T46.4X1	T46.4X2	T46.4X3	T46.4X4	T46.4X5	T46.4X6
Alantolactone	T37.4X1	T37.4X2	T37.4X3	T37.4X4	T37.4X5	T37.4X6
Albamycin	T36.8X1	T36.8X2	T36.8X3	T36.8X4	T36.8X5	T36.8X6
Albendazole	T37.4X1	T37.4X2	T37.4X3	T37.4X4	T37.4X5	T37.4X6
Albumin						
bovine	T45.8X1	T45.8X2	T45.8X3	T45.8X4	T45.8X5	T45.8X6
human serum	T45.8X1	T45.8X2	T45.8X3	T45.8X4	T45.8X5	T45.8X6
salt-poor	T45.8X1	T45.8X2	T45.8X3	T45.8X4	T45.8X5	T45.8X6
normal human serum	T45.8X1	T45.8X2	T45.8X3	T45.8X4	T45.8X5	T45.8X6
Albuterol	T48.6X1	T48.6X2	T48.6X3	T48.6X4	T48.6X5	T48.6X6
Albutoin	T42.0X1	T42.0X2	T42.0X3	T42.0X4	T42.0X5	T42.0X6
Alclometasone	T49.0X1	T49.0X2	T49.0X3	T49.0X4	T49.0X5	T49.0X6
Alcohol	T51.91	T51.92	T51.93	T51.94	—	—
absolute	T51.0X1	T51.0X2	T51.0X3	T51.0X4	—	—
beverage	T51.0X1	T51.0X2	T51.0X3	T51.0X4	—	—
allyl	T51.8X1	T51.8X2	T51.8X3	T51.8X4	—	—
amyl	T51.3X1	T51.3X2	T51.3X3	T51.3X4	—	—
antifreeze	T51.1X1	T51.1X2	T51.1X3	T51.1X4	—	—
beverage	T51.0X1	T51.0X2	T51.0X3	T51.0X4	—	—
butyl	T51.3X1	T51.3X2	T51.3X3	T51.3X4	—	—
dehydrated	T51.0X1	T51.0X2	T51.0X3	T51.0X4	—	—
beverage	T51.0X1	T51.0X2	T51.0X3	T51.0X4	—	—
denatured	T51.0X1	T51.0X2	T51.0X3	T51.0X4	—	—
deterrent NEC	T50.6X1	T50.6X2	T50.6X3	T50.6X4	T50.6X5	T50.6X6
diagnostic (gastric function)	T50.8X1	T50.8X2	T50.8X3	T50.8X4	T50.8X5	T50.8X6
ethyl	T51.0X1	T51.0X2	T51.0X3	T51.0X4	—	—
beverage	T51.0X1	T51.0X2	T51.0X3	T51.0X4	—	—
grain	T51.0X1	T51.0X2	T51.0X3	T51.0X4	—	—
beverage	T51.0X1	T51.0X2	T51.0X3	T51.0X4	—	—
industrial	T51.0X1	T51.0X2	T51.0X3	T51.0X4	—	—
isopropyl	T51.2X1	T51.2X2	T51.2X3	T51.2X4	—	—
methyl	T51.1X1	T51.1X2	T51.1X3	T51.1X4	—	—
preparation for consumption	T51.0X1	T51.0X2	T51.0X3	T51.0X4	—	—
propyl	T51.3X1	T51.3X2	T51.3X3	T51.3X4	—	—
secondary	T51.2X1	T51.2X2	T51.2X3	T51.2X4	—	—
radiator	T51.1X1	T51.1X2	T51.1X3	T51.1X4	—	—
rubbing	T51.2X1	T51.2X2	T51.2X3	T51.2X4	—	—
specified type NEC	T51.8X1	T51.8X2	T51.8X3	T51.8X4	—	—
surgical	T51.0X1	T51.0X2	T51.0X3	T51.0X4	—	—
vapor (from any type of Alcohol)	T59.891	T59.892	T59.893	T59.894	—	—
wood	T51.1X1	T51.1X2	T51.1X3	T51.1X4	—	—
Alcuronium (chloride)	T48.1X1	T48.1X2	T48.1X3	T48.1X4	T48.1X5	T48.1X6
Aldactone	T50.0X1	T50.0X2	T50.0X3	T50.0X4	T50.0X5	T50.0X6
Aldesulfone sodium	T37.1X1	T37.1X2	T37.1X3	T37.1X4	T37.1X5	T37.1X6
Aldicarb	T60.0X1	T60.0X2	T60.0X3	T60.0X4		
Aldomet	T46.5X1	T46.5X2	T46.5X3	T46.5X4	T46.5X5	T46.5X6
Aldosterone	T50.0X1	T50.0X2	T50.0X3	T50.0X4	T50.0X5	T50.0X6
Aldrin (dust)	T60.1X1	T60.1X2	T60.1X3	T60.1X4		
Aleve — *see* Naproxen						

Substance	Poisoning, Accidental (unintentional)	Poisoning, Intentional Self-harm	Poisoning, Assault	Poisoning, Undetermined	Adverse Effect	Under-dosing
Alexitol sodium	T47.1X1	T47.1X2	T47.1X3	T47.1X4	T47.1X5	T47.1X6
Alfacalcidol	T45.2X1	T45.2X2	T45.2X3	T45.2X4	T45.2X5	T45.2X6
Alfadolone	T41.1X1	T41.1X2	T41.1X3	T41.1X4	T41.1X5	T41.1X6
Alfaxalone	T41.1X1	T41.1X2	T41.1X3	T41.1X4	T41.1X5	T41.1X6
Alfentanil	T40.4X1	T40.4X2	T40.4X3	T40.4X4	T40.4X5	T40.4X6
Alfuzosin (hydrochloride)	T44.8X1	T44.8X2	T44.8X3	T44.8X4	T44.8X5	T44.8X6
Algae (harmful) (toxin)	T65.821	T65.822	T65.823	T65.824	—	—
Algeldrate	T47.1X1	T47.1X2	T47.1X3	T47.1X4	T47.1X5	T47.1X6
Algin	T47.8X1	T47.8X2	T47.8X3	T47.8X4	T47.8X5	T47.8X6
Alglucerase	T45.3X1	T45.3X2	T45.3X3	T45.3X4	T45.3X5	T45.3X6
Alidase	T45.3X1	T45.3X2	T45.3X3	T45.3X4	T45.3X5	T45.3X6
Alimemazine	T43.3X1	T43.3X2	T43.3X3	T43.3X4	T43.3X5	T43.3X6
Aliphatic thiocyanates	T65.0X1	T65.0X2	T65.0X3	T65.0X4	—	—
Alizapride	T45.0X1	T45.0X2	T45.0X3	T45.0X4	T45.0X5	T45.0X6
Alkali (caustic)	T54.3X1	T54.3X2	T54.3X3	T54.3X4	—	—
Alkaline antiseptic solution (aromatic)	T49.6X1	T49.6X2	T49.6X3	T49.6X4	T49.6X5	T49.6X6
Alkalinizing agents (medicinal)	T50.901	T50.902	T50.903	T50.904	T50.905	T50.906
Alkalizing agent NEC	T50.901	T50.902	T50.903	T50.904	T50.905	T50.906
Alka-seltzer	T39.011	T39.012	T39.013	T39.014	T39.015	T39.016
Alkavervir	T46.5X1	T46.5X2	T46.5X3	T46.5X4	T46.5X5	T46.5X6
Alkonium (bromide)	T49.0X1	T49.0X2	T49.0X3	T49.0X4	T49.0X5	T49.0X6
Alkylating drug NEC	T45.1X1	T45.1X2	T45.1X3	T45.1X4	T45.1X5	T45.1X6
antimyeloproliferative	T45.1X1	T45.1X2	T45.1X3	T45.1X4	T45.1X5	T45.1X6
lymphatic	T45.1X1	T45.1X2	T45.1X3	T45.1X4	T45.1X5	T45.1X6
Alkylisocyanate	T65.0X1	T65.0X2	T65.0X3	T65.0X4	—	—
Allantoin	T49.4X1	T49.4X2	T49.4X3	T49.4X4	T49.4X5	T49.4X6
Allegron	T43.011	T43.012	T43.013	T43.014	T43.015	T43.016
Allethrin	T49.0X1	T49.0X2	T49.0X3	T49.0X4	T49.0X5	T49.0X6
Allobarbital	T42.3X1	T42.3X2	T42.3X3	T42.3X4	T42.3X5	T42.3X6
Allopurinol	T50.4X1	T50.4X2	T50.4X3	T50.4X4	T50.4X5	T50.4X6
Allyl						
alcohol	T51.8X1	T51.8X2	T51.8X3	T51.8X4	—	—
disulfide	T46.6X1	T46.6X2	T46.6X3	T46.6X4	T46.6X5	T46.6X6
Allylestrenol	T38.5X1	T38.5X2	T38.5X3	T38.5X4	T38.5X5	T38.5X6
Allylisopropylacetylurea	T42.6X1	T42.6X2	T42.6X3	T42.6X4	T42.6X5	T42.6X6
Allylisopropylmalonylurea	T42.3X1	T42.3X2	T42.3X3	T42.3X4	T42.3X5	T42.3X6
Allylthiourea	T49.3X1	T49.3X2	T49.3X3	T49.3X4	T49.3X5	T49.3X6
Allyltribromide	T42.6X1	T42.6X2	T42.6X3	T42.6X4	T42.6X5	T42.6X6
Allypropymal	T42.3X1	T42.3X2	T42.3X3	T42.3X4	T42.3X5	T42.3X6
Almagate	T47.1X1	T47.1X2	T47.1X3	T47.1X4	T47.1X5	T47.1X6
Almasilate	T47.1X1	T47.1X2	T47.1X3	T47.1X4	T47.1X5	T47.1X6
Almitrine	T50.7X1	T50.7X2	T50.7X3	T50.7X4	T50.7X5	T50.7X6
Aloes	T47.2X1	T47.2X2	T47.2X3	T47.2X4	T47.2X5	T47.2X6
Aloglutamol	T47.1X1	T47.1X2	T47.1X3	T47.1X4	T47.1X5	T47.1X6
Aloin	T47.2X1	T47.2X2	T47.2X3	T47.2X4	T47.2X5	T47.2X6
Aloxidone	T42.2X1	T42.2X2	T42.2X3	T42.2X4	T42.2X5	T42.2X6
Alpha						
acetyldigoxin	T46.0X1	T46.0X2	T46.0X3	T46.0X4	T46.0X5	T46.0X6
adrenergic blocking drug	T44.6X1	T44.6X2	T44.6X3	T44.6X4	T44.6X5	T44.6X6
amylase	T45.3X1	T45.3X2	T45.3X3	T45.3X4	T45.3X5	T45.3X6
tocoferol (acetate)	T45.2X1	T45.2X2	T45.2X3	T45.2X4	T45.2X5	T45.2X6
tocopherol	T45.2X1	T45.2X2	T45.2X3	T45.2X4	T45.2X5	T45.2X6
Alphadolone	T41.1X1	T41.1X2	T41.1X3	T41.1X4	T41.1X5	T41.1X6
Alphaprodine	T40.4X1	T40.4X2	T40.4X3	T40.4X4	T40.4X5	T40.4X6
Alphaxalone	T41.1X1	T41.1X2	T41.1X3	T41.1X4	T41.1X5	T41.1X6
Alprazolam	T42.4X1	T42.4X2	T42.4X3	T42.4X4	T42.4X5	T42.4X6
Alprenolol	T44.7X1	T44.7X2	T44.7X3	T44.7X4	T44.7X5	T44.7X6
Alprostadil	T46.7X1	T46.7X2	T46.7X3	T46.7X4	T46.7X5	T46.7X6
Alsactide	T38.811	T38.812	T38.813	T38.814	T38.815	T38.816
Alseroxylon	T46.5X1	T46.5X2	T46.5X3	T46.5X4	T46.5X5	T46.5X6
Alteplase	T45.611	T45.612	T45.613	T45.614	T45.615	T45.616
Altizide	T50.2X1	T50.2X2	T50.2X3	T50.2X4	T50.2X5	T50.2X6
Altretamine	T45.1X1	T45.1X2	T45.1X3	T45.1X4	T45.1X5	T45.1X6
Alum (medicinal)	T49.4X1	T49.4X2	T49.4X3	T49.4X4	T49.4X5	T49.4X6
nonmedicinal (ammonium) (potassium)	T56.891	T56.892	T56.893	T56.894	—	—
Aluminium, aluminum						
acetate	T49.2X1	T49.2X2	T49.2X3	T49.2X4	T49.2X5	T49.2X6
solution	T49.0X1	T49.0X2	T49.0X3	T49.0X4	T49.0X5	T49.0X6
aspirin	T39.011	T39.012	T39.013	T39.014	T39.015	T39.016
bis (acetylsalicylate)	T39.011	T39.012	T39.013	T39.014	T39.015	T39.016
carbonate (gel, basic)	T47.1X1	T47.1X2	T47.1X3	T47.1X4	T47.1X5	T47.1X6
chlorhydroxide-complex	T47.1X1	T47.1X2	T47.1X3	T47.1X4	T47.1X5	T47.1X6
chloride	T49.2X1	T49.2X2	T49.2X3	T49.2X4	T49.2X5	T49.2X6
clofibrate	T46.6X1	T46.6X2	T46.6X3	T46.6X4	T46.6X5	T46.6X6
diacetate	T49.2X1	T49.2X2	T49.2X3	T49.2X4	T49.2X5	T49.2X6
glycinate	T47.1X1	T47.1X2	T47.1X3	T47.1X4	T47.1X5	T47.1X6
hydroxide (gel)	T47.1X1	T47.1X2	T47.1X3	T47.1X4	T47.1X5	T47.1X6
hydroxide-magnesium carb. gel	T47.1X1	T47.1X2	T47.1X3	T47.1X4	T47.1X5	T47.1X6
magnesium silicate	T47.1X1	T47.1X2	T47.1X3	T47.1X4	T47.1X5	T47.1X6

Adrenochrome — Aluminium, aluminum

Table of Drugs and Chemicals

Substance	Poisoning, Accidental (unintentional)	Poisoning, Intentional Self-harm	Poisoning, Assault	Poisoning, Undetermined	Adverse Effect	Under-dosing
Aluminium, aluminum — *continued*						
nicotinate	T46.7X1	T46.7X2	T46.7X3	T46.7X4	T46.7X5	T46.7X6
ointment (surgical) (topical)	T49.3X1	T49.3X2	T49.3X3	T49.3X4	T49.3X5	T49.3X6
phosphate	T47.1X1	T47.1X2	T47.1X3	T47.1X4	T47.1X5	T47.1X6
salicylate	T39.091	T39.092	T39.093	T39.094	T39.095	T39.096
silicate	T47.1X1	T47.1X2	T47.1X3	T47.1X4	T47.1X5	T47.1X6
sodium silicate	T47.1X1	T47.1X2	T47.1X3	T47.1X4	T47.1X5	T47.1X6
subacetate	T49.2X1	T49.2X2	T49.2X3	T49.2X4	T49.2X5	T49.2X6
sulfate	T49.0X1	T49.0X2	T49.0X3	T49.0X4	T49.0X5	T49.0X6
tannate	T47.6X1	T47.6X2	T47.6X3	T47.6X4	T47.6X5	T47.6X6
topical NEC	T49.3X1	T49.3X2	T49.3X3	T49.3X4	T49.3X5	T49.3X6
Alurate	T42.3X1	T42.3X2	T42.3X3	T42.3X4	T42.3X5	T42.3X6
Alverine	T44.3X1	T44.3X2	T44.3X3	T44.3X4	T44.3X5	T44.3X6
Alvodine	T40.2X1	T40.2X2	T40.2X3	T40.2X4	T40.2X5	T40.2X6
Amanita phalloides	T62.0X1	T62.0X2	T62.0X3	T62.0X4	—	—
Amanitine	T62.0X1	T62.0X2	T62.0X3	T62.0X4	—	—
Amantadine	T42.8X1	T42.8X2	T42.8X3	T42.8X4	T42.8X5	T42.8X6
Ambazone	T49.6X1	T49.6X2	T49.6X3	T49.6X4	T49.6X5	T49.6X6
Ambenonium (chloride)	T44.0X1	T44.0X2	T44.0X3	T44.0X4	T44.0X5	T44.0X6
Ambroxol	T48.4X1	T48.4X2	T48.4X3	T48.4X4	T48.4X5	T48.4X6
Ambuphylline	T48.6X1	T48.6X2	T48.6X3	T48.6X4	T48.6X5	T48.6X6
Ambutonium bromide	T44.3X1	T44.3X2	T44.3X3	T44.3X4	T44.3X5	T44.3X6
Amcinonide	T49.0X1	T49.0X2	T49.0X3	T49.0X4	T49.0X5	T49.0X6
Amdinocilline	T36.0X1	T36.0X2	T36.0X3	T36.0X4	T36.0X5	T36.0X6
Ametazole	T50.8X1	T50.8X2	T50.8X3	T50.8X4	T50.8X5	T50.8X6
Amethocaine	T41.3X1	T41.3X2	T41.3X3	T41.3X4	T41.3X5	T41.3X6
regional	T41.3X1	T41.3X2	T41.3X3	T41.3X4	T41.3X5	T41.3X6
spinal	T41.3X1	T41.3X2	T41.3X3	T41.3X4	T41.3X5	T41.3X6
Amethopterin	T45.1X1	T45.1X2	T45.1X3	T45.1X4	T45.1X5	T45.1X6
Amezinium metilsulfate	T44.991	T44.992	T44.993	T44.994	T44.995	T44.996
Amfebutamone	T43.291	T43.292	T43.293	T43.294	T43.295	T43.296
Amfepramone	T50.5X1	T50.5X2	T50.5X3	T50.5X4	T50.5X5	T50.5X6
Amfetamine	T43.621	T43.622	T43.623	T43.624	T43.625	T43.626
Amfetaminil	T43.621	T43.622	T43.623	T43.624	T43.625	T43.626
Amfomycin	T36.8X1	T36.8X2	T36.8X3	T36.8X4	T36.8X5	T36.8X6
Amidefrine mesilate	T48.5X1	T48.5X2	T48.5X3	T48.5X4	T48.5X5	T48.5X6
Amidone	T40.3X1	T40.3X2	T40.3X3	T40.3X4	T40.3X5	T40.3X6
Amidopyrine	T39.2X1	T39.2X2	T39.2X3	T39.2X4	T39.2X5	T39.2X6
Amidotrizoate	T50.8X1	T50.8X2	T50.8X3	T50.8X4	T50.8X5	T50.8X6
Amiflamine	T43.1X1	T43.1X2	T43.1X3	T43.1X4	T43.1X5	T43.1X6
Amikacin	T36.5X1	T36.5X2	T36.5X3	T36.5X4	T36.5X5	T36.5X6
Amikhelline	T46.3X1	T46.3X2	T46.3X3	T46.3X4	T46.3X5	T46.3X6
Amiloride	T50.2X1	T50.2X2	T50.2X3	T50.2X4	T50.2X5	T50.2X6
Aminacrine	T49.0X1	T49.0X2	T49.0X3	T49.0X4	T49.0X5	T49.0X6
Amineptine	T43.011	T43.012	T43.013	T43.014	T43.015	T43.016
Aminitrozole	T37.3X1	T37.3X2	T37.3X3	T37.3X4	T37.3X5	T37.3X6
Aminoacetic acid (derivatives)	T50.3X1	T50.3X2	T50.3X3	T50.3X4	T50.3X5	T50.3X6
Amino acids	T50.3X1	T50.3X2	T50.3X3	T50.3X4	T50.3X5	T50.3X6
Aminoacridine	T49.0X1	T49.0X2	T49.0X3	T49.0X4	T49.0X5	T49.0X6
Aminobenzoic acid (-p)	T49.3X1	T49.3X2	T49.3X3	T49.3X4	T49.3X5	T49.3X6
Aminocaproic acid	T45.621	T45.622	T45.623	T45.624	T45.625	T45.626
Aminoethylisothiourium	T45.8X1	T45.8X2	T45.8X3	T45.8X4	T45.8X5	T45.8X6
Aminofenazone	T39.2X1	T39.2X2	T39.2X3	T39.2X4	T39.2X5	T39.2X6
Aminoglutethimide	T45.1X1	T45.1X2	T45.1X3	T45.1X4	T45.1X5	T45.1X6
Aminohippuric acid	T50.8X1	T50.8X2	T50.8X3	T50.8X4	T50.8X5	T50.8X6
Aminomethylbenzoic acid	T45.691	T45.692	T45.693	T45.694	T45.695	T45.696
Aminometradine	T50.2X1	T50.2X2	T50.2X3	T50.2X4	T50.2X5	T50.2X6
Aminopentamide	T44.3X1	T44.3X2	T44.3X3	T44.3X4	T44.3X5	T44.3X6
Aminophenazone	T39.2X1	T39.2X2	T39.2X3	T39.2X4	T39.2X5	T39.2X6
Aminophenol	T54.0X1	T54.0X2	T54.0X3	T54.0X4	—	—
Aminophenylpyridone	T43.591	T43.592	T43.593	T43.594	T43.595	T43.596
Aminophylline	T48.6X1	T48.6X2	T48.6X3	T48.6X4	T48.6X5	T48.6X6
Aminopterin sodium	T45.1X1	T45.1X2	T45.1X3	T45.1X4	T45.1X5	T45.1X6
Aminopyrine	T39.2X1	T39.2X2	T39.2X3	T39.2X4	T39.2X5	T39.2X6
Aminorex	T50.5X1	T50.5X2	T50.5X3	T50.5X4	T50.5X5	T50.5X6
Aminosalicylic acid	T37.1X1	T37.1X2	T37.1X3	T37.1X4	T37.1X5	T37.1X6
Aminosalylum	T37.1X1	T37.1X2	T37.1X3	T37.1X4	T37.1X5	T37.1X6
Amiodarone	T46.2X1	T46.2X2	T46.2X3	T46.2X4	T46.2X5	T46.2X6
Amiphenazole	T50.7X1	T50.7X2	T50.7X3	T50.7X4	T50.7X5	T50.7X6
Amiquinsin	T46.5X1	T46.5X2	T46.5X3	T46.5X4	T46.5X5	T46.5X6
Amisometradine	T50.2X1	T50.2X2	T50.2X3	T50.2X4	T50.2X5	T50.2X6
Amisulpride	T43.591	T43.592	T43.593	T43.594	T43.595	T43.596
Amitriptyline	T43.011	T43.012	T43.013	T43.014	T43.015	T43.016
Amitriptylinoxide	T43.011	T43.012	T43.013	T43.014	T43.015	T43.016
Amlexanox	T48.6X1	T48.6X2	T48.6X3	T48.6X4	T48.6X5	T48.6X6
Ammonia (fumes) (gas) (vapor)	T59.891	T59.892	T59.893	T59.894	—	—
aromatic spirit	T48.991	T48.992	T48.993	T48.994	T48.995	T48.996
liquid (household)	T54.3X1	T54.3X2	T54.3X3	T54.3X4	—	—
Ammoniated mercury	T49.0X1	T49.0X2	T49.0X3	T49.0X4	T49.0X5	T49.0X6

Substance	Poisoning, Accidental (unintentional)	Poisoning, Intentional Self-harm	Poisoning, Assault	Poisoning, Undetermined	Adverse Effect	Under-dosing
Ammonium						
acid tartrate	T49.5X1	T49.5X2	T49.5X3	T49.5X4	T49.5X5	T49.5X6
bromide	T42.6X1	T42.6X2	T42.6X3	T42.6X4	T42.6X5	T42.6X6
carbonate	T54.3X1	T54.3X2	T54.3X3	T54.3X4	—	—
chloride	T50.991	T50.992	T50.993	T50.994	T50.995	T50.996
expectorant	T48.4X1	T48.4X2	T48.4X3	T48.4X4	T48.4X5	T48.4X6
compounds (household) NEC	T54.3X1	T54.3X2	T54.3X3	T54.3X4	—	—
fumes (any usage)	T59.891	T59.892	T59.893	T59.894	—	—
industrial	T54.3X1	T54.3X2	T54.3X3	T54.3X4	—	—
ichthyosulronate	T49.4X1	T49.4X2	T49.4X3	T49.4X4	T49.4X5	T49.4X6
mandelate	T37.91	T37.92	T37.93	T37.94	T37.95	T37.96
sulfamate	T60.3X1	T60.3X2	T60.3X3	T60.3X4	—	—
sulfonate resin	T47.8X1	T47.8X2	T47.8X3	T47.8X4	T47.8X5	T47.8X6
Amobarbital (sodium)	T42.3X1	T42.3X2	T42.3X3	T42.3X4	T42.3X5	T42.3X6
Amodiaquine	T37.2X1	T37.2X2	T37.2X3	T37.2X4	T37.2X5	T37.2X6
Amopyroquin (e)	T37.2X1	T37.2X2	T37.2X3	T37.2X4	T37.2X5	T37.2X6
Amoxapine	T43.011	T43.012	T43.013	T43.014	T43.015	T43.016
Amoxicillin	T36.0X1	T36.0X2	T36.0X3	T36.0X4	T36.0X5	T36.0X6
Amperozide	T43.591	T43.592	T43.593	T43.594	T43.595	T43.596
Amphenidone	T43.591	T43.592	T43.593	T43.594	T43.595	T43.596
Amphetamine NEC	T43.621	T43.622	T43.623	T43.624	T43.625	T43.626
Amphomycin	T36.8X1	T36.8X2	T36.8X3	T36.8X4	T36.8X5	T36.8X6
Amphotalide	T37.4X1	T37.4X2	T37.4X3	T37.4X4	T37.4X5	T37.4X6
Amphotericin B	T36.7X1	T36.7X2	T36.7X3	T36.7X4	T36.7X5	T36.7X6
topical	T49.0X1	T49.0X2	T49.0X3	T49.0X4	T49.0X5	T49.0X6
Ampicillin	T36.0X1	T36.0X2	T36.0X3	T36.0X4	T36.0X5	T36.0X6
Amprotropine	T44.3X1	T44.3X2	T44.3X3	T44.3X4	T44.3X5	T44.3X6
Amsacrine	T45.1X1	T45.1X2	T45.1X3	T45.1X4	T45.1X5	T45.1X6
Amygdaline	T62.2X1	T62.2X2	T62.2X3	T62.2X4	—	—
Amyl						
acetate	T52.8X1	T52.8X2	T52.8X3	T52.8X4	—	—
vapor	T59.891	T59.892	T59.893	T59.894	—	—
alcohol	T51.3X1	T51.3X2	T51.3X3	T51.3X4	—	—
chloride	T53.6X1	T53.6X2	T53.6X3	T53.6X4	—	—
formate	T52.8X1	T52.8X2	T52.8X3	T52.8X4	—	—
nitrite	T46.3X1	T46.3X2	T46.3X3	T46.3X4	T46.3X5	T46.3X6
propionate	T65.891	T65.892	T65.893	T65.894	—	—
Amylase	T47.5X1	T47.5X2	T47.5X3	T47.5X4	T47.5X5	T47.5X6
Amyleine, regional	T41.3X1	T41.3X2	T41.3X3	T41.3X4	T41.3X5	T41.3X6
Amylene						
dichloride	T53.6X1	T53.6X2	T53.6X3	T53.6X4	—	—
hydrate	T51.3X1	T51.3X2	T51.3X3	T51.3X4	—	—
Amylmetacresol	T49.6X1	T49.6X2	T49.6X3	T49.6X4	T49.6X5	T49.6X6
Amylobarbitone	T42.3X1	T42.3X2	T42.3X3	T42.3X4	T42.3X5	T42.3X6
Amylocaine, regional	T41.3X1	T41.3X2	T41.3X3	T41.3X4	T41.3X5	T41.3X6
infiltration (subcutaneous)	T41.3X1	T41.3X2	T41.3X3	T41.3X4	T41.3X5	T41.3X6
nerve block (peripheral) (plexus)	T41.3X1	T41.3X2	T41.3X3	T41.3X4	T41.3X5	T41.3X6
spinal	T41.3X1	T41.3X2	T41.3X3	T41.3X4	T41.3X5	T41.3X6
topical (surface)	T41.3X1	T41.3X2	T41.3X3	T41.3X4	T41.3X5	T41.3X6
Amylopectin	T47.6X1	T47.6X2	T47.6X3	T47.6X4	T47.6X5	T47.6X6
Amytal (sodium)	T42.3X1	T42.3X2	T42.3X3	T42.3X4	T42.3X5	T42.3X6
Anabolic steroid	T38.7X1	T38.7X2	T38.7X3	T38.7X4	T38.7X5	T38.7X6
Analeptic NEC	T50.7X1	T50.7X2	T50.7X3	T50.7X4	T50.7X5	T50.7X6
Analgesic	T39.91	T39.92	T39.93	T39.94	T39.95	T39.96
anti-inflammatory NEC	T39.91	T39.92	T39.93	T39.94	T39.95	T39.96
propionic acid derivative	T39.311	T39.312	T39.313	T39.314	T39.315	T39.316
antirheumatic NEC	T39.4X1	T39.4X2	T39.4X3	T39.4X4	T39.4X5	T39.4X6
aromatic NEC	T39.1X1	T39.1X2	T39.1X3	T39.1X4	T39.1X5	T39.1X6
narcotic NEC	T40.601	T40.602	T40.603	T40.604	T40.605	T40.606
combination	T40.601	T40.602	T40.603	T40.604	T40.605	T40.606
obstetric	T40.601	T40.602	T40.603	T40.604	T40.605	T40.606
non-narcotic NEC	T39.91	T39.92	T39.93	T39.94	T39.95	T39.96
combination	T39.91	T39.92	T39.93	T39.94	T39.95	T39.96
pyrazole	T39.2X1	T39.2X2	T39.2X3	T39.2X4	T39.2X5	T39.2X6
specified NEC	T39.8X1	T39.8X2	T39.8X3	T39.8X4	T39.8X5	T39.8X6
Analgin	T39.2X1	T39.2X2	T39.2X3	T39.2X4	T39.2X5	T39.2X6
Anamirta cocculus	T62.1X1	T62.1X2	T62.1X3	T62.1X4	—	—
Ancillin	T36.0X1	T36.0X2	T36.0X3	T36.0X4	T36.0X5	T36.0X6
Ancrod	T45.691	T45.692	T45.693	T45.694	T45.695	T45.696
Androgen	T38.7X1	T38.7X2	T38.7X3	T38.7X4	T38.7X5	T38.7X6
Androgen-estrogen mixture	T38.7X1	T38.7X2	T38.7X3	T38.7X4	T38.7X5	T38.7X6
Androstalone	T38.7X1	T38.7X2	T38.7X3	T38.7X4	T38.7X5	T38.7X6
Androstanolone	T38.7X1	T38.7X2	T38.7X3	T38.7X4	T38.7X5	T38.7X6
Androsterone	T38.7X1	T38.7X2	T38.7X3	T38.7X4	T38.7X5	T38.7X6
Anemone pulsatilla	T62.2X1	T62.2X2	T62.2X3	T62.2X4	—	—
Anesthesia						
caudal	T41.3X1	T41.3X2	T41.3X3	T41.3X4	T41.3X5	T41.3X6
endotracheal	T41.0X1	T41.0X2	T41.0X3	T41.0X4	T41.0X5	T41.0X6
epidural	T41.3X1	T41.3X2	T41.3X3	T41.3X4	T41.3X5	T41.3X6
inhalation	T41.0X1	T41.0X2	T41.0X3	T41.0X4	T41.0X5	T41.0X6

Table of Drugs and Chemicals

Substance	Poisoning, Accidental (unintentional)	Poisoning, Intentional Self-harm	Poisoning, Assault	Poisoning, Undetermined	Adverse Effect	Under-dosing
Anesthesia — *continued*						
local	T41.3X1	T41.3X2	T41.3X3	T41.3X4	T41.3X5	T41.3X6
mucosal	T41.3X1	T41.3X2	T41.3X3	T41.3X4	T41.3X5	T41.3X6
muscle relaxation	T48.1X1	T48.1X2	T48.1X3	T48.1X4	T48.1X5	T48.1X6
nerve blocking	T41.3X1	T41.3X2	T41.3X3	T41.3X4	T41.3X5	T41.3X6
plexus blocking	T41.3X1	T41.3X2	T41.3X3	T41.3X4	T41.3X5	T41.3X6
potentiated	T41.201	T41.202	T41.203	T41.204	T41.205	T41.206
rectal	T41.201	T41.202	T41.203	T41.204	T41.205	T41.206
general	T41.201	T41.202	T41.203	T41.204	T41.205	T41.206
local	T41.3X1	T41.3X2	T41.3X3	T41.3X4	T41.3X5	T41.3X6
regional	T41.3X1	T41.3X2	T41.3X3	T41.3X4	T41.3X5	T41.3X6
surface	T41.3X1	T41.3X2	T41.3X3	T41.3X4	T41.3X5	T41.3X6
Anesthetic NEC — *see also* Anesthesia	T41.41	T41.42	T41.43	T41.44	T41.45	T41.46
with muscle relaxant	T41.201	T41.202	T41.203	T41.204	T41.205	T41.206
general	T41.201	T41.202	T41.203	T41.204	T41.205	T41.206
local	T41.3X1	T41.3X2	T41.3X3	T41.3X4	T41.3X5	T41.3X6
gaseous NEC	T41.0X1	T41.0X2	T41.0X3	T41.0X4	T41.0X5	T41.0X6
general NEC	T41.201	T41.202	T41.203	T41.204	T41.205	T41.206
halogenated hydrocarbon derivatives NEC	T41.0X1	T41.0X2	T41.0X3	T41.0X4	T41.0X5	T41.0X6
infiltration NEC	T41.3X1	T41.3X2	T41.3X3	T41.3X4	T41.3X5	T41.3X6
intravenous NEC	T41.1X1	T41.1X2	T41.1X3	T41.1X4	T41.1X5	T41.1X6
local NEC	T41.3X1	T41.3X2	T41.3X3	T41.3X4	T41.3X5	T41.3X6
rectal	T41.201	T41.202	T41.203	T41.204	T41.205	T41.206
general	T41.201	T41.202	T41.203	T41.204	T41.205	T41.206
local	T41.3X1	T41.3X2	T41.3X3	T41.3X4	T41.3X5	T41.3X6
regional NEC	T41.3X1	T41.3X2	T41.3X3	T41.3X4	T41.3X5	T41.3X6
spinal NEC	T41.3X1	T41.3X2	T41.3X3	T41.3X4	T41.3X5	T41.3X6
thiobarbiturate	T41.1X1	T41.1X2	T41.1X3	T41.1X4	T41.1X5	T41.1X6
topical	T41.3X1	T41.3X2	T41.3X3	T41.3X4	T41.3X5	T41.3X6
Aneurine	T45.2X1	T45.2X2	T45.2X3	T45.2X4	T45.2X5	T45.2X6
Angio-Conray	T50.8X1	T50.8X2	T50.8X3	T50.8X4	T50.8X5	T50.8X6
Angiotensin	T44.5X1	T44.5X2	T44.5X3	T44.5X4	T44.5X5	T44.5X6
Angiotensinamide	T44.991	T44.992	T44.993	T44.994	T44.995	T44.996
Anhydrohydroxy-progesterone	T38.5X1	T38.5X2	T38.5X3	T38.5X4	T38.5X5	T38.5X6
Anhydron	T50.2X1	T50.2X2	T50.2X3	T50.2X4	T50.2X5	T50.2X6
Anileridine	T40.4X1	T40.4X2	T40.4X3	T40.4X4	T40.4X5	T40.4X6
Aniline (dye) (liquid)	T65.3X1	T65.3X2	T65.3X3	T65.3X4		
analgesic	T39.1X1	T39.1X2	T39.1X3	T39.1X4	T39.1X5	T39.1X6
derivatives, therapeutic NEC	T39.1X1	T39.1X2	T39.1X3	T39.1X4	T39.1X5	T39.1X6
vapor	T65.3X1	T65.3X2	T65.3X3	T65.3X4	—	—
Aniscoropine	T44.3X1	T44.3X2	T44.3X3	T44.3X4	T44.3X5	T44.3X6
Anise oil	T47.5X1	T47.5X2	T47.5X3	T47.5X4	T47.5X5	T47.5X6
Anisidine	T65.3X1	T65.3X2	T65.3X3	T65.3X4	—	—
Anisindione	T45.511	T45.512	T45.513	T45.514	T45.515	T45.516
Anisotropine methyl-bromide	T44.3X1	T44.3X2	T44.3X3	T44.3X4	T44.3X5	T44.3X6
Anistreplase	T45.611	T45.612	T45.613	T45.614	T45.615	T45.616
Anorexiant (central)	T50.5X1	T50.5X2	T50.5X3	T50.5X4	T50.5X5	T50.5X6
Anorexic agents	T50.5X1	T50.5X2	T50.5X3	T50.5X4	T50.5X5	T50.5X6
Ansamycin	T36.6X1	T36.6X2	T36.6X3	T36.6X4	T36.6X5	T36.6X6
Ant (bite) (sting)	T63.421	T63.422	T63.423	T63.424		
Antabuse	T50.6X1	T50.6X2	T50.6X3	T50.6X4	T50.6X5	T50.6X6
Antacid NEC	T47.1X1	T47.1X2	T47.1X3	T47.1X4	T47.1X5	T47.1X6
Antagonist						
Aldosterone	T50.0X1	T50.0X2	T50.0X3	T50.0X4	T50.0X5	T50.0X6
alpha-adrenoreceptor	T44.6X1	T44.6X2	T44.6X3	T44.6X4	T44.6X5	T44.6X6
anticoagulant	T45.7X1	T45.7X2	T45.7X3	T45.7X4	T45.7X5	T45.7X6
beta-adrenoreceptor	T44.7X1	T44.7X2	T44.7X3	T44.7X4	T44.7X5	T44.7X6
extrapyramidal NEC	T44.3X1	T44.3X2	T44.3X3	T44.3X4	T44.3X5	T44.3X6
folic acid	T45.1X1	T45.1X2	T45.1X3	T45.1X4	T45.1X5	T45.1X6
H2 receptor	T47.0X1	T47.0X2	T47.0X3	T47.0X4	T47.0X5	T47.0X6
heavy metal	T45.8X1	T45.8X2	T45.8X3	T45.8X4	T45.8X5	T45.8X6
narcotic analgesic	T50.7X1	T50.7X2	T50.7X3	T50.7X4	T50.7X5	T50.7X6
opiate	T50.7X1	T50.7X2	T50.7X3	T50.7X4	T50.7X5	T50.7X6
pyrimidine	T45.1X1	T45.1X2	T45.1X3	T45.1X4	T45.1X5	T45.1X6
serotonin	T46.5X1	T46.5X2	T46.5X3	T46.5X4	T46.5X5	T46.5X6
Antazolin (e)	T45.0X1	T45.0X2	T45.0X3	T45.0X4	T45.0X5	T45.0X6
Anterior pituitary hormone NEC	T38.811	T38.812	T38.813	T38.814	T38.815	T38.816
Anthelmintic NEC	T37.4X1	T37.4X2	T37.4X3	T37.4X4	T37.4X5	T37.4X6
Anthiolimine	T37.4X1	T37.4X2	T37.4X3	T37.4X4	T37.4X5	T37.4X6
Anthralin	T49.4X1	T49.4X2	T49.4X3	T49.4X4	T49.4X5	T49.4X6
Anthramycin	T45.1X1	T45.1X2	T45.1X3	T45.1X4	T45.1X5	T45.1X6
Antiadrenergic NEC	T44.8X1	T44.8X2	T44.8X3	T44.8X4	T44.8X5	T44.8X6
Antiallergic NEC	T45.0X1	T45.0X2	T45.0X3	T45.0X4	T45.0X5	T45.0X6
Antiandrogen NEC	T38.6X1	T38.6X2	T38.6X3	T38.6X4	T38.6X5	T38.6X6
Anti-anemic (drug) (preparation)	T45.8X1	T45.8X2	T45.8X3	T45.8X4	T45.8X5	T45.8X6
Antianxiety drug NEC	T43.501	T43.502	T43.503	T43.504	T43.505	T43.506
Antiaris toxicaria	T65.891	T65.892	T65.893	T65.894	—	—

Substance	Poisoning, Accidental (unintentional)	Poisoning, Intentional Self-harm	Poisoning, Assault	Poisoning, Undetermined	Adverse Effect	Under-dosing
Antiarteriosclerotic drug	T46.6X1	T46.6X2	T46.6X3	T46.6X4	T46.6X5	T46.6X6
Antiasthmatic drug NEC	T48.6X1	T48.6X2	T48.6X3	T48.6X4	T48.6X5	T48.6X6
Antibiotic NEC	T36.91	T36.92	T36.93	T36.94	T36.95	T36.96
aminoglycoside	T36.5X1	T36.5X2	T36.5X3	T36.5X4	T36.5X5	T36.5X6
anticancer	T45.1X1	T45.1X2	T45.1X3	T45.1X4	T45.1X5	T45.1X6
antifungal	T36.7X1	T36.7X2	T36.7X3	T36.7X4	T36.7X5	T36.7X6
antimycobacterial	T36.5X1	T36.5X2	T36.5X3	T36.5X4	T36.5X5	T36.5X6
antineoplastic	T45.1X1	T45.1X2	T45.1X3	T45.1X4	T45.1X5	T45.1X6
b-lactam NEC	T36.1X1	T36.1X2	T36.1X3	T36.1X4	T36.1X5	T36.1X6
cephalosporin (group)	T36.1X1	T36.1X2	T36.1X3	T36.1X4	T36.1X5	T36.1X6
chloramphenicol (group)	T36.2X1	T36.2X2	T36.2X3	T36.2X4	T36.2X5	T36.2X6
ENT	T49.6X1	T49.6X2	T49.6X3	T49.6X4	T49.6X5	T49.6X6
eye	T49.5X1	T49.5X2	T49.5X3	T49.5X4	T49.5X5	T49.5X6
fungicidal (local)	T49.0X1	T49.0X2	T49.0X3	T49.0X4	T49.0X5	T49.0X6
intestinal	T36.8X1	T36.8X2	T36.8X3	T36.8X4	T36.8X5	T36.8X6
local	T49.0X1	T49.0X2	T49.0X3	T49.0X4	T49.0X5	T49.0X6
macrolides	T36.3X1	T36.3X2	T36.3X3	T36.3X4	T36.3X5	T36.3X6
polypeptide	T36.8X1	T36.8X2	T36.8X3	T36.8X4	T36.8X5	T36.8X6
specified NEC	T36.8X1	T36.8X2	T36.8X3	T36.8X4	T36.8X5	T36.8X6
tetracycline (group)	T36.4X1	T36.4X2	T36.4X3	T36.4X4	T36.4X5	T36.4X6
throat	T49.6X1	T49.6X2	T49.6X3	T49.6X4	T49.6X5	T49.6X6
Anticancer agents NEC	T45.1X1	T45.1X2	T45.1X3	T45.1X4	T45.1X5	T45.1X6
Anticholesterolemic drug NEC	T46.6X1	T46.6X2	T46.6X3	T46.6X4	T46.6X5	T46.6X6
Anticholinergic NEC	T44.3X1	T44.3X2	T44.3X3	T44.3X4	T44.3X5	T44.3X6
Anticholinesterase						
organophosphorus	T44.0X1	T44.0X2	T44.0X3	T44.0X4	T44.0X5	T44.0X6
insecticide	T60.0X1	T60.0X2	T60.0X3	T60.0X4	—	—
nerve gas	T59.891	T59.892	T59.893	T59.894	—	—
reversible	T44.0X1	T44.0X2	T44.0X3	T44.0X4	T44.0X5	T44.0X6
ophthalmological	T49.5X1	T49.5X2	T49.5X3	T49.5X4	T49.5X5	T49.5X6
Anticoagulant NEC	T45.511	T45.512	T45.513	T45.514	T45.515	T45.516
Antagonist	T45.7X1	T45.7X2	T45.7X3	T45.7X4	T45.7X5	T45.7X6
Anti-common-cold drug NEC	T48.5X1	T48.5X2	T48.5X3	T48.5X4	T48.5X5	T48.5X6
Anticonvulsant	T42.71	T42.72	T42.73	T42.74	T42.75	T42.76
barbiturate	T42.3X1	T42.3X2	T42.3X3	T42.3X4	T42.3X5	T42.3X6
combination (with barbiturate)	T42.3X1	T42.3X2	T42.3X3	T42.3X4	T42.3X5	T42.3X6
hydantoin	T42.0X1	T42.0X2	T42.0X3	T42.0X4	T42.0X5	T42.0X6
hypnotic NEC	T42.6X1	T42.6X2	T42.6X3	T42.6X4	T42.6X5	T42.6X6
oxazolidinedione	T42.2X1	T42.2X2	T42.2X3	T42.2X4	T42.2X5	T42.2X6
pyrimidinedione	T42.6X1	T42.6X2	T42.6X3	T42.6X4	T42.6X5	T42.6X6
specified NEC	T42.6X1	T42.6X2	T42.6X3	T42.6X4	T42.6X5	T42.6X6
succinimide	T42.2X1	T42.2X2	T42.2X3	T42.2X4	T42.2X5	T42.2X6
Antidepressant	T43.201	T43.202	T43.203	T43.204	T43.205	T43.206
monoamine oxidase inhibitor	T43.1X1	T43.1X2	T43.1X3	T43.1X4	T43.1X5	T43.1X6
selective serotonin norepinephrine reuptake inhibitor	T43.211	T43.212	T43.213	T43.214	T43.215	T43.216
selective serotonin reuptake inhibitor	T43.221	T43.222	T43.223	T43.224	T43.225	T43.226
specified NEC	T43.291	T43.292	T43.293	T43.294	T43.295	T43.296
tetracyclic	T43.021	T43.022	T43.023	T43.024	T43.025	T43.026
triazolopyridine	T43.211	T43.212	T43.213	T43.214	T43.215	T43.216
tricyclic	T43.011	T43.012	T43.013	T43.014	T43.015	T43.016
Antidiabetic NEC	T38.3X1	T38.3X2	T38.3X3	T38.3X4	T38.3X5	T38.3X6
biguanide	T38.3X1	T38.3X2	T38.3X3	T38.3X4	T38.3X5	T38.3X6
and sulfonyl combined	T38.3X1	T38.3X2	T38.3X3	T38.3X4	T38.3X5	T38.3X6
combined	T38.3X1	T38.3X2	T38.3X3	T38.3X4	T38.3X5	T38.3X6
sulfonylurea	T38.3X1	T38.3X2	T38.3X3	T38.3X4	T38.3X5	T38.3X6
Antidiarrheal drug NEC	T47.6X1	T47.6X2	T47.6X3	T47.6X4	T47.6X5	T47.6X6
absorbent	T47.6X1	T47.6X2	T47.6X3	T47.6X4	T47.6X5	T47.6X6
Anti-D immunoglobulin (human)	T50.Z11	T50.Z12	T50.Z13	T50.Z14	T50.Z15	T50.Z16
Antidiphtheria serum	T50.Z11	T50.Z12	T50.Z13	T50.Z14	T50.Z15	T50.Z16
Antidiuretic hormone	T38.891	T38.892	T38.893	T38.894	T38.895	T38.896
Antidote NEC	T50.6X1	T50.6X2	T50.6X3	T50.6X4	T50.6X5	T50.6X6
heavy metal	T45.8X1	T45.8X2	T45.8X3	T45.8X4	T45.8X5	T45.8X6
Antidysrhythmic NEC	T46.2X1	T46.2X2	T46.2X3	T46.2X4	T46.2X5	T46.2X6
Antiemetic drug	T45.0X1	T45.0X2	T45.0X3	T45.0X4	T45.0X5	T45.0X6
Antiepilepsy agent	T42.71	T42.72	T42.73	T42.74	T42.75	T42.76
combination	T42.5X1	T42.5X2	T42.5X3	T42.5X4	T42.5X5	T42.5X6
mixed	T42.5X1	T42.5X2	T42.5X3	T42.5X4	T42.5X5	T42.5X6
specified, NEC	T42.6X1	T42.6X2	T42.6X3	T42.6X4	T42.6X5	T42.6X6
Antiestrogen NEC	T38.6X1	T38.6X2	T38.6X3	T38.6X4	T38.6X5	T38.6X6
Antifertility pill	T38.4X1	T38.4X2	T38.4X3	T38.4X4	T38.4X5	T38.4X6
Antifibrinolytic drug	T45.621	T45.622	T45.623	T45.624	T45.625	T45.626
Antifilarial drug	T37.4X1	T37.4X2	T37.4X3	T37.4X4	T37.4X5	T37.4X6
Antiflatulent	T47.5X1	T47.5X2	T47.5X3	T47.5X4	T47.5X5	T47.5X6
Antifreeze	T65.91	T65.92	T65.93	T65.94	—	—
alcohol	T51.1X1	T51.1X2	T51.1X3	T51.1X4		

Anesthesia — Antifreeze

Substance	Poisoning, Accidental (unintentional)	Poisoning, Intentional Self-harm	Poisoning, Assault	Poisoning, Undetermined	Adverse Effect	Under-dosing
Antifreeze — continued						
ethylene glycol	T51.8X1	T51.8X2	T51.8X3	T51.8X4	—	—
Antifungal						
antibiotic (systemic)	T36.7X1	T36.7X2	T36.7X3	T36.7X4	T36.7X5	T36.7X6
anti-infective NEC	T37.91	T37.92	T37.93	T37.94	T37.95	T37.96
disinfectant, local	T49.0X1	T49.0X2	T49.0X3	T49.0X4	T49.0X5	T49.0X6
nonmedicinal (spray)	T60.3X1	T60.3X2	T60.3X3	T60.3X4	—	—
topical	T49.0X1	T49.0X2	T49.0X3	T49.0X4	T49.0X5	T49.0X6
Anti-gastric-secretion drug NEC	T47.1X1	T47.1X2	T47.1X3	T47.1X4	T47.1X5	T47.1X6
Antigonadotrophin NEC	T38.6X1	T38.6X2	T38.6X3	T38.6X4	T38.6X5	T38.6X6
Antihallucinogen	T43.501	T43.502	T43.503	T43.504	T43.505	T43.506
Antihelmintics	T37.4X1	T37.4X2	T37.4X3	T37.4X4	T37.4X5	T37.4X6
Antihemophilic						
factor	T45.8X1	T45.8X2	T45.8X3	T45.8X4	T45.8X5	T45.8X6
fraction	T45.8X1	T45.8X2	T45.8X3	T45.8X4	T45.8X5	T45.8X6
globulin concentrate	T45.7X1	T45.7X2	T45.7X3	T45.7X4	T45.7X5	T45.7X6
human plasma	T45.8X1	T45.8X2	T45.8X3	T45.8X4	T45.8X5	T45.8X6
plasma, dried	T45.7X1	T45.7X2	T45.7X3	T45.7X4	T45.7X5	T45.7X6
Antihemorrhoidal preparation	T49.2X1	T49.2X2	T49.2X3	T49.2X4	T49.2X5	T49.2X6
Antiheparin drug	T45.7X1	T45.7X2	T45.7X3	T45.7X4	T45.7X5	T45.7X6
Antihistamine	T45.0X1	T45.0X2	T45.0X3	T45.0X4	T45.0X5	T45.0X6
Antihookworm drug	T37.4X1	T37.4X2	T37.4X3	T37.4X4	T37.4X5	T37.4X6
Anti-human lymphocytic globulin	T50.Z11	T50.Z12	T50.Z13	T50.Z14	T50.Z15	T50.Z16
Antihyperlipidemic drug	T46.6X1	T46.6X2	T46.6X3	T46.6X4	T46.6X5	T46.6X6
Antihypertensive drug NEC	T46.5X1	T46.5X2	T46.5X3	T46.5X4	T46.5X5	T46.5X6
Anti-infective NEC	T37.91	T37.92	T37.93	T37.94	T37.95	T37.96
anthelmintic	T37.4X1	T37.4X2	T37.4X3	T37.4X4	T37.4X5	T37.4X6
antibiotics	T36.91	T36.92	T36.93	T36.94	T36.95	T36.96
specified NEC	T36.8X1	T36.8X2	T36.8X3	T36.8X4	T36.8X5	T36.8X6
antimalarial	T37.2X1	T37.2X2	T37.2X3	T37.2X4	T37.2X5	T37.2X6
antimycobacterial NEC	T37.1X1	T37.1X2	T37.1X3	T37.1X4	T37.1X5	T37.1X6
antibiotics	T36.5X1	T36.5X2	T36.5X3	T36.5X4	T36.5X5	T36.5X6
antiprotozoal NEC	T37.3X1	T37.3X2	T37.3X3	T37.3X4	T37.3X5	T37.3X6
blood	T37.2X1	T37.2X2	T37.2X3	T37.2X4	T37.2X5	T37.2X6
antiviral	T37.5X1	T37.5X2	T37.5X3	T37.5X4	T37.5X5	T37.5X6
arsenical	T37.8X1	T37.8X2	T37.8X3	T37.8X4	T37.8X5	T37.8X6
bismuth, local	T49.0X1	T49.0X2	T49.0X3	T49.0X4	T49.0X5	T49.0X6
ENT	T49.6X1	T49.6X2	T49.6X3	T49.6X4	T49.6X5	T49.6X6
eye NEC	T49.5X1	T49.5X2	T49.5X3	T49.5X4	T49.5X5	T49.5X6
heavy metals NEC	T37.8X1	T37.8X2	T37.8X3	T37.8X4	T37.8X5	T37.8X6
local NEC	T49.0X1	T49.0X2	T49.0X3	T49.0X4	T49.0X5	T49.0X6
specified NEC	T49.0X1	T49.0X2	T49.0X3	T49.0X4	T49.0X5	T49.0X6
mixed	T37.91	T37.92	T37.93	T37.94	T37.95	T37.96
ophthalmic preparation	T49.5X1	T49.5X2	T49.5X3	T49.5X4	T49.5X5	T49.5X6
topical NEC	T49.0X1	T49.0X2	T49.0X3	T49.0X4	T49.0X5	T49.0X6
Anti-inflammatory drug NEC	T39.391	T39.392	T39.393	T39.394	T39.395	T39.396
local	T49.0X1	T49.0X2	T49.0X3	T49.0X4	T49.0X5	T49.0X6
nonsteroidal NEC	T39.391	T39.392	T39.393	T39.394	T39.395	T39.396
propionic acid derivative	T39.311	T39.312	T39.313	T39.314	T39.315	T39.316
specified NEC	T39.391	T39.392	T39.393	T39.394	T39.395	T39.396
Antikaluretic	T50.3X1	T50.3X2	T50.3X3	T50.3X4	T50.3X5	T50.3X6
Antiknock (tetraethyl lead)	T56.0X1	T56.0X2	T56.0X3	T56.0X4	—	—
Antilipemic drug NEC	T46.6X1	T46.6X2	T46.6X3	T46.6X4	T46.6X5	T46.6X6
Antimalarial	T37.2X1	T37.2X2	T37.2X3	T37.2X4	T37.2X5	T37.2X6
prophylactic NEC	T37.2X1	T37.2X2	T37.2X3	T37.2X4	T37.2X5	T37.2X6
pyrimidine derivative	T37.2X1	T37.2X2	T37.2X3	T37.2X4	T37.2X5	T37.2X6
Antimetabolite	T45.1X1	T45.1X2	T45.1X3	T45.1X4	T45.1X5	T45.1X6
Antimitotic agent	T45.1X1	T45.1X2	T45.1X3	T45.1X4	T45.1X5	T45.1X6
Antimony (compounds) (vapor) NEC	T56.891	T56.892	T56.893	T56.894	—	—
anti-infectives	T37.8X1	T37.8X2	T37.8X3	T37.8X4	T37.8X5	T37.8X6
dimercaptosuccinate	T37.3X1	T37.3X2	T37.3X3	T37.3X4	T37.3X5	T37.3X6
hydride	T56.891	T56.892	T56.893	T56.894	—	—
pesticide (vapor)	T60.8X1	T60.8X2	T60.8X3	T60.8X4	—	—
potassium (sodium) tartrate	T37.8X1	T37.8X2	T37.8X3	T37.8X4	T37.8X5	T37.8X6
sodium	T37.3X1	T37.3X2	T37.3X3	T37.3X4	T37.3X5	T37.3X6
dimercaptosuccinate						
tartrated	T37.8X1	T37.8X2	T37.8X3	T37.8X4	T37.8X5	T37.8X6
Antimuscarinic NEC	T44.3X1	T44.3X2	T44.3X3	T44.3X4	T44.3X5	T44.3X6
Antimycobacterial drug NEC	T37.1X1	T37.1X2	T37.1X3	T37.1X4	T37.1X5	T37.1X6
antibiotics	T36.5X1	T36.5X2	T36.5X3	T36.5X4	T36.5X5	T36.5X6
combination	T37.1X1	T37.1X2	T37.1X3	T37.1X4	T37.1X5	T37.1X6
Antinausea drug	T45.0X1	T45.0X2	T45.0X3	T45.0X4	T45.0X5	T45.0X6
Antinematode drug	T37.4X1	T37.4X2	T37.4X3	T37.4X4	T37.4X5	T37.4X6
Antineoplastic NEC	T45.1X1	T45.1X2	T45.1X3	T45.1X4	T45.1X5	T45.1X6
alkaloidal	T45.1X1	T45.1X2	T45.1X3	T45.1X4	T45.1X5	T45.1X6
Antineoplastic — continued						
antibiotics	T45.1X1	T45.1X2	T45.1X3	T45.1X4	T45.1X5	T45.1X6
combination	T45.1X1	T45.1X2	T45.1X3	T45.1X4	T45.1X5	T45.1X6
estrogen	T38.5X1	T38.5X2	T38.5X3	T38.5X4	T38.5X5	T38.5X6
steroid	T38.7X1	T38.7X2	T38.7X3	T38.7X4	T38.7X5	T38.7X6
Antiparasitic drug (systemic)	T37.91	T37.92	T37.93	T37.94	T37.95	T37.96
local	T49.0X1	T49.0X2	T49.0X3	T49.0X4	T49.0X5	T49.0X6
specified NEC	T37.8X1	T37.8X2	T37.8X3	T37.8X4	T37.8X5	T37.8X6
Antiparkinsonism drug NEC	T42.8X1	T42.8X2	T42.8X3	T42.8X4	T42.8X5	T42.8X6
Antiperspirant NEC	T49.2X1	T49.2X2	T49.2X3	T49.2X4	T49.2X5	T49.2X6
Antiphlogistic NEC	T39.4X1	T39.4X2	T39.4X3	T39.4X4	T39.4X5	T39.4X6
Antiplatyhelmintic drug	T37.4X1	T37.4X2	T37.4X3	T37.4X4	T37.4X5	T37.4X6
Antiprotozoal drug NEC	T37.3X1	T37.3X2	T37.3X3	T37.3X4	T37.3X5	T37.3X6
blood	T37.2X1	T37.2X2	T37.2X3	T37.2X4	T37.2X5	T37.2X6
local	T49.0X1	T49.0X2	T49.0X3	T49.0X4	T49.0X5	T49.0X6
Antipruritic drug NEC	T49.1X1	T49.1X2	T49.1X3	T49.1X4	T49.1X5	T49.1X6
Antipsychotic drug	T43.501	T43.502	T43.503	T43.504	T43.505	T43.506
specified NEC	T43.591	T43.592	T43.593	T43.594	T43.595	T43.596
Antipyretic	T39.91	T39.92	T39.93	T39.94	T39.95	T39.96
specified NEC	T39.8X1	T39.8X2	T39.8X3	T39.8X4	T39.8X5	T39.8X6
Antipyrine	T39.2X1	T39.2X2	T39.2X3	T39.2X4	T39.2X5	T39.2X6
Antirabies hyperimmune serum	T50.Z11	T50.Z12	T50.Z13	T50.Z14	T50.Z15	T50.Z16
Antirheumatic NEC	T39.4X1	T39.4X2	T39.4X3	T39.4X4	T39.4X5	T39.4X6
Antirigidity drug NEC	T42.8X1	T42.8X2	T42.8X3	T42.8X4	T42.8X5	T42.8X6
Antischistosomal drug	T37.4X1	T37.4X2	T37.4X3	T37.4X4	T37.4X5	T37.4X6
Antiscorpion sera	T50.Z11	T50.Z12	T50.Z13	T50.Z14	T50.Z15	T50.Z16
Antiseborrheics	T49.4X1	T49.4X2	T49.4X3	T49.4X4	T49.4X5	T49.4X6
Antiseptics (external) (medicinal)	T49.0X1	T49.0X2	T49.0X3	T49.0X4	T49.0X5	T49.0X6
Antistine	T45.0X1	T45.0X2	T45.0X3	T45.0X4	T45.0X5	T45.0X6
Antitapeworm drug	T37.4X1	T37.4X2	T37.4X3	T37.4X4	T37.4X5	T37.4X6
Antitetanus immunoglobulin	T50.Z11	T50.Z12	T50.Z13	T50.Z14	T50.Z15	T50.Z16
Antithrombotic	T45.521	T45.522	T45.523	T45.524	T45.525	T45.526
Antithyroid drug NEC	T38.2X1	T38.2X2	T38.2X3	T38.2X4	T38.2X5	T38.2X6
Antitoxin	T50.Z11	T50.Z12	T50.Z13	T50.Z14	T50.Z15	T50.Z16
diphtheria	T50.Z11	T50.Z12	T50.Z13	T50.Z14	T50.Z15	T50.Z16
gas gangrene	T50.Z11	T50.Z12	T50.Z13	T50.Z14	T50.Z15	T50.Z16
tetanus	T50.Z11	T50.Z12	T50.Z13	T50.Z14	T50.Z15	T50.Z16
Antitrichomonal drug	T37.3X1	T37.3X2	T37.3X3	T37.3X4	T37.3X5	T37.3X6
Antituberculars	T37.1X1	T37.1X2	T37.1X3	T37.1X4	T37.1X5	T37.1X6
antibiotics	T36.5X1	T36.5X2	T36.5X3	T36.5X4	T36.5X5	T36.5X6
Antitussive NEC	T48.3X1	T48.3X2	T48.3X3	T48.3X4	T48.3X5	T48.3X6
codeine mixture	T40.2X1	T40.2X2	T40.2X3	T40.2X4	T40.2X5	T40.2X6
opiate	T40.2X1	T40.2X2	T40.2X3	T40.2X4	T40.2X5	T40.2X6
Antivaricose drug	T46.8X1	T46.8X2	T46.8X3	T46.8X4	T46.8X5	T46.8X6
Antivenin, antivenom (sera)	T50.Z11	T50.Z12	T50.Z13	T50.Z14	T50.Z15	T50.Z16
crotaline	T50.Z11	T50.Z12	T50.Z13	T50.Z14	T50.Z15	T50.Z16
spider bite	T50.Z11	T50.Z12	T50.Z13	T50.Z14	T50.Z15	T50.Z16
Antivertigo drug	T45.0X1	T45.0X2	T45.0X3	T45.0X4	T45.0X5	T45.0X6
Antiviral drug NEC	T37.5X1	T37.5X2	T37.5X3	T37.5X4	T37.5X5	T37.5X6
eye	T49.5X1	T49.5X2	T49.5X3	T49.5X4	T49.5X5	T49.5X6
Antiwhipworm drug	T37.4X1	T37.4X2	T37.4X3	T37.4X4	T37.4X5	T37.4X6
Ant poison — see Insecticide						
Antrol — see also by specific chemical substance	T60.91	T60.92	T60.93	T60.94	—	—
fungicide	T60.91	T60.92	T60.93	T60.94	—	—
ANTU (alpha naphthylthiourea)	T60.4X1	T60.4X2	T60.4X3	T60.4X4	—	—
Apalcillin	T36.0X1	T36.0X2	T36.0X3	T36.0X4	T36.0X5	T36.0X6
APC	T48.5X1	T48.5X2	T48.5X3	T48.5X4	T48.5X5	T48.5X6
Aplonidine	T44.4X1	T44.4X2	T44.4X3	T44.4X4	T44.4X5	T44.4X6
Apomorphine	T47.7X1	T47.7X2	T47.7X3	T47.7X4	T47.7X5	T47.7X6
Appetite depressants, central	T50.5X1	T50.5X2	T50.5X3	T50.5X4	T50.5X5	T50.5X6
Apraclonidine (hydrochloride)	T44.4X1	T44.4X2	T44.4X3	T44.4X4	T44.4X5	T44.4X6
Apresoline	T46.5X1	T46.5X2	T46.5X3	T46.5X4	T46.5X5	T46.5X6
Aprindine	T46.2X1	T46.2X2	T46.2X3	T46.2X4	T46.2X5	T46.2X6
Aprobarbital	T42.3X1	T42.3X2	T42.3X3	T42.3X4	T42.3X5	T42.3X6
Apronalide	T42.6X1	T42.6X2	T42.6X3	T42.6X4	T42.6X5	T42.6X6
Aprotinin	T45.621	T45.622	T45.623	T45.624	T45.625	T45.626
Aptocaine	T41.3X1	T41.3X2	T41.3X3	T41.3X4	T41.3X5	T41.3X6
Aqua fortis	T54.2X1	T54.2X2	T54.2X3	T54.2X4	—	—
Ara-A	T37.5X1	T37.5X2	T37.5X3	T37.5X4	T37.5X5	T37.5X6
Ara-C	T45.1X1	T45.1X2	T45.1X3	T45.1X4	T45.1X5	T45.1X6
Arachis oil	T49.3X1	T49.3X2	T49.3X3	T49.3X4	T49.3X5	T49.3X6
cathartic	T47.4X1	T47.4X2	T47.4X3	T47.4X4	T47.4X5	T47.4X6
Aralen	T37.2X1	T37.2X2	T37.2X3	T37.2X4	T37.2X5	T37.2X6

Additional Character May Be Required — Refer to the Tabular List for Character Selection ▽ Subterms under main terms may continue to next column or page

Substance	Poisoning, Accidental (unintentional)	Poisoning, Intentional Self-harm	Poisoning, Assault	Poisoning, Undetermined	Adverse Effect	Under-dosing
Arecoline	T44.1X1	T44.1X2	T44.1X3	T44.1X4	T44.1X5	T44.1X6
Arginine	T50.991	T50.992	T50.993	T50.994	T50.995	T50.996
glutamate	T50.991	T50.992	T50.993	T50.994	T50.995	T50.996
Argyrol	T49.0X1	T49.0X2	T49.0X3	T49.0X4	T49.0X5	T49.0X6
ENT agent	T49.6X1	T49.6X2	T49.6X3	T49.6X4	T49.6X5	T49.6X6
ophthalmic preparation	T49.5X1	T49.5X2	T49.5X3	T49.5X4	T49.5X5	T49.5X6
Aristocort	T38.0X1	T38.0X2	T38.0X3	T38.0X4	T38.0X5	T38.0X6
ENT agent	T49.6X1	T49.6X2	T49.6X3	T49.6X4	T49.6X5	T49.6X6
ophthalmic preparation	T49.5X1	T49.5X2	T49.5X3	T49.5X4	T49.5X5	T49.5X6
topical NEC	T49.0X1	T49.0X2	T49.0X3	T49.0X4	T49.0X5	T49.0X6
Aromatics, corrosive	T54.1X1	T54.1X2	T54.1X3	T54.1X4	—	—
disinfectants	T54.1X1	T54.1X2	T54.1X3	T54.1X4	—	—
Arsenate of lead	T57.0X1	T57.0X2	T57.0X3	T57.0X4	—	—
herbicide	T57.0X1	T57.0X2	T57.0X3	T57.0X4	—	—
Arsenic, arsenicals (compounds) (dust) (vapor) NEC	T57.0X1	T57.0X2	T57.0X3	T57.0X4	—	—
anti-infectives	T37.8X1	T37.8X2	T37.8X3	T37.8X4	T37.8X5	T37.8X6
pesticide (dust) (fumes)	T57.0X1	T57.0X2	T57.0X3	T57.0X4	—	—
Arsine (gas)	T57.0X1	T57.0X2	T57.0X3	T57.0X4	—	—
Arsphenamine (silver)	T37.8X1	T37.8X2	T37.8X3	T37.8X4	T37.8X5	T37.8X6
Arsthinol	T37.3X1	T37.3X2	T37.3X3	T37.3X4	T37.3X5	T37.3X6
Artane	T44.3X1	T44.3X2	T44.3X3	T44.3X4	T44.3X5	T44.3X6
Arthropod (venomous) NEC	T63.481	T63.482	T63.483	T63.484	—	—
Articaine	T41.3X1	T41.3X2	T41.3X3	T41.3X4	T41.3X5	T41.3X6
Asbestos	T57.8X1	T57.8X2	T57.8X3	T57.8X4	—	—
Ascaridole	T37.4X1	T37.4X2	T37.4X3	T37.4X4	T37.4X5	T37.4X6
Ascorbic acid	T45.2X1	T45.2X2	T45.2X3	T45.2X4	T45.2X5	T45.2X6
Asiaticoside	T49.0X1	T49.0X2	T49.0X3	T49.0X4	T49.0X5	T49.0X6
Asparaginase	T45.1X1	T45.1X2	T45.1X3	T45.1X4	T45.1X5	T45.1X6
Aspidium (oleoresin)	T37.4X1	T37.4X2	T37.4X3	T37.4X4	T37.4X5	T37.4X6
Aspirin (aluminum)	T39.011	T39.012	T39.013	T39.014	T39.015	T39.016
(soluble)	T39.011	T39.012	T39.013	T39.014	T39.015	T39.016
Aspoxicillin	T36.0X1	T36.0X2	T36.0X3	T36.0X4	T36.0X5	T36.0X6
Astemizole	T45.0X1	T45.0X2	T45.0X3	T45.0X4	T45.0X5	T45.0X6
Astringent (local)	T49.2X1	T49.2X2	T49.2X3	T49.2X4	T49.2X5	T49.2X6
specified NEC	T49.2X1	T49.2X2	T49.2X3	T49.2X4	T49.2X5	T49.2X6
Astromicin	T36.5X1	T36.5X2	T36.5X3	T36.5X4	T36.5X5	T36.5X6
Ataractic drug NEC	T43.501	T43.502	T43.503	T43.504	T43.505	T43.506
Atenolol	T44.7X1	T44.7X2	T44.7X3	T44.7X4	T44.7X5	T44.7X6
Atonia drug, intestinal	T47.4X1	T47.4X2	T47.4X3	T47.4X4	T47.4X5	T47.4X6
Atophan	T50.4X1	T50.4X2	T50.4X3	T50.4X4	T50.4X5	T50.4X6
Atracurium besilate	T48.1X1	T48.1X2	T48.1X3	T48.1X4	T48.1X5	T48.1X6
Atropine	T44.3X1	T44.3X2	T44.3X3	T44.3X4	T44.3X5	T44.3X6
derivative	T44.3X1	T44.3X2	T44.3X3	T44.3X4	T44.3X5	T44.3X6
methonitrate	T44.3X1	T44.3X2	T44.3X3	T44.3X4	T44.3X5	T44.3X6
Attapulgite	T47.6X1	T47.6X2	T47.6X3	T47.6X4	T47.6X5	T47.6X6
Auramine	T65.891	T65.892	T65.893	T65.894	—	—
dye	T65.6X1	T65.6X2	T65.6X3	T65.6X4	—	—
fungicide	T60.3X1	T60.3X2	T60.3X3	T60.3X4	—	—
Auranofin	T39.4X1	T39.4X2	T39.4X3	T39.4X4	T39.4X5	T39.4X6
Aurantiin	T46.991	T46.992	T46.993	T46.994	T46.995	T46.996
Aureomycin	T36.4X1	T36.4X2	T36.4X3	T36.4X4	T36.4X5	T36.4X6
ophthalmic preparation	T49.5X1	T49.5X2	T49.5X3	T49.5X4	T49.5X5	T49.5X6
topical NEC	T49.0X1	T49.0X2	T49.0X3	T49.0X4	T49.0X5	T49.0X6
Aurothioglucose	T39.4X1	T39.4X2	T39.4X3	T39.4X4	T39.4X5	T39.4X6
Aurothioglycanide	T39.4X1	T39.4X2	T39.4X3	T39.4X4	T39.4X5	T39.4X6
Aurothiomalate sodium	T39.4X1	T39.4X2	T39.4X3	T39.4X4	T39.4X5	T39.4X6
Aurotioprol	T39.4X1	T39.4X2	T39.4X3	T39.4X4	T39.4X5	T39.4X6
Automobile fuel	T52.0X1	T52.0X2	T52.0X3	T52.0X4	—	—
Autonomic nervous system agent NEC	T44.901	T44.902	T44.903	T44.904	T44.905	T44.906
Avlosulfon	T37.1X1	T37.1X2	T37.1X3	T37.1X4	T37.1X5	T37.1X6
Avomine	T42.6X1	T42.6X2	T42.6X3	T42.6X4	T42.6X5	T42.6X6
Axerophthol	T45.2X1	T45.2X2	T45.2X3	T45.2X4	T45.2X5	T45.2X6
Azacitidine	T45.1X1	T45.1X2	T45.1X3	T45.1X4	T45.1X5	T45.1X6
Azacyclonol	T43.591	T43.592	T43.593	T43.594	T43.595	T43.596
Azadirachta	T60.2X1	T60.2X2	T60.2X3	T60.2X4	—	—
Azanidazole	T37.3X1	T37.3X2	T37.3X3	T37.3X4	T37.3X5	T37.3X6
Azapetine	T46.7X1	T46.7X2	T46.7X3	T46.7X4	T46.7X5	T46.7X6
Azapropazone	T39.2X1	T39.2X2	T39.2X3	T39.2X4	T39.2X5	T39.2X6
Azaribine	T45.1X1	T45.1X2	T45.1X3	T45.1X4	T45.1X5	T45.1X6
Azaserine	T45.1X1	T45.1X2	T45.1X3	T45.1X4	T45.1X5	T45.1X6
Azatadine	T45.0X1	T45.0X2	T45.0X3	T45.0X4	T45.0X5	T45.0X6
Azatepa	T45.1X1	T45.1X2	T45.1X3	T45.1X4	T45.1X5	T45.1X6
Azathioprine	T45.1X1	T45.1X2	T45.1X3	T45.1X4	T45.1X5	T45.1X6
Azelaic acid	T49.0X1	T49.0X2	T49.0X3	T49.0X4	T49.0X5	T49.0X6
Azelastine	T45.0X1	T45.0X2	T45.0X3	T45.0X4	T45.0X5	T45.0X6
Azidocillin	T36.0X1	T36.0X2	T36.0X3	T36.0X4	T36.0X5	T36.0X6
Azidothymidine	T37.5X1	T37.5X2	T37.5X3	T37.5X4	T37.5X5	T37.5X6
Azinphos (ethyl) (methyl)	T60.0X1	T60.0X2	T60.0X3	T60.0X4	—	—
Aziridine (chelating)	T54.1X1	T54.1X2	T54.1X3	T54.1X4	—	—
Azithromycin	T36.3X1	T36.3X2	T36.3X3	T36.3X4	T36.3X5	T36.3X6
Azlocillin	T36.0X1	T36.0X2	T36.0X3	T36.0X4	T36.0X5	T36.0X6
Azobenzene smoke	T65.3X1	T65.3X2	T65.3X3	T65.3X4	—	—
acaricide	T60.8X1	T60.8X2	T60.8X3	T60.8X4	—	—
Azosulfamide	T37.0X1	T37.0X2	T37.0X3	T37.0X4	T37.0X5	T37.0X6
AZT	T37.5X1	T37.5X2	T37.5X3	T37.5X4	T37.5X5	T37.5X6
Aztreonam	T36.1X1	T36.1X2	T36.1X3	T36.1X4	T36.1X5	T36.1X6
Azulfidine	T37.0X1	T37.0X2	T37.0X3	T37.0X4	T37.0X5	T37.0X6
Azuresin	T50.8X1	T50.8X2	T50.8X3	T50.8X4	T50.8X5	T50.8X6
b-acetyldigoxin	T46.0X1	T46.0X2	T46.0X3	T46.0X4	T46.0X5	T46.0X6
P-Acetamidophenol	T39.1X1	T39.1X2	T39.1X3	T39.1X4	T39.1X5	T39.1X6
Bacampicillin	T36.0X1	T36.0X2	T36.0X3	T36.0X4	T36.0X5	T36.0X6
Bacillus						
lactobacillus	T47.8X1	T47.8X2	T47.8X3	T47.8X4	T47.8X5	T47.8X6
subtilis	T47.6X1	T47.6X2	T47.6X3	T47.6X4	T47.6X5	T47.6X6
Bacimycin	T49.0X1	T49.0X2	T49.0X3	T49.0X4	T49.0X5	T49.0X6
ophthalmic preparation	T49.5X1	T49.5X2	T49.5X3	T49.5X4	T49.5X5	T49.5X6
Bacitracin zinc	T49.0X1	T49.0X2	T49.0X3	T49.0X4	T49.0X5	T49.0X6
with neomycin	T49.0X1	T49.0X2	T49.0X3	T49.0X4	T49.0X5	T49.0X6
ENT agent	T49.6X1	T49.6X2	T49.6X3	T49.6X4	T49.6X5	T49.6X6
ophthalmic preparation	T49.5X1	T49.5X2	T49.5X3	T49.5X4	T49.5X5	T49.5X6
topical NEC	T49.0X1	T49.0X2	T49.0X3	T49.0X4	T49.0X5	T49.0X6
Baclofen	T42.8X1	T42.8X2	T42.8X3	T42.8X4	T42.8X5	T42.8X6
Baking soda	T50.991	T50.992	T50.993	T50.994	T50.995	T50.996
BAL	T45.8X1	T45.8X2	T45.8X3	T45.8X4	T45.8X5	T45.8X6
Bambuterol	T48.6X1	T48.6X2	T48.6X3	T48.6X4	T48.6X5	T48.6X6
Bamethan (sulfate)	T46.7X1	T46.7X2	T46.7X3	T46.7X4	T46.7X5	T46.7X6
Bamifylline	T48.6X1	T48.6X2	T48.6X3	T48.6X4	T48.6X5	T48.6X6
Bamipine	T45.0X1	T45.0X2	T45.0X3	T45.0X4	T45.0X5	T45.0X6
Baneberry — see Actaea spicata						
Banewort — see Belladonna						
Barbenyl	T42.3X1	T42.3X2	T42.3X3	T42.3X4	T42.3X5	T42.3X6
Barbexaclone	T42.6X1	T42.6X2	T42.6X3	T42.6X4	T42.6X5	T42.6X6
Barbital	T42.3X1	T42.3X2	T42.3X3	T42.3X4	T42.3X5	T42.3X6
sodium	T42.3X1	T42.3X2	T42.3X3	T42.3X4	T42.3X5	T42.3X6
Barbitone	T42.3X1	T42.3X2	T42.3X3	T42.3X4	T42.3X5	T42.3X6
Barbiturate NEC	T42.3X1	T42.3X2	T42.3X3	T42.3X4	T42.3X5	T42.3X6
with tranquilizer	T42.3X1	T42.3X2	T42.3X3	T42.3X4	T42.3X5	T42.3X6
anesthetic (intravenous)	T41.1X1	T41.1X2	T41.1X3	T41.1X4	T41.1X5	T41.1X6
Barium (carbonate) (chloride) (sulfite)	T57.8X1	T57.8X2	T57.8X3	T57.8X4	—	—
diagnostic agent	T50.8X1	T50.8X2	T50.8X3	T50.8X4	T50.8X5	T50.8X6
pesticide	T60.4X1	T60.4X2	T60.4X3	T60.4X4	—	—
rodenticide	T60.4X1	T60.4X2	T60.4X3	T60.4X4	—	—
sulfate (medicinal)	T50.8X1	T50.8X2	T50.8X3	T50.8X4	T50.8X5	T50.8X6
Barrier cream	T49.3X1	T49.3X2	T49.3X3	T49.3X4	T49.3X5	T49.3X6
Basic fuchsin	T49.0X1	T49.0X2	T49.0X3	T49.0X4	T49.0X5	T49.0X6
Battery acid or fluid	T54.2X1	T54.2X2	T54.2X3	T54.2X4	—	—
Bay rum	T51.8X1	T51.8X2	T51.8X3	T51.8X4	—	—
b-benzalbutyramide	T46.6X1	T46.6X2	T46.6X3	T46.6X4	T46.6X5	T46.6X6
BCG (vaccine)	T50.A91	T50.A92	T50.A93	T50.A94	T50.A95	T50.A96
BCNU	T45.1X1	T45.1X2	T45.1X3	T45.1X4	T45.1X5	T45.1X6
Bearsfoot	T62.2X1	T62.2X2	T62.2X3	T62.2X4	—	—
Beclamide	T42.6X1	T42.6X2	T42.6X3	T42.6X4	T42.6X5	T42.6X6
Beclomethasone	T44.5X1	T44.5X2	T44.5X3	T44.5X4	T44.5X5	T44.5X6
Bee (sting) (venom)	T63.441	T63.442	T63.443	T63.444	—	—
Befunolol	T49.5X1	T49.5X2	T49.5X3	T49.5X4	T49.5X5	T49.5X6
Bekanamycin	T36.5X1	T36.5X2	T36.5X3	T36.5X4	T36.5X5	T36.5X6
Belladonna — see also Nightshade						
alkaloids	T44.3X1	T44.3X2	T44.3X3	T44.3X4	T44.3X5	T44.3X6
extract	T44.3X1	T44.3X2	T44.3X3	T44.3X4	T44.3X5	T44.3X6
herb	T44.3X1	T44.3X2	T44.3X3	T44.3X4	T44.3X5	T44.3X6
Bemegride	T50.7X1	T50.7X2	T50.7X3	T50.7X4	T50.7X5	T50.7X6
Benactyzine	T44.3X1	T44.3X2	T44.3X3	T44.3X4	T44.3X5	T44.3X6
Benadryl	T45.0X1	T45.0X2	T45.0X3	T45.0X4	T45.0X5	T45.0X6
Benaprizine	T44.3X1	T44.3X2	T44.3X3	T44.3X4	T44.3X5	T44.3X6
Benazepril	T46.4X1	T46.4X2	T46.4X3	T46.4X4	T46.4X5	T46.4X6
Bencyclane	T46.7X1	T46.7X2	T46.7X3	T46.7X4	T46.7X5	T46.7X6
Bendazol	T46.3X1	T46.3X2	T46.3X3	T46.3X4	T46.3X5	T46.3X6
Bendrofluazide	T50.2X1	T50.2X2	T50.2X3	T50.2X4	T50.2X5	T50.2X6
Bendroflumethiazide	T50.2X1	T50.2X2	T50.2X3	T50.2X4	T50.2X5	T50.2X6
Benemid	T50.4X1	T50.4X2	T50.4X3	T50.4X4	T50.4X5	T50.4X6
Benethamine penicillin	T36.0X1	T36.0X2	T36.0X3	T36.0X4	T36.0X5	T36.0X6
Benexate	T47.1X1	T47.1X2	T47.1X3	T47.1X4	T47.1X5	T47.1X6
Benflurex	T46.6X1	T46.6X2	T46.6X3	T46.6X4	T46.6X5	T46.6X6
Benfotiamine	T45.2X1	T45.2X2	T45.2X3	T45.2X4	T45.2X5	T45.2X6
Benisone	T49.0X1	T49.0X2	T49.0X3	T49.0X4	T49.0X5	T49.0X6
Benomyl	T60.0X1	T60.0X2	T60.0X3	T60.0X4	—	—
Benoquin	T49.8X1	T49.8X2	T49.8X3	T49.8X4	T49.8X5	T49.8X6
Benoxinate	T41.3X1	T41.3X2	T41.3X3	T41.3X4	T41.3X5	T41.3X6
Benperidol	T43.4X1	T43.4X2	T43.4X3	T43.4X4	T43.4X5	T43.4X6
Benproperine	T48.3X1	T48.3X2	T48.3X3	T48.3X4	T48.3X5	T48.3X6
Benserazide	T42.8X1	T42.8X2	T42.8X3	T42.8X4	T42.8X5	T42.8X6
Bentazepam	T42.4X1	T42.4X2	T42.4X3	T42.4X4	T42.4X5	T42.4X6

▽ Subterms under main terms may continue to next column or page　　　Additional Character May Be Required — Refer to the Tabular List for Character Selection　　　355

Arecoline — Bentazepam

Table of Drugs and Chemicals

Substance	Poisoning, Accidental (unintentional)	Poisoning, Intentional Self-harm	Poisoning, Assault	Poisoning, Undetermined	Adverse Effect	Under-dosing
Bentiromide	T50.8X1	T50.8X2	T50.8X3	T50.8X4	T50.8X5	T50.8X6
Bentonite	T49.3X1	T49.3X2	T49.3X3	T49.3X4	T49.3X5	T49.3X6
Benzalbutyramide	T46.6X1	T46.6X2	T46.6X3	T46.6X4	T46.6X5	T46.6X6
Benzalkonium (chloride)	T49.0X1	T49.0X2	T49.0X3	T49.0X4	T49.0X5	T49.0X6
ophthalmic preparation	T49.5X1	T49.5X2	T49.5X3	T49.5X4	T49.5X5	T49.5X6
Benzamidosalicylate (calcium)	T37.1X1	T37.1X2	T37.1X3	T37.1X4	T37.1X5	T37.1X6
Benzamine	T41.3X1	T41.3X2	T41.3X3	T41.3X4	T41.3X5	T41.3X6
lactate	T49.1X1	T49.1X2	T49.1X3	T49.1X4	T49.1X5	T49.1X6
Benzamphetamine	T50.5X1	T50.5X2	T50.5X3	T50.5X4	T50.5X5	T50.5X6
Benzapril hydrochloride	T46.5X1	T46.5X2	T46.5X3	T46.5X4	T46.5X5	T46.5X6
Benzathine benzylpenicillin	T36.0X1	T36.0X2	T36.0X3	T36.0X4	T36.0X5	T36.0X6
Benzathine penicillin	T36.0X1	T36.0X2	T36.0X3	T36.0X4	T36.0X5	T36.0X6
Benzatropine	T42.8X1	T42.8X2	T42.8X3	T42.8X4	T42.8X5	T42.8X6
Benzbromarone	T50.4X1	T50.4X2	T50.4X3	T50.4X4	T50.4X5	T50.4X6
Benzcarbimine	T45.1X1	T45.1X2	T45.1X3	T45.1X4	T45.1X5	T45.1X6
Benzedrex	T44.991	T44.992	T44.993	T44.994	T44.995	T44.996
Benzedrine (amphetamine)	T43.621	T43.622	T43.623	T43.624	T43.625	T43.626
Benzenamine	T65.3X1	T65.3X2	T65.3X3	T65.3X4	—	—
Benzene	T52.1X1	T52.1X2	T52.1X3	T52.1X4	—	—
homologues (acetyl) (dimethyl) (methyl) (solvent)	T52.2X1	T52.2X2	T52.2X3	T52.2X4	—	—
Benzethonium (chloride)	T49.0X1	T49.0X2	T49.0X3	T49.0X4	T49.0X5	T49.0X6
Benzfetamine	T50.5X1	T50.5X2	T50.5X3	T50.5X4	T50.5X5	T50.5X6
Benzhexol	T44.3X1	T44.3X2	T44.3X3	T44.3X4	T44.3X5	T44.3X6
Benzhydramine (chloride)	T45.0X1	T45.0X2	T45.0X3	T45.0X4	T45.0X5	T45.0X6
Benzidine	T65.891	T65.892	T65.893	T65.894	—	—
Benzilonium bromide	T44.3X1	T44.3X2	T44.3X3	T44.3X4	T44.3X5	T44.3X6
Benzimidazole	T60.3X1	T60.3X2	T60.3X3	T60.3X4	—	—
Benzin (e) — see Ligroin						
Benziodarone	T46.3X1	T46.3X2	T46.3X3	T46.3X4	T46.3X5	T46.3X6
Benznidazole	T37.3X1	T37.3X2	T37.3X3	T37.3X4	T37.3X5	T37.3X6
Benzocaine	T41.3X1	T41.3X2	T41.3X3	T41.3X4	T41.3X5	T41.3X6
Benzodiapin	T42.4X1	T42.4X2	T42.4X3	T42.4X4	T42.4X5	T42.4X6
Benzodiazepine NEC	T42.4X1	T42.4X2	T42.4X3	T42.4X4	T42.4X5	T42.4X6
Benzoic acid	T49.0X1	T49.0X2	T49.0X3	T49.0X4	T49.0X5	T49.0X6
with salicylic acid	T49.0X1	T49.0X2	T49.0X3	T49.0X4	T49.0X5	T49.0X6
Benzoin (tincture)	T48.5X1	T48.5X2	T48.5X3	T48.5X4	T48.5X5	T48.5X6
Benzol (benzene)	T52.1X1	T52.1X2	T52.1X3	T52.1X4	—	—
vapor	T52.0X1	T52.0X2	T52.0X3	T52.0X4	—	—
Benzomorphan	T40.2X1	T40.2X2	T40.2X3	T40.2X4	T40.2X5	T40.2X6
Benzonatate	T48.3X1	T48.3X2	T48.3X3	T48.3X4	T48.3X5	T48.3X6
Benzophenones	T49.3X1	T49.3X2	T49.3X3	T49.3X4	T49.3X5	T49.3X6
Benzopyrone	T46.991	T46.992	T46.993	T46.994	T46.995	T46.996
Benzothiadiazides	T50.2X1	T50.2X2	T50.2X3	T50.2X4	T50.2X5	T50.2X6
Benzoxonium chloride	T49.0X1	T49.0X2	T49.0X3	T49.0X4	T49.0X5	T49.0X6
Benzoylpas calcium	T37.1X1	T37.1X2	T37.1X3	T37.1X4	T37.1X5	T37.1X6
Benzoyl peroxide	T49.0X1	T49.0X2	T49.0X3	T49.0X4	T49.0X5	T49.0X6
Benzperidin	T43.591	T43.592	T43.593	T43.594	T43.595	T43.596
Benzperidol	T43.591	T43.592	T43.593	T43.594	T43.595	T43.596
Benzphetamine	T50.5X1	T50.5X2	T50.5X3	T50.5X4	T50.5X5	T50.5X6
Benzpyrinium bromide	T44.1X1	T44.1X2	T44.1X3	T44.1X4	T44.1X5	T44.1X6
Benzquinamide	T45.0X1	T45.0X2	T45.0X3	T45.0X4	T45.0X5	T45.0X6
Benzthiazide	T50.2X1	T50.2X2	T50.2X3	T50.2X4	T50.2X5	T50.2X6
Benztropine						
anticholinergic	T44.3X1	T44.3X2	T44.3X3	T44.3X4	T44.3X5	T44.3X6
antiparkinson	T42.8X1	T42.8X2	T42.8X3	T42.8X4	T42.8X5	T42.8X6
Benzydamine	T49.0X1	T49.0X2	T49.0X3	T49.0X4	T49.0X5	T49.0X6
Benzyl						
acetate	T52.8X1	T52.8X2	T52.8X3	T52.8X4	—	—
alcohol	T49.0X1	T49.0X2	T49.0X3	T49.0X4	T49.0X5	T49.0X6
benzoate	T49.0X1	T49.0X2	T49.0X3	T49.0X4	T49.0X5	T49.0X6
Benzoic acid	T49.0X1	T49.0X2	T49.0X3	T49.0X4	T49.0X5	T49.0X6
morphine	T40.2X1	T40.2X2	T40.2X3	T40.2X4	—	—
nicotinate	T46.6X1	T46.6X2	T46.6X3	T46.6X4	T46.6X5	T46.6X6
penicillin	T36.0X1	T36.0X2	T36.0X3	T36.0X4	T36.0X5	T36.0X6
Benzylhydrochlorthiazide	T50.2X1	T50.2X2	T50.2X3	T50.2X4	T50.2X5	T50.2X6
Benzylpenicillin	T36.0X1	T36.0X2	T36.0X3	T36.0X4	T36.0X5	T36.0X6
Benzylthiouracil	T38.2X1	T38.2X2	T38.2X3	T38.2X4	T38.2X5	T38.2X6
Bephenium hydroxynaphthoate	T37.4X1	T37.4X2	T37.4X3	T37.4X4	T37.4X5	T37.4X6
Bepridil	T46.1X1	T46.1X2	T46.1X3	T46.1X4	T46.1X5	T46.1X6
Bergamot oil	T65.891	T65.892	T65.893	T65.894	—	—
Bergapten	T50.991	T50.992	T50.993	T50.994	T50.995	T50.996
Berries, poisonous	T62.1X1	T62.1X2	T62.1X3	T62.1X4	—	—
Beryllium (compounds)	T56.7X1	T56.7X2	T56.7X3	T56.7X4	—	—
beta adrenergic blocking agent, heart	T44.7X1	T44.7X2	T44.7X3	T44.7X4	T44.7X5	T44.7X6
Betacarotene	T45.2X1	T45.2X2	T45.2X3	T45.2X4	T45.2X5	T45.2X6
Beta-Chlor	T42.6X1	T42.6X2	T42.6X3	T42.6X4	T42.6X5	T42.6X6
Betahistine	T46.7X1	T46.7X2	T46.7X3	T46.7X4	T46.7X5	T46.7X6
Betaine	T47.5X1	T47.5X2	T47.5X3	T47.5X4	T47.5X5	T47.5X6

Substance	Poisoning, Accidental (unintentional)	Poisoning, Intentional Self-harm	Poisoning, Assault	Poisoning, Undetermined	Adverse Effect	Under-dosing
Betamethasone	T49.0X1	T49.0X2	T49.0X3	T49.0X4	T49.0X5	T49.0X6
topical	T49.0X1	T49.0X2	T49.0X3	T49.0X4	T49.0X5	T49.0X6
Betamicin	T36.8X1	T36.8X2	T36.8X3	T36.8X4	T36.8X5	T36.8X6
Betanidine	T46.5X1	T46.5X2	T46.5X3	T46.5X4	T46.5X5	T46.5X6
Betaxolol	T44.7X1	T44.7X2	T44.7X3	T44.7X4	T44.7X5	T44.7X6
Betazole	T50.8X1	T50.8X2	T50.8X3	T50.8X4	T50.8X5	T50.8X6
Bethanechol	T44.1X1	T44.1X2	T44.1X3	T44.1X4	T44.1X5	T44.1X6
chloride	T44.1X1	T44.1X2	T44.1X3	T44.1X4	T44.1X5	T44.1X6
Bethanidine	T46.5X1	T46.5X2	T46.5X3	T46.5X4	T46.5X5	T46.5X6
Betoxycaine	T41.3X1	T41.3X2	T41.3X3	T41.3X4	T41.3X5	T41.3X6
Betula oil	T49.3X1	T49.3X2	T49.3X3	T49.3X4	T49.3X5	T49.3X6
Bevantolol	T44.7X1	T44.7X2	T44.7X3	T44.7X4	T44.7X5	T44.7X6
Bevonium metilsulfate	T44.3X1	T44.3X2	T44.3X3	T44.3X4	T44.3X5	T44.3X6
Bezafibrate	T46.6X1	T46.6X2	T46.6X3	T46.6X4	T46.6X5	T46.6X6
Bezitramide	T40.4X1	T40.4X2	T40.4X3	T40.4X4	T40.4X5	T40.4X6
BHA	T50.991	T50.992	T50.993	T50.994	T50.995	T50.996
Bhang	T40.7X1	T40.7X2	T40.7X3	T40.7X4	T40.7X5	T40.7X6
BHC (medicinal)	T49.0X1	T49.0X2	T49.0X3	T49.0X4	T49.0X5	T49.0X6
nonmedicinal (vapor)	T53.6X1	T53.6X2	T53.6X3	T53.6X4	—	—
Bialamicol	T37.3X1	T37.3X2	T37.3X3	T37.3X4	T37.3X5	T37.3X6
Bibenzonium bromide	T48.3X1	T48.3X2	T48.3X3	T48.3X4	T48.3X5	T48.3X6
Bibrocathol	T49.5X1	T49.5X2	T49.5X3	T49.5X4	T49.5X5	T49.5X6
Bichloride of mercury — see Mercury, chloride						
Bichromates (calcium) (potassium)(sodium) (crystals)	T57.8X1	T57.8X2	T57.8X3	T57.8X4	—	
fumes	T56.2X1	T56.2X2	T56.2X3	T56.2X4	—	—
Biclotymol	T49.6X1	T49.6X2	T49.6X3	T49.6X4	T49.6X5	T49.6X6
Bicucculine	T50.7X1	T50.7X2	T50.7X3	T50.7X4	T50.7X5	T50.7X6
Bifemelane	T43.291	T43.292	T43.293	T43.294	T43.295	T43.296
Biguanide derivatives, oral	T38.3X1	T38.3X2	T38.3X3	T38.3X4	T38.3X5	T38.3X6
Bile salts	T47.5X1	T47.5X2	T47.5X3	T47.5X4	T47.5X5	T47.5X6
Biligrafin	T50.8X1	T50.8X2	T50.8X3	T50.8X4	T50.8X5	T50.8X6
Bilopaque	T50.8X1	T50.8X2	T50.8X3	T50.8X4	T50.8X5	T50.8X6
Binifibrate	T46.6X1	T46.6X2	T46.6X3	T46.6X4	T46.6X5	T46.6X6
Binitrobenzol	T65.3X1	T65.3X2	T65.3X3	T65.3X4	—	—
Bioflavonoid(s)	T46.991	T46.992	T46.993	T46.994	T46.995	T46.996
Biological substance NEC	T50.901	T50.902	T50.903	T50.904	T50.905	T50.906
Biotin	T45.2X1	T45.2X2	T45.2X3	T45.2X4	T45.2X5	T45.2X6
Biperiden	T44.3X1	T44.3X2	T44.3X3	T44.3X4	T44.3X5	T44.3X6
Bisacodyl	T47.2X1	T47.2X2	T47.2X3	T47.2X4	T47.2X5	T47.2X6
Bisbentiamine	T45.2X1	T45.2X2	T45.2X3	T45.2X4	T45.2X5	T45.2X6
Bisbutiamine	T45.2X1	T45.2X2	T45.2X3	T45.2X4	T45.2X5	T45.2X6
Bisdequalinium (salts) (diacetate)	T49.6X1	T49.6X2	T49.6X3	T49.6X4	T49.6X5	T49.6X6
Bishydroxycoumarin	T45.511	T45.512	T45.513	T45.514	T45.515	T45.516
Bismarsen	T37.8X1	T37.8X2	T37.8X3	T37.8X4	T37.8X5	T37.8X6
Bismuth salts	T47.6X1	T47.6X2	T47.6X3	T47.6X4	T47.6X5	T47.6X6
aluminate	T47.1X1	T47.1X2	T47.1X3	T47.1X4	T47.1X5	T47.1X6
anti-infectives	T37.8X1	T37.8X2	T37.8X3	T37.8X4	T37.8X5	T37.8X6
formic iodide	T49.0X1	T49.0X2	T49.0X3	T49.0X4	T49.0X5	T49.0X6
glycolylarsenate	T49.0X1	T49.0X2	T49.0X3	T49.0X4	T49.0X5	T49.0X6
nonmedicinal (compounds) NEC	T65.91	T65.92	T65.93	T65.94	—	—
subcarbonate	T47.6X1	T47.6X2	T47.6X3	T47.6X4	T47.6X5	T47.6X6
subsalicylate	T37.8X1	T37.8X2	T37.8X3	T37.8X4	T37.8X5	T37.8X6
sulfarsphenamine	T37.8X1	T37.8X2	T37.8X3	T37.8X4	T37.8X5	T37.8X6
Bisoprolol	T44.7X1	T44.7X2	T44.7X3	T44.7X4	T44.7X5	T44.7X6
Bisoxatin	T47.2X1	T47.2X2	T47.2X3	T47.2X4	T47.2X5	T47.2X6
Bisulepin (hydrochloride)	T45.0X1	T45.0X2	T45.0X3	T45.0X4	T45.0X5	T45.0X6
Bithionol	T37.8X1	T37.8X2	T37.8X3	T37.8X4	T37.8X5	T37.8X6
anthelminthic	T37.4X1	T37.4X2	T37.4X3	T37.4X4	T37.4X5	T37.4X6
Bitolterol	T48.6X1	T48.6X2	T48.6X3	T48.6X4	T48.6X5	T48.6X6
Bitoscanate	T37.4X1	T37.4X2	T37.4X3	T37.4X4	T37.4X5	T37.4X6
Bitter almond oil	T62.8X1	T62.8X2	T62.8X3	T62.8X4	—	—
Bittersweet	T62.2X1	T62.2X2	T62.2X3	T62.2X4	—	—
Black						
flag	T60.91	T60.92	T60.93	T60.94	—	—
henbane	T62.2X1	T62.2X2	T62.2X3	T62.2X4	—	—
leaf (40)	T60.91	T60.92	T60.93	T60.94	—	—
widow spider (bite)	T63.311	T63.312	T63.313	T63.314	—	—
antivenin	T50.Z11	T50.Z12	T50.Z13	T50.Z14	T50.Z15	T50.Z16
Blast furnace gas (carbon monoxide from)	T58.8X1	T58.8X2	T58.8X3	T58.8X4	—	—
Bleach	T54.91	T54.92	T54.93	T54.94	—	—
Bleaching agent (medicinal)	T49.4X1	T49.4X2	T49.4X3	T49.4X4	T49.4X5	T49.4X6
Bleomycin	T45.1X1	T45.1X2	T45.1X3	T45.1X4	T45.1X5	T45.1X6
Blockain	T41.3X1	T41.3X2	T41.3X3	T41.3X4	T41.3X5	T41.3X6
infiltration (subcutaneous)	T41.3X1	T41.3X2	T41.3X3	T41.3X4	T41.3X5	T41.3X6

Additional Character May Be Required — Refer to the Tabular List for Character Selection ▽ Subterms under main terms may continue to next column or page

Bentiromide — Blockain

Substance	Poisoning, Accidental (unintentional)	Poisoning, Intentional Self-harm	Poisoning, Assault	Poisoning, Undetermined	Adverse Effect	Underdosing
Blockain — *continued*						
nerve block (peripheral) (plexus)	T41.3X1	T41.3X2	T41.3X3	T41.3X4	T41.3X5	T41.3X6
topical (surface)	T41.3X1	T41.3X2	T41.3X3	T41.3X4	T41.3X5	T41.3X6
Blockers, calcium channel	T46.1X1	T46.1X2	T46.1X3	T46.1X4	T46.1X5	T46.1X6
Blood (derivatives) (natural) (plasma) (whole)	T45.8X1	T45.8X2	T45.8X3	T45.8X4	T45.8X5	T45.8X6
dried	T45.8X1	T45.8X2	T45.8X3	T45.8X4	T45.8X5	T45.8X6
drug affecting NEC	T45.91	T45.92	T45.93	T45.94	T45.95	T45.96
expander NEC	T45.8X1	T45.8X2	T45.8X3	T45.8X4	T45.8X5	T45.8X6
fraction NEC	T45.8X1	T45.8X2	T45.8X3	T45.8X4	T45.8X5	T45.8X6
substitute (macromolecular)	T45.8X1	T45.8X2	T45.8X3	T45.8X4	T45.8X5	T45.8X6
Blue velvet	T40.2X1	T40.2X2	T40.2X3	T40.2X4	—	—
Bone meal	T62.8X1	T62.8X2	T62.8X3	T62.8X4	—	—
Bonine	T45.0X1	T45.0X2	T45.0X3	T45.0X4	T45.0X5	T45.0X6
Bopindolol	T44.7X1	T44.7X2	T44.7X3	T44.7X4	T44.7X5	T44.7X6
Boracic acid	T49.0X1	T49.0X2	T49.0X3	T49.0X4	T49.0X5	T49.0X6
ENT agent	T49.6X1	T49.6X2	T49.6X3	T49.6X4	T49.6X5	T49.6X6
ophthalmic preparation	T49.5X1	T49.5X2	T49.5X3	T49.5X4	T49.5X5	T49.5X6
Borane complex	T57.8X1	T57.8X2	T57.8X3	T57.8X4	—	—
Borate(s)	T57.8X1	T57.8X2	T57.8X3	T57.8X4	—	—
buffer	T50.991	T50.992	T50.993	T50.994	T50.995	T50.996
cleanser	T54.91	T54.92	T54.93	T54.94	—	—
sodium	T57.8X1	T57.8X2	T57.8X3	T57.8X4	—	—
Borax (cleanser)	T54.91	T54.92	T54.93	T54.94	—	—
Bordeaux mixture	T60.3X1	T60.3X2	T60.3X3	T60.3X4	—	—
Boric acid	T49.0X1	T49.0X2	T49.0X3	T49.0X4	T49.0X5	T49.0X6
ENT agent	T49.6X1	T49.6X2	T49.6X3	T49.6X4	T49.6X5	T49.6X6
ophthalmic preparation	T49.5X1	T49.5X2	T49.5X3	T49.5X4	T49.5X5	T49.5X6
Bornaprine	T44.3X1	T44.3X2	T44.3X3	T44.3X4	T44.3X5	T44.3X6
Boron	T57.8X1	T57.8X2	T57.8X3	T57.8X4	—	—
hydride NEC	T57.8X1	T57.8X2	T57.8X3	T57.8X4	—	—
fumes or gas	T57.8X1	T57.8X2	T57.8X3	T57.8X4	—	—
trifluoride	T59.891	T59.892	T59.893	T59.894	—	—
Botox	T48.291	T48.292	T48.293	T48.294	T48.295	T48.296
Botulinus anti-toxin (type A, B)	T50.Z11	T50.Z12	T50.Z13	T50.Z14	T50.Z15	T50.Z16
Brake fluid vapor	T59.891	T59.892	T59.893	T59.894	—	—
Brallobarbital	T42.3X1	T42.3X2	T42.3X3	T42.3X4	T42.3X5	T42.3X6
Bran (wheat)	T47.4X1	T47.4X2	T47.4X3	T47.4X4	T47.4X5	T47.4X6
Brass (fumes)	T56.891	T56.892	T56.893	T56.894	—	—
Brasso	T52.0X1	T52.0X2	T52.0X3	T52.0X4	—	—
Bretylium tosilate	T46.2X1	T46.2X2	T46.2X3	T46.2X4	T46.2X5	T46.2X6
Brevital (sodium)	T41.1X1	T41.1X2	T41.1X3	T41.1X4	T41.1X5	T41.1X6
Brinase	T45.3X1	T45.3X2	T45.3X3	T45.3X4	T45.3X5	T45.3X6
British antilewisite	T45.8X1	T45.8X2	T45.8X3	T45.8X4	T45.8X5	T45.8X6
Brodifacoum	T60.4X1	T60.4X2	T60.4X3	T60.4X4	—	—
Bromal (hydrate)	T42.6X1	T42.6X2	T42.6X3	T42.6X4	T42.6X5	T42.6X6
Bromazepam	T42.4X1	T42.4X2	T42.4X3	T42.4X4	T42.4X5	T42.4X6
Bromazine	T45.0X1	T45.0X2	T45.0X3	T45.0X4	T45.0X5	T45.0X6
Brombenzylcyanide	T59.3X1	T59.3X2	T59.3X3	T59.3X4	—	—
Bromelains	T45.3X1	T45.3X2	T45.3X3	T45.3X4	T45.3X5	T45.3X6
Bromethalin	T60.4X1	T60.4X2	T60.4X3	T60.4X4	—	—
Bromhexine	T48.4X1	T48.4X2	T48.4X3	T48.4X4	T48.4X5	T48.4X6
Bromide salts	T42.6X1	T42.6X2	T42.6X3	T42.6X4	T42.6X5	T42.6X6
Bromindione	T45.511	T45.512	T45.513	T45.514	T45.515	T45.516
Bromine						
compounds (medicinal)	T42.6X1	T42.6X2	T42.6X3	T42.6X4	T42.6X5	T42.6X6
sedative	T42.6X1	T42.6X2	T42.6X3	T42.6X4	T42.6X5	T42.6X6
vapor	T59.891	T59.892	T59.893	T59.894	—	—
Bromisoval	T42.6X1	T42.6X2	T42.6X3	T42.6X4	T42.6X5	T42.6X6
Bromisovalum	T42.6X1	T42.6X2	T42.6X3	T42.6X4	T42.6X5	T42.6X6
Bromobenzylcyanide	T59.3X1	T59.3X2	T59.3X3	T59.3X4	—	—
Bromochlorosalicylani-lide	T49.0X1	T49.0X2	T49.0X3	T49.0X4	T49.0X5	T49.0X6
Bromocriptine	T42.8X1	T42.8X2	T42.8X3	T42.8X4	T42.8X5	T42.8X6
Bromodiphenhydramine	T45.0X1	T45.0X2	T45.0X3	T45.0X4	T45.0X5	T45.0X6
Bromoform	T42.6X1	T42.6X2	T42.6X3	T42.6X4	T42.6X5	T42.6X6
Bromophenol blue reagent	T50.991	T50.992	T50.993	T50.994	T50.995	T50.996
Bromopride	T47.8X1	T47.8X2	T47.8X3	T47.8X4	T47.8X5	T47.8X6
Bromosalicylchloranitide	T49.0X1	T49.0X2	T49.0X3	T49.0X4	T49.0X5	T49.0X6
Bromosalicylhydroxamic acid	T37.1X1	T37.1X2	T37.1X3	T37.1X4	T37.1X5	T37.1X6
Bromo-seltzer	T39.1X1	T39.1X2	T39.1X3	T39.1X4	T39.1X5	T39.1X6
Bromoxynil	T60.3X1	T60.3X2	T60.3X3	T60.3X4	—	—
Bromperidol	T43.4X1	T43.4X2	T43.4X3	T43.4X4	T43.4X5	T43.4X6
Brompheniramine	T45.0X1	T45.0X2	T45.0X3	T45.0X4	T45.0X5	T45.0X6
Bromsulfophthalein	T50.8X1	T50.8X2	T50.8X3	T50.8X4	T50.8X5	T50.8X6
Bromural	T42.6X1	T42.6X2	T42.6X3	T42.6X4	T42.6X5	T42.6X6
Bromvaletone	T42.6X1	T42.6X2	T42.6X3	T42.6X4	T42.6X5	T42.6X6
Bronchodilator NEC	T48.6X1	T48.6X2	T48.6X3	T48.6X4	T48.6X5	T48.6X6
Brotizolam	T42.4X1	T42.4X2	T42.4X3	T42.4X4	T42.4X5	T42.4X6
Brovincamine	T46.7X1	T46.7X2	T46.7X3	T46.7X4	T46.7X5	T46.7X6
Brown recluse spider (bite) (venom)	T63.331	T63.332	T63.333	T63.334	—	—
Brown spider (bite) (venom)	T63.391	T63.392	T63.393	T63.394	—	—
Broxaterol	T48.6X1	T48.6X2	T48.6X3	T48.6X4	T48.6X5	T48.6X6
Broxuridine	T45.1X1	T45.1X2	T45.1X3	T45.1X4	T45.1X5	T45.1X6
Broxyquinoline	T37.8X1	T37.8X2	T37.8X3	T37.8X4	T37.8X5	T37.8X6
Bruceine	T48.291	T48.292	T48.293	T48.294	T48.295	T48.296
Brucia	T62.2X1	T62.2X2	T62.2X3	T62.2X4	—	—
Brucine	T65.1X1	T65.1X2	T65.1X3	T65.1X4	—	—
Brunswick green — *see* Copper						
Bruten — *see* Ibuprofen						
Bryonia	T47.2X1	T47.2X2	T47.2X3	T47.2X4	T47.2X5	T47.2X6
Buclizine	T45.0X1	T45.0X2	T45.0X3	T45.0X4	T45.0X5	T45.0X6
Buclosamide	T49.0X1	T49.0X2	T49.0X3	T49.0X4	T49.0X5	T49.0X6
Budesonide	T44.5X1	T44.5X2	T44.5X3	T44.5X4	T44.5X5	T44.5X6
Budralazine	T46.5X1	T46.5X2	T46.5X3	T46.5X4	T46.5X5	T46.5X6
Bufferin	T39.011	T39.012	T39.013	T39.014	T39.015	T39.016
Buflomedil	T46.7X1	T46.7X2	T46.7X3	T46.7X4	T46.7X5	T46.7X6
Buformin	T38.3X1	T38.3X2	T38.3X3	T38.3X4	T38.3X5	T38.3X6
Bufotenine	T40.991	T40.992	T40.993	T40.994	—	—
Bufrolin	T48.6X1	T48.6X2	T48.6X3	T48.6X4	T48.6X5	T48.6X6
Bufylline	T48.6X1	T48.6X2	T48.6X3	T48.6X4	T48.6X5	T48.6X6
Bulk filler	T50.5X1	T50.5X2	T50.5X3	T50.5X4	T50.5X5	T50.5X6
cathartic	T47.4X1	T47.4X2	T47.4X3	T47.4X4	T47.4X5	T47.4X6
Bumetanide	T50.1X1	T50.1X2	T50.1X3	T50.1X4	T50.1X5	T50.1X6
Bunaftine	T46.2X1	T46.2X2	T46.2X3	T46.2X4	T46.2X5	T46.2X6
Bunamiodyl	T50.8X1	T50.8X2	T50.8X3	T50.8X4	T50.8X5	T50.8X6
Bunazosin	T44.6X1	T44.6X2	T44.6X3	T44.6X4	T44.6X5	T44.6X6
Bunitrolol	T44.7X1	T44.7X2	T44.7X3	T44.7X4	T44.7X5	T44.7X6
Buphenine	T46.7X1	T46.7X2	T46.7X3	T46.7X4	T46.7X5	T46.7X6
Bupivacaine	T41.3X1	T41.3X2	T41.3X3	T41.3X4	T41.3X5	T41.3X6
infiltration (subcutaneous)	T41.3X1	T41.3X2	T41.3X3	T41.3X4	T41.3X5	T41.3X6
nerve block (peripheral) (plexus)	T41.3X1	T41.3X2	T41.3X3	T41.3X4	T41.3X5	T41.3X6
spinal	T41.3X1	T41.3X2	T41.3X3	T41.3X4	T41.3X5	T41.3X6
Bupranolol	T44.7X1	T44.7X2	T44.7X3	T44.7X4	T44.7X5	T44.7X6
Buprenorphine	T40.4X1	T40.4X2	T40.4X3	T40.4X4	T40.4X5	T40.4X6
Bupropion	T43.291	T43.292	T43.293	T43.294	T43.295	T43.296
Burimamide	T47.1X1	T47.1X2	T47.1X3	T47.1X4	T47.1X5	T47.1X6
Buserelin	T38.891	T38.892	T38.893	T38.894	T38.895	T38.896
Buspirone	T43.591	T43.592	T43.593	T43.594	T43.595	T43.596
Busulfan, busulphan	T45.1X1	T45.1X2	T45.1X3	T45.1X4	T45.1X5	T45.1X6
Butabarbital (sodium)	T42.3X1	T42.3X2	T42.3X3	T42.3X4	T42.3X5	T42.3X6
Butabarbitone	T42.3X1	T42.3X2	T42.3X3	T42.3X4	T42.3X5	T42.3X6
Butabarpal	T42.3X1	T42.3X2	T42.3X3	T42.3X4	T42.3X5	T42.3X6
Butacaine	T41.3X1	T41.3X2	T41.3X3	T41.3X4	T41.3X5	T41.3X6
Butalamine	T46.7X1	T46.7X2	T46.7X3	T46.7X4	T46.7X5	T46.7X6
Butalbital	T42.3X1	T42.3X2	T42.3X3	T42.3X4	T42.3X5	T42.3X6
Butallylonal	T42.3X1	T42.3X2	T42.3X3	T42.3X4	T42.3X5	T42.3X6
Butamben	T41.3X1	T41.3X2	T41.3X3	T41.3X4	T41.3X5	T41.3X6
Butamirate	T48.3X1	T48.3X2	T48.3X3	T48.3X4	T48.3X5	T48.3X6
Butane (distributed in mobile container)	T59.891	T59.892	T59.893	T59.894	—	—
distributed through pipes	T59.891	T59.892	T59.893	T59.894	—	—
incomplete combustion	T58.11	T58.12	T58.13	T58.14	—	—
Butanilicaine	T41.3X1	T41.3X2	T41.3X3	T41.3X4	T41.3X5	T41.3X6
Butanol	T51.3X1	T51.3X2	T51.3X3	T51.3X4	—	—
Butanone, 2-butanone	T52.4X1	T52.4X2	T52.4X3	T52.4X4	—	—
Butantrone	T49.4X1	T49.4X2	T49.4X3	T49.4X4	T49.4X5	T49.4X6
Butaperazine	T43.3X1	T43.3X2	T43.3X3	T43.3X4	T43.3X5	T43.3X6
Butazolidin	T39.2X1	T39.2X2	T39.2X3	T39.2X4	T39.2X5	T39.2X6
Butetamate	T48.6X1	T48.6X2	T48.6X3	T48.6X4	T48.6X5	T48.6X6
Butethal	T42.3X1	T42.3X2	T42.3X3	T42.3X4	T42.3X5	T42.3X6
Butethamate	T44.3X1	T44.3X2	T44.3X3	T44.3X4	T44.3X5	T44.3X6
Buthalitone (sodium)	T41.1X1	T41.1X2	T41.1X3	T41.1X4	T41.1X5	T41.1X6
Butisol (sodium)	T42.3X1	T42.3X2	T42.3X3	T42.3X4	T42.3X5	T42.3X6
Butizide	T50.2X1	T50.2X2	T50.2X3	T50.2X4	T50.2X5	T50.2X6
Butobarbital	T42.3X1	T42.3X2	T42.3X3	T42.3X4	T42.3X5	T42.3X6
sodium	T42.3X1	T42.3X2	T42.3X3	T42.3X4	T42.3X5	T42.3X6
Butobarbitone	T42.3X1	T42.3X2	T42.3X3	T42.3X4	T42.3X5	T42.3X6
Butoconazole (nitrate)	T49.0X1	T49.0X2	T49.0X3	T49.0X4	T49.0X5	T49.0X6
Butorphanol	T40.4X1	T40.4X2	T40.4X3	T40.4X4	T40.4X5	T40.4X6
Butriptyline	T43.011	T43.012	T43.013	T43.014	T43.015	T43.016
Butropium bromide	T44.3X1	T44.3X2	T44.3X3	T44.3X4	—	T44.3X6
Buttercups	T62.2X1	T62.2X2	T62.2X3	T62.2X4	—	—
Butter of antimony — *see* Antimony						
Butyl						
acetate (secondary)	T52.8X1	T52.8X2	T52.8X3	T52.8X4	—	—
alcohol	T51.3X1	T51.3X2	T51.3X3	T51.3X4	—	—
aminobenzoate	T41.3X1	T41.3X2	T41.3X3	T41.3X4	T41.3X5	T41.3X6

Blockain — Butyl

Table of Drugs and Chemicals

Substance	Poisoning, Accidental (unintentional)	Poisoning, Intentional Self-harm	Poisoning, Assault	Poisoning, Undetermined	Adverse Effect	Underdosing
Butyl — *continued*						
butyrate	T52.8X1	T52.8X2	T52.8X3	T52.8X4	—	—
carbinol	T51.3X1	T51.3X2	T51.3X3	T51.3X4	—	—
carbitol	T52.3X1	T52.3X2	T52.3X3	T52.3X4	—	—
cellosolve	T52.3X1	T52.3X2	T52.3X3	T52.3X4	—	—
chloral (hydrate)	T42.6X1	T42.6X2	T42.6X3	T42.6X4	T42.6X5	T42.6X6
formate	T52.8X1	T52.8X2	T52.8X3	T52.8X4	—	—
lactate	T52.8X1	T52.8X2	T52.8X3	T52.8X4	—	—
propionate	T52.8X1	T52.8X2	T52.8X3	T52.8X4	—	—
scopolamine bromide	T44.3X1	T44.3X2	T44.3X3	T44.3X4	T44.3X5	T44.3X6
thiobarbital sodium	T41.1X1	T41.1X2	T41.1X3	T41.1X4	T41.1X5	T41.1X6
Butylated hydroxyanisole	T50.991	T50.992	T50.993	T50.994	T50.995	T50.996
Butylchloral hydrate	T42.6X1	T42.6X2	T42.6X3	T42.6X4	T42.6X5	T42.6X6
Butyltoluene	T52.2X1	T52.2X2	T52.2X3	T52.2X4	—	—
Butyn	T41.3X1	T41.3X2	T41.3X3	T41.3X4	T41.3X5	T41.3X6
Butyrophenone (-based tranquilizers)	T43.4X1	T43.4X2	T43.4X3	T43.4X4	T43.4X5	T43.4X6
Cabergoline	T42.8X1	T42.8X2	T42.8X3	T42.8X4	T42.8X5	T42.8X6
Cacodyl, cacodylic acid	T57.0X1	T57.0X2	T57.0X3	T57.0X4	—	—
Cactinomycin	T45.1X1	T45.1X2	T45.1X3	T45.1X4	T45.1X5	T45.1X6
Cade oil	T49.4X1	T49.4X2	T49.4X3	T49.4X4	T49.4X5	T49.4X6
Cadexomer iodine	T49.0X1	T49.0X2	T49.0X3	T49.0X4	T49.0X5	T49.0X6
Cadmium (chloride) (fumes) (oxide)	T56.3X1	T56.3X2	T56.3X3	T56.3X4	—	—
sulfide (medicinal) NEC	T49.4X1	T49.4X2	T49.4X3	T49.4X4	T49.4X5	T49.4X6
Cadralazine	T46.5X1	T46.5X2	T46.5X3	T46.5X4	T46.5X5	T46.5X6
Caffeine	T43.611	T43.612	T43.613	T43.614	T43.615	T43.616
Calabar bean	T62.2X1	T62.2X2	T62.2X3	T62.2X4	—	—
Caladium seguinum	T62.2X1	T62.2X2	T62.2X3	T62.2X4	—	—
Calamine (lotion)	T49.3X1	T49.3X2	T49.3X3	T49.3X4	T49.3X5	T49.3X6
Calcifediol	T45.2X1	T45.2X2	T45.2X3	T45.2X4	T45.2X5	T45.2X6
Calciferol	T45.2X1	T45.2X2	T45.2X3	T45.2X4	T45.2X5	T45.2X6
Calcitonin	T50.991	T50.992	T50.993	T50.994	T50.995	T50.996
Calcitriol	T45.2X1	T45.2X2	T45.2X3	T45.2X4	T45.2X5	T45.2X6
Calcium	T50.3X1	T50.3X2	T50.3X3	T50.3X4	T50.3X5	T50.3X6
actylsalicylate	T39.011	T39.012	T39.013	T39.014	T39.015	T39.016
benzamidosalicylate	T37.1X1	T37.1X2	T37.1X3	T37.1X4	T37.1X5	T37.1X6
bromide	T42.6X1	T42.6X2	T42.6X3	T42.6X4	T42.6X5	T42.6X6
bromolactobionate	T42.6X1	T42.6X2	T42.6X3	T42.6X4	T42.6X5	T42.6X6
carbaspirin	T39.011	T39.012	T39.013	T39.014	T39.015	T39.016
carbimide	T50.6X1	T50.6X2	T50.6X3	T50.6X4	T50.6X5	T50.6X6
carbonate	T47.1X1	T47.1X2	T47.1X3	T47.1X4	T47.1X5	T47.1X6
chloride	T50.991	T50.992	T50.993	T50.994	T50.995	T50.996
anhydrous	T50.991	T50.992	T50.993	T50.994	T50.995	T50.996
cyanide	T57.8X1	T57.8X2	T57.8X3	T57.8X4	—	—
dioctyl sulfosuccinate	T47.4X1	T47.4X2	T47.4X3	T47.4X4	T47.4X5	T47.4X6
disodium edathamil	T45.8X1	T45.8X2	T45.8X3	T45.8X4	T45.8X5	T45.8X6
disodium edetate	T45.8X1	T45.8X2	T45.8X3	T45.8X4	T45.8X5	T45.8X6
dobesilate	T46.991	T46.992	T46.993	T46.994	T46.995	T46.996
EDTA	T45.8X1	T45.8X2	T45.8X3	T45.8X4	T45.8X5	T45.8X6
ferrous citrate	T45.4X1	T45.4X2	T45.4X3	T45.4X4	T45.4X5	T45.4X6
folinate	T45.8X1	T45.8X2	T45.8X3	T45.8X4	T45.8X5	T45.8X6
glubionate	T50.3X1	T50.3X2	T50.3X3	T50.3X4	T50.3X5	T50.3X6
gluconate	T50.3X1	T50.3X2	T50.3X3	T50.3X4	T50.3X5	T50.3X6
gluconogalactogluconate	T50.3X1	T50.3X2	T50.3X3	T50.3X4	T50.3X5	T50.3X6
hydrate, hydroxide	T54.3X1	T54.3X2	T54.3X3	T54.3X4	—	—
hypochlorite	T54.3X1	T54.3X2	T54.3X3	T54.3X4	—	—
iodide	T48.4X1	T48.4X2	T48.4X3	T48.4X4	T48.4X5	T48.4X6
ipodate	T50.8X1	T50.8X2	T50.8X3	T50.8X4	T50.8X5	T50.8X6
lactate	T50.3X1	T50.3X2	T50.3X3	T50.3X4	T50.3X5	T50.3X6
leucovorin	T45.8X1	T45.8X2	T45.8X3	T45.8X4	T45.8X5	T45.8X6
mandelate	T37.91	T37.92	T37.93	T37.94	T37.95	T37.96
oxide	T54.3X1	T54.3X2	T54.3X3	T54.3X4	—	—
pantothenate	T45.2X1	T45.2X2	T45.2X3	T45.2X4	T45.2X5	T45.2X6
phosphate	T50.3X1	T50.3X2	T50.3X3	T50.3X4	T50.3X5	T50.3X6
salicylate	T39.091	T39.092	T39.093	T39.094	T39.095	T39.096
salts	T50.3X1	T50.3X2	T50.3X3	T50.3X4	T50.3X5	T50.3X6
Calculus-dissolving drug	T50.991	T50.992	T50.993	T50.994	T50.995	T50.996
Calomel	T49.0X1	T49.0X2	T49.0X3	T49.0X4	T49.0X5	T49.0X6
Caloric agent	T50.3X1	T50.3X2	T50.3X3	T50.3X4	T50.3X5	T50.3X6
Calusterone	T38.7X1	T38.7X2	T38.7X3	T38.7X4	T38.7X5	T38.7X6
Camazepam	T42.4X1	T42.4X2	T42.4X3	T42.4X4	T42.4X5	T42.4X6
Camomile	T49.0X1	T49.0X2	T49.0X3	T49.0X4	T49.0X5	T49.0X6
Camoquin	T37.2X1	T37.2X2	T37.2X3	T37.2X4	T37.2X5	T37.2X6
Camphor						
insecticide	T60.2X1	T60.2X2	T60.2X3	T60.2X4	—	—
medicinal	T49.8X1	T49.8X2	T49.8X3	T49.8X4	T49.8X5	T49.8X6
Camylofin	T44.3X1	T44.3X2	T44.3X3	T44.3X4	T44.3X5	T44.3X6
Cancer chemotherapy drug regimen	T45.1X1	T45.1X2	T45.1X3	T45.1X4	T45.1X5	T45.1X6
Candeptin	T49.0X1	T49.0X2	T49.0X3	T49.0X4	T49.0X5	T49.0X6
Candicidin	T49.0X1	T49.0X2	T49.0X3	T49.0X4	T49.0X5	T49.0X6
Cannabinol	T40.7X1	T40.7X2	T40.7X3	T40.7X4	T40.7X5	T40.7X6
Cannabis (derivatives)	T40.7X1	T40.7X2	T40.7X3	T40.7X4	T40.7X5	T40.7X6
Canned heat	T51.1X1	T51.1X2	T51.1X3	T51.1X4	—	—
Canrenoic acid	T50.0X1	T50.0X2	T50.0X3	T50.0X4	T50.0X5	T50.0X6
Canrenone	T50.0X1	T50.0X2	T50.0X3	T50.0X4	T50.0X5	T50.0X6
Cantharides, cantharidin, cantharis	T49.8X1	T49.8X2	T49.8X3	T49.8X4	T49.8X5	T49.8X6
Canthaxanthin	T50.991	T50.992	T50.993	T50.994	T50.995	T50.996
Capillary-active drug NEC	T46.901	T46.902	T46.903	T46.904	T46.905	T46.906
Capreomycin	T36.8X1	T36.8X2	T36.8X3	T36.8X4	T36.8X5	T36.8X6
Capsicum	T49.4X1	T49.4X2	T49.4X3	T49.4X4	T49.4X5	T49.4X6
Captafol	T60.3X1	T60.3X2	T60.3X3	T60.3X4	—	—
Captan	T60.3X1	T60.3X2	T60.3X3	T60.3X4	—	—
Captodiame, captodiamine	T43.591	T43.592	T43.593	T43.594	T43.595	T43.596
Captopril	T46.4X1	T46.4X2	T46.4X3	T46.4X4	T46.4X5	T46.4X6
Caramiphen	T44.3X1	T44.3X2	T44.3X3	T44.3X4	T44.3X5	T44.3X6
Carazolol	T44.7X1	T44.7X2	T44.7X3	T44.7X4	T44.7X5	T44.7X6
Carbachol	T44.1X1	T44.1X2	T44.1X3	T44.1X4	T44.1X5	T44.1X6
Carbacrylamine (resin)	T50.3X1	T50.3X2	T50.3X3	T50.3X4	T50.3X5	T50.3X6
Carbamate (insecticide)	T60.0X1	T60.0X2	T60.0X3	T60.0X4	—	—
Carbamate (sedative)	T42.6X1	T42.6X2	T42.6X3	T42.6X4	T42.6X5	T42.6X6
herbicide	T60.0X1	T60.0X2	T60.0X3	T60.0X4	—	—
insecticide	T60.0X1	T60.0X2	T60.0X3	T60.0X4	—	—
Carbamazepine	T42.1X1	T42.1X2	T42.1X3	T42.1X4	T42.1X5	T42.1X6
Carbamide	T47.3X1	T47.3X2	T47.3X3	T47.3X4	T47.3X5	T47.3X6
peroxide	T49.0X1	T49.0X2	T49.0X3	T49.0X4	T49.0X5	T49.0X6
topical	T49.8X1	T49.8X2	T49.8X3	T49.8X4	T49.8X5	T49.8X6
Carbamylcholine chloride	T44.1X1	T44.1X2	T44.1X3	T44.1X4	T44.1X5	T44.1X6
Carbaril	T60.0X1	T60.0X2	T60.0X3	T60.0X4	—	—
Carbarsone	T37.3X1	T37.3X2	T37.3X3	T37.3X4	T37.3X5	T37.3X6
Carbaryl	T60.0X1	T60.0X2	T60.0X3	T60.0X4	—	—
Carbaspirin	T39.011	T39.012	T39.013	T39.014	T39.015	T39.016
Carbazochrome (salicylate) (sodium sulfonate)	T49.4X1	T49.4X2	T49.4X3	T49.4X4	T49.4X5	T49.4X6
Carbenicillin	T36.0X1	T36.0X2	T36.0X3	T36.0X4	T36.0X5	T36.0X6
Carbenoxolone	T47.1X1	T47.1X2	T47.1X3	T47.1X4	T47.1X5	T47.1X6
Carbetapentane	T48.3X1	T48.3X2	T48.3X3	T48.3X4	T48.3X5	T48.3X6
Carbethyl salicylate	T39.091	T39.092	T39.093	T39.094	T39.095	T39.096
Carbidopa (with levodopa)	T42.8X1	T42.8X2	T42.8X3	T42.8X4	T42.8X5	T42.8X6
Carbimazole	T38.2X1	T38.2X2	T38.2X3	T38.2X4	T38.2X5	T38.2X6
Carbinol	T51.1X1	T51.1X2	T51.1X3	T51.1X4	—	—
Carbinoxamine	T45.0X1	T45.0X2	T45.0X3	T45.0X4	T45.0X5	T45.0X6
Carbiphene	T39.8X1	T39.8X2	T39.8X3	T39.8X4	T39.8X5	T39.8X6
Carbitol	T52.3X1	T52.3X2	T52.3X3	T52.3X4	—	—
Carbocaine	T41.3X1	T41.3X2	T41.3X3	T41.3X4	T41.3X5	T41.3X6
infiltration (subcutaneous)	T41.3X1	T41.3X2	T41.3X3	T41.3X4	T41.3X5	T41.3X6
nerve block (peripheral) (plexus)	T41.3X1	T41.3X2	T41.3X3	T41.3X4	T41.3X5	T41.3X6
topical (surface)	T41.3X1	T41.3X2	T41.3X3	T41.3X4	T41.3X5	T41.3X6
Carbocisteine	T48.4X1	T48.4X2	T48.4X3	T48.4X4	T48.4X5	T48.4X6
Carbocromen	T46.3X1	T46.3X2	T46.3X3	T46.3X4	T46.3X5	T46.3X6
Carbol fuchsin	T49.0X1	T49.0X2	T49.0X3	T49.0X4	T49.0X5	T49.0X6
Carbolic acid — *see also* Phenol	T54.0X1	T54.0X2	T54.0X3	T54.0X4	—	—
Carbolonium (bromide)	T48.1X1	T48.1X2	T48.1X3	T48.1X4	T48.1X5	T48.1X6
Carbo medicinalis	T47.6X1	T47.6X2	T47.6X3	T47.6X4	T47.6X5	T47.6X6
Carbomycin	T36.8X1	T36.8X2	T36.8X3	T36.8X4	T36.8X5	T36.8X6
Carbon						
bisulfide (liquid)	T65.4X1	T65.4X2	T65.4X3	T65.4X4	—	—
vapor	T65.4X1	T65.4X2	T65.4X3	T65.4X4	—	—
dioxide (gas)	T59.7X1	T59.7X2	T59.7X3	T59.7X4	—	—
medicinal	T41.5X1	T41.5X2	T41.5X3	T41.5X4	T41.5X5	T41.5X6
nonmedicinal	T59.7X1	T59.7X2	T59.7X3	T59.7X4	—	—
snow	T49.4X1	T49.4X2	T49.4X3	T49.4X4	T49.4X5	T49.4X6
disulfide (liquid)	T65.4X1	T65.4X2	T65.4X3	T65.4X4	—	—
vapor	T65.4X1	T65.4X2	T65.4X3	T65.4X4	—	—
monoxide (from incomplete combustion)	T58.91	T58.92	T58.93	T58.94	—	—
blast furnace gas	T58.8X1	T58.8X2	T58.8X3	T58.8X4	—	—
butane (distributed in mobile container)	T58.11	T58.12	T58.13	T58.14	—	—
distributed through pipes	T58.11	T58.12	T58.13	T58.14	—	—
charcoal fumes	T58.2X1	T58.2X2	T58.2X3	T58.2X4	—	—
coal	T58.2X1	T58.2X2	T58.2X3	T58.2X4	—	—
coke (in domestic stoves, fireplaces)	T58.2X1	T58.2X2	T58.2X3	T58.2X4	—	—
exhaust gas (motor) not in transit	T58.01	T58.02	T58.03	T58.04	—	—
combustion engine, any not in watercraft	T58.01	T58.02	T58.03	T58.04	—	—
farm tractor, not in transit	T58.01	T58.02	T58.03	T58.04	—	—

Substance	Poisoning, Accidental (unintentional)	Poisoning, Intentional Self-harm	Poisoning, Assault	Poisoning, Undetermined	Adverse Effect	Under-dosing
Carbon — *continued*						
monoxide — *continued*						
exhaust gas not in transit — *continued*						
gas engine	T58.Ø1	T58.Ø2	T58.Ø3	T58.Ø4	—	—
motor pump	T58.Ø1	T58.Ø2	T58.Ø3	T58.Ø4	—	—
motor vehicle, not in transit	T58.Ø1	T58.Ø2	T58.Ø3	T58.Ø4	—	—
fuel (in domestic use)	T58.2X1	T58.2X2	T58.2X3	T58.2X4	—	—
gas (piped)	T58.11	T58.12	T58.13	T58.14	—	—
in mobile container	T58.11	T58.12	T58.13	T58.14	—	—
piped (natural)	T58.11	T58.12	T58.13	T58.14	—	—
utility	T58.11	T58.12	T58.13	T58.14	—	—
in mobile container	T58.11	T58.12	T58.13	T58.14	—	—
gas (piped)	T58.11	T58.12	T58.13	T58.14	—	—
illuminating gas	T58.11	T58.12	T58.13	T58.14	—	—
industrial fuels or gases, any	T58.8X1	T58.8X2	T58.8X3	T58.8X4	—	—
kerosene (in domestic stoves, fireplaces)	T58.2X1	T58.2X2	T58.2X3	T58.2X4	—	—
kiln gas or vapor	T58.8X1	T58.8X2	T58.8X3	T58.8X4	—	—
motor exhaust gas, not in transit	T58.Ø1	T58.Ø2	T58.Ø3	T58.Ø4	—	—
piped gas (manufactured) (natural)	T58.11	T58.12	T58.13	T58.14	—	—
producer gas	T58.8X1	T58.8X2	T58.8X3	T58.8X4	—	—
propane (distributed in mobile container)	T58.11	T58.12	T58.13	T58.14	—	—
distributed through pipes	T58.11	T58.12	T58.13	T58.14	—	—
solid (in domestic stoves, fireplaces)	T58.2X1	T58.2X2	T58.2X3	T58.2X4	—	—
specified source NEC	T58.8X1	T58.8X2	T58.8X3	T58.8X4	—	—
stove gas	T58.11	T58.12	T58.13	T58.14	—	—
piped	T58.11	T58.12	T58.13	T58.14	—	—
utility gas	T58.11	T58.12	T58.13	T58.14	—	—
piped	T58.11	T58.12	T58.13	T58.14	—	—
water gas	T58.11	T58.12	T58.13	T58.14	—	—
wood (in domestic stoves, fireplaces)	T58.2X1	T58.2X2	T58.2X3	T58.2X4	—	—
tetrachloride (vapor) NEC	T53.ØX1	T53.ØX2	T53.ØX3	T53.ØX4	—	—
liquid (cleansing agent) NEC	T53.ØX1	T53.ØX2	T53.ØX3	T53.ØX4	—	—
solvent	T53.ØX1	T53.ØX2	T53.ØX3	T53.ØX4	—	—
Carbonic acid gas	T59.7X1	T59.7X2	T59.7X3	T59.7X4	—	—
anhydrase inhibitor NEC	T50.2X1	T50.2X2	T50.2X3	T50.2X4	T50.2X5	T50.2X6
Carbophenothion	T60.ØX1	T60.ØX2	T60.ØX3	T60.ØX4	—	—
Carboplatin	T45.1X1	T45.1X2	T45.1X3	T45.1X4	T45.1X5	T45.1X6
Carboprost	T48.ØX1	T48.ØX2	T48.ØX3	T48.ØX4	T48.ØX5	T48.ØX6
Carboquone	T45.1X1	T45.1X2	T45.1X3	T45.1X4	T45.1X5	T45.1X6
Carbowax	T49.3X1	T49.3X2	T49.3X3	T49.3X4	T49.3X5	T49.3X6
Carboxymethylcellulose	T47.4X1	T47.4X2	T47.4X3	T47.4X4	T47.4X5	T47.4X6
Carbrital	T42.3X1	T42.3X2	T42.3X3	T42.3X4	T42.3X5	T42.3X6
Carbromal	T42.6X1	T42.6X2	T42.6X3	T42.6X4	T42.6X5	T42.6X6
Carbutamide	T38.3X1	T38.3X2	T38.3X3	T38.3X4	T38.3X5	T38.3X6
Carbuterol	T48.6X1	T48.6X2	T48.6X3	T48.6X4	T48.6X5	T48.6X6
Cardiac						
depressants	T46.2X1	T46.2X2	T46.2X3	T46.2X4	T46.2X5	T46.2X6
rhythm regulator	T46.2X1	T46.2X2	T46.2X3	T46.2X4	T46.2X5	T46.2X6
specified NEC	T46.2X1	T46.2X2	T46.2X3	T46.2X4	T46.2X5	T46.2X6
Cardiografin	T50.8X1	T50.8X2	T50.8X3	T50.8X4	T50.8X5	T50.8X6
Cardiogreen	T50.8X1	T50.8X2	T50.8X3	T50.8X4	T50.8X5	T50.8X6
Cardiotonic (glycoside) **NEC**	T46.ØX1	T46.ØX2	T46.ØX3	T46.ØX4	T46.ØX5	T46.ØX6
Cardiovascular drug NEC	T46.9Ø1	T46.9Ø2	T46.9Ø3	T46.9Ø4	T46.9Ø5	T46.9Ø6
Cardrase	T50.2X1	T50.2X2	T50.2X3	T50.2X4	T50.2X5	T50.2X6
Carfecillin	T36.ØX1	T36.ØX2	T36.ØX3	T36.ØX4	T36.ØX5	T36.ØX6
Carfenazine	T43.3X1	T43.3X2	T43.3X3	T43.3X4	T43.3X5	T43.3X6
Carfusin	T49.ØX1	T49.ØX2	T49.ØX3	T49.ØX4	T49.ØX5	T49.ØX6
Carindacillin	T36.ØX1	T36.ØX2	T36.ØX3	T36.ØX4	T36.ØX5	T36.ØX6
Carisoprodol	T42.8X1	T42.8X2	T42.8X3	T42.8X4	T42.8X5	T42.8X6
Carmellose	T47.4X1	T47.4X2	T47.4X3	T47.4X4	T47.4X5	T47.4X6
Carminative	T47.5X1	T47.5X2	T47.5X3	T47.5X4	T47.5X5	T47.5X6
Carmofur	T45.1X1	T45.1X2	T45.1X3	T45.1X4	T45.1X5	T45.1X6
Carmustine	T45.1X1	T45.1X2	T45.1X3	T45.1X4	T45.1X5	T45.1X6
Carotene	T45.2X1	T45.2X2	T45.2X3	T45.2X4	T45.2X5	T45.2X6
Carphenazine	T43.3X1	T43.3X2	T43.3X3	T43.3X4	T43.3X5	T43.3X6
Carpipramine	T42.4X1	T42.4X2	T42.4X3	T42.4X4	T42.4X5	T42.4X6
Carprofen	T39.311	T39.312	T39.313	T39.314	T39.315	T39.316
Carpronium chloride	T44.3X1	T44.3X2	T44.3X3	T44.3X4	T44.3X5	T44.3X6
Carrageenan	T47.8X1	T47.8X2	T47.8X3	T47.8X4	T47.8X5	T47.8X6
Carteolol	T44.7X1	T44.7X2	T44.7X3	T44.7X4	T44.7X5	T44.7X6
Carter's Little Pills	T47.2X1	T47.2X2	T47.2X3	T47.2X4	T47.2X5	T47.2X6
Cascara (sagrada)	T47.2X1	T47.2X2	T47.2X3	T47.2X4	T47.2X5	T47.2X6
Cassava	T62.2X1	T62.2X2	T62.2X3	T62.2X4	—	—
Castellani's paint	T49.ØX1	T49.ØX2	T49.ØX3	T49.ØX4	T49.ØX5	T49.ØX6
Castor						
bean	T62.2X1	T62.2X2	T62.2X3	T62.2X4	—	—
oil	T47.2X1	T47.2X2	T47.2X3	T47.2X4	T47.2X5	T47.2X6
Catalase	T45.3X1	T45.3X2	T45.3X3	T45.3X4	T45.3X5	T45.3X6
Caterpillar (sting)	T63.431	T63.432	T63.433	T63.434	—	—
Catha (edulis) (tea)	T43.691	T43.692	T43.693	T43.694	—	—
Cathartic NEC	T47.4X1	T47.4X2	T47.4X3	T47.4X4	T47.4X5	T47.4X6
anthacene derivative	T47.2X1	T47.2X2	T47.2X3	T47.2X4	T47.2X5	T47.2X6
bulk	T47.4X1	T47.4X2	T47.4X3	T47.4X4	T47.4X5	T47.4X6
contact	T47.2X1	T47.2X2	T47.2X3	T47.2X4	T47.2X5	T47.2X6
emollient NEC	T47.4X1	T47.4X2	T47.4X3	T47.4X4	T47.4X5	T47.4X6
irritant NEC	T47.2X1	T47.2X2	T47.2X3	T47.2X4	T47.2X5	T47.2X6
mucilage	T47.4X1	T47.4X2	T47.4X3	T47.4X4	T47.4X5	T47.4X6
saline	T47.3X1	T47.3X2	T47.3X3	T47.3X4	T47.3X5	T47.3X6
vegetable	T47.2X1	T47.2X2	T47.2X3	T47.2X4	T47.2X5	T47.2X6
Cathine	T50.5X1	T50.5X2	T50.5X3	T50.5X4	T50.5X5	T50.5X6
Cathomycin	T36.8X1	T36.8X2	T36.8X3	T36.8X4	T36.8X5	T36.8X6
Cation exchange resin	T50.3X1	T50.3X2	T50.3X3	T50.3X4	T50.3X5	T50.3X6
Caustic(s) NEC	T54.91	T54.92	T54.93	T54.94	—	—
alkali	T54.3X1	T54.3X2	T54.3X3	T54.3X4	—	—
hydroxide	T54.3X1	T54.3X2	T54.3X3	T54.3X4	—	—
potash	T54.3X1	T54.3X2	T54.3X3	T54.3X4	—	—
soda	T54.3X1	T54.3X2	T54.3X3	T54.3X4	—	—
specified NEC	T54.91	T54.92	T54.93	T54.94	—	—
Ceepryn	T49.ØX1	T49.ØX2	T49.ØX3	T49.ØX4	T49.ØX5	T49.ØX6
ENT agent	T49.6X1	T49.6X2	T49.6X3	T49.6X4	T49.6X5	T49.6X6
lozenges	T49.6X1	T49.6X2	T49.6X3	T49.6X4	T49.6X5	T49.6X6
Cefacetrile	T36.1X1	T36.1X2	T36.1X3	T36.1X4	T36.1X5	T36.1X6
Cefaclor	T36.1X1	T36.1X2	T36.1X3	T36.1X4	T36.1X5	T36.1X6
Cefadroxil	T36.1X1	T36.1X2	T36.1X3	T36.1X4	T36.1X5	T36.1X6
Cefalexin	T36.1X1	T36.1X2	T36.1X3	T36.1X4	T36.1X5	T36.1X6
Cefaloglycin	T36.1X1	T36.1X2	T36.1X3	T36.1X4	T36.1X5	T36.1X6
Cefaloridine	T36.1X1	T36.1X2	T36.1X3	T36.1X4	T36.1X5	T36.1X6
Cefalosporins	T36.1X1	T36.1X2	T36.1X3	T36.1X4	T36.1X5	T36.1X6
Cefalotin	T36.1X1	T36.1X2	T36.1X3	T36.1X4	T36.1X5	T36.1X6
Cefamandole	T36.1X1	T36.1X2	T36.1X3	T36.1X4	T36.1X5	T36.1X6
Cefamycin antibiotic	T36.1X1	T36.1X2	T36.1X3	T36.1X4	T36.1X5	T36.1X6
Cefapirin	T36.1X1	T36.1X2	T36.1X3	T36.1X4	T36.1X5	T36.1X6
Cefatrizine	T36.1X1	T36.1X2	T36.1X3	T36.1X4	T36.1X5	T36.1X6
Cefazedone	T36.1X1	T36.1X2	T36.1X3	T36.1X4	T36.1X5	T36.1X6
Cefazolin	T36.1X1	T36.1X2	T36.1X3	T36.1X4	T36.1X5	T36.1X6
Cefbuperazone	T36.1X1	T36.1X2	T36.1X3	T36.1X4	T36.1X5	T36.1X6
Cefetamet	T36.1X1	T36.1X2	T36.1X3	T36.1X4	T36.1X5	T36.1X6
Cefixime	T36.1X1	T36.1X2	T36.1X3	T36.1X4	T36.1X5	T36.1X6
Cefmenoxime	T36.1X1	T36.1X2	T36.1X3	T36.1X4	T36.1X5	T36.1X6
Cefmetazole	T36.1X1	T36.1X2	T36.1X3	T36.1X4	T36.1X5	T36.1X6
Cefminox	T36.1X1	T36.1X2	T36.1X3	T36.1X4	T36.1X5	T36.1X6
Cefonicid	T36.1X1	T36.1X2	T36.1X3	T36.1X4	T36.1X5	T36.1X6
Cefoperazone	T36.1X1	T36.1X2	T36.1X3	T36.1X4	T36.1X5	T36.1X6
Ceforanide	T36.1X1	T36.1X2	T36.1X3	T36.1X4	T36.1X5	T36.1X6
Cefotaxime	T36.1X1	T36.1X2	T36.1X3	T36.1X4	T36.1X5	T36.1X6
Cefotetan	T36.1X1	T36.1X2	T36.1X3	T36.1X4	T36.1X5	T36.1X6
Cefotiam	T36.1X1	T36.1X2	T36.1X3	T36.1X4	T36.1X5	T36.1X6
Cefoxitin	T36.1X1	T36.1X2	T36.1X3	T36.1X4	T36.1X5	T36.1X6
Cefpimizole	T36.1X1	T36.1X2	T36.1X3	T36.1X4	T36.1X5	T36.1X6
Cefpiramide	T36.1X1	T36.1X2	T36.1X3	T36.1X4	T36.1X5	T36.1X6
Cefradine	T36.1X1	T36.1X2	T36.1X3	T36.1X4	T36.1X5	T36.1X6
Cefroxadine	T36.1X1	T36.1X2	T36.1X3	T36.1X4	T36.1X5	T36.1X6
Cefsulodin	T36.1X1	T36.1X2	T36.1X3	T36.1X4	T36.1X5	T36.1X6
Ceftazidime	T36.1X1	T36.1X2	T36.1X3	T36.1X4	T36.1X5	T36.1X6
Cefteram	T36.1X1	T36.1X2	T36.1X3	T36.1X4	T36.1X5	T36.1X6
Ceftezole	T36.1X1	T36.1X2	T36.1X3	T36.1X4	T36.1X5	T36.1X6
Ceftizoxime	T36.1X1	T36.1X2	T36.1X3	T36.1X4	T36.1X5	T36.1X6
Ceftriaxone	T36.1X1	T36.1X2	T36.1X3	T36.1X4	T36.1X5	T36.1X6
Cefuroxime	T36.1X1	T36.1X2	T36.1X3	T36.1X4	T36.1X5	T36.1X6
Cefuzonam	T36.1X1	T36.1X2	T36.1X3	T36.1X4	T36.1X5	T36.1X6
Celestone	T38.ØX1	T38.ØX2	T38.ØX3	T38.ØX4	T38.ØX5	T38.ØX6
topical	T49.ØX1	T49.ØX2	T49.ØX3	T49.ØX4	T49.ØX5	T49.ØX6
Celiprolol	T44.7X1	T44.7X2	T44.7X3	T44.7X4	T44.7X5	T44.7X6
Cellosolve	T52.91	T52.92	T52.93	T52.94	—	—
Cell stimulants and proliferants	T49.8X1	T49.8X2	T49.8X3	T49.8X4	T49.8X5	T49.8X6
Cellulose						
cathartic	T47.4X1	T47.4X2	T47.4X3	T47.4X4	T47.4X5	T47.4X6
hydroxyethyl	T47.4X1	T47.4X2	T47.4X3	T47.4X4	T47.4X5	T47.4X6
nitrates (topical)	T49.3X1	T49.3X2	T49.3X3	T49.3X4	T49.3X5	T49.3X6
oxidized	T49.4X1	T49.4X2	T49.4X3	T49.4X4	T49.4X5	T49.4X6
Centipede (bite)	T63.411	T63.412	T63.413	T63.414	—	—
Central nervous system						
depressants	T42.71	T42.72	T42.73	T42.74	T42.75	T42.76
anesthetic (general) NEC	T41.2Ø1	T41.2Ø2	T41.2Ø3	T41.2Ø4	T41.2Ø5	T41.2Ø6

Table of Drugs and Chemicals

Substance	Poisoning, Accidental (unintentional)	Poisoning, Intentional Self-harm	Poisoning, Assault	Poisoning, Undetermined	Adverse Effect	Under-dosing
Central nervous system — *continued*						
depressants — *continued*						
anesthetic — *continued*						
gases NEC	T41.0X1	T41.0X2	T41.0X3	T41.0X4	T41.0X5	T41.0X6
intravenous	T41.1X1	T41.1X2	T41.1X3	T41.1X4	T41.1X5	T41.1X6
barbiturates	T42.3X1	T42.3X2	T42.3X3	T42.3X4	T42.3X5	T42.3X6
benzodiazepines	T42.4X1	T42.4X2	T42.4X3	T42.4X4	T42.4X5	T42.4X6
bromides	T42.6X1	T42.6X2	T42.6X3	T42.6X4	T42.6X5	T42.6X6
cannabis sativa	T40.7X1	T40.7X2	T40.7X3	T40.7X4	T40.7X5	T40.7X6
chloral hydrate	T42.6X1	T42.6X2	T42.6X3	T42.6X4	T42.6X5	T42.6X6
ethanol	T51.0X1	T51.0X2	T51.0X3	T51.0X4	—	—
hallucinogenics	T40.901	T40.902	T40.903	T40.904	T40.905	T40.906
hypnotics	T42.71	T42.72	T42.73	T42.74	T42.75	T42.76
specified NEC	T42.6X1	T42.6X2	T42.6X3	T42.6X4	T42.6X5	T42.6X6
muscle relaxants	T42.8X1	T42.8X2	T42.8X3	T42.8X4	T42.8X5	T42.8X6
paraldehyde	T42.6X1	T42.6X2	T42.6X3	T42.6X4	T42.6X5	T42.6X6
sedatives;	T42.71	T42.72	T42.73	T42.74	T42.75	T42.76
sedative-hypnotics mixed NEC	T42.6X1	T42.6X2	T42.6X3	T42.6X4	T42.6X5	T42.6X6
specified NEC	T42.6X1	T42.6X2	T42.6X3	T42.6X4	T42.6X5	T42.6X6
muscle-tone depressants	T42.8X1	T42.8X2	T42.8X3	T42.8X4	T42.8X5	T42.8X6
stimulants	T43.601	T43.602	T43.603	T43.604	T43.605	T43.606
amphetamines	T43.621	T43.622	T43.623	T43.624	T43.625	T43.626
analeptics	T50.7X1	T50.7X2	T50.7X3	T50.7X4	T50.7X5	T50.7X6
antidepressants	T43.201	T43.202	T43.203	T43.204	T43.205	T43.206
opiate antagonists	T50.7X1	T50.7X2	T50.7X3	T50.7X4	T50.7X5	T50.7X6
specified NEC	T43.691	T43.692	T43.693	T43.694	T43.695	T43.696
Cephalexin	T36.1X1	T36.1X2	T36.1X3	T36.1X4	T36.1X5	T36.1X6
Cephaloglycin	T36.1X1	T36.1X2	T36.1X3	T36.1X4	T36.1X5	T36.1X6
Cephaloridine	T36.1X1	T36.1X2	T36.1X3	T36.1X4	T36.1X5	T36.1X6
Cephalosporins	T36.1X1	T36.1X2	T36.1X3	T36.1X4	T36.1X5	T36.1X6
N (adicillin)	T36.0X1	T36.0X2	T36.0X3	T36.0X4	T36.0X5	T36.0X6
Cephalothin	T36.1X1	T36.1X2	T36.1X3	T36.1X4	T36.1X5	T36.1X6
Cephalotin	T36.1X1	T36.1X2	T36.1X3	T36.1X4	T36.1X5	T36.1X6
Cephradine	T36.1X1	T36.1X2	T36.1X3	T36.1X4	T36.1X5	T36.1X6
Cerbera (odallam)	T62.2X1	T62.2X2	T62.2X3	T62.2X4	—	—
Cerberin	T46.0X1	T46.0X2	T46.0X3	T46.0X4	T46.0X5	T46.0X6
Cerebral stimulants	T43.601	T43.602	T43.603	T43.604	T43.605	T43.606
psychotherapeutic	T43.601	T43.602	T43.603	T43.604	T43.605	T43.606
specified NEC	T43.691	T43.692	T43.693	T43.694	T43.695	T43.696
Cerium oxalate	T45.0X1	T45.0X2	T45.0X3	T45.0X4	T45.0X5	T45.0X6
Cerous oxalate	T45.0X1	T45.0X2	T45.0X3	T45.0X4	T45.0X5	T45.0X6
Ceruletide	T50.8X1	T50.8X2	T50.8X3	T50.8X4	T50.8X5	T50.8X6
Cetalkonium (chloride)	T49.0X1	T49.0X2	T49.0X3	T49.0X4	T49.0X5	T49.0X6
Cethexonium chloride	T49.0X1	T49.0X2	T49.0X3	T49.0X4	T49.0X5	T49.0X6
Cetiedil	T46.7X1	T46.7X2	T46.7X3	T46.7X4	T46.7X5	T46.7X6
Cetirizine	T45.0X1	T45.0X2	T45.0X3	T45.0X4	T45.0X5	T45.0X6
Cetomacrogol	T50.991	T50.992	T50.993	T50.994	T50.995	T50.996
Cetotiamine	T45.2X1	T45.2X2	T45.2X3	T45.2X4	T45.2X5	T45.2X6
Cetoxime	T45.0X1	T45.0X2	T45.0X3	T45.0X4	T45.0X5	T45.0X6
Cetraxate	T47.1X1	T47.1X2	T47.1X3	T47.1X4	T47.1X5	T47.1X6
Cetrimide	T49.0X1	T49.0X2	T49.0X3	T49.0X4	T49.0X5	T49.0X6
Cetrimonium (bromide)	T49.0X1	T49.0X2	T49.0X3	T49.0X4	T49.0X5	T49.0X6
Cetylpyridinium chloride	T49.0X1	T49.0X2	T49.0X3	T49.0X4	T49.0X5	T49.0X6
ENT agent	T49.6X1	T49.6X2	T49.6X3	T49.6X4	T49.6X5	T49.6X6
lozenges	T49.6X1	T49.6X2	T49.6X3	T49.6X4	T49.6X5	T49.6X6
Cevadilla — *see* Sabadilla						
Cevitamic acid	T45.2X1	T45.2X2	T45.2X3	T45.2X4	T45.2X5	T45.2X6
Chalk, precipitated	T47.1X1	T47.1X2	T47.1X3	T47.1X4	T47.1X5	T47.1X6
Chamomile	T49.0X1	T49.0X2	T49.0X3	T49.0X4	T49.0X5	T49.0X6
Ch'an su	T46.0X1	T46.0X2	T46.0X3	T46.0X4	T46.0X5	T46.0X6
Charcoal						
activated — *see also* Charcoal, medicinal	T47.6X1	T47.6X2	T47.6X3	T47.6X4	T47.6X5	T47.6X6
fumes (Carbon monoxide)	T58.2X1	T58.2X2	T58.2X3	T58.2X4	—	—
industrial	T58.8X1	T58.8X2	T58.8X3	T58.8X4	—	—
medicinal (activated)	T47.6X1	T47.6X2	T47.6X3	T47.6X4	T47.6X5	T47.6X6
antidiarrheal	T47.6X1	T47.6X2	T47.6X3	T47.6X4	T47.6X5	T47.6X6
poison control	T47.8X1	T47.8X2	T47.8X3	T47.8X4	T47.8X5	T47.8X6
specified use other than for diarrhea	T47.8X1	T47.8X2	T47.8X3	T47.8X4	T47.8X5	T47.8X6
topical	T49.8X1	T49.8X2	T49.8X3	T49.8X4	T49.8X5	T49.8X6
Chaulmosulfone	T37.1X1	T37.1X2	T37.1X3	T37.1X4	T37.1X5	T37.1X6
Chelating agent NEC	T50.6X1	T50.6X2	T50.6X3	T50.6X4	T50.6X5	T50.6X6
Chelidonium majus	T62.2X1	T62.2X2	T62.2X3	T62.2X4	—	—
Chemical substance NEC	T65.91	T65.92	T65.93	T65.94	—	—
Chenodeoxycholic acid	T47.5X1	T47.5X2	T47.5X3	T47.5X4	T47.5X5	T47.5X6
Chenodiol	T47.5X1	T47.5X2	T47.5X3	T47.5X4	T47.5X5	T47.5X6
Chenopodium	T37.4X1	T37.4X2	T37.4X3	T37.4X4	T37.4X5	T37.4X6
Cherry laurel	T62.2X1	T62.2X2	T62.2X3	T62.2X4	—	—
Chinidin (e)	T46.2X1	T46.2X2	T46.2X3	T46.2X4	T46.2X5	T46.2X6
Chiniofon	T37.8X1	T37.8X2	T37.8X3	T37.8X4	T37.8X5	T37.8X6

Substance	Poisoning, Accidental (unintentional)	Poisoning, Intentional Self-harm	Poisoning, Assault	Poisoning, Undetermined	Adverse Effect	Under-dosing
Chlophedianol	T48.3X1	T48.3X2	T48.3X3	T48.3X4	T48.3X5	T48.3X6
Chloral	T42.6X1	T42.6X2	T42.6X3	T42.6X4	T42.6X5	T42.6X6
derivative	T42.6X1	T42.6X2	T42.6X3	T42.6X4	T42.6X5	T42.6X6
hydrate	T42.6X1	T42.6X2	T42.6X3	T42.6X4	T42.6X5	T42.6X6
Chloralamide	T42.6X1	T42.6X2	T42.6X3	T42.6X4	T42.6X5	T42.6X6
Chloralodol	T42.6X1	T42.6X2	T42.6X3	T42.6X4	T42.6X5	T42.6X6
Chloralose	T60.4X1	T60.4X2	T60.4X3	T60.4X4	—	—
Chlorambucil	T45.1X1	T45.1X2	T45.1X3	T45.1X4	T45.1X5	T45.1X6
Chloramine	T57.8X1	T57.8X2	T57.8X3	T57.8X4	—	—
T	T49.0X1	T49.0X2	T49.0X3	T49.0X4	T49.0X5	T49.0X6
topical	T49.0X1	T49.0X2	T49.0X3	T49.0X4	T49.0X5	T49.0X6
Chloramphenicol	T36.2X1	T36.2X2	T36.2X3	T36.2X4	T36.2X5	T36.2X6
ENT agent	T49.6X1	T49.6X2	T49.6X3	T49.6X4	T49.6X5	T49.6X6
ophthalmic preparation	T49.5X1	T49.5X2	T49.5X3	T49.5X4	T49.5X5	T49.5X6
topical NEC	T49.0X1	T49.0X2	T49.0X3	T49.0X4	T49.0X5	T49.0X6
Chlorate (potassium) (sodium) **NEC**	T60.3X1	T60.3X2	T60.3X3	T60.3X4	—	—
herbicide	T60.3X1	T60.3X2	T60.3X3	T60.3X4	—	—
Chlorazanil	T50.2X1	T50.2X2	T50.2X3	T50.2X4	T50.2X5	T50.2X6
Chlorbenzene, chlorbenzol	T53.7X1	T53.7X2	T53.7X3	T53.7X4	—	—
Chlorbenzoxamine	T44.3X1	T44.3X2	T44.3X3	T44.3X4	T44.3X5	T44.3X6
Chlorbutol	T42.6X1	T42.6X2	T42.6X3	T42.6X4	T42.6X5	T42.6X6
Chlorcyclizine	T45.0X1	T45.0X2	T45.0X3	T45.0X4	T45.0X5	T45.0X6
Chlordan (e) (dust)	T60.1X1	T60.1X2	T60.1X3	T60.1X4	—	—
Chlordantoin	T49.0X1	T49.0X2	T49.0X3	T49.0X4	T49.0X5	T49.0X6
Chlordiazepoxide	T42.4X1	T42.4X2	T42.4X3	T42.4X4	T42.4X5	T42.4X6
Chlordiethyl benzamide	T49.3X1	T49.3X2	T49.3X3	T49.3X4	T49.3X5	T49.3X6
Chloresium	T49.8X1	T49.8X2	T49.8X3	T49.8X4	T49.8X5	T49.8X6
Chlorethiazol	T42.6X1	T42.6X2	T42.6X3	T42.6X4	T42.6X5	T42.6X6
Chlorethyl — *see* Ethyl chloride						
Chloretone	T42.6X1	T42.6X2	T42.6X3	T42.6X4	T42.6X5	T42.6X6
Chlorex	T53.6X1	T53.6X2	T53.6X3	T53.6X4	—	—
insecticide	T60.1X1	T60.1X2	T60.1X3	T60.1X4	—	—
Chlorfenvinphos	T60.0X1	T60.0X2	T60.0X3	T60.0X4	—	—
Chlorhexadol	T42.6X1	T42.6X2	T42.6X3	T42.6X4	T42.6X5	T42.6X6
Chlorhexamide	T45.1X1	T45.1X2	T45.1X3	T45.1X4	T45.1X5	T45.1X6
Chlorhexidine	T49.0X1	T49.0X2	T49.0X3	T49.0X4	T49.0X5	T49.0X6
Chlorhydroxyquinolin	T49.0X1	T49.0X2	T49.0X3	T49.0X4	T49.0X5	T49.0X6
Chloride of lime (bleach)	T54.3X1	T54.3X2	T54.3X3	T54.3X4	—	—
Chlorimipramine	T43.011	T43.012	T43.013	T43.014	T43.015	T43.016
Chlorinated						
camphene	T53.6X1	T53.6X2	T53.6X3	T53.6X4	—	—
diphenyl	T53.7X1	T53.7X2	T53.7X3	T53.7X4	—	—
hydrocarbons NEC	T53.91	T53.92	T53.93	T53.94	—	—
solvents	T53.91	T53.92	T53.93	T53.94	—	—
lime (bleach)	T54.3X1	T54.3X2	T54.3X3	T54.3X4	—	—
and boric acid solution	T49.0X1	T49.0X2	T49.0X3	T49.0X4	T49.0X5	T49.0X6
naphthalene (insecticide)	T60.1X1	T60.1X2	T60.1X3	T60.1X4	—	—
industrial (non-pesticide)	T53.7X1	T53.7X2	T53.7X3	T53.7X4	—	—
pesticide NEC	T60.8X1	T60.8X2	T60.8X3	T60.8X4	—	—
soda — *see also* sodium hypochlorite						
solution	T49.0X1	T49.0X2	T49.0X3	T49.0X4	T49.0X5	T49.0X6
Chlorine (fumes) (gas)	T59.4X1	T59.4X2	T59.4X3	T59.4X4	—	—
bleach	T54.3X1	T54.3X2	T54.3X3	T54.3X4	—	—
compound gas NEC	T59.4X1	T59.4X2	T59.4X3	T59.4X4	—	—
disinfectant	T59.4X1	T59.4X2	T59.4X3	T59.4X4	—	—
releasing agents NEC	T59.4X1	T59.4X2	T59.4X3	T59.4X4	—	—
Chlorisondamine chloride	T46.991	T46.992	T46.993	T46.994	T46.995	T46.996
Chlormadinone	T38.5X1	T38.5X2	T38.5X3	T38.5X4	T38.5X5	T38.5X6
Chlormephos	T60.0X1	T60.0X2	T60.0X3	T60.0X4	—	—
Chlormerodrin	T50.2X1	T50.2X2	T50.2X3	T50.2X4	T50.2X5	T50.2X6
Chlormethiazole	T42.6X1	T42.6X2	T42.6X3	T42.6X4	T42.6X5	T42.6X6
Chlormethine	T45.1X1	T45.1X2	T45.1X3	T45.1X4	T45.1X5	T45.1X6
Chlormethylenecycline	T36.4X1	T36.4X2	T36.4X3	T36.4X4	T36.4X5	T36.4X6
Chlormezanone	T42.6X1	T42.6X2	T42.6X3	T42.6X4	T42.6X5	T42.6X6
Chloroacetic acid	T60.3X1	T60.3X2	T60.3X3	T60.3X4	—	—
Chloroacetone	T59.3X1	T59.3X2	T59.3X3	T59.3X4	—	—
Chloroacetophenone	T59.3X1	T59.3X2	T59.3X3	T59.3X4	—	—
Chloroaniline	T53.7X1	T53.7X2	T53.7X3	T53.7X4	—	—
Chlorobenzene, chlorobenzol	T53.7X1	T53.7X2	T53.7X3	T53.7X4	—	—
Chlorobromomethane (fire extinguisher)	T53.6X1	T53.6X2	T53.6X3	T53.6X4	—	—
Chlorobutanol	T49.0X1	T49.0X2	T49.0X3	T49.0X4	T49.0X5	T49.0X6
Chlorocresol	T49.0X1	T49.0X2	T49.0X3	T49.0X4	T49.0X5	T49.0X6
Chlorodehydromethyltestosterone	T38.7X1	T38.7X2	T38.7X3	T38.7X4	T38.7X5	T38.7X6
Chlorodinitrobenzene	T53.7X1	T53.7X2	T53.7X3	T53.7X4	—	—
dust or vapor	T53.7X1	T53.7X2	T53.7X3	T53.7X4	—	—
Chlorodiphenyl	T53.7X1	T53.7X2	T53.7X3	T53.7X4	—	—

Central nervous system — Chlorodiphenyl

360   Additional Character May Be Required — Refer to the Tabular List for Character Selection   ▽ Subterms under main terms may continue to next column or page

Substance	Poisoning, Accidental (unintentional)	Poisoning, Intentional Self-harm	Poisoning, Assault	Poisoning, Undetermined	Adverse Effect	Under-dosing
Chloroethane — see Ethyl chloride						
Chloroethylene	T53.6X1	T53.6X2	T53.6X3	T53.6X4	—	—
Chlorofluorocarbons	T53.5X1	T53.5X2	T53.5X3	T53.5X4	—	—
Chloroform (fumes) (vapor)	T53.1X1	T53.1X2	T53.1X3	T53.1X4	—	—
anesthetic	T41.0X1	T41.0X2	T41.0X3	T41.0X4	T41.0X5	T41.0X6
solvent	T53.1X1	T53.1X2	T53.1X3	T53.1X4	—	—
water, concentrated	T41.0X1	T41.0X2	T41.0X3	T41.0X4	T41.0X5	T41.0X6
Chloroguanide	T37.2X1	T37.2X2	T37.2X3	T37.2X4	T37.2X5	T37.2X6
Chloromycetin	T36.2X1	T36.2X2	T36.2X3	T36.2X4	T36.2X5	T36.2X6
ENT agent	T49.6X1	T49.6X2	T49.6X3	T49.6X4	T49.6X5	T49.6X6
ophthalmic preparation	T49.5X1	T49.5X2	T49.5X3	T49.5X4	T49.5X5	T49.5X6
otic solution	T49.6X1	T49.6X2	T49.6X3	T49.6X4	T49.6X5	T49.6X6
topical NEC	T49.0X1	T49.0X2	T49.0X3	T49.0X4	T49.0X5	T49.0X6
Chloronitrobenzene	T53.7X1	T53.7X2	T53.7X3	T53.7X4	—	—
dust or vapor	T53.7X1	T53.7X2	T53.7X3	T53.7X4	—	—
Chlorophacinone	T60.4X1	T60.4X2	T60.4X3	T60.4X4	—	—
Chlorophenol	T53.7X1	T53.7X2	T53.7X3	T53.7X4	—	—
Chlorophenothane	T60.1X1	T60.1X2	T60.1X3	T60.1X4	—	—
Chlorophyll	T50.991	T50.992	T50.993	T50.994	T50.995	T50.996
Chloropicrin (fumes)	T53.6X1	T53.6X2	T53.6X3	T53.6X4	—	—
fumigant	T60.8X1	T60.8X2	T60.8X3	T60.8X4	—	—
fungicide	T60.3X1	T60.3X2	T60.3X3	T60.3X4	—	—
pesticide	T60.8X1	T60.8X2	T60.8X3	T60.8X4	—	—
Chloroprocaine	T41.3X1	T41.3X2	T41.3X3	T41.3X4	T41.3X5	T41.3X6
infiltration (subcutaneous)	T41.3X1	T41.3X2	T41.3X3	T41.3X4	T41.3X5	T41.3X6
nerve block (peripheral) (plexus)	T41.3X1	T41.3X2	T41.3X3	T41.3X4	T41.3X5	T41.3X6
spinal	T41.3X1	T41.3X2	T41.3X3	T41.3X4	T41.3X5	T41.3X6
Chloroptic	T49.5X1	T49.5X2	T49.5X3	T49.5X4	T49.5X5	T49.5X6
Chloropurine	T45.1X1	T45.1X2	T45.1X3	T45.1X4	T45.1X5	T45.1X6
Chloropyramine	T45.0X1	T45.0X2	T45.0X3	T45.0X4	T45.0X5	T45.0X6
Chloropyrifos	T60.0X1	T60.0X2	T60.0X3	T60.0X4	—	—
Chloropyrilene	T45.0X1	T45.0X2	T45.0X3	T45.0X4	T45.0X5	T45.0X6
Chloroquine	T37.2X1	T37.2X2	T37.2X3	T37.2X4	T37.2X5	T37.2X6
Chlorothalonil	T60.3X1	T60.3X2	T60.3X3	T60.3X4	—	—
Chlorothen	T45.0X1	T45.0X2	T45.0X3	T45.0X4	T45.0X5	T45.0X6
Chlorothiazide	T50.2X1	T50.2X2	T50.2X3	T50.2X4	T50.2X5	T50.2X6
Chlorothymol	T49.4X1	T49.4X2	T49.4X3	T49.4X4	T49.4X5	T49.4X6
Chlorotrianisene	T38.5X1	T38.5X2	T38.5X3	T38.5X4	T38.5X5	T38.5X6
Chlorovinyldichloroarsine, not in war	T57.0X1	T57.0X2	T57.0X3	T57.0X4	—	—
Chloroxine	T49.4X1	T49.4X2	T49.4X3	T49.4X4	T49.4X5	T49.4X6
Chloroxylenol	T49.0X1	T49.0X2	T49.0X3	T49.0X4	T49.0X5	T49.0X6
Chlorphenamine	T45.0X1	T45.0X2	T45.0X3	T45.0X4	T45.0X5	T45.0X6
Chlorphenesin	T42.8X1	T42.8X2	T42.8X3	T42.8X4	T42.8X5	T42.8X6
topical (antifungal)	T49.0X1	T49.0X2	T49.0X3	T49.0X4	T49.0X5	T49.0X6
Chlorpheniramine	T45.0X1	T45.0X2	T45.0X3	T45.0X4	T45.0X5	T45.0X6
Chlorphenoxamine	T45.0X1	T45.0X2	T45.0X3	T45.0X4	T45.0X5	T45.0X6
Chlorphentermine	T50.5X1	T50.5X2	T50.5X3	T50.5X4	T50.5X5	T50.5X6
Chlorprocaine — see Chloroprocaine						
Chlorproguanil	T37.2X1	T37.2X2	T37.2X3	T37.2X4	T37.2X5	T37.2X6
Chlorpromazine	T43.3X1	T43.3X2	T43.3X3	T43.3X4	T43.3X5	T43.3X6
Chlorpropamide	T38.3X1	T38.3X2	T38.3X3	T38.3X4	T38.3X5	T38.3X6
Chlorprothixene	T43.4X1	T43.4X2	T43.4X3	T43.4X4	T43.4X5	T43.4X6
Chlorquinaldol	T49.0X1	T49.0X2	T49.0X3	T49.0X4	T49.0X5	T49.0X6
Chlorquinol	T49.0X1	T49.0X2	T49.0X3	T49.0X4	T49.0X5	T49.0X6
Chlortalidone	T50.2X1	T50.2X2	T50.2X3	T50.2X4	T50.2X5	T50.2X6
Chlortetracycline	T36.4X1	T36.4X2	T36.4X3	T36.4X4	T36.4X5	T36.4X6
Chlorthalidone	T50.2X1	T50.2X2	T50.2X3	T50.2X4	T50.2X5	T50.2X6
Chlorthion	T60.0X1	T60.0X2	T60.0X3	T60.0X4	—	—
Chlorthiophos	T60.0X1	T60.0X2	T60.0X3	T60.0X4	—	—
Chlortrianisene	T38.5X1	T38.5X2	T38.5X3	T38.5X4	T38.5X5	T38.5X6
Chlor-Trimeton	T45.0X1	T45.0X2	T45.0X3	T45.0X4	T45.0X5	T45.0X6
Chlorzoxazone	T42.8X1	T42.8X2	T42.8X3	T42.8X4	T42.8X5	T42.8X6
Choke damp	T59.7X1	T59.7X2	T59.7X3	T59.7X4	—	—
Cholagogues	T47.5X1	T47.5X2	T47.5X3	T47.5X4	T47.5X5	T47.5X6
Cholebrine	T50.8X1	T50.8X2	T50.8X3	T50.8X4	T50.8X5	T50.8X6
Cholecalciferol	T45.2X1	T45.2X2	T45.2X3	T45.2X4	T45.2X5	T45.2X6
Cholecystokinin	T50.8X1	T50.8X2	T50.8X3	T50.8X4	T50.8X5	T50.8X6
Cholera vaccine	T50.A91	T50.A92	T50.A93	T50.A94	T50.A95	T50.A96
Choleretic	T47.5X1	T47.5X2	T47.5X3	T47.5X4	T47.5X5	T47.5X6
Cholesterol-lowering agents	T46.6X1	T46.6X2	T46.6X3	T46.6X4	T46.6X5	T46.6X6
Cholestyramine (resin)	T46.6X1	T46.6X2	T46.6X3	T46.6X4	T46.6X5	T46.6X6
Cholic acid	T47.5X1	T47.5X2	T47.5X3	T47.5X4	T47.5X5	T47.5X6
Choline	T48.6X1	T48.6X2	T48.6X3	T48.6X4	T48.6X5	T48.6X6
chloride	T50.991	T50.992	T50.993	T50.994	T50.995	T50.996
dihydrogen citrate	T50.991	T50.992	T50.993	T50.994	T50.995	T50.996
salicylate	T39.091	T39.092	T39.093	T39.094	T39.095	T39.096
theophyllinate	T48.6X1	T48.6X2	T48.6X3	T48.6X4	T48.6X5	T48.6X6
Cholinergic (drug) NEC	T44.1X1	T44.1X2	T44.1X3	T44.1X4	T44.1X5	T44.1X6
Cholinergic (drug) NEC — continued						
muscle tone enhancer	T44.1X1	T44.1X2	T44.1X3	T44.1X4	T44.1X5	T44.1X6
organophosphorus	T44.0X1	T44.0X2	T44.0X3	T44.0X4	T44.0X5	T44.0X6
insecticide	T60.0X1	T60.0X2	T60.0X3	T60.0X4	—	—
nerve gas	T59.891	T59.892	T59.893	T59.894	—	—
trimethyl ammonium propanediol	T44.1X1	T44.1X2	T44.1X3	T44.1X4	T44.1X5	T44.1X6
Cholinesterase reactivator	T50.6X1	T50.6X2	T50.6X3	T50.6X4	T50.6X5	T50.6X6
Cholografin	T50.8X1	T50.8X2	T50.8X3	T50.8X4	T50.8X5	T50.8X6
Chorionic gonadotropin	T38.891	T38.892	T38.893	T38.894	T38.895	T38.896
Chromate	T56.2X1	T56.2X2	T56.2X3	T56.2X4	—	—
dust or mist	T56.2X1	T56.2X2	T56.2X3	T56.2X4	—	—
lead — see also lead	T56.0X1	T56.0X2	T56.0X3	T56.0X4	—	—
paint	T56.0X1	T56.0X2	T56.0X3	T56.0X4	—	—
Chromic						
acid	T56.2X1	T56.2X2	T56.2X3	T56.2X4	—	—
dust or mist	T56.2X1	T56.2X2	T56.2X3	T56.2X4	—	—
phosphate 32P	T45.1X1	T45.1X2	T45.1X3	T45.1X4	T45.1X5	T45.1X6
Chromium	T56.2X1	T56.2X2	T56.2X3	T56.2X4	—	—
compounds — see Chromate						
sesquioxide	T50.8X1	T50.8X2	T50.8X3	T50.8X4	T50.8X5	T50.8X6
Chromomycin A3	T45.1X1	T45.1X2	T45.1X3	T45.1X4	T45.1X5	T45.1X6
Chromonar	T46.3X1	T46.3X2	T46.3X3	T46.3X4	T46.3X5	T46.3X6
Chromyl chloride	T56.2X1	T56.2X2	T56.2X3	T56.2X4	—	—
Chrysarobin	T49.4X1	T49.4X2	T49.4X3	T49.4X4	T49.4X5	T49.4X6
Chrysazin	T47.2X1	T47.2X2	T47.2X3	T47.2X4	T47.2X5	T47.2X6
Chymar	T45.3X1	T45.3X2	T45.3X3	T45.3X4	T45.3X5	T45.3X6
ophthalmic preparation	T49.5X1	T49.5X2	T49.5X3	T49.5X4	T49.5X5	T49.5X6
Chymopapain	T45.3X1	T45.3X2	T45.3X3	T45.3X4	T45.3X5	T45.3X6
Chymotrypsin	T45.3X1	T45.3X2	T45.3X3	T45.3X4	T45.3X5	T45.3X6
ophthalmic preparation	T49.5X1	T49.5X2	T49.5X3	T49.5X4	T49.5X5	T49.5X6
Cianidanol	T50.991	T50.992	T50.993	T50.994	T50.995	T50.996
Cianopramine	T43.011	T43.012	T43.013	T43.014	T43.015	T43.016
Cibenzoline	T46.2X1	T46.2X2	T46.2X3	T46.2X4	T46.2X5	T46.2X6
Ciclacillin	T36.0X1	T36.0X2	T36.0X3	T36.0X4	T36.0X5	T36.0X6
Ciclobarbital — see Hexobarbital						
Ciclonicate	T46.7X1	T46.7X2	T46.7X3	T46.7X4	T46.7X5	T46.7X6
Ciclopirox (olamine)	T49.0X1	T49.0X2	T49.0X3	T49.0X4	T49.0X5	T49.0X6
Ciclosporin	T45.1X1	T45.1X2	T45.1X3	T45.1X4	T45.1X5	T45.1X6
Cicuta maculata or virosa	T62.2X1	T62.2X2	T62.2X3	T62.2X4	—	—
Cicutoxin	T62.2X1	T62.2X2	T62.2X3	T62.2X4	—	—
Cigarette lighter fluid	T52.0X1	T52.0X2	T52.0X3	T52.0X4	—	—
Cigarettes (tobacco)	T65.221	T65.222	T65.223	T65.224	—	—
Ciguatoxin	T61.01	T61.02	T61.03	T61.04	—	—
Cilazapril	T46.4X1	T46.4X2	T46.4X3	T46.4X4	T46.4X5	T46.4X6
Cimetidine	T47.0X1	T47.0X2	T47.0X3	T47.0X4	T47.0X5	T47.0X6
Cimetropium bromide	T44.3X1	T44.3X2	T44.3X3	T44.3X4	T44.3X5	T44.3X6
Cinchocaine	T41.3X1	T41.3X2	T41.3X3	T41.3X4	T41.3X5	T41.3X6
topical (surface)	T41.3X1	T41.3X2	T41.3X3	T41.3X4	T41.3X5	T41.3X6
Cinchona	T37.2X1	T37.2X2	T37.2X3	T37.2X4	T37.2X5	T37.2X6
Cinchonine alkaloids	T37.2X1	T37.2X2	T37.2X3	T37.2X4	T37.2X5	T37.2X6
Cinchophen	T50.4X1	T50.4X2	T50.4X3	T50.4X4	T50.4X5	T50.4X6
Cinepazide	T46.7X1	T46.7X2	T46.7X3	T46.7X4	T46.7X5	T46.7X6
Cinnamedrine	T48.5X1	T48.5X2	T48.5X3	T48.5X4	T48.5X5	T48.5X6
Cinnarizine	T45.0X1	T45.0X2	T45.0X3	T45.0X4	T45.0X5	T45.0X6
Cinoxacin	T37.8X1	T37.8X2	T37.8X3	T37.8X4	T37.8X5	T37.8X6
Ciprofibrate	T46.6X1	T46.6X2	T46.6X3	T46.6X4	T46.6X5	T46.6X6
Ciprofloxacin	T36.8X1	T36.8X2	T36.8X3	T36.8X4	T36.8X5	T36.8X6
Cisapride	T47.8X1	T47.8X2	T47.8X3	T47.8X4	T47.8X5	T47.8X6
Cisplatin	T45.1X1	T45.1X2	T45.1X3	T45.1X4	T45.1X5	T45.1X6
Citalopram	T43.221	T43.222	T43.223	T43.224	T43.225	T43.226
Citanest	T41.3X1	T41.3X2	T41.3X3	T41.3X4	T41.3X5	T41.3X6
infiltration (subcutaneous)	T41.3X1	T41.3X2	T41.3X3	T41.3X4	T41.3X5	T41.3X6
nerve block (peripheral) (plexus)	T41.3X1	T41.3X2	T41.3X3	T41.3X4	T41.3X5	T41.3X6
Citric acid	T47.5X1	T47.5X2	T47.5X3	T47.5X4	T47.5X5	T47.5X6
Citrovorum (factor)	T45.8X1	T45.8X2	T45.8X3	T45.8X4	T45.8X5	T45.8X6
Claviceps purpurea	T62.2X1	T62.2X2	T62.2X3	T62.2X4	—	—
Clavulanic acid	T36.1X1	T36.1X2	T36.1X3	T36.1X4	T36.1X5	T36.1X6
Cleaner, cleansing agent, type not specified	T65.891	T65.892	T65.893	T65.894	—	—
of paint or varnish	T52.91	T52.92	T52.93	T52.94	—	—
specified type NEC	T65.891	T65.892	T65.893	T65.894	—	—
Clebopride	T47.8X1	T47.8X2	T47.8X3	T47.8X4	T47.8X5	T47.8X6
Clefamide	T37.3X1	T37.3X2	T37.3X3	T37.3X4	T37.3X5	T37.3X6
Clemastine	T45.0X1	T45.0X2	T45.0X3	T45.0X4	T45.0X5	T45.0X6
Clematis vitalba	T62.2X1	T62.2X2	T62.2X3	T62.2X4	—	—
Clemizole	T45.0X1	T45.0X2	T45.0X3	T45.0X4	T45.0X5	T45.0X6
penicillin	T36.0X1	T36.0X2	T36.0X3	T36.0X4	T36.0X5	T36.0X6
Clenbuterol	T48.6X1	T48.6X2	T48.6X3	T48.6X4	T48.6X5	T48.6X6
Clidinium bromide	T44.3X1	T44.3X2	T44.3X3	T44.3X4	T44.3X5	T44.3X6

Table of Drugs and Chemicals

Clindamycin — Coral

Substance	Poisoning, Accidental (unintentional)	Poisoning, Intentional Self-harm	Poisoning, Assault	Poisoning, Undetermined	Adverse Effect	Under-dosing
Clindamycin	T36.8X1	T36.8X2	T36.8X3	T36.8X4	T36.8X5	T36.8X6
Clinofibrate	T46.6X1	T46.6X2	T46.6X3	T46.6X4	T46.6X5	T46.6X6
Clioquinol	T37.8X1	T37.8X2	T37.8X3	T37.8X4	T37.8X5	T37.8X6
Cliradon	T40.2X1	T40.2X2	T40.2X3	T40.2X4	—	—
Clobazam	T42.4X1	T42.4X2	T42.4X3	T42.4X4	T42.4X5	T42.4X6
Clobenzorex	T50.5X1	T50.5X2	T50.5X3	T50.5X4	T50.5X5	T50.5X6
Clobetasol	T49.0X1	T49.0X2	T49.0X3	T49.0X4	T49.0X5	T49.0X6
Clobetasone	T49.0X1	T49.0X2	T49.0X3	T49.0X4	T49.0X5	T49.0X6
Clobutinol	T48.3X1	T48.3X2	T48.3X3	T48.3X4	T48.3X5	T48.3X6
Clocortolone	T38.0X1	T38.0X2	T38.0X3	T38.0X4	T38.0X5	T38.0X6
Clodantoin	T49.0X1	T49.0X2	T49.0X3	T49.0X4	T49.0X5	T49.0X6
Clodronic acid	T50.991	T50.992	T50.993	T50.994	T50.995	T50.996
Clofazimine	T37.1X1	T37.1X2	T37.1X3	T37.1X4	T37.1X5	T37.1X6
Clofedanol	T48.3X1	T48.3X2	T48.3X3	T48.3X4	T48.3X5	T48.3X6
Clofenamide	T50.2X1	T50.2X2	T50.2X3	T50.2X4	T50.2X5	T50.2X6
Clofenotane	T49.0X1	T49.0X2	T49.0X3	T49.0X4	T49.0X5	T49.0X6
Clofezone	T39.2X1	T39.2X2	T39.2X3	T39.2X4	T39.2X5	T39.2X6
Clofibrate	T46.6X1	T46.6X2	T46.6X3	T46.6X4	T46.6X5	T46.6X6
Clofibride	T46.6X1	T46.6X2	T46.6X3	T46.6X4	T46.6X5	T46.6X6
Cloforex	T50.5X1	T50.5X2	T50.5X3	T50.5X4	T50.5X5	T50.5X6
Clomethiazole	T42.6X1	T42.6X2	T42.6X3	T42.6X4	T42.6X5	T42.6X6
Clometocillin	T36.0X1	T36.0X2	T36.0X3	T36.0X4	T36.0X5	T36.0X6
Clomifene	T38.5X1	T38.5X2	T38.5X3	T38.5X4	T38.5X5	T38.5X6
Clomiphene	T38.5X1	T38.5X2	T38.5X3	T38.5X4	T38.5X5	T38.5X6
Clomipramine	T43.011	T43.012	T43.013	T43.014	T43.015	T43.016
Clomocycline	T36.4X1	T36.4X2	T36.4X3	T36.4X4	T36.4X5	T36.4X6
Clonazepam	T42.4X1	T42.4X2	T42.4X3	T42.4X4	T42.4X5	T42.4X6
Clonidine	T46.5X1	T46.5X2	T46.5X3	T46.5X4	T46.5X5	T46.5X6
Clonixin	T39.8X1	T39.8X2	T39.8X3	T39.8X4	T39.8X5	T39.8X6
Clopamide	T50.2X1	T50.2X2	T50.2X3	T50.2X4	T50.2X5	T50.2X6
Clopenthixol	T43.4X1	T43.4X2	T43.4X3	T43.4X4	T43.4X5	T43.4X6
Cloperastine	T48.3X1	T48.3X2	T48.3X3	T48.3X4	T48.3X5	T48.3X6
Clophedianol	T48.3X1	T48.3X2	T48.3X3	T48.3X4	T48.3X5	T48.3X6
Cloponone	T36.2X1	T36.2X2	T36.2X3	T36.2X4	T36.2X5	T36.2X6
Cloprednol	T38.0X1	T38.0X2	T38.0X3	T38.0X4	T38.0X5	T38.0X6
Cloral betaine	T42.6X1	T42.6X2	T42.6X3	T42.6X4	T42.6X5	T42.6X6
Cloramfenicol	T36.2X1	T36.2X2	T36.2X3	T36.2X4	T36.2X5	T36.2X6
Clorazepate (dipotassium)	T42.4X1	T42.4X2	T42.4X3	T42.4X4	T42.4X5	T42.4X6
Clorexolone	T50.2X1	T50.2X2	T50.2X3	T50.2X4	T50.2X5	T50.2X6
Clorfenamine	T45.0X1	T45.0X2	T45.0X3	T45.0X4	T45.0X5	T45.0X6
Clorgiline	T43.1X1	T43.1X2	T43.1X3	T43.1X4	T43.1X5	T43.1X6
Clorotepine	T44.3X1	T44.3X2	T44.3X3	T44.3X4	T44.3X5	T44.3X6
Clorox (bleach)	T54.91	T54.92	T54.93	T54.94	—	—
Clorprenaline	T48.6X1	T48.6X2	T48.6X3	T48.6X4	T48.6X5	T48.6X6
Clortermine	T50.5X1	T50.5X2	T50.5X3	T50.5X4	T50.5X5	T50.5X6
Clotiapine	T43.591	T43.592	T43.593	T43.594	T43.595	T43.596
Clotiazepam	T42.4X1	T42.4X2	T42.4X3	T42.4X4	T42.4X5	T42.4X6
Clotibric acid	T46.6X1	T46.6X2	T46.6X3	T46.6X4	T46.6X5	T46.6X6
Clotrimazole	T49.0X1	T49.0X2	T49.0X3	T49.0X4	T49.0X5	T49.0X6
Cloxacillin	T36.0X1	T36.0X2	T36.0X3	T36.0X4	T36.0X5	T36.0X6
Cloxazolam	T42.4X1	T42.4X2	T42.4X3	T42.4X4	T42.4X5	T42.4X6
Cloxiquine	T49.0X1	T49.0X2	T49.0X3	T49.0X4	T49.0X5	T49.0X6
Clozapine	T42.4X1	T42.4X2	T42.4X3	T42.4X4	T42.4X5	T42.4X6
Coagulant NEC	T45.7X1	T45.7X2	T45.7X3	T45.7X4	T45.7X5	T45.7X6
Coal (carbon monoxide from) — see also Carbon, monoxide, coal	T58.2X1	T58.2X2	T58.2X3	T58.2X4	—	—
oil — see Kerosene						
tar	T49.1X1	T49.1X2	T49.1X3	T49.1X4	T49.1X5	T49.1X6
fumes	T59.891	T59.892	T59.893	T59.894		
medicinal (ointment)	T49.4X1	T49.4X2	T49.4X3	T49.4X4	T49.4X5	T49.4X6
analgesics NEC	T39.2X1	T39.2X2	T39.2X3	T39.2X4	T39.2X5	T39.2X6
naphtha (solvent)	T52.0X1	T52.0X2	T52.0X3	T52.0X4		
Cobalamine	T45.2X1	T45.2X2	T45.2X3	T45.2X4	T45.2X5	T45.2X6
Cobalt (nonmedicinal) (fumes) (industrial)	T56.891	T56.892	T56.893	T56.894		
medicinal (trace) (chloride)	T45.8X1	T45.8X2	T45.8X3	T45.8X4	T45.8X5	T45.8X6
Cobra (venom)	T63.041	T63.042	T63.043	T63.044	—	—
Coca (leaf)	T40.5X1	T40.5X2	T40.5X3	T40.5X4	T40.5X5	T40.5X6
Cocaine	T40.5X1	T40.5X2	T40.5X3	T40.5X4	T40.5X5	T40.5X6
topical anesthetic	T41.3X1	T41.3X2	T41.3X3	T41.3X4	T41.3X5	T41.3X6
Cocarboxylase	T45.3X1	T45.3X2	T45.3X3	T45.3X4	T45.3X5	T45.3X6
Coccidioidin	T50.8X1	T50.8X2	T50.8X3	T50.8X4	T50.8X5	T50.8X6
Cocculus indicus	T62.1X1	T62.1X2	T62.1X3	T62.1X4	—	—
Cochineal	T65.6X1	T65.6X2	T65.6X3	T65.6X4	—	—
medicinal products	T50.991	T50.992	T50.993	T50.994	T50.995	T50.996
Codeine	T40.2X1	T40.2X2	T40.2X3	T40.2X4	T40.2X5	T40.2X6
Cod-liver oil	T45.2X1	T45.2X2	T45.2X3	T45.2X4	T45.2X5	T45.2X6
Coenzyme A	T50.991	T50.992	T50.993	T50.994	T50.995	T50.996
Coffee	T62.8X1	T62.8X2	T62.8X3	T62.8X4	—	—
Cogalactoisomerase	T50.991	T50.992	T50.993	T50.994	T50.995	T50.996
Cogentin	T44.3X1	T44.3X2	T44.3X3	T44.3X4	T44.3X5	T44.3X6
Coke fumes or gas (carbon monoxide)	T58.2X1	T58.2X2	T58.2X3	T58.2X4	—	—
industrial use	T58.8X1	T58.8X2	T58.8X3	T58.8X4		
Colace	T47.4X1	T47.4X2	T47.4X3	T47.4X4	T47.4X5	T47.4X6
Colaspase	T45.1X1	T45.1X2	T45.1X3	T45.1X4	T45.1X5	T45.1X6
Colchicine	T50.4X1	T50.4X2	T50.4X3	T50.4X4	T50.4X5	T50.4X6
Colchicum	T62.2X1	T62.2X2	T62.2X3	T62.2X4		
Cold cream	T49.3X1	T49.3X2	T49.3X3	T49.3X4	T49.3X5	T49.3X6
Colecalciferol	T45.2X1	T45.2X2	T45.2X3	T45.2X4	T45.2X5	T45.2X6
Colestipol	T46.6X1	T46.6X2	T46.6X3	T46.6X4	T46.6X5	T46.6X6
Colestyramine	T46.6X1	T46.6X2	T46.6X3	T46.6X4	T46.6X5	T46.6X6
Colimycin	T36.8X1	T36.8X2	T36.8X3	T36.8X4	T36.8X5	T36.8X6
Colistimethate	T36.8X1	T36.8X2	T36.8X3	T36.8X4	T36.8X5	T36.8X6
Colistin	T36.8X1	T36.8X2	T36.8X3	T36.8X4	T36.8X5	T36.8X6
sulfate (eye preparation)	T49.5X1	T49.5X2	T49.5X3	T49.5X4	T49.5X5	T49.5X6
Collagen	T50.991	T50.992	T50.993	T50.994	T50.995	T50.996
Collagenase	T49.4X1	T49.4X2	T49.4X3	T49.4X4	T49.4X5	T49.4X6
Collodion	T49.3X1	T49.3X2	T49.3X3	T49.3X4	T49.3X5	T49.3X6
Colocynth	T47.2X1	T47.2X2	T47.2X3	T47.2X4	T47.2X5	T47.2X6
Colophony adhesive	T49.3X1	T49.3X2	T49.3X3	T49.3X4	T49.3X5	T49.3X6
Colorant — see also Dye	T50.991	T50.992	T50.993	T50.994	T50.995	T50.996
Coloring matter — see Dye(s)						
Combustion gas (after combustion) — see Carbon, monoxide						
prior to combustion	T59.891	T59.892	T59.893	T59.894	—	—
Compazine	T43.3X1	T43.3X2	T43.3X3	T43.3X4	T43.3X5	T43.3X6
Compound						
1080 (sodium fluoroacetate)	T60.4X1	T60.4X2	T60.4X3	T60.4X4		
269 (endrin)	T60.1X1	T60.1X2	T60.1X3	T60.1X4		
3422 (parathion)	T60.0X1	T60.0X2	T60.0X3	T60.0X4		
3911 (phorate)	T60.0X1	T60.0X2	T60.0X3	T60.0X4		
3956 (toxaphene)	T60.1X1	T60.1X2	T60.1X3	T60.1X4		
4049 (malathion)	T60.0X1	T60.0X2	T60.0X3	T60.0X4		
4069 (malathion)	T60.0X1	T60.0X2	T60.0X3	T60.0X4		
4124 (dicapthon)	T60.0X1	T60.0X2	T60.0X3	T60.0X4		
42 (warfarin)	T60.4X1	T60.4X2	T60.4X3	T60.4X4		
497 (dieldrin)	T60.1X1	T60.1X2	T60.1X3	T60.1X4		
E (cortisone)	T38.0X1	T38.0X2	T38.0X3	T38.0X4	T38.0X5	T38.0X6
F (hydrocortisone)	T38.0X1	T38.0X2	T38.0X3	T38.0X4	T38.0X5	T38.0X6
Congener, anabolic	T38.7X1	T38.7X2	T38.7X3	T38.7X4	T38.7X5	T38.7X6
Congo red	T50.8X1	T50.8X2	T50.8X3	T50.8X4	T50.8X5	T50.8X6
Coniine, conine	T62.2X1	T62.2X2	T62.2X3	T62.2X4	—	—
Conium (maculatum)	T62.2X1	T62.2X2	T62.2X3	T62.2X4	—	—
Conjugated estrogenic substances	T38.5X1	T38.5X2	T38.5X3	T38.5X4	T38.5X5	T38.5X6
Contac	T48.5X1	T48.5X2	T48.5X3	T48.5X4	T48.5X5	T48.5X6
Contact lens solution	T49.5X1	T49.5X2	T49.5X3	T49.5X4	T49.5X5	T49.5X6
Contraceptive (oral)	T38.4X1	T38.4X2	T38.4X3	T38.4X4	T38.4X5	T38.4X6
vaginal	T49.8X1	T49.8X2	T49.8X3	T49.8X4	T49.8X5	T49.8X6
Contrast medium, radiography	T50.8X1	T50.8X2	T50.8X3	T50.8X4		T50.8X6
Convallaria glycosides	T46.0X1	T46.0X2	T46.0X3	T46.0X4	T46.0X5	T46.0X6
Convallaria majalis	T62.2X1	T62.2X2	T62.2X3	T62.2X4	—	—
berry	T62.1X1	T62.1X2	T62.1X3	T62.1X4	—	—
Copperhead snake (bite) (venom)	T63.061	T63.062	T63.063	T63.064	—	—
Copper (dust) (fumes) (nonmedicinal) NEC	T56.4X1	T56.4X2	T56.4X3	T56.4X4	—	—
arsenate, arsenite	T57.0X1	T57.0X2	T57.0X3	T57.0X4	—	—
insecticide	T60.2X1	T60.2X2	T60.2X3	T60.2X4	—	—
emetic	T47.7X1	T47.7X2	T47.7X3	T47.7X4	T47.7X5	T47.7X6
fungicide	T60.3X1	T60.3X2	T60.3X3	T60.3X4	—	—
gluconate	T49.0X1	T49.0X2	T49.0X3	T49.0X4	T49.0X5	T49.0X6
insecticide	T60.2X1	T60.2X2	T60.2X3	T60.2X4	—	—
medicinal (trace)	T45.8X1	T45.8X2	T45.8X3	T45.8X4	T45.8X5	T45.8X6
oleate	T49.0X1	T49.0X2	T49.0X3	T49.0X4	T49.0X5	T49.0X6
sulfate	T56.4X1	T56.4X2	T56.4X3	T56.4X4	—	—
cupric	T56.4X1	T56.4X2	T56.4X3	T56.4X4	—	—
fungicide	T60.3X1	T60.3X2	T60.3X3	T60.3X4	—	—
medicinal						
ear	T49.6X1	T49.6X2	T49.6X3	T49.6X4	T49.6X5	T49.6X6
emetic	T47.7X1	T47.7X2	T47.7X3	T47.7X4	T47.7X5	T47.7X6
eye	T49.5X1	T49.5X2	T49.5X3	T49.5X4	T49.5X5	T49.5X6
cuprous	T56.4X1	T56.4X2	T56.4X3	T56.4X4	—	—
fungicide	T60.3X1	T60.3X2	T60.3X3	T60.3X4		
medicinal						
ear	T49.6X1	T49.6X2	T49.6X3	T49.6X4	T49.6X5	T49.6X6
emetic	T47.7X1	T47.7X2	T47.7X3	T47.7X4	T47.7X5	T47.7X6
eye	T49.5X1	T49.5X2	T49.5X3	T49.5X4	T49.5X5	T49.5X6
Coral (sting)	T63.691	T63.692	T63.693	T63.694		
snake (bite) (venom)	T63.021	T63.022	T63.023	T63.024		

Substance	Poisoning, Accidental (unintentional)	Poisoning, Intentional Self-harm	Poisoning, Assault	Poisoning, Undetermined	Adverse Effect	Under-dosing
Corbadrine	T49.6X1	T49.6X2	T49.6X3	T49.6X4	T49.6X5	T49.6X6
Cordite	T65.891	T65.892	T65.893	T65.894	—	—
vapor	T59.891	T59.892	T59.893	T59.894	—	—
Cordran	T49.0X1	T49.0X2	T49.0X3	T49.0X4	T49.0X5	T49.0X6
Corn cures	T49.4X1	T49.4X2	T49.4X3	T49.4X4	T49.4X5	T49.4X6
Cornhusker's lotion	T49.3X1	T49.3X2	T49.3X3	T49.3X4	T49.3X5	T49.3X6
Corn starch	T49.3X1	T49.3X2	T49.3X3	T49.3X4	T49.3X5	T49.3X6
Coronary vasodilator NEC	T46.3X1	T46.3X2	T46.3X3	T46.3X4	T46.3X5	T46.3X6
Corrosive NEC	T54.91	T54.92	T54.93	T54.94	—	—
acid NEC	T54.2X1	T54.2X2	T54.2X3	T54.2X4	—	—
aromatics	T54.1X1	T54.1X2	T54.1X3	T54.1X4	—	—
disinfectant	T54.1X1	T54.1X2	T54.1X3	T54.1X4	—	—
fumes NEC	T54.91	T54.92	T54.93	T54.94	—	—
specified NEC	T54.91	T54.92	T54.93	T54.94	—	—
sublimate	T56.1X1	T56.1X2	T56.1X3	T56.1X4	—	—
Cortate	T38.0X1	T38.0X2	T38.0X3	T38.0X4	T38.0X5	T38.0X6
Cort-Dome	T38.0X1	T38.0X2	T38.0X3	T38.0X4	T38.0X5	T38.0X6
ENT agent	T49.6X1	T49.6X2	T49.6X3	T49.6X4	T49.6X5	T49.6X6
ophthalmic preparation	T49.5X1	T49.5X2	T49.5X3	T49.5X4	T49.5X5	T49.5X6
topical NEC	T49.0X1	T49.0X2	T49.0X3	T49.0X4	T49.0X5	T49.0X6
Cortef	T38.0X1	T38.0X2	T38.0X3	T38.0X4	T38.0X5	T38.0X6
ENT agent	T49.6X1	T49.6X2	T49.6X3	T49.6X4	T49.6X5	T49.6X6
ophthalmic preparation	T49.5X1	T49.5X2	T49.5X3	T49.5X4	T49.5X5	T49.5X6
topical NEC	T49.0X1	T49.0X2	T49.0X3	T49.0X4	T49.0X5	T49.0X6
Corticosteroid	T38.0X1	T38.0X2	T38.0X3	T38.0X4	T38.0X5	T38.0X6
ENT agent	T49.6X1	T49.6X2	T49.6X3	T49.6X4	T49.6X5	T49.6X6
mineral	T50.0X1	T50.0X2	T50.0X3	T50.0X4	T50.0X5	T50.0X6
ophthalmic	T49.5X1	T49.5X2	T49.5X3	T49.5X4	T49.5X5	T49.5X6
topical NEC	T49.0X1	T49.0X2	T49.0X3	T49.0X4	T49.0X5	T49.0X6
Corticotropin	T38.811	T38.812	T38.813	T38.814	T38.815	T38.816
Cortisol	T49.0X1	T49.0X2	T49.0X3	T49.0X4	T49.0X5	T49.0X6
ENT agent	T49.6X1	T49.6X2	T49.6X3	T49.6X4	T49.6X5	T49.6X6
ophthalmic preparation	T49.5X1	T49.5X2	T49.5X3	T49.5X4	T49.5X5	T49.5X6
topical NEC	T49.0X1	T49.0X2	T49.0X3	T49.0X4	T49.0X5	T49.0X6
Cortisone (acetate)	T38.0X1	T38.0X2	T38.0X3	T38.0X4	T38.0X5	T38.0X6
ENT agent	T49.6X1	T49.6X2	T49.6X3	T49.6X4	T49.6X5	T49.6X6
ophthalmic preparation	T49.5X1	T49.5X2	T49.5X3	T49.5X4	T49.5X5	T49.5X6
topical NEC	T49.0X1	T49.0X2	T49.0X3	T49.0X4	T49.0X5	T49.0X6
Cortivazol	T38.0X1	T38.0X2	T38.0X3	T38.0X4	T38.0X5	T38.0X6
Cortogen	T38.0X1	T38.0X2	T38.0X3	T38.0X4	T38.0X5	T38.0X6
ENT agent	T49.6X1	T49.6X2	T49.6X3	T49.6X4	T49.6X5	T49.6X6
ophthalmic preparation	T49.5X1	T49.5X2	T49.5X3	T49.5X4	T49.5X5	T49.5X6
Cortone	T38.0X1	T38.0X2	T38.0X3	T38.0X4	T38.0X5	T38.0X6
ENT agent	T49.6X1	T49.6X2	T49.6X3	T49.6X4	T49.6X5	T49.6X6
ophthalmic preparation	T49.5X1	T49.5X2	T49.5X3	T49.5X4	T49.5X5	T49.5X6
Cortril	T38.0X1	T38.0X2	T38.0X3	T38.0X4	T38.0X5	T38.0X6
ENT agent	T49.6X1	T49.6X2	T49.6X3	T49.6X4	T49.6X5	T49.6X6
ophthalmic preparation	T49.5X1	T49.5X2	T49.5X3	T49.5X4	T49.5X5	T49.5X6
topical NEC	T49.0X1	T49.0X2	T49.0X3	T49.0X4	T49.0X5	T49.0X6
Corynebacterium parvum	T45.1X1	T45.1X2	T45.1X3	T45.1X4	T45.1X5	T45.1X6
Cosmetic preparation	T49.8X1	T49.8X2	T49.8X3	T49.8X4	T49.8X5	T49.8X6
Cosmetics	T49.8X1	T49.8X2	T49.8X3	T49.8X4	T49.8X5	T49.8X6
Cosyntropin	T38.811	T38.812	T38.813	T38.814	T38.815	T38.816
Cotarnine	T45.7X1	T45.7X2	T45.7X3	T45.7X4	T45.7X5	T45.7X6
Co-trimoxazole	T36.8X1	T36.8X2	T36.8X3	T36.8X4	T36.8X5	T36.8X6
Cottonseed oil	T49.3X1	T49.3X2	T49.3X3	T49.3X4	T49.3X5	T49.3X6
Cough mixture (syrup)	T48.4X1	T48.4X2	T48.4X3	T48.4X4	T48.4X5	T48.4X6
containing opiates	T40.2X1	T40.2X2	T40.2X3	T40.2X4	T40.2X5	T40.2X6
expectorants	T48.4X1	T48.4X2	T48.4X3	T48.4X4	T48.4X5	T48.4X6
Coumadin	T45.511	T45.512	T45.513	T45.514	T45.515	T45.516
rodenticide	T60.4X1	T60.4X2	T60.4X3	T60.4X4	—	—
Coumaphos	T60.0X1	T60.0X2	T60.0X3	T60.0X4	—	—
Coumarin	T45.511	T45.512	T45.513	T45.514	T45.515	T45.516
Coumetarol	T45.511	T45.512	T45.513	T45.514	T45.515	T45.516
Cowbane	T62.2X1	T62.2X2	T62.2X3	T62.2X4	—	—
Cozyme	T45.2X1	T45.2X2	T45.2X3	T45.2X4	T45.2X5	T45.2X6
Crack	T40.5X1	T40.5X2	T40.5X3	T40.5X4	—	—
Crataegus extract	T46.0X1	T46.0X2	T46.0X3	T46.0X4	T46.0X5	T46.0X6
Creolin	T54.1X1	T54.1X2	T54.1X3	T54.1X4	—	—
disinfectant	T54.1X1	T54.1X2	T54.1X3	T54.1X4	—	—
Creosol (compound)	T49.0X1	T49.0X2	T49.0X3	T49.0X4	T49.0X5	T49.0X6
Creosote (coal tar)	T49.0X1	T49.0X2	T49.0X3	T49.0X4	T49.0X5	T49.0X6
(beechwood)						
medicinal (expectorant)	T48.4X1	T48.4X2	T48.4X3	T48.4X4	T48.4X5	T48.4X6
syrup	T48.4X1	T48.4X2	T48.4X3	T48.4X4	T48.4X5	T48.4X6
Cresol(s)	T49.0X1	T49.0X2	T49.0X3	T49.0X4	T49.0X5	T49.0X6
and soap solution	T49.0X1	T49.0X2	T49.0X3	T49.0X4	T49.0X5	T49.0X6
Cresyl acetate	T49.0X1	T49.0X2	T49.0X3	T49.0X4	T49.0X5	T49.0X6
Cresylic acid	T49.0X1	T49.0X2	T49.0X3	T49.0X4	T49.0X5	T49.0X6
Crimidine	T60.4X1	T60.4X2	T60.4X3	T60.4X4	—	—
Croconazole	T37.8X1	T37.8X2	T37.8X3	T37.8X4	T37.8X5	T37.8X6
Cromoglicic acid	T48.6X1	T48.6X2	T48.6X3	T48.6X4	T48.6X5	T48.6X6
Cromolyn	T48.6X1	T48.6X2	T48.6X3	T48.6X4	T48.6X5	T48.6X6

Substance	Poisoning, Accidental (unintentional)	Poisoning, Intentional Self-harm	Poisoning, Assault	Poisoning, Undetermined	Adverse Effect	Under-dosing
Cromonar	T46.3X1	T46.3X2	T46.3X3	T46.3X4	T46.3X5	T46.3X6
Cropropamide	T39.8X1	T39.8X2	T39.8X3	T39.8X4	T39.8X5	T39.8X6
with crotethamide	T50.7X1	T50.7X2	T50.7X3	T50.7X4	T50.7X5	T50.7X6
Crotamiton	T49.0X1	T49.0X2	T49.0X3	T49.0X4	T49.0X5	T49.0X6
Crotethamide	T39.8X1	T39.8X2	T39.8X3	T39.8X4	T39.8X5	T39.8X6
with cropropamide	T50.7X1	T50.7X2	T50.7X3	T50.7X4	T50.7X5	T50.7X6
Croton (oil)	T47.2X1	T47.2X2	T47.2X3	T47.2X4	T47.2X5	T47.2X6
chloral	T42.6X1	T42.6X2	T42.6X3	T42.6X4	T42.6X5	T42.6X6
Crude oil	T52.0X1	T52.0X2	T52.0X3	T52.0X4	—	—
Cryogenine	T39.8X1	T39.8X2	T39.8X3	T39.8X4	T39.8X5	T39.8X6
Cryolite (vapor)	T60.1X1	T60.1X2	T60.1X3	T60.1X4	—	—
insecticide	T60.1X1	T60.1X2	T60.1X3	T60.1X4	—	—
Cryptenamine (tannates)	T46.5X1	T46.5X2	T46.5X3	T46.5X4	T46.5X5	T46.5X6
Crystal violet	T49.0X1	T49.0X2	T49.0X3	T49.0X4	T49.0X5	T49.0X6
Cuckoopint	T62.2X1	T62.2X2	T62.2X3	T62.2X4	—	—
Cumetharol	T45.511	T45.512	T45.513	T45.514	T45.515	T45.516
Cupric						
acetate	T60.3X1	T60.3X2	T60.3X3	T60.3X4	—	—
acetoarsenite	T57.0X1	T57.0X2	T57.0X3	T57.0X4	—	—
arsenate	T57.0X1	T57.0X2	T57.0X3	T57.0X4	—	—
gluconate	T49.0X1	T49.0X2	T49.0X3	T49.0X4	T49.0X5	T49.0X6
oleate	T49.0X1	T49.0X2	T49.0X3	T49.0X4	T49.0X5	T49.0X6
sulfate	T56.4X1	T56.4X2	T56.4X3	T56.4X4	—	—
Cuprous sulfate — see also Copper sulfate	T56.4X1	T56.4X2	T56.4X3	T56.4X4	—	—
Curare, curarine	T48.1X1	T48.1X2	T48.1X3	T48.1X4	T48.1X5	T48.1X6
Cyamemazine	T43.3X1	T43.3X2	T43.3X3	T43.3X4	T43.3X5	T43.3X6
Cyamopsis tetragonoloba	T46.6X1	T46.6X2	T46.6X3	T46.6X4	T46.6X5	T46.6X6
Cyanacetyl hydrazide	T37.1X1	T37.1X2	T37.1X3	T37.1X4	T37.1X5	T37.1X6
Cyanic acid (gas)	T59.891	T59.892	T59.893	T59.894	—	—
Cyanide(s) (compounds) (potassium) (sodium)	T65.0X1	T65.0X2	T65.0X3	T65.0X4		
NEC						
dust or gas (inhalation)	T57.3X1	T57.3X2	T57.3X3	T57.3X4		
NEC						
fumigant	T65.0X1	T65.0X2	T65.0X3	T65.0X4		
hydrogen	T57.3X1	T57.3X2	T57.3X3	T57.3X4		
mercuric — see Mercury						
pesticide (dust) (fumes)	T65.0X1	T65.0X2	T65.0X3	T65.0X4		
Cyanoacrylate adhesive	T49.3X1	T49.3X2	T49.3X3	T49.3X4	T49.3X5	T49.3X6
Cyanocobalamin	T45.8X1	T45.8X2	T45.8X3	T45.8X4	T45.8X5	T45.8X6
Cyanogen (chloride) (gas)	T59.891	T59.892	T59.893	T59.894	—	—
NEC						
Cyclacillin	T36.0X1	T36.0X2	T36.0X3	T36.0X4	T36.0X5	T36.0X6
Cyclaine	T41.3X1	T41.3X2	T41.3X3	T41.3X4	T41.3X5	T41.3X6
Cyclamate	T50.991	T50.992	T50.993	T50.994	T50.995	T50.996
Cyclamen europaeum	T62.2X1	T62.2X2	T62.2X3	T62.2X4	—	—
Cyclandelate	T46.7X1	T46.7X2	T46.7X3	T46.7X4	T46.7X5	T46.7X6
Cyclazocine	T50.7X1	T50.7X2	T50.7X3	T50.7X4	T50.7X5	T50.7X6
Cyclizine	T45.0X1	T45.0X2	T45.0X3	T45.0X4	T45.0X5	T45.0X6
Cyclobarbital	T42.3X1	T42.3X2	T42.3X3	T42.3X4	T42.3X5	T42.3X6
Cyclobarbitone	T42.3X1	T42.3X2	T42.3X3	T42.3X4	T42.3X5	T42.3X6
Cyclobenzaprine	T48.1X1	T48.1X2	T48.1X3	T48.1X4	T48.1X5	T48.1X6
Cyclodrine	T44.3X1	T44.3X2	T44.3X3	T44.3X4	T44.3X5	T44.3X6
Cycloguanil embonate	T37.2X1	T37.2X2	T37.2X3	T37.2X4	T37.2X5	T37.2X6
Cyclohexane	T52.8X1	T52.8X2	T52.8X3	T52.8X4	—	—
Cyclohexanol	T51.8X1	T51.8X2	T51.8X3	T51.8X4	—	—
Cyclohexanone	T52.4X1	T52.4X2	T52.4X3	T52.4X4	—	—
Cycloheximide	T60.3X1	T60.3X2	T60.3X3	T60.3X4	—	—
Cyclohexyl acetate	T52.8X1	T52.8X2	T52.8X3	T52.8X4	—	—
Cycloleucin	T45.1X1	T45.1X2	T45.1X3	T45.1X4	T45.1X5	T45.1X6
Cyclomethycaine	T41.3X1	T41.3X2	T41.3X3	T41.3X4	T41.3X5	T41.3X6
Cyclopentamine	T44.4X1	T44.4X2	T44.4X3	T44.4X4	T44.4X5	T44.4X6
Cyclopenthiazide	T50.2X1	T50.2X2	T50.2X3	T50.2X4	T50.2X5	T50.2X6
Cyclopentolate	T44.3X1	T44.3X2	T44.3X3	T44.3X4	T44.3X5	T44.3X6
Cyclophosphamide	T45.1X1	T45.1X2	T45.1X3	T45.1X4	T45.1X5	T45.1X6
Cycloplegic drug	T49.5X1	T49.5X2	T49.5X3	T49.5X4	T49.5X5	T49.5X6
Cyclopropane	T41.291	T41.292	T41.293	T41.294	T41.295	T41.296
Cyclopyrabital	T39.8X1	T39.8X2	T39.8X3	T39.8X4	T39.8X5	T39.8X6
Cycloserine	T37.1X1	T37.1X2	T37.1X3	T37.1X4	T37.1X5	T37.1X6
Cyclosporin	T45.1X1	T45.1X2	T45.1X3	T45.1X4	T45.1X5	T45.1X6
Cyclothiazide	T50.2X1	T50.2X2	T50.2X3	T50.2X4	T50.2X5	T50.2X6
Cycrimine	T44.3X1	T44.3X2	T44.3X3	T44.3X4	T44.3X5	T44.3X6
Cyhalothrin	T60.1X1	T60.1X2	T60.1X3	T60.1X4	—	—
Cymarin	T46.0X1	T46.0X2	T46.0X3	T46.0X4	T46.0X5	T46.0X6
Cypermethrin	T60.1X1	T60.1X2	T60.1X3	T60.1X4	—	—
Cyphenothrin	T60.2X1	T60.2X2	T60.2X3	T60.2X4	—	—
Cyproheptadine	T45.0X1	T45.0X2	T45.0X3	T45.0X4	T45.0X5	T45.0X6
Cyproterone	T38.6X1	T38.6X2	T38.6X3	T38.6X4	T38.6X5	T38.6X6
Cysteamine	T50.6X1	T50.6X2	T50.6X3	T50.6X4	T50.6X5	T50.6X6
Cytarabine	T45.1X1	T45.1X2	T45.1X3	T45.1X4	T45.1X5	T45.1X6
Cytisus						
laburnum	T62.2X1	T62.2X2	T62.2X3	T62.2X4		

▽ Subterms under main terms may continue to next column or page   Additional Character May Be Required — Refer to the Tabular List for Character Selection   363

Corbadrine — Cytisus

Substance	Poisoning, Accidental (unintentional)	Poisoning, Intentional Self-harm	Poisoning, Assault	Poisoning, Undetermined	Adverse Effect	Under-dosing
Cytisus — continued						
scoparius	T62.2X1	T62.2X2	T62.2X3	T62.2X4	—	—
Cytochrome C	T47.5X1	T47.5X2	T47.5X3	T47.5X4	T47.5X5	T47.5X6
Cytomel	T38.1X1	T38.1X2	T38.1X3	T38.1X4	T38.1X5	T38.1X6
Cytosine arabinoside	T45.1X1	T45.1X2	T45.1X3	T45.1X4	T45.1X5	T45.1X6
Cytoxan	T45.1X1	T45.1X2	T45.1X3	T45.1X4	T45.1X5	T45.1X6
Cytozyme	T45.7X1	T45.7X2	T45.7X3	T45.7X4	T45.7X5	T45.7X6
S-Carboxymethylcysteine	T48.4X1	T48.4X2	T48.4X3	T48.4X4	T48.4X5	T48.4X6
Dacarbazine	T45.1X1	T45.1X2	T45.1X3	T45.1X4	T45.1X5	T45.1X6
Dactinomycin	T45.1X1	T45.1X2	T45.1X3	T45.1X4	T45.1X5	T45.1X6
DADPS	T37.1X1	T37.1X2	T37.1X3	T37.1X4	T37.1X5	T37.1X6
Dakin's solution	T49.0X1	T49.0X2	T49.0X3	T49.0X4	T49.0X5	T49.0X6
Dalapon (sodium)	T60.3X1	T60.3X2	T60.3X3	T60.3X4	—	—
Dalmane	T42.4X1	T42.4X2	T42.4X3	T42.4X4	T42.4X5	T42.4X6
Danazol	T38.6X1	T38.6X2	T38.6X3	T38.6X4	T38.6X5	T38.6X6
Danilone	T45.511	T45.512	T45.513	T45.514	T45.515	T45.516
Danthron	T47.2X1	T47.2X2	T47.2X3	T47.2X4	T47.2X5	T47.2X6
Dantrolene	T42.8X1	T42.8X2	T42.8X3	T42.8X4	T42.8X5	T42.8X6
Dantron	T47.2X1	T47.2X2	T47.2X3	T47.2X4	T47.2X5	T47.2X6
Daphne (gnidium) (mezereum)	T62.2X1	T62.2X2	T62.2X3	T62.2X4	—	—
berry	T62.1X1	T62.1X2	T62.1X3	T62.1X4	—	—
Dapsone	T37.1X1	T37.1X2	T37.1X3	T37.1X4	T37.1X5	T37.1X6
Daraprim	T37.2X1	T37.2X2	T37.2X3	T37.2X4	T37.2X5	T37.2X6
Darnel	T62.2X1	T62.2X2	T62.2X3	T62.2X4	—	—
Darvon	T39.8X1	T39.8X2	T39.8X3	T39.8X4	T39.8X5	T39.8X6
Daunomycin	T45.1X1	T45.1X2	T45.1X3	T45.1X4	T45.1X5	T45.1X6
Daunorubicin	T45.1X1	T45.1X2	T45.1X3	T45.1X4	T45.1X5	T45.1X6
DBI	T38.3X1	T38.3X2	T38.3X3	T38.3X4	T38.3X5	T38.3X6
D-Con	T60.91	T60.92	T60.93	T60.94	—	—
insecticide	T60.2X1	T60.2X2	T60.2X3	T60.2X4	—	—
rodenticide	T60.4X1	T60.4X2	T60.4X3	T60.4X4	—	—
DDAVP	T38.891	T38.892	T38.893	T38.894	T38.895	T38.896
DDE (bis(chlorophenyl)-dichloroethylene)	T60.2X1	T60.2X2	T60.2X3	T60.2X4	—	—
DDS	T37.1X1	T37.1X2	T37.1X3	T37.1X4	T37.1X5	T37.1X6
DDT (dust)	T60.1X1	T60.1X2	T60.1X3	T60.1X4	—	—
Deadly nightshade — see also Belladonna	T62.2X1	T62.2X2	T62.2X3	T62.2X4	—	—
berry	T62.1X1	T62.1X2	T62.1X3	T62.1X4	—	—
Deamino-D-arginine vasopressin	T38.891	T38.892	T38.893	T38.894	T38.895	T38.896
Deanol (aceglumate)	T50.991	T50.992	T50.993	T50.994	T50.995	T50.996
Debrisoquine	T46.5X1	T46.5X2	T46.5X3	T46.5X4	T46.5X5	T46.5X6
Decaborane	T57.8X1	T57.8X2	T57.8X3	T57.8X4	—	—
fumes	T59.891	T59.892	T59.893	T59.894	—	—
Decadron	T38.0X1	T38.0X2	T38.0X3	T38.0X4	T38.0X5	T38.0X6
ENT agent	T49.6X1	T49.6X2	T49.6X3	T49.6X4	T49.6X5	T49.6X6
ophthalmic preparation	T49.5X1	T49.5X2	T49.5X3	T49.5X4	T49.5X5	T49.5X6
topical NEC	T49.0X1	T49.0X2	T49.0X3	T49.0X4	T49.0X5	T49.0X6
Decahydronaphthalene	T52.8X1	T52.8X2	T52.8X3	T52.8X4	—	—
Decalin	T52.8X1	T52.8X2	T52.8X3	T52.8X4	—	—
Decamethonium (bromide)	T48.1X1	T48.1X2	T48.1X3	T48.1X4	T48.1X5	T48.1X6
Decholin	T47.5X1	T47.5X2	T47.5X3	T47.5X4	T47.5X5	T47.5X6
Declomycin	T36.4X1	T36.4X2	T36.4X3	T36.4X4	T36.4X5	T36.4X6
Decongestant, nasal (mucosa)	T48.5X1	T48.5X2	T48.5X3	T48.5X4	T48.5X5	T48.5X6
combination	T48.5X1	T48.5X2	T48.5X3	T48.5X4	T48.5X5	T48.5X6
Deet	T60.8X1	T60.8X2	T60.8X3	T60.8X4	—	—
Deferoxamine	T45.8X1	T45.8X2	T45.8X3	T45.8X4	T45.8X5	T45.8X6
Deflazacort	T38.0X1	T38.0X2	T38.0X3	T38.0X4	T38.0X5	T38.0X6
Deglycyrrhizinized extract of licorice	T48.4X1	T48.4X2	T48.4X3	T48.4X4	T48.4X5	T48.4X6
Dehydrocholic acid	T47.5X1	T47.5X2	T47.5X3	T47.5X4	T47.5X5	T47.5X6
Dehydroemetine	T37.3X1	T37.3X2	T37.3X3	T37.3X4	T37.3X5	T37.3X6
Dekalin	T52.8X1	T52.8X2	T52.8X3	T52.8X4	—	—
Delalutin	T38.5X1	T38.5X2	T38.5X3	T38.5X4	T38.5X5	T38.5X6
Delorazepam	T42.4X1	T42.4X2	T42.4X3	T42.4X4	T42.4X5	T42.4X6
Delphinium	T62.2X1	T62.2X2	T62.2X3	T62.2X4	—	—
Deltamethrin	T60.1X1	T60.1X2	T60.1X3	T60.1X4	—	—
Deltasone	T38.0X1	T38.0X2	T38.0X3	T38.0X4	T38.0X5	T38.0X6
Deltra	T38.0X1	T38.0X2	T38.0X3	T38.0X4	T38.0X5	T38.0X6
Delvinal	T42.3X1	T42.3X2	T42.3X3	T42.3X4	T42.3X5	T42.3X6
Demecarium (bromide)	T49.5X1	T49.5X2	T49.5X3	T49.5X4	T49.5X5	T49.5X6
Demeclocycline	T36.4X1	T36.4X2	T36.4X3	T36.4X4	T36.4X5	T36.4X6
Demecolcine	T45.1X1	T45.1X2	T45.1X3	T45.1X4	T45.1X5	T45.1X6
Demegestone	T38.5X1	T38.5X2	T38.5X3	T38.5X4	T38.5X5	T38.5X6
Demelanizing agents	T49.8X1	T49.8X2	T49.8X3	T49.8X4	T49.8X5	T49.8X6
Demephion -O and -S	T60.0X1	T60.0X2	T60.0X3	T60.0X4	—	—
Demerol	T40.2X1	T40.2X2	T40.2X3	T40.2X4	T40.2X5	T40.2X6
Demethylchlortetracycline	T36.4X1	T36.4X2	T36.4X3	T36.4X4	T36.4X5	T36.4X6
Demethyltetracycline	T36.4X1	T36.4X2	T36.4X3	T36.4X4	T36.4X5	T36.4X6
Demeton -O and -S	T60.0X1	T60.0X2	T60.0X3	T60.0X4	—	—

Substance	Poisoning, Accidental (unintentional)	Poisoning, Intentional Self-harm	Poisoning, Assault	Poisoning, Undetermined	Adverse Effect	Under-dosing
Demulcent (external)	T49.3X1	T49.3X2	T49.3X3	T49.3X4	T49.3X5	T49.3X6
specified NEC	T49.3X1	T49.3X2	T49.3X3	T49.3X4	T49.3X5	T49.3X6
Demulen	T38.4X1	T38.4X2	T38.4X3	T38.4X4	T38.4X5	T38.4X6
Denatured alcohol	T51.0X1	T51.0X2	T51.0X3	T51.0X4		
Dendrid	T49.5X1	T49.5X2	T49.5X3	T49.5X4	T49.5X5	T49.5X6
Dental drug, topical application NEC	T49.7X1	T49.7X2	T49.7X3	T49.7X4	T49.7X5	T49.7X6
Dentifrice	T49.7X1	T49.7X2	T49.7X3	T49.7X4	T49.7X5	T49.7X6
Deodorant spray (feminine hygiene)	T49.8X1	T49.8X2	T49.8X3	T49.8X4	T49.8X5	T49.8X6
Deoxycortone	T50.0X1	T50.0X2	T50.0X3	T50.0X4	T50.0X5	T50.0X6
Deoxyribonuclease (pancreatic)	T45.3X1	T45.3X2	T45.3X3	T45.3X4	T45.3X5	T45.3X6
Depilatory	T49.4X1	T49.4X2	T49.4X3	T49.4X4	T49.4X5	T49.4X6
Deprenalin	T42.8X1	T42.8X2	T42.8X3	T42.8X4	T42.8X5	T42.8X6
Deprenyl	T42.8X1	T42.8X2	T42.8X3	T42.8X4	T42.8X5	T42.8X6
Depressant						
appetite (central)	T50.5X1	T50.5X2	T50.5X3	T50.5X4	T50.5X5	T50.5X6
cardiac	T46.2X1	T46.2X2	T46.2X3	T46.2X4	T46.2X5	T46.2X6
central nervous system (anesthetic) — see also Central nervous system, depressants	T42.71	T42.72	T42.73	T42.74	T42.75	T42.76
general anesthetic	T41.201	T41.202	T41.203	T41.204	T41.205	T41.206
muscle tone	T42.8X1	T42.8X2	T42.8X3	T42.8X4	T42.8X5	T42.8X6
muscle tone, central	T42.8X1	T42.8X2	T42.8X3	T42.8X4	T42.8X5	T42.8X6
psychotherapeutic	T43.501	T43.502	T43.503	T43.504	T43.505	T43.506
Depressant, appetite	T50.5X1	T50.5X2	T50.5X3	T50.5X4	T50.5X5	T50.5X6
Deptropine	T45.0X1	T45.0X2	T45.0X3	T45.0X4	T45.0X5	T45.0X6
Dequalinium (chloride)	T49.0X1	T49.0X2	T49.0X3	T49.0X4	T49.0X5	T49.0X6
Derris root	T60.2X1	T60.2X2	T60.2X3	T60.2X4	—	—
Deserpidine	T46.5X1	T46.5X2	T46.5X3	T46.5X4	T46.5X5	T46.5X6
Desferrioxamine	T45.8X1	T45.8X2	T45.8X3	T45.8X4	T45.8X5	T45.8X6
Desipramine	T43.011	T43.012	T43.013	T43.014	T43.015	T43.016
Deslanoside	T46.0X1	T46.0X2	T46.0X3	T46.0X4	T46.0X5	T46.0X6
Desloughing agent	T49.4X1	T49.4X2	T49.4X3	T49.4X4	T49.4X5	T49.4X6
Desmethylimipramine	T43.011	T43.012	T43.013	T43.014	T43.015	T43.016
Desmopressin	T38.891	T38.892	T38.893	T38.894	T38.895	T38.896
Desocodeine	T40.2X1	T40.2X2	T40.2X3	T40.2X4	T40.2X5	T40.2X6
Desogestrel	T38.5X1	T38.5X2	T38.5X3	T38.5X4	T38.5X5	T38.5X6
Desomorphine	T40.2X1	T40.2X2	T40.2X3	T40.2X4	—	—
Desonide	T49.0X1	T49.0X2	T49.0X3	T49.0X4	T49.0X5	T49.0X6
Desoximetasone	T49.0X1	T49.0X2	T49.0X3	T49.0X4	T49.0X5	T49.0X6
Desoxycorticosteroid	T50.0X1	T50.0X2	T50.0X3	T50.0X4	T50.0X5	T50.0X6
Desoxycortone	T50.0X1	T50.0X2	T50.0X3	T50.0X4	T50.0X5	T50.0X6
Desoxyephedrine	T43.621	T43.622	T43.623	T43.624	T43.625	T43.626
Detaxtran	T46.6X1	T46.6X2	T46.6X3	T46.6X4	T46.6X5	T46.6X6
Detergent	T49.2X1	T49.2X2	T49.2X3	T49.2X4	T49.2X5	T49.2X6
external medication	T49.2X1	T49.2X2	T49.2X3	T49.2X4	T49.2X5	T49.2X6
local	T49.2X1	T49.2X2	T49.2X3	T49.2X4	T49.2X5	T49.2X6
medicinal	T49.2X1	T49.2X2	T49.2X3	T49.2X4	T49.2X5	T49.2X6
nonmedicinal	T55.1X1	T55.1X2	T55.1X3	T55.1X4	—	—
specified NEC	T55.1X1	T55.1X2	T55.1X3	T55.1X4	—	—
Deterrent, alcohol	T50.6X1	T50.6X2	T50.6X3	T50.6X4	T50.6X5	T50.6X6
Detoxifying agent	T50.6X1	T50.6X2	T50.6X3	T50.6X4	T50.6X5	T50.6X6
Detrothyronine	T38.1X1	T38.1X2	T38.1X3	T38.1X4	T38.1X5	T38.1X6
Dettol (external medication)	T49.0X1	T49.0X2	T49.0X3	T49.0X4	T49.0X5	T49.0X6
Dexamethasone	T38.0X1	T38.0X2	T38.0X3	T38.0X4	T38.0X5	T38.0X6
ENT agent	T49.6X1	T49.6X2	T49.6X3	T49.6X4	T49.6X5	T49.6X6
ophthalmic preparation	T49.5X1	T49.5X2	T49.5X3	T49.5X4	T49.5X5	T49.5X6
topical NEC	T49.0X1	T49.0X2	T49.0X3	T49.0X4	T49.0X5	T49.0X6
Dexamfetamine	T43.621	T43.622	T43.623	T43.624	T43.625	T43.626
Dexamphetamine	T43.621	T43.622	T43.623	T43.624	T43.625	T43.626
Dexbrompheniramine	T45.0X1	T45.0X2	T45.0X3	T45.0X4	T45.0X5	T45.0X6
Dexchlorpheniramine	T45.0X1	T45.0X2	T45.0X3	T45.0X4	T45.0X5	T45.0X6
Dexedrine	T43.621	T43.622	T43.623	T43.624	T43.625	T43.626
Dexetimide	T44.3X1	T44.3X2	T44.3X3	T44.3X4	T44.3X5	T44.3X6
Dexfenfluramine	T50.5X1	T50.5X2	T50.5X3	T50.5X4	T50.5X5	T50.5X6
Dexpanthenol	T45.2X1	T45.2X2	T45.2X3	T45.2X4	T45.2X5	T45.2X6
Dextran (40) (70) (150)	T45.8X1	T45.8X2	T45.8X3	T45.8X4	T45.8X5	T45.8X6
Dextriferron	T45.4X1	T45.4X2	T45.4X3	T45.4X4	T45.4X5	T45.4X6
Dextroamphetamine	T43.621	T43.622	T43.623	T43.624	T43.625	T43.626
Dextro calcium pantothenate	T45.2X1	T45.2X2	T45.2X3	T45.2X4	T45.2X5	T45.2X6
Dextromethorphan	T48.3X1	T48.3X2	T48.3X3	T48.3X4	T48.3X5	T48.3X6
Dextromoramide	T40.4X1	T40.4X2	T40.4X3	T40.4X4		
topical	T49.8X1	T49.8X2	T49.8X3	T49.8X4	T49.8X5	T49.8X6
Dextro pantothenyl alcohol	T45.2X1	T45.2X2	T45.2X3	T45.2X4	T45.2X5	T45.2X6
Dextropropoxyphene	T40.4X1	T40.4X2	T40.4X3	T40.4X4	T40.4X5	T40.4X6
Dextrorphan	T40.2X1	T40.2X2	T40.2X3	T40.2X4	T40.2X5	T40.2X6
Dextrose	T50.3X1	T50.3X2	T50.3X3	T50.3X4	T50.3X5	T50.3X6

Substance	Poisoning, Accidental (unintentional)	Poisoning, Intentional Self-harm	Poisoning, Assault	Poisoning, Undetermined	Adverse Effect	Under-dosing
Dextrose — *continued*						
concentrated solution, intravenous	T46.8X1	T46.8X2	T46.8X3	T46.8X4	T46.8X5	T46.8X6
Dextrothyroxin	T38.1X1	T38.1X2	T38.1X3	T38.1X4	T38.1X5	T38.1X6
Dextrothyroxine sodium	T38.1X1	T38.1X2	T38.1X3	T38.1X4	T38.1X5	T38.1X6
DFP	T44.0X1	T44.0X2	T44.0X3	T44.0X4	T44.0X5	T44.0X6
DHE	T37.3X1	T37.3X2	T37.3X3	T37.3X4	T37.3X5	T37.3X6
45	T46.5X1	T46.5X2	T46.5X3	T46.5X4	T46.5X5	T46.5X6
Diabinese	T38.3X1	T38.3X2	T38.3X3	T38.3X4	T38.3X5	T38.3X6
Diacetone alcohol	T52.4X1	T52.4X2	T52.4X3	T52.4X4	—	—
Diacetyl monoxime	T50.991	T50.992	T50.993	T50.994	—	—
Diacetylmorphine	T40.1X1	T40.1X2	T40.1X3	T40.1X4	—	—
Diachylon plaster	T49.4X1	T49.4X2	T49.4X3	T49.4X4	T49.4X5	T49.4X6
Diaethylstilboestrolum	T38.5X1	T38.5X2	T38.5X3	T38.5X4	T38.5X5	T38.5X6
Diagnostic agent NEC	T50.8X1	T50.8X2	T50.8X3	T50.8X4	T50.8X5	T50.8X6
Dial (soap)	T49.2X1	T49.2X2	T49.2X3	T49.2X4	T49.2X5	T49.2X6
sedative	T42.3X1	T42.3X2	T42.3X3	T42.3X4	T42.3X5	T42.3X6
Dialkyl carbonate	T52.91	T52.92	T52.93	T52.94	—	—
Diallylbarbituric acid	T42.3X1	T42.3X2	T42.3X3	T42.3X4	T42.3X5	T42.3X6
Diallymal	T42.3X1	T42.3X2	T42.3X3	T42.3X4	T42.3X5	T42.3X6
Dialysis solution (intraperitoneal)	T50.3X1	T50.3X2	T50.3X3	T50.3X4	T50.3X5	T50.3X6
Diaminodiphenylsulfone	T37.1X1	T37.1X2	T37.1X3	T37.1X4	T37.1X5	T37.1X6
Diamorphine	T40.1X1	T40.1X2	T40.1X3	T40.1X4	—	—
Diamox	T50.2X1	T50.2X2	T50.2X3	T50.2X4	T50.2X5	T50.2X6
Diamthazole	T49.0X1	T49.0X2	T49.0X3	T49.0X4	T49.0X5	T49.0X6
Dianthone	T47.2X1	T47.2X2	T47.2X3	T47.2X4	T47.2X5	T47.2X6
Diaphenylsulfone	T37.0X1	T37.0X2	T37.0X3	T37.0X4	T37.0X5	T37.0X6
Diasone (sodium)	T37.1X1	T37.1X2	T37.1X3	T37.1X4	T37.1X5	T37.1X6
Diastase	T47.5X1	T47.5X2	T47.5X3	T47.5X4	T47.5X5	T47.5X6
Diatrizoate	T50.8X1	T50.8X2	T50.8X3	T50.8X4	T50.8X5	T50.8X6
Diazepam	T42.4X1	T42.4X2	T42.4X3	T42.4X4	T42.4X5	T42.4X6
Diazinon	T60.0X1	T60.0X2	T60.0X3	T60.0X4	—	—
Diazomethane (gas)	T59.891	T59.892	T59.893	T59.894	—	—
Diazoxide	T46.5X1	T46.5X2	T46.5X3	T46.5X4	T46.5X5	T46.5X6
Dibekacin	T36.5X1	T36.5X2	T36.5X3	T36.5X4	T36.5X5	T36.5X6
Dibenamine	T44.6X1	T44.6X2	T44.6X3	T44.6X4	T44.6X5	T44.6X6
Dibenzepin	T43.011	T43.012	T43.013	T43.014	T43.015	T43.016
Dibenzheptropine	T45.0X1	T45.0X2	T45.0X3	T45.0X4	T45.0X5	T45.0X6
Dibenzyline	T44.6X1	T44.6X2	T44.6X3	T44.6X4	T44.6X5	T44.6X6
Diborane (gas)	T59.891	T59.892	T59.893	T59.894	—	—
Dibromochloropropane	T60.8X1	T60.8X2	T60.8X3	T60.8X4	—	—
Dibromodulcitol	T45.1X1	T45.1X2	T45.1X3	T45.1X4	T45.1X5	T45.1X6
Dibromoethane	T53.6X1	T53.6X2	T53.6X3	T53.6X4	—	—
Dibromomannitol	T45.1X1	T45.1X2	T45.1X3	T45.1X4	T45.1X5	T45.1X6
Dibromopropamidine isethionate	T49.0X1	T49.0X2	T49.0X3	T49.0X4	T49.0X5	T49.0X6
Dibrompropamidine	T49.0X1	T49.0X2	T49.0X3	T49.0X4	T49.0X5	T49.0X6
Dibucaine	T41.3X1	T41.3X2	T41.3X3	T41.3X4	T41.3X5	T41.3X6
topical (surface)	T41.3X1	T41.3X2	T41.3X3	T41.3X4	T41.3X5	T41.3X6
Dibunate sodium	T48.3X1	T48.3X2	T48.3X3	T48.3X4	T48.3X5	T48.3X6
Dibutoline sulfate	T44.3X1	T44.3X2	T44.3X3	T44.3X4	T44.3X5	T44.3X6
Dicamba	T60.3X1	T60.3X2	T60.3X3	T60.3X4	—	—
Dicapthon	T60.0X1	T60.0X2	T60.0X3	T60.0X4	—	—
Dichlobenil	T60.3X1	T60.3X2	T60.3X3	T60.3X4	—	—
Dichlone	T60.3X1	T60.3X2	T60.3X3	T60.3X4	—	—
Dichloralphenozone	T42.6X1	T42.6X2	T42.6X3	T42.6X4	T42.6X5	T42.6X6
Dichlorbenzidine	T65.3X1	T65.3X2	T65.3X3	T65.3X4	—	—
Dichlorhydrin	T52.8X1	T52.8X2	T52.8X3	T52.8X4	—	—
Dichlorhydroxyquinoline	T37.8X1	T37.8X2	T37.8X3	T37.8X4	T37.8X5	T37.8X6
Dichlorobenzene	T53.7X1	T53.7X2	T53.7X3	T53.7X4	—	—
Dichlorobenzyl alcohol	T49.6X1	T49.6X2	T49.6X3	T49.6X4	T49.6X5	T49.6X6
Dichlorodifluoromethane	T53.5X1	T53.5X2	T53.5X3	T53.5X4	—	—
Dichloroethane	T52.8X1	T52.8X2	T52.8X3	T52.8X4	—	—
Dichloroethylene	T53.6X1	T53.6X2	T53.6X3	T53.6X4	—	—
Dichloroethyl sulfide, not in war	T59.891	T59.892	T59.893	T59.894	—	—
Dichloroformoxine, not in war	T59.891	T59.892	T59.893	T59.894	—	—
Dichlorohydrin, alpha-dichlorohydrin	T52.8X1	T52.8X2	T52.8X3	T52.8X4	—	—
Dichloromethane (solvent)	T53.4X1	T53.4X2	T53.4X3	T53.4X4	—	—
vapor	T53.4X1	T53.4X2	T53.4X3	T53.4X4	—	—
Dichloronaphthoquinone	T60.3X1	T60.3X2	T60.3X3	T60.3X4	—	—
Dichlorophen	T37.4X1	T37.4X2	T37.4X3	T37.4X4	T37.4X5	T37.4X6
Dichloropropene	T60.3X1	T60.3X2	T60.3X3	T60.3X4	—	—
Dichloropropionic acid	T60.3X1	T60.3X2	T60.3X3	T60.3X4	—	—
Dichlorphenamide	T50.2X1	T50.2X2	T50.2X3	T50.2X4	T50.2X5	T50.2X6
Dichlorvos	T60.0X1	T60.0X2	T60.0X3	T60.0X4	—	—
Diclofenac	T39.391	T39.392	T39.393	T39.394	T39.395	T39.396
Diclofenamide	T50.2X1	T50.2X2	T50.2X3	T50.2X4	T50.2X5	T50.2X6
Diclofensine	T43.291	T43.292	T43.293	T43.294	T43.295	T43.296
Diclonixine	T39.8X1	T39.8X2	T39.8X3	T39.8X4	T39.8X5	T39.8X6
Dicloxacillin	T36.0X1	T36.0X2	T36.0X3	T36.0X4	T36.0X5	T36.0X6
Dicophane	T49.0X1	T49.0X2	T49.0X3	T49.0X4	T49.0X5	T49.0X6
Dicoumarol, dicoumarin, dicumarol	T45.511	T45.512	T45.513	T45.514	T45.515	T45.516
Dicrotophos	T60.0X1	T60.0X2	T60.0X3	T60.0X4	—	—
Dicyanogen (gas)	T65.0X1	T65.0X2	T65.0X3	T65.0X4	—	—
Dicyclomine	T44.3X1	T44.3X2	T44.3X3	T44.3X4	T44.3X5	T44.3X6
Dicycloverine	T44.3X1	T44.3X2	T44.3X3	T44.3X4	T44.3X5	T44.3X6
Dideoxycytidine	T37.5X1	T37.5X2	T37.5X3	T37.5X4	T37.5X5	T37.5X6
Dideoxyinosine	T37.5X1	T37.5X2	T37.5X3	T37.5X4	T37.5X5	T37.5X6
Dieldrin (vapor)	T60.1X1	T60.1X2	T60.1X3	T60.1X4	—	—
Diemal	T42.3X1	T42.3X2	T42.3X3	T42.3X4	T42.3X5	T42.3X6
Dienestrol	T38.5X1	T38.5X2	T38.5X3	T38.5X4	T38.5X5	T38.5X6
Dienoestrol	T38.5X1	T38.5X2	T38.5X3	T38.5X4	T38.5X5	T38.5X6
Dietetic drug NEC	T50.901	T50.902	T50.903	T50.904	T50.905	T50.906
Diethazine	T42.8X1	T42.8X2	T42.8X3	T42.8X4	T42.8X5	T42.8X6
Diethyl						
barbituric acid	T42.3X1	T42.3X2	T42.3X3	T42.3X4	T42.3X5	T42.3X6
carbamazine	T37.4X1	T37.4X2	T37.4X3	T37.4X4	T37.4X5	T37.4X6
carbinol	T51.3X1	T51.3X2	T51.3X3	T51.3X4	—	—
carbonate	T52.8X1	T52.8X2	T52.8X3	T52.8X4	—	—
ether (vapor) — *see also* ether	T41.0X1	T41.0X2	T41.0X3	T41.0X4	T41.0X5	T41.0X6
oxide	T52.8X1	T52.8X2	T52.8X3	T52.8X4	—	—
propion	T50.5X1	T50.5X2	T50.5X3	T50.5X4	T50.5X5	T50.5X6
stilbestrol	T38.5X1	T38.5X2	T38.5X3	T38.5X4	T38.5X5	T38.5X6
toluamide (nonmedicinal)	T60.8X1	T60.8X2	T60.8X3	T60.8X4	—	—
medicinal	T49.3X1	T49.3X2	T49.3X3	T49.3X4	T49.3X5	T49.3X6
Diethylcarbamazine	T37.4X1	T37.4X2	T37.4X3	T37.4X4	T37.4X5	T37.4X6
Diethylene						
dioxide	T52.8X1	T52.8X2	T52.8X3	T52.8X4	—	—
glycol (monoacetate) (monobutyl ether) (monoethyl ether)	T52.3X1	T52.3X2	T52.3X3	T52.3X4	—	—
Diethylhexylphthalate	T65.891	T65.892	T65.893	T65.894	—	—
Diethylpropion	T50.5X1	T50.5X2	T50.5X3	T50.5X4	T50.5X5	T50.5X6
Diethylstilbestrol	T38.5X1	T38.5X2	T38.5X3	T38.5X4	T38.5X5	T38.5X6
Diethylstilboestrol	T38.5X1	T38.5X2	T38.5X3	T38.5X4	T38.5X5	T38.5X6
Diethylsulfone-diethylmethane	T42.6X1	T42.6X2	T42.6X3	T42.6X4	T42.6X5	T42.6X6
Diethyltoluamide	T49.0X1	T49.0X2	T49.0X3	T49.0X4	T49.0X5	T49.0X6
Diethyltryptamine (DET)	T40.991	T40.992	T40.993	T40.994	—	—
Difebarbamate	T42.3X1	T42.3X2	T42.3X3	T42.3X4	T42.3X5	T42.3X6
Difencloxazine	T40.2X1	T40.2X2	T40.2X3	T40.2X4	T40.2X5	T40.2X6
Difenidol	T45.0X1	T45.0X2	T45.0X3	T45.0X4	T45.0X5	T45.0X6
Difenoxin	T47.6X1	T47.6X2	T47.6X3	T47.6X4	T47.6X5	T47.6X6
Difetarsone	T37.3X1	T37.3X2	T37.3X3	T37.3X4	T37.3X5	T37.3X6
Diffusin	T45.3X1	T45.3X2	T45.3X3	T45.3X4	T45.3X5	T45.3X6
Diflorasone	T49.0X1	T49.0X2	T49.0X3	T49.0X4	T49.0X5	T49.0X6
Diflos	T44.0X1	T44.0X2	T44.0X3	T44.0X4	—	T44.0X6
Diflubenzuron	T60.1X1	T60.1X2	T60.1X3	T60.1X4	—	—
Diflucortolone	T49.0X1	T49.0X2	T49.0X3	T49.0X4	T49.0X5	T49.0X6
Diflunisal	T39.091	T39.092	T39.093	T39.094	T39.095	T39.096
Difluoromethyldopa	T42.8X1	T42.8X2	T42.8X3	T42.8X4	T42.8X5	T42.8X6
Difluorophate	T44.0X1	T44.0X2	T44.0X3	T44.0X4	T44.0X5	T44.0X6
Digestant NEC	T47.5X1	T47.5X2	T47.5X3	T47.5X4	T47.5X5	T47.5X6
Digitalin (e)	T46.0X1	T46.0X2	T46.0X3	T46.0X4	T46.0X5	T46.0X6
Digitalis (leaf)(glycoside)	T46.0X1	T46.0X2	T46.0X3	T46.0X4	T46.0X5	T46.0X6
lanata	T46.0X1	T46.0X2	T46.0X3	T46.0X4	T46.0X5	T46.0X6
purpurea	T46.0X1	T46.0X2	T46.0X3	T46.0X4	T46.0X5	T46.0X6
Digitoxin	T46.0X1	T46.0X2	T46.0X3	T46.0X4	T46.0X5	T46.0X6
Digitoxose	T46.0X1	T46.0X2	T46.0X3	T46.0X4	T46.0X5	T46.0X6
Digoxin	T46.0X1	T46.0X2	T46.0X3	T46.0X4	T46.0X5	T46.0X6
Digoxine	T46.0X1	T46.0X2	T46.0X3	T46.0X4	T46.0X5	T46.0X6
Dihydralazine	T46.5X1	T46.5X2	T46.5X3	T46.5X4	T46.5X5	T46.5X6
Dihydrazine	T46.5X1	T46.5X2	T46.5X3	T46.5X4	T46.5X5	T46.5X6
Dihydrocodeine	T40.2X1	T40.2X2	T40.2X3	T40.2X4	T40.2X5	T40.2X6
Dihydrocodeinone	T40.2X1	T40.2X2	T40.2X3	T40.2X4	T40.2X5	T40.2X6
Dihydroergocornine	T46.7X1	T46.7X2	T46.7X3	T46.7X4	T46.7X5	T46.7X6
Dihydroergocristine (mesilate)	T46.7X1	T46.7X2	T46.7X3	T46.7X4	T46.7X5	T46.7X6
Dihydroergokryptine	T46.7X1	T46.7X2	T46.7X3	T46.7X4	T46.7X5	T46.7X6
Dihydroergotamine	T46.5X1	T46.5X2	T46.5X3	T46.5X4	T46.5X5	T46.5X6
Dihydroergotoxine	T46.7X1	T46.7X2	T46.7X3	T46.7X4	T46.7X5	T46.7X6
mesilate	T46.7X1	T46.7X2	T46.7X3	T46.7X4	T46.7X5	T46.7X6
Dihydrohydroxycodeinone	T40.2X1	T40.2X2	T40.2X3	T40.2X4	T40.2X5	T40.2X6
Dihydrohydroxymorphinone	T40.2X1	T40.2X2	T40.2X3	T40.2X4	T40.2X5	T40.2X6
Dihydroisocodeine	T40.2X1	T40.2X2	T40.2X3	T40.2X4	T40.2X5	T40.2X6
Dihydromorphine	T40.2X1	T40.2X2	T40.2X3	T40.2X4	—	—
Dihydromorphinone	T40.2X1	T40.2X2	T40.2X3	T40.2X4	T40.2X5	T40.2X6
Dihydrostreptomycin	T36.5X1	T36.5X2	T36.5X3	T36.5X4	T36.5X5	T36.5X6
Dihydrotachysterol	T45.2X1	T45.2X2	T45.2X3	T45.2X4	T45.2X5	T45.2X6
Dihydroxyaluminum aminoacetate	T47.1X1	T47.1X2	T47.1X3	T47.1X4	T47.1X5	T47.1X6

▽ Subterms under main terms may continue to next column or page   Additional Character May Be Required — Refer to the Tabular List for Character Selection   365

Dextrose — Dihydroxyaluminum aminoacetate

Table of Drugs and Chemicals

Dihydroxyaluminum sodium carbonate — DNOC

Substance	Poisoning, Accidental (unintentional)	Poisoning, Intentional Self-harm	Poisoning, Assault	Poisoning, Undetermined	Adverse Effect	Under-dosing
Dihydroxyaluminum sodium carbonate	T47.1X1	T47.1X2	T47.1X3	T47.1X4	T47.1X5	T47.1X6
Dihydroxyanthraquinone	T47.2X1	T47.2X2	T47.2X3	T47.2X4	T47.2X5	T47.2X6
Dihydroxycodeinone	T40.2X1	T40.2X2	T40.2X3	T40.2X4	T40.2X5	T40.2X6
Dihydroxypropyl theophylline	T50.2X1	T50.2X2	T50.2X3	T50.2X4	T50.2X5	T50.2X6
Diiodohydroxyquin	T37.8X1	T37.8X2	T37.8X3	T37.8X4	T37.8X5	T37.8X6
topical	T49.0X1	T49.0X2	T49.0X3	T49.0X4	T49.0X5	T49.0X6
Diiodohydroxyquinoline	T37.8X1	T37.8X2	T37.8X3	T37.8X4	T37.8X5	T37.8X6
Diiodotyrosine	T38.2X1	T38.2X2	T38.2X3	T38.2X4	T38.2X5	T38.2X6
Diisopromine	T44.3X1	T44.3X2	T44.3X3	T44.3X4	T44.3X5	T44.3X6
Diisopropylamine	T46.3X1	T46.3X2	T46.3X3	T46.3X4	T46.3X5	T46.3X6
Diisopropylfluorophosphonate	T44.0X1	T44.0X2	T44.0X3	T44.0X4	T44.0X5	T44.0X6
Dilantin	T42.0X1	T42.0X2	T42.0X3	T42.0X4	T42.0X5	T42.0X6
Dilaudid	T40.2X1	T40.2X2	T40.2X3	T40.2X4	T40.2X5	T40.2X6
Dilazep	T46.3X1	T46.3X2	T46.3X3	T46.3X4	T46.3X5	T46.3X6
Dill	T47.5X1	T47.5X2	T47.5X3	T47.5X4	T47.5X5	T47.5X6
Diloxanide	T37.3X1	T37.3X2	T37.3X3	T37.3X4	T37.3X5	T37.3X6
Diltiazem	T46.1X1	T46.1X2	T46.1X3	T46.1X4	T46.1X5	T46.1X6
Dimazole	T49.0X1	T49.0X2	T49.0X3	T49.0X4	T49.0X5	T49.0X6
Dimefline	T50.7X1	T50.7X2	T50.7X3	T50.7X4	T50.7X5	T50.7X6
Dimefox	T60.0X1	T60.0X2	T60.0X3	T60.0X4	—	—
Dimemorfan	T48.3X1	T48.3X2	T48.3X3	T48.3X4	T48.3X5	T48.3X6
Dimenhydrinate	T45.0X1	T45.0X2	T45.0X3	T45.0X4	T45.0X5	T45.0X6
Dimercaprol (British anti-lewisite)	T45.8X1	T45.8X2	T45.8X3	T45.8X4	T45.8X5	T45.8X6
Dimercaptopropanol	T45.8X1	T45.8X2	T45.8X3	T45.8X4	T45.8X5	T45.8X6
Dimestrol	T38.5X1	T38.5X2	T38.5X3	T38.5X4	T38.5X5	T38.5X6
Dimetane	T45.0X1	T45.0X2	T45.0X3	T45.0X4	T45.0X5	T45.0X6
Dimethicone	T47.1X1	T47.1X2	T47.1X3	T47.1X4	T47.1X5	T47.1X6
Dimethindene	T45.0X1	T45.0X2	T45.0X3	T45.0X4	T45.0X5	T45.0X6
Dimethisoquin	T49.1X1	T49.1X2	T49.1X3	T49.1X4	T49.1X5	T49.1X6
Dimethisterone	T38.5X1	T38.5X2	T38.5X3	T38.5X4	T38.5X5	T38.5X6
Dimethoate	T60.0X1	T60.0X2	T60.0X3	T60.0X4	—	—
Dimethocaine	T41.3X1	T41.3X2	T41.3X3	T41.3X4	T41.3X5	T41.3X6
Dimethoxanate	T48.3X1	T48.3X2	T48.3X3	T48.3X4	T48.3X5	T48.3X6
Dimethyl						
arsine, arsinic acid	T57.0X1	T57.0X2	T57.0X3	T57.0X4	—	—
carbinol	T51.2X1	T51.2X2	T51.2X3	T51.2X4	—	—
carbonate	T52.8X1	T52.8X2	T52.8X3	T52.8X4	—	—
diguanide	T38.3X1	T38.3X2	T38.3X3	T38.3X4	T38.3X5	T38.3X6
ketone	T52.4X1	T52.4X2	T52.4X3	T52.4X4	—	—
vapor	T52.4X1	T52.4X2	T52.4X3	T52.4X4	—	—
meperidine	T40.2X1	T40.2X2	T40.2X3	T40.2X4	T40.2X5	T40.2X6
parathion	T60.0X1	T60.0X2	T60.0X3	T60.0X4	—	—
phthlate	T49.3X1	T49.3X2	T49.3X3	T49.3X4	T49.3X5	T49.3X6
polysiloxane	T47.8X1	T47.8X2	T47.8X3	T47.8X4	T47.8X5	T47.8X6
sulfate (fumes)	T59.891	T59.892	T59.893	T59.894	—	—
liquid	T65.891	T65.892	T65.893	T65.894	—	—
sulfoxide (nonmedicinal)	T52.8X1	T52.8X2	T52.8X3	T52.8X4	—	—
medicinal	T49.4X1	T49.4X2	T49.4X3	T49.4X4	T49.4X5	T49.4X6
tryptamine	T40.991	T40.992	T40.993	T40.994	—	—
tubocurarine	T48.1X1	T48.1X2	T48.1X3	T48.1X4	T48.1X5	T48.1X6
Dimethylamine sulfate	T49.4X1	T49.4X2	T49.4X3	T49.4X4	T49.4X5	T49.4X6
Dimethylformamide	T52.8X1	T52.8X2	T52.8X3	T52.8X4	—	—
Dimethyltubocurarinium chloride	T48.1X1	T48.1X2	T48.1X3	T48.1X4	T48.1X5	T48.1X6
Dimeticone	T47.1X1	T47.1X2	T47.1X3	T47.1X4	T47.1X5	T47.1X6
Dimetilan	T60.0X1	T60.0X2	T60.0X3	T60.0X4	—	—
Dimetindene	T45.0X1	T45.0X2	T45.0X3	T45.0X4	T45.0X5	T45.0X6
Dimetotiazine	T43.3X1	T43.3X2	T43.3X3	T43.3X4	T43.3X5	T43.3X6
Dimorpholamine	T50.7X1	T50.7X2	T50.7X3	T50.7X4	T50.7X5	T50.7X6
Dimoxyline	T46.3X1	T46.3X2	T46.3X3	T46.3X4	T46.3X5	T46.3X6
Dinitrobenzene	T65.3X1	T65.3X2	T65.3X3	T65.3X4	—	—
vapor	T59.891	T59.892	T59.893	T59.894	—	—
Dinitrobenzol	T65.3X1	T65.3X2	T65.3X3	T65.3X4	—	—
vapor	T59.891	T59.892	T59.893	T59.894	—	—
Dinitrobutylphenol	T65.3X1	T65.3X2	T65.3X3	T65.3X4	—	—
Dinitro (-ortho-)cresol (pesticide) (spray)	T65.3X1	T65.3X2	T65.3X3	T65.3X4	—	—
Dinitrocyclohexylphenol	T65.3X1	T65.3X2	T65.3X3	T65.3X4	—	—
Dinitrophenol	T65.3X1	T65.3X2	T65.3X3	T65.3X4	—	—
Dinoprost	T48.0X1	T48.0X2	T48.0X3	T48.0X4	T48.0X5	T48.0X6
Dinoprostone	T48.0X1	T48.0X2	T48.0X3	T48.0X4	T48.0X5	T48.0X6
Dinoseb	T60.3X1	T60.3X2	T60.3X3	T60.3X4	—	—
Dioctyl sulfosuccinate (calcium)	T47.4X1	T47.4X2	T47.4X3	T47.4X4	T47.4X5	T47.4X6
(sodium)						
Diodone	T50.8X1	T50.8X2	T50.8X3	T50.8X4	T50.8X5	T50.8X6
Diodoquin	T37.8X1	T37.8X2	T37.8X3	T37.8X4	T37.8X5	T37.8X6
Dionin	T40.2X1	T40.2X2	T40.2X3	T40.2X4	T40.2X5	T40.2X6
Diosmin	T46.991	T46.992	T46.993	T46.994	T46.995	T46.996
Dioxane	T52.8X1	T52.8X2	T52.8X3	T52.8X4	—	—
Dioxathion	T60.0X1	T60.0X2	T60.0X3	T60.0X4	—	—
Dioxin	T53.7X1	T53.7X2	T53.7X3	T53.7X4	—	—
Dioxopromethazine	T43.3X1	T43.3X2	T43.3X3	T43.3X4	T43.3X5	T43.3X6
Dioxyline	T46.3X1	T46.3X2	T46.3X3	T46.3X4	T46.3X5	T46.3X6
Dipentene	T52.8X1	T52.8X2	T52.8X3	T52.8X4	—	—
Diperodon	T41.3X1	T41.3X2	T41.3X3	T41.3X4	T41.3X5	T41.3X6
Diphacinone	T60.4X1	T60.4X2	T60.4X3	T60.4X4	—	—
Diphemanil	T44.3X1	T44.3X2	T44.3X3	T44.3X4	T44.3X5	T44.3X6
metilsulfate	T44.3X1	T44.3X2	T44.3X3	T44.3X4	T44.3X5	T44.3X6
Diphenadione	T45.511	T45.512	T45.513	T45.514	T45.515	T45.516
rodenticide	T60.4X1	T60.4X2	T60.4X3	T60.4X4	—	—
Diphenhydramine	T45.0X1	T45.0X2	T45.0X3	T45.0X4	T45.0X5	T45.0X6
Diphenidol	T45.0X1	T45.0X2	T45.0X3	T45.0X4	T45.0X5	T45.0X6
Diphenoxylate	T47.6X1	T47.6X2	T47.6X3	T47.6X4	T47.6X5	T47.6X6
Diphenylamine	T65.3X1	T65.3X2	T65.3X3	T65.3X4	—	—
Diphenylbutazone	T39.2X1	T39.2X2	T39.2X3	T39.2X4	T39.2X5	T39.2X6
Diphenylchloroarsine, not in war	T57.0X1	T57.0X2	T57.0X3	T57.0X4	—	—
Diphenylhydantoin	T42.0X1	T42.0X2	T42.0X3	T42.0X4	T42.0X5	T42.0X6
Diphenylmethane dye	T52.1X1	T52.1X2	T52.1X3	T52.1X4	—	—
Diphenylpyraline	T45.0X1	T45.0X2	T45.0X3	T45.0X4	T45.0X5	T45.0X6
Diphtheria						
antitoxin	T50.Z11	T50.Z12	T50.Z13	T50.Z14	T50.Z15	T50.Z16
toxoid	T50.A91	T50.A92	T50.A93	T50.A94	T50.A95	T50.A96
with tetanus toxoid	T50.A21	T50.A22	T50.A23	T50.A24	T50.A25	T50.A26
with pertussis component	T50.A11	T50.A12	T50.A13	T50.A14	T50.A15	T50.A16
vaccine	T50.A91	T50.A92	T50.A93	T50.A94	T50.A95	T50.A96
combination						
without pertussis	T50.A21	T50.A22	T50.A23	T50.A24	T50.A25	T50.A26
including pertussis	T50.A11	T50.A12	T50.A13	T50.A14	T50.A15	T50.A16
Diphylline	T50.2X1	T50.2X2	T50.2X3	T50.2X4	T50.2X5	T50.2X6
Dipipanone	T40.4X1	T40.4X2	T40.4X3	T40.4X4	—	—
Dipivefrine	T49.5X1	T49.5X2	T49.5X3	T49.5X4	T49.5X5	T49.5X6
Diplovax	T50.B91	T50.B92	T50.B93	T50.B94	T50.B95	T50.B96
Diprophylline	T50.2X1	T50.2X2	T50.2X3	T50.2X4	T50.2X5	T50.2X6
Dipropyline	T48.291	T48.292	T48.293	T48.294	T48.295	T48.296
Dipyridamole	T46.3X1	T46.3X2	T46.3X3	T46.3X4	T46.3X5	T46.3X6
Dipyrone	T39.2X1	T39.2X2	T39.2X3	T39.2X4	T39.2X5	T39.2X6
Diquat (dibromide)	T60.3X1	T60.3X2	T60.3X3	T60.3X4	—	—
Disinfectant	T65.891	T65.892	T65.893	T65.894	—	—
alkaline	T54.3X1	T54.3X2	T54.3X3	T54.3X4	—	—
aromatic	T54.1X1	T54.1X2	T54.1X3	T54.1X4	—	—
intestinal	T37.8X1	T37.8X2	T37.8X3	T37.8X4	T37.8X5	T37.8X6
Disipal	T42.8X1	T42.8X2	T42.8X3	T42.8X4	T42.8X5	T42.8X6
Disodium edetate	T50.6X1	T50.6X2	T50.6X3	T50.6X4	T50.6X5	T50.6X6
Disoprofol	T41.291	T41.292	T41.293	T41.294	T41.295	T41.296
Disopyramide	T46.2X1	T46.2X2	T46.2X3	T46.2X4	T46.2X5	T46.2X6
Distigmine (bromide)	T44.0X1	T44.0X2	T44.0X3	T44.0X4	T44.0X5	T44.0X6
Disulfamide	T50.2X1	T50.2X2	T50.2X3	T50.2X4	T50.2X5	T50.2X6
Disulfanilamide	T37.0X1	T37.0X2	T37.0X3	T37.0X4	T37.0X5	T37.0X6
Disulfiram	T50.6X1	T50.6X2	T50.6X3	T50.6X4	T50.6X5	T50.6X6
Disulfoton	T60.0X1	T60.0X2	T60.0X3	T60.0X4	—	—
Dithiazanine iodide	T37.4X1	T37.4X2	T37.4X3	T37.4X4	T37.4X5	T37.4X6
Dithiocarbamate	T60.0X1	T60.0X2	T60.0X3	T60.0X4	—	—
Dithranol	T49.4X1	T49.4X2	T49.4X3	T49.4X4	T49.4X5	T49.4X6
Diucardin	T50.2X1	T50.2X2	T50.2X3	T50.2X4	T50.2X5	T50.2X6
Diupres	T50.2X1	T50.2X2	T50.2X3	T50.2X4	T50.2X5	T50.2X6
Diuretic NEC	T50.2X1	T50.2X2	T50.2X3	T50.2X4	T50.2X5	T50.2X6
benzothiadiazine	T50.2X1	T50.2X2	T50.2X3	T50.2X4	T50.2X5	T50.2X6
carbonic acid anhydrase inhibitors	T50.2X1	T50.2X2	T50.2X3	T50.2X4	T50.2X5	T50.2X6
furfuryl NEC	T50.2X1	T50.2X2	T50.2X3	T50.2X4	T50.2X5	T50.2X6
loop (high-ceiling)	T50.1X1	T50.1X2	T50.1X3	T50.1X4	T50.1X5	T50.1X6
mercurial NEC	T50.2X1	T50.2X2	T50.2X3	T50.2X4	T50.2X5	T50.2X6
osmotic	T50.2X1	T50.2X2	T50.2X3	T50.2X4	T50.2X5	T50.2X6
purine NEC	T50.2X1	T50.2X2	T50.2X3	T50.2X4	T50.2X5	T50.2X6
saluretic NEC	T50.2X1	T50.2X2	T50.2X3	T50.2X4	T50.2X5	T50.2X6
sulfonamide	T50.2X1	T50.2X2	T50.2X3	T50.2X4	T50.2X5	T50.2X6
thiazide NEC	T50.2X1	T50.2X2	T50.2X3	T50.2X4	T50.2X5	T50.2X6
xanthine	T50.2X1	T50.2X2	T50.2X3	T50.2X4	T50.2X5	T50.2X6
Diurgin	T50.2X1	T50.2X2	T50.2X3	T50.2X4	T50.2X5	T50.2X6
Diuril	T50.2X1	T50.2X2	T50.2X3	T50.2X4	T50.2X5	T50.2X6
Diuron	T60.3X1	T60.3X2	T60.3X3	T60.3X4	—	—
Divalproex	T42.6X1	T42.6X2	T42.6X3	T42.6X4	T42.6X5	T42.6X6
Divinyl ether	T41.0X1	T41.0X2	T41.0X3	T41.0X4	T41.0X5	T41.0X6
Dixanthogen	T49.0X1	T49.0X2	T49.0X3	T49.0X4	T49.0X5	T49.0X6
Dixyrazine	T43.3X1	T43.3X2	T43.3X3	T43.3X4	T43.3X5	T43.3X6
D-lysergic acid diethylamide	T40.8X1	T40.8X2	T40.8X3	T40.8X4	—	—
DMCT	T36.4X1	T36.4X2	T36.4X3	T36.4X4	T36.4X5	T36.4X6
DMSO — see Dimethyl sulfoxide						
DNBP	T60.3X1	T60.3X2	T60.3X3	T60.3X4	—	—
DNOC	T65.3X1	T65.3X2	T65.3X3	T65.3X4	—	—

Substance	Poisoning, Accidental (unintentional)	Poisoning, Intentional Self-harm	Poisoning, Assault	Poisoning, Undetermined	Adverse Effect	Under-dosing
Dobutamine	T44.5X1	T44.5X2	T44.5X3	T44.5X4	T44.5X5	T44.5X6
DOCA	T38.0X1	T38.0X2	T38.0X3	T38.0X4	T38.0X5	T38.0X6
Docusate sodium	T47.4X1	T47.4X2	T47.4X3	T47.4X4	T47.4X5	T47.4X6
Dodicin	T49.0X1	T49.0X2	T49.0X3	T49.0X4	T49.0X5	T49.0X6
Dofamium chloride	T49.0X1	T49.0X2	T49.0X3	T49.0X4	T49.0X5	T49.0X6
Dolophine	T40.3X1	T40.3X2	T40.3X3	T40.3X4	T40.3X5	T40.3X6
Doloxene	T39.8X1	T39.8X2	T39.8X3	T39.8X4	T39.8X5	T39.8X6
Domestic gas (after combustion) — see Gas, utility						
prior to combustion	T59.891	T59.892	T59.893	T59.894	—	—
Domiodol	T48.4X1	T48.4X2	T48.4X3	T48.4X4	T48.4X5	T48.4X6
Domiphen (bromide)	T49.0X1	T49.0X2	T49.0X3	T49.0X4	T49.0X5	T49.0X6
Domperidone	T45.0X1	T45.0X2	T45.0X3	T45.0X4	T45.0X5	T45.0X6
Dopa	T42.8X1	T42.8X2	T42.8X3	T42.8X4	T42.8X5	T42.8X6
Dopamine	T44.991	T44.992	T44.993	T44.994	T44.995	T44.996
Doriden	T42.6X1	T42.6X2	T42.6X3	T42.6X4	T42.6X5	T42.6X6
Dormiral	T42.3X1	T42.3X2	T42.3X3	T42.3X4	T42.3X5	T42.3X6
Dormison	T42.6X1	T42.6X2	T42.6X3	T42.6X4	T42.6X5	T42.6X6
Dornase	T48.4X1	T48.4X2	T48.4X3	T48.4X4	T48.4X5	T48.4X6
Dorsacaine	T41.3X1	T41.3X2	T41.3X3	T41.3X4	T41.3X5	T41.3X6
Dosulepin	T43.011	T43.012	T43.013	T43.014	T43.015	T43.016
Dothiepin	T43.011	T43.012	T43.013	T43.014	T43.015	T43.016
Doxantrazole	T48.6X1	T48.6X2	T48.6X3	T48.6X4	T48.6X5	T48.6X6
Doxapram	T50.7X1	T50.7X2	T50.7X3	T50.7X4	T50.7X5	T50.7X6
Doxazosin	T44.6X1	T44.6X2	T44.6X3	T44.6X4	T44.6X5	T44.6X6
Doxepin	T43.011	T43.012	T43.013	T43.014	T43.015	T43.016
Doxifluridine	T45.1X1	T45.1X2	T45.1X3	T45.1X4	T45.1X5	T45.1X6
Doxorubicin	T45.1X1	T45.1X2	T45.1X3	T45.1X4	T45.1X5	T45.1X6
Doxycycline	T36.4X1	T36.4X2	T36.4X3	T36.4X4	T36.4X5	T36.4X6
Doxylamine	T45.0X1	T45.0X2	T45.0X3	T45.0X4	T45.0X5	T45.0X6
Dramamine	T45.0X1	T45.0X2	T45.0X3	T45.0X4	T45.0X5	T45.0X6
Drano (drain cleaner)	T54.3X1	T54.3X2	T54.3X3	T54.3X4	—	—
Dressing, live pulp	T49.7X1	T49.7X2	T49.7X3	T49.7X4	T49.7X5	T49.7X6
Drocode	T40.2X1	T40.2X2	T40.2X3	T40.2X4	T40.2X5	T40.2X6
Dromoran	T40.2X1	T40.2X2	T40.2X3	T40.2X4	T40.2X5	T40.2X6
Dromostanolone	T38.7X1	T38.7X2	T38.7X3	T38.7X4	T38.7X5	T38.7X6
Dronabinol	T40.7X1	T40.7X2	T40.7X3	T40.7X4	T40.7X5	T40.7X6
Droperidol	T43.591	T43.592	T43.593	T43.594	T43.595	T43.596
Dropropizine	T48.3X1	T48.3X2	T48.3X3	T48.3X4	T48.3X5	T48.3X6
Drostanolone	T38.7X1	T38.7X2	T38.7X3	T38.7X4	T38.7X5	T38.7X6
Drotaverine	T44.3X1	T44.3X2	T44.3X3	T44.3X4	T44.3X5	T44.3X6
Drotrecogin alfa	T45.511	T45.512	T45.513	T45.514	T45.515	T45.516
Drug NEC	T50.901	T50.902	T50.903	T50.904	T50.905	T50.906
specified NEC	T50.991	T50.992	T50.993	T50.994	T50.995	T50.996
DTIC	T45.1X1	T45.1X2	T45.1X3	T45.1X4	T45.1X5	T45.1X6
Duboisine	T44.3X1	T44.3X2	T44.3X3	T44.3X4	T44.3X5	T44.3X6
Dulcolax	T47.2X1	T47.2X2	T47.2X3	T47.2X4	T47.2X5	T47.2X6
Duponol (C) (EP)	T49.2X1	T49.2X2	T49.2X3	T49.2X4	T49.2X5	T49.2X6
Durabolin	T38.7X1	T38.7X2	T38.7X3	T38.7X4	T38.7X5	T38.7X6
Dyclone	T41.3X1	T41.3X2	T41.3X3	T41.3X4	T41.3X5	T41.3X6
Dyclonine	T41.3X1	T41.3X2	T41.3X3	T41.3X4	T41.3X5	T41.3X6
Dydrogesterone	T38.5X1	T38.5X2	T38.5X3	T38.5X4	T38.5X5	T38.5X6
Dye NEC	T65.6X1	T65.6X2	T65.6X3	T65.6X4	—	—
antiseptic	T49.0X1	T49.0X2	T49.0X3	T49.0X4	T49.0X5	T49.0X6
diagnostic agents	T50.8X1	T50.8X2	T50.8X3	T50.8X4	T50.8X5	T50.8X6
pharmaceutical NEC	T50.901	T50.902	T50.903	T50.904	T50.905	T50.906
Dyflos	T44.0X1	T44.0X2	T44.0X3	T44.0X4	T44.0X5	T44.0X6
Dymelor	T38.3X1	T38.3X2	T38.3X3	T38.3X4	T38.3X5	T38.3X6
Dynamite	T65.3X1	T65.3X2	T65.3X3	T65.3X4	—	—
fumes	T59.891	T59.892	T59.893	T59.894	—	—
Dyphylline	T44.3X1	T44.3X2	T44.3X3	T44.3X4	T44.3X5	T44.3X6
b-eucaine	T49.1X1	T49.1X2	T49.1X3	T49.1X4	T49.1X5	T49.1X6
Ear drug NEC	T49.6X1	T49.6X2	T49.6X3	T49.6X4	T49.6X5	T49.6X6
Ear preparations	T49.6X1	T49.6X2	T49.6X3	T49.6X4	T49.6X5	T49.6X6
Echothiophate, echothiopate, ecothiopate	T49.5X1	T49.5X2	T49.5X3	T49.5X4	T49.5X5	T49.5X6
Econazole	T49.0X1	T49.0X2	T49.0X3	T49.0X4	T49.0X5	T49.0X6
Ecothiopate iodide	T49.5X1	T49.5X2	T49.5X3	T49.5X4	T49.5X5	T49.5X6
Ecstasy	T43.641	T43.642	T43.643	T43.644	—	—
Ectylurea	T42.6X1	T42.6X2	T42.6X3	T42.6X4	T42.6X5	T42.6X6
Edathamil disodium	T45.8X1	T45.8X2	T45.8X3	T45.8X4	T45.8X5	T45.8X6
Edecrin	T50.1X1	T50.1X2	T50.1X3	T50.1X4	T50.1X5	T50.1X6
Edetate, disodium	T45.8X1	T45.8X2	T45.8X3	T45.8X4	T45.8X5	T45.8X6
(calcium)						
Edoxudine	T49.5X1	T49.5X2	T49.5X3	T49.5X4	T49.5X5	T49.5X6
Edrophonium	T44.0X1	T44.0X2	T44.0X3	T44.0X4	T44.0X5	T44.0X6
chloride	T44.0X1	T44.0X2	T44.0X3	T44.0X4	T44.0X5	T44.0X6
EDTA	T50.6X1	T50.6X2	T50.6X3	T50.6X4	T50.6X5	T50.6X6
Eflornithine	T37.2X1	T37.2X2	T37.2X3	T37.2X4	T37.2X5	T37.2X6
Efloxate	T46.3X1	T46.3X2	T46.3X3	T46.3X4	T46.3X5	T46.3X6
Elase	T49.8X1	T49.8X2	T49.8X3	T49.8X4	T49.8X5	T49.8X6
Elastase	T47.5X1	T47.5X2	T47.5X3	T47.5X4	T47.5X5	T47.5X6
Elaterium	T47.2X1	T47.2X2	T47.2X3	T47.2X4	T47.2X5	T47.2X6
Elcatonin	T50.991	T50.992	T50.993	T50.994	T50.995	T50.996
Elder	T62.2X1	T62.2X2	T62.2X3	T62.2X4	—	—
berry, (unripe)	T62.1X1	T62.1X2	T62.1X3	T62.1X4	—	—
Electrolyte balance drug	T50.3X1	T50.3X2	T50.3X3	T50.3X4	T50.3X5	T50.3X6
Electrolytes NEC	T50.3X1	T50.3X2	T50.3X3	T50.3X4	T50.3X5	T50.3X6
Electrolytic agent NEC	T50.3X1	T50.3X2	T50.3X3	T50.3X4	T50.3X5	T50.3X6
Elemental diet	T50.901	T50.902	T50.903	T50.904	T50.905	T50.906
Elliptinium acetate	T45.1X1	T45.1X2	T45.1X3	T45.1X4	T45.1X5	T45.1X6
Embramine	T45.0X1	T45.0X2	T45.0X3	T45.0X4	T45.0X5	T45.0X6
Emepronium (salts)	T44.3X1	T44.3X2	T44.3X3	T44.3X4	T44.3X5	T44.3X6
bromide	T44.3X1	T44.3X2	T44.3X3	T44.3X4	T44.3X5	T44.3X6
Emetic NEC	T47.7X1	T47.7X2	T47.7X3	T47.7X4	T47.7X5	T47.7X6
Emetine	T37.3X1	T37.3X2	T37.3X3	T37.3X4	T37.3X5	T37.3X6
Emollient NEC	T49.3X1	T49.3X2	T49.3X3	T49.3X4	T49.3X5	T49.3X6
Emorfazone	T39.8X1	T39.8X2	T39.8X3	T39.8X4	T39.8X5	T39.8X6
Emylcamate	T43.591	T43.592	T43.593	T43.594	T43.595	T43.596
Enalapril	T46.4X1	T46.4X2	T46.4X3	T46.4X4	T46.4X5	T46.4X6
Enalaprilat	T46.4X1	T46.4X2	T46.4X3	T46.4X4	T46.4X5	T46.4X6
Encainide	T46.2X1	T46.2X2	T46.2X3	T46.2X4	T46.2X5	T46.2X6
Endocaine	T41.3X1	T41.3X2	T41.3X3	T41.3X4	T41.3X5	T41.3X6
Endosulfan	T60.2X1	T60.2X2	T60.2X3	T60.2X4	—	—
Endothall	T60.3X1	T60.3X2	T60.3X3	T60.3X4	—	—
Endralazine	T46.5X1	T46.5X2	T46.5X3	T46.5X4	T46.5X5	T46.5X6
Endrin	T60.1X1	T60.1X2	T60.1X3	T60.1X4	—	—
Enflurane	T41.0X1	T41.0X2	T41.0X3	T41.0X4	T41.0X5	T41.0X6
Enhexymal	T42.3X1	T42.3X2	T42.3X3	T42.3X4	T42.3X5	T42.3X6
Enocitabine	T45.1X1	T45.1X2	T45.1X3	T45.1X4	T45.1X5	T45.1X6
Enovid	T38.4X1	T38.4X2	T38.4X3	T38.4X4	T38.4X5	T38.4X6
Enoxacin	T36.8X1	T36.8X2	T36.8X3	T36.8X4	T36.8X5	T36.8X6
Enoxaparin (sodium)	T45.511	T45.512	T45.513	T45.514	T45.515	T45.516
Enpiprazole	T43.591	T43.592	T43.593	T43.594	T43.595	T43.596
Enprofylline	T48.6X1	T48.6X2	T48.6X3	T48.6X4	T48.6X5	T48.6X6
Enprostil	T47.1X1	T47.1X2	T47.1X3	T47.1X4	T47.1X5	T47.1X6
Enterogastrone	T38.891	T38.892	T38.893	T38.894	T38.895	T38.896
ENT preparations (anti-infectives)	T49.6X1	T49.6X2	T49.6X3	T49.6X4	T49.6X5	T49.6X6
Enviomycin	T36.8X1	T36.8X2	T36.8X3	T36.8X4	T36.8X5	T36.8X6
Enzodase	T45.3X1	T45.3X2	T45.3X3	T45.3X4	T45.3X5	T45.3X6
Enzyme NEC	T45.3X1	T45.3X2	T45.3X3	T45.3X4	T45.3X5	T45.3X6
depolymerizing	T49.8X1	T49.8X2	T49.8X3	T49.8X4	T49.8X5	T49.8X6
fibrolytic	T45.3X1	T45.3X2	T45.3X3	T45.3X4	T45.3X5	T45.3X6
gastric	T47.5X1	T47.5X2	T47.5X3	T47.5X4	T47.5X5	T47.5X6
intestinal	T47.5X1	T47.5X2	T47.5X3	T47.5X4	T47.5X5	T47.5X6
local action	T49.4X1	T49.4X2	T49.4X3	T49.4X4	T49.4X5	T49.4X6
proteolytic	T49.4X1	T49.4X2	T49.4X3	T49.4X4	T49.4X5	T49.4X6
thrombolytic	T45.3X1	T45.3X2	T45.3X3	T45.3X4	T45.3X5	T45.3X6
EPAB	T41.3X1	T41.3X2	T41.3X3	T41.3X4	T41.3X5	T41.3X6
Epanutin	T42.0X1	T42.0X2	T42.0X3	T42.0X4	T42.0X5	T42.0X6
Ephedra	T44.991	T44.992	T44.993	T44.994	T44.995	T44.996
Ephedrine	T44.991	T44.992	T44.993	T44.994	T44.995	T44.996
Epichlorhydrin, epichlorohydrin	T52.8X1	T52.8X2	T52.8X3	T52.8X4	—	—
Epicillin	T36.0X1	T36.0X2	T36.0X3	T36.0X4	T36.0X5	T36.0X6
Epiestriol	T38.5X1	T38.5X2	T38.5X3	T38.5X4	T38.5X5	T38.5X6
Epilim — see Sodium valproate						
Epimestrol	T38.5X1	T38.5X2	T38.5X3	T38.5X4	T38.5X5	T38.5X6
Epinephrine	T44.5X1	T44.5X2	T44.5X3	T44.5X4	T44.5X5	T44.5X6
Epirubicin	T45.1X1	T45.1X2	T45.1X3	T45.1X4	T45.1X5	T45.1X6
Epitiostanol	T38.7X1	T38.7X2	T38.7X3	T38.7X4	T38.7X5	T38.7X6
Epitizide	T50.2X1	T50.2X2	T50.2X3	T50.2X4	T50.2X5	T50.2X6
EPN	T60.0X1	T60.0X2	T60.0X3	T60.0X4	—	—
EPO	T45.8X1	T45.8X2	T45.8X3	T45.8X4	T45.8X5	T45.8X6
Epoetin alpha	T45.8X1	T45.8X2	T45.8X3	T45.8X4	T45.8X5	T45.8X6
Epomediol	T50.991	T50.992	T50.993	T50.994	T50.995	T50.996
Epoprostenol	T45.521	T45.522	T45.523	T45.524	T45.525	T45.526
Epoxy resin	T65.891	T65.892	T65.893	T65.894	—	—
Eprazinone	T48.4X1	T48.4X2	T48.4X3	T48.4X4	T48.4X5	T48.4X6
Epsilon aminocaproic acid	T45.621	T45.622	T45.623	T45.624	T45.625	T45.626
Epsom salt	T47.3X1	T47.3X2	T47.3X3	T47.3X4	T47.3X5	T47.3X6
Eptazocine	T40.4X1	T40.4X2	T40.4X3	T40.4X4	T40.4X5	T40.4X6
Equanil	T43.591	T43.592	T43.593	T43.594	T43.595	T43.596
Equisetum	T62.2X1	T62.2X2	T62.2X3	T62.2X4	—	—
diuretic	T50.2X1	T50.2X2	T50.2X3	T50.2X4	T50.2X5	T50.2X6
Ergobasine	T48.0X1	T48.0X2	T48.0X3	T48.0X4	T48.0X5	T48.0X6
Ergocalciferol	T45.2X1	T45.2X2	T45.2X3	T45.2X4	T45.2X5	T45.2X6
Ergoloid mesylates	T46.7X1	T46.7X2	T46.7X3	T46.7X4	T46.7X5	T46.7X6
Ergometrine	T48.0X1	T48.0X2	T48.0X3	T48.0X4	T48.0X5	T48.0X6
Ergonovine	T48.0X1	T48.0X2	T48.0X3	T48.0X4	T48.0X5	T48.0X6
Ergotamine	T46.5X1	T46.5X2	T46.5X3	T46.5X4	T46.5X5	T46.5X6
Ergotocine	T48.0X1	T48.0X2	T48.0X3	T48.0X4	T48.0X5	T48.0X6
Ergotrate	T48.0X1	T48.0X2	T48.0X3	T48.0X4	T48.0X5	T48.0X6
Ergot NEC	T64.81	T64.82	T64.83	T64.84	—	—
derivative	T48.0X1	T48.0X2	T48.0X3	T48.0X4	T48.0X5	T48.0X6

Substance	Poisoning, Accidental (unintentional)	Poisoning, Intentional Self-harm	Poisoning, Assault	Poisoning, Undetermined	Adverse Effect	Under-dosing
Ergot — *continued*						
medicinal (alkaloids)	T48.0X1	T48.0X2	T48.0X3	T48.0X4	T48.0X5	T48.0X6
prepared	T48.0X1	T48.0X2	T48.0X3	T48.0X4	T48.0X5	T48.0X6
Eritrityl tetranitrate	T46.3X1	T46.3X2	T46.3X3	T46.3X4	T46.3X5	T46.3X6
Erythrityl tetranitrate	T46.3X1	T46.3X2	T46.3X3	T46.3X4	T46.3X5	T46.3X6
Erythrol tetranitrate	T46.3X1	T46.3X2	T46.3X3	T46.3X4	T46.3X5	T46.3X6
Erythromycin (salts)	T36.3X1	T36.3X2	T36.3X3	T36.3X4	T36.3X5	T36.3X6
ophthalmic preparation	T49.5X1	T49.5X2	T49.5X3	T49.5X4	T49.5X5	T49.5X6
topical NEC	T49.0X1	T49.0X2	T49.0X3	T49.0X4	T49.0X5	T49.0X6
Erythropoietin	T45.8X1	T45.8X2	T45.8X3	T45.8X4	T45.8X5	T45.8X6
human	T45.8X1	T45.8X2	T45.8X3	T45.8X4	T45.8X5	T45.8X6
Escin	T46.991	T46.992	T46.993	T46.994	T46.995	T46.996
Esculin	T45.2X1	T45.2X2	T45.2X3	T45.2X4	T45.2X5	T45.2X6
Esculoside	T45.2X1	T45.2X2	T45.2X3	T45.2X4	T45.2X5	T45.2X6
ESDT (ether-soluble tar distillate)	T49.1X1	T49.1X2	T49.1X3	T49.1X4	T49.1X5	T49.1X6
Eserine	T49.5X1	T49.5X2	T49.5X3	T49.5X4	T49.5X5	T49.5X6
Esflurbiprofen	T39.311	T39.312	T39.313	T39.314	T39.315	T39.316
Eskabarb	T42.3X1	T42.3X2	T42.3X3	T42.3X4	T42.3X5	T42.3X6
Eskalith	T43.8X1	T43.8X2	T43.8X3	T43.8X4	T43.8X5	T43.8X6
Esmolol	T44.7X1	T44.7X2	T44.7X3	T44.7X4	T44.7X5	T44.7X6
Estanozolol	T38.7X1	T38.7X2	T38.7X3	T38.7X4	T38.7X5	T38.7X6
Estazolam	T42.4X1	T42.4X2	T42.4X3	T42.4X4	T42.4X5	T42.4X6
Estradiol	T38.5X1	T38.5X2	T38.5X3	T38.5X4	T38.5X5	T38.5X6
with testosterone	T38.7X1	T38.7X2	T38.7X3	T38.7X4	T38.7X5	T38.7X6
benzoate	T38.5X1	T38.5X2	T38.5X3	T38.5X4	T38.5X5	T38.5X6
Estramustine	T45.1X1	T45.1X2	T45.1X3	T45.1X4	T45.1X5	T45.1X6
Estriol	T38.5X1	T38.5X2	T38.5X3	T38.5X4	T38.5X5	T38.5X6
Estrogen	T38.5X1	T38.5X2	T38.5X3	T38.5X4	T38.5X5	T38.5X6
with progesterone	T38.5X1	T38.5X2	T38.5X3	T38.5X4	T38.5X5	T38.5X6
conjugated	T38.5X1	T38.5X2	T38.5X3	T38.5X4	T38.5X5	T38.5X6
Estrone	T38.5X1	T38.5X2	T38.5X3	T38.5X4	T38.5X5	T38.5X6
Estropipate	T38.5X1	T38.5X2	T38.5X3	T38.5X4	T38.5X5	T38.5X6
Etacrynate sodium	T50.1X1	T50.1X2	T50.1X3	T50.1X4	T50.1X5	T50.1X6
Etacrynic acid	T50.1X1	T50.1X2	T50.1X3	T50.1X4	T50.1X5	T50.1X6
Etafedrine	T48.6X1	T48.6X2	T48.6X3	T48.6X4	T48.6X5	T48.6X6
Etafenone	T46.3X1	T46.3X2	T46.3X3	T46.3X4	T46.3X5	T46.3X6
Etambutol	T37.1X1	T37.1X2	T37.1X3	T37.1X4	T37.1X5	T37.1X6
Etamiphyllin	T48.6X1	T48.6X2	T48.6X3	T48.6X4	T48.6X5	T48.6X6
Etamivan	T50.7X1	T50.7X2	T50.7X3	T50.7X4	T50.7X5	T50.7X6
Etamsylate	T45.7X1	T45.7X2	T45.7X3	T45.7X4	T45.7X5	T45.7X6
Etebenecid	T50.4X1	T50.4X2	T50.4X3	T50.4X4	T50.4X5	T50.4X6
Ethacridine	T49.0X1	T49.0X2	T49.0X3	T49.0X4	T49.0X5	T49.0X6
Ethacrynic acid	T50.1X1	T50.1X2	T50.1X3	T50.1X4	T50.1X5	T50.1X6
Ethadione	T42.2X1	T42.2X2	T42.2X3	T42.2X4	T42.2X5	T42.2X6
Ethambutol	T37.1X1	T37.1X2	T37.1X3	T37.1X4	T37.1X5	T37.1X6
Ethamide	T50.2X1	T50.2X2	T50.2X3	T50.2X4	T50.2X5	T50.2X6
Ethamivan	T50.7X1	T50.7X2	T50.7X3	T50.7X4	T50.7X5	T50.7X6
Ethamsylate	T45.7X1	T45.7X2	T45.7X3	T45.7X4	T45.7X5	T45.7X6
Ethanol	T51.0X1	T51.0X2	T51.0X3	T51.0X4	—	—
beverage	T51.0X1	T51.0X2	T51.0X3	T51.0X4	—	—
Ethanolamine oleate	T46.8X1	T46.8X2	T46.8X3	T46.8X4	T46.8X5	T46.8X6
Ethaverine	T44.3X1	T44.3X2	T44.3X3	T44.3X4	T44.3X5	T44.3X6
Ethchlorvynol	T42.6X1	T42.6X2	T42.6X3	T42.6X4	T42.6X5	T42.6X6
Ethebenecid	T50.4X1	T50.4X2	T50.4X3	T50.4X4	T50.4X5	T50.4X6
Ether (vapor)	T41.0X1	T41.0X2	T41.0X3	T41.0X4	T41.0X5	T41.0X6
anesthetic	T41.0X1	T41.0X2	T41.0X3	T41.0X4	T41.0X5	T41.0X6
divinyl	T41.0X1	T41.0X2	T41.0X3	T41.0X4	T41.0X5	T41.0X6
ethyl (medicinal)	T41.0X1	T41.0X2	T41.0X3	T41.0X4	T41.0X5	T41.0X6
nonmedicinal	T52.8X1	T52.8X2	T52.8X3	T52.8X4	—	—
petroleum — *see* Ligroin						
solvent	T52.8X1	T52.8X2	T52.8X3	T52.8X4	—	—
Ethiazide	T50.2X1	T50.2X2	T50.2X3	T50.2X4	T50.2X5	T50.2X6
Ethidium chloride (vapor)	T59.891	T59.892	T59.893	T59.894	—	—
Ethinamate	T42.6X1	T42.6X2	T42.6X3	T42.6X4	T42.6X5	T42.6X6
Ethinylestradiol, ethinyloestradiol	T38.5X1	T38.5X2	T38.5X3	T38.5X4	T38.5X5	T38.5X6
with						
levonorgestrel	T38.4X1	T38.4X2	T38.4X3	T38.4X4	T38.4X5	T38.4X6
norethisterone	T38.4X1	T38.4X2	T38.4X3	T38.4X4	T38.4X5	T38.4X6
Ethiodized oil (131 I)	T50.8X1	T50.8X2	T50.8X3	T50.8X4	T50.8X5	T50.8X6
Ethion	T60.0X1	T60.0X2	T60.0X3	T60.0X4	—	—
Ethionamide	T37.1X1	T37.1X2	T37.1X3	T37.1X4	T37.1X5	T37.1X6
Ethioniamide	T37.1X1	T37.1X2	T37.1X3	T37.1X4	T37.1X5	T37.1X6
Ethisterone	T38.5X1	T38.5X2	T38.5X3	T38.5X4	T38.5X5	T38.5X6
Ethobral	T42.3X1	T42.3X2	T42.3X3	T42.3X4	T42.3X5	T42.3X6
Ethocaine (infiltration) (topical)	T41.3X1	T41.3X2	T41.3X3	T41.3X4	T41.3X5	T41.3X6
nerve block (peripheral) (plexus)	T41.3X1	T41.3X2	T41.3X3	T41.3X4	T41.3X5	T41.3X6
spinal	T41.3X1	T41.3X2	T41.3X3	T41.3X4	T41.3X5	T41.3X6
Ethoheptazine	T40.4X1	T40.4X2	T40.4X3	T40.4X4	T40.4X5	T40.4X6
Ethopropazine	T44.3X1	T44.3X2	T44.3X3	T44.3X4	T44.3X5	T44.3X6

Substance	Poisoning, Accidental (unintentional)	Poisoning, Intentional Self-harm	Poisoning, Assault	Poisoning, Undetermined	Adverse Effect	Under-dosing
Ethosuximide	T42.2X1	T42.2X2	T42.2X3	T42.2X4	T42.2X5	T42.2X6
Ethotoin	T42.0X1	T42.0X2	T42.0X3	T42.0X4	T42.0X5	T42.0X6
Ethoxazene	T37.91	T37.92	T37.93	T37.94	T37.95	T37.96
Ethoxazorutoside	T46.991	T46.992	T46.993	T46.994	T46.995	T46.996
Ethoxzolamide	T50.2X1	T50.2X2	T50.2X3	T50.2X4	T50.2X5	T50.2X6
Ethyl						
acetate	T52.8X1	T52.8X2	T52.8X3	T52.8X4	—	—
alcohol	T51.0X1	T51.0X2	T51.0X3	T51.0X4	—	—
beverage	T51.0X1	T51.0X2	T51.0X3	T51.0X4	—	—
aldehyde (vapor)	T59.891	T59.892	T59.893	T59.894	—	—
liquid	T52.8X1	T52.8X2	T52.8X3	T52.8X4	—	—
aminobenzoate	T41.3X1	T41.3X2	T41.3X3	T41.3X4	T41.3X5	T41.3X6
aminophenothiazine	T43.3X1	T43.3X2	T43.3X3	T43.3X4	T43.3X5	T43.3X6
benzoate	T52.8X1	T52.8X2	T52.8X3	T52.8X4	—	—
biscoumacetate	T45.511	T45.512	T45.513	T45.514	T45.515	T45.516
bromide (anesthetic)	T41.0X1	T41.0X2	T41.0X3	T41.0X4	T41.0X5	T41.0X6
carbamate	T45.1X1	T45.1X2	T45.1X3	T45.1X4	T45.1X5	T45.1X6
carbinol	T51.3X1	T51.3X2	T51.3X3	T51.3X4	—	—
carbonate	T52.8X1	T52.8X2	T52.8X3	T52.8X4	—	—
chaulmoograte	T37.1X1	T37.1X2	T37.1X3	T37.1X4	T37.1X5	T37.1X6
chloride (anesthetic)	T41.0X1	T41.0X2	T41.0X3	T41.0X4	T41.0X5	T41.0X6
anesthetic (local)	T41.3X1	T41.3X2	T41.3X3	T41.3X4	T41.3X5	T41.3X6
inhaled	T41.0X1	T41.0X2	T41.0X3	T41.0X4	T41.0X5	T41.0X6
local	T49.4X1	T49.4X2	T49.4X3	T49.4X4	T49.4X5	T49.4X6
solvent	T53.6X1	T53.6X2	T53.6X3	T53.6X4	—	—
dibunate	T48.3X1	T48.3X2	T48.3X3	T48.3X4	T48.3X5	T48.3X6
dichloroarsine (vapor)	T57.0X1	T57.0X2	T57.0X3	T57.0X4	—	—
estranol	T38.7X1	T38.7X2	T38.7X3	T38.7X4	T38.7X5	T38.7X6
ether — *see also* ether	T52.8X1	T52.8X2	T52.8X3	T52.8X4	—	—
formate NEC (solvent)	T52.0X1	T52.0X2	T52.0X3	T52.0X4	—	—
fumarate	T49.4X1	T49.4X2	T49.4X3	T49.4X4	T49.4X5	T49.4X6
hydroxyisobutyrate NEC (solvent)	T52.8X1	T52.8X2	T52.8X3	T52.8X4	—	—
iodoacetate	T59.3X1	T59.3X2	T59.3X3	T59.3X4		
lactate NEC (solvent)	T52.8X1	T52.8X2	T52.8X3	T52.8X4	—	—
loflazepate	T42.4X1	T42.4X2	T42.4X3	T42.4X4	T42.4X5	T42.4X6
mercuric chloride	T56.1X1	T56.1X2	T56.1X3	T56.1X4	—	—
methylcarbinol	T51.8X1	T51.8X2	T51.8X3	T51.8X4	—	—
morphine	T40.2X1	T40.2X2	T40.2X3	T40.2X4	T40.2X5	T40.2X6
noradrenaline	T48.6X1	T48.6X2	T48.6X3	T48.6X4	T48.6X5	T48.6X6
oxybutyrate NEC (solvent)	T52.8X1	T52.8X2	T52.8X3	T52.8X4	—	—
Ethylene (gas)	T59.891	T59.892	T59.893	T59.894	—	—
anesthetic (general)	T41.0X1	T41.0X2	T41.0X3	T41.0X4	T41.0X5	T41.0X6
chlorohydrin	T52.8X1	T52.8X2	T52.8X3	T52.8X4	—	—
vapor	T53.6X1	T53.6X2	T53.6X3	T53.6X4	—	—
dichloride	T52.8X1	T52.8X2	T52.8X3	T52.8X4	—	—
vapor	T53.6X1	T53.6X2	T53.6X3	T53.6X4	—	—
dinitrate	T52.3X1	T52.3X2	T52.3X3	T52.3X4	—	—
glycol(s)	T52.8X1	T52.8X2	T52.8X3	T52.8X4	—	—
dinitrate	T52.3X1	T52.3X2	T52.3X3	T52.3X4	—	—
monobutyl ether	T52.3X1	T52.3X2	T52.3X3	T52.3X4	—	—
imine	T54.1X1	T54.1X2	T54.1X3	T54.1X4	—	—
oxide (fumigant) (nonmedicinal)	T59.891	T59.892	T59.893	T59.894	—	—
medicinal	T49.0X1	T49.0X2	T49.0X3	T49.0X4	T49.0X5	T49.0X6
Ethylenediaminetetra-acetic acid	T50.6X1	T50.6X2	T50.6X3	T50.6X4	T50.6X5	T50.6X6
Ethylenediamine theophylline	T48.6X1	T48.6X2	T48.6X3	T48.6X4	T48.6X5	T48.6X6
Ethylenedinitrilotetra-acetate	T50.6X1	T50.6X2	T50.6X3	T50.6X4	T50.6X5	T50.6X6
Ethylestrenol	T38.7X1	T38.7X2	T38.7X3	T38.7X4	T38.7X5	T38.7X6
Ethylhydroxycellulose	T47.4X1	T47.4X2	T47.4X3	T47.4X4	T47.4X5	T47.4X6
Ethylidene						
chloride NEC	T53.6X1	T53.6X2	T53.6X3	T53.6X4	—	—
diacetate	T60.3X1	T60.3X2	T60.3X3	T60.3X4	—	—
dicoumarin	T45.511	T45.512	T45.513	T45.514	T45.515	T45.516
dicoumarol	T45.511	T45.512	T45.513	T45.514	T45.515	T45.516
diethyl ether	T52.0X1	T52.0X2	T52.0X3	T52.0X4	—	—
Ethylmorphine	T40.2X1	T40.2X2	T40.2X3	T40.2X4	T40.2X5	T40.2X6
Ethylnorepinephrine	T48.6X1	T48.6X2	T48.6X3	T48.6X4	T48.6X5	T48.6X6
Ethylparachlorophen-oxyisobutyrate	T46.6X1	T46.6X2	T46.6X3	T46.6X4	T46.6X5	T46.6X6
Ethynodiol	T38.4X1	T38.4X2	T38.4X3	T38.4X4	T38.4X5	T38.4X6
with mestranol diacetate	T38.4X1	T38.4X2	T38.4X3	T38.4X4	T38.4X5	T38.4X6
Etidocaine	T41.3X1	T41.3X2	T41.3X3	T41.3X4	T41.3X5	T41.3X6
infiltration (subcutaneous)	T41.3X1	T41.3X2	T41.3X3	T41.3X4	T41.3X5	T41.3X6
nerve (peripheral) (plexus)	T41.3X1	T41.3X2	T41.3X3	T41.3X4	T41.3X5	T41.3X6
Etidronate	T50.991	T50.992	T50.993	T50.994	T50.995	T50.996
Etidronic acid (disodium salt)	T50.991	T50.992	T50.993	T50.994	T50.995	T50.996
Etifoxine	T42.6X1	T42.6X2	T42.6X3	T42.6X4	T42.6X5	T42.6X6
Etilefrine	T44.4X1	T44.4X2	T44.4X3	T44.4X4	T44.4X5	T44.4X6
Etilfen	T42.3X1	T42.3X2	T42.3X3	T42.3X4	T42.3X5	T42.3X6

Substance	Poisoning, Accidental (unintentional)	Poisoning, Intentional Self-harm	Poisoning, Assault	Poisoning, Undetermined	Adverse Effect	Under-dosing
Etinodiol	T38.4X1	T38.4X2	T38.4X3	T38.4X4	T38.4X5	T38.4X6
Etiroxate	T46.6X1	T46.6X2	T46.6X3	T46.6X4	T46.6X5	T46.6X6
Etizolam	T42.4X1	T42.4X2	T42.4X3	T42.4X4	T42.4X5	T42.4X6
Etodolac	T39.391	T39.392	T39.393	T39.394	T39.395	T39.396
Etofamide	T37.3X1	T37.3X2	T37.3X3	T37.3X4	T37.3X5	T37.3X6
Etofibrate	T46.6X1	T46.6X2	T46.6X3	T46.6X4	T46.6X5	T46.6X6
Etofylline	T46.7X1	T46.7X2	T46.7X3	T46.7X4	T46.7X5	T46.7X6
clofibrate	T46.6X1	T46.6X2	T46.6X3	T46.6X4	T46.6X5	T46.6X6
Etoglucid	T45.1X1	T45.1X2	T45.1X3	T45.1X4	T45.1X5	T45.1X6
Etomidate	T41.1X1	T41.1X2	T41.1X3	T41.1X4	T41.1X5	T41.1X6
Etomide	T39.8X1	T39.8X2	T39.8X3	T39.8X4	T39.8X5	T39.8X6
Etomidoline	T44.3X1	T44.3X2	T44.3X3	T44.3X4	T44.3X5	T44.3X6
Etoposide	T45.1X1	T45.1X2	T45.1X3	T45.1X4	T45.1X5	T45.1X6
Etorphine	T40.2X1	T40.2X2	T40.2X3	T40.2X4	T40.2X5	T40.2X6
Etoval	T42.3X1	T42.3X2	T42.3X3	T42.3X4	T42.3X5	T42.3X6
Etozolin	T50.1X1	T50.1X2	T50.1X3	T50.1X4	T50.1X5	T50.1X6
Etretinate	T50.991	T50.992	T50.993	T50.994	T50.995	T50.996
Etryptamine	T43.691	T43.692	T43.693	T43.694	T43.695	T43.696
Etybenzatropine	T44.3X1	T44.3X2	T44.3X3	T44.3X4	T44.3X5	T44.3X6
Etynodiol	T38.4X1	T38.4X2	T38.4X3	T38.4X4	T38.4X5	T38.4X6
Eucaine	T41.3X1	T41.3X2	T41.3X3	T41.3X4	T41.3X5	T41.3X6
Eucalyptus oil	T49.7X1	T49.7X2	T49.7X3	T49.7X4	T49.7X5	T49.7X6
Eucatropine	T49.5X1	T49.5X2	T49.5X3	T49.5X4	T49.5X5	T49.5X6
Eucodal	T40.2X1	T40.2X2	T40.2X3	T40.2X4	T40.2X5	T40.2X6
Euneryl	T42.3X1	T42.3X2	T42.3X3	T42.3X4	T42.3X5	T42.3X6
Euphthalmine	T44.3X1	T44.3X2	T44.3X3	T44.3X4	T44.3X5	T44.3X6
Eurax	T49.0X1	T49.0X2	T49.0X3	T49.0X4	T49.0X5	T49.0X6
Euresol	T49.4X1	T49.4X2	T49.4X3	T49.4X4	T49.4X5	T49.4X6
Euthroid	T38.1X1	T38.1X2	T38.1X3	T38.1X4	T38.1X5	T38.1X6
Evans blue	T50.8X1	T50.8X2	T50.8X3	T50.8X4	T50.8X5	T50.8X6
Evipal	T42.3X1	T42.3X2	T42.3X3	T42.3X4	T42.3X5	T42.3X6
sodium	T41.1X1	T41.1X2	T41.1X3	T41.1X4	T41.1X5	T41.1X6
Evipan	T42.3X1	T42.3X2	T42.3X3	T42.3X4	T42.3X5	T42.3X6
sodium	T41.1X1	T41.1X2	T41.1X3	T41.1X4	T41.1X5	T41.1X6
Exalamide	T49.0X1	T49.0X2	T49.0X3	T49.0X4	T49.0X5	T49.0X6
Exalgin	T39.1X1	T39.1X2	T39.1X3	T39.1X4	T39.1X5	T39.1X6
Excipients, pharmaceutical	T50.901	T50.902	T50.903	T50.904	T50.905	T50.906
Exhaust gas (engine) (motor vehicle)	T58.01	T58.02	T58.03	T58.04	—	—
Ex-Lax (phenolphthalein)	T47.2X1	T47.2X2	T47.2X3	T47.2X4	T47.2X5	T47.2X6
Expectorant NEC	T48.4X1	T48.4X2	T48.4X3	T48.4X4	T48.4X5	T48.4X6
Extended insulin zinc suspension	T38.3X1	T38.3X2	T38.3X3	T38.3X4	T38.3X5	T38.3X6
External medications (skin)	T49.91	T49.92	T49.93	T49.94	T49.95	T49.96
(mucous membrane)						
dental agent	T49.7X1	T49.7X2	T49.7X3	T49.7X4	T49.7X5	T49.7X6
ENT agent	T49.6X1	T49.6X2	T49.6X3	T49.6X4	T49.6X5	T49.6X6
ophthalmic preparation	T49.5X1	T49.5X2	T49.5X3	T49.5X4	T49.5X5	T49.5X6
specified NEC	T49.8X1	T49.8X2	T49.8X3	T49.8X4	T49.8X5	T49.8X6
Extrapyramidal antagonist NEC	T44.3X1	T44.3X2	T44.3X3	T44.3X4	T44.3X5	T44.3X6
Eye agents (anti-infective)	T49.5X1	T49.5X2	T49.5X3	T49.5X4	T49.5X5	T49.5X6
Eye drug NEC	T49.5X1	T49.5X2	T49.5X3	T49.5X4	T49.5X5	T49.5X6
FAC (fluorouracil + doxorubicin + cyclophosphamide)	T45.1X1	T45.1X2	T45.1X3	T45.1X4	T45.1X5	T45.1X6
Factor						
I (fibrinogen)	T45.8X1	T45.8X2	T45.8X3	T45.8X4	T45.8X5	T45.8X6
III (thromboplastin)	T45.8X1	T45.8X2	T45.8X3	T45.8X4	T45.8X5	T45.8X6
IX complex	T45.7X1	T45.7X2	T45.7X3	T45.7X4	T45.7X5	T45.7X6
human	T45.8X1	T45.8X2	T45.8X3	T45.8X4	T45.8X5	T45.8X6
VIII (antihemophilic Factor) (concentrate)	T45.8X1	T45.8X2	T45.8X3	T45.8X4	T45.8X5	T45.8X6
Famotidine	T47.0X1	T47.0X2	T47.0X3	T47.0X4	T47.0X5	T47.0X6
Fat suspension, intravenous	T50.991	T50.992	T50.993	T50.994	T50.995	T50.996
Fazadinium bromide	T48.1X1	T48.1X2	T48.1X3	T48.1X4	T48.1X5	T48.1X6
Febarbamate	T42.3X1	T42.3X2	T42.3X3	T42.3X4	T42.3X5	T42.3X6
Fecal softener	T47.4X1	T47.4X2	T47.4X3	T47.4X4	T47.4X5	T47.4X6
Fedrilate	T48.3X1	T48.3X2	T48.3X3	T48.3X4	T48.3X5	T48.3X6
Felodipine	T46.1X1	T46.1X2	T46.1X3	T46.1X4	T46.1X5	T46.1X6
Felypressin	T38.891	T38.892	T38.893	T38.894	T38.895	T38.896
Femoxetine	T43.221	T43.222	T43.223	T43.224	T43.225	T43.226
Fenalcomine	T46.3X1	T46.3X2	T46.3X3	T46.3X4	T46.3X5	T46.3X6
Fenamisal	T37.1X1	T37.1X2	T37.1X3	T37.1X4	T37.1X5	T37.1X6
Fenazone	T39.2X1	T39.2X2	T39.2X3	T39.2X4	T39.2X5	T39.2X6
Fenbendazole	T37.4X1	T37.4X2	T37.4X3	T37.4X4	T37.4X5	T37.4X6
Fenbutrazate	T50.5X1	T50.5X2	T50.5X3	T50.5X4	T50.5X5	T50.5X6
Fencamfamine	T43.691	T43.692	T43.693	T43.694	T43.695	T43.696
Fendiline	T46.1X1	T46.1X2	T46.1X3	T46.1X4	T46.1X5	T46.1X6
Fenetylline	T43.691	T43.692	T43.693	T43.694	T43.695	T43.696
Fenflumizole	T39.391	T39.392	T39.393	T39.394	T39.395	T39.396
Fenfluramine	T50.5X1	T50.5X2	T50.5X3	T50.5X4	T50.5X5	T50.5X6

Substance	Poisoning, Accidental (unintentional)	Poisoning, Intentional Self-harm	Poisoning, Assault	Poisoning, Undetermined	Adverse Effect	Under-dosing
Fenobarbital	T42.3X1	T42.3X2	T42.3X3	T42.3X4	T42.3X5	T42.3X6
Fenofibrate	T46.6X1	T46.6X2	T46.6X3	T46.6X4	T46.6X5	T46.6X6
Fenoprofen	T39.311	T39.312	T39.313	T39.314	T39.315	T39.316
Fenoterol	T48.6X1	T48.6X2	T48.6X3	T48.6X4	T48.6X5	T48.6X6
Fenoverine	T44.3X1	T44.3X2	T44.3X3	T44.3X4	T44.3X5	T44.3X6
Fenoxazoline	T48.5X1	T48.5X2	T48.5X3	T48.5X4	T48.5X5	T48.5X6
Fenproporex	T50.5X1	T50.5X2	T50.5X3	T50.5X4	T50.5X5	T50.5X6
Fenquizone	T50.2X1	T50.2X2	T50.2X3	T50.2X4	T50.2X5	T50.2X6
Fentanyl	T40.4X1	T40.4X2	T40.4X3	T40.4X4	T40.4X5	T40.4X6
Fentazin	T43.3X1	T43.3X2	T43.3X3	T43.3X4	T43.3X5	T43.3X6
Fenthion	T60.0X1	T60.0X2	T60.0X3	T60.0X4	—	—
Fenticlor	T49.0X1	T49.0X2	T49.0X3	T49.0X4	T49.0X5	T49.0X6
Fenylbutazone	T39.2X1	T39.2X2	T39.2X3	T39.2X4	T39.2X5	T39.2X6
Feprazone	T39.2X1	T39.2X2	T39.2X3	T39.2X4	T39.2X5	T39.2X6
Fer de lance (bite) (venom)	T63.061	T63.062	T63.063	T63.064	—	—
Ferric — *see also* Iron						
chloride	T45.4X1	T45.4X2	T45.4X3	T45.4X4	T45.4X5	T45.4X6
citrate	T45.4X1	T45.4X2	T45.4X3	T45.4X4	T45.4X5	T45.4X6
hydroxide						
colloidal	T45.4X1	T45.4X2	T45.4X3	T45.4X4	T45.4X5	T45.4X6
polymaltose	T45.4X1	T45.4X2	T45.4X3	T45.4X4	T45.4X5	T45.4X6
pyrophosphate	T45.4X1	T45.4X2	T45.4X3	T45.4X4	T45.4X5	T45.4X6
Ferritin	T45.4X1	T45.4X2	T45.4X3	T45.4X4	T45.4X5	T45.4X6
Ferrocholinate	T45.4X1	T45.4X2	T45.4X3	T45.4X4	T45.4X5	T45.4X6
Ferrodextrane	T45.4X1	T45.4X2	T45.4X3	T45.4X4	T45.4X5	T45.4X6
Ferropolimaler	T45.4X1	T45.4X2	T45.4X3	T45.4X4	T45.4X5	T45.4X6
Ferrous — *see also* Iron						
phosphate	T45.4X1	T45.4X2	T45.4X3	T45.4X4	T45.4X5	T45.4X6
salt	T45.4X1	T45.4X2	T45.4X3	T45.4X4	T45.4X5	T45.4X6
with folic acid	T45.4X1	T45.4X2	T45.4X3	T45.4X4	T45.4X5	T45.4X6
Ferrous fumerate, gluconate, lactate, salt NEC, sulfate (medicinal)	T45.4X1	T45.4X2	T45.4X3	T45.4X4	T45.4X5	T45.4X6
Ferrovanadium (fumes)	T59.891	T59.892	T59.893	T59.894	—	—
Ferrum — *see* Iron						
Fertilizers NEC	T65.891	T65.892	T65.893	T65.894	—	—
with herbicide mixture	T60.3X1	T60.3X2	T60.3X3	T60.3X4	—	—
Fetoxilate	T47.6X1	T47.6X2	T47.6X3	T47.6X4	T47.6X5	T47.6X6
Fiber, dietary	T47.4X1	T47.4X2	T47.4X3	T47.4X4	T47.4X5	T47.4X6
Fiberglass	T65.831	T65.832	T65.833	T65.834	—	—
Fibrinogen (human)	T45.8X1	T45.8X2	T45.8X3	T45.8X4	T45.8X5	T45.8X6
Fibrinolysin (human)	T45.691	T45.692	T45.693	T45.694	T45.695	T45.696
Fibrinolysis						
affecting drug	T45.601	T45.602	T45.603	T45.604	T45.605	T45.606
inhibitor NEC	T45.621	T45.622	T45.623	T45.624	T45.625	T45.626
Fibrinolytic drug	T45.611	T45.612	T45.613	T45.614	T45.615	T45.616
Filix mas	T37.4X1	T37.4X2	T37.4X3	T37.4X4	T37.4X5	T37.4X6
Filtering cream	T49.3X1	T49.3X2	T49.3X3	T49.3X4	T49.3X5	T49.3X6
Fiorinal	T39.011	T39.012	T39.013	T39.014	T39.015	T39.016
Firedamp	T59.891	T59.892	T59.893	T59.894	—	—
Fish, noxious, nonbacterial	T61.91	T61.92	T61.93	T61.94	—	—
ciguatera	T61.01	T61.02	T61.03	T61.04	—	—
scombroid	T61.11	T61.12	T61.13	T61.14	—	—
shell	T61.781	T61.782	T61.783	T61.784	—	—
specified NEC	T61.771	T61.772	T61.773	T61.774	—	—
Flagyl	T37.3X1	T37.3X2	T37.3X3	T37.3X4	T37.3X5	T37.3X6
Flavine adenine dinucleotide	T45.2X1	T45.2X2	T45.2X3	T45.2X4	T45.2X5	T45.2X6
Flavodic acid	T46.991	T46.992	T46.993	T46.994	T46.995	T46.996
Flavoxate	T44.3X1	T44.3X2	T44.3X3	T44.3X4	T44.3X5	T44.3X6
Flaxedil	T48.1X1	T48.1X2	T48.1X3	T48.1X4	T48.1X5	T48.1X6
Flaxseed (medicinal)	T49.3X1	T49.3X2	T49.3X3	T49.3X4	T49.3X5	T49.3X6
Flecainide	T46.2X1	T46.2X2	T46.2X3	T46.2X4	T46.2X5	T46.2X6
Fleroxacin	T36.8X1	T36.8X2	T36.8X3	T36.8X4	T36.8X5	T36.8X6
Floctafenine	T39.8X1	T39.8X2	T39.8X3	T39.8X4	T39.8X5	T39.8X6
Flomax	T44.6X1	T44.6X2	T44.6X3	T44.6X4	T44.6X5	T44.6X6
Flomoxef	T36.1X1	T36.1X2	T36.1X3	T36.1X4	T36.1X5	T36.1X6
Flopropione	T44.3X1	T44.3X2	T44.3X3	T44.3X4	T44.3X5	T44.3X6
Florantyrone	T47.5X1	T47.5X2	T47.5X3	T47.5X4	T47.5X5	T47.5X6
Floraquin	T37.8X1	T37.8X2	T37.8X3	T37.8X4	T37.8X5	T37.8X6
Florinef	T38.0X1	T38.0X2	T38.0X3	T38.0X4	T38.0X5	T38.0X6
ENT agent	T49.6X1	T49.6X2	T49.6X3	T49.6X4	T49.6X5	T49.6X6
ophthalmic preparation	T49.5X1	T49.5X2	T49.5X3	T49.5X4	T49.5X5	T49.5X6
topical NEC	T49.0X1	T49.0X2	T49.0X3	T49.0X4	T49.0X5	T49.0X6
Flowers of sulfur	T49.4X1	T49.4X2	T49.4X3	T49.4X4	T49.4X5	T49.4X6
Floxuridine	T45.1X1	T45.1X2	T45.1X3	T45.1X4	T45.1X5	T45.1X6
Fluanisone	T43.4X1	T43.4X2	T43.4X3	T43.4X4	T43.4X5	T43.4X6
Flubendazole	T37.4X1	T37.4X2	T37.4X3	T37.4X4	T37.4X5	T37.4X6
Fluclorolone acetonide	T49.0X1	T49.0X2	T49.0X3	T49.0X4	T49.0X5	T49.0X6
Flucloxacillin	T36.0X1	T36.0X2	T36.0X3	T36.0X4	T36.0X5	T36.0X6
Fluconazole	T37.8X1	T37.8X2	T37.8X3	T37.8X4	T37.8X5	T37.8X6
Flucytosine	T37.8X1	T37.8X2	T37.8X3	T37.8X4	T37.8X5	T37.8X6

Etinodiol — Flucytosine

Substance	Poisoning, Accidental (unintentional)	Poisoning, Intentional Self-harm	Poisoning, Assault	Poisoning, Undetermined	Adverse Effect	Under-dosing
Fludeoxyglucose (18F)	T50.8X1	T50.8X2	T50.8X3	T50.8X4	T50.8X5	T50.8X6
Fludiazepam	T42.4X1	T42.4X2	T42.4X3	T42.4X4	T42.4X5	T42.4X6
Fludrocortisone	T50.0X1	T50.0X2	T50.0X3	T50.0X4	T50.0X5	T50.0X6
ENT agent	T49.6X1	T49.6X2	T49.6X3	T49.6X4	T49.6X5	T49.6X6
ophthalmic preparation	T49.5X1	T49.5X2	T49.5X3	T49.5X4	T49.5X5	T49.5X6
topical NEC	T49.0X1	T49.0X2	T49.0X3	T49.0X4	T49.0X5	T49.0X6
Fludroxycortide	T49.0X1	T49.0X2	T49.0X3	T49.0X4	T49.0X5	T49.0X6
Flufenamic acid	T39.391	T39.392	T39.393	T39.394	T39.395	T39.396
Fluindione	T45.511	T45.512	T45.513	T45.514	T45.515	T45.516
Flumequine	T37.8X1	T37.8X2	T37.8X3	T37.8X4	T37.8X5	T37.8X6
Flumethasone	T49.0X1	T49.0X2	T49.0X3	T49.0X4	T49.0X5	T49.0X6
Flumethiazide	T50.2X1	T50.2X2	T50.2X3	T50.2X4	T50.2X5	T50.2X6
Flumidin	T37.5X1	T37.5X2	T37.5X3	T37.5X4	T37.5X5	T37.5X6
Flunarizine	T46.7X1	T46.7X2	T46.7X3	T46.7X4	T46.7X5	T46.7X6
Flunidazole	T37.8X1	T37.8X2	T37.8X3	T37.8X4	T37.8X5	T37.8X6
Flunisolide	T48.6X1	T48.6X2	T48.6X3	T48.6X4	T48.6X5	T48.6X6
Flunitrazepam	T42.4X1	T42.4X2	T42.4X3	T42.4X4	T42.4X5	T42.4X6
Fluocinolone (acetonide)	T49.0X1	T49.0X2	T49.0X3	T49.0X4	T49.0X5	T49.0X6
Fluocinonide	T49.0X1	T49.0X2	T49.0X3	T49.0X4	T49.0X5	T49.0X6
Fluocortin (butyl)	T49.0X1	T49.0X2	T49.0X3	T49.0X4	T49.0X5	T49.0X6
Fluocortolone	T49.0X1	T49.0X2	T49.0X3	T49.0X4	T49.0X5	T49.0X6
Fluohydrocortisone	T38.0X1	T38.0X2	T38.0X3	T38.0X4	T38.0X5	T38.0X6
ENT agent	T49.6X1	T49.6X2	T49.6X3	T49.6X4	T49.6X5	T49.6X6
ophthalmic preparation	T49.5X1	T49.5X2	T49.5X3	T49.5X4	T49.5X5	T49.5X6
topical NEC	T49.0X1	T49.0X2	T49.0X3	T49.0X4	T49.0X5	T49.0X6
Fluonid	T49.0X1	T49.0X2	T49.0X3	T49.0X4	T49.0X5	T49.0X6
Fluopromazine	T43.3X1	T43.3X2	T43.3X3	T43.3X4	T43.3X5	T43.3X6
Fluoracetate	T60.8X1	T60.8X2	T60.8X3	T60.8X4	—	—
Fluorescein	T50.8X1	T50.8X2	T50.8X3	T50.8X4	T50.8X5	T50.8X6
Fluorhydrocortisone	T50.0X1	T50.0X2	T50.0X3	T50.0X4	T50.0X5	T50.0X6
Fluoride (nonmedicinal) (pesticide) (sodium) **NEC**	T60.8X1	T60.8X2	T60.8X3	T60.8X4	—	—
hydrogen — see Hydrofluoric acid						
medicinal NEC	T50.991	T50.992	T50.993	T50.994	T50.995	T50.996
dental use	T49.7X1	T49.7X2	T49.7X3	T49.7X4	T49.7X5	T49.7X6
not pesticide NEC	T54.91	T54.92	T54.93	T54.94	—	—
stannous	T49.7X1	T49.7X2	T49.7X3	T49.7X4	T49.7X5	T49.7X6
Fluorinated corticosteroids	T38.0X1	T38.0X2	T38.0X3	T38.0X4	T38.0X5	T38.0X6
Fluorine (gas)	T59.5X1	T59.5X2	T59.5X3	T59.5X4	—	—
salt — see Fluoride(s)						
Fluoristan	T49.7X1	T49.7X2	T49.7X3	T49.7X4	T49.7X5	T49.7X6
Fluormetholone	T49.0X1	T49.0X2	T49.0X3	T49.0X4	T49.0X5	T49.0X6
Fluoroacetate	T60.8X1	T60.8X2	T60.8X3	T60.8X4	—	—
Fluorocarbon monomer	T53.6X1	T53.6X2	T53.6X3	T53.6X4	—	—
Fluorocytosine	T37.8X1	T37.8X2	T37.8X3	T37.8X4	T37.8X5	T37.8X6
Fluorodeoxyuridine	T45.1X1	T45.1X2	T45.1X3	T45.1X4	T45.1X5	T45.1X6
Fluorometholone	T49.0X1	T49.0X2	T49.0X3	T49.0X4	T49.0X5	T49.0X6
ophthalmic preparation	T49.5X1	T49.5X2	T49.5X3	T49.5X4	T49.5X5	T49.5X6
Fluorophosphate insecticide	T60.0X1	T60.0X2	T60.0X3	T60.0X4	—	—
Fluorosol	T46.3X1	T46.3X2	T46.3X3	T46.3X4	T46.3X5	T46.3X6
Fluorouracil	T45.1X1	T45.1X2	T45.1X3	T45.1X4	T45.1X5	T45.1X6
Fluorphenylalanine	T49.5X1	T49.5X2	T49.5X3	T49.5X4	T49.5X5	T49.5X6
Fluothane	T41.0X1	T41.0X2	T41.0X3	T41.0X4	T41.0X5	T41.0X6
Fluoxetine	T43.221	T43.222	T43.223	T43.224	T43.225	T43.226
Fluoxymesterone	T38.7X1	T38.7X2	T38.7X3	T38.7X4	T38.7X5	T38.7X6
Flupenthixol	T43.4X1	T43.4X2	T43.4X3	T43.4X4	T43.4X5	T43.4X6
Flupentixol	T43.4X1	T43.4X2	T43.4X3	T43.4X4	T43.4X5	T43.4X6
Fluphenazine	T43.3X1	T43.3X2	T43.3X3	T43.3X4	T43.3X5	T43.3X6
Fluprednidene	T49.0X1	T49.0X2	T49.0X3	T49.0X4	T49.0X5	T49.0X6
Fluprednisolone	T38.0X1	T38.0X2	T38.0X3	T38.0X4	T38.0X5	T38.0X6
Fluradoline	T39.8X1	T39.8X2	T39.8X3	T39.8X4	T39.8X5	T39.8X6
Flurandrenolide	T49.0X1	T49.0X2	T49.0X3	T49.0X4	T49.0X5	T49.0X6
Flurandrenolone	T49.0X1	T49.0X2	T49.0X3	T49.0X4	T49.0X5	T49.0X6
Flurazepam	T42.4X1	T42.4X2	T42.4X3	T42.4X4	T42.4X5	T42.4X6
Flurbiprofen	T39.311	T39.312	T39.313	T39.314	T39.315	T39.316
Flurobate	T49.0X1	T49.0X2	T49.0X3	T49.0X4	T49.0X5	T49.0X6
Fluroxene	T41.0X1	T41.0X2	T41.0X3	T41.0X4	T41.0X5	T41.0X6
Fluspirilene	T43.591	T43.592	T43.593	T43.594	T43.595	T43.596
Flutamide	T38.6X1	T38.6X2	T38.6X3	T38.6X4	T38.6X5	T38.6X6
Flutazolam	T38.0X1	T38.0X2	T38.0X3	T38.0X4	T38.0X5	T38.0X6
Fluticasone propionate	T38.0X1	T38.0X2	T38.0X3	T38.0X4	T38.0X5	T38.0X6
Flutoprazepam	T42.4X1	T42.4X2	T42.4X3	T42.4X4	T42.4X5	T42.4X6
Flutropium bromide	T48.6X1	T48.6X2	T48.6X3	T48.6X4	T48.6X5	T48.6X6
Fluvoxamine	T43.221	T43.222	T43.223	T43.224	T43.225	T43.226
Folacin	T45.8X1	T45.8X2	T45.8X3	T45.8X4	T45.8X5	T45.8X6
Folic acid	T45.8X1	T45.8X2	T45.8X3	T45.8X4	T45.8X5	T45.8X6
with ferrous salt	T45.2X1	T45.2X2	T45.2X3	T45.2X4	T45.2X5	T45.2X6
antagonist	T45.1X1	T45.1X2	T45.1X3	T45.1X4	T45.1X5	T45.1X6
Folinic acid	T45.8X1	T45.8X2	T45.8X3	T45.8X4	T45.8X5	T45.8X6
Folium stramoniae	T48.6X1	T48.6X2	T48.6X3	T48.6X4	T48.6X5	T48.6X6
Follicle-stimulating hormone, human	T38.811	T38.812	T38.813	T38.814	T38.815	T38.816
Folpet	T60.3X1	T60.3X2	T60.3X3	T60.3X4	—	—
Fominoben	T48.3X1	T48.3X2	T48.3X3	T48.3X4	T48.3X5	T48.3X6
Food, foodstuffs, noxious, nonbacterial, NEC	T62.91	T62.92	T62.93	T62.94	—	—
berries	T62.1X1	T62.1X2	T62.1X3	T62.1X4	—	—
fish — see also Fish	T61.91	T61.92	T61.93	T61.94	—	—
mushrooms	T62.0X1	T62.0X2	T62.0X3	T62.0X4	—	—
plants	T62.2X1	T62.2X2	T62.2X3	T62.2X4	—	—
seafood	T61.91	T61.92	T61.93	T61.94	—	—
specified NEC	T61.8X1	T61.8X2	T61.8X3	T61.8X4	—	—
seeds	T62.2X1	T62.2X2	T62.2X3	T62.2X4	—	—
shellfish	T61.781	T61.782	T61.783	T61.784	—	—
specified NEC	T62.8X1	T62.8X2	T62.8X3	T62.8X4	—	—
Fool's parsley	T62.2X1	T62.2X2	T62.2X3	T62.2X4	—	—
Formaldehyde (solution), gas or vapor	T59.2X1	T59.2X2	T59.2X3	T59.2X4	—	—
fungicide	T60.3X1	T60.3X2	T60.3X3	T60.3X4	—	—
Formalin	T59.2X1	T59.2X2	T59.2X3	T59.2X4	—	—
fungicide	T60.3X1	T60.3X2	T60.3X3	T60.3X4	—	—
vapor	T59.2X1	T59.2X2	T59.2X3	T59.2X4	—	—
Formic acid	T54.2X1	T54.2X2	T54.2X3	T54.2X4	—	—
vapor	T59.891	T59.892	T59.893	T59.894	—	—
Foscarnet sodium	T37.5X1	T37.5X2	T37.5X3	T37.5X4	T37.5X5	T37.5X6
Fosfestrol	T38.5X1	T38.5X2	T38.5X3	T38.5X4	T38.5X5	T38.5X6
Fosfomycin	T36.8X1	T36.8X2	T36.8X3	T36.8X4	T36.8X5	T36.8X6
Fosfonet sodium	T37.5X1	T37.5X2	T37.5X3	T37.5X4	T37.5X5	T37.5X6
Fosinopril	T46.4X1	T46.4X2	T46.4X3	T46.4X4	T46.4X5	T46.4X6
sodium	T46.4X1	T46.4X2	T46.4X3	T46.4X4	T46.4X5	T46.4X6
Fowler's solution	T57.0X1	T57.0X2	T57.0X3	T57.0X4	—	—
Foxglove	T62.2X1	T62.2X2	T62.2X3	T62.2X4	—	—
Framycetin	T36.5X1	T36.5X2	T36.5X3	T36.5X4	T36.5X5	T36.5X6
Frangula	T47.2X1	T47.2X2	T47.2X3	T47.2X4	T47.2X5	T47.2X6
extract	T47.2X1	T47.2X2	T47.2X3	T47.2X4	T47.2X5	T47.2X6
Frei antigen	T50.8X1	T50.8X2	T50.8X3	T50.8X4	T50.8X5	T50.8X6
Freon	T53.5X1	T53.5X2	T53.5X3	T53.5X4	—	—
Fructose	T50.3X1	T50.3X2	T50.3X3	T50.3X4	T50.3X5	T50.3X6
Frusemide	T50.1X1	T50.1X2	T50.1X3	T50.1X4	T50.1X5	T50.1X6
FSH	T38.811	T38.812	T38.813	T38.814	T38.815	T38.816
Ftorafur	T45.1X1	T45.1X2	T45.1X3	T45.1X4	T45.1X5	T45.1X6
Fuel						
automobile	T52.0X1	T52.0X2	T52.0X3	T52.0X4	—	—
exhaust gas, not in transit	T58.01	T58.02	T58.03	T58.04	—	—
vapor NEC	T52.0X1	T52.0X2	T52.0X3	T52.0X4	—	—
gas (domestic use) — see also Carbon, monoxide, fuel, utility	T59.891	T59.892	T59.893	T59.894	—	—
utility	T59.891	T59.892	T59.893	T59.894	—	—
incomplete combustion of — see Carbon, monoxide, fuel, utility						
in mobile container	T59.891	T59.892	T59.893	T59.894	—	—
piped (natural)	T59.891	T59.892	T59.893	T59.894	—	—
industrial, incomplete combustion	T58.8X1	T58.8X2	T58.8X3	T58.8X4	—	—
Fugillin	T36.8X1	T36.8X2	T36.8X3	T36.8X4	T36.8X5	T36.8X6
Fulminate of mercury	T56.1X1	T56.1X2	T56.1X3	T56.1X4	—	—
Fulvicin	T36.7X1	T36.7X2	T36.7X3	T36.7X4	T36.7X5	T36.7X6
Fumadil	T36.8X1	T36.8X2	T36.8X3	T36.8X4	T36.8X5	T36.8X6
Fumagillin	T36.8X1	T36.8X2	T36.8X3	T36.8X4	T36.8X5	T36.8X6
Fumaric acid	T49.4X1	T49.4X2	T49.4X3	T49.4X4	T49.4X5	T49.4X6
Fumes (from)	T59.91	T59.92	T59.93	T59.94	—	—
carbon monoxide — see Carbon, monoxide						
charcoal (domestic use) — see Charcoal, fumes						
chloroform — see Chloroform						
coke (in domestic stoves, fireplaces) — see Coke fumes						
corrosive NEC	T54.91	T54.92	T54.93	T54.94	—	—
ether — see ether						
freons	T53.5X1	T53.5X2	T53.5X3	T53.5X4	—	—
hydrocarbons	T59.891	T59.892	T59.893	T59.894	—	—
petroleum (liquefied)	T59.891	T59.892	T59.893	T59.894	—	—
distributed through pipes (pure or mixed with air)	T59.891	T59.892	T59.893	T59.894	—	—
lead — see lead						
metal — see Metals, or the specified metal						

Additional Character May Be Required — Refer to the Tabular List for Character Selection ▶ **Subterms under main terms may continue to next column or page**

Substance	Poisoning, Accidental (unintentional)	Poisoning, Intentional Self-harm	Poisoning, Assault	Poisoning, Undetermined	Adverse Effect	Under-dosing
Fumes — *continued*						
nitrogen dioxide	T59.0X1	T59.0X2	T59.0X3	T59.0X4	—	—
pesticides — *see* Pesticides						
petroleum (liquefied)	T59.891	T59.892	T59.893	T59.894	—	—
distributed through pipes (pure or mixed with air)	T59.891	T59.892	T59.893	T59.894	—	—
polyester	T59.891	T59.892	T59.893	T59.894	—	—
specified source NEC — *see also* substance specified	T59.891	T59.892	T59.893	T59.894	—	—
sulfur dioxide	T59.1X1	T59.1X2	T59.1X3	T59.1X4	—	—
Fumigant NEC	T60.91	T60.92	T60.93	T60.94	—	—
Fungicide NEC	T60.3X1	T60.3X2	T60.3X3	T60.3X4	—	—
(nonmedicinal)						
Fungi, noxious, used as food	T62.0X1	T62.0X2	T62.0X3	T62.0X4	—	—
Fungizone	T36.7X1	T36.7X2	T36.7X3	T36.7X4	T36.7X5	T36.7X6
topical	T49.0X1	T49.0X2	T49.0X3	T49.0X4	T49.0X5	T49.0X6
Furacin	T49.0X1	T49.0X2	T49.0X3	T49.0X4	T49.0X5	T49.0X6
Furadantin	T37.91	T37.92	T37.93	T37.94	T37.95	T37.96
Furazolidone	T37.8X1	T37.8X2	T37.8X3	T37.8X4	T37.8X5	T37.8X6
Furazolium chloride	T49.0X1	T49.0X2	T49.0X3	T49.0X4	T49.0X5	T49.0X6
Furfural	T52.8X1	T52.8X2	T52.8X3	T52.8X4	—	—
Furnace (coal burning) (domestic), gas from	T58.2X1	T58.2X2	T58.2X3	T58.2X4	—	—
industrial	T58.8X1	T58.8X2	T58.8X3	T58.8X4	—	—
Furniture polish	T65.891	T65.892	T65.893	T65.894	—	—
Furosemide	T50.1X1	T50.1X2	T50.1X3	T50.1X4	T50.1X5	T50.1X6
Furoxone	T37.91	T37.92	T37.93	T37.94	T37.95	T37.96
Fursultiamine	T45.2X1	T45.2X2	T45.2X3	T45.2X4	T45.2X5	T45.2X6
Fusafungine	T36.8X1	T36.8X2	T36.8X3	T36.8X4	T36.8X5	T36.8X6
Fusel oil (any) (amyl) (butyl) (propyl), vapor	T51.3X1	T51.3X2	T51.3X3	T51.3X4	—	—
Fusidate (ethanolamine) (sodium)	T36.8X1	T36.8X2	T36.8X3	T36.8X4	T36.8X5	T36.8X6
Fusidic acid	T36.8X1	T36.8X2	T36.8X3	T36.8X4	T36.8X5	T36.8X6
Fytic acid, nonasodium	T50.6X1	T50.6X2	T50.6X3	T50.6X4	T50.6X5	T50.6X6
b-Galactosidase	T47.5X1	T47.5X2	T47.5X3	T47.5X4	T47.5X5	T47.5X6
GABA	T43.8X1	T43.8X2	T43.8X3	T43.8X4	T43.8X5	T43.8X6
Gadopentetic acid	T50.8X1	T50.8X2	T50.8X3	T50.8X4	T50.8X5	T50.8X6
Galactose	T50.3X1	T50.3X2	T50.3X3	T50.3X4	T50.3X5	T50.3X6
Galantamine	T44.0X1	T44.0X2	T44.0X3	T44.0X4	T44.0X5	T44.0X6
Gallamine (triethiodide)	T48.1X1	T48.1X2	T48.1X3	T48.1X4	T48.1X5	T48.1X6
Gallium citrate	T50.991	T50.992	T50.993	T50.994	T50.995	T50.996
Gallopamil	T46.1X1	T46.1X2	T46.1X3	T46.1X4	T46.1X5	T46.1X6
Gamboge	T47.2X1	T47.2X2	T47.2X3	T47.2X4	T47.2X5	T47.2X6
Gamimune	T50.Z11	T50.Z12	T50.Z13	T50.Z14	T50.Z15	T50.Z16
Gamma-aminobutyric acid	T43.8X1	T43.8X2	T43.8X3	T43.8X4	T43.8X5	T43.8X6
Gamma-benzene hexachloride (medicinal)	T49.0X1	T49.0X2	T49.0X3	T49.0X4	T49.0X5	T49.0X6
nonmedicinal, vapor	T53.6X1	T53.6X2	T53.6X3	T53.6X4	—	—
Gamma-BHC (medicinal) — *see also* Gamma-benzene hexachloride	T49.0X1	T49.0X2	T49.0X3	T49.0X4	T49.0X5	T49.0X6
Gamma globulin	T50.Z11	T50.Z12	T50.Z13	T50.Z14	T50.Z15	T50.Z16
Gamulin	T50.Z11	T50.Z12	T50.Z13	T50.Z14	T50.Z15	T50.Z16
Ganciclovir (sodium)	T37.5X1	T37.5X2	T37.5X3	T37.5X4	T37.5X5	T37.5X6
Ganglionic blocking drug NEC	T44.2X1	T44.2X2	T44.2X3	T44.2X4	T44.2X5	T44.2X6
specified NEC	T44.2X1	T44.2X2	T44.2X3	T44.2X4	T44.2X5	T44.2X6
Ganja	T40.7X1	T40.7X2	T40.7X3	T40.7X4	T40.7X5	T40.7X6
Garamycin	T36.5X1	T36.5X2	T36.5X3	T36.5X4	T36.5X5	T36.5X6
ophthalmic preparation	T49.5X1	T49.5X2	T49.5X3	T49.5X4	T49.5X5	T49.5X6
topical NEC	T49.0X1	T49.0X2	T49.0X3	T49.0X4	T49.0X5	T49.0X6
Gardenal	T42.3X1	T42.3X2	T42.3X3	T42.3X4	T42.3X5	T42.3X6
Gardepanyl	T42.3X1	T42.3X2	T42.3X3	T42.3X4	T42.3X5	T42.3X6
Gaseous substance — *see* Gas						
Gasoline	T52.0X1	T52.0X2	T52.0X3	T52.0X4	—	—
vapor	T52.0X1	T52.0X2	T52.0X3	T52.0X4	—	—
Gastric enzymes	T47.5X1	T47.5X2	T47.5X3	T47.5X4	T47.5X5	T47.5X6
Gastrografin	T50.8X1	T50.8X2	T50.8X3	T50.8X4	T50.8X5	T50.8X6
Gastrointestinal drug	T47.91	T47.92	T47.93	T47.94	T47.95	T47.96
biological	T47.8X1	T47.8X2	T47.8X3	T47.8X4	T47.8X5	T47.8X6
specified NEC	T47.8X1	T47.8X2	T47.8X3	T47.8X4	T47.8X5	T47.8X6
Gas NEC	T59.91	T59.92	T59.93	T59.94	—	—
acetylene	T59.891	T59.892	T59.893	T59.894	—	—
incomplete combustion of	T58.11	T58.12	T58.13	T58.14	—	—
air contaminants, source or type not specified	T59.91	T59.92	T59.93	T59.94	—	—
anesthetic	T41.0X1	T41.0X2	T41.0X3	T41.0X4	T41.0X5	T41.0X6
blast furnace	T58.8X1	T58.8X2	T58.8X3	T58.8X4	—	—
butane — *see* butane						

Substance	Poisoning, Accidental (unintentional)	Poisoning, Intentional Self-harm	Poisoning, Assault	Poisoning, Undetermined	Adverse Effect	Under-dosing
Gas — *continued*						
carbon monoxide — *see* Carbon, monoxide						
chlorine	T59.4X1	T59.4X2	T59.4X3	T59.4X4	—	—
coal	T58.2X1	T58.2X2	T58.2X3	T58.2X4	—	—
cyanide	T57.3X1	T57.3X2	T57.3X3	T57.3X4	—	—
dicyanogen	T65.0X1	T65.0X2	T65.0X3	T65.0X4	—	—
domestic — *see* Domestic gas						
exhaust	T58.01	T58.02	T58.03	T58.04	—	—
from utility (for cooking, heating, or lighting) (after combustion) — *see* Carbon, monoxide, fuel, utility						
prior to combustion	T59.891	T59.892	T59.893	T59.894	—	—
from wood- or coal-burning stove or fireplace	T58.2X1	T58.2X2	T58.2X3	T58.2X4	—	—
fuel (domestic use) (after combustion) — *see also* Carbon, monoxide, fuel						
industrial use	T58.8X1	T58.8X2	T58.8X3	T58.8X4	—	—
prior to combustion	T59.891	T59.892	T59.893	T59.894	—	—
utility	T59.891	T59.892	T59.893	T59.894	—	—
incomplete combustion of — *see* Carbon, monoxide, fuel, utility						
in mobile container	T59.891	T59.892	T59.893	T59.894	—	—
piped (natural)	T59.891	T59.892	T59.893	T59.894	—	—
garage	T58.01	T58.02	T58.03	T58.04	—	—
hydrocarbon NEC	T59.891	T59.892	T59.893	T59.894	—	—
incomplete combustion of — *see* Carbon, monoxide, fuel, utility						
liquefied — *see* butane						
piped	T59.891	T59.892	T59.893	T59.894	—	—
hydrocyanic acid	T65.0X1	T65.0X2	T65.0X3	T65.0X4	—	—
illuminating (after combustion)	T58.11	T58.12	T58.13	T58.14	—	—
prior to combustion	T59.891	T59.892	T59.893	T59.894	—	—
incomplete combustion, any — *see* Carbon, monoxide						
kiln	T58.8X1	T58.8X2	T58.8X3	T58.8X4	—	—
lacrimogenic	T59.3X1	T59.3X2	T59.3X3	T59.3X4	—	—
liquefied petroleum — *see* butane						
marsh	T59.891	T59.892	T59.893	T59.894	—	—
motor exhaust, not in transit	T58.01	T58.02	T58.03	T58.04	—	—
mustard, not in war	T59.891	T59.892	T59.893	T59.894	—	—
natural	T59.891	T59.892	T59.893	T59.894	—	—
nerve, not in war	T59.91	T59.92	T59.93	T59.94	—	—
oil	T52.0X1	T52.0X2	T52.0X3	T52.0X4	—	—
petroleum (liquefied) (distributed in mobile containers)	T59.891	T59.892	T59.893	T59.894	—	—
piped (pure or mixed with air)	T59.891	T59.892	T59.893	T59.894	—	—
piped (manufactured) (natural) NEC	T59.891	T59.892	T59.893	T59.894	—	—
producer	T58.8X1	T58.8X2	T58.8X3	T58.8X4	—	—
propane — *see* propane						
refrigerant (chlorofluoro-carbon)	T53.5X1	T53.5X2	T53.5X3	T53.5X4	—	—
not chlorofluoro-carbon	T59.891	T59.892	T59.893	T59.894	—	—
sewer	T59.91	T59.92	T59.93	T59.94	—	—
specified source NEC	T59.91	T59.92	T59.93	T59.94	—	—
stove (after combustion)	T58.11	T58.12	T58.13	T58.14	—	—
prior to combustion	T59.891	T59.892	T59.893	T59.894	—	—
tear	T59.3X1	T59.3X2	T59.3X3	T59.3X4	—	—
therapeutic	T41.5X1	T41.5X2	T41.5X3	T41.5X4	T41.5X5	T41.5X6
utility (for cooking, heating, or lighting) (piped) NEC	T59.891	T59.892	T59.893	T59.894	—	—
incomplete combustion of — *see* Carbon, monoxide, fuel, utilty						
in mobile container	T59.891	T59.892	T59.893	T59.894	—	—
piped (natural)	T59.891	T59.892	T59.893	T59.894	—	—
water	T58.11	T58.12	T58.13	T58.14	—	—
incomplete combustion of — *see* Carbon, monoxide, fuel, utility						
Gaultheria procumbens	T62.2X1	T62.2X2	T62.2X3	T62.2X4	—	—
Gefarnate	T44.3X1	T44.3X2	T44.3X3	T44.3X4	T44.3X5	T44.3X6
Gelatin (intravenous)	T45.8X1	T45.8X2	T45.8X3	T45.8X4	T45.8X5	T45.8X6

Substance	Poisoning, Accidental (unintentional)	Poisoning, Intentional Self-harm	Poisoning, Assault	Poisoning, Undetermined	Adverse Effect	Under-dosing
Gelatin — *continued*						
absorbable (sponge)	T45.7X1	T45.7X2	T45.7X3	T45.7X4	T45.7X5	T45.7X6
Gelfilm	T49.8X1	T49.8X2	T49.8X3	T49.8X4	T49.8X5	T49.8X6
Gelfoam	T45.7X1	T45.7X2	T45.7X3	T45.7X4	T45.7X5	T45.7X6
Gelsemine	T50.991	T50.992	T50.993	T50.994	T50.995	T50.996
Gelsemium (sempervirens)	T62.2X1	T62.2X2	T62.2X3	T62.2X4	—	—
Gemeprost	T48.0X1	T48.0X2	T48.0X3	T48.0X4	T48.0X5	T48.0X6
Gemfibrozil	T46.6X1	T46.6X2	T46.6X3	T46.6X4	T46.6X5	T46.6X6
Gemonil	T42.3X1	T42.3X2	T42.3X3	T42.3X4	T42.3X5	T42.3X6
Gentamicin	T36.5X1	T36.5X2	T36.5X3	T36.5X4	T36.5X5	T36.5X6
ophthalmic preparation	T49.5X1	T49.5X2	T49.5X3	T49.5X4	T49.5X5	T49.5X6
topical NEC	T49.0X1	T49.0X2	T49.0X3	T49.0X4	T49.0X5	T49.0X6
Gentian	T47.5X1	T47.5X2	T47.5X3	T47.5X4	T47.5X5	T47.5X6
violet	T49.0X1	T49.0X2	T49.0X3	T49.0X4	T49.0X5	T49.0X6
Gepefrine	T44.4X1	T44.4X2	T44.4X3	T44.4X4	T44.4X5	T44.4X6
Gestonorone caproate	T38.5X1	T38.5X2	T38.5X3	T38.5X4	T38.5X5	T38.5X6
Gexane	T49.0X1	T49.0X2	T49.0X3	T49.0X4	T49.0X5	T49.0X6
Gila monster (venom)	T63.111	T63.112	T63.113	T63.114	—	—
Ginger	T47.5X1	T47.5X2	T47.5X3	T47.5X4	T47.5X5	T47.5X6
Jamaica — *see* Jamaica, ginger						
Gitalin	T46.0X1	T46.0X2	T46.0X3	T46.0X4	T46.0X5	T46.0X6
amorphous	T46.0X1	T46.0X2	T46.0X3	T46.0X4	T46.0X5	T46.0X6
Gitaloxin	T46.0X1	T46.0X2	T46.0X3	T46.0X4	T46.0X5	T46.0X6
Gitoxin	T46.0X1	T46.0X2	T46.0X3	T46.0X4	T46.0X5	T46.0X6
Glafenine	T39.8X1	T39.8X2	T39.8X3	T39.8X4	T39.8X5	T39.8X6
Glandular extract (medicinal) NEC	T50.Z91	T50.Z92	T50.Z93	T50.Z94	T50.Z95	T50.Z96
Glaucarubin	T37.3X1	T37.3X2	T37.3X3	T37.3X4	T37.3X5	T37.3X6
Glibenclamide	T38.3X1	T38.3X2	T38.3X3	T38.3X4	T38.3X5	T38.3X6
Glibornuride	T38.3X1	T38.3X2	T38.3X3	T38.3X4	T38.3X5	T38.3X6
Gliclazide	T38.3X1	T38.3X2	T38.3X3	T38.3X4	T38.3X5	T38.3X6
Glimidine	T38.3X1	T38.3X2	T38.3X3	T38.3X4	T38.3X5	T38.3X6
Glipizide	T38.3X1	T38.3X2	T38.3X3	T38.3X4	T38.3X5	T38.3X6
Gliquidone	T38.3X1	T38.3X2	T38.3X3	T38.3X4	T38.3X5	T38.3X6
Glisolamide	T38.3X1	T38.3X2	T38.3X3	T38.3X4	T38.3X5	T38.3X6
Glisoxepide	T38.3X1	T38.3X2	T38.3X3	T38.3X4	T38.3X5	T38.3X6
Globin zinc insulin	T38.3X1	T38.3X2	T38.3X3	T38.3X4	T38.3X5	T38.3X6
Globulin						
antilymphocytic	T50.Z11	T50.Z12	T50.Z13	T50.Z14	T50.Z15	T50.Z16
antirhesus	T50.Z11	T50.Z12	T50.Z13	T50.Z14	T50.Z15	T50.Z16
antivenin	T50.Z11	T50.Z12	T50.Z13	T50.Z14	T50.Z15	T50.Z16
antiviral	T50.Z11	T50.Z12	T50.Z13	T50.Z14	T50.Z15	T50.Z16
Glucagon	T38.3X1	T38.3X2	T38.3X3	T38.3X4	T38.3X5	T38.3X6
Glucocorticoids	T38.0X1	T38.0X2	T38.0X3	T38.0X4	T38.0X5	T38.0X6
Glucocorticosteroid	T38.0X1	T38.0X2	T38.0X3	T38.0X4	T38.0X5	T38.0X6
Gluconic acid	T50.991	T50.992	T50.993	T50.994	T50.995	T50.996
Glucosamine sulfate	T39.4X1	T39.4X2	T39.4X3	T39.4X4	T39.4X5	T39.4X6
Glucose	T50.3X1	T50.3X2	T50.3X3	T50.3X4	T50.3X5	T50.3X6
with sodium chloride	T50.3X1	T50.3X2	T50.3X3	T50.3X4	T50.3X5	T50.3X6
Glucosulfone sodium	T37.1X1	T37.1X2	T37.1X3	T37.1X4	T37.1X5	T37.1X6
Glucurolactone	T47.8X1	T47.8X2	T47.8X3	T47.8X4	T47.8X5	T47.8X6
Glue NEC	T52.8X1	T52.8X2	T52.8X3	T52.8X4	—	—
Glutamic acid	T47.5X1	T47.5X2	T47.5X3	T47.5X4	T47.5X5	T47.5X6
Glutaral (medicinal)	T49.0X1	T49.0X2	T49.0X3	T49.0X4	T49.0X5	T49.0X6
nonmedicinal	T65.891	T65.892	T65.893	T65.894	—	—
Glutaraldehyde (nonmedicinal)	T65.891	T65.892	T65.893	T65.894	—	—
medicinal	T49.0X1	T49.0X2	T49.0X3	T49.0X4	T49.0X5	T49.0X6
Glutathione	T50.6X1	T50.6X2	T50.6X3	T50.6X4	T50.6X5	T50.6X6
Glutethimide	T42.6X1	T42.6X2	T42.6X3	T42.6X4	T42.6X5	T42.6X6
Glyburide	T38.3X1	T38.3X2	T38.3X3	T38.3X4	T38.3X5	T38.3X6
Glycerin	T47.4X1	T47.4X2	T47.4X3	T47.4X4	T47.4X5	T47.4X6
Glycerol	T47.4X1	T47.4X2	T47.4X3	T47.4X4	T47.4X5	T47.4X6
borax	T49.6X1	T49.6X2	T49.6X3	T49.6X4	T49.6X5	T49.6X6
intravenous	T50.3X1	T50.3X2	T50.3X3	T50.3X4	T50.3X5	T50.3X6
iodinated	T48.4X1	T48.4X2	T48.4X3	T48.4X4	T48.4X5	T48.4X6
Glycerophosphate	T50.991	T50.992	T50.993	T50.994	T50.995	T50.996
Glyceryl						
gualacolate	T48.4X1	T48.4X2	T48.4X3	T48.4X4	T48.4X5	T48.4X6
nitrate	T46.3X1	T46.3X2	T46.3X3	T46.3X4	T46.3X5	T46.3X6
triacetate (topical)	T49.0X1	T49.0X2	T49.0X3	T49.0X4	T49.0X5	T49.0X6
trinitrate	T46.3X1	T46.3X2	T46.3X3	T46.3X4	T46.3X5	T46.3X6
Glycine	T50.3X1	T50.3X2	T50.3X3	T50.3X4	T50.3X5	T50.3X6
Glyclopyramide	T38.3X1	T38.3X2	T38.3X3	T38.3X4	T38.3X5	T38.3X6
Glycobiarsol	T37.3X1	T37.3X2	T37.3X3	T37.3X4	T37.3X5	T37.3X6
Glycols (ether)	T52.3X1	T52.3X2	T52.3X3	T52.3X4	—	—
Glyconiazide	T37.1X1	T37.1X2	T37.1X3	T37.1X4	T37.1X5	T37.1X6
Glycopyrrolate	T44.3X1	T44.3X2	T44.3X3	T44.3X4	T44.3X5	T44.3X6
Glycopyrronium	T44.3X1	T44.3X2	T44.3X3	T44.3X4	T44.3X5	T44.3X6
bromide	T44.3X1	T44.3X2	T44.3X3	T44.3X4	T44.3X5	T44.3X6
Glycoside, cardiac (stimulant)	T46.0X1	T46.0X2	T46.0X3	T46.0X4	T46.0X5	T46.0X6
Glycyclamide	T38.3X1	T38.3X2	T38.3X3	T38.3X4	T38.3X5	T38.3X6

Substance	Poisoning, Accidental (unintentional)	Poisoning, Intentional Self-harm	Poisoning, Assault	Poisoning, Undetermined	Adverse Effect	Under-dosing
Glycyrrhiza extract	T48.4X1	T48.4X2	T48.4X3	T48.4X4	T48.4X5	T48.4X6
Glycyrrhizic acid	T48.4X1	T48.4X2	T48.4X3	T48.4X4	T48.4X5	T48.4X6
Glycyrrhizinate potassium	T48.4X1	T48.4X2	T48.4X3	T48.4X4	T48.4X5	T48.4X6
Glymidine sodium	T38.3X1	T38.3X2	T38.3X3	T38.3X4	T38.3X5	T38.3X6
Glyphosate	T60.3X1	T60.3X2	T60.3X3	T60.3X4	—	—
Glyphylline	T48.6X1	T48.6X2	T48.6X3	T48.6X4	T48.6X5	T48.6X6
Gold						
colloidal (I98Au)	T45.1X1	T45.1X2	T45.1X3	T45.1X4	T45.1X5	T45.1X6
salts	T39.4X1	T39.4X2	T39.4X3	T39.4X4	T39.4X5	T39.4X6
Golden sulfide of antimony	T56.891	T56.892	T56.893	T56.894		
Goldylocks	T62.2X1	T62.2X2	T62.2X3	T62.2X4	—	—
Gonadal tissue extract	T38.901	T38.902	T38.903	T38.904	T38.905	T38.906
female	T38.5X1	T38.5X2	T38.5X3	T38.5X4	T38.5X5	T38.5X6
male	T38.7X1	T38.7X2	T38.7X3	T38.7X4	T38.7X5	T38.7X6
Gonadorelin	T38.891	T38.892	T38.893	T38.894	T38.895	T38.896
Gonadotropin	T38.891	T38.892	T38.893	T38.894	T38.895	T38.896
chorionic	T38.891	T38.892	T38.893	T38.894	T38.895	T38.896
pituitary	T38.811	T38.812	T38.813	T38.814	T38.815	T38.816
Goserelin	T45.1X1	T45.1X2	T45.1X3	T45.1X4	T45.1X5	T45.1X6
Grain alcohol	T51.0X1	T51.0X2	T51.0X3	T51.0X4	—	—
Gramicidin	T49.0X1	T49.0X2	T49.0X3	T49.0X4	T49.0X5	T49.0X6
Granisetron	T45.0X1	T45.0X2	T45.0X3	T45.0X4	T45.0X5	T45.0X6
Gratiola officinalis	T62.2X1	T62.2X2	T62.2X3	T62.2X4	—	—
Grease	T65.891	T65.892	T65.893	T65.894	—	—
Green hellebore	T62.2X1	T62.2X2	T62.2X3	T62.2X4	—	—
Green soap	T49.2X1	T49.2X2	T49.2X3	T49.2X4	T49.2X5	T49.2X6
Grifulvin	T36.7X1	T36.7X2	T36.7X3	T36.7X4	T36.7X5	T36.7X6
Griseofulvin	T36.7X1	T36.7X2	T36.7X3	T36.7X4	T36.7X5	T36.7X6
Growth hormone	T38.811	T38.812	T38.813	T38.814	T38.815	T38.816
Guaiacol derivatives	T48.4X1	T48.4X2	T48.4X3	T48.4X4	T48.4X5	T48.4X6
Guaiac reagent	T50.991	T50.992	T50.993	T50.994	T50.995	T50.996
Guaifenesin	T48.4X1	T48.4X2	T48.4X3	T48.4X4	T48.4X5	T48.4X6
Guaimesal	T48.4X1	T48.4X2	T48.4X3	T48.4X4	T48.4X5	T48.4X6
Guaiphenesin	T48.4X1	T48.4X2	T48.4X3	T48.4X4	T48.4X5	T48.4X6
Guamecycline	T36.4X1	T36.4X2	T36.4X3	T36.4X4	T36.4X5	T36.4X6
Guanabenz	T46.5X1	T46.5X2	T46.5X3	T46.5X4	T46.5X5	T46.5X6
Guanacline	T46.5X1	T46.5X2	T46.5X3	T46.5X4	T46.5X5	T46.5X6
Guanadrel	T46.5X1	T46.5X2	T46.5X3	T46.5X4	T46.5X5	T46.5X6
Guanatol	T37.2X1	T37.2X2	T37.2X3	T37.2X4	T37.2X5	T37.2X6
Guanethidine	T46.5X1	T46.5X2	T46.5X3	T46.5X4	T46.5X5	T46.5X6
Guanfacine	T46.5X1	T46.5X2	T46.5X3	T46.5X4	T46.5X5	T46.5X6
Guano	T65.891	T65.892	T65.893	T65.894	—	—
Guanochlor	T46.5X1	T46.5X2	T46.5X3	T46.5X4	T46.5X5	T46.5X6
Guanoclor	T46.5X1	T46.5X2	T46.5X3	T46.5X4	T46.5X5	T46.5X6
Guanoctine	T46.5X1	T46.5X2	T46.5X3	T46.5X4	T46.5X5	T46.5X6
Guanoxabenz	T46.5X1	T46.5X2	T46.5X3	T46.5X4	T46.5X5	T46.5X6
Guanoxan	T46.5X1	T46.5X2	T46.5X3	T46.5X4	T46.5X5	T46.5X6
Guar gum (medicinal)	T46.6X1	T46.6X2	T46.6X3	T46.6X4	T46.6X5	T46.6X6
Hachimycin	T36.7X1	T36.7X2	T36.7X3	T36.7X4	T36.7X5	T36.7X6
Hair						
dye	T49.4X1	T49.4X2	T49.4X3	T49.4X4	T49.4X5	T49.4X6
preparation NEC	T49.4X1	T49.4X2	T49.4X3	T49.4X4	T49.4X5	T49.4X6
Halazepam	T42.4X1	T42.4X2	T42.4X3	T42.4X4	T42.4X5	T42.4X6
Halcinolone	T49.0X1	T49.0X2	T49.0X3	T49.0X4	T49.0X5	T49.0X6
Halcinonide	T49.0X1	T49.0X2	T49.0X3	T49.0X4	T49.0X5	T49.0X6
Halethazole	T49.0X1	T49.0X2	T49.0X3	T49.0X4	T49.0X5	T49.0X6
Hallucinogen NEC	T40.901	T40.902	T40.903	T40.904	T40.905	T40.906
Halofantrine	T37.2X1	T37.2X2	T37.2X3	T37.2X4	T37.2X5	T37.2X6
Halofenate	T46.6X1	T46.6X2	T46.6X3	T46.6X4	T46.6X5	T46.6X6
Halometasone	T49.0X1	T49.0X2	T49.0X3	T49.0X4	T49.0X5	T49.0X6
Haloperidol	T43.4X1	T43.4X2	T43.4X3	T43.4X4	T43.4X5	T43.4X6
Haloprogin	T49.0X1	T49.0X2	T49.0X3	T49.0X4	T49.0X5	T49.0X6
Halotex	T49.0X1	T49.0X2	T49.0X3	T49.0X4	T49.0X5	T49.0X6
Halothane	T41.0X1	T41.0X2	T41.0X3	T41.0X4	T41.0X5	T41.0X6
Haloxazolam	T42.4X1	T42.4X2	T42.4X3	T42.4X4	T42.4X5	T42.4X6
Halquinols	T49.0X1	T49.0X2	T49.0X3	T49.0X4	T49.0X5	T49.0X6
Hamamelis	T49.2X1	T49.2X2	T49.2X3	T49.2X4	T49.2X5	T49.2X6
Haptendextran	T45.8X1	T45.8X2	T45.8X3	T45.8X4	T45.8X5	T45.8X6
Harmonyl	T46.5X1	T46.5X2	T46.5X3	T46.5X4	T46.5X5	T46.5X6
Hartmann's solution	T50.3X1	T50.3X2	T50.3X3	T50.3X4	T50.3X5	T50.3X6
Hashish	T40.7X1	T40.7X2	T40.7X3	T40.7X4	T40.7X5	T40.7X6
Hawaiian Woodrose seeds	T40.991	T40.992	T40.993	T40.994	—	—
HCB	T60.3X1	T60.3X2	T60.3X3	T60.3X4	—	—
HCH	T53.6X1	T53.6X2	T53.6X3	T53.6X4	—	—
medicinal	T49.0X1	T49.0X2	T49.0X3	T49.0X4	T49.0X5	T49.0X6
HCN	T57.3X1	T57.3X2	T57.3X3	T57.3X4	—	—
Headache cures, drugs, powders NEC	T50.901	T50.902	T50.903	T50.904	T50.905	T50.906
Heavenly Blue (morning glory)	T40.991	T40.992	T40.993	T40.994	—	—
Heavy metal antidote	T45.8X1	T45.8X2	T45.8X3	T45.8X4	T45.8X5	T45.8X6
Hedaquinium	T49.0X1	T49.0X2	T49.0X3	T49.0X4	T49.0X5	T49.0X6

372

Additional Character May Be Required — Refer to the Tabular List for Character Selection   ▽ Subterms under main terms may continue to next column or page

Substance	Poisoning, Accidental (unintentional)	Poisoning, Intentional Self-harm	Poisoning, Assault	Poisoning, Undetermined	Adverse Effect	Under-dosing
Hedge hyssop	T62.2X1	T62.2X2	T62.2X3	T62.2X4	—	—
Heet	T49.8X1	T49.8X2	T49.8X3	T49.8X4	T49.8X5	T49.8X6
Helenin	T37.4X1	T37.4X2	T37.4X3	T37.4X4	T37.4X5	T37.4X6
Helium (nonmedicinal) **NEC**	T59.891	T59.892	T59.893	T59.894	—	—
medicinal	T48.991	T48.992	T48.993	T48.994	T48.995	T48.996
Hellebore (black) (green) (white)	T62.2X1	T62.2X2	T62.2X3	T62.2X4	—	—
Hematin	T45.8X1	T45.8X2	T45.8X3	T45.8X4	T45.8X5	T45.8X6
Hematinic preparation	T45.8X1	T45.8X2	T45.8X3	T45.8X4	T45.8X5	T45.8X6
Hematological agent	T45.91	T45.92	T45.93	T45.94	T45.95	T45.96
specified NEC	T45.8X1	T45.8X2	T45.8X3	T45.8X4	T45.8X5	T45.8X6
Hemlock	T62.2X1	T62.2X2	T62.2X3	T62.2X4	—	—
Hemostatic	T45.621	T45.622	T45.623	T45.624	T45.625	T45.626
drug, systemic	T45.621	T45.622	T45.623	T45.624	T45.625	T45.626
Hemostyptic	T49.4X1	T49.4X2	T49.4X3	T49.4X4	T49.4X5	T49.4X6
Henbane	T62.2X1	T62.2X2	T62.2X3	T62.2X4	—	—
Heparin (sodium)	T45.511	T45.512	T45.513	T45.514	T45.515	T45.516
action reverser	T45.7X1	T45.7X2	T45.7X3	T45.7X4	T45.7X5	T45.7X6
Heparin-fraction	T45.511	T45.512	T45.513	T45.514	T45.515	T45.516
Heparinoid (systemic)	T45.511	T45.512	T45.513	T45.514	T45.515	T45.516
Hepatic secretion stimulant	T47.8X1	T47.8X2	T47.8X3	T47.8X4	T47.8X5	T47.8X6
Hepatitis B						
immune globulin	T50.Z11	T50.Z12	T50.Z13	T50.Z14	T50.Z15	T50.Z16
vaccine	T50.B91	T50.B92	T50.B93	T50.B94	T50.B95	T50.B96
Hepronicate	T46.7X1	T46.7X2	T46.7X3	T46.7X4	T46.7X5	T46.7X6
Heptabarb	T42.3X1	T42.3X2	T42.3X3	T42.3X4	T42.3X5	T42.3X6
Heptabarbital	T42.3X1	T42.3X2	T42.3X3	T42.3X4	T42.3X5	T42.3X6
Heptabarbitone	T42.3X1	T42.3X2	T42.3X3	T42.3X4	T42.3X5	T42.3X6
Heptachlor	T60.1X1	T60.1X2	T60.1X3	T60.1X4	—	—
Heptalgin	T40.2X1	T40.2X2	T40.2X3	T40.2X4	T40.2X5	T40.2X6
Heptaminol	T46.3X1	T46.3X2	T46.3X3	T46.3X4	T46.3X5	T46.3X6
Herbicide NEC	T60.3X1	T60.3X2	T60.3X3	T60.3X4	—	—
Heroin	T40.1X1	T40.1X2	T40.1X3	T40.1X4	—	—
Herplex	T49.5X1	T49.5X2	T49.5X3	T49.5X4	T49.5X5	T49.5X6
HES	T45.8X1	T45.8X2	T45.8X3	T45.8X4	T45.8X5	T45.8X6
Hesperidin	T46.991	T46.992	T46.993	T46.994	T46.995	T46.996
Hetacillin	T36.0X1	T36.0X2	T36.0X3	T36.0X4	T36.0X5	T36.0X6
Hetastarch	T45.8X1	T45.8X2	T45.8X3	T45.8X4	T45.8X5	T45.8X6
HETP	T60.0X1	T60.0X2	T60.0X3	T60.0X4	—	—
Hexachlorobenzene (vapor)	T60.3X1	T60.3X2	T60.3X3	T60.3X4	—	—
Hexachlorocyclohexane	T53.6X1	T53.6X2	T53.6X3	T53.6X4	—	—
Hexachlorophene	T49.0X1	T49.0X2	T49.0X3	T49.0X4	T49.0X5	T49.0X6
Hexadiline	T46.3X1	T46.3X2	T46.3X3	T46.3X4	T46.3X5	T46.3X6
Hexadimethrine (bromide)	T45.7X1	T45.7X2	T45.7X3	T45.7X4	T45.7X5	T45.7X6
Hexadylamine	T46.3X1	T46.3X2	T46.3X3	T46.3X4	T46.3X5	T46.3X6
Hexaethyl tetraphosphate	T60.0X1	T60.0X2	T60.0X3	T60.0X4	—	—
Hexafluorenium bromide	T48.1X1	T48.1X2	T48.1X3	T48.1X4	T48.1X5	T48.1X6
Hexafluronium (bromide)	T48.1X1	T48.1X2	T48.1X3	T48.1X4	T48.1X5	T48.1X6
Hexa-germ	T49.2X1	T49.2X2	T49.2X3	T49.2X4	T49.2X5	T49.2X6
Hexahydrobenzol	T52.8X1	T52.8X2	T52.8X3	T52.8X4	—	—
Hexahydrocresol(s)	T51.8X1	T51.8X2	T51.8X3	T51.8X4	—	—
arsenide	T57.0X1	T57.0X2	T57.0X3	T57.0X4	—	—
arseniurated	T57.0X1	T57.0X2	T57.0X3	T57.0X4	—	—
cyanide	T57.3X1	T57.3X2	T57.3X3	T57.3X4	—	—
gas	T59.891	T59.892	T59.893	T59.894	—	—
Fluoride (liquid)	T57.8X1	T57.8X2	T57.8X3	T57.8X4	—	—
vapor	T59.891	T59.892	T59.893	T59.894	—	—
phophorated	T60.0X1	T60.0X2	T60.0X3	T60.0X4	—	—
sulfate	T57.8X1	T57.8X2	T57.8X3	T57.8X4	—	—
sulfide (gas)	T59.6X1	T59.6X2	T59.6X3	T59.6X4	—	—
arseniurated	T57.0X1	T57.0X2	T57.0X3	T57.0X4	—	—
sulfurated	T57.8X1	T57.8X2	T57.8X3	T57.8X4	—	—
Hexahydrophenol	T51.8X1	T51.8X2	T51.8X3	T51.8X4	—	—
Hexalen	T51.8X1	T51.8X2	T51.8X3	T51.8X4	—	—
Hexamethonium bromide	T44.2X1	T44.2X2	T44.2X3	T44.2X4	T44.2X5	T44.2X6
Hexamethylene	T52.8X1	T52.8X2	T52.8X3	T52.8X4	—	—
Hexamethylmelamine	T45.1X1	T45.1X2	T45.1X3	T45.1X4	T45.1X5	T45.1X6
Hexamidine	T49.0X1	T49.0X2	T49.0X3	T49.0X4	T49.0X5	T49.0X6
Hexamine (mandelate)	T37.8X1	T37.8X2	T37.8X3	T37.8X4	T37.8X5	T37.8X6
Hexanone, 2-hexanone	T52.4X1	T52.4X2	T52.4X3	T52.4X4	—	—
Hexanuorenium	T48.1X1	T48.1X2	T48.1X3	T48.1X4	T48.1X5	T48.1X6
Hexapropymate	T42.6X1	T42.6X2	T42.6X3	T42.6X4	T42.6X5	T42.6X6
Hexasonium iodide	T44.3X1	T44.3X2	T44.3X3	T44.3X4	T44.3X5	T44.3X6
Hexcarbacholine bromide	T48.1X1	T48.1X2	T48.1X3	T48.1X4	T48.1X5	T48.1X6
Hexemal	T42.3X1	T42.3X2	T42.3X3	T42.3X4	T42.3X5	T42.3X6
Hexestrol	T38.5X1	T38.5X2	T38.5X3	T38.5X4	T38.5X5	T38.5X6
Hexethal (sodium)	T42.3X1	T42.3X2	T42.3X3	T42.3X4	T42.3X5	T42.3X6
Hexetidine	T37.8X1	T37.8X2	T37.8X3	T37.8X4	T37.8X5	T37.8X6
Hexobarbital	T42.3X1	T42.3X2	T42.3X3	T42.3X4	T42.3X5	T42.3X6
rectal	T41.291	T41.292	T41.293	T41.294	T41.295	T41.296
sodium	T41.1X1	T41.1X2	T41.1X3	T41.1X4	T41.1X5	T41.1X6
Hexobendine	T46.3X1	T46.3X2	T46.3X3	T46.3X4	T46.3X5	T46.3X6
Hexocyclium	T44.3X1	T44.3X2	T44.3X3	T44.3X4	T44.3X5	T44.3X6
metilsulfate	T44.3X1	T44.3X2	T44.3X3	T44.3X4	T44.3X5	T44.3X6
Hexoestrol	T38.5X1	T38.5X2	T38.5X3	T38.5X4	T38.5X5	T38.5X6
Hexone	T52.4X1	T52.4X2	T52.4X3	T52.4X4	—	—
Hexoprenaline	T48.6X1	T48.6X2	T48.6X3	T48.6X4	T48.6X5	T48.6X6
Hexylcaine	T41.3X1	T41.3X2	T41.3X3	T41.3X4	T41.3X5	T41.3X6
Hexylresorcinol	T52.2X1	T52.2X2	T52.2X3	T52.2X4	—	—
HGH (human growth hormone)	T38.811	T38.812	T38.813	T38.814	T38.815	T38.816
Hinkle's pills	T47.2X1	T47.2X2	T47.2X3	T47.2X4	T47.2X5	T47.2X6
Histalog	T50.8X1	T50.8X2	T50.8X3	T50.8X4	T50.8X5	T50.8X6
Histamine (phosphate)	T50.8X1	T50.8X2	T50.8X3	T50.8X4	T50.8X5	T50.8X6
Histoplasmin	T50.8X1	T50.8X2	T50.8X3	T50.8X4	T50.8X5	T50.8X6
Holly berries	T62.2X1	T62.2X2	T62.2X3	T62.2X4	—	—
Homatropine	T44.3X1	T44.3X2	T44.3X3	T44.3X4	T44.3X5	T44.3X6
methylbromide	T44.3X1	T44.3X2	T44.3X3	T44.3X4	T44.3X5	T44.3X6
Homochlorcyclizine	T45.0X1	T45.0X2	T45.0X3	T45.0X4	T45.0X5	T45.0X6
Homosalate	T49.3X1	T49.3X2	T49.3X3	T49.3X4	T49.3X5	T49.3X6
Homo-tet	T50.Z11	T50.Z12	T50.Z13	T50.Z14	T50.Z15	T50.Z16
Hormone	T38.801	T38.802	T38.803	T38.804	T38.805	T38.806
adrenal cortical steroids	T38.0X1	T38.0X2	T38.0X3	T38.0X4	T38.0X5	T38.0X6
androgenic	T38.7X1	T38.7X2	T38.7X3	T38.7X4	T38.7X5	T38.7X6
anterior pituitary NEC	T38.811	T38.812	T38.813	T38.814	T38.815	T38.816
antidiabetic agents	T38.3X1	T38.3X2	T38.3X3	T38.3X4	T38.3X5	T38.3X6
antidiuretic	T38.891	T38.892	T38.893	T38.894	T38.895	T38.896
cancer therapy	T45.1X1	T45.1X2	T45.1X3	T45.1X4	T45.1X5	T45.1X6
follicle stimulating	T38.811	T38.812	T38.813	T38.814	T38.815	T38.816
gonadotropic	T38.891	T38.892	T38.893	T38.894	T38.895	T38.896
pituitary	T38.811	T38.812	T38.813	T38.814	T38.815	T38.816
growth	T38.811	T38.812	T38.813	T38.814	T38.815	T38.816
luteinizing	T38.811	T38.812	T38.813	T38.814	T38.815	T38.816
ovarian	T38.5X1	T38.5X2	T38.5X3	T38.5X4	T38.5X5	T38.5X6
oxytocic	T48.0X1	T48.0X2	T48.0X3	T48.0X4	T48.0X5	T48.0X6
parathyroid (derivatives)	T50.991	T50.992	T50.993	T50.994	T50.995	T50.996
pituitary (posterior) NEC	T38.891	T38.892	T38.893	T38.894	T38.895	T38.896
anterior	T38.811	T38.812	T38.813	T38.814	T38.815	T38.816
specified, NEC	T38.891	T38.892	T38.893	T38.894	T38.895	T38.896
thyroid	T38.1X1	T38.1X2	T38.1X3	T38.1X4	T38.1X5	T38.1X6
Hornet (sting)	T63.451	T63.452	T63.453	T63.454	—	—
Horse anti-human lymphocytic serum	T50.Z11	T50.Z12	T50.Z13	T50.Z14	T50.Z15	T50.Z16
Horticulture agent NEC	T65.91	T65.92	T65.93	T65.94	—	—
with pesticide	T60.91	T60.92	T60.93	T60.94	—	—
Human						
albumin	T45.8X1	T45.8X2	T45.8X3	T45.8X4	T45.8X5	T45.8X6
growth hormone (HGH)	T38.811	T38.812	T38.813	T38.814	T38.815	T38.816
immune serum	T50.Z11	T50.Z12	T50.Z13	T50.Z14	T50.Z15	T50.Z16
Hyaluronidase	T45.3X1	T45.3X2	T45.3X3	T45.3X4	T45.3X5	T45.3X6
Hyazyme	T45.3X1	T45.3X2	T45.3X3	T45.3X4	T45.3X5	T45.3X6
Hycodan	T40.2X1	T40.2X2	T40.2X3	T40.2X4	T40.2X5	T40.2X6
Hydantoin derivative NEC	T42.0X1	T42.0X2	T42.0X3	T42.0X4	T42.0X5	T42.0X6
Hydeltra	T38.0X1	T38.0X2	T38.0X3	T38.0X4	T38.0X5	T38.0X6
Hydergine	T44.6X1	T44.6X2	T44.6X3	T44.6X4	T44.6X5	T44.6X6
Hydrabamine penicillin	T36.0X1	T36.0X2	T36.0X3	T36.0X4	T36.0X5	T36.0X6
Hydralazine	T46.5X1	T46.5X2	T46.5X3	T46.5X4	T46.5X5	T46.5X6
Hydrargaphen	T49.0X1	T49.0X2	T49.0X3	T49.0X4	T49.0X5	T49.0X6
Hydrargyri aminochloridum	T49.0X1	T49.0X2	T49.0X3	T49.0X4	T49.0X5	T49.0X6
Hydrastine	T48.291	T48.292	T48.293	T48.294	T48.295	T48.296
Hydrazine	T54.1X1	T54.1X2	T54.1X3	T54.1X4	—	—
monoamine oxidase inhibitors	T43.1X1	T43.1X2	T43.1X3	T43.1X4	T43.1X5	T43.1X6
Hydrazoic acid, azides	T54.2X1	T54.2X2	T54.2X3	T54.2X4	—	—
Hydriodic acid	T48.4X1	T48.4X2	T48.4X3	T48.4X4	T48.4X5	T48.4X6
Hydrocarbon gas	T59.891	T59.892	T59.893	T59.894	—	—
incomplete combustion of — see Carbon, monoxide, fuel, utility						
liquefied (mobile container)	T59.891	T59.892	T59.893	T59.894	—	—
piped (natural)	T59.891	T59.892	T59.893	T59.894	—	—
Hydrochloric acid (liquid)	T54.2X1	T54.2X2	T54.2X3	T54.2X4	—	—
medicinal (digestant)	T47.5X1	T47.5X2	T47.5X3	T47.5X4	T47.5X5	T47.5X6
vapor	T59.891	T59.892	T59.893	T59.894	—	—
Hydrochlorothiazide	T50.2X1	T50.2X2	T50.2X3	T50.2X4	T50.2X5	T50.2X6
Hydrocodone	T40.2X1	T40.2X2	T40.2X3	T40.2X4	T40.2X5	T40.2X6
Hydrocortisone	T38.0X1	T38.0X2	T38.0X3	T38.0X4	T38.0X5	T38.0X6
(derivatives)						
aceponate	T49.0X1	T49.0X2	T49.0X3	T49.0X4	T49.0X5	T49.0X6
ENT agent	T49.6X1	T49.6X2	T49.6X3	T49.6X4	T49.6X5	T49.6X6
ophthalmic preparation	T49.5X1	T49.5X2	T49.5X3	T49.5X4	T49.5X5	T49.5X6
topical NEC	T49.0X1	T49.0X2	T49.0X3	T49.0X4	T49.0X5	T49.0X6

Substance	Poisoning, Accidental (unintentional)	Poisoning, Intentional Self-harm	Poisoning, Assault	Poisoning, Undetermined	Adverse Effect	Under-dosing
Hydrocortone	T38.0X1	T38.0X2	T38.0X3	T38.0X4	T38.0X5	T38.0X6
ENT agent	T49.6X1	T49.6X2	T49.6X3	T49.6X4	T49.6X5	T49.6X6
ophthalmic preparation	T49.5X1	T49.5X2	T49.5X3	T49.5X4	T49.5X5	T49.5X6
topical NEC	T49.0X1	T49.0X2	T49.0X3	T49.0X4	T49.0X5	T49.0X6
Hydrocyanic acid (liquid)	T57.3X1	T57.3X2	T57.3X3	T57.3X4	—	—
gas	T65.0X1	T65.0X2	T65.0X3	T65.0X4	—	—
Hydroflumethiazide	T50.2X1	T50.2X2	T50.2X3	T50.2X4	T50.2X5	T50.2X6
Hydrofluoric acid (liquid)	T54.2X1	T54.2X2	T54.2X3	T54.2X4	—	—
vapor	T59.891	T59.892	T59.893	T59.894	—	—
Hydrogen	T59.891	T59.892	T59.893	T59.894	—	—
arsenide	T57.0X1	T57.0X2	T57.0X3	T57.0X4	—	—
arseniureted	T57.0X1	T57.0X2	T57.0X3	T57.0X4	—	—
chloride	T57.8X1	T57.8X2	T57.8X3	T57.8X4	—	—
cyanide (salts)	T57.3X1	T57.3X2	T57.3X3	T57.3X4	—	—
gas	T57.3X1	T57.3X2	T57.3X3	T57.3X4	—	—
Fluoride	T59.5X1	T59.5X2	T59.5X3	T59.5X4	—	—
vapor	T59.5X1	T59.5X2	T59.5X3	T59.5X4	—	—
peroxide	T49.0X1	T49.0X2	T49.0X3	T49.0X4	T49.0X5	T49.0X6
phosphureted	T57.1X1	T57.1X2	T57.1X3	T57.1X4	—	—
sulfide	T59.6X1	T59.6X2	T59.6X3	T59.6X4	—	—
arseniureted	T57.0X1	T57.0X2	T57.0X3	T57.0X4	—	—
sulfureted	T59.6X1	T59.6X2	T59.6X3	T59.6X4	—	—
Hydromethylpyridine	T46.7X1	T46.7X2	T46.7X3	T46.7X4	T46.7X5	T46.7X6
Hydromorphinol	T40.2X1	T40.2X2	T40.2X3	T40.2X4	—	—
Hydromorphinone	T40.2X1	T40.2X2	T40.2X3	T40.2X4	T40.2X5	T40.2X6
Hydromorphone	T40.2X1	T40.2X2	T40.2X3	T40.2X4	T40.2X5	T40.2X6
Hydromox	T50.2X1	T50.2X2	T50.2X3	T50.2X4	T50.2X5	T50.2X6
Hydrophilic lotion	T49.3X1	T49.3X2	T49.3X3	T49.3X4	T49.3X5	T49.3X6
Hydroquinidine	T46.2X1	T46.2X2	T46.2X3	T46.2X4	T46.2X5	T46.2X6
Hydroquinone	T52.2X1	T52.2X2	T52.2X3	T52.2X4	—	—
vapor	T59.891	T59.892	T59.893	T59.894	—	—
Hydrosulfuric acid (gas)	T59.6X1	T59.6X2	T59.6X3	T59.6X4	—	—
Hydrotalcite	T47.1X1	T47.1X2	T47.1X3	T47.1X4	T47.1X5	T47.1X6
Hydrous wool fat	T49.3X1	T49.3X2	T49.3X3	T49.3X4	T49.3X5	T49.3X6
Hydroxide, caustic	T54.3X1	T54.3X2	T54.3X3	T54.3X4	—	—
Hydroxocobalamin	T45.8X1	T45.8X2	T45.8X3	T45.8X4	T45.8X5	T45.8X6
Hydroxyamphetamine	T49.5X1	T49.5X2	T49.5X3	T49.5X4	T49.5X5	T49.5X6
Hydroxycarbamide	T45.1X1	T45.1X2	T45.1X3	T45.1X4	T45.1X5	T45.1X6
Hydroxychloroquine	T37.8X1	T37.8X2	T37.8X3	T37.8X4	T37.8X5	T37.8X6
Hydroxydihydrocodeinone	T40.2X1	T40.2X2	T40.2X3	T40.2X4	T40.2X5	T40.2X6
Hydroxyestrone	T38.5X1	T38.5X2	T38.5X3	T38.5X4	T38.5X5	T38.5X6
Hydroxyethyl starch	T45.8X1	T45.8X2	T45.8X3	T45.8X4	T45.8X5	T45.8X6
Hydroxymethylpentanone	T52.4X1	T52.4X2	T52.4X3	T52.4X4	—	—
Hydroxyphenamate	T43.591	T43.592	T43.593	T43.594	T43.595	T43.596
Hydroxyphenylbutazone	T39.2X1	T39.2X2	T39.2X3	T39.2X4	T39.2X5	T39.2X6
Hydroxyprogesterone	T38.5X1	T38.5X2	T38.5X3	T38.5X4	T38.5X5	T38.5X6
caproate	T38.5X1	T38.5X2	T38.5X3	T38.5X4	T38.5X5	T38.5X6
Hydroxyquinoline (derivatives) NEC	T37.8X1	T37.8X2	T37.8X3	T37.8X4	T37.8X5	T37.8X6
Hydroxystilbamidine	T37.3X1	T37.3X2	T37.3X3	T37.3X4	T37.3X5	T37.3X6
Hydroxytoluene (nonmedicinal)	T54.0X1	T54.0X2	T54.0X3	T54.0X4	—	—
medicinal	T49.0X1	T49.0X2	T49.0X3	T49.0X4	T49.0X5	T49.0X6
Hydroxyurea	T45.1X1	T45.1X2	T45.1X3	T45.1X4	T45.1X5	T45.1X6
Hydroxyzine	T43.591	T43.592	T43.593	T43.594	T43.595	T43.596
Hyoscine	T44.3X1	T44.3X2	T44.3X3	T44.3X4	T44.3X5	T44.3X6
Hyoscyamine	T44.3X1	T44.3X2	T44.3X3	T44.3X4	T44.3X5	T44.3X6
Hyoscyamus	T44.3X1	T44.3X2	T44.3X3	T44.3X4	T44.3X5	T44.3X6
dry extract	T44.3X1	T44.3X2	T44.3X3	T44.3X4	T44.3X5	T44.3X6
Hypaque	T50.8X1	T50.8X2	T50.8X3	T50.8X4	T50.8X5	T50.8X6
Hypertussis	T50.Z11	T50.Z12	T50.Z13	T50.Z14	T50.Z15	T50.Z16
Hypnotic	T42.71	T42.72	T42.73	T42.74	T42.75	T42.76
anticonvulsant	T42.71	T42.72	T42.73	T42.74	T42.75	T42.76
specified NEC	T42.6X1	T42.6X2	T42.6X3	T42.6X4	T42.6X5	T42.6X6
Hypochlorite	T49.0X1	T49.0X2	T49.0X3	T49.0X4	T49.0X5	T49.0X6
Hypophysis, posterior	T38.891	T38.892	T38.893	T38.894	T38.895	T38.896
Hypotensive NEC	T46.5X1	T46.5X2	T46.5X3	T46.5X4	T46.5X5	T46.5X6
Hypromellose	T49.5X1	T49.5X2	T49.5X3	T49.5X4	T49.5X5	T49.5X6
Ibacitabine	T37.5X1	T37.5X2	T37.5X3	T37.5X4	T37.5X5	T37.5X6
Ibopamine	T44.991	T44.992	T44.993	T44.994	T44.995	T44.996
Ibufenac	T39.311	T39.312	T39.313	T39.314	T39.315	T39.316
Ibuprofen	T39.311	T39.312	T39.313	T39.314	T39.315	T39.316
Ibuproxam	T39.311	T39.312	T39.313	T39.314	T39.315	T39.316
Ibuterol	T48.6X1	T48.6X2	T48.6X3	T48.6X4	T48.6X5	T48.6X6
Ichthammol	T49.0X1	T49.0X2	T49.0X3	T49.0X4	T49.0X5	T49.0X6
Ichthyol	T49.4X1	T49.4X2	T49.4X3	T49.4X4	T49.4X5	T49.4X6
Idarubicin	T45.1X1	T45.1X2	T45.1X3	T45.1X4	T45.1X5	T45.1X6
Idrocilamide	T42.8X1	T42.8X2	T42.8X3	T42.8X4	T42.8X5	T42.8X6
Ifenprodil	T46.7X1	T46.7X2	T46.7X3	T46.7X4	T46.7X5	T46.7X6
Ifosfamide	T45.1X1	T45.1X2	T45.1X3	T45.1X4	T45.1X5	T45.1X6
Iletin	T38.3X1	T38.3X2	T38.3X3	T38.3X4	T38.3X5	T38.3X6
Ilex	T62.2X1	T62.2X2	T62.2X3	T62.2X4	—	—
Illuminating gas (after combustion)	T58.11	T58.12	T58.13	T58.14	—	—
prior to combustion	T59.891	T59.892	T59.893	T59.894	—	—
Ilopan	T45.2X1	T45.2X2	T45.2X3	T45.2X4	T45.2X5	T45.2X6
Iloprost	T46.7X1	T46.7X2	T46.7X3	T46.7X4	T46.7X5	T46.7X6
Ilotycin	T36.3X1	T36.3X2	T36.3X3	T36.3X4	T36.3X5	T36.3X6
ophthalmic preparation	T49.5X1	T49.5X2	T49.5X3	T49.5X4	T49.5X5	T49.5X6
topical NEC	T49.0X1	T49.0X2	T49.0X3	T49.0X4	T49.0X5	T49.0X6
Imidazole-4-carboxamide	T45.1X1	T45.1X2	T45.1X3	T45.1X4	T45.1X5	T45.1X6
Iminostilbene	T42.1X1	T42.1X2	T42.1X3	T42.1X4	T42.1X5	T42.1X6
Imipenem	T36.0X1	T36.0X2	T36.0X3	T36.0X4	T36.0X5	T36.0X6
Imipramine	T43.011	T43.012	T43.013	T43.014	T43.015	T43.016
Immu-G	T50.Z11	T50.Z12	T50.Z13	T50.Z14	T50.Z15	T50.Z16
Immuglobin	T50.Z11	T50.Z12	T50.Z13	T50.Z14	T50.Z15	T50.Z16
Immune						
globulin	T50.Z11	T50.Z12	T50.Z13	T50.Z14	T50.Z15	T50.Z16
serum globulin	T50.Z11	T50.Z12	T50.Z13	T50.Z14	T50.Z15	T50.Z16
Immunoglobin human (intravenous) (normal)	T50.Z11	T50.Z12	T50.Z13	T50.Z14	T50.Z15	T50.Z16
unmodified	T50.Z11	T50.Z12	T50.Z13	T50.Z14	T50.Z15	T50.Z16
Immunosuppressive drug	T45.1X1	T45.1X2	T45.1X3	T45.1X4	T45.1X5	T45.1X6
Immu-tetanus	T50.Z11	T50.Z12	T50.Z13	T50.Z14	T50.Z15	T50.Z16
Indalpine	T43.221	T43.222	T43.223	T43.224	T43.225	T43.226
Indanazoline	T48.5X1	T48.5X2	T48.5X3	T48.5X4	T48.5X5	T48.5X6
Indandione (derivatives)	T45.511	T45.512	T45.513	T45.514	T45.515	T45.516
Indapamide	T46.5X1	T46.5X2	T46.5X3	T46.5X4	T46.5X5	T46.5X6
Indenedione (derivatives)	T45.511	T45.512	T45.513	T45.514	T45.515	T45.516
Indenolol	T44.7X1	T44.7X2	T44.7X3	T44.7X4	T44.7X5	T44.7X6
Inderal	T44.7X1	T44.7X2	T44.7X3	T44.7X4	T44.7X5	T44.7X6
Indian						
hemp	T40.7X1	T40.7X2	T40.7X3	T40.7X4	T40.7X5	T40.7X6
tobacco	T62.2X1	T62.2X2	T62.2X3	T62.2X4	—	—
Indigo carmine	T50.8X1	T50.8X2	T50.8X3	T50.8X4	T50.8X5	T50.8X6
Indobufen	T45.521	T45.522	T45.523	T45.524	T45.525	T45.526
Indocin	T39.2X1	T39.2X2	T39.2X3	T39.2X4	T39.2X5	T39.2X6
Indocyanine green	T50.8X1	T50.8X2	T50.8X3	T50.8X4	T50.8X5	T50.8X6
Indometacin	T39.391	T39.392	T39.393	T39.394	T39.395	T39.396
Indomethacin	T39.391	T39.392	T39.393	T39.394	T39.395	T39.396
farnesil	T39.4X1	T39.4X2	T39.4X3	T39.4X4	T39.4X5	T39.4X6
Indoramin	T44.6X1	T44.6X2	T44.6X3	T44.6X4	T44.6X5	T44.6X6
Industrial						
alcohol	T51.0X1	T51.0X2	T51.0X3	T51.0X4	—	—
fumes	T59.891	T59.892	T59.893	T59.894	—	—
solvents (fumes) (vapors)	T52.91	T52.92	T52.93	T52.94	—	—
Influenza vaccine	T50.B91	T50.B92	T50.B93	T50.B94	T50.B95	T50.B96
Ingested substance NEC	T65.91	T65.92	T65.93	T65.94	—	—
INH	T37.1X1	T37.1X2	T37.1X3	T37.1X4	T37.1X5	T37.1X6
Inhalation, gas (noxious) — see Gas						
Inhibitor						
angiotensin-converting enzyme	T46.4X1	T46.4X2	T46.4X3	T46.4X4	T46.4X5	T46.4X6
carbonic anhydrase	T50.2X1	T50.2X2	T50.2X3	T50.2X4	T50.2X5	T50.2X6
fibrinolysis	T45.621	T45.622	T45.623	T45.624	T45.625	T45.626
monoamine oxidase NEC	T43.1X1	T43.1X2	T43.1X3	T43.1X4	T43.1X5	T43.1X6
hydrazine	T43.1X1	T43.1X2	T43.1X3	T43.1X4	T43.1X5	T43.1X6
postsynaptic	T43.8X1	T43.8X2	T43.8X3	T43.8X4	T43.8X5	T43.8X6
prothrombin synthesis	T45.511	T45.512	T45.513	T45.514	T45.515	T45.516
Ink	T65.891	T65.892	T65.893	T65.894	—	—
Inorganic substance NEC	T57.91	T57.92	T57.93	T57.94	—	—
Inosine pranobex	T37.5X1	T37.5X2	T37.5X3	T37.5X4	T37.5X5	T37.5X6
Inositol	T50.991	T50.992	T50.993	T50.994	T50.995	T50.996
nicotinate	T46.7X1	T46.7X2	T46.7X3	T46.7X4	T46.7X5	T46.7X6
Inproquone	T45.1X1	T45.1X2	T45.1X3	T45.1X4	T45.1X5	T45.1X6
Insecticide NEC	T60.91	T60.92	T60.93	T60.94	—	—
carbamate	T60.0X1	T60.0X2	T60.0X3	T60.0X4	—	—
chlorinated	T60.1X1	T60.1X2	T60.1X3	T60.1X4	—	—
mixed	T60.91	T60.92	T60.93	T60.94	—	—
organochlorine	T60.1X1	T60.1X2	T60.1X3	T60.1X4	—	—
organophosphorus	T60.0X1	T60.0X2	T60.0X3	T60.0X4	—	—
Insect (sting), venomous	T63.481	T63.482	T63.483	T63.484	—	—
ant	T63.421	T63.422	T63.423	T63.424	—	—
bee	T63.441	T63.442	T63.443	T63.444	—	—
caterpillar	T63.431	T63.432	T63.433	T63.434	—	—
hornet	T63.451	T63.452	T63.453	T63.454	—	—
wasp	T63.461	T63.462	T63.463	T63.464	—	—
Insular tissue extract	T38.3X1	T38.3X2	T38.3X3	T38.3X4	T38.3X5	T38.3X6
Insulin (amorphous) (globin) (isophane) (Lente) (NPH) (Semilente) (Ultralente)	T38.3X1	T38.3X2	T38.3X3	T38.3X4	T38.3X5	T38.3X6
defalan	T38.3X1	T38.3X2	T38.3X3	T38.3X4	T38.3X5	T38.3X6
human	T38.3X1	T38.3X2	T38.3X3	T38.3X4	T38.3X5	T38.3X6
injection, soluble	T38.3X1	T38.3X2	T38.3X3	T38.3X4	T38.3X5	T38.3X6

Additional Character May Be Required — Refer to the Tabular List for Character Selection ▼ Subterms under main terms may continue to next column or page

Substance	Poisoning, Accidental (unintentional)	Poisoning, Intentional Self-harm	Poisoning, Assault	Poisoning, Undetermined	Adverse Effect	Under-dosing
Insulin — *continued*						
injection, soluble — *continued*						
biphasic	T38.3X1	T38.3X2	T38.3X3	T38.3X4	T38.3X5	T38.3X6
intermediate acting	T38.3X1	T38.3X2	T38.3X3	T38.3X4	T38.3X5	T38.3X6
protamine zinc	T38.3X1	T38.3X2	T38.3X3	T38.3X4	T38.3X5	T38.3X6
slow acting	T38.3X1	T38.3X2	T38.3X3	T38.3X4	T38.3X5	T38.3X6
zinc						
protamine injection	T38.3X1	T38.3X2	T38.3X3	T38.3X4	T38.3X5	T38.3X6
suspension (amorphous) (crystalline)	T38.3X1	T38.3X2	T38.3X3	T38.3X4	T38.3X5	T38.3X6
Interferon (alpha) (beta) (gamma)	T37.5X1	T37.5X2	T37.5X3	T37.5X4	T37.5X5	T37.5X6
Intestinal motility control drug	T47.6X1	T47.6X2	T47.6X3	T47.6X4	T47.6X5	T47.6X6
biological	T47.8X1	T47.8X2	T47.8X3	T47.8X4	T47.8X5	T47.8X6
Intranarcon	T41.1X1	T41.1X2	T41.1X3	T41.1X4	T41.1X5	T41.1X6
Intravenous						
amino acids	T50.991	T50.992	T50.993	T50.994	T50.995	T50.996
fat suspension	T50.991	T50.992	T50.993	T50.994	T50.995	T50.996
Inulin	T50.8X1	T50.8X2	T50.8X3	T50.8X4	T50.8X5	T50.8X6
Invert sugar	T50.3X1	T50.3X2	T50.3X3	T50.3X4	T50.3X5	T50.3X6
Inza — *see* Naproxen						
Iobenzamic acid	T50.8X1	T50.8X2	T50.8X3	T50.8X4	T50.8X5	T50.8X6
Iocarmic acid	T50.8X1	T50.8X2	T50.8X3	T50.8X4	T50.8X5	T50.8X6
Iocetamic acid	T50.8X1	T50.8X2	T50.8X3	T50.8X4	T50.8X5	T50.8X6
Iodamide	T50.8X1	T50.8X2	T50.8X3	T50.8X4	T50.8X5	T50.8X6
Iodide NEC — *see also* Iodine	T49.0X1	T49.0X2	T49.0X3	T49.0X4	T49.0X5	T49.0X6
mercury (ointment)	T49.0X1	T49.0X2	T49.0X3	T49.0X4	T49.0X5	T49.0X6
methylate	T49.0X1	T49.0X2	T49.0X3	T49.0X4	T49.0X5	T49.0X6
potassium (expectorant) NEC	T48.4X1	T48.4X2	T48.4X3	T48.4X4	T48.4X5	T48.4X6
Iodinated						
contrast medium	T50.8X1	T50.8X2	T50.8X3	T50.8X4	T50.8X5	T50.8X6
glycerol	T48.4X1	T48.4X2	T48.4X3	T48.4X4	T48.4X5	T48.4X6
human serum albumin (131I)	T50.8X1	T50.8X2	T50.8X3	T50.8X4	T50.8X5	T50.8X6
Iodine (antiseptic, external) (tincture) **NEC**	T49.0X1	T49.0X2	T49.0X3	T49.0X4	T49.0X5	T49.0X6
125 — *see also* Radiation sickness, and Exposure to radioactivce isotopes	T50.8X1	T50.8X2	T50.8X3	T50.8X4	T50.8X5	T50.8X6
therapeutic	T50.991	T50.992	T50.993	T50.994	T50.995	T50.996
131 — *see also* Radiation sickness, and Exposure to radioactivce isotopes	T50.8X1	T50.8X2	T50.8X3	T50.8X4	T50.8X5	T50.8X6
therapeutic	T38.2X1	T38.2X2	T38.2X3	T38.2X4	T38.2X5	T38.2X6
diagnostic	T50.8X1	T50.8X2	T50.8X3	T50.8X4	T50.8X5	T50.8X6
for thyroid conditions (antithyroid)	T38.2X1	T38.2X2	T38.2X3	T38.2X4	T38.2X5	T38.2X6
solution	T49.0X1	T49.0X2	T49.0X3	T49.0X4	T49.0X5	T49.0X6
vapor	T59.891	T59.892	T59.893	T59.894	—	—
Iodipamide	T50.8X1	T50.8X2	T50.8X3	T50.8X4	T50.8X5	T50.8X6
Iodized (poppy seed) oil	T50.8X1	T50.8X2	T50.8X3	T50.8X4	T50.8X5	T50.8X6
Iodobismitol	T37.8X1	T37.8X2	T37.8X3	T37.8X4	T37.8X5	T37.8X6
Iodochlorhydroxyquin	T37.8X1	T37.8X2	T37.8X3	T37.8X4	T37.8X5	T37.8X6
topical	T49.0X1	T49.0X2	T49.0X3	T49.0X4	T49.0X5	T49.0X6
Iodochlorhydroxyquinoline	T37.8X1	T37.8X2	T37.8X3	T37.8X4	T37.8X5	T37.8X6
Iodocholesterol (131I)	T50.8X1	T50.8X2	T50.8X3	T50.8X4	T50.8X5	T50.8X6
Iodoform	T49.0X1	T49.0X2	T49.0X3	T49.0X4	T49.0X5	T49.0X6
Iodohippuric acid	T50.8X1	T50.8X2	T50.8X3	T50.8X4	T50.8X5	T50.8X6
Iodopanoic acid	T50.8X1	T50.8X2	T50.8X3	T50.8X4	T50.8X5	T50.8X6
Iodophthalein (sodium)	T50.8X1	T50.8X2	T50.8X3	T50.8X4	T50.8X5	T50.8X6
Iodopyracet	T50.8X1	T50.8X2	T50.8X3	T50.8X4	T50.8X5	T50.8X6
Iodoquinol	T37.8X1	T37.8X2	T37.8X3	T37.8X4	T37.8X5	T37.8X6
Iodoxamic acid	T50.8X1	T50.8X2	T50.8X3	T50.8X4	T50.8X5	T50.8X6
Iofendylate	T50.8X1	T50.8X2	T50.8X3	T50.8X4	T50.8X5	T50.8X6
Ioglycamic acid	T50.8X1	T50.8X2	T50.8X3	T50.8X4	T50.8X5	T50.8X6
Iohexol	T50.8X1	T50.8X2	T50.8X3	T50.8X4	T50.8X5	T50.8X6
Ion exchange resin						
anion	T47.8X1	T47.8X2	T47.8X3	T47.8X4	T47.8X5	T47.8X6
cation	T50.3X1	T50.3X2	T50.3X3	T50.3X4	T50.3X5	T50.3X6
cholestyramine	T46.6X1	T46.6X2	T46.6X3	T46.6X4	T46.6X5	T46.6X6
intestinal	T47.8X1	T47.8X2	T47.8X3	T47.8X4	T47.8X5	T47.8X6
Iopamidol	T50.8X1	T50.8X2	T50.8X3	T50.8X4	T50.8X5	T50.8X6
Iopanoic acid	T50.8X1	T50.8X2	T50.8X3	T50.8X4	T50.8X5	T50.8X6
Iophenoic acid	T50.8X1	T50.8X2	T50.8X3	T50.8X4	T50.8X5	T50.8X6
Iopodate, sodium	T50.8X1	T50.8X2	T50.8X3	T50.8X4	T50.8X5	T50.8X6
Iopodic acid	T50.8X1	T50.8X2	T50.8X3	T50.8X4	T50.8X5	T50.8X6
Iopromide	T50.8X1	T50.8X2	T50.8X3	T50.8X4	T50.8X5	T50.8X6
Iopydol	T50.8X1	T50.8X2	T50.8X3	T50.8X4	T50.8X5	T50.8X6
Iotalamic acid	T50.8X1	T50.8X2	T50.8X3	T50.8X4	T50.8X5	T50.8X6
Iothalamate	T50.8X1	T50.8X2	T50.8X3	T50.8X4	T50.8X5	T50.8X6

Substance	Poisoning, Accidental (unintentional)	Poisoning, Intentional Self-harm	Poisoning, Assault	Poisoning, Undetermined	Adverse Effect	Under-dosing
Iothiouracil	T38.2X1	T38.2X2	T38.2X3	T38.2X4	T38.2X5	T38.2X6
Iotrol	T50.8X1	T50.8X2	T50.8X3	T50.8X4	T50.8X5	T50.8X6
Iotrolan	T50.8X1	T50.8X2	T50.8X3	T50.8X4	T50.8X5	T50.8X6
Iotroxate	T50.8X1	T50.8X2	T50.8X3	T50.8X4	T50.8X5	T50.8X6
Iotroxic acid	T50.8X1	T50.8X2	T50.8X3	T50.8X4	T50.8X5	T50.8X6
Ioversol	T50.8X1	T50.8X2	T50.8X3	T50.8X4	T50.8X5	T50.8X6
Ioxaglate	T50.8X1	T50.8X2	T50.8X3	T50.8X4	T50.8X5	T50.8X6
Ioxaglic acid	T50.8X1	T50.8X2	T50.8X3	T50.8X4	T50.8X5	T50.8X6
Ioxitalamic acid	T50.8X1	T50.8X2	T50.8X3	T50.8X4	T50.8X5	T50.8X6
Ipecac	T47.7X1	T47.7X2	T47.7X3	T47.7X4	T47.7X5	T47.7X6
Ipecacuanha	T48.4X1	T48.4X2	T48.4X3	T48.4X4	T48.4X5	T48.4X6
Ipodate, calcium	T50.8X1	T50.8X2	T50.8X3	T50.8X4	T50.8X5	T50.8X6
Ipral	T42.3X1	T42.3X2	T42.3X3	T42.3X4	T42.3X5	T42.3X6
Ipratropium (bromide)	T48.6X1	T48.6X2	T48.6X3	T48.6X4	T48.6X5	T48.6X6
Ipriflavone	T46.3X1	T46.3X2	T46.3X3	T46.3X4	T46.3X5	T46.3X6
Iprindole	T43.011	T43.012	T43.013	T43.014	T43.015	T43.016
Iproclozide	T43.1X1	T43.1X2	T43.1X3	T43.1X4	T43.1X5	T43.1X6
Iprofenin	T50.8X1	T50.8X2	T50.8X3	T50.8X4	T50.8X5	T50.8X6
Iproheptine	T49.2X1	T49.2X2	T49.2X3	T49.2X4	T49.2X5	T49.2X6
Iproniazid	T43.1X1	T43.1X2	T43.1X3	T43.1X4	T43.1X5	T43.1X6
Iproplatin	T45.1X1	T45.1X2	T45.1X3	T45.1X4	T45.1X5	T45.1X6
Iproveratril	T46.1X1	T46.1X2	T46.1X3	T46.1X4	T46.1X5	T46.1X6
Iron (compounds) (medicinal) **NEC**	T45.4X1	T45.4X2	T45.4X3	T45.4X4	T45.4X5	T45.4X6
ammonium	T45.4X1	T45.4X2	T45.4X3	T45.4X4	T45.4X5	T45.4X6
dextran injection	T45.4X1	T45.4X2	T45.4X3	T45.4X4	T45.4X5	T45.4X6
nonmedicinal	T56.891	T56.892	T56.893	T56.894	—	—
salts	T45.4X1	T45.4X2	T45.4X3	T45.4X4	T45.4X5	T45.4X6
sorbitex	T45.4X1	T45.4X2	T45.4X3	T45.4X4	T45.4X5	T45.4X6
sorbitol citric acid complex	T45.4X1	T45.4X2	T45.4X3	T45.4X4	T45.4X5	T45.4X6
Irrigating fluid (vaginal)	T49.8X1	T49.8X2	T49.8X3	T49.8X4	T49.8X5	T49.8X6
eye	T49.5X1	T49.5X2	T49.5X3	T49.5X4	T49.5X5	T49.5X6
Isepamicin	T36.5X1	T36.5X2	T36.5X3	T36.5X4	T36.5X5	T36.5X6
Isoaminile (citrate)	T48.3X1	T48.3X2	T48.3X3	T48.3X4	T48.3X5	T48.3X6
Isoamyl nitrite	T46.3X1	T46.3X2	T46.3X3	T46.3X4	T46.3X5	T46.3X6
Isobenzan	T60.1X1	T60.1X2	T60.1X3	T60.1X4	—	—
Isobutyl acetate	T52.8X1	T52.8X2	T52.8X3	T52.8X4	—	—
Isocarboxazid	T43.1X1	T43.1X2	T43.1X3	T43.1X4	T43.1X5	T43.1X6
Isoconazole	T49.0X1	T49.0X2	T49.0X3	T49.0X4	T49.0X5	T49.0X6
Isocyanate	T65.0X1	T65.0X2	T65.0X3	T65.0X4	—	—
Isoephedrine	T44.991	T44.992	T44.993	T44.994	T44.995	T44.996
Isoetarine	T48.6X1	T48.6X2	T48.6X3	T48.6X4	T48.6X5	T48.6X6
Isoethadione	T42.2X1	T42.2X2	T42.2X3	T42.2X4	T42.2X5	T42.2X6
Isoetharine	T44.5X1	T44.5X2	T44.5X3	T44.5X4	T44.5X5	T44.5X6
Isoflurane	T41.0X1	T41.0X2	T41.0X3	T41.0X4	T41.0X5	T41.0X6
Isoflurophate	T44.0X1	T44.0X2	T44.0X3	T44.0X4	T44.0X5	T44.0X6
Isomaltose, ferric complex	T45.4X1	T45.4X2	T45.4X3	T45.4X4	T45.4X5	T45.4X6
Isometheptene	T44.3X1	T44.3X2	T44.3X3	T44.3X4	T44.3X5	T44.3X6
Isoniazid	T37.1X1	T37.1X2	T37.1X3	T37.1X4	T37.1X5	T37.1X6
with						
rifampicin	T36.6X1	T36.6X2	T36.6X3	T36.6X4	T36.6X5	T36.6X6
thioacetazone	T37.1X1	T37.1X2	T37.1X3	T37.1X4	T37.1X5	T37.1X6
Isonicotinic acid hydrazide	T37.1X1	T37.1X2	T37.1X3	T37.1X4	T37.1X5	T37.1X6
Isonipecaine	T40.4X1	T40.4X2	T40.4X3	T40.4X4	T40.4X5	T40.4X6
Isopentaquine	T37.2X1	T37.2X2	T37.2X3	T37.2X4	T37.2X5	T37.2X6
Isophane insulin	T38.3X1	T38.3X2	T38.3X3	T38.3X4	T38.3X5	T38.3X6
Isophorone	T65.891	T65.892	T65.893	T65.894	—	—
Isophosphamide	T45.1X1	T45.1X2	T45.1X3	T45.1X4	T45.1X5	T45.1X6
Isopregnenone	T38.5X1	T38.5X2	T38.5X3	T38.5X4	T38.5X5	T38.5X6
Isoprenaline	T48.6X1	T48.6X2	T48.6X3	T48.6X4	T48.6X5	T48.6X6
Isopromethazine	T43.3X1	T43.3X2	T43.3X3	T43.3X4	T43.3X5	T43.3X6
Isopropamide	T44.3X1	T44.3X2	T44.3X3	T44.3X4	T44.3X5	T44.3X6
iodide	T44.3X1	T44.3X2	T44.3X3	T44.3X4	T44.3X5	T44.3X6
Isopropanol	T51.2X1	T51.2X2	T51.2X3	T51.2X4	—	—
Isopropyl						
acetate	T52.8X1	T52.8X2	T52.8X3	T52.8X4	—	—
alcohol	T51.2X1	T51.2X2	T51.2X3	T51.2X4	—	—
medicinal	T49.4X1	T49.4X2	T49.4X3	T49.4X4	T49.4X5	T49.4X6
ether	T52.8X1	T52.8X2	T52.8X3	T52.8X4	—	—
Isopropylaminophenazone	T39.2X1	T39.2X2	T39.2X3	T39.2X4	T39.2X5	T39.2X6
Isoproterenol	T48.6X1	T48.6X2	T48.6X3	T48.6X4	T48.6X5	T48.6X6
Isosorbide dinitrate	T46.3X1	T46.3X2	T46.3X3	T46.3X4	T46.3X5	T46.3X6
Isothipendyl	T45.0X1	T45.0X2	T45.0X3	T45.0X4	T45.0X5	T45.0X6
Isotretinoin	T50.991	T50.992	T50.993	T50.994	T50.995	T50.996
Isoxazolyl penicillin	T36.0X1	T36.0X2	T36.0X3	T36.0X4	T36.0X5	T36.0X6
Isoxicam	T39.391	T39.392	T39.393	T39.394	T39.395	T39.396
Isoxsuprine	T46.7X1	T46.7X2	T46.7X3	T46.7X4	T46.7X5	T46.7X6
Ispagula	T47.4X1	T47.4X2	T47.4X3	T47.4X4	T47.4X5	T47.4X6
husk	T47.4X1	T47.4X2	T47.4X3	T47.4X4	T47.4X5	T47.4X6
Isradipine	T46.1X1	T46.1X2	T46.1X3	T46.1X4	T46.1X5	T46.1X6
I-thyroxine sodium	T38.1X1	T38.1X2	T38.1X3	T38.1X4	T38.1X5	T38.1X6
Itraconazole	T37.8X1	T37.8X2	T37.8X3	T37.8X4	T37.8X5	T37.8X6
Itramin tosilate	T46.3X1	T46.3X2	T46.3X3	T46.3X4	T46.3X5	T46.3X6

Insulin — Itramin tosilate

Table of Drugs and Chemicals

Substance	Poisoning, Accidental (unintentional)	Poisoning, Intentional Self-harm	Poisoning, Assault	Poisoning, Undetermined	Adverse Effect	Under-dosing
Ivermectin	T37.4X1	T37.4X2	T37.4X3	T37.4X4	T37.4X5	T37.4X6
Izoniazid	T37.1X1	T37.1X2	T37.1X3	T37.1X4	T37.1X5	T37.1X6
with thioacetazone	T37.1X1	T37.1X2	T37.1X3	T37.1X4	T37.1X5	T37.1X6
Jalap	T47.2X1	T47.2X2	T47.2X3	T47.2X4	T47.2X5	T47.2X6
Jamaica						
dogwood (bark)	T39.8X1	T39.8X2	T39.8X3	T39.8X4	T39.8X5	T39.8X6
ginger	T65.891	T65.892	T65.893	T65.894	—	—
root	T62.2X1	T62.2X2	T62.2X3	T62.2X4	—	—
Jatropha	T62.2X1	T62.2X2	T62.2X3	T62.2X4	—	—
curcas	T62.2X1	T62.2X2	T62.2X3	T62.2X4	—	—
Jectofer	T45.4X1	T45.4X2	T45.4X3	T45.4X4	T45.4X5	T45.4X6
Jellyfish (sting)	T63.621	T63.622	T63.623	T63.624	—	—
Jequirity (bean)	T62.2X1	T62.2X2	T62.2X3	T62.2X4	—	—
Jimson weed (stramonium)	T62.2X1	T62.2X2	T62.2X3	T62.2X4	—	—
seeds	T62.2X1	T62.2X2	T62.2X3	T62.2X4	—	—
Josamycin	T36.3X1	T36.3X2	T36.3X3	T36.3X4	T36.3X5	T36.3X6
Juniper tar	T49.1X1	T49.1X2	T49.1X3	T49.1X4	T49.1X5	T49.1X6
Kallidinogenase	T46.7X1	T46.7X2	T46.7X3	T46.7X4	T46.7X5	T46.7X6
Kallikrein	T46.7X1	T46.7X2	T46.7X3	T46.7X4	T46.7X5	T46.7X6
Kanamycin	T36.5X1	T36.5X2	T36.5X3	T36.5X4	T36.5X5	T36.5X6
Kantrex	T36.5X1	T36.5X2	T36.5X3	T36.5X4	T36.5X5	T36.5X6
Kaolin	T47.6X1	T47.6X2	T47.6X3	T47.6X4	T47.6X5	T47.6X6
light	T47.6X1	T47.6X2	T47.6X3	T47.6X4	T47.6X5	T47.6X6
Karaya (gum)	T47.4X1	T47.4X2	T47.4X3	T47.4X4	T47.4X5	T47.4X6
Kebuzone	T39.2X1	T39.2X2	T39.2X3	T39.2X4	T39.2X5	T39.2X6
Kelevan	T60.1X1	T60.1X2	T60.1X3	T60.1X4	—	—
Kemithal	T41.1X1	T41.1X2	T41.1X3	T41.1X4	T41.1X5	T41.1X6
Kenacort	T38.0X1	T38.0X2	T38.0X3	T38.0X4	T38.0X5	T38.0X6
Keratolytic drug NEC	T49.4X1	T49.4X2	T49.4X3	T49.4X4	T49.4X5	T49.4X6
anthracene	T49.4X1	T49.4X2	T49.4X3	T49.4X4	T49.4X5	T49.4X6
Keratoplastic NEC	T49.4X1	T49.4X2	T49.4X3	T49.4X4	T49.4X5	T49.4X6
Kerosene, kerosine (fuel) (solvent) NEC	T52.0X1	T52.0X2	T52.0X3	T52.0X4		
insecticide	T52.0X1	T52.0X2	T52.0X3	T52.0X4	—	—
vapor	T52.0X1	T52.0X2	T52.0X3	T52.0X4	—	—
Ketamine	T41.291	T41.292	T41.293	T41.294	T41.295	T41.296
Ketazolam	T42.4X1	T42.4X2	T42.4X3	T42.4X4	T42.4X5	T42.4X6
Ketazon	T39.2X1	T39.2X2	T39.2X3	T39.2X4	T39.2X5	T39.2X6
Ketobemidone	T40.4X1	T40.4X2	T40.4X3	T40.4X4		
Ketoconazole	T49.0X1	T49.0X2	T49.0X3	T49.0X4	T49.0X5	T49.0X6
Ketols	T52.4X1	T52.4X2	T52.4X3	T52.4X4	—	—
Ketone oils	T52.4X1	T52.4X2	T52.4X3	T52.4X4	—	—
Ketoprofen	T39.311	T39.312	T39.313	T39.314	T39.315	T39.316
Ketorolac	T39.8X1	T39.8X2	T39.8X3	T39.8X4	T39.8X5	T39.8X6
Ketotifen	T45.0X1	T45.0X2	T45.0X3	T45.0X4	T45.0X5	T45.0X6
Khat	T43.691	T43.692	T43.693	T43.694		
Khellin	T46.3X1	T46.3X2	T46.3X3	T46.3X4	T46.3X5	T46.3X6
Khelloside	T46.3X1	T46.3X2	T46.3X3	T46.3X4	T46.3X5	T46.3X6
Kiln gas or vapor (carbon monoxide)	T58.8X1	T58.8X2	T58.8X3	T58.8X4	—	—
Kitasamycin	T36.3X1	T36.3X2	T36.3X3	T36.3X4	T36.3X5	T36.3X6
Konsyl	T47.4X1	T47.4X2	T47.4X3	T47.4X4	T47.4X5	T47.4X6
Kosam seed	T62.2X1	T62.2X2	T62.2X3	T62.2X4	—	—
Krait (venom)	T63.091	T63.092	T63.093	T63.094	—	—
Kwell (insecticide)	T60.1X1	T60.1X2	T60.1X3	T60.1X4	—	—
anti-infective (topical)	T49.0X1	T49.0X2	T49.0X3	T49.0X4	T49.0X5	T49.0X6
Labetalol	T44.8X1	T44.8X2	T44.8X3	T44.8X4	T44.8X5	T44.8X6
Laburnum (seeds)	T62.2X1	T62.2X2	T62.2X3	T62.2X4	—	—
leaves	T62.2X1	T62.2X2	T62.2X3	T62.2X4	—	—
Lachesine	T49.5X1	T49.5X2	T49.5X3	T49.5X4	T49.5X5	T49.5X6
Lacidipine	T46.5X1	T46.5X2	T46.5X3	T46.5X4	T46.5X5	T46.5X6
Lacquer	T65.6X1	T65.6X2	T65.6X3	T65.6X4	—	—
Lacrimogenic gas	T59.3X1	T59.3X2	T59.3X3	T59.3X4	—	—
Lactated potassic saline	T50.3X1	T50.3X2	T50.3X3	T50.3X4	T50.3X5	T50.3X6
Lactic acid	T49.8X1	T49.8X2	T49.8X3	T49.8X4	T49.8X5	T49.8X6
Lactobacillus						
acidophilus	T47.6X1	T47.6X2	T47.6X3	T47.6X4	T47.6X5	T47.6X6
compound	T47.6X1	T47.6X2	T47.6X3	T47.6X4	T47.6X5	T47.6X6
bifidus, lyophilized	T47.6X1	T47.6X2	T47.6X3	T47.6X4	T47.6X5	T47.6X6
bulgaricus	T47.6X1	T47.6X2	T47.6X3	T47.6X4	T47.6X5	T47.6X6
sporogenes	T47.6X1	T47.6X2	T47.6X3	T47.6X4	T47.6X5	T47.6X6
Lactoflavin	T45.2X1	T45.2X2	T45.2X3	T45.2X4	T45.2X5	T45.2X6
Lactose (as excipient)	T50.901	T50.902	T50.903	T50.904	T50.905	T50.906
Lactuca (virosa) (extract)	T42.6X1	T42.6X2	T42.6X3	T42.6X4	T42.6X5	T42.6X6
Lactucarium	T42.6X1	T42.6X2	T42.6X3	T42.6X4	T42.6X5	T42.6X6
Lactulose	T47.3X1	T47.3X2	T47.3X3	T47.3X4	T47.3X5	T47.3X6
Laevo — see Levo-						
Lanatosides	T46.0X1	T46.0X2	T46.0X3	T46.0X4	T46.0X5	T46.0X6
Lanolin	T49.3X1	T49.3X2	T49.3X3	T49.3X4	T49.3X5	T49.3X6
Largactil	T43.3X1	T43.3X2	T43.3X3	T43.3X4	T43.3X5	T43.3X6
Larkspur	T62.2X1	T62.2X2	T62.2X3	T62.2X4	—	—
Laroxyl	T43.011	T43.012	T43.013	T43.014	T43.015	T43.016
Lasix	T50.1X1	T50.1X2	T50.1X3	T50.1X4	T50.1X5	T50.1X6
Lassar's paste	T49.4X1	T49.4X2	T49.4X3	T49.4X4	T49.4X5	T49.4X6
Latamoxef	T36.1X1	T36.1X2	T36.1X3	T36.1X4	T36.1X5	T36.1X6
Latex	T65.811	T65.812	T65.813	T65.814	—	—
Lathyrus (seed)	T62.2X1	T62.2X2	T62.2X3	T62.2X4	—	—
Laudanum	T40.0X1	T40.0X2	T40.0X3	T40.0X4	T40.0X5	T40.0X6
Laudexium	T48.1X1	T48.1X2	T48.1X3	T48.1X4	T48.1X5	T48.1X6
Laughing gas	T41.0X1	T41.0X2	T41.0X3	T41.0X4	T41.0X5	T41.0X6
Laurel, black or cherry	T62.2X1	T62.2X2	T62.2X3	T62.2X4	—	—
Laurolinium	T49.0X1	T49.0X2	T49.0X3	T49.0X4	T49.0X5	T49.0X6
Lauryl sulfoacetate	T49.2X1	T49.2X2	T49.2X3	T49.2X4	T49.2X5	T49.2X6
Laxative NEC	T47.4X1	T47.4X2	T47.4X3	T47.4X4	T47.4X5	T47.4X6
osmotic	T47.3X1	T47.3X2	T47.3X3	T47.3X4	T47.3X5	T47.3X6
saline	T47.3X1	T47.3X2	T47.3X3	T47.3X4	T47.3X5	T47.3X6
stimulant	T47.2X1	T47.2X2	T47.2X3	T47.2X4	T47.2X5	T47.2X6
L-dopa	T42.8X1	T42.8X2	T42.8X3	T42.8X4	T42.8X5	T42.8X6
Lead (dust) (fumes) (vapor) NEC	T56.0X1	T56.0X2	T56.0X3	T56.0X4	—	—
acetate	T49.2X1	T49.2X2	T49.2X3	T49.2X4	T49.2X5	T49.2X6
alkyl (fuel additive)	T56.0X1	T56.0X2	T56.0X3	T56.0X4	—	—
anti-infectives	T37.8X1	T37.8X2	T37.8X3	T37.8X4	T37.8X5	T37.8X6
antiknock compound (tetraethyl)	T56.0X1	T56.0X2	T56.0X3	T56.0X4	—	—
arsenate, arsenite (dust)(herbicide) (insecticide) (vapor)	T57.0X1	T57.0X2	T57.0X3	T57.0X4		
carbonate	T56.0X1	T56.0X2	T56.0X3	T56.0X4	—	—
paint	T56.0X1	T56.0X2	T56.0X3	T56.0X4	—	—
chromate	T56.0X1	T56.0X2	T56.0X3	T56.0X4	—	—
paint	T56.0X1	T56.0X2	T56.0X3	T56.0X4	—	—
dioxide	T56.0X1	T56.0X2	T56.0X3	T56.0X4	—	—
inorganic	T56.0X1	T56.0X2	T56.0X3	T56.0X4	—	—
iodide	T56.0X1	T56.0X2	T56.0X3	T56.0X4	—	—
pigment (paint)	T56.0X1	T56.0X2	T56.0X3	T56.0X4	—	—
monoxide (dust)	T56.0X1	T56.0X2	T56.0X3	T56.0X4	—	—
paint	T56.0X1	T56.0X2	T56.0X3	T56.0X4	—	—
organic	T56.0X1	T56.0X2	T56.0X3	T56.0X4	—	—
oxide	T56.0X1	T56.0X2	T56.0X3	T56.0X4	—	—
paint	T56.0X1	T56.0X2	T56.0X3	T56.0X4	—	—
paint	T56.0X1	T56.0X2	T56.0X3	T56.0X4	—	—
salts	T56.0X1	T56.0X2	T56.0X3	T56.0X4	—	—
specified compound NEC	T56.0X1	T56.0X2	T56.0X3	T56.0X4	—	—
tetra-ethyl	T56.0X1	T56.0X2	T56.0X3	T56.0X4	—	—
Lebanese red	T40.7X1	T40.7X2	T40.7X3	T40.7X4	T40.7X5	T40.7X6
Lefetamine	T39.8X1	T39.8X2	T39.8X3	T39.8X4	T39.8X5	T39.8X6
Lenperone	T43.4X1	T43.4X2	T43.4X3	T43.4X4	T43.4X5	T43.4X6
Lente lietin (insulin)	T38.3X1	T38.3X2	T38.3X3	T38.3X4	T38.3X5	T38.3X6
Leptazol	T50.7X1	T50.7X2	T50.7X3	T50.7X4	T50.7X5	T50.7X6
Leptophos	T60.0X1	T60.0X2	T60.0X3	T60.0X4	—	—
Leritine	T40.2X1	T40.2X2	T40.2X3	T40.2X4	T40.2X5	T40.2X6
Letosteine	T48.4X1	T48.4X2	T48.4X3	T48.4X4	T48.4X5	T48.4X6
Letter	T38.1X1	T38.1X2	T38.1X3	T38.1X4	T38.1X5	T38.1X6
Lettuce opium	T42.6X1	T42.6X2	T42.6X3	T42.6X4	T42.6X5	T42.6X6
Leucinocaine	T41.3X1	T41.3X2	T41.3X3	T41.3X4	T41.3X5	T41.3X6
Leucocianidol	T46.991	T46.992	T46.993	T46.994	T46.995	T46.996
Leucovorin (factor)	T45.8X1	T45.8X2	T45.8X3	T45.8X4	T45.8X5	T45.8X6
Leukeran	T45.1X1	T45.1X2	T45.1X3	T45.1X4	T45.1X5	T45.1X6
Leuprolide	T38.891	T38.892	T38.893	T38.894	T38.895	T38.896
Levalbuterol	T48.6X1	T48.6X2	T48.6X3	T48.6X4	T48.6X5	T48.6X6
Levallorphan	T50.7X1	T50.7X2	T50.7X3	T50.7X4	T50.7X5	T50.7X6
Levamisole	T37.4X1	T37.4X2	T37.4X3	T37.4X4	T37.4X5	T37.4X6
Levanil	T42.6X1	T42.6X2	T42.6X3	T42.6X4	T42.6X5	T42.6X6
Levarterenol	T44.4X1	T44.4X2	T44.4X3	T44.4X4	T44.4X5	T44.4X6
Levdropropizine	T48.3X1	T48.3X2	T48.3X3	T48.3X4	T48.3X5	T48.3X6
Levobunolol	T49.5X1	T49.5X2	T49.5X3	T49.5X4	T49.5X5	T49.5X6
Levocabastine (hydrochloride)	T45.0X1	T45.0X2	T45.0X3	T45.0X4	T45.0X5	T45.0X6
Levocarnitine	T50.991	T50.992	T50.993	T50.994	T50.995	T50.996
Levodopa	T42.8X1	T42.8X2	T42.8X3	T42.8X4	T42.8X5	T42.8X6
with carbidopa	T42.8X1	T42.8X2	T42.8X3	T42.8X4	T42.8X5	T42.8X6
Levo-dromoran	T40.2X1	T40.2X2	T40.2X3	T40.2X4	T40.2X5	T40.2X6
Levoglutamide	T50.991	T50.992	T50.993	T50.994	T50.995	T50.996
Levoid	T38.1X1	T38.1X2	T38.1X3	T38.1X4	T38.1X5	T38.1X6
Levo-isomethadone	T40.3X1	T40.3X2	T40.3X3	T40.3X4	T40.3X5	T40.3X6
Levomepromazine	T43.3X1	T43.3X2	T43.3X3	T43.3X4	T43.3X5	T43.3X6
Levonordefrin	T49.6X1	T49.6X2	T49.6X3	T49.6X4	T49.6X5	T49.6X6
Levonorgestrel	T38.4X1	T38.4X2	T38.4X3	T38.4X4	T38.4X5	T38.4X6
with ethinylestradiol	T38.5X1	T38.5X2	T38.5X3	T38.5X4	T38.5X5	T38.5X6
Levopromazine	T43.3X1	T43.3X2	T43.3X3	T43.3X4	T43.3X5	T43.3X6
Levoprome	T42.6X1	T42.6X2	T42.6X3	T42.6X4	T42.6X5	T42.6X6
Levopropoxyphene	T40.4X1	T40.4X2	T40.4X3	T40.4X4	T40.4X5	T40.4X6
Levopropylhexedrine	T50.5X1	T50.5X2	T50.5X3	T50.5X4	T50.5X5	T50.5X6
Levoproxyphylline	T48.6X1	T48.6X2	T48.6X3	T48.6X4	T48.6X5	T48.6X6
Levorphanol	T40.4X1	T40.4X2	T40.4X3	T40.4X4	T40.4X5	T40.4X6

Table of Drugs and Chemicals

Substance	Poisoning, Accidental (unintentional)	Poisoning, Intentional Self-harm	Poisoning, Assault	Poisoning, Undetermined	Adverse Effect	Under-dosing
Levothyroxine	T38.1X1	T38.1X2	T38.1X3	T38.1X4	T38.1X5	T38.1X6
sodium	T38.1X1	T38.1X2	T38.1X3	T38.1X4	T38.1X5	T38.1X6
Levsin	T44.3X1	T44.3X2	T44.3X3	T44.3X4	T44.3X5	T44.3X6
Levulose	T50.3X1	T50.3X2	T50.3X3	T50.3X4	T50.3X5	T50.3X6
Lewisite (gas), not in war	T57.0X1	T57.0X2	T57.0X3	T57.0X4	—	—
Librium	T42.4X1	T42.4X2	T42.4X3	T42.4X4	T42.4X5	T42.4X6
Lidex	T49.0X1	T49.0X2	T49.0X3	T49.0X4	T49.0X5	T49.0X6
Lidocaine	T41.3X1	T41.3X2	T41.3X3	T41.3X4	T41.3X5	T41.3X6
regional	T41.3X1	T41.3X2	T41.3X3	T41.3X4	T41.3X5	T41.3X6
spinal	T41.3X1	T41.3X2	T41.3X3	T41.3X4	T41.3X5	T41.3X6
Lidofenin	T50.8X1	T50.8X2	T50.8X3	T50.8X4	T50.8X5	T50.8X6
Lidoflazine	T46.1X1	T46.1X2	T46.1X3	T46.1X4	T46.1X5	T46.1X6
Lighter fluid	T52.0X1	T52.0X2	T52.0X3	T52.0X4	—	—
Lignin hemicellulose	T47.6X1	T47.6X2	T47.6X3	T47.6X4	T47.6X5	T47.6X6
Lignocaine	T41.3X1	T41.3X2	T41.3X3	T41.3X4	T41.3X5	T41.3X6
regional	T41.3X1	T41.3X2	T41.3X3	T41.3X4	T41.3X5	T41.3X6
spinal	T41.3X1	T41.3X2	T41.3X3	T41.3X4	T41.3X5	T41.3X6
Ligroin (e) (solvent)	T52.0X1	T52.0X2	T52.0X3	T52.0X4	—	—
vapor	T59.891	T59.892	T59.893	T59.894	—	—
Ligustrum vulgare	T62.2X1	T62.2X2	T62.2X3	T62.2X4	—	—
Lily of the valley	T62.2X1	T62.2X2	T62.2X3	T62.2X4	—	—
Lime (chloride)	T54.3X1	T54.3X2	T54.3X3	T54.3X4	—	—
Limonene	T52.8X1	T52.8X2	T52.8X3	T52.8X4	—	—
Lincomycin	T36.8X1	T36.8X2	T36.8X3	T36.8X4	T36.8X5	T36.8X6
Lindane (insecticide) (nonmedicinal) (vapor)	T53.6X1	T53.6X2	T53.6X3	T53.6X4	—	—
medicinal	T49.0X1	T49.0X2	T49.0X3	T49.0X4	T49.0X5	T49.0X6
Liniments NEC	T49.91	T49.92	T49.93	T49.94	T49.95	T49.96
Linoleic acid	T46.6X1	T46.6X2	T46.6X3	T46.6X4	T46.6X5	T46.6X6
Linolenic acid	T46.6X1	T46.6X2	T46.6X3	T46.6X4	T46.6X5	T46.6X6
Linseed	T47.4X1	T47.4X2	T47.4X3	T47.4X4	T47.4X5	T47.4X6
Liothyronine	T38.1X1	T38.1X2	T38.1X3	T38.1X4	T38.1X5	T38.1X6
Liotrix	T38.1X1	T38.1X2	T38.1X3	T38.1X4	T38.1X5	T38.1X6
Lipancreatin	T47.5X1	T47.5X2	T47.5X3	T47.5X4	T47.5X5	T47.5X6
Lipo-alprostadil	T46.7X1	T46.7X2	T46.7X3	T46.7X4	T46.7X5	T46.7X6
Lipo-Lutin	T38.5X1	T38.5X2	T38.5X3	T38.5X4	T38.5X5	T38.5X6
Lipotropic drug NEC	T50.901	T50.902	T50.903	T50.904	T50.905	T50.906
Liquefied petroleum gases	T59.891	T59.892	T59.893	T59.894	—	—
piped (pure or mixed with air)	T59.891	T59.892	T59.893	T59.894	—	—
Liquid						
paraffin	T47.4X1	T47.4X2	T47.4X3	T47.4X4	T47.4X5	T47.4X6
petrolatum	T47.4X1	T47.4X2	T47.4X3	T47.4X4	T47.4X5	T47.4X6
topical	T49.3X1	T49.3X2	T49.3X3	T49.3X4	T49.3X5	T49.3X6
specified NEC	T65.891	T65.892	T65.893	T65.894	—	—
substance	T65.91	T65.92	T65.93	T65.94	—	—
Liquor creosolis compositus	T65.891	T65.892	T65.893	T65.894	—	—
Liquorice	T48.4X1	T48.4X2	T48.4X3	T48.4X4	T48.4X5	T48.4X6
extract	T47.8X1	T47.8X2	T47.8X3	T47.8X4	T47.8X5	T47.8X6
Lisinopril	T46.4X1	T46.4X2	T46.4X3	T46.4X4	T46.4X5	T46.4X6
Lisuride	T42.8X1	T42.8X2	T42.8X3	T42.8X4	T42.8X5	T42.8X6
Lithane	T43.8X1	T43.8X2	T43.8X3	T43.8X4	T43.8X5	T43.8X6
Lithium	T56.891	T56.892	T56.893	T56.894	—	—
gluconate	T43.591	T43.592	T43.593	T43.594	T43.595	T43.596
salts (carbonate)	T43.591	T43.592	T43.593	T43.594	T43.595	T43.596
Lithonate	T43.8X1	T43.8X2	T43.8X3	T43.8X4	T43.8X5	T43.8X6
Liver						
extract	T45.8X1	T45.8X2	T45.8X3	T45.8X4	T45.8X5	T45.8X6
for parenteral use	T45.8X1	T45.8X2	T45.8X3	T45.8X4	T45.8X5	T45.8X6
fraction 1	T45.8X1	T45.8X2	T45.8X3	T45.8X4	T45.8X5	T45.8X6
hydrolysate	T45.8X1	T45.8X2	T45.8X3	T45.8X4	T45.8X5	T45.8X6
Lizard (bite) (venom)	T63.121	T63.122	T63.123	T63.124	—	—
LMD	T45.8X1	T45.8X2	T45.8X3	T45.8X4	T45.8X5	T45.8X6
Lobelia	T62.2X1	T62.2X2	T62.2X3	T62.2X4	—	—
Lobeline	T50.7X1	T50.7X2	T50.7X3	T50.7X4	T50.7X5	T50.7X6
Local action drug NEC	T49.8X1	T49.8X2	T49.8X3	T49.8X4	T49.8X5	T49.8X6
Locorten	T49.0X1	T49.0X2	T49.0X3	T49.0X4	T49.0X5	T49.0X6
Lofepramine	T43.011	T43.012	T43.013	T43.014	T43.015	T43.016
Lolium temulentum	T62.2X1	T62.2X2	T62.2X3	T62.2X4	—	—
Lomotil	T47.6X1	T47.6X2	T47.6X3	T47.6X4	T47.6X5	T47.6X6
Lomustine	T45.1X1	T45.1X2	T45.1X3	T45.1X4	T45.1X5	T45.1X6
Lonidamine	T45.1X1	T45.1X2	T45.1X3	T45.1X4	T45.1X5	T45.1X6
Loperamide	T47.6X1	T47.6X2	T47.6X3	T47.6X4	T47.6X5	T47.6X6
Loprazolam	T42.4X1	T42.4X2	T42.4X3	T42.4X4	T42.4X5	T42.4X6
Lorajmine	T46.2X1	T46.2X2	T46.2X3	T46.2X4	T46.2X5	T46.2X6
Loratidine	T45.0X1	T45.0X2	T45.0X3	T45.0X4	T45.0X5	T45.0X6
Lorazepam	T42.4X1	T42.4X2	T42.4X3	T42.4X4	T42.4X5	T42.4X6
Lorcainide	T46.2X1	T46.2X2	T46.2X3	T46.2X4	T46.2X5	T46.2X6
Lormetazepam	T42.4X1	T42.4X2	T42.4X3	T42.4X4	T42.4X5	T42.4X6
Lotions NEC	T49.91	T49.92	T49.93	T49.94	T49.95	T49.96
Lotusate	T42.3X1	T42.3X2	T42.3X3	T42.3X4	T42.3X5	T42.3X6
Lovastatin	T46.6X1	T46.6X2	T46.6X3	T46.6X4	T46.6X5	T46.6X6
Lowila	T49.2X1	T49.2X2	T49.2X3	T49.2X4	T49.2X5	T49.2X6
Loxapine	T43.591	T43.592	T43.593	T43.594	T43.595	T43.596
Lozenges (throat)	T49.6X1	T49.6X2	T49.6X3	T49.6X4	T49.6X5	T49.6X6
LSD	T40.8X1	T40.8X2	T40.8X3	T40.8X4	—	—
L-Tryptophan — see amino acid						
Lubricant, eye	T49.5X1	T49.5X2	T49.5X3	T49.5X4	T49.5X5	T49.5X6
Lubricating oil NEC	T52.0X1	T52.0X2	T52.0X3	T52.0X4	—	—
Lucanthone	T37.4X1	T37.4X2	T37.4X3	T37.4X4	T37.4X5	T37.4X6
Luminal	T42.3X1	T42.3X2	T42.3X3	T42.3X4	T42.3X5	T42.3X6
Lung irritant (gas) NEC	T59.91	T59.92	T59.93	T59.94	—	—
Luteinizing hormone	T38.811	T38.812	T38.813	T38.814	T38.815	T38.816
Lutocylol	T38.5X1	T38.5X2	T38.5X3	T38.5X4	T38.5X5	T38.5X6
Lutromone	T38.5X1	T38.5X2	T38.5X3	T38.5X4	T38.5X5	T38.5X6
Lututrin	T48.291	T48.292	T48.293	T48.294	T48.295	T48.296
Lye (concentrated)	T54.3X1	T54.3X2	T54.3X3	T54.3X4	—	—
Lygranum (skin test)	T50.8X1	T50.8X2	T50.8X3	T50.8X4	T50.8X5	T50.8X6
Lymecycline	T36.4X1	T36.4X2	T36.4X3	T36.4X4	T36.4X5	T36.4X6
Lymphogranuloma venereum antigen	T50.8X1	T50.8X2	T50.8X3	T50.8X4	T50.8X5	T50.8X6
Lynestrenol	T38.4X1	T38.4X2	T38.4X3	T38.4X4	T38.4X5	T38.4X6
Lyovac Sodium Edecrin	T50.1X1	T50.1X2	T50.1X3	T50.1X4	T50.1X5	T50.1X6
Lypressin	T38.891	T38.892	T38.893	T38.894	T38.895	T38.896
Lysergic acid diethylamide	T40.8X1	T40.8X2	T40.8X3	T40.8X4	—	—
Lysergide	T40.8X1	T40.8X2	T40.8X3	T40.8X4	—	—
Lysine vasopressin	T38.891	T38.892	T38.893	T38.894	T38.895	T38.896
Lysol	T54.1X1	T54.1X2	T54.1X3	T54.1X4	—	—
Lysozyme	T49.0X1	T49.0X2	T49.0X3	T49.0X4	T49.0X5	T49.0X6
Lytta (vitatta)	T49.8X1	T49.8X2	T49.8X3	T49.8X4	T49.8X5	T49.8X6
Mace	T59.3X1	T59.3X2	T59.3X3	T59.3X4	—	—
Macrogol	T50.991	T50.992	T50.993	T50.994	T50.995	T50.996
Macrolide						
anabolic drug	T38.7X1	T38.7X2	T38.7X3	T38.7X4	T38.7X5	T38.7X6
antibiotic	T36.3X1	T36.3X2	T36.3X3	T36.3X4	T36.3X5	T36.3X6
Mafenide	T49.0X1	T49.0X2	T49.0X3	T49.0X4	T49.0X5	T49.0X6
Magaldrate	T47.1X1	T47.1X2	T47.1X3	T47.1X4	T47.1X5	T47.1X6
Magic mushroom	T40.991	T40.992	T40.993	T40.994	—	—
Magnamycin	T36.8X1	T36.8X2	T36.8X3	T36.8X4	T36.8X5	T36.8X6
Magnesia magma	T47.1X1	T47.1X2	T47.1X3	T47.1X4	T47.1X5	T47.1X6
Magnesium NEC	T56.891	T56.892	T56.893	T56.894	—	—
carbonate	T47.1X1	T47.1X2	T47.1X3	T47.1X4	T47.1X5	T47.1X6
citrate	T47.4X1	T47.4X2	T47.4X3	T47.4X4	T47.4X5	T47.4X6
hydroxide	T47.1X1	T47.1X2	T47.1X3	T47.1X4	T47.1X5	T47.1X6
oxide	T47.1X1	T47.1X2	T47.1X3	T47.1X4	T47.1X5	T47.1X6
peroxide	T49.0X1	T49.0X2	T49.0X3	T49.0X4	T49.0X5	T49.0X6
salicylate	T39.091	T39.092	T39.093	T39.094	T39.095	T39.096
silicofluoride	T50.3X1	T50.3X2	T50.3X3	T50.3X4	T50.3X5	T50.3X6
sulfate	T47.4X1	T47.4X2	T47.4X3	T47.4X4	T47.4X5	T47.4X6
thiosulfate	T45.0X1	T45.0X2	T45.0X3	T45.0X4	T45.0X5	T45.0X6
trisilicate	T47.1X1	T47.1X2	T47.1X3	T47.1X4	T47.1X5	T47.1X6
Malathion (medicinal)	T49.0X1	T49.0X2	T49.0X3	T49.0X4	T49.0X5	T49.0X6
insecticide	T60.0X1	T60.0X2	T60.0X3	T60.0X4	—	—
Male fern extract	T37.4X1	T37.4X2	T37.4X3	T37.4X4	T37.4X5	T37.4X6
M-AMSA	T45.1X1	T45.1X2	T45.1X3	T45.1X4	T45.1X5	T45.1X6
Mandelic acid	T37.8X1	T37.8X2	T37.8X3	T37.8X4	T37.8X5	T37.8X6
Manganese (dioxide) (salts)	T57.2X1	T57.2X2	T57.2X3	T57.2X4	—	—
medicinal	T50.991	T50.992	T50.993	T50.994	T50.995	T50.996
Mannitol	T47.3X1	T47.3X2	T47.3X3	T47.3X4	T47.3X5	T47.3X6
hexanitrate	T46.3X1	T46.3X2	T46.3X3	T46.3X4	T46.3X5	T46.3X6
Mannomustine	T45.1X1	T45.1X2	T45.1X3	T45.1X4	T45.1X5	T45.1X6
MAO inhibitors	T43.1X1	T43.1X2	T43.1X3	T43.1X4	T43.1X5	T43.1X6
Mapharsen	T37.8X1	T37.8X2	T37.8X3	T37.8X4	T37.8X5	T37.8X6
Maphenide	T49.0X1	T49.0X2	T49.0X3	T49.0X4	T49.0X5	T49.0X6
Maprotiline	T43.021	T43.022	T43.023	T43.024	T43.025	T43.026
Marcaine	T41.3X1	T41.3X2	T41.3X3	T41.3X4	T41.3X5	T41.3X6
infiltration (subcutaneous)	T41.3X1	T41.3X2	T41.3X3	T41.3X4	T41.3X5	T41.3X6
nerve block (peripheral) (plexus)	T41.3X1	T41.3X2	T41.3X3	T41.3X4	T41.3X5	T41.3X6
Marezine	T45.0X1	T45.0X2	T45.0X3	T45.0X4	T45.0X5	T45.0X6
Marihuana	T40.7X1	T40.7X2	T40.7X3	T40.7X4	T40.7X5	T40.7X6
Marijuana	T40.7X1	T40.7X2	T40.7X3	T40.7X4	T40.7X5	T40.7X6
Marine (sting)	T63.691	T63.692	T63.693	T63.694	—	—
animals (sting)	T63.691	T63.692	T63.693	T63.694	—	—
plants (sting)	T63.711	T63.712	T63.713	T63.714	—	—
Marplan	T43.1X1	T43.1X2	T43.1X3	T43.1X4	T43.1X5	T43.1X6
Marsh gas	T59.891	T59.892	T59.893	T59.894	—	—
Marsilid	T43.1X1	T43.1X2	T43.1X3	T43.1X4	T43.1X5	T43.1X6
Matulane	T45.1X1	T45.1X2	T45.1X3	T45.1X4	T45.1X5	T45.1X6
Mazindol	T50.5X1	T50.5X2	T50.5X3	T50.5X4	T50.5X5	T50.5X6
MCPA	T60.3X1	T60.3X2	T60.3X3	T60.3X4	—	—
MDMA	T43.641	T43.642	T43.643	T43.644	—	—
Meadow saffron	T62.2X1	T62.2X2	T62.2X3	T62.2X4	—	—
Measles virus vaccine (attenuated)	T50.B91	T50.B92	T50.B93	T50.B94	T50.B95	T50.B96

Levothyroxine — Measles virus vaccine

Substance	Poisoning, Accidental (unintentional)	Poisoning, Intentional Self-harm	Poisoning, Assault	Poisoning, Undetermined	Adverse Effect	Under-dosing
Meat, noxious	T62.8X1	T62.8X2	T62.8X3	T62.8X4	—	—
Meballymal	T42.3X1	T42.3X2	T42.3X3	T42.3X4	T42.3X5	T42.3X6
Mebanazine	T43.1X1	T43.1X2	T43.1X3	T43.1X4	T43.1X5	T43.1X6
Mebaral	T42.3X1	T42.3X2	T42.3X3	T42.3X4	T42.3X5	T42.3X6
Mebendazole	T37.4X1	T37.4X2	T37.4X3	T37.4X4	T37.4X5	T37.4X6
Mebeverine	T44.3X1	T44.3X2	T44.3X3	T44.3X4	T44.3X5	T44.3X6
Mebhydrolin	T45.0X1	T45.0X2	T45.0X3	T45.0X4	T45.0X5	T45.0X6
Mebumal	T42.3X1	T42.3X2	T42.3X3	T42.3X4	T42.3X5	T42.3X6
Mebutamate	T43.591	T43.592	T43.593	T43.594	T43.595	T43.596
Mecamylamine	T44.2X1	T44.2X2	T44.2X3	T44.2X4	T44.2X5	T44.2X6
Mechlorethamine	T45.1X1	T45.1X2	T45.1X3	T45.1X4	T45.1X5	T45.1X6
Mecillinam	T36.0X1	T36.0X2	T36.0X3	T36.0X4	T36.0X5	T36.0X6
Meclizine (hydrochloride)	T45.0X1	T45.0X2	T45.0X3	T45.0X4	T45.0X5	T45.0X6
Meclocycline	T36.4X1	T36.4X2	T36.4X3	T36.4X4	T36.4X5	T36.4X6
Meclofenamate	T39.391	T39.392	T39.393	T39.394	T39.395	T39.396
Meclofenamic acid	T39.391	T39.392	T39.393	T39.394	T39.395	T39.396
Meclofenoxate	T43.691	T43.692	T43.693	T43.694	T43.695	T43.696
Meclozine	T45.0X1	T45.0X2	T45.0X3	T45.0X4	T45.0X5	T45.0X6
Mecobalamin	T45.8X1	T45.8X2	T45.8X3	T45.8X4	T45.8X5	T45.8X6
Mecoprop	T60.3X1	T60.3X2	T60.3X3	T60.3X4	—	—
Mecrilate	T49.3X1	T49.3X2	T49.3X3	T49.3X4	T49.3X5	T49.3X6
Mecysteine	T48.4X1	T48.4X2	T48.4X3	T48.4X4	T48.4X5	T48.4X6
Medazepam	T42.4X1	T42.4X2	T42.4X3	T42.4X4	T42.4X5	T42.4X6
Medicament NEC	T50.901	T50.902	T50.903	T50.904	T50.905	T50.906
Medinal	T42.3X1	T42.3X2	T42.3X3	T42.3X4	T42.3X5	T42.3X6
Medomin	T42.3X1	T42.3X2	T42.3X3	T42.3X4	T42.3X5	T42.3X6
Medrogestone	T38.5X1	T38.5X2	T38.5X3	T38.5X4	T38.5X5	T38.5X6
Medroxalol	T44.8X1	T44.8X2	T44.8X3	T44.8X4	T44.8X5	T44.8X6
Medroxyprogesterone acetate (depot)	T38.5X1	T38.5X2	T38.5X3	T38.5X4	T38.5X5	T38.5X6
Medrysone	T49.0X1	T49.0X2	T49.0X3	T49.0X4	T49.0X5	T49.0X6
Mefenamic acid	T39.391	T39.392	T39.393	T39.394	T39.395	T39.396
Mefenorex	T50.5X1	T50.5X2	T50.5X3	T50.5X4	T50.5X5	T50.5X6
Mefloquine	T37.2X1	T37.2X2	T37.2X3	T37.2X4	T37.2X5	T37.2X6
Mefruside	T50.2X1	T50.2X2	T50.2X3	T50.2X4	T50.2X5	T50.2X6
Megahallucinogen	T40.901	T40.902	T40.903	T40.904	T40.905	T40.906
Megestrol	T38.5X1	T38.5X2	T38.5X3	T38.5X4	T38.5X5	T38.5X6
Meglumine						
antimoniate	T37.8X1	T37.8X2	T37.8X3	T37.8X4	T37.8X5	T37.8X6
diatrizoate	T50.8X1	T50.8X2	T50.8X3	T50.8X4	T50.8X5	T50.8X6
iodipamide	T50.8X1	T50.8X2	T50.8X3	T50.8X4	T50.8X5	T50.8X6
iotroxate	T50.8X1	T50.8X2	T50.8X3	T50.8X4	T50.8X5	T50.8X6
MEK (methyl ethyl ketone)	T52.4X1	T52.4X2	T52.4X3	T52.4X4	—	—
Meladinin	T49.3X1	T49.3X2	T49.3X3	T49.3X4	T49.3X5	T49.3X6
Meladrazine	T44.3X1	T44.3X2	T44.3X3	T44.3X4	T44.3X5	T44.3X6
Melaleuca alternifolia oil	T49.0X1	T49.0X2	T49.0X3	T49.0X4	T49.0X5	T49.0X6
Melanizing agents	T49.3X1	T49.3X2	T49.3X3	T49.3X4	T49.3X5	T49.3X6
Melanocyte-stimulating hormone	T38.891	T38.892	T38.893	T38.894	T38.895	T38.896
Melarsonyl potassium	T37.3X1	T37.3X2	T37.3X3	T37.3X4	T37.3X5	T37.3X6
Melarsoprol	T37.3X1	T37.3X2	T37.3X3	T37.3X4	T37.3X5	T37.3X6
Melia azedarach	T62.2X1	T62.2X2	T62.2X3	T62.2X4	—	—
Melitracen	T43.011	T43.012	T43.013	T43.014	T43.015	T43.016
Mellaril	T43.3X1	T43.3X2	T43.3X3	T43.3X4	T43.3X5	T43.3X6
Meloxine	T49.3X1	T49.3X2	T49.3X3	T49.3X4	T49.3X5	T49.3X6
Melperone	T43.4X1	T43.4X2	T43.4X3	T43.4X4	T43.4X5	T43.4X6
Melphalan	T45.1X1	T45.1X2	T45.1X3	T45.1X4	T45.1X5	T45.1X6
Memantine	T43.8X1	T43.8X2	T43.8X3	T43.8X4	T43.8X5	T43.8X6
Menadiol	T45.7X1	T45.7X2	T45.7X3	T45.7X4	T45.7X5	T45.7X6
sodium sulfate	T45.7X1	T45.7X2	T45.7X3	T45.7X4	T45.7X5	T45.7X6
Menadione	T45.7X1	T45.7X2	T45.7X3	T45.7X4	T45.7X5	T45.7X6
sodium bisulfite	T45.7X1	T45.7X2	T45.7X3	T45.7X4	T45.7X5	T45.7X6
Menaphthone	T45.7X1	T45.7X2	T45.7X3	T45.7X4	T45.7X5	T45.7X6
Menaquinone	T45.7X1	T45.7X2	T45.7X3	T45.7X4	T45.7X5	T45.7X6
Menatetrenone	T45.7X1	T45.7X2	T45.7X3	T45.7X4	T45.7X5	T45.7X6
Meningococcal vaccine	T50.A91	T50.A92	T50.A93	T50.A94	T50.A95	T50.A96
Menningovax (-AC) (-C)	T50.A91	T50.A92	T50.A93	T50.A94	T50.A95	T50.A96
Menotropins	T38.811	T38.812	T38.813	T38.814	T38.815	T38.816
Menthol	T48.5X1	T48.5X2	T48.5X3	T48.5X4	T48.5X5	T48.5X6
Mepacrine	T37.2X1	T37.2X2	T37.2X3	T37.2X4	T37.2X5	T37.2X6
Meparfynol	T42.6X1	T42.6X2	T42.6X3	T42.6X4	T42.6X5	T42.6X6
Mepartricin	T36.7X1	T36.7X2	T36.7X3	T36.7X4	T36.7X5	T36.7X6
Mepazine	T43.3X1	T43.3X2	T43.3X3	T43.3X4	T43.3X5	T43.3X6
Mepenzolate	T44.3X1	T44.3X2	T44.3X3	T44.3X4	T44.3X5	T44.3X6
bromide	T44.3X1	T44.3X2	T44.3X3	T44.3X4	T44.3X5	T44.3X6
Meperidine	T40.4X1	T40.4X2	T40.4X3	T40.4X4	T40.4X5	T40.4X6
Mephebarbital	T42.3X1	T42.3X2	T42.3X3	T42.3X4	T42.3X5	T42.3X6
Mephenamin (e)	T42.8X1	T42.8X2	T42.8X3	T42.8X4	T42.8X5	T42.8X6
Mephenesin	T42.8X1	T42.8X2	T42.8X3	T42.8X4	T42.8X5	T42.8X6
Mephenhydramine	T45.0X1	T45.0X2	T45.0X3	T45.0X4	T45.0X5	T45.0X6
Mephenoxalone	T42.8X1	T42.8X2	T42.8X3	T42.8X4	T42.8X5	T42.8X6
Mephentermine	T44.991	T44.992	T44.993	T44.994	T44.995	T44.996
Mephenytoin	T42.0X1	T42.0X2	T42.0X3	T42.0X4	T42.0X5	T42.0X6

Substance	Poisoning, Accidental (unintentional)	Poisoning, Intentional Self-harm	Poisoning, Assault	Poisoning, Undetermined	Adverse Effect	Under-dosing
Mephenytoin — continued						
with phenobarbital	T42.3X1	T42.3X2	T42.3X3	T42.3X4	T42.3X5	T42.3X6
Mephobarbital	T42.3X1	T42.3X2	T42.3X3	T42.3X4	T42.3X5	T42.3X6
Mephosfolan	T60.0X1	T60.0X2	T60.0X3	T60.0X4	—	—
Mepindolol	T44.7X1	T44.7X2	T44.7X3	T44.7X4	T44.7X5	T44.7X6
Mepiperphenidol	T44.3X1	T44.3X2	T44.3X3	T44.3X4	T44.3X5	T44.3X6
Mepitiostane	T38.7X1	T38.7X2	T38.7X3	T38.7X4	T38.7X5	T38.7X6
Mepivacaine	T41.3X1	T41.3X2	T41.3X3	T41.3X4	T41.3X5	T41.3X6
epidural	T41.3X1	T41.3X2	T41.3X3	T41.3X4	T41.3X5	T41.3X6
Meprednisone	T38.0X1	T38.0X2	T38.0X3	T38.0X4	T38.0X5	T38.0X6
Meprobam	T43.591	T43.592	T43.593	T43.594	T43.595	T43.596
Meprobamate	T43.591	T43.592	T43.593	T43.594	T43.595	T43.596
Meproscillarin	T46.0X1	T46.0X2	T46.0X3	T46.0X4	T46.0X5	T46.0X6
Meprylcaine	T41.3X1	T41.3X2	T41.3X3	T41.3X4	T41.3X5	T41.3X6
Meptazinol	T39.8X1	T39.8X2	T39.8X3	T39.8X4	T39.8X5	T39.8X6
Mepyramine	T45.0X1	T45.0X2	T45.0X3	T45.0X4	T45.0X5	T45.0X6
Mequitazine	T43.3X1	T43.3X2	T43.3X3	T43.3X4	T43.3X5	T43.3X6
Meralluride	T50.2X1	T50.2X2	T50.2X3	T50.2X4	T50.2X5	T50.2X6
Merbaphen	T50.2X1	T50.2X2	T50.2X3	T50.2X4	T50.2X5	T50.2X6
Merbromin	T49.0X1	T49.0X2	T49.0X3	T49.0X4	T49.0X5	T49.0X6
Mercaptobenzothiazole salts	T49.0X1	T49.0X2	T49.0X3	T49.0X4	T49.0X5	T49.0X6
Mercaptomerin	T50.2X1	T50.2X2	T50.2X3	T50.2X4	T50.2X5	T50.2X6
Mercaptopurine	T45.1X1	T45.1X2	T45.1X3	T45.1X4	T45.1X5	T45.1X6
Mercumatilin	T50.2X1	T50.2X2	T50.2X3	T50.2X4	T50.2X5	T50.2X6
Mercuramide	T50.2X1	T50.2X2	T50.2X3	T50.2X4	T50.2X5	T50.2X6
Mercurochrome	T49.0X1	T49.0X2	T49.0X3	T49.0X4	T49.0X5	T49.0X6
Mercurophylline	T50.2X1	T50.2X2	T50.2X3	T50.2X4	T50.2X5	T50.2X6
Mercury, mercurial, mercuric, mercurous (compounds) (cyanide) (fumes) (nonmedicinal) (vapor) NEC	T56.1X1	T56.1X2	T56.1X3	T56.1X4	—	—
ammoniated	T49.0X1	T49.0X2	T49.0X3	T49.0X4	T49.0X5	T49.0X6
anti-infective						
local	T49.0X1	T49.0X2	T49.0X3	T49.0X4	T49.0X5	T49.0X6
systemic	T37.8X1	T37.8X2	T37.8X3	T37.8X4	T37.8X5	T37.8X6
topical	T49.0X1	T49.0X2	T49.0X3	T49.0X4	T49.0X5	T49.0X6
chloride (ammoniated)	T49.0X1	T49.0X2	T49.0X3	T49.0X4	T49.0X5	T49.0X6
fungicide	T56.1X1	T56.1X2	T56.1X3	T56.1X4	—	—
diuretic NEC	T50.2X1	T50.2X2	T50.2X3	T50.2X4	T50.2X5	T50.2X6
fungicide	T56.1X1	T56.1X2	T56.1X3	T56.1X4	—	—
organic (fungicide)	T56.1X1	T56.1X2	T56.1X3	T56.1X4	—	—
oxide, yellow	T49.0X1	T49.0X2	T49.0X3	T49.0X4	T49.0X5	T49.0X6
Mersalyl	T50.2X1	T50.2X2	T50.2X3	T50.2X4	T50.2X5	T50.2X6
Merthiolate	T49.0X1	T49.0X2	T49.0X3	T49.0X4	T49.0X5	T49.0X6
ophthalmic preparation	T49.5X1	T49.5X2	T49.5X3	T49.5X4	T49.5X5	T49.5X6
Meruvax	T50.B91	T50.B92	T50.B93	T50.B94	T50.B95	T50.B96
Mesalazine	T47.8X1	T47.8X2	T47.8X3	T47.8X4	T47.8X5	T47.8X6
Mescal buttons	T40.991	T40.992	T40.993	T40.994	—	—
Mescaline	T40.991	T40.992	T40.993	T40.994	—	—
Mesna	T48.4X1	T48.4X2	T48.4X3	T48.4X4	T48.4X5	T48.4X6
Mesoglycan	T46.6X1	T46.6X2	T46.6X3	T46.6X4	T46.6X5	T46.6X6
Mesoridazine	T43.3X1	T43.3X2	T43.3X3	T43.3X4	T43.3X5	T43.3X6
Mestanolone	T38.7X1	T38.7X2	T38.7X3	T38.7X4	T38.7X5	T38.7X6
Mesterolone	T38.7X1	T38.7X2	T38.7X3	T38.7X4	T38.7X5	T38.7X6
Mestranol	T38.5X1	T38.5X2	T38.5X3	T38.5X4	T38.5X5	T38.5X6
Mesulergine	T42.8X1	T42.8X2	T42.8X3	T42.8X4	T42.8X5	T42.8X6
Mesulfen	T49.0X1	T49.0X2	T49.0X3	T49.0X4	T49.0X5	T49.0X6
Mesuximide	T42.2X1	T42.2X2	T42.2X3	T42.2X4	T42.2X5	T42.2X6
Metabutethamine	T41.3X1	T41.3X2	T41.3X3	T41.3X4	T41.3X5	T41.3X6
Metactesylacetate	T49.0X1	T49.0X2	T49.0X3	T49.0X4	T49.0X5	T49.0X6
Metacycline	T36.4X1	T36.4X2	T36.4X3	T36.4X4	T36.4X5	T36.4X6
Metaldehyde (snail killer) NEC	T60.8X1	T60.8X2	T60.8X3	T60.8X4	—	—
Metals (heavy) (nonmedicinal)	T56.91	T56.92	T56.93	T56.94	—	—
dust, fumes, or vapor NEC	T56.91	T56.92	T56.93	T56.94	—	—
light NEC	T56.91	T56.92	T56.93	T56.94	—	—
dust, fumes, or vapor NEC	T56.91	T56.92	T56.93	T56.94	—	—
specified NEC	T56.891	T56.892	T56.893	T56.894	—	—
thallium	T56.811	T56.812	T56.813	T56.814	—	—
Metamfetamine	T43.621	T43.622	T43.623	T43.624	T43.625	T43.626
Metamizole sodium	T39.2X1	T39.2X2	T39.2X3	T39.2X4	T39.2X5	T39.2X6
Metampicillin	T36.0X1	T36.0X2	T36.0X3	T36.0X4	T36.0X5	T36.0X6
Metamucil	T47.4X1	T47.4X2	T47.4X3	T47.4X4	T47.4X5	T47.4X6
Metandienone	T38.7X1	T38.7X2	T38.7X3	T38.7X4	T38.7X5	T38.7X6
Metandrostenolone	T38.7X1	T38.7X2	T38.7X3	T38.7X4	T38.7X5	T38.7X6
Metaphen	T49.0X1	T49.0X2	T49.0X3	T49.0X4	T49.0X5	T49.0X6
Metaphos	T60.0X1	T60.0X2	T60.0X3	T60.0X4	—	—
Metapramine	T43.011	T43.012	T43.013	T43.014	T43.015	T43.016
Metaproterenol	T48.291	T48.292	T48.293	T48.294	T48.295	T48.296

Additional Character May Be Required — Refer to the Tabular List for Character Selection   ▽ Subterms under main terms may continue to next column or page

Substance	Poisoning, Accidental (unintentional)	Poisoning, Intentional Self-harm	Poisoning, Assault	Poisoning, Undetermined	Adverse Effect	Under-dosing
Metaraminol	T44.4X1	T44.4X2	T44.4X3	T44.4X4	T44.4X5	T44.4X6
Metaxalone	T42.8X1	T42.8X2	T42.8X3	T42.8X4	T42.8X5	T42.8X6
Metenolone	T38.7X1	T38.7X2	T38.7X3	T38.7X4	T38.7X5	T38.7X6
Metergoline	T42.8X1	T42.8X2	T42.8X3	T42.8X4	T42.8X5	T42.8X6
Metescufylline	T46.991	T46.992	T46.993	T46.994	T46.995	T46.996
Metetoin	T42.0X1	T42.0X2	T42.0X3	T42.0X4	T42.0X5	T42.0X6
Metformin	T38.3X1	T38.3X2	T38.3X3	T38.3X4	T38.3X5	T38.3X6
Methacholine	T44.1X1	T44.1X2	T44.1X3	T44.1X4	T44.1X5	T44.1X6
Methacycline	T36.4X1	T36.4X2	T36.4X3	T36.4X4	T36.4X5	T36.4X6
Methadone	T40.3X1	T40.3X2	T40.3X3	T40.3X4	T40.3X5	T40.3X6
Methallenestril	T38.5X1	T38.5X2	T38.5X3	T38.5X4	T38.5X5	T38.5X6
Methallenoestril	T38.5X1	T38.5X2	T38.5X3	T38.5X4	T38.5X5	T38.5X6
Methamphetamine	T43.621	T43.622	T43.623	T43.624	T43.625	T43.626
Methampyrone	T39.2X1	T39.2X2	T39.2X3	T39.2X4	T39.2X5	T39.2X6
Methandienone	T38.7X1	T38.7X2	T38.7X3	T38.7X4	T38.7X5	T38.7X6
Methandriol	T38.7X1	T38.7X2	T38.7X3	T38.7X4	T38.7X5	T38.7X6
Methandrostenolone	T38.7X1	T38.7X2	T38.7X3	T38.7X4	T38.7X5	T38.7X6
Methane	T59.891	T59.892	T59.893	T59.894	—	—
Methanethiol	T59.891	T59.892	T59.893	T59.894	—	—
Methaniazide	T37.1X1	T37.1X2	T37.1X3	T37.1X4	T37.1X5	T37.1X6
Methanol (vapor)	T51.1X1	T51.1X2	T51.1X3	T51.1X4	—	—
Methantheline	T44.3X1	T44.3X2	T44.3X3	T44.3X4	T44.3X5	T44.3X6
Methanthelinium bromide	T44.3X1	T44.3X2	T44.3X3	T44.3X4	T44.3X5	T44.3X6
Methaphenilene	T45.0X1	T45.0X2	T45.0X3	T45.0X4	T45.0X5	T45.0X6
Methapyrilene	T45.0X1	T45.0X2	T45.0X3	T45.0X4	T45.0X5	T45.0X6
Methaqualone (compound)	T42.6X1	T42.6X2	T42.6X3	T42.6X4	T42.6X5	T42.6X6
Metharbital	T42.3X1	T42.3X2	T42.3X3	T42.3X4	T42.3X5	T42.3X6
Methazolamide	T50.2X1	T50.2X2	T50.2X3	T50.2X4	T50.2X5	T50.2X6
Methdilazine	T43.3X1	T43.3X2	T43.3X3	T43.3X4	T43.3X5	T43.3X6
Methedrine	T43.621	T43.622	T43.623	T43.624	T43.625	T43.626
Methenamine (mandelate)	T37.8X1	T37.8X2	T37.8X3	T37.8X4	T37.8X5	T37.8X6
Methenolone	T38.7X1	T38.7X2	T38.7X3	T38.7X4	T38.7X5	T38.7X6
Methergine	T48.0X1	T48.0X2	T48.0X3	T48.0X4	T48.0X5	T48.0X6
Methetoin	T42.0X1	T42.0X2	T42.0X3	T42.0X4	T42.0X5	T42.0X6
Methiacil	T38.2X1	T38.2X2	T38.2X3	T38.2X4	T38.2X5	T38.2X6
Methicillin	T36.0X1	T36.0X2	T36.0X3	T36.0X4	T36.0X5	T36.0X6
Methimazole	T38.2X1	T38.2X2	T38.2X3	T38.2X4	T38.2X5	T38.2X6
Methiodal sodium	T50.8X1	T50.8X2	T50.8X3	T50.8X4	T50.8X5	T50.8X6
Methionine	T50.991	T50.992	T50.993	T50.994	T50.995	T50.996
Methisazone	T37.5X1	T37.5X2	T37.5X3	T37.5X4	T37.5X5	T37.5X6
Methisoprinol	T37.5X1	T37.5X2	T37.5X3	T37.5X4	T37.5X5	T37.5X6
Methitural	T42.3X1	T42.3X2	T42.3X3	T42.3X4	T42.3X5	T42.3X6
Methixene	T44.3X1	T44.3X2	T44.3X3	T44.3X4	T44.3X5	T44.3X6
Methobarbital, methobarbitone	T42.3X1	T42.3X2	T42.3X3	T42.3X4	T42.3X5	T42.3X6
Methocarbamol	T42.8X1	T42.8X2	T42.8X3	T42.8X4	T42.8X5	T42.8X6
skeletal muscle relaxant	T48.1X1	T48.1X2	T48.1X3	T48.1X4	T48.1X5	T48.1X6
Methohexital	T41.1X1	T41.1X2	T41.1X3	T41.1X4	T41.1X5	T41.1X6
Methohexitone	T41.1X1	T41.1X2	T41.1X3	T41.1X4	T41.1X5	T41.1X6
Methoin	T42.0X1	T42.0X2	T42.0X3	T42.0X4	T42.0X5	T42.0X6
Methopholine	T39.8X1	T39.8X2	T39.8X3	T39.8X4	T39.8X5	T39.8X6
Methopromazine	T43.3X1	T43.3X2	T43.3X3	T43.3X4	T43.3X5	T43.3X6
Methorate	T48.3X1	T48.3X2	T48.3X3	T48.3X4	T48.3X5	T48.3X6
Methoserpidine	T46.5X1	T46.5X2	T46.5X3	T46.5X4	T46.5X5	T46.5X6
Methotrexate	T45.1X1	T45.1X2	T45.1X3	T45.1X4	T45.1X5	T45.1X6
Methotrimeprazine	T43.3X1	T43.3X2	T43.3X3	T43.3X4	T43.3X5	T43.3X6
Methoxa-Dome	T49.3X1	T49.3X2	T49.3X3	T49.3X4	T49.3X5	T49.3X6
Methoxamine	T44.4X1	T44.4X2	T44.4X3	T44.4X4	T44.4X5	T44.4X6
Methoxsalen	T50.991	T50.992	T50.993	T50.994	T50.995	T50.996
Methoxyaniline	T65.3X1	T65.3X2	T65.3X3	T65.3X4	—	—
Methoxybenzyl penicillin	T36.0X1	T36.0X2	T36.0X3	T36.0X4	T36.0X5	T36.0X6
Methoxychlor	T53.7X1	T53.7X2	T53.7X3	T53.7X4	—	—
Methoxy-DDT	T53.7X1	T53.7X2	T53.7X3	T53.7X4	—	—
Methoxyflurane	T41.0X1	T41.0X2	T41.0X3	T41.0X4	T41.0X5	T41.0X6
Methoxyphenamine	T48.6X1	T48.6X2	T48.6X3	T48.6X4	T48.6X5	T48.6X6
Methoxypromazine	T43.3X1	T43.3X2	T43.3X3	T43.3X4	T43.3X5	T43.3X6
Methscopolamine bromide	T44.3X1	T44.3X2	T44.3X3	T44.3X4	T44.3X5	T44.3X6
Methsuximide	T42.2X1	T42.2X2	T42.2X3	T42.2X4	T42.2X5	T42.2X6
Methyclothiazide	T50.2X1	T50.2X2	T50.2X3	T50.2X4	T50.2X5	T50.2X6
Methyl						
acetate	T52.4X1	T52.4X2	T52.4X3	T52.4X4	—	—
acetone	T52.4X1	T52.4X2	T52.4X3	T52.4X4	—	—
acrylate	T65.891	T65.892	T65.893	T65.894	—	—
alcohol	T51.1X1	T51.1X2	T51.1X3	T51.1X4	—	—
aminophenol	T65.3X1	T65.3X2	T65.3X3	T65.3X4	—	—
amphetamine	T43.621	T43.622	T43.623	T43.624	T43.625	T43.626
androstanolone	T38.7X1	T38.7X2	T38.7X3	T38.7X4	T38.7X5	T38.7X6
atropine	T44.3X1	T44.3X2	T44.3X3	T44.3X4	T44.3X5	T44.3X6
benzene	T52.2X1	T52.2X2	T52.2X3	T52.2X4	—	—
benzoate	T52.8X1	T52.8X2	T52.8X3	T52.8X4	—	—
benzol	T52.2X1	T52.2X2	T52.2X3	T52.2X4	—	—
bromide (gas)	T59.891	T59.892	T59.893	T59.894	—	—

Substance	Poisoning, Accidental (unintentional)	Poisoning, Intentional Self-harm	Poisoning, Assault	Poisoning, Undetermined	Adverse Effect	Under-dosing
Methyl — continued						
bromide — continued						
fumigant	T60.8X1	T60.8X2	T60.8X3	T60.8X4	—	—
butanol	T51.3X1	T51.3X2	T51.3X3	T51.3X4	—	—
carbinol	T51.1X1	T51.1X2	T51.1X3	T51.1X4	—	—
carbonate	T52.8X1	T52.8X2	T52.8X3	T52.8X4	—	—
CCNU	T45.1X1	T45.1X2	T45.1X3	T45.1X4	T45.1X5	T45.1X6
cellosolve	T52.91	T52.92	T52.93	T52.94	—	—
cellulose	T47.4X1	T47.4X2	T47.4X3	T47.4X4	T47.4X5	T47.4X6
chloride (gas)	T59.891	T59.892	T59.893	T59.894	—	—
chloroformate	T59.3X1	T59.3X2	T59.3X3	T59.3X4	—	—
cyclohexane	T52.8X1	T52.8X2	T52.8X3	T52.8X4	—	—
cyclohexanol	T51.8X1	T51.8X2	T51.8X3	T51.8X4	—	—
cyclohexanone	T52.8X1	T52.8X2	T52.8X3	T52.8X4	—	—
cyclohexyl acetate	T52.8X1	T52.8X2	T52.8X3	T52.8X4	—	—
demeton	T60.0X1	T60.0X2	T60.0X3	T60.0X4	—	—
dihydromorphinone	T40.2X1	T40.2X2	T40.2X3	T40.2X4	T40.2X5	T40.2X6
ergometrine	T48.0X1	T48.0X2	T48.0X3	T48.0X4	T48.0X5	T48.0X6
ergonovine	T48.0X1	T48.0X2	T48.0X3	T48.0X4	T48.0X5	T48.0X6
ethyl ketone	T52.4X1	T52.4X2	T52.4X3	T52.4X4	—	—
glucamine antimonate	T37.8X1	T37.8X2	T37.8X3	T37.8X4	T37.8X5	T37.8X6
hydrazine	T65.891	T65.892	T65.893	T65.894	—	—
iodide	T65.891	T65.892	T65.893	T65.894	—	—
isobutyl ketone	T52.4X1	T52.4X2	T52.4X3	T52.4X4	—	—
isothiocyanate	T60.3X1	T60.3X2	T60.3X3	T60.3X4	—	—
mercaptan	T59.891	T59.892	T59.893	T59.894	—	—
morphine NEC	T40.2X1	T40.2X2	T40.2X3	T40.2X4	T40.2X5	T40.2X6
nicotinate	T49.4X1	T49.4X2	T49.4X3	T49.4X4	T49.4X5	T49.4X6
paraben	T49.0X1	T49.0X2	T49.0X3	T49.0X4	T49.0X5	T49.0X6
parafynol	T42.6X1	T42.6X2	T42.6X3	T42.6X4	T42.6X5	T42.6X6
parathion	T60.0X1	T60.0X2	T60.0X3	T60.0X4	—	—
peridol	T43.4X1	T43.4X2	T43.4X3	T43.4X4	T43.4X5	T43.4X6
phenidate	T43.631	T43.632	T43.633	T43.634	T43.635	T43.636
prednisolone	T38.0X1	T38.0X2	T38.0X3	T38.0X4	T38.0X5	T38.0X6
ENT agent	T49.6X1	T49.6X2	T49.6X3	T49.6X4	T49.6X5	T49.6X6
ophthalmic preparation	T49.5X1	T49.5X2	T49.5X3	T49.5X4	T49.5X5	T49.5X6
topical NEC	T49.0X1	T49.0X2	T49.0X3	T49.0X4	T49.0X5	T49.0X6
propylcarbinol	T51.3X1	T51.3X2	T51.3X3	T51.3X4	—	—
rosaniline NEC	T49.0X1	T49.0X2	T49.0X3	T49.0X4	T49.0X5	T49.0X6
salicylate	T49.2X1	T49.2X2	T49.2X3	T49.2X4	T49.2X5	T49.2X6
sulfate (fumes)	T59.891	T59.892	T59.893	T59.894	—	—
liquid	T52.8X1	T52.8X2	T52.8X3	T52.8X4	—	—
sulfonal	T42.6X1	T42.6X2	T42.6X3	T42.6X4	T42.6X5	T42.6X6
testosterone	T38.7X1	T38.7X2	T38.7X3	T38.7X4	T38.7X5	T38.7X6
thiouracil	T38.2X1	T38.2X2	T38.2X3	T38.2X4	T38.2X5	T38.2X6
Methylamphetamine	T43.621	T43.622	T43.623	T43.624	T43.625	T43.626
Methylated spirit	T51.1X1	T51.1X2	T51.1X3	T51.1X4	—	—
Methylatropine nitrate	T44.3X1	T44.3X2	T44.3X3	T44.3X4	T44.3X5	T44.3X6
Methylbenactyzium bromide	T44.3X1	T44.3X2	T44.3X3	T44.3X4	T44.3X5	T44.3X6
Methylbenzethonium chloride	T49.0X1	T49.0X2	T49.0X3	T49.0X4	T49.0X5	T49.0X6
Methylcellulose	T47.4X1	T47.4X2	T47.4X3	T47.4X4	T47.4X5	T47.4X6
laxative	T47.4X1	T47.4X2	T47.4X3	T47.4X4	T47.4X5	T47.4X6
Methylchlorophenoxyacetic acid	T60.3X1	T60.3X2	T60.3X3	T60.3X4	—	—
Methyldopa	T46.5X1	T46.5X2	T46.5X3	T46.5X4	T46.5X5	T46.5X6
Methyldopate	T46.5X1	T46.5X2	T46.5X3	T46.5X4	T46.5X5	T46.5X6
Methylene						
blue	T50.6X1	T50.6X2	T50.6X3	T50.6X4	T50.6X5	T50.6X6
chloride or dichloride (solvent) NEC	T53.4X1	T53.4X2	T53.4X3	T53.4X4	—	—
Methylenedioxyamphetamine	T43.621	T43.622	T43.623	T43.624	T43.625	T43.626
Methylenedioxymeth-amphetamine	T43.641	T43.642	T43.643	T43.644	—	—
Methylergometrine	T48.0X1	T48.0X2	T48.0X3	T48.0X4	T48.0X5	T48.0X6
Methylergonovine	T48.0X1	T48.0X2	T48.0X3	T48.0X4	T48.0X5	T48.0X6
Methylestrenolone	T38.5X1	T38.5X2	T38.5X3	T38.5X4	T38.5X5	T38.5X6
Methylethyl cellulose	T50.991	T50.992	T50.993	T50.994	T50.995	T50.996
Methylhexabital	T42.3X1	T42.3X2	T42.3X3	T42.3X4	T42.3X5	T42.3X6
Methylmorphine	T40.2X1	T40.2X2	T40.2X3	T40.2X4	T40.2X5	T40.2X6
Methylparaben	T49.5X1	T49.5X2	T49.5X3	T49.5X4	T49.5X5	T49.5X6
(ophthalmic)						
Methylparafynol	T42.6X1	T42.6X2	T42.6X3	T42.6X4	T42.6X5	T42.6X6
Methylpentynol, methylpenthynol	T42.6X1	T42.6X2	T42.6X3	T42.6X4	T42.6X5	T42.6X6
Methylphenidate	T43.631	T43.632	T43.633	T43.634	T43.635	T43.636
Methylphenobarbital	T42.3X1	T42.3X2	T42.3X3	T42.3X4	T42.3X5	T42.3X6
Methylpolysiloxane	T47.1X1	T47.1X2	T47.1X3	T47.1X4	T47.1X5	T47.1X6
Methylprednisolone — see Methyl, prednisolone						
Methylrosaniline	T49.0X1	T49.0X2	T49.0X3	T49.0X4	T49.0X5	T49.0X6

⏷ Subterms under main terms may continue to next column or page   Additional Character May Be Required — Refer to the Tabular List for Character Selection   379

Metaraminol — Methylrosaniline

Table of Drugs and Chemicals

Methylrosanilinium chloride — Mustard

Substance	Poisoning, Accidental (unintentional)	Poisoning, Intentional Self-harm	Poisoning, Assault	Poisoning, Undetermined	Adverse Effect	Under-dosing
Methylrosanilinium chloride	T49.0X1	T49.0X2	T49.0X3	T49.0X4	T49.0X5	T49.0X6
Methyltestosterone	T38.7X1	T38.7X2	T38.7X3	T38.7X4	T38.7X5	T38.7X6
Methylthionine chloride	T50.6X1	T50.6X2	T50.6X3	T50.6X4	T50.6X5	T50.6X6
Methylthioninium chloride	T50.6X1	T50.6X2	T50.6X3	T50.6X4	T50.6X5	T50.6X6
Methylthiouracil	T38.2X1	T38.2X2	T38.2X3	T38.2X4	T38.2X5	T38.2X6
Methyprylon	T42.6X1	T42.6X2	T42.6X3	T42.6X4	T42.6X5	T42.6X6
Methysergide	T46.5X1	T46.5X2	T46.5X3	T46.5X4	T46.5X5	T46.5X6
Metiamide	T47.1X1	T47.1X2	T47.1X3	T47.1X4	T47.1X5	T47.1X6
Meticillin	T36.0X1	T36.0X2	T36.0X3	T36.0X4	T36.0X5	T36.0X6
Meticrane	T50.2X1	T50.2X2	T50.2X3	T50.2X4	T50.2X5	T50.2X6
Metildigoxin	T46.0X1	T46.0X2	T46.0X3	T46.0X4	T46.0X5	T46.0X6
Metipranolol	T49.5X1	T49.5X2	T49.5X3	T49.5X4	T49.5X5	T49.5X6
Metirosine	T46.5X1	T46.5X2	T46.5X3	T46.5X4	T46.5X5	T46.5X6
Metisazone	T37.5X1	T37.5X2	T37.5X3	T37.5X4	T37.5X5	T37.5X6
Metixene	T44.3X1	T44.3X2	T44.3X3	T44.3X4	T44.3X5	T44.3X6
Metizoline	T48.5X1	T48.5X2	T48.5X3	T48.5X4	T48.5X5	T48.5X6
Metoclopramide	T45.0X1	T45.0X2	T45.0X3	T45.0X4	T45.0X5	T45.0X6
Metofenazate	T43.3X1	T43.3X2	T43.3X3	T43.3X4	T43.3X5	T43.3X6
Metofoline	T39.8X1	T39.8X2	T39.8X3	T39.8X4	T39.8X5	T39.8X6
Metolazone	T50.2X1	T50.2X2	T50.2X3	T50.2X4	T50.2X5	T50.2X6
Metopon	T40.2X1	T40.2X2	T40.2X3	T40.2X4	T40.2X5	T40.2X6
Metoprine	T45.1X1	T45.1X2	T45.1X3	T45.1X4	T45.1X5	T45.1X6
Metoprolol	T44.7X1	T44.7X2	T44.7X3	T44.7X4	T44.7X5	T44.7X6
Metrifonate	T60.0X1	T60.0X2	T60.0X3	T60.0X4	—	—
Metrizamide	T50.8X1	T50.8X2	T50.8X3	T50.8X4	T50.8X5	T50.8X6
Metrizoic acid	T50.8X1	T50.8X2	T50.8X3	T50.8X4	T50.8X5	T50.8X6
Metronidazole	T37.8X1	T37.8X2	T37.8X3	T37.8X4	T37.8X5	T37.8X6
Metycaine	T41.3X1	T41.3X2	T41.3X3	T41.3X4	T41.3X5	T41.3X6
infiltration (subcutaneous)	T41.3X1	T41.3X2	T41.3X3	T41.3X4	T41.3X5	T41.3X6
nerve block (peripheral) (plexus)	T41.3X1	T41.3X2	T41.3X3	T41.3X4	T41.3X5	T41.3X6
topical (surface)	T41.3X1	T41.3X2	T41.3X3	T41.3X4	T41.3X5	T41.3X6
Metyrapone	T50.8X1	T50.8X2	T50.8X3	T50.8X4	T50.8X5	T50.8X6
Mevinphos	T60.0X1	T60.0X2	T60.0X3	T60.0X4	—	—
Mexazolam	T42.4X1	T42.4X2	T42.4X3	T42.4X4	T42.4X5	T42.4X6
Mexenone	T49.3X1	T49.3X2	T49.3X3	T49.3X4	T49.3X5	T49.3X6
Mexiletine	T46.2X1	T46.2X2	T46.2X3	T46.2X4	T46.2X5	T46.2X6
Mezereon	T62.2X1	T62.2X2	T62.2X3	T62.2X4	—	—
berries	T62.1X1	T62.1X2	T62.1X3	T62.1X4	—	—
Mezlocillin	T36.0X1	T36.0X2	T36.0X3	T36.0X4	T36.0X5	T36.0X6
Mianserin	T43.021	T43.022	T43.023	T43.024	T43.025	T43.026
Micatin	T49.0X1	T49.0X2	T49.0X3	T49.0X4	T49.0X5	T49.0X6
Miconazole	T49.0X1	T49.0X2	T49.0X3	T49.0X4	T49.0X5	T49.0X6
Micronomicin	T36.5X1	T36.5X2	T36.5X3	T36.5X4	T36.5X5	T36.5X6
Midazolam	T42.4X1	T42.4X2	T42.4X3	T42.4X4	T42.4X5	T42.4X6
Midecamycin	T36.3X1	T36.3X2	T36.3X3	T36.3X4	T36.3X5	T36.3X6
Mifepristone	T38.6X1	T38.6X2	T38.6X3	T38.6X4	T38.6X5	T38.6X6
Milk of magnesia	T47.1X1	T47.1X2	T47.1X3	T47.1X4	T47.1X5	T47.1X6
Millipede (tropical) (venomous)	T63.411	T63.412	T63.413	T63.414	—	—
Miltown	T43.591	T43.592	T43.593	T43.594	T43.595	T43.596
Milverine	T44.3X1	T44.3X2	T44.3X3	T44.3X4	T44.3X5	T44.3X6
Minaprine	T43.291	T43.292	T43.293	T43.294	T43.295	T43.296
Minaxolone	T41.291	T41.292	T41.293	T41.294	T41.295	T41.296
Mineral						
acids	T54.2X1	T54.2X2	T54.2X3	T54.2X4	—	—
oil (laxative)(medicinal)	T47.4X1	T47.4X2	T47.4X3	T47.4X4	T47.4X5	T47.4X6
emulsion	T47.2X1	T47.2X2	T47.2X3	T47.2X4	T47.2X5	T47.2X6
nonmedicinal	T52.0X1	T52.0X2	T52.0X3	T52.0X4	—	—
topical	T49.3X1	T49.3X2	T49.3X3	T49.3X4	T49.3X5	T49.3X6
salt NEC	T50.3X1	T50.3X2	T50.3X3	T50.3X4	T50.3X5	T50.3X6
spirits	T52.0X1	T52.0X2	T52.0X3	T52.0X4	—	—
Mineralocorticosteroid	T50.0X1	T50.0X2	T50.0X3	T50.0X4	T50.0X5	T50.0X6
Minocycline	T36.4X1	T36.4X2	T36.4X3	T36.4X4	T36.4X5	T36.4X6
Minoxidil	T46.7X1	T46.7X2	T46.7X3	T46.7X4	T46.7X5	T46.7X6
Miokamycin	T36.3X1	T36.3X2	T36.3X3	T36.3X4	T36.3X5	T36.3X6
Miotic drug	T49.5X1	T49.5X2	T49.5X3	T49.5X4	T49.5X5	T49.5X6
Mipafox	T60.0X1	T60.0X2	T60.0X3	T60.0X4	—	—
Mirex	T60.1X1	T60.1X2	T60.1X3	T60.1X4	—	—
Mirtazapine	T43.021	T43.022	T43.023	T43.024	T43.025	T43.026
Misonidazole	T37.3X1	T37.3X2	T37.3X3	T37.3X4	T37.3X5	T37.3X6
Misoprostol	T47.1X1	T47.1X2	T47.1X3	T47.1X4	T47.1X5	T47.1X6
Mithramycin	T45.1X1	T45.1X2	T45.1X3	T45.1X4	T45.1X5	T45.1X6
Mitobronitol	T45.1X1	T45.1X2	T45.1X3	T45.1X4	T45.1X5	T45.1X6
Mitoguazone	T45.1X1	T45.1X2	T45.1X3	T45.1X4	T45.1X5	T45.1X6
Mitolactol	T45.1X1	T45.1X2	T45.1X3	T45.1X4	T45.1X5	T45.1X6
Mitomycin	T45.1X1	T45.1X2	T45.1X3	T45.1X4	T45.1X5	T45.1X6
Mitopodozide	T45.1X1	T45.1X2	T45.1X3	T45.1X4	T45.1X5	T45.1X6
Mitotane	T45.1X1	T45.1X2	T45.1X3	T45.1X4	T45.1X5	T45.1X6
Mitoxantrone	T45.1X1	T45.1X2	T45.1X3	T45.1X4	T45.1X5	T45.1X6
Mivacurium chloride	T48.1X1	T48.1X2	T48.1X3	T48.1X4	T48.1X5	T48.1X6

Substance	Poisoning, Accidental (unintentional)	Poisoning, Intentional Self-harm	Poisoning, Assault	Poisoning, Undetermined	Adverse Effect	Under-dosing
Miyari bacteria	T47.6X1	T47.6X2	T47.6X3	T47.6X4	T47.6X5	T47.6X6
Moclobemide	T43.1X1	T43.1X2	T43.1X3	T43.1X4	T43.1X5	T43.1X6
Moderil	T46.5X1	T46.5X2	T46.5X3	T46.5X4	T46.5X5	T46.5X6
Mofebutazone	T39.2X1	T39.2X2	T39.2X3	T39.2X4	T39.2X5	T39.2X6
Mogadon — see Nitrazepam						
Molindone	T43.591	T43.592	T43.593	T43.594	T43.595	T43.596
Molsidomine	T46.3X1	T46.3X2	T46.3X3	T46.3X4	T46.3X5	T46.3X6
Mometasone	T49.0X1	T49.0X2	T49.0X3	T49.0X4	T49.0X5	T49.0X6
Monistat	T49.0X1	T49.0X2	T49.0X3	T49.0X4	T49.0X5	T49.0X6
Monkshood	T62.2X1	T62.2X2	T62.2X3	T62.2X4	—	—
Monoamine oxidase inhibitor NEC	T43.1X1	T43.1X2	T43.1X3	T43.1X4	T43.1X5	T43.1X6
hydrazine	T43.1X1	T43.1X2	T43.1X3	T43.1X4	T43.1X5	T43.1X6
Monobenzone	T49.4X1	T49.4X2	T49.4X3	T49.4X4	T49.4X5	T49.4X6
Monochloroacetic acid	T60.3X1	T60.3X2	T60.3X3	T60.3X4	—	—
Monochlorobenzene	T53.7X1	T53.7X2	T53.7X3	T53.7X4	—	—
Monoethanolamine	T46.8X1	T46.8X2	T46.8X3	T46.8X4	T46.8X5	T46.8X6
oleate	T46.8X1	T46.8X2	T46.8X3	T46.8X4	T46.8X5	T46.8X6
Monooctanoin	T50.991	T50.992	T50.993	T50.994	T50.995	T50.996
Monophenylbutazone	T39.2X1	T39.2X2	T39.2X3	T39.2X4	T39.2X5	T39.2X6
Monosodium glutamate	T65.891	T65.892	T65.893	T65.894		
Monosulfiram	T49.0X1	T49.0X2	T49.0X3	T49.0X4	T49.0X5	T49.0X6
Monoxide, carbon — see Carbon, monoxide						
Monoxidine hydrochloride	T46.1X1	T46.1X2	T46.1X3	T46.1X4	T46.1X5	T46.1X6
Monuron	T60.3X1	T60.3X2	T60.3X3	T60.3X4	—	—
Moperone	T43.4X1	T43.4X2	T43.4X3	T43.4X4	T43.4X5	T43.4X6
Mopidamol	T45.1X1	T45.1X2	T45.1X3	T45.1X4	T45.1X5	T45.1X6
MOPP (mechloreth-amine + vincristine + prednisone + procarba-zine)	T45.1X1	T45.1X2	T45.1X3	T45.1X4	T45.1X5	T45.1X6
Morfin	T40.2X1	T40.2X2	T40.2X3	T40.2X4	T40.2X5	T40.2X6
Morinamide	T37.1X1	T37.1X2	T37.1X3	T37.1X4	T37.1X5	T37.1X6
Morning glory seeds	T40.991	T40.992	T40.993	T40.994		
Moroxydine	T37.5X1	T37.5X2	T37.5X3	T37.5X4	T37.5X5	T37.5X6
Morphazinamide	T37.1X1	T37.1X2	T37.1X3	T37.1X4	T37.1X5	T37.1X6
Morphine	T40.2X1	T40.2X2	T40.2X3	T40.2X4	T40.2X5	T40.2X6
antagonist	T50.7X1	T50.7X2	T50.7X3	T50.7X4	T50.7X5	T50.7X6
Morpholinylethylmorphine	T40.2X1	T40.2X2	T40.2X3	T40.2X4		
Morsuximide	T42.2X1	T42.2X2	T42.2X3	T42.2X4	T42.2X5	T42.2X6
Mosapramine	T43.591	T43.592	T43.593	T43.594	T43.595	T43.596
Moth balls — see also Pesticides	T60.2X1	T60.2X2	T60.2X3	T60.2X4		
naphthalene	T60.2X1	T60.2X2	T60.2X3	T60.2X4	—	—
paradichlorobenzene	T60.1X1	T60.1X2	T60.1X3	T60.1X4	—	—
Motor exhaust gas	T58.01	T58.02	T58.03	T58.04	—	—
Mouthwash (antiseptic) (zinc chloride)	T49.6X1	T49.6X2	T49.6X3	T49.6X4	T49.6X5	T49.6X6
Moxastine	T45.0X1	T45.0X2	T45.0X3	T45.0X4	T45.0X5	T45.0X6
Moxaverine	T44.3X1	T44.3X2	T44.3X3	T44.3X4	T44.3X5	T44.3X6
Moxisylyte	T46.7X1	T46.7X2	T46.7X3	T46.7X4	T46.7X5	T46.7X6
Mucilage, plant	T47.4X1	T47.4X2	T47.4X3	T47.4X4	T47.4X5	T47.4X6
Mucolytic drug	T48.4X1	T48.4X2	T48.4X3	T48.4X4	T48.4X5	T48.4X6
Mucomyst	T48.4X1	T48.4X2	T48.4X3	T48.4X4	T48.4X5	T48.4X6
Mucous membrane agents (external)	T49.91	T49.92	T49.93	T49.94	T49.95	T49.96
specified NEC	T49.8X1	T49.8X2	T49.8X3	T49.8X4	T49.8X5	T49.8X6
Mumps						
immune globulin (human)	T50.Z11	T50.Z12	T50.Z13	T50.Z14	T50.Z15	T50.Z16
skin test antigen	T50.8X1	T50.8X2	T50.8X3	T50.8X4	T50.8X5	T50.8X6
vaccine	T50.B91	T50.B92	T50.B93	T50.B94	T50.B95	T50.B96
Mumpsvax	T50.B91	T50.B92	T50.B93	T50.B94	T50.B95	T50.B96
Mupirocin	T49.0X1	T49.0X2	T49.0X3	T49.0X4	T49.0X5	T49.0X6
Muriatic acid — see Hydrochloric acid						
Muromonab-CD3	T45.1X1	T45.1X2	T45.1X3	T45.1X4	T45.1X5	T45.1X6
Muscle-action drug NEC	T48.201	T48.202	T48.203	T48.204	T48.205	T48.206
Muscle affecting agents NEC	T48.201	T48.202	T48.203	T48.204	T48.205	T48.206
oxytocic	T48.0X1	T48.0X2	T48.0X3	T48.0X4	T48.0X5	T48.0X6
relaxants	T48.201	T48.202	T48.203	T48.204	T48.205	T48.206
central nervous system	T42.8X1	T42.8X2	T42.8X3	T42.8X4	T42.8X5	T42.8X6
skeletal	T48.1X1	T48.1X2	T48.1X3	T48.1X4	T48.1X5	T48.1X6
smooth	T44.3X1	T44.3X2	T44.3X3	T44.3X4	T44.3X5	T44.3X6
Muscle relaxant — see Relaxant, muscle						
Muscle-tone depressant, central NEC	T42.8X1	T42.8X2	T42.8X3	T42.8X4	T42.8X5	T42.8X6
specified NEC	T42.8X1	T42.8X2	T42.8X3	T42.8X4	T42.8X5	T42.8X6
Mushroom, noxious	T62.0X1	T62.0X2	T62.0X3	T62.0X4	—	—
Mussel, noxious	T61.781	T61.782	T61.783	T61.784	—	—
Mustard (emetic)	T47.7X1	T47.7X2	T47.7X3	T47.7X4	T47.7X5	T47.7X6
black	T47.7X1	T47.7X2	T47.7X3	T47.7X4	T47.7X5	T47.7X6

Additional Character May Be Required — Refer to the Tabular List for Character Selection   ▼ Subterms under main terms may continue to next column or page

Table of Drugs and Chemicals

Substance	Poisoning, Accidental (unintentional)	Poisoning, Intentional Self-harm	Poisoning, Assault	Poisoning, Undetermined	Adverse Effect	Under-dosing
Mustard — *continued*						
gas, not in war	T59.91	T59.92	T59.93	T59.94	—	—
nitrogen	T45.1X1	T45.1X2	T45.1X3	T45.1X4	T45.1X5	T45.1X6
Mustine	T45.1X1	T45.1X2	T45.1X3	T45.1X4	T45.1X5	T45.1X6
M-vac	T45.1X1	T45.1X2	T45.1X3	T45.1X4	T45.1X5	T45.1X6
Mycifradin	T36.5X1	T36.5X2	T36.5X3	T36.5X4	T36.5X5	T36.5X6
topical	T49.0X1	T49.0X2	T49.0X3	T49.0X4	T49.0X5	T49.0X6
Mycitracin	T36.8X1	T36.8X2	T36.8X3	T36.8X4	T36.8X5	T36.8X6
ophthalmic preparation	T49.5X1	T49.5X2	T49.5X3	T49.5X4	T49.5X5	T49.5X6
Mycostatin	T36.7X1	T36.7X2	T36.7X3	T36.7X4	T36.7X5	T36.7X6
topical	T49.0X1	T49.0X2	T49.0X3	T49.0X4	T49.0X5	T49.0X6
Mycotoxins	T64.81	T64.82	T64.83	T64.84	—	—
aflatoxin	T64.01	T64.02	T64.03	T64.04	—	—
specified NEC	T64.81	T64.82	T64.83	T64.84	—	—
Mydriacyl	T44.3X1	T44.3X2	T44.3X3	T44.3X4	T44.3X5	T44.3X6
Mydriatic drug	T49.5X1	T49.5X2	T49.5X3	T49.5X4	T49.5X5	T49.5X6
Myelobromal	T45.1X1	T45.1X2	T45.1X3	T45.1X4	T45.1X5	T45.1X6
Myleran	T45.1X1	T45.1X2	T45.1X3	T45.1X4	T45.1X5	T45.1X6
Myochrysin (e)	T39.2X1	T39.2X2	T39.2X3	T39.2X4	T39.2X5	T39.2X6
Myoneural blocking agents	T48.1X1	T48.1X2	T48.1X3	T48.1X4	T48.1X5	T48.1X6
Myralact	T49.0X1	T49.0X2	T49.0X3	T49.0X4	T49.0X5	T49.0X6
Myristica fragrans	T62.2X1	T62.2X2	T62.2X3	T62.2X4	—	—
Myristicin	T65.891	T65.892	T65.893	T65.894	—	—
Mysoline	T42.3X1	T42.3X2	T42.3X3	T42.3X4	T42.3X5	T42.3X6
Nabilone	T40.7X1	T40.7X2	T40.7X3	T40.7X4	T40.7X5	T40.7X6
Nabumetone	T39.391	T39.392	T39.393	T39.394	T39.395	T39.396
Nadolol	T44.7X1	T44.7X2	T44.7X3	T44.7X4	T44.7X5	T44.7X6
Nafcillin	T36.0X1	T36.0X2	T36.0X3	T36.0X4	T36.0X5	T36.0X6
Nafoxidine	T38.6X1	T38.6X2	T38.6X3	T38.6X4	T38.6X5	T38.6X6
Naftazone	T46.991	T46.992	T46.993	T46.994	T46.995	T46.996
Naftidrofuryl (oxalate)	T46.7X1	T46.7X2	T46.7X3	T46.7X4	T46.7X5	T46.7X6
Naftifine	T49.0X1	T49.0X2	T49.0X3	T49.0X4	T49.0X5	T49.0X6
Nail polish remover	T52.91	T52.92	T52.93	T52.94	—	—
Nalbuphine	T40.4X1	T40.4X2	T40.4X3	T40.4X4	T40.4X5	T40.4X6
Naled	T60.0X1	T60.0X2	T60.0X3	T60.0X4	—	—
Nalidixic acid	T37.8X1	T37.8X2	T37.8X3	T37.8X4	T37.8X5	T37.8X6
Nalorphine	T50.7X1	T50.7X2	T50.7X3	T50.7X4	T50.7X5	T50.7X6
Naloxone	T50.7X1	T50.7X2	T50.7X3	T50.7X4	T50.7X5	T50.7X6
Naltrexone	T50.7X1	T50.7X2	T50.7X3	T50.7X4	T50.7X5	T50.7X6
Namenda	T43.8X1	T43.8X2	T43.8X3	T43.8X4	T43.8X5	T43.8X6
Nandrolone	T38.7X1	T38.7X2	T38.7X3	T38.7X4	T38.7X5	T38.7X6
Naphazoline	T48.5X1	T48.5X2	T48.5X3	T48.5X4	T48.5X5	T48.5X6
Naphtha (painters') (petroleum)	T52.0X1	T52.0X2	T52.0X3	T52.0X4	—	—
solvent	T52.0X1	T52.0X2	T52.0X3	T52.0X4	—	—
vapor	T52.0X1	T52.0X2	T52.0X3	T52.0X4	—	—
Naphthalene (non-chlorinated)	T60.2X1	T60.2X2	T60.2X3	T60.2X4	—	—
chlorinated	T60.1X1	T60.1X2	T60.1X3	T60.1X4	—	—
vapor	T60.1X1	T60.1X2	T60.1X3	T60.1X4	—	—
insecticide or moth repellent	T60.2X1	T60.2X2	T60.2X3	T60.2X4	—	—
chlorinated	T60.1X1	T60.1X2	T60.1X3	T60.1X4	—	—
vapor	T60.2X1	T60.2X2	T60.2X3	T60.2X4	—	—
chlorinated	T60.1X1	T60.1X2	T60.1X3	T60.1X4	—	—
Naphthol	T65.891	T65.892	T65.893	T65.894	—	—
Naphthylamine	T65.891	T65.892	T65.893	T65.894	—	—
Naphthylthiourea (ANTU)	T60.4X1	T60.4X2	T60.4X3	T60.4X4	—	—
Naprosyn — *see* Naproxen						
Naproxen	T39.311	T39.312	T39.313	T39.314	T39.315	T39.316
Narcotic (drug)	T40.601	T40.602	T40.603	T40.604	T40.605	T40.606
analgesic NEC	T40.601	T40.602	T40.603	T40.604	T40.605	T40.606
antagonist	T50.7X1	T50.7X2	T50.7X3	T50.7X4	T50.7X5	T50.7X6
specified NEC	T40.691	T40.692	T40.693	T40.694	T40.695	T40.696
synthetic	T40.4X1	T40.4X2	T40.4X3	T40.4X4	T40.4X5	T40.4X6
Narcotine	T48.3X1	T48.3X2	T48.3X3	T48.3X4	T48.3X5	T48.3X6
Nardil	T43.1X1	T43.1X2	T43.1X3	T43.1X4	T43.1X5	T43.1X6
Nasal drug NEC	T49.6X1	T49.6X2	T49.6X3	T49.6X4	T49.6X5	T49.6X6
Natamycin	T49.0X1	T49.0X2	T49.0X3	T49.0X4	T49.0X5	T49.0X6
Natrium cyanide — *see* Cyanide(s)						
Natural						
blood (product)	T45.8X1	T45.8X2	T45.8X3	T45.8X4	T45.8X5	T45.8X6
gas (piped)	T59.891	T59.892	T59.893	T59.894	—	—
incomplete combustion	T58.11	T58.12	T58.13	T58.14	—	—
Nealbarbital	T42.3X1	T42.3X2	T42.3X3	T42.3X4	T42.3X5	T42.3X6
Nectadon	T48.3X1	T48.3X2	T48.3X3	T48.3X4	T48.3X5	T48.3X6
Nedocromil	T48.6X1	T48.6X2	T48.6X3	T48.6X4	T48.6X5	T48.6X6
Nefopam	T39.8X1	T39.8X2	T39.8X3	T39.8X4	T39.8X5	T39.8X6
Nematocyst (sting)	T63.691	T63.692	T63.693	T63.694	—	—
Nembutal	T42.3X1	T42.3X2	T42.3X3	T42.3X4	T42.3X5	T42.3X6
Nemonapride	T43.591	T43.592	T43.593	T43.594	T43.595	T43.596
Neoarsphenamine	T37.8X1	T37.8X2	T37.8X3	T37.8X4	T37.8X5	T37.8X6
Neocinchophen	T50.4X1	T50.4X2	T50.4X3	T50.4X4	T50.4X5	T50.4X6
Neomycin (derivatives)	T36.5X1	T36.5X2	T36.5X3	T36.5X4	T36.5X5	T36.5X6
with						
bacitracin	T49.0X1	T49.0X2	T49.0X3	T49.0X4	T49.0X5	T49.0X6
neostigmine	T44.0X1	T44.0X2	T44.0X3	T44.0X4	T44.0X5	T44.0X6
ENT agent	T49.6X1	T49.6X2	T49.6X3	T49.6X4	T49.6X5	T49.6X6
ophthalmic preparation	T49.5X1	T49.5X2	T49.5X3	T49.5X4	T49.5X5	T49.5X6
topical NEC	T49.0X1	T49.0X2	T49.0X3	T49.0X4	T49.0X5	T49.0X6
Neonal	T42.3X1	T42.3X2	T42.3X3	T42.3X4	T42.3X5	T42.3X6
Neoprontosil	T37.0X1	T37.0X2	T37.0X3	T37.0X4	T37.0X5	T37.0X6
Neosalvarsan	T37.8X1	T37.8X2	T37.8X3	T37.8X4	T37.8X5	T37.8X6
Neosilversalvarsan	T37.8X1	T37.8X2	T37.8X3	T37.8X4	T37.8X5	T37.8X6
Neosporin	T36.8X1	T36.8X2	T36.8X3	T36.8X4	T36.8X5	T36.8X6
ENT agent	T49.6X1	T49.6X2	T49.6X3	T49.6X4	T49.6X5	T49.6X6
opthalmic preparation	T49.5X1	T49.5X2	T49.5X3	T49.5X4	T49.5X5	T49.5X6
topical NEC	T49.0X1	T49.0X2	T49.0X3	T49.0X4	T49.0X5	T49.0X6
Neostigmine bromide	T44.0X1	T44.0X2	T44.0X3	T44.0X4	T44.0X5	T44.0X6
Neraval	T42.3X1	T42.3X2	T42.3X3	T42.3X4	T42.3X5	T42.3X6
Neravan	T42.3X1	T42.3X2	T42.3X3	T42.3X4	T42.3X5	T42.3X6
Nerium oleander	T62.2X1	T62.2X2	T62.2X3	T62.2X4	—	—
Nerve gas, not in war	T59.91	T59.92	T59.93	T59.94	—	—
Nesacaine	T41.3X1	T41.3X2	T41.3X3	T41.3X4	T41.3X5	T41.3X6
infiltration (subcutaneous)	T41.3X1	T41.3X2	T41.3X3	T41.3X4	T41.3X5	T41.3X6
nerve block (peripheral) (plexus)	T41.3X1	T41.3X2	T41.3X3	T41.3X4	T41.3X5	T41.3X6
Netilmicin	T36.5X1	T36.5X2	T36.5X3	T36.5X4	T36.5X5	T36.5X6
Neurobarb	T42.3X1	T42.3X2	T42.3X3	T42.3X4	T42.3X5	T42.3X6
Neuroleptic drug NEC	T43.501	T43.502	T43.503	T43.504	T43.505	T43.506
Neuromuscular blocking drug	T48.1X1	T48.1X2	T48.1X3	T48.1X4	T48.1X5	T48.1X6
Neutral insulin injection	T38.3X1	T38.3X2	T38.3X3	T38.3X4	T38.3X5	T38.3X6
Neutral spirits	T51.0X1	T51.0X2	T51.0X3	T51.0X4	—	—
beverage	T51.0X1	T51.0X2	T51.0X3	T51.0X4	—	—
Niacin	T46.7X1	T46.7X2	T46.7X3	T46.7X4	T46.7X5	T46.7X6
Niacinamide	T45.2X1	T45.2X2	T45.2X3	T45.2X4	T45.2X5	T45.2X6
Nialamide	T43.1X1	T43.1X2	T43.1X3	T43.1X4	T43.1X5	T43.1X6
Niaprazine	T42.6X1	T42.6X2	T42.6X3	T42.6X4	T42.6X5	T42.6X6
Nicametate	T46.7X1	T46.7X2	T46.7X3	T46.7X4	T46.7X5	T46.7X6
Nicardipine	T46.1X1	T46.1X2	T46.1X3	T46.1X4	T46.1X5	T46.1X6
Nicergoline	T46.7X1	T46.7X2	T46.7X3	T46.7X4	T46.7X5	T46.7X6
Nickel (carbonyl) (tetra-carbonyl) (fumes) (vapor)	T56.891	T56.892	T56.893	T56.894	—	—
Nickelocene	T56.891	T56.892	T56.893	T56.894	—	—
Niclosamide	T37.4X1	T37.4X2	T37.4X3	T37.4X4	T37.4X5	T37.4X6
Nicofuranose	T46.7X1	T46.7X2	T46.7X3	T46.7X4	T46.7X5	T46.7X6
Nicomorphine	T40.2X1	T40.2X2	T40.2X3	T40.2X4	—	—
Nicorandil	T46.3X1	T46.3X2	T46.3X3	T46.3X4	T46.3X5	T46.3X6
Nicotiana (plant)	T62.2X1	T62.2X2	T62.2X3	T62.2X4	—	—
Nicotinamide	T45.2X1	T45.2X2	T45.2X3	T45.2X4	T45.2X5	T45.2X6
Nicotine (insecticide) (spray) (sulfate) NEC	T60.2X1	T60.2X2	T60.2X3	T60.2X4	—	—
from tobacco	T65.291	T65.292	T65.293	T65.294	—	—
cigarettes	T65.221	T65.222	T65.223	T65.224	—	—
not insecticide	T65.291	T65.292	T65.293	T65.294	—	—
Nicotinic acid	T46.7X1	T46.7X2	T46.7X3	T46.7X4	T46.7X5	T46.7X6
Nicotinyl alcohol	T46.7X1	T46.7X2	T46.7X3	T46.7X4	T46.7X5	T46.7X6
Nicoumalone	T45.511	T45.512	T45.513	T45.514	T45.515	T45.516
Nifedipine	T46.1X1	T46.1X2	T46.1X3	T46.1X4	T46.1X5	T46.1X6
Nifenazone	T39.2X1	T39.2X2	T39.2X3	T39.2X4	T39.2X5	T39.2X6
Nifuraldezone	T37.91	T37.92	T37.93	T37.94	T37.95	T37.96
Nifuratel	T37.8X1	T37.8X2	T37.8X3	T37.8X4	T37.8X5	T37.8X6
Nifurtimox	T37.3X1	T37.3X2	T37.3X3	T37.3X4	T37.3X5	T37.3X6
Nifurtoinol	T37.8X1	T37.8X2	T37.8X3	T37.8X4	T37.8X5	T37.8X6
Nightshade, deadly (solanum) — *see also* Belladonna	T62.2X1	T62.2X2	T62.2X3	T62.2X4	—	—
berry	T62.1X1	T62.1X2	T62.1X3	T62.1X4	—	—
Nikethamide	T50.7X1	T50.7X2	T50.7X3	T50.7X4	T50.7X5	T50.7X6
Nilstat	T36.7X1	T36.7X2	T36.7X3	T36.7X4	T36.7X5	T36.7X6
topical	T49.0X1	T49.0X2	T49.0X3	T49.0X4	T49.0X5	T49.0X6
Nilutamide	T38.6X1	T38.6X2	T38.6X3	T38.6X4	T38.6X5	T38.6X6
Nimesulide	T39.391	T39.392	T39.393	T39.394	T39.395	T39.396
Nimetazepam	T42.4X1	T42.4X2	T42.4X3	T42.4X4	T42.4X5	T42.4X6
Nimodipine	T46.1X1	T46.1X2	T46.1X3	T46.1X4	T46.1X5	T46.1X6
Nimorazole	T37.3X1	T37.3X2	T37.3X3	T37.3X4	T37.3X5	T37.3X6
Nimustine	T45.1X1	T45.1X2	T45.1X3	T45.1X4	T45.1X5	T45.1X6
Niridazole	T37.4X1	T37.4X2	T37.4X3	T37.4X4	T37.4X5	T37.4X6
Nisentil	T40.2X1	T40.2X2	T40.2X3	T40.2X4	T40.2X5	T40.2X6
Nisoldipine	T46.1X1	T46.1X2	T46.1X3	T46.1X4	T46.1X5	T46.1X6
Nitramine	T65.3X1	T65.3X2	T65.3X3	T65.3X4	—	—
Nitrate, organic	T46.3X1	T46.3X2	T46.3X3	T46.3X4	T46.3X5	T46.3X6
Nitrazepam	T42.4X1	T42.4X2	T42.4X3	T42.4X4	T42.4X5	T42.4X6
Nitrefazole	T50.6X1	T50.6X2	T50.6X3	T50.6X4	T50.6X5	T50.6X6

Table of Drugs and Chemicals

Mustard — Nitrefazole

Substance	Poisoning, Accidental (unintentional)	Poisoning, Intentional Self-harm	Poisoning, Assault	Poisoning, Undetermined	Adverse Effect	Under-dosing
Nitrendipine	T46.1X1	T46.1X2	T46.1X3	T46.1X4	T46.1X5	T46.1X6
Nitric						
acid (liquid)	T54.2X1	T54.2X2	T54.2X3	T54.2X4	—	—
vapor	T59.891	T59.892	T59.893	T59.894	—	—
oxide (gas)	T59.0X1	T59.0X2	T59.0X3	T59.0X4	—	—
Nitrimidazine	T37.3X1	T37.3X2	T37.3X3	T37.3X4	T37.3X5	T37.3X6
Nitrite, amyl (medicinal)	T46.3X1	T46.3X2	T46.3X3	T46.3X4	T46.3X5	T46.3X6
(vapor)						
Nitroaniline	T65.3X1	T65.3X2	T65.3X3	T65.3X4	—	—
vapor	T59.891	T59.892	T59.893	T59.894	—	—
Nitrobenzene, nitrobenzol	T65.3X1	T65.3X2	T65.3X3	T65.3X4	—	—
vapor	T65.3X1	T65.3X2	T65.3X3	T65.3X4	—	—
Nitrocellulose	T65.891	T65.892	T65.893	T65.894	—	—
lacquer	T65.891	T65.892	T65.893	T65.894	—	—
Nitrodiphenyl	T65.3X1	T65.3X2	T65.3X3	T65.3X4	—	—
Nitrofural	T49.0X1	T49.0X2	T49.0X3	T49.0X4	T49.0X5	T49.0X6
Nitrofurantoin	T37.8X1	T37.8X2	T37.8X3	T37.8X4	T37.8X5	T37.8X6
Nitrofurazone	T49.0X1	T49.0X2	T49.0X3	T49.0X4	T49.0X5	T49.0X6
Nitrogen	T59.0X1	T59.0X2	T59.0X3	T59.0X4	—	—
mustard	T45.1X1	T45.1X2	T45.1X3	T45.1X4	T45.1X5	T45.1X6
Nitroglycerin, nitroglycerol (medicinal)	T46.3X1	T46.3X2	T46.3X3	T46.3X4	T46.3X5	T46.3X6
nonmedicinal	T65.5X1	T65.5X2	T65.5X3	T65.5X4	—	—
fumes	T65.5X1	T65.5X2	T65.5X3	T65.5X4	—	—
Nitroglycol	T52.3X1	T52.3X2	T52.3X3	T52.3X4	—	—
Nitrohydrochloric acid	T54.2X1	T54.2X2	T54.2X3	T54.2X4	—	—
Nitromersol	T49.0X1	T49.0X2	T49.0X3	T49.0X4	T49.0X5	T49.0X6
Nitronaphthalene	T65.891	T65.892	T65.893	T65.894	—	—
Nitrophenol	T54.0X1	T54.0X2	T54.0X3	T54.0X4	—	—
Nitropropane	T52.8X1	T52.8X2	T52.8X3	T52.8X4	—	—
Nitroprusside	T46.5X1	T46.5X2	T46.5X3	T46.5X4	T46.5X5	T46.5X6
Nitrosodimethylamine	T65.3X1	T65.3X2	T65.3X3	T65.3X4	—	—
Nitrothiazol	T37.4X1	T37.4X2	T37.4X3	T37.4X4	T37.4X5	T37.4X6
Nitrotoluene, nitrotoluol	T65.3X1	T65.3X2	T65.3X3	T65.3X4	—	—
vapor	T65.3X1	T65.3X2	T65.3X3	T65.3X4	—	—
Nitrous						
acid (liquid)	T54.2X1	T54.2X2	T54.2X3	T54.2X4	—	—
fumes	T59.891	T59.892	T59.893	T59.894	—	—
ether spirit	T46.3X1	T46.3X2	T46.3X3	T46.3X4	T46.3X5	T46.3X6
oxide	T41.0X1	T41.0X2	T41.0X3	T41.0X4	T41.0X5	T41.0X6
Nitroxoline	T37.8X1	T37.8X2	T37.8X3	T37.8X4	T37.8X5	T37.8X6
Nitrozone	T49.0X1	T49.0X2	T49.0X3	T49.0X4	T49.0X5	T49.0X6
Nizatidine	T47.0X1	T47.0X2	T47.0X3	T47.0X4	T47.0X5	T47.0X6
Nizofenone	T43.8X1	T43.8X2	T43.8X3	T43.8X4	T43.8X5	T43.8X6
Noctec	T42.6X1	T42.6X2	T42.6X3	T42.6X4	T42.6X5	T42.6X6
Noludar	T42.6X1	T42.6X2	T42.6X3	T42.6X4	T42.6X5	T42.6X6
Nomegestrol	T38.5X1	T38.5X2	T38.5X3	T38.5X4	T38.5X5	T38.5X6
Nomifensine	T43.291	T43.292	T43.293	T43.294	T43.295	T43.296
Nonoxinol	T49.8X1	T49.8X2	T49.8X3	T49.8X4	T49.8X5	T49.8X6
Nonylphenoxy (polyethoxyethanol)	T49.8X1	T49.8X2	T49.8X3	T49.8X4	T49.8X5	T49.8X6
Noptil	T42.3X1	T42.3X2	T42.3X3	T42.3X4	T42.3X5	T42.3X6
Noradrenaline	T44.4X1	T44.4X2	T44.4X3	T44.4X4	T44.4X5	T44.4X6
Noramidopyrine	T39.2X1	T39.2X2	T39.2X3	T39.2X4	T39.2X5	T39.2X6
methanesulfonate sodium	T39.2X1	T39.2X2	T39.2X3	T39.2X4	T39.2X5	T39.2X6
Norbormide	T60.4X1	T60.4X2	T60.4X3	T60.4X4	—	—
Nordazepam	T42.4X1	T42.4X2	T42.4X3	T42.4X4	T42.4X5	T42.4X6
Norepinephrine	T44.4X1	T44.4X2	T44.4X3	T44.4X4	T44.4X5	T44.4X6
Norethandrolone	T38.7X1	T38.7X2	T38.7X3	T38.7X4	T38.7X5	T38.7X6
Norethindrone	T38.4X1	T38.4X2	T38.4X3	T38.4X4	T38.4X5	T38.4X6
Norethisterone (acetate) (enantate)	T38.4X1	T38.4X2	T38.4X3	T38.4X4	T38.4X5	T38.4X6
with ethinylestradiol	T38.5X1	T38.5X2	T38.5X3	T38.5X4	T38.5X5	T38.5X6
Noretynodrel	T38.5X1	T38.5X2	T38.5X3	T38.5X4	T38.5X5	T38.5X6
Norfenefrine	T44.4X1	T44.4X2	T44.4X3	T44.4X4	T44.4X5	T44.4X6
Norfloxacin	T36.8X1	T36.8X2	T36.8X3	T36.8X4	T36.8X5	T36.8X6
Norgestrel	T38.4X1	T38.4X2	T38.4X3	T38.4X4	T38.4X5	T38.4X6
Norgestrienone	T38.4X1	T38.4X2	T38.4X3	T38.4X4	T38.4X5	T38.4X6
Norlestrin	T38.4X1	T38.4X2	T38.4X3	T38.4X4	T38.4X5	T38.4X6
Norlutin	T38.4X1	T38.4X2	T38.4X3	T38.4X4	T38.4X5	T38.4X6
Normal serum albumin (human), salt-poor	T45.8X1	T45.8X2	T45.8X3	T45.8X4	T45.8X5	T45.8X6
Normethandrone	T38.5X1	T38.5X2	T38.5X3	T38.5X4	T38.5X5	T38.5X6
Normison — see Benzodiazepines						
Normorphine	T40.2X1	T40.2X2	T40.2X3	T40.2X4	—	—
Norpseudoephedrine	T50.5X1	T50.5X2	T50.5X3	T50.5X4	T50.5X5	T50.5X6
Nortestosterone (furanpropionate)	T38.7X1	T38.7X2	T38.7X3	T38.7X4	T38.7X5	T38.7X6
Nortriptyline	T43.011	T43.012	T43.013	T43.014	T43.015	T43.016
Noscapine	T48.3X1	T48.3X2	T48.3X3	T48.3X4	T48.3X5	T48.3X6
Nose preparations	T49.6X1	T49.6X2	T49.6X3	T49.6X4	T49.6X5	T49.6X6
Novobiocin	T36.5X1	T36.5X2	T36.5X3	T36.5X4	T36.5X5	T36.5X6
Novocain (infiltration) (topical)	T41.3X1	T41.3X2	T41.3X3	T41.3X4	T41.3X5	T41.3X6
nerve block (peripheral) (plexus)	T41.3X1	T41.3X2	T41.3X3	T41.3X4	T41.3X5	T41.3X6
spinal	T41.3X1	T41.3X2	T41.3X3	T41.3X4	T41.3X5	T41.3X6
Noxious foodstuff	T62.91	T62.92	T62.93	T62.94	—	—
specified NEC	T62.8X1	T62.8X2	T62.8X3	T62.8X4	—	—
Noxiptiline	T43.011	T43.012	T43.013	T43.014	T43.015	T43.016
Noxytiolin	T49.0X1	T49.0X2	T49.0X3	T49.0X4	T49.0X5	T49.0X6
NPH lletin (insulin)	T38.3X1	T38.3X2	T38.3X3	T38.3X4	T38.3X5	T38.3X6
Numorphan	T40.2X1	T40.2X2	T40.2X3	T40.2X4	T40.2X5	T40.2X6
Nunol	T42.3X1	T42.3X2	T42.3X3	T42.3X4	T42.3X5	T42.3X6
Nupercaine (spinal anesthetic)	T41.3X1	T41.3X2	T41.3X3	T41.3X4	T41.3X5	T41.3X6
topical (surface)	T41.3X1	T41.3X2	T41.3X3	T41.3X4	T41.3X5	T41.3X6
Nutmeg oil (liniment)	T49.3X1	T49.3X2	T49.3X3	T49.3X4	T49.3X5	T49.3X6
Nutritional supplement	T50.901	T50.902	T50.903	T50.904	T50.905	T50.906
Nux vomica	T65.1X1	T65.1X2	T65.1X3	T65.1X4	—	—
Nydrazid	T37.1X1	T37.1X2	T37.1X3	T37.1X4	T37.1X5	T37.1X6
Nylidrin	T46.7X1	T46.7X2	T46.7X3	T46.7X4	T46.7X5	T46.7X6
Nystatin	T36.7X1	T36.7X2	T36.7X3	T36.7X4	T36.7X5	T36.7X6
topical	T49.0X1	T49.0X2	T49.0X3	T49.0X4	T49.0X5	T49.0X6
Nytol	T45.0X1	T45.0X2	T45.0X3	T45.0X4	T45.0X5	T45.0X6
Obidoxime chloride	T50.6X1	T50.6X2	T50.6X3	T50.6X4	T50.6X5	T50.6X6
Octafonium (chloride)	T49.3X1	T49.3X2	T49.3X3	T49.3X4	T49.3X5	T49.3X6
Octamethyl pyrophosphoramide	T60.0X1	T60.0X2	T60.0X3	T60.0X4	—	—
Octanoin	T50.991	T50.992	T50.993	T50.994	T50.995	T50.996
Octatropine methylbromide	T44.3X1	T44.3X2	T44.3X3	T44.3X4	T44.3X5	T44.3X6
Octotiamine	T45.2X1	T45.2X2	T45.2X3	T45.2X4	T45.2X5	T45.2X6
Octoxinol (9)	T49.8X1	T49.8X2	T49.8X3	T49.8X4	T49.8X5	T49.8X6
Octreotide	T38.991	T38.992	T38.993	T38.994	T38.995	T38.996
Octyl nitrite	T46.3X1	T46.3X2	T46.3X3	T46.3X4	T46.3X5	T46.3X6
Oestradiol	T38.5X1	T38.5X2	T38.5X3	T38.5X4	T38.5X5	T38.5X6
Oestriol	T38.5X1	T38.5X2	T38.5X3	T38.5X4	T38.5X5	T38.5X6
Oestrogen	T38.5X1	T38.5X2	T38.5X3	T38.5X4	T38.5X5	T38.5X6
Oestrone	T38.5X1	T38.5X2	T38.5X3	T38.5X4	T38.5X5	T38.5X6
Ofloxacin	T36.8X1	T36.8X2	T36.8X3	T36.8X4	T36.8X5	T36.8X6
Oil (of)	T65.891	T65.892	T65.893	T65.894	—	—
bitter almond	T62.8X1	T62.8X2	T62.8X3	T62.8X4	—	—
cloves	T49.7X1	T49.7X2	T49.7X3	T49.7X4	T49.7X5	T49.7X6
colors	T65.6X1	T65.6X2	T65.6X3	T65.6X4	—	—
fumes	T59.891	T59.892	T59.893	T59.894	—	—
lubricating	T52.0X1	T52.0X2	T52.0X3	T52.0X4	—	—
Niobe	T52.8X1	T52.8X2	T52.8X3	T52.8X4	—	—
vitriol (liquid)	T54.2X1	T54.2X2	T54.2X3	T54.2X4	—	—
fumes	T54.2X1	T54.2X2	T54.2X3	T54.2X4	—	—
wintergreen (bitter) NEC	T49.3X1	T49.3X2	T49.3X3	T49.3X4	T49.3X5	T49.3X6
Oily preparation (for skin)	T49.3X1	T49.3X2	T49.3X3	T49.3X4	T49.3X5	T49.3X6
Ointment NEC	T49.3X1	T49.3X2	T49.3X3	T49.3X4	T49.3X5	T49.3X6
Olanzapine	T43.591	T43.592	T43.593	T43.594	T43.595	T43.596
Oleander	T62.2X1	T62.2X2	T62.2X3	T62.2X4	—	—
Oleandomycin	T36.3X1	T36.3X2	T36.3X3	T36.3X4	T36.3X5	T36.3X6
Oleandrin	T46.0X1	T46.0X2	T46.0X3	T46.0X4	T46.0X5	T46.0X6
Oleic acid	T46.6X1	T46.6X2	T46.6X3	T46.6X4	T46.6X5	T46.6X6
Oleovitamin A	T45.2X1	T45.2X2	T45.2X3	T45.2X4	T45.2X5	T45.2X6
Oleum ricini	T47.2X1	T47.2X2	T47.2X3	T47.2X4	T47.2X5	T47.2X6
Olive oil (medicinal) NEC	T47.4X1	T47.4X2	T47.4X3	T47.4X4	T47.4X5	T47.4X6
Olivomycin	T45.1X1	T45.1X2	T45.1X3	T45.1X4	T45.1X5	T45.1X6
Olsalazine	T47.8X1	T47.8X2	T47.8X3	T47.8X4	T47.8X5	T47.8X6
Omeprazole	T47.1X1	T47.1X2	T47.1X3	T47.1X4	T47.1X5	T47.1X6
OMPA	T60.0X1	T60.0X2	T60.0X3	T60.0X4	—	—
Oncovin	T45.1X1	T45.1X2	T45.1X3	T45.1X4	T45.1X5	T45.1X6
Ondansetron	T45.0X1	T45.0X2	T45.0X3	T45.0X4	T45.0X5	T45.0X6
Ophthaine	T41.3X1	T41.3X2	T41.3X3	T41.3X4	T41.3X5	T41.3X6
Ophthetic	T41.3X1	T41.3X2	T41.3X3	T41.3X4	T41.3X5	T41.3X6
Opiate NEC	T40.601	T40.602	T40.603	T40.604	T40.605	T40.606
antagonists	T50.7X1	T50.7X2	T50.7X3	T50.7X4	T50.7X5	T50.7X6
Opioid NEC	T40.2X1	T40.2X2	T40.2X3	T40.2X4	T40.2X5	T40.2X6
Opipramol	T43.011	T43.012	T43.013	T43.014	T43.015	T43.016
Opium alkaloids (total)	T40.0X1	T40.0X2	T40.0X3	T40.0X4	T40.0X5	T40.0X6
standardized powdered	T40.0X1	T40.0X2	T40.0X3	T40.0X4	T40.0X5	T40.0X6
tincture (camphorated)	T40.0X1	T40.0X2	T40.0X3	T40.0X4	T40.0X5	T40.0X6
Oracon	T38.4X1	T38.4X2	T38.4X3	T38.4X4	T38.4X5	T38.4X6
Oragrafin	T50.8X1	T50.8X2	T50.8X3	T50.8X4	T50.8X5	T50.8X6
Oral contraceptives	T38.4X1	T38.4X2	T38.4X3	T38.4X4	T38.4X5	T38.4X6
Oral rehydration salts	T50.3X1	T50.3X2	T50.3X3	T50.3X4	T50.3X5	T50.3X6
Orazamide	T50.991	T50.992	T50.993	T50.994	T50.995	T50.996
Orciprenaline	T48.291	T48.292	T48.293	T48.294	T48.295	T48.296
Organidin	T48.4X1	T48.4X2	T48.4X3	T48.4X4	T48.4X5	T48.4X6
Organonitrate NEC	T46.3X1	T46.3X2	T46.3X3	T46.3X4	T46.3X5	T46.3X6
Organophosphates	T60.0X1	T60.0X2	T60.0X3	T60.0X4		

Additional Character May Be Required — Refer to the Tabular List for Character Selection

▽ Subterms under main terms may continue to next column or page

Table of Drugs and Chemicals

Substance	Poisoning, Accidental (unintentional)	Poisoning, Intentional Self-harm	Poisoning, Assault	Poisoning, Undetermined	Adverse Effect	Under-dosing
Orimune	T50.B91	T50.B92	T50.B93	T50.B94	T50.B95	T50.B96
Orinase	T38.3X1	T38.3X2	T38.3X3	T38.3X4	T38.3X5	T38.3X6
Ormeloxifene	T38.6X1	T38.6X2	T38.6X3	T38.6X4	T38.6X5	T38.6X6
Ornidazole	T37.3X1	T37.3X2	T37.3X3	T37.3X4	T37.3X5	T37.3X6
Ornithine aspartate	T50.992	T50.992	T50.993	T50.994	T50.995	T50.996
Ornoprostil	T47.1X1	T47.1X2	T47.1X3	T47.1X4	T47.1X5	T47.1X6
Orphenadrine	T42.8X1	T42.8X2	T42.8X3	T42.8X4	T42.8X5	T42.8X6
(hydrochloride)						
Ortal	T42.3X1	T42.3X2	T42.3X3	T42.3X4	T42.3X5	T42.3X6
Orthoboric acid	T49.0X1	T49.0X2	T49.0X3	T49.0X4	T49.0X5	T49.0X6
ENT agent	T49.6X1	T49.6X2	T49.6X3	T49.6X4	T49.6X5	T49.6X6
ophthalmic preparation	T49.5X1	T49.5X2	T49.5X3	T49.5X4	T49.5X5	T49.5X6
Orthocaine	T41.3X1	T41.3X2	T41.3X3	T41.3X4	T41.3X5	T41.3X6
Orthodichlorobenzene	T53.7X1	T53.7X2	T53.7X3	T53.7X4	—	—
Ortho-Novum	T38.4X1	T38.4X2	T38.4X3	T38.4X4	T38.4X5	T38.4X6
Orthotolidine (reagent)	T54.2X1	T54.2X2	T54.2X3	T54.2X4	—	—
Osmic acid (liquid)	T54.2X1	T54.2X2	T54.2X3	T54.2X4	—	—
fumes	T54.2X1	T54.2X2	T54.2X3	T54.2X4	—	—
Osmotic diuretics	T50.2X1	T50.2X2	T50.2X3	T50.2X4	T50.2X5	T50.2X6
Otilonium bromide	T44.3X1	T44.3X2	T44.3X3	T44.3X4	T44.3X5	T44.3X6
Otorhinolaryngological drug NEC	T49.6X1	T49.6X2	T49.6X3	T49.6X4	T49.6X5	T49.6X6
Ouabain (e)	T46.0X1	T46.0X2	T46.0X3	T46.0X4	T46.0X5	T46.0X6
Ovarian						
hormone	T38.5X1	T38.5X2	T38.5X3	T38.5X4	T38.5X5	T38.5X6
stimulant	T38.5X1	T38.5X2	T38.5X3	T38.5X4	T38.5X5	T38.5X6
Ovral	T38.4X1	T38.4X2	T38.4X3	T38.4X4	T38.4X5	T38.4X6
Ovulen	T38.4X1	T38.4X2	T38.4X3	T38.4X4	T38.4X5	T38.4X6
Oxacillin	T36.0X1	T36.0X2	T36.0X3	T36.0X4	T36.0X5	T36.0X6
Oxalic acid	T54.2X1	T54.2X2	T54.2X3	T54.2X4	—	—
ammonium salt	T50.991	T50.992	T50.993	T50.994	T50.995	T50.996
Oxamniquine	T37.4X1	T37.4X2	T37.4X3	T37.4X4	T37.4X5	T37.4X6
Oxanamide	T43.591	T43.592	T43.593	T43.594	T43.595	T43.596
Oxandrolone	T38.7X1	T38.7X2	T38.7X3	T38.7X4	T38.7X5	T38.7X6
Oxantel	T37.4X1	T37.4X2	T37.4X3	T37.4X4	T37.4X5	T37.4X6
Oxapium iodide	T44.3X1	T44.3X2	T44.3X3	T44.3X4	T44.3X5	T44.3X6
Oxaprotiline	T43.021	T43.022	T43.023	T43.024	T43.025	T43.026
Oxaprozin	T39.311	T39.312	T39.313	T39.314	T39.315	T39.316
Oxatomide	T45.0X1	T45.0X2	T45.0X3	T45.0X4	T45.0X5	T45.0X6
Oxazepam	T42.4X1	T42.4X2	T42.4X3	T42.4X4	T42.4X5	T42.4X6
Oxazimedrine	T50.5X1	T50.5X2	T50.5X3	T50.5X4	T50.5X5	T50.5X6
Oxazolam	T42.4X1	T42.4X2	T42.4X3	T42.4X4	T42.4X5	T42.4X6
Oxazolidine derivatives	T42.2X1	T42.2X2	T42.2X3	T42.2X4	T42.2X5	T42.2X6
Oxazolidinedione	T42.2X1	T42.2X2	T42.2X3	T42.2X4	T42.2X5	T42.2X6
(derivative)						
Ox bile extract	T47.5X1	T47.5X2	T47.5X3	T47.5X4	T47.5X5	T47.5X6
Oxcarbazepine	T42.1X1	T42.1X2	T42.1X3	T42.1X4	T42.1X5	T42.1X6
Oxedrine	T44.4X1	T44.4X2	T44.4X3	T44.4X4	T44.4X5	T44.4X6
Oxeladin (citrate)	T48.3X1	T48.3X2	T48.3X3	T48.3X4	T48.3X5	T48.3X6
Oxendolone	T38.5X1	T38.5X2	T38.5X3	T38.5X4	T38.5X5	T38.5X6
Oxetacaine	T41.3X1	T41.3X2	T41.3X3	T41.3X4	T41.3X5	T41.3X6
Oxethazine	T41.3X1	T41.3X2	T41.3X3	T41.3X4	T41.3X5	T41.3X6
Oxetorone	T39.8X1	T39.8X2	T39.8X3	T39.8X4	T39.8X5	T39.8X6
Oxiconazole	T49.0X1	T49.0X2	T49.0X3	T49.0X4	T49.0X5	T49.0X6
Oxidizing agent NEC	T54.91	T54.92	T54.93	T54.94	—	—
Oxipurinol	T50.4X1	T50.4X2	T50.4X3	T50.4X4	T50.4X5	T50.4X6
Oxitriptan	T43.291	T43.292	T43.293	T43.294	T43.295	T43.296
Oxitropium bromide	T48.6X1	T48.6X2	T48.6X3	T48.6X4	T48.6X5	T48.6X6
Oxodipine	T46.1X1	T46.1X2	T46.1X3	T46.1X4	T46.1X5	T46.1X6
Oxolamine	T48.3X1	T48.3X2	T48.3X3	T48.3X4	T48.3X5	T48.3X6
Oxolinic acid	T37.8X1	T37.8X2	T37.8X3	T37.8X4	T37.8X5	T37.8X6
Oxomemazine	T43.3X1	T43.3X2	T43.3X3	T43.3X4	T43.3X5	T43.3X6
Oxophenarsine	T37.3X1	T37.3X2	T37.3X3	T37.3X4	T37.3X5	T37.3X6
Oxprenolol	T44.7X1	T44.7X2	T44.7X3	T44.7X4	T44.7X5	T44.7X6
Oxsoralen	T49.3X1	T49.3X2	T49.3X3	T49.3X4	T49.3X5	T49.3X6
Oxtriphylline	T48.6X1	T48.6X2	T48.6X3	T48.6X4	T48.6X5	T48.6X6
Oxybate sodium	T41.291	T41.292	T41.293	T41.294	T41.295	T41.296
Oxybuprocaine	T41.3X1	T41.3X2	T41.3X3	T41.3X4	T41.3X5	T41.3X6
Oxybutynin	T44.3X1	T44.3X2	T44.3X3	T44.3X4	T44.3X5	T44.3X6
Oxychlorosene	T49.0X1	T49.0X2	T49.0X3	T49.0X4	T49.0X5	T49.0X6
Oxycodone	T40.2X1	T40.2X2	T40.2X3	T40.2X4	T40.2X5	T40.2X6
Oxyfedrine	T46.3X1	T46.3X2	T46.3X3	T46.3X4	T46.3X5	T46.3X6
Oxygen	T41.5X1	T41.5X2	T41.5X3	T41.5X4	T41.5X5	T41.5X6
Oxylone	T49.0X1	T49.0X2	T49.0X3	T49.0X4	T49.0X5	T49.0X6
ophthalmic preparation	T49.5X1	T49.5X2	T49.5X3	T49.5X4	T49.5X5	T49.5X6
Oxymesterone	T38.7X1	T38.7X2	T38.7X3	T38.7X4	T38.7X5	T38.7X6
Oxymetazoline	T48.5X1	T48.5X2	T48.5X3	T48.5X4	T48.5X5	T48.5X6
Oxymetholone	T38.7X1	T38.7X2	T38.7X3	T38.7X4	T38.7X5	T38.7X6
Oxymorphone	T40.2X1	T40.2X2	T40.2X3	T40.2X4	T40.2X5	T40.2X6
Oxypertine	T43.591	T43.592	T43.593	T43.594	T43.595	T43.596
Oxyphenbutazone	T39.2X1	T39.2X2	T39.2X3	T39.2X4	T39.2X5	T39.2X6
Oxyphencyclimine	T44.3X1	T44.3X2	T44.3X3	T44.3X4	T44.3X5	T44.3X6
Oxyphenisatine	T47.2X1	T47.2X2	T47.2X3	T47.2X4	T47.2X5	T47.2X6
Oxyphenonium bromide	T44.3X1	T44.3X2	T44.3X3	T44.3X4	T44.3X5	T44.3X6
Oxypolygelatin	T45.8X1	T45.8X2	T45.8X3	T45.8X4	T45.8X5	T45.8X6
Oxyquinoline (derivatives)	T37.8X1	T37.8X2	T37.8X3	T37.8X4	T37.8X5	T37.8X6
Oxytetracycline	T36.4X1	T36.4X2	T36.4X3	T36.4X4	T36.4X5	T36.4X6
Oxytocic drug NEC	T48.0X1	T48.0X2	T48.0X3	T48.0X4	T48.0X5	T48.0X6
Oxytocin (synthetic)	T48.0X1	T48.0X2	T48.0X3	T48.0X4	T48.0X5	T48.0X6
Ozone	T59.891	T59.892	T59.893	T59.894		
PABA	T49.3X1	T49.3X2	T49.3X3	T49.3X4	T49.3X5	T49.3X6
Packed red cells	T45.8X1	T45.8X2	T45.8X3	T45.8X4	T45.8X5	T45.8X6
Padimate	T49.3X1	T49.3X2	T49.3X3	T49.3X4	T49.3X5	T49.3X6
Paint NEC	T65.6X1	T65.6X2	T65.6X3	T65.6X4	—	—
cleaner	T52.91	T52.92	T52.93	T52.94	—	—
fumes NEC	T59.891	T59.892	T59.893	T59.894	—	—
lead (fumes)	T56.0X1	T56.0X2	T56.0X3	T56.0X4	—	—
solvent NEC	T52.8X1	T52.8X2	T52.8X3	T52.8X4	—	—
stripper	T52.8X1	T52.8X2	T52.8X3	T52.8X4	—	—
Palfium	T40.2X1	T40.2X2	T40.2X3	T40.2X4	—	—
Palm kernel oil	T50.991	T50.992	T50.993	T50.994	T50.995	T50.996
Paludrine	T37.2X1	T37.2X2	T37.2X3	T37.2X4	T37.2X5	T37.2X6
PAM (pralidoxime)	T50.6X1	T50.6X2	T50.6X3	T50.6X4	T50.6X5	T50.6X6
Pamaquine (naphthoute)	T37.2X1	T37.2X2	T37.2X3	T37.2X4	T37.2X5	T37.2X6
Panadol	T39.1X1	T39.1X2	T39.1X3	T39.1X4	T39.1X5	T39.1X6
Pancreatic						
digestive secretion stimulant	T47.8X1	T47.8X2	T47.8X3	T47.8X4	T47.8X5	T47.8X6
dornase	T45.3X1	T45.3X2	T45.3X3	T45.3X4	T45.3X5	T45.3X6
Pancreatin	T47.5X1	T47.5X2	T47.5X3	T47.5X4	T47.5X5	T47.5X6
Pancrelipase	T47.5X1	T47.5X2	T47.5X3	T47.5X4	T47.5X5	T47.5X6
Pancuronium (bromide)	T48.1X1	T48.1X2	T48.1X3	T48.1X4	T48.1X5	T48.1X6
Pangamic acid	T45.2X1	T45.2X2	T45.2X3	T45.2X4	T45.2X5	T45.2X6
Panthenol	T45.2X1	T45.2X2	T45.2X3	T45.2X4	T45.2X5	T45.2X6
topical	T49.8X1	T49.8X2	T49.8X3	T49.8X4	T49.8X5	T49.8X6
Pantopon	T40.0X1	T40.0X2	T40.0X3	T40.0X4	T40.0X5	T40.0X6
Pantothenic acid	T45.2X1	T45.2X2	T45.2X3	T45.2X4	T45.2X5	T45.2X6
Panwarfin	T45.511	T45.512	T45.513	T45.514	T45.515	T45.516
Papain	T47.5X1	T47.5X2	T47.5X3	T47.5X4	T47.5X5	T47.5X6
digestant	T47.5X1	T47.5X2	T47.5X3	T47.5X4	T47.5X5	T47.5X6
Papaveretum	T40.0X1	T40.0X2	T40.0X3	T40.0X4	T40.0X5	T40.0X6
Papaverine	T44.3X1	T44.3X2	T44.3X3	T44.3X4	T44.3X5	T44.3X6
Para-acetamidophenol	T39.1X1	T39.1X2	T39.1X3	T39.1X4	T39.1X5	T39.1X6
Para-aminobenzoic acid	T49.3X1	T49.3X2	T49.3X3	T49.3X4	T49.3X5	T49.3X6
Para-aminophenol derivatives	T39.1X1	T39.1X2	T39.1X3	T39.1X4	T39.1X5	T39.1X6
Para-aminosalicylic acid	T37.1X1	T37.1X2	T37.1X3	T37.1X4	T37.1X5	T37.1X6
Paracetaldehyde	T42.6X1	T42.6X2	T42.6X3	T42.6X4	T42.6X5	T42.6X6
Paracetamol	T39.1X1	T39.1X2	T39.1X3	T39.1X4	T39.1X5	T39.1X6
Parachlorophenol	T49.0X1	T49.0X2	T49.0X3	T49.0X4	T49.0X5	T49.0X6
(camphorated)						
Paracodin	T40.2X1	T40.2X2	T40.2X3	T40.2X4	T40.2X5	T40.2X6
Paradione	T42.2X1	T42.2X2	T42.2X3	T42.2X4	T42.2X5	T42.2X6
Paraffin(s) (wax)	T52.0X1	T52.0X2	T52.0X3	T52.0X4	—	—
liquid (medicinal)	T47.4X1	T47.4X2	T47.4X3	T47.4X4	T47.4X5	T47.4X6
nonmedicinal	T52.0X1	T52.0X2	T52.0X3	T52.0X4	—	—
Paraformaldehyde	T60.3X1	T60.3X2	T60.3X3	T60.3X4	—	—
Paraldehyde	T42.6X1	T42.6X2	T42.6X3	T42.6X4	T42.6X5	T42.6X6
Paramethadione	T42.2X1	T42.2X2	T42.2X3	T42.2X4	T42.2X5	T42.2X6
Paramethasone	T38.0X1	T38.0X2	T38.0X3	T38.0X4	T38.0X5	T38.0X6
acetate	T49.0X1	T49.0X2	T49.0X3	T49.0X4	T49.0X5	T49.0X6
Paraoxon	T60.0X1	T60.0X2	T60.0X3	T60.0X4	—	—
Paraquat	T60.3X1	T60.3X2	T60.3X3	T60.3X4	—	—
Parasympatholytic NEC	T44.3X1	T44.3X2	T44.3X3	T44.3X4	T44.3X5	T44.3X6
Parasympathomimetic drug NEC	T44.1X1	T44.1X2	T44.1X3	T44.1X4	T44.1X5	T44.1X6
Parathion	T60.0X1	T60.0X2	T60.0X3	T60.0X4	—	—
Parathormone	T50.991	T50.992	T50.993	T50.994	T50.995	T50.996
Parathyroid extract	T50.991	T50.992	T50.993	T50.994	T50.995	T50.996
Paratyphoid vaccine	T50.A91	T50.A92	T50.A93	T50.A94	T50.A95	T50.A96
Paredrine	T44.4X1	T44.4X2	T44.4X3	T44.4X4	T44.4X5	T44.4X6
Paregoric	T40.0X1	T40.0X2	T40.0X3	T40.0X4	T40.0X5	T40.0X6
Pargyline	T46.5X1	T46.5X2	T46.5X3	T46.5X4	T46.5X5	T46.5X6
Paris green	T57.0X1	T57.0X2	T57.0X3	T57.0X4	—	—
insecticide	T57.0X1	T57.0X2	T57.0X3	T57.0X4	—	—
Parnate	T43.1X1	T43.1X2	T43.1X3	T43.1X4	T43.1X5	T43.1X6
Paromomycin	T36.5X1	T36.5X2	T36.5X3	T36.5X4	T36.5X5	T36.5X6
Paroxypropione	T45.1X1	T45.1X2	T45.1X3	T45.1X4	T45.1X5	T45.1X6
Parzone	T40.2X1	T40.2X2	T40.2X3	T40.2X4	T40.2X5	T40.2X6
PAS	T37.1X1	T37.1X2	T37.1X3	T37.1X4	T37.1X5	T37.1X6
Pasiniazid	T37.1X1	T37.1X2	T37.1X3	T37.1X4	T37.1X5	T37.1X6
PBB (polybrominated biphenyls)	T65.891	T65.892	T65.893	T65.894	—	—
PCB	T65.891	T65.892	T65.893	T65.894	—	—
PCP						

Substance	Poisoning, Accidental (unintentional)	Poisoning, Intentional Self-harm	Poisoning, Assault	Poisoning, Undetermined	Adverse Effect	Under-dosing
PCP — *continued*						
meaning	T60.1X1	T60.1X2	T60.1X3	T60.1X4	—	—
pentachlorophenol						
fungicide	T60.3X1	T60.3X2	T60.3X3	T60.3X4	—	—
herbicide	T60.3X1	T60.3X2	T60.3X3	T60.3X4	—	—
insecticide	T60.1X1	T60.1X2	T60.1X3	T60.1X4	—	—
meaning phencyclidine	T40.991	T40.992	T40.993	T40.994	—	—
Peach kernel oil (emulsion)	T47.4X1	T47.4X2	T47.4X3	T47.4X4	T47.4X5	T47.4X6
Peanut oil (emulsion) **NEC**	T47.4X1	T47.4X2	T47.4X3	T47.4X4	T47.4X5	T47.4X6
topical	T49.3X1	T49.3X2	T49.3X3	T49.3X4	T49.3X5	T49.3X6
Pearly Gates (morning glory seeds)	T40.991	T40.992	T40.993	T40.994		
Pecazine	T43.3X1	T43.3X2	T43.3X3	T43.3X4	T43.3X5	T43.3X6
Pectin	T47.6X1	T47.6X2	T47.6X3	T47.6X4	T47.6X5	T47.6X6
Pefloxacin	T37.8X1	T37.8X2	T37.8X3	T37.8X4	T37.8X5	T37.8X6
Pegademase, bovine	T50.Z91	T50.Z92	T50.Z93	T50.Z94	T50.Z95	T50.Z96
Pelletierine tannate	T37.4X1	T37.4X2	T37.4X3	T37.4X4	T37.4X5	T37.4X6
Pemirolast (potassium)	T48.6X1	T48.6X2	T48.6X3	T48.6X4	T48.6X5	T48.6X6
Pemoline	T50.7X1	T50.7X2	T50.7X3	T50.7X4	T50.7X5	T50.7X6
Pempidine	T44.2X1	T44.2X2	T44.2X3	T44.2X4	T44.2X5	T44.2X6
Penamecillin	T36.0X1	T36.0X2	T36.0X3	T36.0X4	T36.0X5	T36.0X6
Penbutolol	T44.7X1	T44.7X2	T44.7X3	T44.7X4	T44.7X5	T44.7X6
Penethamate	T36.0X1	T36.0X2	T36.0X3	T36.0X4	T36.0X5	T36.0X6
Penfluridol	T43.591	T43.592	T43.593	T43.594	T43.595	T43.596
Penflutizide	T50.2X1	T50.2X2	T50.2X3	T50.2X4	T50.2X5	T50.2X6
Pengitoxin	T46.0X1	T46.0X2	T46.0X3	T46.0X4	T46.0X5	T46.0X6
Penicillamine	T50.6X1	T50.6X2	T50.6X3	T50.6X4	T50.6X5	T50.6X6
Penicillin (any)	T36.0X1	T36.0X2	T36.0X3	T36.0X4	T36.0X5	T36.0X6
Penicillinase	T45.3X1	T45.3X2	T45.3X3	T45.3X4	T45.3X5	T45.3X6
Penicilloyl polylysine	T50.8X1	T50.8X2	T50.8X3	T50.8X4	T50.8X5	T50.8X6
Penimepicycline	T36.4X1	T36.4X2	T36.4X3	T36.4X4	T36.4X5	T36.4X6
Pentachloroethane	T53.6X1	T53.6X2	T53.6X3	T53.6X4	—	—
Pentachloronaphthalene	T53.7X1	T53.7X2	T53.7X3	T53.7X4	—	—
Pentachlorophenol	T60.1X1	T60.1X2	T60.1X3	T60.1X4	—	—
(pesticide)						
fungicide	T60.3X1	T60.3X2	T60.3X3	T60.3X4	—	—
herbicide	T60.3X1	T60.3X2	T60.3X3	T60.3X4	—	—
insecticide	T60.1X1	T60.1X2	T60.1X3	T60.1X4	—	—
Pentaerythritol	T46.3X1	T46.3X2	T46.3X3	T46.3X4	T46.3X5	T46.3X6
chloral	T42.6X1	T42.6X2	T42.6X3	T42.6X4	T42.6X5	T42.6X6
tetranitrate NEC	T46.3X1	T46.3X2	T46.3X3	T46.3X4	T46.3X5	T46.3X6
Pentaerythrityl tetranitrate	T46.3X1	T46.3X2	T46.3X3	T46.3X4	T46.3X5	T46.3X6
Pentagastrin	T50.8X1	T50.8X2	T50.8X3	T50.8X4	T50.8X5	T50.8X6
Pentalin	T53.6X1	T53.6X2	T53.6X3	T53.6X4	—	—
Pentamethonium bromide	T44.2X1	T44.2X2	T44.2X3	T44.2X4	T44.2X5	T44.2X6
Pentamidine	T37.3X1	T37.3X2	T37.3X3	T37.3X4	T37.3X5	T37.3X6
Pentanol	T51.3X1	T51.3X2	T51.3X3	T51.3X4	—	—
Pentapyrrolinium	T44.2X1	T44.2X2	T44.2X3	T44.2X4	T44.2X5	T44.2X6
(bitartrate)						
Pentaquine	T37.2X1	T37.2X2	T37.2X3	T37.2X4	T37.2X5	T37.2X6
Pentazocine	T40.4X1	T40.4X2	T40.4X3	T40.4X4	T40.4X5	T40.4X6
Pentetrazole	T50.7X1	T50.7X2	T50.7X3	T50.7X4	T50.7X5	T50.7X6
Penthienate bromide	T44.3X1	T44.3X2	T44.3X3	T44.3X4	T44.3X5	T44.3X6
Pentifylline	T46.7X1	T46.7X2	T46.7X3	T46.7X4	T46.7X5	T46.7X6
Pentobarbital	T42.3X1	T42.3X2	T42.3X3	T42.3X4	T42.3X5	T42.3X6
sodium	T42.3X1	T42.3X2	T42.3X3	T42.3X4	T42.3X5	T42.3X6
Pentobarbitone	T42.3X1	T42.3X2	T42.3X3	T42.3X4	T42.3X5	T42.3X6
Pentolonium tartrate	T44.2X1	T44.2X2	T44.2X3	T44.2X4	T44.2X5	T44.2X6
Pentosan polysulfate	T39.8X1	T39.8X2	T39.8X3	T39.8X4	T39.8X5	T39.8X6
(sodium)						
Pentostatin	T45.1X1	T45.1X2	T45.1X3	T45.1X4	T45.1X5	T45.1X6
Pentothal	T41.1X1	T41.1X2	T41.1X3	T41.1X4	T41.1X5	T41.1X6
Pentoxifylline	T46.7X1	T46.7X2	T46.7X3	T46.7X4	T46.7X5	T46.7X6
Pentoxyverine	T48.3X1	T48.3X2	T48.3X3	T48.3X4	T48.3X5	T48.3X6
Pentrinat	T46.3X1	T46.3X2	T46.3X3	T46.3X4	T46.3X5	T46.3X6
Pentylenetetrazole	T50.7X1	T50.7X2	T50.7X3	T50.7X4	T50.7X5	T50.7X6
Pentylsalicylamide	T37.1X1	T37.1X2	T37.1X3	T37.1X4	T37.1X5	T37.1X6
Pentymal	T42.3X1	T42.3X2	T42.3X3	T42.3X4	T42.3X5	T42.3X6
Peplomycin	T45.1X1	T45.1X2	T45.1X3	T45.1X4	T45.1X5	T45.1X6
Peppermint (oil)	T47.5X1	T47.5X2	T47.5X3	T47.5X4	T47.5X5	T47.5X6
Pepsin	T47.5X1	T47.5X2	T47.5X3	T47.5X4	T47.5X5	T47.5X6
digestant	T47.5X1	T47.5X2	T47.5X3	T47.5X4	T47.5X5	T47.5X6
Pepstatin	T47.1X1	T47.1X2	T47.1X3	T47.1X4	T47.1X5	T47.1X6
Peptavlon	T50.8X1	T50.8X2	T50.8X3	T50.8X4	T50.8X5	T50.8X6
Perazine	T43.3X1	T43.3X2	T43.3X3	T43.3X4	T43.3X5	T43.3X6
Percaine (spinal)	T41.3X1	T41.3X2	T41.3X3	T41.3X4	T41.3X5	T41.3X6
topical (surface)	T41.3X1	T41.3X2	T41.3X3	T41.3X4	T41.3X5	T41.3X6
Perchloroethylene	T53.3X1	T53.3X2	T53.3X3	T53.3X4	—	—
medicinal	T37.4X1	T37.4X2	T37.4X3	T37.4X4	T37.4X5	T37.4X6
vapor	T53.3X1	T53.3X2	T53.3X3	T53.3X4	—	—
Percodan	T40.2X1	T40.2X2	T40.2X3	T40.2X4	T40.2X5	T40.2X6

Substance	Poisoning, Accidental (unintentional)	Poisoning, Intentional Self-harm	Poisoning, Assault	Poisoning, Undetermined	Adverse Effect	Under-dosing
Percogesic — *see also* acetaminophen	T45.0X1	T45.0X2	T45.0X3	T45.0X4	T45.0X5	T45.0X6
Percorten	T38.0X1	T38.0X2	T38.0X3	T38.0X4	T38.0X5	T38.0X6
Pergolide	T42.8X1	T42.8X2	T42.8X3	T42.8X4	T42.8X5	T42.8X6
Pergonal	T38.811	T38.812	T38.813	T38.814	T38.815	T38.816
Perhexilene	T46.3X1	T46.3X2	T46.3X3	T46.3X4	T46.3X5	T46.3X6
Perhexiline (maleate)	T46.3X1	T46.3X2	T46.3X3	T46.3X4	T46.3X5	T46.3X6
Periactin	T45.0X1	T45.0X2	T45.0X3	T45.0X4	T45.0X5	T45.0X6
Periciazine	T43.3X1	T43.3X2	T43.3X3	T43.3X4	T43.3X5	T43.3X6
Periclor	T42.6X1	T42.6X2	T42.6X3	T42.6X4	T42.6X5	T42.6X6
Perindopril	T46.4X1	T46.4X2	T46.4X3	T46.4X4	T46.4X5	T46.4X6
Perisoxal	T39.8X1	T39.8X2	T39.8X3	T39.8X4	T39.8X5	T39.8X6
Peritoneal dialysis solution	T50.3X1	T50.3X2	T50.3X3	T50.3X4	T50.3X5	T50.3X6
Peritrate	T46.3X1	T46.3X2	T46.3X3	T46.3X4	T46.3X5	T46.3X6
Perlapine	T42.4X1	T42.4X2	T42.4X3	T42.4X4	T42.4X5	T42.4X6
Permanganate	T65.891	T65.892	T65.893	T65.894	—	—
Permethrin	T60.1X1	T60.1X2	T60.1X3	T60.1X4	—	—
Pernocton	T42.3X1	T42.3X2	T42.3X3	T42.3X4	T42.3X5	T42.3X6
Pernoston	T42.3X1	T42.3X2	T42.3X3	T42.3X4	T42.3X5	T42.3X6
Peronine	T40.2X1	T40.2X2	T40.2X3	T40.2X4	—	—
Perphenazine	T43.3X1	T43.3X2	T43.3X3	T43.3X4	T43.3X5	T43.3X6
Pertofrane	T43.011	T43.012	T43.013	T43.014	T43.015	T43.016
Pertussis						
immune serum (human)	T50.Z11	T50.Z12	T50.Z13	T50.Z14	T50.Z15	T50.Z16
vaccine (with diphtheria toxoid) (with tetanus toxoid)	T50.A11	T50.A12	T50.A13	T50.A14	T50.A15	T50.A16
Peruvian balsam	T49.0X1	T49.0X2	T49.0X3	T49.0X4	T49.0X5	T49.0X6
Peruvoside	T46.0X1	T46.0X2	T46.0X3	T46.0X4	T46.0X5	T46.0X6
Pesticide (dust) (fumes) (vapor)	T60.91	T60.92	T60.93	T60.94	—	—
NEC						
arsenic	T57.0X1	T57.0X2	T57.0X3	T57.0X4	—	—
chlorinated	T60.1X1	T60.1X2	T60.1X3	T60.1X4	—	—
cyanide	T65.0X1	T65.0X2	T65.0X3	T65.0X4	—	—
kerosene	T52.0X1	T52.0X2	T52.0X3	T52.0X4	—	—
mixture (of compounds)	T60.91	T60.92	T60.93	T60.94	—	—
naphthalene	T60.2X1	T60.2X2	T60.2X3	T60.2X4	—	—
organochlorine (compounds)	T60.1X1	T60.1X2	T60.1X3	T60.1X4	—	—
petroleum (distillate) (products) NEC	T60.8X1	T60.8X2	T60.8X3	T60.8X4	—	—
specified ingredient NEC	T60.8X1	T60.8X2	T60.8X3	T60.8X4	—	—
strychnine	T65.1X1	T65.1X2	T65.1X3	T65.1X4	—	—
thallium	T60.4X1	T60.4X2	T60.4X3	T60.4X4	—	—
Pethidine	T40.4X1	T40.4X2	T40.4X3	T40.4X4	T40.4X5	T40.4X6
Petrichloral	T42.6X1	T42.6X2	T42.6X3	T42.6X4	T42.6X5	T42.6X6
Petrol	T52.0X1	T52.0X2	T52.0X3	T52.0X4	—	—
vapor	T52.0X1	T52.0X2	T52.0X3	T52.0X4	—	—
Petrolatum	T49.3X1	T49.3X2	T49.3X3	T49.3X4	T49.3X5	T49.3X6
hydrophilic	T49.3X1	T49.3X2	T49.3X3	T49.3X4	T49.3X5	T49.3X6
liquid	T47.4X1	T47.4X2	T47.4X3	T47.4X4	T47.4X5	T47.4X6
topical	T49.3X1	T49.3X2	T49.3X3	T49.3X4	T49.3X5	T49.3X6
nonmedicinal	T52.0X1	T52.0X2	T52.0X3	T52.0X4	—	—
red veterinary	T49.3X1	T49.3X2	T49.3X3	T49.3X4	T49.3X5	T49.3X6
white	T49.3X1	T49.3X2	T49.3X3	T49.3X4	T49.3X5	T49.3X6
Petroleum (products) **NEC**	T52.0X1	T52.0X2	T52.0X3	T52.0X4	—	—
benzine(s) — *see* Ligroin						
ether — *see* Ligroin						
jelly — *see* Petrolatum						
naphtha — *see* Ligroin						
pesticide	T60.8X1	T60.8X2	T60.8X3	T60.8X4	—	—
solids	T52.0X1	T52.0X2	T52.0X3	T52.0X4	—	—
solvents	T52.0X1	T52.0X2	T52.0X3	T52.0X4	—	—
vapor	T52.0X1	T52.0X2	T52.0X3	T52.0X4	—	—
Peyote	T40.991	T40.992	T40.993	T40.994	—	—
Phanodorm, phanodorn	T42.3X1	T42.3X2	T42.3X3	T42.3X4	T42.3X5	T42.3X6
Phanquinone	T37.3X1	T37.3X2	T37.3X3	T37.3X4	T37.3X5	T37.3X6
Phanquone	T37.3X1	T37.3X2	T37.3X3	T37.3X4	T37.3X5	T37.3X6
Pharmaceutical						
adjunct NEC	T50.901	T50.902	T50.903	T50.904	T50.905	T50.906
excipient NEC	T50.901	T50.902	T50.903	T50.904	T50.905	T50.906
sweetener	T50.901	T50.902	T50.903	T50.904	T50.905	T50.906
viscous agent	T50.901	T50.902	T50.903	T50.904	T50.905	T50.906
Phemitone	T42.3X1	T42.3X2	T42.3X3	T42.3X4	T42.3X5	T42.3X6
Phenacaine	T41.3X1	T41.3X2	T41.3X3	T41.3X4	T41.3X5	T41.3X6
Phenacemide	T42.6X1	T42.6X2	T42.6X3	T42.6X4	T42.6X5	T42.6X6
Phenacetin	T39.1X1	T39.1X2	T39.1X3	T39.1X4	T39.1X5	T39.1X6
Phenadoxone	T40.2X1	T40.2X2	T40.2X3	T40.2X4	—	—
Phenaglycodol	T43.591	T43.592	T43.593	T43.594	T43.595	T43.596
Phenantoin	T42.0X1	T42.0X2	T42.0X3	T42.0X4	T42.0X5	T42.0X6
Phenaphthazine reagent	T50.991	T50.992	T50.993	T50.994	T50.995	T50.996
Phenazocine	T40.4X1	T40.4X2	T40.4X3	T40.4X4	T40.4X5	T40.4X6
Phenazone	T39.2X1	T39.2X2	T39.2X3	T39.2X4	T39.2X5	T39.2X6

Additional Character May Be Required — Refer to the Tabular List for Character Selection   ▽ Subterms under main terms may continue to next column or page

Substance	Poisoning, Accidental (unintentional)	Poisoning, Intentional Self-harm	Poisoning, Assault	Poisoning, Undetermined	Adverse Effect	Under-dosing
Phenazopyridine	T39.8X1	T39.8X2	T39.8X3	T39.8X4	T39.8X5	T39.8X6
Phenbenicillin	T36.0X1	T36.0X2	T36.0X3	T36.0X4	T36.0X5	T36.0X6
Phenbutrazate	T50.5X1	T50.5X2	T50.5X3	T50.5X4	T50.5X5	T50.5X6
Phencyclidine	T40.991	T40.992	T40.993	T40.994	T40.995	T40.996
Phendimetrazine	T50.5X1	T50.5X2	T50.5X3	T50.5X4	T50.5X5	T50.5X6
Phenelzine	T43.1X1	T43.1X2	T43.1X3	T43.1X4	T43.1X5	T43.1X6
Phenemal	T42.3X1	T42.3X2	T42.3X3	T42.3X4	T42.3X5	T42.3X6
Phenergan	T42.6X1	T42.6X2	T42.6X3	T42.6X4	T42.6X5	T42.6X6
Pheneticillin	T36.0X1	T36.0X2	T36.0X3	T36.0X4	T36.0X5	T36.0X6
Pheneturide	T42.6X1	T42.6X2	T42.6X3	T42.6X4	T42.6X5	T42.6X6
Phenformin	T38.3X1	T38.3X2	T38.3X3	T38.3X4	T38.3X5	T38.3X6
Phenglutarimide	T44.3X1	T44.3X2	T44.3X3	T44.3X4	T44.3X5	T44.3X6
Phenicarbazide	T39.8X1	T39.8X2	T39.8X3	T39.8X4	T39.8X5	T39.8X6
Phenindamine	T45.0X1	T45.0X2	T45.0X3	T45.0X4	T45.0X5	T45.0X6
Phenindione	T45.511	T45.512	T45.513	T45.514	T45.515	T45.516
Pheniprazine	T43.1X1	T43.1X2	T43.1X3	T43.1X4	T43.1X5	T43.1X6
Pheniramine	T45.0X1	T45.0X2	T45.0X3	T45.0X4	T45.0X5	T45.0X6
Phenisatin	T47.2X1	T47.2X2	T47.2X3	T47.2X4	T47.2X5	T47.2X6
Phenmetrazine	T50.5X1	T50.5X2	T50.5X3	T50.5X4	T50.5X5	T50.5X6
Phenobal	T42.3X1	T42.3X2	T42.3X3	T42.3X4	T42.3X5	T42.3X6
Phenobarbital	T42.3X1	T42.3X2	T42.3X3	T42.3X4	T42.3X5	T42.3X6
with						
mephenytoin	T42.3X1	T42.3X2	T42.3X3	T42.3X4	T42.3X5	T42.3X6
phenytoin	T42.3X1	T42.3X2	T42.3X3	T42.3X4	T42.3X5	T42.3X6
sodium	T42.3X1	T42.3X2	T42.3X3	T42.3X4	T42.3X5	T42.3X6
Phenobarbitone	T42.3X1	T42.3X2	T42.3X3	T42.3X4	T42.3X5	T42.3X6
Phenobutiodil	T50.8X1	T50.8X2	T50.8X3	T50.8X4	T50.8X5	T50.8X6
Phenoctide	T49.0X1	T49.0X2	T49.0X3	T49.0X4	T49.0X5	T49.0X6
Phenol	T49.0X1	T49.0X2	T49.0X3	T49.0X4	T49.0X5	T49.0X6
disinfectant	T54.0X1	T54.0X2	T54.0X3	T54.0X4	—	—
in oil injection	T46.8X1	T46.8X2	T46.8X3	T46.8X4	T46.8X5	T46.8X6
medicinal	T49.1X1	T49.1X2	T49.1X3	T49.1X4	T49.1X5	T49.1X6
nonmedicinal NEC	T54.0X1	T54.0X2	T54.0X3	T54.0X4	—	—
pesticide	T60.8X1	T60.8X2	T60.8X3	T60.8X4	—	—
red	T50.8X1	T50.8X2	T50.8X3	T50.8X4	T50.8X5	T50.8X6
Phenolic preparation	T49.1X1	T49.1X2	T49.1X3	T49.1X4	T49.1X5	T49.1X6
Phenolphthalein	T47.2X1	T47.2X2	T47.2X3	T47.2X4	T47.2X5	T47.2X6
Phenolsulfonphthalein	T50.8X1	T50.8X2	T50.8X3	T50.8X4	T50.8X5	T50.8X6
Phenomorphan	T40.2X1	T40.2X2	T40.2X3	T40.2X4		
Phenonyl	T42.3X1	T42.3X2	T42.3X3	T42.3X4	T42.3X5	T42.3X6
Phenoperidine	T40.4X1	T40.4X2	T40.4X3	T40.4X4	—	—
Phenopyrazone	T46.991	T46.992	T46.993	T46.994	T46.995	T46.996
Phenoquin	T50.4X1	T50.4X2	T50.4X3	T50.4X4	T50.4X5	T50.4X6
Phenothiazine (psychotropic)	T43.3X1	T43.3X2	T43.3X3	T43.3X4	T43.3X5	T43.3X6
NEC						
insecticide	T60.2X1	T60.2X2	T60.2X3	T60.2X4	—	—
Phenothrin	T49.0X1	T49.0X2	T49.0X3	T49.0X4	T49.0X5	T49.0X6
Phenoxybenzamine	T46.7X1	T46.7X2	T46.7X3	T46.7X4	T46.7X5	T46.7X6
Phenoxyethanol	T49.0X1	T49.0X2	T49.0X3	T49.0X4	T49.0X5	T49.0X6
Phenoxymethyl penicillin	T36.0X1	T36.0X2	T36.0X3	T36.0X4	T36.0X5	T36.0X6
Phenprobamate	T42.8X1	T42.8X2	T42.8X3	T42.8X4	T42.8X5	T42.8X6
Phenprocoumon	T45.511	T45.512	T45.513	T45.514	T45.515	T45.516
Phensuximide	T42.2X1	T42.2X2	T42.2X3	T42.2X4	T42.2X5	T42.2X6
Phentermine	T50.5X1	T50.5X2	T50.5X3	T50.5X4	T50.5X5	T50.5X6
Phenthicillin	T36.0X1	T36.0X2	T36.0X3	T36.0X4	T36.0X5	T36.0X6
Phentolamine	T46.7X1	T46.7X2	T46.7X3	T46.7X4	T46.7X5	T46.7X6
Phenyl						
butazone	T39.2X1	T39.2X2	T39.2X3	T39.2X4	T39.2X5	T39.2X6
enediamine	T65.3X1	T65.3X2	T65.3X3	T65.3X4	—	—
hydrazine	T65.3X1	T65.3X2	T65.3X3	T65.3X4	—	—
antineoplastic	T45.1X1	T45.1X2	T45.1X3	T45.1X4	T45.1X5	T45.1X6
mercuric compounds — see						
Mercury						
salicylate	T49.3X1	T49.3X2	T49.3X3	T49.3X4	T49.3X5	T49.3X6
Phenylalanine mustard	T45.1X1	T45.1X2	T45.1X3	T45.1X4	T45.1X5	T45.1X6
Phenylbutazone	T39.2X1	T39.2X2	T39.2X3	T39.2X4	T39.2X5	T39.2X6
Phenylenediamine	T65.3X1	T65.3X2	T65.3X3	T65.3X4	—	—
Phenylephrine	T44.4X1	T44.4X2	T44.4X3	T44.4X4	T44.4X5	T44.4X6
Phenylethylbiguanide	T38.3X1	T38.3X2	T38.3X3	T38.3X4	T38.3X5	T38.3X6
Phenylmercuric						
acetate	T49.0X1	T49.0X2	T49.0X3	T49.0X4	T49.0X5	T49.0X6
borate	T49.0X1	T49.0X2	T49.0X3	T49.0X4	T49.0X5	T49.0X6
nitrate	T49.0X1	T49.0X2	T49.0X3	T49.0X4	T49.0X5	T49.0X6
Phenylmethylbarbitone	T42.3X1	T42.3X2	T42.3X3	T42.3X4	T42.3X5	T42.3X6
Phenylpropanol	T47.5X1	T47.5X2	T47.5X3	T47.5X4	T47.5X5	T47.5X6
Phenylpropanolamine	T44.991	T44.992	T44.993	T44.994	T44.995	T44.996
Phenylsulfthion	T60.0X1	T60.0X2	T60.0X3	T60.0X4	—	—
Phenyltoloxamine	T45.0X1	T45.0X2	T45.0X3	T45.0X4	T45.0X5	T45.0X6
Phenyramidol,	T39.8X1	T39.8X2	T39.8X3	T39.8X4	T39.8X5	T39.8X6
phenyramidon						
Phenytoin	T42.0X1	T42.0X2	T42.0X3	T42.0X4	T42.0X5	T42.0X6
with Phenobarbital	T42.3X1	T42.3X2	T42.3X3	T42.3X4	T42.3X5	T42.3X6
pHisoHex	T49.2X1	T49.2X2	T49.2X3	T49.2X4	T49.2X5	T49.2X6

Substance	Poisoning, Accidental (unintentional)	Poisoning, Intentional Self-harm	Poisoning, Assault	Poisoning, Undetermined	Adverse Effect	Under-dosing
Pholcodine	T48.3X1	T48.3X2	T48.3X3	T48.3X4	T48.3X5	T48.3X6
Pholedrine	T46.991	T46.992	T46.993	T46.994	T46.995	T46.996
Phorate	T60.0X1	T60.0X2	T60.0X3	T60.0X4	—	—
Phosdrin	T60.0X1	T60.0X2	T60.0X3	T60.0X4	—	—
Phosfolan	T60.0X1	T60.0X2	T60.0X3	T60.0X4	—	—
Phosgene (gas)	T59.891	T59.892	T59.893	T59.894	—	—
Phosphamidon	T60.0X1	T60.0X2	T60.0X3	T60.0X4	—	—
Phosphate	T65.891	T65.892	T65.893	T65.894	—	—
laxative	T47.4X1	T47.4X2	T47.4X3	T47.4X4	T47.4X5	T47.4X6
organic	T60.0X1	T60.0X2	T60.0X3	T60.0X4	—	—
solvent	T52.91	T52.92	T52.93	T52.94	—	—
tricresyl	T65.891	T65.892	T65.893	T65.894	—	—
Phosphine	T57.1X1	T57.1X2	T57.1X3	T57.1X4	—	—
fumigant	T57.1X1	T57.1X2	T57.1X3	T57.1X4	—	—
Phospholine	T49.5X1	T49.5X2	T49.5X3	T49.5X4	T49.5X5	T49.5X6
Phosphoric acid	T54.2X1	T54.2X2	T54.2X3	T54.2X4	—	—
Phosphorus (compound)	T57.1X1	T57.1X2	T57.1X3	T57.1X4	—	—
NEC						
	T60.0X1	T60.0X2	T60.0X3	T60.0X4	—	—
pesticide	T60.0X1	T60.0X2	T60.0X3	T60.0X4	—	—
Phthalates	T65.891	T65.892	T65.893	T65.894	—	—
Phthalic anhydride	T65.891	T65.892	T65.893	T65.894	—	—
Phthalimidoglutarimide	T42.6X1	T42.6X2	T42.6X3	T42.6X4	T42.6X5	T42.6X6
Phthalylsulfathiazole	T37.0X1	T37.0X2	T37.0X3	T37.0X4	T37.0X5	T37.0X6
Phylloquinone	T45.7X1	T45.7X2	T45.7X3	T45.7X4	T45.7X5	T45.7X6
Physeptone	T40.3X1	T40.3X2	T40.3X3	T40.3X4	T40.3X5	T40.3X6
Physostigma venenosum	T62.2X1	T62.2X2	T62.2X3	T62.2X4		
Physostigmine	T49.5X1	T49.5X2	T49.5X3	T49.5X4	T49.5X5	T49.5X6
Phytolacca decandra	T62.2X1	T62.2X2	T62.2X3	T62.2X4		
berries	T62.1X1	T62.1X2	T62.1X3	T62.1X4		
Phytomenadione	T45.7X1	T45.7X2	T45.7X3	T45.7X4	T45.7X5	T45.7X6
Phytonadione	T45.7X1	T45.7X2	T45.7X3	T45.7X4	T45.7X5	T45.7X6
Picoperine	T48.3X1	T48.3X2	T48.3X3	T48.3X4	T48.3X5	T48.3X6
Picosulfate (sodium)	T47.2X1	T47.2X2	T47.2X3	T47.2X4	T47.2X5	T47.2X6
Picric (acid)	T54.2X1	T54.2X2	T54.2X3	T54.2X4		
Picrotoxin	T50.7X1	T50.7X2	T50.7X3	T50.7X4	T50.7X5	T50.7X6
Piketoprofen	T49.0X1	T49.0X2	T49.0X3	T49.0X4	T49.0X5	T49.0X6
Pilocarpine	T44.1X1	T44.1X2	T44.1X3	T44.1X4	T44.1X5	T44.1X6
Pilocarpus (jaborandi)	T44.1X1	T44.1X2	T44.1X3	T44.1X4	T44.1X5	T44.1X6
extract						
Pilsicainide (hydrochloride)	T46.2X1	T46.2X2	T46.2X3	T46.2X4	T46.2X5	T46.2X6
Pimaricin	T36.7X1	T36.7X2	T36.7X3	T36.7X4	T36.7X5	T36.7X6
Pimeclone	T50.7X1	T50.7X2	T50.7X3	T50.7X4	T50.7X5	T50.7X6
Pimelic ketone	T52.8X1	T52.8X2	T52.8X3	T52.8X4		
Pimethixene	T45.0X1	T45.0X2	T45.0X3	T45.0X4	T45.0X5	T45.0X6
Piminodine	T40.2X1	T40.2X2	T40.2X3	T40.2X4	T40.2X5	T40.2X6
Pimozide	T43.591	T43.592	T43.593	T43.594	T43.595	T43.596
Pinacidil	T46.5X1	T46.5X2	T46.5X3	T46.5X4	T46.5X5	T46.5X6
Pinaverium bromide	T44.3X1	T44.3X2	T44.3X3	T44.3X4	T44.3X5	T44.3X6
Pinazepam	T42.4X1	T42.4X2	T42.4X3	T42.4X4	T42.4X5	T42.4X6
Pindolol	T44.7X1	T44.7X2	T44.7X3	T44.7X4	T44.7X5	T44.7X6
Pindone	T60.4X1	T60.4X2	T60.4X3	T60.4X4	—	—
Pine oil (disinfectant)	T65.891	T65.892	T65.893	T65.894		
Pinkroot	T37.4X1	T37.4X2	T37.4X3	T37.4X4	T37.4X5	T37.4X6
Pipadone	T40.2X1	T40.2X2	T40.2X3	T40.2X4		
Pipamazine	T45.0X1	T45.0X2	T45.0X3	T45.0X4	T45.0X5	T45.0X6
Pipamperone	T43.4X1	T43.4X2	T43.4X3	T43.4X4	T43.4X5	T43.4X6
Pipazetate	T48.3X1	T48.3X2	T48.3X3	T48.3X4	T48.3X5	T48.3X6
Pipemidic acid	T37.8X1	T37.8X2	T37.8X3	T37.8X4	T37.8X5	T37.8X6
Pipenzolate bromide	T44.3X1	T44.3X2	T44.3X3	T44.3X4	T44.3X5	T44.3X6
Piperacetazine	T43.3X1	T43.3X2	T43.3X3	T43.3X4	T43.3X5	T43.3X6
Piperacillin	T36.0X1	T36.0X2	T36.0X3	T36.0X4	T36.0X5	T36.0X6
Piperazine	T37.4X1	T37.4X2	T37.4X3	T37.4X4	T37.4X5	T37.4X6
estrone sulfate	T38.5X1	T38.5X2	T38.5X3	T38.5X4	T38.5X5	T38.5X6
Piper cubeba	T62.2X1	T62.2X2	T62.2X3	T62.2X4		
Piperidione	T48.3X1	T48.3X2	T48.3X3	T48.3X4	T48.3X5	T48.3X6
Piperidolate	T44.3X1	T44.3X2	T44.3X3	T44.3X4	T44.3X5	T44.3X6
Piperocaine	T41.3X1	T41.3X2	T41.3X3	T41.3X4	T41.3X5	T41.3X6
infiltration (subcutaneous)	T41.3X1	T41.3X2	T41.3X3	T41.3X4	T41.3X5	T41.3X6
nerve block (peripheral)	T41.3X1	T41.3X2	T41.3X3	T41.3X4	T41.3X5	T41.3X6
(plexus)						
topical (surface)	T41.3X1	T41.3X2	T41.3X3	T41.3X4	T41.3X5	T41.3X6
Piperonyl butoxide	T60.8X1	T60.8X2	T60.8X3	T60.8X4	—	—
Pipethanate	T44.3X1	T44.3X2	T44.3X3	T44.3X4	T44.3X5	T44.3X6
Pipobroman	T45.1X1	T45.1X2	T45.1X3	T45.1X4	T45.1X5	T45.1X6
Pipotiazine	T43.3X1	T43.3X2	T43.3X3	T43.3X4	T43.3X5	T43.3X6
Pipoxizine	T45.0X1	T45.0X2	T45.0X3	T45.0X4	T45.0X5	T45.0X6
Pipradrol	T43.691	T43.692	T43.693	T43.694	T43.695	T43.696
Piprinhydrinate	T45.0X1	T45.0X2	T45.0X3	T45.0X4	T45.0X5	T45.0X6
Pirarubicin	T45.1X1	T45.1X2	T45.1X3	T45.1X4	T45.1X5	T45.1X6
Pirazinamide	T37.1X1	T37.1X2	T37.1X3	T37.1X4	T37.1X5	T37.1X6
Pirbuterol	T48.6X1	T48.6X2	T48.6X3	T48.6X4	T48.6X5	T48.6X6
Pirenzepine	T47.1X1	T47.1X2	T47.1X3	T47.1X4	T47.1X5	T47.1X6
Piretanide	T50.1X1	T50.1X2	T50.1X3	T50.1X4	T50.1X5	T50.1X6

Substance	Poisoning, Accidental (unintentional)	Poisoning, Intentional Self-harm	Poisoning, Assault	Poisoning, Undetermined	Adverse Effect	Under-dosing
Piribedil	T42.8X1	T42.8X2	T42.8X3	T42.8X4	T42.8X5	T42.8X6
Piridoxilate	T46.3X1	T46.3X2	T46.3X3	T46.3X4	T46.3X5	T46.3X6
Piritramide	T40.4X1	T40.4X2	T40.4X3	T40.4X4		
Piromidic acid	T37.8X1	T37.8X2	T37.8X3	T37.8X4	T37.8X5	T37.8X6
Piroxicam	T39.391	T39.392	T39.393	T39.394	T39.395	T39.396
beta-cyclodextrin complex	T39.8X1	T39.8X2	T39.8X3	T39.8X4	T39.8X5	T39.8X6
Pirozadil	T46.6X1	T46.6X2	T46.6X3	T46.6X4	T46.6X5	T46.6X6
Piscidia (bark) (erythrina)	T39.8X1	T39.8X2	T39.8X3	T39.8X4	T39.8X5	T39.8X6
Pitch	T65.891	T65.892	T65.893	T65.894		
Pitkin's solution	T41.3X1	T41.3X2	T41.3X3	T41.3X4	T41.3X5	T41.3X6
Pitocin	T48.0X1	T48.0X2	T48.0X3	T48.0X4	T48.0X5	T48.0X6
Pitressin (tannate)	T38.891	T38.892	T38.893	T38.894	T38.895	T38.896
Pituitary extracts	T38.891	T38.892	T38.893	T38.894	T38.895	T38.896
(posterior)						
anterior	T38.811	T38.812	T38.813	T38.814	T38.815	T38.816
Pituitrin	T38.891	T38.892	T38.893	T38.894	T38.895	T38.896
Pivampicillin	T36.0X1	T36.0X2	T36.0X3	T36.0X4	T36.0X5	T36.0X6
Pivmecillinam	T36.0X1	T36.0X2	T36.0X3	T36.0X4	T36.0X5	T36.0X6
Placental hormone	T38.891	T38.892	T38.893	T38.894	T38.895	T38.896
Placidyl	T42.6X1	T42.6X2	T42.6X3	T42.6X4	T42.6X5	T42.6X6
Plague vaccine	T50.A91	T50.A92	T50.A93	T50.A94	T50.A95	T50.A96
Plant						
food or fertilizer NEC	T65.891	T65.892	T65.893	T65.894	—	—
containing herbicide	T60.3X1	T60.3X2	T60.3X3	T60.3X4	—	—
noxious, used as food	T62.2X1	T62.2X2	T62.2X3	T62.2X4	—	—
berries	T62.1X1	T62.1X2	T62.1X3	T62.1X4	—	—
seeds	T62.2X1	T62.2X2	T62.2X3	T62.2X4	—	—
specified type NEC	T62.2X1	T62.2X2	T62.2X3	T62.2X4	—	—
Plasma	T45.8X1	T45.8X2	T45.8X3	T45.8X4	T45.8X5	T45.8X6
expander NEC	T45.8X1	T45.8X2	T45.8X3	T45.8X4	T45.8X5	T45.8X6
protein fraction (human)	T45.8X1	T45.8X2	T45.8X3	T45.8X4	T45.8X5	T45.8X6
Plasmanate	T45.8X1	T45.8X2	T45.8X3	T45.8X4	T45.8X5	T45.8X6
Plasminogen (tissue)	T45.611	T45.612	T45.613	T45.614	T45.615	T45.616
activator						
Plaster dressing	T49.3X1	T49.3X2	T49.3X3	T49.3X4	T49.3X5	T49.3X6
Plastic dressing	T49.3X1	T49.3X2	T49.3X3	T49.3X4	T49.3X5	T49.3X6
Plegicil	T43.3X1	T43.3X2	T43.3X3	T43.3X4	T43.3X5	T43.3X6
Plicamycin	T45.1X1	T45.1X2	T45.1X3	T45.1X4	T45.1X5	T45.1X6
Podophyllotoxin	T49.8X1	T49.8X2	T49.8X3	T49.8X4	T49.8X5	T49.8X6
Podophyllum (resin)	T49.4X1	T49.4X2	T49.4X3	T49.4X4	T49.4X5	T49.4X6
Poisonous berries	T62.1X1	T62.1X2	T62.1X3	T62.1X4	—	—
Poison NEC	T65.91	T65.92	T65.93	T65.94	—	—
Pokeweed (any part)	T62.2X1	T62.2X2	T62.2X3	T62.2X4	—	—
Poldine metilsulfate	T44.3X1	T44.3X2	T44.3X3	T44.3X4	T44.3X5	T44.3X6
Polidexide (sulfate)	T46.6X1	T46.6X2	T46.6X3	T46.6X4	T46.6X5	T46.6X6
Polidocanol	T46.8X1	T46.8X2	T46.8X3	T46.8X4	T46.8X5	T46.8X6
Poliomyelitis vaccine	T50.B91	T50.B92	T50.B93	T50.B94	T50.B95	T50.B96
Polish (car) (floor) (furniture)	T65.891	T65.892	T65.893	T65.894		
(metal) (porcelain)						
(silver)						
abrasive	T65.891	T65.892	T65.893	T65.894	—	—
porcelain	T65.891	T65.892	T65.893	T65.894	—	—
Poloxalkol	T47.4X1	T47.4X2	T47.4X3	T47.4X4	T47.4X5	T47.4X6
Poloxamer	T47.4X1	T47.4X2	T47.4X3	T47.4X4	T47.4X5	T47.4X6
Polyaminostyrene resins	T50.3X1	T50.3X2	T50.3X3	T50.3X4	T50.3X5	T50.3X6
Polycarbophil	T47.4X1	T47.4X2	T47.4X3	T47.4X4	T47.4X5	T47.4X6
Polychlorinated biphenyl	T65.891	T65.892	T65.893	T65.894	—	—
Polycycline	T36.4X1	T36.4X2	T36.4X3	T36.4X4	T36.4X5	T36.4X6
Polyester fumes	T59.891	T59.892	T59.893	T59.894	—	—
Polyester resin hardener	T52.91	T52.92	T52.93	T52.94	—	—
fumes	T59.891	T59.892	T59.893	T59.894	—	—
Polyestradiol phosphate	T38.5X1	T38.5X2	T38.5X3	T38.5X4	T38.5X5	T38.5X6
Polyethanolamine alkyl	T49.2X1	T49.2X2	T49.2X3	T49.2X4	T49.2X5	T49.2X6
sulfate						
Polyethylene adhesive	T49.3X1	T49.3X2	T49.3X3	T49.3X4	T49.3X5	T49.3X6
Polyferose	T45.4X1	T45.4X2	T45.4X3	T45.4X4	T45.4X5	T45.4X6
Polygeline	T45.8X1	T45.8X2	T45.8X3	T45.8X4	T45.8X5	T45.8X6
Polymyxin	T36.8X1	T36.8X2	T36.8X3	T36.8X4	T36.8X5	T36.8X6
B	T36.8X1	T36.8X2	T36.8X3	T36.8X4	T36.8X5	T36.8X6
ENT agent	T49.6X1	T49.6X2	T49.6X3	T49.6X4	T49.6X5	T49.6X6
ophthalmic preparation	T49.5X1	T49.5X2	T49.5X3	T49.5X4	T49.5X5	T49.5X6
topical NEC	T49.0X1	T49.0X2	T49.0X3	T49.0X4	T49.0X5	T49.0X6
E sulfate (eye preparation)	T49.5X1	T49.5X2	T49.5X3	T49.5X4	T49.5X5	T49.5X6
Polynoxylin	T49.0X1	T49.0X2	T49.0X3	T49.0X4	T49.0X5	T49.0X6
Polyoestradiol phosphate	T38.5X1	T38.5X2	T38.5X3	T38.5X4	T38.5X5	T38.5X6
Polyoxymethyleneurea	T49.0X1	T49.0X2	T49.0X3	T49.0X4	T49.0X5	T49.0X6
Polysilane	T47.8X1	T47.8X2	T47.8X3	T47.8X4	T47.8X5	T47.8X6
Polytetrafluoroethylene	T59.891	T59.892	T59.893	T59.894	—	—
(inhaled)						
Polythiazide	T50.2X1	T50.2X2	T50.2X3	T50.2X4	T50.2X5	T50.2X6
Polyvidone	T45.8X1	T45.8X2	T45.8X3	T45.8X4	T45.8X5	T45.8X6
Polyvinylpyrrolidone	T45.8X1	T45.8X2	T45.8X3	T45.8X4	T45.8X5	T45.8X6

Substance	Poisoning, Accidental (unintentional)	Poisoning, Intentional Self-harm	Poisoning, Assault	Poisoning, Undetermined	Adverse Effect	Under-dosing
Pontocaine (hydrochloride) (infiltration) (topical)	T41.3X1	T41.3X2	T41.3X3	T41.3X4	T41.3X5	T41.3X6
nerve block (peripheral) (plexus)	T41.3X1	T41.3X2	T41.3X3	T41.3X4	T41.3X5	T41.3X6
spinal	T41.3X1	T41.3X2	T41.3X3	T41.3X4	T41.3X5	T41.3X6
Porfiromycin	T45.1X1	T45.1X2	T45.1X3	T45.1X4	T45.1X5	T45.1X6
Posterior pituitary hormone NEC	T38.891	T38.892	T38.893	T38.894	T38.895	T38.896
Pot	T40.7X1	T40.7X2	T40.7X3	T40.7X4	T40.7X5	T40.7X6
Potash (caustic)	T54.3X1	T54.3X2	T54.3X3	T54.3X4	—	—
Potassic saline injection (lactated)	T50.3X1	T50.3X2	T50.3X3	T50.3X4	T50.3X5	T50.3X6
Potassium (salts) NEC	T50.3X1	T50.3X2	T50.3X3	T50.3X4	T50.3X5	T50.3X6
aminobenzoate	T45.8X1	T45.8X2	T45.8X3	T45.8X4	T45.8X5	T45.8X6
aminosalicylate	T37.1X1	T37.1X2	T37.1X3	T37.1X4	T37.1X5	T37.1X6
antimony ' tartrate'	T37.8X1	T37.8X2	T37.8X3	T37.8X4	T37.8X5	T37.8X6
arsenite (solution)	T57.0X1	T57.0X2	T57.0X3	T57.0X4	—	—
bichromate	T56.2X1	T56.2X2	T56.2X3	T56.2X4	—	—
bisulfate	T47.3X1	T47.3X2	T47.3X3	T47.3X4	T47.3X5	T47.3X6
bromide	T42.6X1	T42.6X2	T42.6X3	T42.6X4	T42.6X5	T42.6X6
canrenoate	T50.0X1	T50.0X2	T50.0X3	T50.0X4	T50.0X5	T50.0X6
carbonate	T54.3X1	T54.3X2	T54.3X3	T54.3X4	—	—
chlorate NEC	T65.891	T65.892	T65.893	T65.894	—	—
chloride	T50.3X1	T50.3X2	T50.3X3	T50.3X4	T50.3X5	T50.3X6
citrate	T50.991	T50.992	T50.993	T50.994	T50.995	T50.996
cyanide	T65.0X1	T65.0X2	T65.0X3	T65.0X4	—	—
ferric hexacyanoferrate (medicinal)	T50.6X1	T50.6X2	T50.6X3	T50.6X4	T50.6X5	T50.6X6
nonmedicinal	T65.891	T65.892	T65.893	T65.894	—	—
Fluoride	T57.8X1	T57.8X2	T57.8X3	T57.8X4	—	—
glucaldrate	T47.1X1	T47.1X2	T47.1X3	T47.1X4	T47.1X5	T47.1X6
hydroxide	T54.3X1	T54.3X2	T54.3X3	T54.3X4	—	—
iodate	T49.0X1	T49.0X2	T49.0X3	T49.0X4	T49.0X5	T49.0X6
iodide	T48.4X1	T48.4X2	T48.4X3	T48.4X4	T48.4X5	T48.4X6
nitrate	T57.8X1	T57.8X2	T57.8X3	T57.8X4	—	—
oxalate	T65.891	T65.892	T65.893	T65.894	—	—
perchlorate (nonmedicinal) NEC	T65.891	T65.892	T65.893	T65.894	—	—
antithyroid	T38.2X1	T38.2X2	T38.2X3	T38.2X4	T38.2X5	T38.2X6
medicinal	T38.2X1	T38.2X2	T38.2X3	T38.2X4	T38.2X5	T38.2X6
Permanganate (nonmedicinal)	T65.891	T65.892	T65.893	T65.894	—	—
medicinal	T49.0X1	T49.0X2	T49.0X3	T49.0X4	T49.0X5	T49.0X6
sulfate	T47.2X1	T47.2X2	T47.2X3	T47.2X4	T47.2X5	T47.2X6
Potassium-removing resin	T50.3X1	T50.3X2	T50.3X3	T50.3X4	T50.3X5	T50.3X6
Potassium-retaining drug	T50.3X1	T50.3X2	T50.3X3	T50.3X4	T50.3X5	T50.3X6
Povidone	T45.8X1	T45.8X2	T45.8X3	T45.8X4	T45.8X5	T45.8X6
iodine	T49.0X1	T49.0X2	T49.0X3	T49.0X4	T49.0X5	T49.0X6
Practolol	T44.7X1	T44.7X2	T44.7X3	T44.7X4	T44.7X5	T44.7X6
Prajmalium bitartrate	T46.2X1	T46.2X2	T46.2X3	T46.2X4	T46.2X5	T46.2X6
Pralidoxime (iodide)	T50.6X1	T50.6X2	T50.6X3	T50.6X4	T50.6X5	T50.6X6
chloride	T50.6X1	T50.6X2	T50.6X3	T50.6X4	T50.6X5	T50.6X6
Pramiverine	T44.3X1	T44.3X2	T44.3X3	T44.3X4	T44.3X5	T44.3X6
Pramocaine	T49.1X1	T49.1X2	T49.1X3	T49.1X4	T49.1X5	T49.1X6
Pramoxine	T49.1X1	T49.1X2	T49.1X3	T49.1X4	T49.1X5	T49.1X6
Prasterone	T38.7X1	T38.7X2	T38.7X3	T38.7X4	T38.7X5	T38.7X6
Pravastatin	T46.6X1	T46.6X2	T46.6X3	T46.6X4	T46.6X5	T46.6X6
Prazepam	T42.4X1	T42.4X2	T42.4X3	T42.4X4	T42.4X5	T42.4X6
Praziquantel	T37.4X1	T37.4X2	T37.4X3	T37.4X4	T37.4X5	T37.4X6
Prazitone	T43.291	T43.292	T43.293	T43.294	T43.295	T43.296
Prazosin	T44.6X1	T44.6X2	T44.6X3	T44.6X4	T44.6X5	T44.6X6
Prednicarbate	T49.0X1	T49.0X2	T49.0X3	T49.0X4	T49.0X5	T49.0X6
Prednimustine	T45.1X1	T45.1X2	T45.1X3	T45.1X4	T45.1X5	T45.1X6
Prednisolone	T38.0X1	T38.0X2	T38.0X3	T38.0X4	T38.0X5	T38.0X6
ENT agent	T49.6X1	T49.6X2	T49.6X3	T49.6X4	T49.6X5	T49.6X6
ophthalmic preparation	T49.5X1	T49.5X2	T49.5X3	T49.5X4	T49.5X5	T49.5X6
steaglate	T49.0X1	T49.0X2	T49.0X3	T49.0X4	T49.0X5	T49.0X6
topical NEC	T49.0X1	T49.0X2	T49.0X3	T49.0X4	T49.0X5	T49.0X6
Prednisone	T38.0X1	T38.0X2	T38.0X3	T38.0X4	T38.0X5	T38.0X6
Prednylidene	T38.0X1	T38.0X2	T38.0X3	T38.0X4	T38.0X5	T38.0X6
Pregnandiol	T38.5X1	T38.5X2	T38.5X3	T38.5X4	T38.5X5	T38.5X6
Pregneninolone	T38.5X1	T38.5X2	T38.5X3	T38.5X4	T38.5X5	T38.5X6
Preludin	T43.691	T43.692	T43.693	T43.694	T43.695	T43.696
Premarin	T38.5X1	T38.5X2	T38.5X3	T38.5X4	T38.5X5	T38.5X6
Premedication anesthetic	T41.201	T41.202	T41.203	T41.204	T41.205	T41.206
Prenalterol	T44.5X1	T44.5X2	T44.5X3	T44.5X4	T44.5X5	T44.5X6
Prenoxdiazine	T48.3X1	T48.3X2	T48.3X3	T48.3X4	T48.3X5	T48.3X6
Prenylamine	T46.3X1	T46.3X2	T46.3X3	T46.3X4	T46.3X5	T46.3X6
Preparation H	T49.8X1	T49.8X2	T49.8X3	T49.8X4	T49.8X5	T49.8X6
Preparation, local	T49.4X1	T49.4X2	T49.4X3	T49.4X4	T49.4X5	T49.4X6
Preservative (nonmedicinal)	T65.891	T65.892	T65.893	T65.894		
medicinal	T50.901	T50.902	T50.903	T50.904	T50.905	T50.906

Additional Character May Be Required — Refer to the Tabular List for Character Selection   ▽ Subterms under main terms may continue to next column or page

Substance	Poisoning, Accidental (unintentional)	Poisoning, Intentional Self-harm	Poisoning, Assault	Poisoning, Undetermined	Adverse Effect	Under-dosing
Preservative — continued						
wood	T60.91	T60.92	T60.93	T60.94	—	—
Prethcamide	T50.7X1	T50.7X2	T50.7X3	T50.7X4	T50.7X5	T50.7X6
Pride of China	T62.2X1	T62.2X2	T62.2X3	T62.2X4	—	—
Pridinol	T44.3X1	T44.3X2	T44.3X3	T44.3X4	T44.3X5	T44.3X6
Prifinium bromide	T44.3X1	T44.3X2	T44.3X3	T44.3X4	T44.3X5	T44.3X6
Prilocaine	T41.3X1	T41.3X2	T41.3X3	T41.3X4	T41.3X5	T41.3X6
infiltration (subcutaneous)	T41.3X1	T41.3X2	T41.3X3	T41.3X4	T41.3X5	T41.3X6
nerve block (peripheral) (plexus)	T41.3X1	T41.3X2	T41.3X3	T41.3X4	T41.3X5	T41.3X6
regional	T41.3X1	T41.3X2	T41.3X3	T41.3X4	T41.3X5	T41.3X6
Primaquine	T37.2X1	T37.2X2	T37.2X3	T37.2X4	T37.2X5	T37.2X6
Primidone	T42.6X1	T42.6X2	T42.6X3	T42.6X4	T42.6X5	T42.6X6
Primula (veris)	T62.2X1	T62.2X2	T62.2X3	T62.2X4	—	—
Prinadol	T40.2X1	T40.2X2	T40.2X3	T40.2X4	T40.2X5	T40.2X6
Priscol, Priscoline	T44.6X1	T44.6X2	T44.6X3	T44.6X4	T44.6X5	T44.6X6
Pristinamycin	T36.3X1	T36.3X2	T36.3X3	T36.3X4	T36.3X5	T36.3X6
Privet	T62.2X1	T62.2X2	T62.2X3	T62.2X4	—	—
berries	T62.1X1	T62.1X2	T62.1X3	T62.1X4	—	—
Privine	T44.4X1	T44.4X2	T44.4X3	T44.4X4	T44.4X5	T44.4X6
Pro-Banthine	T44.3X1	T44.3X2	T44.3X3	T44.3X4	T44.3X5	T44.3X6
Probarbital	T42.3X1	T42.3X2	T42.3X3	T42.3X4	T42.3X5	T42.3X6
Probenecid	T50.4X1	T50.4X2	T50.4X3	T50.4X4	T50.4X5	T50.4X6
Probucol	T46.6X1	T46.6X2	T46.6X3	T46.6X4	T46.6X5	T46.6X6
Procainamide	T46.2X1	T46.2X2	T46.2X3	T46.2X4	T46.2X5	T46.2X6
Procaine	T41.3X1	T41.3X2	T41.3X3	T41.3X4	T41.3X5	T41.3X6
benzylpenicillin	T36.0X1	T36.0X2	T36.0X3	T36.0X4	T36.0X5	T36.0X6
nerve block (periphreal) (plexus)	T41.3X1	T41.3X2	T41.3X3	T41.3X4	T41.3X5	T41.3X6
penicillin G	T36.0X1	T36.0X2	T36.0X3	T36.0X4	T36.0X5	T36.0X6
regional	T41.3X1	T41.3X2	T41.3X3	T41.3X4	T41.3X5	T41.3X6
spinal	T41.3X1	T41.3X2	T41.3X3	T41.3X4	T41.3X5	T41.3X6
Procalmidol	T43.591	T43.592	T43.593	T43.594	T43.595	T43.596
Procarbazine	T45.1X1	T45.1X2	T45.1X3	T45.1X4	T45.1X5	T45.1X6
Procaterol	T44.5X1	T44.5X2	T44.5X3	T44.5X4	T44.5X5	T44.5X6
Prochlorperazine	T43.3X1	T43.3X2	T43.3X3	T43.3X4	T43.3X5	T43.3X6
Procyclidine	T44.3X1	T44.3X2	T44.3X3	T44.3X4	T44.3X5	T44.3X6
Producer gas	T58.8X1	T58.8X2	T58.8X3	T58.8X4	—	—
Profadol	T40.4X1	T40.4X2	T40.4X3	T40.4X4	T40.4X5	T40.4X6
Profenamine	T44.3X1	T44.3X2	T44.3X3	T44.3X4	T44.3X5	T44.3X6
Profenil	T44.3X1	T44.3X2	T44.3X3	T44.3X4	T44.3X5	T44.3X6
Proflavine	T49.0X1	T49.0X2	T49.0X3	T49.0X4	T49.0X5	T49.0X6
Progabide	T42.6X1	T42.6X2	T42.6X3	T42.6X4	T42.6X5	T42.6X6
Progesterone	T38.5X1	T38.5X2	T38.5X3	T38.5X4	T38.5X5	T38.5X6
Progestin	T38.5X1	T38.5X2	T38.5X3	T38.5X4	T38.5X5	T38.5X6
oral contraceptive	T38.4X1	T38.4X2	T38.4X3	T38.4X4	T38.4X5	T38.4X6
Progestogen NEC	T38.5X1	T38.5X2	T38.5X3	T38.5X4	T38.5X5	T38.5X6
Progestone	T38.5X1	T38.5X2	T38.5X3	T38.5X4	T38.5X5	T38.5X6
Proglumide	T47.1X1	T47.1X2	T47.1X3	T47.1X4	T47.1X5	T47.1X6
Proguanil	T37.2X1	T37.2X2	T37.2X3	T37.2X4	T37.2X5	T37.2X6
Prolactin	T38.811	T38.812	T38.813	T38.814	T38.815	T38.816
Prolintane	T43.691	T43.692	T43.693	T43.694	T43.695	T43.696
Proloid	T38.1X1	T38.1X2	T38.1X3	T38.1X4	T38.1X5	T38.1X6
Proluton	T38.5X1	T38.5X2	T38.5X3	T38.5X4	T38.5X5	T38.5X6
Promacetin	T37.1X1	T37.1X2	T37.1X3	T37.1X4	T37.1X5	T37.1X6
Promazine	T43.3X1	T43.3X2	T43.3X3	T43.3X4	T43.3X5	T43.3X6
Promedol	T40.2X1	T40.2X2	T40.2X3	T40.2X4	—	—
Promegestone	T38.5X1	T38.5X2	T38.5X3	T38.5X4	T38.5X5	T38.5X6
Promethazine (teoclate)	T43.3X1	T43.3X2	T43.3X3	T43.3X4	T43.3X5	T43.3X6
Promin	T37.1X1	T37.1X2	T37.1X3	T37.1X4	T37.1X5	T37.1X6
Pronase	T45.3X1	T45.3X2	T45.3X3	T45.3X4	T45.3X5	T45.3X6
Pronestyl (hydrochloride)	T46.2X1	T46.2X2	T46.2X3	T46.2X4	T46.2X5	T46.2X6
Pronetalol	T44.7X1	T44.7X2	T44.7X3	T44.7X4	T44.7X5	T44.7X6
Prontosil	T37.0X1	T37.0X2	T37.0X3	T37.0X4	T37.0X5	T37.0X6
Propachlor	T60.3X1	T60.3X2	T60.3X3	T60.3X4	—	—
Propafenone	T46.2X1	T46.2X2	T46.2X3	T46.2X4	T46.2X5	T46.2X6
Propallylonal	T42.3X1	T42.3X2	T42.3X3	T42.3X4	T42.3X5	T42.3X6
Propamidine	T49.0X1	T49.0X2	T49.0X3	T49.0X4	T49.0X5	T49.0X6
Propane (distributed in mobile container)	T59.891	T59.892	T59.893	T59.894	—	—
distributed through pipes	T59.891	T59.892	T59.893	T59.894	—	—
incomplete combustion	T58.11	T58.12	T58.13	T58.14	—	—
Propanidid	T41.291	T41.292	T41.293	T41.294	T41.295	T41.296
Propanil	T60.3X1	T60.3X2	T60.3X3	T60.3X4	—	—
Propantheline	T44.3X1	T44.3X2	T44.3X3	T44.3X4	T44.3X5	T44.3X6
bromide	T44.3X1	T44.3X2	T44.3X3	T44.3X4	T44.3X5	T44.3X6
Proparacaine	T41.3X1	T41.3X2	T41.3X3	T41.3X4	T41.3X5	T41.3X6
Propatylnitrate	T46.3X1	T46.3X2	T46.3X3	T46.3X4	T46.3X5	T46.3X6
Propicillin	T36.0X1	T36.0X2	T36.0X3	T36.0X4	T36.0X5	T36.0X6
Propiolactone	T49.0X1	T49.0X2	T49.0X3	T49.0X4	T49.0X5	T49.0X6
Propiomazine	T45.0X1	T45.0X2	T45.0X3	T45.0X4	T45.0X5	T45.0X6
Propionaldehyde (medicinal)	T42.6X1	T42.6X2	T42.6X3	T42.6X4	T42.6X5	T42.6X6

Substance	Poisoning, Accidental (unintentional)	Poisoning, Intentional Self-harm	Poisoning, Assault	Poisoning, Undetermined	Adverse Effect	Under-dosing
Propionate (calcium) (sodium)	T49.0X1	T49.0X2	T49.0X3	T49.0X4	T49.0X5	T49.0X6
Propion gel	T49.0X1	T49.0X2	T49.0X3	T49.0X4	T49.0X5	T49.0X6
Propitocaine	T41.3X1	T41.3X2	T41.3X3	T41.3X4	T41.3X5	T41.3X6
infiltration (subcutaneous)	T41.3X1	T41.3X2	T41.3X3	T41.3X4	T41.3X5	T41.3X6
nerve block (peripheral) (plexus)	T41.3X1	T41.3X2	T41.3X3	T41.3X4	T41.3X5	T41.3X6
Propofol	T41.291	T41.292	T41.293	T41.294	T41.295	T41.296
Propoxur	T60.0X1	T60.0X2	T60.0X3	T60.0X4	—	—
Propoxycaine	T41.3X1	T41.3X2	T41.3X3	T41.3X4	T41.3X5	T41.3X6
infiltration (subcutaneous)	T41.3X1	T41.3X2	T41.3X3	T41.3X4	T41.3X5	T41.3X6
nerve block (peripheral) (plexus)	T41.3X1	T41.3X2	T41.3X3	T41.3X4	T41.3X5	T41.3X6
topical (surface)	T41.3X1	T41.3X2	T41.3X3	T41.3X4	T41.3X5	T41.3X6
Propoxyphene	T40.4X1	T40.4X2	T40.4X3	T40.4X4	T40.4X5	T40.4X6
Propranolol	T44.7X1	T44.7X2	T44.7X3	T44.7X4	T44.7X5	T44.7X6
Propyl						
alcohol	T51.3X1	T51.3X2	T51.3X3	T51.3X4	—	—
carbinol	T51.3X1	T51.3X2	T51.3X3	T51.3X4	—	—
hexadrine	T44.4X1	T44.4X2	T44.4X3	T44.4X4	T44.4X5	T44.4X6
iodone	T50.8X1	T50.8X2	T50.8X3	T50.8X4	T50.8X5	T50.8X6
thiouracil	T38.2X1	T38.2X2	T38.2X3	T38.2X4	T38.2X5	T38.2X6
Propylaminophenothiazine	T43.3X1	T43.3X2	T43.3X3	T43.3X4	T43.3X5	T43.3X6
Propylene	T59.891	T59.892	T59.893	T59.894	—	—
Propylhexedrine	T48.5X1	T48.5X2	T48.5X3	T48.5X4	T48.5X5	T48.5X6
Propyliodone	T50.8X1	T50.8X2	T50.8X3	T50.8X4	T50.8X5	T50.8X6
Propylparaben (ophthalmic)	T49.5X1	T49.5X2	T49.5X3	T49.5X4	T49.5X5	T49.5X6
Propylthiouracil	T38.2X1	T38.2X2	T38.2X3	T38.2X4	T38.2X5	T38.2X6
Propyphenazone	T39.2X1	T39.2X2	T39.2X3	T39.2X4	T39.2X5	T39.2X6
Proquazone	T39.391	T39.392	T39.393	T39.394	T39.395	T39.396
Proscillaridin	T46.0X1	T46.0X2	T46.0X3	T46.0X4	T46.0X5	T46.0X6
Prostacyclin	T45.521	T45.522	T45.523	T45.524	T45.525	T45.526
Prostaglandin (I2)	T45.521	T45.522	T45.523	T45.524	T45.525	T45.526
E1	T46.7X1	T46.7X2	T46.7X3	T46.7X4	T46.7X5	T46.7X6
E2	T48.0X1	T48.0X2	T48.0X3	T48.0X4	T48.0X5	T48.0X6
F2 alpha	T48.0X1	T48.0X2	T48.0X3	T48.0X4	T48.0X5	T48.0X6
Prostigmin	T44.0X1	T44.0X2	T44.0X3	T44.0X4	T44.0X5	T44.0X6
Prosultiamine	T45.2X1	T45.2X2	T45.2X3	T45.2X4	T45.2X5	T45.2X6
Protamine sulfate	T45.7X1	T45.7X2	T45.7X3	T45.7X4	T45.7X5	T45.7X6
zinc insulin	T38.3X1	T38.3X2	T38.3X3	T38.3X4	T38.3X5	T38.3X6
Protease	T47.5X1	T47.5X2	T47.5X3	T47.5X4	T47.5X5	T47.5X6
Protectant, skin NEC	T49.3X1	T49.3X2	T49.3X3	T49.3X4	T49.3X5	T49.3X6
Protein hydrolysate	T50.991	T50.992	T50.993	T50.994	T50.995	T50.996
Prothiaden — see Dothiepin hydrochloride						
Prothionamide	T37.1X1	T37.1X2	T37.1X3	T37.1X4	T37.1X5	T37.1X6
Prothipendyl	T43.591	T43.592	T43.593	T43.594	T43.595	T43.596
Prothoate	T60.0X1	T60.0X2	T60.0X3	T60.0X4	—	—
Prothrombin						
activator	T45.7X1	T45.7X2	T45.7X3	T45.7X4	T45.7X5	T45.7X6
synthesis inhibitor	T45.511	T45.512	T45.513	T45.514	T45.515	T45.516
Protionamide	T37.1X1	T37.1X2	T37.1X3	T37.1X4	T37.1X5	T37.1X6
Protirelin	T38.891	T38.892	T38.893	T38.894	T38.895	T38.896
Protokylol	T48.6X1	T48.6X2	T48.6X3	T48.6X4	T48.6X5	T48.6X6
Protopam	T50.6X1	T50.6X2	T50.6X3	T50.6X4	T50.6X5	T50.6X6
Protoveratrine(s) (A) (B)	T46.5X1	T46.5X2	T46.5X3	T46.5X4	T46.5X5	T46.5X6
Protriptyline	T43.011	T43.012	T43.013	T43.014	T43.015	T43.016
Provera	T38.5X1	T38.5X2	T38.5X3	T38.5X4	T38.5X5	T38.5X6
Provitamin A	T45.2X1	T45.2X2	T45.2X3	T45.2X4	T45.2X5	T45.2X6
Proxibarbal	T42.3X1	T42.3X2	T42.3X3	T42.3X4	T42.3X5	T42.3X6
Proxymetacaine	T41.3X1	T41.3X2	T41.3X3	T41.3X4	T41.3X5	T41.3X6
Proxyphylline	T48.6X1	T48.6X2	T48.6X3	T48.6X4	T48.6X5	T48.6X6
Prozac — see Fluoxetine hydrochloride						
Prunus						
laurocerasus	T62.2X1	T62.2X2	T62.2X3	T62.2X4	—	—
virginiana	T62.2X1	T62.2X2	T62.2X3	T62.2X4	—	—
Prussian blue						
commercial	T65.891	T65.892	T65.893	T65.894	—	—
therapeutic	T50.6X1	T50.6X2	T50.6X3	T50.6X4	T50.6X5	T50.6X6
Prussic acid	T65.0X1	T65.0X2	T65.0X3	T65.0X4	—	—
vapor	T57.3X1	T57.3X2	T57.3X3	T57.3X4	—	—
Pseudoephedrine	T44.991	T44.992	T44.993	T44.994	T44.995	T44.996
Psilocin	T40.991	T40.992	T40.993	T40.994	—	—
Psilocybin	T40.991	T40.992	T40.993	T40.994	—	—
Psilocybine	T40.991	T40.992	T40.993	T40.994	—	—
Psoralene (nonmedicinal)	T65.891	T65.892	T65.893	T65.894	—	—
Psoralens (medicinal)	T50.991	T50.992	T50.993	T50.994	T50.995	T50.996
PSP (phenolsulfonphthalein)	T50.8X1	T50.8X2	T50.8X3	T50.8X4	T50.8X5	T50.8X6
Psychodysleptic drug NEC	T40.901	T40.902	T40.903	T40.904	T40.905	T40.906
Psychostimulant	T43.601	T43.602	T43.603	T43.604	T43.605	T43.606

⬇ Subterms under main terms may continue to next column or page   Additional Character May Be Required — Refer to the Tabular List for Character Selection   387

Preservative — Psychostimulant

Substance	Poisoning, Accidental (unintentional)	Poisoning, Intentional Self-harm	Poisoning, Assault	Poisoning, Undetermined	Adverse Effect	Under-dosing
Psychostimulant — *continued*						
amphetamine	T43.621	T43.622	T43.623	T43.624	T43.625	T43.626
caffeine	T43.611	T43.612	T43.613	T43.614	T43.615	T43.616
methylphenidate	T43.631	T43.632	T43.633	T43.634	T43.635	T43.636
specified NEC	T43.691	T43.692	T43.693	T43.694	T43.695	T43.696
Psychotherapeutic drug NEC	T43.91	T43.92	T43.93	T43.94	T43.95	T43.96
antidepressants — *see also* Antidepressant	T43.201	T43.202	T43.203	T43.204	T43.205	T43.206
specified NEC	T43.8X1	T43.8X2	T43.8X3	T43.8X4	T43.8X5	T43.8X6
tranquilizers NEC	T43.501	T43.502	T43.503	T43.504	T43.505	T43.506
Psychotomimetic agents	T40.901	T40.902	T40.903	T40.904	T40.905	T40.906
Psychotropic drug NEC	T43.91	T43.92	T43.93	T43.94	T43.95	T43.96
specified NEC	T43.8X1	T43.8X2	T43.8X3	T43.8X4	T43.8X5	T43.8X6
Psyllium hydrophilic mucilloid	T47.4X1	T47.4X2	T47.4X3	T47.4X4	T47.4X5	T47.4X6
Pteroylglutamic acid	T45.8X1	T45.8X2	T45.8X3	T45.8X4	T45.8X5	T45.8X6
Pteroyltriglutamate	T45.1X1	T45.1X2	T45.1X3	T45.1X4	T45.1X5	T45.1X6
PTFE — *see* Polytetrafluoroethylene						
Pulp						
devitalizing paste	T49.7X1	T49.7X2	T49.7X3	T49.7X4	T49.7X5	T49.7X6
dressing	T49.7X1	T49.7X2	T49.7X3	T49.7X4	T49.7X5	T49.7X6
Pulsatilla	T62.2X1	T62.2X2	T62.2X3	T62.2X4		
Pumpkin seed extract	T37.4X1	T37.4X2	T37.4X3	T37.4X4	T37.4X5	T37.4X6
Purex (bleach)	T54.91	T54.92	T54.93	T54.94	—	—
Purgative NEC — *see also* Cathartic	T47.4X1	T47.4X2	T47.4X3	T47.4X4	T47.4X5	T47.4X6
Purine analogue (antineoplastic)	T45.1X1	T45.1X2	T45.1X3	T45.1X4	T45.1X5	T45.1X6
Purine diuretics	T50.2X1	T50.2X2	T50.2X3	T50.2X4	T50.2X5	T50.2X6
Purinethol	T45.1X1	T45.1X2	T45.1X3	T45.1X4	T45.1X5	T45.1X6
PVP	T45.8X1	T45.8X2	T45.8X3	T45.8X4	T45.8X5	T45.8X6
Pyrabital	T39.8X1	T39.8X2	T39.8X3	T39.8X4	T39.8X5	T39.8X6
Pyramidon	T39.2X1	T39.2X2	T39.2X3	T39.2X4	T39.2X5	T39.2X6
Pyrantel	T37.4X1	T37.4X2	T37.4X3	T37.4X4	T37.4X5	T37.4X6
Pyrathiazine	T45.0X1	T45.0X2	T45.0X3	T45.0X4	T45.0X5	T45.0X6
Pyrazinamide	T37.1X1	T37.1X2	T37.1X3	T37.1X4	T37.1X5	T37.1X6
Pyrazinoic acid (amide)	T37.1X1	T37.1X2	T37.1X3	T37.1X4	T37.1X5	T37.1X6
Pyrazole (derivatives)	T39.2X1	T39.2X2	T39.2X3	T39.2X4	T39.2X5	T39.2X6
Pyrazolone analgesic NEC	T39.2X1	T39.2X2	T39.2X3	T39.2X4	T39.2X5	T39.2X6
Pyrethrin, pyrethrum (nonmedicinal)	T60.2X1	T60.2X2	T60.2X3	T60.2X4	—	—
Pyrethrum extract	T49.0X1	T49.0X2	T49.0X3	T49.0X4	T49.0X5	T49.0X6
Pyribenzamine	T45.0X1	T45.0X2	T45.0X3	T45.0X4	T45.0X5	T45.0X6
Pyridine	T52.8X1	T52.8X2	T52.8X3	T52.8X4		
aldoxime methiodide	T50.6X1	T50.6X2	T50.6X3	T50.6X4	T50.6X5	T50.6X6
aldoxime methyl chloride	T50.6X1	T50.6X2	T50.6X3	T50.6X4	T50.6X5	T50.6X6
vapor	T59.891	T59.892	T59.893	T59.894		
Pyridium	T39.8X1	T39.8X2	T39.8X3	T39.8X4	T39.8X5	T39.8X6
Pyridostigmine bromide	T44.0X1	T44.0X2	T44.0X3	T44.0X4	T44.0X5	T44.0X6
Pyridoxal phosphate	T45.2X1	T45.2X2	T45.2X3	T45.2X4	T45.2X5	T45.2X6
Pyridoxine	T45.2X1	T45.2X2	T45.2X3	T45.2X4	T45.2X5	T45.2X6
Pyrilamine	T45.0X1	T45.0X2	T45.0X3	T45.0X4	T45.0X5	T45.0X6
Pyrimethamine	T37.2X1	T37.2X2	T37.2X3	T37.2X4	T37.2X5	T37.2X6
with sulfadoxine	T37.2X1	T37.2X2	T37.2X3	T37.2X4	T37.2X5	T37.2X6
Pyrimidine antagonist	T45.1X1	T45.1X2	T45.1X3	T45.1X4	T45.1X5	T45.1X6
Pyriminil	T60.4X1	T60.4X2	T60.4X3	T60.4X4	—	—
Pyrithione zinc	T49.4X1	T49.4X2	T49.4X3	T49.4X4	T49.4X5	T49.4X6
Pyrithyldione	T42.6X1	T42.6X2	T42.6X3	T42.6X4	T42.6X5	T42.6X6
Pyrogallic acid	T49.0X1	T49.0X2	T49.0X3	T49.0X4	T49.0X5	T49.0X6
Pyrogallol	T49.0X1	T49.0X2	T49.0X3	T49.0X4	T49.0X5	T49.0X6
Pyroxylin	T49.3X1	T49.3X2	T49.3X3	T49.3X4	T49.3X5	T49.3X6
Pyrrobutamine	T45.0X1	T45.0X2	T45.0X3	T45.0X4	T45.0X5	T45.0X6
Pyrrolizidine alkaloids	T62.8X1	T62.8X2	T62.8X3	T62.8X4	—	—
Pyrvinium chloride	T37.4X1	T37.4X2	T37.4X3	T37.4X4	T37.4X5	T37.4X6
PZI	T38.3X1	T38.3X2	T38.3X3	T38.3X4	T38.3X5	T38.3X6
Quaalude	T42.6X1	T42.6X2	T42.6X3	T42.6X4	T42.6X5	T42.6X6
Quarternary ammonium						
anti-infective	T49.0X1	T49.0X2	T49.0X3	T49.0X4	T49.0X5	T49.0X6
ganglion blocking	T44.2X1	T44.2X2	T44.2X3	T44.2X4	T44.2X5	T44.2X6
parasympatholytic	T44.3X1	T44.3X2	T44.3X3	T44.3X4	T44.3X5	T44.3X6
Quazepam	T42.4X1	T42.4X2	T42.4X3	T42.4X4	T42.4X5	T42.4X6
Quicklime	T54.3X1	T54.3X2	T54.3X3	T54.3X4	—	—
Quillaja extract	T48.4X1	T48.4X2	T48.4X3	T48.4X4	T48.4X5	T48.4X6
Quinacrine	T37.2X1	T37.2X2	T37.2X3	T37.2X4	T37.2X5	T37.2X6
Quinaglute	T46.2X1	T46.2X2	T46.2X3	T46.2X4	T46.2X5	T46.2X6
Quinalbarbital	T42.3X1	T42.3X2	T42.3X3	T42.3X4	T42.3X5	T42.3X6
Quinalbarbitone sodium	T42.3X1	T42.3X2	T42.3X3	T42.3X4	T42.3X5	T42.3X6
Quinalphos	T60.0X1	T60.0X2	T60.0X3	T60.0X4	—	—
Quinapril	T46.4X1	T46.4X2	T46.4X3	T46.4X4	T46.4X5	T46.4X6
Quinestradiol	T38.5X1	T38.5X2	T38.5X3	T38.5X4	T38.5X5	T38.5X6
Quinestradol	T38.5X1	T38.5X2	T38.5X3	T38.5X4	T38.5X5	T38.5X6

Substance	Poisoning, Accidental (unintentional)	Poisoning, Intentional Self-harm	Poisoning, Assault	Poisoning, Undetermined	Adverse Effect	Under-dosing
Quinestrol	T38.5X1	T38.5X2	T38.5X3	T38.5X4	T38.5X5	T38.5X6
Quinethazone	T50.2X1	T50.2X2	T50.2X3	T50.2X4	T50.2X5	T50.2X6
Quingestanol	T38.4X1	T38.4X2	T38.4X3	T38.4X4	T38.4X5	T38.4X6
Quinidine	T46.2X1	T46.2X2	T46.2X3	T46.2X4	T46.2X5	T46.2X6
Quinine	T37.2X1	T37.2X2	T37.2X3	T37.2X4	T37.2X5	T37.2X6
Quiniobine	T37.8X1	T37.8X2	T37.8X3	T37.8X4	T37.8X5	T37.8X6
Quinisocaine	T49.1X1	T49.1X2	T49.1X3	T49.1X4	T49.1X5	T49.1X6
Quinocide	T37.2X1	T37.2X2	T37.2X3	T37.2X4	T37.2X5	T37.2X6
Quinoline (derivatives) **NEC**	T37.8X1	T37.8X2	T37.8X3	T37.8X4	T37.8X5	T37.8X6
Quinupramine	T43.011	T43.012	T43.013	T43.014	T43.015	T43.016
Quotane	T41.3X1	T41.3X2	T41.3X3	T41.3X4	T41.3X5	T41.3X6
Rabies						
immune globulin (human)	T50.Z11	T50.Z12	T50.Z13	T50.Z14	T50.Z15	T50.Z16
vaccine	T50.B91	T50.B92	T50.B93	T50.B94	T50.B95	T50.B96
Racemoramide	T40.2X1	T40.2X2	T40.2X3	T40.2X4	—	—
Racemorphan	T40.2X1	T40.2X2	T40.2X3	T40.2X4	T40.2X5	T40.2X6
Racepinefrin	T44.5X1	T44.5X2	T44.5X3	T44.5X4	T44.5X5	T44.5X6
Raclopride	T43.591	T43.592	T43.593	T43.594	T43.595	T43.596
Radiator alcohol	T51.1X1	T51.1X2	T51.1X3	T51.1X4		
Radioactive drug NEC	T50.8X1	T50.8X2	T50.8X3	T50.8X4	T50.8X5	T50.8X6
Radio-opaque (drugs) (materials)	T50.8X1	T50.8X2	T50.8X3	T50.8X4	T50.8X5	T50.8X6
Ramifenazone	T39.2X1	T39.2X2	T39.2X3	T39.2X4	T39.2X5	T39.2X6
Ramipril	T46.4X1	T46.4X2	T46.4X3	T46.4X4	T46.4X5	T46.4X6
Ranitidine	T47.0X1	T47.0X2	T47.0X3	T47.0X4	T47.0X5	T47.0X6
Ranunculus	T62.2X1	T62.2X2	T62.2X3	T62.2X4	—	—
Rat poison NEC	T60.4X1	T60.4X2	T60.4X3	T60.4X4	—	—
Rattlesnake (venom)	T63.011	T63.012	T63.013	T63.014		
Raubasine	T46.7X1	T46.7X2	T46.7X3	T46.7X4	T46.7X5	T46.7X6
Raudixin	T46.5X1	T46.5X2	T46.5X3	T46.5X4	T46.5X5	T46.5X6
Rautensin	T46.5X1	T46.5X2	T46.5X3	T46.5X4	T46.5X5	T46.5X6
Rautina	T46.5X1	T46.5X2	T46.5X3	T46.5X4	T46.5X5	T46.5X6
Rautotal	T46.5X1	T46.5X2	T46.5X3	T46.5X4	T46.5X5	T46.5X6
Rauwiloid	T46.5X1	T46.5X2	T46.5X3	T46.5X4	T46.5X5	T46.5X6
Rauwoldin	T46.5X1	T46.5X2	T46.5X3	T46.5X4	T46.5X5	T46.5X6
Rauwolfia (alkaloids)	T46.5X1	T46.5X2	T46.5X3	T46.5X4	T46.5X5	T46.5X6
Razoxane	T45.1X1	T45.1X2	T45.1X3	T45.1X4	T45.1X5	T45.1X6
Realgar	T57.0X1	T57.0X2	T57.0X3	T57.0X4	—	—
Recombinant (R) — *see* specific protein						
Red blood cells, packed	T45.8X1	T45.8X2	T45.8X3	T45.8X4	T45.8X5	T45.8X6
Red squill (scilliroside)	T60.4X1	T60.4X2	T60.4X3	T60.4X4	—	—
Reducing agent, industrial NEC	T65.891	T65.892	T65.893	T65.894	—	—
Refrigerant gas (chlorofluorocarbon)	T53.5X1	T53.5X2	T53.5X3	T53.5X4	—	—
not chlorofluorocarbon	T59.891	T59.892	T59.893	T59.894	—	—
Regroton	T50.2X1	T50.2X2	T50.2X3	T50.2X4	T50.2X5	T50.2X6
Rehydration salts (oral)	T50.3X1	T50.3X2	T50.3X3	T50.3X4	T50.3X5	T50.3X6
Rela	T42.8X1	T42.8X2	T42.8X3	T42.8X4	T42.8X5	T42.8X6
Relaxant, muscle						
anesthetic	T48.1X1	T48.1X2	T48.1X3	T48.1X4	T48.1X5	T48.1X6
central nervous system	T42.8X1	T42.8X2	T42.8X3	T42.8X4	T42.8X5	T42.8X6
skeletal NEC	T48.1X1	T48.1X2	T48.1X3	T48.1X4	T48.1X5	T48.1X6
smooth NEC	T44.3X1	T44.3X2	T44.3X3	T44.3X4	T44.3X5	T44.3X6
Remoxipride	T43.591	T43.592	T43.593	T43.594	T43.595	T43.596
Renese	T50.2X1	T50.2X2	T50.2X3	T50.2X4	T50.2X5	T50.2X6
Renografin	T50.8X1	T50.8X2	T50.8X3	T50.8X4	T50.8X5	T50.8X6
Replacement solution	T50.3X1	T50.3X2	T50.3X3	T50.3X4	T50.3X5	T50.3X6
Reproterol	T48.6X1	T48.6X2	T48.6X3	T48.6X4	T48.6X5	T48.6X6
Rescinnamine	T46.5X1	T46.5X2	T46.5X3	T46.5X4	T46.5X5	T46.5X6
Reserpin (e)	T46.5X1	T46.5X2	T46.5X3	T46.5X4	T46.5X5	T46.5X6
Resorcin, resorcinol (nonmedicinal)	T65.891	T65.892	T65.893	T65.894	—	—
medicinal	T49.4X1	T49.4X2	T49.4X3	T49.4X4	T49.4X5	T49.4X6
Respaire	T48.4X1	T48.4X2	T48.4X3	T48.4X4	T48.4X5	T48.4X6
Respiratory drug NEC	T48.901	T48.902	T48.903	T48.904	T48.905	T48.906
antiasthmatic NEC	T48.6X1	T48.6X2	T48.6X3	T48.6X4	T48.6X5	T48.6X6
anti-common-cold NEC	T48.5X1	T48.5X2	T48.5X3	T48.5X4	T48.5X5	T48.5X6
expectorant NEC	T48.4X1	T48.4X2	T48.4X3	T48.4X4	T48.4X5	T48.4X6
stimulant	T48.901	T48.902	T48.903	T48.904	T48.905	T48.906
Retinoic acid	T49.0X1	T49.0X2	T49.0X3	T49.0X4	T49.0X5	T49.0X6
Retinol	T45.2X1	T45.2X2	T45.2X3	T45.2X4	T45.2X5	T45.2X6
Rh (D) immune globulin (human)	T50.Z11	T50.Z12	T50.Z13	T50.Z14	T50.Z15	T50.Z16
Rhodine	T39.011	T39.012	T39.013	T39.014	T39.015	T39.016
RhoGAM	T50.Z11	T50.Z12	T50.Z13	T50.Z14	T50.Z15	T50.Z16
Rhubarb						
dry extract	T47.2X1	T47.2X2	T47.2X3	T47.2X4	T47.2X5	T47.2X6
tincture, compound	T47.2X1	T47.2X2	T47.2X3	T47.2X4	T47.2X5	T47.2X6
Ribavirin	T37.5X1	T37.5X2	T37.5X3	T37.5X4	T37.5X5	T37.5X6
Riboflavin	T45.2X1	T45.2X2	T45.2X3	T45.2X4	T45.2X5	T45.2X6
Ribostamycin	T36.5X1	T36.5X2	T36.5X3	T36.5X4	T36.5X5	T36.5X6

Additional Character May Be Required — Refer to the Tabular List for Character Selection

Subterms under main terms may continue to next column or page

Substance	Poisoning, Accidental (unintentional)	Poisoning, Intentional Self-harm	Poisoning, Assault	Poisoning, Undetermined	Adverse Effect	Under-dosing
Ricin	T62.2X1	T62.2X2	T62.2X3	T62.2X4	—	—
Ricinus communis	T62.2X1	T62.2X2	T62.2X3	T62.2X4	—	—
Rickettsial vaccine NEC	T50.A91	T50.A92	T50.A93	T50.A94	T50.A95	T50.A96
Rifabutin	T36.6X1	T36.6X2	T36.6X3	T36.6X4	T36.6X5	T36.6X6
Rifamide	T36.6X1	T36.6X2	T36.6X3	T36.6X4	T36.6X5	T36.6X6
Rifampicin	T36.6X1	T36.6X2	T36.6X3	T36.6X4	T36.6X5	T36.6X6
with isoniazid	T37.1X1	T37.1X2	T37.1X3	T37.1X4	T37.1X5	T37.1X6
Rifampin	T36.6X1	T36.6X2	T36.6X3	T36.6X4	T36.6X5	T36.6X6
Rifamycin	T36.6X1	T36.6X2	T36.6X3	T36.6X4	T36.6X5	T36.6X6
Rifaximin	T36.6X1	T36.6X2	T36.6X3	T36.6X4	T36.6X5	T36.6X6
Rimantadine	T37.5X1	T37.5X2	T37.5X3	T37.5X4	T37.5X5	T37.5X6
Rimazolium metilsulfate	T39.8X1	T39.8X2	T39.8X3	T39.8X4	T39.8X5	T39.8X6
Rimifon	T37.1X1	T37.1X2	T37.1X3	T37.1X4	T37.1X5	T37.1X6
Rimiterol	T48.6X1	T48.6X2	T48.6X3	T48.6X4	T48.6X5	T48.6X6
Ringer (lactate) solution	T50.3X1	T50.3X2	T50.3X3	T50.3X4	T50.3X5	T50.3X6
Ristocetin	T36.8X1	T36.8X2	T36.8X3	T36.8X4	T36.8X5	T36.8X6
Ritalin	T43.631	T43.632	T43.633	T43.634	T43.635	T43.636
Ritodrine	T44.5X1	T44.5X2	T44.5X3	T44.5X4	T44.5X5	T44.5X6
Roach killer — *see* Insecticide						
Rociverine	T44.3X1	T44.3X2	T44.3X3	T44.3X4	T44.3X5	T44.3X6
Rocky Mountain spotted fever vaccine	T50.A91	T50.A92	T50.A93	T50.A94	T50.A95	T50.A96
Rodenticide NEC	T60.4X1	T60.4X2	T60.4X3	T60.4X4		
Rohypnol	T42.4X1	T42.4X2	T42.4X3	T42.4X4	T42.4X5	T42.4X6
Rokitamycin	T36.3X1	T36.3X2	T36.3X3	T36.3X4	T36.3X5	T36.3X6
Rolaids	T47.1X1	T47.1X2	T47.1X3	T47.1X4	T47.1X5	T47.1X6
Rolitetracycline	T36.4X1	T36.4X2	T36.4X3	T36.4X4	T36.4X5	T36.4X6
Romilar	T48.3X1	T48.3X2	T48.3X3	T48.3X4	T48.3X5	T48.3X6
Ronifibrate	T46.6X1	T46.6X2	T46.6X3	T46.6X4	T46.6X5	T46.6X6
Rosaprostol	T47.1X1	T47.1X2	T47.1X3	T47.1X4	T47.1X5	T47.1X6
Rose bengal sodium (131I)	T50.8X1	T50.8X2	T50.8X3	T50.8X4	T50.8X5	T50.8X6
Rose water ointment	T49.3X1	T49.3X2	T49.3X3	T49.3X4	T49.3X5	T49.3X6
Rosoxacin	T37.8X1	T37.8X2	T37.8X3	T37.8X4	T37.8X5	T37.8X6
Rotenone	T60.2X1	T60.2X2	T60.2X3	T60.2X4		
Rotoxamine	T45.0X1	T45.0X2	T45.0X3	T45.0X4	T45.0X5	T45.0X6
Rough-on-rats	T60.4X1	T60.4X2	T60.4X3	T60.4X4		
Roxatidine	T47.0X1	T47.0X2	T47.0X3	T47.0X4	T47.0X5	T47.0X6
Roxithromycin	T36.3X1	T36.3X2	T36.3X3	T36.3X4	T36.3X5	T36.3X6
Rt-PA	T45.611	T45.612	T45.613	T45.614	T45.615	T45.616
Rubbing alcohol	T51.2X1	T51.2X2	T51.2X3	T51.2X4	—	—
Rubefacient	T49.4X1	T49.4X2	T49.4X3	T49.4X4	T49.4X5	T49.4X6
Rubella vaccine	T50.B91	T50.B92	T50.B93	T50.B94	T50.B95	T50.B96
Rubeola vaccine	T50.B91	T50.B92	T50.B93	T50.B94	T50.B95	T50.B96
Rubidium chloride Rb82	T50.8X1	T50.8X2	T50.8X3	T50.8X4	T50.8X5	T50.8X6
Rubidomycin	T45.1X1	T45.1X2	T45.1X3	T45.1X4	T45.1X5	T45.1X6
Rue	T62.2X1	T62.2X2	T62.2X3	T62.2X4	—	—
Rufocromomycin	T45.1X1	T45.1X2	T45.1X3	T45.1X4	T45.1X5	T45.1X6
Russel's viper venin	T45.7X1	T45.7X2	T45.7X3	T45.7X4	T45.7X5	T45.7X6
Ruta (graveolens)	T62.2X1	T62.2X2	T62.2X3	T62.2X4	—	—
Rutinum	T46.991	T46.992	T46.993	T46.994	T46.995	T46.996
Rutoside	T46.991	T46.992	T46.993	T46.994	T46.995	T46.996
b-sitosterol(s)	T46.6X1	T46.6X2	T46.6X3	T46.6X4	T46.6X5	T46.6X6
Sabadilla (plant)	T62.2X1	T62.2X2	T62.2X3	T62.2X4	—	—
pesticide	T60.2X1	T60.2X2	T60.2X3	T60.2X4	—	—
Saccharated iron oxide	T45.8X1	T45.8X2	T45.8X3	T45.8X4	T45.8X5	T45.8X6
Saccharin	T50.901	T50.902	T50.903	T50.904	T50.905	T50.906
Saccharomyces boulardii	T47.6X1	T47.6X2	T47.6X3	T47.6X4	T47.6X5	T47.6X6
Safflower oil	T46.6X1	T46.6X2	T46.6X3	T46.6X4	T46.6X5	T46.6X6
Safrazine	T43.1X1	T43.1X2	T43.1X3	T43.1X4	T43.1X5	T43.1X6
Salazosulfapyridine	T37.0X1	T37.0X2	T37.0X3	T37.0X4	T37.0X5	T37.0X6
Salbutamol	T48.6X1	T48.6X2	T48.6X3	T48.6X4	T48.6X5	T48.6X6
Salicylamide	T39.091	T39.092	T39.093	T39.094	T39.095	T39.096
Salicylate NEC	T39.091	T39.092	T39.093	T39.094	T39.095	T39.096
methyl	T49.3X1	T49.3X2	T49.3X3	T49.3X4	T49.3X5	T49.3X6
theobromine calcium	T50.2X1	T50.2X2	T50.2X3	T50.2X4	T50.2X5	T50.2X6
Salicylazosulfapyridine	T37.0X1	T37.0X2	T37.0X3	T37.0X4	T37.0X5	T37.0X6
Salicylhydroxamic acid	T49.0X1	T49.0X2	T49.0X3	T49.0X4	T49.0X5	T49.0X6
Salicylic acid	T49.4X1	T49.4X2	T49.4X3	T49.4X4	T49.4X5	T49.4X6
with benzoic acid	T49.4X1	T49.4X2	T49.4X3	T49.4X4	T49.4X5	T49.4X6
congeners	T39.091	T39.092	T39.093	T39.094	T39.095	T39.096
derivative	T39.091	T39.092	T39.093	T39.094	T39.095	T39.096
salts	T39.091	T39.092	T39.093	T39.094	T39.095	T39.096
Salinazid	T37.1X1	T37.1X2	T37.1X3	T37.1X4	T37.1X5	T37.1X6
Salmeterol	T48.6X1	T48.6X2	T48.6X3	T48.6X4	T48.6X5	T48.6X6
Salol	T49.3X1	T49.3X2	T49.3X3	T49.3X4	T49.3X5	T49.3X6
Salsalate	T39.091	T39.092	T39.093	T39.094	T39.095	T39.096
Salt-replacing drug	T50.901	T50.902	T50.903	T50.904	T50.905	T50.906
Salt-retaining mineralocorticoid	T50.0X1	T50.0X2	T50.0X3	T50.0X4	T50.0X5	T50.0X6
Salt substitute	T50.901	T50.902	T50.903	T50.904	T50.905	T50.906
Saluretic NEC	T50.2X1	T50.2X2	T50.2X3	T50.2X4	T50.2X5	T50.2X6
Saluron	T50.2X1	T50.2X2	T50.2X3	T50.2X4	T50.2X5	T50.2X6

Substance	Poisoning, Accidental (unintentional)	Poisoning, Intentional Self-harm	Poisoning, Assault	Poisoning, Undetermined	Adverse Effect	Under-dosing
Salvarsan 606 (neosilver) (silver)	T37.8X1	T37.8X2	T37.8X3	T37.8X4	T37.8X5	T37.8X6
Sambucus canadensis	T62.2X1	T62.2X2	T62.2X3	T62.2X4	—	—
berry	T62.1X1	T62.1X2	T62.1X3	T62.1X4	—	—
Sandril	T46.5X1	T46.5X2	T46.5X3	T46.5X4	T46.5X5	T46.5X6
Sanguinaria canadensis	T62.2X1	T62.2X2	T62.2X3	T62.2X4	—	—
Saniflush (cleaner)	T54.2X1	T54.2X2	T54.2X3	T54.2X4	—	—
Santonin	T37.4X1	T37.4X2	T37.4X3	T37.4X4	T37.4X5	T37.4X6
Santyl	T49.8X1	T49.8X2	T49.8X3	T49.8X4	T49.8X5	T49.8X6
Saralasin	T46.5X1	T46.5X2	T46.5X3	T46.5X4	T46.5X5	T46.5X6
Sarcolysin	T45.1X1	T45.1X2	T45.1X3	T45.1X4	T45.1X5	T45.1X6
Sarkomycin	T45.1X1	T45.1X2	T45.1X3	T45.1X4	T45.1X5	T45.1X6
Saroten	T43.011	T43.012	T43.013	T43.014	T43.015	T43.016
Saturnine — *see* Lead						
Savin (oil)	T49.4X1	T49.4X2	T49.4X3	T49.4X4	T49.4X5	T49.4X6
Scammony	T47.2X1	T47.2X2	T47.2X3	T47.2X4	T47.2X5	T47.2X6
Scarlet red	T49.8X1	T49.8X2	T49.8X3	T49.8X4	T49.8X5	T49.8X6
Scheele's green	T57.0X1	T57.0X2	T57.0X3	T57.0X4	—	—
insecticide	T57.0X1	T57.0X2	T57.0X3	T57.0X4	—	—
Schizontozide (blood) (tissue)	T37.2X1	T37.2X2	T37.2X3	T37.2X4	T37.2X5	T37.2X6
Schradan	T60.0X1	T60.0X2	T60.0X3	T60.0X4	—	—
Schweinfurth green	T57.0X1	T57.0X2	T57.0X3	T57.0X4	—	—
insecticide	T57.0X1	T57.0X2	T57.0X3	T57.0X4	—	—
Scilla, rat poison	T60.4X1	T60.4X2	T60.4X3	T60.4X4	—	—
Scillaren	T60.4X1	T60.4X2	T60.4X3	T60.4X4	—	—
Sclerosing agent	T46.8X1	T46.8X2	T46.8X3	T46.8X4	T46.8X5	T46.8X6
Scombrotoxin	T61.11	T61.12	T61.13	T61.14	—	—
Scopolamine	T44.3X1	T44.3X2	T44.3X3	T44.3X4	T44.3X5	T44.3X6
Scopolia extract	T44.3X1	T44.3X2	T44.3X3	T44.3X4	T44.3X5	T44.3X6
Scouring powder	T65.891	T65.892	T65.893	T65.894	—	—
Sea						
anemone (sting)	T63.631	T63.632	T63.633	T63.634	—	—
cucumber (sting)	T63.691	T63.692	T63.693	T63.694	—	—
snake (bite) (venom)	T63.091	T63.092	T63.093	T63.094	—	—
urchin spine (puncture)	T63.691	T63.692	T63.693	T63.694	—	—
Seafood	T61.91	T61.92	T61.93	T61.94	—	—
specified NEC	T61.8X1	T61.8X2	T61.8X3	T61.8X4	—	—
Secbutabarbital	T42.3X1	T42.3X2	T42.3X3	T42.3X4	T42.3X5	T42.3X6
Secbutabarbitone	T42.3X1	T42.3X2	T42.3X3	T42.3X4	T42.3X5	T42.3X6
Secnidazole	T37.3X1	T37.3X2	T37.3X3	T37.3X4	T37.3X5	T37.3X6
Secobarbital	T42.3X1	T42.3X2	T42.3X3	T42.3X4	T42.3X5	T42.3X6
Seconal	T42.3X1	T42.3X2	T42.3X3	T42.3X4	T42.3X5	T42.3X6
Secretin	T50.8X1	T50.8X2	T50.8X3	T50.8X4	T50.8X5	T50.8X6
Sedative NEC	T42.71	T42.72	T42.73	T42.74	T42.75	T42.76
mixed NEC	T42.6X1	T42.6X2	T42.6X3	T42.6X4	T42.6X5	T42.6X6
Sedormid	T42.6X1	T42.6X2	T42.6X3	T42.6X4	T42.6X5	T42.6X6
Seed disinfectant or dressing	T60.8X1	T60.8X2	T60.8X3	T60.8X4	—	—
Seeds (poisonous)	T62.2X1	T62.2X2	T62.2X3	T62.2X4	—	—
Selegiline	T42.8X1	T42.8X2	T42.8X3	T42.8X4	T42.8X5	T42.8X6
Selenium NEC	T56.891	T56.892	T56.893	T56.894	—	—
disulfide or sulfide	T49.4X1	T49.4X2	T49.4X3	T49.4X4	T49.4X5	T49.4X6
fumes	T59.891	T59.892	T59.893	T59.894	—	—
sulfide	T49.4X1	T49.4X2	T49.4X3	T49.4X4	T49.4X5	T49.4X6
Selenomethionine (75Se)	T50.8X1	T50.8X2	T50.8X3	T50.8X4	T50.8X5	T50.8X6
Selsun	T49.4X1	T49.4X2	T49.4X3	T49.4X4	T49.4X5	T49.4X6
Semustine	T45.1X1	T45.1X2	T45.1X3	T45.1X4	T45.1X5	T45.1X6
Senega syrup	T48.4X1	T48.4X2	T48.4X3	T48.4X4	T48.4X5	T48.4X6
Senna	T47.2X1	T47.2X2	T47.2X3	T47.2X4	T47.2X5	T47.2X6
Sennoside A+B	T47.2X1	T47.2X2	T47.2X3	T47.2X4	T47.2X5	T47.2X6
Septisol	T49.2X1	T49.2X2	T49.2X3	T49.2X4	T49.2X5	T49.2X6
Seractide	T38.811	T38.812	T38.813	T38.814	T38.815	T38.816
Serax	T42.4X1	T42.4X2	T42.4X3	T42.4X4	T42.4X5	T42.4X6
Serenesil	T42.6X1	T42.6X2	T42.6X3	T42.6X4	T42.6X5	T42.6X6
Serenium (hydrochloride)	T37.91	T37.92	T37.93	T37.94	T37.95	T37.96
Serepax — *see* Oxazepam						
Sermorelin	T38.891	T38.892	T38.893	T38.894	T38.895	T38.896
Sernyl	T41.1X1	T41.1X2	T41.1X3	T41.1X4	T41.1X5	T41.1X6
Serotonin	T50.991	T50.992	T50.993	T50.994	T50.995	T50.996
Serpasil	T46.5X1	T46.5X2	T46.5X3	T46.5X4	T46.5X5	T46.5X6
Serrapeptase	T45.3X1	T45.3X2	T45.3X3	T45.3X4	T45.3X5	T45.3X6
Serum						
antibotulinus	T50.Z11	T50.Z12	T50.Z13	T50.Z14	T50.Z15	T50.Z16
anticytotoxic	T50.Z11	T50.Z12	T50.Z13	T50.Z14	T50.Z15	T50.Z16
antidiphtheria	T50.Z11	T50.Z12	T50.Z13	T50.Z14	T50.Z15	T50.Z16
antimeningococcus	T50.Z11	T50.Z12	T50.Z13	T50.Z14	T50.Z15	T50.Z16
anti-Rh	T50.Z11	T50.Z12	T50.Z13	T50.Z14	T50.Z15	T50.Z16
anti-snake-bite	T50.Z11	T50.Z12	T50.Z13	T50.Z14	T50.Z15	T50.Z16
antitetanic	T50.Z11	T50.Z12	T50.Z13	T50.Z14	T50.Z15	T50.Z16
antitoxic	T50.Z11	T50.Z12	T50.Z13	T50.Z14	T50.Z15	T50.Z16
complement (inhibitor)	T45.8X1	T45.8X2	T45.8X3	T45.8X4	T45.8X5	T45.8X6
convalescent	T50.Z11	T50.Z12	T50.Z13	T50.Z14	T50.Z15	T50.Z16

Table of Drugs and Chemicals

Substance	Poisoning, Accidental (unintentional)	Poisoning, Intentional Self-harm	Poisoning, Assault	Poisoning, Undetermined	Adverse Effect	Under-dosing
Serum — *continued*						
hemolytic complement	T45.8X1	T45.8X2	T45.8X3	T45.8X4	T45.8X5	T45.8X6
immune (human)	T50.Z11	T50.Z12	T50.Z13	T50.Z14	T50.Z15	T50.Z16
protective NEC	T50.Z11	T50.Z12	T50.Z13	T50.Z14	T50.Z15	T50.Z16
Setastine	T45.0X1	T45.0X2	T45.0X3	T45.0X4	T45.0X5	T45.0X6
Setoperone	T43.591	T43.592	T43.593	T43.594	T43.595	T43.596
Sewer gas	T59.91	T59.92	T59.93	T59.94	—	—
Shampoo	T55.0X1	T55.0X2	T55.0X3	T55.0X4	—	—
Shellfish, noxious, nonbacterial	T61.781	T61.782	T61.783	T61.784	—	—
Sildenafil	T46.7X1	T46.7X2	T46.7X3	T46.7X4	T46.7X5	T46.7X6
Silibinin	T50.991	T50.992	T50.993	T50.994	T50.995	T50.996
Silicone NEC	T65.891	T65.892	T65.893	T65.894	—	—
medicinal	T49.3X1	T49.3X2	T49.3X3	T49.3X4	T49.3X5	T49.3X6
Silvadene	T49.0X1	T49.0X2	T49.0X3	T49.0X4	T49.0X5	T49.0X6
Silver	T49.0X1	T49.0X2	T49.0X3	T49.0X4	T49.0X5	T49.0X6
anti-infectives	T49.0X1	T49.0X2	T49.0X3	T49.0X4	T49.0X5	T49.0X6
arsphenamine	T37.8X1	T37.8X2	T37.8X3	T37.8X4	T37.8X5	T37.8X6
colloidal	T49.0X1	T49.0X2	T49.0X3	T49.0X4	T49.0X5	T49.0X6
nitrate	T49.0X1	T49.0X2	T49.0X3	T49.0X4	T49.0X5	T49.0X6
ophthalmic preparation	T49.5X1	T49.5X2	T49.5X3	T49.5X4	T49.5X5	T49.5X6
toughened (keratolytic)	T49.4X1	T49.4X2	T49.4X3	T49.4X4	T49.4X5	T49.4X6
nonmedicinal (dust)	T56.891	T56.892	T56.893	T56.894	—	—
protein	T49.5X1	T49.5X2	T49.5X3	T49.5X4	T49.5X5	T49.5X6
salvarsan	T37.8X1	T37.8X2	T37.8X3	T37.8X4	T37.8X5	T37.8X6
sulfadiazine	T49.4X1	T49.4X2	T49.4X3	T49.4X4	T49.4X5	T49.4X6
Silymarin	T50.991	T50.992	T50.993	T50.994	T50.995	T50.996
Simaldrate	T47.1X1	T47.1X2	T47.1X3	T47.1X4	T47.1X5	T47.1X6
Simazine	T60.3X1	T60.3X2	T60.3X3	T60.3X4	—	—
Simethicone	T47.1X1	T47.1X2	T47.1X3	T47.1X4	T47.1X5	T47.1X6
Simfibrate	T46.6X1	T46.6X2	T46.6X3	T46.6X4	T46.6X5	T46.6X6
Simvastatin	T46.6X1	T46.6X2	T46.6X3	T46.6X4	T46.6X5	T46.6X6
Sincalide	T50.8X1	T50.8X2	T50.8X3	T50.8X4	T50.8X5	T50.8X6
Sinequan	T43.011	T43.012	T43.013	T43.014	T43.015	T43.016
Singoserp	T46.5X1	T46.5X2	T46.5X3	T46.5X4	T46.5X5	T46.5X6
Sintrom	T45.511	T45.512	T45.513	T45.514	T45.515	T45.516
Sisomicin	T36.5X1	T36.5X2	T36.5X3	T36.5X4	T36.5X5	T36.5X6
Sitosterols	T46.6X1	T46.6X2	T46.6X3	T46.6X4	T46.6X5	T46.6X6
Skeletal muscle relaxants	T48.1X1	T48.1X2	T48.1X3	T48.1X4	T48.1X5	T48.1X6
Skin						
agents (external)	T49.91	T49.92	T49.93	T49.94	T49.95	T49.96
specified NEC	T49.8X1	T49.8X2	T49.8X3	T49.8X4	T49.8X5	T49.8X6
test antigen	T50.8X1	T50.8X2	T50.8X3	T50.8X4	T50.8X5	T50.8X6
Sleep-eze	T45.0X1	T45.0X2	T45.0X3	T45.0X4	T45.0X5	T45.0X6
Sleeping draught, pill	T42.71	T42.72	T42.73	T42.74	T42.75	T42.76
Smallpox vaccine	T50.B11	T50.B12	T50.B13	T50.B14	T50.B15	T50.B16
Smelter fumes NEC	T56.91	T56.92	T56.93	T56.94	—	—
Smog	T59.1X1	T59.1X2	T59.1X3	T59.1X4	—	—
Smoke NEC	T59.811	T59.812	T59.813	T59.814	—	—
Smooth muscle relaxant	T44.3X1	T44.3X2	T44.3X3	T44.3X4	T44.3X5	T44.3X6
Snail killer NEC	T60.8X1	T60.8X2	T60.8X3	T60.8X4	—	—
Snake venom or bite	T63.001	T63.002	T63.003	T63.004	—	—
hemocoagulase	T45.7X1	T45.7X2	T45.7X3	T45.7X4	T45.7X5	T45.7X6
Snuff	T65.211	T65.212	T65.213	T65.214	—	—
Soap (powder) (product)	T55.0X1	T55.0X2	T55.0X3	T55.0X4	—	—
enema	T47.4X1	T47.4X2	T47.4X3	T47.4X4	T47.4X5	T47.4X6
medicinal, soft	T49.2X1	T49.2X2	T49.2X3	T49.2X4	T49.2X5	T49.2X6
superfatted	T49.2X1	T49.2X2	T49.2X3	T49.2X4	T49.2X5	T49.2X6
Sobrerol	T48.4X1	T48.4X2	T48.4X3	T48.4X4	T48.4X5	T48.4X6
Soda (caustic)	T54.3X1	T54.3X2	T54.3X3	T54.3X4	—	—
bicarb	T47.1X1	T47.1X2	T47.1X3	T47.1X4	T47.1X5	T47.1X6
chlorinated — *see* Sodium, hypochlorite						
Sodium						
acetosulfone	T37.1X1	T37.1X2	T37.1X3	T37.1X4	T37.1X5	T37.1X6
acetrizoate	T50.8X1	T50.8X2	T50.8X3	T50.8X4	T50.8X5	T50.8X6
acid phosphate	T50.3X1	T50.3X2	T50.3X3	T50.3X4	T50.3X5	T50.3X6
alginate	T47.8X1	T47.8X2	T47.8X3	T47.8X4	T47.8X5	T47.8X6
amidotrizoate	T50.8X1	T50.8X2	T50.8X3	T50.8X4	T50.8X5	T50.8X6
aminopterin	T45.1X1	T45.1X2	T45.1X3	T45.1X4	T45.1X5	T45.1X6
amylosulfate	T47.8X1	T47.8X2	T47.8X3	T47.8X4	T47.8X5	T47.8X6
amytal	T42.3X1	T42.3X2	T42.3X3	T42.3X4	T42.3X5	T42.3X6
antimony gluconate	T37.3X1	T37.3X2	T37.3X3	T37.3X4	T37.3X5	T37.3X6
arsenate	T57.0X1	T57.0X2	T57.0X3	T57.0X4	—	—
aurothiomalate	T39.4X1	T39.4X2	T39.4X3	T39.4X4	T39.4X5	T39.4X6
aurothiosulfate	T39.4X1	T39.4X2	T39.4X3	T39.4X4	T39.4X5	T39.4X6
barbiturate	T42.3X1	T42.3X2	T42.3X3	T42.3X4	T42.3X5	T42.3X6
basic phosphate	T47.4X1	T47.4X2	T47.4X3	T47.4X4	T47.4X5	T47.4X6
bicarbonate	T47.1X1	T47.1X2	T47.1X3	T47.1X4	T47.1X5	T47.1X6
bichromate	T57.8X1	T57.8X2	T57.8X3	T57.8X4	—	—
biphosphate	T50.3X1	T50.3X2	T50.3X3	T50.3X4	T50.3X5	T50.3X6
bisulfate	T65.891	T65.892	T65.893	T65.894	—	—
borate						

Substance	Poisoning, Accidental (unintentional)	Poisoning, Intentional Self-harm	Poisoning, Assault	Poisoning, Undetermined	Adverse Effect	Under-dosing
Sodium — *continued*						
borate — *continued*						
cleanser	T57.8X1	T57.8X2	T57.8X3	T57.8X4	—	—
eye	T49.5X1	T49.5X2	T49.5X3	T49.5X4	T49.5X5	T49.5X6
therapeutic	T49.8X1	T49.8X2	T49.8X3	T49.8X4	T49.8X5	T49.8X6
bromide	T42.6X1	T42.6X2	T42.6X3	T42.6X4	T42.6X5	T42.6X6
cacodylate (nonmedicinal)	T50.8X1	T50.8X2	T50.8X3	T50.8X4	T50.8X5	T50.8X6
NEC						
anti-infective	T37.8X1	T37.8X2	T37.8X3	T37.8X4	T37.8X5	T37.8X6
herbicide	T60.3X1	T60.3X2	T60.3X3	T60.3X4	—	—
calcium edetate	T45.8X1	T45.8X2	T45.8X3	T45.8X4	T45.8X5	T45.8X6
carbonate NEC	T54.3X1	T54.3X2	T54.3X3	T54.3X4	—	—
chlorate NEC	T65.891	T65.892	T65.893	T65.894	—	—
herbicide	T54.91	T54.92	T54.93	T54.94	—	—
chloride	T50.3X1	T50.3X2	T50.3X3	T50.3X4	T50.3X5	T50.3X6
with glucose	T50.3X1	T50.3X2	T50.3X3	T50.3X4	T50.3X5	T50.3X6
chromate	T65.891	T65.892	T65.893	T65.894	—	—
citrate	T50.991	T50.992	T50.993	T50.994	T50.995	T50.996
cromoglicate	T48.6X1	T48.6X2	T48.6X3	T48.6X4	T48.6X5	T48.6X6
cyanide	T65.0X1	T65.0X2	T65.0X3	T65.0X4	—	—
cyclamate	T50.3X1	T50.3X2	T50.3X3	T50.3X4	T50.3X5	T50.3X6
dehydrocholate	T45.8X1	T45.8X2	T45.8X3	T45.8X4	T45.8X5	T45.8X6
diatrizoate	T50.8X1	T50.8X2	T50.8X3	T50.8X4	T50.8X5	T50.8X6
dibunate	T48.4X1	T48.4X2	T48.4X3	T48.4X4	T48.4X5	T48.4X6
dioctyl sulfosuccinate	T47.4X1	T47.4X2	T47.4X3	T47.4X4	T47.4X5	T47.4X6
dipantoyl ferrate	T45.8X1	T45.8X2	T45.8X3	T45.8X4	T45.8X5	T45.8X6
edetate	T45.8X1	T45.8X2	T45.8X3	T45.8X4	T45.8X5	T45.8X6
ethacrynate	T50.1X1	T50.1X2	T50.1X3	T50.1X4	T50.1X5	T50.1X6
feredetate	T45.8X1	T45.8X2	T45.8X3	T45.8X4	T45.8X5	T45.8X6
Fluoride — *see* Fluoride						
fluoroacetate (dust) (pesticide)	T60.4X1	T60.4X2	T60.4X3	T60.4X4	—	—
free salt	T50.3X1	T50.3X2	T50.3X3	T50.3X4	T50.3X5	T50.3X6
fusidate	T36.8X1	T36.8X2	T36.8X3	T36.8X4	T36.8X5	T36.8X6
glucaldrate	T47.1X1	T47.1X2	T47.1X3	T47.1X4	T47.1X5	T47.1X6
glucosulfone	T37.1X1	T37.1X2	T37.1X3	T37.1X4	T37.1X5	T37.1X6
glutamate	T45.8X1	T45.8X2	T45.8X3	T45.8X4	T45.8X5	T45.8X6
hydrogen carbonate	T50.3X1	T50.3X2	T50.3X3	T50.3X4	T50.3X5	T50.3X6
hydroxide	T54.3X1	T54.3X2	T54.3X3	T54.3X4	—	—
hypochlorite (bleach) NEC	T54.3X1	T54.3X2	T54.3X3	T54.3X4	—	—
disinfectant	T54.3X1	T54.3X2	T54.3X3	T54.3X4	—	—
medicinal (anti-infective) (external)	T49.0X1	T49.0X2	T49.0X3	T49.0X4	T49.0X5	T49.0X6
vapor	T54.3X1	T54.3X2	T54.3X3	T54.3X4	—	—
hyposulfite	T49.0X1	T49.0X2	T49.0X3	T49.0X4	T49.0X5	T49.0X6
indigotin disulfonate	T50.8X1	T50.8X2	T50.8X3	T50.8X4	T50.8X5	T50.8X6
iodide	T50.991	T50.992	T50.993	T50.994	T50.995	T50.996
I-131	T50.8X1	T50.8X2	T50.8X3	T50.8X4	T50.8X5	T50.8X6
therapeutic	T38.2X1	T38.2X2	T38.2X3	T38.2X4	T38.2X5	T38.2X6
iodohippurate (131I)	T50.8X1	T50.8X2	T50.8X3	T50.8X4	T50.8X5	T50.8X6
iopodate	T50.8X1	T50.8X2	T50.8X3	T50.8X4	T50.8X5	T50.8X6
iothalamate	T50.8X1	T50.8X2	T50.8X3	T50.8X4	T50.8X5	T50.8X6
iron edetate	T45.4X1	T45.4X2	T45.4X3	T45.4X4	T45.4X5	T45.4X6
lactate (compound solution)	T45.8X1	T45.8X2	T45.8X3	T45.8X4	T45.8X5	T45.8X6
lauryl (sulfate)	T49.2X1	T49.2X2	T49.2X3	T49.2X4	T49.2X5	T49.2X6
L-triiodothyronine	T38.1X1	T38.1X2	T38.1X3	T38.1X4	T38.1X5	T38.1X6
magnesium citrate	T50.991	T50.992	T50.993	T50.994	T50.995	T50.996
mersalate	T50.2X1	T50.2X2	T50.2X3	T50.2X4	T50.2X5	T50.2X6
metasilicate	T65.891	T65.892	T65.893	T65.894	—	—
metrizoate	T50.8X1	T50.8X2	T50.8X3	T50.8X4	T50.8X5	T50.8X6
monofluoroacetate (pesticide)	T60.1X1	T60.1X2	T60.1X3	T60.1X4	—	—
morrhuate	T46.8X1	T46.8X2	T46.8X3	T46.8X4	T46.8X5	T46.8X6
nafcillin	T36.0X1	T36.0X2	T36.0X3	T36.0X4	T36.0X5	T36.0X6
nitrate (oxidizing agent)	T65.891	T65.892	T65.893	T65.894	—	—
nitrite	T50.6X1	T50.6X2	T50.6X3	T50.6X4	T50.6X5	T50.6X6
nitroferricyanide	T46.5X1	T46.5X2	T46.5X3	T46.5X4	T46.5X5	T46.5X6
nitroprusside	T46.5X1	T46.5X2	T46.5X3	T46.5X4	T46.5X5	T46.5X6
oxalate	T65.891	T65.892	T65.893	T65.894	—	—
oxide/peroxide	T65.891	T65.892	T65.893	T65.894	—	—
oxybate	T41.291	T41.292	T41.293	T41.294	T41.295	T41.296
para-aminohippurate	T50.8X1	T50.8X2	T50.8X3	T50.8X4	T50.8X5	T50.8X6
perborate (nonmedicinal) NEC	T65.891	T65.892	T65.893	T65.894	—	—
medicinal	T49.0X1	T49.0X2	T49.0X3	T49.0X4	T49.0X5	T49.0X6
soap	T55.0X1	T55.0X2	T55.0X3	T55.0X4	—	—
percarbonate — *see* Sodium, perborate						
pertechnetate Tc99m	T50.8X1	T50.8X2	T50.8X3	T50.8X4	T50.8X5	T50.8X6
phosphate						
cellulose	T45.8X1	T45.8X2	T45.8X3	T45.8X4	T45.8X5	T45.8X6
dibasic	T47.2X1	T47.2X2	T47.2X3	T47.2X4	T47.2X5	T47.2X6

Additional Character May Be Required — Refer to the Tabular List for Character Selection   ▽ Subterms under main terms may continue to next column or page

Table of Drugs and Chemicals

Substance	Poisoning, Accidental (unintentional)	Poisoning, Intentional Self-harm	Poisoning, Assault	Poisoning, Undetermined	Adverse Effect	Under-dosing
Sodium — continued						
phosphate — continued						
monobasic	T47.2X1	T47.2X2	T47.2X3	T47.2X4	T47.2X5	T47.2X6
phytate	T50.6X1	T50.6X2	T50.6X3	T50.6X4	T50.6X5	T50.6X6
picosulfate	T47.2X1	T47.2X2	T47.2X3	T47.2X4	T47.2X5	T47.2X6
polyhydroxyaluminium monocarbonate	T47.1X1	T47.1X2	T47.1X3	T47.1X4	T47.1X5	T47.1X6
polystyrene sulfonate	T50.3X1	T50.3X2	T50.3X3	T50.3X4	T50.3X5	T50.3X6
propionate	T49.0X1	T49.0X2	T49.0X3	T49.0X4	T49.0X5	T49.0X6
propyl hydroxybenzoate	T50.991	T50.992	T50.993	T50.994	T50.995	T50.996
psylliate	T46.8X1	T46.8X2	T46.8X3	T46.8X4	T46.8X5	T46.8X6
removing resins	T50.3X1	T50.3X2	T50.3X3	T50.3X4	T50.3X5	T50.3X6
salicylate	T39.091	T39.092	T39.093	T39.094	T39.095	T39.096
salt NEC	T50.3X1	T50.3X2	T50.3X3	T50.3X4	T50.3X5	T50.3X6
selenate	T60.2X1	T60.2X2	T60.2X3	T60.2X4	—	—
stibogluconate	T37.3X1	T37.3X2	T37.3X3	T37.3X4	T37.3X5	T37.3X6
sulfate	T47.4X1	T47.4X2	T47.4X3	T47.4X4	T47.4X5	T47.4X6
sulfoxone	T37.1X1	T37.1X2	T37.1X3	T37.1X4	T37.1X5	T37.1X6
tetradecyl sulfate	T46.8X1	T46.8X2	T46.8X3	T46.8X4	T46.8X5	T46.8X6
thiopental	T41.1X1	T41.1X2	T41.1X3	T41.1X4	T41.1X5	T41.1X6
thiosalicylate	T39.091	T39.092	T39.093	T39.094	T39.095	T39.096
thiosulfate	T50.6X1	T50.6X2	T50.6X3	T50.6X4	T50.6X5	T50.6X6
tolbutamide	T38.3X1	T38.3X2	T38.3X3	T38.3X4	T38.3X5	T38.3X6
(L)-triiodothyronine	T38.1X1	T38.1X2	T38.1X3	T38.1X4	T38.1X5	T38.1X6
tyropanoate	T50.8X1	T50.8X2	T50.8X3	T50.8X4	T50.8X5	T50.8X6
valproate	T42.6X1	T42.6X2	T42.6X3	T42.6X4	T42.6X5	T42.6X6
versenate	T50.6X1	T50.6X2	T50.6X3	T50.6X4	T50.6X5	T50.6X6
Sodium-free salt	T50.901	T50.902	T50.903	T50.904	T50.905	T50.906
Sodium-removing resin	T50.3X1	T50.3X2	T50.3X3	T50.3X4	T50.3X5	T50.3X6
Soft soap	T55.0X1	T55.0X2	T55.0X3	T55.0X4	—	—
Solanine	T62.2X1	T62.2X2	T62.2X3	T62.2X4	—	—
berries	T62.1X1	T62.1X2	T62.1X3	T62.1X4	—	—
Solanum dulcamara	T62.2X1	T62.2X2	T62.2X3	T62.2X4	—	—
berries	T62.1X1	T62.1X2	T62.1X3	T62.1X4	—	—
Solapsone	T37.1X1	T37.1X2	T37.1X3	T37.1X4	T37.1X5	T37.1X6
Solar lotion	T49.3X1	T49.3X2	T49.3X3	T49.3X4	T49.3X5	T49.3X6
Solasulfone	T37.1X1	T37.1X2	T37.1X3	T37.1X4	T37.1X5	T37.1X6
Soldering fluid	T65.891	T65.892	T65.893	T65.894	—	—
Solid substance	T65.91	T65.92	T65.93	T65.94	—	—
specified NEC	T65.891	T65.892	T65.893	T65.894	—	—
Solvent, industrial NEC	T52.91	T52.92	T52.93	T52.94	—	—
naphtha	T52.0X1	T52.0X2	T52.0X3	T52.0X4	—	—
petroleum	T52.0X1	T52.0X2	T52.0X3	T52.0X4	—	—
specified NEC	T52.8X1	T52.8X2	T52.8X3	T52.8X4	—	—
Soma	T42.8X1	T42.8X2	T42.8X3	T42.8X4	T42.8X5	T42.8X6
Somatorelin	T38.891	T38.892	T38.893	T38.894	T38.895	T38.896
Somatostatin	T38.991	T38.992	T38.993	T38.994	T38.995	T38.996
Somatotropin	T38.811	T38.812	T38.813	T38.814	T38.815	T38.816
Somatrem	T38.811	T38.812	T38.813	T38.814	T38.815	T38.816
Somatropin	T38.811	T38.812	T38.813	T38.814	T38.815	T38.816
Sominex	T45.0X1	T45.0X2	T45.0X3	T45.0X4	T45.0X5	T45.0X6
Somnos	T42.6X1	T42.6X2	T42.6X3	T42.6X4	T42.6X5	T42.6X6
Somonal	T42.3X1	T42.3X2	T42.3X3	T42.3X4	T42.3X5	T42.3X6
Soneryl	T42.3X1	T42.3X2	T42.3X3	T42.3X4	T42.3X5	T42.3X6
Soothing syrup	T50.901	T50.902	T50.903	T50.904	T50.905	T50.906
Sopor	T42.6X1	T42.6X2	T42.6X3	T42.6X4	T42.6X5	T42.6X6
Soporific	T42.71	T42.72	T42.73	T42.74	T42.75	T42.76
Soporific drug	T42.71	T42.72	T42.73	T42.74	T42.75	T42.76
specified type NEC	T42.6X1	T42.6X2	T42.6X3	T42.6X4	T42.6X5	T42.6X6
Sorbide nitrate	T46.3X1	T46.3X2	T46.3X3	T46.3X4	T46.3X5	T46.3X6
Sorbitol	T47.4X1	T47.4X2	T47.4X3	T47.4X4	T47.4X5	T47.4X6
Sotalol	T44.7X1	T44.7X2	T44.7X3	T44.7X4	T44.7X5	T44.7X6
Sotradecol	T46.8X1	T46.8X2	T46.8X3	T46.8X4	T46.8X5	T46.8X6
Soysterol	T46.6X1	T46.6X2	T46.6X3	T46.6X4	T46.6X5	T46.6X6
Spacoline	T44.3X1	T44.3X2	T44.3X3	T44.3X4	T44.3X5	T44.3X6
Spanish fly	T49.8X1	T49.8X2	T49.8X3	T49.8X4	T49.8X5	T49.8X6
Sparine	T43.3X1	T43.3X2	T43.3X3	T43.3X4	T43.3X5	T43.3X6
Sparteine	T48.0X1	T48.0X2	T48.0X3	T48.0X4	T48.0X5	T48.0X6
Spasmolytic						
anticholinergics	T44.3X1	T44.3X2	T44.3X3	T44.3X4	T44.3X5	T44.3X6
autonomic	T44.3X1	T44.3X2	T44.3X3	T44.3X4	T44.3X5	T44.3X6
bronchial NEC	T48.6X1	T48.6X2	T48.6X3	T48.6X4	T48.6X5	T48.6X6
quaternary ammonium	T44.3X1	T44.3X2	T44.3X3	T44.3X4	T44.3X5	T44.3X6
skeletal muscle NEC	T48.1X1	T48.1X2	T48.1X3	T48.1X4	T48.1X5	T48.1X6
Spectinomycin	T36.5X1	T36.5X2	T36.5X3	T36.5X4	T36.5X5	T36.5X6
Speed	T43.621	T43.622	T43.623	T43.624	T43.625	T43.626
Spermicide	T49.8X1	T49.8X2	T49.8X3	T49.8X4	T49.8X5	T49.8X6
Spider (bite) (venom)	T63.391	T63.392	T63.393	T63.394	—	—
antivenin	T50.Z11	T50.Z12	T50.Z13	T50.Z14	T50.Z15	T50.Z16
Spigelia (root)	T37.4X1	T37.4X2	T37.4X3	T37.4X4	T37.4X5	T37.4X6
Spindle inactivator	T50.4X1	T50.4X2	T50.4X3	T50.4X4	T50.4X5	T50.4X6
Spiperone	T43.4X1	T43.4X2	T43.4X3	T43.4X4	T43.4X5	T43.4X6
Spiramycin	T36.3X1	T36.3X2	T36.3X3	T36.3X4	T36.3X5	T36.3X6

Substance	Poisoning, Accidental (unintentional)	Poisoning, Intentional Self-harm	Poisoning, Assault	Poisoning, Undetermined	Adverse Effect	Under-dosing
Spirapril	T46.4X1	T46.4X2	T46.4X3	T46.4X4	T46.4X5	T46.4X6
Spirilene	T43.591	T43.592	T43.593	T43.594	T43.595	T43.596
Spirit(s) (neutral) **NEC**	T51.0X1	T51.0X2	T51.0X3	T51.0X4	—	—
beverage	T51.0X1	T51.0X2	T51.0X3	T51.0X4	—	—
industrial	T51.0X1	T51.0X2	T51.0X3	T51.0X4	—	—
mineral	T52.0X1	T52.0X2	T52.0X3	T52.0X4	—	—
of salt — see Hydrochloric acid						
surgical	T51.0X1	T51.0X2	T51.0X3	T51.0X4	—	—
Spironolactone	T50.0X1	T50.0X2	T50.0X3	T50.0X4	T50.0X5	T50.0X6
Spiroperidol	T43.4X1	T43.4X2	T43.4X3	T43.4X4	T43.4X5	T43.4X6
Sponge, absorbable	T45.7X1	T45.7X2	T45.7X3	T45.7X4	T45.7X5	T45.7X6
(gelatin)						
Sporostacin	T49.0X1	T49.0X2	T49.0X3	T49.0X4	T49.0X5	T49.0X6
Spray (aerosol)	T65.91	T65.92	T65.93	T65.94	—	—
cosmetic	T65.891	T65.892	T65.893	T65.894	—	—
medicinal NEC	T50.901	T50.902	T50.903	T50.904	T50.905	T50.906
pesticides — see Pesticides						
specified content — see specific substance						
Spurge flax	T62.2X1	T62.2X2	T62.2X3	T62.2X4	—	—
Spurges	T62.2X1	T62.2X2	T62.2X3	T62.2X4	—	—
Sputum viscosity-lowering drug	T48.4X1	T48.4X2	T48.4X3	T48.4X4	T48.4X5	T48.4X6
Squill	T46.0X1	T46.0X2	T46.0X3	T46.0X4	T46.0X5	T46.0X6
rat poison	T60.4X1	T60.4X2	T60.4X3	T60.4X4	—	—
Squirting cucumber	T47.2X1	T47.2X2	T47.2X3	T47.2X4	T47.2X5	T47.2X6
(cathartic)						
Stains	T65.6X1	T65.6X2	T65.6X3	T65.6X4	—	—
Stannous fluoride	T49.7X1	T49.7X2	T49.7X3	T49.7X4	T49.7X5	T49.7X6
Stanolone	T38.7X1	T38.7X2	T38.7X3	T38.7X4	T38.7X5	T38.7X6
Stanozolol	T38.7X1	T38.7X2	T38.7X3	T38.7X4	T38.7X5	T38.7X6
Staphisagria or stavesacre (pediculicide)	T49.0X1	T49.0X2	T49.0X3	T49.0X4	T49.0X5	T49.0X6
Starch	T50.901	T50.902	T50.903	T50.904	T50.905	T50.906
Stelazine	T43.3X1	T43.3X2	T43.3X3	T43.3X4	T43.3X5	T43.3X6
Stemetil	T43.3X1	T43.3X2	T43.3X3	T43.3X4	T43.3X5	T43.3X6
Stepronin	T48.4X1	T48.4X2	T48.4X3	T48.4X4	T48.4X5	T48.4X6
Sterculia	T47.4X1	T47.4X2	T47.4X3	T47.4X4	T47.4X5	T47.4X6
Sternutator gas	T59.891	T59.892	T59.893	T59.894	—	—
Steroid	T38.0X1	T38.0X2	T38.0X3	T38.0X4	T38.0X5	T38.0X6
anabolic	T38.7X1	T38.7X2	T38.7X3	T38.7X4	T38.7X5	T38.7X6
androgenic	T38.7X1	T38.7X2	T38.7X3	T38.7X4	T38.7X5	T38.7X6
antineoplastic, hormone	T38.7X1	T38.7X2	T38.7X3	T38.7X4	T38.7X5	T38.7X6
estrogen	T38.5X1	T38.5X2	T38.5X3	T38.5X4	T38.5X5	T38.5X6
ENT agent	T49.6X1	T49.6X2	T49.6X3	T49.6X4	T49.6X5	T49.6X6
ophthalmic preparation	T49.5X1	T49.5X2	T49.5X3	T49.5X4	T49.5X5	T49.5X6
topical NEC	T49.0X1	T49.0X2	T49.0X3	T49.0X4	T49.0X5	T49.0X6
Stibine	T56.891	T56.892	T56.893	T56.894	—	—
Stibogluconate	T37.3X1	T37.3X2	T37.3X3	T37.3X4	T37.3X5	T37.3X6
Stibophen	T37.4X1	T37.4X2	T37.4X3	T37.4X4	T37.4X5	T37.4X6
Stilbamidine (isetionate)	T37.3X1	T37.3X2	T37.3X3	T37.3X4	T37.3X5	T37.3X6
Stilbestrol	T38.5X1	T38.5X2	T38.5X3	T38.5X4	T38.5X5	T38.5X6
Stilboestrol	T38.5X1	T38.5X2	T38.5X3	T38.5X4	T38.5X5	T38.5X6
Stimulant						
central nervous system — see also Psychostimulant		T43.601	T43.602	T43.603	T43.604	T43.605	T43.606
analeptics	T50.7X1	T50.7X2	T50.7X3	T50.7X4	T50.7X5	T50.7X6
opiate antagonist	T50.7X1	T50.7X2	T50.7X3	T50.7X4	T50.7X5	T50.7X6
psychotherapeutic NEC — see also Psychotherapeutic drug	T43.601	T43.602	T43.603	T43.604	T43.605	T43.606
specified NEC	T43.691	T43.692	T43.693	T43.694	T43.695	T43.696
respiratory	T48.901	T48.902	T48.903	T48.904	T48.905	T48.906
Stone-dissolving drug	T50.901	T50.902	T50.903	T50.904	T50.905	T50.906
Storage battery (cells) (acid)	T54.2X1	T54.2X2	T54.2X3	T54.2X4	—	—
Stovaine	T41.3X1	T41.3X2	T41.3X3	T41.3X4	T41.3X5	T41.3X6
infiltration (subcutaneous)	T41.3X1	T41.3X2	T41.3X3	T41.3X4	T41.3X5	T41.3X6
nerve block (peripheral) (plexus)	T41.3X1	T41.3X2	T41.3X3	T41.3X4	T41.3X5	T41.3X6
spinal	T41.3X1	T41.3X2	T41.3X3	T41.3X4	T41.3X5	T41.3X6
topical (surface)	T41.3X1	T41.3X2	T41.3X3	T41.3X4	T41.3X5	T41.3X6
Stovarsal	T37.8X1	T37.8X2	T37.8X3	T37.8X4	T37.8X5	T37.8X6
Stove gas — see Gas, stove						
Stoxil	T49.5X1	T49.5X2	T49.5X3	T49.5X4	T49.5X5	T49.5X6
Stramonium	T48.6X1	T48.6X2	T48.6X3	T48.6X4	T48.6X5	T48.6X6
natural state	T62.2X1	T62.2X2	T62.2X3	T62.2X4	—	—
Streptodornase	T45.3X1	T45.3X2	T45.3X3	T45.3X4	T45.3X5	T45.3X6
Streptoduocin	T36.5X1	T36.5X2	T36.5X3	T36.5X4	T36.5X5	T36.5X6
Streptokinase	T45.611	T45.612	T45.613	T45.614	T45.615	T45.616
Streptomycin (derivative)	T36.5X1	T36.5X2	T36.5X3	T36.5X4	T36.5X5	T36.5X6
Streptonivicin	T36.5X1	T36.5X2	T36.5X3	T36.5X4	T36.5X5	T36.5X6
Streptovarycin	T36.5X1	T36.5X2	T36.5X3	T36.5X4	T36.5X5	T36.5X6

Sodium — Streptovarycin

Substance	Poisoning, Accidental (unintentional)	Poisoning, Intentional Self-harm	Poisoning, Assault	Poisoning, Undetermined	Adverse Effect	Under-dosing
Streptozocin	T45.1X1	T45.1X2	T45.1X3	T45.1X4	T45.1X5	T45.1X6
Streptozotocin	T45.1X1	T45.1X2	T45.1X3	T45.1X4	T45.1X5	T45.1X6
Stripper (paint) (solvent)	T52.8X1	T52.8X2	T52.8X3	T52.8X4	—	—
Strobane	T60.1X1	T60.1X2	T60.1X3	T60.1X4	—	—
Strofantina	T46.0X1	T46.0X2	T46.0X3	T46.0X4	T46.0X5	T46.0X6
Strophanthin (g) (k)	T46.0X1	T46.0X2	T46.0X3	T46.0X4	T46.0X5	T46.0X6
Strophanthus	T46.0X1	T46.0X2	T46.0X3	T46.0X4	T46.0X5	T46.0X6
Strophantin	T46.0X1	T46.0X2	T46.0X3	T46.0X4	T46.0X5	T46.0X6
Strophantin-g	T46.0X1	T46.0X2	T46.0X3	T46.0X4	T46.0X5	T46.0X6
Strychnine (nonmedicinal) (pesticide) (salts)	T65.1X1	T65.1X2	T65.1X3	T65.1X4	—	—
medicinal	T48.291	T48.292	T48.293	T48.294	T48.295	T48.296
Strychnos (ignatii) — see Strychnine						
Styramate	T42.8X1	T42.8X2	T42.8X3	T42.8X4	T42.8X5	T42.8X6
Styrene	T65.891	T65.892	T65.893	T65.894	—	—
Succinimide, antiepileptic or anticonvulsant	T42.2X1	T42.2X2	T42.2X3	T42.2X4	T42.2X5	T42.2X6
mercuric — see Mercury						
Succinylcholine	T48.1X1	T48.1X2	T48.1X3	T48.1X4	T48.1X5	T48.1X6
Succinylsulfathiazole	T37.0X1	T37.0X2	T37.0X3	T37.0X4	T37.0X5	T37.0X6
Sucralfate	T47.1X1	T47.1X2	T47.1X3	T47.1X4	T47.1X5	T47.1X6
Sucrose	T50.3X1	T50.3X2	T50.3X3	T50.3X4	T50.3X5	T50.3X6
Sufentanil	T40.4X1	T40.4X2	T40.4X3	T40.4X4	T40.4X5	T40.4X6
Sulbactam	T36.0X1	T36.0X2	T36.0X3	T36.0X4	T36.0X5	T36.0X6
Sulbenicillin	T36.0X1	T36.0X2	T36.0X3	T36.0X4	T36.0X5	T36.0X6
Sulbentine	T49.0X1	T49.0X2	T49.0X3	T49.0X4	T49.0X5	T49.0X6
Sulfacetamide	T49.0X1	T49.0X2	T49.0X3	T49.0X4	T49.0X5	T49.0X6
ophthalmic preparation	T49.5X1	T49.5X2	T49.5X3	T49.5X4	T49.5X5	T49.5X6
Sulfachlorpyridazine	T37.0X1	T37.0X2	T37.0X3	T37.0X4	T37.0X5	T37.0X6
Sulfacitine	T37.0X1	T37.0X2	T37.0X3	T37.0X4	T37.0X5	T37.0X6
Sulfadiasulfone sodium	T37.0X1	T37.0X2	T37.0X3	T37.0X4	T37.0X5	T37.0X6
Sulfadiazine	T37.0X1	T37.0X2	T37.0X3	T37.0X4	T37.0X5	T37.0X6
silver (topical)	T49.0X1	T49.0X2	T49.0X3	T49.0X4	T49.0X5	T49.0X6
Sulfadimethoxine	T37.0X1	T37.0X2	T37.0X3	T37.0X4	T37.0X5	T37.0X6
Sulfadimidine	T37.0X1	T37.0X2	T37.0X3	T37.0X4	T37.0X5	T37.0X6
Sulfadoxine	T37.0X1	T37.0X2	T37.0X3	T37.0X4	T37.0X5	T37.0X6
with pyrimethamine	T37.2X1	T37.2X2	T37.2X3	T37.2X4	T37.2X5	T37.2X6
Sulfaethidole	T37.0X1	T37.0X2	T37.0X3	T37.0X4	T37.0X5	T37.0X6
Sulfafurazole	T37.0X1	T37.0X2	T37.0X3	T37.0X4	T37.0X5	T37.0X6
Sulfaguanidine	T37.0X1	T37.0X2	T37.0X3	T37.0X4	T37.0X5	T37.0X6
Sulfalene	T37.0X1	T37.0X2	T37.0X3	T37.0X4	T37.0X5	T37.0X6
Sulfaloxate	T37.0X1	T37.0X2	T37.0X3	T37.0X4	T37.0X5	T37.0X6
Sulfaloxic acid	T37.0X1	T37.0X2	T37.0X3	T37.0X4	T37.0X5	T37.0X6
Sulfamazone	T39.2X1	T39.2X2	T39.2X3	T39.2X4	T39.2X5	T39.2X6
Sulfamerazine	T37.0X1	T37.0X2	T37.0X3	T37.0X4	T37.0X5	T37.0X6
Sulfameter	T37.0X1	T37.0X2	T37.0X3	T37.0X4	T37.0X5	T37.0X6
Sulfamethazine	T37.0X1	T37.0X2	T37.0X3	T37.0X4	T37.0X5	T37.0X6
Sulfamethizole	T37.0X1	T37.0X2	T37.0X3	T37.0X4	T37.0X5	T37.0X6
Sulfamethoxazole	T37.0X1	T37.0X2	T37.0X3	T37.0X4	T37.0X5	T37.0X6
with trimethoprim	T36.8X1	T36.8X2	T36.8X3	T36.8X4	T36.8X5	T36.8X6
Sulfamethoxydiazine	T37.0X1	T37.0X2	T37.0X3	T37.0X4	T37.0X5	T37.0X6
Sulfamethoxypyridazine	T36.0X1	T36.0X2	T36.0X3	T36.0X4	T36.0X5	T36.0X6
Sulfamethylthiazole	T37.0X1	T37.0X2	T37.0X3	T37.0X4	T37.0X5	T37.0X6
Sulfametoxydiazine	T37.0X1	T37.0X2	T37.0X3	T37.0X4	T37.0X5	T37.0X6
Sulfamidopyrine	T39.2X1	T39.2X2	T39.2X3	T39.2X4	T39.2X5	T39.2X6
Sulfamonomethoxine	T37.0X1	T37.0X2	T37.0X3	T37.0X4	T37.0X5	T37.0X6
Sulfamoxole	T37.0X1	T37.0X2	T37.0X3	T37.0X4	T37.0X5	T37.0X6
Sulfamylon	T49.0X1	T49.0X2	T49.0X3	T49.0X4	T49.0X5	T49.0X6
Sulfan blue (diagnostic dye)	T50.8X1	T50.8X2	T50.8X3	T50.8X4	T50.8X5	T50.8X6
Sulfanilamide	T37.0X1	T37.0X2	T37.0X3	T37.0X4	T37.0X5	T37.0X6
Sulfanilylguanidine	T37.0X1	T37.0X2	T37.0X3	T37.0X4	T37.0X5	T37.0X6
Sulfaperin	T37.0X1	T37.0X2	T37.0X3	T37.0X4	T37.0X5	T37.0X6
Sulfaphenazole	T37.0X1	T37.0X2	T37.0X3	T37.0X4	T37.0X5	T37.0X6
Sulfaphenylthiazole	T37.0X1	T37.0X2	T37.0X3	T37.0X4	T37.0X5	T37.0X6
Sulfaproxyline	T37.0X1	T37.0X2	T37.0X3	T37.0X4	T37.0X5	T37.0X6
Sulfapyridine	T37.0X1	T37.0X2	T37.0X3	T37.0X4	T37.0X5	T37.0X6
Sulfapyrimidine	T37.0X1	T37.0X2	T37.0X3	T37.0X4	T37.0X5	T37.0X6
Sulfarsphenamine	T37.8X1	T37.8X2	T37.8X3	T37.8X4	T37.8X5	T37.8X6
Sulfasalazine	T37.0X1	T37.0X2	T37.0X3	T37.0X4	T37.0X5	T37.0X6
Sulfasuxidine	T53.6X1	T53.6X2	T53.6X3	T53.6X4	—	—
Sulfasymazine	T37.0X1	T37.0X2	T37.0X3	T37.0X4	T37.0X5	T37.0X6
Sulfated amylopectin	T47.8X1	T47.8X2	T47.8X3	T47.8X4	T47.8X5	T47.8X6
Sulfathiazole	T37.0X1	T37.0X2	T37.0X3	T37.0X4	T37.0X5	T37.0X6
Sulfatostearate	T49.2X1	T49.2X2	T49.2X3	T49.2X4	T49.2X5	T49.2X6
Sulfinpyrazone	T50.4X1	T50.4X2	T50.4X3	T50.4X4	T50.4X5	T50.4X6
Sulfiram	T49.0X1	T49.0X2	T49.0X3	T49.0X4	T49.0X5	T49.0X6
Sulfisomidine	T37.0X1	T37.0X2	T37.0X3	T37.0X4	T37.0X5	T37.0X6
Sulfisoxazole	T37.0X1	T37.0X2	T37.0X3	T37.0X4	T37.0X5	T37.0X6
ophthalmic preparation	T49.5X1	T49.5X2	T49.5X3	T49.5X4	T49.5X5	T49.5X6
Sulfobromophthalein (sodium)	T50.8X1	T50.8X2	T50.8X3	T50.8X4	T50.8X5	T50.8X6
Sulfobromphthalein	T50.8X1	T50.8X2	T50.8X3	T50.8X4	T50.8X5	T50.8X6
Sulfogaiacol	T48.4X1	T48.4X2	T48.4X3	T48.4X4	T48.4X5	T48.4X6
Sulfomyxin	T36.8X1	T36.8X2	T36.8X3	T36.8X4	T36.8X5	T36.8X6
Sulfonal	T42.6X1	T42.6X2	T42.6X3	T42.6X4	T42.6X5	T42.6X6
Sulfonamide NEC	T37.0X1	T37.0X2	T37.0X3	T37.0X4	T37.0X5	T37.0X6
eye	T49.5X1	T49.5X2	T49.5X3	T49.5X4	T49.5X5	T49.5X6
Sulfonazide	T37.1X1	T37.1X2	T37.1X3	T37.1X4	T37.1X5	T37.1X6
Sulfones	T37.1X1	T37.1X2	T37.1X3	T37.1X4	T37.1X5	T37.1X6
Sulfonethylmethane	T42.6X1	T42.6X2	T42.6X3	T42.6X4	T42.6X5	T42.6X6
Sulfonmethane	T42.6X1	T42.6X2	T42.6X3	T42.6X4	T42.6X5	T42.6X6
Sulfonphthal, sulfonphthol	T50.8X1	T50.8X2	T50.8X3	T50.8X4	T50.8X5	T50.8X6
Sulfonylurea derivatives, oral	T38.3X1	T38.3X2	T38.3X3	T38.3X4	T38.3X5	T38.3X6
Sulforidazine	T43.3X1	T43.3X2	T43.3X3	T43.3X4	T43.3X5	T43.3X6
Sulfoxone	T37.1X1	T37.1X2	T37.1X3	T37.1X4	T37.1X5	T37.1X6
Sulfuric acid	T54.2X1	T54.2X2	T54.2X3	T54.2X4		
Sulfur, sulfurated, sulfuric, sulfurous, sulfuryl (compounds NEC) (medicinal)	T49.4X1	T49.4X2	T49.4X3	T49.4X4	T49.4X5	T49.4X6
acid	T54.2X1	T54.2X2	T54.2X3	T54.2X4	—	—
dioxide (gas)	T59.1X1	T59.1X2	T59.1X3	T59.1X4	—	—
ether — see Ether(s)						
hydrogen	T59.6X1	T59.6X2	T59.6X3	T59.6X4	—	—
medicinal (keratolytic) (ointment) NEC	T49.4X1	T49.4X2	T49.4X3	T49.4X4	T49.4X5	T49.4X6
ointment	T49.0X1	T49.0X2	T49.0X3	T49.0X4	T49.0X5	T49.0X6
pesticide (vapor)	T60.91	T60.92	T60.93	T60.94	—	—
vapor NEC	T59.891	T59.892	T59.893	T59.894	—	—
Sulglicotide	T47.1X1	T47.1X2	T47.1X3	T47.1X4	T47.1X5	T47.1X6
Sulindac	T39.391	T39.392	T39.393	T39.394	T39.395	T39.396
Sulisatin	T47.2X1	T47.2X2	T47.2X3	T47.2X4	T47.2X5	T47.2X6
Sulisobenzone	T49.3X1	T49.3X2	T49.3X3	T49.3X4	T49.3X5	T49.3X6
Sulkowitch's reagent	T50.8X1	T50.8X2	T50.8X3	T50.8X4	T50.8X5	T50.8X6
Sulmetozine	T44.3X1	T44.3X2	T44.3X3	T44.3X4	T44.3X5	T44.3X6
Suloctidil	T46.7X1	T46.7X2	T46.7X3	T46.7X4	T46.7X5	T46.7X6
Sulph- — see also Sulf-						
Sulphadiazine	T37.0X1	T37.0X2	T37.0X3	T37.0X4	T37.0X5	T37.0X6
Sulphadimethoxine	T37.0X1	T37.0X2	T37.0X3	T37.0X4	T37.0X5	T37.0X6
Sulphadimidine	T37.0X1	T37.0X2	T37.0X3	T37.0X4	T37.0X5	T37.0X6
Sulphadione	T37.1X1	T37.1X2	T37.1X3	T37.1X4	T37.1X5	T37.1X6
Sulphafurazole	T37.0X1	T37.0X2	T37.0X3	T37.0X4	T37.0X5	T37.0X6
Sulphamethizole	T37.0X1	T37.0X2	T37.0X3	T37.0X4	T37.0X5	T37.0X6
Sulphamethoxazole	T37.0X1	T37.0X2	T37.0X3	T37.0X4	T37.0X5	T37.0X6
Sulphan blue	T50.8X1	T50.8X2	T50.8X3	T50.8X4	T50.8X5	T50.8X6
Sulphaphenazole	T37.0X1	T37.0X2	T37.0X3	T37.0X4	T37.0X5	T37.0X6
Sulphapyridine	T37.0X1	T37.0X2	T37.0X3	T37.0X4	T37.0X5	T37.0X6
Sulphasalazine	T37.0X1	T37.0X2	T37.0X3	T37.0X4	T37.0X5	T37.0X6
Sulphinpyrazone	T50.4X1	T50.4X2	T50.4X3	T50.4X4	T50.4X5	T50.4X6
Sulpiride	T43.591	T43.592	T43.593	T43.594	T43.595	T43.596
Sulprostone	T48.0X1	T48.0X2	T48.0X3	T48.0X4	T48.0X5	T48.0X6
Sulpyrine	T39.2X1	T39.2X2	T39.2X3	T39.2X4	T39.2X5	T39.2X6
Sultamicillin	T36.0X1	T36.0X2	T36.0X3	T36.0X4	T36.0X5	T36.0X6
Sulthiame	T42.6X1	T42.6X2	T42.6X3	T42.6X4	T42.6X5	T42.6X6
Sultiame	T42.6X1	T42.6X2	T42.6X3	T42.6X4	T42.6X5	T42.6X6
Sultopride	T43.591	T43.592	T43.593	T43.594	T43.595	T43.596
Sumatriptan	T39.8X1	T39.8X2	T39.8X3	T39.8X4	T39.8X5	T39.8X6
Sunflower seed oil	T46.6X1	T46.6X2	T46.6X3	T46.6X4	T46.6X5	T46.6X6
Superinone	T48.4X1	T48.4X2	T48.4X3	T48.4X4	T48.4X5	T48.4X6
Suprofen	T39.311	T39.312	T39.313	T39.314	T39.315	T39.316
Suramin (sodium)	T37.4X1	T37.4X2	T37.4X3	T37.4X4	T37.4X5	T37.4X6
Surfacaine	T41.3X1	T41.3X2	T41.3X3	T41.3X4	T41.3X5	T41.3X6
Surital	T41.1X1	T41.1X2	T41.1X3	T41.1X4	T41.1X5	T41.1X6
Sutilains	T45.3X1	T45.3X2	T45.3X3	T45.3X4	T45.3X5	T45.3X6
Suxamethonium (chloride)	T48.1X1	T48.1X2	T48.1X3	T48.1X4	T48.1X5	T48.1X6
Suxethonium (chloride)	T48.1X1	T48.1X2	T48.1X3	T48.1X4	T48.1X5	T48.1X6
Suxibuzone	T39.2X1	T39.2X2	T39.2X3	T39.2X4	T39.2X5	T39.2X6
Sweetener	T50.901	T50.902	T50.903	T50.904	T50.905	T50.906
Sweet niter spirit	T46.3X1	T46.3X2	T46.3X3	T46.3X4	T46.3X5	T46.3X6
Sweet oil (birch)	T49.3X1	T49.3X2	T49.3X3	T49.3X4	T49.3X5	T49.3X6
Sym-dichloroethyl ether	T53.6X1	T53.6X2	T53.6X3	T53.6X4	—	—
Sympatholytic NEC	T44.8X1	T44.8X2	T44.8X3	T44.8X4	T44.8X5	T44.8X6
haloalkylamine	T44.8X1	T44.8X2	T44.8X3	T44.8X4	T44.8X5	T44.8X6
Sympathomimetic NEC	T44.901	T44.902	T44.903	T44.904	T44.905	T44.906
anti-common-cold	T48.5X1	T48.5X2	T48.5X3	T48.5X4	T48.5X5	T48.5X6
bronchodilator	T48.6X1	T48.6X2	T48.6X3	T48.6X4	T48.6X5	T48.6X6
specified NEC	T44.991	T44.992	T44.993	T44.994	T44.995	T44.996
Synagis	T50.B91	T50.B92	T50.B93	T50.B94	T50.B95	T50.B96
Synalar	T49.0X1	T49.0X2	T49.0X3	T49.0X4	T49.0X5	T49.0X6
Synthroid	T38.1X1	T38.1X2	T38.1X3	T38.1X4	T38.1X5	T38.1X6
Syntocinon	T48.0X1	T48.0X2	T48.0X3	T48.0X4	T48.0X5	T48.0X6
Syrosingopine	T46.5X1	T46.5X2	T46.5X3	T46.5X4	T46.5X5	T46.5X6
Systemic drug	T45.91	T45.92	T45.93	T45.94	T45.95	T45.96

Additional Character May Be Required — Refer to the Tabular List for Character Selection

▽ Subterms under main terms may continue to next column or page

Substance	Poisoning, Accidental (unintentional)	Poisoning, Intentional Self-harm	Poisoning, Assault	Poisoning, Undetermined	Adverse Effect	Under-dosing
Systemic drug — continued						
specified NEC	T45.8X1	T45.8X2	T45.8X3	T45.8X4	T45.8X5	T45.8X6
Tablets — see also specified substance	T50.901	T50.902	T50.903	T50.904	T50.905	T50.906
Tace	T38.5X1	T38.5X2	T38.5X3	T38.5X4	T38.5X5	T38.5X6
Tacrine	T44.0X1	T44.0X2	T44.0X3	T44.0X4	T44.0X5	T44.0X6
Tadalafil	T46.7X1	T46.7X2	T46.7X3	T46.7X4	T46.7X5	T46.7X6
Talampicillin	T36.0X1	T36.0X2	T36.0X3	T36.0X4	T36.0X5	T36.0X6
Talbutal	T42.3X1	T42.3X2	T42.3X3	T42.3X4	T42.3X5	T42.3X6
Talc powder	T49.3X1	T49.3X2	T49.3X3	T49.3X4	T49.3X5	T49.3X6
Talcum	T49.3X1	T49.3X2	T49.3X3	T49.3X4	T49.3X5	T49.3X6
Taleranol	T38.6X1	T38.6X2	T38.6X3	T38.6X4	T38.6X5	T38.6X6
Tamoxifen	T38.6X1	T38.6X2	T38.6X3	T38.6X4	T38.6X5	T38.6X6
Tamsulosin	T44.6X1	T44.6X2	T44.6X3	T44.6X4	T44.6X5	T44.6X6
Tandearil, tanderil	T39.2X1	T39.2X2	T39.2X3	T39.2X4	T39.2X5	T39.2X6
Tannic acid	T49.2X1	T49.2X2	T49.2X3	T49.2X4	T49.2X5	T49.2X6
medicinal (astringent)	T49.2X1	T49.2X2	T49.2X3	T49.2X4	T49.2X5	T49.2X6
Tannin — see Tannic acid						
Tansy	T62.2X1	T62.2X2	T62.2X3	T62.2X4	—	—
TAO	T36.3X1	T36.3X2	T36.3X3	T36.3X4	T36.3X5	T36.3X6
Tapazole	T38.2X1	T38.2X2	T38.2X3	T38.2X4	T38.2X5	T38.2X6
Taractan	T43.591	T43.592	T43.593	T43.594	T43.595	T43.596
Tarantula (venomous)	T63.321	T63.322	T63.323	T63.324	—	—
Tartar emetic	T37.8X1	T37.8X2	T37.8X3	T37.8X4	T37.8X5	T37.8X6
Tartaric acid	T65.891	T65.892	T65.893	T65.894	—	—
Tartrated antimony (anti-infective)	T37.8X1	T37.8X2	T37.8X3	T37.8X4	T37.8X5	T37.8X6
Tartrate, laxative	T47.4X1	T47.4X2	T47.4X3	T47.4X4	T47.4X5	T47.4X6
Tar NEC	T52.0X1	T52.0X2	T52.0X3	T52.0X4	—	—
camphor	T60.1X1	T60.1X2	T60.1X3	T60.1X4	—	—
distillate	T49.1X1	T49.1X2	T49.1X3	T49.1X4	T49.1X5	T49.1X6
fumes	T59.891	T59.892	T59.893	T59.894	—	—
medicinal	T49.1X1	T49.1X2	T49.1X3	T49.1X4	T49.1X5	T49.1X6
ointment	T49.1X1	T49.1X2	T49.1X3	T49.1X4	T49.1X5	T49.1X6
Tauromustine	T45.1X1	T45.1X2	T45.1X3	T45.1X4	T45.1X5	T45.1X6
TCA — see Trichloroacetic acid						
TCDD	T53.7X1	T53.7X2	T53.7X3	T53.7X4	—	—
TDI (vapor)	T65.0X1	T65.0X2	T65.0X3	T65.0X4	—	—
Tear						
gas	T59.3X1	T59.3X2	T59.3X3	T59.3X4	—	—
solution	T49.5X1	T49.5X2	T49.5X3	T49.5X4	T49.5X5	T49.5X6
Teclothiazide	T50.2X1	T50.2X2	T50.2X3	T50.2X4	T50.2X5	T50.2X6
Teclozan	T37.3X1	T37.3X2	T37.3X3	T37.3X4	T37.3X5	T37.3X6
Tegafur	T45.1X1	T45.1X2	T45.1X3	T45.1X4	T45.1X5	T45.1X6
Tegretol	T42.1X1	T42.1X2	T42.1X3	T42.1X4	T42.1X5	T42.1X6
Teicoplanin	T36.8X1	T36.8X2	T36.8X3	T36.8X4	T36.8X5	T36.8X6
Telepaque	T50.8X1	T50.8X2	T50.8X3	T50.8X4	T50.8X5	T50.8X6
Tellurium	T56.891	T56.892	T56.893	T56.894	—	—
fumes	T56.891	T56.892	T56.893	T56.894	—	—
TEM	T45.1X1	T45.1X2	T45.1X3	T45.1X4	T45.1X5	T45.1X6
Temazepam	T42.4X1	T42.4X2	T42.4X3	T42.4X4	T42.4X5	T42.4X6
Temocillin	T36.0X1	T36.0X2	T36.0X3	T36.0X4	T36.0X5	T36.0X6
Tenamfetamine	T43.621	T43.622	T43.623	T43.624	T43.625	T43.626
Teniposide	T45.1X1	T45.1X2	T45.1X3	T45.1X4	T45.1X5	T45.1X6
Tenitramine	T46.3X1	T46.3X2	T46.3X3	T46.3X4	T46.3X5	T46.3X6
Tenoglicin	T48.4X1	T48.4X2	T48.4X3	T48.4X4	T48.4X5	T48.4X6
Tenonitrozole	T37.3X1	T37.3X2	T37.3X3	T37.3X4	T37.3X5	T37.3X6
Tenoxicam	T39.391	T39.392	T39.393	T39.394	T39.395	T39.396
TEPA	T45.1X1	T45.1X2	T45.1X3	T45.1X4	T45.1X5	T45.1X6
TEPP	T60.0X1	T60.0X2	T60.0X3	T60.0X4	—	—
Teprotide	T46.5X1	T46.5X2	T46.5X3	T46.5X4	T46.5X5	T46.5X6
Terazosin	T44.6X1	T44.6X2	T44.6X3	T44.6X4	T44.6X5	T44.6X6
Terbufos	T60.0X1	T60.0X2	T60.0X3	T60.0X4	—	—
Terbutaline	T48.6X1	T48.6X2	T48.6X3	T48.6X4	T48.6X5	T48.6X6
Terconazole	T49.0X1	T49.0X2	T49.0X3	T49.0X4	T49.0X5	T49.0X6
Terfenadine	T45.0X1	T45.0X2	T45.0X3	T45.0X4	T45.0X5	T45.0X6
Teriparatide (acetate)	T50.991	T50.992	T50.993	T50.994	T50.995	T50.996
Terizidone	T37.1X1	T37.1X2	T37.1X3	T37.1X4	T37.1X5	T37.1X6
Terlipressin	T38.891	T38.892	T38.893	T38.894	T38.895	T38.896
Terodiline	T46.3X1	T46.3X2	T46.3X3	T46.3X4	T46.3X5	T46.3X6
Teroxalene	T37.4X1	T37.4X2	T37.4X3	T37.4X4	T37.4X5	T37.4X6
Terpin (cis) hydrate	T48.4X1	T48.4X2	T48.4X3	T48.4X4	T48.4X5	T48.4X6
Terramycin	T36.4X1	T36.4X2	T36.4X3	T36.4X4	T36.4X5	T36.4X6
Tertatolol	T44.7X1	T44.7X2	T44.7X3	T44.7X4	T44.7X5	T44.7X6
Tessalon	T48.3X1	T48.3X2	T48.3X3	T48.3X4	T48.3X5	T48.3X6
Testolactone	T38.7X1	T38.7X2	T38.7X3	T38.7X4	T38.7X5	T38.7X6
Testosterone	T38.7X1	T38.7X2	T38.7X3	T38.7X4	T38.7X5	T38.7X6
Tetanus toxoid or vaccine	T50.A91	T50.A92	T50.A93	T50.A94	T50.A95	T50.A96
antitoxin	T50.Z11	T50.Z12	T50.Z13	T50.Z14	T50.Z15	T50.Z16
immune globulin (human)	T50.Z11	T50.Z12	T50.Z13	T50.Z14	T50.Z15	T50.Z16
toxoid	T50.A91	T50.A92	T50.A93	T50.A94	T50.A95	T50.A96
with diphtheria toxoid	T50.A21	T50.A22	T50.A23	T50.A24	T50.A25	T50.A26
with pertussis	T50.A11	T50.A12	T50.A13	T50.A14	T50.A15	T50.A16
Tetrabenazine	T43.591	T43.592	T43.593	T43.594	T43.595	T43.596
Tetracaine	T41.3X1	T41.3X2	T41.3X3	T41.3X4	T41.3X5	T41.3X6
nerve block (peripheral) (plexus)	T41.3X1	T41.3X2	T41.3X3	T41.3X4	T41.3X5	T41.3X6
regional	T41.3X1	T41.3X2	T41.3X3	T41.3X4	T41.3X5	T41.3X6
spinal	T41.3X1	T41.3X2	T41.3X3	T41.3X4	T41.3X5	T41.3X6
Tetrachlorethylene — see Tetrachloroethylene						
Tetrachlormethiazide	T50.2X1	T50.2X2	T50.2X3	T50.2X4	T50.2X5	T50.2X6
Tetrachloroethane	T53.6X1	T53.6X2	T53.6X3	T53.6X4	—	—
vapor	T53.6X1	T53.6X2	T53.6X3	T53.6X4	—	—
paint or varnish	T53.6X1	T53.6X2	T53.6X3	T53.6X4	—	—
Tetrachloroethylene (liquid)	T53.3X1	T53.3X2	T53.3X3	T53.3X4	—	—
medicinal	T37.4X1	T37.4X2	T37.4X3	T37.4X4	T37.4X5	T37.4X6
vapor	T53.3X1	T53.3X2	T53.3X3	T53.3X4	—	—
Tetrachloromethane — see Carbon tetrachloride						
Tetracosactide	T38.811	T38.812	T38.813	T38.814	T38.815	T38.816
Tetracosactrin	T38.811	T38.812	T38.813	T38.814	T38.815	T38.816
Tetracycline	T36.4X1	T36.4X2	T36.4X3	T36.4X4	T36.4X5	T36.4X6
ophthalmic preparation	T49.5X1	T49.5X2	T49.5X3	T49.5X4	T49.5X5	T49.5X6
topical NEC	T49.0X1	T49.0X2	T49.0X3	T49.0X4	T49.0X5	T49.0X6
Tetradifon	T60.8X1	T60.8X2	T60.8X3	T60.8X4	—	—
Tetradotoxin	T61.771	T61.772	T61.773	T61.774	—	—
Tetraethyl						
lead	T56.0X1	T56.0X2	T56.0X3	T56.0X4	—	—
pyrophosphate	T60.0X1	T60.0X2	T60.0X3	T60.0X4	—	—
Tetraethylammonium chloride	T44.2X1	T44.2X2	T44.2X3	T44.2X4	T44.2X5	T44.2X6
Tetraethylthiuram disulfide	T50.6X1	T50.6X2	T50.6X3	T50.6X4	T50.6X5	T50.6X6
Tetrahydroaminoacridine	T44.0X1	T44.0X2	T44.0X3	T44.0X4	T44.0X5	T44.0X6
Tetrahydrocannabinol	T40.7X1	T40.7X2	T40.7X3	T40.7X4	T40.7X5	T40.7X6
Tetrahydrofuran	T52.8X1	T52.8X2	T52.8X3	T52.8X4	—	—
Tetrahydronaphthalene	T52.8X1	T52.8X2	T52.8X3	T52.8X4	—	—
Tetrahydrozoline	T49.5X1	T49.5X2	T49.5X3	T49.5X4	T49.5X5	T49.5X6
Tetralin	T52.8X1	T52.8X2	T52.8X3	T52.8X4	—	—
Tetramethrin	T60.2X1	T60.2X2	T60.2X3	T60.2X4	—	—
Tetramethylthiuram (disulfide) NEC	T60.3X1	T60.3X2	T60.3X3	T60.3X4	—	—
medicinal	T49.0X1	T49.0X2	T49.0X3	T49.0X4	T49.0X5	T49.0X6
Tetramisole	T37.4X1	T37.4X2	T37.4X3	T37.4X4	T37.4X5	T37.4X6
Tetranicotinoyl fructose	T46.7X1	T46.7X2	T46.7X3	T46.7X4	T46.7X5	T46.7X6
Tetrazepam	T42.4X1	T42.4X2	T42.4X3	T42.4X4	T42.4X5	T42.4X6
Tetronal	T42.6X1	T42.6X2	T42.6X3	T42.6X4	T42.6X5	T42.6X6
Tetryl	T65.3X1	T65.3X2	T65.3X3	T65.3X4	—	—
Tetrylammonium chloride	T44.2X1	T44.2X2	T44.2X3	T44.2X4	T44.2X5	T44.2X6
Tetryzoline	T49.5X1	T49.5X2	T49.5X3	T49.5X4	T49.5X5	T49.5X6
Thalidomide	T45.1X1	T45.1X2	T45.1X3	T45.1X4	T45.1X5	T45.1X6
Thallium (compounds) (dust)	T56.811	T56.812	T56.813	T56.814	—	—
NEC						
pesticide	T60.4X1	T60.4X2	T60.4X3	T60.4X4	—	—
THC	T40.7X1	T40.7X2	T40.7X3	T40.7X4	T40.7X5	T40.7X6
Thebacon	T48.3X1	T48.3X2	T48.3X3	T48.3X4	T48.3X5	T48.3X6
Thebaine	T40.2X1	T40.2X2	T40.2X3	T40.2X4	T40.2X5	T40.2X6
Thenoic acid	T49.6X1	T49.6X2	T49.6X3	T49.6X4	T49.6X5	T49.6X6
Thenyldiamine	T45.0X1	T45.0X2	T45.0X3	T45.0X4	T45.0X5	T45.0X6
Theobromine (calcium salicylate)	T48.6X1	T48.6X2	T48.6X3	T48.6X4	T48.6X5	T48.6X6
sodium salicylate	T48.6X1	T48.6X2	T48.6X3	T48.6X4	T48.6X5	T48.6X6
Theophyllamine	T48.6X1	T48.6X2	T48.6X3	T48.6X4	T48.6X5	T48.6X6
Theophylline	T48.6X1	T48.6X2	T48.6X3	T48.6X4	T48.6X5	T48.6X6
aminobenzoic acid	T48.6X1	T48.6X2	T48.6X3	T48.6X4	T48.6X5	T48.6X6
ethylenediamine	T48.6X1	T48.6X2	T48.6X3	T48.6X4	T48.6X5	T48.6X6
piperazine	T48.6X1	T48.6X2	T48.6X3	T48.6X4	T48.6X5	T48.6X6
p-amino-benzoate						
Thiabendazole	T37.4X1	T37.4X2	T37.4X3	T37.4X4	T37.4X5	T37.4X6
Thialbarbital	T41.1X1	T41.1X2	T41.1X3	T41.1X4	T41.1X5	T41.1X6
Thiamazole	T38.2X1	T38.2X2	T38.2X3	T38.2X4	T38.2X5	T38.2X6
Thiambutosine	T37.1X1	T37.1X2	T37.1X3	T37.1X4	T37.1X5	T37.1X6
Thiamine	T45.2X1	T45.2X2	T45.2X3	T45.2X4	T45.2X5	T45.2X6
Thiamphenicol	T36.2X1	T36.2X2	T36.2X3	T36.2X4	T36.2X5	T36.2X6
Thiamylal	T41.1X1	T41.1X2	T41.1X3	T41.1X4	T41.1X5	T41.1X6
sodium	T41.1X1	T41.1X2	T41.1X3	T41.1X4	T41.1X5	T41.1X6
Thiazesim	T43.291	T43.292	T43.293	T43.294	T43.295	T43.296
Thiazides (diuretics)	T50.2X1	T50.2X2	T50.2X3	T50.2X4	T50.2X5	T50.2X6
Thiazinamium metilsulfate	T43.3X1	T43.3X2	T43.3X3	T43.3X4	T43.3X5	T43.3X6
Thiethylperazine	T43.3X1	T43.3X2	T43.3X3	T43.3X4	T43.3X5	T43.3X6
Thimerosal	T49.0X1	T49.0X2	T49.0X3	T49.0X4	T49.0X5	T49.0X6
ophthalmic preparation	T49.5X1	T49.5X2	T49.5X3	T49.5X4	T49.5X5	T49.5X6
Thioacetazone	T37.1X1	T37.1X2	T37.1X3	T37.1X4	T37.1X5	T37.1X6

Substance	Poisoning, Accidental (unintentional)	Poisoning, Intentional Self-harm	Poisoning, Assault	Poisoning, Undetermined	Adverse Effect	Under-dosing
Thioacetazone — continued						
with isoniazid	T37.1X1	T37.1X2	T37.1X3	T37.1X4	T37.1X5	T37.1X6
Thiobarbital sodium	T41.1X1	T41.1X2	T41.1X3	T41.1X4	T41.1X5	T41.1X6
Thiobarbiturate anesthetic	T41.1X1	T41.1X2	T41.1X3	T41.1X4	T41.1X5	T41.1X6
Thiobismol	T37.8X1	T37.8X2	T37.8X3	T37.8X4	T37.8X5	T37.8X6
Thiobutabarbital sodium	T41.1X1	T41.1X2	T41.1X3	T41.1X4	T41.1X5	T41.1X6
Thiocarbamate (insecticide)	T60.0X1	T60.0X2	T60.0X3	T60.0X4	—	—
Thiocarbamide	T38.2X1	T38.2X2	T38.2X3	T38.2X4	T38.2X5	T38.2X6
Thiocarbarsone	T37.8X1	T37.8X2	T37.8X3	T37.8X4	T37.8X5	T37.8X6
Thiocarlide	T37.1X1	T37.1X2	T37.1X3	T37.1X4	T37.1X5	T37.1X6
Thioctamide	T50.991	T50.992	T50.993	T50.994	T50.995	T50.996
Thioctic acid	T50.991	T50.992	T50.993	T50.994	T50.995	T50.996
Thiofos	T60.0X1	T60.0X2	T60.0X3	T60.0X4	—	—
Thioglycolate	T49.4X1	T49.4X2	T49.4X3	T49.4X4	T49.4X5	T49.4X6
Thioglycolic acid	T65.891	T65.892	T65.893	T65.894	—	—
Thioguanine	T45.1X1	T45.1X2	T45.1X3	T45.1X4	T45.1X5	T45.1X6
Thiomercaptomerin	T50.2X1	T50.2X2	T50.2X3	T50.2X4	T50.2X5	T50.2X6
Thiomerin	T50.2X1	T50.2X2	T50.2X3	T50.2X4	T50.2X5	T50.2X6
Thiomersal	T49.0X1	T49.0X2	T49.0X3	T49.0X4	T49.0X5	T49.0X6
Thionazin	T60.0X1	T60.0X2	T60.0X3	T60.0X4	—	—
Thiopental (sodium)	T41.1X1	T41.1X2	T41.1X3	T41.1X4	T41.1X5	T41.1X6
Thiopentone (sodium)	T41.1X1	T41.1X2	T41.1X3	T41.1X4	T41.1X5	T41.1X6
Thiopropazate	T43.3X1	T43.3X2	T43.3X3	T43.3X4	T43.3X5	T43.3X6
Thioproperazine	T43.3X1	T43.3X2	T43.3X3	T43.3X4	T43.3X5	T43.3X6
Thioridazine	T43.3X1	T43.3X2	T43.3X3	T43.3X4	T43.3X5	T43.3X6
Thiosinamine	T49.3X1	T49.3X2	T49.3X3	T49.3X4	T49.3X5	T49.3X6
Thiotepa	T45.1X1	T45.1X2	T45.1X3	T45.1X4	T45.1X5	T45.1X6
Thiothixene	T43.4X1	T43.4X2	T43.4X3	T43.4X4	T43.4X5	T43.4X6
Thiouracil (benzyl) (methyl) (propyl)	T38.2X1	T38.2X2	T38.2X3	T38.2X4	T38.2X5	T38.2X6
Thiourea	T38.2X1	T38.2X2	T38.2X3	T38.2X4	T38.2X5	T38.2X6
Thiphenamil	T44.3X1	T44.3X2	T44.3X3	T44.3X4	T44.3X5	T44.3X6
Thiram	T60.3X1	T60.3X2	T60.3X3	T60.3X4	—	—
medicinal	T49.2X1	T49.2X2	T49.2X3	T49.2X4	T49.2X5	T49.2X6
Thonzylamine (systemic)	T45.0X1	T45.0X2	T45.0X3	T45.0X4	T45.0X5	T45.0X6
mucosal decongestant	T48.5X1	T48.5X2	T48.5X3	T48.5X4	T48.5X5	T48.5X6
Thorazine	T43.3X1	T43.3X2	T43.3X3	T43.3X4	T43.3X5	T43.3X6
Thorium dioxide suspension	T50.8X1	T50.8X2	T50.8X3	T50.8X4	T50.8X5	T50.8X6
Thornapple	T62.2X1	T62.2X2	T62.2X3	T62.2X4	—	—
Throat drug NEC	T49.6X1	T49.6X2	T49.6X3	T49.6X4	T49.6X5	T49.6X6
Thrombin	T45.7X1	T45.7X2	T45.7X3	T45.7X4	T45.7X5	T45.7X6
Thrombolysin	T45.611	T45.612	T45.613	T45.614	T45.615	T45.616
Thromboplastin	T45.7X1	T45.7X2	T45.7X3	T45.7X4	T45.7X5	T45.7X6
Thurfyl nicotinate	T46.7X1	T46.7X2	T46.7X3	T46.7X4	T46.7X5	T46.7X6
Thymol	T49.0X1	T49.0X2	T49.0X3	T49.0X4	T49.0X5	T49.0X6
Thymopentin	T37.5X1	T37.5X2	T37.5X3	T37.5X4	T37.5X5	T37.5X6
Thymoxamine	T46.7X1	T46.7X2	T46.7X3	T46.7X4	T46.7X5	T46.7X6
Thymus extract	T38.891	T38.892	T38.893	T38.894	T38.895	T38.896
Thyreotrophic hormone	T38.811	T38.812	T38.813	T38.814	T38.815	T38.816
Thyroglobulin	T38.1X1	T38.1X2	T38.1X3	T38.1X4	T38.1X5	T38.1X6
Thyroid (hormone)	T38.1X1	T38.1X2	T38.1X3	T38.1X4	T38.1X5	T38.1X6
Thyrolar	T38.1X1	T38.1X2	T38.1X3	T38.1X4	T38.1X5	T38.1X6
Thyrotrophin	T38.811	T38.812	T38.813	T38.814	T38.815	T38.816
Thyrotropic hormone	T38.811	T38.812	T38.813	T38.814	T38.815	T38.816
Thyroxine	T38.1X1	T38.1X2	T38.1X3	T38.1X4	T38.1X5	T38.1X6
Tiabendazole	T37.4X1	T37.4X2	T37.4X3	T37.4X4	T37.4X5	T37.4X6
Tiamizide	T50.2X1	T50.2X2	T50.2X3	T50.2X4	T50.2X5	T50.2X6
Tianeptine	T43.291	T43.292	T43.293	T43.294	T43.295	T43.296
Tiapamil	T46.1X1	T46.1X2	T46.1X3	T46.1X4	T46.1X5	T46.1X6
Tiapride	T43.591	T43.592	T43.593	T43.594	T43.595	T43.596
Tiaprofenic acid	T39.311	T39.312	T39.313	T39.314	T39.315	T39.316
Tiaramide	T39.8X1	T39.8X2	T39.8X3	T39.8X4	T39.8X5	T39.8X6
Ticarcillin	T36.0X1	T36.0X2	T36.0X3	T36.0X4	T36.0X5	T36.0X6
Ticlatone	T49.0X1	T49.0X2	T49.0X3	T49.0X4	T49.0X5	T49.0X6
Ticlopidine	T45.521	T45.522	T45.523	T45.524	T45.525	T45.526
Ticrynafen	T50.1X1	T50.1X2	T50.1X3	T50.1X4	T50.1X5	T50.1X6
Tidiacic	T50.991	T50.992	T50.993	T50.994	T50.995	T50.996
Tiemonium	T44.3X1	T44.3X2	T44.3X3	T44.3X4	T44.3X5	T44.3X6
iodide	T44.3X1	T44.3X2	T44.3X3	T44.3X4	T44.3X5	T44.3X6
Tienilic acid	T50.1X1	T50.1X2	T50.1X3	T50.1X4	T50.1X5	T50.1X6
Tifenamil	T44.3X1	T44.3X2	T44.3X3	T44.3X4	T44.3X5	T44.3X6
Tigan	T45.0X1	T45.0X2	T45.0X3	T45.0X4	T45.0X5	T45.0X6
Tigloidine	T44.3X1	T44.3X2	T44.3X3	T44.3X4	T44.3X5	T44.3X6
Tilactase	T47.5X1	T47.5X2	T47.5X3	T47.5X4	T47.5X5	T47.5X6
Tiletamine	T41.291	T41.292	T41.293	T41.294	T41.295	T41.296
Tilidine	T40.4X1	T40.4X2	T40.4X3	T40.4X4	—	—
Timepidium bromide	T44.3X1	T44.3X2	T44.3X3	T44.3X4	T44.3X5	T44.3X6
Timiperone	T43.4X1	T43.4X2	T43.4X3	T43.4X4	T43.4X5	T43.4X6
Timolol	T44.7X1	T44.7X2	T44.7X3	T44.7X4	T44.7X5	T44.7X6
Tincture, iodine — see Iodine						
Tindal	T43.3X1	T43.3X2	T43.3X3	T43.3X4	T43.3X5	T43.3X6
Tinidazole	T37.3X1	T37.3X2	T37.3X3	T37.3X4	T37.3X5	T37.3X6
Tin (chloride) (dust) (oxide)	T56.6X1	T56.6X2	T56.6X3	T56.6X4	—	—
NEC						
anti-infectives	T37.8X1	T37.8X2	T37.8X3	T37.8X4	T37.8X5	T37.8X6
Tinoridine	T39.8X1	T39.8X2	T39.8X3	T39.8X4	T39.8X5	T39.8X6
Tiocarlide	T37.1X1	T37.1X2	T37.1X3	T37.1X4	T37.1X5	T37.1X6
Tioclomarol	T45.511	T45.512	T45.513	T45.514	T45.515	T45.516
Tioconazole	T49.0X1	T49.0X2	T49.0X3	T49.0X4	T49.0X5	T49.0X6
Tioguanine	T45.1X1	T45.1X2	T45.1X3	T45.1X4	T45.1X5	T45.1X6
Tiopronin	T50.991	T50.992	T50.993	T50.994	T50.995	T50.996
Tiotixene	T43.4X1	T43.4X2	T43.4X3	T43.4X4	T43.4X5	T43.4X6
Tioxolone	T49.4X1	T49.4X2	T49.4X3	T49.4X4	T49.4X5	T49.4X6
Tipepidine	T48.3X1	T48.3X2	T48.3X3	T48.3X4	T48.3X5	T48.3X6
Tiquizium bromide	T44.3X1	T44.3X2	T44.3X3	T44.3X4	T44.3X5	T44.3X6
Tiratricol	T38.1X1	T38.1X2	T38.1X3	T38.1X4	T38.1X5	T38.1X6
Tisopurine	T50.4X1	T50.4X2	T50.4X3	T50.4X4	T50.4X5	T50.4X6
Titanium (compounds) (vapor)	T56.891	T56.892	T56.893	T56.894	—	—
dioxide	T49.3X1	T49.3X2	T49.3X3	T49.3X4	T49.3X5	T49.3X6
ointment	T49.3X1	T49.3X2	T49.3X3	T49.3X4	T49.3X5	T49.3X6
oxide	T49.3X1	T49.3X2	T49.3X3	T49.3X4	T49.3X5	T49.3X6
tetrachloride	T56.891	T56.892	T56.893	T56.894	—	—
Titanocene	T56.891	T56.892	T56.893	T56.894	—	—
Titroid	T38.1X1	T38.1X2	T38.1X3	T38.1X4	T38.1X5	T38.1X6
Tizanidine	T42.8X1	T42.8X2	T42.8X3	T42.8X4	T42.8X5	T42.8X6
TMTD	T60.3X1	T60.3X2	T60.3X3	T60.3X4	—	—
TNT (fumes)	T65.3X1	T65.3X2	T65.3X3	T65.3X4	—	—
Toadstool	T62.0X1	T62.0X2	T62.0X3	T62.0X4	—	—
Tobacco NEC	T65.291	T65.292	T65.293	T65.294	—	—
cigarettes	T65.221	T65.222	T65.223	T65.224	—	—
Indian	T62.2X1	T62.2X2	T62.2X3	T62.2X4	—	—
smoke, second-hand	T65.221	T65.222	T65.223	T65.224	—	—
Tobramycin	T36.5X1	T36.5X2	T36.5X3	T36.5X4	T36.5X5	T36.5X6
Tocainide	T46.2X1	T46.2X2	T46.2X3	T46.2X4	T46.2X5	T46.2X6
Tocoferol	T45.2X1	T45.2X2	T45.2X3	T45.2X4	T45.2X5	T45.2X6
Tocopherol	T45.2X1	T45.2X2	T45.2X3	T45.2X4	T45.2X5	T45.2X6
acetate	T45.2X1	T45.2X2	T45.2X3	T45.2X4	T45.2X5	T45.2X6
Tocosamine	T48.0X1	T48.0X2	T48.0X3	T48.0X4	T48.0X5	T48.0X6
Todralazine	T46.5X1	T46.5X2	T46.5X3	T46.5X4	T46.5X5	T46.5X6
Tofisopam	T42.4X1	T42.4X2	T42.4X3	T42.4X4	T42.4X5	T42.4X6
Tofranil	T43.011	T43.012	T43.013	T43.014	T43.015	T43.016
Toilet deodorizer	T65.891	T65.892	T65.893	T65.894	—	—
Tolamolol	T44.7X1	T44.7X2	T44.7X3	T44.7X4	T44.7X5	T44.7X6
Tolazamide	T38.3X1	T38.3X2	T38.3X3	T38.3X4	T38.3X5	T38.3X6
Tolazoline	T46.7X1	T46.7X2	T46.7X3	T46.7X4	T46.7X5	T46.7X6
Tolbutamide (sodium)	T38.3X1	T38.3X2	T38.3X3	T38.3X4	T38.3X5	T38.3X6
Tolciclate	T49.0X1	T49.0X2	T49.0X3	T49.0X4	T49.0X5	T49.0X6
Tolmetin	T39.391	T39.392	T39.393	T39.394	T39.395	T39.396
Tolnaftate	T49.0X1	T49.0X2	T49.0X3	T49.0X4	T49.0X5	T49.0X6
Tolonidine	T46.5X1	T46.5X2	T46.5X3	T46.5X4	T46.5X5	T46.5X6
Toloxatone	T42.6X1	T42.6X2	T42.6X3	T42.6X4	T42.6X5	T42.6X6
Tolperisone	T44.3X1	T44.3X2	T44.3X3	T44.3X4	T44.3X5	T44.3X6
Tolserol	T42.8X1	T42.8X2	T42.8X3	T42.8X4	T42.8X5	T42.8X6
Toluene (liquid)	T52.2X1	T52.2X2	T52.2X3	T52.2X4	—	—
diisocyanate	T65.0X1	T65.0X2	T65.0X3	T65.0X4	—	—
Toluidine	T65.891	T65.892	T65.893	T65.894	—	—
vapor	T59.891	T59.892	T59.893	T59.894	—	—
Toluol (liquid)	T52.2X1	T52.2X2	T52.2X3	T52.2X4	—	—
vapor	T52.2X1	T52.2X2	T52.2X3	T52.2X4	—	—
Toluylenediamine	T65.3X1	T65.3X2	T65.3X3	T65.3X4	—	—
Tolylene-2,4-diisocyanate	T65.0X1	T65.0X2	T65.0X3	T65.0X4	—	—
Tonic NEC	T50.901	T50.902	T50.903	T50.904	T50.905	T50.906
Topical action drug NEC	T49.91	T49.92	T49.93	T49.94	T49.95	T49.96
ear, nose or throat	T49.6X1	T49.6X2	T49.6X3	T49.6X4	T49.6X5	T49.6X6
eye	T49.5X1	T49.5X2	T49.5X3	T49.5X4	T49.5X5	T49.5X6
skin	T49.91	T49.92	T49.93	T49.94	T49.95	T49.96
specified NEC	T49.8X1	T49.8X2	T49.8X3	T49.8X4	T49.8X5	T49.8X6
Toquizine	T44.3X1	T44.3X2	T44.3X3	T44.3X4	T44.3X5	T44.3X6
Toremifene	T38.6X1	T38.6X2	T38.6X3	T38.6X4	T38.6X5	T38.6X6
Tosylchloramide sodium	T49.8X1	T49.8X2	T49.8X3	T49.8X4	T49.8X5	T49.8X6
Toxaphene (dust) (spray)	T60.1X1	T60.1X2	T60.1X3	T60.1X4	—	—
Toxin, diphtheria (Schick Test)	T50.8X1	T50.8X2	T50.8X3	T50.8X4	T50.8X5	T50.8X6
Toxoid						
combined	T50.A21	T50.A22	T50.A23	T50.A24	T50.A25	T50.A26
diphtheria	T50.A91	T50.A92	T50.A93	T50.A94	T50.A95	T50.A96
tetanus	T50.A91	T50.A92	T50.A93	T50.A94	T50.A95	T50.A96
Trace element NEC	T45.8X1	T45.8X2	T45.8X3	T45.8X4	T45.8X5	T45.8X6
Tractor fuel NEC	T52.0X1	T52.0X2	T52.0X3	T52.0X4	—	—
Tragacanth	T50.991	T50.992	T50.993	T50.994	T50.995	T50.996
Tramadol	T40.4X1	T40.4X2	T40.4X3	T40.4X4	T40.4X5	T40.4X6
Tramazoline	T48.5X1	T48.5X2	T48.5X3	T48.5X4	T48.5X5	T48.5X6

Additional Character May Be Required — Refer to the Tabular List for Character Selection ▪ Subterms under main terms may continue to next column or page

Substance	Poisoning, Accidental (unintentional)	Poisoning, Intentional Self-harm	Poisoning, Assault	Poisoning, Undetermined	Adverse Effect	Under-dosing
Tranexamic acid	T45.621	T45.622	T45.623	T45.624	T45.625	T45.626
Tranilast	T45.0X1	T45.0X2	T45.0X3	T45.0X4	T45.0X5	T45.0X6
Tranquilizer NEC	T43.501	T43.502	T43.503	T43.504	T43.505	T43.506
with hypnotic or sedative	T42.6X1	T42.6X2	T42.6X3	T42.6X4	T42.6X5	T42.6X6
benzodiazepine NEC	T42.4X1	T42.4X2	T42.4X3	T42.4X4	T42.4X5	T42.4X6
butyrophenone NEC	T43.4X1	T43.4X2	T43.4X3	T43.4X4	T43.4X5	T43.4X6
carbamate	T43.591	T43.592	T43.593	T43.594	T43.595	T43.596
dimethylamine	T43.3X1	T43.3X2	T43.3X3	T43.3X4	T43.3X5	T43.3X6
ethylamine	T43.3X1	T43.3X2	T43.3X3	T43.3X4	T43.3X5	T43.3X6
hydroxyzine	T43.591	T43.592	T43.593	T43.594	T43.595	T43.596
major NEC	T43.501	T43.502	T43.503	T43.504	T43.505	T43.506
penothiazine NEC	T43.3X1	T43.3X2	T43.3X3	T43.3X4	T43.3X5	T43.3X6
phenothiazine-based	T43.3X1	T43.3X2	T43.3X3	T43.3X4	T43.3X5	T43.3X6
piperazine NEC	T43.3X1	T43.3X2	T43.3X3	T43.3X4	T43.3X5	T43.3X6
piperidine	T43.3X1	T43.3X2	T43.3X3	T43.3X4	T43.3X5	T43.3X6
propylamine	T43.3X1	T43.3X2	T43.3X3	T43.3X4	T43.3X5	T43.3X6
specified NEC	T43.591	T43.592	T43.593	T43.594	T43.595	T43.596
thioxanthene NEC	T43.591	T43.592	T43.593	T43.594	T43.595	T43.596
Tranxene	T42.4X1	T42.4X2	T42.4X3	T42.4X4	T42.4X5	T42.4X6
Tranylcypromine	T43.1X1	T43.1X2	T43.1X3	T43.1X4	T43.1X5	T43.1X6
Trapidil	T46.3X1	T46.3X2	T46.3X3	T46.3X4	T46.3X5	T46.3X6
Trasentine	T44.3X1	T44.3X2	T44.3X3	T44.3X4	T44.3X5	T44.3X6
Travert	T50.3X1	T50.3X2	T50.3X3	T50.3X4	T50.3X5	T50.3X6
Trazodone	T43.211	T43.212	T43.213	T43.214	T43.215	T43.216
Trecator	T37.1X1	T37.1X2	T37.1X3	T37.1X4	T37.1X5	T37.1X6
Treosulfan	T45.1X1	T45.1X2	T45.1X3	T45.1X4	T45.1X5	T45.1X6
Tretamine	T45.1X1	T45.1X2	T45.1X3	T45.1X4	T45.1X5	T45.1X6
Tretinoin	T49.0X1	T49.0X2	T49.0X3	T49.0X4	T49.0X5	T49.0X6
Tretoquinol	T48.6X1	T48.6X2	T48.6X3	T48.6X4	T48.6X5	T48.6X6
Triacetin	T49.0X1	T49.0X2	T49.0X3	T49.0X4	T49.0X5	T49.0X6
Triacetoxyanthracene	T49.4X1	T49.4X2	T49.4X3	T49.4X4	T49.4X5	T49.4X6
Triacetyloleandomycin	T36.3X1	T36.3X2	T36.3X3	T36.3X4	T36.3X5	T36.3X6
Triamcinolone	T38.0X1	T38.0X2	T38.0X3	T38.0X4	T38.0X5	T38.0X6
ENT agent	T49.6X1	T49.6X2	T49.6X3	T49.6X4	T49.6X5	T49.6X6
hexacetonide	T49.0X1	T49.0X2	T49.0X3	T49.0X4	T49.0X5	T49.0X6
ophthalmic preparation	T49.5X1	T49.5X2	T49.5X3	T49.5X4	T49.5X5	T49.5X6
topical NEC	T49.0X1	T49.0X2	T49.0X3	T49.0X4	T49.0X5	T49.0X6
Triampyzine	T44.3X1	T44.3X2	T44.3X3	T44.3X4	T44.3X5	T44.3X6
Triamterene	T50.2X1	T50.2X2	T50.2X3	T50.2X4	T50.2X5	T50.2X6
Triazine (herbicide)	T60.3X1	T60.3X2	T60.3X3	T60.3X4	—	—
Triaziquone	T45.1X1	T45.1X2	T45.1X3	T45.1X4	T45.1X5	T45.1X6
Triazolam	T42.4X1	T42.4X2	T42.4X3	T42.4X4	T42.4X5	T42.4X6
Triazole (herbicide)	T60.3X1	T60.3X2	T60.3X3	T60.3X4	—	—
Tribenoside	T46.991	T46.992	T46.993	T46.994	T46.995	T46.996
Tribromacetaldehyde	T42.6X1	T42.6X2	T42.6X3	T42.6X4	T42.6X5	T42.6X6
Tribromoethanol, rectal	T41.291	T41.292	T41.293	T41.294	T41.295	T41.296
Tribromomethane	T42.6X1	T42.6X2	T42.6X3	T42.6X4	T42.6X5	T42.6X6
Trichlorethane	T53.2X1	T53.2X2	T53.2X3	T53.2X4	—	—
Trichlorethylene	T53.2X1	T53.2X2	T53.2X3	T53.2X4	—	—
Trichlorfon	T60.0X1	T60.0X2	T60.0X3	T60.0X4	—	—
Trichlormethiazide	T50.2X1	T50.2X2	T50.2X3	T50.2X4	T50.2X5	T50.2X6
Trichlormethine	T45.1X1	T45.1X2	T45.1X3	T45.1X4	T45.1X5	T45.1X6
Trichloroacetic acid, Trichloracetic acid	T54.2X1	T54.2X2	T54.2X3	T54.2X4	—	—
medicinal	T49.4X1	T49.4X2	T49.4X3	T49.4X4	T49.4X5	T49.4X6
Trichloroethane	T53.2X1	T53.2X2	T53.2X3	T53.2X4	—	—
Trichloroethanol	T42.6X1	T42.6X2	T42.6X3	T42.6X4	T42.6X5	T42.6X6
Trichloroethylene (liquid)	T53.2X1	T53.2X2	T53.2X3	T53.2X4	—	—
(vapor)						
anesthetic (gas)	T41.0X1	T41.0X2	T41.0X3	T41.0X4	T41.0X5	T41.0X6
vapor NEC	T53.2X1	T53.2X2	T53.2X3	T53.2X4	—	—
Trichloroethyl phosphate	T42.6X1	T42.6X2	T42.6X3	T42.6X4	T42.6X5	T42.6X6
Trichlorofluoromethane NEC	T53.5X1	T53.5X2	T53.5X3	T53.5X4	—	—
Trichloronate	T60.0X1	T60.0X2	T60.0X3	T60.0X4	—	—
Trichloropropane	T53.6X1	T53.6X2	T53.6X3	T53.6X4	—	—
Trichlorotriethylamine	T45.1X1	T45.1X2	T45.1X3	T45.1X4	T45.1X5	T45.1X6
Trichomonacides NEC	T37.3X1	T37.3X2	T37.3X3	T37.3X4	T37.3X5	T37.3X6
Trichomycin	T36.7X1	T36.7X2	T36.7X3	T36.7X4	T36.7X5	T36.7X6
Triclobisonium chloride	T49.0X1	T49.0X2	T49.0X3	T49.0X4	T49.0X5	T49.0X6
Triclocarban	T49.0X1	T49.0X2	T49.0X3	T49.0X4	T49.0X5	T49.0X6
Triclofos	T42.6X1	T42.6X2	T42.6X3	T42.6X4	T42.6X5	T42.6X6
Triclosan	T49.0X1	T49.0X2	T49.0X3	T49.0X4	T49.0X5	T49.0X6
Tricresyl phosphate	T65.891	T65.892	T65.893	T65.894	—	—
solvent	T52.91	T52.92	T52.93	T52.94	—	—
Tricyclamol chloride	T44.3X1	T44.3X2	T44.3X3	T44.3X4	T44.3X5	T44.3X6
Tridesilon	T49.0X1	T49.0X2	T49.0X3	T49.0X4	T49.0X5	T49.0X6
Tridihexethyl iodide	T44.3X1	T44.3X2	T44.3X3	T44.3X4	T44.3X5	T44.3X6
Tridione	T42.2X1	T42.2X2	T42.2X3	T42.2X4	T42.2X5	T42.2X6
Trientine	T45.8X1	T45.8X2	T45.8X3	T45.8X4	T45.8X5	T45.8X6
Triethanolamine NEC	T54.3X1	T54.3X2	T54.3X3	T54.3X4	—	—
detergent	T54.3X1	T54.3X2	T54.3X3	T54.3X4	—	—
trinitrate (biphosphate)	T46.3X1	T46.3X2	T46.3X3	T46.3X4	T46.3X5	T46.3X6

Substance	Poisoning, Accidental (unintentional)	Poisoning, Intentional Self-harm	Poisoning, Assault	Poisoning, Undetermined	Adverse Effect	Under-dosing
Triethanomelamine	T45.1X1	T45.1X2	T45.1X3	T45.1X4	T45.1X5	T45.1X6
Triethylenemelamine	T45.1X1	T45.1X2	T45.1X3	T45.1X4	T45.1X5	T45.1X6
Triethylenephosphoramide	T45.1X1	T45.1X2	T45.1X3	T45.1X4	T45.1X5	T45.1X6
Triethylenethiophosphoramide	T45.1X1	T45.1X2	T45.1X3	T45.1X4	T45.1X5	T45.1X6
Trifluoperazine	T43.3X1	T43.3X2	T43.3X3	T43.3X4	T43.3X5	T43.3X6
Trifluoroethyl vinyl ether	T41.0X1	T41.0X2	T41.0X3	T41.0X4	T41.0X5	T41.0X6
Trifluperidol	T43.4X1	T43.4X2	T43.4X3	T43.4X4	T43.4X5	T43.4X6
Triflupromazine	T43.3X1	T43.3X2	T43.3X3	T43.3X4	T43.3X5	T43.3X6
Trifluridine	T37.5X1	T37.5X2	T37.5X3	T37.5X4	T37.5X5	T37.5X6
Triflusal	T45.521	T45.522	T45.523	T45.524	T45.525	T45.526
Trihexyphenidyl	T44.3X1	T44.3X2	T44.3X3	T44.3X4	T44.3X5	T44.3X6
Triiodothyronine	T38.1X1	T38.1X2	T38.1X3	T38.1X4	T38.1X5	T38.1X6
Trilene	T41.0X1	T41.0X2	T41.0X3	T41.0X4	T41.0X5	T41.0X6
Trilostane	T38.991	T38.992	T38.993	T38.994	T38.995	T38.996
Trimebutine	T44.3X1	T44.3X2	T44.3X3	T44.3X4	T44.3X5	T44.3X6
Trimecaine	T41.3X1	T41.3X2	T41.3X3	T41.3X4	T41.3X5	T41.3X6
Trimeprazine (tartrate)	T44.3X1	T44.3X2	T44.3X3	T44.3X4	T44.3X5	T44.3X6
Trimetaphan camsilate	T44.2X1	T44.2X2	T44.2X3	T44.2X4	T44.2X5	T44.2X6
Trimetazidine	T46.7X1	T46.7X2	T46.7X3	T46.7X4	T46.7X5	T46.7X6
Trimethadione	T42.2X1	T42.2X2	T42.2X3	T42.2X4	T42.2X5	T42.2X6
Trimethaphan	T44.2X1	T44.2X2	T44.2X3	T44.2X4	T44.2X5	T44.2X6
Trimethidinium	T44.2X1	T44.2X2	T44.2X3	T44.2X4	T44.2X5	T44.2X6
Trimethobenzamide	T45.0X1	T45.0X2	T45.0X3	T45.0X4	T45.0X5	T45.0X6
Trimethoprim	T37.8X1	T37.8X2	T37.8X3	T37.8X4	T37.8X5	T37.8X6
with sulfamethoxazole	T36.8X1	T36.8X2	T36.8X3	T36.8X4	T36.8X5	T36.8X6
Trimethylcarbinol	T51.3X1	T51.3X2	T51.3X3	T51.3X4	—	—
Trimethylpsoralen	T49.3X1	T49.3X2	T49.3X3	T49.3X4	T49.3X5	T49.3X6
Trimeton	T45.0X1	T45.0X2	T45.0X3	T45.0X4	T45.0X5	T45.0X6
Trimetrexate	T45.1X1	T45.1X2	T45.1X3	T45.1X4	T45.1X5	T45.1X6
Trimipramine	T43.011	T43.012	T43.013	T43.014	T43.015	T43.016
Trimustine	T45.1X1	T45.1X2	T45.1X3	T45.1X4	T45.1X5	T45.1X6
Trinitrine	T46.3X1	T46.3X2	T46.3X3	T46.3X4	T46.3X5	T46.3X6
Trinitrobenzol	T65.3X1	T65.3X2	T65.3X3	T65.3X4	—	—
Trinitrophenol	T65.3X1	T65.3X2	T65.3X3	T65.3X4	—	—
Trinitrotoluene (fumes)	T65.3X1	T65.3X2	T65.3X3	T65.3X4	—	—
Trional	T42.6X1	T42.6X2	T42.6X3	T42.6X4	T42.6X5	T42.6X6
Triorthocresyl phosphate	T65.891	T65.892	T65.893	T65.894	—	—
Trioxide of arsenic	T57.0X1	T57.0X2	T57.0X3	T57.0X4	—	—
Trioxysalen	T49.4X1	T49.4X2	T49.4X3	T49.4X4	T49.4X5	T49.4X6
Tripamide	T50.2X1	T50.2X2	T50.2X3	T50.2X4	T50.2X5	T50.2X6
Triparanol	T46.6X1	T46.6X2	T46.6X3	T46.6X4	T46.6X5	T46.6X6
Tripelennamine	T45.0X1	T45.0X2	T45.0X3	T45.0X4	T45.0X5	T45.0X6
Triperiden	T44.3X1	T44.3X2	T44.3X3	T44.3X4	T44.3X5	T44.3X6
Triperidol	T43.4X1	T43.4X2	T43.4X3	T43.4X4	T43.4X5	T43.4X6
Triphenylphosphate	T65.891	T65.892	T65.893	T65.894	—	—
Triple						
bromides	T42.6X1	T42.6X2	T42.6X3	T42.6X4	T42.6X5	T42.6X6
carbonate	T47.1X1	T47.1X2	T47.1X3	T47.1X4	T47.1X5	T47.1X6
vaccine						
DPT	T50.A11	T50.A12	T50.A13	T50.A14	T50.A15	T50.A16
including pertussis	T50.A11	T50.A12	T50.A13	T50.A14	T50.A15	T50.A16
MMR	T50.B91	T50.B92	T50.B93	T50.B94	T50.B95	T50.B96
Triprolidine	T45.0X1	T45.0X2	T45.0X3	T45.0X4	T45.0X5	T45.0X6
Trisodium hydrogen edetate	T50.6X1	T50.6X2	T50.6X3	T50.6X4	T50.6X5	T50.6X6
Trisoralen	T49.3X1	T49.3X2	T49.3X3	T49.3X4	T49.3X5	T49.3X6
Trisulfapyrimidines	T37.0X1	T37.0X2	T37.0X3	T37.0X4	T37.0X5	T37.0X6
Trithiozine	T44.3X1	T44.3X2	T44.3X3	T44.3X4	T44.3X5	T44.3X6
Tritiozine	T44.3X1	T44.3X2	T44.3X3	T44.3X4	T44.3X5	T44.3X6
Tritoqualine	T45.0X1	T45.0X2	T45.0X3	T45.0X4	T45.0X5	T45.0X6
Trofosfamide	T45.1X1	T45.1X2	T45.1X3	T45.1X4	T45.1X5	T45.1X6
Troleandomycin	T36.3X1	T36.3X2	T36.3X3	T36.3X4	T36.3X5	T36.3X6
Trolnitrate (phosphate)	T46.3X1	T46.3X2	T46.3X3	T46.3X4	T46.3X5	T46.3X6
Tromantadine	T37.5X1	T37.5X2	T37.5X3	T37.5X4	T37.5X5	T37.5X6
Trometamol	T50.2X1	T50.2X2	T50.2X3	T50.2X4	T50.2X5	T50.2X6
Tromethamine	T50.2X1	T50.2X2	T50.2X3	T50.2X4	T50.2X5	T50.2X6
Tronothane	T41.3X1	T41.3X2	T41.3X3	T41.3X4	T41.3X5	T41.3X6
Tropacine	T44.3X1	T44.3X2	T44.3X3	T44.3X4	T44.3X5	T44.3X6
Tropatepine	T44.3X1	T44.3X2	T44.3X3	T44.3X4	T44.3X5	T44.3X6
Tropicamide	T44.3X1	T44.3X2	T44.3X3	T44.3X4	T44.3X5	T44.3X6
Trospium chloride	T44.3X1	T44.3X2	T44.3X3	T44.3X4	T44.3X5	T44.3X6
Troxerutin	T46.991	T46.992	T46.993	T46.994	T46.995	T46.996
Troxidone	T42.2X1	T42.2X2	T42.2X3	T42.2X4	T42.2X5	T42.2X6
Tryparsamide	T37.3X1	T37.3X2	T37.3X3	T37.3X4	T37.3X5	T37.3X6
Trypsin	T45.3X1	T45.3X2	T45.3X3	T45.3X4	T45.3X5	T45.3X6
Tryptizol	T43.011	T43.012	T43.013	T43.014	T43.015	T43.016
TSH	T38.811	T38.812	T38.813	T38.814	T38.815	T38.816
Tuaminoheptane	T48.5X1	T48.5X2	T48.5X3	T48.5X4	T48.5X5	T48.5X6
Tuberculin, purified protein derivative (PPD)	T50.8X1	T50.8X2	T50.8X3	T50.8X4	T50.8X5	T50.8X6
Tubocurare	T48.1X1	T48.1X2	T48.1X3	T48.1X4	T48.1X5	T48.1X6
Tubocurarine (chloride)	T48.1X1	T48.1X2	T48.1X3	T48.1X4	T48.1X5	T48.1X6
Tulobuterol	T48.6X1	T48.6X2	T48.6X3	T48.6X4	T48.6X5	T48.6X6

▽ Subterms under main terms may continue to next column or page   Additional Character May Be Required — Refer to the Tabular List for Character Selection   395

Tranexamic acid — Tulobuterol

Substance	Poisoning, Accidental (unintentional)	Poisoning, Intentional Self-harm	Poisoning, Assault	Poisoning, Undetermined	Adverse Effect	Under-dosing
Turpentine (spirits of)	T52.8X1	T52.8X2	T52.8X3	T52.8X4	—	—
vapor	T52.8X1	T52.8X2	T52.8X3	T52.8X4	—	—
Tybamate	T43.591	T43.592	T43.593	T43.594	T43.595	T43.596
Tyloxapol	T48.4X1	T48.4X2	T48.4X3	T48.4X4	T48.4X5	T48.4X6
Tymazoline	T48.5X1	T48.5X2	T48.5X3	T48.5X4	T48.5X5	T48.5X6
Typhoid-paratyphoid vaccine	T50.A91	T50.A92	T50.A93	T50.A94	T50.A95	T50.A96
Typhus vaccine	T50.A91	T50.A92	T50.A93	T50.A94	T50.A95	T50.A96
Tyropanoate	T50.8X1	T50.8X2	T50.8X3	T50.8X4	T50.8X5	T50.8X6
Tyrothricin	T49.6X1	T49.6X2	T49.6X3	T49.6X4	T49.6X5	T49.6X6
ENT agent	T49.6X1	T49.6X2	T49.6X3	T49.6X4	T49.6X5	T49.6X6
ophthalmic preparation	T49.5X1	T49.5X2	T49.5X3	T49.5X4	T49.5X5	T49.5X6
Ufenamate	T39.391	T39.392	T39.393	T39.394	T39.395	T39.396
Ultraviolet light protectant	T49.3X1	T49.3X2	T49.3X3	T49.3X4	T49.3X5	T49.3X6
Undecenoic acid	T49.0X1	T49.0X2	T49.0X3	T49.0X4	T49.0X5	T49.0X6
Undecoylium	T49.0X1	T49.0X2	T49.0X3	T49.0X4	T49.0X5	T49.0X6
Undecylenic acid	T49.0X1	T49.0X2	T49.0X3	T49.0X4	T49.0X5	T49.0X6
(derivatives)						
Unna's boot	T49.3X1	T49.3X2	T49.3X3	T49.3X4	T49.3X5	T49.3X6
Unsaturated fatty acid	T46.6X1	T46.6X2	T46.6X3	T46.6X4	T46.6X5	T46.6X6
Uracil mustard	T45.1X1	T45.1X2	T45.1X3	T45.1X4	T45.1X5	T45.1X6
Uramustine	T45.1X1	T45.1X2	T45.1X3	T45.1X4	T45.1X5	T45.1X6
Urapidil	T46.5X1	T46.5X2	T46.5X3	T46.5X4	T46.5X5	T46.5X6
Urari	T48.1X1	T48.1X2	T48.1X3	T48.1X4	T48.1X5	T48.1X6
Urate oxidase	T50.4X1	T50.4X2	T50.4X3	T50.4X4	T50.4X5	T50.4X6
Urea	T47.3X1	T47.3X2	T47.3X3	T47.3X4	T47.3X5	T47.3X6
peroxide	T49.0X1	T49.0X2	T49.0X3	T49.0X4	T49.0X5	T49.0X6
stibamine	T37.4X1	T37.4X2	T37.4X3	T37.4X4	T37.4X5	T37.4X6
topical	T49.8X1	T49.8X2	T49.8X3	T49.8X4	T49.8X5	T49.8X6
Urethane	T45.1X1	T45.1X2	T45.1X3	T45.1X4	T45.1X5	T45.1X6
Urginea (maritima) (scilla) — see Squill						
Uric acid metabolism drug NEC	T50.4X1	T50.4X2	T50.4X3	T50.4X4	T50.4X5	T50.4X6
Uricosuric agent	T50.4X1	T50.4X2	T50.4X3	T50.4X4	T50.4X5	T50.4X6
Urinary anti-infective	T37.8X1	T37.8X2	T37.8X3	T37.8X4	T37.8X5	T37.8X6
Urofollitropin	T38.812	T38.812	T38.813	T38.814	T38.815	T38.816
Urokinase	T45.611	T45.612	T45.613	T45.614	T45.615	T45.616
Urokon	T50.8X1	T50.8X2	T50.8X3	T50.8X4	T50.8X5	T50.8X6
Ursodeoxycholic acid	T50.991	T50.992	T50.993	T50.994	T50.995	T50.996
Ursodiol	T50.991	T50.992	T50.993	T50.994	T50.995	T50.996
Urtica	T62.2X1	T62.2X2	T62.2X3	T62.2X4		
Utility gas — see Gas, utility						
Vaccine NEC	T50.Z91	T50.Z92	T50.Z93	T50.Z94	T50.Z95	T50.Z96
antineoplastic	T50.Z91	T50.Z92	T50.Z93	T50.Z94	T50.Z95	T50.Z96
bacterial NEC	T50.A91	T50.A92	T50.A93	T50.A94	T50.A95	T50.A96
with						
other bacterial component	T50.A21	T50.A22	T50.A23	T50.A24	T50.A25	T50.A26
pertussis component	T50.A11	T50.A12	T50.A13	T50.A14	T50.A15	T50.A16
viral-rickettsial component	T50.A21	T50.A22	T50.A23	T50.A24	T50.A25	T50.A26
mixed NEC	T50.A21	T50.A22	T50.A23	T50.A24	T50.A25	T50.A26
BCG	T50.A91	T50.A92	T50.A93	T50.A94	T50.A95	T50.A96
cholera	T50.A91	T50.A92	T50.A93	T50.A94	T50.A95	T50.A96
diphtheria	T50.A91	T50.A92	T50.A93	T50.A94	T50.A95	T50.A96
with tetanus	T50.A21	T50.A22	T50.A23	T50.A24	T50.A25	T50.A26
and pertussis	T50.A11	T50.A12	T50.A13	T50.A14	T50.A15	T50.A16
influenza	T50.B91	T50.B92	T50.B93	T50.B94	T50.B95	T50.B96
measles	T50.B91	T50.B92	T50.B93	T50.B94	T50.B95	T50.B96
with mumps and rubella	T50.B91	T50.B92	T50.B93	T50.B94	T50.B95	T50.B96
meningococcal	T50.A91	T50.A92	T50.A93	T50.A94	T50.A95	T50.A96
mumps	T50.B91	T50.B92	T50.B93	T50.B94	T50.B95	T50.B96
paratyphoid	T50.A91	T50.A92	T50.A93	T50.A94	T50.A95	T50.A96
pertussis	T50.A11	T50.A12	T50.A13	T50.A14	T50.A15	T50.A16
with diphtheria	T50.A11	T50.A12	T50.A13	T50.A14	T50.A15	T50.A16
and tetanus	T50.A11	T50.A12	T50.A13	T50.A14	T50.A15	T50.A16
with other component	T50.A11	T50.A12	T50.A13	T50.A14	T50.A15	T50.A16
plague	T50.A91	T50.A92	T50.A93	T50.A94	T50.A95	T50.A96
poliomyelitis	T50.B91	T50.B92	T50.B93	T50.B94	T50.B95	T50.B96
poliovirus	T50.B91	T50.B92	T50.B93	T50.B94	T50.B95	T50.B96
rabies	T50.B91	T50.B92	T50.B93	T50.B94	T50.B95	T50.B96
respiratory syncytial virus	T50.B91	T50.B92	T50.B93	T50.B94	T50.B95	T50.B96
rickettsial NEC	T50.A91	T50.A92	T50.A93	T50.A94	T50.A95	T50.A96
with						
bacterial component	T50.A21	T50.A22	T50.A23	T50.A24	T50.A25	T50.A26
Rocky Mountain spotted fever	T50.A91	T50.A92	T50.A93	T50.A94	T50.A95	T50.A96
rubella	T50.B91	T50.B92	T50.B93	T50.B94	T50.B95	T50.B96
sabin oral	T50.B91	T50.B92	T50.B93	T50.B94	T50.B95	T50.B96
smallpox	T50.B11	T50.B12	T50.B13	T50.B14	T50.B15	T50.B16
TAB	T50.A91	T50.A92	T50.A93	T50.A94	T50.A95	T50.A96

Substance	Poisoning, Accidental (unintentional)	Poisoning, Intentional Self-harm	Poisoning, Assault	Poisoning, Undetermined	Adverse Effect	Under-dosing
Vaccine — continued						
tetanus	T50.A91	T50.A92	T50.A93	T50.A94	T50.A95	T50.A96
typhoid	T50.A91	T50.A92	T50.A93	T50.A94	T50.A95	T50.A96
typhus	T50.A91	T50.A92	T50.A93	T50.A94	T50.A95	T50.A96
viral NEC	T50.B91	T50.B92	T50.B93	T50.B94	T50.B95	T50.B96
yellow fever	T50.B91	T50.B92	T50.B93	T50.B94	T50.B95	T50.B96
Vaccinia immune globulin	T50.Z11	T50.Z12	T50.Z13	T50.Z14	T50.Z15	T50.Z16
Vaginal contraceptives	T49.8X1	T49.8X2	T49.8X3	T49.8X4	T49.8X5	T49.8X6
Valerian						
root	T42.6X1	T42.6X2	T42.6X3	T42.6X4	T42.6X5	T42.6X6
tincture	T42.6X1	T42.6X2	T42.6X3	T42.6X4	T42.6X5	T42.6X6
Valethamate bromide	T44.3X1	T44.3X2	T44.3X3	T44.3X4	T44.3X5	T44.3X6
Valisone	T49.0X1	T49.0X2	T49.0X3	T49.0X4	T49.0X5	T49.0X6
Valium	T42.4X1	T42.4X2	T42.4X3	T42.4X4	T42.4X5	T42.4X6
Valmid	T42.6X1	T42.6X2	T42.6X3	T42.6X4	T42.6X5	T42.6X6
Valnoctamide	T42.6X1	T42.6X2	T42.6X3	T42.6X4	T42.6X5	T42.6X6
Valproate (sodium)	T42.6X1	T42.6X2	T42.6X3	T42.6X4	T42.6X5	T42.6X6
Valproic acid	T42.6X1	T42.6X2	T42.6X3	T42.6X4	T42.6X5	T42.6X6
Valpromide	T42.6X1	T42.6X2	T42.6X3	T42.6X4	T42.6X5	T42.6X6
Vanadium	T56.891	T56.892	T56.893	T56.894		
Vancomycin	T36.8X1	T36.8X2	T36.8X3	T36.8X4	T36.8X5	T36.8X6
Vapor — see also Gas	T59.91	T59.92	T59.93	T59.94	—	—
kiln (carbon monoxide)	T58.8X1	T58.8X2	T58.8X3	T58.8X4		
lead — see lead						
specified source NEC	T59.891	T59.892	T59.893	T59.894	—	—
Vardenafil	T46.7X1	T46.7X2	T46.7X3	T46.7X4	T46.7X5	T46.7X6
Varicose reduction drug	T46.8X1	T46.8X2	T46.8X3	T46.8X4	T46.8X5	T46.8X6
Varnish	T65.4X1	T65.4X2	T65.4X3	T65.4X4	—	—
cleaner	T52.91	T52.92	T52.93	T52.94	—	—
Vaseline	T49.3X1	T49.3X2	T49.3X3	T49.3X4	T49.3X5	T49.3X6
Vasodilan	T46.7X1	T46.7X2	T46.7X3	T46.7X4	T46.7X5	T46.7X6
Vasodilator						
coronary NEC	T46.3X1	T46.3X2	T46.3X3	T46.3X4	T46.3X5	T46.3X6
peripheral NEC	T46.7X1	T46.7X2	T46.7X3	T46.7X4	T46.7X5	T46.7X6
Vasopressin	T38.891	T38.892	T38.893	T38.894	T38.895	T38.896
Vasopressor drugs	T38.891	T38.892	T38.893	T38.894	T38.895	T38.896
Vecuronium bromide	T48.1X1	T48.1X2	T48.1X3	T48.1X4	T48.1X5	T48.1X6
Vegetable extract, astringent	T49.2X1	T49.2X2	T49.2X3	T49.2X4	T49.2X5	T49.2X6
Venlafaxine	T43.211	T43.212	T43.213	T43.214	T43.215	T43.216
Venom, venomous (bite)	T63.91	T63.92	T63.93	T63.94	—	—
(sting)						
amphibian NEC	T63.831	T63.832	T63.833	T63.834	—	—
animal NEC	T63.891	T63.892	T63.893	T63.894	—	—
ant	T63.421	T63.422	T63.423	T63.424	—	—
arthropod NEC	T63.481	T63.482	T63.483	T63.484	—	—
bee	T63.441	T63.442	T63.443	T63.444	—	—
centipede	T63.411	T63.412	T63.413	T63.414	—	—
fish	T63.591	T63.592	T63.593	T63.594	—	—
frog	T63.811	T63.812	T63.813	T63.814	—	—
hornet	T63.451	T63.452	T63.453	T63.454	—	—
insect NEC	T63.481	T63.482	T63.483	T63.484	—	—
lizard	T63.121	T63.122	T63.123	T63.124	—	—
marine						
animals	T63.691	T63.692	T63.693	T63.694	—	—
bluebottle	T63.611	T63.612	T63.613	T63.614	—	—
jellyfish NEC	T63.621	T63.622	T63.623	T63.624	—	—
Portugese Man-o-war	T63.611	T63.612	T63.613	T63.614	—	—
sea anemone	T63.631	T63.632	T63.633	T63.634	—	—
specified NEC	T63.691	T63.692	T63.693	T63.694	—	—
fish	T63.591	T63.592	T63.593	T63.594	—	—
plants	T63.711	T63.712	T63.713	T63.714	—	—
sting ray	T63.511	T63.512	T63.513	T63.514	—	—
millipede (tropical)	T63.411	T63.412	T63.413	T63.414	—	—
plant NEC	T63.791	T63.792	T63.793	T63.794	—	—
marine	T63.711	T63.712	T63.713	T63.714	—	—
reptile	T63.191	T63.192	T63.193	T63.194	—	—
gila monster	T63.111	T63.112	T63.113	T63.114	—	—
lizard NEC	T63.121	T63.122	T63.123	T63.124	—	—
scorpion	T63.2X1	T63.2X2	T63.2X3	T63.2X4	—	—
snake	T63.001	T63.002	T63.003	T63.004	—	—
African NEC	T63.081	T63.082	T63.083	T63.084	—	—
American (North) (South) NEC	T63.061	T63.062	T63.063	T63.064	—	—
Asian	T63.081	T63.082	T63.083	T63.084	—	—
Australian	T63.071	T63.072	T63.073	T63.074	—	—
cobra	T63.041	T63.042	T63.043	T63.044	—	—
coral snake	T63.021	T63.022	T63.023	T63.024	—	—
rattlesnake	T63.011	T63.012	T63.013	T63.014	—	—
specified NEC	T63.091	T63.092	T63.093	T63.094	—	—
taipan	T63.031	T63.032	T63.033	T63.034	—	—
specified NEC	T63.891	T63.892	T63.893	T63.894	—	—
spider	T63.301	T63.302	T63.303	T63.304	—	—

Additional Character May Be Required — Refer to the Tabular List for Character Selection   ▽ Subterms under main terms may continue to next column or page

Substance	Poisoning, Accidental (unintentional)	Poisoning, Intentional Self-harm	Poisoning, Assault	Poisoning, Undetermined	Adverse Effect	Under-dosing
Venom, venomous — continued						
spider — continued						
black widow	T63.311	T63.312	T63.313	T63.314	—	—
brown recluse	T63.331	T63.332	T63.333	T63.334	—	—
specified NEC	T63.391	T63.392	T63.393	T63.394	—	—
tarantula	T63.321	T63.322	T63.323	T63.324	—	—
sting ray	T63.511	T63.512	T63.513	T63.514	—	—
toad	T63.821	T63.822	T63.823	T63.824	—	—
wasp	T63.461	T63.462	T63.463	T63.464	—	—
Venous sclerosing drug NEC	T46.8X1	T46.8X2	T46.8X3	T46.8X4	T46.8X5	T46.8X6
Ventolin — see Albuterol						
Veramon	T42.3X1	T42.3X2	T42.3X3	T42.3X4	T42.3X5	T42.3X6
Verapamil	T46.1X1	T46.1X2	T46.1X3	T46.1X4	T46.1X5	T46.1X6
Veratrine	T46.5X1	T46.5X2	T46.5X3	T46.5X4	T46.5X5	T46.5X6
Veratrum						
album	T62.2X1	T62.2X2	T62.2X3	T62.2X4	—	—
alkaloids	T46.5X1	T46.5X2	T46.5X3	T46.5X4	T46.5X5	T46.5X6
viride	T62.2X1	T62.2X2	T62.2X3	T62.2X4	—	—
Verdigris	T60.3X1	T60.3X2	T60.3X3	T60.3X4	—	—
Veronal	T42.3X1	T42.3X2	T42.3X3	T42.3X4	T42.3X5	T42.3X6
Veroxil	T37.4X1	T37.4X2	T37.4X3	T37.4X4	T37.4X5	T37.4X6
Versenate	T50.6X1	T50.6X2	T50.6X3	T50.6X4	T50.6X5	T50.6X6
Versidyne	T39.8X1	T39.8X2	T39.8X3	T39.8X4	T39.8X5	T39.8X6
Vetrabutine	T48.0X1	T48.0X2	T48.0X3	T48.0X4	T48.0X5	T48.0X6
Vidarabine	T37.5X1	T37.5X2	T37.5X3	T37.5X4	T37.5X5	T37.5X6
Vienna						
green	T57.0X1	T57.0X2	T57.0X3	T57.0X4	—	—
insecticide	T60.2X1	T60.2X2	T60.2X3	T60.2X4	—	—
red	T57.0X1	T57.0X2	T57.0X3	T57.0X4	—	—
pharmaceutical dye	T50.991	T50.992	T50.993	T50.994	T50.995	T50.996
Vigabatrin	T42.6X1	T42.6X2	T42.6X3	T42.6X4	T42.6X5	T42.6X6
Viloxazine	T43.291	T43.292	T43.293	T43.294	T43.295	T43.296
Viminol	T39.8X1	T39.8X2	T39.8X3	T39.8X4	T39.8X5	T39.8X6
Vinbarbital, vinbarbitone	T42.3X1	T42.3X2	T42.3X3	T42.3X4	T42.3X5	T42.3X6
Vinblastine	T45.1X1	T45.1X2	T45.1X3	T45.1X4	T45.1X5	T45.1X6
Vinburnine	T46.7X1	T46.7X2	T46.7X3	T46.7X4	T46.7X5	T46.7X6
Vincamine	T45.1X1	T45.1X2	T45.1X3	T45.1X4	T45.1X5	T45.1X6
Vincristine	T45.1X1	T45.1X2	T45.1X3	T45.1X4	T45.1X5	T45.1X6
Vindesine	T45.1X1	T45.1X2	T45.1X3	T45.1X4	T45.1X5	T45.1X6
Vinesthene, vinethene	T41.0X1	T41.0X2	T41.0X3	T41.0X4	T41.0X5	T41.0X6
Vinorelbine tartrate	T45.1X1	T45.1X2	T45.1X3	T45.1X4	T45.1X5	T45.1X6
Vinpocetine	T46.7X1	T46.7X2	T46.7X3	T46.7X4	T46.7X5	T46.7X6
Vinyl						
acetate	T65.891	T65.892	T65.893	T65.894	—	—
bital	T42.3X1	T42.3X2	T42.3X3	T42.3X4	T42.3X5	T42.3X6
bromide	T65.891	T65.892	T65.893	T65.894	—	—
chloride	T59.891	T59.892	T59.893	T59.894	—	—
ether	T41.0X1	T41.0X2	T41.0X3	T41.0X4	T41.0X5	T41.0X6
Vinylbital	T42.3X1	T42.3X2	T42.3X3	T42.3X4	T42.3X5	T42.3X6
Vinylidene chloride	T65.891	T65.892	T65.893	T65.894	—	—
Vioform	T37.8X1	T37.8X2	T37.8X3	T37.8X4	T37.8X5	T37.8X6
topical	T49.0X1	T49.0X2	T49.0X3	T49.0X4	T49.0X5	T49.0X6
Viomycin	T36.8X1	T36.8X2	T36.8X3	T36.8X4	T36.8X5	T36.8X6
Viosterol	T45.2X1	T45.2X2	T45.2X3	T45.2X4	T45.2X5	T45.2X6
Viper (venom)	T63.091	T63.092	T63.093	T63.094	—	—
Viprynium	T37.4X1	T37.4X2	T37.4X3	T37.4X4	T37.4X5	T37.4X6
Viquidil	T46.7X1	T46.7X2	T46.7X3	T46.7X4	T46.7X5	T46.7X6
Viral vaccine NEC	T50.B91	T50.B92	T50.B93	T50.B94	T50.B95	T50.B96
Virginiamycin	T36.8X1	T36.8X2	T36.8X3	T36.8X4	T36.8X5	T36.8X6
Virugon	T37.5X1	T37.5X2	T37.5X3	T37.5X4	T37.5X5	T37.5X6
Viscous agent	T50.901	T50.902	T50.903	T50.904	T50.905	T50.906
Visine	T49.5X1	T49.5X2	T49.5X3	T49.5X4	T49.5X5	T49.5X6
Visnadine	T46.3X1	T46.3X2	T46.3X3	T46.3X4	T46.3X5	T46.3X6
Vitamin NEC	T45.2X1	T45.2X2	T45.2X3	T45.2X4	T45.2X5	T45.2X6
A	T45.2X1	T45.2X2	T45.2X3	T45.2X4	T45.2X5	T45.2X6
B1	T45.2X1	T45.2X2	T45.2X3	T45.2X4	T45.2X5	T45.2X6
B2	T45.2X1	T45.2X2	T45.2X3	T45.2X4	T45.2X5	T45.2X6
B6	T45.2X1	T45.2X2	T45.2X3	T45.2X4	T45.2X5	T45.2X6
B12	T45.2X1	T45.2X2	T45.2X3	T45.2X4	T45.2X5	T45.2X6
B15	T45.2X1	T45.2X2	T45.2X3	T45.2X4	T45.2X5	T45.2X6
B NEC	T45.2X1	T45.2X2	T45.2X3	T45.2X4	T45.2X5	T45.2X6
nicotinic acid	T46.7X1	T46.7X2	T46.7X3	T46.7X4	T46.7X5	T46.7X6
C	T45.2X1	T45.2X2	T45.2X3	T45.2X4	T45.2X5	T45.2X6
D	T45.2X1	T45.2X2	T45.2X3	T45.2X4	T45.2X5	T45.2X6
D2	T45.2X1	T45.2X2	T45.2X3	T45.2X4	T45.2X5	T45.2X6
D3	T45.2X1	T45.2X2	T45.2X3	T45.2X4	T45.2X5	T45.2X6
E	T45.2X1	T45.2X2	T45.2X3	T45.2X4	T45.2X5	T45.2X6
E acetate	T45.2X1	T45.2X2	T45.2X3	T45.2X4	T45.2X5	T45.2X6
hematopoietic	T45.8X1	T45.8X2	T45.8X3	T45.8X4	T45.8X5	T45.8X6
K1	T45.7X1	T45.7X2	T45.7X3	T45.7X4	T45.7X5	T45.7X6
K2	T45.7X1	T45.7X2	T45.7X3	T45.7X4	T45.7X5	T45.7X6
K NEC	T45.7X1	T45.7X2	T45.7X3	T45.7X4	T45.7X5	T45.7X6

Substance	Poisoning, Accidental (unintentional)	Poisoning, Intentional Self-harm	Poisoning, Assault	Poisoning, Undetermined	Adverse Effect	Under-dosing
Vitamin — continued						
PP	T45.2X1	T45.2X2	T45.2X3	T45.2X4	T45.2X5	T45.2X6
ulceroprotectant	T47.1X1	T47.1X2	T47.1X3	T47.1X4	T47.1X5	T47.1X6
Vleminckx's solution	T49.4X1	T49.4X2	T49.4X3	T49.4X4	T49.4X5	T49.4X6
Voltaren — see Diclofenac sodium						
Warfarin	T45.511	T45.512	T45.513	T45.514	T45.515	T45.516
rodenticide	T60.4X1-	T60.4X2-	T60.4X3-	T60.4X4-	—	—
sodium	T45.511	T45.512	T45.513	T45.514	T45.515	T45.516
Wasp (sting)	T63.461	T63.462	T63.463	T63.464	—	—
Water						
balance drug	T50.3X1	T50.3X2	T50.3X3	T50.3X4	T50.3X5	T50.3X6
distilled	T50.3X1	T50.3X2	T50.3X3	T50.3X4	T50.3X5	T50.3X6
gas — see Gas, water						
incomplete combustion of — see Carbon, monoxide, fuel, utility						
hemlock	T62.2X1	T62.2X2	T62.2X3	T62.2X4	—	—
moccasin (venom)	T63.061	T63.062	T63.063	T63.064	—	—
purified	T50.3X1	T50.3X2	T50.3X3	T50.3X4	T50.3X5	T50.3X6
Wax (paraffin) (petroleum)	T52.0X1	T52.0X2	T52.0X3	T52.0X4	—	—
automobile	T65.891	T65.892	T65.893	T65.894	—	—
floor	T52.0X1	T52.0X2	T52.0X3	T52.0X4	—	—
Weed killers NEC	T60.3X1	T60.3X2	T60.3X3	T60.3X4	—	—
Welldorm	T42.6X1	T42.6X2	T42.6X3	T42.6X4	T42.6X5	T42.6X6
White						
arsenic	T57.0X1	T57.0X2	T57.0X3	T57.0X4	—	—
hellebore	T62.2X1	T62.2X2	T62.2X3	T62.2X4	—	—
lotion (keratolytic)	T49.4X1	T49.4X2	T49.4X3	T49.4X4	T49.4X5	T49.4X6
spirit	T52.0X1	T52.0X2	T52.0X3	T52.0X4	—	—
Whitewash	T65.891	T65.892	T65.893	T65.894	—	—
Whole blood (human)	T45.8X1	T45.8X2	T45.8X3	T45.8X4	T45.8X5	T45.8X6
Wild						
black cherry	T62.2X1	T62.2X2	T62.2X3	T62.2X4	—	—
poisonous plants NEC	T62.2X1	T62.2X2	T62.2X3	T62.2X4	—	—
Window cleaning fluid	T65.891	T65.892	T65.893	T65.894	—	—
Wintergreen (oil)	T49.3X1	T49.3X2	T49.3X3	T49.3X4	T49.3X5	T49.3X6
Wisterine	T62.2X1	T62.2X2	T62.2X3	T62.2X4	—	—
Witch hazel	T49.2X1	T49.2X2	T49.2X3	T49.2X4	T49.2X5	T49.2X6
Wood alcohol or spirit	T51.1X1	T51.1X2	T51.1X3	T51.1X4	—	—
Wool fat (hydrous)	T49.3X1	T49.3X2	T49.3X3	T49.3X4	T49.3X5	T49.3X6
Woorali	T48.1X1	T48.1X2	T48.1X3	T48.1X4	T48.1X5	T48.1X6
Wormseed, American	T37.4X1	T37.4X2	T37.4X3	T37.4X4	T37.4X5	T37.4X6
Xamoterol	T44.5X1	T44.5X2	T44.5X3	T44.5X4	T44.5X5	T44.5X6
Xanthine diuretics	T50.2X1	T50.2X2	T50.2X3	T50.2X4	T50.2X5	T50.2X6
Xanthinol nicotinate	T46.7X1	T46.7X2	T46.7X3	T46.7X4	T46.7X5	T46.7X6
Xanthotoxin	T49.3X1	T49.3X2	T49.3X3	T49.3X4	T49.3X5	T49.3X6
Xantinol nicotinate	T46.7X1	T46.7X2	T46.7X3	T46.7X4	T46.7X5	T46.7X6
Xantocillin	T36.0X1	T36.0X2	T36.0X3	T36.0X4	T36.0X5	T36.0X6
Xenon (127Xe) (133Xe)	T50.8X1	T50.8X2	T50.8X3	T50.8X4	T50.8X5	T50.8X6
Xenysalate	T49.4X1	T49.4X2	T49.4X3	T49.4X4	T49.4X5	T49.4X6
Xibornol	T37.8X1	T37.8X2	T37.8X3	T37.8X4	T37.8X5	T37.8X6
Xigris	T45.511	T45.512	T45.513	T45.514	T45.515	T45.516
Xipamide	T50.2X1	T50.2X2	T50.2X3	T50.2X4	T50.2X5	T50.2X6
Xylene (vapor)	T52.2X1	T52.2X2	T52.2X3	T52.2X4	—	—
Xylocaine (infiltration) (topical)	T41.3X1	T41.3X2	T41.3X3	T41.3X4	T41.3X5	T41.3X6
nerve block (peripheral) (plexus)	T41.3X1	T41.3X2	T41.3X3	T41.3X4	T41.3X5	T41.3X6
spinal	T41.3X1	T41.3X2	T41.3X3	T41.3X4	T41.3X5	T41.3X6
Xylol (vapor)	T52.2X1	T52.2X2	T52.2X3	T52.2X4	—	—
Xylometazoline	T48.5X1	T48.5X2	T48.5X3	T48.5X4	T48.5X5	T48.5X6
Yeast	T45.2X1	T45.2X2	T45.2X3	T45.2X4	T45.2X5	T45.2X6
dried	T45.2X1	T45.2X2	T45.2X3	T45.2X4	T45.2X5	T45.2X6
Yellow						
fever vaccine	T50.B91	T50.B92	T50.B93	T50.B94	T50.B95	T50.B96
jasmine	T62.2X1	T62.2X2	T62.2X3	T62.2X4	—	—
phenolphthalein	T47.2X1	T47.2X2	T47.2X3	T47.2X4	T47.2X5	T47.2X6
Yew	T62.2X1	T62.2X2	T62.2X3	T62.2X4	—	—
Yohimbic acid	T40.991	T40.992	T40.993	T40.994	T40.995	T40.996
Zactane	T39.8X1	T39.8X2	T39.8X3	T39.8X4	T39.8X5	T39.8X6
Zalcitabine	T37.5X1	T37.5X2	T37.5X3	T37.5X4	T37.5X5	T37.5X6
Zaroxolyn	T50.2X1	T50.2X2	T50.2X3	T50.2X4	T50.2X5	T50.2X6
Zephiran (topical)	T49.0X1	T49.0X2	T49.0X3	T49.0X4	T49.0X5	T49.0X6
ophthalmic preparation	T49.5X1	T49.5X2	T49.5X3	T49.5X4	T49.5X5	T49.5X6
Zeranol	T38.7X1	T38.7X2	T38.7X3	T38.7X4	T38.7X5	T38.7X6
Zerone	T51.1X1	T51.1X2	T51.1X3	T51.1X4	—	—
Zidovudine	T37.5X1	T37.5X2	T37.5X3	T37.5X4	T37.5X5	T37.5X6
Zimeldine	T43.221	T43.222	T43.223	T43.224	T43.225	T43.226
Zinc (compounds) (fumes) (vapor)	T56.5X1	T56.5X2	T56.5X3	T56.5X4	—	—
NEC						
anti-infectives	T49.0X1	T49.0X2	T49.0X3	T49.0X4	T49.0X5	T49.0X6
antivaricose	T46.8X1	T46.8X2	T46.8X3	T46.8X4	T46.8X5	T46.8X6

Table of Drugs and Chemicals

Substance	Poisoning, Accidental (unintentional)	Poisoning, Intentional Self-harm	Poisoning, Assault	Poisoning, Undetermined	Adverse Effect	Under-dosing
Zinc (compounds) (fumes) (vapor) **NEC** — *continued*						
bacitracin	T49.0X1	T49.0X2	T49.0X3	T49.0X4	T49.0X5	T49.0X6
chloride (mouthwash)	T49.6X1	T49.6X2	T49.6X3	T49.6X4	T49.6X5	T49.6X6
chromate	T56.5X1	T56.5X2	T56.5X3	T56.5X4	—	—
gelatin	T49.3X1	T49.3X2	T49.3X3	T49.3X4	T49.3X5	T49.3X6
oxide	T49.3X1	T49.3X2	T49.3X3	T49.3X4	T49.3X5	T49.3X6
plaster	T49.3X1	T49.3X2	T49.3X3	T49.3X4	T49.3X5	T49.3X6
peroxide	T49.0X1	T49.0X2	T49.0X3	T49.0X4	T49.0X5	T49.0X6
pesticides	T56.5X1	T56.5X2	T56.5X3	T56.5X4	—	—
phosphide	T60.4X1	T60.4X2	T60.4X3	T60.4X4	—	—
pyrithionate	T49.4X1	T49.4X2	T49.4X3	T49.4X4	T49.4X5	T49.4X6
stearate	T49.3X1	T49.3X2	T49.3X3	T49.3X4	T49.3X5	T49.3X6
sulfate	T49.5X1	T49.5X2	T49.5X3	T49.5X4	T49.5X5	T49.5X6
ENT agent	T49.6X1	T49.6X2	T49.6X3	T49.6X4	T49.6X5	T49.6X6
ophthalmic solution	T49.5X1	T49.5X2	T49.5X3	T49.5X4	T49.5X5	T49.5X6
topical NEC	T49.0X1	T49.0X2	T49.0X3	T49.0X4	T49.0X5	T49.0X6
undecylenate	T49.0X1	T49.0X2	T49.0X3	T49.0X4	T49.0X5	T49.0X6
Zineb	T60.0X1	T60.0X2	T60.0X3	T60.0X4	—	—
Zinostatin	T45.1X1	T45.1X2	T45.1X3	T45.1X4	T45.1X5	T45.1X6
Zipeprol	T48.3X1	T48.3X2	T48.3X3	T48.3X4	T48.3X5	T48.3X6
Zofenopril	T46.4X1	T46.4X2	T46.4X3	T46.4X4	T46.4X5	T46.4X6
Zolpidem	T42.6X1	T42.6X2	T42.6X3	T42.6X4	T42.6X5	T42.6X6
Zomepirac	T39.391	T39.392	T39.393	T39.394	T39.395	T39.396
Zopiclone	T42.6X1	T42.6X2	T42.6X3	T42.6X4	T42.6X5	T42.6X6
Zorubicin	T45.1X1	T45.1X2	T45.1X3	T45.1X4	T45.1X5	T45.1X6
Zotepine	T43.591	T43.592	T43.593	T43.594	T43.595	T43.596
Zovant	T45.511	T45.512	T45.513	T45.514	T45.515	T45.516
Zoxazolamine	T42.8X1	T42.8X2	T42.8X3	T42.8X4	T42.8X5	T42.8X6
Zuclopenthixol	T43.4X1	T43.4X2	T43.4X3	T43.4X4	T43.4X5	T43.4X6
Zygadenus (venenosus)	T62.2X1	T62.2X2	T62.2X3	T62.2X4	—	—
Zyprexa	T43.591	T43.592	T43.593	T43.594	T43.595	T43.596

Additional Character May Be Required — Refer to the Tabular List for Character Selection ▽ Subterms under main terms may continue to next column or page

Zinc — Zyprexa

A

Abandonment (causing exposure to weather conditions) (with intent to injure or kill) NEC X58 ☑
Abuse (adult) (child) (mental) (physical) (sexual) X58 ☑
Accident (to) X58 ☑
  aircraft (in transit) (powered) (*see also* Accident, transport, aircraft)
    due to, caused by cataclysm — *see* Forces of nature, by type
  animal-drawn vehicle — *see* Accident, transport, animal-drawn vehicle occupant
  animal-rider — *see* Accident, transport, animal-rider
  automobile — *see* Accident, transport, car occupant
  bare foot water skier V94.4 ☑
  boat, boating (*see also* Accident, watercraft)
    striking swimmer
      powered V94.11 ☑
      unpowered V94.12 ☑
  bus — *see* Accident, transport, bus occupant
  cable car, not on rails V98.0 ☑
    on rails — *see* Accident, transport, streetcar occupant
  car — *see* Accident, transport, car occupant
  caused by, due to
    animal NEC W64 ☑
    chain hoist W24.0 ☑
    cold (excessive) — *see* Exposure, cold
    corrosive liquid, substance — *see* Table of Drugs and Chemicals
    cutting or piercing instrument — *see* Contact, with, by type of instrument
    drive belt W24.0 ☑
    electric
      current — *see* Exposure, electric current
      motor (*see also* Contact, with, by type of machine) W31.3 ☑
        current (of) W86.8 ☑
    environmental factor NEC X58 ☑
    explosive material — *see* Explosion
    fire, flames — *see* Exposure, fire
    firearm missile — *see* Discharge, firearm by type
    heat (excessive) — *see* Heat
    hot — *see* Contact, with, hot
    ignition — *see* Ignition
    lifting device W24.0 ☑
    lightning — *see* subcategory T75.0 ☑
      causing fire — *see* Exposure, fire
    machine, machinery — *see* Contact, with, by type of machine
    natural factor NEC X58 ☑
    pulley (block) W24.0 ☑
    radiation — *see* Radiation
    steam X13.1 ☑
      inhalation X13.0 ☑
      pipe X16 ☑
    thunderbolt — *see* subcategory T75.0 ☑
      causing fire — *see* Exposure, fire
    transmission device W24.1 ☑
  coach — *see* Accident, transport, bus occupant
  coal car — *see* Accident, transport, industrial vehicle occupant
  diving (*see also* Fall, into, water)
    with
      drowning or submersion — *see* Drowning
  forklift — *see* Accident, transport, industrial vehicle occupant
  heavy transport vehicle NOS — *see* Accident, transport, truck occupant
  ice yacht V98.2 ☑
  in
    medical, surgical procedure
      as, or due to misadventure — *see* Misadventure
      causing an abnormal reaction or later complication without mention of misadventure (*see also* Complication of or following, by type of procedure) Y84.9
  land yacht V98.1 ☑
  late effect of — *see* W00-X58 with 7th character S
  logging car — *see* Accident, transport, industrial vehicle occupant
  machine, machinery (*see also* Contact, with, by type of machine)
    on board watercraft V93.69 ☑
      explosion — *see* Explosion, in, watercraft

Accident — *continued*
  machine, machinery (*see also* Contact, with, by type of machine) — *continued*
    on board watercraft — *continued*
      fire — *see* Burn, on board watercraft
      powered craft V93.63 ☑
        ferry boat V93.61 ☑
        fishing boat V93.62 ☑
        jetskis V93.63 ☑
        liner V93.61 ☑
        merchant ship V93.60 ☑
        passenger ship V93.61 ☑
        sailboat V93.64 ☑
  mine tram — *see* Accident, transport, industrial vehicle occupant
  mobility scooter (motorized) — *see* Accident, transport, pedestrian, conveyance, specified type NEC
  motor scooter — *see* Accident, transport, motorcyclist
  motor vehicle NOS (traffic) (*see also* Accident, transport) V89.2 ☑
    nontraffic V89.0 ☑
    three-wheeled NOS — *see* Accident, transport, three-wheeled motor vehicle occupant
  motorcycle NOS — *see* Accident, transport, motorcyclist
  nonmotor vehicle NOS (nontraffic) (*see also* Accident, transport) V89.1 ☑
    traffic NOS V89.3 ☑
  nontraffic (victim's mode of transport NOS) V88.9 ☑
    collision (between) V88.7 ☑
      bus and truck V88.5 ☑
      car and:
        bus V88.3 ☑
        pickup V88.2 ☑
        three-wheeled motor vehicle V88.0 ☑
        train V88.6 ☑
        truck V88.4 ☑
        two-wheeled motor vehicle V88.0 ☑
        van V88.2 ☑
      specified vehicle NEC and:
        three-wheeled motor vehicle V88.1 ☑
        two-wheeled motor vehicle V88.1 ☑
    known mode of transport — *see* Accident, transport, by type of vehicle
    noncollision V88.8 ☑
  on board watercraft V93.89 ☑
    powered craft V93.83 ☑
      ferry boat V93.81 ☑
      fishing boat V93.82 ☑
      jetskis V93.83 ☑
      liner V93.81 ☑
      merchant ship V93.80 ☑
      passenger ship V93.81 ☑
    unpowered craft V93.88 ☑
      canoe V93.85 ☑
      inflatable V93.86 ☑
        in tow
          recreational V94.31 ☑
          specified NEC V94.32 ☑
      kayak V93.85 ☑
      sailboat V93.84 ☑
      surf-board V93.88 ☑
      water skis V93.87 ☑
      windsurfer V93.88 ☑
  parachutist V97.29 ☑
    entangled in object V97.21 ☑
    injured on landing V97.22 ☑
  pedal cycle — *see* Accident, transport, pedal cyclist
  pedestrian (on foot)
    with
      another pedestrian W51 ☑
        on pedestrian conveyance NEC V00.09 ☑
      with fall W03 ☑
        due to ice or snow W00.0 ☑
      roller skater (in-line) V00.01 ☑
      skate boarder V00.02 ☑
      transport vehicle — *see* Accident, transport
    on pedestrian conveyance — *see* Accident, transport, pedestrian, conveyance
  pick-up truck or van — *see* Accident, transport, pickup truck occupant
  quarry truck — *see* Accident, transport, industrial vehicle occupant
  railway vehicle (any) (in motion) — *see* Accident, transport, railway vehicle occupant
    due to cataclysm — *see* Forces of nature, by type

Accident — *continued*
  scooter (non-motorized) — *see* Accident, transport, pedestrian, conveyance, scooter
  sequelae of — *see* categories W00-X58 with 7th character S
  skateboard — *see* Accident, transport, pedestrian, conveyance, skateboard
  ski(ing) — *see* Accident, transport, pedestrian, conveyance
    lift V98.3 ☑
  specified cause NEC X58 ☑
  streetcar — *see* Accident, transport, streetcar occupant
  traffic (victim's mode of transport NOS) V87.9 ☑
    collision (between) V87.7 ☑
      bus and truck V87.5 ☑
      car and:
        bus V87.3 ☑
        pickup V87.2 ☑
        three-wheeled motor vehicle V87.0 ☑
        train V87.6 ☑
        truck V87.4 ☑
        two-wheeled motor vehicle V87.0 ☑
        van V87.2 ☑
      specified vehicle NEC and:
        three-wheeled motor vehicle V87.1 ☑
        two-wheeled motor vehicle V87.1 ☑
    known mode of transport — *see* Accident, transport, by type of vehicle
    noncollision V87.8 ☑
  transport (involving injury to) V99 ☑
    18 wheeler — *see* Accident, transport, truck occupant
    agricultural vehicle occupant (nontraffic) V84.9 ☑
      driver V84.5 ☑
      hanger-on V84.7 ☑
      passenger V84.6 ☑
      traffic V84.3 ☑
        driver V84.0 ☑
        hanger-on V84.2 ☑
        passenger V84.1 ☑
      while boarding or alighting V84.4 ☑
    aircraft NEC V97.89 ☑
      military NEC V97.818 ☑
        civilian injured by V97.811 ☑
        with civlian aircraft V97.810 ☑
      occupant injured (in)
        nonpowered craft accident V96.9 ☑
          balloon V96.00 ☑
            collision V96.03 ☑
            crash V96.01 ☑
            explosion V96.05 ☑
            fire V96.04 ☑
            forced landing V96.02 ☑
            specified type NEC V96.09 ☑
          glider V96.20 ☑
            collision V96.23 ☑
            crash V96.21 ☑
            explosion V96.25 ☑
            fire V96.24 ☑
            forced landing V96.22 ☑
            specified type NEC V96.29 ☑
          hang glider V96.10 ☑
            collision V96.13 ☑
            crash V96.11 ☑
            explosion V96.15 ☑
            fire V96.14 ☑
            forced landing V96.12 ☑
            specified type NEC V96.19 ☑
          specified craft NEC V96.8 ☑
        powered craft accident V95.9 ☑
          fixed wing NEC
            commercial V95.30 ☑
              collision V95.33 ☑
              crash V95.31 ☑
              explosion V95.35 ☑
              fire V95.34 ☑
              forced landing V95.32 ☑
              specified type NEC V95.39 ☑
            private V95.20 ☑
              collision V95.23 ☑
              crash V95.21 ☑
              explosion V95.25 ☑
              fire V95.24 ☑
              forced landing V95.22 ☑
              specified type NEC V95.29 ☑
          glider V95.10 ☑

Accident — *continued*
  transport — *continued*
    aircraft — *continued*
      occupant injured — *continued*
        powered craft accident — *continued*
          glider — *continued*
            collision V95.13 ☑
            crash V95.11 ☑
            explosion V95.15 ☑
            fire V95.14 ☑
            forced landing V95.12 ☑
            specified type NEC V95.19 ☑
          helicopter V95.00 ☑
            collision V95.03 ☑
            crash V95.01 ☑
            explosion V95.05 ☑
            fire V95.04 ☑
            forced landing V95.02 ☑
            specified type NEC V95.09 ☑
          spacecraft V95.40 ☑
            collision V95.43 ☑
            crash V95.41 ☑
            explosion V95.45 ☑
            fire V95.44 ☑
            forced landing V95.42 ☑
            specified type NEC V95.49 ☑
          specified craft NEC V95.8 ☑
          ultralight V95.10 ☑
            collision V95.13 ☑
            crash V95.11 ☑
            explosion V95.15 ☑
            fire V95.14 ☑
            forced landing V95.12 ☑
            specified type NEC V95.19 ☑
        specified accident NEC V97.0 ☑
        while boarding or alighting V97.1 ☑
      person (injured by)
        falling from, in or on aircraft V97.0 ☑
        machinery on aircraft V97.89 ☑
        on ground with aircraft involvement
          V97.39 ☑
        rotating propeller V97.32 ☑
        struck by object falling from aircraft V97.31 ☑
        sucked into aircraft jet V97.33 ☑
        while boarding or alighting aircraft V97.1 ☑
    airport (battery-powered) passenger vehicle — *see*
      Accident, transport, industrial vehicle occu-
      pant
    all-terrain vehicle occupant (nontraffic) V86.95 ☑
      driver V86.55 ☑
      dune buggy — *see* Accident, transport, dune
        buggy occupant
      hanger-on V86.75 ☑
      passenger V86.65 ☑
      snowmobile — *see* Accident, transport, snowmo-
        bile occupant
      specified type NEC V86.99 ☑
      traffic V86.35 ☑
        driver V86.05 ☑
        hanger-on V86.25 ☑
        passenger V86.15 ☑
      while boarding or alighting V86.45 ☑
    ambulance occupant (traffic) V86.31 ☑
      driver V86.01 ☑
      hanger-on V86.21 ☑
      nontraffic V86.91 ☑
        driver V86.51 ☑
        hanger-on V86.71 ☑
        passenger V86.61 ☑
      passenger V86.11 ☑
      while boarding or alighting V86.41 ☑
    animal-drawn vehicle occupant (in) V80.929 ☑
      collision (with)
        animal V80.12 ☑
          being ridden V80.711 ☑
        animal-drawn vehicle V80.721 ☑
        bus V80.42 ☑
        car V80.42 ☑
        fixed or stationary object V80.82 ☑
        military vehicle V80.920 ☑
        nonmotor vehicle V80.791 ☑
        pedal cycle V80.22 ☑
        pedestrian V80.12 ☑
        pickup V80.42 ☑
        railway train or vehicle V80.62 ☑
        specified motor vehicle NEC V80.52 ☑

Accident — *continued*
  transport — *continued*
    animal-drawn vehicle occupant — *continued*
      collision — *continued*
        streetcar V80.731 ☑
        truck V80.42 ☑
        two- or three-wheeled motor vehicle
          V80.32 ☑
        van V80.42 ☑
      noncollision V80.02 ☑
      specified circumstance NEC V80.928 ☑
    animal-rider V80.919 ☑
      collision (with)
        animal V80.11 ☑
          being ridden V80.710 ☑
        animal-drawn vehicle V80.720 ☑
        bus V80.41 ☑
        car V80.41 ☑
        fixed or stationary object V80.81 ☑
        military vehicle V80.910 ☑
        nonmotor vehicle V80.790 ☑
        pedal cycle V80.21 ☑
        pedestrian V80.11 ☑
        pickup V80.41 ☑
        railway train or vehicle V80.61 ☑
        specified motor vehicle NEC V80.51 ☑
        streetcar V80.730 ☑
        truck V80.41 ☑
        two- or three-wheeled motor vehicle
          V80.31 ☑
        van V80.41 ☑
      noncollision V80.018 ☑
        specified as horse rider V80.010 ☑
      specified circumstance NEC V80.918 ☑
    armored car — *see* Accident, transport, truck occu-
      pant
    battery-powered truck (baggage) (mail) — *see* Ac-
      cident, transport, industrial vehicle occupant
    bus occupant V79.9 ☑
      collision (with)
        animal (traffic) V70.9 ☑
          being ridden (traffic) V76.9 ☑
            nontraffic V76.3 ☑
            while boarding or alighting V76.4 ☑
          nontraffic V70.3 ☑
          while boarding or alighting V70.4 ☑
        animal-drawn vehicle (traffic) V76.9 ☑
          nontraffic V76.3 ☑
          while boarding or alighting V76.4 ☑
        bus (traffic) V74.9 ☑
          nontraffic V74.3 ☑
          while boarding or alighting V74.4 ☑
        car (traffic) V73.9 ☑
          nontraffic V73.3 ☑
          while boarding or alighting V73.4 ☑
        motor vehicle NOS (traffic) V79.60 ☑
          nontraffic V79.20 ☑
          specified type NEC (traffic) V79.69 ☑
            nontraffic V79.29 ☑
        pedal cycle (traffic) V71.9 ☑
          nontraffic V71.3 ☑
          while boarding or alighting V71.4 ☑
        pickup truck (traffic) V73.9 ☑
          nontraffic V73.3 ☑
          while boarding or alighting V73.4 ☑
        railway vehicle (traffic) V75.9 ☑
          nontraffic V75.3 ☑
          while boarding or alighting V75.4 ☑
        specified vehicle NEC (traffic) V76.9 ☑
          nontraffic V76.3 ☑
          while boarding or alighting V76.4 ☑
        stationary object (traffic) V77.9 ☑
          nontraffic V77.3 ☑
          while boarding or alighting V77.4 ☑
        streetcar (traffic) V76.9 ☑
          nontraffic V76.3 ☑
          while boarding or alighting V76.4 ☑
        three wheeled motor vehicle (traffic) V72.9 ☑
          nontraffic V72.3 ☑
          while boarding or alighting V72.4 ☑
        truck (traffic) V74.9 ☑
          nontraffic V74.3 ☑
          while boarding or alighting V74.4 ☑
        two wheeled motor vehicle (traffic) V72.9 ☑
          nontraffic V72.3 ☑
          while boarding or alighting V72.4 ☑

Accident — *continued*
  transport — *continued*
    bus occupant — *continued*
      collision — *continued*
        van (traffic) V73.9 ☑
          nontraffic V73.3 ☑
          while boarding or alighting V73.4 ☑
      driver
        collision (with)
          animal (traffic) V70.5 ☑
            being ridden (traffic) V76.5 ☑
              nontraffic V76.0 ☑
            nontraffic V70.0 ☑
          animal-drawn vehicle (traffic) V76.5 ☑
            nontraffic V76.0 ☑
          bus (traffic) V74.5 ☑
            nontraffic V74.0 ☑
          car (traffic) V73.5 ☑
            nontraffic V73.0 ☑
          motor vehicle NOS (traffic) V79.40 ☑
            nontraffic V79.00 ☑
            specified type NEC (traffic) V79.49 ☑
              nontraffic V79.09 ☑
          pedal cycle (traffic) V71.5 ☑
            nontraffic V71.0 ☑
          pickup truck (traffic) V73.5 ☑
            nontraffic V73.0 ☑
          railway vehicle (traffic) V75.5 ☑
            nontraffic V75.0 ☑
          specified vehicle NEC (traffic) V76.5 ☑
            nontraffic V76.0 ☑
          stationary object (traffic) V77.5 ☑
            nontraffic V77.0 ☑
          streetcar (traffic) V76.5 ☑
            nontraffic V76.0 ☑
          three wheeled motor vehicle (traffic)
            V72.5 ☑
            nontraffic V72.0 ☑
          truck (traffic) V74.5 ☑
            nontraffic V74.0 ☑
          two wheeled motor vehicle (traffic)
            V72.5 ☑
            nontraffic V72.0 ☑
          van (traffic) V73.5 ☑
            nontraffic V73.0 ☑
        noncollision accident (traffic) V78.5 ☑
          nontraffic V78.0 ☑
      hanger-on
        collision (with)
          animal (traffic) V70.7 ☑
            being ridden (traffic) V76.7 ☑
              nontraffic V76.2 ☑
            nontraffic V70.2 ☑
          animal-drawn vehicle (traffic) V76.7 ☑
            nontraffic V76.2 ☑
          bus (traffic) V74.7 ☑
            nontraffic V74.2 ☑
          car (traffic) V73.7 ☑
            nontraffic V73.2 ☑
          pedal cycle (traffic) V71.7 ☑
            nontraffic V71.2 ☑
          pickup truck (traffic) V73.7 ☑
            nontraffic V73.2 ☑
          railway vehicle (traffic) V75.7 ☑
            nontraffic V75.2 ☑
          specified vehicle NEC (traffic) V76.7 ☑
            nontraffic V76.2 ☑
          stationary object (traffic) V77.7 ☑
            nontraffic V77.2 ☑
          streetcar (traffic) V76.7 ☑
            nontraffic V76.2 ☑
          three wheeled motor vehicle (traffic)
            V72.7 ☑
            nontraffic V72.2 ☑
          truck (traffic) V74.7 ☑
            nontraffic V74.2 ☑
          two wheeled motor vehicle (traffic)
            V72.7 ☑
            nontraffic V72.2 ☑
          van (traffic) V73.7 ☑
            nontraffic V73.2 ☑
        noncollision accident (traffic) V78.7 ☑
          nontraffic V78.2 ☑
      noncollision accident (traffic) V78.9 ☑
        nontraffic V78.3 ☑
        while boarding or alighting ☑78.4 ☑

Accident — *continued*
  transport — *continued*
    bus occupant — *continued*
      nontraffic V79.3 ☑
      passenger
        collision (with)
          animal (traffic) V70.6 ☑
            being ridden (traffic) V76.6 ☑
              nontraffic V76.1 ☑
            nontraffic V70.1 ☑
          animal-drawn vehicle (traffic) V76.6 ☑
            nontraffic V76.1 ☑
          bus (traffic) V74.6 ☑
            nontraffic V74.1 ☑
          car (traffic) V73.6 ☑
            nontraffic V73.1 ☑
          motor vehicle NOS (traffic) V79.50 ☑
            nontraffic V79.10 ☑
            specified type NEC (traffic) V79.59 ☑
              nontraffic V79.19 ☑
          pedal cycle (traffic) V71.6 ☑
            nontraffic V71.1 ☑
          pickup truck (traffic) V73.6 ☑
            nontraffic V73.1 ☑
          railway vehicle (traffic) V75.6 ☑
            nontraffic V75.1 ☑
          specified vehicle NEC (traffic) V76.6 ☑
            nontraffic V76.1 ☑
          stationary object (traffic) V77.6 ☑
            nontraffic V77.1 ☑
          streetcar (traffic) V76.6 ☑
            nontraffic V76.1 ☑
          three wheeled motor vehicle (traffic)
            V72.6 ☑
            nontraffic V72.1 ☑
          truck (traffic) V74.6 ☑
            nontraffic V74.1 ☑
          two wheeled motor vehicle (traffic)
            V72.6 ☑
            nontraffic V72.1 ☑
          van (traffic) V73.6 ☑
            nontraffic V73.1 ☑
        noncollision accident (traffic) V78.6 ☑
          nontraffic V78.1 ☑
        specified type NEC V79.88 ☑
          military vehicle V79.81 ☑
    cable car, not on rails V98.0 ☑
      on rails — *see* Accident, transport, streetcar occupant
    car occupant V49.9 ☑
      ambulance occupant — *see* Accident, transport, ambulance occupant
      collision (with)
        animal (traffic) V40.9 ☑
          being ridden (traffic) V46.9 ☑
            nontraffic V46.3 ☑
            while boarding or alighting V46.4 ☑
          nontraffic V40.3 ☑
          while boarding or alighting V40.4 ☑
        animal-drawn vehicle (traffic) V46.9 ☑
          nontraffic V46.3 ☑
          while boarding or alighting V46.4 ☑
        bus (traffic) V44.9 ☑
          nontraffic V44.3 ☑
          while boarding or alighting V44.4 ☑
        car (traffic) V43.92 ☑
          nontraffic V43.32 ☑
          while boarding or alighting V43.42 ☑
        motor vehicle NOS (traffic) V49.60 ☑
          nontraffic V49.20 ☑
          specified type NEC (traffic) V49.69 ☑
            nontraffic V49.29 ☑
        pedal cycle (traffic) V41.9 ☑
          nontraffic V41.3 ☑
          while boarding or alighting V41.4 ☑
        pickup truck (traffic) V43.93 ☑
          nontraffic V43.33 ☑
          while boarding or alighting V43.43 ☑
        railway vehicle (traffic) V45.9 ☑
          nontraffic V45.3 ☑
          while boarding or alighting V45.4 ☑
        specified vehicle NEC (traffic) V46.9 ☑
          nontraffic V46.3 ☑
          while boarding or alighting V46.4 ☑
        sport utility vehicle (traffic) V43.91 ☑
          nontraffic V43.31 ☑

Accident — *continued*
  transport — *continued*
    car occupant — *continued*
      collision — *continued*
        sport utility vehicle — *continued*
          while boarding or alighting V43.41 ☑
        stationary object (traffic) V47.9 ☑
          nontraffic V47.3 ☑
          while boarding or alighting V47.4 ☑
        streetcar (traffic) V46.9 ☑
          nontraffic V46.3 ☑
          while boarding or alighting V46.4 ☑
        three wheeled motor vehicle (traffic) V42.9 ☑
          nontraffic V42.3 ☑
          while boarding or alighting V42.4 ☑
        truck (traffic) V44.9 ☑
          nontraffic V44.3 ☑
          while boarding or alighting V44.4 ☑
        two wheeled motor vehicle (traffic) V42.9 ☑
          nontraffic V42.3 ☑
          while boarding or alighting V42.4 ☑
        van (traffic) V43.94 ☑
          nontraffic V43.34 ☑
          while boarding or alighting V43.44 ☑
      driver
        collision (with)
          animal (traffic) V40.5 ☑
            being ridden (traffic) V46.5 ☑
              nontraffic V46.0 ☑
            nontraffic V40.0 ☑
          animal-drawn vehicle (traffic) V46.5 ☑
            nontraffic V46.0 ☑
          bus (traffic) V44.5 ☑
            nontraffic V44.0 ☑
          car (traffic) V43.52 ☑
            nontraffic V43.02 ☑
          motor vehicle NOS (traffic) V49.40 ☑
            nontraffic V49.00 ☑
            specified type NEC (traffic) V49.49 ☑
              nontraffic V49.09 ☑
          pedal cycle (traffic) V41.5 ☑
            nontraffic V41.0 ☑
          pickup truck (traffic) V43.53 ☑
            nontraffic V43.03 ☑
          railway vehicle (traffic) V45.5 ☑
            nontraffic V45.0 ☑
          specified vehicle NEC (traffic) V46.5 ☑
            nontraffic V46.0 ☑
          sport utility vehicle (traffic) V43.51 ☑
            nontraffic V43.01 ☑
          stationary object (traffic) V47.5 ☑
            nontraffic V47.0 ☑
          streetcar (traffic) V46.5 ☑
            nontraffic V46.0 ☑
          three wheeled motor vehicle (traffic)
            V42.5 ☑
            nontraffic V42.0 ☑
          truck (traffic) V44.5 ☑
            nontraffic V44.0 ☑
          two wheeled motor vehicle (traffic)
            V42.5 ☑
            nontraffic V42.0 ☑
          van (traffic) V43.54 ☑
            nontraffic V43.04 ☑
        noncollision accident (traffic) V48.5 ☑
          nontraffic V48.0 ☑
      hanger-on
        collision (with)
          animal (traffic) V40.7 ☑
            being ridden (traffic) V46.7 ☑
              nontraffic V46.2 ☑
            nontraffic V40.2 ☑
          animal-drawn vehicle (traffic) V46.7 ☑
            nontraffic V46.2 ☑
          bus (traffic) V44.7 ☑
            nontraffic V44.2 ☑
          car (traffic) V43.72 ☑
            nontraffic V43.22 ☑
          pedal cycle (traffic) V41.7 ☑
            nontraffic V41.2 ☑
          pickup truck (traffic) V43.73 ☑
            nontraffic V43.23 ☑
          railway vehicle (traffic) V45.7 ☑
            nontraffic V45.2 ☑
          specified vehicle NEC (traffic) V46.7 ☑
            nontraffic V46.2 ☑

Accident — *continued*
  transport — *continued*
    car occupant — *continued*
      hanger-on — *continued*
        collision — *continued*
          sport utility vehicle (traffic) V43.71 ☑
            nontraffic V43.21 ☑
          stationary object (traffic) V47.7 ☑
            nontraffic V47.2 ☑
          streetcar (traffic) V46.7 ☑
            nontraffic V46.2 ☑
          three wheeled motor vehicle (traffic)
            V42.7 ☑
            nontraffic V42.2 ☑
          truck (traffic) V44.7 ☑
            nontraffic V44.2 ☑
          two wheeled motor vehicle (traffic)
            V42.7 ☑
            nontraffic V42.2 ☑
          van (traffic) V43.74 ☑
            nontraffic V43.24 ☑
        noncollision accident (traffic) V48.7 ☑
          nontraffic V48.2 ☑
      noncollision accident (traffic) V48.9 ☑
        nontraffic V48.3 ☑
        while boarding or alighting V48.4 ☑
      nontraffic V49.3 ☑
      passenger
        collision (with)
          animal (traffic) V40.6 ☑
            being ridden (traffic) V46.6 ☑
              nontraffic V46.1 ☑
            nontraffic V40.1 ☑
          animal-drawn vehicle (traffic) V46.6 ☑
            nontraffic V46.1 ☑
          bus (traffic) V44.6 ☑
            nontraffic V44.1 ☑
          car (traffic) V43.62 ☑
            nontraffic V43.12 ☑
          motor vehicle NOS (traffic) V49.50 ☑
            nontraffic V49.10 ☑
            specified type NEC (traffic) V49.59 ☑
              nontraffic V49.19 ☑
          pedal cycle (traffic) V41.6 ☑
            nontraffic V41.1 ☑
          pickup truck (traffic) V43.63 ☑
            nontraffic V43.13 ☑
          railway vehicle (traffic) V45.6 ☑
            nontraffic V45.1 ☑
          specified vehicle NEC (traffic) V46.6 ☑
            nontraffic V46.1 ☑
          sport utility vehicle (traffic) V43.61 ☑
            nontraffic V43.11 ☑
          stationary object (traffic) V47.6 ☑
            nontraffic V47.1 ☑
          streetcar (traffic) V46.6 ☑
            nontraffic V46.1 ☑
          three wheeled motor vehicle (traffic)
            V42.6 ☑
            nontraffic V42.1 ☑
          truck (traffic) V44.6 ☑
            nontraffic V44.1 ☑
          two wheeled motor vehicle (traffic)
            V42.6 ☑
            nontraffic V42.1 ☑
          van (traffic) V43.64 ☑
            nontraffic V43.14 ☑
        noncollision accident (traffic) V48.6 ☑
          nontraffic V48.1 ☑
      specified type NEC V49.88 ☑
        military vehicle V49.81 ☑
      coal car — *see* Accident, transport, industrial vehicle occupant
    construction vehicle occupant (nontraffic) V85.9 ☑
      driver V85.5 ☑
      hanger-on V85.7 ☑
      passenger V85.6 ☑
      traffic V85.3 ☑
        driver V85.0 ☑
        hanger-on V85.2 ☑
        passenger V85.1 ☑
      while boarding or alighting V85.4 ☑
    dirt bike rider (nontraffic) V86.96 ☑
      driver V86.56 ☑
      hanger-on V86.76 ☑
      passenger V86.66 ☑

Accident — *continued*
  transport — *continued*
    dirt bike rider — *continued*
      traffic V86.36 ☑
        driver V86.06 ☑
        hanger-on V86.26 ☑
        passenger V86.16 ☑
        while boarding or alighting V86.46 ☑
    due to cataclysm — *see* Forces of nature, by type
    dune buggy occupant (nontraffic) V86.93 ☑
      driver V86.53 ☑
      hanger-on V86.73 ☑
      passenger V86.63 ☑
      traffic V86.33 ☑
        driver V86.03 ☑
        hanger-on V86.23 ☑
        passenger V86.13 ☑
        while boarding or alighting V86.43 ☑
    forklift — *see* Accident, transport, industrial vehicle occupant
    go cart — *see* Accident, transport, all-terrain vehicle occupant
    golf cart — *see* Accident, transport, all-terrain vehicle occupant
    heavy transport vehicle occupant — *see* Accident, transport, truck occupant
    ice yacht V98.2 ☑
    industrial vehicle occupant (nontraffic) V83.9 ☑
      driver V83.5 ☑
      hanger-on V83.7 ☑
      passenger V83.6 ☑
      traffic V83.3 ☑
        driver V83.0 ☑
        hanger-on V83.2 ☑
        passenger V83.1 ☑
      while boarding or alighting V83.4 ☑
    interurban electric car — *see* Accident, transport, streetcar
    land yacht V98.1 ☑
    logging car — *see* Accident, transport, industrial vehicle occupant
    military vehicle occupant (traffic) V86.34 ☑
      driver V86.04 ☑
      hanger-on V86.24 ☑
      nontraffic V86.94 ☑
        driver V86.54 ☑
        hanger-on V86.74 ☑
        passenger V86.64 ☑
      passenger V86.14 ☑
      while boarding or alighting V86.44 ☑
    mine tram — *see* Accident, transport, industrial vehicle occupant
    motor vehicle NEC occupant (traffic) V89.2 ☑
    motorcoach — *see* Accident, transport, bus occupant
    motor/cross bike rider (*see also* Accident, transport, dirt bike rider) V86.96 ☑
    motorcyclist V29.9 ☑
      collision (with)
        animal (traffic) V20.9 ☑
          being ridden (traffic) V26.9 ☑
            nontraffic V26.2 ☑
            while boarding or alighting V26.3 ☑
          nontraffic V20.2 ☑
          while boarding or alighting V20.3 ☑
        animal-drawn vehicle (traffic) V26.9 ☑
          nontraffic V26.2 ☑
          while boarding or alighting V26.3 ☑
        bus (traffic) V24.9 ☑
          nontraffic V24.2 ☑
          while boarding or alighting V24.3 ☑
        car (traffic) V23.9 ☑
          nontraffic V23.2 ☑
          while boarding or alighting V23.3 ☑
        motor vehicle NOS (traffic) V29.60 ☑
          nontraffic V29.20 ☑
          specified type NEC (traffic) V29.69 ☑
            nontraffic V29.29 ☑
        pedal cycle (traffic) V21.9 ☑
          nontraffic V21.2 ☑
          while boarding or alighting V21.3 ☑
        pickup truck (traffic) V23.9 ☑
          nontraffic V23.2 ☑
          while boarding or alighting V23.3 ☑
        railway vehicle (traffic) V25.9 ☑
          nontraffic V25.2 ☑

Accident — *continued*
  transport — *continued*
    motorcyclist — *continued*
      collision — *continued*
        railway vehicle — *continued*
          while boarding or alighting V25.3 ☑
        specified vehicle NEC (traffic) V26.9 ☑
          nontraffic V26.2 ☑
          while boarding or alighting V26.3 ☑
        stationary object (traffic) V27.9 ☑
          nontraffic V27.2 ☑
          while boarding or alighting V27.3 ☑
        streetcar (traffic) V26.9 ☑
          nontraffic V26.2 ☑
          while boarding or alighting V26.3 ☑
        three wheeled motor vehicle (traffic) V22.9 ☑
          nontraffic V22.2 ☑
          while boarding or alighting V22.3 ☑
        truck (traffic) V24.9 ☑
          nontraffic V24.2 ☑
          while boarding or alighting V24.3 ☑
        two wheeled motor vehicle (traffic) V22.9 ☑
          nontraffic V22.2 ☑
          while boarding or alighting V22.3 ☑
        van (traffic) V23.9 ☑
          nontraffic V23.2 ☑
          while boarding or alighting V23.3 ☑
      driver
        collision (with)
          animal (traffic) V20.4 ☑
            being ridden (traffic) V26.4 ☑
              nontraffic V26.0 ☑
            nontraffic V20.0 ☑
          animal-drawn vehicle (traffic) V26.4 ☑
            nontraffic V26.0 ☑
          bus (traffic) V24.4 ☑
            nontraffic V24.0 ☑
          car (traffic) V23.4 ☑
            nontraffic V23.0 ☑
          motor vehicle NOS (traffic) V29.40 ☑
            nontraffic V29.00 ☑
            specified type NEC (traffic) V29.49 ☑
              nontraffic V29.09 ☑
          pedal cycle (traffic) V21.4 ☑
            nontraffic V21.0 ☑
          pickup truck (traffic) V23.4 ☑
            nontraffic V23.0 ☑
          railway vehicle (traffic) V25.4 ☑
            nontraffic V25.0 ☑
          specified vehicle NEC (traffic) V26.4 ☑
            nontraffic V26.0 ☑
          stationary object (traffic) V27.4 ☑
            nontraffic V27.0 ☑
          streetcar (traffic) V26.4 ☑
            nontraffic V26.0 ☑
          three wheeled motor vehicle (traffic) V22.4 ☑
            nontraffic V22.0 ☑
          truck (traffic) V24.4 ☑
            nontraffic V24.0 ☑
          two wheeled motor vehicle (traffic) V22.4 ☑
            nontraffic V22.0 ☑
          van (traffic) V23.4 ☑
            nontraffic V23.0 ☑
        noncollision accident (traffic) V28.4 ☑
          nontraffic V28.0 ☑
      noncollision accident (traffic) V28.9 ☑
        nontraffic V28.2 ☑
        while boarding or alighting V28.3 ☑
      nontraffic V29.3 ☑
      passenger
        collision (with)
          animal (traffic) V20.5 ☑
            being ridden (traffic) V26.5 ☑
              nontraffic V26.1 ☑
            nontraffic V20.1 ☑
          animal-drawn vehicle (traffic) V26.5 ☑
            nontraffic V26.1 ☑
          bus (traffic) V24.5 ☑
            nontraffic V24.1 ☑
          car (traffic) V23.5 ☑
            nontraffic V23.1 ☑
          motor vehicle NOS (traffic) V29.50 ☑
            nontraffic V29.10 ☑
            specified type NEC (traffic) V29.59 ☑

Accident — *continued*
  transport — *continued*
    motorcyclist — *continued*
      passenger — *continued*
        collision — *continued*
          motor vehicle — *continued*
            specified type — *continued*
              nontraffic V29.19 ☑
          pedal cycle (traffic) V21.5 ☑
            nontraffic V21.1 ☑
          pickup truck (traffic) V23.5 ☑
            nontraffic V23.1 ☑
          railway vehicle (traffic) V25.5 ☑
            nontraffic V25.1 ☑
          specified vehicle NEC (traffic) V26.5 ☑
            nontraffic V26.1 ☑
          stationary object (traffic) V27.5 ☑
            nontraffic V27.1 ☑
          streetcar (traffic) V26.5 ☑
            nontraffic V26.1 ☑
          three wheeled motor vehicle (traffic) V22.5 ☑
            nontraffic V22.1 ☑
          truck (traffic) V24.5 ☑
            nontraffic V24.1 ☑
          two wheeled motor vehicle (traffic) V22.5 ☑
            nontraffic V22.1 ☑
          van (traffic) V23.5 ☑
            nontraffic V23.1 ☑
        noncollision accident (traffic) V28.5 ☑
          nontraffic V28.1 ☑
      specified type NEC V29.88 ☑
      military vehicle V29.81 ☑
    occupant (of)
      aircraft (powered) V95.9 ☑
        fixed wing
          commercial — *see* Accident, transport, aircraft, occupant, powered, fixed wing, commercial
          private — *see* Accident, transport, aircraft, occupant, powered, fixed wing, private
        nonpowered V96.9 ☑
        specified NEC V95.8 ☑
      airport battery-powered vehicle — *see* Accident, transport, industrial vehicle occupant
      all-terrain vehicle (ATV) — *see* Accident, transport, all-terrain vehicle occupant
      animal-drawn vehicle — *see* Accident, transport, animal-drawn vehicle occupant
      automobile — *see* Accident, transport, car occupant
      balloon V96.00 ☑
      battery-powered vehicle — *see* Accident, transport, industrial vehicle occupant
      bicycle — *see* Accident, transport, pedal cyclist
        motorized — *see* Accident, transport, motorcycle rider
      boat NEC — *see* Accident, watercraft
      bulldozer — *see* Accident, transport, construction vehicle occupant
      bus — *see* Accident, transport, bus occupant
      cable car (on rails) (*see also* Accident, transport, streetcar occupant)
        not on rails V98.0 ☑
      car (*see also* Accident, transport, car occupant)
        cable (on rails) (*see also* Accident, transport, streetcar occupant)
        not on rails V98.0 ☑
      coach — *see* Accident, transport, bus occupant
      coal-car — *see* Accident, transport, industrial vehicle occupant
      digger — *see* Accident, transport, construction vehicle occupant
      dump truck — *see* Accident, transport, construction vehicle occupant
      earth-leveler — *see* Accident, transport, construction vehicle occupant
      farm machinery (self-propelled) — *see* Accident, transport, agricultural vehicle occupant
      forklift — *see* Accident, transport, industrial vehicle occupant
      glider (unpowered) V96.20 ☑
        hang V96.10 ☑

Accident — *continued*
  transport — *continued*
    occupant — *continued*
      glider — *continued*
        powered (microlight) (ultralight) — *see* Accident, transport, aircraft, occupant, powered, glider
      glider (unpowered) NEC V96.20 ☑
      hang-glider V96.10 ☑
      harvester — *see* Accident, transport, agricultural vehicle occupant
      heavy (transport) vehicle — *see* Accident, transport, truck occupant
      helicopter — *see* Accident, transport, aircraft, occupant, helicopter
      ice-yacht V98.2 ☑
      kite (carrying person) V96.8 ☑
      land-yacht V98.1 ☑
      logging car — *see* Accident, transport, industrial vehicle occupant
      mechanical shovel — *see* Accident, transport, construction vehicle occupant
      microlight — *see* Accident, transport, aircraft, occupant, powered, glider
      minibus — *see* Accident, transport, pickup truck occupant
      minivan — *see* Accident, transport, pickup truck occupant
      moped — *see* Accident, transport, motorcycle
      motor scooter — *see* Accident, transport, motorcycle
      motorcycle (with sidecar) — *see* Accident, transport, motorcycle
      off-road motor-vehicle (*see also* Accident, transport, all-terrain vehicle occupant) V86.99 ☑
      pedal cycle (*see also* Accident, transport, pedal cyclist)
      pick-up (truck) — *see* Accident, transport, pickup truck occupant
      railway (train) (vehicle) (subterranean) (elevated) — *see* Accident, transport, railway vehicle occupant
      rickshaw — *see* Accident, transport, pedal cycle
        motorized — *see* Accident, transport, three-wheeled motor vehicle
        pedal driven — *see* Accident, transport, pedal cyclist
      road-roller — *see* Accident, transport, construction vehicle occupant
      ship NOS V94.9 ☑
      ski-lift (chair) (gondola) V98.3 ☑
      snowmobile — *see* Accident, transport, snowmobile occupant
      spacecraft, spaceship — *see* Accident, transport, aircraft, occupant, spacecraft
      sport utility vehicle — *see* Accident, transport, pickup truck occupant
      streetcar (interurban) (operating on public street or highway) — *see* Accident, transport, streetcar occupant
      SUV — *see* Accident, transport, pickup truck occupant
      téléférique V98.0 ☑
      three-wheeled vehicle (motorized) (*see also* Accident, transport, three-wheeled motor vehicle occupant)
        nonmotorized — *see* Accident, transport, pedal cycle
      tractor (farm) (and trailer) — *see* Accident, transport, agricultural vehicle occupant
      train — *see* Accident, transport, railway vehicle occupant
      tram — *see* Accident, transport, streetcar occupant
        in mine or quarry — *see* Accident, transport, industrial vehicle occupant
      tricycle — *see* Accident, transport, pedal cycle
        motorized — *see* Accident, transport, three-wheeled motor vehicle
      trolley — *see* Accident, transport, streetcar occupant
        in mine or quarry — *see* Accident, transport, industrial vehicle occupant
      tub, in mine or quarry — *see* Accident, transport, industrial vehicle occupant

Accident — *continued*
  transport — *continued*
    occupant — *continued*
      ultralight — *see* Accident, transport, aircraft, occupant, powered, glider
      van — *see* Accident, transport, van occupant
      vehicle NEC V89.9 ☑
        heavy transport — *see* Accident, transport, truck occupant
        motor (traffic) NEC V89.2 ☑
          nontraffic NEC V89.0 ☑
      watercraft NOS V94.9 ☑
        causing drowning — *see* Drowning, resulting from accident to boat
    off-road motor-vehicle (*see also* Accident, transport, all-terrain vehicle occupant) V86.99 ☑
    parachutist V97.29 ☑
      after accident to aircraft — *see* Accident, transport, aircraft
      entangled in object V97.21 ☑
      injured on landing V97.22 ☑
    pedal cyclist V19.9 ☑
      collision (with)
        animal (traffic) V10.9 ☑
          being ridden (traffic) V16.9 ☑
            nontraffic V16.2 ☑
            while boarding or alighting V16.3 ☑
          nontraffic V10.2 ☑
          while boarding or alighting V10.3 ☑
        animal-drawn vehicle (traffic) V16.9 ☑
          nontraffic V16.2 ☑
          while boarding or alighting V16.3 ☑
        bus (traffic) V14.9 ☑
          nontraffic V14.2 ☑
          while boarding or alighting V14.3 ☑
        car (traffic) V13.9 ☑
          nontraffic V13.2 ☑
          while boarding or alighting V13.3 ☑
        motor vehicle NOS (traffic) V19.60 ☑
          nontraffic V19.20 ☑
          specified type NEC (traffic) V19.69 ☑
            nontraffic V19.29 ☑
        pedal cycle (traffic) V11.9 ☑
          nontraffic V11.2 ☑
          while boarding or alighting V11.3 ☑
        pickup truck (traffic) V13.9 ☑
          nontraffic V13.2 ☑
          while boarding or alighting V13.3 ☑
        railway vehicle (traffic) V15.9 ☑
          nontraffic V15.2 ☑
          while boarding or alighting V15.3 ☑
        specified vehicle NEC (traffic) V16.9 ☑
          nontraffic V16.2 ☑
          while boarding or alighting V16.3 ☑
        stationary object (traffic) V17.9 ☑
          nontraffic V17.2 ☑
          while boarding or alighting V17.3 ☑
        streetcar (traffic) V16.9 ☑
          nontraffic V16.2 ☑
          while boarding or alighting V16.3 ☑
        three wheeled motor vehicle (traffic) V12.9 ☑
          nontraffic V12.2 ☑
          while boarding or alighting V12.3 ☑
        truck (traffic) V14.9 ☑
          nontraffic V14.2 ☑
          while boarding or alighting V14.3 ☑
        two wheeled motor vehicle (traffic) V12.9 ☑
          nontraffic V12.2 ☑
          while boarding or alighting V12.3 ☑
        van (traffic) V13.9 ☑
          nontraffic V13.2 ☑
          while boarding or alighting V13.3 ☑
      driver
        collision (with)
          animal (traffic) V10.4 ☑
            being ridden (traffic) V16.4 ☑
              nontraffic V16.0 ☑
            nontraffic V10.0 ☑
          animal-drawn vehicle (traffic) V16.4 ☑
            nontraffic V16.0 ☑
          bus (traffic) V14.4 ☑
            nontraffic V14.0 ☑
          car (traffic) V13.4 ☑
            nontraffic V13.0 ☑
          motor vehicle NOS (traffic) V19.40 ☑
            nontraffic V19.00 ☑

Accident — *continued*
  transport — *continued*
    pedal cyclist — *continued*
      driver — *continued*
        collision — *continued*
          motor vehicle — *continued*
            specified type NEC (traffic) V19.49 ☑
              nontraffic V19.09 ☑
          pedal cycle (traffic) V11.4 ☑
            nontraffic V11.0 ☑
          pickup truck (traffic) V13.4 ☑
            nontraffic V13.0 ☑
          railway vehicle (traffic) V15.4 ☑
            nontraffic V15.0 ☑
          specified vehicle NEC (traffic) V16.4 ☑
            nontraffic V16.0 ☑
          stationary object (traffic) V17.4 ☑
            nontraffic V17.0 ☑
          streetcar (traffic) V16.4 ☑
            nontraffic V16.0 ☑
          three wheeled motor vehicle (traffic) V12.4 ☑
            nontraffic V12.0 ☑
          truck (traffic) V14.4 ☑
            nontraffic V14.0 ☑
          two wheeled motor vehicle (traffic) V12.4 ☑
            nontraffic V12.0 ☑
          van (traffic) V13.4 ☑
            nontraffic V13.0 ☑
        noncollision accident (traffic) V18.4 ☑
          nontraffic V18.0 ☑
      noncollision accident (traffic) V18.9 ☑
        nontraffic V18.2 ☑
        while boarding or alighting V18.3 ☑
      nontraffic V19.3 ☑
      passenger
        collision (with)
          animal (traffic) V10.5 ☑
            being ridden (traffic) V16.5 ☑
              nontraffic V16.1 ☑
            nontraffic V10.1 ☑
          animal-drawn vehicle (traffic) V16.5 ☑
            nontraffic V16.1 ☑
          bus (traffic) V14.5 ☑
            nontraffic V14.1 ☑
          car (traffic) V13.5 ☑
            nontraffic V13.1 ☑
          motor vehicle NOS (traffic) V19.50 ☑
            nontraffic V19.10 ☑
            specified type NEC (traffic) V19.59 ☑
              nontraffic V19.19 ☑
          pedal cycle (traffic) V11.5 ☑
            nontraffic V11.1 ☑
          pickup truck (traffic) V13.5 ☑
            nontraffic V13.1 ☑
          railway vehicle (traffic) V15.5 ☑
            nontraffic V15.1 ☑
          specified vehicle NEC (traffic) V16.5 ☑
            nontraffic V16.1 ☑
          stationary object (traffic) V17.5 ☑
            nontraffic V17.1 ☑
          streetcar (traffic) V16.5 ☑
            nontraffic V16.1 ☑
          three wheeled motor vehicle (traffic) V12.5 ☑
            nontraffic V12.1 ☑
          truck (traffic) V14.5 ☑
            nontraffic V14.1 ☑
          two wheeled motor vehicle (traffic) V12.5 ☑
            nontraffic V12.1 ☑
          van (traffic) V13.5 ☑
            nontraffic V13.1 ☑
        noncollision accident (traffic) V18.5 ☑
          nontraffic V18.1 ☑
      specified type NEC V19.88 ☑
      military vehicle V19.81 ☑
    pedestrian
      conveyance (occupant) V09.9 ☑
        baby stroller V00.828 ☑
        collision (with) V09.9 ☑
          animal being ridden or animal drawn vehicle V06.99 ☑
            nontraffic V06.09 ☑
            traffic V06.19 ☑

Accident — *continued*
  transport — *continued*
    pedestrian — *continued*
      conveyance — *continued*
        baby stroller — *continued*
          collision — *continued*
            bus or heavy transport V04.99 ☑
              nontraffic V04.09 ☑
              traffic V04.19 ☑
            car V03.99 ☑
              nontraffic V03.09 ☑
              traffic V03.19 ☑
            pedal cycle V01.99 ☑
              nontraffic V01.09 ☑
              traffic V01.19 ☑
            pick-up truck or van V03.99 ☑
              nontraffic V03.09 ☑
              traffic V03.19 ☑
            railway (train) (vehicle) V05.99 ☑
              nontraffic V05.09 ☑
              traffic V05.19 ☑
            stationary object V00.822 ☑
            streetcar V06.99 ☑
              nontraffic V06.09 ☑
              traffic V06.19 ☑
            two- or three-wheeled motor vehicle V02.99 ☑
              nontraffic V02.09 ☑
              traffic V02.19 ☑
            vehicle V09.9 ☑
              animal-drawn V06.99 ☑
                nontraffic V06.09 ☑
                traffic V06.19 ☑
              motor
                nontraffic V09.00 ☑
                traffic V09.20 ☑
           fall V00.821 ☑
          nontraffic V09.1 ☑
            involving motor vehicle NEC V09.00 ☑
          traffic V09.3 ☑
            involving motor vehicle NEC V09.20 ☑
        flat-bottomed NEC V00.388 ☑
          collision (with) V09.9 ☑
            animal being ridden or animal drawn vehicle V06.99 ☑
              nontraffic V06.09 ☑
              traffic V06.19 ☑
            bus or heavy transport V04.99 ☑
              nontraffic V04.09 ☑
              traffic V04.19 ☑
            car V03.99 ☑
              nontraffic V03.09 ☑
              traffic V03.19 ☑
            pedal cycle V01.99 ☑
              nontraffic V01.09 ☑
              traffic V01.19 ☑
            pick-up truck or van V03.99 ☑
              nontraffic V03.09 ☑
              traffic V03.19 ☑
            railway (train) (vehicle) V05.99 ☑
              nontraffic V05.09 ☑
              traffic V05.19 ☑
            stationary object V00.382 ☑
            streetcar V06.99 ☑
              nontraffic V06.09 ☑
              traffic V06.19 ☑
            two- or three-wheeled motor vehicle V02.99 ☑
              nontraffic V02.09 ☑
              traffic V02.19 ☑
            vehicle V09.9 ☑
              animal-drawn V06.99 ☑
                nontraffic V06.09 ☑
                traffic V06.19 ☑
              motor
                nontraffic V09.00 ☑
                traffic V09.20 ☑
          fall V00.381 ☑
         nontraffic V09.1 ☑
          involving motor vehicle NEC V09.00 ☑
        snow
          board — *see* Accident, transport, pedestrian, conveyance, snow board
          ski — *see* Accident, transport, pedestrian, conveyance, skis (snow)

Accident — *continued*
  transport — *continued*
    pedestrian — *continued*
      conveyance — *continued*
        flat-bottomed — *continued*
          traffic V09.3 ☑
            involving motor vehicle NEC V09.20 ☑
        gliding type NEC V00.288 ☑
          collision (with) V09.9 ☑
            animal being ridden or animal drawn vehicle V06.99 ☑
              nontraffic V06.09 ☑
              traffic V06.19 ☑
            bus or heavy transport V04.99 ☑
              nontraffic V04.09 ☑
              traffic V04.19 ☑
            car V03.99 ☑
              nontraffic V03.09 ☑
              traffic V03.19 ☑
            pedal cycle V01.99 ☑
              nontraffic V01.09 ☑
              traffic V01.19 ☑
            pick-up truck or van V03.99 ☑
              nontraffic V03.09 ☑
              traffic V03.19 ☑
            railway (train) (vehicle) V05.99 ☑
              nontraffic V05.09 ☑
              traffic V05.19 ☑
            stationary object V00.282 ☑
            streetcar V06.99 ☑
              nontraffic V06.09 ☑
              traffic V02.19 ☑
            two- or three-wheeled motor vehicle V02.99 ☑
              nontraffic V02.09 ☑
              traffic V02.19 ☑
            vehicle V09.9 ☑
              animal-drawn V06.99 ☑
                nontraffic V06.09 ☑
                traffic V06.19 ☑
              motor
                nontraffic V09.00 ☑
                traffic V09.20 ☑
          fall V00.281 ☑
        heelies — *see* Accident, transport, pedestrian, conveyance, heelies
        ice skate — *see* Accident, transport, pedestrian, conveyance, ice skate
        nontraffic V09.1 ☑
          involving motor vehicle NEC V09.00 ☑
        sled — *see* Accident, transport, pedestrian, conveyance, sled
        traffic V09.3 ☑
          involving motor vehicle NEC V09.20 ☑
          wheelies — *see* Accident, transport, pedestrian, conveyance, heelies
        heelies V00.158 ☑
          colliding with stationary object V00.152 ☑
          fall V00.151 ☑
        ice skates V00.218 ☑
          collision (with) V09.9 ☑
            animal being ridden or animal drawn vehicle V06.99 ☑
              nontraffic V06.09 ☑
              traffic V06.19 ☑
            bus or heavy transport V04.99 ☑
              nontraffic V04.09 ☑
              traffic V04.19 ☑
            car V03.99 ☑
              nontraffic V03.09 ☑
              traffic V03.19 ☑
            pedal cycle V01.99 ☑
              nontraffic V01.09 ☑
              traffic V01.19 ☑
            pick-up truck or van V03.99 ☑
              nontraffic V03.09 ☑
              traffic V03.19 ☑
            railway (train) (vehicle) V05.99 ☑
              nontraffic V05.09 ☑
              traffic V05.19 ☑
            stationary object V00.212 ☑
            streetcar V06.99 ☑
              nontraffic V06.09 ☑
              traffic V06.19 ☑

Accident — *continued*
  transport — *continued*
    pedestrian — *continued*
      conveyance — *continued*
        ice skates — *continued*
          collision — *continued*
            two- or three-wheeled motor vehicle V02.99 ☑
              nontraffic V02.09 ☑
              traffic V02.19 ☑
            vehicle V09.9 ☑
              animal-drawn V06.99 ☑
                nontraffic V06.09 ☑
                traffic V06.19 ☑
              motor
                nontraffic V09.00 ☑
                traffic V09.20 ☑
          fall V00.211 ☑
         nontraffic V09.1 ☑
          involving motor vehicle NEC V09.00 ☑
         traffic V09.3 ☑
          involving motor vehicle NEC V09.20 ☑
        motorized mobility scooter V00.838 ☑
          collision with stationary object V00.832 ☑
          fall from V00.831 ☑
        nontraffic V09.1 ☑
          involving motor vehicle V09.00 ☑
            military V09.01 ☑
            specified type NEC V09.09 ☑
        roller skates (non in-line) V00.128 ☑
          collision (with) V09.9 ☑
            animal being ridden or animal drawn vehicle V06.91 ☑
              nontraffic V06.01 ☑
              traffic V06.11 ☑
            bus or heavy transport V04.91 ☑
              nontraffic V04.01 ☑
              traffic V04.11 ☑
            car V03.91 ☑
              nontraffic V03.01 ☑
              traffic V03.11 ☑
            pedal cycle V01.91 ☑
              nontraffic V01.01 ☑
              traffic V01.11 ☑
            pick-up truck or van V03.91 ☑
              nontraffic V03.01 ☑
              traffic V03.11 ☑
            railway (train) (vehicle) V05.91 ☑
              nontraffic V05.01 ☑
              traffic V05.11 ☑
            stationary object V00.122 ☑
            streetcar V06.91 ☑
              nontraffic V06.01 ☑
              traffic V06.11 ☑
            two- or three-wheeled motor vehicle V02.91 ☑
              nontraffic V02.01 ☑
              traffic V02.11 ☑
            vehicle V09.9 ☑
              animal-drawn V06.91 ☑
                nontraffic V06.01 ☑
                traffic V06.11 ☑
              motor
                nontraffic V09.00 ☑
                traffic V09.20 ☑
          fall V00.121 ☑
         in-line V00.118 ☑
          collision — *see also* Accident, transport, pedestrian, conveyance occupant, roller skates, collision with stationary object V00.112 ☑
          fall V00.111 ☑
          nontraffic V09.1 ☑
           involving motor vehicle NEC V09.00 ☑
          traffic V09.3 ☑
           involving motor vehicle NEC V09.20 ☑
        rolling shoes V00.158 ☑
          colliding with stationary object V00.152 ☑
          fall V00.151 ☑
        rolling type NEC V00.188 ☑
          collision (with) V09.9 ☑
            animal being ridden or animal drawn vehicle V06.99 ☑
              nontraffic V06.09 ☑

☑ **Additional Character Required** — Refer to the Tabular List for Character Selection   ⛛ **Subterms under main terms may continue to next column or page**

Accident — *continued*
  transport — *continued*
    pedestrian — *continued*
      conveyance — *continued*
        rolling type — *continued*
          collision — *continued*
            animal being ridden or animal drawn vehicle — *continued*
              traffic V06.19 ☑
            bus or heavy transport V04.99 ☑
              nontraffic V04.09 ☑
              traffic V04.19 ☑
            car V03.99 ☑
              nontraffic V03.09 ☑
              traffic V03.19 ☑
            pedal cycle V01.99 ☑
              nontraffic V01.09 ☑
              traffic V01.19 ☑
            pick-up truck or van V03.99 ☑
              nontraffic V03.09 ☑
              traffic V03.19 ☑
            railway (train) (vehicle) V05.99 ☑
              nontraffic V05.09 ☑
              traffic V05.19 ☑
            stationary object V00.182 ☑
            streetcar V06.99 ☑
              nontraffic V06.09 ☑
              traffic V06.19 ☑
            two- or three-wheeled motor vehicle V02.99 ☑
              nontraffic V02.09 ☑
              traffic V02.19 ☑
            vehicle V09.9 ☑
              animal-drawn V06.99 ☑
                nontraffic V06.09 ☑
                traffic V06.19 ☑
              motor
                nontraffic V09.00 ☑
                traffic V09.20 ☑
          fall V00.181 ☑
          in-line roller skate — *see* Accident, transport, pedestrian, conveyance, roller skate, in-line
          nontraffic V09.1 ☑
            involving motor vehicle NEC V09.00 ☑
          roller skate — *see* Accident, transport, pedestrian, conveyance, roller skate
          scooter (non-motorized) — *see* Accident, transport, pedestrian, conveyance, scooter
          skateboard — *see* Accident, transport, pedestrian, conveyance, skate-board
          traffic V09.3 ☑
            involving motor vehicle NEC V09.20 ☑
        scooter (non-motorized) V00.148 ☑
          collision (with) V09.9 ☑
            animal being ridden or animal drawn vehicle V06.99 ☑
              nontraffic V06.09 ☑
              traffic V06.19 ☑
            bus or heavy transport V04.99 ☑
              nontraffic V04.09 ☑
              traffic V04.19 ☑
            car V03.99 ☑
              nontraffic V03.09 ☑
              traffic V03.19 ☑
            pedal cycle V01.99 ☑
              nontraffic V01.09 ☑
              traffic V01.19 ☑
            pick-up truck or van V03.99 ☑
              nontraffic V03.09 ☑
              traffic V03.19 ☑
            railway (train) (vehicle) V05.99 ☑
              nontraffic V05.09 ☑
              traffic V05.19 ☑
            stationary object V00.142 ☑
            streetcar V06.99 ☑
              nontraffic V06.09 ☑
              traffic V06.19 ☑
            two- or three-wheeled motor vehicle V02.99 ☑
              nontraffic V02.09 ☑
              traffic V02.19 ☑
            vehicle V09.9 ☑

        scooter — *continued*
          collision — *continued*
            vehicle — *continued*
              animal-drawn V06.99 ☑
                nontraffic V06.09 ☑
                traffic V06.19 ☑
              motor
                nontraffic V09.00 ☑
                traffic V09.20 ☑
          fall V00.141 ☑
          nontraffic V09.1 ☑
            involving motor vehicle NEC V09.00 ☑
          traffic V09.3 ☑
            involving motor vehicle NEC V09.20 ☑
        skate board V00.138 ☑
          collision (with) V09.9 ☑
            animal being ridden or animal drawn vehicle V06.92 ☑
              nontraffic V06.02 ☑
              traffic V06.12 ☑
            bus or heavy transport V04.92 ☑
              nontraffic V04.02 ☑
              traffic V04.12 ☑
            car V03.92 ☑
              nontraffic V03.02 ☑
              traffic V03.12 ☑
            pedal cycle V01.92 ☑
              nontraffic V01.02 ☑
              traffic V01.12 ☑
            pick-up truck or van V03.92 ☑
              nontraffic V03.02 ☑
              traffic V03.12 ☑
            railway (train) (vehicle) V05.92 ☑
              nontraffic V05.02 ☑
              traffic V05.12 ☑
            stationary object V00.132 ☑
            streetcar V06.92 ☑
              nontraffic V06.02 ☑
              traffic V06.12 ☑
            two- or three-wheeled motor vehicle V02.92 ☑
              nontraffic V02.02 ☑
              traffic V02.12 ☑
            vehicle V09.9 ☑
              animal-drawn V06.92 ☑
                nontraffic V06.02 ☑
                traffic V06.12 ☑
              motor
                nontraffic V09.00 ☑
                traffic V09.20 ☑
          fall V00.131 ☑
          nontraffic V09.1 ☑
            involving motor vehicle NEC V09.00 ☑
          traffic V09.3 ☑
            involving motor vehicle NEC V09.20 ☑
        skis (snow) V00.328 ☑
          collision (with) V09.9 ☑
            animal being ridden or animal drawn vehicle V06.99 ☑
              nontraffic V06.09 ☑
              traffic V06.19 ☑
            bus or heavy transport V04.99 ☑
              nontraffic V04.09 ☑
              traffic V04.19 ☑
            car V03.99 ☑
              nontraffic V03.09 ☑
              traffic V03.19 ☑
            pedal cycle V01.99 ☑
              nontraffic V01.09 ☑
              traffic V01.19 ☑
            pick-up truck or van V03.99 ☑
              nontraffic V03.09 ☑
              traffic V03.19 ☑
            railway (train) (vehicle) V05.99 ☑
              nontraffic V05.09 ☑
              traffic V05.19 ☑
            stationary object V00.322 ☑
            streetcar V06.99 ☑
              nontraffic V06.09 ☑
              traffic V06.19 ☑
            two- or three-wheeled motor vehicle V02.99 ☑

        skis — *continued*
          collision — *continued*
            two- or three-wheeled motor vehicle — *continued*
              nontraffic V02.09 ☑
              traffic V02.19 ☑
            vehicle V09.9 ☑
              animal-drawn V06.99 ☑
                nontraffic V06.09 ☑
                traffic V06.19 ☑
              motor
                nontraffic V09.00 ☑
                traffic V09.20 ☑
          fall V00.321 ☑
          nontraffic V09.1 ☑
            involving motor vehicle NEC V09.00 ☑
          traffic V09.3 ☑
            involving motor vehicle NEC V09.20 ☑
        sled V00.228 ☑
          collision (with) V09.9 ☑
            animal being ridden or animal drawn vehicle V06.99 ☑
              nontraffic V06.09 ☑
              traffic V06.19 ☑
            bus or heavy transport V04.99 ☑
              nontraffic V04.09 ☑
              traffic V04.19 ☑
            car V03.99 ☑
              nontraffic V03.09 ☑
              traffic V03.19 ☑
            pedal cycle V01.99 ☑
              nontraffic V01.09 ☑
              traffic V01.19 ☑
            pick-up truck or van V03.99 ☑
              nontraffic V03.09 ☑
              traffic V03.19 ☑
            railway (train) (vehicle) V05.99 ☑
              nontraffic V05.09 ☑
              traffic V05.19 ☑
            stationary object V00.222 ☑
            streetcar V06.99 ☑
              nontraffic V06.09 ☑
              traffic V06.19 ☑
            two- or three-wheeled motor vehicle V02.99 ☑
              nontraffic V02.09 ☑
              traffic V02.19 ☑
            vehicle V09.9 ☑
              animal-drawn V06.99 ☑
                nontraffic V06.09 ☑
                traffic V06.19 ☑
              motor
                nontraffic V09.00 ☑
                traffic V09.20 ☑
          fall V00.221 ☑
          nontraffic V09.1 ☑
            involving motor vehicle NEC V09.00 ☑
          traffic V09.3 ☑
            involving motor vehicle NEC V09.20 ☑
        snow board V00.318 ☑
          collision (with) V09.9 ☑
            animal being ridden or animal drawn vehicle V06.99 ☑
              nontraffic V06.09 ☑
              traffic V06.19 ☑
            bus or heavy transport V04.99 ☑
              nontraffic V04.09 ☑
              traffic V04.19 ☑
            car V03.99 ☑
              nontraffic V03.09 ☑
              traffic V03.19 ☑
            pedal cycle V01.99 ☑
              nontraffic V01.09 ☑
              traffic V01.19 ☑
            pick-up truck or van V03.99 ☑
              nontraffic V03.09 ☑
              traffic V03.19 ☑
            railway (train) (vehicle) V05.99 ☑
              nontraffic V05.09 ☑
              traffic V05.19 ☑
            stationary object V00.312 ☑
            streetcar V06.99 ☑

Accident — *continued*
 transport — *continued*
  pedestrian — *continued*
   conveyance — *continued*
    snow board — *continued*
     collision — *continued*
      streetcar — *continued*
       nontraffic V06.09 ☑
       traffic V06.19 ☑
      two- or three-wheeled motor vehicle V02.99 ☑
       nontraffic V02.09 ☑
       traffic V02.19 ☑
      vehicle V09.9 ☑
       animal-drawn V06.99 ☑
        nontraffic V06.09 ☑
        traffic V06.19 ☑
       motor
        nontraffic V09.00 ☑
        traffic V09.20 ☑
     fall V00.311 ☑
     nontraffic V09.1 ☑
      involving motor vehicle NEC V09.00 ☑
     traffic V09.3 ☑
      involving motor vehicle NEC V09.20 ☑
    specified type NEC V00.898 ☑
     collision (with) V09.9 ☑
      animal being ridden or animal drawn vehicle V06.99 ☑
       nontraffic V06.09 ☑
       traffic V06.19 ☑
      bus or heavy transport V04.99 ☑
       nontraffic V04.09 ☑
       traffic V04.19 ☑
      car V03.99 ☑
       nontraffic V03.09 ☑
       traffic V03.19 ☑
      pedal cycle V01.99 ☑
       nontraffic V01.09 ☑
       traffic V01.19 ☑
      pick-up truck or van V03.99 ☑
       nontraffic V03.09 ☑
       traffic V03.19 ☑
      railway (train) (vehicle) V05.99 ☑
       nontraffic V05.09 ☑
       traffic V05.19 ☑
      stationary object V00.892 ☑
      streetcar V06.99 ☑
       nontraffic V06.09 ☑
       traffic V06.19 ☑
      two- or three-wheeled motor vehicle V02.99 ☑
       nontraffic V02.09 ☑
       traffic V02.19 ☑
      vehicle V09.9 ☑
       animal-drawn V06.99 ☑
        nontraffic V06.09 ☑
        traffic V06.19 ☑
       motor
        nontraffic V09.00 ☑
        traffic V09.20 ☑
     fall V00.891 ☑
     nontraffic V09.1 ☑
      involving motor vehicle NEC V09.00 ☑
     traffic V09.3 ☑
      involving motor vehicle NEC V09.20 ☑
    traffic V09.3 ☑
     involving motor vehicle V09.20 ☑
      military V09.21 ☑
     specified type NEC V09.29 ☑
    wheelchair (powered) V00.818 ☑
     collision (with) V09.9 ☑
      animal being ridden or animal drawn vehicle V06.99 ☑
       nontraffic V06.09 ☑
       traffic V06.19 ☑
      bus or heavy transport V04.99 ☑
       nontraffic V04.09 ☑
       traffic V04.19 ☑
      car V03.99 ☑
       nontraffic V03.09 ☑
       traffic V03.19 ☑
      pedal cycle V01.99 ☑
       nontraffic V01.09 ☑
       traffic V01.19 ☑
      pick-up truck or van V03.99 ☑

Accident — *continued*
 transport — *continued*
  pedestrian — *continued*
   conveyance — *continued*
    wheelchair — *continued*
     collision — *continued*
      pick-up truck or van — *continued*
       nontraffic V03.09 ☑
       traffic V03.19 ☑
      railway (train) (vehicle) V05.99 ☑
       nontraffic V05.09 ☑
       traffic V05.19 ☑
      stationary object V00.812 ☑
      streetcar V06.99 ☑
       nontraffic V06.09 ☑
       traffic V06.19 ☑
      two- or three-wheeled motor vehicle V02.99 ☑
       nontraffic V02.09 ☑
       traffic V02.19 ☑
      vehicle V09.9 ☑
       animal-drawn V06.99 ☑
        nontraffic V06.09 ☑
        traffic V06.19 ☑
       motor
        nontraffic V09.00 ☑
        traffic V09.20 ☑
     fall V00.811 ☑
     nontraffic V09.1 ☑
      involving motor vehicle NEC V09.00 ☑
     traffic V09.3 ☑
      involving motor vehicle NEC V09.20 ☑
    wheeled shoe V00.158 ☑
     colliding with stationary object V00.152 ☑
     fall V00.151 ☑
   on foot (*see also* Accident, pedestrian)
    collision (with)
     animal being ridden or animal drawn vehicle V06.90 ☑
      nontraffic V06.00 ☑
      traffic V06.10 ☑
     bus or heavy transport V04.90 ☑
      nontraffic V04.00 ☑
      traffic V04.10 ☑
     car V03.90 ☑
      nontraffic V03.00 ☑
      traffic V03.10 ☑
     pedal cycle V01.90 ☑
      nontraffic V01.00 ☑
      traffic V01.10 ☑
     pick-up truck or van V03.90 ☑
      nontraffic V03.00 ☑
      traffic V03.10 ☑
     railway (train) (vehicle) V05.90 ☑
      nontraffic V05.00 ☑
      traffic V05.10 ☑
     streetcar V06.90 ☑
      nontraffic V06.00 ☑
      traffic V06.10 ☑
     two- or three-wheeled motor vehicle V02.90 ☑
      nontraffic V02.00 ☑
      traffic V02.10 ☑
     vehicle V09.9 ☑
      animal-drawn V06.90 ☑
       nontraffic V06.00 ☑
       traffic V06.10 ☑
      motor
     nontraffic V09.1 ☑
      involving motor vehicle V09.00 ☑
       military V09.01 ☑
       specified type NEC V09.09 ☑
     traffic V09.3 ☑
      involving motor vehicle V09.20 ☑
       military V09.21 ☑
       specified type NEC V09.29 ☑
   person NEC (unknown way or transportation) V99 ☑
    collision (between)
     bus (with)
      heavy transport vehicle (traffic) V87.5 ☑
       nontraffic V88.5 ☑
     car (with)
      bus (traffic) V87.3 ☑
       nontraffic V88.3 ☑
      heavy transport vehicle (traffic) V87.4 ☑

Accident — *continued*
 transport — *continued*
  person — *continued*
   collision — *continued*
    car — *continued*
     heavy transport vehicle — *continued*
      nontraffic V88.4 ☑
     nontraffic V88.5 ☑
     pick-up truck or van (traffic) V87.2 ☑
      nontraffic V88.2 ☑
     train or railway vehicle (traffic) V87.6 ☑
      nontraffic V88.6 ☑
     two-or three-wheeled motor vehicle (traffic) V87.0 ☑
      nontraffic V88.0 ☑
     motor vehicle (traffic) NEC V87.7 ☑
      nontraffic V88.7 ☑
     two-or three-wheeled vehicle (with) (traffic) motor vehicle NEC V87.1 ☑
      nontraffic V88.1 ☑
     nonmotor vehicle (collision) (noncollision) (traffic) V87.9 ☑
      nontraffic V88.9 ☑
   pickup truck occupant V59.9 ☑
    collision (with)
     animal (traffic) V50.9 ☑
      being ridden (traffic) V56.9 ☑
       nontraffic V56.3 ☑
       while boarding or alighting V56.4 ☑
      nontraffic V50.3 ☑
      while boarding or alighting V50.4 ☑
     animal-drawn vehicle (traffic) V56.9 ☑
      nontraffic V56.3 ☑
      while boarding or alighting V56.4 ☑
     bus (traffic) V54.9 ☑
      nontraffic V54.3 ☑
      while boarding or alighting V54.4 ☑
     car (traffic) V53.9 ☑
      nontraffic V53.3 ☑
      while boarding or alighting V53.4 ☑
     motor vehicle NOS (traffic) V59.60 ☑
      nontraffic V59.20 ☑
      specified type NEC (traffic) V59.69 ☑
       nontraffic V59.29 ☑
     pedal cycle (traffic) V51.9 ☑
      nontraffic V51.3 ☑
      while boarding or alighting V51.4 ☑
     pickup truck (traffic) V53.9 ☑
      nontraffic V53.3 ☑
      while boarding or alighting V53.4 ☑
     railway vehicle (traffic) V55.9 ☑
      nontraffic V55.3 ☑
      while boarding or alighting V55.4 ☑
     specified vehicle NEC (traffic) V56.9 ☑
      nontraffic V56.3 ☑
      while boarding or alighting V56.4 ☑
     stationary object (traffic) V57.9 ☑
      nontraffic V57.3 ☑
      while boarding or alighting V57.4 ☑
     streetcar (traffic) V56.9 ☑
      nontraffic V56.3 ☑
      while boarding or alighting V56.4 ☑
     three wheeled motor vehicle (traffic) V52.9 ☑
      nontraffic V52.3 ☑
      while boarding or alighting V52.4 ☑
     truck (traffic) V54.9 ☑
      nontraffic V54.3 ☑
      while boarding or alighting V54.4 ☑
     two wheeled motor vehicle (traffic) V52.9 ☑
      nontraffic V52.3 ☑
      while boarding or alighting V52.4 ☑
     van (traffic) V53.9 ☑
      nontraffic V53.3 ☑
      while boarding or alighting V53.4 ☑
   driver
    collision (with)
     animal (traffic) V50.5 ☑
      being ridden (traffic) V56.5 ☑
       nontraffic V56.0 ☑
      nontraffic V50.0 ☑
     animal-drawn vehicle (traffic) V56.5 ☑
      nontraffic V56.0 ☑
     bus (traffic) V54.5 ☑
      nontraffic V54.0 ☑
     car (traffic) V53.5 ☑
      nontraffic V53.0 ☑

Accident — continued
  transport — continued
    pickup truck occupant — continued
      driver — continued
        collision — continued
          motor vehicle NOS (traffic) V59.40 ☑
            nontraffic V59.00 ☑
            specified type NEC (traffic) V59.49 ☑
              nontraffic V59.09 ☑
          pedal cycle (traffic) V51.5 ☑
            nontraffic V51.0 ☑
          pickup truck (traffic) V53.5 ☑
            nontraffic V53.0 ☑
          railway vehicle (traffic) V55.5 ☑
            nontraffic V55.0 ☑
          specified vehicle NEC (traffic) V56.5 ☑
            nontraffic V56.0 ☑
          stationary object (traffic) V57.5 ☑
            nontraffic V57.0 ☑
          streetcar (traffic) V56.5 ☑
            nontraffic V56.0 ☑
          three wheeled motor vehicle (traffic) V52.5 ☑
            nontraffic V52.0 ☑
          truck (traffic) V54.5 ☑
            nontraffic V54.0 ☑
          two wheeled motor vehicle (traffic) V52.5 ☑
            nontraffic V52.0 ☑
          van (traffic) V53.5 ☑
            nontraffic V53.0 ☑
        noncollision accident (traffic) V58.5 ☑
          nontraffic V58.0 ☑
      hanger-on
        collision (with)
          animal (traffic) V50.7 ☑
            being ridden (traffic) V56.7 ☑
              nontraffic V56.2 ☑
            nontraffic V50.2 ☑
          animal-drawn vehicle (traffic) V56.7 ☑
            nontraffic V56.2 ☑
          bus (traffic) V54.7 ☑
            nontraffic V54.2 ☑
          car (traffic) V53.7 ☑
            nontraffic V53.2 ☑
          pedal cycle (traffic) V51.7 ☑
            nontraffic V51.2 ☑
          pickup truck (traffic) V53.7 ☑
            nontraffic V53.2 ☑
          railway vehicle (traffic) V55.7 ☑
            nontraffic V55.2 ☑
          specified vehicle NEC (traffic) V56.7 ☑
            nontraffic V56.2 ☑
          stationary object (traffic) V57.7 ☑
            nontraffic V57.2 ☑
          streetcar (traffic) V56.7 ☑
            nontraffic V56.2 ☑
          three wheeled motor vehicle (traffic) V52.7 ☑
            nontraffic V52.2 ☑
          truck (traffic) V54.7 ☑
            nontraffic V54.2 ☑
          two wheeled motor vehicle (traffic) V52.7 ☑
            nontraffic V52.2 ☑
          van (traffic) V53.7 ☑
            nontraffic V53.2 ☑
        noncollision accident (traffic) V58.7 ☑
          nontraffic V58.2 ☑
      noncollision accident (traffic) V58.9 ☑
        nontraffic V58.3 ☑
      while boarding or alighting V58.4 ☑
      nontraffic V59.3 ☑
      passenger
        collision (with)
          animal (traffic) V50.6 ☑
            being ridden (traffic) V56.6 ☑
              nontraffic V56.1 ☑
            nontraffic V50.1 ☑
          animal-drawn vehicle (traffic) V56.6 ☑
            nontraffic V56.1 ☑
          bus (traffic) V54.6 ☑
            nontraffic V54.1 ☑
          car (traffic) V53.6 ☑
            nontraffic V53.1 ☑
          motor vehicle NOS (traffic) V59.50 ☑

Accident — continued
  transport — continued
    pickup truck occupant — continued
      passenger — continued
        collision — continued
          motor vehicle — continued
            nontraffic V59.10 ☑
            specified type NEC (traffic) V59.59 ☑
              nontraffic V59.19 ☑
          pedal cycle (traffic) V51.6 ☑
            nontraffic V51.1 ☑
          pickup truck (traffic) V53.6 ☑
            nontraffic V53.1 ☑
          railway vehicle (traffic) V55.6 ☑
            nontraffic V55.1 ☑
          specified vehicle NEC (traffic) V56.6 ☑
            nontraffic V56.1 ☑
          stationary object (traffic) V57.6 ☑
            nontraffic V57.1 ☑
          streetcar (traffic) V56.6 ☑
            nontraffic V56.1 ☑
          three wheeled motor vehicle (traffic) V52.6 ☑
            nontraffic V52.1 ☑
          truck (traffic) V54.6 ☑
            nontraffic V54.1 ☑
          two wheeled motor vehicle (traffic) V52.6 ☑
            nontraffic V52.1 ☑
          van (traffic) V53.6 ☑
            nontraffic V53.1 ☑
        noncollision accident (traffic) V58.6 ☑
          nontraffic V58.1 ☑
      specified type NEC V59.88 ☑
      military vehicle V59.81 ☑
    quarry truck — see Accident, transport, industrial vehicle occupant
    race car — see Accident, transport, motor vehicle NEC occupant
    railway vehicle occupant V81.9 ☑
      collision (with) V81.3 ☑
        motor vehicle (non-military) (traffic) V81.1 ☑
          military V81.83 ☑
          nontraffic V81.0 ☑
        rolling stock V81.2 ☑
        specified object NEC V81.3 ☑
      during derailment V81.7 ☑
        with antecedent collision — see Accident, transport, railway vehicle occupant, collision
      explosion V81.81 ☑
      fall (in railway vehicle) V81.7 ☑
        during derailment V81.7 ☑
          with antecedent collision — see Accident, transport, railway vehicle occupant, collision
        from railway vehicle V81.6 ☑
          during derailment V81.7 ☑
            with antecedent collision — see Accident, transport, railway vehicle occupant, collision
        while boarding or alighting V81.4 ☑
      fire V81.81 ☑
      object falling onto train V81.82 ☑
      specified type NEC V81.89 ☑
      while boarding or alighting V81.4 ☑
    ski lift V98.3 ☑
    snowmobile occupant (nontraffic) V86.92 ☑
      driver V86.52 ☑
      hanger-on V86.72 ☑
      passenger V86.62 ☑
      traffic V86.32 ☑
        driver V86.02 ☑
        hanger-on V86.22 ☑
        passenger V86.12 ☑
      while boarding or alighting V86.42 ☑
    specified NEC V98.8 ☑
    sport utility vehicle occupant (see also Accident, transport, pickup truck occupant)
    streetcar occupant V82.9 ☑
      collision (with) V82.3 ☑
        motor vehicle (traffic) V82.1 ☑
          nontraffic V82.0 ☑
        rolling stock V82.2 ☑
      during derailment V82.7 ☑

Accident — continued
  transport — continued
    streetcar occupant — continued
      during derailment — continued
        with antecedent collision — see Accident, transport, streetcar occupant, collision
      fall (in streetcar) V82.5 ☑
        during derailment V82.7 ☑
          with antecedent collision — see Accident, transport, streetcar occupant, collision
        from streetcar V82.6 ☑
          during derailment V82.7 ☑
            with antecedent collision — see Accident, transport, streetcar occupant, collision
          while boarding or alighting V82.4 ☑
        while boarding or alighting V82.4 ☑
      specified type NEC V82.8 ☑
      while boarding or alighting V82.4 ☑
    three-wheeled motor vehicle occupant V39.9 ☑
      collision (with)
        animal (traffic) V30.9 ☑
          being ridden (traffic) V36.9 ☑
            nontraffic V36.3 ☑
            while boarding or alighting V36.4 ☑
          nontraffic V30.3 ☑
          while boarding or alighting V30.4 ☑
        animal-drawn vehicle (traffic) V36.9 ☑
          nontraffic V36.3 ☑
          while boarding or alighting V36.4 ☑
        bus (traffic) V34.9 ☑
          nontraffic V34.3 ☑
          while boarding or alighting V34.4 ☑
        car (traffic) V33.9 ☑
          nontraffic V33.3 ☑
          while boarding or alighting V33.4 ☑
        motor vehicle NOS (traffic) V39.60 ☑
          nontraffic V39.20 ☑
          specified type NEC (traffic) V39.69 ☑
            nontraffic V39.29 ☑
        pedal cycle (traffic) V31.9 ☑
          nontraffic V31.3 ☑
          while boarding or alighting V31.4 ☑
        pickup truck (traffic) V33.9 ☑
          nontraffic V33.3 ☑
          while boarding or alighting V33.4 ☑
        railway vehicle (traffic) V35.9 ☑
          nontraffic V35.3 ☑
          while boarding or alighting V35.4 ☑
        specified vehicle NEC (traffic) V36.9 ☑
          nontraffic V36.3 ☑
          while boarding or alighting V36.4 ☑
        stationary object (traffic) V37.9 ☑
          nontraffic V37.3 ☑
          while boarding or alighting V37.4 ☑
        streetcar (traffic) V36.9 ☑
          nontraffic V36.3 ☑
          while boarding or alighting V36.4 ☑
        three wheeled motor vehicle (traffic) V32.9 ☑
          nontraffic V32.3 ☑
          while boarding or alighting V32.4 ☑
        truck (traffic) V34.9 ☑
          nontraffic V34.3 ☑
          while boarding or alighting V34.4 ☑
        two wheeled motor vehicle (traffic) V32.9 ☑
          nontraffic V32.3 ☑
          while boarding or alighting V32.4 ☑
        van (traffic) V33.9 ☑
          nontraffic V33.3 ☑
          while boarding or alighting V33.4 ☑
      driver
        collision (with)
          animal (traffic) V30.5 ☑
            being ridden (traffic) V36.5 ☑
              nontraffic V36.0 ☑
            nontraffic V30.0 ☑
          animal-drawn vehicle (traffic) V36.5 ☑
            nontraffic V36.0 ☑
          bus (traffic) V34.5 ☑
            nontraffic V34.0 ☑
          car (traffic) V33.5 ☑
            nontraffic V33.0 ☑
          motor vehicle NOS (traffic) V39.40 ☑
            nontraffic V39.00 ☑
            specified type NEC (traffic) V39.49 ☑

Accident — *continued*
  transport — *continued*
    three-wheeled motor vehicle occupant — *continued*
      driver — *continued*
        collision — *continued*
          motor vehicle — *continued*
            specified type — *continued*
              nontraffic V39.09 ☑
            pedal cycle (traffic) V31.5 ☑
              nontraffic V31.0 ☑
            pickup truck (traffic) V33.5 ☑
              nontraffic V33.0 ☑
            railway vehicle (traffic) V35.5 ☑
              nontraffic V35.0 ☑
            specified vehicle NEC (traffic) V36.5 ☑
              nontraffic V36.0 ☑
            stationary object (traffic) V37.5 ☑
              nontraffic V37.0 ☑
            streetcar (traffic) V36.5 ☑
              nontraffic V36.0 ☑
            three wheeled motor vehicle (traffic) V32.5 ☑
              nontraffic V32.0 ☑
            truck (traffic) V34.5 ☑
              nontraffic V34.0 ☑
            two wheeled motor vehicle (traffic) V32.5 ☑
              nontraffic V32.0 ☑
            van (traffic) V33.5 ☑
              nontraffic V33.0 ☑
          noncollision accident (traffic) V38.5 ☑
            nontraffic V38.0 ☑
      hanger-on
        collision (with)
          animal (traffic) V30.7 ☑
            being ridden (traffic) V36.7 ☑
              nontraffic V36.2 ☑
            nontraffic V30.2 ☑
          animal-drawn vehicle (traffic) V36.7 ☑
            nontraffic V36.2 ☑
          bus (traffic) V34.7 ☑
            nontraffic V34.2 ☑
          car (traffic) V33.7 ☑
            nontraffic V33.2 ☑
          pedal cycle (traffic) V31.7 ☑
            nontraffic V31.2 ☑
          pickup truck (traffic) V33.7 ☑
            nontraffic V33.2 ☑
          railway vehicle (traffic) V35.7 ☑
            nontraffic V35.2 ☑
          specified vehicle NEC (traffic) V36.7 ☑
            nontraffic V36.2 ☑
          stationary object (traffic) V37.7 ☑
            nontraffic V37.2 ☑
          streetcar (traffic) V36.7 ☑
            nontraffic V36.2 ☑
          three wheeled motor vehicle (traffic) V32.7 ☑
            nontraffic V32.2 ☑
          truck (traffic) V34.7 ☑
            nontraffic V34.2 ☑
          two wheeled motor vehicle (traffic) V32.7 ☑
            nontraffic V32.2 ☑
          van (traffic) V33.7 ☑
            nontraffic V33.2 ☑
        noncollision accident (traffic) V38.7 ☑
          nontraffic V38.2 ☑
      noncollision accident (traffic) V38.9 ☑
        nontraffic V38.3 ☑
        while boarding or alighting V38.4 ☑
      nontraffic V39.3 ☑
      passenger
        collision (with)
          animal (traffic) V30.6 ☑
            being ridden (traffic) V36.6 ☑
              nontraffic V36.1 ☑
            nontraffic V30.1 ☑
          animal-drawn vehicle (traffic) V36.6 ☑
            nontraffic V36.1 ☑
          bus (traffic) V34.6 ☑
            nontraffic V34.1 ☑
          car (traffic) V33.6 ☑
            nontraffic V33.1 ☑
          motor vehicle NOS (traffic) V39.50 ☑

Accident — *continued*
  transport — *continued*
    three-wheeled motor vehicle occupant — *continued*
      passenger — *continued*
        collision — *continued*
          motor vehicle — *continued*
            nontraffic V39.10 ☑
            specified type NEC (traffic) V39.59 ☑
              nontraffic V39.19 ☑
          pedal cycle (traffic) V31.6 ☑
            nontraffic V31.1 ☑
          pickup truck (traffic) V33.6 ☑
            nontraffic V33.1 ☑
          railway vehicle (traffic) V35.6 ☑
            nontraffic V35.1 ☑
          specified vehicle NEC (traffic) V36.6 ☑
            nontraffic V36.1 ☑
          stationary object (traffic) V37.6 ☑
            nontraffic V37.1 ☑
          streetcar (traffic) V36.6 ☑
            nontraffic V36.1 ☑
          three wheeled motor vehicle (traffic) V32.6 ☑
            nontraffic V32.1 ☑
          truck (traffic) V34.6 ☑
            nontraffic V34.1 ☑
          two wheeled motor vehicle (traffic) V32.6 ☑
            nontraffic V32.1 ☑
          van (traffic) V33.6 ☑
            nontraffic V33.1 ☑
        noncollision accident (traffic) V38.6 ☑
          nontraffic V38.1 ☑
      specified type NEC V39.89 ☑
      military vehicle V39.81 ☑
    tractor (farm) (and trailer) — *see* Accident, transport, agricultural vehicle occupant
    tram — *see* Accident, transport, streetcar
      in mine or quarry — *see* Accident, transport, industrial vehicle occupant
    trolley — *see* Accident, transport, streetcar
      in mine or quarry — *see* Accident, transport, industrial vehicle occupant
    truck (heavy) occupant V69.9 ☑
      collision (with)
        animal (traffic) V60.9 ☑
          being ridden (traffic) V66.9 ☑
            nontraffic V66.3 ☑
            while boarding or alighting V66.4 ☑
          nontraffic V60.3 ☑
          while boarding or alighting V60.4 ☑
        animal-drawn vehicle (traffic) V66.9 ☑
          nontraffic V66.3 ☑
          while boarding or alighting V66.4 ☑
        bus (traffic) V64.9 ☑
          nontraffic V64.3 ☑
          while boarding or alighting V64.4 ☑
        car (traffic) V63.9 ☑
          nontraffic V63.3 ☑
          while boarding or alighting V63.4 ☑
        motor vehicle NOS (traffic) V69.60 ☑
          nontraffic V69.20 ☑
          specified type NEC (traffic) V69.69 ☑
            nontraffic V69.29 ☑
        pedal cycle (traffic) V61.9 ☑
          nontraffic V61.3 ☑
          while boarding or alighting V61.4 ☑
        pickup truck (traffic) V63.9 ☑
          nontraffic V63.3 ☑
          while boarding or alighting V63.4 ☑
        railway vehicle (traffic) V65.9 ☑
          nontraffic V65.3 ☑
          while boarding or alighting V65.4 ☑
        specified vehicle NEC (traffic) V66.9 ☑
          nontraffic V66.3 ☑
          while boarding or alighting V66.4 ☑
        stationary object (traffic) V67.9 ☑
          nontraffic V67.3 ☑
          while boarding or alighting V67.4 ☑
        streetcar (traffic) V66.9 ☑
          nontraffic V66.3 ☑
          while boarding or alighting V66.4 ☑
        three wheeled motor vehicle (traffic) V62.9 ☑
          nontraffic V62.3 ☑
          while boarding or alighting V62.4 ☑

Accident — *continued*
  transport — *continued*
    truck occupant — *continued*
      collision — *continued*
        truck (traffic) V64.9 ☑
          nontraffic V64.3 ☑
          while boarding or alighting V64.4 ☑
        two wheeled motor vehicle (traffic) V62.9 ☑
          nontraffic V62.3 ☑
          while boarding or alighting V62.4 ☑
        van (traffic) V63.9 ☑
          nontraffic V63.3 ☑
          while boarding or alighting V63.4 ☑
      driver
        collision (with)
          animal (traffic) V60.5 ☑
            being ridden (traffic) V66.5 ☑
              nontraffic V66.0 ☑
            nontraffic V60.0 ☑
          animal-drawn vehicle (traffic) V66.5 ☑
            nontraffic V66.0 ☑
          bus (traffic) V64.5 ☑
            nontraffic V64.0 ☑
          car (traffic) V63.5 ☑
            nontraffic V63.0 ☑
          motor vehicle NOS (traffic) V69.40 ☑
            nontraffic V69.00 ☑
            specified type NEC (traffic) V69.49 ☑
              nontraffic V69.09 ☑
          pedal cycle (traffic) V61.5 ☑
            nontraffic V61.0 ☑
          pickup truck (traffic) V63.5 ☑
            nontraffic V63.0 ☑
          railway vehicle (traffic) V65.5 ☑
            nontraffic V65.0 ☑
          specified vehicle NEC (traffic) V66.5 ☑
            nontraffic V66.0 ☑
          stationary object (traffic) V67.5 ☑
            nontraffic V67.0 ☑
          streetcar (traffic) V66.5 ☑
            nontraffic V66.0 ☑
          three wheeled motor vehicle (traffic) V62.5 ☑
            nontraffic V62.0 ☑
          truck (traffic) V64.5 ☑
            nontraffic V64.0 ☑
          two wheeled motor vehicle (traffic) V62.5 ☑
            nontraffic V62.0 ☑
          van (traffic) V63.5 ☑
            nontraffic V63.0 ☑
        noncollision accident (traffic) V68.5 ☑
          nontraffic V68.0 ☑
      dump — *see* Accident, transport, construction vehicle occupant
      hanger-on
        collision (with)
          animal (traffic) V60.7 ☑
            being ridden (traffic) V66.7 ☑
              nontraffic V66.2 ☑
            nontraffic V60.2 ☑
          animal-drawn vehicle (traffic) V66.7 ☑
            nontraffic V66.2 ☑
          bus (traffic) V64.7 ☑
            nontraffic V64.2 ☑
          car (traffic) V63.7 ☑
            nontraffic V63.2 ☑
          pedal cycle (traffic) V61.7 ☑
            nontraffic V61.2 ☑
          pickup truck (traffic) V63.7 ☑
            nontraffic V63.2 ☑
          railway vehicle (traffic) V65.7 ☑
            nontraffic V65.2 ☑
          specified vehicle NEC (traffic) V66.7 ☑
            nontraffic V66.2 ☑
          stationary object (traffic) V67.7 ☑
            nontraffic V67.2 ☑
          streetcar (traffic) V66.7 ☑
            nontraffic V66.2 ☑
          three wheeled motor vehicle (traffic) V62.7 ☑
            nontraffic V62.2 ☑
          truck (traffic) V64.7 ☑
            nontraffic V64.2 ☑
          two wheeled motor vehicle (traffic) V62.7 ☑

Accident — *continued*
  transport — *continued*
    truck occupant — *continued*
      hanger-on — *continued*
        collision — *continued*
          two wheeled motor vehicle — *continued*
            nontraffic V62.2 ☑
            van (traffic) V63.7 ☑
            nontraffic V63.2 ☑
          noncollision accident (traffic) V68.7 ☑
            nontraffic V68.2 ☑
        noncollision accident (traffic) V68.9 ☑
          nontraffic V68.3 ☑
          while boarding or alighting V68.4 ☑
        nontraffic V69.3 ☑
      passenger
        collision (with)
          animal (traffic) V60.6 ☑
            being ridden (traffic) V66.6 ☑
              nontraffic V66.1- ☑
            nontraffic V60.1 ☑
          animal-drawn vehicle (traffic) V66.6 ☑
            nontraffic V66.1 ☑
          bus (traffic) V64.6 ☑
            nontraffic V64.1 ☑
          car (traffic) V63.6 ☑
            nontraffic V63.1 ☑
          motor vehicle NOS (traffic) V69.50 ☑
            nontraffic V69.10 ☑
            specified type NEC (traffic) V69.59 ☑
              nontraffic V69.19 ☑
          pedal cycle (traffic) V61.6 ☑
            nontraffic V61.1 ☑
          pickup truck (traffic) V63.6 ☑
            nontraffic V63.1 ☑
          railway vehicle (traffic) V65.6 ☑
            nontraffic V65.1 ☑
          specified vehicle NEC (traffic) V66.6 ☑
            nontraffic V66.1 ☑
          stationary object (traffic) V67.6 ☑
            nontraffic V67.1 ☑
          streetcar (traffic) V66.6 ☑
            nontraffic V66.1 ☑
          three wheeled motor vehicle (traffic) V62.6 ☑
            nontraffic V62.1 ☑
          truck (traffic) V64.6 ☑
            nontraffic V64.1 ☑
          two wheeled motor vehicle (traffic) V62.6 ☑
            nontraffic V62.1 ☑
          van (traffic) V63.6 ☑
            nontraffic V63.1 ☑
        noncollision accident (traffic) V68.6 ☑
          nontraffic V68.1 ☑
      pickup — *see* Accident, transport, pickup truck occupant
      specified type NEC V69.88 ☑
      military vehicle V69.81 ☑
    van occupant V59.9 ☑
      collision (with)
        animal (traffic) V50.9 ☑
          being ridden (traffic) V56.9 ☑
            nontraffic V56.3 ☑
            while boarding or alighting V56.4 ☑
          nontraffic V50.3 ☑
          while boarding or alighting V50.4 ☑
        animal-drawn vehicle (traffic) V56.9 ☑
          nontraffic V56.3 ☑
          while boarding or alighting V56.4 ☑
        bus (traffic) V54.9 ☑
          nontraffic V54.3 ☑
          while boarding or alighting V54.4 ☑
        car (traffic) V53.9 ☑
          nontraffic V53.3 ☑
          while boarding or alighting V53.4 ☑
        motor vehicle NOS (traffic) V59.60 ☑
          nontraffic V59.20 ☑
          specified type NEC (traffic) V59.69 ☑
            nontraffic V59.29 ☑
        pedal cycle (traffic) V51.9 ☑
          nontraffic V51.3 ☑
          while boarding or alighting V51.4 ☑
        pickup truck (traffic) V53.9 ☑
          nontraffic V53.3 ☑

Accident — *continued*
  transport — *continued*
    van occupant — *continued*
      collision — *continued*
        pickup truck — *continued*
          while boarding or alighting V53.4 ☑
        railway vehicle (traffic) V55.9 ☑
          nontraffic V55.3 ☑
          while boarding or alighting V55.4 ☑
        specified vehicle NEC (traffic) V56.9 ☑
          nontraffic V56.3 ☑
          while boarding or alighting V56.4 ☑
        stationary object (traffic) V57.9 ☑
          nontraffic V57.3 ☑
          while boarding or alighting V57.4 ☑
        streetcar (traffic) V56.9 ☑
          nontraffic V56.3 ☑
          while boarding or alighting V56.4 ☑
        three wheeled motor vehicle (traffic) V52.9 ☑
          nontraffic V52.3 ☑
          while boarding or alighting V52.4 ☑
        truck (traffic) V54.9 ☑
          nontraffic V54.3 ☑
          while boarding or alighting V54.4 ☑
        two wheeled motor vehicle (traffic) V52.9 ☑
          nontraffic V52.3 ☑
          while boarding or alighting V52.4 ☑
        van (traffic) V53.9 ☑
          nontraffic V53.3 ☑
          while boarding or alighting V53.4 ☑
      driver
        collision (with)
          animal (traffic) V50.5 ☑
            being ridden (traffic) V56.5 ☑
              nontraffic V56.0 ☑
            nontraffic V50.0 ☑
          animal-drawn vehicle (traffic) V56.5 ☑
            nontraffic V56.0 ☑
          bus (traffic) V54.5 ☑
            nontraffic V54.0 ☑
          car (traffic) V53.5 ☑
            nontraffic V53.0 ☑
          motor vehicle NOS (traffic) V59.40 ☑
            nontraffic V59.00 ☑
            specified type NEC (traffic) V59.49 ☑
              nontraffic V59.09 ☑
          pedal cycle (traffic) V51.5 ☑
            nontraffic V51.0 ☑
          pickup truck (traffic) V53.5 ☑
            nontraffic V53.0 ☑
          railway vehicle (traffic) V55.5 ☑
            nontraffic V55.0 ☑
          specified vehicle NEC (traffic) V56.5 ☑
            nontraffic V56.0 ☑
          stationary object (traffic) V57.5 ☑
            nontraffic V57.0 ☑
          streetcar (traffic) V56.5 ☑
            nontraffic V56.0 ☑
          three wheeled motor vehicle (traffic) V52.5 ☑
            nontraffic V52.0 ☑
          truck (traffic) V54.5 ☑
            nontraffic V54.0 ☑
          two wheeled motor vehicle (traffic) V52.5 ☑
            nontraffic V52.0 ☑
          van (traffic) V53.5 ☑
            nontraffic V53.0 ☑
        noncollision accident (traffic) V58.5 ☑
          nontraffic V58.0 ☑
      hanger-on
        collision (with)
          animal (traffic) V50.7 ☑
            being ridden (traffic) V56.7 ☑
              nontraffic V56.2 ☑
            nontraffic V50.2 ☑
          animal-drawn vehicle (traffic) V56.7 ☑
            nontraffic V56.2 ☑
          bus (traffic) V54.7 ☑
            nontraffic V54.2 ☑
          car (traffic) V53.7 ☑
            nontraffic V53.2 ☑
          pedal cycle (traffic) V51.7 ☑
            nontraffic V51.2 ☑
          pickup truck (traffic) V53.7 ☑
            nontraffic V53.2 ☑

Accident — *continued*
  transport — *continued*
    van occupant — *continued*
      hanger-on — *continued*
        collision — *continued*
          railway vehicle (traffic) V55.7 ☑
            nontraffic V55.2 ☑
          specified vehicle NEC (traffic) V56.7 ☑
            nontraffic V56.2 ☑
          stationary object (traffic) V57.7 ☑
            nontraffic V57.2 ☑
          streetcar (traffic) V56.7 ☑
            nontraffic V56.2 ☑
          three wheeled motor vehicle (traffic) V52.7 ☑
            nontraffic V52.2 ☑
          truck (traffic) V54.7 ☑
            nontraffic V54.2 ☑
          two wheeled motor vehicle (traffic) V52.7 ☑
            nontraffic V52.2 ☑
          van (traffic) V53.7 ☑
            nontraffic V53.2 ☑
        noncollision accident (traffic) V58.7 ☑
          nontraffic V58.2 ☑
      noncollision accident (traffic) V58.9 ☑
        nontraffic V58.3 ☑
        while boarding or alighting V58.4 ☑
      nontraffic V59.3 ☑
      passenger
        collision (with)
          animal (traffic) V50.6 ☑
            being ridden (traffic) V56.6 ☑
              nontraffic V56.1 ☑
            nontraffic V50.1 ☑
          animal-drawn vehicle (traffic) V56.6 ☑
            nontraffic V56.1 ☑
          bus (traffic) V54.6 ☑
            nontraffic V54.1 ☑
          car (traffic) V53.6 ☑
            nontraffic V53.1 ☑
          motor vehicle NOS (traffic) V59.50 ☑
            nontraffic V59.10 ☑
            specified type NEC (traffic) V59.59 ☑
              nontraffic V59.19 ☑
          pedal cycle (traffic) V51.6 ☑
            nontraffic V51.1 ☑
          pickup truck (traffic) V53.6 ☑
            nontraffic V53.1 ☑
          railway vehicle (traffic) V55.6 ☑
            nontraffic V55.1 ☑
          specified vehicle NEC (traffic) V56.6 ☑
            nontraffic V56.1 ☑
          stationary object (traffic) V57.6 ☑
            nontraffic V57.1 ☑
          streetcar (traffic) V56.6 ☑
            nontraffic V56.1 ☑
          three wheeled motor vehicle (traffic) V52.6 ☑
            nontraffic V52.1 ☑
          truck (traffic) V54.6 ☑
            nontraffic V54.1 ☑
          two wheeled motor vehicle (traffic) V52.6 ☑
            nontraffic V52.1 ☑
          van (traffic) V53.6 ☑
            nontraffic V53.1 ☑
        noncollision accident (traffic) V58.6 ☑
          nontraffic V58.1 ☑
      specified type NEC V59.88 ☑
      military vehicle V59.81 ☑
    watercraft occupant — *see* Accident, watercraft
  vehicle NEC V89.9 ☑
    animal-drawn NEC — *see* Accident, transport, animal-drawn vehicle occupant
    special
      agricultural — *see* Accident, transport, agricultural vehicle occupant
      construction — *see* Accident, transport, construction vehicle occupant
      industrial — *see* Accident, transport, industrial vehicle occupant
    three-wheeled NEC (motorized) — *see* Accident, transport, three-wheeled motor vehicle occupant
  watercraft V94.9 ☑

Accident — *continued*
  watercraft — *continued*
    causing
      drowning — *see* Drowning, due to, accident to, watercraft
      injury NEC V91.89 ☑
        crushed between craft and object V91.19 ☑
          powered craft V91.13 ☑
            ferry boat V91.11 ☑
            fishing boat V91.12 ☑
            jetskis V91.13 ☑
            liner V91.11 ☑
            merchant ship V91.10 ☑
            passenger ship V91.11 ☑
          unpowered craft V91.18 ☑
            canoe V91.15 ☑
            inflatable V91.16 ☑
            kayak V91.15 ☑
            sailboat V91.14 ☑
            surf-board V91.18 ☑
            windsurfer V91.18 ☑
        fall on board V91.29 ☑
          powered craft V91.23 ☑
            ferry boat V91.21 ☑
            fishing boat V91.22 ☑
            jetskis V91.23 ☑
            liner V91.21 ☑
            merchant ship V91.20 ☑
            passenger ship V91.21 ☑
          unpowered craft
            canoe V91.25 ☑
            inflatable V91.26 ☑
            kayak V91.25 ☑
            sailboat V91.24 ☑
        fire on board causing burn V91.09 ☑
          powered craft V91.03 ☑
            ferry boat V91.01 ☑
            fishing boat V91.02 ☑
            jetskis V91.03 ☑
            liner V91.01 ☑
            merchant ship V91.00 ☑
            passenger ship V91.01 ☑
          unpowered craft V91.08 ☑
            canoe V91.05 ☑
            inflatable V91.06 ☑
            kayak V91.05 ☑
            sailboat V91.04 ☑
            surf-board V91.08 ☑
            water skis V91.07 ☑
            windsurfer V91.08 ☑
        hit by falling object V91.39 ☑
          powered craft V91.33 ☑
            ferry boat V91.31 ☑
            fishing boat V91.32 ☑
            jetskis V91.33 ☑
            liner V91.31 ☑
            merchant ship V91.30 ☑
            passenger ship V91.31 ☑
          unpowered craft V91.38 ☑
            canoe V91.35 ☑
            inflatable V91.36 ☑
            kayak V91.35 ☑
            sailboat V91.34 ☑
            surf-board V91.38 ☑
            water skis V91.37 ☑
            windsurfer V91.38 ☑
        specified type NEC V91.89 ☑
          powered craft V91.83 ☑
            ferry boat V91.81 ☑
            fishing boat V91.82 ☑
            jetskis V91.83 ☑
            liner V91.81 ☑
            merchant ship V91.80 ☑
            passenger ship V91.81 ☑
          unpowered craft V91.88 ☑
            canoe V91.85 ☑
            inflatable V91.86 ☑
            kayak V91.85 ☑
            sailboat V91.84 ☑
            surf-board V91.88 ☑
            water skis V91.87 ☑
            windsurfer V91.88 ☑
    due to, caused by cataclysm — *see* Forces of nature, by type
    military NEC V94.818 ☑
      civilian in water injured by V94.811 ☑

Accident — *continued*
  watercraft — *continued*
    military — *continued*
      with civilian watercraft V94.810 ☑
    nonpowered, struck by
      nonpowered vessel V94.22 ☑
      powered vessel V94.21 ☑
    specified type NEC V94.89 ☑
    striking swimmer
      powered V94.11 ☑
      unpowered V94.12 ☑

Acid throwing (assault) Y08.89 ☑

Activity (involving) (of victim at time of event) Y93.9
  aerobic and step exercise (class) Y93.A3 (*following* Y93.7)
  alpine skiing Y93.23
  animal care NEC Y93.K9 (*following* Y93.7)
  arts and handcrafts NEC Y93.D9 (*following* Y93.7)
  athletics played as a team or group NEC Y93.69
  athletics played individually NEC Y93.59
  athletics NEC Y93.79
  baking Y93.G3 (*following* Y93.7)
  ballet Y93.41
  barbells Y93.B3 (*following* Y93.7)
  BASE (Building, Antenna, Span, Earth) jumping Y93.33
  baseball Y93.64
  basketball Y93.67
  bathing (personal) Y93.E1 (*following* Y93.7)
  beach volleyball Y93.68
  bike riding Y93.55
  blackout game Y93.85
  boogie boarding Y93.18
  bowling Y93.54
  boxing Y93.71
  brass instrument playing Y93.J4 (*following* Y93.7)
  building construction Y93.H3 (*following* Y93.7)
  bungee jumping Y93.34
  calisthenics Y93.A2 (*following* Y93.7)
  canoeing (in calm and turbulent water) Y93.16
  capture the flag Y93.6A
  cardiorespiratory exercise NEC Y93.A9 (*following* Y93.7)
  caregiving (providing) NEC Y93.F9 (*following* Y93.7)
    bathing Y93.F1 (*following* Y93.7)
    lifting Y93.F2 (*following* Y93.7)
  cellular
    communication device Y93.C2 (*following* Y93.7)
    telephone Y93.C2 (*following* Y93.7)
  challenge course Y93.A5 (*following* Y93.7)
  cheerleading Y93.45
  choking game Y93.85
  circuit training Y93.A4 (*following* Y93.7)
  cleaning
    floor Y93.E5 (*following* Y93.7)
  climbing NEC Y93.39
    mountain Y93.31
    rock Y93.31
    wall Y93.31
  clothing care and maintenance NEC Y93.E9 (*following* Y93.7)
  combatives Y93.75
  computer
    keyboarding Y93.C1 (*following* Y93.7)
    technology NEC Y93.C9 (*following* Y93.7)
  confidence course Y93.A5 (*following* Y93.7)
  construction (building) Y93.H3 (*following* Y93.7)
  cooking and baking Y93.G3 (*following* Y93.7)
  cool down exercises Y93.A2 (*following* Y93.7)
  cricket Y93.69
  crocheting Y93.D1 (*following* Y93.7)
  cross country skiing Y93.24
  dancing (all types) Y93.41
  digging
    dirt Y93.H1 (*following* Y93.7)
  dirt digging Y93.H1 (*following* Y93.7)
  dishwashing Y93.G1 (*following* Y93.7)
  diving (platform) (springboard) Y93.12
    underwater Y93.15
  dodge ball Y93.6A
  downhill skiing Y93.23
  drum playing Y93.J2 (*following* Y93.7)
  dumbbells Y93.B3 (*following* Y93.7)
  electronic
    devices NEC Y93.C9 (*following* Y93.7)
      hand held interactive Y93.C2 (*following* Y93.7)
    game playing (using) (with)
      interactive device Y93.C2 (*following* Y93.7)
      keyboard or other stationary device Y93.C1 (*following* Y93.7)

Activity — *continued*
  elliptical machine Y93.A1 (*following* Y93.7)
  exercise(s)
    machines ((primarily) for)
      cardiorespiratory conditioning Y93.A1 (*following* Y93.7)
      muscle strengthening Y93.B1 (*following* Y93.7)
    muscle strengthening (non-machine) NEC Y93.B9 (*following* Y93.7)
  external motion NEC Y93.I9 (*following* Y93.7)
    rollercoaster Y93.I1 (*following* Y93.7)
  fainting game Y93.85
  field hockey Y93.65
  figure skating (pairs) (singles) Y93.21
  flag football Y93.62
  floor mopping and cleaning Y93.E5 (*following* Y93.7)
  food preparation and clean up Y93.G1 (*following* Y93.7)
  football (American) NOS Y93.61
    flag Y93.62
    tackle Y93.61
    touch Y93.62
  four square Y93.6A
  free weights Y93.B3 (*following* Y93.7)
  frisbee (ultimate) Y93.74
  furniture
    building Y93.D3 (*following* Y93.7)
    finishing Y93.D3 (*following* Y93.7)
    repair Y93.D3 (*following* Y93.7)
  game playing (electronic)
    using interactive device Y93.C2 (*following* Y93.7)
    using keyboard or other stationary device Y93.C1 (*following* Y93.7)
  gardening Y93.H2 (*following* Y93.7)
  golf Y93.53
  grass drills Y93.A6 (*following* Y93.7)
  grilling and smoking food Y93.G2 (*following* Y93.7)
  grooming and shearing an animal Y93.K3 (*following* Y93.7)
  guerilla drills Y93.A6 (*following* Y93.7)
  gymnastics (rhythmic) Y93.43
  hand held interactive electronic device Y93.C2 (*following* Y93.7)
  handball Y93.73
  handcrafts NEC Y93.D9 (*following* Y93.7)
  hang gliding Y93.35
  hiking (on level or elevated terrain) Y93.01
  hockey (ice) Y93.22
    field Y93.65
  horseback riding Y93.52
  household (interior) maintenance NEC Y93.E9 (*following* Y93.7)
  ice NEC Y93.29
    dancing Y93.21
    hockey Y93.22
    skating Y93.21
  inline roller skating Y93.51
  ironing Y93.E4 (*following* Y93.7)
  judo Y93.75
  jumping jacks Y93.A2 (*following* Y93.7)
  jumping rope Y93.56
  jumping (off) NEC Y93.39
    BASE (Building, Antenna, Span, Earth) Y93.33
    bungee Y93.34
    jacks Y93.A2 (*following* Y93.7)
    rope Y93.56
  karate Y93.75
  kayaking (in calm and turbulent water) Y93.16
  keyboarding (computer) Y93.C1 (*following* Y93.7)
  kickball Y93.6A
  knitting Y93.D1 (*following* Y93.7)
  lacrosse Y93.65
  land maintenance NEC Y93.H9 (*following* Y93.7)
  landscaping Y93.H2 (*following* Y93.7)
  laundry Y93.E2 (*following* Y93.7)
  machines (exercise)
    primarily for cardiorespiratory conditioning Y93.A1 (*following* Y93.7)
    primarily for muscle strengthening Y93.B1 (*following* Y93.7)
  maintenance
    exterior building NEC Y93.H9 (*following* Y93.7)
    household (interior) NEC Y93.E9 (*following* Y93.7)
    land Y93.H9 (*following* Y93.7)
    property Y93.H9 (*following* Y93.7)
  marching (on level or elevated terrain) Y93.01
  martial arts Y93.75
  microwave oven Y93.G3 (*following* Y93.7)
  milking an animal Y93.K2 (*following* Y93.7)
  mopping (floor) Y93.E5 (*following* Y93.7)

Activity — *continued*
  mountain climbing Y93.31
  muscle strengthening
    exercises (non-machine) NEC Y93.B9 (*following* Y93.7)
    machines Y93.B1 (*following* Y93.7)
  musical keyboard (electronic) playing Y93.J1 (*following* Y93.7)
  nordic skiing Y93.24
  obstacle course Y93.A5 (*following* Y93.7)
  oven (microwave) Y93.G3 (*following* Y93.7)
  packing up and unpacking in moving to a new residence Y93.E6 (*following* Y93.7)
  parasailing Y93.19
  pass out game Y93.85
  percussion instrument playing NEC Y93.J2 (*following* Y93.7)
  personal
    bathing and showering Y93.E1 (*following* Y93.7)
    hygiene NEC Y93.E8 (*following* Y93.7)
    showering Y93.E1 (*following* Y93.7)
  physical games generally associated with school recess, summer camp and children Y93.6A
  physical training NEC Y93.A9 (*following* Y93.7)
  piano playing Y93.J1 (*following* Y93.7)
  pilates Y93.B4 (*following* Y93.7)
  platform diving Y93.12
  playing musical instrument
    brass instrument Y93.J4 (*following* Y93.7)
    drum Y93.J2 (*following* Y93.7)
    musical keyboard (electronic) Y93.J1 (*following* Y93.7)
    percussion instrument NEC Y93.J2 (*following* Y93.7)
    piano Y93.J1 (*following* Y93.7)
    string instrument Y93.J3 (*following* Y93.7)
    winds instrument Y93.J4 (*following* Y93.7)
  property maintenance
    exterior NEC Y93.H9 (*following* Y93.7)
    interior NEC Y93.E9 (*following* Y93.7)
  pruning (garden and lawn) Y93.H2 (*following* Y93.7)
  pull-ups Y93.B2 (*following* Y93.7)
  push-ups Y93.B2 (*following* Y93.7)
  racquetball Y93.73
  rafting (in calm and turbulent water) Y93.16
  raking (leaves) Y93.H1 (*following* Y93.7)
  rappelling Y93.32
  refereeing a sports activity Y93.81
  residential relocation Y93.E6 (*following* Y93.7)
  rhythmic gymnastics Y93.43
  rhythmic movement NEC Y93.49
  riding
    horseback Y93.52
    rollercoaster Y93.I1 (*following* Y93.7)
  rock climbing Y93.31
  roller skating (inline) Y93.51
  rollercoaster riding Y93.I1 (*following* Y93.7)
  rough housing and horseplay Y93.83
  rowing (in calm and turbulent water) Y93.16
  rugby Y93.63
  running Y93.02
  SCUBA diving Y93.15
  sewing Y93.D2 (*following* Y93.7)
  shoveling Y93.H1 (*following* Y93.7)
    dirt Y93.H1 (*following* Y93.7)
    snow Y93.H1 (*following* Y93.7)
  showering (personal) Y93.E1 (*following* Y93.7)
  sit-ups Y93.B2 (*following* Y93.7)
  skateboarding Y93.51
  skating (ice) Y93.21
    roller Y93.51
  skiing (alpine) (downhill) Y93.23
    cross country Y93.24
    nordic Y93.24
    water Y93.17
  sledding (snow) Y93.23
  sleeping (sleep) Y93.84
  smoking and grilling food Y93.G2 (*following* Y93.7)
  snorkeling Y93.15
  snow NEC Y93.29
    boarding Y93.23
    shoveling Y93.H1 (*following* Y93.7)
    sledding Y93.23
    tubing Y93.23
  soccer Y93.66
  softball Y93.64
  specified NEC Y93.89
  spectator at an event Y93.82
  sports NEC Y93.79
    sports played as a team or group NEC Y93.69

Activity — *continued*
  sports — *continued*
    sports played individually NEC Y93.59
  springboard diving Y93.12
  squash Y93.73
  stationary bike Y93.A1 (*following* Y93.7)
  step (stepping) exercise (class) Y93.A3 (*following* Y93.7)
  stepper machine Y93.A1 (*following* Y93.7)
  stove Y93.G3 (*following* Y93.7)
  string instrument playing Y93.J3 (*following* Y93.7)
  surfing Y93.18
    wind Y93.18
  swimming Y93.11
  tackle football Y93.61
  tap dancing Y93.41
  tennis Y93.73
  tobogganing Y93.23
  touch football Y93.62
  track and field events (non-running) Y93.57
    running Y93.02
  trampoline Y93.44
  treadmill Y93.A1 (*following* Y93.7)
  trimming shrubs Y93.H2 (*following* Y93.7)
  tubing (in calm and turbulent water) Y93.16
    snow Y93.23
  ultimate frisbee Y93.74
  underwater diving Y93.15
  unpacking in moving to a new residence Y93.E6 (*following* Y93.7)
  use of stove, oven and microwave oven Y93.G3 (*following* Y93.7)
  vacuuming Y93.E3 (*following* Y93.7)
  volleyball (beach) (court) Y93.68
  wake boarding Y93.17
  walking (on level or elevated terrain) Y93.01
    an animal Y93.K1 (*following* Y93.7)
  walking an animal Y93.K1 (*following* Y93.7)
  wall climbing Y93.31
  warm up and cool down exercises Y93.A2 (*following* Y93.7)
  water NEC Y93.19
    aerobics Y93.14
    craft NEC Y93.19
    exercise Y93.14
    polo Y93.13
    skiing Y93.17
    sliding Y93.18
    survival training and testing Y93.19
  weeding (garden and lawn) Y93.H2 (*following* Y93.7)
  wind instrument playing Y93.J4 (*following* Y93.7)
  windsurfing Y93.18
  wrestling Y93.72
  yoga Y93.42
Adverse effect of drugs — *see* Table of Drugs and Chemicals
Aerosinusitis — *see* Air, pressure
After-effect, late — *see* Sequelae
Air
  blast in war operations — *see* War operations, air blast
  pressure
    change, rapid
      during
        ascent W94.29 ☑
          while (in) (surfacing from)
            aircraft W94.23 ☑
            deep water diving W94.21 ☑
            underground W94.22 ☑
        descent W94.39 ☑
          in
            aircraft W94.31 ☑
            water W94.32 ☑
    high, prolonged W94.0 ☑
    low, prolonged W94.12 ☑
      due to residence or long visit at high altitude W94.11 ☑
Alpine sickness W94.11 ☑
Altitude sickness W94.11 ☑
Anaphylactic shock, anaphylaxis — *see* Table of Drugs and Chemicals
Andes disease W94.11 ☑
Arachnidism, arachnoidism X58 ☑
Arson (with intent to injure or kill) X97 ☑
Asphyxia, asphyxiation
  by
    food (bone) (seed) — *see* categories T17 and T18 ☑
    gas (*see also* Table of Drugs and Chemicals)
      legal
        execution — *see* Legal, intervention, gas

Asphyxia, asphyxiation — *continued*
  by — *continued*
    gas (*see also* Table of Drugs and Chemicals) — *continued*
      legal — *continued*
        intervention — *see* Legal, intervention, gas
  from
    fire (*see also* Exposure, fire)
      in war operations — *see* War operations, fire
    ignition — *see* Ignition
    vomitus T17.81
  in war operations — *see* War operations, restriction of airway
Aspiration
  food (any type) (into respiratory tract) (with asphyxia, obstruction respiratory tract, suffocation) — *see* categories T17 and T18 ☑
  foreign body — *see* Foreign body, aspiration
  vomitus (with asphyxia, obstruction respiratory tract, suffocation) T17.81 ☑
Assassination (attempt) — *see* Assault
Assault (homicidal) (by) (in) Y09
  arson X97 ☑
  bite (of human being) Y04.1 ☑
  bodily force Y04.8 ☑
    bite Y04.1 ☑
    bumping into Y04.2 ☑
    sexual — *see* subcategories T74.0, T76.0 ☑
    unarmed fight Y04.0 ☑
  bomb X96.9 ☑
    antipersonnel X96.0 ☑
    fertilizer X96.3 ☑
    gasoline X96.1 ☑
    letter X96.2 ☑
    petrol X96.1 ☑
    pipe X96.3 ☑
    specified NEC X96.8 ☑
  brawl (hand) (fists) (foot) (unarmed) Y04.0 ☑
  burning, burns (by fire) NEC X97 ☑
    acid Y08.89 ☑
    caustic, corrosive substance Y08.89 ☑
    chemical from swallowing caustic, corrosive substance — *see* Table of Drugs and Chemicals
    cigarette(s) X97 ☑
    hot object X98.9 ☑
      fluid NEC X98.2 ☑
      household appliance X98.3 ☑
      specified NEC X98.8 ☑
      steam X98.0 ☑
      tap water X98.1 ☑
      vapors X98.0 ☑
    scalding — *see* Assault, burning
    steam X98.0 ☑
    vitriol Y08.89 ☑
  caustic, corrosive substance (gas) Y08.89 ☑
  crashing of
    aircraft Y08.81 ☑
    motor vehicle Y03.8 ☑
      pushed in front of Y02.0 ☑
      run over Y03.0 ☑
      specified NEC Y03.8 ☑
  cutting or piercing instrument X99.9 ☑
    dagger X99.2 ☑
    glass X99.0 ☑
    knife X99.1 ☑
    specified NEC X99.8 ☑
    sword X99.2 ☑
  dagger X99.2 ☑
  drowning (in) X92.9 ☑
    bathtub X92.0 ☑
    natural water X92.3 ☑
    specified NEC X92.8 ☑
    swimming pool X92.1 ☑
      following fall X92.2 ☑
  dynamite X96.8 ☑
  explosive(s) (material) X96.9 ☑
  fight (hand) (fists) (foot) (unarmed) Y04.0 ☑
    with weapon — *see* Assault, by type of weapon
  fire X97 ☑
  firearm X95.9 ☑
    airgun X95.01 ☑
    handgun X93 ☑
    hunting rifle X94.1 ☑
    larger X94.9 ☑
      specified NEC X94.8 ☑
    machine gun X94.2 ☑

Assault — *continued*
  firearm — *continued*
    shotgun X94.0 ☑
    specified NEC X95.8 ☑
  from high place Y01 ☑
  gunshot (wound) NEC — *see* Assault, firearm, by type
  incendiary device X97 ☑
  injury Y09
    to child due to criminal abortion attempt NEC
      Y08.89 ☑
  knife X99.1 ☑
  late effect of — *see* categories X92-Y08 with 7th character S
  placing before moving object NEC Y02.8 ☑
    motor vehicle Y02.0 ☑
  poisoning — *see* categories T36-T65 with 7th character S
  puncture, any part of body — *see* Assault, cutting or piercing instrument
  pushing
    before moving object NEC Y02.8 ☑
      motor vehicle Y02.0 ☑
      subway train Y02.1 ☑
      train Y02.1 ☑
    from high place Y01 ☑
  rape T74.2- ☑
  scalding — *see* Assault, burning
  sequelae of — *see* categories X92-Y08 with 7th character S
  sexual (by bodily force) T74.2- ☑
  shooting — *see* Assault, firearm
  specified means NEC Y08.89 ☑
  stab, any part of body — *see* Assault, cutting or piercing instrument
  steam X98.0 ☑
  striking against
    other person Y04.2 ☑
    sports equipment Y08.09 ☑
      baseball bat Y08.02 ☑
      hockey stick Y08.01 ☑
  struck by
    sports equipment Y08.09 ☑
      baseball bat Y08.02 ☑
      hockey stick Y08.01 ☑
  submersion — *see* Assault, drowning
  violence Y09
  weapon Y09
    blunt Y00 ☑
    cutting or piercing — *see* Assault, cutting or piercing instrument
    firearm — *see* Assault, firearm
  wound Y09
    cutting — *see* Assault, cutting or piercing instrument
    gunshot — *see* Assault, firearm
    knife X99.1 ☑
    piercing — *see* Assault, cutting or piercing instrument
    puncture — *see* Assault, cutting or piercing instrument
    stab — *see* Assault, cutting or piercing instrument
Attack by mammals NEC W55.89 ☑
Avalanche — *see* Landslide
Aviator's disease — *see* Air, pressure

B

Barotitis, barodontalgia, barosinusitis, barotrauma
  (otitic) (sinus) — *see* Air, pressure
Battered (baby) (child) (person) (syndrome) X58 ☑
Bayonet wound W26.1 ☑
  in
    legal intervention — *see* Legal, intervention, sharp object, bayonet
    war operations — *see* War operations, combat
  stated as undetermined whether accidental or intentional Y28.8 ☑
  suicide (attempt) X78.2 ☑
Bean in nose — *see* categories T17 and T18 ☑
Bed set on fire NEC — *see* Exposure, fire, uncontrolled, building, bed
Beheading (by guillotine)
  homicide X99.9 ☑
  legal execution — *see* Legal, intervention
Bending, injury in (prolonged) (static) X50.1 ☑
Bends — *see* Air, pressure, change

Bite, bitten by
  alligator W58.01 ☑
  arthropod (nonvenomous) NEC W57 ☑
  bull W55.21 ☑
  cat W55.01 ☑
  cow W55.21 ☑
  crocodile W58.11 ☑
  dog W54.0 ☑
  goat W55.31 ☑
  hoof stock NEC W55.31 ☑
  horse W55.11 ☑
  human being (accidentally) W50.3 ☑
    with intent to injure or kill Y04.1 ☑
    as, or caused by, a crowd or human stampede (with fall) W52 ☑
    assault Y04.1 ☑
    homicide (attempt) Y04.1 ☑
    in
      fight Y04.1 ☑
  insect (nonvenomous) W57 ☑
  lizard (nonvenomous) W59.01 ☑
  mammal NEC W55.81 ☑
    marine W56.31 ☑
  marine animal (nonvenomous) W56.81 ☑
  millipede W57 ☑
  moray eel W56.51 ☑
  mouse W53.01 ☑
  person(s) (accidentally) W50.3 ☑
    with intent to injure or kill Y04.1 ☑
    as, or caused by, a crowd or human stampede (with fall) W52 ☑
    assault Y04.1 ☑
    homicide (attempt) Y04.1 ☑
    in
      fight Y04.1 ☑
  pig W55.41 ☑
  raccoon W55.51 ☑
  rat W53.11 ☑
  reptile W59.81 ☑
    lizard W59.01 ☑
    snake W59.11 ☑
    turtle W59.21 ☑
      terrestrial W59.81 ☑
  rodent W53.81 ☑
    mouse W53.01 ☑
    rat W53.11 ☑
    specified NEC W53.81 ☑
    squirrel W53.21 ☑
  shark W56.41 ☑
  sheep W55.31 ☑
  snake (nonvenomous) W59.11 ☑
  spider (nonvenomous) W57 ☑
  squirrel W53.21 ☑
Blast (air) in war operations — *see* War operations, blast
Blizzard X37.2 ☑
Blood alcohol level Y90.9
  less than 20mg/100ml Y90.0
  presence in blood, level not specified Y90.9
  20-39mg/100ml Y90.1
  40-59mg/100ml Y90.2
  60-79mg/100ml Y90.3
  80-99mg/100ml Y90.4
  100-119mg/100ml Y90.5
  120-199mg/100ml Y90.6
  200-239mg/100ml Y90.7
Blow X58 ☑
  by law-enforcing agent, police (on duty) — *see* Legal, intervention, manhandling
  blunt object — *see* Legal, intervention, blunt object
Blowing up — *see* Explosion
Brawl (hand) (fists) (foot) Y04.0 ☑
Breakage (accidental) (part of)
  ladder (causing fall) W11 ☑
  scaffolding (causing fall) W12 ☑
Broken
  glass, contact with — *see* Contact, with, glass
  power line (causing electric shock) W85 ☑
Bumping against, into (accidentally)
  object NEC W22.8 ☑
    caused by crowd or human stampede (with fall) W52 ☑
    sports equipment W21.9 ☑
    with fall — *see* Fall, due to, bumping against, object
  person(s) W51 ☑
    with fall W03 ☑
      due to ice or snow W00.0 ☑

Bumping against, into — *continued*
  person(s) — *continued*
    assault Y04.2 ☑
    caused by, a crowd or human stampede (with fall) W52 ☑
    homicide (attempt) Y04.2 ☑
  sports equipment W21.9 ☑
Burn, burned, burning (accidental) (by) (from) (on)
  acid NEC — *see* Table of Drugs and Chemicals
  bed linen — *see* Exposure, fire, uncontrolled, in building, bed
  blowtorch X08.8 ☑
    with ignition of clothing NEC X06.2 ☑
      nightwear X05 ☑
  bonfire, campfire (controlled) (*see also* Exposure, fire, controlled, not in building)
    uncontrolled — *see* Exposure, fire, uncontrolled, not in building
  candle X08.8 ☑
    with ignition of clothing NEC X06.2 ☑
      nightwear X05 ☑
  caustic liquid, substance (external) (internal) NEC — *see* Table of Drugs and Chemicals
  chemical (external) (internal) (*see also* Table of Drugs and Chemicals)
    in war operations — *see* War operations, fire
  cigar(s) or cigarette(s) X08.8 ☑
    with ignition of clothing NEC X06.2 ☑
      nightwear X05 ☑
  clothes, clothing NEC (from controlled fire) X06.2 ☑
    with conflagration — *see* Exposure, fire, uncontrolled, building
    not in building or structure — *see* Exposure, fire, uncontrolled, not in building
  cooker (hot) X15.8 ☑
    stated as undetermined whether accidental or intentional Y27.3 ☑
    suicide (attempt) X77.3 ☑
  electric blanket X16 ☑
  engine (hot) X17 ☑
  fire, flames — *see* Exposure, fire
  flare, Very pistol — *see* Discharge, firearm NEC
  heat
    from appliance (electrical) (household) X15.8 ☑
      cooker X15.8 ☑
      hotplate X15.2 ☑
      kettle X15.8 ☑
      light bulb X15.8 ☑
      saucepan X15.3 ☑
      skillet X15.3 ☑
      stated as undetermined whether accidental or intentional Y27.3 ☑
      stove X15.0 ☑
      suicide (attempt) X77.3 ☑
      toaster X15.1 ☑
    in local application or packing during medical or surgical procedure Y63.5
  heating
    appliance, radiator or pipe X16 ☑
  homicide (attempt) — *see* Assault, burning
  hot
    air X14.1 ☑
    cooker X15.8 ☑
    drink X10.0 ☑
    engine X17 ☑
    fat X10.2 ☑
    fluid NEC X12 ☑
    food X10.1 ☑
    gases X14.1 ☑
    heating appliance X16 ☑
    household appliance NEC X15.8 ☑
    kettle X15.8 ☑
    liquid NEC X12 ☑
    machinery X17 ☑
    metal (molten) (liquid) NEC X18 ☑
    object (not producing fire or flames) NEC X19 ☑
    oil (cooking) X10.2 ☑
    pipe(s) X16 ☑
    radiator X16 ☑
    saucepan (glass) (metal) X15.3 ☑
    stove (kitchen) X15.0 ☑
    substance NEC X19 ☑
      caustic or corrosive NEC — *see* Table of Drugs and Chemicals
    toaster X15.1 ☑
    tool X17 ☑

Burn, burned, burning — *continued*
- hot — *continued*
    - vapor X13.1
    - water (tap) — *see* Contact, with, hot, tap water
- hotplate X15.2 ☑
    - suicide (attempt) X77.3 ☑
- ignition — *see* Ignition
- in war operations — *see* War operations, fire
- inflicted by other person X97 ☑
    - by hot objects, hot vapor, and steam — *see* Assault, burning, hot object
- internal, from swallowed caustic, corrosive liquid, substance — *see* Table of Drugs and Chemicals
- iron (hot) X15.8 ☑
    - stated as undetermined whether accidental or intentional Y27.3 ☑
    - suicide (attempt) X77.3 ☑
- kettle (hot) X15.8 ☑
    - stated as undetermined whether accidental or intentional Y27.3 ☑
    - suicide (attempt) X77.3 ☑
- lamp (flame) X08.8 ☑
    - with ignition of clothing NEC X06.2 ☑
        - nightwear X05 ☑
- lighter (cigar) (cigarette) X08.8 ☑
    - with ignition of clothing NEC X06.2 ☑
        - nightwear X05 ☑
- lightning — *see* subcategory T75.0 ☑
    - causing fire — *see* Exposure, fire
- liquid (boiling) (hot) NEC X12 ☑
    - stated as undetermined whether accidental or intentional Y27.2 ☑
    - suicide (attempt) X77.2 ☑
- local application of externally applied substance in medical or surgical care Y63.5
- machinery (hot) X17 ☑
- matches X08.8 ☑
    - with ignition of clothing NEC X06.2 ☑
        - nightwear X05 ☑
- mattress — *see* Exposure, fire, uncontrolled, building, bed
- medicament, externally applied Y63.5
- metal (hot) (liquid) (molten) NEC X18 ☑
- nightwear (nightclothes, nightdress, gown, pajamas, robe) X05 ☑
- object (hot) NEC X19 ☑
- on board watercraft
    - due to
        - accident to watercraft V91.09 ☑
            - powered craft V91.03 ☑
                - ferry boat V91.01 ☑
                - fishing boat V91.02 ☑
                - jetskis V91.03 ☑
                - liner V91.01 ☑
                - merchant ship V91.00 ☑
                - passenger ship V91.01 ☑
            - unpowered craft V91.08 ☑
                - canoe V91.05 ☑
                - inflatable V91.06 ☑
                - kayak V91.05 ☑
                - sailboat V91.04 ☑
                - surf-board V91.08 ☑
                - water skis V91.07 ☑
                - windsurfer V91.08 ☑
        - fire on board V93.09 ☑
            - ferry boat V93.01 ☑
            - fishing boat V93.02 ☑
            - jetskis V93.03 ☑
            - liner V93.01 ☑
            - merchant ship V93.00 ☑
            - passenger ship V93.01 ☑
            - powered craft NEC V93.03 ☑
            - sailboat V93.04 ☑
        - specified heat source NEC on board V93.19 ☑
            - ferry boat V93.11 ☑
            - fishing boat V93.12 ☑
            - jetskis V93.13 ☑
            - liner V93.11 ☑
            - merchant ship V93.10 ☑
            - passenger ship V93.11 ☑
            - powered craft NEC V93.13 ☑
            - sailboat V93.14 ☑
- pipe (hot) X16 ☑
    - smoking X08.8 ☑
        - with ignition of clothing NEC X06.2 ☑
            - nightwear X05 ☑

Burn, burned, burning — *continued*
- powder — *see* Powder burn
- radiator (hot) X16
- saucepan (hot) (glass) (metal) X15.3
    - stated as undetermined whether accidental or intentional Y27.3 ☑
    - suicide (attempt) X77.3 ☑
- self-inflicted X76
    - stated as undetermined whether accidental or intentional Y26 ☑
- stated as undetermined whether accidental or intentional Y27.0 ☑
- steam X13.1 ☑
    - pipe X16
        - stated as undetermined whether accidental or intentional Y27.8 ☑
    - stated as undetermined whether accidental or intentional Y27.0 ☑
    - suicide (attempt) X77.0 ☑
- stove (hot) (kitchen) X15.0 ☑
    - stated as undetermined whether accidental or intentional Y27.3 ☑
    - suicide (attempt) X77.3 ☑
- substance (hot) NEC X19 ☑
    - boiling X12
        - stated as undetermined whether accidental or intentional Y27.2 ☑
        - suicide (attempt) X77.2 ☑
    - molten (metal) X18 ☑
- suicide (attempt) NEC X76 ☑
    - hot
        - household appliance X77.3 ☑
        - object X77.9 ☑
- therapeutic misadventure
    - heat in local application or packing during medical or surgical procedure Y63.5
    - overdose of radiation Y63.2
- toaster (hot) X15.1 ☑
    - stated as undetermined whether accidental or intentional Y27.3 ☑
    - suicide (attempt) X77.3 ☑
- tool (hot) X17 ☑
- torch, welding X08.8 ☑
    - with ignition of clothing NEC X06.2 ☑
        - nightwear X05 ☑
- trash fire (controlled) — *see* Exposure, fire, controlled, not in building
    - uncontrolled — *see* Exposure, fire, uncontrolled, not in building
- vapor (hot) X13.1 ☑
    - stated as undetermined whether accidental or intentional Y27.0 ☑
    - suicide (attempt) X77.0 ☑
- Very pistol — *see* Discharge, firearm NEC

Butted by animal W55.82 ☑
- bull W55.22 ☑
- cow W55.22 ☑
- goat W55.32 ☑
- horse W55.12 ☑
- pig W55.42 ☑
- sheep W55.32 ☑

C

Caisson disease — *see* Air, pressure, change
Campfire (exposure to) (controlled) (*see also* Exposure, fire, controlled, not in building)
- uncontrolled — *see* Exposure, fire, uncontrolled, not in building
Capital punishment (any means) — *see* Legal, intervention
Car sickness T75.3 ☑
Casualty (not due to war) NEC X58 ☑
- war — *see* War operations
Cat
- bite W55.01 ☑
- scratch W55.03 ☑
Cataclysm, cataclysmic (any injury) NEC — *see* Forces of nature
Catching fire — *see* Exposure, fire
Caught
- between
    - folding object W23.0 ☑
    - objects (moving) (stationary and moving) W23.0 ☑
        - and machinery — *see* Contact, with, by type of machine

Caught — *continued*
- between — *continued*
    - objects — *continued*
        - stationary W23.1 ☑
        - sliding door and door frame W23.0 ☑
- by, in
    - machinery (moving parts of) — *see* Contact, with, by type of machine
    - washing-machine wringer W23.0 ☑
- under packing crate (due to losing grip) W23.1 ☑
Cave-in caused by cataclysmic earth surface movement or eruption — *see* Landslide
Change(s) in air pressure — *see* Air, pressure, change
Choked, choking (on) (any object except food or vomitus)
- food (bone) (seed) — *see* categories T17 and T18 ☑
- vomitus T17.81-
Civil insurrection — *see* War operations
Cloudburst (any injury) X37.8 ☑
Cold, exposure to (accidental) (excessive) (extreme) (natural) (place) NEC — *see* Exposure, cold
Collapse
- building W20.1 ☑
    - burning (uncontrolled fire) X00.2 ☑
- dam or man-made structure (causing earth movement) X36.0 ☑
- machinery — *see* Contact, with, by type of machine
- structure W20.1 ☑
    - burning (uncontrolled fire) X00.2 ☑
Collision (accidental) NEC (*see also* Accident, transport) V89.9 ☑
- pedestrian W51 ☑
    - with fall W03 ☑
        - due to ice or snow W00.0 ☑
            - involving pedestrian conveyance — *see* Accident, transport, pedestrian, conveyance
    - and
        - crowd or human stampede (with fall) W52 ☑
        - object W22.8 ☑
            - with fall — *see* Fall, due to, bumping against, object
- person(s) — *see* Collision, pedestrian
- transport vehicle NEC V89.9 ☑
    - and
        - avalanche, fallen or not moving — *see* Accident, transport
            - falling or moving — *see* Landslide
        - landslide, fallen or not moving — *see* Accident, transport
            - falling or moving — *see* Landslide
    - due to cataclysm — *see* Forces of nature, by type
    - intentional, purposeful suicide (attempt) — *see* Suicide, collision
Combustion, spontaneous — *see* Ignition
Complication (delayed) **of or following** (medical or surgical procedure) Y84.9
- with misadventure — *see* Misadventure
- amputation of limb(s) Y83.5
- anastomosis (arteriovenous) (blood vessel) (gastrojejunal) (tendon) (natural or artificial material) Y83.2
- aspiration (of fluid) Y84.4
    - tissue Y84.8
- biopsy Y84.8
- blood
    - sampling Y84.7
    - transfusion
        - procedure Y84.8
- bypass Y83.2
- catheterization (urinary) Y84.6
    - cardiac Y84.0
- colostomy Y83.3
- cystostomy Y83.3
- dialysis (kidney) Y84.1
- drug — *see* Table of Drugs and Chemicals
- due to misadventure — *see* Misadventure
- duodenostomy Y83.3
- electroshock therapy Y84.3
- external stoma, creation of Y83.3
- formation of external stoma Y83.3
- gastrostomy Y83.3
- graft Y83.2
- hypothermia (medically-induced) Y84.8
- implant, implantation (of)
    - artificial
        - internal device (cardiac pacemaker) (electrodes in brain) (heart valve prosthesis) (orthopedic) Y83.1

Complication (delayed) **of or following** — *continued*
  continued
  implant, implantation — *continued*
    artificial — *continued*
      material or tissue (for anastomosis or bypass) Y83.2
        with creation of external stoma Y83.3
      natural tissues (for anastomosis or bypass) Y83.2
        with creation of external stoma Y83.3
  infusion
    procedure Y84.8
  injection — *see* Table of Drugs and Chemicals
    procedure Y84.8
  insertion of gastric or duodenal sound Y84.5
  insulin-shock therapy Y84.3
  paracentesis (abdominal) (thoracic) (aspirative) Y84.4
  procedures other than surgical operation — *see* Complication of or following, by type of procedure
  radiological procedure or therapy Y84.2
  removal of organ (partial) (total) NEC Y83.6
  sampling
    blood Y84.7
    fluid NEC Y84.4
    tissue Y84.8
  shock therapy Y84.3
  surgical operation NEC (*see also* Complication of or following, by type of operation) Y83.9
    reconstructive NEC Y83.4
      with
        anastomosis, bypass or graft Y83.2
        formation of external stoma Y83.3
    specified NEC Y83.8
  transfusion (*see also* Table of Drugs and Chemicals)
    procedure Y84.8
  transplant, transplantation (heart) (kidney) (liver) (whole organ, any) Y83.0
    partial organ Y83.4
  ureterostomy Y83.3
  vaccination (*see also* Table of Drugs and Chemicals)
    procedure Y84.8

Compression
  divers' squeeze — *see* Air, pressure, change
  trachea by
    food (lodged in esophagus) — *see* categories T17 and T18 ☑
    vomitus (lodged in esophagus) T17.81- ☑

Conflagration — *see* Exposure, fire, uncontrolled

Constriction (external)
  hair W49.01 ☑
  jewelry W49.04 ☑
  ring W49.04 ☑
  rubber band W49.03 ☑
  specified item NEC W49.09 ☑
  string W49.02 ☑
  thread W49.02 ☑

Contact (accidental)
  with
    abrasive wheel (metalworking) W31.1 ☑
    alligator W58.09 ☑
      bite W58.01 ☑
      crushing W58.03 ☑
      strike W58.02 ☑
    amphibian W62.9 ☑
      frog W62.0 ☑
      toad W62.1 ☑
    animal (nonvenomous) NEC W64 ☑
      marine W56.89 ☑
        bite W56.81 ☑
        dolphin — *see* Contact, with, dolphin
        fish NEC — *see* Contact, with, fish
        mammal — *see* Contact, with, mammal, marine
        orca — *see* Contact, with, orca
        sea lion — *see* Contact, with, sea lion
        shark — *see* Contact, with, shark
        strike W56.82 ☑
    animate mechanical force NEC W64 ☑
    arrow W21.89 ☑
      not thrown, projected or falling W45.8 ☑
    arthropods (nonvenomous) W57 ☑
    axe W27.0 ☑
    band-saw (industrial) W31.2 ☑
    bayonet — *see* Bayonet wound
    bee(s) X58 ☑
    bench-saw (industrial) W31.2 ☑
    bird W61.99 ☑
      bite W61.91 ☑

Contact — *continued*
  with — *continued*
    bird — *continued*
      chicken — *see* Contact, with, chicken
      duck — *see* Contact, with, duck
      goose — *see* Contact, with, goose
      macaw — *see* Contact, with, macaw
      parrot — *see* Contact, with, parrot
      psittacine — *see* Contact, with, psittacine
      strike W61.92 ☑
      turkey — *see* Contact, with, turkey
    blender W29.0 ☑
    boiling water X12 ☑
      stated as undetermined whether accidental or intentional Y27.2 ☑
      suicide (attempt) X77.2 ☑
    bore, earth-drilling or mining (land) (seabed) W31.0 ☑
    buffalo — *see* Contact, with, hoof stock NEC
    bull W55.29 ☑
      bite W55.21 ☑
      gored W55.22 ☑
      strike W55.22 ☑
    bumper cars W31.81 ☑
    camel — *see* Contact, with, hoof stock NEC
    can
      lid W26.8 ☑
      opener W27.4 ☑
        powered W29.0 ☑
    cat W55.09 ☑
      bite W55.01 ☑
      scratch W55.03 ☑
    caterpillar (venomous) X58 ☑
    centipede (venomous) X58 ☑
    chain
      hoist W24.0 ☑
        agricultural operations W30.89 ☑
      saw W29.3 ☑
    chicken W61.39 ☑
      peck W61.33 ☑
      strike W61.32 ☑
    chisel W27.0 ☑
    circular saw W31.2 ☑
    cobra X58 ☑
    combine (harvester) W30.0 ☑
    conveyer belt W24.1 ☑
    cooker (hot) X15.8 ☑
      stated as undetermined whether accidental or intentional Y27.3 ☑
      suicide (attempt) X77.3 ☑
    coral X58 ☑
    cotton gin W31.82 ☑
    cow W55.29 ☑
      bite W55.21 ☑
      strike W55.22 ☑
    crane W24.0 ☑
      agricultural operations W30.89 ☑
    crocodile W58.19 ☑
      bite W58.11 ☑
      crushing W58.13 ☑
      strike W58.12 ☑
    dagger W26.1 ☑
      stated as undetermined whether accidental or intentional Y28.2 ☑
      suicide (attempt) X78.2 ☑
    dairy equipment W31.82 ☑
    dart W21.89 ☑
      not thrown, projected or falling W45.8 ☑
    deer — *see* Contact, with, hoof stock NEC
    derrick W24.0 ☑
      agricultural operations W30.89 ☑
        hay W30.2 ☑
    dog W54.8 ☑
      bite W54.0 ☑
      strike W54.1 ☑
    dolphin W56.09 ☑
      bite W56.01 ☑
      strike W56.02 ☑
    donkey — *see* Contact, with, hoof stock NEC
    drill (powered) W29.8 ☑
      earth (land) (seabed) W31.0 ☑
      nonpowered W27.8 ☑
    drive belt W24.0 ☑
      agricultural operations W30.89 ☑
    dry ice — *see* Exposure, cold, man-made
    dryer (clothes) (powered) (spin) W29.2 ☑

Contact — *continued*
  with — *continued*
    duck W61.69 ☑
      bite W61.61 ☑
      strike W61.62 ☑
    earth (-)
      drilling machine (industrial) W31.0 ☑
      scraping machine in stationary use W31.83 ☑
    edge of stiff paper W26.2 ☑
    electric
      beater W29.0 ☑
      blanket X16 ☑
      fan W29.2 ☑
        commercial W31.82 ☑
      knife W29.1 ☑
      mixer W29.0 ☑
    elevator (building) W24.0 ☑
      agricultural operations W30.89 ☑
        grain W30.3 ☑
    engine(s), hot NEC X17 ☑
    excavating machine W31.0 ☑
    farm machine W30.9 ☑
    feces — *see* Contact, with, by type of animal
    fer de lance X58 ☑
    fish W56.59 ☑
      bite W56.51 ☑
      shark — *see* Contact, with, shark
      strike W56.52 ☑
    flying horses W31.81 ☑
    forging (metalworking) machine W31.1 ☑
    fork W27.4 ☑
    forklift (truck) W24.0 ☑
      agricultural operations W30.89 ☑
    frog W62.0 ☑
    garden
      cultivator (powered) W29.3 ☑
        riding W30.89 ☑
      fork W27.1 ☑
    gas turbine W31.3 ☑
    Gila monster X58 ☑
    giraffe — *see* Contact, with, hoof stock NEC
    glass (sharp) (broken) W25 ☑
      assault X99.0 ☑
      due to fall — *see* Fall, by type
      stated as undetermined whether accidental or intentional Y28.0 ☑
      suicide (attempt) X78.0 ☑
      with subsequent fall W18.02 ☑
    goat W55.39 ☑
      bite W55.31 ☑
      strike W55.32 ☑
    goose W61.59 ☑
      bite W61.51 ☑
      strike W61.52 ☑
    hand
      saw W27.0 ☑
      tool (not powered) NEC W27.8 ☑
        powered W29.8 ☑
    harvester W30.0 ☑
    hay-derrick W30.2 ☑
    heating
      appliance (hot) X16 ☑
      pad (electric) X16 ☑
    heat NEC X19 ☑
      from appliance (electrical) (household) — *see* Contact, with, hot, household appliance heating appliance X16 ☑
    hedge-trimmer (powered) W29.3 ☑
    hoe W27.1 ☑
    hoist (chain) (shaft) NEC W24.0 ☑
      agricultural W30.89 ☑
    hoof stock NEC W55.39 ☑
      bite W55.31 ☑
      strike W55.32 ☑
    hornet(s) X58 ☑
    horse W55.19 ☑
      bite W55.11 ☑
      strike W55.12 ☑
    hot
      air X14.1 ☑
        inhalation X14.0 ☑
      cooker X15.8 ☑
      drinks X10.0 ☑
      engine X17 ☑
      fats X10.2 ☑
      fluids NEC X12 ☑

Contact — *continued*
  with — *continued*
    hot — *continued*
      fluids — *continued*
        assault X98.2 ☑
        suicide (attempt) X77.2 ☑
        undetermined whether accidental or intentional Y27.2 ☑
      food X10.1 ☑
      gases X14.1 ☑
        inhalation X14.0 ☑
      heating appliance X16 ☑
      household appliance X15.8 ☑
        assault X98.3 ☑
        cooker X15.8 ☑
        hotplate X15.2 ☑
        kettle X15.8 ☑
        light bulb X15.8 ☑
        object NEC X19 ☑
          assault X98.8 ☑
          stated as undetermined whether accidental or intentional Y27.9 ☑
          suicide (attempt) X77.8 ☑
        saucepan X15.3 ☑
        skillet X15.3 ☑
        stated as undetermined whether accidental or intentional Y27.3 ☑
        stove X15.0 ☑
        suicide (attempt) X77.3 ☑
        toaster X15.1 ☑
      kettle X15.8 ☑
      light bulb X15.8 ☑
      liquid NEC (*see also* Burn) X12 ☑
        drinks X10.0 ☑
        stated as undetermined whether accidental or intentional Y27.2 ☑
        suicide (attempt) X77.2 ☑
        tap water X11.8 ☑
          stated as undetermined whether accidental or intentional Y27.1 ☑
          suicide (attempt) X77.1 ☑
      machinery X17 ☑
      metal (molten) (liquid) NEC X18 ☑
      object (not producing fire or flames) NEC X19 ☑
      oil (cooking) X10.2 ☑
      pipe X16 ☑
      plate X15.2 ☑
      radiator X16 ☑
      saucepan (glass) (metal) X15.3 ☑
      skillet X15.3 ☑
      stove (kitchen) X15.0 ☑
      substance NEC X19 ☑
      tap-water X11.8 ☑
        assault X98.1 ☑
        heated on stove X12 ☑
          stated as undetermined whether accidental or intentional Y27.2 ☑
          suicide (attempt) X77.2 ☑
        in bathtub X11.0 ☑
        running X11.1 ☑
        stated as undetermined whether accidental or intentional Y27.1 ☑
        suicide (attempt) X77.1 ☑
      toaster X15.1 ☑
      tool X17 ☑
      vapors X13.1 ☑
        inhalation X13.0 ☑
      water (tap) X11.8 ☑
        boiling X12 ☑
          stated as undetermined whether accidental or intentional Y27.2 ☑
          suicide (attempt) X77.2 ☑
        heated on stove X12 ☑
          stated as undetermined whether accidental or intentional Y27.2 ☑
          suicide (attempt) X77.2 ☑
        in bathtub X11.0 ☑
        running X11.1 ☑
        stated as undetermined whether accidental or intentional Y27.1 ☑
        suicide (attempt) X77.1 ☑
    hotplate X15.2 ☑
    ice-pick W27.4 ☑
    insect (nonvenomous) NEC W57 ☑
    kettle (hot) X15.8 ☑
    knife W26.0 ☑

Contact — *continued*
  with — *continued*
    knife — *continued*
      assault X99.1 ☑
      electric W29.1 ☑
      stated as undetermined whether accidental or intentional Y28.1 ☑
      suicide (attempt) X78.1 ☑
    lathe (metalworking) W31.1 ☑
      turnings W45.8 ☑
      woodworking W31.2 ☑
    lawnmower (powered) (ridden) W28 ☑
      causing electrocution W86.8 ☑
        suicide (attempt) X83.1 ☑
      unpowered W27.1 ☑
    lift, lifting (devices) W24.0 ☑
      agricultural operations W30.89 ☑
      shaft W24.0 ☑
    liquefied gas — *see* Exposure, cold, man-made
    liquid air, hydrogen, nitrogen — *see* Exposure, cold, man-made
    lizard (nonvenomous) W59.09 ☑
      bite W59.01 ☑
      strike W59.02 ☑
    llama — *see* Contact, with, hoof stock NEC
    macaw W61.19 ☑
      bite W61.11 ☑
      strike W61.12 ☑
    machine, machinery W31.9 ☑
      abrasive wheel W31.1 ☑
      agricultural including animal-powered W30.9 ☑
        combine harvester W30.0 ☑
        grain storage elevator W30.3 ☑
        hay derrick W30.2 ☑
        power take-off device W30.1 ☑
        reaper W30.0 ☑
        specified NEC W30.89 ☑
        thresher W30.0 ☑
        transport vehicle, stationary W30.81 ☑
      band saw W31.2 ☑
      bench saw W31.2 ☑
      circular saw W31.2 ☑
      commercial NEC W31.82 ☑
      drilling, metal (industrial) W31.1 ☑
      earth-drilling W31.0 ☑
      earthmoving or scraping W31.89 ☑
      excavating W31.89 ☑
      forging machine W31.1 ☑
      gas turbine W31.3 ☑
      hot X17 ☑
      internal combustion engine W31.3 ☑
      land drill W31.0 ☑
      lathe W31.1 ☑
      lifting (devices) W24.0 ☑
      metal drill W31.1 ☑
      metalworking (industrial) W31.1 ☑
      milling, metal W31.1 ☑
      mining W31.0 ☑
      molding W31.2 ☑
      overhead plane W31.2 ☑
      power press, metal W31.1 ☑
      prime mover W31.3 ☑
      printing W31.89 ☑
      radial saw W31.2 ☑
      recreational W31.81 ☑
      roller-coaster W31.81 ☑
      rolling mill, metal W31.1 ☑
      sander W31.2 ☑
      seabed drill W31.0 ☑
      shaft
        hoist W31.0 ☑
        lift W31.0 ☑
      specified NEC W31.89 ☑
      spinning W31.89 ☑
      steam engine W31.3 ☑
      transmission W24.1 ☑
      undercutter W31.0 ☑
      water driven turbine W31.3 ☑
      weaving W31.89 ☑
      woodworking or forming (industrial) W31.2 ☑
    mammal (feces) (urine) W55.89 ☑
      bull — *see* Contact, with, bull
      cat — *see* Contact, with, cat
      cow — *see* Contact, with, cow
      goat — *see* Contact, with, goat
      hoof stock — *see* Contact, with, hoof stock

Contact — *continued*
  with — *continued*
    mammal — *continued*
      horse — *see* Contact, with, horse
      marine W56.39 ☑
        dolphin — *see* Contact, with, dolphin
        orca — *see* Contact, with, orca
        sea lion — *see* Contact, with, sea lion
        specified NEC W56.39 ☑
          bite W56.31 ☑
          strike W56.32 ☑
      pig — *see* Contact, with, pig
      raccoon — *see* Contact, with, raccoon
      rodent — *see* Contact, with, rodent
      sheep — *see* Contact, with, sheep
      specified NEC W55.89 ☑
        bite W55.81 ☑
        strike W55.82 ☑
    marine
      animal W56.89 ☑
        bite W56.81 ☑
        dolphin — *see* Contact, with, dolphin
        fish NEC — *see* Contact, with, fish
        mammal — *see* Contact, with, mammal, marine
        orca — *see* Contact, with, orca
        sea lion — *see* Contact, with, sea lion
        shark — *see* Contact, with, shark
        strike W56.82 ☑
    meat
      grinder (domestic) W29.0 ☑
        industrial W31.82 ☑
        nonpowered W27.4 ☑
      slicer (domestic) W29.0 ☑
        industrial W31.82 ☑
    merry go round W31.81 ☑
    metal, hot (liquid) (molten) NEC X18 ☑
    millipede W57 ☑
    nail W45.0 ☑
      gun W29.4 ☑
    needle (sewing) W27.3 ☑
      hypodermic W46.0 ☑
        contaminated W46.1 ☑
    object (blunt) NEC
      hot NEC X19 ☑
      legal intervention — *see* Legal, intervention, blunt object
      sharp NEC W45.8 ☑
        inflicted by other person NEC W45.8 ☑
          stated as
            intentional homicide (attempt) — *see* Assault, cutting or piercing instrument
        legal intervention — *see* Legal, intervention, sharp object
        self-inflicted X78.9 ☑
    orca W56.29 ☑
      bite W56.21 ☑
      strike W56.22 ☑
    overhead plane W31.2 ☑
    paper (as sharp object) W26.2 ☑
    paper-cutter W27.5 ☑
    parrot W61.09 ☑
      bite W61.01 ☑
      strike W61.02 ☑
    pig W55.49 ☑
      bite W55.41 ☑
      strike W55.42 ☑
    pipe, hot X16 ☑
    pitchfork W27.1 ☑
    plane (metal) (wood) W27.0 ☑
      overhead W31.2 ☑
    plant thorns, spines, sharp leaves or other mechanisms W60 ☑
    powered
      garden cultivator W29.3 ☑
      household appliance, implement, or machine W29.8 ☑
      saw (industrial) W31.2 ☑
        hand W29.8 ☑
    printing machine W31.89 ☑
    psittacine bird W61.29 ☑
      bite W61.21 ☑
      macaw — *see* Contact, with, macaw
      parrot — *see* Contact, with, parrot
      strike W61.22 ☑

Contact — *continued*
  with — *continued*
    pulley (block) (transmission) W24.0 ☑
      agricultural operations W30.89 ☑
    raccoon W55.59 ☑
      bite W55.51 ☑
      strike W55.52 ☑
    radial-saw (industrial) W31.2 ☑
    radiator (hot) X16 ☑
    rake W27.1 ☑
    rattlesnake X58 ☑
    reaper W30.0 ☑
    reptile W59.89 ☑
      lizard — *see* Contact, with, lizard
      snake — *see* Contact, with, snake
      specified NEC W59.89 ☑
        bite W59.81 ☑
        crushing W59.83 ☑
        strike W59.82 ☑
      turtle — *see* Contact, with, turtle
    rivet gun (powered) W29.4 ☑
    road scraper — *see* Accident, transport, construction
      vehicle
    rodent (feces) (urine) W53.89 ☑
      bite W53.81 ☑
      mouse W53.09 ☑
        bite W53.01 ☑
      rat W53.19 ☑
        bite W53.11 ☑
      specified NEC W53.89 ☑
        bite W53.81 ☑
      squirrel W53.29 ☑
        bite W53.21 ☑
    roller coaster W31.81 ☑
    rope NEC W24.0 ☑
      agricultural operations W30.89 ☑
    saliva — *see* Contact, with, by type of animal
    sander W29.8 ☑
      industrial W31.2 ☑
    saucepan (hot) (glass) (metal) X15.3 ☑
    saw W27.0 ☑
      band (industrial) W31.2 ☑
      bench (industrial) W31.2 ☑
      chain W29.3 ☑
      hand W27.0 ☑
    sawing machine, metal W31.1 ☑
    scissors W27.2 ☑
    scorpion X58 ☑
    screwdriver W27.0 ☑
      powered W29.8 ☑
    sea
      anemone, cucumber or urchin (spine) X58 ☑
      lion W56.19 ☑
        bite W56.11 ☑
        strike W56.12 ☑
    serpent — *see* Contact, with, snake, by type
    sewing-machine (electric) (powered) W29.2 ☑
      not powered W27.8 ☑
    shaft (hoist) (lift) (transmission) NEC W24.0 ☑
      agricultural W30.89 ☑
    shark W56.49 ☑
      bite W56.41 ☑
      strike W56.42 ☑
    sharp object(s) W26.9 ☑
      specified NEC W26.8 ☑
    shears (hand) W27.2 ☑
      powered (industrial) W31.1 ☑
        domestic W29.2 ☑
    sheep W55.39 ☑
      bite W55.31 ☑
      strike W55.32 ☑
    shovel W27.8 ☑
      steam — *see* Accident, transport, construction
        vehicle
    snake (nonvenomous) W59.19 ☑
      bite W59.11 ☑
      crushing W59.13 ☑
      strike W59.12 ☑
    spade W27.1 ☑
    spider (venomous) X58 ☑
    spin-drier W29.2 ☑
    spinning machine W31.89 ☑
    splinter W45.8 ☑
    sports equipment W21.9 ☑
    staple gun (powered) W29.8 ☑
    steam X13.1 ☑

Contact — *continued*
  with — *continued*
    steam — *continued*
      engine W31.3 ☑
      inhalation X13.0 ☑
      pipe X16 ☑
      shovel W31.89 ☑
    stove (hot) (kitchen) X15.0 ☑
    substance, hot NEC X19 ☑
      molten (metal) X18 ☑
    sword W26.1 ☑
      assault X99.2 ☑
      stated as undetermined whether accidental or
        intentional Y28.2 ☑
      suicide (attempt) X78.2 ☑
    tarantula X58 ☑
    thresher W30.0 ☑
    tin can lid W26.8 ☑
    toad W62.1 ☑
    toaster (hot) X15.1 ☑
    tool W27.8 ☑
      hand (not powered) W27.8 ☑
        auger W27.0 ☑
        axe W27.0 ☑
        can opener W27.4 ☑
        chisel W27.0 ☑
        fork W27.4 ☑
        garden W27.1 ☑
        handsaw W27.0 ☑
        hoe W27.1 ☑
        ice-pick W27.4 ☑
        kitchen utensil W27.4 ☑
        manual
          lawn mower W27.1 ☑
          sewing machine W27.8 ☑
        meat grinder W27.4 ☑
        needle (sewing) W27.3 ☑
          hypodermic W46.0 ☑
            contaminated W46.1 ☑
        paper cutter W27.5 ☑
        pitchfork W27.1 ☑
        rake W27.1 ☑
        scissors W27.2 ☑
        screwdriver W27.0 ☑
        specified NEC W27.8 ☑
        workbench W27.0 ☑
      hot X17 ☑
      powered W29.8 ☑
        blender W29.0 ☑
          commercial W31.82 ☑
        can opener W29.0 ☑
          commercial W31.82 ☑
        chainsaw W29.3 ☑
        clothes dryer W29.2 ☑
          commercial W31.82 ☑
        dishwasher W29.2 ☑
          commercial W31.82 ☑
        edger W29.3 ☑
        electric fan W29.2 ☑
          commercial W31.82 ☑
        electric knife W29.1 ☑
        food processor W29.0 ☑
          commercial W31.82 ☑
        garbage disposal W29.0 ☑
          commercial W31.82 ☑
        garden tool W29.3 ☑
        hedge trimmer W29.3 ☑
        ice maker W29.0 ☑
          commercial W31.82 ☑
        kitchen appliance W29.0 ☑
          commercial W31.82 ☑
        lawn mower W28 ☑
        meat grinder W29.0 ☑
          commercial W31.82 ☑
        mixer W29.0 ☑
          commercial W31.82 ☑
        rototiller W29.3 ☑
        sewing machine W29.2 ☑
          commercial W31.82 ☑
        washing machine W29.2 ☑
          commercial W31.82 ☑
    transmission device (belt, cable, chain, gear, pinion,
      shaft) W24.1 ☑
      agricultural operations W30.89 ☑
    turbine (gas) (water-driven) W31.3 ☑
    turkey W61.49 ☑

Contact — *continued*
  with — *continued*
    turkey — *continued*
      peck W61.43 ☑
      strike W61.42 ☑
    turtle (nonvenomous) W59.29 ☑
      bite W59.21 ☑
      strike W59.22 ☑
      terrestrial W59.89 ☑
        bite W59.81 ☑
        crushing W59.83 ☑
        strike W59.82 ☑
    under-cutter W31.0 ☑
    urine — *see* Contact, with, by type of animal
    vehicle
      agricultural use (transport) — *see* Accident,
        transport, agricultural vehicle
        not on public highway W30.81 ☑
      industrial use (transport) — *see* Accident, trans-
        port, industrial vehicle
        not on public highway W31.83 ☑
      off-road use (transport) — *see* Accident, trans-
        port, all-terrain or off-road vehicle
        not on public highway W31.83 ☑
      special construction use (transport) — *see* Acci-
        dent, transport, construction vehicle
        not on public highway W31.83 ☑
    venomous
      animal X58 ☑
      arthropods X58 ☑
      lizard X58 ☑
      marine animal NEC X58 ☑
      marine plant NEC X58 ☑
      millipedes (tropical) X58 ☑
      plant(s) X58 ☑
      snake X58 ☑
      spider X58 ☑
      viper X58 ☑
    washing-machine (powered) W29.2 ☑
    wasp X58 ☑
    weaving-machine W31.89 ☑
    winch W24.0 ☑
      agricultural operations W30.89 ☑
    wire NEC W24.0 ☑
      agricultural operations W30.89 ☑
    wood slivers W45.8 ☑
    yellow jacket X58 ☑
    zebra — *see* Contact, with, hoof stock NEC
  pressure X50.9 ☑
  stress X50.9 ☑
Coup de soleil X32 ☑
Crash
  aircraft (in transit) (powered) V95.9 ☑
    balloon V96.01 ☑
    fixed wing NEC (private) V95.21 ☑
      commercial V95.31 ☑
    glider V96.21 ☑
      hang V96.11 ☑
      powered V95.11 ☑
    helicopter V95.01 ☑
    in war operations — *see* War operations, destruction
      of aircraft
    microlight V95.11 ☑
    nonpowered V96.9 ☑
      specified NEC V96.8 ☑
    powered NEC V95.8 ☑
    stated as
      homicide (attempt) Y08.81 ☑
      suicide (attempt) X83.0 ☑
    ultralight V95.11 ☑
  spacecraft V95.41 ☑
  transport vehicle NEC (*see also* Accident, transport)
    V89.9 ☑
    homicide (attempt) Y03.8 ☑
    motor NEC (traffic) V89.2 ☑
      homicide (attempt) Y03.8 ☑
      suicide (attempt) — *see* Suicide, collision
Cruelty (mental) (physical) (sexual) X58 ☑
Crushed (accidentally) X58 ☑
  between objects (moving) (stationary and moving)
    W23.0 ☑
    stationary W23.1 ☑
  by
    alligator W58.03 ☑
    avalanche NEC — *see* Landslide
    cave-in W20.0 ☑

Crushed — *continued*
  by — *continued*
    cave-in — *continued*
      caused by cataclysmic earth surface movement
        — *see* Landslide
    crocodile W58.13 ☑
    crowd or human stampede W52 ☑
    falling
      aircraft V97.39 ☑
        in war operations — *see* War operations, de-
          struction of aircraft
      earth, material W20.0 ☑
        caused by cataclysmic earth surface move-
          ment — *see* Landslide
      object NEC W20.8 ☑
    landslide NEC — *see* Landslide
    lizard (nonvenomous) W59.09 ☑
    machinery — *see* Contact, with, by type of machine
    reptile NEC W59.89 ☑
    snake (nonvenomous) W59.13 ☑
  in
    machinery — *see* Contact, with, by type of machine
Cut, cutting (any part of body) (accidental) (*see also*
  Contact, with, by object or machine)
  during medical or surgical treatment as misadventure
    — *see* Index to Diseases and Injuries, Complica-
    tions
  homicide (attempt) — *see* Assault, cutting or piercing
    instrument
  inflicted by other person — *see* Assault, cutting or
    piercing instrument
  legal
    execution — *see* Legal, intervention
    intervention — *see* Legal, intervention, sharp object
  machine NEC (*see also* Contact, with, by type of ma-
    chine) W31.9 ☑
  self-inflicted — *see* Suicide, cutting or piercing instru-
    ment
  suicide (attempt) — *see* Suicide, cutting or piercing
    instrument
Cyclone (any injury) X37.1 ☑

D

Decapitation (accidental circumstances) NEC X58 ☑
  homicide X99.9 ☑
  legal execution — *see* Legal, intervention
Dehydration from lack of water X58 ☑
Deprivation X58 ☑
Derailment (accidental)
  railway (rolling stock) (train) (vehicle) (without an-
    tecedent collision) V81.7 ☑
    with antecedent collision — *see* Accident, transport,
      railway vehicle occupant
  streetcar (without antecedent collision) V82.7 ☑
    with antecedent collision — *see* Accident, transport,
      streetcar occupant
Descent
  parachute (voluntary) (without accident to aircraft)
    V97.29 ☑
    due to accident to aircraft — *see* Accident, transport,
      aircraft
Desertion X58 ☑
Destitution X58 ☑
Disability, late effect or sequela of injury — *see* Se-
  quelae
Discharge (accidental)
  airgun W34.010 ☑
    assault X95.01 ☑
    homicide (attempt) X95.01 ☑
    stated as undetermined whether accidental or inten-
      tional Y24.0 ☑
    suicide (attempt) X74.01 ☑
  BB gun — *see* Discharge, airgun
  firearm (accidental) W34.00 ☑
    assault X95.9 ☑
    handgun (pistol) (revolver) W32.0 ☑
      assault X93 ☑
      homicide (attempt) X93 ☑
      legal intervention — *see* Legal, intervention,
        firearm, handgun
      stated as undetermined whether accidental or
        intentional Y22 ☑
      suicide (attempt) X72 ☑
    homicide (attempt) X95.9 ☑
    hunting rifle W33.02 ☑

Discharge — *continued*
  firearm — *continued*
    hunting rifle — *continued*
      assault X94.1 ☑
      homicide (attempt) X94.1 ☑
      legal intervention
        injuring
          bystander Y35.032 ☑
          law enforcement personnel Y35.031 ☑
          suspect Y35.033 ☑
      stated as undetermined whether accidental or
        intentional Y23.1 ☑
      suicide (attempt) X73.1 ☑
    larger W33.00 ☑
      assault X94.9 ☑
      homicide (attempt) X94.9 ☑
      hunting rifle — *see* Discharge, firearm, hunting
        rifle
      legal intervention — *see* Legal, intervention,
        firearm by type of firearm
      machine gun — *see* Discharge, firearm, machine
        gun
      shotgun — *see* Discharge, firearm, shotgun
      specified NEC W33.09 ☑
        assault X94.8 ☑
        homicide (attempt) X94.8 ☑
        legal intervention
          injuring
            bystander Y35.092 ☑
            law enforcement personnel
              Y35.091 ☑
            suspect Y35.093 ☑
        stated as undetermined whether accidental
          or intentional Y23.8 ☑
        suicide (attempt) X73.8 ☑
      stated as undetermined whether accidental or
        intentional Y23.9 ☑
      suicide (attempt) X73.9 ☑
    legal intervention
      injuring
        bystander Y35.002 ☑
        law enforcement personnel Y35.001 ☑
        suspect Y35.03 ☑
      using rubber bullet
        injuring
          bystander Y35.042 ☑
          law enforcement personnel Y35.041 ☑
          suspect Y35.043 ☑
    machine gun W33.03 ☑
      assault X94.2 ☑
      homicide (attempt) X94.2 ☑
      legal intervention — *see* Legal, intervention,
        firearm, machine gun
      stated as undetermined whether accidental or
        intentional Y23.3 ☑
      suicide (attempt) X73.2 ☑
    pellet gun — *see* Discharge, airgun
    shotgun W33.01 ☑
      assault X94.0 ☑
      homicide (attempt) X94.0 ☑
      legal intervention — *see* Legal, intervention,
        firearm, specified NEC
      stated as undetermined whether accidental or
        intentional Y23.0 ☑
      suicide (attempt) X73.0 ☑
    specified NEC W34.09 ☑
      assault X95.8 ☑
      homicide (attempt) X95.8 ☑
      legal intervention — *see* Legal, intervention,
        firearm, specified NEC
      stated as undetermined whether accidental or
        intentional Y24.8 ☑
      suicide (attempt) X74.8 ☑
    stated as undetermined whether accidental or inten-
      tional Y24.9 ☑
    suicide (attempt) X74.9 ☑
    Very pistol W34.09 ☑
      assault X95.8 ☑
      homicide (attempt) X95.8 ☑
      stated as undetermined whether accidental or
        intentional Y24.8 ☑
      suicide (attempt) X74.8 ☑
  firework(s) W39 ☑
    stated as undetermined whether accidental or inten-
      tional Y25 ☑
  gas-operated gun NEC W34.018 ☑

Discharge — *continued*
  gas-operated gun — *continued*
    airgun — *see* Discharge, airgun
    assault X95.09 ☑
    homicide (attempt) X95.09 ☑
    paintball gun — *see* Discharge, paintball gun
    stated as undetermined whether accidental or inten-
      tional Y24.8 ☑
    suicide (attempt) X74.09 ☑
  gun NEC (*see also* Discharge, firearm NEC)
    air — *see* Discharge, airgun
    BB — *see* Discharge, airgun
    for single hand use — *see* Discharge, firearm,
      handgun
    hand — *see* Discharge, firearm, handgun
    machine — *see* Discharge, firearm, machine gun
    other specified — *see* Discharge, firearm NEC
    paintball — *see* Discharge, paintball gun
    pellet — *see* Discharge, airgun
  handgun — *see* Discharge, firearm, handgun
  machine gun — *see* Discharge, firearm, machine gun
  paintball gun W34.011 ☑
    assault X95.02 ☑
    homicide (attempt) X95.02 ☑
    stated as undetermined whether accidental or inten-
      tional Y24.8 ☑
    suicide (attempt) X74.02 ☑
  pistol — *see* Discharge, firearm, handgun
    flare — *see* Discharge, firearm, Very pistol
    pellet — *see* Discharge, airgun
    Very — *see* Discharge, firearm, Very pistol
  revolver — *see* Discharge, firearm, handgun
  rifle (hunting) — *see* Discharge, firearm, hunting rifle
  shotgun — *see* Discharge, firearm, shotgun
  spring-operated gun NEC W34.018 ☑
    assault X95.09 ☑
    homicide (attempt) X95.09 ☑
    stated as undetermined whether accidental or inten-
      tional Y24.8 ☑
    suicide (attempt) X74.09 ☑
Disease
  Andes W94.11 ☑
  aviator's — *see* Air, pressure
  range W94.11 ☑
Diver's disease, palsy, paralysis, squeeze — *see* Air,
  pressure
Diving (into water) — *see* Accident, diving
Dog bite W54.0 ☑
Dragged by transport vehicle NEC (*see also* Accident,
  transport) V09.9 ☑
Drinking poison (accidental) — *see* Table of Drugs and
  Chemicals
Dropped (accidentally) **while being carried or support-
  ed by other person** W04 ☑
Drowning (accidental) W74 ☑
  assault X92.9 ☑
  due to
    accident (to)
      machinery — *see* Contact, with, by type of ma-
        chine
      watercraft V90.89 ☑
        burning V90.29 ☑
          powered V90.23 ☑
            fishing boat V90.22 ☑
            jetskis V90.23 ☑
            merchant ship V90.20 ☑
            passenger ship V90.21 ☑
          unpowered V90.28 ☑
            canoe V90.25 ☑
            inflatable V90.26 ☑
            kayak V90.25 ☑
            sailboat V90.24 ☑
            water skis V90.27 ☑
        crushed V90.39 ☑
          powered V90.33 ☑
            fishing boat V90.32 ☑
            jetskis V90.33 ☑
            merchant ship V90.30 ☑
            passenger ship V90.31 ☑
          unpowered V90.38 ☑
            canoe V90.35 ☑
            inflatable V90.36 ☑
            kayak V90.35 ☑
            sailboat V90.34 ☑
            water skis V90.37 ☑
        overturning V90.09 ☑

Drowning — *continued*
  due to — *continued*
    accident — *continued*
      watercraft — *continued*
        overturning — *continued*
          powered V90.03 ☑
            fishing boat V90.02 ☑
            jetskis V90.03 ☑
            merchant ship V90.00 ☑
            passenger ship V90.01 ☑
          unpowered V90.08 ☑
            canoe V90.05 ☑
            inflatable V90.06 ☑
            kayak V90.05 ☑
            sailboat V90.04 ☑
        sinking V90.19 ☑
          powered V90.13 ☑
            fishing boat V90.12 ☑
            jetskis V90.13 ☑
            merchant ship V90.10 ☑
            passenger ship V90.11 ☑
          unpowered V90.18 ☑
            canoe V90.15 ☑
            inflatable V90.16 ☑
            kayak V90.15 ☑
            sailboat V90.14 ☑
        specified type NEC V90.89 ☑
          powered V90.83 ☑
            fishing boat V90.82 ☑
            jetskis V90.83 ☑
            merchant ship V90.80 ☑
            passenger ship V90.81 ☑
          unpowered V90.88 ☑
            canoe V90.85 ☑
            inflatable V90.86 ☑
            kayak V90.85 ☑
            sailboat V90.84 ☑
            water skis V90.87 ☑
    avalanche — *see* Landslide
    cataclysmic
      earth surface movement NEC — *see* Forces of nature, earth movement
      storm — *see* Forces of nature, cataclysmic storm
    cloudburst X37.8 ☑
    cyclone X37.1 ☑
    fall overboard (from) V92.09 ☑
      powered craft V92.03 ☑
        ferry boat V92.01 ☑
        fishing boat V92.02 ☑
        jetskis V92.03 ☑
        liner V92.01 ☑
        merchant ship V92.00 ☑
        passenger ship V92.01 ☑
      resulting from
        accident to watercraft — *see* Drowning, due to, accident, watercraft
        being washed overboard (from) V92.29 ☑
          powered craft V92.23 ☑
            ferry boat V92.21 ☑
            fishing boat V92.22 ☑
            jetskis V92.23 ☑
            liner V92.21 ☑
            merchant ship V92.20 ☑
            passenger ship V92.21 ☑
          unpowered craft V92.28 ☑
            canoe V92.25 ☑
            inflatable V92.26 ☑
            kayak V92.25 ☑
            sailboat V92.24 ☑
            surf-board V92.28 ☑
            water skis V92.27 ☑
            windsurfer V92.28 ☑
        motion of watercraft V92.19 ☑
          powered craft V92.13 ☑
            ferry boat V92.11 ☑
            fishing boat V92.12 ☑
            jetskis V92.13 ☑
            liner V92.11 ☑
            merchant ship V92.10 ☑
            passenger ship V92.11 ☑
          unpowered craft
            canoe V92.15 ☑
            inflatable V92.16 ☑
            kayak V92.15 ☑
            sailboat V92.14 ☑
      unpowered craft V92.08 ☑

Drowning — *continued*
  due to — *continued*
    fall overboard — *continued*
      unpowered craft — *continued*
        canoe V92.05 ☑
        inflatable V92.06 ☑
        kayak V92.05 ☑
        sailboat V92.04 ☑
        surf-board V92.08 ☑
        water skis V92.07 ☑
        windsurfer V92.08 ☑
    hurricane X37.0 ☑
    jumping into water from watercraft (involved in accident) (*see also* Drowning, due to, accident to, watercraft)
      without accident to or on watercraft W16.711 ☑
    tidal wave NEC — *see* Forces of nature, tidal wave
    torrential rain X37.8 ☑
  following
    fall
      into
        bathtub W16.211 ☑
        bucket W16.221 ☑
        fountain — *see* Drowning, following, fall, into, water, specified NEC
        quarry — *see* Drowning, following, fall, into, water, specified NEC
        reservoir — *see* Drowning, following, fall, into, water, specified NEC
        swimming-pool W16.011 ☑
          stated as undetermined whether accidental or intentional Y21.3 ☑
          striking
            bottom W16.021 ☑
            wall W16.031 ☑
          suicide (attempt) X71.2 ☑
        water NOS W16.41 ☑
          natural (lake) (open sea) (river) (stream) (pond) W16.111 ☑
            striking
              bottom W16.121 ☑
              side W16.131 ☑
          specified NEC W16.311 ☑
            striking
              bottom W16.321 ☑
              wall W16.331 ☑
      overboard NEC — *see* Drowning, due to, fall overboard
    jump or dive
      from boat W16.711 ☑
        striking bottom W16.721 ☑
      into
        fountain — *see* Drowning, following, jump or dive, into, water, specified NEC
        quarry — *see* Drowning, following, jump or dive, into, water, specified NEC
        reservoir — *see* Drowning, following, jump or dive, into, water, specified NEC
        swimming-pool W16.511 ☑
          striking
            bottom W16.521 ☑
            wall W16.531 ☑
          suicide (attempt) X71.2 ☑
        water NOS W16.91 ☑
          natural (lake) (open sea) (river) (stream) (pond) W16.611 ☑
          specified NEC W16.811 ☑
            bottom W16.821 ☑
            striking
              bottom W16.821 ☑
              wall W16.831 ☑
          striking
            bottom W16.821 ☑
            wall W16.831 ☑
          striking bottom W16.621 ☑
    homicide (attempt) X92.9 ☑
    in
      bathtub (accidental) W65 ☑
        assault X92.0 ☑
        following fall W16.211 ☑
          stated as undetermined whether accidental or intentional Y21.1 ☑
        stated as undetermined whether accidental or intentional Y21.0 ☑
        suicide (attempt) X71.0 ☑
      lake — *see* Drowning, in, natural water

Drowning — *continued*
  in — *continued*
    natural water (lake) (open sea) (river) (stream) (pond) W69 ☑
      assault X92.3 ☑
      following
        dive or jump W16.611 ☑
          striking bottom W16.621 ☑
        fall W16.111 ☑
          striking
            bottom W16.121 ☑
            side W16.131 ☑
      stated as undetermined whether accidental or intentional Y21.4 ☑
      suicide (attempt) X71.3 ☑
    quarry — *see* Drowning, in, specified place NEC
    quenching tank — *see* Drowning, in, specified place NEC
    reservoir — *see* Drowning, in, specified place NEC
    river — *see* Drowning, in, natural water
    sea — *see* Drowning, in, natural water
    specified place NEC W73 ☑
      assault X92.8 ☑
      following
        dive or jump W16.811 ☑
          striking
            bottom W16.821 ☑
            wall W16.831 ☑
        fall W16.311 ☑
          striking
            bottom W16.321 ☑
            wall W16.331 ☑
      stated as undetermined whether accidental or intentional Y21.8 ☑
      suicide (attempt) X71.8 ☑
    stream — *see* Drowning, in, natural water
    swimming-pool W67 ☑
      assault X92.1 ☑
        following fall X92.2 ☑
      following
        dive or jump W16.511 ☑
          striking
            bottom W16.521 ☑
            wall W16.531 ☑
        fall W16.011 ☑
          striking
            bottom W16.021 ☑
            wall W16.031 ☑
      stated as undetermined whether accidental or intentional Y21.2 ☑
        following fall Y21.3 ☑
      suicide (attempt) X71.1 ☑
        following fall X71.2 ☑
    war operations — *see* War operations, restriction of airway
  resulting from accident to watercraft — *see* Drowning, due to, accident, watercraft
  self-inflicted X71.9 ☑
  stated as undetermined whether accidental or intentional Y21.9 ☑
  suicide (attempt) X71.9 ☑

E

Earth falling (on) W20.0 ☑
  caused by cataclysmic earth surface movement or eruption — *see* Landslide
Earth (surface) **movement NEC** — *see* Forces of nature, earth movement
Earthquake (any injury) X34 ☑
Effect(s) (adverse) **of**
  air pressure (any) — *see* Air, pressure
  cold, excessive (exposure to) — *see* Exposure, cold
  heat (excessive) — *see* Heat
  hot place (weather) — *see* Heat
  insolation X30 ☑
  late — *see* Sequelae
  motion — *see* Motion
  nuclear explosion or weapon in war operations — *see* War operations, nuclear weapon
  radiation — *see* Radiation
  travel — *see* Travel
Electric shock (accidental) (by) (in) — *see* Exposure, electric current
Electrocution (accidental) — *see* Exposure, electric current

Endotracheal tube wrongly placed during anesthetic procedure
Entanglement
  in
    bed linen, causing suffocation T71 ☑
    wheel of pedal cycle V19.88 ☑
Entry of foreign body or material — *see* Foreign body
Environmental pollution related condition — *see*
  category Z57 ☑
Execution, legal (any method) — *see* Legal, intervention
Exhaustion
  cold — *see* Exposure, cold
  due to excessive exertion (*see also* Overexertion)
    X50.9 ☑
  heat — *see* Heat
Explosion (accidental) (of) (with secondary fire) W40.9 ☑
  acetylene W40.1 ☑
  aerosol can W36.1 ☑
  air tank (compressed) (in machinery) W36.2 ☑
  aircraft (in transit) (powered) NEC V95.9 ☑
    balloon V96.05 ☑
    fixed wing NEC (private) V95.25 ☑
      commercial V95.35 ☑
    glider V96.25 ☑
      hang V96.15 ☑
      powered V95.15 ☑
    helicopter V95.05 ☑
    in war operations — *see* War operations, destruction
      of aircraft
    microlight V95.15 ☑
    nonpowered V96.9 ☑
      specified NEC V96.8 ☑
    powered NEC V95.8 ☑
    stated as
      homicide (attempt) Y03.8 ☑
      suicide (attempt) X83.0 ☑
    ultralight V95.15 ☑
  anesthetic gas in operating room W40.1 ☑
  antipersonnel bomb W40.8 ☑
    assault X96.0 ☑
    homicide (attempt) X96.0 ☑
    suicide (attempt) X75 ☑
  assault X96.9 ☑
  bicycle tire W37.0 ☑
  blasting (cap) (materials) W40.0 ☑
  boiler (machinery), not on transport vehicle W35 ☑
    on watercraft — *see* Explosion, in, watercraft
  butane W40.1 ☑
  caused by other person X96.9 ☑
  coal gas W40.1 ☑
  detonator W40.0 ☑
  dump (munitions) W40.8 ☑
  dynamite W40.0 ☑
    in
      assault X96.8 ☑
      homicide (attempt) X96.8 ☑
      legal intervention
        injuring
          bystander Y35.112 ☑
          law enforcement personnel Y35.111 ☑
          suspect Y35.113 ☑
      suicide (attempt) X75 ☑
  explosive (material) W40.9 ☑
    gas W40.1 ☑
    in blasting operation W40.0 ☑
    specified NEC W40.8 ☑
      in
        assault X96.8 ☑
        homicide (attempt) X96.8 ☑
        legal intervention
          injuring
            bystander Y35.192 ☑
            law enforcement personnel
              Y35.191 ☑
            suspect Y35.193 ☑
        suicide (attempt) X75 ☑
  factory (munitions) W40.8 ☑
  fertilizer bomb W40.8 ☑
    assault X96.3 ☑
    homicide (attempt) X96.3 ☑
    suicide (attempt) X75 ☑
  firearm (parts) NEC W34.19 ☑
    airgun W34.110 ☑
    BB gun W34.110 ☑
    gas, air or spring-operated gun NEC W34.118 ☑
    hangun W32.1 ☑

Explosion — *continued*
  firearm — *continued*
    hunting rifle W33.12 ☑
    larger firearm W33.10 ☑
      specified NEC W33.19 ☑
    machine gun W33.13 ☑
    paintball gun W34.111 ☑
    pellet gun W34.110 ☑
    shotgun W33.11 ☑
    Very pistol [flare] W34.19 ☑
  fire-damp W40.1 ☑
  fireworks W39 ☑
  gas (coal) (explosive) W40.1 ☑
    cylinder W36.9 ☑
      aerosol can W36.1 ☑
      air tank W36.2 ☑
      pressurized W36.3 ☑
      specified NEC W36.8 ☑
  gasoline (fumes) (tank) not in moving motor vehicle
    W40.1 ☑
    bomb W40.8 ☑
      assault X96.1 ☑
      homicide (attempt) X96.1 ☑
      suicide (attempt) X75 ☑
    in motor vehicle — *see* Accident, transport, by type
      of vehicle
  grain store W40.8 ☑
  grenade W40.8 ☑
    in
      assault X96.8 ☑
      homicide (attempt) X96.8 ☑
      legal intervention
        injuring
          bystander Y35.192 ☑
          law enforcement personnel Y35.191 ☑
          suspect Y35.193 ☑
      suicide (attempt) X75 ☑
  handgun (parts) — *see* Explosion, firearm, hangun
    (parts)
  homicide (attempt) X96.9 ☑
    antipersonnel bomb — *see* Explosion, antipersonnel
      bomb
    fertilizer bomb — *see* Explosion, fertilizer bomb
    gasoline bomb — *see* Explosion, gasoline bomb
    letter bomb — *see* Explosion, letter bomb
    pipe bomb — *see* Explosion, pipe bomb
    specified NEC X96.8 ☑
  hose, pressurized W37.8 ☑
  hot water heater, tank (in machinery) W35 ☑
    on watercraft — *see* Explosion, in, watercraft
  in, on
    dump W40.8 ☑
    factory W40.8 ☑
    mine (of explosive gases) NEC W40.1 ☑
    watercraft V93.59 ☑
      powered craft V93.53 ☑
        ferry boat V93.51 ☑
        fishing boat V93.52 ☑
        jetskis V93.53 ☑
        liner V93.51 ☑
        merchant ship V93.50 ☑
        passenger ship V93.51 ☑
        sailboat V93.54 ☑
  letter bomb W40.8 ☑
    assault X96.2 ☑
    homicide (attempt) X96.2 ☑
    suicide (attempt) X75 ☑
  machinery (*see also* Contact, with, by type of machine)
    on board watercraft — *see* Explosion, in, watercraft
    pressure vessel — *see* Explosion, by type of vessel
  methane W40.1 ☑
  mine W40.1 ☑
  missile NEC W40.8 ☑
  mortar bomb W40.8 ☑
    in
      assault X96.8 ☑
      homicide (attempt) X96.8 ☑
      legal intervention
        injuring
          bystander Y35.192 ☑
          law enforcement personnel Y35.191 ☑
          suspect Y35.193 ☑
      suicide (attempt) X75 ☑
  munitions (dump) (factory) W40.8 ☑
  pipe, pressurized W37.8 ☑
    bomb W40.8 ☑

Explosion — *continued*
  pipe, pressurized — *continued*
    bomb — *continued*
      assault X96.4 ☑
      homicide (attempt) X96.4 ☑
      suicide (attempt) X75 ☑
  pressure, pressurized
    cooker W38 ☑
    gas tank (in machinery) W36.3 ☑
    hose W37.8 ☑
    pipe W37.8 ☑
    specified device NEC W38 ☑
    tire W37.8 ☑
      bicycle W37.0 ☑
    vessel (in machinery) W38 ☑
  propane W40.1 ☑
  self-inflicted X75 ☑
  shell (artillery) NEC W40.8 ☑
    during war operations — *see* War operations, explosion
    in
      legal intervention
        injuring
          bystander Y35.122 ☑
          law enforcement personnel Y35.121 ☑
          suspect Y35.123 ☑
      war — *see* War operations, explosion
  spacecraft V95.45 ☑
  stated as undetermined whether accidental or intentional Y25 ☑
  steam or water lines (in machinery) W37.8 ☑
  stove W40.9 ☑
  suicide (attempt) X75 ☑
  tire, pressurized W37.8 ☑
    bicycle W37.0 ☑
  undetermined whether accidental or intentional Y25 ☑
  vehicle tire NEC W37.8 ☑
    bicycle W37.0 ☑
  war operations — *see* War operations, explosion
Exposure (to) X58 ☑
  air pressure change — *see* Air, pressure
  cold (accidental) (excessive) (extreme) (natural) (place)
    X31 ☑
    assault Y08.89 ☑
    due to
      man-made conditions W93.8 ☑
        dry ice (contact) W93.01 ☑
          inhalation W93.02 ☑
        liquid air (contact) (hydrogen) (nitrogen)
          W93.11 ☑
          inhalation W93.12 ☑
        refrigeration unit (deep freeze) W93.2 ☑
        suicide (attempt) X83.2 ☑
      weather (conditions) X31 ☑
    homicide (attempt) Y08.89 ☑
    self-inflicted X83.2 ☑
  due to abandonment or neglect X58 ☑
  electric current W86.8 ☑
    appliance (faulty) W86.8 ☑
      domestic W86.0 ☑
    caused by other person Y08.89 ☑
    conductor (faulty) W86.1 ☑
    control apparatus (faulty) W86.1 ☑
    electric power generating plant, distribution station
      W86.1 ☑
    electroshock gun — *see* Exposure, electric current,
      taser
    high-voltage cable W85 ☑
    homicide (attempt) Y08.89 ☑
    legal execution — *see* Legal, intervention, specified
      means NEC
    lightning — *see* subcategory T75.0 ☑
    live rail W86.8 ☑
    misadventure in medical or surgical procedure in
      electroshock therapy Y63.4
    motor (electric) (faulty) W86.8 ☑
      domestic W86.0 ☑
    self-inflicted X83.1 ☑
    specified NEC W86.8 ☑
      domestic W86.0 ☑
    stun gun — *see* Exposure, electric current, taser
    suicide (attempt) X83.1 ☑
    taser W86.8 ☑
      assault Y08.89 ☑
      legal intervention — *see* category Y35 ☑
      self-harm (intentional) X83.8 ☑

Exposure — continued
  electric current — continued
    taser — continued
      undetermined intent Y33 ☑
    third rail W86.8 ☑
    transformer (faulty) W86.1 ☑
    transmission lines W85 ☑
  environmental tobacco smoke X58 ☑
  excessive
    cold — see Exposure, cold
    heat (natural) NEC X30 ☑
      man-made W92 ☑
  factor(s) NOS X58 ☑
    environmental NEC X58 ☑
      man-made NEC W99 ☑
      natural NEC — see Forces of nature
    specified NEC X58 ☑
  fire, flames (accidental) X08.8 ☑
    assault X97 ☑
    campfire — see Exposure, fire, controlled, not in
        building
    controlled (in)
      with ignition (of) clothing (see also Ignition,
          clothes) X06.2 ☑
        nightwear X05 ☑
      bonfire — see Exposure, fire, controlled, not in
          building
      brazier (in building or structure) (see also Expo-
          sure, fire, controlled, building)
        not in building or structure — see Exposure,
            fire, controlled, not in building
      building or structure X02.0 ☑
        with
          fall from building X02.3 ☑
          from building X02.5 ☑
          injury due to building collapse X02.2 ☑
          smoke inhalation X02.1 ☑
          hit by object from building X02.4 ☑
          specified mode of injury NEC X02.8 ☑
      fireplace, furnace or stove — see Exposure, fire,
          controlled, building
      not in building or structure X03.0 ☑
        with
          fall X03.3 ☑
          smoke inhalation X03.1 ☑
          hit by object X03.4 ☑
          specified mode of injury NEC X03.8 ☑
      trash — see Exposure, fire, controlled, not in
          building
    fireplace — see Exposure, fire, controlled, building
    fittings or furniture (in building or structure) (uncon-
        trolled) — see Exposure, fire, uncontrolled,
        building
    forest (uncontrolled) — see Exposure, fire, uncon-
        trolled, not in building
    grass (uncontrolled) — see Exposure, fire, uncon-
        trolled, not in building
    hay (uncontrolled) — see Exposure, fire, uncon-
        trolled, not in building
    homicide (attempt) X97 ☑
    ignition of highly flammable material X04 ☑
    in, of, on, starting in
      machinery — see Contact, with, by type of ma-
          chine
      motor vehicle (in motion) (see also Accident,
          transport, occupant by type of vehicle)
          V87.8 ☑
        with collision — see Collision
      railway rolling stock, train, vehicle V81.81 ☑
        with collision — see Accident, transport, rail-
            way vehicle occupant
      street car (in motion) V82.8 ☑
        with collision — see Accident, transport,
            streetcar occupant
      transport vehicle NEC (see also Accident, trans-
          port)
        with collision — see Collision
      war operations (see also War operations, fire)
        from nuclear explosion — see War operations,
            nuclear weapons
      watercraft (in transit) (not in transit) V91.09 ☑
        localized — see Burn, on board watercraft,
            due to, fire on board
        powered craft V91.03 ☑
          ferry boat V91.01 ☑
          fishing boat V91.02 ☑
          jet skis V91.03 ☑

Exposure — continued
  fire, flames — continued
    in, of, on, starting in — continued
      watercraft — continued
        powered craft — continued
          liner V91.01 ☑
          merchant ship V91.00 ☑
          passenger ship V91.01 ☑
        unpowered craft V91.08 ☑
          canoe V91.05 ☑
          inflatable V91.06 ☑
          kayak V91.05 ☑
          sailboat V91.04 ☑
          surf-board V91.08 ☑
          waterskis V91.07 ☑
          windsurfer V91.08 ☑
    lumber (uncontrolled) — see Exposure, fire, uncon-
        trolled, not in building
    mine (uncontrolled) — see Exposure, fire, uncon-
        trolled, not in building
    prairie (uncontrolled) — see Exposure, fire, uncon-
        trolled, not in building
    resulting from
      explosion — see Explosion
      lightning X08.8 ☑
    self-inflicted X76 ☑
    specified NEC X08.8 ☑
    started by other person X97 ☑
    stated as undetermined whether accidental or inten-
        tional Y26 ☑
    stove — see Exposure, fire, controlled, building
    suicide (attempt) X76 ☑
    tunnel (uncontrolled) — see Exposure, fire, uncon-
        trolled, not in building
    uncontrolled
      in building or structure X00.0 ☑
        with
          fall from building X00.3 ☑
          injury due to building collapse X00.2 ☑
          jump from building X00.5 ☑
          smoke inhalation X00.1 ☑
        bed X08.00 ☑
          due to
            cigarette X08.01 ☑
            specified material NEC X08.09 ☑
        furniture NEC X08.20 ☑
          due to
            cigarette X08.21 ☑
            specified material NEC X08.29 ☑
        hit by object from building X00.4 ☑
        sofa X08.10 ☑
          due to
            cigarette X08.11 ☑
            specified material NEC X08.19 ☑
        specified mode of injury NEC X00.8 ☑
      not in building or structure (any) X01.0 ☑
        with
          fall X01.3 ☑
          smoke inhalation X01.1 ☑
        hit by object X01.4 ☑
        specified mode of injury NEC X01.8 ☑
    undetermined whether accidental or intentional
        Y26 ☑
  forces of nature NEC — see Forces of nature
  G-forces (abnormal) W49.9 ☑
  gravitational forces (abnormal) W49.9 ☑
  heat (natural) NEC — see Heat
  high-pressure jet (hydraulic) (pneumatic) W49.9 ☑
  hydraulic jet W49.9 ☑
  inanimate mechanical force W49.9 ☑
  jet, high-pressure (hydraulic) (pneumatic) W49.9 ☑
  lightning — see subcategory T75.0 ☑
    causing fire — see Exposure, fire
  mechanical forces NEC W49.9 ☑
    animate NEC W64
    inanimate NEC W49.9 ☑
  noise W42.9 ☑
    supersonic W42.0 ☑
  noxious substance — see Table of Drugs and Chemicals
  pneumatic jet W49.9 ☑
  prolonged in deep-freeze unit or refrigerator W93.2 ☑
  radiation — see Radiation
  smoke (see also Exposure, fire)
    tobacco, second hand Z77.22
  specified factors NEC X58 ☑
  sunlight X32 ☑

Exposure — continued
  sunlight — continued
    man-made (sun lamp) W89.8 ☑
      tanning bed W89.1 ☑
  supersonic waves W42.0 ☑
  transmission line(s), electric W85 ☑
  vibration W49.9 ☑
  waves
    infrasound W49.9 ☑
    sound W42.9 ☑
    supersonic W42.0 ☑
  weather NEC — see Forces of nature
External cause status Y99.9
  child assisting in compensated work for family Y99.8
  civilian activity done for financial or other compensa-
      tion Y99.0
  civilian activity done for income or pay Y99.0
  family member assisting in compensated work for
      other family member Y99.8
  hobby not done for income Y99.8
  leisure activity Y99.8
  military activity Y99.1
  off-duty activity of military personnel Y99.8
  recreation or sport not for income or while a student
      Y99.8
  specified NEC Y99.8
  student activity Y99.8
  volunteer activity Y99.2

F

Factors, supplemental
  alcohol
    blood level
      less than 20mg/100ml Y90.0
      presence in blood, level not specified Y90.9
      20-39mg/100ml Y90.1
      40-59mg/100ml Y90.2
      60-79mg/100ml Y90.3
      80-99mg/100ml Y90.4
      100-119mg/100ml Y90.5
      120-199mg/100ml Y90.6
      200-239mg/100ml Y90.7
      240mg/100ml or more Y90.8
    presence in blood, but level not specified Y90.9
  environmental-pollution-related condition- see Z57 ☑
  nosocomial condition Y95
  work-related condition Y99.0
Failure
  in suture or ligature during surgical procedure Y65.2
  mechanical, of instrument or apparatus (any) (during
      any medical or surgical procedure) Y65.8
  sterile precautions (during medical and surgical care)
      — see Misadventure, failure, sterile precautions,
      by type of procedure
  to
    introduce tube or instrument Y65.4
      endotracheal tube during anesthesia Y65.3
    make curve (transport vehicle) NEC — see Accident,
        transport
    remove tube or instrument Y65.4
Fall, falling (accidental) W19 ☑
  building W20.1 ☑
    burning (uncontrolled fire) X00.3 ☑
  down
    embankment W17.81 ☑
    escalator W10.0 ☑
    hill W17.81 ☑
    ladder W11 ☑
    ramp W10.2 ☑
    stairs, steps W10.9 ☑
  due to
    bumping against
      object W18.00 ☑
        sharp glass W18.02 ☑
        specified NEC W18.09 ☑
        sports equipment W18.01 ☑
      person W03 ☑
        due to ice or snow W00.0 ☑
        on pedestrian conveyance — see Accident,
            transport, pedestrian, conveyance
    collision with another person W03 ☑
      due to ice or snow W00.0 ☑
      involving pedestrian conveyance — see Acci-
          dent, transport, pedestrian, conveyance
    grocery cart tipping over W17.82 ☑
    ice or snow W00.9 ☑

Fall, falling — *continued*
- due to — *continued*
  - ice or snow — *continued*
    - from one level to another W00.2 ☑
      - on stairs or steps W00.1 ☑
    - involving pedestrian conveyance — *see* Accident, transport, pedestrian, conveyance
    - on same level W00.0 ☑
  - slipping (on moving sidewalk) W01.0 ☑
    - with subsequent striking against object W01.10 ☑
      - furniture W01.190 ☑
      - sharp object W01.119 ☑
        - glass W01.110 ☑
        - power tool or machine W01.111 ☑
        - specified NEC W01.118 ☑
      - specified NEC W01.198 ☑
  - striking against
    - object W18.00 ☑
      - sharp glass W18.02 ☑
      - specified NEC W18.09 ☑
      - sports equipment W18.01 ☑
    - person W03 ☑
      - due to ice or snow W00.0 ☑
      - on pedestrian conveyance — *see* Accident, transport, pedestrian, conveyance
- earth (with asphyxia or suffocation (by pressure)) — *see* Earth, falling
- from, off, out of
  - aircraft NEC (with accident to aircraft NEC) V97.0 ☑
    - while boarding or alighting V97.1 ☑
  - balcony W13.0 ☑
  - bed W06 ☑
  - boat, ship, watercraft NEC (with drowning or submersion) — *see* Drowning, due to, fall overboard
    - with hitting bottom or object V94.0 ☑
  - bridge W13.1 ☑
  - building W13.9 ☑
    - burning (uncontrolled fire) X00.3 ☑
  - cavity W17.2 ☑
  - chair W07 ☑
  - cherry picker W17.89 ☑
  - cliff W15 ☑
  - dock W17.4 ☑
  - embankment W17.81 ☑
  - escalator W10.0 ☑
  - flagpole W13.8 ☑
  - furniture NEC W08 ☑
  - grocery cart W17.82 ☑
  - haystack W17.89 ☑
  - high place NEC W17.89 ☑
    - stated as undetermined whether accidental or intentional Y30 ☑
  - hole W17.2 ☑
  - incline W10.2 ☑
  - ladder W11 ☑
  - lifting device W17.89 ☑
  - machine, machinery (*see also* Contact, with, by type of machine)
    - not in operation W17.89 ☑
  - manhole W17.1 ☑
  - mobile elevated work platform [MEWP] W17.89 ☑
  - motorized mobility scooter W05.2 ☑
  - one level to another NEC W17.89 ☑
    - intentional, purposeful, suicide (attempt) X80 ☑
    - stated as undetermined whether accidental or intentional Y30 ☑
  - pit W17.2 ☑
  - playground equipment W09.8 ☑
    - jungle gym W09.2 ☑
    - slide W09.0 ☑
    - swing W09.1 ☑
  - quarry W17.89 ☑
  - railing W13.9 ☑
  - ramp W10.2 ☑
  - roof W13.2 ☑
  - scaffolding W12 ☑
  - scooter (nonmotorized) W05.1 ☑
    - motorized mobility W05.2 ☑
  - sky lift W17.89 ☑
  - stairs, steps W10.9 ☑
    - curb W10.1 ☑
    - due to ice or snow W00.1 ☑
    - escalator W10.0 ☑
    - incline W10.2 ☑

Fall, falling — *continued*
- from, off, out of — *continued*
  - stairs, steps — *continued*
    - ramp W10.2 ☑
    - sidewalk curb W10.1 ☑
    - specified NEC W10.8 ☑
  - stepladder W11 ☑
  - storm drain W17.1 ☑
  - streetcar NEC V82.6 ☑
    - while boarding or alighting V82.4 ☑
    - with antecedent collision — *see* Accident, transport, streetcar occupant
  - structure NEC W13.8 ☑
    - burning (uncontrolled fire) X00.3 ☑
  - table W08 ☑
  - toilet W18.11 ☑
    - with subsequent striking against object W18.12 ☑
  - train NEC V81.6 ☑
    - during derailment (without antecedent collision) V81.7 ☑
      - with antecedent collision — *see* Accident, transport, railway vehicle occupant
    - while boarding or alighting V81.4 ☑
  - transport vehicle after collision — *see* Accident, transport, by type of vehicle, collision
  - tree W14 ☑
  - vehicle (in motion) NEC (*see also* Accident, transport) V89.9 ☑
    - motor NEC (*see also* Accident, transport, occupant, by type of vehicle) V87.8 ☑
    - stationary W17.89 ☑
      - while boarding or alighting — *see* Accident, transport, by type of vehicle, while boarding or alighting
  - viaduct W13.8 ☑
  - wall W13.8 ☑
  - watercraft (*see also* Drowning, due to, fall overboard)
    - with hitting bottom or object V94.0 ☑
  - well W17.0 ☑
  - wheelchair, non-moving W05.0 ☑
    - powered — *see* Accident, transport, pedestrian, conveyance occupant, specified type NEC
  - window W13.4 ☑
- in, on
  - aircraft NEC V97.0 ☑
    - while boarding or alighting V97.1 ☑
    - with accident to aircraft V97.0 ☑
  - bathtub (empty) W18.2 ☑
    - filled W16.212 ☑
      - causing drowning W16.211 ☑
  - escalator W10.0 ☑
  - incline W10.2 ☑
  - ladder W11 ☑
  - machine, machinery — *see* Contact, with, by type of machine
  - object, edged, pointed or sharp (with cut) — *see* Fall, by type
  - playground equipment W09.8 ☑
    - jungle gym W09.2 ☑
    - slide W09.0 ☑
    - swing W09.1 ☑
  - ramp W10.2 ☑
  - scaffolding W12 ☑
  - shower W18.2 ☑
    - causing drowning W16.211 ☑
  - staircase, stairs, steps W10.9 ☑
    - curb W10.1 ☑
    - due to ice or snow W00.1 ☑
    - escalator W10.0 ☑
    - incline W10.2 ☑
    - specified NEC W10.8 ☑
  - streetcar (without antecedent collision) V82.5 ☑
    - with antecedent collision — *see* Accident, transport, streetcar occupant
    - while boarding or alighting V82.4 ☑
  - train (without antecedent collision) V81.5 ☑
    - with antecedent collision — *see* Accident, transport, railway vehicle occupant
    - during derailment (without antecedent collision) V81.7 ☑
      - with antecedent collision — *see* Accident, transport, railway vehicle occupant
    - while boarding or alighting V81.4 ☑

Fall, falling — *continued*
- in, on — *continued*
  - transport vehicle after collision — *see* Accident, transport, by type of vehicle, collision
  - watercraft V93.39 ☑
    - due to
      - accident to craft V91.29 ☑
        - powered craft V91.23 ☑
          - ferry boat V91.21 ☑
          - fishing boat V91.22 ☑
          - jetskis V91.23 ☑
          - liner V91.21 ☑
          - merchant ship V91.20 ☑
          - passenger ship V91.21 ☑
        - unpowered craft
          - canoe V91.25 ☑
          - inflatable V91.26 ☑
          - kayak V91.25 ☑
          - sailboat V91.24 ☑
      - powered craft V93.33 ☑
        - ferry boat V93.31 ☑
        - fishing boat V93.32 ☑
        - jetskis V93.33 ☑
        - liner V93.31 ☑
        - merchant ship V93.30 ☑
        - passenger ship V93.31 ☑
      - unpowered craft V93.38 ☑
        - canoe V93.35 ☑
        - inflatable V93.36 ☑
        - kayak V93.35 ☑
        - sailboat V93.34 ☑
        - surf-board V93.38 ☑
        - windsurfer V93.38 ☑
- into
  - cavity W17.2 ☑
  - dock W17.4 ☑
  - fire — *see* Exposure, fire, by type
  - haystack W17.89 ☑
  - hole W17.2 ☑
  - lake — *see* Fall, into, water
  - manhole W17.1 ☑
  - moving part of machinery — *see* Contact, with, by type of machine
  - ocean — *see* Fall, into, water
  - opening in surface NEC W17.89 ☑
  - pit W17.2 ☑
  - pond — *see* Fall, into, water
  - quarry W17.89 ☑
  - river — *see* Fall, into, water
  - shaft W17.89 ☑
  - storm drain W17.1 ☑
  - stream — *see* Fall, into, water
  - swimming pool (*see also* Fall, into, water, in, swimming pool)
    - empty W17.3 ☑
  - tank W17.89 ☑
  - water W16.42 ☑
    - causing drowning W16.41 ☑
    - from watercraft — *see* Drowning, due to, fall overboard
    - hitting diving board W21.4 ☑
    - in
      - bathtub W16.212 ☑
        - causing drowning W16.211 ☑
      - bucket W16.222 ☑
        - causing drowning W16.221 ☑
      - natural body of water W16.112 ☑
        - causing drowning W16.111 ☑
        - striking
          - bottom W16.122 ☑
            - causing drowning W16.121 ☑
          - side W16.132 ☑
            - causing drowning W16.131 ☑
      - specified water NEC W16.312 ☑
        - causing drowning W16.311 ☑
        - striking
          - bottom W16.322 ☑
            - causing drowning W16.321 ☑
          - wall W16.332 ☑
            - causing drowning W16.331 ☑
      - swimming pool W16.012 ☑
        - causing drowning W16.011 ☑
        - striking
          - bottom W16.022 ☑
            - causing drowning W16.031 ☑
          - wall W16.032 ☑

Fall, falling — *continued*
  into — *continued*
    water — *continued*
      in — *continued*
        swimming pool — *continued*
          striking — *continued*
            wall — *continued*
              causing drowning W16.021 ☑
          utility bucket W16.222 ☑
            causing drowning W16.221 ☑
      well W17.0 ☑
  involving
    bed W06 ☑
    chair W07 ☑
    furniture NEC W08 ☑
    glass — *see* Fall, by type
    playground equipment W09.8 ☑
      jungle gym W09.2 ☑
      slide W09.0 ☑
      swing W09.1 ☑
    roller blades — *see* Accident, transport, pedestrian, conveyance
    skateboard(s) — *see* Accident, transport, pedestrian, conveyance
    skates (ice) (in line) (roller) — *see* Accident, transport, pedestrian, conveyance
    skis — *see* Accident, transport, pedestrian, conveyance
    table W08 ☑
    wheelchair, non-moving W05.0 ☑
      powered — *see* Accident, transport, pedestrian, conveyance, specified type NEC
  object — *see* Struck by, object, falling
  off
    toilet W18.11 ☑
      with subsequent striking against object W18.12 ☑
  on same level W18.30 ☑
    due to
      specified NEC W18.39 ☑
      stepping on an object W18.31 ☑
  out of
    bed W06 ☑
    building NEC W13.8 ☑
    chair W07 ☑
    furniture NEC W08 ☑
    wheelchair, non-moving W05.0 ☑
      powered — *see* Accident, transport, pedestrian, conveyance, specified type NEC
    window W13.4 ☑
  over
    animal W01.0 ☑
    cliff W15 ☑
    embankment W17.81 ☑
    small object W01.0 ☑
  rock W20.8 ☑
  same level W18.30 ☑
    from
      being crushed, pushed, or stepped on by a crowd or human stampede W52 ☑
      collision, pushing, shoving, by or with other person W03 ☑
      slipping, stumbling, tripping W01.0 ☑
      involving ice or snow W00.0 ☑
      involving skates (ice) (roller), skateboard, skis — *see* Accident, transport, pedestrian, conveyance
  snowslide (avalanche) — *see* Landslide
  stone W20.8 ☑
  structure W20.1 ☑
    burning (uncontrolled fire) X00.3 ☑
  through
    bridge W13.1 ☑
    floor W13.3 ☑
    roof W13.2 ☑
    wall W13.8 ☑
    window W13.4 ☑
  timber W20.8 ☑
  tree (caused by lightning) W20.8 ☑
  while being carried or supported by other person(s) W04 ☑
Fallen on by
  animal (not being ridden) NEC W55.89 ☑
Felo-de-se — *see* Suicide
Fight (hand) (fists) (foot) — *see* Assault, fight
Fire (accidental) — *see* Exposure, fire

Firearm discharge — *see* Discharge, firearm
Fireball effects from nuclear explosion in war operations — *see* War operations, nuclear weapons
Fireworks (explosion) W39 ☑
Flash burns from explosion — *see* Explosion
Flood (any injury) (caused by) X38 ☑
  collapse of man-made structure causing earth movement X36.0 ☑
  tidal wave — *see* Forces of nature, tidal wave
Food (any type) **in**
  air passages (with asphyxia, obstruction, or suffocation) — *see* categories T17 and T18 ☑
  alimentary tract causing asphyxia (due to compression of trachea) — *see* categories T17 and T18 ☑
Forces of nature X39.8 ☑
  avalanche X36.1 ☑
    causing transport accident — *see* Accident, transport, by type of vehicle
  blizzard X37.2 ☑
  cataclysmic storm X37.9 ☑
    with flood X38 ☑
    blizzard X37.2 ☑
    cloudburst X37.8 ☑
    cyclone X37.1 ☑
    dust storm X37.3 ☑
    hurricane X37.0 ☑
    specified storm NEC X37.8 ☑
    storm surge X37.0 ☑
    tornado X37.1 ☑
    twister X37.1 ☑
    typhoon X37.0 ☑
  cloudburst X37.8 ☑
  cold (natural) X31 ☑
  cyclone X37.1 ☑
  dam collapse causing earth movement X36.0 ☑
  dust storm X37.3 ☑
  earth movement X36.1 ☑
    caused by dam or structure collapse X36.0 ☑
    earthquake X34 ☑
  earthquake X34 ☑
  flood (caused by) X38 ☑
    dam collapse X36.0 ☑
    tidal wave — *see* Forces of nature, tidal wave
  heat (natural) X30 ☑
  hurricane X37.0 ☑
  landslide X36.1 ☑
    causing transport accident — *see* Accident, transport, by type of vehicle
  lightning — *see* subcategory T75.0 ☑
    causing fire — *see* Exposure, fire
  mudslide X36.1 ☑
    causing transport accident — *see* Accident, transport, by type of vehicle
  radiation (natural) X39.08 ☑
    radon X39.01 ☑
  radon X39.01 ☑
  specified force NEC X39.8 ☑
  storm surge X37.0 ☑
  structure collapse causing earth movement X36.0 ☑
  sunlight X32 ☑
  tidal wave X37.41 ☑
    due to
      earthquake X37.41 ☑
      landslide X37.43 ☑
      storm X37.42 ☑
      volcanic eruption X37.41 ☑
  tornado X37.1 ☑
  tsunami X37.41 ☑
  twister X37.1 ☑
  typhoon X37.0 ☑
  volcanic eruption X35 ☑
Foreign body
  aspiration — *see* Index to Diseases and Injuries, Foreign body, respiratory tract
  embedded in skin W45 ☑
  entering through skin W45.8 ☑
    can lid W26.8 ☑
    nail W45.0 ☑
    paper W26.2 ☑
    specified NEC W45.8 ☑
    splinter W45.8 ☑
Forest fire (exposure to) — *see* Exposure, fire, uncontrolled, not in building
Found injured X58 ☑
  from exposure (to) — *see* Exposure

Found injured — *continued*
  on
    highway, road(way), street V89.9 ☑
    railway right of way V81.9 ☑
Fracture (circumstances unknown or unspecified) X58 ☑
  due to specified cause NEC X58 ☑
Freezing — *see* Exposure, cold
Frostbite X31 ☑
  due to man-made conditions — *see* Exposure, cold, man-made
Frozen — *see* Exposure, cold

G

Gored by bull W55.22 ☑
Gunshot wound W34.00 ☑

H

Hailstones, injured by X39.8 ☑
Hanged herself or himself — *see* Hanging, self-inflicted
Hanging (accidental) (*see also* category) T71 ☑
  legal execution — *see* Legal, intervention, specified means NEC
Heat (effects of) (excessive) X30 ☑
  due to
    man-made conditions W92 ☑
      on board watercraft V93.29 ☑
        fishing boat V93.22 ☑
        merchant ship V93.20 ☑
        passenger ship V93.21 ☑
        sailboat V93.24 ☑
        specified powered craft NEC V93.23 ☑
    weather (conditions) X30 ☑
  from
    electric heating apparatus causing burning X16 ☑
    nuclear explosion in war operations — *see* War operations, nuclear weapons
  inappropriate in local application or packing in medical or surgical procedure Y63.5
Hemorrhage
  delayed following medical or surgical treatment without mention of misadventure — *see* Index to Diseases and Injuries, Complication(s)
  during medical or surgical treatment as misadventure — *see* Index to Diseases and Injuries, Complication(s)
High
  altitude (effects) — *see* Air, pressure, low
  level of radioactivity, effects — *see* Radiation
  pressure (effects) — *see* Air, pressure, high
  temperature, effects — *see* Heat
Hit, hitting (accidental) by — *see* Struck by
Hitting against — *see* Striking against
Homicide (attempt) (justifiable) — *see* Assault
Hot
  place, effects (*see also* Heat)
  weather, effects X30 ☑
House fire (uncontrolled) — *see* Exposure, fire, uncontrolled, building
Humidity, causing problem X39.8 ☑
Hunger X58 ☑
Hurricane (any injury) X37.0 ☑
Hypobarism, hypobaropathy — *see* Air, pressure, low

I

Ictus
  caloris (*see also* Heat)
  solaris X30 ☑
Ignition (accidental) (*see also* Exposure, fire) X08.8 ☑
  anesthetic gas in operating room W40.1 ☑
  apparel X06.2 ☑
    from highly flammable material X04 ☑
    nightwear X05 ☑
  bed linen (sheets) (spreads) (pillows) (mattress) — *see* Exposure, fire, uncontrolled, building, bed
  benzine X04 ☑
  clothes, clothing NEC (from controlled fire) X06.2 ☑
    from
      highly flammable material X04 ☑
  ether X04 ☑
    in operating room W40.1 ☑
  explosive material — *see* Explosion
  gasoline X04 ☑
  jewelry (plastic) (any) X06.0 ☑

Ignition — *continued*
  kerosene X04 ☑
  material
    explosive — *see* Explosion
    highly flammable with secondary explosion X04 ☑
  nightwear X05 ☑
  paraffin X04 ☑
  petrol X04 ☑
Immersion (accidental) (*see also* Drowning)
  hand or foot due to cold (excessive) X31 ☑
Implantation of quills of porcupine W55.89 ☑
Inanition (from) (hunger) X58 ☑
  thirst X58 ☑
Inappropriate operation performed
  correct operation on wrong side or body part (wrong side) (wrong site) Y65.53
  operation intended for another patient done on wrong patient Y65.52
  wrong operation performed on correct patient Y65.51
Inattention after, at birth (homicidal intent) (infanticidal intent) X58 ☑
Incident, adverse
  device
    anesthesiology Y70.8
      accessory Y70.2
      diagnostic Y70.0
      miscellaneous Y70.8
      monitoring Y70.0
      prosthetic Y70.2
      rehabilitative Y70.1
      surgical Y70.3
      therapeutic Y70.1
    cardiovascular Y71.8
      accessory Y71.2
      diagnostic Y71.0
      miscellaneous Y71.8
      monitoring Y71.0
      prosthetic Y71.2
      rehabilitative Y71.1
      surgical Y71.3
      therapeutic Y71.1
    gastroenterology Y73.8
      accessory Y73.2
      diagnostic Y73.0
      miscellaneous Y73.8
      monitoring Y73.0
      prosthetic Y73.2
      rehabilitative Y73.1
      surgical Y73.3
      therapeutic Y73.1
    general
      hospital Y74.8
        accessory Y74.2
        diagnostic Y74.0
        miscellaneous Y74.8
        monitoring Y74.0
        prosthetic Y74.2
        rehabilitative Y74.1
        surgical Y74.3
        therapeutic Y74.1
      surgical Y81.8
        accessory Y81.2
        diagnostic Y81.0
        miscellaneous Y81.8
        monitoring Y81.0
        prosthetic Y81.2
        rehabilitative Y81.1
        surgical Y81.3
        therapeutic Y81.1
    gynecological Y76.8
      accessory Y76.2
      diagnostic Y76.0
      miscellaneous Y76.8
      monitoring Y76.0
      prosthetic Y76.2
      rehabilitative Y76.1
      surgical Y76.3
      therapeutic Y76.1
    medical Y82.9
      specified type NEC Y82.8
    neurological Y75.8
      accessory Y75.2
      diagnostic Y75.0
      miscellaneous Y75.8
      monitoring Y75.0
      prosthetic Y75.2
      rehabilitative Y75.1
      surgical Y75.3

Incident, adverse — *continued*
  device — *continued*
    neurological — *continued*
      therapeutic Y75.1
    obstetrical Y76.8
      accessory Y76.2
      diagnostic Y76.0
      miscellaneous Y76.8
      monitoring Y76.0
      prosthetic Y76.2
      rehabilitative Y76.1
      surgical Y76.3
      therapeutic Y76.1
    ophthalmic Y77.8
      accessory Y77.2
      diagnostic Y77.0
      miscellaneous Y77.8
      monitoring Y77.0
      prosthetic Y77.2
      rehabilitative Y77.1
      surgical Y77.3
      therapeutic Y77.1
    orthopedic Y79.8
      accessory Y79.2
      diagnostic Y79.0
      miscellaneous Y79.8
      monitoring Y79.0
      prosthetic Y79.2
      rehabilitative Y79.1
      surgical Y79.3
      therapeutic Y79.1
    otorhinolaryngological Y72.8
      accessory Y72.2
      diagnostic Y72.0
      miscellaneous Y72.8
      monitoring Y72.0
      prosthetic Y72.2
      rehabilitative Y72.1
      surgical Y72.3
      therapeutic Y72.1
    personal use Y74.8
      accessory Y74.2
      diagnostic Y74.0
      miscellaneous Y74.8
      monitoring Y74.0
      prosthetic Y74.2
      rehabilitative Y74.1
      surgical Y74.3
      therapeutic Y74.1
    physical medicine Y80.8
      accessory Y80.2
      diagnostic Y80.0
      miscellaneous Y80.8
      monitoring Y80.0
      prosthetic Y80.2
      rehabilitative Y80.1
      surgical Y80.3
      therapeutic Y80.1
    plastic surgical Y81.8
      accessory Y81.2
      diagnostic Y81.0
      miscellaneous Y81.8
      monitoring Y81.0
      prosthetic Y81.2
      rehabilitative Y81.1
      surgical Y81.3
      therapeutic Y81.1
    radiological Y78.8
      accessory Y78.2
      diagnostic Y78.0
      miscellaneous Y78.8
      monitoring Y78.0
      prosthetic Y78.2
      rehabilitative Y78.1
      surgical Y78.3
      therapeutic Y78.1
    urology Y73.8
      accessory Y73.2
      diagnostic Y73.0
      miscellaneous Y73.8
      monitoring Y73.0
      prosthetic Y73.2
      rehabilitative Y73.1
      surgical Y73.3
      therapeutic Y73.1
Incineration (accidental) — *see* Exposure, fire
Infanticide — *see* Assault
Infrasound waves (causing injury) W49.9 ☑

Ingestion
  foreign body (causing injury) (with obstruction) — *see* Foreign body, alimentary canal
  poisonous
    plant(s) X58 ☑
    substance NEC — *see* Table of Drugs and Chemicals
Inhalation
  excessively cold substance, man-made — *see* Exposure, cold, man-made
  food (any type) (into respiratory tract) (with asphyxia, obstruction respiratory tract, suffocation) — *see* categories T17 and T18
  foreign body — *see* Foreign body, aspiration
  gastric contents (with asphyxia, obstruction respiratory passage, suffocation) T17.81- ☑
  hot air or gases X14.0 ☑
  liquid air, hydrogen, nitrogen W93.12 ☑
    suicide (attempt) X83.2 ☑
  steam X13.0 ☑
    assault X98.0 ☑
    stated as undetermined whether accidental or intentional Y27.0 ☑
    suicide (attempt) X77.0 ☑
  toxic gas — *see* Table of Drugs and Chemicals
  vomitus (with asphyxia, obstruction respiratory passage, suffocation) T17.81- ☑
Injury, injured (accidental(ly)) NOS X58 ☑
  by, caused by, from
    assault — *see* Assault
    law-enforcing agent, police, in course of legal intervention — *see* Legal intervention
    suicide (attempt) X83.8 ☑
  due to, in
    civil insurrection — *see* War operations
    fight (*see also* Assault, fight) Y04.0 ☑
    war operations — *see* War operations
  homicide (*see also* Assault) Y09
  inflicted (by)
    in course of arrest (attempted), suppression of disturbance, maintenance of order, by law-enforcing agents — *see* Legal intervention
    other person
      stated as
        accidental X58 ☑
        intentional, homicide (attempt) — *see* Assault
        undetermined whether accidental or intentional Y33 ☑
  purposely (inflicted) by other person(s) — *see* Assault
  self-inflicted X83.8 ☑
    stated as accidental X58 ☑
  specified cause NEC X58 ☑
  undetermined whether accidental or intentional Y33 ☑
Insolation, effects X30 ☑
Insufficient nourishment X58 ☑
Interruption of respiration (by)
  food (lodged in esophagus) — *see* categories T17 and T18 ☑
  vomitus (lodged in esophagus) T17.81- ☑
Intervention, legal — *see* Legal intervention
Intoxication
  drug — *see* Table of Drugs and Chemicals
  poison — *see* Table of Drugs and Chemicals

J

Jammed (accidentally)
  between objects (moving) (stationary and moving) W23.0 ☑
    stationary W23.1 ☑
Jumped, jumping
  before moving object NEC X81.8 ☑
    motor vehicle X81.0 ☑
    subway train X81.1 ☑
    train X81.1 ☑
    undetermined whether accidental or intentional Y31 ☑
  from
    boat (into water) voluntarily, without accident (to or on boat) W16.712 ☑
      striking bottom W16.722 ☑
        causing drowning W16.721 ☑
      with
        accident to or on boat — *see* Accident, watercraft
        drowning or submersion W16.711 ☑
          suicide (attempt) X71.3 ☑

Jumped, jumping — continued

from — *continued*
  building (*see also* Jumped, from, high place)
    W13.9 ☑
    burning (uncontrolled fire) X00.5 ☑
  high place NEC W17.89 ☑
    suicide (attempt) X80 ☑
    undetermined whether accidental or intentional
      Y30 ☑
  structure (*see also* Jumped, from, high place)
    W13.9 ☑
    burning (uncontrolled fire) X00.5 ☑
  into water W16.92 ☑
    causing drowning W16.91 ☑
  from, off watercraft — *see* Jumped, from, boat
in
  natural body W16.612 ☑
    causing drowning W16.611 ☑
    striking bottom W16.622 ☑
      causing drowning W16.621 ☑
  specified place NEC W16.812 ☑
    causing drowning W16.811 ☑
    striking
      bottom W16.822 ☑
        causing drowning W16.821 ☑
      wall W16.832 ☑
        causing drowning W16.831 ☑
  swimming pool W16.512 ☑
    causing drowning W16.511 ☑
    striking
      bottom W16.522 ☑
        causing drowning W16.521 ☑
      wall W16.532 ☑
        causing drowning W16.531 ☑
suicide (attempt) X71.3 ☑

K

Kicked by

animal NEC W55.82 ☑
person(s) (accidentally) W50.1 ☑
  with intent to injure or kill Y04.0 ☑
  as, or caused by, a crowd or human stampede (with
    fall) W52 ☑
  assault Y04.0 ☑
  homicide (attempt) Y04.0 ☑
  in
    fight Y04.0 ☑
    legal intervention
      injuring
        bystander Y35.812 ☑
        law enforcement personnel Y35.811 ☑
        suspect Y35.813 ☑

Kicking

against
  object W22.8 ☑
    sports equipment W21.9 ☑
    stationary W22.09 ☑
      sports equipment W21.89 ☑
  person — *see* Striking against, person
  sports equipment W21.9 ☑
carpet stretcher with knee X50.3 ☑

Killed, killing (accidentally) NOS (*see also* Injury) X58 ☑
in
  action — *see* War operations
  brawl, fight (hand) (fists) (foot) Y04.0 ☑
    by weapon (*see also* Assault)
      cutting, piercing — *see* Assault, cutting or
        piercing instrument
      firearm — *see* Discharge, firearm, by type,
        homicide
self
  stated as
    accident NOS X58 ☑
    suicide — *see* Suicide
    undetermined whether accidental or intentional
      Y33 ☑
Kneeling (prolonged) (static) X50.1 ☑
Knocked down (accidentally) (by) NOS X58 ☑
animal (not being ridden) NEC (*see also* Struck by, by
  type of animal)
crowd or human stampede W52 ☑
person W51 ☑
  in brawl, fight Y04.0 ☑
transport vehicle NEC (*see also* Accident, transport)
  V09.9 ☑

L

Laceration NEC — *see* Injury
Lack of
care (helpless person) (infant) (newborn) X58 ☑
food except as result of abandonment or neglect
  X58 ☑
  due to abandonment or neglect X58 ☑
water except as result of transport accident X58 ☑
  due to transport accident — *see* Accident, transport,
    by type
helpless person, infant, newborn X58 ☑
Landslide (falling on transport vehicle) X36.1 ☑
caused by collapse of man-made structure X36.0 ☑
Late effect — *see* Sequelae
Legal
execution (any method) — *see* Legal, intervention
intervention (by)
  baton — *see* Legal, intervention, blunt object, baton
  bayonet — *see* Legal, intervention, sharp object,
    bayonet
  blow — *see* Legal, intervention, manhandling
  blunt object
    baton
      injuring
        bystander Y35.312 ☑
        law enforcement personnel Y35.311 ☑
        suspect Y35.313 ☑
    injuring
      bystander Y35.302 ☑
      law enforcement personnel Y35.301 ☑
      suspect Y35.303 ☑
    specified NEC
      injuring
        bystander Y35.392 ☑
        law enforcement personnel Y35.391 ☑
        suspect Y35.393 ☑
    stave
      injuring
        bystander Y35.392 ☑
        law enforcement personnel Y35.391 ☑
        suspect Y35.393 ☑
  bomb — *see* Legal, intervention, explosive
  cutting or piercing instrument — *see* Legal, inter-
    vention, sharp object
  dynamite — *see* Legal, intervention, explosive, dy-
    namite
  explosive(s)
    dynamite
      injuring
        bystander Y35.112 ☑
        law enforcement personnel Y35.111 ☑
        suspect Y35.113 ☑
    grenade
      injuring
        bystander Y35.192 ☑
        law enforcement personnel Y35.191 ☑
        suspect Y35.193 ☑
    injuring
      bystander Y35.102 ☑
      law enforcement personnel Y35.101 ☑
      suspect Y35.103 ☑
    mortar bomb
      injuring
        bystander Y35.192 ☑
        law enforcement personnel Y35.191 ☑
        suspect Y35.193 ☑
    shell
      injuring
        bystander Y35.122 ☑
        law enforcement personnel Y35.121 ☑
        suspect Y35.123 ☑
    specified NEC
      injuring
        bystander Y35.192 ☑
        law enforcement personnel Y35.191 ☑
        suspect Y35.193 ☑
  firearm(s) (discharge)
    handgun
      injuring
        bystander Y35.022 ☑
        law enforcement personnel Y35.021 ☑
        suspect Y35.023 ☑
    injuring
      bystander Y35.002 ☑
      law enforcement personnel Y35.001 ☑

Legal — continued

intervention — *continued*
  firearm(s) — *continued*
    injuring — *continued*
      suspect Y35.003 ☑
    machine gun
      injuring
        bystander Y35.012 ☑
        law enforcement personnel Y35.011 ☑
        suspect Y35.013 ☑
    rifle pellet
      injuring
        bystander Y35.032 ☑
        law enforcement personnel Y35.031 ☑
        suspect Y35.033 ☑
    rubber bullet
      injuring
        bystander Y35.042 ☑
        law enforcement personnel Y35.041 ☑
        suspect Y35.043 ☑
    shotgun — *see* Legal, intervention, firearm,
      specified NEC
    specified NEC
      injuring
        bystander Y35.092 ☑
        law enforcement personnel Y35.091 ☑
        suspect Y35.093 ☑
  gas (asphyxiation) (poisoning)
    injuring
      bystander Y35.202 ☑
      law enforcement personnel Y35.201 ☑
      suspect Y35.203 ☑
    specified NEC
      injuring
        bystander Y35.292 ☑
        law enforcement personnel Y35.291 ☑
        suspect Y35.293 ☑
    tear gas
      injuring
        bystander Y35.212 ☑
        law enforcement personnel Y35.211 ☑
        suspect Y35.213 ☑
  grenade — *see* Legal, intervention, explosive,
    grenade
  injuring
    bystander Y35.92 ☑
    law enforcement personnel Y35.91 ☑
    suspect Y35.93 ☑
  late effect (of) — *see* with 7th character S Y35 ☑
  manhandling
    injuring
      bystander Y35.812 ☑
      law enforcement personnel Y35.811 ☑
      suspect Y35.813 ☑
  sequelae (of) — *see* with 7th character S Y35 ☑
  sharp objects
    bayonet
      injuring
        bystander Y35.412 ☑
        law enforcement personnel Y35.411 ☑
        suspect Y35.413 ☑
    injuring
      bystander Y35.402 ☑
      law enforcement personnel Y35.401 ☑
      suspect Y35.403 ☑
    specified NEC
      injuring
        bystander Y35.492 ☑
        law enforcement personnel Y35.491 ☑
        suspect Y35.493 ☑
  specified means NEC
    injuring
      bystander Y35.892 ☑
      law enforcement personnel Y35.891 ☑
      suspect Y35.893 ☑
  stabbing — *see* Legal, intervention, sharp object
  stave — *see* Legal, intervention, blunt object, stave
  tear gas — *see* Legal, intervention, gas, tear gas
  truncheon — *see* Legal, intervention, blunt object,
    stave
Lifting — *see also* Overexertion
heavy objects X50.0 ☑
weights X50.0 ☑
Lightning (shock) (stroke) (struck by) — *see* subcategory
  T75.0 ☑
causing fire — *see* Exposure, fire

Loss of control (transport vehicle) NEC — *see* Accident, transport
Lost at sea NOS — *see* Drowning, due to, fall overboard
Low
  pressure (effects) — *see* Air, pressure, low
  temperature (effects) — *see* Exposure, cold
Lying before train, vehicle or other moving object
  X81.8 ☑
  subway train X81.1 ☑
  train X81.1 ☑
  undetermined whether accidental or intentional Y31 ☑
Lynching — *see* Assault

M

Malfunction (mechanism or component) (of)
  firearm W34.10 ☑
    airgun W34.110 ☑
    BB gun W34.110 ☑
    gas, air or spring-operated gun NEC W34.118 ☑
    handgun W32.1 ☑
    hunting rifle W33.12 ☑
    larger firearm W33.10 ☑
      specified NEC W33.19 ☑
    machine gun W33.13 ☑
    paintball gun W34.111 ☑
    pellet gun W34.110 ☑
    shotgun W33.11 ☑
    specified NEC W34.19 ☑
    Very pistol [flare] W34.19 ☑
  handgun — *see* Malfunction, firearm, handgun
Maltreatment — *see* Perpetrator
Mangled (accidentally) NOS X58 ☑
Manhandling (in brawl, fight) Y04.0 ☑
  legal intervention — *see* Legal, intervention, manhandling
Manslaughter (nonaccidental) — *see* Assault
Mauled by animal NEC W55.89 ☑
Medical procedure, complication of (delayed or as an abnormal reaction without mention of misadventure) — *see* Complication of or following, by specified type of procedure
  due to or as a result of misadventure — *see* Misadventure
Melting (due to fire) (*see also* Exposure, fire)
  apparel NEC X06.3 ☑
  clothes, clothing NEC X06.3 ☑
    nightwear X05 ☑
  fittings or furniture (burning building) (uncontrolled fire) X00.8 ☑
  nightwear X05 ☑
  plastic jewelry X06.1 ☑
Mental cruelty X58 ☑
Military operations (injuries to military and civilians occuring during peacetime on military property and during routine military exercises and operations) (by) (from) (involving) Y37.90- ☑
  air blast Y37.20- ☑
  aircraft
    destruction — *see* Military operations, destruction of aircraft
  airway restriction — *see* Military operations, restriction of airways
  asphyxiation — *see* Military operations, restriction of airways
  biological weapons Y37.6X- ☑
  blast Y37.20- ☑
  blast fragments Y37.20- ☑
  blast wave Y37.20- ☑
  blast wind Y37.20- ☑
  bomb Y37.20- ☑
    dirty Y37.50- ☑
    gasoline Y37.31- ☑
    incendiary Y37.31- ☑
    petrol Y37.31- ☑
  bullet Y37.43- ☑
    incendiary Y37.32- ☑
    rubber Y37.41- ☑
  chemical weapons Y37.7X- ☑
  combat
    hand to hand (unarmed) combat Y37.44- ☑
    using blunt or piercing object Y37.45- ☑
  conflagration — *see* Military operations, fire
  conventional warfare NEC Y37.49- ☑
  depth-charge Y37.01- ☑
  destruction of aircraft Y37.10- ☑

Military operations — *continued*
  destruction of aircraft — *continued*
    due to
      air to air missile Y37.11- ☑
      collision with other aircraft Y37.12- ☑
      detonation (accidental) of onboard munitions and explosives Y37.14- ☑
      enemy fire or explosives Y37.11- ☑
      explosive placed on aircraft Y37.11- ☑
      onboard fire Y37.13- ☑
      rocket propelled grenade [RPG] Y37.11- ☑
      small arms fire Y37.11- ☑
      surface to air missile Y37.11- ☑
    specified NEC Y37.19- ☑
  detonation (accidental) of
    onboard marine weapons Y37.05- ☑
    own munitions or munitions launch device Y37.24- ☑
  dirty bomb Y37.50- ☑
  explosion (of) Y37.20- ☑
    aerial bomb Y37.21- ☑
    bomb NOS (*see also* Military operations, bomb(s)) Y37.20- ☑
    fragments Y37.20- ☑
    grenade Y37.29- ☑
    guided missile Y37.22- ☑
    improvised explosive device [IED] (person-borne) (roadside) (vehicle-borne) Y37.23- ☑
    land mine Y37.29- ☑
    marine mine (at sea) (in harbor) Y37.02- ☑
    marine weapon Y37.00- ☑
      specified NEC Y37.09- ☑
    own munitions or munitions launch device (accidental) Y37.24- ☑
    sea-based artillery shell Y37.03- ☑
    specified NEC Y37.29- ☑
    torpedo Y37.04- ☑
  fire Y37.30- ☑
    specified NEC Y37.39- ☑
  firearms
    discharge Y37.43- ☑
    pellets Y37.42- ☑
  flamethrower Y37.33- ☑
  fragments (from) (of)
    improvised explosive device [IED] (person-borne) (roadside) (vehicle-borne) Y37.26- ☑
    munitions Y37.25- ☑
    specified NEC Y37.29- ☑
    weapons Y37.27- ☑
  friendly fire Y37.92- ☑
  hand to hand (unarmed) combat Y37.44- ☑
  hot substances — *see* Military operations, fire
  incendiary bullet Y37.32- ☑
  nuclear weapon (effects of) Y37.50- ☑
    acute radiation exposure Y37.54- ☑
    blast pressure Y37.51- ☑
    direct blast Y37.51- ☑
    direct heat Y37.53- ☑
    fallout exposure Y37.54- ☑
    fireball Y37.53- ☑
    indirect blast (struck or crushed by blast debris) (being thrown by blast) Y37.52- ☑
    ionizing radiation (immediate exposure) Y37.54- ☑
    nuclear radiation Y37.54- ☑
    radiation
      ionizing (immediate exposure) Y37.54- ☑
      nuclear Y37.54- ☑
      thermal Y37.53- ☑
    secondary effects Y37.54- ☑
    specified NEC Y37.59- ☑
    thermal radiation Y37.53- ☑
  restriction of air (airway)
    intentional Y37.46- ☑
    unintentional Y37.47- ☑
  rubber bullets Y37.41- ☑
  shrapnel NOS Y37.29- ☑
  suffocation — *see* Military operations, restriction of airways
  unconventional warfare NEC Y37.7X- ☑
  underwater blast NOS Y37.00- ☑
  warfare
    conventional NEC Y37.49- ☑
    unconventional NEC Y37.7X- ☑
  weapon of mass destruction [WMD] Y37.91- ☑
  weapons
    biological weapons Y37.6X- ☑

Military operations — *continued*
  weapons — *continued*
    chemical Y37.7X- ☑
    nuclear (effects of) Y37.50- ☑
      acute radiation exposure Y37.54- ☑
      blast pressure Y37.51- ☑
      direct blast Y37.51- ☑
      direct heat Y37.53- ☑
      fallout exposure Y37.54- ☑
      fireball Y37.53- ☑
      radiation
        ionizing (immediate exposure) Y37.54- ☑
        nuclear Y37.54- ☑
        thermal Y37.53- ☑
      secondary effects Y37.54- ☑
      specified NEC Y37.59- ☑
    of mass destruction [WMD] Y37.91- ☑
Misadventure(s) **to patient**(s) **during surgical or medical care** Y69
  contaminated medical or biological substance (blood, drug, fluid) Y64.9
    administered (by) NEC Y64.9
      immunization Y64.1
      infusion Y64.0
      injection Y64.1
      specified means NEC Y64.8
      transfusion Y64.0
      vaccination Y64.1
  excessive amount of blood or other fluid during transfusion or infusion Y63.0
  failure
    in dosage Y63.9
      electroshock therapy Y63.4
      inappropriate temperature (too hot or too cold) in local application and packing Y63.5
      infusion
        excessive amount of fluid Y63.0
        incorrect dilution of fluid Y63.1
      insulin-shock therapy Y63.4
      nonadministration of necessary drug or biological substance Y63.6
      overdose — *see* Table of Drugs and Chemicals
      radiation, in therapy Y63.2
      radiation
        overdose Y63.2
      specified procedure NEC Y63.8
      transfusion
        excessive amount of blood Y63.0
    mechanical, of instrument or apparatus (any) (during any procedure) Y65.8
    sterile precautions (during procedure) Y62.9
      aspiration of fluid or tissue (by puncture or catheterization, except heart) Y62.6
      biopsy (except needle aspiration) Y62.8
        needle (aspirating) Y62.6
      blood sampling Y62.6
      catheterization Y62.6
        heart Y62.5
      dialysis (kidney) Y62.2
      endoscopic examination Y62.4
      enema Y62.8
      immunization Y62.3
      infusion Y62.1
      injection Y62.3
      needle biopsy Y62.6
      paracentesis (abdominal) (thoracic) Y62.6
      perfusion Y62.2
      puncture (lumbar) Y62.6
      removal of catheter or packing Y62.8
      specified procedure NEC Y62.8
      surgical operation Y62.0
      transfusion Y62.1
      vaccination Y62.3
    suture or ligature during surgical procedure Y65.2
    to introduce or to remove tube or instrument — *see* Failure, to
  hemorrhage — *see* Index to Diseases and Injuries, Complication(s)
  inadvertent exposure of patient to radiation Y63.3
  inappropriate
    operation performed — *see* Inappropriate operation performed
    temperature (too hot or too cold) in local application or packing Y63.5
  infusion (*see also* Misadventure, by type, infusion) Y69
    excessive amount of fluid Y63.0
    incorrect dilution of fluid Y63.1
    wrong fluid Y65.1

Misadventure(s) **to patient**(s) **during surgical or medical care** — *continued*
  mismatched blood in transfusion Y65.Ø
  nonadministration of necessary drug or biological substance Y63.6
  overdose — *see* Table of Drugs and Chemicals
    radiation (in therapy) Y63.2
  perforation — *see* Index to Diseases and Injuries, Complication(s)
  performance of inappropriate operation — *see* Inappropriate operation performed
  puncture — *see* Index to Diseases and Injuries, Complication(s)
  specified type NEC Y65.8
    failure
      suture or ligature during surgical operation Y65.2
      to introduce or to remove tube or instrument — *see* Failure, to
    infusion of wrong fluid Y65.1
    performance of inappropriate operation — *see* Inappropriate operation performed
    transfusion of mismatched blood Y65.Ø
    wrong
      fluid in infusion Y65.1
      placement of endotracheal tube during anesthetic procedure Y65.3
  transfusion — *see* Misadventure, by type, transfusion
    excessive amount of blood Y63.Ø
    mismatched blood Y65.Ø
  wrong
    drug given in error — *see* Table of Drugs and Chemicals
    fluid in infusion Y65.1
    placement of endotracheal tube during anesthetic procedure Y65.3
Mismatched blood in transfusion Y65.Ø
Motion sickness T75.3 ☑
Mountain sickness W94.11 ☑
Mudslide (of cataclysmic nature) — *see* Landslide
Murder (attempt) — *see* Assault

N

Nail
  contact with W45.Ø ☑
    gun W29.4 ☑
  embedded in skin W45.Ø ☑
Neglect (criminal) (homicidal intent) X58 ☑
Noise (causing injury) (pollution) W42.9 ☑
  supersonic W42.Ø ☑
Nonadministration (of)
  drug or biological substance (necessary) Y63.6
  surgical and medical care Y66
Nosocomial condition Y95

O

Object
  falling
    from, in, on, hitting
      machinery — *see* Contact, with, by type of machine
    set in motion by
      accidental explosion or rupture of pressure vessel W38 ☑
      firearm — *see* Discharge, firearm, by type
      machine(ry) — *see* Contact, with, by type of machine
Overdose (drug) — *see* Table of Drugs and Chemicals
  radiation Y63.2
Overexertion X5Ø.9 ☑
  from
    prolonged static or awkward postures X5Ø.1 ☑
    repetitive movements X5Ø.3 ☑
    specified strenuous movements or postures NEC X5Ø.9 ☑
    strenuous movement or load X5Ø.Ø ☑
Overexposure (accidental) (to)
  cold (*see also* Exposure, cold) X31 ☑
    due to man-made conditions — *see* Exposure, cold, man-made
  heat (*see also* Heat) X3Ø ☑
  radiation — *see* Radiation
  radioactivity W88.Ø ☑
  sun (sunburn) X32 ☑
  weather NEC — *see* Forces of nature
  wind NEC — *see* Forces of nature

Overheated — *see* Heat
Overturning (accidental)
  machinery — *see* Contact, with, by type of machine
  transport vehicle NEC (*see also* Accident, transport) V89.9 ☑
  watercraft (causing drowning, submersion) (*see also* Drowning, due to, accident to, watercraft, overturning)
    causing injury except drowning or submersion — *see* Accident, watercraft, causing, injury NEC

P

Parachute descent (voluntary) (without accident to aircraft) V97.29 ☑
  due to accident to aircraft — *see* Accident, transport, aircraft
Pecked by bird W61.99 ☑
Perforation during medical or surgical treatment as misadventure — *see* Index to Diseases and Injuries, Complication(s)
Perpetrator, perpetration, of assault, maltreatment and neglect (by) YØ7.9
  boyfriend YØ7.Ø3
  brother YØ7.41Ø
    stepbrother YØ7.435
  coach YØ7.53
  cousin
    female YØ7.491
    male YØ7.49Ø
  daycare provider YØ7.519
    at-home
      adult care YØ7.512
      childcare YØ7.51Ø
    care center
      adult care YØ7.513
      childcare YØ7.511
  family member NEC YØ7.499
  father YØ7.11
    adoptive YØ7.13
    foster YØ7.42Ø
    stepfather YØ7.43Ø
  foster father YØ7.42Ø
  foster mother YØ7.421
  girl friend YØ7.Ø4
  healthcare provider YØ7.529
    mental health YØ7.521
    specified NEC YØ7.528
  husband YØ7.Ø1
  instructor YØ7.53
  mother YØ7.12
    adoptive YØ7.14
    foster YØ7.421
    stepmother YØ7.433
  multiple perpetrators YØ7.6
  nonfamily member YØ7.5Ø
    specified NEC YØ7.59
  nurse YØ7.528
  occupational therapist YØ7.528
  partner of parent
    female YØ7.434
    male YØ7.432
  physical therapist YØ7.528
  sister YØ7.411
  speech therapist YØ7.528
  stepbrother YØ7.435
  stepfather YØ7.43Ø
  stepmother YØ7.433
  stepsister YØ7.436
  teacher YØ7.53
  wife YØ7.Ø2
Piercing — *see* Contact, with, by type of object or machine
Pinched
  between objects (moving) (stationary and moving) W23.Ø ☑
    stationary W23.1 ☑
Pinned under machine(ry) — *see* Contact, with, by type of machine
Place of occurrence Y92.9
  abandoned house Y92.89
  airplane Y92.813
  airport Y92.52Ø
  ambulatory health services establishment NEC Y92.538
  ambulatory surgery center Y92.53Ø
  amusement park Y92.831
  apartment (co-op) — *see* Place of occurrence, residence, apartment

Place of occurrence — *continued*
  assembly hall Y92.29
  bank Y92.51Ø
  barn Y92.71
  baseball field Y92.32Ø
  basketball court Y92.31Ø
  beach Y92.832
  boarding house — *see* Place of occurrence, residence, boarding house
  boat Y92.814
  bowling alley Y92.39
  bridge Y92.89
  building under construction Y92.61
  bus Y92.811
    station Y92.521
  cafe Y92.511
  campsite Y92.833
  campus — *see* Place of occurrence, school
  canal Y92.89
  car Y92.81Ø
  casino Y92.59
  children's home — *see* Place of occurrence, residence, institutional, orphanage
  church Y92.22
  cinema Y92.26
  clubhouse Y92.29
  coal pit Y92.64
  college (community) Y92.214
  condominium — *see* Place of occurrence, residence, apartment
  construction area — *see* Place of occurrence, industrial and construction area
  convalescent home — *see* Place of occurrence, residence, institutional, nursing home
  court-house Y92.24Ø
  cricket ground Y92.328
  cultural building Y92.258
    art gallery Y92.25Ø
    museum Y92.251
    music hall Y92.252
    opera house Y92.253
    specified NEC Y92.258
    theater Y92.254
  dancehall Y92.252
  day nursery Y92.21Ø
  dentist office Y92.531
  derelict house Y92.89
  desert Y92.82Ø
  dockyard Y92.62
  dock NOS Y92.89
  doctor's office Y92.531
  dormitory — *see* Place of occurrence, residence, institutional, school dormitory
  dry dock Y92.62
  factory (building) (premises) Y92.63
  farm (land under cultivation) (outbuildings) Y92.79
    barn Y92.71
    chicken coop Y92.72
    field Y92.73
    hen house Y92.72
    house — *see* Place of occurrence, residence, house
    orchard Y92.74
    specified NEC Y92.79
  football field Y92.321
  forest Y92.821
  freeway Y92.411
  gallery Y92.25Ø
  garage (commercial) Y92.59
    boarding house Y92.Ø44
    military base Y92.135
    mobile home Y92.Ø25
    nursing home Y92.124
    orphanage Y92.114
    private house Y92.Ø15
    reform school Y92.155
  gas station Y92.524
  gasworks Y92.69
  golf course Y92.39
  gravel pit Y92.64
  grocery Y92.512
  gymnasium Y92.39
  handball court Y92.318
  harbor Y92.89
  harness racing course Y92.39
  healthcare provider office Y92.531
  highway (interstate) Y92.411
  hill Y92.828
  hockey rink Y92.33Ø

Place of occurrence — *continued*

- home — *see* Place of occurrence, residence
- hospice — *see* Place of occurrence, residence, institutional, nursing home
- hospital Y92.239
  - cafeteria Y92.233
  - corridor Y92.232
  - operating room Y92.234
  - patient
    - bathroom Y92.231
    - room Y92.230
  - specified NEC Y92.238
- hotel Y92.59
- house (*see also* Place of occurrence, residence)
  - abandoned Y92.89
  - under construction Y92.61
- industrial and construction area (yard) Y92.69
  - building under construction Y92.61
  - dock Y92.62
  - dry dock Y92.62
  - factory Y92.63
  - gasworks Y92.69
  - mine Y92.64
  - oil rig Y92.65
  - pit Y92.64
  - power station Y92.69
  - shipyard Y92.62
  - specified NEC Y92.69
  - tunnel under construction Y92.69
  - workshop Y92.69
- kindergarten Y92.211
- lacrosse field Y92.328
- lake Y92.828
- library Y92.241
- mall Y92.59
- market Y92.512
- marsh Y92.828
- military
  - base — *see* Place of occurrence, residence, institutional, military base
  - training ground Y92.84
- mine Y92.64
- mosque Y92.22
- motel Y92.59
- motorway (interstate) Y92.411
- mountain Y92.828
- movie-house Y92.26
- museum Y92.251
- music-hall Y92.252
- not applicable Y92.9
- nuclear power station Y92.69
- nursing home — *see* Place of occurrence, residence, institutional, nursing home
- office building Y92.59
- offshore installation Y92.65
- oil rig Y92.65
- old people's home — *see* Place of occurrence, residence, institutional, specified NEC
- opera-house Y92.253
- orphanage — *see* Place of occurrence, residence, institutional, orphanage
- outpatient surgery center Y92.530
- park (public) Y92.830
  - amusement Y92.831
- parking garage Y92.89
  - lot Y92.481
- pavement Y92.480
- physician office Y92.531
- polo field Y92.328
- pond Y92.828
- post office Y92.242
- power station Y92.69
- prairie Y92.828
- prison — *see* Place of occurrence, residence, institutional, prison
- public
  - administration building Y92.248
    - city hall Y92.243
    - courthouse Y92.240
    - library Y92.241
    - post office Y92.242
    - specified NEC Y92.248
  - building NEC Y92.29
  - hall Y92.29
  - place NOS Y92.89
- race course Y92.39
- radio station Y92.59
- railway line (bridge) Y92.85

Place of occurrence — *continued*

- ranch (outbuildings) — *see* Place of occurrence, farm
- recreation area Y92.838
  - amusement park Y92.831
  - beach Y92.832
  - campsite Y92.833
  - park (public) Y92.830
  - seashore Y92.832
  - specified NEC Y92.838
- reform school - — *see* Place of occurrence, residence, institutional, reform school
- religious institution Y92.22
- residence (non-institutional) (private) Y92.009
  - apartment Y92.039
    - bathroom Y92.031
    - bedroom Y92.032
    - kitchen Y92.030
    - specified NEC Y92.038
  - bathroom Y92.002
  - bedroom Y92.003
  - boarding house Y92.049
    - bathroom Y92.041
    - bedroom Y92.042
    - driveway Y92.043
    - garage Y92.044
    - garden Y92.046
    - kitchen Y92.040
    - specified NEC Y92.048
    - swimming pool Y92.045
    - yard Y92.046
  - dining room Y92.001
  - garden Y92.007
  - home Y92.009
  - house, single family Y92.019
    - bathroom Y92.012
    - bedroom Y92.013
    - dining room Y92.011
    - driveway Y92.014
    - garage Y92.015
    - garden Y92.017
    - kitchen Y92.010
    - specified NEC Y92.018
    - swimming pool Y92.016
    - yard Y92.017
  - institutional Y92.10
    - children's home — *see* Place of occurrence, residence, institutional, orphanage
    - hospice — *see* Place of occurrence, residence, institutional, nursing home
    - military base Y92.139
      - barracks Y92.133
      - garage Y92.135
      - garden Y92.137
      - kitchen Y92.130
      - mess hall Y92.131
      - specified NEC Y92.138
      - swimming pool Y92.136
      - yard Y92.137
    - nursing home Y92.129
      - bathroom Y92.121
      - bedroom Y92.122
      - driveway Y92.123
      - garage Y92.124
      - garden Y92.126
      - kitchen Y92.120
      - specified NEC Y92.128
      - swimming pool Y92.125
      - yard Y92.126
    - orphanage Y92.119
      - bathroom Y92.111
      - bedroom Y92.112
      - driveway Y92.113
      - garage Y92.114
      - garden Y92.116
      - kitchen Y92.110
      - specified NEC Y92.118
      - swimming pool Y92.115
      - yard Y92.116
    - prison Y92.149
      - bathroom Y92.142
      - cell Y92.143
      - courtyard Y92.147
      - dining room Y92.141
      - kitchen Y92.140
      - specified NEC Y92.148
      - swimming pool Y92.146
    - reform school Y92.159
      - bathroom Y92.152
      - bedroom Y92.153

Place of occurrence — *continued*

- residence — *continued*
  - institutional — *continued*
    - reform school — *continued*
      - dining room Y92.151
      - driveway Y92.154
      - garage Y92.155
      - garden Y92.157
      - kitchen Y92.150
      - specified NEC Y92.158
      - swimming pool Y92.156
      - yard Y92.157
    - school dormitory Y92.169
      - bathroom Y92.162
      - bedroom Y92.163
      - dining room Y92.161
      - kitchen Y92.160
      - specified NEC Y92.168
    - specified NEC Y92.199
      - bathroom Y92.192
      - bedroom Y92.193
      - dining room Y92.191
      - driveway Y92.194
      - garage Y92.195
      - garden Y92.197
      - kitchen Y92.190
      - specified NEC Y92.198
      - swimming pool Y92.196
      - yard Y92.197
  - kitchen Y92.000
  - mobile home Y92.029
    - bathroom Y92.022
    - bedroom Y92.023
    - dining room Y92.021
    - driveway Y92.024
    - garage Y92.025
    - garden Y92.027
    - kitchen Y92.020
    - specified NEC Y92.028
    - swimming pool Y92.026
    - yard Y92.027
  - specified place in residence NEC Y92.008
  - specified residence type NEC Y92.099
    - bathroom Y92.091
    - bedroom Y92.092
    - driveway Y92.093
    - garage Y92.094
    - garden Y92.096
    - kitchen Y92.090
    - specified NEC Y92.098
    - swimming pool Y92.095
    - yard Y92.096
- restaurant Y92.511
- riding school Y92.39
- river Y92.828
- road Y92.410
- rodeo ring Y92.39
- rugby field Y92.328
- same day surgery center Y92.530
- sand pit Y92.64
- school (private) (public) (state) Y92.219
  - college Y92.214
  - daycare center Y92.210
  - elementary school Y92.211
  - high school Y92.213
  - kindergarten Y92.211
  - middle school Y92.212
  - specified NEC Y92.218
  - trace school Y92.215
  - university Y92.214
  - vocational school Y92.215
- sea (shore) Y92.832
- senior citizen center Y92.29
- service area
  - airport Y92.520
  - bus station Y92.521
  - gas station Y92.524
  - highway rest stop Y92.523
  - railway station Y92.522
- shipyard Y92.62
- shop (commercial) Y92.513
- sidewalk Y92.480
- silo Y92.79
- skating rink (roller) Y92.331
  - ice Y92.330
- slaughter house Y92.86
- soccer field Y92.322
- specified place NEC Y92.89
- sports area Y92.39

Place of occurrence — *continued*

sports area — *continued*
  athletic
    court Y92.318
      basketball Y92.310
      specified NEC Y92.318
      squash Y92.311
      tennis Y92.312
    field Y92.328
      baseball Y92.320
      cricket ground Y92.328
      football Y92.321
      hockey Y92.328
      soccer Y92.322
      specified NEC Y92.328
    golf course Y92.39
    gymnasium Y92.39
    riding school Y92.39
    skating rink (roller) Y92.331
      ice Y92.330
    stadium Y92.39
    swimming pool Y92.34
  squash court Y92.311
  stadium Y92.39
  steeplechasing course Y92.39
  store Y92.512
  stream Y92.828
  street and highway Y92.410
    bike path Y92.482
    freeway Y92.411
    highway ramp Y92.415
    interstate highway Y92.411
    local residential or business street Y92.414
    motorway Y92.411
    parking lot Y92.481
    parkway Y92.412
    sidewalk Y92.480
    specified NEC Y92.488
    state road Y92.413
  subway car Y92.816
  supermarket Y92.512
  swamp Y92.828
  swimming pool (public) Y92.34
    private (at) Y92.095
      boarding house Y92.045
      military base Y92.136
      mobile home Y92.026
      nursing home Y92.125
      orphanage Y92.115
      prison Y92.146
      reform school Y92.156
      single family residence Y92.016
  synagogue Y92.22
  television station Y92.59
  tennis court Y92.312
  theater Y92.254
  trade area Y92.59
    bank Y92.510
    cafe Y92.511
    casino Y92.59
    garage Y92.59
    hotel Y92.59
    market Y92.512
    office building Y92.59
    radio station Y92.59
    restaurant Y92.511
    shop Y92.513
    shopping mall Y92.59
    store Y92.512
    supermarket Y92.512
    television station Y92.59
    warehouse Y92.59
  trailer park, residential — *see* Place of occurrence, residence, mobile home
  trailer site NOS Y92.89
  train Y92.815
    station Y92.522
  truck Y92.812
  tunnel under construction Y92.69
  university Y92.214
  urgent (health) care center Y92.532
  vehicle (transport) Y92.818
    airplane Y92.813
    boat Y92.814
    bus Y92.811
    car Y92.810
    specified NEC Y92.818
    subway car Y92.816
    train Y92.815

Place of occurrence — *continued*

vehicle — *continued*
    truck Y92.812
  warehouse Y92.59
  water reservoir Y92.89
  wilderness area Y92.828
    desert Y92.820
    forest Y92.821
    marsh Y92.828
    mountain Y92.828
    prairie Y92.828
    specified NEC Y92.828
    swamp Y92.828
  workshop Y92.69
  yard, private Y92.096
    boarding house Y92.046
    mobile home Y92.027
    single family house Y92.017
  youth center Y92.29
  zoo (zoological garden) Y92.834

Plumbism — *see* Table of Drugs and Chemicals, lead

Poisoning (accidental) (by) (*see also* Table of Drugs and Chemicals)

by plant, thorns, spines, sharp leaves or other mechanisms NEC X58 ☑
carbon monoxide
  generated by
    motor vehicle — *see* Accident, transport
    watercraft (in transit) (not in transit) V93.89 ☑
      ferry boat V93.81 ☑
      fishing boat V93.82 ☑
      jet skis V93.83 ☑
      liner V93.81 ☑
      merchant ship V93.80 ☑
      passenger ship V93.81 ☑
      powered craft NEC V93.83 ☑
caused by injection of poisons into skin by plant thorns, spines, sharp leaves X58 ☑
  marine or sea plants (venomous) X58 ☑
execution — *see* Legal, intervention, gas
intervention
  by gas — *see* Legal, intervention, gas
  other specified means — *see* Legal, intervention, specified means NEC
exhaust gas
  generated by
    motor vehicle — *see* Accident, transport
    watercraft (in transit) (not in transit) V93.89 ☑
      ferry boat V93.81 ☑
      fishing boat V93.82 ☑
      jet skis V93.83 ☑
      liner V93.81 ☑
      merchant ship V93.80 ☑
      passenger ship V93.81 ☑
      powered craft NEC V93.83 ☑
fumes or smoke due to
  explosion (*see also* Explosion) W40.9 ☑
  fire — *see* Exposure, fire
  ignition — *see* Ignition
gas
  in legal intervention — *see* Legal, intervention, gas
  legal execution — *see* Legal, intervention, gas
in war operations — *see* War operations
legal

Powder burn (by) (from)
airgun W34.110 ☑
BB gun W34.110 ☑
firearm NEC W34.19 ☑
gas, air or spring-operated gun NEC W34.118 ☑
handgun W32.1 ☑
hunting rifle W33.12 ☑
larger firearm W33.10 ☑
  specified NEC W33.19 ☑
machine gun W33.13 ☑
paintball gun W34.111 ☑
pellet gun W34.110 ☑
shotgun W33.11 ☑
Very pistol [flare] W34.19 ☑

Premature cessation (of) **surgical and medical care** Y66

Privation (food) (water) X58 ☑

Procedure (operation)
correct, on wrong side or body part (wrong side) (wrong site) Y65.53
intended for another patient done on wrong patient Y65.52
performed on patient not scheduled for surgery Y65.52

Procedure — *continued*
performed on wrong patient Y65.52
wrong, performed on correct patient Y65.51

Prolonged
sitting in transport vehicle — *see* Travel, by type of vehicle
stay in
  high altitude as cause of anoxia, barodontalgia, barotitis or hypoxia W94.11 ☑
  weightless environment X52 ☑

Pulling, excessive (*see also* Overexertion) X50.9- ☑

Puncture, puncturing (*see also* Contact, with, by type of object or machine)
by
  plant thorns, spines, sharp leaves or other mechanisms NEC W60 ☑
during medical or surgical treatment as misadventure — *see* Index to Diseases and Injuries, Complication(s)

Pushed, pushing (accidental) (injury in)
by other person(s) (accidental) W51 ☑
  as, or caused by, a crowd or human stampede (with fall) W52 ☑
  before moving object NEC Y02.8 ☑
    motor vehicle Y02.0 ☑
    subway train Y02.1 ☑
    train Y02.1 ☑
  from
    high place NEC
      in accidental circumstances W17.89 ☑
      stated as
        intentional, homicide (attempt) Y01 ☑
        undetermined whether accidental or intentional Y30 ☑
    transport vehicle NEC (*see also* Accident, transport) V89.9 ☑
      stated as
        intentional, homicide (attempt) Y08.89 ☑
  with fall W03 ☑
    due to ice or snow W00.0 ☑
overexertion X50.9 ☑

R

Radiation (exposure to)
arc lamps W89.0 ☑
atomic power plant (malfunction) NEC W88.1 ☑
complication of or abnormal reaction to medical radiotherapy Y84.2
electromagnetic, ionizing W88.0 ☑
gamma rays W88.1 ☑
in
  war operations (from or following nuclear explosion) — *see* War operations
inadvertent exposure of patient (receiving test or therapy) Y63.3
infrared (heaters and lamps) W90.1 ☑
  excessive heat from W92 ☑
ionized, ionizing (particles, artificially accelerated)
  radioisotopes W88.1 ☑
  specified NEC W88.8 ☑
  x-rays W88.0 ☑
isotopes, radioactive — *see* Radiation, radioactive isotopes
laser(s) W90.2 ☑
  in war operations — *see* War operations
  misadventure in medical care Y63.2
light sources (man-made visible and ultraviolet) W89.9 ☑
  natural X32 ☑
  specified NEC W89.8 ☑
  tanning bed W89.1 ☑
  welding light W89.0 ☑
man-made visible light W89.9 ☑
  specified NEC W89.8 ☑
  tanning bed W89.1 ☑
  welding light W89.0 ☑
microwave W90.8 ☑
misadventure in medical or surgical procedure Y63.2
natural NEC X39.08 ☑
  radon X39.01 ☑
overdose (in medical or surgical procedure) Y63.2
radar W90.0 ☑
radioactive isotopes (any) W88.1 ☑
  atomic power plant malfunction W88.1 ☑
  misadventure in medical or surgical treatment Y63.2

Radiation — *continued*
  radiofrequency W90.0 ☑
  radium NEC W88.1 ☑
  sun X32 ☑
  ultraviolet (light) (man-made) W89.9 ☑
    natural X32 ☑
    specified NEC W89.8 ☑
    tanning bed W89.1 ☑
    welding light W89.0 ☑
  welding arc, torch, or light W89.0 ☑
    excessive heat from W92 ☑
  x-rays (hard) (soft) W88.0 ☑
Range disease W94.11 ☑
Rape (attempted) T74.2- ☑
Rat bite W53.11 ☑
Reaching (prolonged) (static) X50.1 ☑
Reaction, abnormal to medical procedure (*see also* Complication of or following, by type of procedure) Y84.9
  biologicals — *see* Table of Drugs and Chemicals
  drugs — *see* Table of Drugs and Chemicals
  vaccine — *see* Table of Drugs and Chemicals
  with misadventure — *see* Misadventure
Recoil
  airgun W34.110 ☑
  BB gun W34.110 ☑
  firearm NEC W34.19 ☑
  gas, air or spring-operated gun NEC W34.118 ☑
  handgun W32.1 ☑
  hunting rifle W33.12 ☑
  larger firearm W33.10 ☑
    specified NEC W33.19 ☑
  machine gun W33.13 ☑
  paintball gun W34.111 ☑
  pellet W34.110 ☑
  shotgun W33.11 ☑
  Very pistol [flare] W34.19 ☑
Reduction in
  atmospheric pressure — *see* Air, pressure, change
Rock falling on or hitting (accidentally) (person) W20.8 ☑
  in cave-in W20.0 ☑
Run over (accidentally) (by)
  animal (not being ridden) NEC W55.89 ☑
  machinery — *see* Contact, with, by specified type of machine
  transport vehicle NEC (*see also* Accident, transport) V09.9 ☑
    intentional homicide (attempt) Y03.0 ☑
    motor NEC V09.20 ☑
      intentional homicide (attempt) Y03.0 ☑
Running
  before moving object X81.8 ☑
    motor vehicle X81.0 ☑
Running off, away
  animal (being ridden) (*see also* Accident, transport) V80.918 ☑
    not being ridden W55.89 ☑
  animal-drawn vehicle NEC (*see also* Accident, transport) V80.928 ☑
  highway, road(way), street
    transport vehicle NEC (*see also* Accident, transport) V89.9 ☑
Rupture pressurized devices — *see* Explosion, by type of device

S

Saturnism — *see* Table of Drugs and Chemicals, lead
Scald, scalding (accidental) (by) (from) (in) X19 ☑
  air (hot) X14.1 ☑
  gases (hot) X14.1 ☑
  homicide (attempt) — *see* Assault, burning, hot object
  inflicted by other person
    stated as intentional, homicide (attempt) — *see* Assault, burning, hot object
  liquid (boiling) (hot) NEC X12 ☑
    stated as undetermined whether accidental or intentional Y27.2 ☑
    suicide (attempt) X77.2 ☑
  local application of externally applied substance in medical or surgical care Y63.5
  metal (molten) (liquid) (hot) NEC X18 ☑
  self-inflicted X77.9 ☑
  stated as undetermined whether accidental or intentional Y27.8 ☑

Scald, scalding — *continued*
  steam X13.1 ☑
    assault X98.0 ☑
    stated as undetermined whether accidental or intentional Y27.0 ☑
    suicide (attempt) X77.0 ☑
  suicide (attempt) X77.9 ☑
  vapor (hot) X13.1 ☑
    assault X98.0 ☑
    stated as undetermined whether accidental or intentional Y27.0 ☑
    suicide (attempt) X77.0 ☑
Scratched by
  cat W55.03 ☑
  person(s) (accidentally) W50.4 ☑
    with intent to injure or kill Y04.0 ☑
    as, or caused by, a crowd or human stampede (with fall) W52 ☑
    assault Y04.0 ☑
    homicide (attempt) Y04.0 ☑
    in
      fight Y04.0 ☑
      legal intervention
        injuring
          bystander Y35.892 ☑
          law enforcement personnel Y35.891 ☑
          suspect Y35.893 ☑
Seasickness T75.3 ☑
Self-harm NEC (*see also* External cause by type, undetermined whether accidental or intentional)
  intentional — *see* Suicide
  poisoning NEC — *see* Table of Drugs and Chemicals, poisoning, accidental
Self-inflicted (injury) **NEC** (*see also* External cause by type, undetermined whether accidental or intentional)
  intentional — *see* Suicide
  poisoning NEC — *see* Table of Drugs and Chemicals, poisoning, accidental
Sequelae (of)
  accident NEC — *see* W00-X58 with 7th character S
  assault (homicidal) (any means) — *see* X92-Y08 with 7th character S
  homicide, attempt (any means) — *see* X92-Y08 with 7th character S
  injury undetermined whether accidentally or purposely inflicted — *see* Y21-Y33 with 7th character S
  intentional self-harm (classifiable to X71-X83) — *see* X71-X83 with 7th character S
  legal intervention — *see* with 7th character S Y35 ☑
  motor vehicle accident — *see* V00-V99 with 7th character S
  suicide, attempt (any means) — *see* X71-X83 with 7th character S
  transport accident — *see* V00-V99 with 7th character S
  war operations — *see* War operations
Shock
  electric — *see* Exposure, electric current
  from electric appliance (any) (faulty) W86.8 ☑
    domestic W86.0 ☑
    suicide (attempt) X83.1 ☑
Shooting, shot (accidental(ly)) (*see also* Discharge, firearm, by type)
  herself or himself — *see* Discharge, firearm by type, self-inflicted
  homicide (attempt) — *see* Discharge, firearm by type, homicide
  in war operations — *see* War operations
  inflicted by other person — *see* Discharge, firearm by type, homicide
    accidental — *see* Discharge, firearm, by type of firearm
  legal
    execution — *see* Legal, intervention, firearm
    intervention — *see* Legal, intervention, firearm
  self-inflicted — *see* Discharge, firearm by type, suicide
    accidental — *see* Discharge, firearm, by type of firearm
  suicide (attempt) — *see* Discharge, firearm by type, suicide
Shoving (accidentally) **by other person** — *see* Pushed, by other person
Sickness
  alpine W94.11 ☑
  motion — *see* Motion
  mountain W94.11 ☑

Sinking (accidental)
  watercraft (causing drowning, submersion) (*see also* Drowning, due to, accident to, watercraft, sinking)
    causing injury except drowning or submersion — *see* Accident, watercraft, causing, injury NEC
Siriasis X32 ☑
Sitting (prolonged) (static) X50.1 ☑
Slashed wrists — *see* Cut, self-inflicted
Slipping (accidental) (on same level) (with fall) W01.0 ☑
  on
    ice W00.0 ☑
      with skates — *see* Accident, transport, pedestrian, conveyance
    mud W01.0 ☑
    oil W01.0 ☑
    snow W00.0 ☑
      with skis — *see* Accident, transport, pedestrian, conveyance
    surface (slippery) (wet) NEC W01.0 ☑
  without fall W18.40 ☑
    due to
      specified NEC W18.49 ☑
      stepping from one level to another W18.43 ☑
      stepping into hole or opening W18.42 ☑
      stepping on object W18.41 ☑
Sliver, wood, contact with W45.8 ☑
Smoldering (due to fire) — *see* Exposure, fire
Sodomy (attempted) **by force** T74.2 ☑
Sound waves (causing injury) W42.9 ☑
  supersonic W42.0 ☑
Splinter, contact with W45.8 ☑
Stab, stabbing — *see* Cut
Standing (prolonged) (static) X50.1 ☑
Starvation X58 ☑
Status of external cause Y99.9
  child assisting in compensated work for family Y99.8
  civilian activity done for financial or other compensation Y99.0
  civilian activity done for income or pay Y99.0
  family member assisting in compensated work for other family member Y99.8
  hobby not done for income Y99.8
  leisure activity Y99.8
  military activity Y99.1
  off-duty activity of military personnel Y99.8
  recreation or sport not for income or while a student Y99.8
  specified NEC Y99.8
  student activity Y99.8
  volunteer activity Y99.2
Stepped on
  by
    animal (not being ridden) NEC W55.89 ☑
    crowd or human stampede W52 ☑
    person W50.0 ☑
Stepping on
  object W22.8 ☑
    sports equipment W21.9 ☑
    stationary W22.09 ☑
      sports equipment W21.89 ☑
    with fall W18.31 ☑
  person W51 ☑
    by crowd or human stampede W52 ☑
  sports equipment W21.9 ☑
Sting
  arthropod, nonvenomous W57 ☑
  insect, nonvenomous W57 ☑
Storm (cataclysmic) — *see* Forces of nature, cataclysmic storm
Straining, excessive (*see also* Overexertion) X50.9 ☑
Strangling — *see* Strangulation
Strangulation (accidental) T71 ☑
Strenuous movements (*see also* Overexertion) X50.9 ☑
Striking against
  airbag (automobile) W22.10 ☑
    driver side W22.11 ☑
    front passenger side W22.12 ☑
    specified NEC W22.19 ☑
  bottom when
    diving or jumping into water (in) W16.822 ☑
      causing drowning W16.821 ☑
      from boat W16.722 ☑
        causing drowning W16.721 ☑
      natural body W16.622 ☑
        causing drowning W16.821 ☑

Striking against — *continued*
  bottom when — *continued*
    diving or jumping into water — *continued*
      swimming pool W16.522 ✓
        causing drowning W16.521 ✓
    falling into water (in) W16.322 ✓
      causing drowning W16.321 ✓
    fountain — *see* Striking against, bottom when, falling into water, specified NEC
    natural body W16.122 ✓
      causing drowning W16.121 ✓
    reservoir — *see* Striking against, bottom when, falling into water, specified NEC
    specified NEC W16.322 ✓
      causing drowning W16.321 ✓
    swimming pool W16.022 ✓
      causing drowning W16.021 ✓
  diving board (swimming-pool) W21.4 ✓
  object W22.8 ✓
    caused by crowd or human stampede (with fall) W52 ✓
    furniture W22.03 ✓
    lamppost W22.02 ✓
    sports equipment W21.9 ✓
    stationary W22.09 ✓
      sports equipment W21.89 ✓
    wall W22.01 ✓
    with
      drowning or submersion — *see* Drowning
      fall — *see* Fall, due to, bumping against, object
  person(s) W51 ✓
    as, or caused by, a crowd or human stampede (with fall) W52 ✓
    assault Y04.2 ✓
    homicide (attempt) Y04.2 ✓
    with fall W03 ✓
      due to ice or snow W00.0 ✓
  sports equipment W21.9 ✓
  wall (when) W22.01 ✓
    diving or jumping into water (in) W16.832 ✓
      causing drowning W16.831 ✓
    swimming pool W16.532 ✓
      causing drowning W16.531 ✓
    falling into water (in) W16.332 ✓
      causing drowning W16.331 ✓
    fountain — *see* Striking against, wall when, falling into water, specified NEC
    natural body W16.132 ✓
      causing drowning W16.131 ✓
    reservoir — *see* Striking against, wall when, falling into water, specified NEC
    specified NEC W16.332 ✓
      causing drowning W16.331 ✓
    swimming pool W16.032 ✓
      causing drowning W16.031 ✓
    swimming pool (when) W22.042 ✓
      causing drowning W22.041 ✓
      diving or jumping into water W16.532 ✓
        causing drowning W16.531 ✓
      falling into water W16.032 ✓
        causing drowning W16.031 ✓

Struck (accidentally) **by**
  airbag (automobile) W22.10 ✓
    driver side W22.11 ✓
    front passenger side W22.12 ✓
    specified NEC W22.19 ✓
  alligator W58.02 ✓
  animal (not being ridden) NEC W55.89 ✓
  avalanche — *see* Landslide
  ball (hit) (thrown) W21.00 ✓
    assault Y08.09 ✓
    baseball W21.03 ✓
    basketball W21.05 ✓
    football W21.01 ✓
    golf ball W21.04 ✓
    soccer W21.02 ✓
    softball W21.07 ✓
    specified NEC W21.09 ✓
    volleyball W21.06 ✓
  bat or racquet
    baseball bat W21.11 ✓
      assault Y08.02 ✓
    golf club W21.13 ✓
      assault Y08.09 ✓
    specified NEC W21.19 ✓
      assault Y08.09 ✓

Struck (accidentally) **by** — *continued*
  bat or racquet — *continued*
    tennis racquet W21.12 ✓
      assault Y08.09 ✓
  bullet (*see also* Discharge, firearm by type)
    in war operations — *see* War operations
  crocodile W58.12 ✓
  dog W54.1 ✓
  flare, Very pistol — *see* Discharge, firearm NEC
  hailstones X39.8 ✓
  hockey (ice)
    field
      puck W21.221 ✓
      stick W21.211 ✓
    puck W21.220 ✓
    stick W21.210 ✓
      assault Y08.01 ✓
  landslide — *see* Landslide
  law-enforcement agent (on duty) — *see* Legal, intervention, manhandling
    with blunt object — *see* Legal, intervention, blunt object
  lightning T75.0 ✓
    causing fire — *see* Exposure, fire
  machine — *see* Contact, with, by type of machine
  mammal NEC W55.89 ✓
    marine W56.32 ✓
  marine animal W56.82 ✓
  missile
    firearm — *see* Discharge, firearm by type
    in war operations — *see* War operations, missile
  object W22.8 ✓
    blunt W22.8 ✓
      assault Y00 ✓
      suicide (attempt) X79 ✓
      undetermined whether accidental or intentional Y29 ✓
    falling W20.8 ✓
      from, in, on
        building W20.1 ✓
          burning (uncontrolled fire) X00.4 ✓
        cataclysmic
          earth surface movement NEC — *see* Landslide
          storm — *see* Forces of nature, cataclysmic storm
        cave-in W20.0 ✓
        earthquake X34 ✓
        machine (in operation) — *see* Contact, with, by type of machine
        structure W20.1 ✓
          burning X00.4 ✓
        transport vehicle (in motion) — *see* Accident, transport, by type of vehicle
        watercraft V93.49 ✓
          due to
            accident to craft V91.39 ✓
              powered craft V91.33 ✓
                ferry boat V91.31 ✓
                fishing boat V91.32 ✓
                jetskis V91.33 ✓
                liner V91.31 ✓
                merchant ship V91.30 ✓
                passenger ship V91.31 ✓
              unpowered craft V91.38 ✓
                canoe V91.35 ✓
                inflatable V91.36 ✓
                kayak V91.35 ✓
                sailboat V91.34 ✓
                surf-board V91.38 ✓
                windsurfer V91.38 ✓
            powered craft V93.43 ✓
              ferry boat V93.41 ✓
              fishing boat V93.42 ✓
              jetskis V93.43 ✓
              liner V93.41 ✓
              merchant ship V93.40 ✓
              passenger ship V93.41 ✓
            unpowered craft V93.48 ✓
              sailboat V93.44 ✓
              surf-board V93.48 ✓
              windsurfer V93.48 ✓
      moving NEC W20.8 ✓
      projected W20.8 ✓
        assault Y00 ✓
        in sports W21.9 ✓

Struck (accidentally) **by** — *continued*
  object — *continued*
    projected — *continued*
      in sports — *continued*
        assault Y08.09 ✓
        ball W21.00 ✓
          baseball W21.03 ✓
          basketball W21.05 ✓
          football W21.01 ✓
          golf ball W21.04 ✓
          soccer W21.02 ✓
          softball W21.07 ✓
          specified NEC W21.09 ✓
          volleyball W21.06 ✓
        bat or racquet
          baseball bat W21.11 ✓
            assault Y08.02 ✓
          golf club W21.13 ✓
            assault Y08.09 ✓
          specified NEC W21.19 ✓
            assault Y08.09 ✓
          tennis racquet W21.12 ✓
            assault Y08.09 ✓
        hockey (ice)
          field
            puck W21.221 ✓
            stick W21.211 ✓
          puck W21.220 ✓
          stick W21.210 ✓
            assault Y08.01 ✓
        specified NEC W21.89 ✓
    set in motion by explosion — *see* Explosion
    thrown W20.8 ✓
      assault Y00 ✓
      in sports W21.9 ✓
        assault Y08.09 ✓
        ball W21.00 ✓
          baseball W21.03 ✓
          basketball W21.05 ✓
          football W21.01 ✓
          golf ball W21.04 ✓
          soccer W21.02 ✓
          soft ball W21.07 ✓
          specified NEC W21.09 ✓
          volleyball W21.06 ✓
        bat or racquet
          baseball bat W21.11 ✓
            assault Y08.02 ✓
          golf club W21.13 ✓
            assault Y08.09 ✓
          specified NEC W21.19 ✓
            assault Y08.09 ✓
          tennis racquet W21.12 ✓
            assault Y08.09 ✓
        hockey (ice)
          field
            puck W21.221 ✓
            stick W21.211 ✓
          puck W21.220 ✓
          stick W21.210 ✓
            assault Y08.01 ✓
        specified NEC W21.89 ✓
  other person(s) W50.0 ✓
    with
      blunt object W22.8 ✓
        intentional, homicide (attempt) Y00 ✓
        sports equipment W21.9 ✓
        undetermined whether accidental or intentional Y29 ✓
      fall W03 ✓
        due to ice or snow W00.0 ✓
    as, or caused by, a crowd or human stampede (with fall) W52 ✓
    assault Y04.2 ✓
    homicide (attempt) Y04.2 ✓
    in legal intervention
      injuring
        bystander Y35.812 ✓
        law enforcement personnel Y35.811 ✓
        suspect Y35.813 ✓
    sports equipment W21.9 ✓
  police (on duty) — *see* Legal, intervention, manhandling
    with blunt object — *see* Legal, intervention, blunt object
  sports equipment W21.9 ✓

✓ **Additional Character Required** — **Refer to the Tabular List for Character Selection**   ⬙ **Subterms under main terms may continue to next column or page**

Struck (accidentally) **by** — continued
  sports equipment — continued
    assault Y08.09 ☑
    ball W21.00 ☑
      baseball W21.03 ☑
      basketball W21.05 ☑
      football W21.01 ☑
      golf ball W21.04 ☑
      soccer W21.02 ☑
      soft ball W21.07 ☑
      specified NEC W21.09 ☑
      volleyball W21.06 ☑
    bat or racquet
      baseball bat W21.11 ☑
        assault Y08.02 ☑
      golf club W21.13 ☑
        assault Y08.09 ☑
      specified NEC W21.19 ☑
      tennis racquet W21.12 ☑
        assault Y08.09 ☑
    cleats (shoe) W21.31 ☑
    foot wear NEC W21.39 ☑
    football helmet W21.81 ☑
    hockey (ice)
      field
        puck W21.221 ☑
        stick W21.211 ☑
      puck W21.220 ☑
      stick W21.210 ☑
        assault Y08.01 ☑
    skate blades W21.32 ☑
    specified NEC W21.89 ☑
      assault Y08.09 ☑
  thunderbolt — see subcategory T75.0 ☑
  causing fire — see Exposure, fire
  transport vehicle NEC (see also Accident, transport)
    V09.9 ☑
    intentional, homicide (attempt) Y03.0 ☑
    motor NEC (see also Accident, transport) V09.20 ☑
      homicide Y03.0 ☑
  vehicle (transport) NEC — see Accident, transport, by
    type of vehicle
    stationary (falling from jack, hydraulic lift, ramp)
      W20.8 ☑
Stumbling
  over
    animal NEC W01.0 ☑
      with fall W18.09 ☑
    carpet, rug or (small) object W22.8 ☑
      with fall W18.09 ☑
    person W51 ☑
      with fall W03 ☑
        due to ice or snow W00.0 ☑
  without fall W18.40 ☑
    due to
      specified NEC W18.49 ☑
      stepping from one level to another W18.43 ☑
      stepping into hole or opening W18.42 ☑
      stepping on object W18.41 ☑
Submersion (accidental) — see Drowning
Suffocation (accidental) (by external means) (by pressure)
  (mechanical) (see also category) T71 ☑
  due to, by
    avalanche — see Landslide
    explosion — see Explosion
    fire — see Exposure, fire
    food, any type (aspiration) (ingestion) (inhalation)
      — see categories T17 and T18 ☑
    ignition — see Ignition
    landslide — see Landslide
    machine(ry) — see Contact, with, by type of ma-
      chine
    vomitus (aspiration) (inhalation) T17.81- ☑
  in
    burning building X00.8 ☑
Suicide, suicidal (attempted) (by) X83.8 ☑
  blunt object X79 ☑
  burning, burns X76 ☑
  hot object X77.9 ☑
    fluid NEC X77.2 ☑
    household appliance X77.3 ☑
    specified NEC X77.8 ☑
    steam X77.0 ☑
    tap water X77.1 ☑
    vapors X77.0 ☑
  caustic substance — see Table of Drugs and Chemicals

Suicide, suicidal — continued
  cold, extreme X83.2 ☑
  collision of motor vehicle with
    motor vehicle X82.0 ☑
    specified NEC X82.8 ☑
    train X82.1 ☑
    tree X82.2 ☑
  crashing of aircraft X83.0 ☑
  cut (any part of body) X78.9 ☑
  cutting or piercing instrument X78.9 ☑
    dagger X78.2 ☑
    glass X78.0 ☑
    knife X78.1 ☑
    specified NEC X78.8 ☑
    sword X78.2 ☑
  drowning (in) X71.9 ☑
    bathtub X71.0 ☑
    natural water X71.3 ☑
    specified NEC X71.8 ☑
    swimming pool X71.1 ☑
      following fall X71.2 ☑
  electrocution X83.1 ☑
  explosive(s) (material) X75 ☑
  fire, flames X76 ☑
  firearm X74.9 ☑
    airgun X74.01 ☑
    handgun X72 ☑
    hunting rifle X73.1 ☑
    larger X73.9 ☑
      specified NEC X73.8 ☑
    machine gun X73.2 ☑
    shotgun X73.0 ☑
    specified NEC X74.8 ☑
  hanging X83.8 ☑
  hot object — see Suicide, burning, hot object
  jumping
    before moving object X81.8 ☑
      motor vehicle X81.0 ☑
      subway train X81.1 ☑
      train X81.1 ☑
    from high place X80 ☑
  late effect of attempt — see X71-X83 with 7th character
    S
  lying before moving object, train, vehicle X81.8 ☑
  poisoning — see Table of Drugs and Chemicals
  puncture (any part of body) — see Suicide, cutting or
    piercing instrument
  scald — see Suicide, burning, hot object
  sequelae of attempt — see X71-X83 with 7th character
    S
  sharp object (any) — see Suicide, cutting or piercing
    instrument
  shooting — see Suicide, firearm
  specified means NEC X83.8 ☑
  stab (any part of body) — see Suicide, cutting or
    piercing instrument
  steam, hot vapors X77.0 ☑
  strangulation X83.8 ☑
  submersion — see Suicide, drowning
  suffocation X83.8 ☑
  wound NEC X83.8 ☑
Sunstroke X32 ☑
Supersonic waves (causing injury) W42.0 ☑
Surgical procedure, complication of (delayed or as an
  abnormal reaction without mention of misadventure) (see also Complication of or following, by type
  of procedure)
  due to or as a result of misadventure — see Misadven-
    ture
Swallowed, swallowing
  foreign body — see Foreign body, alimentary canal
  poison — see Table of Drugs and Chemicals
  substance
    caustic or corrosive — see Table of Drugs and
      Chemicals
    poisonous — see Table of Drugs and Chemicals

T

Tackle in sport W03 ☑
Terrorism (involving) Y38.80 ☑
  biological weapons Y38.6X- ☑
  chemical weapons Y38.7X- ☑
  conflagration Y38.3X- ☑
  drowning and submersion Y38.89- ☑
  explosion Y38.2X- ☑

Terrorism — continued
  explosion — continued
    destruction of aircraft Y38.1X- ☑
    marine weapons Y38.0X- ☑
    fire Y38.3X- ☑
    firearms Y38.4X- ☑
    hot substances Y38.3X- ☑
    lasers Y38.89- ☑
    nuclear weapons Y38.5X- ☑
    piercing or stabbing instruments Y38.89- ☑
    secondary effects Y38.9X- ☑
    specified method NEC Y38.89- ☑
    suicide bomber Y38.81- ☑
Thirst X58 ☑
Threat to breathing
  aspiration — see Aspiration
  due to cave-in, falling earth or substance NEC T71 ☑
Thrown (accidentally)
  against part (any) of or object in transport vehicle (in
    motion) NEC (see also Accident, transport)
  from
    high place, homicide (attempt) Y01 ☑
    machinery — see Contact, with, by type of machine
    transport vehicle NEC (see also Accident, transport)
      V89.9 ☑
  off — see Thrown, from
Thunderbolt — see subcategory T75.0 ☑
  causing fire — see Exposure, fire
Tidal wave (any injury) **NEC** — see Forces of nature, tidal
  wave
Took
  overdose (drug) — see Table of Drugs and Chemicals
  poison — see Table of Drugs and Chemicals
Tornado (any injury) X37.1 ☑
Torrential rain (any injury) X37.8 ☑
Torture X58 ☑
Trampled by animal NEC W55.89 ☑
Trapped (accidentally)
  between objects (moving) (stationary and moving) —
    see Caught
  by part (any) of
    motorcycle V29.88 ☑
    pedal cycle V19.88 ☑
    transport vehicle NEC (see also Accident, transport)
      V89.9 ☑
Travel (effects) (sickness) T75.3 ☑
Tree falling on or hitting (accidentally) (person)
  W20.8 ☑
Tripping
  over
    animal W01.0 ☑
      with fall W01.0 ☑
    carpet, rug or (small) object W22.8 ☑
      with fall W18.09 ☑
    person W51 ☑
      with fall W03 ☑
        due to ice or snow W00.0 ☑
  without fall W18.40 ☑
    due to
      specified NEC W18.49 ☑
      stepping from one level to another W18.43 ☑
      stepping into hole or opening W18.42 ☑
      stepping on object W18.41 ☑
Twisted by person(s) (accidentally) W50.2 ☑
  with intent to injure or kill Y04.0 ☑
  as, or caused by, a crowd or human stampede (with
    fall) W52 ☑
  assault Y04.0 ☑
  homicide (attempt) Y04.0 ☑
  in
    fight Y04.0 ☑
    legal intervention — see Legal, intervention, man-
      handling
Twisting (prolonged) (static) X50.1- ☑

U

Underdosing of necessary drugs, medicaments or
  biological substances Y63.6
Undetermined intent (contact) (exposure)
  automobile collision Y32 ☑
  blunt object Y29 ☑
  drowning (submersion) (in) Y21.9 ☑
    bathtub Y21.0 ☑
      after fall Y21.1 ☑

Undetermined intent — *continued*
  drowning — *continued*
    natural water (lake) (ocean) (pond) (river) (stream)
      Y21.4 ☑
    specified place NEC Y21.8 ☑
    swimming pool Y21.2 ☑
    after fall Y21.3 ☑
  explosive material Y25 ☑
  fall, jump or push from high place Y30 ☑
  falling, lying or running before moving object Y31 ☑
  fire Y26 ☑
  firearm discharge Y24.9 ☑
    airgun (BB) (pellet) Y24.0 ☑
    handgun (pistol) (revolver) Y22 ☑
    hunting rifle Y23.1 ☑
    larger Y23.9 ☑
      hunting rifle Y23.1 ☑
      machine gun Y23.3 ☑
      military Y23.2 ☑
      shotgun Y23.0 ☑
      specified type NEC Y23.8 ☑
    machine gun Y23.3 ☑
    military Y23.2 ☑
    shotgun Y23.0 ☑
    specified type NEC Y24.8 ☑
    Very pistol Y24.8 ☑
  hot object Y27.9 ☑
    fluid NEC Y27.2 ☑
    household appliance Y27.3 ☑
    specified object NEC Y27.8 ☑
    steam Y27.0 ☑
    tap water Y27.1 ☑
    vapor Y27.0 ☑
  jump, fall or push from high place Y30 ☑
  lying, falling or running before moving object Y31 ☑
  motor vehicle crash Y32 ☑
  push, fall or jump from high place Y30 ☑
  running, falling or lying before moving object Y31 ☑
  sharp object Y28.9 ☑
    dagger Y28.2 ☑
    glass Y28.0 ☑
    knife Y28.1 ☑
    specified object NEC Y28.8 ☑
    sword Y28.2 ☑
  smoke Y26
  specified event NEC Y33 ☑
Use of hand as hammer X50.3 ☑

V

Vibration (causing injury) W49.9 ☑
Victim (of)
  avalanche — *see* Landslide
  earth movements NEC — *see* Forces of nature, earth
    movement
  earthquake X34 ☑
  flood — *see* Flood
  landslide — *see* Landslide
  lightning — *see* subcategory T75.0 ☑
    causing fire — *see* Exposure, fire
  storm (cataclysmic) NEC — *see* Forces of nature, cata-
    clysmic storm
  volcanic eruption X35 ☑
Volcanic eruption (any injury) X35 ☑
Vomitus, gastric contents in air passages (with asphyxia, obstruction or suffocation) T17.81- ☑

W

Walked into stationary object (any) W22.09 ☑
  furniture W22.03 ☑
  lamppost W22.02 ☑
  wall W22.01 ☑
War operations (injuries to military personnel and civilians during war, civil insurrection and peacekeeping
  missions) (by) (from) (involving) Y36.90 ☑
  after cessation of hostilities Y36.89- ☑

War operations — *continued*
  after cessation of hostilities — *continued*
    explosion (of)
      bomb placed during war operations Y36.82- ☑
      mine placed during war operations Y36.81- ☑
      specified NEC Y36.88- ☑
  air blast Y36.20- ☑
  aircraft
    destruction — *see* War operations, destruction of
      aircraft
    airway restriction — *see* War operations, restriction of
      airways
    asphyxiation — *see* War operations, restriction of air-
      ways
  biological weapons Y36.6X- ☑
  blast Y36.20- ☑
  blast fragments Y36.20- ☑
  blast wave Y36.20- ☑
  blast wind Y36.20- ☑
  bomb Y36.20- ☑
    dirty Y36.50- ☑
    gasoline Y36.31- ☑
    incendiary Y36.31- ☑
    petrol Y36.31- ☑
  bullet Y36.43- ☑
    incendiary Y36.32- ☑
    rubber Y36.41- ☑
  chemical weapons Y36.7X- ☑
  combat
    hand to hand (unarmed) combat Y36.44- ☑
    using blunt or piercing object Y36.45- ☑
  conflagration — *see* War operations, fire
  conventional warfare NEC Y36.49- ☑
  depth-charge Y36.01- ☑
  destruction of aircraft Y36.10- ☑
    due to
      air to air missile Y36.11- ☑
      collision with other aircraft Y36.12- ☑
      detonation (accidental) of onboard munitions
        and explosives Y36.14- ☑
      enemy fire or explosives Y36.11- ☑
      explosive placed on aircraft Y36.11- ☑
      onboard fire Y36.13- ☑
      rocket propelled grenade [RPG] Y36.11- ☑
      small arms fire Y36.11- ☑
      surface to air missile Y36.11- ☑
    specified NEC Y36.19- ☑
  detonation (accidental) of
    onboard marine weapons Y36.05- ☑
    own munitions or munitions launch device
      Y36.24- ☑
  dirty bomb Y36.50- ☑
  explosion (of) Y36.20- ☑
    aerial bomb Y36.21- ☑
    after cessation of hostilities
      bomb placed during war operations Y36.82- ☑
      mine placed during war operations Y36.81- ☑
    bomb NOS (*see also* War operations, bomb(s))
      Y36.20- ☑
    fragments Y36.20- ☑
    grenade Y36.29- ☑
    guided missile Y36.22- ☑
    improvised explosive device [IED] (person-borne)
      (roadside) (vehicle-borne) Y36.23- ☑
    land mine Y36.29- ☑
    marine mine (at sea) (in harbor) Y36.02- ☑
    marine weapon Y36.00- ☑
      specified NEC Y36.09- ☑
    own munitions or munitions launch device (acciden-
      tal) Y36.24- ☑
    sea-based artillery shell Y36.03- ☑
    specified NEC Y36.29- ☑
    torpedo Y36.04- ☑
  fire Y36.30- ☑
    specified NEC Y36.39- ☑
  firearms
    discharge Y36.43- ☑
    pellets Y36.42- ☑

War operations — *continued*
  flamethrower Y36.33- ☑
  fragments (from) (of)
    improvised explosive device [IED] (person-borne)
      (roadside) (vehicle-borne) Y36.26- ☑
    munitions Y36.25- ☑
    specified NEC Y36.29- ☑
    weapons Y36.27- ☑
  friendly fire Y36.92 ☑
  hand to hand (unarmed) combat Y36.44- ☑
  hot substances — *see* War operations, fire
  incendiary bullet Y36.32- ☑
  nuclear weapon (effects of) Y36.50- ☑
    acute radiation exposure Y36.54- ☑
    blast pressure Y36.51- ☑
    direct blast Y36.51- ☑
    direct heat Y36.53- ☑
    fallout exposure Y36.54- ☑
    fireball Y36.53- ☑
    indirect blast (struck or crushed by blast debris)
      (being thrown by blast) Y36.52- ☑
    ionizing radiation (immediate exposure) Y36.54- ☑
    nuclear radiation Y36.54- ☑
    radiation
      ionizing (immediate exposure) Y36.54- ☑
      nuclear Y36.54- ☑
      thermal Y36.53- ☑
    secondary effects Y36.54- ☑
    specified NEC Y36.59- ☑
    thermal radiation Y36.53- ☑
  restriction of air (airway)
    intentional Y36.46- ☑
    unintentional Y36.47- ☑
  rubber bullets Y36.41- ☑
  shrapnel NOS Y36.29- ☑
  suffocation — *see* War operations, restriction of airways
  unconventional warfare NEC Y36.7X- ☑
  underwater blast NOS Y36.00- ☑
  warfare
    conventional NEC Y36.49- ☑
    unconventional NEC Y36.7X- ☑
  weapon of mass destruction [WMD] Y36.91 ☑
  weapons
    biological weapons Y36.6X- ☑
    chemical Y36.7X- ☑
    nuclear (effects of) Y36.50- ☑
      acute radiation exposure Y36.54- ☑
      blast pressure Y36.51- ☑
      direct blast Y36.51- ☑
      direct heat Y36.53- ☑
      fallout exposure Y36.54- ☑
      fireball Y36.53- ☑
      radiation
        ionizing (immediate exposure) Y36.54- ☑
        nuclear Y36.54- ☑
        thermal Y36.53- ☑
      secondary effects Y36.54- ☑
      specified NEC Y36.59- ☑
    of mass destruction [WMD] Y36.91 ☑
Washed
  away by flood — *see* Flood
  off road by storm (transport vehicle) — *see* Forces of
    nature, cataclysmic storm
Weather exposure NEC — *see* Forces of nature
Weightlessness (causing injury) (effects of) (in spacecraft,
  real or simulated) X52 ☑
Work related condition Y99.0
Wound (accidental) NEC (*see also* Injury) X58 ☑
  battle (*see also* War operations) Y36.90 ☑
  gunshot — *see* Discharge, firearm by type
Wreck transport vehicle NEC (*see also* Accident, transport) V89.9 ☑
Wrong
  device implanted into correct surgical site Y65.51
  fluid in infusion Y65.1
  patient, procedure performed on Y65.52
  procedure (operation) on correct patient Y65.51

☑ **Additional Character Required — Refer to the Tabular List for Character Selection** ▽ **Subterms under main terms may continue to next column or page**

ICD-10-CM Tabular List of Diseases and Injuries

Chapter 1. Certain Infectious and Parasitic Diseases (AØØ–B99)

Chapter Specific Guidelines with Coding Examples

The chapter specific guidelines from the ICD-10-CM Official Guidelines for Coding and Reporting have been provided below. Along with these guidelines are coding examples, contained in the shaded boxes, that have been developed to help illustrate the coding and/or sequencing guidance found in these guidelines.

a. Human immunodeficiency virus (HIV) infections

1) Code only confirmed cases

Code only confirmed cases of HIV infection/illness. This is an exception to the hospital inpatient guideline Section II, H.

In this context, "confirmation" does not require documentation of positive serology or culture for HIV; the provider's diagnostic statement that the patient is HIV positive, or has an HIV-related illness is sufficient.

> Patient admitted with anemia with possible HIV infection
>
> **D64.9   Anemia, unspecified**
>
> *Explanation:* Only the anemia is coded in this scenario because it has not been confirmed that an HIV infection is present. This is an exception to the guideline Section II, H for hospital inpatient coding.

2) Selection and sequencing of HIV codes

(a) Patient admitted for HIV-related condition

If a patient is admitted for an HIV-related condition, the principal diagnosis should be B2Ø, Human immunodeficiency virus [HIV] disease followed by additional diagnosis codes for all reported HIV-related conditions.

> HIV with PCP
>
> **B2Ø   Human immunodeficiency virus [HIV] disease**
>
> **B59   Pneumocystosis**
>
> *Explanation:* Pneumonia due to *Pneumocystis carinii* is an HIV related condition, so the HIV diagnosis code is reported first, followed by the code for the pneumonia.

(b) Patient with HIV disease admitted for unrelated condition

If a patient with HIV disease is admitted for an unrelated condition (such as a traumatic injury), the code for the unrelated condition (e.g., the nature of injury code) should be the principal diagnosis. Other diagnoses would be B2Ø followed by additional diagnosis codes for all reported HIV-related conditions.

> Unstable angina, native coronary artery atherosclerosis, HIV
>
> **I25.11Ø   Atherosclerotic heart disease of native coronary artery with unstable angina pectoris**
>
> **B2Ø   Human immunodeficiency virus [HIV] disease**
>
> *Explanation:* The arteriosclerotic coronary artery disease and the unstable angina are not related to HIV, so those conditions are reported first using a combination code, and HIV is reported secondarily.

(c) Whether the patient is newly diagnosed

Whether the patient is newly diagnosed or has had previous admissions/encounters for HIV conditions is irrelevant to the sequencing decision.

> Newly diagnosed multiple cutaneous Kaposi's sarcoma lesions in previously diagnosed HIV disease
>
> **B2Ø   Human immunodeficiency virus [HIV] disease**
>
> **C46.Ø   Kaposi's sarcoma of skin**
>
> *Explanation:* Even though the HIV was diagnosed on a previous encounter, it is still sequenced first when coded with an HIV related condition. Kaposi's sarcoma is an HIV-related condition.

(d) Asymptomatic human immunodeficiency virus

Z21, Asymptomatic human immunodeficiency virus [HIV] infection status, is to be applied when the patient without any documentation of symptoms is listed as being "HIV positive," "known HIV," "HIV test positive," or similar terminology. Do not use this code if the term "AIDS" is used or if the patient is treated for any HIV-related illness or is described as having any condition(s) resulting from his/her HIV positive status; use B2Ø in these cases.

> Patient admitted with acute appendicitis. Status positive HIV test on Atripla, with no prior symptoms
>
> **K35.8Ø   Unspecified acute appendicitis**
>
> **Z21   Asymptomatic human immunodeficiency virus [HIV] infection status**
>
> *Explanation:* Code Z21 is sequenced second since documentation indicates that the patient has had a positive HIV test but has been asymptomatic. Being on medication for HIV is not an indication that code B2Ø is used instead of Z21. Unless there has been documentation that the patient has had current or prior symptoms or HIV-related complications, code B2Ø is not used. The appendicitis is not an AIDS-related complication and is sequenced first.

(e) Patients with inconclusive HIV serology

Patients with inconclusive HIV serology, but no definitive diagnosis or manifestations of the illness, may be assigned code R75, Inconclusive laboratory evidence of human immunodeficiency virus [HIV].

(f) Previously diagnosed HIV-related illness

Patients with any known prior diagnosis of an HIV-related illness should be coded to B2Ø. Once a patient has developed an HIV-related illness, the patient should always be assigned code B2Ø on every subsequent admission/encounter. Patients previously diagnosed with any HIV illness (B2Ø) should never be assigned to R75 or Z21, Asymptomatic human immunodeficiency virus [HIV] infection status.

(g) HIV infection in pregnancy, childbirth and the puerperium

During pregnancy, childbirth or the puerperium, a patient admitted (or presenting for a health care encounter) because of an HIV-related illness should receive a principal diagnosis code of O98.7-, Human immunodeficiency [HIV] disease complicating pregnancy, childbirth and the puerperium, followed by B2Ø and the code(s) for the HIV-related illness(es). Codes from Chapter 15 always take sequencing priority.

Patients with asymptomatic HIV infection status admitted (or presenting for a health care encounter) during pregnancy, childbirth, or the puerperium should receive codes of O98.7- and Z21.

(h) Encounters for testing for HIV

If a patient is being seen to determine his/her HIV status, use code Z11.4, Encounter for screening for human immunodeficiency virus [HIV]. Use additional codes for any associated high risk behavior.

If a patient with signs or symptoms is being seen for HIV testing, code the signs and symptoms. An additional counseling code Z71.7, Human immunodeficiency virus [HIV] counseling, may be used if counseling is provided during the encounter for the test.

When a patient returns to be informed of his/her HIV test results and the test result is negative, use code Z71.7, Human immunodeficiency virus [HIV] counseling.

If the results are positive, see previous guidelines and assign codes as appropriate.

b. Infectious agents as the cause of diseases classified to other chapters

Certain infections are classified in chapters other than Chapter 1 and no organism is identified as part of the infection code. In these instances, it is necessary to use an additional code from Chapter 1 to identify the organism. A code from category B95, Streptococcus, Staphylococcus, and Enterococcus as the cause of diseases classified to other chapters, B96, Other bacterial agents as the cause of diseases classified to other chapters, or B97, Viral agents as the cause of diseases classified to other chapters, is to be used as an additional code to identify the organism. An instructional note will be found at the infection code advising that an additional organism code is required.

E. coli UTI

N39.Ø	**Urinary tract infection, site not specified**
B96.2Ø	**Unspecified Escherichia coli [E.coli] as the cause of diseases classified elsewhere**

Explanation: An instructional note under the code for the urinary tract infection indicates to code also the specific organism.

c. Infections resistant to antibiotics

Many bacterial infections are resistant to current antibiotics. It is necessary to identify all infections documented as antibiotic resistant. Assign a code from category Z16, Resistance to antimicrobial drugs, following the infection code only if the infection code does not identify drug resistance.

d. Sepsis, severe sepsis, and septic shock

1) Coding of sepsis and severe sepsis

(a) Sepsis

For a diagnosis of sepsis, assign the appropriate code for the underlying systemic infection. If the type of infection or causal organism is not further specified, assign code A41.9, Sepsis, unspecified organism.

A code from subcategory R65.2, Severe sepsis, should not be assigned unless severe sepsis or an associated acute organ dysfunction is documented.

Gram-negative sepsis

A41.5Ø	**Gram-negative sepsis, unspecified**

Staphylococcal sepsis

A41.2	**Sepsis due to unspecified staphylococcus**

Explanation: In both examples above the organism causing the sepsis is identified, therefore A41.9 Sepsis, unspecified organism, would not be appropriate as this code would not capture the highest degree of specificity found in the documentation. Do not use an additional code for severe sepsis unless an acute organ dysfunction was also documented as "associated with" or "due to" the sepsis or the sepsis was documented as "severe."

(i) Negative or inconclusive blood cultures and sepsis

Negative or inconclusive blood cultures do not preclude a diagnosis of sepsis in patients with clinical evidence of the condition; however, the provider should be queried.

(ii) Urosepsis

The term urosepsis is a nonspecific term. It is not to be considered synonymous with sepsis. It has no default code in the Alphabetic Index. Should a provider use this term, he/she must be queried for clarification.

(iii) Sepsis with organ dysfunction

If a patient has sepsis and associated acute organ dysfunction or multiple organ dysfunction (MOD), follow the instructions for coding severe sepsis.

(iv) Acute organ dysfunction that is not clearly associated with the sepsis

If a patient has sepsis and an acute organ dysfunction, but the medical record documentation indicates that the acute organ dysfunction is related to a medical condition other than the sepsis, do not assign a code from subcategory R65.2, Severe sepsis. An acute organ dysfunction must be associated with the sepsis in order to assign the severe sepsis code. If the documentation is not clear as to whether an acute organ dysfunction is related to the sepsis or another medical condition, query the provider.

Sepsis and acute respiratory failure due to COPD exacerbation

A41.9	**Sepsis, unspecified organism**
J44.1	**Chronic obstructive pulmonary disease with (acute) exacerbation**
J96.ØØ	**Acute respiratory failure, unspecified whether with hypoxia or hypercapnia**

Explanation: Although acute organ dysfunction is present in the form of acute respiratory failure, severe sepsis (R65.2) is not coded in this example, as the acute respiratory failure is attributed to the COPD exacerbation rather than the sepsis. Sequencing of these codes would be determined by the circumstances of the admission.

(b) Severe sepsis

The coding of severe sepsis requires a minimum of 2 codes: first a code for the underlying systemic infection, followed by a code from subcategory R65.2, Severe sepsis. If the causal organism is not documented, assign code A41.9, Sepsis, unspecified organism, for the infection. Additional code(s) for the associated acute organ dysfunction are also required.

Due to the complex nature of severe sepsis, some cases may require querying the provider prior to assignment of the codes.

2) Septic shock

(a) Septic shock generally refers to circulatory failure associated with severe sepsis, and therefore, it represents a type of acute organ dysfunction.

For cases of septic shock, the code for the systemic infection should be sequenced first, followed by code R65.21, Severe sepsis with septic shock or code T81.12, Postprocedural septic shock. Any additional codes for the other acute organ dysfunctions should also be assigned. As noted in the sequencing instructions in the Tabular List, the code for septic shock cannot be assigned as a principal diagnosis.

Sepsis with septic shock

A41.9	**Sepsis, unspecified organism**
R65.21	**Severe sepsis with septic shock**

Explanation: Documentation of septic shock automatically implies severe sepsis as it is a form of acute organ dysfunction. Septic shock is not coded as the principal diagnosis; it is always preceded by the code for the systemic infection.

3) Sequencing of severe sepsis

If severe sepsis is present on admission, and meets the definition of principal diagnosis, the underlying systemic infection should be assigned as principal diagnosis followed by the appropriate code from subcategory R65.2 as required by the sequencing rules in the Tabular List. A code from subcategory R65.2 can never be assigned as a principal diagnosis.

When severe sepsis develops during an encounter (it was not present on admission), the underlying systemic infection and the appropriate code from subcategory R65.2 should be assigned as secondary diagnoses.

Severe sepsis may be present on admission, but the diagnosis may not be confirmed until sometime after admission. If the documentation is not clear whether severe sepsis was present on admission, the provider should be queried.

4) Sepsis and severe sepsis with a localized infection

If the reason for admission is both sepsis or severe sepsis and a localized infection, such as pneumonia or cellulitis, a code(s) for the underlying systemic infection should be assigned first and the code for the localized infection should be assigned as a secondary diagnosis. If the patient has severe sepsis, a code from subcategory R65.2 should also be assigned as a secondary diagnosis. If the patient is admitted with a localized infection, such as pneumonia, and sepsis/severe sepsis doesn't develop until after admission, the localized infection should be assigned first, followed by the appropriate sepsis/severe sepsis codes.

Patient presents with acute renal failure due to severe sepsis from *Pseudomonas* pneumonia

A41.9	**Sepsis, unspecified organism**
J15.1	**Pneumonia due to Pseudomonas**
R65.2Ø	**Severe sepsis without septic shock**
N17.9	**Acute kidney failure, unspecified**

Explanation: If all conditions are present on admission, the systemic infection (sepsis) is sequenced first followed by the codes for the localized infection (pneumonia), severe sepsis and any organ dysfunction. If only the pneumonia was present on admission with the sepsis and resulting renal failure developing later in the admission, then the pneumonia would be sequenced first.

5) Sepsis due to a postprocedural infection

(a) Documentation of causal relationship

As with all postprocedural complications, code assignment is based on the provider's documentation of the relationship between the infection and the procedure.

(b) Sepsis due to a postprocedural infection

For **infections following a procedure, a code from** T81.4Ø, to **T81.43** Infection following a procedure, or **a code from O86.ØØ to O86.Ø3,** Infection of obstetric surgical wound, **that identifies the site of the infection** should be coded first, **if known. Assign an**

additional code for sepsis following a procedure (T81.44) or sepsis following an obstetrical procedure (O86.04). **Use an additional code to identify the infectious agent.** If the patient has severe sepsis, the appropriate code from subcategory R65.2 should also be assigned with the additional code(s) for any acute organ dysfunction.

For infections following infusion, transfusion, therapeutic injection, or immunization, a code from subcategory T80.2, Infections following infusion, transfusion, and therapeutic injection, or code T88.0-, Infection following immunization, should be coded first, followed by the code for the specific infection. If the patient has severe sepsis, the appropriate code from subcategory R65.2 should also be assigned, with the additional codes(s) for any acute organ dysfunction.

(c) **Postprocedural infection and postprocedural septic shock**

If a postprocedural infection has resulted in postprocedural septic shock, **assign the codes indicated above for sepsis due to a postprocedural infection, followed by code T81.12-, Postprocedural septic shock. Do not assign code R65.21, Severe sepsis with septic shock. Additional code(s) should be assigned for any acute organ dysfunction.**

6) **Sepsis and severe sepsis associated with a noninfectious process (condition)**

In some cases a noninfectious process (condition), such as trauma, may lead to an infection which can result in sepsis or severe sepsis. If sepsis or severe sepsis is documented as associated with a noninfectious condition, such as a burn or serious injury, and this condition meets the definition for principal diagnosis, the code for the noninfectious condition should be sequenced first, followed by the code for the resulting infection. If severe sepsis is present, a code from subcategory R65.2 should also be assigned with any associated organ dysfunction(s) codes. It is not necessary to assign a code from subcategory R65.1, Systemic inflammatory response syndrome (SIRS) of non-infectious origin, for these cases.

If the infection meets the definition of principal diagnosis, it should be sequenced before the non-infectious condition. When both the associated non-infectious condition and the infection meet the definition of principal diagnosis, either may be assigned as principal diagnosis.

Only one code from category R65, Symptoms and signs specifically associated with systemic inflammation and infection, should be assigned. Therefore, when a non-infectious condition leads to an infection resulting in severe sepsis, assign the appropriate code from subcategory R65.2, Severe sepsis. Do not additionally assign a code from subcategory R65.1, Systemic inflammatory response syndrome (SIRS) of non-infectious origin.

See Section I.C.18. SIRS due to non-infectious process

> Patient admitted with multiple third-degree burns of right upper arm develops severe MSSA sepsis with septic shock, three days into admission
>
> | **T22.391A** | **Burn of third degree of multiple sites of right shoulder and upper arm limb, except wrist and hand, initial encounter** |
> |---|---|
> | **A41.01** | **Sepsis due to Methicillin susceptible Staphylococcus aureus** |
> | **R65.21** | **Severe sepsis with septic shock** |
>
> *Explanation:* Severe sepsis is coded rather than SIRS from R65 because it is documented as a severe systemic infectious response with septic shock to a noninfectious condition. The code for the systemic infection is not used as the principal diagnosis because it was not present on admission. The patient was admitted for the burn injury.

7) **Sepsis and septic shock complicating abortion, pregnancy, childbirth, and the puerperium**

See Section I.C.15. Sepsis and septic shock complicating abortion, pregnancy, childbirth and the puerperium

8) **Newborn sepsis**

See Section I.C.16. f. Bacterial sepsis of Newborn

e. **Methicillin resistant Staphylococcus aureus (MRSA) conditions**

1) **Selection and sequencing of MRSA codes**

(a) **Combination codes for MRSA infection**

When a patient is diagnosed with an infection that is due to methicillin resistant *Staphylococcus aureus* (MRSA), and that infection has a combination code that includes the causal organism (e.g., sepsis, pneumonia) assign the appropriate combination code for the

condition (e.g., code A41.02, Sepsis due to Methicillin resistant Staphylococcus aureus or code J15.212, Pneumonia due to Methicillin resistant Staphylococcus aureus). Do not assign code B95.62, Methicillin resistant Staphylococcus aureus infection as the cause of diseases classified elsewhere, as an additional code, because the combination code includes the type of infection and the MRSA organism. Do not assign a code from subcategory Z16.11, Resistance to penicillins, as an additional diagnosis.

See Section C.1. for instructions on coding and sequencing of sepsis and severe sepsis.

(b) **Other codes for MRSA infection**

When there is documentation of a current infection (e.g., wound infection, stitch abscess, urinary tract infection) due to MRSA, and that infection does not have a combination code that includes the causal organism, assign the appropriate code to identify the condition along with code B95.62, Methicillin resistant Staphylococcus aureus infection as the cause of diseases classified elsewhere for the MRSA infection. Do not assign a code from subcategory Z16.11, Resistance to penicillins.

(c) **Methicillin susceptible Staphylococcus aureus (MSSA) and MRSA colonization**

The condition or state of being colonized or carrying MSSA or MRSA is called colonization or carriage, while an individual person is described as being colonized or being a carrier. Colonization means that MSSA or MSRA is present on or in the body without necessarily causing illness. A positive MRSA colonization test might be documented by the provider as "MRSA screen positive" or "MRSA nasal swab positive".

Assign code Z22.322, Carrier or suspected carrier of Methicillin resistant Staphylococcus aureus, for patients documented as having MRSA colonization. Assign code Z22.321, Carrier or suspected carrier of Methicillin susceptible Staphylococcus aureus, for patient documented as having MSSA colonization. Colonization is not necessarily indicative of a disease process or as the cause of a specific condition the patient may have unless documented as such by the provider.

(d) **MRSA colonization and infection**

If a patient is documented as having both MRSA colonization and infection during a hospital admission, code Z22.322, Carrier or suspected carrier of Methicillin resistant Staphylococcus aureus, and a code for the MRSA infection may both be assigned.

f. **Zika virus infections**

1) **Code only confirmed cases**

Code only a confirmed diagnosis of Zika virus (A92.5, Zika virus disease) as documented by the provider. This is an exception to the hospital inpatient guideline Section II, H. In this context, "confirmation" does not require documentation of the type of test performed; the physician's diagnostic statement that the condition is confirmed is sufficient. This code should be assigned regardless of the stated mode of transmission.

If the provider documents "suspected", "possible" or "probable" Zika, do not assign code A92.5. Assign a code(s) explaining the reason for encounter (such as fever, rash, or joint pain) or Z20.821, Contact with and (suspected) exposure to **Zika virus.**

> A 45-year-old female recently returned from a Caribbean vacation complaining of fever, headache, joint and muscle aches and is admitted for suspected influenza. Infectious Disease consult diagnoses Zika virus. Patient discharged with Zika virus disease and instructions for hydration, rest, acetaminophen, and follow-up with Infectious Disease.
>
> | **A92.5** | **Zika virus disease** |
> |---|---|
>
> *Explanation:* Although only a confirmed diagnosis of Zika virus, code A92.5 Zika virus disease, is reported whether or not there is any indication of the type of tests performed. If the patient is pregnant, code first a code from category O98.5- Other viral diseases complicating pregnancy, childbirth and the puerperium, followed by code (A92.5) for the confirmed Zika virus. See also guideline 1.C.15.a.1.

Chapter 1. Certain Infectious and Parasitic Diseases (A00–B99)

INCLUDES diseases generally recognized as communicable or transmissible

Use additional code to identify resistance to antimicrobial drugs (Z16.-)

EXCLUDES 1 certain localized infections—see body system-related chapters

EXCLUDES 2 carrier or suspected carrier of infectious disease (Z22.-)

infectious and parasitic diseases complicating pregnancy, childbirth and the puerperium (O98.-)

infectious and parasitic diseases specific to the perinatal period (P35-P39)

influenza and other acute respiratory infections (J00-J22)

This chapter contains the following blocks:

A00-A09   Intestinal infectious diseases
A15-A19   Tuberculosis
A20-A28   Certain zoonotic bacterial diseases
A30-A49   Other bacterial diseases
A50-A64   Infections with a predominantly sexual mode of transmission
A65-A69   Other spirochetal diseases
A70-A74   Other diseases caused by chlamydiae
A75-A79   Rickettsioses
A80-A89   Viral and prion infections of the central nervous system
A90-A99   Arthropod-borne viral fevers and viral hemorrhagic fevers
B00-B09   Viral infections characterized by skin and mucous membrane lesions
B10   Other human herpesviruses
B15-B19   Viral hepatitis
B20   Human immunodeficiency virus [HIV] disease
B25-B34   Other viral diseases
B35-B49   Mycoses
B50-B64   Protozoal diseases
B65-B83   Helminthiases
B85-B89   Pediculosis, acariasis and other infestations
B90-B94   Sequelae of infectious and parasitic diseases
B95-B97   Bacterial and viral infectious agents
B99   Other infectious diseases

Intestinal Infectious Diseases (A00-A09)

✓4th A00 Cholera

DEF: Acute infection of the bowel due to vibrio cholerae that presents with profuse diarrhea, cramps, and vomiting, resulting in severe dehydration, electrolyte imbalance, and death. It is spread through ingestion of food or water contaminated with feces of infected persons.

CC Excl: For CC codes in category A00: PDX collection 2

A00.0 Cholera due to Vibrio cholerae 01, biovar cholerae `CC`
Classical cholera

A00.1 Cholera due to Vibrio cholerae 01, biovar eltor `CC`
Cholera eltor

A00.9 Cholera, unspecified `CC`

✓4th A01 Typhoid and paratyphoid fevers

DEF: Typhoid fever: Acute generalized illness caused by Salmonella typhi. Clinical features include fever, headache, abdominal pain, cough, toxemia, leukopenia, abnormal pulse, rose spots on the skin, bacteremia, hyperplasia of intestinal lymph nodes, mesenteric lymphadenopathy, and Peyer's patches in the intestines.

DEF: Paratyphoid fever: Prolonged febrile illness, caused by Salmonella serotypes other than S. typhi, especially S. enterica serotypes paratyphi A, B, and C.

CC Excl: For CC codes in category A01: PDX collection 3

✓5th A01.0 Typhoid fever
Infection due to Salmonella typhi

     A01.00 Typhoid fever, unspecified `CC`
     A01.01 Typhoid meningitis `CC`
     A01.02 Typhoid fever with heart involvement `CC`
         Typhoid endocarditis   Typhoid myocarditis
     A01.03 Typhoid pneumonia `CC` `HCC`
     A01.04 Typhoid arthritis `CC` `HCC`
     A01.05 Typhoid osteomyelitis `CC` `HCC`
     A01.09 Typhoid fever with other complications `CC`

A01.1 Paratyphoid fever A `CC`
A01.2 Paratyphoid fever B `CC`
A01.3 Paratyphoid fever C `CC`
A01.4 Paratyphoid fever, unspecified `CC`
Infection due to Salmonella paratyphi NOS

✓4th A02 Other salmonella infections

INCLUDES infection or foodborne intoxication due to any Salmonella species other than S. typhi and S. paratyphi

A02.0 Salmonella enteritis `CC`
Salmonellosis
TIP: Dehydration (E86.0) is a complication of salmonella enteritis and may be reported separately.
CC Excl: PDX collection 4

A02.1 Salmonella sepsis `HIV` `MCC` `HCC`
CC Excl: PDX collection 5

✓5th A02.2 Localized salmonella infections

     A02.20 Localized salmonella infection, unspecified `HIV`
     A02.21 Salmonella meningitis `HIV` `MCC`
         CC Excl: PDX collection 6
     A02.22 Salmonella pneumonia `HIV` `MCC` `HCC`
         CC Excl: PDX collection 7
     A02.23 Salmonella arthritis `HIV` `CC` `HCC`
         CC Excl: PDX collection 8
     A02.24 Salmonella osteomyelitis `HIV` `CC` `HCC`
         CC Excl: PDX collection 9
     A02.25 Salmonella pyelonephritis `HIV` `CC`
         Salmonella tubulo-interstitial nephropathy
         CC Excl: PDX collection 10
     A02.29 Salmonella with other localized infection `HIV` `CC`
         CC Excl: PDX collection 10

A02.8 Other specified salmonella infections `HIV` `CC`
     CC Excl: PDX collection 11

A02.9 Salmonella infection, unspecified `HIV` `CC`
     CC Excl: PDX collection 12

✓4th A03 Shigellosis

DEF: Infection caused by the genus the Shigella, of the family Enterobacteriaceae that is known to cause an acute dysenteric infection of the bowel with fever, drowsiness, anorexia, nausea, vomiting, bloody diarrhea, abdominal cramps, and distention.

A03.0 Shigellosis due to Shigella dysenteriae `CC`
Group A shigellosis [Shiga-Kruse dysentery]
CC Excl: PDX collection 13

A03.1 Shigellosis due to Shigella flexneri
Group B shigellosis

A03.2 Shigellosis due to Shigella boydii
Group C shigellosis

A03.3 Shigellosis due to Shigella sonnei
Group D shigellosis

A03.8 Other shigellosis

A03.9 Shigellosis, unspecified
Bacillary dysentery NOS

✓4th A04 Other bacterial intestinal infections

EXCLUDES 1 bacterial foodborne intoxications, NEC (A05.-)
tuberculous enteritis (A18.32)

DEF: Escherichia coli: Gram negative, anaerobic of the family Enterobacteriaceae found in the large intestine of warm-blooded animals, generally as a nonpathologic entity aiding in digestion. They become pathogenic when an opportunity to grow somewhere outside this relationship presents itself, such as ingestion of fecal contaminated food or water.

CC Excl: For CC codes in category A04, unless otherwise noted:
For codes A04.0-A04.4: PDX collection 14
For codes A04.5-A04.8: PDX collection 15

A04.0 Enteropathogenic Escherichia coli infection `CC`

A04.1 Enterotoxigenic Escherichia coli infection `CC`

A04.2 Enteroinvasive Escherichia coli infection `CC`

A04.3 Enterohemorrhagic Escherichia coli infection `CC`
DEF: E. coli infection penetrating the intestinal mucosa, producing microscopic ulceration and bleeding.

A04.4 Other intestinal Escherichia coli infections `CC`
Escherichia coli enteritis NOS

A04.5 Campylobacter enteritis `CC`
TIP: For Guillain-Barre syndrome occurring as a sequela of Campylobacter enteritis, assign code G61.0 as the first-listed diagnosis, followed by B94.8 for the sequelae.

A04.6 Enteritis due to Yersinia enterocolitica `CC`
EXCLUDES 1 extraintestinal yersiniosis (A28.2)

N Newborn: 0   **P** Pediatric: 0-17   **M** Maternity: 12-55   **A** Adult: 15-124   **MCC** Major Complication/Comorbidity   **CC** Complication/Comorbidity   **SW** Severe Wound Dx

436   ICD-10-CM 2019

☑5ᵗʰ **A04.7 Enterocolitis due to Clostridium difficile**
Foodborne intoxication by Clostridium difficile
Pseudomembraneous colitis
AHA: 2017, 4Q, 4

    A04.71 Enterocolitis due to Clostridium difficile, `CC`
recurrent

    A04.72 Enterocolitis due to Clostridium difficile, `CC`
not specified as recurrent

A04.8 Other specified bacterial intestinal infections `CC`

A04.9 Bacterial intestinal infection, unspecified `CC`
Bacterial enteritis NOS
CC Excl: PDX collection 16

☑4ᵗʰ **A05 Other bacterial foodborne intoxications, not elsewhere classified**
EXCLUDES 1   *Clostridium difficile foodborne intoxication and infection (A04.7-)*
Escherichia coli infection (A04.0-A04.4)
listeriosis (A32.-)
salmonella foodborne intoxication and infection (A02.-)
toxic effect of noxious foodstuffs (T61-T62)

CC Excl: For CC codes in category A05, unless otherwise noted:
PDX collection 17

A05.0 Foodborne staphylococcal intoxication `CC`
TIP: Assign code A04.8 to report a staphylococcal infection when it is caused by the ingestion of contaminated food but not caused by *S. aureus* toxins.

A05.1 Botulism food poisoning `CC`
Botulism NOS
Classical foodborne intoxication due to Clostridium botulinum
EXCLUDES 1   *infant botulism (A48.51)*
wound botulism (A48.52)
DEF: Muscle-paralyzing neurotoxic disease caused by ingesting pre-formed toxin from the bacterium *Clostridium botulinum*. It causes vomiting and diarrhea, vision problems, slurred speech, difficulty swallowing, paralysis, and death.
CC Excl: PDX collection 18

A05.2 Foodborne Clostridium perfringens [Clostridium welchii] `CC`
intoxication
Enteritis necroticans
Pig-bel
CC Excl: PDX collection 19

A05.3 Foodborne Vibrio parahaemolyticus intoxication `CC`

A05.4 Foodborne Bacillus cereus intoxication `CC`

A05.5 Foodborne Vibrio vulnificus intoxication `CC`

A05.8 Other specified bacterial foodborne intoxications `CC`

A05.9 Bacterial foodborne intoxication, unspecified

☑4ᵗʰ **A06 Amebiasis**
INCLUDES   infection due to Entamoeba histolytica
EXCLUDES 1   *other protozoal intestinal diseases (A07.-)*
EXCLUDES 2   *acanthamebiasis (B60.1-)*
Naegleriasis (B60.2)
DEF: Infection with a single cell protozoan known as the amoeba. Transmission occurs through ingestion of feces, contaminated food or water, use of human feces as fertilizer, or person-to-person contact.

A06.0 Acute amebic dysentery `CC`
Acute amebiasis
Intestinal amebiasis NOS
CC Excl: PDX collection 20

A06.1 Chronic intestinal amebiasis `CC`
CC Excl: PDX collection 20

A06.2 Amebic nondysenteric colitis `CC`
CC Excl: PDX collection 21

A06.3 Ameboma of intestine `CC`
Ameboma NOS
CC Excl: PDX collection 22

A06.4 Amebic liver abscess `MCC`
Hepatic amebiasis
CC Excl: PDX collection 23

A06.5 Amebic lung abscess `MCC` `HCC`
Amebic abscess of lung (and liver)
CC Excl: PDX collection 24

A06.6 Amebic brain abscess `MCC`
Amebic abscess of brain (and liver) (and lung)
CC Excl: PDX collection 25

A06.7 Cutaneous amebiasis

☑5ᵗʰ **A06.8 Amebic infection of other sites**

CC Excl: For CC codes in subcategory A06.8:
PDX collection 22

    A06.81 Amebic cystitis `CC`

    A06.82 Other amebic genitourinary infections `CC`
Amebic balanitis
Amebic vesiculitis
Amebic vulvovaginitis

    A06.89 Other amebic infections `CC`
Amebic appendicitis
Amebic splenic abscess

A06.9 Amebiasis, unspecified

☑4ᵗʰ **A07 Other protozoal intestinal diseases**
DEF: Protozoa: Group comprised of the simplest, single celled organisms, ranging in size from micro to macroscopic. They can live alone or in colonies, and do not show any differentiation in tissues. Most are motile and can live free in nature, but some are parasitic, causing disease in the variety of hosts they inhabit.

CC Excl: For CC codes in category A07, unless otherwise noted:
PDX collection 26

A07.0 Balantidiasis
Balantidial dysentery

A07.1 Giardiasis [lambliasis] `CC`
DEF: Infection caused by the flagellate protozoan *Giardia lamblia* causing gastrointestinal problems such as vomiting, chronic diarrhea, and weight loss. The most common parasite in the US, this is usually transmitted by ingesting contaminated water while in the cyst state and latches onto the wall of the small intestine.

A07.2 Cryptosporidiosis `CC` `HCC`
DEF: Microscopic parasite found in water and one of the most common causes of waterborne gastrointestinal infectious disease in the United States. It is usually transmitted by ingesting contaminated drinking water or recreational water and causes profuse watery diarrhea, flatulence, abdominal pain, and cramping.

A07.3 Isosporiasis `HIV` `CC`
Infection due to Isospora belli and Isospora hominis
Intestinal coccidiosis
Isosporosis

A07.4 Cyclosporiasis `CC`
CC Excl: PDX collection 27

A07.8 Other specified protozoal intestinal diseases `CC`
Intestinal microsporidiosis   Sarcocystosis
Intestinal trichomoniasis   Sarcosporidiosis

A07.9 Protozoal intestinal disease, unspecified `CC`
Flagellate diarrhea   Protozoal diarrhea
Protozoal colitis   Protozoal dysentery

☑4ᵗʰ **A08 Viral and other specified intestinal infections**
EXCLUDES 1   *influenza with involvement of gastrointestinal tract (J09.X3, J10.2, J11.2)*

CC Excl: For CC codes in category A08: PDX collection 28

A08.0 Rotaviral enteritis `CC`

☑5ᵗʰ **A08.1 Acute gastroenteropathy due to Norwalk agent and other small round viruses**

    A08.11 Acute gastroenteropathy due to Norwalk agent `CC`
Acute gastroenteropathy due to Norovirus
Acute gastroenteropathy due to Norwalk-like agent

    A08.19 Acute gastroenteropathy due to other small `CC`
round viruses
Acute gastroenteropathy due to small round virus [SRV] NOS

A08.2 Adenoviral enteritis `CC`

☑5ᵗʰ **A08.3 Other viral enteritis**

    A08.31 Calicivirus enteritis `CC`

    A08.32 Astrovirus enteritis `CC`

    A08.39 Other viral enteritis `CC`
Coxsackie virus enteritis
Echovirus enteritis
Enterovirus enteritis NEC
Torovirus enteritis

A08.4 Viral intestinal infection, unspecified
Viral enteritis NOS
Viral gastroenteritis NOS
Viral gastroenteropathy NOS
AHA: 2016, 3Q, 12

A08.8 Other specified intestinal infections

☑ Additional Character Required   ☑x7ᵗʰ Placeholder   Unacceptable PDx   Questionable PDx   Manifestation   `H1`-`H14` HAC   `HCC` CMS-HCC Dx   `HIV` HIV Dx

ICD-10-CM 2019   437

A09   **Infectious gastroenteritis and colitis, unspecified**   `CC`
  Infectious colitis NOS
  Infectious enteritis NOS
  Infectious gastroenteritis NOS
  EXCLUDES 1   *colitis NOS (K52.9)*
       diarrhea NOS (R19.7)
       enteritis NOS (K52.9)
       gastroenteritis NOS (K52.9)
       noninfective gastroenteritis and colitis, unspecified (K52.9)
  DEF: Colitis: Inflammation of mucous membranes of the colon.
  DEF: Enteritis: Inflammation of mucous membranes of the small intestine.
  DEF: Gastroenteritis: Inflammation of mucous membranes of the stomach and intestines.
  CC Excl: PDX collection 17

Tuberculosis (A15-A19)

INCLUDES   infections due to Mycobacterium tuberculosis and Mycobacterium bovis
EXCLUDES 1   *congenital tuberculosis (P37.0)*
     nonspecific reaction to test for tuberculosis without active tuberculosis (R76.1-)
     pneumoconiosis associated with tuberculosis, any type in A15 (J65)
     positive PPD (R76.11)
     positive tuberculin skin test without active tuberculosis (R76.11)
     sequelae of tuberculosis (B90.-)
     silicotuberculosis (J65)
DEF: Bacterial infection that typically spreads by inhalation of an airborne agent that usually attacks the lungs, but may also affect other organs.

√4ᵗʰ A15   **Respiratory tuberculosis**

> **CC Excl:** For CC codes in category A15, unless otherwise noted: PDX collection 29

  A15.0   **Tuberculosis of lung**   `HIV` `CC`
  Tuberculous bronchiectasis
  Tuberculous fibrosis of lung
  Tuberculous pneumonia
  Tuberculous pneumothorax

  A15.4   **Tuberculosis of intrathoracic lymph nodes**   `HIV` `CC`
  Tuberculosis of hilar lymph nodes
  Tuberculosis of mediastinal lymph nodes
  Tuberculosis of tracheobronchial lymph nodes
  EXCLUDES 1   *tuberculosis specified as primary (A15.7)*

  A15.5   **Tuberculosis of larynx, trachea and bronchus**   `HIV` `CC`
  Tuberculosis of bronchus
  Tuberculosis of glottis
  Tuberculosis of larynx
  Tuberculosis of trachea

  A15.6   **Tuberculous pleurisy**   `HIV` `CC`
  Tuberculous of pleura Tuberculous empyema
  EXCLUDES 1   *primary respiratory tuberculosis (A15.7)*

  A15.7   **Primary respiratory tuberculosis**   `HIV` `CC`
  CC Excl: PDX collection 30

Tuberculosis of Lung

Granulomas from Mycobacterium tuberculosis

A15.8   **Other respiratory tuberculosis**   `HIV` `CC`
  Mediastinal tuberculosis
  Nasopharyngeal tuberculosis
  Tuberculosis of nose
  Tuberculosis of sinus [any nasal]
  CC Excl: PDX collection 31

A15.9   **Respiratory tuberculosis unspecified**   `HIV` `CC`
  CC Excl: PDX collection 31

√4ᵗʰ A17   **Tuberculosis of nervous system**

  A17.0   **Tuberculous meningitis**   `HIV` `MCC`
  Tuberculosis of meninges (cerebral)(spinal)
  Tuberculous leptomeningitis
  EXCLUDES 1   *tuberculous meningoencephalitis (A17.82)*
  CC Excl: PDX collection 32

  A17.1   **Meningeal tuberculoma**   `HIV` `MCC`
  Tuberculoma of meninges (cerebral) (spinal)
  EXCLUDES 2   *tuberculoma of brain and spinal cord (A17.81)*
  CC Excl: PDX collection 32

  √5ᵗʰ A17.8   **Other tuberculosis of nervous system**
    A17.81   **Tuberculoma of brain and spinal cord**   `HIV` `MCC`
    Tuberculous abscess of brain and spinal cord
    CC Excl: PDX collection 33

    A17.82   **Tuberculous meningoencephalitis**   `HIV` `MCC`
    Tuberculous myelitis
    CC Excl: PDX collection 33

    A17.83   **Tuberculous neuritis**   `HIV` `MCC`
    Tuberculous mononeuropathy
    CC Excl: No Excl

    A17.89   **Other tuberculosis of nervous system**   `HIV` `MCC`
    Tuberculous polyneuropathy
    CC Excl: PDX collection 34

  A17.9   **Tuberculosis of nervous system, unspecified**   `HIV` `CC`
  CC Excl: PDX collection 35

√4ᵗʰ A18   **Tuberculosis of other organs**

  √5ᵗʰ A18.0   **Tuberculosis of bones and joints**
    A18.01   **Tuberculosis of spine**   `HIV` `CC`
    Pott's disease or curvature of spine
    Tuberculous arthritis
    Tuberculous osteomyelitis of spine
    Tuberculous spondylitis
    CC Excl: PDX collection 36

    A18.02   **Tuberculous arthritis of other joints**   `HIV` `CC`
    Tuberculosis of hip (joint)
    Tuberculosis of knee (joint)
    CC Excl: PDX collection 37

    A18.03   **Tuberculosis of other bones**   `HIV` `CC`
    Tuberculous mastoiditis
    Tuberculous osteomyelitis
    CC Excl: PDX collection 38

    A18.09   **Other musculoskeletal tuberculosis**   `HIV` `CC`
    Tuberculous myositis
    Tuberculous synovitis
    Tuberculous tenosynovitis
    CC Excl: PDX collection 39

  √5ᵗʰ A18.1   **Tuberculosis of genitourinary system**
    A18.10   **Tuberculosis of genitourinary system, unspecified**   `HIV` `CC`
    CC Excl: PDX collection 40

    A18.11   **Tuberculosis of kidney and ureter**   `HIV` `CC`
    CC Excl: PDX collection 41

    A18.12   **Tuberculosis of bladder**   `HIV` `CC`
    CC Excl: PDX collection 41

    A18.13   **Tuberculosis of other urinary organs**   `HIV` `CC`
    Tuberculous urethritis
    CC Excl: PDX collection 41

    A18.14   **Tuberculosis of prostate**   `HIV` `CC` `A` ♂
    CC Excl: PDX collection 42

    A18.15   **Tuberculosis of other male genital organs**   `HIV` `CC` ♂
    CC Excl: PDX collection 42

    A18.16   **Tuberculosis of cervix**   `HIV` `CC` ♀
    CC Excl: PDX collection 43

    A18.17   **Tuberculous female pelvic inflammatory disease**   `HIV` `CC` ♀
    Tuberculous endometritis
    Tuberculous oophoritis and salpingitis
    CC Excl: PDX collection 43

N Newborn: 0   **P** Pediatric: 0-17   **M** Maternity: 12-55   **A** Adult: 15-124   **MCC** Major Complication/Comorbidity   **CC** Complication/Comorbidity   **SW** Severe Wound Dx

438   ICD-10-CM 2019

A18.18 Tuberculosis of other female genital organs `HIV` `CC` ♀
Tuberculous ulceration of vulva
CC Excl: PDX collection 43

A18.2 Tuberculous peripheral lymphadenopathy `HIV` `CC`
Tuberculous adenitis
EXCLUDES 2   tuberculosis of bronchial and mediastinal lymph nodes
(A15.4)
tuberculosis of mesenteric and retroperitoneal lymph
nodes (A18.39)
tuberculous tracheobronchial adenopathy (A15.4)
CC Excl: PDX collection 44

✓5ᵗʰ **A18.3 Tuberculosis of** intestines, peritoneum and mesenteric glands

CC Excl: For CC/MCC codes in subcategory A18.3:
PDX collection 45

A18.31 Tuberculous peritonitis `HIV` `MCC`
Tuberculous ascites
DEF: Tuberculous inflammation of the membrane lining
the abdomen.

A18.32 Tuberculous enteritis `HIV` `CC`
Tuberculosis of anus and rectum
Tuberculosis of intestine (large) (small)

A18.39 Retroperitoneal tuberculosis `HIV` `CC`
Tuberculosis of mesenteric glands
Tuberculosis of retroperitoneal (lymph glands)

A18.4 Tuberculosis of skin and subcutaneous tissue `HIV` `CC`
Erythema induratum, tuberculous
Lupus excedens
Lupus vulgaris NOS
Lupus vulgaris of eyelid
Scrofuloderma
Tuberculosis of external ear
EXCLUDES 2   lupus erythematosus (L93.-)
lupus NOS (M32.9)
systemic (M32.-)
CC Excl: PDX collection 30

✓5ᵗʰ **A18.5 Tuberculosis of** eye
EXCLUDES 2   lupus vulgaris of eyelid (A18.4)

CC Excl: For CC codes in subcategory A18.5:
PDX collection 46

A18.50 Tuberculosis of eye, unspecified `HIV` `CC`
A18.51 Tuberculous episcleritis `HIV` `CC`
A18.52 Tuberculous keratitis `HIV` `CC`
Tuberculous interstitial keratitis
Tuberculous keratoconjunctivitis (interstitial)
(phlyctenular)
A18.53 Tuberculous chorioretinitis `HIV` `CC`
A18.54 Tuberculous iridocyclitis `HIV` `CC`
A18.59 Other tuberculosis of eye `HIV` `CC`
Tuberculous conjunctivitis

A18.6 Tuberculosis of (inner) (middle) ear `HIV` `CC`
Tuberculous otitis media
EXCLUDES 2   tuberculosis of external ear (A18.4)
tuberculous mastoiditis (A18.03)
CC Excl: PDX collection 47

A18.7 Tuberculosis of adrenal glands `HIV` `CC`
Tuberculous Addison's disease
CC Excl: PDX collection 48

✓5ᵗʰ **A18.8 Tuberculosis of** other specified organs
A18.81 Tuberculosis of thyroid gland `HIV` `CC`
CC Excl: PDX collection 49

A18.82 Tuberculosis of other endocrine glands `HIV` `CC`
Tuberculosis of pituitary gland
Tuberculosis of thymus gland
CC Excl: PDX collection 35

A18.83 Tuberculosis of digestive tract organs, not `HIV` `CC`
elsewhere classified
EXCLUDES 1   tuberculosis of intestine (A18.32)
CC Excl: PDX collection 45

A18.84 Tuberculosis of heart `HIV` `CC`
Tuberculous cardiomyopathy
Tuberculous endocarditis
Tuberculous myocarditis
Tuberculous pericarditis
CC Excl: PDX collection 35

A18.85 Tuberculosis of spleen `HIV` `CC`
CC Excl: PDX collection 50

A18.89 Tuberculosis of other sites `HIV` `CC`
Tuberculosis of muscle
Tuberculous cerebral arteritis
CC Excl: PDX collection 35

✓4ᵗʰ **A19 Miliary tuberculosis**
INCLUDES   disseminated tuberculosis
generalized tuberculosis
tuberculous polyserositis

CC Excl: For MCC codes in category A19: PDX collection 51

A19.0 Acute miliary tuberculosis of a single specified site `HIV` `MCC`
A19.1 Acute miliary tuberculosis of multiple sites `HIV` `MCC`
A19.2 Acute miliary tuberculosis, unspecified `HIV` `MCC`
A19.8 Other miliary tuberculosis `HIV` `MCC`
A19.9 Miliary tuberculosis, unspecified `HIV` `MCC`

Certain zoonotic bacterial diseases (A20-A28)

✓4ᵗʰ **A20 Plague**
INCLUDES   infection due to Yersinia pestis

A20.0 Bubonic plague `MCC`
CC Excl: PDX collection 52
A20.1 Cellulocutaneous plague `MCC`
CC Excl: PDX collection 52
A20.2 Pneumonic plague `MCC` `HCC`
CC Excl: PDX collection 53
A20.3 Plague meningitis `MCC`
CC Excl: PDX collection 54
A20.7 Septicemic plague `MCC` `HCC`
CC Excl: PDX collection 55
A20.8 Other forms of plague `MCC`
Abortive plague
Asymptomatic plague
Pestis minor
CC Excl: PDX collection 54
A20.9 Plague, unspecified `MCC`
CC Excl: PDX collection 56

✓4ᵗʰ **A21 Tularemia**
INCLUDES   deer-fly fever
infection due to Francisella tularensis
rabbit fever
DEF: Febrile disease transmitted to humans by the bites of deer flies, fleas,
and ticks, by inhaling aerosolized *F. tularensis*, or by ingesting
contaminated food or water. Patients quickly develop fever, chills,
weakness, headache, backache, and malaise.

A21.0 Ulceroglandular tularemia `CC`
CC Excl: PDX collection 57
A21.1 Oculoglandular tularemia `CC`
Ophthalmic tularemia
CC Excl: PDX collection 58
A21.2 Pulmonary tularemia `CC` `HCC`
CC Excl: PDX collection 59
A21.3 Gastrointestinal tularemia `CC`
Abdominal tularemia
CC Excl: PDX collection 60
A21.7 Generalized tularemia `CC`
CC Excl: PDX collection 61
A21.8 Other forms of tularemia `CC`
CC Excl: PDX collection 61
A21.9 Tulamirea, unspecified `CC`
CC Excl: PDX collection 61

✓4ᵗʰ **A22 Anthrax**
INCLUDES   infection due to Bacillus anthracis
A22.0 Cutaneous anthrax `CC`
Malignant carbuncle
Malignant pustule
CC Excl: PDX collection 62
A22.1 Pulmonary anthrax `MCC` `HCC`
Inhalation anthrax
Ragpicker's disease
Woolsorter's disease
CC Excl: PDX collection 63
A22.2 Gastrointestinal anthrax `CC`
CC Excl: PDX collection 64
A22.7 Anthrax sepsis `MCC` `HCC`
CC Excl: PDX collection 5

A22.8 Other forms of anthrax `CC`
    Anthrax meningitis
    CC Excl: PDX collection 65

A22.9 Anthrax, unspecified `CC`
    CC Excl: PDX collection 66

✓4ᵗʰ **A23 Brucellosis**
    INCLUDES   Malta fever
                   Mediterranean fever
                    undulant fever

    A23.0 Brucellosis due to Brucella melitensis

    A23.1 Brucellosis due to Brucella abortus

    A23.2 Brucellosis due to Brucella suis

    A23.3 Brucellosis due to Brucella canis

    A23.8 Other brucellosis `CC`
        CC Excl: PDX collection 67

    A23.9 Brucellosis, unspecified `CC`
        CC Excl: PDX collection 67

✓4ᵗʰ **A24 Glanders and melioidosis**

    CC Excl: For CC codes in category A24, unless otherwise noted: PDX collection 69

    A24.0 Glanders `CC`
        Infection due to Pseudomonas mallei
        Malleus
        CC Excl: PDX collection 68

    A24.1 Acute and fulminating melioidosis `CC`
        Melioidosis pneumonia
        Melioidosis sepsis

    A24.2 Subacute and chronic melioidosis `CC`

    A24.3 Other melioidosis `CC`

    A24.9 Melioidosis, unspecified `CC`
        Infection due to Pseudomonas pseudomallei NOS
        Whitmore's disease

✓4ᵗʰ **A25 Rat-bite fevers**

    CC Excl: For CC codes in category A25: PDX collection 70

    A25.0 Spirillosis `CC`
        Sodoku

    A25.1 Streptobacillosis `CC`
        Epidemic arthritic erythema   Streptobacillary rat-bite fever
        Haverhill fever

    A25.9 Rat-bite fever, unspecified `CC`

✓4ᵗʰ **A26 Erysipeloid**
    DEF: Acute cutaneous infection typically caused by trauma to the skin. Presenting as cellulitis, it may become systemic affecting other organs. It is gram positive bacillus and mainly acquired by those who routinely handle meat.

    A26.0 Cutaneous erysipeloid
        Erythema migrans

    A26.7 Erysipelothrix sepsis `MCC` `HCC`
        CC Excl: PDX collection 71

    A26.8 Other forms of erysipeloid

    A26.9 Erysipeloid, unspecified

✓4ᵗʰ **A27 Leptospirosis**

    CC Excl: For CC/MCC codes in category A27: PDX collection 72

    A27.0 Leptospirosis icterohemorrhagica `CC`
        Leptospiral or spirochetal jaundice (hemorrhagic)
        Weil's disease

    ✓5ᵗʰ **A27.8 Other forms of leptospirosis**
        A27.81 Aseptic meningitis in leptospirosis `MCC`
            CC Excl: PDX collection 73
        A27.89 Other forms of leptospirosis `CC`

    A27.9 Leptospirosis, unspecified `CC`

✓4ᵗʰ **A28 Other zoonotic bacterial diseases, not elsewhere classified**

    CC Excl: For CC codes in category A28, unless otherwise noted: PDX collection 74

    A28.0 Pasteurellosis `CC`

    A28.1 Cat-scratch disease `CC`
        Cat-scratch fever
        CC Excl: PDX collection 75

    A28.2 Extraintestinal yersiniosis `CC`
        EXCLUDES 1   enteritis due to Yersinia enterocolitica (A04.6)
                     plague (A20.-)

A28.8 Other specified zoonotic bacterial diseases, not elsewhere classified `CC`

A28.9 Zoonotic bacterial disease, unspecified `CC`

Other bacterial diseases (A30-A49)

AHA: 2016, 3Q, 8-14

✓4ᵗʰ **A30 Leprosy [Hansen's disease]**
    INCLUDES   infection due to Mycobacterium leprae
    EXCLUDES 1   sequelae of leprosy (B92)

    A30.0 Indeterminate leprosy `CC`
        I leprosy
        CC Excl: PDX collection 76

    A30.1 Tuberculoid leprosy `CC`
        TT leprosy
        CC Excl: PDX collection 77

    A30.2 Borderline tuberculoid leprosy `CC`
        BT leprosy
        CC Excl: PDX collection 78

    A30.3 Borderline leprosy `CC`
        BB leprosy
        CC Excl: PDX collection 78

    A30.4 Borderline lepromatous leprosy `CC`
        BL leprosy
        CC Excl: PDX collection 78

    A30.5 Lepromatous leprosy `CC`
        LL leprosy
        CC Excl: PDX collection 79

    A30.8 Other forms of leprosy `CC`
        CC Excl: PDX collection 80

    A30.9 Leprosy, unspecified `CC`
        CC Excl: PDX collection 81

✓4ᵗʰ **A31 Infection due to other mycobacteria**
    EXCLUDES 2   leprosy (A30.-)
                 tuberculosis (A15-A19)

    CC Excl: For CC codes in category A31, unless otherwise noted: PDX collection 83

    A31.0 Pulmonary mycobacterial infection `CC` `HCC`
        Infection due to Mycobacterium avium
        Infection due to Mycobacterium intracellulare [Battey bacillus]
        Infection due to Mycobacterium kansasii
        CC Excl: PDX collection 82

    A31.1 Cutaneous mycobacterial infection `CC`
        Buruli ulcer
        Infection due to Mycobacterium marinum
        Infection due to Mycobacterium ulcerans

    A31.2 Disseminated mycobacterium avium-intracellulare complex (DMAC) `HIV` `CC` `HCC`
        MAC sepsis

    A31.8 Other mycobacterial infections `HIV` `CC`

    A31.9 Mycobacterial infection, unspecified `HIV` `CC`
        Atypical mycobacterial infection NOS
        Mycobacteriosis NOS

✓4ᵗʰ **A32 Listeriosis**
    INCLUDES   listerial foodborne infection
    EXCLUDES 1   neonatal (disseminated) listeriosis (P37.2)

    CC Excl: For CC/MCC codes in category A32, unless otherwise noted: PDX collection 74

    A32.0 Cutaneous listeriosis `CC`

    ✓5ᵗʰ **A32.1 Listerial meningitis and meningoencephalitis**
        A32.11 Listerial meningitis `CC`
        A32.12 Listerial meningoencephalitis `CC`

    A32.7 Listerial sepsis `MCC` `HCC`
        CC Excl: PDX collection 71

    ✓5ᵗʰ **A32.8 Other forms of listeriosis**
        A32.81 Oculoglandular listeriosis `CC`
        A32.82 Listerial endocarditis `CC`
        A32.89 Other forms of listeriosis `CC`
            Listerial cerebral arteritis

    A32.9 Listeriosis, unspecified `CC`

A33 Tetanus neonatorum `MCC` `N`
    CC Excl: PDX collection 84

A34 Obstetrical tetanus `CC` `M` `♀`
    CC Excl: PDX collection 85

`N` Newborn: 0   `P` Pediatric: 0-17   `M` Maternity: 12-55   `A` Adult: 15-124   `MCC` Major Complication/Comorbidity   `CC` Complication/Comorbidity   `SW` Severe Wound Dx

440   ICD-10-CM 2019

A35 Other tetanus `MCC`
    Tetanus NOS
    `EXCLUDES 1`   *obstetrical tetanus (A34)*
       tetanus neonatorum (A33)
    DEF: Tetanus: Acute, often fatal, infectious disease caused by the anaerobic, spore-forming bacillus *Clostridium tetani*. The bacillus enters the body through a contaminated wound, burns, surgical wounds, or cutaneous ulcers. Symptoms include lockjaw, spasms, seizures, and paralysis.
    CC Excl: PDX collection 86

`✓4ᵗʰ` **A36 Diphtheria**

    CC Excl: For CC codes in category A36, unless otherwise noted: PDX collection 87

    A36.0 Pharyngeal diphtheria `CC`
       Diphtheritic membranous angina
       Tonsillar diphtheria
    A36.1 Nasopharyngeal diphtheria `CC`
    A36.2 Laryngeal diphtheria `CC`
       Diphtheritic laryngotracheitis
    A36.3 Cutaneous diphtheria `CC`
       `EXCLUDES 2`   *erythrasma (L08.1)*
`✓5ᵗʰ`   **A36.8 Other diphtheria**
       A36.81 Diphtheritic cardiomyopathy `CC` `HCC`
          Diphtheritic myocarditis
          CC Excl: PDX collection 88
       A36.82 Diphtheritic radiculomyelitis `CC`
       A36.83 Diphtheritic polyneuritis `CC`
       A36.84 Diphtheritic tubulo-interstitial nephropathy `CC`
       A36.85 Diphtheritic cystitis `CC`
       A36.86 Diphtheritic conjunctivitis `CC`
       A36.89 Other diphtheritic complications `CC`
          Diphtheritic peritonitis
    A36.9 Diphtheria, unspecified `CC`

`✓4ᵗʰ` **A37 Whooping cough**
    DEF: Acute, highly contagious respiratory tract infection caused by *Bordetella pertussis* and *B. bronchiseptica*. Whooping cough is known by its characteristic paroxysmal cough.

    CC Excl: For CC codes in category A37: PDX collection 89
    For MCC codes in category A37: PDX collection 90

`✓5ᵗʰ`   **A37.0 Whooping cough due to Bordetella pertussis**
       A37.00 Whooping cough due to Bordetella pertussis without pneumonia `CC`
       A37.01 Whooping cough due to Bordetella pertussis with pneumonia `MCC`
`✓5ᵗʰ`   **A37.1 Whooping cough due to Bordetella parapertussis**
       A37.10 Whooping cough due to Bordetella parapertussis without pneumonia `CC`
       A37.11 Whooping cough due to Bordetella parapertussis with pneumonia `MCC`
`✓5ᵗʰ`   **A37.8 Whooping cough due to other Bordetella species**
       A37.80 Whooping cough due to other Bordetella species without pneumonia `CC`
       A37.81 Whooping cough due to other Bordetella species with pneumonia `MCC`
`✓5ᵗʰ`   **A37.9 Whooping cough, unspecified species**
       A37.90 Whooping cough, unspecified species without pneumonia `CC`
       A37.91 Whooping cough, unspecified species with pneumonia `MCC`

`✓4ᵗʰ` **A38 Scarlet fever**
    `INCLUDES`   scarlatina
    `EXCLUDES 2`   *streptococcal sore throat (J02.0)*
    DEF: Acute contagious disease caused by Group A bacteria, the same bacterium that causes strep throat. Individuals with strep throat can develop scarlet fever particularly if the infection is not treated with antibiotics. It is characterized by a red blush to the skin of the chest and abdomen and swelling of the nose, throat, and mouth.

    CC Excl: For CC codes in category A38: PDX collection 91

    A38.0 Scarlet fever with otitis media `CC`
    A38.1 Scarlet fever with myocarditis `CC`
    A38.8 Scarlet fever with other complications `CC`
    A38.9 Scarlet fever, uncomplicated `CC`
       Scarlet fever, NOS

`✓4ᵗʰ` **A39 Meningococcal infection**
    DEF: Condition caused by *Neisseria meningitidis*, a bacteria that may invade the spinal cord, brain, heart, joints, optic nerve, or bloodstream.
    A39.0 Meningococcal meningitis `MCC`
       CC Excl: PDX collection 92
    A39.1 Waterhouse-Friderichsen syndrome `MCC` `HCC`
       Meningococcal hemorrhagic adrenalitis
       Meningococcic adrenal syndrome
       CC Excl: PDX collection 93
    A39.2 Acute meningococcemia `MCC` `HCC`
       CC Excl: PDX collection 94
    A39.3 Chronic meningococcemia `MCC` `HCC`
       CC Excl: PDX collection 94
    A39.4 Meningococcemia, unspecified `MCC` `HCC`
       CC Excl: PDX collection 94
`✓5ᵗʰ`   **A39.5 Meningococcal heart disease**
       A39.50 Meningococcal carditis, unspecified `MCC`
          CC Excl: PDX collection 95
       A39.51 Meningococcal endocarditis `MCC`
          CC Excl: PDX collection 96
       A39.52 Meningococcal myocarditis `MCC`
          CC Excl: PDX collection 97
       A39.53 Meningococcal pericarditis `MCC`
          CC Excl: PDX collection 98
`✓5ᵗʰ`   **A39.8 Other meningococcal infections**
       A39.81 Meningococcal encephalitis `MCC`
          CC Excl: PDX collection 99
       A39.82 Meningococcal retrobulbar neuritis `CC`
          CC Excl: PDX collection 100
       A39.83 Meningococcal arthritis `CC` `HCC`
          CC Excl: PDX collection 101
       A39.84 Postmeningococcal arthritis `CC` `HCC`
          CC Excl: PDX collection 101
       A39.89 Other meningococcal infections `CC`
          Meningococcal conjunctivitis
          CC Excl: PDX collection 102
    A39.9 Meningococcal infection, unspecified `CC`
       Meningococcal disease NOS
       CC Excl: PDX collection 102

`✓4ᵗʰ` **A40 Streptococcal sepsis**
    Code first: postprocedural streptococcal sepsis (T81.4-)
       streptococcal sepsis during labor (O75.3)
       streptococcal sepsis following abortion or ectopic or molar pregnancy (O03-O07, O08.0)
       streptococcal sepsis following immunization (T88.0)
       streptococcal sepsis following infusion, transfusion or therapeutic injection (T80.2-)
    `EXCLUDES 1`   *neonatal (P36.0-P36.1)*
       puerperal sepsis (O85)
       sepsis due to Streptococcus, group D (A41.81)
    AHA: 2018, 1Q, 16; 2016, 1Q, 32

    CC Excl: For MCC codes in category A40, unless otherwise noted: PDX collection 71

    A40.0 Sepsis due to streptococcus, group A `MCC` `HCC`
    A40.1 Sepsis due to streptococcus, group B `MCC` `HCC`
    A40.3 Sepsis due to Streptococcus pneumoniae `MCC` `HCC`
       Pneumococcal sepsis
       CC Excl: No Excl
    A40.8 Other streptococcal sepsis `MCC` `HCC`
    A40.9 Streptococcal sepsis, unspecified `HIV` `MCC` `HCC`

`✓` Additional Character Required   `√x7ᵗʰ` Placeholder   Unacceptable PDx   Questionable PDx   Manifestation   `H1`-`H14` HAC   `HCC` CMS-HCC Dx   `HIV` HIV Dx

☑4th A41 Other sepsis

Code first: postprocedural sepsis (T81.4-)
sepsis during labor (O75.3)
sepsis following abortion, ectopic or molar pregnancy
(O03-O07, O08.0)
sepsis following immunization (T88.0)
sepsis following infusion, transfusion or therapeutic injection
(T80.2-)

EXCLUDES 1 bacteremia NOS (R78.81)
neonatal (P36.-)
puerperal sepsis (O85)
streptococcal sepsis (A40.-)

EXCLUDES 2 sepsis (due to) (in) actinomycotic (A42.7)
sepsis (due to) (in) anthrax (A22.7)
sepsis (due to) (in) candidal (B37.7)
sepsis (due to) (in) Erysipelothrix (A26.7)
sepsis (due to) (in) extraintestinal yersiniosis (A28.2)
sepsis (due to) (in) gonococcal (A54.86)
sepsis (due to) (in) herpesviral (B00.7)
sepsis (due to) (in) listerial (A32.7)
sepsis (due to) (in) melioidosis (A24.1)
sepsis (due to) (in) meningococcal (A39.2-A39.4)
sepsis (due to) (in) plague (A20.7)
sepsis (due to) (in) tularemia (A21.7)
toxic shock syndrome (A48.3)

AHA: 2018, 1Q, 16; 2016, 1Q, 32; 2014, 2Q, 13

CC Excl: For MCC codes in category A41: PDX collection 71

☑5th A41.0 Sepsis due to Staphylococcus aureus

A41.01 Sepsis due to Methicillin susceptible `HIV` `MCC` `HCC`
Staphylococcus aureus
MSSA sepsis
Staphylococcus aureus sepsis NOS

A41.02 Sepsis due to Methicillin resistant `HIV` `MCC` `HCC`
Staphylococcus aureus

A41.1 Sepsis due to other specified staphylococcus `HIV` `MCC` `HCC`
Coagulase negative staphylococcus sepsis

A41.2 Sepsis due to unspecified staphylococcus `HIV` `MCC` `HCC`

A41.3 Sepsis due to Hemophilus influenzae `HIV` `MCC` `HCC`

A41.4 Sepsis due to anaerobes `HIV` `MCC` `HCC`
EXCLUDES 1 gas gangrene (A48.0)

☑5th A41.5 Sepsis due to other Gram-negative organisms

A41.50 Gram-negative sepsis, unspecified `HIV` `MCC` `HCC`
Gram-negative sepsis NOS

A41.51 Sepsis due to Escherichia coli [E. coli] `HIV` `MCC` `HCC`

A41.52 Sepsis due to Pseudomonas `HIV` `MCC` `HCC`
Pseudomonas aeroginosa

A41.53 Sepsis due to Serratia `HIV` `MCC` `HCC`

A41.59 Other Gram-negative sepsis `HIV` `MCC` `HCC`

☑5th A41.8 Other specified sepsis

A41.81 Sepsis due to Enterococcus `HIV` `MCC` `HCC`
TIP: E. faecium is a species of Enterococcus that is highly
resistant to multiple antibiotics. Assign a code from
category Z16 when resistance to antimicrobial drugs is
documented.

A41.89 Other specified sepsis `HIV` `MCC` `HCC`
AHA: 2017, 1Q, 51; 2016, 3Q, 8-14
TIP: Viral sepsis is coded here; assign an additional code
to identify the specific viral agent or illness.

A41.9 Sepsis, unspecified organism `HIV` `MCC` `HCC`
Septicemia NOS

☑4th A42 Actinomycosis

EXCLUDES 1 actinomycetoma (B47.1)

A42.0 Pulmonary actinomycosis `HIV` `CC` `HCC`
CC Excl: PDX collection 103

A42.1 Abdominal actinomycosis `HIV` `CC`
CC Excl: PDX collection 104

A42.2 Cervicofacial actinomycosis `HIV` `CC`
CC Excl: PDX collection 105

A42.7 Actinomycotic sepsis `HIV` `MCC` `HCC`
CC Excl: PDX collection 71

☑5th A42.8 Other forms of actinomycosis

CC Excl: For CC codes in subcategory A42.8:
PDX collection 106

A42.81 Actinomycotic meningitis `HIV` `CC`

A42.82 Actinomycotic encephalitis `HIV` `CC`

A42.89 Other forms of actinomycosis `HIV` `CC`

A42.9 Actinomycosis, unspecified `HIV` `CC`
CC Excl: PDX collection 106

☑4th A43 Nocardiosis

DEF: Rare bacterial infection occurring most often in those with weakened
immune systems. Can be acquired in soil, decaying plants, or standing
water. It typically begins in the lungs and has a tendency to spread to other
body systems.

A43.0 Pulmonary nocardiosis `HIV` `CC` `HCC`
CC Excl: PDX collection 103

A43.1 Cutaneous nocardiosis `HIV` `CC`
CC Excl: PDX collection 107

A43.8 Other forms of nocardiosis `HIV` `CC`
CC Excl: PDX collection 106

A43.9 Nocardiosis, unspecified `HIV` `CC`
CC Excl: PDX collection 106

☑4th A44 Bartonellosis

CC Excl: For CC codes in category A44: PDX collection 108

A44.0 Systemic bartonellosis `CC`
Oroya fever

A44.1 Cutaneous and mucocutaneous bartonellosis `CC`
Verruga peruana

A44.8 Other forms of bartonellosis `CC`

A44.9 Bartonellosis, unspecified `CC`

A46 Erysipelas

EXCLUDES 1 postpartum or puerperal erysipelas (O86.89)
DEF: Skin infection affecting the upper dermis and superficial dermal
lymphatics. Lesion edges are well-demarcated with distinct raised borders.
It is often caused by group A Streptococci.

☑4th A48 Other bacterial diseases, not elsewhere classified

EXCLUDES 1 actinomycetoma (B47.1)

A48.0 Gas gangrene `MCC` `HCC`
Clostridial cellulitis
Clostridial myonecrosis
AHA: 2017, 4Q, 102
CC Excl: PDX collection 109

A48.1 Legionnaires' disease `HIV` `MCC` `HCC`
DEF: Severe and often fatal infection by Legionella pneumophila.
Symptoms include high fever, gastrointestinal pain, headache,
myalgia, dry cough, and pneumonia and it is usually transmitted
through airborne water droplets via air conditioning systems or
hot tubs.
CC Excl: PDX collection 110

A48.2 Nonpneumonic Legionnaires' disease [Pontiac fever]

A48.3 Toxic shock syndrome `MCC` `HCC`
Use additional code to identify the organism (B95, B96)
EXCLUDES 1 endotoxic shock NOS (R57.8)
sepsis NOS (A41.9)
DEF: Bacteria producing an endotoxin, such as Staphylococci,
flood the body with the toxins producing a high fever, vomiting
and diarrhea, decreasing blood pressure, a skin rash, and shock.
Synonym(s): TSS.
CC Excl: PDX collection 111

A48.4 Brazilian purpuric fever
Systemic Hemophilus aegyptius infection

☑5th A48.5 Other specified botulism

Non-foodborne intoxication due to toxins of Clostridium
botulinum [C. botulinum]
EXCLUDES 1 food poisoning due to toxins of Clostridium botulinum
(A05.1)

CC Excl: For CC codes in subcategory A48.5:
PDX collection 18

A48.51 Infant botulism `CC` `P`

A48.52 Wound botulism `CC`
Non-foodborne botulism NOS
Use additional code for associated wound

A48.8 Other specified bacterial diseases

`N` Newborn: 0 `P` Pediatric: 0-17 `M` Maternity: 12-55 `A` Adult: 15-124 `MCC` Major Complication/Comorbidity `CC` Complication/Comorbidity `SW` Severe Wound Dx

442

ICD-10-CM 2019

☑4ᵗʰ A49   Bacterial infection of unspecified site

     EXCLUDES 1   bacterial agents as the cause of diseases classified elsewhere (B95-B96)
          chlamydial infection NOS (A74.9)
          meningococcal infection NOS (A39.9)
          rickettsial infection NOS (A79.9)
          spirochetal infection NOS (A69.9)

   ☑5ᵗʰ A49.0   Staphylococcal infection, unspecified site

      A49.01   Methicillin susceptible Staphylococcus aureus infection, unspecified site
         Methicillin susceptible Staphylococcus aureus (MSSA) infection
         Staphylococcus aureus infection NOS

      A49.02   Methicillin resistant Staphylococcus aureus infection, unspecified site
         Methicillin resistant Staphylococcus aureus (MRSA) infection

   A49.1   Streptococcal infection, unspecified site

   A49.2   Hemophilus influenzae infection, unspecified site

   A49.3   Mycoplasma infection, unspecified site

   A49.8   Other bacterial infections of unspecified site

   A49.9   Bacterial infection, unspecified
      EXCLUDES 1   bacteremia NOS (R78.81)

Infections with a predominantly sexual mode of transmission (A50-A64)

     EXCLUDES 1   human immunodeficiency virus [HIV] disease (B20)
          nonspecific and nongonococcal urethritis (N34.1)
          Reiter's disease (M02.3-)

☑4ᵗʰ A50   Congenital syphilis

     CC Excl: For CC/MCC codes in category A50, unless otherwise noted: PDX collection 112

   ☑5ᵗʰ A50.0   Early congenital syphilis, symptomatic
     Any congenital syphilitic condition specified as early or manifest less than two years after birth.

      A50.01   Early congenital syphilitic oculopathy   `CC`

      A50.02   Early congenital syphilitic osteochondropathy   `CC`

      A50.03   Early congenital syphilitic pharyngitis   `CC`
         Early congenital syphilitic laryngitis

      A50.04   Early congenital syphilitic pneumonia   `CC`

      A50.05   Early congenital syphilitic rhinitis   `CC`

      A50.06   Early cutaneous congenital syphilis   `CC`

      A50.07   Early mucocutaneous congenital syphilis   `CC`

      A50.08   Early visceral congenital syphilis   `CC`

      A50.09   Other early congenital syphilis, symptomatic   `CC`

   A50.1   Early congenital syphilis, latent
     Congenital syphilis without clinical manifestations, with positive serological reaction and negative spinal fluid test, less than two years after birth.

   A50.2   Early congenital syphilis, unspecified   `CC`
     Congenital syphilis NOS less than two years after birth.
     CC Excl: PDX collection 113

   ☑5ᵗʰ A50.3   Late congenital syphilitic oculopathy
      EXCLUDES 1   Hutchinson's triad (A50.53)

      A50.30   Late congenital syphilitic oculopathy, unspecified   `CC`

      A50.31   Late congenital syphilitic interstitial keratitis   `CC`

      A50.32   Late congenital syphilitic chorioretinitis   `CC`

      A50.39   Other late congenital syphilitic oculopathy   `CC`

   ☑5ᵗʰ A50.4   Late congenital neurosyphilis [juvenile neurosyphilis]
     Use additional code to identify any associated mental disorder
      EXCLUDES 1   Hutchinson's triad (A50.53)

     CC Excl: For CC codes in subcategory A50.4, unless otherwise noted: PDX collection 114

      A50.40   Late congenital neurosyphilis, unspecified   `CC`
         Juvenile neurosyphilis NOS

      A50.41   Late congenital syphilitic meningitis   `MCC`
         CC Excl: PDX collection 115

      A50.42   Late congenital syphilitic encephalitis   `MCC`

      A50.43   Late congenital syphilitic polyneuropathy   `CC`

      A50.44   Late congenital syphilitic optic nerve atrophy   `CC`
         CC Excl: PDX collection 112

      A50.45   Juvenile general paresis   `CC`
         Dementia paralytica juvenilis
         Juvenile tabetoparetic neurosyphilis

      A50.49   Other late congenital neurosyphilis   `CC`
         Juvenile tabes dorsalis

   ☑5ᵗʰ A50.5   Other late congenital syphilis, symptomatic
     Any congenital syphilitic condition specified as late or manifest two years or more after birth.

      A50.51   Clutton's joints   `CC`

      A50.52   Hutchinson's teeth   `CC`

      A50.53   Hutchinson's triad   `CC`

      A50.54   Late congenital cardiovascular syphilis   `CC`

      A50.55   Late congenital syphilitic arthropathy   `CC` `HCC`

      A50.56   Late congenital syphilitic osteochondropathy   `CC`

      A50.57   Syphilitic saddle nose   `CC`

      A50.59   Other late congenital syphilis, symptomatic   `CC`

   A50.6   Late congenital syphilis, latent
     Congenital syphilis without clinical manifestations, with positive serological reaction and negative spinal fluid test, two years or more after birth.

   A50.7   Late congenital syphilis, unspecified
     Congenital syphilis NOS two years or more after birth.

   A50.9   Congenital syphilis, unspecified

☑4ᵗʰ A51   Early syphilis
     DEF: Syphilis: Sexually transmitted disease caused by the treponema pallidum spirochete. Syphilis usually exhibits cutaneous manifestations and may exist for years without symptoms.

   A51.0   Primary genital syphilis
     Syphilitic chancre NOS

   A51.1   Primary anal syphilis

   A51.2   Primary syphilis of other sites

   ☑5ᵗʰ A51.3   Secondary syphilis of skin and mucous membranes
     DEF: Transitory or chronic cutaneous eruptions that present within two to 10 weeks following an initial syphilis infection that may include nontender lymphadenopathy along with alopecia and condylomata lata.

      A51.31   Condyloma latum   `CC`
         CC Excl: PDX collection 112

      A51.32   Syphilitic alopecia   `CC`
         CC Excl: PDX collection 116

      A51.39   Other secondary syphilis of skin   `CC`
         Syphilitic leukoderma
         Syphilitic mucous patch
         EXCLUDES 1   late syphilitic leukoderma (A52.79)
         CC Excl: PDX collection 112

   ☑5ᵗʰ A51.4   Other secondary syphilis

      A51.41   Secondary syphilitic meningitis   `MCC`
         CC Excl: PDX collection 117

      A51.42   Secondary syphilitic female pelvic disease   `CC♀`
         CC Excl: PDX collection 113

      A51.43   Secondary syphilitic oculopathy   `CC`
         Secondary syphilitic chorioretinitis
         Secondary syphilitic iridocyclitis, iritis
         Secondary syphilitic uveitis
         CC Excl: PDX collection 112

      A51.44   Secondary syphilitic nephritis   `CC`
         CC Excl: PDX collection 113

      A51.45   Secondary syphilitic hepatitis   `CC`
         CC Excl: PDX collection 118

      A51.46   Secondary syphilitic osteopathy   `CC`
         CC Excl: PDX collection 119

      A51.49   Other secondary syphilitic conditions   `CC`
         Secondary syphilitic lymphadenopathy
         Secondary syphilitic myositis
         CC Excl: No Excl

   A51.5   Early syphilis, latent
     Syphilis (acquired) without clinical manifestations, with positive serological reaction and negative spinal fluid test, less than two years after infection.

   A51.9   Early syphilis, unspecified

✔ Additional Character Required   ✔x7ᵗʰ Placeholder   Unacceptable PDx   Questionable PDx   Manifestation   **H1**-**H14** HAC   **HCC** CMS-HCC Dx   **HIV** HIV Dx

ICD-10-CM 2019   **443**

✓4ᵗʰ **A52 Late syphilis**

  ✓5ᵗʰ **A52.0 Cardiovascular and cerebrovascular syphilis**

> **CC Excl: For CC codes in subcategory A52.0:**
> PDX collection 114

    A52.00 Cardiovascular syphilis, unspecified `CC`

    A52.01 Syphilitic aneurysm of aorta `CC`

    A52.02 Syphilitic aortitis `CC`

    A52.03 Syphilitic endocarditis `CC`
      Syphilitic aortic valve incompetence or stenosis
      Syphilitic mitral valve stenosis
      Syphilitic pulmonary valve regurgitation

    A52.04 Syphilitic cerebral arteritis `CC`

    A52.05 Other cerebrovascular syphilis `CC`
      Syphilitic cerebral aneurysm (ruptured) (non-ruptured)
      Syphilitic cerebral thrombosis

    A52.06 Other syphilitic heart involvement `CC`
      Syphilitic coronary artery disease
      Syphilitic myocarditis
      Syphilitic pericarditis

    A52.09 Other cardiovascular syphilis `CC`

  ✓5ᵗʰ **A52.1 Symptomatic neurosyphilis**

> **CC Excl: For CC/MCC codes in subcategory A52.1, unless otherwise noted:** PDX collection 114

    A52.10 Symptomatic neurosyphilis, unspecified `CC`

    A52.11 Tabes dorsalis `CC`
      Locomotor ataxia (progressive)
      Tabetic neurosyphilis

    A52.12 Other cerebrospinal syphilis `CC`

    A52.13 Late syphilitic meningitis `MCC`
      CC Excl: PDX collection 115

    A52.14 Late syphilitic encephalitis `MCC`

    A52.15 Late syphilitic neuropathy `CC`
      Late syphilitic acoustic neuritis
      Late syphilitic optic (nerve) atrophy
      Late syphilitic polyneuropathy
      Late syphilitic retrobulbar neuritis

    A52.16 Charcôt's arthropathy (tabetic) `CC`
      DEF: Progressive neurologic arthropathy in which chronic degeneration of joints in the weight-bearing areas with peripheral hypertrophy occurs as a complication of a neuropathy disorder. Supporting structures relax from a loss of sensation resulting in chronic joint instability.

    A52.17 General paresis `CC`
      Dementia paralytica

    A52.19 Other symptomatic neurosyphilis `CC`
      Syphilitic parkinsonism

  A52.2 Asymptomatic neurosyphilis `CC`
    CC Excl: PDX collection 114

  A52.3 Neurosyphilis, unspecified `CC`
    Gumma (syphilitic)
    Syphilis (late)
    Syphiloma
    CC Excl: PDX collection 114

  ✓5ᵗʰ **A52.7 Other symptomatic late syphilis**

> **CC Excl: For CC codes in subcategory A52.7, unless otherwise noted:** PDX collection 116

    A52.71 Late syphilitic oculopathy `CC`
      Late syphilitic chorioretinitis
      Late syphilitic episcleritis
      CC Excl: PDX collection 120

    A52.72 Syphilis of lung and bronchus `CC`

    A52.73 Symptomatic late syphilis of other respiratory organs `CC`

    A52.74 Syphilis of liver and other viscera `CC`
      Late syphilitic peritonitis

    A52.75 Syphilis of kidney and ureter `CC`
      Syphilitic glomerular disease

    A52.76 Other genitourinary symptomatic late syphilis `CC`
      Late syphilitic female pelvic inflammatory disease

    A52.77 Syphilis of bone and joint `CC`

    A52.78 Syphilis of other musculoskeletal tissue `CC`
      Late syphilitic bursitis
      Syphilis [stage unspecified] of bursa
      Syphilis [stage unspecified] of muscle
      Syphilis [stage unspecified] of synovium
      Syphilis [stage unspecified] of tendon

    A52.79 Other symptomatic late syphilis `CC`
      Late syphilitic leukoderma
      Syphilis of adrenal gland
      Syphilis of pituitary gland
      Syphilis of thyroid gland
      Syphilic splenomegaly
      EXCLUDES 1 *syphilitic leukoderma (secondary) (A51.39)*

  A52.8 Late syphilis, latent
    Syphilis (acquired) without clinical manifestations, with positive serological reaction and negative spinal fluid test, two years or more after infection

  A52.9 Late syphilis, unspecified

✓4ᵗʰ **A53 Other and unspecified syphilis**

  A53.0 Latent syphilis, unspecified as early or late
    Latent syphilis NOS   Positive serological reaction for syphilis

  A53.9 Syphilis, unspecified
    Infection due to Treponema pallidum NOS
    Syphilis (acquired) NOS
    EXCLUDES 1 *syphilis NOS under two years of age (A50.2)*

✓4ᵗʰ **A54 Gonococcal infection**
  DEF: Sexually transmitted bacterial infection caused by *Neisseria gonorrhoeae.* Women are often asymptomatic, while men tend to develop urinary symptoms quickly.

  ✓5ᵗʰ **A54.0 Gonococcal infection of lower genitourinary tract without periurethral or accessory gland abscess**
    EXCLUDES 1 *gonococcal infection with genitourinary gland abscess (A54.1)*
            gonococcal infection with periurethral abscess (A54.1)

> **CC Excl: For CC codes in subcategory A54.0:**
> PDX collection 121

    A54.00 Gonococcal infection of lower genitourinary tract, unspecified `CC`

    A54.01 Gonococcal cystitis and urethritis, unspecified `CC`

    A54.02 Gonococcal vulvovaginitis, unspecified `CC` ♀

    A54.03 Gonococcal cervicitis, unspecified `CC` ♀

    A54.09 Other gonococcal infection of lower genitourinary tract `CC`

  A54.1 Gonococcal infection of lower genitourinary tract with periurethral and accessory gland abscess `CC`
    Gonococcal Bartholin's gland abscess
    CC Excl: PDX collection 121

  ✓5ᵗʰ **A54.2 Gonococcal pelviperitonitis and other gonococcal genitourinary infection**

> **CC Excl: For CC codes in subcategory A54.2:**
> PDX collection 121

    A54.21 Gonococcal infection of kidney and ureter `CC`

    A54.22 Gonococcal prostatitis `CC` ♂

    A54.23 Gonococcal infection of other male genital organs `CC` ♂
      Gonococcal epididymitis   Gonococcal orchitis

    A54.24 Gonococcal female pelvic inflammatory disease `CC` ♀
      Gonococcal pelviperitonitis
      EXCLUDES 1 *gonococcal peritonitis (A54.85)*

    A54.29 Other gonococcal genitourinary infections `CC`

  ✓5ᵗʰ **A54.3 Gonococcal infection of eye**

> **CC Excl: For CC codes in subcategory A54.3:**
> PDX collection 116

    A54.30 Gonococcal infection of eye, unspecified `CC`

    A54.31 Gonococcal conjunctivitis `CC`
      Ophthalmia neonatorum due to gonococcus

    A54.32 Gonococcal iridocyclitis `CC`

    A54.33 Gonococcal keratitis `CC`

    A54.39 Other gonococcal eye infection `CC`
      Gonococcal endophthalmia

  ✓5ᵗʰ **A54.4 Gonococcal infection of musculoskeletal system**

> **CC Excl: For CC codes in subcategory A54.4:**
> PDX collection 122

    A54.40 Gonococcal infection of musculoskeletal system, unspecified `CC` `HCC`

Ⓝ Newborn: 0 　Ⓟ Pediatric: 0-17 　Ⓜ Maternity: 12-55 　Ⓐ Adult: 15-124 　`MCC` Major Complication/Comorbidity 　`CC` Complication/Comorbidity 　`SW` Severe Wound Dx

444　　　　ICD-10-CM 2019

A54.41 **Gonococcal** spondylopathy   `CC` `HCC`

A54.42 **Gonococcal** arthritis   `CC` `HCC`
     EXCLUDES 2   *gonococcal infection of spine (A54.41)*

A54.43 **Gonococcal** osteomyelitis   `CC` `HCC`
     EXCLUDES 2   *gonococcal infection of spine (A54.41)*

A54.49 **Gonococcal infection of** other musculoskeletal tissue   `CC` `HCC`
     Gonococcal bursitis
     Gonococcal myositis
     Gonococcal synovitis
     Gonococcal tenosynovitis

A54.5 **Gonococcal** pharyngitis

A54.6 **Gonococcal infection of** anus and rectum

✓5ᵗʰ A54.8 **Other gonococcal infections**

A54.81 **Gonococcal** meningitis   `MCC`
     CC Excl: PDX collection 117

A54.82 **Gonococcal** brain abscess   `CC`
     CC Excl: PDX collection 123

A54.83 **Gonococcal** heart infection   `CC`
     Gonococcal endocarditis
     Gonococcal myocarditis
     Gonococcal pericarditis
     CC Excl: PDX collection 124

A54.84 **Gonococcal** pneumonia   `CC` `HCC`
     CC Excl: PDX collection 123

A54.85 **Gonococcal** peritonitis   `CC` `HCC`
     EXCLUDES 1   *gonococcal pelviperitonitis (A54.24)*
     CC Excl: PDX collection 125

A54.86 **Gonococcal** sepsis   `MCC` `HCC`
     CC Excl: PDX collection 71

A54.89 **Other gonococcal infections**   `CC`
     Gonococcal keratoderma
     Gonococcal lymphadenitis
     CC Excl: PDX collection 123

A54.9 **Gonococcal infection,** unspecified   `CC`
     CC Excl: PDX collection 123

A55 Chlamydial lymphogranuloma (venereum)
     Climatic or tropical bubo
     Durand-Nicolas-Favre disease
     Esthiomene
     Lymphogranuloma inguinale

✓4ᵗʰ **A56 Other sexually transmitted chlamydial diseases**
     INCLUDES   sexually transmitted diseases due to Chlamydia trachomatis
     EXCLUDES 1   *neonatal chlamydial conjunctivitis (P39.1)*
             neonatal chlamydial pneumonia (P23.1)
     EXCLUDES 2   *chlamydial lymphogranuloma (A55)*
             conditions classified to A74-

✓5ᵗʰ A56.0 **Chlamydial infection of** lower genitourinary tract

A56.00 **Chlamydial infection of lower genitourinary tract,** unspecified

A56.01 **Chlamydial** cystitis and urethritis

A56.02 **Chlamydial** vulvovaginitis   ♀

A56.09 **Other chlamydial infection of lower genitourinary tract**
     Chlamydial cervicitis

✓5ᵗʰ A56.1 **Chlamydial infection of** pelviperitoneum and other genitourinary organs

A56.11 **Chlamydial** female pelvic inflammatory disease   ♀

A56.19 **Other chlamydial genitourinary infection**
     Chlamydial epididymitis
     Chlamydial orchitis

A56.2 **Chlamydial infection of genitourinary tract,** unspecified

A56.3 **Chlamydial infection of** anus and rectum

A56.4 **Chlamydial infection of** pharynx

A56.8 **Sexually transmitted chlamydial infection of** other sites

A57 Chancroid
     Ulcus molle
     DEF: Localized infection by *Haemophilus ducreyi,* causing genital ulcers and infecting the inguinal lymph nodes.

A58 Granuloma inguinale
     Donovanosis

✓4ᵗʰ **A59 Trichomoniasis**
     EXCLUDES 2   *intestinal trichomoniasis (A07.8)*
     DEF: Infection with the parasitic, flagellated protozoa of the genus *Trichomonas.* This protozoon is found in the intestinal and genitourinary tracts of humans and in the mouth around tartar, cavities, and areas of periodontal disease.

✓5ᵗʰ A59.0 **Urogenital** trichomoniasis

A59.00 **Urogenital trichomoniasis,** unspecified
     Fluor (vaginalis) due to Trichomonas
     Leukorrhea (vaginalis) due to Trichomonas

A59.01 **Trichomonal** vulvovaginitis   ♀

A59.02 **Trichomonal** prostatitis   ♂

A59.03 **Trichomonal** cystitis and urethritis

A59.09 **Other** urogenital trichomoniasis
     Trichomonas cervicitis

A59.8 **Trichomoniasis of** other sites

A59.9 **Trichomoniasis,** unspecified

✓4ᵗʰ **A60 Anogenital herpesviral [herpes simplex] infections**

✓5ᵗʰ A60.0 **Herpesviral infection of** genitalia and urogenital tract

A60.00 **Herpesviral infection of urogenital system,** unspecified   `HIV`

A60.01 **Herpesviral infection of** penis   `HIV` ♂

A60.02 **Herpesviral infection of** other male genital organs   ♂

A60.03 **Herpesviral** cervicitis   ♀

A60.04 **Herpesviral** vulvovaginitis   `HIV` ♀
     Herpesviral [herpes simplex] ulceration
     Herpesviral [herpes simplex] vaginitis
     Herpesviral [herpes simplex] vulvitis

A60.09 **Herpesviral infection of other** urogenital tract   `HIV`

A60.1 **Herpesviral infection of** perianal skin and rectum   `HIV`

A60.9 **Anogenital herpesviral infection,** unspecified   `HIV`

✓4ᵗʰ **A63 Other predominantly sexually transmitted diseases, not elsewhere classified**
     EXCLUDES 2   *molluscum contagiosum (B08.1)*
             papilloma of cervix (D26.0)

A63.0 **Anogenital (venereal) warts**
     Anogenital warts due to (human) papillomavirus [HPV]
     Condyloma acuminatum

A63.8 **Other specified predominantly sexually transmitted diseases**

A64 Unspecified sexually transmitted disease

Other spirochetal diseases (A65-A69)

     EXCLUDES 2   *leptospirosis (A27.-)*
             syphilis (A50-A53)

A65 Nonvenereal syphilis
     Bejel
     Endemic syphilis
     Njovera

✓4ᵗʰ **A66 Yaws**
     INCLUDES   bouba
              frambesia (tropica)
              pian

A66.0 **Initial lesions of yaws**
     Chancre of yaws
     Frambesia, initial or primary
     Initial frambesial ulcer
     Mother yaw

A66.1 **Multiple papillomata and wet crab yaws**
     Frambesioma
     Pianoma
     Plantar or palmar papilloma of yaws

A66.2 **Other early skin lesions of yaws**
     Cutaneous yaws, less than five years after infection
     Early yaws (cutaneous) (macular) (maculopapular) (micropapular) (papular)
     Frambeside of early yaws

A66.3 **Hyperkeratosis of yaws**
     Ghoul hand
     Hyperkeratosis, palmar or plantar (early) (late) due to yaws
     Worm-eaten soles

A66.4 **Gummata and ulcers of yaws**
     Gummatous frambeside
     Nodular late yaws (ulcerated)

A66.5 **Gangosa**
     Rhinopharyngitis mutilans

Chapter 1. Certain Infectious and Parasitic Diseases

A66.6 Bone and joint lesions of yaws `HCC`
- Yaws ganglion
- Yaws goundou
- Yaws gumma, bone
- Yaws gummatous osteitis or periostitis
- Yaws hydrarthrosis
- Yaws osteitis
- Yaws periostitis (hypertrophic)

A66.7 Other manifestations of yaws
- Juxta-articular nodules of yaws
- Mucosal yaws

A66.8 Latent yaws
- Yaws without clinical manifestations, with positive serology

A66.9 Yaws, unspecified

✓4ᵗʰ **A67 Pinta [carate]**

A67.0 Primary lesions of pinta
- Chancre (primary) of pinta
- Papule (primary) of pinta

A67.1 Intermediate lesions of pinta
- Erythematous plaques of pinta
- Hyperchromic lesions of pinta
- Hyperkeratosis of pinta
- Pintids

A67.2 Late lesions of pinta
- Achromic skin lesions of pinta
- Cicatricial skin lesions of pinta
- Dyschromic skin lesions of pinta

A67.3 Mixed lesions of pinta
- Achromic with hyperchromic skin lesions of pinta [carate]

A67.9 Pinta, unspecified

✓4ᵗʰ **A68 Relapsing fevers**
- INCLUDES recurrent fever
- EXCLUDES 2 Lyme disease (A69.2-)

CC Excl: For CC codes in category A68: PDX collection 108

A68.0 Louse-borne relapsing fever `CC`
- Relapsing fever due to Borrelia recurrentis

A68.1 Tick-borne relapsing fever `CC`
- Relapsing fever due to any Borrelia species other than Borrelia recurrentis

A68.9 Relapsing fever, unspecified `CC`

✓4ᵗʰ **A69 Other spirochetal infections**

A69.0 Necrotizing ulcerative stomatitis
- Cancrum oris
- Fusospirochetal gangrene
- Noma
- Stomatitis gangrenosa

A69.1 Other Vincent's infections `CC`
- Fusospirochetal pharyngitis
- Necrotizing ulcerative (acute) gingivitis
- Necrotizing ulcerative (acute) gingivostomatitis
- Spirochetal stomatitis
- Trench mouth
- Vincent's angina
- Vincent's gingivitis
- CC Excl: PDX collection 126

✓5ᵗʰ **A69.2 Lyme disease**
- Erythema chronicum migrans due to Borrelia burgdorferi
- **DEF:** Recurrent multisystem disorder through tick bites that begins with lesions of erythema chronicum migrans and is followed by arthritis of the large joints, myalgia, malaise, and neurological and cardiac manifestations.

CC Excl: For CC codes in subcategory A69.2: PDX collection 108

A69.20 Lyme disease, unspecified `CC`
A69.21 Meningitis due to Lyme disease `CC`
A69.22 Other neurologic disorders in Lyme disease `CC`
- Cranial neuritis
- Meningoencephalitis
- Polyneuropathy
A69.23 Arthritis due to Lyme disease `CC` `HCC`
A69.29 Other conditions associated with Lyme disease `CC`
- Myopericarditis due to Lyme disease
- AHA: 2016, 3Q, 12

A69.8 Other specified spirochetal infections

A69.9 Spirochetal infection, unspecified

Other diseases caused by chlamydiae (A70-A74)

EXCLUDES 1 *sexually transmitted chlamydial diseases (A55-A56)*

A70 Chlamydia psittaci infections `CC`
- Ornithosis
- Parrot fever
- Psittacosis
- CC Excl: PDX collection 127

✓4ᵗʰ **A71 Trachoma**
- EXCLUDES 1 *sequelae of trachoma (B94.0)*

A71.0 Initial stage of trachoma
- Trachoma dubium

A71.1 Active stage of trachoma
- Granular conjunctivitis (trachomatous)
- Trachomatous follicular conjunctivitis
- Trachomatous pannus

A71.9 Trachoma, unspecified

✓4ᵗʰ **A74 Other diseases caused by chlamydiae**
- EXCLUDES 1 *neonatal chlamydial conjunctivitis (P39.1)*
  neonatal chlamydial pneumonia (P23.1)
  Reiter's disease (M02.3-)
  sexually transmitted chlamydial diseases (A55-A56)
- EXCLUDES 2 *chlamydial pneumonia (J16.0)*

A74.0 Chlamydial conjunctivitis
- Paratrachoma

✓5ᵗʰ **A74.8 Other chlamydial diseases**
A74.81 Chlamydial peritonitis
A74.89 Other chlamydial diseases

A74.9 Chlamydial infection, unspecified
- Chlamydiosis NOS

Rickettsioses (A75-A79)

✓4ᵗʰ **A75 Typhus fever**
- EXCLUDES 1 *rickettsiosis due to Ehrlichia sennetsu (A79.81)*

CC Excl: For CC codes in category A75, unless otherwise noted: PDX collection 108

A75.0 Epidemic louse-borne typhus fever due to Rickettsia prowazekii `CC`
- Classical typhus (fever)
- Epidemic (louse-borne) typhus

A75.1 Recrudescent typhus [Brill's disease] `CC`
- Brill-Zinsser disease

A75.2 Typhus fever due to Rickettsia typhi `CC`
- Murine (flea-borne) typhus

A75.3 Typhus fever due to Rickettsia tsutsugamushi `CC`
- Scrub (mite-borne) typhus
- Tsutsugamushi fever

A75.9 Typhus fever, unspecified `CC`
- Typhus (fever) NOS
- CC Excl: PDX collection 128

✓4ᵗʰ **A77 Spotted fever [tick-borne rickettsioses]**

CC Excl: For CC codes in category A77: PDX collection 108

A77.0 Spotted fever due to Rickettsia rickettsii `CC`
- Rocky Mountain spotted fever
- Sao Paulo fever

A77.1 Spotted fever due to Rickettsia conorii `CC`
- African tick typhus
- Boutonneuse fever
- India tick typhus
- Kenya tick typhus
- Marseilles fever
- Mediterranean tick fever

A77.2 Spotted fever due to Rickettsia siberica `CC`
- North Asian tick fever
- Siberian tick typhus

A77.3 Spotted fever due to Rickettsia australis `CC`
- Queensland tick typhus

✓5ᵗʰ **A77.4 Ehrlichiosis**
- EXCLUDES 1 *Rickettsiosis due to Ehrlichia sennetsu (A79.81)*

A77.40 Ehrlichiosis, unspecified `CC`
A77.41 Ehrlichiosis chaffeensis [E. chaffeensis] `CC`
A77.49 Other ehrlichiosis `CC`

A77.8 Other spotted fevers `CC`

A77.9 Spotted fever, unspecified `CC`
- Tick-borne typhus NOS

N Newborn: 0   P Pediatric: 0-17   M Maternity: 12-55   A Adult: 15-124   MCC Major Complication/Comorbidity   CC Complication/Comorbidity   SW Severe Wound Dx

A78   **Q fever** `CC`
    Infection due to Coxiella burnetii
    Nine Mile fever
    Quadrilateral fever
    CC Excl: PDX collection 108

✓4ᵗʰ **A79**   **Other rickettsioses**

> **CC Excl: For CC codes in category A79, unless otherwise noted:** PDX collection 129

    A79.0   **Trench fever** `CC`
       Quintan fever
       Wolhynian fever
       CC Excl: PDX collection 108

    A79.1   **Rickettsialpox due to Rickettsia akari** `CC`
       Kew Garden fever
       Vesicular rickettsiosis

    ✓5ᵗʰ **A79.8**   **Other specified rickettsioses**
       A79.81   **Rickettsiosis due to Ehrlichia sennetsu** `CC`
       A79.89   **Other specified rickettsioses** `CC`

    A79.9   **Rickettsiosis, unspecified** `CC`
       Rickettsial infection NOS

Viral and prion infections of the central nervous system (A80-A89)

> EXCLUDES 1   postpolio syndrome (G14)
>   sequelae of poliomyelitis (B91)
>   sequelae of viral encephalitis (B94.1)

✓4ᵗʰ **A80**   **Acute poliomyelitis**

> **CC Excl: For MCC codes in category A80:** PDX collection 130

    A80.0   **Acute paralytic poliomyelitis, vaccine-associated** `MCC`
    A80.1   **Acute paralytic poliomyelitis, wild virus, imported** `MCC`
    A80.2   **Acute paralytic poliomyelitis, wild virus, indigenous** `MCC`

    ✓5ᵗʰ **A80.3**   **Acute paralytic poliomyelitis, other and unspecified**
       A80.30   **Acute paralytic poliomyelitis, unspecified** `MCC`
       A80.39   **Other acute paralytic poliomyelitis** `MCC`

    A80.4   **Acute nonparalytic poliomyelitis**
    A80.9   **Acute poliomyelitis, unspecified**

✓4ᵗʰ **A81**   **Atypical virus infections of central nervous system**
    INCLUDES   diseases of the central nervous system caused by prions
    Use additional code to identify:
       dementia with behavioral disturbance (F02.81)
       dementia without behavioral disturbance (F02.80)

    ✓5ᵗʰ **A81.0**   **Creutzfeldt-Jakob disease**
       DEF: Communicable, rare spongiform encephalopathy occurring later in life with progressive destruction of the pyramidal and extrapyramidal systems eventually leading to death. Progressive dementia, wasting of muscles, tremor, and other symptoms are present.

> **CC Excl: For CC codes in subcategory A81.0:** PDX collection 131

       A81.00   **Creutzfeldt-Jakob disease, unspecified** `CC`
          Jakob-Creutzfeldt disease, unspecified

       A81.01   **Variant Creutzfeldt-Jakob disease** `CC`
          vCJD

       A81.09   **Other Creutzfeldt-Jakob disease** `CC`
          CJD
          Familial Creutzfeldt-Jakob disease
          Iatrogenic Creutzfeldt-Jakob disease
          Sporadic Creutzfeldt-Jakob disease
          Subacute spongiform encephalopathy (with dementia)

    A81.1   **Subacute sclerosing panencephalitis** `CC`
       Dawson's inclusion body encephalitis
       Van Bogaert's sclerosing leukoencephalopathy
       CC Excl: PDX collection 132

    A81.2   **Progressive multifocal leukoencephalopathy** `HIV` `CC`
       Multifocal leukoencephalopathy NOS
       CC Excl: PDX collection 133

    ✓5ᵗʰ **A81.8**   **Other atypical virus infections of central nervous system**

> **CC Excl: For CC codes in subcategory A81.8, unless otherwise noted:** PDX collection 135

       A81.81   **Kuru** `CC`
          CC Excl: PDX collection 134

       A81.82   **Gerstmann-Sträussler-Scheinker syndrome** `HIV` `CC`
          GSS syndrome

       A81.83   **Fatal familial insomnia** `HIV` `CC`
          FFI

       A81.89   **Other atypical virus infections of central nervous system** `HIV` `CC`

    A81.9   **Atypical virus infection of central nervous system, unspecified** `HIV` `CC`
       Prion diseases of the central nervous system NOS
       CC Excl: PDX collection 134

✓4ᵗʰ **A82**   **Rabies**

> **CC Excl: For CC codes in category A82:** PDX collection 136

    A82.0   **Sylvatic rabies** `CC`
    A82.1   **Urban rabies** `CC`
    A82.9   **Rabies, unspecified** `CC`

✓4ᵗʰ **A83**   **Mosquito-borne viral encephalitis**
    INCLUDES   mosquito-borne viral meningoencephalitis
    EXCLUDES 2   Venezuelan equine encephalitis (A92.2)
          West Nile fever (A92.3-)
          West Nile virus (A92.3-)

> **CC Excl: For MCC codes in category A83:** PDX collection 137

    A83.0   **Japanese encephalitis** `MCC`
    A83.1   **Western equine encephalitis** `MCC`
    A83.2   **Eastern equine encephalitis** `MCC`
    A83.3   **St Louis encephalitis** `MCC`
    A83.4   **Australian encephalitis** `MCC`
       Kunjin virus disease

    A83.5   **California encephalitis** `MCC`
       California meningoencephalitis
       La Crosse encephalitis

    A83.6   **Rocio virus disease** `MCC`
    A83.8   **Other mosquito-borne viral encephalitis** `MCC`
    A83.9   **Mosquito-borne viral encephalitis, unspecified** `MCC`

✓4ᵗʰ **A84**   **Tick-borne viral encephalitis**
    INCLUDES   tick-borne viral meningoencephalitis

> **CC Excl: For MCC codes in category A84:** PDX collection 137

    A84.0   **Far Eastern tick-borne encephalitis [Russian spring-summer encephalitis]** `MCC`
    A84.1   **Central European tick-borne encephalitis** `MCC`
    A84.8   **Other tick-borne viral encephalitis** `MCC`
       Louping ill
       Powassan virus disease

    A84.9   **Tick-borne viral encephalitis, unspecified** `MCC`

✓4ᵗʰ **A85**   **Other viral encephalitis, not elsewhere classified**
    INCLUDES   specified viral encephalomyelitis NEC
          specified viral meningoencephalitis NEC
    EXCLUDES 1   benign myalgic encephalomyelitis (G93.3)
          encephalitis due to cytomegalovirus (B25.8)
          encephalitis due to herpesvirus NEC (B10.0-)
          encephalitis due to herpesvirus [herpes simplex] (B00.4)
          encephalitis due to measles virus (B05.0)
          encephalitis due to mumps virus (B26.2)
          encephalitis due to poliomyelitis virus (A80.-)
          encephalitis due to zoster (B02.0)
          lymphocytic choriomeningitis (A87.2)

> **CC Excl: For CC/MCC codes in category A85, unless otherwise noted:** PDX collection 138

    A85.0   **Enteroviral encephalitis** `HIV` `CC`
       Enteroviral encephalomyelitis

    A85.1   **Adenoviral encephalitis** `HIV` `CC`
       Adenoviral meningoencephalitis

    A85.2   **Arthropod-borne viral encephalitis, unspecified** `MCC`
       EXCLUDES 1   West nile virus with encephalitis (A92.31)
       CC Excl: PDX collection 137

    A85.8   **Other specified viral encephalitis** `HIV` `CC`
       Encephalitis lethargica
       Von Economo-Cruchet disease

A86   **Unspecified viral encephalitis** `HIV` `CC`
    Viral encephalomyelitis NOS
    Viral meningoencephalitis NOS
    CC Excl: PDX collection 139

✓ Additional Character Required   ✓x7ᵗʰ Placeholder   Unacceptable PDx   Questionable PDx   Manifestation   H1 - H14 HAC   HCC CMS-HCC Dx   HIV HIV Dx

ICD-10-CM 2019   447

✓4ᵗʰ **A87 Viral meningitis**
> **EXCLUDES 1**   meningitis due to herpesvirus [herpes simplex] (B00.3)
>   meningitis due to measles virus (B05.1)
>   meningitis due to mumps virus (B26.1)
>   meningitis due to poliomyelitis virus (A80.-)
>   meningitis due to zoster (B02.1)

DEF: Meningitis: Inflammation of the meningeal layers of the brain and spine.

> **CC Excl: For CC codes in category A87, unless otherwise noted:** PDX collection 140

A87.0 Enteroviral meningitis   `CC`
     Coxsackievirus meningitis
     Echovirus meningitis

A87.1 Adenoviral meningitis   `CC`

A87.2 Lymphocytic choriomeningitis   `CC`
     Lymphocytic meningoencephalitis
     CC Excl: PDX collection 141

A87.8 Other viral meningitis   `CC`

A87.9 Viral meningitis, unspecified   `CC`

✓4ᵗʰ **A88 Other viral infections of central nervous system, not elsewhere classified**
> **EXCLUDES 1**   viral encephalitis NOS (A86)
>   viral meningitis NOS (A87.9)

A88.0 Enteroviral exanthematous fever [Boston exanthem]   `CC`
     CC Excl: PDX collection 137

A88.1 Epidemic vertigo

A88.8 Other specified viral infections of central nervous system   `HIV` `CC`
     CC Excl: PDX collection 138

A89 Unspecified viral infection of central nervous system   `HIV` `CC`
     CC Excl: PDX collection 139

Arthropod-borne viral fevers and viral hemorrhagic fevers (A90-A99)

A90 Dengue fever [classical dengue]   `CC`
> **EXCLUDES 1**   dengue hemorrhagic fever (A91)

AHA: 2016, 3Q, 13
CC Excl: PDX collection 142

A91 Dengue hemorrhagic fever   `CC`
     CC Excl: PDX collection 143

✓4ᵗʰ **A92 Other mosquito-borne viral fevers**
> **EXCLUDES 1**   Ross River disease (B33.1)

> **CC Excl: For CC/MCC codes in category A92, unless otherwise noted:** PDX collection 144

A92.0 Chikungunya virus disease   `CC`
     Chikungunya (hemorrhagic) fever
     CC Excl: PDX collection 143

A92.1 O'nyong-nyong fever   `CC`

A92.2 Venezuelan equine fever   `CC`
     Venezuelan equine encephalitis
     Venezuelan equine encephalomyelitis virus disease

✓5ᵗʰ **A92.3 West Nile virus infection**
     West Nile fever
     AHA: 2016, 3Q, 12

> **CC Excl: For MCC codes in subcategory A92.3:** PDX collection 145

A92.30 West Nile virus infection, unspecified   `MCC`
     West Nile fever NOS
     West Nile fever without complications
     West Nile virus NOS

A92.31 West Nile virus infection with encephalitis   `MCC`
     West Nile encephalitis
     West Nile encephalomyelitis

A92.32 West Nile virus infection with other neurologic manifestation   `MCC`
     Use additional code to specify the neurologic manifestation

A92.39 West Nile virus infection with other complications   `MCC`
     Use additional code to specify the other conditions

A92.4 Rift Valley fever   `CC`

A92.5 Zika virus disease   `CC`
     Zika virus fever
     Zika virus infection
     Zika NOS
> **EXCLUDES 1** ▶ congenital Zika virus disease (P35.4)◄

AHA: 2016, 4Q, 4-7
DEF: Virus transmitted via a bite from an infected Aedes species mosquito. Common symptoms of the virus include fever, rash, joint pain, and conjunctivitis; they are usually mild in nature and may last from several days to a week. Most people who have the Zika virus do not require medical attention; however, in pregnant women, the Zika virus can cause a serious birth defect called microcephaly, as well as other severe fetal brain defects.

A92.8 Other specified mosquito-borne viral fevers   `CC`

A92.9 Mosquito-borne viral fever, unspecified   `CC`
     CC Excl: PDX collection 143

✓4ᵗʰ **A93 Other arthropod-borne viral fevers, not elsewhere classified**

> **CC Excl: For CC codes in category A93, unless otherwise noted:** PDX collection 143

A93.0 Oropouche virus disease   `CC`
     Oropouche fever
     CC Excl: PDX collection 144

A93.1 Sandfly fever   `CC`
     Pappataci fever
     Phlebotomus fever

A93.2 Colorado tick fever   `CC`

A93.8 Other specified arthropod-borne viral fevers   `CC`
     Piry virus disease
     Vesicular stomatitis virus disease [Indiana fever]

A94 Unspecified arthropod-borne viral fever   `CC`
     Arboviral fever NOS
     Arbovirus infection NOS
     CC Excl: PDX collection 143

✓4ᵗʰ **A95 Yellow fever**

> **CC Excl: For CC codes in category A95:** PDX collection 146

A95.0 Sylvatic yellow fever   `CC`
     Jungle yellow fever

A95.1 Urban yellow fever   `CC`

A95.9 Yellow fever, unspecified   `CC`

✓4ᵗʰ **A96 Arenaviral hemorrhagic fever**

> **CC Excl: For CC codes in category A96:** PDX collection 147

A96.0 Junin hemorrhagic fever   `CC`
     Argentinian hemorrhagic fever

A96.1 Machupo hemorrhagic fever   `CC`
     Bolivian hemorrhagic fever

A96.2 Lassa fever

A96.8 Other arenaviral hemorrhagic fevers   `CC`

A96.9 Arenaviral hemorrhagic fever, unspecified   `CC`

✓4ᵗʰ **A98 Other viral hemorrhagic fevers, not elsewhere classified**
> **EXCLUDES 1**   chikungunya hemorrhagic fever (A92.0)
>   dengue hemorrhagic fever (A91)

> **CC Excl: For CC codes in category A98, unless otherwise noted:** PDX collection 143

A98.0 Crimean-Congo hemorrhagic fever   `CC`
     Central Asian hemorrhagic fever

A98.1 Omsk hemorrhagic fever   `CC`

A98.2 Kyasanur Forest disease   `CC`

A98.3 Marburg virus disease

A98.4 Ebola virus disease

A98.5 Hemorrhagic fever with renal syndrome   `CC`
     Epidemic hemorrhagic fever
     Korean hemorrhagic fever
     Russian hemorrhagic fever
     Hantaan virus disease
     Hantavirus disease with renal manifestations
     Nephropathia epidemica
     Songo fever
> **EXCLUDES 1**   hantavirus (cardio)-pulmonary syndrome (B33.4)

     CC Excl: PDX collection 148

A98.8 Other specified viral hemorrhagic fevers   `CC`

A99 Unspecified viral hemorrhagic fever   `CC`
     CC Excl: PDX collection 143

`N` Newborn: 0   `P` Pediatric: 0-17   `M` Maternity: 12-55   `A` Adult: 15-124   `MCC` Major Complication/Comorbidity   `CC` Complication/Comorbidity   `SW` Severe Wound Dx

448   ICD-10-CM 2019

Viral infections characterized by skin and mucous membrane lesions (B00-B09)

✓4ᵗʰ B00 Herpesviral [herpes simplex] infections
- EXCLUDES 1   congenital herpesviral infections (P35.2)
- EXCLUDES 2   anogenital herpesviral infection (A60.-)
  - gammaherpesviral mononucleosis (B27.0-)
  - herpangina (B08.5)

B00.0 Eczema herpeticum   HIV
- Kaposi's varicelliform eruption

B00.1 Herpesviral vesicular dermatitis   HIV
- Herpes simplex facialis
- Herpes simplex labialis
- Herpes simplex otitis externa
- Vesicular dermatitis of ear
- Vesicular dermatitis of lip

B00.2 Herpesviral gingivostomatitis and pharyngotonsillitis   HIV CC
- Herpesviral pharyngitis
- **CC Excl:** PDX collection 149

B00.3 Herpesviral meningitis   HIV MCC
- **CC Excl:** PDX collection 150

B00.4 Herpesviral encephalitis   HIV MCC
- Herpesviral meningoencephalitis
- Simian B disease
- EXCLUDES 1   herpesviral encephalitis due to herpesvirus 6 and 7 (B10.01, B10.09)
  - non-simplex herpesviral encephalitis (B10.0-)
- **CC Excl:** PDX collection 151

✓5ᵗʰ B00.5 Herpesviral ocular disease

CC Excl: For CC codes in subcategory B00.5: PDX collection 152

- **B00.50 Herpesviral ocular disease, unspecified**   HIV CC
- **B00.51 Herpesviral iridocyclitis**   HIV CC
  - Herpesviral iritis
  - Herpesviral uveitis, anterior
- **B00.52 Herpesviral keratitis**   HIV CC
  - Herpesviral keratoconjunctivitis
- **B00.53 Herpesviral conjunctivitis**   HIV CC
- **B00.59 Other herpesviral disease of eye**   HIV CC
  - Herpesviral dermatitis of eyelid

B00.7 Disseminated herpesviral disease   HIV MCC HCC
- Herpesviral sepsis
- **CC Excl:** PDX collection 153

✓5ᵗʰ B00.8 Other forms of herpesviral infections
- **B00.81 Herpesviral hepatitis**   HIV CC
  - **CC Excl:** PDX collection 154
- **B00.82 Herpes simplex myelitis**   MCC HCC
  - **CC Excl:** PDX collection 155
- **B00.89 Other herpesviral infection**   HIV CC
  - Herpesviral whitlow
  - **CC Excl:** PDX collection 156

B00.9 Herpesviral infection, unspecified   HIV
- Herpes simplex infection NOS

✓4ᵗʰ B01 Varicella [chickenpox]

CC Excl: For CC/MCC codes in category B01, unless otherwise noted: PDX collection 157

B01.0 Varicella meningitis   CC

✓5ᵗʰ B01.1 Varicella encephalitis, myelitis and encephalomyelitis
- Postchickenpox encephalitis, myelitis and encephalomyelitis
- **B01.11 Varicella encephalitis and encephalomyelitis**   MCC
  - Postchickenpox encephalitis and encephalomyelitis
  - **CC Excl:** PDX collection 158
- **B01.12 Varicella myelitis**   MCC HCC
  - Postchickenpox myelitis
  - **CC Excl:** PDX collection 159

B01.2 Varicella pneumonia   MCC
- **CC Excl:** PDX collection 160

✓5ᵗʰ B01.8 Varicella with other complications
- **B01.81 Varicella keratitis**   CC
- **B01.89 Other varicella complications**   CC

B01.9 Varicella without complication   CC
- Varicella NOS

✓4ᵗʰ B02 Zoster [herpes zoster]
- INCLUDES   shingles
  - zona

B02.0 Zoster encephalitis   HIV CC
- Zoster meningoencephalitis
- **CC Excl:** PDX collection 161

B02.1 Zoster meningitis   HIV MCC
- **CC Excl:** PDX collection 162

✓5ᵗʰ B02.2 Zoster with other nervous system involvement

CC Excl: For CC/MCC codes in subcategory B02.2, unless otherwise noted: PDX collection 161

- **B02.21 Postherpetic geniculate ganglionitis**   HIV CC
- **B02.22 Postherpetic trigeminal neuralgia**   HIV CC
- **B02.23 Postherpetic polyneuropathy**   HIV CC
- **B02.24 Postherpetic myelitis**   MCC HCC
  - Herpes zoster myelitis
  - **CC Excl:** PDX collection 163
- **B02.29 Other postherpetic nervous system involvement**   HIV CC
  - Postherpetic radiculopathy

✓5ᵗʰ B02.3 Zoster ocular disease

CC Excl: For CC codes in subcategory B02.3: PDX collection 164

- **B02.30 Zoster ocular disease, unspecified**   HIV CC
- **B02.31 Zoster conjunctivitis**   HIV CC
- **B02.32 Zoster iridocyclitis**   HIV CC
- **B02.33 Zoster keratitis**   HIV CC
  - Herpes zoster keratoconjunctivitis
- **B02.34 Zoster scleritis**   HIV CC
- **B02.39 Other herpes zoster eye disease**   HIV CC
  - Zoster blepharitis

B02.7 Disseminated zoster   HIV CC
- **CC Excl:** PDX collection 165

B02.8 Zoster with other complications   HIV CC
- Herpes zoster otitis externa
- **CC Excl:** PDX collection 165

B02.9 Zoster without complications   HIV
- Zoster NOS

B03 Smallpox   CC
- NOTE   In 1980 the 33rd World Health Assembly declared that smallpox had been eradicated. The classification is maintained for surveillance purposes.
- **CC Excl:** PDX collection 166

B04 Monkeypox   CC
- **CC Excl:** PDX collection 167

✓4ᵗʰ B05 Measles
- INCLUDES   morbilli
- EXCLUDES 1   subacute sclerosing panencephalitis (A81.1)

B05.0 Measles complicated by encephalitis   MCC
- Postmeasles encephalitis
- **CC Excl:** PDX collection 168

B05.1 Measles complicated by meningitis   CC
- Postmeasles meningitis
- **CC Excl:** PDX collection 169

B05.2 Measles complicated by pneumonia   MCC
- Postmeasles pneumonia
- **CC Excl:** PDX collection 170

B05.3 Measles complicated by otitis media
- Postmeasles otitis media

B05.4 Measles with intestinal complications   CC
- **CC Excl:** PDX collection 169

✓5ᵗʰ B05.8 Measles with other complications
- **B05.81 Measles keratitis and keratoconjunctivitis**   CC
  - **CC Excl:** PDX collection 171
- **B05.89 Other measles complications**   CC
  - **CC Excl:** PDX collection 169

B05.9 Measles without complication
- Measles NOS

✓ Additional Character Required   ✓x7ᵗʰ Placeholder   Unacceptable PDx   Questionable PDx   Manifestation   H1-H14 HAC   HCC CMS-HCC Dx   HIV HIV Dx

ICD-10-CM 2019   449

B00–B05.9

✓4th **B06   Rubella [German measles]**
> **EXCLUDES 1**   congenital rubella (P35.0)
>
> **DEF:** Highly contagious virus in which the symptoms are mild and short-lived in most people. Rubella during pregnancy, however, can result in abortion, stillbirth, or congenital defects.
>
> **CC Excl: For CC/MCC codes in category B06, unless otherwise noted:** PDX collection 172

✓5th **B06.0   Rubella with neurological complications**

    B06.00   Rubella with neurological complication, unspecified   `CC`

    B06.01   Rubella encephalitis   `MCC`
        Rubella meningoencephalitis

    B06.02   Rubella meningitis   `CC`

    B06.09   Other neurological complications of rubella   `CC`

✓5th **B06.8   Rubella with other complications**

    B06.81   Rubella pneumonia   `CC`

    B06.82   Rubella arthritis   `CC` `HCC`
        CC Excl: PDX collection 173

    B06.89   Other rubella complications   `CC`

  B06.9   Rubella without complication
    Rubella NOS

✓4th **B07   Viral warts**
> **INCLUDES**   verruca simplex
>   verruca vulgaris
>   viral warts due to human papillomavirus
>
> **EXCLUDES 2**   anogenital (venereal) warts (A63.0)
>   papilloma of bladder (D41.4)
>   papilloma of cervix (D26.0)
>   papilloma larynx (D14.1)

  B07.0   Plantar wart
    Verruca plantaris

  B07.8   Other viral warts
    Common wart
    Flat wart
    Verruca plana

  B07.9   Viral wart, unspecified

✓4th **B08   Other viral infections characterized by skin and mucous membrane lesions, not elsewhere classified**
> **EXCLUDES 1**   vesicular stomatitis virus disease (A93.8)

✓5th **B08.0   Other orthopoxvirus infections**
> **EXCLUDES 2**   monkeypox (B04)

✓6th **B08.01   Cowpox and vaccinia not from vaccine**

    B08.010   Cowpox
        DEF: Disease contracted by milking infected cows. The vesicles usually appear on the fingers, hands, and adjacent areas and usually disappear without scarring. Other symptoms include local edema, lymphangitis, and regional lymphadenitis with or without fever.

    B08.011   Vaccinia not from vaccine
        EXCLUDES 1   vaccinia (from vaccination) (generalized) (T88.1)

  B08.02   Orf virus disease
    Contagious pustular dermatitis
    Ecthyma contagiosum

  B08.03   Pseudocowpox [milker's node]

  B08.04   Paravaccinia, unspecified

  B08.09   Other orthopoxvirus infections
    Orthopoxvirus infection NOS

  B08.1   Molluscum contagiosum
    DEF: Benign poxvirus infection causing small bumps on the skin or conjunctiva and is transmitted by close contact.

✓5th **B08.2   Exanthema subitum [sixth disease]**
    Roseola infantum

    B08.20   Exanthema subitum [sixth disease], unspecified   `P`
        Roseola infantum, unspecified

    B08.21   Exanthema subitum [sixth disease] due to human herpesvirus 6   `P`
        Roseola infantum due to human herpesvirus 6

    B08.22   Exanthema subitum [sixth disease] due to human herpesvirus 7   `P`
        Roseola infantum due to human herpesvirus 7

  B08.3   Erythema infectiosum [fifth disease]   `CC`
    DEF: Infection with human parvovirus B19, mainly occurring in children. Symptoms include a low-grade fever, malaise, or a "cold" a few days before the appearance of a mild rash illness that presents as a "slapped-cheek" rash on the face and a lacy red rash on the trunk and limbs.
    CC Excl: PDX collection 174

  B08.4   Enteroviral vesicular stomatitis with exanthem
    Hand, foot and mouth disease

  B08.5   Enteroviral vesicular pharyngitis
    Herpangina
    DEF: Acute infectious Coxsackie virus infection causing throat lesions, fever, and vomiting that generally affects children in the summer.

✓5th **B08.6   Parapoxvirus infections**

    B08.60   Parapoxvirus infection, unspecified

    B08.61   Bovine stomatitis

    B08.62   Sealpox

    B08.69   Other parapoxvirus infections

✓5th **B08.7   Yatapoxvirus infections**

    B08.70   Yatapoxvirus infection, unspecified

    B08.71   Tanapox virus disease   `CC`
        CC Excl: PDX collection 167

    B08.72   Yaba pox virus disease
        Yaba monkey tumor disease

    B08.79   Other yatapoxvirus infections

  B08.8   Other specified viral infections characterized by skin and mucous membrane lesions
    Enteroviral lymphonodular pharyngitis
    Foot-and-mouth disease
    Poxvirus NEC

B09   Unspecified viral infection characterized by skin and mucous membrane lesions
    Viral enanthema NOS
    Viral exanthema NOS

Other human herpesviruses (B10)

✓4th **B10   Other human herpesviruses**
> **EXCLUDES 2**   cytomegalovirus (B25.9)
>   Epstein-Barr virus (B27.0-)
>   herpes NOS (B00.9)
>   herpes simplex (B00.-)
>   herpes zoster (B02.-)
>   human herpesvirus NOS (B00.-)
>   human herpesvirus 1 and 2 (B00.-)
>   human herpesvirus 3 (B01.-, B02.-)
>   human herpesvirus 4 (B27.0-)
>   human herpesvirus 5 (B25.-)
>   varicella (B01.-)
>   zoster (B02.-)

✓5th **B10.0   Other human herpesvirus encephalitis**
> **EXCLUDES 2**   herpes encephalitis NOS (B00.4)
>   herpes simplex encephalitis (B00.4)
>   human herpesvirus encephalitis (B00.4)
>   simian B herpes virus encephalitis (B00.4)

    B10.01   Human herpesvirus 6 encephalitis   `HIV` `MCC`
        CC Excl: PDX collection 151

    B10.09   Other human herpesvirus encephalitis   `HIV` `MCC`
        Human herpesvirus 7 encephalitis
        CC Excl: PDX collection 151

✓5th **B10.8   Other human herpesvirus infection**

    B10.81   Human herpesvirus 6 infection

    B10.82   Human herpesvirus 7 infection

    B10.89   Other human herpesvirus infection
        Human herpesvirus 8 infection
        Kaposi's sarcoma-associated herpesvirus infection

`N` Newborn: 0   `P` Pediatric: 0-17   `M` Maternity: 12-55   `A` Adult: 15-124   `MCC` Major Complication/Comorbidity   `CC` Complication/Comorbidity   `SW` Severe Wound Dx

450   ICD-10-CM 2019

Viral hepatitis (B15-B19)

EXCLUDES 1   sequelae of viral hepatitis (B94.2)
EXCLUDES 2   cytomegaloviral hepatitis (B25.1)
        herpesviral [herpes simplex] hepatitis (B00.81)

DEF: Hepatitis A: HAV infection that is self-limiting with flulike symptoms. Transmission is fecal-oral.
DEF: Hepatitis B: HBV infection that can be chronic and systemic. Transmission is bodily fluids.
DEF: Hepatitis C: HCV infection that can be chronic and systemic. Transmission is blood transfusion and unidentified agents.
DEF: Hepatitis D (delta): HDV that occurs only in the presence of hepatitis B virus. Transmission is contaminated blood in contact with mucous membranes.
DEF: Hepatitis E: HEV is an epidemic form. Transmission is fecal-oral, most often from contaminated water.

CC Excl: For CC/MCC codes in categories B15-B19: PDX collection 175

✓4ᵗʰ **B15**   **Acute hepatitis A**
     B15.0   **Hepatitis A** with hepatic coma   MCC
     B15.9   **Hepatitis A** without hepatic coma   CC
         Hepatitis A (acute)(viral) NOS

✓4ᵗʰ **B16**   **Acute hepatitis B**
     AHA: 2016, 3Q, 13
     B16.0   **Acute hepatitis B** with delta-agent with hepatic coma   MCC
     B16.1   **Acute hepatitis B** with delta-agent without hepatic coma   CC
     B16.2   **Acute hepatitis B** without delta-agent with hepatic coma   MCC
     B16.9   **Acute hepatitis B** without delta-agent and without hepatic coma   CC
         Hepatitis B (acute) (viral) NOS

✓4ᵗʰ **B17**   **Other acute viral hepatitis**
     B17.0   **Acute delta-(super) infection of hepatitis B carrier**   CC
     ✓5ᵗʰ **B17.1**   **Acute hepatitis C**
         B17.10   **Acute hepatitis C** without hepatic coma   CC
             Acute hepatitis C NOS
         B17.11   **Acute hepatitis C** with hepatic coma   MCC
     B17.2   **Acute hepatitis E**   CC
     B17.8   **Other specified acute viral hepatitis**   CC
         Hepatitis non-A non-B (acute) (viral) NEC
     B17.9   **Acute viral hepatitis, unspecified**   CC
         Acute hepatitis NOS
         Acute infectious hepatitis NOSb

✓4ᵗʰ **B18**   **Chronic viral hepatitis**
     INCLUDES   carrier of viral hepatitis
     AHA: 2017, 1Q, 41
     B18.0   **Chronic viral hepatitis B** with delta-agent   CC HCC
     B18.1   **Chronic viral hepatitis B** without delta-agent   CC HCC
         Carrier of viral hepatitis B
         Chronic (viral) hepatitis B
     B18.2   **Chronic viral hepatitis C**   HCC
         Carrier of viral hepatitis C
         AHA: 2018, 1Q, 4
     B18.8   **Other chronic viral hepatitis**   CC HCC
         Carrier of other viral hepatitis
     B18.9   **Chronic viral hepatitis, unspecified**   CC HCC
         Carrier of unspecified viral hepatitis

✓4ᵗʰ **B19**   **Unspecified viral hepatitis**
     B19.0   **Unspecified viral hepatitis** with hepatic coma   MCC
     ✓5ᵗʰ **B19.1**   **Unspecified viral hepatitis B**
         B19.10   **Unspecified viral hepatitis B** without hepatic coma   CC
             Unspecified viral hepatitis B NOS
         B19.11   **Unspecified viral hepatitis B** with hepatic coma   MCC
     ✓5ᵗʰ **B19.2**   **Unspecified viral hepatitis C**
         B19.20   **Unspecified viral hepatitis C** without hepatic coma   CC
             Viral hepatitis C NOS
         B19.21   **Unspecified viral hepatitis C** with hepatic coma   MCC
     B19.9   **Unspecified viral hepatitis** without hepatic coma   CC
         Viral hepatitis NOS

Human immunodeficiency virus [HIV] disease (B20)

✓4ᵗʰ **B20**   **Human immunodeficiency virus [HIV] disease**   CC HCC
     INCLUDES   acquired immune deficiency syndrome [AIDS]
         AIDS-related complex [ARC]
         HIV infection, symptomatic
     Code first human immunodeficiency virus [HIV] disease complicating pregnancy, childbirth and the puerperium, if applicable (O98.7-)
     Use additional code(s) to identify all manifestations of HIV infection
     EXCLUDES 1   asymptomatic human immunodeficiency virus [HIV] infection status (Z21)
            exposure to HIV virus (Z20.6)
            inconclusive serologic evidence of HIV (R75)
     CC Excl: PDX collection 176

Other viral diseases (B25-B34)

✓4ᵗʰ **B25**   **Cytomegaloviral disease**
     EXCLUDES 1   congenital cytomegalovirus infection (P35.1)
            cytomegaloviral mononucleosis (B27.1-)
     B25.0   **Cytomegaloviral** pneumonitis   MCC HCC
         CC Excl: PDX collection 110
     B25.1   **Cytomegaloviral** hepatitis   CC HCC
         CC Excl: No Excl
     B25.2   **Cytomegaloviral** pancreatitis   MCC HCC
         CC Excl: PDX collection 177
     B25.8   **Other cytomegaloviral diseases**   HIV CC HCC
         Cytomegaloviral encephalitis
         CC Excl: PDX collection 178
     B25.9   **Cytomegaloviral disease, unspecified**   HIV CC HCC
         CC Excl: PDX collection 178

✓4ᵗʰ **B26**   **Mumps**
     INCLUDES   epidemic parotitis
         infectious parotitis
     B26.0   **Mumps** orchitis   CC ♂
         CC Excl: PDX collection 179
     B26.1   **Mumps** meningitis   MCC
         CC Excl: PDX collection 180
     B26.2   **Mumps** encephalitis   MCC
         CC Excl: PDX collection 181
     B26.3   **Mumps** pancreatitis   CC
         CC Excl: PDX collection 182
     ✓5ᵗʰ **B26.8**   **Mumps with other complications**

         CC Excl: For CC codes in subcategory B26.8, unless otherwise noted: PDX collection 184

         B26.81   **Mumps** hepatitis   CC
             CC Excl: PDX collection 183
         B26.82   **Mumps** myocarditis   CC
         B26.83   **Mumps** nephritis   CC
         B26.84   **Mumps** polyneuropathy   CC
             CC Excl: PDX collection 185
         B26.85   **Mumps** arthritis   CC HCC
         B26.89   **Other mumps complications**   CC
     B26.9   **Mumps without complication**
         Mumps NOS
         Mumps parotitis NOS

✓4ᵗʰ **B27**   **Infectious mononucleosis**
     INCLUDES   glandular fever
         monocytic angina
         Pfeiffer's disease
     ✓5ᵗʰ **B27.0**   **Gammaherpesviral mononucleosis**
         Mononucleosis due to Epstein-Barr virus
         B27.00   **Gammaherpesviral mononucleosis** without complication
         B27.01   **Gammaherpesviral mononucleosis** with polyneuropathy
         B27.02   **Gammaherpesviral mononucleosis** with meningitis
         B27.09   **Gammaherpesviral mononucleosis** with other complications
             Hepatomegaly in gammaherpesviral mononucleosis
     ✓5ᵗʰ **B27.1**   **Cytomegaloviral mononucleosis**
         B27.10   **Cytomegaloviral mononucleosis** without complications
         B27.11   **Cytomegaloviral mononucleosis** with polyneuropathy
         B27.12   **Cytomegaloviral mononucleosis** with meningitis

✓ Additional Character Required   ✓7ᵗʰ Placeholder   Unacceptable PDx   Questionable PDx   Manifestation   H1-H14 HAC   HCC CMS-HCC Dx   HIV HIV Dx

ICD-10-CM 2019   **451**

B27.19   **Cytomegaloviral mononucleosis** with other complication
Hepatomegaly in cytomegaloviral mononucleosis

☑5ᵗʰ B27.8   Other **infectious mononucleosis**

B27.80   **Other infectious mononucleosis** without complication

B27.81   **Other infectious mononucleosis** with **polyneuropathy**

B27.82   **Other infectious mononucleosis** with **meningitis**

B27.89   **Other infectious mononucleosis with** other complication
Hepatomegaly in other infectious mononucleosis

☑5ᵗʰ B27.9   **Infectious mononucleosis,** unspecified

B27.90   **Infectious mononucleosis, unspecified** without complication

B27.91   **Infectious mononucleosis, unspecified** with **polyneuropathy**

B27.92   **Infectious mononucleosis, unspecified** with **meningitis**

B27.99   **Infectious mononucleosis, unspecified** with other complication
Hepatomegaly in unspecified infectious mononucleosis

Viral Conjunctivitis

Normal conjunctiva

Inflamed conjunctiva

☑4ᵗʰ **B30   Viral conjunctivitis**
EXCLUDES 1   *herpesviral [herpes simplex] ocular disease (B00.5)*
ocular zoster (B02.3)

B30.0   **Keratoconjunctivitis due to adenovirus**
Epidemic keratoconjunctivitis
Shipyard eye

B30.1   **Conjunctivitis due to adenovirus**
Acute adenoviral follicular conjunctivitis
Swimming-pool conjunctivitis

B30.2   **Viral pharyngoconjunctivitis**

B30.3   **Acute epidemic hemorrhagic conjunctivitis (enteroviral)**
Conjunctivitis due to coxsackievirus 24
Conjunctivitis due to enterovirus 70
Hemorrhagic conjunctivitis (acute)(epidemic)

B30.8   **Other viral conjunctivitis**
Newcastle conjunctivitis

B30.9   **Viral conjunctivitis,** unspecified

☑4ᵗʰ **B33   Other viral diseases, not elsewhere classified**

B33.0   **Epidemic myalgia**
Bornholm disease

B33.1   **Ross River disease**   CC
Epidemic polyarthritis and exanthema
Ross River fever
CC Excl: PDX collection 144

☑5ᵗʰ B33.2   **Viral carditis**
Coxsackie (virus) carditis

B33.20   **Viral carditis,** unspecified   CC
CC Excl: PDX collection 186

B33.21   **Viral endocarditis**   CC
CC Excl: PDX collection 187

B33.22   **Viral myocarditis**   CC
CC Excl: PDX collection 186

B33.23   **Viral pericarditis**   CC
CC Excl: PDX collection 188

B33.24   **Viral cardiomyopathy**   HCC

B33.3   **Retrovirus infections, not elsewhere classified**
Retrovirus infection NOS

B33.4   **Hantavirus (cardio)-pulmonary syndrome [HPS] [HCPS]**   CC
Hantavirus disease with pulmonary manifestations
Sin nombre virus disease
Use additional code to identify any associated acute kidney failure (N17.9)
EXCLUDES 1   *hantavirus disease with renal manifestations (A98.5)*
hemorrhagic fever with renal manifestations (A98.5)
CC Excl: PDX collection 189

B33.8   **Other specified viral diseases**
EXCLUDES 1   *anogenital human papillomavirus infection (A63.0)*
viral warts due to human papillomavirus infection (B07)

☑4ᵗʰ **B34   Viral infection of unspecified site**
EXCLUDES 1   *anogenital human papillomavirus infection (A63.0)*
cytomegaloviral disease NOS (B25.9)
herpesvirus [herpes simplex] infection NOS (B00.9)
retrovirus infection NOS (B33.3)
viral agents as the cause of diseases classified elsewhere (B97.-)
viral warts due to human papillomavirus infection (B07)

B34.0   **Adenovirus infection, unspecified**

B34.1   **Enterovirus infection, unspecified**
Coxsackievirus infection NOS
Echovirus infection NOS

B34.2   **Coronavirus infection, unspecified**
EXCLUDES 1   *pneumonia due to SARS-associated coronavirus (J12.81)*

B34.3   **Parvovirus infection, unspecified**   CC
CC Excl: PDX collection 174

B34.4   **Papovavirus infection, unspecified**

B34.8   **Other viral infections of unspecified site**

B34.9   **Viral infection,** unspecified
Viremia NOS
AHA: 2016, 3Q, 10

Mycoses (B35-B49)

EXCLUDES 2   *hypersensitivity pneumonitis due to organic dust (J67.-)*
mycosis fungoides (C84.0-)

☑4ᵗʰ **B35   Dermatophytosis**
INCLUDES   favus
infections due to species of Epidermophyton, Micro-sporum and Trichophyton
tinea, any type except those in B36-
DEF: Contagious superficial fungal infection of the skin that invades and grows in dead keratin.

B35.0   **Tinea barbae and tinea capitis**
Beard ringworm
Kerion
Scalp ringworm
Sycosis, mycotic

B35.1   **Tinea unguium**
Dermatophytic onychia
Dermatophytosis of nail
Onychomycosis
Ringworm of nails

B35.2   **Tinea manuum**
Dermatophytosis of hand
Hand ringworm

B35.3   **Tinea pedis**
Athlete's foot
Dermatophytosis of foot
Foot ringworm

B35.4   **Tinea corporis**
Ringworm of the body

B35.5   **Tinea imbricata**
Tokelau

B35.6   **Tinea cruris**
Dhobi itch
Groin ringworm
Jock itch

B35.8   **Other dermatophytoses**
Disseminated dermatophytosis
Granulomatous dermatophytosis

B35.9   **Dermatophytosis,** unspecified
Ringworm NOS

Ⓝ Newborn: 0   Ⓟ Pediatric: 0-17   Ⓜ Maternity: 12-55   Ⓐ Adult: 15-124   ᴹᶜᶜ Major Complication/Comorbidity   ᶜᶜ Complication/Comorbidity   ˢʷ Severe Wound Dx

452   ICD-10-CM 2019

✓4th **B36 Other superficial mycoses**

  B36.0 Pityriasis versicolor
    Tinea flava
    Tinea versicolor

  B36.1 Tinea nigra
    Keratomycosis nigricans palmaris
    Microsporosis nigra
    Pityriasis nigra

  B36.2 White piedra
    Tinea blanca

  B36.3 Black piedra

  B36.8 Other specified superficial mycoses

  B36.9 Superficial mycosis, unspecified

✓4th **B37 Candidiasis**
  INCLUDES candidosis
          moniliasis
  EXCLUDES 1 *neonatal candidiasis (P37.5)*

  B37.0 Candidal stomatitis   HIV CC
    Oral thrush
    CC Excl: PDX collection 190

  B37.1 Pulmonary candidiasis   HIV MCC HCC
    Candidal bronchitis
    Candidal pneumonia
    CC Excl: PDX collection 190

  B37.2 Candidiasis of skin and nail   HIV
    Candidal onychia
    Candidal paronychia
    EXCLUDES 2 *diaper dermatitis (L22)*

  B37.3 Candidiasis of vulva and vagina   ♀
    Candidal vulvovaginitis
    Monilial vulvovaginitis
    Vaginal thrush

✓5th   **B37.4 Candidiasis of other urogenital sites**

    B37.41 Candidal cystitis and urethritis   CC H6
        CC Excl: PDX collection 191

    B37.42 Candidal balanitis   ♂

    B37.49 Other urogenital candidiasis   CC H6
        Candidal pyelonephritis
        CC Excl: PDX collection 191

  B37.5 Candidal meningitis   HIV MCC
    CC Excl: PDX collection 192

  B37.6 Candidal endocarditis   HIV MCC
    CC Excl: PDX collection 190

  B37.7 Candidal sepsis   MCC HCC
    Disseminated candidiasis
    Systemic candidiasis
    AHA: 2014, 4Q, 46
    CC Excl: PDX collection 193

✓5th   **B37.8 Candidiasis of other sites**

    CC Excl: For CC codes in subcategory B37.8, unless otherwise noted: PDX collection 190

    B37.81 Candidal esophagitis   HIV CC HCC

    B37.82 Candidal enteritis   HIV CC
        Candidal proctitis

    B37.83 Candidal cheilitis   HIV CC

    B37.84 Candidal otitis externa   HIV CC

    B37.89 Other sites of candidiasis   HIV CC
        Candidal osteomyelitis
        CC Excl: PDX collection 194

  B37.9 Candidiasis, unspecified   HIV
    Thrush NOS

✓4th **B38 Coccidioidomycosis**

  B38.0 Acute pulmonary coccidioidomycosis   HIV CC HCC
    CC Excl: PDX collection 195

  B38.1 Chronic pulmonary coccidioidomycosis   HIV CC HCC
    CC Excl: PDX collection 196

  B38.2 Pulmonary coccidioidomycosis, unspecified   HIV CC HCC
    CC Excl: PDX collection 196

  B38.3 Cutaneous coccidioidomycosis   HIV CC
    CC Excl: PDX collection 197

  B38.4 Coccidioidomycosis meningitis   HIV MCC
    DEF: *Coccidioides immitis* infection of the lining of the brain and/or spinal cord.
    CC Excl: PDX collection 198

  B38.7 Disseminated coccidioidomycosis   HIV CC
    Generalized coccidioidomycosis
    CC Excl: PDX collection 199

✓5th   **B38.8 Other forms of coccidioidomycosis**

    B38.81 Prostatic coccidioidomycosis   HIV CC ♂
        CC Excl: PDX collection 197

    B38.89 Other forms of coccidioidomycosis   HIV CC
        CC Excl: PDX collection 199

  B38.9 Coccidioidomycosis, unspecified   HIV CC
    CC Excl: PDX collection 199

Histoplasmosis

Histoplasma capsulatum spores

Spores

✓4th **B39 Histoplasmosis**
  Code first associated AIDS (B20)
  Use additional code for any associated manifestations, such as:
    endocarditis (I39)
    meningitis (G02)
    pericarditis (I32)
    ▶retinitis◄ (H32)
  DEF: Type of lung infection caused by breathing in fungal spores often found in the droppings of bats and birds or soil contaminated by their droppings.

  CC Excl: For CC/MCC codes in category B39, unless otherwise noted: PDX collection 200

  B39.0 Acute pulmonary histoplasmosis capsulati   HIV MCC HCC

  B39.1 Chronic pulmonary histoplasmosis capsulati   HIV MCC HCC

  B39.2 Pulmonary histoplasmosis capsulati, unspecified   HIV MCC HCC

  B39.3 Disseminated histoplasmosis capsulati   HIV CC
    Generalized histoplasmosis capsulati
    CC Excl: PDX collection 201

  B39.4 Histoplasmosis capsulati, unspecified   HIV
    American histoplasmosis

  B39.5 Histoplasmosis duboisii   HIV
    African histoplasmosis

  B39.9 Histoplasmosis, unspecified   HIV

✓4th **B40 Blastomycosis**
  EXCLUDES 1 *Brazilian blastomycosis (B41.-)*
          keloidal blastomycosis (B48.0)

  CC Excl: For CC codes in category B40: PDX collection 202

  B40.0 Acute pulmonary blastomycosis   CC HCC

  B40.1 Chronic pulmonary blastomycosis   CC HCC

  B40.2 Pulmonary blastomycosis, unspecified   CC HCC

  B40.3 Cutaneous blastomycosis   CC

  B40.7 Disseminated blastomycosis   CC
    Generalized blastomycosis

✓5th   **B40.8 Other forms of blastomycosis**

    B40.81 Blastomycotic meningoencephalitis   CC
        Meningomyelitis due to blastomycosis

    B40.89 Other forms of blastomycosis   CC

  B40.9 Blastomycosis, unspecified   CC

☑ Additional Character Required   ✓7th Placeholder   Unacceptable PDx   Questionable PDx   Manifestation   H1-H14 HAC   HCC CMS-HCC Dx   HIV HIV Dx

ICD-10-CM 2019   453

Chapter 1. Certain Infectious and Parasitic Diseases

√4ᵗʰ B41 Paracoccidioidomycosis
    INCLUDES   Brazilian blastomycosis
          Lutz' disease

    CC Excl: For CC codes in category B41: PDX collection 203

    B41.0 Pulmonary paracoccidioidomycosis   **CC HCC**
    B41.7 Disseminated paracoccidioidomycosis   **CC**
          Generalized paracoccidioidomycosis
    B41.8 Other forms of paracoccidioidomycosis   **CC**
    B41.9 Paracoccidioidomycosis, unspecified   **CC**

√4ᵗʰ B42 Sporotrichosis
    B42.0 Pulmonary sporotrichosis
    B42.1 Lymphocutaneous sporotrichosis
    B42.7 Disseminated sporotrichosis
          Generalized sporotrichosis
    √5ᵗʰ B42.8 Other forms of sporotrichosis
         B42.81 Cerebral sporotrichosis
              Meningitis due to sporotrichosis
         B42.82 Sporotrichosis arthritis   **HCC**
         B42.89 Other forms of sporotrichosis
    B42.9 Sporotrichosis, unspecified

√4ᵗʰ B43 Chromomycosis and pheomycotic abscess
    B43.0 Cutaneous chromomycosis
          Dermatitis verrucosa
    B43.1 Pheomycotic brain abscess
          Cerebral chromomycosis
    B43.2 Subcutaneous pheomycotic abscess and cyst
    B43.8 Other forms of chromomycosis
    B43.9 Chromomycosis, unspecified

√4ᵗʰ B44 Aspergillosis
    INCLUDES   aspergilloma

    CC Excl: For CC/MCC codes in category B44, unless otherwise noted: PDX collection 204

    B44.0 Invasive pulmonary aspergillosis   **MCC HCC**
          CC Excl: PDX collection 110
    B44.1 Other pulmonary aspergillosis   **CC HCC**
    B44.2 Tonsillar aspergillosis   **CC HCC**
    B44.7 Disseminated aspergillosis   **CC HCC**
          Generalized aspergillosis
    √5ᵗʰ B44.8 Other forms of aspergillosis
         B44.81 Allergic bronchopulmonary aspergillosis   **CC HCC**
              CC Excl: PDX collection 205
         B44.89 Other forms of aspergillosis   **CC HCC**
    B44.9 Aspergillosis, unspecified   **CC HCC**

√4ᵗʰ B45 Cryptococcosis

    CC Excl: For CC/MCC codes in category B45, unless otherwise noted: PDX collection 206

    B45.0 Pulmonary cryptococcosis   **HIV CC HCC**
    B45.1 Cerebral cryptococcosis   **MCC HCC**
          Cryptococcal meningitis
          Cryptococcosis meningocerebralis
          CC Excl: PDX collection 207
    B45.2 Cutaneous cryptococcosis   **HIV CC HCC**
    B45.3 Osseous cryptococcosis   **HIV CC HCC**
    B45.7 Disseminated cryptococcosis   **HIV CC HCC**
          Generalized cryptococcosis
    B45.8 Other forms of cryptococcosis   **HIV CC HCC**
    B45.9 Cryptococcosis, unspecified   **HIV CC HCC**

√4ᵗʰ B46 Zygomycosis

    CC Excl: For MCC codes in category B46: PDX collection 208

    B46.0 Pulmonary mucormycosis   **MCC HCC**
    B46.1 Rhinocerebral mucormycosis   **MCC HCC**
    B46.2 Gastrointestinal mucormycosis   **MCC HCC**
    B46.3 Cutaneous mucormycosis   **MCC HCC**
          Subcutaneous mucormycosis
    B46.4 Disseminated mucormycosis   **MCC HCC**
          Generalized mucormycosis
    B46.5 Mucormycosis, unspecified   **MCC HCC**
    B46.8 Other zygomycoses   **MCC HCC**
          Entomophthoromycosis

B46.9 Zygomycosis, unspecified   **MCC HCC**
     Phycomycosis NOS

√4ᵗʰ B47 Mycetoma
    B47.0 Eumycetoma   **CC**
          Madura foot, mycotic
          Maduromycosis
          CC Excl: PDX collection 209
    B47.1 Actinomycetoma   **HIV CC**
          CC Excl: PDX collection 106
    B47.9 Mycetoma, unspecified   **HIV CC**
          Madura foot NOS
          CC Excl: PDX collection 210

√4ᵗʰ B48 Other mycoses, not elsewhere classified
    B48.0 Lobomycosis
          Keloidal blastomycosis
          Lobo's disease
    B48.1 Rhinosporidiosis
    B48.2 Allescheriasis   **CC**
          Infection due to Pseudallescheria boydii
          EXCLUDES 1   eumycetoma (B47.0)
          CC Excl: PDX collection 211
    B48.3 Geotrichosis   **CC**
          Geotrichum stomatitis
          CC Excl: PDX collection 212
    B48.4 Penicillosis   **CC HCC**
          CC Excl: PDX collection 204
    B48.8 Other specified mycoses   **HIV CC HCC**
          Adiaspiromycosis
          Infection of tissue and organs by Alternaria
          Infection of tissue and organs by Drechslera
          Infection of tissue and organs by Fusarium
          Infection of tissue and organs by saprophytic fungi NEC
          AHA: 2014, 4Q, 46; 2014, 2Q, 13
          CC Excl: PDX collection 213

B49 Unspecified mycosis   **CC**
     Fungemia NOS
     CC Excl: PDX collection 212

Protozoal diseases (B50-B64)
    EXCLUDES 1   amebiasis (A06.-)
          other protozoal intestinal diseases (A07.-)

√4ᵗʰ B50 Plasmodium falciparum malaria
    INCLUDES   mixed infections of Plasmodium falciparum with any other Plasmodium species

    CC Excl: For CC/MCC codes in category B50: PDX collection 214

    B50.0 Plasmodium falciparum malaria with cerebral complications   **CC**
          Cerebral malaria NOS
    B50.8 Other severe and complicated Plasmodium falciparum malaria   **CC**
          Severe or complicated Plasmodium falciparum malaria NOS
    B50.9 Plasmodium falciparum malaria, unspecified   **MCC**

√4ᵗʰ B51 Plasmodium vivax malaria
    INCLUDES   mixed infections of Plasmodium vivax with other Plasmodium species, except Plasmodium falciparum
    EXCLUDES 1 ▶Plasmodium vivax with Plasmodium falciparum◀ (B50.-)

    CC Excl: For CC codes in category B51, unless otherwise noted: PDX collection 214

    B51.0 Plasmodium vivax malaria with rupture of spleen   **CC**
    B51.8 Plasmodium vivax malaria with other complications   **CC**
    B51.9 Plasmodium vivax malaria without complication   **CC**
          Plasmodium vivax malaria NOS
          CC Excl: PDX collection 215

√4ᵗʰ B52 Plasmodium malariae malaria
    INCLUDES   mixed infections of Plasmodium malariae with other Plasmodium species, except Plasmodium falciparum and Plasmodium vivax
    EXCLUDES 1   Plasmodium falciparum (B50.-)
          Plasmodium vivax (B51.-)

    CC Excl: For CC codes in category B52, unless otherwise noted: PDX collection 214

    B52.0 Plasmodium malariae malaria with nephropathy   **CC**
          CC Excl: PDX collection 216
    B52.8 Plasmodium malariae malaria with other complications   **CC**

N Newborn: 0   **P** Pediatric: 0-17   **M** Maternity: 12-55   **A** Adult: 15-124   **MCC** Major Complication/Comorbidity   **CC** Complication/Comorbidity   **SW** Severe Wound Dx

454   ICD-10-CM 2019

B52.9   **Plasmodium malariae malaria** without complication   `CC`
Plasmodium malariae malaria NOS

✓4ᵗʰ B53   **Other** specified **malaria**

> CC Excl: For CC codes in subcategory B53: PDX collection 214

     B53.0   **Plasmodium ovale malaria**   `CC`
         EXCLUDES 1   *Plasmodium ovale with Plasmodium falciparum (B50.-)*
            Plasmodium ovale with Plasmodium malariae (B52.-)
            Plasmodium ovale with Plasmodium vivax (B51.-)

     B53.1   **Malaria due to simian plasmodia**   `CC`
         EXCLUDES 1   *malaria due to simian plasmodia with Plasmodium falciparum (B50.-)*
            malaria due to simian plasmodia with Plasmodium malariae (B52.-)
            malaria due to simian plasmodia with Plasmodium ovale (B53.0)
            malaria due to simian plasmodia with Plasmodium vivax (B51.-)

     B53.8   **Other malaria**, not elsewhere classified   `CC`

B54   **Unspecified malaria**   `CC`
     CC Excl: PDX collection 217

✓4ᵗʰ B55   **Leishmaniasis**

> CC Excl: For CC codes in category B55: PDX collection 218

     B55.0   **Visceral leishmaniasis**   `CC`
         Kala-azar
         Post-kala-azar dermal leishmaniasis

     B55.1   **Cutaneous leishmaniasis**   `CC`
     B55.2   **Mucocutaneous leishmaniasis**   `CC`
     B55.9   **Leishmaniasis**, unspecified   `CC`

✓4ᵗʰ B56   **African trypanosomiasis**

> CC Excl: For CC codes in category B56: PDX collection 218

     B56.0   **Gambiense trypanosomiasis**   `CC`
         Infection due to Trypanosoma brucei gambiense
         West African sleeping sickness

     B56.1   **Rhodesiense trypanosomiasis**   `CC`
         East African sleeping sickness
         Infection due to Trypanosoma brucei rhodesiense

     B56.9   **African trypanosomiasis**, unspecified   `CC`
         Sleeping sickness NOS

✓4ᵗʰ B57   **Chagas' disease**
     INCLUDES   American trypanosomiasis
            infection due to Trypanosoma cruzi

> CC Excl: For CC codes in category B57, unless otherwise noted: PDX collection 218

     B57.0   **Acute Chagas' disease with heart involvement**   `CC`
         Acute Chagas' disease with myocarditis
         CC Excl: PDX collection 219

     B57.1   **Acute Chagas' disease without heart involvement**   `CC`
         Acute Chagas' disease NOS

     B57.2   **Chagas' disease** (chronic) **with heart involvement**   `CC`
         American trypanosomiasis NOS
         Chagas' disease (chronic) NOS
         Chagas' disease (chronic) with myocarditis
         Trypanosomiasis NOS
         CC Excl: PDX collection 219

     ✓5ᵗʰ B57.3   **Chagas' disease** (chronic) **with digestive system involvement**
         B57.30   **Chagas' disease with digestive system involvement,** unspecified   `CC`
         B57.31   **Megaesophagus in Chagas' disease**   `CC`
         B57.32   **Megacolon in Chagas' disease**   `CC`
         B57.39   **Other digestive system involvement in Chagas' disease**   `CC`

     ✓5ᵗʰ B57.4   **Chagas' disease** (chronic) **with nervous system involvement**
         B57.40   **Chagas' disease with nervous system involvement,** unspecified   `CC`
         B57.41   **Meningitis in Chagas' disease**   `CC`
         B57.42   **Meningoencephalitis in Chagas' disease**   `CC`
         B57.49   **Other nervous system involvement in Chagas' disease**   `CC`

     B57.5   **Chagas' disease** (chronic) **with other organ involvement**   `CC`

✓4ᵗʰ B58   **Toxoplasmosis**
     INCLUDES   infection due to Toxoplasma gondii
     EXCLUDES 1   *congenital toxoplasmosis (P37.1)*

     ✓5ᵗʰ B58.0   **Toxoplasma oculopathy**
         B58.00   **Toxoplasma oculopathy,** unspecified   `HIV` `CC`
            CC Excl: PDX collection 220
         B58.01   **Toxoplasma chorioretinitis**   `HIV` `CC`
            CC Excl: PDX collection 221
         B58.09   **Other toxoplasma oculopathy**   `HIV` `CC`
            Toxoplasma uveitis
            CC Excl: PDX collection 222

     B58.1   **Toxoplasma hepatitis**   `HIV` `CC`
         CC Excl: PDX collection 223

     B58.2   **Toxoplasma meningoencephalitis**   `HIV` `MCC` `HCC`
         CC Excl: PDX collection 224

     B58.3   **Pulmonary toxoplasmosis**   `HIV` `MCC` `HCC`
         CC Excl: PDX collection 225

     ✓5ᵗʰ B58.8   **Toxoplasmosis with other organ involvement**

> CC Excl: For CC/MCC codes in subcategory B58.8, unless otherwise noted: PDX collection 220

         B58.81   **Toxoplasma myocarditis**   `HIV` `MCC`
            CC Excl: PDX collection 226
         B58.82   **Toxoplasma myositis**   `HIV` `CC`
         B58.83   **Toxoplasma tubulo-interstitial nephropathy**   `HIV` `CC`
            Toxoplasma pyelonephritis
         B58.89   **Toxoplasmosis with other organ involvement**   `HIV` `CC`

     B58.9   **Toxoplasmosis,** unspecified   `HIV` `CC`
         CC Excl: PDX collection 227

B59   **Pneumocystosis**   `HIV` `MCC` `HCC`
     Pneumonia due to Pneumocystis carinii
     Pneumonia due to Pneumocystis jiroveci
     CC Excl: PDX collection 228

✓4ᵗʰ B60   **Other protozoal diseases, not elsewhere classified**
     EXCLUDES 1   *cryptosporidiosis (A07.2)*
            intestinal microsporidiosis (A07.8)
            isosporiasis (A07.3)

> CC Excl: For CC codes in category B60, unless otherwise noted: PDX collection 229

     B60.0   **Babesiosis**   `CC`
         Piroplasmosis
         CC Excl: PDX collection 218

     ✓5ᵗʰ B60.1   **Acanthamebiasis**
         B60.10   **Acanthamebiasis,** unspecified   `CC`
         B60.11   **Meningoencephalitis due to Acanthamoeba (culbertsoni)**
         B60.12   **Conjunctivitis due to Acanthamoeba**
         B60.13   **Keratoconjunctivitis due to Acanthamoeba**
         B60.19   **Other acanthamebic disease**   `CC`

     B60.2   **Naegleriasis**
         Primary amebic meningoencephalitis

     B60.8   **Other specified protozoal diseases**   `HIV`
         Microsporidiosis

B64   **Unspecified protozoal disease**

Helminthiases (B65-B83)

✓4ᵗʰ B65   **Schistosomiasis [bilharziasis]**
     INCLUDES   snail fever

> CC Excl: For CC codes in category B65: PDX collection 230

     B65.0   **Schistosomiasis due to Schistosoma haematobium [urinary schistosomiasis]**   `CC`

     B65.1   **Schistosomiasis due to Schistosoma mansoni [intestinal schistosomiasis]**   `CC`

     B65.2   **Schistosomiasis due to Schistosoma japonicum**   `CC`
         Asiatic schistosomiasis

     B65.3   **Cercarial dermatitis**   `CC`
         Swimmer's itch

     B65.8   **Other schistosomiasis**   `CC`
         Infection due to Schistosoma intercalatum
         Infection due to Schistosoma mattheei
         Infection due to Schistosoma mekongi

     B65.9   **Schistosomiasis,** unspecified   `CC`

✓ Additional Character Required   ✓x7ᵗʰ Placeholder   Unacceptable PDx   Questionable PDx   Manifestation   `H1`-`H14` HAC   `HCC` CMS-HCC Dx   `HIV` HIV Dx

ICD-10-CM 2019   455

✓4th **B66 Other fluke infections**

> **CC Excl: For CC codes in category B66:** PDX collection 231

B66.0 Opisthorchiasis   CC
Infection due to cat liver fluke
Infection due to Opisthorchis (felineus)(viverrini)

B66.1 Clonorchiasis   CC
Chinese liver fluke disease
Infection due to Clonorchis sinensis
Oriental liver fluke disease

B66.2 Dicroceliasis   CC
Infection due to Dicrocoelium dendriticum
Lancet fluke infection

B66.3 Fascioliasis   CC
Infection due to Fasciola gigantica
Infection due to Fasciola hepatica
Infection due to Fasciola indica
Sheep liver fluke disease

B66.4 Paragonimiasis   CC HCC
Infection due to Paragonimus species
Lung fluke disease
Pulmonary distomiasis

B66.5 Fasciolopsiasis   CC
Infection due to Fasciolopsis buski
Intestinal distomiasis

B66.8 Other specified fluke infections   CC
Echinostomiasis
Heterophyiasis
Metagonimiasis
Nanophyetiasis
Watsoniasis

B66.9 Fluke infection, unspecified

✓4th **B67 Echinococcosis**
> **INCLUDES** hydatidosis

B67.0 Echinococcus granulosus infection of liver   CC
CC Excl: PDX collection 232

B67.1 Echinococcus granulosus infection of lung   CC HCC
CC Excl: PDX collection 233

B67.2 Echinococcus granulosus infection of bone   CC
CC Excl: PDX collection 234

✓5th **B67.3 Echinococcus granulosus infection, other and multiple sites**

B67.31 Echinococcus granulosus infection, thyroid gland CC
CC Excl: PDX collection 235

B67.32 Echinococcus granulosus infection, multiple sites CC
CC Excl: PDX collection 234

B67.39 Echinococcus granulosus infection, other sites   CC
CC Excl: PDX collection 234

B67.4 Echinococcus granulosus infection, unspecified   CC
Dog tapeworm (infection)
CC Excl: PDX collection 236

B67.5 Echinococcus multilocularis infection of liver   CC
CC Excl: PDX collection 237

✓5th **B67.6 Echinococcus multilocularis infection, other and multiple sites**

B67.61 Echinococcus multilocularis infection, multiple sites CC
CC Excl: PDX collection 238

B67.69 Echinococcus multilocularis infection, other sites CC
CC Excl: PDX collection 238

B67.7 Echinococcus multilocularis infection, unspecified   CC
CC Excl: PDX collection 239

B67.8 Echinococcosis, unspecified, of liver   CC
CC Excl: PDX collection 240

✓5th **B67.9 Echinococcosis, other and unspecified**

B67.90 Echinococcosis, unspecified   CC
Echinococcosis NOS
CC Excl: PDX collection 240

B67.99 Other echinococcosis   CC
CC Excl: PDX collection 240

✓4th **B68 Taeniasis**
> **EXCLUDES 1** cysticercosis (B69.-)

B68.0 Taenia solium taeniasis   CC
Pork tapeworm (infection)
CC Excl: PDX collection 241

B68.1 Taenia saginata taeniasis   CC
Beef tapeworm (infection)
Infection due to adult tapeworm Taenia saginata
CC Excl: PDX collection 242

B68.9 Taeniasis, unspecified   CC
CC Excl: PDX collection 242

✓4th **B69 Cysticercosis**
> **INCLUDES** cysticerciasis infection due to larval form of Taenia solium

DEF: Condition that is developed when larvae or eggs of the tapeworm *Taenia solium* are ingested, most commonly in fecally contaminated water or undercooked pork.

> **CC Excl: For CC codes in category B69:** PDX collection 242

B69.0 Cysticercosis of central nervous system   CC

B69.1 Cysticercosis of eye   CC

✓5th **B69.8 Cysticercosis of other sites**

B69.81 Myositis in cysticercosis   CC

B69.89 Cysticercosis of other sites   CC

B69.9 Cysticercosis, unspecified   CC

✓4th **B70 Diphyllobothriasis and sparganosis**

B70.0 Diphyllobothriasis   CC
Diphyllobothrium (adult) (latum) (pacificum) infection
Fish tapeworm (infection)
> **EXCLUDES 2** larval diphyllobothriasis (B70.1)
CC Excl: PDX collection 242

B70.1 Sparganosis   CC
Infection due to Sparganum (mansoni) (proliferum)
Infection due to Spirometra larva
Larval diphyllobothriasis
Spirometrosis
CC Excl: PDX collection 242

✓4th **B71 Other cestode infections**

> **CC Excl: For CC codes in category B71:** PDX collection 242

B71.0 Hymenolepiasis   CC
Dwarf tapeworm infection
Rat tapeworm (infection)

B71.1 Dipylidiasis   CC

B71.8 Other specified cestode infections   CC
Coenurosis

B71.9 Cestode infection, unspecified
Tapeworm (infection) NOS

B72 Dracunculiasis   CC
> **INCLUDES** guinea worm infection
infection due to Dracunculus medinensis
CC Excl: PDX collection 243

✓4th **B73 Onchocerciasis**
> **INCLUDES** onchocerca volvulus infection
onchocercosis
river blindness

> **CC Excl: For CC codes in category B73:** PDX collection 243

✓5th **B73.0 Onchocerciasis with eye disease**

B73.00 Onchocerciasis with eye involvement, unspecified CC

B73.01 Onchocerciasis with endophthalmitis   CC

B73.02 Onchocerciasis with glaucoma   CC

B73.09 Onchocerciasis with other eye involvement   CC
Infestation of eyelid due to onchocerciasis

B73.1 Onchocerciasis without eye disease   CC

✓4th **B74 Filariasis**
> **EXCLUDES 2** onchocerciasis (B73)
tropical (pulmonary) eosinophilia NOS (J82)

> **CC Excl: For CC codes in category B74:** PDX collection 243

B74.0 Filariasis due to Wuchereria bancrofti   CC
Bancroftian elephantiasis
Bancroftian filariasis

B74.1 Filariasis due to Brugia malayi   CC

B74.2 Filariasis due to Brugia timori   CC

B74.3 Loiasis   CC
Calabar swelling
Eyeworm disease of Africa
Loa loa infection

B74.4 Mansonelliasis `CC`
Infection due to Mansonella ozzardi
Infection due to Mansonella perstans
Infection due to Mansonella streptocerca

B74.8 Other filariases `CC`
Dirofilariasis

B74.9 Filariasis, unspecified `CC`

B75 Trichinellosis `CC`
INCLUDES infection due to Trichinella species
trichiniasis
DEF: Infection by *Trichinella spiralis,* the smallest of the parasitic nematodes, that is transmitted by eating undercooked pork or bear meat. *Synonym(s):Trichinosis.*
CC Excl: PDX collection 244

✓4ᵗʰ B76 Hookworm diseases
INCLUDES uncinariasis

    CC Excl: For CC codes in category B76: PDX collection 245

B76.0 Ancylostomiasis `CC`
Infection due to Ancylostoma species

B76.1 Necatoriasis `CC`
Infection due to Necator americanus

B76.8 Other hookworm diseases `CC`

B76.9 Hookworm disease, unspecified `CC`
Cutaneous larva migrans NOS

✓4ᵗʰ B77 Ascariasis
INCLUDES ascaridiasis
roundworm infection

    CC Excl: For CC /MCC codes in category B77, unless otherwise noted: PDX collection 246

B77.0 Ascariasis with intestinal complications `CC`

✓5ᵗʰ B77.8 Ascariasis with other complications
  B77.81 Ascariasis pneumonia `MCC`
    CC Excl: PDX collection 247
  B77.89 Ascariasis with other complications `CC`

B77.9 Ascariasis, unspecified `CC`

✓4ᵗʰ B78 Strongyloidiasis
EXCLUDES 1 trichostrongyliasis (B81.2)

    CC Excl: For CC codes in category B78: PDX collection 246

B78.0 Intestinal strongyloidiasis `HIV` `CC`
B78.1 Cutaneous strongyloidiasis
B78.7 Disseminated strongyloidiasis `HIV` `CC`
B78.9 Strongyloidiasis, unspecified `HIV` `CC`

B79 Trichuriasis `CC`
INCLUDES trichocephaliasis
whipworm (disease)(infection)
CC Excl: PDX collection 246

B80 Enterobiasis `CC`
INCLUDES oxyuriasis
pinworm infection
threadworm infection
CC Excl: PDX collection 246

✓4ᵗʰ B81 Other intestinal helminthiases, not elsewhere classified
EXCLUDES 1 angiostrongyliasis due to:
angiostrongylus cantonensis (B83.2)
parastrongylus cantonensis (B83.2)

B81.0 Anisakiasis `CC`
Infection due to Anisakis larva
CC Excl: PDX collection 246

B81.1 Intestinal capillariasis `CC`
Capillariasis NOS
Infection due to Capillaria philippinensis
EXCLUDES 2 hepatic capillariasis (B83.8)
CC Excl: PDX collection 246

B81.2 Trichostrongyliasis `CC`
CC Excl: PDX collection 246

B81.3 Intestinal angiostrongyliasis `CC`
Angiostrongyliasis due to:
angiostrongylus costaricensis
parastrongylus costaricensis
CC Excl: PDX collection 248

B81.4 Mixed intestinal helminthiases
Infection due to intestinal helminths classified to more than one of the categories B65.0-B81.3 and B81.8
Mixed helminthiasis NOS
CC Excl: PDX collection 248

B81.8 Other specified intestinal helminthiases `CC`
Infection due to Oesophagostomum species [esophagostomiasis]
Infection due to Ternidens diminutus [ternidensiasis]
CC Excl: PDX collection 248

✓4ᵗʰ B82 Unspecified intestinal parasitism

B82.0 Intestinal helminthiasis, unspecified `CC`
CC Excl: PDX collection 248

B82.9 Intestinal parasitism, unspecified

✓4ᵗʰ B83 Other helminthiases
EXCLUDES 1 capillariasis NOS (B81.1)
EXCLUDES 2 intestinal capillariasis (B81.1)

B83.0 Visceral larva migrans
Toxocariasis

B83.1 Gnathostomiasis
Wandering swelling

B83.2 Angiostrongyliasis due to Parastrongylus cantonensis
Eosinophilic meningoencephalitis due to Parastrongylus cantonensis
EXCLUDES 2 intestinal angiostrongyliasis (B81.3)

B83.3 Syngamiasis
Syngamosis

B83.4 Internal hirudiniasis
EXCLUDES 2 external hirudiniasis (B88.3)

B83.8 Other specified helminthiases
Acanthocephaliasis   Metastrongyliasis
Gongylonemiasis   Thelaziasis
Hepatic capillariasis

B83.9 Helminthiasis, unspecified
Worms NOS
EXCLUDES 1 intestinal helminthiasis NOS (B82.0)

Pediculosis, acariasis and other infestations (B85-B89)

✓4ᵗʰ B85 Pediculosis and phthiriasis

B85.0 Pediculosis due to Pediculus humanus capitis
Head-louse infestation

B85.1 Pediculosis due to Pediculus humanus corporis
Body-louse infestation

B85.2 Pediculosis, unspecified

B85.3 Phthiriasis
Infestation by crab-louse
Infestation by Phthirus pubis

B85.4 Mixed pediculosis and phthiriasis
Infestation classifiable to more than one of the categories B85.0-B85.3

B86 Scabies
Sarcoptic itch
DEF: Mite infestation that is caused by *Sarcoptes scabiei.* Scabies causes intense itching and sometimes secondary infection.

✓4ᵗʰ B87 Myiasis
INCLUDES infestation by larva of flies

B87.0 Cutaneous myiasis
Creeping myiasis

B87.1 Wound myiasis
Traumatic myiasis

B87.2 Ocular myiasis

B87.3 Nasopharyngeal myiasis
Laryngeal myiasis

B87.4 Aural myiasis

✓5ᵗʰ B87.8 Myiasis of other sites
  B87.81 Genitourinary myiasis
  B87.82 Intestinal myiasis
  B87.89 Myiasis of other sites

B87.9 Myiasis, unspecified

✓ Additional Character Required   ✓x7ᵗʰ Placeholder   Unacceptable PDx   Questionable PDx   Manifestation   **H1**-**H14** HAC   **HCC** CMS-HCC Dx   **HIV** HIV Dx

ICD-10-CM 2019   457

☑4ᵗʰ **B88 Other infestations**

    B88.0 Other acariasis
        Acarine dermatitis
        Dermatitis due to Demodex species
        Dermatitis due to Dermanyssus gallinae
        Dermatitis due to Liponyssoides sanguineus
        Trombiculosis
        EXCLUDES 2   scabies (B86)

    B88.1 Tungiasis [sandflea infestation]

    B88.2 Other arthropod infestations
        Scarabiasis

    B88.3 External hirudiniasis
        Leech infestation NOS
        EXCLUDES 2   internal hirudiniasis (B83.4)

    B88.8 Other specified infestations
        Ichthyoparasitism due to Vandellia cirrhosa
        Linguatulosis
        Porocephaliasis

    B88.9 Infestation, unspecified
        Infestation (skin) NOS   Skin parasites NOS
        Infestation by mites NOS

B89 Unspecified parasitic disease

Sequelae of infectious and parasitic diseases (B90-B94)

    NOTE   Categories B90-B94 are to be used to indicate conditions in categories A00-B89 as the cause of sequelae, which are themselves classified elsewhere. The "sequelae" include conditions specified as such; they also include residuals of diseases classifiable to the above categories if there is evidence that the disease itself is no longer present. Codes from these categories are not to be used for chronic infections. Code chronic current infections to active infectious disease as appropriate.

    Code first condition resulting from (sequela) the infectious or parasitic disease

☑4ᵗʰ **B90 Sequelae of tuberculosis**

    B90.0 Sequelae of central nervous system tuberculosis

    B90.1 Sequelae of genitourinary tuberculosis

    B90.2 Sequelae of tuberculosis of bones and joints

    B90.8 Sequelae of tuberculosis of other organs
        EXCLUDES 2   sequelae of respiratory tuberculosis (B90.9)

    B90.9 Sequelae of respiratory and unspecified tuberculosis
        Sequelae of tuberculosis NOS

B91 Sequelae of poliomyelitis
    EXCLUDES 1   postpolio syndrome (G14)

B92 Sequelae of leprosy

☑4ᵗʰ **B94 Sequelae of other and unspecified infectious and parasitic diseases**

    B94.0 Sequelae of trachoma

    B94.1 Sequelae of viral encephalitis

    B94.2 Sequelae of viral hepatitis

    B94.8 Sequelae of other specified infectious and parasitic diseases
        AHA: 2017, 4Q, 109

    B94.9 Sequelae of unspecified infectious and parasitic disease

Bacterial and viral infectious agents (B95-B97)

    NOTE   These categories are provided for use as supplementary or additional codes to identify the infectious agent(s) in diseases classified elsewhere.

    AHA: 2018, 1Q, 16

☑4ᵗʰ **B95 Streptococcus, Staphylococcus, and Enterococcus as the cause of diseases classified elsewhere**

    B95.0 Streptococcus, group A, as the cause of diseases classified elsewhere

    B95.1 Streptococcus, group B, as the cause of diseases classified elsewhere

    B95.2 Enterococcus as the cause of diseases classified elsewhere

    B95.3 Streptococcus pneumoniae as the cause of diseases classified elsewhere

    B95.4 Other streptococcus as the cause of diseases classified elsewhere

    B95.5 Unspecified streptococcus as the cause of diseases classified elsewhere

☑5ᵗʰ **B95.6 Staphylococcus aureus as the cause of diseases classified elsewhere**

    B95.61 Methicillin susceptible Staphylococcus aureus infection as the cause of diseases classified elsewhere
        Methicillin susceptible Staphylococcus aureus (MSSA) infection as the cause of diseases classified elsewhere
        Staphylococcus aureus infection NOS as the cause of diseases classified elsewhere

    B95.62 Methicillin resistant Staphylococcus aureus infection as the cause of diseases classified elsewhere
        Methicillin resistant Staphylococcus aureus (MRSA) infection as the cause of diseases classified elsewhere
        AHA: 2016, 1Q, 12

    B95.7 Other staphylococcus as the cause of diseases classified elsewhere

    B95.8 Unspecified staphylococcus as the cause of diseases classified elsewhere

☑4ᵗʰ **B96 Other bacterial agents as the cause of diseases classified elsewhere**

    B96.0 Mycoplasma pneumoniae [M. pneumoniae] as the cause of diseases classified elsewhere
        Pleuro-pneumonia-like-organism [PPLO]

    B96.1 Klebsiella pneumoniae [K. pneumoniae] as the cause of diseases classified elsewhere

☑5ᵗʰ **B96.2 Escherichia coli [E. coli] as the cause of diseases classified elsewhere**

    B96.20 Unspecified Escherichia coli [E. coli] as the cause of diseases classified elsewhere
        Escherichia coli [E. coli] NOS

    B96.21 Shiga toxin-producing Escherichia coli [E. coli] (STEC) O157 as the cause of diseases classified elsewhere
        E. coli O157:H- (nonmotile) with confirmation of Shiga toxin
        E. coli O157 with confirmation of Shiga toxin when H antigen is unknown, or is not H7
        O157:H7 Escherichia coli [E.coli] with or without confirmation of Shiga toxin-production
        Shiga toxin-producing Escherichia coli [E.coli] O157:H7 with or without confirmation of Shiga toxin-production
        STEC O157:H7 with or without confirmation of Shiga toxin-production

    B96.22 Other specified Shiga toxin-producing Escherichia coli [E. coli] (STEC) as the cause of diseases classified elsewhere
        Non-O157 Shiga toxin-producing Escherichia coli [E.coli]
        Non-O157 Shiga toxin-producing Escherichia coli [E.coli] with known O group

    B96.23 Unspecified Shiga toxin-producing Escherichia coli [E. coli] (STEC) as the cause of diseases classified elsewhere
        Shiga toxin-producing Escherichia coli [E. coli] with unspecified O group
        STEC NOS

    B96.29 Other Escherichia coli [E. coli] as the cause of diseases classified elsewhere
        Non-Shiga toxin-producing E. coli

    B96.3 Hemophilus influenzae [H. influenzae] as the cause of diseases classified elsewhere

    B96.4 Proteus (mirabilis) (morganii) as the cause of diseases classified elsewhere

    B96.5 Pseudomonas (aeruginosa) (mallei) (pseudomallei) as the cause of diseases classified elsewhere
        AHA: 2015, 1Q, 18

    B96.6 Bacteroides fragilis [B. fragilis] as the cause of diseases classified elsewhere

    B96.7 Clostridium perfringens [C. perfringens] as the cause of diseases classified elsewhere

☑5ᵗʰ **B96.8 Other specified bacterial agents as the cause of diseases classified elsewhere**

    B96.81 Helicobacter pylori [H. pylori] as the cause of diseases classified elsewhere

    B96.82 Vibrio vulnificus as the cause of diseases classified elsewhere

N Newborn: 0   **P** Pediatric: 0-17   **M** Maternity: 12-55   **A** Adult: 15-124   **MCC** Major Complication/Comorbidity   **CC** Complication/Comorbidity   **SW** Severe Wound Dx

458   ICD-10-CM 2019

B88–B96.82

    B96.89   Other specified bacterial agents as the cause of diseases classified elsewhere

✓4ᵗʰ **B97 Viral agents as the cause of diseases classified elsewhere**
    AHA: 2016, 3Q, 8-10, 14

    B97.0   Adenovirus as the cause of diseases classified elsewhere

✓5ᵗʰ   B97.1   Enterovirus as the cause of diseases classified elsewhere

    B97.10   Unspecified enterovirus as the cause of diseases classified elsewhere

    B97.11   Coxsackievirus as the cause of diseases classified elsewhere

    B97.12   Echovirus as the cause of diseases classified elsewhere

    B97.19   Other enterovirus as the cause of diseases classified elsewhere

✓5ᵗʰ   B97.2   Coronavirus as the cause of diseases classified elsewhere

    B97.21   SARS-associated coronavirus as the cause of diseases classified elsewhere   **CC**

         EXCLUDES 1   pneumonia due to SARS-associated coronavirus (J12.81)

         CC Excl: PDX collection 249

    B97.29   Other coronavirus as the cause of diseases classified elsewhere

✓5ᵗʰ   B97.3   Retrovirus as the cause of diseases classified elsewhere

         EXCLUDES 1   human immunodeficiency virus [HIV] disease (B20)

    B97.30   Unspecified retrovirus as the cause of diseases classified elsewhere

    B97.31   Lentivirus as the cause of diseases classified elsewhere

    B97.32   Oncovirus as the cause of diseases classified elsewhere

    B97.33   Human T-cell lymphotrophic virus, type I [HTLV-I] as the cause of diseases classified elsewhere   **CC**

         CC Excl: PDX collection 250

    B97.34   Human T-cell lymphotrophic virus, type II [HTLV-II] as the cause of diseases classified elsewhere   **CC**

         CC Excl: PDX collection 251

    B97.35   Human immunodeficiency virus, type 2 [HIV 2] as the cause of diseases classified elsewhere   **CC** **HCC**

         CC Excl: PDX collection 252

    B97.39   Other retrovirus as the cause of diseases classified elsewhere

    B97.4   Respiratory syncytial virus as the cause of diseases classified elsewhere

    B97.5   Reovirus as the cause of diseases classified elsewhere

    B97.6   Parvovirus as the cause of diseases classified elsewhere

    B97.7   Papillomavirus as the cause of diseases classified elsewhere

✓5ᵗʰ   B97.8   Other viral agents as the cause of diseases classified elsewhere

    B97.81   Human metapneumovirus as the cause of diseases classified elsewhere

    B97.89   Other viral agents as the cause of diseases classified elsewhere

Other infectious diseases (B99)

✓4ᵗʰ **B99 Other and unspecified infectious diseases**

    B99.8   Other infectious disease   **HIV**

    B99.9   Unspecified infectious disease

☑ Additional Character Required   ✓x7ᵗʰ Placeholder   Unacceptable PDx   Questionable PDx   Manifestation   **H1 - H14** HAC   **HCC** CMS-HCC Dx   **HIV** HIV Dx

ICD-10-CM 2019   459

Chapter 2. Neoplasms (C00–D49)

Chapter Specific Guidelines with Coding Examples

The chapter specific guidelines from the ICD-10-CM Official Guidelines for Coding and Reporting have been provided below. Along with these guidelines are coding examples, contained in the shaded boxes, that have been developed to help illustrate the coding and/or sequencing guidance found in these guidelines.

General guidelines

Chapter 2 of the ICD-10-CM contains the codes for most benign and all malignant neoplasms. Certain benign neoplasms, such as prostatic adenomas, may be found in the specific body system chapters. To properly code a neoplasm it is necessary to determine from the record if the neoplasm is benign, in-situ, malignant, or of uncertain histologic behavior. If malignant, any secondary (metastatic) sites should also be determined.

Primary malignant neoplasms overlapping site boundaries

A primary malignant neoplasm that overlaps two or more contiguous (next to each other) sites should be classified to the subcategory/code .8 ('overlapping lesion'), unless the combination is specifically indexed elsewhere. For multiple neoplasms of the same site that are not contiguous such as tumors in different quadrants of the same breast, codes for each site should be assigned.

A 73-year-old white female with a large rapidly growing malignant tumor in the left breast extending from the upper outer quadrant into the axillary tail

C50.812   **Malignant neoplasm of overlapping sites of left female breast**

Explanation: Because this is a single large tumor that overlaps two contiguous sites, a single code for overlapping sites is assigned.

A 52-year old white female with two distinct lesions of the right breast, one (0.5 cm) in the upper outer quadrant and a second (1.5 cm) in the lower outer quadrant; path report indicates both lesions are malignant

C50.411   **Malignant neoplasm of upper-outer quadrant of right female breast**

C50.511   **Malignant neoplasm of lower-outer quadrant of right female breast**

Explanation: This patient has two distinct malignant lesions of right breast in adjacent quadrants. Because the lesions are not contiguous, two codes are reported.

Malignant neoplasm of ectopic tissue

Malignant neoplasms of ectopic tissue are to be coded to the site of origin mentioned, e.g., ectopic pancreatic malignant neoplasms involving the stomach are coded to malignant neoplasm of pancreas, unspecified (C25.9).

The neoplasm table in the Alphabetic Index should be referenced first. However, if the histological term is documented, that term should be referenced first, rather than going immediately to the Neoplasm Table, in order to determine which column in the Neoplasm Table is appropriate. For example, if the documentation indicates "adenoma," refer to the term in the Alphabetic Index to review the entries under this term and the instructional note to "see also neoplasm, by site, benign." The table provides the proper code based on the type of neoplasm and the site. It is important to select the proper column in the table that corresponds to the type of neoplasm. The Tabular List should then be referenced to verify that the correct code has been selected from the table and that a more specific site code does not exist.

See Section I.C.21. Factors influencing health status and contact with health services, Status, for information regarding Z15.0, codes for genetic susceptibility to cancer.

a. Treatment directed at the malignancy

If the treatment is directed at the malignancy, designate the malignancy as the principal diagnosis.

The only exception to this guideline is if a patient admission/encounter is solely for the administration of chemotherapy, immunotherapy or external beam radiation therapy, assign the appropriate Z51.-- code as the first-listed or principal diagnosis, and the diagnosis or problem for which the service is being performed as a secondary diagnosis.

b. Treatment of secondary site

When a patient is admitted because of a primary neoplasm with metastasis and treatment is directed toward the secondary site only, the secondary neoplasm is designated as the principal diagnosis even though the primary malignancy is still present.

Patient with primary prostate cancer with metastasis to lungs admitted for wedge resection of mass in right lung

C78.01   **Secondary malignant neoplasm of right lung**

C61   **Malignant neoplasm of prostate**

Explanation: Since the admission is for treatment of the lung metastasis, the secondary lung metastasis is sequenced before the primary prostate cancer.

---

c. Coding and sequencing of complications

Coding and sequencing of complications associated with the malignancies or with the therapy thereof are subject to the following guidelines:

1) Anemia associated with malignancy

When admission/encounter is for management of an anemia associated with the malignancy, and the treatment is only for anemia, the appropriate code for the malignancy is sequenced as the principal or first-listed diagnosis followed by the appropriate code for the anemia (such as code D63.0, Anemia in neoplastic disease).

Patient is admitted for treatment of anemia in advanced colon cancer

C18.9   **Malignant neoplasm of colon, unspecified**

D63.0   **Anemia in neoplastic disease**

Explanation: Even though the admission was solely to treat the anemia, this guideline indicates that the code for the malignancy is sequenced first.

---

2) Anemia associated with chemotherapy, immunotherapy and radiation therapy

When the admission/encounter is for management of an anemia associated with an adverse effect of the administration of chemotherapy or immunotherapy and the only treatment is for the anemia, the anemia code is sequenced first followed by the appropriate codes for the neoplasm and the adverse effect (T45.1X5, Adverse effect of antineoplastic and immunosuppressive drugs).

A 56-year-old Hispanic male with grade II follicular lymphoma involving multiple lymph node sites referred for blood transfusion to treat anemia due to chemotherapy

D64.81   **Anemia due to antineoplastic chemotherapy**

C82.18   **Follicular lymphoma grade II, lymph nodes of multiple sites**

T45.1X5A   **Adverse effect of antineoplastic and immunosuppressive drugs, initial encounter**

Explanation: The code for the anemia is sequenced first followed by the code for the malignant neoplasm and lastly the code for the adverse effect.

When the admission/encounter is for management of an anemia associated with an adverse effect of radiotherapy, the anemia code should be sequenced first, followed by the appropriate neoplasm code and code Y84.2, Radiological procedure and radiotherapy as the cause of abnormal reaction of the patient, or of later complication, without mention of misadventure at the time of the procedure.

A 55-year-old male with a large malignant rectal tumor has been receiving external radiation therapy to shrink the tumor prior to planned surgery. He is admitted today for a blood transfusion to treat anemia related to radiation therapy.

D64.89	Other specified anemias
C20	Malignant neoplasm of rectum
Y84.2	Radiological procedure and radiotherapy as the cause of abnormal reaction of the patient, or of later complication, without mention of misadventure at the time of the procedure

Explanation: The code for the anemia is sequenced first, followed by the code for the malignancy, and lastly the code for the abnormal reaction due to radiotherapy.

3) Management of dehydration due to the malignancy

When the admission/encounter is for management of dehydration due to the malignancy and only the dehydration is being treated (intravenous rehydration), the dehydration is sequenced first, followed by the code(s) for the malignancy.

4) Treatment of a complication resulting from a surgical procedure

When the admission/encounter is for treatment of a complication resulting from a surgical procedure, designate the complication as the principal or first-listed diagnosis if treatment is directed at resolving the complication.

d. Primary malignancy previously excised

When a primary malignancy has been previously excised or eradicated from its site and there is no further treatment directed to that site and there is no evidence of any existing primary malignancy **at that site**, a code from category Z85, Personal history of malignant neoplasm, should be used to indicate the former site of the malignancy. Any mention of extension, invasion, or metastasis to another site is coded as a secondary malignant neoplasm to that site. The secondary site may be the principal or first-listed with the Z85 code used as a secondary code.

History of breast cancer, left radical mastectomy 18 months ago with no current treatment; bronchoscopy with lung biopsy shows metastatic disease in the right lung

C78.01	Secondary malignant neoplasm of right lung
Z85.3	Personal history of malignant neoplasm of breast

Explanation: The patient has undergone a diagnostic procedure that revealed metastatic breast cancer in the right lung. The code for the secondary (metastatic) site is sequenced first followed by a personal history code to identify the former site of the primary malignancy.

e. Admissions/encounters involving chemotherapy, immunotherapy and radiation therapy

1) Episode of care involves surgical removal of neoplasm

When an episode of care involves the surgical removal of a neoplasm, primary or secondary site, followed by adjunct chemotherapy or radiation treatment during the same episode of care, the code for the neoplasm should be assigned as principal or first-listed diagnosis.

2) Patient admission/encounter solely for administration of chemotherapy, immunotherapy and radiation therapy

If a patient admission/encounter is solely for the administration of chemotherapy, immunotherapy or external beam radiation therapy assign code Z51.0, Encounter for antineoplastic radiation therapy, or Z51.11, Encounter for antineoplastic chemotherapy, or Z51.12, Encounter for antineoplastic immunotherapy as the first-listed or principal diagnosis. If a patient receives more than one of these therapies during the same admission more than one of these codes may be assigned, in any sequence.

The malignancy for which the therapy is being administered should be assigned as a secondary diagnosis.

If a patient admission/encounter is for the insertion or implantation of radioactive elements (e.g., brachytherapy) the appropriate code for the malignancy is sequenced as the principal or first-listed diagnosis. Code Z51.0 should not be assigned.

3) Patient admitted for radiation therapy, chemotherapy or immunotherapy and develops complications

When a patient is admitted for the purpose of external beam radiotherapy, immunotherapy or chemotherapy and develops complications such as uncontrolled nausea and vomiting or dehydration, the principal or first-listed diagnosis is Z51.0, Encounter for antineoplastic radiation therapy, or Z51.11, Encounter for antineoplastic chemotherapy, or Z51.12, Encounter for antineoplastic immunotherapy followed by any codes for the complications.

When a patient is admitted for the purpose of insertion or implantation of radioactive elements (e.g., brachytherapy) and develops complications such as uncontrolled nausea and vomiting or dehydration, the principal or first-listed diagnosis is the appropriate code for the malignancy followed by any codes for the complications.

A patient with prostate cancer was admitted for brachytherapy seed implantation and consequently developed urinary retention.

C61	Malignant neoplasm of prostate
R33.9	Retention of urine, unspecified

Explanation: A code for the malignancy should be listed as the principal diagnosis when insertion of a radioactive element is the reason for admission, even when a complication related to that radioactive element occurs. Codes describing the complications should be listed as secondary codes.

f. Admission/encounter to determine extent of malignancy

When the reason for admission/encounter is to determine the extent of the malignancy, or for a procedure such as paracentesis or thoracentesis, the primary malignancy or appropriate metastatic site is designated as the principal or first-listed diagnosis, even though chemotherapy or radiotherapy is administered.

Patient with left lung cancer with malignant pleural effusion admitted for paracentesis and initiation/administration of chemotherapy

C34.92	Malignant neoplasm of unspecified part of left bronchus or lung
J91.0	Malignant pleural effusion
Z51.11	Encounter for antineoplastic chemotherapy

Explanation: The lung cancer is sequenced before the chemotherapy in this instance because the paracentesis for the malignant effusion is also being performed. An instructional note under the malignant effusion instructs that the lung cancer be sequenced first.

g. Symptoms, signs, and abnormal findings listed in Chapter 18 associated with neoplasms

Symptoms, signs, and ill-defined conditions listed in Chapter 18 characteristic of, or associated with, an existing primary or secondary site malignancy cannot be used to replace the malignancy as principal or first-listed diagnosis, regardless of the number of admissions or encounters for treatment and care of the neoplasm.

See Section I.C.21. Factors influencing health status and contact with health services, Encounter for prophylactic organ removal.

h. Admission/encounter for pain control/management

See Section I.C.6. for information on coding admission/encounter for pain control/management.

i. Malignancy in two or more noncontiguous sites

A patient may have more than one malignant tumor in the same organ. These tumors may represent different primaries or metastatic disease, depending on the site. Should the documentation be unclear, the provider should be queried as to the status of each tumor so that the correct codes can be assigned.

j. Disseminated malignant neoplasm, unspecified

Code C80.0, Disseminated malignant neoplasm, unspecified, is for use only in those cases where the patient has advanced metastatic disease and no known primary or secondary sites are specified. It should not be used in place of assigning codes for the primary site and all known secondary sites.

Patient who has had no medical care for many years is seen today and diagnosed with carcinomatosis

C80.0	Disseminated malignant neoplasm, unspecified

Explanation: Carcinomatosis NOS is an "includes" note under this code. Should seldom be used but is available for use in cases such as this.

Chapter 2. Neoplasms

k. Malignant neoplasm without specification of site

Code C80.1, Malignant (primary) neoplasm, unspecified, equates to Cancer, unspecified. This code should only be used when no determination can be made as to the primary site of a malignancy. This code should rarely be used in the inpatient setting.

> Evaluation of painful hip leads to diagnosis of a metastatic bone lesion from an unknown primary neoplasm source
>
> **C79.51**   **Secondary malignant neoplasm of bone**
>
> **C80.1**   **Malignant (primary) neoplasm, unspecified**
>
> *Explanation*: If only the secondary site is known, use code C80.1 for the unknown primary site.

l. Sequencing of neoplasm codes

1) Encounter for treatment of primary malignancy

If the reason for the encounter is for treatment of a primary malignancy, assign the malignancy as the principal/first-listed diagnosis. The primary site is to be sequenced first, followed by any metastatic sites.

2) Encounter for treatment of secondary malignancy

When an encounter is for a primary malignancy with metastasis and treatment is directed toward the metastatic (secondary) site(s) only, the metastatic site(s) is designated as the principal/first-listed diagnosis. The primary malignancy is coded as an additional code.

> Patient has primary colon cancer with metastasis to rib and is evaluated for possible excision of portion of rib bone
>
> **C79.51**   **Secondary malignant neoplasm of bone**
>
> **C18.9**   **Malignant neoplasm of colon, unspecified**
>
> *Explanation*: The treatment for this encounter is focused on the metastasis to the rib bone rather than the primary colon cancer, thus indicating that the bone metastasis is sequenced as the first-listed code.

3) Malignant neoplasm in a pregnant patient

When a pregnant woman has a malignant neoplasm, a code from subcategory O9A.1-, Malignant neoplasm complicating pregnancy, childbirth, and the puerperium, should be sequenced first, followed by the appropriate code from Chapter 2 to indicate the type of neoplasm.

> A 30-year-old pregnant female in second trimester evaluated for thyroid malignancy
>
> **O9A.112**   **Malignant neoplasm complicating pregnancy, second trimester**
>
> **C73**   **Malignant neoplasm of thyroid gland**
>
> *Explanation*: Codes from chapter 15 describing complications of pregnancy are sequenced as first-listed codes, further specified by codes from other chapters such as neoplastic, unless the pregnancy is documented as incidental to the condition. See also guideline 1.C.15.a.1.

4) Encounter for complication associated with a neoplasm

When an encounter is for management of a complication associated with a neoplasm, such as dehydration, and the treatment is only for the complication, the complication is coded first, followed by the appropriate code(s) for the neoplasm.

The exception to this guideline is anemia. When the admission/encounter is for management of an anemia associated with the malignancy, and the treatment is only for anemia, the appropriate code for the malignancy is sequenced as the principal or first-listed diagnosis followed by code D63.0, Anemia in neoplastic disease.

> Patient with pancreatic cancer is seen for initiation of TPN for cancer-related moderate protein-calorie malnutrition
>
> **E44.0**   **Moderate protein-calorie malnutrition**
>
> **C25.9**   **Malignant neoplasm of pancreas, unspecified**
>
> *Explanation*: The encounter is to initiate treatment for malnutrition, a common complication of many types of neoplasms, and is sequenced first.

5) Complication from surgical procedure for treatment of a neoplasm

When an encounter is for treatment of a complication resulting from a surgical procedure performed for the treatment of the neoplasm, designate the complication as the principal/first-listed diagnosis. See guideline regarding the coding of a current malignancy versus personal history to determine if the code for the neoplasm should also be assigned.

6) Pathologic fracture due to a neoplasm

When an encounter is for a pathological fracture due to a neoplasm, and the focus of treatment is the fracture, a code from subcategory M84.5, Pathological fracture in neoplastic disease, should be sequenced first, followed by the code for the neoplasm.

If the focus of treatment is the neoplasm with an associated pathological fracture, the neoplasm code should be sequenced first, followed by a code from M84.5 for the pathological fracture.

m. Current malignancy versus personal history of malignancy

When a primary malignancy has been excised but further treatment, such as an additional surgery for the malignancy, radiation therapy or chemotherapy is directed to that site, the primary malignancy code should be used until treatment is completed.

When a primary malignancy has been previously excised or eradicated from its site, there is no further treatment (of the malignancy) directed to that site, and there is no evidence of any existing primary malignancy **at that site**, a code from category Z85, Personal history of malignant neoplasm, should be used to indicate the former site of the malignancy.

Subcategories Z85.0 – Z85.7 should only be assigned for the former site of a primary malignancy, not the site of a secondary malignancy. Codes from subcategory Z85.8-, may be assigned for the former site(s) of either a primary or secondary malignancy included in this subcategory.

See Section I.C.21. Factors influencing health status and contact with health services, History (of)

> Female patient with ongoing chemotherapy after right mastectomy for breast cancer
>
> **C50.911**   **Malignant neoplasm of unspecified site of right female breast**
>
> **Z90.11**   **Acquired absence of right breast and nipple**
>
> *Explanation*: Even though the breast has been removed, the breast cancer is still being treated with chemotherapy and therefore is still coded as a current condition rather than personal history.

n. Leukemia, multiple myeloma, and malignant plasma cell neoplasms in remission versus personal history

The categories for leukemia, and category C90, Multiple myeloma and malignant plasma cell neoplasms, have codes indicating whether or not the leukemia has achieved remission. There are also codes Z85.6, Personal history of leukemia, and Z85.79, Personal history of other malignant neoplasms of lymphoid, hematopoietic and related tissues. If the documentation is unclear as to whether the leukemia has achieved remission, the provider should be queried.

See Section I.C.21. Factors influencing health status and contact with health services, History (of)

o. Aftercare following surgery for neoplasm

See Section I.C.21. Factors influencing health status and contact with health services, Aftercare

p. Follow-up care for completed treatment of a malignancy

See Section I.C.21. Factors influencing health status and contact with health services, Follow-up

q. Prophylactic organ removal for prevention of malignancy

See Section I.C. 21, Factors influencing health status and contact with health services, Prophylactic organ removal

r. Malignant neoplasm associated with transplanted organ

A malignant neoplasm of a transplanted organ should be coded as a transplant complication. Assign first the appropriate code from category T86.-, Complications of transplanted organs and tissue, followed by code C80.2, Malignant neoplasm associated with transplanted organ. Use an additional code for the specific malignancy.

Chapter 2. Neoplasms *(sidebar)*

C00–C02.4 *(sidebar)*

Chapter 2. Neoplasms (C00-D49)

NOTE

Functional activity
All neoplasms are classified in this chapter, whether they are functionally active or not. An additional code from Chapter 4 may be used, to identify functional activity associated with any neoplasm.

Morphology [Histology]
Chapter 2 classifies neoplasms primarily by site (topography), with broad groupings for behavior, malignant, in situ, benign, etc. The Table of Neoplasms should be used to identify the correct topography code. In a few cases, such as for malignant melanoma and certain neuroendocrine tumors, the morphology (histologic type) is included in the category and codes.

Primary malignant neoplasms overlapping site boundaries
A primary malignant neoplasm that overlaps two or more contiguous (next to each other) sites should be classified to the subcategory/code 8 ("overlapping lesion"), unless the combination is specifically indexed elsewhere. For multiple neoplasms of the same site that are not contiguous, such as tumors in different quadrants of the same breast, codes for each site should be assigned.

Malignant neoplasm of ectopic tissue
Malignant neoplasms of ectopic tissue are to be coded to the site mentioned, e.g., ectopic pancreatic malignant neoplasms are coded to pancreas, unspecified (C25.9).

AHA: 2017, 4Q, 103; 2017, 1Q, 4, 5-6, 8

This chapter contains the following blocks:

C00-C14	Malignant neoplasms of lip, oral cavity and pharynx
C15-C26	Malignant neoplasms of digestive organs
C30-C39	Malignant neoplasms of respiratory and intrathoracic organs
C40-C41	Malignant neoplasms of bone and articular cartilage
C43-C44	Melanoma and other malignant neoplasms of skin
C45-C49	Malignant neoplasms of mesothelial and soft tissue
C50	Malignant neoplasms of breast
C51-C58	Malignant neoplasms of female genital organs
C60-C63	Malignant neoplasms of male genital organs
C64-C68	Malignant neoplasms of urinary tract
C69-C72	Malignant neoplasms of eye, brain and other parts of central nervous system
C73-C75	Malignant neoplasms of thyroid and other endocrine glands
C7A	Malignant neuroendocrine tumors
C7B	Secondary neuroendocrine tumors
C76-C80	Malignant neoplasms of ill-defined, other secondary and unspecified sites
C81-C96	Malignant neoplasms of lymphoid, hematopoietic and related tissue
D00-D09	In situ neoplasms
D10-D36	Benign neoplasms, except benign neuroendocrine tumors
D3A	Benign neuroendocrine tumors
D37-D48	Neoplasms of uncertain behavior, polycythemia vera and myelodysplastic syndromes
D49	Neoplasms of unspecified behavior

MALIGNANT NEOPLASMS (C00-C96)

Malignant neoplasms, stated or presumed to be primary (of specified sites), and certain specified histologies, except neuroendocrine, and of lymphoid, hematopoietic and related tissue (C00-C75)

Malignant neoplasms of lip, oral cavity and pharynx (C00-C14)

☑4ᵗʰ C00 Malignant neoplasm of lip

Use additional code to identify:
- alcohol abuse and dependence (F10.-)
- history of tobacco dependence (Z87.891)
- tobacco dependence (F17.-)
- tobacco use (Z72.0)

EXCLUDES 1 malignant melanoma of lip (C43.0)
Merkel cell carcinoma of lip (C4A.0)
other and unspecified malignant neoplasm of skin of lip (C44.0-)

C00.0 Malignant neoplasm of external upper lip
Malignant neoplasm of lipstick area of upper lip
Malignant neoplasm of upper lip NOS
Malignant neoplasm of vermilion border of upper lip

C00.1 Malignant neoplasm of external lower lip
Malignant neoplasm of lower lip NOS
Malignant neoplasm of lipstick area of lower lip
Malignant neoplasm of vermilion border of lower lip

C00.2 Malignant neoplasm of external lip, unspecified
Malignant neoplasm of vermilion border of lip NOS

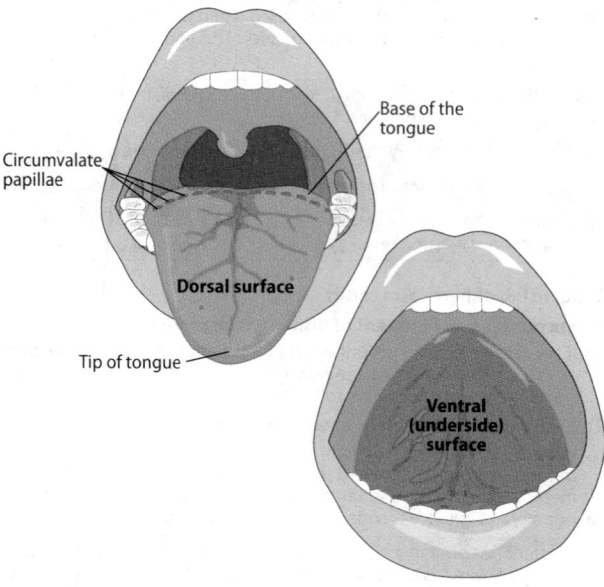

Malignant Neoplasm of Tongue

(Labels: Base of the tongue; Circumvalate papillae; Dorsal surface; Tip of tongue; Ventral (underside) surface)

C00.3 Malignant neoplasm of upper lip, inner aspect
Malignant neoplasm of buccal aspect of upper lip
Malignant neoplasm of frenulum of upper lip
Malignant neoplasm of mucosa of upper lip
Malignant neoplasm of oral aspect of upper lip

C00.4 Malignant neoplasm of lower lip, inner aspect
Malignant neoplasm of buccal aspect of lower lip
Malignant neoplasm of frenulum of lower lip
Malignant neoplasm of mucosa of lower lip
Malignant neoplasm of oral aspect of lower lip

C00.5 Malignant neoplasm of lip, unspecified, inner aspect
Malignant neoplasm of buccal aspect of lip, unspecified
Malignant neoplasm of frenulum of lip, unspecified
Malignant neoplasm of mucosa of lip, unspecified
Malignant neoplasm of oral aspect of lip, unspecified

C00.6 Malignant neoplasm of commissure of lip, unspecified

C00.8 Malignant neoplasm of overlapping sites of lip

C00.9 Malignant neoplasm of lip, unspecified

C01 Malignant neoplasm of base of tongue   HCC
Malignant neoplasm of dorsal surface of base of tongue
Malignant neoplasm of fixed part of tongue NOS
Malignant neoplasm of posterior third of tongue
Use additional code to identify:
- alcohol abuse and dependence (F10.-)
- history of tobacco dependence (Z87.891)
- tobacco dependence (F17.-)
- tobacco use (Z72.0)

☑4ᵗʰ C02 Malignant neoplasm of other and unspecified parts of tongue
Use additional code to identify:
- alcohol abuse and dependence (F10.-)
- history of tobacco dependence (Z87.891)
- tobacco dependence (F17.-)
- tobacco use (Z72.0)

C02.0 Malignant neoplasm of dorsal surface of tongue   HCC
Malignant neoplasm of anterior two-thirds of tongue, dorsal surface
EXCLUDES 2 malignant neoplasm of dorsal surface of base of tongue (C01)

C02.1 Malignant neoplasm of border of tongue   HCC
Malignant neoplasm of tip of tongue

C02.2 Malignant neoplasm of ventral surface of tongue   HCC
Malignant neoplasm of anterior two-thirds of tongue, ventral surface
Malignant neoplasm of frenulum linguae

C02.3 Malignant neoplasm of anterior two-thirds of tongue, part unspecified   HCC
Malignant neoplasm of middle third of tongue NOS
Malignant neoplasm of mobile part of tongue NOS

C02.4 Malignant neoplasm of lingual tonsil   HCC
EXCLUDES 2 malignant neoplasm of tonsil NOS (C09.9)

Ⓝ Newborn: 0   Ⓟ Pediatric: 0-17   Ⓜ Maternity: 12-55   Ⓐ Adult: 15-124   MCC Major Complication/Comorbidity   CC Complication/Comorbidity   SW Severe Wound Dx

464

ICD-10-CM 2019

C02.8 Malignant neoplasm of overlapping sites **of tongue** `HCC`
: Malignant neoplasm of two or more contiguous sites of tongue

C02.9 Malignant neoplasm of tongue, unspecified `HCC`

✓4ᵗʰ **C03 Malignant neoplasm of** gum
: `INCLUDES` malignant neoplasm of alveolar (ridge) mucosa
malignant neoplasm of gingiva

Use additional code to identify:
: alcohol abuse and dependence (F10.-)
history of tobacco dependence (Z87.891)
tobacco dependence (F17.-)
tobacco use (Z72.0)

`EXCLUDES 2` *malignant odontogenic neoplasms (C41.0-C41.1)*

C03.0 Malignant neoplasm of upper gum `HCC`

C03.1 Malignant neoplasm of lower gum `HCC`

C03.9 Malignant neoplasm of gum, unspecified `HCC`

✓4ᵗʰ **C04 Malignant neoplasm of** floor of mouth
: Use additional code to identify:
alcohol abuse and dependence (F10.-)
history of tobacco dependence (Z87.891)
tobacco dependence (F17.-)
tobacco use (Z72.0)

C04.0 Malignant neoplasm of anterior **floor of mouth** `HCC`
: Malignant neoplasm of anterior to the premolar-canine junction

C04.1 Malignant neoplasm of lateral **floor of mouth** `HCC`

C04.8 Malignant neoplasm of overlapping sites **of floor of mouth** `HCC`

C04.9 Malignant neoplasm of floor of mouth, unspecified `HCC`

✓4ᵗʰ **C05 Malignant neoplasm of** palate
: Use additional code to identify:
alcohol abuse and dependence (F10.-)
history of tobacco dependence (Z87.891)
tobacco dependence (F17.-)
tobacco use (Z72.0)

`EXCLUDES 1` *Kaposi's sarcoma of palate (C46.2)*

C05.0 Malignant neoplasm of hard **palate** `HCC`

C05.1 Malignant neoplasm of soft **palate** `HCC`
: `EXCLUDES 2` *malignant neoplasm of nasopharyngeal surface of soft palate (C11.3)*

C05.2 Malignant neoplasm of uvula `HCC`

C05.8 Malignant neoplasm of overlapping sites **of palate** `HCC`

C05.9 Malignant neoplasm of palate, unspecified `HCC`
: Malignant neoplasm of roof of mouth

✓4ᵗʰ **C06 Malignant neoplasm of** other and unspecified parts of mouth
: Use additional code to identify:
alcohol abuse and dependence (F10.-)
history of tobacco dependence (Z87.891)
tobacco dependence (F17.-)
tobacco use (Z72.0)

C06.0 Malignant neoplasm of cheek mucosa `HCC`
: Malignant neoplasm of buccal mucosa NOS
Malignant neoplasm of internal cheek

C06.1 Malignant neoplasm of vestibule **of mouth** `HCC`
: Malignant neoplasm of buccal sulcus (upper) (lower)
Malignant neoplasm of labial sulcus (upper) (lower)

C06.2 Malignant neoplasm of retromolar area `HCC`

✓5ᵗʰ **C06.8 Malignant neoplasm of** overlapping sites of other and unspecified **parts of mouth**

C06.80 Malignant neoplasm of overlapping sites of unspecified **parts of mouth** `HCC`

C06.89 Malignant neoplasm of overlapping sites of other **parts of mouth** `HCC`
: "book leaf" neoplasm [ventral surface of tongue and floor of mouth]

C06.9 Malignant neoplasm of mouth, unspecified `HCC`
: Malignant neoplasm of minor salivary gland, unspecified site
Malignant neoplasm of oral cavity NOS

C07 Malignant neoplasm of parotid gland `HCC`
: Use additional code to identify:
alcohol abuse and dependence (F10.-)
exposure to environmental tobacco smoke (Z77.22)
exposure to tobacco smoke in the perinatal period (P96.81)
history of tobacco dependence (Z87.891)
occupational exposure to environmental tobacco smoke (Z57.31)
tobacco dependence (F17.-)
tobacco use (Z72.0)

✓4ᵗʰ **C08 Malignant neoplasm of** other and unspecified major salivary glands
: `INCLUDES` malignant neoplasm of salivary ducts

Use additional code to identify:
: alcohol abuse and dependence (F10.-)
exposure to environmental tobacco smoke (Z77.22)
exposure to tobacco smoke in the perinatal period (P96.81)
history of tobacco dependence (Z87.891)
occupational exposure to environmental tobacco smoke (Z57.31)
tobacco dependence (F17.-)
tobacco use (Z72.0)

`EXCLUDES 1` *malignant neoplasms of specified minor salivary glands which are classified according to their anatomical location*

`EXCLUDES 2` *malignant neoplasms of minor salivary glands NOS (C06.9)*
malignant neoplasm of parotid gland (C07)

C08.0 Malignant neoplasm of submandibular **gland** `HCC`
: Malignant neoplasm of submaxillary gland

C08.1 Malignant neoplasm of sublingual **gland** `HCC`

C08.9 Malignant neoplasm of major salivary gland, **unspecified** `HCC`
: Malignant neoplasm of salivary gland (major) NOS

✓4ᵗʰ **C09 Malignant neoplasm of** tonsil
: Use additional code to identify:
alcohol abuse and dependence (F10.-)
exposure to environmental tobacco smoke (Z77.22)
exposure to tobacco smoke in the perinatal period (P96.81)
history of tobacco dependence (Z87.891)
occupational exposure to environmental tobacco smoke (Z57.31)
tobacco dependence (F17.-)
tobacco use (Z72.0)

`EXCLUDES 2` *malignant neoplasm of lingual tonsil (C02.4)*
malignant neoplasm of pharyngeal tonsil (C11.1)

C09.0 Malignant neoplasm of tonsillar fossa `HCC`

C09.1 Malignant neoplasm of tonsillar pillar **(anterior) (posterior)** `HCC`

C09.8 Malignant neoplasm of overlapping sites **of tonsil** `HCC`

C09.9 Malignant neoplasm of tonsil, unspecified `HCC`
: Malignant neoplasm of tonsil NOS
Malignant neoplasm of faucial tonsils
Malignant neoplasm of palatine tonsils

✓4ᵗʰ **C10 Malignant neoplasm of** oropharynx
: Use additional code to identify:
alcohol abuse and dependence (F10.-)
exposure to environmental tobacco smoke (Z77.22)
exposure to tobacco smoke in the perinatal period (P96.81)
history of tobacco dependence (Z87.891)
occupational exposure to environmental tobacco smoke (Z57.31)
tobacco dependence (F17.-)
tobacco use (Z72.0)

`EXCLUDES 2` *malignant neoplasm of tonsil (C09.-)*

C10.0 Malignant neoplasm of vallecula `HCC`

C10.1 Malignant neoplasm of anterior surface of epiglottis `HCC`
: Malignant neoplasm of epiglottis, free border [margin]
Malignant neoplasm of glossoepiglottic fold(s)
: `EXCLUDES 2` *malignant neoplasm of epiglottis (suprahyoid portion) NOS (C32.1)*

C10.2 Malignant neoplasm of lateral wall **of oropharynx** `HCC`

C10.3 Malignant neoplasm of posterior wall **of oropharynx** `HCC`

C10.4 Malignant neoplasm of branchial cleft `HCC`
: Malignant neoplasm of branchial cyst [site of neoplasm]

C10.8 Malignant neoplasm of overlapping sites **of oropharynx** `HCC`
: Malignant neoplasm of junctional region of oropharynx

C10.9 Malignant neoplasm of oropharynx, unspecified `HCC`

✓4ᵗʰ **C11 Malignant neoplasm of** nasopharynx
: Use additional code to identify:
exposure to environmental tobacco smoke (Z77.22)
exposure to tobacco smoke in the perinatal period (P96.81)
history of tobacco dependence (Z87.891)
occupational exposure to environmental tobacco smoke (Z57.31)
tobacco dependence (F17.-)
tobacco use (Z72.0)

C11.0 Malignant neoplasm of superior wall **of nasopharynx** `HCC`
: Malignant neoplasm of roof of nasopharynx

C11.1 Malignant neoplasm of posterior wall **of nasopharynx** `HCC`
: Malignant neoplasm of adenoid
Malignant neoplasm of pharyngeal tonsil

C11.2 Malignant neoplasm of lateral wall **of nasopharynx** `HCC`
: Malignant neoplasm of fossa of Rosenmüller
Malignant neoplasm of opening of auditory tube
Malignant neoplasm of pharyngeal recess

✓Additional Character Required   ✓×7ᵗʰ Placeholder   Unacceptable PDx   Questionable PDx   Manifestation   **H1** - **H14** HAC   `HCC` CMS-HCC Dx   `HIV` HIV Dx

ICD-10-CM 2019   **465**

C02.8–C11.2

Chapter 2. Neoplasms (side)

C11.3 Malignant neoplasm of anterior wall of nasopharynx `HCC`
Malignant neoplasm of floor of nasopharynx
Malignant neoplasm of nasopharyngeal (anterior) (posterior) surface of soft palate
Malignant neoplasm of posterior margin of nasal choana
Malignant neoplasm of posterior margin of nasal septum

C11.8 Malignant neoplasm of overlapping sites of nasopharynx `HCC`

C11.9 Malignant neoplasm of nasopharynx, unspecified `HCC`
Malignant neoplasm of nasopharyngeal wall NOS

C12 Malignant neoplasm of pyriform sinus `HCC`
Malignant neoplasm of pyriform fossa
Use additional code to identify:
exposure to environmental tobacco smoke (Z77.22)
exposure to tobacco smoke in the perinatal period (P96.81)
history of tobacco dependence (Z87.891)
occupational exposure to environmental tobacco smoke (Z57.31)
tobacco dependence (F17.-)
tobacco use (Z72.0)

✓4ᵗʰ C13 Malignant neoplasm of hypopharynx
Use additional code to identify:
exposure to environmental tobacco smoke (Z77.22)
exposure to tobacco smoke in the perinatal period (P96.81)
history of tobacco dependence (Z87.891)
occupational exposure to environmental tobacco smoke (Z57.31)
tobacco dependence (F17.-)
tobacco use (Z72.0)
EXCLUDES 2 malignant neoplasm of pyriform sinus (C12)

C13.0 Malignant neoplasm of postcricoid region `HCC`

C13.1 Malignant neoplasm of aryepiglottic fold, hypopharyngeal aspect `HCC`
Malignant neoplasm of aryepiglottic fold, marginal zone
Malignant neoplasm of aryepiglottic fold NOS
Malignant neoplasm of interarytenoid fold, marginal zone
Malignant neoplasm of interarytenoid fold NOS
EXCLUDES 2 malignant neoplasm of aryepiglottic fold or interarytenoid fold, laryngeal aspect (C32.1)

C13.2 Malignant neoplasm of posterior wall of hypopharynx `HCC`

C13.8 Malignant neoplasm of overlapping sites of hypopharynx `HCC`

C13.9 Malignant neoplasm of hypopharynx, unspecified `HCC`
Malignant neoplasm of hypopharyngeal wall NOS

✓4ᵗʰ C14 Malignant neoplasm of other and ill-defined sites in the lip, oral cavity and pharynx
Use additional code to identify:
alcohol abuse and dependence (F10.-)
exposure to environmental tobacco smoke (Z77.22)
exposure to tobacco smoke in the perinatal period (P96.81)
history of tobacco dependence (Z87.891)
occupational exposure to environmental tobacco smoke (Z57.31)
tobacco dependence (F17.-)
tobacco use (Z72.0)
EXCLUDES 1 malignant neoplasm of oral cavity NOS (C06.9)

C14.0 Malignant neoplasm of pharynx, unspecified `HCC`

C14.2 Malignant neoplasm of Waldeyer's ring `HCC`
DEF: Waldeyer's ring: Ring of lymphoid tissue that is made up of the two palatine tonsils, the pharyngeal tonsil (adenoid), and the lingual tonsil. It functions as the defense against infection and assists with the development of the immune system.

C14.8 Malignant neoplasm of overlapping sites of lip, oral cavity and pharynx `HCC`
Primary malignant neoplasm of two or more contiguous sites of lip, oral cavity and pharynx
EXCLUDES 1 "book leaf" neoplasm [ventral surface of tongue and floor of mouth] (C06.89)

Malignant neoplasms of digestive organs (C15-C26)
EXCLUDES 1 Kaposi's sarcoma of gastrointestinal sites (C46.4)
EXCLUDES 2 gastrointestinal stromal tumors (C49.A-)

✓4ᵗʰ C15 Malignant neoplasm of esophagus
Use additional code to identify:
alcohol abuse and dependence (F10.-)

CC Excl: For CC codes in category C15: PDX collection 253

C15.3 Malignant neoplasm of upper third of esophagus `CC` `HCC`

C15.4 Malignant neoplasm of middle third of esophagus `CC` `HCC`

C15.5 Malignant neoplasm of lower third of esophagus `CC` `HCC`
EXCLUDES 1 malignant neoplasm of cardio-esophageal junction (C16.0)

C15.8 Malignant neoplasm of overlapping sites of esophagus `CC` `HCC`

C15.9 Malignant neoplasm of esophagus, unspecified `CC` `HCC`

✓4ᵗʰ C16 Malignant neoplasm of stomach
Use additional code to identify:
alcohol abuse and dependence (F10.-)
EXCLUDES 2 malignant carcinoid tumor of the stomach (C7A.092)

CC Excl: For CC codes in category C16: PDX collection 254

C16.0 Malignant neoplasm of cardia `CC` `HCC`
Malignant neoplasm of cardiac orifice
Malignant neoplasm of cardio-esophageal junction
Malignant neoplasm of esophagus and stomach
Malignant neoplasm of gastro-esophageal junction

C16.1 Malignant neoplasm of fundus of stomach `CC` `HCC`

C16.2 Malignant neoplasm of body of stomach `CC` `HCC`

C16.3 Malignant neoplasm of pyloric antrum `CC` `HCC`
Malignant neoplasm of gastric antrum

C16.4 Malignant neoplasm of pylorus `CC` `HCC`
Malignant neoplasm of prepylorus
Malignant neoplasm of pyloric canal

C16.5 Malignant neoplasm of lesser curvature of stomach, unspecified `CC` `HCC`
Malignant neoplasm of lesser curvature of stomach, not classifiable to C16.1-C16.4

C16.6 Malignant neoplasm of greater curvature of stomach, unspecified `CC` `HCC`
Malignant neoplasm of greater curvature of stomach, not classifiable to C16.0-C16.4

C16.8 Malignant neoplasm of overlapping sites of stomach `CC` `HCC`

C16.9 Malignant neoplasm of stomach, unspecified `CC` `HCC`
Gastric cancer NOS

✓4ᵗʰ C17 Malignant neoplasm of small intestine
EXCLUDES 1 malignant carcinoid tumors of the small intestine (C7A.01)
AHA: 2016, 1Q, 19

C17.0 Malignant neoplasm of duodenum `CC` `HCC`
CC Excl: PDX collection 255

C17.1 Malignant neoplasm of jejunum `CC` `HCC`
CC Excl: PDX collection 256

C17.2 Malignant neoplasm of ileum `CC` `HCC`
EXCLUDES 1 malignant neoplasm of ileocecal valve (C18.0)
CC Excl: PDX collection 257

C17.3 Meckel's diverticulum, malignant `CC` `HCC`
EXCLUDES 1 Meckel's diverticulum, congenital (Q43.0)
DEF: Congenital, abnormal remnant of embryonic digestive system development that leaves a sacculation or outpouching from the wall of the small intestine near the terminal part of the ileum made of acid-secreting tissue as in the stomach.
CC Excl: PDX collection 258

C17.8 Malignant neoplasm of overlapping sites of small intestine `CC` `HCC`
CC Excl: PDX collection 259

C17.9 Malignant neoplasm of small intestine, unspecified `CC` `HCC`
CC Excl: PDX collection 259

✓4ᵗʰ C18 Malignant neoplasm of colon
EXCLUDES 1 malignant carcinoid tumors of the colon (C7A.02-)

C18.0 Malignant neoplasm of cecum `CC` `HCC`
Malignant neoplasm of ileocecal valve
CC Excl: PDX collection 260

Colon

Anatomical distribution of large bowel cancers

C18.1 Malignant neoplasm of appendix   `CC` `HCC`
CC Excl: PDX collection 261

C18.2 Malignant neoplasm of ascending colon   `CC` `HCC`
CC Excl: PDX collection 262

C18.3 Malignant neoplasm of hepatic flexure   `CC` `HCC`
CC Excl: PDX collection 263

C18.4 Malignant neoplasm of transverse colon   `CC` `HCC`
CC Excl: PDX collection 264

C18.5 Malignant neoplasm of splenic flexure   `CC` `HCC`
CC Excl: PDX collection 265

C18.6 Malignant neoplasm of descending colon   `CC` `HCC`
CC Excl: PDX collection 266

C18.7 Malignant neoplasm of sigmoid colon   `CC` `HCC`
Malignant neoplasm of sigmoid (flexure)
EXCLUDES 1   *malignant neoplasm of rectosigmoid junction (C19)*
CC Excl: PDX collection 267

C18.8 Malignant neoplasm of overlapping sites **of colon**   `CC` `HCC`
CC Excl: PDX collection 268

C18.9 Malignant neoplasm of colon, unspecified   `CC` `HCC`
Malignant neoplasm of large intestine NOS
CC Excl: PDX collection 268

C19 Malignant neoplasm of rectosigmoid junction   `CC` `HCC`
Malignant neoplasm of colon with rectum
Malignant neoplasm of rectosigmoid (colon)
EXCLUDES 1   *malignant carcinoid tumors of the colon (C7A.02-)*
CC Excl: PDX collection 269

C20 Malignant neoplasm of rectum   `CC` `HCC`
Malignant neoplasm of rectal ampulla
EXCLUDES 1   *malignant carcinoid tumor of the rectum (C7A.026)*
CC Excl: PDX collection 270

✅4ᵗʰ **C21 Malignant neoplasm of** anus and anal canal
EXCLUDES 2   *malignant carcinoid tumors of the colon (C7A.02-)*
malignant melanoma of anal margin (C43.51)
malignant melanoma of anal skin (C43.51)
malignant melanoma of perianal skin (C43.51)
other and unspecified malignant neoplasm of anal margin
(C44.500, C44.510, C44.520, C44.590)
other and unspecified malignant neoplasm of anal skin
(C44.500, C44.510, C44.520, C44.590)
other and unspecified malignant neoplasm of perianal skin
(C44.500, C44.510, C44.520, C44.590)

C21.0 Malignant neoplasm of anus, unspecified   `CC` `HCC`
CC Excl: PDX collection 271

C21.1 Malignant neoplasm of anal canal   `CC` `HCC`
Malignant neoplasm of anal sphincter
CC Excl: PDX collection 271

C21.2 Malignant neoplasm of cloacogenic zone   `CC` `HCC`
CC Excl: PDX collection 272

C21.8 Malignant neoplasm of overlapping sites **of rectum, anus and anal canal**   `CC` `HCC`
Malignant neoplasm of anorectal junction
Malignant neoplasm of anorectum
Primary malignant neoplasm of two or more contiguous sites of rectum, anus and anal canal
CC Excl: PDX collection 272

✅4ᵗʰ **C22 Malignant neoplasm of** liver and intrahepatic bile ducts
Use additional code to identify:
alcohol abuse and dependence (F10.-)
hepatitis B (B16.-, B18.0-B18.1)
hepatitis C (B17.1-, B18.2)
EXCLUDES 1   *malignant neoplasm of biliary tract NOS (C24.9)*
secondary malignant neoplasm of liver and intrahepatic bile duct (C78.7)

CC Excl: For CC codes in category C22: PDX collection 273

C22.0 Liver cell carcinoma   `CC` `HCC`
Hepatocellular carcinoma
Hepatoma
AHA: 2016, 1Q, 18

C22.1 Intrahepatic bile duct carcinoma   `CC` `HCC`
Cholangiocarcinoma
EXCLUDES 1   *malignant neoplasm of hepatic duct (C24.0)*

C22.2 Hepatoblastoma   `CC` `HCC`

C22.3 Angiosarcoma of liver   `CC` `HCC`
Kupffer cell sarcoma

C22.4 Other sarcomas of liver   `CC` `HCC`

C22.7 Other specified carcinomas of liver   `CC` `HCC`

C22.8 Malignant neoplasm of liver, primary, unspecified as to type   `CC` `HCC`

C22.9 Malignant neoplasm of liver, not specified as primary or secondary   `CC` `HCC`

C23 Malignant neoplasm of gallbladder   `CC` `HCC`
CC Excl: PDX collection 274

✅4ᵗʰ **C24 Malignant neoplasm of** other and unspecified parts of biliary tract
EXCLUDES 1   *malignant neoplasm of intrahepatic bile duct (C22.1)*

C24.0 Malignant neoplasm of extrahepatic bile duct   `CC` `HCC`
Malignant neoplasm of biliary duct or passage NOS
Malignant neoplasm of common bile duct
Malignant neoplasm of cystic duct
Malignant neoplasm of hepatic duct
CC Excl: PDX collection 275

C24.1 Malignant neoplasm of ampulla of Vater   `CC` `HCC`
DEF: Malignant neoplasm in the area of dilation at the juncture of the common bile and pancreatic ducts near the opening into the lumen of the duodenum.
CC Excl: PDX collection 276

C24.8 Malignant neoplasm of overlapping sites **of biliary tract**   `CC` `HCC`
Malignant neoplasm involving both intrahepatic and extrahepatic bile ducts
Primary malignant neoplasm of two or more contiguous sites of biliary tract
CC Excl: PDX collection 277

C24.9 Malignant neoplasm of biliary tract, unspecified   `CC` `HCC`
CC Excl: PDX collection 277

✅4ᵗʰ **C25 Malignant neoplasm of** pancreas
Code also exocrine pancreatic insufficiency (K86.81)
Use additional code to identify:
alcohol abuse and dependence (F10.-)

CC Excl: For CC codes in category C25: PDX collection 278

C25.0 Malignant neoplasm of head **of pancreas**   `CC` `HCC`

C25.1 Malignant neoplasm of body **of pancreas**   `CC` `HCC`

C25.2 Malignant neoplasm of tail **of pancreas**   `CC` `HCC`

C25.3 Malignant neoplasm of pancreatic duct   `CC` `HCC`

C25.4 Malignant neoplasm of endocrine pancreas
Malignant neoplasm of islets of Langerhans
Use additional code to identify any functional activity

C25.7 Malignant neoplasm of other parts **of pancreas**   `CC` `HCC`
Malignant neoplasm of neck of pancreas

C25.8 Malignant neoplasm of overlapping sites **of pancreas**   `CC` `HCC`

C25.9 Malignant neoplasm of pancreas, unspecified   `CC` `HCC`

Pancreas

✅4ᵗʰ **C26 Malignant neoplasm of** other and ill-defined digestive organs
EXCLUDES 1   *malignant neoplasm of peritoneum and retroperitoneum (C48.-)*

C26.0 Malignant neoplasm of intestinal tract, **part unspecified**   `HCC`
Malignant neoplasm of intestine NOS

C26.1 Malignant neoplasm of spleen   `HCC`
EXCLUDES 1   *Hodgkin lymphoma (C81.-)*
non-Hodgkin lymphoma (C82-C85)

☑ Additional Character Required   ✓x7ᵗʰ Placeholder   Unacceptable PDx   Questionable PDx   Manifestation   **H1**-**H14** HAC   `HCC` CMS-HCC Dx   **HIV** HIV Dx

ICD-10-CM 2019   **467**

C26.9   **Malignant neoplasm of ill-defined sites within the digestive system**   `HCC`
- Malignant neoplasm of alimentary canal or tract NOS
- Malignant neoplasm of gastrointestinal tract NOS
- **EXCLUDES 1**   *malignant neoplasm of abdominal NOS (C76.2)*
  - *malignant neoplasm of intra-abdominal NOS (C76.2)*

Malignant neoplasms of respiratory and intrathoracic organs (C30-C39)

INCLUDES   malignant neoplasm of middle ear
EXCLUDES 1   *mesothelioma (C45.-)*

✓4th C30   Malignant neoplasm of nasal cavity and middle ear

C30.0   **Malignant neoplasm of nasal cavity**   `HCC`
- Malignant neoplasm of cartilage of nose
- Malignant neoplasm of nasal concha
- Malignant neoplasm of internal nose
- Malignant neoplasm of septum of nose
- Malignant neoplasm of vestibule of nose
- **EXCLUDES 1**   *malignant melanoma of skin of nose (C43.31)*
  - *malignant neoplasm of nasal bone (C41.0)*
  - *malignant neoplasm of nose NOS (C76.0)*
  - *malignant neoplasm of olfactory bulb (C72.2-)*
  - *malignant neoplasm of posterior margin of nasal septum and choana (C11.3)*
  - *malignant neoplasm of turbinates (C41.0)*
  - *other and unspecified malignant neoplasm of skin of nose (C44.301, C44.311, C44.321, C44.391)*

C30.1   **Malignant neoplasm of middle ear**   `HCC`
- Malignant neoplasm of antrum tympanicum
- Malignant neoplasm of auditory tube
- Malignant neoplasm of eustachian tube
- Malignant neoplasm of inner ear
- Malignant neoplasm of mastoid air cells
- Malignant neoplasm of tympanic cavity
- **EXCLUDES 1**   *malignant melanoma of skin of (external) ear (C43.2-)*
  - *malignant neoplasm of auricular canal (external) (C43.2-,C44.2-)*
  - *malignant neoplasm of bone of ear (meatus) (C41.0)*
  - *malignant neoplasm of cartilage of ear (C49.0)*
  - *other and unspecified malignant neoplasm of skin of (external) ear (C44.2-)*

✓4th C31   Malignant neoplasm of accessory sinuses

C31.0   **Malignant neoplasm of maxillary sinus**   `HCC`
- Malignant neoplasm of antrum (Highmore) (maxillary)

C31.1   **Malignant neoplasm of ethmoidal sinus**   `HCC`

C31.2   **Malignant neoplasm of frontal sinus**   `HCC`

C31.3   **Malignant neoplasm of sphenoid sinus**   `HCC`

C31.8   **Malignant neoplasm of overlapping sites of accessory sinuses**   `HCC`

C31.9   **Malignant neoplasm of accessory sinus, unspecified**   `HCC`

✓4th C32   Malignant neoplasm of larynx

Use additional code to identify:
- alcohol abuse and dependence (F10.-)
- exposure to environmental tobacco smoke (Z77.22)
- exposure to tobacco smoke in the perinatal period (P96.81)
- history of tobacco dependence (Z87.891)
- occupational exposure to environmental tobacco smoke (Z57.31)
- tobacco dependence (F17.-)
- tobacco use (Z72.0)

C32.0   **Malignant neoplasm of glottis**   `HCC`
- Malignant neoplasm of intrinsic larynx
- Malignant neoplasm of laryngeal commissure (anterior)(posterior)
- Malignant neoplasm of vocal cord (true) NOS

C32.1   **Malignant neoplasm of supraglottis**   `HCC`
- Malignant neoplasm of aryepiglottic fold or interarytenoid fold, laryngeal aspect
- Malignant neoplasm of epiglottis (suprahyoid portion) NOS
- Malignant neoplasm of extrinsic larynx
- Malignant neoplasm of false vocal cord
- Malignant neoplasm of posterior (laryngeal) surface of epiglottis
- Malignant neoplasm of ventricular bands
- **EXCLUDES 2**   *malignant neoplasm of anterior surface of epiglottis (C10.1)*
  - *malignant neoplasm of aryepiglottic fold or interarytenoid fold, hypopharyngeal aspect (C13.1)*
  - *malignant neoplasm of aryepiglottic fold or interarytenoid fold, marginal zone (C13.1)*
  - *malignant neoplasm of aryepiglottic fold or interarytenoid fold NOS (C13.1)*

C32.2   **Malignant neoplasm of subglottis**   `HCC`

C32.3   **Malignant neoplasm of laryngeal cartilage**   `HCC`

C32.8   **Malignant neoplasm of overlapping sites of larynx**   `HCC`

C32.9   **Malignant neoplasm of larynx, unspecified**   `HCC`

C33   Malignant neoplasm of trachea   `CC` `HCC`

Use additional code to identify:
- exposure to environmental tobacco smoke (Z77.22)
- exposure to tobacco smoke in the perinatal period (P96.81)
- history of tobacco dependence (Z87.891)
- occupational exposure to environmental tobacco smoke (Z57.31)
- tobacco dependence (F17.-)
- tobacco use (Z72.0)

CC Excl: PDX collection 279

✓4th C34   Malignant neoplasm of bronchus and lung

Use additional code to identify:
- exposure to environmental tobacco smoke (Z77.22)
- exposure to tobacco smoke in the perinatal period (P96.81)
- history of tobacco dependence (Z87.891)
- occupational exposure to environmental tobacco smoke (Z57.31)
- tobacco dependence (F17.-)
- tobacco use (Z72.0)
- **EXCLUDES 1**   *Kaposi's sarcoma of lung (C46.5-)*
  - *malignant carcinoid tumor of the bronchus and lung (C7A.090)*

✓5th C34.0   **Malignant neoplasm of main bronchus**
- Malignant neoplasm of carina
- Malignant neoplasm of hilus (of lung)

> **CC Excl: For CC codes in subcategory C34.0:** PDX collection 280

   C34.00   **Malignant neoplasm of unspecified main bronchus**   `CC` `HCC`

   C34.01   **Malignant neoplasm of right main bronchus**   `CC` `HCC`

   C34.02   **Malignant neoplasm of left main bronchus**   `CC` `HCC`

✓5th C34.1   **Malignant neoplasm of upper lobe, bronchus or lung**

> **CC Excl: For CC codes in subcategory C34.1:** PDX collection 281

   C34.10   **Malignant neoplasm of upper lobe, unspecified bronchus or lung**   `CC` `HCC`

   C34.11   **Malignant neoplasm of upper lobe, right bronchus or lung**   `CC` `HCC`

   C34.12   **Malignant neoplasm of upper lobe, left bronchus or lung**   `CC` `HCC`

C34.2   **Malignant neoplasm of middle lobe, bronchus or lung**   `CC` `HCC`
   CC Excl: PDX collection 282

✓5th C34.3   **Malignant neoplasm of lower lobe, bronchus or lung**

> **CC Excl: For CC codes in subcategory C34.3:** PDX collection 283

   C34.30   **Malignant neoplasm of lower lobe, unspecified bronchus or lung**   `CC` `HCC`

   C34.31   **Malignant neoplasm of lower lobe, right bronchus or lung**   `CC` `HCC`

   C34.32   **Malignant neoplasm of lower lobe, left bronchus or lung**   `CC` `HCC`

✓5th C34.8   **Malignant neoplasm of overlapping sites of bronchus and lung**

> **CC Excl: For CC codes in subcategory C34.8:** PDX collection 284

   C34.80   **Malignant neoplasm of overlapping sites of unspecified bronchus and lung**   `CC` `HCC`

   C34.81   **Malignant neoplasm of overlapping sites of right bronchus and lung**   `CC` `HCC`

   C34.82   **Malignant neoplasm of overlapping sites of left bronchus and lung**   `CC` `HCC`

✓5th C34.9   **Malignant neoplasm of unspecified part of bronchus or lung**

> **CC Excl: For CC codes in subcategory C34.9:** PDX collection 284

   C34.90   **Malignant neoplasm of unspecified part of unspecified bronchus or lung**   `CC` `HCC`
     Lung cancer NOS

   C34.91   **Malignant neoplasm of unspecified part of right bronchus or lung**   `CC` `HCC`

   C34.92   **Malignant neoplasm of unspecified part of left bronchus or lung**   `CC` `HCC`

C37   **Malignant neoplasm of** thymus   `CC` `HCC`
> *EXCLUDES1*   *malignant carcinoid tumor of the thymus (C7A.Ø91)*
> **CC Excl:** PDX collection 285

✓4ᵗʰ **C38**   **Malignant neoplasm of** heart, mediastinum and pleura
> *EXCLUDES1*   *mesothelioma (C45.-)*

> **CC Excl: For CC codes in category C38, unless otherwise noted:**
> PDX collection 287

    C38.Ø   **Malignant neoplasm of** heart
> Malignant neoplasm of pericardium
> *EXCLUDES1*   *malignant neoplasm of great vessels (C49.3)*
> **CC Excl:** PDX collection 286

    C38.1   **Malignant neoplasm of** anterior mediastinum   `CC` `HCC`

    C38.2   **Malignant neoplasm of** posterior mediastinum   `CC` `HCC`

    C38.3   **Malignant neoplasm of** mediastinum, part unspecified   `CC` `HCC`

    C38.4   **Malignant neoplasm of** pleura   `CC` `HCC`
> **CC Excl:** PDX collection 288

    C38.8   **Malignant neoplasm of** overlapping sites of heart, mediastinum and pleura   `CC` `HCC`

✓4ᵗʰ **C39**   **Malignant neoplasm of** other and ill-defined sites in the respiratory system and intrathoracic organs
> Use additional code to identify:
> exposure to environmental tobacco smoke (Z77.22)
> exposure to tobacco smoke in the perinatal period (P96.81)
> history of tobacco dependence (Z87.891)
> occupational exposure to environmental tobacco smoke (Z57.31)
> tobacco dependence (F17.-)
> tobacco use (Z72.Ø)
> *EXCLUDES1*   *intrathoracic malignant neoplasm NOS (C76.1)*
>   *thoracic malignant neoplasm NOS (C76.1)*

    C39.Ø   **Malignant neoplasm of** upper respiratory tract, part unspecified   `HCC`

    C39.9   **Malignant neoplasm of** lower respiratory tract, part unspecified   `HCC`
> Malignant neoplasm of respiratory tract NOS

Malignant neoplasms of bone and articular cartilage (C40-C41)

> `INCLUDES`   malignant neoplasm of cartilage (articular) (joint)
>   malignant neoplasm of periosteum
> *EXCLUDES1*   *malignant neoplasm of bone marrow NOS (C96.9)*
>   *malignant neoplasm of synovia (C49.-)*

✓4ᵗʰ **C40**   **Malignant neoplasm of** bone and articular cartilage of limbs
> Use additional code to identify major osseous defect, if applicable
> (M89.7-)

✓5ᵗʰ   **C40.Ø**   **Malignant neoplasm of** scapula and long bones of upper limb

> **CC Excl: For CC codes in subcategory C40.Ø:**
> PDX collection 289

      C40.00   **Malignant neoplasm of** scapula and long bones of unspecified upper limb   `CC` `HCC`

      C40.01   **Malignant neoplasm of** scapula and long bones of right upper limb   `CC` `HCC`

      C40.02   **Malignant neoplasm of** scapula and long bones of left upper limb   `CC` `HCC`

✓5ᵗʰ   **C40.1**   **Malignant neoplasm of** short bones of upper limb

> **CC Excl: For CC codes in subcategory C40.1:**
> PDX collection 290

      C40.10   **Malignant neoplasm of** short bones of unspecified upper limb   `CC` `HCC`

      C40.11   **Malignant neoplasm of** short bones of right upper limb   `CC` `HCC`

      C40.12   **Malignant neoplasm of** short bones of left upper limb   `CC` `HCC`

✓5ᵗʰ   **C40.2**   **Malignant neoplasm of** long bones of lower limb

> **CC Excl: For CC codes in subcategory C40.2:**
> PDX collection 291

      C40.20   **Malignant neoplasm of** long bones of unspecified lower limb   `CC` `HCC`

      C40.21   **Malignant neoplasm of** long bones of right lower limb   `CC` `HCC`

      C40.22   **Malignant neoplasm of** long bones of left lower limb   `CC` `HCC`

✓5ᵗʰ   **C40.3**   **Malignant neoplasm of** short bones of lower limb

> **CC Excl: For CC codes in subcategory C40.3:**
> PDX collection 292

      C40.30   **Malignant neoplasm of** short bones of unspecified lower limb   `CC` `HCC`

      C40.31   **Malignant neoplasm of** short bones of right lower limb   `CC` `HCC`

      C40.32   **Malignant neoplasm of** short bones of left lower limb   `CC` `HCC`

✓5ᵗʰ   **C40.8**   **Malignant neoplasm of** overlapping sites of bone and articular cartilage of limb

> **CC Excl: For CC codes in subcategory C40.8:**
> PDX collection 293

      C40.80   **Malignant neoplasm of** overlapping sites of bone and articular cartilage of unspecified limb   `CC` `HCC`

      C40.81   **Malignant neoplasm of** overlapping sites of bone and articular cartilage of right limb   `CC` `HCC`

      C40.82   **Malignant neoplasm of** overlapping sites of bone and articular cartilage of left limb   `CC` `HCC`

✓5ᵗʰ   **C40.9**   **Malignant neoplasm of** unspecified bones and articular cartilage of limb

> **CC Excl: For CC codes in subcategory C40.9:**
> PDX collection 293

      C40.90   **Malignant neoplasm of** unspecified bones and articular cartilage of unspecified limb   `CC` `HCC`

      C40.91   **Malignant neoplasm of** unspecified bones and articular cartilage of right limb   `CC` `HCC`

      C40.92   **Malignant neoplasm of** unspecified bones and articular cartilage of left limb   `CC` `HCC`

✓4ᵗʰ **C41**   **Malignant neoplasm of bone and articular cartilage of other and unspecified sites**
> *EXCLUDES1*   *malignant neoplasm of bones of limbs (C40.-)*
>   *malignant neoplasm of cartilage of ear (C49.Ø)*
>   *malignant neoplasm of cartilage of eyelid (C49.Ø)*
>   *malignant neoplasm of cartilage of larynx (C32.3)*
>   *malignant neoplasm of cartilage of limbs (C40.-)*
>   *malignant neoplasm of cartilage of nose (C30.Ø)*

    C41.Ø   **Malignant neoplasm of bones of** skull and face   `CC` `HCC`
> Malignant neoplasm of maxilla (superior)
> Malignant neoplasm of orbital bone
> *EXCLUDES2*   *carcinoma, any type except intraosseous or*
>   *odontogenic of:*
>   *maxillary sinus (C31.Ø)*
>   *upper jaw (C03.Ø)*
>   *malignant neoplasm of jaw bone (lower) (C41.1)*
> **CC Excl:** PDX collection 294

    C41.1   **Malignant neoplasm of** mandible   `CC` `HCC`
> Malignant neoplasm of inferior maxilla
> Malignant neoplasm of lower jaw bone
> *EXCLUDES2*   *carcinoma, any type except intraosseous or*
>   *odontogenic of:*
>   *jaw NOS (C03.9)*
>   *lower (C03.1)*
>   *malignant neoplasm of upper jaw bone (C41.Ø)*
> **CC Excl:** PDX collection 295

    C41.2   **Malignant neoplasm of** vertebral column   `CC` `HCC`
> *EXCLUDES1*   *malignant neoplasm of sacrum and coccyx (C41.4)*
> **CC Excl:** PDX collection 296

    C41.3   **Malignant neoplasm of** ribs, sternum and clavicle   `CC` `HCC`
> **CC Excl:** PDX collection 297

    C41.4   **Malignant neoplasm of** pelvic bones, sacrum and coccyx   `CC` `HCC`
> **CC Excl:** PDX collection 298

    C41.9   **Malignant neoplasm of** bone and articular cartilage, unspecified   `CC` `HCC`
> **CC Excl:** PDX collection 293

✓ Additional Character Required   ✓7ᵗʰ Placeholder   Unacceptable PDx   Questionable PDx   Manifestation   `H1`-`H14` HAC   `HCC` CMS-HCC Dx   `HIV` HIV Dx

ICD-10-CM 2019   469

Chapter 2. Neoplasms *(side tab)*

C43–C44.Ø9 *(side tab)*

Melanoma and other malignant neoplasms of skin (C43-C44)

✓4ᵗʰ **C43 Malignant melanoma of skin**
- EXCLUDES 1   *melanoma in situ (DØ3.-)*
- EXCLUDES 2   *malignant melanoma of skin of genital organs (C51-C52, C6Ø.-, C63.-)*
  - *Merkel cell carcinoma (C4A.-)*
  - *sites other than skin—code to malignant neoplasm of the site*

C43.Ø Malignant melanoma of lip   HCC
- EXCLUDES 1   *malignant neoplasm of vermilion border of lip (CØØ.Ø-CØØ.2)*

✓5ᵗʰ **C43.1 Malignant melanoma of eyelid, including canthus**
- **C43.1Ø Malignant melanoma of unspecified eyelid, including canthus**   HCC
- ✓6ᵗʰ **C43.11 Malignant melanoma of right eyelid, including canthus**
  - **C43.111 Malignant melanoma of right upper eyelid, including canthus**
  - **C43.112 Malignant melanoma of right lower eyelid, including canthus**
- ✓6ᵗʰ **C43.12 Malignant melanoma of left eyelid, including canthus**
  - **C43.121 Malignant melanoma of left upper eyelid, including canthus**
  - **C43.122 Malignant melanoma of left lower eyelid, including canthus**

✓5ᵗʰ **C43.2 Malignant melanoma of ear and external auricular canal**
- **C43.2Ø Malignant melanoma of unspecified ear and external auricular canal**   HCC
- **C43.21 Malignant melanoma of right ear and external auricular canal**   HCC
- **C43.22 Malignant melanoma of left ear and external auricular canal**   HCC

✓5ᵗʰ **C43.3 Malignant melanoma of other and unspecified parts of face**
- **C43.3Ø Malignant melanoma of unspecified part of face**   HCC
- **C43.31 Malignant melanoma of nose**   HCC
- **C43.39 Malignant melanoma of other parts of face**   HCC

C43.4 Malignant melanoma of scalp and neck   HCC

✓5ᵗʰ **C43.5 Malignant melanoma of trunk**
- EXCLUDES 2   *malignant neoplasm of anus NOS (C21.Ø)*
  - *malignant neoplasm of scrotum (C63.2)*
- **C43.51 Malignant melanoma of anal skin**   HCC
  - Malignant melanoma of anal margin
  - Malignant melanoma of perianal skin
- **C43.52 Malignant melanoma of skin of breast**   HCC
- **C43.59 Malignant melanoma of other part of trunk**   HCC

✓5ᵗʰ **C43.6 Malignant melanoma of upper limb, including shoulder**
- **C43.6Ø Malignant melanoma of unspecified upper limb, including shoulder**   HCC
- **C43.61 Malignant melanoma of right upper limb, including shoulder**   HCC
- **C43.62 Malignant melanoma of left upper limb, including shoulder**   HCC

✓5ᵗʰ **C43.7 Malignant melanoma of lower limb, including hip**
- **C43.7Ø Malignant melanoma of unspecified lower limb, including hip**   HCC
- **C43.71 Malignant melanoma of right lower limb, including hip**   HCC
- **C43.72 Malignant melanoma of left lower limb, including hip**   HCC

C43.8 Malignant melanoma of overlapping sites of skin   HCC

C43.9 Malignant melanoma of skin, unspecified   HCC
- Malignant melanoma of unspecified site of skin
- Melanoma (malignant) NOS

✓4ᵗʰ **C4A Merkel cell carcinoma**
- DEF: Malignant cutaneous cancer predominantly found in elderly patients with sun exposure that usually presents as a flesh-colored or bluish-red lump typically seen on the neck, head, and face.

C4A.Ø Merkel cell carcinoma of lip   HCC
- EXCLUDES 1   *malignant neoplasm of vermilion border of lip (CØØ.Ø-CØØ.2)*

✓5ᵗʰ **C4A.1 Merkel cell carcinoma of eyelid, including canthus**
- **C4A.1Ø Merkel cell carcinoma of unspecified eyelid, including canthus**   HCC

- ✓6ᵗʰ **C4A.11 Merkel cell carcinoma of right eyelid, including canthus**
  - **C4A.111 Merkel cell carcinoma of right upper eyelid, including canthus**
  - **C4A.112 Merkel cell carcinoma of right lower eyelid, including canthus**
- ✓6ᵗʰ **C4A.12 Merkel cell carcinoma of left eyelid, including canthus**
  - **C4A.121 Merkel cell carcinoma of left upper eyelid, including canthus**
  - **C4A.122 Merkel cell carcinoma of left lower eyelid, including canthus**

✓5ᵗʰ **C4A.2 Merkel cell carcinoma of ear and external auricular canal**
- **C4A.2Ø Merkel cell carcinoma of unspecified ear and external auricular canal**   HCC
- **C4A.21 Merkel cell carcinoma of right ear and external auricular canal**   HCC
- **C4A.22 Merkel cell carcinoma of left ear and external auricular canal**   HCC

✓5ᵗʰ **C4A.3 Merkel cell carcinoma of other and unspecified parts of face**
- **C4A.3Ø Merkel cell carcinoma of unspecified part of face**   HCC
- **C4A.31 Merkel cell carcinoma of nose**   HCC
- **C4A.39 Merkel cell carcinoma of other parts of face**   HCC

C4A.4 Merkel cell carcinoma of scalp and neck   HCC

✓5ᵗʰ **C4A.5 Merkel cell carcinoma of trunk**
- EXCLUDES 2   *malignant neoplasm of anus NOS (C21.Ø)*
  - *malignant neoplasm of scrotum (C63.2)*
- **C4A.51 Merkel cell carcinoma of anal skin**   HCC
  - Merkel cell carcinoma of anal margin
  - Merkel cell carcinoma of perianal skin
- **C4A.52 Merkel cell carcinoma of skin of breast**   HCC
- **C4A.59 Merkel cell carcinoma of other part of trunk**   HCC

✓5ᵗʰ **C4A.6 Merkel cell carcinoma of upper limb, including shoulder**
- **C4A.6Ø Merkel cell carcinoma of unspecified upper limb, including shoulder**   HCC
- **C4A.61 Merkel cell carcinoma of right upper limb, including shoulder**   HCC
- **C4A.62 Merkel cell carcinoma of left upper limb, including shoulder**   HCC

✓5ᵗʰ **C4A.7 Merkel cell carcinoma of lower limb, including hip**
- **C4A.7Ø Merkel cell carcinoma of unspecified lower limb, including hip**   HCC
- **C4A.71 Merkel cell carcinoma of right lower limb, including hip**   HCC
- **C4A.72 Merkel cell carcinoma of left lower limb, including hip**   HCC

C4A.8 Merkel cell carcinoma of overlapping sites   HCC

C4A.9 Merkel cell carcinoma, unspecified   HCC
- Merkel cell carcinoma of unspecified site
- Merkel cell carcinoma (NOS)

✓4ᵗʰ **C44 Other and unspecified malignant neoplasm of skin**
- INCLUDES   malignant neoplasm of sebaceous glands
  - malignant neoplasm of sweat glands
- EXCLUDES 1   *Kaposi's sarcoma of skin (C46.Ø)*
  - *malignant melanoma of skin (C43.-)*
  - *malignant neoplasm of skin of genital organs (C51-C52, C6Ø-, C63.2)*
  - *Merkel cell carcinoma (C4A.-)*

DEF: Basal cell carcinoma: Abnormal growth of skin cells that arises from the deepest layer of the epidermis and may present as an open sore, red patches, pink growth, or scar. Typically caused by sun exposure, it is one of the most common forms of skin cancer.

DEF: Squamous cell carcinoma: Uncontrolled growth of abnormal skin cells that arises from the outer layers of the skin (epidermis) and may present as an open sore. It is characterized by a firm, red nodule, elevated growth with a central depression, or a flat sore with a scaly crust.

✓5ᵗʰ **C44.Ø Other and unspecified malignant neoplasm of skin of lip**
- EXCLUDES 1   *malignant neoplasm of lip (CØØ.-)*
- **C44.ØØ Unspecified malignant neoplasm of skin of lip**
- **C44.Ø1 Basal cell carcinoma of skin of lip**
- **C44.Ø2 Squamous cell carcinoma of skin of lip**
- **C44.Ø9 Other specified malignant neoplasm of skin of lip**

N Newborn: 0   P Pediatric: 0-17   M Maternity: 12-55   A Adult: 15-124   MCC Major Complication/Comorbidity   CC Complication/Comorbidity   SW Severe Wound Dx

470   ICD-10-CM 2019

✓5ᵗʰ **C44.1** Other and unspecified malignant neoplasm of skin of eyelid, including canthus

    EXCLUDES 1   connective tissue of eyelid (C49.0)

✓6ᵗʰ **C44.10** Unspecified malignant neoplasm of skin of eyelid, including canthus

    C44.101 Unspecified malignant neoplasm of skin of unspecified eyelid, including canthus

✓7ᵗʰ **C44.102** Unspecified malignant neoplasm of skin of right eyelid, including canthus

        C44.1021 Unspecified malignant neoplasm of skin of right upper eyelid, including canthus

        C44.1022 Unspecified malignant neoplasm of skin of right lower eyelid, including canthus

✓7ᵗʰ **C44.109** Unspecified malignant neoplasm of skin of left eyelid, including canthus

        C44.1091 Unspecified malignant neoplasm of skin of left upper eyelid, including canthus

        C44.1092 Unspecified malignant neoplasm of skin of left lower eyelid, including canthus

✓6ᵗʰ **C44.11** Basal cell carcinoma of skin of eyelid, including canthus

    C44.111 Basal cell carcinoma of skin of unspecified eyelid, including canthus

✓7ᵗʰ **C44.112** Basal cell carcinoma of skin of right eyelid, including canthus

        C44.1121 Basal cell carcinoma of skin of right upper eyelid, including canthus

        C44.1122 Basal cell carcinoma of skin of right lower eyelid, including canthus

✓7ᵗʰ **C44.119** Basal cell carcinoma of skin of left eyelid, including canthus

        C44.1191 Basal cell carcinoma of skin of left upper eyelid, including canthus

        C44.1192 Basal cell carcinoma of skin of left lower eyelid, including canthus

✓6ᵗʰ **C44.12** Squamous cell carcinoma of skin of eyelid, including canthus

    C44.121 Squamous cell carcinoma of skin of unspecified eyelid, including canthus

✓7ᵗʰ **C44.122** Squamous cell carcinoma of skin of right eyelid, including canthus

        C44.1221 Squamous cell carcinoma of skin of right upper eyelid, including canthus

        C44.1222 Squamous cell carcinoma of skin of right lower eyelid, including canthus

✓7ᵗʰ **C44.129** Squamous cell carcinoma of skin of left eyelid, including canthus

        C44.1291 Squamous cell carcinoma of skin of left upper eyelid, including canthus

        C44.1292 Squamous cell carcinoma of skin of left lower eyelid, including canthus

✓6ᵗʰ **C44.13** Sebaceous cell carcinoma of skin of eyelid, including canthus

    C44.131 Sebaceous cell carcinoma of skin of unspecified eyelid, including canthus

✓7ᵗʰ **C44.132** Sebaceous cell carcinoma of skin of right eyelid, including canthus

        C44.1321 Sebaceous cell carcinoma of skin of right upper eyelid, including canthus

        C44.1322 Sebaceous cell carcinoma of skin of right lower eyelid, including canthus

✓7ᵗʰ **C44.139** Sebaceous cell carcinoma of skin of left eyelid, including canthus

        C44.1391 Sebaceous cell carcinoma of skin of left upper eyelid, including canthus

        C44.1392 Sebaceous cell carcinoma of skin of left lower eyelid, including canthus

✓6ᵗʰ **C44.19** Other specified malignant neoplasm of skin of eyelid, including canthus

    C44.191 Other specified malignant neoplasm of skin of unspecified eyelid, including canthus

✓7ᵗʰ **C44.192** Other specified malignant neoplasm of skin of right eyelid, including canthus

        C44.1921 Other specified malignant neoplasm of skin of right upper eyelid, including canthus

        C44.1922 Other specified malignant neoplasm of skin of right lower eyelid, including canthus

✓7ᵗʰ **C44.199** Other specified malignant neoplasm of skin of left eyelid, including canthus

        C44.1991 Other specified malignant neoplasm of skin of left upper eyelid, including canthus

        C44.1992 Other specified malignant neoplasm of skin of left lower eyelid, including canthus

✓5ᵗʰ **C44.2** Other and unspecified malignant neoplasm of skin of ear and external auricular canal

    EXCLUDES 1   connective tissue of ear (C49.0)

✓6ᵗʰ **C44.20** Unspecified malignant neoplasm of skin of ear and external auricular canal

    C44.201 Unspecified malignant neoplasm of skin of unspecified ear and external auricular canal

    C44.202 Unspecified malignant neoplasm of skin of right ear and external auricular canal

    C44.209 Unspecified malignant neoplasm of skin of left ear and external auricular canal

✓6ᵗʰ **C44.21** Basal cell carcinoma of skin of ear and external auricular canal

    C44.211 Basal cell carcinoma of skin of unspecified ear and external auricular canal

    C44.212 Basal cell carcinoma of skin of right ear and external auricular canal

    C44.219 Basal cell carcinoma of skin of left ear and external auricular canal

✓6ᵗʰ **C44.22** Squamous cell carcinoma of skin of ear and external auricular canal

    C44.221 Squamous cell carcinoma of skin of unspecified ear and external auricular canal

    C44.222 Squamous cell carcinoma of skin of right ear and external auricular canal

    C44.229 Squamous cell carcinoma of skin of left ear and external auricular canal

✓6ᵗʰ **C44.29** Other specified malignant neoplasm of skin of ear and external auricular canal

    C44.291 Other specified malignant neoplasm of skin of unspecified ear and external auricular canal

    C44.292 Other specified malignant neoplasm of skin of right ear and external auricular canal

    C44.299 Other specified malignant neoplasm of skin of left ear and external auricular canal

✓5ᵗʰ **C44.3** Other and unspecified malignant neoplasm of skin of other and unspecified parts of face

✓6ᵗʰ **C44.30** Unspecified malignant neoplasm of skin of other and unspecified parts of face

    C44.300 Unspecified malignant neoplasm of skin of unspecified part of face

    C44.301 Unspecified malignant neoplasm of skin of nose

✓ Additional Character Required   ✓x7ᵗʰ Placeholder   Unacceptable PDx   Questionable PDx   Manifestation   H1 - H14 HAC   HCC CMS-HCC Dx   HIV HIV Dx

ICD-10-CM 2019   471

Chapter 2. Neoplasms

    C44.309 Unspecified malignant neoplasm of skin of other parts of face

✓6ᵗʰ C44.31 Basal cell carcinoma of skin of other and unspecified parts of face

    C44.310 Basal cell carcinoma of skin of unspecified parts of face

    C44.311 Basal cell carcinoma of skin of nose

    C44.319 Basal cell carcinoma of skin of other parts of face

✓6ᵗʰ C44.32 Squamous cell carcinoma of skin of other and unspecified parts of face

    C44.320 Squamous cell carcinoma of skin of unspecified parts of face

    C44.321 Squamous cell carcinoma of skin of nose

    C44.329 Squamous cell carcinoma of skin of other parts of face

✓6ᵗʰ C44.39 Other specified malignant neoplasm of skin of other and unspecified parts of face

    C44.390 Other specified malignant neoplasm of skin of unspecified parts of face

    C44.391 Other specified malignant neoplasm of skin of nose

    C44.399 Other specified malignant neoplasm of skin of other parts of face

✓5ᵗʰ C44.4 Other and unspecified malignant neoplasm of skin of scalp and neck

    C44.40 Unspecified malignant neoplasm of skin of scalp and neck

    C44.41 Basal cell carcinoma of skin of scalp and neck

    C44.42 Squamous cell carcinoma of skin of scalp and neck

    C44.49 Other specified malignant neoplasm of skin of scalp and neck

✓5ᵗʰ C44.5 Other and unspecified malignant neoplasm of skin of trunk

    EXCLUDES 1 anus NOS (C21.0)
                   scrotum (C63.2)

✓6ᵗʰ C44.50 Unspecified malignant neoplasm of skin of trunk

    C44.500 Unspecified malignant neoplasm of anal skin
          Unspecified malignant neoplasm of anal margin
          Unspecified malignant neoplasm of perianal skin

    C44.501 Unspecified malignant neoplasm of skin of breast

    C44.509 Unspecified malignant neoplasm of skin of other part of trunk

✓6ᵗʰ C44.51 Basal cell carcinoma of skin of trunk

    C44.510 Basal cell carcinoma of anal skin
          Basal cell carcinoma of anal margin
          Basal cell carcinoma of perianal skin

    C44.511 Basal cell carcinoma of skin of breast

    C44.519 Basal cell carcinoma of skin of other part of trunk

✓6ᵗʰ C44.52 Squamous cell carcinoma of skin of trunk

    C44.520 Squamous cell carcinoma of anal skin
          Squamous cell carcinoma of anal margin
          Squamous cell carcinoma of perianal skin

    C44.521 Squamous cell carcinoma of skin of breast

    C44.529 Squamous cell carcinoma of skin of other part of trunk

✓6ᵗʰ C44.59 Other specified malignant neoplasm of skin of trunk

    C44.590 Other specified malignant neoplasm of anal skin
          Other specified malignant neoplasm of anal margin
          Other specified malignant neoplasm of perianal skin

    C44.591 Other specified malignant neoplasm of skin of breast

    C44.599 Other specified malignant neoplasm of skin of other part of trunk

✓5ᵗʰ C44.6 Other and unspecified malignant neoplasm of skin of upper limb, including shoulder

✓6ᵗʰ C44.60 Unspecified malignant neoplasm of skin of upper limb, including shoulder

    C44.601 Unspecified malignant neoplasm of skin of unspecified upper limb, including shoulder

    C44.602 Unspecified malignant neoplasm of skin of right upper limb, including shoulder

    C44.609 Unspecified malignant neoplasm of skin of left upper limb, including shoulder

✓6ᵗʰ C44.61 Basal cell carcinoma of skin of upper limb, including shoulder

    C44.611 Basal cell carcinoma of skin of unspecified upper limb, including shoulder

    C44.612 Basal cell carcinoma of skin of right upper limb, including shoulder

    C44.619 Basal cell carcinoma of skin of left upper limb, including shoulder

✓6ᵗʰ C44.62 Squamous cell carcinoma of skin of upper limb, including shoulder

    C44.621 Squamous cell carcinoma of skin of unspecified upper limb, including shoulder

    C44.622 Squamous cell carcinoma of skin of right upper limb, including shoulder

    C44.629 Squamous cell carcinoma of skin of left upper limb, including shoulder

✓6ᵗʰ C44.69 Other specified malignant neoplasm of skin of upper limb, including shoulder

    C44.691 Other specified malignant neoplasm of skin of unspecified upper limb, including shoulder

    C44.692 Other specified malignant neoplasm of skin of right upper limb, including shoulder

    C44.699 Other specified malignant neoplasm of skin of left upper limb, including shoulder

✓5ᵗʰ C44.7 Other and unspecified malignant neoplasm of skin of lower limb, including hip

✓6ᵗʰ C44.70 Unspecified malignant neoplasm of skin of lower limb, including hip

    C44.701 Unspecified malignant neoplasm of skin of unspecified lower limb, including hip

    C44.702 Unspecified malignant neoplasm of skin of right lower limb, including hip

    C44.709 Unspecified malignant neoplasm of skin of left lower limb, including hip

✓6ᵗʰ C44.71 Basal cell carcinoma of skin of lower limb, including hip

    C44.711 Basal cell carcinoma of skin of unspecified lower limb, including hip

    C44.712 Basal cell carcinoma of skin of right lower limb, including hip

    C44.719 Basal cell carcinoma of skin of left lower limb, including hip

✓6ᵗʰ C44.72 Squamous cell carcinoma of skin of lower limb, including hip

    C44.721 Squamous cell carcinoma of skin of unspecified lower limb, including hip

    C44.722 Squamous cell carcinoma of skin of right lower limb, including hip

    C44.729 Squamous cell carcinoma of skin of left lower limb, including hip

✓6ᵗʰ C44.79 Other specified malignant neoplasm of skin of lower limb, including hip

    C44.791 Other specified malignant neoplasm of skin of unspecified lower limb, including hip

    C44.792 Other specified malignant neoplasm of skin of right lower limb, including hip

    C44.799 Other specified malignant neoplasm of skin of left lower limb, including hip

✓5ᵗʰ C44.8 Other and unspecified malignant neoplasm of overlapping sites of skin

    C44.80 Unspecified malignant neoplasm of overlapping sites of skin

    C44.81 Basal cell carcinoma of overlapping sites of skin

    C44.82 Squamous cell carcinoma of overlapping sites of skin

    C44.89 Other specified malignant neoplasm of overlapping sites of skin

Ⓝ Newborn: 0   Ⓟ Pediatric: 0-17   Ⓜ Maternity: 12-55   Ⓐ Adult: 15-124   **MCC** Major Complication/Comorbidity   **CC** Complication/Comorbidity   **SW** Severe Wound Dx

472   ICD-10-CM 2019

✓5ᵗʰ **C44.9 Other and unspecified malignant neoplasm of skin, unspecified**

    C44.90 Unspecified malignant neoplasm of skin, unspecified
        Malignant neoplasm of unspecified site of skin

    C44.91 Basal cell carcinoma of skin, unspecified

    C44.92 Squamous cell carcinoma of skin, unspecified

    C44.99 Other specified malignant neoplasm of skin, unspecified

Malignant neoplasms of mesothelial and soft tissue (C45-C49)

✓4ᵗʰ **C45 Mesothelioma**

    DEF: Rare type of cancer that forms in the thin layer of protective tissue that covers the majority of internal organs (mesothelium).

    C45.0 Mesothelioma of pleura   CC HCC
        EXCLUDES 1   *other malignant neoplasm of pleura (C38.4)*
        AHA: 2017, 2Q, 11
        CC Excl: PDX collection 288

    C45.1 Mesothelioma of peritoneum   CC HCC
        Mesothelioma of cul-de-sac
        Mesothelioma of mesentery
        Mesothelioma of mesocolon
        Mesothelioma of omentum
        Mesothelioma of peritoneum (parietal) (pelvic)
        EXCLUDES 1   *other malignant neoplasm of soft tissue of peritoneum (C48.-)*
        CC Excl: PDX collection 299

    C45.2 Mesothelioma of pericardium   CC HCC
        EXCLUDES 1   *other malignant neoplasm of pericardium (C38.0)*
        CC Excl: PDX collection 286

    C45.7 Mesothelioma of other sites   HCC

    C45.9 Mesothelioma, unspecified   HCC

✓4ᵗʰ **C46 Kaposi's sarcoma**

    Code first any human immunodeficiency virus [HIV] disease (B20)
    DEF: Malignant neoplasm that causes patches of abnormal tissue to grow under the skin, in the lining of the mouth, nose, and throat, in lymph nodes, or in other visceral organs. Kaposi's sarcoma is caused by human herpesvirus8 (HHV8).

    C46.0 Kaposi's sarcoma of skin   HIV CC HCC
        CC Excl: PDX collection 300

    C46.1 Kaposi's sarcoma of soft tissue   HIV CC HCC
        Kaposi's sarcoma of blood vessel
        Kaposi's sarcoma of connective tissue
        Kaposi's sarcoma of fascia
        Kaposi's sarcoma of ligament
        Kaposi's sarcoma of lymphatic(s) NEC
        Kaposi's sarcoma of muscle
        EXCLUDES 2   *Kaposi's sarcoma of lymph glands and nodes (C46.3)*
        CC Excl: PDX collection 301

    C46.2 Kaposi's sarcoma of palate   HIV CC HCC
        CC Excl: PDX collection 302

    C46.3 Kaposi's sarcoma of lymph nodes   HIV CC HCC
        CC Excl: PDX collection 303

    C46.4 Kaposi's sarcoma of gastrointestinal sites   HIV CC HCC
        CC Excl: PDX collection 304

    ✓5ᵗʰ **C46.5 Kaposi's sarcoma of lung**

        CC Excl: For CC codes in subcategory C46.5: PDX collection 284

        C46.50 Kaposi's sarcoma of unspecified lung   HIV CC HCC
        C46.51 Kaposi's sarcoma of right lung   HIV CC HCC
        C46.52 Kaposi's sarcoma of left lung   HIV CC HCC

    C46.7 Kaposi's sarcoma of other sites   HIV CC HCC
        CC Excl: PDX collection 305

    C46.9 Kaposi's sarcoma, unspecified   HIV CC HCC
        Kaposi's sarcoma of unspecified site
        CC Excl: PDX collection 306

✓4ᵗʰ **C47 Malignant neoplasm of peripheral nerves and autonomic nervous system**

    INCLUDES   malignant neoplasm of sympathetic and parasympathetic nerves and ganglia
    EXCLUDES 1   *Kaposi's sarcoma of soft tissue (C46.1)*

    CC Excl: For CC codes in category C47: PDX collection 307

    C47.0 Malignant neoplasm of peripheral nerves of head, face and neck   CC HCC
        EXCLUDES 1   *malignant neoplasm of peripheral nerves of orbit (C69.6-)*

✓5ᵗʰ **C47.1 Malignant neoplasm of peripheral nerves of upper limb, including shoulder**

    C47.10 Malignant neoplasm of peripheral nerves of unspecified upper limb, including shoulder   CC HCC

    C47.11 Malignant neoplasm of peripheral nerves of right upper limb, including shoulder   CC HCC

    C47.12 Malignant neoplasm of peripheral nerves of left upper limb, including shoulder   CC HCC

✓5ᵗʰ **C47.2 Malignant neoplasm of peripheral nerves of lower limb, including hip**

    C47.20 Malignant neoplasm of peripheral nerves of unspecified lower limb, including hip   CC HCC

    C47.21 Malignant neoplasm of peripheral nerves of right lower limb, including hip   CC HCC

    C47.22 Malignant neoplasm of peripheral nerves of left lower limb, including hip   CC HCC

C47.3 Malignant neoplasm of peripheral nerves of thorax   CC HCC

C47.4 Malignant neoplasm of peripheral nerves of abdomen   CC HCC

C47.5 Malignant neoplasm of peripheral nerves of pelvis   CC HCC

C47.6 Malignant neoplasm of peripheral nerves of trunk, unspecified   CC HCC
    Malignant neoplasm of peripheral nerves of unspecified part of trunk

C47.8 Malignant neoplasm of overlapping sites of peripheral nerves and autonomic nervous system   CC HCC

C47.9 Malignant neoplasm of peripheral nerves and nervous autonomic system, unspecified   CC HCC
    Malignant neoplasm of unspecified site of peripheral nerves and autonomic nervous system

✓4ᵗʰ **C48 Malignant neoplasm of retroperitoneum and peritoneum**

    EXCLUDES 1   *Kaposi's sarcoma of connective tissue (C46.1)*
           mesothelioma (C45.-)

    CC Excl: For CC codes in category C48, unless otherwise noted: PDX collection 299

    C48.0 Malignant neoplasm of retroperitoneum   CC HCC
        CC Excl: PDX collection 308

    C48.1 Malignant neoplasm of specified parts of peritoneum   CC HCC
        Malignant neoplasm of cul-de-sac
        Malignant neoplasm of mesentery
        Malignant neoplasm of mesocolon
        Malignant neoplasm of omentum
        Malignant neoplasm of parietal peritoneum
        Malignant neoplasm of pelvic peritoneum

    C48.2 Malignant neoplasm of peritoneum, unspecified   CC HCC

    C48.8 Malignant neoplasm of overlapping sites of retroperitoneum and peritoneum   CC HCC

✓4ᵗʰ **C49 Malignant neoplasm of other connective and soft tissue**

    INCLUDES   malignant neoplasm of blood vessel
           malignant neoplasm of bursa
           malignant neoplasm of cartilage
           malignant neoplasm of fascia
           malignant neoplasm of fat
           malignant neoplasm of ligament, except uterine
           malignant neoplasm of lymphatic vessel
           malignant neoplasm of muscle
           malignant neoplasm of synovia
           malignant neoplasm of tendon (sheath)
    EXCLUDES 1   *malignant neoplasm of cartilage (of):*
           articular (C40-C41)   larynx (C32.3)   nose (C30.0)
           malignant neoplasm of connective tissue of breast (C50.-)
    EXCLUDES 2   *Kaposi's sarcoma of soft tissue (C46.1)*
           malignant neoplasm of heart (C38.0)
           malignant neoplasm of peripheral nerves and autonomic nervous system (C47.-)
           malignant neoplasm of peritoneum (C48.2)
           malignant neoplasm of retroperitoneum (C48.0)
           malignant neoplasm of uterine ligament (C57.3)
           mesothelioma (C45.-)

    CC Excl: For CC codes in category C49, unless otherwise noted: PDX collection 307

    C49.0 Malignant neoplasm of connective and soft tissue of head, face and neck   CC HCC
        Malignant neoplasm of connective tissue of ear
        Malignant neoplasm of connective tissue of eyelid
        EXCLUDES 1   *connective tissue of orbit (C69.6-)*

Chapter 2. Neoplasms

✓5ᵗʰ **C49.1 Malignant neoplasm of connective and soft tissue of** upper limb, including shoulder

     C49.10 Malignant neoplasm of connective and soft tissue of unspecified **upper limb, including shoulder** CC HCC

     C49.11 Malignant neoplasm of connective and soft tissue of right **upper limb, including shoulder** CC HCC

     C49.12 Malignant neoplasm of connective and soft tissue of left **upper limb, including shoulder** CC HCC

✓5ᵗʰ **C49.2 Malignant neoplasm of connective and soft tissue of** lower limb, including hip

     C49.20 Malignant neoplasm of connective and soft tissue of unspecified **lower limb, including hip** CC HCC

     C49.21 Malignant neoplasm of connective and soft tissue of right **lower limb, including hip** CC HCC

     C49.22 Malignant neoplasm of connective and soft tissue of left **lower limb, including hip** CC HCC

C49.3 Malignant neoplasm of connective and soft tissue of thorax CC HCC
     Malignant neoplasm of axilla
     Malignant neoplasm of diaphragm
     Malignant neoplasm of great vessels
     EXCLUDES 1 *malignant neoplasm of breast (C50.-)*
              malignant neoplasm of heart (C38.0)
              malignant neoplasm of mediastinum (C38.1-C38.3)
              malignant neoplasm of thymus (C37)
     AHA: 2015, 3Q, 19

C49.4 Malignant neoplasm of connective and soft tissue of abdomen CC HCC
     Malignant neoplasm of abdominal wall
     Malignant neoplasm of hypochondrium

C49.5 Malignant neoplasm of connective and soft tissue of pelvis CC HCC
     Malignant neoplasm of buttock
     Malignant neoplasm of groin
     Malignant neoplasm of perineum

C49.6 Malignant neoplasm of connective and soft tissue of trunk, unspecified CC HCC
     Malignant neoplasm of back NOS

C49.8 Malignant neoplasm of overlapping sites **of connective and soft tissue** CC HCC
     Primary malignant neoplasm of two or more contiguous sites of connective and soft tissue

C49.9 Malignant neoplasm of connective and soft tissue, unspecified CC HCC

✓5ᵗʰ **C49.A Gastrointestinal stromal tumor**
     AHA: 2016, 4Q, 8
     DEF: Uncommon malignant tumor found in the GI tract that originates from interstitial cells of the autonomic nervous system. Most occur in the stomach or small intestine but can originate anywhere in the GI tract.

     C49.A0 Gastrointestinal stromal tumor, unspecified site CC HCC

     C49.A1 Gastrointestinal stromal tumor of esophagus CC HCC

     C49.A2 Gastrointestinal stromal tumor of stomach CC HCC
         CC Excl: PDX collection 511

     C49.A3 Gastrointestinal stromal tumor of small intestine CC HCC

     C49.A4 Gastrointestinal stromal tumor of large intestine CC HCC

     C49.A5 Gastrointestinal stromal tumor of rectum CC HCC

     C49.A9 Gastrointestinal stromal tumor of other sites CC HCC

Malignant neoplasms of breast (C50)

✓4ᵗʰ **C50 Malignant neoplasm of** breast
     INCLUDES   connective tissue of breast
               Paget's disease of breast
               Paget's disease of nipple
     Use additional code to identify estrogen receptor status (Z17.0, Z17.1)
     EXCLUDES 1 *skin of breast (C44.501, C44.511, C44.521, C44.591)*
     AHA: 2017, 4Q, 19

✓5ᵗʰ **C50.0 Malignant neoplasm of** nipple and areola

     ✓6ᵗʰ **C50.01 Malignant neoplasm of nipple and areola,** female

         C50.011 Malignant neoplasm of nipple and areola, right **female breast** HCC ♀

         C50.012 Malignant neoplasm of nipple and areola, left **female breast** HCC ♀

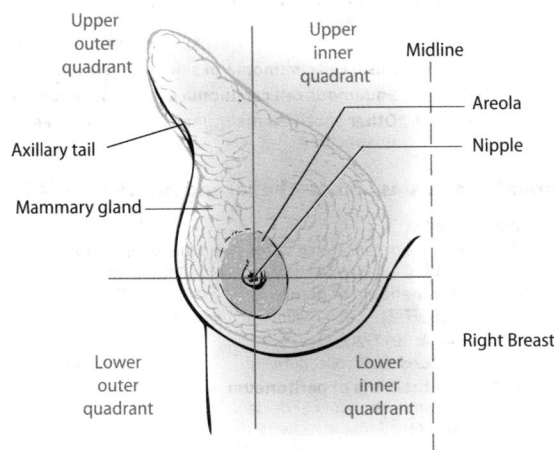

Female Breast

Upper outer quadrant · Upper inner quadrant · Midline · Areola · Axillary tail · Nipple · Mammary gland · Lower outer quadrant · Lower inner quadrant · Right Breast

         C50.019 Malignant neoplasm of nipple and areola, unspecified **female breast** HCC ♀

     ✓6ᵗʰ **C50.02 Malignant neoplasm of nipple and areola,** male

         C50.021 Malignant neoplasm of nipple and areola, right **male breast** HCC ♂

         C50.022 Malignant neoplasm of nipple and areola, left **male breast** HCC ♂

         C50.029 Malignant neoplasm of nipple and areola, unspecified **male breast** HCC ♂

✓5ᵗʰ **C50.1 Malignant neoplasm of** central portion **of breast**

     ✓6ᵗʰ **C50.11 Malignant neoplasm of central portion of breast,** female

         C50.111 Malignant neoplasm of central portion of right **female breast** HCC ♀

         C50.112 Malignant neoplasm of central portion of left **female breast** HCC ♀

         C50.119 Malignant neoplasm of central portion of unspecified **female breast** HCC ♀

     ✓6ᵗʰ **C50.12 Malignant neoplasm of central portion of breast,** male

         C50.121 Malignant neoplasm of central portion of right **male breast** HCC ♂

         C50.122 Malignant neoplasm of central portion of left **male breast** HCC ♂

         C50.129 Malignant neoplasm of central portion of unspecified **male breast** HCC ♂

✓5ᵗʰ **C50.2 Malignant neoplasm of** upper-inner quadrant **of breast**

     ✓6ᵗʰ **C50.21 Malignant neoplasm of upper-inner quadrant of breast,** female

         C50.211 Malignant neoplasm of upper-inner quadrant of right **female breast** HCC ♀

         C50.212 Malignant neoplasm of upper-inner quadrant of left **female breast** HCC ♀

         C50.219 Malignant neoplasm of upper-inner quadrant of unspecified **female breast** HCC ♀

     ✓6ᵗʰ **C50.22 Malignant neoplasm of upper-inner quadrant of breast,** male

         C50.221 Malignant neoplasm of upper-inner quadrant of right **male breast** HCC ♂

         C50.222 Malignant neoplasm of upper-inner quadrant of left **male breast** HCC ♂

         C50.229 Malignant neoplasm of upper-inner quadrant of unspecified **male breast** HCC ♂

✓5ᵗʰ **C50.3 Malignant neoplasm of** lower-inner quadrant **of breast**

     ✓6ᵗʰ **C50.31 Malignant neoplasm of lower-inner quadrant of breast,** female

         C50.311 Malignant neoplasm of lower-inner quadrant of right **female breast** HCC ♀

         C50.312 Malignant neoplasm of lower-inner quadrant of left **female breast** HCC ♀

         C50.319 Malignant neoplasm of lower-inner quadrant of unspecified **female breast** HCC ♀

N Newborn: 0   P Pediatric: 0-17   M Maternity: 12-55   A Adult: 15-124   MCC Major Complication/Comorbidity   CC Complication/Comorbidity   SW Severe Wound Dx

474   ICD-10-CM 2019

☑6th C50.32 Malignant neoplasm of lower-inner quadrant of breast, male

    C50.321 Malignant neoplasm of lower-inner quadrant of right male breast **HCC ♂**

    C50.322 Malignant neoplasm of lower-inner quadrant of left male breast **HCC ♂**

    C50.329 Malignant neoplasm of lower-inner quadrant of unspecified male breast **HCC ♂**

☑5th C50.4 Malignant neoplasm of upper-outer quadrant of breast

  ☑6th C50.41 Malignant neoplasm of upper-outer quadrant of breast, female

    C50.411 Malignant neoplasm of upper-outer quadrant of right female breast **HCC ♀**

    C50.412 Malignant neoplasm of upper-outer quadrant of left female breast **HCC ♀**

    C50.419 Malignant neoplasm of upper-outer quadrant of unspecified female breast **HCC ♀**

  ☑6th C50.42 Malignant neoplasm of upper-outer quadrant of breast, male

    C50.421 Malignant neoplasm of upper-outer quadrant of right male breast **HCC ♂**

    C50.422 Malignant neoplasm of upper-outer quadrant of left male breast **HCC ♂**

    C50.429 Malignant neoplasm of upper-outer quadrant of unspecified male breast **HCC ♂**

☑5th C50.5 Malignant neoplasm of lower-outer quadrant of breast

  ☑6th C50.51 Malignant neoplasm of lower-outer quadrant of breast, female

    C50.511 Malignant neoplasm of lower-outer quadrant of right female breast **HCC ♀**

    C50.512 Malignant neoplasm of lower-outer quadrant of left female breast **HCC ♀**

    C50.519 Malignant neoplasm of lower-outer quadrant of unspecified female breast **HCC ♀**

  ☑6th C50.52 Malignant neoplasm of lower-outer quadrant of breast, male

    C50.521 Malignant neoplasm of lower-outer quadrant of right male breast **HCC ♂**

    C50.522 Malignant neoplasm of lower-outer quadrant of left male breast **HCC ♂**

    C50.529 Malignant neoplasm of lower-outer quadrant of unspecified male breast **HCC ♂**

☑5th C50.6 Malignant neoplasm of axillary tail of breast

  ☑6th C50.61 Malignant neoplasm of axillary tail of breast, female

    C50.611 Malignant neoplasm of axillary tail of right female breast **HCC ♀**

    C50.612 Malignant neoplasm of axillary tail of left female breast **HCC ♀**

    C50.619 Malignant neoplasm of axillary tail of unspecified female breast **HCC ♀**

  ☑6th C50.62 Malignant neoplasm of axillary tail of breast, male

    C50.621 Malignant neoplasm of axillary tail of right male breast **HCC ♂**

    C50.622 Malignant neoplasm of axillary tail of left male breast **HCC ♂**

    C50.629 Malignant neoplasm of axillary tail of unspecified male breast **HCC ♂**

☑5th C50.8 Malignant neoplasm of overlapping sites of breast

  ☑6th C50.81 Malignant neoplasm of overlapping sites of breast, female

    C50.811 Malignant neoplasm of overlapping sites of right female breast **HCC ♀**

    C50.812 Malignant neoplasm of overlapping sites of left female breast **HCC ♀**

    C50.819 Malignant neoplasm of overlapping sites of unspecified female breast **HCC ♀**

  ☑6th C50.82 Malignant neoplasm of overlapping sites of breast, male

    C50.821 Malignant neoplasm of overlapping sites of right male breast **HCC ♂**

    C50.822 Malignant neoplasm of overlapping sites of left male breast **HCC ♂**

    C50.829 Malignant neoplasm of overlapping sites of unspecified male breast **HCC ♂**

☑5th C50.9 Malignant neoplasm of breast of unspecified site

  ☑6th C50.91 Malignant neoplasm of breast of unspecified site, female

    C50.911 Malignant neoplasm of unspecified site of right female breast **HCC ♀**

    C50.912 Malignant neoplasm of unspecified site of left female breast **HCC ♀**

    C50.919 Malignant neoplasm of unspecified site of unspecified female breast **HCC ♀**

  ☑6th C50.92 Malignant neoplasm of breast of unspecified site, male

    C50.921 Malignant neoplasm of unspecified site of right male breast **HCC ♂**

    C50.922 Malignant neoplasm of unspecified site of left male breast **HCC ♂**

    C50.929 Malignant neoplasm of unspecified site of unspecified male breast **HCC ♂**

Malignant neoplasms of female genital organs (C51-C58)

INCLUDES malignant neoplasm of skin of female genital organs

☑4th C51 Malignant neoplasm of vulva

  EXCLUDES 1 carcinoma in situ of vulva (D07.1)

  C51.0 Malignant neoplasm of labium majus **HCC ♀**
    Malignant neoplasm of Bartholin's [greater vestibular] gland

  C51.1 Malignant neoplasm of labium minus **HCC ♀**

  C51.2 Malignant neoplasm of clitoris **HCC ♀**

  C51.8 Malignant neoplasm of overlapping sites of vulva **HCC ♀**

  C51.9 Malignant neoplasm of vulva, unspecified **HCC ♀**
    Malignant neoplasm of external female genitalia NOS
    Malignant neoplasm of pudendum

C52 Malignant neoplasm of vagina **HCC ♀**

  EXCLUDES 1 carcinoma in situ of vagina (D07.2)

☑4th C53 Malignant neoplasm of cervix uteri

  EXCLUDES 1 carcinoma in situ of cervix uteri (D06.-)

  AHA: 2017, 4Q, 103

  C53.0 Malignant neoplasm of endocervix **HCC ♀**

  C53.1 Malignant neoplasm of exocervix **HCC ♀**

  C53.8 Malignant neoplasm of overlapping sites of cervix uteri **HCC ♀**

  C53.9 Malignant neoplasm of cervix uteri, unspecified **HCC ♀**

☑4th C54 Malignant neoplasm of corpus uteri

  C54.0 Malignant neoplasm of isthmus uteri **HCC ♀**
    Malignant neoplasm of lower uterine segment

  C54.1 Malignant neoplasm of endometrium **HCC ♀**

  C54.2 Malignant neoplasm of myometrium **HCC ♀**

  C54.3 Malignant neoplasm of fundus uteri **HCC ♀**

  C54.8 Malignant neoplasm of overlapping sites of corpus uteri **HCC ♀**

  C54.9 Malignant neoplasm of corpus uteri, unspecified **HCC ♀**

C55 Malignant neoplasm of uterus, part unspecified **HCC ♀**

☑4th C56 Malignant neoplasm of ovary

  Use additional code to identify any functional activity

  CC Excl: For CC codes in category C56: PDX collection 309

  C56.1 Malignant neoplasm of right ovary **CC HCC ♀**

  C56.2 Malignant neoplasm of left ovary **CC HCC ♀**

  C56.9 Malignant neoplasm of unspecified ovary **CC HCC ♀**

☑4th C57 Malignant neoplasm of other and unspecified female genital organs

  ☑5th C57.0 Malignant neoplasm of fallopian tube
    Malignant neoplasm of oviduct
    Malignant neoplasm of uterine tube

    C57.00 Malignant neoplasm of unspecified fallopian tube **HCC ♀**

    C57.01 Malignant neoplasm of right fallopian tube **HCC ♀**

    C57.02 Malignant neoplasm of left fallopian tube **HCC ♀**

  ☑5th C57.1 Malignant neoplasm of broad ligament

    C57.10 Malignant neoplasm of unspecified broad ligament **HCC ♀**

    C57.11 Malignant neoplasm of right broad ligament **HCC ♀**

    C57.12 Malignant neoplasm of left broad ligament **HCC ♀**

☑ Additional Character Required   x7th Placeholder   Unacceptable PDx   Questionable PDx   Manifestation   H1-H14 HAC   HCC CMS-HCC Dx   HIV HIV Dx

ICD-10-CM 2019   475

Chapter 2. Neoplasms *(left margin)*

C57.2   Malignant neoplasm of round ligament
- **C57.20**   Malignant neoplasm of unspecified round ligament   HCC ♀
- **C57.21**   Malignant neoplasm of right round ligament   HCC ♀
- **C57.22**   Malignant neoplasm of left round ligament   HCC ♀

C57.3   Malignant neoplasm of parametrium   HCC ♀
  Malignant neoplasm of uterine ligament NOS

C57.4   Malignant neoplasm of uterine adnexa, unspecified   HCC ♀

C57.7   Malignant neoplasm of other specified female genital organs   HCC ♀
  Malignant neoplasm of wolffian body or duct

C57.8   Malignant neoplasm of overlapping sites of female genital organs   HCC ♀
  Primary malignant neoplasm of two or more contiguous sites of the female genital organs whose point of origin cannot be determined
  Primary tubo-ovarian malignant neoplasm whose point of origin cannot be determined
  Primary utero-ovarian malignant neoplasm whose point of origin cannot be determined

C57.9   Malignant neoplasm of female genital organ, unspecified   HCC ♀
  Malignant neoplasm of female genitourinary tract NOS

C58   Malignant neoplasm of placenta   HCC M ♀
  INCLUDES   choriocarcinoma NOS
  chorionepithelioma NOS
  EXCLUDES 1   chorioadenoma (destruens) (D39.2)
  hydatidiform mole NOS (O01.9)
  invasive hydatidiform mole (D39.2)
  male choriocarcinoma NOS (C62.9-)
  malignant hydatidiform mole (D39.2)

Malignant neoplasms of male genital organs (C60-C63)

INCLUDES   malignant neoplasm of skin of male genital organs

C60   Malignant neoplasm of penis
- **C60.0**   Malignant neoplasm of prepuce   HCC ♂
  Malignant neoplasm of foreskin
- **C60.1**   Malignant neoplasm of glans penis   HCC ♂
- **C60.2**   Malignant neoplasm of body of penis   HCC ♂
  Malignant neoplasm of corpus cavernosum
- **C60.8**   Malignant neoplasm of overlapping sites of penis   HCC ♂
- **C60.9**   Malignant neoplasm of penis, unspecified   HCC ♂
  Malignant neoplasm of skin of penis NOS

C61   Malignant neoplasm of prostate   HCC ♂
  Use additional code to identify:
  hormone sensitivity status (Z19.1-Z19.2)
  rising PSA following treatment for malignant neoplasm of prostate (R97.21)
  EXCLUDES 1   malignant neoplasm of seminal vesicle (C63.7)
  AHA: 2017, 1Q, 17

C62   Malignant neoplasm of testis
  Use additional code to identify any functional activity
- **C62.0**   Malignant neoplasm of undescended testis
  Malignant neoplasm of ectopic testis
  Malignant neoplasm of retained testis
  - **C62.00**   Malignant neoplasm of unspecified undescended testis   HCC ♂
  - **C62.01**   Malignant neoplasm of undescended right testis   HCC ♂
  - **C62.02**   Malignant neoplasm of undescended left testis   HCC ♂
- **C62.1**   Malignant neoplasm of descended testis
  Malignant neoplasm of scrotal testis
  - **C62.10**   Malignant neoplasm of unspecified descended testis   HCC ♂
  - **C62.11**   Malignant neoplasm of descended right testis   HCC ♂
  - **C62.12**   Malignant neoplasm of descended left testis   HCC ♂
- **C62.9**   Malignant neoplasm of testis, unspecified whether descended or undescended
  - **C62.90**   Malignant neoplasm of unspecified testis, unspecified whether descended or undescended   HCC ♂
    Malignant neoplasm of testis NOS
  - **C62.91**   Malignant neoplasm of right testis, unspecified whether descended or undescended   HCC ♂
  - **C62.92**   Malignant neoplasm of left testis, unspecified whether descended or undescended   HCC ♂

C63   Malignant neoplasm of other and unspecified male genital organs
- **C63.0**   Malignant neoplasm of epididymis
  - **C63.00**   Malignant neoplasm of unspecified epididymis   HCC ♂
  - **C63.01**   Malignant neoplasm of right epididymis   HCC ♂
  - **C63.02**   Malignant neoplasm of left epididymis   HCC ♂
- **C63.1**   Malignant neoplasm of spermatic cord
  - **C63.10**   Malignant neoplasm of unspecified spermatic cord   HCC ♂
  - **C63.11**   Malignant neoplasm of right spermatic cord   HCC ♂
  - **C63.12**   Malignant neoplasm of left spermatic cord   HCC ♂
- **C63.2**   Malignant neoplasm of scrotum   HCC ♂
  Malignant neoplasm of skin of scrotum
- **C63.7**   Malignant neoplasm of other specified male genital organs   HCC ♂
  Malignant neoplasm of seminal vesicle
  Malignant neoplasm of tunica vaginalis
- **C63.8**   Malignant neoplasm of overlapping sites of male genital organs   HCC ♂
  Primary malignant neoplasm of two or more contiguous sites of male genital organs whose point of origin cannot be determined
- **C63.9**   Malignant neoplasm of male genital organ, unspecified   HCC ♂
  Malignant neoplasm of male genitourinary tract NOS

Malignant neoplasms of urinary tract (C64-C68)

C64   Malignant neoplasm of kidney, except renal pelvis
  EXCLUDES 1   malignant carcinoid tumor of the kidney (C7A.093)
  malignant neoplasm of renal calyces (C65.-)
  malignant neoplasm of renal pelvis (C65.-)

CC Excl: For CC codes in category C64: PDX collection 310
- **C64.1**   Malignant neoplasm of right kidney, except renal pelvis   HCC CC
- **C64.2**   Malignant neoplasm of left kidney, except renal pelvis   HCC CC
- **C64.9**   Malignant neoplasm of unspecified kidney, except renal pelvis   HCC CC

C65   Malignant neoplasm of renal pelvis
  INCLUDES   malignant neoplasm of pelviureteric junction
  malignant neoplasm of renal calyces

CC Excl: For CC codes in category C65: PDX collection 310
- **C65.1**   Malignant neoplasm of right renal pelvis   CC HCC
- **C65.2**   Malignant neoplasm of left renal pelvis   CC HCC
- **C65.9**   Malignant neoplasm of unspecified renal pelvis   CC HCC

C66   Malignant neoplasm of ureter
  EXCLUDES 1   malignant neoplasm of ureteric orifice of bladder (C67.6)

CC Excl: For CC codes in category C66: PDX collection 311
- **C66.1**   Malignant neoplasm of right ureter   CC HCC
- **C66.2**   Malignant neoplasm of left ureter   CC HCC
- **C66.9**   Malignant neoplasm of unspecified ureter   CC HCC

C67   Malignant neoplasm of bladder
- **C67.0**   Malignant neoplasm of trigone of bladder   HCC
- **C67.1**   Malignant neoplasm of dome of bladder   HCC
- **C67.2**   Malignant neoplasm of lateral wall of bladder   HCC
- **C67.3**   Malignant neoplasm of anterior wall of bladder   HCC
- **C67.4**   Malignant neoplasm of posterior wall of bladder   HCC
- **C67.5**   Malignant neoplasm of bladder neck   HCC
  Malignant neoplasm of internal urethral orifice
- **C67.6**   Malignant neoplasm of ureteric orifice   HCC
- **C67.7**   Malignant neoplasm of urachus   HCC
- **C67.8**   Malignant neoplasm of overlapping sites of bladder   HCC
- **C67.9**   Malignant neoplasm of bladder, unspecified   HCC
  AHA: 2016, 1Q, 19

C68   Malignant neoplasm of other and unspecified urinary organs
  EXCLUDES 1   malignant neoplasm of female genitourinary tract NOS (C57.9)
  malignant neoplasm of male genitourinary tract NOS (C63.9)
- **C68.0**   Malignant neoplasm of urethra   CC HCC
  EXCLUDES 1   malignant neoplasm of urethral orifice of bladder (C67.5)
  CC Excl: PDX collection 312

N Newborn: 0   P Pediatric: 0-17   M Maternity: 12-55   A Adult: 15-124   MCC Major Complication/Comorbidity   CC Complication/Comorbidity   SW Severe Wound Dx

C68.1 Malignant neoplasm of paraurethral glands   `CC` `HCC`
     CC Excl: PDX collection 312

C68.8 Malignant neoplasm of overlapping sites **of urinary organs**   `CC` `HCC`
     Primary malignant neoplasm of two or more contiguous sites of urinary organs whose point of origin cannot be determined
     CC Excl: PDX collection 313

C68.9 Malignant neoplasm of urinary organ, unspecified   `CC` `HCC`
     Malignant neoplasm of urinary system NOS
     CC Excl: PDX collection 313

Malignant neoplasms of eye, brain and other parts of central nervous system (C69-C72)

✓4ᵗʰ C69 Malignant neoplasm of eye and adnexa
     EXCLUDES 1   *malignant neoplasm of connective tissue of eyelid (C49.0)*
          malignant neoplasm of eyelid (skin) (C43.1-, C44.1-)
          malignant neoplasm of optic nerve (C72.3-)

   ✓5ᵗʰ C69.0 Malignant neoplasm of conjunctiva
     C69.00 Malignant neoplasm of unspecified **conjunctiva**   `HCC`
     C69.01 Malignant neoplasm of right **conjunctiva**   `HCC`
     C69.02 Malignant neoplasm of left **conjunctiva**   `HCC`

   ✓5ᵗʰ C69.1 Malignant neoplasm of cornea
     C69.10 Malignant neoplasm of unspecified **cornea**   `HCC`
     C69.11 Malignant neoplasm of right **cornea**   `HCC`
     C69.12 Malignant neoplasm of left **cornea**   `HCC`

   ✓5ᵗʰ C69.2 Malignant neoplasm of retina
     EXCLUDES 1   *dark area on retina (D49.81)*
          neoplasm of unspecified behavior of retina and choroid (D49.81)
          retinal freckle (D49.81)
     C69.20 Malignant neoplasm of unspecified **retina**   `HCC`
     C69.21 Malignant neoplasm of right **retina**   `HCC`
     C69.22 Malignant neoplasm of left **retina**   `HCC`

   ✓5ᵗʰ C69.3 Malignant neoplasm of choroid
     C69.30 Malignant neoplasm of unspecified **choroid**   `HCC`
     C69.31 Malignant neoplasm of right **choroid**   `HCC`
     C69.32 Malignant neoplasm of left **choroid**   `HCC`

   ✓5ᵗʰ C69.4 Malignant neoplasm of ciliary body
     C69.40 Malignant neoplasm of unspecified **ciliary body**   `HCC`
     C69.41 Malignant neoplasm of right **ciliary body**   `HCC`
     C69.42 Malignant neoplasm of left **ciliary body**   `HCC`

   ✓5ᵗʰ C69.5 Malignant neoplasm of lacrimal gland and duct
     Malignant neoplasm of lacrimal sac
     Malignant neoplasm of nasolacrimal duct
     C69.50 Malignant neoplasm of unspecified **lacrimal gland and duct**   `HCC`
     C69.51 Malignant neoplasm of right **lacrimal gland and duct**   `HCC`
     C69.52 Malignant neoplasm of left **lacrimal gland and duct**   `HCC`

   ✓5ᵗʰ C69.6 Malignant neoplasm of orbit
     Malignant neoplasm of connective tissue of orbit
     Malignant neoplasm of extraocular muscle
     Malignant neoplasm of peripheral nerves of orbit
     Malignant neoplasm of retrobulbar tissue
     Malignant neoplasm of retro-ocular tissue
     EXCLUDES 1   *malignant neoplasm of orbital bone (C41.0)*
     C69.60 Malignant neoplasm of unspecified **orbit**   `HCC`
     C69.61 Malignant neoplasm of right **orbit**   `HCC`
     C69.62 Malignant neoplasm of left **orbit**   `HCC`

   ✓5ᵗʰ C69.8 Malignant neoplasm of overlapping sites **of eye and adnexa**
     C69.80 Malignant neoplasm of overlapping sites of unspecified **eye and adnexa**   `HCC`
     C69.81 Malignant neoplasm of overlapping sites of right **eye and adnexa**   `HCC`
     C69.82 Malignant neoplasm of overlapping sites of left **eye and adnexa**   `HCC`

   ✓5ᵗʰ C69.9 Malignant neoplasm of unspecified **site of eye**
     Malignant neoplasm of eyeball
     C69.90 Malignant neoplasm of unspecified site of unspecified **eye**   `HCC`
     C69.91 Malignant neoplasm of unspecified site of right **eye**   `HCC`

C69.92 Malignant neoplasm of unspecified site of left **eye**   `HCC`

✓4ᵗʰ C70 Malignant neoplasm of meninges
   C70.0 Malignant neoplasm of cerebral **meninges**   `CC` `HCC`
     CC Excl: PDX collection 314
   C70.1 Malignant neoplasm of spinal **meninges**   `CC` `HCC`
     CC Excl: PDX collection 315
   C70.9 Malignant neoplasm of meninges, unspecified   `CC` `HCC`
     CC Excl: PDX collection 314

✓4ᵗʰ C71 Malignant neoplasm of brain
   EXCLUDES 1   *malignant neoplasm of cranial nerves (C72.2-C72.5)*
          retrobulbar malignant neoplasm (C69.6-)

   CC Excl: For CC codes in category C71: PDX collection 316

   C71.0 Malignant neoplasm of cerebrum, except lobes and ventricles   `CC` `HCC`
     Malignant neoplasm of supratentorial NOS
   C71.1 Malignant neoplasm of frontal **lobe**   `CC` `HCC`
   C71.2 Malignant neoplasm of temporal **lobe**   `CC` `HCC`
   C71.3 Malignant neoplasm of parietal **lobe**   `CC` `HCC`
   C71.4 Malignant neoplasm of occipital **lobe**   `CC` `HCC`
   C71.5 Malignant neoplasm of cerebral **ventricle**   `CC` `HCC`
     EXCLUDES 1   *malignant neoplasm of fourth cerebral ventricle (C71.7)*
   C71.6 Malignant neoplasm of cerebellum   `CC` `HCC`
   C71.7 Malignant neoplasm of brain stem   `CC` `HCC`
     Malignant neoplasm of fourth cerebral ventricle
     Infratentorial malignant neoplasm NOS
   C71.8 Malignant neoplasm of overlapping sites **of brain**   `CC` `HCC`
   C71.9 Malignant neoplasm of brain, unspecified   `CC` `HCC`
     AHA: 2014, 3Q, 3

Lobes of the Brain

Frontal lobe • Parietal lobe • Occipital lobe • Temporal lobe • Brain stem • Cerebellum

✓4ᵗʰ C72 Malignant neoplasm of spinal cord, cranial nerves and other parts of central nervous system
   EXCLUDES 1   *malignant neoplasm of meninges (C70.-)*
          malignant neoplasm of peripheral nerves and autonomic nervous system (C47.-)

   CC Excl: For CC codes in category C72, unless otherwise noted: PDX collection 318

   C72.0 Malignant neoplasm of spinal cord   `CC` `HCC`
     CC Excl: PDX collection 317
   C72.1 Malignant neoplasm of cauda equina   `CC` `HCC`
     CC Excl: PDX collection 317
   ✓5ᵗʰ C72.2 Malignant neoplasm of olfactory nerve
     Malignant neoplasm of olfactory bulb
     C72.20 Malignant neoplasm of unspecified olfactory **nerve**   `CC` `HCC`
     C72.21 Malignant neoplasm of right olfactory nerve   `CC` `HCC`
     C72.22 Malignant neoplasm of left olfactory nerve   `CC` `HCC`
   ✓5ᵗʰ C72.3 Malignant neoplasm of optic nerve
     C72.30 Malignant neoplasm of unspecified optic **nerve**   `CC` `HCC`
     C72.31 Malignant neoplasm of right optic nerve   `CC` `HCC`
     C72.32 Malignant neoplasm of left optic nerve   `CC` `HCC`

✓5ᵗʰ C72.4 Malignant neoplasm of acoustic nerve

    C72.4Ø Malignant neoplasm of unspecified acoustic nerve `CC` `HCC`

    C72.41 Malignant neoplasm of right acoustic nerve `CC` `HCC`

    C72.42 Malignant neoplasm of left acoustic nerve `CC` `HCC`

✓5ᵗʰ C72.5 Malignant neoplasm of other and unspecified cranial nerves

    C72.5Ø Malignant neoplasm of unspecified cranial nerve `CC` `HCC`

        Malignant neoplasm of cranial nerve NOS

    C72.59 Malignant neoplasm of other cranial nerves `CC` `HCC`

  C72.9 Malignant neoplasm of central nervous system, unspecified `CC` `HCC`

    Malignant neoplasm of unspecified site of central nervous system

    Malignant neoplasm of nervous system NOS

    CC Excl: PDX collection 319

Malignant neoplasms of thyroid and other endocrine glands (C73-C75)

C73 Malignant neoplasm of thyroid gland `HCC`

  Use additional code to identify any functional activity

✓4ᵗʰ C74 Malignant neoplasm of adrenal gland

  TIP: If an adrenal gland tumor is described as functional (producing too much of a hormone), additional codes should be assigned to report the functional activity.

  CC Excl: For CC codes in category C74: PDX collection 32Ø

✓5ᵗʰ C74.Ø Malignant neoplasm of cortex of adrenal gland

    C74.ØØ Malignant neoplasm of cortex of unspecified adrenal gland `CC` `HCC`

    C74.Ø1 Malignant neoplasm of cortex of right adrenal gland `CC` `HCC`

    C74.Ø2 Malignant neoplasm of cortex of left adrenal gland `CC` `HCC`

✓5ᵗʰ C74.1 Malignant neoplasm of medulla of adrenal gland

    C74.1Ø Malignant neoplasm of medulla of unspecified adrenal gland `CC` `HCC`

    C74.11 Malignant neoplasm of medulla of right adrenal gland `CC` `HCC`

    C74.12 Malignant neoplasm of medulla of left adrenal gland `CC` `HCC`

✓5ᵗʰ C74.9 Malignant neoplasm of unspecified part of adrenal gland

    C74.9Ø Malignant neoplasm of unspecified part of unspecified adrenal gland `CC` `HCC`

    C74.91 Malignant neoplasm of unspecified part of right adrenal gland `CC` `HCC`

    C74.92 Malignant neoplasm of unspecified part of left adrenal gland `CC` `HCC`

✓4ᵗʰ C75 Malignant neoplasm of other endocrine glands and related structures

  EXCLUDES 1 malignant carcinoid tumors (C7A.Ø-)
        malignant neoplasm of adrenal gland (C74.-)
        malignant neoplasm of endocrine pancreas (C25.4)
        malignant neoplasm of islets of Langerhans (C25.4)
        malignant neoplasm of ovary (C56.-)
        malignant neoplasm of testis (C62.-)
        malignant neoplasm of thymus (C37)
        malignant neoplasm of thyroid gland (C73)
        malignant neuroendocrine tumors (C7A.-)

  C75.Ø Malignant neoplasm of parathyroid gland `CC` `HCC`
    CC Excl: PDX collection 321

  C75.1 Malignant neoplasm of pituitary gland `CC` `HCC`
    CC Excl: PDX collection 322

  C75.2 Malignant neoplasm of craniopharyngeal duct `CC` `HCC`
    CC Excl: PDX collection 322

  C75.3 Malignant neoplasm of pineal gland `CC` `HCC`
    CC Excl: PDX collection 323

  C75.4 Malignant neoplasm of carotid body `CC` `HCC`
    CC Excl: PDX collection 324

  C75.5 Malignant neoplasm of aortic body and other paraganglia `CC` `HCC`
    CC Excl: PDX collection 325

  C75.8 Malignant neoplasm with pluriglandular involvement, unspecified `CC` `HCC`
    CC Excl: PDX collection 326

C75.9 Malignant neoplasm of endocrine gland, unspecified `CC` `HCC`
  CC Excl: PDX collection 326

Malignant neuroendocrine tumors (C7A)

✓4ᵗʰ C7A Malignant neuroendocrine tumors

  Code also any associated multiple endocrine neoplasia [MEN] syndromes (E31.2-)

  Use additional code to identify any associated endocrine syndrome, such as:

    carcinoid syndrome (E34.Ø)

  EXCLUDES 2 malignant pancreatic islet cell tumors (C25.4)
        Merkel cell carcinoma (C4A.-)

  DEF: Tumors comprised of cells that are capable of producing hormonal syndromes in which the normal hormonal balance required to support body system functions is adversely affected.

✓5ᵗʰ C7A.Ø Malignant carcinoid tumors

  DEF: Specific type of slow-growing benign or malignant neuroendocrine tumors. Carcinoid tumors occur most commonly in the hormone producing cells of the gastrointestinal tracts and can also occur in the pancreas, testes, ovaries, or lungs.

  C7A.ØØ Malignant carcinoid tumor of unspecified site `CC` `HCC`
    CC Excl: PDX collection 346

✓6ᵗʰ C7A.Ø1 Malignant carcinoid tumors of the small intestine

    C7A.Ø1Ø Malignant carcinoid tumor of the duodenum `CC` `HCC`
        CC Excl: PDX collection 347

    C7A.Ø11 Malignant carcinoid tumor of the jejunum `CC` `HCC`
        CC Excl: PDX collection 348

    C7A.Ø12 Malignant carcinoid tumor of the ileum `CC` `HCC`
        CC Excl: PDX collection 349

    C7A.Ø19 Malignant carcinoid tumor of the small intestine, unspecified portion `CC` `HCC`
        CC Excl: PDX collection 35Ø

✓6ᵗʰ C7A.Ø2 Malignant carcinoid tumors of the appendix, large intestine, and rectum

    C7A.Ø2Ø Malignant carcinoid tumor of the appendix `CC` `HCC`
        CC Excl: PDX collection 351

    C7A.Ø21 Malignant carcinoid tumor of the cecum `CC` `HCC`
        CC Excl: PDX collection 352

    C7A.Ø22 Malignant carcinoid tumor of the ascending colon `CC` `HCC`
        CC Excl: PDX collection 353

    C7A.Ø23 Malignant carcinoid tumor of the transverse colon `CC` `HCC`
        CC Excl: PDX collection 354

    C7A.Ø24 Malignant carcinoid tumor of the descending colon `CC` `HCC`
        CC Excl: PDX collection 355

    C7A.Ø25 Malignant carcinoid tumor of the sigmoid colon `CC` `HCC`
        CC Excl: PDX collection 356

    C7A.Ø26 Malignant carcinoid tumor of the rectum `CC` `HCC`
        CC Excl: PDX collection 357

    C7A.Ø29 Malignant carcinoid tumor of the large, intestine, unspecified portion `CC` `HCC`
        Malignant carcinoid tumor of the colon NOS
        CC Excl: PDX collection 358

✓6ᵗʰ C7A.Ø9 Malignant carcinoid tumors of other sites

    C7A.Ø9Ø Malignant carcinoid tumor of the bronchus and lung `CC` `HCC`
        CC Excl: PDX collection 359

    C7A.Ø91 Malignant carcinoid tumor of the thymus `CC` `HCC`
        CC Excl: PDX collection 36Ø

    C7A.Ø92 Malignant carcinoid tumor of the stomach `CC` `HCC`
        CC Excl: PDX collection 361

    C7A.Ø93 Malignant carcinoid tumor of the kidney `CC` `HCC`
        CC Excl: PDX collection 362

    C7A.Ø94 Malignant carcinoid tumor of the foregut, unspecified `CC` `HCC`
        CC Excl: PDX collection 361

C7A.Ø95 **Malignant carcinoid tumor of the** `CC` `HCC`
midgut, unspecified
    CC Excl: PDX collection 361

C7A.Ø96 **Malignant carcinoid tumor of the** `CC` `HCC`
hindgut, unspecified
    CC Excl: PDX collection 361

C7A.Ø98 **Malignant carcinoid tumors of** `CC` `HCC`
other sites
    CC Excl: PDX collection 346

C7A.1 **Malignant poorly differentiated neuroendocrine** `CC` `HCC`
tumors
    High grade neuroendocrine carcinoma, any site
    Malignant poorly differentiated neuroendocrine tumor NOS
    Malignant poorly differentiated neuroendocrine carcinoma, any
    site
    CC Excl: PDX collection 346

C7A.8 **Other malignant neuroendocrine tumors** `CC` `HCC`
    CC Excl: PDX collection 346

Secondary neuroendocrine tumors (C7B)

✓4ᵗʰ **C7B** **Secondary neuroendocrine tumors**
    Use additional code to identify any functional activity

✓5ᵗʰ **C7B.Ø** **Secondary carcinoid tumors**

C7B.ØØ **Secondary carcinoid tumors, unspecified site** `HCC`

C7B.Ø1 **Secondary carcinoid tumors of distant lymph** `CC` `HCC`
nodes
    CC Excl: PDX collection 363

C7B.Ø2 **Secondary carcinoid tumors of liver** `CC` `HCC`
    CC Excl: PDX collection 364

C7B.Ø3 **Secondary carcinoid tumors of bone** `CC` `HCC`
    CC Excl: PDX collection 365

C7B.Ø4 **Secondary carcinoid tumors of peritoneum** `CC` `HCC`
    Mesentery metastasis of carcinoid tumor
    CC Excl: PDX collection 366

C7B.Ø9 **Secondary carcinoid tumors of other sites** `CC` `HCC`
    CC Excl: PDX collection 367

C7B.1 **Secondary Merkel cell carcinoma** `HCC`
    Merkel cell carcinoma nodal presentation
    Merkel cell carcinoma visceral metastatic presentation

C7B.8 **Other secondary neuroendocrine tumors** `CC` `HCC`
    CC Excl: PDX collection 367

Malignant neoplasms of ill-defined, other secondary and unspecified sites (C76-C8Ø)

✓4ᵗʰ **C76** **Malignant neoplasm of other and ill-defined sites**
    EXCLUDES 1 malignant neoplasm of female genitourinary tract NOS (C57.9)
        malignant neoplasm of male genitourinary tract NOS (C63.9)
        malignant neoplasm of lymphoid, hematopoietic and related
          tissue (C81-C96)
        malignant neoplasm of skin (C44.-)
        malignant neoplasm of unspecified site NOS (C8Ø.1)

C76.Ø **Malignant neoplasm of head, face and neck** `HCC`
    Malignant neoplasm of cheek NOS
    Malignant neoplasm of nose NOS

C76.1 **Malignant neoplasm of thorax** `HCC`
    Intrathoracic malignant neoplasm NOS
    Malignant neoplasm of axilla NOS
    Thoracic malignant neoplasm NOS

C76.2 **Malignant neoplasm of abdomen** `HCC`

C76.3 **Malignant neoplasm of pelvis** `HCC`
    Malignant neoplasm of groin NOS
    Malignant neoplasm of sites overlapping systems within the
       pelvis
    Rectovaginal (septum) malignant neoplasm
    Rectovesical (septum) malignant neoplasm

✓5ᵗʰ **C76.4** **Malignant neoplasm of upper limb**

C76.4Ø **Malignant neoplasm of unspecified upper limb** `HCC`

C76.41 **Malignant neoplasm of right upper limb** `HCC`

C76.42 **Malignant neoplasm of left upper limb** `HCC`

✓5ᵗʰ **C76.5** **Malignant neoplasm of lower limb**

C76.5Ø **Malignant neoplasm of unspecified lower limb** `HCC`

C76.51 **Malignant neoplasm of right lower limb** `HCC`

C76.52 **Malignant neoplasm of left lower limb** `HCC`

C76.8 **Malignant neoplasm of other specified ill-defined sites** `HCC`
    Malignant neoplasm of overlapping ill-defined sites

✓4ᵗʰ **C77** **Secondary and unspecified malignant neoplasm of lymph nodes**
    EXCLUDES 1 malignant neoplasm of lymph nodes, specified as primary (C81-
          C86, C88, C96.-)
        mesentery metastasis of carcinoid tumor (C7B.Ø4)
        secondary carcinoid tumors of distant lymph nodes (C7B.Ø1)

    CC Excl: For CC codes in category C77: PDX collection 3Ø3

C77.Ø **Secondary and unspecified malignant neoplasm of** `CC` `HCC`
lymph nodes of head, face and neck
    Secondary and unspecified malignant neoplasm of
       supraclavicular lymph nodes

C77.1 **Secondary and unspecified malignant neoplasm of** `CC` `HCC`
intrathoracic lymph nodes

C77.2 **Secondary and unspecified malignant neoplasm of** `CC` `HCC`
intra-abdominal lymph nodes

C77.3 **Secondary and unspecified malignant neoplasm of** `CC` `HCC`
axilla and upper limb lymph nodes
    Secondary and unspecified malignant neoplasm of pectoral
       lymph nodes

C77.4 **Secondary and unspecified malignant neoplasm of** `CC` `HCC`
inguinal and lower limb lymph nodes

C77.5 **Secondary and unspecified malignant neoplasm of** `CC` `HCC`
intrapelvic lymph nodes

C77.8 **Secondary and unspecified malignant neoplasm of** `CC` `HCC`
lymph nodes of multiple regions

C77.9 **Secondary and unspecified malignant neoplasm of** `CC` `HCC`
lymph node, unspecified

✓4ᵗʰ **C78** **Secondary malignant neoplasm of respiratory and digestive organs**
    EXCLUDES 1 secondary carcinoid tumors of liver (C7B.Ø2)
        secondary carcinoid tumors of peritoneum (C7B.Ø4)
    EXCLUDES 2 lymph node metastases (C77.Ø)

✓5ᵗʰ **C78.Ø** **Secondary malignant neoplasm of lung**

    CC Excl: For CC codes in subcategory C78.Ø:
    PDX collection 327

C78.ØØ **Secondary malignant neoplasm of** `CC` `HCC`
unspecified lung

C78.Ø1 **Secondary malignant neoplasm of right lung** `CC` `HCC`

C78.Ø2 **Secondary malignant neoplasm of left lung** `CC` `HCC`

C78.1 **Secondary malignant neoplasm of mediastinum** `CC` `HCC`
    CC Excl: PDX collection 328

C78.2 **Secondary malignant neoplasm of pleura** `CC` `HCC`
    CC Excl: PDX collection 329

✓5ᵗʰ **C78.3** **Secondary malignant neoplasm of other and unspecified respiratory organs**

C78.3Ø **Secondary malignant neoplasm of** `CC` `HCC`
unspecified respiratory organ
    CC Excl: PDX collection 33Ø

C78.39 **Secondary malignant neoplasm of other** `CC` `HCC`
respiratory organs
    CC Excl: PDX collection 33Ø

C78.4 **Secondary malignant neoplasm of small intestine** `CC` `HCC`
    CC Excl: PDX collection 331

C78.5 **Secondary malignant neoplasm of large intestine and** `CC` `HCC`
rectum
    CC Excl: PDX collection 332

C78.6 **Secondary malignant neoplasm of retroperitoneum** `CC` `HCC`
and peritoneum
    AHA: 2017, 2Q, 12
    CC Excl: PDX collection 333

C78.7 **Secondary malignant neoplasm of liver and** `CC` `HCC`
intrahepatic bile duct
    CC Excl: PDX collection 334

✓5ᵗʰ **C78.8** **Secondary malignant neoplasm of other and unspecified digestive organs**

C78.8Ø **Secondary malignant neoplasm of** `CC` `HCC`
digestive unspecified organ
    CC Excl: PDX collection 335

C78.89 **Secondary malignant neoplasm of other** `CC` `HCC`
digestive organs
    Code also exocrine pancreatic insufficiency (K86.81)
    CC Excl: PDX collection 335

✓ Additional Character Required   ✓x7ᵗʰ Placeholder   Unacceptable PDx   Questionable PDx   Manifestation   H1 - H14 HAC   HCC CMS-HCC Dx   HIV HIV Dx

ICD-10-CM 2019   479

Chapter 2. Neoplasms

C7A.Ø95–C78.89

✓4ᵗʰ **C79 Secondary malignant neoplasm of other and unspecified sites**
> EXCLUDES 1   *secondary carcinoid tumors (C7B.-)*
> *secondary neuroendocrine tumors (C7B.-)*

✓5ᵗʰ **C79.Ø Secondary malignant neoplasm of kidney and renal pelvis**

> **CC Excl: For CC codes in subcategory C79.Ø:**
> PDX collection 336

     C79.ØØ Secondary malignant neoplasm of CC HCC
                unspecified kidney and renal pelvis

     C79.Ø1 Secondary malignant neoplasm of right CC HCC
                kidney and renal pelvis

     C79.Ø2 Secondary malignant neoplasm of left CC HCC
                kidney and renal pelvis

✓5ᵗʰ **C79.1 Secondary malignant neoplasm of bladder and other and unspecified urinary organs**

> **CC Excl: For CC codes in subcategory C79.1:**
> PDX collection 336

     C79.1Ø Secondary malignant neoplasm of CC HCC
                unspecified urinary organs

     C79.11 Secondary malignant neoplasm of bladder CC HCC
> EXCLUDES 2   *lymph node metastases (C77.Ø)*

     C79.19 Secondary malignant neoplasm of other CC HCC
                urinary organs

C79.2 Secondary malignant neoplasm of skin CC HCC
> EXCLUDES 1   *secondary Merkel cell carcinoma (C7B.1)*
> **CC Excl:** PDX collection 337

✓5ᵗʰ **C79.3 Secondary malignant neoplasm of brain and cerebral meninges**

     C79.31 Secondary malignant neoplasm of brain CC HCC
                CC Excl: PDX collection 338

     C79.32 Secondary malignant neoplasm of cerebral CC HCC
                meninges
                CC Excl: PDX collection 339

✓5ᵗʰ **C79.4 Secondary malignant neoplasm of other and unspecified parts of nervous system**

     C79.4Ø Secondary malignant neoplasm of CC HCC
                unspecified part of nervous system
                CC Excl: PDX collection 339

     C79.49 Secondary malignant neoplasm of other CC HCC
                parts of nervous system
                CC Excl: PDX collection 339

✓5ᵗʰ **C79.5 Secondary malignant neoplasm of bone and bone marrow**
> EXCLUDES 1   *secondary carcinoid tumors of bone (C7B.Ø3)*

     C79.51 Secondary malignant neoplasm of bone CC HCC
                TIP: Do not assign in addition to a code from subcategory C9Ø.Ø when multiple myeloma is described as metastatic to the bone; bone involvement is integral to multiple myeloma.
                CC Excl: PDX collection 34Ø

     C79.52 Secondary malignant neoplasm of bone CC HCC
                marrow
                CC Excl: PDX collection 34Ø

✓5ᵗʰ **C79.6 Secondary malignant neoplasm of ovary**

> **CC Excl: For CC codes in subcategory C79.6:**
> PDX collection 341

     C79.6Ø Secondary malignant neoplasm of CC HCC ♀
                unspecified ovary

     C79.61 Secondary malignant neoplasm of right CC HCC ♀
                ovary

     C79.62 Secondary malignant neoplasm of left CC HCC ♀
                ovary

✓5ᵗʰ **C79.7 Secondary malignant neoplasm of adrenal gland**

> **CC Excl: For CC codes in subcategory C79.7:**
> PDX collection 342

     C79.7Ø Secondary malignant neoplasm of CC HCC
                unspecified adrenal gland

     C79.71 Secondary malignant neoplasm of right CC HCC
                adrenal gland

     C79.72 Secondary malignant neoplasm of left CC HCC
                adrenal gland

✓5ᵗʰ **C79.8 Secondary malignant neoplasm of other specified sites**

     C79.81 Secondary malignant neoplasm of breast CC HCC
                CC Excl: PDX collection 343

     C79.82 Secondary malignant neoplasm of CC HCC
                genital organs
                CC Excl: PDX collection 344

     C79.89 Secondary malignant neoplasm of other CC HCC
                specified sites
                AHA: 2017, 2Q, 11
                CC Excl: PDX collection 345

C79.9 Secondary malignant neoplasm of unspecified site CC HCC
     Metastatic cancer NOS
     Metastatic disease NOS
> EXCLUDES 1   *carcinomatosis NOS (C8Ø.Ø)*
> *generalized cancer NOS (C8Ø.Ø)*
> *malignant (primary) neoplasm of unspecified site (C8Ø.1)*
> **CC Excl:** PDX collection 345

✓4ᵗʰ **C8Ø Malignant neoplasm without specification of site**
> EXCLUDES 1   *malignant carcinoid tumor of unspecified site (C7A.ØØ)*
> *malignant neoplasm of specified multiple sites—code to each site*

C8Ø.Ø Disseminated malignant neoplasm, unspecified CC HCC
     Carcinomatosis NOS
     Generalized cancer, unspecified site (primary) (secondary)
     Generalized malignancy, unspecified site (primary) (secondary)
     CC Excl: PDX collection 345

C8Ø.1 Malignant (primary) neoplasm, unspecified HCC
     Cancer NOS
     Cancer unspecified site (primary)
     Carcinoma unspecified site (primary)
     Malignancy unspecified site (primary)
> EXCLUDES 1   *secondary malignant neoplasm of unspecified site (C79.9)*

C8Ø.2 Malignant neoplasm associated with transplanted organ CC HCC
     Code first complication of transplanted organ (T86.-)
     Use additional code to identify the specific malignancy
     CC Excl: PDX collection 345

Malignant neoplasms of lymphoid, hematopoietic and related tissue (C81-C96)

> EXCLUDES 2   *Kaposi's sarcoma of lymph nodes (C46.3)*
> *secondary and unspecified neoplasm of lymph nodes (C77.-)*
> *secondary neoplasm of bone marrow (C79.52)*
> *secondary neoplasm of spleen (C78.89)*

✓4ᵗʰ **C81 Hodgkin lymphoma**
> EXCLUDES 1   *personal history of Hodgkin lymphoma (Z85.71)*
> **DEF:** Malignant disorder of lymphoid cells characterized by the presence of progressively swollen lymph nodes and spleen that may also involve the liver. A diagnosis of Hodgkin's lymphoma can be confirmed by the presence of Reed-Sternberg cells. ***Synonym(s):*** *Hodgkin disease.*

✓5ᵗʰ **C81.Ø Nodular lymphocyte predominant Hodgkin lymphoma**

     C81.ØØ Nodular lymphocyte predominant Hodgkin CC HCC
                lymphoma, unspecified site
                CC Excl: PDX collection 368

     C81.Ø1 Nodular lymphocyte predominant Hodgkin CC HCC
                lymphoma, lymph nodes of head, face, and neck
                CC Excl: PDX collection 369

     C81.Ø2 Nodular lymphocyte predominant Hodgkin CC HCC
                lymphoma, intrathoracic lymph nodes
                CC Excl: PDX collection 37Ø

     C81.Ø3 Nodular lymphocyte predominant Hodgkin CC HCC
                lymphoma, intra-abdominal lymph nodes
                CC Excl: PDX collection 371

     C81.Ø4 Nodular lymphocyte predominant Hodgkin CC HCC
                lymphoma, lymph nodes of axilla and upper limb
                CC Excl: PDX collection 372

     C81.Ø5 Nodular lymphocyte predominant Hodgkin CC HCC
                lymphoma, lymph nodes of inguinal region and lower limb
                CC Excl: PDX collection 373

     C81.Ø6 Nodular lymphocyte predominant Hodgkin CC HCC
                lymphoma, intrapelvic lymph nodes
                CC Excl: PDX collection 374

     C81.Ø7 Nodular lymphocyte predominant Hodgkin CC HCC
                lymphoma, spleen
                CC Excl: PDX collection 375

     C81.Ø8 Nodular lymphocyte predominant Hodgkin CC HCC
                lymphoma, lymph nodes of multiple sites
                CC Excl: PDX collection 368

N Newborn: 0   P Pediatric: 0-17   M Maternity: 12-55   A Adult: 15-124   MCC Major Complication/Comorbidity   CC Complication/Comorbidity   SW Severe Wound Dx

C81.09 **Nodular lymphocyte predominant Hodgkin lymphoma,** extranodal and solid organ sites   CC HCC
CC Excl: PDX collection 368

☑5ᵗʰ **C81.1** Nodular sclerosis **Hodgkin lymphoma**
Nodular sclerosis classical Hodgkin lymphoma

C81.10 **Nodular sclerosis Hodgkin lymphoma,** unspecified site   CC HCC
CC Excl: PDX collection 376

C81.11 **Nodular sclerosis Hodgkin lymphoma, lymph nodes of** head, face, and neck   CC HCC
CC Excl: PDX collection 377

C81.12 **Nodular sclerosis Hodgkin lymphoma,** intrathoracic **lymph nodes**   CC HCC
CC Excl: PDX collection 378

C81.13 **Nodular sclerosis Hodgkin lymphoma,** intra-abdominal **lymph nodes**   CC HCC
CC Excl: PDX collection 379

C81.14 **Nodular sclerosis Hodgkin lymphoma, lymph nodes of** axilla and upper limb   CC HCC
CC Excl: PDX collection 380

C81.15 **Nodular sclerosis Hodgkin lymphoma, lymph nodes of** inguinal region and lower limb   CC HCC
CC Excl: PDX collection 381

C81.16 **Nodular sclerosis Hodgkin lymphoma,** intrapelvic **lymph nodes**   CC HCC
CC Excl: PDX collection 382

C81.17 **Nodular sclerosis Hodgkin lymphoma,** spleen   CC HCC
CC Excl: PDX collection 383

C81.18 **Nodular sclerosis Hodgkin lymphoma, lymph nodes of** multiple sites   CC HCC
CC Excl: PDX collection 376

C81.19 **Nodular sclerosis Hodgkin lymphoma,** extranodal and solid organ sites   CC HCC
CC Excl: PDX collection 376

☑5ᵗʰ **C81.2** Mixed cellularity **Hodgkin lymphoma**
Mixed cellularity classical Hodgkin lymphoma

C81.20 **Mixed cellularity Hodgkin lymphoma,** unspecified site   CC HCC
CC Excl: PDX collection 384

C81.21 **Mixed cellularity Hodgkin lymphoma, lymph nodes of** head, face, and neck   CC HCC
CC Excl: PDX collection 385

C81.22 **Mixed cellularity Hodgkin lymphoma,** intrathoracic **lymph nodes**   CC HCC
CC Excl: PDX collection 386

C81.23 **Mixed cellularity Hodgkin lymphoma,** intra-abdominal **lymph nodes**   CC HCC
CC Excl: PDX collection 387

C81.24 **Mixed cellularity Hodgkin lymphoma, lymph nodes of** axilla and upper limb   CC HCC
CC Excl: PDX collection 388

C81.25 **Mixed cellularity Hodgkin lymphoma, lymph nodes of** inguinal region and lower limb   CC HCC
CC Excl: PDX collection 389

C81.26 **Mixed cellularity Hodgkin lymphoma,** intrapelvic **lymph nodes**   CC HCC
CC Excl: CPDX collection 390

C81.27 **Mixed cellularity Hodgkin lymphoma,** spleen   CC HCC
CC Excl: PDX collection 391

C81.28 **Mixed cellularity Hodgkin lymphoma, lymph nodes of** multiple sites   CC HCC
CC Excl: PDX collection 384

C81.29 **Mixed cellularity Hodgkin lymphoma,** extranodal and solid organ sites   CC HCC
CC Excl: PDX collection 384

☑5ᵗʰ **C81.3** Lymphocyte depleted **Hodgkin lymphoma**
Lymphocyte depleted classical Hodgkin lymphoma

C81.30 **Lymphocyte depleted Hodgkin lymphoma,** unspecified site   CC HCC
CC Excl: PDX collection 392

C81.31 **Lymphocyte depleted Hodgkin lymphoma, lymph nodes of** head, face, and neck   CC HCC
CC Excl: PDX collection 393

C81.32 **Lymphocyte depleted Hodgkin lymphoma,** intrathoracic **lymph nodes**   CC HCC
CC Excl: PDX collection 394

C81.33 **Lymphocyte depleted Hodgkin lymphoma,** intra-abdominal **lymph nodes**   CC HCC
CC Excl: PDX collection 395

C81.34 **Lymphocyte depleted Hodgkin lymphoma, lymph nodes of** axilla and upper limb   CC HCC
CC Excl: PDX collection 396

C81.35 **Lymphocyte depleted Hodgkin lymphoma, lymph nodes of** inguinal region and lower limb   CC HCC
CC Excl: PDX collection 397

C81.36 **Lymphocyte depleted Hodgkin lymphoma,** intrapelvic **lymph nodes**   CC HCC
CC Excl: PDX collection 398

C81.37 **Lymphocyte depleted Hodgkin lymphoma,** spleen   CC HCC
CC Excl: PDX collection 399

C81.38 **Lymphocyte depleted Hodgkin lymphoma, lymph nodes of** multiple sites   CC HCC
CC Excl: PDX collection 400

C81.39 **Lymphocyte depleted Hodgkin lymphoma,** extranodal and solid organ sites   CC HCC
CC Excl: PDX collection 392

☑5ᵗʰ **C81.4** Lymphocyte-rich **Hodgkin lymphoma**
Lymphocyte-rich classical Hodgkin lymphoma
EXCLUDES 1   nodular lymphocyte predominant Hodgkin lymphoma (C81.0-)

C81.40 **Lymphocyte-rich Hodgkin lymphoma,** unspecified site   CC HCC
CC Excl: PDX collection 368

C81.41 **Lymphocyte-rich Hodgkin lymphoma, lymph nodes of** head, face, and neck   CC HCC
CC Excl: PDX collection 369

C81.42 **Lymphocyte-rich Hodgkin lymphoma,** intrathoracic **lymph nodes**   CC HCC
CC Excl: PDX collection 370

C81.43 **Lymphocyte-rich Hodgkin lymphoma,** intra-abdominal **lymph nodes**   CC HCC
CC Excl: PDX collection 371

C81.44 **Lymphocyte-rich Hodgkin lymphoma, lymph nodes of** axilla and upper limb   CC HCC
CC Excl: PDX collection 372

C81.45 **Lymphocyte-rich Hodgkin lymphoma, lymph nodes of** inguinal region and lower limb   CC HCC
CC Excl: PDX collection 373

C81.46 **Lymphocyte-rich Hodgkin lymphoma,** intrapelvic **lymph nodes**   CC HCC
CC Excl: PDX collection 374

C81.47 **Lymphocyte-rich Hodgkin lymphoma,** spleen   CC HCC
CC Excl: CPDX collection 375

C81.48 **Lymphocyte-rich Hodgkin lymphoma, lymph nodes of** multiple sites   CC HCC
CC Excl: PDX collection 368

C81.49 **Lymphocyte-rich Hodgkin lymphoma,** extranodal and solid organ sites   CC HCC
CC Excl: PDX collection 368

☑5ᵗʰ **C81.7** Other **Hodgkin lymphoma**
Classical Hodgkin lymphoma NOS
Other classical Hodgkin lymphoma

C81.70 **Other Hodgkin lymphoma,** unspecified site   CC HCC
CC Excl: PDX collection 401

C81.71 **Other Hodgkin lymphoma, lymph nodes of** head, face, and neck   CC HCC
CC Excl: PDX collection 402

C81.72 **Other Hodgkin lymphoma,** intrathoracic **lymph nodes**   CC HCC
CC Excl: PDX collection 403

C81.73 **Other Hodgkin lymphoma,** intra-abdominal **lymph nodes**   CC HCC
CC Excl: PDX collection 404

C81.74 **Other Hodgkin lymphoma, lymph nodes of** axilla and upper limb   CC HCC
CC Excl: PDX collection 405

C81.75 **Other Hodgkin lymphoma, lymph nodes of** inguinal region and lower limb   CC HCC
CC Excl: PDX collection 406

C81.76 **Other Hodgkin lymphoma,** intrapelvic **lymph nodes**   CC HCC
CC Excl: PDX collection 407

Chapter 2. Neoplasms

C81.09–C81.76

Chapter 2. Neoplasms

C81.77   **Other Hodgkin lymphoma,** spleen   CC HCC
CC Excl: PDX collection 408

C81.78   **Other Hodgkin lymphoma, lymph nodes of** multiple sites   CC HCC
CC Excl: PDX collection 401

C81.79   **Other Hodgkin lymphoma,** extranodal and solid organ sites   CC HCC
CC Excl: PDX collection 401

✓5th **C81.9**   **Hodgkin lymphoma,** unspecified

C81.90   **Hodgkin lymphoma, unspecified,** unspecified site   CC HCC
CC Excl: PDX collection 409

C81.91   **Hodgkin lymphoma, unspecified, lymph nodes of** head, face, and neck   CC HCC
CC Excl: PDX collection 410

C81.92   **Hodgkin lymphoma, unspecified,** intrathoracic lymph nodes   CC HCC
CC Excl: PDX collection 411

C81.93   **Hodgkin lymphoma, unspecified,** intra-abdominal lymph nodes   CC HCC
CC Excl: PDX collection 412

C81.94   **Hodgkin lymphoma, unspecified, lymph nodes of** axilla and upper limb   CC HCC
CC Excl: PDX collection 413

C81.95   **Hodgkin lymphoma, unspecified, lymph nodes of** inguinal region and lower limb   CC HCC
CC Excl: PDX collection 414

C81.96   **Hodgkin lymphoma, unspecified,** intrapelvic lymph nodes   CC HCC
CC Excl: PDX collection 415

C81.97   **Hodgkin lymphoma, unspecified,** spleen   CC HCC
CC Excl: PDX collection 416

C81.98   **Hodgkin lymphoma, unspecified, lymph nodes of** multiple sites   CC HCC
CC Excl: PDX collection 409

C81.99   **Hodgkin lymphoma, unspecified,** extranodal and solid organ sites   CC HCC
CC Excl: No Excl

✓4th **C82**   **Follicular** lymphoma
INCLUDES follicular lymphoma with or without diffuse areas
EXCLUDES 1 mature T/NK-cell lymphomas (C84.-)
personal history of non-Hodgkin lymphoma (Z85.72)
DEF: Most common subgroup of non-Hodgkin lymphomas (NHL), accounting for 20 to 30 percent of all NHLs. NHL is a B-cell lymphoma that is slow growing and characterized by the circular pattern of malignant cell growth with the cells clustered into identifiable nodules or follicles.

✓5th **C82.0**   **Follicular lymphoma** grade I

C82.00   **Follicular lymphoma grade I,** unspecified site   CC HCC
CC Excl: PDX collection 417

C82.01   **Follicular lymphoma grade I, lymph nodes of** head, face, and neck   CC HCC
CC Excl: PDX collection 418

C82.02   **Follicular lymphoma grade I,** intrathoracic lymph nodes   CC HCC
CC Excl: PDX collection 419

C82.03   **Follicular lymphoma grade I,** intra-abdominal lymph nodes   CC HCC
CC Excl: PDX collection 420

C82.04   **Follicular lymphoma grade I, lymph nodes of** axilla and upper limb   CC HCC
CC Excl: PDX collection 421

C82.05   **Follicular lymphoma grade I, lymph nodes of** inguinal region and lower limb   CC HCC
CC Excl: PDX collection 422

C82.06   **Follicular lymphoma grade I,** intrapelvic lymph nodes   CC HCC
CC Excl: PDX collection 423

C82.07   **Follicular lymphoma grade I,** spleen   CC HCC
CC Excl: PDX collection 424

C82.08   **Follicular lymphoma grade I, lymph nodes of** multiple sites   CC HCC
CC Excl: PDX collection 425

C82.09   **Follicular lymphoma grade I,** extranodal and solid organ sites   CC HCC
CC Excl: PDX collection 417

✓5th **C82.1**   **Follicular lymphoma** grade II

C82.10   **Follicular lymphoma grade II,** unspecified site   CC HCC
CC Excl: PDX collection 417

C82.11   **Follicular lymphoma grade II, lymph nodes of** head, face, and neck   CC HCC
CC Excl: PDX collection 418

C82.12   **Follicular lymphoma grade II,** intrathoracic lymph nodes   CC HCC
CC Excl: PDX collection 419

C82.13   **Follicular lymphoma grade II,** intra-abdominal lymph nodes   CC HCC
CC Excl: PDX collection 420

C82.14   **Follicular lymphoma grade II, lymph nodes of** axilla and upper limb   CC HCC
CC Excl: PDX collection 421

C82.15   **Follicular lymphoma grade II, lymph nodes of** inguinal region and lower limb   CC HCC
CC Excl: PDX collection 422

C82.16   **Follicular lymphoma grade II,** intrapelvic lymph nodes   CC HCC
CC Excl: PDX collection 423

C82.17   **Follicular lymphoma grade II,** spleen   CC HCC
CC Excl: PDX collection 424

C82.18   **Follicular lymphoma grade II, lymph nodes of** multiple sites   CC HCC
CC Excl: PDX collection 425

C82.19   **Follicular lymphoma grade II,** extranodal and solid organ sites   CC HCC
CC Excl: PDX collection 417

✓5th **C82.2**   **Follicular lymphoma** grade III, unspecified

C82.20   **Follicular lymphoma grade III, unspecified,** unspecified site   CC HCC
CC Excl: PDX collection 417

C82.21   **Follicular lymphoma grade III, unspecified, lymph nodes of** head, face, and neck   CC HCC
CC Excl: PDX collection 418

C82.22   **Follicular lymphoma grade III, unspecified,** intrathoracic lymph nodes   CC HCC
CC Excl: PDX collection 419

C82.23   **Follicular lymphoma grade III, unspecified,** intra-abdominal lymph nodes   CC HCC
CC Excl: PDX collection 420

C82.24   **Follicular lymphoma grade III, unspecified, lymph nodes of** axilla and upper limb   CC HCC
CC Excl: PDX collection 421

C82.25   **Follicular lymphoma grade III, unspecified, lymph nodes of** inguinal region and lower limb   CC HCC
CC Excl: PDX collection 422

C82.26   **Follicular lymphoma grade III, unspecified,** intrapelvic lymph nodes   CC HCC
CC Excl: PDX collection 423

C82.27   **Follicular lymphoma grade III, unspecified,** spleen   CC HCC
CC Excl: PDX collection 424

C82.28   **Follicular lymphoma grade III, unspecified, lymph nodes of** multiple sites   CC HCC
CC Excl: PDX collection 425

C82.29   **Follicular lymphoma grade III, unspecified,** extranodal and solid organ sites   CC HCC
CC Excl: PDX collection 417

✓5th **C82.3**   **Follicular lymphoma** grade IIIa

C82.30   **Follicular lymphoma grade IIIa,** unspecified site   CC HCC
CC Excl: PDX collection 417

C82.31   **Follicular lymphoma grade IIIa, lymph nodes of** head, face, and neck   CC HCC
CC Excl: PDX collection 418

C82.32   **Follicular lymphoma grade IIIa,** intrathoracic lymph nodes   CC HCC
CC Excl: PDX collection 419

C82.33   **Follicular lymphoma grade IIIa,** intra-abdominal lymph nodes   CC HCC
CC Excl: PDX collection 420

C82.34   **Follicular lymphoma grade IIIa, lymph nodes of** axilla and upper limb   CC HCC
CC Excl: PDX collection 421

C82.35   **Follicular lymphoma grade IIIa, lymph nodes of** inguinal region and lower limb   CC HCC
CC Excl: PDX collection 422

C82.36 Follicular lymphoma grade IIIa, intrapelvic `CC` `HCC`
lymph nodes
CC Excl: PDX collection 423

C82.37 Follicular lymphoma grade IIIa, spleen `CC` `HCC`
CC Excl: PDX collection 424

C82.38 Follicular lymphoma grade IIIa, lymph nodes `CC` `HCC`
of multiple sites
CC Excl: PDX collection 425

C82.39 Follicular lymphoma grade IIIa, extranodal `CC` `HCC`
and solid organ sites
CC Excl: PDX collection 417

✓5th **C82.4** **Follicular lymphoma** grade IIIb

C82.40 Follicular lymphoma grade IIIb, `CC` `HCC`
unspecified site
CC Excl: PDX collection 417

C82.41 Follicular lymphoma grade IIIb, lymph nodes `CC` `HCC`
of head, face, and neck
CC Excl: PDX collection 418

C82.42 Follicular lymphoma grade IIIb, intrathoracic `CC` `HCC`
lymph nodes
CC Excl: PDX collection 419

C82.43 Follicular lymphoma grade IIIb, `CC` `HCC`
intra-abdominal lymph nodes
CC Excl: PDX collection 420

C82.44 Follicular lymphoma grade IIIb, lymph nodes `CC` `HCC`
of axilla and upper limb
CC Excl: PDX collection 421

C82.45 Follicular lymphoma grade IIIb, lymph `CC` `HCC`
nodes of inguinal region and lower limb
CC Excl: PDX collection 422

C82.46 Follicular lymphoma grade IIIb, intrapelvic `CC` `HCC`
lymph nodes
CC Excl: PDX collection 423

C82.47 Follicular lymphoma grade IIIb, spleen `CC` `HCC`
CC Excl: PDX collection 424

C82.48 Follicular lymphoma grade IIIb, lymph nodes `CC` `HCC`
of multiple sites
CC Excl: PDX collection 425

C82.49 Follicular lymphoma grade IIIb, extranodal `CC` `HCC`
and solid organ sites
CC Excl: PDX collection 417

✓5th **C82.5** **Diffuse follicle center** lymphoma

C82.50 Diffuse follicle center lymphoma, `HIV` `CC` `HCC`
unspecified site
CC Excl: PDX collection 426

C82.51 Diffuse follicle center lymphoma, lymph `HIV` `CC` `HCC`
nodes of head, face, and neck
CC Excl: PDX collection 427

C82.52 Diffuse follicle center lymphoma, `HIV` `CC` `HCC`
intrathoracic lymph nodes
CC Excl: PDX collection 428

C82.53 Diffuse follicle center lymphoma, intra- `HIV` `CC` `HCC`
abdominal lymph nodes
CC Excl: PDX collection 429

C82.54 Diffuse follicle center lymphoma, lymph `HIV` `CC` `HCC`
nodes of axilla and upper limb
CC Excl: PDX collection 430

C82.55 Diffuse follicle center lymphoma, lymph `HIV` `CC` `HCC`
nodes of inguinal region and lower limb
CC Excl: PDX collection 431

C82.56 Diffuse follicle center lymphoma, `HIV` `CC` `HCC`
intrapelvic lymph nodes
CC Excl: PDX collection 432

C82.57 Diffuse follicle center lymphoma, spleen `HIV` `CC` `HCC`
CC Excl: PDX collection 433

C82.58 Diffuse follicle center lymphoma, lymph `HIV` `CC` `HCC`
nodes of multiple sites
CC Excl: PDX collection 434

C82.59 Diffuse follicle center lymphoma, `HIV` `CC` `HCC`
extranodal and solid organ sites
CC Excl: PDX collection 426

✓5th **C82.6** **Cutaneous follicle center** lymphoma

C82.60 Cutaneous follicle center lymphoma, `CC` `HCC`
unspecified site
CC Excl: PDX collection 417

C82.61 Cutaneous follicle center lymphoma, lymph `CC` `HCC`
nodes of head, face, and neck
CC Excl: PDX collection 418

C82.62 Cutaneous follicle center lymphoma, `CC` `HCC`
intrathoracic lymph nodes
CC Excl: PDX collection 419

C82.63 Cutaneous follicle center lymphoma, `CC` `HCC`
intra-abdominal lymph nodes
CC Excl: PDX collection 420

C82.64 Cutaneous follicle center lymphoma, lymph `CC` `HCC`
nodes of axilla and upper limb
CC Excl: PDX collection 421

C82.65 Cutaneous follicle center lymphoma, lymph `CC` `HCC`
nodes of inguinal region and lower limb
CC Excl: PDX collection 422

C82.66 Cutaneous follicle center lymphoma, `CC` `HCC`
intrapelvic lymph nodes
CC Excl: PDX collection 423

C82.67 Cutaneous follicle center lymphoma, spleen `CC` `HCC`
CC Excl: PDX collection 424

C82.68 Cutaneous follicle center lymphoma, lymph `CC` `HCC`
nodes of multiple sites
CC Excl: PDX collection 425

C82.69 Cutaneous follicle center lymphoma, `CC` `HCC`
extranodal and solid organ sites
CC Excl: PDX collection 417

✓5th **C82.8** **Other types** of follicular lymphoma

C82.80 Other types of follicular lymphoma, `CC` `HCC`
unspecified site
CC Excl: PDX collection 417

C82.81 Other types of follicular lymphoma, lymph `CC` `HCC`
nodes of head, face, and neck
CC Excl: PDX collection 418

C82.82 Other types of follicular lymphoma, `CC` `HCC`
intrathoracic lymph nodes
CC Excl: PDX collection 419

C82.83 Other types of follicular lymphoma, `CC` `HCC`
intra-abdominal lymph nodes
CC Excl: PDX collection 420

C82.84 Other types of follicular lymphoma, lymph `CC` `HCC`
nodes of axilla and upper limb
CC Excl: PDX collection 421

C82.85 Other types of follicular lymphoma, lymph `CC` `HCC`
nodes of inguinal region and lower limb
CC Excl: PDX collection 422

C82.86 Other types of follicular lymphoma, `CC` `HCC`
intrapelvic lymph nodes
CC Excl: PDX collection 423

C82.87 Other types of follicular lymphoma, spleen `CC` `HCC`
CC Excl: PDX collection 424

C82.88 Other types of follicular lymphoma, lymph `CC` `HCC`
nodes of multiple sites
CC Excl: PDX collection 425

C82.89 Other types of follicular lymphoma, `CC` `HCC`
extranodal and solid organ sites
CC Excl: PDX collection 417

✓5th **C82.9** **Follicular lymphoma,** unspecified

C82.90 Follicular lymphoma, unspecified, `CC` `HCC`
unspecified site
CC Excl: PDX collection 417

C82.91 Follicular lymphoma, unspecified, lymph `CC` `HCC`
nodes of head, face, and neck
CC Excl: PDX collection 418

C82.92 Follicular lymphoma, unspecified, `CC` `HCC`
intrathoracic lymph nodes
CC Excl: PDX collection 419

C82.93 Follicular lymphoma, unspecified, intra- `CC` `HCC`
abdominal lymph nodes
CC Excl: PDX collection 420

C82.94 Follicular lymphoma, unspecified, lymph `CC` `HCC`
nodes of axilla and upper limb
CC Excl: PDX collection 421

C82.95 Follicular lymphoma, unspecified, lymph `CC` `HCC`
nodes of inguinal region and lower limb
CC Excl: PDX collection 422

C82.96 Follicular lymphoma, unspecified, `CC` `HCC`
intrapelvic lymph nodes
CC Excl: PDX collection 423

C82.97 Follicular lymphoma, unspecified, spleen `CC` `HCC`
CC Excl: PDX collection 424

✓ Additional Character Required   ✓x 7th Placeholder   Unacceptable PDx   Questionable PDx   Manifestation   `H1`-`H14` HAC   `HCC` CMS-HCC Dx   `HIV` HIV Dx

ICD-10-CM 2019   483

Chapter 2. Neoplasms

C82.98   **Follicular lymphoma, unspecified, lymph nodes of multiple sites**   `CC` `HCC`
     CC Excl: PDX collection 425

C82.99   **Follicular lymphoma, unspecified, extranodal and solid organ sites**   `CC` `HCC`
     CC Excl: PDX collection 417

✓4ᵗʰ **C83**   **Non-follicular lymphoma**
   `EXCLUDES 1`   *personal history of non-Hodgkin lymphoma (Z85.72)*

   ✓5ᵗʰ **C83.0**   **Small cell B-cell lymphoma**
     Lymphoplasmacytic lymphoma
     Nodal marginal zone lymphoma
     Non-leukemic variant of B-CLL
     Splenic marginal zone lymphoma
     `EXCLUDES 1`   *chronic lymphocytic leukemia (C91.1)*
              mature T/NK-cell lymphomas (C84.-)
              Waldenström macroglubulinemia (C88.0)
     DEF: Nonfollicular lymphoma that is rare, slow growing, and usually found in the older population.

     C83.00   **Small cell B-cell lymphoma, unspecified site**   `HIV` `CC` `HCC`
       CC Excl: PDX collection 435

     C83.01   **Small cell B-cell lymphoma, lymph nodes of head, face, and neck**   `HIV` `CC` `HCC`
       CC Excl: PDX collection 436

     C83.02   **Small cell B-cell lymphoma, intrathoracic lymph nodes**   `HIV` `CC` `HCC`
       CC Excl: PDX collection 437

     C83.03   **Small cell B-cell lymphoma, intra-abdominal lymph nodes**   `HIV` `CC` `HCC`
       CC Excl: PDX collection 438

     C83.04   **Small cell B-cell lymphoma, lymph nodes of axilla and upper limb**   `HIV` `CC` `HCC`
       CC Excl: PDX collection 439

     C83.05   **Small cell B-cell lymphoma, lymph nodes of inguinal region and lower limb**   `HIV` `CC` `HCC`
       CC Excl: CPDX collection 440

     C83.06   **Small cell B-cell lymphoma, intrapelvic lymph nodes**   `HIV` `CC` `HCC`
       CC Excl: PDX collection 441

     C83.07   **Small cell B-cell lymphoma, spleen**   `HIV` `CC` `HCC`
       CC Excl: PDX collection 442

     C83.08   **Small cell B-cell lymphoma, lymph nodes of multiple sites**   `HIV` `CC` `HCC`
       CC Excl: PDX collection 435

     C83.09   **Small cell B-cell lymphoma, extranodal and solid organ sites**   `HIV` `CC` `HCC`
       CC Excl: PDX collection 435

   ✓5ᵗʰ **C83.1**   **Mantle cell lymphoma**
     Centrocytic lymphoma
     Malignant lymphomatous polyposis
     DEF: Rare form of B-cell non-Hodgkin lymphoma named for the location of the tumor cell production, the mantle zone of the lymph nodes.

     C83.10   **Mantle cell lymphoma, unspecified site**   `HIV` `CC` `HCC`
       CC Excl: PDX collection 426

     C83.11   **Mantle cell lymphoma, lymph nodes of head, face, and neck**   `HIV` `CC` `HCC`
       CC Excl: PDX collection 427

     C83.12   **Mantle cell lymphoma, intrathoracic lymph nodes**   `HIV` `CC` `HCC`
       CC Excl: PDX collection 428

     C83.13   **Mantle cell lymphoma, intra-abdominal lymph nodes**   `HIV` `CC` `HCC`
       CC Excl: PDX collection 429

     C83.14   **Mantle cell lymphoma, lymph nodes of axilla and upper limb**   `HIV` `CC` `HCC`
       CC Excl: PDX collection 430

     C83.15   **Mantle cell lymphoma, lymph nodes of inguinal region and lower limb**   `HIV` `CC` `HCC`
       CC Excl: PDX collection 431

     C83.16   **Mantle cell lymphoma, intrapelvic lymph nodes**   `HIV` `CC` `HCC`
       CC Excl: PDX collection 432

     C83.17   **Mantle cell lymphoma, spleen**   `HIV` `CC` `HCC`
       CC Excl: PDX collection 433

     C83.18   **Mantle cell lymphoma, lymph nodes of multiple sites**   `HIV` `CC` `HCC`
       CC Excl: PDX collection 434

     C83.19   **Mantle cell lymphoma, extranodal and solid organ sites**   `HIV` `CC` `HCC`
       CC Excl: PDX collection 426

   ✓5ᵗʰ **C83.3**   **Diffuse large B-cell lymphoma**
     Anaplastic diffuse large B-cell lymphoma
     CD30-positive diffuse large B-cell lymphoma
     Centroblastic diffuse large B-cell lymphoma
     Diffuse large B-cell lymphoma, subtype not specified
     Immunoblastic diffuse large B-cell lymphoma
     Plasmablastic diffuse large B-cell lymphoma
     T-cell rich diffuse large B-cell lymphoma
     `EXCLUDES 1`   *mature T/NK-cell lymphomas (C84.-)*
              mediastinal (thymic) large B-cell lymphoma (C85.2-)
     DEF: Nonfollicular lymphoma that is one of the more common types of lymphoma. This cancer is fast growing and affects any age but is found mostly in the older population.

     C83.30   **Diffuse large B-cell lymphoma, unspecified site**   `HIV` `CC` `HCC`
       CC Excl: PDX collection 443

     C83.31   **Diffuse large B-cell lymphoma, lymph nodes of head, face, and neck**   `HIV` `CC` `HCC`
       CC Excl: PDX collection 444

     C83.32   **Diffuse large B-cell lymphoma, intrathoracic lymph nodes**   `HIV` `CC` `HCC`
       CC Excl: PDX collection 445

     C83.33   **Diffuse large B-cell lymphoma, intra-abdominal lymph nodes**   `HIV` `CC` `HCC`
       CC Excl: PDX collection 446

     C83.34   **Diffuse large B-cell lymphoma, lymph nodes of axilla and upper limb**   `HIV` `CC` `HCC`
       CC Excl: PDX collection 447

     C83.35   **Diffuse large B-cell lymphoma, lymph nodes of inguinal region and lower limb**   `HIV` `CC` `HCC`
       CC Excl: PDX collection 448

     C83.36   **Diffuse large B-cell lymphoma, intrapelvic lymph nodes**   `HIV` `CC` `HCC`
       CC Excl: PDX collection 449

     C83.37   **Diffuse large B-cell lymphoma, spleen**   `HIV` `CC` `HCC`
       CC Excl: PDX collection 450

     C83.38   **Diffuse large B-cell lymphoma, lymph nodes of multiple sites**   `HIV` `CC` `HCC`
       CC Excl: PDX collection 443

     C83.39   **Diffuse large B-cell lymphoma, extranodal and solid organ sites**   `HIV` `CC` `HCC`
       CC Excl: PDX collection 443

   ✓5ᵗʰ **C83.5**   **Lymphoblastic (diffuse) lymphoma**
     B-precursor lymphoma
     Lymphoblastic B-cell lymphoma
     Lymphoblastic lymphoma NOS
     Lymphoblastic T-cell lymphoma
     T-precursor lymphoma
     DEF: Type of non-Hodgkin lymphoma considered lymphoma or leukemia—the determination is made based on the amount of bone marrow involvement. The cells are small to medium immature T-cells that often originate in the thymus where many of the T-cells are made.

     C83.50   **Lymphoblastic (diffuse) lymphoma, unspecified site**   `CC` `HCC`
       CC Excl: PDX collection 451

     C83.51   **Lymphoblastic (diffuse) lymphoma, lymph nodes of head, face, and neck**   `CC` `HCC`
       CC Excl: PDX collection 452

     C83.52   **Lymphoblastic (diffuse) lymphoma, intrathoracic lymph nodes**   `CC` `HCC`
       CC Excl: PDX collection 453

     C83.53   **Lymphoblastic (diffuse) lymphoma, intra-abdominal lymph nodes**   `CC` `HCC`
       CC Excl: PDX collection 454

     C83.54   **Lymphoblastic (diffuse) lymphoma, lymph nodes of axilla and upper limb**   `CC` `HCC`
       CC Excl: PDX collection 455

     C83.55   **Lymphoblastic (diffuse) lymphoma, lymph nodes of inguinal region and lower limb**   `CC` `HCC`
       CC Excl: PDX collection 456

     C83.56   **Lymphoblastic (diffuse) lymphoma, intrapelvic lymph nodes**   `CC` `HCC`
       CC Excl: PDX collection 457

     C83.57   **Lymphoblastic (diffuse) lymphoma, spleen**   `CC` `HCC`
       CC Excl: PDX collection 458

Ⓝ Newborn: 0   Ⓟ Pediatric: 0-17   Ⓜ Maternity: 12-55   Ⓐ Adult: 15-124   `MCC` Major Complication/Comorbidity   `CC` Complication/Comorbidity   `SW` Severe Wound Dx

484   ICD-10-CM 2019

C83.58   **Lymphoblastic (diffuse) lymphoma, lymph nodes of multiple sites**   `CC` `HCC`
CC Excl: PDX collection 451

C83.59   **Lymphoblastic (diffuse) lymphoma, extranodal and solid organ sites**   `CC` `HCC`
CC Excl: PDX collection 451

√5th **C83.7**   **Burkitt lymphoma**
Atypical Burkitt lymphoma
Burkitt-like lymphoma
EXCLUDES 1   *mature B-cell leukemia Burkitt type (C91.A-)*
DEF: Malignancy of the lymphatic system, most often seen as a large bone-deteriorating lesion within the jaw or as an abdominal mass. It is a form of non-Hodgkin's lymphoma and is recognized as the fastest growing human tumor.

C83.70   **Burkitt lymphoma, unspecified site**   `HIV` `CC` `HCC`
CC Excl: PDX collection 459

C83.71   **Burkitt lymphoma, lymph nodes of head, face, and neck**   `HIV` `CC` `HCC`
CC Excl: PDX collection 460

C83.72   **Burkitt lymphoma, intrathoracic lymph nodes**   `HIV` `CC` `HCC`
CC Excl: PDX collection 461

C83.73   **Burkitt lymphoma, intra-abdominal lymph nodes**   `HIV` `CC` `HCC`
CC Excl: PDX collection 462

C83.74   **Burkitt lymphoma, lymph nodes of axilla and upper limb**   `HIV` `CC` `HCC`
CC Excl: PDX collection 463

C83.75   **Burkitt lymphoma, lymph nodes of inguinal region and lower limb**   `HIV` `CC` `HCC`
CC Excl: PDX collection 464

C83.76   **Burkitt lymphoma, intrapelvic lymph nodes**   `HIV` `CC` `HCC`
CC Excl: PDX collection 465

C83.77   **Burkitt lymphoma, spleen**   `HIV` `CC` `HCC`
CC Excl: PDX collection 466

C83.78   **Burkitt lymphoma, lymph nodes of multiple sites**   `HIV` `CC` `HCC`
CC Excl: PDX collection 459

C83.79   **Burkitt lymphoma, extranodal and solid organ sites**   `HIV` `CC` `HCC`
CC Excl: PDX collection 459

√5th **C83.8**   **Other non-follicular lymphoma**
Intravascular large B-cell lymphoma
Lymphoid granulomatosis
Primary effusion B-cell lymphoma
EXCLUDES 1   *mediastinal (thymic) large B-cell lymphoma (C85.2-)*
T-cell rich B-cell lymphoma (C83.3-)

C83.80   **Other non-follicular lymphoma, unspecified site**   `HIV` `CC` `HCC`
CC Excl: PDX collection 435

C83.81   **Other non-follicular lymphoma, lymph nodes of head, face, and neck**   `HIV` `CC` `HCC`
CC Excl: PDX collection 436

C83.82   **Other non-follicular lymphoma, intrathoracic lymph nodes**   `HIV` `CC` `HCC`
CC Excl: PDX collection 437

C83.83   **Other non-follicular lymphoma, intra-abdominal lymph nodes**   `HIV` `CC` `HCC`
CC Excl: PDX collection 438

C83.84   **Other non-follicular lymphoma, lymph nodes of axilla and upper limb**   `HIV` `CC` `HCC`
CC Excl: PDX collection 439

C83.85   **Other non-follicular lymphoma, lymph nodes of inguinal region and lower limb**   `HIV` `CC` `HCC`
CC Excl: PDX collection 440

C83.86   **Other non-follicular lymphoma, intrapelvic lymph nodes**   `HIV` `CC` `HCC`
CC Excl: PDX collection 441

C83.87   **Other non-follicular lymphoma, spleen**   `HIV` `CC` `HCC`
CC Excl: PDX collection 442

C83.88   **Other non-follicular lymphoma, lymph nodes of multiple sites**   `HIV` `CC` `HCC`
CC Excl: PDX collection 435

C83.89   **Other non-follicular lymphoma, extranodal and solid organ sites**   `HIV` `CC` `HCC`
CC Excl: SPDX collection 435

√5th **C83.9**   **Non-follicular (diffuse) lymphoma, unspecified**

C83.90   **Non-follicular (diffuse) lymphoma, unspecified, unspecified site**   `HIV` `CC` `HCC`
CC Excl: PDX collection 435

C83.91   **Non-follicular (diffuse) lymphoma, unspecified, lymph nodes of head, face, and neck**   `HIV` `CC` `HCC`
CC Excl: PDX collection 436

C83.92   **Non-follicular (diffuse) lymphoma, unspecified, intrathoracic lymph nodes**   `HIV` `CC` `HCC`
CC Excl: PDX collection 437

C83.93   **Non-follicular (diffuse) lymphoma, unspecified, intra-abdominal lymph nodes**   `HIV` `CC` `HCC`
CC Excl: PDX collection 438

C83.94   **Non-follicular (diffuse) lymphoma, unspecified, lymph nodes of axilla and upper limb**   `HIV` `CC` `HCC`
CC Excl: PDX collection 439

C83.95   **Non-follicular (diffuse) lymphoma, unspecified, lymph nodes of inguinal region and lower limb**   `HIV` `CC` `HCC`
CC Excl: PDX collection 440

C83.96   **Non-follicular (diffuse) lymphoma, unspecified, intrapelvic lymph nodes**   `HIV` `CC` `HCC`
CC Excl: PDX collection 441

C83.97   **Non-follicular (diffuse) lymphoma, unspecified, spleen**   `HIV` `CC` `HCC`
CC Excl: PDX collection 442

C83.98   **Non-follicular (diffuse) lymphoma, unspecified, lymph nodes of multiple sites**   `HIV` `CC` `HCC`
CC Excl: PDX collection 435

C83.99   **Non-follicular (diffuse) lymphoma, unspecified, extranodal and solid organ sites**   `HIV` `CC` `HCC`
CC Excl: PDX collection 435

√4th **C84**   **Mature T/NK-cell lymphomas**
EXCLUDES 1   *personal history of non-Hodgkin lymphoma (Z85.72)*

√5th **C84.0**   **Mycosis fungoides**
EXCLUDES 1   *peripheral T-cell lymphoma, not classified (C84.4-)*
DEF: Most common form of cutaneous T-cell lymphoma. A type of non-Hodgkin lymphoma in which white blood cells become cancerous and affect the skin and sometimes internal organs. Synonym(s): Alibert-Bazin syndrome.

C84.00   **Mycosis fungoides, unspecified site**   `CC` `HCC`
CC Excl: PDX collection 467

C84.01   **Mycosis fungoides, lymph nodes of head, face, and neck**   `CC` `HCC`
CC Excl: PDX collection 468

C84.02   **Mycosis fungoides, intrathoracic lymph nodes**   `CC` `HCC`
CC Excl: PDX collection 469

C84.03   **Mycosis fungoides, intra-abdominal lymph nodes**   `CC` `HCC`
CC Excl: PDX collection 470

C84.04   **Mycosis fungoides, lymph nodes of axilla and upper limb**   `CC` `HCC`
CC Excl: PDX collection 471

C84.05   **Mycosis fungoides, lymph nodes of inguinal region and lower limb**   `CC` `HCC`
CC Excl: PDX collection 472

C84.06   **Mycosis fungoides, intrapelvic lymph nodes**   `CC` `HCC`
CC Excl: PDX collection 473

C84.07   **Mycosis fungoides, spleen**   `CC` `HCC`
CC Excl: PDX collection 474

C84.08   **Mycosis fungoides, lymph nodes of multiple sites**   `CC` `HCC`
CC Excl: PDX collection 475

C84.09   **Mycosis fungoides, extranodal and solid organ sites**   `CC` `HCC`
CC Excl: PDX collection 467

√5th **C84.1**   **Sézary disease**
DEF: Extension of mycosis fungoides that affects the blood and all of the skin, appearing as sunburn, rather than patches. It spreads to the lymph nodes and is often linked to a weakened immune system.

C84.10   **Sézary disease, unspecified site**   `CC` `HCC`
CC Excl: PDX collection 476

C84.11   **Sézary disease, lymph nodes of head, face, and neck**   `CC` `HCC`
CC Excl: PDX collection 477

C84.12 Sézary disease, intrathoracic lymph nodes `CC` `HCC`
    CC Excl: PDX collection 478

C84.13 Sézary disease, intra-abdominal lymph nodes `CC` `HCC`
    CC Excl: PDX collection 479

C84.14 Sézary disease, lymph nodes of axilla and upper limb `CC` `HCC`
    CC Excl: PDX collection 480

C84.15 Sézary disease, lymph nodes of inguinal region and lower limb `CC` `HCC`
    CC Excl: PDX collection 481

C84.16 Sézary disease, intrapelvic lymph nodes `CC` `HCC`
    CC Excl: PDX collection 482

C84.17 Sézary disease, spleen `CC` `HCC`
    CC Excl: PDX collection 483

C84.18 Sézary disease, lymph nodes of multiple sites `CC` `HCC`
    CC Excl: PDX collection 484

C84.19 Sézary disease, extranodal and solid organ sites `CC` `HCC`
    CC Excl: PDX collection 476

✓5th **C84.4 Peripheral T-cell lymphoma, not classified**
Lennert's lymphoma
Lymphoepithelioid lymphoma
Mature T-cell lymphoma, not elsewhere classified

C84.40 Peripheral T-cell lymphoma, not classified, unspecified site `HIV` `CC` `HCC`
    CC Excl: PDX collection 426

C84.41 Peripheral T-cell lymphoma, not classified, lymph nodes of head, face, and neck `HIV` `CC` `HCC`
    CC Excl: PDX collection 427

C84.42 Peripheral T-cell lymphoma, not classified, intrathoracic lymph nodes `HIV` `CC` `HCC`
    CC Excl: PDX collection 428

C84.43 Peripheral T-cell lymphoma, not classified, intra-abdominal lymph nodes `HIV` `CC` `HCC`
    CC Excl: PDX collection 429

C84.44 Peripheral T-cell lymphoma, not classified, lymph nodes of axilla and upper limb `HIV` `CC` `HCC`
    CC Excl: PDX collection 430

C84.45 Peripheral T-cell lymphoma, not classified, lymph nodes of inguinal region and lower limb `HIV` `CC` `HCC`
    CC Excl: PDX collection 431

C84.46 Peripheral T-cell lymphoma, not classified, intrapelvic lymph nodes `HIV` `CC` `HCC`
    CC Excl: PDX collection 432

C84.47 Peripheral T-cell lymphoma, not classified, spleen `HIV` `CC` `HCC`
    CC Excl: PDX collection 433

C84.48 Peripheral T-cell lymphoma, not classified, lymph nodes of multiple sites `HIV` `CC` `HCC`
    CC Excl: PDX collection 434

C84.49 Peripheral T-cell lymphoma, not classified, extranodal and solid organ sites `HIV` `CC` `HCC`
    CC Excl: PDX collection 426

✓5th **C84.6 Anaplastic large cell lymphoma, ALK-positive**
Anaplastic large cell lymphoma, CD30-positive

C84.60 Anaplastic large cell lymphoma, ALK-positive, unspecified site `HIV` `CC` `HCC`
    CC Excl: PDX collection 426

C84.61 Anaplastic large cell lymphoma, ALK-positive, lymph nodes of head, face, and neck `HIV` `CC` `HCC`
    CC Excl: PDX collection 427

C84.62 Anaplastic large cell lymphoma, ALK-positive, intrathoracic lymph nodes `HIV` `CC` `HCC`
    CC Excl: PDX collection 428

C84.63 Anaplastic large cell lymphoma, ALK-positive, intra-abdominal lymph nodes `HIV` `CC` `HCC`
    CC Excl: PDX collection 429

C84.64 Anaplastic large cell lymphoma, ALK-positive, lymph nodes of axilla and upper limb `HIV` `CC` `HCC`
    CC Excl: PDX collection 430

C84.65 Anaplastic large cell lymphoma, ALK-positive, lymph nodes of inguinal region and lower limb `HIV` `CC` `HCC`
    CC Excl: PDX collection 431

C84.66 Anaplastic large cell lymphoma, ALK-positive, intrapelvic lymph nodes `HIV` `CC` `HCC`
    CC Excl: PDX collection 432

C84.67 Anaplastic large cell lymphoma, ALK-positive, spleen `HIV` `CC` `HCC`
    CC Excl: PDX collection 433

C84.68 Anaplastic large cell lymphoma, ALK-positive, lymph nodes of multiple sites `HIV` `CC` `HCC`
    CC Excl: PDX collection 434

C84.69 Anaplastic large cell lymphoma, ALK-positive, extranodal and solid organ sites `HIV` `CC` `HCC`
    CC Excl: PDX collection 426

✓5th **C84.7 Anaplastic large cell lymphoma, ALK-negative**
EXCLUDES 1 *primary cutaneous CD30-positive T-cell proliferations (C86.6-)*

C84.70 Anaplastic large cell lymphoma, ALK-negative, unspecified site `HIV` `CC` `HCC`
    CC Excl: PDX collection 426

C84.71 Anaplastic large cell lymphoma, ALK-negative, lymph nodes of head, face, and neck `HIV` `CC` `HCC`
    CC Excl: PDX collection 427

C84.72 Anaplastic large cell lymphoma, ALK-negative, intrathoracic lymph nodes `HIV` `CC` `HCC`
    CC Excl: PDX collection 428

C84.73 Anaplastic large cell lymphoma, ALK-negative, intra-abdominal lymph nodes `HIV` `CC` `HCC`
    CC Excl: PDX collection 429

C84.74 Anaplastic large cell lymphoma, ALK-negative, lymph nodes of axilla and upper limb `HIV` `CC` `HCC`
    CC Excl: PDX collection 430

C84.75 Anaplastic large cell lymphoma, ALK-negative, lymph nodes of inguinal region and lower limb `HIV` `CC` `HCC`
    CC Excl: PDX collection 431

C84.76 Anaplastic large cell lymphoma, ALK-negative, intrapelvic lymph nodes `HIV` `CC` `HCC`
    CC Excl: PDX collection 432

C84.77 Anaplastic large cell lymphoma, ALK-negative, spleen `HIV` `CC` `HCC`
    CC Excl: PDX collection 433

C84.78 Anaplastic large cell lymphoma, ALK-negative, lymph nodes of multiple sites `HIV` `CC` `HCC`
    CC Excl: PDX collection 434

C84.79 Anaplastic large cell lymphoma, ALK-negative, extranodal and solid organ sites `HIV` `CC` `HCC`
    CC Excl: PDX collection 426

✓5th **C84.A Cutaneous T-cell lymphoma, unspecified**

C84.A0 Cutaneous T-cell lymphoma, unspecified, unspecified site `HIV` `CC` `HCC`
    CC Excl: PDX collection 426

C84.A1 Cutaneous T-cell lymphoma, unspecified, lymph nodes of head, face, and neck `HIV` `CC` `HCC`
    CC Excl: PDX collection 427

C84.A2 Cutaneous T-cell lymphoma, unspecified, intrathoracic lymph nodes `HIV` `CC` `HCC`
    CC Excl: PDX collection 428

C84.A3 Cutaneous T-cell lymphoma, unspecified, intra-abdominal lymph nodes `HIV` `CC` `HCC`
    CC Excl: PDX collection 429

C84.A4 Cutaneous T-cell lymphoma, unspecified, lymph nodes of axilla and upper limb `HIV` `CC` `HCC`
    CC Excl: PDX collection 430

C84.A5 Cutaneous T-cell lymphoma, unspecified, lymph nodes of inguinal region and lower limb `HIV` `CC` `HCC`
    CC Excl: PDX collection 431

C84.A6 Cutaneous T-cell lymphoma, unspecified, intrapelvic lymph nodes `HIV` `CC` `HCC`
    CC Excl: PDX collection 432

C84.A7 Cutaneous T-cell lymphoma, unspecified, spleen `HIV` `CC` `HCC`
    CC Excl: PDX collection 433

C84.A8 Cutaneous T-cell lymphoma, unspecified, lymph nodes of multiple sites `HIV` `CC` `HCC`
    CC Excl: PDX collection 434

C84.A9 Cutaneous T-cell lymphoma, unspecified, extranodal and solid organ sites `HIV` `CC` `HCC`
    CC Excl: PDX collection 426

N Newborn: 0   P Pediatric: 0-17   M Maternity: 12-55   A Adult: 15-124   MCC Major Complication/Comorbidity   CC Complication/Comorbidity   SW Severe Wound Dx

486   ICD-10-CM 2019

☑5ᵗʰ **C84.Z** **Other mature T/NK-cell lymphomas**

> **NOTE** If T-cell lineage or involvement is mentioned in conjunction with a specific lymphoma, code to the more specific description.
>
> **EXCLUDES 1** angioimmunoblastic T-cell lymphoma (C86.5)
> blastic NK-cell lymphoma (C86.4)
> enteropathy-type T-cell lymphoma (C86.2)
> extranodal NK-cell lymphoma, nasal type (C86.0)
> hepatosplenic T-cell lymphoma (C86.1)
> primary cutaneous CD30-positive T-cell proliferations (C86.6)
> subcutaneous panniculitis-like T-cell lymphoma (C86.3)
> T-cell leukemia (C91.1-)

C84.Z0 **Other mature T/NK-cell lymphomas, unspecified site** HIV CC HCC
> CC Excl: PDX collection 426

C84.Z1 **Other mature T/NK-cell lymphomas, lymph nodes of** head, face, and neck HIV CC HCC
> CC Excl: PDX collection 427

C84.Z2 **Other mature T/NK-cell lymphomas, intrathoracic lymph nodes** HIV CC HCC
> CC Excl: PDX collection 428

C84.Z3 **Other mature T/NK-cell lymphomas, intra-abdominal lymph nodes** HIV CC HCC
> CC Excl: PDX collection 429

C84.Z4 **Other mature T/NK-cell lymphomas, lymph nodes of** axilla and upper limb HIV CC HCC
> CC Excl: PDX collection 430

C84.Z5 **Other mature T/NK-cell lymphomas, lymph nodes of** inguinal region and lower limb HIV CC HCC
> CC Excl: PDX collection 431

C84.Z6 **Other mature T/NK-cell lymphomas, intrapelvic lymph nodes** HIV CC HCC
> CC Excl: PDX collection 432

C84.Z7 **Other mature T/NK-cell lymphomas, spleen** HIV CC HCC
> CC Excl: PDX collection 433

C84.Z8 **Other mature T/NK-cell lymphomas, lymph ndoes of** multiple sites HIV CC HCC
> CC Excl: PDX collection 434

C84.Z9 **Other mature T/NK-cell lymphomas, extranodal and solid organ sites** HIV CC HCC
> CC Excl: PDX collection 426

☑5ᵗʰ **C84.9** **Mature T/NK-cell lymphomas, unspecified**
NK/T cell lymphoma NOS
> **EXCLUDES 1** mature T-cell lymphoma, not elsewhere classified (C84.4-)

C84.90 **Mature T/NK-cell lymphomas, unspecified, unspecified site** HIV CC HCC
> CC Excl: PDX collection 426

C84.91 **Mature T/NK-cell lymphomas, unspecified, lymph nodes of** head, face, and neck HIV CC HCC
> CC Excl: PDX collection 427

C84.92 **Mature T/NK-cell lymphomas, unspecified, intrathoracic lymph nodes** HIV CC HCC
> CC Excl: PDX collection 428

C84.93 **Mature T/NK-cell lymphomas, unspecified, intra-abdominal lymph nodes** HIV CC HCC
> CC Excl: PDX collection 429

C84.94 **Mature T/NK-cell lymphomas, unspecified, lymph nodes of** axilla and upper limb HIV CC HCC
> CC Excl: PDX collection 430

C84.95 **Mature T/NK-cell lymphomas, unspecified, lymph nodes of** inguinal region and lower limb HIV CC HCC
> CC Excl: PDX collection 431

C84.96 **Mature T/NK-cell lymphomas, unspecified, intrapelvic lymph nodes** HIV CC HCC
> CC Excl: PDX collection 432

C84.97 **Mature T/NK-cell lymphomas, unspecified, spleen** HIV CC HCC
> CC Excl: PDX collection 433

C84.98 **Mature T/NK-cell lymphomas, unspecified, lymph nodes of** multiple sites HIV CC HCC
> CC Excl: PDX collection 434

C84.99 **Mature T/NK-cell lymphomas, unspecified, extranodal and solid organ sites** HIV CC HCC
> CC Excl: PDX collection 426

☑4ᵗʰ **C85** **Other specified and unspecified types of non-Hodgkin lymphoma**
> **EXCLUDES 1** other specified types of T/NK-cell lymphoma (C86.-)
> personal history of non-Hodgkin lymphoma (Z85.72)

☑5ᵗʰ **C85.1** **Unspecified B-cell lymphoma**
> **NOTE** If B-cell lineage or involvement is mentioned in conjunction with a specific lymphoma, code to the more specific description.

C85.10 **Unspecified B-cell lymphoma, unspecified site** HIV CC HCC
> CC Excl: PDX collection 426

C85.11 **Unspecified B-cell lymphoma, lymph nodes of** head, face, and neck HIV CC HCC
> CC Excl: PDX collection 427

C85.12 **Unspecified B-cell lymphoma, intrathoracic lymph nodes** HIV CC HCC
> CC Excl: PDX collection 428

C85.13 **Unspecified B-cell lymphoma, intra-abdominal lymph nodes** HIV CC HCC
> CC Excl: PDX collection 429

C85.14 **Unspecified B-cell lymphoma, lymph nodes of** axilla and upper limb HIV CC HCC
> CC Excl: PDX collection 430

C85.15 **Unspecified B-cell lymphoma, lymph nodes of** inguinal region and lower limb HIV CC HCC
> CC Excl: PDX collection 431

C85.16 **Unspecified B-cell lymphoma, intrapelvic lymph nodes** HIV CC HCC
> CC Excl: PDX collection 432

C85.17 **Unspecified B-cell lymphoma, spleen** HIV CC HCC
> CC Excl: PDX collection 433

C85.18 **Unspecified B-cell lymphoma, lymph nodes of** multiple sites HIV CC HCC
> CC Excl: PDX collection 434

C85.19 **Unspecified B-cell lymphoma, extranodal and solid organ sites** HIV CC HCC
> CC Excl: PDX collection 426

☑5ᵗʰ **C85.2** **Mediastinal (thymic) large B-cell lymphoma**

C85.20 **Mediastinal (thymic) large B-cell lymphoma, unspecified site** HIV CC HCC
> CC Excl: PDX collection 426

C85.21 **Mediastinal (thymic) large B-cell lymphoma, lymph nodes of** head, face, and neck HIV CC HCC
> CC Excl: PDX collection 427

C85.22 **Mediastinal (thymic) large B-cell lymphoma, intrathoracic lymph nodes** HIV CC HCC
> CC Excl: PDX collection 428

C85.23 **Mediastinal (thymic) large B-cell lymphoma, intra-abdominal lymph nodes** HIV CC HCC
> CC Excl: PDX collection 429

C85.24 **Mediastinal (thymic) large B-cell lymphoma, lymph nodes of** axilla and upper limb HIV CC HCC
> CC Excl: PDX collection 430

C85.25 **Mediastinal (thymic) large B-cell lymphoma, lymph nodes of** inguinal region and lower limb HIV CC HCC
> CC Excl: PDX collection 431

C85.26 **Mediastinal (thymic) large B-cell lymphoma, intrapelvic lymph nodes** HIV CC HCC
> CC Excl: PDX collection 432

C85.27 **Mediastinal (thymic) large B-cell lymphoma, spleen** HIV CC HCC
> CC Excl: PDX collection 433

C85.28 **Mediastinal (thymic) large B-cell lymphoma, lymph nodes of** multiple sites HIV CC HCC
> CC Excl: PDX collection 434

C85.29 **Mediastinal (thymic) large B-cell lymphoma, extranodal and solid organ sites** HIV CC HCC
> CC Excl: PDX collection 426

☑5ᵗʰ **C85.8** **Other specified types of non-Hodgkin lymphoma**

C85.80 **Other specified types of non-Hodgkin lymphoma, unspecified site** HIV CC HCC
> CC Excl: PDX collection 426

C85.81 **Other specified types of non-Hodgkin lymphoma, lymph nodes of** head, face, and neck HIV CC HCC
> CC Excl: PDX collection 427

Chapter 2. Neoplasms

C85.82 Other specified types of non-Hodgkin lymphoma, **intrathoracic** lymph nodes `HIV` `CC` `HCC`
    CC Excl: PDX collection 428

C85.83 Other specified types of non-Hodgkin lymphoma, **intra-abdominal** lymph nodes `HIV` `CC` `HCC`
    CC Excl: PDX collection 429

C85.84 Other specified types of non-Hodgkin lymphoma, lymph nodes of **axilla and upper limb** `HIV` `CC` `HCC`
    CC Excl: PDX collection 430

C85.85 Other specified types of non-Hodgkin lymphoma, lymph nodes of **inguinal region and lower limb** `HIV` `CC` `HCC`
    CC Excl: PDX collection 431

C85.86 Other specified types of non-Hodgkin lymphoma, **intrapelvic** lymph nodes `HIV` `CC` `HCC`
    CC Excl: PDX collection 432

C85.87 Other specified types of non-Hodgkin lymphoma, **spleen** `HIV` `CC` `HCC`
    CC Excl: PDX collection 433

C85.88 Other specified types of non-Hodgkin lymphoma, lymph nodes of **multiple sites** `HIV` `CC` `HCC`
    CC Excl: PDX collection 434

C85.89 Other specified types of non-Hodgkin lymphoma, **extranodal and solid organ sites** `HIV` `CC` `HCC`
    CC Excl: PDX collection 426

✓5ᵗʰ C85.9 Non-Hodgkin lymphoma, unspecified
Lymphoma NOS
Malignant lymphoma NOS
Non-Hodgkin lymphoma NOS

C85.90 Non-Hodgkin lymphoma, unspecified, **unspecified site** `HIV` `CC` `HCC`
    CC Excl: PDX collection 426

C85.91 Non-Hodgkin lymphoma, unspecified, lymph nodes of **head, face, and neck** `HIV` `CC` `HCC`
    CC Excl: PDX collection 427

C85.92 Non-Hodgkin lymphoma, unspecified, **intrathoracic** lymph nodes `HIV` `CC` `HCC`
    CC Excl: PDX collection 428

C85.93 Non-Hodgkin lymphoma, unspecified, **intra-abdominal** lymph nodes `HIV` `CC` `HCC`
    CC Excl: PDX collection 429

C85.94 Non-Hodgkin lymphoma, unspecified, lymph nodes of **axilla and upper limb** `HIV` `CC` `HCC`
    CC Excl: PDX collection 430

C85.95 Non-Hodgkin lymphoma, unspecified, lymph nodes of **inguinal region and lower limb** `HIV` `CC` `HCC`
    CC Excl: PDX collection 431

C85.96 Non-Hodgkin lymphoma, unspecified, **intrapelvic** lymph nodes `HIV` `CC` `HCC`
    CC Excl: PDX collection 432

C85.97 Non-Hodgkin lymphoma, unspecified, **spleen** `HIV` `CC` `HCC`
    CC Excl: PDX collection 433

C85.98 Non-Hodgkin lymphoma, unspecified, lymph nodes of **multiple sites** `HIV` `CC` `HCC`
    CC Excl: PDX collection 434

C85.99 Non-Hodgkin lymphoma, unspecified, **extranodal and solid organ sites** `HIV` `CC` `HCC`
    CC Excl: PDX collection 426

✓4ᵗʰ C86 Other specified types of T/NK-cell lymphoma
    EXCLUDES 1   *anaplastic large cell lymphoma, ALK negative (C84.7-)*
    anaplastic large cell lymphoma, ALK positive (C84.6-)
    mature T/NK-cell lymphomas (C84.-)
    other specified types of non-Hodgkin lymphoma (C85.8-)

C86.0 Extranodal NK/T-cell lymphoma, nasal type `HIV` `CC` `HCC`
    CC Excl: PDX collection 427

C86.1 Hepatosplenic T-cell lymphoma `HIV` `CC` `HCC`
Alpha-beta and gamma delta types
    CC Excl: PDX collection 433

C86.2 Enteropathy-type (intestinal) T-cell lymphoma `HIV` `CC` `HCC`
Enteropathy associated T-cell lymphoma
    CC Excl: PDX collection 429

C86.3 Subcutaneous panniculitis-like T-cell lymphoma `HIV` `CC` `HCC`
    CC Excl: PDX collection 429

C86.4 Blastic NK-cell lymphoma `HIV` `CC` `HCC`
Blastic plasmacytoid dendritic cell neoplasm (BPDCN)
    CC Excl: PDX collection 426

C86.5 Angioimmunoblastic T-cell lymphoma `HIV` `CC` `HCC`
Angioimmunoblastic lymphadenopathy with dysproteinemia [AILD]
    CC Excl: PDX collection 435

C86.6 Primary cutaneous CD30-positive T-cell proliferations `HIV` `CC` `HCC`
Lymphomatoid papulosis
Primary cutaneous anaplastic large cell lymphoma
Primary cutaneous CD30-positive large T-cell lymphoma
    CC Excl: PDX collection 435

✓4ᵗʰ C88 Malignant immunoproliferative diseases and certain other B-cell lymphomas
    EXCLUDES 1   *B-cell lymphoma, unspecified (C85.1-)*
    personal history of other malignant neoplasms of lymphoid, hematopoietic and related tissues (Z85.79)

CC Excl: For CC codes in category C88, unless otherwise noted: PDX collection 485

C88.0 Waldenström macroglobulinemia `HCC`
Lymphoplasmacytic lymphoma with IgM-production
Macroglobulinemia (idiopathic) (primary)
    EXCLUDES 1   *small cell B-cell lymphoma (C83.0)*

C88.2 Heavy chain disease `CC` `HCC`
Franklin disease
Gamma heavy chain disease
Mu heavy chain disease

C88.3 Immunoproliferative small intestinal disease `CC` `HCC`
Alpha heavy chain disease
Mediterranean lymphoma

C88.4 Extranodal marginal zone B-cell lymphoma of mucosa-associated lymphoid tissue [MALT-lymphoma] `HIV` `CC` `HCC`
Lymphoma of skin-associated lymphoid tissue [SALT-lymphoma]
Lymphoma of bronchial-associated lymphoid tissue [BALT-lymphoma]
    EXCLUDES 1   *high malignant (diffuse large B-cell) lymphoma (C83.3-)*
    CC Excl: PDX collection 426

C88.8 Other malignant immunoproliferative diseases `CC` `HCC`
    CC Excl: PDX collection 486

C88.9 Malignant immunoproliferative disease, unspecified `CC` `HCC`
Immunoproliferative disease NOS

✓4ᵗʰ C90 Multiple myeloma and malignant plasma cell neoplasms
    EXCLUDES 1   *personal history of other malignant neoplasms of lymphoid, hematopoietic and related tissues (Z85.79)*

CC Excl: For CC codes in category C90: PDX collection 485

✓5ᵗʰ C90.0 Multiple myeloma
Kahler's disease   Myelomatosis
Medullary plasmacytoma   Plasma cell myeloma
    EXCLUDES 1   *solitary myeloma (C90.3-)*
    solitary plasmactyoma (C90.3-)
    TIP: Do not assign an additional code for bone metastasis (C79.51) when multiple myeloma is described as metastatic to the bone; bone involvement is integral to this disease process.

C90.00 Multiple myeloma **not having achieved remission** `CC` `HCC`
Multiple myeloma with failed remission
Multiple myeloma NOS

C90.01 Multiple myeloma **in remission** `CC` `HCC`

C90.02 Multiple myeloma **in relapse** `CC` `HCC`

✓5ᵗʰ C90.1 Plasma cell leukemia
Plasmacytic leukemia

C90.10 Plasma cell leukemia **not having achieved remission** `CC` `HCC`
Plasma cell leukemia with failed remission
Plasma cell leukemia NOS

C90.11 Plasma cell leukemia **in remission** `CC` `HCC`

C90.12 Plasma cell leukemia **in relapse** `CC` `HCC`

✓5ᵗʰ C90.2 Extramedullary plasmacytoma

C90.20 Extramedullary plasmacytoma **not having achieved remission** `CC` `HCC`
Extramedullary plasmacytoma with failed remission
Extramedullary plasmacytoma NOS

C90.21 Extramedullary plasmacytoma **in remission** `CC` `HCC`

C90.22 Extramedullary plasmacytoma **in relapse** `CC` `HCC`

`N` Newborn: 0   `P` Pediatric: 0-17   `M` Maternity: 12-55   `A` Adult: 15-124   `MCC` Major Complication/Comorbidity   `CC` Complication/Comorbidity   `SW` Severe Wound Dx

488   ICD-10-CM 2019

✓5ᵗʰ **C90.3 Solitary plasmacytoma**
Localized malignant plasma cell tumor NOS
Plasmacytoma NOS
Solitary myeloma

    C90.30 Solitary plasmacytoma not having achieved remission `CC` `HCC`
        Solitary plasmacytoma with failed remission
        Solitary plasmacytoma NOS

    C90.31 Solitary plasmacytoma in remission `CC` `HCC`

    C90.32 Solitary plasmacytoma in relapse `CC` `HCC`

✓4ᵗʰ **C91 Lymphoid leukemia**
    EXCLUDES 1   personal history of leukemia (Z85.6)
    DEF: Malignant proliferation of immature lymphocytes (white blood cells that make up lymphoid tissue), called lymphoblasts, that originate in the bone marrow. Can be acute (ALL) or chronic (CLL).

    CC Excl: For CC codes in category C91, unless otherwise noted:
    PDX collection 485

✓5ᵗʰ **C91.0 Acute lymphoblastic leukemia [ALL]**
      NOTE   Code C91.0 should only be used for T-cell and B-cell precursor leukemia

    C91.00 Acute lymphoblastic leukemia not having achieved remission `CC` `HCC`
        Acute lymphoblastic leukemia with failed remission
        Acute lymphoblastic leukemia NOS

    C91.01 Acute lymphoblastic leukemia, in remission `CC` `HCC`

    C91.02 Acute lymphoblastic leukemia, in relapse `CC` `HCC`

✓5ᵗʰ **C91.1 Chronic lymphocytic leukemia of B-cell type**
Lymphoplasmacytic leukemia
Richter syndrome
    EXCLUDES 1   lymphoplasmacytic lymphoma (C83.0-)

    C91.10 Chronic lymphocytic leukemia of B-cell type not having achieved remission `CC` `HCC`
        Chronic lymphocytic leukemia of B-cell type with failed remission
        Chronic lymphocytic leukemia of B-cell type NOS

    C91.11 Chronic lymphocytic leukemia of B-cell type in remission `CC` `HCC`

    C91.12 Chronic lymphocytic leukemia of B-cell type in relapse `CC` `HCC`

✓5ᵗʰ **C91.3 Prolymphocytic leukemia of B-cell type**

    C91.30 Prolymphocytic leukemia of B-cell type not having achieved remission `CC` `HCC`
        Prolymphocytic leukemia of B-cell type with failed remission
        Prolymphocytic leukemia of B-cell type NOS

    C91.31 Prolymphocytic leukemia of B-cell type, in remission `CC` `HCC`

    C91.32 Prolymphocytic leukemia of B-cell type, in relapse `CC` `HCC`

✓5ᵗʰ **C91.4 Hairy cell leukemia**
Leukemic reticuloendotheliosis
    DEF: Rare type of leukemia that is slow growing and often also considered a type of lymphoma. The small B-cell lymphocytes appear with "hairy" projections under a microscope and are found mostly in the bone marrow, spleen, and blood.

    CC Excl: For CC codes in subcategory C91.4:
    PDX collection 487

    C91.40 Hairy cell leukemia not having achieved remission `CC` `HCC`
        Hairy cell leukemia with failed remission
        Hairy cell leukemia NOS

    C91.41 Hairy cell leukemia, in remission `CC` `HCC`

    C91.42 Hairy cell leukemia, in relapse `CC` `HCC`

✓5ᵗʰ **C91.5 Adult T-cell lymphoma/leukemia (HTLV-1-associated)**
Acute variant of adult T-cell lymphoma/leukemia (HTLV-1-associated)
Chronic variant of adult T-cell lymphoma/leukemia (HTLV-1-associated)
Lymphomatoid variant of adult T-cell lymphoma/leukemia (HTLV-1-associated)
Smouldering variant of adult T-cell lymphoma/leukemia (HTLV-1-associated)

    C91.50 Adult T-cell lymphoma/leukemia (HTLV-1-associated) not having achieved remission `CC` `HCC` `A`
        Adult T-cell lymphoma/leukemia (HTLV-1-associated) with failed remission
        Adult T-cell lymphoma/leukemia (HTLV-1-associated) NOS

    C91.51 Adult T-cell lymphoma/leukemia (HTLV-1-associated), in remission `CC` `HCC` `A`

    C91.52 Adult T-cell lymphoma/leukemia (HTLV-1-associated), in relapse `CC` `HCC` `A`

✓5ᵗʰ **C91.6 Prolymphocytic leukemia of T-cell type**

    C91.60 Prolymphocytic leukemia of T-cell type not having achieved remission `CC` `HCC`
        Prolymphocytic leukemia of T-cell type with failed remission
        Prolymphocytic leukemia of T-cell type NOS

    C91.61 Prolymphocytic leukemia of T-cell type, in remission `CC` `HCC`

    C91.62 Prolymphocytic leukemia of T-cell type, in relapse `CC` `HCC`

✓5ᵗʰ **C91.A Mature B-cell leukemia Burkitt-type**
    EXCLUDES 1   Burkitt lymphoma (C83.7-)

    C91.A0 Mature B-cell leukemia Burkitt-type not having achieved remission `CC` `HCC`
        Mature B-cell leukemia Burkitt-type with failed remission
        Mature B-cell leukemia Burkitt-type NOS

    C91.A1 Mature B-cell leukemia Burkitt-type, in remission `CC` `HCC`

    C91.A2 Mature B-cell leukemia Burkitt-type, in relapse `CC` `HCC`

✓5ᵗʰ **C91.Z Other lymphoid leukemia**
T-cell large granular lymphocytic leukemia (associated with rheumatoid arthritis)

    C91.Z0 Other lymphoid leukemia not having achieved remission `CC` `HCC`
        Other lymphoid leukemia with failed remission
        Other lymphoid leukemia NOS

    C91.Z1 Other lymphoid leukemia, in remission `CC` `HCC`

    C91.Z2 Other lymphoid leukemia, in relapse `CC` `HCC`

✓5ᵗʰ **C91.9 Lymphoid leukemia, unspecified**

    C91.90 Lymphoid leukemia, unspecified not having achieved remission `CC` `HCC`
        Lymphoid leukemia with failed remission
        Lymphoid leukemia NOS

    C91.91 Lymphoid leukemia, unspecified, in remission `CC` `HCC`

    C91.92 Lymphoid leukemia, unspecified, in relapse `CC` `HCC`

✓4ᵗʰ **C92 Myeloid leukemia**
    INCLUDES   granulocytic leukemia
                 myelogenous leukemia
    EXCLUDES 1   personal history of leukemia (Z85.6)
    DEF: Cancer that develops in immature myelocytes called myeloblasts. These are the cells that become white blood cells (except lymphocytes), red blood cells, or platelet making cells. Can be acute (AML) or chronic (CML).

    CC Excl: For CC codes in category C92: PDX collection 485

✓5ᵗʰ **C92.0 Acute myeloblastic leukemia**
Acute myeloblastic leukemia, minimal differentiation
Acute myeloblastic leukemia (with maturation)
Acute myeloblastic leukemia 1/ETO
Acute myeloblastic leukemia M0
Acute myeloblastic leukemia M1
Acute myeloblastic leukemia M2
Acute myeloblastic leukemia with t(8;21)
Acute myeloblastic leukemia (without a FAB classification) NOS
Refractory anemia with excess blasts in transformation [RAEB T]
    EXCLUDES 1   acute exacerbation of chronic myeloid leukemia (C92.10)
               refractory anemia with excess of blasts not in transformation (D46.2-)

    C92.00 Acute myeloblastic leukemia, not having achieved remission `CC` `HCC`
        Acute myeloblastic leukemia with failed remission
        Acute myeloblastic leukemia NOS

    C92.01 Acute myeloblastic leukemia, in remission `CC` `HCC`

    C92.02 Acute myeloblastic leukemia, in relapse `CC` `HCC`

☑ Additional Character Required   ✓x7ᵗʰ Placeholder   Unacceptable PDx   Questionable PDx   Manifestation   `H1`-`H14` HAC   `HCC` CMS-HCC Dx   `HIV` HIV Dx

ICD-10-CM 2019   489

Chapter 2. Neoplasms (side tab)

C92.1–C93.92 (side tab)

✓5ᵗʰ **C92.1** Chronic **myeloid leukemia, BCR/ABL-positive**
Chronic myelogenous leukemia, Philadelphia chromosome (Ph1) positive
Chronic myelogenous leukemia, t(9;22) (q34;q11)
Chronic myelogenous leukemia with crisis of blast cells
  EXCLUDES 1   atypical chronic myeloid leukemia BCR/ABL-negative (C92.2-)
  chronic myelomonocytic leukemia (C93.1-)
  chronic myeloproliferative disease (D47.1)

    C92.10 **Chronic myeloid leukemia, BCR/ABL-positive,** CC HCC
       not having achieved remission
       Chronic myeloid leukemia, BCR/ABL-positive with failed remission
       Chronic myeloid leukemia, BCR/ABL-positive NOS

    C92.11 **Chronic myeloid leukemia, BCR/ABL-positive,** CC HCC
       in remission

    C92.12 **Chronic myeloid leukemia, BCR/ABL-positive,** CC HCC
       in relapse

✓5ᵗʰ **C92.2** **Atypical chronic myeloid leukemia,** BCR/ABL-negative

    C92.20 **Atypical chronic myeloid leukemia,** CC HCC
       BCR/ABL-negative, not having achieved remission
       Atypical chronic myeloid leukemia, BCR/ABL-negative with failed remission
       Atypical chronic myeloid leukemia, BCR/ABL-negative NOS

    C92.21 **Atypical chronic myeloid leukemia,** CC HCC
       BCR/ABL-negative, in remission

    C92.22 **Atypical chronic myeloid leukemia,** CC HCC
       BCR/ABL-negative, in relapse

✓5ᵗʰ **C92.3** **Myeloid sarcoma**
A malignant tumor of immature myeloid cells
Chloroma
Granulocytic sarcoma

    C92.30 **Myeloid sarcoma, not having achieved** CC HCC
       remission
       Myeloid sarcoma with failed remission
       Myeloid sarcoma NOS

    C92.31 **Myeloid sarcoma, in remission** CC HCC

    C92.32 **Myeloid sarcoma, in relapse** CC HCC

✓5ᵗʰ **C92.4** **Acute promyelocytic leukemia**
AML M3   AML Me with t(15;17) and variants

    C92.40 **Acute promyelocytic leukemia, not having** CC HCC
       achieved remission
       Acute promyelocytic leukemia with failed remission
       Acute promyelocytic leukemia NOS

    C92.41 **Acute promyelocytic leukemia, in remission** CC HCC

    C92.42 **Acute promyelocytic leukemia, in relapse** CC HCC

✓5ᵗʰ **C92.5** **Acute myelomonocytic leukemia**
AML M4   AML M4 Eo with inv(16) or t(16;16)

    C92.50 **Acute myelomonocytic leukemia, not having** CC HCC
       achieved remission
       Acute myelomonocytic leukemia with failed remission
       Acute myelomonocytic leukemia NOS

    C92.51 **Acute myelomonocytic leukemia, in** CC HCC
       remission

    C92.52 **Acute myelomonocytic leukemia, in relapse** CC HCC

✓5ᵗʰ **C92.6** **Acute myeloid leukemia with 11q23-abnormality**
Acute myeloid leukemia with variation of MLL-gene

    C92.60 **Acute myeloid leukemia with** CC HCC
       11q23-abnormality not having achieved remission
       Acute myeloid leukemia with 11q23-abnormality with failed remission
       Acute myeloid leukemia with 11q23-abnormality NOS

    C92.61 **Acute myeloid leukemia with** CC HCC
       11q23-abnormality in remission

    C92.62 **Acute myeloid leukemia with** CC HCC
       11q23-abnormality in relapse

✓5ᵗʰ **C92.A** **Acute myeloid leukemia with multilineage dysplasia**
Acute myeloid leukemia with dysplasia of remaining hematopoesis and/or myelodysplastic disease in its history

    C92.A0 **Acute myeloid leukemia with multilineage** CC HCC
       dysplasia, not having achieved remission
       Acute myeloid leukemia with multilineage dysplasia with failed remission
       Acute myeloid leukemia with multilineage dysplasia NOS

    C92.A1 **Acute myeloid leukemia with multilineage** CC HCC
       dysplasia, in remission

    C92.A2 **Acute myeloid leukemia with multilineage** CC HCC
       dysplasia, in relapse

✓5ᵗʰ **C92.Z** **Other myeloid leukemia**

    C92.Z0 **Other myeloid leukemia not having achieved** CC HCC
       remission
       Myeloid leukemia NEC with failed remission
       Myeloid leukemia NEC

    C92.Z1 **Other myeloid leukemia, in remission** CC HCC

    C92.Z2 **Other myeloid leukemia, in relapse** CC HCC

✓5ᵗʰ **C92.9** **Myeloid leukemia, unspecified**

    C92.90 **Myeloid leukemia, unspecified, not having** CC HCC
       achieved remission
       Myeloid leukemia, unspecified with failed remission
       Myeloid leukemia, unspecified NOS

    C92.91 **Myeloid leukemia, unspecified in remission** CC HCC

    C92.92 **Myeloid leukemia, unspecified in relapse** CC HCC

✓4ᵗʰ **C93** **Monocytic leukemia**
  INCLUDES   monocytoid leukemia
  EXCLUDES 1   personal history of leukemia (Z85.6))

  CC Excl: For CC codes in category C93: PDX collection 485

✓5ᵗʰ **C93.0** **Acute monoblastic/monocytic leukemia**
    AML M5   AML M5b
    AML M5a

    C93.00 **Acute monoblastic/monocytic leukemia, not** CC HCC
       having achieved remission
       Acute monoblastic/monocytic leukemia with failed remission
       Acute monoblastic/monocytic leukemia NOS

    C93.01 **Acute monoblastic/monocytic leukemia, in** CC HCC
       remission

    C93.02 **Acute monoblastic/monocytic leukemia, in** CC HCC
       relapse

✓5ᵗʰ **C93.1** **Chronic myelomonocytic leukemia**
Chronic monocytic leukemia
CMML-1
CMML-2
CMML with eosinophilia

    C93.10 **Chronic myelomonocytic leukemia not** CC HCC
       having achieved remission
       Chronic myelomonocytic leukemia with failed remission
       Chronic myelomonocytic leukemia NOS

    C93.11 **Chronic myelomonocytic leukemia, in** CC HCC
       remission

    C93.12 **Chronic myelomonocytic leukemia,** CC HCC
       in relapse

✓5ᵗʰ **C93.3** **Juvenile myelomonocytic leukemia**

    C93.30 **Juvenile myelomonocytic leukemia, not** CC HCC P
       having achieved remission
       Juvenile myelomonocytic leukemia with failed remission
       Juvenile myelomonocytic leukemia NOS

    C93.31 **Juvenile myelomonocytic leukemia, in** CC HCC P
       remission

    C93.32 **Juvenile myelomonocytic leukemia, in** CC HCC P
       relapse

✓5ᵗʰ **C93.Z** **Other monocytic leukemia**

    C93.Z0 **Other monocytic leukemia, not having** CC HCC
       achieved remission
       Other monocytic leukemia NOS

    C93.Z1 **Other monocytic leukemia, in remission** CC HCC

    C93.Z2 **Other monocytic leukemia, in relapse** CC HCC

✓5ᵗʰ **C93.9** **Monocytic leukemia, unspecified**

    C93.90 **Monocytic leukemia, unspecified, not having** CC HCC
       achieved remission
       Monocytic leukemia, unspecified with failed remission
       Monocytic leukemia, unspecified NOS

    C93.91 **Monocytic leukemia, unspecified in** CC HCC
       remission

    C93.92 **Monocytic leukemia, unspecified in relapse** CC HCC

N Newborn: 0   P Pediatric: 0-17   M Maternity: 12-55   A Adult: 15-124   MCC Major Complication/Comorbidity   CC Complication/Comorbidity   SW Severe Wound Dx

490   ICD-10-CM 2019

✓4ᵗʰ **C94** Other **leukemias of** specified cell type

> *EXCLUDES 1*   *leukemic reticuloendotheliosis (C91.4-)*
> *myelodysplastic syndromes (D46.-)*
> *personal history of leukemia (Z85.6)*
> *plasma cell leukemia (C90.1-)*

> **CC Excl: For CC codes in category C94, unless otherwise noted:** PDX collection 485

✓5ᵗʰ **C94.0** Acute erythroid leukemia
Acute myeloid leukemia M6(a)(b)
Erythroleukemia
DEF: Erythroleukemia: Malignant blood dyscrasia (a myeloproliferative disorder).

     C94.00 **Acute erythroid leukemia,** not having achieved remission   `CC` `HCC`
Acute erythroid leukemia with failed remission
Acute erythroid leukemia NOS

     C94.01 **Acute erythroid leukemia,** in remission   `CC` `HCC`

     C94.02 **Acute erythroid leukemia,** in relapse   `CC` `HCC`

✓5ᵗʰ **C94.2** Acute megakaryoblastic leukemia
Acute myeloid leukemia M7
Acute megakaryocytic leukemia

     C94.20 **Acute megakaryoblastic leukemia** not having achieved remission   `CC` `HCC`
Acute megakaryoblastic leukemia with failed remission
Acute megakaryoblastic leukemia NOS

     C94.21 **Acute megakaryoblastic leukemia,** in remission   `CC` `HCC`

     C94.22 **Acute megakaryoblastic leukemia,** in relapse   `CC` `HCC`

✓5ᵗʰ **C94.3** Mast cell leukemia
AHA: 2017, 4Q, 5

     C94.30 **Mast cell leukemia** not having achieved remission   `CC` `HCC`
Mast cell leukemia with failed remission
Mast cell leukemia NOS

     C94.31 **Mast cell leukemia,** in remission   `CC` `HCC`

     C94.32 **Mast cell leukemia,** in relapse   `CC` `HCC`

✓5ᵗʰ **C94.4** Acute panmyelosis with myelofibrosis
Acute myelofibrosis

> *EXCLUDES 1*   *myelofibrosis NOS (D75.81)*
> *secondary myelofibrosis NOS (D75.81)*

> **CC Excl: For CC codes in subcategory C94.4:** PDX collection 488

     C94.40 **Acute panmyelosis with myelofibrosis** not having achieved remission   `CC` `HCC`
Acute myelofibrosis NOS
Acute panmyelosis with myelofibrosis with failed remission
Acute panmyelosis NOS

     C94.41 **Acute panmyelosis with myelofibrosis,** in remission   `CC` `HCC`

     C94.42 **Acute panmyelosis with myelofibrosis,** in relapse   `CC` `HCC`

C94.6 **Myelodysplastic disease, not classified**   `CC` `HCC`
Myeloproliferative disease, not classified
CC Excl: PDX collection 488

✓5ᵗʰ **C94.8** Other specified leukemias
Aggressive NK-cell leukemia
Acute basophilic leukemia

     C94.80 **Other specified leukemias** not having achieved remission   `CC` `HCC`
Other specified leukemia with failed remission
Other specified leukemias NOS

     C94.81 **Other specified leukemias,** in remission   `CC` `HCC`

     C94.82 **Other specified leukemias,** in relapse   `CC` `HCC`

✓4ᵗʰ **C95** Leukemia of unspecified cell type

> *EXCLUDES 1*   *personal history of leukemia (Z85.6)*

> **CC Excl: For CC codes in category C95:** PDX collection 485

✓5ᵗʰ **C95.0** Acute leukemia of unspecified cell type
Acute bilineal leukemia
Acute mixed lineage leukemia
Biphenotypic acute leukemia
Stem cell leukemia of unclear lineage

> *EXCLUDES 1*   *acute exacerbation of unspecified chronic leukemia (C95.10)*

     C95.00 **Acute leukemia of unspecified cell type** not having achieved remission   `CC` `HCC`
Acute leukemia of unspecified cell type with failed remission
Acute leukemia NOS

     C95.01 **Acute leukemia of unspecified cell type,** in remission   `CC` `HCC`

     C95.02 **Acute leukemia of unspecified cell type,** in relapse   `CC` `HCC`

✓5ᵗʰ **C95.1** Chronic leukemia of unspecified cell type

     C95.10 **Chronic leukemia of unspecified cell type** not having achieved remission   `CC` `HCC`
Chronic leukemia of unspecified cell type with failed remission
Chronic leukemia NOS

     C95.11 **Chronic leukemia of unspecified cell type,** in remission   `CC` `HCC`

     C95.12 **Chronic leukemia of unspecified cell type,** in relapse   `CC` `HCC`

✓5ᵗʰ **C95.9** Leukemia, unspecified

     C95.90 **Leukemia, unspecified** not having achieved remission   `CC` `HCC`
Leukemia, unspecified with failed remission
Leukemia NOS

     C95.91 **Leukemia, unspecified,** in remission   `CC` `HCC`

     C95.92 **Leukemia, unspecified,** in relapse   `CC` `HCC`

✓4ᵗʰ **C96** Other and unspecified malignant neoplasms of lymphoid, hematopoietic and related tissue

> *EXCLUDES 1*   *personal history of other malignant neoplasms of lymphoid, hematopoietic and related tissues (Z85.79)*

C96.0 **Multifocal and multisystemic (disseminated) Langerhans-cell histiocytosis**   `CC` `HCC`
Histiocytosis X, multisystemic
Letterer-Siwe disease

> *EXCLUDES 1*   *adult pulmonary Langerhans cell histiocytosis (J84.82)*
> *multifocal and unisystemic Langerhans-cell histiocytosis (C96.5)*
> *unifocal Langerhans-cell histiocytosis (C96.6)*

CC Excl: PDX collection 489

✓5ᵗʰ **C96.2** Malignant mast cell neoplasm

> *EXCLUDES 1*   *indolent mastocytosis (D47.02)*
> *mast cell leukemia (C94.30)*
> *mastocytosis (congenital) (cutaneous) (Q82.2)*

AHA: 2017, 4Q, 5
DEF: Mast cell: Type of white blood cell found in the loose connective tissue of blood vessels and bronchioles responsible for acute hypersensitivity reactions, including anaphylactic shock. The IgE receptors on these cells bind with allergens causing cell degranulation and diffuse, widespread histamine release that results in airway constriction and vasodilation with decreased systemic blood pressure.

> **CC Excl: For CC codes in subcategory C96.2:** PDX collection 490

     C96.20 **Malignant mast cell neoplasm, unspecified**   `CC` `HCC`

     C96.21 **Aggressive systemic mastocytosis**   `CC` `HCC`

     C96.22 **Mast cell sarcoma**   `CC` `HCC`

     C96.29 **Other malignant mast cell neoplasm**   `CC` `HCC`

C96.4 **Sarcoma of dendritic cells (accessory cells)**   `CC` `HCC`
Follicular dendritic cell sarcoma
Interdigitating dendritic cell sarcoma
Langerhans cell sarcoma
CC Excl: PDX collection 491

C96.5 **Multifocal and unisystemic Langerhans-cell histiocytosis** `CC` `HCC`
Hand-Schüller-Christian disease
Histiocytosis X, multifocal
> EXCLUDES 1   multifocal and multisystemic (disseminated) Langerhans-cell histiocytosis (C96.0)
> unifocal Langerhans-cell histiocytosis (C96.6)

CC Excl: PDX collection 492

C96.6 **Unifocal Langerhans-cell histiocytosis** `CC` `HCC`
Eosinophilic granuloma
Histiocytosis X, unifocal
Histiocytosis X NOS
Langerhans-cell histiocytosis NOS
> EXCLUDES 1   multifocal and multisystemic (disseminated) Langerhans-cell histiocytosis (C96.0)
> multifocal and unisystemic Langerhans-cell histiocytosis (C96.5)

CC Excl: PDX collection 492

C96.A **Histiocytic sarcoma** `CC` `HCC`
Malignant histiocytosis
CC Excl: PDX collection 493

C96.Z **Other specified malignant neoplasms of lymphoid, hematopoietic and related tissue** `CC` `HCC`
CC Excl: PDX collection 491

C96.9 **Malignant neoplasm of lymphoid, hematopoietic and related tissue, unspecified** `CC` `HCC`
CC Excl: PDX collection 491

In situ neoplasms (D00-D09)

> INCLUDES   Bowen's disease
> erythroplasia
> grade III intraepithelial neoplasia
> Queyrat's erythroplasia

✓4ᵗʰ **D00** **Carcinoma in situ of oral cavity, esophagus and stomach**
> EXCLUDES 1   melanoma in situ (D03.-)

  ✓5ᵗʰ **D00.0** **Carcinoma in situ of lip, oral cavity and pharynx**
Use additional code to identify:
exposure to environmental tobacco smoke (Z77.22)
exposure to tobacco smoke in the perinatal period (P96.81)
history of tobacco dependence (Z87.891)
occupational exposure to environmental tobacco smoke (Z57.31)
tobacco dependence (F17.-)
tobacco use (Z72.0)
> EXCLUDES 1   carcinoma in situ of aryepiglottic fold or interarytenoid fold, laryngeal aspect (D02.0)
> carcinoma in situ of epiglottis NOS (D02.0)
> carcinoma in situ of epiglottis suprahyoid portion (D02.0)
> carcinoma in situ of skin of lip (D03.0, D04.0)

    D00.00 **Carcinoma in situ of oral cavity, unspecified site**

    D00.01 **Carcinoma in situ of labial mucosa and vermilion border**

    D00.02 **Carcinoma in situ of buccal mucosa**

    D00.03 **Carcinoma in situ of gingiva and edentulous alveolar ridge**

    D00.04 **Carcinoma in situ of soft palate**

    D00.05 **Carcinoma in situ of hard palate**

    D00.06 **Carcinoma in situ of floor of mouth**

    D00.07 **Carcinoma in situ of tongue**

    D00.08 **Carcinoma in situ of pharynx**
Carcinoma in situ of aryepiglottic fold NOS
Carcinoma in situ of hypopharyngeal aspect of aryepiglottic fold
Carcinoma in situ of marginal zone of aryepiglottic fold

  D00.1 **Carcinoma in situ of esophagus**

  D00.2 **Carcinoma in situ of stomach**

✓4ᵗʰ **D01** **Carcinoma in situ of other and unspecified digestive organs**
> EXCLUDES 1   melanoma in situ (D03.-)

  D01.0 **Carcinoma in situ of colon**
> EXCLUDES 1   carcinoma in situ of rectosigmoid junction (D01.1)

  D01.1 **Carcinoma in situ of rectosigmoid junction**

  D01.2 **Carcinoma in situ of rectum**

D01.3 **Carcinoma in situ of anus and anal canal**
Anal intraepithelial neoplasia III [AIN III]
Severe dysplasia of anus
> EXCLUDES 1   anal intraepithelial neoplasia I and II [AIN I and AIN II] (K62.82)
> carcinoma in situ of anal margin (D04.5)
> carcinoma in situ of anal skin (D04.5)
> carcinoma in situ of perianal skin (D04.5)

  ✓5ᵗʰ **D01.4** **Carcinoma in situ of other and unspecified parts of intestine**
> EXCLUDES 1   carcinoma in situ of ampulla of Vater (D01.5)

    D01.40 **Carcinoma in situ of unspecified part of intestine**

    D01.49 **Carcinoma in situ of other parts of intestine**

  D01.5 **Carcinoma in situ of liver, gallbladder and bile ducts**
Carcinoma in situ of ampulla of Vater

  D01.7 **Carcinoma in situ of other specified digestive organs**
Carcinoma in situ of pancreas

  D01.9 **Carcinoma in situ of digestive organ, unspecified**

✓4ᵗʰ **D02** **Carcinoma in situ of middle ear and respiratory system**
Use additional code to identify:
exposure to environmental tobacco smoke (Z77.22)
exposure to tobacco smoke in the perinatal period (P96.81)
history of tobacco dependence (Z87.891)
occupational exposure to environmental tobacco smoke (Z57.31)
tobacco dependence (F17.-)
tobacco use (Z72.0)
> EXCLUDES 1   melanoma in situ (D03.-)

  D02.0 **Carcinoma in situ of larynx**
Carcinoma in situ of aryepiglottic fold or interarytenoid fold, laryngeal aspect
Carcinoma in situ of epiglottis (suprahyoid portion)
> EXCLUDES 1   carcinoma in situ of aryepiglottic fold or interarytenoid fold NOS (D00.08)
> carcinoma in situ of hypopharyngeal aspect (D00.08)
> carcinoma in situ of marginal zone (D00.08)

  D02.1 **Carcinoma in situ of trachea**

  ✓5ᵗʰ **D02.2** **Carcinoma in situ of bronchus and lung**

    D02.20 **Carcinoma in situ of unspecified bronchus and lung**

    D02.21 **Carcinoma in situ of right bronchus and lung**

    D02.22 **Carcinoma in situ of left bronchus and lung**

  D02.3 **Carcinoma in situ of other parts of respiratory system**
Carcinoma in situ of accessory sinuses
Carcinoma in situ of middle ear
Carcinoma in situ of nasal cavities
> EXCLUDES 1   carcinoma in situ of ear (external) (skin) (D04.2-)
> carcinoma in situ of nose NOS (D09.8)
> carcinoma in situ of skin of nose (D04.3)

  D02.4 **Carcinoma in situ of respiratory system, unspecified**

✓4ᵗʰ **D03** **Melanoma in situ**

  D03.0 **Melanoma in situ of lip** `HCC`

  ✓5ᵗʰ **D03.1** **Melanoma in situ of eyelid, including canthus**

    D03.10 **Melanoma in situ of unspecified eyelid, including canthus** `HCC`

    ✓6ᵗʰ **D03.11** **Melanoma in situ of right eyelid, including canthus**

      D03.111 **Melanoma in situ of right upper eyelid, including canthus**

      D03.112 **Melanoma in situ of right lower eyelid, including canthus**

    ✓6ᵗʰ **D03.12** **Melanoma in situ of left eyelid, including canthus**

      D03.121 **Melanoma in situ of left upper eyelid, including canthus**

      D03.122 **Melanoma in situ of left lower eyelid, including canthus**

  ✓5ᵗʰ **D03.2** **Melanoma in situ of ear and external auricular canal**

    D03.20 **Melanoma in situ of unspecified ear and external auricular canal** `HCC`

    D03.21 **Melanoma in situ of right ear and external auricular canal** `HCC`

    D03.22 **Melanoma in situ of left ear and external auricular canal** `HCC`

  ✓5ᵗʰ **D03.3** **Melanoma in situ of other and unspecified parts of face**

    D03.30 **Melanoma in situ of unspecified part of face** `HCC`

    D03.39 **Melanoma in situ of other parts of face** `HCC`

  D03.4 **Melanoma in situ of scalp and neck** `HCC`

✓5ᵗʰ **D03.5** **Melanoma in situ of** trunk

     D03.51 **Melanoma in situ of** anal skin   `HCC`
           Melanoma in situ of anal margin
           Melanoma in situ of perianal skin

     D03.52 **Melanoma in situ of** breast (skin) (soft tissue)   `HCC`

     D03.59 **Melanoma in situ of** other part of trunk   `HCC`

✓5ᵗʰ **D03.6** **Melanoma in situ of** upper limb, including shoulder

     D03.60 **Melanoma in situ of** unspecified upper limb, including shoulder   `HCC`

     D03.61 **Melanoma in situ of** right upper limb, including shoulder   `HCC`

     D03.62 **Melanoma in situ of** left upper limb, including shoulder   `HCC`

✓5ᵗʰ **D03.7** **Melanoma in situ of** lower limb, including hip

     D03.70 **Melanoma in situ of** unspecified lower limb, including hip   `HCC`

     D03.71 **Melanoma in situ of** right lower limb, including hip   `HCC`

     D03.72 **Melanoma in situ of** left lower limb, including hip   `HCC`

D03.8 **Melanoma in situ of** other sites   `HCC`
     Melanoma in situ of scrotum
     EXCLUDES 1   *carcinoma in situ of scrotum (D07.61)*

D03.9 **Melanoma in situ,** unspecified   `HCC`

✓4ᵗʰ **D04** **Carcinoma in situ of** skin
     EXCLUDES 1   *erythroplasia of Queyrat (penis) NOS (D07.4)*
                melanoma in situ (D03.-)

D04.0 **Carcinoma in situ of skin of** lip
     EXCLUDES 1   *carcinoma in situ of vermilion border of lip (D00.01)*

✓5ᵗʰ **D04.1** **Carcinoma in situ of skin of** eyelid, including canthus

     D04.10 **Carcinoma in situ of skin of** unspecified eyelid, including canthus

     ✓6ᵗʰ **D04.11** **Carcinoma in situ of skin of** right eyelid, including canthus

●   **D04.111** **Carcinoma in situ of skin of right** upper eyelid, including canthus

●   **D04.112** **Carcinoma in situ of skin of right** lower eyelid, including canthus

     ✓6ᵗʰ **D04.12** **Carcinoma in situ of skin of** left eyelid, including canthus

●   **D04.121** **Carcinoma in situ of skin of left** upper eyelid, including canthus

●   **D04.122** **Carcinoma in situ of skin of left** lower eyelid, including canthus

✓5ᵗʰ **D04.2** **Carcinoma in situ of skin of** ear and external auricular canal

     D04.20 **Carcinoma in situ of skin of** unspecified ear and external auricular canal

     D04.21 **Carcinoma in situ of skin of** right ear and external auricular canal

     D04.22 **Carcinoma in situ of skin of** left ear and external auricular canal

✓5ᵗʰ **D04.3** **Carcinoma in situ of skin of** other and unspecified parts of face

     D04.30 **Carcinoma in situ of skin of** unspecified part of face

     D04.39 **Carcinoma in situ of skin of** other parts of face

D04.4 **Carcinoma in situ of skin of** scalp and neck

D04.5 **Carcinoma in situ of skin of** trunk
     Carcinoma in situ of anal margin
     Carcinoma in situ of anal skin
     Carcinoma in situ of perianal skin
     Carcinoma in situ of skin of breast
     EXCLUDES 1   *carcinoma in situ of anus NOS (D01.3)*
                carcinoma in situ of scrotum (D07.61)
                carcinoma in situ of skin of genital organs (D07.-)

✓5ᵗʰ **D04.6** **Carcinoma in situ of skin of** upper limb, including shoulder

     D04.60 **Carcinoma in situ of skin of** unspecified upper limb, including shoulder

     D04.61 **Carcinoma in situ of skin of** right upper limb, including shoulder

     D04.62 **Carcinoma in situ of skin of** left upper limb, including shoulder

✓5ᵗʰ **D04.7** **Carcinoma in situ of skin of** lower limb, including hip

     D04.70 **Carcinoma in situ of skin of** unspecified lower limb, including hip

     D04.71 **Carcinoma in situ of skin of** right lower limb, including hip

     D04.72 **Carcinoma in situ of skin of** left lower limb, including hip

D04.8 **Carcinoma in situ of skin of** other sites

D04.9 **Carcinoma in situ of skin,** unspecified

✓4ᵗʰ **D05** **Carcinoma in situ of** breast
     EXCLUDES 1   *carcinoma in situ of skin of breast (D04.5)*
                melanoma in situ of breast (skin) (D03.5)
                Paget's disease of breast or nipple (C50.-)

✓5ᵗʰ **D05.0** **Lobular carcinoma in situ of breast**

     D05.00 **Lobular carcinoma in situ of** unspecified breast

     D05.01 **Lobular carcinoma in situ of** right breast

     D05.02 **Lobular carcinoma in situ of** left breast

✓5ᵗʰ **D05.1** **Intraductal carcinoma in situ of breast**

     D05.10 **Intraductal carcinoma in situ of** unspecified breast

     D05.11 **Intraductal carcinoma in situ of** right breast

     D05.12 **Intraductal carcinoma in situ of** left breast

✓5ᵗʰ **D05.8** **Other specified type of carcinoma in situ of breast**

     D05.80 **Other specified type of carcinoma in situ of** unspecified breast

     D05.81 **Other specified type of carcinoma in situ of** right breast

     D05.82 **Other specified type of carcinoma in situ of** left breast

✓5ᵗʰ **D05.9** **Unspecified type of carcinoma in situ of breast**

     D05.90 **Unspecified type of carcinoma in situ of** unspecified breast

     D05.91 **Unspecified type of carcinoma in situ of** right breast

     D05.92 **Unspecified type of carcinoma in situ of** left breast

✓4ᵗʰ **D06** **Carcinoma in situ of** cervix uteri
     `INCLUDES`   cervical adenocarcinoma in situ
              cervical intraepithelial glandular neoplasia
              cervical intraepithelial neoplasia III [CIN III]
              severe dysplasia of cervix uteri
     EXCLUDES 1   *cervical intraepithelial neoplasia II [CIN II] (N87.1)*
                cytologic evidence of malignancy of cervix without histologic confirmation (R87.614)
                high grade squamous intraepithelial lesion (HGSIL) of cervix (R87.613)
                melanoma in situ of cervix (D03.5)
                moderate cervical dysplasia (N87.1)

D06.0 **Carcinoma in situ of** endocervix   ♀

D06.1 **Carcinoma in situ of** exocervix   ♀

D06.7 **Carcinoma in situ of** other parts of cervix   ♀

D06.9 **Carcinoma in situ of** cervix, unspecified   ♀

✓4ᵗʰ **D07** **Carcinoma in situ of** other and unspecified genital organs
     EXCLUDES 1   *melanoma in situ of trunk (D03.5)*

D07.0 **Carcinoma in situ of** endometrium   ♀

D07.1 **Carcinoma in situ of** vulva   ♀
     Severe dysplasia of vulva
     Vulvar intraepithelial neoplasia III [VIN III]
     EXCLUDES 1   *moderate dysplasia of vulva (N90.1)*
                vulvar intraepithelial neoplasia II [VIN II] (N90.1)

D07.2 **Carcinoma in situ of** vagina   ♀
     Severe dysplasia of vagina
     Vaginal intraepithelial neoplasia III [VAIN III]
     EXCLUDES 1   *moderate dysplasia of vagina (N89.1)*
                vaginal intraepithelial neoplasia II [VIN II] (N89.1)

✓5ᵗʰ **D07.3** **Carcinoma in situ of** other and unspecified female genital organs

     D07.30 **Carcinoma in situ of** unspecified female genital organs   ♀

     D07.39 **Carcinoma in situ of** other female genital organs   ♀

D07.4 **Carcinoma in situ of** penis   ♂
     Erythroplasia of Queyrat NOS

D07.5 **Carcinoma in situ of** prostate   ♂
     Prostatic intraepithelial neoplasia III (PIN III)
     Severe dysplasia of prostate
     EXCLUDES 1   *dysplasia (mild) (moderate) of prostate (N42.3-)*
                prostatic intraepithelial neoplasia II [PIN II] (N42.3-)

☑ Additional Character Required   ✓x7ᵗʰ Placeholder   Unacceptable PDx   Questionable PDx   Manifestation   H1 - H14 HAC   HCC CMS-HCC Dx   HIV HIV Dx

ICD-10-CM 2019   493

☑5ᵗʰ **D07.6 Carcinoma in situ of** other and unspecified male genital organs

    D07.60 Carcinoma in situ of unspecified **male genital organs** ♂

    D07.61 Carcinoma in situ of scrotum ♂

    D07.69 Carcinoma in situ of other **male genital organs** ♂

☑4ᵗʰ **D09 Carcinoma in situ of** other and unspecified sites

    EXCLUDES 1 *melanoma in situ (D03.-)*

    D09.0 Carcinoma in situ of bladder

☑5ᵗʰ **D09.1 Carcinoma in situ of other and unspecified** urinary organs

    D09.10 Carcinoma in situ of unspecified **urinary organ**

    D09.19 Carcinoma in situ of other **urinary organs**

☑5ᵗʰ **D09.2 Carcinoma in situ of** eye

    EXCLUDES 1 *carcinoma in situ of skin of eyelid (D04.1-)*

    D09.20 Carcinoma in situ of unspecified **eye**

    D09.21 Carcinoma in situ of right **eye**

    D09.22 Carcinoma in situ of left **eye**

    D09.3 Carcinoma in situ of thyroid and other endocrine glands

        EXCLUDES 1 *carcinoma in situ of endocrine pancreas (D01.7)*
             carcinoma in situ of ovary (D07.39)
             carcinoma in situ of testis (D07.69)

    D09.8 Carcinoma in situ of other specified sites

    D09.9 Carcinoma in situ, unspecified

Benign neoplasms, except benign neuroendocrine tumors (D10-D36)

☑4ᵗʰ **D10 Benign neoplasm of** mouth and pharynx

    D10.0 Benign neoplasm of lip
        Benign neoplasm of lip (frenulum) (inner aspect) (mucosa) (vermilion border)
        EXCLUDES 1 *benign neoplasm of skin of lip (D22.0, D23.0)*

    D10.1 Benign neoplasm of tongue
        Benign neoplasm of lingual tonsil

    D10.2 Benign neoplasm of floor of mouth

☑5ᵗʰ **D10.3 Benign neoplasm of other and unspecified parts of mouth**

        D10.30 Benign neoplasm of unspecified **part of mouth**

        D10.39 Benign neoplasm of other **parts of mouth**
            Benign neoplasm of minor salivary gland NOS
            EXCLUDES 1 *benign odontogenic neoplasms (D16.4-D16.5)*
               benign neoplasm of mucosa of lip (D10.0)
               benign neoplasm of nasopharyngeal surface of soft palate (D10.6)

    D10.4 Benign neoplasm of tonsil
        Benign neoplasm of tonsil (faucial) (palatine)
        EXCLUDES 1 *benign neoplasm of lingual tonsil (D10.1)*
            benign neoplasm of pharyngeal tonsil (D10.6)
            benign neoplasm of tonsillar fossa (D10.5)
            benign neoplasm of tonsillar pillars (D10.5)

    D10.5 Benign neoplasm of other parts of oropharynx
        Benign neoplasm of epiglottis, anterior aspect
        Benign neoplasm of tonsillar fossa
        Benign neoplasm of tonsillar pillars
        Benign neoplasm of vallecula
        EXCLUDES 1 *benign neoplasm of epiglottis NOS (D14.1)*
            benign neoplasm of epiglottis, suprahyoid portion (D14.1)

    D10.6 Benign neoplasm of nasopharynx
        Benign neoplasm of pharyngeal tonsil
        Benign neoplasm of posterior margin of septum and choanae

    D10.7 Benign neoplasm of hypopharynx

    D10.9 Benign neoplasm of pharynx, unspecified

☑4ᵗʰ **D11 Benign neoplasm of** major salivary glands

    EXCLUDES 1 *benign neoplasms of specified minor salivary glands which are classified according to their anatomical location*
        benign neoplasms of minor salivary glands NOS (D10.39)

    D11.0 Benign neoplasm of parotid gland

    D11.7 Benign neoplasm of other **major salivary glands**
        Benign neoplasm of sublingual salivary gland
        Benign neoplasm of submandibular salivary gland

    D11.9 Benign neoplasm of major salivary gland, unspecified

☑4ᵗʰ **D12 Benign neoplasm of** colon, rectum, anus and anal canal

    EXCLUDES 1 *benign carcinoid tumors of the large intestine, and rectum (D3A.02-)*

    AHA: 2018, 2Q, 14; 2017, 1Q, 15; 2015, 2Q, 14

    D12.0 Benign neoplasm of cecum
        Benign neoplasm of ileocecal valve

    D12.1 Benign neoplasm of appendix
        EXCLUDES 1 *benign carcinoid tumor of the appendix (D3A.020)*

    D12.2 Benign neoplasm of ascending colon

    D12.3 Benign neoplasm of transverse colon
        Benign neoplasm of hepatic flexure
        Benign neoplasm of splenic flexure
        AHA: 2017, 1Q, 16

    D12.4 Benign neoplasm of descending colon

    D12.5 Benign neoplasm of sigmoid colon

    D12.6 Benign neoplasm of colon, unspecified
        Adenomatosis of colon
        Benign neoplasm of large intestine NOS
        Polyposis (hereditary) of colon
        EXCLUDES 1 *inflammatory polyp of colon (K51.4-)*
            polyp of colon NOS (K63.5)

    D12.7 Benign neoplasm of rectosigmoid junction

    D12.8 Benign neoplasm of rectum
        EXCLUDES 1 *benign carcinoid tumor of the rectum (D3A.026)*
        AHA: 2018, 1Q, 6

    D12.9 Benign neoplasm of anus and anal canal
        Benign neoplasm of anus NOS
        EXCLUDES 1 *benign neoplasm of anal margin (D22.5, D23.5)*
            benign neoplasm of anal skin (D22.5, D23.5)
            benign neoplasm of perianal skin (D22.5, D23.5)

☑4ᵗʰ **D13 Benign neoplasm of** other and ill-defined parts of digestive system

    EXCLUDES 1 *benign stromal tumors of digestive system (D21.4)*

    D13.0 Benign neoplasm of esophagus

    D13.1 Benign neoplasm of stomach
        EXCLUDES 1 *benign carcinoid tumor of the stomach (D3A.092)*

    D13.2 Benign neoplasm of duodenum
        EXCLUDES 1 *benign carcinoid tumor of the duodenum (D3A.010)*

☑5ᵗʰ **D13.3 Benign neoplasm of other and unspecified parts of** small intestine

        EXCLUDES 1 *benign carcinoid tumors of the small intestine (D3A.01)*
            benign neoplasm of ileocecal valve (D12.0)

        D13.30 Benign neoplasm of unspecified **part of small intestine**

        D13.39 Benign neoplasm of other parts **of small intestine**

    D13.4 Benign neoplasm of liver
        Benign neoplasm of intrahepatic bile ducts

    D13.5 Benign neoplasm of extrahepatic bile ducts

    D13.6 Benign neoplasm of pancreas
        EXCLUDES 1 *benign neoplasm of endocrine pancreas (D13.7)*

    D13.7 Benign neoplasm of endocrine pancreas
        Islet cell tumor
        Benign neoplasm of islets of Langerhans
        Use additional code to identify any functional activity

    D13.9 Benign neoplasm of ill-defined sites **within the digestive system**
        Benign neoplasm of digestive system NOS
        Benign neoplasm of intestine NOS
        Benign neoplasm of spleen

☑4ᵗʰ **D14 Benign neoplasm of** middle ear and respiratory system

    D14.0 Benign neoplasm of middle ear, nasal cavity and accessory sinuses
        Benign neoplasm of cartilage of nose
        EXCLUDES 1 *benign neoplasm of auricular canal (external) (D22.2-, D23.2-)*
            benign neoplasm of bone of ear (D16.4)
            benign neoplasm of bone of nose (D16.4)
            benign neoplasm of cartilage of ear (D21.0)
            benign neoplasm of ear (external)(skin) (D22.2-, D23.2-)
            benign neoplasm of nose NOS (D36.7)
            benign neoplasm of skin of nose (D22.39, D23.39)
            benign neoplasm of olfactory bulb (D33.3)
            benign neoplasm of posterior margin of septum and choanae (D10.6)
            polyp of accessory sinus (J33.8)
            polyp of ear (middle) (H74.4)
            polyp of nasal (cavity) (J33.-)

Ⓝ Newborn: 0   Ⓟ Pediatric: 0-17   Ⓜ Maternity: 12-55   Ⓐ Adult: 15-124   MCC Major Complication/Comorbidity   CC Complication/Comorbidity   SW Severe Wound Dx

494   ICD-10-CM 2019

D14.1 Benign neoplasm of larynx
Adenomatous polyp of larynx
Benign neoplasm of epiglottis (suprahyoid portion)
> EXCLUDES 1   *benign neoplasm of epiglottis, anterior aspect (D10.5)*
> *polyp (nonadenomatous) of vocal cord or larynx*
> *(J38.1)*

D14.2 Benign neoplasm of trachea

✓5th **D14.3 Benign neoplasm of** bronchus and lung
> EXCLUDES 1   *benign carcinoid tumor of the bronchus and lung*
> *(D3A.090)*

     D14.30 Benign neoplasm of unspecified **bronchus and lung**

     D14.31 Benign neoplasm of right **bronchus and lung**

     D14.32 Benign neoplasm of left **bronchus and lung**

D14.4 Benign neoplasm of respiratory system, unspecified

✓4th **D15 Benign neoplasm of** other and unspecified intrathoracic organs
> EXCLUDES 1   *benign neoplasm of mesothelial tissue (D19.-)*

D15.0 Benign neoplasm of thymus
> EXCLUDES 1   *benign carcinoid tumor of the thymus (D3A.091)*

D15.1 Benign neoplasm of heart
> EXCLUDES 1   *benign neoplasm of great vessels (D21.3)*

D15.2 Benign neoplasm of mediastinum

D15.7 Benign neoplasm of other specified **intrathoracic organs**

D15.9 Benign neoplasm of intrathoracic organ, unspecified

✓4th **D16 Benign neoplasm of** bone and articular cartilage
> EXCLUDES 1   *benign neoplasm of connective tissue of ear (D21.0)*
> *benign neoplasm of connective tissue of eyelid (D21.0)*
> *benign neoplasm of connective tissue of larynx (D14.1)*
> *benign neoplasm of connective tissue of nose (D14.0)*
> *benign neoplasm of synovia (D21.-)*

✓5th **D16.0 Benign neoplasm of** scapula and long bones of upper limb

     D16.00 Benign neoplasm of scapula and long bones of unspecified **upper limb**

     D16.01 Benign neoplasm of scapula and long bones of right **upper limb**

     D16.02 Benign neoplasm of scapula and long bones of left **upper limb**

✓5th **D16.1 Benign neoplasm of** short bones of upper limb

     D16.10 Benign neoplasm of short bones of unspecified **upper limb**

     D16.11 Benign neoplasm of short bones of right **upper limb**

     D16.12 Benign neoplasm of short bones of left **upper limb**

✓5th **D16.2 Benign neoplasm of** long bones of lower limb

     D16.20 Benign neoplasm of long bones of unspecified **lower limb**

     D16.21 Benign neoplasm of long bones of right **lower limb**

     D16.22 Benign neoplasm of long bones of left **lower limb**

✓5th **D16.3 Benign neoplasm of** short bones of lower limb

     D16.30 Benign neoplasm of short bones of unspecified **lower limb**

     D16.31 Benign neoplasm of short bones of right **lower limb**

     D16.32 Benign neoplasm of short bones of left **lower limb**

D16.4 Benign neoplasm of bones of skull and face
Benign neoplasm of maxilla (superior)
Benign neoplasm of orbital bone
Keratocyst of maxilla
Keratocystic odontogenic tumor of maxilla
> EXCLUDES 2   *benign neoplasm of lower jaw bone (D16.5)*

D16.5 Benign neoplasm of lower jaw bone
Keratocyst of mandible
Keratocystic odontogenic tumor of mandible

D16.6 Benign neoplasm of vertebral column
> EXCLUDES 1   *benign neoplasm of sacrum and coccyx (D16.8)*

D16.7 Benign neoplasm of ribs, sternum and clavicle

D16.8 Benign neoplasm of pelvic bones, sacrum and coccyx

D16.9 Benign neoplasm of bone and articular cartilage, unspecified

✓4th **D17 Benign** lipomatous **neoplasm**

D17.0 Benign lipomatous neoplasm of skin and subcutaneous tissue of head, face and neck

D17.1 Benign lipomatous neoplasm of skin and subcutaneous tissue of trunk

✓5th **D17.2 Benign lipomatous neoplasm of** skin and subcutaneous tissue of limb

     D17.20 Benign lipomatous neoplasm of skin and subcutaneous tissue of unspecified **limb**

D17.21 Benign lipomatous neoplasm of skin and subcutaneous tissue of right arm

D17.22 Benign lipomatous neoplasm of skin and subcutaneous tissue of left arm

D17.23 Benign lipomatous neoplasm of skin and subcutaneous tissue of right leg

D17.24 Benign lipomatous neoplasm of skin and subcutaneous tissue of left leg

✓5th **D17.3 Benign lipomatous neoplasm of** skin and subcutaneous tissue of other and unspecified sites

     D17.30 Benign lipomatous neoplasm of skin and subcutaneous tissue of unspecified **sites**

     D17.39 Benign lipomatous neoplasm of skin and subcutaneous tissue of other **sites**

D17.4 Benign lipomatous neoplasm of intrathoracic organs

D17.5 Benign lipomatous neoplasm of intra-abdominal organs
> EXCLUDES 1   *benign lipomatous neoplasm of peritoneum and*
> *retroperitoneum (D17.79)*

D17.6 Benign lipomatous neoplasm of spermatic cord   ♂

✓5th **D17.7 Benign lipomatous neoplasm of** other sites

     D17.71 Benign lipomatous neoplasm of kidney

     D17.72 Benign lipomatous neoplasm of other genitourinary organ

     D17.79 Benign lipomatous neoplasm of other sites
Benign lipomatous neoplasm of peritoneum
Benign lipomatous neoplasm of retroperitoneum

D17.9 Benign lipomatous neoplasm, unspecified
Lipoma NOS

✓4th **D18 Hemangioma and lymphangioma, any site**
> EXCLUDES 1   *benign neoplasm of glomus jugulare (D35.6)*
> *blue or pigmented nevus (D22.-)*
> *nevus NOS (D22.-)*
> *vascular nevus (Q82.5)*

✓5th **D18.0 Hemangioma**
Angioma NOS
Cavernous nevus
DEF: Common benign tumor usually occurring in infancy that is composed of newly formed blood vessels due to malformation of the angioblastic tissue.

     D18.00 Hemangioma unspecified site

     D18.01 Hemangioma of skin and subcutaneous tissue

     D18.02 Hemangioma of intracranial structures   HCC

     D18.03 Hemangioma of intra-abdominal structures

     D18.09 Hemangioma of other sites

D18.1 Lymphangioma, any site
AHA: 2018, 2Q, 13

✓4th **D19 Benign neoplasm of** mesothelial tissue

D19.0 Benign neoplasm of mesothelial tissue of pleura

D19.1 Benign neoplasm of mesothelial tissue of peritoneum

D19.7 Benign neoplasm of mesothelial tissue of other sites

D19.9 Benign neoplasm of mesothelial tissue, unspecified
Benign mesothelioma NOS

✓4th **D20 Benign neoplasm of soft tissue of** retroperitoneum and peritoneum
> EXCLUDES 1   *benign lipomatous neoplasm of peritoneum and*
> *retroperitoneum (D17.79)*
> *benign neoplasm of mesothelial tissue (D19.-)*

D20.0 Benign neoplasm of soft tissue of retroperitoneum

D20.1 Benign neoplasm of soft tissue of peritoneum

✔ Additional Character Required   ✓x7th Placeholder   Unacceptable PDx   Questionable PDx   Manifestation   H1 - H14 HAC   HCC CMS-HCC Dx   HIV HIV Dx

ICD-10-CM 2019   495

Chapter 2. Neoplasms

✓4ᵗʰ **D21 Other benign neoplasms of connective and other soft tissue**

INCLUDES   benign neoplasm of blood vessel
benign neoplasm of bursa
benign neoplasm of cartilage
benign neoplasm of fascia
benign neoplasm of fat
benign neoplasm of ligament, except uterine
benign neoplasm of lymphatic channel
benign neoplasm of muscle
benign neoplasm of synovia
benign neoplasm of tendon (sheath)
benign stromal tumors

EXCLUDES 1   *benign neoplasm of articular cartilage (D16.-)*
benign neoplasm of cartilage of larynx (D14.1)
benign neoplasm of cartilage of nose (D14.0)
benign neoplasm of connective tissue of breast (D24.-)
benign neoplasm of peripheral nerves and autonomic nervous system (D36.1-)
benign neoplasm of peritoneum (D20.1)
benign neoplasm of retroperitoneum (D20.0)
benign neoplasm of uterine ligament, any (D28.2)
benign neoplasm of vascular tissue (D18.-)
hemangioma (D18.0-)
lipomatous neoplasm (D17.-)
lymphangioma (D18.1)
uterine leiomyoma (D25.-)

D21.0 Benign neoplasm of connective and other soft tissue of head, face and neck
Benign neoplasm of connective tissue of ear
Benign neoplasm of connective tissue of eyelid
EXCLUDES 1   *benign neoplasm of connective tissue of orbit (D31.6-)*

✓5ᵗʰ **D21.1 Benign neoplasm of connective and other soft tissue of** upper limb, including shoulder

  D21.10 Benign neoplasm of connective and other soft tissue of unspecified **upper limb, including shoulder**

  D21.11 Benign neoplasm of connective and other soft tissue of right **upper limb, including shoulder**

  D21.12 Benign neoplasm of connective and other soft tissue of left **upper limb, including shoulder**

✓5ᵗʰ **D21.2 Benign neoplasm of connective and other soft tissue of** lower limb, including hip

  D21.20 Benign neoplasm of connective and other soft tissue of unspecified **lower limb, including hip**

  D21.21 Benign neoplasm of connective and other soft tissue of right **lower limb, including hip**

  D21.22 Benign neoplasm of connective and other soft tissue of left **lower limb, including hip**

D21.3 Benign neoplasm of connective and other soft tissue of thorax
Benign neoplasm of axilla
Benign neoplasm of diaphragm
Benign neoplasm of great vessels
EXCLUDES 1   *benign neoplasm of heart (D15.1)*
benign neoplasm of mediastinum (D15.2)
benign neoplasm of thymus (D15.0)

D21.4 Benign neoplasm of connective and other soft tissue of abdomen
Benign stromal tumors of abdomen

D21.5 Benign neoplasm of connective and other soft tissue of pelvis
EXCLUDES 1   *benign neoplasm of any uterine ligament (D28.2)*
uterine leiomyoma (D25.-)

D21.6 Benign neoplasm of connective and other soft tissue of trunk, unspecified
Benign neoplasm of back NOS

D21.9 Benign neoplasm of connective and other soft tissue, unspecified

✓4ᵗʰ **D22 Melanocytic nevi**

INCLUDES   atypical nevus
blue hairy pigmented nevus
nevus NOS

D22.0 Melanocytic nevi of lip

✓5ᵗʰ **D22.1 Melanocytic nevi of** eyelid, including canthus

  D22.10 Melanocytic nevi of unspecified **eyelid, including canthus**

  ✓6ᵗʰ **D22.11 Melanocytic nevi of** right **eyelid, including canthus**

    ● **D22.111 Melanocytic nevi of right** upper **eyelid, including canthus**

    ● **D22.112 Melanocytic nevi of right** lower **eyelid, including canthus**

  ✓6ᵗʰ **D22.12 Melanocytic nevi of** left **eyelid, including canthus**

    ● **D22.121 Melanocytic nevi of left** upper **eyelid, including canthus**

    ● **D22.122 Melanocytic nevi of left** lower **eyelid, including canthus**

✓5ᵗʰ **D22.2 Melanocytic nevi of** ear and external auricular canal

  D22.20 Melanocytic nevi of unspecified **ear and external auricular canal**

  D22.21 Melanocytic nevi of right **ear and external auricular canal**

  D22.22 Melanocytic nevi of left **ear and external auricular canal**

✓5ᵗʰ **D22.3 Melanocytic nevi of** other and unspecified parts of face

  D22.30 Melanocytic nevi of unspecified **part of face**

  D22.39 Melanocytic nevi of other **parts of face**

D22.4 Melanocytic nevi of scalp and neck

D22.5 Melanocytic nevi of trunk
Melanocytic nevi of anal margin
Melanocytic nevi of anal skin
Melanocytic nevi of perianal skin
Melanocytic nevi of skin of breast

✓5ᵗʰ **D22.6 Melanocytic nevi of** upper limb, including shoulder

  D22.60 Melanocytic nevi of unspecified **upper limb, including shoulder**

  D22.61 Melanocytic nevi of right **upper limb, including shoulder**

  D22.62 Melanocytic nevi of left **upper limb, including shoulder**

✓5ᵗʰ **D22.7 Melanocytic nevi of** lower limb, including hip

  D22.70 Melanocytic nevi of unspecified **lower limb, including hip**

  D22.71 Melanocytic nevi of right **lower limb, including hip**

  D22.72 Melanocytic nevi of left **lower limb, including hip**

D22.9 Melanocytic nevi, unspecified

✓4ᵗʰ **D23 Other benign neoplasms of** skin

INCLUDES   benign neoplasm of hair follicles
benign neoplasm of sebaceous glands
benign neoplasm of sweat glands

EXCLUDES 1   *benign lipomatous neoplasms of skin (D17.0-D17.3)*
melanocytic nevi (D22.-)

D23.0 Other benign neoplasm of skin of lip
EXCLUDES 1   *benign neoplasm of vermilion border of lip (D10.0)*

✓5ᵗʰ **D23.1 Other benign neoplasm of skin of** eyelid, including canthus

  D23.10 Other benign neoplasm of skin of unspecified **eyelid, including canthus**

  ✓6ᵗʰ **D23.11 Other benign neoplasm of skin of** right **eyelid, including canthus**

    ● **D23.111 Other benign neoplasm of skin of right** upper **eyelid, including canthus**

    ● **D23.112 Other benign neoplasm of skin of right** lower **eyelid, including canthus**

  ✓6ᵗʰ **D23.12 Other benign neoplasm of skin of** left **eyelid, including canthus**

    ● **D23.121 Other benign neoplasm of skin of left** upper **eyelid, including canthus**

    ● **D23.122 Other benign neoplasm of skin of left** lower **eyelid, including canthus**

✓5ᵗʰ **D23.2 Other benign neoplasm of skin of** ear and external auricular canal

  D23.20 Other benign neoplasm of skin of unspecified **ear and external auricular canal**

  D23.21 Other benign neoplasm of skin of right **ear and external auricular canal**

  D23.22 Other benign neoplasm of skin of left **ear and external auricular canal**

✓5ᵗʰ **D23.3 Other benign neoplasm of skin of** other and unspecified parts of face

  D23.30 Other benign neoplasm of skin of unspecified **part of face**

  D23.39 Other benign neoplasm of skin of other **parts of face**

D23.4 Other benign neoplasm of skin of scalp and neck

D23.5   **Other benign neoplasm of skin of** trunk
     Other benign neoplasm of anal margin
     Other benign neoplasm of anal skin
     Other benign neoplasm of perianal skin
     Other benign neoplasm of skin of breast
     EXCLUDES 1   *benign neoplasm of anus NOS (D12.9)*

✓5th **D23.6**   **Other benign neoplasm of skin of** upper limb, including shoulder

     D23.60   **Other benign neoplasm of skin of** unspecified **upper limb, including shoulder**

     D23.61   **Other benign neoplasm of skin of** right **upper limb, including shoulder**

     D23.62   **Other benign neoplasm of skin of** left **upper limb, including shoulder**

✓5th **D23.7**   **Other benign neoplasm of skin of** lower limb, including hip

     D23.70   **Other benign neoplasm of skin of** unspecified **lower limb, including hip**

     D23.71   **Other benign neoplasm of skin of** right **lower limb, including hip**

     D23.72   **Other benign neoplasm of skin of** left **lower limb, including hip**

D23.9   **Other benign neoplasm of skin,** unspecified

✓4th **D24**   **Benign neoplasm of** breast
     INCLUDES   benign neoplasm of connective tissue of breast
     benign neoplasm of soft parts of breast
     fibroadenoma of breast
     EXCLUDES 2   *adenofibrosis of breast (N60.2)*
     benign cyst of breast (N60.-)
     benign mammary dysplasia (N60.-)
     benign neoplasm of skin of breast (D22.5, D23.5)
     fibrocystic disease of breast (N60.-)

     D24.1   **Benign neoplasm of** right **breast**

     D24.2   **Benign neoplasm of** left **breast**

     D24.9   **Benign neoplasm of** unspecified **breast**

✓4th **D25**   **Leiomyoma of uterus**
     INCLUDES   uterine fibroid
     uterine fibromyoma
     uterine myoma

     D25.0   **Submucous leiomyoma of uterus**   ♀

     D25.1   **Intramural leiomyoma of uterus**   ♀
         Interstitial leiomyoma of uterus

     D25.2   **Subserosal leiomyoma of uterus**   ♀
         Subperitoneal leiomyoma of uterus

     D25.9   **Leiomyoma of uterus,** unspecified

Uterine Leiomyomas (Fibroids)

✓4th **D26**   **Other benign neoplasms of** uterus
     D26.0   **Other benign neoplasm of** cervix uteri   ♀
     D26.1   **Other benign neoplasm of** corpus uteri   ♀
     D26.7   **Other benign neoplasm of** other parts **of uterus**   ♀
     D26.9   **Other benign neoplasm of uterus,** unspecified   ♀

✓4th **D27**   **Benign neoplasm of** ovary
     Use additional code to identify any functional activity
     EXCLUDES 2   *corpus albicans cyst (N83.2-)*
     corpus luteum cyst (N83.1-)
     endometrial cyst (N80.1)
     follicular (atretic) cyst (N83.0-)
     graafian follicle cyst (N83.0-)
     ovarian cyst NEC (N83.2-)
     ovarian retention cyst (N83.2-)

     D27.0   **Benign neoplasm of** right **ovary**   ♀
     D27.1   **Benign neoplasm of** left **ovary**   ♀
     D27.9   **Benign neoplasm of** unspecified **ovary**   ♀

✓4th **D28**   **Benign neoplasm of** other and unspecified female genital organs
     INCLUDES   adenomatous polyp
     benign neoplasm of skin of female genital organs
     benign teratoma
     EXCLUDES 1   *epoophoron cyst (Q50.5)*
     fimbrial cyst (Q50.4)
     Gartner's duct cyst (Q52.4)
     parovarian cyst (Q50.5)

     D28.0   **Benign neoplasm of** vulva   ♀
     D28.1   **Benign neoplasm of** vagina   ♀
     D28.2   **Benign neoplasm of** uterine tubes and ligaments   ♀
         Benign neoplasm of fallopian tube
         Benign neoplasm of uterine ligament (broad) (round)

     D28.7   **Benign neoplasm of** other specified female genital organs   ♀
     D28.9   **Benign neoplasm of** female genital organ, unspecified   ♀

✓4th **D29**   **Benign neoplasm of** male genital organs
     INCLUDES   benign neoplasm of skin of male genital organs

     D29.0   **Benign neoplasm of** penis   ♂
     D29.1   **Benign neoplasm of** prostate   ♂
         EXCLUDES 1   *enlarged prostate (N40.-)*

     ✓5th **D29.2**   **Benign neoplasm of** testis
         Use additional code to identify any functional activity
         D29.20   **Benign neoplasm of** unspecified **testis**   ♂
         D29.21   **Benign neoplasm of** right **testis**   ♂
         D29.22   **Benign neoplasm of** left **testis**   ♂

     ✓5th **D29.3**   **Benign neoplasm of** epididymis
         D29.30   **Benign neoplasm of** unspecified **epididymis**   ♂
         D29.31   **Benign neoplasm of** right **epididymis**   ♂
         D29.32   **Benign neoplasm of** left **epididymis**   ♂

     D29.4   **Benign neoplasm of** scrotum   ♂
         Benign neoplasm of skin of scrotum

     D29.8   **Benign neoplasm of** other specified male genital organs   ♂
         Benign neoplasm of seminal vesicle
         Benign neoplasm of spermatic cord
         Benign neoplasm of tunica vaginalis

     D29.9   **Benign neoplasm of** male genital organ, unspecified   ♂

✓4th **D30**   **Benign neoplasm of** urinary organs
     ✓5th **D30.0**   **Benign neoplasm of** kidney
         EXCLUDES 1   *benign carcinoid tumor of the kidney (D3A.093)*
         benign neoplasm of renal calyces (D30.1-)
         benign neoplasm of renal pelvis (D30.1-)
         D30.00   **Benign neoplasm of** unspecified **kidney**
         D30.01   **Benign neoplasm of** right **kidney**
         D30.02   **Benign neoplasm of** left **kidney**

     ✓5th **D30.1**   **Benign neoplasm of** renal pelvis
         D30.10   **Benign neoplasm of** unspecified **renal pelvis**
         D30.11   **Benign neoplasm of** right **renal pelvis**
         D30.12   **Benign neoplasm of** left **renal pelvis**

     ✓5th **D30.2**   **Benign neoplasm of** ureter
         EXCLUDES 1   *benign neoplasm of ureteric orifice of bladder (D30.3)*
         D30.20   **Benign neoplasm of** unspecified **ureter**
         D30.21   **Benign neoplasm of** right **ureter**
         D30.22   **Benign neoplasm of** left **ureter**

     D30.3   **Benign neoplasm of** bladder
         Benign neoplasm of ureteric orifice of bladder
         Benign neoplasm of urethral orifice of bladder

     D30.4   **Benign neoplasm of** urethra
         EXCLUDES 1   *benign neoplasm of urethral orifice of bladder (D30.3)*

     D30.8   **Benign neoplasm of** other specified urinary organs
         Benign neoplasm of paraurethral glands

✓Additional Character Required   ✓x7th Placeholder   Unacceptable PDx   Questionable PDx   Manifestation   H1-H14 HAC   HCC CMS-HCC Dx   HIV HIV Dx

ICD-10-CM 2019   497

Chapter 2. Neoplasms

D30.9   **Benign neoplasm of urinary organ,** unspecified
     Benign neoplasm of urinary system NOS

✓4ᵗʰ **D31**   **Benign neoplasm of** eye and adnexa
     EXCLUDES 1   *benign neoplasm of connective tissue of eyelid (D21.0)*
             benign neoplasm of optic nerve (D33.3)
             benign neoplasm of skin of eyelid (D22.1-, D23.1-)

✓5ᵗʰ **D31.0**   **Benign neoplasm of** conjunctiva

     D31.00   **Benign neoplasm of** unspecified **conjunctiva**

     D31.01   **Benign neoplasm of** right **conjunctiva**

     D31.02   **Benign neoplasm of** left **conjunctiva**

✓5ᵗʰ **D31.1**   **Benign neoplasm of** cornea

     D31.10   **Benign neoplasm of** unspecified **cornea**

     D31.11   **Benign neoplasm of** right **cornea**

     D31.12   **Benign neoplasm of** left **cornea**

✓5ᵗʰ **D31.2**   **Benign neoplasm of** retina
     EXCLUDES 1   *dark area on retina (D49.81)*
             hemangioma of retina (D49.81)
             neoplasm of unspecified behavior of retina and choroid (D49.81)
             retinal freckle (D49.81)

     D31.20   **Benign neoplasm of** unspecified **retina**

     D31.21   **Benign neoplasm of** right **retina**

     D31.22   **Benign neoplasm of** left **retina**

✓5ᵗʰ **D31.3**   **Benign neoplasm of** choroid

     D31.30   **Benign neoplasm of** unspecified **choroid**

     D31.31   **Benign neoplasm of** right **choroid**

     D31.32   **Benign neoplasm of** left **choroid**

✓5ᵗʰ **D31.4**   **Benign neoplasm of** ciliary body

     D31.40   **Benign neoplasm of** unspecified **ciliary body**

     D31.41   **Benign neoplasm of** right **ciliary body**

     D31.42   **Benign neoplasm of** left **ciliary body**

✓5ᵗʰ **D31.5**   **Benign neoplasm of** lacrimal gland and duct
     Benign neoplasm of lacrimal sac
     Benign neoplasm of nasolacrimal duct

     D31.50   **Benign neoplasm of** unspecified **lacrimal gland and duct**

     D31.51   **Benign neoplasm of** right **lacrimal gland and duct**

     D31.52   **Benign neoplasm of** left **lacrimal gland and duct**

✓5ᵗʰ **D31.6**   **Benign neoplasm of unspecified site of** orbit
     Benign neoplasm of connective tissue of orbit
     Benign neoplasm of extraocular muscle
     Benign neoplasm of peripheral nerves of orbit
     Benign neoplasm of retrobulbar tissue
     Benign neoplasm of retro-ocular tissue
     EXCLUDES 1   *benign neoplasm of orbital bone (D16.4)*

     D31.60   **Benign neoplasm of unspecified site of** unspecified **orbit**

     D31.61   **Benign neoplasm of unspecified site of** right **orbit**

     D31.62   **Benign neoplasm of unspecified site of** left **orbit**

✓5ᵗʰ **D31.9**   **Benign neoplasm of** unspecified part of eye
     Benign neoplasm of eyeball

     D31.90   **Benign neoplasm of unspecified part of** unspecified **eye**

     D31.91   **Benign neoplasm of unspecified part of** right **eye**

     D31.92   **Benign neoplasm of unspecified part of** left **eye**

✓4ᵗʰ **D32**   **Benign neoplasm of** meninges

     D32.0   **Benign neoplasm of** cerebral **meninges**   HCC

     D32.1   **Benign neoplasm of** spinal **meninges**   HCC

     D32.9   **Benign neoplasm of meninges,** unspecified   HCC
            Meningioma NOS

✓4ᵗʰ **D33**   **Benign neoplasm of** brain and other parts of central nervous system
     EXCLUDES 1   *angioma (D18.0-)*
             benign neoplasm of meninges (D32.-)
             benign neoplasm of peripheral nerves and autonomic nervous system (D36.1-)
             hemangioma (D18.0-)
             neurofibromatosis (Q85.0-)
             retro-ocular benign neoplasm (D31.6-)

     D33.0   **Benign neoplasm of** brain, supratentorial   HCC
            Benign neoplasm of cerebral ventricle
            Benign neoplasm of cerebrum
            Benign neoplasm of frontal lobe
            Benign neoplasm of occipital lobe
            Benign neoplasm of parietal lobe
            Benign neoplasm of temporal lobe
            EXCLUDES 1   *benign neoplasm of fourth ventricle (D33.1)*

     D33.1   **Benign neoplasm of** brain, infratentorial   HCC
            Benign neoplasm of brain stem
            Benign neoplasm of cerebellum
            Benign neoplasm of fourth ventricle

     D33.2   **Benign neoplasm of** brain, unspecified   HCC

     D33.3   **Benign neoplasm of** cranial nerves   HCC
            Benign neoplasm of olfactory bulb

     D33.4   **Benign neoplasm of** spinal cord   HCC

     D33.7   **Benign neoplasm of** other **specified parts of central nervous system**   HCC

     D33.9   **Benign neoplasm of central nervous system,** unspecified   HCC
            Benign neoplasm of nervous system (central) NOS

D34   **Benign neoplasm of** thyroid gland
     Use additional code to identify any functional activity

✓4ᵗʰ **D35**   **Benign neoplasm of** other and unspecified endocrine glands
     Use additional code to identify any functional activity
     EXCLUDES 1   *benign neoplasm of endocrine pancreas (D13.7)*
             benign neoplasm of ovary (D27.-)
             benign neoplasm of testis (D29.2-)
             benign neoplasm of thymus (D15.0)

✓5ᵗʰ **D35.0**   **Benign neoplasm of** adrenal gland

     D35.00   **Benign neoplasm of** unspecified **adrenal gland**

     D35.01   **Benign neoplasm of** right **adrenal gland**

     D35.02   **Benign neoplasm of** left **adrenal gland**

     D35.1   **Benign neoplasm of** parathyroid gland

     D35.2   **Benign neoplasm of** pituitary gland   HCC
            AHA: 2014, 3Q, 22

     D35.3   **Benign neoplasm of** craniopharyngeal duct   HCC

     D35.4   **Benign neoplasm of** pineal gland   HCC

     D35.5   **Benign neoplasm of** carotid body

     D35.6   **Benign neoplasm of** aortic body and other paraganglia
            Benign tumor of glomus jugulare

     D35.7   **Benign neoplasm of** other **specified endocrine glands**

     D35.9   **Benign neoplasm of endocrine gland,** unspecified
            Benign neoplasm of unspecified endocrine gland

✓4ᵗʰ **D36**   **Benign neoplasm of** other and unspecified sites

     D36.0   **Benign neoplasm of** lymph nodes
            EXCLUDES 1   *lymphangioma (D18.1)*

✓5ᵗʰ **D36.1**   **Benign neoplasm of** peripheral nerves and autonomic nervous system
            EXCLUDES 1   *benign neoplasm of peripheral nerves of orbit (D31.6-)*
                  neurofibromatosis (Q85.0-)

     D36.10   **Benign neoplasm of peripheral nerves and autonomic nervous system,** unspecified

     D36.11   **Benign neoplasm of peripheral nerves and autonomic nervous system of** face, head, and neck

     D36.12   **Benign neoplasm of peripheral nerves and autonomic nervous system, upper limb, including shoulder**

     D36.13   **Benign neoplasm of peripheral nerves and autonomic nervous system of** lower limb, including hip

     D36.14   **Benign neoplasm of peripheral nerves and autonomic nervous system of** thorax

     D36.15   **Benign neoplasm of peripheral nerves and autonomic nervous system of** abdomen

     D36.16   **Benign neoplasm of peripheral nerves and autonomic nervous system of** pelvis

Ⓝ Newborn: 0   Ⓟ Pediatric: 0-17   Ⓜ Maternity: 12-55   Ⓐ Adult: 15-124   **MCC** Major Complication/Comorbidity   **CC** Complication/Comorbidity   **SW** Severe Wound Dx

498   ICD-10-CM 2019

D36.17   **Benign neoplasm of peripheral nerves and autonomic nervous system of** trunk, unspecified

D36.7   **Benign neoplasm of** other **specified sites**
Benign neoplasm of nose NOS

D36.9   **Benign neoplasm,** unspecified site

Benign neuroendocrine tumors (D3A)

✓4ᵗʰ **D3A**   **Benign neuroendocrine tumors**
Code also any associated multiple endocrine neoplasia [MEN] syndromes (E31.2-)
Use additional code to identify any associated endocrine syndrome, such as:
carcinoid syndrome (E34.Ø)
EXCLUDES 2   *benign pancreatic islet cell tumors (D13.7)*

✓5ᵗʰ **D3A.Ø**   **Benign** carcinoid tumors

D3A.ØØ   **Benign carcinoid tumor of** unspecified site
Carcinoid tumor NOS

✓6ᵗʰ **D3A.Ø1**   **Benign carcinoid tumors of the** small intestine
D3A.Ø1Ø   **Benign carcinoid tumor of the** duodenum
D3A.Ø11   **Benign carcinoid tumor of the** jejunum
D3A.Ø12   **Benign carcinoid tumor of the** ileum
D3A.Ø19   **Benign carcinoid tumor of the small intestine,** unspecified portion

✓6ᵗʰ **D3A.Ø2**   **Benign carcinoid tumors of the** appendix, large intestine, and rectum
D3A.Ø2Ø   **Benign carcinoid tumor of the** appendix
D3A.Ø21   **Benign carcinoid tumor of the** cecum
D3A.Ø22   **Benign carcinoid tumor of the** ascending colon
D3A.Ø23   **Benign carcinoid tumor of the** transverse colon
D3A.Ø24   **Benign carcinoid tumor of the** descending colon
D3A.Ø25   **Benign carcinoid tumor of the** sigmoid colon
D3A.Ø26   **Benign carcinoid tumor of the** rectum
D3A.Ø29   **Benign carcinoid tumor of the** large intestine, unspecified portion
Benign carcinoid tumor of the colon NOS

✓6ᵗʰ **D3A.Ø9**   **Benign carcinoid tumors of** other **sites**
D3A.Ø9Ø   **Benign carcinoid tumor of the** bronchus and lung
D3A.Ø91   **Benign carcinoid tumor of the** thymus
D3A.Ø92   **Benign carcinoid tumor of the** stomach
D3A.Ø93   **Benign carcinoid tumor of the** kidney
D3A.Ø94   **Benign carcinoid tumor of the** foregut, unspecified
D3A.Ø95   **Benign carcinoid tumor of the** midgut, unspecified
D3A.Ø96   **Benign carcinoid tumor of the** hindgut, unspecified
D3A.Ø98   **Benign carcinoid tumors of** other sites

D3A.8   Other **benign neuroendocrine tumors**
Neuroendocrine tumor NOS

Neoplasms of uncertain behavior, polycythemia vera and myelodysplastic syndromes (D37-D48)

NOTE   Categories D37-D44, and D48 classify by site neoplasms of uncertain behavior, i.e., histologic confirmation whether the neoplasm is malignant or benign cannot be made.
EXCLUDES 1   *neoplasms of unspecified behavior (D49.-)*

✓4ᵗʰ **D37**   **Neoplasm of uncertain behavior of** oral cavity and digestive organs
EXCLUDES 1   *stromal tumors of uncertain behavior of digestive system (D48.1)*

✓5ᵗʰ **D37.Ø**   **Neoplasm of uncertain behavior of** lip, oral cavity and pharynx
EXCLUDES 1   *neoplasm of uncertain behavior of aryepiglottic fold or interarytenoid fold, laryngeal aspect (D38.Ø)*
neoplasm of uncertain behavior of epiglottis NOS (D38.Ø)
neoplasm of uncertain behavior of skin of lip (D48.5)
neoplasm of uncertain behavior of suprahyoid portion of epiglottis (D38.Ø)

D37.Ø1   **Neoplasm of uncertain behavior of** lip
Neoplasm of uncertain behavior of vermilion border of lip

D37.Ø2   **Neoplasm of uncertain behavior of** tongue

✓6ᵗʰ **D37.Ø3**   **Neoplasm of uncertain behavior of the** major salivary glands
D37.Ø3Ø   **Neoplasm of uncertain behavior of the** parotid **salivary glands**
D37.Ø31   **Neoplasm of uncertain behavior of the** sublingual **salivary glands**
D37.Ø32   **Neoplasm of uncertain behavior of the** submandibular **salivary glands**
D37.Ø39   **Neoplasm of uncertain behavior of the** major salivary glands, unspecified

D37.Ø4   **Neoplasm of uncertain behavior of the** minor salivary glands
Neoplasm of uncertain behavior of submucosal salivary glands of lip
Neoplasm of uncertain behavior of submucosal salivary glands of cheek
Neoplasm of uncertain behavior of submucosal salivary glands of hard palate
Neoplasm of uncertain behavior of submucosal salivary glands of soft palate

D37.Ø5   **Neoplasm of uncertain behavior of** pharynx
Neoplasm of uncertain behavior of aryepiglottic fold of pharynx NOS
Neoplasm of uncertain behavior of hypopharyngeal aspect of aryepiglottic fold of pharynx
Neoplasm of uncertain behavior of marginal zone of aryepiglottic fold of pharynx

D37.Ø9   **Neoplasm of uncertain behavior of** other **specified sites of the oral cavity**

D37.1   **Neoplasm of uncertain behavior of** stomach

D37.2   **Neoplasm of uncertain behavior of** small intestine

D37.3   **Neoplasm of uncertain behavior of** appendix

D37.4   **Neoplasm of uncertain behavior of** colon

D37.5   **Neoplasm of uncertain behavior of** rectum
Neoplasm of uncertain behavior of rectosigmoid junction

D37.6   **Neoplasm of uncertain behavior of** liver, gallbladder and bile ducts
Neoplasm of uncertain behavior of ampulla of Vater

D37.8   **Neoplasm of uncertain behavior of** other **specified digestive organs**
Neoplasm of uncertain behavior of anal canal
Neoplasm of uncertain behavior of anal sphincter
Neoplasm of uncertain behavior of anus NOS
Neoplasm of uncertain behavior of esophagus
Neoplasm of uncertain behavior of intestine NOS
Neoplasm of uncertain behavior of pancreas
EXCLUDES 1   *neoplasm of uncertain behavior of anal margin (D48.5)*
neoplasm of uncertain behavior of anal skin (D48.5)
neoplasm of uncertain behavior of perianal skin (D48.5)

D37.9   **Neoplasm of uncertain behavior of digestive organ,** unspecified

✓4ᵗʰ **D38**   **Neoplasm of uncertain behavior of** middle ear and respiratory and intrathoracic organs
EXCLUDES 1   *neoplasm of uncertain behavior of heart (D48.7)*

D38.Ø   **Neoplasm of uncertain behavior of** larynx
Neoplasm of uncertain behavior of aryepiglottic fold or interarytenoid fold, laryngeal aspect
Neoplasm of uncertain behavior of epiglottis (suprahyoid portion)
EXCLUDES 1   *neoplasm of uncertain behavior of aryepiglottic fold or interarytenoid fold NOS (D37.Ø5)*
neoplasm of uncertain behavior of hypopharyngeal aspect of aryepiglottic fold (D37.Ø5)
neoplasm of uncertain behavior of marginal zone of aryepiglottic fold (D37.Ø5)

D38.1   **Neoplasm of uncertain behavior of** trachea, bronchus and lung

D38.2   **Neoplasm of uncertain behavior of** pleura

D38.3   **Neoplasm of uncertain behavior of** mediastinum

D38.4   **Neoplasm of uncertain behavior of** thymus

✔ Additional Character Required   ✓x7ᵗʰ Placeholder   Unacceptable PDx   Questionable PDx   Manifestation   H1-H14 HAC   HCC CMS-HCC Dx   HIV HIV Dx

ICD-10-CM 2019   499

D36.17–D38.4

Chapter 2. Neoplasms *(left margin)*

D38.5   **Neoplasm of uncertain behavior of** other **respiratory organs**
Neoplasm of uncertain behavior of accessory sinuses
Neoplasm of uncertain behavior of cartilage of nose
Neoplasm of uncertain behavior of middle ear
Neoplasm of uncertain behavior of nasal cavities
> **EXCLUDES 1**   *neoplasm of uncertain behavior of ear (external) (skin) (D48.5)*
> *neoplasm of uncertain behavior of nose NOS (D48.7)*
> *neoplasm of uncertain behavior of skin of nose (D48.5)*

D38.6   **Neoplasm of uncertain behavior of respiratory organ, unspecified**

✓4ᵗʰ **D39**   **Neoplasm of uncertain behavior of** female genital organs

    D39.0   **Neoplasm of uncertain behavior of** uterus   ♀

✓5ᵗʰ   **D39.1**   **Neoplasm of uncertain behavior of** ovary
       Use additional code to identify any functional activity

        D39.10   **Neoplasm of uncertain behavior of** unspecified **ovary**   ♀

        D39.11   **Neoplasm of uncertain behavior of** right **ovary**   ♀

        D39.12   **Neoplasm of uncertain behavior of** left **ovary**   ♀

    D39.2   **Neoplasm of uncertain behavior of** placenta   Ⓜ♀
Chorioadenoma destruens
Invasive hydatidiform mole
Malignant hydatidiform mole
> **EXCLUDES 1**   *hydatidiform mole NOS (O01.9)*

    D39.8   **Neoplasm of uncertain behavior of** other **specified female genital organs**   ♀
Neoplasm of uncertain behavior of skin of female genital organs

    D39.9   **Neoplasm of uncertain behavior of female genital organ, unspecified**   ♀

✓4ᵗʰ **D40**   **Neoplasm of uncertain behavior of** male genital organs

    D40.0   **Neoplasm of uncertain behavior of** prostate   ♂

✓5ᵗʰ   **D40.1**   **Neoplasm of uncertain behavior of** testis

        D40.10   **Neoplasm of uncertain behavior of** unspecified **testis**   ♂

        D40.11   **Neoplasm of uncertain behavior of** right **testis**   ♂

        D40.12   **Neoplasm of uncertain behavior of** left **testis**   ♂

    D40.8   **Neoplasm of uncertain behavior of** other **specified male genital organs**   ♂
Neoplasm of uncertain behavior of skin of male genital organs

    D40.9   **Neoplasm of uncertain behavior of male genital organ, unspecified**   ♂

✓4ᵗʰ **D41**   **Neoplasm of uncertain behavior of** urinary organs

✓5ᵗʰ   **D41.0**   **Neoplasm of uncertain behavior of** kidney
> **EXCLUDES 1**   *neoplasm of uncertain behavior of renal pelvis (D41.1-)*

        D41.00   **Neoplasm of uncertain behavior of** unspecified **kidney**

        D41.01   **Neoplasm of uncertain behavior of** right **kidney**

        D41.02   **Neoplasm of uncertain behavior of** left **kidney**

✓5ᵗʰ   **D41.1**   **Neoplasm of uncertain behavior of** renal pelvis

        D41.10   **Neoplasm of uncertain behavior of** unspecified **renal pelvis**

        D41.11   **Neoplasm of uncertain behavior of** right **renal pelvis**

        D41.12   **Neoplasm of uncertain behavior of** left **renal pelvis**

✓5ᵗʰ   **D41.2**   **Neoplasm of uncertain behavior of** ureter

        D41.20   **Neoplasm of uncertain behavior of** unspecified **ureter**

        D41.21   **Neoplasm of uncertain behavior of** right **ureter**

        D41.22   **Neoplasm of uncertain behavior of** left **ureter**

    D41.3   **Neoplasm of uncertain behavior of** urethra

    D41.4   **Neoplasm of uncertain behavior of** bladder

    D41.8   **Neoplasm of uncertain behavior of** other **specified urinary organs**

    D41.9   **Neoplasm of uncertain behavior of** unspecified **urinary organ**

✓4ᵗʰ **D42**   **Neoplasm of uncertain behavior of** meninges

    D42.0   **Neoplasm of uncertain behavior of** cerebral **meninges**   HCC

    D42.1   **Neoplasm of uncertain behavior of** spinal **meninges**   HCC

    D42.9   **Neoplasm of uncertain behavior of meninges, unspecified**   HCC

✓4ᵗʰ **D43**   **Neoplasm of uncertain behavior of** brain and central nervous system
> **EXCLUDES 1**   *neoplasm of uncertain behavior of peripheral nerves and autonomic nervous system (D48.2)*

    D43.0   **Neoplasm of uncertain behavior of** brain, supratentorial   HCC
Neoplasm of uncertain behavior of cerebral ventricle
Neoplasm of uncertain behavior of cerebrum
Neoplasm of uncertain behavior of frontal lobe
Neoplasm of uncertain behavior of occipital lobe
Neoplasm of uncertain behavior of parietal lobe
Neoplasm of uncertain behavior of temporal lobe
> **EXCLUDES 1**   *neoplasm of uncertain behavior of fourth ventricle (D43.1)*

    D43.1   **Neoplasm of uncertain behavior of** brain, infratentorial   HCC
Neoplasm of uncertain behavior of brain stem
Neoplasm of uncertain behavior of cerebellum
Neoplasm of uncertain behavior of fourth ventricle

    D43.2   **Neoplasm of uncertain behavior of** brain, unspecified   HCC

    D43.3   **Neoplasm of uncertain behavior of** cranial nerves   HCC

    D43.4   **Neoplasm of uncertain behavior of** spinal cord   HCC

    D43.8   **Neoplasm of uncertain behavior of** other specified parts **of central nervous system**   HCC

    D43.9   **Neoplasm of uncertain behavior of** central nervous **system, unspecified**   HCC
Neoplasm of uncertain behavior of nervous system (central) NOS

✓4ᵗʰ **D44**   **Neoplasm of uncertain behavior of** endocrine glands
> **EXCLUDES 1**   *multiple endocrine adenomatosis (E31.2-)*
> *multiple endocrine neoplasia (E31.2-)*
> *neoplasm of uncertain behavior of endocrine pancreas (D37.8)*
> *neoplasm of uncertain behavior of ovary (D39.1-)*
> *neoplasm of uncertain behavior of testis (D40.1-)*
> *neoplasm of uncertain behavior of thymus (D38.4)*

    D44.0   **Neoplasm of uncertain behavior of** thyroid gland

✓5ᵗʰ   **D44.1**   **Neoplasm of uncertain behavior of** adrenal gland
       Use additional code to identify any functional activity

        D44.10   **Neoplasm of uncertain behavior of** unspecified **adrenal gland**

        D44.11   **Neoplasm of uncertain behavior of** right **adrenal gland**

        D44.12   **Neoplasm of uncertain behavior of** left **adrenal gland**

    D44.2   **Neoplasm of uncertain behavior of** parathyroid gland

    D44.3   **Neoplasm of uncertain behavior of** pituitary gland   HCC
       Use additional code to identify any functional activity

    D44.4   **Neoplasm of uncertain behavior of** craniopharyngeal **duct**   HCC

    D44.5   **Neoplasm of uncertain behavior of** pineal gland   HCC

    D44.6   **Neoplasm of uncertain behavior of** carotid body   HCC

    D44.7   **Neoplasm of uncertain behavior of** aortic body and **other paraganglia**   HCC
       AHA: 2016, 4Q, 26

    D44.9   **Neoplasm of uncertain behavior of** unspecified endocrine **gland**

D45   **Polycythemia vera**   HCC
> **EXCLUDES 1**   *familial polycythemia (D75.0)*
> *secondary polycythemia (D75.1)*

DEF: Abnormal proliferation of all bone marrow elements, increased red cell mass, and total blood volume. The etiology is unknown, but it is frequently associated with splenomegaly, leukocytosis, and thrombocythemia.

✓4ᵗʰ **D46**   **Myelodysplastic syndromes**
     Use additional code for adverse effect, if applicable, to identify drug (T36-T50 with fifth or sixth character 5)
> **EXCLUDES 2**   *drug-induced aplastic anemia (D61.1)*

    D46.0   **Refractory anemia** without ring sideroblasts, so stated   HCC
Refractory anemia without sideroblasts, without excess of blasts

    D46.1   **Refractory anemia** with ring sideroblasts   HCC
RARS

✓5ᵗʰ   **D46.2**   **Refractory anemia** with excess of blasts [RAEB]

        D46.20   **Refractory anemia with excess of blasts, unspecified**   HCC
RAEB NOS

        D46.21   **Refractory anemia with excess of** blasts 1   HCC
RAEB 1

*(left margin)* D38.5–D46.21

Ⓝ Newborn: 0   Ⓟ Pediatric: 0-17   Ⓜ Maternity: 12-55   Ⓐ Adult: 15-124   MCC Major Complication/Comorbidity   CC Complication/Comorbidity   SW Severe Wound Dx

500   ICD-10-CM 2019

D46.22 Refractory anemia with excess of blasts 2   `CC` `HCC`
RAEB 2
CC Excl: PDX collection 488

D46.A Refractory cytopenia with multilineage dysplasia   `HCC`

D46.B Refractory cytopenia with multilineage dysplasia   `HCC`
and ring sideroblasts
RCMD RS

D46.C Myelodysplastic syndrome with isolated del(5q)   `CC` `HCC`
chromosomal abnormality
Myelodysplastic syndrome with 5q deletion
5q minus syndrome NOS
CC Excl: PDX collection 488

D46.4 Refractory anemia, unspecified   `HCC`

D46.Z Other myelodysplastic syndromes   `HCC`
EXCLUDES 1   *chronic myelomonocytic leukemia (C93.1-)*

D46.9 Myelodysplastic syndrome, unspecified   `HCC`
Myelodysplasia NOS

☑4ᵗʰ **D47 Other neoplasms of uncertain behavior of** lymphoid,
hematopoietic and related tissue

> **CC Excl: For CC codes in category D47, unless otherwise noted:**
> PDX collection 488

☑5ᵗʰ **D47.0 Mast cell neoplasms of uncertain behavior**
EXCLUDES 1   *congenital cutaneous mastocytosis ▶(Q82.2)◀*
histiocytic neoplasms of uncertain behavior (D47.Z9)
malignant mast cell neoplasm (C96.2-)
AHA: 2017, 4Q, 5

> **CC Excl: For CC codes in subcategory D47.0:**
> PDX collection 494

D47.01 Cutaneous mastocytosis   `CC`
Diffuse cutaneous mastocytosis
Maculopapular cutaneous mastocytosis
Solitary mastocytoma
Telangiectasia macularis eruptiva perstans
Urticaria pigmentosa
EXCLUDES 1   *congenital (diffuse) (maculopapular)*
cutaneous mastocytosis (Q82.2)
congenital urticaria pigmentosa (Q82.2)
extracutaneous mastocytoma (D47.09)

D47.02 Systemic mastocytosis   `CC`
Indolent systemic mastocytosis
Isolated bone marrow mastocytosis
Smoldering systemic mastocytosis
Systemic mastocytosis, with an associated
hematological non-mast cell lineage disease
(SM-AHNMD)
Code also, if applicable, any associated hematological
non-mast cell lineage disease, such as:
acute myeloid leukemia (C92.6-, C92.A-)
chronic myelomonocytic leukemia (C93.1-)
essential thrombocytosis (D47.3)
hypereosinophilic syndrome (D72.1)
myelodysplastic syndrome (D46.9)
myeloproliferative syndrome (D47.1)
non-Hodgkin lymphoma (C82-C85)
plasma cell myeloma (C90.0-)
polycythemia vera (D45)
EXCLUDES 1   *aggressive systemic mastocytosis (C96.21)*
mast cell leukemia (C94.3-)

D47.09 Other mast cell neoplasms of uncertain behavior   `CC`
Extracutaneous mastocytoma
Mast cell tumor NOS
Mastocytoma NOS
Mastocytosis NOS

D47.1 Chronic myeloproliferative disease   `CC` `HCC`
Chronic neutrophilic leukemia
Myeloproliferative disease, unspecified
EXCLUDES 1   *atypical chronic myeloid leukemia BCR/ABL-negative*
(C92.2-)
chronic myeloid leukemia BCR/ABL-positive (C92.1-)
myelofibrosis NOS (D75.81)
myelophthisic anemia (D61.82)
myelophthisis (D61.82)
secondary myelofibrosis NOS (D75.81)

D47.2 Monoclonal gammopathy
Monoclonal gammopathy of undetermined significance [MGUS]

D47.3 Essential (hemorrhagic) thrombocythemia   `HCC`
Essential thrombocytosis
Idiopathic hemorrhagic thrombocythemia
DEF: Chronic myeloproliferative neoplasm involving production
of excess blood platelets that may result in abnormal clotting or
hemorrhaging.

D47.4 Osteomyelofibrosis   `HCC`
Chronic idiopathic myelofibrosis
Myelofibrosis (idiopathic) (with myeloid metaplasia)
Myelosclerosis (megakaryocytic) with myeloid metaplasia
Secondary myelofibrosis in myeloproliferative disease
EXCLUDES 1   *acute myelofibrosis (C94.4-)*

☑5ᵗʰ **D47.Z Other** specified neoplasms of uncertain behavior of
lymphoid, hematopoietic and related tissue
AHA: 2016, 4Q, 8

D47.Z1 Post-transplant lymphoproliferative disorder   `CC` `HCC`
(PTLD)
Code first complications of transplanted organs and
tissue (T86.-)
DEF: Excessive proliferation of B-cell lymphocytes
following Epstein-Barr virus infection in organ
transplant patients. It may progress to non-Hodgkin
lymphoma.
CC Excl: PDX collection 495

D47.Z2 Castleman disease   `CC` `HCC`
Code also if applicable human herpesvirus 8 infection
(B10.89)
EXCLUDES 2   *Kaposi's sarcoma (C46-)*
DEF: Rare disease of the lymph nodes and lymphoid
tissues that closely mimics lymphoma.

D47.Z9 Other specified neoplasms of uncertain   `CC` `HCC`
behavior of lymphoid, hematopoietic and
related tissue
Histiocytic tumors of uncertain behavior

D47.9 Neoplasm of uncertain behavior of lymphoid,   `CC` `HCC`
hematopoietic and related tissue, unspecified
Lymphoproliferative disease NOS

☑4ᵗʰ **D48 Neoplasm of uncertain behavior of other and unspecified sites**
EXCLUDES 1   *neurofibromatosis (nonmalignant) (Q85.0-)*

D48.0 Neoplasm of uncertain behavior of bone and articular
cartilage
EXCLUDES 1   *neoplasm of uncertain behavior of cartilage of ear*
(D48.1)
neoplasm of uncertain behavior of cartilage of larynx
(D38.0)
neoplasm of uncertain behavior of cartilage of nose
(D38.5)
neoplasm of uncertain behavior of connective tissue of
eyelid (D48.1)
neoplasm of uncertain behavior of synovia (D48.1)

D48.1 Neoplasm of uncertain behavior of connective and other soft
tissue
Neoplasm of uncertain behavior of connective tissue of ear
Neoplasm of uncertain behavior of connective tissue of eyelid
Stromal tumors of uncertain behavior of digestive system
EXCLUDES 1   *neoplasm of uncertain behavior of articular cartilage*
(D48.0)
neoplasm of uncertain behavior of cartilage of larynx
(D38.0)
neoplasm of uncertain behavior of cartilage of nose
(D38.5)
neoplasm of uncertain behavior of connective tissue of
breast (D48.6-)

D48.2 Neoplasm of uncertain behavior of peripheral nerves and
autonomic nervous system
EXCLUDES 1   *neoplasm of uncertain behavior of peripheral nerves of*
orbit (D48.7)

D48.3 Neoplasm of uncertain behavior of retroperitoneum

D48.4 Neoplasm of uncertain behavior of peritoneum

D48.5 Neoplasm of uncertain behavior of skin
Neoplasm of uncertain behavior of anal margin
Neoplasm of uncertain behavior of anal skin
Neoplasm of uncertain behavior of perianal skin
Neoplasm of uncertain behavior of skin of breast
EXCLUDES 1   *neoplasm of uncertain behavior of anus NOS (D37.8)*
neoplasm of uncertain behavior of skin of genital
organs (D39.8, D40.8)
neoplasm of uncertain behavior of vermilion border of
lip (D37.0)

☑ Additional Character Required   ☑x7ᵗʰ Placeholder   Unacceptable PDx   Questionable PDx   Manifestation   `H1`-`H14` HAC   `HCC` CMS-HCC Dx   `HIV` HIV Dx

ICD-10-CM 2019   **501**

Chapter 2. Neoplasms (side margin)

✓5ᵗʰ **D48.6 Neoplasm of uncertain behavior of** breast
Neoplasm of uncertain behavior of connective tissue of breast
Cystosarcoma phyllodes
EXCLUDES 1   *neoplasm of uncertain behavior of skin of breast (D48.5)*

   D48.60 Neoplasm of uncertain behavior of unspecified **breast**

   D48.61 Neoplasm of uncertain behavior of right **breast**

   D48.62 Neoplasm of uncertain behavior of left **breast**

D48.7 Neoplasm of uncertain behavior of other **specified sites**
Neoplasm of uncertain behavior of eye
Neoplasm of uncertain behavior of heart
Neoplasm of uncertain behavior of peripheral nerves of orbit
EXCLUDES 1   *neoplasm of uncertain behavior of connective tissue (D48.1)*
           neoplasm of uncertain behavior of skin of eyelid (D48.5)

D48.9 Neoplasm of uncertain behavior, unspecified

Neoplasms of unspecified behavior (D49)

✓4ᵗʰ **D49 Neoplasms of unspecified behavior**
NOTE   Category D49 classifies by site neoplasms of unspecified morphology and behavior. The term "mass", unless otherwise stated, is not to be regarded as a neoplastic growth.
INCLUDES   "growth" NOS
neoplasm NOS
new growth NOS
tumor NOS
EXCLUDES 1   *neoplasms of uncertain behavior (D37-D44, D48)*

D49.0 Neoplasm of unspecified behavior of digestive system
EXCLUDES 1   *neoplasm of unspecified behavior of margin of anus (D49.2)*
           neoplasm of unspecified behavior of perianal skin (D49.2)
           neoplasm of unspecified behavior of skin of anus (D49.2)

D49.1 Neoplasm of unspecified behavior of respiratory system

D49.2 Neoplasm of unspecified behavior of bone, soft tissue, and skin
EXCLUDES 1   *neoplasm of unspecified behavior of anal canal (D49.0)*
           neoplasm of unspecified behavior of anus NOS (D49.0)
           neoplasm of unspecified behavior of bone marrow (D49.89)
           neoplasm of unspecified behavior of cartilage of larynx (D49.1)
           neoplasm of unspecified behavior of cartilage of nose (D49.1)
           neoplasm of unspecified behavior of connective tissue of breast (D49.3)
           neoplasm of unspecified behavior of skin of genital organs (D49.59)
           neoplasm of unspecified behavior of vermilion border of lip (D49.0)

D49.3 Neoplasm of unspecified behavior of breast
EXCLUDES 1   *neoplasm of unspecified behavior of skin of breast (D49.2)*

D49.4 Neoplasm of unspecified behavior of bladder

✓5ᵗʰ **D49.5 Neoplasm of unspecified behavior of** other genitourinary organs
AHA: 2016, 4Q, 9

   ✓6ᵗʰ **D49.51 Neoplasm of unspecified behavior of** kidney

     D49.511 Neoplasm of unspecified behavior of right **kidney**

     D49.512 Neoplasm of unspecified behavior of left **kidney**

     D49.519 Neoplasm of unspecified behavior of unspecified **kidney**

   D49.59 Neoplasm of unspecified behavior of other genitourinary organ

D49.6 Neoplasm of unspecified behavior of brain   HCC
EXCLUDES 1   *neoplasm of unspecified behavior of cerebral meninges (D49.7)*
           neoplasm of unspecified behavior of cranial nerves (D49.7)

D49.7 Neoplasm of unspecified behavior of endocrine glands and other parts of nervous system
EXCLUDES 1   *neoplasm of unspecified behavior of peripheral, sympathetic, and parasympathetic nerves and ganglia (D49.2)*

✓5ᵗʰ **D49.8 Neoplasm of unspecified behavior of** other specified sites
EXCLUDES 1   *neoplasm of unspecified behavior of eyelid (skin) (D49.2)*
           neoplasm of unspecified behavior of eyelid cartilage (D49.2)
           neoplasm of unspecified behavior of great vessels (D49.2)
           neoplasm of unspecified behavior of optic nerve (D49.7)

   D49.81 Neoplasm of unspecified behavior of retina and choroid
Dark area on retina
Retinal freckle

   D49.89 Neoplasm of unspecified behavior of other specified sites

D49.9 Neoplasm of unspecified behavior of unspecified site

Chapter 3. Diseases of the Blood and Blood-forming Organs and Certain Disorders Involving the Immune Mechanism (D50–D89)

Chapter Specific Coding Guidelines and Examples
Reserved for future guideline expansion

Chapter 3. Diseases of the Blood and Blood-forming Organs

D50–D56.1

Chapter 3. Diseases of the Blood and Blood-forming Organs and Certain Disorders Involving the Immune Mechanism (D50-D89)

EXCLUDES 2 *autoimmune disease (systemic) NOS (M35.9)*
certain conditions originating in the perinatal period (P00-P96)
complications of pregnancy, childbirth and the puerperium (O00-O9A)
congenital malformations, deformations and chromosomal abnormalities (Q00-Q99)
endocrine, nutritional and metabolic diseases (E00-E88)
human immunodeficiency virus [HIV] disease (B20)
injury, poisoning and certain other consequences of external causes (S00-T88)
neoplasms (C00-D49)
symptoms, signs and abnormal clinical and laboratory findings, not elsewhere classified (R00-R94)

This chapter contains the following blocks:

D50-D53	Nutritional anemias
D55-D59	Hemolytic anemias
D60-D64	Aplastic and other anemias and other bone marrow failure syndromes
D65-D69	Coagulation defects, purpura and other hemorrhagic conditions
D70-D77	Other disorders of blood and blood-forming organs
D78	Intraoperative and postprocedural complications of the spleen
D80-D89	Certain disorders involving the immune mechanism

Nutritional anemias (D50-D53)

DEF: Nutritional anemia: The result of inadequate intake or absorption of a vitamin or mineral that impacts the production of red blood cells or causes them to develop abnormally affecting the size and shape.

TIP: Documentation must identify a link between anemia and the nutritional deficiency; low levels of a particular nutrient may occur concurrently with anemia but not be the cause of the anemia.

✓4ᵗʰ D50   Iron deficiency anemia
     INCLUDES   asiderotic anemia
                hypochromic anemia

D50.0   **Iron deficiency anemia secondary to blood loss (chronic)**
     Posthemorrhagic anemia (chronic)
     EXCLUDES 1   *acute posthemorrhagic anemia (D62)*
                congenital anemia from fetal blood loss (P61.3)

D50.1   **Sideropenic dysphagia**
     Kelly-Paterson syndrome   Plummer-Vinson syndrome

D50.8   **Other iron deficiency anemias**
     Iron deficiency anemia due to inadequate dietary iron intake

D50.9   **Iron deficiency anemia, unspecified**

✓4ᵗʰ D51   Vitamin B12 deficiency anemia
     EXCLUDES 1   *vitamin B12 deficiency (E53.8)*

D51.0   **Vitamin B12 deficiency anemia due to intrinsic factor deficiency**
     Addison anemia   Pernicious (congenital) anemia
     Biermer anemia   Congenital intrinsic factor deficiency
     DEF: Chronic progressive anemia due to vitamin B12 malabsorption, caused by lack of secretion of intrinsic factor, which is produced by the gastric mucosa of the stomach.

D51.1   **Vitamin B12 deficiency anemia due to selective vitamin B12 malabsorption with proteinuria**
     Imerslund (Gräsbeck) syndrome
     Megaloblastic hereditary anemia

D51.2   **Transcobalamin II deficiency**

D51.3   **Other dietary vitamin B12 deficiency anemia**
     Vegan anemia

D51.8   **Other vitamin B12 deficiency anemias**

D51.9   **Vitamin B12 deficiency anemia, unspecified**

✓4ᵗʰ D52   Folate deficiency anemia
     EXCLUDES 1   *folate deficiency without anemia (E53.8)*
     DEF: Deficiency in a B complex vitamin needed for the production of healthy red blood cells. Lack of folate, or folic acid, and other absorption conditions can cause anemia resulting in large, misshapen red blood cells called megaloblasts.

D52.0   **Dietary folate deficiency anemia**
     Nutritional megaloblastic anemia
     DEF: Result of a poor diet with inadequate intake of folate, which is needed to produce healthy red blood cells.

D52.1   **Drug-induced folate deficiency anemia**
     Use additional code for adverse effect, if applicable, to identify drug (T36-T50 with fifth or sixth character 5)

D52.8   **Other folate deficiency anemias**

D52.9   **Folate deficiency anemia, unspecified**
     Folic acid deficiency anemia NOS

✓4ᵗʰ D53   Other nutritional anemias
     INCLUDES   megaloblastic anemia unresponsive to vitamin B12 or folate therapy

D53.0   **Protein deficiency anemia**
     Amino-acid deficiency anemia
     Orotaciduric anemia
     EXCLUDES 1   *Lesch-Nyhan syndrome (E79.1)*

D53.1   **Other megaloblastic anemias, not elsewhere classified**
     Megaloblastic anemia NOS
     EXCLUDES 1   *Di Guglielmo's disease (C94.0)*

D53.2   **Scorbutic anemia**
     EXCLUDES 1   *scurvy (E54)*

D53.8   **Other specified nutritional anemias**
     Anemia associated with deficiency of copper
     Anemia associated with deficiency of molybdenum
     Anemia associated with deficiency of zinc
     EXCLUDES 1   *nutritional deficiencies without anemia, such as:*
                copper deficiency NOS (E61.0)
                molybdenum deficiency NOS (E61.5)
                zinc deficiency NOS (E60)

D53.9   **Nutritional anemia, unspecified**
     Simple chronic anemia
     EXCLUDES 1   *anemia NOS (D64.9)*

Hemolytic anemias (D55-D59)

✓4ᵗʰ D55   Anemia due to enzyme disorders
     EXCLUDES 1   *drug-induced enzyme deficiency anemia (D59.2)*

D55.0   **Anemia due to glucose-6-phosphate dehydrogenase [G6PD] deficiency**   HCC
     Favism
     G6PD deficiency anemia

D55.1   **Anemia due to other disorders of glutathione metabolism**   HCC
     Anemia (due to) enzyme deficiencies, except G6PD, related to the hexose monophosphate [HMP] shunt pathway
     Anemia (due to) hemolytic nonspherocytic (hereditary), type I

D55.2   **Anemia due to disorders of glycolytic enzymes**   HCC
     Hemolytic nonspherocytic (hereditary) anemia, type II
     Hexokinase deficiency anemia
     Pyruvate kinase [PK] deficiency anemia
     Triose-phosphate isomerase deficiency anemia
     EXCLUDES 1   *disorders of glycolysis not associated with anemia (E74.8)*

D55.3   **Anemia due to disorders of nucleotide metabolism**   HCC

D55.8   **Other anemias due to enzyme disorders**   HCC

D55.9   **Anemia due to enzyme disorder, unspecified**   HCC

✓4ᵗʰ D56   Thalassemia
     EXCLUDES 1   *sickle-cell thalassemia (D57.4-)*
     DEF: Group of inherited disorders of hemoglobin metabolism causing mild to severe anemia. It is usually found in people of Mediterranean, African, Chinese, or Asian descent.

D56.0   **Alpha thalassemia**   HCC
     Alpha thalassemia major
     Hemoglobin H Constant Spring
     Hemoglobin H disease
     Hydrops fetalis due to alpha thalassemia
     Severe alpha thalassemia
     Triple gene defect alpha thalassemia
     Use additional code, if applicable, for hydrops fetalis due to alpha thalassemia (P56.99)
     EXCLUDES 1   *alpha thalassemia trait or minor (D56.3)*
                asymptomatic alpha thalassemia (D56.3)
                hydrops fetalis due to isoimmunization (P56.0)
                hydrops fetalis not due to immune hemolysis (P83.2)
     DEF: HBA1 and HBA2 genetic variant of chromosome 16 prevalent among those of African and Southeast Asian descent. Alpha thalassemia is associated with a wide spectrum of anemic presentation and includes hemoglobin H disease subtypes.

D56.1   **Beta thalassemia**   HCC
     Beta thalassemia major   Severe beta thalassemia
     Cooley's anemia   Thalassemia intermedia
     Homozygous beta thalassemia   Thalassemia major
     EXCLUDES 1   *beta thalassemia minor (D56.3)*
                beta thalassemia trait (D56.3)
                delta-beta thalassemia (D56.2)
                hemoglobin E-beta thalassemia (D56.5)
                sickle-cell beta thalassemia (D57.4-)

N Newborn: 0   P Pediatric: 0-17   M Maternity: 12-55   A Adult: 15-124   MCC Major Complication/Comorbidity   CC Complication/Comorbidity   SW Severe Wound Dx

504   ICD-10-CM 2019

Thalassemia

Misshapen RBC

Misshapen RBC

Healthy RBC

D56.2 Delta-beta thalassemia `HCC`
Homozygous delta-beta thalassemia
> **EXCLUDES 1**   *delta-beta thalassemia minor (D56.3)*
> *delta-beta thalassemia trait (D56.3)*

D56.3 Thalassemia minor
Alpha thalassemia minor
Alpha thalassemia silent carrier
Alpha thalassemia trait
Beta thalassemia minor
Beta thalassemia trait
Delta-beta thalassemia minor
Delta-beta thalassemia trait
Thalassemia trait NOS
> **EXCLUDES 1**   *alpha thalassemia (D56.Ø)*
> *beta thalassemia (D56.1)*
> *delta-beta thalassemia (D56.2)*
> *hemoglobin E-beta thalassemia (D56.5)*
> *sickle-cell trait (D57.3)*

DEF: Solitary abnormal gene that identifies a carrier of the disease, yet with an absence of symptoms or a clinically mild anemic presentation.

D56.4 Hereditary persistence of fetal hemoglobin [HPFH] `HCC`

D56.5 Hemoglobin E-beta thalassemia `HCC`
> **EXCLUDES 1**   *beta thalassemia (D56.1)*
> *beta thalassemia minor (D56.3)*
> *beta thalassemia trait (D56.3)*
> *delta-beta thalassemia (D56.2)*
> *delta-beta thalassemia trait (D56.3)*
> *hemoglobin E disease (D58.2)*
> *other hemoglobinopathies (D58.2)*
> *sickle-cell beta thalassemia (D57.4-)*

D56.8 Other thalassemias `HCC`
Dominant thalassemia
Hemoglobin C thalassemia
Mixed thalassemia
Thalassemia with other hemoglobinopathy
> **EXCLUDES 1**   *hemoglobin C disease (D58.2)*
> *hemoglobin E disease (D58.2)*
> *other hemoglobinopathies (D58.2)*
> *sickle-cell anemia (D57.-)*
> *sickle-cell thalassemia (D57.4)*

D56.9 Thalassemia, unspecified
Mediterranean anemia (with other hemoglobinopathy)

✓4ᵗʰ D57 Sickle-cell disorders
Use additional code for any associated fever (R5Ø.81)
> **EXCLUDES 1**   *other hemoglobinopathies (D58.-)*

DEF: Severe, chronic inherited diseases caused by a genetic variation in hemoglobin protein of the red blood cell. The gene mutation causes the red blood cell to become hard, sticky, and crescent or sickle shaped making it harder for red blood cells to travel through the bloodstream disrupting blood flow and decreasing oxygen transport to tissues.

CC Excl: For MCC codes in category D57: PDX collection 496

✓5ᵗʰ D57.Ø Hb-SS disease with crisis
Sickle-cell disease NOS with crisis
Hb-SS disease with vasoocclusive pain
   D57.ØØ Hb-SS disease with crisis, unspecified `MCC` `HCC`
   D57.Ø1 Hb-SS disease with acute chest syndrome `MCC` `HCC`
   D57.Ø2 Hb-SS disease with splenic sequestration `MCC` `HCC`

Sickle cell

Sickle cells

Normal RBCs

D57.1 Sickle-cell disease without crisis `HCC`
Hb-SS disease without crisis
Sickle-cell anemia NOS
Sickle-cell disease NOS
Sickle-cell disorder NOS

✓5ᵗʰ D57.2 Sickle-cell/Hb-C disease
Hb-SC disease
Hb-S/Hb-C disease
   D57.2Ø Sickle-cell/Hb-C disease without crisis `HCC`
   ✓6ᵗʰ D57.21 Sickle-cell/Hb-C disease with crisis
     D57.211 Sickle-cell/Hb-C disease with acute chest syndrome `MCC` `HCC`
     D57.212 Sickle-cell/Hb-C disease with splenic sequestration `MCC` `HCC`
     D57.219 Sickle-cell/Hb-C disease with crisis, unspecified `MCC` `HCC`
      Sickle-cell/Hb-C disease with crisis NOS

D57.3 Sickle-cell trait `HCC`
Hb-S trait
Heterozygous hemoglobin S
DEF: Heterozygous genetic makeup characterized by one gene for normal hemoglobin and one for sickle-cell hemoglobin. The clinical disease is rarely present.

✓5ᵗʰ D57.4 Sickle-cell thalassemia
Sickle-cell beta thalassemia
Thalassemia Hb-S disease
   D57.4Ø Sickle-cell thalassemia without crisis `HCC`
     Microdrepanocytosis
     Sickle-cell thalassemia NOS
   ✓6ᵗʰ D57.41 Sickle-cell thalassemia with crisis
     Sickle-cell thalassemia with vasoocclusive pain
     D57.411 Sickle-cell thalassemia with acute chest syndrome `MCC` `HCC`
     D57.412 Sickle-cell thalassemia with splenic sequestration `MCC` `HCC`
     D57.419 Sickle-cell thalassemia with crisis, unspecified `MCC` `HCC`
      Sickle-cell thalassemia with crisis NOS

✓5ᵗʰ D57.8 Other sickle-cell disorders
Hb-SD disease
Hb-SE disease
   D57.8Ø Other sickle-cell disorders without crisis `HCC`
   ✓6ᵗʰ D57.81 Other sickle-cell disorders with crisis
     D57.811 Other sickle-cell disorders with acute chest syndrome `MCC` `HCC`
     D57.812 Other sickle-cell disorders with splenic sequestration `MCC` `HCC`
     D57.819 Other sickle-cell disorders with crisis, unspecified `MCC` `HCC`
      Other sickle-cell disorders with crisis NOS

✓4ᵗʰ D58 Other hereditary hemolytic anemias
> **EXCLUDES 1**   *hemolytic anemia of the newborn (P55.-)*

D58.Ø Hereditary spherocytosis `HCC`
Acholuric (familial) jaundice
Congenital (spherocytic) hemolytic icterus
Minkowski-Chauffard syndrome
DEF: Inherited condition caused by mutations to genes responsible for the production of proteins that form the membranes of red blood cells. The shape and flexibility of the red blood cell membrane is altered diminishing the cells ability to traverse the spleen, therefore becoming trapped and destroyed before the red blood cell has reached maturity.

☑ Additional Character Required   ✓x7ᵗʰ Placeholder   Unacceptable PDx   Questionable PDx   Manifestation   `H1`-`H14` HAC   `HCC` CMS-HCC Dx   `HIV` HIV Dx

ICD-10-CM 2019   **505**

Chapter 3. Diseases of the Blood and Blood-forming Organs

D56.2–D58.Ø

D58.1   **Hereditary elliptocytosis**   `HCC`
Elliptocytosis (congenital)
Ovalocytosis (congenital) (hereditary)

D58.2   **Other hemoglobinopathies**   `HCC`
Abnormal hemoglobin NOS
Congenital Heinz body anemia
Hb-C disease
Hb-D disease
Hb-E disease
Hemoglobinopathy NOS
Unstable hemoglobin hemolytic disease
   EXCLUDES 1   *familial polycythemia (D75.0)*
        Hb-M disease (D74.0)
        hemoglobin E-beta thalassemia (D56.5)
        hereditary persistence of fetal hemoglobin [HPFH]
          (D56.4)
        high-altitude polycythemia (D75.1)
        methemoglobinemia (D74.-)
        other hemoglobinopathies with thalassemia (D56.8)

D58.8   **Other specified hereditary hemolytic anemias**   `CC` `HCC`
Stomatocytosis
   CC Excl: PDX collection 497

D58.9   **Hereditary hemolytic anemia, unspecified**   `CC` `HCC`
   CC Excl: PDX collection 497

✓4ᵗʰ **D59**   **Acquired hemolytic anemia**
   DEF: Non-hereditary anemia characterized by premature destruction of red blood cells caused by infectious organisms, poisons, and physical agents.

   CC Excl: For CC/MCC codes in category D59: PDX collection 496

D59.0   **Drug-induced autoimmune hemolytic anemia**   `CC` `HCC`
Use additional code for adverse effect, if applicable, to identify drug (T36-T50 with fifth or sixth character 5)

D59.1   **Other autoimmune hemolytic anemias**   `CC` `HCC`
Autoimmune hemolytic disease (cold type) (warm type)
Chronic cold hemagglutinin disease
Cold agglutinin disease
Cold agglutinin hemoglobinuria
Cold type (secondary) (symptomatic) hemolytic anemia
Warm type (secondary) (symptomatic) hemolytic anemia
   EXCLUDES 1   *Evans syndrome (D69.41)*
        hemolytic disease of newborn (P55.-)
        paroxysmal cold hemoglobinuria (D59.6)

D59.2   **Drug-induced nonautoimmune hemolytic anemia**   `CC` `HCC`
Drug-induced enzyme deficiency anemia
Use additional code for adverse effect, if applicable, to identify drug (T36-T50 with fifth or sixth character 5)

D59.3   **Hemolytic-uremic syndrome**   `MCC` `HCC`
Use additional code to identify associated:
   E. coli infection (B96.2-)
   Pneumococcal pneumonia (J13)
   Shigella dysenteriae (A03.9)
   DEF: Condition typically precipitated by infection causing low platelets and destruction of red blood cells resulting in hemolytic anemia. This cell damage and blockage of renal capillaries lead to kidney failure. Mainly affects children.

D59.4   **Other nonautoimmune hemolytic anemias**   `CC` `HCC`
Mechanical hemolytic anemia
Microangiopathic hemolytic anemia
Toxic hemolytic anemia

D59.5   **Paroxysmal nocturnal hemoglobinuria [Marchiafava-Micheli]**   `HCC`
   EXCLUDES 1   *hemoglobinuria NOS (R82.3)*

D59.6   **Hemoglobinuria due to hemolysis from other external causes**   `HCC`
Hemoglobinuria from exertion
March hemoglobinuria
Paroxysmal cold hemoglobinuria
Use additional code (Chapter 20) to identify external cause
   EXCLUDES 1   *hemoglobinuria NOS (R82.3)*

D59.8   **Other acquired hemolytic anemias**   `HCC`

D59.9   **Acquired hemolytic anemia, unspecified**   `CC` `HCC`
Idiopathic hemolytic anemia, chronic

Aplastic and other anemias and other bone marrow failure syndromes (D60-D64)

✓4ᵗʰ **D60**   **Acquired pure red cell aplasia [erythroblastopenia]**
   `INCLUDES`   red cell aplasia (acquired) (adult) (with thymoma)
   EXCLUDES 1   *congenital red cell aplasia (D61.01)*

   CC Excl: For MCC codes in category D60: PDX collection 496

D60.0   **Chronic acquired pure red cell aplasia**   `MCC` `HCC`

D60.1   **Transient acquired pure red cell aplasia**   `MCC` `HCC`

D60.8   **Other acquired pure red cell aplasias**   `MCC` `HCC`

D60.9   **Acquired pure red cell aplasia, unspecified**   `MCC` `HCC`

✓4ᵗʰ **D61**   **Other aplastic anemias and other bone marrow failure syndromes**
   EXCLUDES 1   *neutropenia (D70.-)*
   AHA: 2014, 4Q, 22

   CC Excl: For CC/MCC codes in category D61, unless otherwise noted: PDX collection 496

✓5ᵗʰ **D61.0**   **Constitutional aplastic anemia**

   D61.01   **Constitutional (pure) red blood cell aplasia**   `CC` `HCC`
     Blackfan-Diamond syndrome
     Congenital (pure) red cell aplasia
     Familial hypoplastic anemia
     Primary (pure) red cell aplasia
     Red cell (pure) aplasia of infants
      EXCLUDES 1   *acquired red cell aplasia (D60.9)*
      CC Excl: PDX collection 498

   D61.09   **Other constitutional aplastic anemia**   `CC` `HCC`
     Fanconi's anemia
     Pancytopenia with malformations
      CC Excl: PDX collection 499

D61.1   **Drug-induced aplastic anemia**   `MCC` `HCC`
Use additional code for adverse effect, if applicable, to identify drug (T36-T50 with fifth or sixth character 5)

D61.2   **Aplastic anemia due to other external agents**   `MCC` `HCC`
Code first, if applicable, toxic effects of substances chiefly nonmedicinal as to source (T51-T65)

D61.3   **Idiopathic aplastic anemia**   `MCC` `HCC`

✓5ᵗʰ **D61.8**   **Other specified aplastic anemias and other bone marrow failure syndromes**

   CC Excl: For CC/MCC codes in subcategory D61.8, unless otherwise noted: PDX collection 500

   ✓6ᵗʰ **D61.81**   **Pancytopenia**
      EXCLUDES 1   *pancytopenia (due to) (with) aplastic anemia*
         (D61.9)
        pancytopenia (due to) (with) bone marrow
         infiltration (D61.82)
        pancytopenia (due to) (with) congenital
         (pure) red cell aplasia (D61.01)
        pancytopenia (due to) (with) hairy cell
         leukemia (C91.4-)
        pancytopenia (due to) (with) human
         immunodeficiency virus disease (B20)
        pancytopenia (due to) (with)
         leukoerythroblastic anemia (D61.82)
        pancytopenia (due to) (with)
         myeloproliferative disease (D47.1)
      EXCLUDES 2   *pancytopenia (due to) (with) myelodysplastic*
         syndromes (D46.-)
      DEF: Shortage of all three blood cells: white, red, and platelets.

     D61.810   **Antineoplastic chemotherapy induced pancytopenia**   `MCC` `HCC`
       EXCLUDES 2   *aplastic anemia due to*
         antineoplastic
         chemotherapy (D61.1)

     D61.811   **Other drug-induced pancytopenia**   `MCC` `HCC`
       EXCLUDES 2   *aplastic anemia due to drugs*
         (D61.1)

     D61.818   **Other pancytopenia**   `CC` `HCC`

N Newborn: 0   P Pediatric: 0-17   M Maternity: 12-55   A Adult: 15-124   `MCC` Major Complication/Comorbidity   `CC` Complication/Comorbidity   `SW` Severe Wound Dx

506   ICD-10-CM 2019

D61.82 Myelophthisis `CC` `HCC`
Leukoerythroblastic anemia
Myelophthisic anemia
Panmyelophthisis
Code also the underlying disorder, such as:
   malignant neoplasm of breast (C50.-)
   tuberculosis (A15.-)
   EXCLUDES 1 *idiopathic myelofibrosis (D47.1)*
      myelofibrosis NOS (D75.81)
      myelofibrosis with myeloid metaplasia
       (D47.4)
      primary myelofibrosis (D47.1)
      secondary myelofibrosis (D75.81)

DEF: Condition that occurs when normal hematopoietic tissue in the bone marrow is replaced with abnormal tissue, such as fibrous tissue or tumors. Most commonly seen during the advanced stages of cancer.

D61.89 Other specified aplastic anemias and other `MCC` `HCC`
bone marrow failure syndromes
CC Excl: PDX collection 496

D61.9 Aplastic anemia, unspecified `CC` `HCC`
Hypoplastic anemia NOS
Medullary hypoplasia

D62 Acute posthemorrhagic anemia `CC`
EXCLUDES 1 *anemia due to chronic blood loss (D50.0)*
   blood loss anemia NOS (D50.0)
   congenital anemia from fetal blood loss (P61.3)
CC Excl: PDX collection 501

✓4ᵗʰ D63 Anemia in chronic diseases classified elsewhere

D63.0 Anemia in neoplastic disease
Code first neoplasm (C00-D49)
EXCLUDES 1 *aplastic anemia due to antineoplastic chemotherapy (D61.1)*
EXCLUDES 2 *anemia due to antineoplastic chemotherapy (D64.81)*

D63.1 Anemia in chronic kidney disease
Erythropoietin resistant anemia (EPO resistant anemia)
Code first underlying chronic kidney disease (CKD) (N18.-)

D63.8 Anemia in other chronic diseases classified elsewhere
Code first underlying disease, such as:
   diphyllobothriasis (B70.0)
   hookworm disease (B76.0-B76.9)
   hypothyroidism (E00.0-E03.9)
   malaria (B50.0-B54)
   symptomatic late syphilis (A52.79)
   tuberculosis (A18.89)

✓4ᵗʰ D64 Other anemias
EXCLUDES 1 *refractory anemia (D46.-)*
   refractory anemia with excess blasts in transformation [RAEB T] (C92.0-)

DEF: Sideroblastic anemia: Hereditary or secondary disorder in which the red blood cells cannot effectively use iron, a nutrient needed to make hemoglobin. Although the iron can enter the red blood cell it is not assimilated into the hemoglobin molecule and builds up ringed sideroblasts around the cell nucleus.

D64.0 Hereditary sideroblastic anemia `HCC`
Sex-linked hypochromic sideroblastic anemia

D64.1 Secondary sideroblastic anemia due to disease `HCC`
Code first underlying disease

D64.2 Secondary sideroblastic anemia due to drugs and toxins `HCC`
Code first poisoning due to drug or toxin, if applicable (T36-T65 with fifth or sixth character 1-4 or 6)
Use additional code for adverse effect, if applicable, to identify drug (T36-T50 with fifth or sixth character 5)

D64.3 Other sideroblastic anemias `HCC`
Sideroblastic anemia NOS
Pyridoxine-responsive sideroblastic anemia NEC

D64.4 Congenital dyserythropoietic anemia
Dyshematopoietic anemia (congenital)
EXCLUDES 1 *Blackfan-Diamond syndrome (D61.01)*
   Di Guglielmo's disease (C94.0)

✓5ᵗʰ D64.8 Other specified anemias

D64.81 Anemia due to antineoplastic chemotherapy
Antineoplastic chemotherapy induced anemia
EXCLUDES 1 *aplastic anemia due to antineoplastic chemotherapy (D61.1)*
EXCLUDES 2 *anemia in neoplastic disease (D63.0)*
AHA: 2014, 4Q, 22
DEF: Reversible adverse effect of chemotherapy, causing inhibition of bone marrow production. A decrease in red blood cell production prevents adequate oxygenation of the tissues and organs causing fatigue, shortness of breath (SOB), and exacerbation of other medical conditions.

D64.89 Other specified anemias
Infantile pseudoleukemia

D64.9 Anemia, unspecified
AHA: 2017, 1Q, 7

Coagulation defects, purpura and other hemorrhagic conditions (D65-D69)

D65 Disseminated intravascular coagulation [defibrination `MCC` `HCC`
syndrome]
Afibrinogenemia, acquired
Consumption coagulopathy
Diffuse or disseminated intravascular coagulation [DIC]
Fibrinolytic hemorrhage, acquired
Fibrinolytic purpura
Purpura fulminans
EXCLUDES 1 *disseminated intravascular coagulation (complicating):*
   abortion or ectopic or molar pregnancy (O00-O07, O08.1)
   in newborn (P60)
   pregnancy, childbirth and the puerperium (O45.0, O46.0, O67.0, O72.3)
CC Excl: PDX collection 502

Coagulation

White blood cell
Fibrin
Red blood cells
Platelets
Injury site

D66 Hereditary factor VIII deficiency `MCC` `HCC`
Classical hemophilia
Deficiency factor VIII (with functional defect)
Hemophilia A
Hemophilia NOS
EXCLUDES 1 *factor VIII deficiency with vascular defect (D68.0)*

DEF: Hereditary, sex-linked lack of antihemophilic globulin (AHG) (factor VIII) that causes abnormal coagulation characterized by increased bleeding; large bruises of skin; bleeding in the mouth, nose, and gastrointestinal tract; and hemorrhages into joints, resulting in swelling and impaired function.
CC Excl: PDX collection 502

D67 Hereditary factor IX deficiency `MCC` `HCC`
Christmas disease
Factor IX deficiency (with functional defect)
Hemophilia B
Plasma thromboplastin component [PTC] deficiency
CC Excl: PDX collection 502

✓ Additional Character Required   √x 7ᵗʰ Placeholder   Unacceptable PDx   Questionable PDx   Manifestation   H1 -H14 HAC   HCC CMS-HCC Dx   HIV HIV Dx

ICD-10-CM 2019   507

Chapter 3. Diseases of the Blood and Blood-forming Organs

D68-D68.61

✓4ᵗʰ **D68 Other coagulation defects**

    EXCLUDES1   *abnormal coagulation profile (R79.1)*
       coagulation defects complicating abortion or ectopic or molar pregnancy (O00-O07, O08.1)
       coagulation defects complicating pregnancy, childbirth and the puerperium (O45.0, O46.0, O67.0, O72.3)

    AHA: 2016, 1Q, 14

    CC Excl: For CC codes in category D68, unless otherwise noted: PDX collection 502

    D68.0 Von Willebrand's disease `CC` `HCC`
      Angiohemophilia
      Factor VIII deficiency with vascular defect
      Vascular hemophilia
      EXCLUDES1   *capillary fragility (hereditary) (D69.8)*
         factor VIII deficiency NOS (D66)
         factor VIII deficiency with functional defect (D66)
      DEF: Congenital, abnormal blood coagulation caused by deficient blood factor VII. Symptoms include excess or prolonged bleeding.

    D68.1 Hereditary factor XI deficiency `CC` `HCC`
      Hemophilia C
      Plasma thromboplastin antecedent [PTA] deficiency
      Rosenthal's disease

    D68.2 Hereditary deficiency of other clotting factors `CC` `HCC`
      AC globulin deficiency
      Congenital afibrinogenemia
      Deficiency of factor I [fibrinogen]
      Deficiency of factor II [prothrombin]
      Deficiency of factor V [labile]
      Deficiency of factor VII [stable]
      Deficiency of factor X [Stuart-Prower]
      Deficiency of factor XII [Hageman]
      Deficiency of factor XIII [fibrin stabilizing]
      Dysfibrinogenemia (congenital)
      Hypoproconvertinemia
      Owren's disease
      Proaccelerin deficiency

✓5ᵗʰ   **D68.3 Hemorrhagic disorder due to circulating anticoagulants**

    ✓6ᵗʰ   **D68.31 Hemorrhagic disorder due to intrinsic circulating anticoagulants, antibodies, or inhibitors**

      D68.311 Acquired hemophilia `CC` `HCC`
        Autoimmune hemophilia
        Autoimmune inhibitors to clotting factors
        Secondary hemophilia
        CC Excl: PDX collection 503

      D68.312 Antiphospholipid antibody with hemorrhagic disorder `CC` `HCC`
        Lupus anticoagulant (LAC) with hemorrhagic disorder
        Systemic lupus erythematosus [SLE] inhibitor with hemorrhagic disorder
        EXCLUDES1   *antiphospholipid antibody, finding without diagnosis (R76.0)*
          antiphospholipid antibody syndrome (D68.61)
          antiphospholipid antibody with hypercoagulable state (D68.61)
          lupus anticoagulant (LAC) finding without diagnosis (R76.0)
          lupus anticoagulant (LAC) with hypercoagulable state (D68.62)
          systemic lupus erythematosus [SLE] inhibitor finding without diagnosis (R76.0)
          systemic lupus erythematosus [SLE] inhibitor with hypercoagulable state (D68.62)
        CC Excl: PDX collection 504

      D68.318 Other hemorrhagic disorder due to `CC` `HCC` **intrinsic circulating anticoagulants, antibodies, or inhibitors**
        Antithromboplastinemia
        Antithromboplastinogenemia
        Hemorrhagic disorder due to intrinsic increase in antithrombin
        Hemorrhagic disorder due to intrinsic increase in anti-VIIIa
        Hemorrhagic disorder due to intrinsic increase in anti-IXa
        Hemorrhagic disorder due to intrinsic increase in anti-XIa
        CC Excl: PDX collection 503

    D68.32 Hemorrhagic disorder due to extrinsic circulating anticoagulants `CC` `HCC`
      Drug-induced hemorrhagic disorder
      Hemorrhagic disorder due to increase in anti-IIa
      Hemorrhagic disorder due to increase in anti-Xa
      Hyperheparinemia
      Use additional code for adverse effect, if applicable, to identify drug (T45.515, T45.525)
      AHA: 2016, 1Q, 14-15
      TIP: Do not assign to identify routine therapeutic anticoagulation effects; assign only for documented adverse effects.

    D68.4 Acquired coagulation factor deficiency `CC` `HCC`
      Deficiency of coagulation factor due to liver disease
      Deficiency of coagulation factor due to vitamin K deficiency
      EXCLUDES1   *vitamin K deficiency of newborn (P53)*

✓5ᵗʰ   **D68.5 Primary thrombophilia**
      Primary hypercoagulable states
      EXCLUDES1   *antiphospholipid syndrome (D68.61)*
        lupus anticoagulant (D68.62)
        secondary activated protein C resistance (D68.69)
        secondary antiphospholipid antibody syndrome (D68.69)
        secondary lupus anticoagulant with hypercoagulable state (D68.69)
        secondary systemic lupus erythematosus [SLE] inhibitor with hypercoagulable state (D68.69)
        systemic lupus erythematosus [SLE] inhibitor finding without diagnosis (R76.0)
        systemic lupus erythematosus [SLE] inhibitor with hemorrhagic disorder (D68.312)
        thrombotic thrombocytopenic purpura (M31.1)
      DEF: Thrombophilia: Increased tendency of the blood to clot, which can lead to thrombus or embolus formation.

      CC Excl: For CC codes in subcategory D68.5: PDX collection 505

    D68.51 Activated protein C resistance `CC` `HCC`
      Factor V Leiden mutation

    D68.52 Prothrombin gene mutation `CC` `HCC`

    D68.59 Other primary thrombophilia `CC` `HCC`
      Antithrombin III deficiency
      Hypercoagulable state NOS
      Primary hypercoagulable state NEC
      Primary thrombophilia NEC
      Protein C deficiency
      Protein S deficiency
      Thrombophilia NOS

✓5ᵗʰ   **D68.6 Other thrombophilia**
      Other hypercoagulable states
      EXCLUDES1   *diffuse or disseminated intravascular coagulation [DIC] (D65)*
        heparin induced thrombocytopenia (HIT) (D75.82)
        hyperhomocysteinemia (E72.11)

      CC Excl: For CC codes in subcategory D68.6: PDX collection 505

    D68.61 Antiphospholipid syndrome `CC` `HCC`
      Anticardiolipin syndrome
      Antiphospholipid antibody syndrome
      EXCLUDES1   *antiphospholipid antibody, finding without diagnosis (R76.0)*
        antiphospholipid antibody with hemorrhagic disorder (D68.312)
        lupus anticoagulant syndrome (D68.62)

N Newborn: 0   **P** Pediatric: 0-17   **M** Maternity: 12-55   **A** Adult: 15-124   **MCC** Major Complication/Comorbidity   **CC** Complication/Comorbidity   **SW** Severe Wound Dx

508   ICD-10-CM 2019

D68.62   **Lupus anticoagulant syndrome**   `CC` `HCC`
Lupus anticoagulant
Presence of systemic lupus erythematosus [SLE]
    inhibitor
EXCLUDES 1   *anticardiolipin syndrome (D68.61)*
    antiphospholipid syndrome (D68.61)
    lupus anticoagulant (LAC) finding without
      diagnosis (R76.0)
    lupus anticoagulant (LAC) with hemorrhagic
      disorder (D68.312)

D68.69   **Other thrombophilia**   `CC` `HCC`
Hypercoagulable states NEC
Secondary hypercoagulable state NOS

D68.8   **Other specified coagulation defects**   `CC` `HCC`
EXCLUDES 1   *hemorrhagic disease of newborn (P53)*

D68.9   **Coagulation defect, unspecified**   `CC` `HCC`

✓4ᵗʰ   **D69**   **Purpura and other hemorrhagic conditions**
EXCLUDES 1   *benign hypergammaglobulinemic purpura (D89.0)*
    cryoglobulinemic purpura (D89.1)
    essential (hemorrhagic) thrombocythemia (D47.3)
    hemorrhagic thrombocythemia (D47.3)
    purpura fulminans (D65)
    thrombotic thrombocytopenic purpura (M31.1)
    Waldenström hypergammaglobulinemic purpura (D89.0)

CC Excl: For CC codes in category D69: PDX collection 502

D69.0   **Allergic purpura**   `CC` `HCC`
Allergic vasculitis
Nonthrombocytopenic hemorrhagic purpura
Nonthrombocytopenic idiopathic purpura
Purpura anaphylactoid
Purpura Henoch(-Schönlein)
Purpura rheumatica
Vascular purpura
EXCLUDES 1   *thrombocytopenic hemorrhagic purpura (D69.3)*
DEF: Any hemorrhagic condition, thrombocytic or
nonthrombocytopenic in origin, caused by a presumed allergic
reaction.

D69.1   **Qualitative platelet defects**   `HCC`
Bernard-Soulier [giant platelet] syndrome
Glanzmann's disease
Grey platelet syndrome
Thromboasthenia (hemorrhagic) (hereditary)
Thrombocytopathy
EXCLUDES 1   *von Willebrand's disease (D68.0)*

D69.2   **Other nonthrombocytopenic purpura**   `HCC`
Purpura NOS
Purpura simplex
Senile purpura

D69.3   **Immune thrombocytopenic purpura**   `CC` `HCC`
Hemorrhagic (thrombocytopenic) purpura
Idiopathic thrombocytopenic purpura
Tidal platelet dysgenesis
DEF: Tidal platelet dysgenesis: Fluctuation of platelet counts from
normal to very low within periods of 20 to 40 days and may
involve autoimmune platelet destruction.

✓5ᵗʰ   **D69.4**   **Other primary thrombocytopenia**
EXCLUDES 1   *transient neonatal thrombocytopenia (P61.0)*
    Wiskott-Aldrich syndrome (D82.0)

D69.41   **Evans syndrome**   `CC` `HCC`

D69.42   **Congenital and hereditary**   `CC` `HCC`
thrombocytopenia purpura
Congenital thrombocytopenia
Hereditary thrombocytopenia
Code first congenital or hereditary disorder, such as:
    thrombocytopenia with absent radius (TAR
    syndrome) (Q87.2)

D69.49   **Other primary thrombocytopenia**   `HCC`
Megakaryocytic hypoplasia
Primary thrombocytopenia NOS

✓5ᵗʰ   **D69.5**   **Secondary thrombocytopenia**
EXCLUDES 1   *heparin induced thrombocytopenia (HIT) (D75.82)*
    transient thrombocytopenia of newborn (P61.0)

D69.51   **Posttransfusion purpura**
Posttransfusion purpura from whole blood (fresh) or
    blood products
PTP

D69.59   **Other secondary thrombocytopenia**
AHA: 2014, 4Q, 22

D69.6   **Thrombocytopenia, unspecified**   `HCC`

D69.8   **Other specified hemorrhagic conditions**   `HCC`
Capillary fragility (hereditary)
Vascular pseudohemophilia

D69.9   **Hemorrhagic condition, unspecified**   `HCC`

Other disorders of blood and blood-forming organs (D70-D77)

✓4ᵗʰ   **D70**   **Neutropenia**
INCLUDES   agranulocytosis
    decreased absolute neurophile count (ANC)
Use additional code for any associated:
    fever (R50.81)
    mucositis (J34.81, K12.3-, K92.81, N76.81)
EXCLUDES 1   *neutropenic splenomegaly (D73.81)*
    transient neonatal neutropenia (P61.5)
DEF: Abnormally low number of neutrophils. Neutrophils are phagocytic,
meaning they surround and consume harmful pathogens, primarily
bacteria. When neutrophil counts decrease the risk of infection increases.

D70.0   **Congenital agranulocytosis**   `HCC`
Congenital neutropenia
Infantile genetic agranulocytosis
Kostmann's disease

D70.1   **Agranulocytosis secondary to cancer chemotherapy**   `HCC`
Code also underlying neoplasm
Use additional code for adverse effect, if applicable, to identify
    drug (T45.1X5)
AHA: 2014, 4Q, 22

D70.2   **Other drug-induced agranulocytosis**   `HCC`
Use additional code for adverse effect, if applicable, to identify
    drug (T36-T50 with fifth or sixth character 5)

D70.3   **Neutropenia due to infection**   `HCC`

D70.4   **Cyclic neutropenia**   `HCC`
Cyclic hematopoiesis
Periodic neutropenia

D70.8   **Other neutropenia**   `HCC`

D70.9   **Neutropenia, unspecified**   `HCC`

D71   **Functional disorders of polymorphonuclear neutrophils**   `HCC`
Cell membrane receptor complex [CR3] defect
Chronic (childhood) granulomatous disease
Congenital dysphagocytosis
Progressive septic granulomatosis

✓4ᵗʰ   **D72**   **Other disorders of white blood cells**
EXCLUDES 1   *basophilia (D72.824)*
    immunity disorders (D80-D89)
    neutropenia (D70)
    preleukemia (syndrome) (D46.9)

D72.0   **Genetic anomalies of leukocytes**   `HCC`
Alder (granulation) (granulocyte) anomaly
Alder syndrome
Hereditary leukocytic hypersegmentation
Hereditary leukocytic hyposegmentation
Hereditary leukomelanopathy
May-Hegglin (granulation) (granulocyte) anomaly
May-Hegglin syndrome
Pelger-Huët (granulation) (granulocyte) anomaly
Pelger-Huët syndrome
EXCLUDES 1   *Chédiak (-Steinbrinck)-Higashi syndrome (E70.330)*

D72.1   **Eosinophilia**
Allergic eosinophilia
Hereditary eosinophilia
EXCLUDES 1   *Löffler's syndrome (J82)*
    pulmonary eosinophilia (J82)

✓5ᵗʰ   **D72.8**   **Other specified disorders of white blood cells**
EXCLUDES 1   *leukemia (C91-C95)*

✓6ᵗʰ   **D72.81**   **Decreased white blood cell count**
EXCLUDES 1   *neutropenia (D70.-)*

D72.810   **Lymphocytopenia**
Decreased lymphocytes

D72.818   **Other decreased white blood cell count**
Basophilic leukopenia
Eosinophilic leukopenia
Monocytopenia
Other decreased leukocytes
Plasmacytopenia

D72.819   **Decreased white blood cell count,**
unspecified
Decreased leukocytes, unspecified
Leukocytopenia, unspecified
Leukopenia
EXCLUDES 1   *malignant leukopenia (D70.9)*

☑ Additional Character Required   ✓×7ᵗʰ Placeholder   Unacceptable PDx   Questionable PDx   Manifestation   `H1`-`H14` HAC   `HCC` CMS-HCC Dx   `HIV` HIV Dx

ICD-10-CM 2019   509

✓6ᵗʰ D72.82 Elevated white blood cell count
     EXCLUDES 1   eosinophilia (D72.1)

     D72.820 Lymphocytosis (symptomatic)
       Elevated lymphocytes

     D72.821 Monocytosis (symptomatic)
       EXCLUDES 1   infectious mononucleosis (B27.-)

     D72.822 Plasmacytosis

     D72.823 Leukemoid reaction
       Basophilic leukemoid reaction
       Leukemoid reaction NOS
       Lymphocytic leukemoid reaction
       Monocytic leukemoid reaction
       Myelocytic leukemoid reaction
       Neutrophilic leukemoid reaction

     D72.824 Basophilia
       DEF: Increase in the basophils of the blood, a type of white blood cell, often seen in conjunction with neoplastic disorders.

     D72.825 Bandemia
       Bandemia without diagnosis of specific infection
       EXCLUDES 1   confirmed infection—code to infection
         leukemia (C91.-, C92.-, C93.-, C94.-, C95.-)
       DEF: Increase in early neutrophil cells, called band cells that may indicate infection.

     D72.828 Other elevated white blood cell count

     D72.829 Elevated white blood cell count, unspecified
       Elevated leukocytes, unspecified
       Leukocytosis, unspecified

   D72.89 Other specified disorders of white blood cells
     Abnormality of white blood cells NEC

   D72.9 Disorder of white blood cells, unspecified
     Abnormal leukocyte differential NOS

✓4ᵗʰ D73 Diseases of spleen

   D73.0 Hyposplenism
     Atrophy of spleen
     EXCLUDES 1   asplenia (congenital) (Q89.01)
       postsurgical absence of spleen (Z90.81)

   D73.1 Hypersplenism
     EXCLUDES 1   neutropenic splenomegaly (D73.81)
       primary splenic neutropenia (D73.81)
       splenitis, splenomegaly in late syphilis (A52.79)
       splenitis, splenomegaly in tuberculosis (A18.85)
       splenomegaly NOS (R16.1)
       splenomegaly congenital (Q89.0)

   D73.2 Chronic congestive splenomegaly

   D73.3 Abscess of spleen

   D73.4 Cyst of spleen

   D73.5 Infarction of spleen
     Splenic rupture, nontraumatic
     Torsion of spleen
     EXCLUDES 1   rupture of spleen due to Plasmodium vivax malaria (B51.0)
       traumatic rupture of spleen (S36.03-)

   ✓5ᵗʰ D73.8 Other diseases of spleen

     D73.81 Neutropenic splenomegaly
       Werner-Schultz disease

     D73.89 Other diseases of spleen
       Fibrosis of spleen NOS
       Perisplenitis
       Splenitis NOS

   D73.9 Disease of spleen, unspecified

✓4ᵗʰ D74 Methemoglobinemia

   CC Excl: For CC codes in category D74: PDX collection 506

   D74.0 Congenital methemoglobinemia   `CC`
     Congenital NADH-methemoglobin reductase deficiency
     Hemoglobin-M [Hb-M] disease
     Methemoglobinemia, hereditary

   D74.8 Other methemoglobinemias   `CC`
     Acquired methemoglobinemia (with sulfhemoglobinemia)
     Toxic methemoglobinemia

   D74.9 Methemoglobinemia, unspecified   `CC`

✓4ᵗʰ D75 Other and unspecified diseases of blood and blood-forming organs
     EXCLUDES 2   acute lymphadenitis (L04.-)
       chronic lymphadenitis (I88.1)
       enlarged lymph nodes (R59.-)
       hypergammaglobulinemia NOS (D89.2)
       lymphadenitis NOS (I88.9)
       mesenteric lymphadenitis (acute) (chronic) (I88.0)

   D75.0 Familial erythrocytosis
     Benign polycythemia
     Familial polycythemia
     EXCLUDES 1   hereditary ovalocytosis (D58.1)

   D75.1 Secondary polycythemia
     Acquired polycythemia
     Emotional polycythemia
     Erythrocytosis NOS
     Hypoxemic polycythemia
     Nephrogenous polycythemia
     Polycythemia due to erythropoietin
     Polycythemia due to fall in plasma volume
     Polycythemia due to high altitude
     Polycythemia due to stress
     Polycythemia NOS
     Relative polycythemia
     EXCLUDES 1   polycythemia neonatorum (P61.1)
       polycythemia vera (D45)
     DEF: Elevated number of red blood cells in circulating blood as a result of reduced oxygen supply to the tissues.

   ✓5ᵗʰ D75.8 Other specified diseases of blood and blood-forming organs

     D75.81 Myelofibrosis   `CC` `HCC`
       Myelofibrosis NOS
       Secondary myelofibrosis NOS
       Code first the underlying disorder, such as:
         malignant neoplasm of breast (C50.-)
       Use additional code, if applicable, for associated therapy-related myelodysplastic syndrome (D46.-)
       Use additional code for adverse effect, if applicable, to identify drug (T45.1X5)
       EXCLUDES 1   acute myelofibrosis (C94.4-)
         idiopathic myelofibrosis (D47.1)
         leukoerythroblastic anemia (D61.82)
         myelofibrosis with myeloid metaplasia (D47.4)
         myelophthisic anemia (D61.82)
         myelophthisis (D61.82)
         primary myelofibrosis (D47.1)
       CC Excl: PDX collection 488

     D75.82 Heparin induced thrombocytopenia (HIT)   `HCC`
       DEF: Immune-mediated reaction to heparin therapy causing an abrupt fall in platelet count and serious complications such as pulmonary embolism, stroke, AMI, or DVT.

     D75.89 Other specified diseases of blood and blood-forming organs

   D75.9 Disease of blood and blood-forming organs, unspecified

✓4ᵗʰ D76 Other specified diseases with participation of lymphoreticular and reticulohistiocytic tissue
     EXCLUDES 1   (Abt-) Letterer-Siwe disease (C96.0)
       eosinophilic granuloma (C96.6)
       Hand-Schüller-Christian disease (C96.5)
       histiocytic medullary reticulosis (C96.9)
       histiocytic sarcoma (C96.A)
       histiocytosis X, multifocal (C96.5)
       histiocytosis X, unifocal (C96.6)
       Langerhans-cell histiocytosis, multifocal (C96.5)
       Langerhans-cell histiocytosis NOS (C96.6)
       Langerhans-cell histiocytosis, unifocal (C96.6)
       leukemic reticuloendotheliosis (C91.4-)
       lipomelanotic reticulosis (I89.8)
       malignant histiocytosis (C96.A)
       malignant reticulosis (C86.0)
       nonlipid reticuloendotheliosis (C96.0)

   CC Excl: For CC codes in category D76: PDX collection 507

   D76.1 Hemophagocytic lymphohistiocytosis   `CC` `HCC`
     Familial hemophagocytic reticulosis
     Histiocytoses of mononuclear phagocytes

   D76.2 Hemophagocytic syndrome, infection-associated   `CC` `HCC`
     Use additional code to identify infectious agent or disease

---

N Newborn: 0   **P** Pediatric: 0-17   **M** Maternity: 12-55   **A** Adult: 15-124   **MCC** Major Complication/Comorbidity   **CC** Complication/Comorbidity   **SW** Severe Wound Dx

D76.3 Other histiocytosis syndromes `CC` `HCC`
Reticulohistiocytoma (giant-cell)
Sinus histiocytosis with massive lymphadenopathy
Xanthogranuloma

D77 *Other disorders of blood and blood-forming organs in diseases classified elsewhere*
Code first underlying disease, such as:
amyloidosis (E85.-)
congenital early syphilis (A50.Ø)
echinococcosis (B67.Ø-B67.9)
malaria (B5Ø.Ø-B54)
schistosomiasis [bilharziasis] (B65.Ø-B65.9)
vitamin C deficiency (E54)
EXCLUDES 1 *rupture of spleen due to Plasmodium vivax malaria (B51.Ø)*
splenitis, splenomegaly in late syphilis (A52.79)
splenitis, splenomegaly in tuberculosis (A18.85)

Intraoperative and postprocedural complications of the spleen (D78)

✓4th D78 Intraoperative and postprocedural complications of the spleen
AHA: 2016, 4Q, 9-10

CC Excl: For CC codes in category D78, unless otherwise noted:
PDX collection 5Ø8

✓5th D78.Ø Intraoperative hemorrhage and hematoma of the spleen complicating a procedure
EXCLUDES 1 *intraoperative hemorrhage and hematoma of the spleen due to accidental puncture or laceration during a procedure (D78.1-)*

D78.Ø1 Intraoperative hemorrhage and hematoma of the spleen complicating a procedure on the spleen `CC`

D78.Ø2 Intraoperative hemorrhage and hematoma of the spleen complicating other procedure `CC`

✓5th D78.1 Accidental puncture and laceration of the spleen during a procedure

D78.11 Accidental puncture and laceration of the spleen during a procedure on the spleen `CC`
CC Excl: PDX collection 5Ø9

D78.12 Accidental puncture and laceration of the spleen during other procedure `CC`
CC Excl: PDX collection 5Ø9

✓5th D78.2 Postprocedural hemorrhage of the spleen following a procedure

D78.21 Postprocedural hemorrhage of the spleen following a procedure on the spleen `CC`

D78.22 Postprocedural hemorrhage of the spleen following other procedure `CC`

✓5th D78.3 Postprocedural hematoma and seroma of the spleen following a procedure

D78.31 Postprocedural hematoma **of the spleen following a** procedure on the spleen `HCC`

D78.32 Postprocedural hematoma **of the spleen following** other procedure `CC`

D78.33 Postprocedural seroma **of the spleen following a** procedure on the spleen `CC`

D78.34 Postprocedural seroma **of the spleen following** other procedure `CC`

✓5th D78.8 Other intraoperative and postprocedural complications of the spleen
Use additional code, if applicable, to further specify disorder

D78.81 Other intraoperative **complications of the spleen** `CC`
CC Excl: PDX collection 51Ø

D78.89 Other postprocedural **complications of the spleen** `CC`
CC Excl: PDX collection 51Ø

Certain disorders involving the immune mechanism (D8Ø-D89)

INCLUDES defects in the complement system
immunodeficiency disorders, except human immunodeficiency virus [HIV] disease
sarcoidosis
EXCLUDES 1 *autoimmune disease (systemic) NOS (M35.9)*
functional disorders of polymorphonuclear neutrophils (D71)
human immunodeficiency virus [HIV] disease (B2Ø)

✓4th D80 Immunodeficiency with predominantly antibody defects

CC Excl: For CC codes in category D80, unless otherwise noted:
PDX collection 511

D80.Ø Hereditary hypogammaglobulinemia `CC` `HCC`
Autosomal recessive agammaglobulinemia (Swiss type)
X-linked agammaglobulinemia [Bruton] (with growth hormone deficiency)

D80.1 Nonfamilial hypogammaglobulinemia `CC` `HCC`
Agammaglobulinemia with immunoglobulin-bearing B-lymphocytes
Common variable agammaglobulinemia [CVAgamma]
Hypogammaglobulinemia NOS
CC Excl: PDX collection 512

D80.2 Selective deficiency of immunoglobulin A [IgA] `CC` `HCC`
CC Excl: PDX collection 512

D80.3 Selective deficiency of immunoglobulin G [IgG] subclasses `CC` `HCC`

D80.4 Selective deficiency of immunoglobulin M [IgM] `CC` `HCC`

D80.5 Immunodeficiency with increased immunoglobulin M [IgM] `CC` `HCC`

D80.6 Antibody deficiency with near-normal immunoglobulins or with hyperimmunoglobulinemia `CC` `HCC`

D80.7 Transient hypogammaglobulinemia of infancy `CC` `HCC`

D80.8 Other immunodeficiencies with predominantly antibody defects `CC` `HCC`
Kappa light chain deficiency

D80.9 Immunodeficiency with predominantly antibody defects, unspecified `CC` `HCC`

✓4th D81 Combined immunodeficiencies
EXCLUDES 1 *autosomal recessive agammaglobulinemia (Swiss type) (D8Ø.Ø)*

CC Excl: For CC codes in category D81, unless otherwise noted:
PDX collection 511

D81.Ø Severe combined immunodeficiency [SCID] with reticular dysgenesis `CC` `HCC`

D81.1 Severe combined immunodeficiency [SCID] with low T- and B-cell numbers `CC` `HCC`

D81.2 Severe combined immunodeficiency [SCID] with low or normal B-cell numbers `CC` `HCC`

D81.3 Adenosine deaminase [ADA] deficiency `CC` `HCC`
CC Excl: PDX collection 513

D81.4 Nezelof's syndrome `CC` `HCC`

D81.5 Purine nucleoside phosphorylase [PNP] deficiency `CC` `HCC`
CC Excl: PDX collection 513

D81.6 Major histocompatibility complex class I deficiency `CC` `HCC`
Bare lymphocyte syndrome

D81.7 Major histocompatibility complex class II deficiency `CC` `HCC`

✓5th D81.8 Other combined immunodeficiencies

✓6th D81.81 Biotin-dependent carboxylase deficiency
Multiple carboxylase deficiency
EXCLUDES 1 *biotin-dependent carboxylase deficiency due to dietary deficiency of biotin (E53.8)*

D81.81Ø Biotinidase deficiency

D81.818 Other biotin-dependent carboxylase deficiency
Holocarboxylase synthetase deficiency
Other multiple carboxylase deficiency

D81.819 Biotin-dependent carboxylase deficiency, unspecified
Multiple carboxylase deficiency, unspecified

D81.89 Other combined immunodeficiencies `CC` `HCC`

D81.9 Combined immunodeficiency, unspecified `CC` `HCC`
Severe combined immunodeficiency disorder [SCID] NOS

☑ Additional Character Required   ✓x7th Placeholder   Unacceptable PDx   Questionable PDx   Manifestation   **H1**-**H14** HAC   `HCC` CMS-HCC Dx   **HIV** HIV Dx

ICD-10-CM 2019   **511**

Chapter 3. Diseases of the Blood and Blood-forming Organs

D76.3–D81.9

Chapter 3. Diseases of the Blood and Blood-forming Organs

☑4ᵗʰ **D82 Immunodeficiency associated with other major defects**
> *EXCLUDES 1*   *ataxia telangiectasia [Louis-Bar] (G11.3)*

D82.0 Wiskott-Aldrich syndrome   CC HCC
> Immunodeficiency with thrombocytopenia and eczema
> **CC Excl:** PDX collection 511

D82.1 Di George's syndrome   CC HCC
> Pharyngeal pouch syndrome
> Thymic alymphoplasia
> Thymic aplasia or hypoplasia with immunodeficiency
> **CC Excl:** PDX collection 511

D82.2 Immunodeficiency with short-limbed stature   HCC

D82.3 Immunodeficiency following hereditary defective response to Epstein-Barr virus   HCC
> X-linked lymphoproliferative disease

D82.4 Hyperimmunoglobulin E [IgE] syndrome   HCC

D82.8 Immunodeficiency associated with other specified major defects   HCC

D82.9 Immunodeficiency associated with major defect, unspecified   HCC

☑4ᵗʰ **D83 Common variable immunodeficiency**

> **CC Excl: For CC codes in category D83:** PDX collection 511

D83.0 Common variable immunodeficiency with predominant abnormalities of B-cell numbers and function   CC HCC

D83.1 Common variable immunodeficiency with predominant immunoregulatory T-cell disorders   CC HCC

D83.2 Common variable immunodeficiency with autoantibodies to B- or T-cells   CC HCC

D83.8 Other common variable immunodeficiencies   CC HCC

D83.9 Common variable immunodeficiency, unspecified   CC HCC

☑4ᵗʰ **D84 Other immunodeficiencies**

D84.0 Lymphocyte function antigen-1 [LFA-1] defect   HCC

D84.1 Defects in the complement system   HCC
> C1 esterase inhibitor [C1-INH] deficiency

D84.8 Other specified immunodeficiencies   CC HCC
> **CC Excl:** PDX collection 511

D84.9 Immunodeficiency, unspecified   CC HCC
> **CC Excl:** PDX collection 511

☑4ᵗʰ **D86 Sarcoidosis**

D86.0 Sarcoidosis of lung   HCC

D86.1 Sarcoidosis of lymph nodes

D86.2 Sarcoidosis of lung with sarcoidosis of lymph nodes   HCC

D86.3 Sarcoidosis of skin

☑5ᵗʰ **D86.8 Sarcoidosis of other sites**

> **D86.81 Sarcoid meningitis**

> **D86.82 Multiple cranial nerve palsies in sarcoidosis**   HCC

> **D86.83 Sarcoid iridocyclitis**

> **D86.84 Sarcoid pyelonephritis**
> > Tubulo-interstitial nephropathy in sarcoidosis

> **D86.85 Sarcoid myocarditis**

> **D86.86 Sarcoid arthropathy**
> > Polyarthritis in sarcoidosis

> **D86.87 Sarcoid myositis**

> **D86.89 Sarcoidosis of other sites**
> > Hepatic granuloma
> > Uveoparotid fever [Heerfordt]

D86.9 Sarcoidosis, unspecified

☑4ᵗʰ **D89 Other disorders involving the immune mechanism, not elsewhere classified**
> *EXCLUDES 1*   *hyperglobulinemia NOS (R77.1)*
> > *monoclonal gammopathy (of undetermined significance) (D47.2)*
>
> *EXCLUDES 2*   *transplant failure and rejection (T86.-)*

D89.0 Polyclonal hypergammaglobulinemia
> Benign hypergammaglobulinemic purpura
> Polyclonal gammopathy NOS

D89.1 Cryoglobulinemia   HCC
> Cryoglobulinemic purpura
> Cryoglobulinemic vasculitis
> Essential cryoglobulinemia
> Idiopathic cryoglobulinemia
> Mixed cryoglobulinemia
> Primary cryoglobulinemia
> Secondary cryoglobulinemia

D89.2 Hypergammaglobulinemia, unspecified

D89.3 Immune reconstitution syndrome   HCC
> Immune reconstitution inflammatory syndrome [IRIS]
> Use additional code for adverse effect, if applicable, to identify drug (T36-T50 with fifth or sixth character 5)

☑5ᵗʰ **D89.4 Mast cell activation syndrome and related disorders**
> *EXCLUDES 1*   *aggressive systemic mastocytosis (C96.21)*
> > *congenital cutaneous mastocytosis (Q82.2)*
> > *(non-congenital) cutaneous mastocytosis (D47.01)*
> > *(indolent) systemic mastocytosis (D47.02)*
> > *malignant mast cell neoplasm (C96.2-)*
> > *malignant mastocytoma (C96.29)*
> > *mast cell leukemia (C94.3-)*
> > *mast cell sarcoma (C96.22)*
> > *mastocytoma NOS (D47.09)*
> > *other mast cell neoplasms of uncertain behavior (D47.09)*
> > *systemic mastocytosis associated with a clonal hematologic non-mast cell lineage disease (SM-AHNMD)(D47.02)*
>
> **AHA:** 2016, 4Q, 11

> **D89.40 Mast cell activation, unspecified**   HCC
> > Mast cell activation disorder, unspecified
> > Mast cell activation syndrome, NOS

> **D89.41 Monoclonal mast cell activation syndrome**   HCC

> **D89.42 Idiopathic mast cell activation syndrome**   HCC

> **D89.43 Secondary mast cell activation**   HCC
> > Secondary mast cell activation syndrome
> > Code also underlying etiology, if known

> **D89.49 Other mast cell activation disorder**   HCC
> > Other mast cell activation syndrome

☑5ᵗʰ **D89.8 Other specified disorders involving the immune mechanism, not elsewhere classified**

☑6ᵗʰ **D89.81 Graft-versus-host disease**
> > Code first underlying cause, such as:
> > > complications of transplanted organs and tissue (T86.-)
> > > complications of blood transfusion (T80.89)
> > Use additional code to identify associated manifestations, such as:
> > > desquamative dermatitis (L30.8)
> > > diarrhea (R19.7)
> > > elevated bilirubin (R17)
> > > hair loss (L65.9)

> > **CC Excl: For CC codes in subcategory D89.81:** PDX collection 514

> > **D89.810 Acute graft-versus-host disease**   CC HCC

> > **D89.811 Chronic graft-versus-host disease**   CC HCC

> > **D89.812 Acute on chronic graft-versus-host disease**   CC HCC

> > **D89.813 Graft-versus-host disease, unspecified**   CC HCC

> **D89.82 Autoimmune lymphoproliferative syndrome [ALPS]**   HCC
> > **DEF:** Rare genetic alteration of the Fas protein that impairs normal cellular apoptosis (normal cell death), causing abnormal accumulation of lymphocytes in the lymph glands, liver, and spleen. Symptoms include neutropenia, anemia, and thrombocytopenia.

> **D89.89 Other specified disorders involving the immune mechanism, not elsewhere classified**   HCC
> > *EXCLUDES 1*   *human immunodeficiency virus disease (B20)*
> > **AHA:** 2017, 4Q, 109

D89.9 Disorder involving the immune mechanism, unspecified   HCC
> Immune disease NOS
> **AHA:** 2015, 3Q, 22

N Newborn: 0   **P** Pediatric: 0-17   **M** Maternity: 12-55   **A** Adult: 15-124   **MCC** Major Complication/Comorbidity   **CC** Complication/Comorbidity   **SW** Severe Wound Dx

512   ICD-10-CM 2019

Chapter 4. Endocrine, Nutritional and Metabolic Diseases (E00–E89)

Chapter Specific Guidelines with Coding Examples

The chapter specific guidelines from the ICD-10-CM Official Guidelines for Coding and Reporting have been provided below. Along with these guidelines are coding examples, contained in the shaded boxes, that have been developed to help illustrate the coding and/or sequencing guidance found in these guidelines.

a. Diabetes mellitus

The diabetes mellitus codes are combination codes that include the type of diabetes mellitus, the body system affected, and the complications affecting that body system. As many codes within a particular category as are necessary to describe all of the complications of the disease may be used. They should be sequenced based on the reason for a particular encounter. Assign as many codes from categories E08–E13 as needed to identify all of the associated conditions that the patient has.

> Patient is seen for poorly controlled diabetes, type 2, with diabetic polyneuropathy and diabetic retinopathy with macular edema
>
> **E11.65**   **Type 2 diabetes mellitus with hyperglycemia**
>
> **E11.311**   **Type 2 diabetes mellitus with unspecified diabetic retinopathy with macular edema**
>
> **E11.42**   **Type 2 diabetes mellitus with diabetic polyneuropathy**
>
> *Explanation*: Use as many codes to describe the diabetic complications as needed. Many are combination codes that describe more than one condition. Code first the reason for the encounter. "Poorly controlled" is described as "with hyperglycemia." Diabetes documented as "uncontrolled" is not assumed to be hyperglycemic but can be classified to either hyperglycemia or hypoglycemia. If documentation is not clear, the provider must be queried so that the appropriate code can be reported.

1) Type of diabetes

The age of a patient is not the sole determining factor, though most type 1 diabetics develop the condition before reaching puberty. For this reason type 1 diabetes mellitus is also referred to as juvenile diabetes.

> A 45-year-old patient is diagnosed with type 1 diabetes
>
> **E10.9**   **Type 1 diabetes mellitus without complications**
>
> *Explanation*: Although most type 1 diabetics are diagnosed in childhood or adolescence, it can also begin in adults.

2) Type of diabetes mellitus not documented

If the type of diabetes mellitus is not documented in the medical record the default is E11.-, Type 2 diabetes mellitus.

> H & P lists diabetes and hypertension on patient problem list
>
> **E11.9**   **Type 2 diabetes mellitus without complications**
>
> **I10**   **Essential (primary) hypertension**
>
> *Explanation*: Since the type of diabetes was not documented and no complications were noted, the default code is E11.9.

3) Diabetes mellitus and the use of insulin and oral hypoglycemics

If the documentation in a medical record does not indicate the type of diabetes but does indicate that the patient uses insulin, code E11-, Type 2 diabetes mellitus, should be assigned. An additional code should be assigned from category Z79 to identify the long-term (current) use of insulin or oral hypoglycemic drugs. If the patient is treated with both oral medications and insulin, only the code for long-term (current) use of insulin should be assigned. Code Z79.4 should not be assigned if insulin is given temporarily to bring a type 2 patient's blood sugar under control during an encounter.

> Diabetic patient on daily metformin is admitted in ketoacidosis; insulin given to stabilize blood sugars and discontinued at discharge
>
> **E11.10**   **Type 2 diabetes mellitus with ketoacidosis without coma**
>
> **Z79.84**   **Long term (current) use of oral hypoglycemic drugs**
>
> *Explanation*: Type 2 is the default for diabetes when not further specified in the documentation. Although insulin was given to the patient during the encounter, it was discontinued at discharge, indicating that the patient does not regularly use insulin. Applying code Z79.4 to represent long-term use of insulin would be inappropriate.

4) Diabetes mellitus in pregnancy and gestational diabetes

See Section I.C.15. Diabetes mellitus in pregnancy.

See Section I.C.15. Gestational (pregnancy induced) diabetes

5) Complications due to insulin pump malfunction

(a) Underdose of insulin due to insulin pump failure

An underdose of insulin due to an insulin pump failure should be assigned to a code from subcategory T85.6, Mechanical complication of other specified internal and external prosthetic devices, implants and grafts, that specifies the type of pump malfunction, as the principal or first-listed code, followed by code T38.3X6-, Underdosing of insulin and oral hypoglycemic [antidiabetic] drugs. Additional codes for the type of diabetes mellitus and any associated complications due to the underdosing should also be assigned.

> A 24-year-old type 1 diabetic male treated in ED for hyperglycemia; insulin pump found to be malfunctioning and underdosing
>
> **T85.614A**   **Breakdown (mechanical) of insulin pump, initial encounter**
>
> **T38.3X6A**   **Underdosing of insulin and oral hypoglycemic [antidiabetic] drugs, initial encounter**
>
> **E10.65**   **Type 1 diabetes mellitus with hyperglycemia**
>
> *Explanation*: The complication code for the mechanical breakdown of the pump is sequenced first, followed by the underdosing code and type of diabetes with complication. Code all other diabetic complication codes necessary to describe the patient's condition.

(b) Overdose of insulin due to insulin pump failure

The principal or first-listed code for an encounter due to an insulin pump malfunction resulting in an overdose of insulin, should also be T85.6-, Mechanical complication of other specified internal and external prosthetic devices, implants and grafts, followed by code T38.3X1-, Poisoning by insulin and oral hypoglycemic [antidiabetic] drugs, accidental (unintentional).

> A 24-year-old type 1 diabetic male found down with diabetic coma, brought into ED and treated for hypoglycemia; insulin pump found to be malfunctioning and overdosing
>
> **T85.614A**   **Breakdown (mechanical) of insulin pump, initial encounter**
>
> **T38.3X1A**   **Poisoning by insulin and oral hypoglycemic [antidiabetic] drugs, accidental (unintentional), initial encounter**
>
> **E10.641**   **Type 1 diabetes mellitus with hypoglycemia with coma**
>
> *Explanation*: The complication code for the mechanical breakdown of the pump is sequenced first, followed by the poisoning code and type of diabetes with complication. All the characters in the combination code must be used to form a valid code and to fully describe the type of diabetes, the hypoglycemia, and the coma.

6) Secondary diabetes mellitus

Codes under categories E08, Diabetes mellitus due to underlying condition, E09, Drug or chemical induced diabetes mellitus, and E13, Other specified diabetes mellitus, identify complications/manifestations associated with secondary diabetes mellitus. Secondary diabetes is always caused by another condition or event (e.g., cystic fibrosis, malignant neoplasm of pancreas, pancreatectomy, adverse effect of drug, or poisoning).

(a) Secondary diabetes mellitus and the use of insulin or oral hypoglycemic drugs

For patients with secondary diabetes mellitus who routinely use insulin or oral hypoglycemic drugs, an additional code from category Z79 should be assigned to identify the long-term (current) use of insulin or oral hypoglycemic drugs. If the patient is treated with both oral medications and insulin, only the code for long-term (current) use of insulin should be assigned. Code Z79.4 should not be assigned if insulin is given temporarily to bring a secondary diabetic patient's blood sugar under control during an encounter.

> The patient, maintained on metformin and insulin, was admitted for treatment of diabetic gangrene. The patient developed diabetes secondary to Nelson's syndrome.
>
> | E24.1 | Nelson's syndrome |
> |---|---|
> | E08.52 | Diabetes mellitus due to underlying condition with diabetic peripheral angiopathy with gangrene |
> | Z79.4 | Long term (current) use of insulin |
>
> *Explanation*: When diabetes is caused by an underlying condition, the underlying condition should always be sequenced before any codes representing the diabetes. Patients with secondary diabetes may be maintained on both insulin and an oral hypoglycemic. Report only the code for the long-term use of insulin when both oral hypoglycemic and insulin are prescribed.

(b) Assigning and sequencing secondary diabetes codes and its causes

The sequencing of the secondary diabetes codes in relationship to codes for the cause of the diabetes is based on the Tabular List instructions for categories E08, E09 and E13.

(i) Secondary diabetes mellitus due to pancreatectomy

For postpancreatectomy diabetes mellitus (lack of insulin due to the surgical removal of all or part of the pancreas), assign code E89.1, Postprocedural hypoinsulinemia. Assign a code from category E13 and a code from subcategory Z90.41, Acquired absence of pancreas, as additional codes.

> Patient with newly diagnosed diabetes after surgical removal of part of pancreas is discharged with referral for consult to initiate insulin.
>
> | E89.1 | Postprocedural hypoinsulinemia |
> |---|---|
> | E13.9 | Other specified diabetes mellitus without complications |
> | Z90.411 | Acquired partial absence of pancreas |
>
> *Explanation*: Sequence the postprocedural complication of the hypoinsulinemia due to the partial removal of the pancreas as the first-listed code, followed by the other specified diabetes (NEC) with or without complications and the partial or total acquired absence of the pancreas. Code Z79.4 Long term (current) use of insulin, is not added because the insulin has not yet been started.

(ii) Secondary diabetes due to drugs

Secondary diabetes may be caused by an adverse effect of correctly administered medications, poisoning or sequela of poisoning.

See section I.C.19.e for coding of adverse effects and poisoning, and section I.C.20 for external cause code reporting.

> Initial encounter for corticosteroid-induced diabetes mellitus
>
> | E09.9 | Drug or chemical induced diabetes mellitus without complications |
> |---|---|
> | T38.0X5A | Adverse effect of glucocorticoids and synthetic analogues, initial encounter |
>
> *Explanation*: If the diabetes is caused by an adverse effect of a drug, the diabetic condition is coded first. If it occurs from a poisoning or overdose, the poisoning code causing the diabetes is sequenced first.

Chapter 4. Endocrine, Nutritional and Metabolic Diseases (E00-E89)

NOTE All neoplasms, whether functionally active or not, are classified in Chapter 2. Appropriate codes in this chapter (i.e. E05.8, E07.0, E16-E31, E34-) may be used as additional codes to indicate either functional activity by neoplasms and ectopic endocrine tissue or hyperfunction and hypofunction of endocrine glands associated with neoplasms and other conditions classified elsewhere.

EXCLUDES 1 *transitory endocrine and metabolic disorders specific to newborn (P70-P74)*

AHA: 2018, 2Q, 6

This chapter contains the following blocks:

E00-E07　Disorders of thyroid gland
E08-E13　Diabetes mellitus
E15-E16　Other disorders of glucose regulation and pancreatic internal secretion
E20-E35　Disorders of other endocrine glands
E36　Intraoperative complications of endocrine system
E40-E46　Malnutrition
E50-E64　Other nutritional deficiencies
E65-E68　Overweight, obesity and other hyperalimentation
E70-E88　Metabolic disorders
E89　Postprocedural endocrine and metabolic complications and disorders, not elsewhere classified

Disorders of thyroid gland (E00-E07)

√4th **E00** **Congenital iodine-deficiency syndrome**
Use additional code (F70-F79) to identify associated intellectual disabilities
EXCLUDES 1 *subclinical iodine-deficiency hypothyroidism (E02)*

E00.0 **Congenital iodine-deficiency syndrome, neurological type**
Endemic cretinism, neurological type

E00.1 **Congenital iodine-deficiency syndrome, myxedematous type**
Endemic hypothyroid cretinism
Endemic cretinism, myxedematous type

E00.2 **Congenital iodine-deficiency syndrome, mixed type**
Endemic cretinism, mixed type

E00.9 **Congenital iodine-deficiency syndrome, unspecified**
Congenital iodine-deficiency hypothyroidism NOS
Endemic cretinism NOS

√4th **E01** **Iodine-deficiency related thyroid disorders and allied conditions**
EXCLUDES 1 *congenital iodine-deficiency syndrome (E00.-)*
subclinical iodine-deficiency hypothyroidism (E02)

E01.0 **Iodine-deficiency related diffuse (endemic) goiter**

E01.1 **Iodine-deficiency related multinodular (endemic) goiter**
Iodine-deficiency related nodular goiter

E01.2 **Iodine-deficiency related (endemic) goiter, unspecified**
Endemic goiter NOS

E01.8 **Other iodine-deficiency related thyroid disorders and allied conditions**
Acquired iodine-deficiency hypothyroidism NOS

E02 **Subclinical iodine-deficiency hypothyroidism**

√4th **E03** **Other hypothyroidism**
EXCLUDES 1 *iodine-deficiency related hypothyroidism (E00-E02)*
postprocedural hypothyroidism (E89.0)

E03.0 **Congenital hypothyroidism with diffuse goiter**
Congenital parenchymatous goiter (nontoxic)
Congenital goiter (nontoxic) NOS
EXCLUDES 1 *transitory congenital goiter with normal function (P72.0)*

E03.1 **Congenital hypothyroidism without goiter**
Aplasia of thyroid (with myxedema)
Congenital atrophy of thyroid
Congenital hypothyroidism NOS

E03.2 **Hypothyroidism due to medicaments and other exogenous substances**
Code first poisoning due to drug or toxin, if applicable (T36-T65 with fifth or sixth character 1-4 or 6)
Use additional code for adverse effect, if applicable, to identify drug (T36-T50 with fifth or sixth character 5)

E03.3 **Postinfectious hypothyroidism**

E03.4 **Atrophy of thyroid (acquired)**
EXCLUDES 1 *congenital atrophy of thyroid (E03.1)*

E03.5 **Myxedema coma** `MCC` `HCC`
CC Excl: PDX collection 515

E03.8 **Other specified hypothyroidism**

E03.9 **Hypothyroidism, unspecified**
Myxedema NOS

√4th **E04** **Other nontoxic goiter**
EXCLUDES 1 *congenital goiter (NOS) (diffuse) (parenchymatous) (E03.0)*
iodine-deficiency related goiter (E00-E02)

E04.0 **Nontoxic diffuse goiter**
Diffuse (colloid) nontoxic goiter
Simple nontoxic goiter

E04.1 **Nontoxic single thyroid nodule**
Colloid nodule (cystic) (thyroid)　Thyroid (cystic) nodule NOS
Nontoxic uninodular goiter
DEF: Enlarged thyroid, commonly due to decreased thyroid production, with a single nodule. No clinical hypothyroidism.

E04.2 **Nontoxic multinodular goiter**
Cystic goiter NOS
Multinodular (cystic) goiter NOS
DEF: Enlarged thyroid, commonly due to decreased thyroid production with multiple nodules. No clinical hypothyroidism.

E04.8 **Other specified nontoxic goiter**

E04.9 **Nontoxic goiter, unspecified**
Goiter NOS
Nodular goiter (nontoxic) NOS

√4th **E05** **Thyrotoxicosis [hyperthyroidism]**
EXCLUDES 1 *chronic thyroiditis with transient thyrotoxicosis (E06.2)*
neonatal thyrotoxicosis (P72.1)
DEF: Excessive quantities of hormones from the thyroid gland caused by overproduction or loss of storage ability.

CC Excl: For MCC codes in category E05: PDX collection 516

√5th **E05.0** **Thyrotoxicosis with diffuse goiter**
Exophthalmic or toxic goiter NOS
Graves' disease
Toxic diffuse goiter
DEF: Diffuse thyroid enlargement accompanied by hyperthyroidism, bulging eyes, and dermopathy.

E05.00 **Thyrotoxicosis with diffuse goiter without thyrotoxic crisis or storm**

E05.01 **Thyrotoxicosis with diffuse goiter with thyrotoxic crisis or storm** `MCC`

Goiter

√5th **E05.1** **Thyrotoxicosis with toxic single thyroid nodule**
Thyrotoxicosis with toxic uninodular goiter
DEF: Symptomatic hyperthyroidism with a single nodule on the enlarged thyroid gland. Onset of symptoms can be abrupt and include extreme nervousness, insomnia, weight loss, tremors, and psychosis or coma.

E05.10 **Thyrotoxicosis with toxic single thyroid nodule without thyrotoxic crisis or storm**

E05.11 **Thyrotoxicosis with toxic single thyroid nodule with thyrotoxic crisis or storm** `MCC`

√5th **E05.2** **Thyrotoxicosis with toxic multinodular goiter**
Toxic nodular goiter NOS

E05.20 **Thyrotoxicosis with toxic multinodular goiter without thyrotoxic crisis or storm**

E05.21 **Thyrotoxicosis with toxic multinodular goiter with thyrotoxic crisis or storm** `MCC`

√5th **E05.3** **Thyrotoxicosis from ectopic thyroid tissue**

E05.30 **Thyrotoxicosis from ectopic thyroid tissue without thyrotoxic crisis or storm**

E05.31 **Thyrotoxicosis from ectopic thyroid tissue with thyrotoxic crisis or storm** `MCC`

☑Additional Character Required　　√x7th Placeholder　　Unacceptable PDx　　Questionable PDx　　Manifestation　　H1-H14 HAC　　HCC CMS-HCC Dx　　HIV HIV Dx

ICD-10-CM 2019　　　　　　　　　　515

Chapter 4. Endocrine, Nutritional and Metabolic Diseases

E05.4–E08.311

✓5th **E05.4** Thyrotoxicosis factitia

    E05.40 **Thyrotoxicosis factitia** without thyrotoxic crisis or storm

    E05.41 **Thyrotoxicosis factitia** with thyrotoxic crisis or storm   MCC

✓5th **E05.8** Other thyrotoxicosis

    Overproduction of thyroid-stimulating hormone

    E05.80 **Other thyrotoxicosis** without thyrotoxic crisis or storm

    E05.81 **Other thyrotoxicosis** with thyrotoxic crisis or storm   MCC

✓5th **E05.9** Thyrotoxicosis, unspecified

    Hyperthyroidism NOS

    E05.90 **Thyrotoxicosis, unspecified** without thyrotoxic crisis or storm

    E05.91 **Thyrotoxicosis, unspecified** with thyrotoxic crisis or storm   MCC

✓4th **E06** Thyroiditis

    EXCLUDES 1   postpartum thyroiditis (O90.5)

    DEF: Inflammation of the thyroid gland.

    E06.0 Acute thyroiditis   CC

        Abscess of thyroid

        Pyogenic thyroiditis

        Suppurative thyroiditis

        Use additional code (B95-B97) to identify infectious agent

        CC Excl: PDX collection 517

    E06.1 Subacute thyroiditis

        de Quervain thyroiditis

        Giant-cell thyroiditis

        Granulomatous thyroiditis

        Nonsuppurative thyroiditis

        Viral thyroiditis

        EXCLUDES 1   autoimmune thyroiditis (E06.3)

    E06.2 Chronic thyroiditis with transient thyrotoxicosis

        EXCLUDES 1   autoimmune thyroiditis (E06.3)

    E06.3 Autoimmune thyroiditis

        Hashimoto's thyroiditis

        Hashitoxicosis (transient)

        Lymphadenoid goiter

        Lymphocytic thyroiditis

        Struma lymphomatosa

    E06.4 Drug-induced thyroiditis

        Use additional code for adverse effect, if applicable, to identify drug (T36-T50 with fifth or sixth character 5)

    E06.5 Other chronic thyroiditis

        Chronic fibrous thyroiditis

        Chronic thyroiditis NOS

        Ligneous thyroiditis

        Riedel thyroiditis

    E06.9 Thyroiditis, unspecified

✓4th **E07** Other disorders of thyroid

    E07.0 Hypersecretion of calcitonin

        C-cell hyperplasia of thyroid

        Hypersecretion of thyrocalcitonin

    E07.1 Dyshormogenetic goiter

        Familial dyshormogenetic goiter

        Pendred's syndrome

        EXCLUDES 1   transitory congenital goiter with normal function (P72.0)

✓5th **E07.8** Other specified disorders of thyroid

    E07.81 **Sick-euthyroid syndrome**

        Euthyroid sick-syndrome

        DEF: Thyroid dysfunction caused by abnormal levels of thyroid hormones T3 and/or T4. This syndrome is often associated with starvation or critical illness.

    E07.89 **Other specified disorders of thyroid**

        Abnormality of thyroid-binding globulin

        Hemorrhage of thyroid

        Infarction of thyroid

    E07.9 Disorder of thyroid, unspecified

Diabetes mellitus (E08-E13)

AHA: 2018, 2Q, 6; 2017, 4Q, 6; 2017, 1Q, 42; 2016, 4Q, 11-13; 2016, 2Q, 36; 2016, 1Q, 11-13

✓4th **E08** Diabetes mellitus due to underlying condition

    Code first the underlying condition, such as:

        congenital rubella (P35.0)

        cushing's syndrome (E24.-)

        cystic fibrosis (E84.-)

        malignant neoplasm (C00-C96)

        malnutrition (E40-E46)

        pancreatitis and other diseases of the pancreas (K85.-, K86.-)

    Use additional code to identify control using:

        insulin (Z79.4)

        oral antidiabetic drugs (Z79.84)

        oral hypoglycemic drugs (Z79.84)

    EXCLUDES 1   drug or chemical induced diabetes mellitus (E09.-)

        gestational diabetes (O24.4-)

        neonatal diabetes mellitus (P70.2)

        postpancreatectomy diabetes mellitus (E13.-)

        postprocedural diabetes mellitus (E13.-)

        secondary diabetes mellitus NEC (E13.-)

        type 1 diabetes mellitus (E10.-)\

        type 2 diabetes mellitus (E11.-)

    AHA: 2013, 4Q, 114; 2013, 3Q, 20

    CC Excl: For CC/MCC codes in category E08, unless otherwise noted: PDX collection 518

✓5th **E08.0** Diabetes mellitus due to underlying condition with hyperosmolarity

    DEF: Diabetic hyperosmolarity: Extremely high levels of glucose in the blood without ketones.

    E08.00 *Diabetes mellitus due to underlying condition with hyperosmolarity without nonketotic hyperglycemic-hyperosmolar coma (NKHHC)*   MCC   H9   HCC

    E08.01 *Diabetes mellitus due to underlying condition with hyperosmolarity with coma*   MCC   H9   HCC

✓5th **E08.1** Diabetes mellitus due to underlying condition with ketoacidosis

    DEF: Diabetic ketoacidosis: Potentially life-threatening complication due to a shortage of insulin in which the body switches to burning fatty acids and producing acidic ketone bodies.

    E08.10 *Diabetes mellitus due to underlying condition with ketoacidosis without coma*   MCC   H9   HCC

    E08.11 *Diabetes mellitus due to underlying condition with ketoacidosis with coma*   MCC   HCC

✓5th **E08.2** Diabetes mellitus due to underlying condition with kidney complications

    E08.21 *Diabetes mellitus due to underlying condition with diabetic nephropathy*   HCC

        Diabetes mellitus due to underlying condition with intercapillary glomerulosclerosis

        Diabetes mellitus due to underlying condition with intracapillary glomerulonephrosis

        Diabetes mellitus due to underlying condition with Kimmelstiel-Wilson disease

    E08.22 *Diabetes mellitus due to underlying condition with diabetic chronic kidney disease*   HCC

        Use additional code to identify stage of chronic kidney disease (N18.1-N18.6)

    E08.29 *Diabetes mellitus due to underlying condition with other diabetic kidney complication*   HCC

        Renal tubular degeneration in diabetes mellitus due to underlying condition

✓5th **E08.3** Diabetes mellitus due to underlying condition with ophthalmic complications

    One of the following 7th characters is to be assigned to codes in subcategories E08.32, E08.33, E08.34, E08.35, and E08.37 to designate laterality of the disease:

    1   right eye

    2   left eye

    3   bilateral

    9   unspecified eye

✓6th **E08.31** Diabetes mellitus due to underlying condition with unspecified diabetic retinopathy

    DEF: Diabetic retinopathy: Diabetic complication from damage to the retinal vessels resulting in vision problems that can progress to blindness.

    E08.311 *Diabetes mellitus due to underlying condition with unspecified diabetic retinopathy with macular edema*   HCC

N Newborn: 0   P Pediatric: 0-17   M Maternity: 12-55   A Adult: 15-124   MCC Major Complication/Comorbidity   CC Complication/Comorbidity   SW Severe Wound Dx

516   ICD-10-CM 2019

E08.319   *Diabetes mellitus due to underlying condition with unspecified diabetic retinopathy without macular edema*   `HCC`

✓6th **E08.32**   Diabetes mellitus due to underlying condition with mild nonproliferative diabetic retinopathy

> Diabetes mellitus due to underlying condition with nonproliferative diabetic retinopathy NOS

     ✓7th **E08.321**   *Diabetes mellitus due to underlying condition with mild nonproliferative diabetic retinopathy with macular edema*   `HCC`

     ✓7th **E08.329**   *Diabetes mellitus due to underlying condition with mild nonproliferative diabetic retinopathy without macular edema*   `HCC`

✓6th **E08.33**   Diabetes mellitus due to underlying condition with moderate nonproliferative diabetic retinopathy

     ✓7th **E08.331**   *Diabetes mellitus due to underlying condition with moderate nonproliferative diabetic retinopathy with macular edema*   `HCC`

     ✓7th **E08.339**   *Diabetes mellitus due to underlying condition with moderate nonproliferative diabetic retinopathy without macular edema*   `HCC`

✓6th **E08.34**   Diabetes mellitus due to underlying condition with severe nonproliferative diabetic retinopathy

     ✓7th **E08.341**   *Diabetes mellitus due to underlying condition with severe nonproliferative diabetic retinopathy with macular edema*   `HCC`

     ✓7th **E08.349**   *Diabetes mellitus due to underlying condition with severe nonproliferative diabetic retinopathy without macular edema*   `HCC`

✓6th **E08.35**   Diabetes mellitus due to underlying condition with proliferative diabetic retinopathy

     ✓7th **E08.351**   *Diabetes mellitus due to underlying condition with proliferative diabetic retinopathy with macular edema*   `HCC`

     ✓7th **E08.352**   *Diabetes mellitus due to underlying condition with proliferative diabetic retinopathy with traction retinal detachment involving the macula*   `HCC`

     ✓7th **E08.353**   *Diabetes mellitus due to underlying condition with proliferative diabetic retinopathy with traction retinal detachment not involving the macula*   `HCC`

     ✓7th **E08.354**   *Diabetes mellitus due to underlying condition with proliferative diabetic retinopathy with combined traction retinal detachment and rhegmatogenous retinal detachment*   `HCC`

     ✓7th **E08.355**   *Diabetes mellitus due to underlying condition with stable proliferative diabetic retinopathy*   `HCC`

     ✓7th **E08.359**   *Diabetes mellitus due to underlying condition with proliferative diabetic retinopathy without macular edema*   `HCC`

E08.36   *Diabetes mellitus due to underlying condition with diabetic cataract*   `HCC`
> **AHA:** 2016, 4Q, 142

✓x7th **E08.37**   *Diabetes mellitus due to underlying condition with diabetic macular edema, resolved following treatment*   `HCC`

E08.39   *Diabetes mellitus due to underlying condition with other diabetic ophthalmic complication*   `HCC`
> Use additional code to identify manifestation, such as: diabetic glaucoma (H40-H42)

✓5th **E08.4**   Diabetes mellitus due to underlying condition with neurological complications

     E08.40   *Diabetes mellitus due to underlying condition with diabetic neuropathy, unspecified*   `HCC`

     E08.41   *Diabetes mellitus due to underlying condition with diabetic mononeuropathy*   `HCC`

     E08.42   *Diabetes mellitus due to underlying condition with diabetic polyneuropathy*   `HCC`
> Diabetes mellitus due to underlying condition with diabetic neuralgia

E08.43   *Diabetes mellitus due to underlying condition with diabetic autonomic (poly)neuropathy*   `HCC`
> Diabetes mellitus due to underlying condition with diabetic gastroparesis
> **AHA:** 2013, 4Q, 114

E08.44   *Diabetes mellitus due to underlying condition with diabetic amyotrophy*   `HCC`

E08.49   *Diabetes mellitus due to underlying condition with other diabetic neurological complication*   `HCC`

✓5th **E08.5**   Diabetes mellitus due to underlying condition with circulatory complications

     E08.51   *Diabetes mellitus due to underlying condition with diabetic peripheral angiopathy without gangrene*   `HCC`
> **AHA:** 2018, 2Q, 7

     E08.52   *Diabetes mellitus due to underlying condition with diabetic peripheral angiopathy with gangrene*   `CC` `HCC`
> Diabetes mellitus due to underlying condition with diabetic gangrene
> **AHA:** 2018, 2Q, 7; 2017, 4Q, 102
> **CC Excl:** PDX collection 519

     E08.59   *Diabetes mellitus due to underlying condition with other circulatory complications*   `HCC`

✓5th **E08.6**   Diabetes mellitus due to underlying condition with other specified complications

     ✓6th **E08.61**   Diabetes mellitus due to underlying condition with diabetic arthropathy

       E08.610   *Diabetes mellitus due to underlying condition with diabetic neuropathic arthropathy*   `HCC`
> Diabetes mellitus due to underlying condition with Charcôt's joints
> **DEF:** Charcot's joint: Progressive neurologic arthropathy in which chronic degeneration of joints in the weight-bearing areas with peripheral hypertrophy occurs as a complication of a neuropathy disorder. Supporting structures relax from a loss of sensation resulting in chronic joint instability.

       E08.618   *Diabetes mellitus due to underlying condition with other diabetic arthropathy*   `HCC`
> **AHA:** 2018, 2Q, 6

     ✓6th **E08.62**   Diabetes mellitus due to underlying condition with skin complications

       E08.620   *Diabetes mellitus due to underlying condition with diabetic dermatitis*   `HCC`
> Diabetes mellitus due to underlying condition with diabetic necrobiosis lipoidica

       E08.621   *Diabetes mellitus due to underlying condition with foot ulcer*   `HCC`
> Use additional code to identify site of ulcer (L97.4-, L97.5-)

       E08.622   *Diabetes mellitus due to underlying condition with other skin ulcer*   `HCC`
> Use additional code to identify site of ulcer (L97.1-L97.9, L98.41-L98.49)
> **AHA:** 2017, 4Q, 17

       E08.628   *Diabetes mellitus due to underlying condition with other skin complications*   `HCC`
> **AHA:** 2017, 4Q, 100-101

     ✓6th **E08.63**   Diabetes mellitus due to underlying condition with oral complications

       E08.630   *Diabetes mellitus due to underlying condition with periodontal disease*   `HCC`

       E08.638   *Diabetes mellitus due to underlying condition with other oral complications*   `HCC`

     ✓6th **E08.64**   Diabetes mellitus due to underlying condition with hypoglycemia

       E08.641   *Diabetes mellitus due to underlying condition with hypoglycemia with coma*   `MCC` `HCC`

       E08.649   *Diabetes mellitus due to underlying condition with hypoglycemia without coma*   `HCC`
> **AHA:** 2016, 3Q, 42; 2015, 3Q, 21

     E08.65   *Diabetes mellitus due to underlying condition with hyperglycemia*   `HCC`

     E08.69   *Diabetes mellitus due to underlying condition with other specified complication*   `HCC`
> Use additional code to identify complication
> **AHA:** 2016, 4Q, 141; 2016, 1Q, 13

✓ Additional Character Required   ✓x7th Placeholder   Unacceptable PDx   Questionable PDx   Manifestation   `H1`-`H14` HAC   `HCC` CMS-HCC Dx   `HIV` HIV Dx

ICD-10-CM 2019   517

E08.8   *Diabetes mellitus due to underlying condition with unspecified complications*   `HCC`

E08.9   *Diabetes mellitus due to underlying condition without complications*   `HCC`

✓4ᵗʰ **E09**   **Drug or chemical induced diabetes mellitus**

Code first poisoning due to drug or toxin, if applicable (T36-T65 with fifth or sixth character 1-4 or 6)

Use additional code for adverse effect, if applicable, to identify drug (T36-T50 with fifth or sixth character 5)

Use additional code to identify control using:
insulin (Z79.4)
oral antidiabetic drugs (Z79.84)
oral hypoglycemic drugs (Z79.84)

> **EXCLUDES 1**   diabetes mellitus due to underlying condition (E08.-)
> gestational diabetes (O24.4-)
> neonatal diabetes mellitus (P70.2)
> postpancreatectomy diabetes mellitus (E13.-)
> postprocedural diabetes mellitus (E13.-)
> secondary diabetes mellitus NEC (E13.-)
> type 1 diabetes mellitus (E10.-)
> type 2 diabetes mellitus (E11.-)

AHA: 2016, 1Q, 11-13; 2013, 4Q, 114; 2013, 3Q, 20

CC Excl: For CC/MCC codes in category E09, unless otherwise noted: PDX collection 518

✓5ᵗʰ **E09.0**   **Drug or chemical induced diabetes mellitus with hyperosmolarity**

DEF: Diabetic hyperosmolarity: Extremely high levels of glucose in the blood without ketones.

E09.00   **Drug or chemical induced diabetes mellitus with hyperosmolarity without nonketotic hyperglycemic-hyperosmolar coma (NKHHC)**   `MCC` `H9` `HCC`

E09.01   **Drug or chemical induced diabetes mellitus with hyperosmolarity with coma**   `MCC` `H9` `HCC`

✓5ᵗʰ **E09.1**   **Drug or chemical induced diabetes mellitus with ketoacidosis**

DEF: Diabetic ketoacidosis: Potentially life-threatening complication due to a shortage of insulin in which the body switches to burning fatty acids and producing acidic ketone bodies.

E09.10   **Drug or chemical induced diabetes mellitus with ketoacidosis without coma**   `MCC` `H9` `HCC`

E09.11   **Drug or chemical induced diabetes mellitus with ketoacidosis with coma**   `MCC` `HCC`

✓5ᵗʰ **E09.2**   **Drug or chemical induced diabetes mellitus with kidney complications**

E09.21   **Drug or chemical induced diabetes mellitus with diabetic nephropathy**   `HCC`
Drug or chemical induced diabetes mellitus with intercapillary glomerulosclerosis
Drug or chemical induced diabetes mellitus with intracapillary glomerulonephrosis
Drug or chemical induced diabetes mellitus with Kimmelstiel-Wilson disease

E09.22   **Drug or chemical induced diabetes mellitus with diabetic chronic kidney disease**   `HCC`
Use additional code to identify stage of chronic kidney disease (N18.1-N18.6)

E09.29   **Drug or chemical induced diabetes mellitus with other diabetic kidney complication**   `HCC`
Drug or chemical induced diabetes mellitus with renal tubular degeneration

✓5ᵗʰ **E09.3**   **Drug or chemical induced diabetes mellitus with ophthalmic complications**

One of the following 7th characters is to be assigned to codes in subcategories E09.32, E09.33, E09.34, E09.35, and E09.37 to designate laterality of the disease:
1   right eye
2   left eye
3   bilateral
9   unspecified eye

✓6ᵗʰ **E09.31**   **Drug or chemical induced diabetes mellitus with unspecified diabetic retinopathy**

DEF: Diabetic retinopathy: Diabetic complication from damage to the retinal vessels resulting in vision problems that can progress to blindness.

E09.311   **Drug or chemical induced diabetes mellitus with unspecified diabetic retinopathy with macular edema**   `HCC`

E09.319   **Drug or chemical induced diabetes mellitus with unspecified diabetic retinopathy without macular edema**   `HCC`

✓6ᵗʰ **E09.32**   **Drug or chemical induced diabetes mellitus with mild nonproliferative diabetic retinopathy**
Drug or chemical induced diabetes mellitus with nonproliferative diabetic retinopathy NOS

✓7ᵗʰ **E09.321**   **Drug or chemical induced diabetes mellitus with mild nonproliferative diabetic retinopathy with macular edema**   `HCC`

✓7ᵗʰ **E09.329**   **Drug or chemical induced diabetes mellitus with mild nonproliferative diabetic retinopathy without macular edema**   `HCC`

✓6ᵗʰ **E09.33**   **Drug or chemical induced diabetes mellitus with moderate nonproliferative diabetic retinopathy**

✓7ᵗʰ **E09.331**   **Drug or chemical induced diabetes mellitus with moderate nonproliferative diabetic retinopathy with macular edema**   `HCC`

✓7ᵗʰ **E09.339**   **Drug or chemical induced diabetes mellitus with moderate nonproliferative diabetic retinopathy without macular edema**   `HCC`

✓6ᵗʰ **E09.34**   **Drug or chemical induced diabetes mellitus with severe nonproliferative diabetic retinopathy**

✓7ᵗʰ **E09.341**   **Drug or chemical induced diabetes mellitus with severe nonproliferative diabetic retinopathy with macular edema**   `HCC`

✓7ᵗʰ **E09.349**   **Drug or chemical induced diabetes mellitus with severe nonproliferative diabetic retinopathy without macular edema**   `HCC`

✓6ᵗʰ **E09.35**   **Drug or chemical induced diabetes mellitus with proliferative diabetic retinopathy**

✓7ᵗʰ **E09.351**   **Drug or chemical induced diabetes mellitus with proliferative diabetic retinopathy with macular edema**   `HCC`

✓7ᵗʰ **E09.352**   **Drug or chemical induced diabetes mellitus with proliferative diabetic retinopathy with traction retinal detachment involving the macula**   `HCC`

✓7ᵗʰ **E09.353**   **Drug or chemical induced diabetes mellitus with proliferative diabetic retinopathy with traction retinal detachment not involving the macula**   `HCC`

✓7ᵗʰ **E09.354**   **Drug or chemical induced diabetes mellitus with proliferative diabetic retinopathy with combined traction retinal detachment and rhegmatogenous retinal detachment**   `HCC`

✓7ᵗʰ **E09.355**   **Drug or chemical induced diabetes mellitus with stable proliferative diabetic retinopathy**   `HCC`

✓7ᵗʰ **E09.359**   **Drug or chemical induced diabetes mellitus with proliferative diabetic retinopathy without macular edema**   `HCC`

E09.36   **Drug or chemical induced diabetes mellitus with diabetic cataract**   `HCC`
AHA: 2016, 4Q, 142

✓x7ᵗʰ **E09.37**   **Drug or chemical induced diabetes mellitus with diabetic macular edema, resolved following treatment**   `HCC`

E09.39   **Drug or chemical induced diabetes mellitus with other diabetic ophthalmic complication**   `HCC`
Use additional code to identify manifestation, such as:
diabetic glaucoma (H40-H42)

✓5ᵗʰ **E09.4**   **Drug or chemical induced diabetes mellitus with neurological complications**

E09.40   **Drug or chemical induced diabetes mellitus with neurological complications with diabetic neuropathy, unspecified**   `HCC`

E09.41   **Drug or chemical induced diabetes mellitus with neurological complications with diabetic mononeuropathy**   `HCC`

E09.42   **Drug or chemical induced diabetes mellitus with neurological complications with diabetic polyneuropathy**   `HCC`
Drug or chemical induced diabetes mellitus with diabetic neuralgia

N Newborn: 0   P Pediatric: 0-17   M Maternity: 12-55   A Adult: 15-124   MCC Major Complication/Comorbidity   CC Complication/Comorbidity   SW Severe Wound Dx

518   ICD-10-CM 2019

E09.43 Drug or chemical induced diabetes mellitus with neurological complications with diabetic autonomic (poly)neuropathy `HCC`
> Drug or chemical induced diabetes mellitus with diabetic gastroparesis
> **AHA:** 2013, 4Q, 114

E09.44 Drug or chemical induced diabetes mellitus with neurological complications with diabetic amyotrophy `HCC`

E09.49 Drug or chemical induced diabetes mellitus with neurological complications with other diabetic neurological complication `HCC`

✓5ᵗʰ **E09.5** Drug or chemical induced diabetes mellitus with circulatory complications

E09.51 Drug or chemical induced diabetes mellitus with diabetic peripheral angiopathy without gangrene `HCC`
> **AHA:** 2018, 2Q, 7

E09.52 Drug or chemical induced diabetes mellitus with diabetic peripheral angiopathy with gangrene `CC` `HCC`
> Drug or chemical induced diabetes mellitus with diabetic gangrene
> **AHA:** 2018, 2Q, 7; 2017, 4Q, 102
> **CC Excl:** PDX collection 519

E09.59 Drug or chemical induced diabetes mellitus with other circulatory complications `HCC`

✓5ᵗʰ **E09.6** Drug or chemical induced diabetes mellitus with other specified complications

✓6ᵗʰ **E09.61** Drug or chemical induced diabetes mellitus with diabetic arthropathy

E09.610 Drug or chemical induced diabetes mellitus with diabetic neuropathic arthropathy `HCC`
> Drug or chemical induced diabetes mellitus with Charcôt's joints
> **DEF:** Charcot's joint: Progressive neurologic arthropathy in which chronic degeneration of joints in the weight-bearing areas with peripheral hypertrophy occurs as a complication of a neuropathy disorder. Supporting structures relax from a loss of sensation resulting in chronic joint instability.

E09.618 Drug or chemical induced diabetes mellitus with other diabetic arthropathy `HCC`
> **AHA:** 2018, 2Q, 6

✓6ᵗʰ **E09.62** Drug or chemical induced diabetes mellitus with skin complications

E09.620 Drug or chemical induced diabetes mellitus with diabetic dermatitis `HCC`
> Drug or chemical induced diabetes mellitus with diabetic necrobiosis lipoidica

E09.621 Drug or chemical induced diabetes mellitus with foot ulcer `HCC`
> Use additional code to identify site of ulcer (L97.4-, L97.5-)

E09.622 Drug or chemical induced diabetes mellitus with other skin ulcer `HCC`
> Use additional code to identify site of ulcer (L97.1-L97.9, L98.41-L98.49)
> **AHA:** 2017, 4Q, 17

E09.628 Drug or chemical induced diabetes mellitus with other skin complications `HCC`
> **AHA:** 2017, 4Q, 100-101

✓6ᵗʰ **E09.63** Drug or chemical induced diabetes mellitus with oral complications

E09.630 Drug or chemical induced diabetes mellitus with periodontal disease `HCC`

E09.638 Drug or chemical induced diabetes mellitus with other oral complications `HCC`

✓6ᵗʰ **E09.64** Drug or chemical induced diabetes mellitus with hypoglycemia

E09.641 Drug or chemical induced diabetes mellitus with hypoglycemia with coma `MCC` `HCC`

E09.649 Drug or chemical induced diabetes mellitus with hypoglycemia without coma `HCC`
> **AHA:** 2016, 3Q, 42; 2015, 3Q, 21

E09.65 Drug or chemical induced diabetes mellitus with hyperglycemia `HCC`

E09.69 Drug or chemical induced diabetes mellitus with other specified complication `HCC`
> Use additional code to identify complication
> **AHA:** 2016, 4Q, 141; 2016, 1Q, 13

E09.8 Drug or chemical induced diabetes mellitus with unspecified complications `HCC`

E09.9 Drug or chemical induced diabetes mellitus without complications `HCC`

✓4ᵗʰ **E10** Type 1 diabetes mellitus
> **INCLUDES** brittle diabetes (mellitus)
> diabetes (mellitus) due to autoimmune process
> diabetes (mellitus) due to immune mediated pancreatic islet beta-cell destruction
> idiopathic diabetes (mellitus)
> juvenile onset diabetes (mellitus)
> ketosis-prone diabetes (mellitus)
> **EXCLUDES 1** *diabetes mellitus due to underlying condition (E08.-)*
> *drug or chemical induced diabetes mellitus (E09.-)*
> *gestational diabetes (O24.4-)*
> *hyperglycemia NOS (R73.9)*
> *neonatal diabetes mellitus (P70.2)*
> *postpancreatectomy diabetes mellitus (E13.-)*
> *postprocedural diabetes mellitus (E13.-)*
> *secondary diabetes mellitus NEC (E13.-)*
> *type 2 diabetes mellitus (E11.-)*
> **AHA:** 2016, 1Q, 11-13; 2013, 4Q, 114; 2013, 3Q, 20

> **CC Excl:** For CC/MCC codes in category E10, unless otherwise noted: PDX collection 520

✓5ᵗʰ **E10.1** Type 1 diabetes mellitus with ketoacidosis
> **AHA:** 2013, 3Q, 20
> **DEF:** Diabetic ketoacidosis: Potentially life-threatening complication due to a shortage of insulin in which the body switches to burning fatty acids and producing acidic ketone bodies.

E10.10 Type 1 diabetes mellitus with ketoacidosis without coma `MCC` `H9` `HCC`

E10.11 Type 1 diabetes mellitus with ketoacidosis with coma `MCC` `HCC`

✓5ᵗʰ **E10.2** Type 1 diabetes mellitus with kidney complications

E10.21 Type 1 diabetes mellitus with diabetic nephropathy `HCC`
> Type 1 diabetes mellitus with intercapillary glomerulosclerosis
> Type 1 diabetes mellitus with intracapillary glomerulonephrosis
> Type 1 diabetes mellitus with Kimmelstiel-Wilson disease

E10.22 Type 1 diabetes mellitus with diabetic chronic kidney disease `HCC`
> Use additional code to identify stage of chronic kidney disease (N18.1-N18.6)

E10.29 Type 1 diabetes mellitus with other diabetic kidney complication `HCC`
> Type 1 diabetes mellitus with renal tubular degeneration
> **AHA:** 2016, 1Q, 13

✓5ᵗʰ **E10.3** Type 1 diabetes mellitus with ophthalmic complications

> One of the following 7th characters is to be assigned to codes in subcategories E10.32, E10.33, E10.34, E10.35, and E10.37 to designate laterality of the disease:
> 1   right eye
> 2   left eye
> 3   bilateral
> 9   unspecified eye

✓6ᵗʰ **E10.31** Type 1 diabetes mellitus with unspecified diabetic retinopathy
> **DEF:** Diabetic retinopathy: Diabetic complication from damage to the retinal vessels resulting in vision problems that can progress to blindness.

E10.311 Type 1 diabetes mellitus with unspecified diabetic retinopathy with macular edema `HCC`

E10.319 Type 1 diabetes mellitus with unspecified diabetic retinopathy without macular edema `HCC`

| ✔ Additional Character Required | ✓x7ᵗʰ Placeholder | Unacceptable PDx | Questionable PDx | Manifestation | `H1`-`H14` HAC | `HCC` CMS-HCC Dx | `HIV` HIV Dx |

ICD-10-CM 2019   519

✓6ᵗʰ **E10.32 Type 1 diabetes mellitus with mild nonproliferative diabetic retinopathy**
Type 1 diabetes mellitus with nonproliferative diabetic retinopathy NOS

✓7ᵗʰ **E10.321 Type 1 diabetes mellitus with mild nonproliferative diabetic retinopathy with macular edema** HCC

✓7ᵗʰ **E10.329 Type 1 diabetes mellitus with mild nonproliferative diabetic retinopathy without macular edema** HCC

✓6ᵗʰ **E10.33 Type 1 diabetes mellitus with moderate nonproliferative diabetic retinopathy**

✓7ᵗʰ **E10.331 Type 1 diabetes mellitus with moderate nonproliferative diabetic retinopathy with macular edema** HCC

✓7ᵗʰ **E10.339 Type 1 diabetes mellitus with moderate nonproliferative diabetic retinopathy without macular edema** HCC

✓6ᵗʰ **E10.34 Type 1 diabetes mellitus with severe nonproliferative diabetic retinopathy**

✓7ᵗʰ **E10.341 Type 1 diabetes mellitus with severe nonproliferative diabetic retinopathy with macular edema** HCC

✓7ᵗʰ **E10.349 Type 1 diabetes mellitus with severe nonproliferative diabetic retinopathy without macular edema** HCC

✓6ᵗʰ **E10.35 Type 1 diabetes mellitus with proliferative diabetic retinopathy**

✓7ᵗʰ **E10.351 Type 1 diabetes mellitus with proliferative diabetic retinopathy with macular edema** HCC

✓7ᵗʰ **E10.352 Type 1 diabetes mellitus with proliferative diabetic retinopathy with traction retinal detachment involving the macula** HCC

✓7ᵗʰ **E10.353 Type 1 diabetes mellitus with proliferative diabetic retinopathy with traction retinal detachment not involving the macula** HCC

✓7ᵗʰ **E10.354 Type 1 diabetes mellitus with proliferative diabetic retinopathy with combined traction retinal detachment and rhegmatogenous retinal detachment** HCC

✓7ᵗʰ **E10.355 Type 1 diabetes mellitus with stable proliferative diabetic retinopathy** HCC

✓7ᵗʰ **E10.359 Type 1 diabetes mellitus with proliferative diabetic retinopathy without macular edema** HCC

E10.36 Type 1 diabetes mellitus with diabetic cataract HCC
AHA: 2016, 4Q, 142

✓x7ᵗʰ **E10.37 Type 1 diabetes mellitus with diabetic macular edema, resolved following treatment** HCC

E10.39 Type 1 diabetes mellitus with other diabetic ophthalmic complication HCC
Use additional code to identify manifestation, such as: diabetic glaucoma (H40-H42)

✓5ᵗʰ **E10.4 Type 1 diabetes mellitus with neurological complications**

E10.40 Type 1 diabetes mellitus with diabetic neuropathy, unspecified HCC

E10.41 Type 1 diabetes mellitus with diabetic mononeuropathy HCC

E10.42 Type 1 diabetes mellitus with diabetic polyneuropathy HCC
Type 1 diabetes mellitus with diabetic neuralgia

E10.43 Type 1 diabetes mellitus with diabetic autonomic (poly)neuropathy HCC
Type 1 diabetes mellitus with diabetic gastroparesis
AHA: 2013, 4Q, 114

E10.44 Type 1 diabetes mellitus with diabetic amyotrophy HCC

E10.49 Type 1 diabetes mellitus with other diabetic neurological complication HCC

✓5ᵗʰ **E10.5 Type 1 diabetes mellitus with circulatory complications**

E10.51 Type 1 diabetes mellitus with diabetic peripheral angiopathy without gangrene HCC
AHA: 2018, 2Q, 7

E10.52 Type 1 diabetes mellitus with diabetic peripheral angiopathy with gangrene CC HCC
Type 1 diabetes mellitus with diabetic gangrene
AHA: 2018, 2Q, 7; 2017, 4Q, 102
CC Excl: PDX collection 519

E10.59 Type 1 diabetes mellitus with other circulatory complications HCC

✓5ᵗʰ **E10.6 Type 1 diabetes mellitus with other specified complications**

✓6ᵗʰ **E10.61 Type 1 diabetes mellitus with diabetic arthropathy**

E10.610 Type 1 diabetes mellitus with diabetic neuropathic arthropathy HCC
Type 1 diabetes mellitus with Charcôt's joints
DEF: Charcot's joint: Progressive neurologic arthropathy in which chronic degeneration of joints in the weight-bearing areas with peripheral hypertrophy occurs as a complication of a neuropathy disorder. Supporting structures relax from a loss of sensation resulting in chronic joint instability.

E10.618 Type 1 diabetes mellitus with other diabetic arthropathy HCC
AHA: 2018, 2Q, 6

✓6ᵗʰ **E10.62 Type 1 diabetes mellitus with skin complications**

E10.620 Type 1 diabetes mellitus with diabetic dermatitis HCC
Type 1 diabetes mellitus with diabetic necrobiosis lipoidica

E10.621 Type 1 diabetes mellitus with foot ulcer HCC
Use additional code to identify site of ulcer (L97.4-, L97.5-)

E10.622 Type 1 diabetes mellitus with other skin ulcer HCC
Use additional code to identify site of ulcer (L97.1-L97.9, L98.41-L98.49)
AHA: 2017, 4Q, 17

E10.628 Type 1 diabetes mellitus with other skin complications HCC
AHA: 2017, 4Q, 100-101

✓6ᵗʰ **E10.63 Type 1 diabetes mellitus with oral complications**

E10.630 Type 1 diabetes mellitus with periodontal disease HCC

E10.638 Type 1 diabetes mellitus with other oral complications HCC

✓6ᵗʰ **E10.64 Type 1 diabetes mellitus with hypoglycemia**

E10.641 Type 1 diabetes mellitus with hypoglycemia with coma MCC HCC

E10.649 Type 1 diabetes mellitus with hypoglycemia without coma HCC
AHA: 2016, 3Q, 42; 2016, 1Q, 13; 2015, 3Q, 21

E10.65 Type 1 diabetes mellitus with hyperglycemia HCC
AHA: 2013, 3Q, 20

E10.69 Type 1 diabetes mellitus with other specified complication HCC
Use additional code to identify complication
AHA: 2016, 4Q, 141; 2016, 1Q, 13

E10.8 Type 1 diabetes mellitus with unspecified complications HCC

E10.9 Type 1 diabetes mellitus without complications HCC

✓4ᵗʰ **E11 Type 2 diabetes mellitus**
INCLUDES diabetes (mellitus) due to insulin secretory defect
diabetes NOS
insulin resistant diabetes (mellitus)
Use additional code to identify control using:
insulin (Z79.4)
oral antidiabetic drugs (Z79.84)
oral hypoglycemic drugs (Z79.84)
EXCLUDES 1 diabetes mellitus due to underlying condition (E08.-)
drug or chemical induced diabetes mellitus (E09.-)
gestational diabetes (O24.4-)
neonatal diabetes mellitus (P70.2)
postpancreatectomy diabetes mellitus (E13.-)
postprocedural diabetes mellitus (E13.-)
secondary diabetes mellitus NEC (E13.-)
type 1 diabetes mellitus (E10.-)
AHA: 2016, 2Q, 10; 2016, 1Q, 11-13; 2013, 4Q, 114; 2013, 3Q, 20; 2013, 1Q, 26

CC Excl: For CC/MCC codes in category E11, unless otherwise noted: PDX collection 518

√5ᵗʰ **E11.0　Type 2 diabetes mellitus with** hyperosmolarity

> **DEF:** Diabetic hyperosmolarity: Extremely high levels of glucose in the blood without ketones.

E11.00　Type 2 diabetes mellitus with hyperosmolarity without nonketotic hyperglycemic-hyperosmolar coma (NKHHC)　`MCC` `H9` `HCC`

E11.01　Type 2 diabetes mellitus with hyperosmolarity with coma　`MCC` `H9` `HCC`

√5ᵗʰ **E11.1　Type 2 diabetes mellitus with** ketoacidosis

> **DEF:** Diabetic ketoacidosis: Potentially life-threatening complication due to a shortage of insulin in which the body switches to burning fatty acids and producing acidic ketone bodies.

E11.10　Type 2 diabetes mellitus with ketoacidosis without coma　`MCC` `HCC`

E11.11　Type 2 diabetes mellitus with ketoacidosis with coma　`MCC` `HCC`

√5ᵗʰ **E11.2　Type 2 diabetes mellitus with** kidney complications

E11.21　Type 2 diabetes mellitus with diabetic nephropathy

> Type 2 diabetes mellitus with intercapillary glomerulosclerosis
> Type 2 diabetes mellitus with intracapillary glomerulonephrosis
> Type 2 diabetes mellitus with Kimmelstiel-Wilson disease

E11.22　Type 2 diabetes mellitus with diabetic chronic kidney disease　`HCC`

> Use additional code to identify stage of chronic kidney disease (N18.1-N18.6)
> **AHA:** 2016, 1Q, 12

E11.29　Type 2 diabetes mellitus with other **diabetic kidney complication**　`HCC`

> Type 2 diabetes mellitus with renal tubular degeneration

√5ᵗʰ **E11.3　Type 2 diabetes mellitus with** ophthalmic complications

> One of the following 7th characters is to be assigned to codes in subcategories E11.32, E11.33, E11.34, E11.35, and E11.37 to designate laterality of the disease:
> 1　right eye
> 2　left eye
> 3　bilateral
> 9　unspecified eye

√6ᵗʰ **E11.31　Type 2 diabetes mellitus with** unspecified diabetic retinopathy

> **DEF:** Diabetic retinopathy: Diabetic complication from damage to the retinal vessels resulting in vision problems that can progress to blindness.

E11.311　Type 2 diabetes mellitus with unspecified diabetic retinopathy with macular edema　`HCC`

E11.319　Type 2 diabetes mellitus with unspecified diabetic retinopathy without macular edema　`HCC`

√6ᵗʰ **E11.32　Type 2 diabetes mellitus with** mild nonproliferative **diabetic** retinopathy

> Type 2 diabetes mellitus with nonproliferative diabetic retinopathy NOS

√7ᵗʰ **E11.321　Type 2 diabetes mellitus with mild nonproliferative diabetic retinopathy with macular edema**　`HCC`

√7ᵗʰ **E11.329　Type 2 diabetes mellitus with mild nonproliferative diabetic retinopathy** without macular edema　`HCC`

√6ᵗʰ **E11.33　Type 2 diabetes mellitus with** moderate nonproliferative **diabetic** retinopathy

√7ᵗʰ **E11.331　Type 2 diabetes mellitus with moderate nonproliferative diabetic retinopathy** with macular edema　`HCC`

√7ᵗʰ **E11.339　Type 2 diabetes mellitus with moderate nonproliferative diabetic retinopathy** without macular edema　`HCC`

√6ᵗʰ **E11.34　Type 2 diabetes mellitus with** severe nonproliferative **diabetic** retinopathy

√7ᵗʰ **E11.341　Type 2 diabetes mellitus with severe nonproliferative diabetic retinopathy** with macular edema　`HCC`

√7ᵗʰ **E11.349　Type 2 diabetes mellitus with severe nonproliferative diabetic retinopathy** without macular edema　`HCC`

√6ᵗʰ **E11.35　Type 2 diabetes mellitus with** proliferative diabetic retinopathy

√7ᵗʰ **E11.351　Type 2 diabetes mellitus with proliferative diabetic retinopathy with macular edema**　`HCC`

√7ᵗʰ **E11.352　Type 2 diabetes mellitus with proliferative diabetic retinopathy with traction retinal detachment involving the macula**　`HCC`

√7ᵗʰ **E11.353　Type 2 diabetes mellitus with proliferative diabetic retinopathy** with traction retinal detachment not involving the macula　`HCC`

√7ᵗʰ **E11.354　Type 2 diabetes mellitus with proliferative diabetic retinopathy with combined traction retinal detachment and rhegmatogenous retinal detachment**　`HCC`

√7ᵗʰ **E11.355　Type 2 diabetes mellitus** with stable proliferative diabetic retinopathy　`HCC`

√7ᵗʰ **E11.359　Type 2 diabetes mellitus with proliferative diabetic retinopathy** without macular edema　`HCC`

E11.36　Type 2 diabetes mellitus with diabetic cataract　`HCC`

> **AHA:** 2016, 4Q, 142

√x7ᵗʰ **E11.37　Type 2 diabetes mellitus with diabetic** macular edema, resolved following treatment　`HCC`

E11.39　Type 2 diabetes mellitus with other **diabetic ophthalmic complication**　`HCC`

> Use additional code to identify manifestation, such as: diabetic glaucoma (H40-H42)

√5ᵗʰ **E11.4　Type 2 diabetes mellitus with** neurological complications

E11.40　Type 2 diabetes mellitus with diabetic neuropathy, unspecified　`HCC`

> **AHA:** 2013, 4Q, 129

E11.41　Type 2 diabetes mellitus with diabetic mononeuropathy　`HCC`

E11.42　Type 2 diabetes mellitus with diabetic polyneuropathy　`HCC`

> Type 2 diabetes mellitus with diabetic neuralgia
> **AHA:** 2016, 1Q, 12

E11.43　Type 2 diabetes mellitus with diabetic autonomic (poly)neuropathy　`HCC`

> Type 2 diabetes mellitus with diabetic gastroparesis
> **AHA:** 2013, 4Q, 114

E11.44　Type 2 diabetes mellitus with diabetic amyotrophy　`HCC`

E11.49　Type 2 diabetes mellitus with other **diabetic neurological complication**　`HCC`

√5ᵗʰ **E11.5　Type 2 diabetes mellitus with** circulatory complications

E11.51　Type 2 diabetes mellitus with diabetic peripheral angiopathy without gangrene　`HCC`

> **AHA:** 2018, 2Q, 7

E11.52　Type 2 diabetes mellitus with diabetic peripheral angiopathy with gangrene　`CC` `HCC`

> Type 2 diabetes mellitus with diabetic gangrene
> **AHA:** 2018, 2Q, 7; 2017, 4Q, 102
> **CC Excl:** PDX collection 519

E11.59　Type 2 diabetes mellitus with other **circulatory complications**　`HCC`

√5ᵗʰ **E11.6　Type 2 diabetes mellitus with** other specified complications

√6ᵗʰ **E11.61　Type 2 diabetes mellitus with** diabetic arthropathy

E11.610　Type 2 diabetes mellitus with diabetic neuropathic arthropathy　`HCC`

> Type 2 diabetes mellitus with Charcôt's joints
>
> **DEF:** Charcot's joint: Progressive neurologic arthropathy in which chronic degeneration of joints in the weight-bearing areas with peripheral hypertrophy occurs as a complication of a neuropathy disorder. Supporting structures relax from a loss of sensation resulting in chronic joint instability.

E11.618　Type 2 diabetes mellitus with other **diabetic arthropathy**　`HCC`

> **AHA:** 2018, 2Q, 6

Chapter 4. Endocrine, Nutritional and Metabolic Diseases

E11.62–E13.354

✓6ᵗʰ **E11.62   Type 2 diabetes mellitus with** skin complications

     E11.620   Type 2 diabetes mellitus with diabetic HCC
         dermatitis

         Type 2 diabetes mellitus with diabetic
         necrobiosis lipoidica

     E11.621   Type 2 diabetes mellitus with foot HCC
         ulcer

         Use additional code to identify site of ulcer
         (L97.4-, L97.5-)

         AHA: 2016, 1Q, 12

     E11.622   Type 2 diabetes mellitus with other HCC
         skin ulcer

         Use additional code to identify site of ulcer
         (L97.1-L97.9, L98.41-L98.49)

         AHA: 2017, 4Q, 17

     E11.628   Type 2 diabetes mellitus with other HCC
         skin complications

         AHA: 2017, 4Q, 100-101

✓6ᵗʰ **E11.63   Type 2 diabetes mellitus with** oral complications

     E11.630   Type 2 diabetes mellitus with HCC
         periodontal disease

     E11.638   Type 2 diabetes mellitus with other HCC
         oral complications

✓6ᵗʰ **E11.64   Type 2 diabetes mellitus with** hypoglycemia

     E11.641   Type 2 diabetes mellitus with MCC HCC
         hypoglycemia with coma

     E11.649   Type 2 diabetes mellitus with HCC
         hypoglycemia without coma

         AHA: 2016, 3Q, 42; 2015, 3Q, 21

     E11.65   Type 2 diabetes mellitus with hyperglycemia HCC

         AHA: 2013, 3Q, 20

     E11.69   Type 2 diabetes mellitus with other **specified** HCC
         complication

         Use additional code to identify complication

         AHA: 2016, 4Q, 141; 2016, 1Q, 13

   E11.8   Type 2 diabetes mellitus with unspecified complications HCC

   E11.9   Type 2 diabetes mellitus without complications HCC

✓4ᵗʰ **E13   Other specified diabetes mellitus**

   INCLUDES   diabetes mellitus due to genetic defects of beta-cell function
         diabetes mellitus due to genetic defects in insulin action
         postpancreatectomy diabetes mellitus
         postprocedural diabetes mellitus
         secondary diabetes mellitus NEC

   Use additional code to identify control using:
     insulin (Z79.4)
     oral antidiabetic drugs (Z79.84)
     oral hypoglycemic drugs (Z79.84)

   EXCLUDES 1   *diabetes (mellitus) due to autoimmune process (E10.-)*
         diabetes (mellitus) due to immune mediated pancreatic islet
         beta-cell destruction (E10.-)
         diabetes mellitus due to underlying condition (E08.-)
         drug or chemical induced diabetes mellitus (E09.-)
         gestational diabetes (O24.4-)
         neonatal diabetes mellitus (P70.2)
         type 1 diabetes mellitus (E10.-)

   AHA: 2016, 1Q, 11-13; 2013, 4Q, 114; 2013, 3Q, 20

   TIP: When postprocedural or postpancreatectomy hypoinsulinemia
   (E89.1) is documented with postprocedural or postpancreatectomy
   diabetes mellitus (E13.-), code E89.1 should be sequenced first.

   **CC Excl: For CC/MCC codes in category E13, unless otherwise
   noted:** PDX collection 518

✓5ᵗʰ **E13.0   Other specified diabetes mellitus with** hyperosmolarity

     DEF: Diabetic hyperosmolarity: Extremely high levels of glucose in
     the blood without ketones.

     E13.00   Other specified diabetes mellitus with MCC H9 HCC
         hyperosmolarity without nonketotic
         hyperglycemic-hyperosmolar coma (NKHHC)

         EXCLUDES 2   *type 2 diabetes mellitus (E11.-)*

     E13.01   Other specified diabetes mellitus with MCC H9 HCC
         hyperosmolarity with coma

✓5ᵗʰ **E13.1   Other specified diabetes mellitus with** ketoacidosis

     AHA: 2016, 2Q, 10; 2013, 1Q, 26

     DEF: Diabetic ketoacidosis: Potentially life-threatening
     complication due to a shortage of insulin in which the body
     switches to burning fatty acids and producing acidic ketone
     bodies.

     E13.10   Other specified diabetes mellitus with MCC H9 HCC
         ketoacidosis without coma

     E13.11   Other specified diabetes mellitus with MCC HCC
         ketoacidosis with coma

✓5ᵗʰ **E13.2   Other specified diabetes mellitus with** kidney complications

   E13.21   Other specified diabetes mellitus with diabetic HCC
         nephropathy

         Other specified diabetes mellitus with intercapillary
         glomerulosclerosis

         Other specified diabetes mellitus with intracapillary
         glomerulonephrosis

         Other specified diabetes mellitus with Kimmelstiel-
         Wilson disease

   E13.22   Other specified diabetes mellitus with diabetic HCC
         chronic kidney disease

         Use additional code to identify stage of chronic kidney
         disease (N18.1-N18.6)

   E13.29   Other specified diabetes mellitus with other HCC
         diabetic kidney complication

         Other specified diabetes mellitus with renal tubular
         degeneration

✓5ᵗʰ **E13.3   Other specified diabetes mellitus with** ophthalmic complications

   One of the following 7th characters is to be assigned to codes
   in subcategories E13.32, E13.33, E13.34, E13.35, and E13.37 to
   designate laterality of the disease:
   1   right eye
   2   left eye
   3   bilateral
   9   unspecified eye

✓6ᵗʰ **E13.31   Other specified diabetes mellitus with** unspecified
         diabetic retinopathy

         DEF: Diabetic retinopathy: Diabetic complication from
         damage to the retinal vessels resulting in vision
         problems that can progress to blindness.

     E13.311   Other specified diabetes mellitus with HCC
         unspecified diabetic retinopathy with
         macular edema

     E13.319   Other specified diabetes mellitus with HCC
         unspecified diabetic retinopathy
         without macular edema

✓6ᵗʰ **E13.32   Other specified diabetes mellitus with** mild
         nonproliferative diabetic retinopathy

         Other specified diabetes mellitus with nonproliferative
         diabetic retinopathy NOS

     ✓7ᵗʰ **E13.321   Other specified diabetes mellitus with** HCC
         **mild nonproliferative diabetic
         retinopathy** with macular edema

     ✓7ᵗʰ **E13.329   Other specified diabetes mellitus with** HCC
         **mild nonproliferative diabetic
         retinopathy** without macular edema

✓6ᵗʰ **E13.33   Other specified diabetes mellitus with** moderate
         nonproliferative diabetic retinopathy

     ✓7ᵗʰ **E13.331   Other specified diabetes mellitus with** HCC
         **moderate nonproliferative diabetic
         retinopathy** with macular edema

     ✓7ᵗʰ **E13.339   Other specified diabetes mellitus with** HCC
         **moderate nonproliferative diabetic
         retinopathy** without macular edema

✓6ᵗʰ **E13.34   Other specified diabetes mellitus with** severe
         nonproliferative diabetic retinopathy

     ✓7ᵗʰ **E13.341   Other specified diabetes mellitus with** HCC
         **severe nonproliferative diabetic
         retinopathy** with macular edema

     ✓7ᵗʰ **E13.349   Other specified diabetes mellitus with** HCC
         **severe nonproliferative diabetic
         retinopathy** without macular edema

✓6ᵗʰ **E13.35   Other specified diabetes mellitus with** proliferative
         diabetic retinopathy

     ✓7ᵗʰ **E13.351   Other specified diabetes mellitus with** HCC
         proliferative diabetic retinopathy with
         macular edema

     ✓7ᵗʰ **E13.352   Other specified diabetes mellitus with** HCC
         proliferative diabetic retinopathy with
         **traction retinal detachment involving the
         macula**

     ✓7ᵗʰ **E13.353   Other specified diabetes mellitus with** HCC
         proliferative diabetic retinopathy with
         **traction retinal detachment not involving
         the macula**

     ✓7ᵗʰ **E13.354   Other specified diabetes mellitus with** HCC
         proliferative diabetic retinopathy with
         **combined traction retinal detachment and
         rhegmatogenous retinal detachment**

N Newborn: 0   P Pediatric: 0-17   M Maternity: 12-55   A Adult: 15-124   MCC Major Complication/Comorbidity   CC Complication/Comorbidity   SW Severe Wound Dx

522   ICD-10-CM 2019

☑7ᵗʰ **E13.355 Other specified diabetes mellitus with** HCC **stable proliferative diabetic retinopathy**

☑7ᵗʰ **E13.359 Other specified diabetes mellitus with** HCC **proliferative diabetic retinopathy** without **macular edema**

E13.36 Other specified diabetes mellitus with diabetic HCC **cataract**
AHA: 2016, 4Q, 142

☑x7ᵗʰ **E13.37 Other specified diabetes mellitus with diabetic** HCC **macular edema, resolved following treatment**

E13.39 Other specified diabetes mellitus with other HCC **diabetic ophthalmic complication**
Use additional code to identify manifestation, such as: diabetic glaucoma (H40-H42)

☑5ᵗʰ **E13.4 Other specified diabetes mellitus with** neurological **complications**

E13.40 Other specified diabetes mellitus with diabetic HCC **neuropathy, unspecified**

E13.41 Other specified diabetes mellitus with diabetic HCC **mononeuropathy**

E13.42 Other specified diabetes mellitus with diabetic HCC **polyneuropathy**
Other specified diabetes mellitus with diabetic neuralgia

E13.43 Other specified diabetes mellitus with diabetic HCC **autonomic (poly)neuropathy**
Other specified diabetes mellitus with diabetic gastroparesis
AHA: 2013, 4Q, 114

E13.44 Other specified diabetes mellitus with diabetic HCC **amyotrophy**

E13.49 Other specified diabetes mellitus with other HCC **diabetic neurological complication**

☑5ᵗʰ **E13.5 Other specified diabetes mellitus with** circulatory **complications**

E13.51 Other specified diabetes mellitus with diabetic HCC **peripheral angiopathy without gangrene**
AHA: 2018, 2Q, 7

E13.52 Other specified diabetes mellitus with CC HCC **diabetic peripheral angiopathy with gangrene**
Other specified diabetes mellitus with diabetic gangrene
AHA: 2018, 2Q, 7; 2017, 4Q, 102
CC Excl: PDX collection 519

E13.59 Other specified diabetes mellitus with other HCC **circulatory complications**

☑5ᵗʰ **E13.6 Other specified diabetes mellitus with** other specified **complications**

☑6ᵗʰ **E13.61 Other specified diabetes mellitus with diabetic** **arthropathy**

E13.610 Other specified diabetes mellitus with HCC **diabetic** neuropathic **arthropathy**
Other specified diabetes mellitus with Charcôt's joints
DEF: Charcôt's joint: Progressive neurologic arthropathy in which chronic degeneration of joints in the weight-bearing areas with peripheral hypertrophy occurs as a complication of a neuropathy disorder. Supporting structures relax from a loss of sensation resulting in chronic joint instability.

E13.618 Other specified diabetes mellitus with HCC **other diabetic arthropathy**
AHA: 2018, 2Q, 6

☑6ᵗʰ **E13.62 Other specified diabetes mellitus with** skin **complications**

E13.620 Other specified diabetes mellitus with HCC **diabetic** dermatitis
Other specified diabetes mellitus with diabetic necrobiosis lipoidica

E13.621 Other specified diabetes mellitus with HCC **foot ulcer**
Use additional code to identify site of ulcer (L97.4-, L97.5-)

E13.622 Other specified diabetes mellitus with HCC **other skin ulcer**
Use additional code to identify site of ulcer (L97.1-L97.9, L98.41-L98.49)
AHA: 2017, 4Q, 17

E13.628 Other specified diabetes mellitus with HCC **other skin complications**
AHA: 2017, 4Q, 100-101

☑6ᵗʰ **E13.63 Other specified diabetes mellitus with** oral **complications**

E13.630 Other specified diabetes mellitus with HCC **periodontal disease**

E13.638 Other specified diabetes mellitus with HCC **other oral complications**

☑6ᵗʰ **E13.64 Other specified diabetes mellitus with** **hypoglycemia**

E13.641 Other specified diabetes mellitus MCC HCC **with hypoglycemia** with **coma**

E13.649 Other specified diabetes mellitus with HCC **hypoglycemia** without **coma**
AHA: 2016, 3Q, 42; 2015, 3Q, 21

E13.65 Other specified diabetes mellitus with HCC **hyperglycemia**

E13.69 Other specified diabetes mellitus with other HCC **specified complication**
Use additional code to identify complication
AHA: 2016, 4Q, 141; 2016, 1Q, 13

E13.8 Other specified diabetes mellitus with unspecified HCC **complications**

E13.9 Other specified diabetes mellitus without complications HCC

Other disorders of glucose regulation and pancreatic internal secretion (E15-E16)

E15 Nondiabetic hypoglycemic coma CC H9 HCC
INCLUDES drug-induced insulin coma in nondiabetic
hyperinsulinism with hypoglycemic coma
hypoglycemic coma NOS
CC Excl: PDX collection 520

☑4ᵗʰ **E16 Other disorders of pancreatic internal secretion**

E16.0 Drug-induced hypoglycemia without coma
Use additional code for adverse effect, if applicable, to identify drug (T36-T50 with fifth or sixth character 5)
EXCLUDES 1 diabetes with hypoglycemia without coma (E09.649)

E16.1 Other hypoglycemia
Functional hyperinsulinism
Functional nonhyperinsulinemic hypoglycemia
Hyperinsulinism NOS
Hyperplasia of pancreatic islet beta cells NOS
EXCLUDES 1 diabetes with hypoglycemia (E08.649, E10.649, E11.649, E13.649)
hypoglycemia in infant of diabetic mother (P70.1)
neonatal hypoglycemia (P70.4)

E16.2 Hypoglycemia, unspecified
EXCLUDES 1 diabetes with hypoglycemia (E08.649, E10.649, E11.649, E13.649)
AHA: 2016, 3Q, 42
TIP: Assign for nondiabetic hypoglycemic encephalopathy not further clarified in the documentation.

E16.3 Increased secretion of glucagon
Hyperplasia of pancreatic endocrine cells with glucagon excess

E16.4 Increased secretion of gastrin
Hypergastrinemia
Hyperplasia of pancreatic endocrine cells with gastrin excess
Zollinger-Ellison syndrome

E16.8 Other specified disorders of pancreatic internal secretion
Increased secretion from endocrine pancreas of growth hormone-releasing hormone
Increased secretion from endocrine pancreas of pancreatic polypeptide
Increased secretion from endocrine pancreas of somatostatin
Increased secretion from endocrine pancreas of vasoactive-intestinal polypeptide

E16.9 Disorder of pancreatic internal secretion, unspecified
Islet-cell hyperplasia NOS
Pancreatic endocrine cell hyperplasia NOS

Disorders of other endocrine glands (E20-E35)

EXCLUDES 1   galactorrhea (N64.3)
        gynecomastia (N62)

✓4ᵗʰ E20   Hypoparathyroidism

EXCLUDES 1   Di George's syndrome (D82.1)
        postprocedural hypoparathyroidism (E89.2)
        tetany NOS (R29.0)
        transitory neonatal hypoparathyroidism (P71.4)

E20.0   **Idiopathic** hypoparathyroidism   HCC
     DEF: Abnormally low secretion of parathyroid hormones, with unknown cause, which causes decreased calcium and increased phosphorus in the blood, resulting in muscle cramps, tetany, tingling, or burning in the lips, fingers, and toes, and cataracts.

E20.1   **Pseudohypoparathyroidism**

E20.8   **Other** hypoparathyroidism   HCC

E20.9   **Hypoparathyroidism, unspecified**   HCC
     Parathyroid tetany

✓4ᵗʰ E21   Hyperparathyroidism and other disorders of parathyroid gland

EXCLUDES 1   adult osteomalacia (M83.-)
        ectopic hyperparathyroidism (E34.2)
        familial hypocalciuric hypercalcemia (E83.52)
        hungry bone syndrome (E83.81)
        infantile and juvenile osteomalacia (E55.0)

E21.0   **Primary** hyperparathyroidism   HCC
     Hyperplasia of parathyroid
     Osteitis fibrosa cystica generalisata [von Recklinghausen's disease of bone]
     DEF: Parathyroid dysfunction commonly caused by hyperplasia of two or more glands. Symptoms include hypercalcemia and increased parathyroid hormone levels.

E21.1   **Secondary** hyperparathyroidism, not elsewhere classified   HCC
     EXCLUDES 1   secondary hyperparathyroidism of renal origin (N25.81)

E21.2   **Other** hyperparathyroidism   HCC
     Tertiary hyperparathyroidism
     EXCLUDES 1   familial hypocalciuric hypercalcemia (E83.52)

E21.3   **Hyperparathyroidism, unspecified**   HCC

E21.4   **Other** specified disorders of parathyroid gland   HCC

E21.5   **Disorder of parathyroid gland, unspecified**   HCC

✓4ᵗʰ E22   Hyperfunction of pituitary gland

EXCLUDES 1   Cushing's syndrome (E24.-)
        Nelson's syndrome (E24.1)
        overproduction of ACTH not associated with Cushing's disease (E27.0)
        overproduction of pituitary ACTH (E24.0)
        overproduction of thyroid-stimulating hormone (E05.8-)

CC Excl: For CC codes in category E22, unless otherwise noted: PDX collection 521

E22.0   **Acromegaly and pituitary gigantism**   HCC
     Overproduction of growth hormone
     EXCLUDES 1   constitutional gigantism (E34.4)
           constitutional tall stature (E34.4)
           increased secretion from endocrine pancreas of growth hormone-releasing hormone (E16.8)
     DEF: Acromegaly: Chronic condition caused by overproduction of the pituitary growth hormone resulting in enlarged skeletal parts and facial features.

E22.1   **Hyperprolactinemia**   CC HCC
     Use additional code for adverse effect, if applicable, to identify drug (T36-T50 with fifth or sixth character 5)

E22.2   **Syndrome of inappropriate secretion of antidiuretic hormone**   CC HCC
     CC Excl: PDX collection 522

E22.8   **Other hyperfunction of pituitary gland**   CC HCC
     Central precocious puberty

E22.9   **Hyperfunction of pituitary gland, unspecified**   CC HCC

✓4ᵗʰ E23   Hypofunction and other disorders of the pituitary gland

INCLUDES   the listed conditions whether the disorder is in the pituitary or the hypothalamus

EXCLUDES 1   postprocedural hypopituitarism (E89.3)

E23.0   **Hypopituitarism**   CC HCC
     Fertile eunuch syndrome
     Hypogonadotropic hypogonadism
     Idiopathic growth hormone deficiency
     Isolated deficiency of gonadotropin
     Isolated deficiency of growth hormone
     Isolated deficiency of pituitary hormone
     Kallmann's syndrome
     Lorain-Levi short stature
     Necrosis of pituitary gland (postpartum)
     Panhypopituitarism
     Pituitary cachexia
     Pituitary insufficiency NOS
     Pituitary short stature
     Sheehan's syndrome
     Simmonds' disease
     CC Excl: PDX collection 523

E23.1   **Drug-induced hypopituitarism**   HCC
     Use additional code for adverse effect, if applicable, to identify drug (T36-T50 with fifth or sixth character 5)

E23.2   **Diabetes insipidus**   CC HCC
     EXCLUDES 1   nephrogenic diabetes insipidus (N25.1)
     CC Excl: PDX collection 524

E23.3   **Hypothalamic dysfunction, not elsewhere classified**   HCC
     EXCLUDES 1   Prader-Willi syndrome (Q87.1)
           Russell-Silver syndrome (Q87.1)

E23.6   **Other disorders of pituitary gland**   HCC
     Abscess of pituitary
     Adiposogenital dystrophy

E23.7   **Disorder of pituitary gland, unspecified**   HCC

✓4ᵗʰ E24   Cushing's syndrome

EXCLUDES 1   congenital adrenal hyperplasia (E25.0)

DEF: Abdominal striae, acne, hypertension, decreased carbohydrate tolerance, moon face, obesity, protein catabolism, and psychiatric disturbances resulting from increased adrenocortical secretion of cortisol caused by ACTH-dependent adrenocortical hyperplasia or tumor, or by steroid effects.

CC Excl: For CC codes in category E24: PDX collection 525

E24.0   **Pituitary-dependent Cushing's disease**   CC HCC
     Overproduction of pituitary ACTH
     Pituitary-dependent hypercorticalism

E24.1   **Nelson's syndrome**   HCC

E24.2   **Drug-induced Cushing's syndrome**   CC HCC
     Use additional code for adverse effect, if applicable, to identify drug (T36-T50 with fifth or sixth character 5)

E24.3   **Ectopic ACTH syndrome**   CC HCC

E24.4   **Alcohol-induced pseudo-Cushing's syndrome**   CC HCC

E24.8   **Other Cushing's syndrome**   CC HCC

E24.9   **Cushing's syndrome, unspecified**   CC HCC

✓4ᵗʰ E25   Adrenogenital disorders

INCLUDES   adrenogenital syndromes, virilizing or feminizing, whether acquired or due to adrenal hyperplasia consequent on inborn enzyme defects in hormone synthesis
        female adrenal pseudohermaphroditism
        female heterosexual precocious pseudopuberty
        male isosexual precocious pseudopuberty
        male macrogenitosomia praecox
        male sexual precocity with adrenal hyperplasia
        male virilization (female)

EXCLUDES 1   indeterminate sex and pseudohermaphroditism (Q56)
        chromosomal abnormalities (Q90-Q99)

E25.0   **Congenital adrenogenital disorders associated with enzyme deficiency**   HCC
     Congenital adrenal hyperplasia
     21-Hydroxylase deficiency
     Salt-losing congenital adrenal hyperplasia

E25.8   **Other adrenogenital disorders**   HCC
     Idiopathic adrenogenital disorder
     Use additional code for adverse effect, if applicable, to identify drug (T36-T50 with fifth or sixth character 5)

E25.9   **Adrenogenital disorder, unspecified**   HCC
     Adrenogenital syndrome NOS

N Newborn: 0   P Pediatric: 0-17   M Maternity: 12-55   A Adult: 15-124   MCC Major Complication/Comorbidity   CC Complication/Comorbidity   SW Severe Wound Dx

524   ICD-10-CM 2019

✓4ᵗʰ **E26   Hyperaldosteronism**

✓5ᵗʰ **E26.0   Primary hyperaldosteronism**

    E26.01   Conn's syndrome   HCC
        Code also adrenal adenoma (D35.0-)

    E26.02   Glucocorticoid-remediable aldosteronism   HCC
        Familial aldosteronism type I
        DEF: Rare autosomal dominant familial form of primary aldosteronism in which the secretion of aldosterone is under the influence of adrenocorticotrophic hormone (ACTH) rather than the renin-angiotensin mechanism. Moderate hypersecretion of aldosterone and suppressed plasma renin activity that are rapidly reversed by administration of glucosteroids. Symptoms include hypertension and mild hypokalemia.

    E26.09   Other primary hyperaldosteronism   HCC
        Primary aldosteronism due to adrenal hyperplasia (bilateral)

  E26.1   Secondary hyperaldosteronism   HCC

✓5ᵗʰ **E26.8   Other hyperaldosteronism**

    E26.81   Bartter's syndrome   HCC

    E26.89   Other hyperaldosteronism   HCC

  E26.9   Hyperaldosteronism, unspecified   HCC
    Aldosteronism NOS
    Hyperaldosteronism NOS

✓4ᵗʰ **E27   Other disorders of adrenal gland**

  CC Excl: For CC codes in category E27: PDX collection 526

  E27.0   Other adrenocortical overactivity   CC HCC
    Overproduction of ACTH, not associated with Cushing's disease
    Premature adrenarche
    EXCLUDES 1   *Cushing's syndrome (E24.-)*

  E27.1   Primary adrenocortical insufficiency   CC HCC
    Addison's disease
    Autoimmune adrenalitis
    EXCLUDES 1   *Addison only phenotype adrenoleukodystrophy (E71.528)*
        amyloidosis (E85.-)
        tuberculous Addison's disease (A18.7)
        Waterhouse-Friderichsen syndrome (A39.1)

  E27.2   Addisonian crisis   CC HCC
    Adrenal crisis
    Adrenocortical crisis
    DEF: Life-threatening condition that occurs when there is not enough cortisol excreted from the adrenal glands. This condition may be due to injury to the adrenal glands or to the pituitary gland, which controls adrenal hormone secretion, or when a patient stops hydrocortisone treatment too quickly or too early.

  E27.3   Drug-induced adrenocortical insufficiency   CC HCC
    Use additional code for adverse effect, if applicable, to identify drug (T36-T50 with fifth or sixth character 5)

✓5ᵗʰ **E27.4   Other and unspecified adrenocortical insufficiency**
    EXCLUDES 1   *adrenoleukodystrophy [Addison-Schilder] (E71.528)*
        Waterhouse-Friderichsen syndrome (A39.1)

    E27.40   Unspecified adrenocortical insufficiency   CC HCC
        Adrenocortical insufficiency NOS
        Hypoaldosteronism

    E27.49   Other adrenocortical insufficiency   CC HCC
        Adrenal hemorrhage
        Adrenal infarction

  E27.5   Adrenomedullary hyperfunction   CC HCC
    Adrenomedullary hyperplasia
    Catecholamine hypersecretion

  E27.8   Other specified disorders of adrenal gland   HCC
    Abnormality of cortisol-binding globulin

  E27.9   Disorder of adrenal gland, unspecified   HCC

✓4ᵗʰ **E28   Ovarian dysfunction**
  EXCLUDES 1   *isolated gonadotropin deficiency (E23.0)*
      postprocedural ovarian failure (E89.4-)

  E28.0   Estrogen excess   ♀
    Use additional code for adverse effect, if applicable, to identify drug (T36-T50 with fifth or sixth character 5)

  E28.1   Androgen excess   ♀
    Hypersecretion of ovarian androgens
    Use additional code for adverse effect, if applicable, to identify drug (T36-T50 with fifth or sixth character 5)

  E28.2   Polycystic ovarian syndrome   ♀
    Sclerocystic ovary syndrome
    Stein-Leventhal syndrome
    DEF: Common hormonal disorder among women of reproductive age that involves enlarged ovaries with numerous small cysts located along the outer ovarian edge.

✓5ᵗʰ **E28.3   Primary ovarian failure**
    EXCLUDES 1   *pure gonadal dysgenesis (Q99.1)*
        Turner's syndrome (Q96.-)

  ✓6ᵗʰ **E28.31   Premature menopause**

    E28.310   Symptomatic premature menopause   A ♀
        Symptoms such as flushing, sleeplessness, headache, lack of concentration, associated with premature menopause

    E28.319   Asymptomatic premature menopause   A ♀
        Premature menopause NOS

    E28.39   Other primary ovarian failure   ♀
        Decreased estrogen
        Resistant ovary syndrome

  E28.8   Other ovarian dysfunction   ♀
    Ovarian hyperfunction NOS
    EXCLUDES 1   *postprocedural ovarian failure (E89.4-)*

  E28.9   Ovarian dysfunction, unspecified   ♀

✓4ᵗʰ **E29   Testicular dysfunction**
  EXCLUDES 1   *androgen insensitivity syndrome (E34.5-)*
      azoospermia or oligospermia NOS (N46.0-N46.1)
      isolated gonadotropin deficiency (E23.0)
      Klinefelter's syndrome (Q98.0-Q98.1, Q98.4)

  E29.0   Testicular hyperfunction   ♂
    Hypersecretion of testicular hormones

  E29.1   Testicular hypofunction   ♂
    Defective biosynthesis of testicular androgen NOS
    5-delta-Reductase deficiency (with male pseudohermaphroditism)
    Testicular hypogonadism NOS
    Use additional code for adverse effect, if applicable, to identify drug (T36-T50 with fifth or sixth character 5)
    EXCLUDES 1   *postprocedural testicular hypofunction (E89.5)*

  E29.8   Other testicular dysfunction   ♂

  E29.9   Testicular dysfunction, unspecified   ♂

✓4ᵗʰ **E30   Disorders of puberty, not elsewhere classified**

  E30.0   Delayed puberty
    Constitutional delay of puberty
    Delayed sexual development

  E30.1   Precocious puberty   P
    Precocious menstruation
    EXCLUDES 1   *Albright (-McCune) (-Sternberg) syndrome (Q78.1)*
        central precocious puberty (E22.8)
        congenital adrenal hyperplasia (E25.0)
        female heterosexual precocious pseudopuberty (E25.-)
        male isosexual precocious pseudopuberty (E25.-)

  E30.8   Other disorders of puberty   P
    Premature thelarche

  E30.9   Disorder of puberty, unspecified

✓4ᵗʰ **E31   Polyglandular dysfunction**
  EXCLUDES 1   *ataxia telangiectasia [Louis-Bar] (G11.3)*
      dystrophia myotonica [Steinert] (G71.11)
      pseudohypoparathyroidism (E20.1)

  E31.0   Autoimmune polyglandular failure   HCC
    Schmidt's syndrome

  E31.1   Polyglandular hyperfunction   HCC
    EXCLUDES 1   *multiple endocrine adenomatosis (E31.2-)*
        multiple endocrine neoplasia (E31.2-)

✓5ᵗʰ **E31.2   Multiple endocrine neoplasia [MEN] syndromes**
    Multiple endocrine adenomatosis
    Code also any associated malignancies and other conditions associated with the syndromes

    E31.20   Multiple endocrine neoplasia [MEN] syndrome, unspecified   HCC
        Multiple endocrine adenomatosis NOS
        Multiple endocrine neoplasia [MEN] syndrome NOS

    E31.21   Multiple endocrine neoplasia [MEN] type I   HCC
        Wermer's syndrome

    E31.22   Multiple endocrine neoplasia [MEN] type IIA   HCC
        Sipple's syndrome

    E31.23   Multiple endocrine neoplasia [MEN] type IIB   HCC

  E31.8   Other polyglandular dysfunction   HCC

✓ Additional Character Required   ✓7ᵗʰ Placeholder   Unacceptable PDx   Questionable PDx   Manifestation   H1-H14 HAC   HCC CMS-HCC Dx   HIV HIV Dx

E31.9   **Polyglandular dysfunction,** unspecified   `HCC`

☑4ᵗʰ **E32**   **Diseases of thymus**
     EXCLUDES 1   *aplasia or hypoplasia of thymus with immunodeficiency (D82.1)*
               myasthenia gravis (G70.0)

E32.0   **Persistent hyperplasia of thymus**   `HCC`
        Hypertrophy of thymus

E32.1   **Abscess of thymus**   `CC` `HCC`
        CC Excl: PDX collection 527

E32.8   **Other diseases of thymus**   `HCC`
     EXCLUDES 1   *aplasia or hypoplasia with immunodeficiency (D82.1)*
               thymoma (D15.0)

E32.9   **Disease of thymus,** unspecified   `HCC`

☑4ᵗʰ **E34**   **Other endocrine disorders**
     EXCLUDES 1   *pseudohypoparathyroidism (E20.1)*

E34.0   **Carcinoid syndrome**   `CC` `HCC`
        NOTE   May be used as an additional code to identify functional activity associated with a carcinoid tumor.
        CC Excl: PDX collection 528

E34.1   **Other hypersecretion of intestinal hormones**

E34.2   **Ectopic hormone secretion, not elsewhere classified**
     EXCLUDES 1   *ectopic ACTH syndrome (E24.3)*

E34.3   **Short stature due to endocrine disorder**
        Constitutional short stature
        Laron-type short stature
     EXCLUDES 1   *achondroplastic short stature (Q77.4)*
               hypochondroplastic short stature (Q77.4)
               nutritional short stature (E45)
               pituitary short stature (E23.0)
               progeria (E34.8)
               renal short stature (N25.0)
               Russell-Silver syndrome (Q87.1)
               short-limbed stature with immunodeficiency (D82.2)
               short stature in specific dysmorphic syndromes— code to syndrome—see Alphabetical Index
               short stature NOS (R62.52)

E34.4   **Constitutional tall stature**   `HCC`
        Constitutional gigantism

☑5ᵗʰ **E34.5**   **Androgen insensitivity syndrome**
        DEF: X-linked recessive condition in which individuals that are chromosomally male fail to develop normal male external genitalia due to an abnormality on the X chromosome that prohibits the body, completely or in part, from recognizing the androgens produced. *Synonym(s):* AIS.

        E34.50   **Androgen insensitivity syndrome,** unspecified
               Androgen insensitivity NOS

        E34.51   **Complete androgen insensitivity syndrome**
               Complete androgen insensitivity
               de Quervain syndrome
               Goldberg-Maxwell syndrome

        E34.52   **Partial androgen insensitivity syndrome**
               Partial androgen insensitivity
               Reifenstein syndrome

E34.8   **Other specified endocrine disorders**
        Pineal gland dysfunction
        Progeria
     EXCLUDES 2   *pseudohypoparathyroidism (E20.1)*

E34.9   **Endocrine disorder,** unspecified
        Endocrine disturbance NOS
        Hormone disturbance NOS

E35   *Disorders of endocrine glands in diseases classified elsewhere*
        Code first underlying disease, such as:
            late congenital syphilis of thymus gland [Dubois disease] (A50.5)
        Use additional code, if applicable, to identify:
            sequelae of tuberculosis of other organs (B90.8)
     EXCLUDES 1   *Echinococcus granulosus infection of thyroid gland (B67.3)*
               meningococcal hemorrhagic adrenalitis (A39.1)
               syphilis of endocrine gland (A52.79)
               tuberculosis of adrenal gland, except calcification (A18.7)
               tuberculosis of endocrine gland NEC (A18.82)
               tuberculosis of thyroid gland (A18.81)
               Waterhouse-Friderichsen syndrome (A39.1)

Intraoperative Complications of Endocrine System (E36)

☑4ᵗʰ **E36**   **Intraoperative complications of endocrine system**
     EXCLUDES 2   *postprocedural endocrine and metabolic complications and disorders, not elsewhere classified (E89.-)*

☑5ᵗʰ **E36.0**   **Intraoperative hemorrhage and hematoma** of an endocrine system organ or structure complicating a procedure
     EXCLUDES 1   *intraoperative hemorrhage and hematoma of an endocrine system organ or structure due to accidental puncture or laceration during a procedure (E36.1-)*

        E36.01   **Intraoperative hemorrhage and hematoma of an endocrine system organ or structure complicating an** endocrine system procedure   `CC`
               CC Excl: PDX collection 529

        E36.02   **Intraoperative hemorrhage and hematoma of an endocrine system organ or structure complicating** other procedure   `CC`
               CC Excl: PDX collection 529

☑5ᵗʰ **E36.1**   **Accidental puncture and laceration** of an endocrine system organ or structure during a procedure

        E36.11   **Accidental puncture and laceration of an endocrine system organ or structure during an** endocrine system procedure   `CC`
               CC Excl: PDX collection 509

        E36.12   **Accidental puncture and laceration of an endocrine system organ or structure during** other procedure   `CC`
               CC Excl: PDX collection 509

E36.8   **Other intraoperative complications of endocrine system**
        Use additional code, if applicable, to further specify disorder

Malnutrition (E40-E46)

     EXCLUDES 1   *intestinal malabsorption (K90.-)*
               sequelae of protein-calorie malnutrition (E64.0)
     EXCLUDES 2   *nutritional anemias (D50-D53)*
               starvation (T73.0)
     AHA: 2017, 4Q, 108; 2017, 3Q, 25
     TIP: Assign an additional code for BMI from category Z68, when documented. BMI can be based on documentation from clinicians who are not the patient's provider.

     CC Excl: For CC/MCC codes in categories E40-E46: PDX collection 530

E40   **Kwashiorkor**   `MCC` `HCC`
        Severe malnutrition with nutritional edema with dyspigmentation of skin and hair
     EXCLUDES 1   *marasmic kwashiorkor (E42)*

E41   **Nutritional marasmus**   `MCC` `HCC`
        Severe malnutrition with marasmus
     EXCLUDES 1   *marasmic kwashiorkor (E42)*
     AHA: 2017, 3Q, 24
     DEF: Protein-calorie malabsorption or malnutrition in children characterized by tissue wasting, dehydration, and subcutaneous fat depletion. It may occur with infectious disease.

E42   **Marasmic kwashiorkor**   `MCC` `HCC`
        Intermediate form severe protein-calorie malnutrition
        Severe protein-calorie malnutrition with signs of both kwashiorkor and marasmus

E43   **Unspecified severe protein-calorie malnutrition**   `MCC` `HCC`
        Starvation edema
     AHA: 2017, 4Q, 108

☑4ᵗʰ **E44**   **Protein-calorie malnutrition of moderate and mild degree**
        E44.0   **Moderate protein-calorie malnutrition**   `CC` `HCC`
        E44.1   **Mild protein-calorie malnutrition**   `CC` `HCC`

E45   **Retarded development following protein-calorie malnutrition**   `CC` `HCC`
        Nutritional short stature
        Nutritional stunting
        Physical retardation due to malnutrition

E46   **Unspecified protein-calorie malnutrition**   `CC` `HCC`
        Malnutrition NOS
        Protein-calorie imbalance NOS
     EXCLUDES 1   *nutritional deficiency NOS (E63.9)*

ℕ Newborn: 0   ℙ Pediatric: 0-17   Ⓜ Maternity: 12-55   Ⓐ Adult: 15-124   `MCC` Major Complication/Comorbidity   `CC` Complication/Comorbidity   `SW` Severe Wound Dx

526   ICD-10-CM 2019

Other nutritional deficiencies (E50-E64)

EXCLUDES 2 *nutritional anemias (D50-D53)*

✓4th E50   Vitamin A deficiency

EXCLUDES 1 *sequelae of vitamin A deficiency (E64.1)*

E50.0   Vitamin A deficiency with conjunctival xerosis

E50.1   Vitamin A deficiency with Bitot's spot and conjunctival xerosis

Bitot's spot in the young child

DEF: Vitamin A deficiency with conjunctival dryness and superficial spots of keratinized epithelium.

E50.2   Vitamin A deficiency with corneal xerosis

E50.3   Vitamin A deficiency with corneal ulceration and xerosis

E50.4   Vitamin A deficiency with keratomalacia

DEF: Vitamin A deficiency creating corneal dryness that progresses to corneal insensitivity, softness, and necrosis. It is usually bilateral.

E50.5   Vitamin A deficiency with night blindness

E50.6   Vitamin A deficiency with xerophthalmic scars of cornea

E50.7   Other ocular manifestations of vitamin A deficiency

Xerophthalmia NOS

E50.8   Other manifestations of vitamin A deficiency

Follicular keratosis
Xeroderma

E50.9   Vitamin A deficiency, unspecified

Hypovitaminosis A NOS

✓4th E51   Thiamine deficiency

EXCLUDES 1 *sequelae of thiamine deficiency (E64.8)*

CC Excl: For CC codes in category E51: PDX collection 531

✓5th E51.1   Beriberi

E51.11   Dry beriberi   CC

Beriberi NOS
Beriberi with polyneuropathy

E51.12   Wet beriberi   CC

Beriberi with cardiovascular manifestations
Cardiovascular beriberi
Shoshin disease

E51.2   Wernicke's encephalopathy   CC

DEF: Deficiency of vitamin B1 resulting in a triad of acute mental confusion, ataxia, and ophthalmoplegia. The vast majority of affected patients are alcoholics.

E51.8   Other manifestations of thiamine deficiency   CC

E51.9   Thiamine deficiency, unspecified   CC

E52   Niacin deficiency [pellagra]

Niacin (-tryptophan) deficiency
Nicotinamide deficiency
Pellagra (alcoholic)

EXCLUDES 1 *sequelae of niacin deficiency (E64.8)*

✓4th E53   Deficiency of other B group vitamins

EXCLUDES 1 *sequelae of vitamin B deficiency (E64.8)*

E53.0   Riboflavin deficiency   CC

Ariboflavinosis
Vitamin B2 deficiency

CC Excl: PDX collection 531

E53.1   Pyridoxine deficiency

Vitamin B6 deficiency

EXCLUDES 1 *pyridoxine-responsive sideroblastic anemia (D64.3)*

E53.8   Deficiency of other specified B group vitamins

Biotin deficiency
Cyanocobalamin deficiency
Folate deficiency
Folic acid deficiency
Pantothenic acid deficiency
Vitamin B12 deficiency

EXCLUDES 1 *folate deficiency anemia (D52.-)*
vitamin B12 deficiency anemia (D51.-)

E53.9   Vitamin B deficiency, unspecified

E54   Ascorbic acid deficiency

Deficiency of vitamin C
Scurvy

EXCLUDES 1 *scorbutic anemia (D53.2)*
sequelae of vitamin C deficiency (E64.2)

DEF: Vitamin C deficiency causing swollen gums, myalgia, weight loss, and weakness.

✓4th E55   Vitamin D deficiency

EXCLUDES 1 *adult osteomalacia (M83.-)*
osteoporosis (M80.-)
sequelae of rickets (E64.3)

E55.0   Rickets, active   CC

Infantile osteomalacia
Juvenile osteomalacia

EXCLUDES 1 *celiac rickets (K90.0)*
Crohn's rickets (K50.-)
hereditary vitamin D-dependent rickets (E83.32)
inactive rickets (E64.3)
renal rickets (N25.0)
sequelae of rickets (E64.3)
vitamin D-resistant rickets (E83.31)

DEF: Rickets: Softening or weakening of the bones due to a lack of vitamin D, calcium, and phosphate.

CC Excl: PDX collection 532

E55.9   Vitamin D deficiency, unspecified

Avitaminosis D

✓4th E56   Other vitamin deficiencies

EXCLUDES 1 *sequelae of other vitamin deficiencies (E64.8)*

E56.0   Deficiency of vitamin E

E56.1   Deficiency of vitamin K

EXCLUDES 1 *deficiency of coagulation factor due to vitamin K deficiency (D68.4)*
vitamin K deficiency of newborn (P53)

E56.8   Deficiency of other vitamins

E56.9   Vitamin deficiency, unspecified

E58   Dietary calcium deficiency

EXCLUDES 1 *disorders of calcium metabolism (E83.5-)*
sequelae of calcium deficiency (E64.8)

E59   Dietary selenium deficiency

Keshan disease

EXCLUDES 1 *sequelae of selenium deficiency (E64.8)*

E60   Dietary zinc deficiency

✓4th E61   Deficiency of other nutrient elements

Use additional code for adverse effect, if applicable, to identify drug (T36-T50 with fifth or sixth character 5)

EXCLUDES 1 *disorders of mineral metabolism (E83.-)*
iodine deficiency related thyroid disorders (E00-E02)
sequelae of malnutrition and other nutritional deficiencies (E64.-)

E61.0   Copper deficiency

E61.1   Iron deficiency

EXCLUDES 1 *iron deficiency anemia (D50.-)*

E61.2   Magnesium deficiency

E61.3   Manganese deficiency

E61.4   Chromium deficiency

E61.5   Molybdenum deficiency

E61.6   Vanadium deficiency

E61.7   Deficiency of multiple nutrient elements

E61.8   Deficiency of other specified nutrient elements

E61.9   Deficiency of nutrient element, unspecified

✓4th E63   Other nutritional deficiencies

EXCLUDES 1 *dehydration (E86.0)*
failure to thrive, adult (R62.7)
failure to thrive, child (R62.51)
feeding problems in newborn (P92.-)
sequelae of malnutrition and other nutritional deficiencies (E64.-)

E63.0   Essential fatty acid [EFA] deficiency

E63.1   Imbalance of constituents of food intake

E63.8   Other specified nutritional deficiencies

E63.9   Nutritional deficiency, unspecified

✔ Additional Character Required   ✔x7th Placeholder   Unacceptable PDx   Questionable PDx   Manifestation   H1 - H14 HAC   HCC CMS-HCC Dx   HIV HIV Dx

ICD-10-CM 2019   **527**

Chapter 4. Endocrine, Nutritional and Metabolic Diseases

☑4ᵗʰ **E64 Sequelae of malnutrition and other nutritional deficiencies**

> **NOTE** This category is to be used to indicate conditions in categories E43, E44, E46, E50-E63 as the cause of sequelae, which are themselves classified elsewhere. The 'sequelae' include conditions specified as such; they also include the late effects of diseases classifiable to the above categories if the disease itself is no longer present

Code first condition resulting from (sequela) of malnutrition and other nutritional deficiencies

E64.0 Sequelae of protein-calorie malnutrition CC HCC

> **EXCLUDES 2** retarded development following protein-calorie malnutrition (E45)

> **CC Excl:** PDX collection 530

E64.1 Sequelae of vitamin A deficiency

E64.2 Sequelae of vitamin C deficiency

E64.3 Sequelae of rickets

E64.8 Sequelae of other nutritional deficiencies

E64.9 Sequelae of unspecified nutritional deficiency

Overweight, obesity and other hyperalimentation (E65-E68)

E65 Localized adiposity
> Fat pad

☑4ᵗʰ **E66 Overweight and obesity**

> Code first obesity complicating pregnancy, childbirth and the puerperium, if applicable (O99.21-)
> Use additional code to identify body mass index (BMI), if known (Z68.-)
> **EXCLUDES 1** adiposogenital dystrophy (E23.6)
> lipomatosis NOS (E88.2)
> lipomatosis dolorosa [Dercum] (E88.2)
> Prader-Willi syndrome (Q87.1)

☑5ᵗʰ **E66.0 Obesity due to excess calories**

E66.01 Morbid (severe) obesity due to excess calories H11 HCC

> **EXCLUDES 1** morbid (severe) obesity with alveolar hypoventilation (E66.2)

E66.09 Other obesity due to excess calories

E66.1 Drug-induced obesity

> Use additional code for adverse effect, if applicable, to identify drug (T36-T50 with fifth or sixth character 5)

E66.2 Morbid (severe) obesity with alveolar hypoventilation CC HCC

> Obesity hypoventilation syndrome (OHS)
> Pickwickian syndrome
> **CC Excl:** PDX collection 533

E66.3 Overweight

E66.8 Other obesity

E66.9 Obesity, unspecified
> Obesity NOS

☑4ᵗʰ **E67 Other hyperalimentation**

> **EXCLUDES 1** hyperalimentation NOS (R63.2)
> sequelae of hyperalimentation (E68)

E67.0 Hypervitaminosis A

▲ **E67.1 Hypercarotenemia**

> **DEF:** Elevated blood carotene level as a result of excessive carotenoid ingestion or an inability to convert carotenoids to vitamin A. Characteristics often include yellow discoloration of the skin, which may follow overeating of carotenoid-rich foods such as carrots, sweet potatoes, or squash.

E67.2 Megavitamin-B6 syndrome

E67.3 Hypervitaminosis D

E67.8 Other specified hyperalimentation

E68 Sequelae of hyperalimentation

> Code first condition resulting from (sequela) of hyperalimentation

Metabolic disorders (E70-E88)

> **EXCLUDES 1** androgen insensitivity syndrome (E34.5-)
> congenital adrenal hyperplasia (E25.0)
> Ehlers-Danlos syndrome (Q79.6)
> hemolytic anemias attributable to enzyme disorders (D55.-)
> Marfan's syndrome (Q87.4)
> 5-alpha-reductase deficiency (E29.1)
> **AHA:** 2018, 2Q, 6

☑4ᵗʰ **E70 Disorders of aromatic amino-acid metabolism**

> **CC Excl: For CC codes in category E70:** PDX collection 534

E70.0 Classical phenylketonuria CC HCC

E70.1 Other hyperphenylalaninemias CC HCC

☑5ᵗʰ **E70.2 Disorders of tyrosine metabolism**

> **EXCLUDES 1** transitory tyrosinemia of newborn (P74.5)

E70.20 Disorder of tyrosine metabolism, unspecified CC HCC

E70.21 Tyrosinemia CC HCC
> Hypertyrosinemia

E70.29 Other disorders of tyrosine metabolism CC HCC
> Alkaptonuria
> Ochronosis

☑5ᵗʰ **E70.3 Albinism**

> **DEF:** Absence of pigment in skin, hair, and eyes. This genetic condition is often accompanied by astigmatism, photophobia, and nystagmus.

E70.30 Albinism, unspecified CC HCC

☑6ᵗʰ **E70.31 Ocular albinism**

E70.310 X-linked ocular albinism CC HCC

E70.311 Autosomal recessive ocular albinism CC HCC

E70.318 Other ocular albinism CC HCC

E70.319 Ocular albinism, unspecified CC HCC

☑6ᵗʰ **E70.32 Oculocutaneous albinism**

> **EXCLUDES 1** Chediak-Higashi syndrome (E70.330)
> Hermansky-Pudlak syndrome (E70.331)

E70.320 Tyrosinase negative oculocutaneous albinism CC HCC
> Albinism I
> Oculocutaneous albinism ty-neg

E70.321 Tyrosinase positive oculocutaneous albinism CC HCC
> Albinism II
> Oculocutaneous albinism ty-pos

E70.328 Other oculocutaneous albinism CC HCC
> Cross syndrome

E70.329 Oculocutaneous albinism, unspecified CC HCC

☑6ᵗʰ **E70.33 Albinism with hematologic abnormality**

E70.330 Chediak-Higashi syndrome CC HCC

E70.331 Hermansky-Pudlak syndrome CC HCC

E70.338 Other albinism with hematologic abnormality CC HCC

E70.339 Albinism with hematologic abnormality, unspecified CC HCC

E70.39 Other specified albinism CC HCC
> Piebaldism

☑5ᵗʰ **E70.4 Disorders of histidine metabolism**

E70.40 Disorders of histidine metabolism, unspecified CC HCC

E70.41 Histidinemia CC HCC

E70.49 Other disorders of histidine metabolism CC HCC

E70.5 Disorders of tryptophan metabolism CC HCC

E70.8 Other disorders of aromatic amino-acid metabolism CC HCC

E70.9 Disorder of aromatic amino-acid metabolism, unspecified CC HCC

☑4ᵗʰ **E71 Disorders of branched-chain amino-acid metabolism and fatty-acid metabolism**

E71.0 Maple-syrup-urine disease CC HCC
> **CC Excl:** PDX collection 534

☑5ᵗʰ **E71.1 Other disorders of branched-chain amino-acid metabolism**

> **CC Excl: For CC codes in subcategory E71.1:** PDX collection 534

☑6ᵗʰ **E71.11 Branched-chain organic acidurias**

E71.110 Isovaleric acidemia CC HCC

E71.111 3-methylglutaconic aciduria CC HCC

E71.118 Other branched-chain organic acidurias CC HCC

☑6ᵗʰ **E71.12 Disorders of propionate metabolism**

E71.120 Methylmalonic acidemia CC HCC

E71.121 Propionic acidemia CC HCC

E71.128 Other disorders of propionate metabolism CC HCC

E71.19 Other disorders of branched-chain amino-acid metabolism CC HCC
> Hyperleucine-isoleucinemia
> Hypervalinemia

☑ Newborn: 0   ☑ Pediatric: 0-17   ☑ Maternity: 12-55   ☑ Adult: 15-124   **MCC** Major Complication/Comorbidity   **CC** Complication/Comorbidity   **SW** Severe Wound Dx

528   ICD-10-CM 2019

E71.2 Disorder of branched-chain amino-acid metabolism, unspecified CC HCC
CC Excl: PDX collection 534

✓5th **E71.3 Disorders of fatty-acid metabolism**
EXCLUDES 1 peroxisomal disorders (E71.5)
Refsum's disease (G60.1)
Schilder's disease (G37.0)
EXCLUDES 2 carnitine deficiency due to inborn error of metabolism (E71.42)

CC Excl: For CC codes in subcategory E71.3, unless otherwise noted: PDX collection 535

E71.30 Disorder of fatty-acid metabolism, unspecified

✓6th **E71.31 Disorders of fatty-acid oxidation**
E71.310 Long chain/very long chain acyl CoA dehydrogenase deficiency CC HCC
LCAD
VLCAD
E71.311 Medium chain acyl CoA dehydrogenase deficiency CC HCC
MCAD
E71.312 Short chain acyl CoA dehydrogenase deficiency CC HCC
SCAD
E71.313 Glutaric aciduria type II CC HCC
Glutaric aciduria type II A
Glutaric aciduria type II B
Glutaric aciduria type II C
EXCLUDES 1 glutaric aciduria (type 1) NOS (E72.3)
E71.314 Muscle carnitine palmitoyltransferase deficiency CC HCC
E71.318 Other disorders of fatty-acid oxidation CC HCC

E71.32 Disorders of ketone metabolism CC HCC
E71.39 Other disorders of fatty-acid metabolism CC HCC
CC Excl: PDX collection 492

✓5th **E71.4 Disorders of carnitine metabolism**
EXCLUDES 1 muscle carnitine palmitoyltransferase deficiency (E71.314)

E71.40 Disorder of carnitine metabolism, unspecified HCC
E71.41 Primary carnitine deficiency HCC
E71.42 Carnitine deficiency due to inborn errors of metabolism HCC
Code also associated inborn error or metabolism
E71.43 Iatrogenic carnitine deficiency HCC
Carnitine deficiency due to hemodialysis
Carnitine deficiency due to Valproic acid therapy
✓6th **E71.44 Other secondary carnitine deficiency**
E71.440 Ruvalcaba-Myhre-Smith syndrome HCC
E71.448 Other secondary carnitine deficiency HCC

✓5th **E71.5 Peroxisomal disorders**
EXCLUDES 1 Schilder's disease (G37.0)

CC Excl: For CC codes in subcategory E71.5: PDX collection 536

E71.50 Peroxisomal disorder, unspecified CC HCC
✓6th **E71.51 Disorders of peroxisome biogenesis**
Group 1 peroxisomal disorders
EXCLUDES 1 Refsum's disease (G60.1)
E71.510 Zellweger syndrome CC HCC
E71.511 Neonatal adrenoleukodystrophy CC HCC
EXCLUDES 1 X-linked adrenoleukodystrophy (E71.52-)
E71.518 Other disorders of peroxisome biogenesis CC HCC

✓6th **E71.52 X-linked adrenoleukodystrophy**
E71.520 Childhood cerebral X-linked adrenoleukodystrophy CC HCC
E71.521 Adolescent X-linked adrenoleukodystrophy CC HCC
E71.522 Adrenomyeloneuropathy CC HCC
E71.528 Other X-linked adrenoleukodystrophy CC HCC
Addison only phenotype adrenoleukodystrophy
Addison-Schilder adrenoleukodystrophy
E71.529 X-linked adrenoleukodystrophy, unspecified type CC HCC

E71.53 Other group 2 peroxisomal disorders CC HCC
✓6th **E71.54 Other peroxisomal disorders**
E71.540 Rhizomelic chondrodysplasia punctata
EXCLUDES 1 chondrodysplasia punctata NOS (Q77.3)
E71.541 Zellweger-like syndrome CC HCC
E71.542 Other group 3 peroxisomal disorders CC HCC
E71.548 Other peroxisomal disorders CC HCC

✓4th **E72 Other disorders of amino-acid metabolism**
EXCLUDES 1 disorders of:
aromatic amino-acid metabolism (E70.-)
branched-chain amino-acid metabolism (E71.0-E71.2)
fatty-acid metabolism (E71.3)
purine and pyrimidine metabolism (E79.-)
gout (M1A.-, M10.-)

CC Excl: For CC codes in category E72, unless otherwise noted: PDX collection 534

✓5th **E72.0 Disorders of amino-acid transport**
EXCLUDES 1 disorders of tryptophan metabolism (E70.5)
E72.00 Disorders of amino-acid transport, unspecified CC HCC
E72.01 Cystinuria CC HCC
E72.02 Hartnup's disease CC HCC
E72.03 Lowe's syndrome CC HCC
Use additional code for associated glaucoma (H42)
CC Excl: No Excl
E72.04 Cystinosis CC HCC
Fanconi (-de Toni) (-Debré) syndrome with cystinosis
EXCLUDES 1 Fanconi (-de Toni) (-Debré) syndrome without cystinosis (E72.09)
E72.09 Other disorders of amino-acid transport CC HCC
Fanconi (-de Toni) (-Debré) syndrome, unspecified

✓5th **E72.1 Disorders of sulfur-bearing amino-acid metabolism**
EXCLUDES 1 cystinosis (E72.04)
cystinuria (E72.01)
transcobalamin II deficiency (D51.2)
E72.10 Disorders of sulfur-bearing amino-acid metabolism, unspecified CC HCC
E72.11 Homocystinuria CC HCC
Cystathionine synthase deficiency
E72.12 Methylenetetrahydrofolate reductase deficiency CC HCC
E72.19 Other disorders of sulfur-bearing amino-acid metabolism CC HCC
Cystathioninuria
Methioninemia
Sulfite oxidase deficiency

✓5th **E72.2 Disorders of urea cycle metabolism**
EXCLUDES 1 disorders of ornithine metabolism (E72.4)
E72.20 Disorder of urea cycle metabolism, unspecified CC HCC
Hyperammonemia
EXCLUDES 1 hyperammonemia- hyperornithinemia-homocitrullinemia syndrome (E72.4)
transient hyperammonemia of newborn (P74.6)
E72.21 Argininemia CC HCC
E72.22 Arginosuccinic aciduria CC HCC
E72.23 Citrullinemia CC HCC
E72.29 Other disorders of urea cycle metabolism CC HCC
E72.3 Disorders of lysine and hydroxylysine metabolism
Glutaric aciduria NOS
Glutaric aciduria (type I)
Hydroxylysinemia
Hyperlysinemia
EXCLUDES 1 glutaric aciduria type II (E71.313)
Refsum's disease (G60.1)
Zellweger syndrome (E71.510)
E72.4 Disorders of ornithine metabolism CC HCC
Hyperammonemia-hyperornithinemia-homocitrullinemia syndrome
Ornithinemia (types I, II)
Ornithine transcarbamylase deficiency
EXCLUDES 1 hereditary choroidal dystrophy (H31.2-)

Chapter 4. Endocrine, Nutritional and Metabolic Diseases

E72.5–E75.19

√5th **E72.5 Disorders of glycine metabolism**

     E72.50 Disorder of glycine metabolism, unspecified `CC` `HCC`

     E72.51 Non-ketotic hyperglycinemia `CC` `HCC`

     E72.52 Trimethylaminuria `CC` `HCC`

▲   **E72.53 Primary hyperoxaluria** `CC` `HCC`
         Oxalosis
         Oxaluria

     E72.59 Other disorders of glycine metabolism `CC` `HCC`
         D-glycericacidemia
         Hyperhydroxyprolinemia
         Hyperprolinemia (types I, II)
         Sarcosinemia

√5th **E72.8 Other specified disorders of amino-acid metabolism**
~~Disorders of beta-amino-acid metabolism~~
~~Disorders of gamma-glutamyl cycle~~

●   **E72.81 Disorders of gamma aminobutyric acid metabolism** `CC`
         4-hydroxybutyric aciduria
         Disorders of GABA metabolism
         GABA metabolic defect
         GABA transaminase deficiency
         GABA-T deficiency
         Gamma-hydroxybutyric aciduria
         SSADHD
         Succinic semialdehyde dehydrogenase deficiency

●   **E72.89 Other specified disorders of amino-acid metabolism** `CC`
         Disorders of beta-amino-acid metabolism
         Disorders of gamma-glutamyl cycle

     E72.9 Disorder of amino-acid metabolism, unspecified `CC` `HCC`

√4th **E73 Lactose intolerance**
     DEF: Inability to break down sugar in dairy products due to a deficiency in the enzyme lactase.

     E73.0 Congenital lactase deficiency

     E73.1 Secondary lactase deficiency

     E73.8 Other lactose intolerance

     E73.9 Lactose intolerance, unspecified

√4th **E74 Other disorders of carbohydrate metabolism**
     EXCLUDES 1   *diabetes mellitus (E08-E13)*
                hypoglycemia NOS (E16.2)
                increased secretion of glucagon (E16.3)
                mucopolysaccharidosis (E76.0-E76.3)

     CC Excl: For CC codes in category E74: PDX collection 534

√5th **E74.0 Glycogen storage disease**

     E74.00 Glycogen storage disease, unspecified `CC` `HCC`

     E74.01 von Gierke disease `CC` `HCC`
         Type I glycogen storage disease

     E74.02 Pompe disease `CC` `HCC`
         Cardiac glycogenosis
         Type II glycogen storage disease

     E74.03 Cori disease `CC` `HCC`
         Forbes disease
         Type III glycogen storage disease

     E74.04 McArdle disease `CC` `HCC`
         Type V glycogen storage disease

     E74.09 Other glycogen storage disease `CC` `HCC`
         Andersen disease
         Hers disease
         Tauri disease
         Glycogen storage disease, types 0, IV, VI-XI
         Liver phosphorylase deficiency
         Muscle phosphofructokinase deficiency

√5th **E74.1 Disorders of fructose metabolism**
     EXCLUDES 1   *muscle phosphofructokinase deficiency (E74.09)*

     E74.10 Disorder of fructose metabolism, unspecified

     E74.11 Essential fructosuria
         Fructokinase deficiency

     E74.12 Hereditary fructose intolerance
         Fructosemia

     E74.19 Other disorders of fructose metabolism
         Fructose-1, 6-diphosphatase deficiency

√5th **E74.2 Disorders of galactose metabolism**

     E74.20 Disorders of galactose metabolism, unspecified `CC` `HCC`

     E74.21 Galactosemia `CC` `HCC`
         DEF: Any of three genetic disorders caused by a defective galactose metabolism. Symptoms include failure to thrive in infancy, jaundice, liver and spleen damage, cataracts, and mental retardation.

     E74.29 Other disorders of galactose metabolism `CC` `HCC`
         Galactokinase deficiency

√5th **E74.3 Other disorders of intestinal carbohydrate absorption**
     EXCLUDES 2   *lactose intolerance (E73.-)*

     E74.31 Sucrase-isomaltase deficiency

     E74.39 Other disorders of intestinal carbohydrate absorption
         Disorder of intestinal carbohydrate absorption NOS
         Glucose-galactose malabsorption
         Sucrase deficiency

     E74.4 Disorders of pyruvate metabolism and gluconeogenesis `CC` `HCC`
         Deficiency of phosphoenolpyruvate carboxykinase
         Deficiency of pyruvate carboxylase
         Deficiency of pyruvate dehydrogenase
     EXCLUDES 1   *disorders of pyruvate metabolism and gluconeogenesis with anemia (D55.-)*
                Leigh's syndrome (G31.82)

     E74.8 Other specified disorders of carbohydrate metabolism `CC` `HCC`
         Essential pentosuria
         Renal glycosuria

     E74.9 Disorder of carbohydrate metabolism, unspecified `HCC`

√4th **E75 Disorders of sphingolipid metabolism and other lipid storage disorders**
     EXCLUDES 1   *mucolipidosis, types I-III (E77.0-E77.1)*
                Refsum's disease (G60.1)

     CC Excl: For CC codes in category E75, unless otherwise noted: PDX collection 537

√5th **E75.0 GM2 gangliosidosis**

     E75.00 GM2 gangliosidosis, unspecified `CC`

     E75.01 Sandhoff disease `CC`

     E75.02 Tay-Sachs disease `CC`
         DEF: Genetic mutation of the HEXA gene that inhibits the breakdown of a toxic substance called ganglioside. The accumulation of ganglioside results in destruction of the neurons in the brain and spinal cord.

Tay-Sachs Disease

Healthy neuron
Lysosome
Neuron affected by Tay-Sachs
Bulging lysosome

     E75.09 Other GM2 gangliosidosis `CC`
         Adult GM2 gangliosidosis
         Juvenile GM2 gangliosidosis

√5th **E75.1 Other and unspecified gangliosidosis**

     E75.10 Unspecified gangliosidosis `CC`
         Gangliosidosis NOS

     E75.11 Mucolipidosis IV `CC`

     E75.19 Other gangliosidosis `CC`
         GM1 gangliosidosis
         GM3 gangliosidosis

N Newborn: 0   P Pediatric: 0-17   M Maternity: 12-55   A Adult: 15-124   MCC Major Complication/Comorbidity   CC Complication/Comorbidity   SW Severe Wound Dx

530   ICD-10-CM 2019

✓5th **E75.2 Other sphingolipidosis**

> EXCLUDES 1   adrenoleukodystrophy [Addison-Schilder] (E71.528)

> **CC Excl: For CC codes in subcategory E75.2:**
> PDX collection 538

     E75.21 Fabry (-Anderson) disease `HCC`

     E75.22 Gaucher disease `HCC`

     E75.23 Krabbe disease `CC`

✓6th   **E75.24 Niemann-Pick disease**

       E75.240 Niemann-Pick disease type A `HCC`

       E75.241 Niemann-Pick disease type B `HCC`

       E75.242 Niemann-Pick disease type C `HCC`

       E75.243 Niemann-Pick disease type D `HCC`

       E75.248 Other Niemann-Pick disease `HCC`

       E75.249 Niemann-Pick disease, unspecified `HCC`

     E75.25 Metachromatic leukodystrophy `CC`

●   **E75.26 Sulfatase deficiency** `CC`
       Multiple sulfatase deficiency (MSD)

     E75.29 Other sphingolipidosis `CC`
       Farber's syndrome
       ~~Sulfatase deficiency~~
       Sulfatide lipidosis

E75.3 Sphingolipidosis, unspecified `HCC`

E75.4 Neuronal ceroid lipofuscinosis `CC`
     Batten disease
     Bielschowsky-Jansky disease
     Kufs disease
     Spielmeyer-Vogt disease

E75.5 Other lipid storage disorders
     Cerebrotendinous cholesterosis [van Bogaert-Scherer-Epstein]
     Wolman's disease

E75.6 Lipid storage disorder, unspecified

✓4th **E76 Disorders of glycosaminoglycan metabolism**

> **CC Excl: For CC codes in category E76:** PDX collection 539

✓5th **E76.0 Mucopolysaccharidosis, type I**

     E76.01 Hurler's syndrome `CC` `HCC`

     E76.02 Hurler-Scheie syndrome `CC` `HCC`

     E76.03 Scheie's syndrome `CC` `HCC`

E76.1 Mucopolysaccharidosis, type II `CC` `HCC`
     Hunter's syndrome

✓5th **E76.2 Other mucopolysaccharidoses**

✓6th   **E76.21 Morquio mucopolysaccharidoses**

       E76.210 Morquio A mucopolysaccharidoses `CC` `HCC`
         Classic Morquio syndrome
         Morquio syndrome A
         Mucopolysaccharidosis, type IVA

       E76.211 Morquio B mucopolysaccharidoses `CC` `HCC`
         Morquio-like mucopolysaccharidoses
         Morquio-like syndrome
         Morquio syndrome B
         Mucopolysaccharidosis, type IVB

       E76.219 Morquio mucopolysaccharidoses, unspecified `CC` `HCC`
         Morquio syndrome
         Mucopolysaccharidosis, type IV

     E76.22 Sanfilippo mucopolysaccharidoses `CC` `HCC`
       Mucopolysaccharidosis, type III (A) (B) (C) (D)
       Sanfilippo A syndrome
       Sanfilippo B syndrome
       Sanfilippo C syndrome
       Sanfilippo D syndrome

     E76.29 Other mucopolysaccharidoses `CC` `HCC`
       beta-Glucuronidase deficiency
       Maroteaux-Lamy (mild) (severe) syndrome
       Mucopolysaccharidosis, types VI, VII

E76.3 Mucopolysaccharidosis, unspecified `CC` `HCC`

E76.8 Other disorders of glucosaminoglycan metabolism `CC` `HCC`

E76.9 Glucosaminoglycan metabolism disorder, unspecified `CC` `HCC`

✓4th **E77 Disorders of glycoprotein metabolism**

E77.0 Defects in post-translational modification of lysosomal enzymes `HCC`
     Mucolipidosis II [I-cell disease]
     Mucolipidosis III [pseudo-Hurler polydystrophy]

E77.1 Defects in glycoprotein degradation `HCC`
     Aspartylglucosaminuria
     Fucosidosis
     Mannosidosis
     Sialidosis [mucolipidosis I]

E77.8 Other disorders of glycoprotein metabolism `HCC`

E77.9 Disorder of glycoprotein metabolism, unspecified `HCC`

✓4th **E78 Disorders of lipoprotein metabolism and other lipidemias**

> EXCLUDES 1   sphingolipidosis (E75.0-E75.3)

✓5th **E78.0 Pure hypercholesterolemia**
     AHA: 2016, 4Q, 13-14

     E78.00 Pure hypercholesterolemia, unspecified
       Fredrickson's hyperlipoproteinemia, type IIa
       Hyperbetalipoproteinemia
       Low-density-lipoprotein-type [LDL] hyperlipoproteinemia
       (Pure) hypercholesterolemia NOS

     E78.01 Familial hypercholesterolemia

E78.1 Pure hyperglyceridemia
     Elevated fasting triglycerides
     Endogenous hyperglyceridemia
     Fredrickson's hyperlipoproteinemia, type IV
     Hyperlipidemia, group B
     Hyperprebetalipoproteinemia
     Very-low-density-lipoprotein-type [VLDL] hyperlipoproteinemia

E78.2 Mixed hyperlipidemia
     Broad- or floating-betalipoproteinemia
     Combined hyperlipidemia NOS
     Elevated cholesterol with elevated triglycerides NEC
     Fredrickson's hyperlipoproteinemia, type IIb or III
     Hyperbetalipoproteinemia with prebetalipoproteinemia
     Hypercholesteremia with endogenous hyperglyceridemia
     Hyperlipidemia, group C
     Tubo-eruptive xanthoma
     Xanthoma tuberosum

> EXCLUDES 1   cerebrotendinous cholesterosis [van Bogaert-Scherer-Epstein] (E75.5)
>   familial combined hyperlipidemia ▶(E78.49)◀

E78.3 Hyperchylomicronemia
     Chylomicron retention disease
     Fredrickson's hyperlipoproteinemia, type I or V
     Hyperlipidemia, group D
     Mixed hyperglyceridemia

✓5th **E78.4 Other hyperlipidemia**
     ~~Familial combined hyperlipidemia~~

●   **E78.41 Elevated Lipoprotein(a)**
       Elevated Lp(a)

●   **E78.49 Other hyperlipidemia**
       Familial combined hyperlipidemia

E78.5 Hyperlipidemia, unspecified

E78.6 Lipoprotein deficiency
     Abetalipoproteinemia
     Depressed HDL cholesterol
     High-density lipoprotein deficiency
     Hypoalphalipoproteinemia
     Hypobetalipoproteinemia (familial)
     Lecithin cholesterol acyltransferase deficiency
     Tangier disease

✓5th **E78.7 Disorders of bile acid and cholesterol metabolism**

> EXCLUDES 1   Niemann-Pick disease type C (E75.242)

     E78.70 Disorder of bile acid and cholesterol metabolism, unspecified

     E78.71 Barth syndrome `CC`
       CC Excl: PDX collection 540

     E78.72 Smith-Lemli-Opitz syndrome `CC`
       CC Excl: PDX collection 540

     E78.79 Other disorders of bile acid and cholesterol metabolism

✓5th **E78.8 Other disorders of lipoprotein metabolism**

     E78.81 Lipoid dermatoarthritis

     E78.89 Other lipoprotein metabolism disorders

E78.9 Disorder of lipoprotein metabolism, unspecified

✓ Additional Character Required   ✓x7th Placeholder   Unacceptable PDx   Questionable PDx   Manifestation   **H1** - **H14** HAC   `HCC` CMS-HCC Dx   **HIV** HIV Dx

✓4ᵗʰ E79   Disorders of purine and pyrimidine metabolism

> EXCLUDES 1   Ataxia-telangiectasia (Q87.1)
> Bloom's syndrome (Q82.8)
> Cockayne's syndrome (Q87.1)
> calculus of kidney (N20.0)
> combined immunodeficiency disorders (D81.-)
> Fanconi's anemia (D61.09)
> gout (M1A.-, M10.-)
> orotaciduric anemia (D53.0)
> progeria (E34.8)
> Werner's syndrome (E34.8)
> xeroderma pigmentosum (Q82.1)

> CC Excl: For CC codes in category E79: PDX collection 513

E79.0   **Hyperuricemia without signs of inflammatory arthritis and tophaceous disease**
> Asymptomatic hyperuricemia

E79.1   **Lesch-Nyhan syndrome**   CC HCC
> HGPRT deficiency

E79.2   **Myoadenylate deaminase deficiency**   CC HCC

E79.8   **Other disorders of purine and pyrimidine metabolism**   CC HCC
> Hereditary xanthinuria

E79.9   **Disorder of purine and pyrimidine metabolism, unspecified**   CC HCC

✓4ᵗʰ E80   Disorders of porphyrin and bilirubin metabolism

> INCLUDES   defects of catalase and peroxidase

> CC Excl: For CC codes in category E80, unless otherwise noted: PDX collection 513

E80.0   **Hereditary erythropoietic porphyria**   CC HCC
> Congenital erythropoietic porphyria
> Erythropoietic protoporphyria

E80.1   **Porphyria cutanea tarda**   CC HCC

✓5ᵗʰ **E80.2**   **Other and unspecified porphyria**

     E80.20   **Unspecified porphyria**   CC HCC
> Porphyria NOS

     E80.21   **Acute intermittent (hepatic) porphyria**   CC HCC

     E80.29   **Other porphyria**   CC HCC
> Hereditary coproporphyria

E80.3   **Defects of catalase and peroxidase**   CC HCC
> Acatalasia [Takahara]
> CC Excl: PDX collection 492

E80.4   **Gilbert syndrome**

E80.5   **Crigler-Najjar syndrome**

E80.6   **Other disorders of bilirubin metabolism**
> Dubin-Johnson syndrome
> Rotor's syndrome

E80.7   **Disorder of bilirubin metabolism, unspecified**

✓4ᵗʰ E83   Disorders of mineral metabolism

> EXCLUDES 1   dietary mineral deficiency (E58-E61)
> parathyroid disorders (E20-E21)
> vitamin D deficiency (E55.-)

✓5ᵗʰ **E83.0**   **Disorders of copper metabolism**

     E83.00   **Disorder of copper metabolism, unspecified**

     E83.01   **Wilson's disease**
> Code also associated Kayser Fleischer ring (H18.04-)

     E83.09   **Other disorders of copper metabolism**
> Menkes' (kinky hair) (steely hair) disease

✓5ᵗʰ **E83.1**   **Disorders of iron metabolism**
> EXCLUDES 1   iron deficiency anemia (D50.-)
> sideroblastic anemia (D64.0-D64.3)

     E83.10   **Disorder of iron metabolism, unspecified**

     ✓6ᵗʰ **E83.11**   **Hemochromatosis**
> EXCLUDES 1   GALD (P78.84)
> gestational alloimmune liver disease (P78.84)
> neonatal hemochromatosis (P78.84)

         E83.110   **Hereditary hemochromatosis**   HCC
> Bronzed diabetes
> Pigmentary cirrhosis (of liver)
> Primary (hereditary) hemochromatosis

         E83.111   **Hemochromatosis due to repeated red blood cell transfusions**
> Iron overload due to repeated red blood cell transfusions
> Transfusion (red blood cell) associated hemochromatosis

         E83.118   **Other hemochromatosis**

         E83.119   **Hemochromatosis, unspecified**

     E83.19   **Other disorders of iron metabolism**
> Use additional code, if applicable, for idiopathic pulmonary hemosiderosis (J84.03)

E83.2   **Disorders of zinc metabolism**
> Acrodermatitis enteropathica

✓5ᵗʰ **E83.3**   **Disorders of phosphorus metabolism and phosphatases**
> EXCLUDES 1   adult osteomalacia (M83.-)
> osteoporosis (M80.-)

     E83.30   **Disorder of phosphorus metabolism, unspecified**

     E83.31   **Familial hypophosphatemia**
> Vitamin D-resistant osteomalacia
> Vitamin D-resistant rickets
> EXCLUDES 1   vitamin D-deficiency rickets (E55.0)

     E83.32   **Hereditary vitamin D-dependent rickets (type 1) (type 2)**
> 25-hydroxyvitamin D 1-alpha-hydroxylase deficiency
> Pseudovitamin D deficiency
> Vitamin D receptor defect

     E83.39   **Other disorders of phosphorus metabolism**
> Acid phosphatase deficiency
> Hypophosphatasia

✓5ᵗʰ **E83.4**   **Disorders of magnesium metabolism**

     E83.40   **Disorders of magnesium metabolism, unspecified**

     E83.41   **Hypermagnesemia**
> AHA: 2016, 4Q, 54

     E83.42   **Hypomagnesemia**

     E83.49   **Other disorders of magnesium metabolism**

✓5ᵗʰ **E83.5**   **Disorders of calcium metabolism**
> EXCLUDES 1   chondrocalcinosis (M11.1-M11.2)
> hungry bone syndrome (E83.81)
> hyperparathyroidism (E21.0-E21.3)

     E83.50   **Unspecified disorder of calcium metabolism**

     E83.51   **Hypocalcemia**

     E83.52   **Hypercalcemia**
> Familial hypocalciuric hypercalcemia

     E83.59   **Other disorders of calcium metabolism**
> Idiopathic hypercalciuria

✓5ᵗʰ **E83.8**   **Other disorders of mineral metabolism**

     E83.81   **Hungry bone syndrome**

     E83.89   **Other disorders of mineral metabolism**

E83.9   **Disorder of mineral metabolism, unspecified**

✓4ᵗʰ E84   Cystic fibrosis

> INCLUDES   mucoviscidosis

> Code also exocrine pancreatic insufficiency (K86.81)

> **DEF:** Genetic disorder affecting the respiratory, digestive, and reproductive systems in infants to young adults by disturbing exocrine gland function and causing chronic pulmonary disease with excess mucus production and pancreatic deficiency.

> CC Excl: For CC/MCC codes in category E84: PDX collection 541

E84.0   **Cystic fibrosis with pulmonary manifestations**   MCC HCC
> Use additional code to identify any infectious organism present, such as:
> Pseudomonas (B96.5)

✓5ᵗʰ **E84.1**   **Cystic fibrosis with intestinal manifestations**

     E84.11   **Meconium ileus in cystic fibrosis**   MCC HCC N
> EXCLUDES 1   meconium ileus not due to cystic fibrosis (P76.0)

     E84.19   **Cystic fibrosis with other intestinal manifestations**   CC HCC
> Distal intestinal obstruction syndrome

E84.8   **Cystic fibrosis with other manifestations**   CC HCC

E84.9   **Cystic fibrosis, unspecified**   CC HCC

✓4ᵗʰ E85   Amyloidosis

> EXCLUDES 2   Alzheimer's disease (G30.0-)

> **DEF:** Conditions of diverse etiologies characterized by the accumulation of insoluble fibrillar proteins (amyloid) in various organs and tissues of the body, compromising vital functions.

E85.0   **Non-neuropathic heredofamilial amyloidosis**   CC HCC
> Hereditary amyloid nephropathy
> Code also associated disorders, such as:
> autoinflammatory syndromes (M04.-)
> EXCLUDES 2   transthyretin-related (ATTR) familial amyloid cardiomyopathy (E85.4)

N Newborn: 0   P Pediatric: 0-17   M Maternity: 12-55   A Adult: 15-124   MCC Major Complication/Comorbidity   CC Complication/Comorbidity   SW Severe Wound Dx

532   ICD-10-CM 2019

E85.1 **Neuropathic heredofamilial amyloidosis** `CC` `HCC`
Amyloid polyneuropathy (Portuguese)
Transthyretin-related (ATTR) familial amyloid polyneuropathy
AHA: 2012, 4Q, 99

E85.2 **Heredofamilial amyloidosis, unspecified** `CC` `HCC`

E85.3 **Secondary systemic amyloidosis** `CC` `HCC`
Hemodialysis-associated amyloidosis

E85.4 **Organ-limited amyloidosis** `CC` `HCC`
Localized amyloidosis
Transthyretin-related (ATTR) familial amyloid cardiomyopathy

✓5ᵗʰ **E85.8** **Other amyloidosis**
AHA: 2017, 4Q, 7

    E85.81 **Light chain (AL) amyloidosis** `CC` `HCC`

    E85.82 **Wild-type transthyretin-related (ATTR)** `CC` `HCC`
amyloidosis
Senile systemic amyloidosis (SSA)

    E85.89 **Other amyloidosis** `CC` `HCC`

E85.9 **Amyloidosis, unspecified** `CC` `HCC`

✓4ᵗʰ **E86** **Volume depletion**
Use additional code(s) for any associated disorders of electrolyte and acid-base balance (E87.-)
EXCLUDES 1 *dehydration of newborn (P74.1)*
hypovolemic shock NOS (R57.1)
postprocedural hypovolemic shock (T81.19)
traumatic hypovolemic shock (T79.4)
AHA: 2018, 2Q, 6

E86.0 **Dehydration**
AHA: 2014, 1Q, 7
TIP: Can be assigned in addition to hypernatremia (E87.0) or hyponatremia (E87.1), when documented.

E86.1 **Hypovolemia**
Depletion of volume of plasma

E86.9 **Volume depletion, unspecified**
DEF: Depletion of total body water (dehydration) and/or contraction of total intravascular plasma (hypovolemia).

✓4ᵗʰ **E87** **Other disorders of fluid, electrolyte and acid-base balance**
EXCLUDES 1 *diabetes insipidus (E23.2)*
electrolyte imbalance associated with hyperemesis gravidarum (O21.1)
electrolyte imbalance following ectopic or molar pregnancy (O08.5)
familial periodic paralysis (G72.3)
AHA: 2018, 2Q, 6

CC Excl: For CC codes in category E87: PDX collection 543

E87.0 **Hyperosmolality and hypernatremia** `CC`
Sodium [Na] excess
Sodium [Na] overload
AHA: 2014, 1Q, 7
TIP: Assign an additional code for dehydration (E86.0), when documented.

E87.1 **Hypo-osmolality and hyponatremia** `CC`
Sodium [Na] deficiency
EXCLUDES 1 *syndrome of inappropriate secretion of antidiuretic hormone (E22.2)*
AHA: 2014, 1Q, 7
TIP: Assign an additional code for dehydration (E86.0), when documented.

E87.2 **Acidosis** `CC`
Acidosis NOS
Lactic acidosis
Metabolic acidosis
Respiratory acidosis
EXCLUDES 1 *diabetic acidosis see categories E08-E10, E13 with ketoacidosis*
DEF: Reduction of alkaline in the blood and tissues caused by an increase in acid and decrease in bicarbonate.

E87.3 **Alkalosis** `CC`
Alkalosis NOS
Metabolic alkalosis
Respiratory alkalosis

E87.4 **Mixed disorder of acid-base balance** `CC`

E87.5 **Hyperkalemia**
Potassium [K] excess
Potassium [K] overload

E87.6 **Hypokalemia**
Potassium [K] deficiency

✓5ᵗʰ **E87.7** **Fluid overload**
EXCLUDES 1 *edema NOS (R60.9)*
fluid retention (R60.9)

    E87.70 **Fluid overload, unspecified**

    E87.71 **Transfusion associated circulatory overload**
Fluid overload due to transfusion (blood) (blood components)
TACO

    E87.79 **Other fluid overload**

E87.8 **Other disorders of electrolyte and fluid balance, not elsewhere classified**
Electrolyte imbalance NOS
Hyperchloremia
Hypochloremia

✓4ᵗʰ **E88** **Other and unspecified metabolic disorders**
Use additional codes for associated conditions
EXCLUDES 1 *histiocytosis X (chronic) (C96.6)*

✓5ᵗʰ **E88.0** **Disorders of plasma-protein metabolism, not elsewhere classified**
EXCLUDES 1 *disorder of lipoprotein metabolism (E78.-)*
monoclonal gammopathy (of undetermined significance) (D47.2)
polyclonal hypergammaglobulinemia (D89.0)
Waldenström's macroglobulinemia (C88.0)

    E88.01 **Alpha-1-antitrypsin deficiency** `HCC`
AAT deficiency

●   **E88.02** **Plasminogen deficiency** `CC`
Dysplasminogenemia
Hypoplasminogenemia
Type 1 plasminogen deficiency
Type 2 plasminogen deficiency
Code also, if applicable, ligneous conjunctivitis (H10.51)
Use additional code for associated findings, such as:
hydrocephalus (G91.4)
ligneous conjunctivitis (H10.51)
otitis media (H67.-)
respiratory disorder related to plasminogen deficiency (J99)

    E88.09 **Other disorders of plasma-protein metabolism, not elsewhere classified**
Bisalbuminemia

E88.1 **Lipodystrophy, not elsewhere classified**
Lipodystrophy NOS
EXCLUDES 1 *Whipple's disease (K90.81)*

E88.2 **Lipomatosis, not elsewhere classified**
Lipomatosis NOS
Lipomatosis (Check) dolorosa [Dercum]

E88.3 **Tumor lysis syndrome** `MCC`
Tumor lysis syndrome (spontaneous)
Tumor lysis syndrome following antineoplastic drug chemotherapy
Use additional code for adverse effect, if applicable, to identify drug (T45.1X5)
DEF: Potentially fatal metabolic complication of tumor necrosis caused by spontaneous or treatment-related accumulation of byproducts from dying cancer cells. Symptoms include hyperkalemia, hyperphosphatemia, hypocalcemia, hyperuricemia, and hyperuricosuria.
CC Excl: PDX collection 544

✓5ᵗʰ **E88.4** **Mitochondrial metabolism disorders**
EXCLUDES 1 *disorders of pyruvate metabolism (E74.4)*
Kearns-Sayre syndrome (H49.81)
Leber's disease (H47.22)
Leigh's encephalopathy (G31.82)
Mitochondrial myopathy, NEC (G71.3)
Reye's syndrome (G93.7)

CC Excl: For CC codes in subcategory E88.4: PDX collection 545

    E88.40 **Mitochondrial metabolism disorder, unspecified** `CC` `HCC`

    E88.41 **MELAS syndrome** `CC` `HCC`
Mitochondrial myopathy, encephalopathy, lactic acidosis and stroke-like episodes

    E88.42 **MERRF syndrome** `CC` `HCC`
Myoclonic epilepsy associated with ragged-red fibers
Code also progressive myoclonic epilepsy (G40.3-)

    E88.49 **Other mitochondrial metabolism disorders** `CC` `HCC`

✓ Additional Character Required   ✓7ᵗʰ Placeholder   Unacceptable PDx   Questionable PDx   Manifestation   H1 - H14 HAC   HCC CMS-HCC Dx   HIV HIV Dx

ICD-10-CM 2019   533

Chapter 4. Endocrine, Nutritional and Metabolic Diseases

✓5ᵗʰ **E88.8**   **Other specified metabolic disorders**

    E88.81   **Metabolic syndrome**
        Dysmetabolic syndrome X
        Use additional codes for associated manifestations,
            such as:
            obesity (E66.-)
        DEF: Group of health risks that increase the likelihood of
        developing heart disease, stroke, and diabetes. These
        risks include certain parameters for blood pressure,
        cholesterol, and glucose levels.

    E88.89   **Other specified metabolic disorders**   `HCC`
        Launois-Bensaude adenolipomatosis
        `EXCLUDES 1`   *adult pulmonary Langerhans cell*
                  histiocytosis (J84.82)

  E88.9   **Metabolic disorder, unspecified**

Postprocedural endocrine and metabolic complications and disorders, not elsewhere classified (E89)

✓4ᵗʰ **E89**   **Postprocedural endocrine and metabolic complications and disorders, not elsewhere classified**
    `EXCLUDES 2`   *intraoperative complications of endocrine system organ or structure (E36.0-, E36.1-, E36.8)*

  E89.0   **Postprocedural hypothyroidism**
    Postirradiation hypothyroidism
    Postsurgical hypothyroidism

  E89.1   **Postprocedural hypoinsulinemia**   `CC`
    Postpancreatectomy hyperglycemia
    Postsurgical hypoinsulinemia
    Use additional code, if applicable, to identify:
      acquired absence of pancreas (Z90.41-)
      diabetes mellitus (postpancreatectomy) (postprocedural)
        (E13.-)
      insulin use (Z79.4)
    `EXCLUDES 1`   *transient postprocedural hyperglycemia (R73.9)*
                transient postprocedural hypoglycemia (E16.2)
    CC Excl: PDX collection 520

  E89.2   **Postprocedural hypoparathyroidism**   `HCC`
    Parathyroprival tetany

  E89.3   **Postprocedural hypopituitarism**   `HCC`
    Postirradiation hypopituitarism

✓5ᵗʰ **E89.4**   **Postprocedural ovarian failure**

    E89.40   **Asymptomatic postprocedural ovarian failure**   ♀
        Postprocedural ovarian failure NOS

    E89.41   **Symptomatic postprocedural ovarian failure**   ♀
        Symptoms such as flushing, sleeplessness, headache,
           lack of concentration, associated with
           postprocedural menopause

  E89.5   **Postprocedural testicular hypofunction**   ♂

  E89.6   **Postprocedural adrenocortical (-medullary) hypofunction**   `CC` `HCC`
    CC Excl: PDX collection 526

✓5ᵗʰ **E89.8**   **Other postprocedural endocrine and metabolic complications and disorders**
    AHA: 2016, 4Q, 9-10

    CC Excl: For CC codes in subcategory E89.8:
    PDX collection 546

✓6ᵗʰ **E89.81**   **Postprocedural hemorrhage of an endocrine system organ or structure following a procedure**

    E89.810   **Postprocedural hemorrhage of an**   `CC`
        endocrine system organ or structure
        following an endocrine system procedure

    E89.811   **Postprocedural hemorrhage of an**   `CC`
        endocrine system organ or structure
        following other procedure

✓6ᵗʰ **E89.82**   **Postprocedural hematoma and seroma of an endocrine system organ or structure**

    E89.820   **Postprocedural hematoma of an**   `CC`
        endocrine system organ or structure
        following an endocrine system procedure

    E89.821   **Postprocedural hematoma of an**   `CC`
        endocrine system organ or structure
        following other procedure

    E89.822   **Postprocedural seroma of an**   `CC`
        endocrine system organ or structure
        following an endocrine system procedure

    E89.823   **Postprocedural seroma of an**   `CC`
        endocrine system organ or structure
        following other procedure

  E89.89   **Other postprocedural endocrine and metabolic**   `CC`
    complications and disorders
      Use additional code, if applicable, to further specify
        disorder

N Newborn: 0   P Pediatric: 0-17   M Maternity: 12-55   A Adult: 15-124   `MCC` Major Complication/Comorbidity   `CC` Complication/Comorbidity   `SW` Severe Wound Dx

534   ICD-10-CM 2019

Chapter 5. Mental, Behavioral and Neurodevelopmental Disorders (F01–F99)

Chapter Specific Guidelines with Coding Examples

The chapter specific guidelines from the ICD-10-CM Official Guidelines for Coding and Reporting have been provided below. Along with these guidelines are coding examples, contained in the shaded boxes, that have been developed to help illustrate the coding and/or sequencing guidance found in these guidelines.

a. Pain disorders related to psychological factors

Assign code F45.41, for pain that is exclusively related to psychological disorders. As indicated by the Excludes 1 note under category G89, a code from category G89 should not be assigned with code F45.41.

> Perceived abdominal pain determined to be persistent somatoform pain disorder
>
> **F45.41   Pain disorder exclusively related to psychological factors**
>
> *Explanation*: This pain was diagnosed as being exclusively psychological; therefore, no code from category G89 is added.

Code F45.42, Pain disorders with related psychological factors, should be used with a code from category G89, Pain, not elsewhere classified, if there is documentation of a psychological component for a patient with acute or chronic pain.

See Section I.C.6. Pain

b. Mental and behavioral disorders due to psychoactive substance use

1) In remission

Selection of codes for "in remission" for categories F10-F19, Mental and behavioral disorders due to psychoactive substance use (categories F10-F19 with -11, -.21) requires the provider's clinical judgment. The appropriate codes for "in remission" are assigned only on the basis of provider documentation (as defined in the Official Guidelines for Coding and Reporting), unless otherwise instructed by the classification.

Mild substance use disorders in early or sustained remission are classified to the appropriate codes for substance abuse in remission, and moderate or severe substance use disorders in early or sustained remission are classified to the appropriate codes for substance dependence in remission.

> Insomnia in patient with history of methamphetamine abuse; lab results indicate no current drug use
>
> **G47.00   Insomnia, unspecified**
>
> **F15.10   Other stimulant abuse, uncomplicated**
>
> *Explanation*: Insomnia is a common side-effect of stimulant use, such as methamphetamines. Although lab tests do not indicate that the patient is currently using methamphetamines, there is no specific documentation stating that the stimulant abuse is in remission. "History of" abuse does not equate to "in remission" in this instance.

2) Psychoactive substance use, abuse and dependence

When the provider documentation refers to use, abuse and dependence of the same substance (e.g. alcohol, opioid, cannabis, etc.), only one code should be assigned to identify the pattern of use based on the following hierarchy:

- If both use and abuse are documented, assign only the code for abuse
- If both abuse and dependence are documented, assign only the code for dependence
- If use, abuse and dependence are all documented, assign only the code for dependence
- If both use and dependence are documented, assign only the code for dependence.

> History and physical notes cannabis dependence; progress note says cannabis abuse
>
> **F12.20   Cannabis dependence, uncomplicated**
>
> *Explanation*: In the hierarchy, the dependence code is used if both abuse and dependence are documented.

> Discharge summary says cocaine abuse; progress notes list cocaine use
>
> **F14.10   Cocaine abuse, uncomplicated**
>
> *Explanation*: In the hierarchy, the abuse code is used if both abuse and use are documented.

3) Psychoactive substance use, *unspecified*

As with all other **unspecified** diagnoses, the codes for **unspecified** psychoactive substance use disorders (F10.9-, F11.9-, F12.9-, F13.9-, F14.9-, F15.9-, F16.9-, **F18.9-, F19.9-**) should only be assigned based on provider documentation and when they meet the definition of a reportable diagnosis (see Section III, Reporting Additional Diagnoses). The**se** codes are to be used only when the psychoactive substance use is associated with a physical, mental or behavioral disorder, and such a relationship is documented by the provider.

c. Factitious disorder

Factitious disorder imposed on self or Munchausen's syndrome is a disorder in which a person falsely reports or causes his or her own physical or psychological signs or symptoms. For patients with documented factitious disorder on self or Munchausen's syndrome, assign the appropriate code from subcategory F68.1-, Factitious disorder imposed on self.

Munchausen's syndrome by proxy (MSBP) is a disorder in which a caregiver (perpetrator) falsely reports or causes an illness or injury in another person (victim) under his or her care, such as a child, an elderly adult, or a person who has a disability. The condition is also referred to as "factitious disorder imposed on another" or "factitious disorder by proxy." The perpetrator, not the victim, receives this diagnosis. Assign code F68.A, Factitious disorder imposed on another, to the perpetrator's record. For the victim of a patient suffering from MSBP, assign the appropriate code from categories T74, Adult and child abuse, neglect and other maltreatment, confirmed, or T76, Adult and child abuse, neglect and other maltreatment, suspected.

See Section I.C.19.f. Adult and child abuse, neglect and other maltreatment

Chapter 5. Mental, Behavioral and Neurodevelopmental Disorders (F01-F99)

INCLUDES   disorders of psychological development
EXCLUDES 2   *symptoms, signs and abnormal clinical laboratory findings, not elsewhere classified (R00-R99)*

This chapter contains the following blocks:

F01-F09   Mental disorders due to known physiological conditions
F10-F19   Mental and behavioral disorders due to psychoactive substance use
F20-F29   Schizophrenia, schizotypal, delusional, and other non-mood psychotic disorders
F30-F39   Mood [affective] disorders
F40-F48   Anxiety, dissociative, stress-related, somatoform and other nonpsychotic mental disorders
F50-F59   Behavioral syndromes associated with physiological disturbances and physical factors
F60-F69   Disorders of adult personality and behavior
F70-F79   Intellectual disabilities
F80-F89   Pervasive and specific developmental disorders
F90-F98   Behavioral and emotional disorders with onset usually occurring in childhood and adolescence
F99   Unspecified mental disorder

Mental disorders due to known physiological conditions (F01-F09)

NOTE   This block comprises a range of mental disorders grouped together on the basis of their having in common a demonstrable etiology in cerebral disease, brain injury, or other insult leading to cerebral dysfunction. The dysfunction may be primary, as in diseases, injuries, and insults that affect the brain directly and selectively; or secondary, as in systemic diseases and disorders that attack the brain only as one of the multiple organs or systems of the body that are involved.

✓4ᵗʰ F01   Vascular dementia

Vascular dementia as a result of infarction of the brain due to vascular disease, including hypertensive cerebrovascular disease.
INCLUDES   arteriosclerotic dementia
Code first the underlying physiological condition or sequelae of cerebrovascular disease.

✓5ᵗʰ F01.5   Vascular dementia

F01.50   **Vascular dementia** without behavioral disturbance   Ⓐ
     Major neurocognitive disorder without behavioral disturbance

F01.51   **Vascular dementia** with behavioral disturbance   CC Ⓐ
     Major neurocognitive disorder due to vascular disease, with behavioral disturbance
     Major neurocognitive disorder with aggressive behavior
     Major neurocognitive disorder with combative behavior
     Major neurocognitive disorder with violent behavior
     Vascular dementia with aggressive behavior
     Vascular dementia with combative behavior
     Vascular dementia with violent behavior
     Use additional code, if applicable, to identify wandering in vascular dementia (Z91.83)
     CC Excl: PDX collection 547

✓4ᵗʰ F02   Dementia in other diseases classified elsewhere

INCLUDES   major neurocognitive disorder in other diseases classified elsewhere
Code first the underlying physiological condition, such as:
   Alzheimer's (G30.-)
   cerebral lipidosis (E75.4)
   Creutzfeldt-Jakob disease (A81.0-)
   dementia with Lewy bodies (G31.83)
   dementia with Parkinsonism (G31.83)
   epilepsy and recurrent seizures (G40.-)
   frontotemporal dementia (G31.09)
   hepatolenticular degeneration (E83.0)
   human immunodeficiency virus [HIV] disease (B20)
   Huntington's disease (G10)
   hypercalcemia (E83.52)
   hypothyroidism, acquired (E00-E03.-)
   intoxications (T36-T65)
   Jakob-Creutzfeldt disease (A81.0-)
   multiple sclerosis (G35)
   neurosyphilis (A52.17)
   niacin deficiency [pellagra] (E52)
   Parkinson's disease (G20)
   Pick's disease (G31.01)
   polyarteritis nodosa (M30.0)
   prion disease (A81.9)
   systemic lupus erythematosus (M32.-)
   traumatic brain injury (S06.-)
   trypanosomiasis (B56.-, B57.-)
   vitamin B deficiency (E53.8)
EXCLUDES 2   *dementia in alcohol and psychoactive substance disorders (F10-F19, with .17, .27, .97)*
     vascular dementia (F01.5-)

✓5ᵗʰ F02.8   Dementia in other diseases classified elsewhere

AHA: 2017, 2Q, 7; 2016, 4Q, 141; 2016, 2Q, 6
TIP: A code from this subcategory should always be assigned with a code from category G30 when Alzheimer's disease is documented, even in the absence of documented dementia.

F02.80   *Dementia in other diseases classified elsewhere without behavioral disturbance*
     Dementia in other diseases classified elsewhere NOS
     Major neurocognitive disorder in other diseases classified elsewhere

F02.81   *Dementia in other diseases classified elsewhere with behavioral disturbance*   CC
     Dementia in other diseases classified elsewhere with aggressive behavior
     Dementia in other diseases classified elsewhere with combative behavior
     Dementia in other diseases classified elsewhere with violent behavior
     Major neurocognitive disorder in other diseases classified elsewhere with aggressive behavior
     Major neurocognitive disorder in other diseases classified elsewhere with combative behavior
     Major neurocognitive disorder in other diseases classified elsewhere with violent behavior
     Use additional code, if applicable, to identify wandering in dementia in conditions classified elsewhere (Z91.83)
     CC Excl: PDX collection 548

✓4ᵗʰ F03   Unspecified dementia

Presenile dementia NOS   Senile dementia NOS
Presenile psychosis NOS   Senile dementia depressed
Primary degenerative dementia NOS   or paranoid type
Senile dementia NOS   Senile psychosis NOS
EXCLUDES 1   *senility NOS (R41.81)*
EXCLUDES 2   *mild memory disturbance due to known physiological condition (F06.8)*
     senile dementia with delirium or acute confusional state (F05)

✓5ᵗʰ F03.9   Unspecified dementia

F03.90   **Unspecified dementia** without behavioral disturbance   HIV Ⓐ
     Dementia NOS
     AHA: 2012, 4Q, 92

F03.91   **Unspecified dementia** with behavioral disturbance   CC Ⓐ
     Unspecified dementia with aggressive behavior
     Unspecified dementia with combative behavior
     Unspecified dementia with violent behavior
     Use additional code, if applicable, to identify wandering in unspecified dementia (Z91.83)
     CC Excl: PDX collection 548

F04   Amnestic disorder due to known physiological condition

Korsakov's psychosis or syndrome, nonalcoholic

Code first the underlying physiological condition

> *EXCLUDES 1*   *amnesia NOS (R41.3)*
> *anterograde amnesia (R41.1)*
> *dissociative amnesia (F44.0)*
> *retrograde amnesia (R41.2)*
>
> *EXCLUDES 2*   *alcohol-induced or unspecified Korsakov's syndrome (F10.26, F10.96)*
> *Korsakov's syndrome induced by other psychoactive substances (F13.26, F13.96, F19.16, F19.26, F19.96)*

F05   Delirium due to known physiological condition   `CC`

Acute or subacute brain syndrome

Acute or subacute confusional state (nonalcoholic)

Acute or subacute infective psychosis

Acute or subacute organic reaction

Acute or subacute psycho-organic syndrome

Delirium of mixed etiology

Delirium superimposed on dementia

Sundowning

Code first the underlying physiological condition

> *EXCLUDES 1*   *delirium NOS (R41.0)*
>
> *EXCLUDES 2*   *delirium tremens alcohol-induced or unspecified (F10.231, F10.921)*

CC Excl: PDX collection 549

✓4ᵗʰ F06   Other mental disorders due to known physiological condition

> *INCLUDES*   mental disorders due to endocrine disorder
> mental disorders due to exogenous hormone
> mental disorders due to exogenous toxic substance
> mental disorders due to primary cerebral disease
> mental disorders due to somatic illness
> mental disorders due to systemic disease affecting the brain

Code first the underlying physiological condition

> *EXCLUDES 1*   *unspecified dementia (F03)*
>
> *EXCLUDES 2*   *delirium due to known physiological condition (F05)*
> *dementia as classified in F01-F02*
> *other mental disorders associated with alcohol and other psychoactive substances (F10-F19)*

F06.0   Psychotic disorder with hallucinations due to known physiological condition   `CC`

Organic hallucinatory state (nonalcoholic)

> *EXCLUDES 2*   *hallucinations and perceptual disturbance induced by alcohol and other psychoactive substances (F10-F19 with .151, .251, .951)*
> *schizophrenia (F20.-)*

CC Excl: PDX collection 550

F06.1   Catatonic disorder due to known physiological condition

Catatonia associated with another mental disorder

Catatonia NOS

> *EXCLUDES 1*   *catatonic stupor (R40.1)*
> *stupor NOS (R40.1)*
>
> *EXCLUDES 2*   *catatonic schizophrenia (F20.2)*
> *dissociative stupor (F44.2)*

DEF: Catatonic: Abnormal neuropsychiatric state characterized by stupor, immobility or purposeless movements, or unresponsiveness in a person who otherwise appears awake.

F06.2   Psychotic disorder with delusions due to known physiological condition   `CC`

Paranoid and paranoid-hallucinatory organic states

Schizophrenia-like psychosis in epilepsy

> *EXCLUDES 2*   *alcohol and drug-induced psychotic disorder (F10-F19 with .150, .250, .950)*
> *brief psychotic disorder (F23)*
> *delusional disorder (F22)*
> *schizophrenia (F20.-)*

CC Excl: PDX collection 550

✓5ᵗʰ F06.3   Mood disorder due to known physiological condition

> *EXCLUDES 2*   *mood disorders due to alcohol and other psychoactive substances (F10-F19 with .14, .24, .94)*
> *mood disorders, not due to known physiological condition or unspecified (F30-F39)*

F06.30   Mood disorder due to known physiological condition, unspecified

F06.31   Mood disorder due to known physiological condition with depressive features

Depressive disorder due to known physiological condition, with depressive features

F06.32   Mood disorder due to known physiological condition with major depressive-like episode

Depressive disorder due to known physiological condition, with major depressive–like episode

F06.33   Mood disorder due to known physiological condition with manic features

Bipolar and related disorder due to a known physiological condition, with manic features

Bipolar and related disorder due to known physiological condition, with manic- or hypomanic-like episodes

F06.34   Mood disorder due to known physiological condition with mixed features

Bipolar and related disorder due to known physiological condition, with mixed features

Depressive disorder due to known physiological condition, with mixed features

F06.4   Anxiety disorder due to known physiological condition

> *EXCLUDES 2*   *anxiety disorders due to alcohol and other psychoactive substances (F10-F19 with .180, .280, .980)*
> *anxiety disorders, not due to known physiological condition or unspecified (F40.-, F41.-)*

F06.8   Other specified mental disorders due to known physiological condition   `HIV`

Epileptic psychosis NOS

Obsessive-compulsive and related disorder due to a known physiological condition

Organic dissociative disorder

Organic emotionally labile [asthenic] disorder

✓4ᵗʰ F07   Personality and behavioral disorders due to known physiological condition

Code first the underlying physiological condition

F07.0   Personality change due to known physiological condition

Frontal lobe syndrome

Limbic epilepsy personality syndrome

Lobotomy syndrome

Organic personality disorder

Organic pseudopsychopathic personality

Organic pseudoretarded personality

Postleucotomy syndrome

Code first underlying physiological condition

> *EXCLUDES 1*   *mild cognitive impairment (G31.84)*
> *postconcussional syndrome (F07.81)*
> *postencephalitic syndrome (F07.89)*
> *signs and symptoms involving emotional state (R45.-)*
>
> *EXCLUDES 2*   *specific personality disorder (F60.-)*

✓5ᵗʰ F07.8   Other personality and behavioral disorders due to known physiological condition

F07.81   Postconcussional syndrome

Postcontusional syndrome (encephalopathy)

Post-traumatic brain syndrome, nonpsychotic

Use additional code to identify associated post-traumatic headache, if applicable (G44.3-)

> *EXCLUDES 1*   *current concussion (brain) (S06.0-)*
> *postencephalitic syndrome (F07.89)*

DEF: Concussion symptoms that persist for weeks or months after a head injury. These symptoms may include headache, giddiness, fatigue, insomnia, mood fluctuation, and a subjective feeling of impaired intellectual function with extreme reaction to normal stressors.

F07.89   Other personality and behavioral disorders due to known physiological condition

Postencephalitic syndrome

Right hemispheric organic affective disorder

F07.9   Unspecified personality and behavioral disorder due to known physiological condition   `HIV`

Organic psychosyndrome

F09   Unspecified mental disorder due to known physiological condition   `HIV`

Mental disorder NOS due to known physiological condition

Organic brain syndrome NOS

Organic mental disorder NOS

Organic psychosis NOS

Symptomatic psychosis NOS

Code first the underlying physiological condition

> *EXCLUDES 1*   *psychosis NOS (F29)*

☑ Additional Character Required   ✓x7ᵗʰ Placeholder   Unacceptable PDx   Questionable PDx   Manifestation   `H1`-`H14` HAC   `HCC` CMS-HCC Dx   `HIV` HIV Dx

ICD-10-CM 2019   537

Chapter 5. Mental, Behavioral and Neurodevelopmental Disorders

Mental and behavioral disorders due to psychoactive substance use (F10-F19)

AHA: 2017, 4Q, 8; 2017, 2Q, 27

√4th **F10**   Alcohol **related disorders**

Use additional code for blood alcohol level, if applicable (Y90.-)

CC Excl: For CC codes in category F10: PDX collection 550

√5th **F10.1**   **Alcohol** abuse

     EXCLUDES 1   alcohol dependence (F10.2-)
                alcohol use, unspecified (F10.9-)

AHA: 2018, 1Q, 16; 2015, 2Q, 15
TIP: Alcohol withdrawal is classified to dependence only (F10.23-); there is no combination code for alcohol abuse with withdrawal. When alcohol abuse and alcohol withdrawal are documented for the same encounter, query the provider for clarification.
TIP: Assign when documentation indicates alcohol withdrawal without dependence; do not assign an additional code for withdrawal.

F10.10   **Alcohol abuse,** uncomplicated
        Alcohol use disorder, mild

F10.11   **Alcohol abuse,** in remission
        Alcohol use disorder, mild, in early remission
        Alcohol use disorder, mild, in sustained remission

√6th **F10.12**   **Alcohol abuse with** intoxication

     F10.120   **Alcohol abuse with intoxication,** uncomplicated   `HCC`

     F10.121   **Alcohol abuse with intoxication** delirium   `CC` `HCC`

     F10.129   **Alcohol abuse with intoxication,** unspecified   `HCC`

F10.14   **Alcohol abuse with alcohol-induced** mood disorder   `CC` `HCC`
        Alcohol use disorder, mild, with alcohol-induced bipolar or related disorder
        Alcohol use disorder, mild, with alcohol-induced depressive disorder

√6th **F10.15**   **Alcohol abuse with alcohol-induced** psychotic disorder

     F10.150   **Alcohol abuse with alcohol-induced psychotic disorder with** delusions   `HCC`

     F10.151   **Alcohol abuse with alcohol-induced psychotic disorder with** hallucinations   `CC` `HCC`
        DEF: Psychosis lasting less than six months with slight or no clouding of consciousness in which auditory hallucinations predominate.

     F10.159   **Alcohol abuse with alcohol-induced psychotic disorder,** unspecified   `CC` `HCC`

√6th **F10.18**   **Alcohol abuse with** other **alcohol-induced disorders**

     F10.180   **Alcohol abuse with alcohol-induced** anxiety disorder   `CC` `HCC`

     F10.181   **Alcohol abuse with alcohol-induced** sexual dysfunction

     F10.182   **Alcohol abuse with alcohol-induced** sleep disorder   `CC` `HCC`

     F10.188   **Alcohol abuse with** other **alcohol-induced disorder**   `CC` `HCC`

F10.19   **Alcohol abuse with** unspecified **alcohol-induced disorder**   `CC` `HCC`

√5th **F10.2**   **Alcohol** dependence

     EXCLUDES 1   alcohol abuse (F10.1-)
                alcohol use, unspecified (F10.9-)
     EXCLUDES 2   toxic effect of alcohol (T51.0-)

F10.20   **Alcohol dependence,** uncomplicated   `HCC`
        Alcohol use disorder, moderate
        Alcohol use disorder, severe

F10.21   **Alcohol dependence,** in remission   `HCC`
        Alcohol use disorder, moderate, in early remission
        Alcohol use disorder, moderate, in sustained remission
        Alcohol use disorder, severe, in early remission
        Alcohol use disorder, severe, in sustained remission

√6th **F10.22**   **Alcohol dependence with** intoxication
        Acute drunkenness (in alcoholism)
     EXCLUDES 2   alcohol dependence with withdrawal (F10.23-)

     F10.220   **Alcohol dependence with intoxication,** uncomplicated   `HCC`

     F10.221   **Alcohol dependence with intoxication** delirium   `CC` `HCC`

     F10.229   **Alcohol dependence with intoxication,** unspecified   `HCC`

√6th **F10.23**   **Alcohol dependence with** withdrawal

     EXCLUDES 2   alcohol dependence with intoxication (F10.22-)

AHA: 2018, 1Q, 16; 2015, 2Q, 15
TIP: Do not assign a code from this subcategory when documentation indicates alcohol withdrawal without dependence.

     F10.230   **Alcohol dependence with withdrawal,** uncomplicated   `CC` `HCC`

     F10.231   **Alcohol dependence with withdrawal** delirium   `CC` `HCC`

     F10.232   **Alcohol dependence with withdrawal with** perceptual disturbance   `CC` `HCC`

     F10.239   **Alcohol dependence with withdrawal,** unspecified   `CC` `HCC`

F10.24   **Alcohol dependence with alcohol-induced** mood disorder   `CC` `HCC`
        Alcohol use disorder, moderate, with alcohol-induced bipolar or related disorder
        Alcohol use disorder, moderate, with alcohol-induced depressive disorder
        Alcohol use disorder, severe, with alcohol-induced bipolar or related disorder
        Alcohol use disorder, severe, with alcohol-induced depressive disorder

√6th **F10.25**   **Alcohol dependence with alcohol-induced** psychotic disorder

     F10.250   **Alcohol dependence with alcohol-induced psychotic disorder with** delusions   `HCC`

     F10.251   **Alcohol dependence with alcohol-induced psychotic disorder with** hallucinations   `CC` `HCC`

     F10.259   **Alcohol dependence with alcohol-induced psychotic disorder,** unspecified   `CC` `HCC`

F10.26   **Alcohol dependence with alcohol-induced** persisting amnestic disorder   `HCC`
        Alcohol use disorder, moderate, with alcohol-induced major neurocognitive disorder, amnestic-confabulatory type
        Alcohol use disorder, severe, with alcohol-induced major neurocognitive disorder, amnestic-confabulatory type
        DEF: Prominent and lasting reduced memory span and disordered time appreciation and confabulation that occurs in alcoholics as sequel to acute alcoholic psychosis.

F10.27   **Alcohol dependence with alcohol-induced** persisting dementia   `CC` `HCC`
        Alcohol use disorder, moderate, with alcohol-induced major neurocognitive disorder, nonamnestic-confabulatory type
        Alcohol use disorder, severe, with alcohol-induced major neurocognitive disorder, nonamnestic-confabulatory type

√6th **F10.28**   **Alcohol dependence with** other **alcohol-induced disorders**

     F10.280   **Alcohol dependence with alcohol-induced** anxiety disorder   `CC` `HCC`

     F10.281   **Alcohol dependence with alcohol-induced** sexual dysfunction   `CC` `HCC`

     F10.282   **Alcohol dependence with alcohol-induced** sleep disorder   `HCC`

     F10.288   **Alcohol dependence with** other **alcohol-induced disorder**   `CC` `HCC`
        Alcohol use disorder, moderate, with alcohol-induced mild neurocognitive disorder
        Alcohol use disorder, severe, with alcohol-induced mild neurocognitive disorder

F10.29   **Alcohol dependence with** unspecified **alcohol-induced disorder**   `CC` `HCC`

`N` Newborn: 0   `P` Pediatric: 0-17   `M` Maternity: 12-55   `A` Adult: 15-124   `MCC` Major Complication/Comorbidity   `CC` Complication/Comorbidity   `SW` Severe Wound Dx

538   ICD-10-CM 2019

✓5th **F10.9** **Alcohol** use, unspecified
     EXCLUDES 1   *alcohol abuse (F10.1-)*
                 alcohol dependence (F10.2-)
     AHA: 2018, 2Q, 10-11

   ✓6th **F10.92** **Alcohol use, unspecified with** intoxication

     F10.920 **Alcohol use, unspecified with**   HCC
                 intoxication, **uncomplicated**
                 AHA: 2018, 2Q, 10-11

     F10.921 **Alcohol use, unspecified with**   CC HCC
                 intoxication delirium

     F10.929 **Alcohol use, unspecified with**   HCC
                 intoxication, **unspecified**

   F10.94 **Alcohol use, unspecified with**   CC HCC
     alcohol-induced mood disorder
       Alcohol induced bipolar or related disorder, without
         use disorder
       Alcohol induced depressive disorder, without use
         disorder

   ✓6th **F10.95** **Alcohol use, unspecified with alcohol-induced**
     psychotic disorder

     F10.950 **Alcohol use, unspecified with**   HCC
                 alcohol-induced psychotic disorder
                 with delusions

     F10.951 **Alcohol use, unspecified with**   CC HCC
                 alcohol-induced psychotic disorder
                 with hallucinations

     F10.959 **Alcohol use, unspecified with**   CC HCC
                 alcohol-induced psychotic disorder,
                 unspecified
                   Alcohol-induced psychotic disorder
                     without use disorder

   F10.96 **Alcohol use, unspecified with alcohol-induced**   HCC
     persisting amnestic disorder
       Alcohol-induced major neurocognitive disorder,
         amnestic-confabulatory type, without use
         disorder

   F10.97 **Alcohol use, unspecified with alcohol-induced**   HCC
     persisting dementia
       Alcohol-induced major neurocognitive disorder,
         nonamnestic-confabulatory type, without use
         disorder

   ✓6th **F10.98** **Alcohol use,** unspecified **with other alcohol-induced**
     disorders

     F10.980 **Alcohol use, unspecified with**   CC HCC
                 alcohol-induced anxiety disorder
                   Alcohol induced anxiety disorder, without
                     use disorder

     F10.981 **Alcohol use, unspecified with**   CC HCC
                 alcohol-induced sexual dysfunction
                   Alcohol induced sexual dysfunction,
                     without use disorder

     F10.982 **Alcohol use, unspecified with**   HCC
                 alcohol-induced sleep disorder
                   Alcohol induced sleep disorder, without
                     use disorder

     F10.988 **Alcohol use, unspecified with**   CC HCC
                 other alcohol-induced disorder
                   Alcohol induced mild neurocognitive
                     disorder, without use disorder

   F10.99 **Alcohol use, unspecified with** unspecified   CC HCC
     alcohol-induced disorder

✓4th **F11** **Opioid** related disorders

   CC Excl: For CC codes in category F11, unless otherwise noted:
   PDX collection 550

✓5th **F11.1** **Opioid** abuse
     EXCLUDES 1   *opioid dependence (F11.2-)*
                 opioid use, unspecified (F11.9-)

   F11.10 **Opioid abuse,** uncomplicated
     Opioid use disorder, mild

   F11.11 **Opioid abuse,** in remission
     Opioid use disorder, mild, in early remission
     Opioid use disorder, mild, in sustained remission

   ✓6th **F11.12** **Opioid abuse with** intoxication

     F11.120 **Opioid abuse with intoxication,**   HCC
                 uncomplicated

     F11.121 **Opioid abuse with intoxication**   CC HCC
                 delirium

     F11.122 **Opioid abuse with intoxication with**   HCC
                 perceptual disturbance

     F11.129 **Opioid abuse with intoxication,**   HCC
                 unspecified

   F11.14 **Opioid abuse with opioid-induced** mood   HCC
     disorder
       Opioid use disorder, mild, with opioid-induced
         depressive disorder

   ✓6th **F11.15** **Opioid abuse with opioid-induced** psychotic
     disorder

     F11.150 **Opioid abuse with opioid-induced**   CC HCC
                 psychotic disorder with delusions

     F11.151 **Opioid abuse with opioid-induced**   CC HCC
                 psychotic disorder with hallucinations

     F11.159 **Opioid abuse with opioid-induced**   HCC
                 psychotic disorder, unspecified

   ✓6th **F11.18** **Opioid abuse with** other **opioid-induced disorder**

     F11.181 **Opioid abuse with opioid-induced**   HCC
                 sexual dysfunction

     F11.182 **Opioid abuse with opioid-induced**   HCC
                 sleep disorder

     F11.188 **Opioid abuse with** other   HCC
                 opioid-induced disorder

   F11.19 **Opioid abuse with** unspecified **opioid-induced**   HCC
     disorder

✓5th **F11.2** **Opioid** dependence
     EXCLUDES 1   *opioid abuse (F11.1-)*
                 opioid use, unspecified (F11.9-)
     EXCLUDES 2   *opioid poisoning (T40.0-T40.2-)*

   F11.20 **Opioid dependence,** uncomplicated   CC HCC
     Opioid use disorder, moderate
     Opioid use disorder, severe
     CC Excl: No Excl

   F11.21 **Opioid dependence,** in remission   HCC
     Opioid use disorder, moderate, in early remission
     Opioid use disorder, moderate, in sustained remission
     Opioid use disorder, severe, in early remission
     Opioid use disorder, severe, in sustained remission

   ✓6th **F11.22** **Opioid dependence with** intoxication
     EXCLUDES 1   *opioid dependence with withdrawal (F11.23)*

     F11.220 **Opioid dependence with intoxication,** HCC
                 uncomplicated

     F11.221 **Opioid dependence with**   CC HCC
                 intoxication delirium

     F11.222 **Opioid dependence with**   CC HCC
                 intoxication with perceptual
                 disturbance
                 CC Excl: No Excl

     F11.229 **Opioid dependence with intoxication,** HCC
                 unspecified

   F11.23 **Opioid dependence with** withdrawal   CC HCC
     EXCLUDES 1   *opioid dependence with intoxication*
                 (F11.22-)

   F11.24 **Opioid dependence with opioid-induced**   HCC
     mood disorder
       Opioid use disorder, moderate, with opioid induced
         depressive disorder

   ✓6th **F11.25** **Opioid dependence with opioid-induced**
     psychotic disorder

     F11.250 **Opioid dependence with**   CC HCC
                 opioid-induced psychotic disorder
                 with delusions

     F11.251 **Opioid dependence with opioid-**   CC HCC
                 induced psychotic disorder
                 with hallucinations

     F11.259 **Opioid dependence with opioid-**   CC HCC
                 induced psychotic disorder, unspecified
                 CC Excl: No Excl

   ✓6th **F11.28** **Opioid dependence with** other **opioid-induced**
     disorder

     F11.281 **Opioid dependence with opioid-**   CC HCC
                 induced sexual dysfunction
                 CC Excl: No Excl

     F11.282 **Opioid dependence with**   CC HCC
                 opioid-induced sleep disorder
                 CC Excl: No Excl

     F11.288 **Opioid dependence with** other   CC HCC
                 opioid-induced disorder
                 CC Excl: No Excl

   F11.29 **Opioid dependence with** unspecified   HCC
     opioid-induced disorder

✔ Additional Character Required   ✓x7th Placeholder   Unacceptable PDx   Questionable PDx   Manifestation   H1 - H14 HAC   HCC CMS-HCC Dx   HIV HIV Dx

ICD-10-CM 2019   539

Chapter 5. Mental, Behavioral and Neurodevelopmental Disorders

✓5ᵗʰ **F11.9 Opioid use, unspecified**
- EXCLUDES 1   *opioid abuse (F11.1-)*
       opioid dependence (F11.2-)

   F11.90 Opioid use, unspecified, uncomplicated
     AHA: 2018, 2Q, 10-11

✓6ᵗʰ **F11.92 Opioid use, unspecified with intoxication**
- EXCLUDES 1   *opioid use, unspecified with withdrawal (F11.93)*

     F11.920 Opioid use, unspecified with intoxication, uncomplicated HCC
     F11.921 Opioid use, unspecified with intoxication delirium CC HCC
       Opioid-induced delirium
     F11.922 Opioid use, unspecified with intoxication with perceptual disturbance HCC
     F11.929 Opioid use, unspecified with intoxication, unspecified HCC

   F11.93 Opioid use, unspecified with withdrawal CC HCC
- EXCLUDES 1   *opioid use, unspecified with intoxication (F11.92-)*

   F11.94 Opioid use, unspecified with opioid-induced mood disorder HCC
     Opioid induced depressive disorder, without use disorder

✓6ᵗʰ **F11.95 Opioid use, unspecified with opioid-induced psychotic disorder**
     F11.950 Opioid use, unspecified with opioid-induced psychotic disorder with delusions CC HCC
     F11.951 Opioid use, unspecified with opioid-induced psychotic disorder with hallucinations CC HCC
     F11.959 Opioid use, unspecified with opioid-induced psychotic disorder, unspecified HCC

✓6ᵗʰ **F11.98 Opioid use, unspecified with other specified opioid-induced disorder**
     F11.981 Opioid use, unspecified with opioid-induced sexual dysfunction HCC
       Opioid induced sexual dysfunction, without use disorder
     F11.982 Opioid use, unspecified with opioid-induced sleep disorder HCC
       Opioid induced sleep disorder, without use disorder
     F11.988 Opioid use, unspecified with other opioid-induced disorder HCC
       Opioid induced anxiety disorder, without use disorder

   F11.99 Opioid use, unspecified with unspecified opioid-induced disorder HCC

✓4ᵗʰ **F12 Cannabis related disorders**
- INCLUDES   marijuana

CC Excl: For CC codes in category F12: PDX collection 550

✓5ᵗʰ **F12.1 Cannabis abuse**
- EXCLUDES 1   *cannabis dependence (F12.2-)*
       cannabis use, unspecified (F12.9-)

   F12.10 Cannabis abuse, uncomplicated
     Cannabis use disorder, mild

   F12.11 Cannabis abuse, in remission
     Cannabis use disorder, mild, in early remission
     Cannabis use disorder, mild, in sustained remission

✓6ᵗʰ **F12.12 Cannabis abuse with intoxication**
     F12.120 Cannabis abuse with intoxication, uncomplicated HCC
     F12.121 Cannabis abuse with intoxication delirium CC HCC
     F12.122 Cannabis abuse with intoxication with perceptual disturbance HCC
     F12.129 Cannabis abuse with intoxication, unspecified HCC

✓6ᵗʰ **F12.15 Cannabis abuse with psychotic disorder**
     F12.150 Cannabis abuse with psychotic disorder with delusions CC HCC
     F12.151 Cannabis abuse with psychotic disorder with hallucinations CC HCC
     F12.159 Cannabis abuse with psychotic disorder, unspecified HCC

✓6ᵗʰ **F12.18 Cannabis abuse with other cannabis-induced disorder**
     F12.180 Cannabis abuse with cannabis-induced anxiety disorder HCC
     F12.188 Cannabis abuse with other cannabis-induced disorder HCC
       Cannabis use disorder, mild, with cannabis-induced sleep disorder

   F12.19 Cannabis abuse with unspecified cannabis-induced disorder HCC

✓5ᵗʰ **F12.2 Cannabis dependence**
- EXCLUDES 1   *cannabis abuse (F12.1-)*
       cannabis use, unspecified (F12.9-)
- EXCLUDES 2   *cannabis poisoning (T40.7-)*

   F12.20 Cannabis dependence, uncomplicated HCC
     Cannabis use disorder, moderate
     Cannabis use disorder, severe

   F12.21 Cannabis dependence, in remission HCC
     Cannabis use disorder, moderate, in early remission
     Cannabis use disorder, moderate, in sustained remission
     Cannabis use disorder, severe, in early remission
     Cannabis use disorder, severe, in sustained remission

✓6ᵗʰ **F12.22 Cannabis dependence with intoxication**
     F12.220 Cannabis dependence with intoxication, uncomplicated HCC
     F12.221 Cannabis dependence with intoxication delirium CC HCC
     F12.222 Cannabis dependence with intoxication with perceptual disturbance HCC
     F12.229 Cannabis dependence with intoxication, unspecified HCC

   ● **F12.23 Cannabis dependence with withdrawal**

✓6ᵗʰ **F12.25 Cannabis dependence with psychotic disorder**
     F12.250 Cannabis dependence with psychotic disorder with delusions CC HCC
     F12.251 Cannabis dependence with psychotic disorder with hallucinations CC HCC
     F12.259 Cannabis dependence with psychotic disorder, unspecified HCC

✓6ᵗʰ **F12.28 Cannabis dependence with other cannabis-induced disorder**
     F12.280 Cannabis dependence with cannabis-induced anxiety disorder HCC
     F12.288 Cannabis dependence with other cannabis-induced disorder HCC
       Cannabis use disorder, moderate, with cannabis-induced sleep disorder
       Cannabis use disorder, severe, with cannabis-induced sleep disorder
       ~~Cannabis withdrawal~~

   F12.29 Cannabis dependence with unspecified cannabis-induced disorder HCC

✓5ᵗʰ **F12.9 Cannabis use, unspecified**
- EXCLUDES 1   *cannabis abuse (F12.1-)*
       cannabis dependence (F12.2-)

   F12.90 Cannabis use, unspecified, uncomplicated
     AHA: 2018, 2Q, 10-11

✓6ᵗʰ **F12.92 Cannabis use, unspecified with intoxication**
     F12.920 Cannabis use, unspecified with intoxication, uncomplicated HCC
     F12.921 Cannabis use, unspecified with intoxication delirium CC HCC
     F12.922 Cannabis use, unspecified with intoxication with perceptual disturbance HCC
     F12.929 Cannabis use, unspecified with intoxication, unspecified HCC

   ● **F12.93 Cannabis use, unspecified with withdrawal**

✓6ᵗʰ **F12.95 Cannabis use, unspecified with psychotic disorder**
     F12.950 Cannabis use, unspecified with psychotic disorder with delusions CC HCC
     F12.951 Cannabis use, unspecified with psychotic disorder with hallucinations CC HCC
     F12.959 Cannabis use, unspecified with psychotic disorder, unspecified HCC
       Cannabis induced psychotic disorder, without use disorder

---

N Newborn: 0   P Pediatric: 0-17   M Maternity: 12-55   A Adult: 15-124   MCC Major Complication/Comorbidity   CC Complication/Comorbidity   SW Severe Wound Dx

✓6th **F12.98** **Cannabis use, unspecified with** other **cannabis-induced disorder**

    F12.980 **Cannabis use, unspecified with** `HCC` **anxiety disorder**
        Cannabis induced anxiety disorder, without use disorder

    F12.988 **Cannabis use, unspecified with** other `HCC` **cannabis-induced disorder**
        Cannabis induced sleep disorder, without use disorder

    F12.99 **Cannabis use, unspecified with** unspecified `HCC` **cannabis-induced disorder**

✓4th **F13** Sedative, hypnotic, or anxiolytic **related disorders**

    CC Excl: For CC codes in category F13, unless otherwise noted: PDX collection 550

✓5th **F13.1** **Sedative, hypnotic or anxiolytic-related** abuse

    EXCLUDES 1 *sedative, hypnotic or anxiolytic-related dependence (F13.2-)*
        sedative, hypnotic, or anxiolytic use, unspecified (F13.9-)

    F13.10 **Sedative, hypnotic or anxiolytic abuse,** uncomplicated
        Sedative, hypnotic, or anxiolytic use disorder, mild

    F13.11 **Sedative, hypnotic or anxiolytic abuse,** in remission
        Sedative, hypnotic or anxiolytic use disorder, mild, in early remission
        Sedative, hypnotic or anxiolytic use disorder, mild, in sustained remission

✓6th **F13.12** **Sedative, hypnotic or anxiolytic abuse with** intoxication

    F13.120 **Sedative, hypnotic or anxiolytic abuse** `HCC` **with intoxication,** uncomplicated

    F13.121 **Sedative, hypnotic or anxiolytic** `CC` `HCC` **abuse with intoxication** delirium

    F13.129 **Sedative, hypnotic or anxiolytic abuse** `HCC` **with intoxication,** unspecified

    F13.14 **Sedative, hypnotic or anxiolytic abuse with** `HCC` **sedative, hypnotic or anxiolytic-induced** mood disorder
        Sedative, hypnotic, or anxiolytic use disorder, mild, with sedative, hypnotic, or anxiolytic-induced bipolar or related disorder
        Sedative, hypnotic, or anxiolytic use disorder, mild, with sedative, hypnotic, or anxiolytic-induced depressive disorder

✓6th **F13.15** **Sedative, hypnotic or anxiolytic abuse with sedative, hypnotic or anxiolytic-induced** psychotic disorder

    F13.150 **Sedative, hypnotic or anxiolytic** `CC` `HCC` **abuse with sedative, hypnotic or anxiolytic-induced psychotic disorder with** delusions

    F13.151 **Sedative, hypnotic or anxiolytic** `CC` `HCC` **abuse with sedative, hypnotic or anxiolytic-induced psychotic disorder with** hallucinations

    F13.159 **Sedative, hypnotic or anxiolytic abuse** `HCC` **with sedative, hypnotic or anxiolytic-induced psychotic disorder,** unspecified

✓6th **F13.18** **Sedative, hypnotic or anxiolytic abuse with** other **sedative, hypnotic or anxiolytic-induced disorders**

    F13.180 **Sedative, hypnotic or anxiolytic** `HCC` **abuse with sedative, hypnotic or anxiolytic-induced** anxiety disorder

    F13.181 **Sedative, hypnotic or anxiolytic** `HCC` **abuse with sedative, hypnotic or anxiolytic-induced** sexual dysfunction

    F13.182 **Sedative, hypnotic or anxiolytic** `HCC` **abuse with sedative, hypnotic or anxiolytic-induced** sleep disorder

    F13.188 **Sedative, hypnotic or anxiolytic** `HCC` **abuse with** other **sedative, hypnotic or anxiolytic-induced disorder**

    F13.19 **Sedative, hypnotic or anxiolytic abuse with** `HCC` unspecified **sedative, hypnotic or anxiolytic-induced disorder**

✓5th **F13.2** **Sedative, hypnotic or anxiolytic-related** dependence

    EXCLUDES 1 *sedative, hypnotic or anxiolytic-related abuse (F13.1-)*
        sedative, hypnotic, or anxiolytic use, unspecified (F13.9-)
    EXCLUDES 2 *sedative, hypnotic, or anxiolytic poisoning (T42.-)*

    F13.20 **Sedative, hypnotic or anxiolytic dependence,** `CC` `HCC` **uncomplicated**
        CC Excl: No Excl

    F13.21 **Sedative, hypnotic or anxiolytic dependence, in** `HCC` **remission**
        Sedative, hypnotic or anxiolytic use disorder, moderate, in early remission
        Sedative, hypnotic or anxiolytic use disorder, moderate, in sustained remission
        Sedative, hypnotic or anxiolytic use disorder, severe, in early remission
        Sedative, hypnotic or anxiolytic use disorder, severe, in sustained remission

✓6th **F13.22** **Sedative, hypnotic or anxiolytic dependence with** intoxication

    EXCLUDES 1 *sedative, hypnotic or anxiolytic dependence with withdrawal (F13.23-)*

    F13.220 **Sedative, hypnotic or anxiolytic** `HCC` **dependence with intoxication,** uncomplicated

    F13.221 **Sedative, hypnotic or anxiolytic** `CC` `HCC` **dependence with intoxication** delirium

    F13.229 **Sedative, hypnotic or anxiolytic** `HCC` **dependence with intoxication,** unspecified

✓6th **F13.23** **Sedative, hypnotic or anxiolytic dependence with** withdrawal
        Sedative, hypnotic, or anxiolytic use disorder, moderate
        Sedative, hypnotic, or anxiolytic use disorder, severe

    EXCLUDES 1 *sedative, hypnotic or anxiolytic dependence with intoxication (F13.22-)*

    F13.230 **Sedative, hypnotic or anxiolytic** `CC` `HCC` **dependence with withdrawal,** uncomplicated

    F13.231 **Sedative, hypnotic or anxiolytic** `CC` `HCC` **dependence with withdrawal** delirium

    F13.232 **Sedative, hypnotic or anxiolytic** `CC` `HCC` **dependence with withdrawal with** perceptual disturbance
        Sedative, hypnotic, or anxiolytic withdrawal with perceptual disturbances

    F13.239 **Sedative, hypnotic or anxiolytic** `CC` `HCC` **dependence with withdrawal,** unspecified
        Sedative, hypnotic, or anxiolytic withdrawal without perceptual disturbances

    F13.24 **Sedative, hypnotic or anxiolytic dependence** `HCC` **with sedative, hypnotic or anxiolytic-induced** mood disorder
        Sedative, hypnotic, or anxiolytic use disorder, moderate, with sedative, hypnotic, or anxiolytic-induced bipolar or related disorder
        Sedative, hypnotic, or anxiolytic use disorder, moderate, with sedative, hypnotic, or anxiolytic-induced depressive disorder
        Sedative, hypnotic, or anxiolytic use disorder, severe, with sedative, hypnotic, or anxiolytic-induced bipolar or related disorder
        Sedative, hypnotic, or anxiolytic use disorder, severe, with sedative, hypnotic, or anxiolytic-induced depressive disorder

✓6th **F13.25** **Sedative, hypnotic or anxiolytic dependence with sedative, hypnotic or anxiolytic-induced** psychotic disorder

    F13.250 **Sedative, hypnotic or anxiolytic** `CC` `HCC` **dependence with sedative, hypnotic or anxiolytic-induced psychotic disorder with** delusions

    F13.251 **Sedative, hypnotic or anxiolytic** `CC` `HCC` **dependence with sedative, hypnotic or anxiolytic-induced psychotic disorder with** hallucinations

✓ Additional Character Required   ✓x7th Placeholder   Unacceptable PDx   Questionable PDx   Manifestation   `H1`-`H14` HAC   `HCC` CMS-HCC Dx   `HIV` HIV Dx

ICD-10-CM 2019   **541**

F13.259   Sedative, hypnotic or anxiolytic   `CC` `HCC`
dependence with sedative, hypnotic or
anxiolytic-induced psychotic disorder,
unspecified
    CC Excl: No Excl

F13.26   Sedative, hypnotic or anxiolytic dependence   `CC` `HCC`
with sedative, hypnotic or anxiolytic-induced
persisting amnestic disorder
    CC Excl: No Excl

F13.27   Sedative, hypnotic or anxiolytic dependence   `CC` `HCC`
with sedative, hypnotic or anxiolytic-induced
persisting dementia
    Sedative, hypnotic, or anxiolytic use disorder,
moderate, with sedative, hypnotic, or anxiolytic-
induced major neurocognitive disorder
    Sedative, hypnotic, or anxiolytic use disorder, severe,
with sedative, hypnotic, or anxiolytic-induced
major neurocognitive disorder

✓6ᵗʰ **F13.28**   Sedative, hypnotic or anxiolytic dependence with
other sedative, hypnotic or anxiolytic-induced
disorders

    F13.280   Sedative, hypnotic or anxiolytic   `CC` `HCC`
dependence with sedative, hypnotic or
anxiolytic-induced anxiety disorder
       CC Excl: No Excl

    F13.281   Sedative, hypnotic or anxiolytic   `CC` `HCC`
dependence with sedative, hypnotic or
anxiolytic-induced sexual dysfunction
       CC Excl: No Excl

    F13.282   Sedative, hypnotic or anxiolytic   `CC` `HCC`
dependence with sedative, hypnotic or
anxiolytic-induced sleep disorder
       CC Excl: No Excl

    F13.288   Sedative, hypnotic or anxiolytic   `CC` `HCC`
dependence with other sedative,
hypnotic or anxiolytic-induced disorder
       Sedative, hypnotic, or anxiolytic use
disorder, moderate, with sedative,
hypnotic, or anxiolytic-induced mild
neurocognitive disorder
       Sedative, hypnotic, or anxiolytic use
disorder, severe, with sedative,
hypnotic, or anxiolytic-induced mild
neurocognitive disorder
       CC Excl: No Excl

F13.29   Sedative, hypnotic or anxiolytic dependence   `HCC`
with unspecified sedative, hypnotic or anxiolytic-
induced disorder

✓5ᵗʰ **F13.9**   Sedative, hypnotic or anxiolytic-related use, unspecified
    `EXCLUDES 1`   sedative, hypnotic or anxiolytic-related abuse (F13.1-)
              sedative, hypnotic or anxiolytic-related dependence
(F13.2-)

    F13.90   Sedative, hypnotic, or anxiolytic use, unspecified,
uncomplicated
       AHA: 2018, 2Q, 10-11

✓6ᵗʰ **F13.92**   Sedative, hypnotic or anxiolytic use, unspecified
with intoxication
    `EXCLUDES 1`   sedative, hypnotic or anxiolytic use,
unspecified with withdrawal (F13.93-)

    F13.920   Sedative, hypnotic or anxiolytic use,   `HCC`
unspecified with intoxication,
uncomplicated

    F13.921   Sedative, hypnotic or anxiolytic   `CC` `HCC`
use, unspecified with intoxication
delirium
       Sedative, hypnotic, or anxiolytic-induced
delirium

    F13.929   Sedative, hypnotic or anxiolytic use,   `HCC`
unspecified with intoxication,
unspecified

✓6ᵗʰ **F13.93**   Sedative, hypnotic or anxiolytic use, unspecified
with withdrawal
    `EXCLUDES 1`   sedative, hypnotic or anxiolytic use,
unspecified with intoxication (F13.92-)

    F13.930   Sedative, hypnotic or anxiolytic   `CC` `HCC`
use, unspecified with withdrawal,
uncomplicated

    F13.931   Sedative, hypnotic or anxiolytic   `CC` `HCC`
use, unspecified with withdrawal
delirium

F13.932   Sedative, hypnotic or anxiolytic   `CC` `HCC`
use, unspecified with withdrawal
with perceptual disturbances

F13.939   Sedative, hypnotic or anxiolytic   `CC` `HCC`
use, unspecified with withdrawal,
unspecified

F13.94   Sedative, hypnotic or anxiolytic use,   `HCC`
unspecified with sedative, hypnotic or
anxiolytic-induced mood disorder
    Sedative, hypnotic, or anxiolytic-induced bipolar or
related disorder, without use disorder
    Sedative, hypnotic, or anxiolytic-induced depressive
disorder, without use disorder

✓6ᵗʰ **F13.95**   Sedative, hypnotic or anxiolytic use, unspecified
with sedative, hypnotic or anxiolytic-induced
psychotic disorder

    F13.950   Sedative, hypnotic or anxiolytic   `CC` `HCC`
use, unspecified with sedative, hypnotic
or anxiolytic-induced psychotic disorder
with delusions

    F13.951   Sedative, hypnotic or anxiolytic   `CC` `HCC`
use, unspecified with sedative, hypnotic
or anxiolytic-induced psychotic disorder
with hallucinations

    F13.959   Sedative, hypnotic or anxiolytic use,   `HCC`
unspecified with sedative, hypnotic or
anxiolytic-induced psychotic disorder,
unspecified
       Sedative, hypnotic, or anxiolytic-induced
psychotic disorder, without use
disorder

F13.96   Sedative, hypnotic or anxiolytic use, unspecified   `HCC`
with sedative, hypnotic or anxiolytic-induced
persisting amnestic disorder

F13.97   Sedative, hypnotic or anxiolytic use,   `CC` `HCC`
unspecified with sedative, hypnotic or anxiolytic-
induced persisting dementia
    Sedative, hypnotic, or anxiolytic-induced major
neurocognitive disorder, without use disorder

✓6ᵗʰ **F13.98**   Sedative, hypnotic or anxiolytic use, unspecified
with other sedative, hypnotic or anxiolytic-induced
disorders

    F13.980   Sedative, hypnotic or anxiolytic use,   `HCC`
unspecified with sedative, hypnotic or
anxiolytic-induced anxiety disorder
       Sedative, hypnotic, or anxiolytic-induced
anxiety disorder, without use disorder

    F13.981   Sedative, hypnotic or anxiolytic use,   `HCC`
unspecified with sedative, hypnotic or
anxiolytic-induced sexual dysfunction
       Sedative, hypnotic, or anxiolytic-induced
sexual dysfunction disorder, without
use disorder

    F13.982   Sedative, hypnotic or anxiolytic use,   `HCC`
unspecified with sedative, hypnotic or
anxiolytic-induced sleep disorder
       Sedative, hypnotic, or anxiolytic-induced
sleep disorder, without use disorder

    F13.988   Sedative, hypnotic or anxiolytic use,   `HCC`
unspecified with other sedative,
hypnotic or anxiolytic-induced disorder
       Sedative, hypnotic, or anxiolytic-induced
mild neurocognitive disorder

F13.99   Sedative, hypnotic or anxiolytic use, unspecified   `HCC`
with unspecified sedative, hypnotic or anxiolytic-
induced disorder

✓4ᵗʰ **F14**   **Cocaine related disorders**
    `EXCLUDES 2`   other stimulant-related disorders (F15.-)

    CC Excl: For CC codes in category F14, unless otherwise noted:
PDX collection 550

✓5ᵗʰ **F14.1**   **Cocaine abuse**
    `EXCLUDES 1`   cocaine dependence (F14.2-)
              cocaine use, unspecified (F14.9-)

    F14.10   Cocaine abuse, uncomplicated
       Cocaine use disorder, mild

    F14.11   Cocaine abuse, in remission
       Cocaine use disorder, mild, in early remission
       Cocaine use disorder, mild, in sustained remission

✓6ᵗʰ **F14.12**   **Cocaine abuse with** intoxication

     F14.120   **Cocaine abuse with intoxication,** HCC
            uncomplicated

     F14.121   **Cocaine abuse with intoxication** CC HCC
            with delirium

     F14.122   **Cocaine abuse with intoxication** HCC
            with perceptual disturbance

     F14.129   **Cocaine abuse with intoxication,** HCC
            unspecified

F14.14   **Cocaine abuse with cocaine-induced** mood HCC
     disorder
     Cocaine use disorder, mild, with cocaine-induced
     bipolar or related disorder
     Cocaine use disorder, mild, with cocaine-induced
     depressive disorder

✓6ᵗʰ **F14.15**   **Cocaine abuse with cocaine-induced** psychotic
     disorder

     F14.150   **Cocaine abuse with cocaine-** CC HCC
            induced psychotic disorder with delusions

     F14.151   **Cocaine abuse with cocaine-** CC HCC
            induced psychotic disorder with
            hallucinations

     F14.159   **Cocaine abuse with cocaine-induced** HCC
            psychotic disorder, unspecified

✓6ᵗʰ **F14.18**   **Cocaine abuse with** other **cocaine-induced disorder**

     F14.180   **Cocaine abuse with cocaine-induced** HCC
            anxiety disorder

     F14.181   **Cocaine abuse with cocaine-induced** HCC
            sexual dysfunction

     F14.182   **Cocaine abuse with cocaine-induced** HCC
            sleep disorder

     F14.188   **Cocaine abuse with** other **cocaine-** HCC
            induced disorder
            Cocaine use disorder, mild, with cocaine-
            induced obsessive compulsive or
            related disorder

F14.19   **Cocaine abuse with** unspecified **cocaine-** HCC
     induced disorder

✓5ᵗʰ **F14.2**   **Cocaine** dependence

     EXCLUDES 1   *cocaine abuse (F14.1-)*
                cocaine use, unspecified (F14.9-)

     EXCLUDES 2   *cocaine poisoning (T40.5-)*

     F14.20   **Cocaine dependence,** uncomplicated CC HCC
            Cocaine use disorder, moderate
            Cocaine use disorder, severe
            CC Excl: No Excl

     F14.21   **Cocaine dependence, in remission** HCC
            Cocaine use disorder, moderate, in early remission
            Cocaine use disorder, moderate, in sustained
            remission
            Cocaine use disorder, severe, in early remission
            Cocaine use disorder, severe, in sustained remission

✓6ᵗʰ **F14.22**   **Cocaine dependence with** intoxication

     EXCLUDES 1   *cocaine dependence with withdrawal*
                (F14.23)

     F14.220   **Cocaine dependence with** HCC
            intoxication, uncomplicated

     F14.221   **Cocaine dependence with** CC HCC
            intoxication delirium

     F14.222   **Cocaine dependence with** CC HCC
            intoxication with perceptual
            disturbance
            CC Excl: No Excl

     F14.229   **Cocaine dependence with** CC HCC
            intoxication, unspecified
            CC Excl: No Excl

     F14.23   **Cocaine dependence with** withdrawal CC HCC
            EXCLUDES 1   *cocaine dependence with intoxication*
                    (F14.22-)

     F14.24   **Cocaine dependence with cocaine-induced** HCC
         mood disorder
         Cocaine use disorder, moderate, with cocaine-induced
         bipolar or related disorder
         Cocaine use disorder, moderate, with cocaine-induced
         depressive disorder
         Cocaine use disorder, severe, with cocaine-induced
         bipolar or related disorder
         Cocaine use disorder, severe, with cocaine-induced
         depressive disorder

✓6ᵗʰ **F14.25**   **Cocaine dependence with cocaine-induced**
     psychotic disorder

     F14.250   **Cocaine dependence with** CC HCC
            cocaine-induced psychotic disorder
            with delusions

     F14.251   **Cocaine dependence with** CC HCC
            cocaine-induced psychotic disorder
            with hallucinations

     F14.259   **Cocaine dependence with** CC HCC
            cocaine-induced psychotic disorder,
            unspecified
            CC Excl: No Excl

✓6ᵗʰ **F14.28**   **Cocaine dependence with** other **cocaine-induced**
     disorder

     F14.280   **Cocaine dependence with** CC HCC
            cocaine-induced anxiety disorder
            CC Excl: No Excl

     F14.281   **Cocaine dependence with** CC HCC
            cocaine-induced sexual dysfunction
            CC Excl: No Excl

     F14.282   **Cocaine dependence with** CC HCC
            cocaine-induced sleep disorder
            CC Excl: No Excl

     F14.288   **Cocaine dependence with** other CC HCC
            cocaine-induced disorder
            Cocaine use disorder, moderate, with
            cocaine-induced obsessive
            compulsive or related disorder
            Cocaine use disorder, severe, with cocaine-
            induced obsessive compulsive or
            related disorder
            CC Excl: No Excl

     F14.29   **Cocaine dependence with** unspecified HCC
         cocaine-induced disorder

✓5ᵗʰ **F14.9**   **Cocaine use,** unspecified

     EXCLUDES 1   *cocaine abuse (F14.1-)*
                cocaine dependence (F14.2-)

     F14.90   **Cocaine use, unspecified,** uncomplicated
            AHA: 2018, 2Q, 10-11

✓6ᵗʰ **F14.92**   **Cocaine use, unspecified with** intoxication

     F14.920   **Cocaine use, unspecified with** HCC
            intoxication, uncomplicated

     F14.921   **Cocaine use, unspecified with** CC HCC
            intoxication delirium

     F14.922   **Cocaine use, unspecified with** HCC
            intoxication with perceptual
            disturbance

     F14.929   **Cocaine use, unspecified with** HCC
            intoxication, unspecified

     F14.94   **Cocaine use, unspecified with cocaine-induced** HCC
         mood disorder
         Cocaine induced bipolar or related disorder, without
         use disorder
         Cocaine induced depressive disorder, without use
         disorder

✓6ᵗʰ **F14.95**   **Cocaine use, unspecified with cocaine-induced**
     psychotic disorder

     F14.950   **Cocaine use, unspecified with** CC HCC
            cocaine-induced psychotic disorder
            with delusions

     F14.951   **Cocaine use, unspecified with** CC HCC
            cocaine-induced psychotic disorder
            with hallucinations

     F14.959   **Cocaine use, unspecified with** HCC
            cocaine-induced psychotic disorder,
            unspecified
            Cocaine induced psychotic disorder,
            without use disorder

✓6ᵗʰ **F14.98**   **Cocaine use, unspecified with** other **specified**
     cocaine-induced disorder

     F14.980   **Cocaine use, unspecified with** HCC
            cocaine-induced anxiety disorder
            Cocaine induced anxiety disorder, without
            use disorder

     F14.981   **Cocaine use, unspecified with** HCC
            cocaine-induced sexual dysfunction
            Cocaine induced sexual dysfunction,
            without use disorder

✓ Additional Character Required   ✓×7ᵗʰ Placeholder   Unacceptable PDx   Questionable PDx   Manifestation   H1 - H14 HAC   HCC CMS-HCC Dx   HIV HIV Dx

ICD-10-CM 2019   **543**

F14.982 Cocaine use, unspecified with [HCC]
cocaine-induced sleep disorder
Cocaine induced sleep disorder, without
use disorder

F14.988 Cocaine use, unspecified with other [HCC]
cocaine-induced disorder
Cocaine induced obsessive compulsive or
related disorder

F14.99 Cocaine use, unspecified with unspecified [HCC]
cocaine-induced disorder

✓4th **F15 Other stimulant related disorders**
INCLUDES amphetamine-related disorders
caffeine
EXCLUDES 2 cocaine-related disorders (F14.-)

CC Excl: For CC codes in category F15, unless otherwise noted:
PDX collection 550

✓5th **F15.1 Other stimulant abuse**
EXCLUDES 1 other stimulant dependence (F15.2-)
other stimulant use, unspecified (F15.9-)

F15.10 Other stimulant abuse, uncomplicated
Amphetamine type substance use disorder, mild
Other or unspecified stimulant use disorder, mild

F15.11 Other stimulant abuse, in remission
Amphetamine type substance use disorder, mild, in
early remission
Amphetamine type substance use disorder, mild, in
sustained remission
Other or unspecified stimulant use disorder, mild, in
early remission
Other or unspecified stimulant use disorder, mild, in
sustained remission

✓6th **F15.12 Other stimulant abuse with intoxication**
F15.120 Other stimulant abuse with [HCC]
intoxication, uncomplicated
F15.121 Other stimulant abuse with [CC] [HCC]
intoxication delirium
F15.122 Other stimulant abuse with [HCC]
intoxication with perceptual disturbance
Amphetamine or other stimulant use
disorder, mild, with amphetamine or
other stimulant intoxication, with
perceptual disturbances
F15.129 Other stimulant abuse with [HCC]
intoxication, unspecified
Amphetamine or other stimulant use
disorder, mild, with amphetamine or
other stimulant intoxication, without
perceptual disturbances

F15.14 Other stimulant abuse with stimulant-induced [HCC]
mood disorder
Amphetamine or other stimulant use disorder, mild,
with amphetamine or other stimulant induced
bipolar or related disorder
Amphetamine or other stimulant use disorder, mild,
with amphetamine or other stimulant induced
depressive disorder

✓6th **F15.15 Other stimulant abuse with stimulant-induced**
psychotic disorder
F15.150 Other stimulant abuse with [CC] [HCC]
stimulant-induced psychotic disorder
with delusions
F15.151 Other stimulant abuse with [CC] [HCC]
stimulant-induced psychotic disorder
with hallucinations
F15.159 Other stimulant abuse with [HCC]
stimulant-induced psychotic disorder,
unspecified

✓6th **F15.18 Other stimulant abuse with other stimulant-induced**
disorder
F15.180 Other stimulant abuse with [HCC]
stimulant-induced anxiety disorder
F15.181 Other stimulant abuse with [HCC]
stimulant-induced sexual dysfunction
F15.182 Other stimulant abuse with [HCC]
stimulant-induced sleep disorder

F15.188 Other stimulant abuse with other [HCC]
stimulant-induced disorder
Amphetamine or other stimulant use
disorder, mild, with amphetamine or
other stimulant induced obsessive-
compulsive or related disorder

F15.19 Other stimulant abuse with unspecified [HCC]
stimulant-induced disorder

✓5th **F15.2 Other stimulant dependence**
EXCLUDES 1 other stimulant abuse (F15.1-)
other stimulant use, unspecified (F15.9-)

F15.20 Other stimulant dependence, uncomplicated [CC] [HCC]
Amphetamine type substance use disorder, moderate
Amphetamine type substance use disorder, severe
Other or unspecified stimulant use disorder, moderate
Other or unspecified stimulant use disorder, severe
CC Excl: No Excl

F15.21 Other stimulant dependence, in remission [HCC]
Amphetamine type substance use disorder, moderate,
in early remission
Amphetamine type substance use disorder, moderate,
in sustained remission
Amphetamine type substance use disorder, severe, in
early remission
Amphetamine type substance use disorder, severe, in
sustained remission
Other or unspecified stimulant use disorder,
moderate, in early remission
Other or unspecified stimulant use disorder,
moderate, in sustained remission
Other or unspecified stimulant use disorder, severe, in
early remission
Other or unspecified stimulant use disorder, severe, in
sustained remission

✓6th **F15.22 Other stimulant dependence with intoxication**
EXCLUDES 1 other stimulant dependence with withdrawal
(F15.23)
F15.220 Other stimulant dependence with [HCC]
intoxication, uncomplicated
F15.221 Other stimulant dependence with [CC] [HCC]
intoxication delirium
F15.222 Other stimulant dependence with [CC] [HCC]
intoxication with perceptual disturbance
Amphetamine or other stimulant use
disorder, moderate, with
amphetamine or other stimulant
intoxication, with perceptual
disturbances
Amphetamine or other stimulant use
disorder, severe, with amphetamine or
other stimulant intoxication, with
perceptual disturbances
CC Excl: No Excl
F15.229 Other stimulant dependence with [HCC]
intoxication, unspecified
Amphetamine or other stimulant use
disorder, moderate, with
amphetamine or other stimulant
intoxication, without perceptual
disturbances
Amphetamine or other stimulant use
disorder, severe, with amphetamine or
other stimulant intoxication, without
perceptual disturbances

F15.23 Other stimulant dependence with [CC] [HCC]
withdrawal
Amphetamine or other stimulant withdrawal
EXCLUDES 1 other stimulant dependence with
intoxication (F15.22-)

F15.24 Other stimulant dependence with stimulant- [HCC]
induced mood disorder
Amphetamine or other stimulant use disorder,
moderate, with amphetamine or other stimulant-
induced bipolar or related disorder
Amphetamine or other stimulant use disorder,
moderate, with amphetamine or other stimulant
induced depressive disorder
Amphetamine or other stimulant use disorder, severe,
with amphetamine or other stimulant-induced
bipolar or related disorder
Amphetamine or other stimulant use disorder, severe,
with amphetamine or other stimulant-induced
depressive disorder

✓6th **F15.25　Other stimulant dependence with stimulant-induced** psychotic disorder

　F15.250　Other stimulant dependence with CC HCC **stimulant-induced psychotic disorder with** delusions

　F15.251　Other stimulant dependence with CC HCC **stimulant-induced psychotic disorder with** hallucinations

　F15.259　Other stimulant dependence with CC HCC **stimulant-induced psychotic disorder,** unspecified
　　　CC Excl: No Excl

✓6th **F15.28　Other stimulant dependence with** other stimulant-induced disorder

　F15.280　Other stimulant dependence with CC HCC **stimulant-induced** anxiety disorder
　　　CC Excl: No Excl

　F15.281　Other stimulant dependence with CC HCC **stimulant-induced** sexual dysfunction
　　　CC Excl: No Excl

　F15.282　Other stimulant dependence with CC HCC **stimulant-induced** sleep disorder
　　　CC Excl: No Excl

　F15.288　Other stimulant dependence with CC HCC other **stimulant-induced disorder**
　　　Amphetamine or other stimulant use disorder, moderate, with amphetamine or other stimulant induced obsessive compulsive or related disorder
　　　Amphetamine or other stimulant use disorder, severe, with amphetamine or other stimulant induced obsessive compulsive or related disorder
　　　CC Excl: No Excl

　F15.29　Other stimulant dependence with unspecified HCC **stimulant-induced disorder**

✓5th **F15.9　Other stimulant use,** unspecified
　　EXCLUDES 1　other stimulant abuse (F15.1-)
　　　　　　　other stimulant dependence (F15.2-)

　F15.90　Other stimulant use, unspecified, uncomplicated
　　　AHA: 2018, 2Q, 10-11

✓6th **F15.92　Other stimulant use, unspecified** with intoxication
　　EXCLUDES 1　other stimulant use, unspecified with withdrawal (F15.93)

　F15.920　Other stimulant use, unspecified with HCC **intoxication,** uncomplicated

　F15.921　Other stimulant use, unspecified CC HCC **with intoxication** delirium
　　　Amphetamine or other stimulant-induced delirium

　F15.922　Other stimulant use, unspecified with HCC **intoxication with** perceptual disturbance

　F15.929　Other stimulant use, unspecified with HCC **intoxication,** unspecified
　　　Caffeine intoxication

　F15.93　Other stimulant use, unspecified with CC HCC withdrawal
　　　Caffeine withdrawal
　　　EXCLUDES 1　other stimulant use, unspecified with intoxication (F15.92-)

　F15.94　Other stimulant use, unspecified with HCC **stimulant-induced** mood disorder
　　　Amphetamine or other stimulant-induced bipolar or related disorder, without use disorder
　　　Amphetamine or other stimulant-induced depressive disorder, without use disorder

✓6th **F15.95　Other stimulant use, unspecified with stimulant-induced** psychotic disorder

　F15.950　Other stimulant use, unspecified CC HCC **with stimulant-induced psychotic disorder with** delusions

　F15.951　Other stimulant use, unspecified CC HCC **with stimulant-induced psychotic disorder with** hallucinations

　F15.959　Other stimulant use, unspecified with HCC **stimulant-induced psychotic disorder,** unspecified
　　　Amphetamine or other stimulant-induced psychotic disorder, without use disorder

✓6th **F15.98　Other stimulant use, unspecified with** other stimulant-induced disorder

　F15.980　Other stimulant use, unspecified HCC **with stimulant-induced** anxiety disorder
　　　Amphetamine or other stimulant-induced anxiety disorder, without use disorder
　　　Caffeine induced anxiety disorder, without use disorder

　F15.981　Other stimulant use, unspecified HCC **with stimulant-induced** sexual dysfunction
　　　Amphetamine or other stimulant-induced sexual dysfunction, without use disorder

　F15.982　Other stimulant use, unspecified HCC **with stimulant-induced** sleep disorder
　　　Amphetamine or other stimulant-induced sleep disorder, without use disorder
　　　Caffeine induced sleep disorder, without use disorder

　F15.988　Other stimulant use, unspecified with HCC other **stimulant-induced disorder**
　　　Amphetamine or other stimulant-induced obsessive compulsive or related disorder, without use disorder

　F15.99　Other stimulant use, unspecified with HCC unspecified **stimulant-induced disorder**

✓4th **F16　Hallucinogen related disorders**
　　INCLUDES　ecstasy
　　　　　　PCP
　　　　　　phencyclidine

　　CC Excl: For CC codes in category F16, unless otherwise noted:
　　PDX collection 550

✓5th **F16.1　Hallucinogen** abuse
　　EXCLUDES 1　hallucinogen dependence (F16.2-)
　　　　　　hallucinogen use, unspecified (F16.9-)

　F16.10　Hallucinogen abuse, uncomplicated
　　　Other hallucinogen use disorder, mild
　　　Phencyclidine use disorder, mild

　F16.11　Hallucinogen abuse, in remission
　　　Other hallucinogen use disorder, mild, in early remission
　　　Other hallucinogen use disorder, mild, in sustained remission
　　　Phencyclidine use disorder, mild, in early remission
　　　Phencyclidine use disorder, mild, in sustained remission

✓6th **F16.12　Hallucinogen abuse with** intoxication

　F16.120　Hallucinogen abuse with intoxication, HCC uncomplicated

　F16.121　Hallucinogen abuse with CC HCC **intoxication with** delirium

　F16.122　Hallucinogen abuse with intoxication HCC **with** perceptual disturbance

　F16.129　Hallucinogen abuse with intoxication, HCC unspecified

　F16.14　Hallucinogen abuse with hallucinogen-induced HCC mood disorder
　　　Other hallucinogen use disorder, mild, with other hallucinogen induced bipolar or related disorder
　　　Other hallucinogen use disorder, mild, with other hallucinogen induced depressive disorder
　　　Phencyclidine use disorder, mild, with phencyclidine induced bipolar or related disorder
　　　Phencyclidine use disorder, mild, with phencyclidine induced depressive disorder

✓6th **F16.15　Hallucinogen abuse with hallucinogen-induced** psychotic disorder

　F16.150　Hallucinogen abuse with CC HCC **hallucinogen-induced psychotic disorder with** delusions

　F16.151　Hallucinogen abuse with CC HCC **hallucinogen-induced psychotic disorder with** hallucinations

　F16.159　Hallucinogen abuse with HCC **hallucinogen-induced psychotic disorder,** unspecified

✓6ᵗʰ **F16.18** **Hallucinogen abuse with** other **hallucinogen-induced disorder**

     F16.180 **Hallucinogen abuse with hallucinogen-induced** anxiety disorder   HCC

     F16.183 **Hallucinogen abuse with hallucinogen-induced** persisting perception disorder (flashbacks)   HCC

     F16.188 **Hallucinogen abuse with** other **hallucinogen-induced disorder**   HCC

     F16.19 **Hallucinogen abuse with** unspecified **hallucinogen-induced disorder**   HCC

✓5ᵗʰ **F16.2** **Hallucinogen** dependence

     EXCLUDES 1   *hallucinogen abuse (F16.1-)*
                   hallucinogen use, unspecified (F16.9-)

     F16.20 **Hallucinogen dependence,** uncomplicated   CC HCC
         Other hallucinogen use disorder, moderate
         Other hallucinogen use disorder, severe
         Phencyclidine use disorder, moderate
         Phencyclidine use disorder, severe
         CC Excl: No Excl

     F16.21 **Hallucinogen dependence,** in remission   HCC
         Other hallucinogen use disorder, moderate, in early remission
         Other hallucinogen use disorder, moderate, in sustained remission
         Other hallucinogen use disorder, severe, in early remission
         Other hallucinogen use disorder, severe, in sustained remission
         Phencyclidine use disorder, moderate, in early remission
         Phencyclidine use disorder, moderate, in sustained remission
         Phencyclidine use disorder, severe, in early remission
         Phencyclidine use disorder, severe, in sustained remission

✓6ᵗʰ   **F16.22** **Hallucinogen dependence with** intoxication

     F16.220 **Hallucinogen dependence with intoxication,** uncomplicated   HCC

     F16.221 **Hallucinogen dependence with intoxication with** delirium   CC HCC

     F16.229 **Hallucinogen dependence with intoxication,** unspecified   HCC

     F16.24 **Hallucinogen dependence with hallucinogen-induced** mood disorder   HCC
         Other hallucinogen use disorder, moderate, with other hallucinogen induced bipolar or related disorder
         Other hallucinogen use disorder, moderate, with other hallucinogen induced depressive disorder
         Other hallucinogen use disorder, severe, with other hallucinogen-induced bipolar or related disorder
         Other hallucinogen use disorder, severe, with other hallucinogen-induced depressive disorder
         Phencyclidine use disorder, moderate, with phencyclidine induced bipolar or related disorder
         Phencyclidine use disorder, moderate, with phencyclidine induced depressive disorder
         Phencyclidine use disorder, severe, with phencyclidine induced bipolar or related disorder
         Phencyclidine use disorder, severe, with phencyclidine-induced depressive disorder

✓6ᵗʰ   **F16.25** **Hallucinogen dependence with hallucinogen-induced** psychotic disorder

     F16.250 **Hallucinogen dependence with hallucinogen-induced psychotic disorder with** delusions   CC HCC

     F16.251 **Hallucinogen dependence with hallucinogen-induced psychotic disorder with** hallucinations   CC HCC

     F16.259 **Hallucinogen dependence with hallucinogen-induced psychotic disorder,** unspecified   CC HCC
         CC Excl: No Excl

✓6ᵗʰ   **F16.28** **Hallucinogen dependence with** other **hallucinogen-induced disorder**

     F16.280 **Hallucinogen dependence with hallucinogen-induced** anxiety disorder   CC HCC
         CC Excl: No Excl

     F16.283 **Hallucinogen dependence with hallucinogen** persisting perception disorder (flashbacks)   CC HCC
         CC Excl: No Excl

     F16.288 **Hallucinogen dependence with** other **hallucinogen-induced disorder**   CC HCC
         CC Excl: No Excl

     F16.29 **Hallucinogen dependence with** unspecified **hallucinogen-induced disorder**   HCC

✓5ᵗʰ **F16.9** **Hallucinogen use,** unspecified

     EXCLUDES 1   *hallucinogen abuse (F16.1-)*
                   hallucinogen dependence (F16.2-)

     F16.90 **Hallucinogen use, unspecified,** uncomplicated
         AHA: 2018, 2Q, 10-11

✓6ᵗʰ   **F16.92** **Hallucinogen use, unspecified with** intoxication

     F16.920 **Hallucinogen use, unspecified with intoxication,** uncomplicated   HCC

     F16.921 **Hallucinogen use, unspecified with intoxication with** delirium   CC HCC
         Other hallucinogen intoxication delirium

     F16.929 **Hallucinogen use, unspecified with intoxication,** unspecified   HCC

     F16.94 **Hallucinogen use, unspecified with hallucinogen-induced** mood disorder   HCC
         Other hallucinogen induced bipolar or related disorder, without use disorder
         Other hallucinogen induced depressive disorder, without use disorder
         Phencyclidine induced bipolar or related disorder, without use disorder
         Phencyclidine induced depressive disorder, without use disorder

✓6ᵗʰ   **F16.95** **Hallucinogen use, unspecified with hallucinogen-induced** psychotic disorder

     F16.950 **Hallucinogen use, unspecified with hallucinogen-induced psychotic disorder with** delusions   CC HCC

     F16.951 **Hallucinogen use, unspecified with hallucinogen-induced psychotic disorder with** hallucinations   CC HCC

     F16.959 **Hallucinogen use, unspecified with hallucinogen-induced psychotic disorder,** unspecified   HCC
         Other hallucinogen induced psychotic disorder, without use disorder
         Phencyclidine induced psychotic disorder, without use disorder

✓6ᵗʰ   **F16.98** **Hallucinogen use, unspecified with** other **specified hallucinogen-induced disorder**

     F16.980 **Hallucinogen use, unspecified with hallucinogen-induced** anxiety disorder   HCC
         Other hallucinogen-induced anxiety disorder, without use disorder
         Phencyclidine induced anxiety disorder, without use disorder

     F16.983 **Hallucinogen use, unspecified with hallucinogen** persisting perception disorder (flashbacks)   HCC

     F16.988 **Hallucinogen use, unspecified with** other **hallucinogen-induced disorder**   HCC

     F16.99 **Hallucinogen use, unspecified with** unspecified **hallucinogen-induced disorder**   HCC

✓4ᵗʰ **F17** **Nicotine** dependence

     EXCLUDES 1   *history of tobacco dependence (Z87.891)*
                   tobacco use NOS (Z72.0)

     EXCLUDES 2   *tobacco use (smoking) during pregnancy, childbirth and the puerperium (O99.33-)*
                   toxic effect of nicotine (T65.2-)

     AHA: 2013, 4Q, 108-109

     CC Excl: For CC codes in category F17: PDX collection 550

✓5ᵗʰ **F17.2** **Nicotine** dependence

✓6ᵗʰ   **F17.20** **Nicotine dependence,** unspecified

     F17.200 **Nicotine dependence, unspecified, uncomplicated**
         Tobacco use disorder, mild
         Tobacco use disorder, moderate
         Tobacco use disorder, severe
         AHA: 2016, 1Q, 36
         TIP: Assign when provider documentation indicates "smoker" without further specification.

N Newborn: 0   **P** Pediatric: 0-17   **M** Maternity: 12-55   **A** Adult: 15-124   **MCC** Major Complication/Comorbidity   **CC** Complication/Comorbidity   **SW** Severe Wound Dx

546   ICD-10-CM 2019

F17.201 **Nicotine dependence, unspecified, in remission**
  Tobacco use disorder, mild, in early remission
  Tobacco use disorder, mild, in sustained remission
  Tobacco use disorder, moderate, in early remission
  Tobacco use disorder, moderate, in sustained remission
  Tobacco use disorder, severe, in early remission
  Tobacco use disorder, severe, in sustained remission

F17.203 **Nicotine dependence unspecified, withdrawal** `CC`
  Tobacco withdrawal

F17.208 **Nicotine dependence, unspecified, with other nicotine-induced disorders**

F17.209 **Nicotine dependence, unspecified, with unspecified nicotine-induced disorders**

✓6th **F17.21 Nicotine dependence, cigarettes**

F17.210 **Nicotine dependence, cigarettes, uncomplicated**
  AHA: 2017, 2Q, 28-29

F17.211 **Nicotine dependence, cigarettes, in remission**
  Tobacco use disorder, cigarettes, mild, in early remission
  Tobacco use disorder, cigarettes, mild, in sustained remission
  Tobacco use disorder, cigarettes, moderate, in early remission
  Tobacco use disorder, cigarettes, moderate, in sustained remission
  Tobacco use disorder, cigarettes, severe, in early remission
  Tobacco use disorder, cigarettes, severe, in sustained remission

F17.213 **Nicotine dependence, cigarettes, with withdrawal** `CC`

F17.218 **Nicotine dependence, cigarettes, with other nicotine-induced disorders**

F17.219 **Nicotine dependence, cigarettes, with unspecified nicotine-induced disorders**

✓6th **F17.22 Nicotine dependence, chewing tobacco**

F17.220 **Nicotine dependence, chewing tobacco, uncomplicated**

F17.221 **Nicotine dependence, chewing tobacco, in remission**
  Tobacco use disorder, chewing tobacco, mild, in early remission
  Tobacco use disorder, chewing tobacco, mild, in sustained remission
  Tobacco use disorder, chewing tobacco, moderate, in early remission
  Tobacco use disorder, chewing tobacco, moderate, in sustained remission
  Tobacco use disorder, chewing tobacco, severe, in early remission
  Tobacco use disorder, chewing tobacco, severe, in sustained remission

F17.223 **Nicotine dependence, chewing tobacco, with withdrawal** `CC`

F17.228 **Nicotine dependence, chewing tobacco, with other nicotine-induced disorders**

F17.229 **Nicotine dependence, chewing tobacco, with unspecified nicotine-induced disorders**

✓6th **F17.29 Nicotine dependence, other tobacco product**

F17.290 **Nicotine dependence, other tobacco product, uncomplicated**
  AHA: 2017, 2Q, 28-29

F17.291 **Nicotine dependence, other tobacco product, in remission**
  Tobacco use disorder, other tobacco product, mild, in early remission
  Tobacco use disorder, other tobacco product, mild, in sustained remission
  Tobacco use disorder, other tobacco product, moderate, in early remission
  Tobacco use disorder, other tobacco product, moderate, in sustained remission
  Tobacco use disorder, other tobacco product, severe, in early remission
  Tobacco use disorder, other tobacco product, severe, in sustained remission

F17.293 **Nicotine dependence, other tobacco product, with withdrawal** `CC`

F17.298 **Nicotine dependence, other tobacco product, with other nicotine-induced disorders**

F17.299 **Nicotine dependence, other tobacco product, with unspecified nicotine-induced disorders**

✓4th **F18 Inhalant related disorders**
  `INCLUDES` volatile solvents

  CC Excl: For CC codes in category F18, unless otherwise noted: PDX collection 550

✓5th **F18.1 Inhalant abuse**
  `EXCLUDES 1` *inhalant dependence (F18.2-)*
  inhalant use, unspecified (F18.9-)

F18.10 **Inhalant abuse, uncomplicated**
  Inhalant use disorder, mild

F18.11 **Inhalant abuse, in remission**
  Inhalant use disorder, mild, in early remission
  Inhalant use disorder, mild, in sustained remission

✓6th **F18.12 Inhalant abuse with intoxication**

F18.120 **Inhalant abuse with intoxication, uncomplicated** `HCC`

F18.121 **Inhalant abuse with intoxication delirium** `CC` `HCC`

F18.129 **Inhalant abuse with intoxication, unspecified** `HCC`

F18.14 **Inhalant abuse with inhalant-induced mood disorder** `HCC`
  Inhalant use disorder, mild, with inhalant induced depressive disorder

✓6th **F18.15 Inhalant abuse with inhalant-induced psychotic disorder**

F18.150 **Inhalant abuse with inhalant-induced psychotic disorder with delusions** `CC` `HCC`

F18.151 **Inhalant abuse with inhalant-induced psychotic disorder with hallucinations** `CC` `HCC`

F18.159 **Inhalant abuse with inhalant-induced psychotic disorder, unspecified** `HCC`

F18.17 **Inhalant abuse with inhalant-induced dementia** `CC` `HCC`
  Inhalant use disorder, mild, with inhalant induced major neurocognitive disorder

✓6th **F18.18 Inhalant abuse with other inhalant-induced disorders**

F18.180 **Inhalant abuse with inhalant-induced anxiety disorder** `HCC`

F18.188 **Inhalant abuse with other inhalant-induced disorder** `HCC`
  Inhalant use disorder, mild, with inhalant induced mild neurocognitive disorder

F18.19 **Inhalant abuse with unspecified inhalant-induced disorder** `HCC`

✓5th **F18.2 Inhalant dependence**
  `EXCLUDES 1` *inhalant abuse (F18.1-)*
  inhalant use, unspecified (F18.9-)

F18.20 **Inhalant dependence, uncomplicated** `CC` `HCC`
  Inhalant use disorder, moderate
  Inhalant use disorder, severe
  CC Excl: No Excl

✓ Additional Character Required   ✓x7th Placeholder   Unacceptable PDx   Questionable PDx   Manifestation   H1 - H14 HAC   HCC CMS-HCC Dx   HIV HIV Dx

ICD-10-CM 2019   547

Chapter 5. Mental, Behavioral and Neurodevelopmental Disorders

F18.21 **Inhalant dependence, in remission** `HCC`
   Inhalant use disorder, moderate, in early remission
   Inhalant use disorder, moderate, in sustained remission
   Inhalant use disorder, severe, in early remission
   Inhalant use disorder, severe, in sustained remission

✓6ᵗʰ **F18.22** **Inhalant dependence with intoxication**

   F18.220 **Inhalant dependence with intoxication, uncomplicated** `HCC`

   F18.221 **Inhalant dependence with intoxication delirium** `CC` `HCC`

   F18.229 **Inhalant dependence with intoxication, unspecified** `HCC`

F18.24 **Inhalant dependence with inhalant-induced mood disorder** `HCC`
   Inhalant use disorder, moderate, with inhalant induced depressive disorder
   Inhalant use disorder, severe, with inhalant induced depressive disorder

✓6ᵗʰ **F18.25** **Inhalant dependence with inhalant-induced psychotic disorder**

   F18.250 **Inhalant dependence with inhalant-induced psychotic disorder with delusions** `CC` `HCC`

   F18.251 **Inhalant dependence with inhalant-induced psychotic disorder with hallucinations** `CC` `HCC`

   F18.259 **Inhalant dependence with inhalant-induced psychotic disorder, unspecified** `CC` `HCC`
      CC Excl: No Excl

F18.27 **Inhalant dependence with inhalant-induced dementia** `CC` `HCC`
   Inhalant use disorder, moderate, with inhalant induced major neurocognitive disorder
   Inhalant use disorder, severe, with inhalant induced major neurocognitive disorder

✓6ᵗʰ **F18.28** **Inhalant dependence with other inhalant-induced disorders**

   F18.280 **Inhalant dependence with inhalant-induced anxiety disorder** `CC` `HCC`
      CC Excl: No Excl

   F18.288 **Inhalant dependence with other inhalant-induced disorder** `CC` `HCC`
      Inhalant use disorder, moderate, with inhalant-induced mild neurocognitive disorder
      Inhalant use disorder, severe, with inhalant-induced mild neurocognitive disorder
      CC Excl: No Excl

F18.29 **Inhalant dependence with unspecified inhalant-induced disorder** `HCC`

✓5ᵗʰ **F18.9** **Inhalant use, unspecified**
      EXCLUDES 1 inhalant abuse (F18.1-)
                  inhalant dependence (F18.2-)

F18.90 **Inhalant use, unspecified, uncomplicated**
      AHA: 2018, 2Q, 10-11

✓6ᵗʰ **F18.92** **Inhalant use, unspecified with intoxication**

   F18.920 **Inhalant use, unspecified with intoxication, uncomplicated** `HCC`

   F18.921 **Inhalant use, unspecified with intoxication with delirium** `CC` `HCC`

   F18.929 **Inhalant use, unspecified with intoxication, unspecified** `HCC`

F18.94 **Inhalant use, unspecified with inhalant-induced mood disorder** `HCC`
   Inhalant induced depressive disorder

✓6ᵗʰ **F18.95** **Inhalant use, unspecified with inhalant-induced psychotic disorder**

   F18.950 **Inhalant use, unspecified with inhalant-induced psychotic disorder with delusions** `CC` `HCC`

   F18.951 **Inhalant use, unspecified with inhalant-induced psychotic disorder with hallucinations** `CC` `HCC`

   F18.959 **Inhalant use, unspecified with inhalant-induced psychotic disorder, unspecified** `HCC`

F18.97 **Inhalant use, unspecified with inhalant-induced persisting dementia** `CC` `HCC`
   Inhalant-induced major neurocognitive disorder

✓6ᵗʰ **F18.98** **Inhalant use, unspecified with other inhalant-induced disorders**

   F18.980 **Inhalant use, unspecified with inhalant-induced anxiety disorder** `HCC`

   F18.988 **Inhalant use, unspecified with other inhalant-induced disorder** `HCC`
      Inhalant-induced mild neurocognitive disorder

F18.99 **Inhalant use, unspecified with unspecified inhalant-induced disorder** `HCC`

✓4ᵗʰ **F19** **Other psychoactive substance related disorders**
      INCLUDES polysubstance drug use (indiscriminate drug use)

   CC Excl: For CC codes in category F19, unless otherwise noted: PDX collection 550

✓5ᵗʰ **F19.1** **Other psychoactive substance abuse**
      EXCLUDES 1 other psychoactive substance dependence (F19.2-)
                  other psychoactive substance use, unspecified (F19.9-)

F19.10 **Other psychoactive substance abuse, uncomplicated**
   Other (or unknown) substance use disorder, mild

F19.11 **Other psychoactive substance abuse, in remission**
   Other (or unknown) substance use disorder, mild, in early remission
   Other (or unknown) substance use disorder, mild, in sustained remission

✓6ᵗʰ **F19.12** **Other psychoactive substance abuse with intoxication**

   F19.120 **Other psychoactive substance abuse with intoxication, uncomplicated** `HCC`

   F19.121 **Other psychoactive substance abuse with intoxication delirium** `CC` `HCC`

   F19.122 **Other psychoactive substance abuse with intoxication with perceptual disturbances** `HCC`

   F19.129 **Other psychoactive substance abuse with intoxication, unspecified** `HCC`

F19.14 **Other psychoactive substance abuse with psychoactive substance-induced mood disorder** `HCC`
   Other (or unknown) substance use disorder, mild, with other (or unknown) substance-induced bipolar or related disorder
   Other (or unknown) substance use disorder, mild, with other (or unknown) substance-induced depressive disorder

✓6ᵗʰ **F19.15** **Other psychoactive substance abuse with psychoactive substance-induced psychotic disorder**

   F19.150 **Other psychoactive substance abuse with psychoactive substance-induced psychotic disorder with delusions** `CC` `HCC`

   F19.151 **Other psychoactive substance abuse with psychoactive substance-induced psychotic disorder with hallucinations** `CC` `HCC`

   F19.159 **Other psychoactive substance abuse with psychoactive substance-induced psychotic disorder, unspecified** `HCC`

F19.16 **Other psychoactive substance abuse with psychoactive substance-induced persisting amnestic disorder** `HCC`

F19.17 **Other psychoactive substance abuse with psychoactive substance-induced persisting dementia** `CC` `HCC`
   Other (or unknown) substance use disorder, mild, with other (or unknown) substance-induced major neurocognitive disorder

✓6ᵗʰ **F19.18** **Other psychoactive substance abuse with other psychoactive substance-induced disorders**

   F19.180 **Other psychoactive substance abuse with psychoactive substance-induced anxiety disorder** `HCC`

   F19.181 **Other psychoactive substance abuse with psychoactive substance-induced sexual dysfunction** `HCC`

   F19.182 **Other psychoactive substance abuse with psychoactive substance-induced sleep disorder** `HCC`

F19.188   **Other psychoactive substance abuse** `HCC` **with other psychoactive substance-induced disorder**
Other (or unknown) substance use disorder, mild, with other (or unknown) substance induced mild neurocognitive disorder
Other (or unknown) substance use disorder, mild, with other (or unknown) substance induced obsessive-compulsive or related disorder

F19.19   **Other psychoactive substance abuse with** `HCC` **unspecified psychoactive substance-induced disorder**

✓5th   **F19.2**   **Other psychoactive substance dependence**
> *EXCLUDES 1*   *other psychoactive substance abuse (F19.1-)*
> *other psychoactive substance use, unspecified (F19.9-)*

F19.20   **Other psychoactive substance dependence,** `CC` `HCC` **uncomplicated**
Other (or unknown) substance use disorder, moderate
Other (or unknown) substance use disorder, severe
CC Excl: No Excl

F19.21   **Other psychoactive substance dependence, in** `HCC` **remission**
Other (or unknown) substance use disorder, moderate, in early remission
Other (or unknown) substance use disorder, moderate, in sustained remission
Other (or unknown) substance use disorder, severe, in early remission
▶Other (or unknown) substance use disorder, severe, in sustained remission◀

✓6th   **F19.22**   **Other psychoactive substance dependence with intoxication**
> *EXCLUDES 1*   *other psychoactive substance dependence with withdrawal (F19.23-)*

F19.220   **Other psychoactive substance** `HCC` **dependence with intoxication, uncomplicated**

F19.221   **Other psychoactive substance** `CC` `HCC` **dependence with intoxication delirium**

F19.222   **Other psychoactive substance** `CC` `HCC` **dependence with intoxication with perceptual disturbance**
CC Excl: No Excl

F19.229   **Other psychoactive substance** `HCC` **dependence with intoxication, unspecified**

✓6th   **F19.23**   **Other psychoactive substance dependence with withdrawal**
> *EXCLUDES 1*   *other psychoactive substance dependence with intoxication (F19.22-)*

F19.230   **Other psychoactive substance** `CC` `HCC` **dependence with withdrawal, uncomplicated**

F19.231   **Other psychoactive substance** `CC` `HCC` **dependence with withdrawal delirium**

F19.232   **Other psychoactive substance** `CC` `HCC` **dependence with withdrawal with perceptual disturbance**

F19.239   **Other psychoactive substance** `CC` `HCC` **dependence with withdrawal, unspecified**

F19.24   **Other psychoactive substance dependence** `HCC` **with psychoactive substance-induced mood disorder**
Other (or unknown) substance use disorder, moderate, with other (or unknown) substance induced bipolar or related disorder
Other (or unknown) substance use disorder, moderate, with other (or unknown) substance induced depressive disorder
Other (or unknown) substance use disorder, severe, with other (or unknown) substance induced bipolar or related disorder
Other (or unknown) substance use disorder, severe, with other (or unknown) substance induced depressive disorder

✓6th   **F19.25**   **Other psychoactive substance dependence with psychoactive substance-induced psychotic disorder**

F19.250   **Other psychoactive substance** `CC` `HCC` **dependence with psychoactive substance-induced psychotic disorder with delusions**

F19.251   **Other psychoactive substance** `CC` `HCC` **dependence with psychoactive substance-induced psychotic disorder with hallucinations**

F19.259   **Other psychoactive substance** `CC` `HCC` **dependence with psychoactive substance-induced psychotic disorder, unspecified**
CC Excl: No Excl

F19.26   **Other psychoactive substance dependence** `CC` `HCC` **with psychoactive substance-induced persisting amnestic disorder**
CC Excl: No Excl

F19.27   **Other psychoactive substance dependence** `CC` `HCC` **with psychoactive substance-induced persisting dementia**
Other (or unknown) substance use disorder, moderate, with other (or unknown) substance induced major neurocognitive disorder
Other (or unknown) substance use disorder, severe, with other (or unknown) substance induced major neurocognitive disorder

✓6th   **F19.28**   **Other psychoactive substance dependence with other psychoactive substance-induced disorders**

F19.280   **Other psychoactive substance** `CC` `HCC` **dependence with psychoactive substance-induced anxiety disorder**
CC Excl: No Excl

F19.281   **Other psychoactive substance** `CC` `HCC` **dependence with psychoactive substance-induced sexual dysfunction**
CC Excl: No Excl

F19.282   **Other psychoactive substance** `CC` `HCC` **dependence with psychoactive substance-induced sleep disorder**
CC Excl: No Excl

F19.288   **Other psychoactive substance** `CC` `HCC` **dependence with other psychoactive substance-induced disorder**
Other (or unknown) substance use disorder, moderate, with other (or unknown) substance induced mild neurocognitive disorder
Other (or unknown) substance use disorder, severe, with other (or unknown) substance induced mild neurocognitive disorder
Other (or unknown) substance use disorder, moderate, with other (or unknown) substance induced obsessive compulsive or related disorder
Other (or unknown) substance use disorder, severe, with other (or unknown) substance induced obsessive-compulsive or related disorder
CC Excl: No Excl

F19.29   **Other psychoactive substance dependence** `HCC` **with unspecified psychoactive substance-induced disorder**

✓5th   **F19.9**   **Other psychoactive substance use, unspecified**
> *EXCLUDES 1*   *other psychoactive substance abuse (F19.1-)*
> *other psychoactive substance dependence (F19.2-)*

F19.90   **Other psychoactive substance use, unspecified, uncomplicated**
AHA: 2018, 2Q, 10-11

✓6th   **F19.92**   **Other psychoactive substance use, unspecified with intoxication**
> *EXCLUDES 1*   *other psychoactive substance use, unspecified with withdrawal (F19.93)*

F19.920   **Other psychoactive substance use,** `HCC` **unspecified with intoxication, uncomplicated**

✓ Additional Character Required   ✓x7th Placeholder   Unacceptable PDx   Questionable PDx   Manifestation   `H1`-`H14` HAC   `HCC` CMS-HCC Dx   `HIV` HIV Dx

ICD-10-CM 2019   **549**

F19.921   **Other psychoactive substance use,** `CC` `HCC` **unspecified with intoxication with** delirium
Other (or unknown) substance-induced delirium

F19.922   **Other psychoactive substance use,** `HCC` **unspecified with intoxication with** perceptual disturbance

F19.929   **Other psychoactive substance use,** `HCC` **unspecified with intoxication,** unspecified

✓6ᵗʰ **F19.93**   **Other psychoactive substance use, unspecified with** withdrawal
> EXCLUDES 1   *other psychoactive substance use, unspecified with intoxication (F19.92-)*

F19.930   **Other psychoactive substance use,** `CC` `HCC` **unspecified with withdrawal,** uncomplicated

F19.931   **Other psychoactive substance use,** `CC` `HCC` **unspecified with withdrawal** delirium

F19.932   **Other psychoactive substance use,** `CC` `HCC` **unspecified with withdrawal with** perceptual disturbance

F19.939   **Other psychoactive substance use,** `CC` `HCC` **unspecified with withdrawal,** unspecified

F19.94   **Other psychoactive substance use, unspecified** `HCC` **with psychoactive substance-induced** mood disorder
Other (or unknown) substance-induced bipolar or related disorder, without use disorder
Other (or unknown) substance-induced depressive disorder, without use disorder

✓6ᵗʰ **F19.95**   **Other psychoactive substance use, unspecified with psychoactive substance-induced** psychotic disorder

F19.950   **Other psychoactive substance use,** `CC` `HCC` **unspecified with psychoactive substance-induced psychotic disorder with** delusions

F19.951   **Other psychoactive substance use,** `CC` `HCC` **unspecified with psychoactive substance-induced psychotic disorder with** hallucinations

F19.959   **Other psychoactive substance use,** `HCC` **unspecified with psychoactive substance-induced psychotic disorder,** unspecified
Other or unknown substance-induced psychotic disorder, without use disorder

F19.96   **Other psychoactive substance use, unspecified** `HCC` **with psychoactive substance-induced** persisting amnestic disorder

F19.97   **Other psychoactive substance use,** `CC` `HCC` **unspecified with psychoactive substance-induced** persisting dementia
Other (or unknown) substance-induced major neurocognitive disorder, without use disorder

✓6ᵗʰ **F19.98**   **Other psychoactive substance use, unspecified with** other **psychoactive substance-induced disorders**

F19.980   **Other psychoactive substance use,** `HCC` **unspecified with psychoactive substance-induced** anxiety disorder
Other (or unknown) substance-induced anxiety disorder, without use disorder

F19.981   **Other psychoactive substance use,** `HCC` **unspecified with psychoactive substance-induced** sexual dysfunction
Other (or unknown) substance-induced sexual dysfunction, without use disorder

F19.982   **Other psychoactive substance use,** `HCC` **unspecified with psychoactive substance-induced** sleep disorder
Other (or unknown) substance-induced sleep disorder, without use disorder

F19.988   **Other psychoactive substance use,** `HCC` **unspecified with** other **psychoactive substance-induced disorder**
Other (or unknown) substance-induced mild neurocognitive disorder, without use disorder
Other (or unknown) substance-induced obsessive-compulsive or related disorder, without use disorder

F19.99   **Other psychoactive substance use, unspecified** `HCC` **with** unspecified **psychoactive substance-induced disorder**

Schizophrenia, schizotypal, delusional, and other non-mood psychotic disorders (F20-F29)

✓4ᵗʰ **F20**   **Schizophrenia**
> EXCLUDES 1   *brief psychotic disorder (F23)*
> *cyclic schizophrenia (F25.0)*
> *mood [affective] disorders with psychotic symptoms (F30.2, F31.2, F31.5, F31.64, F32.3, F33.3)*
> *schizoaffective disorder (F25.-)*
> *schizophrenic reaction NOS (F23)*
> EXCLUDES 2   *schizophrenic reaction in:*
> *alcoholism (F10.15-, F10.25-, F10.95-)*
> *brain disease (F06.2)*
> *epilepsy (F06.2)*
> *psychoactive drug use (F11-F19 with .15. .25, .95)*
> *schizotypal disorder (F21)*

DEF: Group of disorders with disturbances in thought (delusions, hallucinations), mood (blunted, flattened, inappropriate affect), and sense of self. Schizophrenia also includes bizarre, purposeless behavior, repetitive activity, or inactivity.

CC Excl: For CC codes in category F20: PDX collection 551

F20.0   **Paranoid schizophrenia** `CC` `HCC`
Paraphrenic schizophrenia
> EXCLUDES 1   *involutional paranoid state (F22)*
> *paranoia (F22)*

DEF: Preoccupied with delusional suspicions and auditory hallucinations related to a single theme. This type of schizophrenia is usually hostile, grandiose, threatening, persecutory, and occasionally hypochondriacal.

F20.1   **Disorganized schizophrenia** `CC` `HCC`
Hebephrenic schizophrenia
Hebephrenia

F20.2   **Catatonic schizophrenia** `CC` `HCC`
Schizophrenic catalepsy
Schizophrenic catatonia
Schizophrenic flexibilitas cerea
> EXCLUDES 1   *catatonic stupor (R40.1)*

DEF: Extreme changes in motor activity. One extreme is a decreased response or reaction to the environment and the other is spontaneous activity.

F20.3   **Undifferentiated schizophrenia** `HCC`
Atypical schizophrenia
> EXCLUDES 1   *acute schizophrenia-like psychotic disorder (F23)*
> EXCLUDES 2   *post-schizophrenic depression (F32.89)*

F20.5   **Residual schizophrenia** `CC` `HCC`
Restzustand (schizophrenic)
Schizophrenic residual state

✓5ᵗʰ **F20.8**   **Other schizophrenia**

F20.81   **Schizophreniform disorder** `CC` `HCC`
Schizophreniform psychosis NOS

F20.89   **Other schizophrenia** `CC` `HCC`
Cenesthopathic schizophrenia
Simple schizophrenia

F20.9   **Schizophrenia,** unspecified `HCC`

F21   **Schizotypal disorder**
Borderline schizophrenia
Latent schizophrenia
Latent schizophrenic reaction
Prepsychotic schizophrenia
Prodromal schizophrenia
Pseudoneurotic schizophrenia
Pseudopsychopathic schizophrenia
Schizotypal personality disorder
> EXCLUDES 2   *Asperger's syndrome (F84.5)*
> *schizoid personality disorder (F60.1)*

DEF: Disorder characterized by various oddities of thinking, perception, communication, and behavior that may be manifested as magical thinking, ideas of reference, paranoid ideation, recurrent illusions and derealization (depersonalization), or social isolation.

F22 Delusional disorders   `HCC`

Delusional dysmorphophobia
Involutional paranoid state
Paranoia
Paranoia querulans
Paranoid psychosis
Paranoid state
Paraphrenia (late)
Sensitiver Beziehungswahn

> **EXCLUDES 1**   *mood [affective] disorders with psychotic symptoms (F30.2, F31.2, F31.5, F31.64, F32.3, F33.3)*
> *paranoid schizophrenia (F20.0)*

> **EXCLUDES 2**   *paranoid personality disorder (F60.0)*
> *paranoid psychosis, psychogenic (F23)*
> *paranoid reaction (F23)*

F23 Brief psychotic disorder   `CC`

Paranoid reaction
Psychogenic paranoid psychosis

> **EXCLUDES 2**   *mood [affective] disorders with psychotic symptoms (F30.2, F31.2, F31.5, F31.64, F32.3, F33.3)*

CC Excl: No Excl

F24 Shared psychotic disorder   `HCC`

Folie à deux
Induced paranoid disorder
Induced psychotic disorder

✓4ᵗʰ F25 Schizoaffective disorders

> **EXCLUDES 1**   *mood [affective] disorders with psychotic symptoms (F30.2, F31.2, F31.5, F31.64, F32.3, F33.3)*
> *schizophrenia (F20.-)*

F25.0 Schizoaffective disorder, bipolar type   `HCC`
Cyclic schizophrenia
Schizoaffective disorder, manic type
Schizoaffective disorder, mixed type
Schizoaffective psychosis, bipolar type

F25.1 Schizoaffective disorder, depressive type   `HCC`
Schizoaffective psychosis, depressive type

F25.8 Other schizoaffective disorders   `HCC`

F25.9 Schizoaffective disorder, unspecified   `HCC`
Schizoaffective psychosis NOS

F28 Other psychotic disorder not due to a substance or known physiological condition   `HIV`

Chronic hallucinatory psychosis
Other specified schizophrenia spectrum and other psychotic disorder

F29 Unspecified psychosis not due to a substance or known physiological condition   `HIV`

Chronic hallucinatory psychosis
Unspecified schizophrenia spectrum and other psychotic disorder

> **EXCLUDES 1**   *mental disorder NOS (F99)*
> *unspecified mental disorder due to known physiological condition (F09)*

Mood [affective] disorders (F30-F39)

✓4ᵗʰ F30 Manic episode

> **INCLUDES**   bipolar disorder, single manic episode
> mixed affective episode

> **EXCLUDES 1**   *bipolar disorder (F31.-)*
> *major depressive disorder, recurrent (F33.-)*
> *major depressive disorder, single episode (F32.-)*

DEF: Mania: Characterized by abnormal states of elation or excitement out of keeping with the individual's circumstances and varying from enhanced liveliness (hypomania) to violent, almost uncontrollable, excitement. Aggression and anger, flight of ideas, distractibility, impaired judgment, and grandiose ideas are common.

CC Excl: For CC codes in category F30, unless otherwise noted: PDX collection 551

✓5ᵗʰ F30.1 Manic episode without psychotic symptoms

F30.10 Manic episode without psychotic symptoms, unspecified   `CC` `HCC`

F30.11 Manic episode without psychotic symptoms, mild   `CC` `HCC`

F30.12 Manic episode without psychotic symptoms, moderate   `CC` `HCC`

F30.13 Manic episode, severe, without psychotic symptoms   `CC` `HCC`
     CC Excl: PDX collection 552

F30.2 Manic episode, severe with psychotic symptoms   `CC` `HCC`
Manic stupor
Mania with mood-congruent psychotic symptoms
Mania with mood-incongruent psychotic symptoms

F30.3 Manic episode in partial remission   `HCC`

F30.4 Manic episode in full remission   `HCC`

F30.8 Other manic episodes   `HCC`
Hypomania

F30.9 Manic episode, unspecified   `CC` `HCC`
Mania NOS

✓4ᵗʰ F31 Bipolar disorder

> **INCLUDES**   bipolar I disorder
> bipolar type I disorder
> manic-depressive illness
> manic-depressive psychosis
> manic-depressive reaction

> **EXCLUDES 1**   *bipolar disorder, single manic episode (F30.-)*
> *major depressive disorder, single episode (F32.-)*
> *major depressive disorder, recurrent (F33.-)*

> **EXCLUDES 2**   *cyclothymia (F34.0)*

CC Excl: For CC codes in category F31, unless otherwise noted: PDX collection 551

F31.0 Bipolar disorder, current episode hypomanic   `CC` `HCC`

✓5ᵗʰ F31.1 Bipolar disorder, current episode manic without psychotic features

F31.10 Bipolar disorder, current episode manic without psychotic features, unspecified   `CC` `HCC`

F31.11 Bipolar disorder, current episode manic without psychotic features, mild   `CC` `HCC`

F31.12 Bipolar disorder, current episode manic without psychotic features, moderate   `CC` `HCC`

F31.13 Bipolar disorder, current episode manic without psychotic features, severe   `CC` `HCC`
     CC Excl: PDX collection 553

F31.2 Bipolar disorder, current episode manic severe with psychotic features   `CC` `HCC`
Bipolar disorder, current episode manic with mood-congruent psychotic symptoms
Bipolar disorder, current episode manic with mood-incongruent psychotic symptoms
Bipolar I disorder, current or most recent episode manic with psychotic features

✓5ᵗʰ F31.3 Bipolar disorder, current episode depressed, mild or moderate severity

F31.30 Bipolar disorder, current episode depressed, mild or moderate severity, unspecified   `CC` `HCC`

F31.31 Bipolar disorder, current episode depressed, mild   `CC` `HCC`

F31.32 Bipolar disorder, current episode depressed, moderate   `CC` `HCC`

F31.4 Bipolar disorder, current episode depressed, severe, without psychotic features   `CC` `HCC`
     CC Excl: PDX collection 554

F31.5 Bipolar disorder, current episode depressed, severe, with psychotic features   `CC` `HCC`
Bipolar disorder, current episode depressed with mood-incongruent psychotic symptoms
Bipolar disorder, current episode depressed with mood-congruent psychotic symptoms
Bipolar I disorder, current or most recent episode depressed, with psychotic features

✓5ᵗʰ F31.6 Bipolar disorder, current episode mixed

F31.60 Bipolar disorder, current episode mixed, unspecified   `CC` `HCC`

F31.61 Bipolar disorder, current episode mixed, mild   `CC` `HCC`

F31.62 Bipolar disorder, current episode mixed, moderate   `CC` `HCC`

F31.63 Bipolar disorder, current episode mixed, severe, without psychotic features   `CC` `HCC`
     CC Excl: PDX collection 554

F31.64 Bipolar disorder, current episode mixed, severe, with psychotic features   `CC` `HCC`
Bipolar disorder, current episode mixed with mood-congruent psychotic symptoms
Bipolar disorder, current episode mixed with mood-incongruent psychotic symptoms

✓5ᵗʰ F31.7 Bipolar disorder, currently in remission

F31.70 Bipolar disorder, currently in remission, most recent episode unspecified   `HCC`

F31.71 Bipolar disorder, in partial remission, most recent episode hypomanic   `HCC`

✓ Additional Character Required	✓x7ᵗʰ Placeholder	Unacceptable PDx	Questionable PDx	Manifestation	H1 – H14 HAC	HCC CMS-HCC Dx	HIV HIV Dx

ICD-10-CM 2019   551

F31.72   **Bipolar disorder, in full remission, most recent episode hypomanic**   HCC

F31.73   **Bipolar disorder, in partial remission, most recent episode manic**   HCC

F31.74   **Bipolar disorder, in full remission, most recent episode manic**   HCC

F31.75   **Bipolar disorder, in partial remission, most recent episode depressed**   HCC

F31.76   **Bipolar disorder, in full remission, most recent episode depressed**   HCC

F31.77   **Bipolar disorder, in partial remission, most recent episode mixed**   HCC

F31.78   **Bipolar disorder, in full remission, most recent episode mixed**   HCC

✓5ᵗʰ **F31.8**   **Other bipolar disorders**

     F31.81   **Bipolar II disorder**   CC HCC
         Bipolar disorder, type 2

     F31.89   **Other bipolar disorder**   CC HCC
         Recurrent manic episodes NOS

F31.9   **Bipolar disorder, unspecified**   HCC
     Manic depression

F32   **Major depressive disorder, single episode**

     INCLUDES   single episode of agitated depression
               single episode of depressive reaction
               single episode of major depression
               single episode of psychogenic depression
               single episode of reactive depression
               single episode of vital depression

     EXCLUDES 1   bipolar disorder (F31.-)
                manic episode (F30.-)
                recurrent depressive disorder (F33.-)
     EXCLUDES 2   adjustment disorder (F43.2)

DEF: Mood disorder that produces depression that may exhibit as sadness, low self-esteem, or guilt feelings. Other manifestations may be withdrawal from friends and family and interrupted sleep.

CC Excl: For CC codes in category F32: PDX collection 555

F32.0   **Major depressive disorder, single episode, mild**   CC HCC

F32.1   **Major depressive disorder, single episode, moderate**   CC HCC

F32.2   **Major depressive disorder, single episode, severe without psychotic features**   CC HCC

F32.3   **Major depressive disorder, single episode, severe with psychotic features**   CC HCC
     Single episode of major depression with mood-congruent psychotic symptoms
     Single episode of major depression with mood-incongruent psychotic symptoms
     Single episode of major depression with psychotic symptoms
     Single episode of psychogenic depressive psychosis
     Single episode of psychotic depression
     Single episode of reactive depressive psychosis

F32.4   **Major depressive disorder, single episode, in partial remission**   HCC

F32.5   **Major depressive disorder, single episode, in full remission**   HCC

✓5ᵗʰ **F32.8**   **Other depressive episodes**
     AHA: 2016, 4Q, 14

     F32.81   **Premenstrual dysphoric disorder**   ♀
         EXCLUDES 1   premenstrual tension syndrome (N94.3)
         DEF: Severe manifestation of premenstrual syndrome (PMS) that can be disabling and destructive to day-to-day activities. It can exacerbate pre-existing emotional disorders, like depression and anxiety, and cause feelings of loss of control, fatigue, and irritability.

     F32.89   **Other specified depressive episodes**
         Atypical depression
         Post-schizophrenic depression
         Single episode of 'masked' depression NOS

F32.9   **Major depressive disorder, single episode, unspecified**
     Depression NOS
     Depressive disorder NOS
     Major depression NOS
     AHA: 2013, 4Q, 107

✓4ᵗʰ **F33**   **Major depressive disorder, recurrent**
     INCLUDES   recurrent episodes of depressive reaction
               recurrent episodes of endogenous depression
               recurrent episodes of major depression
               recurrent episodes of psychogenic depression
               recurrent episodes of reactive depression
               recurrent episodes of seasonal depressive disorder
               recurrent episodes of vital depression

     EXCLUDES 1   bipolar disorder (F31.-)
                manic episode (F30.-)

CC Excl: For CC codes in category F33, unless otherwise noted: PDX collection 555

F33.0   **Major depressive disorder, recurrent, mild**   CC HCC

F33.1   **Major depressive disorder, recurrent, moderate**   CC HCC

F33.2   **Major depressive disorder, recurrent, severe without psychotic features**   CC HCC

F33.3   **Major depressive disorder, recurrent, severe with psychotic symptoms**   CC HCC
     Endogenous depression with psychotic symptoms
     Major depressive disorder, recurrent, with psychotic features
     Recurrent severe episodes of major depression with mood-congruent psychotic symptoms
     Recurrent severe episodes of major depression with mood-incongruent psychotic symptoms
     Recurrent severe episodes of major depression with psychotic symptoms
     Recurrent severe episodes of psychogenic depressive psychosis
     Recurrent severe episodes of psychotic depression
     Recurrent severe episodes of reactive depressive psychosis
     CC Excl: PDX collection 551

✓5ᵗʰ **F33.4**   **Major depressive disorder, recurrent, in remission**

     F33.40   **Major depressive disorder, recurrent, in remission, unspecified**   CC HCC

     F33.41   **Major depressive disorder, recurrent, in partial remission**   HCC

     F33.42   **Major depressive disorder, recurrent, in full remission**   HCC

F33.8   **Other recurrent depressive disorders**   HCC
     Recurrent brief depressive episodes
     CC Excl: PDX collection 551

F33.9   **Major depressive disorder, recurrent, unspecified**   CC HCC
     Monopolar depression NOS

✓4ᵗʰ **F34**   **Persistent mood [affective] disorders**

F34.0   **Cyclothymic disorder**
     Affective personality disorder
     Cycloid personality
     Cyclothymia
     Cyclothymic personality
     DEF: Mood disorder characterized by fast and repeated alterations between hypomanic and depressed moods.

F34.1   **Dysthymic disorder**
     Depressive neurosis
     Depressive personality disorder
     Dysthymia
     Neurotic depression
     Persistent anxiety depression
     Persistent depressive disorder
     EXCLUDES 2   anxiety depression (mild or not persistent) (F41.8)
     DEF: Depression without psychosis. It is a less severe but persistent depression and is considered a mild to moderate chronic form of depression.

✓5ᵗʰ **F34.8**   **Other persistent mood [affective] disorders**
     AHA: 2016, 4Q, 14

     F34.81   **Disruptive mood dysregulation disorder**   CC HCC
         CC Excl: PDX collection 551

     F34.89   **Other specified persistent mood disorders**   CC HCC
         CC Excl: PDX collection 551

F34.9   **Persistent mood [affective] disorder, unspecified**   CC HCC
     CC Excl: PDX collection 551

F39   **Unspecified mood [affective] disorder**   HCC
     Affective psychosis NOS

N Newborn: 0   P Pediatric: 0-17   M Maternity: 12-55   A Adult: 15-124   MCC Major Complication/Comorbidity   CC Complication/Comorbidity   SW Severe Wound Dx

Anxiety, dissociative, stress-related, somatoform and other nonpsychotic mental disorders (F4Ø-F48)

✅4ᵗʰ **F4Ø   Phobic anxiety disorders**

✅5ᵗʰ **F4Ø.Ø   Agoraphobia**
> **DEF:** Profound anxiety or fear of leaving familiar settings like home, or being in unfamiliar locations or with strangers or crowds. Agoraphobia may or may not be preceded by recurrent panic attacks.

F4Ø.ØØ   Agoraphobia, unspecified

F4Ø.Ø1   Agoraphobia with panic disorder
> Panic disorder with agoraphobia
> *EXCLUDES 1*   panic disorder without agoraphobia (F41.Ø)

F4Ø.Ø2   Agoraphobia without panic disorder

✅5ᵗʰ **F4Ø.1   Social phobias**
> Anthropophobia
> Social anxiety disorder
> Social anxiety disorder of childhood
> Social neurosis

F4Ø.1Ø   Social phobia, unspecified

F4Ø.11   Social phobia, generalized

✅5ᵗʰ **F4Ø.2   Specific (isolated) phobias**
> *EXCLUDES 2*   dysmorphophobia (nondelusional) (F45.22)
> nosophobia (F45.22)

✅6ᵗʰ **F4Ø.21   Animal type phobia**
> **F4Ø.21Ø   Arachnophobia**
> > Fear of spiders
> **F4Ø.218   Other animal type phobia**

✅6ᵗʰ **F4Ø.22   Natural environment type phobia**
> **F4Ø.22Ø   Fear of thunderstorms**
> **F4Ø.228   Other natural environment type phobia**

✅6ᵗʰ **F4Ø.23   Blood, injection, injury type phobia**
> **F4Ø.23Ø   Fear of blood**
> **F4Ø.231   Fear of injections and transfusions**
> **F4Ø.232   Fear of other medical care**
> **F4Ø.233   Fear of injury**

✅6ᵗʰ **F4Ø.24   Situational type phobia**
> **F4Ø.24Ø   Claustrophobia**
> **F4Ø.241   Acrophobia**
> **F4Ø.242   Fear of bridges**
> **F4Ø.243   Fear of flying**
> **F4Ø.248   Other situational type phobia**

✅6ᵗʰ **F4Ø.29   Other specified phobia**
> **F4Ø.29Ø   Androphobia**
> > Fear of men
> **F4Ø.291   Gynephobia**
> > Fear of women
> **F4Ø.298   Other specified phobia**

F4Ø.8   Other phobic anxiety disorders
> Phobic anxiety disorder of childhood

F4Ø.9   Phobic anxiety disorder, unspecified
> Phobia NOS
> Phobic state NOS

✅4ᵗʰ **F41   Other anxiety disorders**
> *EXCLUDES 2*   anxiety in:
> > acute stress reaction (F43.Ø)
> > transient adjustment reaction (F43.2)
> > neurasthenia (F48.8)
> > psychophysiologic disorders (F45.-)
> > separation anxiety (F93.Ø)

F41.Ø   Panic disorder [episodic paroxysmal anxiety]
> Panic attack
> Panic state
> *EXCLUDES 1*   panic disorder with agoraphobia (F4Ø.Ø1)
> **DEF:** Neurotic disorder characterized by recurrent panic or anxiety, apprehension, fear, or terror. Symptoms include shortness of breath, palpitations, dizziness, and shakiness; fear of dying may persist.

F41.1   Generalized anxiety disorder
> Anxiety neurosis
> Anxiety reaction
> Anxiety state
> Overanxious disorder
> *EXCLUDES 2*   neurasthenia (F48.8)

F41.3   Other mixed anxiety disorders

F41.8   Other specified anxiety disorders
> Anxiety depression (mild or not persistent)
> Anxiety hysteria
> Mixed anxiety and depressive disorder

F41.9   Anxiety disorder, unspecified
> Anxiety NOS

✅4ᵗʰ **F42   Obsessive-compulsive disorder**
> *EXCLUDES 2*   obsessive-compulsive personality (disorder) (F6Ø.5)
> obsessive-compulsive symptoms occurring in depression (F32-F33)
> obsessive-compulsive symptoms occurring in schizophrenia (F2Ø.-)
> **AHA:** 2016, 4Q, 14-15

F42.2   Mixed obsessional thoughts and acts

F42.3   Hoarding disorder

F42.4   Excoriation (skin-picking) disorder
> *EXCLUDES 1*   factitial dermatitis (L98.1)
> other specified behavioral and emotional disorders with onset usually occurring in early childhood and adolescence (F98.8)

F42.8   Other obsessive-compulsive disorder
> Anancastic neurosis
> Obsessive-compulsive neurosis

F42.9   Obsessive-compulsive disorder, unspecified

✅4ᵗʰ **F43   Reaction to severe stress, and adjustment disorders**

F43.Ø   Acute stress reaction
> Acute crisis reaction
> Acute reaction to stress
> Combat and operational stress reaction
> Combat fatigue
> Crisis state
> Psychic shock

✅5ᵗʰ **F43.1   Post-traumatic stress disorder (PTSD)**
> Traumatic neurosis
> **DEF:** Preoccupation with traumatic events beyond normal experience (i.e., rape, personal assault, etc.) that may also include recurring flashbacks of the trauma. Symptoms include difficulty remembering, sleeping, or concentrating, and guilt feelings for surviving.

F43.1Ø   Post-traumatic stress disorder, unspecified

F43.11   Post-traumatic stress disorder, acute

F43.12   Post-traumatic stress disorder, chronic

✅5ᵗʰ **F43.2   Adjustment disorders**
> Culture shock
> Grief reaction
> Hospitalism in children
> *EXCLUDES 2*   separation anxiety disorder of childhood (F93.Ø)

F43.2Ø   Adjustment disorder, unspecified

F43.21   Adjustment disorder with depressed mood
> **AHA:** 2014, 1Q, 25

F43.22   Adjustment disorder with anxiety

F43.23   Adjustment disorder with mixed anxiety and depressed mood

F43.24   Adjustment disorder with disturbance of conduct

F43.25   Adjustment disorder with mixed disturbance of emotions and conduct

F43.29   Adjustment disorder with other symptoms

F43.8   Other reactions to severe stress
> Other specified trauma and stressor-related disorder

F43.9   Reaction to severe stress, unspecified
> Trauma and stressor-related disorder, NOS

✅4ᵗʰ **F44   Dissociative and conversion disorders**
> *INCLUDES*   conversion hysteria
> conversion reaction
> hysteria
> hysterical psychosis
> *EXCLUDES 2*   malingering [conscious simulation] (Z76.5)

F44.Ø   Dissociative amnesia
> *EXCLUDES 1*   amnesia NOS (R41.3)
> anterograde amnesia (R41.1)
> dissociative amnesia with dissociative fugue (F44.1)
> retrograde amnesia (R41.2)
> *EXCLUDES 2*   alcohol-or other psychoactive substance-induced amnestic disorder (F1Ø, F13, F19 with .26, .96)
> amnestic disorder due to known physiological condition (FØ4)
> postictal amnesia in epilepsy (G4Ø.-)

☑ Additional Character Required   ✅7ᵗʰ Placeholder   Unacceptable PDx   Questionable PDx   Manifestation   **H1**-**H14** HAC   **HCC** CMS-HCC Dx   **HIV** HIV Dx

ICD-10-CM 2019   **553**

Chapter 5. Mental, Behavioral and Neurodevelopmental Disorders

F4Ø–F44.Ø

F44.1　Dissociative fugue
　　　Dissociative amnesia with dissociative fugue
　　　EXCLUDES 2　*postictal fugue in epilepsy (G40.-)*
　　　DEF: Dissociative hysteria identified by memory loss and flight
　　　from familiar surroundings to a completely separate environment.
　　　Episodes may last hours or days. Conscious activity is not
　　　associated with perception of surroundings and there is no later
　　　memory of the episode.

F44.2　Dissociative stupor
　　　EXCLUDES 1　*catatonic stupor (R40.1)*
　　　　　　　　stupor NOS (R40.1)
　　　EXCLUDES 2　*catatonic disorder due to known physiological*
　　　　　　　　　　condition (F06.1)
　　　　　　　　depressive stupor (F32, F33)
　　　　　　　　manic stupor (F30, F31)

F44.4　Conversion disorder with motor symptom or deficit
　　　Conversion disorder with abnormal movement
　　　Conversion disorder with speech symptoms
　　　Conversion disorder with swallowing symptoms
　　　Conversion disorder with weakness/paralysis
　　　Dissociative motor disorders
　　　Psychogenic aphonia
　　　Psychogenic dysphonia

F44.5　Conversion disorder with seizures or convulsions
　　　Conversion disorder with attacks or seizures
　　　Dissociative convulsions

F44.6　Conversion disorder with sensory symptom or deficit
　　　Conversion disorder with anesthesia or sensory loss
　　　Conversion disorder with special sensory symptoms
　　　Dissociative anesthesia and sensory loss
　　　Psychogenic deafness

F44.7　Conversion disorder with mixed symptom presentation

√5ᵗʰ **F44.8　Other dissociative and conversion disorders**
　　　F44.81　Dissociative identity **disorder**
　　　　　　Multiple personality disorder
　　　F44.89　Other dissociative and conversion disorders
　　　　　　Ganser's syndrome
　　　　　　Psychogenic confusion
　　　　　　Psychogenic twilight state
　　　　　　Trance and possession disorders

F44.9　Dissociative and conversion disorder, unspecified
　　　Dissociative disorder NOS

√4ᵗʰ **F45　Somatoform disorders**
　　　EXCLUDES 2　*dissociative and conversion disorders (F44.-)*
　　　　　　　　factitious disorders ▸(F68.1-, F68.A)◂
　　　　　　　　hair-plucking (F63.3)
　　　　　　　　lalling (F80.0)
　　　　　　　　lisping (F80.0)
　　　　　　　　malingering [conscious simulation] (Z76.5)
　　　　　　　　nail-biting (F98.8)
　　　　　　　　psychological or behavioral factors associated with disorders or
　　　　　　　　　　diseases classified elsewhere (F54)
　　　　　　　　sexual dysfunction, not due to a substance or known
　　　　　　　　　　physiological condition (F52.-)
　　　　　　　　thumb-sucking (F98.8)
　　　　　　　　tic disorders (in childhood and adolescence) (F95.-)
　　　　　　　　Tourette's syndrome (F95.2)
　　　　　　　　trichotillomania (F63.3)
　　　　　　DEF: Types of disorders causing inconsistent physical symptoms that
　　　　　　cannot be explained.
　　　F45.0　Somatization disorder
　　　　　　Briquet's disorder
　　　　　　Multiple psychosomatic disorder
　　　F45.1　Undifferentiated somatoform disorder
　　　　　　Somatic symptom disorder
　　　　　　Undifferentiated psychosomatic disorder
　　√5ᵗʰ **F45.2　Hypochondriacal disorders**
　　　　　EXCLUDES 2　*delusional dysmorphophobia (F22)*
　　　　　　　　　　fixed delusions about bodily functions or shape (F22)
　　　　　F45.20　Hypochondriacal disorder, unspecified
　　　　　F45.21　Hypochondriasis
　　　　　　　Hypochondriacal neurosis
　　　　　　　Illness anxiety disorder
　　　　　F45.22　Body dysmorphic disorder
　　　　　　　Dysmorphophobia (nondelusional)
　　　　　　　Nosophobia
　　　　　F45.29　Other hypochondriacal disorders

√5ᵗʰ **F45.4　Pain disorders related to psychological factors**
　　　EXCLUDES 1　*pain NOS (R52)*
　　　F45.41　Pain disorder exclusively related to psychological
　　　　　　factors
　　　　　　Somatoform pain disorder (persistent)
　　　F45.42　Pain disorder with related psychological factors
　　　　　　Code also associated acute or chronic pain (G89.-)
F45.8　Other somatoform disorders
　　　Psychogenic dysmenorrhea
　　　Psychogenic dysphagia, including "globus hystericus"
　　　Psychogenic pruritus
　　　Psychogenic torticollis
　　　Somatoform autonomic dysfunction
　　　Teeth grinding
　　　EXCLUDES 1　*sleep related teeth grinding (G47.63)*
F45.9　Somatoform disorder, unspecified
　　　Psychosomatic disorder NOS

√4ᵗʰ **F48　Other nonpsychotic mental disorders**
　　　F48.1　Depersonalization-derealization syndrome
　　　F48.2　Pseudobulbar affect
　　　　　　Involuntary emotional expression disorder
　　　　　　Code first underlying cause, if known, such as:
　　　　　　　amyotrophic lateral sclerosis (G12.21)
　　　　　　　multiple sclerosis (G35)
　　　　　　　sequelae of cerebrovascular disease (I69.-)
　　　　　　　sequelae of traumatic intracranial injury (S06.-)
　　　F48.8　Other specified nonpsychotic mental disorders
　　　　　　Dhat syndrome
　　　　　　Neurasthenia
　　　　　　Occupational neurosis, including writer's cramp
　　　　　　Psychasthenia
　　　　　　Psychasthenic neurosis
　　　　　　Psychogenic syncope
　　　F48.9　Nonpsychotic mental disorder, unspecified
　　　　　　Neurosis NOS

Behavioral syndromes associated with physiological disturbances and physical factors (F50-F59)

√4ᵗʰ **F50　Eating disorders**
　　　EXCLUDES 1　*anorexia NOS (R63.0)*
　　　　　　　　feeding difficulties (R63.3)
　　　　　　　　feeding problems of newborn (P92.-)
　　　　　　　　polyphagia (R63.2)
　　　EXCLUDES 2　*feeding disorder in infancy or childhood (F98.2-)*
　　　TIP: Assign an additional code for BMI from category Z68, when
　　　documented. BMI can be based on documentation from clinicians who are
　　　not the patient's provider.

　　　CC Excl: For CC codes in category F50, unless otherwise noted:
　　　PDX collection 556

　　√5ᵗʰ **F50.0　Anorexia nervosa**
　　　　　EXCLUDES 1　*loss of appetite (R63.0)*
　　　　　　　　　　psychogenic loss of appetite (F50.89)
　　　　　DEF: Psychological eating disorder characterized by an intense
　　　　　fear of gaining weight and an unrealistic perception of body
　　　　　image that perpetuates the feeling of being fat or having too
　　　　　much fat. Avoidance of food and restrictive or unhealthy eating
　　　　　are common.
　　　　　F50.00　Anorexia nervosa, unspecified　　　　　CC
　　　　　F50.01　Anorexia nervosa, restricting type　　　CC
　　　　　F50.02　Anorexia nervosa, binge eating/purging type　CC
　　　　　　　EXCLUDES 1　*bulimia nervosa (F50.2)*
　　　F50.2　Bulimia nervosa　　　　　　　　　　　　CC
　　　　　Bulimia NOS
　　　　　Hyperorexia nervosa
　　　　　EXCLUDES 1　*anorexia nervosa, binge eating/purging type (F50.02)*
　　　　　DEF: Episodic pattern of overeating (binge eating) followed by
　　　　　purging or extreme exercise accompanied by an awareness of the
　　　　　abnormal eating pattern with a fear of not being able to stop
　　　　　eating.
　　　　　CC Excl: PDX collection 557
　　√5ᵗʰ **F50.8　Other eating disorders**
　　　　　EXCLUDES 2　*pica of infancy and childhood (F98.3)*
　　　　　AHA: 2017, 4Q, 9; 2016, 4Q, 15-16
　　　　　F50.81　Binge eating disorder
　　　　　F50.82　Avoidant/restrictive food intake disorder
　　　　　F50.89　Other specified eating disorder
　　　　　　　Pica in adults
　　　　　　　Psychogenic loss of appetite

F50.9 Eating disorder, unspecified
Atypical anorexia nervosa
Atypical bulimia nervosa
Feeding or eating disorder, unspecified
Other specified feeding disorder

√4ᵗʰ **F51 Sleep disorders not due to a substance or known physiological condition**
EXCLUDES 2 *organic sleep disorders (G47.-)*

√5ᵗʰ **F51.0 Insomnia not due to a substance or known physiological condition**
EXCLUDES 2 *alcohol related insomnia (F10.182, F10.282, F10.982)*
drug-related insomnia (F11.182, F11.282, F11.982, F13.182, F13.282, F13.982, F14.182, F14.282, F14.982, F15.182, F15.282, F15.982, F19.182, F19.282, F19.982)
insomnia NOS (G47.0-)
insomnia due to known physiological condition (G47.0-)
organic insomnia (G47.0-)
sleep deprivation (Z72.820)

F51.01 Primary insomnia
Idiopathic insomnia

F51.02 Adjustment insomnia

F51.03 Paradoxical insomnia

F51.04 Psychophysiologic insomnia

F51.05 Insomnia due to other mental disorder
Code also associated mental disorder

F51.09 Other insomnia not due to a substance or known physiological condition

√5ᵗʰ **F51.1 Hypersomnia not due to a substance or known physiological condition**
EXCLUDES 2 *alcohol related hypersomnia (F10.182, F10.282, F10.982)*
drug-related hypersomnia (F11.182, F11.282, F11.982, F13.182, F13.282, F13.982, F14.182, F14.282, F14.982, F15.182, F15.282, F15.982, F19.182, F19.282, F19.982)
hypersomnia NOS (G47.10)
hypersomnia due to known physiological condition (G47.10)
idiopathic hypersomnia (G47.11, G47.12)
narcolepsy (G47.4-)

F51.11 Primary hypersomnia

F51.12 Insufficient sleep syndrome
EXCLUDES 1 *sleep deprivation (Z72.820)*

F51.13 Hypersomnia due to other mental disorder
Code also associated mental disorder

F51.19 Other hypersomnia not due to a substance or known physiological condition

F51.3 Sleepwalking [somnambulism]
Non–rapid eye movement sleep arousal disorders, sleepwalking type

F51.4 Sleep terrors [night terrors]
Non–rapid eye movement sleep arousal disorders, sleep terror type

F51.5 Nightmare disorder
Dream anxiety disorder

F51.8 Other sleep disorders not due to a substance or known physiological condition

F51.9 Sleep disorder not due to a substance or known physiological condition, unspecified
Emotional sleep disorder NOS

√4ᵗʰ **F52 Sexual dysfunction not due to a substance or known physiological condition**
EXCLUDES 2 *Dhat syndrome (F48.8)*

F52.0 Hypoactive sexual desire disorder
Lack or loss of sexual desire
Male hypoactive sexual desire disorder
Sexual anhedonia
EXCLUDES 1 *decreased libido (R68.82)*

F52.1 Sexual aversion disorder
Sexual aversion and lack of sexual enjoyment

√5ᵗʰ **F52.2 Sexual arousal disorders**
Failure of genital response

F52.21 Male erectile disorder ♂
Erectile disorder
Psychogenic impotence
EXCLUDES 1 *impotence of organic origin (N52.-)*
impotence NOS (N52.-)

F52.22 Female sexual arousal disorder ♀
Female sexual interest/arousal disorder

√5ᵗʰ **F52.3 Orgasmic disorder**
Inhibited orgasm
Psychogenic anorgasmy

F52.31 Female orgasmic disorder ♀

F52.32 Male orgasmic disorder ♂
Delayed ejaculation

F52.4 Premature ejaculation ♂

F52.5 Vaginismus not due to a substance or known physiological condition ♀
Psychogenic vaginismus
EXCLUDES 2 *vaginismus (due to a known physiological condition) (N94.2)*

DEF: Psychogenic response resulting in painful contractions of the vaginal canal muscles. This condition can be severe enough to prevent sexual intercourse.

F52.6 Dyspareunia not due to a substance or known physiological condition
Genito-pelvic pain penetration disorderPsychogenic dyspareunia
EXCLUDES 2 *dyspareunia (due to a known physiological condition) (N94.1-)*

F52.8 Other sexual dysfunction not due to a substance or known physiological condition
Excessive sexual drive
Nymphomania
Satyriasis

F52.9 Unspecified sexual dysfunction not due to a substance or known physiological condition
Sexual dysfunction NOS

▲√4ᵗʰ **F53 Mental and behavioral disorders associated with the puerperium, not elsewhere classified**
~~Postpartum depression~~
EXCLUDES 1 *mood disorders with psychotic features (F30.2, F31.2, F31.5, F31.64, F32.3, F33.3)*
postpartum dysphoria (O90.6)
psychosis in schizophrenia, schizotypal, delusional, and other psychotic disorders (F20-F29)

● **F53.0 Postpartum depression** MQ
Postnatal depression, NOS
Postpartum depression, NOS

● **F53.1 Puerperal psychosis** MQ
Postpartum psychosis
Puerperal psychosis, NOS

F54 *Psychological and behavioral factors associated with disorders or diseases classified elsewhere*
Psychological factors affecting physical conditions
Code first the associated physical disorder, such as:
asthma (J45.-)
dermatitis (L23-L25)
gastric ulcer (K25.-)
mucous colitis (K58.-)
ulcerative colitis (K51.-)
urticaria (L50.-)
EXCLUDES 2 *tension-type headache (G44.2)*

√4ᵗʰ **F55 Abuse of non-psychoactive substances**
EXCLUDES 2 *abuse of psychoactive substances (F10-F19)*

F55.0 Abuse of antacids

F55.1 Abuse of herbal or folk remedies

F55.2 Abuse of laxatives

F55.3 Abuse of steroids or hormones

F55.4 Abuse of vitamins

F55.8 Abuse of other non-psychoactive substances

F59 Unspecified behavioral syndromes associated with physiological disturbances and physical factors
Psychogenic physiological dysfunction NOS

Disorders of adult personality and behavior (F60-F69)

✓4ᵗʰ **F60   Specific personality disorders**

F60.0   Paranoid personality disorder
Expansive paranoid personality (disorder)
Fanatic personality (disorder)
Paranoid personality (disorder)
Querulant personality (disorder)
Sensitive paranoid personality (disorder)
   EXCLUDES 2   *paranoia (F22)*
          paranoia querulans (F22)
          paranoid psychosis (F22)
          paranoid schizophrenia (F20.0)
          paranoid state (F22)

F60.1   Schizoid personality disorder
   EXCLUDES 2   *Asperger's syndrome (F84.5)*
          delusional disorder (F22)
          schizoid disorder of childhood (F84.5)
          schizophrenia (F20.-)
          schizotypal disorder (F21)

F60.2   Antisocial personality disorder
Amoral personality (disorder)
Asocial personality (disorder)
Dissocial personality disorder
Psychopathic personality (disorder)
Sociopathic personality (disorder)
   EXCLUDES 1   *conduct disorders (F91.-)*
   EXCLUDES 2   *borderline personality disorder (F60.3)*

F60.3   Borderline personality disorder
Aggressive personality (disorder)
Emotionally unstable personality disorder
Explosive personality (disorder)
   EXCLUDES 2   *antisocial personality disorder (F60.2)*

F60.4   Histrionic personality disorder
Hysterical personality (disorder)
Psychoinfantile personality (disorder)

F60.5   Obsessive-compulsive personality disorder
Anankastic personality (disorder)
Compulsive personality (disorder)
Obsessional personality (disorder)
   EXCLUDES 2   *obsessive-compulsive disorder (F42-)*

F60.6   Avoidant personality disorder
Anxious personality disorder

F60.7   Dependent personality disorder
Asthenic personality (disorder)
Inadequate personality (disorder)
Passive personality (disorder)
   DEF: Lack of self-confidence, fear of abandonment, and an obsessive need to be taken care of.

✓5ᵗʰ **F60.8   Other specific personality disorders**
   F60.81   Narcissistic personality disorder
   F60.89   Other specific personality disorders
       Eccentric personality disorder
       "Haltlose" type personality disorder
       Immature personality disorder
       Passive-aggressive personality disorder
       Psychoneurotic personality disorder
       Self-defeating personality disorder

F60.9   Personality disorder, unspecified
Character disorder NOS
Character neurosis NOS
Pathological personality NOS

✓4ᵗʰ **F63   Impulse disorders**
   EXCLUDES 2   *habitual excessive use of alcohol or psychoactive substances (F10-F19)*
          impulse disorders involving sexual behavior (F65.-)

F63.0   Pathological gambling
Compulsive gambling
Gambling disorder
   EXCLUDES 1   *gambling and betting NOS (Z72.6)*
   EXCLUDES 2   *excessive gambling by manic patients (F30, F31)*
          gambling in antisocial personality disorder (F60.2)

F63.1   Pyromania
Pathological fire-setting
   EXCLUDES 2   *fire-setting (by) (in):*
          adult with antisocial personality disorder (F60.2)
          alcohol or psychoactive substance intoxication (F10-F19)
          conduct disorders (F91.-)
          mental disorders due to known physiological condition (F01-F09)
          schizophrenia (F20.-)

F63.2   Kleptomania
Pathological stealing
   EXCLUDES 1   *shoplifting as the reason for observation for suspected mental disorder (Z03.8)*
   EXCLUDES 2   *depressive disorder with stealing (F31-F33)*
          stealing due to underlying mental condition—code to mental condition
          stealing in mental disorders due to known physiological condition (F01-F09)

F63.3   Trichotillomania
Hair plucking
   EXCLUDES 2   *other stereotyped movement disorder (F98.4)*

✓5ᵗʰ **F63.8   Other impulse disorders**
   F63.81   Intermittent explosive disorder
   F63.89   Other impulse disorders

F63.9   Impulse disorder, unspecified
Impulse control disorder NOS

✓4ᵗʰ **F64   Gender identity disorders**
   AHA: 2016, 4Q, 16

F64.0   Transsexualism
Gender identity disorder in adolescence and adulthood
Gender dysphoria in adolescents and adults

F64.1   Dual role transvestism
Use additional code to identify sex reassignment status (Z87.890)
   EXCLUDES 1   *gender identity disorder in childhood (F64.2)*
   EXCLUDES 2   *fetishistic transvestism (F65.1)*

F64.2   Gender identity disorder of childhood   ℗
Gender dysphoria in children
   EXCLUDES 1   *gender identity disorder in adolescence and adulthood (F64.0)*
   EXCLUDES 2   *sexual maturation disorder (F66)*

F64.8   Other gender identity disorders
Other specified gender dysphoria

F64.9   Gender identity disorder, unspecified
Gender dysphoria, unspecified
Gender-role disorder NOS

✓4ᵗʰ **F65   Paraphilias**

F65.0   Fetishism
Fetishistic disorder

F65.1   Transvestic fetishism
Fetishistic transvestism
Transvestic disorder

F65.2   Exhibitionism
Exhibitionistic disorder

F65.3   Voyeurism
Voyeuristic disorder

F65.4   Pedophilia
Pedophilic disorder

✓5ᵗʰ **F65.5   Sadomasochism**
   F65.50   Sadomasochism, unspecified
   F65.51   Sexual masochism
       Sexual masochism disorder
   F65.52   Sexual sadism
       Sexual sadism disorder

✓5ᵗʰ **F65.8   Other paraphilias**
   F65.81   Frotteurism
       Frotteuristic disorder
   F65.89   Other paraphilias
       Necrophilia
       Other specified paraphilic disorder

F65.9   Paraphilia, unspecified
Paraphilic disorder, unspecified
Sexual deviation NOS

F66   Other sexual disorders
Sexual maturation disorder
Sexual relationship disorder

☑️4ᵗʰ **F68 Other disorders of adult personality and behavior**

▲ ☑️5ᵗʰ **F68.1 Factitious disorder** imposed on self
Compensation neurosis
Elaboration of physical symptoms for psychological reasons
Hospital hopper syndrome
Münchhausen's syndrome
Peregrinating patient
EXCLUDES 2   factitial dermatitis (L98.1)
       person feigning illness (with obvious motivation) (Z76.5)

▲   **F68.10 Factitious disorder imposed on self, unspecified** `CC`
     CC Excl: PDX collection 551

▲   **F68.11 Factitious disorder imposed on self, with predominantly psychological signs and symptoms**

▲   **F68.12 Factitious disorder imposed on self, with predominantly physical signs and symptoms** `CC`
     CC Excl: PDX collection 551

▲   **F68.13 Factitious disorder imposed on self, with combined psychological and physical signs and symptoms**

●   **F68.A Factitious disorder** imposed on another `CC`
Factitious disorder by proxy
Münchhausen's by proxy

     F68.8 Other specified disorders of adult personality and behavior

F69 Unspecified disorder of adult personality and behavior `A`

Intellectual Disabilities (F70-F79)

Code first any associated physical or developmental disorders
EXCLUDES 1   borderline intellectual functioning, IQ above 70 to 84 (R41.83)

F70 Mild intellectual disabilities
IQ level 50-55 to approximately 70
Mild mental subnormality

F71 Moderate intellectual disabilities
IQ level 35-40 to 50-55
Moderate mental subnormality

F72 Severe intellectual disabilities `CC`
IQ 20-25 to 35-40
Severe mental subnormality
CC Excl: PDX collection 558

F73 Profound intellectual disabilities `CC`
IQ level below 20-25
Profound mental subnormality
CC Excl: PDX collection 558

F78 Other intellectual disabilities

F79 Unspecified intellectual disabilities
Mental deficiency NOS
Mental subnormality NOS

Pervasive and specific developmental disorders (F80-F89)

☑️4ᵗʰ **F80 Specific developmental disorders of speech and language**

     F80.0 Phonological disorder
Dyslalia
Functional speech articulation disorder
Lalling
Lisping
Phonological developmental disorder
Speech articulation developmental disorder
Speech-sound disorder
EXCLUDES 1   speech articulation impairment due to aphasia NOS (R47.01)
       speech articulation impairment due to apraxia (R48.2)
EXCLUDES 2   speech articulation impairment due to hearing loss (F80.4)
       speech articulation impairment due to intellectual disabilities (F70-F79)
       speech articulation impairment with expressive language developmental disorder (F80.1)
       speech articulation impairment with mixed receptive expressive language developmental disorder (F80.2)

     F80.1 Expressive language disorder
Developmental dysphasia or aphasia, expressive type
EXCLUDES 1   dysphasia and aphasia NOS (R47.-)
       mixed receptive-expressive language disorder (F80.2)
EXCLUDES 2   acquired aphasia with epilepsy [Landau-Kleffner] (G40.80-)
       intellectual disabilities (F70-F79)
       pervasive developmental disorders (F84.-)
       selective mutism (F94.0)

     F80.2 Mixed receptive-expressive language disorder
Developmental dysphasia or aphasia, receptive type
Developmental Wernicke's aphasia
EXCLUDES 1   central auditory processing disorder (H93.25)
       dysphasia or aphasia NOS (R47.-)
       expressive language disorder (F80.1)
       expressive type dysphasia or aphasia (F80.1)
       word deafness (H93.25)
EXCLUDES 2   acquired aphasia with epilepsy [Landau-Kleffner] (G40.80-)
       intellectual disabilities (F70-F79)
       pervasive developmental disorders (F84.-)
       selective mutism (F94.0)

     F80.4 Speech and language development delay due to hearing loss
Code also type of hearing loss (H90.-, H91.-)

☑️5ᵗʰ **F80.8 Other** developmental disorders of speech and language
AHA: 2017, 1Q, 27

     F80.81 Childhood onset fluency disorder
Cluttering NOS
Stuttering NOS
EXCLUDES 1   adult onset fluency disorder (F98.5)
       fluency disorder in conditions classified elsewhere (R47.82)
       fluency disorder (stuttering) following cerebrovascular disease (I69. with final characters-23)

     F80.82 Social pragmatic communication disorder
EXCLUDES 1   Asperger's syndrome (F84.5)
       autistic disorder (F84.0)
AHA: 2016, 4Q, 16

     F80.89 Other developmental disorders of speech and language

     F80.9 Developmental disorder of speech and language, unspecified
Communication disorder NOS
Language disorder NOS

☑️4ᵗʰ **F81 Specific developmental disorders of scholastic skills**

     F81.0 Specific reading disorder
"Backward reading"
Developmental dyslexia
Specific learning disorder, with impairment in reading
Specific reading retardation
EXCLUDES 1   alexia NOS (R48.0)
       dyslexia NOS (R48.0)
DEF: Serious impairment of reading skills unexplained in relation to general intelligence and teaching processes.

     F81.2 Mathematics disorder
Developmental acalculia
Developmental arithmetical disorder
Developmental Gerstmann's syndrome
Specific learning disorder, with impairment in mathmatics
EXCLUDES 1   acalculia NOS (R48.8)
EXCLUDES 2   arithmetical difficulties associated with a reading disorder (F81.0)
       arithmetical difficulties associated with a spelling disorder (F81.81)
       arithmetical difficulties due to inadequate teaching (Z55.8)

☑️5ᵗʰ **F81.8 Other developmental disorders of scholastic skills**

     F81.81 Disorder of written expression
Specific learning disorder, with impairment in written expression
Specific spelling disorder

     F81.89 Other developmental disorders of scholastic skills

     F81.9 Developmental disorder of scholastic skills, unspecified
Knowledge acquisition disability NOS
Learning disability NOS
Learning disorder NOS

F82 Specific developmental disorder of motor function
Clumsy child syndrome
Developmental coordination disorder
Developmental dyspraxia
EXCLUDES 1   abnormalities of gait and mobility (R26.-)
       lack of coordination (R27.-)
EXCLUDES 2   lack of coordination secondary to intellectual disabilities (F70-F79)

☑️ Additional Character Required   ☑️x7ᵗʰ Placeholder   Unacceptable PDx   Questionable PDx   Manifestation   `H1`-`H14` HAC   `HCC` CMS-HCC Dx   `HIV` HIV Dx

✓4ᵗʰ F84 Pervasive developmental disorders

Use additional code to identify any associated medical condition and intellectual disabilities

CC Excl: For CC codes in category F84, unless otherwise noted: PDX collection 551

F84.0 Autistic disorder   CC
Autism spectrum disorder
Infantile autism
Infantile psychosis
Kanner's syndrome
EXCLUDES 1   *Asperger's syndrome (F84.5)*
AHA: 2017, 1Q, 27

F84.2 Rett's syndrome   CC
EXCLUDES 1   *Asperger's syndrome (F84.5)*
autistic disorder (F84.0)
other childhood disintegrative disorder (F84.3)
CC Excl: PDX collection 537

F84.3 Other childhood disintegrative disorder   CC P
Dementia infantilis
Disintegrative psychosis
Heller's syndrome
Symbiotic psychosis
Use additional code to identify any associated neurological condition
EXCLUDES 1   *Asperger's syndrome (F84.5)*
autistic disorder (F84.0)
Rett's syndrome (F84.2)

F84.5 Asperger's syndrome   CC
Asperger's disorder
Autistic psychopathy
Schizoid disorder of childhood
DEF: High-functioning form of autism. Children with this syndrome usually develop speech on schedule, are generally very intelligent, and communicate well, but have considerable social shortcomings. ***Synonym(s):*** *AS.*

F84.8 Other pervasive developmental disorders   CC
Overactive disorder associated with intellectual disabilities and stereotyped movements

F84.9 Pervasive developmental disorder, unspecified   CC
Atypical autism

F88 Other disorders of psychological development

Developmental agnosia
Global development delay
Other specified neurodevelopmental disorder

F89 Unspecified disorder of psychological development

Developmental disorder NOS
Neurodevelopmental disorder NOS

Behavioral and emotional disorders with onset usually occurring in childhood and adolescence (F90-F98)

NOTE   Codes within categories F90-F98 may be used regardless of the age of a patient. These disorders generally have onset within the childhood or adolescent years, but may continue throughout life or not be diagnosed until adulthood

✓4ᵗʰ F90 Attention-deficit hyperactivity disorders

INCLUDES   attention deficit disorder with hyperactivity
attention deficit syndrome with hyperactivity
EXCLUDES 2   *anxiety disorders (F40.-, F41.-)*
mood [affective] disorders (F30-F39)
pervasive developmental disorders (F84.-)
schizophrenia (F20.-)

F90.0 Attention-deficit hyperactivity disorder, predominantly inattentive type
Attention-deficit/hyperactivity disorder, predominantly inattentive presentation

F90.1 Attention-deficit hyperactivity disorder, predominantly hyperactive type
Attention-deficit/hyperactivity disorder, predominantly hyperactive impulsive presentation

F90.2 Attention-deficit hyperactivity disorder, combined type
Attention-deficit/hyperactivity disorder, combined presentation

F90.8 Attention-deficit hyperactivity disorder, other type

F90.9 Attention-deficit hyperactivity disorder, unspecified type
Attention-deficit hyperactivity disorder of childhood or adolescence NOS
Attention-deficit hyperactivity disorder NOS

✓4ᵗʰ F91 Conduct disorders

EXCLUDES 1   *antisocial behavior (Z72.81-)*
antisocial personality disorder (F60.2)
EXCLUDES 2   *conduct problems associated with attention-deficit hyperactivity disorder (F90.-)*
mood [affective] disorders (F30-F39)
pervasive developmental disorders (F84.-)
schizophrenia (F20.-)

F91.0 Conduct disorder confined to family context

F91.1 Conduct disorder, childhood-onset type
Unsocialized conduct disorder
Conduct disorder, solitary aggressive type
Unsocialized aggressive disorder

F91.2 Conduct disorder, adolescent-onset type
Socialized conduct disorder
Conduct disorder, group type

F91.3 Oppositional defiant disorder

F91.8 Other conduct disorders
Other specified conduct disorder
Other specified disruptive disorder

F91.9 Conduct disorder, unspecified
Behavioral disorder NOS
Conduct disorder NOS
Disruptive behavior disorder NOS
Disruptive disorder NOS

✓4ᵗʰ F93 Emotional disorders with onset specific to childhood

F93.0 Separation anxiety disorder of childhood
EXCLUDES 2   *mood [affective] disorders (F30-F39)*
nonpsychotic mental disorders (F40-F48)
phobic anxiety disorder of childhood (F40.8)
social phobia (F40.1)

F93.8 Other childhood emotional disorders
Identity disorder
EXCLUDES 2   *gender identity disorder of childhood (F64.2)*

F93.9 Childhood emotional disorder, unspecified

✓4ᵗʰ F94 Disorders of social functioning with onset specific to childhood and adolescence

F94.0 Selective mutism
Elective mutism
EXCLUDES 2   *pervasive developmental disorders (F84.-)*
schizophrenia (F20.-)
specific developmental disorders of speech and language (F80.-)
transient mutism as part of separation anxiety in young children (F93.0)

F94.1 Reactive attachment disorder of childhood
Use additional code to identify any associated failure to thrive or growth retardation
EXCLUDES 1   *disinhibited attachment disorder of childhood (F94.1)*
normal variation in pattern of selective attachment
EXCLUDES 2   *Asperger's syndrome (F84.5)*
maltreatment syndromes (T74.-)
sexual or physical abuse in childhood, resulting in psychosocial problems (Z62.81-)

F94.2 Disinhibited attachment disorder of childhood
Affectionless psychopathy
Institutional syndrome
EXCLUDES 1   *reactive attachment disorder of childhood (F94.1)*
EXCLUDES 2   *Asperger's syndrome (F84.5)*
attention-deficit hyperactivity disorders (F90.-)
hospitalism in children (F43.2-)

F94.8 Other childhood disorders of social functioning

F94.9 Childhood disorder of social functioning, unspecified

✓4ᵗʰ F95 Tic disorder

F95.0 Transient tic disorder
Provisional tic disorder

F95.1 Chronic motor or vocal tic disorder

F95.2 Tourette's disorder
Combined vocal and multiple motor tic disorder [de la Tourette]
Tourette's syndrome

F95.8 Other tic disorders

F95.9 Tic disorder, unspecified
Tic NOS

☑4ᵗʰ **F98 Other behavioral and emotional disorders with onset usually occurring in childhood and adolescence**

> EXCLUDES 2   *breath-holding spells (R06.89)*
> *gender identity disorder of childhood (F64.2)*
> *Kleine-Levin syndrome (G47.13)*
> *obsessive-compulsive disorder (F42-)*
> *sleep disorders not due to a substance or known physiological condition (F51.-)*

F98.0 Enuresis not due to a substance or known physiological condition

Enuresis (primary) (secondary) of nonorganic origin
Functional enuresis
Psychogenic enuresis
Urinary incontinence of nonorganic origin

> EXCLUDES 1   *enuresis NOS (R32)*

F98.1 Encopresis not due to a substance or known physiological condition

Functional encopresis
Incontinence of feces of nonorganic origin
Psychogenic encopresis
Use additional code to identify the cause of any coexisting constipation

> EXCLUDES 1   *encopresis NOS (R15.-)*

☑5ᵗʰ **F98.2 Other feeding disorders of infancy and childhood**

> EXCLUDES 1   *feeding difficulties (R63.3)*
> EXCLUDES 2   *anorexia nervosa and other eating disorders (F50.-)*
> *feeding problems of newborn (P92.-)*
> *pica of infancy or childhood (F98.3)*

F98.21 Rumination disorder of infancy

F98.29 Other feeding disorders of infancy and early childhood

F98.3 Pica of infancy and childhood

F98.4 Stereotyped movement disorders

Stereotype/habit disorder

> EXCLUDES 1   *abnormal involuntary movements (R25.-)*
> EXCLUDES 2   *compulsions in obsessive-compulsive disorder (F42-)*
> *hair plucking (F63.3)*
> *movement disorders of organic origin (G20-G25)*
> *nail-biting (F98.8)*
> *nose-picking (F98.8)*
> *stereotypies that are part of a broader psychiatric condition (F01-F95)*
> *thumb-sucking (F98.8)*
> *tic disorders (F95.-)*
> *trichotillomania (F63.3)*

F98.5 Adult onset fluency disorder

> EXCLUDES 1   *childhood onset fluency disorder (F80.81)*
> *dysphasia (R47.02)*
> *fluency disorder in conditions classified elsewhere (R47.82)*
> *fluency disorder (stuttering) following cerebrovascular disease (I69. with final characters -23)*
> *tic disorders (F95.-)*

F98.8 Other specified behavioral and emotional disorders with onset usually occurring in childhood and adolescence

Excessive masturbation
Nail-biting
Nose-picking
Thumb-sucking

F98.9 Unspecified behavioral and emotional disorders with onset usually occurring in childhood and adolescence

Unspecified mental disorder (F99)

F99 Mental disorder, not otherwise specified

Mental illness NOS

> EXCLUDES 1   *unspecified mental disorder due to known physiological condition (F09)*

☑ Additional Character Required   √x7ᵗʰ Placeholder   Unacceptable PDx   Questionable PDx   Manifestation   H1 - H14 HAC   HCC CMS-HCC Dx   HIV HIV Dx

ICD-10-CM 2019   559

Chapter 6. Diseases of the Nervous System (G00-G99)

Chapter Specific Guidelines with Coding Examples

The chapter specific guidelines from the ICD-10-CM Official Guidelines for Coding and Reporting have been provided below. Along with these guidelines are coding examples, contained in the shaded boxes, that have been developed to help illustrate the coding and/or sequencing guidance found in these guidelines.

a. Dominant/nondominant side

Codes from category G81, Hemiplegia and hemiparesis, and subcategories G83.1, Monoplegia of lower limb, G83.2, Monoplegia of upper limb, and G83.3, Monoplegia, unspecified, identify whether the dominant or nondominant side is affected. Should the affected side be documented, but not specified as dominant or nondominant, and the classification system does not indicate a default, code selection is as follows:

- For ambidextrous patients, the default should be dominant.
- If the left side is affected, the default is non-dominant.
- If the right side is affected, the default is dominant.

> Hemiplegia affecting left side of ambidextrous patient
>
> **G81.92**   **Hemiplegia, unspecified affecting left dominant side**
>
> *Explanation*: Documentation states that the left side is affected and dominant is used for ambidextrous persons.

> Right spastic hemiplegia, unknown whether patient is right- or left-handed
>
> **G81.11**   **Spastic hemiplegia affecting right dominant side**
>
> *Explanation*: Since it is unknown whether the patient is right- or left-handed, if the right side is affected, the default is dominant.

b. Pain—category G89

1) General coding information

Codes in category G89, Pain, not elsewhere classified, may be used in conjunction with codes from other categories and chapters to provide more detail about acute or chronic pain and neoplasm-related pain, unless otherwise indicated below.

If the pain is not specified as acute or chronic, post-thoracotomy, postprocedural, or neoplasm-related, do not assign codes from category G89.

A code from category G89 should not be assigned if the underlying (definitive) diagnosis is known, unless the reason for the encounter is pain control/ management and not management of the underlying condition.

When an admission or encounter is for a procedure aimed at treating the underlying condition (e.g., spinal fusion, kyphoplasty), a code for the underlying condition (e.g., vertebral fracture, spinal stenosis) should be assigned as the principal diagnosis. No code from category G89 should be assigned.

> Elderly patient with back pain is admitted for kyphoplasty for age-related osteopathic compression fracture at vertebra T3
>
> **M80.08XA**   **Age-related osteoporosis with current pathological fracture, vertebra(e), initial encounter for fracture**
>
> *Explanation*: No code is assigned for the pain as it is inherent in the underlying condition being treated.

(a) Category G89 codes as principal or first-listed diagnosis

Category G89 codes are acceptable as principal diagnosis or the first-listed code:

- When pain control or pain management is the reason for the admission/encounter (e.g., a patient with displaced intervertebral disc, nerve impingement and severe back pain presents for injection of steroid into the spinal canal). The underlying cause of the pain should be reported as an additional diagnosis, if known.

- When a patient is admitted for the insertion of a neurostimulator for pain control, assign the appropriate pain code as the principal or first-listed diagnosis. When an admission or encounter is for a procedure aimed at treating the underlying condition and a neurostimulator is inserted for pain control during the same admission/encounter, a code for the underlying condition should be assigned as the principal diagnosis and the appropriate pain code should be assigned as a secondary diagnosis.

> Patient with chronic pain from lumbar spondylosis with radiculopathy not relieved by surgery is admitted for insertion of neurostimulator.
>
> **G89.29**   **Other chronic pain**
>
> **M47.26**   **Other spondylosis with radiculopathy, lumbar region**
>
> *Explanation*: Since the patient is admitted specifically for a neurostimulator implantation for pain management and not to treat the underlying spondylosis, the chronic pain code is sequenced first, followed by the underlying condition. Neither code M54.16 nor M54.5 is necessary because M47.26 describes the radiculopathy and the site.

(b) Use of category G89 codes in conjunction with site specific pain codes

(i) Assigning category G89 and site-specific pain codes

Codes from category G89 may be used in conjunction with codes that identify the site of pain (including codes from chapter 18) if the category G89 code provides additional information. For example, if the code describes the site of the pain, but does not fully describe whether the pain is acute or chronic, then both codes should be assigned.

> During hospital stay, patient is seen by orthopaedics to evaluate chronic left shoulder pain.
>
> **M25.512**   **Pain in left shoulder**
>
> **G89.29**   **Other chronic pain**
>
> *Explanation*: No underlying condition has been determined yet so the pain would be the reason for the visit. The M25 pain code in this instance does not fully describe the condition as it does not represent that the pain is chronic. The G89 chronic pain code is assigned to provide specificity.

(ii) Sequencing of category G89 codes with site-specific pain codes

The sequencing of category G89 codes with site-specific pain codes (including chapter 18 codes), is dependent on the circumstances of the encounter/admission as follows:

- If the encounter is for pain control or pain management, assign the code from category G89 followed by the code identifying the specific site of pain (e.g., encounter for pain management for acute neck pain from trauma is assigned code G89.11, Acute pain due to trauma, followed by code M54.2, Cervicalgia, to identify the site of pain).

> Management of acute, traumatic right knee pain
>
> **G89.11**   **Acute pain due to trauma**
>
> **M25.561**   **Pain in right knee**
>
> *Explanation*: The reason for the encounter is to manage or control the pain, not to treat or evaluate an underlying condition. The G89 pain code is assigned as the principal diagnosis but in this instance does not fully describe the condition as it does not include the site and laterality. The M25 pain code is added to provide this information.

- If the encounter is for any other reason except pain control or pain management, and a related definitive diagnosis has not been established (confirmed) by the provider, assign the code for the specific site of pain first, followed by the appropriate code from category G89.

> Tests are performed to investigate the source of the patient's chronic epigastric abdominal pain
>
> **R10.13**   **Epigastric pain**
>
> **G89.29**   **Other chronic pain**
>
> *Explanation*: In this instance the patient's epigastric pain is not being treated; rather the source of the pain is being investigated. A code from chapter 18 for epigastric pain is sequenced before the additional specificity of the G89 code for the chronic pain.

2) Pain due to devices, implants and grafts

See Section I.C.19. Pain due to medical devices

3) Postoperative pain

The provider's documentation should be used to guide the coding of postoperative pain, as well as *Section III. Reporting Additional Diagnoses* and *Section IV. Diagnostic Coding and Reporting in the Outpatient Setting.*

The default for post-thoracotomy and other postoperative pain not specified as acute or chronic is the code for the acute form.

Routine or expected postoperative pain immediately after surgery should not be coded.

> Pain pump dose is increased for the patient's unexpected, extreme pain post-thoracotomy
>
> **G89.12**   **Acute post-thoracotomy pain**
>
> *Explanation*: When acute or chronic is not documented, default to acute. The use of "unexpected, extreme" and the increase of medication dosage indicate that the pain was more than routine or expected.

(a) Postoperative pain not associated with specific postoperative complication

Postoperative pain not associated with a specific postoperative complication is assigned to the appropriate postoperative pain code in category G89.

(b) Postoperative pain associated with specific postoperative complication

Postoperative pain associated with a specific postoperative complication (such as painful wire sutures) is assigned to the appropriate code(s) found in Chapter 19, Injury, poisoning, and certain other consequences of external causes. If appropriate, use additional code(s) from category G89 to identify acute or chronic pain (G89.18 or G89.28).

4) Chronic pain

Chronic pain is classified to subcategory G89.2. There is no time frame defining when pain becomes chronic pain. The provider's documentation should be used to guide use of these codes.

5) Neoplasm related pain

Code G89.3 is assigned to pain documented as being related, associated or due to cancer, primary or secondary malignancy, or tumor. This code is assigned regardless of whether the pain is acute or chronic.

This code may be assigned as the principal or first-listed code when the stated reason for the admission/encounter is documented as pain control/pain management. The underlying neoplasm should be reported as an additional diagnosis.

> Pain medication adjustment for chronic pain from bone metastasis
>
> **G89.3**   **Neoplasm related pain (acute)(chronic)**
>
> **C79.51**   **Secondary malignant neoplasm of bone**
>
> *Explanation*: Since the encounter was for pain medication management, the pain, rather than the neoplasm, was the reason for the encounter and is sequenced first. This "neoplasm-related pain" code includes both acute and chronic pain.

When the reason for the admission/encounter is management of the neoplasm and the pain associated with the neoplasm is also documented, code G89.3 may be assigned as an additional diagnosis. It is not necessary to assign an additional code for the site of the pain.

See Section I.C.2 for instructions on the sequencing of neoplasms for all other stated reasons for the admission/encounter (except for pain control/pain management).

> Patient with lung cancer presents with acute hip pain and is evaluated and found to have iliac bone metastasis
>
> **C79.51**   **Secondary malignant neoplasm of bone**
>
> **C34.90**   **Malignant neoplasm of unspecified part of unspecified bronchus or lung**
>
> **G89.3**   **Neoplasm related pain (acute)(chronic)**
>
> *Explanation*: The reason for the encounter was the evaluation and diagnosis of the bone metastasis, whose code would be assigned as first-listed, followed by codes for the primary neoplasm and the pain due to the iliac bone metastasis.

6) Chronic pain syndrome

Central pain syndrome (G89.0) and chronic pain syndrome (G89.4) are different than the term "chronic pain," and therefore codes should only be used when the provider has specifically documented this condition.

See Section I.C.5. Pain disorders related to psychological factors

Chapter 6. Diseases of the Nervous System (G00-G99)

EXCLUDES 2   certain conditions originating in the perinatal period (P04-P96)
certain infectious and parasitic diseases (A00-B99)
complications of pregnancy, childbirth and the puerperium (O00-O9A)
congenital malformations, deformations, and chromosomal abnormalities (Q00-Q99)
endocrine, nutritional and metabolic diseases (E00-E88)
injury, poisoning and certain other consequences of external causes (S00-T88)
neoplasms (C00-D49)
symptoms, signs and abnormal clinical and laboratory findings, not elsewhere classified (R00-R94)

This chapter contains the following blocks:

G00-G09   Inflammatory diseases of the central nervous system
G10-G14   Systemic atrophies primarily affecting the central nervous system
G20-G26   Extrapyramidal and movement disorders
G30-G32   Other degenerative diseases of the nervous system
G35-G37   Demyelinating diseases of the central nervous system
G40-G47   Episodic and paroxysmal disorders
G50-G59   Nerve, nerve root and plexus disorders
G60-G65   Polyneuropathies and other disorders of the peripheral nervous system
G70-G73   Diseases of myoneural junction and muscle
G80-G83   Cerebral palsy and other paralytic syndromes
G89-G99   Other disorders of the nervous system

Inflammatory diseases of the central nervous system (G00-G09)

✓4th G00   Bacterial meningitis, not elsewhere classified
INCLUDES   bacterial arachnoiditis
bacterial leptomeningitis
bacterial meningitis
bacterial pachymeningitis
EXCLUDES 1   bacterial meningoencephalitis (G04.2)
bacterial meningomyelitis (G04.2)
DEF: Inflammation of meningeal layers of the brain and spinal cord due to a bacterial infection.

CC Excl: For MCC codes in category G00: PDX collection 207

G00.0   Hemophilus meningitis   MCC
Meningitis due to Hemophilus influenzae

G00.1   Pneumococcal meningitis   MCC
Meningitis due to Streptococcal pneumoniae

G00.2   Streptococcal meningitis   MCC
Use additional code to further identify organism (B95.0-B95.5)

G00.3   Staphylococcal meningitis   MCC
Use additional code to further identify organism (B95.61-B95.8)

G00.8   Other bacterial meningitis   MCC
Meningitis due to Escherichia coli
Meningitis due to Friedländer's bacillus
Meningitis due to Klebsiella
Use additional code to further identify organism (B96.-)

G00.9   Bacterial meningitis, unspecified   MCC
Meningitis due to gram-negative bacteria, unspecified
Purulent meningitis NOS
Pyogenic meningitis NOS
Suppurative meningitis NOS

G01   Meningitis in bacterial diseases classified elsewhere   MCC
Code first underlying disease
EXCLUDES 1   meningitis (in):
gonococcal (A54.81)
leptospirosis (A27.81)
listeriosis (A32.11)
Lyme disease (A69.21)
meningococcal (A39.0)
neurosyphilis (A52.13)
tuberculosis (A17.0)
meningoencephalitis and meningomyelitis in bacterial diseases classified elsewhere (G05)
CC Excl: PDX collection 207

G02   Meningitis in other infectious and parasitic diseases classified elsewhere   MCC
Code first underlying disease, such as:
African trypanosomiasis (B56.-)
poliovirus infection (A80.-)
EXCLUDES 1   candidal meningitis (B37.5)
coccidioidomycosis meningitis (B38.4)
cryptococcal meningitis (B45.1)
herpesviral [herpes simplex] meningitis (B00.3)
infectious mononucleosis complicated by meningitis (B27.- with fourth character 2)
measles complicated by meningitis (B05.1)
meningoencephalitis and meningomyelitis in other infectious and parasitic diseases classified elsewhere (G05)
mumps meningitis (B26.1)
rubella meningitis (B06.02)
varicella [chickenpox] meningitis (B01.0)
zoster meningitis (B02.1)
CC Excl: PDX collection 559

✓4th G03   Meningitis due to other and unspecified causes
INCLUDES   arachnoiditis NOS
leptomeningitis NOS
meningitis NOS
pachymeningitis NOS
EXCLUDES 1   meningoencephalitis (G04.-)
meningomyelitis (G04.-)

CC Excl: For CC/MCC codes in category G03, unless otherwise noted: PDX collection 207

G03.0   Nonpyogenic meningitis   MCC
Aseptic meningitis
Nonbacterial meningitis
DEF: Type of meningitis where no bacterial, viral, or other infectious source exists that explains the meningitis symptomology.

G03.1   Chronic meningitis   CC

G03.2   Benign recurrent meningitis [Mollaret]   CC
DEF: Aseptic or noninfectious inflammation of the meninges with the presence of Mollaret cells in the spinal fluid. The patient experiences recurrent bouts of inflammation, lasting anywhere from two to five days.
CC Excl: PDX collection 140

G03.8   Meningitis due to other specified causes   MCC

G03.9   Meningitis, unspecified   MCC
Arachnoiditis (spinal) NOS

✓4th G04   Encephalitis, myelitis and encephalomyelitis
INCLUDES   acute ascending myelitis
meningoencephalitis
meningomyelitis
EXCLUDES 1   encephalopathy NOS (G93.40)
EXCLUDES 2   acute transverse myelitis (G37.3-)
alcoholic encephalopathy (G31.2)
benign myalgic encephalomyelitis (G93.3)
multiple sclerosis (G35)
subacute necrotizing myelitis (G37.4)
toxic encephalitis (G92)
toxic encephalopathy (G92)
DEF: Encephalitis: Inflammation of the brain, often caused by viral or bacterial infection.
DEF: Encephalomyelitis: Inflammatory disease, often viral in nature, that affects the brain and spinal cord.
DEF: Myelitis: Inflammation of the spinal cord.

CC Excl: For CC/MCC codes in category G04, unless otherwise noted: PDX collection 560

✓5th G04.0   Acute disseminated encephalitis and encephalomyelitis (ADEM)
EXCLUDES 1   acute necrotizing hemorrhagic encephalopathy (G04.3-)
other noninfectious acute disseminated encephalomyelitis (noninfectious ADEM) (G04.81)

G04.00   Acute disseminated encephalitis and encephalomyelitis, unspecified   MCC

G04.01   Postinfectious acute disseminated encephalitis and encephalomyelitis (postinfectious ADEM)   MCC
EXCLUDES 1   post chickenpox encephalitis (B01.1)
post measles encephalitis (B05.0)
post measles myelitis (B05.1)

Chapter 6. Diseases of the Nervous System

G04.02   **Postimmunization acute disseminated encephalitis, myelitis and encephalomyelitis**   `MCC`
Encephalitis, postimmunization
Encephalomyelitis, postimmunization
Use additional code to identify the vaccine (T50.A-, T50.B-, T50Z-)
CC Excl: No Excl

G04.1   **Tropical spastic paraplegia**   `CC` `HCC`
CC Excl: PDX collection 561

G04.2   **Bacterial meningoencephalitis and meningomyelitis, not elsewhere classified**   `MCC`
CC Excl: PDX collection 207

✓5th **G04.3**   **Acute necrotizing hemorrhagic encephalopathy**
EXCLUDES 1   *acute disseminated encephalitis and encephalomyelitis (G04.0-)*

G04.30   **Acute necrotizing hemorrhagic encephalopathy, unspecified**   `MCC`
CC Excl: No Excl

G04.31   **Postinfectious acute necrotizing hemorrhagic encephalopathy**   `MCC`

G04.32   **Postimmunization acute necrotizing hemorrhagic encephalopathy**   `MCC`
Use additional code to identify the vaccine (T50.A-, T50.B-, T50Z-)
CC Excl: No Excl

G04.39   **Other acute necrotizing hemorrhagic encephalopathy**   `MCC`
Code also underlying etiology, if applicable
CC Excl: No Excl

✓5th **G04.8**   **Other encephalitis, myelitis and encephalomyelitis**
Code also any associated seizure (G40.-, R56.9)

G04.81   **Other encephalitis and encephalomyelitis**   `HIV` `MCC`
Noninfectious acute disseminated encephalomyelitis (noninfectious ADEM)

G04.89   **Other myelitis**   `HIV` `MCC` `HCC`

✓5th **G04.9**   **Encephalitis, myelitis and encephalomyelitis, unspecified**

G04.90   **Encephalitis and encephalomyelitis, unspecified**   `HIV` `MCC`
Ventriculitis (cerebral) NOS
CC Excl: PDX collection 562

G04.91   **Myelitis, unspecified**   `HIV` `MCC` `HCC`
CC Excl: PDX collection 562

✓4th **G05**   **Encephalitis, myelitis and encephalomyelitis in diseases classified elsewhere**
Code first underlying disease, such as:
human immunodeficiency virus [HIV] disease (B20)
poliovirus (A80.-)
suppurative otitis media (H66.01-H66.4)
trichinellosis (B75)
EXCLUDES 1   *adenoviral encephalitis, myelitis and encephalomyelitis (A85.1)*
congenital toxoplasmosis encephalitis, myelitis and encephalomyelitis (P37.1)
cytomegaloviral encephalitis, myelitis and encephalomyelitis (B25.8)
encephalitis, myelitis and encephalomyelitis (in) measles (B05.0)
encephalitis, myelitis and encephalomyelitis (in) systemic lupus erythematosus (M32.19)
enteroviral encephalitis, myelitis and encephalomyelitis (A85.0)
eosinophilic meningoencephalitis (B83.2)
herpesviral [herpes simplex] encephalitis, myelitis and encephalomyelitis (B00.4)
listerial encephalitis, myelitis and encephalomyelitis (A32.12)
meningococcal encephalitis, myelitis and encephalomyelitis (A39.81)
mumps encephalitis, myelitis and encephalomyelitis (B26.2)
postchickenpox encephalitis, myelitis and encephalomyelitis (B01.1-)
rubella encephalitis, myelitis and encephalomyelitis (B06.01)
toxoplasmosis encephalitis, myelitis and encephalomyelitis (B58.2)
zoster encephalitis, myelitis and encephalomyelitis (B02.0)

G05.3   *Encephalitis and encephalomyelitis in diseases classified elsewhere*   `MCC`
Meningoencephalitis in diseases classified elsewhere
CC Excl: PDX collection 560

G05.4   *Myelitis in diseases classified elsewhere*   `MCC` `HCC`
Meningomyelitis in diseases classified elsewhere
CC Excl: PDX collection 560

✓4th **G06**   **Intracranial and intraspinal abscess and granuloma**
Use additional code (B95-B97) to identify infectious agent
DEF: Abscess: Circumscribed collection of pus resulting from bacteria, frequently associated with swelling and other signs of inflammation.
DEF: Granuloma: Abnormal, dense collections or cells forming a mass or nodule of chronically inflamed tissue with granulations that is usually associated with an infective process.

G06.0   **Intracranial abscess and granuloma**   `MCC`
Brain [any part] abscess (embolic)
Cerebellar abscess (embolic)
Cerebral abscess (embolic)
Intracranial epidural abscess or granuloma
Intracranial extradural abscess or granuloma
Intracranial subdural abscess or granuloma
Otogenic abscess (embolic)
EXCLUDES 1   *tuberculous intracranial abscess and granuloma (A17.81)*
CC Excl: PDX collection 563

G06.1   **Intraspinal abscess and granuloma**   `MCC`
Abscess (embolic) of spinal cord [any part]
Intraspinal epidural abscess or granuloma
Intraspinal extradural abscess or granuloma
Intraspinal subdural abscess or granuloma
EXCLUDES 1   *tuberculous intraspinal abscess and granuloma (A17.81)*
CC Excl: PDX collection 564.

G06.2   **Extradural and subdural abscess, unspecified**   `MCC`
CC Excl: PDX collection 565

G07   *Intracranial and intraspinal abscess and granuloma in diseases classified elsewhere*   `MCC`
Code first underlying disease, such as:
schistosomiasis granuloma of brain (B65.-)
EXCLUDES 1   *abscess of brain:*
amebic (A06.6)
chromomycotic (B43.1)
gonococcal (A54.82)
tuberculous (A17.81)
tuberculoma of meninges (A17.1)
CC Excl: PDX collection 565

G08   **Intracranial and intraspinal phlebitis and thrombophlebitis**   `MCC`
Septic embolism of intracranial or intraspinal venous sinuses and veins
Septic endophlebitis of intracranial or intraspinal venous sinuses and veins
Septic phlebitis of intracranial or intraspinal venous sinuses and veins
Septic thrombophlebitis of intracranial or intraspinal venous sinuses and veins
Septic thrombosis of intracranial or intraspinal venous sinuses and veins
EXCLUDES 1   *intracranial phlebitis and thrombophlebitis complicating:*
abortion, ectopic or molar pregnancy (O00-O07, O08.7)
pregnancy, childbirth and the puerperium (O22.5, O87.3)
nonpyogenic intracranial phlebitis and thrombophlebitis (I67.6)
EXCLUDES 2   *intracranial phlebitis and thrombophlebitis complicating nonpyogenic intraspinal phlebitis and thrombophlebitis (G95.1)*
DEF: Inflammation and formation of a blood clot in a vein within the brain or spine, or their linings.
CC Excl: PDX collection 565

G09   **Sequelae of inflammatory diseases of central nervous system**
`NOTE`   Category G09 is to be used to indicate conditions whose primary classification is to G00-G08 as the cause of sequelae, themselves classifiable elsewhere. The "sequelae" include conditions specified as residuals.
Code first condition resulting from (sequela) of inflammatory diseases of central nervous system

Systemic atrophies primarily affecting the central nervous system (G10-G14)

G10   **Huntington's disease**   `CC` `HCC`
Huntington's chorea
Huntington's dementia
Code also dementia in other diseases classified elsewhere without behavioral disturbance (F02.80)
DEF: Genetic disease caused by degeneration of nerve cells in the brain, characterized by chronic progressive mental deterioration. Dementia and death occur within 15 to 20 years of onset.
CC Excl: PDX collection 566

`N` Newborn: 0   `P` Pediatric: 0-17   `M` Maternity: 12-55   `A` Adult: 15-124   `MCC` Major Complication/Comorbidity   `CC` Complication/Comorbidity   `SW` Severe Wound Dx

564   ICD-10-CM 2019

✓4th **G11 Hereditary ataxia**

> EXCLUDES 2   cerebral palsy (G80.-)
> hereditary and idiopathic neuropathy (G60.-)
> metabolic disorders (E70-E88)

DEF: Ataxia: Defect in muscular control or coordination due to a central nervous system disorder, particularly when voluntary muscular movements are attempted.

> **CC Excl: For CC codes in category G11, unless otherwise noted:** PDX collection 567

G11.0   **Congenital nonprogressive ataxia**   CC HCC

G11.1   **Early-onset cerebellar ataxia**   CC HCC
Early-onset cerebellar ataxia with essential tremor
Early-onset cerebellar ataxia with myoclonus [Hunt's ataxia]
Early-onset cerebellar ataxia with retained tendon reflexes
Friedreich's ataxia (autosomal recessive)
X-linked recessive spinocerebellar ataxia

G11.2   **Late-onset cerebellar ataxia**   CC HCC A

G11.3   **Cerebellar ataxia with defective DNA repair**   CC HCC
Ataxia telangiectasia [Louis-Bar]
> EXCLUDES 2   Cockayne's syndrome (Q87.1)
> other disorders of purine and pyrimidine metabolism (E79.-)
> xeroderma pigmentosum (Q82.1)

G11.4   **Hereditary spastic paraplegia**   CC HCC
CC Excl: PDX collection 568

G11.8   **Other hereditary ataxias**   CC HCC

G11.9   **Hereditary ataxia, unspecified**   CC HCC
Hereditary cerebellar ataxia NOS
Hereditary cerebellar degeneration
Hereditary cerebellar disease
Hereditary cerebellar syndrome
CC Excl: PDX collection 569

✓4th **G12 Spinal muscular atrophy and related syndromes**

> **CC Excl: For CC codes in category G12:** PDX collection 570

G12.0   **Infantile spinal muscular atrophy, type I [Werdnig-Hoffman]**   CC HCC

G12.1   **Other inherited spinal muscular atrophy**   CC HCC
Adult form spinal muscular atrophy
Childhood form, type II spinal muscular atrophy
Distal spinal muscular atrophy
Juvenile form, type III spinal muscular atrophy [Kugelberg-Welander]
Progressive bulbar palsy of childhood [Fazio-Londe]
Scapuloperoneal form spinal muscular atrophy

✓5th **G12.2**   **Motor neuron disease**
AHA: 2017, 4Q, 9-10

     G12.20   **Motor neuron disease, unspecified**   CC HCC

     G12.21   **Amyotrophic lateral sclerosis**   CC HCC A

     G12.22   **Progressive bulbar palsy**   CC HCC

     G12.23   **Primary lateral sclerosis**   CC HCC

     G12.24   **Familial motor neuron disease**   CC HCC

     G12.25   **Progressive spinal muscle atrophy**   CC HCC

     G12.29   **Other motor neuron disease**   CC HCC

G12.8   **Other spinal muscular atrophies and related syndromes**   CC HCC

G12.9   **Spinal muscular atrophy, unspecified**   CC HCC

✓4th **G13 Systemic atrophies primarily affecting central nervous system in diseases classified elsewhere**

G13.0   *Paraneoplastic neuromyopathy and neuropathy*   HCC
Carcinomatous neuromyopathy
Sensorial paraneoplastic neuropathy [Denny Brown]
Code first underlying neoplasm (C00-D49)

G13.1   *Other systemic atrophy primarily affecting central nervous system in neoplastic disease*   HCC
Paraneoplastic limbic encephalopathy
Code first underlying neoplasm (C00-D49)

G13.2   *Systemic atrophy primarily affecting the central nervous system in myxedema*
Code first underlying disease, such as:
hypothyroidism (E03.-)
myxedematous congenital iodine deficiency (E00.1)

G13.8   *Systemic atrophy primarily affecting central nervous system in other diseases classified elsewhere*
Code first underlying disease

G14 Postpolio syndrome

> INCLUDES   postpolio myelitic syndrome
> EXCLUDES 1   sequelae of poliomyelitis (B91)

Extrapyramidal and movement disorders (G20-G26)

G20 Parkinson's disease   HCC
Hemiparkinsonism
Idiopathic Parkinsonism or Parkinson's disease
Paralysis agitans
Parkinsonism or Parkinson's disease NOS
Primary Parkinsonism or Parkinson's disease
> EXCLUDES 1   dementia with Parkinsonism (G31.83)

AHA: 2017, 2Q, 7; 2016, 2Q, 6
TIP: Repeated falls (R29.6) are not integral to Parkinson's disease and can be separately coded.

✓4th **G21 Secondary parkinsonism**

> EXCLUDES 1   dementia with Parkinsonism (G31.83)
> Huntington's disease (G10)
> Shy-Drager syndrome (G90.3)
> syphilitic Parkinsonism (A52.19)

> **CC Excl: For CC/MCC codes in category G21, unless otherwise noted:** PDX collection 572

G21.0   **Malignant neuroleptic syndrome**   MCC
Use additional code for adverse effect, if applicable, to identify drug (T43.3X5, T43.4X5, T43.505, T43.595)
> EXCLUDES 1   neuroleptic induced parkinsonism (G21.11)
CC Excl: PDX collection 571

✓5th **G21.1**   **Other drug-induced secondary parkinsonism**

     G21.11   **Neuroleptic induced parkinsonism**   CC HCC
Use additional code for adverse effect, if applicable, to identify drug (T43.3X5, T43.4X5, T43.505, T43.595)
> EXCLUDES 1   malignant neuroleptic syndrome (G21.0)

     G21.19   **Other drug induced secondary parkinsonism**   CC HCC
Other medication-induced parkinsonism
Use additional code for adverse effect, if applicable, to identify drug (T36-T50 with fifth or sixth character 5)

G21.2   **Secondary parkinsonism due to other external agents**   CC HCC
Code first (T51-T65) to identify external agent

G21.3   **Postencephalitic parkinsonism**   CC HCC

G21.4   **Vascular parkinsonism**   HCC

G21.8   **Other secondary parkinsonism**   CC HCC

G21.9   **Secondary parkinsonism, unspecified**   CC HCC

✓4th **G23 Other degenerative diseases of basal ganglia**

> EXCLUDES 2   multi-system degeneration of the autonomic nervous system (G90.3)

> **CC Excl: For CC codes in category G23:** PDX collection 573

G23.0   **Hallervorden-Spatz disease**   CC HCC
Pigmentary pallidal degeneration

G23.1   **Progressive supranuclear ophthalmoplegia [Steele-Richardson-Olszewski]**   CC HCC
Progressive supranuclear palsy

G23.2   **Striatonigral degeneration**   CC HCC

G23.8   **Other specified degenerative diseases of basal ganglia**   CC HCC
Calcification of basal ganglia

G23.9   **Degenerative disease of basal ganglia, unspecified**   CC HCC

✓4th **G24 Dystonia**

> INCLUDES   dyskinesia
> EXCLUDES 2   athetoid cerebral palsy (G80.3)

DEF: Disorder of abnormal muscle tone, excessive or inadequate. Involuntary movements and prolonged muscle contractions result in tremors, abnormalities in posture, and twisting body motions that affect an isolated area or the whole body.

> **CC Excl: For CC codes in category G24:** PDX collection 574

✓5th **G24.0**   **Drug induced dystonia**
Use additional code for adverse effect, if applicable, to identify drug (T36-T50 with fifth or sixth character 5)

     G24.01   **Drug induced subacute dyskinesia**
Drug induced blepharospasm
Drug induced orofacial dyskinesia
Neuroleptic induced tardive dyskinesia
Tardive dyskinesia

✓ Additional Character Required   ✓x7th Placeholder   Unacceptable PDx   Questionable PDx   Manifestation   H1 - H14 HAC   HCC CMS-HCC Dx   HIV HIV Dx

ICD-10-CM 2019   **565**

G24.02 Drug induced acute dystonia `CC`
Acute dystonic reaction to drugs
Neuroleptic induced acute dystonia

G24.09 Other drug induced dystonia `CC`

G24.1 Genetic torsion dystonia
Dystonia deformans progressiva
Dystonia musculorum deformans
Familial torsion dystonia
Idiopathic familial dystonia
Idiopathic (torsion) dystonia NOS
(Schwalbe-) Ziehen-Oppenheim disease

G24.2 Idiopathic nonfamilial dystonia `CC`

G24.3 Spasmodic torticollis
EXCLUDES 1 *congenital torticollis (Q68.0)*
hysterical torticollis (F44.4)
ocular torticollis (R29.891)
psychogenic torticollis (F45.8)
torticollis NOS (M43.6)
traumatic recurrent torticollis (S13.4)
·**DEF:** Twisted, unnatural position of the neck due to contracted cervical muscles that pull the head to one side or cause involuntary shaking of the head.

G24.4 Idiopathic orofacial dystonia
Orofacial dyskinesia
EXCLUDES 1 *drug induced orofacial dyskinesia (G24.01)*

G24.5 Blepharospasm
EXCLUDES 1 *drug induced blepharospasm (G24.01)*
DEF: Involuntary contraction of the orbicularis oculi muscle, resulting in the eyelids being completely closed.

G24.8 Other dystonia `CC`
Acquired torsion dystonia NOS

G24.9 Dystonia, unspecified
Dyskinesia NOS

✓4ᵗʰ G25 Other extrapyramidal and movement disorders
EXCLUDES 2 *sleep related movement disorders (G47.6-)*

G25.0 Essential tremor
Familial tremor
EXCLUDES 1 *tremor NOS (R25.1)*

G25.1 Drug-induced tremor
Use additional code for adverse effect, if applicable, to identify drug (T36-T50 with fifth or sixth character 5)

G25.2 Other specified forms of tremor
Intention tremor

G25.3 Myoclonus
Drug-induced myoclonus
Palatal myoclonus
Use additional code for adverse effect, if applicable, to identify drug (T36-T50 with fifth or sixth character 5)
EXCLUDES 1 *facial myokymia (G51.4)*
myoclonic epilepsy (G40.-)
DEF: Spasmodic, brief, involuntary muscle contractions that can be due to an undetermined etiology, drug-induced, or caused by a disease process.

G25.4 Drug-induced chorea
Use additional code for adverse effect, if applicable, to identify drug (T36-T50 with fifth or sixth character 5)

G25.5 Other chorea
Chorea NOS
EXCLUDES 1 *chorea NOS with heart involvement (I02.0)*
Huntington's chorea (G10)
rheumatic chorea (I02.-)
Sydenham's chorea (I02.-)

✓5ᵗʰ G25.6 Drug induced tics and other tics of organic origin

G25.61 Drug induced tics
Use additional code for adverse effect, if applicable, to identify drug (T36-T50 with fifth or sixth character 5)

G25.69 Other tics of organic origin
EXCLUDES 1 *habit spasm (F95.9)*
tic NOS (F95.9)
Tourette's syndrome (F95.2)

✓5ᵗʰ G25.7 Other and unspecified drug induced movement disorders
Use additional code for adverse effect, if applicable, to identify drug (T36-T50 with fifth or sixth character 5)

G25.70 Drug induced movement disorder, unspecified

G25.71 Drug induced akathisia
Drug induced acathisia
Neuroleptic induced acute akathisia
Tardive akathisia

G25.79 Other drug induced movement disorders

✓5ᵗʰ G25.8 Other specified extrapyramidal and movement disorders

G25.81 Restless legs syndrome
DEF: Neurological disorder of unknown etiology creating an irresistible urge to move the legs, which may temporarily relieve the symptoms. This syndrome is accompanied by motor restlessness and sensations of pain, burning, prickling, or tingling.

G25.82 Stiff-man syndrome `CC`
CC Excl: PDX collection 575

G25.83 Benign shuddering attacks

G25.89 Other specified extrapyramidal and movement disorders

G25.9 Extrapyramidal and movement disorder, unspecified `CC`
CC Excl: PDX collection 575

G26 *Extrapyramidal and movement disorders in diseases classified elsewhere*
Code first underlying disease

Other degenerative diseases of the nervous system (G30-G32)

✓4ᵗʰ G30 Alzheimer's disease
INCLUDES Alzheimer's dementia senile and presenile forms
Use additional code to identify:
delirium, if applicable (F05)
dementia with behavioral disturbance (F02.81)
dementia without behavioral disturbance (F02.80)
EXCLUDES 1 *senile degeneration of brain NEC (G31.1)*
senile dementia NOS (F03)
senility NOS (R41.81)
AHA: 2017, 1Q, 43
TIP: A code from subcategory F02.8 should always be assigned with a code from this category, even in the absence of documented dementia.
TIP: Functional quadriplegia (R53.2) is not integral to Alzheimer's disease and can be coded in addition to codes from category G30.

G30.0 Alzheimer's disease with early onset

G30.1 Alzheimer's disease with late onset `A`

G30.8 Other Alzheimer's disease

G30.9 Alzheimer's disease, unspecified
AHA: 2016, 2Q, 6; 2012, 4Q, 95

✓4ᵗʰ G31 Other degenerative diseases of nervous system, not elsewhere classified
Use additional code to identify:
dementia with behavioral disturbance (F02.81)
dementia without behavioral disturbance (F02.80)
EXCLUDES 2 *Reye's syndrome (G93.7)*

✓5ᵗʰ G31.0 Frontotemporal dementia

G31.01 Pick's disease
Primary progressive aphasia
Progressive isolated aphasia
DEF: Progressive frontotemporal dementia with asymmetrical atrophy of the frontal and temporal regions of the cerebral cortex and abnormal rounded brain cells called Pick cells with the presence of abnormal staining of protein (called tau). Symptoms include prominent apathy, behavioral changes such as disinhibition and restlessness, echolalia, impairment of language, memory, and intellect, increased carelessness, poor personal hygiene, and decreased attention span.

G31.09 Other frontotemporal dementia
Frontal dementia

G31.1 Senile degeneration of brain, not elsewhere classified
EXCLUDES 1 *Alzheimer's disease (G30.-)*
senility NOS (R41.81)

G31.2 Degeneration of nervous system due to alcohol
Alcoholic cerebellar ataxia
Alcoholic cerebellar degeneration
Alcoholic cerebral degeneration
Alcoholic encephalopathy
Dysfunction of the autonomic nervous system due to alcohol
Code also associated alcoholism (F10.-)

✓5ᵗʰ G31.8 Other specified degenerative diseases of nervous system

G31.81 Alpers disease `CC`
Grey-matter degeneration
CC Excl: PDX collection 537

G31.82 Leigh's disease `CC`
Subacute necrotizing encephalopathy
CC Excl: PDX collection 537

G31.83 Dementia with Lewy bodies
Dementia with Parkinsonism
Lewy body disease
Lewy body dementia
AHA: 2017, 2Q, 7; 2016, 4Q, 141
DEF: Cerebral dementia with neurophysiologic changes, increased hippocampal volume, hypoperfusion in the occipital lobes, beta amyloid deposits with neurofibrillary tangles, and atrophy of the cortex and brainstem. Hallmark neuropsychological characteristics include fluctuating cognition with pronounced variation in attention and alertness, recurrent hallucinations, and Parkinsonism.

G31.84 Mild cognitive impairment, so stated
Mild neurocognitive disorder
EXCLUDES 1   *age related cognitive decline (R41.81)*
altered mental status (R41.82)
cerebral degeneration (G31.9)
change in mental status (R41.82)
cognitive deficits following (sequelae of) cerebral hemorrhage or infarction (I69.01-, I69.11-, I69.21-, I69.31-, I69.81-, I69.91-)
cognitive impairment due to intracranial or head injury (S06.-)
dementia (F01.-, F02.-, F03)
mild memory disturbance (F06.8)
neurologic neglect syndrome (R41.4)
personality change, nonpsychotic (F68.8)

G31.85 Corticobasal degeneration

G31.89 Other specified degenerative diseases of nervous system

G31.9 Degenerative disease of nervous system, unspecified

✓4ᵗʰ G32 Other degenerative disorders of nervous system in diseases classified elsewhere

G32.0 Subacute combined degeneration of spinal cord in diseases classified elsewhere   CC HCC
Dana-Putnam syndrome
Sclerosis of spinal cord (combined) (dorsolateral) (posterolateral)
Code first underlying disease, such as:
anemia (D51.9)
dietary (D51.3)
pernicious (D51.0)
vitamin B12 deficiency (E53.8)
EXCLUDES 1   *syphilitic combined degeneration of spinal cord (A52.11)*
CC Excl: PDX collection 576

✓5ᵗʰ G32.8 Other specified degenerative disorders of nervous system in diseases classified elsewhere
Code first underlying disease, such as:
amyloidosis cerebral degeneration (E85.-)
cerebral degeneration (due to) hypothyroidism (E00.0-E03.9)
cerebral degeneration (due to) neoplasm (C00-D49)
cerebral degeneration (due to) vitamin B deficiency, except thiamine (E52-E53.-)
EXCLUDES 1   *superior hemorrhagic polioencephalitis [Wernicke's encephalopathy] (E51.2)*

G32.81 Cerebellar ataxia in diseases classified elsewhere   CC HCC
Code first underlying disease, such as:
celiac disease (with gluten ataxia) (K90.0)
cerebellar ataxia (in) neoplastic disease (paraneoplastic cerebellar degeneration) (C00-D49)
non-celiac gluten ataxia (M35.9)
EXCLUDES 1   *systemic atrophy primarily affecting the central nervous system in alcoholic cerebellar ataxia (G31.2)*
systemic atrophy primarily affecting the central nervous system in myxedema (G13.2)
CC Excl: PDX collection 567

G32.89 Other specified degenerative disorders of nervous system in diseases classified elsewhere
Degenerative encephalopathy in diseases classified elsewhere

Demyelinating diseases of the central nervous system (G35-G37)

G35 Multiple sclerosis   HCC
Disseminated multiple sclerosis
Generalized multiple sclerosis
Multiple sclerosis NOS
Multiple sclerosis of brain stem
Multiple sclerosis of cord

✓4ᵗʰ G36 Other acute disseminated demyelination
EXCLUDES 1   *postinfectious encephalitis and encephalomyelitis NOS (G04.01)*
DEF: Demyelination: Abnormal loss of myelin, the protective white matter that insulates nerve endings and facilitates neuroreception and neurotransmission. When this substance is damaged, the nerve is short-circuited, resulting in impaired or loss of function.

CC Excl: For CC codes in category G36, unless otherwise noted: PDX collection 578

G36.0 Neuromyelitis optica [Devic]   CC HCC
Demyelination in optic neuritis
EXCLUDES 1   *optic neuritis NOS (H46)*
CC Excl: PDX collection 577

G36.1 Acute and subacute hemorrhagic leukoencephalitis [Hurst]   CC HCC

G36.8 Other specified acute disseminated demyelination   CC HCC

G36.9 Acute disseminated demyelination, unspecified   HIV CC HCC

✓4ᵗʰ G37 Other demyelinating diseases of central nervous system

CC Excl: For CC/MCC codes in category G37, unless otherwise noted: PDX collection 578

G37.0 Diffuse sclerosis of central nervous system   CC HCC
Periaxial encephalitis
Schilder's disease
EXCLUDES 1   *X linked adrenoleukodystrophy (E71.52-)*
CC Excl: PDX collection 579

G37.1 Central demyelination of corpus callosum   CC HCC

G37.2 Central pontine myelinolysis   CC HCC

G37.3 Acute transverse myelitis in demyelinating disease of central nervous system   CC HCC
Acute transverse myelitis NOS
Acute transverse myelopathy
EXCLUDES 1   *multiple sclerosis (G35)*
neuromyelitis optica [Devic] (G36.0)
CC Excl: PDX collection 580

G37.4 Subacute necrotizing myelitis of central nervous system   HIV MCC HCC
CC Excl: PDX collection 562

G37.5 Concentric sclerosis [Balo] of central nervous system   CC HCC
CC Excl: PDX collection 579

G37.8 Other specified demyelinating diseases of central nervous system   CC HCC

G37.9 Demyelinating disease of central nervous system, unspecified   HIV CC HCC

✓Additional Character Required   ✓x7ᵗʰ Placeholder   Unacceptable PDx   Questionable PDx   Manifestation   H1-H14 HAC   HCC CMS-HCC Dx   HIV HIV Dx

ICD-10-CM 2019   **567**

Chapter 6. Diseases of the Nervous System

Episodic and paroxysmal disorders (G40-G47)

✓4th **G40 Epilepsy and recurrent seizures**

> **NOTE** The following terms are to be considered equivalent to intractable: pharmacoresistant (pharmacologically resistant), treatment resistant, refractory (medically) and poorly controlled

> **EXCLUDES 1** conversion disorder with seizures (F44.5)
> convulsions NOS (R56.9)
> post traumatic seizures (R56.1)
> seizure (convulsive) NOS (R56.9)
> seizure of newborn (P90)

> **EXCLUDES 2** hippocampal sclerosis (G93.81)
> mesial temporal sclerosis (G93.81)
> temporal sclerosis (G93.81)
> Todd's paralysis (G83.84)

> **CC Excl: For CC/MCC codes in category G40, unless otherwise noted:** PDX collection 582

✓5th **G40.0 Localization-related (focal) (partial) idiopathic epilepsy and epileptic syndromes with** seizures of localized onset
> Benign childhood epilepsy with centrotemporal EEG spikes
> Childhood epilepsy with occipital EEG paroxysms
> > **EXCLUDES 1** adult onset localization-related epilepsy (G40.1-, G40.2-)

> ✓6th **G40.00 Localization-related (focal) (partial) idiopathic epilepsy and epileptic syndromes with seizures of localized onset,** not intractable
> > Localization-related (focal) (partial) idiopathic epilepsy and epileptic syndromes with seizures of localized onset without intractability

> > **G40.001 Localization-related (focal) (partial) idiopathic epilepsy and epileptic syndromes with seizures of localized onset, not intractable, with status epilepticus** `CC` `HCC`
> > > **CC Excl:** PDX collection 581

> > **G40.009 Localization-related (focal) (partial) idiopathic epilepsy and epileptic syndromes with seizures of localized onset, not intractable, without status epilepticus** `CC` `HCC`
> > > Localization-related (focal) (partial) idiopathic epilepsy and epileptic syndromes with seizures of localized onset NOS
> > > **CC Excl:** PDX collection 581

> ✓6th **G40.01 Localization-related (focal) (partial) idiopathic epilepsy and epileptic syndromes with seizures of localized onset,** intractable

> > **G40.011 Localization-related (focal) (partial) idiopathic epilepsy and epileptic syndromes with seizures of localized onset, intractable, with status epilepticus** `CC` `HCC`

> > **G40.019 Localization-related (focal) (partial) idiopathic epilepsy and epileptic syndromes with seizures of localized onset, intractable, without status epilepticus** `CC` `HCC`

✓5th **G40.1 Localization-related (focal) (partial) symptomatic epilepsy and epileptic syndromes** with simple partial seizures
> Attacks without alteration of consciousness
> Epilepsia partialis continua [Kozhevnikof]
> Simple partial seizures developing into secondarily generalized seizures

> ✓6th **G40.10 Localization-related (focal) (partial) symptomatic epilepsy and epileptic syndromes with simple partial seizures,** not intractable
> > Localization-related (focal) (partial) symptomatic epilepsy and epileptic syndromes with simple partial seizures without intractability

> > **G40.101 Localization-related (focal) (partial) symptomatic epilepsy and epileptic syndromes with simple partial seizures, not intractable, with status epilepticus** `CC` `HCC`
> > > **CC Excl:** PDX collection 581

> **G40.109 Localization-related (focal) (partial) symptomatic epilepsy and epileptic syndromes with simple partial seizures, not intractable, without status epilepticus** `CC` `HCC`
> > Localization-related (focal) (partial) symptomatic epilepsy and epileptic syndromes with simple partial seizures NOS
> > **CC Excl:** PDX collection 581

> ✓6th **G40.11 Localization-related (focal) (partial) symptomatic epilepsy and epileptic syndromes with simple partial seizures,** intractable

> > **G40.111 Localization-related (focal) (partial) symptomatic epilepsy and epileptic syndromes with simple partial seizures, intractable, with status epilepticus** `CC` `HCC`

> > **G40.119 Localization-related (focal) (partial) symptomatic epilepsy and epileptic syndromes with simple partial seizures, intractable, without status epilepticus** `CC` `HCC`

✓5th **G40.2 Localization-related (focal) (partial) symptomatic epilepsy and epileptic syndromes** with complex partial seizures
> Attacks with alteration of consciousness, often with automatisms
> Complex partial seizures developing into secondarily generalized seizures

> ✓6th **G40.20 Localization-related (focal) (partial) symptomatic epilepsy and epileptic syndromes with complex partial seizures,** not intractable
> > Localization-related (focal) (partial) symptomatic epilepsy and epileptic syndromes with complex partial seizures without intractability

> > **G40.201 Localization-related (focal) (partial) symptomatic epilepsy and epileptic syndromes with complex partial seizures, not intractable, with status epilepticus** `CC` `HCC`
> > > **CC Excl:** PDX collection 581

> > **G40.209 Localization-related (focal) (partial) symptomatic epilepsy and epileptic syndromes with complex partial seizures, not intractable, without status epilepticus** `CC` `HCC`
> > > Localization-related (focal) (partial) symptomatic epilepsy and epileptic syndromes with complex partial seizures NOS
> > > **CC Excl:** PDX collection 581

> ✓6th **G40.21 Localization-related (focal) (partial) symptomatic epilepsy and epileptic syndromes with complex partial seizures,** intractable

> > **G40.211 Localization-related (focal) (partial) symptomatic epilepsy and epileptic syndromes with complex partial seizures, intractable, with status epilepticus** `CC` `HCC`

> > **G40.219 Localization-related (focal) (partial) symptomatic epilepsy and epileptic syndromes with complex partial seizures, intractable, without status epilepticus** `CC` `HCC`

✓5th **G40.3 Generalized idiopathic epilepsy and epileptic syndromes**
> Code also MERRF syndrome, if applicable (E88.42)

> **CC Excl: For MCC codes in subcategory G40.3:** PDX collection 583

> ✓6th **G40.30 Generalized idiopathic epilepsy and epileptic syndromes,** not intractable
> > Generalized idiopathic epilepsy and epileptic syndromes without intractability

> > **G40.301 Generalized idiopathic epilepsy and epileptic syndromes, not intractable, with status epilepticus** `MCC` `HCC`

> > **G40.309 Generalized idiopathic epilepsy and epileptic syndromes, not intractable, without status epilepticus** `HCC`
> > > Generalized idiopathic epilepsy and epileptic syndromes NOS

N Newborn: 0   P Pediatric: 0-17   M Maternity: 12-55   A Adult: 15-124   MCC Major Complication/Comorbidity   CC Complication/Comorbidity   SW Severe Wound Dx

568   ICD-10-CM 2019

√6th **G40.31** **Generalized idiopathic epilepsy and epileptic syndromes,** intractable

    G40.311 **Generalized idiopathic epilepsy and epileptic syndromes, intractable, with status epilepticus** `MCC` `HCC`

    G40.319 **Generalized idiopathic epilepsy and epileptic syndromes, intractable, without status epilepticus** `MCC` `HCC`

√5th **G40.A** **Absence epileptic syndrome**
    Childhood absence epilepsy [pyknolepsy]
    Juvenile absence epilepsy
    Absence epileptic syndrome, NOS

  √6th **G40.A0** **Absence epileptic syndrome,** not intractable

    G40.A01 **Absence epileptic syndrome, not intractable, with status epilepticus** `HCC`

    G40.A09 **Absence epileptic syndrome, not intractable, without status epilepticus** `HCC`

  √6th **G40.A1** **Absence epileptic syndrome,** intractable

    G40.A11 **Absence epileptic syndrome, intractable, with status epilepticus** `CC` `HCC`

    G40.A19 **Absence epileptic syndrome, intractable, without status epilepticus** `CC` `HCC`

√5th **G40.B** **Juvenile myoclonic epilepsy [impulsive petit mal]**

  √6th **G40.B0** **Juvenile myoclonic epilepsy,** not intractable

    G40.B01 **Juvenile myoclonic epilepsy, not intractable, with status epilepticus** `CC` `HCC`

    G40.B09 **Juvenile myoclonic epilepsy, not intractable, without status epilepticus** `CC` `HCC`

  √6th **G40.B1** **Juvenile myoclonic epilepsy,** intractable

    G40.B11 **Juvenile myoclonic epilepsy, intractable, with status epilepticus** `CC` `HCC`

    G40.B19 **Juvenile myoclonic epilepsy, intractable, without status epilepticus** `CC` `HCC`

√5th **G40.4** **Other generalized epilepsy and epileptic syndromes**
    Epilepsy with grand mal seizures on awakening
    Epilepsy with myoclonic absences
    Epilepsy with myoclonic-astatic seizures
    Grand mal seizure NOS
    Nonspecific atonic epileptic seizures
    Nonspecific clonic epileptic seizures
    Nonspecific myoclonic epileptic seizures
    Nonspecific tonic epileptic seizures
    Nonspecific tonic-clonic epileptic seizures
    Symptomatic early myoclonic encephalopathy

  √6th **G40.40** **Other generalized epilepsy and epileptic syndromes,** not intractable
    Other generalized epilepsy and epileptic syndromes without intractability
    Other generalized epilepsy and epileptic syndromes NOS

    G40.401 **Other generalized epilepsy and epileptic syndromes, not intractable, with status epilepticus** `HCC`

    G40.409 **Other generalized epilepsy and epileptic syndromes, not intractable, without status epilepticus** `HCC`

  √6th **G40.41** **Other generalized epilepsy and epileptic syndromes,** intractable

    G40.411 **Other generalized epilepsy and epileptic syndromes, intractable, with status epilepticus** `CC` `HCC`

    G40.419 **Other generalized epilepsy and epileptic syndromes, intractable, without status epilepticus** `CC` `HCC`

√5th **G40.5** **Epileptic seizures related to** external causes
    Epileptic seizures related to alcohol
    Epileptic seizures related to drugs
    Epileptic seizures related to hormonal changes
    Epileptic seizures related to sleep deprivation
    Epileptic seizures related to stress
    Use additional code for adverse effect, if applicable, to identify drug (T36-T50 with fifth or sixth character 5)
    Code also, if applicable, associated epilepsy and recurrent seizures (G40.-)

  √6th **G40.50** **Epileptic seizures related to external causes,** not intractable

    G40.501 **Epileptic seizures related to external causes, not intractable, with status epilepticus** `CC` `HCC`

    G40.509 **Epileptic seizures related to external causes, not intractable,** without status epilepticus `CC` `HCC`
      Epileptic seizures related to external causes, NOS

√5th **G40.8** **Other epilepsy and recurrent seizures**
    Epilepsies and epileptic syndromes undetermined as to whether they are focal or generalized
    Landau-Kleffner syndrome

  √6th **G40.80** **Other epilepsy**

    G40.801 **Other epilepsy, not intractable, with status epilepticus** `CC` `HCC`
      Other epilepsy without intractability with status epilepticus

    G40.802 **Other epilepsy, not intractable, without status epilepticus** `CC` `HCC`
      Other epilepsy without intractability without status epilepticus

    G40.803 **Other epilepsy, intractable, with status epilepticus** `CC` `HCC`

    G40.804 **Other epilepsy, intractable, without status epilepticus** `CC` `HCC`

  √6th **G40.81** **Lennox-Gastaut syndrome**
    DEF: Severe form of epilepsy with usual onset in early childhood. Seizures are frequent and difficult to treat, causing falls and intellectual impairment.

    G40.811 **Lennox-Gastaut syndrome,** not intractable, with status epilepticus `CC` `HCC`

    G40.812 **Lennox-Gastaut syndrome,** not intractable, without status epilepticus `CC` `HCC`

    G40.813 **Lennox-Gastaut syndrome, intractable, with status epilepticus** `CC` `HCC`

    G40.814 **Lennox-Gastaut syndrome,** intractable, without status epilepticus `CC` `HCC`

  √6th **G40.82** **Epileptic spasms**
    Infantile spasms
    Salaam attacks
    West's syndrome

    G40.821 **Epileptic spasms, not intractable, with status epilepticus** `CC` `HCC`
      CC Excl: PDX collection 581

    G40.822 **Epileptic spasms, not intractable, without status epilepticus** `CC` `HCC`
      CC Excl: PDX collection 581

    G40.823 **Epileptic spasms, intractable, with status epilepticus** `CC` `HCC`

    G40.824 **Epileptic spasms, intractable, without status epilepticus** `CC` `HCC`

  G40.89 **Other seizures** `CC` `HCC`
    `EXCLUDES 1` *post traumatic seizures (R56.1)*
      recurrent seizures NOS (G40.909)
      seizure NOS (R56.9)

√5th **G40.9** **Epilepsy,** unspecified

  √6th **G40.90** **Epilepsy, unspecified,** not intractable
    Epilepsy, unspecified, without intractability

    G40.901 **Epilepsy, unspecified, not intractable,** with status epilepticus `HCC`

    G40.909 **Epilepsy, unspecified, not intractable,** without status epilepticus `HCC`
      Epilepsy NOS
      Epileptic convulsions NOS
      Epileptic fits NOS
      Epileptic seizures NOS
      Recurrent seizures NOS
      Seizure disorder NOS

  √6th **G40.91** **Epilepsy, unspecified,** intractable
    Intractable seizure disorder NOS

    G40.911 **Epilepsy, unspecified, intractable,** with status epilepticus `CC` `HCC`

    G40.919 **Epilepsy, unspecified, intractable,** without status epilepticus `CC` `HCC`

☑ Additional Character Required   √x7th Placeholder   Unacceptable PDx   Questionable PDx   Manifestation   `H1`-`H14` HAC   `HCC` CMS-HCC Dx   `HIV` HIV Dx

ICD-10-CM 2019   569

✓4th G43 Migraine

NOTE The following terms are to be considered equivalent to intractable: pharmacoresistant (pharmacologically resistant), treatment resistant, refractory (medically) and poorly controlled

Use additional code for adverse effect, if applicable, to identify drug (T36-T50 with fifth or sixth character 5)

EXCLUDES 1 headache NOS (R51)
lower half migraine (G44.00)

EXCLUDES 2 headache syndromes (G44.-)

DEF: Headaches that occur periodically on one or both sides of the head that may be associated with nausea and vomiting, sensitivity to light and sound, dizziness, distorted vision, and cognitive disturbances.

✓5th G43.0 Migraine without aura
Common migraine

EXCLUDES 1 chronic migraine without aura (G43.7-)

✓6th G43.00 Migraine without aura, not intractable
Migraine without aura without mention of refractory migraine

G43.001 Migraine without aura, not intractable, with status migrainosus

G43.009 Migraine without aura, not intractable, without status migrainosus
Migraine without aura NOS

✓6th G43.01 Migraine without aura, intractable
Migraine without aura with refractory migraine

G43.011 Migraine without aura, intractable, with status migrainosus

G43.019 Migraine without aura, intractable, without status migrainosus

✓5th G43.1 Migraine with aura
Basilar migraine
Classical migraine
Migraine equivalents
Migraine preceded or accompanied by transient focal neurological phenomena
Migraine triggered seizures
Migraine with acute-onset aura
Migraine with aura without headache (migraine equivalents)
Migraine with prolonged aura
Migraine with typical aura
Retinal migraine

Code also any associated seizure (G40.-, R56.9)

EXCLUDES 1 persistent migraine aura (G43.5-, G43.6-)

✓6th G43.10 Migraine with aura, not intractable
Migraine with aura without mention of refractory migraine

G43.101 Migraine with aura, not intractable, with status migrainosus

G43.109 Migraine with aura, not intractable, without status migrainosus
Migraine with aura NOS

✓6th G43.11 Migraine with aura, intractable
Migraine with aura with refractory migraine

G43.111 Migraine with aura, intractable, with status migrainosus

G43.119 Migraine with aura, intractable, without status migrainosus

✓5th G43.4 Hemiplegic migraine
Familial migraine
Sporadic migraine

✓6th G43.40 Hemiplegic migraine, not intractable
Hemiplegic migraine without refractory migraine

G43.401 Hemiplegic migraine, not intractable, with status migrainosus

G43.409 Hemiplegic migraine, not intractable, without status migrainosus
Hemiplegic migraine NOS

✓6th G43.41 Hemiplegic migraine, intractable
Hemiplegic migraine with refractory migraine

G43.411 Hemiplegic migraine, intractable, with status migrainosus

G43.419 Hemiplegic migraine, intractable, without status migrainosus

✓5th G43.5 Persistent migraine aura without cerebral infarction

✓6th G43.50 Persistent migraine aura without cerebral infarction, not intractable
Persistent migraine aura without cerebral infarction, without refractory migraine

G43.501 Persistent migraine aura without cerebral infarction, not intractable, with status migrainosus

G43.509 Persistent migraine aura without cerebral infarction, not intractable, without status migrainosus
Persistent migraine aura NOS

✓6th G43.51 Persistent migraine aura without cerebral infarction, intractable
Persistent migraine aura without cerebral infarction, with refractory migraine

G43.511 Persistent migraine aura without cerebral infarction, intractable, with status migrainosus

G43.519 Persistent migraine aura without cerebral infarction, intractable, without status migrainosus

✓5th G43.6 Persistent migraine aura with cerebral infarction
Code also the type of cerebral infarction (I63.-)

CC Excl: For CC codes in subcategory G43.6, unless otherwise noted: PDX collection 584

✓6th G43.60 Persistent migraine aura with cerebral infarction, not intractable
Persistent migraine aura with cerebral infarction, without refractory migraine

G43.601 Persistent migraine aura with cerebral infarction, not intractable, with status migrainosus CC

G43.609 Persistent migraine aura with cerebral infarction, not intractable, without status migrainosus CC
CC Excl: PDX collection 585

✓6th G43.61 Persistent migraine aura with cerebral infarction, intractable
Persistent migraine aura with cerebral infarction, with refractory migraine

G43.611 Persistent migraine aura with cerebral infarction, intractable, with status migrainosus CC

G43.619 Persistent migraine aura with cerebral infarction, intractable, without status migrainosus CC

✓5th G43.7 Chronic migraine without aura
Transformed migraine

EXCLUDES 1 migraine without aura (G43.0-)

✓6th G43.70 Chronic migraine without aura, not intractable
Chronic migraine without aura, without refractory migraine

G43.701 Chronic migraine without aura, not intractable, with status migrainosus

G43.709 Chronic migraine without aura, not intractable, without status migrainosus
Chronic migraine without aura NOS

✓6th G43.71 Chronic migraine without aura, intractable
Chronic migraine without aura, with refractory migraine

G43.711 Chronic migraine without aura, intractable, with status migrainosus

G43.719 Chronic migraine without aura, intractable, without status migrainosus

✓5th G43.A Cyclical vomiting
TIP: Assign K31.89 Other diseases of stomach and duodenum, along with the appropriate code from category R11 Nausea and vomiting, to identify cyclical vomiting not related to migraine.

G43.A0 Cyclical vomiting, not intractable
Cyclical vomiting, without refractory migraine

G43.A1 Cyclical vomiting, intractable
Cyclical vomiting, with refractory migraine

✓5th G43.B Ophthalmoplegic migraine

G43.B0 Ophthalmoplegic migraine, not intractable
Ophthalmoplegic migraine, without refractory migraine

G43.B1 Ophthalmoplegic migraine, intractable
Ophthalmoplegic migraine, with refractory migraine

N Newborn: 0   P Pediatric: 0-17   M Maternity: 12-55   A Adult: 15-124   MCC Major Complication/Comorbidity   CC Complication/Comorbidity   SW Severe Wound Dx

570   ICD-10-CM 2019

Chapter 6. Diseases of the Nervous System

☑5th **G43.C** Periodic headache syndromes in child or adult

    G43.C0 **Periodic headache syndromes in child or adult,** not intractable

         Periodic headache syndromes in child or adult, without refractory migraine

    G43.C1 **Periodic headache syndromes in child or adult,** intractable

         Periodic headache syndromes in child or adult, with refractory migraine

☑5th **G43.D** Abdominal migraine

    G43.D0 **Abdominal migraine,** not intractable

         Abdominal migraine, without refractory migraine

    G43.D1 **Abdominal migraine,** intractable

         Abdominal migraine, with refractory migraine

☑5th **G43.8** Other migraine

  ☑6th **G43.80** **Other migraine,** not intractable

         Other migraine, without refractory migraine

    G43.801 **Other migraine, not intractable,** with status migrainosus

    G43.809 **Other migraine, not intractable,** without status migrainosus

  ☑6th **G43.81** **Other migraine,** intractable

         Other migraine, with refractory migraine

    G43.811 **Other migraine, intractable,** with status migrainosus

    G43.819 **Other migraine, intractable,** without status migrainosus

  ☑6th **G43.82** **Menstrual migraine,** not intractable

         Menstrual headache, not intractable
         Menstrual migraine, without refractory migraine
         Menstrually related migraine, not intractable
         Pre-menstrual headache, not intractable
         Pre-menstrual migraine, not intractable
         Pure menstrual migraine, not intractable
         Code also associated premenstrual tension syndrome (N94.3)

    G43.821 **Menstrual migraine, not intractable, with status migrainosus** ♀

    G43.829 **Menstrual migraine, not intractable, without status migrainosus** ♀

         Menstrual migraine NOS

  ☑6th **G43.83** **Menstrual migraine,** intractable

         Menstrual headache, intractable
         Menstrual migraine, with refractory migraine
         Menstrually related migraine, intractable
         Pre-menstrual headache, intractable
         Pre-menstrual migraine, intractable
         Pure menstrual migraine, intractable
         Code also associated premenstrual tension syndrome (N94.3)

    G43.831 **Menstrual migraine, intractable, with status migrainosus** ♀

    G43.839 **Menstrual migraine, intractable, without status migrainosus** ♀

☑5th **G43.9** Migraine, unspecified

  ☑6th **G43.90** **Migraine, unspecified,** not intractable

         Migraine, unspecified, without refractory migraine

    G43.901 **Migraine, unspecified, not intractable, with status migrainosus**

         Status migrainosus NOS

    G43.909 **Migraine, unspecified, not intractable, without status migrainosus**

         Migraine NOS

  ☑6th **G43.91** **Migraine, unspecified,** intractable

         Migraine, unspecified, with refractory migraine

    G43.911 **Migraine, unspecified, intractable, with status migrainosus**

    G43.919 **Migraine, unspecified, intractable, without status migrainosus**

☑4th **G44** Other headache syndromes

  EXCLUDES 1   *headache NOS (R51)*

  EXCLUDES 2   *atypical facial pain (G50.1)*
          headache due to lumbar puncture (G97.1)
          migraines (G43.-)
          trigeminal neuralgia (G50.0)

☑5th **G44.0** Cluster headaches and other trigeminal autonomic cephalgias (TAC)

    DEF: Cluster headache: Characteristic grouping or clustering of headaches that can last for a number of weeks or months and then completely disappear for months or years. They are typically not associated with gastrointestinal upset or light sensitivity as experienced in migraines.

  ☑6th **G44.00** **Cluster headache syndrome,** unspecified

       Ciliary neuralgia   Lower half migraine
       Cluster headache NOS   Migrainous neuralgia
       Histamine cephalgia

    G44.001 **Cluster headache syndrome, unspecified, intractable**

    G44.009 **Cluster headache syndrome, unspecified, not intractable**

         Cluster headache syndrome NOS

  ☑6th **G44.01** **Episodic cluster headache**

    G44.011 **Episodic cluster headache,** intractable

    G44.019 **Episodic cluster headache,** not intractable

         Episodic cluster headache NOS

  ☑6th **G44.02** **Chronic cluster headache**

    G44.021 **Chronic cluster headache,** intractable

    G44.029 **Chronic cluster headache,** not intractable

         Chronic cluster headache NOS

  ☑6th **G44.03** **Episodic paroxysmal hemicrania**

         Paroxysmal hemicrania NOS

    G44.031 **Episodic paroxysmal hemicrania, intractable**

    G44.039 **Episodic paroxysmal hemicrania,** not intractable

         Episodic paroxysmal hemicrania NOS

  ☑6th **G44.04** **Chronic paroxysmal hemicrania**

    G44.041 **Chronic paroxysmal hemicrania, intractable**

    G44.049 **Chronic paroxysmal hemicrania,** not intractable

         Chronic paroxysmal hemicrania NOS

  ☑6th **G44.05** **Short lasting unilateral neuralgiform headache with conjunctival injection and tearing (SUNCT)**

    G44.051 **Short lasting unilateral neuralgiform headache with conjunctival injection and tearing (SUNCT),** intractable

    G44.059 **Short lasting unilateral neuralgiform headache with conjunctival injection and tearing (SUNCT),** not intractable

         Short lasting unilateral neuralgiform headache with conjunctival injection and tearing (SUNCT) NOS

  ☑6th **G44.09** **Other** trigeminal autonomic cephalgias (TAC)

    G44.091 **Other trigeminal autonomic cephalgias (TAC),** intractable

    G44.099 **Other trigeminal autonomic cephalgias syndrome (TAC),** not intractable

  G44.1 Vascular headache, not elsewhere classified

    EXCLUDES 2   *cluster headache (G44.0)*
          complicated headache syndromes (G44.5-)
          drug-induced headache (G44.4-)
          migraine (G43.-)
          other specified headache syndromes (G44.8-)
          post-traumatic headache (G44.3-)
          tension-type headache (G44.2-)

☑5th **G44.2** Tension-type headache

  ☑6th **G44.20** **Tension-type headache,** unspecified

    G44.201 **Tension-type headache, unspecified,** intractable

    G44.209 **Tension-type headache, unspecified,** not intractable

         Tension headache NOS

  ☑6th **G44.21** **Episodic** tension-type headache

    G44.211 **Episodic tension-type headache,** intractable

✔ Additional Character Required   ✔x7th Placeholder   Unacceptable PDx   Questionable PDx   Manifestation   H1 - H14 HAC   HCC CMS-HCC Dx   HIV HIV Dx

ICD-10-CM 2019   571

G44.219 **Episodic tension-type headache,** not **intractable**
Episodic tension-type headache NOS

✓6th **G44.22** **Chronic tension-type headache**

G44.221 **Chronic tension-type headache, intractable**

G44.229 **Chronic tension-type headache,** not **intractable**
Chronic tension-type headache NOS

✓5th **G44.3** **Post-traumatic headache**

✓6th **G44.30** **Post-traumatic headache,** unspecified

G44.301 **Post-traumatic headache, unspecified, intractable**

G44.309 **Post-traumatic headache, unspecified,** not **intractable**
Post-traumatic headache NOS

✓6th **G44.31** **Acute post-traumatic headache**

G44.311 **Acute post-traumatic headache, intractable**

G44.319 **Acute post-traumatic headache,** not **intractable**
Acute post-traumatic headache NOS

✓6th **G44.32** **Chronic post-traumatic headache**

G44.321 **Chronic post-traumatic headache, intractable**

G44.329 **Chronic post-traumatic headache,** not **intractable**
Chronic post-traumatic headache NOS

✓5th **G44.4** **Drug-induced headache, not elsewhere classified**
Medication overuse headache
Use additional code for adverse effect, if applicable, to identify drug (T36-T50 with fifth or sixth character 5)

G44.40 **Drug-induced headache, not elsewhere classified,** not **intractable**

G44.41 **Drug-induced headache, not elsewhere classified, intractable**

✓5th **G44.5** **Complicated headache syndromes**

G44.51 **Hemicrania continua**
DEF: Persistent primary headache of unknown causation occurring on one side of the face and head. May last for more than three months, with daily and continuous pain of moderate intensity with severe exacerbations.

G44.52 **New daily persistent headache (NDPH)**

G44.53 **Primary thunderclap headache**

G44.59 **Other complicated headache syndrome**

✓5th **G44.8** **Other specified headache syndromes**

G44.81 **Hypnic headache**

G44.82 **Headache associated with** sexual activity
Orgasmic headache
Preorgasmic headache

G44.83 **Primary cough headache**

G44.84 **Primary exertional headache**

G44.85 **Primary stabbing headache**

G44.89 **Other headache syndrome**

✓4th **G45** **Transient cerebral ischemic attacks and related syndromes**
EXCLUDES 1 neonatal cerebral ischemia (P91.0)
transient retinal artery occlusion (H34.0-)
AHA: 2018, 2Q, 9
DEF: Transient cerebral ischemic attack: Intermittent or brief cerebral dysfunction from lack of oxygenation with no persistent neurological deficits associated with occlusive vascular disease. TIA may denote an impending cerebrovascular accident.

CC Excl: For CC codes in category G45, unless otherwise noted: PDX collection 586

G45.0 **Vertebro-basilar artery syndrome** CC

G45.1 **Carotid artery syndrome (hemispheric)** CC

G45.2 **Multiple and bilateral precerebral artery syndromes** CC

G45.3 **Amaurosis fugax** CC
CC Excl: PDX collection 587

G45.4 **Transient global amnesia**
EXCLUDES 1 amnesia NOS (R41.3)

G45.8 **Other transient cerebral ischemic attacks and related syndromes** CC

G45.9 **Transient cerebral ischemic attack, unspecified** CC
Spasm of cerebral artery
TIA
Transient cerebral ischemia NOS

✓4th **G46** **Vascular syndromes of brain in cerebrovascular diseases**
Code first underlying cerebrovascular disease (I60-I69)

CC Excl: For CC codes in category G46: PDX collection 586

G46.0 **Middle cerebral artery syndrome** CC

G46.1 **Anterior cerebral artery syndrome** CC

G46.2 **Posterior cerebral artery syndrome** CC

G46.3 **Brain stem stroke syndrome**
Benedikt syndrome
Claude syndrome
Foville syndrome
Millard-Gubler syndrome
Wallenberg syndrome
Weber syndrome

G46.4 **Cerebellar stroke syndrome**

G46.5 **Pure motor lacunar syndrome**

G46.6 **Pure sensory lacunar syndrome**

G46.7 **Other lacunar syndromes**

G46.8 **Other vascular syndromes of brain in cerebrovascular diseases**

✓4th **G47** **Sleep disorders**
EXCLUDES 2 nightmares (F51.5)
nonorganic sleep disorders (F51.-)
sleep terrors (F51.4)
sleepwalking (F51.3)

✓5th **G47.0** **Insomnia**
EXCLUDES 2 alcohol related insomnia (F10.182, F10.282, F10.982)
drug-related insomnia (F11.182, F11.282, F11.982, F13.182, F13.282, F13.982, F14.182, F14.282, F14.982, F15.182, F15.282, F15.982, F19.182, F19.282, F19.982)
idiopathic insomnia (F51.01)
insomnia due to a mental disorder (F51.05)
insomnia not due to a substance or known physiological condition (F51.0-)
nonorganic insomnia (F51.0-)
primary insomnia (F51.01)
sleep apnea (G47.3-)

G47.00 **Insomnia,** unspecified
Insomnia NOS

G47.01 **Insomnia** due to medical condition
Code also associated medical condition

G47.09 **Other insomnia**

✓5th **G47.1** **Hypersomnia**
EXCLUDES 2 alcohol-related hypersomnia (F10.182, F10.282, F10.982)
drug-related hypersomnia (F11.182, F11.282, F11.982, F13.182, F13.282, F13.982, F14.182, F14.282, F14.982, F15.182, F15.282, F15.982, F19.182, F19.282, F19.982)
hypersomnia due to a mental disorder (F51.13)
hypersomnia not due to a substance or known physiological condition (F51.1-)
primary hypersomnia (F51.11)
sleep apnea (G47.3-)

G47.10 **Hypersomnia,** unspecified
Hypersomnia NOS

G47.11 **Idiopathic hypersomnia with long sleep time**
Idiopathic hypersomnia NOS

G47.12 **Idiopathic hypersomnia without long sleep time**

G47.13 **Recurrent hypersomnia**
Kleine-Levin syndrome
Menstrual related hypersomnia

G47.14 **Hypersomnia due to medical condition**
Code also associated medical condition

G47.19 **Other hypersomnia**

✓5th **G47.2** **Circadian rhythm sleep disorders**
Disorders of the sleep wake schedule
Inversion of nyctohemeral rhythm
Inversion of sleep rhythm

G47.20 **Circadian rhythm sleep disorder,** unspecified **type**
Sleep wake schedule disorder NOS

G47.21 **Circadian rhythm sleep disorder,** delayed sleep phase **type**
Delayed sleep phase syndrome

G47.22 **Circadian rhythm sleep disorder,** advanced sleep phase **type**

G47.23 **Circadian rhythm sleep disorder,** irregular sleep wake **type**
Irregular sleep-wake pattern

G47.24 **Circadian rhythm sleep disorder,** free running **type**
Circadian rhythm sleep disorder, non-24-hour sleep-wake type

G47.25 **Circadian rhythm sleep disorder,** jet lag **type**

G47.26 **Circadian rhythm sleep disorder,** shift work **type**

G47.27 Circadian rhythm sleep disorder in conditions classified elsewhere
Code first underlying condition

G47.29 **Other** circadian rhythm sleep disorder

✓5ᵗʰ **G47.3 Sleep apnea**
Code also any associated underlying condition
EXCLUDES 1   apnea NOS (R06.81)
Cheyne-Stokes breathing (R06.3)
pickwickian syndrome (E66.2)
sleep apnea of newborn (P28.3)

G47.30 **Sleep apnea,** unspecified
Sleep apnea NOS

G47.31 **Primary central sleep apnea**
Idiopathic central sleep apnea

G47.32 **High altitude periodic breathing**

G47.33 Obstructive **sleep apnea** (adult) (pediatric)
Obstructive sleep apnea hypopnea
EXCLUDES 1   obstructive sleep apnea of newborn (P28.3)

G47.34 **Idiopathic sleep related nonobstructive alveolar hypoventilation**
Sleep related hypoxia

G47.35 **Congenital central alveolar hypoventilation syndrome**

G47.36 Sleep related hypoventilation in conditions classified elsewhere
Sleep related hypoxemia in conditions classified elsewhere
Code first underlying condition

G47.37 Central sleep apnea in conditions classified elsewhere
Code first underlying condition

G47.39 **Other sleep apnea**

✓5ᵗʰ **G47.4 Narcolepsy and cataplexy**

✓6ᵗʰ **G47.41 Narcolepsy**
G47.411 **Narcolepsy** with cataplexy
G47.419 **Narcolepsy** without cataplexy
Narcolepsy NOS

✓6ᵗʰ **G47.42 Narcolepsy in conditions classified elsewhere**
Code first underlying condition
G47.421 Narcolepsy in conditions classified elsewhere with cataplexy
G47.429 Narcolepsy in conditions classified elsewhere without cataplexy

✓5ᵗʰ **G47.5 Parasomnia**
EXCLUDES 1   alcohol induced parasomnia (F10.182, F10.282, F10.982)
drug induced parasomnia (F11.182, F11.282, F11.982, F13.182, F13.282, F13.982, F14.182, F14.282, F14.982, F15.182, F15.282, F15.982, F19.182, F19.282, F19.982)
parasomnia not due to a substance or known physiological condition (F51.8)

G47.50 **Parasomnia,** unspecified
Parasomnia NOS

G47.51 **Confusional arousals**

G47.52 **REM sleep behavior disorder**

G47.53 **Recurrent isolated sleep paralysis**

G47.54 Parasomnia in conditions classified elsewhere
Code first underlying condition

G47.59 **Other parasomnia**

✓5ᵗʰ **G47.6 Sleep related movement disorders**
EXCLUDES 2   restless legs syndrome (G25.81)

G47.61 **Periodic limb movement disorder**

G47.62 **Sleep related** leg cramps

G47.63 **Sleep related** bruxism
EXCLUDES 1   psychogenic bruxism (F45.8)

G47.69 **Other sleep related movement disorders**

G47.8 **Other sleep disorders**
Other specified sleep-wake disorder

G47.9 **Sleep disorder,** unspecified
Sleep disorder NOS
Unspecified sleep-wake disorder

Nerve, nerve root and plexus disorders (G50-G59)

EXCLUDES 1   current traumatic nerve, nerve root and plexus disorders—see Injury, nerve by body region
neuralgia NOS (M79.2)
neuritis NOS (M79.2)
peripheral neuritis in pregnancy (O26.82-)
radiculitis NOS (M54.1-)

✓4ᵗʰ **G50 Disorders of** trigeminal nerve
INCLUDES   disorders of 5th cranial nerve

G50.0 **Trigeminal neuralgia**
Syndrome of paroxysmal facial pain
Tic douloureux

G50.1 **Atypical facial pain**

G50.8 **Other disorders of trigeminal nerve**

G50.9 **Disorder of trigeminal nerve,** unspecified

Trigeminal and Facial Nerve Branches

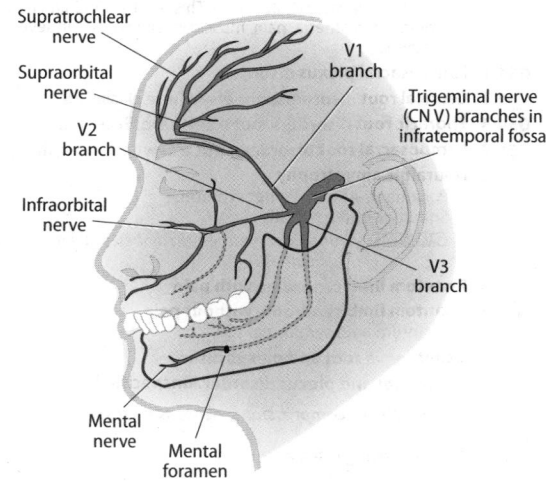

Supratrochlear nerve
Supraorbital nerve
V2 branch
Infraorbital nerve
V1 branch
Trigeminal nerve (CN V) branches in infratemporal fossa
V3 branch
Mental nerve
Mental foramen

✓4ᵗʰ **G51 Facial nerve disorders**
INCLUDES   disorders of 7th cranial nerve

G51.0 **Bell's palsy**
Facial palsy

G51.1 **Geniculate ganglionitis**
EXCLUDES 1   postherpetic geniculate ganglionitis (B02.21)

G51.2 **Melkersson's syndrome**
Melkersson-Rosenthal syndrome

✓5ᵗʰ **G51.3 Clonic hemifacial spasm**
●   G51.31 **Clonic hemifacial spasm,** right
●   G51.32 **Clonic hemifacial spasm,** left
●   G51.33 **Clonic hemifacial spasm,** bilateral
●   G51.39 **Clonic hemifacial spasm,** unspecified

G51.4 **Facial myokymia**

G51.8 **Other disorders of facial nerve**

G51.9 **Disorder of facial nerve, unspecified**

✓4ᵗʰ **G52 Disorders of** other cranial nerves
EXCLUDES 2   disorders of acoustic [8th] nerve (H93.3)
disorders of optic [2nd] nerve (H46, H47.0)
paralytic strabismus due to nerve palsy (H49.0-H49.2)

G52.0 **Disorders of** olfactory **nerve**
Disorders of 1st cranial nerve

G52.1 **Disorders of** glossopharyngeal **nerve**
Disorder of 9th cranial nerve
Glossopharyngeal neuralgia

G52.2 **Disorders of** vagus **nerve**
Disorders of pneumogastric [10th] nerve

G52.3 **Disorders of** hypoglossal **nerve**
Disorders of 12th cranial nerve

G52.7 **Disorders of** multiple cranial **nerves**
Polyneuritis cranialis

✓ Additional Character Required   ✓7ᵗʰ Placeholder   Unacceptable PDx   Questionable PDx   Manifestation   H1-H14 HAC   HCC CMS-HCC Dx   HIV HIV Dx

ICD-10-CM 2019   573

G52.8 Disorders of other specified **cranial nerves**

G52.9 Cranial nerve disorder, unspecified

G53 *Cranial nerve disorders in diseases classified elsewhere*

Code first underlying disease, such as:
neoplasm (C00-D49)

> EXCLUDES 1 *multiple cranial nerve palsy in sarcoidosis (D86.82)*
> *multiple cranial nerve palsy in syphilis (A52.15)*
> *postherpetic geniculate ganglionitis (B02.21)*
> *postherpetic trigeminal neuralgia (B02.22)*

✓4th G54 Nerve root and plexus **disorders**

> EXCLUDES 1 *current traumatic nerve root and plexus disorders—see nerve injury by body region*
> *intervertebral disc disorders (M50-M51)*
> *neuritis or radiculitis brachial NOS (M54.13)*
> *neuritis or radiculitis lumbar NOS (M54.16)*
> *neuritis or radiculitis lumbosacral NOS (M54.17)*
> *neuritis or radiculitis thoracic NOS (M54.14)*
> *radiculitis NOS (M54.10)*
> *radiculopathy NOS (M54.10)*
> *spondylosis (M47.-)*

G54.0 Brachial plexus disorders
Thoracic outlet syndrome
DEF: Acquired disorder affecting the spinal nerves that send signals to the shoulder, arm, and hand, causing corresponding motor and sensory dysfunction. This disorder is characterized by regional paresthesia, pain, muscle weakness, and in severe cases paralysis.

G54.1 Lumbosacral plexus disorders

G54.2 Cervical root disorders, not elsewhere classified

G54.3 Thoracic root disorders, not elsewhere classified

G54.4 Lumbosacral root disorders, not elsewhere classified

G54.5 Neuralgic amyotrophy
Parsonage-Aldren-Turner syndrome
Shoulder-girdle neuritis

> EXCLUDES 1 *neuralgic amyotrophy in diabetes mellitus (E08-E13 with .44)*

G54.6 Phantom limb syndrome with pain HCC

G54.7 Phantom limb syndrome without pain HCC
Phantom limb syndrome NOS

G54.8 Other nerve root and plexus disorders

G54.9 Nerve root and plexus disorder, unspecified

G55 *Nerve root and plexus compressions in diseases classified elsewhere*

Code first underlying disease, such as:
neoplasm (C00-D49)

> EXCLUDES 1 *nerve root compression (due to) (in) ankylosing spondylitis (M45.-)*
> *nerve root compression (due to) (in) dorsopathies (M53.-, M54.-)*
> *nerve root compression (due to) (in) intervertebral disc disorders (M50.1-, M51.1-)*
> *nerve root compression (due to) (in) spondylopathies (M46.-, M48.-)*

✓4th G56 Mononeuropathies of upper limb

> EXCLUDES 1 *current traumatic nerve disorder—see nerve injury by body region*

AHA: 2016, 4Q, 17-18

✓5th G56.0 Carpal tunnel **syndrome**

G56.00 Carpal tunnel syndrome, unspecified **upper limb**

G56.01 Carpal tunnel syndrome, right **upper limb**

G56.02 Carpal tunnel syndrome, left **upper limb**

G56.03 Carpal tunnel syndrome, bilateral **upper limbs**

✓5th G56.1 Other lesions of median nerve

G56.10 Other lesions of median nerve, unspecified **upper limb**

G56.11 Other lesions of median nerve, right **upper limb**

G56.12 Other lesions of median nerve, left **upper limb**

G56.13 Other lesions of median nerve, bilateral **upper limbs**

✓5th G56.2 Lesion of ulnar nerve
Tardy ulnar nerve palsy

G56.20 Lesion of ulnar nerve, unspecified **upper limb**

G56.21 Lesion of ulnar nerve, right **upper limb**

G56.22 Lesion of ulnar nerve, left **upper limb**

G56.23 Lesion of ulnar nerve, bilateral **upper limbs**

✓5th G56.3 Lesion of radial nerve

G56.30 Lesion of radial nerve, unspecified **upper limb**

G56.31 Lesion of radial nerve, right **upper limb**

G56.32 Lesion of radial nerve, left **upper limb**

G56.33 Lesion of radial nerve, bilateral **upper limbs**

✓5th G56.4 Causalgia of upper limb
Complex regional pain syndrome II of upper limb

> EXCLUDES 1 *complex regional pain syndrome I of lower limb (G90.52-)*
> *complex regional pain syndrome I of upper limb (G90.51-)*
> *complex regional pain syndrome II of lower limb (G57.7-)*
> *reflex sympathetic dystrophy of lower limb (G90.52-)*
> *reflex sympathetic dystrophy of upper limb (G90.51-)*

G56.40 Causalgia of unspecified **upper limb**

G56.41 Causalgia of right **upper limb**

G56.42 Causalgia of left **upper limb**

G56.43 Causalgia of bilateral **upper limbs**

✓5th G56.8 Other specified mononeuropathies of upper limb
Interdigital neuroma of upper limb

G56.80 Other specified mononeuropathies of unspecified **upper limb**

G56.81 Other specified mononeuropathies of right **upper limb**

G56.82 Other specified mononeuropathies of left **upper limb**

G56.83 Other specified mononeuropathies of bilateral **upper limbs**

Nerves of Upper Limb

Radial

Deep branch of radial
Ulnar
Superficial branch of radial
Median

✓5th G56.9 Unspecified mononeuropathy of upper limb

G56.90 Unspecified mononeuropathy of unspecified upper **limb**

G56.91 Unspecified mononeuropathy of right **upper limb**

G56.92 Unspecified mononeuropathy of left **upper limb**

G56.93 Unspecified mononeuropathy of bilateral **upper limbs**

✓4th G57 Mononeuropathies of lower limb

> EXCLUDES 1 *current traumatic nerve disorder—see nerve injury by body region*

AHA: 2016, 4Q, 17-18

✓5th G57.0 Lesion of sciatic nerve

> EXCLUDES 1 *sciatica NOS (M54.3-)*
> EXCLUDES 2 *sciatica attributed to intervertebral disc disorder (M51.1-)*

G57.00 Lesion of sciatic nerve, unspecified **lower limb**

G57.01 Lesion of sciatic nerve, right **lower limb**

G57.02 Lesion of sciatic nerve, left **lower limb**

G57.03 Lesion of sciatic nerve, bilateral **lower limbs**

N Newborn: 0 P Pediatric: 0-17 M Maternity: 12-55 A Adult: 15-124 MCC Major Complication/Comorbidity CC Complication/Comorbidity SW Severe Wound Dx

574 ICD-10-CM 2019

Nerves of Lower Limb

- Obturator nerve
- Sciatic nerve
- Femoral nerve
- Saphenous nerve
- Common fibular (peroneal) nerve
- Deep fibular (peroneal) nerve
- Tibial nerve
- Superficial fibular (peroneal) nerve

✓5ᵗʰ **G57.1 Meralgia paresthetica**
   Lateral cutaneous nerve of thigh syndrome
   G57.10 Meralgia paresthetica, unspecified lower limb
   G57.11 Meralgia paresthetica, right lower limb
   G57.12 Meralgia paresthetica, left lower limb
   G57.13 Meralgia paresthetica, bilateral lower limbs

✓5ᵗʰ **G57.2 Lesion of femoral nerve**
   G57.20 Lesion of femoral nerve, unspecified lower limb
   G57.21 Lesion of femoral nerve, right lower limb
   G57.22 Lesion of femoral nerve, left lower limb
   G57.23 Lesion of femoral nerve, bilateral lower limbs

✓5ᵗʰ **G57.3 Lesion of lateral popliteal nerve**
   Peroneal nerve palsy
   G57.30 Lesion of lateral popliteal nerve, unspecified lower limb
   G57.31 Lesion of lateral popliteal nerve, right lower limb
   G57.32 Lesion of lateral popliteal nerve, left lower limb
   G57.33 Lesion of lateral popliteal nerve, bilateral lower limbs

✓5ᵗʰ **G57.4 Lesion of medial popliteal nerve**
   G57.40 Lesion of medial popliteal nerve, unspecified lower limb
   G57.41 Lesion of medial popliteal nerve, right lower limb
   G57.42 Lesion of medial popliteal nerve, left lower limb
   G57.43 Lesion of medial popliteal nerve, bilateral lower limbs

✓5ᵗʰ **G57.5 Tarsal tunnel syndrome**
   G57.50 Tarsal tunnel syndrome, unspecified lower limb
   G57.51 Tarsal tunnel syndrome, right lower limb
   G57.52 Tarsal tunnel syndrome, left lower limb
   G57.53 Tarsal tunnel syndrome, bilateral lower limbs

✓5ᵗʰ **G57.6 Lesion of plantar nerve**
   Morton's metatarsalgia
   G57.60 Lesion of plantar nerve, unspecified lower limb
   G57.61 Lesion of plantar nerve, right lower limb
   G57.62 Lesion of plantar nerve, left lower limb
   G57.63 Lesion of plantar nerve, bilateral lower limbs

✓5ᵗʰ **G57.7 Causalgia of lower limb**
   Complex regional pain syndrome II of lower limb
   EXCLUDES 1   *complex regional pain syndrome I of lower limb (G90.52-)*
     complex regional pain syndrome I of upper limb (G90.51-)
     complex regional pain syndrome II of upper limb (G56.4-)
     reflex sympathetic dystrophy of lower limb (G90.52-)
     reflex sympathetic dystrophy of upper limb (G90.51-)
   G57.70 Causalgia of unspecified lower limb
   G57.71 Causalgia of right lower limb
   G57.72 Causalgia of left lower limb
   G57.73 Causalgia of bilateral lower limbs

✓5ᵗʰ **G57.8 Other specified mononeuropathies of lower limb**
   Interdigital neuroma of lower limb
   G57.80 Other specified mononeuropathies of unspecified lower limb
   G57.81 Other specified mononeuropathies of right lower limb
   G57.82 Other specified mononeuropathies of left lower limb
   G57.83 Other specified mononeuropathies of bilateral lower limbs

✓5ᵗʰ **G57.9 Unspecified mononeuropathy of lower limb**
   G57.90 Unspecified mononeuropathy of unspecified lower limb
   G57.91 Unspecified mononeuropathy of right lower limb
   G57.92 Unspecified mononeuropathy of left lower limb
   G57.93 Unspecified mononeuropathy of bilateral lower limbs

✓4ᵗʰ **G58 Other mononeuropathies**
   G58.0 Intercostal neuropathy
   G58.7 Mononeuritis multiplex
   G58.8 Other specified mononeuropathies
   G58.9 Mononeuropathy, unspecified

G59 *Mononeuropathy in diseases classified elsewhere*
   Code first underlying disease
   EXCLUDES 1   *diabetic mononeuropathy (E08-E13 with .41)*
     syphilitic nerve paralysis (A52.19)
     syphilitic neuritis (A52.15)
     tuberculous mononeuropathy (A17.83)

Polyneuropathies and other disorders of the peripheral nervous system (G60-G65)

EXCLUDES 1   *neuralgia NOS (M79.2)*
     neuritis NOS (M79.2)
     peripheral neuritis in pregnancy (O26.82-)
     radiculitis NOS (M54.10)

✓4ᵗʰ **G60 Hereditary and idiopathic neuropathy**
   G60.0 Hereditary motor and sensory neuropathy
     Charcôt-Marie-Tooth disease
     Déjérine-Sottas disease
     Hereditary motor and sensory neuropathy, types I-IV
     Hypertrophic neuropathy of infancy
     Peroneal muscular atrophy (axonal type) (hypertrophic type)
     Roussy-Levy syndrome
   G60.1 Refsum's disease   CC
     Infantile Refsum disease
     AHA: 2014, 2Q, 4
     DEF: Genetic disorder of the lipid metabolism characterized by retinitis pigmentosa, degenerative nerve disease, ataxia, and dry, rough, scaly skin.
     CC Excl: PDX collection 588
   G60.2 Neuropathy in association with hereditary ataxia
   G60.3 Idiopathic progressive neuropathy
   G60.8 Other hereditary and idiopathic neuropathies
     Dominantly inherited sensory neuropathy
     Morvan's disease
     Nelaton's syndrome
     Recessively inherited sensory neuropathy
   G60.9 Hereditary and idiopathic neuropathy, unspecified

✓ Additional Character Required   ✓×7ᵗʰ Placeholder   Unacceptable PDx   Questionable PDx   Manifestation   **H1**-**H14** HAC   **HCC** CMS-HCC Dx   **HIV** HIV Dx

ICD-10-CM 2019   575

G57.1–G60.9

Chapter 6. Diseases of the Nervous System

✓4ᵗʰ G61   Inflammatory polyneuropathy

G61.0   Guillain-Barre syndrome `CC` `HCC`
Acute (post-)infective polyneuritis
Miller Fisher syndrome
AHA: 2014, 2Q, 4
DEF: Autoimmune disorder due to an immune response to foreign antigens with paraplegia of limbs, flaccid paralysis, ophthalmoplegia, ataxia, and areflexia. In most cases, this disorder is triggered by a mild viral infection, surgery, or following an immunization.
TIP: Guillain-Barre syndrome can occur as a sequela of *Campylobacter enteritis.* Assign code B94.8 for the sequelae as an additional diagnosis.
CC Excl: PDX collection 92

G61.1   Serum neuropathy `HCC`
Use additional code for adverse effect, if applicable, to identify serum (T50.-)

✓5ᵗʰ G61.8   Other inflammatory polyneuropathies

G61.81   Chronic inflammatory demyelinating polyneuritis `CC` `HCC`
CC Excl: PDX collection 589

G61.82   Multifocal motor neuropathy `HCC`
MMN
AHA: 2016, 4Q, 18

G61.89   Other inflammatory polyneuropathies `HCC`

G61.9   Inflammatory polyneuropathy, unspecified `HCC`

✓4ᵗʰ G62   Other and unspecified polyneuropathies

G62.0   Drug-induced polyneuropathy `HCC`
Use additional code for adverse effect, if applicable, to identify drug (T36-T50 with fifth or sixth character 5)

G62.1   Alcoholic polyneuropathy `HCC`

G62.2   Polyneuropathy due to other toxic agents `HCC`
Code first (T51-T65) to identify toxic agent

✓5ᵗʰ G62.8   Other specified polyneuropathies

G62.81   Critical illness polyneuropathy `CC` `HCC`
Acute motor neuropathy
CC Excl: PDX collection 590

G62.82   Radiation-induced polyneuropathy `HCC`
Use additional external cause code (W88-W90, X39.0-) to identify cause

G62.89   Other specified polyneuropathies
AHA: 2016, 2Q, 11

G62.9   Polyneuropathy, unspecified
Neuropathy NOS

G63   *Polyneuropathy in diseases classified elsewhere* `HCC`
Code first underlying disease, such as:
amyloidosis (E85.-)
endocrine disease, except diabetes (E00-E07, E15-E16, E20-E34)
metabolic diseases (E70-E88)
neoplasm (C00-D49)
nutritional deficiency (E40-E64)
EXCLUDES 1   *polyneuropathy (in):*
diabetes mellitus (E08-E13 with .42)
diphtheria (A36.83)
infectious mononucleosis (B27.0-B27.9 with 1)
Lyme disease (A69.22)
mumps (B26.84)
postherpetic (B02.23)
rheumatoid arthritis (M05.33)
scleroderma (M34.83)
systemic lupus erythematosus (M32.19)
AHA: 2012, 4Q, 99

G64   Other disorders of peripheral nervous system
Disorder of peripheral nervous system NOS

✓4ᵗʰ G65   Sequelae of inflammatory and toxic polyneuropathies
Code first condition resulting from (sequela) of inflammatory and toxic polyneuropathies

G65.0   Sequelae of Guillain-Barré syndrome `HCC`

G65.1   Sequelae of other inflammatory polyneuropathy `HCC`

G65.2   Sequelae of toxic polyneuropathy `HCC`

Diseases of myoneural junction and muscle (G70-G73)

✓4ᵗʰ G70   Myasthenia gravis and other myoneural disorders
EXCLUDES 1   *botulism (A05.1, A48.51-A48.52)*
transient neonatal myasthenia gravis (P94.0)

CC Excl: For CC/MCC codes in category G70: PDX collection 591

✓5ᵗʰ G70.0   Myasthenia gravis
DEF: Autoimmune neuromuscular disorder caused by antibodies to the acetylcholine receptors at the neuromuscular junction, interfering with proper binding of the neurotransmitter from the neuron to the target muscle, causing muscle weakness, fatigue, and exhaustion, without pain or atrophy.

G70.00   Myasthenia gravis without (acute) exacerbation `HCC`
Myasthenia gravis NOS

G70.01   Myasthenia gravis with (acute) exacerbation `MCC` `HCC`
Myasthenia gravis in crisis

G70.1   Toxic myoneural disorders `HCC`
Code first (T51-T65) to identify toxic agent

G70.2   Congenital and developmental myasthenia `HCC`

✓5ᵗʰ G70.8   Other specified myoneural disorders

G70.80   Lambert-Eaton syndrome, unspecified `CC` `HCC`
Lambert-Eaton syndrome NOS

G70.81   *Lambert-Eaton syndrome in disease classified elsewhere* `CC` `HCC`
Code first underlying disease
EXCLUDES 1   *Lambert-Eaton syndrome in neoplastic disease (G73.1)*

G70.89   Other specified myoneural disorders `HCC`

G70.9   Myoneural disorder, unspecified `HCC`

✓4ᵗʰ G71   Primary disorders of muscles
EXCLUDES 2   *arthrogryposis multiplex congenita (Q74.3)*
metabolic disorders (E70-E88)
myositis (M60.-)

✓5ᵗʰ G71.0   Muscular dystrophy
~~Autosomal recessive, childhood type, muscular dystrophy resembling Duchenne or Becker muscular dystrophy~~
~~Benign [Becker] muscular dystrophy~~
~~Benign scapuloperoneal muscular dystrophy with early contractures [Emery-Dreifuss]~~
~~Congenital muscular dystrophy NOS~~
~~Congenital muscular dystrophy with specific morphological abnormalities of the muscle fiber~~
~~Distal muscular dystrophy~~
~~Facioscapulohumeral muscular dystrophy~~
~~Limb-girdle muscular dystrophy~~
~~Ocular muscular dystrophy~~
~~Oculopharyngeal muscular dystrophy~~
~~Scapuloperoneal muscular dystrophy~~
~~Severe [Duchenne] muscular dystrophy~~

•   **G71.00   Muscular dystrophy, unspecified**

•   **G71.01   Duchenne or Becker muscular dystrophy**
Autosomal recessive, childhood type, muscular dystrophy resembling Duchenne or Becker muscular dystrophy
Benign [Becker] muscular dystrophy
Severe [Duchenne] muscular dystrophy

•   **G71.02   Facioscapulohumeral muscular dystrophy**
Scapulohumeral muscular dystrophy

•   **G71.09   Other specified muscular dystrophies**
Benign scapuloperoneal muscular dystrophy with early contractures [Emery-Dreifuss]
Congenital muscular dystrophy NOS
Congenital muscular dystrophy with specific morphological abnormalities of the muscle fiber
Distal muscular dystrophy
Limb-girdle muscular dystrophy
Ocular muscular dystrophy
Oculopharyngeal muscular dystrophy
Scapuloperoneal muscular dystrophy

✓5ᵗʰ G71.1   Myotonic disorders

G71.11   Myotonic muscular dystrophy `HCC`
Dystrophia myotonica [Steinert]
Myotonia atrophica
Myotonic dystrophy
Proximal myotonic myopathy (PROMM)
Steinert disease

N Newborn: 0   P Pediatric: 0-17   M Maternity: 12-55   A Adult: 15-124   MCC Major Complication/Comorbidity   CC Complication/Comorbidity   SW Severe Wound Dx

576   ICD-10-CM 2019

G71.12 Myotonia congenita
Acetazolamide responsive myotonia congenita
Dominant myotonia congenita [Thomsen disease]
Myotonia levior
Recessive myotonia congenita [Becker disease]

G71.13 Myotonic chondrodystrophy
Chondrodystrophic myotonia
Congenital myotonic chondrodystrophy
Schwartz-Jampel disease

G71.14 Drug induced myotonia
Use additional code for adverse effect, if applicable, to identify drug (T36-T50 with fifth or sixth character 5)

G71.19 Other specified myotonic disorders
Myotonia fluctuans
Myotonia permanens
Neuromyotonia [Isaacs]
Paramyotonia congenita (of von Eulenburg)
Pseudomyotonia
Symptomatic myotonia

G71.2 Congenital myopathies   `CC` `HCC`
Central core disease
Fiber-type disproportion
Minicore disease
Multicore disease
Myotubular (centronuclear) myopathy
Nemaline myopathy
EXCLUDES 1 arthrogryposis multiplex congenita (Q74.3)
CC Excl: PDX collection 592

G71.3 Mitochondrial myopathy, not elsewhere classified
EXCLUDES 1 Kearns-Sayre syndrome (H49.81)
Leber's disease (H47.21)
Leigh's encephalopathy (G31.82)
mitochondrial metabolism disorders (E88.4-)
Reye's syndrome (G93.7)

G71.8 Other primary disorders of muscles

G71.9 Primary disorder of muscle, unspecified
Hereditary myopathy NOS

✓4th **G72 Other and unspecified myopathies**
EXCLUDES 1 arthrogryposis multiplex congenita (Q74.3)
dermatopolymyositis (M33.-)
ischemic infarction of muscle (M62.2-)
myositis (M60.-)
polymyositis (M33.2-)

CC Excl: For CC codes in category G72, unless otherwise noted: PDX collection 593

G72.0 Drug-induced myopathy   `CC`
Use additional code for adverse effect, if applicable, to identify drug (T36-T50 with fifth or sixth character 5)

G72.1 Alcoholic myopathy   `CC`
Use additional code to identify alcoholism (F10.-)

G72.2 Myopathy due to other toxic agents   `CC`
Code first (T51-T65) to identify toxic agent

G72.3 Periodic paralysis
Familial periodic paralysis
Hyperkalemic periodic paralysis (familial)
Hypokalemic periodic paralysis (familial)
Myotonic periodic paralysis (familial)
Normokalemic paralysis (familial)
Potassium sensitive periodic paralysis
EXCLUDES 1 paramyotonia congenita (of von Eulenburg) (G71.19)

✓5th **G72.4 Inflammatory and immune myopathies, not elsewhere classified**

G72.41 Inclusion body myositis [IBM]

G72.49 Other inflammatory and immune myopathies, not elsewhere classified
Inflammatory myopathy NOS

✓5th **G72.8 Other specified myopathies**

G72.81 Critical illness myopathy   `CC`
Acute necrotizing myopathy
Acute quadriplegic myopathy
Intensive care (ICU) myopathy
Myopathy of critical illness
CC Excl: PDX collection 594

G72.89 Other specified myopathies

G72.9 Myopathy, unspecified

✓4th **G73 Disorders of myoneural junction and muscle in diseases classified elsewhere**

G73.1 Lambert-Eaton syndrome in neoplastic disease   `CC` `HCC`
Code first underlying neoplasm (C00-D49)
EXCLUDES 1 Lambert-Eaton syndrome not associated with neoplasm (G70.80-G70.81)
CC Excl: PDX collection 591

G73.3 Myasthenic syndromes in other diseases classified elsewhere   `CC` `HCC`
Code first underlying disease, such as:
neoplasm (C00-D49)
thyrotoxicosis (E05.-)
CC Excl: PDX collection 591

G73.7 Myopathy in diseases classified elsewhere
Code first underlying disease, such as:
hyperparathyroidism (E21.0, E21.3)
hypoparathyroidism (E20.-)
glycogen storage disease (E74.0)
lipid storage disorders (E75.-)
EXCLUDES 1 myopathy in:
rheumatoid arthritis (M05.4-)
sarcoidosis (D86.87)
scleroderma (M34.82)
sicca syndrome [Sjögren] (M35.03)
systemic lupus erythematosus (M32.19)

Cerebral palsy and other paralytic syndromes (G80-G83)

✓4th **G80 Cerebral palsy**
EXCLUDES 1 hereditary spastic paraplegia (G11.4)

G80.0 Spastic quadriplegic cerebral palsy   `MCC` `HCC`
Congenital spastic paralysis (cerebral)
CC Excl: PDX collection 595

G80.1 Spastic diplegic cerebral palsy   `CC` `HCC`
Spastic cerebral palsy NOS
CC Excl: PDX collection 596

G80.2 Spastic hemiplegic cerebral palsy   `CC` `HCC`
CC Excl: PDX collection 597

G80.3 Athetoid cerebral palsy   `CC` `HCC`
Double athetosis (syndrome)
Dyskinetic cerebral palsy
Dystonic cerebral palsy
Vogt disease
CC Excl: PDX collection 598

G80.4 Ataxic cerebral palsy   `HCC`

G80.8 Other cerebral palsy   `HCC`
Mixed cerebral palsy syndromes

G80.9 Cerebral palsy, unspecified   `HCC`
Cerebral palsy NOS

✓4th **G81 Hemiplegia and hemiparesis**
NOTE This category is to be used only when hemiplegia (complete)(incomplete) is reported without further specification, or is stated to be old or longstanding but of unspecified cause. The category is also for use in multiple coding to identify these types of hemiplegia resulting from any cause.
EXCLUDES 1 congenital cerebral palsy (G80.-)
hemiplegia and hemiparesis due to sequela of cerebrovascular disease (I69.05-, I69.15-, I69.25-, I69.35-, I69.85-, I69.95-)
AHA: 2015, 1Q, 25
TIP: If the documentation specifies the affected side but not whether it is the dominant or nondominant side, the default is as follows: for ambidextrous patients, the default is dominant; when the left side is affected, the default is nondominant; and when the right side is affected, the default is dominant.

CC Excl: For CC codes in category G81: PDX collection 561

✓5th **G81.0 Flaccid hemiplegia**

G81.00 Flaccid hemiplegia affecting unspecified side   `CC` `HCC`

G81.01 Flaccid hemiplegia affecting right dominant side   `CC` `HCC`

G81.02 Flaccid hemiplegia affecting left dominant side   `CC` `HCC`

G81.03 Flaccid hemiplegia affecting right nondominant side   `CC` `HCC`

G81.04 Flaccid hemiplegia affecting left nondominant side   `CC` `HCC`

✔ Additional Character Required   ✔x7th Placeholder   Unacceptable PDx   Questionable PDx   Manifestation   `H1`-`H14` HAC   `HCC` CMS-HCC Dx   `HIV` HIV Dx

ICD-10-CM 2019   **577**

Chapter 6. Diseases of the Nervous System

G71.12–G81.04

Chapter 6. Diseases of the Nervous System

√5ᵗʰ **G81.1 Spastic hemiplegia**

G81.10 Spastic hemiplegia affecting unspecified side `CC` `HCC`

G81.11 Spastic hemiplegia affecting right dominant side `CC` `HCC`

G81.12 Spastic hemiplegia affecting left dominant side `CC` `HCC`

G81.13 Spastic hemiplegia affecting right nondominant side `CC` `HCC`

G81.14 Spastic hemiplegia affecting left nondominant side `CC` `HCC`

√5ᵗʰ **G81.9 Hemiplegia, unspecified**
AHA: 2014, 1Q, 23

G81.90 Hemiplegia, unspecified affecting unspecified side `CC` `HCC`

G81.91 Hemiplegia, unspecified affecting right dominant side `CC` `HCC`

G81.92 Hemiplegia, unspecified affecting left dominant side `CC` `HCC`

G81.93 Hemiplegia, unspecified affecting right nondominant side `CC` `HCC`

G81.94 Hemiplegia, unspecified affecting left nondominant side `CC` `HCC`

√4ᵗʰ **G82 Paraplegia (paraparesis) and quadriplegia (quadriparesis)**
NOTE This category is to be used only when the listed conditions are reported without further specification, or are stated to be old or longstanding but of unspecified cause. The category is also for use in multiple coding to identify these conditions resulting from any cause

EXCLUDES 1 *congenital cerebral palsy (G80.-)*
functional quadriplegia (R53.2)
hysterical paralysis (F44.4)

√5ᵗʰ **G82.2 Paraplegia**
Paralysis of both lower limbs NOS
Paraparesis (lower) NOS
Paraplegia (lower) NOS
AHA: 2017, 3Q, 3

CC Excl: For CC codes in subcategory G82.2:
PDX collection 561

G82.20 Paraplegia, unspecified `CC` `HCC`

G82.21 Paraplegia, complete `CC` `HCC`

G82.22 Paraplegia, incomplete `CC` `HCC`

√5ᵗʰ **G82.5 Quadriplegia**

CC Excl: For MCC codes in subcategory G82.5:
PDX collection 595

G82.50 Quadriplegia, unspecified `MCC` `HCC`

G82.51 Quadriplegia, C1-C4 complete `MCC` `HCC`

G82.52 Quadriplegia, C1-C4 incomplete `MCC` `HCC`

G82.53 Quadriplegia, C5-C7 complete `MCC` `HCC`

G82.54 Quadriplegia, C5-C7 incomplete `MCC` `HCC`

√4ᵗʰ **G83 Other paralytic syndromes**
NOTE This category is to be used only when the listed conditions are reported without further specification, or are stated to be old or longstanding but of unspecified cause. The category is also for use in multiple coding to identify these conditions resulting from any cause.
INCLUDES paralysis (complete) (incomplete), except as in G80-G82

G83.0 Diplegia of upper limbs `CC` `HCC`
Diplegia (upper)
Paralysis of both upper limbs
CC Excl: PDX collection 599

√5ᵗʰ **G83.1 Monoplegia of lower limb**
Paralysis of lower limb
EXCLUDES 1 *monoplegia of lower limbs due to sequela of cerebrovascular disease (I69.04-, I69.14-, I69.24-, I69.34-, I69.84-, I69.94-)*

TIP: If the documentation specifies the affected side but not whether it is the dominant or nondominant side, the default is as follows: for ambidextrous patients, the default is dominant; when the left side is affected, the default is nondominant; and when the right side is affected, the default is dominant.

G83.10 Monoplegia of lower limb affecting unspecified side `HCC`

G83.11 Monoplegia of lower limb affecting right dominant side `HCC`

G83.12 Monoplegia of lower limb affecting left dominant side `HCC`

G83.13 Monoplegia of lower limb affecting right nondominant side `HCC`

G83.14 Monoplegia of lower limb affecting left nondominant side `HCC`

√5ᵗʰ **G83.2 Monoplegia of upper limb**
Paralysis of upper limb
EXCLUDES 1 *monoplegia of upper limbs due to sequela of cerebrovascular disease (I69.03-, I69.13-, I69.23-, I69.33-, I69.83-, I69.93-)*

TIP: If the documentation specifies the affected side but not whether it is the dominant or nondominant side, the default is as follows: for ambidextrous patients, the default is dominant; when the left side is affected, the default is nondominant; and when the right side is affected, the default is dominant.

G83.20 Monoplegia of upper limb affecting unspecified side `HCC`

G83.21 Monoplegia of upper limb affecting right dominant side `HCC`

G83.22 Monoplegia of upper limb affecting left dominant side `HCC`

G83.23 Monoplegia of upper limb affecting right nondominant side `HCC`

G83.24 Monoplegia of upper limb affecting left nondominant side `HCC`

√5ᵗʰ **G83.3 Monoplegia, unspecified**
TIP: If the documentation specifies the affected side but not whether it is the dominant or nondominant side, the default is as follows: for ambidextrous patients, the default is dominant; when the left side is affected, the default is nondominant; and when the right side is affected, the default is dominant.

G83.30 Monoplegia, unspecified affecting unspecified side `HCC`

G83.31 Monoplegia, unspecified affecting right dominant side `HCC`

G83.32 Monoplegia, unspecified affecting left dominant side `HCC`

G83.33 Monoplegia, unspecified affecting right nondominant side `HCC`

G83.34 Monoplegia, unspecified affecting left nondominant side `HCC`

G83.4 Cauda equina syndrome `CC` `HCC`
Neurogenic bladder due to cauda equina syndrome
EXCLUDES 1 *cord bladder NOS (G95.89)*
neurogenic bladder NOS (N31.9)

DEF: Compression of the spinal nerve roots presenting with pain and tingling radiating down the buttocks, back of the thigh and calf, and into the foot in a sciatic manner with aching in the bladder, perineum, and sacrum. Loss of bowel and bladder control may also occur.
CC Excl: PDX collection 600

G83.5 Locked-in state `MCC` `HCC`
CC Excl: PDX collection 601

√5ᵗʰ **G83.8 Other specified paralytic syndromes**
EXCLUDES 1 *paralytic syndromes due to current spinal cord injury—code to spinal cord injury (S14, S24, S34)*

G83.81 Brown-Séquard syndrome `HCC`

G83.82 Anterior cord syndrome `HCC`

G83.83 Posterior cord syndrome `HCC`

G83.84 Todd's paralysis (postepileptic) `HCC`

G83.89 Other specified paralytic syndromes `HCC`

G83.9 Paralytic syndrome, unspecified `HCC`

Ⓝ Newborn: 0   Ⓟ Pediatric: 0-17   Ⓜ Maternity: 12-55   Ⓐ Adult: 15-124   `MCC` Major Complication/Comorbidity   `CC` Complication/Comorbidity   `SW` Severe Wound Dx

Other disorders of the nervous system (G89-G99)

✓4ᵗʰ G89   Pain, not elsewhere classified
Code also related psychological factors associated with pain (F45.42)
EXCLUDES 1   *generalized pain NOS (R52)*
pain disorders exclusively related to psychological factors
    (F45.41)
pain NOS (R52)
EXCLUDES 2   *atypical face pain (G50.1)*
headache syndromes (G44.-)
localized pain, unspecified type—code to pain by site, such as:
    abdomen pain (R10.-)
    back pain (M54.9)
    breast pain (N64.4)
    chest pain (R07.1-R07.9)
    ear pain (H92.0-)
    eye pain (H57.1)
    headache (R51)
    joint pain (M25.5-)
    limb pain (M79.6-)
    lumbar region pain (M54.5)
    painful urination (R30.9)
    pelvic and perineal pain (R10.2)
    renal colic (N23)
    shoulder pain (M25.51-)
    spine pain (M54.-)
    throat pain (R07.0)
    tongue pain (K14.6)
    tooth pain (K08.8)
migraines (G43.-)
myalgia ▶(M79.1-)◀
pain from prosthetic devices, implants, and grafts (T82.84,
    T83.84, T84.84, T85.84-)
phantom limb syndrome with pain (G54.6)
vulvar vestibulitis (N94.810)
vulvodynia (N94.81-)

G89.0   Central pain syndrome
Déjérine-Roussy syndrome
Myelopathic pain syndrome
Thalamic pain syndrome (hyperesthetic)

✓5ᵗʰ G89.1   Acute pain, not elsewhere classified
G89.11   Acute pain due to trauma
G89.12   Acute post-thoracotomy pain
Post-thoracotomy pain NOS
G89.18   Other acute postprocedural pain
Postoperative pain NOS
Postprocedural pain NOS

✓5ᵗʰ G89.2   Chronic pain, not elsewhere classified
EXCLUDES 1   *causalgia, lower limb (G57.7-)*
causalgia, upper limb (G56.4-)
central pain syndrome (G89.0)
chronic pain syndrome (G89.4)
complex regional pain syndrome II, lower limb (G57.7-)
complex regional pain syndrome II, upper limb (G56.4-)
neoplasm related chronic pain (G89.3)
reflex sympathetic dystrophy (G90.5-)
G89.21   Chronic pain due to trauma
G89.22   Chronic post-thoracotomy pain
G89.28   Other chronic postprocedural pain
Other chronic postoperative pain
G89.29   Other chronic pain

G89.3   Neoplasm related pain (acute) (chronic)
Cancer associated pain
Pain due to malignancy (primary) (secondary)
Tumor associated pain

G89.4   Chronic pain syndrome
Chronic pain associated with significant psychosocial
    dysfunction

✓4ᵗʰ G90   Disorders of autonomic nervous system
EXCLUDES 1   *dysfunction of the autonomic nervous system due to alcohol*
    (G31.2)

✓5ᵗʰ G90.0   Idiopathic peripheral autonomic neuropathy
G90.01   Carotid sinus syncope
Carotid sinus syndrome
DEF: Vagal activation caused by pressure on the carotid
sinus baroreceptors. Sympathetic nerve impulses may
cause sinus arrest or AV block.
G90.09   Other idiopathic peripheral autonomic neuropathy
Idiopathic peripheral autonomic neuropathy NOS

G90.1   Familial dysautonomia [Riley-Day]   **HCC**
G90.2   Horner's syndrome
Bernard(-Horner) syndrome
Cervical sympathetic dystrophy or paralysis
G90.3   Multi-system degeneration of the autonomic nervous   **CC** **HCC**
system
Neurogenic orthostatic hypotension [Shy-Drager]
EXCLUDES 1   *orthostatic hypotension NOS (I95.1)*
CC Excl: PDX collection 573

G90.4   Autonomic dysreflexia
Use additional code to identify the cause, such as:
    fecal impaction (K56.41)
    pressure ulcer (pressure area) (L89.-)
    urinary tract infection (N39.0)

✓5ᵗʰ G90.5   Complex regional pain syndrome I (CRPS I)
Reflex sympathetic dystrophy
EXCLUDES 1   *causalgia of lower limb (G57.7-)*
causalgia of upper limb (G56.4-)
complex regional pain syndrome II of lower limb
    (G57.7-)
complex regional pain syndrome II of upper limb
    (G56.4-)

CC Excl: For CC codes in subcategory G90.5, unless
otherwise noted: PDX collection 603

G90.50   Complex regional pain syndrome I, unspecified   **CC**
CC Excl: PDX collection 602
✓6ᵗʰ G90.51   Complex regional pain syndrome I of upper limb
G90.511   Complex regional pain syndrome I of   **CC**
right upper limb
G90.512   Complex regional pain syndrome I of   **CC**
left upper limb
G90.513   Complex regional pain syndrome I of   **CC**
upper limb, bilateral
G90.519   Complex regional pain syndrome I of   **CC**
unspecified upper limb
✓6ᵗʰ G90.52   Complex regional pain syndrome I of lower limb
G90.521   Complex regional pain syndrome I of   **CC**
right lower limb
G90.522   Complex regional pain syndrome I of   **CC**
left lower limb
G90.523   Complex regional pain syndrome I of   **CC**
lower limb, bilateral
G90.529   Complex regional pain syndrome I of   **CC**
unspecified lower limb
G90.59   Complex regional pain syndrome I of other   **CC**
specified site

G90.8   Other disorders of autonomic nervous system
G90.9   Disorder of the autonomic nervous system, unspecified

✓4ᵗʰ G91   Hydrocephalus
INCLUDES   acquired hydrocephalus
EXCLUDES 1   *Arnold-Chiari syndrome with hydrocephalus (Q07.-)*
congenital hydrocephalus (Q03.-)
spina bifida with hydrocephalus (Q05.-)

CC Excl: For CC codes in category G91, unless otherwise noted:
PDX collection 605

G91.0   Communicating hydrocephalus   **CC**
Secondary normal pressure hydrocephalus
CC Excl: PDX collection 604
G91.1   Obstructive hydrocephalus   **CC**
DEF: Obstruction of the cerebrospinal fluid passage from the brain
into the spinal canal characterized by headaches, drowsiness, poor
coordination, urinary incontinence, nausea, vomiting, and
papilledema.
G91.2   (Idiopathic) normal pressure hydrocephalus   **CC**
Normal pressure hydrocephalus NOS
CC Excl: PDX collection 604
G91.3   Post-traumatic hydrocephalus, unspecified   **CC**
G91.4   *Hydrocephalus in diseases classified elsewhere*
Code first underlying condition, such as:
    congenital syphilis (A50.4-)
    neoplasm (C00-D49)
    ▶plasminogen deficiency (E88.02)◀
EXCLUDES 1   *hydrocephalus due to congenital toxoplasmosis*
    (P37.1)

AHA: 2014, 3Q, 3

✓ Additional Character Required   ✓×7ᵗʰ Placeholder   Unacceptable PDx   Questionable PDx   Manifestation   H1-H14 HAC   HCC CMS-HCC Dx   HIV HIV Dx

ICD-10-CM 2019   579

Chapter 6. Diseases of the Nervous System

Hydrocephalus (Acquired)

Normal ventricles   Hydrocephalic ventricles

G91.8   Other hydrocephalus   `CC`

G91.9   Hydrocephalus, unspecified   `CC`

G92   **Toxic encephalopathy**   `MCC`
Toxic encephalitis
Toxic metabolic encephalopathy
Code first, if applicable, drug induced (T36-T50)
Code first (T51-T65) to identify toxic agent
AHA: 2017, 1Q, 39-40
DEF: Brain tissue degeneration due to a toxic substance.
CC Excl: PDX collection 606

`✓4ᵗʰ` **G93**   **Other disorders of brain**

G93.0   **Cerebral cysts**
Arachnoid cyst
Porencephalic cyst, acquired
EXCLUDES 1   *acquired periventricular cysts of newborn (P91.1)*
congenital cerebral cysts (Q04.6)

G93.1   **Anoxic brain damage, not elsewhere classified**   `CC` `HCC`
EXCLUDES 1   *cerebral anoxia due to anesthesia during labor and delivery (O74.3)*
cerebral anoxia due to anesthesia during the puerperium (O89.2)
neonatal anoxia (P84)
DEF: Brain injury not resulting from birth trauma that is due to lack of oxygen. Brain cells, when deprived of oxygen, begin to expire after 4 minutes.
CC Excl: PDX collection 607

G93.2   **Benign intracranial hypertension**
EXCLUDES 1   *hypertensive encephalopathy (I67.4)*

G93.3   **Postviral fatigue syndrome**
Benign myalgic encephalomyelitis
EXCLUDES 1   *chronic fatigue syndrome NOS (R53.82)*

`✓5ᵗʰ` **G93.4**   **Other and unspecified encephalopathy**
EXCLUDES 1   *alcoholic encephalopathy (G31.2)*
encephalopathy in diseases classified elsewhere (G94)
hypertensive encephalopathy (I67.4)
toxic (metabolic) encephalopathy (G92)

   G93.40   **Encephalopathy, unspecified**   `HIV` `MCC`
AHA: 2017, 2Q, 8
CC Excl: PDX collection 608

   G93.41   **Metabolic encephalopathy**   `HIV` `MCC`
Septic encephalopathy
AHA: 2017, 2Q, 8; 2016, 3Q, 42; 2015, 3Q, 21
TIP: Assign separately when documented with diabetic hypoglycemia (E08.649, E09.649, E10.649, E11.649, E13.649).
CC Excl: PDX collection 609

   G93.49   **Other encephalopathy**   `HIV` `MCC`
Encephalopathy NEC
AHA: 2018, 2Q, 22, 24; 2017, 2Q, 9
CC Excl: PDX collection 610

G93.5   **Compression of brain**   `MCC` `HCC`
Arnold-Chiari type 1 compression of brain
Compression of brain (stem)
Herniation of brain (stem)
EXCLUDES 1   *diffuse traumatic compression of brain (S06.2-)*
focal traumatic compression of brain (S06.3-)
CC Excl: PDX collection 611

G93.6   **Cerebral edema**   `MCC` `HCC`
EXCLUDES 1   *cerebral edema due to birth injury (P11.0)*
traumatic cerebral edema (S06.1-)
CC Excl: PDX collection 612

G93.7   **Reye's syndrome**   `MCC` `P`
Code first poisoning due to salicylates, if applicable (T39.0-, with sixth character 1-4)
Use additional code for adverse effect due to salicylates, if applicable (T39.0-, with sixth character 5)
DEF: Rare childhood illness often developed after a viral upper respiratory infection. Symptoms include vomiting, elevated serum transaminase, brain swelling, disturbances of consciousness, seizures, and changes in liver and other viscera and it can be fatal.
CC Excl: PDX collection 613

`✓5ᵗʰ` **G93.8**   **Other specified disorders of brain**

   G93.81   **Temporal sclerosis**
Hippocampal sclerosis
Mesial temporal sclerosis

   G93.82   **Brain death**   `MCC`
CC Excl: PDX collection 515

   G93.89   **Other specified disorders of brain**
Postradiation encephalopathy

G93.9   **Disorder of brain, unspecified**   `HIV`

G94   *Other disorders of brain in diseases classified elsewhere*
Code first underlying disease
EXCLUDES 1   *encephalopathy in congenital syphilis (A50.49)*
encephalopathy in influenza (J09.X9, J10.81, J11.81)
encephalopathy in syphilis (A52.19)
hydrocephalus in diseases classified elsewhere (G91.4)
AHA: 2018, 2Q, 22; 2017, 2Q, 8-9

`✓4ᵗʰ` **G95**   **Other and unspecified diseases of spinal cord**
EXCLUDES 2   *myelitis (G04.-)*

G95.0   **Syringomyelia and syringobulbia**   `CC` `HCC`
CC Excl: PDX collection 614

`✓5ᵗʰ` **G95.1**   **Vascular myelopathies**
EXCLUDES 2   *intraspinal phlebitis and thrombophlebitis, except non-pyogenic (G08)*

   G95.11   **Acute infarction of spinal cord (embolic) (nonembolic)**   `MCC` `HCC`
Anoxia of spinal cord
Arterial thrombosis of spinal cord
CC Excl: PDX collection 603

   G95.19   **Other vascular myelopathies**   `MCC` `HCC`
Edema of spinal cord
Hematomyelia
Nonpyogenic intraspinal phlebitis and thrombophlebitis
Subacute necrotic myelopathy
CC Excl: PDX collection 603

`✓5ᵗʰ` **G95.2**   **Other and unspecified cord compression**

   G95.20   **Unspecified cord compression**   `HIV` `CC` `HCC`
CC Excl: PDX collection 615

   G95.29   **Other cord compression**   `HIV` `CC` `HCC`
CC Excl: PDX collection 615

`✓5ᵗʰ` **G95.8**   **Other specified diseases of spinal cord**
EXCLUDES 1   *neurogenic bladder NOS (N31.9)*
neurogenic bladder due to cauda equina syndrome (G83.4)
neuromuscular dysfunction of bladder without spinal cord lesion (N31.-)

   G95.81   **Conus medullaris syndrome**   `CC` `HCC`
CC Excl: PDX collection 603

   G95.89   **Other specified diseases of spinal cord**   `CC` `HCC`
Cord bladder NOS
Drug-induced myelopathy
Radiation-induced myelopathy
EXCLUDES 1   *myelopathy NOS (G95.9)*
CC Excl: PDX collection 603

G95.9   **Disease of spinal cord, unspecified**   `HIV` `CC` `HCC`
Myelopathy NOS
CC Excl: PDX collection 615

`N` Newborn: 0   `P` Pediatric: 0-17   `M` Maternity: 12-55   `A` Adult: 15-124   `MCC` Major Complication/Comorbidity   `CC` Complication/Comorbidity   `SW` Severe Wound Dx

580   ICD-10-CM 2019

✓4th **G96 Other disorders of central nervous system**

G96.0 Cerebrospinal fluid leak `CC`

EXCLUDES 1 *cerebrospinal fluid leak from spinal puncture (G97.0)*

AHA: 2018, 2Q, 13

DEF: Cerebrospinal fluid discharging from the nose or the ear caused by a fracture of the frontal bone with tearing of dura mater and arachnoid. It is characterized by watery drainage usually from only one side of the nose or one ear, headache, vision changes, and hearing loss.

CC Excl: PDX collection 616

✓5th **G96.1 Disorders of meninges, not elsewhere classified**

G96.11 Dural tear `CC`

EXCLUDES 1 *accidental puncture or laceration of dura during a procedure (G97.41)*

AHA: 2014, 4Q, 24

CC Excl: PDX collection 509

G96.12 Meningeal adhesions (cerebral) (spinal)

G96.19 Other disorders of meninges, not elsewhere classified

G96.8 Other specified disorders of central nervous system

G96.9 Disorder of central nervous system, unspecified `HIV`

✓4th **G97 Intraoperative and postprocedural complications and disorders of nervous system, not elsewhere classified**

EXCLUDES 2 *intraoperative and postprocedural cerebrovascular infarction (I97.81-, I97.82-)*

AHA: 2016, 4Q, 9-10

G97.0 Cerebrospinal fluid leak from spinal puncture `CC`

CC Excl: PDX collection 617

G97.1 Other reaction to spinal and lumbar puncture

Headache due to lumbar puncture

G97.2 Intracranial hypotension following ventricular shunting `CC`

CC Excl: PDX collection 617

✓5th **G97.3 Intraoperative hemorrhage and hematoma of a nervous system organ or structure complicating a procedure**

EXCLUDES 1 *intraoperative hemorrhage and hematoma of a nervous system organ or structure due to accidental puncture and laceration during a procedure (G97.4-)*

G97.31 Intraoperative hemorrhage and hematoma of a nervous system organ or structure complicating a nervous system procedure `CC`

CC Excl: PDX collection 618

G97.32 Intraoperative hemorrhage and hematoma of a nervous system organ or structure complicating other procedure `CC`

CC Excl: PDX collection 618

✓5th **G97.4 Accidental puncture and laceration of a nervous system organ or structure during a procedure**

CC Excl: For CC codes in subcategory G97.4:
PDX collection 509

G97.41 Accidental puncture or laceration of dura during a procedure `CC`

Incidental (inadvertent) durotomy

AHA: 2014, 4Q, 24

Spinal Puncture

- Spinal cord
- Epidural space
- Subarachnoid space
- Vertebra
- Spinal needle
- Lumbar area

G97.48 Accidental puncture and laceration of other nervous system organ or structure during a nervous system procedure `CC`

G97.49 Accidental puncture and laceration of other nervous system organ or structure during other procedure `CC`

✓5th **G97.5 Postprocedural hemorrhage of a nervous system organ or structure following a procedure**

G97.51 Postprocedural hemorrhage of a nervous system organ or structure following a nervous system procedure `CC`

CC Excl: PDX collection 619

G97.52 Postprocedural hemorrhage of a nervous system organ or structure following other procedure `CC`

CC Excl: PDX collection 619

✓5th **G97.6 Postprocedural hematoma and seroma of a nervous system organ or structure following a procedure**

CC Excl: For CC codes in subcategory G97.6:
PDX collection 619

G97.61 Postprocedural hematoma of a nervous system organ or structure following a nervous system procedure `CC`

G97.62 Postprocedural hematoma of a nervous system organ or structure following other procedure `CC`

G97.63 Postprocedural seroma of a nervous system organ or structure following a nervous system procedure `CC`

G97.64 Postprocedural seroma of a nervous system organ or structure following other procedure `CC`

✓5th **G97.8 Other intraoperative and postprocedural complications and disorders of nervous system**

Use additional code to further specify disorder

G97.81 Other intraoperative complications of nervous system `CC`

CC Excl: PDX collection 617

G97.82 Other postprocedural complications and disorders of nervous system `CC`

CC Excl: PDX collection 617

✓4th **G98 Other disorders of nervous system not elsewhere classified**

INCLUDES nervous system disorder NOS

G98.0 Neurogenic arthritis, not elsewhere classified

Nonsyphilitic neurogenic arthropathy NEC

Nonsyphilitic neurogenic spondylopathy NEC

EXCLUDES 1 *spondylopathy (in):*
syringomyelia and syringobulbia (G95.0)
tabes dorsalis (A52.11)

G98.8 Other disorders of nervous system `HIV`

Nervous system disorder NOS

✓4th **G99 Other disorders of nervous system in diseases classified elsewhere**

G99.0 *Autonomic neuropathy in diseases classified elsewhere* `CC`

Code first underlying disease, such as:
amyloidosis (E85.-)
gout (M1A.-, M10.-)
hyperthyroidism (E05.-)

EXCLUDES 1 *diabetic autonomic neuropathy (E08-E13 with .43)*

CC Excl: PDX collection 620

G99.2 *Myelopathy in diseases classified elsewhere* `CC` `HCC`

Code first underlying disease, such as:
neoplasm (C00-D49)

EXCLUDES 1 *myelopathy in:*
intervertebral disease (M50.0-, M51.0-)
spondylosis (M47.0-, M47.1-)

CC Excl: PDX collection 603

G99.8 *Other specified disorders of nervous system in diseases classified elsewhere*

Code first underlying disorder, such as:
amyloidosis (E85.-)
avitaminosis (E56.9)

EXCLUDES 1 *nervous system involvement in:*
cysticercosis (B69.0)
rubella (B06.0-)
syphilis (A52.1-)

Chapter 7. Diseases of the Eye and Adnexa (H00–H59)

Chapter Specific Guidelines with Coding Examples

The chapter specific guidelines from the ICD-10-CM Official Guidelines for Coding and Reporting have been provided below. Along with these guidelines are coding examples, contained in the shaded boxes, that have been developed to help illustrate the coding and/or sequencing guidance found in these guidelines.

a. Glaucoma

1) Assigning glaucoma codes

Assign as many codes from category H40, Glaucoma, as needed to identify the type of glaucoma, the affected eye, and the glaucoma stage.

2) Bilateral glaucoma with same type and stage

When a patient has bilateral glaucoma and both eyes are documented as being the same type and stage, and there is a code for bilateral glaucoma, report only the code for the type of glaucoma, bilateral, with the seventh character for the stage.

> Bilateral severe stage pigmentary glaucoma
>
> **H40.1333   Pigmentary glaucoma, bilateral, severe stage**
>
> *Explanation*: In this scenario, the patient has the same type and stage of glaucoma in both eyes. As this type of glaucoma has a code for bilateral, assign only the code for the bilateral glaucoma with the seventh character for the stage.

When a patient has bilateral glaucoma and both eyes are documented as being the same type and stage, and the classification does not provide a code for bilateral glaucoma (i.e. subcategories H40.10 and H40.20) report only one code for the type of glaucoma with the appropriate seventh character for the stage.

> Bilateral open-angle glaucoma; not specified as to type and stage indeterminate in both eyes
>
> **H40.10X4   Unspecified open-angle glaucoma, indeterminate stage**
>
> *Explanation*: In this scenario, the patient has glaucoma of the same type and stage of both eyes, but there is no code specifically for bilateral glaucoma. Only one code is assigned with the appropriate seventh character for the stage.

3) Bilateral glaucoma stage with different types or stages

When a patient has bilateral glaucoma and each eye is documented as having a different type or stage, and the classification distinguishes laterality, assign the appropriate code for each eye rather than the code for bilateral glaucoma.

When a patient has bilateral glaucoma and each eye is documented as having a different type, and the classification does not distinguish laterality (i.e. subcategories H40.10 and H40.20), assign one code for each type of glaucoma with the appropriate seventh character for the stage.

> Documentation relates mild, unspecified primary angle-closure glaucoma of the left eye with mild unspecified open-angle glaucoma of the right eye
>
> **H40.20X1   Unspecified primary angle-closure glaucoma, mild stage**
>
> **H40.10X1   Unspecified open-angle glaucoma, mild stage**
>
> *Explanation*: In this scenario the patient has a different type of glaucoma in each eye and the classification does not distinguish laterality. A code for each type of glaucoma is assigned, each with the appropriate seventh character for the stage.

When a patient has bilateral glaucoma and each eye is documented as having the same type, but different stage, and the classification does not distinguish laterality (i.e. subcategories H40.10 and H40.20), assign a code for the type of glaucoma for each eye with the seventh character for the specific glaucoma stage documented for each eye.

> Bilateral open-angle glaucoma, not specified as to type; the right eye is documented to be in mild stage and the left eye as being in moderate stage
>
> **H40.10X1   Unspecified open-angle glaucoma, mild stage**
>
> **H40.10X2   Unspecified open-angle glaucoma, moderate stage**
>
> *Explanation*: In this scenario the patient has the same type of glaucoma in each eye but each eye is at a different stage, and the classification does not distinguish laterality at this subcategory level. Two codes are assigned; both codes represent the same type of glaucoma but each has a different seventh character identifying the appropriate stage for each eye.

4) Patient admitted with glaucoma and stage evolves during the admission

If a patient is admitted with glaucoma and the stage progresses during the admission, assign the code for highest stage documented.

> Patient admitted with mild low-tension glaucoma of the right eye, which progresses to moderate stage during the patient's stay
>
> **H40.1212   Low-tension glaucoma, right eye, moderate stage**
>
> *Explanation*: When the glaucoma stage progresses during an admission, assign only the code for the highest stage documented.

5) Indeterminate stage glaucoma

Assignment of the seventh character "4" for "indeterminate stage" should be based on the clinical documentation. The seventh character "4" is used for glaucomas whose stage cannot be clinically determined. This seventh character should not be confused with the seventh character "0", unspecified, which should be assigned when there is no documentation regarding the stage of the glaucoma.

b. Blindness

If "blindness" or "low vision" of both eyes is documented but the visual impairment category is not documented, assign code H54.3, Unqualified visual loss, both eyes. If "blindness" or "low vision" in one eye is documented but the visual impairment category is not documented, assign a code from H54.6-, Unqualified visual loss, one eye. If "blindness" or "visual loss" is documented without any information about whether one or both eyes are affected, assign code H54.7, Unspecified visual loss.

> Blindness in 89-year-old male
>
> **H54.7   Unspecified visual loss**
>
> *Explanation*: Blindness is stated, but there is no mention of whether one or both eyes are affected or the severity of this visual impairment.

Chapter 7. Diseases of the Eye and Adnexa (H00-H59)

NOTE Use an external cause code following the code for the eye condition, if applicable, to identify the cause of the eye condition.

EXCLUDES 2 certain conditions originating in the perinatal period (P04-P96)
certain infectious and parasitic diseases (A00-B99)
complications of pregnancy, childbirth and the puerperium (O00-O9A)
congenital malformations, deformations, and chromosomal abnormalities (Q00-Q99)
diabetes mellitus related eye conditions (E09.3-, E10.3-, E11.3-, E13.3-)
endocrine, nutritional and metabolic diseases (E00-E88)
injury (trauma) of eye and orbit (S05.-)
injury, poisoning and certain other consequences of external causes (S00-T88)
neoplasms (C00-D49)
symptoms, signs and abnormal clinical and laboratory findings, not elsewhere classified (R00-R94)
syphilis related eye disorders (A50.01, A50.3-, A51.43, A52.71)

This chapter contains the following blocks:

H00-H05	Disorders of eyelid, lacrimal system and orbit
H10-H11	Disorders of conjunctiva
H15-H22	Disorders of sclera, cornea, iris and ciliary body
H25-H28	Disorders of lens
H30-H36	Disorders of choroid and retina
H40-H42	Glaucoma
H43-H44	Disorders of vitreous body and globe
H46-H47	Disorders of optic nerve and visual pathways
H49-H52	Disorders of ocular muscles, binocular movement, accommodation and refraction
H53-H54	Visual disturbances and blindness
H55-H57	Other disorders of eye and adnexa
H59	Intraoperative and postprocedural complications and disorders of eye and adnexa, not elsewhere classified

Disorders of eyelid, lacrimal system and orbit (H00-H05)

EXCLUDES 2 open wound of eyelid (S01.1-)
superficial injury of eyelid (S00.1-, S00.2-)

✓4th H00 **Hordeolum and chalazion**

✓5th H00.0 **Hordeolum (externum) (internum) of eyelid**
DEF: Acute localized infection of the gland of Zeis (external hordeolum) or Molt or of the meibomian glands (internal hordeolum) of the orbit.

✓6th H00.01 **Hordeolum** externum
Hordeolum NOS
Stye
H00.011 **Hordeolum externum** right upper eyelid
H00.012 **Hordeolum externum** right lower eyelid
H00.013 **Hordeolum externum** right eye, unspecified eyelid
H00.014 **Hordeolum externum** left upper eyelid
H00.015 **Hordeolum externum** left lower eyelid
H00.016 **Hordeolum externum** left eye, unspecified eyelid
H00.019 **Hordeolum externum** unspecified eye, unspecified eyelid

✓6th H00.02 **Hordeolum** internum
Infection of meibomian gland
H00.021 **Hordeolum internum** right upper eyelid
H00.022 **Hordeolum internum** right lower eyelid
H00.023 **Hordeolum internum** right eye, unspecified eyelid
H00.024 **Hordeolum internum** left upper eyelid
H00.025 **Hordeolum internum** left lower eyelid
H00.026 **Hordeolum internum** left eye, unspecified eyelid
H00.029 **Hordeolum internum** unspecified eye, unspecified eyelid

✓6th H00.03 **Abscess** of eyelid
Furuncle of eyelid
H00.031 **Abscess of** right upper eyelid
H00.032 **Abscess of** right lower eyelid
H00.033 **Abscess of eyelid** right eye, unspecified eyelid
H00.034 **Abscess of** left upper eyelid
H00.035 **Abscess of** left lower eyelid
H00.036 **Abscess of eyelid** left eye, unspecified eyelid
H00.039 **Abscess of eyelid** unspecified eye, unspecified eyelid

✓5th H00.1 **Chalazion**
Meibomian (gland) cyst
EXCLUDES 2 infected meibomian gland (H00.02-)
DEF: Noninfectious, obstructive mass in the oil gland of the eyelid that results in a small chronic lump or inflammation.
H00.11 **Chalazion** right upper eyelid
H00.12 **Chalazion** right lower eyelid
H00.13 **Chalazion** right eye, unspecified eyelid
H00.14 **Chalazion** left upper eyelid
H00.15 **Chalazion** left lower eyelid
H00.16 **Chalazion** left eye, unspecified eyelid
H00.19 **Chalazion** unspecified eye, unspecified eyelid

✓4th H01 **Other inflammation of eyelid**

✓5th H01.0 **Blepharitis**
EXCLUDES 1 blepharoconjunctivitis (H10.5-)

✓6th H01.00 **Unspecified blepharitis**
H01.001 **Unspecified blepharitis** right upper eyelid
H01.002 **Unspecified blepharitis** right lower eyelid
H01.003 **Unspecified blepharitis** right eye, unspecified eyelid
H01.004 **Unspecified blepharitis** left upper eyelid
H01.005 **Unspecified blepharitis** left lower eyelid
H01.006 **Unspecified blepharitis** left eye, unspecified eyelid
H01.009 **Unspecified blepharitis** unspecified eye, unspecified eyelid
● **H01.00A** **Unspecified blepharitis** right eye, upper and lower eyelids
● **H01.00B** **Unspecified blepharitis** left eye, upper and lower eyelids

✓6th H01.01 **Ulcerative blepharitis**
H01.011 **Ulcerative blepharitis** right upper eyelid
H01.012 **Ulcerative blepharitis** right lower eyelid
H01.013 **Ulcerative blepharitis** right eye, unspecified eyelid
H01.014 **Ulcerative blepharitis** left upper eyelid
H01.015 **Ulcerative blepharitis** left lower eyelid
H01.016 **Ulcerative blepharitis** left eye, unspecified eyelid
H01.019 **Ulcerative blepharitis** unspecified eye, unspecified eyelid
● **H01.01A** **Ulcerative blepharitis** right eye, upper and lower eyelids
● **H01.01B** **Ulcerative blepharitis** left eye, upper and lower eyelids

✓6th H01.02 **Squamous blepharitis**
H01.021 **Squamous blepharitis** right upper eyelid
H01.022 **Squamous blepharitis** right lower eyelid
H01.023 **Squamous blepharitis** right eye, unspecified eyelid
H01.024 **Squamous blepharitis** left upper eyelid
H01.025 **Squamous blepharitis** left lower eyelid
H01.026 **Squamous blepharitis** left eye, unspecified eyelid
H01.029 **Squamous blepharitis** unspecified eye, unspecified eyelid
● **H01.02A** **Squamous blepharitis** right eye, upper and lower eyelids
● **H01.02B** **Squamous blepharitis** left eye, upper and lower eyelids

✓5th H01.1 **Noninfectious dermatoses of eyelid**

✓6th H01.11 **Allergic dermatitis of eyelid**
Contact dermatitis of eyelid
H01.111 **Allergic dermatitis of** right upper eyelid
H01.112 **Allergic dermatitis of** right lower eyelid
H01.113 **Allergic dermatitis of** right eye, unspecified eyelid
H01.114 **Allergic dermatitis of** left upper eyelid
H01.115 **Allergic dermatitis of** left lower eyelid
H01.116 **Allergic dermatitis of** left eye, unspecified eyelid
H01.119 **Allergic dermatitis of** unspecified eye, unspecified eyelid

N Newborn: 0   P Pediatric: 0-17   M Maternity: 12-55   A Adult: 15-124   **MCC** Major Complication/Comorbidity   **CC** Complication/Comorbidity   **SW** Severe Wound Dx

584

ICD-10-CM 2019

✓6ᵗʰ **H01.12 Discoid lupus erythematosus of eyelid**
     H01.121 Discoid lupus erythematosus of right upper **eyelid**
     H01.122 Discoid lupus erythematosus of right lower **eyelid**
     H01.123 Discoid lupus erythematosus of right eye, unspecified **eyelid**
     H01.124 Discoid lupus erythematosus of left upper **eyelid**
     H01.125 Discoid lupus erythematosus of left lower **eyelid**
     H01.126 Discoid lupus erythematosus of left eye, unspecified **eyelid**
     H01.129 Discoid lupus erythematosus of unspecified eye, unspecified **eyelid**

✓6ᵗʰ **H01.13 Eczematous dermatitis of eyelid**
     H01.131 Eczematous dermatitis of right upper **eyelid**
     H01.132 Eczematous dermatitis of right lower **eyelid**
     H01.133 Eczematous dermatitis of right eye, unspecified **eyelid**
     H01.134 Eczematous dermatitis of left upper **eyelid**
     H01.135 Eczematous dermatitis of left lower **eyelid**
     H01.136 Eczematous dermatitis of left eye, unspecified **eyelid**
     H01.139 Eczematous dermatitis of unspecified eye, unspecified **eyelid**

✓6ᵗʰ **H01.14 Xeroderma of eyelid**
     H01.141 Xeroderma of right upper **eyelid**
     H01.142 Xeroderma of right lower **eyelid**
     H01.143 Xeroderma of right eye, unspecified **eyelid**
     H01.144 Xeroderma of left upper **eyelid**
     H01.145 Xeroderma of left lower **eyelid**
     H01.146 Xeroderma of left eye, unspecified **eyelid**
     H01.149 Xeroderma of unspecified eye, unspecified **eyelid**

H01.8 Other specified inflammations of eyelid

H01.9 Unspecified inflammation of eyelid
     Inflammation of eyelid NOS

✓4ᵗʰ **H02 Other disorders of eyelid**
     EXCLUDES 1   congenital malformations of eyelid (Q10.0-Q10.3)

✓5ᵗʰ **H02.0 Entropion and trichiasis of eyelid**
     DEF: Entropion: Inversion of the eyelid, turning the edge in toward the eyeball and causing irritation from contact of the lashes with the surface of the eye.
     DEF: Trichiasis: Condition wherein the eyelid is in a normal position but lashes are ingrown or misdirected in their growth so that they irritate the tissues of the eye.

✓6ᵗʰ **H02.00 Unspecified entropion of eyelid**
     H02.001 Unspecified entropion of right upper **eyelid**
     H02.002 Unspecified entropion of right lower **eyelid**
     H02.003 Unspecified entropion of right eye, unspecified **eyelid**
     H02.004 Unspecified entropion of left upper **eyelid**
     H02.005 Unspecified entropion of left lower **eyelid**
     H02.006 Unspecified entropion of left eye, unspecified **eyelid**
     H02.009 Unspecified entropion of unspecified eye, unspecified **eyelid**

✓6ᵗʰ **H02.01 Cicatricial entropion of eyelid**
     H02.011 Cicatricial entropion of right upper **eyelid**
     H02.012 Cicatricial entropion of right lower **eyelid**
     H02.013 Cicatricial entropion of right eye, unspecified **eyelid**
     H02.014 Cicatricial entropion of left upper **eyelid**
     H02.015 Cicatricial entropion of left lower **eyelid**
     H02.016 Cicatricial entropion of left eye, unspecified **eyelid**
     H02.019 Cicatricial entropion of unspecified eye, unspecified **eyelid**

Entropion and Ectropion

Normal eyelid   Entropion   Ectropion

✓6ᵗʰ **H02.02 Mechanical entropion of eyelid**
     H02.021 Mechanical entropion of right upper **eyelid**
     H02.022 Mechanical entropion of right lower **eyelid**
     H02.023 Mechanical entropion of right eye, unspecified **eyelid**
     H02.024 Mechanical entropion of left upper **eyelid**
     H02.025 Mechanical entropion of left lower **eyelid**
     H02.026 Mechanical entropion of left eye, unspecified **eyelid**
     H02.029 Mechanical entropion of unspecified eye, unspecified **eyelid**

✓6ᵗʰ **H02.03 Senile entropion of eyelid**
     H02.031 Senile entropion of right upper **eyelid** 🅰
     H02.032 Senile entropion of right lower **eyelid** 🅰
     H02.033 Senile entropion of right eye, unspecified **eyelid** 🅰
     H02.034 Senile entropion of left upper **eyelid** 🅰
     H02.035 Senile entropion of left lower **eyelid** 🅰
     H02.036 Senile entropion of left eye, unspecified **eyelid** 🅰
     H02.039 Senile entropion of unspecified eye, unspecified **eyelid** 🅰

✓6ᵗʰ **H02.04 Spastic entropion of eyelid**
     H02.041 Spastic entropion of right upper **eyelid**
     H02.042 Spastic entropion of right lower **eyelid**
     H02.043 Spastic entropion of right eye, unspecified **eyelid**
     H02.044 Spastic entropion of left upper **eyelid**
     H02.045 Spastic entropion of left lower **eyelid**
     H02.046 Spastic entropion of left eye, unspecified **eyelid**
     H02.049 Spastic entropion of unspecified eye, unspecified **eyelid**

✓6ᵗʰ **H02.05 Trichiasis without entropion**
     H02.051 Trichiasis without entropion right upper **eyelid**
     H02.052 Trichiasis without entropion right lower **eyelid**
     H02.053 Trichiasis without entropion right eye, unspecified **eyelid**
     H02.054 Trichiasis without entropion left upper **eyelid**
     H02.055 Trichiasis without entropion left lower **eyelid**
     H02.056 Trichiasis without entropion left eye, unspecified **eyelid**
     H02.059 Trichiasis without entropion unspecified eye, unspecified **eyelid**

✓5ᵗʰ **H02.1 Ectropion of eyelid**
     DEF: Drooping of the lower eyelid away from the eye or outward turning or eversion of the edge of the eyelid, exposing the palpebral conjunctiva and causing irritation.

✓6ᵗʰ **H02.10 Unspecified ectropion of eyelid**
     H02.101 Unspecified ectropion of right upper **eyelid**
     H02.102 Unspecified ectropion of right lower **eyelid**
     H02.103 Unspecified ectropion of right eye, unspecified **eyelid**
     H02.104 Unspecified ectropion of left upper **eyelid**
     H02.105 Unspecified ectropion of left lower **eyelid**

✓ Additional Character Required   ✓x7ᵗʰ Placeholder   Unacceptable PDx   Questionable PDx   Manifestation   H1 - H14 HAC   HCC CMS-HCC Dx   HIV HIV Dx

ICD-10-CM 2019   585

Chapter 7. Diseases of the Eye and Adnexa

H01.12-H02.105

Chapter 7. Diseases of the Eye and Adnexa (side tab)

H02.106   Unspecified ectropion of left eye, unspecified eyelid

H02.109   Unspecified ectropion of unspecified eye, unspecified eyelid

✓6ᵗʰ **H02.11**   Cicatricial ectropion of eyelid

H02.111   Cicatricial ectropion of right upper eyelid

H02.112   Cicatricial ectropion of right lower eyelid

H02.113   Cicatricial ectropion of right eye, unspecified eyelid

H02.114   Cicatricial ectropion of left upper eyelid

H02.115   Cicatricial ectropion of left lower eyelid

H02.116   Cicatricial ectropion of left eye, unspecified eyelid

H02.119   Cicatricial ectropion of unspecified eye, unspecified eyelid

✓6ᵗʰ **H02.12**   Mechanical ectropion of eyelid

H02.121   Mechanical ectropion of right upper eyelid

H02.122   Mechanical ectropion of right lower eyelid

H02.123   Mechanical ectropion of right eye, unspecified eyelid

H02.124   Mechanical ectropion of left upper eyelid

H02.125   Mechanical ectropion of left lower eyelid

H02.126   Mechanical ectropion of left eye, unspecified eyelid

H02.129   Mechanical ectropion of unspecified eye, unspecified eyelid

✓6ᵗʰ **H02.13**   Senile ectropion of eyelid

H02.131   Senile ectropion of right upper eyelid   A

H02.132   Senile ectropion of right lower eyelid   A

H02.133   Senile ectropion of right eye, unspecified eyelid   A

H02.134   Senile ectropion of left upper eyelid   A

H02.135   Senile ectropion of left lower eyelid   A

H02.136   Senile ectropion of left eye, unspecified eyelid   A

H02.139   Senile ectropion of unspecified eye, unspecified eyelid   A

✓6ᵗʰ **H02.14**   Spastic ectropion of eyelid

H02.141   Spastic ectropion of right upper eyelid

H02.142   Spastic ectropion of right lower eyelid

H02.143   Spastic ectropion of right eye, unspecified eyelid

H02.144   Spastic ectropion of left upper eyelid

H02.145   Spastic ectropion of left lower eyelid

H02.146   Spastic ectropion of left eye, unspecified eyelid

H02.149   Spastic ectropion of unspecified eye, unspecified eyelid

● ✓6ᵗʰ **H02.15**   Paralytic ectropion of eyelid

● H02.151   Paralytic ectropion of right upper eyelid

● H02.152   Paralytic ectropion of right lower eyelid

● H02.153   Paralytic ectropion of right eye, unspecified eyelid

● H02.154   Paralytic ectropion of left upper eyelid

● H02.155   Paralytic ectropion of left lower eyelid

● H02.156   Paralytic ectropion of left eye, unspecified eyelid

● H02.159   Paralytic ectropion of unspecified eye, unspecified eyelid

✓5ᵗʰ **H02.2**   **Lagophthalmos**

DEF: Condition of the eye that prevents it from closing completely.

✓6ᵗʰ **H02.20**   Unspecified lagophthalmos

H02.201   Unspecified lagophthalmos right upper eyelid

H02.202   Unspecified lagophthalmos right lower eyelid

H02.203   Unspecified lagophthalmos right eye, unspecified eyelid

H02.204   Unspecified lagophthalmos left upper eyelid

H02.205   Unspecified lagophthalmos left lower eyelid

H02.206   Unspecified lagophthalmos left eye, unspecified eyelid

H02.209   Unspecified lagophthalmos unspecified eye, unspecified eyelid

● H02.20A   Unspecified lagophthalmos right eye, upper and lower eyelids

● H02.20B   Unspecified lagophthalmos left eye, upper and lower eyelids

● H02.20C   Unspecified lagophthalmos, bilateral, upper and lower eyelids

✓6ᵗʰ **H02.21**   Cicatricial lagophthalmos

H02.211   Cicatricial lagophthalmos right upper eyelid

H02.212   Cicatricial lagophthalmos right lower eyelid

H02.213   Cicatricial lagophthalmos right eye, unspecified eyelid

H02.214   Cicatricial lagophthalmos left upper eyelid

H02.215   Cicatricial lagophthalmos left lower eyelid

H02.216   Cicatricial lagophthalmos left eye, unspecified eyelid

H02.219   Cicatricial lagophthalmos unspecified eye, unspecified eyelid

● H02.21A   Cicatricial lagophthalmos right eye, upper and lower eyelids

● H02.21B   Cicatricial lagophthalmos left eye, upper and lower eyelids

● H02.21C   Cicatricial lagophthalmos, bilateral, upper and lower eyelids

✓6ᵗʰ **H02.22**   Mechanical lagophthalmos

H02.221   Mechanical lagophthalmos right upper eyelid

H02.222   Mechanical lagophthalmos right lower eyelid

H02.223   Mechanical lagophthalmos right eye, unspecified eyelid

H02.224   Mechanical lagophthalmos left upper eyelid

H02.225   Mechanical lagophthalmos left lower eyelid

H02.226   Mechanical lagophthalmos left eye, unspecified eyelid

H02.229   Mechanical lagophthalmos unspecified eye, unspecified eyelid

● H02.22A   Mechanical lagophthalmos right eye, upper and lower eyelids

● H02.22B   Mechanical lagophthalmos left eye, upper and lower eyelids

● H02.22C   Mechanical lagophthalmos, bilateral, upper and lower eyelids

✓6ᵗʰ **H02.23**   Paralytic lagophthalmos

H02.231   Paralytic lagophthalmos right upper eyelid

H02.232   Paralytic lagophthalmos right lower eyelid

H02.233   Paralytic lagophthalmos right eye, unspecified eyelid

H02.234   Paralytic lagophthalmos left upper eyelid

H02.235   Paralytic lagophthalmos left lower eyelid

H02.236   Paralytic lagophthalmos left eye, unspecified eyelid

H02.239   Paralytic lagophthalmos unspecified eye, unspecified eyelid

● H02.23A   Paralytic lagophthalmos right eye, upper and lower eyelids

● H02.23B   Paralytic lagophthalmos left eye, upper and lower eyelids

● H02.23C   Paralytic lagophthalmos, bilateral, upper and lower eyelids

✓5ᵗʰ **H02.3**   **Blepharochalasis**

Pseudoptosis

DEF: Loss of elasticity and relaxation of skin of the eyelid, thickened or indurated skin on the eyelid associated with recurrent episodes of edema, and intracellular atrophy.

H02.30   Blepharochalasis unspecified eye, unspecified eyelid

H02.31   Blepharochalasis right upper eyelid

H02.32   Blepharochalasis right lower eyelid

H02.33   Blepharochalasis right eye, unspecified eyelid

H02.34   Blepharochalasis left upper eyelid

N Newborn: 0   P Pediatric: 0-17   M Maternity: 12-55   A Adult: 15-124   MCC Major Complication/Comorbidity   CC Complication/Comorbidity   SW Severe Wound Dx

586   ICD-10-CM 2019

H02.35   **Blepharochalasis** left lower **eyelid**

H02.36   **Blepharochalasis** left eye, unspecified **eyelid**

✓5ᵗʰ **H02.4   Ptosis of eyelid**

   ✓6ᵗʰ **H02.40   Unspecified ptosis of eyelid**

       H02.401   **Unspecified ptosis of** right **eyelid**

       H02.402   **Unspecified ptosis of** left **eyelid**

       H02.403   **Unspecified ptosis of** bilateral **eyelids**

       H02.409   **Unspecified ptosis of** unspecified **eyelid**

   ✓6ᵗʰ **H02.41   Mechanical ptosis of eyelid**

       H02.411   **Mechanical ptosis of** right **eyelid**

       H02.412   **Mechanical ptosis of** left **eyelid**

       H02.413   **Mechanical ptosis of** bilateral **eyelids**

       H02.419   **Mechanical ptosis of** unspecified **eyelid**

   ✓6ᵗʰ **H02.42   Myogenic ptosis of eyelid**

       H02.421   **Myogenic ptosis of** right **eyelid**

       H02.422   **Myogenic ptosis of** left **eyelid**

       H02.423   **Myogenic ptosis of** bilateral **eyelids**

       H02.429   **Myogenic ptosis of** unspecified **eyelid**

   ✓6ᵗʰ **H02.43   Paralytic ptosis of eyelid**

       Neurogenic ptosis of eyelid

       H02.431   **Paralytic ptosis of** right **eyelid**

       H02.432   **Paralytic ptosis of** left **eyelid**

       H02.433   **Paralytic ptosis of** bilateral **eyelids**

       H02.439   **Paralytic ptosis** unspecified **eyelid**

✓5ᵗʰ **H02.5   Other disorders affecting eyelid function**

       EXCLUDES 2   *blepharospasm (G24.5)*

              organic tic (G25.69)

              psychogenic tic (F95.-)

   ✓6ᵗʰ **H02.51   Abnormal innervation syndrome**

       H02.511   **Abnormal innervation syndrome** right upper **eyelid**

       H02.512   **Abnormal innervation syndrome** right lower **eyelid**

       H02.513   **Abnormal innervation syndrome** right eye, unspecified **eyelid**

       H02.514   **Abnormal innervation syndrome** left upper **eyelid**

       H02.515   **Abnormal innervation syndrome** left lower **eyelid**

       H02.516   **Abnormal innervation syndrome** left eye, unspecified **eyelid**

       H02.519   **Abnormal innervation syndrome** unspecified eye, unspecified **eyelid**

   ✓6ᵗʰ **H02.52   Blepharophimosis**

       Ankyloblepharon

       H02.521   **Blepharophimosis** right upper **eyelid**

       H02.522   **Blepharophimosis** right lower **eyelid**

       H02.523   **Blepharophimosis** right eye, unspecified **eyelid**

       H02.524   **Blepharophimosis** left upper **eyelid**

       H02.525   **Blepharophimosis** left lower **eyelid**

       H02.526   **Blepharophimosis** left eye, unspecified **eyelid**

       H02.529   **Blepharophimosis** unspecified eye, unspecified **lid**

   ✓6ᵗʰ **H02.53   Eyelid retraction**

       Eyelid lag

       H02.531   **Eyelid retraction** right upper **eyelid**

       H02.532   **Eyelid retraction** right lower **eyelid**

       H02.533   **Eyelid retraction** right eye, unspecified **eyelid**

       H02.534   **Eyelid retraction** left upper **eyelid**

       H02.535   **Eyelid retraction** left lower **eyelid**

       H02.536   **Eyelid retraction** left eye, unspecified **eyelid**

       H02.539   **Eyelid retraction** unspecified eye, unspecified **lid**

     H02.59   **Other disorders affecting eyelid function**

       Deficient blink reflex

       Sensory disorders

✓5ᵗʰ **H02.6   Xanthelasma of eyelid**

       DEF: Condition in which there are small yellow tumors that occur on the eyelid, usually appearing near the nose.

     H02.60   **Xanthelasma of** unspecified eye, unspecified **eyelid**

     H02.61   **Xanthelasma of** right upper **eyelid**

H02.62   **Xanthelasma of** right lower **eyelid**

H02.63   **Xanthelasma of** right eye, unspecified **eyelid**

H02.64   **Xanthelasma of** left upper **eyelid**

H02.65   **Xanthelasma of** left lower **eyelid**

H02.66   **Xanthelasma of** left eye, unspecified **eyelid**

✓5ᵗʰ **H02.7   Other and unspecified degenerative disorders of eyelid and periocular area**

     H02.70   **Unspecified degenerative disorders of eyelid and periocular area**

   ✓6ᵗʰ **H02.71   Chloasma of eyelid and periocular area**

       Dyspigmentation of eyelid

       Hyperpigmentation of eyelid

       H02.711   **Chloasma of** right upper **eyelid and periocular area**

       H02.712   **Chloasma of** right lower **eyelid and periocular area**

       H02.713   **Chloasma of** right eye, unspecified **eyelid and periocular area**

       H02.714   **Chloasma of** left upper **eyelid and periocular area**

       H02.715   **Chloasma of** left lower **eyelid and periocular area**

       H02.716   **Chloasma of** left eye, unspecified **eyelid and periocular area**

       H02.719   **Chloasma of** unspecified eye, unspecified **eyelid and periocular area**

   ✓6ᵗʰ **H02.72   Madarosis of eyelid and periocular area**

       Hypotrichosis of eyelid

       H02.721   **Madarosis of** right upper **eyelid and periocular area**

       H02.722   **Madarosis of** right lower **eyelid and periocular area**

       H02.723   **Madarosis of** right eye, unspecified **eyelid and periocular area**

       H02.724   **Madarosis of** left upper **eyelid and periocular area**

       H02.725   **Madarosis of** left lower **eyelid and periocular area**

       H02.726   **Madarosis of** left eye, unspecified **eyelid and periocular area**

       H02.729   **Madarosis of** unspecified eye, unspecified **eyelid and periocular area**

   ✓6ᵗʰ **H02.73   Vitiligo of eyelid and periocular area**

       Hypopigmentation of eyelid

       H02.731   **Vitiligo of** right upper **eyelid and periocular area**

       H02.732   **Vitiligo of** right lower **eyelid and periocular area**

       H02.733   **Vitiligo of** right eye, unspecified **eyelid and periocular area**

       H02.734   **Vitiligo of** left upper **eyelid and periocular area**

       H02.735   **Vitiligo of** left lower **eyelid and periocular area**

       H02.736   **Vitiligo of** left eye, unspecified **eyelid and periocular area**

       H02.739   **Vitiligo of** unspecified eye, unspecified **eyelid and periocular area**

     H02.79   **Other degenerative disorders of eyelid and periocular area**

✓5ᵗʰ **H02.8   Other specified disorders of eyelid**

   ✓6ᵗʰ **H02.81   Retained foreign body in eyelid**

       Use additional code to identify the type of retained foreign body (Z18.-)

       EXCLUDES 1   *laceration of eyelid with foreign body (S01.12-)*

              retained intraocular foreign body (H44.6-, H44.7-)

              superficial foreign body of eyelid and periocular area (S00.25-)

       H02.811   **Retained foreign body in** right upper **eyelid**

       H02.812   **Retained foreign body in** right lower **eyelid**

       H02.813   **Retained foreign body in** right eye, unspecified **eyelid**

       H02.814   **Retained foreign body in** left upper **eyelid**

       H02.815   **Retained foreign body in** left lower **eyelid**

✔ Additional Character Required   ✓x7ᵗʰ Placeholder   Unacceptable PDx   Questionable PDx   Manifestation   H1-H14 HAC   HCC CMS-HCC Dx   HIV HIV Dx

ICD-10-CM 2019   587

Chapter 7. Diseases of the Eye and Adnexa

H02.816   **Retained foreign body in** left **eye,** unspecified **eyelid**

H02.819   **Retained foreign body in** unspecified **eye,** unspecified **eyelid**

✓6ᵗʰ   **H02.82**   **Cysts of eyelid**
Sebaceous cyst of eyelid

H02.821   **Cysts of** right upper **eyelid**

H02.822   **Cysts of** right lower **eyelid**

H02.823   **Cysts of** right eye, unspecified **eyelid**

H02.824   **Cysts of** left upper **eyelid**

H02.825   **Cysts of** left lower **eyelid**

H02.826   **Cysts of** left eye, unspecified **eyelid**

H02.829   **Cysts of** unspecified eye, unspecified **eyelid**

✓6ᵗʰ   **H02.83**   **Dermatochalasis of eyelid**
DEF: Acquired form of connective tissue disorder associated with decreased elastic tissue and abnormal elastin formation, resulting in loss of elasticity of the skin of the eyelid. It is generally associated with aging.

H02.831   **Dermatochalasis of** right upper **eyelid**

H02.832   **Dermatochalasis of** right lower **eyelid**

H02.833   **Dermatochalasis of** right eye, unspecified **eyelid**

H02.834   **Dermatochalasis of** left upper **eyelid**

H02.835   **Dermatochalasis of** left lower **eyelid**

H02.836   **Dermatochalasis of** left eye, unspecified **eyelid**

H02.839   **Dermatochalasis of** unspecified eye, unspecified **eyelid**

✓6ᵗʰ   **H02.84**   **Edema of eyelid**
Hyperemia of eyelid

H02.841   **Edema of** right upper **eyelid**

H02.842   **Edema of** right lower **eyelid**

H02.843   **Edema of** right eye, unspecified **eyelid**

H02.844   **Edema of** left upper **eyelid**

H02.845   **Edema of** left lower **eyelid**

H02.846   **Edema of** left eye, unspecified **eyelid**

H02.849   **Edema of** unspecified eye, unspecified **eyelid**

✓6ᵗʰ   **H02.85**   **Elephantiasis of eyelid**

H02.851   **Elephantiasis of** right upper **eyelid**

H02.852   **Elephantiasis of** right lower **eyelid**

H02.853   **Elephantiasis of** right eye, unspecified **eyelid**

H02.854   **Elephantiasis of** left upper **eyelid**

H02.855   **Elephantiasis of** left lower **eyelid**

H02.856   **Elephantiasis of** left eye, unspecified **eyelid**

H02.859   **Elephantiasis of** unspecified eye, unspecified **eyelid**

✓6ᵗʰ   **H02.86**   **Hypertrichosis of eyelid**

H02.861   **Hypertrichosis of** right upper **eyelid**

H02.862   **Hypertrichosis of** right lower **eyelid**

H02.863   **Hypertrichosis of** right eye, unspecified **eyelid**

H02.864   **Hypertrichosis of** left upper **eyelid**

H02.865   **Hypertrichosis of** left lower **eyelid**

H02.866   **Hypertrichosis of** left eye, unspecified **eyelid**

H02.869   **Hypertrichosis of** unspecified eye, unspecified **eyelid**

✓6ᵗʰ   **H02.87**   **Vascular anomalies of eyelid**

H02.871   **Vascular anomalies of** right upper **eyelid**

H02.872   **Vascular anomalies of** right lower **eyelid**

H02.873   **Vascular anomalies of** right eye, unspecified **eyelid**

H02.874   **Vascular anomalies of** left upper **eyelid**

H02.875   **Vascular anomalies of** left lower **eyelid**

H02.876   **Vascular anomalies of** left eye, unspecified **eyelid**

H02.879   **Vascular anomalies of** unspecified eye, unspecified **eyelid**

● ✓6ᵗʰ   **H02.88**   **Meibomian gland dysfunction of eyelid**

●   H02.881   **Meibomian gland dysfunction** right upper **eyelid**

●   H02.882   **Meibomian gland dysfunction** right lower **eyelid**

●   H02.883   **Meibomian gland dysfunction of** right eye, unspecified **eyelid**

●   H02.884   **Meibomian gland dysfunction** left upper **eyelid**

●   H02.885   **Meibomian gland dysfunction** left lower **eyelid**

●   H02.886   **Meibomian gland dysfunction of** left eye, unspecified **eyelid**

●   H02.889   **Meibomian gland dysfunction of** unspecified eye, unspecified **eyelid**

●   H02.88A   **Meibomian gland dysfunction** right eye, upper and lower **eyelids**

●   H02.88B   **Meibomian gland dysfunction** left eye, upper and lower **eyelids**

H02.89   **Other specified disorders of eyelid**
Hemorrhage of eyelid

H02.9   **Unspecified disorder of eyelid**
Disorder of eyelid NOS

✓4ᵗʰ   **H04**   **Disorders of lacrimal system**
EXCLUDES 1   *congenital malformations of lacrimal system (Q10.4-Q10.6)*

✓5ᵗʰ   **H04.0**   **Dacryoadenitis**
DEF: Inflammation of the lacrimal gland.

✓6ᵗʰ   **H04.00**   Unspecified **dacryoadenitis**

H04.001   **Unspecified dacryoadenitis,** right **lacrimal gland**

H04.002   **Unspecified dacryoadenitis,** left **lacrimal gland**

H04.003   **Unspecified dacryoadenitis,** bilateral **lacrimal glands**

H04.009   **Unspecified dacryoadenitis,** unspecified **lacrimal gland**

✓6ᵗʰ   **H04.01**   Acute **dacryoadenitis**

H04.011   **Acute dacryoadenitis,** right **lacrimal gland**

H04.012   **Acute dacryoadenitis,** left **lacrimal gland**

H04.013   **Acute dacryoadenitis,** bilateral **lacrimal glands**

H04.019   **Acute dacryoadenitis,** unspecified **lacrimal gland**

✓6ᵗʰ   **H04.02**   Chronic **dacryoadenitis**

H04.021   **Chronic dacryoadenitis,** right **lacrimal gland**

H04.022   **Chronic dacryoadenitis,** left **lacrimal gland**

H04.023   **Chronic dacryoadenitis,** bilateral **lacrimal glands**

H04.029   **Chronic dacryoadenitis,** unspecified **lacrimal gland**

✓6ᵗʰ   **H04.03**   **Chronic enlargement of lacrimal gland**

H04.031   **Chronic enlargement of** right **lacrimal gland**

H04.032   **Chronic enlargement of** left **lacrimal gland**

H04.033   **Chronic enlargement of** bilateral **lacrimal glands**

H04.039   **Chronic enlargement of** unspecified **lacrimal gland**

✓5ᵗʰ   **H04.1**   **Other disorders of lacrimal gland**

✓6ᵗʰ   **H04.11**   **Dacryops**

H04.111   **Dacryops of** right **lacrimal gland**

H04.112   **Dacryops of** left **lacrimal gland**

H04.113   **Dacryops of** bilateral **lacrimal glands**

H04.119   **Dacryops of** unspecified **lacrimal gland**

✓6ᵗʰ   **H04.12**   **Dry eye syndrome**
Tear film insufficiency, NOS

H04.121   **Dry eye syndrome of** right **lacrimal gland**

H04.122   **Dry eye syndrome of** left **lacrimal gland**

H04.123   **Dry eye syndrome of** bilateral **lacrimal glands**

H04.129   **Dry eye syndrome of** unspecified **lacrimal gland**

N Newborn: 0   **P** Pediatric: 0-17   **M** Maternity: 12-55   **A** Adult: 15-124   **MCC** Major Complication/Comorbidity   **CC** Complication/Comorbidity   **SW** Severe Wound Dx

588   ICD-10-CM 2019

✓6ᵗʰ H04.13 Lacrimal cyst
    Lacrimal cystic degeneration
    H04.131 Lacrimal cyst, right lacrimal gland
    H04.132 Lacrimal cyst, left lacrimal gland
    H04.133 Lacrimal cyst, bilateral lacrimal glands
    H04.139 Lacrimal cyst, unspecified lacrimal gland

✓6ᵗʰ H04.14 Primary lacrimal gland atrophy
    H04.141 Primary lacrimal gland atrophy, right lacrimal gland
    H04.142 Primary lacrimal gland atrophy, left lacrimal gland
    H04.143 Primary lacrimal gland atrophy, bilateral lacrimal glands
    H04.149 Primary lacrimal gland atrophy, unspecified lacrimal gland

✓6ᵗʰ H04.15 Secondary lacrimal gland atrophy
    H04.151 Secondary lacrimal gland atrophy, right lacrimal gland
    H04.152 Secondary lacrimal gland atrophy, left lacrimal gland
    H04.153 Secondary lacrimal gland atrophy, bilateral lacrimal glands
    H04.159 Secondary lacrimal gland atrophy, unspecified lacrimal gland

✓6ᵗʰ H04.16 Lacrimal gland dislocation
    H04.161 Lacrimal gland dislocation, right lacrimal gland
    H04.162 Lacrimal gland dislocation, left lacrimal gland
    H04.163 Lacrimal gland dislocation, bilateral lacrimal glands
    H04.169 Lacrimal gland dislocation, unspecified lacrimal gland

    H04.19 Other specified disorders of lacrimal gland

✓5ᵗʰ H04.2 Epiphora
    DEF: Excessive tearing or overflow of tears down the cheeks often due to a stricture in the lacrimal passages but can be caused by other conditions.

✓6ᵗʰ H04.20 Unspecified epiphora
▲   **H04.201 Unspecified epiphora, right side**
▲   **H04.202 Unspecified epiphora, left side**
▲   **H04.203 Unspecified epiphora, bilateral**
▲   **H04.209 Unspecified epiphora, unspecified side**

✓6ᵗʰ H04.21 Epiphora due to excess lacrimation
    H04.211 Epiphora due to excess lacrimation, right lacrimal gland
    H04.212 Epiphora due to excess lacrimation, left lacrimal gland
    H04.213 Epiphora due to excess lacrimation, bilateral lacrimal glands
    H04.219 Epiphora due to excess lacrimation, unspecified lacrimal gland

✓6ᵗʰ H04.22 Epiphora due to insufficient drainage
▲   **H04.221 Epiphora due to insufficient drainage, right side**
▲   **H04.222 Epiphora due to insufficient drainage, left side**
▲   **H04.223 Epiphora due to insufficient drainage, bilateral**
▲   **H04.229 Epiphora due to insufficient drainage, unspecified side**

✓5ᵗʰ H04.3 Acute and unspecified inflammation of lacrimal passages
    EXCLUDES 1 neonatal dacryocystitis (P39.1)

✓6ᵗʰ H04.30 Unspecified dacryocystitis
    H04.301 Unspecified dacryocystitis of right lacrimal passage
    H04.302 Unspecified dacryocystitis of left lacrimal passage
    H04.303 Unspecified dacryocystitis of bilateral lacrimal passages
    H04.309 Unspecified dacryocystitis of unspecified lacrimal passage

✓6ᵗʰ H04.31 Phlegmonous dacryocystitis
    H04.311 Phlegmonous dacryocystitis of right lacrimal passage

    H04.312 Phlegmonous dacryocystitis of left lacrimal passage
    H04.313 Phlegmonous dacryocystitis of bilateral lacrimal passages
    H04.319 Phlegmonous dacryocystitis of unspecified lacrimal passage

✓6ᵗʰ H04.32 Acute dacryocystitis
    Acute dacryopericystitis
    H04.321 Acute dacryocystitis of right lacrimal passage
    H04.322 Acute dacryocystitis of left lacrimal passage
    H04.323 Acute dacryocystitis of bilateral lacrimal passages
    H04.329 Acute dacryocystitis of unspecified lacrimal passage

✓6ᵗʰ H04.33 Acute lacrimal canaliculitis
    H04.331 Acute lacrimal canaliculitis of right lacrimal passage
    H04.332 Acute lacrimal canaliculitis of left lacrimal passage
    H04.333 Acute lacrimal canaliculitis of bilateral lacrimal passages
    H04.339 Acute lacrimal canaliculitis of unspecified lacrimal passage

✓5ᵗʰ H04.4 Chronic inflammation of lacrimal passages

✓6ᵗʰ H04.41 Chronic dacryocystitis
    H04.411 Chronic dacryocystitis of right lacrimal passage
    H04.412 Chronic dacryocystitis of left lacrimal passage
    H04.413 Chronic dacryocystitis of bilateral lacrimal passages
    H04.419 Chronic dacryocystitis of unspecified lacrimal passage

✓6ᵗʰ H04.42 Chronic lacrimal canaliculitis
    H04.421 Chronic lacrimal canaliculitis of right lacrimal passage
    H04.422 Chronic lacrimal canaliculitis of left lacrimal passage
    H04.423 Chronic lacrimal canaliculitis of bilateral lacrimal passages
    H04.429 Chronic lacrimal canaliculitis of unspecified lacrimal passage

✓6ᵗʰ H04.43 Chronic lacrimal mucocele
    H04.431 Chronic lacrimal mucocele of right lacrimal passage
    H04.432 Chronic lacrimal mucocele of left lacrimal passage
    H04.433 Chronic lacrimal mucocele of bilateral lacrimal passages
    H04.439 Chronic lacrimal mucocele of unspecified lacrimal passage

✓5ᵗʰ H04.5 Stenosis and insufficiency of lacrimal passages

✓6ᵗʰ H04.51 Dacryolith
    H04.511 Dacryolith of right lacrimal passage
    H04.512 Dacryolith of left lacrimal passage
    H04.513 Dacryolith of bilateral lacrimal passages
    H04.519 Dacryolith of unspecified lacrimal passage

✓6ᵗʰ H04.52 Eversion of lacrimal punctum
    H04.521 Eversion of right lacrimal punctum
    H04.522 Eversion of left lacrimal punctum
    H04.523 Eversion of bilateral lacrimal punctum
    H04.529 Eversion of unspecified lacrimal punctum

✓6ᵗʰ H04.53 Neonatal obstruction of nasolacrimal duct
    EXCLUDES 1 congenital stenosis and stricture of lacrimal duct (Q10.5)
    H04.531 Neonatal obstruction of right nasolacrimal duct ▯N
    H04.532 Neonatal obstruction of left nasolacrimal duct ▯N
    H04.533 Neonatal obstruction of bilateral nasolacrimal duct ▯N
    H04.539 Neonatal obstruction of unspecified nasolacrimal duct ▯N

☑ Additional Character Required   ✓x7ᵗʰ Placeholder   Unacceptable PDx   Questionable PDx   Manifestation   H1–H14 HAC   HCC CMS-HCC Dx   HIV HIV Dx

ICD-10-CM 2019   589

Chapter 7. Diseases of the Eye and Adnexa

H04.13–H04.539

Chapter 7. Diseases of the Eye and Adnexa

√6th **H04.54** Stenosis of lacrimal canaliculi
    H04.541 Stenosis of right lacrimal canaliculi
    H04.542 Stenosis of left lacrimal canaliculi
    H04.543 Stenosis of bilateral lacrimal canaliculi
    H04.549 Stenosis of unspecified lacrimal canaliculi

√6th **H04.55** Acquired stenosis of nasolacrimal duct
    H04.551 Acquired stenosis of right nasolacrimal duct
    H04.552 Acquired stenosis of left nasolacrimal duct
    H04.553 Acquired stenosis of bilateral nasolacrimal duct
    H04.559 Acquired stenosis of unspecified nasolacrimal duct

√6th **H04.56** Stenosis of lacrimal punctum
    H04.561 Stenosis of right lacrimal punctum
    H04.562 Stenosis of left lacrimal punctum
    H04.563 Stenosis of bilateral lacrimal punctum
    H04.569 Stenosis of unspecified lacrimal punctum

√6th **H04.57** Stenosis of lacrimal sac
    H04.571 Stenosis of right lacrimal sac
    H04.572 Stenosis of left lacrimal sac
    H04.573 Stenosis of bilateral lacrimal sac
    H04.579 Stenosis of unspecified lacrimal sac

√5th **H04.6** Other changes of lacrimal passages
  √6th **H04.61** Lacrimal fistula
    H04.611 Lacrimal fistula right lacrimal passage `SW`
    H04.612 Lacrimal fistula left lacrimal passage `SW`
    H04.613 Lacrimal fistula bilateral lacrimal passages `SW`
    H04.619 Lacrimal fistula unspecified lacrimal passage `SW`
    H04.69 Other changes of lacrimal passages

√5th **H04.8** Other disorders of lacrimal system
  √6th **H04.81** Granuloma of lacrimal passages
    H04.811 Granuloma of right lacrimal passage
    H04.812 Granuloma of left lacrimal passage
    H04.813 Granuloma of bilateral lacrimal passages
    H04.819 Granuloma of unspecified lacrimal passage
    H04.89 Other disorders of lacrimal system
  H04.9 Disorder of lacrimal system, unspecified

√4th **H05 Disorders of orbit**
  EXCLUDES 1 congenital malformation of orbit (Q10.7)

√5th **H05.0** Acute inflammation of orbit
  H05.00 Unspecified acute inflammation of orbit
  √6th **H05.01** Cellulitis of orbit
    Abscess of orbit

> **CC Excl: For CC codes in subcategory H05.01:**
> PDX collection 621

    H05.011 Cellulitis of right orbit `CC`
    H05.012 Cellulitis of left orbit `CC`
    H05.013 Cellulitis of bilateral orbits `CC`
    H05.019 Cellulitis of unspecified orbit `CC`

  √6th **H05.02** Osteomyelitis of orbit

> **CC Excl: For CC codes in subcategory H05.02:**
> PDX collection 622

    H05.021 Osteomyelitis of right orbit `CC`
    H05.022 Osteomyelitis of left orbit `CC`
    H05.023 Osteomyelitis of bilateral orbits `CC`
    H05.029 Osteomyelitis of unspecified orbit `CC`

  √6th **H05.03** Periostitis of orbit

> **CC Excl: For CC codes in subcategory H05.03:**
> PDX collection 623

    H05.031 Periostitis of right orbit `CC`
    H05.032 Periostitis of left orbit `CC`
    H05.033 Periostitis of bilateral orbits `CC`
    H05.039 Periostitis of unspecified orbit `CC`

  √6th **H05.04** Tenonitis of orbit
    H05.041 Tenonitis of right orbit
    H05.042 Tenonitis of left orbit

    H05.043 Tenonitis of bilateral orbits
    H05.049 Tenonitis of unspecified orbit

√5th **H05.1** Chronic inflammatory disorders of orbit
  H05.10 Unspecified chronic inflammatory disorders of orbit
  √6th **H05.11** Granuloma of orbit
    Pseudotumor (inflammatory) of orbit
    H05.111 Granuloma of right orbit
    H05.112 Granuloma of left orbit
    H05.113 Granuloma of bilateral orbits
    H05.119 Granuloma of unspecified orbit
  √6th **H05.12** Orbital myositis
    H05.121 Orbital myositis, right orbit
    H05.122 Orbital myositis, left orbit
    H05.123 Orbital myositis, bilateral
    H05.129 Orbital myositis, unspecified orbit

√5th **H05.2** Exophthalmic conditions
  H05.20 Unspecified exophthalmos
  √6th **H05.21** Displacement (lateral) of globe
    H05.211 Displacement (lateral) of globe, right eye
    H05.212 Displacement (lateral) of globe, left eye
    H05.213 Displacement (lateral) of globe, bilateral
    H05.219 Displacement (lateral) of globe, unspecified eye
  √6th **H05.22** Edema of orbit
    Orbital congestion
    H05.221 Edema of right orbit
    H05.222 Edema of left orbit
    H05.223 Edema of bilateral orbit
    H05.229 Edema of unspecified orbit
  √6th **H05.23** Hemorrhage of orbit
    H05.231 Hemorrhage of right orbit
    H05.232 Hemorrhage of left orbit
    H05.233 Hemorrhage of bilateral orbit
    H05.239 Hemorrhage of unspecified orbit
  √6th **H05.24** Constant exophthalmos
    H05.241 Constant exophthalmos, right eye
    H05.242 Constant exophthalmos, left eye
    H05.243 Constant exophthalmos, bilateral
    H05.249 Constant exophthalmos, unspecified eye
  √6th **H05.25** Intermittent exophthalmos
    H05.251 Intermittent exophthalmos, right eye
    H05.252 Intermittent exophthalmos, left eye
    H05.253 Intermittent exophthalmos, bilateral
    H05.259 Intermittent exophthalmos, unspecified eye
  √6th **H05.26** Pulsating exophthalmos
    H05.261 Pulsating exophthalmos, right eye
    H05.262 Pulsating exophthalmos, left eye
    H05.263 Pulsating exophthalmos, bilateral
    H05.269 Pulsating exophthalmos, unspecified eye

√5th **H05.3** Deformity of orbit
  EXCLUDES 1 congenital deformity of orbit (Q10.7)
            hypertelorism (Q75.2)
  H05.30 Unspecified deformity of orbit
  √6th **H05.31** Atrophy of orbit
    H05.311 Atrophy of right orbit
    H05.312 Atrophy of left orbit
    H05.313 Atrophy of bilateral orbit
    H05.319 Atrophy of unspecified orbit
  √6th **H05.32** Deformity of orbit due to bone disease
    Code also associated bone disease
    H05.321 Deformity of right orbit due to bone disease
    H05.322 Deformity of left orbit due to bone disease
    H05.323 Deformity of bilateral orbits due to bone disease
    H05.329 Deformity of unspecified orbit due to bone disease
  √6th **H05.33** Deformity of orbit due to trauma or surgery
    H05.331 Deformity of right orbit due to trauma or surgery
    H05.332 Deformity of left orbit due to trauma or surgery

N Newborn: 0   P Pediatric: 0-17   M Maternity: 12-55   A Adult: 15-124   MCC Major Complication/Comorbidity   CC Complication/Comorbidity   SW Severe Wound Dx

590   ICD-10-CM 2019

H05.333   **Deformity of** bilateral **orbits due to trauma or surgery**

H05.339   **Deformity of** unspecified **orbit due to trauma or surgery**

✓6th   **H05.34**   Enlargement **of orbit**

H05.341   **Enlargement of** right **orbit**

H05.342   **Enlargement of** left **orbit**

H05.343   **Enlargement of** bilateral **orbits**

H05.349   **Enlargement of** unspecified **orbit**

✓6th   **H05.35**   Exostosis **of orbit**

H05.351   **Exostosis of** right **orbit**

H05.352   **Exostosis of** left **orbit**

H05.353   **Exostosis of** bilateral **orbits**

H05.359   **Exostosis of** unspecified **orbit**

✓5th   **H05.4**   **Enophthalmos**

✓6th   **H05.40**   Unspecified **enophthalmos**

H05.401   **Unspecified enophthalmos,** right **eye**

H05.402   **Unspecified enophthalmos,** left **eye**

H05.403   **Unspecified enophthalmos,** bilateral

H05.409   **Unspecified enophthalmos,** unspecified **eye**

✓6th   **H05.41**   **Enophthalmos** due to atrophy of orbital tissue

H05.411   **Enophthalmos due to atrophy of orbital tissue,** right **eye**

H05.412   **Enophthalmos due to atrophy of orbital tissue,** left **eye**

H05.413   **Enophthalmos due to atrophy of orbital tissue,** bilateral

H05.419   **Enophthalmos due to atrophy of orbital tissue,** unspecified **eye**

✓6th   **H05.42**   **Enophthalmos** due to trauma or surgery

H05.421   **Enophthalmos due to trauma or surgery,** right **eye**

H05.422   **Enophthalmos due to trauma or surgery,** left **eye**

H05.423   **Enophthalmos due to trauma or surgery,** bilateral

H05.429   **Enophthalmos due to trauma or surgery,** unspecified **eye**

✓5th   **H05.5**   **Retained (old) foreign body following penetrating wound of orbit**

Retrobulbar foreign body

Use additional code to identify the type of retained foreign body (Z18.-)

EXCLUDES 1   *current penetrating wound of orbit (S05.4-)*

EXCLUDES 2   *retained foreign body of eyelid (H02.81-)*
                retained intraocular foreign body (H44.6-, H44.7-)

H05.50   **Retained (old) foreign body following penetrating wound of** unspecified **orbit**

H05.51   **Retained (old) foreign body following penetrating wound of** right **orbit**

H05.52   **Retained (old) foreign body following penetrating wound of** left **orbit**

H05.53   **Retained (old) foreign body following penetrating wound of** bilateral **orbits**

✓5th   **H05.8**   **Other disorders of orbit**

✓6th   **H05.81**   **Cyst of orbit**

Encephalocele of orbit

H05.811   **Cyst of** right **orbit**

H05.812   **Cyst of** left **orbit**

H05.813   **Cyst of** bilateral **orbits**

H05.819   **Cyst of** unspecified **orbit**

✓6th   **H05.82**   **Myopathy of extraocular muscles**

H05.821   **Myopathy of extraocular muscles,** right **orbit**

H05.822   **Myopathy of extraocular muscles,** left **orbit**

H05.823   **Myopathy of extraocular muscles,** bilateral

H05.829   **Myopathy of extraocular muscles,** unspecified **orbit**

H05.89   **Other disorders of orbit**

H05.9   **Unspecified disorder of orbit**

Disorders of conjunctiva (H10-H11)

✓4th   **H10**   **Conjunctivitis**

EXCLUDES 1   *keratoconjunctivitis (H16.2-)*

✓5th   **H10.0**   Mucopurulent **conjunctivitis**

✓6th   **H10.01**   **Acute follicular conjunctivitis**

H10.011   **Acute follicular conjunctivitis,** right **eye**

H10.012   **Acute follicular conjunctivitis,** left **eye**

H10.013   **Acute follicular conjunctivitis,** bilateral

H10.019   **Acute follicular conjunctivitis,** unspecified **eye**

✓6th   **H10.02**   **Other mucopurulent conjunctivitis**

H10.021   **Other mucopurulent conjunctivitis,** right **eye**

H10.022   **Other mucopurulent conjunctivitis,** left **eye**

H10.023   **Other mucopurulent conjunctivitis,** bilateral

H10.029   **Other mucopurulent conjunctivitis,** unspecified **eye**

✓5th   **H10.1**   Acute atopic **conjunctivitis**

Acute papillary conjunctivitis

H10.10   **Acute atopic conjunctivitis,** unspecified **eye**

H10.11   **Acute atopic conjunctivitis,** right **eye**

H10.12   **Acute atopic conjunctivitis,** left **eye**

H10.13   **Acute atopic conjunctivitis,** bilateral

✓5th   **H10.2**   Other acute **conjunctivitis**

✓6th   **H10.21**   **Acute** toxic **conjunctivitis**

Acute chemical conjunctivitis

Code first (T51-T65) to identify chemical and intent

EXCLUDES 1   *burn and corrosion of eye and adnexa (T26.-)*

H10.211   **Acute toxic conjunctivitis,** right **eye**

H10.212   **Acute toxic conjunctivitis,** left **eye**

H10.213   **Acute toxic conjunctivitis,** bilateral

H10.219   **Acute toxic conjunctivitis,** unspecified **eye**

✓6th   **H10.22**   Pseudomembranous **conjunctivitis**

H10.221   **Pseudomembranous conjunctivitis,** right **eye**

H10.222   **Pseudomembranous conjunctivitis,** left **eye**

H10.223   **Pseudomembranous conjunctivitis,** bilateral

H10.229   **Pseudomembranous conjunctivitis,** unspecified **eye**

✓6th   **H10.23**   Serous **conjunctivitis, except viral**

EXCLUDES 1   *viral conjunctivitis (B30.-)*

H10.231   **Serous conjunctivitis, except viral,** right **eye**

H10.232   **Serous conjunctivitis, except viral,** left **eye**

H10.233   **Serous conjunctivitis, except viral,** bilateral

H10.239   **Serous conjunctivitis, except viral,** unspecified **eye**

✓5th   **H10.3**   Unspecified acute **conjunctivitis**

EXCLUDES 1   *ophthalmia neonatorum NOS (P39.1)*

H10.30   **Unspecified acute conjunctivitis,** unspecified **eye**

H10.31   **Unspecified acute conjunctivitis,** right **eye**

H10.32   **Unspecified acute conjunctivitis,** left **eye**

H10.33   **Unspecified acute conjunctivitis,** bilateral

✓5th   **H10.4**   Chronic **conjunctivitis**

✓6th   **H10.40**   Unspecified **chronic conjunctivitis**

H10.401   **Unspecified chronic conjunctivitis,** right **eye**

H10.402   **Unspecified chronic conjunctivitis,** left **eye**

H10.403   **Unspecified chronic conjunctivitis,** bilateral

H10.409   **Unspecified chronic conjunctivitis,** unspecified **eye**

✓6th   **H10.41**   **Chronic** giant papillary **conjunctivitis**

H10.411   **Chronic giant papillary conjunctivitis,** right **eye**

H10.412   **Chronic giant papillary conjunctivitis,** left **eye**

H10.413   **Chronic giant papillary conjunctivitis,** bilateral

✓ Additional Character Required   ✓x7th Placeholder   Unacceptable PDx   Questionable PDx   Manifestation   H1-H14 HAC   HCC CMS-HCC Dx   HIV HIV Dx

ICD-10-CM 2019   591

H10.419   Chronic giant papillary conjunctivitis, unspecified eye

✓6th H10.42   Simple chronic conjunctivitis
- H10.421   Simple chronic conjunctivitis, right eye
- H10.422   Simple chronic conjunctivitis, left eye
- H10.423   Simple chronic conjunctivitis, bilateral
- H10.429   Simple chronic conjunctivitis, unspecified eye

✓6th H10.43   Chronic follicular conjunctivitis
- H10.431   Chronic follicular conjunctivitis, right eye
- H10.432   Chronic follicular conjunctivitis, left eye
- H10.433   Chronic follicular conjunctivitis, bilateral
- H10.439   Chronic follicular conjunctivitis, unspecified eye

H10.44   Vernal conjunctivitis
- EXCLUDES 1   vernal keratoconjunctivitis with limbar and corneal involvement (H16.26-)

H10.45   Other chronic allergic conjunctivitis

✓5th H10.5   Blepharoconjunctivitis

✓6th H10.50   Unspecified blepharoconjunctivitis
- H10.501   Unspecified blepharoconjunctivitis, right eye
- H10.502   Unspecified blepharoconjunctivitis, left eye
- H10.503   Unspecified blepharoconjunctivitis, bilateral
- H10.509   Unspecified blepharoconjunctivitis, unspecified eye

✓6th H10.51   Ligneous conjunctivitis
- ▶Code also underlying condition if known, such as: plasminogen deficiency (E88.02)◀
- H10.511   Ligneous conjunctivitis, right eye
- H10.512   Ligneous conjunctivitis, left eye
- H10.513   Ligneous conjunctivitis, bilateral
- H10.519   Ligneous conjunctivitis, unspecified eye

✓6th H10.52   Angular blepharoconjunctivitis
- H10.521   Angular blepharoconjunctivitis, right eye
- H10.522   Angular blepharoconjunctivitis, left eye
- H10.523   Angular blepharoconjunctivitis, bilateral
- H10.529   Angular blepharoconjunctivitis, unspecified eye

✓6th H10.53   Contact blepharoconjunctivitis
- H10.531   Contact blepharoconjunctivitis, right eye
- H10.532   Contact blepharoconjunctivitis, left eye
- H10.533   Contact blepharoconjunctivitis, bilateral
- H10.539   Contact blepharoconjunctivitis, unspecified eye

✓5th H10.8   Other conjunctivitis

✓6th H10.81   Pingueculitis
- EXCLUDES 1   pinguecula (H11.15-)
- H10.811   Pingueculitis, right eye
- H10.812   Pingueculitis, left eye
- H10.813   Pingueculitis, bilateral
- H10.819   Pingueculitis, unspecified eye

● ✓6th H10.82   Rosacea conjunctivitis
- Code first underlying rosacea dermatitis (L71.-)
- ● H10.821   Rosacea conjunctivitis, right eye
- ● H10.822   Rosacea conjunctivitis, left eye
- ● H10.823   Rosacea conjunctivitis, bilateral
- ● H10.829   Rosacea conjunctivitis, unspecified eye

H10.89   Other conjunctivitis

H10.9   Unspecified conjunctivitis

✓4th H11   Other disorders of conjunctiva
- EXCLUDES 1   keratoconjunctivitis (H16.2-)

✓5th H11.0   Pterygium of eye
- EXCLUDES 1   pseudopterygium (H11.81-)

✓6th H11.00   Unspecified pterygium of eye
- H11.001   Unspecified pterygium of right eye
- H11.002   Unspecified pterygium of left eye
- H11.003   Unspecified pterygium of eye, bilateral
- H11.009   Unspecified pterygium of unspecified eye

✓6th H11.01   Amyloid pterygium
- H11.011   Amyloid pterygium of right eye
- H11.012   Amyloid pterygium of left eye
- H11.013   Amyloid pterygium of eye, bilateral
- H11.019   Amyloid pterygium of unspecified eye

Pterygium

Pterygium

✓6th H11.02   Central pterygium of eye
- H11.021   Central pterygium of right eye
- H11.022   Central pterygium of left eye
- H11.023   Central pterygium of eye, bilateral
- H11.029   Central pterygium of unspecified eye

✓6th H11.03   Double pterygium of eye
- H11.031   Double pterygium of right eye
- H11.032   Double pterygium of left eye
- H11.033   Double pterygium of eye, bilateral
- H11.039   Double pterygium of unspecified eye

✓6th H11.04   Peripheral pterygium of eye, stationary
- H11.041   Peripheral pterygium, stationary, right eye
- H11.042   Peripheral pterygium, stationary, left eye
- H11.043   Peripheral pterygium, stationary, bilateral
- H11.049   Peripheral pterygium, stationary, unspecified eye

✓6th H11.05   Peripheral pterygium of eye, progressive
- H11.051   Peripheral pterygium, progressive, right eye
- H11.052   Peripheral pterygium, progressive, left eye
- H11.053   Peripheral pterygium, progressive, bilateral
- H11.059   Peripheral pterygium, progressive, unspecified eye

✓6th H11.06   Recurrent pterygium of eye
- H11.061   Recurrent pterygium of right eye
- H11.062   Recurrent pterygium of left eye
- H11.063   Recurrent pterygium of eye, bilateral
- H11.069   Recurrent pterygium of unspecified eye

✓5th H11.1   Conjunctival degenerations and deposits
- EXCLUDES 2   pseudopterygium (H11.81)

H11.10   Unspecified conjunctival degenerations

✓6th H11.11   Conjunctival deposits
- H11.111   Conjunctival deposits, right eye
- H11.112   Conjunctival deposits, left eye
- H11.113   Conjunctival deposits, bilateral
- H11.119   Conjunctival deposits, unspecified eye

✓6th H11.12   Conjunctival concretions
- H11.121   Conjunctival concretions, right eye
- H11.122   Conjunctival concretions, left eye
- H11.123   Conjunctival concretions, bilateral
- H11.129   Conjunctival concretions, unspecified eye

✓6th H11.13   Conjunctival pigmentations
- Conjunctival argyrosis [argyria]
- H11.131   Conjunctival pigmentations, right eye
- H11.132   Conjunctival pigmentations, left eye
- H11.133   Conjunctival pigmentations, bilateral
- H11.139   Conjunctival pigmentations, unspecified eye

N Newborn: 0   P Pediatric: 0-17   M Maternity: 12-55   A Adult: 15-124   MCC Major Complication/Comorbidity   CC Complication/Comorbidity   SW Severe Wound Dx

592   ICD-10-CM 2019

✓6ᵗʰ **H11.14** **Conjunctival xerosis,** unspecified
     EXCLUDES 1 *xerosis of conjunctiva due to vitamin A deficiency (E50.0, E50.1)*
     DEF: Abnormal dryness of the conjunctiva due to lack of insufficient tears or conjunctival secretions.
     H11.141 **Conjunctival xerosis, unspecified,** right eye
     H11.142 **Conjunctival xerosis, unspecified,** left eye
     H11.143 **Conjunctival xerosis, unspecified,** bilateral
     H11.149 **Conjunctival xerosis, unspecified,** unspecified eyed

✓6ᵗʰ **H11.15** Pinguecula
     EXCLUDES 1 *pingueculitis (H10.81-)*
     H11.151 **Pinguecula,** right eye
     H11.152 **Pinguecula,** left eye
     H11.153 **Pinguecula,** bilateral
     H11.159 **Pinguecula,** unspecified eye

Pinguecula

Pinguecula

✓5ᵗʰ **H11.2** **Conjunctival scars**
     ✓6ᵗʰ **H11.21** Conjunctival adhesions and strands **(localized)**
         H11.211 **Conjunctival adhesions and strands (localized),** right eye
         H11.212 **Conjunctival adhesions and strands (localized),** left eye
         H11.213 **Conjunctival adhesions and strands (localized),** bilateral
         H11.219 **Conjunctival adhesions and strands (localized),** unspecified eye
     ✓6ᵗʰ **H11.22** Conjunctival granuloma
         H11.221 **Conjunctival granuloma,** right eye
         H11.222 **Conjunctival granuloma,** left eye
         H11.223 **Conjunctival granuloma,** bilateral
         H11.229 **Conjunctival granuloma,** unspecified
     ✓6ᵗʰ **H11.23** Symblepharon
         H11.231 **Symblepharon,** right eye
         H11.232 **Symblepharon,** left eye
         H11.233 **Symblepharon,** bilateral
         H11.239 **Symblepharon,** unspecified eye
     ✓6ᵗʰ **H11.24** Scarring of conjunctiva
         H11.241 **Scarring of conjunctiva,** right eye
         H11.242 **Scarring of conjunctiva,** left eye
         H11.243 **Scarring of conjunctiva,** bilateral
         H11.249 **Scarring of conjunctiva,** unspecified eye

✓5ᵗʰ **H11.3** **Conjunctival hemorrhage**
     Subconjunctival hemorrhage
     H11.30 **Conjunctival hemorrhage,** unspecified eye
     H11.31 **Conjunctival hemorrhage,** right eye
     H11.32 **Conjunctival hemorrhage,** left eye
     H11.33 **Conjunctival hemorrhage,** bilateral

✓5ᵗʰ **H11.4** **Other conjunctival vascular disorders and cysts**
     ✓6ᵗʰ **H11.41** Vascular abnormalities of conjunctiva
     Conjunctival aneurysm
         H11.411 **Vascular abnormalities of conjunctiva,** right eye
         H11.412 **Vascular abnormalities of conjunctiva,** left eye
         H11.413 **Vascular abnormalities of conjunctiva,** bilateral
         H11.419 **Vascular abnormalities of conjunctiva,** unspecified eye

✓6ᵗʰ **H11.42** **Conjunctival** edema
     H11.421 **Conjunctival edema,** right eye
     H11.422 **Conjunctival edema,** left eye
     H11.423 **Conjunctival edema,** bilateral
     H11.429 **Conjunctival edema,** unspecified eye

✓6ᵗʰ **H11.43** **Conjunctival** hyperemia
     H11.431 **Conjunctival hyperemia,** right eye
     H11.432 **Conjunctival hyperemia,** left eye
     H11.433 **Conjunctival hyperemia,** bilateral
     H11.439 **Conjunctival hyperemia,** unspecified eye

✓6ᵗʰ **H11.44** **Conjunctival** cysts
     H11.441 **Conjunctival cysts,** right eye
     H11.442 **Conjunctival cysts,** left eye
     H11.443 **Conjunctival cysts,** bilateral
     H11.449 **Conjunctival cysts,** unspecified eye

✓5ᵗʰ **H11.8** **Other specified disorders of conjunctiva**
     ✓6ᵗʰ **H11.81** **Pseudopterygium of conjunctiva**
         H11.811 **Pseudopterygium of conjunctiva,** right eye
         H11.812 **Pseudopterygium of conjunctiva,** left eye
         H11.813 **Pseudopterygium of conjunctiva,** bilateral
         H11.819 **Pseudopterygium of conjunctiva,** unspecified eye
     ✓6ᵗʰ **H11.82** **Conjunctivochalasis**
         H11.821 **Conjunctivochalasis,** right eye
         H11.822 **Conjunctivochalasis,** left eye
         H11.823 **Conjunctivochalasis,** bilateral
         H11.829 **Conjunctivochalasis,** unspecified eye
     H11.89 **Other specified disorders of conjunctiva**
     H11.9 **Unspecified disorder of conjunctiva**

Disorders of sclera, cornea, iris and ciliary body (H15-H22)

✓4ᵗʰ **H15** **Disorders of sclera**
     ✓5ᵗʰ **H15.0** **Scleritis**
         ✓6ᵗʰ **H15.00** Unspecified scleritis
             H15.001 **Unspecified scleritis,** right eye
             H15.002 **Unspecified scleritis,** left eye
             H15.003 **Unspecified scleritis,** bilateral
             H15.009 **Unspecified scleritis,** unspecified eye
         ✓6ᵗʰ **H15.01** Anterior scleritis
             H15.011 **Anterior scleritis,** right eye
             H15.012 **Anterior scleritis,** left eye
             H15.013 **Anterior scleritis,** bilateral
             H15.019 **Anterior scleritis,** unspecified eye
         ✓6ᵗʰ **H15.02** Brawny scleritis
             H15.021 **Brawny scleritis,** right eye
             H15.022 **Brawny scleritis,** left eye
             H15.023 **Brawny scleritis,** bilateral
             H15.029 **Brawny scleritis,** unspecified eye
         ✓6ᵗʰ **H15.03** Posterior scleritis
         Sclerotenonitis
             H15.031 **Posterior scleritis,** right eye
             H15.032 **Posterior scleritis,** left eye
             H15.033 **Posterior scleritis,** bilateral
             H15.039 **Posterior scleritis,** unspecified eye
         ✓6ᵗʰ **H15.04** **Scleritis with** corneal involvement
             H15.041 **Scleritis with corneal involvement,** right eye
             H15.042 **Scleritis with corneal involvement,** left eye
             H15.043 **Scleritis with corneal involvement,** bilateral
             H15.049 **Scleritis with corneal involvement,** unspecified eye
         ✓6ᵗʰ **H15.05** Scleromalacia perforans
             H15.051 **Scleromalacia perforans,** right eye
             H15.052 **Scleromalacia perforans,** left eye
             H15.053 **Scleromalacia perforans,** bilateral
             H15.059 **Scleromalacia perforans,** unspecified eye
         ✓6ᵗʰ **H15.09** Other scleritis
         Scleral abscess
             H15.091 **Other scleritis,** right eye
             H15.092 **Other scleritis,** left eye

✓ Additional Character Required   ✓x7ᵗʰ Placeholder   Unacceptable PDx   Questionable PDx   Manifestation   H1 - H14 HAC   HCC CMS-HCC Dx   HIV HIV Dx

ICD-10-CM 2019   593

Chapter 7. Diseases of the Eye and Adnexa

H11.14–H15.092

H15.093   Other scleritis, bilateral
H15.099   Other scleritis, unspecified eye

√5ᵗʰ **H15.1**   **Episcleritis**

√6ᵗʰ **H15.10**   Unspecified episcleritis
    H15.101   Unspecified episcleritis, right eye
    H15.102   Unspecified episcleritis, left eye
    H15.103   Unspecified episcleritis, bilateral
    H15.109   Unspecified episcleritis, unspecified eye

√6ᵗʰ **H15.11**   Episcleritis periodica fugax
    H15.111   Episcleritis periodica fugax, right eye
    H15.112   Episcleritis periodica fugax, left eye
    H15.113   Episcleritis periodica fugax, bilateral
    H15.119   Episcleritis periodica fugax, unspecified eye

√6ᵗʰ **H15.12**   Nodular episcleritis
    H15.121   Nodular episcleritis, right eye
    H15.122   Nodular episcleritis, left eye
    H15.123   Nodular episcleritis, bilateral
    H15.129   Nodular episcleritis, unspecified eye

√5ᵗʰ **H15.8**   **Other disorders of sclera**
    EXCLUDES 2   blue sclera (Q13.5)
            degenerative myopia (H44.2-)

√6ᵗʰ **H15.81**   Equatorial staphyloma
    H15.811   Equatorial staphyloma, right eye
    H15.812   Equatorial staphyloma, left eye
    H15.813   Equatorial staphyloma, bilateral
    H15.819   Equatorial staphyloma, unspecified eye

√6ᵗʰ **H15.82**   Localized anterior staphyloma
    H15.821   Localized anterior staphyloma, right eye
    H15.822   Localized anterior staphyloma, left eye
    H15.823   Localized anterior staphyloma, bilateral
    H15.829   Localized anterior staphyloma, unspecified eye

√6ᵗʰ **H15.83**   Staphyloma posticum
    H15.831   Staphyloma posticum, right eye
    H15.832   Staphyloma posticum, left eye
    H15.833   Staphyloma posticum, bilateral
    H15.839   Staphyloma posticum, unspecified eye

√6ᵗʰ **H15.84**   Scleral ectasia
    H15.841   Scleral ectasia, right eye
    H15.842   Scleral ectasia, left eye
    H15.843   Scleral ectasia, bilateral
    H15.849   Scleral ectasia, unspecified eye

√6ᵗʰ **H15.85**   Ring staphyloma
    H15.851   Ring staphyloma, right eye
    H15.852   Ring staphyloma, left eye
    H15.853   Ring staphyloma, bilateral
    H15.859   Ring staphyloma, unspecified eye

    H15.89   Other disorders of sclera
    H15.9   Unspecified disorder of sclera

√4ᵗʰ **H16**   **Keratitis**
    DEF: Condition in which the cornea becomes inflamed and irritated.

√5ᵗʰ **H16.0**   **Corneal ulcer**

√6ᵗʰ **H16.00**   Unspecified corneal ulcer
    H16.001   Unspecified corneal ulcer, right eye
    H16.002   Unspecified corneal ulcer, left eye
    H16.003   Unspecified corneal ulcer, bilateral
    H16.009   Unspecified corneal ulcer, unspecified eye

√6ᵗʰ **H16.01**   Central corneal ulcer
    H16.011   Central corneal ulcer, right eye
    H16.012   Central corneal ulcer, left eye
    H16.013   Central corneal ulcer, bilateral
    H16.019   Central corneal ulcer, unspecified eye

√6ᵗʰ **H16.02**   Ring corneal ulcer
    H16.021   Ring corneal ulcer, right eye
    H16.022   Ring corneal ulcer, left eye
    H16.023   Ring corneal ulcer, bilateral
    H16.029   Ring corneal ulcer, unspecified eye

√6ᵗʰ **H16.03**   Corneal ulcer with hypopyon
    H16.031   Corneal ulcer with hypopyon, right eye
    H16.032   Corneal ulcer with hypopyon, left eye

H16.033   Corneal ulcer with hypopyon, bilateral
H16.039   Corneal ulcer with hypopyon, unspecified eye

√6ᵗʰ **H16.04**   Marginal corneal ulcer
    H16.041   Marginal corneal ulcer, right eye
    H16.042   Marginal corneal ulcer, left eye
    H16.043   Marginal corneal ulcer, bilateral
    H16.049   Marginal corneal ulcer, unspecified eye

√6ᵗʰ **H16.05**   Mooren's corneal ulcer
    H16.051   Mooren's corneal ulcer, right eye
    H16.052   Mooren's corneal ulcer, left eye
    H16.053   Mooren's corneal ulcer, bilateral
    H16.059   Mooren's corneal ulcer, unspecified eye

√6ᵗʰ **H16.06**   Mycotic corneal ulcer
    H16.061   Mycotic corneal ulcer, right eye
    H16.062   Mycotic corneal ulcer, left eye
    H16.063   Mycotic corneal ulcer, bilateral
    H16.069   Mycotic corneal ulcer, unspecified eye

√6ᵗʰ **H16.07**   Perforated corneal ulcer
    H16.071   Perforated corneal ulcer, right eye
    H16.072   Perforated corneal ulcer, left eye
    H16.073   Perforated corneal ulcer, bilateral
    H16.079   Perforated corneal ulcer, unspecified eye

√5ᵗʰ **H16.1**   **Other and unspecified superficial keratitis without conjunctivitis**

√6ᵗʰ **H16.10**   Unspecified superficial keratitis
    H16.101   Unspecified superficial keratitis, right eye
    H16.102   Unspecified superficial keratitis, left eye
    H16.103   Unspecified superficial keratitis, bilateral
    H16.109   Unspecified superficial keratitis, unspecified eye

√6ᵗʰ **H16.11**   Macular keratitis
    Areolar keratitis
    Nummular keratitis
    Stellate keratitis
    Striate keratitis
    H16.111   Macular keratitis, right eye
    H16.112   Macular keratitis, left eye
    H16.113   Macular keratitis, bilateral
    H16.119   Macular keratitis, unspecified eye

√6ᵗʰ **H16.12**   Filamentary keratitis
    H16.121   Filamentary keratitis, right eye
    H16.122   Filamentary keratitis, left eye
    H16.123   Filamentary keratitis, bilateral
    H16.129   Filamentary keratitis, unspecified eye

√6ᵗʰ **H16.13**   Photokeratitis
    Snow blindness
    Welders keratitis
    H16.131   Photokeratitis, right eye
    H16.132   Photokeratitis, left eye
    H16.133   Photokeratitis, bilateral
    H16.139   Photokeratitis, unspecified eye

√6ᵗʰ **H16.14**   Punctate keratitis
    H16.141   Punctate keratitis, right eye
    H16.142   Punctate keratitis, left eye
    H16.143   Punctate keratitis, bilateral
    H16.149   Punctate keratitis, unspecified eye

√5ᵗʰ **H16.2**   **Keratoconjunctivitis**

√6ᵗʰ **H16.20**   Unspecified keratoconjunctivitis
    Superficial keratitis with conjunctivitis NOS
    H16.201   Unspecified keratoconjunctivitis, right eye
    H16.202   Unspecified keratoconjunctivitis, left eye
    H16.203   Unspecified keratoconjunctivitis, bilateral
    H16.209   Unspecified keratoconjunctivitis, unspecified eye

√6ᵗʰ **H16.21**   Exposure keratoconjunctivitis
    H16.211   Exposure keratoconjunctivitis, right eye
    H16.212   Exposure keratoconjunctivitis, left eye
    H16.213   Exposure keratoconjunctivitis, bilateral
    H16.219   Exposure keratoconjunctivitis, unspecified eye

N Newborn: 0   P Pediatric: 0-17   M Maternity: 12-55   A Adult: 15-124   MCC Major Complication/Comorbidity   CC Complication/Comorbidity   SW Severe Wound Dx

594   ICD-10-CM 2019

✓6th H16.22 Keratoconjunctivitis sicca, not specified as Sjögren's
> **EXCLUDES 1** *Sjögren's syndrome (M35.01)*

- **H16.221 Keratoconjunctivitis sicca, not specified as Sjögren's, right eye**
- **H16.222 Keratoconjunctivitis sicca, not specified as Sjögren's, left eye**
- **H16.223 Keratoconjunctivitis sicca, not specified as Sjögren's, bilateral**
- **H16.229 Keratoconjunctivitis sicca, not specified as Sjögren's, unspecified eye**

✓6th H16.23 Neurotrophic keratoconjunctivitis
- **H16.231 Neurotrophic keratoconjunctivitis, right eye**
- **H16.232 Neurotrophic keratoconjunctivitis, left eye**
- **H16.233 Neurotrophic keratoconjunctivitis, bilateral**
- **H16.239 Neurotrophic keratoconjunctivitis, unspecified eye**

✓6th H16.24 Ophthalmia nodosa
- **H16.241 Ophthalmia nodosa, right eye**
- **H16.242 Ophthalmia nodosa, left eye**
- **H16.243 Ophthalmia nodosa, bilateral**
- **H16.249 Ophthalmia nodosa, unspecified eye**

✓6th H16.25 Phlyctenular keratoconjunctivitis
- **H16.251 Phlyctenular keratoconjunctivitis, right eye**
- **H16.252 Phlyctenular keratoconjunctivitis, left eye**
- **H16.253 Phlyctenular keratoconjunctivitis, bilateral**
- **H16.259 Phlyctenular keratoconjunctivitis, unspecified eye**

✓6th H16.26 Vernal keratoconjunctivitis, with limbar and corneal involvement
> **EXCLUDES 1** *vernal conjunctivitis without limbar and corneal involvement (H10.44)*

- **H16.261 Vernal keratoconjunctivitis, with limbar and corneal involvement, right eye**
- **H16.262 Vernal keratoconjunctivitis, with limbar and corneal involvement, left eye**
- **H16.263 Vernal keratoconjunctivitis, with limbar and corneal involvement, bilateral**
- **H16.269 Vernal keratoconjunctivitis, with limbar and corneal involvement, unspecified eye**

✓6th H16.29 Other keratoconjunctivitis
- **H16.291 Other keratoconjunctivitis, right eye**
- **H16.292 Other keratoconjunctivitis, left eye**
- **H16.293 Other keratoconjunctivitis, bilateral**
- **H16.299 Other keratoconjunctivitis, unspecified eye**

✓5th H16.3 Interstitial and deep keratitis

✓6th H16.30 Unspecified interstitial keratitis
- **H16.301 Unspecified interstitial keratitis, right eye**
- **H16.302 Unspecified interstitial keratitis, left eye**
- **H16.303 Unspecified interstitial keratitis, bilateral**
- **H16.309 Unspecified interstitial keratitis, unspecified eye**

✓6th H16.31 Corneal abscess
- **H16.311 Corneal abscess, right eye**
- **H16.312 Corneal abscess, left eye**
- **H16.313 Corneal abscess, bilateral**
- **H16.319 Corneal abscess, unspecified eye**

✓6th H16.32 Diffuse interstitial keratitis
> Cogan's syndrome
- **H16.321 Diffuse interstitial keratitis, right eye**
- **H16.322 Diffuse interstitial keratitis, left eye**
- **H16.323 Diffuse interstitial keratitis, bilateral**
- **H16.329 Diffuse interstitial keratitis, unspecified eye**

✓6th H16.33 Sclerosing keratitis
- **H16.331 Sclerosing keratitis, right eye**
- **H16.332 Sclerosing keratitis, left eye**
- **H16.333 Sclerosing keratitis, bilateral**
- **H16.339 Sclerosing keratitis, unspecified eye**

✓6th H16.39 Other interstitial and deep keratitis
- **H16.391 Other interstitial and deep keratitis, right eye**
- **H16.392 Other interstitial and deep keratitis, left eye**
- **H16.393 Other interstitial and deep keratitis, bilateral**
- **H16.399 Other interstitial and deep keratitis, unspecified eye**

✓5th H16.4 Corneal neovascularization

✓6th H16.40 Unspecified corneal neovascularization
- **H16.401 Unspecified corneal neovascularization, right eye**
- **H16.402 Unspecified corneal neovascularization, left eye**
- **H16.403 Unspecified corneal neovascularization, bilateral**
- **H16.409 Unspecified corneal neovascularization, unspecified eye**

✓6th H16.41 Ghost vessels (corneal)
- **H16.411 Ghost vessels (corneal), right eye**
- **H16.412 Ghost vessels (corneal), left eye**
- **H16.413 Ghost vessels (corneal), bilateral**
- **H16.419 Ghost vessels (corneal), unspecified eye**

✓6th H16.42 Pannus (corneal)
- **H16.421 Pannus (corneal), right eye**
- **H16.422 Pannus (corneal), left eye**
- **H16.423 Pannus (corneal), bilateral**
- **H16.429 Pannus (corneal), unspecified eye**

✓6th H16.43 Localized vascularization of cornea
- **H16.431 Localized vascularization of cornea, right eye**
- **H16.432 Localized vascularization of cornea, left eye**
- **H16.433 Localized vascularization of cornea, bilateral**
- **H16.439 Localized vascularization of cornea, unspecified eye**

✓6th H16.44 Deep vascularization of cornea
- **H16.441 Deep vascularization of cornea, right eye**
- **H16.442 Deep vascularization of cornea, left eye**
- **H16.443 Deep vascularization of cornea, bilateral**
- **H16.449 Deep vascularization of cornea, unspecified eye**

H16.8 Other keratitis

H16.9 Unspecified keratitis

✓4th H17 Corneal scars and opacities

✓5th H17.0 Adherent leukoma
- **H17.00 Adherent leukoma, unspecified eye**
- **H17.01 Adherent leukoma, right eye**
- **H17.02 Adherent leukoma, left eye**
- **H17.03 Adherent leukoma, bilateral**

✓5th H17.1 Central corneal opacity
- **H17.10 Central corneal opacity, unspecified eye**
- **H17.11 Central corneal opacity, right eye**
- **H17.12 Central corneal opacity, left eye**
- **H17.13 Central corneal opacity, bilateral**

✓5th H17.8 Other corneal scars and opacities

✓6th H17.81 Minor opacity of cornea
> Corneal nebula
- **H17.811 Minor opacity of cornea, right eye**
- **H17.812 Minor opacity of cornea, left eye**
- **H17.813 Minor opacity of cornea, bilateral**
- **H17.819 Minor opacity of cornea, unspecified eye**

✓6th H17.82 Peripheral opacity of cornea
- **H17.821 Peripheral opacity of cornea, right eye**
- **H17.822 Peripheral opacity of cornea, left eye**
- **H17.823 Peripheral opacity of cornea, bilateral**
- **H17.829 Peripheral opacity of cornea, unspecified eye**

H17.89 Other corneal scars and opacities

H17.9 Unspecified corneal scar and opacity

✓ Additional Character Required   ✓x7th Placeholder   Unacceptable PDx   Questionable PDx   Manifestation   H1-H14 HAC   HCC CMS-HCC Dx   HIV HIV Dx

ICD-10-CM 2019   595

✓4th **H18 Other disorders of cornea**

  ✓5th **H18.0 Corneal pigmentations and deposits**

    ✓6th **H18.00 Unspecified corneal deposit**
- **H18.001 Unspecified corneal deposit, right eye**
- **H18.002 Unspecified corneal deposit, left eye**
- **H18.003 Unspecified corneal deposit, bilateral**
- **H18.009 Unspecified corneal deposit, unspecified eye**

    ✓6th **H18.01 Anterior corneal pigmentations**
Staehli's line
- **H18.011 Anterior corneal pigmentations, right eye**
- **H18.012 Anterior corneal pigmentations, left eye**
- **H18.013 Anterior corneal pigmentations, bilateral**
- **H18.019 Anterior corneal pigmentations, unspecified eye**

    ✓6th **H18.02 Argentous corneal deposits**
- **H18.021 Argentous corneal deposits, right eye**
- **H18.022 Argentous corneal deposits, left eye**
- **H18.023 Argentous corneal deposits, bilateral**
- **H18.029 Argentous corneal deposits, unspecified eye**

    ✓6th **H18.03 Corneal deposits in metabolic disorders**
Code also associated metabolic disorder
- **H18.031 Corneal deposits in metabolic disorders, right eye**
- **H18.032 Corneal deposits in metabolic disorders, left eye**
- **H18.033 Corneal deposits in metabolic disorders, bilateral**
- **H18.039 Corneal deposits in metabolic disorders, unspecified eye**

    ✓6th **H18.04 Kayser-Fleischer ring**
Code also associated Wilson's disease (E83.01)
- **H18.041 Kayser-Fleischer ring, right eye**
- **H18.042 Kayser-Fleischer ring, left eye**
- **H18.043 Kayser-Fleischer ring, bilateral**
- **H18.049 Kayser-Fleischer ring, unspecified eye**

    ✓6th **H18.05 Posterior corneal pigmentations**
Krukenberg's spindle
- **H18.051 Posterior corneal pigmentations, right eye**
- **H18.052 Posterior corneal pigmentations, left eye**
- **H18.053 Posterior corneal pigmentations, bilateral**
- **H18.059 Posterior corneal pigmentations, unspecified eye**

    ✓6th **H18.06 Stromal corneal pigmentations**
Hematocornea
- **H18.061 Stromal corneal pigmentations, right eye**
- **H18.062 Stromal corneal pigmentations, left eye**
- **H18.063 Stromal corneal pigmentations, bilateral**
- **H18.069 Stromal corneal pigmentations, unspecified eye**

  ✓5th **H18.1 Bullous keratopathy**
DEF: Corneal swelling due to a damaged corneal endothelium. Bullous keratopathy is characterized by recurring, rupturing epithelial blisters causing glaucoma, iridocyclitis, and Fuchs dystrophy.
- **H18.10 Bullous keratopathy, unspecified eye**
- **H18.11 Bullous keratopathy, right eye**
- **H18.12 Bullous keratopathy, left eye**
- **H18.13 Bullous keratopathy, bilateral**

  ✓5th **H18.2 Other and unspecified corneal edema**
- **H18.20 Unspecified corneal edema**

    ✓6th **H18.21 Corneal edema secondary to contact lens**
EXCLUDES 2 other corneal disorders due to contact lens (H18.82-)
- **H18.211 Corneal edema secondary to contact lens, right eye**
- **H18.212 Corneal edema secondary to contact lens, left eye**
- **H18.213 Corneal edema secondary to contact lens, bilateral**
- **H18.219 Corneal edema secondary to contact lens, unspecified eye**

    ✓6th **H18.22 Idiopathic corneal edema**
- **H18.221 Idiopathic corneal edema, right eye**
- **H18.222 Idiopathic corneal edema, left eye**
- **H18.223 Idiopathic corneal edema, bilateral**
- **H18.229 Idiopathic corneal edema, unspecified eye**

    ✓6th **H18.23 Secondary corneal edema**
- **H18.231 Secondary corneal edema, right eye**
- **H18.232 Secondary corneal edema, left eye**
- **H18.233 Secondary corneal edema, bilateral**
- **H18.239 Secondary corneal edema, unspecified eye**

  ✓5th **H18.3 Changes of corneal membranes**
- **H18.30 Unspecified corneal membrane change**

    ✓6th **H18.31 Folds and rupture in Bowman's membrane**
- **H18.311 Folds and rupture in Bowman's membrane, right eye**
- **H18.312 Folds and rupture in Bowman's membrane, left eye**
- **H18.313 Folds and rupture in Bowman's membrane, bilateral**
- **H18.319 Folds and rupture in Bowman's membrane, unspecified eye**

    ✓6th **H18.32 Folds in Descemet's membrane**
- **H18.321 Folds in Descemet's membrane, right eye**
- **H18.322 Folds in Descemet's membrane, left eye**
- **H18.323 Folds in Descemet's membrane, bilateral**
- **H18.329 Folds in Descemet's membrane, unspecified eye**

    ✓6th **H18.33 Rupture in Descemet's membrane**
- **H18.331 Rupture in Descemet's membrane, right eye**
- **H18.332 Rupture in Descemet's membrane, left eye**
- **H18.333 Rupture in Descemet's membrane, bilateral**
- **H18.339 Rupture in Descemet's membrane, unspecified eye**

  ✓5th **H18.4 Corneal degeneration**
EXCLUDES 1 Mooren's ulcer (H16.0-)
recurrent erosion of cornea (H18.83-)
- **H18.40 Unspecified corneal degeneration**

    ✓6th **H18.41 Arcus senilis**
Senile corneal changes
- **H18.411 Arcus senilis, right eye**
- **H18.412 Arcus senilis, left eye**
- **H18.413 Arcus senilis, bilateral**
- **H18.419 Arcus senilis, unspecified eye**

    ✓6th **H18.42 Band keratopathy**
- **H18.421 Band keratopathy, right eye**
- **H18.422 Band keratopathy, left eye**
- **H18.423 Band keratopathy, bilateral**
- **H18.429 Band keratopathy, unspecified eye**
- **H18.43 Other calcerous corneal degeneration**

    ✓6th **H18.44 Keratomalacia**
EXCLUDES 1 keratomalacia due to vitamin A deficiency (E50.4)
- **H18.441 Keratomalacia, right eye**
- **H18.442 Keratomalacia, left eye**
- **H18.443 Keratomalacia, bilateral**
- **H18.449 Keratomalacia, unspecified eye**

    ✓6th **H18.45 Nodular corneal degeneration**
- **H18.451 Nodular corneal degeneration, right eye**
- **H18.452 Nodular corneal degeneration, left eye**
- **H18.453 Nodular corneal degeneration, bilateral**
- **H18.459 Nodular corneal degeneration, unspecified eye**

    ✓6th **H18.46 Peripheral corneal degeneration**
- **H18.461 Peripheral corneal degeneration, right eye**
- **H18.462 Peripheral corneal degeneration, left eye**
- **H18.463 Peripheral corneal degeneration, bilateral**
- **H18.469 Peripheral corneal degeneration, unspecified eye**
- **H18.49 Other corneal degeneration**

  ✓5th **H18.5 Hereditary corneal dystrophies**
- **H18.50 Unspecified hereditary corneal dystrophies**
- **H18.51 Endothelial corneal dystrophy**
Fuchs' dystrophy

H18.52   Epithelial (juvenile) corneal dystrophy

H18.53   Granular corneal dystrophy

H18.54   Lattice corneal dystrophy

H18.55   Macular corneal dystrophy

H18.59   Other hereditary corneal dystrophies

√5th **H18.6   Keratoconus**

√6th   **H18.60   Keratoconus, unspecified**

     H18.601   Keratoconus, unspecified, right eye

     H18.602   Keratoconus, unspecified, left eye

     H18.603   Keratoconus, unspecified, bilateral

     H18.609   Keratoconus, unspecified, unspecified eye

√6th   **H18.61   Keratoconus, stable**

     H18.611   Keratoconus, stable, right eye

     H18.612   Keratoconus, stable, left eye

     H18.613   Keratoconus, stable, bilateral

     H18.619   Keratoconus, stable, unspecified eye

√6th   **H18.62   Keratoconus, unstable**

     Acute hydrops

     H18.621   Keratoconus, unstable, right eye

     H18.622   Keratoconus, unstable, left eye

     H18.623   Keratoconus, unstable, bilateral

     H18.629   Keratoconus, unstable, unspecified eye

√5th **H18.7   Other and unspecified corneal deformities**

   EXCLUDES 1   *congenital malformations of cornea (Q13.3-Q13.4)*

    H18.70   Unspecified corneal deformity

√6th   **H18.71   Corneal ectasia**

     H18.711   Corneal ectasia, right eye

     H18.712   Corneal ectasia, left eye

     H18.713   Corneal ectasia, bilateral

     H18.719   Corneal ectasia, unspecified eye

√6th   **H18.72   Corneal staphyloma**

     H18.721   Corneal staphyloma, right eye

     H18.722   Corneal staphyloma, left eye

     H18.723   Corneal staphyloma, bilateral

     H18.729   Corneal staphyloma, unspecified eye

√6th   **H18.73   Descemetocele**

     H18.731   Descemetocele, right eye

     H18.732   Descemetocele, left eye

     H18.733   Descemetocele, bilateral

     H18.739   Descemetocele, unspecified eye

√6th   **H18.79   Other corneal deformities**

     H18.791   Other corneal deformities, right eye

     H18.792   Other corneal deformities, left eye

     H18.793   Other corneal deformities, bilateral

     H18.799   Other corneal deformities, unspecified eye

√5th **H18.8   Other specified disorders of cornea**

√6th   **H18.81   Anesthesia and hypoesthesia of cornea**

     H18.811   Anesthesia and hypoesthesia of cornea, right eye

     H18.812   Anesthesia and hypoesthesia of cornea, left eye

     H18.813   Anesthesia and hypoesthesia of cornea, bilateral

     H18.819   Anesthesia and hypoesthesia of cornea, unspecified eye

√6th   **H18.82   Corneal disorder due to contact lens**

   EXCLUDES 2   *corneal edema due to contact lens (H18.21-)*

     H18.821   Corneal disorder due to contact lens, right eye

     H18.822   Corneal disorder due to contact lens, left eye

     H18.823   Corneal disorder due to contact lens, bilateral

     H18.829   Corneal disorder due to contact lens, unspecified eye

√6th   **H18.83   Recurrent erosion of cornea**

     H18.831   Recurrent erosion of cornea, right eye

     H18.832   Recurrent erosion of cornea, left eye

     H18.833   Recurrent erosion of cornea, bilateral

     H18.839   Recurrent erosion of cornea, unspecified eye

√6th   **H18.89   Other specified disorders of cornea**

     H18.891   Other specified disorders of cornea, right eye

     H18.892   Other specified disorders of cornea, left eye

     H18.893   Other specified disorders of cornea, bilateral

     H18.899   Other specified disorders of cornea, unspecified eye

   H18.9   Unspecified disorder of cornea

√4th **H20   Iridocyclitis**

   CC Excl: For CC codes in category H20: PDX collection 624

√5th   **H20.0   Acute and subacute iridocyclitis**

     Acute anterior uveitis

     Acute cyclitis

     Acute iritis

     Subacute anterior uveitis

     Subacute cyclitis

     Subacute iritis

     EXCLUDES 1   *iridocyclitis, iritis, uveitis (due to) (in) diabetes mellitus (E08-E13 with .39)*

          iridocyclitis, iritis, uveitis (due to) (in) diphtheria (A36.89)

          iridocyclitis, iritis, uveitis (due to) (in) gonococcal (A54.32)

          iridocyclitis, iritis, uveitis (due to) (in) herpes (simplex) (B00.51)

          iridocyclitis, iritis, uveitis (due to) (in) herpes zoster (B02.32)

          iridocyclitis, iritis, uveitis (due to) (in) late congenital syphilis (A50.39)

          iridocyclitis, iritis, uveitis (due to) (in) late syphilis (A52.71)

          iridocyclitis, iritis, uveitis (due to) (in) sarcoidosis (D86.83)

          iridocyclitis, iritis, uveitis (due to) (in) syphilis (A51.43)

          iridocyclitis, iritis, uveitis (due to) (in) toxoplasmosis (B58.09)

          iridocyclitis, iritis, uveitis (due to) (in) tuberculosis (A18.54)

    H20.00   Unspecified acute and subacute iridocyclitis   `CC`

√6th   **H20.01   Primary iridocyclitis**

     H20.011   Primary iridocyclitis, right eye   `CC`

     H20.012   Primary iridocyclitis, left eye   `CC`

     H20.013   Primary iridocyclitis, bilateral   `CC`

     H20.019   Primary iridocyclitis, unspecified eye   `CC`

√6th   **H20.02   Recurrent acute iridocyclitis**

     H20.021   Recurrent acute iridocyclitis, right eye   `CC`

     H20.022   Recurrent acute iridocyclitis, left eye   `CC`

     H20.023   Recurrent acute iridocyclitis, bilateral   `CC`

     H20.029   Recurrent acute iridocyclitis, unspecified eye   `CC`

√6th   **H20.03   Secondary infectious iridocyclitis**

     H20.031   Secondary infectious iridocyclitis, right eye   `CC`

     H20.032   Secondary infectious iridocyclitis, left eye   `CC`

     H20.033   Secondary infectious iridocyclitis, bilateral   `CC`

     H20.039   Secondary infectious iridocyclitis, unspecified eye   `CC`

√6th   **H20.04   Secondary noninfectious iridocyclitis**

     H20.041   Secondary noninfectious iridocyclitis, right eye

     H20.042   Secondary noninfectious iridocyclitis, left eye

     H20.043   Secondary noninfectious iridocyclitis, bilateral

     H20.049   Secondary noninfectious iridocyclitis, unspecified eye

√6th   **H20.05   Hypopyon**

     H20.051   Hypopyon, right eye

     H20.052   Hypopyon, left eye

     H20.053   Hypopyon, bilateral

     H20.059   Hypopyon, unspecified eye

✔ Additional Character Required   √7th Placeholder   Unacceptable PDx   Questionable PDx   Manifestation   H1 - H14 HAC   HCC CMS-HCC Dx   HIV HIV Dx

ICD-10-CM 2019   597

Chapter 7. Diseases of the Eye and Adnexa

H20.1–H21.329

√5th **H20.1** Chronic **iridocyclitis**
Use additional code for any associated cataract (H26.21-)
EXCLUDES 2   *posterior cyclitis (H30.2-)*
    H20.10 Chronic iridocyclitis, unspecified eye
    H20.11 Chronic iridocyclitis, right eye
    H20.12 Chronic iridocyclitis, left eye
    H20.13 Chronic iridocyclitis, bilateral

√5th **H20.2** Lens-induced **iridocyclitis**
    H20.20 Lens-induced iridocyclitis, unspecified eye
    H20.21 Lens-induced iridocyclitis, right eye
    H20.22 Lens-induced iridocyclitis, left eye
    H20.23 Lens-induced iridocyclitis, bilateral

√5th **H20.8** Other **iridocyclitis**
EXCLUDES 2   *glaucomatocyclitis crises (H40.4-)*
         posterior cyclitis (H30.2-)
         sympathetic uveitis (H44.13-)

√6th **H20.81** Fuchs' heterochromic cyclitis
    H20.811 Fuchs' heterochromic cyclitis, right eye
    H20.812 Fuchs' heterochromic cyclitis, left eye
    H20.813 Fuchs' heterochromic cyclitis, bilateral
    H20.819 Fuchs' heterochromic cyclitis, unspecified eye

√6th **H20.82** Vogt-Koyanagi syndrome
    H20.821 Vogt-Koyanagi syndrome, right eye
    H20.822 Vogt-Koyanagi syndrome, left eye
    H20.823 Vogt-Koyanagi syndrome, bilateral
    H20.829 Vogt-Koyanagi syndrome, unspecified eye

H20.9 Unspecified **iridocyclitis**   CC
Uveitis NOS

√4th **H21** **Other disorders of iris and ciliary body**
EXCLUDES 2   *sympathetic uveitis (H44.1-)*

√5th **H21.0** Hyphema
EXCLUDES 1   *traumatic hyphema (S05.1-)*
    H21.00 Hyphema, unspecified eye
    H21.01 Hyphema, right eye
    H21.02 Hyphema, left eye
    H21.03 Hyphema, bilateral

Hyphema

Iris — Cornea — Hyphema

√5th **H21.1** Other vascular disorders of iris and ciliary body
Neovascularization of iris or ciliary body
Rubeosis iridis
Rubeosis of iris

√6th **H21.1X** Other vascular disorders of iris and ciliary body
    H21.1X1 Other vascular disorders of iris and ciliary body, right eye
    H21.1X2 Other vascular disorders of iris and ciliary body, left eye
    H21.1X3 Other vascular disorders of iris and ciliary body, bilateral
    H21.1X9 Other vascular disorders of iris and ciliary body, unspecified eye

√5th **H21.2** Degeneration of iris and ciliary body
√6th **H21.21** Degeneration of chamber angle
    H21.211 Degeneration of chamber angle, right eye
    H21.212 Degeneration of chamber angle, left eye
    H21.213 Degeneration of chamber angle, bilateral
    H21.219 Degeneration of chamber angle, unspecified eye

√6th **H21.22** Degeneration of ciliary body
    H21.221 Degeneration of ciliary body, right eye
    H21.222 Degeneration of ciliary body, left eye
    H21.223 Degeneration of ciliary body, bilateral
    H21.229 Degeneration of ciliary body, unspecified eye

√6th **H21.23** Degeneration of iris (pigmentary)
Translucency of iris
    H21.231 Degeneration of iris (pigmentary), right eye
    H21.232 Degeneration of iris (pigmentary), left eye
    H21.233 Degeneration of iris (pigmentary), bilateral
    H21.239 Degeneration of iris (pigmentary), unspecified eye

√6th **H21.24** Degeneration of pupillary margin
    H21.241 Degeneration of pupillary margin, right eye
    H21.242 Degeneration of pupillary margin, left eye
    H21.243 Degeneration of pupillary margin, bilateral
    H21.249 Degeneration of pupillary margin, unspecified eye

√6th **H21.25** Iridoschisis
    H21.251 Iridoschisis, right eye
    H21.252 Iridoschisis, left eye
    H21.253 Iridoschisis, bilateral
    H21.259 Iridoschisis, unspecified eye

√6th **H21.26** Iris atrophy (essential) (progressive)
    H21.261 Iris atrophy (essential) (progressive), right eye
    H21.262 Iris atrophy (essential) (progressive), left eye
    H21.263 Iris atrophy (essential) (progressive), bilateral
    H21.269 Iris atrophy (essential) (progressive), unspecified eye

√6th **H21.27** Miotic pupillary cyst
    H21.271 Miotic pupillary cyst, right eye
    H21.272 Miotic pupillary cyst, left eye
    H21.273 Miotic pupillary cyst, bilateral
    H21.279 Miotic pupillary cyst, unspecified eye

    H21.29 Other iris atrophy

√5th **H21.3** Cyst of iris, ciliary body and anterior chamber
EXCLUDES 2   *miotic pupillary cyst (H21.27-)*

√6th **H21.30** Idiopathic cysts of iris, ciliary body or anterior chamber
Cyst of iris, ciliary body or anterior chamber NOS
    H21.301 Idiopathic cysts of iris, ciliary body or anterior chamber, right eye
    H21.302 Idiopathic cysts of iris, ciliary body or anterior chamber, left eye
    H21.303 Idiopathic cysts of iris, ciliary body or anterior chamber, bilateral
    H21.309 Idiopathic cysts of iris, ciliary body or anterior chamber, unspecified eye

√6th **H21.31** Exudative cysts of iris or anterior chamber
    H21.311 Exudative cysts of iris or anterior chamber, right eye
    H21.312 Exudative cysts of iris or anterior chamber, left eye
    H21.313 Exudative cysts of iris or anterior chamber, bilateral
    H21.319 Exudative cysts of iris or anterior chamber, unspecified eye

√6th **H21.32** Implantation cysts of iris, ciliary body or anterior chamber
    H21.321 Implantation cysts of iris, ciliary body or anterior chamber, right eye
    H21.322 Implantation cysts of iris, ciliary body or anterior chamber, left eye
    H21.323 Implantation cysts of iris, ciliary body or anterior chamber, bilateral
    H21.329 Implantation cysts of iris, ciliary body or anterior chamber, unspecified eye

√6ᵗʰ **H21.33** Parasitic **cyst of iris, ciliary body or anterior chamber**

    CC Excl: For CC codes in subcategory H21.33:
    PDX collection 625

    H21.331 **Parasitic cyst of iris, ciliary body or anterior chamber,** right **eye** `CC`

    H21.332 **Parasitic cyst of iris, ciliary body or anterior chamber,** left **eye** `CC`

    H21.333 **Parasitic cyst of iris, ciliary body or anterior chamber,** bilateral `CC`

    H21.339 **Parasitic cyst of iris, ciliary body or anterior chamber,** unspecified **eye** `CC`

√6ᵗʰ **H21.34** Primary **cyst of pars plana**

    H21.341 **Primary cyst of pars plana,** right **eye**

    H21.342 **Primary cyst of pars plana,** left **eye**

    H21.343 **Primary cyst of pars plana,** bilateral

    H21.349 **Primary cyst of pars plana,** unspecified **eye**

√6ᵗʰ **H21.35** Exudative **cyst of pars plana**

    DEF: Protein, fatty-filled bullous elevation of the nonpigmented outermost ciliary epithelium of pars plana, due to fluid leak from blood vessels.

    H21.351 **Exudative cyst of pars plana,** right **eye**

    H21.352 **Exudative cyst of pars plana,** left **eye**

    H21.353 **Exudative cyst of pars plana,** bilateral

    H21.359 **Exudative cyst of pars plana,** unspecified **eye**

√5ᵗʰ **H21.4** **Pupillary membranes**
    Iris bombé   Pupillary seclusion
    Pupillary occlusion
    EXCLUDES 1   congenital pupillary membranes (Q13.8)

    H21.40 **Pupillary membranes,** unspecified **eye**

    H21.41 **Pupillary membranes,** right **eye**

    H21.42 **Pupillary membranes,** left **eye**

    H21.43 **Pupillary membranes,** bilateral

√5ᵗʰ **H21.5** **Other and unspecified adhesions and disruptions of iris and ciliary body**
    EXCLUDES 1   corectopia (Q13.2)

    √6ᵗʰ **H21.50** **Unspecified adhesions of iris**
        Synechia (iris) NOS

        H21.501 **Unspecified adhesions of iris,** right **eye**

        H21.502 **Unspecified adhesions of iris,** left **eye**

        H21.503 **Unspecified adhesions of iris,** bilateral

        H21.509 **Unspecified adhesions of iris and ciliary body,** unspecified **eye**

    √6ᵗʰ **H21.51** **Anterior synechiae (iris)**

        H21.511 **Anterior synechiae (iris),** right **eye**

        H21.512 **Anterior synechiae (iris),** left **eye**

        H21.513 **Anterior synechiae (iris),** bilateral

        H21.519 **Anterior synechiae (iris),** unspecified **eye**

    √6ᵗʰ **H21.52** **Goniosynechiae**

        H21.521 **Goniosynechiae,** right **eye**

        H21.522 **Goniosynechiae,** left **eye**

        H21.523 **Goniosynechiae,** bilateral

        H21.529 **Goniosynechiae,** unspecified **eye**

    √6ᵗʰ **H21.53** **Iridodialysis**

        H21.531 **Iridodialysis,** right **eye**

        H21.532 **Iridodialysis,** left **eye**

        H21.533 **Iridodialysis,** bilateral

        H21.539 **Iridodialysis,** unspecified **eye**

    √6ᵗʰ **H21.54** **Posterior synechiae (iris)**

        H21.541 **Posterior synechiae (iris),** right **eye**

        H21.542 **Posterior synechiae (iris),** left **eye**

        H21.543 **Posterior synechiae (iris),** bilateral

        H21.549 **Posterior synechiae (iris),** unspecified **eye**

    √6ᵗʰ **H21.55** **Recession of chamber angle**

        H21.551 **Recession of chamber angle,** right **eye**

        H21.552 **Recession of chamber angle,** left **eye**

        H21.553 **Recession of chamber angle,** bilateral

        H21.559 **Recession of chamber angle,** unspecified **eye**

√6ᵗʰ **H21.56** **Pupillary abnormalities**
    Deformed pupil   Rupture of sphincter, pupil
    Ectopic pupil
    EXCLUDES 1   congenital deformity of pupil (Q13.2-)

    H21.561 **Pupillary abnormality,** right **eye**

    H21.562 **Pupillary abnormality,** left **eye**

    H21.563 **Pupillary abnormality,** bilateral

    H21.569 **Pupillary abnormality,** unspecified **eye**

√5ᵗʰ **H21.8** **Other specified disorders of iris and ciliary body**

    H21.81 **Floppy iris syndrome**
        Intraoperative floppy iris syndrome (IFIS)
        Use additional code for adverse effect, if applicable, to identify drug (T36-T50 with fifth or sixth character 5)

    H21.82 **Plateau iris syndrome (post-iridectomy) (postprocedural)**

    H21.89 **Other specified disorders of iris and ciliary body**

    H21.9 **Unspecified disorder of iris and ciliary body**

H22 Disorders of iris and ciliary body in diseases classified elsewhere

    Code first underlying disease, such as:
        gout (M1A.-, M10.-)
        leprosy (A30.-)
        parasitic disease (B89)

Disorders of lens (H25-H28)

√4ᵗʰ **H25** **Age-related cataract**
    Senile cataract
    EXCLUDES 2   capsular glaucoma with pseudoexfoliation of lens (H40.1-)

    √5ᵗʰ **H25.0** **Age-related** incipient **cataract**

      √6ᵗʰ **H25.01** Cortical **age-related cataract**

        H25.011 **Cortical age-related cataract,** right **eye** `A`

        H25.012 **Cortical age-related cataract,** left **eye** `A`

        H25.013 **Cortical age-related cataract,** bilateral `A`

        H25.019 **Cortical age-related cataract,** unspecified **eye** `A`

      √6ᵗʰ **H25.03** Anterior subcapsular polar **age-related cataract**

        H25.031 **Anterior subcapsular polar age-related cataract,** right **eye** `A`

        H25.032 **Anterior subcapsular polar age-related cataract,** left **eye** `A`

        H25.033 **Anterior subcapsular polar age-related cataract,** bilateral `A`

        H25.039 **Anterior subcapsular polar age-related cataract,** unspecified **eye** `A`

      √6ᵗʰ **H25.04** Posterior subcapsular polar **age-related cataract**

        H25.041 **Posterior subcapsular polar age-related cataract,** right **eye** `A`

        H25.042 **Posterior subcapsular polar age-related cataract,** left **eye** `A`

        H25.043 **Posterior subcapsular polar age-related cataract,** bilateral `A`

        H25.049 **Posterior subcapsular polar age-related cataract,** unspecified **eye** `A`

      √6ᵗʰ **H25.09** Other **age-related incipient cataract**
        Coronary age-related cataract
        Punctate age-related cataract
        Water clefts

        H25.091 **Other age-related incipient cataract,** right **eye** `A`

        H25.092 **Other age-related incipient cataract,** left **eye** `A`

        H25.093 **Other age-related incipient cataract,** bilateral `A`

        H25.099 **Other age-related incipient cataract,** unspecified **eye** `A`

    √5ᵗʰ **H25.1** **Age-related** nuclear **cataract**
      Cataracta brunescens
      Nuclear sclerosis cataract
      AHA: 2016, 1Q, 32

      H25.10 **Age-related nuclear cataract,** unspecified **eye** `A`

      H25.11 **Age-related nuclear cataract,** right **eye** `A`

      H25.12 **Age-related nuclear cataract,** left **eye** `A`

      H25.13 **Age-related nuclear cataract,** bilateral `A`

☑ Additional Character Required   √x7ᵗʰ Placeholder   Unacceptable PDx   Questionable PDx   Manifestation   **H1**-**H14** HAC   **HCC** CMS-HCC Dx   **HIV** HIV Dx

ICD-10-CM 2019   **599**

Chapter 7. Diseases of the Eye and Adnexa

H21.33–H25.13

Chapter 7. Diseases of the Eye and Adnexa

H25.2–H26.221

Cataracts

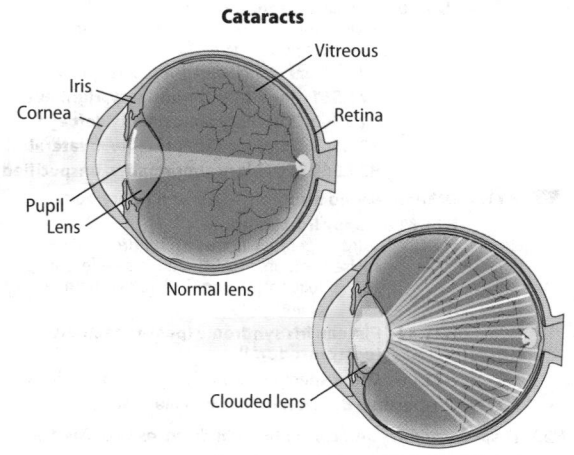

Normal lens

Clouded lens

Lens affected by cataracts

✓5th **H25.2 Age-related cataract,** morgagnian type
Age-related hypermature cataract

    H25.20 Age-related cataract, morgagnian type, unspecified eye [A]

    H25.21 Age-related cataract, morgagnian type, right eye [A]

    H25.22 Age-related cataract, morgagnian type, left eye [A]

    H25.23 Age-related cataract, morgagnian type, bilateral [A]

✓5th **H25.8 Other age-related cataract**

    ✓6th **H25.81 Combined forms of age-related cataract**

        H25.811 Combined forms of age-related cataract, right eye [A]

        H25.812 Combined forms of age-related cataract, left eye [A]

        H25.813 Combined forms of age-related cataract, bilateral [A]

        H25.819 Combined forms of age-related cataract, unspecified eye [A]

    H25.89 Other age-related cataract [A]

  H25.9 Unspecified age-related cataract [A]

✓4th **H26 Other cataract**

    EXCLUDES 1 *congenital cataract (Q12.0)*

  ✓5th **H26.0 Infantile and juvenile cataract**

    ✓6th **H26.00 Unspecified infantile and juvenile cataract**

        H26.001 Unspecified infantile and juvenile cataract, right eye [P]

        H26.002 Unspecified infantile and juvenile cataract, left eye [P]

        H26.003 Unspecified infantile and juvenile cataract, bilateral [P]

        H26.009 Unspecified infantile and juvenile cataract, unspecified eye [P]

    ✓6th **H26.01 Infantile and juvenile** cortical, lamellar, or zonular cataract

        H26.011 Infantile and juvenile cortical, lamellar, or zonular cataract, right eye [P]

        H26.012 Infantile and juvenile cortical, lamellar, or zonular cataract, left eye [P]

        H26.013 Infantile and juvenile cortical, lamellar, or zonular cataract, bilateral [P]

        H26.019 Infantile and juvenile cortical, lamellar, or zonular cataract, unspecified eye [P]

    ✓6th **H26.03 Infantile and juvenile** nuclear cataract

        H26.031 Infantile and juvenile nuclear cataract, right eye [P]

        H26.032 Infantile and juvenile nuclear cataract, left eye [P]

        H26.033 Infantile and juvenile nuclear cataract, bilateral [P]

        H26.039 Infantile and juvenile nuclear cataract, unspecified eye [P]

    ✓6th **H26.04 Anterior subcapsular polar infantile and juvenile cataract**

        H26.041 Anterior subcapsular polar infantile and juvenile cataract, right eye [P]

        H26.042 Anterior subcapsular polar infantile and juvenile cataract, left eye [P]

        H26.043 Anterior subcapsular polar infantile and juvenile cataract, bilateral [P]

        H26.049 Anterior subcapsular polar infantile and juvenile cataract, unspecified eye [P]

    ✓6th **H26.05 Posterior subcapsular polar infantile and juvenile cataract**

        H26.051 Posterior subcapsular polar infantile and juvenile cataract, right eye [P]

        H26.052 Posterior subcapsular polar infantile and juvenile cataract, left eye [P]

        H26.053 Posterior subcapsular polar infantile and juvenile cataract, bilateral [P]

        H26.059 Posterior subcapsular polar infantile and juvenile cataract, unspecified eye [P]

    ✓6th **H26.06 Combined forms of infantile and juvenile cataract**

        H26.061 Combined forms of infantile and juvenile cataract, right eye [P]

        H26.062 Combined forms of infantile and juvenile cataract, left eye [P]

        H26.063 Combined forms of infantile and juvenile cataract, bilateral [P]

        H26.069 Combined forms of infantile and juvenile cataract, unspecified eye [P]

    H26.09 Other infantile and juvenile cataract [P]

  ✓5th **H26.1 Traumatic cataract**
    Use additional code (Chapter 20) to identify external cause

    ✓6th **H26.10 Unspecified traumatic cataract**

        H26.101 Unspecified traumatic cataract, right eye

        H26.102 Unspecified traumatic cataract, left eye

        H26.103 Unspecified traumatic cataract, bilateral

        H26.109 Unspecified traumatic cataract, unspecified eye

    ✓6th **H26.11 Localized traumatic opacities**

        H26.111 Localized traumatic opacities, right eye

        H26.112 Localized traumatic opacities, left eye

        H26.113 Localized traumatic opacities, bilateral

        H26.119 Localized traumatic opacities, unspecified eye

    ✓6th **H26.12 Partially resolved traumatic cataract**

        H26.121 Partially resolved traumatic cataract, right eye

        H26.122 Partially resolved traumatic cataract, left eye

        H26.123 Partially resolved traumatic cataract, bilateral

        H26.129 Partially resolved traumatic cataract, unspecified eye

    ✓6th **H26.13 Total traumatic cataract**

        H26.131 Total traumatic cataract, right eye

        H26.132 Total traumatic cataract, left eye

        H26.133 Total traumatic cataract, bilateral

        H26.139 Total traumatic cataract, unspecified eye

  ✓5th **H26.2 Complicated cataract**

    H26.20 Unspecified complicated cataract
        Cataracta complicata NOS

    ✓6th **H26.21 Cataract with neovascularization**
        Code also associated condition, such as:
          chronic iridocyclitis (H20.1-)

        H26.211 Cataract with neovascularization, right eye

        H26.212 Cataract with neovascularization, left eye

        H26.213 Cataract with neovascularization, bilateral

        H26.219 Cataract with neovascularization, unspecified eye

    ✓6th **H26.22 Cataract secondary to ocular disorders (degenerative) (inflammatory)**
        Code also associated ocular disorder

        H26.221 Cataract secondary to ocular disorders (degenerative) (inflammatory), right eye

[N] Newborn: 0   [P] Pediatric: 0-17   [M] Maternity: 12-55   [A] Adult: 15-124   [MCC] Major Complication/Comorbidity   [CC] Complication/Comorbidity   [SW] Severe Wound Dx

600   ICD-10-CM 2019

H26.222   **Cataract secondary to ocular disorders (degenerative) (inflammatory), left eye**

H26.223   **Cataract secondary to ocular disorders (degenerative) (inflammatory), bilateral**

H26.229   **Cataract secondary to ocular disorders (degenerative) (inflammatory), unspecified eye**

✓6th **H26.23**   **Glaucomatous flecks (subcapsular)**
Code first underlying glaucoma (H40-H42)

H26.231   **Glaucomatous flecks (subcapsular), right eye**

H26.232   **Glaucomatous flecks (subcapsular), left eye**

H26.233   **Glaucomatous flecks (subcapsular), bilateral**

H26.239   **Glaucomatous flecks (subcapsular), unspecified eye**

✓5th **H26.3**   **Drug-induced cataract**
Toxic cataract
Use additional code for adverse effect, if applicable, to identify drug (T36-T50 with fifth or sixth character 5)

H26.30   **Drug-induced cataract, unspecified eye**

H26.31   **Drug-induced cataract, right eye**

H26.32   **Drug-induced cataract, left eye**

H26.33   **Drug-induced cataract, bilateral**

✓5th **H26.4**   **Secondary cataract**

H26.40   **Unspecified secondary cataract**

✓6th **H26.41**   **Soemmering's ring**

H26.411   **Soemmering's ring, right eye**

H26.412   **Soemmering's ring, left eye**

H26.413   **Soemmering's ring, bilateral**

H26.419   **Soemmering's ring, unspecified eye**

✓6th **H26.49**   **Other secondary cataract**
AHA: 2018, 2Q, 14

H26.491   **Other secondary cataract, right eye**

H26.492   **Other secondary cataract, left eye**

H26.493   **Other secondary cataract, bilateral**

H26.499   **Other secondary cataract, unspecified eye**

H26.8   **Other specified cataract**

H26.9   **Unspecified cataract**

✓4th **H27**   **Other disorders of lens**
EXCLUDES 1   *congenital lens malformations (Q12.-)*
mechanical complications of intraocular lens implant (T85.2)
pseudophakia (Z96.1)

✓5th **H27.0**   **Aphakia**
Acquired absence of lens
Acquired aphakia
Aphakia due to trauma
EXCLUDES 1   *cataract extraction status (Z98.4-)*
congenital absence of lens (Q12.3)
congenital aphakia (Q12.3)

H27.00   **Aphakia, unspecified eye**

H27.01   **Aphakia, right eye**

H27.02   **Aphakia, left eye**

H27.03   **Aphakia, bilateral**

✓5th **H27.1**   **Dislocation of lens**

H27.10   **Unspecified dislocation of lens**

✓6th **H27.11**   **Subluxation of lens**

H27.111   **Subluxation of lens, right eye**

H27.112   **Subluxation of lens, left eye**

H27.113   **Subluxation of lens, bilateral**

H27.119   **Subluxation of lens, unspecified eye**

✓6th **H27.12**   **Anterior dislocation of lens**

H27.121   **Anterior dislocation of lens, right eye**

H27.122   **Anterior dislocation of lens, left eye**

H27.123   **Anterior dislocation of lens, bilateral**

H27.129   **Anterior dislocation of lens, unspecified eye**

✓6th **H27.13**   **Posterior dislocation of lens**

H27.131   **Posterior dislocation of lens, right eye**

H27.132   **Posterior dislocation of lens, left eye**

H27.133   **Posterior dislocation of lens, bilateral**

H27.139   **Posterior dislocation of lens, unspecified eye**

H27.8   **Other specified disorders of lens**

H27.9   **Unspecified disorder of lens**

H28   ***Cataract in diseases classified elsewhere***
Code first underlying disease, such as:
hypoparathyroidism (E20.-)
myotonia (G71.1-)
myxedema (E03.-)
protein-calorie malnutrition (E40-E46)
EXCLUDES 1   *cataract in diabetes mellitus (E08.36, E09.36, E10.36, E11.36, E13.36)*

Disorders of choroid and retina (H30-H36)

✓4th **H30**   **Chorioretinal inflammation**

CC Excl: For CC codes in category H30: PDX collection 626

✓5th **H30.0**   **Focal chorioretinal inflammation**
Focal chorioretinitis
Focal choroiditis
Focal retinitis
Focal retinochoroiditis

✓6th **H30.00**   **Unspecified focal chorioretinal inflammation**
Focal chorioretinitis NOS
Focal choroiditis NOS
Focal retinitis NOS
Focal retinochoroiditis NOS

H30.001   **Unspecified focal chorioretinal inflammation, right eye**

H30.002   **Unspecified focal chorioretinal inflammation, left eye**

H30.003   **Unspecified focal chorioretinal inflammation, bilateral**

H30.009   **Unspecified focal chorioretinal inflammation, unspecified eye**

✓6th **H30.01**   **Focal chorioretinal inflammation, juxtapapillary**

H30.011   **Focal chorioretinal inflammation, juxtapapillary, right eye**

H30.012   **Focal chorioretinal inflammation, juxtapapillary, left eye**

H30.013   **Focal chorioretinal inflammation, juxtapapillary, bilateral**

H30.019   **Focal chorioretinal inflammation, juxtapapillary, unspecified eye**

✓6th **H30.02**   **Focal chorioretinal inflammation of posterior pole**

H30.021   **Focal chorioretinal inflammation of posterior pole, right eye**

H30.022   **Focal chorioretinal inflammation of posterior pole, left eye**

H30.023   **Focal chorioretinal inflammation of posterior pole, bilateral**

H30.029   **Focal chorioretinal inflammation of posterior pole, unspecified eye**

✓6th **H30.03**   **Focal chorioretinal inflammation, peripheral**

H30.031   **Focal chorioretinal inflammation, peripheral, right eye**

H30.032   **Focal chorioretinal inflammation, peripheral, left eye**

H30.033   **Focal chorioretinal inflammation, peripheral, bilateral**

H30.039   **Focal chorioretinal inflammation, peripheral, unspecified eye**

✓6th **H30.04**   **Focal chorioretinal inflammation, macular or paramacular**

H30.041   **Focal chorioretinal inflammation, macular or paramacular, right eye**

H30.042   **Focal chorioretinal inflammation, macular or paramacular, left eye**

H30.043   **Focal chorioretinal inflammation, macular or paramacular, bilateral**

H30.049   **Focal chorioretinal inflammation, macular or paramacular, unspecified eye**

✓ Additional Character Required   ✓x7th Placeholder   Unacceptable PDx   Questionable PDx   Manifestation   H1 - H14 HAC   HCC CMS-HCC Dx   HIV HIV Dx

ICD-10-CM 2019   601

Chapter 7. Diseases of the Eye and Adnexa

H30.1–H31.112

✓5ᵗʰ **H30.1** **Disseminated chorioretinal inflammation**
Disseminated chorioretinitis
Disseminated choroiditis
Disseminated retinitis
Disseminated retinochoroiditis
EXCLUDES 2   *exudative retinopathy (H35.02-)*

   ✓6ᵗʰ **H30.10** **Unspecified disseminated chorioretinal inflammation**
Disseminated chorioretinitis NOS
Disseminated choroiditis NOS
Disseminated retinitis NOS
Disseminated retinochoroiditis NOS

      H30.101 **Unspecified disseminated chorioretinal inflammation, right eye**   CC

      H30.102 **Unspecified disseminated chorioretinal inflammation, left eye**   CC

      H30.103 **Unspecified disseminated chorioretinal inflammation, bilateral**   CC

      H30.109 **Unspecified disseminated chorioretinal inflammation, unspecified eye**   CC

   ✓6ᵗʰ **H30.11** **Disseminated chorioretinal inflammation of posterior pole**

      H30.111 **Disseminated chorioretinal inflammation of posterior pole, right eye**   CC

      H30.112 **Disseminated chorioretinal inflammation of posterior pole, left eye**   CC

      H30.113 **Disseminated chorioretinal inflammation of posterior pole, bilateral**   CC

      H30.119 **Disseminated chorioretinal inflammation of posterior pole, unspecified eye**   CC

   ✓6ᵗʰ **H30.12** **Disseminated chorioretinal inflammation, peripheral**

      H30.121 **Disseminated chorioretinal inflammation, peripheral right eye**   CC

      H30.122 **Disseminated chorioretinal inflammation, peripheral, left eye**   CC

      H30.123 **Disseminated chorioretinal inflammation, peripheral, bilateral**   CC

      H30.129 **Disseminated chorioretinal inflammation, peripheral, unspecified eye**   CC

   ✓6ᵗʰ **H30.13** **Disseminated chorioretinal inflammation, generalized**

      H30.131 **Disseminated chorioretinal inflammation, generalized, right eye**   CC

      H30.132 **Disseminated chorioretinal inflammation, generalized, left eye**   CC

      H30.133 **Disseminated chorioretinal inflammation, generalized, bilateral**   CC

      H30.139 **Disseminated chorioretinal inflammation, generalized, unspecified eye**   CC

   ✓6ᵗʰ **H30.14** **Acute posterior multifocal placoid pigment epitheliopathy**

      H30.141 **Acute posterior multifocal placoid pigment epitheliopathy, right eye**   CC

      H30.142 **Acute posterior multifocal placoid pigment epitheliopathy, left eye**   CC

      H30.143 **Acute posterior multifocal placoid pigment epitheliopathy, bilateral**   CC

      H30.149 **Acute posterior multifocal placoid pigment epitheliopathy, unspecified eye**   CC

✓5ᵗʰ **H30.2** **Posterior cyclitis**
Pars planitis

      H30.20 **Posterior cyclitis, unspecified eye**

      H30.21 **Posterior cyclitis, right eye**

      H30.22 **Posterior cyclitis, left eye**

      H30.23 **Posterior cyclitis, bilateral**

✓5ᵗʰ **H30.8** **Other chorioretinal inflammations**

   ✓6ᵗʰ **H30.81** **Harada's disease**

      H30.811 **Harada's disease, right eye**

      H30.812 **Harada's disease, left eye**

      H30.813 **Harada's disease, bilateral**

      H30.819 **Harada's disease, unspecified eye**

   ✓6ᵗʰ **H30.89** **Other chorioretinal inflammations**

      H30.891 **Other chorioretinal inflammations, right eye**   CC

      H30.892 **Other chorioretinal inflammations, left eye**   CC

      H30.893 **Other chorioretinal inflammations, bilateral**   CC

      H30.899 **Other chorioretinal inflammations, unspecified eye**   CC

✓5ᵗʰ **H30.9** **Unspecified chorioretinal inflammation**
Chorioretinitis NOS
Choroiditis NOS
Neuroretinitis NOS
Retinitis NOS
Retinochoroiditis NOS

      H30.90 **Unspecified chorioretinal inflammation, unspecified eye**   CC

      H30.91 **Unspecified chorioretinal inflammation, right eye**   CC

      H30.92 **Unspecified chorioretinal inflammation, left eye**   CC

      H30.93 **Unspecified chorioretinal inflammation, bilateral**   CC

✓4ᵗʰ **H31** **Other disorders of choroid**

   CC Excl: For CC codes in category H31: PDX collection 627

✓5ᵗʰ **H31.0** **Chorioretinal scars**
EXCLUDES 2   *postsurgical chorioretinal scars (H59.81-)*

   ✓6ᵗʰ **H31.00** **Unspecified chorioretinal scars**

      H31.001 **Unspecified chorioretinal scars, right eye**

      H31.002 **Unspecified chorioretinal scars, left eye**

      H31.003 **Unspecified chorioretinal scars, bilateral**

      H31.009 **Unspecified chorioretinal scars, unspecified eye**

   ✓6ᵗʰ **H31.01** **Macula scars of posterior pole (postinflammatory) (post-traumatic)**
EXCLUDES 1   *postprocedural chorioretinal scar (H59.81-)*

      H31.011 **Macula scars of posterior pole (postinflammatory) (post-traumatic), right eye**

      H31.012 **Macula scars of posterior pole (postinflammatory) (post-traumatic), left eye**

      H31.013 **Macula scars of posterior pole (postinflammatory) (post-traumatic), bilateral**

      H31.019 **Macula scars of posterior pole (postinflammatory) (post-traumatic), unspecified eye**

   ✓6ᵗʰ **H31.02** **Solar retinopathy**

      H31.021 **Solar retinopathy, right eye**

      H31.022 **Solar retinopathy, left eye**

      H31.023 **Solar retinopathy, bilateral**

      H31.029 **Solar retinopathy, unspecified eye**

   ✓6ᵗʰ **H31.09** **Other chorioretinal scars**

      H31.091 **Other chorioretinal scars, right eye**

      H31.092 **Other chorioretinal scars, left eye**

      H31.093 **Other chorioretinal scars, bilateral**

      H31.099 **Other chorioretinal scars, unspecified eye**

✓5ᵗʰ **H31.1** **Choroidal degeneration**
EXCLUDES 2   *angioid streaks of macula (H35.33)*

   ✓6ᵗʰ **H31.10** **Unspecified choroidal degeneration**
Choroidal sclerosis NOS

      H31.101 **Choroidal degeneration, unspecified, right eye**

      H31.102 **Choroidal degeneration, unspecified, left eye**

      H31.103 **Choroidal degeneration, unspecified, bilateral**

      H31.109 **Choroidal degeneration, unspecified, unspecified eye**

   ✓6ᵗʰ **H31.11** **Age-related choroidal atrophy**

      H31.111 **Age-related choroidal atrophy, right eye**   A

      H31.112 **Age-related choroidal atrophy, left eye**   A

N Newborn: 0   P Pediatric: 0-17   M Maternity: 12-55   A Adult: 15-124   MCC Major Complication/Comorbidity   CC Complication/Comorbidity   SW Severe Wound Dx

602   ICD-10-CM 2019

H31.113   **Age-related choroidal atrophy, bilateral**   A

H31.119   **Age-related choroidal atrophy, unspecified eye**   A

✓6th **H31.12**   Diffuse secondary **atrophy of choroid**

H31.121   **Diffuse secondary atrophy of choroid, right eye**

H31.122   **Diffuse secondary atrophy of choroid, left eye**

H31.123   **Diffuse secondary atrophy of choroid, bilateral**

H31.129   **Diffuse secondary atrophy of choroid, unspecified eye**

✓5th **H31.2**   **Hereditary choroidal dystrophy**

     EXCLUDES 2   hyperornithinemia (E72.4)
                 ornithinemia (E72.4)

H31.20   **Hereditary choroidal dystrophy, unspecified**

H31.21   **Choroideremia**

H31.22   **Choroidal dystrophy (central areolar) (generalized) (peripapillary)**

H31.23   **Gyrate atrophy, choroid**

H31.29   **Other hereditary choroidal dystrophy**

✓5th **H31.3**   **Choroidal** hemorrhage and rupture

✓6th **H31.30**   Unspecified **choroidal hemorrhage**

H31.301   **Unspecified choroidal hemorrhage, right eye**

H31.302   **Unspecified choroidal hemorrhage, left eye**

H31.303   **Unspecified choroidal hemorrhage, bilateral**

H31.309   **Unspecified choroidal hemorrhage, unspecified eye**

✓6th **H31.31**   Expulsive **choroidal hemorrhage**

H31.311   **Expulsive choroidal hemorrhage, right eye**

H31.312   **Expulsive choroidal hemorrhage, left eye**

H31.313   **Expulsive choroidal hemorrhage, bilateral**

H31.319   **Expulsive choroidal hemorrhage, unspecified eye**

✓6th **H31.32**   **Choroidal** rupture

H31.321   **Choroidal rupture, right eye**   CC

H31.322   **Choroidal rupture, left eye**   CC

H31.323   **Choroidal rupture, bilateral**   CC

H31.329   **Choroidal rupture, unspecified eye**   CC

✓5th **H31.4**   **Choroidal** detachment

✓6th **H31.40**   Unspecified **choroidal detachment**

H31.401   **Unspecified choroidal detachment, right eye**   CC

H31.402   **Unspecified choroidal detachment, left eye**   CC

H31.403   **Unspecified choroidal detachment, bilateral**   CC

H31.409   **Unspecified choroidal detachment, unspecified eye**   CC

✓6th **H31.41**   Hemorrhagic **choroidal detachment**

H31.411   **Hemorrhagic choroidal detachment, right eye**   CC

H31.412   **Hemorrhagic choroidal detachment, left eye**   CC

H31.413   **Hemorrhagic choroidal detachment, bilateral**   CC

H31.419   **Hemorrhagic choroidal detachment, unspecified eye**   CC

✓6th **H31.42**   Serous **choroidal detachment**

H31.421   **Serous choroidal detachment, right eye**   CC

H31.422   **Serous choroidal detachment, left eye**   CC

H31.423   **Serous choroidal detachment, bilateral**   CC

H31.429   **Serous choroidal detachment, unspecified eye**   CC

H31.8   Other **specified disorders of choroid**

H31.9   Unspecified **disorder of choroid**

H32   *Chorioretinal disorders in diseases classified elsewhere*

Code first underlying disease, such as:
     congenital toxoplasmosis (P37.1)
     histoplasmosis (B39.-)
     leprosy (A30.-)

     EXCLUDES 1   chorioretinitis (in):
                 toxoplasmosis (acquired) (B58.01)
                 tuberculosis (A18.53)

✓4th **H33**   **Retinal detachments and breaks**

     EXCLUDES 1   detachment of retinal pigment epithelium (H35.72-, H35.73-)

     CC Excl: For CC codes in category H33, unless otherwise noted:
     PDX collection 628

✓5th **H33.0**   **Retinal detachment** with retinal break
     Rhegmatogenous retinal detachment

     EXCLUDES 1   serous retinal detachment (without retinal break) (H33.2-)

✓6th **H33.00**   Unspecified **retinal detachment with retinal break**

H33.001   **Unspecified retinal detachment with retinal break, right eye**

H33.002   **Unspecified retinal detachment with retinal break, left eye**

H33.003   **Unspecified retinal detachment with retinal break, bilateral**

H33.009   **Unspecified retinal detachment with retinal break, unspecified eye**

Retinal Detachment

Lens   Vitreous   Choroid   Area of detachment   Iris   Cornea   Retina   Sclera

✓6th **H33.01**   **Retinal detachment with** single break

H33.011   **Retinal detachment with single break, right eye**

H33.012   **Retinal detachment with single break, left eye**

H33.013   **Retinal detachment with single break, bilateral**

H33.019   **Retinal detachment with single break, unspecified eye**

✓6th **H33.02**   **Retinal detachment with** multiple breaks

H33.021   **Retinal detachment with multiple breaks, right eye**

H33.022   **Retinal detachment with multiple breaks, left eye**

H33.023   **Retinal detachment with multiple breaks, bilateral**

H33.029   **Retinal detachment with multiple breaks, unspecified eye**

✓6th **H33.03**   **Retinal detachment with** giant retinal tear

H33.031   **Retinal detachment with giant retinal tear, right eye**

H33.032   **Retinal detachment with giant retinal tear, left eye**

H33.033   **Retinal detachment with giant retinal tear, bilateral**

H33.039   **Retinal detachment with giant retinal tear, unspecified eye**

✓6th **H33.04**   **Retinal detachment with** retinal dialysis

H33.041   **Retinal detachment with retinal dialysis, right eye**

H33.042   **Retinal detachment with retinal dialysis, left eye**

     H33.043   **Retinal detachment with retinal dialysis,** bilateral

     H33.049   **Retinal detachment with retinal dialysis,** unspecified **eye**

✓6ᵗʰ **H33.05   Total retinal detachment**

     H33.051   **Total retinal detachment,** right **eye**

     H33.052   **Total retinal detachment,** left **eye**

     H33.053   **Total retinal detachment,** bilateral

     H33.059   **Total retinal detachment,** unspecified **eye**

✓5ᵗʰ **H33.1   Retinoschisis and retinal cysts**

   EXCLUDES 1   *congenital retinoschisis (Q14.1)*
            microcystoid degeneration of retina (H35.42-)

✓6ᵗʰ **H33.10   Unspecified retinoschisis**

     H33.101   **Unspecified retinoschisis,** right **eye**

     H33.102   **Unspecified retinoschisis,** left **eye**

     H33.103   **Unspecified retinoschisis,** bilateral

     H33.109   **Unspecified retinoschisis,** unspecified **eye**

✓6ᵗʰ **H33.11   Cyst of ora serrata**

     H33.111   **Cyst of ora serrata,** right **eye**

     H33.112   **Cyst of ora serrata,** left **eye**

     H33.113   **Cyst of ora serrata,** bilateral

     H33.119   **Cyst of ora serrata,** unspecified **eye**

✓6ᵗʰ **H33.12   Parasitic cyst of retina**

> **CC Excl: For CC codes in subcategory H33.12:** PDX collection 625

     H33.121   **Parasitic cyst of retina,** right **eye** `CC`

     H33.122   **Parasitic cyst of retina,** left **eye** `CC`

     H33.123   **Parasitic cyst of retina,** bilateral `CC`

     H33.129   **Parasitic cyst of retina,** unspecified **eye** `CC`

✓6ᵗʰ **H33.19   Other retinoschisis and retinal cysts**
     Pseudocyst of retina

     H33.191   **Other retinoschisis and retinal cysts,** right **eye**

     H33.192   **Other retinoschisis and retinal cysts,** left **eye**

     H33.193   **Other retinoschisis and retinal cysts,** bilateral

     H33.199   **Other retinoschisis and retinal cysts,** unspecified **eye**

✓5ᵗʰ **H33.2   Serous retinal detachment**
     Retinal detachment NOS
     Retinal detachment without retinal break

   EXCLUDES 1   *central serous chorioretinopathy (H35.71-)*

     H33.20   **Serous retinal detachment,** unspecified **eye** `CC`

     H33.21   **Serous retinal detachment,** right **eye** `CC`

     H33.22   **Serous retinal detachment,** left **eye** `CC`

     H33.23   **Serous retinal detachment,** bilateral `CC`

✓5ᵗʰ **H33.3   Retinal breaks without detachment**

   EXCLUDES 1   *chorioretinal scars after surgery for detachment (H59.81-)*
            peripheral retinal degeneration without break (H35.4-)

✓6ᵗʰ **H33.30   Unspecified retinal break**

     H33.301   **Unspecified retinal break,** right **eye**

     H33.302   **Unspecified retinal break,** left **eye**

     H33.303   **Unspecified retinal break,** bilateral

     H33.309   **Unspecified retinal break,** unspecified **eye**

✓6ᵗʰ **H33.31   Horseshoe tear of retina without detachment**
     Operculum of retina without detachment

     H33.311   **Horseshoe tear of retina without detachment,** right **eye**

     H33.312   **Horseshoe tear of retina without detachment,** left **eye**

     H33.313   **Horseshoe tear of retina without detachment,** bilateral

     H33.319   **Horseshoe tear of retina without detachment,** unspecified **eye**

✓6ᵗʰ **H33.32   Round hole of retina without detachment**

     H33.321   **Round hole,** right **eye**

     H33.322   **Round hole,** left **eye**

     H33.323   **Round hole,** bilateral

     H33.329   **Round hole,** unspecified **eye**

✓6ᵗʰ **H33.33   Multiple defects of retina without detachment**

     H33.331   **Multiple defects of retina without detachment,** right **eye**

     H33.332   **Multiple defects of retina without detachment,** left **eye**

     H33.333   **Multiple defects of retina without detachment,** bilateral

     H33.339   **Multiple defects of retina without detachment,** unspecified **eye**

✓5ᵗʰ **H33.4   Traction detachment of retina**
     Proliferative vitreo-retinopathy with retinal detachment

     H33.40   **Traction detachment of retina,** unspecified **eye** `CC`

     H33.41   **Traction detachment of retina,** right **eye** `CC`

     H33.42   **Traction detachment of retina,** left **eye** `CC`

     H33.43   **Traction detachment of retina,** bilateral `CC`

   H33.8   Other retinal detachments `CC`

✓4ᵗʰ **H34   Retinal vascular occlusions**

   EXCLUDES 1   *amaurosis fugax (G45.3)*

> **CC Excl: For CC codes in category H34:** PDX collection 587

✓5ᵗʰ **H34.0   Transient retinal artery occlusion**

     H34.00   **Transient retinal artery occlusion,** unspecified **eye** `CC`

     H34.01   **Transient retinal artery occlusion,** right **eye** `CC`

     H34.02   **Transient retinal artery occlusion,** left **eye** `CC`

     H34.03   **Transient retinal artery occlusion,** bilateral `CC`

✓5ᵗʰ **H34.1   Central retinal artery occlusion**

     H34.10   **Central retinal artery occlusion,** unspecified **eye** `CC`

     H34.11   **Central retinal artery occlusion,** right **eye** `CC`

     H34.12   **Central retinal artery occlusion,** left **eye** `CC`

     H34.13   **Central retinal artery occlusion,** bilateral `CC`

✓5ᵗʰ **H34.2   Other retinal artery occlusions**

✓6ᵗʰ **H34.21   Partial retinal artery occlusion**
     Hollenhorst's plaque
     Retinal microembolism

     H34.211   **Partial retinal artery occlusion,** right **eye** `CC`

     H34.212   **Partial retinal artery occlusion,** left **eye** `CC`

     H34.213   **Partial retinal artery occlusion,** bilateral `CC`

     H34.219   **Partial retinal artery occlusion,** unspecified **eye** `CC`

✓6ᵗʰ **H34.23   Retinal artery branch occlusion**

     H34.231   **Retinal artery branch occlusion,** right **eye** `CC`

     H34.232   **Retinal artery branch occlusion,** left **eye** `CC`

     H34.233   **Retinal artery branch occlusion,** bilateral `CC`

     H34.239   **Retinal artery branch occlusion,** unspecified **eye** `CC`

✓5ᵗʰ **H34.8   Other retinal vascular occlusions**
     AHA: 2016, 4Q, 19

✓6ᵗʰ **H34.81   Central retinal vein occlusion**

> One of the following 7th characters is to be assigned to codes in subcategory H34.81 to designate the severity of the occlusion:
> 0   with macular edema
> 1   with retinal neovascularization
> 2   stable
>   old central retinal vein occlusion

     ✓7ᵗʰ H34.811   **Central retinal vein occlusion,** right **eye** `CC`

     ✓7ᵗʰ H34.812   **Central retinal vein occlusion,** left **eye** `CC`

     ✓7ᵗʰ H34.813   **Central retinal vein occlusion,** bilateral `CC`

     ✓7ᵗʰ H34.819   **Central retinal vein occlusion,** unspecified **eye** `CC`

✓6ᵗʰ **H34.82   Venous engorgement**
     Incipient retinal vein occlusion
     Partial retinal vein occlusion

     H34.821   **Venous engorgement,** right **eye**

     H34.822   **Venous engorgement,** left **eye**

     H34.823   **Venous engorgement,** bilateral

     H34.829   **Venous engorgement,** unspecified **eye**

Ⓝ Newborn: 0   Ⓟ Pediatric: 0-17   Ⓜ Maternity: 12-55   Ⓐ Adult: 15-124   `MCC` Major Complication/Comorbidity   `CC` Complication/Comorbidity   `SW` Severe Wound Dx

604   ICD-10-CM 2019

Chapter 7. Diseases of the Eye and Adnexa

√6ᵗʰ **H34.83** **Tributary (branch) retinal vein occlusion**

> One of the following 7th characters is to be assigned to codes in subcategory H34.83 to designate the severity of the occlusion:
> Ø   with macular edema
> 1   with retinal neovascularization
> 2   stable
>   old tributary (branch) retinal vein occlusion

√7ᵗʰ **H34.831** **Tributary (branch) retinal vein occlusion, right eye**

√7ᵗʰ **H34.832** **Tributary (branch) retinal vein occlusion, left eye**

√7ᵗʰ **H34.833** **Tributary (branch) retinal vein occlusion, bilateral**

√7ᵗʰ **H34.839** **Tributary (branch) retinal vein occlusion, unspecified eye**

H34.9 **Unspecified retinal vascular occlusion**   CC

√4ᵗʰ **H35** **Other retinal disorders**

EXCLUDES 2   *diabetic retinal disorders (E08.311- E08.359, E09.311- E09.359, E10.311- E10.359, E11.311- E11.359, E13.311- E13.359)*

√5ᵗʰ **H35.Ø** **Background retinopathy and retinal vascular changes**
Code also any associated hypertension (I10.-)

H35.ØØ Unspecified background retinopathy

√6ᵗʰ **H35.Ø1** **Changes in retinal vascular appearance**
Retinal vascular sheathing

H35.Ø11 **Changes in retinal vascular appearance, right eye**

H35.Ø12 **Changes in retinal vascular appearance, left eye**

H35.Ø13 **Changes in retinal vascular appearance, bilateral**

H35.Ø19 **Changes in retinal vascular appearance, unspecified eye**

√6ᵗʰ **H35.Ø2** **Exudative retinopathy**
Coats retinopathy

H35.Ø21 **Exudative retinopathy, right eye**

H35.Ø22 **Exudative retinopathy, left eye**

H35.Ø23 **Exudative retinopathy, bilateral**

H35.Ø29 **Exudative retinopathy, unspecified eye**

√6ᵗʰ **H35.Ø3** **Hypertensive retinopathy**

H35.Ø31 **Hypertensive retinopathy, right eye**

H35.Ø32 **Hypertensive retinopathy, left eye**

H35.Ø33 **Hypertensive retinopathy, bilateral**

H35.Ø39 **Hypertensive retinopathy, unspecified eye**

√6ᵗʰ **H35.Ø4** **Retinal micro-aneurysms, unspecified**

H35.Ø41 **Retinal micro-aneurysms, unspecified, right eye**

H35.Ø42 **Retinal micro-aneurysms, unspecified, left eye**

H35.Ø43 **Retinal micro-aneurysms, unspecified, bilateral**

H35.Ø49 **Retinal micro-aneurysms, unspecified, unspecified eye**

√6ᵗʰ **H35.Ø5** **Retinal neovascularization, unspecified**

H35.Ø51 **Retinal neovascularization, unspecified, right eye**

H35.Ø52 **Retinal neovascularization, unspecified, left eye**

H35.Ø53 **Retinal neovascularization, unspecified, bilateral**

H35.Ø59 **Retinal neovascularization, unspecified, unspecified eye**

√6ᵗʰ **H35.Ø6** **Retinal vasculitis**
Eales disease
Retinal perivasculitis
DEF: Sight-threatening intraocular inflammation of the retinal blood vessels that causes minimal, partial, or even complete blindness.

H35.Ø61 **Retinal vasculitis, right eye**

H35.Ø62 **Retinal vasculitis, left eye**

H35.Ø63 **Retinal vasculitis, bilateral**

H35.Ø69 **Retinal vasculitis, unspecified eye**

√6ᵗʰ **H35.Ø7** **Retinal telangiectasis**

H35.Ø71 **Retinal telangiectasis, right eye**

H35.Ø72 **Retinal telangiectasis, left eye**

H35.Ø73 **Retinal telangiectasis, bilateral**

H35.Ø79 **Retinal telangiectasis, unspecified eye**

H35.Ø9 **Other intraretinal microvascular abnormalities**
Retinal varices

√5ᵗʰ **H35.1** **Retinopathy of prematurity**

√6ᵗʰ **H35.1Ø** **Retinopathy of prematurity, unspecified**
Retinopathy of prematurity NOS

H35.1Ø1 **Retinopathy of prematurity, unspecified, right eye**

H35.1Ø2 **Retinopathy of prematurity, unspecified, left eye**

H35.1Ø3 **Retinopathy of prematurity, unspecified, bilateral**

H35.1Ø9 **Retinopathy of prematurity, unspecified, unspecified eye**

√6ᵗʰ **H35.11** **Retinopathy of prematurity, stage Ø**

H35.111 **Retinopathy of prematurity, stage Ø, right eye**

H35.112 **Retinopathy of prematurity, stage Ø, left eye**

H35.113 **Retinopathy of prematurity, stage Ø, bilateral**

H35.119 **Retinopathy of prematurity, stage Ø, unspecified eye**

√6ᵗʰ **H35.12** **Retinopathy of prematurity, stage 1**

H35.121 **Retinopathy of prematurity, stage 1, right eye**

H35.122 **Retinopathy of prematurity, stage 1, left eye**

H35.123 **Retinopathy of prematurity, stage 1, bilateral**

H35.129 **Retinopathy of prematurity, stage 1, unspecified eye**

√6ᵗʰ **H35.13** **Retinopathy of prematurity, stage 2**

H35.131 **Retinopathy of prematurity, stage 2, right eye**

H35.132 **Retinopathy of prematurity, stage 2, left eye**

H35.133 **Retinopathy of prematurity, stage 2, bilateral**

H35.139 **Retinopathy of prematurity, stage 2, unspecified eye**

√6ᵗʰ **H35.14** **Retinopathy of prematurity, stage 3**

H35.141 **Retinopathy of prematurity, stage 3, right eye**

H35.142 **Retinopathy of prematurity, stage 3, left eye**

H35.143 **Retinopathy of prematurity, stage 3, bilateral**

H35.149 **Retinopathy of prematurity, stage 3, unspecified eye**

√6ᵗʰ **H35.15** **Retinopathy of prematurity, stage 4**

H35.151 **Retinopathy of prematurity, stage 4, right eye**

H35.152 **Retinopathy of prematurity, stage 4, left eye**

H35.153 **Retinopathy of prematurity, stage 4, bilateral**

H35.159 **Retinopathy of prematurity, stage 4, unspecified eye**

√6ᵗʰ **H35.16** **Retinopathy of prematurity, stage 5**

H35.161 **Retinopathy of prematurity, stage 5, right eye**

H35.162 **Retinopathy of prematurity, stage 5, left eye**

H35.163 **Retinopathy of prematurity, stage 5, bilateral**

H35.169 **Retinopathy of prematurity, stage 5, unspecified eye**

√6ᵗʰ **H35.17** **Retrolental fibroplasia**

H35.171 **Retrolental fibroplasia, right eye**

H35.172 **Retrolental fibroplasia, left eye**

H35.173 **Retrolental fibroplasia, bilateral**

H35.179 **Retrolental fibroplasia, unspecified eye**

☑ Additional Character Required   √x7ᵗʰ Placeholder   Unacceptable PDx   Questionable PDx   Manifestation   H1 - H14 HAC   HCC CMS-HCC Dx   HIV HIV Dx

ICD-10-CM 2019   605

Chapter 7. Diseases of the Eye and Adnexa

H35.2–H35.459

✓5ᵗʰ **H35.2 Other non-diabetic proliferative retinopathy**
Proliferative vitreo-retinopathy
EXCLUDES 1 *proliferative vitreo-retinopathy with retinal detachment (H33.4-)*

H35.20 Other non-diabetic proliferative retinopathy, unspecified eye

H35.21 Other non-diabetic proliferative retinopathy, right eye

H35.22 Other non-diabetic proliferative retinopathy, left eye

H35.23 Other non-diabetic proliferative retinopathy, bilateral

✓5ᵗʰ **H35.3 Degeneration of macula and posterior pole**

H35.30 Unspecified macular degeneration   A
Age-related macular degeneration

✓6ᵗʰ **H35.31** Nonexudative age-related macular degeneration
Atrophic age-related macular degeneration
Dry age-related macular degeneration
AHA: 2016, 4Q, 20-21

> One of the following 7th characters is to be assigned to codes in subcategory H35.31 to designate the stage of the disease:
> Ø   stage unspecified
> 1   early dry stage
> 2   intermediate dry stage
> 3   advanced atrophic without subfoveal involvement
>   advanced dry stage
> 4   advanced atrophic with subfoveal involvement

  ✓7ᵗʰ **H35.311** Nonexudative age-related macular degeneration, right eye   A

  ✓7ᵗʰ **H35.312** Nonexudative age-related macular degeneration, left eye   A

  ✓7ᵗʰ **H35.313** Nonexudative age-related macular degeneration, bilateral   A

  ✓7ᵗʰ **H35.319** Nonexudative age-related macular degeneration, unspecified eye   A

✓6ᵗʰ **H35.32** Exudative age-related macular degeneration
Wet age-related macular degeneration
AHA: 2016, 4Q, 20-21

> One of the following 7th characters is to be assigned to codes in subcategory H35.32 to designate the stage of the disease:
> Ø   stage unspecified
> 1   with active choroidal neovascularization
> 2   with inactive choroidal neovascularization
>   with involuted or regressed neovascularization
> 3   with inactive scar

  ✓7ᵗʰ **H35.321** Exudative age-related macular degeneration, right eye   HCC A

  ✓7ᵗʰ **H35.322** Exudative age-related macular degeneration, left eye   HCC A

  ✓7ᵗʰ **H35.323** Exudative age-related macular degeneration, bilateral   HCC A

  ✓7ᵗʰ **H35.329** Exudative age-related macular degeneration, unspecified eye   HCC A

H35.33 Angioid streaks of macula
DEF: Degeneration of the choroid; characterized by broad, irregular, dark brown streaks radiating from optic disc; occurs with pseudoxanthoma elasticum or Paget's disease.

✓6ᵗʰ **H35.34** Macular cyst, hole, or pseudohole
H35.341 Macular cyst, hole, or pseudohole, right eye
H35.342 Macular cyst, hole, or pseudohole, left eye
H35.343 Macular cyst, hole, or pseudohole, bilateral
H35.349 Macular cyst, hole, or pseudohole, unspecified eye

✓6ᵗʰ **H35.35** Cystoid macular degeneration
EXCLUDES 1 *cystoid macular edema following cataract surgery (H59.Ø3-)*
H35.351 Cystoid macular degeneration, right eye
H35.352 Cystoid macular degeneration, left eye
H35.353 Cystoid macular degeneration, bilateral

H35.359 Cystoid macular degeneration, unspecified eye

✓6ᵗʰ **H35.36** Drusen (degenerative) of macula
AHA: 2017, 1Q, 51; 2016, 4Q, 21
H35.361 Drusen (degenerative) of macula, right eye
H35.362 Drusen (degenerative) of macula, left eye
H35.363 Drusen (degenerative) of macula, bilateral
H35.369 Drusen (degenerative) of macula, unspecified eye

✓6ᵗʰ **H35.37** Puckering of macula
H35.371 Puckering of macula, right eye
H35.372 Puckering of macula, left eye
H35.373 Puckering of macula, bilateral
H35.379 Puckering of macula, unspecified eye

✓6ᵗʰ **H35.38** Toxic maculopathy
Code first poisoning due to drug or toxin, if applicable (T36-T65 with fifth or sixth character 1-4 or 6)
Use additional code for adverse effect, if applicable, to identify drug (T36-T50 with fifth or sixth character 5)
H35.381 Toxic maculopathy, right eye
H35.382 Toxic maculopathy, left eye
H35.383 Toxic maculopathy, bilateral
H35.389 Toxic maculopathy, unspecified eye

✓5ᵗʰ **H35.4 Peripheral retinal degeneration**
EXCLUDES 1 *hereditary retinal degeneration (dystrophy) (H35.5-)*
peripheral retinal degeneration with retinal break (H33.3-)

H35.40 Unspecified peripheral retinal degeneration

✓6ᵗʰ **H35.41** Lattice degeneration of retina
Palisade degeneration of retina
DEF: Degeneration of the retina, often bilateral, that is usually benign. It is characterized by lines intersecting at irregular intervals in the peripheral retina. Retinal thinning and retinal holes may occur.
H35.411 Lattice degeneration of retina, right eye
H35.412 Lattice degeneration of retina, left eye
H35.413 Lattice degeneration of retina, bilateral
H35.419 Lattice degeneration of retina, unspecified eye

✓6ᵗʰ **H35.42** Microcystoid degeneration of retina
H35.421 Microcystoid degeneration of retina, right eye
H35.422 Microcystoid degeneration of retina, left eye
H35.423 Microcystoid degeneration of retina, bilateral
H35.429 Microcystoid degeneration of retina, unspecified eye

✓6ᵗʰ **H35.43** Paving stone degeneration of retina
H35.431 Paving stone degeneration of retina, right eye
H35.432 Paving stone degeneration of retina, left eye
H35.433 Paving stone degeneration of retina, bilateral
H35.439 Paving stone degeneration of retina, unspecified eye

✓6ᵗʰ **H35.44** Age-related reticular degeneration of retina
H35.441 Age-related reticular degeneration of retina, right eye   A
H35.442 Age-related reticular degeneration of retina, left eye   A
H35.443 Age-related reticular degeneration of retina, bilateral   A
H35.449 Age-related reticular degeneration of retina, unspecified eye   A

✓6ᵗʰ **H35.45** Secondary pigmentary degeneration
H35.451 Secondary pigmentary degeneration, right eye
H35.452 Secondary pigmentary degeneration, left eye
H35.453 Secondary pigmentary degeneration, bilateral
H35.459 Secondary pigmentary degeneration, unspecified eye

N Newborn: 0   P Pediatric: 0-17   M Maternity: 12-55   A Adult: 15-124   MCC Major Complication/Comorbidity   CC Complication/Comorbidity   SW Severe Wound Dx

606   ICD-10-CM 2019

✓6ᵗʰ H35.46 Secondary vitreoretinal degeneration
- H35.461 Secondary vitreoretinal degeneration, right eye
- H35.462 Secondary vitreoretinal degeneration, left eye
- H35.463 Secondary vitreoretinal degeneration, bilateral
- H35.469 Secondary vitreoretinal degeneration, unspecified eye

✓5ᵗʰ H35.5 Hereditary retinal dystrophy
> EXCLUDES 1   dystrophies primarily involving Bruch's membrane (H31.1-)

- H35.50 Unspecified hereditary retinal dystrophy
- H35.51 Vitreoretinal dystrophy
- H35.52 Pigmentary retinal dystrophy
  Albipunctate retinal dystrophy
  Retinitis pigmentosa
  Tapetoretinal dystrophy
- H35.53 Other dystrophies primarily involving the sensory retina
  Stargardt's disease
- H35.54 Dystrophies primarily involving the retinal pigment epithelium
  Vitelliform retinal dystrophy

✓5ᵗʰ H35.6 Retinal hemorrhage
- H35.60 Retinal hemorrhage, unspecified eye
- H35.61 Retinal hemorrhage, right eye
- H35.62 Retinal hemorrhage, left eye
- H35.63 Retinal hemorrhage, bilateral

✓5ᵗʰ H35.7 Separation of retinal layers
> EXCLUDES 1   retinal detachment (serous) (H33.2-)
> rhegmatogenous retinal detachment (H33.0-)

> CC Excl: For CC codes in subcategory H35.7:
> PDX collection 628

- H35.70 Unspecified separation of retinal layers   CC
- **✓6ᵗʰ H35.71 Central serous chorioretinopathy**
  - H35.711 Central serous chorioretinopathy, right eye
  - H35.712 Central serous chorioretinopathy, left eye
  - H35.713 Central serous chorioretinopathy, bilateral
  - H35.719 Central serous chorioretinopathy, unspecified eye
- **✓6ᵗʰ H35.72 Serous detachment of retinal pigment epithelium**
  - H35.721 Serous detachment of retinal pigment epithelium, right eye   CC
  - H35.722 Serous detachment of retinal pigment epithelium, left eye   CC
  - H35.723 Serous detachment of retinal pigment epithelium, bilateral   CC
  - H35.729 Serous detachment of retinal pigment epithelium, unspecified eye   CC
- **✓6ᵗʰ H35.73 Hemorrhagic detachment of retinal pigment epithelium**
  - H35.731 Hemorrhagic detachment of retinal pigment epithelium, right eye   CC
  - H35.732 Hemorrhagic detachment of retinal pigment epithelium, left eye   CC
  - H35.733 Hemorrhagic detachment of retinal pigment epithelium, bilateral   CC
  - H35.739 Hemorrhagic detachment of retinal pigment epithelium, unspecified eye   CC

✓5ᵗʰ H35.8 Other specified retinal disorders
> EXCLUDES 2   retinal hemorrhage (H35.6-)

- H35.81 Retinal edema
  Retinal cotton wool spots
- H35.82 Retinal ischemia   CC
  CC Excl: PDX collection 629
- H35.89 Other specified retinal disorders
- H35.9 Unspecified retinal disorder

H36 *Retinal disorders in diseases classified elsewhere*
Code first underlying disease, such as:
lipid storage disorders (E75.-)
sickle-cell disorders (D57.-)
> EXCLUDES 1   arteriosclerotic retinopathy (H35.0-)
> diabetic retinopathy (E08.3-, E09.3-, E10.3-, E11.3-, E13.3-)

Glaucoma (H40-H42)

✓4ᵗʰ H40 Glaucoma
> EXCLUDES 1   absolute glaucoma (H44.51-)
> congenital glaucoma (Q15.0)
> traumatic glaucoma due to birth injury (P15.3)

✓5ᵗʰ H40.0 Glaucoma suspect
- **✓6ᵗʰ H40.00 Preglaucoma, unspecified**
  - H40.001 Preglaucoma, unspecified, right eye
  - H40.002 Preglaucoma, unspecified, left eye
  - H40.003 Preglaucoma, unspecified, bilateral
  - H40.009 Preglaucoma, unspecified, unspecified eye
- **✓6ᵗʰ H40.01 Open angle with borderline findings, low risk**
  Open angle, low risk
  - H40.011 Open angle with borderline findings, low risk, right eye
  - H40.012 Open angle with borderline findings, low risk, left eye
  - H40.013 Open angle with borderline findings, low risk, bilateral
  - H40.019 Open angle with borderline findings, low risk, unspecified eye
- **✓6ᵗʰ H40.02 Open angle with borderline findings, high risk**
  Open angle, high risk
  - H40.021 Open angle with borderline findings, high risk, right eye
  - H40.022 Open angle with borderline findings, high risk, left eye
  - H40.023 Open angle with borderline findings, high risk, bilateral
  - H40.029 Open angle with borderline findings, high risk, unspecified eye
- **✓6ᵗʰ H40.03 Anatomical narrow angle**
  Primary angle closure suspect
  - H40.031 Anatomical narrow angle, right eye
  - H40.032 Anatomical narrow angle, left eye
  - H40.033 Anatomical narrow angle, bilateral
  - H40.039 Anatomical narrow angle, unspecified eye
- **✓6ᵗʰ H40.04 Steroid responder**
  - H40.041 Steroid responder, right eye
  - H40.042 Steroid responder, left eye
  - H40.043 Steroid responder, bilateral
  - H40.049 Steroid responder, unspecified eye
- **✓6ᵗʰ H40.05 Ocular hypertension**
  - H40.051 Ocular hypertension, right eye
  - H40.052 Ocular hypertension, left eye
  - H40.053 Ocular hypertension, bilateral
  - H40.059 Ocular hypertension, unspecified eye
- **✓6ᵗʰ H40.06 Primary angle closure without glaucoma damage**
  - H40.061 Primary angle closure without glaucoma damage, right eye
  - H40.062 Primary angle closure without glaucoma damage, left eye
  - H40.063 Primary angle closure without glaucoma damage, bilateral
  - H40.069 Primary angle closure without glaucoma damage, unspecified eye

✓5ᵗʰ H40.1 Open-angle glaucoma

> One of the following 7th characters is to be assigned to each code in subcategories H40.10, H40.11-, H40.12-, H40.13-, and H40.14- to designate the stage of glaucoma.
> 0   stage unspecified
> 1   mild stage
> 2   moderate stage
> 3   severe stage
> 4   indeterminate stage

- **✓x7ᵗʰ H40.10 Unspecified open-angle glaucoma**
  TIP: Only one code from this subcategory should be assigned when both left and right eyes are the same stage.

✓ Additional Character Required   ✓x7ᵗʰ Placeholder   Unacceptable PDx   Questionable PDx   Manifestation   H1-H14 HAC   HCC CMS-HCC Dx   HIV HIV Dx

ICD-10-CM 2019   607

Chapter 7. Diseases of the Eye and Adnexa

H35.46-H40.10

Open Angle/Angle Closure Glaucoma

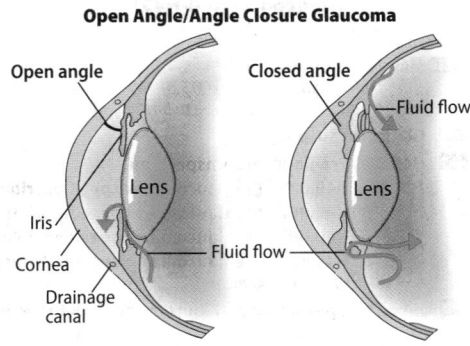

✓6ᵗʰ H40.11 Primary open-angle glaucoma
Chronic simple glaucoma
AHA: 2016, 4Q, 22

    ✓7ᵗʰ H40.111 Primary open-angle glaucoma, right eye
    ✓7ᵗʰ H40.112 Primary open-angle glaucoma, left eye
    ✓7ᵗʰ H40.113 Primary open-angle glaucoma, bilateral
    ✓7ᵗʰ H40.119 Primary open-angle glaucoma, unspecified eye

✓6ᵗʰ H40.12 Low-tension glaucoma
    ✓7ᵗʰ H40.121 Low-tension glaucoma, right eye
    ✓7ᵗʰ H40.122 Low-tension glaucoma, left eye
    ✓7ᵗʰ H40.123 Low-tension glaucoma, bilateral
    ✓7ᵗʰ H40.129 Low-tension glaucoma, unspecified eye

✓6ᵗʰ H40.13 Pigmentary glaucoma
    ✓7ᵗʰ H40.131 Pigmentary glaucoma, right eye
    ✓7ᵗʰ H40.132 Pigmentary glaucoma, left eye
    ✓7ᵗʰ H40.133 Pigmentary glaucoma, bilateral
    ✓7ᵗʰ H40.139 Pigmentary glaucoma, unspecified eye

✓6ᵗʰ H40.14 Capsular glaucoma with pseudoexfoliation of lens
    ✓7ᵗʰ H40.141 Capsular glaucoma with pseudoexfoliation of lens, right eye
    ✓7ᵗʰ H40.142 Capsular glaucoma with pseudoexfoliation of lens, left eye
    ✓7ᵗʰ H40.143 Capsular glaucoma with pseudoexfoliation of lens, bilateral
    ✓7ᵗʰ H40.149 Capsular glaucoma with pseudoexfoliation of lens, unspecified eye

✓6ᵗʰ H40.15 Residual stage of open-angle glaucoma
    H40.151 Residual stage of open-angle glaucoma, right eye
    H40.152 Residual stage of open-angle glaucoma, left eye
    H40.153 Residual stage of open-angle glaucoma, bilateral
    H40.159 Residual stage of open-angle glaucoma, unspecified eye

✓5ᵗʰ H40.2 Primary angle-closure glaucoma
    EXCLUDES 1 aqueous misdirection (H40.83-)
                malignant glaucoma (H40.83-)

    One of the following 7th characters is to be assigned to each code in subcategories H40.20 and H40.22- to designate the stage of glaucoma.
    Ø   stage unspecified
    1   mild stage
    2   moderate stage
    3   severe stage
    4   indeterminate stage

    ✓x7ᵗʰ H40.20 Unspecified primary angle-closure glaucoma
        TIP: Only one code from this subcategory should be assigned when both left and right eyes are the same stage.

    ✓6ᵗʰ H40.21 Acute angle-closure glaucoma
        Acute angle-closure glaucoma attack
        Acute angle-closure glaucoma crisis

        CC Excl: For CC codes in subcategory H40.21:
        PDX collection 630

        H40.211 Acute angle-closure glaucoma, right eye   **CC**

H40.212 Acute angle-closure glaucoma, left eye   **CC**
H40.213 Acute angle-closure glaucoma, bilateral   **CC**
H40.219 Acute angle-closure glaucoma, unspecified eye   **CC**

✓6ᵗʰ H40.22 Chronic angle-closure glaucoma
Chronic primary angle-closure glaucoma
    ✓7ᵗʰ H40.221 Chronic angle-closure glaucoma, right eye
    ✓7ᵗʰ H40.222 Chronic angle-closure glaucoma, left eye
    ✓7ᵗʰ H40.223 Chronic angle-closure glaucoma, bilateral
    ✓7ᵗʰ H40.229 Chronic angle-closure glaucoma, unspecified eye

✓6ᵗʰ H40.23 Intermittent angle-closure glaucoma
    H40.231 Intermittent angle-closure glaucoma, right eye
    H40.232 Intermittent angle-closure glaucoma, left eye
    H40.233 Intermittent angle-closure glaucoma, bilateral
    H40.239 Intermittent angle-closure glaucoma, unspecified eye

✓6ᵗʰ H40.24 Residual stage of angle-closure glaucoma
    H40.241 Residual stage of angle-closure glaucoma, right eye
    H40.242 Residual stage of angle-closure glaucoma, left eye
    H40.243 Residual stage of angle-closure glaucoma, bilateral
    H40.249 Residual stage of angle-closure glaucoma, unspecified eye

✓5ᵗʰ H40.3 Glaucoma secondary to eye trauma
Code also underlying condition

    One of the following 7th characters is to be assigned to each code in subcategory H40.3- to designate the stage of glaucoma.
    Ø   stage unspecified
    1   mild stage
    2   moderate stage
    3   severe stage
    4   indeterminate stage

    ✓x7ᵗʰ H40.30 Glaucoma secondary to eye trauma, unspecified eye
    ✓x7ᵗʰ H40.31 Glaucoma secondary to eye trauma, right eye
    ✓x7ᵗʰ H40.32 Glaucoma secondary to eye trauma, left eye
    ✓x7ᵗʰ H40.33 Glaucoma secondary to eye trauma, bilateral

✓5ᵗʰ H40.4 Glaucoma secondary to eye inflammation
Code also underlying condition

    One of the following 7th characters is to be assigned to each code in subcategory H40.4- to designate the stage of glaucoma.
    Ø   stage unspecified
    1   mild stage
    2   moderate stage
    3   severe stage
    4   indeterminate stage

    ✓x7ᵗʰ H40.40 Glaucoma secondary to eye inflammation, unspecified eye
    ✓x7ᵗʰ H40.41 Glaucoma secondary to eye inflammation, right eye
    ✓x7ᵗʰ H40.42 Glaucoma secondary to eye inflammation, left eye
    ✓x7ᵗʰ H40.43 Glaucoma secondary to eye inflammation, bilateral

✓5ᵗʰ H40.5 Glaucoma secondary to other eye disorders
Code also underlying eye disorder

    One of the following 7th characters is to be assigned to each code in subcategory H40.5- to designate the stage of glaucoma.
    Ø   stage unspecified
    1   mild stage
    2   moderate stage
    3   severe stage
    4   indeterminate stage

    ✓x7ᵗʰ H40.50 Glaucoma secondary to other eye disorders, unspecified eye
    ✓x7ᵗʰ H40.51 Glaucoma secondary to other eye disorders, right eye

N Newborn: 0   **P** Pediatric: 0-17   **M** Maternity: 12-55   **A** Adult: 15-124   **MCC** Major Complication/Comorbidity   **CC** Complication/Comorbidity   **SW** Severe Wound Dx

608   ICD-10-CM 2019

✓x7ᵗʰ **H40.52** Glaucoma secondary to other eye disorders, left eye

✓x7ᵗʰ **H40.53** Glaucoma secondary to other eye disorders, bilateral

✓5ᵗʰ **H40.6** Glaucoma secondary to drugs
Use additional code for adverse effect, if applicable, to identify drug (T36-T50 with fifth or sixth character 5)

> One of the following 7th characters is to be assigned to each code in subcategory H40.6- to designate the stage of glaucoma.
> 0   stage unspecified
> 1   mild stage
> 2   moderate stage
> 3   severe stage
> 4   indeterminate stage

✓x7ᵗʰ **H40.60** Glaucoma secondary to drugs, unspecified eye

✓x7ᵗʰ **H40.61** Glaucoma secondary to drugs, right eye

✓x7ᵗʰ **H40.62** Glaucoma secondary to drugs, left eye

✓x7ᵗʰ **H40.63** Glaucoma secondary to drugs, bilateral

✓5ᵗʰ **H40.8** Other glaucoma

  ✓6ᵗʰ **H40.81** Glaucoma with increased episcleral venous pressure
      H40.811 Glaucoma with increased episcleral venous pressure, right eye
      H40.812 Glaucoma with increased episcleral venous pressure, left eye
      H40.813 Glaucoma with increased episcleral venous pressure, bilateral
      H40.819 Glaucoma with increased episcleral venous pressure, unspecified eye

  ✓6ᵗʰ **H40.82** Hypersecretion glaucoma
      H40.821 Hypersecretion glaucoma, right eye
      H40.822 Hypersecretion glaucoma, left eye
      H40.823 Hypersecretion glaucoma, bilateral
      H40.829 Hypersecretion glaucoma, unspecified eye

  ✓6ᵗʰ **H40.83** Aqueous misdirection
      Malignant glaucoma
      H40.831 Aqueous misdirection, right eye
      H40.832 Aqueous misdirection, left eye
      H40.833 Aqueous misdirection, bilateral
      H40.839 Aqueous misdirection, unspecified eye

  H40.89 Other specified glaucoma

H40.9 Unspecified glaucoma

H42 *Glaucoma in diseases classified elsewhere*
Code first underlying condition, such as:
  amyloidosis (E85.-)
  aniridia (Q13.1)
  glaucoma (in) diabetes mellitus (E08.39, E09.39, E10.39, E11.39, E13.39)
  Lowe's syndrome (E72.03)
  Reiger's anomaly (Q13.81)
  specified metabolic disorder (E70-E88)

  EXCLUDES 1   glaucoma (in) onchocerciasis (B73.02)
             glaucoma (in) syphilis (A52.71)
             glaucoma (in) tuberculous (A18.59)

Disorders of vitreous body and globe (H43-H44)

✓4ᵗʰ **H43** Disorders of vitreous body

  ✓5ᵗʰ **H43.0** Vitreous prolapse
    EXCLUDES 1   traumatic vitreous prolapse (S05.2-)
             vitreous syndrome following cataract surgery (H59.0-)
    H43.00 Vitreous prolapse, unspecified eye
    H43.01 Vitreous prolapse, right eye
    H43.02 Vitreous prolapse, left eye
    H43.03 Vitreous prolapse, bilateral

  ✓5ᵗʰ **H43.1** Vitreous hemorrhage
    H43.10 Vitreous hemorrhage, unspecified eye   HCC
    H43.11 Vitreous hemorrhage, right eye   HCC
    H43.12 Vitreous hemorrhage, left eye   HCC
    H43.13 Vitreous hemorrhage, bilateral   HCC

  ✓5ᵗʰ **H43.2** Crystalline deposits in vitreous body
    H43.20 Crystalline deposits in vitreous body, unspecified eye
    H43.21 Crystalline deposits in vitreous body, right eye
    H43.22 Crystalline deposits in vitreous body, left eye

    H43.23 Crystalline deposits in vitreous body, bilateral

  ✓5ᵗʰ **H43.3** Other vitreous opacities
    ✓6ᵗʰ **H43.31** Vitreous membranes and strands
      H43.311 Vitreous membranes and strands, right eye
      H43.312 Vitreous membranes and strands, left eye
      H43.313 Vitreous membranes and strands, bilateral
      H43.319 Vitreous membranes and strands, unspecified eye

    ✓6ᵗʰ **H43.39** Other vitreous opacities
      Vitreous floaters
      H43.391 Other vitreous opacities, right eye
      H43.392 Other vitreous opacities, left eye
      H43.393 Other vitreous opacities, bilateral
      H43.399 Other vitreous opacities, unspecified eye

  ✓5ᵗʰ **H43.8** Other disorders of vitreous body
    EXCLUDES 1   proliferative vitreo-retinopathy with retinal detachment (H33.4-)
    EXCLUDES 2   vitreous abscess (H44.02-)
    ✓6ᵗʰ **H43.81** Vitreous degeneration
      Vitreous detachment
      H43.811 Vitreous degeneration, right eye
      H43.812 Vitreous degeneration, left eye
      H43.813 Vitreous degeneration, bilateral
      H43.819 Vitreous degeneration, unspecified eye

    ✓6ᵗʰ **H43.82** Vitreomacular adhesion
      Vitreomacular traction
      H43.821 Vitreomacular adhesion, right eye   A
      H43.822 Vitreomacular adhesion, left eye   A
      H43.823 Vitreomacular adhesion, bilateral   A
      H43.829 Vitreomacular adhesion, unspecified eye   A

    H43.89 Other disorders of vitreous body

  H43.9 Unspecified disorder of vitreous body

✓4ᵗʰ **H44** Disorders of globe
  INCLUDES   disorders affecting multiple structures of eye

  ✓5ᵗʰ **H44.0** Purulent endophthalmitis
    Use additional code to identify organism
    EXCLUDES 1   bleb associated endophthalmitis (H59.4-)

    ✓6ᵗʰ **H44.00** Unspecified purulent endophthalmitis

> **CC Excl: For CC codes in subcategory H44.00:** PDX collection 625

      H44.001 Unspecified purulent endophthalmitis, right eye   CC
      H44.002 Unspecified purulent endophthalmitis, left eye   CC
      H44.003 Unspecified purulent endophthalmitis, bilateral   CC
      H44.009 Unspecified purulent endophthalmitis, unspecified eye   CC

    ✓6ᵗʰ **H44.01** Panophthalmitis (acute)

> **CC Excl: For CC codes in subcategory H44.01:** PDX collection 625

      H44.011 Panophthalmitis (acute), right eye   CC
      H44.012 Panophthalmitis (acute), left eye   CC
      H44.013 Panophthalmitis (acute), bilateral   CC
      H44.019 Panophthalmitis (acute), unspecified eye   CC

    ✓6ᵗʰ **H44.02** Vitreous abscess (chronic)

> **CC Excl: For CC codes in subcategory H44.02:** PDX collection 631

      H44.021 Vitreous abscess (chronic), right eye   CC
      H44.022 Vitreous abscess (chronic), left eye   CC
      H44.023 Vitreous abscess (chronic), bilateral   CC
      H44.029 Vitreous abscess (chronic), unspecified eye   CC

✓ Additional Character Required   ✓x7ᵗʰ Placeholder   Unacceptable PDx   Questionable PDx   Manifestation   H1 - H14 HAC   HCC CMS-HCC Dx   HIV HIV Dx

ICD-10-CM 2019   609

√5ᵗʰ H44.1 Other endophthalmitis

EXCLUDES 1   bleb associated endophthalmitis (H59.4-)

EXCLUDES 2   ophthalmia nodosa (H16.2-)

√6ᵗʰ H44.11 Panuveitis

DEF: Inflammation of all layers of the uvea of the eye, including the choroid, iris, and ciliary body. It also typically involves the lens, retina, optic nerve, and vitreous and causes reduced vision or blindness.

CC Excl: For CC codes in subcategory H44.11: PDX collection 632

H44.111   Panuveitis, right eye   CC

H44.112   Panuveitis, left eye   CC

H44.113   Panuveitis, bilateral   CC

H44.119   Panuveitis, unspecified eye   CC

√6ᵗʰ H44.12 Parasitic endophthalmitis, unspecified

CC Excl: For CC codes in subcategory H44.12: PDX collection 625

H44.121   Parasitic endophthalmitis, unspecified, right eye   CC

H44.122   Parasitic endophthalmitis, unspecified, left eye   CC

H44.123   Parasitic endophthalmitis, unspecified, bilateral   CC

H44.129   Parasitic endophthalmitis, unspecified, unspecified eye   CC

√6ᵗʰ H44.13 Sympathetic uveitis

CC Excl: For CC codes in subcategory H44.13: PDX collection 632

H44.131   Sympathetic uveitis, right eye   CC

H44.132   Sympathetic uveitis, left eye   CC

H44.133   Sympathetic uveitis, bilateral   CC

H44.139   Sympathetic uveitis, unspecified eye   CC

H44.19   Other endophthalmitis   CC

CC Excl: PDX collection 625

√5ᵗʰ H44.2 Degenerative myopia

Malignant myopia

AHA: 2017, 4Q, 10-11

H44.20   Degenerative myopia, unspecified eye

H44.21   Degenerative myopia, right eye

H44.22   Degenerative myopia, left eye

H44.23   Degenerative myopia, bilateral

√6ᵗʰ H44.2A Degenerative myopia with choroidal neovascularization

Use additional code for any associated choroid disorders (H31.-)

H44.2A1   Degenerative myopia with choroidal neovascularization, right eye

H44.2A2   Degenerative myopia with choroidal neovascularization, left eye

H44.2A3   Degenerative myopia with choroidal neovascularization, bilateral eye

H44.2A9   Degenerative myopia with choroidal neovascularization, unspecified eye

√6ᵗʰ H44.2B Degenerative myopia with macular hole

H44.2B1   Degenerative myopia with macular hole, right eye

H44.2B2   Degenerative myopia with macular hole, left eye

H44.2B3   Degenerative myopia with macular hole, bilateral eye

H44.2B9   Degenerative myopia with macular hole, unspecified eye

√6ᵗʰ H44.2C Degenerative myopia with retinal detachment

Use additional code to identify the retinal detachment (H33.-)

H44.2C1   Degenerative myopia with retinal detachment, right eye

H44.2C2   Degenerative myopia with retinal detachment, left eye

H44.2C3   Degenerative myopia with retinal detachment, bilateral eye

H44.2C9   Degenerative myopia with retinal detachment, unspecified eye

√6ᵗʰ H44.2D Degenerative myopia with foveoschisis

H44.2D1   Degenerative myopia with foveoschisis, right eye

H44.2D2   Degenerative myopia with foveoschisis, left eye

H44.2D3   Degenerative myopia with foveoschisis, bilateral eye

H44.2D9   Degenerative myopia with foveoschisis, unspecified eye

√6ᵗʰ H44.2E Degenerative myopia with other maculopathy

H44.2E1   Degenerative myopia with other maculopathy, right eye

H44.2E2   Degenerative myopia with other maculopathy, left eye

H44.2E3   Degenerative myopia with other maculopathy, bilateral eye

H44.2E9   Degenerative myopia with other maculopathy, unspecified eye

√5ᵗʰ H44.3 Other and unspecified degenerative disorders of globe

H44.30   Unspecified degenerative disorder of globe

√6ᵗʰ H44.31 Chalcosis

H44.311   Chalcosis, right eye

H44.312   Chalcosis, left eye

H44.313   Chalcosis, bilateral

H44.319   Chalcosis, unspecified eye

√6ᵗʰ H44.32 Siderosis of eye

DEF: Iron pigment deposits within tissue of the eyeball caused by high iron content of the blood. Symptoms include cataracts, rust-colored anterior subcapsular deposits, iris heterochromia, pupillary mydriasis, and depressed electroretinogram amplitudes.

H44.321   Siderosis of eye, right eye

H44.322   Siderosis of eye, left eye

H44.323   Siderosis of eye, bilateral

H44.329   Siderosis of eye, unspecified eye

√6ᵗʰ H44.39 Other degenerative disorders of globe

H44.391   Other degenerative disorders of globe, right eye

H44.392   Other degenerative disorders of globe, left eye

H44.393   Other degenerative disorders of globe, bilateral

H44.399   Other degenerative disorders of globe, unspecified eye

√5ᵗʰ H44.4 Hypotony of eye

H44.40   Unspecified hypotony of eye

√6ᵗʰ H44.41 Flat anterior chamber hypotony of eye

H44.411   Flat anterior chamber hypotony of right eye

H44.412   Flat anterior chamber hypotony of left eye

H44.413   Flat anterior chamber hypotony of eye, bilateral

H44.419   Flat anterior chamber hypotony of unspecified eye

√6ᵗʰ H44.42 Hypotony of eye due to ocular fistula

H44.421   Hypotony of right eye due to ocular fistula

H44.422   Hypotony of left eye due to ocular fistula

H44.423   Hypotony of eye due to ocular fistula, bilateral

H44.429   Hypotony of unspecified eye due to ocular fistula

√6ᵗʰ H44.43 Hypotony of eye due to other ocular disorders

H44.431   Hypotony of eye due to other ocular disorders, right eye

H44.432   Hypotony of eye due to other ocular disorders, left eye

H44.433   Hypotony of eye due to other ocular disorders, bilateral

H44.439   Hypotony of eye due to other ocular disorders, unspecified eye

√6ᵗʰ H44.44 Primary hypotony of eye

H44.441   Primary hypotony of right eye

H44.442   Primary hypotony of left eye

H44.443   Primary hypotony of eye, bilateral

H44.449   Primary hypotony of unspecified eye

N Newborn: 0   P Pediatric: 0-17   M Maternity: 12-55   A Adult: 15-124   MCC Major Complication/Comorbidity   CC Complication/Comorbidity   SW Severe Wound Dx

610   ICD-10-CM 2019

H44.5 Degenerated conditions of globe
- H44.50 Unspecified degenerated conditions of globe
- H44.51 Absolute glaucoma
  - H44.511 Absolute glaucoma, right eye
  - H44.512 Absolute glaucoma, left eye
  - H44.513 Absolute glaucoma, bilateral
  - H44.519 Absolute glaucoma, unspecified eye
- H44.52 Atrophy of globe
  - Phthisis bulbi
  - H44.521 Atrophy of globe, right eye
  - H44.522 Atrophy of globe, left eye
  - H44.523 Atrophy of globe, bilateral
  - H44.529 Atrophy of globe, unspecified eye
- H44.53 Leucocoria
  - H44.531 Leucocoria, right eye
  - H44.532 Leucocoria, left eye
  - H44.533 Leucocoria, bilateral
  - H44.539 Leucocoria, unspecified eye

H44.6 Retained (old) intraocular foreign body, magnetic
Use additional code to identify magnetic foreign body (Z18.11)
EXCLUDES 1 current intraocular foreign body (S05.-)
EXCLUDES 2 retained foreign body in eyelid (H02.81-)
retained (old) foreign body following penetrating wound of orbit (H05.5-)
retained (old) intraocular foreign body, nonmagnetic (H44.7-)
- H44.60 Unspecified retained (old) intraocular foreign body, magnetic
  - H44.601 Unspecified retained (old) intraocular foreign body, magnetic, right eye
  - H44.602 Unspecified retained (old) intraocular foreign body, magnetic, left eye
  - H44.603 Unspecified retained (old) intraocular foreign body, magnetic, bilateral
  - H44.609 Unspecified retained (old) intraocular foreign body, magnetic, unspecified eye
- H44.61 Retained (old) magnetic foreign body in anterior chamber
  - H44.611 Retained (old) magnetic foreign body in anterior chamber, right eye
  - H44.612 Retained (old) magnetic foreign body in anterior chamber, left eye
  - H44.613 Retained (old) magnetic foreign body in anterior chamber, bilateral
  - H44.619 Retained (old) magnetic foreign body in anterior chamber, unspecified eye
- H44.62 Retained (old) magnetic foreign body in iris or ciliary body
  - H44.621 Retained (old) magnetic foreign body in iris or ciliary body, right eye
  - H44.622 Retained (old) magnetic foreign body in iris or ciliary body, left eye
  - H44.623 Retained (old) magnetic foreign body in iris or ciliary body, bilateral
  - H44.629 Retained (old) magnetic foreign body in iris or ciliary body, unspecified eye
- H44.63 Retained (old) magnetic foreign body in lens
  - H44.631 Retained (old) magnetic foreign body in lens, right eye
  - H44.632 Retained (old) magnetic foreign body in lens, left eye
  - H44.633 Retained (old) magnetic foreign body in lens, bilateral
  - H44.639 Retained (old) magnetic foreign body in lens, unspecified eye
- H44.64 Retained (old) magnetic foreign body in posterior wall of globe
  - H44.641 Retained (old) magnetic foreign body in posterior wall of globe, right eye
  - H44.642 Retained (old) magnetic foreign body in posterior wall of globe, left eye
  - H44.643 Retained (old) magnetic foreign body in posterior wall of globe, bilateral
  - H44.649 Retained (old) magnetic foreign body in posterior wall of globe, unspecified eye

- H44.65 Retained (old) magnetic foreign body in vitreous body
  - H44.651 Retained (old) magnetic foreign body in vitreous body, right eye
  - H44.652 Retained (old) magnetic foreign body in vitreous body, left eye
  - H44.653 Retained (old) magnetic foreign body in vitreous body, bilateral
  - H44.659 Retained (old) magnetic foreign body in vitreous body, unspecified eye
- H44.69 Retained (old) intraocular foreign body, magnetic, in other or multiple sites
  - H44.691 Retained (old) intraocular foreign body, magnetic, in other or multiple sites, right eye
  - H44.692 Retained (old) intraocular foreign body, magnetic, in other or multiple sites, left eye
  - H44.693 Retained (old) intraocular foreign body, magnetic, in other or multiple sites, bilateral
  - H44.699 Retained (old) intraocular foreign body, magnetic, in other or multiple sites, unspecified eye

H44.7 Retained (old) intraocular foreign body, nonmagnetic
Use additional code to identify nonmagnetic foreign body (Z18.01-Z18.10, Z18.12, Z18.2-Z18.9)
EXCLUDES 1 current intraocular foreign body (S05.-)
EXCLUDES 2 retained foreign body in eyelid (H02.81-)
retained (old) foreign body following penetrating wound of orbit (H05.5-)
retained (old) intraocular foreign body, magnetic (H44.6-)
- H44.70 Unspecified retained (old) intraocular foreign body, nonmagnetic
  - H44.701 Unspecified retained (old) intraocular foreign body, nonmagnetic, right eye
  - H44.702 Unspecified retained (old) intraocular foreign body, nonmagnetic, left eye
  - H44.703 Unspecified retained (old) intraocular foreign body, nonmagnetic, bilateral
  - H44.709 Unspecified retained (old) intraocular foreign body, nonmagnetic, unspecified eye
    - Retained (old) intraocular foreign body NOS
- H44.71 Retained (nonmagnetic) (old) foreign body in anterior chamber
  - H44.711 Retained (nonmagnetic) (old) foreign body in anterior chamber, right eye
  - H44.712 Retained (nonmagnetic) (old) foreign body in anterior chamber, left eye
  - H44.713 Retained (nonmagnetic) (old) foreign body in anterior chamber, bilateral
  - H44.719 Retained (nonmagnetic) (old) foreign body in anterior chamber, unspecified eye
- H44.72 Retained (nonmagnetic) (old) foreign body in iris or ciliary body
  - H44.721 Retained (nonmagnetic) (old) foreign body in iris or ciliary body, right eye
  - H44.722 Retained (nonmagnetic) (old) foreign body in iris or ciliary body, left eye
  - H44.723 Retained (nonmagnetic) (old) foreign body in iris or ciliary body, bilateral
  - H44.729 Retained (nonmagnetic) (old) foreign body in iris or ciliary body, unspecified eye
- H44.73 Retained (nonmagnetic) (old) foreign body in lens
  - H44.731 Retained (nonmagnetic) (old) foreign body in lens, right eye
  - H44.732 Retained (nonmagnetic) (old) foreign body in lens, left eye
  - H44.733 Retained (nonmagnetic) (old) foreign body in lens, bilateral
  - H44.739 Retained (nonmagnetic) (old) foreign body in lens, unspecified eye
- H44.74 Retained (nonmagnetic) (old) foreign body in posterior wall of globe
  - H44.741 Retained (nonmagnetic) (old) foreign body in posterior wall of globe, right eye

    H44.742 Retained (nonmagnetic) (old) foreign body in posterior wall of globe, left eye

    H44.743 Retained (nonmagnetic) (old) foreign body in posterior wall of globe, bilateral

    H44.749 Retained (nonmagnetic) (old) foreign body in posterior wall of globe, unspecified eye

✓6ᵗʰ **H44.75** Retained (nonmagnetic) (old) foreign body in vitreous body

    H44.751 Retained (nonmagnetic) (old) foreign body in vitreous body, right eye

    H44.752 Retained (nonmagnetic) (old) foreign body in vitreous body, left eye

    H44.753 Retained (nonmagnetic) (old) foreign body in vitreous body, bilateral

    H44.759 Retained (nonmagnetic) (old) foreign body in vitreous body, unspecified eye

✓6ᵗʰ **H44.79** Retained (old) intraocular foreign body, nonmagnetic, in other or multiple sites

    H44.791 Retained (old) intraocular foreign body, nonmagnetic, in other or multiple sites, right eye

    H44.792 Retained (old) intraocular foreign body, nonmagnetic, in other or multiple sites, left eye

    H44.793 Retained (old) intraocular foreign body, nonmagnetic, in other or multiple sites, bilateral

    H44.799 Retained (old) intraocular foreign body, nonmagnetic, in other or multiple sites, unspecified eye

✓5ᵗʰ **H44.8** Other disorders of globe

  ✓6ᵗʰ **H44.81** Hemophthalmos

    DEF: Pool of blood within the eyeball, not from a current injury.

    H44.811 Hemophthalmos, right eye

    H44.812 Hemophthalmos, left eye

    H44.813 Hemophthalmos, bilateral

    H44.819 Hemophthalmos, unspecified eye

  ✓6ᵗʰ **H44.82** Luxation of globe

    H44.821 Luxation of globe, right eye

    H44.822 Luxation of globe, left eye

    H44.823 Luxation of globe, bilateral

    H44.829 Luxation of globe, unspecified eye

  H44.89 Other disorders of globe

H44.9 Unspecified disorder of globe

Disorders of optic nerve and visual pathways (H46-H47)

✓4ᵗʰ **H46** Optic neuritis

  EXCLUDES 2   ischemic optic neuropathy (H47.01-)
             neuromyelitis optica [Devic] (G36.0)

  CC Excl: For CC codes in category H46: PDX collection 633

  ✓5ᵗʰ **H46.0** Optic papillitis

    H46.00 Optic papillitis, unspecified eye   CC

    H46.01 Optic papillitis, right eye   CC

    H46.02 Optic papillitis, left eye   CC

    H46.03 Optic papillitis, bilateral   CC

  ✓5ᵗʰ **H46.1** Retrobulbar neuritis

    Retrobulbar neuritis NOS

    EXCLUDES 1   syphilitic retrobulbar neuritis (A52.15)

    H46.10 Retrobulbar neuritis, unspecified eye   CC

    H46.11 Retrobulbar neuritis, right eye   CC

    H46.12 Retrobulbar neuritis, left eye   CC

    H46.13 Retrobulbar neuritis, bilateral   CC

  H46.2 Nutritional optic neuropathy

  H46.3 Toxic optic neuropathy

    Code first (T51-T65) to identify cause

  H46.8 Other optic neuritis   CC

  H46.9 Unspecified optic neuritis   CC

✓4ᵗʰ **H47** Other disorders of optic [2nd] nerve and visual pathways

  ✓5ᵗʰ **H47.0** Disorders of optic nerve, not elsewhere classified

    ✓6ᵗʰ **H47.01** Ischemic optic neuropathy

      H47.011 Ischemic optic neuropathy, right eye

      H47.012 Ischemic optic neuropathy, left eye

      H47.013 Ischemic optic neuropathy, bilateral

      H47.019 Ischemic optic neuropathy, unspecified eye

    ✓6ᵗʰ **H47.02** Hemorrhage in optic nerve sheath

      H47.021 Hemorrhage in optic nerve sheath, right eye

      H47.022 Hemorrhage in optic nerve sheath, left eye

      H47.023 Hemorrhage in optic nerve sheath, bilateral

      H47.029 Hemorrhage in optic nerve sheath, unspecified eye

    ✓6ᵗʰ **H47.03** Optic nerve hypoplasia

      H47.031 Optic nerve hypoplasia, right eye

      H47.032 Optic nerve hypoplasia, left eye

      H47.033 Optic nerve hypoplasia, bilateral

      H47.039 Optic nerve hypoplasia, unspecified eye

    ✓6ᵗʰ **H47.09** Other disorders of optic nerve, not elsewhere classified

      Compression of optic nerve

      H47.091 Other disorders of optic nerve, not elsewhere classified, right eye

      H47.092 Other disorders of optic nerve, not elsewhere classified, left eye

      H47.093 Other disorders of optic nerve, not elsewhere classified, bilateral

      H47.099 Other disorders of optic nerve, not elsewhere classified, unspecified eye

  ✓5ᵗʰ **H47.1** Papilledema

    DEF: Swelling of the optic papilla, the raised area connected to the optic disk made up of nerves that enter the eyeball. It may be caused by increased intracranial pressure, decreased ocular pressure, or a retinal disorder.

    H47.10 Unspecified papilledema   CC

      CC Excl: PDX collection 634

    H47.11 Papilledema associated with increased intracranial pressure   CC

      CC Excl: PDX collection 634

    H47.12 Papilledema associated with decreased ocular pressure

    H47.13 Papilledema associated with retinal disorder

    ✓6ᵗʰ **H47.14** Foster-Kennedy syndrome

      H47.141 Foster-Kennedy syndrome, right eye

      H47.142 Foster-Kennedy syndrome, left eye

      H47.143 Foster-Kennedy syndrome, bilateral

      H47.149 Foster-Kennedy syndrome, unspecified eye

  ✓5ᵗʰ **H47.2** Optic atrophy

    H47.20 Unspecified optic atrophy

    ✓6ᵗʰ **H47.21** Primary optic atrophy

      H47.211 Primary optic atrophy, right eye

      H47.212 Primary optic atrophy, left eye

      H47.213 Primary optic atrophy, bilateral

      H47.219 Primary optic atrophy, unspecified eye

    H47.22 Hereditary optic atrophy

      Leber's optic atrophy

    ✓6ᵗʰ **H47.23** Glaucomatous optic atrophy

      H47.231 Glaucomatous optic atrophy, right eye

      H47.232 Glaucomatous optic atrophy, left eye

      H47.233 Glaucomatous optic atrophy, bilateral

      H47.239 Glaucomatous optic atrophy, unspecified eye

    ✓6ᵗʰ **H47.29** Other optic atrophy

      Temporal pallor of optic disc

      H47.291 Other optic atrophy, right eye

      H47.292 Other optic atrophy, left eye

      H47.293 Other optic atrophy, bilateral

      H47.299 Other optic atrophy, unspecified eye

  ✓5ᵗʰ **H47.3** Other disorders of optic disc

    ✓6ᵗʰ **H47.31** Coloboma of optic disc

      H47.311 Coloboma of optic disc, right eye

      H47.312 Coloboma of optic disc, left eye

      H47.313 Coloboma of optic disc, bilateral

      H47.319 Coloboma of optic disc, unspecified eye

N Newborn: 0   P Pediatric: 0-17   M Maternity: 12-55   A Adult: 15-124   MCC Major Complication/Comorbidity   CC Complication/Comorbidity   SW Severe Wound Dx

612   ICD-10-CM 2019

✓6th **H47.32** Drusen of optic disc
     H47.321   Drusen of optic disc, right eye
     H47.322   Drusen of optic disc, left eye
     H47.323   Drusen of optic disc, bilateral
     H47.329   Drusen of optic disc, unspecified eye

✓6th **H47.33** Pseudopapilledema of optic disc
     H47.331   Pseudopapilledema of optic disc, right eye
     H47.332   Pseudopapilledema of optic disc, left eye
     H47.333   Pseudopapilledema of optic disc, bilateral
     H47.339   Pseudopapilledema of optic disc, unspecified eye

✓6th **H47.39** Other disorders of optic disc
     H47.391   Other disorders of optic disc, right eye
     H47.392   Other disorders of optic disc, left eye
     H47.393   Other disorders of optic disc, bilateral
     H47.399   Other disorders of optic disc, unspecified eye

✓5th **H47.4** **Disorders of optic chiasm**
     Code also underlying condition

> **CC Excl: For CC codes in subcategory H47.4:**
> PDX collection 635

     H47.41   Disorders of optic chiasm in (due to) inflammatory disorders   `CC`
     H47.42   Disorders of optic chiasm in (due to) neoplasm   `CC`
     H47.43   Disorders of optic chiasm in (due to) vascular disorders   `CC`
     H47.49   Disorders of optic chiasm in (due to) other disorders   `CC`

✓5th **H47.5** **Disorders of other visual pathways**
     Disorders of optic tracts, geniculate nuclei and optic radiations
     Code also underlying condition

> **CC Excl: For CC codes in subcategory H47.5:**
> PDX collection 635

✓6th **H47.51** Disorders of visual pathways in (due to) inflammatory disorders
     H47.511   Disorders of visual pathways in (due to) inflammatory disorders, right side   `CC`
     H47.512   Disorders of visual pathways in (due to) inflammatory disorders, left side   `CC`
     H47.519   Disorders of visual pathways in (due to) inflammatory disorders, unspecified side   `CC`

✓6th **H47.52** Disorders of visual pathways in (due to) neoplasm
     H47.521   Disorders of visual pathways in (due to) neoplasm, right side   `CC`
     H47.522   Disorders of visual pathways in (due to) neoplasm, left side   `CC`
     H47.529   Disorders of visual pathways in (due to) neoplasm, unspecified side   `CC`

✓6th **H47.53** Disorders of visual pathways in (due to) vascular disorders
     H47.531   Disorders of visual pathways in (due to) vascular disorders, right side   `CC`
     H47.532   Disorders of visual pathways in (due to) vascular disorders, left side   `CC`
     H47.539   Disorders of visual pathways in (due to) vascular disorders, unspecified side   `CC`

✓5th **H47.6** **Disorders of visual cortex**
     Code also underlying condition
     EXCLUDES 1   injury to visual cortex S04.04

> **CC Excl: For CC codes in subcategory H47.6:**
> PDX collection 636

✓6th **H47.61** Cortical blindness
     H47.611   Cortical blindness, right side of brain
     H47.612   Cortical blindness, left side of brain
     H47.619   Cortical blindness, unspecified side of brain

✓6th **H47.62** Disorders of visual cortex in (due to) inflammatory disorders
     H47.621   Disorders of visual cortex in (due to) inflammatory disorders, right side of brain   `CC`
     H47.622   Disorders of visual cortex in (due to) inflammatory disorders, left side of brain   `CC`
     H47.629   Disorders of visual cortex in (due to) inflammatory disorders, unspecified side of brain   `CC`

✓6th **H47.63** Disorders of visual cortex in (due to) neoplasm
     H47.631   Disorders of visual cortex in (due to) neoplasm, right side of brain   `CC`
     H47.632   Disorders of visual cortex in (due to) neoplasm, left side of brain   `CC`
     H47.639   Disorders of visual cortex in (due to) neoplasm, unspecified side of brain   `CC`

✓6th **H47.64** Disorders of visual cortex in (due to) vascular disorders
     H47.641   Disorders of visual cortex in (due to) vascular disorders, right side of brain   `CC`
     H47.642   Disorders of visual cortex in (due to) vascular disorders, left side of brain   `CC`
     H47.649   Disorders of visual cortex in (due to) vascular disorders, unspecified side of brain   `CC`

H47.9   Unspecified disorder of visual pathways

Disorders of ocular muscles, binocular movement, accommodation and refraction (H49-H52)
     EXCLUDES 2   nystagmus and other irregular eye movements (H55)

✓4th **H49** **Paralytic strabismus**
     EXCLUDES 2   internal ophthalmoplegia (H52.51-)
                 internuclear ophthalmoplegia (H51.2-)
                 progressive supranuclear ophthalmoplegia (G23.1)
     DEF: Strabismus: Misalignment of the eyes with the inability to move and focus in the same direction due to conditions affecting the muscles controlling them.

✓5th **H49.0** Third [oculomotor] nerve palsy
     H49.00   Third [oculomotor] nerve palsy, unspecified eye
     H49.01   Third [oculomotor] nerve palsy, right eye
     H49.02   Third [oculomotor] nerve palsy, left eye
     H49.03   Third [oculomotor] nerve palsy, bilateral

✓5th **H49.1** Fourth [trochlear] nerve palsy
     H49.10   Fourth [trochlear] nerve palsy, unspecified eye
     H49.11   Fourth [trochlear] nerve palsy, right eye
     H49.12   Fourth [trochlear] nerve palsy, left eye
     H49.13   Fourth [trochlear] nerve palsy, bilateral

✓5th **H49.2** Sixth [abducent] nerve palsy
     H49.20   Sixth [abducent] nerve palsy, unspecified eye
     H49.21   Sixth [abducent] nerve palsy, right eye
     H49.22   Sixth [abducent] nerve palsy, left eye
     H49.23   Sixth [abducent] nerve palsy, bilateral

✓5th **H49.3** Total (external) ophthalmoplegia
     H49.30   Total (external) ophthalmoplegia, unspecified eye
     H49.31   Total (external) ophthalmoplegia, right eye
     H49.32   Total (external) ophthalmoplegia, left eye
     H49.33   Total (external) ophthalmoplegia, bilateral

✓5th **H49.4** Progressive external ophthalmoplegia
     EXCLUDES 1   Kearns-Sayre syndrome (H49.81-)
     H49.40   Progressive external ophthalmoplegia, unspecified eye
     H49.41   Progressive external ophthalmoplegia, right eye
     H49.42   Progressive external ophthalmoplegia, left eye
     H49.43   Progressive external ophthalmoplegia, bilateral

---

✔ Additional Character Required   ✓x7th Placeholder   Unacceptable PDx   Questionable PDx   Manifestation   **H1**-**H14** HAC   **HCC** CMS-HCC Dx   **HIV** HIV Dx

✓5th **H49.8 Other paralytic strabismus**

  ✓6th **H49.81 Kearns-Sayre syndrome**
      Progressive external ophthalmoplegia with pigmentary retinopathy
      Use additional code for other manifestation, such as: heart block (I45.9)

      CC Excl: For CC codes in subcategory H49.81: PDX collection 545

      H49.811 **Kearns-Sayre syndrome, right eye** `CC` `HCC`
      H49.812 **Kearns-Sayre syndrome, left eye** `CC` `HCC`
      H49.813 **Kearns-Sayre syndrome, bilateral** `CC` `HCC`
      H49.819 **Kearns-Sayre syndrome, unspecified eye** `CC` `HCC`

  ✓6th **H49.88 Other paralytic strabismus**
      External ophthalmoplegia NOS
      H49.881 **Other paralytic strabismus, right eye**
      H49.882 **Other paralytic strabismus, left eye**
      H49.883 **Other paralytic strabismus, bilateral**
      H49.889 **Other paralytic strabismus, unspecified eye**

H49.9 Unspecified paralytic strabismus

✓4th **H50 Other strabismus**
  DEF: Strabismus: Misalignment of the eyes with the inability to move and focus in the same direction due to conditions affecting the muscles controlling them.

  ✓5th **H50.0 Esotropia**
    Convergent concomitant strabismus
    EXCLUDES 1 *intermittent esotropia (H50.31-, H50.32)*

    H50.00 **Unspecified esotropia**

    ✓6th **H50.01 Monocular esotropia**
      H50.011 **Monocular esotropia, right eye**
      H50.012 **Monocular esotropia, left eye**

    ✓6th **H50.02 Monocular esotropia with A pattern**
      H50.021 **Monocular esotropia with A pattern, right eye**
      H50.022 **Monocular esotropia with A pattern, left eye**

    ✓6th **H50.03 Monocular esotropia with V pattern**
      H50.031 **Monocular esotropia with V pattern, right eye**
      H50.032 **Monocular esotropia with V pattern, left eye**

    ✓6th **H50.04 Monocular esotropia with other noncomitancies**
      H50.041 **Monocular esotropia with other noncomitancies, right eye**
      H50.042 **Monocular esotropia with other noncomitancies, left eye**

    H50.05 **Alternating esotropia**
    H50.06 **Alternating esotropia with A pattern**
    H50.07 **Alternating esotropia with V pattern**
    H50.08 **Alternating esotropia with other noncomitancies**

Eye Muscle Diseases

R.   L.
Monocular (one eye only) esotropia (inward)

Monocular exotropia (outward)

Monocular hypertropia (upward)

✓5th **H50.1 Exotropia**
  Divergent concomitant strabismus
  EXCLUDES 1 *intermittent exotropia (H50.33-, H50.34)*

  H50.10 **Unspecified exotropia**

  ✓6th **H50.11 Monocular exotropia**
    H50.111 **Monocular exotropia, right eye**
    H50.112 **Monocular exotropia, left eye**

  ✓6th **H50.12 Monocular exotropia with A pattern**
    H50.121 **Monocular exotropia with A pattern, right eye**
    H50.122 **Monocular exotropia with A pattern, left eye**

  ✓6th **H50.13 Monocular exotropia with V pattern**
    H50.131 **Monocular exotropia with V pattern, right eye**
    H50.132 **Monocular exotropia with V pattern, left eye**

  ✓6th **H50.14 Monocular exotropia with other noncomitancies**
    H50.141 **Monocular exotropia with other noncomitancies, right eye**
    H50.142 **Monocular exotropia with other noncomitancies, left eye**

  H50.15 **Alternating exotropia**
  H50.16 **Alternating exotropia with A pattern**
  H50.17 **Alternating exotropia with V pattern**
  H50.18 **Alternating exotropia with other noncomitancies**

✓5th **H50.2 Vertical strabismus**
  Hypertropia
  H50.21 **Vertical strabismus, right eye**
  H50.22 **Vertical strabismus, left eye**

✓5th **H50.3 Intermittent heterotropia**
  H50.30 **Unspecified intermittent heterotropia**

  ✓6th **H50.31 Intermittent monocular esotropia**
    H50.311 **Intermittent monocular esotropia, right eye**
    H50.312 **Intermittent monocular esotropia, left eye**

  H50.32 **Intermittent alternating esotropia**

  ✓6th **H50.33 Intermittent monocular exotropia**
    H50.331 **Intermittent monocular exotropia, right eye**
    H50.332 **Intermittent monocular exotropia, left eye**

  H50.34 **Intermittent alternating exotropia**

✓5th **H50.4 Other and unspecified heterotropia**
  H50.40 **Unspecified heterotropia**

  ✓6th **H50.41 Cyclotropia**
    H50.411 **Cyclotropia, right eye**
    H50.412 **Cyclotropia, left eye**

  H50.42 **Monofixation syndrome**
  H50.43 **Accommodative component in esotropia**

✓5th **H50.5 Heterophoria**
  H50.50 **Unspecified heterophoria**
  H50.51 **Esophoria**
  H50.52 **Exophoria**
  H50.53 **Vertical heterophoria**
  H50.54 **Cyclophoria**
  H50.55 **Alternating heterophoria**

✓5th **H50.6 Mechanical strabismus**
  H50.60 **Mechanical strabismus, unspecified**

  ✓6th **H50.61 Brown's sheath syndrome**
    H50.611 **Brown's sheath syndrome, right eye**
    H50.612 **Brown's sheath syndrome, left eye**

  H50.69 **Other mechanical strabismus**
    Strabismus due to adhesions
    Traumatic limitation of duction of eye muscle

✓5th **H50.8 Other specified strabismus**

  ✓6th **H50.81 Duane's syndrome**
    H50.811 **Duane's syndrome, right eye**
    H50.812 **Duane's syndrome, left eye**

  H50.89 **Other specified strabismus**

H50.9 Unspecified strabismus

N Newborn: 0   **P** Pediatric: 0-17   **M** Maternity: 12-55   **A** Adult: 15-124   **MCC** Major Complication/Comorbidity   **CC** Complication/Comorbidity   **SW** Severe Wound Dx

614   ICD-10-CM 2019

✓4ᵗʰ **H51 Other disorders of binocular movement**
    H51.0 Palsy (spasm) of conjugate gaze
    ✓5ᵗʰ **H51.1 Convergence insufficiency and excess**
        H51.11 Convergence insufficiency
        H51.12 Convergence excess
    ✓5ᵗʰ **H51.2 Internuclear ophthalmoplegia**
        H51.20 Internuclear ophthalmoplegia, unspecified eye
        H51.21 Internuclear ophthalmoplegia, right eye
        H51.22 Internuclear ophthalmoplegia, left eye
        H51.23 Internuclear ophthalmoplegia, bilateral
    H51.8 Other specified disorders of binocular movement
    H51.9 Unspecified disorder of binocular movement

✓4ᵗʰ **H52 Disorders of refraction and accommodation**
    ✓5ᵗʰ **H52.0 Hypermetropia**
        H52.00 Hypermetropia, unspecified eye
        H52.01 Hypermetropia, right eye
        H52.02 Hypermetropia, left eye
        H52.03 Hypermetropia, bilateral
    ✓5ᵗʰ **H52.1 Myopia**
        EXCLUDES 1   degenerative myopia (H44.2-)
        H52.10 Myopia, unspecified eye
        H52.11 Myopia, right eye
        H52.12 Myopia, left eye
        H52.13 Myopia, bilateral
    ✓5ᵗʰ **H52.2 Astigmatism**
        ✓6ᵗʰ **H52.20 Unspecified astigmatism**
            H52.201 Unspecified astigmatism, right eye
            H52.202 Unspecified astigmatism, left eye
            H52.203 Unspecified astigmatism, bilateral
            H52.209 Unspecified astigmatism, unspecified eye
        ✓6ᵗʰ **H52.21 Irregular astigmatism**
            H52.211 Irregular astigmatism, right eye
            H52.212 Irregular astigmatism, left eye
            H52.213 Irregular astigmatism, bilateral
            H52.219 Irregular astigmatism, unspecified eye
        ✓6ᵗʰ **H52.22 Regular astigmatism**
            H52.221 Regular astigmatism, right eye
            H52.222 Regular astigmatism, left eye
            H52.223 Regular astigmatism, bilateral
            H52.229 Regular astigmatism, unspecified eye
    ✓5ᵗʰ **H52.3 Anisometropia and aniseikonia**
        H52.31 Anisometropia
        H52.32 Aniseikonia
    H52.4 Presbyopia
    ✓5ᵗʰ **H52.5 Disorders of accommodation**
        ✓6ᵗʰ **H52.51 Internal ophthalmoplegia (complete) (total)**
            H52.511 Internal ophthalmoplegia (complete) (total), right eye
            H52.512 Internal ophthalmoplegia (complete) (total), left eye
            H52.513 Internal ophthalmoplegia (complete) (total), bilateral
            H52.519 Internal ophthalmoplegia (complete) (total), unspecified eye
        ✓6ᵗʰ **H52.52 Paresis of accommodation**
            H52.521 Paresis of accommodation, right eye
            H52.522 Paresis of accommodation, left eye
            H52.523 Paresis of accommodation, bilateral
            H52.529 Paresis of accommodation, unspecified eye
        ✓6ᵗʰ **H52.53 Spasm of accommodation**
            H52.531 Spasm of accommodation, right eye
            H52.532 Spasm of accommodation, left eye
            H52.533 Spasm of accommodation, bilateral
            H52.539 Spasm of accommodation, unspecified eye
    H52.6 Other disorders of refraction
    H52.7 Unspecified disorder of refraction

Visual disturbances and blindness (H53-H54)

✓4ᵗʰ **H53 Visual disturbances**
    ✓5ᵗʰ **H53.0 Amblyopia ex anopsia**
        EXCLUDES 1   amblyopia due to vitamin A deficiency (E50.5)
        ✓6ᵗʰ **H53.00 Unspecified amblyopia**
            H53.001 Unspecified amblyopia, right eye
            H53.002 Unspecified amblyopia, left eye
            H53.003 Unspecified amblyopia, bilateral
            H53.009 Unspecified amblyopia, unspecified eye
        ✓6ᵗʰ **H53.01 Deprivation amblyopia**
            H53.011 Deprivation amblyopia, right eye
            H53.012 Deprivation amblyopia, left eye
            H53.013 Deprivation amblyopia, bilateral
            H53.019 Deprivation amblyopia, unspecified eye
        ✓6ᵗʰ **H53.02 Refractive amblyopia**
            H53.021 Refractive amblyopia, right eye
            H53.022 Refractive amblyopia, left eye
            H53.023 Refractive amblyopia, bilateral
            H53.029 Refractive amblyopia, unspecified eye
        ✓6ᵗʰ **H53.03 Strabismic amblyopia**
            EXCLUDES 1   strabismus (H50.-)
            H53.031 Strabismic amblyopia, right eye
            H53.032 Strabismic amblyopia, left eye
            H53.033 Strabismic amblyopia, bilateral
            H53.039 Strabismic amblyopia, unspecified eye
        ✓6ᵗʰ **H53.04 Amblyopia suspect**
            AHA: 2016, 4Q, 22-23
            H53.041 Amblyopia suspect, right eye
            H53.042 Amblyopia suspect, left eye
            H53.043 Amblyopia suspect, bilateral
            H53.049 Amblyopia suspect, unspecified eye
    ✓5ᵗʰ **H53.1 Subjective visual disturbances**
        EXCLUDES 1   subjective visual disturbances due to vitamin A deficiency (E50.5)
                 visual hallucinations (R44.1)

        CC Excl: For CC codes in subcategory H53.1:
        PDX collection 637

        H53.10 Unspecified subjective visual disturbances
        H53.11 Day blindness
            Hemeralopia
        ✓6ᵗʰ **H53.12 Transient visual loss**
            Scintillating scotoma
            EXCLUDES 1   amaurosis fugax (G45.3-)
                      transient retinal artery occlusion (H34.0-)
            H53.121 Transient visual loss, right eye   CC
            H53.122 Transient visual loss, left eye   CC
            H53.123 Transient visual loss, bilateral   CC
            H53.129 Transient visual loss, unspecified eye   CC
        ✓6ᵗʰ **H53.13 Sudden visual loss**
            H53.131 Sudden visual loss, right eye   CC
            H53.132 Sudden visual loss, left eye   CC
            H53.133 Sudden visual loss, bilateral   CC
            H53.139 Sudden visual loss, unspecified eye   CC
        ✓6ᵗʰ **H53.14 Visual discomfort**
            Asthenopia
            Photophobia
            H53.141 Visual discomfort, right eye
            H53.142 Visual discomfort, left eye
            H53.143 Visual discomfort, bilateral
            H53.149 Visual discomfort, unspecified
        H53.15 Visual distortions of shape and size
            Metamorphopsia
        H53.16 Psychophysical visual disturbances
        H53.19 Other subjective visual disturbances
            Visual halos
    H53.2 Diplopia
        Double vision
    ✓5ᵗʰ **H53.3 Other and unspecified disorders of binocular vision**
        H53.30 Unspecified disorder of binocular vision
        H53.31 Abnormal retinal correspondence
        H53.32 Fusion with defective stereopsis
        H53.33 Simultaneous visual perception without fusion

✓Additional Character Required   ✓x7ᵗʰ Placeholder   Unacceptable PDx   Questionable PDx   Manifestation   H1-H14 HAC   HCC CMS-HCC Dx   HIV HIV Dx

ICD-10-CM 2019   615

Chapter 7. Diseases of the Eye and Adnexa

H51–H53.33

H53.34 **Suppression of binocular vision**

✓5ᵗʰ **H53.4 Visual field defects**

H53.40 **Unspecified visual field defects**

✓6ᵗʰ H53.41 **Scotoma involving central area**
Central scotoma

     H53.411 **Scotoma involving central area, right eye**

     H53.412 **Scotoma involving central area, left eye**

     H53.413 **Scotoma involving central area, bilateral**

     H53.419 **Scotoma involving central area, unspecified eye**

✓6ᵗʰ H53.42 **Scotoma of blind spot area**
Enlarged blind spot

     H53.421 **Scotoma of blind spot area, right eye**

     H53.422 **Scotoma of blind spot area, left eye**

     H53.423 **Scotoma of blind spot area, bilateral**

     H53.429 **Scotoma of blind spot area, unspecified eye**

✓6ᵗʰ H53.43 **Sector or arcuate defects**
Arcuate scotoma
Bjerrum scotoma

     H53.431 **Sector or arcuate defects, right eye**

     H53.432 **Sector or arcuate defects, left eye**

     H53.433 **Sector or arcuate defects, bilateral**

     H53.439 **Sector or arcuate defects, unspecified eye**

✓6ᵗʰ H53.45 **Other localized visual field defect**
Peripheral visual field defect
Ring scotoma NOS
Scotoma NOS

     H53.451 **Other localized visual field defect, right eye**

     H53.452 **Other localized visual field defect, left eye**

     H53.453 **Other localized visual field defect, bilateral**

     H53.459 **Other localized visual field defect, unspecified eye**

✓6ᵗʰ H53.46 **Homonymous bilateral field defects**
Homonymous hemianopia
Homonymous hemianopsia
Quadrant anopia
Quadrant anopsia

     H53.461 **Homonymous bilateral field defects, right side**

     H53.462 **Homonymous bilateral field defects, left side**

     H53.469 **Homonymous bilateral field defects, unspecified side**
Homonymous bilateral field defects NOS

H53.47 **Heteronymous bilateral field defects**
Heteronymous hemianop(s)ia

✓6ᵗʰ H53.48 **Generalized contraction of visual field**

     H53.481 **Generalized contraction of visual field, right eye**

     H53.482 **Generalized contraction of visual field, left eye**

     H53.483 **Generalized contraction of visual field, bilateral**

     H53.489 **Generalized contraction of visual field, unspecified eye**

✓5ᵗʰ **H53.5 Color vision deficiencies**
Color blindness
EXCLUDES 2 *day blindness (H53.11)*

H53.50 **Unspecified color vision deficiencies**
Color blindness NOS

H53.51 **Achromatopsia**
DEF: Nonprogressive genetic visual disorder characterized by complete color blindness, decreased vision, and light sensitivity.

H53.52 **Acquired color vision deficiency**

H53.53 **Deuteranomaly**
Deuteranopia
DEF: Male-only genetic disorder causing difficulty in distinguishing green and red; no shortened spectrum.

H53.54 **Protanomaly**
Protanopia

H53.55 **Tritanomaly**
Tritanopia

H53.59 **Other color vision deficiencies**

✓5ᵗʰ **H53.6 Night blindness**
EXCLUDES 1 *night blindness due to vitamin A deficiency (E50.5)*

H53.60 **Unspecified night blindness**

H53.61 **Abnormal dark adaptation curve**

H53.62 **Acquired night blindness**

H53.63 **Congenital night blindness**

H53.69 **Other night blindness**

✓5ᵗʰ **H53.7 Vision sensitivity deficiencies**

H53.71 **Glare sensitivity**

H53.72 **Impaired contrast sensitivity**

H53.8 **Other visual disturbances**

H53.9 **Unspecified visual disturbance**

✓4ᵗʰ **H54 Blindness and low vision**
NOTE For definition of visual impairment categories see table below
Code first any associated underlying cause of the blindness
EXCLUDES 1 *amaurosis fugax (G45.3)*
AHA: 2017, 4Q, 11-12

✓5ᵗʰ **H54.0 Blindness, both eyes**
Visual impairment categories 3, 4, 5 in both eyes.

✓6ᵗʰ H54.0X **Blindness, both eyes, different category levels**

✓7ᵗʰ H54.0X3 **Blindness right eye, category 3**

     H54.0X33 **Blindness right eye category 3, blindness left eye category 3**

     H54.0X34 **Blindness right eye category 3, blindness left eye category 4**

     H54.0X35 **Blindness right eye category 3, blindness left eye category 5**

✓7ᵗʰ H54.0X4 **Blindness right eye, category 4**

     H54.0X43 **Blindness right eye category 4, blindness left eye category 3**

     H54.0X44 **Blindness right eye category 4, blindness left eye category 4**

     H54.0X45 **Blindness right eye category 4, blindness left eye category 5**

✓7ᵗʰ H54.0X5 **Blindness right eye, category 5**

     H54.0X53 **Blindness right eye category 5, blindness left eye category 3**

     H54.0X54 **Blindness right eye category 5, blindness left eye category 4**

     H54.0X55 **Blindness right eye category 5, blindness left eye category 5**

✓5ᵗʰ **H54.1 Blindness, one eye, low vision other eye**
Visual impairment categories 3, 4, 5 in one eye, with categories 1 or 2 in the other eye.

H54.10 **Blindness, one eye, low vision other eye, unspecified eyes**

✓6ᵗʰ H54.11 **Blindness, right eye, low vision left eye**

✓7ᵗʰ H54.113 **Blindness right eye category 3, low vision left eye**

     H54.1131 **Blindness right eye category 3, low vision left eye category 1**

     H54.1132 **Blindness right eye category 3, low vision left eye category 2**

✓7ᵗʰ H54.114 **Blindness right eye category 4, low vision left eye**

     H54.1141 **Blindness right eye category 4, low vision left eye category 1**

     H54.1142 **Blindness right eye category 4, low vision left eye category 2**

✓7ᵗʰ H54.115 **Blindness right eye category 5, low vision left eye**

     H54.1151 **Blindness right eye category 5, low vision left eye category 1**

     H54.1152 **Blindness right eye category 5, low vision left eye category 2**

N Newborn: 0   P Pediatric: 0-17   M Maternity: 12-55   A Adult: 15-124   MCC Major Complication/Comorbidity   CC Complication/Comorbidity   SW Severe Wound Dx

616   ICD-10-CM 2019

✓6ᵗʰ **H54.12**   Blindness, left, low vision right eye

    ✓7ᵗʰ **H54.121**   Low vision right eye category 1, blindness left eye

      H54.1213   Low vision right eye category 1, blindness left eye category 3

      H54.1214   Low vision right eye category 1, blindness left eye category 4

      H54.1215   Low vision right eye category 1, blindness left eye category 5

    ✓7ᵗʰ **H54.122**   Low vision right eye category 2, blindness left eye

      H54.1223   Low vision right eye category 2, blindness left eye category 3

      H54.1224   Low vision right eye category 2, blindness left eye category 4

      H54.1225   Low vision right eye category 2, blindness left eye category 5

✓5ᵗʰ **H54.2**   Low vision, both eyes

    Visual impairment categories 1 or 2 in both eyes.

    ✓6ᵗʰ **H54.2X**   Low vision, both eyes, different category levels

      ✓7ᵗʰ **H54.2X1**   Low vision, right eye, category 1

        H54.2X11   Low vision right eye category 1, low vision left eye category 1

        H54.2X12   Low vision right eye category 1, low vision left eye category 2

      ✓7ᵗʰ **H54.2X2**   Low vision, right eye, category 2

        H54.2X21   Low vision right eye category 2, low vision left eye category 1

        H54.2X22   Low vision right eye category 2, low vision left eye category 2

H54.3   Unqualified visual loss, both eyes

    Visual impairment category 9 in both eyes.

    TIP: Assign only when both eyes are documented as affected by blindness or low vision but the visual impairment category is not documented.

✓5ᵗʰ **H54.4**   Blindness, one eye

    Visual impairment categories 3, 4, 5 in one eye [normal vision in other eye].

    H54.40   Blindness, one eye, unspecified eye

    ✓6ᵗʰ **H54.41**   Blindness, right eye, normal vision left eye

      ✓7ᵗʰ **H54.413**   Blindness, right eye, category 3

        H54.413A   Blindness right eye category 3, normal vision left eye

      ✓7ᵗʰ **H54.414**   Blindness, right eye, category 4

        H54.414A   Blindness right eye category 4, normal vision left eye

      ✓7ᵗʰ **H54.415**   Blindness, right eye, category 5

        H54.415A   Blindness right eye category 5, normal vision left eye

    ✓6ᵗʰ **H54.42**   Blindness, left eye, normal vision right eye

      ✓7ᵗʰ **H54.42A**   Blindness, left eye, category 3-5

        H54.42A3   Blindness left eye category 3, normal vision right eye

        H54.42A4   Blindness left eye category 4, normal vision right eye

        H54.42A5   Blindness left eye category 5, normal vision right eye

✓5ᵗʰ **H54.5**   Low vision, one eye

    Visual impairment categories 1 or 2 in one eye [normal vision in other eye].

    H54.50   Low vision, one eye, unspecified eye

    ✓6ᵗʰ **H54.51**   Low vision, right eye, normal vision left eye

      ✓7ᵗʰ **H54.511**   Low vision, right eye, category 1-2

        H54.511A   Low vision right eye category 1, normal vision left eye

        H54.512A   Low vision right eye category 2, normal vision left eye

    ✓6ᵗʰ **H54.52**   Low vision, left eye, normal vision right eye

      ✓7ᵗʰ **H54.52A**   Low vision, left eye, category 1-2

        H54.52A1   Low vision left eye category 1, normal vision right eye

        H54.52A2   Low vision left eye category 2, normal vision right eye

✓5ᵗʰ **H54.6**   Unqualified visual loss, one eye

    Visual impairment category 9 in one eye [normal vision in other eye].

    TIP: Assign a code from this category only when one eye is documented as affected by blindness or low vision but the visual impairment category is not documented.

    H54.60   Unqualified visual loss, one eye, unspecified

    H54.61   Unqualified visual loss, right eye, normal vision left eye

    H54.62   Unqualified visual loss, left eye, normal vision right eye

H54.7   Unspecified visual loss

    Visual impairment category 9 NOS

    TIP: Assign only when documentation notes blindness, visual loss, or low vision but does not specify whether one or both eyes are affected and the visual impairment category is not documented.

H54.8   Legal blindness, as defined in USA

    Blindness NOS according to USA definition

    EXCLUDES 1   legal blindness with specification of impairment level (H54.0-H54.7)

NOTE   The table below gives a classification of severity of visual impairment recommended by a WHO Study Group on the Prevention of Blindness, Geneva, 6-10 November 1972.

The term "low vision" in category H54 comprises categories 1 and 2 of the table, the term "blindness" categories 3, 4 and 5, and the term "unqualified visual loss" category 9.

If the extent of the visual field is taken into account, patients with a field no greater than 10 but greater than 5 around central fixation should be placed in category 3 and patients with a field no greater than 5 around central fixation should be placed in category 4, even if the central acuity is not impaired.

Category of visual impairment	Visual acuity with best possible correction	
	Maximum less than:	**Minimum equal to or better than:**
1	6/18 3/10 (0.3) 20/70	6/60 1/10 (0.1) 20/200
2	6/60 1/10 (0.1) 20/200	3/60 1/20 (0.05) 20/400
3	3/60 1/20 (0.05) 20/400	1/60 (finger counting at one meter) 1/50 (0.02) 5/300 (20/1200)
4	1/60 (finger counting at one meter) 1/50 (0.02) 5/300	Light perception
5	No light perception	
9	Undetermined or unspecified	

Other disorders of eye and adnexa (H55-H57)

✓4ᵗʰ **H55**   Nystagmus and other irregular eye movements

    ✓5ᵗʰ **H55.0**   Nystagmus

      DEF: Rapid, rhythmic, involuntary movements of the eyeball in vertical, horizontal, rotational, or mixed directions.

      H55.00   Unspecified nystagmus

      H55.01   Congenital nystagmus

    H55.02   Latent **nystagmus**

    H55.03   Visual deprivation **nystagmus**

    H55.04   Dissociated **nystagmus**

    H55.09   Other forms of nystagmus

✓5th **H55.8   Other irregular eye movements**

    H55.81   Saccadic **eye movements**

    H55.89   Other **irregular eye movements**

✓4th **H57   Other disorders of eye and adnexa**

  ✓5th **H57.0   Anomalies of pupillary function**

    H57.00   Unspecified anomaly of pupillary function

    H57.01   Argyll Robertson pupil, atypical
         EXCLUDES 1   *syphilitic Argyll Robertson pupil (A52.19)*

    H57.02   Anisocoria

    H57.03   Miosis

    H57.04   Mydriasis

  ✓6th **H57.05   Tonic pupil**

       H57.051   Tonic pupil, **right** eye

       H57.052   Tonic pupil, **left** eye

       H57.053   Tonic pupil, **bilateral**

       H57.059   Tonic pupil, **unspecified** eye

    H57.09   Other **anomalies of pupillary function**

  ✓5th **H57.1   Ocular pain**

    H57.10   Ocular pain, **unspecified** eye

    H57.11   Ocular pain, **right** eye

    H57.12   Ocular pain, **left** eye

    H57.13   Ocular pain, **bilateral**

  ✓5th **H57.8   Other specified disorders of eye and adnexa**

  ●   ✓6th **H57.81   Brow ptosis**

  ●   H57.811   Brow ptosis, **right**

  ●   H57.812   Brow ptosis, **left**

  ●   H57.813   Brow ptosis, **bilateral**

  ●   H57.819   Brow ptosis, **unspecified**

  ●   H57.89   Other **specified disorders of eye and adnexa**

    H57.9   Unspecified disorder of eye and adnexa

Intraoperative and postprocedural complications and disorders of eye and adnexa, not elsewhere classified (H59)

✓4th **H59   Intraoperative and postprocedural complications and disorders of eye and adnexa, not elsewhere classified**
     EXCLUDES 1   *mechanical complication of intraocular lens (T85.2)*
               mechanical complication of other ocular prosthetic devices, implants and grafts (T85.3)
               pseudophakia (Z96.1)
               secondary cataracts (H26.4-)

  ✓5th **H59.0   Disorders of the eye following cataract surgery**

    CC Excl: For CC codes in subcategory H59.0: PDX collection 638

  ✓6th **H59.01   Keratopathy (bullous aphakic) following cataract surgery**
       Vitreal corneal syndrome
       Vitreous (touch) syndrome

       H59.011   Keratopathy (bullous aphakic) following cataract surgery, **right eye**   CC

       H59.012   Keratopathy (bullous aphakic) following cataract surgery, **left eye**   CC

       H59.013   Keratopathy (bullous aphakic) following cataract surgery, **bilateral**   CC

       H59.019   Keratopathy (bullous aphakic) following cataract surgery, **unspecified eye**   CC

  ✓6th **H59.02   Cataract (lens) fragments in eye following cataract surgery**

       H59.021   Cataract (lens) fragments in eye following cataract surgery, **right eye**

       H59.022   Cataract (lens) fragments in eye following cataract surgery, **left eye**

       H59.023   Cataract (lens) fragments in eye following cataract surgery, **bilateral**

       H59.029   Cataract (lens) fragments in eye following cataract surgery, **unspecified eye**

  ✓6th **H59.03   Cystoid macular edema following cataract surgery**

       H59.031   Cystoid macular edema following cataract surgery, **right eye**   CC

       H59.032   Cystoid macular edema following cataract surgery, **left eye**   CC

       H59.033   Cystoid macular edema following cataract surgery, **bilateral**   CC

       H59.039   Cystoid macular edema following cataract surgery, **unspecified** eye   CC

  ✓6th **H59.09   Other disorders of the eye following cataract surgery**

       H59.091   Other disorders of the **right** eye following cataract surgery   CC

       H59.092   Other disorders of the **left** eye following cataract surgery   CC

       H59.093   Other disorders of the eye following cataract surgery, **bilateral**   CC

       H59.099   Other disorders of **unspecified** eye following cataract surgery   CC

  ✓5th **H59.1   Intraoperative hemorrhage and hematoma of eye and adnexa complicating a procedure**
     EXCLUDES 1   *intraoperative hemorrhage and hematoma of eye and adnexa due to accidental puncture or laceration during a procedure (H59.2-)*

    CC Excl: For CC codes in subcategory H59.1: PDX collection 639

  ✓6th **H59.11   Intraoperative hemorrhage and hematoma of eye and adnexa complicating an ophthalmic procedure**

       H59.111   Intraoperative hemorrhage and hematoma of **right** eye and adnexa complicating an ophthalmic procedure   CC

       H59.112   Intraoperative hemorrhage and hematoma of **left** eye and adnexa complicating an ophthalmic procedure   CC

       H59.113   Intraoperative hemorrhage and hematoma of eye and adnexa complicating an ophthalmic procedure, **bilateral**   CC

       H59.119   Intraoperative hemorrhage and hematoma of **unspecified** eye and adnexa complicating an ophthalmic procedure   CC

  ✓6th **H59.12   Intraoperative hemorrhage and hematoma of eye and adnexa complicating other procedure**

       H59.121   Intraoperative hemorrhage and hematoma of **right** eye and adnexa complicating other procedure   CC

       H59.122   Intraoperative hemorrhage and hematoma of **left** eye and adnexa complicating other procedure   CC

       H59.123   Intraoperative hemorrhage and hematoma of eye and adnexa complicating other procedure, **bilateral**   CC

       H59.129   Intraoperative hemorrhage and hematoma of **unspecified** eye and adnexa complicating other procedure   CC

  ✓5th **H59.2   Accidental puncture and laceration of eye and adnexa during a procedure**

    CC Excl: For CC codes in subcategory H59.2: PDX collection 509

  ✓6th **H59.21   Accidental puncture and laceration of eye and adnexa during an ophthalmic procedure**

       H59.211   Accidental puncture and laceration of **right** eye and adnexa during an ophthalmic procedure   CC

       H59.212   Accidental puncture and laceration of **left** eye and adnexa during an ophthalmic procedure   CC

       H59.213   Accidental puncture and laceration of eye and adnexa during an ophthalmic procedure, **bilateral**   CC

       H59.219   Accidental puncture and laceration of **unspecified** eye and adnexa during an ophthalmic procedure   CC

N Newborn: 0   P Pediatric: 0-17   M Maternity: 12-55   A Adult: 15-124   MCC Major Complication/Comorbidity   CC Complication/Comorbidity   SW Severe Wound Dx

618   ICD-10-CM 2019

✓6th **H59.22** **Accidental puncture and laceration of eye and adnexa during** other procedure

     H59.221   **Accidental puncture and laceration of** right **eye and adnexa during other procedure** CC

     H59.222   **Accidental puncture and laceration of** left **eye and adnexa during other procedure** CC

     H59.223   **Accidental puncture and laceration of eye and adnexa during other procedure, bilateral** CC

     H59.229   **Accidental puncture and laceration of** unspecified **eye and adnexa during other procedure** CC

✓5th **H59.3** **Postprocedural hemorrhage, hematoma, and seroma of eye and adnexa following a procedure**

     AHA: 2016, 4Q, 9-10

> **CC Excl: For CC codes in subcategory H59.3:**
> PDX collection 639

✓6th **H59.31** **Postprocedural** hemorrhage **of eye and adnexa following an** ophthalmic procedure

     H59.311   **Postprocedural hemorrhage of** right **eye and adnexa following an ophthalmic procedure** CC

     H59.312   **Postprocedural hemorrhage of** left **eye and adnexa following an ophthalmic procedure** CC

     H59.313   **Postprocedural hemorrhage of eye and adnexa following an ophthalmic procedure,** bilateral CC

     H59.319   **Postprocedural hemorrhage of** unspecified **eye and adnexa following an ophthalmic procedure** CC

✓6th **H59.32** **Postprocedural** hemorrhage **of eye and adnexa following** other procedure

     H59.321   **Postprocedural hemorrhage of** right **eye and adnexa following other procedure** CC

     H59.322   **Postprocedural hemorrhage of** left **eye and adnexa following other procedure** CC

     H59.323   **Postprocedural hemorrhage of eye and adnexa following other procedure,** bilateral CC

     H59.329   **Postprocedural hemorrhage of** unspecified **eye and adnexa following other procedure** CC

✓6th **H59.33** **Postprocedural** hematoma **of eye and adnexa following an** ophthalmic procedure

     H59.331   **Postprocedural hematoma of** right **eye and adnexa following an ophthalmic procedure** CC

     H59.332   **Postprocedural hematoma of** left **eye and adnexa following an ophthalmic procedure** CC

     H59.333   **Postprocedural hematoma of eye and adnexa following an ophthalmic procedure,** bilateral CC

     H59.339   **Postprocedural hematoma of** unspecified **eye and adnexa following an ophthalmic procedure** CC

✓6th **H59.34** **Postprocedural** hematoma **of eye and adnexa following** other procedure

     H59.341   **Postprocedural hematoma of** right **eye and adnexa following other procedure** CC

     H59.342   **Postprocedural hematoma of** left **eye and adnexa following other procedure** CC

     H59.343   **Postprocedural hematoma of eye and adnexa following other procedure,** bilateral CC

     H59.349   **Postprocedural hematoma of** unspecified **eye and adnexa following other procedure** CC

✓6th **H59.35** **Postprocedural** seroma **of eye and adnexa following an** ophthalmic procedure

     H59.351   **Postprocedural seroma of** right **eye and adnexa following an ophthalmic procedure** CC

     H59.352   **Postprocedural seroma of** left **eye and adnexa following an ophthalmic procedure** CC

     H59.353   **Postprocedural seroma of eye and adnexa following an ophthalmic procedure,** bilateral CC

     H59.359   **Postprocedural seroma of** unspecified **eye and adnexa following an ophthalmic procedure** CC

✓6th **H59.36** **Postprocedural** seroma **of eye and adnexa following** other procedure

     H59.361   **Postprocedural seroma of** right **eye and adnexa following other procedure** CC

     H59.362   **Postprocedural seroma of** left **eye and adnexa following other procedure** CC

     H59.363   **Postprocedural seroma of eye and adnexa following other procedure,** bilateral CC

     H59.369   **Postprocedural seroma of** unspecified **eye and adnexa following other procedurec** CC

✓5th **H59.4** **Inflammation (infection) of** postprocedural bleb

     Postprocedural blebitis

     EXCLUDES 1   *filtering (vitreous) bleb after glaucoma surgery status (Z98.83)*

     H59.40 **Inflammation (infection) of postprocedural bleb,** unspecified

     H59.41 **Inflammation (infection) of postprocedural bleb, stage 1**

     H59.42 **Inflammation (infection) of postprocedural bleb, stage 2**

     H59.43 **Inflammation (infection) of postprocedural bleb, stage 3**

         Bleb endophthalmitis

✓5th **H59.8** **Other intraoperative and postprocedural complications and disorders of eye and adnexa, not elsewhere classified**

> **CC Excl: For CC codes in subcategory H59.8:**
> PDX collection 638

✓6th **H59.81** **Chorioretinal scars after surgery for detachment**

     H59.811   **Chorioretinal scars after surgery for detachment,** right **eye** CC

     H59.812   **Chorioretinal scars after surgery for detachment,** left **eye** CC

     H59.813   **Chorioretinal scars after surgery for detachment,** bilateral CC

     H59.819   **Chorioretinal scars after surgery for detachment,** unspecified **eye** CC

     H59.88 Other intraoperative **complications of eye and adnexa, not elsewhere classified** CC

     H59.89 Other postprocedural **complications and disorders of eye and adnexa, not elsewhere classified** CC

✔ Additional Character Required   ✓x7th Placeholder   Unacceptable PDx   Questionable PDx   Manifestation   H1 - H14 HAC   HCC CMS-HCC Dx   HIV HIV Dx

ICD-10-CM 2019   619

Chapter 8. Diseases of the Ear and Mastoid Process (H60–H95)

Chapter Specific Coding Guidelines and Examples
Reserved for future guideline expansion.

Chapter 8. Diseases of the Ear and Mastoid Process (H60–H95)

NOTE Use an external cause code following the code for the ear condition, if applicable, to identify the cause of the ear condition.

EXCLUDES 2 *certain conditions originating in the perinatal period (P04-P96)*
certain infectious and parasitic diseases (A00-B99)
complications of pregnancy, childbirth and the puerperium (O00-O9A)
congenital malformations, deformations and chromosomal abnormalities (Q00-Q99)
endocrine, nutritional and metabolic diseases (E00-E88)
injury, poisoning and certain other consequences of external causes (S00-T88)
neoplasms (C00-D49)
symptoms, signs and abnormal clinical and laboratory findings, not elsewhere classified (R00-R94)

This chapter contains the following blocks:

H60-H62	Diseases of external ear
H65-H75	Diseases of middle ear and mastoid
H80-H83	Diseases of inner ear
H90-H94	Other disorders of ear
H95	Intraoperative and postprocedural complications and disorders of ear and mastoid process, not elsewhere classified

Diseases of external ear (H60-H62)

✓4ᵗʰ H60 Otitis externa

TIP: When the specific infectious agent is identified, a code from chapter 1 is assigned instead of a code from this category.

✓5ᵗʰ H60.0 Abscess of external ear
Boil of external ear
Carbuncle of auricle or external auditory canal
Furuncle of external ear

    H60.00 Abscess of external ear, unspecified ear
    H60.01 Abscess of right external ear
    H60.02 Abscess of left external ear
    H60.03 Abscess of external ear, bilateral

✓5ᵗʰ H60.1 Cellulitis of external ear
Cellulitis of auricle
Cellulitis of external auditory canal

    H60.10 Cellulitis of external ear, unspecified ear
    H60.11 Cellulitis of right external ear
    H60.12 Cellulitis of left external ear
    H60.13 Cellulitis of external ear, bilateral

✓5ᵗʰ H60.2 Malignant otitis externa

> **CC Excl: For CC codes in subcategory H60.2:**
> PDX collection 640

    H60.20 Malignant otitis externa, unspecified ear `CC`
    H60.21 Malignant otitis externa, right ear `CC`
    H60.22 Malignant otitis externa, left ear `CC`
    H60.23 Malignant otitis externa, bilateral `CC`

✓5ᵗʰ H60.3 Other infective otitis externa

    ✓6ᵗʰ H60.31 Diffuse otitis externa
        H60.311 Diffuse otitis externa, right ear
        H60.312 Diffuse otitis externa, left ear
        H60.313 Diffuse otitis externa, bilateral
        H60.319 Diffuse otitis externa, unspecified ear

    ✓6ᵗʰ H60.32 Hemorrhagic otitis externa
        H60.321 Hemorrhagic otitis externa, right ear
        H60.322 Hemorrhagic otitis externa, left ear
        H60.323 Hemorrhagic otitis externa, bilateral
        H60.329 Hemorrhagic otitis externa, unspecified ear

    ✓6ᵗʰ H60.33 Swimmer's ear
        DEF: Commonly occurs when water gets trapped in the ear after swimming.
        H60.331 Swimmer's ear, right ear
        H60.332 Swimmer's ear, left ear
        H60.333 Swimmer's ear, bilateral
        H60.339 Swimmer's ear, unspecified ear

    ✓6ᵗʰ H60.39 Other infective otitis externa
        H60.391 Other infective otitis externa, right ear
        H60.392 Other infective otitis externa, left ear
        H60.393 Other infective otitis externa, bilateral

        H60.399 Other infective otitis externa, unspecified ear

✓5ᵗʰ H60.4 Cholesteatoma of external ear
Keratosis obturans of external ear (canal)

    EXCLUDES 2 *cholesteatoma of middle ear (H71.-)*
        recurrent cholesteatoma of postmastoidectomy cavity (H95.0-)

DEF: Cholesteatoma: Noncancerous cyst-like mass of cell debris, including cholesterol and epithelial cells resulting from trauma, repeated or improperly healed infections, and congenital enclosure of epidermal cells.

    H60.40 Cholesteatoma of external ear, unspecified ear
    H60.41 Cholesteatoma of right external ear
    H60.42 Cholesteatoma of left external ear
    H60.43 Cholesteatoma of external ear, bilateral

✓5ᵗʰ H60.5 Acute noninfective otitis externa

    ✓6ᵗʰ H60.50 Unspecified acute noninfective otitis externa
        Acute otitis externa NOS
        H60.501 Unspecified acute noninfective otitis externa, right ear
        H60.502 Unspecified acute noninfective otitis externa, left ear
        H60.503 Unspecified acute noninfective otitis externa, bilateral
        H60.509 Unspecified acute noninfective otitis externa, unspecified ear

    ✓6ᵗʰ H60.51 Acute actinic otitis externa
        H60.511 Acute actinic otitis externa, right ear
        H60.512 Acute actinic otitis externa, left ear
        H60.513 Acute actinic otitis externa, bilateral
        H60.519 Acute actinic otitis externa, unspecified ear

    ✓6ᵗʰ H60.52 Acute chemical otitis externa
        H60.521 Acute chemical otitis externa, right ear
        H60.522 Acute chemical otitis externa, left ear
        H60.523 Acute chemical otitis externa, bilateral
        H60.529 Acute chemical otitis externa, unspecified ear

    ✓6ᵗʰ H60.53 Acute contact otitis externa
        H60.531 Acute contact otitis externa, right ear
        H60.532 Acute contact otitis externa, left ear
        H60.533 Acute contact otitis externa, bilateral
        H60.539 Acute contact otitis externa, unspecified ear

    ✓6ᵗʰ H60.54 Acute eczematoid otitis externa
        H60.541 Acute eczematoid otitis externa, right ear
        H60.542 Acute eczematoid otitis externa, left ear
        H60.543 Acute eczematoid otitis externa, bilateral
        H60.549 Acute eczematoid otitis externa, unspecified ear

    ✓6ᵗʰ H60.55 Acute reactive otitis externa
        H60.551 Acute reactive otitis externa, right ear
        H60.552 Acute reactive otitis externa, left ear
        H60.553 Acute reactive otitis externa, bilateral
        H60.559 Acute reactive otitis externa, unspecified ear

    ✓6ᵗʰ H60.59 Other noninfective acute otitis externa
        H60.591 Other noninfective acute otitis externa, right ear
        H60.592 Other noninfective acute otitis externa, left ear
        H60.593 Other noninfective acute otitis externa, bilateral
        H60.599 Other noninfective acute otitis externa, unspecified ear

✓5ᵗʰ H60.6 Unspecified chronic otitis externa
    H60.60 Unspecified chronic otitis externa, unspecified ear
    H60.61 Unspecified chronic otitis externa, right ear
    H60.62 Unspecified chronic otitis externa, left ear
    H60.63 Unspecified chronic otitis externa, bilateral

✓5ᵗʰ H60.8 Other otitis externa
    ✓6ᵗʰ H60.8X Other otitis externa
        H60.8X1 Other otitis externa, right ear
        H60.8X2 Other otitis externa, left ear
        H60.8X3 Other otitis externa, bilateral

N Newborn: 0   P Pediatric: 0-17   M Maternity: 12-55   A Adult: 15-124   MCC Major Complication/Comorbidity   CC Complication/Comorbidity   SW Severe Wound Dx

622

ICD-10-CM 2019

H60.8X9   **Other otitis externa,** unspecified **ear**

√5th **H60.9 Unspecified otitis externa**

     H60.90   **Unspecified otitis externa,** unspecified **ear**

     H60.91   **Unspecified otitis externa,** right **ear**

     H60.92   **Unspecified otitis externa,** left **ear**

     H60.93   **Unspecified otitis externa,** bilateral

√4th **H61   Other disorders of external ear**

√5th **H61.0   Chondritis and perichondritis of external ear**
     Chondrodermatitis nodularis chronica helicis
     Perichondritis of auricle
     Perichondritis of pinna

     √6th **H61.00   Unspecified perichondritis of external ear**

       H61.001   **Unspecified perichondritis of** right **external ear**

       H61.002   **Unspecified perichondritis of** left **external ear**

       H61.003   **Unspecified perichondritis of external ear,** bilateral

       H61.009   **Unspecified perichondritis of external ear,** unspecified **ear**

     √6th **H61.01   Acute perichondritis of external ear**

       H61.011   **Acute perichondritis of** right **external ear**

       H61.012   **Acute perichondritis of** left **external ear**

       H61.013   **Acute perichondritis of external ear,** bilateral

       H61.019   **Acute perichondritis of external ear,** unspecified **ear**

     √6th **H61.02   Chronic perichondritis of external ear**

       H61.021   **Chronic perichondritis of** right **external ear**

       H61.022   **Chronic perichondritis of** left **external ear**

       H61.023   **Chronic perichondritis of external ear,** bilateral

       H61.029   **Chronic perichondritis of external ear,** unspecified **ear**

     √6th **H61.03   Chondritis of external ear**
       Chondritis of auricle   Chondritis of pinna
       AHA: 2015, 1Q, 18
       DEF: Infection that has progressed into the cartilage and presents as indurated and edematous skin over the pinna. Vascular compromise occurs with tissue necrosis and deformity.

       H61.031   **Chondritis of** right **external ear**

       H61.032   **Chondritis of** left **external ear**

       H61.033   **Chondritis of external ear,** bilateral

       H61.039   **Chondritis of external ear,** unspecified **ear**

√5th **H61.1   Noninfective disorders of pinna**
     EXCLUDES 2   *cauliflower ear (M95.1-)*
              gouty tophi of ear (M1A.-)

     √6th **H61.10   Unspecified noninfective disorders of pinna**
       Disorder of pinna NOS

       H61.101   **Unspecified noninfective disorders of pinna,** right **ear**

       H61.102   **Unspecified noninfective disorders of pinna,** left **ear**

       H61.103   **Unspecified noninfective disorders of pinna,** bilateral

       H61.109   **Unspecified noninfective disorders of pinna,** unspecified **ear**

     √6th **H61.11   Acquired deformity of pinna**
       Acquired deformity of auricle
       EXCLUDES 2   *cauliflower ear (M95.1-)*

       H61.111   **Acquired deformity of pinna,** right **ear**

       H61.112   **Acquired deformity of pinna,** left **ear**

       H61.113   **Acquired deformity of pinna,** bilateral

       H61.119   **Acquired deformity of pinna,** unspecified **ear**

     √6th **H61.12   Hematoma of pinna**
       Hematoma of auricle

       H61.121   **Hematoma of pinna,** right **ear**

       H61.122   **Hematoma of pinna,** left **ear**

       H61.123   **Hematoma of pinna,** bilateral

       H61.129   **Hematoma of pinna,** unspecified **ear**

     √6th **H61.19   Other noninfective disorders of pinna**

       H61.191   **Noninfective disorders of pinna,** right **ear**

       H61.192   **Noninfective disorders of pinna,** left **ear**

       H61.193   **Noninfective disorders of pinna,** bilateral

       H61.199   **Noninfective disorders of pinna,** unspecified **ear**

√5th **H61.2   Impacted cerumen**
     Wax in ear

     H61.20   **Impacted cerumen,** unspecified **ear**

     H61.21   **Impacted cerumen,** right **ear**

     H61.22   **Impacted cerumen,** left **ear**

     H61.23   **Impacted cerumen,** bilateral

√5th **H61.3   Acquired stenosis of external ear canal**
     Collapse of external ear canal
     EXCLUDES 1   *postprocedural stenosis of external ear canal (H95.81-)*

     √6th **H61.30   Acquired stenosis of external ear canal,** unspecified

       H61.301   **Acquired stenosis of** right **external ear canal, unspecified**

       H61.302   **Acquired stenosis of** left **external ear canal, unspecified**

       H61.303   **Acquired stenosis of external ear canal, unspecified,** bilateral

       H61.309   **Acquired stenosis of external ear canal, unspecified,** unspecified **ear**

     √6th **H61.31   Acquired stenosis of external ear canal** secondary to trauma

       H61.311   **Acquired stenosis of** right **external ear canal secondary to trauma**

       H61.312   **Acquired stenosis of** left **external ear canal secondary to trauma**

       H61.313   **Acquired stenosis of external ear canal secondary to trauma,** bilateral

       H61.319   **Acquired stenosis of external ear canal secondary to trauma,** unspecified **ear**

     √6th **H61.32   Acquired stenosis of external ear canal** secondary to inflammation and infection
       DEF: Narrowing of the external ear canal due to chronic inflammation or infection.

       H61.321   **Acquired stenosis of** right **external ear canal secondary to inflammation and infection**

       H61.322   **Acquired stenosis of** left **external ear canal secondary to inflammation and infection**

       H61.323   **Acquired stenosis of external ear canal secondary to inflammation and infection,** bilateral

       H61.329   **Acquired stenosis of external ear canal secondary to inflammation and infection,** unspecified **ear**

     √6th **H61.39   Other acquired stenosis of external ear canal**

       H61.391   **Other acquired stenosis of** right **external ear canal**

       H61.392   **Other acquired stenosis of** left **external ear canal**

       H61.393   **Other acquired stenosis of external ear canal,** bilateral

       H61.399   **Other acquired stenosis of external ear canal,** unspecified **ear**

√5th **H61.8   Other specified disorders of external ear**

     √6th **H61.81   Exostosis of external canal**

       H61.811   **Exostosis of** right **external canal**

       H61.812   **Exostosis of** left **external canal**

       H61.813   **Exostosis of external canal,** bilateral

       H61.819   **Exostosis of external canal,** unspecified **ear**

     √6th **H61.89   Other specified disorders of external ear**

       H61.891   **Other specified disorders of** right **external ear**

       H61.892   **Other specified disorders of** left **external ear**

       H61.893   **Other specified disorders of external ear,** bilateral

       H61.899   **Other specified disorders of external ear,** unspecified **ear**

☑ Additional Character Required   √x7th Placeholder   Unacceptable PDx   Questionable PDx   Manifestation   H1–H14 HAC   HCC CMS-HCC Dx   HIV HIV Dx

ICD-10-CM 2019   **623**

H60.8X9–H61.899

✓5ᵗʰ **H61.9** **Disorder of external ear, unspecified**

    H61.90 Disorder of external ear, unspecified, unspecified ear

    H61.91 Disorder of right external ear, unspecified

    H61.92 Disorder of left external ear, unspecified

    H61.93 Disorder of external ear, unspecified, bilateral

✓4ᵗʰ **H62** **Disorders of external ear in diseases classified elsewhere**

  ✓5ᵗʰ **H62.4** **Otitis externa in other diseases classified elsewhere**

    Code first underlying disease, such as:
      erysipelas (A46)
      impetigo (LØ1.Ø)

    EXCLUDES 1 *otitis externa (in):*
      candidiasis (B37.84)
      herpes viral [herpes simplex] (BØØ.1)
      herpes zoster (BØ2.8)

    H62.40 *Otitis externa in other diseases classified elsewhere, unspecified ear*

    H62.41 *Otitis externa in other diseases classified elsewhere, right ear*

    H62.42 *Otitis externa in other diseases classified elsewhere, left ear*

    H62.43 *Otitis externa in other diseases classified elsewhere, bilateral*

  ✓5ᵗʰ **H62.8** **Other disorders of external ear in diseases classified elsewhere**

    Code first underlying disease, such as:
      gout (M1A.-, M1Ø.-)

   ✓6ᵗʰ **H62.8X** **Other disorders of external ear in diseases classified elsewhere**

    H62.8X1 *Other disorders of right external ear in diseases classified elsewhere*

    H62.8X2 *Other disorders of left external ear in diseases classified elsewhere*

    H62.8X3 *Other disorders of external ear in diseases classified elsewhere, bilateral*

    H62.8X9 *Other disorders of external ear in diseases classified elsewhere, unspecified ear*

Diseases of middle ear and mastoid (H65-H75)

✓4ᵗʰ **H65** **Nonsuppurative otitis media**

    INCLUDES nonsuppurative otitis media with myringitis

    Use additional code for any associated perforated tympanic membrane (H72.-)

    Use additional code to identify:
      exposure to environmental tobacco smoke (Z77.22)
      exposure to tobacco smoke in the perinatal period (P96.81)
      history of tobacco dependence (Z87.891)
      occupational exposure to environmental tobacco smoke (Z57.31)
      tobacco dependence (F17.-)
      tobacco use (Z72.Ø)

  ✓5ᵗʰ **H65.Ø** **Acute serous otitis media**

    Acute and subacute secretory otitis

    H65.ØØ Acute serous otitis media, unspecified ear

    H65.Ø1 Acute serous otitis media, right ear

    H65.Ø2 Acute serous otitis media, left ear

    H65.Ø3 Acute serous otitis media, bilateral

    H65.Ø4 Acute serous otitis media, recurrent, right ear

    H65.Ø5 Acute serous otitis media, recurrent, left ear

    H65.Ø6 Acute serous otitis media, recurrent, bilateral

    H65.Ø7 Acute serous otitis media, recurrent, unspecified ear

  ✓5ᵗʰ **H65.1** **Other acute nonsuppurative otitis media**

    EXCLUDES 1 *otitic barotrauma (T7Ø.Ø)*
      otitis media (acute) NOS (H66.9)

   ✓6ᵗʰ **H65.11** **Acute and subacute allergic otitis media (mucoid) (sanguinous) (serous)**

    H65.111 Acute and subacute allergic otitis media (mucoid) (sanguinous) (serous), right ear

    H65.112 Acute and subacute allergic otitis media (mucoid) (sanguinous) (serous), left ear

    H65.113 Acute and subacute allergic otitis media (mucoid) (sanguinous) (serous), bilateral

    H65.114 Acute and subacute allergic otitis media (mucoid) (sanguinous) (serous), recurrent, right ear

    H65.115 Acute and subacute allergic otitis media (mucoid) (sanguinous) (serous), recurrent, left ear

    H65.116 Acute and subacute allergic otitis media (mucoid) (sanguinous) (serous), recurrent, bilateral

    H65.117 Acute and subacute allergic otitis media (mucoid) (sanguinous) (serous), recurrent, unspecified ear

    H65.119 Acute and subacute allergic otitis media (mucoid) (sanguinous) (serous), unspecified ear

   ✓6ᵗʰ **H65.19** **Other acute nonsuppurative otitis media**

    Acute and subacute mucoid otitis media
    Acute and subacute nonsuppurative otitis media NOS
    Acute and subacute sanguinous otitis media
    Acute and subacute seromucinous otitis media

    H65.191 Other acute nonsuppurative otitis media, right ear

    H65.192 Other acute nonsuppurative otitis media, left ear

    H65.193 Other acute nonsuppurative otitis media, bilateral

    H65.194 Other acute nonsuppurative otitis media, recurrent, right ear

    H65.195 Other acute nonsuppurative otitis media, recurrent, left ear

    H65.196 Other acute nonsuppurative otitis media, recurrent, bilateral

    H65.197 Other acute nonsuppurative otitis media recurrent, unspecified ear

    H65.199 Other acute nonsuppurative otitis media, unspecified ear

  ✓5ᵗʰ **H65.2** **Chronic serous otitis media**

    Chronic tubotympanal catarrh

    H65.2Ø Chronic serous otitis media, unspecified ear

    H65.21 Chronic serous otitis media, right ear

    H65.22 Chronic serous otitis media, left ear

    H65.23 Chronic serous otitis media, bilateral

  ✓5ᵗʰ **H65.3** **Chronic mucoid otitis media**

    Chronic mucinous otitis media
    Chronic secretory otitis media
    Chronic transudative otitis media
    Glue ear

    EXCLUDES 1 *adhesive middle ear disease (H74.1)*

    H65.3Ø Chronic mucoid otitis media, unspecified ear

    H65.31 Chronic mucoid otitis media, right ear

    H65.32 Chronic mucoid otitis media, left ear

    H65.33 Chronic mucoid otitis media, bilateral

  ✓5ᵗʰ **H65.4** **Other chronic nonsuppurative otitis media**

   ✓6ᵗʰ **H65.41** **Chronic allergic otitis media**

    H65.411 Chronic allergic otitis media, right ear

    H65.412 Chronic allergic otitis media, left ear

    H65.413 Chronic allergic otitis media, bilateral

    H65.419 Chronic allergic otitis media, unspecified ear

   ✓6ᵗʰ **H65.49** **Other chronic nonsuppurative otitis media**

    Chronic exudative otitis media
    Chronic nonsuppurative otitis media NOS
    Chronic otitis media with effusion (nonpurulent)
    Chronic seromucinous otitis media

    H65.491 Other chronic nonsuppurative otitis media, right ear

    H65.492 Other chronic nonsuppurative otitis media, left ear

    H65.493 Other chronic nonsuppurative otitis media, bilateral

    H65.499 Other chronic nonsuppurative otitis media, unspecified ear

N Newborn: 0   **P** Pediatric: 0-17   **M** Maternity: 12-55   **A** Adult: 15-124   **MCC** Major Complication/Comorbidity   **CC** Complication/Comorbidity   **SW** Severe Wound Dx

624   ICD-10-CM 2019

☑5th **H65.9** Unspecified **nonsuppurative otitis media**
- Allergic otitis media NOS
- Catarrhal otitis media NOS
- Exudative otitis media NOS
- Mucoid otitis media NOS
- Otitis media with effusion (nonpurulent) NOS
- Secretory otitis media NOS
- Seromucinous otitis media NOS
- Serous otitis media NOS
- Transudative otitis media NOS

H65.90 Unspecified nonsuppurative otitis media, unspecified ear

H65.91 Unspecified nonsuppurative otitis media, right ear

H65.92 Unspecified nonsuppurative otitis media, left ear

H65.93 Unspecified nonsuppurative otitis media, bilateral

☑4th **H66** **Suppurative and unspecified otitis media**
> INCLUDES suppurative and unspecified otitis media with myringitis
> Use additional code to identify:
> exposure to environmental tobacco smoke (Z77.22)
> exposure to tobacco smoke in the perinatal period (P96.81)
> history of tobacco dependence (Z87.891)
> occupational exposure to environmental tobacco smoke (Z57.31)
> tobacco dependence (F17.-)
> tobacco use (Z72.0)
> AHA: 2016, 1Q, 34

☑5th **H66.0** Acute suppurative **otitis media**

☑6th **H66.00** Acute suppurative otitis media without spontaneous rupture of ear drum

H66.001 Acute suppurative otitis media without spontaneous rupture of ear drum, right ear

H66.002 Acute suppurative otitis media without spontaneous rupture of ear drum, left ear

H66.003 Acute suppurative otitis media without spontaneous rupture of ear drum, bilateral

H66.004 Acute suppurative otitis media without spontaneous rupture of ear drum, recurrent, right ear

H66.005 Acute suppurative otitis media without spontaneous rupture of ear drum, recurrent, left ear

H66.006 Acute suppurative otitis media without spontaneous rupture of ear drum, recurrent, bilateral

H66.007 Acute suppurative otitis media without spontaneous rupture of ear drum, recurrent, unspecified ear

H66.009 Acute suppurative otitis media without spontaneous rupture of ear drum, unspecified ear

☑6th **H66.01** Acute suppurative otitis media with spontaneous rupture of ear drum
> **DEF:** Sudden, severe inflammation of the middle ear, causing pressure that perforates the ear drum tissue.

H66.011 Acute suppurative otitis media with spontaneous rupture of ear drum, right ear

H66.012 Acute suppurative otitis media with spontaneous rupture of ear drum, left ear

H66.013 Acute suppurative otitis media with spontaneous rupture of ear drum, bilateral

H66.014 Acute suppurative otitis media with spontaneous rupture of ear drum, recurrent, right ear

H66.015 Acute suppurative otitis media with spontaneous rupture of ear drum, recurrent, left ear

H66.016 Acute suppurative otitis media with spontaneous rupture of ear drum, recurrent, bilateral

H66.017 Acute suppurative otitis media with spontaneous rupture of ear drum, recurrent, unspecified ear

H66.019 Acute suppurative otitis media with spontaneous rupture of ear drum, unspecified ear

☑5th **H66.1** Chronic tubotympanic **suppurative otitis media**
- Benign chronic suppurative otitis media
- Chronic tubotympanic disease
> Use additional code for any associated perforated tympanic membrane (H72.-)

H66.10 Chronic tubotympanic suppurative otitis media, unspecified

H66.11 Chronic tubotympanic suppurative otitis media, right ear

H66.12 Chronic tubotympanic suppurative otitis media, left ear

H66.13 Chronic tubotympanic suppurative otitis media, bilateral

☑5th **H66.2** Chronic atticoantral **suppurative otitis media**
- Chronic atticoantral disease
> Use additional code for any associated perforated tympanic membrane (H72.-)

H66.20 Chronic atticoantral suppurative otitis media, unspecified ear

H66.21 Chronic atticoantral suppurative otitis media, right ear

H66.22 Chronic atticoantral suppurative otitis media, left ear

H66.23 Chronic atticoantral suppurative otitis media, bilateral

☑5th **H66.3** Other **chronic suppurative otitis media**
- Chronic suppurative otitis media NOS
> Use additional code for any associated perforated tympanic membrane (H72.-)
> EXCLUDES 1 tuberculous otitis media (A18.6)

☑6th **H66.3X** Other chronic suppurative otitis media

H66.3X1 Other chronic suppurative otitis media, right ear

H66.3X2 Other chronic suppurative otitis media, left ear

H66.3X3 Other chronic suppurative otitis media, bilateral

H66.3X9 Other chronic suppurative otitis media, unspecified ear

☑5th **H66.4** Suppurative otitis media, unspecified
- Purulent otitis media NOS
> Use additional code for any associated perforated tympanic membrane (H72.-)

H66.40 Suppurative otitis media, unspecified, unspecified ear

H66.41 Suppurative otitis media, unspecified, right ear

H66.42 Suppurative otitis media, unspecified, left ear

H66.43 Suppurative otitis media, unspecified, bilateral

☑5th **H66.9** Otitis media, unspecified
- Otitis media NOS
- Acute otitis media NOS
- Chronic otitis media NOS
> Use additional code for any associated perforated tympanic membrane (H72.-)

H66.90 Otitis media, unspecified, unspecified ear

H66.91 Otitis media, unspecified, right ear

H66.92 Otitis media, unspecified, left ear

H66.93 Otitis media, unspecified, bilateral

☑4th **H67** **Otitis media in diseases classified elsewhere**
> Code first underlying disease, such as:
> ▶plasminogen deficiency (E88.02)◀
> viral disease NEC (B00-B34)
> Use additional code for any associated perforated tympanic membrane (H72.-)
> EXCLUDES 1 otitis media in:
> influenza (J09.X9, J10.83, J11.83)
> measles (B05.3)
> scarlet fever (A38.0)
> tuberculosis (A18.6)

H67.1 *Otitis media in diseases classified elsewhere, right ear*

H67.2 *Otitis media in diseases classified elsewhere, left ear*

H67.3 *Otitis media in diseases classified elsewhere, bilateral*

H67.9 *Otitis media in diseases classified elsewhere, unspecified ear*

☑Additional Character Required   ☑x7th Placeholder   Unacceptable PDx   Questionable PDx   Manifestation   H1-H14 HAC   HCC CMS-HCC Dx   HIV HIV Dx

ICD-10-CM 2019   625

Chapter 8. Diseases of the Ear and Mastoid Process

✓4ᵗʰ **H68 Eustachian salpingitis and obstruction**

✓5ᵗʰ **H68.0 Eustachian** salpingitis

✓6ᵗʰ **H68.00 Unspecified** Eustachian salpingitis

H68.001 Unspecified Eustachian salpingitis, right ear

H68.002 Unspecified Eustachian salpingitis, left ear

H68.003 Unspecified Eustachian salpingitis, bilateral

H68.009 Unspecified Eustachian salpingitis, unspecified **ear**

✓6ᵗʰ **H68.01 Acute** Eustachian salpingitis

H68.011 Acute Eustachian salpingitis, right **ear**

H68.012 Acute Eustachian salpingitis, left **ear**

H68.013 Acute Eustachian salpingitis, bilateral

H68.019 Acute Eustachian salpingitis, unspecified **ear**

✓6ᵗʰ **H68.02 Chronic** Eustachian salpingitis

H68.021 Chronic Eustachian salpingitis, right **ear**

H68.022 Chronic Eustachian salpingitis, left **ear**

H68.023 Chronic Eustachian salpingitis, bilateral

H68.029 Chronic Eustachian salpingitis, unspecified **ear**

✓5ᵗʰ **H68.1 Obstruction of Eustachian tube**
Stenosis of Eustachian tube
Stricture of Eustachian tube

✓6ᵗʰ **H68.10 Unspecified** obstruction of Eustachian tube

H68.101 Unspecified obstruction of Eustachian tube, right ear

H68.102 Unspecified obstruction of Eustachian tube, left ear

H68.103 Unspecified obstruction of Eustachian tube, bilateral

H68.109 Unspecified obstruction of Eustachian tube, unspecified ear

✓6ᵗʰ **H68.11 Osseous obstruction of Eustachian tube**

H68.111 Osseous obstruction of Eustachian tube, right ear

H68.112 Osseous obstruction of Eustachian tube, left ear

H68.113 Osseous obstruction of Eustachian tube, bilateral

H68.119 Osseous obstruction of Eustachian tube, unspecified **ear**

✓6ᵗʰ **H68.12 Intrinsic cartilagenous obstruction of Eustachian tube**

H68.121 Intrinsic cartilagenous obstruction of Eustachian tube, right **ear**

H68.122 Intrinsic cartilagenous obstruction of Eustachian tube, left **ear**

H68.123 Intrinsic cartilagenous obstruction of Eustachian tube, bilateral

H68.129 Intrinsic cartilagenous obstruction of Eustachian tube, unspecified **ear**

✓6ᵗʰ **H68.13 Extrinsic cartilagenous obstruction of Eustachian tube**
Compression of Eustachian tube

H68.131 Extrinsic cartilagenous obstruction of Eustachian tube, right **ear**

H68.132 Extrinsic cartilagenous obstruction of Eustachian tube, left **ear**

H68.133 Extrinsic cartilagenous obstruction of Eustachian tube, bilateral

H68.139 Extrinsic cartilagenous obstruction of Eustachian tube, unspecified **ear**

✓4ᵗʰ **H69 Other and unspecified disorders of Eustachian tube**

✓5ᵗʰ **H69.0 Patulous** Eustachian tube

H69.00 Patulous Eustachian tube, unspecified ear

H69.01 Patulous Eustachian tube, right **ear**

H69.02 Patulous Eustachian tube, left **ear**

H69.03 Patulous Eustachian tube, bilateral

✓5ᵗʰ **H69.8 Other specified disorders of Eustachian tube**

H69.80 Other specified disorders of Eustachian tube, unspecified **ear**

H69.81 Other specified disorders of Eustachian tube, right ear

H69.82 Other specified disorders of Eustachian tube, left ear

H69.83 Other specified disorders of Eustachian tube, bilateral

✓5ᵗʰ **H69.9 Unspecified** Eustachian tube disorder

H69.90 Unspecified Eustachian tube disorder, unspecified ear

H69.91 Unspecified Eustachian tube disorder, right **ear**

H69.92 Unspecified Eustachian tube disorder, left **ear**

H69.93 Unspecified Eustachian tube disorder, bilateral

✓4ᵗʰ **H70 Mastoiditis and related conditions**

✓5ᵗʰ **H70.0 Acute mastoiditis**
Abscess of mastoid
Empyema of mastoid

CC Excl: For CC codes in subcategory H70.0:
PDX collection 641

✓6ᵗʰ **H70.00 Acute mastoiditis** without complications

H70.001 Acute mastoiditis without complications, right ear `CC`

H70.002 Acute mastoiditis without complications, left ear `CC`

H70.003 Acute mastoiditis without complications, bilateral `CC`

H70.009 Acute mastoiditis without complications, unspecified **ear** `CC`

✓6ᵗʰ **H70.01 Subperiosteal abscess** of mastoid

H70.011 Subperiosteal abscess of mastoid, right **ear** `CC`

H70.012 Subperiosteal abscess of mastoid, left **ear** `CC`

H70.013 Subperiosteal abscess of mastoid, bilateral `CC`

H70.019 Subperiosteal abscess of mastoid, unspecified **ear** `CC`

✓6ᵗʰ **H70.09 Acute mastoiditis** with other complications

H70.091 Acute mastoiditis with other complications, right **ear** `CC`

H70.092 Acute mastoiditis with other complications, left **ear** `CC`

H70.093 Acute mastoiditis with other complications, bilateral `CC`

H70.099 Acute mastoiditis with other complications, unspecified **ear** `CC`

✓5ᵗʰ **H70.1 Chronic mastoiditis**
Caries of mastoid
Fistula of mastoid
EXCLUDES 1　tuberculous mastoiditis (A18.03)

H70.10 Chronic mastoiditis, unspecified ear

H70.11 Chronic mastoiditis, right ear

H70.12 Chronic mastoiditis, left ear

H70.13 Chronic mastoiditis, bilateral

✓5ᵗʰ **H70.2 Petrositis**
Inflammation of petrous bone

✓6ᵗʰ **H70.20 Unspecified** petrositis

H70.201 Unspecified petrositis, right **ear**

H70.202 Unspecified petrositis, left **ear**

H70.203 Unspecified petrositis, bilateral

H70.209 Unspecified petrositis, unspecified **ear**

✓6ᵗʰ **H70.21 Acute** petrositis

DEF: Sudden, severe inflammation of the petrous temporal bone behind the ear, associated with a middle ear infection.

H70.211 Acute petrositis, right **ear**

H70.212 Acute petrositis, left **ear**

H70.213 Acute petrositis, bilateral

H70.219 Acute petrositis, unspecified **ear**

✓6ᵗʰ **H70.22 Chronic** petrositis

H70.221 Chronic petrositis, right **ear**

H70.222 Chronic petrositis, left **ear**

H70.223 Chronic petrositis, bilateral

H70.229 Chronic petrositis, unspecified **ear**

N Newborn: 0　　**P** Pediatric: 0-17　　**M** Maternity: 12-55　　**A** Adult: 15-124　　**MCC** Major Complication/Comorbidity　　**CC** Complication/Comorbidity　　**SW** Severe Wound Dx

626

ICD-10-CM 2019

✓5ᵗʰ H70.8 Other mastoiditis and related conditions
    EXCLUDES 1   *preauricular sinus and cyst (Q18.1)*
          sinus, fistula, and cyst of branchial cleft (Q18.0)

  ✓6ᵗʰ H70.81 Postauricular fistula
    H70.811 Postauricular fistula, right ear   SW
    H70.812 Postauricular fistula, left ear   SW
    H70.813 Postauricular fistula, bilateral   SW
    H70.819 Postauricular fistula, unspecified ear   SW

  ✓6ᵗʰ H70.89 Other mastoiditis and related conditions
    H70.891 Other mastoiditis and related conditions, right ear
    H70.892 Other mastoiditis and related conditions, left ear
    H70.893 Other mastoiditis and related conditions, bilateral
    H70.899 Other mastoiditis and related conditions, unspecified ear

✓5ᵗʰ H70.9 Unspecified mastoiditis
    H70.90 Unspecified mastoiditis, unspecified ear
    H70.91 Unspecified mastoiditis, right ear
    H70.92 Unspecified mastoiditis, left ear
    H70.93 Unspecified mastoiditis, bilateral

✓4ᵗʰ H71 Cholesteatoma of middle ear
    EXCLUDES 2   *cholesteatoma of external ear (H60.4-)*
          recurrent cholesteatoma of postmastoidectomy cavity (H95.0-)
    DEF: Cholesteatoma: Noncancerous cyst-like mass of cell debris, including cholesterol and epithelial cells resulting from trauma, repeated or improperly healed infections, and congenital enclosure of epidermal cells.

✓5ᵗʰ H71.0 Cholesteatoma of attic
    H71.00 Cholesteatoma of attic, unspecified ear
    H71.01 Cholesteatoma of attic, right ear
    H71.02 Cholesteatoma of attic, left ear
    H71.03 Cholesteatoma of attic, bilateral

✓5ᵗʰ H71.1 Cholesteatoma of tympanum
    H71.10 Cholesteatoma of tympanum, unspecified ear
    H71.11 Cholesteatoma of tympanum, right ear
    H71.12 Cholesteatoma of tympanum, left ear
    H71.13 Cholesteatoma of tympanum, bilateral

✓5ᵗʰ H71.2 Cholesteatoma of mastoid
    H71.20 Cholesteatoma of mastoid, unspecified ear
    H71.21 Cholesteatoma of mastoid, right ear
    H71.22 Cholesteatoma of mastoid, left ear
    H71.23 Cholesteatoma of mastoid, bilateral

✓5ᵗʰ H71.3 Diffuse cholesteatosis
    H71.30 Diffuse cholesteatosis, unspecified ear
    H71.31 Diffuse cholesteatosis, right ear
    H71.32 Diffuse cholesteatosis, left ear
    H71.33 Diffuse cholesteatosis, bilateral

✓5ᵗʰ H71.9 Unspecified cholesteatoma
    H71.90 Unspecified cholesteatoma, unspecified ear
    H71.91 Unspecified cholesteatoma, right ear
    H71.92 Unspecified cholesteatoma, left ear
    H71.93 Unspecified cholesteatoma, bilateral

Cholesteatoma of Middle Ear

Middle ear chamber

Ear drum

Cholesteatoma sac

✓4ᵗʰ H72 Perforation of tympanic membrane
    INCLUDES   persistent post-traumatic perforation of ear drum
          postinflammatory perforation of ear drum
    Code first any associated otitis media (H65.-, H66.1-, H66.2-, H66.3-, H66.4-, H66.9-, H67.-)
    EXCLUDES 1   *acute suppurative otitis media with rupture of the tympanic membrane (H66.01-)*
          traumatic rupture of ear drum (S09.2-)

✓5ᵗʰ H72.0 Central perforation of tympanic membrane
    H72.00 Central perforation of tympanic membrane, unspecified ear
    H72.01 Central perforation of tympanic membrane, right ear
    H72.02 Central perforation of tympanic membrane, left ear
    H72.03 Central perforation of tympanic membrane, bilateral

✓5ᵗʰ H72.1 Attic perforation of tympanic membrane
    Perforation of pars flaccida
    H72.10 Attic perforation of tympanic membrane, unspecified ear
    H72.11 Attic perforation of tympanic membrane, right ear
    H72.12 Attic perforation of tympanic membrane, left ear
    H72.13 Attic perforation of tympanic membrane, bilateral

✓5ᵗʰ H72.2 Other marginal perforations of tympanic membrane
  ✓6ᵗʰ H72.2X Other marginal perforations of tympanic membrane
    H72.2X1 Other marginal perforations of tympanic membrane, right ear
    H72.2X2 Other marginal perforations of tympanic membrane, left ear
    H72.2X3 Other marginal perforations of tympanic membrane, bilateral
    H72.2X9 Other marginal perforations of tympanic membrane, unspecified ear

✓5ᵗʰ H72.8 Other perforations of tympanic membrane
  ✓6ᵗʰ H72.81 Multiple perforations of tympanic membrane
    H72.811 Multiple perforations of tympanic membrane, right ear
    H72.812 Multiple perforations of tympanic membrane, left ear
    H72.813 Multiple perforations of tympanic membrane, bilateral
    H72.819 Multiple perforations of tympanic membrane, unspecified ear
  ✓6ᵗʰ H72.82 Total perforations of tympanic membrane
    H72.821 Total perforations of tympanic membrane, right ear
    H72.822 Total perforations of tympanic membrane, left ear
    H72.823 Total perforations of tympanic membrane, bilateral
    H72.829 Total perforations of tympanic membrane, unspecified ear

✓5ᵗʰ H72.9 Unspecified perforation of tympanic membrane
    H72.90 Unspecified perforation of tympanic membrane, unspecified ear
    H72.91 Unspecified perforation of tympanic membrane, right ear
    H72.92 Unspecified perforation of tympanic membrane, left ear
    H72.93 Unspecified perforation of tympanic membrane, bilateral

✓4ᵗʰ H73 Other disorders of tympanic membrane
  ✓5ᵗʰ H73.0 Acute myringitis
    EXCLUDES 1   *acute myringitis with otitis media (H65, H66)*
   ✓6ᵗʰ H73.00 Unspecified acute myringitis
    Acute tympanitis NOS
    H73.001 Acute myringitis, right ear
    H73.002 Acute myringitis, left ear
    H73.003 Acute myringitis, bilateral
    H73.009 Acute myringitis, unspecified ear
   ✓6ᵗʰ H73.01 Bullous myringitis
    DEF: Bacterial or viral otitis media that is characterized by the appearance of serous or hemorrhagic blebs on the ear drum and sudden onset of severe pain in ear.
    H73.011 Bullous myringitis, right ear

✔ Additional Character Required   ✓ 7ᵗʰ Placeholder   Unacceptable PDx   Questionable PDx   Manifestation   H1-H14 HAC   HCC CMS-HCC Dx   HIV HIV Dx

ICD-10-CM 2019   627

        H73.012   **Bullous myringitis,** left **ear**
        H73.013   **Bullous myringitis,** bilateral
        H73.019   **Bullous myringitis,** unspecified **ear**

✓6th **H73.09**   Other **acute myringitis**
        H73.091   **Other acute myringitis,** right **ear**
        H73.092   **Other acute myringitis,** left **ear**
        H73.093   **Other acute myringitis,** bilateral
        H73.099   **Other acute myringitis,** unspecified **ear**

✓5th **H73.1**   Chronic **myringitis**
    Chronic tympanitis
      EXCLUDES 1   *chronic myringitis with otitis media (H65, H66)*
    H73.10   **Chronic myringitis,** unspecified **ear**
    H73.11   **Chronic myringitis,** right **ear**
    H73.12   **Chronic myringitis,** left **ear**
    H73.13   **Chronic myringitis,** bilateral

✓5th **H73.2**   Unspecified **myringitis**
    H73.20   **Unspecified myringitis,** unspecified **ear**
    H73.21   **Unspecified myringitis,** right **ear**
    H73.22   **Unspecified myringitis,** left **ear**
    H73.23   **Unspecified myringitis,** bilateral

✓5th **H73.8**   **Other specified disorders of tympanic membrane**
    ✓6th **H73.81**   Atrophic flaccid **tympanic membrane**
        H73.811   **Atrophic flaccid tympanic membrane,** right **ear**
        H73.812   **Atrophic flaccid tympanic membrane,** left **ear**
        H73.813   **Atrophic flaccid tympanic membrane,** bilateral
        H73.819   **Atrophic flaccid tympanic membrane,** unspecified **ear**

    ✓6th **H73.82**   Atrophic nonflaccid **tympanic membrane**
        H73.821   **Atrophic nonflaccid tympanic membrane,** right **ear**
        H73.822   **Atrophic nonflaccid tympanic membrane,** left **ear**
        H73.823   **Atrophic nonflaccid tympanic membrane,** bilateral
        H73.829   **Atrophic nonflaccid tympanic membrane,** unspecified **ear**

    ✓6th **H73.89**   Other **specified disorders of tympanic membrane**
        H73.891   **Other specified disorders of tympanic membrane,** right **ear**
        H73.892   **Other specified disorders of tympanic membrane,** left **ear**
        H73.893   **Other specified disorders of tympanic membrane,** bilateral
        H73.899   **Other specified disorders of tympanic membrane,** unspecified **ear**

✓5th **H73.9**   Unspecified **disorder of tympanic membrane**
    H73.90   **Unspecified disorder of tympanic membrane,** unspecified **ear**
    H73.91   **Unspecified disorder of tympanic membrane,** right **ear**
    H73.92   **Unspecified disorder of tympanic membrane,** left **ear**
    H73.93   **Unspecified disorder of tympanic membrane,** bilateral

✓4th **H74**   **Other disorders of middle ear mastoid**
    EXCLUDES 2   *mastoiditis (H70.-)*

✓5th **H74.0**   Tympanosclerosis
    DEF: Calcification of tissue in the ear drum, middle ear bones, and middle ear canal.
    H74.01   **Tympanosclerosis,** right **ear**
    H74.02   **Tympanosclerosis,** left **ear**
    H74.03   **Tympanosclerosis,** bilateral
    H74.09   **Tympanosclerosis,** unspecified **ear**

✓5th **H74.1**   Adhesive **middle ear disease**
    Adhesive otitis
      EXCLUDES 1   *glue ear (H65.3-)*
    H74.11   **Adhesive** right **middle ear disease**
    H74.12   **Adhesive** left **middle ear disease**
    H74.13   **Adhesive middle ear disease,** bilateral
    H74.19   **Adhesive middle ear disease,** unspecified **ear**

✓5th **H74.2**   **Discontinuity and dislocation of ear ossicles**
    H74.20   **Discontinuity and dislocation of ear ossicles,** unspecified **ear**
    H74.21   **Discontinuity and dislocation of** right **ear ossicles**
    H74.22   **Discontinuity and dislocation of** left **ear ossicles**
    H74.23   **Discontinuity and dislocation of ear ossicles,** bilateral

✓5th **H74.3**   **Other acquired abnormalities of ear ossicles**
    ✓6th **H74.31**   Ankylosis **of ear ossicles**
        H74.311   **Ankylosis of ear ossicles,** right **ear**
        H74.312   **Ankylosis of ear ossicles,** left **ear**
        H74.313   **Ankylosis of ear ossicles,** bilateral
        H74.319   **Ankylosis of ear ossicles,** unspecified **ear**

    ✓6th **H74.32**   Partial loss **of ear ossicles**
        H74.321   **Partial loss of ear ossicles,** right **ear**
        H74.322   **Partial loss of ear ossicles,** left **ear**
        H74.323   **Partial loss of ear ossicles,** bilateral
        H74.329   **Partial loss of ear ossicles,** unspecified **ear**

    ✓6th **H74.39**   Other **acquired abnormalities of ear ossicles**
        H74.391   **Other acquired abnormalities of** right **ear ossicles**
        H74.392   **Other acquired abnormalities of** left **ear ossicles**
        H74.393   **Other acquired abnormalities of ear ossicles,** bilateral
        H74.399   **Other acquired abnormalities of ear ossicles,** unspecified **ear**

✓5th **H74.4**   **Polyp of middle ear**
    H74.40   **Polyp of middle ear,** unspecified **ear**
    H74.41   **Polyp of** right **middle ear**
    H74.42   **Polyp of** left **middle ear**
    H74.43   **Polyp of middle ear,** bilateral

✓5th **H74.8**   **Other specified disorders of middle ear and mastoid**
    ✓6th **H74.8X**   **Other specified disorders of middle ear and mastoid**
        H74.8X1   **Other specified disorders of** right **middle ear and mastoid**
        H74.8X2   **Other specified disorders of** left **middle ear and mastoid**
        H74.8X3   **Other specified disorders of middle ear and mastoid,** bilateral
        H74.8X9   **Other specified disorders of middle ear and mastoid,** unspecified **ear**

✓5th **H74.9**   **Unspecified disorder of middle ear and mastoid**
    H74.90   **Unspecified disorder of middle ear and mastoid,** unspecified **ear**
    H74.91   **Unspecified disorder of** right **middle ear and mastoid**
    H74.92   **Unspecified disorder of** left **middle ear and mastoid**
    H74.93   **Unspecified disorder of middle ear and mastoid,** bilateral

✓4th **H75**   **Other disorders of middle ear and mastoid in diseases classified elsewhere**
    Code first underlying disease

    ✓5th **H75.0**   **Mastoiditis in infectious and parasitic diseases classified elsewhere**
      EXCLUDES 1   *mastoiditis (in):*
        syphilis (A52.77)
        tuberculosis (A18.03)
    H75.00   *Mastoiditis in infectious and parasitic diseases classified elsewhere, unspecified ear*
    H75.01   *Mastoiditis in infectious and parasitic diseases classified elsewhere, right ear*
    H75.02   *Mastoiditis in infectious and parasitic diseases classified elsewhere, left ear*
    H75.03   *Mastoiditis in infectious and parasitic diseases classified elsewhere, bilateral*

    ✓5th **H75.8**   **Other specified disorders of middle ear and mastoid in diseases classified elsewhere**
    H75.80   *Other specified disorders of middle ear and mastoid in diseases classified elsewhere, unspecified ear*
    H75.81   *Other specified disorders of right middle ear and mastoid in diseases classified elsewhere*
    H75.82   *Other specified disorders of left middle ear and mastoid in diseases classified elsewhere*

N Newborn: 0   P Pediatric: 0-17   M Maternity: 12-55   A Adult: 15-124   MCC Major Complication/Comorbidity   CC Complication/Comorbidity   SW Severe Wound Dx

628   ICD-10-CM 2019

H75.83   *Other specified disorders of middle ear and mastoid in diseases classified elsewhere, bilateral*

Diseases of inner ear (H80–H83)

√4ᵗʰ H80   Otosclerosis
     INCLUDES   otospongiosis

√5ᵗʰ H80.0   Otosclerosis involving oval window, nonobliterative
- **H80.00**   Otosclerosis involving oval window, nonobliterative, unspecified ear
- **H80.01**   Otosclerosis involving oval window, nonobliterative, right ear
- **H80.02**   Otosclerosis involving oval window, nonobliterative, left ear
- **H80.03**   Otosclerosis involving oval window, nonobliterative, bilateral

√5ᵗʰ H80.1   Otosclerosis involving oval window, obliterative
- **H80.10**   Otosclerosis involving oval window, obliterative, unspecified ear
- **H80.11**   Otosclerosis involving oval window, obliterative, right ear
- **H80.12**   Otosclerosis involving oval window, obliterative, left ear
- **H80.13**   Otosclerosis involving oval window, obliterative, bilateral

√5ᵗʰ H80.2   Cochlear otosclerosis
     Otosclerosis involving otic capsule
     Otosclerosis involving round window
- **H80.20**   Cochlear otosclerosis, unspecified ear
- **H80.21**   Cochlear otosclerosis, right ear
- **H80.22**   Cochlear otosclerosis, left ear
- **H80.23**   Cochlear otosclerosis, bilateral

√5ᵗʰ H80.8   Other otosclerosis
- **H80.80**   Other otosclerosis, unspecified ear
- **H80.81**   Other otosclerosis, right ear
- **H80.82**   Other otosclerosis, left ear
- **H80.83**   Other otosclerosis, bilateral

√5ᵗʰ H80.9   Unspecified otosclerosis
- **H80.90**   Unspecified otosclerosis, unspecified ear
- **H80.91**   Unspecified otosclerosis, right ear
- **H80.92**   Unspecified otosclerosis, left ear
- **H80.93**   Unspecified otosclerosis, bilateral

√4ᵗʰ H81   Disorders of vestibular function
     EXCLUDES 1   epidemic vertigo (A88.1)
                 vertigo NOS (R42)

√5ᵗʰ H81.0   Ménière's disease
     Labyrinthine hydrops
     Ménière's syndrome or vertigo
     DEF: Distended membranous labyrinth of the middle ear from fluctuating pressure of fluid (hydrops) that causes vertigo, tinnitus, pressure, and hearing loss that may last on and off for several hours. Episodes may occur in clusters or may subside for weeks, months, or even years.
- **H81.01**   Ménière's disease, right ear
- **H81.02**   Ménière's disease, left ear
- **H81.03**   Ménière's disease, bilateral
- **H81.09**   Ménière's disease, unspecified ear

√5ᵗʰ H81.1   Benign paroxysmal vertigo
- **H81.10**   Benign paroxysmal vertigo, unspecified ear
- **H81.11**   Benign paroxysmal vertigo, right ear
- **H81.12**   Benign paroxysmal vertigo, left ear
- **H81.13**   Benign paroxysmal vertigo, bilateral

√5ᵗʰ H81.2   Vestibular neuronitis
     DEF: Transient benign vertigo caused by inflammation of the vestibular nerve. It is characterized by response to caloric stimulation on one side and nystagmus with rhythmic movement of the eyes. Normal auditory function is present.
- **H81.20**   Vestibular neuronitis, unspecified ear
- **H81.21**   Vestibular neuronitis, right ear
- **H81.22**   Vestibular neuronitis, left ear
- **H81.23**   Vestibular neuronitis, bilateral

√5ᵗʰ H81.3   Other peripheral vertigo
     √6ᵗʰ H81.31   Aural vertigo
         H81.311   Aural vertigo, right ear

         H81.312   Aural vertigo, left ear
         H81.313   Aural vertigo, bilateral
         H81.319   Aural vertigo, unspecified ear

     √6ᵗʰ H81.39   Other peripheral vertigo
         Lermoyez' syndrome
         Otogenic vertigo
         Peripheral vertigo NOS
         H81.391   Other peripheral vertigo, right ear
         H81.392   Other peripheral vertigo, left ear
         H81.393   Other peripheral vertigo, bilateral
         H81.399   Other peripheral vertigo, unspecified ear

√5ᵗʰ H81.4   Vertigo of central origin
     Central positional nystagmus
- **H81.41**   Vertigo of central origin, right ear
- **H81.42**   Vertigo of central origin, left ear
- **H81.43**   Vertigo of central origin, bilateral
- **H81.49**   Vertigo of central origin, unspecified ear

√5ᵗʰ H81.8   Other disorders of vestibular function
     √6ᵗʰ H81.8X   Other disorders of vestibular function
         H81.8X1   Other disorders of vestibular function, right ear
         H81.8X2   Other disorders of vestibular function, left ear
         H81.8X3   Other disorders of vestibular function, bilateral
         H81.8X9   Other disorders of vestibular function, unspecified ear

√5ᵗʰ H81.9   Unspecified disorder of vestibular function
     Vertiginous syndrome NOS
- **H81.90**   Unspecified disorder of vestibular function, unspecified ear
- **H81.91**   Unspecified disorder of vestibular function, right ear
- **H81.92**   Unspecified disorder of vestibular function, left ear
- **H81.93**   Unspecified disorder of vestibular function, bilateral

√4ᵗʰ H82   Vertiginous syndromes in diseases classified elsewhere
     Code first underlying disease
     EXCLUDES 1   epidemic vertigo (A88.1)

- **H82.1**   *Vertiginous syndromes in diseases classified elsewhere, right ear*
- **H82.2**   *Vertiginous syndromes in diseases classified elsewhere, left ear*
- **H82.3**   *Vertiginous syndromes in diseases classified elsewhere, bilateral*
- **H82.9**   *Vertiginous syndromes in diseases classified elsewhere, unspecified ear*

√4ᵗʰ H83   Other diseases of inner ear
     √5ᵗʰ H83.0   Labyrinthitis
         DEF: Inflammation of the inner ear, or labyrinth, characterized by pus, vertigo, dizziness, nausea, and hearing loss.
- **H83.01**   Labyrinthitis, right ear
- **H83.02**   Labyrinthitis, left ear
- **H83.03**   Labyrinthitis, bilateral
- **H83.09**   Labyrinthitis, unspecified ear

     √5ᵗʰ H83.1   Labyrinthine fistula
- **H83.11**   Labyrinthine fistula, right ear
- **H83.12**   Labyrinthine fistula, left ear   `SW`
- **H83.13**   Labyrinthine fistula, bilateral   `SW`
- **H83.19**   Labyrinthine fistula, unspecified ear   `SW`

     √5ᵗʰ H83.2   Labyrinthine dysfunction
         Labyrinthine hypersensitivity
         Labyrinthine hypofunction
         Labyrinthine loss of function
         DEF: Decreased function of the labyrinth sensors.
     √6ᵗʰ H83.2X   Labyrinthine dysfunction
         H83.2X1   Labyrinthine dysfunction, right ear
         H83.2X2   Labyrinthine dysfunction, left ear
         H83.2X3   Labyrinthine dysfunction, bilateral
         H83.2X9   Labyrinthine dysfunction, unspecified ear

     √5ᵗʰ H83.3   Noise effects on inner ear
         Acoustic trauma of inner ear
         Noise-induced hearing loss of inner ear
     √6ᵗʰ H83.3X   Noise effects on inner ear
         H83.3X1   Noise effects on right inner ear

Chapter 8. Diseases of the Ear and Mastoid Process *(side margin)*

H83.3X2   Noise effects on left inner ear
H83.3X3   Noise effects on inner ear, bilateral
H83.3X9   Noise effects on inner ear, unspecified ear

✓5ᵗʰ **H83.8**   Other specified diseases of inner ear
    ✓6ᵗʰ **H83.8X**   Other specified diseases of inner ear
       H83.8X1   Other specified diseases of right inner ear
       H83.8X2   Other specified diseases of left inner ear
       H83.8X3   Other specified diseases of inner ear, bilateral
       H83.8X9   Other specified diseases of inner ear, unspecified ear

✓5ᵗʰ **H83.9**   Unspecified disease of inner ear
    H83.90   Unspecified disease of inner ear, unspecified ear
    H83.91   Unspecified disease of right inner ear
    H83.92   Unspecified disease of left inner ear
    H83.93   Unspecified disease of inner ear, bilateral

Other disorders of ear (H90-H94)

✓4ᵗʰ **H90**   **Conductive and sensorineural hearing loss**
    EXCLUDES 1   *deaf nonspeaking NEC (H91.3)*
       deafness NOS (H91.9-)
       hearing loss NOS (H91.9-)
       noise-induced hearing loss (H83.3-)
       ototoxic hearing loss (H91.0-)
       sudden (idiopathic) hearing loss (H91.2-)
    AHA: 2015, 2Q, 7
    DEF: Conductive hearing loss: Hearing Loss due to the inability of sound waves to move from the outer (external ear) to the inner ear.
    DEF: Sensorineural hearing loss: Hearing loss that occurs from damage to the hair cells of the inner ear or problems with the nerve pathways from the inner ear to the brain.

    H90.0   Conductive hearing loss, bilateral
✓5ᵗʰ **H90.1**   Conductive hearing loss, unilateral with unrestricted hearing on the contralateral side
       H90.11   Conductive hearing loss, unilateral, right ear, with unrestricted hearing on the contralateral side
       H90.12   Conductive hearing loss, unilateral, left ear, with unrestricted hearing on the contralateral side
    H90.2   Conductive hearing loss, unspecified
       Conductive deafness NOS
    H90.3   Sensorineural hearing loss, bilateral
✓5ᵗʰ **H90.4**   Sensorineural hearing loss, unilateral with unrestricted hearing on the contralateral side
       H90.41   Sensorineural hearing loss, unilateral, right ear, with unrestricted hearing on the contralateral side
       H90.42   Sensorineural hearing loss, unilateral, left ear, with unrestricted hearing on the contralateral side
    H90.5   Unspecified sensorineural hearing loss
       Central hearing loss NOS   Perceptive hearing loss NOS
       Congenital deafness NOS   Sensorineural deafness NOS
       Neural hearing loss NOS   Sensory hearing loss NOS
       EXCLUDES 1   *abnormal auditory perception (H93.2-)*
          psychogenic deafness (F44.6)
    H90.6   Mixed conductive and sensorineural hearing loss, bilateral
       AHA: 2015, 2Q, 7
✓5ᵗʰ **H90.7**   Mixed conductive and sensorineural hearing loss, unilateral with unrestricted hearing on the contralateral side
       H90.71   Mixed conductive and sensorineural hearing loss, unilateral, right ear, with unrestricted hearing on the contralateral side
       H90.72   Mixed conductive and sensorineural hearing loss, unilateral, left ear, with unrestricted hearing on the contralateral side
    H90.8   Mixed conductive and sensorineural hearing loss, unspecified
✓5ᵗʰ **H90.A**   Conductive and sensorineural hearing loss with restricted hearing on the contralateral side
       AHA: 2016, 4Q, 23-25
    ✓6ᵗʰ **H90.A1**   Conductive hearing loss, unilateral, with restricted hearing on the contralateral side
          H90.A11   Conductive hearing loss, unilateral, right ear with restricted hearing on the contralateral side
          H90.A12   Conductive hearing loss, unilateral, left ear with restricted hearing on the contralateral side

    ✓6ᵗʰ **H90.A2**   Sensorineural hearing loss, unilateral, with restricted hearing on the contralateral side
          H90.A21   Sensorineural hearing loss, unilateral, right ear, with restricted hearing on the contralateral side
          H90.A22   Sensorineural hearing loss, unilateral, left ear, with restricted hearing on the contralateral side
    ✓6ᵗʰ **H90.A3**   Mixed conductive and sensorineural hearing loss, unilateral with restricted hearing on the contralateral side
          H90.A31   Mixed conductive and sensorineural hearing loss, unilateral, right ear with restricted hearing on the contralateral side
          H90.A32   Mixed conductive and sensorineural hearing loss, unilateral, left ear with restricted hearing on the contralateral side

✓4ᵗʰ **H91**   **Other and unspecified hearing loss**
    EXCLUDES 1   *abnormal auditory perception (H93.2-)*
       hearing loss as classified in H90-
       impacted cerumen (H61.2-)
       noise-induced hearing loss (H83.3-)
       psychogenic deafness (F44.6)
       transient ischemic deafness (H93.01-)

✓5ᵗʰ **H91.0**   Ototoxic hearing loss
       Code first poisoning due to drug or toxin, if applicable (T36-T65 with fifth or sixth character 1-4 or 6)
       Use additional code for adverse effect, if applicable, to identify drug (T36-T50 with fifth or sixth character 5)
    H91.01   Ototoxic hearing loss, right ear
    H91.02   Ototoxic hearing loss, left ear
    H91.03   Ototoxic hearing loss, bilateral
    H91.09   Ototoxic hearing loss, unspecified ear
✓5ᵗʰ **H91.1**   Presbycusis
       Presbyacusia
    H91.10   Presbycusis, unspecified ear
    H91.11   Presbycusis, right ear
    H91.12   Presbycusis, left ear
    H91.13   Presbycusis, bilateral
✓5ᵗʰ **H91.2**   Sudden idiopathic hearing loss
       Sudden hearing loss NOS
    H91.20   Sudden idiopathic hearing loss, unspecified ear
    H91.21   Sudden idiopathic hearing loss, right ear
    H91.22   Sudden idiopathic hearing loss, left ear
    H91.23   Sudden idiopathic hearing loss, bilateral
    H91.3   Deaf nonspeaking, not elsewhere classified
✓5ᵗʰ **H91.8**   Other specified hearing loss
    ✓6ᵗʰ **H91.8X**   Other specified hearing loss
       H91.8X1   Other specified hearing loss, right ear
       H91.8X2   Other specified hearing loss, left ear
       H91.8X3   Other specified hearing loss, bilateral
       H91.8X9   Other specified hearing loss, unspecified ear
✓5ᵗʰ **H91.9**   Unspecified hearing loss
       Deafness NOS
       High frequency deafness
       Low frequency deafness
    H91.90   Unspecified hearing loss, unspecified ear
    H91.91   Unspecified hearing loss, right ear
    H91.92   Unspecified hearing loss, left ear
    H91.93   Unspecified hearing loss, bilateral

✓4ᵗʰ **H92**   **Otalgia and effusion of ear**
✓5ᵗʰ **H92.0**   Otalgia
    H92.01   Otalgia, right ear
    H92.02   Otalgia, left ear
    H92.03   Otalgia, bilateral
    H92.09   Otalgia, unspecified ear
✓5ᵗʰ **H92.1**   Otorrhea
       EXCLUDES 1   *leakage of cerebrospinal fluid through ear (G96.0)*
    H92.10   Otorrhea, unspecified ear
    H92.11   Otorrhea, right ear
    H92.12   Otorrhea, left ear

N Newborn: 0   P Pediatric: 0-17   M Maternity: 12-55   A Adult: 15-124   MCC Major Complication/Comorbidity   CC Complication/Comorbidity   SW Severe Wound Dx

630   ICD-10-CM 2019

H83.3X2–H92.12 *(side margin)*

H92.13   **Otorrhea,** bilateral

✓5ᵗʰ H92.2 Otorrhagia

    EXCLUDES 1   traumatic otorrhagia—code to injury

H92.20   **Otorrhagia,** unspecified **ear**

H92.21   **Otorrhagia,** right **ear**

H92.22   **Otorrhagia,** left **ear**

H92.23   **Otorrhagia,** bilateral

✓4ᵗʰ H93 Other disorders of ear, not elsewhere classified

✓5ᵗʰ H93.0 Degenerative and vascular disorders of ear

    EXCLUDES 1   presbycusis (H91.1)

✓6ᵗʰ H93.01 Transient ischemic deafness

H93.011   **Transient ischemic deafness,** right **ear**

H93.012   **Transient ischemic deafness,** left **ear**

H93.013   **Transient ischemic deafness,** bilateral

H93.019   **Transient ischemic deafness,** unspecified **ear**

✓6ᵗʰ H93.09 Unspecified degenerative and vascular disorders of ear

H93.091   **Unspecified degenerative and vascular disorders of** right **ear**

H93.092   **Unspecified degenerative and vascular disorders of** left **ear**

H93.093   **Unspecified degenerative and vascular disorders of ear,** bilateral

H93.099   **Unspecified degenerative and vascular disorders of** unspecified **ear**

✓5ᵗʰ H93.1 Tinnitus

H93.11   **Tinnitus,** right **ear**

H93.12   **Tinnitus,** left **ear**

H93.13   **Tinnitus,** bilateral

H93.19   **Tinnitus,** unspecified **ear**

✓5ᵗʰ H93.A Pulsatile Tinnitus

    AHA: 2016, 4Q, 25-26

H93.A1   **Pulsatile tinnitus,** right **ear**

H93.A2   **Pulsatile tinnitus,** left **ear**

H93.A3   **Pulsatile tinnitus,** bilateral

H93.A9   **Pulsatile tinnitus,** unspecified **ear**

✓5ᵗʰ H93.2 Other abnormal auditory perceptions

    EXCLUDES 2   auditory hallucinations (R44.0)

✓6ᵗʰ H93.21 Auditory recruitment

H93.211   **Auditory recruitment,** right **ear**

H93.212   **Auditory recruitment,** left **ear**

H93.213   **Auditory recruitment,** bilateral

H93.219   **Auditory recruitment,** unspecified **ear**

✓6ᵗʰ H93.22 Diplacusis

H93.221   **Diplacusis,** right **ear**

H93.222   **Diplacusis,** left **ear**

H93.223   **Diplacusis,** bilateral

H93.229   **Diplacusis,** unspecified **ear**

✓6ᵗʰ H93.23 Hyperacusis

    DEF: Exceptionally acute sense of hearing caused by such conditions as Bell's palsy. This term may also refer to painful sensitivity to sounds.

H93.231   **Hyperacusis,** right **ear**

H93.232   **Hyperacusis,** left **ear**

H93.233   **Hyperacusis,** bilateral

H93.239   **Hyperacusis,** unspecified **ear**

✓6ᵗʰ H93.24 Temporary auditory threshold shift

H93.241   **Temporary auditory threshold shift,** right **ear**

H93.242   **Temporary auditory threshold shift,** left **ear**

H93.243   **Temporary auditory threshold shift,** bilateral

H93.249   **Temporary auditory threshold shift,** unspecified **ear**

H93.25   **Central auditory processing disorder**

    Congenital auditory imperception

    Word deafness

    EXCLUDES 1   mixed receptive-expressive language disorder (F80.2)

✓6ᵗʰ H93.29 Other abnormal auditory perceptions

H93.291   **Other abnormal auditory perceptions,** right **ear**

H93.292   **Other abnormal auditory perceptions,** left **ear**

H93.293   **Other abnormal auditory perceptions,** bilateral

H93.299   **Other abnormal auditory perceptions,** unspecified **ear**

✓5ᵗʰ H93.3 Disorders of acoustic nerve

    Disorder of 8th cranial nerve

    EXCLUDES 1   acoustic neuroma (D33.3)

                syphilitic acoustic neuritis (A52.15)

✓6ᵗʰ H93.3X Disorders of acoustic nerve

H93.3X1   **Disorders of** right **acoustic nerve**

H93.3X2   **Disorders of** left **acoustic nerve**

H93.3X3   **Disorders of** bilateral **acoustic nerves**

H93.3X9   **Disorders of** unspecified **acoustic nerve**

✓5ᵗʰ H93.8 Other specified disorders of ear

✓6ᵗʰ H93.8X Other specified disorders of ear

H93.8X1   **Other specified disorders of** right **ear**

H93.8X2   **Other specified disorders of** left **ear**

H93.8X3   **Other specified disorders of ear,** bilateral

H93.8X9   **Other specified disorders of ear,** unspecified **ear**

✓5ᵗʰ H93.9 Unspecified disorder of ear

H93.90   **Unspecified disorder of ear,** unspecified **ear**

H93.91   **Unspecified disorder of** right **ear**

H93.92   **Unspecified disorder of** left **ear**

H93.93   **Unspecified disorder of ear,** bilateral

✓4ᵗʰ H94 Other disorders of ear in diseases classified elsewhere

✓5ᵗʰ H94.0 Acoustic neuritis in infectious and parasitic diseases classified elsewhere

    Code first underlying disease, such as:

      parasitic disease (B65-B89)

    EXCLUDES 1   acoustic neuritis (in):

                herpes zoster (B02.29)

                syphilis (A52.15)

H94.00   ***Acoustic neuritis in infectious and parasitic diseases classified elsewhere,** unspecified **ear***

H94.01   ***Acoustic neuritis in infectious and parasitic diseases classified elsewhere,** right **ear***

H94.02   ***Acoustic neuritis in infectious and parasitic diseases classified elsewhere,** left **ear***

H94.03   ***Acoustic neuritis in infectious and parasitic diseases classified elsewhere,** bilateral*

✓5ᵗʰ H94.8 Other specified disorders of ear in diseases classified elsewhere

    Code first underlying disease, such as:

      congenital syphilis (A50.0)

    EXCLUDES 1   aural myiasis (B87.4)

                syphilitic labyrinthitis (A52.79)

H94.80   ***Other specified disorders of ear in diseases classified elsewhere,** unspecified **ear***

H94.81   ***Other specified disorders of** right **ear in diseases classified elsewhere***

H94.82   ***Other specified disorders of** left **ear in diseases classified elsewhere***

H94.83   ***Other specified disorders of ear in diseases classified elsewhere,** bilateral*

Intraoperative and postprocedural complications and disorders of ear and mastoid process, not elsewhere classified (H95)

✓4ᵗʰ H95 Intraoperative and postprocedural complications and disorders of ear and mastoid process, not elsewhere classified

    AHA: 2016, 4Q, 9-10

✓5ᵗʰ H95.0 Recurrent cholesteatoma of postmastoidectomy cavity

H95.00   **Recurrent cholesteatoma of postmastoidectomy cavity,** unspecified **ear**

H95.01   **Recurrent cholesteatoma of postmastoidectomy cavity,** right **ear**

H95.02   **Recurrent cholesteatoma of postmastoidectomy cavity,** left **ear**

H95.03   **Recurrent cholesteatoma of postmastoidectomy cavity,** bilateral **ears**

✓ Additional Character Required   ✓x7ᵗʰ Placeholder   Unacceptable PDx   Questionable PDx   Manifestation   **H1**-**H14** HAC   **HCC** CMS-HCC Dx   **HIV** HIV Dx

ICD-10-CM 2019   631

Chapter 8. Diseases of the Ear and Mastoid Process

✓5ᵗʰ **H95.1** **Other disorders of ear and mastoid process following mastoidectomy**

✓6ᵗʰ **H95.11** **Chronic inflammation of postmastoidectomy cavity**

H95.111 **Chronic inflammation of postmastoidectomy cavity,** right **ear**

H95.112 **Chronic inflammation of postmastoidectomy cavity,** left **ear**

H95.113 **Chronic inflammation of postmastoidectomy cavity,** bilateral **ears**

H95.119 **Chronic inflammation of postmastoidectomy cavity,** unspecified **ear**

✓6ᵗʰ **H95.12** **Granulation of postmastoidectomy cavity**

H95.121 **Granulation of postmastoidectomy cavity,** right **ear**

H95.122 **Granulation of postmastoidectomy cavity,** left **ear**

H95.123 **Granulation of postmastoidectomy cavity,** bilateral **ears**

H95.129 **Granulation of postmastoidectomy cavity,** unspecified **ear**

✓6ᵗʰ **H95.13** **Mucosal cyst of postmastoidectomy cavity**

H95.131 **Mucosal cyst of postmastoidectomy cavity,** right **ear**

H95.132 **Mucosal cyst of postmastoidectomy cavity,** left **ear**

H95.133 **Mucosal cyst of postmastoidectomy cavity,** bilateral **ears**

H95.139 **Mucosal cyst of postmastoidectomy cavity,** unspecified **ear**

✓6ᵗʰ **H95.19** **Other disorders following mastoidectomy**

H95.191 **Other disorders following mastoidectomy,** right **ear**

H95.192 **Other disorders following mastoidectomy,** left **ear**

H95.193 **Other disorders following mastoidectomy,** bilateral **ears**

H95.199 **Other disorders following mastoidectomy,** unspecified **ear**

✓5ᵗʰ **H95.2** Intraoperative hemorrhage and hematoma **of ear and mastoid process complicating a procedure**

> EXCLUDES 1   *intraoperative hemorrhage and hematoma of ear and mastoid process due to accidental puncture or laceration during a procedure (H95.3-)*

H95.21 **Intraoperative hemorrhage and hematoma of ear and mastoid process complicating a procedure on the ear and mastoid process**   CC
> CC Excl: PDX collection 642

H95.22 **Intraoperative hemorrhage and hematoma of of ear and mastoid process complicating** other procedure   CC
> CC Excl: PDX collection 642

✓5ᵗʰ **H95.3** Accidental puncture and laceration **of ear and mastoid process during a procedure**

H95.31 **Accidental puncture and laceration of the ear and mastoid process** during a procedure on the ear and mastoid process   CC
> CC Excl: PDX collection 509

H95.32 **Accidental puncture and laceration of the ear and mastoid process** during other procedure   CC
> CC Excl: PDX collection 509

✓5ᵗʰ **H95.4** Postprocedural hemorrhage **of ear and mastoid process following a procedure**

H95.41 **Postprocedural hemorrhage of ear and mastoid process following a** procedure on the ear and mastoid process   CC
> CC Excl: PDX collection 642

H95.42 **Postprocedural hemorrhage of ear and mastoid process following** other procedure   CC
> CC Excl: PDX collection 642

✓5ᵗʰ **H95.5** Postprocedural hematoma and seroma **of ear and mastoid process following a procedure**

> **CC Excl: For CC codes in subcategory H95.5:**
> PDX collection 642

H95.51 **Postprocedural** hematoma **of ear and mastoid process following a** procedure on the ear and mastoid process   CC

H95.52 **Postprocedural** hematoma **of ear and mastoid process following** other procedure   CC

H95.53 **Postprocedural** seroma **of ear and mastoid process following a** procedure on the ear and mastoid process   CC

H95.54 **Postprocedural** seroma **of ear and mastoid process following** other procedure   CC

✓5ᵗʰ **H95.8** Other intraoperative and postprocedural complications and disorders of the ear and mastoid process, not elsewhere classified

> EXCLUDES 2   *postprocedural complications and disorders following mastoidectomy (H95.0-, H95.1-)*

> **CC Excl: For CC codes in subcategory H95.8:**
> PDX collection 643

✓6ᵗʰ **H95.81** Postprocedural stenosis **of external ear canal**

H95.811 **Postprocedural stenosis of** right **external ear canal**   CC

H95.812 **Postprocedural stenosis of** left **external ear canal**   CC

H95.813 **Postprocedural stenosis of external ear canal,** bilateral   CC

H95.819 **Postprocedural stenosis of** unspecified **external ear canal**   CC

H95.88 **Other intraoperative complications and disorders of the ear and mastoid process, not elsewhere classified**   CC
> Use additional code, if applicable, to further specify disorder

H95.89 **Other postprocedural complications and disorders of the ear and mastoid process, not elsewhere classified**   CC
> Use additional code, if applicable, to further specify disorder

---

N Newborn: 0   P Pediatric: 0-17   M Maternity: 12-55   A Adult: 15-124   MCC Major Complication/Comorbidity   CC Complication/Comorbidity   SW Severe Wound Dx

Chapter 9. Diseases of the Circulatory System (I00–I99)

Chapter Specific Guidelines with Coding Examples

The chapter specific guidelines from the ICD-10-CM Official Guidelines for Coding and Reporting have been provided below. Along with these guidelines are coding examples, contained in the shaded boxes, that have been developed to help illustrate the coding and/or sequencing guidance found in these guidelines.

a. Hypertension

The classification presumes a causal relationship between hypertension and heart involvement and between hypertension and kidney involvement, as the two conditions are linked by the term "with" in the Alphabetic Index. These conditions should be coded as related even in the absence of provider documentation explicitly linking them, unless the documentation clearly states the conditions are unrelated.

For hypertension and conditions not specifically linked by relational terms such as "with," "associated with" or "due to" in the classification, provider documentation must link the conditions in order to code them as related.

1) Hypertension with heart disease

Hypertension with heart conditions classified to I50.- or **I51.4-I51.7, I51.89, I51.9,** are assigned to a code from category I11, Hypertensive heart disease. Use additional code(s) from category I50, Heart failure, to identify the type(s) of heart failure in those patients with heart failure.

The same heart conditions (I50.-, **I51.4-I51.7, I51.89, I51.9**) with hypertension are coded separately if the provider has **documented they are unrelated to the hypertension.** Sequence according to the circumstances of the admission/encounter.

> Patient is admitted in left heart failure. Patient also has a history of hypertension managed by medication.
>
> | | |
> |---|---|
> | 11.0 | **Hypertensive heart disease with heart failure** |
> | I50.1 | **Left ventricular failure, unspecified** |
>
> *Explanation*: Without a diagnostic statement to the contrary, hypertension and heart failure have an assumed causal relationship, and a combination code should be used. An additional code to identify the type of heart failure (I50.-) should also be provided.

2) Hypertensive chronic kidney disease

Assign codes from category I12, Hypertensive chronic kidney disease, when both hypertension and a condition classifiable to category N18, Chronic kidney disease (CKD), are present. CKD should not be coded as hypertensive if the **provider indicates the CKD is not related to the hypertension.**

The appropriate code from category N18 should be used as a secondary code with a code from category I12 to identify the stage of chronic kidney disease.

See Section I.C.14. Chronic kidney disease.

If a patient has hypertensive chronic kidney disease and acute renal failure, an additional code for the acute renal failure is required.

> Patient is admitted with stage IV chronic kidney disease (CKD). The patient also has documented hypertension secondary to primary hyperparathyroidism.
>
> | | |
> |---|---|
> | N18.4 | **Chronic kidney disease, stage 4 (severe)** |
> | I10 | **Essential (primary) hypertension** |
> | E21.0 | **Primary hyperparathyroidism** |
>
> *Explanation*: A combination code describing a relationship between hypertension and CKD is not used due to the physician documentation identifying the primary hyperparathyroidism as the cause for the hypertension.

3) Hypertensive heart and chronic kidney disease

Assign codes from combination category I13, Hypertensive heart and chronic kidney disease, when there is hypertension with both heart and kidney involvement. If heart failure is present, assign an additional code from category I50 to identify the type of heart failure.

The appropriate code from category N18, Chronic kidney disease, should be used as a secondary code with a code from category I13 to identify the stage of chronic kidney disease.

See Section I.C.14. Chronic kidney disease.

The codes in category I13, Hypertensive heart and chronic kidney disease, are combination codes that include hypertension, heart disease and chronic kidney disease. The Includes note at I13 specifies that the conditions included at I11 and I12 are included together in I13. If a patient

has hypertension, heart disease and chronic kidney disease, then a code from I13 should be used, not individual codes for hypertension, heart disease and chronic kidney disease, or codes from I11 or I12.

For patients with both acute renal failure and chronic kidney disease, an additional code for acute renal failure is required.

> Hypertensive heart and kidney disease with congestive heart failure and stage 2 chronic kidney disease
>
> | | |
> |---|---|
> | I13.0 | **Hypertensive heart and chronic kidney disease with heart failure and stage 1 through stage 4 chronic kidney disease, or unspecified chronic kidney disease** |
> | I50.9 | **Heart failure, unspecified** |
> | N18.2 | **Chronic kidney disease, stage 2 (mild)** |
>
> *Explanation*: Combination codes in category I13 are used to report conditions classifiable to *both* categories I11 and I12. Do not report conditions classifiable to I11 and I12 separately. Use additional codes to report type of heart failure and stage of CKD.

4) Hypertensive cerebrovascular disease

For hypertensive cerebrovascular disease, first assign the appropriate code from categories I60-I69, followed by the appropriate hypertension code.

> Rupture of cerebral aneurysm caused by malignant hypertension
>
> | | |
> |---|---|
> | I60.7 | **Nontraumatic subarachnoid hemorrhage from unspecified intracranial artery** |
> | I10 | **Essential (primary) hypertension** |
>
> *Explanation*: Hypertensive cerebrovascular disease requires two codes: the appropriate I60–I69 code followed by the appropriate hypertension code.

5) Hypertensive retinopathy

Subcategory H35.0, Background retinopathy and retinal vascular changes, should be used with a code from category I10 – I15, Hypertensive disease to include the systemic hypertension. The sequencing is based on the reason for the encounter.

6) Hypertension, secondary

Secondary hypertension is due to an underlying condition. Two codes are required: one to identify the underlying etiology and one from category I15 to identify the hypertension. Sequencing of codes is determined by the reason for admission/encounter.

> Renovascular hypertension due to renal artery atherosclerosis
>
> | | |
> |---|---|
> | I15.0 | **Renovascular hypertension** |
> | I70.1 | **Atherosclerosis of renal artery** |
>
> *Explanation*: Secondary hypertension requires two codes: a code to identify the etiology and the appropriate I15 code.

7) Hypertension, transient

Assign code R03.0, Elevated blood pressure reading without diagnosis of hypertension, unless patient has an established diagnosis of hypertension. Assign code O13.-, Gestational [pregnancy-induced] hypertension without significant proteinuria, or O14.-, Pre-eclampsia, for transient hypertension of pregnancy.

8) Hypertension, controlled

This diagnostic statement usually refers to an existing state of hypertension under control by therapy. Assign the appropriate code from categories I10-I15, Hypertensive diseases.

9) Hypertension, uncontrolled

Uncontrolled hypertension may refer to untreated hypertension or hypertension not responding to current therapeutic regimen. In either case, assign the appropriate code from categories I10-I15, Hypertensive diseases.

10) Hypertensive crisis

Assign a code from category I16, Hypertensive crisis, for documented hypertensive urgency, hypertensive emergency or unspecified hypertensive crisis. Code also any identified hypertensive disease (I10-I15). The sequencing is based on the reason for the encounter.

11) Pulmonary hypertension

Pulmonary hypertension is classified to category I27, Other pulmonary heart diseases. For secondary pulmonary hypertension (I27.1, I27.2-), code also any associated conditions or adverse effects of drugs or toxins.

The sequencing is based on the reason for the encounter, **except for adverse effects of drugs (See Section I.C.19.e.).**

b. Atherosclerotic coronary artery disease and angina

ICD-10-CM has combination codes for atherosclerotic heart disease with angina pectoris. The subcategories for these codes are I25.11, Atherosclerotic heart disease of native coronary artery with angina pectoris and I25.7, Atherosclerosis of coronary artery bypass graft(s) and coronary artery of transplanted heart with angina pectoris.

When using one of these combination codes it is not necessary to use an additional code for angina pectoris. A causal relationship can be assumed in a patient with both atherosclerosis and angina pectoris, unless the documentation indicates the angina is due to something other than the atherosclerosis.

If a patient with coronary artery disease is admitted due to an acute myocardial infarction (AMI), the AMI should be sequenced before the coronary artery disease.

See Section I.C.9. Acute myocardial infarction (AMI)

c. Intraoperative and postprocedural cerebrovascular accident

Medical record documentation should clearly specify the cause- and- effect relationship between the medical intervention and the cerebrovascular accident in order to assign a code for intraoperative or postprocedural cerebrovascular accident.

Proper code assignment depends on whether it was an infarction or hemorrhage and whether it occurred intraoperatively or postoperatively. If it was a cerebral hemorrhage, code assignment depends on the type of procedure performed.

Embolic cerebral infarction of the right middle cerebral artery that occurred during hip replacement surgery. The surgeon documented as due to the surgery.

| I97.811 | Intraoperative cerebrovascular infarction during other surgery |
| I63.411 | Cerebral infarction due to embolism of right middle cerebral artery |

Explanation: Code assignment for intraoperative or postprocedural cerebrovascular accident is based on the provider's documentation of a cause-and-effect relationship between the condition and the procedure. Proper code assignment also depends on whether the cerebrovascular accident was an infarction or hemorrhage, occurred intraoperatively or postoperatively, and the type of procedure performed.

d. Sequelae of cerebrovascular disease

1) Category I69, Sequelae of cerebrovascular disease

Category I69 is used to indicate conditions classifiable to categories I60-I67 as the causes of sequela (neurologic deficits), themselves classified elsewhere. These "late effects" include neurologic deficits that persist after initial onset of conditions classifiable to categories I60-I67. The neurologic deficits caused by cerebrovascular disease may be present from the onset or may arise at any time after the onset of the condition classifiable to categories I60-I67.

Codes from category I69, Sequelae of cerebrovascular disease, that specify hemiplegia, hemiparesis and monoplegia identify whether the dominant or nondominant side is affected. Should the affected side be documented, but not specified as dominant or nondominant, and the classification system does not indicate a default, code selection is as follows:

- For ambidextrous patients, the default should be dominant.
- If the left side is affected, the default is non-dominant.
- If the right side is affected, the default is dominant.

2) Codes from category I69 with codes from I60–I67

Codes from category I69 may be assigned on a health care record with codes from I60-I67, if the patient has a current cerebrovascular disease and deficits from an old cerebrovascular disease.

3) Codes from category I69 and personal history of transient ischemic attack (TIA) and cerebral infarction (Z86.73)

Codes from category I69 should not be assigned if the patient does not have neurologic deficits.

See Section I.C.21. 4. History (of) for use of personal history codes

e. Acute myocardial infarction (AMI)

1) Type 1 ST elevation myocardial infarction (STEMI) and non ST elevation myocardial infarction (NSTEMI)

The ICD-10-CM codes for type 1 acute myocardial infarction (AMI) identify the site, such as anterolateral wall or true posterior wall. Subcategories I21.0-I21.2 and code I21.3 are used for type 1 ST elevation myocardial infarction (STEMI). Code I21.4, Non-ST elevation (NSTEMI) myocardial

infarction, is used for type 1 non ST elevation myocardial infarction (NSTEMI) and nontransmural MIs.

If a type 1 NSTEMI evolves to STEMI, assign the STEMI code. If a type 1 STEMI converts to NSTEMI due to thrombolytic therapy, it is still coded as STEMI.

For encounters occurring while the myocardial infarction is equal to, or less than, four weeks old, including transfers to another acute setting or a postacute setting, and the myocardial infarction meets the definition for "other diagnoses" (see Section III, Reporting Additional Diagnoses), codes from category I21 may continue to be reported. For encounters after the 4 week time frame and the patient is still receiving care related to the myocardial infarction, the appropriate aftercare code should be assigned, rather than a code from category I21. For old or healed myocardial infarctions not requiring further care, code I25.2, Old myocardial infarction, may be assigned.

2) Acute myocardial infarction, unspecified

Code I21.9, Acute myocardial infarction, unspecified, is the default for unspecified acute myocardial infarction or unspecified type. If only type 1 STEMI or transmural MI without the site is documented, assign code I21.3, ST elevation (STEMI) myocardial infarction of unspecified site.

3) AMI documented as nontransmural or subendocardial but site provided

If an AMI is documented as nontransmural or subendocardial, but the site is provided, it is still coded as a subendocardial AMI.

See Section I.C.21.3 for information on coding status post administration of tPA in a different facility within the last 24 hours.

4) Subsequent acute myocardial infarction

A code from category I22, Subsequent ST elevation (STEMI) and non-ST elevation (NSTEMI) myocardial infarction, is to be used when a patient who has suffered a type 1 or unspecified AMI has a new AMI within the 4 week time frame of the initial AMI. A code from category I22 must be used in conjunction with a code from category I21. The sequencing of the I22 and I21 codes depends on the circumstances of the encounter.

Do not assign code I22 for subsequent myocardial infarctions other than type 1 or unspecified. For subsequent type 2 AMI assign only code I21.A1. For subsequent type 4 or type 5 AMI, assign only code I21.A9.

If a subsequent myocardial infarction of one type occurs within 4 weeks of a myocardial infarction of a different type, assign the appropriate codes from category I21 to identify each type. Do not assign a code from I22. Codes from category I22 should only be assigned if both the initial and subsequent myocardial infarctions are type 1 or unspecified.

5) Other types of myocardial infarction

The ICD-10-CM provides codes for different types of myocardial infarction. Type 1 myocardial infarctions are assigned to codes I21.0-I21.4 **and I21.9**.

Type 2 myocardial infarction (myocardial infarction due to demand ischemia or secondary to ischemic balance) is assigned to code I21.A1, Myocardial infarction type 2 with a code for the underlying cause. Do not assign code I24.8, Other forms of acute ischemic heart disease for the demand ischemia. Sequencing of type 2 AMI or the underlying cause is dependent on the circumstances of admission. When a type 2 AMI code is described as NSTEMI or STEMI, only assign code I21.A1. Codes I21.01-I21.4 should only be assigned for type 1 AMIs.

Acute myocardial infarctions type 3, 4a, 4b, 4c and 5 are assigned to code I21.A9, Other myocardial infarction type.

The "Code also" and "Code first" notes should be followed related to complications, and for coding of postprocedural myocardial infarctions during or following cardiac surgery.

Myocardial infarction involving the left circumflex artery occurring during PTCA with stent insertion to treat coronary artery disease

I25.10	Atherosclerotic heart disease of native coronary artery without angina pectoris
I97.790	Other intraoperative cardiac functional disturbances during cardiac surgery
I21.A9	Other myocardial infarction type

Explanation: A myocardial infarction occurring during a revascularization procedure is not considered a type 1 myocardial infarction (MI) and should not be coded to a type 1 MI code (I21.0-, I21.1-, I21.2-, I21.3) even when the specific site of the MI is documented. According to the code first instruction at I21.A9, the complication code (I97.790) should be sequenced before code I21.A9.

Chapter 9. Diseases of the Circulatory System (I00-I99)

EXCLUDES 2 certain conditions originating in the perinatal period (P04-P96)
certain infectious and parasitic diseases (A00-B99)
complications of pregnancy, childbirth and the puerperium (O00-O9A)
congenital malformations, deformations, and chromosomal abnormalities (Q00-Q99)
endocrine, nutritional and metabolic diseases (E00-E88)
injury, poisoning and certain other consequences of external causes (S00-T88)
neoplasms (C00-D49)
symptoms, signs and abnormal clinical and laboratory findings, not elsewhere classified (R00-R94)
systemic connective tissue disorders (M30-M36)
transient cerebral ischemic attacks and related syndromes (G45.-)

This chapter contains the following blocks:

I00-I02	Acute rheumatic fever
I05-I09	Chronic rheumatic heart diseases
I10-I16	Hypertensive diseases
I20-I25	Ischemic heart diseases
I26-I28	Pulmonary heart disease and diseases of pulmonary circulation
I30-I52	Other forms of heart disease
I60-I69	Cerebrovascular diseases
I70-I79	Diseases of arteries, arterioles and capillaries
I80-I89	Diseases of veins, lymphatic vessels and lymph nodes, not elsewhere classified
I95-I99	Other and unspecified disorders of the circulatory system

Acute rheumatic fever (I00-I02)
DEF: Inflammatory disease that can follow a throat infection by group A streptococci. Complications can involve the joints (arthritis), subcutaneous tissue (nodules), skin (erythema marginatum), heart (carditis), or brain (chorea).

I00 **Rheumatic fever without heart involvement**
INCLUDES arthritis, rheumatic, acute or subacute
EXCLUDES 1 rheumatic fever with heart involvement (I01.0-I01.9)

I01 **Rheumatic fever with heart involvement**
EXCLUDES 1 chronic diseases of rheumatic origin (I05-I09) unless rheumatic fever is also present or there is evidence of reactivation or activity of the rheumatic process.

I01.0 **Acute rheumatic pericarditis** CC
Any condition in I00 with pericarditis
Rheumatic pericarditis (acute)
EXCLUDES 1 acute pericarditis not specified as rheumatic (I30.-)
CC Excl: PDX collection 188

I01.1 **Acute rheumatic endocarditis** CC
Any condition in I00 with endocarditis or valvulitis
Acute rheumatic valvulitis
CC Excl: PDX collection 644

I01.2 **Acute rheumatic myocarditis** CC
Any condition in I00 with myocarditis
CC Excl: PDX collection 186

I01.8 **Other acute rheumatic heart disease** CC
Any condition in I00 with other or multiple types of heart involvement
Acute rheumatic pancarditis
CC Excl: PDX collection 645

I01.9 **Acute rheumatic heart disease, unspecified** CC
Any condition in I00 with unspecified type of heart involvement
Rheumatic carditis, acute
Rheumatic heart disease, active or acute
CC Excl: PDX collection 646

I02 **Rheumatic chorea**
INCLUDES Sydenham's chorea
EXCLUDES 1 chorea NOS (G25.5)
Huntington's chorea (G10)

I02.0 **Rheumatic chorea with heart involvement** CC
Chorea NOS with heart involvement
Rheumatic chorea with heart involvement of any type classifiable under I01-
CC Excl: PDX collection 645

I02.9 **Rheumatic chorea without heart involvement** CC
Rheumatic chorea NOS
CC Excl: PDX collection 646

Chronic rheumatic heart diseases (I05-I09)

I05 **Rheumatic mitral valve diseases**
INCLUDES conditions classifiable to both I05.0 and I05.2-I05.9, whether specified as rheumatic or not
EXCLUDES 1 mitral valve disease specified as nonrheumatic (I34.-)
mitral valve disease with aortic and/or tricuspid valve involvement (I08.-)

I05.0 **Rheumatic mitral stenosis**
Mitral (valve) obstruction (rheumatic)
DEF: Narrowing of the mitral valve between the left atrium and left ventricle due to rheumatic fever. Symptoms include shortness of breath during or after exercise, fatigue, palpitations, chest discomfort, and swelling of feet or legs.

I05.1 **Rheumatic mitral insufficiency**
Rheumatic mitral incompetence
Rheumatic mitral regurgitation
EXCLUDES 1 mitral insufficiency not specified as rheumatic (I34.0)

I05.2 **Rheumatic mitral stenosis with insufficiency**
Rheumatic mitral stenosis with incompetence or regurgitation

I05.8 **Other rheumatic mitral valve diseases**
Rheumatic mitral (valve) failure

I05.9 **Rheumatic mitral valve disease, unspecified**
Rheumatic mitral (valve) disorder (chronic) NOS

I06 **Rheumatic aortic valve diseases**
EXCLUDES 1 aortic valve disease not specified as rheumatic (I35.-)
aortic valve disease with mitral and/or tricuspid valve involvement (I08.-)

I06.0 **Rheumatic aortic stenosis**
Rheumatic aortic (valve) obstruction

I06.1 **Rheumatic aortic insufficiency**
Rheumatic aortic incompetence
Rheumatic aortic regurgitation

I06.2 **Rheumatic aortic stenosis with insufficiency**
Rheumatic aortic stenosis with incompetence or regurgitation

I06.8 **Other rheumatic aortic valve diseases**

I06.9 **Rheumatic aortic valve disease, unspecified**
Rheumatic aortic (valve) disease NOS

I07 **Rheumatic tricuspid valve diseases**
INCLUDES rheumatic tricuspid valve diseases specified as rheumatic or unspecified
EXCLUDES 1 tricuspid valve disease specified as nonrheumatic (I36.-)
tricuspid valve disease with aortic and/or mitral valve involvement (I08.-)

I07.0 **Rheumatic tricuspid stenosis**
Tricuspid (valve) stenosis (rheumatic)

I07.1 **Rheumatic tricuspid insufficiency**
Tricuspid (valve) insufficiency (rheumatic)

I07.2 **Rheumatic tricuspid stenosis and insufficiency**

I07.8 **Other rheumatic tricuspid valve diseases**

I07.9 **Rheumatic tricuspid valve disease, unspecified**
Rheumatic tricuspid valve disorder NOS

I08 **Multiple valve diseases**
INCLUDES multiple valve diseases specified as rheumatic or unspecified
EXCLUDES 1 endocarditis, valve unspecified (I38)
multiple valve disease specified a nonrheumatic (I34.-, I35.-, I36.-, I37.-, I38.-, Q22.-, Q23.-, Q24.8-)
rheumatic valve disease NOS (I09.1)

I08.0 **Rheumatic disorders of both mitral and aortic valves**
Involvement of both mitral and aortic valves specified as rheumatic or unspecified

I08.1 **Rheumatic disorders of both mitral and tricuspid valves**

I08.2 **Rheumatic disorders of both aortic and tricuspid valves**

I08.3 **Combined rheumatic disorders of mitral, aortic and tricuspid valves**

I08.8 **Other rheumatic multiple valve diseases**

I08.9 **Rheumatic multiple valve disease, unspecified**

I09 **Other rheumatic heart diseases**

I09.0 **Rheumatic myocarditis** CC
EXCLUDES 1 myocarditis not specified as rheumatic (I51.4)
CC Excl: PDX collection 647

I09.1 **Rheumatic diseases of endocardium, valve unspecified**
Rheumatic endocarditis (chronic)
Rheumatic valvulitis (chronic)
EXCLUDES 1 endocarditis, valve unspecified (I38)

I09.2   Chronic rheumatic pericarditis   `CC`
Adherent pericardium, rheumatic
Chronic rheumatic mediastinopericarditis
Chronic rheumatic myopericarditis
> *EXCLUDES 1*   *chronic pericarditis not specified as rheumatic (I31.-)*
CC Excl: PDX collection 188

✓5ᵗʰ **I09.8   Other specified rheumatic heart diseases**

I09.81   Rheumatic heart failure   `CC` `HCC`
Use additional code to identify type of heart failure
(I50.-)
DEF: Decreased cardiac output, edema, and
hypertension due to rheumatic heart disease.
CC Excl: PDX collection 648

I09.89   Other specified rheumatic heart diseases
Rheumatic disease of pulmonary valve

I09.9   Rheumatic heart disease, unspecified
Rheumatic carditis
> *EXCLUDES 1*   *rheumatoid carditis (M05.31)*

Hypertensive diseases (I10-I16)

Use additional code to identify:
exposure to environmental tobacco smoke (Z77.22)
history of tobacco dependence (Z87.891)
occupational exposure to environmental tobacco smoke (Z57.31)
tobacco dependence (F17.-)
tobacco use (Z72.0)
> *EXCLUDES 1*   *neonatal hypertension (P29.2)*
> *primary pulmonary hypertension (I27.0)*
> *EXCLUDES 2*   *hypertensive disease complicating pregnancy, childbirth and the*
> *puerperium (O10-O11, O13-O16)*

I10   Essential (primary) hypertension
> *INCLUDES*   high blood pressure
> hypertension (arterial) (benign) (essential) (malignant)
> (primary) (systemic)
> *EXCLUDES 1*   *hypertensive disease complicating pregnancy, childbirth and*
> *the puerperium (O10-O11, O13-O16)*
> *EXCLUDES 2*   *essential (primary) hypertension involving vessels of brain*
> *(I60-I69)*
> *essential (primary) hypertension involving vessels of eye*
> *(H35.0-)*
AHA: 2018, 2Q, 9; 2016, 4Q, 27

✓4ᵗʰ **I11   Hypertensive heart disease**
> *INCLUDES*   any condition in I50.-, I51.4-I51.9 due to hypertension
AHA: 2018, 2Q, 9
TIP: Do not assign a code from this category when provider
documentation indicates the heart disease is attributable to another
cause.

I11.0   Hypertensive heart disease with heart failure   `HCC`
Hypertensive heart failure
Use additional code to identify type of heart failure (I50.-)
AHA: 2017, 1Q, 47

I11.9   Hypertensive heart disease without heart failure
Hypertensive heart disease NOS

✓4ᵗʰ **I12   Hypertensive chronic kidney disease**
> *INCLUDES*   any condition in N18 and N26- due to hypertension
> arteriosclerosis of kidney
> arteriosclerotic nephritis (chronic) (interstitial)
> hypertensive nephropathy
> nephrosclerosis
> *EXCLUDES 1*   *hypertension due to kidney disease (I15.0, I15.1)*
> *renovascular hypertension (I15.0)*
> *secondary hypertension (I15.-)*
> *EXCLUDES 2*   *acute kidney failure (N17.-)*
AHA: 2016, 3Q, 22
TIP: Do not assign a code from this category when provider
documentation indicates the chronic kidney disease (CKD) is attributable
to another cause.

I12.0   Hypertensive chronic kidney disease with stage 5   `CC` `HCC`
chronic kidney disease or end stage renal disease
Use additional code to identify the stage of chronic kidney
disease (N18.5, N18.6)
CC Excl: PDX collection 649

I12.9   Hypertensive chronic kidney disease with stage 1 through
stage 4 chronic kidney disease, or unspecified chronic kidney
disease
Hypertensive chronic kidney disease NOS
Hypertensive renal disease NOS
Use additional code to identify the stage of chronic kidney
disease (N18.1-N18.4, N18.9)

✓4ᵗʰ **I13   Hypertensive heart and chronic kidney disease**
> *INCLUDES*   any condition in I11.- with any condition in I12.-
> cardiorenal disease
> cardiovascular renal disease
TIP: Do not assign a code from this category when provider
documentation indicates the heart and/or chronic kidney disease is
attributable to another cause.

CC Excl: For CC codes in category I13: PDX collection 650

I13.0   Hypertensive heart and chronic kidney disease with   `CC` `HCC`
heart failure and stage 1 through stage 4 chronic kidney
disease, or unspecified chronic kidney disease
Use additional code to identify type of heart failure (I50.-)
Use additional code to identify stage of chronic kidney disease
(N18.1-N18.4, N18.9)

✓5ᵗʰ **I13.1   Hypertensive heart and chronic kidney disease without heart**
failure

I13.10   Hypertensive heart and chronic kidney disease
without heart failure, with stage 1 through stage 4
chronic kidney disease, or unspecified chronic
kidney disease
Hypertensive heart disease and hypertensive chronic
kidney disease NOS
Use additional code to identify the stage of chronic
kidney disease (N18.1-N18.4, N18.9)

I13.11   Hypertensive heart and chronic kidney   `CC` `HCC`
disease without heart failure, with stage 5
chronic kidney disease, or end stage renal disease
Use additional code to identify the stage of chronic
kidney disease (N18.5, N18.6)

I13.2   Hypertensive heart and chronic kidney disease   `CC` `HCC`
with heart failure and with stage 5 chronic kidney
disease, or end stage renal disease
Use additional code to identify type of heart failure (I50.-)
Use additional code to identify the stage of chronic kidney
disease (N18.5, N18.6)

✓4ᵗʰ **I15   Secondary hypertension**
Code also underlying condition
> *EXCLUDES 1*   *postprocedural hypertension (I97.3)*
> *EXCLUDES 2*   *secondary hypertension involving vessels of brain (I60-I69)*
> *secondary hypertension involving vessels of eye (H35.0-)*

I15.0   Renovascular hypertension

I15.1   Hypertension secondary to other renal disorders
AHA: 2016, 3Q, 22

I15.2   Hypertension secondary to endocrine disorders

I15.8   Other secondary hypertension

I15.9   Secondary hypertension, unspecified

✓4ᵗʰ **I16   Hypertensive crisis**
Code also any identified hypertensive disease (I10-I15)
AHA: 2016, 4Q, 26-28

I16.0   Hypertensive urgency

I16.1   Hypertensive emergency   `CC`
CC Excl: No Excl

I16.9   Hypertensive crisis, unspecified   `CC`
CC Excl: No Excl

Ischemic heart diseases (I20-I25)

Use additional code to identify presence of hypertension (I10-I16)

✓4ᵗʰ **I20   Angina pectoris**
Use additional code to identify:
exposure to environmental tobacco smoke (Z77.22)
history of tobacco dependence (Z87.891)
occupational exposure to environmental tobacco smoke (Z57.31)
tobacco dependence (F17.-)
tobacco use (Z72.0)
> *EXCLUDES 1*   *angina pectoris with atherosclerotic heart disease of native*
> *coronary arteries (I25.1-)*
> *atherosclerosis of coronary artery bypass graft(s) and coronary*
> *artery of transplanted heart with angina pectoris (I25.7-)*
> *postinfarction angina (I23.7)*
DEF: Chest pain due to reduced blood flow resulting in a lack of oxygen to
the heart muscles.

I20.0   **Unstable angina**   `CC` `HCC`
Accelerated angina
Crescendo angina
De novo effort angina
Intermediate coronary syndrome
Preinfarction syndrome
Worsening effort angina
DEF: Condition representing an intermediate stage between
angina of effort and acute myocardial infarction.
CC Excl: PDX collection 651

I20.1   **Angina pectoris with documented spasm**   `CC` `HCC`
Angiospastic angina
Prinzmetal angina
Spasm-induced angina
Variant angina
CC Excl: PDX collection 652

I20.8   **Other forms of angina pectoris**   `HCC`
Angina equivalent
Angina of effort
Coronary slow flow syndrome
Stable angina
Stenocardia
Use additional code(s) for symptoms associated with angina
equivalent

I20.9   **Angina pectoris, unspecified**   `HCC`
Angina NOS
Anginal syndrome
Cardiac angina
Ischemic chest pain

✓4ᵗʰ I21   **Acute myocardial infarction**
`INCLUDES`   cardiac infarction
coronary (artery) embolism
coronary (artery) occlusion
coronary (artery) rupture
coronary (artery) thrombosis
infarction of heart, myocardium, or ventricle
myocardial infarction specified as acute or with a stated
duration of 4 weeks (28 days) or less from onset
Use additional code, if applicable, to identify:
exposure to environmental tobacco smoke (Z77.22)
history of tobacco dependence (Z87.891)
occupational exposure to environmental tobacco smoke (Z57.31)
status post administration of tPA (rtPA) in a different facility within
the last 24 hours prior to admission to current facility (Z92.82)
tobacco dependence (F17.-)
tobacco use (Z72.0)
`EXCLUDES 2`   old myocardial infarction (I25.2)
postmyocardial infarction syndrome (I24.1)
subsequent type 1 myocardial infarction (I22.-)
AHA: 2017, 4Q, 12-14; 2017, 1Q, 44–45; 2016, 4Q, 140; 2015, 2Q, 16; 2013,
1Q, 25; 2012, 4Q, 96, 102-103

CC Excl: For MCC codes in category I21: PDX collection 653

✓5ᵗʰ I21.0   **ST elevation (STEMI) myocardial infarction of anterior wall**
Type 1 ST elevation myocardial infarction of anterior wall
DEF: ST elevation myocardial infarction: Complete obstruction of
one or more coronary arteries causing decreased blood flow
(ischemia) and necrosis of myocardial muscle cells.

I21.01   **ST elevation (STEMI) myocardial infarction**   `MCC` `HCC`
involving left main coronary artery

I21.02   **ST elevation (STEMI) myocardial infarction**   `MCC` `HCC`
involving left anterior descending coronary artery
ST elevation (STEMI) myocardial infarction involving
diagonal coronary artery
AHA: 2013, 1Q, 25

I21.09   **ST elevation (STEMI) myocardial infarction**   `MCC` `HCC`
involving other coronary artery of anterior wall
Acute transmural myocardial infarction of anterior wall
Anteroapical transmural (Q wave) infarction (acute)
Anterolateral transmural (Q wave) infarction (acute)
Anteroseptal transmural (Q wave) infarction (acute)
Transmural (Q wave) infarction (acute) (of) anterior
(wall) NOS
AHA: 2012, 4Q, 102-103

✓5ᵗʰ I21.1   **ST elevation (STEMI) myocardial infarction of inferior wall**
Type 1 ST elevation myocardial infarction of inferior wall
DEF: ST elevation myocardial infarction: Complete obstruction of
one or more coronary arteries causing decreased blood flow
(ischemia) and necrosis of myocardial muscle cells.

I21.11   **ST elevation (STEMI) myocardial infarction**   `MCC` `HCC`
involving right coronary artery
Inferoposterior transmural (Q wave) infarction (acute)

I21.19   **ST elevation (STEMI) myocardial infarction**   `MCC` `HCC`
involving other coronary artery of inferior wall
Acute transmural myocardial infarction of inferior wall
Inferolateral transmural (Q wave) infarction (acute)
Transmural (Q wave) infarction (acute) (of)
diaphragmatic wall
Transmural (Q wave) infarction (acute) (of) inferior
(wall) NOS
`EXCLUDES 2`   ST elevation (STEMI) myocardial infarction
involving left circumflex coronary artery
(I21.21)
AHA: 2012, 4Q, 96

✓5ᵗʰ I21.2   **ST elevation (STEMI) myocardial infarction of other sites**
Type 1 ST elevation myocardial infarction of other sites
DEF: ST elevation myocardial infarction: Complete obstruction of
one or more coronary arteries causing decreased blood flow
(ischemia) and necrosis of myocardial muscle cells.

I21.21   **ST elevation (STEMI) myocardial infarction**   `MCC` `HCC`
involving left circumflex coronary artery
ST elevation (STEMI) myocardial infarction involving
oblique marginal coronary artery

I21.29   **ST elevation (STEMI) myocardial infarction**   `MCC` `HCC`
involving other sites
Acute transmural myocardial infarction of other sites
Apical-lateral transmural (Q wave) infarction (acute)
Basal-lateral transmural (Q wave) infarction (acute)
High lateral transmural (Q wave) infarction (acute)
Lateral (wall) NOS transmural (Q wave) infarction
(acute)
Posterior (true) transmural (Q wave) infarction (acute)
Posterobasal transmural (Q wave) infarction (acute)
Posterolateral transmural (Q wave) infarction (acute)
Posteroseptal transmural (Q wave) infarction (acute)
Septal transmural (Q wave) infarction (acute) NOS

I21.3   **ST elevation (STEMI) myocardial infarction of**   `MCC` `HCC`
unspecified site
Acute transmural myocardial infarction of unspecified site
Transmural (Q wave) myocardial infarction NOS
Type 1 ST elevation myocardial infarction of unspecified site
DEF: ST elevation myocardial infarction: Complete obstruction of
one or more coronary arteries causing decreased blood flow
(ischemia) and necrosis of myocardial muscle cells.

I21.4   **Non-ST elevation (NSTEMI) myocardial infarction**   `MCC` `HCC`
Acute subendocardial myocardial infarction
Non-Q wave myocardial infarction NOS
Nontransmural myocardial infarction NOS
Type 1 non-ST elevation myocardial infarction
AHA: 2017, 1Q, 44-45
DEF: Partial obstruction of one or more coronary arteries that
causes decreased blood flow (ischemia) and may cause partial
thickness necrosis of myocardial muscle cells.

I21.9   **Acute myocardial infarction, unspecified**   `MCC` `HCC`
Myocardial infarction (acute) NOS

✓5ᵗʰ I21.A   **Other type of myocardial infarction**

I21.A1   **Myocardial infarction type 2**   `MCC` `HCC`
Myocardial infarction due to demand ischemia
Myocardial infarction secondary to ischemic
imbalance
Code also the underlying cause, if known and
applicable, such as:
anemia (D50.0-D64.9)
chronic obstructive pulmonary disease (J44.-)
heart failure (I50.-)
paroxysmal tachycardia (I47.0-I47.9)
renal failure (N17.0-N19)
shock (R57.0-R57.9)
AHA: 2017, 4Q, 13-14
DEF: Often referred to as due to demand ischemia,
myocardial infarction (MI) type 2 refers to an MI due to
ischemia and necrosis resulting from an oxygen
imbalance to the heart. This mismatch between oxygen
decreased supply and increased demand is caused by
conditions other than coronary artery disease such as
vasospasm, embolism, anemia, hypertension,
hypotension, or arrhythmias.

✓Additional Character Required   ✓x7ᵗʰ Placeholder   Unacceptable PDx   Questionable PDx   Manifestation   `H1`-`H14` HAC   `HCC` CMS-HCC Dx   `HIV` HIV Dx

ICD-10-CM 2019   637

I21.A9   **Other myocardial infarction type**   `MCC` `HCC`
Myocardial infarction associated with revascularization procedure
Myocardial infarction type 3
Myocardial infarction type 4a
Myocardial infarction type 4b
Myocardial infarction type 4c
Myocardial infarction type 5
Code first, if applicable, postprocedural myocardial infarction following cardiac surgery (I97.190), or postprocedural myocardial infarction during cardiac surgery (I97.790)
Code also complication, if known and applicable, such as:
  (acute) stent occlusion (T82.897-)
  (acute) stent stenosis (T82.857-)
  (acute) stent thrombosis (T82.867-)
  cardiac arrest due to underlying cardiac condition (I46.2)
  complication of percutaneous coronary intervention (PCI) (I97.89)
  occlusion of coronary artery bypass graft (T82.218-)

✓4ᵗʰ **I22**   **Subsequent ST elevation (STEMI) and non-ST elevation (NSTEMI) myocardial infarction**
   INCLUDES   acute myocardial infarction occurring within four weeks (28 days) of a previous acute myocardial infarction, regardless of site
     cardiac infarction
     coronary (artery) embolism
     coronary (artery) occlusion
     coronary (artery) rupture
     coronary (artery) thrombosis
     infarction of heart, myocardium, or ventricle
     recurrent myocardial infarction
     reinfarction of myocardium
     rupture of heart, myocardium, or ventricle
     subsequent type 1 myocardial infarction
Use additional code, if applicable, to identify:
  exposure to environmental tobacco smoke (Z77.22)
  history of tobacco dependence (Z87.891)
  occupational exposure to environmental tobacco smoke (Z57.31)
  status post administration of tPA (rtPA) in a different facility within the last 24 hours prior to admission to current facility (Z92.82)
  tobacco dependence (F17.-)
  tobacco use (Z72.0)
   EXCLUDES 1   subsequent myocardial infarction, type 2 (I21.A1)
      subsequent myocardial infarction of other type (type 3) (type 4) (type 5) (I21.A9)
AHA: 2017, 4Q, 12-13; 2017, 2Q, 11; 2013, 1Q, 25; 2012, 4Q, 97, 102-103
DEF: Non-ST elevation myocardial infarction: Partial obstruction of one or more coronary arteries that causes decreased blood flow (ischemia) and may cause partial thickness necrosis of myocardial muscle cells.
DEF: ST elevation myocardial infarction: Complete obstruction of one or more coronary arteries causing decreased blood flow (ischemia) and necrosis of myocardial muscle cells.

> **CC Excl: For MCC codes in category I22:** PDX collection 653

I22.0   **Subsequent ST elevation (STEMI) myocardial infarction of** anterior wall   `MCC` `HCC`
Subsequent acute transmural myocardial infarction of anterior wall
Subsequent transmural (Q wave) infarction (acute)(of) anterior (wall) NOS
Subsequent anteroapical transmural (Q wave) infarction (acute)
Subsequent anterolateral transmural (Q wave) infarction (acute)
Subsequent anteroseptal transmural (Q wave) infarction (acute)

I22.1   **Subsequent ST elevation (STEMI) myocardial infarction of** inferior wall   `MCC` `HCC`
Subsequent acute transmural myocardial infarction of inferior wall
Subsequent transmural (Q wave) infarction (acute)(of) diaphragmatic wall
Subsequent transmural (Q wave) infarction (acute)(of) inferior (wall) NOS
Subsequent inferolateral transmural (Q wave) infarction (acute)
Subsequent inferoposterior transmural (Q wave) infarction (acute)
AHA: 2012, 4Q, 102

I22.2   **Subsequent** non-ST elevation (NSTEMI) **myocardial infarction**   `MCC` `HCC`
Subsequent acute subendocardial myocardial infarction
Subsequent non-Q wave myocardial infarction NOS
Subsequent nontransmural myocardial infarction NOS

I22.8   **Subsequent ST elevation (STEMI) myocardial infarction of** other sites   `MCC` `HCC`
Subsequent acute transmural myocardial infarction of other sites
Subsequent apical-lateral transmural (Q wave) myocardial infarction (acute)
Subsequent basal-lateral transmural (Q wave) myocardial infarction (acute)
Subsequent high lateral transmural (Q wave) myocardial infarction (acute)
Subsequent transmural (Q wave) myocardial infarction (acute)(of) lateral (wall) NOS
Subsequent posterior (true) transmural (Q wave) myocardial infarction (acute)
Subsequent posterobasal transmural (Q wave) myocardial infarction (acute)
Subsequent posterolateral transmural (Q wave) myocardial infarction (acute)
Subsequent posteroseptal transmural (Q wave) myocardial infarction (acute)
Subsequent septal NOS transmural (Q wave) myocardial infarction (acute)

I22.9   **Subsequent ST elevation (STEMI) myocardial infarction of** unspecified site   `MCC` `HCC`
Subsequent acute myocardial infarction of unspecified site
Subsequent myocardial infarction (acute) NOS

✓4ᵗʰ **I23**   **Certain current complications following ST elevation (STEMI) and non-ST elevation (NSTEMI) myocardial infarction (within the 28 day period)**
AHA: 2017, 2Q, 11
DEF: Non-ST elevation myocardial infarction: Partial obstruction of one or more coronary arteries that causes decreased blood flow (ischemia) and may cause partial thickness necrosis of myocardial muscle cells.
DEF: ST elevation myocardial infarction: Complete obstruction of one or more coronary arteries causing decreased blood flow (ischemia) and necrosis of myocardial muscle cells.

> **CC Excl: For CC/MCC codes in category I23, unless otherwise noted:** PDX collection 654

I23.0   **Hemopericardium as current complication following acute myocardial infarction**   `CC` `HCC` `A`
   EXCLUDES 1   hemopericardium not specified as current complication following acute myocardial infarction (I31.2)

I23.1   **Atrial septal defect as current complication following acute myocardial infarction**   `CC` `HCC` `A`
   EXCLUDES 1   acquired atrial septal defect not specified as current complication following acute myocardial infarction (I51.0)

I23.2   **Ventricular septal defect as current complication following acute myocardial infarction**   `CC` `HCC` `A`
   EXCLUDES 1   acquired ventricular septal defect not specified as current complication following acute myocardial infarction (I51.0)

I23.3   **Rupture of cardiac wall without hemopericardium as current complication following acute myocardial infarction**   `CC` `HCC` `A`

I23.4   **Rupture of chordae tendineae as current complication following acute myocardial infarction**   `MCC` `HCC`
   EXCLUDES 1   rupture of chordae tendineae not specified as current complication following acute myocardial infarction (I51.1)
   CC Excl: PDX collection 655

I23.5   **Rupture of papillary muscle as current complication following acute myocardial infarction**   `MCC` `HCC`
   EXCLUDES 1   rupture of papillary muscle not specified as current complication following acute myocardial infarction (I51.2)
   CC Excl: PDX collection 656

I23.6   **Thrombosis of atrium, auricular appendage, and ventricle as current complications following acute myocardial infarction**   `CC` `HCC` `A`
   EXCLUDES 1   thrombosis of atrium, auricular appendage, and ventricle not specified as current complication following acute myocardial infarction (I51.3)

I23.7   **Postinfarction angina**   `CC` `HCC` `A`
   AHA: 2015, 2Q, 16

I23.8   **Other current complications following acute myocardial infarction**   `CC` `HCC` `A`

N Newborn: 0   **P** Pediatric: 0-17   **M** Maternity: 12-55   **A** Adult: 15-124   **MCC** Major Complication/Comorbidity   **CC** Complication/Comorbidity   **SW** Severe Wound Dx

638   ICD-10-CM 2019

☑4ᵗʰ **I24** **Other acute ischemic heart diseases**

EXCLUDES 1   *angina pectoris (I20.-)*
              transient myocardial ischemia in newborn (P29.4)

CC Excl: For CC codes in category I24, unless otherwise noted:
PDX collection 657

I24.0 **Acute coronary thrombosis not resulting in myocardial infarction** `CC` `HCC`
Acute coronary (artery) (vein) embolism not resulting in myocardial infarction
Acute coronary (artery) (vein) occlusion not resulting in myocardial infarction
Acute coronary (artery) (vein) thromboembolism not resulting in myocardial infarction
EXCLUDES 1   *atherosclerotic heart disease (I25.1-)*
AHA: 2013, 1Q, 24

I24.1 **Dressler's syndrome** `CC` `HCC`
Postmyocardial infarction syndrome
EXCLUDES 1   *postinfarction angina (I23.7)*
DEF: Fever, leukocytosis, chest pain, evidence of pericarditis, pleurisy, and pneumonia occurring days or weeks after a myocardial infarction.
CC Excl: PDX collection 658

I24.8 **Other forms of acute ischemic heart disease** `CC` `HCC`
EXCLUDES 1   *myocardial infarction due to demand ischemia (I21.A1)*
AHA: 2017, 4Q, 13

I24.9 **Acute ischemic heart disease, unspecified** `CC` `HCC`
EXCLUDES 1   *ischemic heart disease (chronic) NOS (I25.9)*

☑4ᵗʰ **I25** **Chronic ischemic heart disease**
Use additional code to identify:
chronic total occlusion of coronary artery (I25.82)
exposure to environmental tobacco smoke (Z77.22)
history of tobacco dependence (Z87.891)
occupational exposure to environmental tobacco smoke (Z57.31)
tobacco dependence (F17.-)
tobacco use (Z72.0)

☑5ᵗʰ **I25.1** **Atherosclerotic heart disease of native coronary artery**
Atherosclerotic cardiovascular disease
Coronary (artery) atheroma
Coronary (artery) atherosclerosis
Coronary (artery) disease
Coronary (artery) sclerosis
Use additional code, if applicable, to identify:
coronary atherosclerosis due to calcified coronary lesion (I25.84)
coronary atherosclerosis due to lipid rich plaque (I25.83)
EXCLUDES 2   *atheroembolism (I75.-)*
              atherosclerosis of coronary artery bypass graft(s) and transplanted heart (I25.7-)

I25.10 **Atherosclerotic heart disease of native coronary artery without angina pectoris** `A`
Atherosclerotic heart disease NOS
AHA: 2015, 2Q, 16; 2012, 4Q, 92

☑6ᵗʰ **I25.11** **Atherosclerotic heart disease of native coronary artery with angina pectoris**

I25.110 **Atherosclerotic heart disease of native coronary artery with unstable angina pectoris** `CC` `HCC` `A`
EXCLUDES 1   *unstable angina without atherosclerotic heart disease (I20.0)*
CC Excl: PDX collection 651

I25.111 **Atherosclerotic heart disease of native coronary artery with angina pectoris with documented spasm** `HCC` `A`
EXCLUDES 1   *angina pectoris with documented spasm without atherosclerotic heart disease (I20.1)*

I25.118 **Atherosclerotic heart disease of native coronary artery with other forms of angina pectoris** `HCC` `A`
EXCLUDES 1   *other forms of angina pectoris without atherosclerotic heart disease (I20.8)*
AHA: 2015, 2Q, 16

Atheromas

Atheromas (fatty tissue and/or plaque)   Lumen

I25.119 **Atherosclerotic heart disease of native coronary artery with unspecified angina pectoris** `HCC` `A`
Atherosclerotic heart disease with angina NOS
Atherosclerotic heart disease with ischemic chest pain
EXCLUDES 1   *unspecified angina pectoris without atherosclerotic heart disease (I20.9)*

I25.2 **Old myocardial infarction**
Healed myocardial infarction
Past myocardial infarction diagnosed by ECG or other investigation, but currently presenting no symptoms

I25.3 **Aneurysm of heart** `CC`
Mural aneurysm
Ventricular aneurysm
CC Excl: PDX collection 659

☑5ᵗʰ **I25.4** **Coronary artery aneurysm and dissection**

I25.41 **Coronary artery aneurysm**
Coronary arteriovenous fistula, acquired
EXCLUDES 1   *congenital coronary (artery) aneurysm (Q24.5)*

I25.42 **Coronary artery dissection** `MCC`
DEF: Tear in the intimal arterial wall of a coronary artery resulting in the sudden intrusion of blood within the layers of the wall.
CC Excl: PDX collection 660

I25.5 **Ischemic cardiomyopathy**
EXCLUDES 2   *coronary atherosclerosis (I25.1-, I25.7-)*

I25.6 **Silent myocardial ischemia**

☑5ᵗʰ **I25.7** **Atherosclerosis of coronary artery bypass graft(s) and coronary artery of transplanted heart with angina pectoris**
Use additional code, if applicable, to identify:
coronary atherosclerosis due to calcified coronary lesion (I25.84)
coronary atherosclerosis due to lipid rich plaque (I25.83)
EXCLUDES 1   *atherosclerosis of bypass graft(s) of transplanted heart without angina pectoris (I25.812)*
              atherosclerosis of coronary artery bypass graft(s) without angina pectoris (I25.810)
              atherosclerosis of native coronary artery of transplanted heart without angina pectoris (I25.811)

☑6ᵗʰ **I25.70** **Atherosclerosis of coronary artery bypass graft(s), unspecified, with angina pectoris**

I25.700 **Atherosclerosis of coronary artery bypass graft(s), unspecified, with unstable angina pectoris** `CC` `HCC` `A`
EXCLUDES 1   *unstable angina pectoris without atherosclerosis of coronary artery bypass graft (I20.0)*
CC Excl: PDX collection 651

I25.701 **Atherosclerosis of coronary artery bypass graft(s), unspecified, with angina pectoris with documented spasm** `HCC` `A`
EXCLUDES 1   *angina pectoris with documented spasm without atherosclerosis of coronary artery bypass graft (I20.1)*

I25.708 **Atherosclerosis of coronary artery bypass graft(s), unspecified, with other forms of angina pectoris** `HCC` `A`
EXCLUDES 1   *other forms of angina pectoris without atherosclerosis of coronary artery bypass graft (I20.8)*

Chapter 9. Diseases of the Circulatory System

I25.709–I25.768

I25.709   **Atherosclerosis of coronary artery bypass graft(s), unspecified, with unspecified angina pectoris** HCC A
> *EXCLUDES 1*   *unspecified angina pectoris without atherosclerosis of coronary artery bypass graft (I20.9)*

✓6th **I25.71**   **Atherosclerosis of autologous vein coronary artery bypass graft(s) with angina pectoris**

> **CC Excl: For CC codes in subcategory I25.71, unless otherwise noted:** PDX collection 662

I25.710   **Atherosclerosis of autologous vein coronary artery bypass graft(s) with unstable angina pectoris** CC HCC A
> *EXCLUDES 1*   *unstable angina without atherosclerosis of autologous vein coronary artery bypass graft(s) (I20.0)*
> *EXCLUDES 2*   *embolism or thrombus of coronary artery bypass graft(s) (T82.8-)*
> **CC Excl:** PDX collection 661

I25.711   **Atherosclerosis of autologous vein coronary artery bypass graft(s) with angina pectoris with documented spasm** CC HCC A
> *EXCLUDES 1*   *angina pectoris with documented spasm without atherosclerosis of autologous vein coronary artery bypass graft(s) (I20.1)*

I25.718   **Atherosclerosis of autologous vein coronary artery bypass graft(s) with other forms of angina pectoris** CC HCC A
> *EXCLUDES 1*   *other forms of angina pectoris without atherosclerosis of autologous vein coronary artery bypass graft(s) (I20.8)*

I25.719   **Atherosclerosis of autologous vein coronary artery bypass graft(s) with unspecified angina pectoris** CC HCC A
> *EXCLUDES 1*   *unspecified angina pectoris without atherosclerosis of autologous vein coronary artery bypass graft(s) (I20.9)*

✓6th **I25.72**   **Atherosclerosis of autologous artery coronary artery bypass graft(s) with angina pectoris**
Atherosclerosis of internal mammary artery graft with angina pectoris

> **CC Excl: For CC codes in subcategories I25.72, unless otherwise noted:** PDX collection 662

I25.720   **Atherosclerosis of autologous artery coronary artery bypass graft(s) with unstable angina pectoris** CC HCC A
> *EXCLUDES 1*   *unstable angina without atherosclerosis of autologous artery coronary artery bypass graft(s) (I20.0)*
> **CC Excl:** PDX collection 661

I25.721   **Atherosclerosis of autologous artery coronary artery bypass graft(s) with angina pectoris with documented spasm** CC HCC A
> *EXCLUDES 1*   *angina pectoris with documented spasm without atherosclerosis of autologous artery coronary artery bypass graft(s) (I20.1)*

I25.728   **Atherosclerosis of autologous artery coronary artery bypass graft(s) with other forms of angina pectoris** CC HCC A
> *EXCLUDES 1*   *other forms of angina pectoris without atherosclerosis of autologous artery coronary artery bypass graft(s) (I20.8)*

I25.729   **Atherosclerosis of autologous artery coronary artery bypass graft(s) with unspecified angina pectoris** CC HCC A
> *EXCLUDES 1*   *unspecified angina pectoris without atherosclerosis of autologous artery coronary artery bypass graft(s) (I20.9)*

✓6th **I25.73**   **Atherosclerosis of nonautologous biological coronary artery bypass graft(s) with angina pectoris**

> **CC Excl: For CC codes in subcategories I25.73, unless otherwise noted:** PDX collection 662

I25.730   **Atherosclerosis of nonautologous biological coronary artery bypass graft(s) with unstable angina pectoris** CC HCC A
> *EXCLUDES 1*   *unstable angina without atherosclerosis of nonautologous biological coronary artery bypass graft(s) (I20.0)*
> **CC Excl:** PDX collection 661

I25.731   **Atherosclerosis of nonautologous biological coronary artery bypass graft(s) with angina pectoris with documented spasm** CC HCC A
> *EXCLUDES 1*   *angina pectoris with documented spasm without atherosclerosis of nonautologous biological coronary artery bypass graft(s) (I20.1)*

I25.738   **Atherosclerosis of nonautologous biological coronary artery bypass graft(s) with other forms of angina pectoris** CC HCC A
> *EXCLUDES 1*   *other forms of angina pectoris without atherosclerosis of nonautologous biological coronary artery bypass graft(s) (I20.8)*

I25.739   **Atherosclerosis of nonautologous biological coronary artery bypass graft(s) with unspecified angina pectoris** CC HCC A
> *EXCLUDES 1*   *unspecified angina pectoris without atherosclerosis of nonautologous biological coronary artery bypass graft(s) (I20.9)*

✓6th **I25.75**   **Atherosclerosis of native coronary artery of transplanted heart with angina pectoris**
> *EXCLUDES 1*   *atherosclerosis of native coronary artery of transplanted heart without angina pectoris (I25.811)*

> **CC Excl: For CC codes in subcategory I25.75, unless otherwise noted:** PDX collection 664

I25.750   **Atherosclerosis of native coronary artery of transplanted heart with unstable angina** CC HCC
> **CC Excl:** PDX collection 663

I25.751   **Atherosclerosis of native coronary artery of transplanted heart with angina pectoris with documented spasm** CC HCC

I25.758   **Atherosclerosis of native coronary artery of transplanted heart with other forms of angina pectoris** CC HCC

I25.759   **Atherosclerosis of native coronary artery of transplanted heart with unspecified angina pectoris** CC HCC

✓6th **I25.76**   **Atherosclerosis of bypass graft of coronary artery of transplanted heart with angina pectoris**
> *EXCLUDES 1*   *atherosclerosis of bypass graft of coronary artery of transplanted heart without angina pectoris (I25.812)*

> **CC Excl: For CC codes in subcategory I25.76, unless otherwise noted:** PDX collection 666

I25.760   **Atherosclerosis of bypass graft of coronary artery of transplanted heart with unstable angina** CC HCC A
> **CC Excl:** PDX collection 665

I25.761   **Atherosclerosis of bypass graft of coronary artery of transplanted heart with angina pectoris with documented spasm** CC HCC A

I25.768   **Atherosclerosis of bypass graft of coronary artery of transplanted heart with other forms of angina pectoris** CC HCC A

N Newborn: 0   P Pediatric: 0-17   M Maternity: 12-55   A Adult: 15-124   HCC Major Complication/Comorbidity   CC Complication/Comorbidity   SW Severe Wound Dx

I25.769   **Atherosclerosis of bypass graft** `CC` `HCC` `A` **of coronary artery of transplanted heart with** unspecified **angina pectoris**

✓6ᵗʰ   **I25.79**   **Atherosclerosis of** other **coronary artery bypass graft(s) with angina pectoris**

     I25.790   **Atherosclerosis of other** `CC` `HCC` `A` **coronary artery bypass graft(s) with** unstable **angina pectoris**

         EXCLUDES 1   *unstable angina without atherosclerosis of other coronary artery bypass graft(s) (I20.0)*

         CC Excl: PDX collection 651

     I25.791   **Atherosclerosis of other** `CC` `HCC` `A` **coronary artery bypass graft(s) with angina pectoris with** documented spasm

         EXCLUDES 1   *angina pectoris with documented spasm without atherosclerosis of other coronary artery bypass graft(s) (I20.1)*

         CC Excl: No Excl

     I25.798   **Atherosclerosis of other** `CC` `HCC` `A` **coronary artery bypass graft(s) with** other forms **of angina pectoris**

         EXCLUDES 1   *other forms of angina pectoris without atherosclerosis of other coronary artery bypass graft(s) (I20.8)*

         CC Excl: No Excl

     I25.799   **Atherosclerosis of other** `CC` `HCC` `A` **coronary artery bypass graft(s) with** unspecified **angina pectoris**

         EXCLUDES 1   *unspecified angina pectoris without atherosclerosis of other coronary artery bypass graft(s) (I20.9)*

         CC Excl: No Excl

✓5ᵗʰ   **I25.8**   **Other forms of chronic ischemic heart disease**

✓6ᵗʰ   **I25.81**   **Atherosclerosis of** other **coronary vessels** without angina pectoris

     Use additional code, if applicable, to identify:
         coronary atherosclerosis due to calcified coronary lesion (I25.84)
         coronary atherosclerosis due to lipid rich plaque (I25.83)

     EXCLUDES 1   *atherosclerotic heart disease of native coronary artery without angina pectoris (I25.10)*

     I25.810   **Atherosclerosis of coronary artery** `CC` `A` **bypass graft(s) without angina pectoris**

         Atherosclerosis of coronary artery bypass graft NOS

         EXCLUDES 1   *atherosclerosis of coronary bypass graft(s) with angina pectoris (I25.70--I25.73-, I25.79-)*

         CC Excl: No Excl

     I25.811   **Atherosclerosis of** native **coronary** `CC` **artery of** transplanted heart **without angina pectoris**

         Atherosclerosis of native coronary artery of transplanted heart NOS

         EXCLUDES 1   *atherosclerosis of native coronary artery of transplanted heart with angina pectoris (I25.75-)*

         CC Excl: PDX collection 664

     I25.812   **Atherosclerosis of** bypass graft **of** `CC` `A` **coronary artery of** transplanted heart **without angina pectoris**

         Atherosclerosis of bypass graft of transplanted heart NOS

         EXCLUDES 1   *atherosclerosis of bypass graft of transplanted heart with angina pectoris (I25.76)*

         CC Excl: PDX collection 666

     I25.82   Chronic total occlusion **of coronary artery**

         Complete occlusion of coronary artery
         Total occlusion of coronary artery
         Code first coronary atherosclerosis (I25.1-, I25.7-, I25.81-)

         EXCLUDES 1   *acute coronary occlusion with myocardial infarction (I21.0-I21.9, I22.-)*
            acute coronary occlusion without myocardial infarction (I24.0)

         DEF: Complete blockage of the coronary artery due to plaque accumulation over an extended period of time, resulting in substantial reduction of blood flow. Symptoms include angina or chest pain.

     I25.83   **Coronary atherosclerosis due to** lipid rich plaque `A`

         Code first coronary atherosclerosis (I25.1-, I25.7-, I25.81-)

     I25.84   **Coronary atherosclerosis due to** calcified coronary lesion

         Coronary atherosclerosis due to severely calcified coronary lesion
         Code first coronary atherosclerosis (I25.1-, I25.7-, I25.81-)

     I25.89   Other **forms of chronic ischemic heart disease**

     I25.9   **Chronic ischemic heart disease,** unspecified

         Ischemic heart disease (chronic) NOS

Pulmonary heart disease and diseases of pulmonary circulation (I26-I28)

✓4ᵗʰ   **I26**   **Pulmonary embolism**

     INCLUDES   pulmonary (acute) (artery)(vein) infarction
         pulmonary (acute) (artery)(vein) thromboembolism
         pulmonary (acute) (artery)(vein) thrombosis

     EXCLUDES 2   *chronic pulmonary embolism (I27.82)*
         personal history of pulmonary embolism (Z86.711)
         pulmonary embolism due to trauma (T79.0, T79.1)
         pulmonary embolism due to complications of surgical and medical care (T80.0, T81.7-, T82.8-)
         pulmonary embolism complicating abortion, ectopic or molar pregnancy (O00-O07, O08.2)
         pulmonary embolism complicating pregnancy, childbirth and the puerperium (O88.-)
         septic (non-pulmonary) arterial embolism (I76)

✓5ᵗʰ   **I26.0**   **Pulmonary embolism** with acute cor pulmonale

     CC Excl: For MCC codes in subcategory I26.0: PDX collection 667

     I26.01   Septic **pulmonary embolism with** `MCC` `HCC` **acute cor pulmonale**

         Code first underlying infection

     I26.02   Saddle **embolus of pulmonary** `MCC` `H10` `HCC` **artery with acute cor pulmonale**

     I26.09   Other **pulmonary embolism with** `MCC` `H10` `HCC` **acute cor pulmonale**

         Acute cor pulmonale NOS
         AHA: 2014, 4Q, 21

✓5ᵗʰ   **I26.9**   **Pulmonary embolism** without acute cor pulmonale

     I26.90   Septic **pulmonary embolism without acute** `MCC` `HCC` **cor pulmonale**

         Code first underlying infection
         CC Excl: PDX collection 668

     I26.92   Saddle **embolus of pulmonary artery** `MCC` `H10` `HCC` **without acute cor pulmonale**

         CC Excl: PDX collection 669

     I26.99   Other **pulmonary embolism without** `MCC` `H10` `HCC` **acute cor pulmonale**

         Acute pulmonary embolism NOS
         Pulmonary embolism NOS
         CC Excl: PDX collection 670

✓ Additional Character Required   ✓x7ᵗʰ Placeholder   Unacceptable PDx   Questionable PDx   Manifestation   `H1`-`H14` HAC   `HCC` CMS-HCC Dx   `HIV` HIV Dx

ICD-10-CM 2019   641

Chapter 9. Diseases of the Circulatory System

✓4ᵗʰ I27   Other pulmonary heart diseases

I27.0   Primary pulmonary hypertension   `CC` `HCC`
     Heritable pulmonary arterial hypertension
     Idiopathic pulmonary arterial hypertension
     Primary group 1 pulmonary hypertension
     Primary pulmonary arterial hypertension
     EXCLUDES 1   *persistent pulmonary hypertension of newborn (P29.30)*
         pulmonary hypertension NOS (I27.20)
         secondary pulmonary arterial hypertension (I27.21)
         secondary pulmonary hypertension (I27.29)
     DEF: Condition that occurs when pressure within the pulmonary artery is elevated and vascular resistance is observed in the lungs.
     CC Excl: PDX collection 671

I27.1   Kyphoscoliotic heart disease   `CC` `HCC`
     CC Excl: PDX collection 533

✓5ᵗʰ I27.2   Other secondary pulmonary hypertension
     Code also associated underlying condition
     EXCLUDES 1   *Eisenmenger's syndrome (I27.83)*
     AHA: 2017, 4Q, 14-15; 2014, 4Q, 21
     DEF: Condition that occurs when pressure within the pulmonary artery is elevated and vascular resistance is observed in the lungs.

I27.20   Pulmonary hypertension, unspecified   `HCC`
     Pulmonary hypertension NOS

I27.21   Secondary pulmonary arterial hypertension   `HCC`
     (Associated) (drug-induced) (toxin-induced) pulmonary arterial hypertension NOS
     (Associated) (drug-induced) (toxin-induced) (secondary) group 1 pulmonary hypertension
     Code also associated conditions if applicable, or adverse effects of drugs or toxins, such as:
         adverse effect of appetite depressants (T50.5X5)
         congenital heart disease (Q20-Q28)
         human immunodeficiency virus [HIV] disease (B20)
         polymyositis (M33.2-)
         portal hypertension (K76.6)
         rheumatoid arthritis (M05.-)
         schistosomiasis (B65.-)
         Sjögren syndrome (M35.0-)
         systemic sclerosis (M34.-)

I27.22   Pulmonary hypertension due to left heart disease   `HCC`
     Group 2 pulmonary hypertension
     Code also associated left heart disease, if known, such as:
         multiple valve disease (I08.-)
         rheumatic mitral valve diseases (I05.-)
         rheumatic aortic valve diseases (I06.-)

I27.23   Pulmonary hypertension due to lung diseases and hypoxia   `HCC`
     Group 3 pulmonary hypertension
     Code also associated lung disease, if known, such as:
         bronchiectasis (J47.-)
         cystic fibrosis with pulmonary manifestations (E84.0)
         interstitial lung disease (J84.-)
         pleural effusion (J90)
         sleep apnea (G47.3-)

I27.24   Chronic thromboembolic pulmonary hypertension   `HCC`
     Group 4 pulmonary hypertension
     Code also associated pulmonary embolism, if applicable (I26.-, I27.82)

I27.29   Other secondary pulmonary hypertension   `HCC`
     Group 5 pulmonary hypertension
     Pulmonary hypertension with unclear multifactorial mechanisms
     Pulmonary hypertension due to hematologic disorders
     Pulmonary hypertension due to metabolic disorders
     Pulmonary hypertension due to other systemic disorders
     Code also other associated disorders, if known, such as:
         chronic myeloid leukemia (C92.10- C92.22)
         essential thrombocythemia (D47.3)
         Gaucher disease (E75.22)
         hypertensive chronic kidney disease with end stage renal disease ▶(I12.0, I13.11, I13.2)◀
         hyperthyroidism (E05.-)
         hypothyroidism (E00-E03)
         polycythemia vera (D45)
         sarcoidosis (D86.-)
     AHA: 2016, 2Q, 8

✓5ᵗʰ I27.8   Other specified pulmonary heart diseases

I27.81   Cor pulmonale (chronic)   `HCC`
     Cor pulmonale NOS
     EXCLUDES 1   *acute cor pulmonale (I26.0-)*
     AHA: 2014, 4Q, 21

I27.82   Chronic pulmonary embolism   `CC` `HCC`
     Use additional code, if applicable, for associated long-term (current) use of anticoagulants (Z79.01)
     EXCLUDES 1   *personal history of pulmonary embolism (Z86.711)*
     DEF: Long-standing condition commonly associated with pulmonary hypertension in which small blood clots travel to the lungs repeatedly over many weeks, months, or years, requiring continuation of established anticoagulant or thrombolytic therapy.
     CC Excl: PDX collection 669

I27.83   Eisenmenger's syndrome   `HCC`
     Eisenmenger's complex
     (Irreversible) Eisenmenger's disease
     Pulmonary hypertension with right to left shunt related to congenital heart disease
     Code also underlying heart defect, if known, such as:
         atrial septal defect (Q21.1)
         Eisenmenger's defect (Q21.8)
         patent ductus arteriosus (Q25.0)
         ventricular septal defect (Q21.0)
     DEF: Pulmonary hypertension with congenital communication between two circulations resulting in a right to left shunt. This causes reduced oxygen saturation in the arterial blood, leading to cyanosis and organ damage. Once it develops, this life-threating condition is irreversible.

I27.89   Other specified pulmonary heart diseases   `HCC`

I27.9   Pulmonary heart disease, unspecified   `HCC`

✓4ᵗʰ I28   Other diseases of pulmonary vessels

I28.0   Arteriovenous fistula of pulmonary vessels   `CC` `HCC`
     EXCLUDES 1   *congenital arteriovenous fistula (Q25.72)*
     CC Excl: PDX collection 672

I28.1   Aneurysm of pulmonary artery   `CC` `HCC`
     EXCLUDES 1   *congenital aneurysm (Q25.79)*
         congenital arteriovenous aneurysm (Q25.72)
     CC Excl: PDX collection 672

I28.8   Other diseases of pulmonary vessels   `HCC`
     Pulmonary arteritis
     Pulmonary endarteritis
     Rupture of pulmonary vessels
     Stenosis of pulmonary vessels
     Stricture of pulmonary vessels

I28.9   Disease of pulmonary vessels, unspecified   `HCC`

Other forms of heart disease (I30-I52)

✓4ᵗʰ I30   Acute pericarditis
     INCLUDES   acute mediastinopericarditis
         acute myopericarditis
         acute pericardial effusion
         acute pleuropericarditis
         acute pneumopericarditis
     EXCLUDES 1   *Dressler's syndrome (I24.1)*
         rheumatic pericarditis (acute) (I01.0)
         viral pericarditis due to Coxsakie virus (B33.23)
     DEF: Pericarditis: Inflammation affecting the pericardium, the fibroserous membrane that surrounds the heart.

     CC Excl: For CC codes in category I30: PDX collection 673

I30.0   Acute nonspecific idiopathic pericarditis   `CC`

I30.1   Infective pericarditis   `CC`
     Pneumococcal pericarditis
     Pneumopyopericardium
     Purulent pericarditis
     Pyopericarditis
     Pyopericardium
     Pyopneumopericardium
     Staphylococcal pericarditis
     Streptococcal pericarditis
     Suppurative pericarditis
     Viral pericarditis
     Use additional code (B95-B97) to identify infectious agent

I30.8   Other forms of acute pericarditis   `CC`

I30.9   Acute pericarditis, unspecified   `CC`

N Newborn: 0   **P** Pediatric: 0-17   **M** Maternity: 12-55   **A** Adult: 15-124   **MCC** Major Complication/Comorbidity   **CC** Complication/Comorbidity   **SW** Severe Wound Dx

642   ICD-10-CM 2019

✓4ᵗʰ **I31 Other diseases of pericardium**

     EXCLUDES 1 *diseases of pericardium specified as rheumatic (I09.2)*
                          postcardiotomy syndrome (I97.0)
                          traumatic injury to pericardium (S26.-)

I31.0 Chronic adhesive pericarditis   `CC`
     Accretio cordis
     Adherent pericardium
     Adhesive mediastinopericarditis
     CC Excl: PDX collection 674

I31.1 Chronic constrictive pericarditis   `CC`
     Concretio cordis
     Pericardial calcification
     CC Excl: PDX collection 674

I31.2 Hemopericardium, not elsewhere classified   `CC`
     EXCLUDES 1 *hemopericardium as current complication following*
                          acute myocardial infarction (I23.0)
     DEF: Presence of blood in the pericardial sac (pericardium). It can
     lead to potentially fatal cardiac tamponade if enough blood enters
     the pericardial cavity.
     CC Excl: PDX collection 674

I31.3 Pericardial effusion (noninflammatory)   `CC`
     Chylopericardium
     EXCLUDES 1 *acute pericardial effusion (I30.9)*
     CC Excl: PDX collection 188

I31.4 Cardiac tamponade   `CC`
     Code first underlying cause
     DEF: Life-threatening condition in which fluid or blood
     accumulates in the space between the muscle of the heart
     (myocardium) and the outer sac that covers the heart
     (pericardium), resulting in compression of the heart.
     CC Excl: PDX collection 188

Cardiac Tamponade

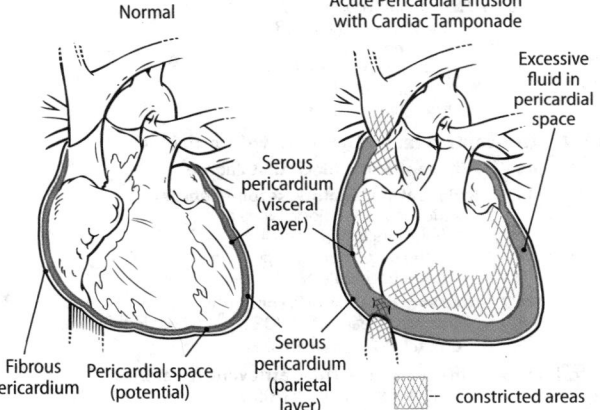

Normal   Acute Pericardial Effusion with Cardiac Tamponade

Excessive fluid in pericardial space

Serous pericardium (visceral layer)

Serous pericardium (parietal layer)

Fibrous pericardium   Pericardial space (potential)

constricted areas

I31.8 Other specified diseases of pericardium   `CC`
     Epicardial plaques   Focal pericardial adhesions
     CC Excl: PDX collection 188

I31.9 Disease of pericardium, unspecified   `CC`
     Pericarditis (chronic) NOS
     CC Excl: PDX collection 188

I32 *Pericarditis in diseases classified elsewhere*   `CC`
     Code first underlying disease
     EXCLUDES 1 *pericarditis (in):*
                  coxsackie (virus) (B33.23)
                  gonococcal (A54.83)
                  meningococcal (A39.53)
                  rheumatoid (arthritis) (M05.31)
                  syphilitic (A52.06)
                  systemic lupus erythematosus (M32.12)
                  tuberculosis (A18.84)
     DEF: Pericarditis: Inflammation affecting the pericardium, the fibroserous
     membrane that surrounds the heart.
     CC Excl: PDX collection 673

✓4ᵗʰ **I33 Acute and subacute endocarditis**

     EXCLUDES 1 *acute rheumatic endocarditis (I01.1)*
                          endocarditis NOS (I38)
     DEF: Endocarditis: Inflammatory disease of the interior lining of the heart
     chamber and heart valves.

I33.0 Acute and subacute infective endocarditis   `HIV` `MCC`
     Bacterial endocarditis (acute) (subacute)
     Infective endocarditis (acute) (subacute) NOS
     Endocarditis lenta (acute) (subacute)
     Malignant endocarditis (acute) (subacute)
     Purulent endocarditis (acute) (subacute)
     Septic endocarditis (acute) (subacute)
     Ulcerative endocarditis (acute) (subacute)
     Vegetative endocarditis (acute) (subacute)
     Use additional code (B95-B97) to identify infectious agent
     CC Excl: PDX collection 675

I33.9 Acute and subacute endocarditis, unspecified   `HIV` `MCC`
     Acute endocarditis NOS
     Acute myoendocarditis NOS
     Acute periendocarditis NOS
     Subacute endocarditis NOS
     Subacute myoendocarditis NOS
     Subacute periendocarditis NOS
     CC Excl: PDX collection 675

✓4ᵗʰ **I34 Nonrheumatic mitral valve disorders**

     EXCLUDES 1 *mitral valve disease (I05.9)*
                          mitral valve failure (I05.8)
                          mitral valve stenosis (I05.0)
                          mitral valve disorder of unspecified cause with diseases of aortic
                                 and/or tricuspid valve(s) (I08.-)
                          mitral valve disorder of unspecified cause with mitral stenosis or
                                 obstruction (I05.0)
                          mitral valve disorder specified as congenital (Q23.2, Q23.9)
                          mitral valve disorder specified as rheumatic (I05.-)

I34.0 Nonrheumatic mitral (valve) insufficiency
     Nonrheumatic mitral (valve) incompetence NOS
     Nonrheumatic mitral (valve) regurgitation NOS

I34.1 Nonrheumatic mitral (valve) prolapse
     Floppy nonrheumatic mitral valve syndrome
     EXCLUDES 1 *Marfan's syndrome (Q87.4-)*

I34.2 Nonrheumatic mitral (valve) stenosis

I34.8 Other nonrheumatic mitral valve disorders

I34.9 Nonrheumatic mitral valve disorder, unspecified

✓4ᵗʰ **I35 Nonrheumatic aortic valve disorders**

     EXCLUDES 1 *aortic valve disorder of unspecified cause but with diseases of*
                                 mitral and/or tricuspid valve(s) (I08.-)
                          aortic valve disorder specified as congenital (Q23.0, Q23.1)
                          aortic valve disorder specified as rheumatic (I06.-)
                          hypertrophic subaortic stenosis (I42.1)

I35.0 Nonrheumatic aortic (valve) stenosis

I35.1 Nonrheumatic aortic (valve) insufficiency
     Nonrheumatic aortic (valve) incompetence NOS
     Nonrheumatic aortic (valve) regurgitation NOS

I35.2 Nonrheumatic aortic (valve) stenosis with insufficiency

I35.8 Other nonrheumatic aortic valve disorders

I35.9 Nonrheumatic aortic valve disorder, unspecified

✓4ᵗʰ **I36 Nonrheumatic tricuspid valve disorders**

     EXCLUDES 1 *tricuspid valve disorders of unspecified cause (I07.-)*
                          tricuspid valve disorders specified as congenital (Q22.4, Q22.8,
                                 Q22.9)
                          tricuspid valve disorders specified as rheumatic (I07.-)
                          tricuspid valve disorders with aortic and/or mitral valve
                               involvement (I08.-)

I36.0 Nonrheumatic tricuspid (valve) stenosis

I36.1 Nonrheumatic tricuspid (valve) insufficiency
     Nonrheumatic tricuspid (valve) incompetence
     Nonrheumatic tricuspid (valve) regurgitation

I36.2 Nonrheumatic tricuspid (valve) stenosis with insufficiency

I36.8 Other nonrheumatic tricuspid valve disorders

I36.9 Nonrheumatic tricuspid valve disorder, unspecified

✓4ᵗʰ **I37 Nonrheumatic pulmonary valve disorders**

     EXCLUDES 1 *pulmonary valve disorder specified as congenital (Q22.1, Q22.2,*
                                 Q22.3)
                          pulmonary valve disorder specified as rheumatic (I09.89)

I37.0 Nonrheumatic pulmonary valve stenosis

I37.1 Nonrheumatic pulmonary valve insufficiency
     Nonrheumatic pulmonary valve incompetence
     Nonrheumatic pulmonary valve regurgitation

✅ Additional Character Required   ✓x7ᵗʰ Placeholder   Unacceptable PDx   Questionable PDx   Manifestation   `H1`-`H14` HAC   `HCC` CMS-HCC Dx   `HIV` HIV Dx

ICD-10-CM 2019   **643**

I37.2   **Nonrheumatic pulmonary valve** stenosis with insufficiency

I37.8   Other **nonrheumatic pulmonary valve disorders**

I37.9   **Nonrheumatic pulmonary valve disorder,** unspecified

I38   **Endocarditis, valve unspecified**   `CC`

> INCLUDES   endocarditis (chronic) NOS
> valvular incompetence NOS
> valvular insufficiency NOS
> valvular regurgitation NOS
> valvular stenosis NOS
> valvulitis (chronic) NOS
>
> EXCLUDES 1   congenital insufficiency of cardiac valve NOS (Q24.8)
> congenital stenosis of cardiac valve NOS (Q24.8)
> endocardial fibroelastosis (I42.4)
> endocarditis specified as rheumatic (I09.1)
>
> **DEF:** Endocarditis: Inflammatory disease of the interior lining of the heart chamber and heart valves.
> **CC Excl:** PDX collection 676

I39   *Endocarditis and heart valve disorders in diseases classified elsewhere*   `CC`

> Code first underlying disease, such as:
> Q fever (A78)
>
> EXCLUDES 1   endocardial involvement in:
> candidiasis (B37.6)
> gonococcal infection (A54.83)
> Libman-Sacks disease (M32.11)
> listerosis (A32.82)
> meningococcal infection (A39.51)
> rheumatoid arthritis (M05.31)
> syphilis (A52.03)
> tuberculosis (A18.84)
> typhoid fever (A01.02)
>
> **DEF:** Endocarditis: Inflammatory disease of the interior lining of the heart chamber and heart valves.
> **CC Excl:** PDX collection 676

✓4ᵗʰ I40   **Acute myocarditis**

> INCLUDES   subacute myocarditis
> EXCLUDES 1   acute rheumatic myocarditis (I01.2)
> **DEF:** Myocarditis: Inflammation of the middle layer of the heart, which is composed of muscle tissue.
>
> CC Excl: For MCC codes in category I40: PDX collection 677

I40.0   **Infective myocarditis**   `HIV` `MCC`
> Septic myocarditis
> Use additional code (B95-B97) to identify infectious agent

I40.1   **Isolated myocarditis**   `HIV` `MCC`
> Fiedler's myocarditis
> Giant cell myocarditis
> Idiopathic myocarditis

I40.8   Other **acute myocarditis**   `HIV` `MCC`

I40.9   **Acute myocarditis,** unspecified   `HIV` `MCC`

I41   *Myocarditis in diseases classified elsewhere*   `MCC`

> Code first underlying disease, such as:
> typhus (A75.0-A75.9)
>
> EXCLUDES 1   myocarditis (in):
> Chagas' disease (chronic) (B57.2)
> acute (B57.0)
> coxsackie (virus) infection (B33.22)
> diphtheritic (A36.81)
> gonococcal (A54.83)
> influenzal (J09.X9, J10.82, J11.82)
> meningococcal (A39.52)
> mumps (B26.82)
> rheumatoid arthritis (M05.31)
> sarcoid (D86.85)
> syphilis (A52.06)
> toxoplasmosis (B58.81)
> tuberculous (A18.84)
>
> **DEF:** Myocarditis: Inflammation of the middle layer of the heart, which is composed of muscle tissue.
> **CC Excl:** PDX collection 677

✓4ᵗʰ I42   **Cardiomyopathy**

> INCLUDES   myocardiopathy
> Code first pre-existing cardiomyopathy complicating pregnancy and puerperium (O99.4)
>
> EXCLUDES 2   ischemic cardiomyopathy (I25.5)
> peripartum cardiomyopathy (O90.3)
> ventricular hypertrophy (I51.7)
>
> CC Excl: For CC codes in category I42: PDX collection 678

I42.0   **Dilated cardiomyopathy**   `CC` `HCC`
> Congestive cardiomyopathy

I42.1   **Obstructive hypertrophic cardiomyopathy**   `CC` `HCC`
> Hypertrophic subaortic stenosis (idiopathic)
> **DEF:** Cardiomyopathy marked by left ventricle hypertrophy and an enlarged septum that result in obstructed blood flow, arrhythmias, mitral regurgitation, and sudden cardiac death.
> **TIP:** When this condition is described as inherited, assign code Q24.8.

I42.2   Other hypertrophic **cardiomyopathy**   `CC` `HCC`
> Nonobstructive hypertrophic cardiomyopathy

I42.3   Endomyocardial (eosinophilic) disease   `CC` `HCC`
> Endomyocardial (tropical) fibrosis
> Löffler's endocarditis

I42.4   Endocardial fibroelastosis   `CC` `HCC`
> Congenital cardiomyopathy
> Elastomyofibrosis

I42.5   Other restrictive **cardiomyopathy**   `CC` `HCC`
> Constrictive cardiomyopathy NOS

I42.6   Alcoholic **cardiomyopathy**   `CC` `HCC`
> Code also presence of alcoholism (F10.-)

I42.7   **Cardiomyopathy** due to drug and external agent   `CC` `HCC`
> Code first poisoning due to drug or toxin, if applicable (T36-T65 with fifth or sixth character 1-4 or 6)
> Use additional code for adverse effect, if applicable, to identify drug (T36-T50 with fifth or sixth character 5)

I42.8   Other **cardiomyopathies**   `CC` `HCC`

I42.9   **Cardiomyopathy,** unspecified   `CC` `HCC`
> Cardiomyopathy (primary) (secondary) NOS

I43   *Cardiomyopathy in diseases classified elsewhere*   `CC` `HCC`

> Code first underlying disease, such as:
> amyloidosis (E85.-)
> glycogen storage disease (E74.0)
> gout (M10.0-)
> thyrotoxicosis (E05.0-E05.9-)
>
> EXCLUDES 1   cardiomyopathy (in):
> coxsackie (virus) (B33.24)
> diphtheria (A36.81)
> sarcoidosis (D86.85)
> tuberculosis (A18.84)
>
> **CC Excl:** PDX collection 678

✓4ᵗʰ I44   **Atrioventricular and left bundle-branch block**

I44.0   **Atrioventricular block,** first degree

I44.1   **Atrioventricular block,** second degree
> Atrioventricular block, type I and II
> Möbitz block, type I and II
> Second degree block, type I and II
> Wenckebach's block

I44.2   **Atrioventricular block,** complete   `CC` `HCC`
> Complete heart block NOS   Third degree block
> **CC Excl:** PDX collection 679

✓5ᵗʰ I44.3   **Other and unspecified** atrioventricular **block**
> Atrioventricular block NOS

I44.30   Unspecified **atrioventricular block**

I44.39   Other **atrioventricular block**

I44.4   Left anterior fascicular **block**

I44.5   Left posterior fascicular **block**

✓5ᵗʰ I44.6   **Other and unspecified** fascicular **block**

I44.60   Unspecified **fascicular block**
> Left bundle-branch hemiblock NOS

I44.69   Other **fascicular block**

I44.7   **Left bundle-branch block,** unspecified

✓4ᵗʰ I45   **Other conduction disorders**

> CC Excl: For CC codes in category I45: PDX collection 679

I45.0   **Right fascicular block**

✓5ᵗʰ I45.1   **Other and unspecified right bundle-branch block**

I45.10   Unspecified **right bundle-branch block**
> Right bundle-branch block NOS

I45.19   Other **right bundle-branch block**

I45.2   **Bifascicular block**   `CC`

I45.3   **Trifascicular block**   `CC`

I45.4   **Nonspecific intraventricular block**
> Bundle-branch block NOS

N Newborn: 0   P Pediatric: 0-17   M Maternity: 12-55   A Adult: 15-124   MCC Major Complication/Comorbidity   CC Complication/Comorbidity   SW Severe Wound Dx

644   ICD-10-CM 2019

Conduction Disorders

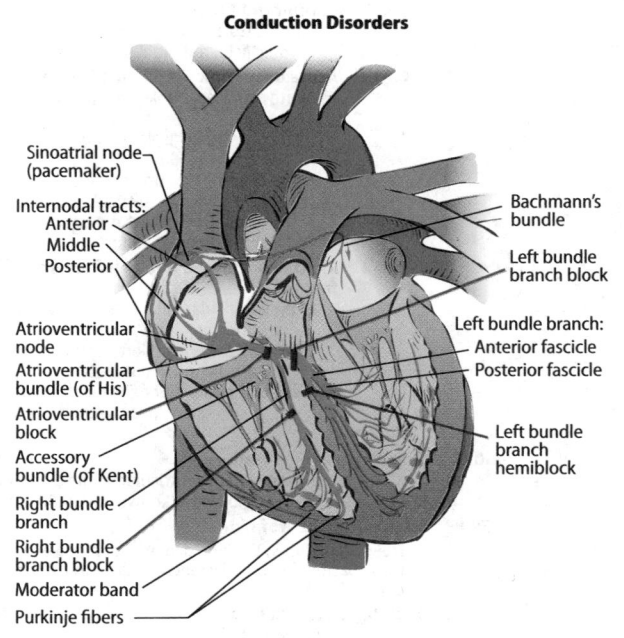

Sinoatrial node (pacemaker)
Internodal tracts:
  Anterior
  Middle
  Posterior
Atrioventricular node
Atrioventricular bundle (of His)
Atrioventricular block
Accessory bundle (of Kent)
Right bundle branch
Right bundle branch block
Moderator band
Purkinje fibers

Bachmann's bundle
Left bundle branch block
Left bundle branch:
  Anterior fascicle
  Posterior fascicle
Left bundle branch hemiblock

I45.5   **Other specified heart block**
Sinoatrial block
Sinoauricular block
   EXCLUDES 1   heart block NOS (I45.9)

I45.6   **Pre-excitation syndrome**
Accelerated atrioventricular conduction
Accessory atrioventricular conduction
Anomalous atrioventricular excitation
Lown-Ganong-Levine syndrome
Pre-excitation atrioventricular conduction
Wolff-Parkinson-White syndrome

✓5ᵗʰ **I45.8**   **Other specified conduction disorders**

   I45.81   **Long QT syndrome**
     DEF: Condition characterized by recurrent syncope, malignant arrhythmias, and sudden death. This syndrome has a characteristic prolonged Q-T interval on an electrocardiogram.

   I45.89   **Other specified conduction disorders**   `CC`
     Atrioventricular [AV] dissociation
     Interference dissociation
     Isorhythmic dissociation
     Nonparoxysmal AV nodal tachycardia
     AHA: 2013, 2Q, 31

I45.9   **Conduction disorder, unspecified**
Heart block NOS
Stokes-Adams syndrome

✓4ᵗʰ **I46**   **Cardiac arrest**
   EXCLUDES 1   cardiogenic shock (R57.0)

   CC Excl: For MCC codes in category I46: PDX collection 680

¹ **I46.2**   **Cardiac arrest due to underlying cardiac condition**   `MCC` `HCC`
   Code first underlying cardiac condition

¹ **I46.8**   **Cardiac arrest due to other underlying condition**   `MCC` `HCC`
   Code first underlying condition

¹ **I46.9**   **Cardiac arrest, cause unspecified**   `MCC` `HCC`

✓4ᵗʰ **I47**   **Paroxysmal tachycardia**
Code first tachycardia complicating:
  abortion or ectopic or molar pregnancy (O00-O07, O08.8)
  obstetric surgery and procedures (O75.4)
   EXCLUDES 1   tachycardia NOS (R00.0)
     sinoauricular tachycardia NOS (R00.0)
     sinus [sinusal] tachycardia NOS (R00.0)

   CC Excl: For CC codes in category I47: PDX collection 679

I47.0   **Re-entry ventricular arrhythmia**   `CC` `HCC`

I47.1   **Supraventricular tachycardia**   `CC` `HCC`
Atrial (paroxysmal) tachycardia
Atrioventricular [AV] (paroxysmal) tachycardia
Atrioventricular re-entrant (nodal) tachycardia [AVNRT] [AVRT]
Junctional (paroxysmal) tachycardia
Nodal (paroxysmal) tachycardia

I47.2   **Ventricular tachycardia**   `CC` `HCC`
   AHA: 2013, 3Q, 23

I47.9   **Paroxysmal tachycardia, unspecified**   `HCC`
Bouveret (-Hoffman) syndrome

✓4ᵗʰ **I48**   **Atrial fibrillation and flutter**

   CC Excl: For CC codes in category I48: PDX collection 679

I48.0   **Paroxysmal atrial fibrillation**   `HCC`

I48.1   **Persistent atrial fibrillation**   `CC` `HCC`

I48.2   **Chronic atrial fibrillation**   `HCC`
Permanent atrial fibrillation

I48.3   **Typical atrial flutter**   `CC` `HCC`
Type I atrial flutter

I48.4   **Atypical atrial flutter**   `CC` `HCC`
Type II atrial flutter

✓5ᵗʰ **I48.9**   **Unspecified atrial fibrillation and atrial flutter**

   I48.91   **Unspecified atrial fibrillation**   `HCC`

   I48.92   **Unspecified atrial flutter**   `CC` `HCC`

✓4ᵗʰ **I49**   **Other cardiac arrhythmias**
Code first cardiac arrhythmia complicating:
  abortion or ectopic or molar pregnancy (O00-O07, O08.8)
  obstetric surgery and procedures (O75.4)
   EXCLUDES 1   neonatal dysrhythmia (P29.1-)
     sinoatrial bradycardia (R00.1)
     sinus bradycardia (R00.1)
     vagal bradycardia (R00.1)
   EXCLUDES 2   bradycardia NOS (R00.1)

   CC Excl: For CC/MCC codes in category I49: PDX collection 679

✓5ᵗʰ **I49.0**   **Ventricular fibrillation and flutter**

   ¹ **I49.01**   **Ventricular fibrillation**   `MCC` `HCC`

   I49.02   **Ventricular flutter**   `MCC` `HCC`

I49.1   **Atrial premature depolarization**
Atrial premature beats

I49.2   **Junctional premature depolarization**   `CC` `HCC`

I49.3   **Ventricular premature depolarization**

✓5ᵗʰ **I49.4**   **Other and unspecified premature depolarization**

   I49.40   **Unspecified premature depolarization**
     Premature beats NOS

   I49.49   **Other premature depolarization**
     Ectopic beats
     Extrasystoles
     Extrasystolic arrhythmias
     Premature contractions

I49.5   **Sick sinus syndrome**   `HCC`
Tachycardia-bradycardia syndrome
TIP: Do not assign when sick sinus syndrome (SSS) is controlled by a pacemaker and no management of the condition is required during the encounter; assign only code Z95.0 Presence of cardiac pacemaker.

I49.8   **Other specified cardiac arrhythmias**
Brugada syndrome
Coronary sinus rhythm disorder
Ectopic rhythm disorder
Nodal rhythm disorder

I49.9   **Cardiac arrhythmia, unspecified**
Arrhythmia (cardiac) NOS

✓ Additional Character Required   🔲 Placeholder   Unacceptable PDx   Questionable PDx   Manifestation   `H1`-`H14` HAC   `HCC` CMS-HCC Dx   `HIV` HIV Dx

ICD-10-CM 2019   **645**

Chapter 9. Diseases of the Circulatory System

✓4ᵗʰ **I50 Heart failure**
Code first:
   heart failure complicating abortion or ectopic or molar pregnancy (O00-O07, O08.8)
   heart failure following surgery (I97.13-)
   heart failure due to hypertension (I11.0)
   heart failure due to hypertension with chronic kidney disease (I13.-)
   obstetric surgery and procedures (O75.4)
   rheumatic heart failure (I09.81)
   EXCLUDES 1   *neonatal cardiac failure (P29.0)*
   EXCLUDES 2   *cardiac arrest (I46.-)*
   AHA: 2018, 2Q, 9; 2017, 1Q, 47; 2014, 1Q, 25; 2013, 2Q, 33

> **CC Excl:** For CC/MCC codes in category I50, unless otherwise noted: PDX collection 682

I50.1 Left ventricular failure, unspecified   CC HCC
   Cardiac asthma
   Edema of lung with heart disease NOS
   Edema of lung with heart failure
   Left heart failure
   Pulmonary edema with heart disease NOS
   Pulmonary edema with heart failure
   EXCLUDES 1   *edema of lung without heart disease or heart failure (J81.-)*
              pulmonary edema without heart disease or failure (J81.-)
   CC Excl: PDX collection 681

✓5ᵗʰ **I50.2 Systolic (congestive) heart failure**
   Heart failure with reduced ejection fraction [HFrEF]
   Systolic left ventricular heart failure
   Code also end stage heart failure, if applicable (I50.84)
   EXCLUDES 1   *combined systolic (congestive) and diastolic (congestive) heart failure (I50.4-)*
   AHA: 2017, 1Q, 46; 2016, 1Q, 10

  I50.20 Unspecified systolic (congestive) heart failure   CC HCC
  I50.21 Acute systolic (congestive) heart failure   MCC HCC
  I50.22 Chronic systolic (congestive) heart failure   CC HCC
  I50.23 Acute on chronic systolic (congestive) heart failure   MCC HCC

✓5ᵗʰ **I50.3 Diastolic (congestive) heart failure**
   Diastolic left ventricular heart failure
   Heart failure with normal ejection fraction
   Heart failure with preserved ejection fraction [HFpEF]
   Code also end stage heart failure, if applicable (I50.84)
   EXCLUDES 1   *combined systolic (congestive) and diastolic (congestive) heart failure (I50.4-)*
   AHA: 2017, 1Q, 46; 2016, 1Q, 10

  I50.30 Unspecified diastolic (congestive) heart failure   CC HCC
  I50.31 Acute diastolic (congestive) heart failure   MCC HCC
  I50.32 Chronic diastolic (congestive) heart failure   CC HCC
  I50.33 Acute on chronic diastolic (congestive) heart failure   MCC HCC

✓5ᵗʰ **I50.4 Combined systolic (congestive) and diastolic (congestive) heart failure**
   Combined systolic and diastolic left ventricular heart failure
   Heart failure with reduced ejection fraction and diastolic dysfunction
   Code also end stage heart failure, if applicable (I50.84)
   AHA: 2017, 1Q, 46; 2016, 1Q, 10

  I50.40 Unspecified combined systolic (congestive) and diastolic (congestive) heart failure   CC HCC
  I50.41 Acute combined systolic (congestive) and diastolic (congestive) heart failure   MCC HCC
  I50.42 Chronic combined systolic (congestive) and diastolic (congestive) heart failure   CC HCC
  I50.43 Acute on chronic combined systolic (congestive) and diastolic (congestive) heart failure   MCC HCC

✓5ᵗʰ **I50.8 Other heart failure**
   AHA: 2017, 4Q, 15-16

  ✓6ᵗʰ **I50.81 Right heart failure**
    Right ventricular failure
    I50.810 Right heart failure, unspecified   HCC
      Right heart failure without mention of left heart failure
      Right ventricular failure NOS
    I50.811 Acute right heart failure   HCC
      Acute isolated right heart failure
      Acute (isolated) right ventricular failure

    I50.812 Chronic right heart failure   HCC
      Chronic isolated right heart failure
      Chronic (isolated) right ventricular failure
    I50.813 Acute on chronic right heart failure   HCC
      Acute on chronic isolated right heart failure
      Acute on chronic (isolated) right ventricular failure
      Acute decompensation of chronic (isolated) right ventricular failure
      Acute exacerbation of chronic (isolated) right ventricular failure
    I50.814 Right heart failure due to left heart failure   HCC
      Right ventricular failure secondary to left ventricular failure
      Code also the type of left ventricular failure, if known (I50.2-I50.43)
      EXCLUDES 1   *right heart failure with but not due to left heart failure (I50.82)*

  I50.82 Biventricular heart failure   HCC
   Code also the type of left ventricular failure as systolic, diastolic, or combined, if known (I50.2-I50.43)
  I50.83 High output heart failure   HCC
   DEF: Occurs when the high demand for blood exceeds the capacity of a normally functioning heart to meet the demand.
  I50.84 End stage heart failure   HCC
   Stage D heart failure
   Code also the type of heart failure as systolic, diastolic, or combined, if known (I50.2-I50.43)
  I50.89 Other heart failure   HCC

I50.9 Heart failure, unspecified   HCC
   Cardiac, heart or myocardial failure NOS
   Congestive heart disease
   Congestive heart failure NOS
   EXCLUDES 2   *fluid overload (E87.70)*
   AHA: 2017, 4Q, 15-16; 2017, 1Q, 45-46; 2014, 4Q, 21; 2012, 4Q, 92

✓4ᵗʰ **I51 Complications and ill-defined descriptions of heart disease**
   EXCLUDES 1   *any condition in I51.4-I51.9 due to hypertension (I11.-)*
         any condition in I51.4-I51.9 due to hypertension and chronic kidney disease (I13.-)
         heart disease specified as rheumatic (I00-I09)

I51.0 Cardiac septal defect, acquired   CC A
   Acquired septal atrial defect (old)
   Acquired septal auricular defect (old)
   Acquired septal ventricular defect (old)
   EXCLUDES 1   *cardiac septal defect as current complication following acute myocardial infarction (I23.1, I23.2)*
   DEF: Abnormal communication between opposite heart chambers due to a defect of the septum. It is not present at birth.
   CC Excl: PDX collection 654

I51.1 Rupture of chordae tendineae, not elsewhere classified   MCC HCC
   EXCLUDES 1   *rupture of chordae tendineae as current complication following acute myocardial infarction (I23.4)*
   CC Excl: PDX collection 655

I51.2 Rupture of papillary muscle, not elsewhere classified   MCC HCC
   EXCLUDES 1   *rupture of papillary muscle as current complication following acute myocardial infarction (I23.5)*
   CC Excl: PDX collection 656

I51.3 Intracardiac thrombosis, not elsewhere classified
   Apical thrombosis (old)
   Atrial thrombosis (old)
   Auricular thrombosis (old)
   Mural thrombosis (old)
   Ventricular thrombosis (old)
   EXCLUDES 1   *intracardiac thrombosis as current complication following acute myocardial infarction (I23.6)*
   AHA: 2013, 1Q, 24

I51.4 Myocarditis, unspecified   HCC
   Chronic (interstitial) myocarditis
   Myocardial fibrosis
   Myocarditis NOS
   EXCLUDES 1   *acute or subacute myocarditis (I40.-)*
   AHA: 2018, 2Q, 9

I51.5 Myocardial degeneration   HCC
   Fatty degeneration of heart or myocardium
   Myocardial disease
   Senile degeneration of heart or myocardium
   AHA: 2018, 2Q, 9

I51.7   **Cardiomegaly**
Cardiac dilatation
Cardiac hypertrophy
Ventricular dilatation
AHA: 2018, 2Q, 9

√5ᵗʰ **I51.8**   **Other ill-defined heart diseases**
AHA: 2018, 2Q, 9

     I51.81   **Takotsubo syndrome**   CC
Reversible left ventricular dysfunction following
sudden emotional stress
Stress induced cardiomyopathy
Takotsubo cardiomyopathy
Transient left ventricular apical ballooning syndrome
DEF: Complex of symptoms mimicking myocardial
infarct in absence of heart disease, with the majority of
cases occurring in postmenopausal women. Heart
muscles are temporarily weakened, and a sudden,
massive surge of adrenalin stuns the heart, greatly
reducing the ability to pump blood.
CC Excl: PDX collection 683

     I51.89   **Other ill-defined heart diseases**
Carditis (acute)(chronic)
Pancarditis (acute)(chronic)

I51.9   **Heart disease, unspecified**
AHA: 2018, 2Q, 9

I52   *Other heart disorders in diseases classified elsewhere*
Code first underlying disease, such as:
congenital syphilis (A50.5)
mucopolysaccharidosis (E76.3)
schistosomiasis (B65.0-B65.9)
EXCLUDES 1   heart disease (in):
gonococcal infection (A54.83)
meningococcal infection (A39.50)
rheumatoid arthritis (M05.31)
syphilis (A52.06)

Cerebrovascular diseases (I60-I69)

Use additional code to identify presence of:
alcohol abuse and dependence (F10.-)
exposure to environmental tobacco smoke (Z77.22)
history of tobacco dependence (Z87.891)
hypertension ▶(I10-I16)◀
occupational exposure to environmental tobacco smoke (Z57.31)
tobacco dependence (F17.-)
tobacco use (Z72.0)
EXCLUDES 1   traumatic intracranial hemorrhage (S06.-)
AHA: 2014, 3Q, 5; 2012, 4Q, 91-92

√4ᵗʰ **I60**   **Nontraumatic subarachnoid hemorrhage**
EXCLUDES 1   syphilitic ruptured cerebral aneurysm (A52.05)
EXCLUDES 2   sequelae of subarachnoid hemorrhage (I69.0-)

CC Excl: For MCC codes in category I60: PDX collection 684

√5ᵗʰ **I60.0**   **Nontraumatic subarachnoid hemorrhage from carotid siphon and bifurcation**

     I60.00   **Nontraumatic subarachnoid hemorrhage from unspecified carotid siphon and bifurcation**   MCC HCC

     I60.01   **Nontraumatic subarachnoid hemorrhage from right carotid siphon and bifurcation**   MCC HCC

     I60.02   **Nontraumatic subarachnoid hemorrhage from left carotid siphon and bifurcation**   MCC HCC

√5ᵗʰ **I60.1**   **Nontraumatic subarachnoid hemorrhage from middle cerebral artery**

     I60.10   **Nontraumatic subarachnoid hemorrhage from unspecified middle cerebral artery**   MCC HCC

     I60.11   **Nontraumatic subarachnoid hemorrhage from right middle cerebral artery**   MCC HCC

     I60.12   **Nontraumatic subarachnoid hemorrhage from left middle cerebral artery**   MCC HCC

I60.2   **Nontraumatic subarachnoid hemorrhage from anterior communicating artery**   MCC HCC

√5ᵗʰ **I60.3**   **Nontraumatic subarachnoid hemorrhage from posterior communicating artery**

     I60.30   **Nontraumatic subarachnoid hemorrhage from unspecified posterior communicating artery**   MCC HCC

     I60.31   **Nontraumatic subarachnoid hemorrhage from right posterior communicating artery**   MCC HCC

     I60.32   **Nontraumatic subarachnoid hemorrhage from left posterior communicating artery**   MCC HCC

I60.4   **Nontraumatic subarachnoid hemorrhage from basilar artery**   MCC HCC

√5ᵗʰ **I60.5**   **Nontraumatic subarachnoid hemorrhage from vertebral artery**

     I60.50   **Nontraumatic subarachnoid hemorrhage from unspecified vertebral artery**   MCC HCC

     I60.51   **Nontraumatic subarachnoid hemorrhage from right vertebral artery**   MCC HCC

     I60.52   **Nontraumatic subarachnoid hemorrhage from left vertebral artery**   MCC HCC

I60.6   **Nontraumatic subarachnoid hemorrhage from other intracranial arteries**   MCC HCC

I60.7   **Nontraumatic subarachnoid hemorrhage from unspecified intracranial artery**   MCC HCC
Ruptured (congenital) berry aneurysm
Ruptured (congenital) cerebral aneurysm
Subarachnoid hemorrhage (nontraumatic) from cerebral artery NOS
Subarachnoid hemorrhage (nontraumatic) from communicating artery NOS
EXCLUDES 1   berry aneurysm, nonruptured (I67.1)

I60.8   **Other nontraumatic subarachnoid hemorrhage**   MCC HCC
Meningeal hemorrhage
Rupture of cerebral arteriovenous malformation

I60.9   **Nontraumatic subarachnoid hemorrhage, unspecified**   MCC HCC

√4ᵗʰ **I61**   **Nontraumatic intracerebral hemorrhage**
EXCLUDES 2   sequelae of intracerebral hemorrhage (I69.1-)
AHA: 2017, 2Q, 9-10

CC Excl: For MCC codes in category I61: PDX collection 684

I61.0   **Nontraumatic intracerebral hemorrhage in hemisphere, subcortical**   MCC HCC
Deep intracerebral hemorrhage (nontraumatic)
AHA: 2016, 4Q, 27

I61.1   **Nontraumatic intracerebral hemorrhage in hemisphere, cortical**   MCC HCC
Cerebral lobe hemorrhage (nontraumatic)
Superficial intracerebral hemorrhage (nontraumatic)

I61.2   **Nontraumatic intracerebral hemorrhage in hemisphere, unspecified**   MCC HCC

I61.3   **Nontraumatic intracerebral hemorrhage in brain stem**   MCC HCC

I61.4   **Nontraumatic intracerebral hemorrhage in cerebellum**   MCC HCC

I61.5   **Nontraumatic intracerebral hemorrhage, intraventricular**   MCC HCC

I61.6   **Nontraumatic intracerebral hemorrhage, multiple localized**   MCC HCC

I61.8   **Other nontraumatic intracerebral hemorrhage**   MCC HCC

I61.9   **Nontraumatic intracerebral hemorrhage, unspecified**   MCC HCC

√4ᵗʰ **I62**   **Other and unspecified nontraumatic intracranial hemorrhage**
EXCLUDES 2   sequelae of intracranial hemorrhage (I69.2)

CC Excl: For CC/MCC codes in category I62: PDX collection 684

√5ᵗʰ **I62.0**   **Nontraumatic subdural hemorrhage**

     I62.00   **Nontraumatic subdural hemorrhage, unspecified**   MCC HCC

     I62.01   **Nontraumatic acute subdural hemorrhage**   MCC HCC

     I62.02   **Nontraumatic subacute subdural hemorrhage**   MCC HCC

     I62.03   **Nontraumatic chronic subdural hemorrhage**   MCC HCC

I62.1   **Nontraumatic extradural hemorrhage**   MCC HCC
Nontraumatic epidural hemorrhage

I62.9   **Nontraumatic intracranial hemorrhage, unspecified**   CC HCC

✓4th **I63** **Cerebral infarction**

INCLUDES occlusion and stenosis of cerebral and precerebral arteries, resulting in cerebral infarction

Use additional code, if applicable, to identify status post administration of tPA (rtPA) in a different facility within the last 24 hours prior to admission to current facility (Z92.82)

Use additional code, if known, to indicate National Institutes of Health Stroke Scale (NIHSS) score (R29.7-)

EXCLUDES 2 *sequelae of cerebral infarction (I69.3-)*

AHA: 2017, 2Q, 9-10; 2016, 4Q, 28, 61-62; 2014, 1Q, 23

TIP: Weakness on one side of the body documented as secondary to stroke is synonymous with hemiparesis/hemiplegia (G81.-). Weakness of one limb documented as secondary to stroke is synonymous with monoplegia (G83.1-, G83.2-, G83.3-).

✓5th **I63.0** **Cerebral infarction due to thrombosis of precerebral arteries**

I63.00 **Cerebral infarction due to thrombosis of unspecified precerebral artery** MCC HCC

CC Excl: PDX collection 685

✓6th **I63.01** **Cerebral infarction due to thrombosis of vertebral artery**

CC Excl: For MCC codes in subcategory I63.01: PDX collection 686

I63.011 **Cerebral infarction due to thrombosis of right vertebral artery** MCC HCC

I63.012 **Cerebral infarction due to thrombosis of left vertebral artery** MCC HCC

I63.013 **Cerebral infarction due to thrombosis of bilateral vertebral arteries** MCC HCC

I63.019 **Cerebral infarction due to thrombosis of unspecified vertebral artery** MCC HCC

I63.02 **Cerebral infarction due to thrombosis of basilar artery** MCC HCC

CC Excl: PDX collection 685

✓6th **I63.03** **Cerebral infarction due to thrombosis of carotid artery**

CC Excl: For MCC codes in subcategory I63.03: PDX collection 687

I63.031 **Cerebral infarction due to thrombosis of right carotid artery** MCC HCC

I63.032 **Cerebral infarction due to thrombosis of left carotid artery** MCC HCC

I63.033 **Cerebral infarction due to thrombosis of bilateral carotid arteries** MCC HCC

I63.039 **Cerebral infarction due to thrombosis of unspecified carotid artery** MCC HCC

I63.09 **Cerebral infarction due to thrombosis of other precerebral artery** MCC HCC

CC Excl: PDX collection 685

✓5th **I63.1** **Cerebral infarction due to embolism of precerebral arteries**

I63.10 **Cerebral infarction due to embolism of unspecified precerebral artery** MCC HCC

CC Excl: PDX collection 685

✓6th **I63.11** **Cerebral infarction due to embolism of vertebral artery**

CC Excl: For MCC codes in subcategory I63.11: PDX collection 686

I63.111 **Cerebral infarction due to embolism of right vertebral artery** MCC HCC

I63.112 **Cerebral infarction due to embolism of left vertebral artery** MCC HCC

I63.113 **Cerebral infarction due to embolism of bilateral vertebral arteries** MCC HCC

I63.119 **Cerebral infarction due to embolism of unspecified vertebral artery** MCC HCC

I63.12 **Cerebral infarction due to embolism of basilar artery** MCC HCC

CC Excl: PDX collection 685

✓6th **I63.13** **Cerebral infarction due to embolism of carotid artery**

CC Excl: For MCC codes in subcategory I63.13: PDX collection 687

I63.131 **Cerebral infarction due to embolism of right carotid artery** MCC HCC

I63.132 **Cerebral infarction due to embolism of left carotid artery** MCC HCC

I63.133 **Cerebral infarction due to embolism of bilateral carotid arteries** MCC HCC

I63.139 **Cerebral infarction due to embolism of unspecified carotid artery** MCC HCC

I63.19 **Cerebral infarction due to embolism of other precerebral artery** MCC HCC

CC Excl: PDX collection 685

✓5th **I63.2** **Cerebral infarction due to unspecified occlusion or stenosis of precerebral arteries**

I63.20 **Cerebral infarction due to unspecified occlusion or stenosis of unspecified precerebral arteries** MCC HCC

CC Excl: PDX collection 685

✓6th **I63.21** **Cerebral infarction due to unspecified occlusion or stenosis of vertebral arteries**

CC Excl: For MCC codes in subcategory I63.21: PDX collection 686

I63.211 **Cerebral infarction due to unspecified occlusion or stenosis of right vertebral artery** MCC HCC

I63.212 **Cerebral infarction due to unspecified occlusion or stenosis of left vertebral artery** MCC HCC

I63.213 **Cerebral infarction due to unspecified occlusion or stenosis of bilateral vertebral arteries** MCC HCC

I63.219 **Cerebral infarction due to unspecified occlusion or stenosis of unspecified vertebral artery** MCC HCC

I63.22 **Cerebral infarction due to unspecified occlusion or stenosis of basilar artery** MCC HCC

CC Excl: PDX collection 685

✓6th **I63.23** **Cerebral infarction due to unspecified occlusion or stenosis of carotid arteries**

CC Excl: For MCC codes in subcategory I63.23: PDX collection 687

I63.231 **Cerebral infarction due to unspecified occlusion or stenosis of right carotid arteries** MCC HCC

I63.232 **Cerebral infarction due to unspecified occlusion or stenosis of left carotid arteries** MCC HCC

I63.233 **Cerebral infarction due to unspecified occlusion or stenosis of bilateral carotid arteries** MCC HCC

I63.239 **Cerebral infarction due to unspecified occlusion or stenosis of unspecified carotid artery** MCC HCC

I63.29 **Cerebral infarction due to unspecified occlusion or stenosis of other precerebral arteries** MCC HCC

CC Excl: PDX collection 685

✓5th **I63.3** **Cerebral infarction due to thrombosis of cerebral arteries**

CC Excl: For MCC codes in subcategory I63.3: PDX collection 688

I63.30 **Cerebral infarction due to thrombosis of unspecified cerebral artery** MCC HCC

✓6th **I63.31** **Cerebral infarction due to thrombosis of middle cerebral artery**

I63.311 **Cerebral infarction due to thrombosis of right middle cerebral artery** MCC HCC

I63.312 **Cerebral infarction due to thrombosis of left middle cerebral artery** MCC HCC

I63.313 **Cerebral infarction due to thrombosis of bilateral middle cerebral arteries** MCC HCC

I63.319 **Cerebral infarction due to thrombosis of unspecified middle cerebral artery** MCC HCC

✓6th **I63.32** **Cerebral infarction due to thrombosis of anterior cerebral artery**

I63.321 **Cerebral infarction due to thrombosis of right anterior cerebral artery** MCC HCC

I63.322 **Cerebral infarction due to thrombosis of left anterior cerebral artery** MCC HCC

N Newborn: 0   P Pediatric: 0-17   M Maternity: 12-55   A Adult: 15-124   MCC Major Complication/Comorbidity   CC Complication/Comorbidity   SW Severe Wound Dx

648   ICD-10-CM 2019

I63.323   **Cerebral infarction due to thrombosis of bilateral anterior cerebral arteries** `MCC` `HCC`

I63.329   **Cerebral infarction due to thrombosis of unspecified anterior cerebral artery** `MCC` `HCC`

✓6ᵗʰ   **I63.33**   **Cerebral infarction due to thrombosis of posterior cerebral artery**

I63.331   **Cerebral infarction due to thrombosis of right posterior cerebral artery** `MCC` `HCC`

I63.332   **Cerebral infarction due to thrombosis of left posterior cerebral artery** `MCC` `HCC`

▲ I63.333   **Cerebral infarction due to thrombosis of bilateral posterior cerebral arteries** `MCC` `HCC`

I63.339   **Cerebral infarction due to thrombosis of unspecified posterior cerebral artery** `MCC` `HCC`

✓6ᵗʰ   **I63.34**   **Cerebral infarction due to thrombosis of cerebellar artery**

I63.341   **Cerebral infarction due to thrombosis of right cerebellar artery** `MCC` `HCC`

I63.342   **Cerebral infarction due to thrombosis of left cerebellar artery** `MCC` `HCC`

▲ I63.343   **Cerebral infarction due to thrombosis of bilateral cerebellar arteries** `MCC` `HCC`

I63.349   **Cerebral infarction due to thrombosis of unspecified cerebellar artery** `MCC` `HCC`

I63.39   **Cerebral infarction due to thrombosis of other cerebral artery** `MCC` `HCC`

✓5ᵗʰ   **I63.4**   **Cerebral infarction due to embolism of cerebral arteries**

> **CC Excl: For MCC codes in subcategory I63.4:**
> PDX collection 688

I63.40   **Cerebral infarction due to embolism of unspecified cerebral artery** `MCC` `HCC`

✓6ᵗʰ   **I63.41**   **Cerebral infarction due to embolism of middle cerebral artery**

I63.411   **Cerebral infarction due to embolism of right middle cerebral artery** `MCC` `HCC`

I63.412   **Cerebral infarction due to embolism of left middle cerebral artery** `MCC` `HCC`

I63.413   **Cerebral infarction due to embolism of bilateral middle cerebral arteries** `MCC` `HCC`

I63.419   **Cerebral infarction due to embolism of unspecified middle cerebral artery** `MCC` `HCC`

✓6ᵗʰ   **I63.42**   **Cerebral infarction due to embolism of anterior cerebral artery**

I63.421   **Cerebral infarction due to embolism of right anterior cerebral artery** `MCC` `HCC`

I63.422   **Cerebral infarction due to embolism of left anterior cerebral artery** `MCC` `HCC`

I63.423   **Cerebral infarction due to embolism of bilateral anterior cerebral arteries** `MCC` `HCC`

I63.429   **Cerebral infarction due to embolism of unspecified anterior cerebral artery** `MCC` `HCC`

✓6ᵗʰ   **I63.43**   **Cerebral infarction due to embolism of posterior cerebral artery**

I63.431   **Cerebral infarction due to embolism of right posterior cerebral artery** `MCC` `HCC`

I63.432   **Cerebral infarction due to embolism of left posterior cerebral artery** `MCC` `HCC`

I63.433   **Cerebral infarction due to embolism of bilateral posterior cerebral arteries** `MCC` `HCC`

I63.439   **Cerebral infarction due to embolism of unspecified posterior cerebral artery** `MCC` `HCC`

✓6ᵗʰ   **I63.44**   **Cerebral infarction due to embolism of cerebellar artery**

I63.441   **Cerebral infarction due to embolism of right cerebellar artery** `MCC` `HCC`

I63.442   **Cerebral infarction due to embolism of left cerebellar artery** `MCC` `HCC`

I63.443   **Cerebral infarction due to embolism of bilateral cerebellar arteries** `MCC` `HCC`

I63.449   **Cerebral infarction due to embolism of unspecified cerebellar artery** `MCC` `HCC`

I63.49   **Cerebral infarction due to embolism of other cerebral artery** `MCC` `HCC`

✓5ᵗʰ   **I63.5**   **Cerebral infarction due to unspecified occlusion or stenosis of cerebral arteries**

> **CC Excl: For MCC codes in subcategory I63.5:**
> PDX collection 688

I63.50   **Cerebral infarction due to unspecified occlusion or stenosis of unspecified cerebral artery** `MCC` `HCC`

✓6ᵗʰ   **I63.51**   **Cerebral infarction due to unspecified occlusion or stenosis of middle cerebral artery**

I63.511   **Cerebral infarction due to unspecified occlusion or stenosis of right middle cerebral artery** `MCC` `HCC`

I63.512   **Cerebral infarction due to unspecified occlusion or stenosis of left middle cerebral artery** `MCC` `HCC`

I63.513   **Cerebral infarction due to unspecified occlusion or stenosis of bilateral middle cerebral arteries** `MCC` `HCC`

I63.519   **Cerebral infarction due to unspecified occlusion or stenosis of unspecified middle cerebral artery** `MCC` `HCC`

✓6ᵗʰ   **I63.52**   **Cerebral infarction due to unspecified occlusion or stenosis of anterior cerebral artery**

I63.521   **Cerebral infarction due to unspecified occlusion or stenosis of right anterior cerebral artery** `MCC` `HCC`

I63.522   **Cerebral infarction due to unspecified occlusion or stenosis of left anterior cerebral artery** `MCC` `HCC`

I63.523   **Cerebral infarction due to unspecified occlusion or stenosis of bilateral anterior cerebral arteries** `MCC` `HCC`

I63.529   **Cerebral infarction due to unspecified occlusion or stenosis of unspecified anterior cerebral artery** `MCC` `HCC`

✓6ᵗʰ   **I63.53**   **Cerebral infarction due to unspecified occlusion or stenosis of posterior cerebral artery**

I63.531   **Cerebral infarction due to unspecified occlusion or stenosis of right posterior cerebral artery** `MCC` `HCC`

I63.532   **Cerebral infarction due to unspecified occlusion or stenosis of left posterior cerebral artery** `MCC` `HCC`

I63.533   **Cerebral infarction due to unspecified occlusion or stenosis of bilateral posterior cerebral arteries** `MCC` `HCC`

I63.539   **Cerebral infarction due to unspecified occlusion or stenosis of unspecified posterior cerebral artery** `MCC` `HCC`

✓6ᵗʰ   **I63.54**   **Cerebral infarction due to unspecified occlusion or stenosis of cerebellar artery**

I63.541   **Cerebral infarction due to unspecified occlusion or stenosis of right cerebellar artery** `MCC` `HCC`

I63.542   **Cerebral infarction due to unspecified occlusion or stenosis of left cerebellar artery** `MCC` `HCC`

✓ Additional Character Required   ✓×7ᵗʰ Placeholder   Unacceptable PDx   Questionable PDx   Manifestation   H1 - H14 HAC   HCC CMS-HCC Dx   HIV HIV Dx

ICD-10-CM 2019   649

Chapter 9. Diseases of the Circulatory System

      I63.543   Cerebral infarction due to unspecified occlusion or stenosis of bilateral cerebellar arteries `MCC` `HCC`

      I63.549   Cerebral infarction due to unspecified occlusion or stenosis of unspecified cerebellar artery `MCC` `HCC`

   I63.59   Cerebral infarction due to unspecified occlusion or stenosis of other cerebral artery `MCC` `HCC`

   I63.6   Cerebral infarction due to cerebral venous thrombosis, nonpyogenic `MCC` `HCC`
      CC Excl: PDX collection 688

  ✓5ᵗʰ **I63.8**   Other cerebral infarction

 ●   **I63.81**   Other cerebral infarction due to occlusion or stenosis of small artery `MCC`
      Lacunar infarction

 ●   **I63.89**   Other cerebral infarction `MCC`

   I63.9   Cerebral infarction, unspecified `MCC` `HCC`
      Stroke NOS
      EXCLUDES 2   transient cerebral ischemic attacks and related syndromes (G45.-)
      AHA: 2015, 1Q, 25
      TIP: Imaging reports can be used to determine the location of an infarction and therefore a more specific infarction code, when provider documentation does not identify the location.
      CC Excl: PDX collection 688

✓4ᵗʰ **I65**   **Occlusion and stenosis of precerebral arteries, not resulting in cerebral infarction**
    INCLUDES   embolism of precerebral artery
             narrowing of precerebral artery
             obstruction (complete) (partial) of precerebral artery
             thrombosis of precerebral artery
    EXCLUDES 1   insufficiency, NOS, of precerebral artery (G45.-)
             insufficiency of precerebral arteries causing cerebral infarction (I63.0-I63.2)
    AHA: 2018, 2Q, 9

  ✓5ᵗʰ **I65.0**   Occlusion and stenosis of vertebral artery
   I65.01   Occlusion and stenosis of right vertebral artery
   I65.02   Occlusion and stenosis of left vertebral artery
   I65.03   Occlusion and stenosis of bilateral vertebral arteries
   I65.09   Occlusion and stenosis of unspecified vertebral artery

   I65.1   Occlusion and stenosis of basilar artery

  ✓5ᵗʰ **I65.2**   Occlusion and stenosis of carotid artery
   I65.21   Occlusion and stenosis of right carotid artery
   I65.22   Occlusion and stenosis of left carotid artery
   I65.23   Occlusion and stenosis of bilateral carotid arteries
   I65.29   Occlusion and stenosis of unspecified carotid artery

   I65.8   Occlusion and stenosis of other precerebral arteries

   I65.9   Occlusion and stenosis of unspecified precerebral artery
      Occlusion and stenosis of precerebral artery NOS

✓4ᵗʰ **I66**   **Occlusion and stenosis of cerebral arteries, not resulting in cerebral infarction**
    INCLUDES   embolism of cerebral artery
             narrowing of cerebral artery
             obstruction (complete) (partial) of cerebral artery
             thrombosis of cerebral artery
    EXCLUDES 1   occlusion and stenosis of cerebral artery causing cerebral infarction (I63.3-I63.5)

  ✓5ᵗʰ **I66.0**   Occlusion and stenosis of middle cerebral artery
   I66.01   Occlusion and stenosis of right middle cerebral artery
   I66.02   Occlusion and stenosis of left middle cerebral artery
   I66.03   Occlusion and stenosis of bilateral middle cerebral arteries
   I66.09   Occlusion and stenosis of unspecified middle cerebral artery

  ✓5ᵗʰ **I66.1**   Occlusion and stenosis of anterior cerebral artery
   I66.11   Occlusion and stenosis of right anterior cerebral artery
   I66.12   Occlusion and stenosis of left anterior cerebral artery
   I66.13   Occlusion and stenosis of bilateral anterior cerebral arteries
   I66.19   Occlusion and stenosis of unspecified anterior cerebral artery

  ✓5ᵗʰ **I66.2**   Occlusion and stenosis of posterior cerebral artery
   I66.21   Occlusion and stenosis of right posterior cerebral artery
   I66.22   Occlusion and stenosis of left posterior cerebral artery
   I66.23   Occlusion and stenosis of bilateral posterior cerebral arteries
   I66.29   Occlusion and stenosis of unspecified posterior cerebral artery

   I66.3   Occlusion and stenosis of cerebellar arteries

   I66.8   Occlusion and stenosis of other cerebral arteries
      Occlusion and stenosis of perforating arteries

   I66.9   Occlusion and stenosis of unspecified cerebral artery

✓4ᵗʰ **I67**   **Other cerebrovascular diseases**
    EXCLUDES 2   sequelae of the listed conditions (I69.8)

   I67.0   Dissection of cerebral arteries, nonruptured `MCC` `HCC`
      EXCLUDES 1   ruptured cerebral arteries (I60.7)
      CC Excl: PDX collection 689

   I67.1   Cerebral aneurysm, nonruptured
      Cerebral aneurysm NOS
      Cerebral arteriovenous fistula, acquired
      Internal carotid artery aneurysm, intracranial portion
      Internal carotid artery aneurysm, NOS
      EXCLUDES 1   congenital cerebral aneurysm, nonruptured (Q28.-)
             ruptured cerebral aneurysm (I60.7)

Berry Aneurysm

Berry aneurysms form at the site of a weakness in an arterial wall, often at a junction

Berry aneurysm

Anterior communicating artery
40%
34%
20%
4%
Anterior cerebral artery
Internal carotid
Middle cerebral artery
Posterior cerebral artery
Posterior communicating artery
Basilar artery

Common sites of berry aneurysms in the circle of Willis arteries

   I67.2   Cerebral atherosclerosis `A`
      Atheroma of cerebral and precerebral arteries

   I67.3   Progressive vascular leukoencephalopathy `HIV` `CC`
      Binswanger's disease
      CC Excl: PDX collection 133

   I67.4   Hypertensive encephalopathy `CC`
      EXCLUDES 2   insufficiency, NOS, of precerebral arteries (G45.2)
      CC Excl: PDX collection 690

   I67.5   Moyamoya disease `CC`
      DEF: Cerebrovascular ischemia. Vessels occlude and rupture, causing tiny hemorrhages at the base of brain. It affects predominantly Japanese people.
      CC Excl: PDX collection 691

   I67.6   Nonpyogenic thrombosis of intracranial venous system `CC`
      Nonpyogenic thrombosis of cerebral vein
      Nonpyogenic thrombosis of intracranial venous sinus
      EXCLUDES 1   nonpyogenic thrombosis of intracranial venous system causing infarction (I63.6)
      CC Excl: PDX collection 692

`N` Newborn: 0   `P` Pediatric: 0-17   `M` Maternity: 12-55   `A` Adult: 15-124   `MCC` Major Complication/Comorbidity   `CC` Complication/Comorbidity   `SW` Severe Wound Dx

650   ICD-10-CM 2019

I63.543–I67.6

Chapter 9. Diseases of the Circulatory System

I67.7   **Cerebral arteritis, not elsewhere classified**   `CC`
Granulomatous angiitis of the nervous system
EXCLUDES 1   *allergic granulomatous angiitis (M30.1)*
CC Excl: PDX collection 693

√5th **I67.8**   **Other specified cerebrovascular diseases**

I67.81   **Acute cerebrovascular insufficiency**   `CC`
Acute cerebrovascular insufficiency unspecified as to location or reversibility
CC Excl: PDX collection 694

I67.82   **Cerebral ischemia**   `CC`
Chronic cerebral ischemia
CC Excl: PDX collection 694

I67.83   **Posterior reversible encephalopathy syndrome**   `HIV` `MCC`
PRES
CC Excl: PDX collection 610

√6th **I67.84**   **Cerebral vasospasm and vasoconstriction**

I67.841   **Reversible cerebrovascular vasoconstriction syndrome**   `CC`
Call-Fleming syndrome
Code first underlying condition, if applicable, such as eclampsia (O15.00-O15.9)
CC Excl: PDX collection 586

I67.848   **Other cerebrovascular vasospasm and vasoconstriction**   `CC`
CC Excl: PDX collection 586

●   √6th **I67.85**   **Hereditary cerebrovascular diseases**
●

I67.850   **Cerebral autosomal dominant arteriopathy with subcortical infarcts and leukoencephalopathy**   `CC`
CADASIL
Code also any associated diagnoses, such as:
epilepsy (G40.-)
stroke (I63.-)
vascular dementia (F01.-)

●   **I67.858**   **Other hereditary cerebrovascular disease**   `CC`

I67.89   **Other cerebrovascular disease**   `CC`
CC Excl: PDX collection 694

I67.9   **Cerebrovascular disease, unspecified**

√4th **I68**   **Cerebrovascular disorders in diseases classified elsewhere**

I68.0   *Cerebral amyloid angiopathy*
Code first underlying amyloidosis (E85.-)

I68.2   *Cerebral arteritis in other diseases classified elsewhere*   `CC`
Code first underlying disease
EXCLUDES 1   *cerebral arteritis (in):*
listerosis (A32.89)
systemic lupus erythematosus (M32.19)
syphilis (A52.04)
tuberculosis (A18.89)
CC Excl: PDX collection 693

I68.8   *Other cerebrovascular disorders in diseases classified elsewhere*
Code first underlying disease
EXCLUDES 1   *syphilitic cerebral aneurysm (A52.05)*

√4th **I69**   **Sequelae of cerebrovascular disease**
`NOTE`   Category I69 is to be used to indicate conditions in I60-I67 as the cause of sequelae. The "sequelae" include conditions specified as such or as residuals which may occur at any time after the onset of the causal condition
EXCLUDES 1   *personal history of cerebral infarction without residual deficit (Z86.73)*
personal history of prolonged reversible ischemic neurologic deficit (PRIND) (Z86.73)
personal history of reversible ischemic neurologcial deficit (RIND) (Z86.73)
sequelae of traumatic intracranial injury (S06.-)
AHA: 2017, 1Q, 47; 2016, 4Q, 28; 2015, 1Q, 25; 2012, 4Q, 106
TIP: Weakness on one side of the body (unilateral weakness) documented as secondary to old cerebrovascular disease is synonymous with hemiparesis/hemiplegia. Weakness of one limb documented as secondary to old cerebrovascular disease is synonymous with monoplegia.
TIP: For codes describing hemiplegia, hemiparesis, and monoplegia, if documentation specifies the affected side but not whether it is the dominant or nondominant side, the default is as follows: for ambidextrous patients, the default is dominant; when the left side is affected, the default is nondominant, and when the right side is affected, the default is dominant.

√5th **I69.0**   **Sequelae of nontraumatic subarachnoid hemorrhage**

I69.00   **Unspecified sequelae of nontraumatic subarachnoid hemorrhage**

√6th **I69.01**   **Cognitive deficits following nontraumatic subarachnoid hemorrhage**

I69.010   **Attention and concentration deficit following nontraumatic subarachnoid hemorrhage**

I69.011   **Memory deficit following nontraumatic subarachnoid hemorrhage**

I69.012   **Visuospatial deficit and spatial neglect following nontraumatic subarachnoid hemorrhage**

I69.013   **Psychomotor deficit following nontraumatic subarachnoid hemorrhage**

I69.014   **Frontal lobe and executive function deficit following nontraumatic subarachnoid hemorrhage**

I69.015   **Cognitive social or emotional deficit following nontraumatic subarachnoid hemorrhage**

I69.018   **Other symptoms and signs involving cognitive functions following nontraumatic subarachnoid hemorrhage**

I69.019   **Unspecified symptoms and signs involving cognitive functions following nontraumatic subarachnoid hemorrhage**

√6th **I69.02**   **Speech and language deficits following nontraumatic subarachnoid hemorrhage**

I69.020   **Aphasia following nontraumatic subarachnoid hemorrhage**

I69.021   **Dysphasia following nontraumatic subarachnoid hemorrhage**

I69.022   **Dysarthria following nontraumatic subarachnoid hemorrhage**

I69.023   **Fluency disorder following nontraumatic subarachnoid hemorrhage**
Stuttering following nontraumatic subarachnoid hemorrhage

I69.028   **Other speech and language deficits following nontraumatic subarachnoid hemorrhage**

√6th **I69.03**   **Monoplegia of upper limb following nontraumatic subarachnoid hemorrhage**
AHA: 2017, 1Q, 47

I69.031   **Monoplegia of upper limb following nontraumatic subarachnoid hemorrhage affecting right dominant side**   `HCC`

I69.032   **Monoplegia of upper limb following nontraumatic subarachnoid hemorrhage affecting left dominant side**   `HCC`

I69.033   **Monoplegia of upper limb following nontraumatic subarachnoid hemorrhage affecting right non-dominant side**   `HCC`

I69.034   **Monoplegia of upper limb following nontraumatic subarachnoid hemorrhage affecting left non-dominant side**   `HCC`

I69.039   **Monoplegia of upper limb following nontraumatic subarachnoid hemorrhage affecting unspecified side**   `HCC`

√6th **I69.04**   **Monoplegia of lower limb following nontraumatic subarachnoid hemorrhage**
AHA: 2017, 1Q, 47

I69.041   **Monoplegia of lower limb following nontraumatic subarachnoid hemorrhage affecting right dominant side**   `HCC`

I69.042   **Monoplegia of lower limb following nontraumatic subarachnoid hemorrhage affecting left dominant side**   `HCC`

I69.043   **Monoplegia of lower limb following nontraumatic subarachnoid hemorrhage affecting right non-dominant side**   `HCC`

I69.044   **Monoplegia of lower limb following nontraumatic subarachnoid hemorrhage affecting left non-dominant side**   `HCC`

I69.049   **Monoplegia of lower limb following nontraumatic subarachnoid hemorrhage affecting unspecified side**   `HCC`

✔ Additional Character Required	√x7th Placeholder	Unacceptable PDx	Questionable PDx	Manifestation	`H1`-`H14` HAC	`HCC` CMS-HCC Dx	`HIV` HIV Dx

ICD-10-CM 2019   651

Chapter 9. Diseases of the Circulatory System

I67.7–I69.049

✓6ᵗʰ **I69.05** **Hemiplegia** and **hemiparesis following nontraumatic subarachnoid hemorrhage**
AHA: 2015, 1Q, 25

I69.051 **Hemiplegia and hemiparesis following nontraumatic subarachnoid hemorrhage affecting** right dominant **side** `CC` `HCC`
CC Excl: PDX collection 695

I69.052 **Hemiplegia and hemiparesis following nontraumatic subarachnoid hemorrhage affecting** left dominant **side** `CC` `HCC`
CC Excl: PDX collection 695

I69.053 **Hemiplegia and hemiparesis following nontraumatic subarachnoid hemorrhage affecting** right non-dominant **side** `CC` `HCC`
CC Excl: PDX collection 696

I69.054 **Hemiplegia and hemiparesis following nontraumatic subarachnoid hemorrhage affecting** left non-dominant **side** `CC` `HCC`
CC Excl: PDX collection 696

I69.059 **Hemiplegia and hemiparesis following nontraumatic subarachnoid hemorrhage affecting** unspecified **side** `CC` `HCC`
CC Excl: PDX collection 697

✓6ᵗʰ **I69.06** **Other paralytic syndrome following nontraumatic subarachnoid hemorrhage**
Use additional code to identify type of paralytic syndrome, such as:
    locked-in state (G83.5)
    quadriplegia (G82.5-)
EXCLUDES 1   *hemiplegia/hemiparesis following nontraumatic subarachnoid hemorrhage (I69.05-)*
    monoplegia of lower limb following nontraumatic subarachnoid hemorrhage (I69.04-)
    monoplegia of upper limb following nontraumatic subarachnoid hemorrhage (I69.03-)

I69.061 **Other paralytic syndrome following nontraumatic subarachnoid hemorrhage affecting** right dominant **side** `HCC`

I69.062 **Other paralytic syndrome following nontraumatic subarachnoid hemorrhage affecting** left dominant **side** `HCC`

I69.063 **Other paralytic syndrome following nontraumatic subarachnoid hemorrhage affecting** right non-dominant **side** `HCC`

I69.064 **Other paralytic syndrome following nontraumatic subarachnoid hemorrhage affecting** left non-dominant **side** `HCC`

I69.065 **Other paralytic syndrome following nontraumatic subarachnoid hemorrhage, bilateral** `HCC`

I69.069 **Other paralytic syndrome following nontraumatic subarachnoid hemorrhage affecting** unspecified **side** `HCC`

✓6ᵗʰ **I69.09** **Other sequelae of nontraumatic subarachnoid hemorrhage**

I69.090 **Apraxia following nontraumatic subarachnoid hemorrhage**

I69.091 **Dysphagia following nontraumatic subarachnoid hemorrhage**
Use additional code to identify the type of dysphagia, if known (R13.1-)

I69.092 **Facial weakness following nontraumatic subarachnoid hemorrhage**
Facial droop following nontraumatic subarachnoid hemorrhage

I69.093 **Ataxia following nontraumatic subarachnoid hemorrhage**

I69.098 **Other sequelae following nontraumatic subarachnoid hemorrhage**
Alterations of sensation following nontraumatic subarachnoid hemorrhage
Disturbance of vision following nontraumatic subarachnoid hemorrhage
Use additional code to identify the sequelae

✓6ᵗʰ **I69.1** **Sequelae of nontraumatic** intracerebral **hemorrhage**

I69.10 Unspecified **sequelae of nontraumatic intracerebral hemorrhage**

✓6ᵗʰ **I69.11** Cognitive deficits **following nontraumatic intracerebral hemorrhage**

I69.110 Attention and concentration **deficit following nontraumatic intracerebral hemorrhage**

I69.111 Memory **deficit following nontraumatic intracerebral hemorrhage**

I69.112 Visuospatial **deficit and** spatial neglect **following nontraumatic intracerebral hemorrhage**

I69.113 Psychomotor **deficit following nontraumatic intracerebral hemorrhage**

I69.114 Frontal lobe and executive function **deficit following nontraumatic intracerebral hemorrhage**

I69.115 Cognitive social or emotional **deficit following nontraumatic intracerebral hemorrhage**

I69.118 Other **symptoms and signs involving cognitive functions following nontraumatic intracerebral hemorrhage**

I69.119 Unspecified **symptoms and signs involving cognitive functions following nontraumatic intracerebral hemorrhage**

✓6ᵗʰ **I69.12** Speech and language deficits **following nontraumatic intracerebral hemorrhage**

I69.120 Aphasia **following nontraumatic intracerebral hemorrhage**

I69.121 Dysphasia **following nontraumatic intracerebral hemorrhage**

I69.122 Dysarthria **following nontraumatic intracerebral hemorrhage**

I69.123 Fluency disorder **following nontraumatic intracerebral hemorrhage**
Stuttering following nontraumatic intracerebral hemorrhage

I69.128 Other **speech and language deficits following nontraumatic intracerebral hemorrhage**

✓6ᵗʰ **I69.13** Monoplegia of upper limb **following nontraumatic intracerebral hemorrhage**
AHA: 2017, 1Q, 47

I69.131 **Monoplegia of upper limb following nontraumatic intracerebral hemorrhage affecting** right dominant **side** `HCC`

I69.132 **Monoplegia of upper limb following nontraumatic intracerebral hemorrhage affecting** left dominant **side** `HCC`

I69.133 **Monoplegia of upper limb following nontraumatic intracerebral hemorrhage affecting** right non-dominant **side** `HCC`

I69.134 **Monoplegia of upper limb following nontraumatic intracerebral hemorrhage affecting** left non-dominant **side** `HCC`

I69.139 **Monoplegia of upper limb following nontraumatic intracerebral hemorrhage affecting** unspecified **side** `HCC`

✓6ᵗʰ **I69.14** Monoplegia of lower limb **following nontraumatic intracerebral hemorrhage**
AHA: 2017, 1Q, 47

I69.141 **Monoplegia of lower limb following nontraumatic intracerebral hemorrhage affecting** right dominant **side** `HCC`

I69.142 **Monoplegia of lower limb following nontraumatic intracerebral hemorrhage affecting** left dominant **side** `HCC`

I69.143 **Monoplegia of lower limb following nontraumatic intracerebral hemorrhage affecting** right non-dominant **side** `HCC`

I69.144 **Monoplegia of lower limb following nontraumatic intracerebral hemorrhage affecting** left non-dominant **side** `HCC`

I69.149 **Monoplegia of lower limb following nontraumatic intracerebral hemorrhage affecting** unspecified **side** `HCC`

✓6ᵗʰ **I69.15** Hemiplegia and hemiparesis following nontraumatic intracerebral hemorrhage
> AHA: 2015, 1Q, 25

  I69.151 Hemiplegia and hemiparesis following nontraumatic intracerebral hemorrhage affecting right dominant side   CC HCC
> CC Excl: PDX collection 695

  I69.152 Hemiplegia and hemiparesis following nontraumatic intracerebral hemorrhage affecting left dominant side   CC HCC
> CC Excl: PDX collection 695

  I69.153 Hemiplegia and hemiparesis following nontraumatic intracerebral hemorrhage affecting right non-dominant side   CC HCC
> CC Excl: PDX collection 696

  I69.154 Hemiplegia and hemiparesis following nontraumatic intracerebral hemorrhage affecting left non-dominant side   CC HCC
> CC Excl: PDX collection 696

  I69.159 Hemiplegia and hemiparesis following nontraumatic intracerebral hemorrhage affecting unspecified side   CC HCC
> CC Excl: PDX collection 697

✓6ᵗʰ **I69.16** Other paralytic syndrome following nontraumatic intracerebral hemorrhage
> Use additional code to identify type of paralytic syndrome, such as:
> locked-in state (G83.5)
> quadriplegia (G82.5-)
>
> EXCLUDES 1   *hemiplegia/hemiparesis following nontraumatic intracerebral hemorrhage (I69.15-)*
> *monoplegia of lower limb following nontraumatic intracerebral hemorrhage (I69.14-)*
> *monoplegia of upper limb following nontraumatic intracerebral hemorrhage (I69.13-)*

  I69.161 Other paralytic syndrome following nontraumatic intracerebral hemorrhage affecting right dominant side   HCC

  I69.162 Other paralytic syndrome following nontraumatic intracerebral hemorrhage affecting left dominant side   HCC

  I69.163 Other paralytic syndrome following nontraumatic intracerebral hemorrhage affecting right non-dominant side   HCC

  I69.164 Other paralytic syndrome following nontraumatic intracerebral hemorrhage affecting left non-dominant side   HCC

  I69.165 Other paralytic syndrome following nontraumatic intracerebral hemorrhage, bilateral   HCC

  I69.169 Other paralytic syndrome following nontraumatic intracerebral hemorrhage affecting unspecified side   HCC

✓6ᵗʰ **I69.19** Other sequelae of nontraumatic intracerebral hemorrhage

  I69.190 Apraxia following nontraumatic intracerebral hemorrhage

  I69.191 Dysphagia following nontraumatic intracerebral hemorrhage
> Use additional code to identify the type of dysphagia, if known (R13.1-)

  I69.192 Facial weakness following nontraumatic intracerebral hemorrhage
> Facial droop following nontraumatic intracerebral hemorrhage

  I69.193 Ataxia following nontraumatic intracerebral hemorrhage

  I69.198 Other sequelae of nontraumatic intracerebral hemorrhage
> Alteration of sensations following nontraumatic intracerebral hemorrhage
> Disturbance of vision following nontraumatic intracerebral hemorrhage
> Use additional code to identify the sequelae

✓5ᵗʰ **I69.2** Sequelae of other nontraumatic intracranial hemorrhage

  I69.20 Unspecified sequelae of other nontraumatic intracranial hemorrhage

✓6ᵗʰ **I69.21** Cognitive deficits following other nontraumatic intracranial hemorrhage

  I69.210 Attention and concentration deficit following other nontraumatic intracranial hemorrhage

  I69.211 Memory deficit following other nontraumatic intracranial hemorrhage

  I69.212 Visuospatial deficit and spatial neglect following other nontraumatic intracranial hemorrhage

  I69.213 Psychomotor deficit following other nontraumatic intracranial hemorrhage

  I69.214 Frontal lobe and executive function deficit following other nontraumatic intracranial hemorrhage

  I69.215 Cognitive social or emotional deficit following other nontraumatic intracranial hemorrhage

  I69.218 Other symptoms and signs involving cognitive functions following other nontraumatic intracranial hemorrhage

  I69.219 Unspecified symptoms and signs involving cognitive functions following other nontraumatic intracranial hemorrhage

✓6ᵗʰ **I69.22** Speech and language deficits following other nontraumatic intracranial hemorrhage

  I69.220 Aphasia following other nontraumatic intracranial hemorrhage

  I69.221 Dysphasia following other nontraumatic intracranial hemorrhage

  I69.222 Dysarthria following other nontraumatic intracranial hemorrhage

  I69.223 Fluency disorder following other nontraumatic intracranial hemorrhage
> Stuttering following other nontraumatic intracranial hemorrhage

  I69.228 Other speech and language deficits following other nontraumatic intracranial hemorrhage

✓6ᵗʰ **I69.23** Monoplegia of upper limb following other nontraumatic intracranial hemorrhage
> AHA: 2017, 1Q, 47

  I69.231 Monoplegia of upper limb following other nontraumatic intracranial hemorrhage affecting right dominant side   HCC

  I69.232 Monoplegia of upper limb following other nontraumatic intracranial hemorrhage affecting left dominant side   HCC

  I69.233 Monoplegia of upper limb following other nontraumatic intracranial hemorrhage affecting right non-dominant side   HCC

  I69.234 Monoplegia of upper limb following other nontraumatic intracranial hemorrhage affecting left non-dominant side   HCC

  I69.239 Monoplegia of upper limb following other nontraumatic intracranial hemorrhage affecting unspecified side   HCC

✓6ᵗʰ **I69.24** Monoplegia of lower limb following other nontraumatic intracranial hemorrhage
> AHA: 2017, 1Q, 47

  I69.241 Monoplegia of lower limb following other nontraumatic intracranial hemorrhage affecting right dominant side   HCC

  I69.242 Monoplegia of lower limb following other nontraumatic intracranial hemorrhage affecting left dominant side   HCC

  I69.243 Monoplegia of lower limb following other nontraumatic intracranial hemorrhage affecting right non-dominant side   HCC

✔ Additional Character Required   ✓x7ᵗʰ Placeholder   Unacceptable PDx   Questionable PDx   Manifestation   H1-H14 HAC   HCC CMS-HCC Dx   HIV HIV Dx

ICD-10-CM 2019   653

I69.244 Monoplegia of lower limb following other nontraumatic intracranial hemorrhage affecting left non-dominant side `HCC`

I69.249 Monoplegia of lower limb following other nontraumatic intracranial hemorrhage affecting unspecified side `HCC`

√6th **I69.25** Hemiplegia and hemiparesis following other nontraumatic intracranial hemorrhage
     AHA: 2015, 1Q, 25

I69.251 Hemiplegia and hemiparesis following other nontraumatic intracranial hemorrhage affecting right dominant side `CC` `HCC`
     CC Excl: PDX collection 695

I69.252 Hemiplegia and hemiparesis following other nontraumatic intracranial hemorrhage affecting left dominant side `CC` `HCC`
     CC Excl: PDX collection 695

I69.253 Hemiplegia and hemiparesis following other nontraumatic intracranial hemorrhage affecting right non-dominant side `CC` `HCC`
     CC Excl: PDX collection 696

I69.254 Hemiplegia and hemiparesis following other nontraumatic intracranial hemorrhage affecting left non-dominant side `CC` `HCC`
     CC Excl: PDX collection 696

I69.259 Hemiplegia and hemiparesis following other nontraumatic intracranial hemorrhage affecting unspecified side `CC` `HCC`
     CC Excl: PDX collection 697

√6th **I69.26** Other paralytic syndrome following other nontraumatic intracranial hemorrhage
     Use additional code to identify type of paralytic syndrome, such as:
         locked-in state (G83.5)
         quadriplegia (G82.5-)
     `EXCLUDES 1` *hemiplegia/hemiparesis following other nontraumatic intracranial hemorrhage (I69.25-)*
         monoplegia of lower limb following other nontraumatic intracranial hemorrhage (I69.24-)
         monoplegia of upper limb following other nontraumatic intracranial hemorrhage (I69.23-)

I69.261 Other paralytic syndrome following other nontraumatic intracranial hemorrhage affecting right dominant side `HCC`

I69.262 Other paralytic syndrome following other nontraumatic intracranial hemorrhage affecting left dominant side `HCC`

I69.263 Other paralytic syndrome following other nontraumatic intracranial hemorrhage affecting right non-dominant side `HCC`

I69.264 Other paralytic syndrome following other nontraumatic intracranial hemorrhage affecting left non-dominant side `HCC`

I69.265 Other paralytic syndrome following other nontraumatic intracranial hemorrhage, bilateral `HCC`

I69.269 Other paralytic syndrome following other nontraumatic intracranial hemorrhage affecting unspecified side `HCC`

√6th **I69.29** Other sequelae of other nontraumatic intracranial hemorrhage

I69.290 Apraxia following other nontraumatic intracranial hemorrhage

I69.291 Dysphagia following other nontraumatic intracranial hemorrhage
     Use additional code to identify the type of dysphagia, if known (R13.1-)

I69.292 Facial weakness following other nontraumatic intracranial hemorrhage
     Facial droop following other nontraumatic intracranial hemorrhage

I69.293 Ataxia following other nontraumatic intracranial hemorrhage

I69.298 Other sequelae of other nontraumatic intracranial hemorrhage
     Alteration of sensation following other nontraumatic intracranial hemorrhage
     Disturbance of vision following other nontraumatic intracranial hemorrhage
     Use additional code to identify the sequelae

√5th **I69.3** Sequelae of cerebral infarction
     Sequelae of stroke NOS
     AHA: 2013, 4Q, 127-128; 2012, 4Q, 92, 94

I69.30 Unspecified sequelae of cerebral infarction

√6th **I69.31** Cognitive deficits following cerebral infarction

I69.310 Attention and concentration deficit following cerebral infarction

I69.311 Memory deficit following cerebral infarction

I69.312 Visuospatial deficit and spatial neglect following cerebral infarction

I69.313 Psychomotor deficit following cerebral infarction

I69.314 Frontal lobe and executive function deficit following cerebral infarction

I69.315 Cognitive social or emotional deficit following cerebral infarction

I69.318 Other symptoms and signs involving cognitive functions following cerebral infarction

I69.319 Unspecified symptoms and signs involving cognitive functions following cerebral infarction

√6th **I69.32** Speech and language deficits following cerebral infarction

I69.320 Aphasia following cerebral infarction

I69.321 Dysphasia following cerebral infarction
     AHA: 2012, 4Q, 91

I69.322 Dysarthria following cerebral infarction
     `EXCLUDES 2` *transient ischemic attack (TIA) (G45.9)*

I69.323 Fluency disorder following cerebral infarction
     Stuttering following cerebral infarction

I69.328 Other speech and language deficits following cerebral infarction

√6th **I69.33** Monoplegia of upper limb following cerebral infarction
     AHA: 2017, 1Q, 47

I69.331 Monoplegia of upper limb following cerebral infarction affecting right dominant side `HCC`

I69.332 Monoplegia of upper limb following cerebral infarction affecting left dominant side `HCC`

I69.333 Monoplegia of upper limb following cerebral infarction affecting right non-dominant side `HCC`

I69.334 Monoplegia of upper limb following cerebral infarction affecting left non-dominant side `HCC`

I69.339 Monoplegia of upper limb following cerebral infarction affecting unspecified side `HCC`

√6th **I69.34** Monoplegia of lower limb following cerebral infarction
     AHA: 2017, 1Q, 47

I69.341 Monoplegia of lower limb following cerebral infarction affecting right dominant side `HCC`

I69.342 Monoplegia of lower limb following cerebral infarction affecting left dominant side `HCC`

I69.343 Monoplegia of lower limb following cerebral infarction affecting right non-dominant side `HCC`

N Newborn: 0   P Pediatric: 0-17   M Maternity: 12-55   A Adult: 15-124   `MCC` Major Complication/Comorbidity   `CC` Complication/Comorbidity   `SW` Severe Wound Dx

654   ICD-10-CM 2019

I69.344 **Monoplegia of lower limb following** `HCC`
cerebral infarction affecting left non-
dominant **side**

I69.349 **Monoplegia of lower limb following** `HCC`
cerebral infarction affecting unspecified
side

✓6ᵗʰ **I69.35** Hemiplegia and hemiparesis **following cerebral**
infarction
AHA: 2015, 1Q, 25

I69.351 **Hemiplegia and hemiparesis** `CC` `HCC`
following cerebral infarction
affecting right dominant **side**
EXCLUDES 2 transient ischemic attack (TIA)
(G45.9)
CC Excl: PDX collection 695

I69.352 **Hemiplegia and hemiparesis** `CC` `HCC`
following cerebral infarction
affecting left dominant **side**
CC Excl: PDX collection 695

I69.353 **Hemiplegia and hemiparesis** `CC` `HCC`
following cerebral infarction
affecting right non-dominant **side**
CC Excl: PDX collection 696

I69.354 **Hemiplegia and hemiparesis** `CC` `HCC`
following cerebral infarction
affecting left non-dominant **side**
AHA: 2012, 4Q, 91
CC Excl: PDX collection 696

I69.359 **Hemiplegia and hemiparesis** `CC` `HCC`
following cerebral infarction
affecting unspecified **side**
CC Excl: PDX collection 697

✓6ᵗʰ **I69.36** Other paralytic syndrome **following cerebral**
infarction
Use additional code to identify type of paralytic
syndrome, such as:
locked-in state (G83.5)
quadriplegia (G82.5-)
EXCLUDES 1 hemiplegia/hemiparesis following cerebral
infarction (I69.35-)
monoplegia of lower limb following cerebral
infarction (I69.34-)
monoplegia of upper limb following cerebral
infarction (I69.33-)

I69.361 **Other paralytic syndrome following** `HCC`
cerebral infarction affecting right
dominant **side**

I69.362 **Other paralytic syndrome following** `HCC`
cerebral infarction affecting left
dominant **side**

I69.363 **Other paralytic syndrome following** `HCC`
cerebral infarction affecting right
non-dominant **side**

I69.364 **Other paralytic syndrome following** `HCC`
cerebral infarction affecting left
non-dominant **side**

I69.365 **Other paralytic syndrome following** `HCC`
cerebral infarction, bilateral

I69.369 **Other paralytic syndrome following** `HCC`
cerebral infarction affecting
unspecified **side**

✓6ᵗʰ **I69.39** Other sequelae of cerebral infarction

I69.390 Apraxia **following cerebral infarction**

I69.391 Dysphagia **following cerebral infarction**
Use additional code to identify the type of
dysphagia, if known (R13.1-)

I69.392 Facial weakness **following cerebral**
infarction
Facial droop following cerebral infarction

I69.393 Ataxia **following cerebral infarction**

I69.398 Other **sequelae of cerebral infarction**
Alteration of sensation following cerebral
infarction
Disturbance of vision following cerebral
infarction
Use additional code to identify the
sequelae

✓5ᵗʰ **I69.8** **Sequelae of** other cerebrovascular diseases
EXCLUDES 1 sequelae of traumatic intracranial injury (S06.-)

I69.80 Unspecified sequelae of other cerebrovascular
disease

✓6ᵗʰ **I69.81** Cognitive deficits **following other cerebrovascular**
disease

I69.810 Attention and concentration **deficit**
following other cerebrovascular disease

I69.811 Memory **deficit following other**
cerebrovascular disease

I69.812 Visuospatial **deficit and** spatial neglect
following other cerebrovascular disease

I69.813 Psychomotor **deficit following other**
cerebrovascular disease

I69.814 Frontal lobe and executive function **deficit**
following other cerebrovascular disease

I69.815 Cognitive social or emotional **deficit**
following other cerebrovascular disease

I69.818 Other **symptoms and signs involving**
cognitive functions following other
cerebrovascular disease

I69.819 Unspecified **symptoms and signs**
involving cognitive functions following
other cerebrovascular disease

✓6ᵗʰ **I69.82** Speech and language deficits **following other**
cerebrovascular disease

I69.820 Aphasia **following other cerebrovascular**
disease

I69.821 Dysphasia **following other**
cerebrovascular disease

I69.822 Dysarthria **following other**
cerebrovascular disease

I69.823 Fluency **disorder following other**
cerebrovascular disease
Stuttering following other cerebrovascular
disease

I69.828 Other **speech and language deficits**
following other cerebrovascular disease

✓6ᵗʰ **I69.83** Monoplegia of upper limb **following other**
cerebrovascular disease
AHA: 2017, 1Q, 47

I69.831 **Monoplegia of upper limb following** `HCC`
other cerebrovascular disease affecting
right dominant **side**

I69.832 **Monoplegia of upper limb following** `HCC`
other cerebrovascular disease affecting
left dominant **side**

I69.833 **Monoplegia of upper limb following** `HCC`
other cerebrovascular disease affecting
right non-dominant **side**

I69.834 **Monoplegia of upper limb following** `HCC`
other cerebrovascular disease affecting
left non-dominant **side**

I69.839 **Monoplegia of upper limb following** `HCC`
other cerebrovascular disease affecting
unspecified **side**

✓6ᵗʰ **I69.84** Monoplegia of lower limb **following other**
cerebrovascular disease
AHA: 2017, 1Q, 47

I69.841 **Monoplegia of lower limb following** `HCC`
other cerebrovascular disease affecting
right dominant **side**

I69.842 **Monoplegia of lower limb following** `HCC`
other cerebrovascular disease affecting
left dominant **side**

I69.843 **Monoplegia of lower limb following** `HCC`
other cerebrovascular disease affecting
right non-dominant **side**

I69.844 **Monoplegia of lower limb following** `HCC`
other cerebrovascular disease affecting
left non-dominant **side**

I69.849 **Monoplegia of lower limb following** `HCC`
other cerebrovascular disease affecting
unspecified **side**

✓6ᵗʰ **I69.85** Hemiplegia and hemiparesis **following other**
cerebrovascular disease
AHA: 2015, 1Q, 25

I69.851 **Hemiplegia and hemiparesis** `CC` `HCC`
following other cerebrovascular
disease affecting right dominant **side**
CC Excl: PDX collection 695

✓ Additional Character Required   ✓x7ᵗʰ Placeholder   Unacceptable PDx   Questionable PDx   Manifestation   `H1`-`H14` HAC   `HCC` CMS-HCC Dx   `HIV` HIV Dx

I69.852   **Hemiplegia and hemiparesis** `CC` `HCC`
**following other cerebrovascular
disease affecting** left dominant **side**
    CC Excl: PDX collection 695

I69.853   **Hemiplegia and hemiparesis** `CC` `HCC`
**following other cerebrovascular
disease affecting** right non-dominant **side**
    CC Excl: PDX collection 696

I69.854   **Hemiplegia and hemiparesis** `CC` `HCC`
**following other cerebrovascular
disease affecting** left non-dominant **side**
    CC Excl: PDX collection 696

I69.859   **Hemiplegia and hemiparesis** `CC` `HCC`
**following other cerebrovascular
disease affecting** unspecified **side**
    CC Excl: PDX collection 697

✓6ᵗʰ **I69.86**   Other paralytic syndrome **following other
cerebrovascular disease**
    Use additional code to identify type of paralytic
syndrome, such as:
    locked-in state (G83.5)
    quadriplegia (G82.5-)
    EXCLUDES 1   hemiplegia/hemiparesis following other
         cerebrovascular disease (I69.85-)
         monoplegia of lower limb following other
         cerebrovascular disease (I69.84-)
         monoplegia of upper limb following other
         cerebrovascular disease (I69.83-)

I69.861   **Other paralytic syndrome following** `HCC`
other cerebrovascular disease affecting
right dominant **side**

I69.862   **Other paralytic syndrome following** `HCC`
other cerebrovascular disease affecting
left dominant **side**

I69.863   **Other paralytic syndrome following** `HCC`
other cerebrovascular disease affecting
right non-dominant **side**

I69.864   **Other paralytic syndrome following** `HCC`
other cerebrovascular disease affecting
left non-dominant **side**

I69.865   **Other paralytic syndrome following** `HCC`
other cerebrovascular disease, bilateral

I69.869   **Other paralytic syndrome following** `HCC`
other cerebrovascular disease affecting
unspecified **side**

✓6ᵗʰ **I69.89**   Other sequelae of other cerebrovascular disease

I69.890   Apraxia **following other cerebrovascular
disease**

I69.891   Dysphagia **following other
cerebrovascular disease**
    Use additional code to identify the type of
dysphagia, if known (R13.1-)

I69.892   Facial weakness **following other
cerebrovascular disease**
    Facial droop following other
cerebrovascular disease

I69.893   Ataxia **following other cerebrovascular
disease**

I69.898   Other **sequelae of other cerebrovascular
disease**
    Alteration of sensation following other
cerebrovascular disease
    Disturbance of vision following other
cerebrovascular disease
    Use additional code to identify the
sequelae

✓5ᵗʰ **I69.9**   Sequelae of unspecified cerebrovascular diseases
    EXCLUDES 1   sequelae of stroke (I69.3)
         sequelae of traumatic intracranial injury (S06.-)

I69.90   Unspecified **sequelae of unspecified cerebrovascular
disease**

✓6ᵗʰ **I69.91**   Cognitive deficits **following unspecified
cerebrovascular disease**

I69.910   Attention and concentration **deficit
following unspecified cerebrovascular
disease**

I69.911   Memory **deficit following unspecified
cerebrovascular disease**

I69.912   Visuospatial **deficit and** spatial neglect
**following unspecified cerebrovascular
disease**

I69.913   Psychomotor **deficit following unspecified
cerebrovascular disease**

I69.914   Frontal lobe and executive function **deficit
following unspecified cerebrovascular
disease**

I69.915   Cognitive social or emotional **deficit
following unspecified cerebrovascular
disease**

I69.918   Other **symptoms and signs involving
cognitive functions following unspecified
cerebrovascular disease**

I69.919   Unspecified **symptoms and signs
involving cognitive functions following
unspecified cerebrovascular disease**

✓6ᵗʰ **I69.92**   Speech and language deficits **following unspecified
cerebrovascular disease**

I69.920   Aphasia **following unspecified
cerebrovascular disease**

I69.921   Dysphasia **following unspecified
cerebrovascular disease**

I69.922   Dysarthria **following unspecified
cerebrovascular disease**

I69.923   Fluency disorder **following unspecified
cerebrovascular disease**
    Stuttering following unspecified
cerebrovascular disease

I69.928   Other **speech and language deficits
following unspecified cerebrovascular
disease**

✓6ᵗʰ **I69.93**   Monoplegia of upper limb **following unspecified
cerebrovascular disease**
    AHA: 2017, 1Q, 47

I69.931   **Monoplegia of upper limb following** `HCC`
**unspecified cerebrovascular disease
affecting** right dominant **side**

I69.932   **Monoplegia of upper limb following** `HCC`
**unspecified cerebrovascular disease
affecting** left dominant **side**

I69.933   **Monoplegia of upper limb following** `HCC`
**unspecified cerebrovascular disease
affecting** right non-dominant **side**

I69.934   **Monoplegia of upper limb following** `HCC`
**unspecified cerebrovascular disease
affecting** left non-dominant **side**

I69.939   **Monoplegia of upper limb following** `HCC`
**unspecified cerebrovascular disease
affecting** unspecified **side**

✓6ᵗʰ **I69.94**   Monoplegia of lower limb **following unspecified
cerebrovascular disease**
    AHA: 2017, 1Q, 47

I69.941   **Monoplegia of lower limb following** `HCC`
**unspecified cerebrovascular disease
affecting** right dominant **side**

I69.942   **Monoplegia of lower limb following** `HCC`
**unspecified cerebrovascular disease
affecting** left dominant **side**

I69.943   **Monoplegia of lower limb following** `HCC`
**unspecified cerebrovascular disease
affecting** right non-dominant **side**

I69.944   **Monoplegia of lower limb following** `HCC`
**unspecified cerebrovascular disease
affecting** left non-dominant **side**

I69.949   **Monoplegia of lower limb following** `HCC`
**unspecified cerebrovascular disease
affecting** unspecified **side**

✓6ᵗʰ **I69.95**   Hemiplegia and hemiparesis **following unspecified
cerebrovascular disease**
    AHA: 2015, 1Q, 25

I69.951   **Hemiplegia and hemiparesis** `CC` `HCC`
**following unspecified cerebrovascular
disease affecting** right dominant **side**
    CC Excl: PDX collection 695

I69.952   **Hemiplegia and hemiparesis** `CC` `HCC`
**following unspecified cerebrovascular
disease affecting** left dominant **side**
    CC Excl: PDX collection 695

I69.953   **Hemiplegia and hemiparesis** `CC` `HCC`
**following unspecified cerebrovascular
disease affecting** right non-dominant **side**
    CC Excl: PDX collection 696

`N` Newborn: 0   `P` Pediatric: 0-17   `M` Maternity: 12-55   `A` Adult: 15-124   `MCC` Major Complication/Comorbidity   `CC` Complication/Comorbidity   `SW` Severe Wound Dx

ICD-10-CM 2019

Chapter 9. Diseases of the Circulatory System

I69.954 Hemiplegia and hemiparesis `CC` `HCC` following unspecified cerebrovascular disease affecting left non-dominant side
    CC Excl: PDX collection 696

I69.959 Hemiplegia and hemiparesis `CC` `HCC` following unspecified cerebrovascular disease affecting unspecified side
    CC Excl: PDX collection 697

√6ᵗʰ **I69.96** Other paralytic syndrome following unspecified cerebrovascular disease
    Use additional code to identify type of paralytic syndrome, such as:
      locked-in state (G83.5)
      quadriplegia (G82.5-)
    EXCLUDES 1 hemiplegia/hemiparesis following unspecified cerebrovascular disease (I69.95-)
      monoplegia of lower limb following unspecified cerebrovascular disease (I69.94-)
      monoplegia of upper limb following unspecified cerebrovascular disease (I69.93-)

I69.961 Other paralytic syndrome following `HCC` unspecified cerebrovascular disease affecting right dominant side

I69.962 Other paralytic syndrome following `HCC` unspecified cerebrovascular disease affecting left dominant side

I69.963 Other paralytic syndrome following `HCC` unspecified cerebrovascular disease affecting right non-dominant side

I69.964 Other paralytic syndrome following `HCC` unspecified cerebrovascular disease affecting left non-dominant side

I69.965 Other paralytic syndrome following `HCC` unspecified cerebrovascular disease, bilateral

I69.969 Other paralytic syndrome following `HCC` unspecified cerebrovascular disease affecting unspecified side

√6ᵗʰ **I69.99** Other sequelae of unspecified cerebrovascular disease

I69.990 Apraxia following unspecified cerebrovascular disease

I69.991 Dysphagia following unspecified cerebrovascular disease
    Use additional code to identify the type of dysphagia, if known (R13.1-)

I69.992 Facial weakness following unspecified cerebrovascular disease
    Facial droop following unspecified cerebrovascular disease

I69.993 Ataxia following unspecified cerebrovascular disease

I69.998 Other sequelae following unspecified cerebrovascular disease
    Alteration in sensation following unspecified cerebrovascular disease
    Disturbance of vision following unspecified cerebrovascular disease
    Use additional code to identify the sequelae

Diseases of arteries, arterioles and capillaries (I70-I79)

√4ᵗʰ **I70** **Atherosclerosis**
  INCLUDES arteriolosclerosis
    arterial degeneration
    arteriosclerosis
    arteriosclerotic vascular disease
    arteriovascular degeneration
    atheroma
    endarteritis deformans or obliterans
    senile arteritis
    senile endarteritis
    vascular degeneration
  Use additional code to identify:
    exposure to environmental tobacco smoke (Z77.22)
    history of tobacco dependence (Z87.891)
    occupational exposure to environmental tobacco smoke (Z57.31)
    tobacco dependence (F17.-)
    tobacco use (Z72.0)
  EXCLUDES 2 arteriosclerotic cardiovascular disease (I25.1-)
    arteriosclerotic heart disease (I25.1-)
    atheroembolism (I75.-)
    cerebral atherosclerosis (I67.2)
    coronary atherosclerosis (I25.1-)
    mesenteric atherosclerosis (K55.1)
    precerebral atherosclerosis (I67.2)
    primary pulmonary atherosclerosis (I27.0)

I70.0 Atherosclerosis of aorta `HCC` `A`

I70.1 Atherosclerosis of renal artery `HCC` `A`
    Goldblatt's kidney
    EXCLUDES 2 atherosclerosis of renal arterioles (I12.-)

√5ᵗʰ **I70.2** Atherosclerosis of native arteries of the extremities
    Mönckeberg's (medial) sclerosis
    Use additional code, if applicable, to identify chronic total occlusion of artery of extremity (I70.92)
    EXCLUDES 2 atherosclerosis of bypass graft of extremities (I70.30-I70.79)
    AHA: 2018, 2Q, 7

√6ᵗʰ **I70.20** Unspecified atherosclerosis of native arteries of extremities

I70.201 Unspecified atherosclerosis of `HCC` `A` native arteries of extremities, right leg

I70.202 Unspecified atherosclerosis of `HCC` `A` native arteries of extremities, left leg

I70.203 Unspecified atherosclerosis of `HCC` `A` native arteries of extremities, bilateral legs

I70.208 Unspecified atherosclerosis of `HCC` `A` native arteries of extremities, other extremity

I70.209 Unspecified atherosclerosis of `HCC` `A` native arteries of extremities, unspecified extremity

√6ᵗʰ **I70.21** Atherosclerosis of native arteries of extremities with intermittent claudication

I70.211 Atherosclerosis of native arteries of `HCC` `A` extremities with intermittent claudication, right leg

I70.212 Atherosclerosis of native arteries of `HCC` `A` extremities with intermittent claudication, left leg

I70.213 Atherosclerosis of native arteries of `HCC` `A` extremities with intermittent claudication, bilateral legs

I70.218 Atherosclerosis of native arteries of `HCC` `A` extremities with intermittent claudication, other extremity

I70.219 Atherosclerosis of native arteries of `HCC` `A` extremities with intermittent claudication, unspecified extremity

√6ᵗʰ **I70.22** Atherosclerosis of native arteries of extremities with rest pain
    INCLUDES any condition classifiable to I70.21-

I70.221 Atherosclerosis of native arteries of `HCC` `A` extremities with rest pain, right leg

I70.222 Atherosclerosis of native arteries of `HCC` `A` extremities with rest pain, left leg

I70.223 Atherosclerosis of native arteries of `HCC` `A` extremities with rest pain, bilateral legs

I70.228 Atherosclerosis of native arteries of `HCC` `A` extremities with rest pain, other extremity

✓Additional Character Required   √x7ᵗʰ Placeholder   Unacceptable PDx   Questionable PDx   Manifestation   `H1`-`H14` HAC   `HCC` CMS-HCC Dx   `HIV` HIV Dx

ICD-10-CM 2019   657

I70.229　**Atherosclerosis of native arteries of** `HCC` `A` **extremities with rest pain,** unspecified extremity

✓6ᵗʰ **I70.23**　**Atherosclerosis of native arteries of** right leg **with** ulceration
　　INCLUDES　any condition classifiable to I70.211 and I70.221
　　Use additional code to identify severity of ulcer (L97.-)

I70.231　**Atherosclerosis of native arteries of** `HCC` `A` **right leg with ulceration of** thigh

I70.232　**Atherosclerosis of native arteries of** `HCC` `A` **right leg with ulceration of** calf

I70.233　**Atherosclerosis of native arteries of** `HCC` `A` **right leg with ulceration of** ankle

I70.234　**Atherosclerosis of native arteries of** `HCC` `A` **right leg with ulceration of** heel and midfoot
　　Atherosclerosis of native arteries of right leg with ulceration of plantar surface of midfoot

I70.235　**Atherosclerosis of native arteries of** `HCC` `A` **right leg with ulceration of** other part of foot
　　Atherosclerosis of native arteries of right leg extremities with ulceration of toe

I70.238　**Atherosclerosis of native arteries of** `HCC` `A` **right leg with ulceration of** other part of lower right leg

I70.239　**Atherosclerosis of native arteries of** `HCC` `A` **right leg with ulceration of** unspecified site

✓6ᵗʰ **I70.24**　**Atherosclerosis of native arteries of** left leg **with** ulceration
　　INCLUDES　any condition classifiable to I70.212 and I70.222
　　Use additional code to identify severity of ulcer (L97.-)

I70.241　**Atherosclerosis of native arteries of** `HCC` `A` **left leg with ulceration of** thigh

I70.242　**Atherosclerosis of native arteries of** `HCC` `A` **left leg with ulceration of** calf

I70.243　**Atherosclerosis of native arteries of** `HCC` `A` **left leg with ulceration of** ankle

I70.244　**Atherosclerosis of native arteries of** `HCC` `A` **left leg with ulceration of** heel and midfoot
　　Atherosclerosis of native arteries of left leg with ulceration of plantar surface of midfoot

I70.245　**Atherosclerosis of native arteries** `HCC` `A` **of left leg with ulceration of** other part of foot
　　Atherosclerosis of native arteries of left leg extremities with ulceration of toe

I70.248　**Atherosclerosis of native arteries of** `HCC` `A` **left leg with ulceration of** other part of lower left leg

I70.249　**Atherosclerosis of native arteries of** `HCC` `A` **left leg with ulceration of** unspecified site

I70.25　**Atherosclerosis of native arteries of** other `HCC` `A` **extremities with** ulceration
　　INCLUDES　any condition classifiable to I70.218 and I70.228
　　Use additional code to identify the severity of the ulcer (L98.49-)

✓6ᵗʰ **I70.26**　**Atherosclerosis of native arteries of extremities with** gangrene
　　INCLUDES　any condition classifiable to I70.21-, I70.22-, I70.23-, I70.24-, and I70.25-
　　Use additional code to identify the severity of any ulcer (L97.-, L98.49-), if applicable

　　CC Excl: For CC codes in subcategory I70.26:
　　PDX collection 519

I70.261　**Atherosclerosis of native** `CC` `HCC` `A` **arteries of extremities with gangrene,** right leg

I70.262　**Atherosclerosis of native** `CC` `HCC` `A` **arteries of extremities with gangrene,** left leg

I70.263　**Atherosclerosis of native** `CC` `HCC` `A` **arteries of extremities with gangrene,** bilateral legs

I70.268　**Atherosclerosis of native** `CC` `HCC` `A` **arteries of extremities with gangrene,** other extremity

I70.269　**Atherosclerosis of native** `CC` `HCC` `A` **arteries of extremities with gangrene,** unspecified extremity

✓5ᵗʰ **I70.29**　Other **atherosclerosis of native arteries of extremities**

I70.291　**Other atherosclerosis of native** `HCC` `A` **arteries of extremities,** right leg

I70.292　**Other atherosclerosis of native** `HCC` `A` **arteries of extremities,** left leg

I70.293　**Other atherosclerosis of native** `HCC` `A` **arteries of extremities,** bilateral legs

I70.298　**Other atherosclerosis of native** `HCC` `A` **arteries of extremities,** other extremity

I70.299　**Other atherosclerosis of native** `HCC` `A` **arteries of extremities,** unspecified extremity

✓5ᵗʰ **I70.3**　**Atherosclerosis of** unspecified type of bypass graft(s) **of the** extremities
　　Use additional code, if applicable, to identify chronic total occlusion of artery of extremity (I70.92)
　　EXCLUDES 1　embolism or thrombus of bypass graft(s) of extremities (T82.8-)

✓6ᵗʰ **I70.30**　Unspecified **atherosclerosis of unspecified type of bypass graft(s) of the extremities**

I70.301　**Unspecified atherosclerosis of** `HCC` `A` **unspecified type of bypass graft(s) of the extremities,** right leg

I70.302　**Unspecified atherosclerosis of** `HCC` `A` **unspecified type of bypass graft(s) of the extremities,** left leg

I70.303　**Unspecified atherosclerosis of** `HCC` `A` **unspecified type of bypass graft(s) of the extremities,** bilateral legs

I70.308　**Unspecified atherosclerosis of** `HCC` `A` **unspecified type of bypass graft(s) of the extremities,** other extremity

I70.309　**Unspecified atherosclerosis of** `HCC` `A` **unspecified type of bypass graft(s) of the extremities,** unspecified extremity

✓6ᵗʰ **I70.31**　**Atherosclerosis of unspecified type of bypass graft(s) of the extremities with** intermittent claudication

I70.311　**Atherosclerosis of unspecified type** `HCC` `A` **of bypass graft(s) of the extremities with intermittent claudication,** right leg

I70.312　**Atherosclerosis of unspecified type** `HCC` `A` **of bypass graft(s) of the extremities with intermittent claudication,** left leg

I70.313　**Atherosclerosis of unspecified type** `HCC` `A` **of bypass graft(s) of the extremities with intermittent claudication,** bilateral legs

I70.318　**Atherosclerosis of unspecified type** `HCC` `A` **of bypass graft(s) of the extremities with intermittent claudication,** other extremity

I70.319　**Atherosclerosis of unspecified type** `HCC` `A` **of bypass graft(s) of the extremities with intermittent claudication,** unspecified extremity

✓6ᵗʰ **I70.32**　**Atherosclerosis of unspecified type of bypass graft(s) of the extremities with** rest pain
　　INCLUDES　any condition classifiable to I70.31-

I70.321　**Atherosclerosis of unspecified type** `HCC` `A` **of bypass graft(s) of the extremities with rest pain,** right leg

I70.322　**Atherosclerosis of unspecified type** `HCC` `A` **of bypass graft(s) of the extremities with rest pain,** left leg

I70.323　**Atherosclerosis of unspecified type** `HCC` `A` **of bypass graft(s) of the extremities with rest pain,** bilateral legs

I70.328　**Atherosclerosis of unspecified type** `HCC` `A` **of bypass graft(s) of the extremities with rest pain,** other extremity

`N` Newborn: 0　`P` Pediatric: 0-17　`M` Maternity: 12-55　`A` Adult: 15-124　`MCC` Major Complication/Comorbidity　`CC` Complication/Comorbidity　`SW` Severe Wound Dx

658　　　　　　　　　　　　　　　　　　　　　　　　　　　　　　　　　　ICD-10-CM 2019

I70.329   **Atherosclerosis of unspecified type** HCC A **of bypass graft(s) of the extremities with rest pain, unspecified extremity**

√6th **I70.33**   **Atherosclerosis of unspecified type of bypass graft(s) of the right leg with ulceration**

INCLUDES   any condition classifiable to I70.311 and I70.321

Use additional code to identify severity of ulcer (L97.-)

CC Excl: For CC codes in subcategory I70.33: PDX collection 698

I70.331   **Atherosclerosis of unspecified** CC HCC A **type of bypass graft(s) of the right leg with ulceration of thigh**

I70.332   **Atherosclerosis of unspecified** CC HCC A **type of bypass graft(s) of the right leg with ulceration of calf**

I70.333   **Atherosclerosis of type of bypass** CC HCC A **graft(s) of the unspecified right leg with ulceration of ankle**

I70.334   **Atherosclerosis of unspecified** CC HCC A **type of bypass graft(s) of the right leg with ulceration of heel and midfoot**

Atherosclerosis of unspecified type of bypass graft(s) of right leg with ulceration of plantar surface of midfoot

I70.335   **Atherosclerosis of unspecified type** HCC A **of bypass graft(s) of the right leg with ulceration of other part of foot**

Atherosclerosis of unspecified type of bypass graft(s) of the right leg with ulceration of toe

I70.338   **Atherosclerosis of unspecified** CC HCC A **type of bypass graft(s) of the right leg with ulceration of other part of lower leg**

I70.339   **Atherosclerosis of unspecified** CC HCC A **type of bypass graft(s) of the right leg with ulceration of unspecified site**

√6th **I70.34**   **Atherosclerosis of unspecified type of bypass graft(s) of the left leg with ulceration**

INCLUDES   any condition classifiable to I70.312 and I70.322

Use additional code to identify severity of ulcer (L97.-)

CC Excl: For CC codes in subcategory I70.34: PDX collection 698

I70.341   **Atherosclerosis of unspecified** CC HCC A **type of bypass graft(s) of the left leg with ulceration of thigh**

I70.342   **Atherosclerosis of unspecified** CC HCC A **type of bypass graft(s) of the left leg with ulceration of calf**

I70.343   **Atherosclerosis of unspecified** CC HCC A **type of bypass graft(s) of the left leg with ulceration of ankle**

I70.344   **Atherosclerosis of unspecified** CC HCC A **type of bypass graft(s) of the left leg with ulceration of heel and midfoot**

Atherosclerosis of unspecified type of bypass graft(s) of left leg with ulceration of plantar surface of midfoot

I70.345   **Atherosclerosis of unspecified** HCC A **type of bypass graft(s) of the left leg with ulceration of other part of foot**

Atherosclerosis of unspecified type of bypass graft(s) of the left leg with ulceration of toe

I70.348   **Atherosclerosis of unspecified** CC HCC A **type of bypass graft(s) of the left leg with ulceration of other part of lower leg**

I70.349   **Atherosclerosis of unspecified** CC HCC A **type of bypass graft(s) of the left leg with ulceration of unspecified site**

I70.35   **Atherosclerosis of unspecified type of bypass** HCC A **graft(s) of other extremity with ulceration**

INCLUDES   any condition classifiable to I70.318 and I70.328

Use additional code to identify severity of ulcer (L98.49-)

√6th **I70.36**   **Atherosclerosis of unspecified type of bypass graft(s) of the extremities with gangrene**

INCLUDES   any condition classifiable to I70.31-, I70.32-, I70.33-, I70.34-, I70.35

Use additional code to identify the severity of any ulcer (L97.-, L98.49-), if applicable

CC Excl: For CC codes in subcategory I70.36: PDX collection 519

I70.361   **Atherosclerosis of unspecified** CC HCC A **type of bypass graft(s) of the extremities with gangrene, right leg**

I70.362   **Atherosclerosis of unspecified** CC HCC A **type of bypass graft(s) of the extremities with gangrene, left leg**

I70.363   **Atherosclerosis of unspecified** CC HCC A **type of bypass graft(s) of the extremities with gangrene, bilateral legs**

I70.368   **Atherosclerosis of unspecified** CC HCC A **type of bypass graft(s) of the extremities with gangrene, other extremity**

I70.369   **Atherosclerosis of unspecified** CC HCC A **type of bypass graft(s) of the extremities with gangrene, unspecified extremity**

√6th **I70.39**   **Other atherosclerosis of unspecified type of bypass graft(s) of the extremities**

I70.391   **Other atherosclerosis of** HCC A **unspecified type of bypass graft(s) of the extremities, right leg**

I70.392   **Other atherosclerosis of** HCC A **unspecified type of bypass graft(s) of the extremities, left leg**

I70.393   **Other atherosclerosis of** HCC A **unspecified type of bypass graft(s) of the extremities, bilateral legs**

I70.398   **Other atherosclerosis of** HCC A **unspecified type of bypass graft(s) of the extremities, other extremity**

I70.399   **Other atherosclerosis of** HCC A **unspecified type of bypass graft(s) of the extremities, unspecified extremity**

√5th **I70.4**   **Atherosclerosis of autologous vein bypass graft(s) of the extremities**

Use additional code, if applicable, to identify chronic total occlusion of artery of extremity (I70.92)

√6th **I70.40**   **Unspecified atherosclerosis of autologous vein bypass graft(s) of the extremities**

I70.401   **Unspecified atherosclerosis of** HCC A **autologous vein bypass graft(s) of the extremities, right leg**

I70.402   **Unspecified atherosclerosis of** HCC A **autologous vein bypass graft(s) of the extremities, left leg**

I70.403   **Unspecified atherosclerosis of** HCC A **autologous vein bypass graft(s) of the extremities, bilateral legs**

I70.408   **Unspecified atherosclerosis of** HCC A **autologous vein bypass graft(s) of the extremities, other extremity**

I70.409   **Unspecified atherosclerosis of** HCC A **autologous vein bypass graft(s) of the extremities, unspecified extremity**

√6th **I70.41**   **Atherosclerosis of autologous vein bypass graft(s) of the extremities with intermittent claudication**

I70.411   **Atherosclerosis of autologous vein** HCC A **bypass graft(s) of the extremities with intermittent claudication, right leg**

I70.412   **Atherosclerosis of autologous vein** HCC A **bypass graft(s) of the extremities with intermittent claudication, left leg**

I70.413   **Atherosclerosis of autologous vein** HCC A **bypass graft(s) of the extremities with intermittent claudication, bilateral legs**

I70.418   **Atherosclerosis of autologous vein** HCC A **bypass graft(s) of the extremities with intermittent claudication, other extremity**

✔ Additional Character Required   √x7th Placeholder   Unacceptable PDx   Questionable PDx   Manifestation   H1–H14 HAC   HCC CMS-HCC Dx   HIV HIV Dx

ICD-10-CM 2019   659

I70.419　Atherosclerosis of autologous vein `HCC` `A`
bypass graft(s) of the extremities with
intermittent claudication, unspecified
extremity

✓6th I70.42　Atherosclerosis of autologous vein bypass graft(s) of
the extremities with rest pain
　`INCLUDES`　any condition classifiable to I70.41-

I70.421　Atherosclerosis of autologous vein `HCC` `A`
bypass graft(s) of the extremities
with rest pain, right leg

I70.422　Atherosclerosis of autologous vein `HCC` `A`
bypass graft(s) of the extremities
with rest pain, left leg

I70.423　Atherosclerosis of autologous vein `HCC` `A`
bypass graft(s) of the extremities
with rest pain, bilateral legs

I70.428　Atherosclerosis of autologous vein `HCC` `A`
bypass graft(s) of the extremities
with rest pain, other extremity

I70.429　Atherosclerosis of autologous vein `HCC` `A`
bypass graft(s) of the extremities
with rest pain, unspecified extremity

✓6th I70.43　Atherosclerosis of autologous vein bypass graft(s) of
the right leg with ulceration
　`INCLUDES`　any condition classifiable to I70.411 and
　　　　　　I70.421
　Use additional code to identify severity of ulcer (L97.-)

`CC Excl: For CC codes in subcategory I70.43:`
`PDX collection 698`

I70.431　Atherosclerosis of autologous `CC` `HCC` `A`
vein bypass graft(s) of the right
leg with ulceration of thigh

I70.432　Atherosclerosis of autologous `CC` `HCC` `A`
vein bypass graft(s) of the right
leg with ulceration of calf

I70.433　Atherosclerosis of autologous `CC` `HCC` `A`
vein bypass graft(s) of the right
leg with ulceration of ankle

I70.434　Atherosclerosis of autologous `CC` `HCC` `A`
vein bypass graft(s) of the right
leg with ulceration of heel and midfoot
　Atherosclerosis of autologous vein bypass
　graft(s) of right leg with ulceration of
　plantar surface of midfoot

I70.435　Atherosclerosis of autologous vein `HCC` `A`
bypass graft(s) of the right leg with
ulceration of other part of foot
　Atherosclerosis of autologous vein bypass
　graft(s) of right leg with ulceration of
　toe

I70.438　Atherosclerosis of autologous `CC` `HCC` `A`
vein bypass graft(s) of the right
leg with ulceration of
other part of lower leg

I70.439　Atherosclerosis of autologous `CC` `HCC` `A`
vein bypass graft(s) of the right
leg with ulceration of unspecified site

✓6th I70.44　Atherosclerosis of autologous vein bypass graft(s) of
the left leg with ulceration
　`INCLUDES`　any condition classifiable to I70.412 and
　　　　　　I70.422
　Use additional code to identify severity of ulcer (L97.-)

`CC Excl: For CC codes in subcategory I70.44:`
`PDX collection 698`

I70.441　Atherosclerosis of autologous `CC` `HCC` `A`
vein bypass graft(s) of the left
leg with ulceration of thigh

I70.442　Atherosclerosis of autologous `CC` `HCC` `A`
vein bypass graft(s) of the left
leg with ulceration of calf

I70.443　Atherosclerosis of autologous `CC` `HCC` `A`
vein bypass graft(s) of the left
leg with ulceration of ankle

I70.444　Atherosclerosis of autologous `CC` `HCC` `A`
vein bypass graft(s) of the left
leg with ulceration of
heel and midfoot
　Atherosclerosis of autologous vein bypass
　graft(s) of left leg with ulceration of
　plantar surface of midfoot

I70.445　Atherosclerosis of autologous vein `HCC` `A`
bypass graft(s) of the left leg with
ulceration of other part of foot
　Atherosclerosis of autologous vein bypass
　graft(s) of left leg with ulceration of
　toe

I70.448　Atherosclerosis of autologous `CC` `HCC` `A`
vein bypass graft(s) of the left
leg with ulceration of
other part of lower leg

I70.449　Atherosclerosis of autologous `CC` `HCC` `A`
vein bypass graft(s) of the left
leg with ulceration of
unspecified site

I70.45　Atherosclerosis of autologous vein bypass `HCC` `A`
graft(s) of other extremity with ulceration
　`INCLUDES`　any condition classifiable to I70.418,
　　　　　　I70.428, and I70.438
　Use additional code to identify severity of ulcer
　(L98.49)

✓6th I70.46　Atherosclerosis of autologous vein bypass graft(s) of
the extremities with gangrene
　`INCLUDES`　any condition classifiable to I70.41-, I70.42-,
　　　　　　and I70.43-, I70.44-, I70.45
　Use additional code to identify the severity of any
　ulcer (L97.-, L98.49-), if applicable

`CC Excl: For CC codes in subcategory I70.46:`
`PDX collection 519`

I70.461　Atherosclerosis of autologous `CC` `HCC` `A`
vein bypass graft(s) of the
extremities with gangrene, right leg

I70.462　Atherosclerosis of autologous `CC` `HCC` `A`
vein bypass graft(s) of the
extremities with gangrene, left leg

I70.463　Atherosclerosis of autologous `CC` `HCC` `A`
vein bypass graft(s) of the
extremities with gangrene, bilateral legs

I70.468　Atherosclerosis of autologous `CC` `HCC` `A`
vein bypass graft(s) of the
extremities with gangrene,
other extremity

I70.469　Atherosclerosis of autologous `CC` `HCC` `A`
vein bypass graft(s) of the
extremities with gangrene,
unspecified extremity

✓6th I70.49　Other atherosclerosis of autologous vein bypass
graft(s) of the extremities

I70.491　Other atherosclerosis of `HCC` `A`
autologous vein bypass graft(s)
of the extremities, right leg

I70.492　Other atherosclerosis of `HCC` `A`
autologous vein bypass graft(s)
of the extremities, left leg

I70.493　Other atherosclerosis of `HCC` `A`
autologous vein bypass graft(s)
of the extremities, bilateral legs

I70.498　Other atherosclerosis of `HCC` `A`
autologous vein bypass graft(s)
of the extremities, other extremity

I70.499　Other atherosclerosis of `HCC` `A`
autologous vein bypass graft(s) of the
extremities, unspecified extremity

✓5th I70.5　Atherosclerosis of nonautologous biological bypass graft(s)
of the extremities
　Use additional code, if applicable, to identify chronic total
　occlusion of artery of extremity (I70.92)

✓6th I70.50　Unspecified atherosclerosis of nonautologous
biological bypass graft(s) of the extremities

I70.501　Unspecified atherosclerosis of `HCC` `A`
nonautologous biological bypass
graft(s) of the extremities, right leg

I70.502　Unspecified atherosclerosis of `HCC` `A`
nonautologous biological bypass
graft(s) of the extremities, left leg

I70.503　Unspecified atherosclerosis of `HCC` `A`
nonautologous biological bypass
graft(s) of the extremities, bilateral legs

I70.508　Unspecified atherosclerosis of `HCC` `A`
nonautologous biological bypass
graft(s) of the extremities, other extremity

I70.509　**Unspecified atherosclerosis of** `HCC` `A`
nonautologous biological bypass
graft(s) of the extremities, unspecified
extremity

✓6ᵗʰ **I70.51**　**Atherosclerosis of nonautologous biological bypass**
graft(s) of the extremities with intermittent
claudication

I70.511　**Atherosclerosis of nonautologous** `HCC` `A`
biological bypass graft(s) of the
extremities with intermittent
claudication, right leg

I70.512　**Atherosclerosis of nonautologous** `HCC` `A`
biological bypass graft(s) of the
extremities with intermittent
claudication, left leg

I70.513　**Atherosclerosis of nonautologous** `HCC` `A`
biological bypass graft(s) of the
extremities with intermittent
claudication, bilateral legs

I70.518　**Atherosclerosis of nonautologous** `HCC` `A`
biological bypass graft(s) of the
extremities with intermittent
claudication, other extremity

I70.519　**Atherosclerosis of nonautologous** `HCC` `A`
biological bypass graft(s) of the
extremities with intermittent
claudication, unspecified extremity

✓6ᵗʰ **I70.52**　**Atherosclerosis of nonautologous biological bypass**
graft(s) of the extremities with rest pain
　　INCLUDES　any condition classifiable to I70.51-

I70.521　**Atherosclerosis of nonautologous** `HCC` `A`
biological bypass graft(s) of the
extremities with rest pain, right leg

I70.522　**Atherosclerosis of nonautologous** `HCC` `A`
biological bypass graft(s) of the
extremities with rest pain, left leg

I70.523　**Atherosclerosis of nonautologous** `HCC` `A`
biological bypass graft(s) of the
extremities with rest pain, bilateral legs

I70.528　**Atherosclerosis of nonautologous** `HCC` `A`
biological bypass graft(s) of the
extremities with rest pain, other extremity

I70.529　**Atherosclerosis of nonautologous** `HCC` `A`
biological bypass graft(s) of the
extremities with rest pain, unspecified
extremity

✓6ᵗʰ **I70.53**　**Atherosclerosis of nonautologous biological bypass**
graft(s) of the right leg **with** ulceration
　　INCLUDES　any condition classifiable to I70.511 and
　　　　　　　I70.521
　Use additional code to identify severity of ulcer (L97.-)

> **CC Excl: For CC codes in subcategory I70.53:**
> PDX collection 698

I70.531　**Atherosclerosis of biological** `CC` `HCC` `A`
nonautologous bypass graft(s) of the
right leg with ulceration of thigh

I70.532　**Atherosclerosis of bilological** `CC` `HCC` `A`
nonautologous bypass graft(s) of
the right leg with ulceration of calf

I70.533　**Atherosclerosis of** `CC` `HCC` `A`
nonautologous biological bypass graft(s)
of the right leg with ulceration of ankle

I70.534　**Atherosclerosis of** `CC` `HCC` `A`
nonautologous biological bypass
graft(s) of the right leg with
ulceration of heel and midfoot
　Atherosclerosis of nonautologous
　　biological bypass graft(s) of right leg
　　with ulceration of plantar surface of
　　midfoot

I70.535　**Atherosclerosis of nonautologous** `HCC` `A`
biological bypass graft(s) of the
right leg with ulceration of other
part of foot
　Atherosclerosis of nonautologous
　　biological bypass graft(s) of the right
　　leg with ulceration of toe

I70.538　**Atherosclerosis of** `CC` `HCC` `A`
nonautologous biological bypass
graft(s) of the right leg with ulceration
of other part of lower leg

I70.539　**Atherosclerosis of** `CC` `HCC` `A`
nonautologous biological bypass
graft(s) of the right leg with ulceration
of unspecified **site**

✓6ᵗʰ **I70.54**　**Atherosclerosis of nonautologous biological bypass**
graft(s) of the left leg **with** ulceration
　　INCLUDES　any condition classifiable to I70.512 and
　　　　　　　I70.522
　Use additional code to identify severity of ulcer (L97.-)

> **CC Excl: For CC codes in subcategory I70.54:**
> PDX collection 698

I70.541　**Atherosclerosis of** `CC` `HCC` `A`
nonautologous biological bypass
graft(s) of the left leg with ulceration
of thigh

I70.542　**Atherosclerosis of** `CC` `HCC` `A`
nonautologous biological bypass
graft(s) of the left leg with ulceration
of calf

I70.543　**Atherosclerosis of** `CC` `HCC` `A`
nonautologous biological bypass
graft(s) of the left leg with ulceration
of ankle

I70.544　**Atherosclerosis of** `CC` `HCC` `A`
nonautologous biological bypass
graft(s) of the left leg with ulceration
of heel and midfoot
　Atherosclerosis of nonautologous
　　biological bypass graft(s) of left leg
　　with ulceration of plantar surface of
　　midfoot

I70.545　**Atherosclerosis of nonautologous** `HCC` `A`
biological bypass graft(s) of the left leg
with ulceration of other part of foot
　Atherosclerosis of nonautologous
　　biological bypass graft(s) of the left leg
　　with ulceration of toe

I70.548　**Atherosclerosis of** `CC` `HCC` `A`
nonautologous biological bypass
graft(s) of the left leg with ulceration
of other part of lower leg

I70.549　**Atherosclerosis of** `CC` `HCC` `A`
nonautologous biological bypass
graft(s) of the left leg with ulceration
of unspecified **site**

I70.55　**Atherosclerosis of nonautologous biological** `HCC` `A`
bypass graft(s) of other extremity **with** ulceration
　　INCLUDES　any condition classifiable to I70.518,
　　　　　　　I70.528, and I70.538
　Use additional code to identify severity of ulcer
　　(L98.49)

✓6ᵗʰ **I70.56**　**Atherosclerosis of nonautologous biological bypass**
graft(s) of the extremities with gangrene
　　INCLUDES　any condition classifiable to I70.51-, I70.52-,
　　　　　　　and I70.53-, I70.54-, I70.55
　Use additional code to identify the severity of any
　　ulcer (L97.-, L98.49-), if applicable

> **CC Excl: For CC codes in subcategory I70.56:**
> PDX collection 519

I70.561　**Atherosclerosis of** `CC` `HCC` `A`
nonautologous biological bypass
graft(s) of the extremities with
gangrene, right leg

I70.562　**Atherosclerosis of** `CC` `HCC` `A`
nonautologous biological bypass
graft(s) of the extremities with
gangrene, left leg

I70.563　**Atherosclerosis of** `CC` `HCC` `A`
nonautologous biological bypass
graft(s) of the extremities with
gangrene, bilateral legs

I70.568　**Atherosclerosis of** `CC` `HCC` `A`
nonautologous biological bypass
graft(s) of the extremities with
gangrene, other extremity

I70.569　**Atherosclerosis of** `CC` `HCC` `A`
nonautologous biological bypass
graft(s) of the extremities with
gangrene, unspecified extremity

✅ Additional Character Required　　✓x7ᵗʰ Placeholder　　Unacceptable PDx　　Questionable PDx　　Manifestation　　`H1`-`H14` HAC　　`HCC` CMS-HCC Dx　　`HIV` HIV Dx

ICD-10-CM 2019　　　　　　　　　　　　　　　　　　　　　　　　　　　　　　　　　　　　**661**

✓6ᵗʰ I70.59 Other atherosclerosis of nonautologous biological bypass graft(s) of the extremities

- **I70.591 Other atherosclerosis of biological nonautologous bypass graft(s) of the extremities, right leg** HCC A
- **I70.592 Other atherosclerosis of nonautologous biological bypass graft(s) of the extremities, left leg** HCC A
- **I70.593 Other atherosclerosis of nonautologous biological bypass graft(s) of the extremities, bilateral legs** HCC A
- **I70.598 Other atherosclerosis of nonautologous biological bypass graft(s) of the extremities, other extremity** HCC A
- **I70.599 Other atherosclerosis of nonautologous biological bypass graft(s) of the extremities, unspecified extremity** HCC A

✓5ᵗʰ I70.6 Atherosclerosis of nonbiological bypass graft(s) of the extremities

Use additional code, if applicable, to identify chronic total occlusion of artery of extremity (I70.92)

✓6ᵗʰ I70.60 Unspecified atherosclerosis of nonbiological bypass graft(s) of the extremities

- **I70.601 Unspecified atherosclerosis of nonbiological bypass graft(s) of the extremities, right leg** HCC A
- **I70.602 Unspecified atherosclerosis of nonbiological bypass graft(s) of the extremities, left leg** HCC A
- **I70.603 Unspecified atherosclerosis of nonbiological bypass graft(s) of the extremities, bilateral legs** HCC A
- **I70.608 Unspecified atherosclerosis of nonbiological bypass graft(s) of the extremities, other extremity** HCC A
- **I70.609 Unspecified atherosclerosis of nonbiological bypass graft(s) of the extremities, unspecified extremity** HCC A

✓6ᵗʰ I70.61 Atherosclerosis of nonbiological bypass graft(s) of the extremities with intermittent claudication

- **I70.611 Atherosclerosis of nonbiological bypass graft(s) of the extremities with intermittent claudication, right leg** HCC A
- **I70.612 Atherosclerosis of nonbiological bypass graft(s) of the extremities with intermittent claudication, left leg** HCC A
- **I70.613 Atherosclerosis of nonbiological bypass graft(s) of the extremities with intermittent claudication, bilateral legs** HCC A
- **I70.618 Atherosclerosis of nonbiological bypass graft(s) of the extremities with intermittent claudication, other extremity** HCC A
- **I70.619 Atherosclerosis of nonbiological bypass graft(s) of the extremities with intermittent claudication, unspecified extremity** HCC A

✓6ᵗʰ I70.62 Atherosclerosis of nonbiological bypass graft(s) of the extremities with rest pain

INCLUDES any condition classifiable to I70.61-

- **I70.621 Atherosclerosis of nonbiological bypass graft(s) of the extremities with rest pain, right leg** HCC A
- **I70.622 Atherosclerosis of nonbiological bypass graft(s) of the extremities with rest pain, left leg** HCC A
- **I70.623 Atherosclerosis of nonbiological bypass graft(s) of the extremities with rest pain, bilateral legs** HCC A
- **I70.628 Atherosclerosis of nonbiological bypass graft(s) of the extremities with rest pain, other extremity** HCC A
- **I70.629 Atherosclerosis of nonbiological bypass graft(s) of the extremities with rest pain, unspecified extremity** HCC A

✓6ᵗʰ I70.63 Atherosclerosis of nonbiological bypass graft(s) of the right leg with ulceration

INCLUDES any condition classifiable to I70.611 and I70.621

Use additional code to identify severity of ulcer (L97.-)

CC Excl: For CC codes in subcategory I70.63: PDX collection 698

- **I70.631 Atherosclerosis of nonbiological bypass graft(s) of the right leg with ulceration of thigh** CC HCC A
- **I70.632 Atherosclerosis of nonbiological bypass graft(s) of the right leg with ulceration of calf** CC HCC A
- **I70.633 Atherosclerosis of nonbiological bypass graft(s) of the right leg with ulceration of ankle** CC HCC A
- **I70.634 Atherosclerosis of nonbiological bypass graft(s) of the right leg with ulceration of heel and midfoot** CC HCC A
  Atherosclerosis of nonbiological bypass graft(s) of right leg with ulceration of plantar surface of midfoot
- **I70.635 Atherosclerosis of nonbiological bypass graft(s) of the right leg with ulceration of other part of foot** HCC A
  Atherosclerosis of nonbiological bypass graft(s) of the right leg with ulceration of toe
- **I70.638 Atherosclerosis of nonbiological bypass graft(s) of the right leg with ulceration of other part of lower leg** CC HCC A
- **I70.639 Atherosclerosis of nonbiological bypass graft(s) of the right leg with ulceration of unspecified site** CC HCC A

✓6ᵗʰ I70.64 Atherosclerosis of nonbiological bypass graft(s) of the left leg with ulceration

INCLUDES any condition classifiable to I70.612 and I70.622

Use additional code to identify severity of ulcer (L97.-)

CC Excl: For CC codes in subcategory I70.64: PDX collection 698

- **I70.641 Atherosclerosis of nonbiological bypass graft(s) of the left leg with ulceration of thigh** CC HCC A
- **I70.642 Atherosclerosis of nonbiological bypass graft(s) of the left leg with ulceration of calf** CC HCC A
- **I70.643 Atherosclerosis of nonbiological bypass graft(s) of the left leg with ulceration of ankle** CC HCC A
- **I70.644 Atherosclerosis of nonbiological bypass graft(s) of the left leg with ulceration of heel and midfoot** CC HCC A
  Atherosclerosis of nonbiological bypass graft(s) of left leg with ulceration of plantar surface of midfoot
- **I70.645 Atherosclerosis of nonbiological bypass graft(s) of the left leg with ulceration of other part of foot** HCC A
  Atherosclerosis of nonbiological bypass graft(s) of the left leg with ulceration of toe
- **I70.648 Atherosclerosis of nonbiological bypass graft(s) of the left leg with ulceration of other part of lower leg** CC HCC A
- **I70.649 Atherosclerosis of nonbiological bypass graft(s) o f the left leg with ulceration of unspecified site** CC HCC A

N Newborn: 0   P Pediatric: 0-17   M Maternity: 12-55   A Adult: 15-124   MCC Major Complication/Comorbidity   CC Complication/Comorbidity   SW Severe Wound Dx

662   ICD-10-CM 2019

I70.65   **Atherosclerosis of nonbiological bypass graft(s) of** other extremity **with** ulceration   HCC A
     INCLUDES   any condition classifiable to I70.618 and I70.628
     Use additional code to identify severity of ulcer (L98.49)

√6ᵗʰ **I70.66**   **Atherosclerosis of nonbiological bypass graft(s) of the extremities with** gangrene
     INCLUDES   any condition classifiable to I70.61-, I70.62-, I70.63-, I70.64-, I70.65
     Use additional code to identify the severity of any ulcer (L97.-, L98.49-), if applicable

     CC Excl: For CC codes in subcategory I70.66: PDX collection 519

     I70.661   **Atherosclerosis of nonbiological bypass graft(s) of the extremities with gangrene,** right leg   CC HCC A

     I70.662   **Atherosclerosis of nonbiological bypass graft(s) of the extremities with gangrene,** left leg   CC HCC A

     I70.663   **Atherosclerosis of nonbiological bypass graft(s) of the extremities with gangrene,** bilateral legs   CC HCC A

     I70.668   **Atherosclerosis of nonbiological bypass graft(s) of the extremities with gangrene,** other extremity   CC HCC A

     I70.669   **Atherosclerosis of nonbiological bypass graft(s) of the extremities with gangrene,** unspecified extremity   CC HCC A

√6ᵗʰ **I70.69**   **Other atherosclerosis of nonbiological bypass graft(s) of the extremities**

     I70.691   **Other atherosclerosis of nonbiological bypass graft(s) of the extremities,** right leg   HCC A

     I70.692   **Other atherosclerosis of nonbiological bypass graft(s) of the extremities,** left leg   HCC A

     I70.693   **Other atherosclerosis of nonbiological bypass graft(s) of the extremities,** bilateral legs   HCC A

     I70.698   **Other atherosclerosis of nonbiological bypass graft(s) of the extremities,** other extremity   HCC A

     I70.699   **Other atherosclerosis of nonbiological bypass graft(s) of the extremities,** unspecified extremity   HCC A

√5ᵗʰ **I70.7**   **Atherosclerosis of** other **type of** bypass graft(s) **of the extremities**
     Use additional code, if applicable, to identify chronic total occlusion of artery of extremity (I70.92)

√6ᵗʰ **I70.70**   Unspecified **atherosclerosis of other type of bypass graft(s) of the extremities**

     I70.701   **Unspecified atherosclerosis of other type of bypass graft(s) of the extremities,** right leg   HCC A

     I70.702   **Unspecified atherosclerosis of other type of bypass graft(s) of the extremities,** left leg   HCC A

     I70.703   **Unspecified atherosclerosis of other type of bypass graft(s) of the extremities,** bilateral legs   HCC A

     I70.708   **Unspecified atherosclerosis of other type of bypass graft(s) of the extremities,** other extremity   HCC A

     I70.709   **Unspecified atherosclerosis of other type of bypass graft(s) of the extremities,** unspecified extremity   HCC A

√6ᵗʰ **I70.71**   **Atherosclerosis of other type of bypass graft(s) of the extremities with** intermittent claudication

     I70.711   **Atherosclerosis of other type of bypass graft(s) of the extremities with intermittent claudication,** right leg   HCC A

     I70.712   **Atherosclerosis of other type of bypass graft(s) of the extremities with intermittent claudication,** left leg   HCC A

     I70.713   **Atherosclerosis of other type of bypass graft(s) of the extremities with intermittent claudication,** bilateral legs   HCC A

     I70.718   **Atherosclerosis of other type of bypass graft(s) of the extremities with intermittent claudication,** other extremity   HCC A

     I70.719   **Atherosclerosis of other type of bypass graft(s) of the extremities with intermittent claudication,** unspecified extremity   HCC A

√6ᵗʰ **I70.72**   **Atherosclerosis of other type of bypass graft(s) of the extremities with** rest pain
     INCLUDES   any condition classifiable to I70.71-

     I70.721   **Atherosclerosis of other type of bypass graft(s) of the extremities with rest pain,** right leg   HCC A

     I70.722   **Atherosclerosis of other type of bypass graft(s) of the extremities with rest pain,** left leg   HCC A

     I70.723   **Atherosclerosis of other type of bypass graft(s) of the extremities with rest pain,** bilateral legs   HCC A

     I70.728   **Atherosclerosis of other type of bypass graft(s) of the extremities with rest pain,** other extremity   HCC A

     I70.729   **Atherosclerosis of other type of bypass graft(s) of the extremities with rest pain,** unspecified extremity   HCC A

√6ᵗʰ **I70.73**   **Atherosclerosis of other type of bypass graft(s) of the** right leg **with** ulceration
     INCLUDES   any condition classifiable to I70.711 and I70.721
     Use additional code to identify severity of ulcer (L97.-)

     CC Excl: For CC codes in subcategory I70.73: PDX collection 698

     I70.731   **Atherosclerosis of other type of bypass graft(s) of the right leg with ulceration of** thigh   CC HCC A

     I70.732   **Atherosclerosis of other type of bypass graft(s) of the right leg with ulceration of** calf   CC HCC A

     I70.733   **Atherosclerosis of other type of bypass graft(s) of the right leg with ulceration of** ankle   CC HCC A

     I70.734   **Atherosclerosis of other type of bypass graft(s) of the right leg with ulceration of** heel and midfoot   CC HCC A
         Atherosclerosis of other type of bypass graft(s) of right leg with ulceration of plantar surface of midfoot

     I70.735   **Atherosclerosis of other type of bypass graft(s) of the right leg with ulceration of** other part of foot   HCC A
         Atherosclerosis of other type of bypass graft(s) of right leg with ulceration of toe

     I70.738   **Atherosclerosis of other type of bypass graft(s) of the right leg with ulceration of** other part of lower leg   CC HCC A

     I70.739   **Atherosclerosis of other type of bypass graft(s) of the right leg with ulceration of** unspecified site   CC HCC A

√6ᵗʰ **I70.74**   **Atherosclerosis of other type of bypass graft(s) of the** left leg **with** ulceration
     INCLUDES   any condition classifiable to I70.712 and I70.722
     Use additional code to identify severity of ulcer (L97.-)

     CC Excl: For CC codes in subcategory I70.74: PDX collection 698

     I70.741   **Atherosclerosis of other type of bypass graft(s) of the left leg with ulceration of** thigh   CC HCC A

     I70.742   **Atherosclerosis of other type of bypass graft(s) of the left leg with ulceration of** calf   CC HCC A

     I70.743   **Atherosclerosis of other type of bypass graft(s) of the left leg with ulceration of** ankle   CC HCC A

☑ Additional Character Required   √7ᵗʰ Placeholder   Unacceptable PDx   Questionable PDx   Manifestation   H1 - H14 HAC   HCC CMS-HCC Dx   HIV HIV Dx

ICD-10-CM 2019   663

Chapter 9. Diseases of the Circulatory System

I70.744   Atherosclerosis of other type of `CC` `HCC` `A`
bypass graft(s) of the left leg
with ulceration of heel and midfoot
Atherosclerosis of other type of bypass
graft(s) of left leg with ulceration of
plantar surface of midfoot

I70.745   Atherosclerosis of other type of `HCC` `A`
bypass graft(s) of the left leg with
ulceration of other part of foot
Atherosclerosis of other type of bypass
graft(s) of left leg with ulceration of
toe

I70.748   Atherosclerosis of other type of `CC` `HCC` `A`
bypass graft(s) of the left leg
with ulceration of other part
of lower leg

I70.749   Atherosclerosis of other type of `CC` `HCC` `A`
bypass graft(s) of the left leg
with ulceration of unspecified site

I70.75   Atherosclerosis of other type of bypass `HCC` `A`
graft(s) of other extremity with ulceration
INCLUDES any condition classifiable to I70.718 and
I70.728
Use additional code to identify severity of ulcer
(L98.49)

✓6ᵗʰ **I70.76   Atherosclerosis of other type of bypass graft(s) of**
the extremities with gangrene
INCLUDES any condition classifiable to I70.71-, I70.72-,
I70.73-, I70.74-, I70.75
Use additional code to identify the severity of any
ulcer (L97.-, L98.49-), if applicable

CC Excl: For CC codes in subcategory I70.76:
PDX collection 519

I70.761   Atherosclerosis of other type of `CC` `HCC` `A`
bypass graft(s) of the extremities
with gangrene, right leg

I70.762   Atherosclerosis of other type of `CC` `HCC` `A`
bypass graft(s) of the extremities
with gangrene, left leg

I70.763   Atherosclerosis of other type of `CC` `HCC` `A`
bypass graft(s) of the extremities
with gangrene, bilateral legs

I70.768   Atherosclerosis of other type of `CC` `HCC` `A`
bypass graft(s) of the extremities
with gangrene, other extremity

I70.769   Atherosclerosis of other type of `CC` `HCC` `A`
bypass graft(s) of the extremities
with gangrene, unspecified extremity

✓6ᵗʰ **I70.79   Other atherosclerosis of other type of bypass graft(s)**
of the extremities

I70.791   Other atherosclerosis of other type `HCC` `A`
of bypass graft(s) of the extremities,
right leg

I70.792   Other atherosclerosis of other type `HCC` `A`
of bypass graft(s) of the extremities,
left leg

I70.793   Other atherosclerosis of other type `HCC` `A`
of bypass graft(s) of the extremities,
bilateral legs

I70.798   Other atherosclerosis of other type `HCC` `A`
of bypass graft(s) of the extremities,
other extremity

I70.799   Other atherosclerosis of other type `HCC` `A`
of bypass graft(s) of the extremities,
unspecified extremity

I70.8   Atherosclerosis of other arteries `A`
TIP: Arteriosclerosis of the iliac arteries is coded here.

✓5ᵗʰ **I70.9   Other and unspecified atherosclerosis**
AHA: 2018, 2Q, 7

I70.90   Unspecified atherosclerosis `A`

I70.91   Generalized atherosclerosis `A`

I70.92   Chronic total occlusion of artery of the `CC` `HCC` `A`
extremities
Complete occlusion of artery of the extremities
Total occlusion of artery of the extremities
Code first atherosclerosis of arteries of the extremities
(I70.2-, I70.3-, I70.4-, I70.5-, I70.6-, I70.7-)
CC Excl: PDX collection 699

✓4ᵗʰ **I71   Aortic aneurysm and dissection**
EXCLUDES 1 aortic ectasia (I77.81-)
syphilitic aortic aneurysm (A52.01)
traumatic aortic aneurysm (S25.09, S35.09)

CC Excl: For MCC codes in category I71: PDX collection 700

✓5ᵗʰ **I71.0   Dissection of aorta**

I71.00   Dissection of unspecified site of aorta `MCC` `HCC`

I71.01   Dissection of thoracic aorta `MCC` `HCC`

I71.02   Dissection of abdominal aorta `MCC` `HCC`

I71.03   Dissection of thoracoabdominal aorta `MCC` `HCC`

I71.1   Thoracic aortic aneurysm, ruptured `MCC` `HCC`

I71.2   Thoracic aortic aneurysm, without rupture `HCC`

I71.3   Abdominal aortic aneurysm, ruptured `MCC` `HCC`

I71.4   Abdominal aortic aneurysm, without rupture `HCC`

I71.5   Thoracoabdominal aortic aneurysm, ruptured `MCC` `HCC`

I71.6   Thoracoabdominal aortic aneurysm, without rupture `HCC`

I71.8   Aortic aneurysm of unspecified site, ruptured `MCC` `HCC`
Rupture of aorta NOS

I71.9   Aortic aneurysm of unspecified site, without rupture `HCC`
Aneurysm of aorta
Dilatation of aorta
Hyaline necrosis of aorta

Aneurysm

Layers of muscular
and elastic tissue

Outer layer

Inner layer

Aneurysm

✓4ᵗʰ **I72   Other aneurysm**
INCLUDES aneurysm (cirsoid) (false) (ruptured)
EXCLUDES 2 acquired aneurysm (I77.0)
aneurysm (of) aorta (I71.-)
aneurysm (of) arteriovenous NOS (Q27.3-)
carotid artery dissection (I77.71)
cerebral (nonruptured) aneurysm (I67.1)
coronary aneurysm (I25.4)
coronary artery dissection (I25.42)
dissection of artery NEC (I77.79)
dissection of precerebral artery, congenital (nonruptured)
(Q28.1)
heart aneurysm (I25.3)
iliac artery dissection (I77.72)
precerebral artery, congenital (nonruptured) (Q28.1)
pulmonary artery aneurysm (I28.1)
renal artery dissection (I77.73)
retinal aneurysm (H35.0)
ruptured cerebral aneurysm (I60.7)
varicose aneurysm (I77.0)
vertebral artery dissection (I77.74)
AHA: 2016, 4Q, 28-29

I72.0   Aneurysm of carotid artery `HCC`
Aneurysm of common carotid artery
Aneurysm of external carotid artery
Aneurysm of internal carotid artery, extracranial portion
EXCLUDES 1 aneurysm of internal carotid artery, intracranial
portion (I67.1)
aneurysm of internal carotid artery NOS (I67.1)

I72.1   Aneurysm of artery of upper extremity `HCC`

I72.2   Aneurysm of renal artery `HCC`

I72.3   Aneurysm of iliac artery `HCC`

I72.4   Aneurysm of artery of lower extremity `HCC`

I72.5   **Aneurysm of** other precerebral **arteries**   `HCC`
Aneurysm of basilar artery (trunk)
    EXCLUDES 2   aneurysm of carotid artery (I72.0)
                    aneurysm of vertebral artery (I72.6)
                    dissection of carotid artery (I77.71)
                    dissection of other precerebral arteries (I77.75)
                    dissection of vertebral artery (I77.74)

I72.6   **Aneurysm of** vertebral **artery**   `HCC`
    EXCLUDES 2   dissection of vertebral artery (I77.74)

I72.8   **Aneurysm of** other specified **arteries**   `HCC`

I72.9   **Aneurysm of** unspecified **site**   `HCC`

✓4ᵗʰ **I73**   **Other peripheral vascular diseases**
    EXCLUDES 2   chilblains (T69.1)
                frostbite (T33- T34)
                immersion hand or foot (T69.0-)
                spasm of cerebral artery (G45.9)

✓5ᵗʰ **I73.0**   **Raynaud's syndrome**
Raynaud's disease
Raynaud's phenomenon (secondary)
DEF: Constriction of the arteries of the digits caused by cold or by nerve or arterial damage and can be prompted by stress or emotion. Blood cannot reach the skin and soft tissues and the skin turns white with blue mottling.

   I73.00   **Raynaud's syndrome** without gangrene

   I73.01   **Raynaud's syndrome** with gangrene   `CC` `HCC`
       CC Excl: PDX collection 519

I73.1   **Thromboangiitis obliterans [Buerger's disease]**   `HCC`
DEF: Inflammatory disease of the extremity blood vessels, mainly the lower blood vessels. This disease is associated with heavy tobacco use. The arteries are more affected than veins. It occurs primarily in young men and leads to tissue ischemia and gangrene.

✓5ᵗʰ **I73.8**   **Other specified peripheral vascular diseases**
    EXCLUDES 1   diabetic (peripheral) angiopathy (E08-E13 with .51-.52)

   I73.81   **Erythromelalgia**   `HCC`

   I73.89   **Other specified peripheral vascular diseases**   `HCC`
Acrocyanosis
Erythrocyanosis
Simple acroparesthesia [Schultze's type]
Vasomotor acroparesthesia [Nothnagel's type]

I73.9   **Peripheral vascular disease, unspecified**   `HCC`
Intermittent claudication
Peripheral angiopathy NOS
Spasm of artery
    EXCLUDES 1   atherosclerosis of the extremities (I70.2--I70.7-)
    AHA: 2018, 2Q, 7

✓4ᵗʰ **I74**   **Arterial embolism and thrombosis**
    INCLUDES   embolic infarction
               embolic occlusion
               thrombotic infarction
               thrombotic occlusion
Code first:
   embolism and thrombosis complicating abortion or ectopic or molar pregnancy (O00-O07, O08.2)
   embolism and thrombosis complicating pregnancy, childbirth and the puerperium (O88.-)
    EXCLUDES 2   atheroembolism (I75.-)
                basilar embolism and thrombosis (I63.0-I63.2, I65.1)
                carotid embolism and thrombosis (I63.0-I63.2, I65.2)
                cerebral embolism and thrombosis (I63.3-I63.5, I66-)
                coronary embolism and thrombosis (I21-I25)
                mesenteric embolism and thrombosis (K55.0-)
                ophthalmic embolism and thrombosis (H34.-)
                precerebral embolism and thrombosis NOS (I63.0-I63.2, I65.9)
                pulmonary embolism and thrombosis (I26.-)
                renal embolism and thrombosis (N28.0)
                retinal embolism and thrombosis (H34.-)
                septic embolism and thrombosis (I76)
                vertebral embolism and thrombosis (I63.0-I63.2, I65.0)

✓5ᵗʰ **I74.0**   **Embolism and thrombosis of** abdominal aorta

   I74.01   **Saddle embolus of abdominal aorta**   `MCC` `HCC`
       CC Excl: PDX collection 669

   I74.09   **Other arterial embolism and thrombosis of abdominal aorta**   `CC` `HCC`
Aortic bifurcation syndrome   Leriche's syndrome
Aortoiliac obstruction
       CC Excl: PDX collection 669

✓5ᵗʰ **I74.1**   **Embolism and thrombosis of** other and unspecified parts **of aorta**

   I74.10   **Embolism and thrombosis of** unspecified **parts of aorta**   `CC` `HCC`
       CC Excl: PDX collection 669

   I74.11   **Embolism and thrombosis of** thoracic **aorta**   `CC` `HCC`
       CC Excl: PDX collection 701

   I74.19   **Embolism and thrombosis of** other parts **of aorta**   `CC` `HCC`
       CC Excl: PDX collection 669

I74.2   **Embolism and thrombosis of arteries of the** upper extremities   `CC` `HCC`
       CC Excl: PDX collection 702

I74.3   **Embolism and thrombosis of arteries of the** lower extremities   `CC` `HCC`
       CC Excl: PDX collection 703

I74.4   **Embolism and thrombosis of arteries of** extremities, unspecified   `CC` `HCC`
Peripheral arterial embolism NOS
       CC Excl: PDX collection 703

I74.5   **Embolism and thrombosis of** iliac **artery**   `CC` `HCC`
       CC Excl: PDX collection 704

I74.8   **Embolism and thrombosis of** other **arteries**   `CC` `HCC`
       CC Excl: PDX collection 705

I74.9   **Embolism and thrombosis of** unspecified **artery**   `CC` `HCC`
       CC Excl: PDX collection 705

✓4ᵗʰ **I75**   **Atheroembolism**
    INCLUDES   atherothrombotic microembolism
               cholesterol embolism

✓5ᵗʰ **I75.0**   **Atheroembolism of** extremities

   ✓6ᵗʰ **I75.01**   **Atheroembolism of** upper **extremity**

       CC Excl: For CC codes in subcategory I75.01: PDX collection 706

     I75.011   **Atheroembolism of** right upper **extremity**   `CC` `HCC`

     I75.012   **Atheroembolism of** left upper **extremity**   `CC` `HCC`

     I75.013   **Atheroembolism of** bilateral **upper extremities**   `CC` `HCC`

     I75.019   **Atheroembolism of** unspecified **upper extremity**   `CC` `HCC`

   ✓6ᵗʰ **I75.02**   **Atheroembolism of** lower **extremity**

       CC Excl: For CC codes in subcategory I75.02: PDX collection 707

     I75.021   **Atheroembolism of** right lower **extremity**   `CC` `HCC`

     I75.022   **Atheroembolism of** left lower **extremity**   `CC` `HCC`

     I75.023   **Atheroembolism of** bilateral lower **extremities**   `CC` `HCC`

     I75.029   **Atheroembolism of** unspecified **lower extremity**   `CC` `HCC`

✓5ᵗʰ **I75.8**   **Atheroembolism of** other sites

   I75.81   **Atheroembolism of** kidney   `CC` `HCC`
Use additional code for any associated acute kidney failure and chronic kidney disease (N17.-, N18.-)
       CC Excl: PDX collection 708

   I75.89   **Atheroembolism of** other site   `CC` `HCC`
       CC Excl: PDX collection 709

I76   **Septic arterial embolism**   `CC` `HCC`
Code first underlying infection, such as:
   infective endocarditis (I33.0)
   lung abscess (J85.-)
Use additional code to identify the site of the embolism (I74.-)
    EXCLUDES 2   septic pulmonary embolism (I26.01, I26.90)
    CC Excl: PDX collection 705

✓ Additional Character Required   ✓x7ᵗʰ Placeholder   Unacceptable PDx   Questionable PDx   Manifestation   **H1**-**H14** HAC   **HCC** CMS-HCC Dx   **HIV** HIV Dx

ICD-10-CM 2019   **665**

√4ᵗʰ **I77   Other disorders of arteries and arterioles**
  EXCLUDES 2   *collagen (vascular) diseases (M30-M36)*
      hypersensitivity angiitis (M31.0)
      pulmonary artery (I28.-)

I77.0   Arteriovenous fistula, acquired   HCC
  Aneurysmal varix
  Arteriovenous aneurysm, acquired
    EXCLUDES 1   *arteriovenous aneurysm NOS (Q27.3-)*
        presence of arteriovenous shunt (fistula) for dialysis
          (Z99.2)
        traumatic—see injury of blood vessel by body region
    EXCLUDES 2   *cerebral (I67.1)*
        coronary (I25.4)
  DEF: Communication between an artery and vein caused by
  trauma or invasive procedures.

I77.1   Stricture of artery   HCC
  Narrowing of artery

I77.2   Rupture of artery   CC HCC
  Erosion of artery
  Fistula of artery
  Ulcer of artery
    EXCLUDES 1   *traumatic rupture of artery—see injury of blood vessel*
        by body region
  CC Excl: PDX collection 710

I77.3   Arterial fibromuscular dysplasia   HCC
  Fibromuscular hyperplasia (of) carotid artery
  Fibromuscular hyperplasia (of) renal artery

I77.4   Celiac artery compression syndrome   CC HCC
  CC Excl: PDX collection 711

I77.5   Necrosis of artery   CC HCC
  CC Excl: PDX collection 712

I77.6   Arteritis, unspecified   HCC
  Aortitis NOS
  Endarteritis NOS
    EXCLUDES 1   *arteritis or endarteritis:*
        aortic arch (M31.4)
        cerebral NEC (I67.7)
        coronary (I25.89)
        deformans (I70.-)
        giant cell (M31.5, M31.6)
        obliterans (I70.-)
        senile (I70.-)

√5ᵗʰ **I77.7   Other arterial dissection**
    EXCLUDES 2   *dissection of aorta (I71.0-)*
        dissection of coronary artery (I25.42)
  AHA: 2016, 4Q, 28-29

  CC Excl: For MCC codes in subcategory I77.7:
  PDX collection 689

  I77.70   Dissection of unspecified **artery**   MCC HCC
  I77.71   Dissection of carotid **artery**   MCC HCC
  I77.72   Dissection of iliac **artery**   MCC HCC
  I77.73   Dissection of renal **artery**   MCC HCC
  I77.74   Dissection of vertebral **artery**   MCC HCC
      EXCLUDES 2   *aneurysm of vertebral artery (I72.6)*
  I77.75   Dissection of other precerebral **arteries**   MCC HCC
      Dissection of basilar artery (trunk)
      EXCLUDES 2   *aneurysm of carotid artery (I72.0)*
          aneurysm of other precerebral arteries (I72.5)
          aneurysm of vertebral artery (I72.6)
          dissection of carotid artery (I77.71)
          dissection of vertebral artery (I77.74)
  I77.76   Dissection of artery of upper extremity   MCC HCC
  I77.77   Dissection of artery of lower extremity   MCC HCC
  I77.79   Dissection of other specified **artery**   MCC HCC

√5ᵗʰ **I77.8   Other specified disorders of arteries and arterioles**
  √6ᵗʰ **I77.81   Aortic ectasia**
      Ectasis aorta
      EXCLUDES 1   *aortic aneurysm and dissection (I71.0-)*
      I77.810   Thoracic aortic ectasia   HCC
      I77.811   Abdominal aortic ectasia   HCC
      I77.812   Thoracoabdominal aortic ectasia   HCC
      I77.819   Aortic ectasia, unspecified site   HCC
  I77.89   Other specified disorders of arteries and   HCC
      arterioles

I77.9   Disorder of arteries and arterioles, unspecified   HCC
  AHA: 2018, 2Q, 7

√4ᵗʰ **I78   Diseases of capillaries**
I78.0   Hereditary hemorrhagic telangiectasia   HCC
  Rendu-Osler-Weber disease

I78.1   Nevus, non-neoplastic
  Araneus nevus   Spider nevus
  Senile nevus   Stellar nevus
    EXCLUDES 1   *nevus NOS (D22.-)*
        vascular NOS (Q82.5)
    EXCLUDES 2   *blue nevus (D22.-)*
        flammeus nevus (Q82.5)
        hairy nevus (D22.-)
        melanocytic nevus (D22.-)
        pigmented nevus (D22.-)
        portwine nevus (Q82.5)
        sanguineous nevus (Q82.5)
        strawberry nevus (Q82.5)
        verrucous nevus (Q82.5)

I78.8   Other diseases of capillaries
I78.9   Disease of capillaries, unspecified

√4ᵗʰ **I79   Disorders of arteries, arterioles and capillaries in diseases**
    classified elsewhere
I79.0   Aneurysm of aorta in diseases classified elsewhere   HCC
  Code first underlying disease
    EXCLUDES 1   *syphilitic aneurysm (A52.01)*

I79.1   Aortitis in diseases classified elsewhere   HCC
  Code first underlying disease
    EXCLUDES 1   *syphilitic aortitis (A52.02)*

I79.8   Other disorders of arteries, arterioles and capillaries   HCC
    in diseases classified elsewhere
  Code first underlying disease, such as:
    amyloidosis (E85.-)
    EXCLUDES 1   *diabetic (peripheral) angiopathy (E08-E13 with .51-*
        .52)
        syphilitic endarteritis (A52.09)
        tuberculous endarteritis (A18.89)

Diseases of veins, lymphatic vessels and lymph nodes, not elsewhere classified (I80-I89)

√4ᵗʰ **I80   Phlebitis and thrombophlebitis**
  INCLUDES   endophlebitis
      inflammation, vein
      periphlebitis
      suppurative phlebitis
  Code first:
    phlebitis and thrombophlebitis complicating abortion, ectopic or
      molar pregnancy (O00-O07, O08.7)
    phlebitis and thrombophlebitis complicating pregnancy, childbirth
      and the puerperium (O22.-, O87.-)
    EXCLUDES 1   *venous embolism and thrombosis of lower extremities (I82.4-,*
        I82.5-, I82.81-)

  CC Excl: For CC codes in category I80: PDX collection 713

√5ᵗʰ **I80.0   Phlebitis and thrombophlebitis of** superficial vessels **of** lower
    extremities
  Phlebitis and thrombophlebitis of femoropopliteal vein
  I80.00   Phlebitis and thrombophlebitis of superficial vessels
      of unspecified **lower extremity**
  I80.01   Phlebitis and thrombophlebitis of superficial vessels
      of right **lower extremity**
  I80.02   Phlebitis and thrombophlebitis of superficial vessels
      of left **lower extremity**
  I80.03   Phlebitis and thrombophlebitis of superficial vessels
      of lower extremities, bilateral

√5ᵗʰ **I80.1   Phlebitis and thrombophlebitis of** femoral vein
  I80.10   Phlebitis and thrombophlebitis of   CC HCC
      unspecified **femoral vein**
  I80.11   Phlebitis and thrombophlebitis of right   CC HCC
      femoral vein
  I80.12   Phlebitis and thrombophlebitis of left   CC HCC
      femoral vein
  I80.13   Phlebitis and thrombophlebitis of femoral   CC HCC
      vein, bilateral

☑5ᵗʰ **I8Ø.2** **Phlebitis and thrombophlebitis of** other and unspecified deep vessels **of** lower extremities

☑6ᵗʰ **I8Ø.2Ø** **Phlebitis and thrombophlebitis of** unspecified **deep vessels of lower extremities**

I8Ø.2Ø1 **Phlebitis and thrombophlebitis of** CC HCC **unspecified deep vessels of** right **lower extremity**

I8Ø.2Ø2 **Phlebitis and thrombophlebitis of** CC HCC **unspecified deep vessels of** left **lower extremity**

I8Ø.2Ø3 **Phlebitis and thrombophlebitis of** CC HCC **unspecified deep vessels of lower extremities,** bilateral

I8Ø.2Ø9 **Phlebitis and thrombophlebitis of** CC HCC **unspecified deep vessels of** unspecified **lower extremity**

☑6ᵗʰ **I8Ø.21** **Phlebitis and thrombophlebitis of** iliac vein

I8Ø.211 **Phlebitis and thrombophlebitis of** CC HCC **right iliac vein**

I8Ø.212 **Phlebitis and thrombophlebitis of** CC HCC **left iliac vein**

I8Ø.213 **Phlebitis and thrombophlebitis of** CC HCC **iliac vein, bilateral**

I8Ø.219 **Phlebitis and thrombophlebitis of** CC HCC **unspecified iliac vein**

☑6ᵗʰ **I8Ø.22** **Phlebitis and thrombophlebitis of** popliteal vein

I8Ø.221 **Phlebitis and thrombophlebitis of** CC HCC **right popliteal vein**

I8Ø.222 **Phlebitis and thrombophlebitis of** CC HCC **left popliteal vein**

I8Ø.223 **Phlebitis and thrombophlebitis of** CC HCC **popliteal vein, bilateral**

I8Ø.229 **Phlebitis and thrombophlebitis of** CC HCC **unspecified popliteal vein**

☑6ᵗʰ **I8Ø.23** **Phlebitis and thrombophlebitis of** tibial vein

I8Ø.231 **Phlebitis and thrombophlebitis of** CC HCC **right tibial vein**

I8Ø.232 **Phlebitis and thrombophlebitis of** CC HCC **left tibial vein**

I8Ø.233 **Phlebitis and thrombophlebitis of** CC HCC **tibial vein, bilateral**

I8Ø.239 **Phlebitis and thrombophlebitis of** CC HCC **unspecified tibial vein**

☑6ᵗʰ **I8Ø.29** **Phlebitis and thrombophlebitis of** other **deep vessels of lower extremities**

I8Ø.291 **Phlebitis and thrombophlebitis of** CC HCC **other deep vessels of** right **lower extremity**

I8Ø.292 **Phlebitis and thrombophlebitis of** CC HCC **other deep vessels of** left **lower extremity**

I8Ø.293 **Phlebitis and thrombophlebitis of** CC HCC **other deep vessels of lower extremity,** bilateral

I8Ø.299 **Phlebitis and thrombophlebitis of** CC HCC **other deep vessels of** unspecified **lower extremity**

I8Ø.3 **Phlebitis and thrombophlebitis of lower extremities,** unspecified

I8Ø.8 **Phlebitis and thrombophlebitis of** other **sites**

I8Ø.9 **Phlebitis and thrombophlebitis of** unspecified **site**

I81 **Portal vein thrombosis** MCC
Portal (vein) obstruction
EXCLUDES 2 *hepatic vein thrombosis (I82.Ø)*
phlebitis of portal vein (K75.1)
CC Excl: PDX collection 714

☑4ᵗʰ **I82** **Other venous embolism and thrombosis**
Code first venous embolism and thrombosis complicating:
abortion, ectopic or molar pregnancy (OØØ-OØ7, OØ8.7)
pregnancy, childbirth and the puerperium (O22.-, O87.-)
EXCLUDES 2 *venous embolism and thrombosis (of):*
cerebral (I63.6, I67.6)
coronary (I21-I25)
intracranial and intraspinal, septic or NOS (GØ8)
intracranial, nonpyogenic (I67.6)
intraspinal, nonpyogenic (G95.1)
mesenteric (K55.Ø-)
portal (I81)
pulmonary (I26.-)

CC Excl: For CC/MCC codes in category I82, unless otherwise noted: PDX collection 717

I82.Ø **Budd-Chiari syndrome** MCC HCC
Hepatic vein thrombosis
DEF: Thrombosis or other obstruction of the hepatic veins. Symptoms include an enlarged liver, extensive collateral vessels, intractable ascites, and severe portal hypertension.
CC Excl: PDX collection 715

I82.1 **Thrombophlebitis migrans** CC
CC Excl: PDX collection 716

☑5ᵗʰ **I82.2** **Embolism and thrombosis of** vena cava **and** other thoracic veins

☑6ᵗʰ **I82.21** **Embolism and thrombosis of** superior vena cava

I82.21Ø **Acute embolism and thrombosis** CC HCC **of superior vena cava**
Embolism and thrombosis of superior vena cava NOS

I82.211 **Chronic embolism and thrombosis** CC HCC **of superior vena cava**

☑6ᵗʰ **I82.22** **Embolism and thrombosis of** inferior vena cava

I82.22Ø **Acute embolism and thrombosis** MCC HCC **of inferior vena cava**
Embolism and thrombosis of inferior vena cava NOS
CC Excl: PDX collection 718

I82.221 **Chronic embolism and thrombosis of inferior vena cava** MCC HCC
CC Excl: PDX collection 718

☑6ᵗʰ **I82.29** **Embolism and thrombosis of** other thoracic veins
Embolism and thrombosis of brachiocephalic (innominate) vein

I82.29Ø **Acute embolism and thrombosis** CC HCC **of other thoracic veins**

I82.291 **Chronic embolism and thrombosis** CC HCC **of other thoracic veins**

I82.3 **Embolism and thrombosis of** renal vein CC HCC
CC Excl: PDX collection 719

☑5ᵗʰ **I82.4** **Acute embolism and thrombosis of** deep veins of lower extremity

☑6ᵗʰ **I82.4Ø** **Acute embolism and thrombosis of** unspecified **deep veins of** lower extremity
Deep vein thrombosis NOS
DVT NOS
EXCLUDES 1 *acute embolism and thrombosis of unspecified deep veins of distal lower extremity (I82.4Z-)*
acute embolism and thrombosis of unspecified deep veins of proximal lower extremity (I82.4Y-)

I82.4Ø1 **Acute embolism and thrombosis of unspecified deep veins of** right **lower extremity** CC H10 HCC

I82.4Ø2 **Acute embolism and thrombosis of unspecified deep veins of** left **lower extremity** CC H10 HCC

I82.4Ø3 **Acute embolism and thrombosis of unspecified deep veins of lower extremity,** bilateral CC H10 HCC

I82.4Ø9 **Acute embolism and thrombosis of unspecified deep veins of** unspecified **lower extremity** CC H10 HCC

☑6ᵗʰ **I82.41** **Acute embolism and thrombosis of** femoral vein

I82.411 **Acute embolism and thrombosis of** right **femoral vein** CC H10 HCC

I82.412 **Acute embolism and thrombosis of** left **femoral vein** CC H10 HCC

Chapter 9. Diseases of the Circulatory System

I82.413   Acute embolism and `CC` `H10` `HCC`
thrombosis of femoral vein, bilateral

I82.419   Acute embolism and `CC` `H10` `HCC`
thrombosis of unspecified femoral vein

✓6ᵗʰ **I82.42**   **Acute embolism and thrombosis of iliac vein**

I82.421   Acute embolism and `CC` `H10` `HCC`
thrombosis of right iliac vein

I82.422   Acute embolism and `CC` `H10` `HCC`
thrombosis of left iliac vein

I82.423   Acute embolism and `CC` `H10` `HCC`
thrombosis of iliac vein, bilateral

I82.429   Acute embolism and `CC` `H10` `HCC`
thrombosis of unspecified iliac vein

✓6ᵗʰ **I82.43**   **Acute embolism and thrombosis of popliteal vein**

I82.431   Acute embolism and `CC` `H10` `HCC`
thrombosis of right popliteal vein

I82.432   Acute embolism and `CC` `H10` `HCC`
thrombosis of left popliteal vein

I82.433   Acute embolism and `CC` `H10` `HCC`
thrombosis of popliteal vein, bilateral

I82.439   Acute embolism and `CC` `H10` `HCC`
thrombosis of unspecified popliteal vein

✓6ᵗʰ **I82.44**   **Acute embolism and thrombosis of tibial vein**

I82.441   Acute embolism and `CC` `H10` `HCC`
thrombosis of right tibial vein

I82.442   Acute embolism and `CC` `H10` `HCC`
thrombosis of left tibial vein

I82.443   Acute embolism and `CC` `H10` `HCC`
thrombosis of tibial vein, bilateral

I82.449   Acute embolism and `CC` `H10` `HCC`
unspecified tibial vein

✓6ᵗʰ **I82.49**   **Acute embolism and thrombosis of other specified deep vein of lower extremity**

I82.491   Acute embolism and `CC` `H10` `HCC`
thrombosis of other specified
deep vein of right lower extremity

I82.492   Acute embolism and `CC` `H10` `HCC`
thrombosis of other specified
deep vein of left lower extremity

I82.493   Acute embolism and `CC` `H10` `HCC`
thrombosis of other specified deep
vein of lower extremity, bilateral

I82.499   Acute embolism and `CC` `H10` `HCC`
thrombosis of other specified deep vein of
unspecified lower extremity

✓6ᵗʰ **I82.4Y**   **Acute embolism and thrombosis of unspecified deep veins of proximal lower extremity**

Acute embolism and thrombosis of deep vein of thigh NOS

Acute embolism and thrombosis of deep vein of upper leg NOS

I82.4Y1   Acute embolism and `CC` `H10` `HCC`
thrombosis of unspecified deep
veins of right proximal lower extremity

I82.4Y2   Acute embolism and `CC` `H10` `HCC`
thrombosis of unspecified deep
veins of left proximal lower extremity

I82.4Y3   Acute embolism and `CC` `H10` `HCC`
thrombosis of unspecified deep veins of
proximal lower extremity, bilateral

I82.4Y9   Acute embolism and `CC` `H10` `HCC`
thrombosis of unspecified deep veins of
unspecified proximal lower extremity

✓6ᵗʰ **I82.4Z**   **Acute embolism and thrombosis of unspecified deep veins of distal lower extremity**

Acute embolism and thrombosis of deep vein of calf NOS

Acute embolism and thrombosis of deep vein of lower leg NOS

I82.4Z1   Acute embolism and `CC` `H10` `HCC`
thrombosis of unspecified deep
veins of right distal lower extremity

I82.4Z2   Acute embolism and `CC` `H10` `HCC`
thrombosis of unspecified deep
veins of left distal lower extremity

I82.4Z3   Acute embolism and `CC` `H10` `HCC`
thrombosis of unspecified deep
veins of distal lower extremity, bilateral

I82.4Z9   Acute embolism and `CC` `H10` `HCC`
thrombosis of unspecified deep
veins of unspecified distal lower extremity

✓5ᵗʰ **I82.5**   **Chronic embolism and thrombosis of deep veins of lower extremity**

Use additional code, if applicable, for associated long-term (current) use of anticoagulants (Z79.01)

EXCLUDES 1   *personal history of venous embolism and thrombosis (Z86.718)*

✓6ᵗʰ **I82.50**   **Chronic embolism and thrombosis of unspecified deep veins of lower extremity**

EXCLUDES 1   *chronic embolism and thrombosis of unspecified deep veins of distal lower extremity (I82.5Z-)*
chronic embolism and thrombosis of unspecified deep veins of proximal lower extremity (I82.5Y-)

I82.501   Chronic embolism and thrombosis `CC` `HCC`
of unspecified deep veins of right lower
extremity

I82.502   Chronic embolism and thrombosis `CC` `HCC`
of unspecified deep veins of left lower
extremity

I82.503   Chronic embolism and thrombosis `CC` `HCC`
of unspecified deep veins of lower
extremity, bilateral

I82.509   Chronic embolism and thrombosis `CC` `HCC`
of unspecified deep veins of unspecified
lower extremity

✓6ᵗʰ **I82.51**   **Chronic embolism and thrombosis of femoral vein**

I82.511   Chronic embolism and thrombosis `CC` `HCC`
of right femoral vein

I82.512   Chronic embolism and thrombosis `CC` `HCC`
left femoral vein

I82.513   Chronic embolism and thrombosis `CC` `HCC`
of femoral vein, bilateral

I82.519   Chronic embolism and thrombosis `CC` `HCC`
of unspecified femoral vein

✓6ᵗʰ **I82.52**   **Chronic embolism and thrombosis of iliac vein**

I82.521   Chronic embolism and thrombosis `CC` `HCC`
of right iliac vein

I82.522   Chronic embolism and thrombosis `CC` `HCC`
of left iliac vein

I82.523   Chronic embolism and thrombosis `CC` `HCC`
of iliac vein, bilateral

I82.529   Chronic embolism and thrombosis `CC` `HCC`
of unspecified iliac vein

✓6ᵗʰ **I82.53**   **Chronic embolism and thrombosis of popliteal vein**

I82.531   Chronic embolism and thrombosis `CC` `HCC`
of right popliteal vein

I82.532   Chronic embolism and thrombosis `CC` `HCC`
of left popliteal vein

I82.533   Chronic embolism and thrombosis `CC` `HCC`
of popliteal vein, bilateral

I82.539   Chronic embolism and thrombosis `CC` `HCC`
of unspecified popliteal vein

✓6ᵗʰ **I82.54**   **Chronic embolism and thrombosis of tibial vein**

I82.541   Chronic embolism and thrombosis `CC` `HCC`
of right tibial vein

I82.542   Chronic embolism and thrombosis `CC` `HCC`
of left tibial vein

I82.543   Chronic embolism and thrombosis `CC` `HCC`
of tibial vein, bilateral

I82.549   Chronic embolism and thrombosis `CC` `HCC`
unspecified tibial vein

✓6ᵗʰ **I82.59**   **Chronic embolism and thrombosis of other specified deep vein of lower extremity**

I82.591   Chronic embolism and thrombosis `CC` `HCC`
of other specified deep vein of right lower
extremity

I82.592   Chronic embolism and thrombosis `CC` `HCC`
of other specified deep vein of left lower
extremity

I82.593   Chronic embolism and thrombosis `CC` `HCC`
of other specified deep vein of lower
extremity, bilateral

I82.599   Chronic embolism and thrombosis `CC` `HCC`
of other specified deep vein of unspecified
lower extremity

N Newborn: 0   P Pediatric: 0-17   M Maternity: 12-55   A Adult: 15-124   `MCC` Major Complication/Comorbidity   `CC` Complication/Comorbidity   `SW` Severe Wound Dx

668   ICD-10-CM 2019

☑6ᵗʰ **I82.5Y** **Chronic embolism and thrombosis of** unspecified **deep veins of** proximal lower extremity

Chronic embolism and thrombosis of deep veins of thigh NOS

Chronic embolism and thrombosis of deep veins of upper leg NOS

     I82.5Y1 **Chronic embolism and thrombosis** CC HCC **of unspecified deep veins of** right **proximal lower extremity**

     I82.5Y2 **Chronic embolism and thrombosis** CC HCC **of unspecified deep veins of** left **proximal lower extremity**

     I82.5Y3 **Chronic embolism and thrombosis** CC HCC **of unspecified deep veins of proximal lower extremity, bilateral**

     I82.5Y9 **Chronic embolism and thrombosis** CC HCC **of unspecified deep veins of** unspecified **proximal lower extremity**

☑6ᵗʰ **I82.5Z** **Chronic embolism and thrombosis of** unspecified **deep veins of** distal lower extremity

Chronic embolism and thrombosis of deep veins of calf NOS

Chronic embolism and thrombosis of deep veins of lower leg NOS

     I82.5Z1 **Chronic embolism and thrombosis** CC HCC **of unspecified deep veins of** right **distal lower extremity**

     I82.5Z2 **Chronic embolism and thrombosis** CC HCC **of unspecified deep veins of** left **distal lower extremity**

     I82.5Z3 **Chronic embolism and thrombosis** CC HCC **of unspecified deep veins of distal lower extremity, bilateral**

     I82.5Z9 **Chronic embolism and thrombosis** CC HCC **of unspecified deep veins of** unspecified **distal lower extremity**

☑5ᵗʰ **I82.6** Acute **embolism and thrombosis of veins of** upper extremity

☑6ᵗʰ **I82.60** **Acute embolism and thrombosis of** unspecified **veins of upper extremity**

     I82.601 **Acute embolism and thrombosis of** CC **unspecified veins of** right **upper extremity**

     I82.602 **Acute embolism and thrombosis of** CC **unspecified veins of** left **upper extremity**

     I82.603 **Acute embolism and thrombosis of** CC **unspecified veins of upper extremity, bilateral**

     I82.609 **Acute embolism and thrombosis of** CC **unspecified veins of** unspecified **upper extremity**

☑6ᵗʰ **I82.61** **Acute embolism and thrombosis of** superficial veins **of** upper extremity

Acute embolism and thrombosis of antecubital vein

Acute embolism and thrombosis of basilic vein

Acute embolism and thrombosis of cephalic vein

     I82.611 **Acute embolism and thrombosis of** CC **superficial veins of** right **upper extremity**

     I82.612 **Acute embolism and thrombosis of** CC **superficial veins of** left **upper extremity**

     I82.613 **Acute embolism and thrombosis of** CC **superficial veins of upper extremity, bilateral**

     I82.619 **Acute embolism and thrombosis of** CC **superficial veins of** unspecified **upper extremity**

☑6ᵗʰ **I82.62** **Acute embolism and thrombosis of** deep veins **of** upper extremity

Acute embolism and thrombosis of brachial vein

Acute embolism and thrombosis of radial vein

Acute embolism and thrombosis of ulnar vein

     I82.621 **Acute embolism and thrombosis of** CC HCC **deep veins of** right **upper extremity**

     I82.622 **Acute embolism and thrombosis of** CC HCC **deep veins of** left **upper extremity**

     I82.623 **Acute embolism and thrombosis of** CC HCC **deep veins of upper extremity, bilateral**

     I82.629 **Acute embolism and thrombosis of** CC HCC **deep veins of** unspecified **upper extremity**

☑5ᵗʰ **I82.7** Chronic **embolism and thrombosis of veins of** upper extremity

Use additional code, if applicable, for associated long-term (current) use of anticoagulants (Z79.01)

EXCLUDES 1   *personal history of venous embolism and thrombosis (Z86.718)*

☑6ᵗʰ **I82.70** **Chronic embolism and thrombosis of** unspecified **veins of upper extremity**

     I82.701 **Chronic embolism and thrombosis of** CC **unspecified veins of** right **upper extremity**

     I82.702 **Chronic embolism and thrombosis of** CC **unspecified veins of** left **upper extremity**

     I82.703 **Chronic embolism and thrombosis of** CC **unspecified veins of upper extremity, bilateral**

     I82.709 **Chronic embolism and thrombosis of** CC **unspecified veins of** unspecified **upper extremity**

☑6ᵗʰ **I82.71** **Chronic embolism and thrombosis of** superficial veins **of upper extremity**

Chronic embolism and thrombosis of antecubital vein

Chronic embolism and thrombosis of basilic vein

Chronic embolism and thrombosis of cephalic vein

     I82.711 **Chronic embolism and thrombosis of** CC **superficial veins of** right **upper extremity**

     I82.712 **Chronic embolism and thrombosis of** CC **superficial veins of** left **upper extremity**

     I82.713 **Chronic embolism and thrombosis of** CC **superficial veins of upper extremity, bilateral**

     I82.719 **Chronic embolism and thrombosis of** CC **superficial veins of** unspecified **upper extremity**

☑6ᵗʰ **I82.72** **Chronic embolism and thrombosis of** deep veins **of upper extremity**

Chronic embolism and thrombosis of brachial vein

Chronic embolism and thrombosis of radial vein

Chronic embolism and thrombosis of ulnar vein

     I82.721 **Chronic embolism and thrombosis** CC HCC **of deep veins of** right **upper extremity**

     I82.722 **Chronic embolism and thrombosis** CC HCC **of deep veins of** left **upper extremity**

     I82.723 **Chronic embolism and thrombosis** CC HCC **of deep veins of** upper **extremity, bilateral**

     I82.729 **Chronic embolism and thrombosis** CC HCC **of deep veins of** unspecified **upper extremity**

☑5ᵗʰ **I82.A** **Embolism and thrombosis of** axillary vein

☑6ᵗʰ **I82.A1** Acute **embolism and thrombosis of axillary vein**

     I82.A11 **Acute embolism and thrombosis** CC HCC **of** right **axillary vein**

     I82.A12 **Acute embolism and thrombosis** CC HCC **of** left **axillary vein**

     I82.A13 **Acute embolism and thrombosis** CC HCC **of axillary vein,** bilateral

     I82.A19 **Acute embolism and thrombosis** CC HCC **of** unspecified **axillary vein**

☑6ᵗʰ **I82.A2** Chronic **embolism and thrombosis of axillary vein**

     I82.A21 **Chronic embolism and thrombosis** CC HCC **of** right **axillary vein**

     I82.A22 **Chronic embolism and thrombosis** CC HCC **of** left **axillary vein**

     I82.A23 **Chronic embolism and thrombosis** CC HCC **of axillary vein,** bilateral

     I82.A29 **Chronic embolism and thrombosis** CC HCC **of** unspecified **axillary vein**

☑5ᵗʰ **I82.B** **Embolism and thrombosis of** subclavian vein

☑6ᵗʰ **I82.B1** Acute **embolism and thrombosis of subclavian vein**

     I82.B11 **Acute embolism and thrombosis** CC HCC **of** right **subclavian vein**

     I82.B12 **Acute embolism and thrombosis** CC HCC **of** left **subclavian vein**

☑Additional Character Required   ◼T◼ Placeholder   Unacceptable PDx   Questionable PDx   Manifestation   H1-H14 HAC   HCC CMS-HCC Dx   HIV HIV Dx

I82.B13 **Acute embolism and thrombosis** `CC` `HCC`
of subclavian vein, bilateral

I82.B19 **Acute embolism and thrombosis** `CC` `HCC`
of unspecified subclavian vein

✓6ᵗʰ I82.B2 **Chronic** embolism and thrombosis of subclavian vein

I82.B21 **Chronic embolism and thrombosis** `CC` `HCC`
of right subclavian vein

I82.B22 **Chronic embolism and thrombosis** `CC` `HCC`
of left subclavian vein

I82.B23 **Chronic embolism and thrombosis** `CC` `HCC`
of subclavian vein, bilateral

I82.B29 **Chronic embolism and thrombosis** `CC` `HCC`
of unspecified subclavian vein

✓5ᵗʰ I82.C **Embolism and thrombosis of** internal jugular vein

✓6ᵗʰ I82.C1 **Acute** embolism and thrombosis of internal jugular vein

I82.C11 **Acute embolism and thrombosis** `CC` `HCC`
of right internal jugular vein

I82.C12 **Acute embolism and thrombosis** `CC` `HCC`
of left internal jugular vein

I82.C13 **Acute embolism and thrombosis** `CC` `HCC`
of internal jugular vein, bilateral

I82.C19 **Acute embolism and thrombosis** `CC` `HCC`
of unspecified internal jugular vein

✓6ᵗʰ I82.C2 **Chronic** embolism and thrombosis of internal jugular vein

I82.C21 **Chronic embolism and thrombosis** `CC` `HCC`
of right internal jugular vein

I82.C22 **Chronic embolism and thrombosis** `CC` `HCC`
of left internal jugular vein

I82.C23 **Chronic embolism and thrombosis** `CC` `HCC`
of internal jugular vein, bilateral

I82.C29 **Chronic embolism and thrombosis** `CC` `HCC`
of unspecified internal jugular vein

✓5ᵗʰ I82.8 **Embolism and thrombosis of other** specified veins
Use additional code, if applicable, for associated long-term (current) use of anticoagulants (Z79.01)

✓6ᵗʰ I82.81 **Embolism and thrombosis of superficial veins of** lower extremities
Embolism and thrombosis of saphenous vein (greater) (lesser)

I82.811 **Embolism and thrombosis of** `CC`
superficial veins of right lower extremity

I82.812 **Embolism and thrombosis of** `CC`
superficial veins of left lower extremity

I82.813 **Embolism and thrombosis of** `CC`
superficial veins of lower extremities, bilateral

I82.819 **Embolism and thrombosis of** `CC`
superficial veins of unspecified lower extremity

✓6ᵗʰ I82.89 **Embolism and thrombosis of** other specified veins

I82.890 **Acute embolism and thrombosis of** `CC`
other specified veins

I82.891 **Chronic embolism and thrombosis of** `CC`
other specified veins

✓5ᵗʰ I82.9 **Embolism and thrombosis of** unspecified vein

I82.90 **Acute embolism and thrombosis of unspecified** `CC`
vein
Embolism of vein NOS
Thrombosis (vein) NOS

I82.91 **Chronic embolism and thrombosis of** `CC`
unspecified vein

✓4ᵗʰ I83 **Varicose veins of lower extremities**
EXCLUDES 1 varicose veins complicating pregnancy (O22.0-)
varicose veins complicating the puerperium (O87.4)

✓5ᵗʰ I83.0 **Varicose veins of lower extremities with** ulcer
Use additional code to identify severity of ulcer (L97.-)

✓6ᵗʰ I83.00 **Varicose veins of** unspecified **lower extremity with** ulcer

I83.001 **Varicose veins of unspecified lower** `HCC` `A`
extremity with ulcer of thigh

I83.002 **Varicose veins of unspecified lower** `HCC` `A`
extremity with ulcer of calf

I83.003 **Varicose veins of unspecified lower** `HCC` `A`
extremity with ulcer of ankle

I83.004 **Varicose veins of unspecified lower** `HCC` `A`
extremity with ulcer of heel and midfoot
Varicose veins of unspecified lower extremity with ulcer of plantar surface of midfoot

I83.005 **Varicose veins of unspecified lower** `HCC` `A`
extremity with ulcer other part of foot
Varicose veins of unspecified lower extremity with ulcer of toe

I83.008 **Varicose veins of unspecified lower** `HCC` `A`
extremity with ulcer other part of lower leg

I83.009 **Varicose veins of unspecified lower** `HCC` `A`
extremity with ulcer of unspecified site

✓6ᵗʰ I83.01 **Varicose veins of** right **lower extremity with ulcer**

I83.011 **Varicose veins of right lower** `HCC` `A`
extremity with ulcer of thigh

I83.012 **Varicose veins of right lower** `HCC` `A`
extremity with ulcer of calf

I83.013 **Varicose veins of right lower** `HCC` `A`
extremity with ulcer of ankle

I83.014 **Varicose veins of right lower** `HCC` `A`
extremity with ulcer of heel and midfoot
Varicose veins of right lower extremity with ulcer of plantar surface of midfoot

I83.015 **Varicose veins of right lower** `HCC` `A`
extremity with ulcer other part of foot
Varicose veins of right lower extremity with ulcer of toe

I83.018 **Varicose veins of right lower** `HCC` `A`
extremity with ulcer other part of lower leg

I83.019 **Varicose veins of right lower** `HCC` `A`
extremity with ulcer of unspecified site

✓6ᵗʰ I83.02 **Varicose veins of** left **lower extremity with ulcer**

I83.021 **Varicose veins of left lower** `HCC` `A`
extremity with ulcer of thigh

I83.022 **Varicose veins of left lower** `HCC` `A`
extremity with ulcer of calf

I83.023 **Varicose veins of left lower** `HCC` `A`
extremity with ulcer of ankle

I83.024 **Varicose veins of left lower** `HCC` `A`
extremity with ulcer of heel and midfoot
Varicose veins of left lower extremity with ulcer of plantar surface of midfoot

I83.025 **Varicose veins of left lower** `HCC` `A`
extremity with ulcer other part of foot
Varicose veins of left lower extremity with ulcer of toe

I83.028 **Varicose veins of left lower** `HCC` `A`
extremity with ulcer other part of lower leg

I83.029 **Varicose veins of left lower** `HCC` `A`
extremity with ulcer of unspecified site

✓5ᵗʰ I83.1 **Varicose veins of lower extremities with** inflammation

I83.10 **Varicose veins of** unspecified **lower extremity** `A`
with inflammation

I83.11 **Varicose veins of** right **lower extremity with** `A`
inflammation

I83.12 **Varicose veins of** left **lower extremity with** `A`
inflammation

✓5ᵗʰ I83.2 **Varicose veins of lower extremities with both** ulcer and inflammation
Use additional code to identify severity of ulcer (L97.-)

CC Excl: For CC codes in subcategory I83.2:
PDX collection 720

✓6ᵗʰ I83.20 **Varicose veins of** unspecified **lower extremity with both ulcer and inflammation**

I83.201 **Varicose veins of unspecified** `CC` `HCC` `A`
lower extremity with both ulcer of thigh and inflammation

I83.202 **Varicose veins of unspecified** `CC` `HCC` `A`
lower extremity with both ulcer of calf and inflammation

I83.203 **Varicose veins of unspecified** `CC` `HCC` `A`
lower extremity with both ulcer of ankle and inflammation

I83.204   Varicose veins of unspecified `CC` `HCC` `A`
lower extremity with both ulcer of heel
and midfoot and inflammation
> Varicose veins of unspecified lower
> extremity with both ulcer of plantar
> surface of midfoot and inflammation

I83.205   Varicose veins of unspecified `CC` `HCC` `A`
lower extremity with both ulcer of other
part of foot and inflammation
> Varicose veins of unspecified lower
> extremity with both ulcer of toe and
> inflammation

I83.208   Varicose veins of unspecified `CC` `HCC` `A`
lower extremity with both ulcer
of other part of lower extremity and
inflammation

I83.209   Varicose veins of unspecified `CC` `HCC` `A`
lower extremity with both ulcer of
unspecified site and inflammation

✓6ᵗʰ **I83.21**   Varicose veins of right lower extremity with both
ulcer and inflammation

I83.211   Varicose veins of right lower `CC` `HCC` `A`
extremity with both ulcer of thigh
and inflammation

I83.212   Varicose veins of right lower `CC` `HCC` `A`
extremity with both ulcer of calf
and inflammation

I83.213   Varicose veins of right lower `CC` `HCC` `A`
extremity with both ulcer of ankle
and inflammation

I83.214   Varicose veins of right lower `CC` `HCC` `A`
extremity with both ulcer of heel
and midfoot and inflammation
> Varicose veins of right lower extremity with
> both ulcer of plantar surface of
> midfoot and inflammation

I83.215   Varicose veins of right lower `CC` `HCC` `A`
extremity with both ulcer other
part of foot and inflammation
> Varicose veins of right lower extremity with
> both ulcer of toe and inflammation

I83.218   Varicose veins of right lower `CC` `HCC` `A`
extremity with both ulcer of other
part of lower extremity and
inflammation

I83.219   Varicose veins of right lower `CC` `HCC` `A`
extremity with both ulcer of
unspecified site and inflammation

✓6ᵗʰ **I83.22**   Varicose veins of left lower extremity with both ulcer
and inflammation

I83.221   Varicose veins of left lower `CC` `HCC` `A`
extremity with both ulcer of thigh
and inflammation

I83.222   Varicose veins of left lower `CC` `HCC` `A`
extremity with both ulcer of calf
and inflammation

I83.223   Varicose veins of left lower `CC` `HCC` `A`
extremity with both ulcer of ankle
and inflammation

I83.224   Varicose veins of left lower `CC` `HCC` `A`
extremity with both ulcer of heel and
midfoot and inflammation
> Varicose veins of left lower extremity with
> both ulcer of plantar surface of
> midfoot and inflammation

I83.225   Varicose veins of left lower `CC` `HCC` `A`
extremity with both ulcer other
part of foot and inflammation
> Varicose veins of left lower extremity with
> both ulcer of toe and inflammation

I83.228   Varicose veins of left lower `CC` `HCC` `A`
extremity with both ulcer of other
part of lower extremity and
inflammation

I83.229   Varicose veins of left lower `CC` `HCC` `A`
extremity with both ulcer of
unspecified site and inflammation

✓5ᵗʰ **I83.8**   Varicose veins of lower extremities with other complications

✓6ᵗʰ **I83.81**   Varicose veins of lower extremities with pain

I83.811   Varicose veins of right lower `A`
extremity with pain

I83.812   Varicose veins of left lower extremity `A`
with pain

I83.813   Varicose veins of bilateral lower `A`
extremities with pain

I83.819   Varicose veins of unspecified lower `A`
extremity with pain

✓6ᵗʰ **I83.89**   Varicose veins of lower extremities with other
complications
> Varicose veins of lower extremities with edema
> Varicose veins of lower extremities with swelling

I83.891   Varicose veins of right lower `A`
extremity with other complications

I83.892   Varicose veins of left lower extremity `A`
with other complications

I83.893   Varicose veins of bilateral lower `A`
extremities with other complications

I83.899   Varicose veins of unspecified lower `A`
extremity with other complications

✓5ᵗʰ **I83.9**   Asymptomatic varicose veins of lower extremities
> Phlebectasia of lower extremities
> Varicose veins of lower extremities
> Varix of lower extremities

I83.90   Asymptomatic varicose veins of unspecified `A`
lower extremity
> Varicose veins NOS

I83.91   Asymptomatic varicose veins of right lower `A`
extremity

I83.92   Asymptomatic varicose veins of left lower `A`
extremity

I83.93   Asymptomatic varicose veins of bilateral lower `A`
extremities

✓4ᵗʰ **I85**   **Esophageal varices**
> Use additional code to identify:
> alcohol abuse and dependence (F10.-)

✓5ᵗʰ **I85.0**   Esophageal varices
> Idiopathic esophageal varices
> Primary esophageal varices

I85.00   Esophageal varices without bleeding `CC` `HCC`
> Esophageal varices NOS
> **CC Excl:** PDX collection 721

I85.01   Esophageal varices with bleeding `MCC` `HCC`
> **CC Excl:** PDX collection 722

✓5ᵗʰ **I85.1**   Secondary esophageal varices
> Esophageal varices secondary to alcoholic liver disease
> Esophageal varices secondary to cirrhosis of liver
> Esophageal varices secondary to schistosomiasis
> Esophageal varices secondary to toxic liver disease
> Code first underlying disease

I85.10   Secondary esophageal varices without `CC` `HCC`
bleeding
> **CC Excl:** PDX collection 723

I85.11   Secondary esophageal varices with `MCC` `HCC`
bleeding
> **CC Excl:** PDX collection 724

✓4ᵗʰ **I86**   **Varicose veins of other sites**
> *EXCLUDES 1*   varicose veins of unspecified site (I83.9-)
> *EXCLUDES 2*   retinal varices (H35.0-)

I86.0   Sublingual varices
> **DEF:** Distended, tortuous veins beneath the tongue.

I86.1   Scrotal varices   ♂
> Varicocele

I86.2   Pelvic varices

I86.3   Vulval varices   ♀
> *EXCLUDES 1*   vulval varices complicating childbirth and the
> puerperium (O87.8)
> vulval varices complicating pregnancy (O22.1-)

I86.4   Gastric varices

I86.8   Varicose veins of other specified sites `A`
> Varicose ulcer of nasal septum

✓ Additional Character Required   ✓x 7ᵗʰ Placeholder   Unacceptable PDx   Questionable PDx   Manifestation   `H1`-`H14` HAC   `HCC` CMS-HCC Dx   `HIV` HIV Dx

ICD-10-CM 2019   671

Chapter 9. Diseases of the Circulatory System

I87–I87.393

√4ᵗʰ **I87 Other disorders of veins**

√5ᵗʰ **I87.0 Postthrombotic syndrome**
Chronic venous hypertension due to deep vein thrombosis
Postphlebitic syndrome
EXCLUDES 1   *chronic venous hypertension without deep vein thrombosis (I87.3-)*

CC Excl: For CC codes in subcategory I87.0:
PDX collection 725

√6ᵗʰ **I87.00 Postthrombotic syndrome without complications**
Asymptomatic postthrombotic syndrome

     I87.001 Postthrombotic syndrome without complications of right lower extremity

     I87.002 Postthrombotic syndrome without complications of left lower extremity

     I87.003 Postthrombotic syndrome without complications of bilateral lower extremity

     I87.009 Postthrombotic syndrome without complications of unspecified extremity
Postthrombotic syndrome NOS

√6ᵗʰ **I87.01 Postthrombotic syndrome with ulcer**
Use additional code to specify site and severity of ulcer (L97.-)

     I87.011 Postthrombotic syndrome with ulcer of right lower extremity `CC` `HCC`

     I87.012 Postthrombotic syndrome with ulcer of left lower extremity `CC` `HCC`

     I87.013 Postthrombotic syndrome with ulcer of bilateral lower extremity `CC` `HCC`

     I87.019 Postthrombotic syndrome with ulcer of unspecified lower extremity `CC` `HCC`

√6ᵗʰ **I87.02 Postthrombotic syndrome with inflammation**

     I87.021 Postthrombotic syndrome with inflammation of right lower extremity

     I87.022 Postthrombotic syndrome with inflammation of left lower extremity

     I87.023 Postthrombotic syndrome with inflammation of bilateral lower extremity

     I87.029 Postthrombotic syndrome with inflammation of unspecified lower extremity

√6ᵗʰ **I87.03 Postthrombotic syndrome with ulcer and inflammation**
Use additional code to specify site and severity of ulcer (L97.-)

     I87.031 Postthrombotic syndrome with ulcer and inflammation of right lower extremity `CC` `HCC`

     I87.032 Postthrombotic syndrome with ulcer and inflammation of left lower extremity `CC` `HCC`

     I87.033 Postthrombotic syndrome with ulcer and inflammation of bilateral lower extremity `CC` `HCC`

     I87.039 Postthrombotic syndrome with ulcer and inflammation of unspecified lower extremity `CC` `HCC`

√6ᵗʰ **I87.09 Postthrombotic syndrome with other complications**

     I87.091 Postthrombotic syndrome with other complications of right lower extremity

     I87.092 Postthrombotic syndrome with other complications of left lower extremity

     I87.093 Postthrombotic syndrome with other complications of bilateral lower extremity

     I87.099 Postthrombotic syndrome with other complications of unspecified lower extremity

I87.1 Compression of vein `CC`
Stricture of vein
Vena cava syndrome (inferior) (superior)
EXCLUDES 2   *compression of pulmonary vein (I28.8)*
CC Excl: PDX collection 726

I87.2 Venous insufficiency (chronic) (peripheral)
Stasis dermatitis
EXCLUDES 1   *stasis dermatitis with varicose veins of lower extremities (I83.1-, I83.2-)*
DEF: Insufficient drainage of venous blood in any part of the body that results in edema or dermatosis.

√5ᵗʰ **I87.3 Chronic venous hypertension (idiopathic)**
Stasis edema
EXCLUDES 1   *chronic venous hypertension due to deep vein thrombosis (I87.0-)*
      varicose veins of lower extremities (I83.-)

CC Excl: For CC codes in subcategory I87.3:
PDX collection 727

√6ᵗʰ **I87.30 Chronic venous hypertension (idiopathic) without complications**
Asymptomatic chronic venous hypertension (idiopathic)

     I87.301 Chronic venous hypertension (idiopathic) without complications of right lower extremity

     I87.302 Chronic venous hypertension (idiopathic) without complications of left lower extremity

     I87.303 Chronic venous hypertension (idiopathic) without complications of bilateral lower extremity

     I87.309 Chronic venous hypertension (idiopathic) without complications of unspecified lower extremity
Chronic venous hypertension NOS

√6ᵗʰ **I87.31 Chronic venous hypertension (idiopathic) with ulcer**
Use additional code to specify site and severity of ulcer (L97.-)

     I87.311 Chronic venous hypertension (idiopathic) with ulcer of right lower extremity `CC` `HCC`

     I87.312 Chronic venous hypertension (idiopathic) with ulcer of left lower extremity `CC` `HCC`

     I87.313 Chronic venous hypertension (idiopathic) with ulcer of bilateral lower extremity `CC` `HCC`

     I87.319 Chronic venous hypertension (idiopathic) with ulcer of unspecified lower extremity `CC` `HCC`

√6ᵗʰ **I87.32 Chronic venous hypertension (idiopathic) with inflammation**

     I87.321 Chronic venous hypertension (idiopathic) with inflammation of right lower extremity

     I87.322 Chronic venous hypertension (idiopathic) with inflammation of left lower extremity

     I87.323 Chronic venous hypertension (idiopathic) with inflammation of bilateral lower extremity

     I87.329 Chronic venous hypertension (idiopathic) with inflammation of unspecified lower extremity

√6ᵗʰ **I87.33 Chronic venous hypertension (idiopathic) with ulcer and inflammation**
Use additional code to specify site and severity of ulcer (L97.-)

     I87.331 Chronic venous hypertension (idiopathic) with ulcer and inflammation of right lower extremity `CC` `HCC`

     I87.332 Chronic venous hypertension (idiopathic) with ulcer and inflammation of left lower extremity `CC` `HCC`

     I87.333 Chronic venous hypertension (idiopathic) with ulcer and inflammation of bilateral lower extremity `CC` `HCC`

     I87.339 Chronic venous hypertension (idiopathic) with ulcer and inflammation of unspecified lower extremity `CC` `HCC`

√6ᵗʰ **I87.39 Chronic venous hypertension (idiopathic) with other complications**

     I87.391 Chronic venous hypertension (idiopathic) with other complications of right lower extremity

     I87.392 Chronic venous hypertension (idiopathic) with other complications of left lower extremity

     I87.393 Chronic venous hypertension (idiopathic) with other complications of bilateral lower extremity

N Newborn: 0   P Pediatric: 0-17   M Maternity: 12-55   A Adult: 15-124   MCC Major Complication/Comorbidity   CC Complication/Comorbidity   SW Severe Wound Dx

672   ICD-10-CM 2019

I87.399   **Chronic venous hypertension (idiopathic) with other complications of unspecified lower extremity**

I87.8   **Other specified disorders of veins**
Phlebosclerosis
Venofibrosis

I87.9   **Disorder of vein, unspecified**

✓4ᵗʰ **I88**   **Nonspecific lymphadenitis**
> *EXCLUDES 1*   *acute lymphadenitis, except mesenteric (L04.-)*
> *enlarged lymph nodes NOS (R59.-)*
> *human immunodeficiency virus [HIV] disease resulting in generalized lymphadenopathy (B20)*

I88.0   **Nonspecific mesenteric lymphadenitis**
Mesenteric lymphadenitis (acute)(chronic)

I88.1   **Chronic lymphadenitis, except mesenteric**
Adenitis
Lymphadenitis

I88.8   **Other nonspecific lymphadenitis**

I88.9   **Nonspecific lymphadenitis, unspecified**
Lymphadenitis NOS

✓4ᵗʰ **I89**   **Other noninfective disorders of lymphatic vessels and lymph nodes**
> *EXCLUDES 1*   *chylocele, tunica vaginalis (nonfilarial) NOS (N50.89)*
> *enlarged lymph nodes NOS (R59.-)*
> *filarial chylocele (B74.-)*
> *hereditary lymphedema (Q82.0)*

I89.0   **Lymphedema, not elsewhere classified**
Elephantiasis (nonfilarial) NOS
Lymphangiectasis
Obliteration, lymphatic vessel
Praecox lymphedema
Secondary lymphedema
> *EXCLUDES 1*   *postmastectomy lymphedema (I97.2)*

I89.1   **Lymphangitis**
Chronic lymphangitis
Lymphangitis NOS
Subacute lymphangitis
> *EXCLUDES 1*   *acute lymphangitis (L03.-)*

I89.8   **Other specified noninfective disorders of lymphatic vessels and lymph nodes**
Chylocele (nonfilarial)
Chylous ascites
Chylous cyst
Lipomelanotic reticulosis
Lymph node or vessel fistula
Lymph node or vessel infarction
Lymph node or vessel rupture

I89.9   **Noninfective disorder of lymphatic vessels and lymph nodes, unspecified**
Disease of lymphatic vessels NOS

Other and unspecified disorders of the circulatory system (I95-I99)

✓4ᵗʰ **I95**   **Hypotension**
> *EXCLUDES 1*   *cardiovascular collapse (R57.9)*
> *maternal hypotension syndrome (O26.5-)*
> *nonspecific low blood pressure reading NOS (R03.1)*

I95.0   **Idiopathic hypotension**

I95.1   **Orthostatic hypotension**
Hypotension, postural
> *EXCLUDES 1*   *neurogenic orthostatic hypotension [Shy-Drager] (G90.3)*
> *orthostatic hypotension due to drugs (I95.2)*

I95.2   **Hypotension due to drugs**
Orthostatic hypotension due to drugs
Use additional code for adverse effect, if applicable, to identify drug (T36-T50 with fifth or sixth character 5)

I95.3   **Hypotension of hemodialysis**
Intra-dialytic hypotension

✓5ᵗʰ **I95.8**   **Other hypotension**

   I95.81   **Postprocedural hypotension**

   I95.89   **Other hypotension**
Chronic hypotension

I95.9   **Hypotension, unspecified**

I96   **Gangrene, not elsewhere classified**   `CC` `HCC`
Gangrenous cellulitis
> *EXCLUDES 1*   *gangrene in atherosclerosis of native arteries of the extremities (I70.26)*
> *gangrene in hernia (K40.1, K40.4, K41.1, K41.4, K42.1, K43.1-, K44.1, K45.1, K46.1)*
> *gangrene in other peripheral vascular diseases (I73.-)*
> *gangrene of certain specified sites—see Alphabetical Index*
> *gas gangrene (A48.0)*
> *pyoderma gangrenosum (L88)*
> *EXCLUDES 2*   *gangrene in diabetes mellitus (E08-E13 with .52)*

AHA: 2017, 3Q, 6; 2013, 2Q, 34
CC Excl: PDX collection 519

✓4ᵗʰ **I97**   **Intraoperative and postprocedural complications and disorders of circulatory system, not elsewhere classified**
> *EXCLUDES 2*   *postprocedural shock (T81.1-)*

I97.0   **Postcardiotomy syndrome**

✓5ᵗʰ **I97.1**   **Other postprocedural cardiac functional disturbances**
> *EXCLUDES 2*   *acute pulmonary insufficiency following thoracic surgery (J95.1)*
> *intraoperative cardiac functional disturbances (I97.7-)*

> **CC Excl: For CC codes in subcategory I97.1:**
> PDX collection 728

✓6ᵗʰ **I97.11**   **Postprocedural cardiac insufficiency**

   I97.110   **Postprocedural cardiac insufficiency following cardiac surgery**   `CC`

   I97.111   **Postprocedural cardiac insufficiency following other surgery**   `CC`

✓6ᵗʰ **I97.12**   **Postprocedural cardiac arrest**

   I97.120   **Postprocedural cardiac arrest following cardiac surgery**   `CC`

   I97.121   **Postprocedural cardiac arrest following other surgery**   `CC`

✓6ᵗʰ **I97.13**   **Postprocedural heart failure**
Use additional code to identify the heart failure (I50.-)

   I97.130   **Postprocedural heart failure following cardiac surgery**   `CC`

   I97.131   **Postprocedural heart failure following other surgery**   `CC`

✓6ᵗʰ **I97.19**   **Other postprocedural cardiac functional disturbances**
Use additional code, if applicable, to further specify disorder

   I97.190   **Other postprocedural cardiac functional disturbances following cardiac surgery**   `CC`
Use additional code, if applicable, for type 4 or type 5 myocardial infarction, to further specify disorder

   I97.191   **Other postprocedural cardiac functional disturbances following other surgery**   `CC`

I97.2   **Postmastectomy lymphedema syndrome**   `A`
Elephantiasis due to mastectomy
Obliteration of lymphatic vessels

I97.3   **Postprocedural hypertension**

✓5ᵗʰ **I97.4**   **Intraoperative hemorrhage and hematoma of a circulatory system organ or structure complicating a procedure**
> *EXCLUDES 1*   *intraoperative hemorrhage and hematoma of a circulatory system organ or structure due to accidental puncture and laceration during a procedure (I97.5-)*
> *EXCLUDES 2*   *intraoperative cerebrovascular hemorrhage complicating a procedure (G97.3-)*

> **CC Excl: For CC codes in subcategory I97.4:**
> PDX collection 729

✓6ᵗʰ **I97.41**   **Intraoperative hemorrhage and hematoma of a circulatory system organ or structure complicating a circulatory system procedure**

   I97.410   **Intraoperative hemorrhage and hematoma of a circulatory system organ or structure complicating a cardiac catheterization**   `CC`

   I97.411   **Intraoperative hemorrhage and hematoma of a circulatory system organ or structure complicating a cardiac bypass**   `CC`

☑ Additional Character Required   ✓x7ᵗʰ Placeholder   Unacceptable PDx   Questionable PDx   Manifestation   H1 - H14 HAC   HCC CMS-HCC Dx   HIV HIV Dx

ICD-10-CM 2019   673

Chapter 9. Diseases of the Circulatory System

I97.418   **Intraoperative hemorrhage and hematoma of a circulatory system organ or structure complicating** other **circulatory system procedure** `CC`

I97.42   **Intraoperative hemorrhage and hematoma of a circulatory system organ or structure complicating** other procedure `CC`

✓5th **I97.5**   **Accidental puncture and laceration of a circulatory system organ or structure during a procedure**

> EXCLUDES 2   accidental puncture and laceration of brain during a procedure (G97.4-)

I97.51   **Accidental puncture and laceration of a circulatory system organ or structure during a circulatory system procedure** `CC`
> **CC Excl:** PDX collection 509

I97.52   **Accidental puncture and laceration of a circulatory system organ or structure during** other procedure `CC`
> **CC Excl:** PDX collection 509

✓5th **I97.6**   **Postprocedural hemorrhage, hematoma and seroma of a circulatory system organ or structure following a procedure**

> EXCLUDES 2   postprocedural cerebrovascular hemorrhage complicating a procedure (G97.5-)

> **AHA:** 2016, 4Q, 9-10

> **CC Excl: For CC codes in subcategory I97.6:** PDX collection 729

✓6th **I97.61**   **Postprocedural** hemorrhage **of a circulatory system organ or structure following a** circulatory system procedure

I97.610   **Postprocedural hemorrhage of a circulatory system organ or structure following a** cardiac catheterization `CC`

I97.611   **Postprocedural hemorrhage of a circulatory system organ or structure following** cardiac bypass `CC`

I97.618   **Postprocedural hemorrhage of a circulatory system organ or structure following** other circulatory system procedure `CC`

✓6th **I97.62**   **Postprocedural hemorrhage, hematoma and seroma of a circulatory system organ or structure following** other procedure

I97.620   **Postprocedural** hemorrhage **of a circulatory system organ or structure following** other procedure `CC`

I97.621   **Postprocedural** hematoma **of a circulatory system organ or structure following** other procedure `CC`

I97.622   **Postprocedural** seroma **of a circulatory system organ or structure following** procedure `CC`

✓6th **I97.63**   **Postprocedural** hematoma **of a circulatory system organ or structure following a** circulatory system procedure

I97.630   **Postprocedural hematoma of a circulatory system organ or structure following a** cardiac catheterization `CC`

I97.631   **Postprocedural hematoma of a circulatory system organ or structure following** cardiac bypass `CC`

I97.638   **Postprocedural hematoma of a circulatory system organ or structure following** other circulatory system procedure `CC`

✓6th **I97.64**   **Postprocedural seroma of a circulatory system organ or structure following a circulatory system procedure**

I97.640   **Postprocedural seroma of a circulatory system organ or structure following a** cardiac catheterization `CC`

I97.641   **Postprocedural seroma of a circulatory system organ or structure following** cardiac bypass `CC`

I97.648   **Postprocedural seroma of a circulatory system organ or structure following** other circulatory system procedure `CC`

✓5th **I97.7**   **Intraoperative** cardiac **functional disturbances**

> EXCLUDES 2   acute pulmonary insufficiency following thoracic surgery (J95.1)
> postprocedural cardiac functional disturbances (I97.1-)

> **CC Excl: For CC codes in subcategory I97.7:** PDX collection 728

✓6th **I97.71**   **Intraoperative** cardiac arrest

I97.710   **Intraoperative cardiac arrest during** cardiac surgery `CC`

I97.711   **Intraoperative cardiac arrest during** other surgery `CC`

✓6th **I97.79**   **Other** intraoperative cardiac functional disturbances
> Use additional code, if applicable, to further specify disorder

I97.790   **Other intraoperative cardiac functional disturbances during** cardiac surgery `CC`

I97.791   **Other intraoperative cardiac functional disturbances during** other surgery `CC`

✓5th **I97.8**   **Other** intraoperative and postprocedural complications and disorders of the circulatory system, not elsewhere classified
> Use additional code, if applicable, to further specify disorder

> **CC Excl: For CC codes in subcategory I97.8, unless otherwise noted:** PDX collection 617

✓6th **I97.81**   **Intraoperative** cerebrovascular infarction

I97.810   **Intraoperative cerebrovascular infarction during** cardiac surgery `CC` `HCC`

I97.811   **Intraoperative cerebrovascular infarction during** other surgery `CC` `HCC`

✓6th **I97.82**   **Postprocedural** cerebrovascular infarction

I97.820   **Postprocedural cerebrovascular infarction following** cardiac surgery `CC` `HCC`

I97.821   **Postprocedural cerebrovascular infarction following** other surgery `CC` `HCC`

I97.88   **Other intraoperative complications of the circulatory system, not elsewhere classified** `CC`
> **CC Excl:** PDX collection 728

I97.89   **Other postprocedural complications and disorders of the circulatory system, not elsewhere classified** `CC`
> **CC Excl:** PDX collection 728

✓4th **I99**   **Other and unspecified disorders of circulatory system**

I99.8   **Other disorder of circulatory system**

I99.9   **Unspecified disorder of circulatory system**

`N` Newborn: 0   `P` Pediatric: 0-17   `M` Maternity: 12-55   `A` Adult: 15-124   `MCC` Major Complication/Comorbidity   `CC` Complication/Comorbidity   `SW` Severe Wound Dx

674   ICD-10-CM 2019

Chapter 10. Diseases of the Respiratory System (J00–J99)

Chapter Specific Guidelines with Coding Examples

The chapter specific guidelines from the ICD-10-CM Official Guidelines for Coding and Reporting have been provided below. Along with these guidelines are coding examples, contained in the shaded boxes, that have been developed to help illustrate the coding and/or sequencing guidance found in these guidelines.

a. Chronic obstructive pulmonary disease [COPD] and asthma

1) Acute exacerbation of chronic obstructive bronchitis and asthma

The codes in categories J44 and J45 distinguish between uncomplicated cases and those in acute exacerbation. An acute exacerbation is a worsening or a decompensation of a chronic condition. An acute exacerbation is not equivalent to an infection superimposed on a chronic condition, though an exacerbation may be triggered by an infection.

> Vancomycin IV was started to treat a patient with acute pneumonia due to *Streptococcus pneumoniae*. Patient also with acute exacerbation of COPD continued on home meds.
>
> **J13**   **Pneumonia due to Streptococcus pneumoniae**
>
> **J44.0**   **Chronic obstructive pulmonary disease with acute lower respiratory infection**
>
> **J44.1**   **Chronic obstructive pulmonary disease with (acute) exacerbation**
>
> *Explanation*: ICD-10-CM uses combination codes to create organism-specific classifications for acute pneumonia. Category J44 codes include combination codes with severity components, which differentiate between COPD with acute lower respiratory infection (acute pneumonia), COPD with acute exacerbation, and COPD without mention of a complication (unspecified).
>
> An acute exacerbation is a worsening or a decompensation of a chronic condition. An acute exacerbation is not equivalent to an infection superimposed on a chronic condition, though an exacerbation may be triggered by an infection, as in this example. Treatment of the pneumonia necessitated the inpatient admission. Instructional notes at J44.0 say to "code also to identify the infection," which informs the coder that another code must be assigned if applicable. Sequencing of the pneumonia and COPD exacerbation are governed by the Section II, "Selection of Principal Diagnosis," guidelines. In this case it was the pneumonia that was "chiefly responsible for occasioning the admission" with the IV vancomycin treatment.

> Exacerbation of moderate persistent asthma with status asthmaticus
>
> **J45.42**   **Moderate persistent asthma with status asthmaticus**
>
> *Explanation*: Category J45 Asthma includes severity-specific subcategories and fifth-character codes to distinguish between uncomplicated cases, those in acute exacerbation, and those with status asthmaticus.

b. Acute respiratory failure

1) Acute respiratory failure as principal diagnosis

A code from subcategory J96.0, Acute respiratory failure, or subcategory J96.2, Acute and chronic respiratory failure, may be assigned as a principal diagnosis when it is the condition established after study to be chiefly responsible for occasioning the admission to the hospital, and the selection is supported by the Alphabetic Index and Tabular List. However, chapter-specific coding guidelines (such as obstetrics, poisoning, HIV, newborn) that provide sequencing direction take precedence.

> Acute hypoxic respiratory failure due to COPD exacerbation
>
> **J96.01**   **Acute respiratory failure with hypoxia**
>
> **J44.1**   **Chronic obstructive pulmonary disease with (acute) exacerbation**
>
> *Explanation*: Category J96 classifies respiratory failure with combination codes that designate the severity and the presence of hypoxia and hypercapnia. Code J96.01 is sequenced as the first-listed diagnosis, as the reason for the admission. Respiratory failure may be assigned as a principal diagnosis when it is the condition established after study to be chiefly responsible for occasioning the admission to the hospital and the selection is supported by the Alphabetic Index and Tabular List.

2) Acute respiratory failure as secondary diagnosis

Respiratory failure may be listed as a secondary diagnosis if it occurs after admission, or if it is present on admission, but does not meet the definition of principal diagnosis.

> Acute respiratory failure due to accidental oxycodone overdose
>
> **T40.2X1A**   **Poisoning by other opioids, accidental (unintentional), initial encounter**
>
> **J96.00**   **Acute respiratory failure, unspecified whether with hypoxia or hypercapnia**
>
> *Explanation*: Respiratory failure may be assigned as a principal diagnosis when it is the condition established after study to be chiefly responsible for occasioning the admission to the hospital, and the selection is supported by the Alphabetic Index and Tabular List. However, chapter-specific coding guidelines, such as poisoning, that provide sequencing direction take precedence. When coding a poisoning or reaction to the improper use of a medication (e.g. overdose, wrong substance given or taken in error, wrong route of administration), first assign the appropriate code from categories T36–T50. Use additional code(s) for all manifestations of the poisoning. In this instance, the respiratory failure is a manifestation of the poisoning and is sequenced as a secondary diagnosis.

> Acute pneumococcal pneumonia with subsequent development of acute respiratory failure
>
> **J13**   **Pneumonia due to Streptococcus pneumoniae**
>
> **J96.00**   **Acute respiratory failure, unspecified whether with hypoxia or hypercapnia**
>
> *Explanation*: Acute respiratory failure may be listed as a secondary diagnosis if it occurs after admission, or if it is present on admission but does not meet the definition of principal diagnosis.

3) Sequencing of acute respiratory failure and another acute condition

When a patient is admitted with respiratory failure and another acute condition, (e.g., myocardial infarction, cerebrovascular accident, aspiration pneumonia), the principal diagnosis will not be the same in every situation. This applies whether the other acute condition is a respiratory or nonrespiratory condition. Selection of the principal diagnosis will be dependent on the circumstances of admission. If both the respiratory failure and the other acute condition are equally responsible for occasioning the admission to the hospital, and there are no chapter-specific sequencing rules, the guideline regarding two or more diagnoses that equally meet the definition for principal diagnosis (*Section II, C.*) may be applied in these situations.

If the documentation is not clear as to whether acute respiratory failure and another condition are equally responsible for occasioning the admission, query the provider for clarification.

> Acute pneumococcal pneumonia and acute respiratory failure, both present on admission
>
> **J96.00**   **Acute respiratory failure, unspecified whether with hypoxia or hypercapnia**
>
> **J13**   **Pneumonia due to Streptococcus pneumoniae**
>
> *Explanation*: When a patient is admitted with respiratory failure and another acute condition, such as a bacterial pneumonia, the principal diagnosis is not the same in every situation. This applies whether the other acute condition is a respiratory or nonrespiratory condition. The principal diagnosis depends on the circumstances of admission.

c. Influenza due to certain identified influenza viruses

Code only confirmed cases of influenza due to certain identified influenza viruses (category J09), and due to other identified influenza virus (category J10). This is an exception to the hospital inpatient guideline Section II, H. (Uncertain Diagnosis).

In this context, "confirmation" does not require documentation of positive laboratory testing specific for avian or other novel influenza A or other identified influenza virus. However, coding should be based on the provider's diagnostic statement that the patient has avian influenza, or other novel influenza A, for category J09, or has another particular identified strain of influenza, such as H1N1 or H3N2, but not identified as novel or variant, for category J10.

If the provider records "suspected" or "possible" or "probable" avian influenza, or novel influenza, or other identified influenza, then the appropriate influenza code from category J11, Influenza due to unidentified influenza virus, should be assigned. A code from category J09, Influenza due to certain identified influenza viruses, should not be assigned nor should a code from category J10, Influenza due to other identified

---

Influenza due to avian influenza virus with pneumonia

J09.X1   **Influenza due to identified novel influenza A virus with pneumonia**

Explanation: Codes in category J09 Influenza due to certain identified influenza viruses should be assigned only for confirmed cases. "Confirmation" does not require positive laboratory testing of a specific influenza virus but does need to be based on the provider's diagnostic statement, which should not include terms such as "possible," "probable," or "suspected."

---

d. Ventilator associated pneumonia

1) Documentation of ventilator associated pneumonia

As with all procedural or postprocedural complications, code assignment is based on the provider's documentation of the relationship between the condition and the procedure.

Code J95.851, Ventilator associated pneumonia, should be assigned only when the provider has documented ventilator associated pneumonia (VAP). An additional code to identify the organism (e.g., Pseudomonas aeruginosa, code B96.5) should also be assigned. Do not assign an additional code from categories J12-J18 to identify the type of pneumonia.

Code J95.851 should not be assigned for cases where the patient has pneumonia and is on a mechanical ventilator and the provider has not specifically stated that the pneumonia is ventilator-associated pneumonia. If the documentation is unclear as to whether the patient has a pneumonia that is a complication attributable to the mechanical ventilator, query the provider.

2) Ventilator associated pneumonia develops after admission

A patient may be admitted with one type of pneumonia (e.g., code J13, Pneumonia due to Streptococcus pneumonia) and subsequently develop VAP. In this instance, the principal diagnosis would be the appropriate code from categories J12-J18 for the pneumonia diagnosed at the time of admission. Code J95.851, Ventilator associated pneumonia, would be assigned as an additional diagnosis when the provider has also documented the presence of ventilator associated pneumonia.

Patient with pneumonia due to *Klebsiella pneumoniae* develops superimposed MRSA ventilator-associated pneumonia

J15.0   **Pneumonia due to Klebsiella pneumoniae**

J95.851   **Ventilator associated pneumonia**

B95.62   **Methicillin resistant Staphylococcus aureus infection as the cause of diseases classified elsewhere**

Explanation: Code assignment for ventilator-associated pneumonia is based on the provider's documentation of the relationship between the condition and the procedure and is reported only when the provider has documented ventilator-associated pneumonia (VAP).

A patient may be admitted with one type of pneumonia and subsequently develop VAP. In this example, the principal diagnosis code describes the pneumonia diagnosed at the time of admission, with code J95.851 Ventilator associated pneumonia, assigned as secondary.

Chapter 10. Diseases of the Respiratory System (J00-J99)

NOTE When a respiratory condition is described as occurring in more than one site and is not specifically indexed, it should be classified to the lower anatomic site (e.g. tracheobronchitis to bronchitis in J40).

Use additional code, where applicable, to identify:
  exposure to environmental tobacco smoke (Z77.22)
  exposure to tobacco smoke in the perinatal period (P96.81)
  history of tobacco dependence (Z87.891)
  occupational exposure to environmental tobacco smoke (Z57.31)
  tobacco dependence (F17.-)
  tobacco use (Z72.0)

EXCLUDES 2 *certain conditions originating in the perinatal period (P04-P96)*
  certain infectious and parasitic diseases (A00-B99)
  complications of pregnancy, childbirth and the puerperium (O00-O9A)
  congenital malformations, deformations and chromosomal abnormalities (Q00-Q99)
  endocrine, nutritional and metabolic diseases (E00-E88)
  injury, poisoning and certain other consequences of external causes (S00-T88)
  neoplasms (C00-D49)
  smoke inhalation (T59.81-)
  symptoms, signs and abnormal clinical and laboratory findings, not elsewhere classified (R00-R94)

This chapter contains the following blocks:

J00-J06	Acute upper respiratory infections
J09-J18	Influenza and pneumonia
J20-J22	Other acute lower respiratory infections
J30-J39	Other diseases of upper respiratory tract
J40-J47	Chronic lower respiratory diseases
J60-J70	Lung diseases due to external agents
J80-J84	Other respiratory diseases principally affecting the interstitium
J85-J86	Suppurative and necrotic conditions of the lower respiratory tract
J90-J94	Other diseases of the pleura
J95	Intraoperative and postprocedural complications and disorders of respiratory system, not elsewhere classified
J96-J99	Other diseases of the respiratory system

Acute upper respiratory infections (J00-J06)

EXCLUDES 1 *chronic obstructive pulmonary disease with acute lower respiratory infection (J44.0)*
  influenza virus with other respiratory manifestations (J09.X2, J10.1, J11.1)

J00   Acute nasopharyngitis (common cold)
  Acute rhinitis   Infective rhinitis
  Coryza (acute)   Nasal catarrh, acute
  Infective nasopharyngitis NOS   Nasopharyngitis NOS

  EXCLUDES 1 *acute pharyngitis (J02.-)*
    acute sore throat NOS (J02.9)
    pharyngitis NOS (J02.9)
    rhinitis NOS (J31.0)
    sore throat NOS (J02.9)

  EXCLUDES 2 *allergic rhinitis (J30.1-J30.9)*
    chronic pharyngitis (J31.2)
    chronic rhinitis (J31.0)
    chronic sore throat (J31.2)
    nasopharyngitis, chronic (J31.1)
    vasomotor rhinitis (J30.0)

  DEF: Acute inflammation of the mucous membranes that extends from the nares to the pharynx. It is characterized by nasal obstruction, sneezing, runny nose, and sore throat.

✓4th J01   Acute sinusitis
  INCLUDES acute abscess of sinus
    acute empyema of sinus
    acute infection of sinus
    acute inflammation of sinus
    acute suppuration of sinus

  Use additional code (B95-B97) to identify infectious agent
  EXCLUDES 1 *sinusitis NOS (J32.9)*
  EXCLUDES 2 *chronic sinusitis (J32.0-J32.8)*

  ✓5th J01.0   Acute maxillary sinusitis
    Acute antritis
    J01.00   Acute maxillary sinusitis, unspecified
    J01.01   Acute recurrent maxillary sinusitis

  ✓5th J01.1   Acute frontal sinusitis
    J01.10   Acute frontal sinusitis, unspecified
    J01.11   Acute recurrent frontal sinusitis

  ✓5th J01.2   Acute ethmoidal sinusitis
    J01.20   Acute ethmoidal sinusitis, unspecified
    J01.21   Acute recurrent ethmoidal sinusitis

  ✓5th J01.3   Acute sphenoidal sinusitis
    J01.30   Acute sphenoidal sinusitis, unspecified
    J01.31   Acute recurrent sphenoidal sinusitis

  ✓5th J01.4   Acute pansinusitis
    J01.40   Acute pansinusitis, unspecified
    J01.41   Acute recurrent pansinusitis

  ✓5th J01.8   Other acute sinusitis
    J01.80   Other acute sinusitis
      Acute sinusitis involving more than one sinus but not pansinusitis
    J01.81   Other acute recurrent sinusitis
      Acute recurrent sinusitis involving more than one sinus but not pansinusitis

  ✓5th J01.9   Acute sinusitis, unspecified
    J01.90   Acute sinusitis, unspecified
    J01.91   Acute recurrent sinusitis, unspecified

✓4th J02   Acute pharyngitis
  INCLUDES acute sore throat
  EXCLUDES 1 *acute laryngopharyngitis (J06.0)*
    peritonsillar abscess (J36)
    pharyngeal abscess (J39.1)
    retropharyngeal abscess (J39.0)
  EXCLUDES 2 *chronic pharyngitis (J31.2)*

  J02.0   Streptococcal pharyngitis
    Septic pharyngitis
    Streptococcal sore throat
    EXCLUDES 2 *scarlet fever (A38.-)*

  J02.8   Acute pharyngitis due to other specified organisms
    Use additional code (B95-B97) to identify infectious agent
    EXCLUDES 1 *acute pharyngitis due to coxsackie virus (B08.5)*
      acute pharyngitis due to gonococcus (A54.5)
      acute pharyngitis due to herpes [simplex] virus (B00.2)
      acute pharyngitis due to infectious mononucleosis (B27.-)
      enteroviral vesicular pharyngitis (B08.5)

  J02.9   Acute pharyngitis, unspecified
    Gangrenous pharyngitis (acute)
    Infective pharyngitis (acute) NOS
    Pharyngitis (acute) NOS
    Sore throat (acute) NOS
    Suppurative pharyngitis (acute)
    Ulcerative pharyngitis (acute)

✓4th J03   Acute tonsillitis
  EXCLUDES 1 *acute sore throat (J02.-)*
    hypertrophy of tonsils (J35.1)
    peritonsillar abscess (J36)
    sore throat NOS (J02.9)
    streptococcal sore throat (J02.0)
  EXCLUDES 2 *chronic tonsillitis (J35.0)*

  ✓5th J03.0   Streptococcal tonsillitis
    J03.00   Acute streptococcal tonsillitis, unspecified
    J03.01   Acute recurrent streptococcal tonsillitis

  ✓5th J03.8   Acute tonsillitis due to other specified organisms
    Use additional code (B95-B97) to identify infectious agent
    EXCLUDES 1 *diphtheritic tonsillitis (A36.0)*
      herpesviral pharyngotonsillitis (B00.2)
      streptococcal tonsillitis (J03.0)
      tuberculous tonsillitis (A15.8)
      Vincent's tonsillitis (A69.1)
    J03.80   Acute tonsillitis due to other specified organisms
    J03.81   Acute recurrent tonsillitis due to other specified organisms

  ✓5th J03.9   Acute tonsillitis, unspecified
    Follicular tonsillitis (acute)
    Gangrenous tonsillitis (acute)
    Infective tonsillitis (acute)
    Tonsillitis (acute) NOS
    Ulcerative tonsillitis (acute)
    J03.90   Acute tonsillitis, unspecified
    J03.91   Acute recurrent tonsillitis, unspecified

✓ Additional Character Required   ✓x7th Placeholder   Unacceptable PDx   Questionable PDx   Manifestation   H1 - H14 HAC   HCC CMS-HCC Dx   HIV HIV Dx

ICD-10-CM 2019   677

✓4ᵗʰ J04   Acute laryngitis and tracheitis

Use additional code (B95-B97) to identify infectious agent

EXCLUDES 1   acute obstructive laryngitis [croup] and epiglottitis (J05.-)

EXCLUDES 2   laryngismus (stridulus) (J38.5)

J04.Ø   Acute laryngitis

Edematous laryngitis (acute)
Laryngitis (acute) NOS
Subglottic laryngitis (acute)
Suppurative laryngitis (acute)
Ulcerative laryngitis (acute)

EXCLUDES 1   acute obstructive laryngitis (J05.Ø)

EXCLUDES 2   chronic laryngitis (J37.Ø)

✓5ᵗʰ J04.1   Acute tracheitis

Acute viral tracheitis
Catarrhal tracheitis (acute)
Tracheitis (acute) NOS

EXCLUDES 2   chronic tracheitis (J42)

J04.10   Acute tracheitis without obstruction

J04.11   Acute tracheitis with obstruction   `MCC`

CC Excl: PDX collection 730

J04.2   Acute laryngotracheitis

Laryngotracheitis NOS
Tracheitis (acute) with laryngitis (acute)

EXCLUDES 1   acute obstructive laryngotracheitis (J05.Ø)

EXCLUDES 2   chronic laryngotracheitis (J37.1)

✓5ᵗʰ J04.3   Supraglottitis, unspecified

J04.30   Supraglottitis, unspecified, without obstruction

J04.31   Supraglottitis, unspecified, with obstruction   `MCC`

CC Excl: PDX collection 731

✓4ᵗʰ J05   Acute obstructive laryngitis [croup] and epiglottitis

Use additional code (B95-B97) to identify infectious agent

J05.Ø   Acute obstructive laryngitis [croup]

Obstructive laryngitis (acute) NOS
Obstructive laryngotracheitis NOS

DEF: Acute laryngeal obstruction due to allergies, foreign bodies, or in the majority of cases a viral infection. Symptoms include a harsh, barking cough, hoarseness, and a persistent, high-pitched respiratory sound (stridor).

✓5ᵗʰ J05.1   Acute epiglottitis

EXCLUDES 2   epiglottitis, chronic (J37.Ø)

J05.10   Acute epiglottitis without obstruction   `CC`

Epiglottitis NOS

CC Excl: PDX collection 732

J05.11   Acute epiglottitis with obstruction   `MCC`

CC Excl: PDX collection 730

✓4ᵗʰ J06   Acute upper respiratory infections of multiple and unspecified sites

EXCLUDES 1   acute respiratory infection NOS (J22)
streptococcal pharyngitis (J02.Ø)

J06.Ø   Acute laryngopharyngitis

J06.9   Acute upper respiratory infection, unspecified

Upper respiratory disease, acute
Upper respiratory infection NOS

Influenza and pneumonia (J09-J18)

EXCLUDES 2   allergic or eosinophilic pneumonia (J82)
aspiration pneumonia NOS (J69.Ø)
congenital pneumonia (P23.9)
lipid pneumonia (J69.1)
meconium pneumonia (P24.Ø1)
neonatal aspiration pneumonia (P24.-)
pneumonia due to solids and liquids (J69.-)
rheumatic pneumonia (IØØ)
ventilator associated pneumonia (J95.851)

AHA: 2017, 4Q, 96

TIP: Hemoptysis (RØ4.2) is not customarily associated with pneumonia and may be reported separately.

✓4ᵗʰ J09   Influenza due to certain identified influenza viruses

EXCLUDES 1   influenza A/H1N1 (J10.-)
influenza due to other identified influenza virus (J10.-)
influenza due to unidentified influenza virus (J11.-)
seasonal influenza due to other identified influenza virus (J10.-)
seasonal influenza due to unidentified influenza virus (J11.-)

✓5ᵗʰ J09.X   Influenza due to identified novel influenza A virus

Avian influenza
Bird influenza
Influenza A/H5N1
Influenza of other animal origin, not bird or swine
Swine influenza virus (viruses that normally cause infections in pigs)

AHA: 2016, 3Q, 10

J09.X1   Influenza due to identified novel influenza A virus with pneumonia   `HIV` `MCC`

Code also, if applicable, associated:
lung abscess (J85.1)
other specified type of pneumonia

CC Excl: PDX collection 110

J09.X2   Influenza due to identified novel influenza A virus with other respiratory manifestations

Influenza due to identified novel influenza A virus NOS
Influenza due to identified novel influenza A virus with laryngitis
Influenza due to identified novel influenza A virus with pharyngitis
Influenza due to identified novel influenza A virus with upper respiratory symptoms

Use additional code, if applicable, for associated:
pleural effusion (J91.8)
sinusitis (J01.-)

J09.X3   Influenza due to identified novel influenza A virus with gastrointestinal manifestations

Influenza due to identified novel influenza A virus gastroenteritis

EXCLUDES 1   'intestinal flu' [viral gastroenteritis] (AØ8.-)

J09.X9   Influenza due to identified novel influenza A virus with other manifestations

Influenza due to identified novel influenza A virus with encephalopathy
Influenza due to identified novel influenza A virus with myocarditis
Influenza due to identified novel influenza A virus with otitis media

Use additional code to identify manifestation

✓4ᵗʰ J10   Influenza due to other identified influenza virus

EXCLUDES 1   influenza due to avian influenza virus (J09.X-)
influenza due to swine flu (J09.X-)
influenza due to unidentifed influenza virus (J11.-)

✓5ᵗʰ J10.Ø   Influenza due to other identified influenza virus with pneumonia

Code also associated lung abscess, if applicable (J85.1)

J10.ØØ   Influenza due to other identified influenza virus with unspecified type of pneumonia   `MCC`

CC Excl: PDX collection 110

J10.Ø1   Influenza due to other identified influenza virus with the same other identified influenza virus pneumonia   `MCC`

CC Excl: PDX collection 110

J10.Ø8   Influenza due to other identified influenza virus with other specified pneumonia   `HIV` `MCC`

Code also other specified type of pneumonia

CC Excl: PDX collection 733

N Newborn: 0   P Pediatric: 0-17   M Maternity: 12-55   A Adult: 15-124   MCC Major Complication/Comorbidity   CC Complication/Comorbidity   SW Severe Wound Dx

678   ICD-10-CM 2019

J10.1　Influenza due to other identified influenza virus with other respiratory manifestations
　　Influenza due to other identified influenza virus NOS
　　Influenza due to other identified influenza virus with laryngitis
　　Influenza due to other identified influenza virus with pharyngitis
　　Influenza due to other identified influenza virus with upper respiratory symptoms
　　Use additional code for associated pleural effusion, if applicable (J91.8)
　　Use additional code for associated sinusitis, if applicable (J01.-)
　　AHA: 2016, 3Q, 10-11

J10.2　Influenza due to other identified influenza virus with gastrointestinal manifestations
　　Influenza due to other identified influenza virus gastroenteritis
　　EXCLUDES 1　'intestinal flu' [viral gastroenteritis] (A08.-)

✓5ᵗʰ J10.8　Influenza due to other identified influenza virus with other manifestations

　　J10.81　Influenza due to other identified influenza virus with encephalopathy

　　J10.82　Influenza due to other identified influenza virus with myocarditis

　　J10.83　Influenza due to other identified influenza virus with otitis media
　　　　Use additional code for any associated perforated tympanic membrane (H72.-)

　　J10.89　Influenza due to other identified influenza virus with other manifestations
　　　　Use additional codes to identify the manifestations

✓4ᵗʰ J11　Influenza due to unidentified influenza virus

✓5ᵗʰ J11.0　Influenza due to unidentified influenza virus with pneumonia
　　Code also associated lung abscess, if applicable (J85.1)
　　AHA: 2016, 3Q, 11

　　J11.00　Influenza due to unidentified influenza virus with unspecified type of pneumonia　MCC
　　　　Influenza with pneumonia NOS
　　　　CC Excl: PDX collection 110

　　J11.08　Influenza due to unidentified influenza virus with specified pneumonia　MCC
　　　　Code also other specified type of pneumonia
　　　　CC Excl: PDX collection 110

J11.1　Influenza due to unidentified influenza virus with other respiratory manifestations
　　Influenza NOS
　　Influenzal laryngitis NOS
　　Influenzal pharyngitis NOS
　　Influenza with upper respiratory symptoms NOS
　　Use additional code for associated pleural effusion, if applicable (J91.8)
　　Use additional code for associated sinusitis, if applicable (J01.-)

J11.2　Influenza due to unidentified influenza virus with gastrointestinal manifestations
　　Influenza gastroenteritis NOS
　　EXCLUDES 1　'intestinal flu' [viral gastroenteritis] (A08.-)

✓5ᵗʰ J11.8　Influenza due to unidentified influenza virus with other manifestations

　　J11.81　Influenza due to unidentified influenza virus with encephalopathy
　　　　Influenzal encephalopathy NOS

　　J11.82　Influenza due to unidentified influenza virus with myocarditis
　　　　Influenzal myocarditis NOS

　　J11.83　Influenza due to unidentified influenza virus with otitis media
　　　　Influenzal otitis media NOS
　　　　Use additional code for any associated perforated tympanic membrane (H72.-)

　　J11.89　Influenza due to unidentified influenza virus with other manifestations
　　　　Use additional codes to identify the manifestations

✓4ᵗʰ J12　Viral pneumonia, not elsewhere classified
　　INCLUDES　bronchopneumonia due to viruses other than influenza viruses
　　Code first associated influenza, if applicable (J09.X1, J10.0-, J11.0-)
　　Code also associated abscess, if applicable (J85.1)
　　EXCLUDES 1　aspiration pneumonia due to anesthesia during labor and delivery (O74.0)
　　　　aspiration pneumonia due to anesthesia during pregnancy (O29)
　　　　aspiration pneumonia due to anesthesia during puerperium (O89.0)
　　　　aspiration pneumonia due to solids and liquids (J69.-)
　　　　aspiration pneumonia NOS (J69.0)
　　　　congenital pneumonia (P23.0)
　　　　congenital rubella pneumonitis (P35.0)
　　　　interstitial pneumonia NOS (J84.9)
　　　　lipid pneumonia (J69.1)
　　　　neonatal aspiration pneumonia (P24.-)
　　AHA: 2016, 3Q, 15; 2013, 4Q, 118

　　CC Excl: For MCC codes in category J12, unless otherwise noted: PDX collection 734

J12.0　Adenoviral pneumonia　MCC

J12.1　Respiratory syncytial virus pneumonia　MCC

J12.2　Parainfluenza virus pneumonia　MCC

J12.3　Human metapneumovirus pneumonia　HIV MCC

✓5ᵗʰ J12.8　Other viral pneumonia

　　J12.81　Pneumonia due to SARS-associated coronavirus　HIV MCC
　　　　Severe acute respiratory syndrome NOS
　　　　DEF: Severe adult respiratory syndrome caused by the coronavirus, specified as inflammation of the lungs with consolidation.
　　　　CC Excl: PDX collection 735

　　J12.89　Other viral pneumonia　HIV MCC

J12.9　Viral pneumonia, unspecified　HIV MCC

J13　Pneumonia due to Streptococcus pneumoniae　HIV MCC HCC
　　Bronchopneumonia due to S. pneumoniae
　　Code first associated influenza, if applicable (J09.X1, J10.0-, J11.0-)
　　Code also associated lung abscess, if applicable (J85.1)
　　EXCLUDES 1　congenital pneumonia due to S. pneumoniae (P23.6)
　　　　lobar pneumonia, unspecified organism (J18.1)
　　　　pneumonia due to other streptococci (J15.3-J15.4)
　　AHA: 2016, 3Q, 15; 2013, 4Q, 118
　　CC Excl: PDX collection 110

J14　Pneumonia due to Hemophilus influenzae　HIV MCC HCC
　　Bronchopneumonia due to H. influenzae
　　Code first associated influenza, if applicable (J09.X1, J10.0-, J11.0-)
　　Code also associated lung abscess, if applicable (J85.1)
　　EXCLUDES 1　congenital pneumonia due to H. influenzae (P23.6)
　　AHA: 2016, 3Q, 15; 2013, 4Q, 118
　　CC Excl: PDX collection 110

✓4ᵗʰ J15　Bacterial pneumonia, not elsewhere classified
　　INCLUDES　bronchopneumonia due to bacteria other than S. pneumoniae and H. influenzae
　　Code first associated influenza, if applicable (J09.X1, J10.0-, J11.0-)
　　Code also associated lung abscess, if applicable (J85.1)
　　EXCLUDES 1　chlamydial pneumonia (J16.0)
　　　　congenital pneumonia (P23.-)
　　　　Legionnaires' disease (A48.1)
　　　　spirochetal pneumonia (A69.8)
　　AHA: 2016, 3Q, 15; 2013, 4Q, 118

　　CC Excl: For MCC codes in category J15: PDX collection 110

J15.0　Pneumonia due to Klebsiella pneumoniae　HIV MCC HCC

J15.1　Pneumonia due to Pseudomonas　HIV MCC HCC

✓5ᵗʰ J15.2　Pneumonia due to staphylococcus

　　J15.20　Pneumonia due to staphylococcus, unspecified　HIV MCC HCC

　　✓6ᵗʰ J15.21　Pneumonia due to Staphylococcus aureus

　　　　J15.211　Pneumonia due to Methicillin susceptible Staphylococcus aureus　HIV MCC HCC
　　　　　　MSSA pneumonia
　　　　　　Pneumonia due to Staphylococcus aureus NOS

　　　　J15.212　Pneumonia due to Methicillin resistant Staphylococcus aureus　HIV MCC HCC

　　　　J15.29　Pneumonia due to other staphylococcus　HIV MCC HCC

J15.3   **Pneumonia due to streptococcus,** group B   `HIV` `MCC` `HCC`

J15.4   **Pneumonia due to** other **streptococci**   `HIV` `MCC` `HCC`
> **EXCLUDES 1**   pneumonia due to streptococcus, group B (J15.3)
> pneumonia due to Streptococcus pneumoniae (J13)

J15.5   **Pneumonia due to** Escherichia coli   `HIV` `MCC` `HCC`

J15.6   **Pneumonia due to** other Gram-negative bacteria   `HIV` `MCC` `HCC`
> Pneumonia due to other aerobic Gram-negative bacteria
> Pneumonia due to Serratia marcescens

J15.7   **Pneumonia due to** Mycoplasma pneumoniae   `MCC`

J15.8   **Pneumonia due to** other specified bacteria   `HIV` `MCC` `HCC`

J15.9   **Unspecified** bacterial pneumonia   `HIV` `MCC`
> Pneumonia due to gram-positive bacteria

✓4ᵗʰ J16   Pneumonia due to other infectious organisms, not elsewhere classified

Code first associated influenza, if applicable (J09.X1, J10.0-, J11.0-)
Code also associated lung abscess, if applicable (J85.1)
> **EXCLUDES 1**   congenital pneumonia (P23.-)
> ornithosis (A70)
> pneumocystosis (B59)
> pneumonia NOS (J18.9)

AHA: 2016, 3Q, 15; 2013, 4Q, 118

J16.0   Chlamydial pneumonia   `MCC`
> **CC Excl:** PDX collection 110

J16.8   **Pneumonia due to** other specified infectious organisms   `MCC`
> **CC Excl:** PDX collection 110

J17   *Pneumonia in diseases classified elsewhere*   `MCC`

Code first underlying disease, such as:
> Q fever (A78)
> rheumatic fever (I00)
> schistosomiasis (B65.0-B65.9)
> **EXCLUDES 1**   candidial pneumonia (B37.1)
> chlamydial pneumonia (J16.0)
> gonorrheal pneumonia (A54.84)
> histoplasmosis pneumonia (B39.0-B39.2)
> measles pneumonia (B05.2)
> nocardiosis pneumonia (A43.0)
> pneumocystosis (B59)
> pneumonia due to Pneumocystis carinii (B59)
> pneumonia due to Pneumocystis jiroveci (B59)
> pneumonia in actinomycosis (A42.0)
> pneumonia in anthrax (A22.1)
> pneumonia in ascariasis (B77.81)
> pneumonia in aspergillosis (B44.0-B44.1)
> pneumonia in coccidioidomycosis (B38.0-B38.2)
> pneumonia in cytomegalovirus disease (B25.0)
> pneumonia in toxoplasmosis (B58.3)
> rubella pneumonia (B06.81)
> salmonella pneumonia (A02.22)
> spirochetal infection NEC with pneumonia (A69.8)
> tularemia pneumonia (A21.2)
> typhoid fever with pneumonia (A01.03)
> varicella pneumonia (B01.2)
> whooping cough with pneumonia (A37 with fifth-character 1)

AHA: 2016, 3Q, 15; 2013, 4Q, 118
CC Excl: PDX collection 110

✓4ᵗʰ J18   Pneumonia, unspecified organism

Code first associated influenza, if applicable (J09.X1, J10.0-, J11.0-)
> **EXCLUDES 1**   abscess of lung with pneumonia (J85.1)
> aspiration pneumonia due to anesthesia during labor and delivery (O74.0)
> aspiration pneumonia due to anesthesia during pregnancy (O29)
> aspiration pneumonia due to anesthesia during puerperium (O89.0)
> aspiration pneumonia due to solids and liquids (J69.-)
> aspiration pneumonia NOS (J69.0)
> congenital pneumonia (P23.0)
> drug-induced interstitial lung disorder (J70.2-J70.4)
> interstitial pneumonia NOS (J84.9)
> lipid pneumonia (J69.1)
> neonatal aspiration pneumonia (P24.-)
> pneumonitis due to external agents (J67-J70)
> pneumonitis due to fumes and vapors (J68.0)
> usual interstitial pneumonia (J84.17)

AHA: 2016, 3Q, 15; 2013, 4Q, 118

> **CC Excl:** For CC/MCC codes in category J18, unless otherwise noted: PDX collection 110

J18.0   **Bronchopneumonia,** unspecified organism   `MCC`
> **EXCLUDES 1**   hypostatic bronchopneumonia (J18.2)
> lipid pneumonia (J69.1)
> **EXCLUDES 2**   acute bronchiolitis (J21.-)
> chronic bronchiolitis (J44.9)

J18.1   **Lobar** pneumonia, unspecified organism   `HIV` `MCC` `HCC`

J18.2   **Hypostatic** pneumonia, unspecified organism   `CC`
> Hypostatic bronchopneumonia
> Passive pneumonia
> **CC Excl:** PDX collection 736

J18.8   **Other** pneumonia, unspecified organism   `HIV` `MCC`

J18.9   **Pneumonia,** unspecified organism   `HIV` `MCC`
> **AHA:** 2014, 3Q, 4; 2013, 4Q, 119; 2012, 4Q, 94

Other acute lower respiratory infections (J20-J22)

> **EXCLUDES 2**   chronic obstructive pulmonary disease with acute lower respiratory infection (J44.0)

✓4ᵗʰ J20   Acute bronchitis

> **INCLUDES**   acute and subacute bronchitis (with) bronchospasm
> acute and subacute bronchitis (with) tracheitis
> acute and subacute bronchitis (with) tracheobronchitis, acute
> acute and subacute fibrinous bronchitis
> acute and subacute membranous bronchitis
> acute and subacute purulent bronchitis
> acute and subacute septic bronchitis
> **EXCLUDES 1**   bronchitis NOS (J40)
> tracheobronchitis NOS (J40)
> **EXCLUDES 2**   acute bronchitis with bronchiectasis (J47.0)
> acute bronchitis with chronic obstructive asthma (J44.0)
> acute bronchitis with chronic obstructive pulmonary disease (J44.0)
> allergic bronchitis NOS (J45.909)
> bronchitis due to chemicals, fumes and vapors (J68.0)
> chronic bronchitis NOS (J42)
> chronic mucopurulent bronchitis (J41.1)
> chronic obstructive bronchitis (J44.-)
> chronic obstructive tracheobronchitis (J44.-)
> chronic simple bronchitis (J41.0)
> chronic tracheobronchitis (J42)

AHA: 2016, 3Q, 10, 16
DEF: Acute inflammation of the main branches of the bronchial tree due to infectious or irritant agents. Symptoms include cough with a varied production of sputum, fever, substernal soreness, and lung rales. Bronchitis usually lasts three to 10 days.

J20.0   **Acute bronchitis due to** Mycoplasma pneumoniae

J20.1   **Acute bronchitis due to** Hemophilus influenzae

J20.2   **Acute bronchitis due to** streptococcus

J20.3   **Acute bronchitis due to** coxsackievirus

J20.4   **Acute bronchitis due to** parainfluenza virus

J20.5   **Acute bronchitis due to** respiratory syncytial virus

J20.6   **Acute bronchitis due to** rhinovirus

J20.7   **Acute bronchitis due to** echovirus

J20.8   **Acute bronchitis due to** other specified organisms

J20.9   **Acute bronchitis,** unspecified

`N` Newborn: 0   `P` Pediatric: 0-17   `M` Maternity: 12-55   `A` Adult: 15-124   `MCC` Major Complication/Comorbidity   `CC` Complication/Comorbidity   `SW` Severe Wound Dx

680   ICD-10-CM 2019

✓4ᵗʰ **J21 Acute bronchiolitis**
> INCLUDES acute bronchiolitis with bronchospasm
> EXCLUDES 2 *respiratory bronchiolitis interstitial lung disease (J84.115)*

> **CC Excl: For CC codes in category J21, unless otherwise noted:**
> PDX collection 738

J21.0 Acute bronchiolitis due to respiratory syncytial virus   CC
> CC Excl: PDX collection 737

J21.1 Acute bronchiolitis due to human metapneumovirus   CC

J21.8 Acute bronchiolitis due to other specified organisms   CC

J21.9 Acute bronchiolitis, unspecified   CC
> Bronchiolitis (acute)
> EXCLUDES 1 *chronic bronchiolitis (J44.-)*

J22 Unspecified acute lower respiratory infection
> Acute (lower) respiratory (tract) infection NOS
> EXCLUDES 1 *upper respiratory infection (acute) (J06.9)*

Other diseases of upper respiratory tract (J30-J39)

✓4ᵗʰ **J30 Vasomotor and allergic rhinitis**
> INCLUDES spasmodic rhinorrhea
> EXCLUDES 1 *allergic rhinitis with asthma (bronchial) (J45.909)*
>   *rhinitis NOS (J31.0)*

J30.0 Vasomotor rhinitis
> **DEF:** Noninfectious and nonallergic type of rhinitis for which the cause is often unknown. Symptoms often mimic those of allergic rhinitis with a diagnosis of vasomotor rhinitis typically made after ruling out allergens as the cause.

J30.1 Allergic rhinitis due to pollen
> Allergy NOS due to pollen
> Hay fever
> Pollinosis

J30.2 Other seasonal allergic rhinitis

J30.5 Allergic rhinitis due to food

✓5ᵗʰ **J30.8 Other allergic rhinitis**

J30.81 Allergic rhinitis due to animal (cat) (dog) hair and dander

J30.89 Other allergic rhinitis
> Perennial allergic rhinitis

J30.9 Allergic rhinitis, unspecified

✓4ᵗʰ **J31 Chronic rhinitis, nasopharyngitis and pharyngitis**
> Use additional code to identify:
> exposure to environmental tobacco smoke (Z77.22)
> exposure to tobacco smoke in the perinatal period (P96.81)
> history of tobacco dependence (Z87.891)
> occupational exposure to environmental tobacco smoke (Z57.31)
> tobacco dependence (F17.-)
> tobacco use (Z72.0)

J31.0 Chronic rhinitis
> Atrophic rhinitis (chronic)
> Granulomatous rhinitis (chronic)
> Hypertrophic rhinitis (chronic)
> Obstructive rhinitis (chronic)
> Ozena
> Purulent rhinitis (chronic)
> Rhinitis (chronic) NOS
> Ulcerative rhinitis (chronic)
> EXCLUDES 1 *allergic rhinitis (J30.1-J30.9)*
>   *vasomotor rhinitis (J30.0)*
> **DEF:** Persistent inflammation of the mucous membranes of the nose, characterized by a postnasal drip.

J31.1 Chronic nasopharyngitis
> EXCLUDES 2 *acute nasopharyngitis (J00)*
> **DEF:** Persistent inflammation of the mucous membranes extending from the nares to the pharynx. It is characterized by constant irritation in the nasopharynx and postnasal drip.

J31.2 Chronic pharyngitis
> Atrophic pharyngitis (chronic)
> Chronic sore throat
> Granular pharyngitis (chronic)
> Hypertrophic pharyngitis (chronic)
> EXCLUDES 2 *acute pharyngitis (J02.9)*

✓4ᵗʰ **J32 Chronic sinusitis**
> INCLUDES sinus abscess
>   sinus empyema
>   sinus infection
>   sinus suppuration
> Use additional code to identify:
> exposure to environmental tobacco smoke (Z77.22)
> exposure to tobacco smoke in the perinatal period (P96.81)
> history of tobacco dependence (Z87.891)
> infectious agent (B95-B97)
> occupational exposure to environmental tobacco smoke (Z57.31)
> tobacco dependence (F17.-)
> tobacco use (Z72.0)
> EXCLUDES 2 *acute sinusitis (J01.-)*

J32.0 Chronic maxillary sinusitis
> Antritis (chronic)
> Maxillary sinusitis NOS

J32.1 Chronic frontal sinusitis
> Frontal sinusitis NOS

J32.2 Chronic ethmoidal sinusitis
> Ethmoidal sinusitis NOS
> EXCLUDES 1 *Woakes' ethmoiditis (J33.1)*

J32.3 Chronic sphenoidal sinusitis
> Sphenoidal sinusitis NOS

J32.4 Chronic pansinusitis
> Pansinusitis NOS

J32.8 Other chronic sinusitis
> Sinusitis (chronic) involving more than one sinus but not pansinusitis

J32.9 Chronic sinusitis, unspecified
> Sinusitis (chronic) NOS

✓4ᵗʰ **J33 Nasal polyp**
> Use additional code to identify:
> exposure to environmental tobacco smoke (Z77.22)
> exposure to tobacco smoke in the perinatal period (P96.81)
> history of tobacco dependence (Z87.891)
> occupational exposure to environmental tobacco smoke (Z57.31)
> tobacco dependence (F17.-)
> tobacco use (Z72.0)
> EXCLUDES 1 *adenomatous polyps (D14.0)*

J33.0 Polyp of nasal cavity
> Choanal polyp
> Nasopharyngeal polyp

J33.1 Polypoid sinus degeneration
> Woakes' syndrome or ethmoiditis

J33.8 Other polyp of sinus
> Accessory polyp of sinus
> Ethmoidal polyp of sinus
> Maxillary polyp of sinus
> Sphenoidal polyp of sinus

J33.9 Nasal polyp, unspecified

✓4ᵗʰ **J34 Other and unspecified disorders of nose and nasal sinuses**
> EXCLUDES 2 *varicose ulcer of nasal septum (I86.8)*

J34.0 Abscess, furuncle and carbuncle of nose
> Cellulitis of nose   Ulceration of nose
> Necrosis of nose

J34.1 Cyst and mucocele of nose and nasal sinus

J34.2 Deviated nasal septum
> Deflection or deviation of septum (nasal) (acquired)
> EXCLUDES 1 *congenital deviated nasal septum (Q67.4)*
> **DEF:** Condition in which the nasal septum, a thin wall composed of cartilage and bone that separates the two nostrils, is crooked or displaced from the midline.

J34.3 Hypertrophy of nasal turbinate
> **DEF:** Overgrowth of bones within the nasal turbinate, which are ridges of bone and soft tissue that project from the sidewalls of the nasal passages. Hypertrophy can cause obstruction of the nasal passages.

✓5ᵗʰ **J34.8 Other specified disorders of nose and nasal sinuses**

J34.81 Nasal mucositis (ulcerative)
> Code also type of associated therapy, such as:
> antineoplastic and immunosuppressive drugs (T45.1X-)
> radiological procedure and radiotherapy (Y84.2)
> EXCLUDES 2 *gastrointestinal mucositis (ulcerative) (K92.81)*
>   *mucositis (ulcerative) of vagina and vulva (N76.81)*
>   *oral mucositis (ulcerative) (K12.3-)*

☑ Additional Character Required   ✓x7ᵗʰ Placeholder   Unacceptable PDx   Questionable PDx   Manifestation   H1–H14 HAC   HCC CMS-HCC Dx   HIV HIV Dx

ICD-10-CM 2019   681

J34.89   Other specified disorders of nose and nasal sinuses
Perforation of nasal septum NOS
Rhinolith

J34.9   Unspecified disorder of nose and nasal sinuses

✓4th **J35   Chronic diseases of tonsils and adenoids**
Use additional code to identify:
exposure to environmental tobacco smoke (Z77.22)
exposure to tobacco smoke in the perinatal period (P96.81)
history of tobacco dependence (Z87.891)
occupational exposure to environmental tobacco smoke (Z57.31)
tobacco dependence (F17.-)
tobacco use (Z72.0)

✓5th **J35.0   Chronic tonsillitis and adenoiditis**
EXCLUDES 2   *acute tonsillitis (J03.-)*

J35.01   Chronic tonsillitis

J35.02   Chronic adenoiditis

J35.03   Chronic tonsillitis and adenoiditis

J35.1   Hypertrophy of tonsils
Enlargement of tonsils
EXCLUDES 1   *hypertrophy of tonsils with tonsillitis (J35.0-)*

J35.2   Hypertrophy of adenoids
Enlargement of adenoids
EXCLUDES 1   *hypertrophy of adenoids with adenoiditis (J35.0-)*

J35.3   Hypertrophy of tonsils with hypertrophy of adenoids
EXCLUDES 1   *hypertrophy of tonsils and adenoids with tonsillitis and adenoiditis (J35.03)*

J35.8   Other chronic diseases of tonsils and adenoids
Adenoid vegetations   Tonsillar tag
Amygdalolith   Ulcer of tonsil
Calculus, tonsil
Cicatrix of tonsil (and adenoid)

J35.9   Chronic disease of tonsils and adenoids, unspecified
Disease (chronic) of tonsils and adenoids NOS

J36   Peritonsillar abscess   CC
INCLUDES   abscess of tonsil
peritonsillar cellulitis
quinsy
Use additional code (B95-B97) to identify infectious agent
EXCLUDES 1   *acute tonsillitis (J03.-)*
chronic tonsillitis (J35.0)
retropharyngeal abscess (J39.0)
tonsillitis NOS (J03.9-)
CC Excl: PDX collection 739

✓4th **J37   Chronic laryngitis and laryngotracheitis**
Use additional code to identify:
exposure to environmental tobacco smoke (Z77.22)
exposure to tobacco smoke in the perinatal period (P96.81)
history of tobacco dependence (Z87.891)
infectious agent (B95-B97)
occupational exposure to environmental tobacco smoke (Z57.31)
tobacco dependence (F17.-)
tobacco use (Z72.0)

J37.0   Chronic laryngitis
Catarrhal laryngitis
Hypertrophic laryngitis
Sicca laryngitis
EXCLUDES 2   *acute laryngitis (J04.0)*
obstructive (acute) laryngitis (J05.0)

J37.1   Chronic laryngotracheitis
Laryngitis, chronic, with tracheitis (chronic)
Tracheitis, chronic, with laryngitis
EXCLUDES 1   *chronic tracheitis (J42)*
EXCLUDES 2   *acute laryngotracheitis (J04.2)*
acute tracheitis (J04.1)

✓4th **J38   Diseases of vocal cords and larynx, not elsewhere classified**
Use additional code to identify:
exposure to environmental tobacco smoke (Z77.22)
exposure to tobacco smoke in the perinatal period (P96.81)
history of tobacco dependence (Z87.891)
occupational exposure to environmental tobacco smoke (Z57.31)
tobacco dependence (F17.-)
tobacco use (Z72.0)
EXCLUDES 1   *congenital laryngeal stridor (P28.89)*
obstructive laryngitis (acute) (J05.0)
postprocedural subglottic stenosis (J95.5)
stridor (R06.1)
ulcerative laryngitis (J04.0)

✓5th **J38.0   Paralysis of vocal cords and larynx**
Laryngoplegia
Paralysis of glottis

J38.00   Paralysis of vocal cords and larynx, unspecified

J38.01   Paralysis of vocal cords and larynx, unilateral

J38.02   Paralysis of vocal cords and larynx, bilateral

J38.1   Polyp of vocal cord and larynx
EXCLUDES 1   *adenomatous polyps (D14.1)*

J38.2   Nodules of vocal cords
Chorditis (fibrinous)(nodosa)(tuberosa)
Singer's nodes
Teacher's nodes

J38.3   Other diseases of vocal cords
Abscess of vocal cords
Cellulitis of vocal cords
Granuloma of vocal cords
Leukokeratosis of vocal cords
Leukoplakia of vocal cords

J38.4   Edema of larynx
Edema (of) glottis
Subglottic edema
Supraglottic edema
EXCLUDES 1   *acute obstructive laryngitis [croup] (J05.0)*
edematous laryngitis (J04.0)

J38.5   Laryngeal spasm
Laryngismus (stridulus)

J38.6   Stenosis of larynx

J38.7   Other diseases of larynx
Abscess of larynx
Cellulitis of larynx
Disease of larynx NOS
Necrosis of larynx
Pachyderma of larynx
Perichondritis of larynx
Ulcer of larynx

✓4th **J39   Other diseases of upper respiratory tract**
EXCLUDES 1   *acute respiratory infection NOS (J22)*
acute upper respiratory infection (J06.9)
upper respiratory inflammation due to chemicals, gases, fumes or vapors (J68.2)

J39.0   Retropharyngeal and parapharyngeal abscess   CC
Peripharyngeal abscess
EXCLUDES 1   *peritonsillar abscess (J36)*
DEF: Purulent infection behind the pharynx and the front of the precerebral fascia, characterized by neck stiffness, cervical lymphadenopathy, sore throat, fever, and stridor.
CC Excl: PDX collection 740

J39.1   Other abscess of pharynx   CC
Cellulitis of pharynx
Nasopharyngeal abscess
CC Excl: PDX collection 740

J39.2   Other diseases of pharynx
Cyst of pharynx
Edema of pharynx
EXCLUDES 2   *chronic pharyngitis (J31.2)*
ulcerative pharyngitis (J02.9)

J39.3   Upper respiratory tract hypersensitivity reaction, site unspecified
EXCLUDES 1   *hypersensitivity reaction of upper respiratory tract, such as:*
extrinsic allergic alveolitis (J67.9)
pneumoconiosis (J60-J67.9)

J39.8   Other specified diseases of upper respiratory tract

J39.9   Disease of upper respiratory tract, unspecified

Chronic lower respiratory diseases (J40-J47)

EXCLUDES 1   *bronchitis due to chemicals, gases, fumes and vapors (J68.0)*
EXCLUDES 2   *cystic fibrosis (E84.-)*

J40   Bronchitis, not specified as acute or chronic
Bronchitis NOS
Bronchitis with tracheitis NOS
Catarrhal bronchitis
Tracheobronchitis NOS
Use additional code to identify:
  exposure to environmental tobacco smoke (Z77.22)
  exposure to tobacco smoke in the perinatal period (P96.81)
  history of tobacco dependence (Z87.891)
  occupational exposure to environmental tobacco smoke (Z57.31)
  tobacco dependence (F17.-)
  tobacco use (Z72.0)
  EXCLUDES 1   *acute bronchitis (J20.-)*
     allergic bronchitis NOS (J45.909)
     asthmatic bronchitis NOS (J45.9-)
     bronchitis due to chemicals, gases, fumes and vapors (J68.0)

✓4ᵗʰ J41   Simple and mucopurulent chronic bronchitis
Use additional code to identify:
  exposure to environmental tobacco smoke (Z77.22)
  exposure to tobacco smoke in the perinatal period (P96.81)
  history of tobacco dependence (Z87.891)
  occupational exposure to environmental tobacco smoke (Z57.31)
  tobacco dependence (F17.-)
  tobacco use (Z72.0)
  EXCLUDES 1   *chronic bronchitis NOS (J42)*
     chronic obstructive bronchitis (J44.-)

J41.0   Simple **chronic bronchitis** `HCC`

J41.1   Mucopurulent **chronic bronchitis** `HCC`

J41.8   Mixed **simple and mucopurulent chronic bronchitis** `HCC`

J42   Unspecified chronic bronchitis `HCC`
Chronic bronchitis NOS
Chronic tracheitis
Chronic tracheobronchitis
Use additional code to identify:
  exposure to environmental tobacco smoke (Z77.22)
  exposure to tobacco smoke in the perinatal period (P96.81)
  history of tobacco dependence (Z87.891)
  occupational exposure to environmental tobacco smoke (Z57.31)
  tobacco dependence (F17.-)
  tobacco use (Z72.0)
  EXCLUDES 1   *chronic asthmatic bronchitis (J44.-)*
     chronic bronchitis with airways obstruction (J44.-)
     chronic emphysematous bronchitis (J44.-)
     chronic obstructive pulmonary disease NOS (J44.9)
     simple and mucopurulent chronic bronchitis (J41.-)

✓4ᵗʰ J43   Emphysema
Use additional code to identify:
  exposure to environmental tobacco smoke (Z77.22)
  history of tobacco dependence (Z87.891)
  occupational exposure to environmental tobacco smoke (Z57.31)
  tobacco dependence (F17.-)
  tobacco use (Z72.0)
  EXCLUDES 1   *compensatory emphysema (J98.3)*
     emphysema due to inhalation of chemicals, gases, fumes or
       vapors (J68.4)
     emphysema with chronic (obstructive) bronchitis (J44.-)
     emphysematous (obstructive) bronchitis (J44.-)
     interstitial emphysema (J98.2)
     mediastinal emphysema (J98.2)
     neonatal interstitial emphysema (P25.0)
     surgical (subcutaneous) emphysema (T81.82)
     traumatic subcutaneous emphysema (T79.7)

DEF: Pathological condition in which there is destructive enlargement of the air sacs in the lungs resulting in damage and lack of elasticity to the alveolar walls, commonly seen in long-term smokers.

J43.0   Unilateral **pulmonary emphysema [MacLeod's syndrome]** `HCC`
  Swyer-James syndrome
  Unilateral emphysema
  Unilateral hyperlucent lung
  Unilateral pulmonary artery functional hypoplasia
  Unilateral transparency of lung

J43.1   Panlobular **emphysema** `HCC`
  Panacinar emphysema

J43.2   Centrilobular **emphysema** `HCC`

J43.8   Other **emphysema** `HCC`

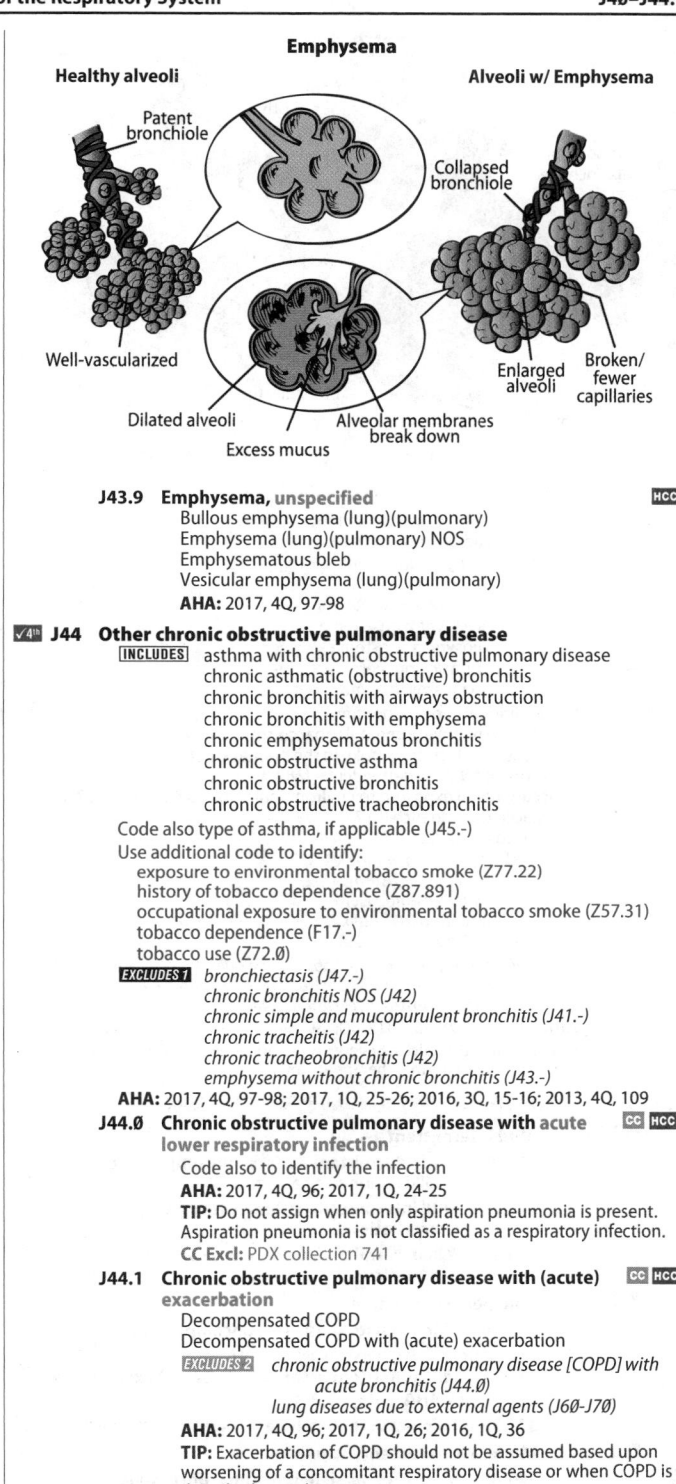

Emphysema

Healthy alveoli   Alveoli w/ Emphysema

Patent bronchiole — Collapsed bronchiole — Well-vascularized — Dilated alveoli — Excess mucus — Alveolar membranes break down — Enlarged alveoli — Broken/fewer capillaries

J43.9   Emphysema, unspecified `HCC`
  Bullous emphysema (lung)(pulmonary)
  Emphysema (lung)(pulmonary) NOS
  Emphysematous bleb
  Vesicular emphysema (lung)(pulmonary)
  AHA: 2017, 4Q, 97-98

✓4ᵗʰ J44   Other chronic obstructive pulmonary disease
INCLUDES   asthma with chronic obstructive pulmonary disease
     chronic asthmatic (obstructive) bronchitis
     chronic bronchitis with airways obstruction
     chronic bronchitis with emphysema
     chronic emphysematous bronchitis
     chronic obstructive asthma
     chronic obstructive bronchitis
     chronic obstructive tracheobronchitis
Code also type of asthma, if applicable (J45.-)
Use additional code to identify:
  exposure to environmental tobacco smoke (Z77.22)
  history of tobacco dependence (Z87.891)
  occupational exposure to environmental tobacco smoke (Z57.31)
  tobacco dependence (F17.-)
  tobacco use (Z72.0)
  EXCLUDES 1   *bronchiectasis (J47.-)*
     chronic bronchitis NOS (J42)
     chronic simple and mucopurulent bronchitis (J41.-)
     chronic tracheitis (J42)
     chronic tracheobronchitis (J42)
     emphysema without chronic bronchitis (J43.-)
AHA: 2017, 4Q, 97-98; 2017, 1Q, 25-26; 2016, 3Q, 15-16; 2013, 4Q, 109

J44.0   Chronic obstructive pulmonary disease with acute `CC` `HCC`
lower respiratory infection
  Code also to identify the infection
  AHA: 2017, 4Q, 96; 2017, 1Q, 24-25
  TIP: Do not assign when only aspiration pneumonia is present. Aspiration pneumonia is not classified as a respiratory infection.
  CC Excl: PDX collection 741

J44.1   Chronic obstructive pulmonary disease with (acute) `CC` `HCC`
exacerbation
  Decompensated COPD
  Decompensated COPD with (acute) exacerbation
  EXCLUDES 2   *chronic obstructive pulmonary disease [COPD] with*
      acute bronchitis (J44.0)
     lung diseases due to external agents (J60-J70)
  AHA: 2017, 4Q, 96; 2017, 1Q, 26; 2016, 1Q, 36
  TIP: Exacerbation of COPD should not be assumed based upon worsening of a concomitant respiratory disease or when COPD is described as end-stage.
  TIP: Assign J43.9 when COPD exacerbation with emphysema is documented.
  CC Excl: PDX collection 741

J44.9   Chronic obstructive pulmonary disease, unspecified `HCC`
  Chronic obstructive airway disease NOS
  Chronic obstructive lung disease NOS
  EXCLUDES 2   *lung diseases due to external agents (J60-J70)*
  AHA: 2017, 4Q, 96-97; 2016, 1Q, 36; 2014, 4Q, 21; 2013, 4Q, 109

✓ Additional Character Required   ✓x7ᵗʰ Placeholder   Unacceptable PDx   Questionable PDx   Manifestation   H1 - H14 HAC   HCC CMS-HCC Dx   HIV HIV Dx

ICD-10-CM 2019   683

Asthma

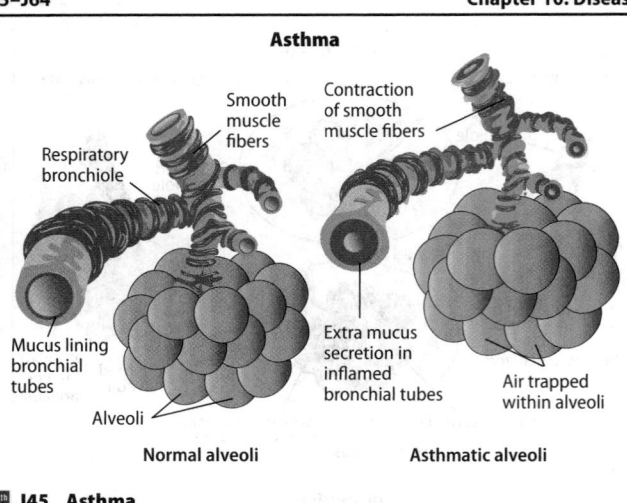

Normal alveoli   Asthmatic alveoli

Labels: Smooth muscle fibers; Contraction of smooth muscle fibers; Respiratory bronchiole; Mucus lining bronchial tubes; Alveoli; Extra mucus secretion in inflamed bronchial tubes; Air trapped within alveoli

✓4th J45 Asthma

INCLUDES
allergic (predominantly) asthma
allergic bronchitis NOS
allergic rhinitis with asthma
atopic asthma
extrinsic allergic asthma
hay fever with asthma
idiosyncratic asthma
intrinsic nonallergic asthma
nonallergic asthma

Use additional code to identify:
exposure to environmental tobacco smoke (Z77.22)
exposure to tobacco smoke in the perinatal period (P96.81)
history of tobacco dependence (Z87.891)
occupational exposure to environmental tobacco smoke (Z57.31)
tobacco dependence (F17.-)
tobacco use (Z72.0)

EXCLUDES 1
detergent asthma (J69.8)
eosinophilic asthma (J82)
miner's asthma (J60)
wheezing NOS (R06.2)
wood asthma (J67.8)

EXCLUDES 2
asthma with chronic obstructive pulmonary disease (J44.9)
chronic asthmatic (obstructive) bronchitis (J44.9)
chronic obstructive asthma (J44.9)

AHA: 2017, 1Q, 25-26; 2012, 4Q, 99

DEF: Status asthmaticus: Severe, intractable episode of asthma that is unresponsive to normal therapeutic measures.

CC Excl: For CC codes in category J45: PDX collection 742

✓5th J45.2 Mild intermittent asthma
J45.20   Mild intermittent asthma, uncomplicated
     Mild intermittent asthma NOS
J45.21   Mild intermittent asthma with (acute) exacerbation   [CC]
J45.22   Mild intermittent asthma with status asthmaticus   [CC]

✓5th J45.3 Mild persistent asthma
J45.30   Mild persistent asthma, uncomplicated
     Mild persistent asthma NOS
J45.31   Mild persistent asthma with (acute) exacerbation [CC]
     AHA: 2016, 1Q, 35
J45.32   Mild persistent asthma with status asthmaticus   [CC]

✓5th J45.4 Moderate persistent asthma
J45.40   Moderate persistent asthma, uncomplicated
     Moderate persistent asthma NOS
J45.41   Moderate persistent asthma with (acute) exacerbation   [CC]
     AHA: 2017, 1Q, 26
J45.42   Moderate persistent asthma with status asthmaticus   [CC]

✓5th J45.5 Severe persistent asthma
J45.50   Severe persistent asthma, uncomplicated
     Severe persistent asthma NOS
J45.51   Severe persistent asthma with (acute) exacerbation   [CC]
J45.52   Severe persistent asthma with status asthmaticus   [CC]

✓5th J45.9 Other and unspecified asthma
✓6th J45.90 Unspecified asthma
Asthmatic bronchitis NOS
Childhood asthma NOS
Late onset asthma
AHA: 2017, 4Q, 96; 2017, 1Q, 25
J45.901   Unspecified asthma with (acute) exacerbation   [CC]
J45.902   Unspecified asthma with status asthmaticus   [CC]
J45.909   Unspecified asthma, uncomplicated
     Asthma NOS
     EXCLUDES 2   lung diseases due to external agents (J60-J70)
     AHA: 2017, 1Q, 25

✓6th J45.99 Other asthma
J45.990   Exercise induced bronchospasm
J45.991   Cough variant asthma
J45.998   Other asthma

✓4th J47 Bronchiectasis
INCLUDES   bronchiolectasis
Use additional code to identify:
exposure to environmental tobacco smoke (Z77.22)
exposure to tobacco smoke in the perinatal period (P96.81)
history of tobacco dependence (Z87.891)
occupational exposure to environmental tobacco smoke (Z57.31)
tobacco dependence (F17.-)
tobacco use (Z72.0)

EXCLUDES 1   congenital bronchiectasis (Q33.4)
     tuberculous bronchiectasis (current disease) (A15.0)

DEF: Dilation of the bronchi with mucus production and persistent cough due to infection or chronic conditions that causes diminished lung capacity and frequent infections of the lung.

J47.0   Bronchiectasis with acute lower respiratory infection   [CC] [HCC]
Bronchiectasis with acute bronchitis
Use additional code to identify the infection
CC Excl: PDX collection 743

J47.1   Bronchiectasis with (acute) exacerbation   [CC] [HCC]
CC Excl: PDX collection 743

J47.9   Bronchiectasis, uncomplicated   [HCC]
Bronchiectasis NOS

Lung diseases due to external agents (J60-J70)
EXCLUDES 2   asthma (J45.-)
     malignant neoplasm of bronchus and lung (C34.-)

DEF: Pneumoconiosis: Condition caused by inhaling inorganic dust particles, typically associated with occupations that require regular exposure to mineral dusts. A form of interstitial lung disease that contributes to the inflammation of the air sacs, causing the lung tissue to harden.

J60   Coalworker's pneumoconiosis   [A] [HCC]
Anthracosilicosis
Anthracosis
Black lung disease
Coalworker's lung
EXCLUDES 1   coalworker pneumoconiosis with tuberculosis, any type in A15 (J65)

J61   Pneumoconiosis due to asbestos and other mineral fibers   [A] [HCC]
Asbestosis
EXCLUDES 1   pleural plaque with asbestosis (J92.0)
     pneumoconiosis with tuberculosis, any type in A15 (J65)

✓4th J62 Pneumoconiosis due to dust containing silica
INCLUDES   silicotic fibrosis (massive) of lung
EXCLUDES 1   pneumoconiosis with tuberculosis, any type in A15 (J65)
J62.0   Pneumoconiosis due to talc dust   [HCC]
J62.8   Pneumoconiosis due to other dust containing silica   [HCC]
Silicosis NOS

✓4th J63 Pneumoconiosis due to other inorganic dusts
EXCLUDES 1   pneumoconiosis with tuberculosis, any type in A15 (J65)
J63.0   Aluminosis (of lung)   [HCC]
J63.1   Bauxite fibrosis (of lung)   [HCC]
J63.2   Berylliosis   [HCC]
J63.3   Graphite fibrosis (of lung)   [HCC]
J63.4   Siderosis   [HCC]
J63.5   Stannosis   [HCC]
J63.6   Pneumoconiosis due to other specified inorganic dusts   [HCC]

J64 Unspecified pneumoconiosis   [HCC]
EXCLUDES 1   pneumonoconiosis with tuberculosis, any type in A15 (J65)

[N] Newborn: 0   [P] Pediatric: 0-17   [M] Maternity: 12-55   [A] Adult: 15-124   [MCC] Major Complication/Comorbidity   [CC] Complication/Comorbidity   [SW] Severe Wound Dx

684   ICD-10-CM 2019

Chapter 10. Diseases of the Respiratory System

J65   **Pneumoconiosis** associated with tuberculosis   `HCC`
Any condition in J60-J64 with tuberculosis, any type in A15
Silicotuberculosis

`✓4th` **J66**   **Airway disease due to specific organic dust**
> `EXCLUDES 2`   *allergic alveolitis (J67.-)*
> *asbestosis (J61)*
> *bagassosis (J67.1)*
> *farmer's lung (J67.0)*
> *hypersensitivity pneumonitis due to organic dust (J67.-)*
> *reactive airways dysfunction syndrome (J68.3)*

   J66.0   **Byssinosis**   `HCC`
     Airway disease due to cotton dust

   J66.1   **Flax-dressers' disease**   `HCC`

   J66.2   **Cannabinosis**   `HCC`

   J66.8   **Airway disease due to other specific organic dusts**   `HCC`

`✓4th` **J67**   **Hypersensitivity pneumonitis due to organic dust**
> `INCLUDES`   allergic alveolitis and pneumonitis due to inhaled organic dust and particles of fungal, actinomycetic or other origin
> `EXCLUDES 1`   *pneumonitis due to inhalation of chemicals, gases, fumes or vapors (J68.0)*

> **CC Excl: For CC codes in category J67:** PDX collection 110

   J67.0   **Farmer's lung**   `HCC`
     Harvester's lung
     Haymaker's lung
     Moldy hay disease

   J67.1   **Bagassosis**   `HCC`
     Bagasse disease
     Bagasse pneumonitis

   J67.2   **Bird fancier's lung**   `HCC`
     Budgerigar fancier's disease or lung
     Pigeon fancier's disease or lung

   J67.3   **Suberosis**   `HCC`
     Corkhandler's disease or lung
     Corkworker's disease or lung

   J67.4   **Maltworker's lung**   `HCC`
     Alveolitis due to Aspergillus clavatus

   J67.5   **Mushroom-worker's lung**   `HCC`

   J67.6   **Maple-bark-stripper's lung**   `HCC`
     Alveolitis due to Cryptostroma corticale
     Cryptostromosis

   J67.7   **Air conditioner and humidifier lung**   `CC` `HCC`
     Allergic alveolitis due to fungal, thermophilic actinomycetes and other organisms growing in ventilation [air conditioning] systems

   J67.8   **Hypersensitivity pneumonitis due to other organic dusts**   `CC` `HCC`
     Cheese-washer's lung
     Coffee-worker's lung
     Fish-meal worker's lung
     Furrier's lung
     Sequoiosis

   J67.9   **Hypersensitivity pneumonitis due to unspecified organic dust**   `CC` `HCC`
     Allergic alveolitis (extrinsic) NOS
     Hypersensitivity pneumonitis NOS

`✓4th` **J68**   **Respiratory conditions due to inhalation of chemicals, gases, fumes and vapors**
> Code first (T51-T65) to identify cause
> Use additional code to identify associated respiratory conditions, such as:
> acute respiratory failure (J96.0-)

> **CC Excl: For CC/MCC codes in category J68:** PDX collection 110

   J68.0   **Bronchitis and pneumonitis** due to chemicals, gases, fumes and vapors   `CC` `HCC`
     Chemical bronchitis (acute)

   J68.1   **Pulmonary edema** due to chemicals, gases, fumes and vapors   `MCC` `HCC`
     Chemical pulmonary edema (acute) (chronic)
      `EXCLUDES 1`   *pulmonary edema (acute) (chronic) NOS (J81.-)*

   J68.2   **Upper respiratory inflammation** due to chemicals, gases, fumes and vapors, not elsewhere classified   `HCC`

   J68.3   **Other acute and subacute respiratory conditions** due to chemicals, gases, fumes and vapors   `HCC`
     Reactive airways dysfunction syndrome

   J68.4   **Chronic respiratory conditions** due to chemicals, gases, fumes and vapors   `HCC`
     Emphysema (diffuse) (chronic) due to inhalation of chemicals, gases and vapors
     Obliterative bronchiolitis (chronic) (subacute) due to inhalation of chemicals, gases, fumes and vapors
     Pulmonary fibrosis (chronic) due to inhalation of chemicals, gases, fumes and vapors
      `EXCLUDES 1`   *chronic pulmonary edema due to chemicals, gases, fumes and vapors (J68.1)*

   J68.8   **Other respiratory conditions** due to chemicals, gases, fumes and vapors   `HCC`

   J68.9   **Unspecified respiratory condition** due to chemicals, gases, fumes and vapors   `HCC`

`✓4th` **J69**   **Pneumonitis due to solids and liquids**
> `EXCLUDES 1`   *neonatal aspiration syndromes (P24.-)*
> *postprocedural pneumonitis (J95.4)*
> **AHA:** 2017, 1Q, 24
> **DEF:** Pneumonitis: Noninfectious inflammation of the walls of the alveoli in the lung tissue due to inhalation of food, vomit, oils, essences, or other solids or liquids.

> **CC Excl: For MCC codes in category J69:** PDX collection 110

   J69.0   **Pneumonitis due to inhalation of food and vomit**   `MCC` `HCC`
     Aspiration pneumonia NOS
     Aspiration pneumonia (due to) food (regurgitated)
     Aspiration pneumonia (due to) gastric secretions
     Aspiration pneumonia (due to) milk
     Aspiration pneumonia (due to) vomit
     Code also any associated foreign body in respiratory tract (T17.-)
      `EXCLUDES 1`   *chemical pneumonia due to anesthesia (J95.4)*
       obstetric aspiration pneumonitis (O74.0)

   J69.1   **Pneumonitis due to inhalation of oils and essences**   `MCC` `HCC`
     Exogenous lipoid pneumonia
     Lipid pneumonia NOS
     Code first (T51-T65) to identify substance
      `EXCLUDES 1`   *endogenous lipoid pneumonia (J84.89)*

   J69.8   **Pneumonitis due to inhalation of other solids and liquids**   `MCC` `HCC`
     Pneumonitis due to aspiration of blood
     Pneumonitis due to aspiration of detergent
     Code first (T51-T65) to identify substance

`✓4th` **J70**   **Respiratory conditions due to other external agents**

> **CC Excl: For CC codes in category J70:** PDX collection 110

   J70.0   **Acute pulmonary manifestations** due to radiation   `CC` `HCC`
     Radiation pneumonitis
     Use additional code (W88-W90, X39.0-) to identify the external cause

   J70.1   **Chronic and other pulmonary manifestations** due to radiation   `CC` `HCC`
     Fibrosis of lung following radiation
     Use additional code (W88-W90, X39.0-) to identify the external cause

   J70.2   **Acute drug-induced interstitial lung disorders**   `HCC`
     Use additional code for adverse effect, if applicable, to identify drug (T36-T50 with fifth or sixth character 5)
      `EXCLUDES 1`   *interstitial pneumonia NOS (J84.9)*
       lymphoid interstitial pneumonia (J84.2)

   J70.3   **Chronic drug-induced interstitial lung disorders**   `HCC`
     Use additional code for adverse effect, if applicable, to identify drug (T36-T50 with fifth or sixth character 5)
      `EXCLUDES 1`   *interstitial pneumonia NOS (J84.9)*
       lymphoid interstitial pneumonia (J84.2)

   J70.4   **Drug-induced interstitial lung disorders, unspecified**   `HCC`
     Use additional code for adverse effect, if applicable, to identify drug (T36-T50 with fifth or sixth character 5)
      `EXCLUDES 1`   *interstitial pneumonia NOS (J84.9)*
       lymphoid interstitial pneumonia (J84.2)

   J70.5   **Respiratory conditions due to smoke inhalation**   `HCC`
     Smoke inhalation NOS
      `EXCLUDES 1`   *smoke inhalation due to chemicals, gases, fumes and vapors (J68.9)*
     AHA: 2013, 4Q, 121

   J70.8   **Respiratory conditions due to other specified external agents**   `HCC`
     Code first (T51-T65) to identify the external agent

   J70.9   **Respiratory conditions due to unspecified external agent**   `HCC`
     Code first (T51-T65) to identify the external agent

✔ Additional Character Required   ✓x7th Placeholder   Unacceptable PDx   Questionable PDx   Manifestation   H1 - H14 HAC   HCC CMS-HCC Dx   HIV HIV Dx

ICD-10-CM 2019   685

Chapter 10. Diseases of the Respiratory System

Other respiratory diseases principally affecting the interstitium (J80-J84)

J80   Acute respiratory distress syndrome `MCC` `HCC`
Acute respiratory distress syndrome in adult or child
Adult hyaline membrane disease
EXCLUDES 1   *respiratory distress syndrome in newborn (perinatal) (P22.0)*
AHA: 2017, 1Q, 26
CC Excl: PDX collection 744

✓4th J81   Pulmonary edema
Use additional code to identify:
exposure to environmental tobacco smoke (Z77.22)
history of tobacco dependence (Z87.891)
occupational exposure to environmental tobacco smoke (Z57.31)
tobacco dependence (F17.-)
tobacco use (Z72.0)
EXCLUDES 1   *chemical (acute) pulmonary edema (J68.1)*
hypostatic pneumonia (J18.2)
passive pneumonia (J18.2)
pulmonary edema due to external agents (J60-J70)
pulmonary edema with heart disease NOS (I50.1)
pulmonary edema with heart failure (I50.1)
DEF: Accumulation of fluid in the air sacs of the lungs, making it difficult to breath.

    J81.0   Acute pulmonary edema `MCC` `HCC`
Acute edema of lung
CC Excl: PDX collection 745

    J81.1   Chronic pulmonary edema `CC`
Pulmonary congestion (chronic) (passive)
Pulmonary edema NOS
CC Excl: PDX collection 736

J82   Pulmonary eosinophilia, not elsewhere classified `CC` `HCC`
Allergic pneumonia
Eosinophilic asthma
Eosinophilic pneumonia
Löffler's pneumonia
Tropical (pulmonary) eosinophilia NOS
EXCLUDES 1   *pulmonary eosinophilia due to aspergillosis (B44.-)*
pulmonary eosinophilia due to drugs (J70.2-J70.4)
pulmonary eosinophilia due to specified parasitic infection (B50-B83)
pulmonary eosinophilia due to systemic connective tissue disorders (M30-M36)
pulmonary infiltrate NOS (R91.8)
DEF: Infiltration of eosinophils (white blood cells of the immune system) into the parenchyma of the lungs, resulting in cough, fever, and dyspnea.
CC Excl: PDX collection 746

✓4th J84   Other interstitial pulmonary diseases
EXCLUDES 1   *drug-induced interstitial lung disorders (J70.2-J70.4)*
interstitial emphysema (J98.2)
EXCLUDES 2   *lung diseases due to external agents (J60-J70)*

    CC Excl: For CC/MCC codes in category J84, unless otherwise noted: PDX collection 747

    ✓5th J84.0   Alveolar and parieto-alveolar conditions
       J84.01   Alveolar proteinosis `CC` `HCC`
DEF: Reduced ventilation due to proteinaceous deposits on alveoli. Symptoms include dyspnea, cough, chest pain, weakness, weight loss, and hemoptysis.

       J84.02   Pulmonary alveolar microlithiasis `CC` `HCC`

       J84.03   Idiopathic pulmonary hemosiderosis `CC` `HCC`
Essential brown induration of lung
Code first underlying disease, such as:
disorders of iron metabolism (E83.1-)
EXCLUDES 1   *acute idiopathic pulmonary hemorrhage in infants [AIPHI] (R04.81)*
DEF: Fibrosis of the alveolar walls marked by abnormal accumulation of iron as hemosiderin in the lungs. It primarily affects children and symptoms include anemia, fluid in the lungs, and blood in the sputum. Etiology is unknown.

       J84.09   Other alveolar and parieto-alveolar conditions `CC` `HCC`

✓5th J84.1   Other interstitial pulmonary diseases with fibrosis
EXCLUDES 1   *pulmonary fibrosis (chronic) due to inhalation of chemicals, gases, fumes or vapors (J68.4)*
pulmonary fibrosis (chronic) following radiation (J70.1)

    J84.10   Pulmonary fibrosis, unspecified `HCC`
Capillary fibrosis of lung
Cirrhosis of lung (chronic) NOS
Fibrosis of lung (atrophic) (chronic) (confluent) (massive) (perialveolar) (peribronchial) NOS
Induration of lung (chronic) NOS
Postinflammatory pulmonary fibrosis

    ✓6th J84.11   Idiopathic interstitial pneumonia
EXCLUDES 1   *lymphoid interstitial pneumonia (J84.2)*
pneumocystis pneumonia (B59)

       J84.111   Idiopathic interstitial pneumonia, not otherwise specified `HCC`

       J84.112   Idiopathic pulmonary fibrosis `HCC`
Cryptogenic fibrosing alveolitis
Idiopathic fibrosing alveolitis

       J84.113   Idiopathic non-specific interstitial pneumonitis `HCC`
EXCLUDES 1   *non-specific interstitial pneumonia NOS, or due to known underlying cause (J84.89)*

       J84.114   Acute interstitial pneumonitis `CC` `HCC`
Hamman-Rich syndrome
EXCLUDES 1   *pneumocystis pneumonia (B59)*

       J84.115   Respiratory bronchiolitis interstitial lung disease `HCC`

       J84.116   Cryptogenic organizing pneumonia `CC` `HCC`
EXCLUDES 1   *organizing pneumonia NOS, or due to known underlying cause (J84.89)*

       J84.117   Desquamative interstitial pneumonia `CC` `HCC`

    J84.17   Other interstitial pulmonary diseases with fibrosis in diseases classified elsewhere `HCC`
Interstitial pneumonia (nonspecific) (usual) due to collagen vascular disease
Interstitial pneumonia (nonspecific) (usual) in diseases classified elsewhere
Organizing pneumonia due to collagen vascular disease
Organizing pneumonia in diseases classified elsewhere
Code first underlying disease, such as:
progressive systemic sclerosis (M34.0)
rheumatoid arthritis (M05.00-M06.9)
systemic lupus erythematosis (M32.0-M32.9)

    J84.2   Lymphoid interstitial pneumonia `CC` `HCC`
Lymphoid interstitial pneumonitis

✓5th J84.8   Other specified interstitial pulmonary diseases
EXCLUDES 1   *exogenous lipoid pneumonia (J69.1)*
unspecified lipoid pneumonia (J69.1)

    J84.81   Lymphangioleiomyomatosis `MCC` `HCC`
Lymphangiomyomatosis

    J84.82   Adult pulmonary Langerhans cell histiocytosis `CC` `HCC` `A`
Adult PLCH

    J84.83   Surfactant mutations of the lung `MCC` `HCC`
DEF: Genetic disorder resulting in insufficient secretion of a complex mixture of phospholipids and proteins that reduce surface tension in the alveoli following the onset of breathing to facilitate lung expansion in the newborn. It is the leading indication for pediatric lung transplantation.
CC Excl: PDX collection 748

    ✓6th J84.84   Other interstitial lung diseases of childhood

       CC Excl: For MCC codes in subcategory J84.84: PDX collection 748

       J84.841   Neuroendocrine cell hyperplasia of infancy `MCC` `HCC`

       J84.842   Pulmonary interstitial glycogenosis `MCC` `HCC`

       J84.843   Alveolar capillary dysplasia with vein misalignment `MCC` `HCC`

       J84.848   Other interstitial lung diseases of childhood `MCC` `HCC`

N Newborn: 0   **P** Pediatric: 0-17   **M** Maternity: 12-55   **A** Adult: 15-124   `MCC` Major Complication/Comorbidity   `CC` Complication/Comorbidity   `SW` Severe Wound Dx

686   ICD-10-CM 2019

J84.89   **Other specified interstitial pulmonary diseases** `HCC`
Endogenous lipoid pneumonia
Interstitial pneumonitis
Non-specific interstitial pneumonitis NOS
Organizing pneumonia NOS
Code first, if applicable:
  poisoning due to drug or toxin (T51-T65 with fifth or
    sixth character to indicate intent), for toxic
    pneumonopathy
  underlying cause of pneumonopathy, if known
Use additional code, for adverse effect, to identify
    drug (T36-T50 with fifth or sixth character 5), if
    drug-induced
  EXCLUDES 1   *cryptogenic organizing pneumonia (J84.116)*
      idiopathic non-specific interstitial
        pneumonitis (J84.113)
      lipoid pneumonia, exogenous or unspecified
        (J69.1)
      lymphoid interstitial pneumonia (J84.2)

J84.9   **Interstitial pulmonary disease, unspecified** `CC` `HCC`
Interstitial pneumonia NOS

Suppurative and necrotic conditions of the lower respiratory tract (J85-J86)

✓4ᵗʰ **J85**   **Abscess of lung and mediastinum**
Use additional code (B95-B97) to identify infectious agent

> **CC Excl: For MCC codes in category J85, unless otherwise noted:**
> PDX collection 749

J85.0   **Gangrene and necrosis of lung** `MCC` `HCC`
J85.1   **Abscess of lung with pneumonia** `MCC` `HCC`
Code also the type of pneumonia
J85.2   **Abscess of lung without pneumonia** `MCC` `HCC`
Abscess of lung NOS
J85.3   **Abscess of mediastinum** `MCC` `HCC`
CC Excl: PDX collection 750

✓4ᵗʰ **J86**   **Pyothorax**
Use additional code (B95-B97) to identify infectious agent
EXCLUDES 1   *abscess of lung (J85.-)*
      pyothorax due to tuberculosis (A15.6)
DEF: Collection of pus in the pleural space that is commonly caused by an
infection that spreads from the lung, such as bacterial pneumonia or a
lung abscess.

J86.0   **Pyothorax with fistula** `MCC` `HCC` `SW`
Bronchocutaneous fistula
Bronchopleural fistula
Hepatopleural fistula
Mediastinal fistula
Pleural fistula
Thoracic fistula
Any condition classifiable to J86.9 with fistula
DEF: Purulent infection of the respiratory cavity, with
communication from a cavity to another structure.
CC Excl: PDX collection 751

J86.9   **Pyothorax without fistula** `MCC` `HCC`
Abscess of pleura   Pyopneumothorax
Abscess of thorax   Septic pleurisy
Empyema (chest) (lung) (pleura) Seropurulent pleurisy
Fibrinopurulent pleurisy   Suppurative pleurisy
Purulent pleurisy
CC Excl: PDX collection 751

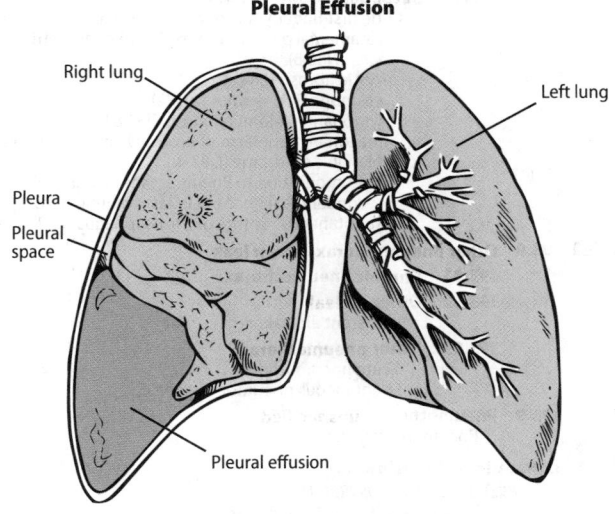

Pleural Effusion

Right lung   Left lung

Pleura

Pleural
space

Pleural effusion

Other diseases of the pleura (J90-J94)

J90   **Pleural effusion, not elsewhere classified** `CC`
Encysted pleurisy
Pleural effusion NOS
Pleurisy with effusion (exudative) (serous)
EXCLUDES 1   *chylous (pleural) effusion (J94.0)*
      malignant pleural effusion (J91.0))
      pleurisy NOS (R09.1)
      tuberculous pleural effusion (A15.6)
DEF: Collection of lymph and other fluid within the pleural space.
CC Excl: PDX collection 752

✓4ᵗʰ **J91**   **Pleural effusion in conditions classified elsewhere**
EXCLUDES 2   *pleural effusion in heart failure (I50.-)*
      pleural effusion in systemic lupus erythematosus (M32.13)
DEF: Collection of lymph and other fluid within the pleural space.

J91.0   ***Malignant pleural effusion*** `CC`
Code first underlying neoplasm
CC Excl: PDX collection 753

J91.8   ***Pleural effusion in other conditions classified elsewhere*** `CC`
Code first underlying disease, such as:
  filariasis (B74.0-B74.9)
  influenza (J09.X2, J10.1, J11.1)
AHA: 2015, 2Q, 15
CC Excl: PDX collection 752

✓4ᵗʰ **J92**   **Pleural plaque**
INCLUDES   pleural thickening
DEF: Areas of fibrous thickening that form on the parietal or visceral
pleura, the membranes that line the ribs and lungs.

J92.0   **Pleural plaque with presence of asbestos**
J92.9   **Pleural plaque without asbestos**
Pleural plaque NOS

✓4ᵗʰ **J93**   **Pneumothorax and air leak**
EXCLUDES 1   *congenital or perinatal pneumothorax (P25.1)*
      postprocedural air leak (J95.812)
      postprocedural pneumothorax (J95.811)
      traumatic pneumothorax (S27.0)
      tuberculous (current disease) pneumothorax (A15.-)
      pyopneumothorax (J86.-)
DEF: Pneumothorax: Lung displacement due to abnormal leakage of air or
gas that is trapped in the pleural space formed by the membrane that
encloses the lungs and lines the thoracic cavity.

> **CC Excl: For CC/MCC codes in category J93:** PDX collection 754

J93.0   **Spontaneous tension pneumothorax** `MCC`
DEF: Leaking air from the lung into the lining, causing collapse.

✓5ᵗʰ **J93.1**   **Other spontaneous pneumothorax**
J93.11   **Primary spontaneous pneumothorax** `CC`

J93.12   Secondary spontaneous pneumothorax   `CC`
Code first underlying condition, such as:
catamenial pneumothorax due to endometriosis
(N80.8)
cystic fibrosis (E84.-)
eosinophilic pneumonia (J82)
lymphangioleiomyomatosis (J84.81)
malignant neoplasm of bronchus and lung (C34.-)
Marfan's syndrome (Q87.4)
pneumonia due to Pneumocystis carinii (B59)
secondary malignant neoplasm of lung (C78.0-)
spontaneous rupture of the esophagus (K22.3)

√5ᵗʰ **J93.8**   Other pneumothorax and air leak

J93.81   Chronic pneumothorax   `CC`

J93.82   Other air leak   `CC`
Persistent air leak

J93.83   Other pneumothorax   `CC`
Acute pneumothorax
Spontaneous pneumothorax NOS

J93.9   Pneumothorax, unspecified   `CC`
Pneumothorax NOS

√4ᵗʰ **J94**   **Other pleural conditions**
EXCLUDES 1   pleurisy NOS (R09.1)
traumatic hemopneumothorax (S27.2)
traumatic hemothorax (S27.1)
tuberculous pleural conditions (current disease) (A15.-)

J94.0   Chylous effusion   `CC`
Chyliform effusion
DEF: Fluid within the pleural space due to the leaking of lymph contents into the space, usually as a result of thoracic duct damage or injury or mediastinal lymphoma.
CC Excl: PDX collection 752

J94.1   Fibrothorax
DEF: Fibrosis within the pleural lining of the lungs commonly seen as a stiff layer surrounding the lung typically attributed to traumatic hemothorax or pleural effusion.

J94.2   Hemothorax   `CC`
Hemopneumothorax
CC Excl: PDX collection 752

J94.8   Other specified pleural conditions   `CC`
Hydropneumothorax
Hydrothorax
CC Excl: No Excl

J94.9   Pleural condition, unspecified

Intraoperative and postprocedural complications and disorders of respiratory system, not elsewhere classified (J95)

√4ᵗʰ **J95**   **Intraoperative and postprocedural complications and disorders of respiratory system, not elsewhere classified**
EXCLUDES 2   aspiration pneumonia (J69.-)
emphysema (subcutaneous) resulting from a procedure (T81.82)
hypostatic pneumonia (J18.2)
pulmonary manifestations due to radiation (J70.0- J70.1)

√5ᵗʰ **J95.0**   Tracheostomy complications

CC Excl: For CC codes in subcategory J95.0:
PDX collection 755

J95.00   Unspecified tracheostomy complication   `CC` `HCC`

J95.01   Hemorrhage from tracheostomy stoma   `CC` `HCC`

J95.02   Infection of tracheostomy stoma   `CC` `HCC`
Use additional code to identify type of infection, such as:
cellulitis of neck (L03.221)
sepsis (A40, A41-)

J95.03   Malfunction of tracheostomy stoma   `CC` `HCC`
Mechanical complication of tracheostomy stoma
Obstruction of tracheostomy airway
Tracheal stenosis due to tracheostomy

Tracheostomy

Tracheostomy in place

Incision in trachea
Trachea
Tracheostomy tube

J95.04   Tracheo-esophageal fistula following tracheostomy   `CC` `HCC`

J95.09   Other tracheostomy complication   `CC` `HCC`

J95.1   Acute pulmonary insufficiency following thoracic surgery   `MCC` `HCC`
EXCLUDES 2   functional disturbances following cardiac surgery (I97.0, I97.1-)
CC Excl: PDX collection 756

J95.2   Acute pulmonary insufficiency following nonthoracic surgery   `MCC` `HCC`
EXCLUDES 2   functional disturbances following cardiac surgery (I97.0, I97.1-)
CC Excl: PDX collection 756

J95.3   Chronic pulmonary insufficiency following surgery   `MCC` `HCC`
EXCLUDES 2   functional disturbances following cardiac surgery (I97.0, I97.1-)
CC Excl: PDX collection 756

J95.4   Chemical pneumonitis due to anesthesia   `CC`
Mendelson's syndrome
Postprocedural aspiration pneumonia
Use additional code for adverse effect, if applicable, to identify drug (T41.- with fifth or sixth character 5)
EXCLUDES 1   aspiration pneumonitis due to anesthesia complicating labor and delivery (O74.0)
aspiration pneumonitis due to anesthesia complicating pregnancy (O29)
aspiration pneumonitis due to anesthesia complicating the puerperium (O89.01)
CC Excl: PDX collection 757

J95.5   Postprocedural subglottic stenosis   `CC`
CC Excl: PDX collection 757

√5ᵗʰ **J95.6**   Intraoperative hemorrhage and hematoma of a respiratory system organ or structure complicating a procedure
EXCLUDES 1   intraoperative hemorrhage and hematoma of a respiratory system organ or structure due to accidental puncture and laceration during procedure (J95.7-)

J95.61   Intraoperative hemorrhage and hematoma of a respiratory system organ or structure complicating a respiratory system procedure   `CC`
CC Excl: PDX collection 758

J95.62   Intraoperative hemorrhage and hematoma of a respiratory system organ or structure complicating other procedure   `CC`
CC Excl: PDX collection 758

Ⓝ Newborn: 0   Ⓟ Pediatric: 0-17   Ⓜ Maternity: 12-55   Ⓐ Adult: 15-124   `MCC` Major Complication/Comorbidity   `CC` Complication/Comorbidity   `SW` Severe Wound Dx

688   ICD-10-CM 2019

✓5ᵗʰ **J95.7** Accidental puncture and laceration of a respiratory system organ or structure during a procedure
> *EXCLUDES 2*   *postprocedural pneumothorax (J95.811)*

J95.71 Accidental puncture and laceration of a respiratory system organ or structure during a respiratory system procedure   `CC`
> CC Excl: PDX collection 509

J95.72 Accidental puncture and laceration of a respiratory system organ or structure during other procedure   `CC`
> CC Excl: PDX collection 509

✓5ᵗʰ **J95.8** Other intraoperative and postprocedural complications and disorders of respiratory system, not elsewhere classified
> AHA: 2016, 4Q, 9-10

✓6ᵗʰ **J95.81** Postprocedural pneumothorax and air leak

J95.811 Postprocedural pneumothorax   `CC` `H14`
> CC Excl: PDX collection 754

J95.812 Postprocedural air leak   `CC`
> CC Excl: PDX collection 754

✓6ᵗʰ **J95.82** Postprocedural respiratory failure
> *EXCLUDES 1*   *respiratory failure in other conditions (J96.-)*

J95.821 Acute postprocedural respiratory failure   `MCC` `HCC`
> Postprocedural respiratory failure NOS
> CC Excl: PDX collection 756

J95.822 Acute and chronic postprocedural respiratory failure   `MCC` `HCC`
> CC Excl: PDX collection 756

✓6ᵗʰ **J95.83** Postprocedural hemorrhage of a respiratory system organ or structure following a procedure

J95.830 Postprocedural hemorrhage of a respiratory system organ or structure following a respiratory system procedure   `CC`
> CC Excl: PDX collection 758

J95.831 Postprocedural hemorrhage of a respiratory system organ or structure following other procedure   `CC`
> CC Excl: PDX collection 758

J95.84 Transfusion-related acute lung injury (TRALI)   `CC`
> **DEF:** Relatively rare, but serious, pulmonary complication of blood transfusion, with acute respiratory distress, noncardiogenic pulmonary edema, cyanosis, hypoxemia, hypotension, fever, and chills.
> CC Excl: PDX collection 757

✓6ᵗʰ **J95.85** Complication of respirator [ventilator]

J95.850 Mechanical complication of respirator   `CC` `HCC`
> *EXCLUDES 1*   *encounter for respirator [ventilator] dependence during power failure (Z99.12)*
> CC Excl: PDX collection 759

J95.851 Ventilator associated pneumonia   `CC` `HCC`
> Ventilator associated pneumonitis
> Use additional code to identify the organism, if known (B95.-, B96.-, B97.-)
> *EXCLUDES 1*   *ventilator lung in newborn (P27.8)*
> AHA: 2017, 1Q, 25
> CC Excl: PDX collection 757

J95.859 Other complication of respirator [ventilator]   `CC` `HCC`
> CC Excl: PDX collection 757

✓6ᵗʰ **J95.86** Postprocedural hematoma and seroma of a respiratory system organ or structure following a procedure

> **CC Excl: For CC codes in subcategory J95.86:** PDX collection 758

J95.860 Postprocedural hematoma of a respiratory system organ or structure following a respiratory system procedure   `CC`

J95.861 Postprocedural hematoma of a respiratory system organ or structure following other procedure   `CC`

J95.862 Postprocedural seroma of a respiratory system organ or structure following a respiratory system procedure   `CC`

J95.863 Postprocedural seroma of a respiratory system organ or structure following other procedure   `CC`

J95.88 Other intraoperative complications of respiratory system, not elsewhere classified   `CC`
> CC Excl: PDX collection 757

J95.89 Other postprocedural complications and disorders of respiratory system, not elsewhere classified   `CC`
> Use additional code to identify disorder, such as:
> aspiration pneumonia (J69.-)
> bacterial or viral pneumonia (J12-J18)
> *EXCLUDES 2*   *acute pulmonary insufficiency following thoracic surgery (J95.1)*
> *postprocedural subglottic stenosis (J95.5)*
> CC Excl: PDX collection 757

Other diseases of the respiratory system (J96-J99)

✓4ᵗʰ **J96** Respiratory failure, not elsewhere classified
> *EXCLUDES 1*   *acute respiratory distress syndrome (J80)*
> *cardiorespiratory failure (R09.2)*
> *newborn respiratory distress syndrome (P22.0)*
> *postprocedural respiratory failure (J95.82-)*
> *respiratory arrest (R09.2)*
> *respiratory arrest of newborn (P28.81)*
> *respiratory failure of newborn (P28.5)*

> **CC Excl: For CC/MCC codes in category J96:** PDX collection 744

✓5ᵗʰ **J96.0** Acute respiratory failure

J96.00 Acute respiratory failure, unspecified whether with hypoxia or hypercapnia   `MCC` `HCC`
> AHA: 2016, 3Q, 14; 2013, 4Q, 121

J96.01 Acute respiratory failure with hypoxia   `MCC` `HCC`

J96.02 Acute respiratory failure with hypercapnia   `MCC` `HCC`

✓5ᵗʰ **J96.1** Chronic respiratory failure

J96.10 Chronic respiratory failure, unspecified whether with hypoxia or hypercapnia   `CC` `HCC`
> AHA: 2016, 1Q, 38; 2015, 1Q, 21

J96.11 Chronic respiratory failure with hypoxia   `CC` `HCC`
> AHA: 2013, 4Q, 129

J96.12 Chronic respiratory failure with hypercapnia   `CC` `HCC`

✓5ᵗʰ **J96.2** Acute and chronic respiratory failure
> Acute on chronic respiratory failure

J96.20 Acute and chronic respiratory failure, unspecified whether with hypoxia or hypercapnia   `MCC` `HCC`

J96.21 Acute and chronic respiratory failure with hypoxia   `MCC` `HCC`

J96.22 Acute and chronic respiratory failure with hypercapnia   `MCC` `HCC`

✓5ᵗʰ **J96.9** Respiratory failure, unspecified

J96.90 Respiratory failure, unspecified, unspecified whether with hypoxia or hypercapnia   `MCC` `HCC`

J96.91 Respiratory failure, unspecified with hypoxia   `MCC` `HCC`

J96.92 Respiratory failure, unspecified with hypercapnia   `MCC` `HCC`

✓4ᵗʰ **J98** Other respiratory disorders
> Use additional code to identify:
> exposure to environmental tobacco smoke (Z77.22)
> exposure to tobacco smoke in the perinatal period (P96.81)
> history of tobacco dependence (Z87.891)
> occupational exposure to environmental tobacco smoke (Z57.31)
> tobacco dependence (F17.-)
> tobacco use (Z72.0)
> *EXCLUDES 1*   *newborn apnea (P28.4)*
> *newborn sleep apnea (P28.3)*
> *EXCLUDES 2*   *apnea NOS (R06.81)*
> *sleep apnea (G47.3-)*

✓5ᵗʰ **J98.0** Diseases of bronchus, not elsewhere classified

J98.01 Acute bronchospasm
> *EXCLUDES 1*   *acute bronchiolitis with bronchospasm (J21.-)*
> *acute bronchitis with bronchospasm (J20.-)*
> *asthma (J45.-)*
> *exercise induced bronchospasm (J45.990)*

Chapter 10. Diseases of the Respiratory System

J98.Ø9   **Other diseases of bronchus, not elsewhere classified**
Broncholithiasis
Calcification of bronchus
Stenosis of bronchus
Tracheobronchial collapse
Tracheobronchial dyskinesia
Ulcer of bronchus

✓5ᵗʰ J98.1   **Pulmonary collapse**
EXCLUDES 1   *therapeutic collapse of lung status (Z98.3)*

J98.11   **Atelectasis**   CC
EXCLUDES 1   *newborn atelectasis*
tuberculous atelectasis (current disease) (A15)
DEF: Collapse of lung tissue affecting part or all of one lung, preventing normal oxygen absorption to healthy tissues.
CC Excl: PDX collection 76Ø

J98.19   **Other pulmonary collapse**   CC
CC Excl: PDX collection 76Ø

J98.2   **Interstitial emphysema**   HCC
Mediastinal emphysema
EXCLUDES 1   *emphysema NOS (J43.9)*
emphysema in newborn (P25.Ø)
surgical emphysema (subcutaneous) (T81.82)
traumatic subcutaneous emphysema (T79.7)

J98.3   **Compensatory emphysema**   HCC
DEF: Distention of all or part of the lung caused by disease processes or surgical intervention that decreased volume in another part of the lung, causing an overcompensation reaction. Compensatory emphysema occurs in association with pneumonias, pleural effusions, atelectasis, empyema, and pneumothorax.

J98.4   **Other disorders of lung**
Calcification of lung
Cystic lung disease (acquired)
Lung disease NOS
Pulmolithiasis
EXCLUDES 1   *acute interstitial pneumonitis (J84.114)*
pulmonary insufficiency following surgery (J95.1-J95.2)

✓5ᵗʰ J98.5   **Diseases of mediastinum, not elsewhere classified**
EXCLUDES 2   *abscess of mediastinum (J85.3)*
AHA: 2016, 4Q, 29

J98.51   **Mediastinitis**   MCC HB
Code first:
underlying condition, if applicable, such as postoperative mediastinitis (T81.-)
CC Excl: No Excl

J98.59   **Other diseases of mediastinum, not elsewhere classified**   MCC HB
Fibrosis of mediastinum
Hernia of mediastinum
Retraction of mediastinum
CC Excl: No Excl

J98.6   **Disorders of diaphragm**
Diaphragmatitis
Paralysis of diaphragm
Relaxation of diaphragm
EXCLUDES 1   *congenital malformation of diaphragm NEC (Q79.1)*
congenital diaphragmatic hernia (Q79.Ø)
EXCLUDES 2   *diaphragmatic hernia (K44.-)*

J98.8   **Other specified respiratory disorders**

J98.9   **Respiratory disorder, unspecified**
Respiratory disease (chronic) NOS

J99   ***Respiratory disorders in diseases classified elsewhere***   HCC
Code first underlying disease, such as:
amyloidosis (E85.-)
ankylosing spondylitis (M45)
congenital syphilis (A5Ø.5)
cryoglobulinemia (D89.1)
early congenital syphilis (A5Ø.Ø)
▶plasminogen deficiency (E88.Ø2)◀
schistosomiasis (B65.Ø-B65.9)
EXCLUDES 1   *respiratory disorders in:*
amebiasis (AØ6.5)
blastomycosis (B4Ø.Ø-B4Ø.2)
candidiasis (B37.1)
coccidioidomycosis (B38.Ø-B38.2)
cystic fibrosis with pulmonary manifestations (E84.Ø)
dermatomyositis (M33.Ø1, M33.11)
histoplasmosis (B39.Ø-B39.2)
late syphilis (A52.72, A52.73)
polymyositis (M33.21)
sicca syndrome (M35.Ø2)
systemic lupus erythematosus (M32.13)
systemic sclerosis (M34.81)
Wegener's granulomatosis (M31.3Ø-M31.31)

Chapter 11. Diseases of the Digestive System (K00–K95)

Chapter Specific Coding Guidelines and Examples
Reserved for future guideline expansion.

Chapter 11. Diseases of the Digestive System (K00-K95)

> EXCLUDES 2   certain conditions originating in the perinatal period (P04-P96)
> certain infectious and parasitic diseases (A00-B99)
> complications of pregnancy, childbirth and the puerperium (O00-O9A)
> congenital malformations, deformations and chromosomal abnormalities (Q00-Q99)
> endocrine, nutritional and metabolic diseases (E00-E88)
> injury, poisoning and certain other consequences of external causes (S00-T88)
> neoplasms (C00-D49)
> symptoms, signs and abnormal clinical and laboratory findings, not elsewhere classified (R00-R94)

This chapter contains the following blocks:

K00-K14	Diseases of oral cavity and salivary glands
K20-K31	Diseases of esophagus, stomach and duodenum
K35-K38	Diseases of appendix
K40-K46	Hernia
K50-K52	Noninfective enteritis and colitis
K55-K64	Other diseases of intestines
K65-K68	Diseases of peritoneum and retroperitoneum
K70-K77	Diseases of liver
K80-K87	Disorders of gallbladder, biliary tract and pancreas
K90-K95	Other diseases of the digestive system

Diseases of oral cavity and salivary glands (K00-K14)

✓4ᵗʰ K00 Disorders of tooth development and eruption

> EXCLUDES 2   embedded and impacted teeth (K01.-)

K00.0 Anodontia
Hypodontia
Oligodontia
> EXCLUDES 1   acquired absence of teeth (K08.1-)

DEF: Partial or complete absence of teeth due to a congenital defect involving the tooth bud.

K00.1 Supernumerary teeth
Distomolar
Fourth molar
Mesiodens
Paramolar
Supplementary teeth
> EXCLUDES 2   supernumerary roots (K00.2)

K00.2 Abnormalities of size and form of teeth
Concrescence of teeth
Dens evaginatus
Dens in dente
Dens invaginatus
Enamel pearls
Fusion of teeth
Gemination of teeth
Macrodontia
Microdontia
Peg-shaped [conical] teeth
Supernumerary roots
Taurodontism
Tuberculum paramolare
> EXCLUDES 1   abnormalities of teeth due to congenital syphilis (A50.5)
> tuberculum Carabelli, which is regarded as a normal variation and should not be coded

K00.3 Mottled teeth
Dental fluorosis
Mottling of enamel
Nonfluoride enamel opacities
> EXCLUDES 2   deposits [accretions] on teeth (K03.6)

K00.4 Disturbances in tooth formation
Aplasia and hypoplasia of cementum
Dilaceration of tooth
Enamel hypoplasia (neonatal) (postnatal) (prenatal)
Regional odontodysplasia
Turner's tooth
> EXCLUDES 1   Hutchinson's teeth and mulberry molars in congenital syphilis (A50.5)
> EXCLUDES 2   mottled teeth (K00.3)

K00.5 Hereditary disturbances in tooth structure, not elsewhere classified
Amelogenesis imperfecta
Dentinogenesis imperfecta
Odontogenesis imperfecta
Dentinal dysplasia
Shell teeth

K00.6 Disturbances in tooth eruption
Dentia praecox
Natal tooth
Neonatal tooth
Premature eruption of tooth
Premature shedding of primary [deciduous] tooth
Prenatal teeth
Retained [persistent] primary tooth
> EXCLUDES 2   embedded and impacted teeth (K01.-)

K00.7 Teething syndrome

K00.8 Other disorders of tooth development
Color changes during tooth formation
Intrinsic staining of teeth NOS
> EXCLUDES 2   posteruptive color changes (K03.7)

K00.9 Disorder of tooth development, unspecified
Disorder of odontogenesis NOS

✓4ᵗʰ K01 Embedded and impacted teeth

> EXCLUDES 1   abnormal position of fully erupted teeth (M26.3-)

K01.0 Embedded teeth

K01.1 Impacted teeth

✓4ᵗʰ K02 Dental caries

> INCLUDES   caries of dentine
> dental cavities
> early childhood caries
> pre-eruptive caries
> recurrent caries (dentino enamel junction) (enamel) (to the pulp)
> tooth decay

K02.3 Arrested dental caries
Arrested coronal and root caries

✓5ᵗʰ K02.5 Dental caries on pit and fissure surface
Dental caries on chewing surface of tooth

    K02.51 Dental caries on pit and fissure surface limited to enamel
White spot lesions [initial caries] on pit and fissure surface of tooth

    K02.52 Dental caries on pit and fissure surface penetrating into dentin
Primary dental caries, cervical origin

    K02.53 Dental caries on pit and fissure surface penetrating into pulp

✓5ᵗʰ K02.6 Dental caries on smooth surface

    K02.61 Dental caries on smooth surface limited to enamel
White spot lesions [initial caries] on smooth surface of tooth

    K02.62 Dental caries on smooth surface penetrating into dentin

    K02.63 Dental caries on smooth surface penetrating into pulp

K02.7 Dental root caries

K02.9 Dental caries, unspecified

Tooth Anatomy

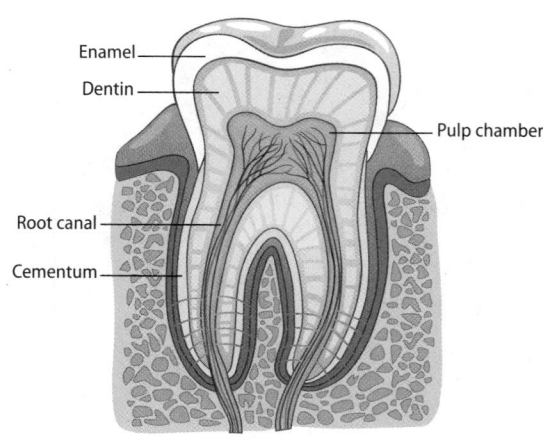

Enamel
Dentin
Pulp chamber
Root canal
Cementum

Ⓝ Newborn: 0   Ⓟ Pediatric: 0-17   Ⓜ Maternity: 12-55   Ⓐ Adult: 15-124   MCC Major Complication/Comorbidity   CC Complication/Comorbidity   SW Severe Wound Dx

692   ICD-10-CM 2019

✓4ᵗʰ **K03 Other diseases of hard tissues of teeth**

     EXCLUDES 2   *bruxism (F45.8)*
               dental caries (K02.-)
               teeth-grinding NOS (F45.8)

K03.0   Excessive attrition of teeth
     Approximal wear of teeth
     Occlusal wear of teeth
     DEF: Attrition: In dentistry, wearing away or erosion of tooth surface from abrasive food or grinding teeth.

K03.1   Abrasion of teeth
     Dentifrice abrasion of teeth
     Habitual abrasion of teeth
     Occupational abrasion of teeth
     Ritual abrasion of teeth
     Traditional abrasion of teeth
     Wedge defect NOS

K03.2   Erosion of teeth
     Erosion of teeth due to diet
     Erosion of teeth due to drugs and medicaments
     Erosion of teeth due to persistent vomiting
     Erosion of teeth NOS
     Idiopathic erosion of teeth
     Occupational erosion of teeth

K03.3   Pathological resorption of teeth
     Internal granuloma of pulp
     Resorption of teeth (external)

K03.4   Hypercementosis
     Cementation hyperplasia

K03.5   Ankylosis of teeth

K03.6   Deposits [accretions] on teeth
     Betel deposits [accretions] on teeth
     Black deposits [accretions] on teeth
     Extrinsic staining of teeth NOS
     Green deposits [accretions] on teeth
     Materia alba deposits [accretions] on teeth
     Orange deposits [accretions] on teeth
     Staining of teeth NOS
     Subgingival dental calculus
     Supragingival dental calculus
     Tobacco deposits [accretions] on teeth

K03.7   Posteruptive color changes of dental hard tissues
     EXCLUDES 2   *deposits [accretions] on teeth (K03.6)*

✓5ᵗʰ **K03.8   Other specified diseases of hard tissues of teeth**

     K03.81   Cracked tooth
         EXCLUDES 1   *asymptomatic craze lines in enamel—omit code*
                   broken or fractured tooth due to trauma (S02.5)

     K03.89   Other specified diseases of hard tissues of teeth

K03.9   Disease of hard tissues of teeth, unspecified

✓4ᵗʰ **K04 Diseases of pulp and periapical tissues**
     AHA: 2016, 4Q, 29-30

     CC Excl: For CC codes in category K04: PDX collection 761

✓5ᵗʰ **K04.0   Pulpitis**
     Acute pulpitis
     Chronic (hyperplastic) (ulcerative) pulpitis

     K04.01   Reversible pulpitis   `CC`

     K04.02   Irreversible pulpitis   `CC`

K04.1   Necrosis of pulp
     Pulpal gangrene

K04.2   Pulp degeneration
     Denticles
     Pulpal calcifications
     Pulpal stones

K04.3   Abnormal hard tissue formation in pulp
     Secondary or irregular dentine

K04.4   Acute apical periodontitis of pulpal origin   `CC`
     Acute apical periodontitis NOS
     EXCLUDES 1   *acute periodontitis (K05.2)*
     DEF: Severe inflammation of the area surrounding the tip of a tooth's root that is often secondary to infection or trauma.

K04.5   Chronic apical periodontitis
     Apical or periapical granuloma
     Apical periodontitis NOS
     EXCLUDES 1   *chronic periodontitis (K05.3-)*

K04.6   Periapical abscess with sinus   `SW`
     Dental abscess with sinus
     Dentoalveolar abscess with sinus

K04.7   Periapical abscess without sinus
     Dental abscess without sinus
     Dentoalveolar abscess without sinus

K04.8   Radicular cyst
     Apical (periodontal) cyst
     Periapical cyst
     Residual radicular cyst
     EXCLUDES 2   *lateral periodontal cyst (K09.0)*
     DEF: Most common odontogenic cyst in tissue around the tooth apex due to chronic inflammation of dental pulp.

✓5ᵗʰ **K04.9   Other and unspecified diseases of pulp and periapical tissues**

     K04.90   Unspecified diseases of pulp and periapical tissues

     K04.99   Other diseases of pulp and periapical tissues

✓4ᵗʰ **K05 Gingivitis and periodontal diseases**
     Use additional code to identify:
         alcohol abuse and dependence (F10.-)
         exposure to environmental tobacco smoke (Z77.22)
         exposure to tobacco smoke in the perinatal period (P96.81)
         history of tobacco dependence (Z87.891)
         occupational exposure to environmental tobacco smoke (Z57.31)
         tobacco dependence (F17.-)
         tobacco use (Z72.0)
     AHA: 2016, 4Q, 29-30

✓5ᵗʰ **K05.0   Acute gingivitis**
     EXCLUDES 1   *acute necrotizing ulcerative gingivitis (A69.1)*
                herpesviral [herpes simplex] gingivostomatitis (B00.2)

     K05.00   Acute gingivitis, plaque induced
         Acute gingivitis NOS
         Plaque induced gingival disease

     K05.01   Acute gingivitis, non-plaque induced

✓5ᵗʰ **K05.1   Chronic gingivitis**
     Desquamative gingivitis (chronic)
     Gingivitis (chronic) NOS
     Hyperplastic gingivitis (chronic)
     Pregnancy associated gingivitis
     Simple marginal gingivitis (chronic)
     Ulcerative gingivitis (chronic)
     Code first, if applicable, diseases of the digestive system complicating pregnancy (O99.61-)

     K05.10   Chronic gingivitis, plaque induced
         Chronic gingivitis NOS
         Gingivitis NOS

     K05.11   Chronic gingivitis, non-plaque induced

✓5ᵗʰ **K05.2   Aggressive periodontitis**
     Acute pericoronitis
     EXCLUDES 1   *acute apical periodontitis (K04.4)*
                periapical abscess (K04.7)
                periapical abscess with sinus (K04.6)

     K05.20   Aggressive periodontitis, unspecified

     ✓6ᵗʰ **K05.21   Aggressive periodontitis, localized**
         Periodontal abscess

         K05.211   Aggressive periodontitis, localized, slight

         K05.212   Aggressive periodontitis, localized, moderate

         K05.213   Aggressive periodontitis, localized, severe

         K05.219   Aggressive periodontitis, localized, unspecified severity

     ✓6ᵗʰ **K05.22   Aggressive periodontitis, generalized**

         K05.221   Aggressive periodontitis, generalized, slight

         K05.222   Aggressive periodontitis, generalized, moderate

         K05.223   Aggressive periodontitis, generalized, severe

         K05.229   Aggressive periodontitis, generalized, unspecified severity

✓5ᵗʰ **K05.3   Chronic periodontitis**
     Chronic pericoronitis   Periodontitis NOS
     Complex periodontitis   Simplex periodontitis
     EXCLUDES 1   *chronic apical periodontitis (K04.5)*

     K05.30   Chronic periodontitis, unspecified

     ✓6ᵗʰ **K05.31   Chronic periodontitis, localized**

         K05.311   Chronic periodontitis, localized, slight

         K05.312   Chronic periodontitis, localized, moderate

✓ Additional Character Required   ✓x7ᵗʰ Placeholder   Unacceptable PDx   Questionable PDx   Manifestation   H1 - H14 HAC   HCC CMS-HCC Dx   HIV HIV Dx

ICD-10-CM 2019   693

      K05.313   **Chronic periodontitis, localized, severe**

      K05.319   **Chronic periodontitis, localized, unspecified severity**

   ✓6ᵗʰ **K05.32**   **Chronic periodontitis, generalized**

      K05.321   **Chronic periodontitis, generalized, slight**

      K05.322   **Chronic periodontitis, generalized, moderate**

      K05.323   **Chronic periodontitis, generalized, severe**

      K05.329   **Chronic periodontitis, generalized, unspecified severity**

K05.4   **Periodontosis**
Juvenile periodontosis

K05.5   **Other periodontal diseases**
Combined periodontic-endodontic lesion
Narrow gingival width (of periodontal soft tissue)
   EXCLUDES 2   leukoplakia of gingiva (K13.21)

K05.6   **Periodontal disease, unspecified**

✓4ᵗʰ **K06**   **Other disorders of gingiva and edentulous alveolar ridge**
   EXCLUDES 2   acute gingivitis (K05.0)
           atrophy of edentulous alveolar ridge (K08.2)
           chronic gingivitis (K05.1)
           gingivitis NOS (K05.1)
   AHA: 2016, 4Q, 29-30

✓5ᵗʰ **K06.0**   **Gingival recession**
Gingival recession (postinfective) (postprocedural)
   AHA: 2017, 4Q, 16

   ✓6ᵗʰ **K06.01**   **Gingival recession, localized**

      K06.010   **Localized gingival recession, unspecified**
Localized gingival recession, NOS

      K06.011   **Localized gingival recession, minimal**

      K06.012   **Localized gingival recession, moderate**

      K06.013   **Localized gingival recession, severe**

   ✓6ᵗʰ **K06.02**   **Gingival recession, generalized**

      K06.020   **Generalized gingival recession, unspecified**
Generalized gingival recession, NOS

      K06.021   **Generalized gingival recession, minimal**

      K06.022   **Generalized gingival recession, moderate**

      K06.023   **Generalized gingival recession, severe**

K06.1   **Gingival enlargement**
Gingival fibromatosis

K06.2   **Gingival and edentulous alveolar ridge lesions associated with trauma**
Irritative hyperplasia of edentulous ridge [denture hyperplasia]
Use additional code (Chapter 20) to identify external cause or denture status (Z97.2)

K06.3   **Horizontal alveolar bone loss**

K06.8   **Other specified disorders of gingiva and edentulous alveolar ridge**
Fibrous epulis
Flabby alveolar ridge
Giant cell epulis
Peripheral giant cell granuloma of gingiva
Pyogenic granuloma of gingiva
Vertical ridge deficiency
   EXCLUDES 2   gingival cyst (K09.0)

K06.9   **Disorder of gingiva and edentulous alveolar ridge, unspecified**

✓4ᵗʰ **K08**   **Other disorders of teeth and supporting structures**
   EXCLUDES 2   dentofacial anomalies [including malocclusion] (M26.-)
           disorders of jaw (M27.-)
   AHA: 2016, 4Q, 29-30

K08.0   **Exfoliation of teeth due to systemic causes**
Code also underlying systemic condition

✓5ᵗʰ **K08.1**   **Complete loss of teeth**
Acquired loss of teeth, complete
   EXCLUDES 1   congenital absence of teeth (K00.0)
           exfoliation of teeth due to systemic causes (K08.0)
           partial loss of teeth (K08.4-)
   DEF: Loss of all teeth as a result of caries, trauma, extraction, periodontal disease, or other specified or unspecified causes.
   Synonym(s): complete edentulism.

   ✓6ᵗʰ **K08.10**   **Complete loss of teeth, unspecified cause**

      K08.101   **Complete loss of teeth, unspecified cause, class I**

      K08.102   **Complete loss of teeth, unspecified cause, class II**

      K08.103   **Complete loss of teeth, unspecified cause, class III**

      K08.104   **Complete loss of teeth, unspecified cause, class IV**

      K08.109   **Complete loss of teeth, unspecified cause, unspecified class**
Edentulism NOS

   ✓6ᵗʰ **K08.11**   **Complete loss of teeth due to trauma**

      K08.111   **Complete loss of teeth due to trauma, class I**

      K08.112   **Complete loss of teeth due to trauma, class II**

      K08.113   **Complete loss of teeth due to trauma, class III**

      K08.114   **Complete loss of teeth due to trauma, class IV**

      K08.119   **Complete loss of teeth due to trauma, unspecified class**

   ✓6ᵗʰ **K08.12**   **Complete loss of teeth due to periodontal diseases**

      K08.121   **Complete loss of teeth due to periodontal diseases, class I**

      K08.122   **Complete loss of teeth due to periodontal diseases, class II**

      K08.123   **Complete loss of teeth due to periodontal diseases, class III**

      K08.124   **Complete loss of teeth due to periodontal diseases, class IV**

      K08.129   **Complete loss of teeth due to periodontal diseases, unspecified class**

   ✓6ᵗʰ **K08.13**   **Complete loss of teeth due to caries**

      K08.131   **Complete loss of teeth due to caries, class I**

      K08.132   **Complete loss of teeth due to caries, class II**

      K08.133   **Complete loss of teeth due to caries, class III**

      K08.134   **Complete loss of teeth due to caries, class IV**

      K08.139   **Complete loss of teeth due to caries, unspecified class**

   ✓6ᵗʰ **K08.19**   **Complete loss of teeth due to other specified cause**

      K08.191   **Complete loss of teeth due to other specified cause, class I**

      K08.192   **Complete loss of teeth due to other specified cause, class II**

      K08.193   **Complete loss of teeth due to other specified cause, class III**

      K08.194   **Complete loss of teeth due to other specified cause, class IV**

      K08.199   **Complete loss of teeth due to other specified cause, unspecified class**

✓5ᵗʰ **K08.2**   **Atrophy of edentulous alveolar ridge**

   K08.20   **Unspecified atrophy of edentulous alveolar ridge**
Atrophy of the mandible NOS
Atrophy of the maxilla NOS

   K08.21   **Minimal atrophy of the mandible**
Minimal atrophy of the edentulous mandible

   K08.22   **Moderate atrophy of the mandible**
Moderate atrophy of the edentulous mandible

   K08.23   **Severe atrophy of the mandible**
Severe atrophy of the edentulous mandible

   K08.24   **Minimal atrophy of maxilla**
Minimal atrophy of the edentulous maxilla

   K08.25   **Moderate atrophy of the maxilla**
Moderate atrophy of the edentulous maxilla

   K08.26   **Severe atrophy of the maxilla**
Severe atrophy of the edentulous maxilla

K08.3   **Retained dental root**

✓5ᵗʰ **K08.4**   **Partial loss of teeth**
Acquired loss of teeth, partial
   EXCLUDES 1   complete loss of teeth (K08.1-)
           congenital absence of teeth (K00.0)
   EXCLUDES 2   exfoliation of teeth due to systemic causes (K08.0)

   ✓6ᵗʰ **K08.40**   **Partial loss of teeth, unspecified cause**

      K08.401   **Partial loss of teeth, unspecified cause, class I**

N Newborn: 0   P Pediatric: 0-17   M Maternity: 12-55   A Adult: 15-124   MCC Major Complication/Comorbidity   CC Complication/Comorbidity   SW Severe Wound Dx

694   ICD-10-CM 2019

K08.402   **Partial loss of teeth, unspecified cause, class II**

K08.403   **Partial loss of teeth, unspecified cause, class III**

K08.404   **Partial loss of teeth, unspecified cause, class IV**

K08.409   **Partial loss of teeth, unspecified cause, unspecified class**
Tooth extraction status NOS

✓6th **K08.41 Partial loss of teeth due to trauma**

K08.411   **Partial loss of teeth due to trauma, class I**

K08.412   **Partial loss of teeth due to trauma, class II**

K08.413   **Partial loss of teeth due to trauma, class III**

K08.414   **Partial loss of teeth due to trauma, class IV**

K08.419   **Partial loss of teeth due to trauma, unspecified class**

✓6th **K08.42 Partial loss of teeth due to periodontal diseases**

K08.421   **Partial loss of teeth due to periodontal diseases, class I**

K08.422   **Partial loss of teeth due to periodontal diseases, class II**

K08.423   **Partial loss of teeth due to periodontal diseases, class III**

K08.424   **Partial loss of teeth due to periodontal diseases, class IV**

K08.429   **Partial loss of teeth due to periodontal diseases, unspecified class**

✓6th **K08.43 Partial loss of teeth due to caries**

K08.431   **Partial loss of teeth due to caries, class I**

K08.432   **Partial loss of teeth due to caries, class II**

K08.433   **Partial loss of teeth due to caries, class III**

K08.434   **Partial loss of teeth due to caries, class IV**

K08.439   **Partial loss of teeth due to caries, unspecified class**

✓6th **K08.49 Partial loss of teeth due to other specified cause**

K08.491   **Partial loss of teeth due to other specified cause, class I**

K08.492   **Partial loss of teeth due to other specified cause, class II**

K08.493   **Partial loss of teeth due to other specified cause, class III**

K08.494   **Partial loss of teeth due to other specified cause, class IV**

K08.499   **Partial loss of teeth due to other specified cause, unspecified class**

✓5th **K08.5 Unsatisfactory restoration of tooth**
Defective bridge, crown, filling
Defective dental restoration
EXCLUDES 1   *dental restoration status (Z98.811)*
EXCLUDES 2   *endosseous dental implant failure (M27.6-)*
                   unsatisfactory endodontic treatment (M27.5-)

K08.50   **Unsatisfactory restoration of tooth, unspecified**
Defective dental restoration NOS

K08.51   **Open restoration margins of tooth**
Dental restoration failure of marginal integrity
Open margin on tooth restoration
Poor gingival margin to tooth restoration

K08.52   **Unrepairable overhanging of dental restorative materials**
Overhanging of tooth restoration

✓6th **K08.53 Fractured dental restorative material**
EXCLUDES 1   *cracked tooth (K03.81)*
                   traumatic fracture of tooth (S02.5)

K08.530   **Fractured dental restorative material without loss of material**

K08.531   **Fractured dental restorative material with loss of material**

K08.539   **Fractured dental restorative material, unspecified**

K08.54   **Contour of existing restoration of tooth biologically incompatible with oral health**
Dental restoration failure of periodontal anatomical integrity
Unacceptable contours of existing restoration of tooth
Unacceptable morphology of existing restoration of tooth

K08.55   **Allergy to existing dental restorative material**
Use additional code to identify the specific type of allergy

K08.56   **Poor aesthetic of existing restoration of tooth**
Dental restoration aesthetically inadequate or displeasing

K08.59   **Other unsatisfactory restoration of tooth**
Other defective dental restoration

✓5th **K08.8 Other specified disorders of teeth and supporting structures**

K08.81   **Primary occlusal trauma**

K08.82   **Secondary occlusal trauma**

K08.89   **Other specified disorders of teeth and supporting structures**
Enlargement of alveolar ridge NOS
Insufficient anatomic crown height
Insufficient clinical crown length
Irregular alveolar process
Toothache NOS

K08.9   **Disorder of teeth and supporting structures, unspecified**

✓4th **K09   Cysts of oral region, not elsewhere classified**
INCLUDES   lesions showing histological features both of aneurysmal cyst and of another fibro-osseous lesion
EXCLUDES 2   *cysts of jaw (M27.0-, M27.4-)*
                   radicular cyst (K04.8)

K09.0   **Developmental odontogenic cysts**
Dentigerous cyst
Eruption cyst
Follicular cyst
Gingival cyst
Lateral periodontal cyst
Primordial cyst
EXCLUDES 2   *keratocysts (D16.4, D16.5)*
                   odontogenic keratocystic tumors (D16.4, D16.5)

K09.1   **Developmental (nonodontogenic) cysts of oral region**
Cyst (of) incisive canal
Cyst (of) palatine of papilla
Globulomaxillary cyst
Median palatal cyst
Nasoalveolar cyst
Nasolabial cyst
Nasopalatine duct cyst

K09.8   **Other cysts of oral region, not elsewhere classified**
Dermoid cyst
Epidermoid cyst
Lymphoepithelial cyst
Epstein's pearl

K09.9   **Cyst of oral region, unspecified**

✓4th **K11   Diseases of salivary glands**
Use additional code to identify:
alcohol abuse and dependence (F10.-)
exposure to environmental tobacco smoke (Z77.22)
exposure to tobacco smoke in the perinatal period (P96.81)
history of tobacco dependence (Z87.891)
occupational exposure to environmental tobacco smoke (Z57.31)
tobacco dependence (F17.-)
tobacco use (Z72.0)

K11.0   **Atrophy of salivary gland**

K11.1   **Hypertrophy of salivary gland**
DEF: Overgrowth of or enlarged salivary gland tissue caused by infection, salivary duct blockage, autoimmune diseases, and benign and malignant tumors.

✓5th **K11.2 Sialoadenitis**
Parotitis
EXCLUDES 1   *epidemic parotitis (B26.-)*
                   mumps (B26.-)
                   uveoparotid fever [Heerfordt] (D86.89)
DEF: Inflammation of the salivary gland.

K11.20   **Sialoadenitis, unspecified**

K11.21   **Acute sialoadenitis**
EXCLUDES 1   *acute recurrent sialoadenitis (K11.22)*

K11.22   **Acute recurrent sialoadenitis**

K11.23   **Chronic sialoadenitis**

✓ Additional Character Required   ✓x7th Placeholder   Unacceptable PDx   Questionable PDx   Manifestation   H1 - H14 HAC   HCC CMS-HCC Dx   HIV HIV Dx

ICD-10-CM 2019   695

K11.3 **Abscess** of salivary gland　　　　　`CC`
　　CC Excl: PDX collection 762

K11.4 **Fistula** of salivary gland　　　　　`CC` `SW`
　　　EXCLUDES 1　congenital fistula of salivary gland (Q38.4)
　　CC Excl: PDX collection 762

K11.5 **Sialolithiasis**
　　Calculus of salivary gland or duct
　　Stone of salivary gland or duct

K11.6 **Mucocele** of salivary gland
　　Mucous extravasation cyst of salivary gland
　　Mucous retention cyst of salivary gland
　　Ranula

K11.7 **Disturbances** of salivary **secretion**
　　Hypoptyalism
　　Ptyalism
　　Xerostomia
　　　EXCLUDES 2　dry mouth NOS (R68.2)

K11.8 **Other** diseases of salivary glands
　　Benign lymphoepithelial lesion of salivary gland
　　Mikulicz' disease
　　Necrotizing sialometaplasia
　　Sialectasia
　　Stenosis of salivary duct
　　Stricture of salivary duct
　　　EXCLUDES 1　sicca syndrome [Sjögren] (M35.0-)

K11.9 **Disease** of salivary gland, **unspecified**
　　Sialoadenopathy NOS

`√4ᵗʰ` **K12** **Stomatitis and related lesions**
　　Use additional code to identify:
　　　alcohol abuse and dependence (F10.-)
　　　exposure to environmental tobacco smoke (Z77.22)
　　　exposure to tobacco smoke in the perinatal period (P96.81)
　　　history of tobacco dependence (Z87.891)
　　　occupational exposure to environmental tobacco smoke (Z57.31)
　　　tobacco dependence (F17.-)
　　　tobacco use (Z72.0)
　　　EXCLUDES 1　cancrum oris (A69.0)
　　　　　　　　　cheilitis (K13.0)
　　　　　　　　　gangrenous stomatitis (A69.0)
　　　　　　　　　herpesviral [herpes simplex] gingivostomatitis (B00.2)
　　　　　　　　　noma (A69.0)

K12.0 **Recurrent oral aphthae**
　　Aphthous stomatitis (major) (minor)
　　Bednar's aphthae
　　Periadenitis mucosa necrotica recurrens
　　Recurrent aphthous ulcer
　　Stomatitis herpetiformis
　　DEF: Disorder of unknown etiology with small oval or round painful ulcers of the mouth marked by a grayish exudate and a red halo effect.

K12.1 **Other forms of stomatitis**
　　Stomatitis NOS
　　Denture stomatitis
　　Ulcerative stomatitis
　　Vesicular stomatitis
　　　EXCLUDES 1　acute necrotizing ulcerative stomatitis (A69.1)
　　　　　　　　　Vincent's stomatitis (A69.1)

K12.2 **Cellulitis and abscess of mouth**　　　　`CC`
　　Cellulitis of mouth (floor)
　　Submandibular abscess
　　　EXCLUDES 2　abscess of salivary gland (K11.3)
　　　　　　　　　abscess of tongue (K14.0)
　　　　　　　　　periapical abscess (K04.6-K04.7)
　　　　　　　　　periodontal abscess (K05.21)
　　　　　　　　　peritonsillar abscess (J36)
　　CC Excl: PDX collection 763

`√5ᵗʰ` **K12.3** **Oral mucositis (ulcerative)**
　　Mucositis (oral) (oropharyneal)
　　　EXCLUDES 2　gastrointestinal mucositis (ulcerative) (K92.81)
　　　　　　　　　mucositis (ulcerative) of vagina and vulva (N76.81)
　　　　　　　　　nasal mucositis (ulcerative) (J34.81)

　　K12.30 **Oral mucositis (ulcerative), unspecified**

　　K12.31 **Oral mucositis (ulcerative) due to antineoplastic therapy**
　　　　Use additional code for adverse effect, if applicable, to identify antineoplastic and immunosuppressive drugs (T45.1X5)
　　　　Use additional code for other antineoplastic therapy, such as:
　　　　　radiological procedure and radiotherapy (Y84.2)

K12.32 **Oral mucositis (ulcerative) due to other drugs**
　　Use additional code for adverse effect, if applicable, to identify drug (T36-T50 with fifth or sixth character 5)

K12.33 **Oral mucositis (ulcerative) due to radiation**
　　Use additional external cause code (W88-W90, X39.0-) to identify cause

K12.39 **Other** oral mucositis (ulcerative)
　　Viral oral mucositis (ulcerative)

`√4ᵗʰ` **K13** **Other diseases of lip and oral mucosa**
　　　`INCLUDES`　epithelial disturbances of tongue
　　Use additional code to identify:
　　　alcohol abuse and dependence (F10.-)
　　　exposure to environmental tobacco smoke (Z77.22)
　　　exposure to tobacco smoke in the perinatal period (P96.81)
　　　history of tobacco dependence (Z87.891)
　　　occupational exposure to environmental tobacco smoke (Z57.31)
　　　tobacco dependence (F17.-)
　　　tobacco use (Z72.0)
　　　EXCLUDES 2　certain disorders of gingiva and edentulous alveolar ridge (K05-K06)
　　　　　　　　　cysts of oral region (K09.-)
　　　　　　　　　diseases of tongue (K14.-)
　　　　　　　　　stomatitis and related lesions (K12.-)

K13.0 **Diseases of lips**
　　Abscess of lips
　　Angular cheilitis
　　Cellulitis of lips
　　Cheilitis NOS
　　Cheilodynia
　　Cheilosis
　　Exfoliative cheilitis
　　Fistula of lips
　　Glandular cheilitis
　　Hypertrophy of lips
　　Perlèche NEC
　　　EXCLUDES 1　ariboflavinosis (E53.0)
　　　　　　　　　cheilitis due to radiation-related disorders (L55-L59)
　　　　　　　　　congenital fistula of lips (Q38.0)
　　　　　　　　　congenital hypertrophy of lips (Q18.6)
　　　　　　　　　Perlèche due to candidiasis (B37.83)
　　　　　　　　　Perlèche due to riboflavin deficiency (E53.0)

K13.1 **Cheek and lip biting**

`√5ᵗʰ` **K13.2** **Leukoplakia and other disturbances of oral epithelium, including tongue**
　　　EXCLUDES 1　carcinoma in situ of oral epithelium (D00.0-)
　　　　　　　　　hairy leukoplakia (K13.3)
　　DEF: Leukoplakia: Thickened white patches or lesions appearing on a mucous membrane, such as oral mucosa or tongue.

　　K13.21 **Leukoplakia of oral mucosa, including tongue**
　　　　Leukokeratosis of oral mucosa
　　　　Leukoplakia of gingiva, lips, tongue
　　　　　EXCLUDES 1　hairy leukoplakia (K13.3)
　　　　　　　　　　　leukokeratosis nicotina palati (K13.24)

　　K13.22 **Minimal keratinized residual ridge mucosa**
　　　　Minimal keratinization of alveolar ridge mucosa

　　K13.23 **Excessive keratinized residual ridge mucosa**
　　　　Excessive keratinization of alveolar ridge mucosa

　　K13.24 **Leukokeratosis nicotina palati**
　　　　Smoker's palate

　　K13.29 **Other disturbances of oral epithelium, including tongue**
　　　　Erythroplakia of mouth or tongue
　　　　Focal epithelial hyperplasia of mouth or tongue
　　　　Leukoedema of mouth or tongue
　　　　Other oral epithelium disturbances

K13.3 **Hairy leukoplakia**

K13.4 **Granuloma and granuloma-like lesions of oral mucosa**
　　Eosinophilic granuloma
　　Granuloma pyogenicum
　　Verrucous xanthoma

K13.5 **Oral submucous fibrosis**
　　Submucous fibrosis of tongue

K13.6 **Irritative hyperplasia of oral mucosa**
　　　EXCLUDES 2　irritative hyperplasia of edentulous ridge [denture hyperplasia] (K06.2)

`√5ᵗʰ` **K13.7** **Other and unspecified lesions of oral mucosa**
　　K13.70 **Unspecified lesions of oral mucosa**
　　K13.79 **Other lesions of oral mucosa**
　　　　Focal oral mucinosis

✓4ᵗʰ K14 Diseases of tongue

Use additional code to identify:
  alcohol abuse and dependence (F10.-)
  exposure to environmental tobacco smoke (Z77.22)
  history of tobacco dependence (Z87.891)
  occupational exposure to environmental tobacco smoke (Z57.31)
  tobacco dependence (F17.-)
  tobacco use (Z72.0)
  EXCLUDES 2   erythroplakia (K13.29)
       focal epithelial hyperplasia (K13.29)
       leukedema of tongue (K13.29)
       leukoplakia of tongue (K13.21)
       hairy leukoplakia (K13.3)
       macroglossia (congenital) (Q38.2)
       submucous fibrosis of tongue (K13.5)

K14.0 Glossitis
Abscess of tongue
Ulceration (traumatic) of tongue
EXCLUDES 1   atrophic glossitis (K14.4)
DEF: Inflammation and swelling of the tongue that may be associated with infection, adverse drug reactions, smoking, or injury.

K14.1 Geographic tongue
Benign migratory glossitis
Glossitis areata exfoliativa

K14.2 Median rhomboid glossitis

K14.3 Hypertrophy of tongue papillae
Black hairy tongue
Coated tongue
Hypertrophy of foliate papillae
Lingua villosa nigra

K14.4 Atrophy of tongue papillae
Atrophic glossitis

K14.5 Plicated tongue
Fissured tongue
Furrowed tongue
Scrotal tongue
EXCLUDES 1   fissured tongue, congenital (Q38.3)

K14.6 Glossodynia
Glossopyrosis
Painful tongue

K14.8 Other diseases of tongue
Atrophy of tongue
Crenated tongue
Enlargement of tongue
Glossocele
Glossoptosis
Hypertrophy of tongue

K14.9 Disease of tongue, unspecified
Glossopathy NOS

Diseases of esophagus, stomach and duodenum (K20-K31)

EXCLUDES 2   hiatus hernia (K44.-)

✓4ᵗʰ K20 Esophagitis

Use additional code to identify:
  alcohol abuse and dependence (F10.-)
EXCLUDES 1   erosion of esophagus (K22.1-)
       esophagitis with gastro-esophageal reflux disease (K21.0)
       reflux esophagitis (K21.0)
       ulcerative esophagitis (K22.1-)
EXCLUDES 2   eosinophilic gastritis or gastroenteritis (K52.81)

K20.0 Eosinophilic esophagitis

K20.8 Other esophagitis
Abscess of esophagus

K20.9 Esophagitis, unspecified
Esophagitis NOS

✓4ᵗʰ K21 Gastro-esophageal reflux disease

EXCLUDES 1   newborn esophageal reflux (P78.83)

K21.0 Gastro-esophageal reflux disease with esophagitis
Reflux esophagitis

K21.9 Gastro-esophageal reflux disease without esophagitis
Esophageal reflux NOS
AHA: 2016, 1Q, 18

✓4ᵗʰ K22 Other diseases of esophagus

EXCLUDES 2   esophageal varices (I85.-)

K22.0 Achalasia of cardia
Achalasia NOS
Cardiospasm
EXCLUDES 1   congenital cardiospasm (Q39.5)
DEF: Esophageal motility disorder that is caused by absence of the esophageal peristalsis and impaired relaxation of the lower esophageal sphincter. It is characterized by dysphagia, regurgitation, and heartburn.

✓5ᵗʰ K22.1 Ulcer of esophagus
Barrett's ulcer
Erosion of esophagus
Fungal ulcer of esophagus
Peptic ulcer of esophagus
Ulcer of esophagus due to ingestion of chemicals
Ulcer of esophagus due to ingestion of drugs and medicaments
Ulcerative esophagitis
Code first poisoning due to drug or toxin, if applicable (T36-T65 with fifth or sixth character 1-4 or 6)
Use additional code for adverse effect, if applicable, to identify drug (T36-T50 with fifth or sixth character 5)
EXCLUDES 1   Barrett's esophagus (K22.7-)
AHA: 2017, 3Q, 27
TIP: For bleeding ulcers resulting from anticoagulant therapy, code D68.32 Hemorrhagic disorder due to extrinsic circulating anticoagulant, and an adverse-effect code from subcategory T45.5- should also be assigned. Either the bleeding ulcer code or code D68.32 may be sequenced first, depending on the circumstances of admission.

K22.10 Ulcer of esophagus without bleeding   `CC`
Ulcer of esophagus NOS
CC Excl: PDX collection 764

K22.11 Ulcer of esophagus with bleeding   `MCC`
EXCLUDES 2   bleeding esophageal varices (I85.01, I85.11)
CC Excl: PDX collection 765

K22.2 Esophageal obstruction
Compression of esophagus
Constriction of esophagus
Stenosis of esophagus
Stricture of esophagus
EXCLUDES 1   congenital stenosis or stricture of esophagus (Q39.3)

K22.3 Perforation of esophagus   `MCC`
Rupture of esophagus
EXCLUDES 1   traumatic perforation of (thoracic) esophagus (S27.8-)
CC Excl: PDX collection 766

K22.4 Dyskinesia of esophagus
Corkscrew esophagus
Diffuse esophageal spasm
Spasm of esophagus
EXCLUDES 1   cardiospasm (K22.0)

K22.5 Diverticulum of esophagus, acquired
Esophageal pouch, acquired
EXCLUDES 1   diverticulum of esophagus (congenital) (Q39.6)

K22.6 Gastro-esophageal laceration-hemorrhage syndrome   `MCC`
Mallory-Weiss syndrome
CC Excl: PDX collection 767

✓5ᵗʰ K22.7 Barrett's esophagus
Barrett's disease
Barrett's syndrome
EXCLUDES 1   Barrett's ulcer (K22.1)
       malignant neoplasm of esophagus (C15.)
DEF: Metaplastic disorder in which specialized columnar epithelial cells replace the normal squamous epithelial cells. Secondary to chronic gastroesophageal reflux damage to the mucosa, this disorder increases the risk of developing adenocarcinoma.

K22.70 Barrett's esophagus without dysplasia
Barrett's esophagus NOS

✓6ᵗʰ K22.71 Barrett's esophagus with dysplasia

K22.710 Barrett's esophagus with low grade dysplasia

K22.711 Barrett's esophagus with high grade dysplasia

K22.719 Barrett's esophagus with dysplasia, unspecified

K22.8 Other specified diseases of esophagus
Hemorrhage of esophagus NOS
EXCLUDES 2   esophageal varices (I85.-)
       Paterson-Kelly syndrome (D50.1)

K22.9 Disease of esophagus, unspecified

✓ Additional Character Required   ✓x7ᵗʰ Placeholder   Unacceptable PDx   Questionable PDx   Manifestation   H1 - H14 HAC   HCC CMS-HCC Dx   HIV HIV Dx

ICD-10-CM 2019   697

Chapter 11. Diseases of the Digestive System

K23   *Disorders of esophagus in diseases classified elsewhere*

Code first underlying disease, such as:
    congenital syphilis (A50.5)

EXCLUDES 1   *late syphilis (A52.79)*
             megaesophagus due to Chagas' disease (B57.31)
             tuberculosis (A18.83)

✓4th K25   Gastric **ulcer**

INCLUDES   erosion (acute) of stomach
           pylorus ulcer (peptic)
           stomach ulcer (peptic)

Use additional code to identify:
    alcohol abuse and dependence (F10.-)

EXCLUDES 1   *acute gastritis (K29.0-)*
             peptic ulcer NOS (K27.-)

AHA: 2017, 3Q, 27

TIP: For bleeding ulcers resulting from anticoagulant therapy, code D68.32 Hemorrhagic disorder due to extrinsic circulating anticoagulant, and an adverse-effect code from subcategory T45.5- should also be assigned. Either the bleeding ulcer code or code D68.32 may be sequenced first, depending on the circumstances of admission.

> **CC Excl: For CC/MCC codes in category K25:** PDX collection 765

K25.0   Acute **gastric ulcer** with hemorrhage   MCC

K25.1   Acute **gastric ulcer** with perforation   MCC HCC

K25.2   Acute **gastric ulcer** with both hemorrhage and perforation   MCC HCC

K25.3   Acute **gastric ulcer** without hemorrhage or perforation   CC

K25.4   Chronic or unspecified **gastric ulcer** with hemorrhage   MCC

K25.5   Chronic or unspecified **gastric ulcer** with perforation   MCC HCC

K25.6   Chronic or unspecified **gastric ulcer** with both hemorrhage and perforation   MCC HCC

K25.7   Chronic **gastric ulcer** without hemorrhage or perforation

K25.9   **Gastric ulcer, unspecified** as acute or chronic, without hemorrhage or perforation

✓4th K26   Duodenal **ulcer**

INCLUDES   erosion (acute) of duodenum
           duodenum ulcer (peptic)
           postpyloric ulcer (peptic)

Use additional code to identify:
    alcohol abuse and dependence (F10.-)

EXCLUDES 1   *peptic ulcer NOS (K27.-)*

AHA: 2017, 3Q, 27

TIP: For bleeding ulcers resulting from anticoagulant therapy, code D68.32 Hemorrhagic disorder due to extrinsic circulating anticoagulant, and an adverse-effect code from subcategory T45.5- should also be assigned. Either the bleeding ulcer code or code D68.32 may be sequenced first, depending on the circumstances of admission.

> **CC Excl: For CC/MCC codes in category K26, unless otherwise noted:** PDX collection 768

K26.0   Acute **duodenal ulcer** with hemorrhage   MCC

K26.1   Acute **duodenal ulcer** with perforation   MCC HCC

K26.2   Acute **duodenal ulcer** with both hemorrhage and perforation   MCC HCC

K26.3   Acute **duodenal ulcer** without hemorrhage or perforation   CC
         CC Excl: PDX collection 769

K26.4   Chronic or unspecified **duodenal ulcer** with hemorrhage   MCC
         AHA: 2016, 1Q, 14

K26.6   Chronic or unspecified **duodenal ulcer** with both hemorrhage and perforation   MCC HCC

K26.5   Chronic or unspecified **duodenal ulcer** with perforation   MCC HCC

K26.7   Chronic **duodenal ulcer** without hemorrhage or perforation

K26.9   **Duodenal ulcer, unspecified** as acute or chronic, without hemorrhage or perforation

✓4th K27   Peptic **ulcer, site unspecified**

INCLUDES   gastroduodenal ulcer NOS
           peptic ulcer NOS

Use additional code to identify:
    alcohol abuse and dependence (F10.-)

EXCLUDES 1   *peptic ulcer of newborn (P78.82)*

AHA: 2017, 3Q, 27

TIP: For bleeding ulcers resulting from anticoagulant therapy, code D68.32 Hemorrhagic disorder due to extrinsic circulating anticoagulant, and an adverse-effect code from subcategory T45.5- should also be assigned. Either the bleeding ulcer code or code D68.32 may be sequenced first, depending on the circumstances of admission.

> **CC Excl: For CC/MCC codes in category K27:** PDX collection 768

K27.0   Acute **peptic ulcer, site unspecified,** with hemorrhage   MCC

K27.1   Acute **peptic ulcer, site unspecified,** with perforation   MCC HCC

K27.2   Acute **peptic ulcer, site unspecified,** with both hemorrhage and perforation   MCC HCC

K27.3   Acute **peptic ulcer, site unspecified,** without hemorrhage or perforation   CC

K27.4   Chronic or unspecified **peptic ulcer, site unspecified,** with hemorrhage   MCC

K27.5   Chronic or unspecified **peptic ulcer, site unspecified,** with perforation   MCC HCC

K27.6   Chronic or unspecified **peptic ulcer, site unspecified,** with both hemorrhage and perforation   MCC HCC

K27.7   Chronic **peptic ulcer, site unspecified,** without hemorrhage or perforation

K27.9   **Peptic ulcer, site unspecified, unspecified** as acute or chronic, without hemorrhage or perforation

✓4th K28   Gastrojejunal **ulcer**

INCLUDES   anastomotic ulcer (peptic) or erosion
           gastrocolic ulcer (peptic) or erosion
           gastrointestinal ulcer (peptic) or erosion
           gastrojejunal ulcer (peptic) or erosion
           jejunal ulcer (peptic) or erosion
           marginal ulcer (peptic) or erosion
           stomal ulcer (peptic) or erosion

Use additional code to identify:
    alcohol abuse and dependence (F10.-)

EXCLUDES 1   *primary ulcer of small intestine (K63.3)*

AHA: 2017, 3Q, 27

TIP: For bleeding ulcers resulting from anticoagulant therapy, code D68.32 Hemorrhagic disorder due to extrinsic circulating anticoagulant, and an adverse-effect code from subcategory T45.5- should also be assigned. Either the bleeding ulcer code or code D68.32 may be sequenced first, depending on the circumstances of admission.

> **CC Excl: For CC/MCC codes in category K28:** PDX collection 765

K28.0   Acute **gastrojejunal ulcer** with hemorrhage   MCC

K28.1   Acute **gastrojejunal ulcer** with perforation   MCC HCC

K28.2   Acute **gastrojejunal ulcer** with both hemorrhage and perforation   MCC HCC

K28.3   Acute **gastrojejunal ulcer** without hemorrhage or perforation   CC

K28.4   Chronic or unspecified **gastrojejunal ulcer** with hemorrhage   MCC

K28.5   Chronic or unspecified **gastrojejunal ulcer** with perforation   MCC HCC

K28.6   Chronic or unspecified **gastrojejunal ulcer** with both hemorrhage and perforation   MCC HCC

K28.7   Chronic **gastrojejunal ulcer** without hemorrhage or perforation

K28.9   **Gastrojejunal ulcer, unspecified** as acute or chronic, without hemorrhage or perforation

Gastrointestinal Ulcers

Esophagus
Esophageal ulcer
Stomach
Duodenal ulcer
Gastric ulcer
Small intestine

N Newborn: 0   P Pediatric: 0-17   M Maternity: 12-55   A Adult: 15-124   MCC Major Complication/Comorbidity   CC Complication/Comorbidity   SW Severe Wound Dx

698   ICD-10-CM 2019

K23–K28.9

Chapter 11. Diseases of the Digestive System

✓4th **K29** **Gastritis and duodenitis**

    EXCLUDES 1   eosinophilic gastritis or gastroenteritis (K52.81)
                     Zollinger-Ellison syndrome (E16.4)

    TIP: For bleeding resulting from anticoagulant therapy, code D68.32 Hemorrhagic disorder due to extrinsic circulating anticoagulant, and an adverse effect code from subcategory T45.5- should also be assigned. Either code K29 or code D68.32 may be sequenced first, depending on the circumstances of admission.

    CC Excl: For MCC codes in category K29: PDX collection 770

✓5th **K29.0**   Acute **gastritis**
     Use additional code to identify:
       alcohol abuse and dependence (F10.-)
     EXCLUDES 1   erosion (acute) of stomach (K25.-)

     K29.00   **Acute gastritis** without bleeding
     K29.01   **Acute gastritis** with bleeding   `MCC`

✓5th **K29.2**   Alcoholic **gastritis**
     Use additional code to identify:
       alcohol abuse and dependence (F10.-)
     K29.20   **Alcoholic gastritis** without bleeding
     K29.21   **Alcoholic gastritis** with bleeding   `MCC`

✓5th **K29.3**   Chronic superficial **gastritis**
     K29.30   **Chronic superficial gastritis** without bleeding
     K29.31   **Chronic superficial gastritis** with bleeding   `MCC`

✓5th **K29.4**   Chronic atrophic **gastritis**
     Gastric atrophy
     K29.40   **Chronic atrophic gastritis** without bleeding
     K29.41   **Chronic atrophic gastritis** with bleeding   `MCC`

✓5th **K29.5**   Unspecified chronic **gastritis**
     Chronic antral gastritis
     Chronic fundal gastritis
     K29.50   **Unspecified chronic gastritis** without bleeding
     K29.51   **Unspecified chronic gastritis** with bleeding   `MCC`

✓5th **K29.6**   Other **gastritis**
     Giant hypertrophic gastritis
     Granulomatous gastritis
     Ménétrier's disease
     K29.60   **Other gastritis** without bleeding
     K29.61   **Other gastritis** with bleeding   `MCC`

✓5th **K29.7**   Gastritis, **unspecified**
     K29.70   **Gastritis, unspecified,** without bleeding
     K29.71   **Gastritis, unspecified,** with bleeding   `MCC`

✓5th **K29.8**   Duodenitis
     K29.80   **Duodenitis** without bleeding
     K29.81   **Duodenitis** with bleeding   `MCC`

✓5th **K29.9**   Gastroduodenitis, **unspecified**
     K29.90   **Gastroduodenitis, unspecified,** without bleeding
     K29.91   **Gastroduodenitis, unspecified,** with bleeding   `MCC`

K30   **Functional dyspepsia**
     Indigestion
     EXCLUDES 1   dyspepsia NOS (R10.13)
               heartburn (R12)
               nervous dyspepsia (F45.8)
               neurotic dyspepsia (F45.8)
               psychogenic dyspepsia (F45.8)

✓4th **K31** **Other diseases of stomach and duodenum**
     INCLUDES   functional disorders of stomach
     EXCLUDES 2   diabetic gastroparesis (E08.43, E09.43, E10.43, E11.43, E13.43)
               diverticulum of duodenum (K57.00-K57.13)

     K31.0   **Acute dilatation of stomach**   `CC`
       Acute distention of stomach
       CC Excl: PDX collection 771

     K31.1   **Adult hypertrophic pyloric stenosis**   `CC` `A`
       Pyloric stenosis NOS
       EXCLUDES 1   congenital or infantile pyloric stenosis (Q40.0)
       CC Excl: PDX collection 772

     K31.2   **Hourglass stricture and stenosis of stomach**
       EXCLUDES 1   congenital hourglass stomach (Q40.2)
                 hourglass contraction of stomach (K31.89)

     K31.3   **Pylorospasm, not elsewhere classified**
       EXCLUDES 1   congenital or infantile pylorospasm (Q40.0)
                 neurotic pylorospasm (F45.8)
                 psychogenic pylorospasm (F45.8)

     K31.4   **Gastric diverticulum**
       EXCLUDES 1   congenital diverticulum of stomach (Q40.2)

     K31.5   **Obstruction of duodenum**   `CC`
       Constriction of duodenum
       Duodenal ileus (chronic)
       Stenosis of duodenum
       Stricture of duodenum
       Volvulus of duodenum
       EXCLUDES 1   congenital stenosis of duodenum (Q41.0)
       CC Excl: PDX collection 773

     K31.6   **Fistula of stomach and duodenum**   `CC` `SW`
       Gastrocolic fistula
       Gastrojejunocolic fistula
       CC Excl: PDX collection 774

     K31.7   **Polyp of stomach and duodenum**
       EXCLUDES 1   adenomatous polyp of stomach (D13.1)

✓5th **K31.8**   **Other specified diseases of stomach and duodenum**

     ✓6th **K31.81**   **Angiodysplasia of stomach and duodenum**
       K31.811   **Angiodysplasia of stomach and duodenum** with bleeding   `MCC`
           CC Excl: PDX collection 770
       K31.819   **Angiodysplasia of stomach and duodenum** without bleeding
           Angiodysplasia of stomach and duodenum NOS

     K31.82   **Dieulafoy lesion (hemorrhagic) of stomach and**   `MCC` **duodenum**
       EXCLUDES 2   Dieulafoy lesion of intestine (K63.81)
       DEF: Abnormally large submucosal artery protruding through a defect in the stomach mucosa or intestines that can cause massive and life-threatening hemorrhaging.
       CC Excl: PDX collection 775

     K31.83   **Achlorhydria**
       DEF: Absence of hydrochloric acid in gastric secretions due to gastric mucosa atrophy. Achlorhydria is unresponsive to histamines.

     K31.84   **Gastroparesis**
       Gastroparalysis
       Code first underlying disease, if known, such as:
         anorexia nervosa (F50.0-)
         diabetes mellitus (E08.43, E09.43, E10.43, E11.43, E13.43)
         scleroderma (M34.-)
       AHA: 2013, 4Q, 114

     K31.89   **Other diseases of stomach and duodenum**
       AHA: 2017, 1Q, 28
       TIP: Assign for cyclical vomiting not related to migraine, along with a code from category R11 Nausea and vomiting.

     K31.9   **Disease of stomach and duodenum, unspecified**

Diseases of appendix (K35-K38)

✓4th **K35**   Acute **appendicitis**

     CC Excl: For CC/MCC codes in category K35: PDX collection 776

✓5th **K35.2**   **Acute appendicitis** with generalized peritonitis
     Appendicitis (acute) with generalized (diffuse) peritonitis following rupture or perforation of appendix
     ~~Perforated appendix NOS~~
     ~~Ruptured appendix NOS~~

   ●   **K35.20**   **Acute appendicitis with generalized peritonitis,** `CC` **without abscess**
       (Acute) appendicitis with generalized peritonitis NOS

   ●   **K35.21**   **Acute appendicitis with generalized peritonitis,** `MCC` **with abscess**

✓5th **K35.3**   **Acute appendicitis** with localized peritonitis
     ~~Acute appendicitis with or without perforation or rupture with peritonitis NOS~~
     ~~Acute appendicitis with or without perforation or rupture with localized peritonitis~~
     ~~Acute appendicitis with peritoneal abscess~~

   ●   **K35.30**   **Acute appendicitis with localized peritonitis,** `CC` **without perforation or gangrene**
       Acute appendicitis with localized peritonitis NOS

   ●   **K35.31**   **Acute appendicitis with localized peritonitis and** `CC` **gangrene, without perforation**

   ●   **K35.32**   **Acute appendicitis with perforation and** `MCC` **localized peritonitis, without abscess**
       (Acute) appendicitis with perforation NOS
       Perforated appendix NOS
       Ruptured appendix (with localized peritonitis) NOS

✓ Additional Character Required   ✓x7th Placeholder   Unacceptable PDx   Questionable PDx   Manifestation   **H1 - H14** HAC   **HCC** CMS-HCC Dx   **HIV** HIV Dx

ICD-10-CM 2019   **699**

Chapter 11. Diseases of the Digestive System

● **K35.33 Acute appendicitis with perforation and localized peritonitis,** with abscess   `MCC`
(Acute) appendicitis with (peritoneal) abscess NOS
Ruptured appendix with localized peritonitis and abscess

✓5ᵗʰ **K35.8** Other **and unspecified acute appendicitis**

     K35.80 Unspecified **acute appendicitis**   `CC`
Acute appendicitis NOS
Acute appendicitis without (localized) (generalized) peritonitis

     ✓6ᵗʰ **K35.89** Other **acute appendicitis**

●   **K35.890 Other acute appendicitis** without **perforation or gangrene**   `CC`

●   **K35.891 Other acute appendicitis** without **perforation, with gangrene**   `CC`
(Acute) appendicitis with gangrene NOS

K36 Other appendicitis
Chronic appendicitis
Recurrent appendicitis

K37 Unspecified appendicitis
   `EXCLUDES 1`   unspecified appendicitis with peritonitis ▶(K35.2-, K35.3-)◀

✓4ᵗʰ **K38 Other diseases of appendix**

K38.0 Hyperplasia of appendix

K38.1 Appendicular concretions
Fecalith of appendix
Stercolith of appendix

K38.2 Diverticulum of appendix

K38.3 Fistula of appendix

K38.8 Other specified diseases of appendix
Intussusception of appendix

K38.9 Disease of appendix, unspecified

Hernia (K40-K46)

   `NOTE`   Hernia with both gangrene and obstruction is classified to hernia with gangrene.

   `INCLUDES`   acquired hernia
congenital [except diaphragmatic or hiatus] hernia
recurrent hernia

✓4ᵗʰ **K40 Inguinal hernia**

   `INCLUDES`   bubonocele
direct inguinal hernia
double inguinal hernia
indirect inguinal hernia
inguinal hernia NOS
oblique inguinal hernia
scrotal hernia

   CC Excl: For CC/MCC codes in category K40: PDX collection 777

✓5ᵗʰ **K40.0** Bilateral **inguinal hernia, with obstruction, without gangrene**
Inguinal hernia (bilateral) causing obstruction without gangrene
Incarcerated inguinal hernia (bilateral) without gangrene
Irreducible inguinal hernia (bilateral) without gangrene
Strangulated inguinal hernia (bilateral) without gangrene

     K40.00 Bilateral inguinal hernia, with obstruction, without gangrene, not specified as recurrent
Bilateral inguinal hernia, with obstruction, without gangrene NOS

     K40.01 Bilateral inguinal hernia, with obstruction, without gangrene, recurrent   `CC`

✓5ᵗʰ **K40.1** Bilateral **inguinal hernia, with gangrene**

     K40.10 Bilateral inguinal hernia, with gangrene, not specified as recurrent   `MCC`
Bilateral inguinal hernia, with gangrene NOS

     K40.11 Bilateral inguinal hernia, with gangrene, recurrent   `MCC`

✓5ᵗʰ **K40.2** Bilateral **inguinal hernia, without obstruction or gangrene**

     K40.20 Bilateral inguinal hernia, without obstruction or gangrene, not specified as recurrent
Bilateral inguinal hernia NOS

     K40.21 Bilateral inguinal hernia, without obstruction or gangrene, recurrent

✓5ᵗʰ **K40.3** Unilateral **inguinal hernia, with obstruction, without gangrene**
Inguinal hernia (unilateral) causing obstruction without gangrene
Incarcerated inguinal hernia (unilateral) without gangrene
Irreducible inguinal hernia (unilateral) without gangrene
Strangulated inguinal hernia (unilateral) without gangrene

     K40.30 Unilateral inguinal hernia, with obstruction, without gangrene, not specified as recurrent   `CC`
Inguinal hernia, with obstruction NOS
Unilateral inguinal hernia, with obstruction, without gangrene NOS

     K40.31 Unilateral inguinal hernia, with obstruction, without gangrene, recurrent   `CC`

✓5ᵗʰ **K40.4** Unilateral **inguinal hernia, with gangrene**

     K40.40 Unilateral inguinal hernia, with gangrene, not specified as recurrent   `MCC`
Inguinal hernia with gangrene NOS
Unilateral inguinal hernia with gangrene NOS

     K40.41 Unilateral inguinal hernia, with gangrene, recurrent   `MCC`

✓5ᵗʰ **K40.9** Unilateral **inguinal hernia, without obstruction or gangrene**

     K40.90 Unilateral inguinal hernia, without obstruction or gangrene, not specified as recurrent
Inguinal hernia NOS
Unilateral inguinal hernia NOS

     K40.91 Unilateral inguinal hernia, without obstruction or gangrene, recurrent

Hernia Sites

Abdominal ring
Indirect inguinal hernia
Anterior inguinal wall
Direct inguinal hernia
Spermatic cord
Femoral hernia
Inguinal ligament
Femoral sheath
Epigastric hernia
Paraumbilical hernia
Inguinal hernias
Femoral hernia

✓4ᵗʰ **K41 Femoral hernia**

   CC Excl: For CC/MCC codes in category K41, unless otherwise noted: PDX collection 778

✓5ᵗʰ **K41.0** Bilateral **femoral hernia, with obstruction, without gangrene**
Femoral hernia (bilateral) causing obstruction, without gangrene
Incarcerated femoral hernia (bilateral), without gangrene
Irreducible femoral hernia (bilateral), without gangrene
Strangulated femoral hernia (bilateral), without gangrene

     K41.00 Bilateral femoral hernia, with obstruction, without gangrene, not specified as recurrent   `CC`
Bilateral femoral hernia, with obstruction, without gangrene NOS

     K41.01 Bilateral femoral hernia, with obstruction, without gangrene, recurrent   `CC`

✓5ᵗʰ **K41.1** Bilateral **femoral hernia, with gangrene**

     K41.10 Bilateral femoral hernia, with gangrene, not specified as recurrent   `MCC`
Bilateral femoral hernia, with gangrene NOS
       CC Excl: PDX collection 779

     K41.11 Bilateral femoral hernia, with gangrene, recurrent   `MCC`
       CC Excl: PDX collection 779

✓5ᵗʰ **K41.2** Bilateral **femoral hernia, without obstruction or gangrene**

     K41.20 Bilateral femoral hernia, without obstruction or gangrene, not specified as recurrent
Bilateral femoral hernia NOS

     K41.21 Bilateral femoral hernia, without obstruction or gangrene, recurrent

N Newborn: 0   P Pediatric: 0-17   M Maternity: 12-55   A Adult: 15-124   `MCC` Major Complication/Comorbidity   `CC` Complication/Comorbidity   `SW` Severe Wound Dx

700   ICD-10-CM 2019

√5ᵗʰ K41.3 Unilateral **femoral hernia,** with obstruction, without gangrene

Femoral hernia (unilateral) causing obstruction, without gangrene
Incarcerated femoral hernia (unilateral), without gangrene
Irreducible femoral hernia (unilateral), without gangrene
Strangulated femoral hernia (unilateral), without gangrene

K41.30 Unilateral **femoral hernia, with obstruction, without gangrene,** not specified as recurrent   `CC`
Femoral hernia, with obstruction NOS
Unilateral femoral hernia, with obstruction NOS

K41.31 Unilateral **femoral hernia, with obstruction, without gangrene,** recurrent   `CC`

√5ᵗʰ K41.4 Unilateral **femoral hernia,** with gangrene

K41.40 Unilateral **femoral hernia, with gangrene,** not specified as recurrent   `MCC`
Femoral hernia, with gangrene NOS
Unilateral femoral hernia, with gangrene NOS
CC Excl: PDX collection 779

K41.41 Unilateral **femoral hernia, with gangrene,** recurrent   `MCC`
CC Excl: PDX collection 779

√5ᵗʰ K41.9 Unilateral **femoral hernia,** without obstruction or gangrene

K41.90 Unilateral **femoral hernia, without obstruction or gangrene,** not specified as recurrent
Femoral hernia NOS
Unilateral femoral hernia NOS

K41.91 Unilateral **femoral hernia, without obstruction or gangrene,** recurrent

√4ᵗʰ K42 Umbilical **hernia**
INCLUDES paraumbilical hernia
EXCLUDES 1 omphalocele (Q79.2)

K42.0 Umbilical **hernia** with obstruction, without gangrene   `CC`
Umbilical hernia causing obstruction, without gangrene
Incarcerated umbilical hernia, without gangrene
Irreducible umbilical hernia, without gangrene
Strangulated umbilical hernia, without gangrene
CC Excl: PDX collection 780

K42.1 Umbilical **hernia** with gangrene   `MCC`
Gangrenous umbilical hernia
CC Excl: PDX collection 781

K42.9 Umbilical **hernia** without obstruction or gangrene
Umbilical hernia NOS

√4ᵗʰ K43 Ventral **hernia**
DEF: Condition in which a loop of bowel protrudes through a weakness in the abdominal wall muscles that may occur as a birth defect, past surgical site (incisional), or form at a stomal site (parastomal).

K43.0 Incisional **hernia** with obstruction, without gangrene   `CC`
Incisional hernia causing obstruction, without gangrene
Incarcerated incisional hernia, without gangrene
Irreducible incisional hernia, without gangrene
Strangulated incisional hernia, without gangrene
CC Excl: PDX collection 780

K43.1 Incisional **hernia** with gangrene   `MCC`
Gangrenous incisional hernia
CC Excl: PDX collection 781

K43.2 Incisional **hernia** without obstruction or gangrene
Incisional hernia NOS

K43.3 Parastomal **hernia** with obstruction, without gangrene   `CC`
Incarcerated parastomal hernia, without gangrene
Irreducible parastomal hernia, without gangrene
Parastomal hernia causing obstruction, without gangrene
Strangulated parastomal hernia, without gangrene
CC Excl: PDX collection 780

K43.4 Parastomal **hernia** with gangrene   `MCC`
Gangrenous parastomal hernia
CC Excl: PDX collection 781

▲ **K43.5** Parastomal **hernia** without obstruction or gangrene
Parastomal hernia NOS

K43.6 Other and unspecified **ventral hernia** with obstruction, without gangrene   `CC`
Epigastric hernia causing obstruction, without gangrene
Hypogastric hernia causing obstruction, without gangrene
Incarcerated epigastric hernia without gangrene
Incarcerated hypogastric hernia without gangrene
Incarcerated midline hernia without gangrene
Incarcerated spigelian hernia without gangrene
Incarcerated subxiphoid hernia without gangrene
Irreducible epigastric hernia without gangrene
Irreducible hypogastric hernia without gangrene
Irreducible midline hernia without gangrene
Irreducible spigelian hernia without gangrene
Irreducible subxiphoid hernia without gangrene
Midline hernia causing obstruction, without gangrene
Spigelian hernia causing obstruction, without gangrene
Strangulated epigastric hernia without gangrene
Strangulated hypogastric hernia without gangrene
Strangulated midline hernia without gangrene
Strangulated spigelian hernia without gangrene
Strangulated subxiphoid hernia without gangrene
Subxiphoid hernia causing obstruction, without gangrene
CC Excl: PDX collection 780

K43.7 Other and unspecified **ventral hernia** with gangrene   `MCC`
Any condition listed under K43.6 specified as gangrenous
CC Excl: PDX collection 781

K43.9 Ventral **hernia** without obstruction or gangrene
Epigastric hernia
Ventral hernia NOS

√4ᵗʰ K44 Diaphragmatic **hernia**
INCLUDES hiatus hernia (esophageal) (sliding)
paraesophageal hernia
EXCLUDES 1 congenital diaphragmatic hernia (Q79.0)
congenital hiatus hernia (Q40.1)
DEF: Protrusion of an abdominal organ, usually the stomach, through the esophageal opening within the diaphragm and occurring in two types: the sliding hiatal hernia and the paraesophageal hernia.

Hiatal Hernia

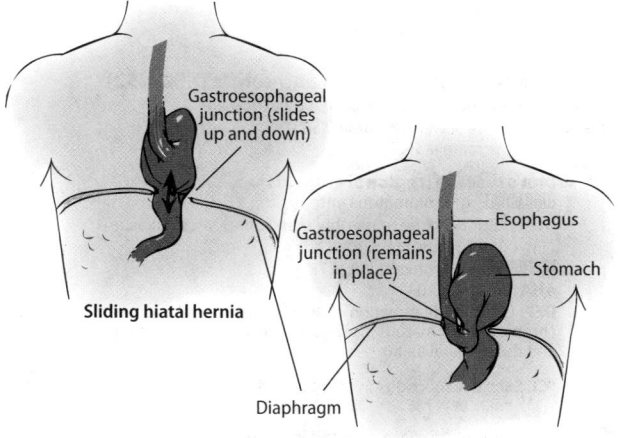

Gastroesophageal junction (slides up and down)

Sliding hiatal hernia

Gastroesophageal junction (remains in place)

Esophagus

Stomach

Diaphragm

Paraesophageal hiatal hernia

K44.0 Diaphragmatic **hernia** with obstruction, without gangrene   `CC`
Diaphragmatic hernia causing obstruction
Incarcerated diaphragmatic hernia
Irreducible diaphragmatic hernia
Strangulated diaphragmatic hernia
CC Excl: PDX collection 782

K44.1 Diaphragmatic **hernia** with gangrene   `MCC`
Gangrenous diaphragmatic hernia
CC Excl: PDX collection 782

K44.9 Diaphragmatic **hernia** without obstruction or gangrene
Diaphragmatic hernia NOS

✓4ᵗʰ **K45** **Other abdominal hernia**
   INCLUDES   abdominal hernia, specified site NEC
           lumbar hernia
           obturator hernia
           pudendal hernia
           retroperitoneal hernia
           sciatic hernia

      K45.0 **Other specified abdominal hernia with obstruction,** CC
      without gangrene
          Other specified abdominal hernia causing obstruction
          Other specified incarcerated abdominal hernia
          Other specified irreducible abdominal hernia
          Other specified strangulated abdominal hernia
          CC Excl: PDX collection 783

      K45.1 **Other specified abdominal hernia with gangrene** MCC
          Any condition listed under K45 specified as gangrenous
          CC Excl: PDX collection 784

      K45.8 **Other specified abdominal hernia without obstruction or**
      gangrene

✓4ᵗʰ **K46** **Unspecified abdominal hernia**
   INCLUDES   enterocele
           epiplocele
           hernia NOS
           interstitial hernia
           intestinal hernia
           intra-abdominal hernia
   EXCLUDES 1   *vaginal enterocele (N81.5)*

      K46.0 **Unspecified abdominal hernia with obstruction, without** CC
      gangrene
          Unspecified abdominal hernia causing obstruction
          Unspecified incarcerated abdominal hernia
          Unspecified irreducible abdominal hernia
          Unspecified strangulated abdominal hernia
          CC Excl: PDX collection 783

      K46.1 **Unspecified abdominal hernia with gangrene** MCC
          Any condition listed under K46 specified as gangrenous
          CC Excl: PDX collection 784

      K46.9 **Unspecified abdominal hernia without obstruction or**
      gangrene
          Abdominal hernia NOS

Noninfective enteritis and colitis (K50-K52)

   INCLUDES   noninfective inflammatory bowel disease
   EXCLUDES 1   *irritable bowel syndrome (K58.-)*
                 megacolon (K59.3-)

✓4ᵗʰ **K50** **Crohn's disease [regional enteritis]**
   INCLUDES   granulomatous enteritis
      Use additional code to identify manifestations, such as:
        pyoderma gangrenosum (L88)
   EXCLUDES 1   *ulcerative colitis (K51.-)*
      AHA: 2012, 4Q, 104
      DEF: Chronic inflammation of the gastrointestinal tract characterized by chronic granulomatous disease, most commonly affecting the intestines and the terminal ileum.

      CC Excl: For CC codes in category K50, unless otherwise noted: PDX collection 785

    ✓5ᵗʰ **K50.0** **Crohn's disease of small intestine**
          Crohn's disease [regional enteritis] of duodenum
          Crohn's disease [regional enteritis] of ileum
          Crohn's disease [regional enteritis] of jejunum
          Regional ileitis
          Terminal ileitis
      EXCLUDES 1   *Crohn's disease of both small and large intestine (K50.8-)*

      K50.00 **Crohn's disease of small intestine** without CC HCC
      complications

   ✓6ᵗʰ **K50.01** **Crohn's disease of small intestine** with complications
        K50.011 **Crohn's disease of small intestine** CC HCC
             with rectal bleeding
        K50.012 **Crohn's disease of small intestine** CC HCC
             with intestinal obstruction
        K50.013 **Crohn's disease of small** CC HCC SW
             intestine with fistula
        K50.014 **Crohn's disease of small** CC HCC
             intestine with abscess
             AHA: 2012, 4Q, 104
        K50.018 **Crohn's disease of small intestine** CC HCC
             with other complication
        K50.019 **Crohn's disease of small intestine** CC HCC
             with unspecified complications

    ✓5ᵗʰ **K50.1** **Crohn's disease of** large intestine
          Crohn's disease [regional enteritis] of colon
          Crohn's disease [regional enteritis] of large bowel
          Crohn's disease [regional enteritis] of rectum
          Granulomatous colitis
          Regional colitis
      EXCLUDES 1   *Crohn's disease of both small and large intestine (K50.8)*

      K50.10 **Crohn's disease of large intestine** without CC HCC
      complications

   ✓6ᵗʰ **K50.11** **Crohn's disease of large intestine** with complications
        K50.111 **Crohn's disease of large intestine** CC HCC
             with rectal bleeding
        K50.112 **Crohn's disease of large intestine** CC HCC
             with intestinal obstruction
        K50.113 **Crohn's disease of large** CC HCC SW
             intestine with fistula
        K50.114 **Crohn's disease of large intestine** CC HCC
             with abscess
        K50.118 **Crohn's disease of large intestine** CC HCC
             with other complication
        K50.119 **Crohn's disease of large intestine** CC HCC
             with unspecified complications

    ✓5ᵗʰ **K50.8** **Crohn's disease of** both small and large intestine

      K50.80 **Crohn's disease of both small and large** CC HCC
      intestine without complications

   ✓6ᵗʰ **K50.81** **Crohn's disease of both small and large intestine**
      with complications
        K50.811 **Crohn's disease of both small and** CC HCC
             large intestine with rectal bleeding
        K50.812 **Crohn's disease of both small and** CC HCC
             large intestine with intestinal
             obstruction
        K50.813 **Crohn's disease of both small** CC HCC SW
             and large intestine with fistula
        K50.814 **Crohn's disease of both small** CC HCC
             large intestine with abscess
        K50.818 **Crohn's disease of both small and** CC HCC
             large intestine with other complication
        ·K50.819 **Crohn's disease of both small and** CC HCC
             large intestine with unspecified
             complications

    ✓5ᵗʰ **K50.9** **Crohn's disease, unspecified**

      CC Excl: For CC codes in subcategory K50.9: PDX collection 786

      K50.90 **Crohn's disease, unspecified,** without CC HCC
      complications
          Crohn's disease NOS
          Regional enteritis NOS

   ✓6ᵗʰ **K50.91** **Crohn's disease, unspecified,** with complications
        K50.911 **Crohn's disease, unspecified, with** CC HCC
             rectal bleeding
        K50.912 **Crohn's disease, unspecified, with** CC HCC
             intestinal obstruction
        K50.913 **Crohn's disease, unspecified,** CC HCC SW
             with fistula
        K50.914 **Crohn's disease, unspecified, with** CC HCC
             abscess
        K50.918 **Crohn's disease, unspecified, with** CC HCC
             other complication
        K50.919 **Crohn's disease, unspecified, with** CC HCC
             unspecified complications

✓4ᵗʰ **K51** **Ulcerative colitis**
      Use additional code to identify manifestations, such as:
        pyoderma gangrenosum (L88)
   EXCLUDES 1   *Crohn's disease [regional enteritis] (K50.-)*

      CC Excl: For CC codes in category K51, unless otherwise noted: PDX collection 785

    ✓5ᵗʰ **K51.0** **Ulcerative (chronic)** pancolitis
          Backwash ileitis

      K51.00 **Ulcerative (chronic) pancolitis** without CC HCC
      complications
          Ulcerative (chronic) pancolitis NOS

   ✓6ᵗʰ **K51.01** **Ulcerative (chronic) pancolitis** with complications
        K51.011 **Ulcerative (chronic) pancolitis** CC HCC
             with rectal bleeding

K51.Ø12 **Ulcerative (chronic) pancolitis with intestinal obstruction** `CC` `HCC`

K51.Ø13 **Ulcerative (chronic) pancolitis with fistula** `CC` `HCC` `SW`

K51.Ø14 **Ulcerative (chronic) pancolitis with abscess** `CC` `HCC`

K51.Ø18 **Ulcerative (chronic) pancolitis with other complication** `CC` `HCC`

K51.Ø19 **Ulcerative (chronic) pancolitis with unspecified complications** `CC` `HCC`

✓6th **K51.2 Ulcerative (chronic) proctitis**

K51.2Ø **Ulcerative (chronic) proctitis without complications** `CC` `HCC`
Ulcerative (chronic) proctitis NOS

✓6th **K51.21 Ulcerative (chronic) proctitis with complications**

K51.211 **Ulcerative (chronic) proctitis with rectal bleeding** `CC` `HCC`

K51.212 **Ulcerative (chronic) proctitis with intestinal obstruction** `CC` `HCC`

K51.213 **Ulcerative (chronic) proctitis with fistula** `CC` `HCC` `SW`

K51.214 **Ulcerative (chronic) proctitis with abscess** `CC` `HCC`

K51.218 **Ulcerative (chronic) proctitis with other complication** `CC` `HCC`

K51.219 **Ulcerative (chronic) proctitis with unspecified complications** `CC` `HCC`

✓6th **K51.3 Ulcerative (chronic) rectosigmoiditis**

K51.3Ø **Ulcerative (chronic) rectosigmoiditis without complications** `CC` `HCC`
Ulcerative (chronic) rectosigmoiditis NOS

✓6th **K51.31 Ulcerative (chronic) rectosigmoiditis with complications**

K51.311 **Ulcerative (chronic) rectosigmoiditis with rectal bleeding** `CC` `HCC`

K51.312 **Ulcerative (chronic) rectosigmoiditis with intestinal obstruction** `CC` `HCC`

K51.313 **Ulcerative (chronic) rectosigmoiditis with fistula** `CC` `HCC` `SW`

K51.314 **Ulcerative (chronic) rectosigmoiditis with abscess** `CC` `HCC`

K51.318 **Ulcerative (chronic) rectosigmoiditis with other complication** `CC` `HCC`

K51.319 **Ulcerative (chronic) rectosigmoiditis with unspecified complications** `CC` `HCC`

✓5th **K51.4 Inflammatory polyps of colon**
EXCLUDES 1   adenomatous polyp of colon (D12.6)
polyposis of colon (D12.6)
polyps of colon NOS (K63.5)

K51.4Ø **Inflammatory polyps of colon without complications** `CC` `HCC`
Inflammatory polyps of colon NOS

✓6th **K51.41 Inflammatory polyps of colon with complications**

K51.411 **Inflammatory polyps of colon with rectal bleeding** `CC` `HCC`

K51.412 **Inflammatory polyps of colon with intestinal obstruction** `CC` `HCC`

K51.413 **Inflammatory polyps of colon with fistula** `CC` `HCC` `SW`

K51.414 **Inflammatory polyps of colon with abscess** `CC` `HCC`

K51.418 **Inflammatory polyps of colon with other complication** `CC` `HCC`

K51.419 **Inflammatory polyps of colon with unspecified complications** `CC` `HCC`

✓5th **K51.5 Left sided colitis**
Left hemicolitis

K51.5Ø **Left sided colitis without complications** `CC` `HCC`
Left sided colitis NOS

✓6th **K51.51 Left sided colitis with complications**

K51.511 **Left sided colitis with rectal bleeding** `CC` `HCC`

K51.512 **Left sided colitis with intestinal obstruction** `CC` `HCC`

K51.513 **Left sided colitis with fistula** `CC` `HCC` `SW`

K51.514 **Left sided colitis with abscess** `CC` `HCC`

K51.518 **Left sided colitis with other complication** `CC` `HCC`

K51.519 **Left sided colitis with unspecified complications** `CC` `HCC`

✓5th **K51.8 Other ulcerative colitis**

K51.8Ø **Other ulcerative colitis without complications** `CC` `HCC`

✓6th **K51.81 Other ulcerative colitis with complications**

K51.811 **Other ulcerative colitis with rectal bleeding** `CC` `HCC`

K51.812 **Other ulcerative colitis with intestinal obstruction** `CC` `HCC`

K51.813 **Other ulcerative colitis with fistula** `CC` `HCC` `SW`

K51.814 **Other ulcerative colitis with abscess** `CC` `HCC`

K51.818 **Other ulcerative colitis with other complication** `CC` `HCC`

K51.819 **Other ulcerative colitis with unspecified complications** `CC` `HCC`

✓5th **K51.9 Ulcerative colitis, unspecified**

CC Excl: For CC codes in subcategory K51.9:
PDX collection 787

K51.9Ø **Ulcerative colitis, unspecified, without complications** `CC` `HCC`

✓6th **K51.91 Ulcerative colitis, unspecified, with complications**

K51.911 **Ulcerative colitis, unspecified with rectal bleeding** `CC` `HCC`

K51.912 **Ulcerative colitis, unspecified with intestinal obstruction** `CC` `HCC`

K51.913 **Ulcerative colitis, unspecified with fistula** `CC` `HCC` `SW`

K51.914 **Ulcerative colitis, unspecified with abscess** `CC` `HCC`

K51.918 **Ulcerative colitis, unspecified with other complication** `CC` `HCC`

K51.919 **Ulcerative colitis, unspecified with unspecified complications** `CC` `HCC`

✓4th **K52 Other and unspecified noninfective gastroenteritis and colitis**
AHA: 2016, 4Q, 30-31

K52.Ø **Gastroenteritis and colitis due to radiation** `CC`
CC Excl: PDX collection 788

K52.1 **Toxic gastroenteritis and colitis** `CC`
Drug-induced gastroenteritis and colitis
Code first (T51-T65) to identify toxic agent
Use additional code for adverse effect, if applicable, to identify drug (T36-T5Ø with fifth or sixth character 5)
CC Excl: PDX collection 789

✓5th **K52.2 Allergic and dietetic gastroenteritis and colitis**
Use additional code to identify type of food allergy (Z91.Ø1-, Z91.Ø2-)
EXCLUDES 2   allergic eosinophilic colitis (K52.82)
allergic eosinophilic esophagitis (K2Ø.Ø)
allergic eosinophilic gastritis (K52.81)
allergic eosinophilic gastroenteritis (K52.81)
food protein-induced proctocolitis (K52.82)

DEF: True immunoglobulin E (IgE)-mediated allergic reaction of the lining of the stomach, intestines, or colon to food proteins. It causes nausea, vomiting, diarrhea, and abdominal cramping.

K52.21 **Food protein-induced enterocolitis syndrome**
▶FPIES◄
Use additional code for hypovolemic shock, if present (R57.1)

K52.22 **Food protein-induced enteropathy**

K52.29 **Other allergic and dietetic gastroenteritis and colitis**
Food hypersensitivity gastroenteritis or colitis
Immediate gastrointestinal hypersensitivity

K52.3 **Indeterminate colitis**
Colonic inflammatory bowel disease unclassified (IBDU)
EXCLUDES 1   unspecified colitis (K52.9)

✓5ᵗʰ K52.8 Other specified noninfective gastroenteritis and colitis

K52.81 Eosinophilic gastritis or gastroenteritis
Eosinophilic enteritis
EXCLUDES 2   *eosinophilic esophagitis (K20.0)*
DEF: Disorder involving the accumulation of eosinophil in the lining of the stomach or multiple levels of the gastrointestinal tract, but without a known cause such as connective tissue disease, drug reaction, malignancy, or parasitic infection.

K52.82 Eosinophilic colitis
Allergic proctocolitis
Food-induced eosinophilic proctocolitis
Food protein-induced proctocolitis
Milk protein-induced proctocolitis
DEF: Disorder involving the accumulation of eosinophil in the tissues lining the colon, but without a known cause such as connective tissue disease, drug reaction, malignancy, or parasitic infection. The resultant inflammation may cause extreme abdominal pain, diarrhea, or bloody stool.

✓6ᵗʰ K52.83 Microscopic colitis
K52.831 Collagenous colitis
K52.832 Lymphocytic colitis
K52.838 Other microscopic colitis
K52.839 Microscopic colitis, unspecified

K52.89 Other specified noninfective gastroenteritis and colitis

K52.9 Noninfective gastroenteritis and colitis, unspecified
Colitis NOS   Ileitis NOS
Enteritis NOS   Jejunitis NOS
Gastroenteritis NOS   Sigmoiditis NOS
EXCLUDES 1   *diarrhea NOS (R19.7)*
functional diarrhea (K59.1)
infectious gastroenteritis and colitis NOS (A09)
neonatal diarrhea (noninfective) (P78.3)
psychogenic diarrhea (F45.8)

Other diseases of intestines (K55-K64)

✓4ᵗʰ K55 Vascular disorders of intestine
EXCLUDES 1   *necrotizing enterocolitis of newborn (P77.-)*
AHA: 2016, 4Q, 32

CC Excl: For CC/MCC codes in category K55, unless otherwise noted: PDX collection 790

✓5ᵗʰ K55.0 Acute vascular disorders of intestine
Infarction of appendices epiploicae
Mesenteric (artery) (vein) embolism
Mesenteric (artery) (vein) infarction
Mesenteric (artery) (vein) thrombosis

✓6ᵗʰ K55.01 Acute (reversible) ischemia of small intestine
K55.011 Focal (segmental) acute (reversible) ischemia of small intestine MCC HCC
K55.012 Diffuse acute (reversible) ischemia of small intestine MCC HCC
K55.019 Acute (reversible) ischemia of small intestine, extent unspecified MCC HCC

✓6ᵗʰ K55.02 Acute infarction of small intestine
Gangrene of small intestine
Necrosis of small intestine
K55.021 Focal (segmental) acute infarction of small intestine MCC HCC
K55.022 Diffuse acute infarction of small intestine MCC HCC
K55.029 Acute infarction of small intestine, extent unspecified MCC HCC

✓6ᵗʰ K55.03 Acute (reversible) ischemia of large intestine
Acute fulminant ischemic colitis
Subacute ischemic colitis
K55.031 Focal (segmental) acute (reversible) ischemia of large intestine MCC HCC
K55.032 Diffuse acute (reversible) ischemia of large intestine MCC HCC
K55.039 Acute (reversible) ischemia of large intestine, extent unspecified MCC HCC

✓6ᵗʰ K55.04 Acute infarction of large intestine
Gangrene of large intestine
Necrosis of large intestine
K55.041 Focal (segmental) acute infarction of large intestine MCC HCC

K55.042 Diffuse acute infarction of large intestine MCC HCC
K55.049 Acute infarction of large intestine, extent unspecified MCC HCC

✓6ᵗʰ K55.05 Acute (reversible) ischemia of intestine, part unspecified
K55.051 Focal (segmental) acute (reversible) ischemia of intestine, part unspecified MCC HCC
K55.052 Diffuse acute (reversible) ischemiaof intestine, part unspecified MCC HCC
K55.059 Acute (reversible) ischemia of intestine, part and extent unspecified MCC HCC

✓6ᵗʰ K55.06 Acute infarction of intestine, part unspecified
Acute intestinal infarction
Gangrene of intestine
Necrosis of intestine
K55.061 Focal (segmental) acute infarction of intestine, part unspecified MCC HCC
K55.062 Diffuse acute infarction of intestine, part unspecified MCC HCC
K55.069 Acute infarction of intestine, part and extent unspecified MCC HCC

K55.1 Chronic vascular disorders of intestine CC HCC
Chronic ischemic colitis
Chronic ischemic enteritis
Chronic ischemic enterocolitis
Ischemic stricture of intestine
Mesenteric atherosclerosis
Mesenteric vascular insufficiency
CC Excl: PDX collection 791

✓5ᵗʰ K55.2 Angiodysplasia of colon
K55.20 Angiodysplasia of colon without hemorrhage
K55.21 Angiodysplasia of colon with hemorrhage MCC
DEF: Small vascular abnormalities due to fragile blood vessels in the colon, resulting in blood loss from the gastrointestinal (GI) tract.
CC Excl: PDX collection 770

✓5ᵗʰ K55.3 Necrotizing enterocolitis
EXCLUDES 1   *necrotizing enterocolitis of newborn (P77.-)*
EXCLUDES 2   *necrotizing enterocolitis due to Clostridium difficile (A04.7-)*
K55.30 Necrotizing enterocolitis, unspecified MCC HCC
Necrotizing enterocolitis, NOS
K55.31 Stage 1 necrotizing enterocolitis MCC HCC
Necrotizing enterocolitis without pneumatosis, without perforation
K55.32 Stage 2 necrotizing enterocolitis MCC HCC
Necrotizing enterocolitis with pneumatosis, without perforation
K55.33 Stage 3 necrotizing enterocolitis MCC HCC
Necrotizing enterocolitis with perforation
Necrotizing enterocolitis with pneumatosis and perforation

K55.8 Other vascular disorders of intestine CC HCC
CC Excl: PDX collection 791

K55.9 Vascular disorder of intestine, unspecified CC HCC
Ischemic colitis
Ischemic enteritis
Ischemic enterocolitis
CC Excl: PDX collection 791

✓4ᵗʰ K56 Paralytic ileus and intestinal obstruction without hernia
EXCLUDES 1   *congenital stricture or stenosis of intestine (Q41-Q42)*
cystic fibrosis with meconium ileus (E84.11)
ischemic stricture of intestine (K55.1)
meconium ileus NOS (P76.0)
neonatal intestinal obstructions classifiable to P76-
obstruction of duodenum (K31.5)
postprocedural intestinal obstruction (K91.3-)
stenosis of anus or rectum (K62.4)

CC Excl: For CC/MCC codes in category K56: PDX collection 792

K56.0 Paralytic ileus `CC` `HCC`
Paralysis of bowel
Paralysis of intestine
Paralysis of colon
> *EXCLUDES 1*   gallstone ileus (K56.3)
> ileus NOS (K56.7)
> obstructive ileus NOS (K56.69-)

DEF: Intestinal obstruction due to paralysis of bowel motility or peristalsis.

K56.1 Intussusception `CC` `HCC`
Intussusception or invagination of bowel
Intussusception or invagination of colon
Intussusception or invagination of intestine
Intussusception or invagination of rectum
> *EXCLUDES 2*   intussusception of appendix (K38.8)

DEF: Intestinal obstruction due to prolapse of a bowel section into an adjacent section. It occurs primarily in children and symptoms include acute abdominal pain, vomiting, and passage of blood and mucus from the rectum.

K56.2 Volvulus `MCC` `HCC`
Strangulation of colon or intestine
Torsion of colon or intestine
Twist of colon or intestine
> *EXCLUDES 2*   volvulus of duodenum (K31.5)

DEF: Twisting, knotting, or entanglement of the bowel on itself that may quickly compromise oxygen supply to the intestinal tissues. A volvulus usually occurs at the sigmoid and ileocecal areas of the intestines.

Volvulus

Knotted intestine (volvulus)

K56.3 Gallstone ileus `CC` `HCC`
Obstruction of intestine by gallstone

✓5ᵗʰ **K56.4 Other impaction of intestine**
    K56.41 Fecal impaction `HCC`
> *EXCLUDES 1*   constipation (K59.0-)
> incomplete defecation (R15.0)

    K56.49 Other impaction of intestine `CC` `HCC`

✓5ᵗʰ **K56.5 Intestinal adhesions [bands] with obstruction (postinfection)**
Abdominal hernia due to adhesions with obstruction
Peritoneal adhesions [bands] with intestinal obstruction (postinfection)
AHA: 2017, 4Q, 16-17

    K56.50 Intestinal adhesions [bands], unspecified as `CC` `HCC`
to partial versus complete obstruction
Intestinal adhesions with obstruction NOS

    K56.51 Intestinal adhesions [bands], with partial `CC` `HCC`
obstruction
Intestinal adhesions with incomplete obstruction

    K56.52 Intestinal adhesions [bands] with complete `CC` `HCC`
obstruction

✓5ᵗʰ **K56.6 Other and unspecified intestinal obstruction**
AHA: 2017, 4Q, 16-17; 2017, 2Q, 12

   ✓6ᵗʰ **K56.60 Unspecified intestinal obstruction**
> *EXCLUDES 1*   intestinal obstruction due to specified condition—code to condition

       K56.600 Partial intestinal obstruction, `CC` `HCC`
unspecified as to cause
Incomplete intestinal obstruction, NOS

       K56.601 Complete intestinal obstruction, `CC` `HCC`
unspecified as to cause

       K56.609 Unspecified intestinal obstruction, `CC` `HCC`
unspecified as to partial versus complete obstruction
Intestinal obstruction NOS

   ✓6ᵗʰ **K56.69 Other intestinal obstruction**
Enterostenosis NOS
Obstructive ileus NOS
Occlusion of colon or intestine NOS
Stenosis of colon or intestine NOS
Stricture of colon or intestine NOS
> *EXCLUDES 1*   intestinal obstruction due to specified condition—code to condition

       K56.690 Other partial intestinal obstruction `CC` `HCC`
Other incomplete intestinal obstruction

       K56.691 Other complete intestinal `CC` `HCC`
obstruction

       K56.699 Other intestinal obstruction `CC` `HCC`
unspecified as to partial versus complete obstruction
Other intestinal obstruction, NEC

K56.7 Ileus, unspecified `CC` `HCC`
> *EXCLUDES 1*   obstructive ileus (K56.69-)
> *EXCLUDES 2*   intestinal obstruction with hernia (K40-K46)

AHA: 2017, 1Q, 40

✓4ᵗʰ **K57 Diverticular disease of intestine**
▶Code also if applicable peritonitis K65.-◀
> *EXCLUDES 1*   congenital diverticulum of intestine (Q43.8)
> Meckel's diverticulum (Q43.0)
> *EXCLUDES 2*   diverticulum of appendix (K38.2)

CC Excl: For CC/MCC codes in category K57, unless otherwise noted: PDX collection 770

✓5ᵗʰ **K57.0 Diverticulitis of small intestine with perforation and abscess**
Diverticulitis of small intestine with peritonitis
> *EXCLUDES 1*   diverticulitis of both small and large intestine with perforation and abscess (K57.4-)

    K57.00 Diverticulitis of small intestine with `CC`
perforation and abscess without bleeding
CC Excl: PDX collection 793

    K57.01 Diverticulitis of small intestine with `MCC`
perforation and abscess with bleeding

✓5ᵗʰ **K57.1 Diverticular disease of small intestine without perforation or abscess**
> *EXCLUDES 1*   diverticular disease of both small and large intestine without perforation or abscess (K57.5-)

    K57.10 Diverticulosis of small intestine without perforation or abscess without bleeding
Diverticular disease of small intestine NOS

    K57.11 Diverticulosis of small intestine without `MCC`
perforation or abscess with bleeding

    K57.12 Diverticulitis of small intestine without `CC`
perforation or abscess without bleeding
CC Excl: PDX collection 793

    K57.13 Diverticulitis of small intestine without `MCC`
perforation or abscess with bleeding

✓5ᵗʰ **K57.2 Diverticulitis of large intestine with perforation and abscess**
Diverticulitis of colon with peritonitis
> *EXCLUDES 1*   diverticulitis of both small and large intestine with perforation and abscess (K57.4-)

    K57.20 Diverticulitis of large intestine with `CC`
perforation and abscess without bleeding
CC Excl: PDX collection 794

    K57.21 Diverticulitis of large intestine with `MCC`
perforation and abscess with bleeding

✓5ᵗʰ **K57.3 Diverticular disease of large intestine without perforation or abscess**
> *EXCLUDES 1*   diverticular disease of both small and large intestine without perforation or abscess (K57.5-)

    K57.30 Diverticulosis of large intestine without perforation or abscess without bleeding
Diverticular disease of colon NOS

    K57.31 Diverticulosis of large intestine without `MCC`
perforation or abscess with bleeding

    K57.32 Diverticulitis of large intestine without `CC`
perforation or abscess without bleeding
CC Excl: PDX collection 794

✓ Additional Character Required   ✓x7ᵗʰ Placeholder   Unacceptable PDx   Questionable PDx   Manifestation   `H1`-`H14` HAC   `HCC` CMS-HCC Dx   `HIV` HIV Dx

ICD-10-CM 2019   **705**

Chapter 11. Diseases of the Digestive System

K56.0–K57.32

K57.33   Diverticulitis of large intestine without perforation or abscess with bleeding   `MCC`

✓5ᵗʰ **K57.4**   **Diverticulitis of both** small and large intestine with perforation and abscess
     Diverticulitis of both small and large intestine with peritonitis

K57.40   Diverticulitis of both small and large intestine with perforation and abscess without bleeding   `CC`
     CC Excl: PDX collection 794

K57.41   Diverticulitis of both small and large intestine with perforation and abscess with bleeding   `MCC`

✓5ᵗʰ **K57.5**   **Diverticular disease of** both small and large intestine without perforation or abscess

K57.50   Diverticulosis of both small and large intestine without perforation or abscess without bleeding
     Diverticular disease of both small and large intestine NOS

K57.51   Diverticulosis of both small and large intestine without perforation or abscess with bleeding   `MCC`

K57.52   Diverticulitis of both small and large intestine without perforation or abscess without bleeding   `CC`
     CC Excl: PDX collection 794

K57.53   Diverticulitis of both small and large intestine without perforation or abscess with bleeding   `MCC`

✓5ᵗʰ **K57.8**   **Diverticulitis of intestine,** part unspecified, with perforation and abscess
     Diverticulitis of intestine NOS with peritonitis

K57.80   Diverticulitis of intestine, part unspecified, with perforation and abscess without bleeding   `CC`
     CC Excl: PDX collection 794

K57.81   Diverticulitis of intestine, part unspecified, with perforation and abscess with bleeding   `MCC`

✓5ᵗʰ **K57.9**   **Diverticular disease of intestine,** part unspecified, without perforation or abscess

K57.90   Diverticulosis of intestine, part unspecified, without perforation or abscess without bleeding
     Diverticular disease of intestine NOS

K57.91   Diverticulosis of intestine, part unspecified, without perforation or abscess with bleeding   `MCC`

K57.92   Diverticulitis of intestine, part unspecified, without perforation or abscess without bleeding   `CC`
     CC Excl: PDX collection 794

K57.93   Diverticulitis of intestine, part unspecified, without perforation or abscess with bleeding   `MCC`

✓4ᵗʰ **K58**   **Irritable bowel syndrome**
     `INCLUDES`   irritable colon
           spastic colon
     AHA: 2016, 4Q, 32-33

K58.0   **Irritable bowel syndrome** with diarrhea

K58.1   **Irritable bowel syndrome** with constipation

K58.2   Mixed **irritable bowel syndrome**

K58.8   Other **irritable bowel syndrome**

K58.9   **Irritable bowel syndrome** without diarrhea
     Irritable bowel syndrome NOS

✓4ᵗʰ **K59**   **Other functional intestinal disorders**
     `EXCLUDES 1`   change in bowel habit NOS (R19.4)
            intestinal malabsorption (K90.-)
            psychogenic intestinal disorders (F45.8)
     `EXCLUDES 2`   functional disorders of stomach (K31.-)

✓5ᵗʰ **K59.0**   **Constipation**
     Use additional code for adverse effect, if applicable, to identify drug (T36-T50 with fifth or sixth character 5)
     `EXCLUDES 1`   fecal impaction (K56.41)
            incomplete defecation (R15.0)
     AHA: 2016, 4Q, 33

K59.00   **Constipation,** unspecified

K59.01   Slow transit **constipation**
     DEF: Delay in the transit of fecal material through the colon secondary to smooth muscle dysfunction or decreased peristaltic contractions along the colon.

K59.02   Outlet dysfunction **constipation**

K59.03   Drug induced **constipation**
     Use additional code for adverse effect, if applicable, to identify drug (T36-T50 with fifth or sixth character 5)

K59.04   Chronic idiopathic **constipation**
     Functional constipation

K59.09   Other **constipation**
     Chronic constipation

K59.1   **Functional diarrhea**
     `EXCLUDES 1`   diarrhea NOS (R19.7)
            irritable bowel syndrome with diarrhea (K58.0)

K59.2   **Neurogenic bowel, not elsewhere classified**   `CC`
     DEF: Disorder of bowel due to a spinal cord lesion due to injury or as a complication of conditions such as multiple sclerosis (MS) or spina bifida. Loss of bowel control is the primary symptom, manifested as constipation or bowel incontinence.
     CC Excl: PDX collection 795

✓5ᵗʰ **K59.3**   **Megacolon, not elsewhere classified**
     Dilatation of colon
     Code first, if applicable (T51-T65) to identify toxic agent
     `EXCLUDES 1`   congenital megacolon (aganglionic) (Q43.1)
            megacolon (due to) (in) Chagas' disease (B57.32)
            megacolon (due to) (in) Clostridium difficile (A04.7-)
            megacolon (due to) (in) Hirschsprung's disease (Q43.1)
     AHA: 2016, 4Q, 33-34

     CC Excl: For CC codes in subcategory K59.3: PDX collection 795

K59.31   Toxic megacolon   `CC` `HCC`

K59.39   Other megacolon   `CC`
     Megacolon NOS

K59.4   **Anal spasm**
     Proctalgia fugax

K59.8   **Other specified functional intestinal disorders**
     Atony of colon
     Pseudo-obstruction (acute) (chronic) of intestine

K59.9   **Functional intestinal disorder, unspecified**

✓4ᵗʰ **K60**   **Fissure and fistula of anal and rectal regions**
     `EXCLUDES 1`   fissure and fistula of anal and rectal regions with abscess or cellulitis (K61.-)
     `EXCLUDES 2`   anal sphincter tear (healed) (nontraumatic) (old) (K62.81)

K60.0   Acute **anal fissure**

K60.1   Chronic **anal fissure**

K60.2   **Anal fissure,** unspecified

K60.3   Anal **fistula**   `SW`

K60.4   Rectal **fistula**   `SW`
     Fistula of rectum to skin
     `EXCLUDES 1`   rectovaginal fistula (N82.3)
            vesicorectal fistual (N32.1)

K60.5   Anorectal **fistula**   `SW`

✓4ᵗʰ **K61**   **Abscess of anal and rectal regions**
     `INCLUDES`   abscess of anal and rectal regions
            cellulitis of anal and rectal regions

     CC Excl: For CC codes in category K61: PDX collection 796

K61.0   Anal **abscess**   `CC`
     Perianal abscess
     `EXCLUDES 1`   ~~intrasphincteric abscess (K61.4)~~
     `EXCLUDES 2`   ▶intrasphincteric abscess (K61.4)◀

K61.1   Rectal **abscess**   `CC`
     Perirectal abscess
     `EXCLUDES 1`   ischiorectal abscess ▶(K61.39)◀
     AHA: 2012, 4Q, 104

K61.2   Anorectal **abscess**   `CC`

✓5ᵗʰ **K61.3**   Ischiorectal **abscess**
     ~~Abscess of ischiorectal fossa~~

●   **K61.31**   Horseshoe **abscess**

●   **K61.39**   Other ischiorectal **abscess**
     Abscess of ischiorectal fossa
     Ischiorectal abscess, NOS

K61.4   Intrasphincteric **abscess**   `CC`
     ▶Intersphincteric abscess◀

● **K61.5**   Supralevator **abscess**   `CC`

N Newborn: 0   **P** Pediatric: 0-17   **M** Maternity: 12-55   **A** Adult: 15-124   `MCC` Major Complication/Comorbidity   `CC` Complication/Comorbidity   `SW` Severe Wound Dx

706   ICD-10-CM 2019

✓4ᵗʰ **K62   Other diseases of anus and rectum**
   INCLUDES   anal canal
   EXCLUDES 2 colostomy and enterostomy malfunction (K94.0-, K94.1-)
         fecal incontinence (R15.-)
         hemorrhoids (K64.-)

   K62.0   Anal polyp
   K62.1   Rectal polyp
      EXCLUDES 1 adenomatous polyp (D12.8)
      AHA: 2018, 1Q, 6
   K62.2   Anal prolapse
         Prolapse of anal canal
   K62.3   Rectal prolapse
         Prolapse of rectal mucosa
   K62.4   Stenosis of anus and rectum
         Stricture of anus (sphincter)
   K62.5   Hemorrhage of anus and rectum   CC
      EXCLUDES 1 gastrointestinal bleeding NOS (K92.2)
            melena (K92.1)
            neonatal rectal hemorrhage (P54.2)
      CC Excl: PDX collection 770
   K62.6   Ulcer of anus and rectum   CC
         Solitary ulcer of anus and rectum
         Stercoral ulcer of anus and rectum
      EXCLUDES 1 fissure and fistula of anus and rectum (K60.-)
            ulcerative colitis (K51.-)
      CC Excl: PDX collection 797
   K62.7   Radiation proctitis
         Use additional code to identify the type of radiation (W90.-)

✓5ᵗʰ **K62.8   Other specified diseases of anus and rectum**
      EXCLUDES 2 ulcerative proctitis (K51.2)
      K62.81   Anal sphincter tear (healed) (nontraumatic) (old)
            Tear of anus, nontraumatic
            Use additional code for any associated fecal
               incontinence (R15.-)
         EXCLUDES 2 anal fissure (K60.-)
               anal sphincter tear (healed) (old)
                  complicating delivery (O34.7-)
               traumatic tear of anal sphincter (S31.831)

      K62.82   Dysplasia of anus
            Anal intraepithelial neoplasia I and II (AIN I and II)
               (histologically confirmed)
            Dysplasia of anus NOS
            Mild and moderate dysplasia of anus (histologically
               confirmed)
         EXCLUDES 1 abnormal results from anal cytologic
               examination without histologic
               confirmation (R85.61-)
            anal intraepithelial neoplasia III (D01.3)
            carcinoma in situ of anus (D01.3)
            HGSIL of anus (R85.613)
            severe dysplasia of anus (D01.3)

      K62.89   Other specified diseases of anus and rectum
            Proctitis NOS
            Use additional code for any associated fecal
               incontinence (R15.-)

   K62.9   Disease of anus and rectum, unspecified

✓4ᵗʰ **K63   Other diseases of intestine**
   K63.0   Abscess of intestine   CC
      EXCLUDES 1 abscess of intestine with Crohn's disease (K50.014,
               K50.114, K50.814, K50.914)
            abscess of intestine with diverticular disease (K57.0,
               K57.2, K57.4, K57.8)
            abscess of intestine with ulcerative colitis (K51.014,
               K51.214, K51.314, K51.414, K51.514, K51.814,
               K51.914)
      EXCLUDES 2 abscess of anal and rectal regions (K61.-)
            abscess of appendix ▶(K35.3-)◀
      CC Excl: PDX collection 798
   K63.1   Perforation of intestine (nontraumatic)   MCC HCC
         Perforation (nontraumatic) of rectum
      EXCLUDES 1 perforation (nontraumatic) of duodenum (K26.-)
            perforation (nontraumatic) of intestine with
               diverticular disease (K57.0, K57.2, K57.4, K57.8)
      EXCLUDES 2 perforation (nontraumatic) of appendix ▶(K35.2-,
               K35.3-)◀
      CC Excl: PDX collection 799

   K63.2   Fistula of intestine   CC SW
      EXCLUDES 1 fistula of duodenum (K31.6)
            fistula of intestine with Crohn's disease (K50.013,
               K50.113, K50.813, K50.913)
            fistula of intestine with ulcerative colitis (K51.013,
               K51.213, K51.313, K51.413, K51.513, K51.813,
               K51.913)
      EXCLUDES 2 fistula of anal and rectal regions (K60.-)
            fistula of appendix (K38.3)
            intestinal-genital fistula, female (N82.2-N82.4)
            vesicointestinal fistula (N32.1)
      AHA: 2017, 3Q, 4
      CC Excl: PDX collection 800
   K63.3   Ulcer of intestine   CC
         Primary ulcer of small intestine
      EXCLUDES 1 duodenal ulcer (K26.-)
            gastrointestinal ulcer (K28.-)
            gastrojejunal ulcer (K28.-)
            jejunal ulcer (K28.-)
            peptic ulcer, site unspecified (K27.-)
            ulcer of intestine with perforation (K63.1)
            ulcer of anus or rectum (K62.6)
            ulcerative colitis (K51.-)
      CC Excl: PDX collection 801
   K63.4   Enteroptosis
   K63.5   Polyp of colon
      EXCLUDES 1 adenomatous polyp of colon (D12.6)
            inflammatory polyp of colon (K51.4-)
            polyposis of colon (D12.6)
      AHA: 2018, 2Q, 14; 2017, 1Q, 15; 2015, 2Q, 14

✓5ᵗʰ **K63.8   Other specified diseases of intestine**
      K63.81   Dieulafoy lesion of intestine   MCC
         EXCLUDES 2 Dieulafoy lesion of stomach and duodenum
               (K31.82)
         DEF: Abnormally large submucosal artery protruding
            through a defect in the stomach mucosa or intestines
            that can cause massive and life-threatening
            hemorrhaging.
         CC Excl: PDX collection 802
      K63.89   Other specified diseases of intestine
         AHA: 2013, 2Q, 31
   K63.9   Disease of intestine, unspecified

✓4ᵗʰ **K64   Hemorrhoids and perianal venous thrombosis**
   INCLUDES   piles
   EXCLUDES 1 hemorrhoids complicating childbirth and the puerperium (O87.2)
         hemorrhoids complicating pregnancy (O22.4)

   K64.0   First degree hemorrhoids
         Grade/stage I hemorrhoids
         Hemorrhoids (bleeding) without prolapse outside of anal canal
   K64.1   Second degree hemorrhoids
         Grade/stage II hemorrhoids
         Hemorrhoids (bleeding) that prolapse with straining, but retract
            spontaneously
   K64.2   Third degree hemorrhoids
         Grade/stage III hemorrhoids
         Hemorrhoids (bleeding) that prolapse with straining and require
            manual replacement back inside anal canal

Hemorrhoids

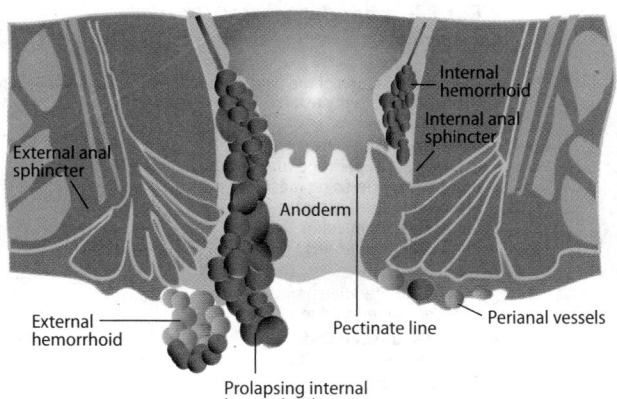

Internal hemorrhoid
Internal anal sphincter
External anal sphincter
Anoderm
Pectinate line
Perianal vessels
External hemorrhoid
Prolapsing internal hemorrhoid

K64.3 Fourth degree **hemorrhoids**
Grade/stage IV hemorrhoids
Hemorrhoids (bleeding) with prolapsed tissue that cannot be manually replaced

K64.4 Residual **hemorrhoidal skin tags**
External hemorrhoids, NOS
Skin tags of anus

K64.5 Perianal venous thrombosis
External hemorrhoids with thrombosis
Perianal hematoma
Thrombosed hemorrhoids NOS

K64.8 Other **hemorrhoids**
Internal hemorrhoids, without mention of degree
Prolapsed hemorrhoids, degree not specified

K64.9 Unspecified **hemorrhoids**
Hemorrhoids (bleeding) NOS
Hemorrhoids (bleeding) without mention of degree

Diseases of peritoneum and retroperitoneum (K65-K68)

√4th **K65** **Peritonitis**
▶Use additional code (B95-B97), to identify infectious agent, if known◀
▶Code also if applicable diverticular disease of intestine (K57.-)◀
EXCLUDES 1 *acute appendicitis with generalized peritonitis ▶(K35.2-)◀*
aseptic peritonitis (T81.6)
benign paroxysmal peritonitis (E85.0)
chemical peritonitis (T81.6)
~~diverticulitis of both small and large intestine with peritonitis (K57.4-)~~
~~diverticulitis of colon with peritonitis (K57.2-)~~
~~diverticulitis of intestine, NOS, with peritonitis (K57.8-)~~
~~diverticulitis of small intestine with peritonitis (K57.0-)~~
gonococcal peritonitis (A54.85)
neonatal peritonitis (P78.0-P78.1)
pelvic peritonitis, female (N73.3-N73.5)
periodic familial peritonitis (E85.0)
peritonitis due to talc or other foreign substance (T81.6)
peritonitis in chlamydia (A74.81)
peritonitis in diphtheria (A36.89)
peritonitis in syphilis (late) (A52.74)
peritonitis in tuberculosis (A18.31)
peritonitis with or following abortion or ectopic or molar pregnancy (O00-O07, O08.0)
peritonitis with or following appendicitis (K35.-)
~~peritonitis with or following diverticular disease of intestine (K57.-)~~
puerperal peritonitis (O85)
retroperitoneal infections (K68.-)

CC Excl: For CC/MCC codes in category K65: PDX collection 803

K65.0 Generalized (acute) **peritonitis**   MCC HCC
Pelvic peritonitis (acute), male
Subphrenic peritonitis (acute)
Suppurative peritonitis (acute)

K65.1 **Peritoneal** abscess   MCC HCC
Abdominopelvic abscess   Subdiaphragmatic abscess
Abscess (of) omentum   Subhepatic abscess
Abscess (of) peritoneum   Subphrenic abscess
Mesenteric abscess
Retrocecal abscess

K65.2 Spontaneous bacterial **peritonitis**   MCC HCC
EXCLUDES 1   *bacterial peritonitis NOS (K65.9)*

K65.3 **Choleperitonitis**   MCC HCC
Peritonitis due to bile
DEF: Inflammation of the peritoneum due to leakage of bile into the peritoneal cavity resulting from rupture of the bile passages or gallbladder.

K65.4 **Sclerosing mesenteritis**   CC HCC
Fat necrosis of peritoneum
(Idiopathic) sclerosing mesenteric fibrosis
Mesenteric lipodystrophy
Mesenteric panniculitis
Retractile mesenteritis

K65.8 Other **peritonitis**   MCC HCC
Chronic proliferative peritonitis
Peritonitis due to urine

K65.9 **Peritonitis,** unspecified   MCC HCC
Bacterial peritonitis NOS
AHA: 2013, 2Q, 31

√4th **K66** **Other disorders of peritoneum**
EXCLUDES 2   *ascites (R18.-)*
peritoneal effusion (chronic) (R18.8)

K66.0 **Peritoneal adhesions (postprocedural) (postinfection)**
Adhesions (of) abdominal (wall)   Adhesions (of) omentum
Adhesions (of) diaphragm   Adhesions (of) stomach
Adhesions (of) intestine   Adhesive bands
Adhesions (of) male pelvis   Mesenteric adhesions
EXCLUDES 1   *female pelvic adhesions [bands] (N73.6)*
peritoneal adhesions with intestinal obstruction (K56.5-)

K66.1 **Hemoperitoneum**   MCC
EXCLUDES 1   *traumatic hemoperitoneum (S36.8-)*
CC Excl: PDX collection 804

K66.8 **Other specified disorders of peritoneum**

K66.9 **Disorder of peritoneum, unspecified**

K67 *Disorders of peritoneum in infectious diseases classified elsewhere*   MCC HCC
Code first underlying disease, such as:
congenital syphilis (A50.0)
helminthiasis (B65.0-B83.9)
EXCLUDES 1   *peritonitis in chlamydia (A74.81)*
peritonitis in diphtheria (A36.89)
peritonitis in gonococcal (A54.85)
peritonitis in syphilis (late) (A52.74)
peritonitis in tuberculosis (A18.31)
CC Excl: PDX collection 803

√4th **K68** **Disorders of retroperitoneum**

√5th **K68.1** **Retroperitoneal abscess**
K68.11 Postprocedural **retroperitoneal abscess**   CC H11 H12 H13
EXCLUDES 2   ▶*infection following procedure (T81.4-)*◀
CC Excl: PDX collection 805

K68.12 Psoas muscle **abscess**   MCC HCC
CC Excl: PDX collection 806

K68.19 Other **retroperitoneal abscess**   MCC HCC
CC Excl: PDX collection 803

K68.9 **Other disorders of retroperitoneum**   MCC
CC Excl: PDX collection 803

Diseases of liver (K70-K77)

EXCLUDES 1   *jaundice NOS (R17)*
EXCLUDES 2   *hemochromatosis (E83.11-)*
Reye's syndrome (G93.7)
viral hepatitis (B15-B19)
Wilson's disease (E83.0)

√4th **K70** **Alcoholic liver disease**
Use additional code to identify:
alcohol abuse and dependence (F10.-)

K70.0 **Alcoholic** fatty liver   A

√5th **K70.1** **Alcoholic** hepatitis
K70.10 **Alcoholic hepatitis** without ascites   A
K70.11 **Alcoholic hepatitis** with ascites   A

K70.2 **Alcoholic** fibrosis and sclerosis **of liver**   A

√5th **K70.3** **Alcoholic** cirrhosis **of liver**
Alcoholic cirrhosis NOS
K70.30 **Alcoholic cirrhosis of liver** without ascites   HCC A
K70.31 **Alcoholic cirrhosis of liver** with ascites   HCC A
AHA: 2018, 1Q, 4

√5th **K70.4** **Alcoholic** hepatic failure
Acute alcoholic hepatic failure
Alcoholic hepatic failure NOS
Chronic alcoholic hepatic failure
Subacute alcoholic hepatic failure
K70.40 **Alcoholic hepatic failure** without coma   HCC A
K70.41 **Alcoholic hepatic failure** with coma   MCC HCC A
CC Excl: PDX collection 807

K70.9 **Alcoholic liver disease, unspecified**   HCC A

N Newborn: 0   P Pediatric: 0-17   M Maternity: 12-55   A Adult: 15-124   MCC Major Complication/Comorbidity   CC Complication/Comorbidity   SW Severe Wound Dx

708   ICD-10-CM 2019

Chapter 11. Diseases of the Digestive System

☑4ᵗʰ **K71 Toxic liver disease**
  INCLUDES   drug-induced idiosyncratic (unpredictable) liver disease
                 drug-induced toxic (predictable) liver disease
  Code first poisoning due to drug or toxin, if applicable (T36-T65 with fifth or sixth character 1-4 or 6)
  Use additional code for adverse effect, if applicable, to identify drug (T36-T50 with fifth or sixth character 5)
  EXCLUDES 2   alcoholic liver disease (K70.-)
                Budd-Chiari syndrome (I82.0)

  K71.0 Toxic liver disease with cholestasis
       Cholestasis with hepatocyte injury
       "Pure" cholestasis

☑5ᵗʰ **K71.1 Toxic liver disease with hepatic necrosis**
       Hepatic failure (acute) (chronic) due to drugs

      K71.10 Toxic liver disease with hepatic necrosis, without coma

      K71.11 Toxic liver disease with hepatic necrosis, with coma   MCC HCC
          CC Excl: PDX collection 807

  K71.2 Toxic liver disease with acute hepatitis
  K71.3 Toxic liver disease with chronic persistent hepatitis
  K71.4 Toxic liver disease with chronic lobular hepatitis

☑5ᵗʰ **K71.5 Toxic liver disease with chronic active hepatitis**
       Toxic liver disease with lupoid hepatitis

      K71.50 Toxic liver disease with chronic active hepatitis without ascites

      K71.51 Toxic liver disease with chronic active hepatitis with ascites
          AHA: 2018, 1Q, 4

  K71.6 Toxic liver disease with hepatitis, not elsewhere classified
  K71.7 Toxic liver disease with fibrosis and cirrhosis of liver
  K71.8 Toxic liver disease with other disorders of liver
       Toxic liver disease with focal nodular hyperplasia
       Toxic liver disease with hepatic granulomas
       Toxic liver disease with peliosis hepatis
       Toxic liver disease with veno-occlusive disease of liver

  K71.9 Toxic liver disease, unspecified

☑4ᵗʰ **K72 Hepatic failure, not elsewhere classified**
  INCLUDES   fulminant hepatitis NEC, with hepatic failure
                hepatic encephalopathy NOS
                liver (cell) necrosis with hepatic failure
                malignant hepatitis NEC, with hepatic failure
                yellow liver atrophy or dystrophy
  EXCLUDES 1   alcoholic hepatic failure (K70.4)
                hepatic failure with toxic liver disease (K71.1-)
                icterus of newborn (P55-P59)
                postprocedural hepatic failure (K91.82)
  EXCLUDES 2   hepatic failure complicating abortion or ectopic or molar pregnancy (O00-O07, O08.8)
                hepatic failure complicating pregnancy, childbirth and the puerperium (O26.6-)
                viral hepatitis with hepatic coma (B15-B19)
  AHA: 2017, 1Q, 41

☑5ᵗʰ **K72.0 Acute and subacute hepatic failure**
       Acute non-viral hepatitis NOS
       AHA: 2015, 2Q, 17; 2014, 2Q, 13

      K72.00 Acute and subacute hepatic failure without coma   MCC
          CC Excl: PDX collection 808

      K72.01 Acute and subacute hepatic failure with coma   MCC HCC
          CC Excl: PDX collection 808

☑5ᵗʰ **K72.1 Chronic hepatic failure**
      K72.10 Chronic hepatic failure without coma   HCC
      K72.11 Chronic hepatic failure with coma   MCC HCC
          CC Excl: PDX collection 807

☑5ᵗʰ **K72.9 Hepatic failure, unspecified**
      K72.90 Hepatic failure, unspecified without coma   HCC
          AHA: 2016, 2Q, 35
      K72.91 Hepatic failure, unspecified with coma   MCC HCC
          Hepatic coma NOS
          CC Excl: PDX collection 807

☑4ᵗʰ **K73 Chronic hepatitis, not elsewhere classified**
  EXCLUDES 1   alcoholic hepatitis (chronic) (K70.1-)
                drug-induced hepatitis (chronic) (K71.-)
                granulomatous hepatitis (chronic) NEC (K75.3)
                reactive, nonspecific hepatitis (chronic) (K75.2)
                viral hepatitis (chronic) (B15-B19)

  K73.0 Chronic persistent hepatitis, not elsewhere classified   HCC
  K73.1 Chronic lobular hepatitis, not elsewhere classified   HCC
  K73.2 Chronic active hepatitis, not elsewhere classified   HCC
  K73.8 Other chronic hepatitis, not elsewhere classified   HCC
  K73.9 Chronic hepatitis, unspecified   HCC

☑4ᵗʰ **K74 Fibrosis and cirrhosis of liver**
  Code also, if applicable, viral hepatitis (acute) (chronic) (B15-B19)
  EXCLUDES 1   alcoholic cirrhosis (of liver) (K70.3)
                alcoholic fibrosis of liver (K70.2)
                cardiac sclerosis of liver (K76.1)
                cirrhosis (of liver) with toxic liver disease (K71.7)
                congenital cirrhosis (of liver) (P78.81)
                pigmentary cirrhosis (of liver) (E83.110)

  K74.0 Hepatic fibrosis
  K74.1 Hepatic sclerosis
  K74.2 Hepatic fibrosis with hepatic sclerosis
  K74.3 Primary biliary cirrhosis   HCC
       Chronic nonsuppurative destructive cholangitis
       ▶Primary biliary cholangitis◀
       EXCLUDES 2 ▶primary sclerosing cholangitis (K83.01)◀
  K74.4 Secondary biliary cirrhosis   HCC
  K74.5 Biliary cirrhosis, unspecified   HCC

☑5ᵗʰ **K74.6 Other and unspecified cirrhosis of liver**
      K74.60 Unspecified cirrhosis of liver   HCC
          Cirrhosis (of liver) NOS
          AHA: 2018, 1Q, 4
      K74.69 Other cirrhosis of liver   HCC
          Cryptogenic cirrhosis (of liver)
          Macronodular cirrhosis (of liver)
          Micronodular cirrhosis (of liver)
          Mixed type cirrhosis (of liver)
          Portal cirrhosis (of liver)
          Postnecrotic cirrhosis (of liver)

☑4ᵗʰ **K75 Other inflammatory liver diseases**
  EXCLUDES 2   toxic liver disease (K71.-)

  K75.0 Abscess of liver   MCC
       Cholangitic hepatic abscess
       Hematogenic hepatic abscess
       Hepatic abscess NOS
       Lymphogenic hepatic abscess
       Pylephlebitic hepatic abscess
       EXCLUDES 1   amebic liver abscess (A06.4)
                cholangitis without liver abscess ▶(K83.09)◀
                pylephlebitis without liver abscess (K75.1)
       EXCLUDES 2   acute or subacute hepatitis NOS (B17.9)
                acute or subacute non-viral hepatitis (K72.0)
                chronic hepatitis NEC (K73.8)
       CC Excl: PDX collection 809

  K75.1 Phlebitis of portal vein   MCC
       Pylephlebitis
       EXCLUDES 1   pylephlebitic liver abscess (K75.0)
       DEF: Inflammation of the portal vein or branches due to diverticulitis, perforated appendicitis, or peritonitis. Symptoms include fever, chills, jaundice, sweating, and abscess in various body parts.
       CC Excl: PDX collection 809

  K75.2 Nonspecific reactive hepatitis
       EXCLUDES 1   acute or subacute hepatitis (K72.0-)
                chronic hepatitis NEC (K73.-)
                viral hepatitis (B15-B19)

  K75.3 Granulomatous hepatitis, not elsewhere classified
       EXCLUDES 1   acute or subacute hepatitis (K72.0-)
                chronic hepatitis NEC (K73.-)
                viral hepatitis (B15-B19)

  K75.4 Autoimmune hepatitis   HCC
       Lupoid hepatitis NEC

☑5ᵗʰ **K75.8 Other specified inflammatory liver diseases**
      K75.81 Nonalcoholic steatohepatitis (NASH)
      K75.89 Other specified inflammatory liver diseases

☑ Additional Character Required   ✓x7ᵗʰ Placeholder   Unacceptable PDx   Questionable PDx   Manifestation   H1-H14 HAC   HCC CMS-HCC Dx   HIV HIV Dx

ICD-10-CM 2019   709

K75.9 Inflammatory liver disease, unspecified
Hepatitis NOS
EXCLUDES 1   *acute or subacute hepatitis (K72.0-)*
chronic hepatitis NEC (K73.-)
viral hepatitis (B15-B19)
AHA: 2015, 2Q, 17

✓4ᵗʰ K76 Other diseases of liver
EXCLUDES 2   *alcoholic liver disease (K70.-)*
amyloid degeneration of liver (E85.-)
cystic disease of liver (congenital) (Q44.6)
hepatic vein thrombosis (I82.0)
hepatomegaly NOS (R16.0)
pigmentary cirrhosis (of liver) (E83.110)
portal vein thrombosis (I81)
toxic liver disease (K71.-)

K76.0 Fatty (change of) liver, not elsewhere classified
Nonalcoholic fatty liver disease (NAFLD)
EXCLUDES 1   *nonalcoholic steatohepatitis (NASH) (K75.81)*

K76.1 Chronic passive congestion of liver
Cardiac cirrhosis
Cardiac sclerosis

K76.2 Central hemorrhagic necrosis of liver   `MCC`
EXCLUDES 1   *liver necrosis with hepatic failure (K72.-)*
CC Excl: PDX collection 808

K76.3 Infarction of liver   `MCC`
CC Excl: PDX collection 808

K76.4 Peliosis hepatis
Hepatic angiomatosis

K76.5 Hepatic veno-occlusive disease
EXCLUDES 1   *Budd-Chiari syndrome (I82.0)*

K76.6 Portal hypertension   `CC` `HCC`
Use additional code for any associated complications, such as:
portal hypertensive gastropathy (K31.89)
CC Excl: PDX collection 810

K76.7 Hepatorenal syndrome   `MCC` `HCC`
EXCLUDES 1   *hepatorenal syndrome following labor and delivery*
(O90.4)
postprocedural hepatorenal syndrome (K91.83)
CC Excl: PDX collection 811

✓5ᵗʰ K76.8 Other specified diseases of liver
K76.81 Hepatopulmonary syndrome   `HCC`
Code first underlying liver disease, such as:
alcoholic cirrhosis of liver (K70.3-)
cirrhosis of liver without mention of alcohol (K74.6-)

K76.89 Other specified diseases of liver
Cyst (simple) of liver
Focal nodular hyperplasia of liver
Hepatoptosis

K76.9 Liver disease, unspecified

K77 *Liver disorders in diseases classified elsewhere*   `CC`
Code first underlying disease, such as:
amyloidosis (E85.-)
congenital syphilis (A50.0, A50.5)
congenital toxoplasmosis (P37.1)
schistosomiasis (B65.0-B65.9)
EXCLUDES 1   *alcoholic hepatitis (K70.1-)*
alcoholic liver disease (K70-.)
cytomegaloviral hepatitis (B25.1)
herpesviral [herpes simplex] hepatitis (B00.81)
infectious mononucleosis with liver disease
(B27.0-B27.9 with .9)
mumps hepatitis (B26.81)
sarcoidosis with liver disease (D86.89)
secondary syphilis with liver disease (A51.45)
syphilis (late) with liver disease (A52.74)
toxoplasmosis (acquired) hepatitis (B58.1)
tuberculosis with liver disease (A18.83)
CC Excl: No Excl

Disorders of gallbladder, biliary tract and pancreas (K80-K87)

✓4ᵗʰ K80 Cholelithiasis
EXCLUDES 1   *retained cholelithiasis following cholecystectomy (K91.86)*
DEF: Presence or formation of concretions (calculi or "gallstones") in the gallbladder. The stones contain cholesterol, calcium carbonate, or calcium bilirubinate in pure forms or in various combinations.

✓5ᵗʰ K80.0 Calculus of gallbladder with acute cholecystitis
Any condition listed in K80.2 with acute cholecystitis
▶Use additional code if applicable for associated gangrene of gallbladder (K82.A1), or perforation of gallbladder (K82.A2)◀

K80.00 Calculus of gallbladder with acute cholecystitis   `CC`
without obstruction
CC Excl: PDX collection 812

Cholelithiasis

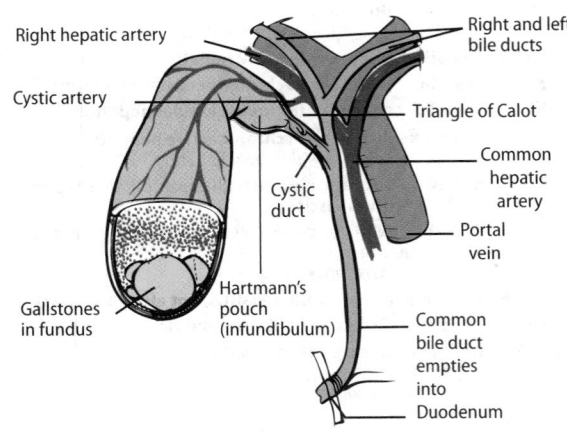

Right hepatic artery
Cystic artery
Cystic duct
Gallstones in fundus
Hartmann's pouch (infundibulum)
Right and left bile ducts
Triangle of Calot
Common hepatic artery
Portal vein
Common bile duct empties into Duodenum

K80.01 Calculus of gallbladder with acute cholecystitis   `CC`
with obstruction
CC Excl: PDX collection 813

✓5ᵗʰ K80.1 Calculus of gallbladder with other cholecystitis
▶Use additional code if applicable for associated gangrene of gallbladder (K82.A1), or perforation of gallbladder (K82.A2)◀

CC Excl: For CC codes in subcategory K80.1, unless otherwise noted: PDX collection 813

K80.10 Calculus of gallbladder with chronic   `CC`
cholecystitis without obstruction
Cholelithiasis with cholecystitis NOS

K80.11 Calculus of gallbladder with chronic   `CC`
cholecystitis with obstruction

K80.12 Calculus of gallbladder with acute and chronic   `CC`
cholecystitis without obstruction
CC Excl: PDX collection 812

K80.13 Calculus of gallbladder with acute and chronic   `CC`
cholecystitis with obstruction

K80.18 Calculus of gallbladder with other cholecystitis   `CC`
without obstruction

K80.19 Calculus of gallbladder with other cholecystitis   `CC`
with obstruction

✓5ᵗʰ K80.2 Calculus of gallbladder without cholecystitis
Cholecystolithiasis without cholecystitis
Cholelithiasis (without cholecystitis)
Colic (recurrent) of gallbladder (without cholecystitis)
Gallstone (impacted) of cystic duct (without cholecystitis)
Gallstone (impacted) of gallbladder (without cholecystitis)

K80.20 Calculus of gallbladder without cholecystitis without obstruction

K80.21 Calculus of gallbladder without cholecystitis   `CC`
with obstruction
CC Excl: PDX collection 813

✓5ᵗʰ K80.3 Calculus of bile duct with cholangitis
Any condition listed in K80.5 with cholangitis
DEF: Cholangitis: Inflammation of the bile ducts.

CC Excl: For CC codes in subcategory K80.3, unless otherwise noted: PDX collection 814

K80.30 Calculus of bile duct with cholangitis,   `CC`
unspecified, without obstruction

`N` Newborn: 0   `P` Pediatric: 0-17   `M` Maternity: 12-55   `A` Adult: 15-124   `MCC` Major Complication/Comorbidity   `CC` Complication/Comorbidity   `SW` Severe Wound Dx

710   ICD-10-CM 2019

K80.31   **Calculus of bile duct with cholangitis, unspecified, with obstruction**   `CC`
    CC Excl: PDX collection 815

K80.32   **Calculus of bile duct with** acute **cholangitis without obstruction**   `CC`

K80.33   **Calculus of bile duct with** acute **cholangitis with obstruction**   `CC`

K80.34   **Calculus of bile duct with** chronic **cholangitis without obstruction**   `CC`

K80.35   **Calculus of bile duct with** chronic **cholangitis with obstruction**   `CC`
    CC Excl: PDX collection 815

K80.36   **Calculus of bile duct with** acute and chronic **cholangitis without obstruction**   `CC`

K80.37   **Calculus of bile duct with** acute and chronic **cholangitis with obstruction**   `CC`
    CC Excl: PDX collection 815

✓5ᵗʰ **K80.4   Calculus of** bile duct with cholecystitis
    Any condition listed in K80.5 with cholecystitis (with cholangitis)
    ▶Use additional code if applicable for associated gangrene of gallbladder (K82.A1), or perforation of gallbladder (K82.A2)◀

    CC Excl: For CC codes in subcategory K80.4: PDX collection 815

K80.40   **Calculus of bile duct with cholecystitis, unspecified, without obstruction**   `CC`

K80.41   **Calculus of bile duct with cholecystitis, unspecified, with obstruction**   `CC`

K80.42   **Calculus of bile duct with** acute **cholecystitis without obstruction**   `CC`

K80.43   **Calculus of bile duct with** acute **cholecystitis with obstruction**   `CC`

K80.44   **Calculus of bile duct with** chronic **cholecystitis without obstruction**   `CC`

K80.45   **Calculus of bile duct with** chronic **cholecystitis with obstruction**   `CC`

K80.46   **Calculus of bile duct with** acute and chronic **cholecystitis without obstruction**   `CC`

K80.47   **Calculus of bile duct with** acute and chronic **cholecystitis with obstruction**   `CC`

✓5ᵗʰ **K80.5   Calculus of** bile duct without cholangitis or cholecystitis
    Choledocholithiasis (without cholangitis or cholecystitis)
    Gallstone (impacted) of bile duct NOS (without cholangitis or cholecystitis)
    Gallstone (impacted) of common duct (without cholangitis or cholecystitis)
    Gallstone (impacted) of hepatic duct (without cholangitis or cholecystitis)
    Hepatic cholelithiasis (without cholangitis or cholecystitis)
    Hepatic colic (recurrent) (without cholangitis or cholecystitis)
    DEF: Cholangitis: Inflammation of the bile ducts.

K80.50   **Calculus of bile duct without cholangitis or cholecystitis without obstruction**

K80.51   **Calculus of bile duct without cholangitis or cholecystitis with obstruction**   `CC`
    CC Excl: PDX collection 815

✓5ᵗʰ **K80.6   Calculus of** gallbladder and bile duct with cholecystitis
    ▶Use additional code if applicable for associated gangrene of gallbladder (K82.A1), or perforation of gallbladder (K82.A2)◀

    CC Excl: For CC codes in subcategory K80.6, unless otherwise noted: PDX collection 815

K80.60   **Calculus of gallbladder and bile duct with cholecystitis, unspecified, without obstruction**   `CC`

K80.61   **Calculus of gallbladder and bile duct with cholecystitis, unspecified, with obstruction**   `CC`

K80.62   **Calculus of gallbladder and bile duct with** acute **cholecystitis without obstruction**   `CC`
    CC Excl: PDX collection 816

K80.63   **Calculus of gallbladder and bile duct with** acute **cholecystitis with obstruction**   `CC`
    CC Excl: PDX collection 816

K80.64   **Calculus of gallbladder and bile duct with** chronic **cholecystitis without obstruction**   `CC`

K80.65   **Calculus of gallbladder and bile duct with** chronic **cholecystitis with obstruction**   `CC`

K80.66   **Calculus of gallbladder and bile duct with** acute and chronic **cholecystitis without obstruction**   `CC`
    CC Excl: PDX collection 817

K80.67   **Calculus of gallbladder and bile duct with** acute and chronic **cholecystitis with obstruction**   `MCC`
    CC Excl: PDX collection 817

✓5ᵗʰ **K80.7   Calculus of** gallbladder and bile duct without cholecystitis

K80.70   **Calculus of gallbladder and bile duct without cholecystitis without obstruction**

K80.71   **Calculus of gallbladder and bile duct without cholecystitis with obstruction**   `CC`
    CC Excl: PDX collection 815

✓5ᵗʰ **K80.8   Other** cholelithiasis

K80.80   **Other cholelithiasis** without obstruction

K80.81   **Other cholelithiasis** with obstruction   `CC`
    CC Excl: PDX collection 815

✓4ᵗʰ **K81   Cholecystitis**
    ▶Use additional code if applicable for associated gangrene of gallbladder (K82.A1), or perforation of gallbladder (K82.A2)◀
    EXCLUDES 1   cholecystitis with cholelithiasis (K80.-)

K81.0   **Acute cholecystitis**   `CC`
    Abscess of gallbladder
    Angiocholecystitis
    Emphysematous (acute) cholecystitis
    Empyema of gallbladder
    Gangrene of gallbladder
    Gangrenous cholecystitis
    Suppurative cholecystitis
    CC Excl: PDX collection 818

K81.1   **Chronic cholecystitis**

K81.2   **Acute cholecystitis** with chronic **cholecystitis**   `CC`
    CC Excl: PDX collection 819

K81.9   **Cholecystitis, unspecified**

✓4ᵗʰ **K82   Other diseases of gallbladder**
    EXCLUDES 1   nonvisualization of gallbladder (R93.2)
              postcholecystectomy syndrome (K91.5)

    CC Excl: For CC/MCC codes in category K82: PDX collection 820

K82.0   **Obstruction of gallbladder**   `CC`
    Occlusion of cystic duct or gallbladder without cholelithiasis
    Stenosis of cystic duct or gallbladder without cholelithiasis
    Stricture of cystic duct or gallbladder without cholelithiasis
    EXCLUDES 1   obstruction of gallbladder with cholelithiasis (K80.-)

K82.1   **Hydrops of gallbladder**   `CC`
    Mucocele of gallbladder

K82.2   **Perforation of gallbladder**   `MCC`
    Rupture of cystic duct or gallbladder
    EXCLUDES 1   ▶perforation of gallbladder in cholecystitis (K82.A2)◀

K82.3   **Fistula of gallbladder**   `CC`
    Cholecystocolic fistula
    Cholecystoduodenal fistula

K82.4   **Cholesterolosis of gallbladder**
    Strawberry gallbladder
    EXCLUDES 1   cholesterolosis of gallbladder with cholecystitis (K81.-)
              cholesterolosis of gallbladder with cholelithiasis (K80.-)

K82.8   **Other specified diseases of gallbladder**
    Adhesions of cystic duct or gallbladder
    Atrophy of cystic duct or gallbladder
    Cyst of cystic duct or gallbladder
    Dyskinesia of cystic duct or gallbladder
    Hypertrophy of cystic duct or gallbladder
    Nonfunctioning of cystic duct or gallbladder
    Ulcer of cystic duct or gallbladder

K82.9   **Disease of gallbladder, unspecified**

● ✓5ᵗʰ **K82.A   Disorders of gallbladder in diseases classified elsewhere**
    Code first the type of cholecystitis (K81.-), or cholelithiasis with cholecystitis (K80.00-K80.19, K80.40-K80.47, K80.60-K80.67)

●   *K82.A1*   *Gangrene of gallbladder in cholecystitis*

●   *K82.A2*   *Perforation of gallbladder in cholecystitis*   `CC`

☑ Additional Character Required   ✓x7ᵗʰ Placeholder   Unacceptable PDx   Questionable PDx   Manifestation   **H1**-**H14** HAC   **HCC** CMS-HCC Dx   **HIV** HIV Dx

ICD-10-CM 2019   711

Chapter 11. Diseases of the Digestive System (side margin)

✓4ᵗʰ **K83 Other diseases of biliary tract**
> EXCLUDES 1   *postcholecystectomy syndrome (K91.5)*
> EXCLUDES 2   *conditions involving the gallbladder (K81-K82)*
> *conditions involving the cystic duct (K81-K82)*

✓5ᵗʰ **K83.0 Cholangitis**

Ascending cholangitis	Sclerosing cholangitis
Cholangitis NOS	Secondary cholangitis
Primary cholangitis	Stenosing cholangitis
Recurrent cholangitis	Suppurative cholangitis

> EXCLUDES 1   *cholangitic liver abscess (K75.0)*
> *cholangitis with choledocholithiasis (K80.3-, K80.4-)*
> *chronic nonsuppurative destructive cholangitis (K74.3)*
> EXCLUDES 2   ▶*chronic nonsuppurative destructive cholangitis (K74.3)*
> *primary biliary cholangitis (K74.3)*
> *primary biliary cirrhosis (K74.3)*◄

●   **K83.01 Primary sclerosing cholangitis**
●   **K83.09 Other cholangitis**
> Ascending cholangitis
> Cholangitis NOS
> Primary cholangitis
> Recurrent cholangitis
> Sclerosing cholangitis
> Secondary cholangitis
> Stenosing cholangitis
> Suppurative cholangitis

K83.1 Obstruction of bile duct   MCC
> Occlusion of bile duct without cholelithiasis
> Stenosis of bile duct without cholelithiasis
> Stricture of bile duct without cholelithiasis
> EXCLUDES 1   *congenital obstruction of bile duct (Q44.3)*
> *obstruction of bile duct with cholelithiasis (K80.-)*
> **AHA:** 2016, 1Q, 18
> **CC Excl:** PDX collection 821

K83.2 Perforation of bile duct   MCC
> Rupture of bile duct
> **CC Excl:** PDX collection 822

K83.3 Fistula of bile duct   CC
> Choledochoduodenal fistula
> **CC Excl:** PDX collection 822

K83.4 Spasm of sphincter of Oddi

K83.5 Biliary cyst

K83.8 Other specified diseases of biliary tract
Adhesions of biliary tract	Hypertrophy of biliary tract
Atrophy of biliary tract	Ulcer of biliary tract

K83.9 Disease of biliary tract, unspecified

✓4ᵗʰ **K85 Acute pancreatitis**
> INCLUDES   acute (recurrent) pancreatitis
> subacute pancreatitis
> **AHA:** 2016, 4Q, 34

CC Excl: For MCC codes in category K85: PDX collection 177

✓5ᵗʰ **K85.0 Idiopathic acute pancreatitis**

    K85.00 Idiopathic acute pancreatitis without necrosis or infection   MCC

    K85.01 Idiopathic acute pancreatitis with uninfected necrosis   MCC

    K85.02 Idiopathic acute pancreatitis with infected necrosis   MCC

✓5ᵗʰ **K85.1 Biliary acute pancreatitis**
> Gallstone pancreatitis

    K85.10 Biliary acute pancreatitis without necrosis or infection   MCC

    K85.11 Biliary acute pancreatitis with uninfected necrosis   MCC

    K85.12 Biliary acute pancreatitis with infected necrosis   MCC

✓5ᵗʰ **K85.2 Alcohol induced acute pancreatitis**
> EXCLUDES 2   *alcohol induced chronic pancreatitis (K86.0)*

    K85.20 Alcohol induced acute pancreatitis without necrosis or infection   MCC

    K85.21 Alcohol induced acute pancreatitis with uninfected necrosis   MCC

    K85.22 Alcohol induced acute pancreatitis with infected necrosis   MCC

✓5ᵗʰ **K85.3 Drug induced acute pancreatitis**
> Use additional code for adverse effect, if applicable, to identify drug (T36-T50 with fifth or sixth character 5)
> Use additional code to identify drug abuse and dependence (F11. – F17.-)

    K85.30 Drug induced acute pancreatitis without necrosis or infection   MCC

    K85.31 Drug induced acute pancreatitis with uninfected necrosis   MCC

    K85.32 Drug induced acute pancreatitis with infected necrosis   MCC

✓5ᵗʰ **K85.8 Other acute pancreatitis**

    K85.80 Other acute pancreatitis without necrosis or infection   MCC

    K85.81 Other acute pancreatitis with uninfected necrosis   MCC

    K85.82 Other acute pancreatitis with infected necrosis   MCC

✓5ᵗʰ **K85.9 Acute pancreatitis, unspecified**
> Pancreatitis NOS

    K85.90 Acute pancreatitis without necrosis or infection, unspecified   MCC

    K85.91 Acute pancreatitis with uninfected necrosis, unspecified   MCC

    K85.92 Acute pancreatitis with infected necrosis, unspecified   MCC

✓4ᵗʰ **K86 Other diseases of pancreas**
> EXCLUDES 2   *fibrocystic disease of pancreas (E84.-)*
> *islet cell tumor (of pancreas) (D13.7)*
> *pancreatic steatorrhea (K90.3)*

K86.0 Alcohol-induced chronic pancreatitis   CC HCC
> Code also exocrine pancreatic insufficiency (K86.81)
> Use additional code to identify:
> alcohol abuse and dependence (F10.-)
> EXCLUDES 2   *alcohol induced acute pancreatitis (K85.2-)*
> **CC Excl:** PDX collection 823

K86.1 Other chronic pancreatitis   CC HCC
> Chronic pancreatitis NOS
> Infectious chronic pancreatitis
> Recurrent chronic pancreatitis
> Relapsing chronic pancreatitis
> Code also exocrine pancreatic insufficiency (K86.81)
> **CC Excl:** PDX collection 823

K86.2 Cyst of pancreas   CC
> **CC Excl:** PDX collection 824

K86.3 Pseudocyst of pancreas   CC
> **CC Excl:** PDX collection 824

✓5ᵗʰ **K86.8 Other specified diseases of pancreas**
> **AHA:** 2016, 4Q, 34-35

    K86.81 Exocrine pancreatic insufficiency

    K86.89 Other specified diseases of pancreas
> Aseptic pancreatic necrosis, unrelated to acute pancreatitis
> Atrophy of pancreas
> Calculus of pancreas
> Cirrhosis of pancreas
> Fibrosis of pancreas
> Pancreatic fat necrosis, unrelated to acute pancreatitis
> Pancreatic infantilism
> Pancreatic necrosis NOS, unrelated to acute pancreatitis

K86.9 Disease of pancreas, unspecified

K87 Disorders of gallbladder, biliary tract and pancreas in diseases classified elsewhere
> Code first underlying disease
> EXCLUDES 1   *cytomegaloviral pancreatitis (B25.2)*
> *mumps pancreatitis (B26.3)*
> *syphilitic gallbladder (A52.74)*
> *syphilitic pancreas (A52.74)*
> *tuberculosis of gallbladder (A18.83)*
> *tuberculosis of pancreas (A18.83)*

N Newborn: 0   P Pediatric: 0-17   M Maternity: 12-55   A Adult: 15-124   MCC Major Complication/Comorbidity   CC Complication/Comorbidity   SW Severe Wound Dx

Other diseases of the digestive system (K90-K95)

✓4th K90 Intestinal malabsorption
EXCLUDES 1   intestinal malabsorption following gastrointestinal surgery (K91.2)

AHA: 2017, 4Q, 108

CC Excl: For CC codes in category K90, unless otherwise noted: PDX collection 825

K90.0 Celiac disease
Celiac disease with steatorrhea
Celiac gluten-sensitive enteropathy
Nontropical sprue
Use additional code for associated disorders including:
dermatitis herpetiformis (L13.0)
gluten ataxia (G32.81)
Code also exocrine pancreatic insufficiency (K86.81)
DEF: Malabsorption syndrome due to gluten consumption. Symptoms include fetid, bulky, frothy, oily stools; a distended abdomen; gas; asthenia; electrolyte depletion; and vitamin B, D, and K deficiency.

K90.1 Tropical sprue [CC]
Sprue NOS
Tropical steatorrhea

K90.2 Blind loop syndrome, not elsewhere classified [CC]
Blind loop syndrome NOS
EXCLUDES 1   congenital blind loop syndrome (Q43.8)
postsurgical blind loop syndrome (K91.2)

K90.3 Pancreatic steatorrhea [CC]

✓5th K90.4 Other malabsorption due to intolerance
EXCLUDES 2   celiac gluten-sensitive enteropathy (K90.0)
lactose intolerance (E73.-)
AHA: 2016, 4Q, 35-36

K90.41 Non-celiac gluten sensitivity [CC]
Gluten sensitivity NOS
Non-celiac gluten sensitive enteropathy

K90.49 Malabsorption due to intolerance, not elsewhere classified [CC]
Malabsorption due to intolerance to carbohydrate
Malabsorption due to intolerance to fat
Malabsorption due to intolerance to protein
Malabsorption due to intolerance to starch

✓5th K90.8 Other intestinal malabsorption

K90.81 Whipple's disease [CC]
CC Excl: PDX collection 826

K90.89 Other intestinal malabsorption [CC]

K90.9 Intestinal malabsorption, unspecified [CC]

✓4th K91 Intraoperative and postprocedural complications and disorders of digestive system, not elsewhere classified
EXCLUDES 2   complications of artificial opening of digestive system (K94.-)
complications of bariatric procedures (K95.-)
gastrojejunal ulcer (K28.-)
postprocedural (radiation) retroperitoneal abscess (K68.11)
radiation colitis (K52.0)
radiation gastroenteritis (K52.0)
radiation proctitis (K62.7)

AHA: 2016, 4Q, 9-10

K91.0 Vomiting following gastrointestinal surgery

K91.1 Postgastric surgery syndromes
Dumping syndrome
Postgastrectomy syndrome
Postvagotomy syndrome

K91.2 Postsurgical malabsorption, not elsewhere classified [CC]
Postsurgical blind loop syndrome
EXCLUDES 1   malabsorption osteomalacia in adults (M83.2)
malabsorption osteoporosis, postsurgical (M80.8-, M81.8)
CC Excl: PDX collection 827

✓5th K91.3 Postprocedural intestinal obstruction
AHA: 2017, 4Q, 16-17; 2017, 1Q, 40

CC Excl: For CC codes in subcategory K91.3: PDX collection 792

K91.30 Postprocedural intestinal obstruction, unspecified as to partial versus complete [CC]
Postprocedural intestinal obstruction NOS

K91.31 Postprocedural partial intestinal obstruction [CC]
Postprocedural incomplete intestinal obstruction

K91.32 Postprocedural complete intestinal obstruction [CC]

K91.5 Postcholecystectomy syndrome

✓5th K91.6 Intraoperative hemorrhage and hematoma of a digestive system organ or structure complicating a procedure
EXCLUDES 1   intraoperative hemorrhage and hematoma of a digestive system organ or structure due to accidental puncture and laceration during a procedure (K91.7-)

K91.61 Intraoperative hemorrhage and hematoma of a digestive system organ or structure complicating a digestive system procedure [CC]
CC Excl: PDX collection 829

K91.62 Intraoperative hemorrhage and hematoma of a digestive system organ or structure complicating other procedure [CC]
CC Excl: PDX collection 829

✓5th K91.7 Accidental puncture and laceration of a digestive system organ or structure during a procedure
K91.71 Accidental puncture and laceration of a digestive system organ or structure during a digestive system procedure [CC]
CC Excl: PDX collection 509

K91.72 Accidental puncture and laceration of a digestive system organ or structure during other procedure [CC]
CC Excl: PDX collection 509

✓5th K91.8 Other intraoperative and postprocedural complications and disorders of digestive system

CC Excl: For CC codes in subcategory K91.8, unless otherwise noted: PDX collection 828

K91.81 Other intraoperative complications of digestive system [CC]

K91.82 Postprocedural hepatic failure [CC]

K91.83 Postprocedural hepatorenal syndrome [CC]

✓6th K91.84 Postprocedural hemorrhage of a digestive system organ or structure following a procedure
K91.840 Postprocedural hemorrhage of a digestive system organ or structure following a digestive system procedure [CC]
AHA: 2016, 1Q, 15
CC Excl: PDX collection 829

K91.841 Postprocedural hemorrhage of a digestive system organ or structure following other procedure [CC]
CC Excl: PDX collection 829

✓6th K91.85 Complications of intestinal pouch
K91.850 Pouchitis [CC HCC]
Inflammation of internal ileoanal pouch
DEF: Inflammatory complication of an existing surgically created ileoanal pouch, resulting in multiple GI complaints, including diarrhea, abdominal pain, rectal bleeding, fecal urgency, or incontinence.

K91.858 Other complications of intestinal pouch [CC HCC]

K91.86 Retained cholelithiasis following cholecystectomy [CC]

✓6th K91.87 Postprocedural hematoma and seroma of a digestive system organ or structure following a procedure

CC Excl: For CC codes in subcategory K91.87: PDX collection 829

K91.870 Postprocedural hematoma of a digestive system organ or structure following a digestive system procedure [CC]

K91.871 Postprocedural hematoma of a digestive system organ or structure following other procedure [CC]

K91.872 Postprocedural seroma of a digestive system organ or structure following a digestive system procedure [CC]

K91.873 Postprocedural seroma of a digestive system organ or structure following other procedure [CC]

K91.89 Other postprocedural complications and disorders of digestive system [CC]
Use additional code, if applicable, to further specify disorder
EXCLUDES 2   postprocedural retroperitoneal abscess (K68.11)
AHA: 2017, 1Q, 40

Chapter 11. Diseases of the Digestive System

✓4ᵗʰ K92   Other diseases of digestive system

> **EXCLUDES 1**   *neonatal gastrointestinal hemorrhage (P54.0-P54.3)*

> **CC Excl: For CC codes in category K92, unless otherwise noted:**
> PDX collection 770

K92.0   Hematemesis   `CC`

K92.1   Melena   `CC`
> **EXCLUDES 1**   *occult blood in feces (R19.5)*

K92.2   Gastrointestinal hemorrhage, unspecified   `CC`
Gastric hemorrhage NOS
Intestinal hemorrhage NOS
> **EXCLUDES 1**   *acute hemorrhagic gastritis (K29.01)*
> *hemorrhage of anus and rectum (K62.5)*
> *angiodysplasia of stomach with hemorrhage (K31.811)*
> *diverticular disease with hemorrhage (K57.-)*
> *gastritis and duodenitis with hemorrhage (K29.-)*
> *peptic ulcer with hemorrhage (K25-K28)*

✓5ᵗʰ K92.8   Other specified diseases of the digestive system

K92.81   Gastrointestinal mucositis (ulcerative)   `CC`
Code also type of associated therapy, such as:
   antineoplastic and immunosuppressive drugs
   (T45.1X-)
   radiological procedure and radiotherapy (Y84.2)
> **EXCLUDES 2**   *mucositis (ulcerative) of vagina and vulva*
> *(N76.81)*
> *nasal mucositis (ulcerative) (J34.81)*
> *oral mucositis (ulcerative) (K12.3-)*
> **CC Excl:** PDX collection 765

K92.89   Other specified diseases of the digestive system

K92.9   Disease of digestive system, unspecified

✓4ᵗʰ K94   Complications of artificial openings of the digestive system

> **CC Excl: For CC codes in category K94, unless otherwise noted:**
> PDX collection 830

✓5ᵗʰ K94.0   Colostomy complications

K94.00   Colostomy complication, unspecified   `HCC`

K94.01   Colostomy hemorrhage   `CC` `HCC`

K94.02   Colostomy infection   `CC` `HCC`
Use additional code to specify type of infection, such
   as:
     cellulitis of abdominal wall (L03.311)
     sepsis (A40-, A41-)

K94.03   Colostomy malfunction   `CC` `HCC`
Mechanical complication of colostomy
> **CC Excl:** PDX collection 831

K94.09   Other complications of colostomy   `CC` `HCC`

✓5ᵗʰ K94.1   Enterostomy complications

K94.10   Enterostomy complication, unspecified   `HCC`

K94.11   Enterostomy hemorrhage   `CC` `HCC`

K94.12   Enterostomy infection   `CC` `HCC`
Use additional code to specify type of infection, such
   as:
     cellulitis of abdominal wall (L03.311)
     sepsis (A40-, A41-)

K94.13   Enterostomy malfunction   `CC` `HCC`
Mechanical complication of enterostomy
> **CC Excl:** PDX collection 831

K94.19   Other complications of enterostomy   `CC` `HCC`

✓5ᵗʰ K94.2   Gastrostomy complications

K94.20   Gastrostomy complication, unspecified   `HCC`

K94.21   Gastrostomy hemorrhage   `HCC`

K94.22   Gastrostomy infection   `CC` `HCC`
Use additional code to specify type of infection, such
   as:
     cellulitis of abdominal wall (L03.311)
     sepsis (A40, A41)
> **CC Excl:** PDX collection 828

K94.23   Gastrostomy malfunction   `CC` `HCC`
Mechanical complication of gastrostomy
> **CC Excl:** PDX collection 828

K94.29   Other complications of gastrostomy   `HCC`

✓5ᵗʰ K94.3   Esophagostomy complications

> **CC Excl: For CC codes in subcategory K94.3:**
> PDX collection 828

K94.30   Esophagostomy complications, unspecified   `CC` `HCC`

K94.31   Esophagostomy hemorrhage   `CC` `HCC`

K94.32   Esophagostomy infection   `CC` `HCC`
Use additional code to identify the infection

K94.33   Esophagostomy malfunction   `CC` `HCC`
Mechanical complication of esophagostomy

K94.39   Other complications of esophagostomy   `CC` `HCC`

✓4ᵗʰ K95   Complications of bariatric procedures

> **CC Excl: For CC codes in category K95:** PDX collection 828

✓5ᵗʰ K95.0   Complications of gastric band procedure

K95.01   Infection due to gastric band procedure   `CC` `H11`
Use additional code to specify type of infection or
   organism, such as:
     bacterial and viral infectious agents (B95.-, B96.-)
     cellulitis of abdominal wall (L03.311)
     sepsis (A40.-, A41.-)

K95.09   Other complications of gastric band procedure   `CC`
Use additional code, if applicable, to further specify
   complication

✓5ᵗʰ K95.8   Complications of other bariatric procedure
> **EXCLUDES 1**   *complications of gastric band surgery (K95.0-)*

K95.81   Infection due to other bariatric procedure   `CC` `H11`
Use additional code to specify type of infection or
   organism, such as:
     bacterial and viral infectious agents (B95.-, B96.-)
     cellulitis of abdominal wall (L03.311)
     sepsis (A40.-, A41.-)

K95.89   Other complications of other bariatric procedure   `CC`
Use additional code, if applicable, to further specify
   complication

N Newborn: 0   **P** Pediatric: 0-17   **M** Maternity: 12-55   **A** Adult: 15-124   **MCC** Major Complication/Comorbidity   **CC** Complication/Comorbidity   **SW** Severe Wound Dx

714   ICD-10-CM 2019

Chapter 12. Diseases of the Skin and Subcutaneous Tissue (LØØ–L99)

Chapter Specific Guidelines with Coding Examples

The chapter specific guidelines from the ICD-10-CM Official Guidelines for Coding and Reporting have been provided below. Along with these guidelines are coding examples, contained in the shaded boxes, that have been developed to help illustrate the coding and/or sequencing guidance found in these guidelines.

a. Pressure ulcer stage codes

1) Pressure ulcer stages

Codes from category L89, Pressure ulcer, identify the site of the pressure ulcer as well as the stage of the ulcer.

The ICD-10-CM classifies pressure ulcer stages based on severity, which is designated by stages 1-4, unspecified stage and unstageable.

Assign as many codes from category L89 as needed to identify all the pressure ulcers the patient has, if applicable.

See Section I.B.14 for pressure ulcer stage documentation by clinicians other than patient's provider

> Stage 4 pressure ulcer right heel, 9 x 1Ø cm that invades the muscle and fascia; stage 2 pressure ulcer of left elbow
>
> **L89.614   Pressure ulcer of right heel, stage 4**
>
> **L89.Ø22   Pressure ulcer of left elbow, stage 2**
>
> *Explanation:* Patient has a right heel pressure ulcer documented as stage 4 and a left elbow pressure ulcer documented as stage 2. Combination codes from category L89 Pressure ulcer, identify the site of the pressure ulcer as well as the stage. Assign as many codes from category L89 as needed to identify all the pressure ulcers the patient has.

2) Unstageable pressure ulcers

Assignment of the code for unstageable pressure ulcer (L89.--Ø) should be based on the clinical documentation. These codes are used for pressure ulcers whose stage cannot be clinically determined (e.g., the ulcer is covered by eschar or has been treated with a skin or muscle graft) and pressure ulcers that are documented as deep tissue injury but not documented as due to trauma. This code should not be confused with the codes for unspecified stage (L89.--9). When there is no documentation regarding the stage of the pressure ulcer, assign the appropriate code for unspecified stage (L89.--9).

> Pressure ulcer of the right lower back documented as unstageable due to the presence of thick eschar covering the ulcer
>
> **L89.13Ø   Pressure ulcer of right lower back, unstageable**
>
> *Explanation:* Codes for unstageable pressure ulcers are assigned when the stage cannot be clinically determined (e.g., the ulcer is covered by eschar or has been treated with a skin or muscle graft).

3) Documented pressure ulcer stage

Assignment of the pressure ulcer stage code should be guided by clinical documentation of the stage or documentation of the terms found in the Alphabetic Index. For clinical terms describing the stage that are not found in the Alphabetic Index, and there is no documentation of the stage, the provider should be queried.

> Left heel pressure ulcer with partial thickness skin loss involving the dermis
>
> **L89.622   Pressure ulcer of left heel, stage 2**
>
> *Explanation:* Code assignment for the pressure ulcer stage should be guided by either the clinical documentation of the stage or the documentation of terms found in the Alphabetic Index. The clinical documentation describing the left heel pressure ulcer "partial thickness skin loss involving the dermis" matches the ICD-10-CM index parenthetical description for stage 2 "(abrasion, blister, partial thickness skin loss involving epidermis and/or dermis)."

4) Patients admitted with pressure ulcers documented as healed

No code is assigned if the documentation states that the pressure ulcer is completely healed.

5) Patients admitted with pressure ulcers documented as healing

Pressure ulcers described as healing should be assigned the appropriate pressure ulcer stage code based on the documentation in the medical record. If the documentation does not provide information about the stage of the healing pressure ulcer, assign the appropriate code for unspecified stage.

If the documentation is unclear as to whether the patient has a current (new) pressure ulcer or if the patient is being treated for a healing pressure ulcer, query the provider.

For ulcers that were present on admission but healed at the time of discharge, assign the code for the site and stage of the pressure ulcer at the time of admission.

> H & P noted healing stage 2 sacral pressure ulcer. Resolved at time of discharge summary.
>
> **L89.152   Pressure ulcer of sacral region, stage 2**
>
> *Explanation:* Although completely healed upon discharge, the pressure ulcer required observation and/or treatment and should be coded based on the site and stage upon admission.

6) Patient admitted with pressure ulcer evolving into another stage during the admission

If a patient is admitted to an inpatient hospital with a pressure ulcer at one stage and it progresses to a higher stage, two separate codes should be assigned: one code for the site and stage of the ulcer on admission and a second code for the same ulcer site and the highest stage reported during the stay.

> Stage 3 right hip pressure ulcer worsened during admission to a stage 4
>
> **L89.213   Pressure ulcer of right hip, stage 3**
>
> **L89.214   Pressure ulcer of right hip, stage 4**
>
> *Explanation:* A pressure ulcer that progresses from a lower stage to a higher stage is assigned two codes, one for the documented stage upon admission and one for the documented stage at discharge.

b. Non-pressure chronic ulcers

1) Patients admitted with non-pressure ulcers documented as healed

No code is assigned if the documentation states that the non-pressure ulcer is completely healed.

2) Patients admitted with non-pressure ulcers documented as healing

Non-pressure ulcers described as healing should be assigned the appropriate non-pressure ulcer code based on the documentation in the medical record. If the documentation does not provide information about the severity of the healing non-pressure ulcer, assign the appropriate code for unspecified severity.

If the documentation is unclear as to whether the patient has a current (new) non-pressure ulcer or if the patient is being treated for a healing non-pressure ulcer, query the provider.

For ulcers that were present on admission but healed at the time of discharge, assign the code for the site and severity of the non-pressure ulcer at the time of admission.

> Admission diagnosis: Chronic ulcer, fat layer exposed, on left ankle
>
> Discharge diagnosis: Resolution of ulcer on the left ankle
>
> **L97.322   Non-pressure chronic ulcer of left ankle with fat layer exposed**
>
> *Explanation:* Although the ulcer was documented as resolved (healed) at discharge, a code representing the site and severity of the ulcer upon admission should be appended.

3) Patient admitted with non-pressure ulcer that progresses to another severity level during the admission

If a patient is admitted to an inpatient hospital with a non-pressure ulcer at one severity level and it progresses to a higher severity level, two separate codes should be assigned: one code for the site and severity level of the ulcer on admission and a second code for the same ulcer site and the highest severity level reported during the stay.

See Section I.B.14 for pressure ulcer stage documentation by clinicians other than patient's provider

Chapter 12. Diseases of the Skin and Subcutaneous Tissue (L00-L99)

EXCLUDES 2   *certain conditions originating in the perinatal period (P04-P96)*
certain infectious and parasitic diseases (A00-B99)
complications of pregnancy, childbirth and the puerperium (O00-O9A)
congenital malformations, deformations, and chromosomal abnormalities (Q00-Q99)
endocrine, nutritional and metabolic diseases (E00-E88)
lipomelanotic reticulosis (I89.8)
neoplasms (C00-D49)
symptoms, signs and abnormal clinical and laboratory findings, not elsewhere classified (R00-R94)
systemic connective tissue disorders (M30-M36)
viral warts (B07.-)

This chapter contains the following blocks:

L00-L08	Infections of the skin and subcutaneous tissue
L10-L14	Bullous disorders
L20-L30	Dermatitis and eczema
L40-L45	Papulosquamous disorders
L49-L54	Urticaria and erythema
L55-L59	Radiation-related disorders of the skin and subcutaneous tissue
L60-L75	Disorders of skin appendages
L76	Intraoperative and postprocedural complications of skin and subcutaneous tissue
L80-L99	Other disorders of the skin and subcutaneous tissue

Infections of the skin and subcutaneous tissue (L00-L08)

Use additional code (B95-B97) to identify infectious agent

EXCLUDES 2   *hordeolum (H00.0)*
infective dermatitis (L30.3)
local infections of skin classified in Chapter 1
lupus panniculitis (L93.2)
panniculitis NOS (M79.3)
panniculitis of neck and back (M54.0-)
Perlèche NOS (K13.0)
Perlèche due to candidiasis (B37.0)
Perlèche due to riboflavin deficiency (E53.0)
pyogenic granuloma (L98.0)
relapsing panniculitis [Weber-Christian] (M35.6)
viral warts (B07.-)
zoster (B02.-)

L00 **Staphylococcal scalded skin syndrome**
Ritter's disease
Use additional code to identify percentage of skin exfoliation (L49.-)
EXCLUDES 1   *bullous impetigo (L01.03)*
pemphigus neonatorum (L01.03)
toxic epidermal necrolysis [Lyell] (L51.2)
DEF: Infectious skin disease of children younger than 5 years marked by eruptions ranging from a few localized blisters to widespread, easily ruptured, fine vesicles and bullae affecting almost the entire body. It results in exfoliation of large planes of skin and leaves raw areas.

✓4th **L01** **Impetigo**
EXCLUDES 1   *impetigo herpetiformis (L40.1)*
DEF: Acute, superficial, highly contagious skin infection commonly occurring in children. Skin lesions usually appear on the face and consist of vesicles and bullae that burst and form yellow crusts.

✓5th **L01.0** **Impetigo**
Impetigo contagiosa
Impetigo vulgaris

    L01.00 **Impetigo, unspecified**
Impetigo NOS

    L01.01 **Non-bullous impetigo**

    L01.02 **Bockhart's impetigo**
Impetigo follicularis
Perifolliculitis NOS
Superficial pustular perifolliculitis
DEF: Superficial inflammation of the hair follicles most commonly caused by staph aureus that manifests as rounded, sphere-shaped, pustular eruptions in the areas of the scalp, beard, underarms, extremities, and buttocks.

    L01.03 **Bullous impetigo**
Impetigo neonatorum
Pemphigus neonatorum

    L01.09 **Other impetigo**
Ulcerative impetigo

  L01.1 **Impetiginization of other dermatoses**

✓4th **L02** **Cutaneous abscess, furuncle and carbuncle**
Use additional code to identify organism (B95-B96)
EXCLUDES 2   *abscess of anus and rectal regions (K61.-)*
abscess of female genital organs (external) (N76.4)
abscess of male genital organs (external) (N48.2, N49-)
DEF: Carbuncle: Infection of the skin that arises from a collection of interconnected infected boils or furuncles, usually from hair follicles infected by *Staphylococcus*. This condition can produce pus and form drainage cavities.
DEF: Furuncle: Inflamed, painful abscess, cyst, or nodule on the skin caused by bacteria, often *Staphylococcus,* entering along the hair follicle.

✓5th **L02.0** **Cutaneous abscess, furuncle and carbuncle of face**
EXCLUDES 2   *abscess of ear, external (H60.0)*
abscess of eyelid (H00.0)
abscess of head [any part, except face] (L02.8)
abscess of lacrimal gland (H04.0)
abscess of lacrimal passages (H04.3)
abscess of mouth (K12.2)
abscess of nose (J34.0)
abscess of orbit (H05.0)
submandibular abscess (K12.2)

  L02.01 **Cutaneous abscess of face**   `CC`
CC Excl: No Excl

  L02.02 **Furuncle of face**
Boil of face
Folliculitis of face

  L02.03 **Carbuncle of face**

✓5th **L02.1** **Cutaneous abscess, furuncle and carbuncle of neck**

  L02.11 **Cutaneous abscess of neck**   `CC`
CC Excl: PDX collection 832

  L02.12 **Furuncle of neck**
Boil of neck
Folliculitis of neck

  L02.13 **Carbuncle of neck**

✓5th **L02.2** **Cutaneous abscess, furuncle and carbuncle of trunk**
EXCLUDES 1   *non-newborn omphalitis (L08.82)*
omphalitis of newborn (P38.-)
EXCLUDES 2   *abscess of breast (N61.1)*
abscess of buttocks (L02.3)
abscess of female external genital organs (N76.4)
abscess of hip (L02.4)
abscess of male external genital organs (N48.2, N49-)

CC Excl: For CC codes in subcategory L02.2:
PDX collection 833

✓6th **L02.21** **Cutaneous abscess of trunk**

    L02.211 **Cutaneous abscess of abdominal wall** `CC`
    L02.212 **Cutaneous abscess of back** [any part, except buttock] `CC`
    L02.213 **Cutaneous abscess of chest wall** `CC`
    L02.214 **Cutaneous abscess of groin** `CC`
    L02.215 **Cutaneous abscess of perineum** `CC`
    L02.216 **Cutaneous abscess of umbilicus** `CC`
    L02.219 **Cutaneous abscess of trunk, unspecified** `CC`

✓6th **L02.22** **Furuncle of trunk**
Boil of trunk   Folliculitis of trunk

    L02.221 **Furuncle of abdominal wall**
    L02.222 **Furuncle of back** [any part, except buttock]
    L02.223 **Furuncle of chest wall**
    L02.224 **Furuncle of groin**
    L02.225 **Furuncle of perineum**
    L02.226 **Furuncle of umbilicus**
    L02.229 **Furuncle of trunk, unspecified**

✓6th **L02.23** **Carbuncle of trunk**

    L02.231 **Carbuncle of abdominal wall**
    L02.232 **Carbuncle of back** [any part, except buttock]
    L02.233 **Carbuncle of chest wall**
    L02.234 **Carbuncle of groin**
    L02.235 **Carbuncle of perineum**
    L02.236 **Carbuncle of umbilicus**
    L02.239 **Carbuncle of trunk, unspecified**

√5ᵗʰ **L02.3** **Cutaneous abscess, furuncle and carbuncle of** buttock

     EXCLUDES 1   *pilonidal cyst with abscess (L05.01)*

     L02.31   **Cutaneous abscess of buttock**   CC

         Cutaneous abscess of gluteal region

         CC Excl: PDX collection 834

     L02.32   **Furuncle of buttock**

         Boil of buttock

         Folliculitis of buttock

         Furuncle of gluteal region

     L02.33   **Carbuncle of buttock**

         Carbuncle of gluteal region

√5ᵗʰ **L02.4** **Cutaneous abscess, furuncle and carbuncle of** limb

     EXCLUDES 2   *cutaneous abscess, furuncle and carbuncle of groin (L02.214, L02.224, L02.234)*

               cutaneous abscess, furuncle and carbuncle of hand (L02.5-)

               cutaneous abscess, furuncle and carbuncle of foot (L02.6-)

     CC Excl: For CC codes in subcategory L02.4, unless otherwise noted: PDX collection 835

     √6ᵗʰ **L02.41**   **Cutaneous abscess of** limb

         L02.411   **Cutaneous abscess of** right axilla   CC

         L02.412   **Cutaneous abscess of** left axilla   CC

         L02.413   **Cutaneous abscess of** right upper **limb**   CC

         L02.414   **Cutaneous abscess of** left upper **limb**   CC

         L02.415   **Cutaneous abscess of** right lower **limb**   CC

               CC Excl: PDX collection 836

         L02.416   **Cutaneous abscess of** left lower **limb**   CC

               CC Excl: PDX collection 836

         L02.419   **Cutaneous abscess of limb,** unspecified   CC

               CC Excl: PDX collection 836

     √6ᵗʰ **L02.42**   **Furuncle of limb**

         Boil of limb

         Folliculitis of limb

         L02.421   **Furuncle of** right axilla

         L02.422   **Furuncle of** left axilla

         L02.423   **Furuncle of** right upper **limb**

         L02.424   **Furuncle of** left upper **limb**

         L02.425   **Furuncle of** right lower **limb**

         L02.426   **Furuncle of** left lower **limb**

         L02.429   **Furuncle of limb,** unspecified

     √6ᵗʰ **L02.43**   **Carbuncle of limb**

         L02.431   **Carbuncle of** right axilla

         L02.432   **Carbuncle of** left axilla

         L02.433   **Carbuncle of** right upper **limb**

         L02.434   **Carbuncle of** left upper **limb**

         L02.435   **Carbuncle of** right lower **limb**

         L02.436   **Carbuncle of** left lower **limb**

         L02.439   **Carbuncle of limb,** unspecified

√5ᵗʰ **L02.5** **Cutaneous abscess, furuncle and carbuncle of** hand

     CC Excl: For CC codes in subcategory L02.5: PDX collection 837

     √6ᵗʰ **L02.51**   **Cutaneous abscess of hand**

         L02.511   **Cutaneous abscess of** right hand   CC

         L02.512   **Cutaneous abscess of** left hand   CC

         L02.519   **Cutaneous abscess of** unspecified **hand**   CC

     √6ᵗʰ **L02.52**   **Furuncle hand**

         Boil of hand

         Folliculitis of hand

         L02.521   **Furuncle** right **hand**

         L02.522   **Furuncle** left **hand**

         L02.529   **Furuncle** unspecified **hand**

     √6ᵗʰ **L02.53**   **Carbuncle of hand**

         L02.531   **Carbuncle of** right **hand**

         L02.532   **Carbuncle of** left **hand**

         L02.539   **Carbuncle of** unspecified **hand**

√5ᵗʰ **L02.6** **Cutaneous abscess, furuncle and carbuncle of** foot

     CC Excl: For CC codes in subcategory L02.6: PDX collection 838

     √6ᵗʰ **L02.61**   **Cutaneous abscess of foot**

         L02.611   **Cutaneous abscess of** right **foot**   CC

         L02.612   **Cutaneous abscess of** left **foot**   CC

         L02.619   **Cutaneous abscess of** unspecified **foot**   CC

     √6ᵗʰ **L02.62**   **Furuncle of foot**

         Boil of foot   Folliculitis of foot

         L02.621   **Furuncle of** right **foot**

         L02.622   **Furuncle of** left **foot**

         L02.629   **Furuncle of** unspecified **foot**

     √6ᵗʰ **L02.63**   **Carbuncle of foot**

         L02.631   **Carbuncle of** right **foot**

         L02.632   **Carbuncle of** left **foot**

         L02.639   **Carbuncle of** unspecified **foot**

√5ᵗʰ **L02.8** **Cutaneous abscess, furuncle and carbuncle of** other sites

     √6ᵗʰ **L02.81**   **Cutaneous abscess of** other sites

         L02.811   **Cutaneous abscess of** head **[any part, except face]**   CC

               CC Excl: PDX collection 839

         L02.818   **Cutaneous abscess of** other sites   CC

               CC Excl: PDX collection 839

     √6ᵗʰ **L02.82**   **Furuncle of** other sites

         Boil of other sites   Folliculitis of other sites

         L02.821   **Furuncle of** head **[any part, except face]**

         L02.828   **Furuncle of** other sites

     √6ᵗʰ **L02.83**   **Carbuncle of** other sites

         L02.831   **Carbuncle of** head **[any part, except face]**

         L02.838   **Carbuncle of** other sites

√5ᵗʰ **L02.9** **Cutaneous abscess, furuncle and carbuncle,** unspecified

     L02.91   **Cutaneous abscess,** unspecified   CC

         CC Excl: PDX collection 839

     L02.92   **Furuncle,** unspecified

         Boil NOS   Furunculosis NOS

     L02.93   **Carbuncle,** unspecified

√4ᵗʰ **L03** **Cellulitis and acute lymphangitis**

     EXCLUDES 2   *cellulitis of anal and rectal region (K61.-)*

               cellulitis of external auditory canal (H60.1)

               cellulitis of eyelid (H00.03-)

               cellulitis of female external genital organs (N76.4)

               cellulitis of lacrimal apparatus (H04.3)

               cellulitis of male external genital organs (N48.2, N49-)

               cellulitis of mouth (K12.2)

               cellulitis of nose (J34.0)

               eosinophilic cellulitis [Wells] (L98.3)

               febrile neutrophilic dermatosis [Sweet] (L98.2)

               lymphangitis (chronic) (subacute) (I89.1)

     AHA: 2017, 4Q, 100

     DEF: Cellulitis: Infection of the skin and subcutaneous tissues, most often caused by *Staphylococcus* or *Streptococcus* bacteria secondary to a cutaneous lesion. Progression of the inflammation may lead to abscess and tissue death, or even systemic infection-like bacteremia.

     DEF: Lymphangitis: Inflammation of the lymph channels most often caused by *Streptococcus*.

√5ᵗʰ **L03.0** **Cellulitis and acute lymphangitis of** finger and toe

     Infection of nail

     Onychia

     Paronychia

     Perionychia

     √6ᵗʰ **L03.01**   **Cellulitis of** finger

         Felon

         Whitlow

         EXCLUDES 1   *herpetic whitlow (B00.89)*

         DEF: Felon: Superficial bacterial skin infection at the tip of the finger.

         L03.011   **Cellulitis of** right **finger**

         L03.012   **Cellulitis of** left **finger**

         L03.019   **Cellulitis of** unspecified **finger**

     √6ᵗʰ **L03.02**   **Acute lymphangitis of** finger

         Hangnail with lymphangitis of finger

         L03.021   **Acute lymphangitis of** right **finger**

         L03.022   **Acute lymphangitis of** left **finger**

         L03.029   **Acute lymphangitis of** unspecified **finger**

     √6ᵗʰ **L03.03**   **Cellulitis of** toe

         L03.031   **Cellulitis of** right **toe**

         L03.032   **Cellulitis of** left **toe**

         L03.039   **Cellulitis of** unspecified **toe**

✓ Additional Character Required   √7ᵗʰ Placeholder   Unacceptable PDx   Questionable PDx   Manifestation   H1 - H14 HAC   HCC CMS-HCC Dx   HIV HIV Dx

ICD-10-CM 2019   **717**

L02.3–L03.039

Chapter 12. Diseases of the Skin and Subcutaneous Tissue

✓6th L03.04 Acute lymphangitis of toe
Hangnail with lymphangitis of toe
   L03.041 Acute lymphangitis of right toe
   L03.042 Acute lymphangitis of left toe
   L03.049 Acute lymphangitis of unspecified toe

✓5th L03.1 Cellulitis and acute lymphangitis of other parts of limb

> CC Excl: For CC codes in subcategory L03.1, unless otherwise noted: PDX collection 835

✓6th L03.11 Cellulitis of other parts of limb
   EXCLUDES 2 cellulitis of fingers (L03.01-)
   cellulitis of toes (L03.03-)
   groin (L03.314)
   L03.111 Cellulitis of right axilla CC
   L03.112 Cellulitis of left axilla CC
   L03.113 Cellulitis of right upper limb CC
   L03.114 Cellulitis of left upper limb CC
   L03.115 Cellulitis of right lower limb CC
      CC Excl: PDX collection 836
   L03.116 Cellulitis of left lower limb CC
      CC Excl: PDX collection 836
   L03.119 Cellulitis of unspecified part of limb CC
      CC Excl: PDX collection 836

✓6th L03.12 Acute lymphangitis of other parts of limb
   EXCLUDES 2 acute lymphangitis of fingers (L03.02-)
   acute lymphangitis of groin (L03.324)
   acute lymphangitis of toes (L03.04-)
   L03.121 Acute lymphangitis of right axilla CC
   L03.122 Acute lymphangitis of left axilla CC
   L03.123 Acute lymphangitis of right upper limb CC
   L03.124 Acute lymphangitis of left upper limb CC
   L03.125 Acute lymphangitis of right lower limb CC
      CC Excl: PDX collection 836
   L03.126 Acute lymphangitis of left lower limb CC
      CC Excl: PDX collection 836
   L03.129 Acute lymphangitis of unspecified part of limb CC
      CC Excl: PDX collection 836

✓5th L03.2 Cellulitis and acute lymphangitis of face and neck

✓6th L03.21 Cellulitis and acute lymphangitis of face
   L03.211 Cellulitis of face CC
      EXCLUDES 2 abscess of orbit (H05.01-)
      cellulitis of ear (H60.1-)
      cellulitis of eyelid (H00.03-)
      cellulitis of head (L03.811)
      cellulitis of lacrimal apparatus (H04.3)
      cellulitis of lip (K13.0)
      cellulitis of mouth (K12.2)
      cellulitis of nose (internal) (J34.0)
      cellulitis of orbit (H05.01-)
      cellulitis of scalp (L03.811)
      AHA: 2013, 4Q, 123
      CC Excl: PDX collection 840
   L03.212 Acute lymphangitis of face CC
      CC Excl: No Excl
   L03.213 Periorbital cellulitis CC
      Preseptal cellulitis
      AHA: 2016, 4Q, 36
      CC Excl: PDX collection 840

✓6th L03.22 Cellulitis and acute lymphangitis of neck
   L03.221 Cellulitis of neck CC
      CC Excl: PDX collection 832
   L03.222 Acute lymphangitis of neck CC
      CC Excl: PDX collection 832

✓5th L03.3 Cellulitis and acute lymphangitis of trunk

> CC Excl: For CC codes in subcategory L03.3, unless otherwise noted: PDX collection 833

✓6th L03.31 Cellulitis of trunk
   EXCLUDES 2 cellulitis of anal and rectal regions (K61.-)
   cellulitis of breast NOS (N61.0)
   cellulitis of female external genital organs (N76.4)
   cellulitis of male external genital organs (N48.2, N49-)
   omphalitis of newborn (P38.-)
   puerperal cellulitis of breast (O91.2)
   L03.311 Cellulitis of abdominal wall CC
      EXCLUDES 2 cellulitis of umbilicus (L03.316)
      cellulitis of groin (L03.314)
   L03.312 Cellulitis of back [any part except buttock] CC
   L03.313 Cellulitis of chest wall CC
   L03.314 Cellulitis of groin CC
   L03.315 Cellulitis of perineum CC
   L03.316 Cellulitis of umbilicus CC
   L03.317 Cellulitis of buttock CC
      CC Excl: PDX collection 834
   L03.319 Cellulitis of trunk, unspecified CC

✓6th L03.32 Acute lymphangitis of trunk
   L03.321 Acute lymphangitis of abdominal wall CC
   L03.322 Acute lymphangitis of back [any part except buttock] CC
   L03.323 Acute lymphangitis of chest wall CC
   L03.324 Acute lymphangitis of groin CC
   L03.325 Acute lymphangitis of perineum CC
   L03.326 Acute lymphangitis of umbilicus CC
   L03.327 Acute lymphangitis of buttock CC
      CC Excl: PDX collection 834
   L03.329 Acute lymphangitis of trunk, unspecified CC

✓5th L03.8 Cellulitis and acute lymphangitis of other sites

> CC Excl: For CC codes in subcategory L03.8: PDX collection 839

✓6th L03.81 Cellulitis of other sites
   L03.811 Cellulitis of head [any part, except face] CC
      Cellulitis of scalp
      EXCLUDES 2 cellulitis of face (L03.211)
   L03.818 Cellulitis of other sites CC

✓6th L03.89 Acute lymphangitis of other sites
   L03.891 Acute lymphangitis of head [any part, except face] CC
   L03.898 Acute lymphangitis of other sites CC

✓5th L03.9 Cellulitis and acute lymphangitis, unspecified
   L03.90 Cellulitis, unspecified CC
      CC Excl: PDX collection 839
   L03.91 Acute lymphangitis, unspecified CC
      EXCLUDES 1 lymphangitis NOS (I89.1)
      CC Excl: PDX collection 839

✓4th L04 Acute lymphadenitis
   INCLUDES abscess (acute) of lymph nodes, except mesenteric
   acute lymphadenitis, except mesenteric
   EXCLUDES 1 chronic or subacute lymphadenitis, except mesenteric (I88.1)
   enlarged lymph nodes (R59.-)
   human immunodeficiency virus [HIV] disease resulting in generalized lymphadenopathy (B20)
   lymphadenitis NOS (I88.9)
   nonspecific mesenteric lymphadenitis (I88.0)
   DEF: Inflammation or enlargement of the lymph nodes.
   L04.0 Acute lymphadenitis of face, head and neck
   L04.1 Acute lymphadenitis of trunk
   L04.2 Acute lymphadenitis of upper limb
      Acute lymphadenitis of axilla   Acute lymphadenitis of shoulder
   L04.3 Acute lymphadenitis of lower limb
      Acute lymphadenitis of hip
      EXCLUDES 2 acute lymphadenitis of groin (L04.1)
   L04.8 Acute lymphadenitis of other sites
   L04.9 Acute lymphadenitis, unspecified

✓4th **L05   Pilonidal cyst and sinus**

  ✓5th **L05.0   Pilonidal cyst and sinus** with abscess

    L05.01   Pilonidal cyst with abscess   `CC` `SW`
      Pilonidal abscess
      Pilonidal dimple with abscess
      Postanal dimple with abscess
      EXCLUDES 2   congenital sacral dimple (Q82.6)
               parasacral dimple (Q82.6)
      CC Excl: PDX collection 841

    L05.02   Pilonidal sinus with abscess   `CC` `SW`
      Coccygeal fistula with abscess
      Coccygeal sinus with abscess
      Pilonidal fistula with abscess
      CC Excl: PDX collection 841

  ✓5th **L05.9   Pilonidal cyst and sinus** without abscess

    L05.91   Pilonidal cyst without abscess
      Pilonidal dimple
      Postanal dimple
      Pilonidal cyst NOS
      EXCLUDES 2   congenital sacral dimple (Q82.6)
               parasacral dimple (Q82.6)

    L05.92   Pilonidal sinus without abscess   `SW`
      Coccygeal fistula
      Coccygeal sinus without abscess
      Pilonidal fistula

Pilonidal Cyst

Skin
Fistula
Pilonidal cyst
Fat
Bone

✓4th **L08   Other local infections of skin and subcutaneous tissue**

  L08.0   Pyoderma
    Dermatitis gangrenosa
    Purulent dermatitis
    Septic dermatitis
    Suppurative dermatitis
    EXCLUDES 1   pyoderma gangrenosum (L88)
             pyoderma vegetans (L08.81)
    DEF: Any superficial skin disease commonly characterized by the discharging of pus not attributed to another condition.

  L08.1   Erythrasma   `HIV` `CC`
    DEF: Chronic, superficial skin infection of brown scaly patches, commonly found in skin folds most prevalent in the overweight or diabetic population.
    CC Excl: PDX collection 107

  ✓5th **L08.8   Other specified local infections of the skin and subcutaneous tissue**

    L08.81   Pyoderma vegetans
      EXCLUDES 1   pyoderma gangrenosum (L88)
             pyoderma NOS (L08.0)

    L08.82   Omphalitis not of newborn
      EXCLUDES 1   omphalitis of newborn (P38.-)

    L08.89   Other specified local infections of the skin and subcutaneous tissue

  L08.9   Local infection of the skin and subcutaneous tissue, unspecified

Bullous disorders (L10-L14)

  EXCLUDES 1   benign familial pemphigus [Hailey-Hailey] (Q82.8)
           staphylococcal scalded skin syndrome (L00)
           toxic epidermal necrolysis [Lyell] (L51.2)

✓4th **L10   Pemphigus**

  EXCLUDES 1   pemphigus neonatorum (L01.03)

  CC Excl: For CC codes in category L10: PDX collection 842

  L10.0   Pemphigus vulgaris   `CC`
  L10.1   Pemphigus vegetans   `CC`
  L10.2   Pemphigus foliaceous   `CC`
  L10.3   Brazilian pemphigus [fogo selvagem]   `CC`
  L10.4   Pemphigus erythematosus   `CC`
    Senear-Usher syndrome
  L10.5   Drug-induced pemphigus   `CC`
    Use additional code for adverse effect, if applicable, to identify drug (T36-T50 with fifth or sixth character 5)

  ✓5th **L10.8   Other pemphigus**
    L10.81   Paraneoplastic pemphigus   `CC`
    L10.89   Other pemphigus   `CC`
  L10.9   Pemphigus, unspecified   `CC`

✓4th **L11   Other acantholytic disorders**

  L11.0   Acquired keratosis follicularis
    EXCLUDES 1   keratosis follicularis (congenital) [Darier-White] (Q82.8)

  L11.1   Transient acantholytic dermatosis [Grover]
  L11.8   Other specified acantholytic disorders
  L11.9   Acantholytic disorder, unspecified

✓4th **L12   Pemphigoid**

  EXCLUDES 1   herpes gestationis (O26.4-)
           impetigo herpetiformis (L40.1)

  CC Excl: For CC codes in category L12, unless otherwise noted: PDX collection 842

  L12.0   Bullous pemphigoid   `CC`
  L12.1   Cicatricial pemphigoid
    Benign mucous membrane pemphigoid
    DEF: Chronic autoimmune disease characterized by subepidermal blistering lesions of the mucosa, including the conjunctiva. It is seen predominantly in the elderly and produces adhesions and scarring.

  L12.2   Chronic bullous disease of childhood   `P`
    Juvenile dermatitis herpetiformis

  ✓5th **L12.3   Acquired epidermolysis bullosa**
    EXCLUDES 1   epidermolysis bullosa (congenital) (Q81.-)

    CC Excl: For CC codes in subcategory L12.3: PDX collection 843

    L12.30   Acquired epidermolysis bullosa, unspecified   `CC` `HCC`
    L12.31   Epidermolysis bullosa due to drug   `CC` `HCC`
      Use additional code for adverse effect, if applicable, to identify drug (T36-T50 with fifth or sixth character 5)
    L12.35   Other acquired epidermolysis bullosa   `CC` `HCC`

  L12.8   Other pemphigoid   `CC`
  L12.9   Pemphigoid, unspecified   `CC`

✓4th **L13   Other bullous disorders**

  L13.0   Dermatitis herpetiformis
    Duhring's disease
    Hydroa herpetiformis
    EXCLUDES 1   juvenile dermatitis herpetiformis (L12.2)
           senile dermatitis herpetiformis (L13.0)
    DEF: Skin disease to which people are genetically predisposed resulting from an immunological response to gluten. Dermatitis herpetiformis is an extremely pruritic eruption of various lesions that frequently heal, leaving hyperpigmentation or hypopigmentation and occasionally scarring. It is usually associated with asymptomatic gluten-sensitive enteropathy.

  L13.1   Subcorneal pustular dermatitis
    Sneddon-Wilkinson disease

  L13.8   Other specified bullous disorders
  L13.9   Bullous disorder, unspecified

  L14   Bullous disorders in diseases classified elsewhere
    Code first underlying disease

Chapter 12. Diseases of the Skin and Subcutaneous Tissue

Dermatitis and eczema (L2Ø-L3Ø)

NOTE   In this block the terms dermatitis and eczema are used synonymously and interchangeably.

EXCLUDES 2   chronic (childhood) granulomatous disease (D71)
dermatitis gangrenosa (LØ8.Ø)
dermatitis herpetiformis (L13.Ø)
dry skin dermatitis (L85.3)
factitial dermatitis (L98.1)
perioral dermatitis (L71.Ø)
radiation-related disorders of the skin and subcutaneous tissue (L55-L59)
stasis dermatitis (I87.2)

√4th **L2Ø   Atopic dermatitis**
- **L2Ø.Ø   Besnier's prurigo**
- √5th **L2Ø.8   Other atopic dermatitis**
  - EXCLUDES 2   circumscribed neurodermatitis (L28.Ø)
  - **L2Ø.81   Atopic neurodermatitis**
    - Diffuse neurodermatitis
  - **L2Ø.82   Flexural eczema**
  - **L2Ø.83   Infantile (acute) (chronic) eczema**   P
  - **L2Ø.84   Intrinsic (allergic) eczema**
  - **L2Ø.89   Other atopic dermatitis**
- **L2Ø.9   Atopic dermatitis, unspecified**

√4th **L21   Seborrheic dermatitis**
- EXCLUDES 2   infective dermatitis (L3Ø.3)
  seborrheic keratosis (L82.-)
- **L21.Ø   Seborrhea capitis**
  - Cradle cap
  - **AHA:** 2018, 1Q, 6
  - **TIP:** Assign for dandruff in an adult patient.
- **L21.1   Seborrheic infantile dermatitis**   P
- **L21.8   Other seborrheic dermatitis**
- **L21.9   Seborrheic dermatitis, unspecified**
  - Seborrhea NOS

L22   Diaper dermatitis
- Diaper erythema
- Diaper rash
- Psoriasiform diaper rash

√4th **L23   Allergic contact dermatitis**
- EXCLUDES 1   allergy NOS (T78.4Ø)
  contact dermatitis NOS (L25.9)
  dermatitis NOS (L3Ø.9)
- EXCLUDES 2   dermatitis due to substances taken internally (L27.-)
  dermatitis of eyelid (HØ1.1-)
  diaper dermatitis (L22)
  eczema of external ear (H6Ø.5-)
  irritant contact dermatitis (L24.-)
  perioral dermatitis (L71.Ø)
  radiation-related disorders of the skin and subcutaneous tissue (L55-L59)
- **L23.Ø   Allergic contact dermatitis due to metals**
  - Allergic contact dermatitis due to chromium
  - Allergic contact dermatitis due to nickel
- **L23.1   Allergic contact dermatitis due to adhesives**
- **L23.2   Allergic contact dermatitis due to cosmetics**
- **L23.3   Allergic contact dermatitis due to drugs in contact with skin**
  - Use additional code for adverse effect, if applicable, to identify drug (T36-T5Ø with fifth or sixth character 5)
  - EXCLUDES 2   dermatitis due to ingested drugs and medicaments (L27.Ø-L27.1)
- **L23.4   Allergic contact dermatitis due to dyes**
- **L23.5   Allergic contact dermatitis due to other chemical products**
  - Allergic contact dermatitis due to cement
  - Allergic contact dermatitis due to insecticide
  - Allergic contact dermatitis due to plastic
  - Allergic contact dermatitis due to rubber
- **L23.6   Allergic contact dermatitis due to food in contact with the skin**
  - EXCLUDES 2   dermatitis due to ingested food (L27.2)
- **L23.7   Allergic contact dermatitis due to plants, except food**
  - EXCLUDES 2   allergy NOS due to pollen (J3Ø.1)
- √5th **L23.8   Allergic contact dermatitis due to other agents**
  - **L23.81   Allergic contact dermatitis due to animal (cat) (dog) dander**
    - Allergic contact dermatitis due to animal (cat) (dog) hair

- **L23.89   Allergic contact dermatitis due to other agents**
- **L23.9   Allergic contact dermatitis, unspecified cause**
  - Allergic contact eczema NOS

√4th **L24   Irritant contact dermatitis**
- EXCLUDES 1   allergy NOS (T78.4Ø)
  contact dermatitis NOS (L25.9)
  dermatitis NOS (L3Ø.9)
- EXCLUDES 2   allergic contact dermatitis (L23.-)
  dermatitis due to substances taken internally (L27.-)
  dermatitis of eyelid (HØ1.1-)
  diaper dermatitis (L22)
  eczema of external ear (H6Ø.5-)
  perioral dermatitis (L71.Ø)
  radiation-related disorders of the skin and subcutaneous tissue (L55-L59)
- **L24.Ø   Irritant contact dermatitis due to detergents**
- **L24.1   Irritant contact dermatitis due to oils and greases**
- **L24.2   Irritant contact dermatitis due to solvents**
  - Irritant contact dermatitis due to chlorocompound
  - Irritant contact dermatitis due to cyclohexane
  - Irritant contact dermatitis due to ester
  - Irritant contact dermatitis due to glycol
  - Irritant contact dermatitis due to hydrocarbon
  - Irritant contact dermatitis due to ketone
- **L24.3   Irritant contact dermatitis due to cosmetics**
- **L24.4   Irritant contact dermatitis due to drugs in contact with skin**
  - Use additional code for adverse effect, if applicable, to identify drug (T36-T5Ø with fifth or sixth character 5)
- **L24.5   Irritant contact dermatitis due to other chemical products**
  - Irritant contact dermatitis due to cement
  - Irritant contact dermatitis due to insecticide
  - Irritant contact dermatitis due to plastic
  - Irritant contact dermatitis due to rubber
- **L24.6   Irritant contact dermatitis due to food in contact with skin**
  - EXCLUDES 2   dermatitis due to ingested food (L27.2)
- **L24.7   Irritant contact dermatitis due to plants, except food**
  - EXCLUDES 2   allergy NOS to pollen (J3Ø.1)
- √5th **L24.8   Irritant contact dermatitis due to other agents**
  - **L24.81   Irritant contact dermatitis due to metals**
    - Irritant contact dermatitis due to chromium
    - Irritant contact dermatitis due to nickel
  - **L24.89   Irritant contact dermatitis due to other agents**
    - Irritant contact dermatitis due to dyes
- **L24.9   Irritant contact dermatitis, unspecified cause**
  - Irritant contact eczema NOS

√4th **L25   Unspecified contact dermatitis**
- EXCLUDES 1   allergic contact dermatitis (L23.-)
  allergy NOS (T78.4Ø)
  dermatitis NOS (L3Ø.9)
  irritant contact dermatitis (L24.-)
- EXCLUDES 2   dermatitis due to ingested substances (L27.-)
  dermatitis of eyelid (HØ1.1-)
  eczema of external ear (H6Ø.5-)
  perioral dermatitis (L71.Ø)
  radiation-related disorders of the skin and subcutaneous tissue (L55-L59)
- **L25.Ø   Unspecified contact dermatitis due to cosmetics**
- **L25.1   Unspecified contact dermatitis due to drugs in contact with skin**
  - Use additional code for adverse effect, if applicable, to identify drug (T36-T5Ø with fifth or sixth character 5)
  - EXCLUDES 2   dermatitis due to ingested drugs and medicaments (L27.Ø-L27.1)
- **L25.2   Unspecified contact dermatitis due to dyes**
- **L25.3   Unspecified contact dermatitis due to other chemical products**
  - Unspecified contact dermatitis due to cement
  - Unspecified contact dermatitis due to insecticide
- **L25.4   Unspecified contact dermatitis due to food in contact with skin**
  - EXCLUDES 2   dermatitis due to ingested food (L27.2)
- **L25.5   Unspecified contact dermatitis due to plants, except food**
  - EXCLUDES 1   nettle rash (L5Ø.9)
  - EXCLUDES 2   allergy NOS due to pollen (J3Ø.1)
- **L25.8   Unspecified contact dermatitis due to other agents**
- **L25.9   Unspecified contact dermatitis, unspecified cause**
  - Contact dermatitis (occupational) NOS
  - Contact eczema (occupational) NOS

N Newborn: 0   P Pediatric: 0-17   M Maternity: 12-55   A Adult: 15-124   MCC Major Complication/Comorbidity   CC Complication/Comorbidity   SW Severe Wound Dx

720   ICD-10-CM 2019

L26 **Exfoliative dermatitis**
     Hebra's pityriasis
     EXCLUDES 1   *Ritter's disease (L00)*

✓4th L27 **Dermatitis due to substances taken internally**
     EXCLUDES 1   *allergy NOS (T78.40)*
     EXCLUDES 2   *adverse food reaction, except dermatitis (T78.0-T78.1)*
                       contact dermatitis (L23-L25)
                       drug photoallergic response (L56.1)
                       drug phototoxic response (L56.0)
                       urticaria (L50.-)

     L27.0 **Generalized skin eruption due to drugs and medicaments taken internally**
         Use additional code for adverse effect, if applicable, to identify drug (T36-T50 with fifth or sixth character 5)

     L27.1 **Localized skin eruption due to drugs and medicaments taken internally**
         Use additional code for adverse effect, if applicable, to identify drug (T36-T50 with fifth or sixth character 5)

     L27.2 **Dermatitis due to ingested food**
         EXCLUDES 2   *dermatitis due to food in contact with skin (L23.6, L24.6, L25.4)*

     L27.8 **Dermatitis due to other substances taken internally**

     L27.9 **Dermatitis due to unspecified substance taken internally**

✓4th L28 **Lichen simplex chronicus and prurigo**
     L28.0 **Lichen simplex chronicus**
         Circumscribed neurodermatitis
         Lichen NOS

     L28.1 **Prurigo nodularis**

     L28.2 **Other prurigo**
         Prurigo NOS   Prurigo mitis
         Prurigo Hebra   Urticaria papulosa

✓4th L29 **Pruritus**
     EXCLUDES 1   *neurotic excoriation (L98.1)*
                       psychogenic pruritus (F45.8)

     L29.0 **Pruritus ani**

     L29.1 **Pruritus scroti**   ♂

     L29.2 **Pruritus vulvae**   ♀

     L29.3 **Anogenital pruritus, unspecified**

     L29.8 **Other pruritus**

     L29.9 **Pruritus, unspecified**
         Itch NOS

✓4th L30 **Other and unspecified dermatitis**
     EXCLUDES 2   *contact dermatitis (L23-L25)*
                       dry skin dermatitis (L85.3)
                       small plaque parapsoriasis (L41.3)
                       stasis dermatitis (I87.2)

     L30.0 **Nummular dermatitis**

     L30.1 **Dyshidrosis [pompholyx]**

     L30.2 **Cutaneous autosensitization**
         Candidid [levurid]
         Dermatophytid
         Eczematid

     L30.3 **Infective dermatitis**
         Infectious eczematoid dermatitis

     L30.4 **Erythema intertrigo**

     L30.5 **Pityriasis alba**
         AHA: 2018, 1Q, 6

     L30.8 **Other specified dermatitis**

     L30.9 **Dermatitis, unspecified**
         Eczema NOS

Papulosquamous disorders (L40-L45)

✓4th L40 **Psoriasis**
     DEF: Chronic autoimmune condition that speeds up skin cell growth, causing excessive immature skin cells to form raised, rounded erythematous lesions covered by dry, silvery scaling patches. Most commonly found on the scalp, elbows, knees, hands, feet, and genitals, it can also affect the joints with stiffness and swelling.

     L40.0 **Psoriasis vulgaris**
         Nummular psoriasis
         Plaque psoriasis

     L40.1 **Generalized pustular psoriasis**
         Impetigo herpetiformis
         Von Zumbusch's disease

     L40.2 **Acrodermatitis continua**

     L40.3 **Pustulosis palmaris et plantaris**

     L40.4 **Guttate psoriasis**

✓5th L40.5 **Arthropathic psoriasis**
         L40.50 **Arthropathic psoriasis, unspecified**   HCC
         L40.51 **Distal interphalangeal psoriatic arthropathy**   HCC
         L40.52 **Psoriatic arthritis mutilans**   HCC
         L40.53 **Psoriatic spondylitis**   HCC
         L40.54 **Psoriatic juvenile arthropathy**   HCC
         L40.59 **Other psoriatic arthropathy**   HCC

     L40.8 **Other psoriasis**
         Flexural psoriasis

     L40.9 **Psoriasis, unspecified**

✓4th L41 **Parapsoriasis**
     EXCLUDES 1   *poikiloderma vasculare atrophicans (L94.5)*

     L41.0 **Pityriasis lichenoides et varioliformis acuta**
         Mucha-Habermann disease

     L41.1 **Pityriasis lichenoides chronica**

     L41.3 **Small plaque parapsoriasis**

     L41.4 **Large plaque parapsoriasis**

     L41.5 **Retiform parapsoriasis**

     L41.8 **Other parapsoriasis**

     L41.9 **Parapsoriasis, unspecified**

     L42 **Pityriasis rosea**

✓4th L43 **Lichen planus**
     EXCLUDES 1   *lichen planopilaris (L66.1)*

     L43.0 **Hypertrophic lichen planus**

     L43.1 **Bullous lichen planus**

     L43.2 **Lichenoid drug reaction**
         Use additional code for adverse effect, if applicable, to identify drug (T36-T50 with fifth or sixth character 5)

     L43.3 **Subacute (active) lichen planus**
         Lichen planus tropicus

     L43.8 **Other lichen planus**

     L43.9 **Lichen planus, unspecified**

✓4th L44 **Other papulosquamous disorders**
     L44.0 **Pityriasis rubra pilaris**

     L44.1 **Lichen nitidus**
         DEF: Chronic, inflammatory, asymptomatic skin disorder, characterized by numerous glistening, flat-topped, discrete, skin-colored micropapules, most often on the penis, lower abdomen, inner thighs, wrists, forearms, breasts, and buttocks.

     L44.2 **Lichen striatus**

     L44.3 **Lichen ruber moniliformis**

     L44.4 **Infantile papular acrodermatitis [Gianotti-Crosti]**   P

     L44.8 **Other specified papulosquamous disorders**

     L44.9 **Papulosquamous disorder, unspecified**

     L45 ***Papulosquamous disorders in diseases classified elsewhere***
         Code first underlying disease

Urticaria and erythema (L49-L54)

     EXCLUDES 1   *Lyme disease (A69.2-)*
                       rosacea (L71.-)

✓4th L49 **Exfoliation due to erythematous conditions according to extent of body surface involved**
     Code first erythematous condition causing exfoliation, such as:
         Ritter's disease (L00)
         (Staphylococcal) scalded skin syndrom (L00)
         Stevens-Johnson syndrome (L51.1)
         Stevens-Johnson syndrome-toxic epidermal necrolysis overlap syndrome (L51.3)
         toxic epidermal necrolysis (L51.2)
     DEF: Exfoliation: Falling or sloughing off skin in layers.

     L49.0 **Exfoliation due to erythematous condition involving less than 10 percent of body surface**
         Exfoliation due to erythematous condition NOS

     L49.1 **Exfoliation due to erythematous condition involving 10-19 percent of body surface**

     L49.2 **Exfoliation due to erythematous condition involving 20-29 percent of body surface**

     L49.3 **Exfoliation due to erythematous condition involving 30-39 percent of body surface**   CC
         CC Excl: PDX collection 844

✓ Additional Character Required   ✓x7th Placeholder   Unacceptable PDx   Questionable PDx   Manifestation   H1 - H14 HAC   HCC CMS-HCC Dx   HIV HIV Dx

ICD-10-CM 2019   721

Chapter 12. Diseases of the Skin and Subcutaneous Tissue

L49.4 **Exfoliation due to erythematous condition involving 40-49 percent of body surface** `CC`
    CC Excl: PDX collection 845

L49.5 **Exfoliation due to erythematous condition involving 50-59 percent of body surface** `CC`
    CC Excl: PDX collection 846

L49.6 **Exfoliation due to erythematous condition involving 60-69 percent of body surface** `CC`
    CC Excl: PDX collection 847

L49.7 **Exfoliation due to erythematous condition involving 70-79 percent of body surface** `CC`
    CC Excl: PDX collection 848

L49.8 **Exfoliation due to erythematous condition involving 80-89 percent of body surface** `CC`
    CC Excl: PDX collection 849

L49.9 **Exfoliation due to erythematous condition involving 90 or more percent of body surface** `CC`
    CC Excl: PDX collection 850

✓4th **L50** **Urticaria**
    EXCLUDES 1   allergic contact dermatitis (L23.-)
         angioneurotic edema (T78.3)
         giant urticaria (T78.3)
         hereditary angio-edema (D84.1)
         Quincke's edema (T78.3)
         serum urticaria (T80.6-)
         solar urticaria (L56.3)
         urticaria neonatorum (P83.8)
         urticaria papulosa (L28.2)
         urticaria pigmentosa (Q82.2)
    DEF: Eruption of itching edema of the skin. **Synonym(s):** hives.

L50.0 **Allergic urticaria**

L50.1 **Idiopathic urticaria**

L50.2 **Urticaria due to cold and heat**
    EXCLUDES 2   familial cold urticaria (M04.2)

L50.3 **Dermatographic urticaria**

L50.4 **Vibratory urticaria**

L50.5 **Cholinergic urticaria**

L50.6 **Contact urticaria**

L50.8 **Other urticaria**
    Chronic urticaria
    Recurrent periodic urticaria

L50.9 **Urticaria, unspecified**

✓4th **L51** **Erythema multiforme**
    Use additional code for adverse effect, if applicable, to identify drug (T36-T50 with fifth or sixth character 5)
    Use additional code to identify associated manifestations, such as:
    arthropathy associated with dermatological disorders (M14.8-)
    conjunctival edema (H11.42)
    conjunctivitis (H10.22-)
    corneal scars and opacities (H17.-)
    corneal ulcer (H16.0-)
    edema of eyelid ▶(H02.84-)◀
    inflammation of eyelid (H01.8)
    keratoconjunctivitis sicca (H16.22-)
    mechanical lagophthalmos (H02.22-)
    stomatitis (K12.-)
    symblepharon (H11.23-)
    Use additional code to identify percentage of skin exfoliation (L49.-)
    EXCLUDES 1   staphylococcal scalded skin syndrome (L00)
         Ritter's disease (L00)
    DEF: Acute complex of symptoms with a varied pattern of skin eruptions, such as macular, bullous, popular, nodose, or vesicular lesions on the neck, face, and legs. Erythema (redness of skin and mucous membranes) multiforme (multiple forms) is a hypersensitivity (allergic) reaction that can occur at any age but primarily affects children or young adults.

    CC Excl: For CC codes in category L51: PDX collection 843

L51.0 **Nonbullous erythema multiforme**

L51.1 **Stevens-Johnson syndrome** `CC` `HCC`

L51.2 **Toxic epidermal necrolysis [Lyell]** `CC` `HCC`

L51.3 **Stevens-Johnson syndrome-toxic epidermal necrolysis overlap syndrome** `CC` `HCC`
    SJS-TEN overlap syndrome

L51.8 **Other erythema multiforme**

L51.9 **Erythema multiforme, unspecified**
    Erythema iris
    Erythema multiforme major NOS
    Erythema multiforme minor NOS
    Herpes iris

L52 **Erythema nodosum**
    EXCLUDES 1   tuberculous erythema nodosum (A18.4)
    DEF: Form of panniculitis (inflammation of the fat layer beneath the skin) most often occurring in women. Commonly seen as a hypersensitivity reaction to infections, drugs, sarcoidosis, and specific enteropathies. The acute stage is associated with fever, malaise, and arthralgia. The lesions are pink to blue in color as tender nodules and are found on the front of the legs below the knees.

✓4th **L53** **Other erythematous conditions**
    EXCLUDES 1   erythema ab igne (L59.0)
         erythema due to external agents in contact with skin (L23-L25)
         erythema intertrigo (L30.4)

    CC Excl: For CC codes in category L53: PDX collection 851

L53.0 **Toxic erythema** `CC`
    Code first poisoning due to drug or toxin, if applicable (T36-T65 with fifth or sixth character 1-4 or 6)
    Use additional code for adverse effect, if applicable, to identify drug (T36-T50 with fifth or sixth character 5)
    EXCLUDES 1   neonatal erythema toxicum (P83.1)

L53.1 **Erythema annulare centrifugum** `CC`

L53.2 **Erythema marginatum** `CC`

L53.3 **Other chronic figurate erythema** `CC`

L53.8 **Other specified erythematous conditions**

L53.9 **Erythematous condition, unspecified**
    Erythema NOS
    Erythroderma NOS

L54 ***Erythema in diseases classified elsewhere***
    Code first underlying disease

Radiation-related disorders of the skin and subcutaneous tissue (L55-L59)

✓4th **L55** **Sunburn**

L55.0 **Sunburn of first degree**

L55.1 **Sunburn of second degree**

L55.2 **Sunburn of third degree**

L55.9 **Sunburn, unspecified**

✓4th **L56** **Other acute skin changes due to ultraviolet radiation**
    Use additional code to identify the source of the ultraviolet radiation (W89, X32)

L56.0 **Drug phototoxic response**
    Use additional code for adverse effect, if applicable, to identify drug (T36-T50 with fifth or sixth character 5)

L56.1 **Drug photoallergic response**
    Use additional code for adverse effect, if applicable, to identify drug (T36-T50 with fifth or sixth character 5)

L56.2 **Photocontact dermatitis [berloque dermatitis]**

L56.3 **Solar urticaria**

L56.4 **Polymorphous light eruption**

L56.5 **Disseminated superficial actinic porokeratosis (DSAP)**
    DEF: Autosomal dominant skin condition occurring in sun-exposed areas of the skin (particularly the arms and legs), characterized by superficial annular, keratotic, brownish-red spots or thickenings with depressed centers and sharp, ridged borders. It may evolve into squamous cell carcinoma.

L56.8 **Other specified acute skin changes due to ultraviolet radiation**

L56.9 **Acute skin change due to ultraviolet radiation, unspecified**

✓4th **L57** **Skin changes due to chronic exposure to nonionizing radiation**
    Use additional code to identify the source of the ultraviolet radiation (W89)

L57.0 **Actinic keratosis**
    Keratosis NOS   Solar keratosis
    Senile keratosis

L57.1 **Actinic reticuloid**

L57.2 **Cutis rhomboidalis nuchae**

L57.3 **Poikiloderma of Civatte**

L57.4 **Cutis laxa senilis**
    Elastosis senilis

L57.5 **Actinic granuloma**

L57.8 **Other skin changes due to chronic exposure to nonionizing radiation**
    Farmer's skin   Solar dermatitis
    Sailor's skin

L57.9 **Skin changes due to chronic exposure to nonionizing radiation, unspecified**

N Newborn: 0   P Pediatric: 0-17   M Maternity: 12-55   A Adult: 15-124   MCC Major Complication/Comorbidity   CC Complication/Comorbidity   SW Severe Wound Dx

722   ICD-10-CM 2019

L49.4–L57.9

☑4ᵗʰ **L58 Radiodermatitis**
Use additional code to identify the source of the radiation (W88, W90)

L58.0 Acute **radiodermatitis**

L58.1 Chronic **radiodermatitis**

L58.9 Radiodermatitis, unspecified

☑4ᵗʰ **L59 Other disorders of skin and subcutaneous tissue related to radiation**

L59.0 Erythema ab igne [dermatitis ab igne]

L59.8 Other specified disorders of the skin and subcutaneous tissue related to radiation
AHA: 2017, 1Q, 33

L59.9 Disorder of the skin and subcutaneous tissue related to radiation, unspecified

Disorders of skin appendages (L60-L75)

EXCLUDES 1　*congenital malformations of integument (Q84.-)*

☑4ᵗʰ **L60 Nail disorders**
EXCLUDES 2　*clubbing of nails (R68.3)*
onychia and paronychia (L03.0-)

L60.0 Ingrowing nail

L60.1 Onycholysis

L60.2 Onychogryphosis

L60.3 Nail dystrophy

L60.4 Beau's lines

L60.5 Yellow nail syndrome

L60.8 Other nail disorders

L60.9 Nail disorder, unspecified

Nail Disorders

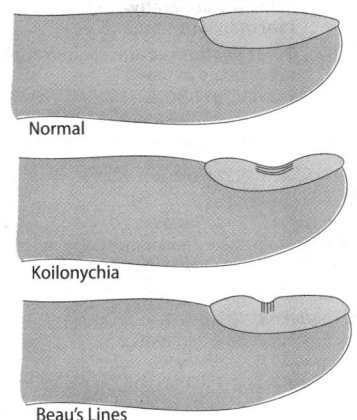

Normal

Koilonychia

Beau's Lines

L62 *Nail disorders in diseases classified elsewhere*
Code first underlying disease, such as:
pachydermoperiostosis (M89.4-)

☑4ᵗʰ **L63 Alopecia areata**

L63.0 Alopecia (capitis) totalis

L63.1 Alopecia universalis

L63.2 Ophiasis

L63.8 Other **alopecia areata**

L63.9 Alopecia areata, unspecified

☑4ᵗʰ **L64 Androgenic alopecia**
INCLUDES　male-pattern baldness

L64.0 Drug-induced **androgenic alopecia**
Use additional code for adverse effect, if applicable, to identify drug (T36-T50 with fifth or sixth character 5)

L64.8 Other **androgenic alopecia**

L64.9 Androgenic alopecia, unspecified

☑4ᵗʰ **L65 Other nonscarring hair loss**
Use additional code for adverse effect, if applicable, to identify drug (T36-T50 with fifth or sixth character 5)
EXCLUDES 1　*trichotillomania (F63.3)*

L65.0 Telogen effluvium
DEF: Form of nonscarring alopecia characterized by shedding of hair from premature telogen development in follicles due to stress, including shock, childbirth, surgery, drugs, or weight loss.

L65.1 Anagen effluvium

L65.2 Alopecia mucinosa

L65.8 Other specified nonscarring hair loss

L65.9 Nonscarring hair loss, unspecified
Alopecia NOS

☑4ᵗʰ **L66 Cicatricial alopecia [scarring hair loss]**

L66.0 Pseudopelade

L66.1 Lichen planopilaris
Follicular lichen planus

L66.2 Folliculitis decalvans

L66.3 Perifolliculitis capitis abscedens

L66.4 Folliculitis ulerythematosa reticulata

L66.8 Other cicatricial alopecia
AHA: 2015, 1Q, 19

L66.9 Cicatricial alopecia, unspecified

☑4ᵗʰ **L67 Hair color and hair shaft abnormalities**
EXCLUDES 1　*monilethrix (Q84.1)*
pili annulati (Q84.1)
telogen effluvium (L65.0)

L67.0 Trichorrhexis nodosa

L67.1 Variations in hair color
Canities
Greyness, hair (premature)
Heterochromia of hair
Poliosis circumscripta, acquired
Poliosis NOS

L67.8 Other hair color and hair shaft abnormalities
Fragilitas crinium

L67.9 Hair color and hair shaft abnormality, unspecified

☑4ᵗʰ **L68 Hypertrichosis**
INCLUDES　excess hair
EXCLUDES 1　*congenital hypertrichosis (Q84.2)*
persistent lanugo (Q84.2)

L68.0 Hirsutism

L68.1 Acquired hypertrichosis lanuginosa

L68.2 Localized hypertrichosis

L68.3 Polytrichia

L68.8 Other hypertrichosis

L68.9 Hypertrichosis, unspecified

☑4ᵗʰ **L70 Acne**
EXCLUDES 2　*acne keloid (L73.0)*

L70.0 Acne vulgaris

L70.1 Acne conglobata

L70.2 Acne varioliformis
Acne necrotica miliaris
DEF: Rare form of acne characterized by development of persistent brown papulopustules followed by scar formation. This type of acne usually presents on the brow and temporoparietal part of the scalp.

L70.3 Acne tropica

L70.4 Infantile **acne**　　　　　　　　　　　　　　Ⓟ

L70.5 Acné excoriée
Acné excoriée des jeunes filles
Picker's acne

L70.8 Other **acne**

L70.9 Acne, unspecified

☑4ᵗʰ **L71 Rosacea**
Use additional code for adverse effect, if applicable, to identify drug (T36-T50 with fifth or sixth character 5)

L71.0 Perioral dermatitis

L71.1 Rhinophyma

L71.8 Other rosacea

L71.9 Rosacea, unspecified

☑4ᵗʰ **L72 Follicular cysts of skin and subcutaneous tissue**

L72.0 Epidermal cyst

☑5ᵗʰ **L72.1 Pilar and trichodermal cyst**

L72.11 Pilar cyst

L72.12 Trichodermal cyst
Trichilemmal (proliferating) cyst

L72.2 Steatocystoma multiplex

L72.3 Sebaceous cyst
EXCLUDES 2　*pilar cyst (L72.11)*
trichilemmal (proliferating) cyst (L72.12)

L72.8 Other follicular cysts of the skin and subcutaneous tissue

☑ Additional Character Required　　☑x7ᵗʰ Placeholder　　Unacceptable PDx　　Questionable PDx　　Manifestation　　H1–H14 HAC　　HCC CMS-HCC Dx　　HIV HIV Dx

ICD-10-CM 2019　　　　　　　　　　　　　　　　　　　　　　　　　　　　　　　　　　　　　　723

L72.9   **Follicular cyst of the skin and subcutaneous tissue, unspecified**

✓4th **L73**   **Other follicular disorders**

L73.0   **Acne keloid**

L73.1   **Pseudofolliculitis barbae**

L73.2   **Hidradenitis suppurativa**

L73.8   **Other specified follicular disorders**
Sycosis barbae

L73.9   **Follicular disorder, unspecified**

✓4th **L74**   **Eccrine sweat disorders**
EXCLUDES 2   *generalized hyperhidrosis (R61)*
DEF: Eccrine sweat glands: Glands found in the dermal and hypodermal layer of the skin throughout the body, particularly on the forehead, scalp, axillae, palms, and soles. These glands produce watery and neutral or slightly acidic sweat.

L74.0   **Miliaria** rubra

L74.1   **Miliaria** crystallina

L74.2   **Miliaria** profunda
Miliaria tropicalis

L74.3   **Miliaria, unspecified**

L74.4   **Anhidrosis**
Hypohidrosis
DEF: Inability to sweat normally. When the body can't cool itself through perspiration it can lead to heatstroke, a life-threatening condition.

✓5th **L74.5**   **Focal hyperhidrosis**

    ✓6th **L74.51**   **Primary focal hyperhidrosis**

       L74.510   **Primary focal hyperhidrosis, axilla**

       L74.511   **Primary focal hyperhidrosis, face**

       L74.512   **Primary focal hyperhidrosis, palms**

       L74.513   **Primary focal hyperhidrosis, soles**

       L74.519   **Primary focal hyperhidrosis, unspecified**

    L74.52   **Secondary focal hyperhidrosis**
Frey's syndrome

L74.8   **Other eccrine sweat disorders**

L74.9   **Eccrine sweat disorder, unspecified**
Sweat gland disorder NOS

✓4th **L75**   **Apocrine sweat disorders**
EXCLUDES 1   *dyshidrosis (L30.1)*
hidradenitis suppurativa (L73.2)
DEF: Apocrine sweat glands: Found in the axilla, areola, and circumanal region, these glands begin to function in puberty and produce viscid milky secretions in response to external stimuli.

L75.0   **Bromhidrosis**

L75.1   **Chromhidrosis**

L75.2   **Apocrine miliaria**
Fox-Fordyce disease
DEF: Chronic, usually pruritic disease evidenced by small follicular papular eruptions, especially in the axillary and pubic areas. Apocrine miliaria develops from the closure and rupture of the affected apocrine glands' intraepidermal portion of the ducts.

L75.8   **Other apocrine sweat disorders**

L75.9   **Apocrine sweat disorder, unspecified**

Intraoperative and postprocedural complications of skin and subcutaneous tissue (L76)

✓4th **L76**   **Intraoperative and postprocedural complications of skin and subcutaneous tissue**
AHA: 2016, 4Q, 9-10

> **CC Excl: For CC codes in category L76, unless otherwise noted:** PDX collection 852

✓5th **L76.0**   **Intraoperative hemorrhage and hematoma of skin and subcutaneous tissue complicating a procedure**
EXCLUDES 1   *intraoperative hemorrhage and hematoma of skin and subcutaneous tissue due to accidental puncture and laceration during a procedure (L76.1-)*

    L76.01   **Intraoperative hemorrhage and hematoma of skin and subcutaneous tissue complicating a dermatologic procedure**   CC

    L76.02   **Intraoperative hemorrhage and hematoma of skin and subcutaneous tissue complicating other procedure**   CC

✓5th **L76.1**   **Accidental puncture and laceration of skin and subcutaneous tissue during a procedure**

    L76.11   **Accidental puncture and laceration of skin and subcutaneous tissue during a dermatologic procedure**   CC
       CC Excl: PDX collection 509

    L76.12   **Accidental puncture and laceration of skin and subcutaneous tissue during other procedure**   CC
       CC Excl: PDX collection 509

✓5th **L76.2**   **Postprocedural hemorrhage of skin and subcutaneous tissue following a procedure**

    L76.21   **Postprocedural hemorrhage of skin and subcutaneous tissue following a dermatologic procedure**   CC

    L76.22   **Postprocedural hemorrhage of skin and subcutaneous tissue following other procedure**   CC

✓5th **L76.3**   **Postprocedural hematoma and seroma of skin and subcutaneous tissue following a procedure**

    L76.31   **Postprocedural hematoma of skin and subcutaneous tissue following a dermatologic procedure**   CC

    L76.32   **Postprocedural hematoma of skin and subcutaneous tissue following other procedure**   CC

    L76.33   **Postprocedural seroma of skin and subcutaneous tissue following a dermatologic procedure**   CC

    L76.34   **Postprocedural seroma of skin and subcutaneous tissue following other procedure**   CC

✓5th **L76.8**   **Other intraoperative and postprocedural complications of skin and subcutaneous tissue**
Use additional code, if applicable, to further specify disorder

    L76.81   **Other intraoperative complications of skin and subcutaneous tissue**

    L76.82   **Other postprocedural complications of skin and subcutaneous tissue**
       AHA: 2017, 3Q, 6

Other disorders of the skin and subcutaneous tissue (L80-L99)

L80   **Vitiligo**
EXCLUDES 2   *vitiligo of eyelids (H02.73-)*
vitiligo of vulva (N90.89)
DEF: Persistent, progressive development of nonpigmented white patches on otherwise normal skin.

✓4th **L81**   **Other disorders of pigmentation**
EXCLUDES 1   *birthmark NOS (Q82.5)*
Peutz-Jeghers syndrome (Q85.8)
EXCLUDES 2   *nevus—see Alphabetical Index*

L81.0   **Postinflammatory hyperpigmentation**

L81.1   **Chloasma**

L81.2   **Freckles**

L81.3   **Café au lait spots**

L81.4   **Other melanin hyperpigmentation**
Lentigo

L81.5   **Leukoderma, not elsewhere classified**

L81.6   **Other disorders of diminished melanin formation**

L81.7   **Pigmented purpuric dermatosis**
Angioma serpiginosum

L81.8   **Other specified disorders of pigmentation**
Iron pigmentation
Tattoo pigmentation

L81.9   **Disorder of pigmentation, unspecified**

✓4th **L82**   **Seborrheic keratosis**
INCLUDES   basal cell papilloma
dermatosis papulosa nigra
Leser-Trélat disease
EXCLUDES 2   *seborrheic dermatitis (L21.-)*
DEF: Common, benign, noninvasive, lightly pigmented, warty growth composed of basaloid cells that usually appear at middle age as soft, easily crumbling plaques on the face, trunk, and extremities.

L82.0   **Inflamed seborrheic keratosis**

L82.1   **Other seborrheic keratosis**
Seborrheic keratosis NOS

N Newborn: 0   P Pediatric: 0-17   M Maternity: 12-55   A Adult: 15-124   MCC Major Complication/Comorbidity   CC Complication/Comorbidity   SW Severe Wound Dx

724   ICD-10-CM 2019

L83   Acanthosis nigricans

Confluent and reticulated papillomatosis

DEF: Diffuse, velvety hyperplasia of the spinous skin layer of the axilla and other body folds marked by gray, brown, or black pigmentation. In adult form, it is often associated with malignant acanthosis nigricans in a benign, nevoid form relatively generalized.

L84   Corns and callosities

Callus

Clavus

✓4ᵗʰ   L85   Other epidermal thickening

EXCLUDES 2   hypertrophic disorders of the skin (L91.-)

L85.0   Acquired ichthyosis

EXCLUDES 1   congenital ichthyosis (Q80.-)

L85.1   Acquired keratosis [keratoderma] palmaris et plantaris

EXCLUDES 1   inherited keratosis palmaris et plantaris (Q82.8)

L85.2   Keratosis punctata (palmaris et plantaris)

L85.3   Xerosis cutis

Dry skin dermatitis

L85.8   Other specified epidermal thickening

Cutaneous horn

L85.9   Epidermal thickening, unspecified

L86   *Keratoderma in diseases classified elsewhere*

Code first underlying disease, such as:

Reiter's disease (M02.3-)

EXCLUDES 1   gonococcal keratoderma (A54.89)

gonococcal keratosis (A54.89)

keratoderma due to vitamin A deficiency (E50.8)

keratosis due to vitamin A deficiency (E50.8)

xeroderma due to vitamin A deficiency (E50.8)

✓4ᵗʰ   L87   Transepidermal elimination disorders

EXCLUDES 1   granuloma annulare (perforating) (L92.0)

L87.0   Keratosis follicularis et parafollicularis in cutem penetrans

Hyperkeratosis follicularis penetrans

Kyrle disease

L87.1   Reactive perforating collagenosis

L87.2   Elastosis perforans serpiginosa

L87.8   Other transepidermal elimination disorders

L87.9   Transepidermal elimination disorder, unspecified

L88   Pyoderma gangrenosum   CC

Phagedenic pyoderma

EXCLUDES 1   dermatitis gangrenosa (L08.0)

DEF: Persistent debilitating skin disease characterized by irregular, boggy, blue-red ulcerations, with central healing and undermined edges.

CC Excl: PDX collection 853

✓4ᵗʰ   L89   Pressure ulcer

INCLUDES   bed sore

decubitus ulcer

plaster ulcer

pressure area

pressure sore

Code first any associated gangrene (I96)

EXCLUDES 2   decubitus (trophic) ulcer of cervix (uteri) (N86)

diabetic ulcers (E08.621, E08.622, E09.621, E09.622, E10.621, E10.622, E11.621, E11.622, E13.621, E13.622)

non-pressure chronic ulcer of skin (L97.-)

skin infections (L00-L08)

varicose ulcer (I83.0, I83.2)

AHA: 2018, 2Q, 21; 2017, 4Q, 109; 2017, 1Q, 49; 2016, 4Q, 143

TIP: The stage of a diagnosed pressure ulcer can be based on documentation from clinicians who are not the patient's provider.

CC Excl: For MCC codes in category L89: PDX collection 854

✓5ᵗʰ   L89.0   Pressure ulcer of elbow

✓6ᵗʰ   L89.00   Pressure ulcer of unspecified elbow

L89.000   Pressure ulcer of unspecified elbow, unstageable   HCC SW

L89.001   Pressure ulcer of unspecified elbow, stage 1

Healing pressure ulcer of unspecified elbow, stage 1

Pressure pre-ulcer skin changes limited to persistent focal edema, unspecified elbow

---

Four Stages of Pressure Ulcer

Stage 1
Persistent focal edema

Stage 2
Abrasion, blister, partial thickness skin loss involving epidermis and/or dermis

Stage 3
Full thickness skin loss involving damage or necrosis of subcutaneous tissue

Stage 4
Necrosis of soft tissues through to underlying muscle, tendon, or bone

Epidermis
Dermis
Subcutaneous tissue
Superficial fascia
Muscle
Deep fascia
Bone

L89.002   Pressure ulcer of unspecified elbow, stage 2

Healing pressure ulcer of unspecified elbow, stage 2

Pressure ulcer with abrasion, blister, partial thickness skin loss involving epidermis and/or dermis, unspecified elbow

L89.003   Pressure ulcer of unspecified elbow, stage 3   MCC H4 HCC SW

Healing pressure ulcer of unspecified elbow, stage 3

Pressure ulcer with full thickness skin loss involving damage or necrosis of subcutaneous tissue, unspecified elbow

L89.004   Pressure ulcer of unspecified elbow, stage 4   MCC H4 HCC SW

Healing pressure ulcer of unspecified elbow, stage 4

Pressure ulcer with necrosis of soft tissues through to underlying muscle, tendon, or bone, unspecified elbow

L89.009   Pressure ulcer of unspecified elbow, unspecified stage

Healing pressure ulcer of elbow NOS

Healing pressure ulcer of unspecified elbow, unspecified stage

✓6ᵗʰ   L89.01   Pressure ulcer of right elbow

L89.010   Pressure ulcer of right elbow, unstageable   HCC SW

L89.011   Pressure ulcer of right elbow, stage 1

Healing pressure ulcer of right elbow, stage 1

Pressure pre-ulcer skin changes limited to persistent focal edema, right elbow

L89.012   Pressure ulcer of right elbow, stage 2

Healing pressure ulcer of right elbow, stage 2

Pressure ulcer with abrasion, blister, partial thickness skin loss involving epidermis and/or dermis, right elbow

L89.013   Pressure ulcer of right elbow, stage 3   MCC H4 HCC SW

Healing pressure ulcer of right elbow, stage 3

Pressure ulcer with full thickness skin loss involving damage or necrosis of subcutaneous tissue, right elbow

L89.014   Pressure ulcer of right elbow, stage 4   MCC H4 HCC SW

Healing pressure ulcer of right elbow, stage 4

Pressure ulcer with necrosis of soft tissues through to underlying muscle, tendon, or bone, right elbow

---

✔ Additional Character Required   ✓x7ᵗʰ Placeholder   Unacceptable PDx   Questionable PDx   Manifestation   H1-H14 HAC   HCC CMS-HCC Dx   HIV HIV Dx

ICD-10-CM 2019   725

L89.Ø19 Pressure ulcer of right elbow, unspecified stage
   Healing pressure right of elbow NOS
   Healing pressure ulcer of right elbow, unspecified stage

✓6ᵗʰ **L89.Ø2 Pressure ulcer of left elbow**

L89.Ø2Ø Pressure ulcer of left elbow, unstageable `HCC` `SW`

L89.Ø21 Pressure ulcer of left elbow, stage 1
   Healing pressure ulcer of left elbow, stage 1
   Pressure pre-ulcer skin changes limited to persistent focal edema, left elbow

L89.Ø22 Pressure ulcer of left elbow, stage 2
   Healing pressure ulcer of left elbow, stage 2
   Pressure ulcer with abrasion, blister, partial thickness skin loss involving epidermis and/or dermis, left elbow

L89.Ø23 Pressure ulcer of left elbow, stage 3 `MCC` `H4` `HCC` `SW`
   Healing pressure ulcer of left elbow, stage 3
   Pressure ulcer with full thickness skin loss involving damage or necrosis of subcutaneous tissue, left elbow

L89.Ø24 Pressure ulcer of left elbow, stage 4 `MCC` `H4` `HCC` `SW`
   Healing pressure ulcer of left elbow, stage 4
   Pressure ulcer with necrosis of soft tissues through to underlying muscle, tendon, or bone, left elbow

L89.Ø29 Pressure ulcer of left elbow, unspecified stage
   Healing pressure ulcer of left of elbow NOS
   Healing pressure ulcer of left elbow, unspecified stage

✓5ᵗʰ **L89.1 Pressure ulcer of back**

✓6ᵗʰ **L89.1Ø Pressure ulcer of unspecified part of back**

L89.1ØØ Pressure ulcer of unspecified part of back, unstageable `HCC` `SW`

L89.1Ø1 Pressure ulcer of unspecified part of back, stage 1
   Healing pressure ulcer of unspecified part of back, stage 1
   Pressure pre-ulcer skin changes limited to persistent focal edema, unspecified part of back

L89.1Ø2 Pressure ulcer of unspecified part of back, stage 2
   Healing pressure ulcer of unspecified part of back, stage 2
   Pressure ulcer with abrasion, blister, partial thickness skin loss involving epidermis and/or dermis, unspecified part of back

L89.1Ø3 Pressure ulcer of unspecified part of back, stage 3 `MCC` `H4` `HCC` `SW`
   Healing pressure ulcer of unspecified part of back, stage 3
   Pressure ulcer with full thickness skin loss involving damage or necrosis of subcutaneous tissue, unspecified part of back

L89.1Ø4 Pressure ulcer of unspecified part of back, stage 4 `MCC` `H4` `HCC` `SW`
   Healing pressure ulcer of unspecified part of back, stage 4
   Pressure ulcer with necrosis of soft tissues through to underlying muscle, tendon, or bone, unspecified part of back

L89.1Ø9 Pressure ulcer of unspecified part of back, unspecified stage
   Healing pressure ulcer of unspecified part of back NOS
   Healing pressure ulcer of unspecified part of back, unspecified stage

✓6ᵗʰ **L89.11 Pressure ulcer of right upper back**
   Pressure ulcer of right shoulder blade

L89.11Ø Pressure ulcer of right upper back, unstageable `HCC` `SW`

L89.111 Pressure ulcer of right upper back, stage 1
   Healing pressure ulcer of right upper back, stage 1
   Pressure pre-ulcer skin changes limited to persistent focal edema, right upper back

L89.112 Pressure ulcer of right upper back, stage 2
   Healing pressure ulcer of right upper back, stage 2
   Pressure ulcer with abrasion, blister, partial thickness skin loss involving epidermis and/or dermis, right upper back

L89.113 Pressure ulcer of right upper back, stage 3 `MCC` `H4` `HCC` `SW`
   Healing pressure ulcer of right upper back, stage 3
   Pressure ulcer with full thickness skin loss involving damage or necrosis of subcutaneous tissue, right upper back

L89.114 Pressure ulcer of right upper back, stage 4 `MCC` `H4` `HCC` `SW`
   Healing pressure ulcer of right upper back, stage 4
   Pressure ulcer with necrosis of soft tissues through to underlying muscle, tendon, or bone, right upper back

L89.119 Pressure ulcer of right upper back, unspecified stage
   Healing pressure ulcer of right upper back NOS
   Healing pressure ulcer of right upper back, unspecified stage

✓6ᵗʰ **L89.12 Pressure ulcer of left upper back**
   Pressure ulcer of left shoulder blade

L89.12Ø Pressure ulcer of left upper back, unstageable `HCC` `SW`

L89.121 Pressure ulcer of left upper back, stage 1
   Healing pressure ulcer of left upper back, stage 1
   Pressure pre-ulcer skin changes limited to persistent focal edema, left upper back

L89.122 Pressure ulcer of left upper back, stage 2
   Healing pressure ulcer of left upper back, stage 2
   Pressure ulcer with abrasion, blister, partial thickness skin loss involving epidermis and/or dermis, left upper back

L89.123 Pressure ulcer of left upper back, stage 3 `MCC` `H4` `HCC` `SW`
   Healing pressure ulcer of left upper back, stage 3
   Pressure ulcer with full thickness skin loss involving damage or necrosis of subcutaneous tissue, left upper back

L89.124 Pressure ulcer of left upper back, stage 4 `MCC` `H4` `HCC` `SW`
   Healing pressure ulcer of left upper back, stage 4
   Pressure ulcer with necrosis of soft tissues through to underlying muscle, tendon, or bone, left upper back

L89.129 Pressure ulcer of left upper back, unspecified stage
   Healing pressure ulcer of left upper back NOS
   Healing pressure ulcer of left upper back, unspecified stage

✓6ᵗʰ **L89.13 Pressure ulcer of right lower back**

L89.13Ø Pressure ulcer of right lower back, unstageable `HCC` `SW`

L89.131 Pressure ulcer of right lower back, stage 1
   Healing pressure ulcer of right lower back, stage 1
   Pressure pre-ulcer skin changes limited to persistent focal edema, right lower back

L89.132 Pressure ulcer of right lower back, stage 2
   Healing pressure ulcer of right lower back, stage 2
   Pressure ulcer with abrasion, blister, partial thickness skin loss involving epidermis and/or dermis, right lower back

N Newborn: 0   P Pediatric: 0-17   M Maternity: 12-55   A Adult: 15-124   `MCC` Major Complication/Comorbidity   `CC` Complication/Comorbidity   `SW` Severe Wound Dx

726   ICD-10-CM 2019

L89.133   **Pressure ulcer of right lower back, stage 3**   `MCC` `H4` `HCC` `SW`
     Healing pressure ulcer of right lower back, stage 3
     Pressure ulcer with full thickness skin loss involving damage or necrosis of subcutaneous tissue, right lower back

L89.134   **Pressure ulcer of right lower back, stage 4**   `MCC` `H4` `HCC` `SW`
     Healing pressure ulcer of right lower back, stage 4
     Pressure ulcer with necrosis of soft tissues through to underlying muscle, tendon, or bone, right lower back

L89.139   **Pressure ulcer of right lower back, unspecified stage**
     Healing pressure ulcer of right lower back NOS
     Healing pressure ulcer of right lower back, unspecified stage

✓6ᵗʰ **L89.14**   **Pressure ulcer of left lower back**

L89.140   **Pressure ulcer of left lower back, unstageable**   `HCC` `SW`

L89.141   **Pressure ulcer of left lower back, stage 1**
     Healing pressure ulcer of left lower back, stage 1
     Pressure pre-ulcer skin changes limited to persistent focal edema, left lower back

L89.142   **Pressure ulcer of left lower back, stage 2**
     Healing pressure ulcer of left lower back, stage 2
     Pressure ulcer with abrasion, blister, partial thickness skin loss involving epidermis and/or dermis, left lower back

L89.143   **Pressure ulcer of left lower back, stage 3**   `MCC` `H4` `HCC` `SW`
     Healing pressure ulcer of left lower back, stage 3
     Pressure ulcer with full thickness skin loss involving damage or necrosis of subcutaneous tissue, left lower back

L89.144   **Pressure ulcer of left lower back, stage 4**   `MCC` `H4` `HCC` `SW`
     Healing pressure ulcer of left lower back, stage 4
     Pressure ulcer with necrosis of soft tissues through to underlying muscle, tendon, or bone, left lower back

L89.149   **Pressure ulcer of left lower back, unspecified stage**
     Healing pressure ulcer of left lower back NOS
     Healing pressure ulcer of left lower back, unspecified stage

✓6ᵗʰ **L89.15**   **Pressure ulcer of sacral region**
     Pressure ulcer of coccyx
     Pressure ulcer of tailbone

L89.150   **Pressure ulcer of sacral region, unstageable**   `HCC` `SW`

L89.151   **Pressure ulcer of sacral region, stage 1**
     Healing pressure ulcer of sacral region, stage 1
     Pressure pre-ulcer skin changes limited to persistent focal edema, sacral region

L89.152   **Pressure ulcer of sacral region, stage 2**
     Healing pressure ulcer of sacral region, stage 2
     Pressure ulcer with abrasion, blister, partial thickness skin loss involving epidermis and/or dermis, sacral region

L89.153   **Pressure ulcer of sacral region, stage 3**   `MCC` `H4` `HCC` `SW`
     Healing pressure ulcer of sacral region, stage 3
     Pressure ulcer with full thickness skin loss involving damage or necrosis of subcutaneous tissue, sacral region

L89.154   **Pressure ulcer of sacral region, stage 4**   `MCC` `H4` `HCC` `SW`
     Healing pressure ulcer of sacral region, stage 4
     Pressure ulcer with necrosis of soft tissues through to underlying muscle, tendon, or bone, sacral region

L89.159   **Pressure ulcer of sacral region, unspecified stage**
     Healing pressure ulcer of sacral region NOS
     Healing pressure ulcer of sacral region, unspecified stage

✓5ᵗʰ **L89.2**   **Pressure ulcer of hip**

✓6ᵗʰ **L89.20**   **Pressure ulcer of unspecified hip**

L89.200   **Pressure ulcer of unspecified hip, unstageable**   `HCC` `SW`

L89.201   **Pressure ulcer of unspecified hip, stage 1**
     Healing pressure ulcer of unspecified hip back, stage 1
     Pressure pre-ulcer skin changes limited to persistent focal edema, unspecified hip

L89.202   **Pressure ulcer of unspecified hip, stage 2**
     Healing pressure ulcer of unspecified hip, stage 2
     Pressure ulcer with abrasion, blister, partial thickness skin loss involving epidermis and/or dermis, unspecified hip

L89.203   **Pressure ulcer of unspecified hip, stage 3**   `MCC` `H4` `HCC` `SW`
     Healing pressure ulcer of unspecified hip, stage 3
     Pressure ulcer with full thickness skin loss involving damage or necrosis of subcutaneous tissue, unspecified hip

L89.204   **Pressure ulcer of unspecified hip, stage 4**   `MCC` `H4` `HCC` `SW`
     Healing pressure ulcer of unspecified hip, stage 4
     Pressure ulcer with necrosis of soft tissues through to underlying muscle, tendon, or bone, unspecified hip

L89.209   **Pressure ulcer of unspecified hip, unspecified stage**
     Healing pressure ulcer of unspecified hip NOS
     Healing pressure ulcer of unspecified hip, unspecified stage

✓6ᵗʰ **L89.21**   **Pressure ulcer of right hip**

L89.210   **Pressure ulcer of right hip, unstageable**   `HCC` `SW`

L89.211   **Pressure ulcer of right hip, stage 1**
     Healing pressure ulcer of right hip back, stage 1
     Pressure pre-ulcer skin changes limited to persistent focal edema, right hip

L89.212   **Pressure ulcer of right hip, stage 2**
     Healing pressure ulcer of right hip, stage 2
     Pressure ulcer with abrasion, blister, partial thickness skin loss involving epidermis and/or dermis, right hip

L89.213   **Pressure ulcer of right hip, stage 3**   `MCC` `H4` `HCC` `SW`
     Healing pressure ulcer of right hip, stage 3
     Pressure ulcer with full thickness skin loss involving damage or necrosis of subcutaneous tissue, right hip

L89.214   **Pressure ulcer of right hip, stage 4**   `MCC` `H4` `HCC` `SW`
     Healing pressure ulcer of right hip, stage 4
     Pressure ulcer with necrosis of soft tissues through to underlying muscle, tendon, or bone, right hip

L89.219   **Pressure ulcer of right hip, unspecified stage**
     Healing pressure ulcer of right hip NOS
     Healing pressure ulcer of right hip, unspecified stage

✓6ᵗʰ **L89.22**   **Pressure ulcer of left hip**

L89.220   **Pressure ulcer of left hip, unstageable**   `HCC` `SW`

L89.221   **Pressure ulcer of left hip, stage 1**
     Healing pressure ulcer of left hip back, stage 1
     Pressure pre-ulcer skin changes limited to persistent focal edema, left hip

L89.222   **Pressure ulcer of left hip, stage 2**
     Healing pressure ulcer of left hip, stage 2
     Pressure ulcer with abrasion, blister, partial thickness skin loss involving epidermis and/or dermis, left hip

✔ Additional Character Required   ✓x7ᵗʰ Placeholder   Unacceptable PDx   Questionable PDx   Manifestation   `H1`-`H14` HAC   `HCC` CMS-HCC Dx   `HIV` HIV Dx

ICD-10-CM 2019   727

Chapter 12. Diseases of the Skin and Subcutaneous Tissue

L89.133–L89.222

L89.223 **Pressure ulcer of left hip, stage 3** `MCC` `H4` `HCC` `SW`
Healing pressure ulcer of left hip, stage 3
Pressure ulcer with full thickness skin loss involving damage or necrosis of subcutaneous tissue, left hip

L89.224 **Pressure ulcer of left hip, stage 4** `MCC` `H4` `HCC` `SW`
Healing pressure ulcer of left hip, stage 4
Pressure ulcer with necrosis of soft tissues through to underlying muscle, tendon, or bone, left hip

L89.229 **Pressure ulcer of left hip, unspecified stage**
Healing pressure ulcer of left hip NOS
Healing pressure ulcer of left hip, unspecified stage

✓5ᵗʰ **L89.3** **Pressure ulcer of buttock**

  ✓6ᵗʰ **L89.30** **Pressure ulcer of unspecified buttock**

L89.300 **Pressure ulcer of unspecified buttock, unstageable** `HCC` `SW`

L89.301 **Pressure ulcer of unspecified buttock, stage 1**
Healing pressure ulcer of unspecified buttock, stage 1
Pressure pre-ulcer skin changes limited to persistent focal edema, unspecified buttock

L89.302 **Pressure ulcer of unspecified buttock, stage 2**
Healing pressure ulcer of unspecified buttock, stage 2
Pressure ulcer with abrasion, blister, partial thickness skin loss involving epidermis and/or dermis, unspecified buttock

L89.303 **Pressure ulcer of unspecified buttock, stage 3** `MCC` `H4` `HCC` `SW`
Healing pressure ulcer of unspecified buttock, stage 3
Pressure ulcer with full thickness skin loss involving damage or necrosis of subcutaneous tissue, unspecified buttock

L89.304 **Pressure ulcer of unspecified buttock, stage 4** `MCC` `H4` `HCC` `SW`
Healing pressure ulcer of unspecified buttock, stage 4
Pressure ulcer with necrosis of soft tissues through to underlying muscle, tendon, or bone, unspecified buttock

L89.309 **Pressure ulcer of unspecified buttock, unspecified stage**
Healing pressure ulcer of unspecified buttock NOS
Healing pressure ulcer of unspecified buttock, unspecified stage

  ✓6ᵗʰ **L89.31** **Pressure ulcer of right buttock**

L89.310 **Pressure ulcer of right buttock, unstageable** `HCC` `SW`

L89.311 **Pressure ulcer of right buttock, stage 1**
Healing pressure ulcer of right buttock, stage 1
Pressure pre-ulcer skin changes limited to persistent focal edema, right buttock

L89.312 **Pressure ulcer of right buttock, stage 2**
Healing pressure ulcer of right buttock, stage 2
Pressure ulcer with abrasion, blister, partial thickness skin loss involving epidermis and/or dermis, right buttock

L89.313 **Pressure ulcer of right buttock, unspecified stage 3** `MCC` `H4` `HCC` `SW`
Healing pressure ulcer of right buttock, stage 3
Pressure ulcer with full thickness skin loss involving damage or necrosis of subcutaneous tissue, right buttock

L89.314 **Pressure ulcer of right buttock, unspecified stage 4** `MCC` `H4` `HCC` `SW`
Healing pressure ulcer of right buttock, stage 4
Pressure ulcer with necrosis of soft tissues through to underlying muscle, tendon, or bone, right buttock

L89.319 **Pressure ulcer of right buttock, unspecified stage**
Healing pressure ulcer of right buttock NOS
Healing pressure ulcer of right buttock, unspecified stage

✓6ᵗʰ **L89.32** **Pressure ulcer of left buttock**

L89.320 **Pressure ulcer of left buttock, unstageable** `HCC` `SW`

L89.321 **Pressure ulcer of left buttock, stage 1**
Healing pressure ulcer of left buttock, stage 1
Pressure pre-ulcer skin changes limited to persistent focal edema, left buttock

L89.322 **Pressure ulcer of left buttock, stage 2**
Healing pressure ulcer of left buttock, stage 2
Pressure ulcer with abrasion, blister, partial thickness skin loss involving epidermis and/or dermis, left buttock

L89.323 **Pressure ulcer of left buttock, stage 3** `MCC` `H4` `HCC` `SW`
Healing pressure ulcer of left buttock, stage 3
Pressure ulcer with full thickness skin loss involving damage or necrosis of subcutaneous tissue, left buttock

L89.324 **Pressure ulcer of left buttock, stage 4** `MCC` `H4` `HCC` `SW`
Healing pressure ulcer of left buttock, stage 4
Pressure ulcer with necrosis of soft tissues through to underlying muscle, tendon, or bone, left buttock

L89.329 **Pressure ulcer of left buttock, unspecified stage**
Healing pressure ulcer of left buttock NOS
Healing pressure ulcer of left buttock, unspecified stage

✓5ᵗʰ **L89.4** **Pressure ulcer of contiguous site of back, buttock and hip**

L89.40 **Pressure ulcer of contiguous site of back, buttock and hip, unspecified stage**
Healing pressure ulcer of contiguous site of back, buttock and hip NOS
Healing pressure ulcer of contiguous site of back, buttock and hip, unspecified stage

L89.41 **Pressure ulcer of contiguous site of back, buttock and hip, stage 1**
Healing pressure ulcer of contiguous site of back, buttock and hip, stage 1
Pressure pre-ulcer skin changes limited to persistent focal edema, contiguous site of back, buttock and hip

L89.42 **Pressure ulcer of contiguous site of back, buttock and hip, stage 2**
Healing pressure ulcer of contiguous site of back, buttock and hip, stage 2
Pressure ulcer with abrasion, blister, partial thickness skin loss involving epidermis and/or dermis, contiguous site of back, buttock and hip

L89.43 **Pressure ulcer of contiguous site of back, buttock and hip, stage 3** `MCC` `H4` `HCC` `SW`
Healing pressure ulcer of contiguous site of back, buttock and hip, stage 3
Pressure ulcer with full thickness skin loss involving damage or necrosis of subcutaneous tissue, contiguous site of back, buttock and hip

L89.44 **Pressure ulcer of contiguous site of back, buttock and hip, stage 4** `MCC` `H4` `HCC` `SW`
Healing pressure ulcer of contiguous site of back, buttock and hip, stage 4
Pressure ulcer with necrosis of soft tissues through to underlying muscle, tendon, or bone, contiguous site of back, buttock and hip

L89.45 **Pressure ulcer of contiguous site of back, buttock and hip, unstageable** `HCC` `SW`

N Newborn: 0   **P** Pediatric: 0-17   **M** Maternity: 12-55   **A** Adult: 15-124   `MCC` Major Complication/Comorbidity   `CC` Complication/Comorbidity   `SW` Severe Wound Dx

728   ICD-10-CM 2019

Chapter 12. Diseases of the Skin and Subcutaneous Tissue

✓5th **L89.5** **Pressure ulcer of** ankle

  ✓6th **L89.50** **Pressure ulcer of** unspecified ankle

    L89.500 **Pressure ulcer of unspecified ankle,** unstageable   `HCC` `SW`

    L89.501 **Pressure ulcer of unspecified ankle,** stage 1
      Healing pressure ulcer of unspecified ankle, stage 1
      Pressure pre-ulcer skin changes limited to persistent focal edema, unspecified ankle

    L89.502 **Pressure ulcer of unspecified ankle,** stage 2
      Healing pressure ulcer of unspecified ankle, stage 2
      Pressure ulcer with abrasion, blister, partial thickness skin loss involving epidermis and/or dermis, unspecified ankle

    L89.503 **Pressure ulcer of unspecified ankle,** stage 3   `MCC` `H4` `HCC` `SW`
      Healing pressure ulcer of unspecified ankle, stage 3
      Pressure ulcer with full thickness skin loss involving damage or necrosis of subcutaneous tissue, unspecified ankle

    L89.504 **Pressure ulcer of unspecified ankle,** stage 4   `MCC` `H4` `HCC` `SW`
      Healing pressure ulcer of unspecified ankle, stage 4
      Pressure ulcer with necrosis of soft tissues through to underlying muscle, tendon, or bone, unspecified ankle

    L89.509 **Pressure ulcer of unspecified ankle,** unspecified stage
      Healing pressure ulcer of unspecified ankle NOS
      Healing pressure ulcer of unspecified ankle, unspecified stage

  ✓6th **L89.51** **Pressure ulcer of** right ankle

    L89.510 **Pressure ulcer of right ankle,** unstageable   `HCC` `SW`

    L89.511 **Pressure ulcer of right ankle,** stage 1
      Healing pressure ulcer of right ankle, stage 1
      Pressure pre-ulcer skin changes limited to persistent focal edema, right ankle

    L89.512 **Pressure ulcer of right ankle,** stage 2
      Healing pressure ulcer of right ankle, stage 2
      Pressure pre-ulcer skin changes limited to persistent focal edema, right ankle

    L89.513 **Pressure ulcer of right ankle,** stage 3   `MCC` `H4` `HCC` `SW`
      Healing pressure ulcer of right ankle, stage 3
      Pressure ulcer with full thickness skin loss involving damage or necrosis of subcutaneous tissue, right ankle

    L89.514 **Pressure ulcer of right ankle,** stage 4   `MCC` `H4` `HCC` `SW`
      Healing pressure ulcer of right ankle, stage 4
      Pressure ulcer with necrosis of soft tissues through to underlying muscle, tendon, or bone, right ankle

    L89.519 **Pressure ulcer of right ankle,** unspecified stage
      Healing pressure ulcer of right ankle NOS
      Healing pressure ulcer of right ankle, unspecified stage

  ✓6th **L89.52** **Pressure ulcer of** left ankle

    L89.520 **Pressure ulcer of left ankle,** unstageable   `HCC` `SW`

    L89.521 **Pressure ulcer of left ankle,** stage 1
      Healing pressure ulcer of left ankle, stage 1
      Pressure pre-ulcer skin changes limited to persistent focal edema, left ankle

    L89.522 **Pressure ulcer of left ankle,** stage 2
      Healing pressure ulcer of left ankle, stage 2
      Pressure ulcer with abrasion, blister, partial thickness skin loss involving epidermis and/or dermis, left ankle

    L89.523 **Pressure ulcer of left ankle,** stage 3   `MCC` `H4` `HCC` `SW`
      Healing pressure ulcer of left ankle, stage 3
      Pressure ulcer with full thickness skin loss involving damage or necrosis of subcutaneous tissue, left ankle

    L89.524 **Pressure ulcer of left ankle,** stage 4   `MCC` `H4` `HCC` `SW`
      Healing pressure ulcer of left ankle, stage 4
      Pressure ulcer with necrosis of soft tissues through to underlying muscle, tendon, or bone, left ankle

    L89.529 **Pressure ulcer of left ankle,** unspecified stage
      Healing pressure ulcer of left ankle NOS
      Healing pressure ulcer of left ankle, unspecified stage

✓5th **L89.6** **Pressure ulcer of** heel

  ✓6th **L89.60** **Pressure ulcer of** unspecified heel

    L89.600 **Pressure ulcer of unspecified heel,** unstageable   `HCC` `SW`

    L89.601 **Pressure ulcer of unspecified heel,** stage 1
      Healing pressure ulcer of unspecified heel, stage 1
      Pressure pre-ulcer skin changes limited to persistent focal edema, unspecified heel

    L89.602 **Pressure ulcer of unspecified heel,** stage 2
      Healing pressure ulcer of unspecified heel, stage 2
      Pressure ulcer with abrasion, blister, partial thickness skin loss involving epidermis and/or dermis, unspecified heel

    L89.603 **Pressure ulcer of unspecified heel,** stage 3   `MCC` `H4` `HCC` `SW`
      Healing pressure ulcer of unspecified heel, stage 3
      Pressure ulcer with full thickness skin loss involving damage or necrosis of subcutaneous tissue, unspecified heel

    L89.604 **Pressure ulcer of unspecified heel,** stage 4   `MCC` `H4` `HCC` `SW`
      Healing pressure ulcer of unspecified heel, stage 4
      Pressure ulcer with necrosis of soft tissues through to underlying muscle, tendon, or bone, unspecified heel

    L89.609 **Pressure ulcer of unspecified heel,** unspecified stage
      Healing pressure ulcer of unspecified heel NOS
      Healing pressure ulcer of unspecified heel, unspecified stage

  ✓6th **L89.61** **Pressure ulcer of** right heel

    L89.610 **Pressure ulcer of right heel,** unstageable   `HCC` `SW`

    L89.611 **Pressure ulcer of right heel,** stage 1
      Healing pressure ulcer of right heel, stage 1
      Pressure pre-ulcer skin changes limited to persistent focal edema, right heel

    L89.612 **Pressure ulcer of right heel,** stage 2
      Healing pressure ulcer of right heel, stage 2
      Pressure ulcer with abrasion, blister, partial thickness skin loss involving epidermis and/or dermis, right heel

    L89.613 **Pressure ulcer of right heel,** stage 3   `MCC` `H4` `HCC` `SW`
      Healing pressure ulcer of right heel, stage 3
      Pressure ulcer with full thickness skin loss involving damage or necrosis of subcutaneous tissue, right heel

    L89.614 **Pressure ulcer of right heel,** stage 4   `MCC` `H4` `HCC` `SW`
      Healing pressure ulcer of right heel, stage 4
      Pressure ulcer with necrosis of soft tissues through to underlying muscle, tendon, or bone, right heel

    L89.619 **Pressure ulcer of right heel,** unspecified stage
      Healing pressure ulcer of right heel NOS
      Healing pressure ulcer of right heel, unspecified stage

✔ Additional Character Required   ✓x7th Placeholder   Unacceptable PDx   Questionable PDx   Manifestation   `H1`-`H14` HAC   `HCC` CMS-HCC Dx   `HIV` HIV Dx

ICD-10-CM 2019   729

Chapter 12. Diseases of the Skin and Subcutaneous Tissue (side margin)

L89.62–L92.1 (side margin)

✓6ᵗʰ **L89.62 Pressure ulcer of** left heel

L89.620 Pressure ulcer of left heel, unstageable `HCC` `SW`

L89.621 Pressure ulcer of left heel, stage 1
Healing pressure ulcer of left heel, stage 1
Pressure pre-ulcer skin changes limited to persistent focal edema, left heel

L89.622 Pressure ulcer of left heel, stage 2
Healing pressure ulcer of left heel, stage 2
Pressure ulcer with abrasion, blister, partial thickness skin loss involving epidermis and/or dermis, left heel

L89.623 Pressure ulcer of left heel, stage 3 `MCC` `H4` `HCC` `SW`
Healing pressure ulcer of left heel, stage 3
Pressure ulcer with full thickness skin loss involving damage or necrosis of subcutaneous tissue, left heel

L89.624 Pressure ulcer of left heel, stage 4 `MCC` `H4` `HCC` `SW`
Healing pressure ulcer of left heel, stage 4
Pressure ulcer with necrosis of soft tissues through to underlying muscle, tendon, or bone, left heel

L89.629 Pressure ulcer of left heel, unspecified stage
Healing pressure ulcer of left heel NOS
Healing pressure ulcer of left heel, unspecified stage

✓5ᵗʰ **L89.8 Pressure ulcer of** other site

✓6ᵗʰ **L89.81 Pressure ulcer of** head
Pressure ulcer of face

L89.810 Pressure ulcer of head, unstageable `HCC` `SW`

L89.811 Pressure ulcer of head, stage 1
Healing pressure ulcer of head, stage 1
Pressure pre-ulcer skin changes limited to persistent focal edema, head

L89.812 Pressure ulcer of head, stage 2
Healing pressure ulcer of head, stage 2
Pressure ulcer with abrasion, blister, partial thickness skin loss involving epidermis and/or dermis, head

L89.813 Pressure ulcer of head, stage 3 `MCC` `H4` `HCC` `SW`
Healing pressure ulcer of head, stage 3
Pressure ulcer with full thickness skin loss involving damage or necrosis of subcutaneous tissue, head

L89.814 Pressure ulcer of head, stage 4 `MCC` `H4` `HCC` `SW`
Healing pressure ulcer of head, stage 4
Pressure ulcer with necrosis of soft tissues through to underlying muscle, tendon, or bone, head

L89.819 Pressure ulcer of head, unspecified stage
Healing pressure ulcer of head NOS
Healing pressure ulcer of head, unspecified stage

✓6ᵗʰ **L89.89 Pressure ulcer of** other site

L89.890 Pressure ulcer of other site, unstageable `HCC` `SW`

L89.891 Pressure ulcer of other site, stage 1
Healing pressure ulcer of other site, stage 1
Pressure pre-ulcer skin changes limited to persistent focal edema, other site

L89.892 Pressure ulcer of other site, stage 2
Healing pressure ulcer of other site, stage 2
Pressure ulcer with abrasion, blister, partial thickness skin loss involving epidermis and/or dermis, other site

L89.893 Pressure ulcer of other site, stage 3 `MCC` `H4` `HCC` `SW`
Healing pressure ulcer of other site, stage 3
Pressure ulcer with full thickness skin loss involving damage or necrosis of subcutaneous tissue, other site

L89.894 Pressure ulcer of other site, stage 4 `MCC` `H4` `HCC` `SW`
Healing pressure ulcer of other site, stage 4
Pressure ulcer with necrosis of soft tissues through to underlying muscle, tendon, or bone, other site

L89.899 Pressure ulcer of other site, unspecified stage
Healing pressure ulcer of other site NOS
Healing pressure ulcer of other site, unspecified stage

✓5ᵗʰ **L89.9 Pressure ulcer of** unspecified site

L89.90 Pressure ulcer of unspecified site, unspecified stage
Healing pressure ulcer of unspecified site NOS
Healing pressure ulcer of unspecified site, unspecified stage

L89.91 Pressure ulcer of unspecified site, stage 1
Healing pressure ulcer of unspecified site, stage 1
Pressure pre-ulcer skin changes limited to persistent focal edema, unspecified site

L89.92 Pressure ulcer of unspecified site, stage 2
Healing pressure ulcer of unspecified site, stage 2
Pressure ulcer with abrasion, blister, partial thickness skin loss involving epidermis and/or dermis, unspecified site

L89.93 Pressure ulcer of unspecified site, stage 3 `MCC` `H4` `HCC` `SW`
Healing pressure ulcer of unspecified site, stage 3
Pressure ulcer with full thickness skin loss involving damage or necrosis of subcutaneous tissue, unspecified site

L89.94 Pressure ulcer of unspecified site, stage 4 `MCC` `H4` `HCC` `SW`
Healing pressure ulcer of unspecified site, stage 4
Pressure ulcer with necrosis of soft tissues through to underlying muscle, tendon, or bone, unspecified site

L89.95 Pressure ulcer of unspecified site, unstageable `HCC` `SW`

✓4ᵗʰ **L90 Atrophic disorders of skin**

L90.0 Lichen sclerosus et atrophicus
EXCLUDES 2   lichen sclerosus of external female genital organs (N90.4)
lichen sclerosus of external male genital organs (N48.0)

L90.1 Anetoderma of Schweninger-Buzzi

L90.2 Anetoderma of Jadassohn-Pellizzari

L90.3 Atrophoderma of Pasini and Pierini

L90.4 Acrodermatitis chronica atrophicans

L90.5 Scar conditions and fibrosis of skin
Adherent scar (skin)
Cicatrix
Disfigurement of skin due to scar
Fibrosis of skin NOS
Scar NOS
EXCLUDES 2   hypertrophic scar (L91.0)
keloid scar (L91.0)
AHA: 2016, 2Q, 5; 2015, 1Q, 19

L90.6 Striae atrophicae

L90.8 Other atrophic disorders of skin

L90.9 Atrophic disorder of skin, unspecified

✓4ᵗʰ **L91 Hypertrophic disorders of skin**

L91.0 Hypertrophic scar
Keloid
Keloid scar
EXCLUDES 2   acne keloid (L73.0)
scar NOS (L90.5)
DEF: Overgrowth of scar tissue due to excess amounts of collagen during connective tissue repair, occurring mainly on the upper trunk and face.

L91.8 Other hypertrophic disorders of the skin

L91.9 Hypertrophic disorder of the skin, unspecified

✓4ᵗʰ **L92 Granulomatous disorders of skin and subcutaneous tissue**
EXCLUDES 2   actinic granuloma (L57.5)

L92.0 Granuloma annulare
Perforating granuloma annulare

L92.1 Necrobiosis lipoidica, not elsewhere classified
EXCLUDES 1   necrobiosis lipoidica associated with diabetes mellitus (E08-E13 with .620)

N Newborn: 0   P Pediatric: 0-17   M Maternity: 12-55   A Adult: 15-124   `MCC` Major Complication/Comorbidity   `CC` Complication/Comorbidity   `SW` Severe Wound Dx

730   ICD-10-CM 2019

L92.2   Granuloma faciale [eosinophilic granuloma of skin]

L92.3   Foreign body granuloma of the skin and subcutaneous tissue
> Use additional code to identify the type of retained foreign body (Z18.-)

L92.8   Other granulomatous disorders of the skin and subcutaneous tissue

L92.9   Granulomatous disorder of the skin and subcutaneous tissue, unspecified
> EXCLUDES 2   *umbilical granuloma (P83.81)*
>
> **AHA:** 2017, 4Q, 21-22

✔4ᵗʰ L93   Lupus erythematosus
> Use additional code for adverse effect, if applicable, to identify drug (T36-T50 with fifth or sixth character 5)
> EXCLUDES 1   *lupus exedens (A18.4)*
> *lupus vulgaris (A18.4)*
> *scleroderma (M34.-)*
> *systemic lupus erythematosus (M32.-)*
>
> **DEF:** Inflammatory, autoimmune skin condition in which the body's autoimmune system attacks healthy tissue of the integumentary system.

L93.0   Discoid lupus erythematosus
> Lupus erythematosus NOS

L93.1   Subacute cutaneous lupus erythematosus

L93.2   Other local lupus erythematosus
> Lupus erythematosus profundus
> Lupus panniculitis

✔4ᵗʰ L94   Other localized connective tissue disorders
> EXCLUDES 1   *systemic connective tissue disorders (M30-M36)*

L94.0   Localized scleroderma [morphea]
> Circumscribed scleroderma

L94.1   Linear scleroderma
> En coup de sabre lesion

L94.2   Calcinosis cutis

L94.3   Sclerodactyly

L94.4   Gottron's papules

L94.5   Poikiloderma vasculare atrophicans

L94.6   Ainhum

L94.8   Other specified localized connective tissue disorders

L94.9   Localized connective tissue disorder, unspecified

✔4ᵗʰ L95   Vasculitis limited to skin, not elsewhere classified
> EXCLUDES 1   *angioma serpiginosum (L81.7)*
> *Henoch(-Schönlein) purpura (D69.0)*
> *hypersensitivity angiitis (M31.0)*
> *lupus panniculitis (L93.2)*
> *panniculitis NOS (M79.3)*
> *panniculitis of neck and back (M54.0-)*
> *polyarteritis nodosa (M30.0)*
> *relapsing panniculitis (M35.6)*
> *rheumatoid vasculitis (M05.2)*
> *serum sickness (T80.6-)*
> *urticaria (L50.-)*
> *Wegener's granulomatosis (M31.3-)*

L95.0   Livedoid vasculitis
> Atrophie blanche (en plaque)

L95.1   Erythema elevatum diutinum

L95.8   Other vasculitis limited to the skin

L95.9   Vasculitis limited to the skin, unspecified

✔4ᵗʰ L97   Non-pressure chronic ulcer of lower limb, not elsewhere classified
> INCLUDES   chronic ulcer of skin of lower limb NOS
> non-healing ulcer of skin
> non-infected sinus of skin
> trophic ulcer NOS
> tropical ulcer NOS
> ulcer of skin of lower limb NOS

Code first any associated underlying condition, such as:
> any associated gangrene (I96)
> atherosclerosis of the lower extremities (I70.23-, I70.24-, I70.33-, I70.34-, I70.43-, I70.44-, I70.53-, I70.54-, I70.63-, I70.64-, I70.73-, I70.74-)
> chronic venous hypertension (I87.31-, I87.33-)
> diabetic ulcers (E08.621, E08.622, E09.621, E09.622, E10.621, E10.622, E11.621, E11.622, E13.621, E13.622)
> postphlebitic syndrome (I87.01-, I87.03-)
> postthrombotic syndrome (I87.01-, I87.03-)
> varicose ulcer (I83.0-, I83.2-)
> EXCLUDES 2   *pressure ulcer (pressure area) (L89.-)*
> *skin infections (L00-L08)*
> *specific infections classified to A00-B99*

AHA: 2017, 4Q, 17
TIP: The depth and/or severity of a diagnosed nonpressure ulcer can be determined based on medical record documentation from clinicians who are not the patient's provider.
TIP: Assign a code from this category/subcategory for nonpressure ulcers documented as acute.

> **CC Excl: For CC codes in category L97:** PDX collection 698

✔5ᵗʰ L97.1   Non-pressure chronic ulcer of thigh

✔6ᵗʰ L97.10   Non-pressure chronic ulcer of unspecified thigh

L97.101   Non-pressure chronic ulcer of unspecified thigh limited to breakdown of skin   CC HCC

L97.102   Non-pressure chronic ulcer of unspecified thigh with fat layer exposed   CC HCC SW

L97.103   Non-pressure chronic ulcer of unspecified thigh with necrosis of muscle   CC HCC SW

L97.104   Non-pressure chronic ulcer of unspecified thigh with necrosis of bone   CC HCC SW

L97.105   Non-pressure chronic ulcer of unspecified thigh with muscle involvement without evidence of necrosis   CC HCC

L97.106   Non-pressure chronic ulcer of unspecified thigh with bone involvement without evidence of necrosis   CC HCC

L97.108   Non-pressure chronic ulcer of unspecified thigh with other specified severity   CC HCC

L97.109   Non-pressure chronic ulcer of unspecified thigh with unspecified severity   CC HCC

✔6ᵗʰ L97.11   Non-pressure chronic ulcer of right thigh

L97.111   Non-pressure chronic ulcer of right thigh limited to breakdown of skin   CC HCC

L97.112   Non-pressure chronic ulcer of right thigh with fat layer exposed   CC HCC SW

L97.113   Non-pressure chronic ulcer of right thigh with necrosis of muscle   CC HCC SW

L97.114   Non-pressure chronic ulcer of right thigh with necrosis of bone   CC HCC SW

L97.115   Non-pressure chronic ulcer of right thigh with muscle involvement without evidence of necrosis   CC HCC

L97.116   Non-pressure chronic ulcer of right thigh with bone involvement without evidence of necrosis   CC HCC

L97.118   Non-pressure chronic ulcer of right thigh with other specified severity   CC HCC

L97.119   Non-pressure chronic ulcer of right thigh with unspecified severity   CC HCC

✔6ᵗʰ L97.12   Non-pressure chronic ulcer of left thigh

L97.121   Non-pressure chronic ulcer of left thigh limited to breakdown of skin   CC HCC

L97.122   Non-pressure chronic ulcer of left thigh with fat layer exposed   CC HCC SW

L97.123   Non-pressure chronic ulcer of left thigh with necrosis of muscle   CC HCC SW

☑ Additional Character Required   ✓x7ᵗʰ Placeholder   Unacceptable PDx   Questionable PDx   Manifestation   H1-H14 HAC   HCC CMS-HCC Dx   HIV HIV Dx

ICD-10-CM 2019   731

L97.124   Non-pressure chronic ulcer of `CC` `HCC` `SW` left thigh with necrosis of bone

L97.125   Non-pressure chronic ulcer of left `CC` `HCC` thigh with muscle involvement without evidence of necrosis

L97.126   Non-pressure chronic ulcer of left `CC` `HCC` thigh with bone involvement without evidence of necrosis

L97.128   Non-pressure chronic ulcer of left `CC` `HCC` thigh with other specified severity

L97.129   Non-pressure chronic ulcer of left `CC` `HCC` thigh with unspecified severity

√5th **L97.2**   **Non-pressure chronic ulcer of** calf

    √6th **L97.20**   **Non-pressure chronic ulcer of** unspecified calf

L97.201   Non-pressure chronic ulcer of `CC` `HCC` unspecified calf limited to breakdown of skin

L97.202   Non-pressure chronic ulcer of `CC` `HCC` `SW` unspecified calf with fat layer exposed

L97.203   Non-pressure chronic ulcer of `CC` `HCC` `SW` unspecified calf with necrosis of muscle

L97.204   Non-pressure chronic ulcer of `CC` `HCC` `SW` unspecified calf with necrosis of bone

L97.205   Non-pressure chronic ulcer of `CC` `HCC` unspecified calf with muscle involvement without evidence of necrosis

L97.206   Non-pressure chronic ulcer of `CC` `HCC` unspecified calf with bone involvement without evidence of necrosis

L97.208   Non-pressure chronic ulcer of `CC` `HCC` unspecified calf with other specified severity

L97.209   Non-pressure chronic ulcer of `CC` `HCC` unspecified calf with unspecified severity

    √6th **L97.21**   **Non-pressure chronic ulcer of** right calf

L97.211   Non-pressure chronic ulcer of right `CC` `HCC` calf limited to breakdown of skin

L97.212   Non-pressure chronic ulcer of `CC` `HCC` `SW` right calf with fat layer exposed

L97.213   Non-pressure chronic ulcer of `CC` `HCC` `SW` right calf with necrosis of muscle

L97.214   Non-pressure chronic ulcer of `CC` `HCC` `SW` right calf with necrosis of bone

L97.215   Non-pressure chronic ulcer of right `CC` `HCC` calf with muscle involvement without evidence of necrosis

L97.216   Non-pressure chronic ulcer of right `CC` `HCC` calf with bone involvement without evidence of necrosis

L97.218   Non-pressure chronic ulcer of right `CC` `HCC` calf with other specified severity

L97.219   Non-pressure chronic ulcer of right `CC` `HCC` calf with unspecified severity

    √6th **L97.22**   **Non-pressure chronic ulcer of** left calf

L97.221   Non-pressure chronic ulcer of left `CC` `HCC` calf limited to breakdown of skin

L97.222   Non-pressure chronic ulcer of `CC` `HCC` `SW` left calf with fat layer exposed

L97.223   Non-pressure chronic ulcer of `CC` `HCC` `SW` left calf with necrosis of muscle

L97.224   Non-pressure chronic ulcer of `CC` `HCC` `SW` left calf with necrosis of bone

L97.225   Non-pressure chronic ulcer of left `CC` `HCC` calf with muscle involvement without evidence of necrosis

L97.226   Non-pressure chronic ulcer of left `CC` `HCC` calf with bone involvement without evidence of necrosis

L97.228   Non-pressure chronic ulcer of left `CC` `HCC` calf with other specified severity

L97.229   Non-pressure chronic ulcer of left `CC` `HCC` calf with unspecified severity

√5th **L97.3**   **Non-pressure chronic ulcer of** ankle

    √6th **L97.30**   **Non-pressure chronic ulcer of** unspecified ankle

L97.301   Non-pressure chronic ulcer of `CC` `HCC` unspecified ankle limited to breakdown of skin

L97.302   Non-pressure chronic ulcer of `CC` `HCC` `SW` unspecified ankle with fat layer exposed

L97.303   Non-pressure chronic ulcer of `CC` `HCC` `SW` unspecified ankle with necrosis of muscle

L97.304   Non-pressure chronic ulcer of `CC` `HCC` `SW` unspecified ankle with necrosis of bone

L97.305   Non-pressure chronic ulcer of `CC` `HCC` unspecified ankle with muscle involvement without evidence of necrosis

L97.306   Non-pressure chronic ulcer of `CC` `HCC` unspecified ankle with bone involvement without evidence of necrosis

L97.308   Non-pressure chronic ulcer of `CC` `HCC` unspecified ankle with other specified severity

L97.309   Non-pressure chronic ulcer of `CC` `HCC` unspecified ankle with unspecified severity

    √6th **L97.31**   **Non-pressure chronic ulcer of** right ankle

L97.311   Non-pressure chronic ulcer of right `CC` `HCC` ankle limited to breakdown of skin

L97.312   Non-pressure chronic ulcer of `CC` `HCC` `SW` right ankle with fat layer exposed

L97.313   Non-pressure chronic ulcer of `CC` `HCC` `SW` right ankle with necrosis of muscle

L97.314   Non-pressure chronic ulcer of `CC` `HCC` `SW` right ankle with necrosis of bone

L97.315   Non-pressure chronic ulcer of right `CC` `HCC` ankle with muscle involvement without evidence of necrosis

L97.316   Non-pressure chronic ulcer of right `CC` `HCC` ankle with bone involvement without evidence of necrosis

L97.318   Non-pressure chronic ulcer of right `CC` `HCC` ankle with other specified severity

L97.319   Non-pressure chronic ulcer of right `CC` `HCC` ankle with unspecified severity

    √6th **L97.32**   **Non-pressure chronic ulcer of** left ankle

L97.321   Non-pressure chronic ulcer of left `CC` `HCC` ankle limited to breakdown of skin

L97.322   Non-pressure chronic ulcer of `CC` `HCC` `SW` left ankle with fat layer exposed

L97.323   Non-pressure chronic ulcer of `CC` `HCC` `SW` left ankle with necrosis of muscle

L97.324   Non-pressure chronic ulcer of `CC` `HCC` `SW` left ankle with necrosis of bone

L97.325   Non-pressure chronic ulcer of left `CC` `HCC` ankle with muscle involvement without evidence of necrosis

L97.326   Non-pressure chronic ulcer of left `CC` `HCC` ankle with bone involvement without evidence of necrosis

L97.328   Non-pressure chronic ulcer of left `CC` `HCC` ankle with other specified severity

L97.329   Non-pressure chronic ulcer of left `CC` `HCC` ankle with unspecified severity

√5th **L97.4**   **Non-pressure chronic ulcer of** heel and midfoot
Non-pressure chronic ulcer of plantar surface of midfoot

    √6th **L97.40**   **Non-pressure chronic ulcer of** unspecified heel and midfoot

L97.401   Non-pressure chronic ulcer of `CC` `HCC` unspecified heel and midfoot limited to breakdown of skin

L97.402   Non-pressure chronic ulcer of `CC` `HCC` `SW` unspecified heel and midfoot with fat layer exposed

L97.403   Non-pressure chronic ulcer of `CC` `HCC` `SW` unspecified heel and midfoot with necrosis of muscle

L97.404   Non-pressure chronic ulcer of `CC` `HCC` `SW` unspecified heel and midfoot with necrosis of bone

L97.405   Non-pressure chronic ulcer of `CC` `HCC` unspecified heel and midfoot with muscle involvement without evidence of necrosis

N Newborn: 0   P Pediatric: 0-17   M Maternity: 12-55   A Adult: 15-124   MCC Major Complication/Comorbidity   CC Complication/Comorbidity   SW Severe Wound Dx

732   ICD-10-CM 2019

L97.406   **Non-pressure chronic ulcer of** `CC` `HCC`
unspecified heel and midfoot with
bone involvement without evidence
of necrosis

L97.408   **Non-pressure chronic ulcer of** `CC` `HCC`
unspecified heel and midfoot with
other specified severity

L97.409   **Non-pressure chronic ulcer of** `CC` `HCC`
unspecified heel and midfoot with
unspecified severity

✓6ᵗʰ **L97.41**   **Non-pressure chronic ulcer of** right heel and midfoot

L97.411   **Non-pressure chronic ulcer of** `CC` `HCC`
right heel and midfoot limited
to breakdown of skin

L97.412   **Non-pressure chronic ulcer of** `CC` `HCC` `SW`
right heel and midfoot with fat
layer exposed

L97.413   **Non-pressure chronic ulcer of** `CC` `HCC` `SW`
right heel and midfoot with
necrosis of muscle

L97.414   **Non-pressure chronic ulcer of** `CC` `HCC` `SW`
right heel and midfoot with
necrosis of bone

L97.415   **Non-pressure chronic ulcer of right** `CC` `HCC`
heel and midfoot with muscle
involvement without evidence of necrosis

L97.416   **Non-pressure chronic ulcer of right** `CC` `HCC`
heel and midfoot with bone involvement
without evidence of necrosis

L97.418   **Non-pressure chronic ulcer of right** `CC` `HCC`
heel and midfoot with other specified
severity

L97.419   **Non-pressure chronic ulcer of** `CC` `HCC`
right heel and midfoot with
unspecified severity

✓6ᵗʰ **L97.42**   **Non-pressure chronic ulcer of** left heel and midfoot

L97.421   **Non-pressure chronic ulcer of left** `CC` `HCC`
heel and midfoot limited to
breakdown of skin
     AHA: 2016, 1Q, 12

L97.422   **Non-pressure chronic ulcer of** `CC` `HCC` `SW`
left heel and midfoot with fat layer
exposed

L97.423   **Non-pressure chronic ulcer of** `CC` `HCC` `SW`
left heel and midfoot with necrosis
of muscle

L97.424   **Non-pressure chronic ulcer of** `CC` `HCC` `SW`
left heel and midfoot with necrosis
of bone

L97.425   **Non-pressure chronic ulcer of left** `CC` `HCC`
heel and midfoot with muscle
involvement without evidence of necrosis

L97.426   **Non-pressure chronic ulcer of left** `CC` `HCC`
heel and midfoot with bone involvement
without evidence of necrosis

L97.428   **Non-pressure chronic ulcer of left** `CC` `HCC`
heel and midfoot with other specified
severity

L97.429   **Non-pressure chronic ulcer of left** `CC` `HCC`
heel and midfoot with unspecified
severity

✓5ᵗʰ **L97.5**   **Non-pressure chronic ulcer of** other part of foot
Non-pressure chronic ulcer of toe

✓6ᵗʰ **L97.50**   **Non-pressure chronic ulcer of** other part of
unspecified foot

L97.501   **Non-pressure chronic ulcer of other** `HCC`
part of unspecified foot limited to
breakdown of skin

L97.502   **Non-pressure chronic ulcer of** `HCC` `SW`
other part of unspecified foot
with fat layer exposed

L97.503   **Non-pressure chronic ulcer of** `HCC` `SW`
otherpart of unspecified foot
with necrosis of muscle

L97.504   **Non-pressure chronic ulcer of** `HCC` `SW`
otherpart of unspecified foot
with necrosis of bone

L97.505   **Non-pressure chronic ulcer of** `CC` `HCC`
other part of unspecified foot
with muscle involvement without
evidence of necrosis

L97.506   **Non-pressure chronic ulcer of** `CC` `HCC`
other part of unspecified foot with bone
involvement without evidence of necrosis

L97.508   **Non-pressure chronic ulcer of** `CC` `HCC`
other part of unspecified foot with other
specified severity

L97.509   **Non-pressure chronic ulcer of other** `HCC`
part of unspecified foot with unspecified
severity

✓6ᵗʰ **L97.51**   **Non-pressure chronic ulcer of** other part of right foot

L97.511   **Non-pressure chronic ulcer of other** `HCC`
part of right foot limited to breakdown of
skin

L97.512   **Non-pressure chronic ulcer of** `HCC` `SW`
other part of right foot with fat layer
exposed

L97.513   **Non-pressure chronic ulcer of** `HCC` `SW`
other part of right foot with necrosis
of muscle

L97.514   **Non-pressure chronic ulcer of** `HCC` `SW`
other part of right foot with necrosis
of bone

L97.515   **Non-pressure chronic ulcer of other** `CC` `HCC`
part of right foot with muscle
involvement without evidence
of necrosis

L97.516   **Non-pressure chronic ulcer of** `CC` `HCC`
other part of right foot with bone
involvement without evidence of necrosis

L97.518   **Non-pressure chronic ulcer of** `CC` `HCC`
other part of right foot with other
specified severity

L97.519   **Non-pressure chronic ulcer of other** `HCC`
part of right foot with unspecified severity

✓6ᵗʰ **L97.52**   **Non-pressure chronic ulcer of** other part of left foot

L97.521   **Non-pressure chronic ulcer of other** `HCC`
part of left foot limited to breakdown
of skin

L97.522   **Non-pressure chronic ulcer of** `HCC` `SW`
other part of left foot with fat layer
exposed

L97.523   **Non-pressure chronic ulcer of** `HCC` `SW`
other part of left foot with necrosis
of muscle

L97.524   **Non-pressure chronic ulcer of** `HCC` `SW`
other part of left foot with necrosis
of bone

L97.525   **Non-pressure chronic ulcer of** `CC` `HCC`
other part of left foot with muscle
involvement without evidence of necrosis

L97.526   **Non-pressure chronic ulcer of** `CC` `HCC`
other part of left foot with bone
involvement without evidence of necrosis

L97.528   **Non-pressure chronic ulcer of** `CC` `HCC`
other part of left foot with other specified
severity

L97.529   **Non-pressure chronic ulcer of other** `HCC`
part of left foot with unspecified severity

✓5ᵗʰ **L97.8**   **Non-pressure chronic ulcer of** other part of lower leg

✓6ᵗʰ **L97.80**   **Non-pressure chronic ulcer of** other part of
unspecified lower leg

L97.801   **Non-pressure chronic ulcer of other** `CC` `HCC`
part of unspecified lower leg limited to
breakdown of skin

L97.802   **Non-pressure chronic ulcer of** `CC` `HCC` `SW`
other part of unspecified lower leg
with fat layer exposed

L97.803   **Non-pressure chronic ulcer of** `CC` `HCC` `SW`
other part of unspecified lower leg
with necrosis of muscle

L97.804   **Non-pressure chronic ulcer of** `CC` `HCC` `SW`
other part of unspecified lower leg
with necrosis of bone

L97.805   **Non-pressure chronic ulcer of other** `CC` `HCC`
part of unspecified lower leg with
muscle involvement without evidence
of necrosis

L97.806   **Non-pressure chronic ulcer of other** `CC` `HCC`
part of unspecified lower leg with
bone involvement without evidence
of necrosis

☑ Additional Character Required   ✓x7ᵗʰ Placeholder   Unacceptable PDx   Questionable PDx   Manifestation   `H1`-`H14` HAC   `HCC` CMS-HCC Dx   `HIV` HIV Dx

ICD-10-CM 2019   733

L97.808   Non-pressure chronic ulcer of other `CC` `HCC` part of unspecified lower leg with other specified severity

L97.809   Non-pressure chronic ulcer of other `CC` `HCC` part of unspecified lower leg with unspecified severity

✓6th L97.81   Non-pressure chronic ulcer of other part of right lower leg

L97.811   Non-pressure chronic ulcer of other `CC` `HCC` part of right lower leg limited to breakdown of skin

L97.812   Non-pressure chronic ulcer of `CC` `HCC` `SW` other part of right lower leg with fat layer exposed

L97.813   Non-pressure chronic ulcer of `CC` `HCC` `SW` other part of right lower leg with necrosis of muscle

L97.814   Non-pressure chronic ulcer of `CC` `HCC` `SW` other part of right lower leg with necrosis of bone

L97.815   Non-pressure chronic ulcer of other `CC` `HCC` part of right lower leg with muscle involvement without evidence of necrosis

L97.816   Non-pressure chronic ulcer of other `CC` `HCC` part of right lower leg with bone involvement without evidence of necrosis

L97.818   Non-pressure chronic ulcer of other `CC` `HCC` part of right lower leg with other specified severity

L97.819   Non-pressure chronic ulcer of other `CC` `HCC` part of right lower leg with unspecified severity

✓6th L97.82   Non-pressure chronic ulcer of other part of left lower leg

L97.821   Non-pressure chronic ulcer of `CC` `HCC` other part of left lower leg limited to breakdown of skin

L97.822   Non-pressure chronic ulcer of `CC` `HCC` `SW` other part of left lower leg with fat layer exposed

L97.823   Non-pressure chronic ulcer of `CC` `HCC` `SW` other part of left lower leg with necrosis of muscle

L97.824   Non-pressure chronic ulcer of `CC` `HCC` `SW` other part of left lower leg with necrosis of bone

L97.825   Non-pressure chronic ulcer of other `CC` `HCC` part of left lower leg with muscle involvement without evidence of necrosis

L97.826   Non-pressure chronic ulcer of other `CC` `HCC` part of left lower leg with bone involvement without evidence of necrosis

L97.828   Non-pressure chronic ulcer of other `CC` `HCC` part of left lower leg with other specified severity

L97.829   Non-pressure chronic ulcer of other `CC` `HCC` part of left lower leg with unspecified severity

✓5th L97.9   Non-pressure chronic ulcer of unspecified part of lower leg

✓6th L97.90   Non-pressure chronic ulcer of unspecified part of unspecified lower leg

L97.901   Non-pressure chronic ulcer of `CC` `HCC` unspecified part of unspecified lower leg limited to breakdown of skin

L97.902   Non-pressure chronic ulcer of `CC` `HCC` `SW` unspecified part of unspecified lower leg with fat layer exposed

L97.903   Non-pressure chronic ulcer of `CC` `HCC` `SW` unspecified part of unspecified lower leg with necrosis of muscle

L97.904   Non-pressure chronic ulcer of `CC` `HCC` `SW` unspecified part of unspecified lower leg with necrosis of bone

L97.905   Non-pressure chronic ulcer of `CC` `HCC` unspecified part of unspecified lower leg with muscle involvement without evidence of necrosis

L97.906   Non-pressure chronic ulcer of `CC` `HCC` unspecified part of unspecified lower leg with bone involvement without evidence of necrosis

L97.908   Non-pressure chronic ulcer of `CC` `HCC` unspecified part of unspecified lower leg with other specified severity

L97.909   Non-pressure chronic ulcer of `CC` `HCC` unspecified part of unspecified lower leg with unspecified severity

✓6th L97.91   Non-pressure chronic ulcer of unspecified part of right lower leg

L97.911   Non-pressure chronic ulcer of `CC` `HCC` unspecified part of right lower leg limited to breakdown of skin

L97.912   Non-pressure chronic ulcer of `CC` `HCC` `SW` unspecified part of right lower leg with fat layer exposed

L97.913   Non-pressure chronic ulcer of `CC` `HCC` `SW` unspecified part of right lower leg with necrosis of muscle

L97.914   Non-pressure chronic ulcer of `CC` `HCC` `SW` unspecified part of right lower leg with necrosis of bone

L97.915   Non-pressure chronic ulcer of `CC` `HCC` unspecified part of right lower leg with muscle involvement without evidence of necrosis

L97.916   Non-pressure chronic ulcer of `CC` `HCC` unspecified part of right lower leg with bone involvement without evidence of necrosis

L97.918   Non-pressure chronic ulcer of `CC` `HCC` unspecified part of right lower leg with other specified severity

L97.919   Non-pressure chronic ulcer of `CC` `HCC` unspecified part of right lower leg with unspecified severity

✓6th L97.92   Non-pressure chronic ulcer of unspecified part of left lower leg

L97.921   Non-pressure chronic ulcer of `CC` `HCC` `SW` unspecified part of left lower leg limited to breakdown of skin

L97.922   Non-pressure chronic ulcer of `CC` `HCC` `SW` unspecified part of left lower leg with fat layer exposed

L97.923   Non-pressure chronic ulcer of `CC` `HCC` `SW` unspecified part of left lower leg with necrosis of muscle

L97.924   Non-pressure chronic ulcer of `CC` `HCC` `SW` unspecified part of left lower leg with necrosis of bone

L97.925   Non-pressure chronic ulcer of `CC` `HCC` unspecified part of left lower leg with muscle involvement without evidence of necrosis

L97.926   Non-pressure chronic ulcer of `CC` `HCC` unspecified part of left lower leg with bone involvement without evidence of necrosis

L97.928   Non-pressure chronic ulcer of `CC` `HCC` unspecified part of left lower leg with other specified severity

L97.929   Non-pressure chronic ulcer of `CC` `HCC` unspecified part of left lower leg with unspecified severity

✓4th L98   Other disorders of skin and subcutaneous tissue, not elsewhere classified

L98.0   Pyogenic granuloma

EXCLUDES 2   pyogenic granuloma of gingiva (K06.8)
pyogenic granuloma of maxillary alveolar ridge (K04.5)
pyogenic granuloma of oral mucosa (K13.4)

DEF: Solitary polypoid capillary hemangioma often associated with local irritation, trauma, and superimposed inflammation. Located on the skin and gingival or oral mucosa, they bleed easily and may ulcerate and form crusted sores.

L98.1   **Factitial dermatitis**
Neurotic excoriation
EXCLUDES 1   *excoriation (skin-picking) disorder (F42.4)*
AHA: 2016, 4Q, 15
DEF: Self-inflicted skin lesions to satisfy an unconscious psychological or emotional need. Methods used to injure the skin include deep excoriations with a sharp instrument, scarification with a knife, or the application of caustic chemicals and burning, sometimes with a cigarette.

L98.2   **Febrile neutrophilic dermatosis [Sweet]**

L98.3   **Eosinophilic cellulitis [Wells]**   `CC`
CC Excl: PDX collection 839

√5ᵗʰ **L98.4**   **Non-pressure chronic ulcer of skin, not elsewhere classified**
Chronic ulcer of skin NOS
Tropical ulcer NOS
Ulcer of skin NOS
EXCLUDES 2   *pressure ulcer (pressure area) (L89.-)*
gangrene (I96)
skin infections (L00-L08)
specific infections classified to A00-B99
ulcer of lower limb NEC (L97.-)
varicose ulcer (I83.0-I82.2)
AHA: 2017, 4Q, 17
TIP: The depth and/or severity of a diagnosed nonpressure ulcer can be determined based on medical record documentation from clinicians who are not the patient's provider.
TIP: Assign a code from this category/subcategory for nonpressure ulcers documented as acute.

CC Excl: For CC codes in subcategory L98.4:
PDX collection 698

√6ᵗʰ **L98.41**   **Non-pressure chronic ulcer of** buttock
   L98.411   **Non-pressure chronic ulcer of**   `HCC`
     buttock limited to breakdown of skin
   L98.412   **Non-pressure chronic ulcer of**   `HCC` `SW`
     buttock with fat layer exposed
   L98.413   **Non-pressure chronic ulcer of**   `HCC` `SW`
     buttock with necrosis of muscle
   L98.414   **Non-pressure chronic ulcer of**   `HCC` `SW`
     buttock with necrosis of bone
   L98.415   **Non-pressure chronic ulcer of**   `CC` `HCC`
     buttock with muscle involvement without evidence of necrosis
   L98.416   **Non-pressure chronic ulcer of**   `CC` `HCC`
     buttock with bone involvement without evidence of necrosis
   L98.418   **Non-pressure chronic ulcer of**   `CC` `HCC`
     buttock with other specified severity
   L98.419   **Non-pressure chronic ulcer of**   `HCC`
     buttock with unspecified severity

√6ᵗʰ **L98.42**   **Non-pressure chronic ulcer of** back
   L98.421   **Non-pressure chronic ulcer of back**   `HCC`
     limited to breakdown of skin
   L98.422   **Non-pressure chronic ulcer of back**   `HCC` `SW`
     with fat layer exposed
   L98.423   **Non-pressure chronic ulcer of back**   `HCC` `SW`
     with necrosis of muscle
   L98.424   **Non-pressure chronic ulcer of back**   `HCC` `SW`
     with necrosis of bone
   L98.425   **Non-pressure chronic ulcer of back**   `CC` `HCC`
     with muscle involvement without evidence of necrosis
   L98.426   **Non-pressure chronic ulcer of back**   `CC` `HCC`
     with bone involvement without evidence of necrosis

   L98.428   **Non-pressure chronic ulcer of back**   `CC` `HCC`
     with other specified severity
   L98.429   **Non-pressure chronic ulcer of back**   `HCC`
     with unspecified severity

√6ᵗʰ **L98.49**   **Non-pressure chronic ulcer of** skin of other sites
Non-pressure chronic ulcer of skin NOS
   L98.491   **Non-pressure chronic ulcer of skin**   `HCC`
     of other sites limited to breakdown of skin
   L98.492   **Non-pressure chronic ulcer of skin**   `HCC` `SW`
     of other sites with fat layer exposed
   L98.493   **Non-pressure chronic ulcer of skin**   `HCC` `SW`
     of other sites with necrosis of muscle
   L98.494   **Non-pressure chronic ulcer of skin**   `HCC` `SW`
     of other sites with necrosis of bone
   L98.495   **Non-pressure chronic ulcer of skin**   `CC` `HCC`
     of other sites with muscle involvement without evidence of necrosis
   L98.496   **Non-pressure chronic ulcer of skin**   `CC` `HCC`
     of other sites with bone involvement without evidence of necrosis
   L98.498   **Non-pressure chronic ulcer of skin**   `CC` `HCC`
     of other sites with other specified severity
   L98.499   **Non-pressure chronic ulcer of skin**   `HCC`
     of other sites with unspecified severity

L98.5   **Mucinosis of the skin**
Focal mucinosis
Lichen myxedematosus
Reticular erythematous mucinosis
EXCLUDES 1   *focal oral mucinosis (K13.79)*
myxedema (E03.9)

L98.6   **Other infiltrative disorders of the skin and subcutaneous tissue**
EXCLUDES 1   *hyalinosis cutis et mucosae (E78.89)*

L98.7   **Excessive and redundant skin and subcutaneous tissue**
Loose or sagging skin following bariatric surgery weight loss
Loose or sagging skin following dietary weight loss
Loose or sagging skin, NOS
EXCLUDES 2   *acquired excess or redundant skin of eyelid (H02.3-)*
congenital excess or redundant skin of eyelid (Q10.3)
skin changes due to chronic exposure to nonionizing radiation (L57.-)
AHA: 2016, 4Q, 36

L98.8   **Other specified disorders of the skin and subcutaneous tissue**
AHA: 2013, 2Q, 32

L98.9   **Disorder of the skin and subcutaneous tissue, unspecified**

L99   ***Other disorders of skin and subcutaneous tissue in diseases classified elsewhere***
Code first underlying disease, such as:
amyloidosis (E85.-)
EXCLUDES 1   *skin disorders in diabetes (E08-E13 with .62)*
skin disorders in gonorrhea (A54.89)
skin disorders in syphilis (A51.31, A52.79)

Chapter 13. Diseases of the Musculoskeletal System and Connective Tissue (MØØ–M99)

Chapter Specific Guidelines with Coding Examples

The chapter specific guidelines from the ICD-10-CM Official Guidelines for Coding and Reporting have been provided below. Along with these guidelines are coding examples, contained in the shaded boxes, that have been developed to help illustrate the coding and/or sequencing guidance found in these guidelines.

a. Site and laterality

Most of the codes within Chapter 13 have site and laterality designations. The site represents the bone, joint or the muscle involved. For some conditions where more than one bone, joint or muscle is usually involved, such as osteoarthritis, there is a "multiple sites" code. For categories where no multiple site code is provided and more than one bone, joint or muscle is involved, multiple codes should be used to indicate the different sites involved.

Rheumatoid arthritis of multiple sites without rheumatoid factor

MØ6.Ø9   **Rheumatoid arthritis without rheumatoid factor, multiple sites**

Explanation: For some conditions where more than one bone, joint or muscle is usually involved, such as rheumatoid arthritis, there is a "multiple sites" code available.

Osteomyelitis of the fourth thoracic and second lumbar vertebrae

M46.24   **Osteomyelitis of vertebra, thoracic region**

M46.26   **Osteomyelitis of vertebra, lumbar region**

Explanation: For categories without a multiple site code and more than one bone, joint, or muscle is involved, multiple codes should be used to indicate the different sites involved.

---

1) Bone versus joint

For certain conditions, the bone may be affected at the upper or lower end, (e.g., avascular necrosis of bone, M87, Osteoporosis, M8Ø, M81). Though the portion of the bone affected may be at the joint, the site designation will be the bone, not the joint.

Idiopathic avascular necrosis of the femoral head of the left hip joint

M87.Ø52   **Idiopathic aseptic necrosis of left femur**

Explanation: For certain conditions such as avascular necrosis, the bone may be affected at the joint, but the site designation is the bone, not the joint.

---

b. Acute traumatic versus chronic or recurrent musculoskeletal conditions

Many musculoskeletal conditions are a result of previous injury or trauma to a site, or are recurrent conditions. Bone, joint or muscle conditions that are the result of a healed injury are usually found in chapter 13. Recurrent bone, joint or muscle conditions are also usually found in chapter 13. Any current, acute injury should be coded to the appropriate injury code from chapter 19. Chronic or recurrent conditions should generally be coded with a code from chapter 13. If it is difficult to determine from the documentation in the record which code is best to describe a condition, query the provider.

Acute traumatic bucket handle tear of right medial meniscus

S83.211A   **Bucket-handle tear of medial meniscus, current injury, right knee, initial encounter**

Explanation: Any current, acute injury is not coded in chapter 13. It should instead be coded to the appropriate injury code from chapter 19.

Old bucket handle tear of right medial meniscus

M23.2Ø3   **Derangement of unspecified medial meniscus due to old tear or injury, right knee**

Explanation: Chronic or recurrent conditions should generally be coded with a code from chapter 13.

---

c. Coding of pathologic fractures

7th character A is for use as long as the patient is receiving active treatment for the fracture. Examples of active treatment are: surgical treatment, emergency department encounter, evaluation and continuing treatment by the same or a different physician. While the patient may be seen by a new or different provider over the course of treatment for a pathological fracture, assignment of the 7th character is based on whether the patient is

undergoing active treatment and not whether the provider is seeing the patient for the first time.

Patient admitted for repair of pathologic fracture of left foot, unknown cause. The surgery will be performed by his orthopedic specialist who he has been seeing for this fracture for the past month.

M84.475A   **Pathological fracture, left foot, initial encounter for fracture**

Explanation: Seventh character A is for use as long as the patient is receiving active treatment for a pathologic fracture. Examples of active treatment are surgical treatment, emergency department encounter, evaluation, and continuing treatment by the same or a different physician.

The seventh character is based on whether the patient is undergoing active treatment such as surgery, and not whether the provider is seeing the patient for the first time.

7th character D is to be used for encounters after the patient has completed active treatment for the fracture and is receiving routine care for the fracture during the healing or recovery phase. The other 7th characters, listed under each subcategory in the Tabular List, are to be used for subsequent encounters for treatment of problems associated with the healing, such as malunions, nonunions, and sequelae.

Care for complications of surgical treatment for fracture repairs during the healing or recovery phase should be coded with the appropriate complication codes.

See Section I.C.19. Coding of traumatic fractures.

d. Osteoporosis

Osteoporosis is a systemic condition, meaning that all bones of the musculoskeletal system are affected. Therefore, site is not a component of the codes under category M81, Osteoporosis without current pathological fracture. The site codes under category M8Ø, Osteoporosis with current pathological fracture, identify the site of the fracture, not the osteoporosis.

1) Osteoporosis without pathological fracture

Category M81, Osteoporosis without current pathological fracture, is for use for patients with osteoporosis who do not currently have a pathologic fracture due to the osteoporosis, even if they have had a fracture in the past. For patients with a history of osteoporosis fractures, status code Z87.31Ø, Personal history of (healed) osteoporosis fracture, should follow the code from M81.

Age-related osteoporosis with healed osteoporotic fracture of the lumbar vertebra

M81.Ø   **Age-related osteoporosis without current pathological fracture**

Z87.31Ø   **Personal history of (healed) osteoporosis fracture**

Explanation: Category M81 is used for patients with osteoporosis who do not currently have a pathologic fracture due to the osteoporosis. To report a previous (healed) fracture, status code Z87.31Ø Personal history of (healed) osteoporosis fracture, should follow the code from M81.

---

2) Osteoporosis with current pathological fracture

Category M8Ø, Osteoporosis with current pathological fracture, is for patients who have a current pathologic fracture at the time of an encounter. The codes under M8Ø identify the site of the fracture. A code from category M8Ø, not a traumatic fracture code, should be used for any patient with known osteoporosis who suffers a fracture, even if the patient had a minor fall or trauma, if that fall or trauma would not usually break a normal, healthy bone.

Disuse osteoporosis with current fracture of right shoulder sustained lifting a grocery bag, initial encounter

M8Ø.811A   **Other osteoporosis with current pathological fracture, right shoulder, initial encounter for fracture**

Explanation: A code from category M8Ø, not a traumatic fracture code, should be used for any patient with known osteoporosis who suffers a fracture, even if the patient had a minor fall or trauma, if that fall or trauma would not usually break a normal, healthy bone.

Muscle/Tendon Table

ICD-10-CM categorizes certain muscles and tendons in the upper and lower extremities by their action (e.g., extension, flexion), their anatomical location (e.g., posterior, anterior), and/or whether they are intrinsic or extrinsic to a certain anatomical area. The Muscle/Tendon Table is provided at the beginning of chapters 13 and 19 as a resource to help users when code selection depends on one or more of these characteristics. Please note that this table is not all-inclusive, and proper code assignment should be based on the provider's documentation.

Body Region	Muscle	Extensor Tendon	Flexor Tendon	Other Tendon
Shoulder				
	Deltoid	Posterior deltoid	Anterior deltoid	
	Rotator cuff			
	Infraspinatus			Infraspinatus
	Subscapularis			Subscapularis
	Supraspinatus			Supraspinatus
	Teres minor			Teres minor
	Teres major	Teres major		
Upper arm				
	Anterior muscles			
	Biceps brachii — long head		Biceps brachii — long head	
	Biceps brachii — short head		Biceps brachii — short head	
	Brachialis		Brachialis	
	Coracobrachialis		Coracobrachialis	
	Posterior muscles			
	Triceps brachii	Triceps brachii		
Forearm				
	Anterior muscles			
	Flexors			
	Deep			
	Flexor digitorum profundus		Flexor digitorum profundus	
	Flexor pollicis longus		Flexor pollicis longus	
	Intermediate			
	Flexor digitorum superficialis		Flexor digitorum superficialis	
	Superficial			
	Flexor carpi radialis		Flexor carpi radialis	
	Flexor carpi ulnaris		Flexor carpi ulnaris	
	Palmaris longus		Palmaris longus	
	Pronators			
	Pronator quadratus			Pronator quadratus
	Pronator teres			Pronator teres
	Posterior muscles			
	Extensors			
	Deep			
	Abductor pollicis longus			Abductor pollicis longus
	Extensor indicis	Extensor indicis		
	Extensor pollicis brevis	Extensor pollicis brevis		
	Extensor pollicis longus	Extensor pollicis longus		
	Superficial			
	Brachioradialis			Brachioradialis
	Extensor carpi radialis brevis	Extensor carpi radialis brevis		
	Extensor carpi radialis longus	Extensor carpi radialis longus		
	Extensor carpi ulnaris	Extensor carpi ulnaris		
	Extensor digiti minimi	Extensor digiti minimi		
	Extensor digitorum	Extensor digitorum		
	Anconeus	Anconeus		
	Supinator			Supinator

Body Region	Muscle	Extensor Tendon	Flexor Tendon	Other Tendon
Hand				
Extrinsic — attach to a site in the forearm as well as a site in the hand with action related to hand movement at the wrist				
	Extensor carpi radialis brevis	Extensor carpi radialis brevis		
	Extensor carpi radialis longus	Extensor carpie radialis longus		
	Extensor carpi ulnaris	Extensor carpi ulnaris		
	Flexor carpi radialis		Flexor carpi radialis	
	Flexor carpi ulnaris		Flexor carpi ulnaris	
	Flexor digitorum superficialis		Flexor digitorum superficialis	
	Palmaris longus		Palmaris longus	
Extrinsic — attach to a site in the forearm as well as a site in the hand with action in the hand related to finger movement				
	Adductor pollicis longus			Adductor pollicis longus
	Extensor digiti minimi	Extensor digiti minimi		
	Extensor digitorum	Extensor digitorum		
	Extensor indicis	Extensor indicis		
	Flexor digitorum profundus		Flexor digitorum profundus	
	Flexor digitorum superficialis		Flexor digitorum superficialis	
Extrinsic — attach to a site in the forearm as well as a site in the hand with action in the hand related to thumb movement				
	Extensor pollicis brevis	Extensor pollicis brevis		
	Extensor pollicis longus	Extensor pollicis longus		
	Flexor pollicis longus		Flexor pollicis longus	
Intrinsic — found within the hand only				
	Adductor pollicis			Adductor pollicis
	Dorsal interossei	Dorsal interossei	Dorsal interossei	
	Lumbricals	Lumbricals	Lumbricals	
	Palmaris brevis			Palmaris brevis
	Palmar interossei	Palmar interossei	Palmar interossei	
	Hypothenar muscles			
	Abductor digiti minimi			Abductor digiti minimi
	Flexor digiti minimi brevis		Flexor digiti minimi brevis	
	Oppenens digiti minimi		Oppenens digiti minimi	
	Thenar muscles			
	Abductor pollicis brevis			Abductor pollicis brevis
	Flexor pollicis brevis		Flexor pollicis brevis	
	Oppenens pollicis		Oppenens pollicis	
Thigh				
	Anterior muscles			
	Iliopsoas		Iliopsoas	
	Pectineus		Pectineus	
	Quadriceps	Quadriceps		
	Rectus femoris	Rectus femoris — Extends knee	Rectus femoris — Flexes hip	
	Vastus intermedius	Vastus intermedius		
	Vastus lateralis	Vastus lateralis		
	Vastus medialis	Vastus medialis		
	Sartorius		Sartorius	
	Medial muscles			
	Adductor brevis			Adductor brevis
	Adductor longus			Adductor longus
	Adductor magnus			Adductor magnus
	Gracilis			Gracilis
	Obturator externus			Obturator externus
	Posterior muscles			
	Hamstring	Hamstring — Extends hip	Hamstring — Flexes knee	
	Biceps femoris	Biceps femoris	Biceps femoris	
	Semimembranosus	Semimembranosus	Semimembranosus	
	Semitendinosus	Semitendinosus	Semitendinosus	

Body Region	Muscle	Extensor Tendon	Flexor Tendon	Other Tendon
Lower leg				
	Anterior muscles			
	Extensor digitorum longus	Extensor digitorum longus		
	Extensor hallucis longus	Extensor hallucis longus		
	Fibularis (peroneus) tertius	Fibularis (peroneus) tertius		
	Tibialis anterior	Tibialis anterior		Tibialis anterior
	Lateral muscles			
	Fibularis (peroneus) brevis		Fibularis (peroneus) brevis	
	Fibularis (peroneus) longus		Fibularis (peroneus) longus	
	Posterior muscles			
	Deep			
	Flexor digitorum longus		Flexor digitorum longus	
	Flexor hallucis longus		Flexor hallucis longus	
	Popliteus		Popliteus	
	Tibialis posterior		Tibialis posterior	
	Superficial			
	Gastrocnemius		Gastrocnemius	
	Plantaris		Plantaris	
	Soleus		Soleus	
				Calcaneal (Achilles)
Ankle/Foot				
Extrinsic — attach to a site in the lower leg as well as a site in the foot with action related to foot movement at the ankle				
	Plantaris		Plantaris	
	Soleus		Soleus	
	Tibialis anterior	Tibialis anterior		
	Tibialis posterior		Tibialis posterior	
Extrinsic — attach to a site in the lower leg as well as a site in the foot with action in the foot related to toe movement				
	Extensor digitorum longus	Extensor digitorum longus		
	Extensor hallicus longus	Extensor hallicus longus		
	Flexor digitorum longus		Flexor digitorum longus	
	Flexor hallucis longus		Flexor hallucis longus	
Intrinsic — found within the ankle/foot only				
	Dorsal muscles			
	Extensor digitorum brevis	Extensor digitorum brevis		
	Extensor hallucis brevis	Extensor hallucis brevis		
	Plantar muscles			
	Abductor digiti minimi		Abductor digiti minimi	
	Abductor hallucis		Abductor hallucis	
	Dorsal interossei	Dorsal interossei	Dorsal interossei	
	Flexor digiti minimi brevis		Flexor digiti minimi brevis	
	Flexor digitorum brevis		Flexor digitorum brevis	
	Flexor hallucis brevis		Flexor hallucis brevis	
	Lumbricals	Lumbricals	Lumbricals	
	Quadratus plantae		Quadratus plantae	
	Plantar interossei	Plantar interossei	Plantar interossei	

Chapter 13. Diseases of the Musculoskeletal System and Connective Tissue (M00–M99)

NOTE   Use an external cause code following the code for the musculoskeletal condition, if applicable, to identify the cause of the musculoskeletal condition.

EXCLUDES 2   arthropathic psoriasis (L40.5-)
certain conditions originating in the perinatal period (P04-P96)
certain infectious and parasitic diseases (A00-B99)
compartment syndrome (traumatic) (T79.A-)
complications of pregnancy, childbirth and the puerperium (O00-O9A)
congenital malformations, deformations, and chromosomal abnormalities (Q00-Q99)
endocrine, nutritional and metabolic diseases (E00-E88)
injury, poisoning and certain other consequences of external causes (S00-T88)
neoplasms (C00-D49)
symptoms, signs and abnormal clinical and laboratory findings, not elsewhere classified (R00-R94)

This chapter contains the following blocks:

M00-M02	Infectious arthropathies
▶M04	Autoinflammatory syndromes◀
M05-M14	Inflammatory polyarthropathies
M15-M19	Osteoarthritis
M20-M25	Other joint disorders
M26-M27	Dentofacial anomalies [including malocclusion] and other disorders of jaw
M30-M36	Systemic connective tissue disorders
M40-M43	Deforming dorsopathies
M45-M49	Spondylopathies
M50-M54	Other dorsopathies
M60-M63	Disorders of muscles
M65-M67	Disorders of synovium and tendon
M70-M79	Other soft tissue disorders
M80-M85	Disorders of bone density and structure
M86-M90	Other osteopathies
M91-M94	Chondropathies
M95	Other disorders of the musculoskeletal system and connective tissue
M96	Intraoperative and postprocedural complications and disorders of musculoskeletal system, not elsewhere classified
▶M97	Periprosthetic fracture around internal prosthetic joint◀
M99	Biomechanical lesions, not elsewhere classified

ARTHROPATHIES (M00-M25)

INCLUDES   disorders affecting predominantly peripheral (limb) joints

Infectious arthropathies (M00-M02)

NOTE   This block comprises arthropathies due to microbiological agents. Distinction is made between the following types of etiological relationship:
   a)   direct infection of joint, where organisms invade synovial tissue and microbial antigen is present in the joint;
   b)   indirect infection, which may be of two types: a reactive arthropathy, where microbial infection of the body is established but neither organisms nor antigens can be identified in the joint, and a postinfective arthropathy, where microbial antigen is present but recovery of an organism is inconstant and evidence of local multiplication is lacking.

✓4ᵗʰ **M00 Pyogenic arthritis**
   DEF: Pyogenic: Relating to or involving pus production, often referred to as suppurative or purulent.

✓5ᵗʰ **M00.0 Staphylococcal arthritis and polyarthritis**
   Use additional code (B95.61-B95.8) to identify bacterial agent
   EXCLUDES 2   infection and inflammatory reaction due to internal joint prosthesis (T84.5-)

   M00.00 Staphylococcal arthritis, unspecified joint `CC` `HCC`
     CC Excl: PDX collection 855

✓6ᵗʰ **M00.01 Staphylococcal arthritis, shoulder**

     CC Excl: For CC codes in subcategory M00.01:
     PDX collection 856

     M00.011 Staphylococcal arthritis, right shoulder `CC` `HCC`
     M00.012 Staphylococcal arthritis, left shoulder `CC` `HCC`
     M00.019 Staphylococcal arthritis, unspecified shoulder `CC` `HCC`

   M00.02 Staphylococcal arthritis, elbow

     CC Excl: For CC codes in subcategory M00.02:
     PDX collection 857

     M00.021 Staphylococcal arthritis, right elbow `CC` `HCC`
     M00.022 Staphylococcal arthritis, left elbow `CC` `HCC`
     M00.029 Staphylococcal arthritis, unspecified elbow `CC` `HCC`

✓6ᵗʰ **M00.03 Staphylococcal arthritis, wrist**
   Staphylococcal arthritis of carpal bones

     CC Excl: For CC codes in subcategory M00.03:
     PDX collection 858

     M00.031 Staphylococcal arthritis, right wrist `CC` `HCC`
     M00.032 Staphylococcal arthritis, left wrist `CC` `HCC`
     M00.039 Staphylococcal arthritis, unspecified wrist `CC` `HCC`

✓6ᵗʰ **M00.04 Staphylococcal arthritis, hand**
   Staphylococcal arthritis of metacarpus and phalanges

     CC Excl: For CC codes in subcategory M00.04:
     PDX collection 859

     M00.041 Staphylococcal arthritis, right hand `CC` `HCC`
     M00.042 Staphylococcal arthritis, left hand `CC` `HCC`
     M00.049 Staphylococcal arthritis, unspecified hand `CC` `HCC`

✓6ᵗʰ **M00.05 Staphylococcal arthritis, hip**

     CC Excl: For CC codes in subcategory M00.05:
     PDX collection 860

     M00.051 Staphylococcal arthritis, right hip `CC` `HCC`
     M00.052 Staphylococcal arthritis, left hip `CC` `HCC`
     M00.059 Staphylococcal arthritis, unspecified hip `CC` `HCC`

✓6ᵗʰ **M00.06 Staphylococcal arthritis, knee**

     CC Excl: For CC codes in subcategory M00.06:
     PDX collection 861

     M00.061 Staphylococcal arthritis, right knee `CC` `HCC`
     M00.062 Staphylococcal arthritis, left knee `CC` `HCC`
     M00.069 Staphylococcal arthritis, unspecified knee `CC` `HCC`

✓6ᵗʰ **M00.07 Staphylococcal arthritis, ankle and foot**
   Staphylococcal arthritis, tarsus, metatarsus and phalanges

     CC Excl: For CC codes in subcategory M00.07:
     PDX collection 862

     M00.071 Staphylococcal arthritis, right ankle and foot `CC` `HCC`
     M00.072 Staphylococcal arthritis, left ankle and foot `CC` `HCC`
     M00.079 Staphylococcal arthritis, unspecified ankle and foot `CC` `HCC`

   M00.08 Staphylococcal arthritis, vertebrae `CC` `HCC`
     CC Excl: PDX collection 855

   M00.09 Staphylococcal polyarthritis `CC` `HCC`
     CC Excl: PDX collection 855

✓5ᵗʰ **M00.1 Pneumococcal arthritis and polyarthritis**
   M00.10 Pneumococcal arthritis, unspecified joint `CC` `HCC`
     CC Excl: PDX collection 855

✓6ᵗʰ **M00.11 Pneumococcal arthritis, shoulder**

     CC Excl: For CC codes in subcategory M00.11:
     PDX collection 856

     M00.111 Pneumococcal arthritis, right shoulder `CC` `HCC`
     M00.112 Pneumococcal arthritis, left shoulder `CC` `HCC`
     M00.119 Pneumococcal arthritis, unspecified shoulder `CC` `HCC`

☑ Additional Character Required   ✓7ᵗʰ Placeholder   Unacceptable PDx   Questionable PDx   Manifestation   **H1**-**H14** HAC   **HCC** CMS-HCC Dx   **HIV** HIV Dx

ICD-10-CM 2019   **741**

✓6ᵗʰ M00.12 Pneumococcal arthritis, elbow

> **CC Excl: For CC codes in subcategory M00.12:**
> PDX collection 857

    M00.121 Pneumococcal arthritis, right elbow `CC` `HCC`

    M00.122 Pneumococcal arthritis, left elbow `CC` `HCC`

    M00.129 Pneumococcal arthritis, unspecified elbow `CC` `HCC`

✓6ᵗʰ M00.13 Pneumococcal arthritis, wrist
Pneumococcal arthritis of carpal bones

> **CC Excl: For CC codes in subcategory M00.13:**
> PDX collection 858

    M00.131 Pneumococcal arthritis, right wrist `CC` `HCC`
    M00.132 Pneumococcal arthritis, left wrist `CC` `HCC`
    M00.139 Pneumococcal arthritis, unspecified wrist `CC` `HCC`

✓6ᵗʰ M00.14 Pneumococcal arthritis, hand
Pneumococcal arthritis of metacarpus and phalanges

> **CC Excl: For CC codes in subcategory M00.14:**
> PDX collection 859

    M00.141 Pneumococcal arthritis, right hand `CC` `HCC`
    M00.142 Pneumococcal arthritis, left hand `CC` `HCC`
    M00.149 Pneumococcal arthritis, unspecified hand `CC` `HCC`

✓6ᵗʰ M00.15 Pneumococcal arthritis, hip

> **CC Excl: For CC codes in subcategory M00.15:**
> PDX collection 860

    M00.151 Pneumococcal arthritis, right hip `CC` `HCC`
    M00.152 Pneumococcal arthritis, left hip `CC` `HCC`
    M00.159 Pneumococcal arthritis, unspecified hip `CC` `HCC`

✓6ᵗʰ M00.16 Pneumococcal arthritis, knee

> **CC Excl: For CC codes in subcategory M00.16:**
> PDX collection 861

    M00.161 Pneumococcal arthritis, right knee `CC` `HCC`
    M00.162 Pneumococcal arthritis, left knee `CC` `HCC`
    M00.169 Pneumococcal arthritis, unspecified knee `CC` `HCC`

✓6ᵗʰ M00.17 Pneumococcal arthritis, ankle and foot
Pneumococcal arthritis, tarsus, metatarsus and phalanges

> **CC Excl: For CC codes in subcategory M00.17:**
> PDX collection 862

    M00.171 Pneumococcal arthritis, right ankle and foot `CC` `HCC`
    M00.172 Pneumococcal arthritis, left ankle and foot `CC` `HCC`
    M00.179 Pneumococcal arthritis, unspecified ankle and foot `CC` `HCC`

M00.18 Pneumococcal arthritis, vertebrae `CC` `HCC`
CC Excl: PDX collection 855

M00.19 Pneumococcal polyarthritis `CC` `HCC`
CC Excl: PDX collection 855

✓5ᵗʰ M00.2 Other streptococcal arthritis and polyarthritis
Use additional code (B95.0-B95.2, B95.4-B95.5) to identify bacterial agent

M00.20 Other streptococcal arthritis, unspecified joint `CC` `HCC`
CC Excl: PDX collection 855

✓6ᵗʰ M00.21 Other streptococcal arthritis, shoulder

> **CC Excl: For CC codes in subcategory M00.21:**
> PDX collection 856

    M00.211 Other streptococcal arthritis, right shoulder `CC` `HCC`

    M00.212 Other streptococcal arthritis, left shoulder `CC` `HCC`

    M00.219 Other streptococcal arthritis, unspecified shoulder `CC` `HCC`

✓6ᵗʰ M00.22 Other streptococcal arthritis, elbow

> **CC Excl: For CC codes in subcategory M00.22:**
> PDX collection 857

    M00.221 Other streptococcal arthritis, right elbow `CC` `HCC`

    M00.222 Other streptococcal arthritis, left elbow `CC` `HCC`

    M00.229 Other streptococcal arthritis, unspecified elbow `CC` `HCC`

✓6ᵗʰ M00.23 Other streptococcal arthritis, wrist
Other streptococcal arthritis of carpal bones

> **CC Excl: For CC codes in subcategory M00.23:**
> PDX collection 858

    M00.231 Other streptococcal arthritis, right wrist `CC` `HCC`

    M00.232 Other streptococcal arthritis, left wrist `CC` `HCC`

    M00.239 Other streptococcal arthritis, unspecified wrist `CC` `HCC`

✓6ᵗʰ M00.24 Other streptococcal arthritis, hand
Other streptococcal arthritis metacarpus and phalanges

> **CC Excl: For CC codes in subcategory M00.24:**
> PDX collection 859

    M00.241 Other streptococcal arthritis, right hand `CC` `HCC`

    M00.242 Other streptococcal arthritis, left hand `CC` `HCC`

    M00.249 Other streptococcal arthritis, unspecified hand `CC` `HCC`

✓6ᵗʰ M00.25 Other streptococcal arthritis, hip

> **CC Excl: For CC codes in subcategory M00.25:**
> PDX collection 860

    M00.251 Other streptococcal arthritis, right hip `CC` `HCC`

    M00.252 Other streptococcal arthritis, left hip `CC` `HCC`

    M00.259 Other streptococcal arthritis, unspecified hip `CC` `HCC`

✓6ᵗʰ M00.26 Other streptococcal arthritis, knee

> **CC Excl: For CC codes in subcategory M00.26:**
> PDX collection 861

    M00.261 Other streptococcal arthritis, right knee `CC` `HCC`

    M00.262 Other streptococcal arthritis, left knee `CC` `HCC`

    M00.269 Other streptococcal arthritis, unspecified knee `CC` `HCC`

✓6ᵗʰ M00.27 Other streptococcal arthritis, ankle and foot
Other streptococcal arthritis, tarsus, metatarsus and phalanges

> **CC Excl: For CC codes in subcategory M00.27:**
> PDX collection 862

    M00.271 Other streptococcal arthritis, right ankle and foot `CC` `HCC`

    M00.272 Other streptococcal arthritis, left ankle and foot `CC` `HCC`

    M00.279 Other streptococcal arthritis, unspecified ankle and foot `CC` `HCC`

M00.28 Other streptococcal arthritis, vertebrae `CC` `HCC`
CC Excl: PDX collection 855

M00.29 Other streptococcal polyarthritis `CC` `HCC`
CC Excl: PDX collection 855

✓5ᵗʰ M00.8 Arthritis and polyarthritis due to other bacteria
Use additional code (B96) to identify bacteria

M00.80 Arthritis due to other bacteria, unspecified joint `CC` `HCC`
CC Excl: PDX collection 855

✓6ᵗʰ M00.81 Arthritis due to other bacteria, shoulder

> **CC Excl: For CC codes in subcategory M00.81:**
> PDX collection 856

    M00.811 Arthritis due to other bacteria, right shoulder `CC` `HCC`

M00.812 Arthritis due to other bacteria, left **shoulder** `CC` `HCC`

M00.819 Arthritis due to other bacteria, unspecified **shoulder** `CC` `HCC`

✓6ᵗʰ **M00.82** Arthritis due to other bacteria, **elbow**

> **CC Excl: For CC codes in subcategory M00.82:** PDX collection 857

M00.821 Arthritis due to other bacteria, right **elbow** `CC` `HCC`

M00.822 Arthritis due to other bacteria, left **elbow** `CC` `HCC`

M00.829 Arthritis due to other bacteria, unspecified **elbow** `CC` `HCC`

✓6ᵗʰ **M00.83** Arthritis due to other bacteria, **wrist**
Arthritis due to other bacteria, carpal bones

> **CC Excl: For CC codes in subcategory M00.83:** PDX collection 858

M00.831 Arthritis due to other bacteria, right **wrist** `CC` `HCC`

M00.832 Arthritis due to other bacteria, left **wrist** `CC` `HCC`

M00.839 Arthritis due to other bacteria, unspecified **wrist** `CC` `HCC`

✓6ᵗʰ **M00.84** Arthritis due to other bacteria, **hand**
Arthritis due to other bacteria, metacarpus and phalanges

> **CC Excl: For CC codes in subcategory M00.84:** PDX collection 859

M00.841 Arthritis due to other bacteria, right **hand** `CC` `HCC`

M00.842 Arthritis due to other bacteria, left **hand** `CC` `HCC`

M00.849 Arthritis due to other bacteria, unspecified **hand** `CC` `HCC`

✓6ᵗʰ **M00.85** Arthritis due to other bacteria, **hip**

> **CC Excl: For CC codes in subcategory M00.85:** PDX collection 860

M00.851 Arthritis due to other bacteria, right **hip** `CC` `HCC`

M00.852 Arthritis due to other bacteria, left **hip** `CC` `HCC`

M00.859 Arthritis due to other bacteria, unspecified **hip** `CC` `HCC`

✓6ᵗʰ **M00.86** Arthritis due to other bacteria, **knee**

> **CC Excl: For CC codes in subcategory M00.86:** PDX collection 861

M00.861 Arthritis due to other bacteria, right **knee** `CC` `HCC`

M00.862 Arthritis due to other bacteria, left **knee** `CC` `HCC`

M00.869 Arthritis due to other bacteria, unspecified **knee** `CC` `HCC`

✓6ᵗʰ **M00.87** Arthritis due to other bacteria, **ankle and foot**
Arthritis due to other bacteria, tarsus, metatarsus, and phalanges

> **CC Excl: For CC codes in subcategory M00.87:** PDX collection 862

M00.871 Arthritis due to other bacteria, right **ankle and foot** `CC` `HCC`

M00.872 Arthritis due to other bacteria, left **ankle and foot** `CC` `HCC`

M00.879 Arthritis due to other bacteria, unspecified **ankle and foot** `CC` `HCC`

M00.88 Arthritis due to other bacteria, **vertebrae** `CC` `HCC`
CC Excl: PDX collection 855

M00.89 **Polyarthritis** due to other bacteria `CC` `HCC`
CC Excl: PDX collection 855

M00.9 Pyogenic arthritis, unspecified `CC` `HCC`
Infective arthritis NOS
CC Excl: PDX collection 855

✓4ᵗʰ **M01** **Direct infections of joint in infectious and parasitic diseases classified elsewhere**
Code first underlying disease, such as:
leprosy [Hansen's disease] (A30.-)
mycoses (B35-B49)
O'nyong-nyong fever (A92.1)
paratyphoid fever (A01.1-A01.4)
EXCLUDES 1   arthropathy in Lyme disease (A69.23)
gonococcal arthritis (A54.42)
meningococcal arthritis (A39.83)
mumps arthritis (B26.85)
postinfective arthropathy (M02.-)
postmeningococcal arthritis (A39.84)
reactive arthritis (M02.3)
rubella arthritis (B06.82)
sarcoidosis arthritis (D86.86)
typhoid fever arthritis (A01.04)
tuberculosis arthritis (A18.01-A18.02)

> **CC Excl: For CC codes in category M01, unless otherwise noted:** PDX collection 863

✓5ᵗʰ **M01.X** **Direct infection of joint in infectious and parasitic diseases classified elsewhere**

M01.X0 *Direct infection of unspecified joint in infectious and parasitic diseases classified elsewhere* `CC` `HCC`

✓6ᵗʰ **M01.X1** **Direct infection of shoulder joint in infectious and parasitic diseases classified elsewhere**

> **CC Excl: For CC codes in subcategory M01.X1:** PDX collection 864

M01.X11 *Direct infection of right shoulder in infectious and parasitic diseases classified elsewhere* `CC` `HCC`

M01.X12 *Direct infection of left shoulder in infectious and parasitic diseases classified elsewhere* `CC` `HCC`

M01.X19 *Direct infection of unspecified shoulder in infectious and parasitic diseases classified elsewhere* `CC` `HCC`

✓6ᵗʰ **M01.X2** **Direct infection of elbow in infectious and parasitic diseases classified elsewhere**

M01.X21 *Direct infection of right elbow in infectious and parasitic diseases classified elsewhere* `CC` `HCC`

M01.X22 *Direct infection of left elbow in infectious and parasitic diseases classified elsewhere* `CC` `HCC`

M01.X29 *Direct infection of unspecified elbow in infectious and parasitic diseases classified elsewhere* `CC` `HCC`

✓6ᵗʰ **M01.X3** **Direct infection of wrist in infectious and parasitic diseases classified elsewhere**
Direct infection of carpal bones in infectious and parasitic diseases classified elsewhere

M01.X31 *Direct infection of right wrist in infectious and parasitic diseases classified elsewhere* `CC` `HCC`

M01.X32 *Direct infection of left wrist in infectious and parasitic diseases classified elsewhere* `CC` `HCC`

M01.X39 *Direct infection of unspecified wrist in infectious and parasitic diseases classified elsewhere* `CC` `HCC`

✓6ᵗʰ **M01.X4** **Direct infection of hand in infectious and parasitic diseases classified elsewhere**
Direct infection of metacarpus and phalanges in infectious and parasitic diseases classified elsewhere

M01.X41 *Direct infection of right hand in infectious and parasitic diseases classified elsewhere* `CC` `HCC`

M01.X42 *Direct infection of left hand in infectious and parasitic diseases classified elsewhere* `CC` `HCC`

M01.X49 *Direct infection of unspecified hand in infectious and parasitic diseases classified elsewhere* `CC` `HCC`

✓6ᵗʰ **M01.X5** **Direct infection of hip in infectious and parasitic diseases classified elsewhere**

M01.X51 *Direct infection of right hip in infectious and parasitic diseases classified elsewhere* `CC` `HCC`

☑ Additional Character Required   ✓ₓ7ᵗʰ Placeholder   Unacceptable PDx   Questionable PDx   Manifestation   `H1`-`H14` HAC   `HCC` CMS-HCC Dx   `HIV` HIV Dx

ICD-10-CM 2019   **743**

        M01.X52   *Direct infection of left hip in infectious and parasitic diseases classified elsewhere*   CC HCC

        M01.X59   *Direct infection of unspecified hip in infectious and parasitic diseases classified elsewhere*   CC HCC

✓6ᵗʰ **M01.X6** **Direct infection of knee in infectious and parasitic diseases classified elsewhere**

        M01.X61   *Direct infection of right knee in infectious and parasitic diseases classified elsewhere*   CC HCC

        M01.X62   *Direct infection of left knee in infectious and parasitic diseases classified elsewhere*   CC HCC

        M01.X69   *Direct infection of unspecified knee in infectious and parasitic diseases classified elsewhere*   CC HCC

✓6ᵗʰ **M01.X7** **Direct infection of ankle and foot in infectious and parasitic diseases classified elsewhere**
    Direct infection of tarsus, metatarsus and phalanges in infectious and parasitic diseases classified elsewhere

        M01.X71   *Direct infection of right ankle and foot in infectious and parasitic diseases classified elsewhere*   CC HCC

        M01.X72   *Direct infection of left ankle and foot in infectious and parasitic diseases classified elsewhere*   CC HCC

        M01.X79   *Direct infection of unspecified ankle and foot in infectious and parasitic diseases classified elsewhere*   CC HCC

        M01.X8   *Direct infection of vertebrae in infectious and parasitic diseases classified elsewhere*   CC HCC

        M01.X9   *Direct infection of multiple joints in infectious and parasitic diseases classified elsewhere*   CC HCC

✓4ᵗʰ **M02** **Postinfective and reactive arthropathies**
    Code first underlying disease, such as:
      congenital syphilis [Clutton's joints] (A50.5)
      enteritis due to Yersinia enterocolitica (A04.6)
      infective endocarditis (I33.0)
      viral hepatitis (B15-B19)

    EXCLUDES 1 *Behçet's disease (M35.2)*
        direct infections of joint in infectious and parasitic diseases classified elsewhere (M01.-)
        mumps arthritis (B26.85)
        postmeningococcal arthritis (A39.84)
        rheumatic fever (I00)
        rubella arthritis (B06.82)
        syphilis arthritis (late) (A52.77)
        tabetic arthropathy [Charcôt's] (A52.16)

✓5ᵗʰ **M02.0** **Arthropathy following intestinal bypass**

    M02.00 **Arthropathy following intestinal bypass, unspecified site**

✓6ᵗʰ **M02.01** **Arthropathy following intestinal bypass, shoulder**

        M02.011 **Arthropathy following intestinal bypass, right shoulder**

        M02.012 **Arthropathy following intestinal bypass, left shoulder**

        M02.019 **Arthropathy following intestinal bypass, unspecified shoulder**

✓6ᵗʰ **M02.02** **Arthropathy following intestinal bypass, elbow**

        M02.021 **Arthropathy following intestinal bypass, right elbow**

        M02.022 **Arthropathy following intestinal bypass, left elbow**

        M02.029 **Arthropathy following intestinal bypass, unspecified elbow**

✓6ᵗʰ **M02.03** **Arthropathy following intestinal bypass, wrist**
    Arthropathy following intestinal bypass, carpal bones

        M02.031 **Arthropathy following intestinal bypass, right wrist**

        M02.032 **Arthropathy following intestinal bypass, left wrist**

        M02.039 **Arthropathy following intestinal bypass, unspecified wrist**

✓6ᵗʰ **M02.04** **Arthropathy following intestinal bypass, hand**
    Arthropathy following intestinal bypass, metacarpals and phalanges

        M02.041 **Arthropathy following intestinal bypass, right hand**

        M02.042 **Arthropathy following intestinal bypass, left hand**

        M02.049 **Arthropathy following intestinal bypass, unspecified hand**

✓6ᵗʰ **M02.05** **Arthropathy following intestinal bypass, hip**

        M02.051 **Arthropathy following intestinal bypass, right hip**

        M02.052 **Arthropathy following intestinal bypass, left hip**

        M02.059 **Arthropathy following intestinal bypass, unspecified hip**

✓6ᵗʰ **M02.06** **Arthropathy following intestinal bypass, knee**

        M02.061 **Arthropathy following intestinal bypass, right knee**

        M02.062 **Arthropathy following intestinal bypass, left knee**

        M02.069 **Arthropathy following intestinal bypass, unspecified knee**

✓6ᵗʰ **M02.07** **Arthropathy following intestinal bypass, ankle and foot**
    Arthropathy following intestinal bypass, tarsus, metatarsus and phalanges

        M02.071 **Arthropathy following intestinal bypass, right ankle and foot**

        M02.072 **Arthropathy following intestinal bypass, left ankle and foot**

        M02.079 **Arthropathy following intestinal bypass, unspecified ankle and foot**

    M02.08 **Arthropathy following intestinal bypass, vertebrae**

    M02.09 **Arthropathy following intestinal bypass, multiple sites**

✓5ᵗʰ **M02.1** **Postdysenteric arthropathy**

    CC Excl: For CC codes in subcategory M02.1, unless otherwise noted: PDX collection 863

    M02.10 **Postdysenteric arthropathy, unspecified site**   CC HCC

✓6ᵗʰ **M02.11** **Postdysenteric arthropathy, shoulder**

        M02.111 **Postdysenteric arthropathy, right shoulder**   CC HCC

        M02.112 **Postdysenteric arthropathy, left shoulder**   CC HCC

        M02.119 **Postdysenteric arthropathy, unspecified shoulder**   CC HCC

✓6ᵗʰ **M02.12** **Postdysenteric arthropathy, elbow**

        M02.121 **Postdysenteric arthropathy, right elbow**   CC HCC

        M02.122 **Postdysenteric arthropathy, left elbow**   CC HCC

        M02.129 **Postdysenteric arthropathy, unspecified elbow**   CC HCC

✓6ᵗʰ **M02.13** **Postdysenteric arthropathy, wrist**
    Postdysenteric arthropathy, carpal bones

        M02.131 **Postdysenteric arthropathy, right wrist**   CC HCC

        M02.132 **Postdysenteric arthropathy, left wrist**   CC HCC

        M02.139 **Postdysenteric arthropathy, unspecified wrist**   CC HCC

✓6ᵗʰ **M02.14** **Postdysenteric arthropathy, hand**
    Postdysenteric arthropathy, metacarpus and phalanges

        M02.141 **Postdysenteric arthropathy, right hand**   CC HCC

        M02.142 **Postdysenteric arthropathy, left hand**   CC HCC

        M02.149 **Postdysenteric arthropathy, unspecified hand**   CC HCC

✓6ᵗʰ **M02.15** **Postdysenteric arthropathy, hip**

        M02.151 **Postdysenteric arthropathy, right hip**   CC HCC

        M02.152 **Postdysenteric arthropathy, left hip**   CC HCC

        M02.159 **Postdysenteric arthropathy, unspecified hip**   CC HCC

✓6ᵗʰ **M02.16** Postdysenteric arthropathy, knee

CC Excl: For CC codes in subcategory M02.16: PDX collection 865

    M02.161 Postdysenteric arthropathy, right knee   `CC` `HCC`

    M02.162 Postdysenteric arthropathy, left knee   `CC` `HCC`

    M02.169 Postdysenteric arthropathy, unspecified knee   `CC` `HCC`

✓6ᵗʰ **M02.17** Postdysenteric arthropathy, ankle and foot
Postdysenteric arthropathy, tarsus, metatarsus and phalanges

    M02.171 Postdysenteric arthropathy, right ankle and foot   `CC` `HCC`

    M02.172 Postdysenteric arthropathy, left ankle and foot   `CC` `HCC`

    M02.179 Postdysenteric arthropathy, unspecified ankle and foot   `CC` `HCC`

    M02.18 Postdysenteric arthropathy, vertebrae   `CC` `HCC`
CC Excl: PDX collection 866

    M02.19 Postdysenteric arthropathy, multiple sites   `CC` `HCC`

✓5ᵗʰ **M02.2** Postimmunization arthropathy

    M02.20 Postimmunization arthropathy, unspecified site

✓6ᵗʰ **M02.21** Postimmunization arthropathy, shoulder

    M02.211 Postimmunization arthropathy, right shoulder

    M02.212 Postimmunization arthropathy, left shoulder

    M02.219 Postimmunization arthropathy, unspecified shoulder

✓6ᵗʰ **M02.22** Postimmunization arthropathy, elbow

    M02.221 Postimmunization arthropathy, right elbow

    M02.222 Postimmunization arthropathy, left elbow

    M02.229 Postimmunization arthropathy, unspecified elbow

✓6ᵗʰ **M02.23** Postimmunization arthropathy, wrist
Postimmunization arthropathy, carpal bones

    M02.231 Postimmunization arthropathy, right wrist

    M02.232 Postimmunization arthropathy, left wrist

    M02.239 Postimmunization arthropathy, unspecified wrist

✓6ᵗʰ **M02.24** Postimmunization arthropathy, hand
Postimmunization arthropathy, metacarpus and phalanges

    M02.241 Postimmunization arthropathy, right hand

    M02.242 Postimmunization arthropathy, left hand

    M02.249 Postimmunization arthropathy, unspecified hand

✓6ᵗʰ **M02.25** Postimmunization arthropathy, hip

    M02.251 Postimmunization arthropathy, right hip

    M02.252 Postimmunization arthropathy, left hip

    M02.259 Postimmunization arthropathy, unspecified hip

✓6ᵗʰ **M02.26** Postimmunization arthropathy, knee

    M02.261 Postimmunization arthropathy, right knee

    M02.262 Postimmunization arthropathy, left knee

    M02.269 Postimmunization arthropathy, unspecified knee

✓6ᵗʰ **M02.27** Postimmunization arthropathy, ankle and foot
Postimmunization arthropathy, tarsus, metatarsus and phalanges

    M02.271 Postimmunization arthropathy, right ankle and foot

    M02.272 Postimmunization arthropathy, left ankle and foot

    M02.279 Postimmunization arthropathy, unspecified ankle and foot

    M02.28 Postimmunization arthropathy, vertebrae

    M02.29 Postimmunization arthropathy, multiple sites

✓5ᵗʰ **M02.3** Reiter's disease
Reactive arthritis
DEF: Arthritis, iridocyclitis, and urethritis, sometimes with diarrhea. While symptoms may recur, arthritis is constant.

CC Excl: For CC codes in subcategory M02.3: PDX collection 863

    M02.30 Reiter's disease, unspecified site   `CC` `HCC`

✓6ᵗʰ **M02.31** Reiter's disease, shoulder

    M02.311 Reiter's disease, right shoulder   `CC` `HCC`

    M02.312 Reiter's disease, left shoulder   `CC` `HCC`

    M02.319 Reiter's disease, unspecified shoulder   `CC` `HCC`

✓6ᵗʰ **M02.32** Reiter's disease, elbow

    M02.321 Reiter's disease, right elbow   `CC` `HCC`

    M02.322 Reiter's disease, left elbow   `CC` `HCC`

    M02.329 Reiter's disease, unspecified elbow   `CC` `HCC`

✓6ᵗʰ **M02.33** Reiter's disease, wrist
Reiter's disease, carpal bones

    M02.331 Reiter's disease, right wrist   `CC` `HCC`

    M02.332 Reiter's disease, left wrist   `CC` `HCC`

    M02.339 Reiter's disease, unspecified wrist   `CC` `HCC`

✓6ᵗʰ **M02.34** Reiter's disease, hand
Reiter's disease, metacarpus and phalanges

    M02.341 Reiter's disease, right hand   `CC` `HCC`

    M02.342 Reiter's disease, left hand   `CC` `HCC`

    M02.349 Reiter's disease, unspecified hand   `CC` `HCC`

✓6ᵗʰ **M02.35** Reiter's disease, hip

    M02.351 Reiter's disease, right hip   `CC` `HCC`

    M02.352 Reiter's disease, left hip   `CC` `HCC`

    M02.359 Reiter's disease, unspecified hip   `CC` `HCC`

✓6ᵗʰ **M02.36** Reiter's disease, knee

    M02.361 Reiter's disease, right knee   `CC` `HCC`

    M02.362 Reiter's disease, left knee   `CC` `HCC`

    M02.369 Reiter's disease, unspecified knee   `CC` `HCC`

✓6ᵗʰ **M02.37** Reiter's disease, ankle and foot
Reiter's disease, tarsus, metatarsus and phalanges

    M02.371 Reiter's disease, right ankle and foot   `CC` `HCC`

    M02.372 Reiter's disease, left ankle and foot   `CC` `HCC`

    M02.379 Reiter's disease, unspecified ankle and foot   `CC` `HCC`

    M02.38 Reiter's disease, vertebrae   `CC` `HCC`

    M02.39 Reiter's disease, multiple sites   `CC` `HCC`

✓5ᵗʰ **M02.8** Other reactive arthropathies

CC Excl: For CC codes in subcategory M02.8, unless otherwise noted: PDX collection 863

    M02.80 *Other reactive arthropathies, unspecified site*   `CC` `HCC`

✓6ᵗʰ **M02.81** Other reactive arthropathies, shoulder

CC Excl: For CC codes in subcategory M02.81: PDX collection 864

    M02.811 *Other reactive arthropathies, right shoulder*   `CC` `HCC`

    M02.812 *Other reactive arthropathies, left shoulder*   `CC` `HCC`

    M02.819 *Other reactive arthropathies, unspecified shoulder*   `CC` `HCC`

✓6ᵗʰ **M02.82** Other reactive arthropathies, elbow

    M02.821 *Other reactive arthropathies, right elbow*   `CC` `HCC`

    M02.822 *Other reactive arthropathies, left elbow*   `CC` `HCC`

    M02.829 *Other reactive arthropathies, unspecified elbow*   `CC` `HCC`

✓6ᵗʰ **M02.83** Other reactive arthropathies, wrist
Other reactive arthropathies, carpal bones

    M02.831 *Other reactive arthropathies, right wrist*   `CC` `HCC`

    M02.832 *Other reactive arthropathies, left wrist*   `CC` `HCC`

    M02.839 *Other reactive arthropathies, unspecified wrist*   `CC` `HCC`

✓6ᵗʰ M02.84 Other reactive arthropathies, hand
Other reactive arthropathies, metacarpus and phalanges

    M02.841 Other reactive arthropathies, right hand `CC` `HCC`

    M02.842 Other reactive arthropathies, left hand `CC` `HCC`

    M02.849 Other reactive arthropathies, unspecified hand `CC` `HCC`

✓6ᵗʰ M02.85 Other reactive arthropathies, hip

    M02.851 Other reactive arthropathies, right hip `CC` `HCC`

    M02.852 Other reactive arthropathies, left hip `CC` `HCC`

    M02.859 Other reactive arthropathies, unspecified hip `CC` `HCC`

✓6ᵗʰ M02.86 Other reactive arthropathies, knee

    M02.861 Other reactive arthropathies, right knee `CC` `HCC`

    M02.862 Other reactive arthropathies, left knee `CC` `HCC`

    M02.869 Other reactive arthropathies, unspecified knee `CC` `HCC`

✓6ᵗʰ M02.87 Other reactive arthropathies, ankle and foot
Other reactive arthropathies, tarsus, metatarsus and phalanges

    M02.871 Other reactive arthropathies, right ankle and foot `CC` `HCC`

    M02.872 Other reactive arthropathies, left ankle and foot `CC` `HCC`

    M02.879 Other reactive arthropathies, unspecified ankle and foot `CC` `HCC`

  M02.88 Other reactive arthropathies, vertebrae `CC` `HCC`

  M02.89 Other reactive arthropathies, multiple sites `CC` `HCC`

  M02.9 Reactive arthropathy, unspecified `HCC`

Autoinflammatory syndromes (M04)

✓4ᵗʰ M04 Autoinflammatory syndromes
  `EXCLUDES 2` Crohn's disease (K50.-)
  AHA: 2016, 4Q, 37

M04.1 Periodic fever syndromes `HCC`
Familial Mediterranean fever
Hyperimmunoglobin D syndrome
Mevalonate kinase deficiency
Tumor necrosis factor receptor associated periodic syndrome [TRAPS]

M04.2 Cryopyrin-associated periodic syndromes `HCC`
Chronic infantile neurological, cutaneous and articular syndrome [CINCA]
Familial cold autoinflammatory syndrome
Familial cold urticaria
Muckle-Wells syndrome
Neonatal onset multisystemic inflammatory disorder [NOMID]

M04.8 Other autoinflammatory syndromes `HCC`
Blau syndrome
Deficiency of interleukin 1 receptor antagonist [DIRA]
Majeed syndrome
Periodic fever, aphthous stomatitis, pharyngitis, and adenopathy syndrome [PFAPA]
Pyogenic arthritis, pyoderma gangrenosum, and acne syndrome [PAPA]

M04.9 Autoinflammatory syndrome, unspecified `HCC`

Inflammatory polyarthropathies (M05-M14)

✓4ᵗʰ M05 Rheumatoid arthritis with rheumatoid factor
  `EXCLUDES 1` rheumatic fever (I00)
           juvenile rheumatoid arthritis (M08.-)
           rheumatoid arthritis of spine (M45.-)
  DEF: Rheumatoid arthritis: Autoimmune systemic disease that causes chronic inflammation of the joints and other areas of the body, manifested by inflammatory changes in articular structures and synovial membranes, atrophy, and loss in bone density.

✓5ᵗʰ M05.0 Felty's syndrome
Rheumatoid arthritis with splenoadenomegaly and leukopenia

  M05.00 Felty's syndrome, unspecified site `HCC`

  ✓6ᵗʰ M05.01 Felty's syndrome, shoulder
    M05.011 Felty's syndrome, right shoulder `HCC`
    M05.012 Felty's syndrome, left shoulder `HCC`
    M05.019 Felty's syndrome, unspecified shoulder `HCC`

  ✓6ᵗʰ M05.02 Felty's syndrome, elbow
    M05.021 Felty's syndrome, right elbow `HCC`
    M05.022 Felty's syndrome, left elbow `HCC`
    M05.029 Felty's syndrome, unspecified elbow `HCC`

  ✓6ᵗʰ M05.03 Felty's syndrome, wrist
Felty's syndrome, carpal bones
    M05.031 Felty's syndrome, right wrist `HCC`
    M05.032 Felty's syndrome, left wrist `HCC`
    M05.039 Felty's syndrome, unspecified wrist `HCC`

  ✓6ᵗʰ M05.04 Felty's syndrome, hand
Felty's syndrome, metacarpus and phalanges
    M05.041 Felty's syndrome, right hand `HCC`
    M05.042 Felty's syndrome, left hand `HCC`
    M05.049 Felty's syndrome, unspecified hand `HCC`

  ✓6ᵗʰ M05.05 Felty's syndrome, hip
    M05.051 Felty's syndrome, right hip `HCC`
    M05.052 Felty's syndrome, left hip `HCC`
    M05.059 Felty's syndrome, unspecified hip `HCC`

  ✓6ᵗʰ M05.06 Felty's syndrome, knee
    M05.061 Felty's syndrome, right knee `HCC`
    M05.062 Felty's syndrome, left knee `HCC`
    M05.069 Felty's syndrome, unspecified knee `HCC`

  ✓6ᵗʰ M05.07 Felty's syndrome, ankle and foot
Felty's syndrome, tarsus, metatarsus and phalanges
    M05.071 Felty's syndrome, right ankle and foot `HCC`
    M05.072 Felty's syndrome, left ankle and foot `HCC`
    M05.079 Felty's syndrome, unspecified ankle and foot `HCC`

  M05.09 Felty's syndrome, multiple sites `HCC`

✓5ᵗʰ M05.1 Rheumatoid lung disease with rheumatoid arthritis
  DEF: Lung disorders associated with rheumatoid arthritis.

  M05.10 Rheumatoid lung disease with rheumatoid arthritis of unspecified site `HCC`

  ✓6ᵗʰ M05.11 Rheumatoid lung disease with rheumatoid arthritis of shoulder
    M05.111 Rheumatoid lung disease with rheumatoid arthritis of right shoulder `HCC`
    M05.112 Rheumatoid lung disease with rheumatoid arthritis of left shoulder `HCC`
    M05.119 Rheumatoid lung disease with rheumatoid arthritis of unspecified shoulder `HCC`

  ✓6ᵗʰ M05.12 Rheumatoid lung disease with rheumatoid arthritis of elbow
    M05.121 Rheumatoid lung disease with rheumatoid arthritis of right elbow `HCC`
    M05.122 Rheumatoid lung disease with rheumatoid arthritis of left elbow `HCC`
    M05.129 Rheumatoid lung disease with rheumatoid arthritis of unspecified elbow `HCC`

`N` Newborn: 0   `P` Pediatric: 0-17   `M` Maternity: 12-55   `A` Adult: 15-124   `MCC` Major Complication/Comorbidity   `CC` Complication/Comorbidity   `SW` Severe Wound Dx

746   ICD-10-CM 2019

✓6ᵗʰ **M05.13 Rheumatoid lung disease with rheumatoid arthritis of** wrist
Rheumatoid lung disease with rheumatoid arthritis, carpal bones

M05.131 Rheumatoid lung disease with rheumatoid arthritis of right **wrist**   HCC

M05.132 Rheumatoid lung disease with rheumatoid arthritis of left **wrist**   HCC

M05.139 Rheumatoid lung disease with rheumatoid arthritis of unspecified **wrist**   HCC

✓6ᵗʰ **M05.14 Rheumatoid lung disease with rheumatoid arthritis of** hand
Rheumatoid lung disease with rheumatoid arthritis, metacarpus and phalanges

M05.141 Rheumatoid lung disease with rheumatoid arthritis of right **hand**   HCC

M05.142 Rheumatoid lung disease with rheumatoid arthritis of left **hand**   HCC

M05.149 Rheumatoid lung disease with rheumatoid arthritis of unspecified **hand**   HCC

✓6ᵗʰ **M05.15 Rheumatoid lung disease with rheumatoid arthritis of** hip

M05.151 Rheumatoid lung disease with rheumatoid arthritis of right **hip**   HCC

M05.152 Rheumatoid lung disease with rheumatoid arthritis of left **hip**   HCC

M05.159 Rheumatoid lung disease with rheumatoid arthritis of unspecified **hip**   HCC

✓6ᵗʰ **M05.16 Rheumatoid lung disease with rheumatoid arthritis of** knee

M05.161 Rheumatoid lung disease with rheumatoid arthritis of right **knee**   HCC

M05.162 Rheumatoid lung disease with rheumatoid arthritis of left **knee**   HCC

M05.169 Rheumatoid lung disease with rheumatoid arthritis of unspecified **knee**   HCC

✓6ᵗʰ **M05.17 Rheumatoid lung disease with rheumatoid arthritis of** ankle and foot
Rheumatoid lung disease with rheumatoid arthritis, tarsus, metatarsus and phalanges

M05.171 Rheumatoid lung disease with rheumatoid arthritis of right **ankle and foot**   HCC

M05.172 Rheumatoid lung disease with rheumatoid arthritis of left **ankle and foot**   HCC

M05.179 Rheumatoid lung disease with rheumatoid arthritis of unspecified **ankle and foot**   HCC

M05.19 Rheumatoid lung disease with rheumatoid arthritis of multiple sites   HCC

✓5ᵗʰ **M05.2 Rheumatoid** vasculitis with rheumatoid arthritis

M05.20 Rheumatoid vasculitis with rheumatoid arthritis of unspecified **site**   HCC

✓6ᵗʰ **M05.21 Rheumatoid vasculitis with rheumatoid arthritis of** shoulder

M05.211 Rheumatoid vasculitis with rheumatoid arthritis of right **shoulder**   HCC

M05.212 Rheumatoid vasculitis with rheumatoid arthritis of left **shoulder**   HCC

M05.219 Rheumatoid vasculitis with rheumatoid arthritis of unspecified **shoulder**   HCC

✓6ᵗʰ **M05.22 Rheumatoid vasculitis with rheumatoid arthritis of** elbow

M05.221 Rheumatoid vasculitis with rheumatoid arthritis of right **elbow**   HCC

M05.222 Rheumatoid vasculitis with rheumatoid arthritis of left **elbow**   HCC

M05.229 Rheumatoid vasculitis with rheumatoid arthritis of unspecified **elbow**   HCC

✓6ᵗʰ **M05.23 Rheumatoid vasculitis with rheumatoid arthritis of** wrist
Rheumatoid vasculitis with rheumatoid arthritis, carpal bones

M05.231 Rheumatoid vasculitis with rheumatoid arthritis of right **wrist**   HCC

M05.232 Rheumatoid vasculitis with rheumatoid arthritis of left **wrist**   HCC

M05.239 Rheumatoid vasculitis with rheumatoid arthritis of unspecified **wrist**   HCC

✓6ᵗʰ **M05.24 Rheumatoid vasculitis with rheumatoid arthritis of** hand
Rheumatoid vasculitis with rheumatoid arthritis, metacarpus and phalanges

M05.241 Rheumatoid vasculitis with rheumatoid arthritis of right **hand**   HCC

M05.242 Rheumatoid vasculitis with rheumatoid arthritis of left **hand**   HCC

M05.249 Rheumatoid vasculitis with rheumatoid arthritis of unspecified **hand**   HCC

✓6ᵗʰ **M05.25 Rheumatoid vasculitis with rheumatoid arthritis of** hip

M05.251 Rheumatoid vasculitis with rheumatoid arthritis of right **hip**   HCC

M05.252 Rheumatoid vasculitis with rheumatoid arthritis of left **hip**   HCC

M05.259 Rheumatoid vasculitis with rheumatoid arthritis of unspecified **hip**   HCC

✓6ᵗʰ **M05.26 Rheumatoid vasculitis with rheumatoid arthritis of** knee

M05.261 Rheumatoid vasculitis with rheumatoid arthritis of right **knee**   HCC

M05.262 Rheumatoid vasculitis with rheumatoid arthritis of left **knee**   HCC

M05.269 Rheumatoid vasculitis with rheumatoid arthritis of unspecified **knee**   HCC

✓6ᵗʰ **M05.27 Rheumatoid vasculitis with rheumatoid arthritis of** ankle and foot
Rheumatoid vasculitis with rheumatoid arthritis, tarsus, metatarsus and phalanges

M05.271 Rheumatoid vasculitis with rheumatoid arthritis of right **ankle and foot**   HCC

M05.272 Rheumatoid vasculitis with rheumatoid arthritis of left **ankle and foot**   HCC

M05.279 Rheumatoid vasculitis with rheumatoid arthritis of unspecified **ankle and foot**   HCC

M05.29 Rheumatoid vasculitis with rheumatoid arthritis of multiple sites   HCC

✓5ᵗʰ **M05.3 Rheumatoid** heart disease with rheumatoid arthritis
Rheumatoid carditis   Rheumatoid myocarditis
Rheumatoid endocarditis   Rheumatoid pericarditis

M05.30 Rheumatoid heart disease with rheumatoid arthritis of unspecified **site**   HCC

✓6ᵗʰ **M05.31 Rheumatoid heart disease with rheumatoid arthritis of** shoulder

M05.311 Rheumatoid heart disease with rheumatoid arthritis of right **shoulder**   HCC

M05.312 Rheumatoid heart disease with rheumatoid arthritis of left **shoulder**   HCC

M05.319 Rheumatoid heart disease with rheumatoid arthritis of unspecified **shoulder**   HCC

✓6ᵗʰ **M05.32 Rheumatoid heart disease with rheumatoid arthritis of** elbow

M05.321 Rheumatoid heart disease with rheumatoid arthritis of right **elbow**   HCC

M05.322 Rheumatoid heart disease with rheumatoid arthritis of left **elbow**   HCC

M05.329 Rheumatoid heart disease with rheumatoid arthritis of unspecified **elbow**   HCC

✓6ᵗʰ **M05.33 Rheumatoid heart disease with rheumatoid arthritis of** wrist
Rheumatoid heart disease with rheumatoid arthritis, carpal bones

M05.331 Rheumatoid heart disease with rheumatoid arthritis of right **wrist**   HCC

M05.332 Rheumatoid heart disease with rheumatoid arthritis of left **wrist**   HCC

M05.339 Rheumatoid heart disease with rheumatoid arthritis of unspecified **wrist**   HCC

✓ Additional Character Required   ✓x7ᵗʰ Placeholder   Unacceptable PDx   Questionable PDx   Manifestation   H1 - H14 HAC   HCC CMS-HCC Dx   HIV HIV Dx

ICD-10-CM 2019   **747**

Chapter 13. Diseases of the Musculoskeletal System and Connective Tissue

M05.13–M05.339

✓6th **M05.34 Rheumatoid heart disease with rheumatoid arthritis of** hand
> Rheumatoid heart disease with rheumatoid arthritis, metacarpus and phalanges

    M05.341 Rheumatoid heart disease with rheumatoid arthritis of right **hand** `HCC`

    M05.342 Rheumatoid heart disease with rheumatoid arthritis of left **hand** `HCC`

    M05.349 Rheumatoid heart disease with rheumatoid arthritis of unspecified **hand** `HCC`

✓6th **M05.35 Rheumatoid heart disease with rheumatoid arthritis of** hip

    M05.351 Rheumatoid heart disease with rheumatoid arthritis of right **hip** `HCC`

    M05.352 Rheumatoid heart disease with rheumatoid arthritis of left **hip** `HCC`

    M05.359 Rheumatoid heart disease with rheumatoid arthritis of unspecified **hip** `HCC`

✓6th **M05.36 Rheumatoid heart disease with rheumatoid arthritis of** knee

    M05.361 Rheumatoid heart disease with rheumatoid arthritis of right **knee** `HCC`

    M05.362 Rheumatoid heart disease with rheumatoid arthritis of left **knee** `HCC`

    M05.369 Rheumatoid heart disease with rheumatoid arthritis of unspecified **knee** `HCC`

✓6th **M05.37 Rheumatoid heart disease with rheumatoid arthritis of** ankle and foot
> Rheumatoid heart disease with rheumatoid arthritis, tarsus, metatarsus and phalanges

    M05.371 Rheumatoid heart disease with rheumatoid arthritis of right **ankle and foot** `HCC`

    M05.372 Rheumatoid heart disease with rheumatoid arthritis of left **ankle and foot** `HCC`

    M05.379 Rheumatoid heart disease with rheumatoid arthritis of unspecified **ankle and foot** `HCC`

  M05.39 Rheumatoid heart disease with rheumatoid arthritis of multiple sites `HCC`

✓5th **M05.4 Rheumatoid** myopathy with rheumatoid arthritis

> **CC Excl: For CC codes in subcategory M05.4:**
> PDX collection 867

  M05.40 Rheumatoid myopathy with rheumatoid arthritis of unspecified **site** `CC` `HCC`

✓6th **M05.41 Rheumatoid myopathy with rheumatoid arthritis of** shoulder

    M05.411 Rheumatoid myopathy with rheumatoid arthritis of right **shoulder** `CC` `HCC`

    M05.412 Rheumatoid myopathy with rheumatoid arthritis of left **shoulder** `CC` `HCC`

    M05.419 Rheumatoid myopathy with rheumatoid arthritis of unspecified **shoulder** `CC` `HCC`

✓6th **M05.42 Rheumatoid myopathy with rheumatoid arthritis of** elbow

    M05.421 Rheumatoid myopathy with rheumatoid arthritis of right **elbow** `CC` `HCC`

    M05.422 Rheumatoid myopathy with rheumatoid arthritis of left **elbow** `CC` `HCC`

    M05.429 Rheumatoid myopathy with rheumatoid arthritis of unspecified **elbow** `CC` `HCC`

✓6th **M05.43 Rheumatoid myopathy with rheumatoid arthritis of** wrist
> Rheumatoid myopathy with rheumatoid arthritis, carpal bones

    M05.431 Rheumatoid myopathy with rheumatoid arthritis of right **wrist** `CC` `HCC`

    M05.432 Rheumatoid myopathy with rheumatoid arthritis of left **wrist** `CC` `HCC`

  M05.439 Rheumatoid myopathy with rheumatoid arthritis of unspecified **wrist** `CC` `HCC`

✓6th **M05.44 Rheumatoid myopathy with rheumatoid arthritis of** hand
> Rheumatoid myopathy with rheumatoid arthritis, metacarpus and phalanges

    M05.441 Rheumatoid myopathy with rheumatoid arthritis of right **hand** `CC` `HCC`

    M05.442 Rheumatoid myopathy with rheumatoid arthritis of left **hand** `CC` `HCC`

    M05.449 Rheumatoid myopathy with rheumatoid arthritis of unspecified **hand** `CC` `HCC`

✓6th **M05.45 Rheumatoid myopathy with rheumatoid arthritis of** hip

    M05.451 Rheumatoid myopathy with rheumatoid arthritis of right **hip** `CC` `HCC`

    M05.452 Rheumatoid myopathy with rheumatoid arthritis of left **hip** `CC` `HCC`

    M05.459 Rheumatoid myopathy with rheumatoid arthritis of unspecified **hip** `CC` `HCC`

✓6th **M05.46 Rheumatoid myopathy with rheumatoid arthritis of** knee

    M05.461 Rheumatoid myopathy with rheumatoid arthritis of right **knee** `CC` `HCC`

    M05.462 Rheumatoid myopathy with rheumatoid arthritis of left **knee** `CC` `HCC`

    M05.469 Rheumatoid myopathy with rheumatoid arthritis of unspecified **knee** `CC` `HCC`

✓6th **M05.47 Rheumatoid myopathy with rheumatoid arthritis of** ankle and foot
> Rheumatoid myopathy with rheumatoid arthritis, tarsus, metatarsus and phalanges

    M05.471 Rheumatoid myopathy with rheumatoid arthritis of right **ankle and foot** `CC` `HCC`

    M05.472 Rheumatoid myopathy with rheumatoid arthritis of left **ankle and foot** `CC` `HCC`

    M05.479 Rheumatoid myopathy with rheumatoid arthritis of unspecified **ankle and foot** `CC` `HCC`

  M05.49 Rheumatoid myopathy with rheumatoid arthritis of multiple sites `CC` `HCC`

✓5th **M05.5 Rheumatoid** polyneuropathy with rheumatoid arthritis

  M05.50 Rheumatoid polyneuropathy with rheumatoid arthritis of unspecified **site** `HCC`

✓6th **M05.51 Rheumatoid polyneuropathy with rheumatoid arthritis of** shoulder

    M05.511 Rheumatoid polyneuropathy with rheumatoid arthritis of right **shoulder** `HCC`

    M05.512 Rheumatoid polyneuropathy with rheumatoid arthritis of left **shoulder** `HCC`

    M05.519 Rheumatoid polyneuropathy with rheumatoid arthritis of unspecified **shoulder** `HCC`

✓6th **M05.52 Rheumatoid polyneuropathy with rheumatoid arthritis of** elbow

    M05.521 Rheumatoid polyneuropathy with rheumatoid arthritis of right **elbow** `HCC`

    M05.522 Rheumatoid polyneuropathy with rheumatoid arthritis of left **elbow** `HCC`

    M05.529 Rheumatoid polyneuropathy with rheumatoid arthritis of unspecified **elbow** `HCC`

✓6th **M05.53 Rheumatoid polyneuropathy with rheumatoid arthritis of** wrist
> Rheumatoid polyneuropathy with rheumatoid arthritis, carpal bones

    M05.531 Rheumatoid polyneuropathy with rheumatoid arthritis of right **wrist** `HCC`

    M05.532 Rheumatoid polyneuropathy with rheumatoid arthritis of left **wrist** `HCC`

    M05.539 Rheumatoid polyneuropathy with rheumatoid arthritis of unspecified **wrist** `HCC`

N Newborn: 0 **P** Pediatric: 0-17 **M** Maternity: 12-55 **A** Adult: 15-124 `MCC` Major Complication/Comorbidity `CC` Complication/Comorbidity `SW` Severe Wound Dx

748   ICD-10-CM 2019

✓6th **M05.54 Rheumatoid polyneuropathy with rheumatoid arthritis of** hand
Rheumatoid polyneuropathy with rheumatoid arthritis, metacarpus and phalanges

M05.541 Rheumatoid polyneuropathy with rheumatoid arthritis of right **hand** HCC

M05.542 Rheumatoid polyneuropathy with rheumatoid arthritis of left **hand** HCC

M05.549 Rheumatoid polyneuropathy with rheumatoid arthritis of unspecified **hand** HCC

✓6th **M05.55 Rheumatoid polyneuropathy with rheumatoid arthritis of** hip

M05.551 Rheumatoid polyneuropathy with rheumatoid arthritis of right **hip** HCC

M05.552 Rheumatoid polyneuropathy with rheumatoid arthritis of left **hip** HCC

M05.559 Rheumatoid polyneuropathy with rheumatoid arthritis of unspecified **hip** HCC

✓6th **M05.56 Rheumatoid polyneuropathy with rheumatoid arthritis of** knee

M05.561 Rheumatoid polyneuropathy with rheumatoid arthritis of right **knee** HCC

M05.562 Rheumatoid polyneuropathy with rheumatoid arthritis of left **knee** HCC

M05.569 Rheumatoid polyneuropathy with rheumatoid arthritis of unspecified **knee** HCC

✓6th **M05.57 Rheumatoid polyneuropathy with rheumatoid arthritis of** ankle and foot
Rheumatoid polyneuropathy with rheumatoid arthritis, tarsus, metatarsus and phalanges

M05.571 Rheumatoid polyneuropathy with rheumatoid arthritis of right **ankle and foot** HCC

M05.572 Rheumatoid polyneuropathy with rheumatoid arthritis of left **ankle and foot** HCC

M05.579 Rheumatoid polyneuropathy with rheumatoid arthritis of unspecified **ankle and foot** HCC

M05.59 Rheumatoid polyneuropathy with rheumatoid arthritis of multiple sites HCC

✓5th **M05.6 Rheumatoid arthritis** with involvement of other organs and systems

M05.60 Rheumatoid arthritis of unspecified site **with involvement of other organs and systems** HCC

✓6th **M05.61 Rheumatoid arthritis of** shoulder **with involvement of other organs and systems**

M05.611 Rheumatoid arthritis of right **shoulder with involvement of other organs and systems** HCC

M05.612 Rheumatoid arthritis of left **shoulder with involvement of other organs and systems** HCC

M05.619 Rheumatoid arthritis of unspecified **shoulder with involvement of other organs and systems** HCC

✓6th **M05.62 Rheumatoid arthritis of** elbow **with involvement of other organs and systems**

M05.621 Rheumatoid arthritis of right **elbow with involvement of other organs and systems** HCC

M05.622 Rheumatoid arthritis of left **elbow with involvement of other organs and systems** HCC

M05.629 Rheumatoid arthritis of unspecified **elbow with involvement of other organs and systems** HCC

✓6th **M05.63 Rheumatoid arthritis of** wrist **with involvement of other organs and systems**
Rheumatoid arthritis of carpal bones with involvement of other organs and systems

M05.631 Rheumatoid arthritis of right **wrist with involvement of other organs and systems** HCC

M05.632 Rheumatoid arthritis of left **wrist with involvement of other organs and systems** HCC

M05.639 Rheumatoid arthritis of unspecified **wrist with involvement of other organs and systems** HCC

✓6th **M05.64 Rheumatoid arthritis of** hand **with involvement of other organs and systems**
Rheumatoid arthritis of metacarpus and phalanges with involvement of other organs and systems

M05.641 Rheumatoid arthritis of right **hand with involvement of other organs and systems** HCC

M05.642 Rheumatoid arthritis of left **hand with involvement of other organs and systems** HCC

M05.649 Rheumatoid arthritis of unspecified **hand with involvement of other organs and systems** HCC

✓6th **M05.65 Rheumatoid arthritis of** hip **with involvement of other organs and systems**

M05.651 Rheumatoid arthritis of right **hip with involvement of other organs and systems** HCC

M05.652 Rheumatoid arthritis of left **hip with involvement of other organs and systems** HCC

M05.659 Rheumatoid arthritis of unspecified **hip with involvement of other organs and systems** HCC

✓6th **M05.66 Rheumatoid arthritis of** knee **with involvement of other organs and systems**

M05.661 Rheumatoid arthritis of right **knee with involvement of other organs and systems** HCC

M05.662 Rheumatoid arthritis of left **knee with involvement of other organs and systems** HCC

M05.669 Rheumatoid arthritis of unspecified **knee with involvement of other organs and systems** HCC

✓6th **M05.67 Rheumatoid arthritis of** ankle and foot **with involvement of other organs and systems**
Rheumatoid arthritis of tarsus, metatarsus and phalanges with involvement of other organs and systems

M05.671 Rheumatoid arthritis of right **ankle and foot with involvement of other organs and systems** HCC

M05.672 Rheumatoid arthritis of left **ankle and foot with involvement of other organs and systems** HCC

M05.679 Rheumatoid arthritis of unspecified **ankle and foot with involvement of other organs and systems** HCC

M05.69 Rheumatoid arthritis of multiple sites **with involvement of other organs and systems** HCC

✓5th **M05.7 Rheumatoid arthritis** with rheumatoid factor without organ or systems involvement

M05.70 Rheumatoid arthritis with rheumatoid factor of unspecified site **without organ or systems involvement** HCC

✓6th **M05.71 Rheumatoid arthritis with rheumatoid factor of** shoulder **without organ or systems involvement**

M05.711 Rheumatoid arthritis with rheumatoid factor of right **shoulder without organ or systems involvement** HCC

M05.712 Rheumatoid arthritis with rheumatoid factor of left **shoulder without organ or systems involvement** HCC

M05.719 Rheumatoid arthritis with rheumatoid factor of unspecified **shoulder without organ or systems involvement** HCC

✓6th **M05.72 Rheumatoid arthritis with rheumatoid factor of** elbow **without organ or systems involvement**

M05.721 Rheumatoid arthritis with rheumatoid factor of right **elbow without organ or systems involvement** HCC

M05.722 Rheumatoid arthritis with rheumatoid factor of left **elbow without organ or systems involvement** HCC

✓ Additional Character Required   ✓x7th Placeholder   Unacceptable PDx   Questionable PDx   Manifestation   H1-H14 HAC   HCC CMS-HCC Dx   HIV HIV Dx

ICD-10-CM 2019   749

M05.729   Rheumatoid arthritis with rheumatoid factor of unspecified elbow without organ or systems involvement   `HCC`

✓6th **M05.73**   Rheumatoid arthritis with rheumatoid factor of wrist without organ or systems involvement

M05.731   Rheumatoid arthritis with rheumatoid factor of right wrist without organ or systems involvement   `HCC`

M05.732   Rheumatoid arthritis with rheumatoid factor of left wrist without organ or systems involvement   `HCC`

M05.739   Rheumatoid arthritis with rheumatoid factor of unspecified wrist without organ or systems involvement   `HCC`

✓6th **M05.74**   Rheumatoid arthritis with rheumatoid factor of hand without organ or systems involvement

M05.741   Rheumatoid arthritis with rheumatoid factor of right hand without organ or systems involvement   `HCC`

M05.742   Rheumatoid arthritis with rheumatoid factor of left hand without organ or systems involvement   `HCC`

M05.749   Rheumatoid arthritis with rheumatoid factor of unspecified hand without organ or systems involvement   `HCC`

✓6th **M05.75**   Rheumatoid arthritis with rheumatoid factor of hip without organ or systems involvement

M05.751   Rheumatoid arthritis with rheumatoid factor of right hip without organ or systems involvement   `HCC`

M05.752   Rheumatoid arthritis with rheumatoid factor of left hip without organ or systems involvement   `HCC`

M05.759   Rheumatoid arthritis with rheumatoid factor of unspecified hip without organ or systems involvement   `HCC`

✓6th **M05.76**   Rheumatoid arthritis with rheumatoid factor of knee without organ or systems involvement

M05.761   Rheumatoid arthritis with rheumatoid factor of right knee without organ or systems involvement   `HCC`

M05.762   Rheumatoid arthritis with rheumatoid factor of left knee without organ or systems involvement   `HCC`

M05.769   Rheumatoid arthritis with rheumatoid factor of unspecified knee without organ or systems involvement   `HCC`

✓6th **M05.77**   Rheumatoid arthritis with rheumatoid factor of ankle and foot without organ or systems involvement

M05.771   Rheumatoid arthritis with rheumatoid factor of right ankle and foot without organ or systems involvement   `HCC`

M05.772   Rheumatoid arthritis with rheumatoid factor of left ankle and foot without organ or systems involvement   `HCC`

M05.779   Rheumatoid arthritis with rheumatoid factor of unspecified ankle and foot without organ or systems involvement   `HCC`

M05.79   Rheumatoid arthritis with rheumatoid factor of multiple sites without organ or systems involvement   `HCC`

✓5th **M05.8**   Other rheumatoid arthritis with rheumatoid factor

M05.80   Other rheumatoid arthritis with rheumatoid actor of unspecified site   `HCC`

✓6th **M05.81**   Other rheumatoid arthritis with rheumatoid factor of shoulder

M05.811   Other rheumatoid arthritis with rheumatoid factor of right shoulder   `HCC`

M05.812   Other rheumatoid arthritis with rheumatoid factor of left shoulder   `HCC`

M05.819   Other rheumatoid arthritis with rheumatoid factor of unspecified shoulder   `HCC`

✓6th **M05.82**   Other rheumatoid arthritis with rheumatoid factor of elbow

M05.821   Other rheumatoid arthritis with rheumatoid factor of right elbow   `HCC`

M05.822   Other rheumatoid arthritis with rheumatoid factor of left elbow   `HCC`

M05.829   Other rheumatoid arthritis with rheumatoid factor of unspecified elbow   `HCC`

✓6th **M05.83**   Other rheumatoid arthritis with rheumatoid factor of wrist

M05.831   Other rheumatoid arthritis with rheumatoid factor of right wrist   `HCC`

M05.832   Other rheumatoid arthritis with rheumatoid factor of left wrist   `HCC`

M05.839   Other rheumatoid arthritis with rheumatoid factor of unspecified wrist   `HCC`

✓6th **M05.84**   Other rheumatoid arthritis with rheumatoid factor of hand

M05.841   Other rheumatoid arthritis with rheumatoid factor of right hand   `HCC`

M05.842   Other rheumatoid arthritis with rheumatoid factor of left hand   `HCC`

M05.849   Other rheumatoid arthritis with rheumatoid factor of unspecified hand   `HCC`

✓6th **M05.85**   Other rheumatoid arthritis with rheumatoid factor of hip

M05.851   Other rheumatoid arthritis with rheumatoid factor of right hip   `HCC`

M05.852   Other rheumatoid arthritis with rheumatoid factor of left hip   `HCC`

M05.859   Other rheumatoid arthritis with rheumatoid factor of unspecified hip   `HCC`

✓6th **M05.86**   Other rheumatoid arthritis with rheumatoid factor of knee

M05.861   Other rheumatoid arthritis with rheumatoid factor of right knee   `HCC`

M05.862   Other rheumatoid arthritis with rheumatoid factor of left knee   `HCC`

M05.869   Other rheumatoid arthritis with rheumatoid factor of unspecified knee   `HCC`

✓6th **M05.87**   Other rheumatoid arthritis with rheumatoid factor of ankle and foot

M05.871   Other rheumatoid arthritis with rheumatoid factor of right ankle and foot   `HCC`

M05.872   Other rheumatoid arthritis with rheumatoid factor of left ankle and foot   `HCC`

M05.879   Other rheumatoid arthritis with rheumatoid factor of unspecified ankle and foot   `HCC`

M05.89   Other rheumatoid arthritis with rheumatoid factor of multiple sites   `HCC`

M05.9   Rheumatoid arthritis with rheumatoid factor, unspecified   `HCC`

✓4th **M06**   **Other rheumatoid arthritis**

DEF: Rheumatoid arthritis: Autoimmune systemic disease that causes chronic inflammation of the joints and other areas of the body, manifested by inflammatory changes in articular structures and synovial membranes, atrophy, and loss in bone density.

✓5th **M06.0**   Rheumatoid arthritis without rheumatoid factor

M06.00   Rheumatoid arthritis without rheumatoid factor, unspecified site   `HCC`

✓6th **M06.01**   Rheumatoid arthritis without rheumatoid factor, shoulder

M06.011   Rheumatoid arthritis without rheumatoid factor, right shoulder   `HCC`

M06.012   Rheumatoid arthritis without rheumatoid factor, left shoulder   `HCC`

M06.019   Rheumatoid arthritis without rheumatoid factor, unspecified shoulder   `HCC`

✓6th **M06.02**   Rheumatoid arthritis without rheumatoid factor, elbow

M06.021   Rheumatoid arthritis without rheumatoid factor, right elbow   `HCC`

M06.022   Rheumatoid arthritis without rheumatoid factor, left elbow   `HCC`

M06.029   Rheumatoid arthritis without rheumatoid factor, unspecified elbow   `HCC`

N Newborn: 0   **P** Pediatric: 0-17   **M** Maternity: 12-55   **A** Adult: 15-124   **MCC** Major Complication/Comorbidity   **CC** Complication/Comorbidity   **SW** Severe Wound Dx

750   ICD-10-CM 2019

✓6ᵗʰ **M06.03** Rheumatoid arthritis without rheumatoid factor, wrist
    M06.031 Rheumatoid arthritis without rheumatoid factor, right wrist `HCC`
    M06.032 Rheumatoid arthritis without rheumatoid factor, left wrist `HCC`
    M06.039 Rheumatoid arthritis without rheumatoid factor, unspecified wrist `HCC`

✓6ᵗʰ **M06.04** Rheumatoid arthritis without rheumatoid factor, hand
    M06.041 Rheumatoid arthritis without rheumatoid factor, right hand `HCC`
    M06.042 Rheumatoid arthritis without rheumatoid factor, left hand `HCC`
    M06.049 Rheumatoid arthritis without rheumatoid factor, unspecified hand `HCC`

✓6ᵗʰ **M06.05** Rheumatoid arthritis without rheumatoid factor, hip
    M06.051 Rheumatoid arthritis without rheumatoid factor, right hip `HCC`
    M06.052 Rheumatoid arthritis without rheumatoid factor, left hip `HCC`
    M06.059 Rheumatoid arthritis without rheumatoid factor, unspecified hip `HCC`

✓6ᵗʰ **M06.06** Rheumatoid arthritis without rheumatoid factor, knee
    M06.061 Rheumatoid arthritis without rheumatoid factor, right knee `HCC`
    M06.062 Rheumatoid arthritis without rheumatoid factor, left knee `HCC`
    M06.069 Rheumatoid arthritis without rheumatoid factor, unspecified knee `HCC`

✓6ᵗʰ **M06.07** Rheumatoid arthritis without rheumatoid factor, ankle and foot
    M06.071 Rheumatoid arthritis without rheumatoid factor, right ankle and foot `HCC`
    M06.072 Rheumatoid arthritis without rheumatoid factor, left ankle and foot `HCC`
    M06.079 Rheumatoid arthritis without rheumatoid factor, unspecified ankle and foot `HCC`

M06.08 Rheumatoid arthritis without rheumatoid factor, vertebrae `HCC`

M06.09 Rheumatoid arthritis without rheumatoid factor, multiple sites `HCC`

M06.1 Adult-onset Still's disease `HCC` `A`
    EXCLUDES 1   Still's disease NOS (M08.2-)
    DEF: Type of systemic arthritis characterized by a transient rash and spiking fevers. This condition may resolve or develop into a chronic condition and may affect internal organs, as well as joints. **Synonym(s):** AOSD.

✓5ᵗʰ **M06.2** Rheumatoid bursitis
    M06.20 Rheumatoid bursitis, unspecified site `HCC`

✓6ᵗʰ **M06.21** Rheumatoid bursitis, shoulder
    M06.211 Rheumatoid bursitis, right shoulder `HCC`
    M06.212 Rheumatoid bursitis, left shoulder `HCC`
    M06.219 Rheumatoid bursitis, unspecified shoulder `HCC`

✓6ᵗʰ **M06.22** Rheumatoid bursitis, elbow
    M06.221 Rheumatoid bursitis, right elbow `HCC`
    M06.222 Rheumatoid bursitis, left elbow `HCC`
    M06.229 Rheumatoid bursitis, unspecified elbow `HCC`

✓6ᵗʰ **M06.23** Rheumatoid bursitis, wrist
    M06.231 Rheumatoid bursitis, right wrist `HCC`
    M06.232 Rheumatoid bursitis, left wrist `HCC`
    M06.239 Rheumatoid bursitis, unspecified wrist `HCC`

✓6ᵗʰ **M06.24** Rheumatoid bursitis, hand
    M06.241 Rheumatoid bursitis, right hand `HCC`
    M06.242 Rheumatoid bursitis, left hand `HCC`
    M06.249 Rheumatoid bursitis, unspecified hand `HCC`

✓6ᵗʰ **M06.25** Rheumatoid bursitis, hip
    M06.251 Rheumatoid bursitis, right hip `HCC`
    M06.252 Rheumatoid bursitis, left hip `HCC`
    M06.259 Rheumatoid bursitis, unspecified hip `HCC`

✓6ᵗʰ **M06.26** Rheumatoid bursitis, knee
    M06.261 Rheumatoid bursitis, right knee `HCC`
    M06.262 Rheumatoid bursitis, left knee `HCC`
    M06.269 Rheumatoid bursitis, unspecified knee `HCC`

✓6ᵗʰ **M06.27** Rheumatoid bursitis, ankle and foot
    M06.271 Rheumatoid bursitis, right ankle and foot `HCC`
    M06.272 Rheumatoid bursitis, left ankle and foot `HCC`
    M06.279 Rheumatoid bursitis, unspecified ankle and foot `HCC`

M06.28 Rheumatoid bursitis, vertebrae `HCC`

M06.29 Rheumatoid bursitis, multiple sites `HCC`

✓5ᵗʰ **M06.3** Rheumatoid nodule
    M06.30 Rheumatoid nodule, unspecified site `HCC`

✓6ᵗʰ **M06.31** Rheumatoid nodule, shoulder
    M06.311 Rheumatoid nodule, right shoulder `HCC`
    M06.312 Rheumatoid nodule, left shoulder `HCC`
    M06.319 Rheumatoid nodule, unspecified shoulder `HCC`

✓6ᵗʰ **M06.32** Rheumatoid nodule, elbow
    M06.321 Rheumatoid nodule, right elbow `HCC`
    M06.322 Rheumatoid nodule, left elbow `HCC`
    M06.329 Rheumatoid nodule, unspecified elbow `HCC`

✓6ᵗʰ **M06.33** Rheumatoid nodule, wrist
    M06.331 Rheumatoid nodule, right wrist `HCC`
    M06.332 Rheumatoid nodule, left wrist `HCC`
    M06.339 Rheumatoid nodule, unspecified wrist `HCC`

✓6ᵗʰ **M06.34** Rheumatoid nodule, hand
    M06.341 Rheumatoid nodule, right hand `HCC`
    M06.342 Rheumatoid nodule, left hand `HCC`
    M06.349 Rheumatoid nodule, unspecified hand `HCC`

✓6ᵗʰ **M06.35** Rheumatoid nodule, hip
    M06.351 Rheumatoid nodule, right hip `HCC`
    M06.352 Rheumatoid nodule, left hip `HCC`
    M06.359 Rheumatoid nodule, unspecified hip `HCC`

✓6ᵗʰ **M06.36** Rheumatoid nodule, knee
    M06.361 Rheumatoid nodule, right knee `HCC`
    M06.362 Rheumatoid nodule, left knee `HCC`
    M06.369 Rheumatoid nodule, unspecified knee `HCC`

✓6ᵗʰ **M06.37** Rheumatoid nodule, ankle and foot
    M06.371 Rheumatoid nodule, right ankle and foot `HCC`
    M06.372 Rheumatoid nodule, left ankle and foot `HCC`
    M06.379 Rheumatoid nodule, unspecified ankle and foot `HCC`

M06.38 Rheumatoid nodule, vertebrae `HCC`

M06.39 Rheumatoid nodule, multiple sites `HCC`

M06.4 Inflammatory polyarthropathy `HCC`
    EXCLUDES 1   polyarthritis NOS (M13.0)

✓5ᵗʰ **M06.8** Other specified rheumatoid arthritis
    M06.80 Other specified rheumatoid arthritis, unspecified site `HCC`

✓6ᵗʰ **M06.81** Other specified rheumatoid arthritis, shoulder
    M06.811 Other specified rheumatoid arthritis, right shoulder `HCC`
    M06.812 Other specified rheumatoid arthritis, left shoulder `HCC`
    M06.819 Other specified rheumatoid arthritis, unspecified shoulder `HCC`

✓6ᵗʰ **M06.82** Other specified rheumatoid arthritis, elbow
    M06.821 Other specified rheumatoid arthritis, right elbow `HCC`
    M06.822 Other specified rheumatoid arthritis, left elbow `HCC`
    M06.829 Other specified rheumatoid arthritis, unspecified elbow `HCC`

✓ Additional Character Required   ✓x7ᵗʰ Placeholder   Unacceptable PDx   Questionable PDx   Manifestation   `H1`-`H14` HAC   `HCC` CMS-HCC Dx   `HIV` HIV Dx

Chapter 13. Diseases of the Musculoskeletal System and Connective Tissue

✓6ᵗʰ **M06.83 Other specified rheumatoid arthritis, wrist**
    M06.831 Other specified rheumatoid arthritis, right wrist `HCC`
    M06.832 Other specified rheumatoid arthritis, left wrist `HCC`
    M06.839 Other specified rheumatoid arthritis, unspecified wrist `HCC`

✓6ᵗʰ **M06.84 Other specified rheumatoid arthritis, hand**
    M06.841 Other specified rheumatoid arthritis, right hand `HCC`
    M06.842 Other specified rheumatoid arthritis, left hand `HCC`
    M06.849 Other specified rheumatoid arthritis, unspecified hand `HCC`

✓6ᵗʰ **M06.85 Other specified rheumatoid arthritis, hip**
    M06.851 Other specified rheumatoid arthritis, right hip `HCC`
    M06.852 Other specified rheumatoid arthritis, left hip `HCC`
    M06.859 Other specified rheumatoid arthritis, unspecified hip `HCC`

✓6ᵗʰ **M06.86 Other specified rheumatoid arthritis, knee**
    M06.861 Other specified rheumatoid arthritis, right knee `HCC`
    M06.862 Other specified rheumatoid arthritis, left knee `HCC`
    M06.869 Other specified rheumatoid arthritis, unspecified knee `HCC`

✓6ᵗʰ **M06.87 Other specified rheumatoid arthritis, ankle and foot**
    M06.871 Other specified rheumatoid arthritis, right ankle and foot `HCC`
    M06.872 Other specified rheumatoid arthritis, left ankle and foot `HCC`
    M06.879 Other specified rheumatoid arthritis, unspecified ankle and foot `HCC`

    M06.88 Other specified rheumatoid arthritis, vertebrae `HCC`
    M06.89 Other specified rheumatoid arthritis, multiple sites `HCC`

M06.9 Rheumatoid arthritis, unspecified `HCC`

✓4ᵗʰ **M07 Enteropathic arthropathies**
Code also associated enteropathy, such as:
    regional enteritis [Crohn's disease] (K50.-)
    ulcerative colitis (K51.-)
EXCLUDES 1 *psoriatic arthropathies (L40.5-)*

✓5ᵗʰ **M07.6 Enteropathic arthropathies**
    M07.60 Enteropathic arthropathies, unspecified site

✓6ᵗʰ **M07.61 Enteropathic arthropathies, shoulder**
    M07.611 Enteropathic arthropathies, right shoulder
    M07.612 Enteropathic arthropathies, left shoulder
    M07.619 Enteropathic arthropathies, unspecified shoulder

✓6ᵗʰ **M07.62 Enteropathic arthropathies, elbow**
    M07.621 Enteropathic arthropathies, right elbow
    M07.622 Enteropathic arthropathies, left elbow
    M07.629 Enteropathic arthropathies, unspecified elbow

✓6ᵗʰ **M07.63 Enteropathic arthropathies, wrist**
    M07.631 Enteropathic arthropathies, right wrist
    M07.632 Enteropathic arthropathies, left wrist
    M07.639 Enteropathic arthropathies, unspecified wrist

✓6ᵗʰ **M07.64 Enteropathic arthropathies, hand**
    M07.641 Enteropathic arthropathies, right hand
    M07.642 Enteropathic arthropathies, left hand
    M07.649 Enteropathic arthropathies, unspecified hand

✓6ᵗʰ **M07.65 Enteropathic arthropathies, hip**
    M07.651 Enteropathic arthropathies, right hip
    M07.652 Enteropathic arthropathies, left hip
    M07.659 Enteropathic arthropathies, unspecified hip

✓6ᵗʰ **M07.66 Enteropathic arthropathies, knee**
    M07.661 Enteropathic arthropathies, right knee
    M07.662 Enteropathic arthropathies, left knee

    M07.669 Enteropathic arthropathies, unspecified knee

✓6ᵗʰ **M07.67 Enteropathic arthropathies, ankle and foot**
    M07.671 Enteropathic arthropathies, right ankle and foot
    M07.672 Enteropathic arthropathies, left ankle and foot
    M07.679 Enteropathic arthropathies, unspecified ankle and foot

    M07.68 Enteropathic arthropathies, vertebrae
    M07.69 Enteropathic arthropathies, multiple sites

✓4ᵗʰ **M08 Juvenile arthritis**
Code also any associated underlying condition, such as:
    regional enteritis [Crohn's disease] (K50.-)
    ulcerative colitis (K51.-)
EXCLUDES 1 *arthropathy in Whipple's disease (M14.8)*
    Felty's syndrome (M05.0)
    juvenile dermatomyositis (M33.0-)
    psoriatic juvenile arthropathy (L40.54)

✓5ᵗʰ **M08.0 Unspecified juvenile rheumatoid arthritis**
Juvenile rheumatoid arthritis with or without rheumatoid factor
    M08.00 Unspecified juvenile rheumatoid arthritis of unspecified site `HCC`

✓6ᵗʰ **M08.01 Unspecified juvenile rheumatoid arthritis, shoulder**
    M08.011 Unspecified juvenile rheumatoid arthritis, right shoulder `HCC`
    M08.012 Unspecified juvenile rheumatoid arthritis, left shoulder `HCC`
    M08.019 Unspecified juvenile rheumatoid arthritis, unspecified shoulder `HCC`

✓6ᵗʰ **M08.02 Unspecified juvenile rheumatoid arthritis of elbow**
    M08.021 Unspecified juvenile rheumatoid arthritis, right elbow `HCC`
    M08.022 Unspecified juvenile rheumatoid arthritis, left elbow `HCC`
    M08.029 Unspecified juvenile rheumatoid arthritis, unspecified elbow `HCC`

✓6ᵗʰ **M08.03 Unspecified juvenile rheumatoid arthritis, wrist**
    M08.031 Unspecified juvenile rheumatoid arthritis, right wrist `HCC`
    M08.032 Unspecified juvenile rheumatoid arthritis, left wrist `HCC`
    M08.039 Unspecified juvenile rheumatoid arthritis, unspecified wrist `HCC`

✓6ᵗʰ **M08.04 Unspecified juvenile rheumatoid arthritis, hand**
    M08.041 Unspecified juvenile rheumatoid arthritis, right hand `HCC`
    M08.042 Unspecified juvenile rheumatoid arthritis, left hand `HCC`
    M08.049 Unspecified juvenile rheumatoid arthritis, unspecified hand `HCC`

✓6ᵗʰ **M08.05 Unspecified juvenile rheumatoid arthritis, hip**
    M08.051 Unspecified juvenile rheumatoid arthritis, right hip `HCC`
    M08.052 Unspecified juvenile rheumatoid arthritis, left hip `HCC`
    M08.059 Unspecified juvenile rheumatoid arthritis, unspecified hip `HCC`

✓6ᵗʰ **M08.06 Unspecified juvenile rheumatoid arthritis, knee**
    M08.061 Unspecified juvenile rheumatoid arthritis, right knee `HCC`
    M08.062 Unspecified juvenile rheumatoid arthritis, left knee `HCC`
    M08.069 Unspecified juvenile rheumatoid arthritis, unspecified knee `HCC`

✓6ᵗʰ **M08.07 Unspecified juvenile rheumatoid arthritis, ankle and foot**
    M08.071 Unspecified juvenile rheumatoid arthritis, right ankle and foot `HCC`
    M08.072 Unspecified juvenile rheumatoid arthritis, left ankle and foot `HCC`
    M08.079 Unspecified juvenile rheumatoid arthritis, unspecified ankle and foot `HCC`

    M08.08 Unspecified juvenile rheumatoid arthritis, vertebrae `HCC`
    M08.09 Unspecified juvenile rheumatoid arthritis, multiple sites `HCC`

M08.1 **Juvenile** ankylosing spondylitis   `HCC`
> EXCLUDES 1   *ankylosing spondylitis in adults (M45.0-)*

☑5th M08.2 **Juvenile rheumatoid arthritis** with systemic onset
> Still's disease NOS
> EXCLUDES 1   *adult-onset Still's disease (M06.1-)*
> **DEF:** Systemic juvenile rheumatoid arthritis characterized by a transient rash and spiking fevers that may affect internal organs, as well as joints.

    M08.20   **Juvenile rheumatoid arthritis with systemic onset,** unspecified site   `HCC`

    ☑6th M08.21   **Juvenile rheumatoid arthritis with systemic onset,** shoulder
       M08.211   **Juvenile rheumatoid arthritis with** systemic onset, right shoulder   `HCC`
       M08.212   **Juvenile rheumatoid arthritis with** systemic onset, left shoulder   `HCC`
       M08.219   **Juvenile rheumatoid arthritis with** systemic onset, unspecified shoulder   `HCC`

    ☑6th M08.22   **Juvenile rheumatoid arthritis with systemic onset,** elbow
       M08.221   **Juvenile rheumatoid arthritis with** systemic onset, right elbow   `HCC`
       M08.222   **Juvenile rheumatoid arthritis with** systemic onset, left elbow   `HCC`
       M08.229   **Juvenile rheumatoid arthritis with** systemic onset, unspecified elbow   `HCC`

    ☑6th M08.23   **Juvenile rheumatoid arthritis with systemic onset,** wrist
       M08.231   **Juvenile rheumatoid arthritis with** systemic onset, right wrist   `HCC`
       M08.232   **Juvenile rheumatoid arthritis with** systemic onset, left wrist   `HCC`
       M08.239   **Juvenile rheumatoid arthritis with** systemic onset, unspecified wrist   `HCC`

    ☑6th M08.24   **Juvenile rheumatoid arthritis with systemic onset,** hand
       M08.241   **Juvenile rheumatoid arthritis with** systemic onset, right hand   `HCC`
       M08.242   **Juvenile rheumatoid arthritis with** systemic onset, left hand   `HCC`
       M08.249   **Juvenile rheumatoid arthritis with** systemic onset, unspecified hand   `HCC`

    ☑6th M08.25   **Juvenile rheumatoid arthritis with systemic onset,** hip
       M08.251   **Juvenile rheumatoid arthritis with** systemic onset, right hip   `HCC`
       M08.252   **Juvenile rheumatoid arthritis with** systemic onset, left hip   `HCC`
       M08.259   **Juvenile rheumatoid arthritis with** systemic onset, unspecified hip   `HCC`

    ☑6th M08.26   **Juvenile rheumatoid arthritis with systemic onset,** knee
       M08.261   **Juvenile rheumatoid arthritis with** systemic onset, right knee   `HCC`
       M08.262   **Juvenile rheumatoid arthritis with** systemic onset, left knee   `HCC`
       M08.269   **Juvenile rheumatoid arthritis with** systemic onset, unspecified knee   `HCC`

    ☑6th M08.27   **Juvenile rheumatoid arthritis with systemic onset,** ankle and foot
       M08.271   **Juvenile rheumatoid arthritis with** systemic onset, right ankle and foot   `HCC`
       M08.272   **Juvenile rheumatoid arthritis with** systemic onset, left ankle and foot   `HCC`
       M08.279   **Juvenile rheumatoid arthritis with** systemic onset, unspecified ankle and foot   `HCC`

    M08.28   **Juvenile rheumatoid arthritis with systemic** onset, vertebrae   `HCC`

    M08.29   **Juvenile rheumatoid arthritis with systemic** onset, multiple sites   `HCC`

M08.3 **Juvenile rheumatoid** polyarthritis (seronegative)   `HCC`

☑5th M08.4 **Pauciarticular** juvenile rheumatoid arthritis
    M08.40   **Pauciarticular juvenile rheumatoid arthritis,** unspecified site   `HCC`

    ☑6th M08.41   **Pauciarticular juvenile rheumatoid arthritis,** shoulder
       M08.411   **Pauciarticular juvenile rheumatoid arthritis,** right shoulder   `HCC`
       M08.412   **Pauciarticular juvenile rheumatoid arthritis,** left shoulder   `HCC`
       M08.419   **Pauciarticular juvenile rheumatoid arthritis,** unspecified shoulder   `HCC`

    ☑6th M08.42   **Pauciarticular juvenile rheumatoid arthritis,** elbow
       M08.421   **Pauciarticular juvenile rheumatoid arthritis,** right elbow   `HCC`
       M08.422   **Pauciarticular juvenile rheumatoid arthritis,** left elbow   `HCC`
       M08.429   **Pauciarticular juvenile rheumatoid arthritis,** unspecified elbow   `HCC`

    ☑6th M08.43   **Pauciarticular juvenile rheumatoid arthritis,** wrist
       M08.431   **Pauciarticular juvenile rheumatoid arthritis,** right wrist   `HCC`
       M08.432   **Pauciarticular juvenile rheumatoid arthritis,** left wrist   `HCC`
       M08.439   **Pauciarticular juvenile rheumatoid arthritis,** unspecified wrist   `HCC`

    ☑6th M08.44   **Pauciarticular juvenile rheumatoid arthritis,** hand
       M08.441   **Pauciarticular juvenile rheumatoid arthritis,** right hand   `HCC`
       M08.442   **Pauciarticular juvenile rheumatoid arthritis,** left hand   `HCC`
       M08.449   **Pauciarticular juvenile rheumatoid arthritis,** unspecified hand   `HCC`

    ☑6th M08.45   **Pauciarticular juvenile rheumatoid arthritis,** hip
       M08.451   **Pauciarticular juvenile rheumatoid arthritis,** right hip   `HCC`
       M08.452   **Pauciarticular juvenile rheumatoid arthritis,** left hip   `HCC`
       M08.459   **Pauciarticular juvenile rheumatoid arthritis,** unspecified hip   `HCC`

    ☑6th M08.46   **Pauciarticular juvenile rheumatoid arthritis,** knee
       M08.461   **Pauciarticular juvenile rheumatoid arthritis,** right knee   `HCC`
       M08.462   **Pauciarticular juvenile rheumatoid arthritis,** left knee   `HCC`
       M08.469   **Pauciarticular juvenile rheumatoid arthritis,** unspecified knee   `HCC`

    ☑6th M08.47   **Pauciarticular juvenile rheumatoid arthritis,** ankle and foot
       M08.471   **Pauciarticular juvenile rheumatoid arthritis,** right ankle and foot   `HCC`
       M08.472   **Pauciarticular juvenile rheumatoid arthritis,** left ankle and foot   `HCC`
       M08.479   **Pauciarticular juvenile rheumatoid arthritis,** unspecified ankle and foot   `HCC`

    M08.48   **Pauciarticular juvenile rheumatoid arthritis,** vertebrae   `HCC`

☑5th M08.8 **Other** juvenile arthritis
    M08.80   **Other juvenile arthritis,** unspecified site   `HCC`

    ☑6th M08.81   **Other juvenile arthritis,** shoulder
       M08.811   **Other juvenile arthritis,** right shoulder   `HCC`
       M08.812   **Other juvenile arthritis,** left shoulder   `HCC`
       M08.819   **Other juvenile arthritis,** unspecified shoulder   `HCC`

    ☑6th M08.82   **Other juvenile arthritis,** elbow
       M08.821   **Other juvenile arthritis,** right elbow   `HCC`
       M08.822   **Other juvenile arthritis,** left elbow   `HCC`
       M08.829   **Other juvenile arthritis,** unspecified elbow   `HCC`

    ☑6th M08.83   **Other juvenile arthritis,** wrist
       M08.831   **Other juvenile arthritis,** right wrist   `HCC`
       M08.832   **Other juvenile arthritis,** left wrist   `HCC`
       M08.839   **Other juvenile arthritis,** unspecified wrist   `HCC`

    ☑6th M08.84   **Other juvenile arthritis,** hand
       M08.841   **Other juvenile arthritis,** right hand   `HCC`
       M08.842   **Other juvenile arthritis,** left hand   `HCC`
       M08.849   **Other juvenile arthritis,** unspecified hand   `HCC`

☑ Additional Character Required   ✓x7th Placeholder   Unacceptable PDx   Questionable PDx   Manifestation   `H1`-`H14` HAC   `HCC` CMS-HCC Dx   `HIV` HIV Dx

√6ᵗʰ **M08.85** Other juvenile arthritis, hip
     M08.851 Other juvenile arthritis, right hip `HCC`
     M08.852 Other juvenile arthritis, left hip `HCC`
     M08.859 Other juvenile arthritis, unspecified hip `HCC`

√6ᵗʰ **M08.86** Other juvenile arthritis, knee
     M08.861 Other juvenile arthritis, right knee `HCC`
     M08.862 Other juvenile arthritis, left knee `HCC`
     M08.869 Other juvenile arthritis, unspecified knee `HCC`

√6ᵗʰ **M08.87** Other juvenile arthritis, ankle and foot
     M08.871 Other juvenile arthritis, right ankle and foot `HCC`
     M08.872 Other juvenile arthritis, left ankle and foot `HCC`
     M08.879 Other juvenile arthritis, unspecified ankle and foot `HCC`

M08.88 Other juvenile arthritis, other specified site `HCC`
     Other juvenile arthritis, vertebrae

M08.89 Other juvenile arthritis, multiple sites `HCC`

√5ᵗʰ **M08.9** Juvenile arthritis, unspecified
     EXCLUDES 1 *juvenile rheumatoid arthritis, unspecified (M08.0-)*

M08.90 Juvenile arthritis, unspecified, unspecified site `HCC`

√6ᵗʰ **M08.91** Juvenile arthritis, unspecified, shoulder
     M08.911 Juvenile arthritis, unspecified, right shoulder `HCC`
     M08.912 Juvenile arthritis, unspecified, left shoulder `HCC`
     M08.919 Juvenile arthritis, unspecified, unspecified shoulder `HCC`

√6ᵗʰ **M08.92** Juvenile arthritis, unspecified, elbow
     M08.921 Juvenile arthritis, unspecified, right elbow `HCC`
     M08.922 Juvenile arthritis, unspecified, left elbow `HCC`
     M08.929 Juvenile arthritis, unspecified, unspecified elbow `HCC`

√6ᵗʰ **M08.93** Juvenile arthritis, unspecified, wrist
     M08.931 Juvenile arthritis, unspecified, right wrist `HCC`
     M08.932 Juvenile arthritis, unspecified, left wrist `HCC`
     M08.939 Juvenile arthritis, unspecified, unspecified wrist `HCC`

√6ᵗʰ **M08.94** Juvenile arthritis, unspecified, hand
     M08.941 Juvenile arthritis, unspecified, right hand `HCC`
     M08.942 Juvenile arthritis, unspecified, left hand `HCC`
     M08.949 Juvenile arthritis, unspecified, unspecified hand `HCC`

√6ᵗʰ **M08.95** Juvenile arthritis, unspecified, hip
     M08.951 Juvenile arthritis, unspecified, right hip `HCC`
     M08.952 Juvenile arthritis, unspecified, left hip `HCC`
     M08.959 Juvenile arthritis, unspecified, unspecified hip `HCC`

√6ᵗʰ **M08.96** Juvenile arthritis, unspecified, knee
     M08.961 Juvenile arthritis, unspecified, right knee `HCC`
     M08.962 Juvenile arthritis, unspecified, left knee `HCC`
     M08.969 Juvenile arthritis, unspecified, unspecified knee `HCC`

√6ᵗʰ **M08.97** Juvenile arthritis, unspecified, ankle and foot
     M08.971 Juvenile arthritis, unspecified, right ankle and foot `HCC`
     M08.972 Juvenile arthritis, unspecified, left ankle and foot `HCC`
     M08.979 Juvenile arthritis, unspecified, unspecified ankle and foot `HCC`

M08.98 Juvenile arthritis, unspecified, vertebrae `HCC`

M08.99 Juvenile arthritis, unspecified, multiple sites `HCC`

√4ᵗʰ **M1A Chronic gout**
Use additional code to identify:
     autonomic neuropathy in diseases classified elsewhere (G99.0)
     calculus of urinary tract in diseases classified elsewhere (N22)
     cardiomyopathy in diseases classified elsewhere (I43)
     disorders of external ear in diseases classified elsewhere (H61.1-, H62.8-)
     disorders of iris and ciliary body in diseases classified elsewhere (H22)
     glomerular disorders in diseases classified elsewhere (N08)
     EXCLUDES 1 *gout NOS (M10.-)*
     EXCLUDES 2 *acute gout (M10.-)*

> The appropriate 7th character is to be added to each code from category M1A.
> 0   without tophus (tophi)
> 1   with tophus (tophi)

√5ᵗʰ **M1A.0** Idiopathic chronic gout
     Chronic gouty bursitis
     Primary chronic gout

√x7ᵗʰ **M1A.00** Idiopathic chronic gout, unspecified site

√6ᵗʰ **M1A.01** Idiopathic chronic gout, shoulder
     √7ᵗʰ **M1A.011** Idiopathic chronic gout, right shoulder
     √7ᵗʰ **M1A.012** Idiopathic chronic gout, left shoulder
     √7ᵗʰ **M1A.019** Idiopathic chronic gout, unspecified shoulder

√6ᵗʰ **M1A.02** Idiopathic chronic gout, elbow
     √7ᵗʰ **M1A.021** Idiopathic chronic gout, right elbow
     √7ᵗʰ **M1A.022** Idiopathic chronic gout, left elbow
     √7ᵗʰ **M1A.029** Idiopathic chronic gout, unspecified elbow

√6ᵗʰ **M1A.03** Idiopathic chronic gout, wrist
     √7ᵗʰ **M1A.031** Idiopathic chronic gout, right wrist
     √7ᵗʰ **M1A.032** Idiopathic chronic gout, left wrist
     √7ᵗʰ **M1A.039** Idiopathic chronic gout, unspecified wrist

√6ᵗʰ **M1A.04** Idiopathic chronic gout, hand
     √7ᵗʰ **M1A.041** Idiopathic chronic gout, right hand
     √7ᵗʰ **M1A.042** Idiopathic chronic gout, left hand
     √7ᵗʰ **M1A.049** Idiopathic chronic gout, unspecified hand

√6ᵗʰ **M1A.05** Idiopathic chronic gout, hip
     √7ᵗʰ **M1A.051** Idiopathic chronic gout, right hip
     √7ᵗʰ **M1A.052** Idiopathic chronic gout, left hip
     √7ᵗʰ **M1A.059** Idiopathic chronic gout, unspecified hip

√6ᵗʰ **M1A.06** Idiopathic chronic gout, knee
     √7ᵗʰ **M1A.061** Idiopathic chronic gout, right knee
     √7ᵗʰ **M1A.062** Idiopathic chronic gout, left knee
     √7ᵗʰ **M1A.069** Idiopathic chronic gout, unspecified knee

√6ᵗʰ **M1A.07** Idiopathic chronic gout, ankle and foot
     √7ᵗʰ **M1A.071** Idiopathic chronic gout, right ankle and foot
     √7ᵗʰ **M1A.072** Idiopathic chronic gout, left ankle and foot
     √7ᵗʰ **M1A.079** Idiopathic chronic gout, unspecified ankle and foot

√x7ᵗʰ **M1A.08** Idiopathic chronic gout, vertebrae

√x7ᵗʰ **M1A.09** Idiopathic chronic gout, multiple sites

√5ᵗʰ **M1A.1** Lead-induced chronic gout
     Code first toxic effects of lead and its compounds (T56.0-)

√x7ᵗʰ **M1A.10** Lead-induced chronic gout, unspecified site

√6ᵗʰ **M1A.11** Lead-induced chronic gout, shoulder
     √7ᵗʰ **M1A.111** Lead-induced chronic gout, right shoulder
     √7ᵗʰ **M1A.112** Lead-induced chronic gout, left shoulder
     √7ᵗʰ **M1A.119** Lead-induced chronic gout, unspecified shoulder

√6ᵗʰ **M1A.12** Lead-induced chronic gout, elbow
     √7ᵗʰ **M1A.121** Lead-induced chronic gout, right elbow
     √7ᵗʰ **M1A.122** Lead-induced chronic gout, left elbow
     √7ᵗʰ **M1A.129** Lead-induced chronic gout, unspecified elbow

√6ᵗʰ **M1A.13** Lead-induced chronic gout, wrist
     √7ᵗʰ **M1A.131** Lead-induced chronic gout, right wrist
     √7ᵗʰ **M1A.132** Lead-induced chronic gout, left wrist

N Newborn: 0   **P** Pediatric: 0-17   **M** Maternity: 12-55   **A** Adult: 15-124   **MCC** Major Complication/Comorbidity   **CC** Complication/Comorbidity   **SW** Severe Wound Dx

754   ICD-10-CM 2019

✓7ᵗʰ **M1A.139 Lead-induced chronic gout,** unspecified wrist

✓6ᵗʰ **M1A.14 Lead-induced chronic gout,** hand

✓7ᵗʰ **M1A.141 Lead-induced chronic gout,** right **hand**

✓7ᵗʰ **M1A.142 Lead-induced chronic gout,** left **hand**

✓7ᵗʰ **M1A.149 Lead-induced chronic gout,** unspecified **hand**

✓6ᵗʰ **M1A.15 Lead-induced chronic gout,** hip

✓7ᵗʰ **M1A.151 Lead-induced chronic gout,** right **hip**

✓7ᵗʰ **M1A.152 Lead-induced chronic gout,** left **hip**

✓7ᵗʰ **M1A.159 Lead-induced chronic gout,** unspecified **hip**

✓6ᵗʰ **M1A.16 Lead-induced chronic gout,** knee

✓7ᵗʰ **M1A.161 Lead-induced chronic gout,** right **knee**

✓7ᵗʰ **M1A.162 Lead-induced chronic gout,** left **knee**

✓7ᵗʰ **M1A.169 Lead-induced chronic gout,** unspecified **knee**

✓6ᵗʰ **M1A.17 Lead-induced chronic gout,** ankle and foot

✓7ᵗʰ **M1A.171 Lead-induced chronic gout,** right **ankle and foot**

✓7ᵗʰ **M1A.172 Lead-induced chronic gout,** left **ankle and foot**

✓7ᵗʰ **M1A.179 Lead-induced chronic gout,** unspecified **ankle and foot**

✓x7ᵗʰ **M1A.18 Lead-induced chronic gout,** vertebrae

✓x7ᵗʰ **M1A.19 Lead-induced chronic gout,** multiple sites

✓5ᵗʰ **M1A.2 Drug-induced chronic gout**
Use additional code for adverse effect, if applicable, to identify drug (T36-T50 with fifth or sixth character 5)

✓x7ᵗʰ **M1A.20 Drug-induced chronic gout,** unspecified site

✓6ᵗʰ **M1A.21 Drug-induced chronic gout,** shoulder

✓7ᵗʰ **M1A.211 Drug-induced chronic gout,** right **shoulder**

✓7ᵗʰ **M1A.212 Drug-induced chronic gout,** left **shoulder**

✓7ᵗʰ **M1A.219 Drug-induced chronic gout,** unspecified **shoulder**

✓6ᵗʰ **M1A.22 Drug-induced chronic gout,** elbow

✓7ᵗʰ **M1A.221 Drug-induced chronic gout,** right **elbow**

✓7ᵗʰ **M1A.222 Drug-induced chronic gout,** left **elbow**

✓7ᵗʰ **M1A.229 Drug-induced chronic gout,** unspecified **elbow**

✓6ᵗʰ **M1A.23 Drug-induced chronic gout,** wrist

✓7ᵗʰ **M1A.231 Drug-induced chronic gout,** right **wrist**

✓7ᵗʰ **M1A.232 Drug-induced chronic gout,** left **wrist**

✓7ᵗʰ **M1A.239 Drug-induced chronic gout,** unspecified **wrist**

✓6ᵗʰ **M1A.24 Drug-induced chronic gout,** hand

✓7ᵗʰ **M1A.241 Drug-induced chronic gout,** right **hand**

✓7ᵗʰ **M1A.242 Drug-induced chronic gout,** left **hand**

✓7ᵗʰ **M1A.249 Drug-induced chronic gout,** unspecified **hand**

✓6ᵗʰ **M1A.25 Drug-induced chronic gout,** hip

✓7ᵗʰ **M1A.251 Drug-induced chronic gout,** right **hip**

✓7ᵗʰ **M1A.252 Drug-induced chronic gout,** left **hip**

✓7ᵗʰ **M1A.259 Drug-induced chronic gout,** unspecified **hip**

✓6ᵗʰ **M1A.26 Drug-induced chronic gout,** knee

✓7ᵗʰ **M1A.261 Drug-induced chronic gout,** right **knee**

✓7ᵗʰ **M1A.262 Drug-induced chronic gout,** left **knee**

✓7ᵗʰ **M1A.269 Drug-induced chronic gout,** unspecified **knee**

✓6ᵗʰ **M1A.27 Drug-induced chronic gout,** ankle and foot

✓7ᵗʰ **M1A.271 Drug-induced chronic gout,** right **ankle and foot**

✓7ᵗʰ **M1A.272 Drug-induced chronic gout,** left **ankle and foot**

✓7ᵗʰ **M1A.279 Drug-induced chronic gout,** unspecified **ankle and foot**

✓x7ᵗʰ **M1A.28 Drug-induced chronic gout,** vertebrae

✓x7ᵗʰ **M1A.29 Drug-induced chronic gout,** multiple sites

✓5ᵗʰ **M1A.3 Chronic gout** due to renal impairment
Code first associated renal disease

✓x7ᵗʰ **M1A.30 Chronic gout due to renal impairment,** unspecified site

✓6ᵗʰ **M1A.31 Chronic gout due to renal impairment,** shoulder

✓7ᵗʰ **M1A.311 Chronic gout due to renal impairment,** right **shoulder**

✓7ᵗʰ **M1A.312 Chronic gout due to renal impairment,** left **shoulder**

✓7ᵗʰ **M1A.319 Chronic gout due to renal impairment,** unspecified **shoulder**

✓6ᵗʰ **M1A.32 Chronic gout due to renal impairment,** elbow

✓7ᵗʰ **M1A.321 Chronic gout due to renal impairment,** right **elbow**

✓7ᵗʰ **M1A.322 Chronic gout due to renal impairment,** left **elbow**

✓7ᵗʰ **M1A.329 Chronic gout due to renal impairment,** unspecified **elbow**

✓6ᵗʰ **M1A.33 Chronic gout due to renal impairment,** wrist

✓7ᵗʰ **M1A.331 Chronic gout due to renal impairment,** right **wrist**

✓7ᵗʰ **M1A.332 Chronic gout due to renal impairment,** left **wrist**

✓7ᵗʰ **M1A.339 Chronic gout due to renal impairment,** unspecified **wrist**

✓6ᵗʰ **M1A.34 Chronic gout due to renal impairment,** hand

✓7ᵗʰ **M1A.341 Chronic gout due to renal impairment,** right **hand**

✓7ᵗʰ **M1A.342 Chronic gout due to renal impairment,** left **hand**

✓7ᵗʰ **M1A.349 Chronic gout due to renal impairment,** unspecified **hand**

✓6ᵗʰ **M1A.35 Chronic gout due to renal impairment,** hip

✓7ᵗʰ **M1A.351 Chronic gout due to renal impairment,** right **hip**

✓7ᵗʰ **M1A.352 Chronic gout due to renal impairment,** left **hip**

✓7ᵗʰ **M1A.359 Chronic gout due to renal impairment,** unspecified **hip**

✓6ᵗʰ **M1A.36 Chronic gout due to renal impairment,** knee

✓7ᵗʰ **M1A.361 Chronic gout due to renal impairment,** right **knee**

✓7ᵗʰ **M1A.362 Chronic gout due to renal impairment,** left **knee**

✓7ᵗʰ **M1A.369 Chronic gout due to renal impairment,** unspecified **knee**

✓6ᵗʰ **M1A.37 Chronic gout due to renal impairment,** ankle and foot

✓7ᵗʰ **M1A.371 Chronic gout due to renal impairment,** right **ankle and foot**

✓7ᵗʰ **M1A.372 Chronic gout due to renal impairment,** left **ankle and foot**

✓7ᵗʰ **M1A.379 Chronic gout due to renal impairment,** unspecified **ankle and foot**

✓x7ᵗʰ **M1A.38 Chronic gout due to renal impairment,** vertebrae

✓x7ᵗʰ **M1A.39 Chronic gout due to renal impairment,** multiple sites

✓5ᵗʰ **M1A.4 Other secondary chronic gout**
Code first associated condition

✓x7ᵗʰ **M1A.40 Other secondary chronic gout,** unspecified site

✓6ᵗʰ **M1A.41 Other secondary chronic gout,** shoulder

✓7ᵗʰ **M1A.411 Other secondary chronic gout,** right **shoulder**

✓7ᵗʰ **M1A.412 Other secondary chronic gout,** left **shoulder**

✓7ᵗʰ **M1A.419 Other secondary chronic gout,** unspecified **shoulder**

✓6ᵗʰ **M1A.42 Other secondary chronic gout,** elbow

✓7ᵗʰ **M1A.421 Other secondary chronic gout,** right **elbow**

✓7ᵗʰ **M1A.422 Other secondary chronic gout,** left **elbow**

✓7ᵗʰ **M1A.429 Other secondary chronic gout,** unspecified **elbow**

✓ Additional Character Required   ✓x7ᵗʰ Placeholder   Unacceptable PDx   Questionable PDx   Manifestation   **H1**–**H14** HAC   **HCC** CMS-HCC Dx   **HIV** HIV Dx

√6ᵗʰ **M1A.43 Other secondary chronic gout,** wrist
- √7ᵗʰ **M1A.431 Other secondary chronic gout,** right wrist
- √7ᵗʰ **M1A.432 Other secondary chronic gout,** left wrist
- √7ᵗʰ **M1A.439 Other secondary chronic gout,** unspecified wrist

√6ᵗʰ **M1A.44 Other secondary chronic gout,** hand
- √7ᵗʰ **M1A.441 Other secondary chronic gout,** right hand
- √7ᵗʰ **M1A.442 Other secondary chronic gout,** left hand
- √7ᵗʰ **M1A.449 Other secondary chronic gout,** unspecified hand

√6ᵗʰ **M1A.45 Other secondary chronic gout,** hip
- √7ᵗʰ **M1A.451 Other secondary chronic gout,** right hip
- √7ᵗʰ **M1A.452 Other secondary chronic gout,** left hip
- √7ᵗʰ **M1A.459 Other secondary chronic gout,** unspecified hip

√6ᵗʰ **M1A.46 Other secondary chronic gout,** knee
- √7ᵗʰ **M1A.461 Other secondary chronic gout,** right knee
- √7ᵗʰ **M1A.462 Other secondary chronic gout,** left knee
- √7ᵗʰ **M1A.469 Other secondary chronic gout,** unspecified knee

√6ᵗʰ **M1A.47 Other secondary chronic gout,** ankle and foot
- √7ᵗʰ **M1A.471 Other secondary chronic gout,** right ankle and foot
- √7ᵗʰ **M1A.472 Other secondary chronic gout,** left ankle and foot
- √7ᵗʰ **M1A.479 Other secondary chronic gout,** unspecified ankle and foot

√x7ᵗʰ **M1A.48 Other secondary chronic gout,** vertebrae
√x7ᵗʰ **M1A.49 Other secondary chronic gout,** multiple sites

√x7ᵗʰ **M1A.9 Chronic gout,** unspecified

√4ᵗʰ **M10 Gout**
Acute gout
Gout attack
Gout flare
Podagra
Use additional code to identify:
  autonomic neuropathy in diseases classified elsewhere (G99.0)
  calculus of urinary tract in diseases classified elsewhere (N22)
  cardiomyopathy in diseases classified elsewhere (I43)
  disorders of external ear in diseases classified elsewhere (H61.1-, H62.8-)
  disorders of iris and ciliary body in diseases classified elsewhere (H22)
  glomerular disorders in diseases classified elsewhere (N08)
EXCLUDES 2   chronic gout (M1A.-)
DEF: Purine and pyrimidine metabolic disorders, manifested by hyperuricemia and recurrent acute inflammatory arthritis. Monosodium urate or monohydrate crystals may be deposited in and around the joints, leading to joint destruction and severe crippling.

√5ᵗʰ **M10.0 Idiopathic gout**
Gouty bursitis
Primary gout
- **M10.00 Idiopathic gout,** unspecified site
- √6ᵗʰ **M10.01 Idiopathic gout,** shoulder
  - **M10.011 Idiopathic gout,** right shoulder
  - **M10.012 Idiopathic gout,** left shoulder
  - **M10.019 Idiopathic gout,** unspecified shoulder
- √6ᵗʰ **M10.02 Idiopathic gout,** elbow
  - **M10.021 Idiopathic gout,** right elbow
  - **M10.022 Idiopathic gout,** left elbow
  - **M10.029 Idiopathic gout,** unspecified elbow
- √6ᵗʰ **M10.03 Idiopathic gout,** wrist
  - **M10.031 Idiopathic gout,** right wrist
  - **M10.032 Idiopathic gout,** left wrist
  - **M10.039 Idiopathic gout,** unspecified wrist
- √6ᵗʰ **M10.04 Idiopathic gout,** hand
  - **M10.041 Idiopathic gout,** right hand
  - **M10.042 Idiopathic gout,** left hand
  - **M10.049 Idiopathic gout,** unspecified hand
- √6ᵗʰ **M10.05 Idiopathic gout,** hip
  - **M10.051 Idiopathic gout,** right hip
  - **M10.052 Idiopathic gout,** left hip
  - **M10.059 Idiopathic gout,** unspecified hip

√6ᵗʰ **M10.06 Idiopathic gout,** knee
- **M10.061 Idiopathic gout,** right knee
- **M10.062 Idiopathic gout,** left knee
- **M10.069 Idiopathic gout,** unspecified knee

√6ᵗʰ **M10.07 Idiopathic gout,** ankle and foot
- **M10.071 Idiopathic gout,** right ankle and foot
- **M10.072 Idiopathic gout,** left ankle and foot
- **M10.079 Idiopathic gout,** unspecified ankle and foot

M10.08 Idiopathic gout, vertebrae
M10.09 Idiopathic gout, multiple sites

√5ᵗʰ **M10.1 Lead-induced gout**
Code first toxic effects of lead and its compounds (T56.0-)
- **M10.10 Lead-induced gout,** unspecified site
- √6ᵗʰ **M10.11 Lead-induced gout,** shoulder
  - **M10.111 Lead-induced gout,** right shoulder
  - **M10.112 Lead-induced gout,** left shoulder
  - **M10.119 Lead-induced gout,** unspecified shoulder
- √6ᵗʰ **M10.12 Lead-induced gout,** elbow
  - **M10.121 Lead-induced gout,** right elbow
  - **M10.122 Lead-induced gout,** left elbow
  - **M10.129 Lead-induced gout,** unspecified elbow
- √6ᵗʰ **M10.13 Lead-induced gout,** wrist
  - **M10.131 Lead-induced gout,** right wrist
  - **M10.132 Lead-induced gout,** left wrist
  - **M10.139 Lead-induced gout,** unspecified wrist
- √6ᵗʰ **M10.14 Lead-induced gout,** hand
  - **M10.141 Lead-induced gout,** right hand
  - **M10.142 Lead-induced gout,** left hand
  - **M10.149 Lead-induced gout,** unspecified hand
- √6ᵗʰ **M10.15 Lead-induced gout,** hip
  - **M10.151 Lead-induced gout,** right hip
  - **M10.152 Lead-induced gout,** left hip
  - **M10.159 Lead-induced gout,** unspecified hip
- √6ᵗʰ **M10.16 Lead-induced gout,** knee
  - **M10.161 Lead-induced gout,** right knee
  - **M10.162 Lead-induced gout,** left knee
  - **M10.169 Lead-induced gout,** unspecified knee
- √6ᵗʰ **M10.17 Lead-induced gout,** ankle and foot
  - **M10.171 Lead-induced gout,** right ankle and foot
  - **M10.172 Lead-induced gout,** left ankle and foot
  - **M10.179 Lead-induced gout,** unspecified ankle and foot
- **M10.18 Lead-induced gout,** vertebrae
- **M10.19 Lead-induced gout,** multiple sites

√5ᵗʰ **M10.2 Drug-induced gout**
Use additional code for adverse effect, if applicable, to identify drug (T36-T50 with fifth or sixth character 5)
- **M10.20 Drug-induced gout,** unspecified site
- √6ᵗʰ **M10.21 Drug-induced gout,** shoulder
  - **M10.211 Drug-induced gout,** right shoulder
  - **M10.212 Drug-induced gout,** left shoulder
  - **M10.219 Drug-induced gout,** unspecified shoulder
- √6ᵗʰ **M10.22 Drug-induced gout,** elbow
  - **M10.221 Drug-induced gout,** right elbow
  - **M10.222 Drug-induced gout,** left elbow
  - **M10.229 Drug-induced gout,** unspecified elbow
- √6ᵗʰ **M10.23 Drug-induced gout,** wrist
  - **M10.231 Drug-induced gout,** right wrist
  - **M10.232 Drug-induced gout,** left wrist
  - **M10.239 Drug-induced gout,** unspecified wrist
- √6ᵗʰ **M10.24 Drug-induced gout,** hand
  - **M10.241 Drug-induced gout,** right hand
  - **M10.242 Drug-induced gout,** left hand
  - **M10.249 Drug-induced gout,** unspecified hand
- √6ᵗʰ **M10.25 Drug-induced gout,** hip
  - **M10.251 Drug-induced gout,** right hip
  - **M10.252 Drug-induced gout,** left hip
  - **M10.259 Drug-induced gout,** unspecified hip

✓6ᵗʰ **M10.26 Drug-induced gout,** knee
     M10.261 **Drug-induced gout,** right **knee**
     M10.262 **Drug-induced gout,** left **knee**
     M10.269 **Drug-induced gout,** unspecified **knee**

✓6ᵗʰ **M10.27 Drug-induced gout,** ankle and foot
     M10.271 **Drug-induced gout,** right **ankle and foot**
     M10.272 **Drug-induced gout,** left **ankle and foot**
     M10.279 **Drug-induced gout,** unspecified **ankle and foot**

M10.28 Drug-induced gout, vertebrae
M10.29 Drug-induced gout, multiple sites

✓5ᵗʰ **M10.3 Gout due to** renal impairment
     Code first associated renal disease

M10.30 Gout due to renal impairment, unspecified site

✓6ᵗʰ **M10.31 Gout due to renal impairment,** shoulder
     M10.311 **Gout due to renal impairment,** right **shoulder**
     M10.312 **Gout due to renal impairment,** left **shoulder**
     M10.319 **Gout due to renal impairment,** unspecified **shoulder**

✓6ᵗʰ **M10.32 Gout due to renal impairment,** elbow
     M10.321 **Gout due to renal impairment,** right **elbow**
     M10.322 **Gout due to renal impairment,** left **elbow**
     M10.329 **Gout due to renal impairment,** unspecified **elbow**

✓6ᵗʰ **M10.33 Gout due to renal impairment,** wrist
     M10.331 **Gout due to renal impairment,** right **wrist**
     M10.332 **Gout due to renal impairment,** left **wrist**
     M10.339 **Gout due to renal impairment,** unspecified **wrist**

✓6ᵗʰ **M10.34 Gout due to renal impairment,** hand
     M10.341 **Gout due to renal impairment,** right **hand**
     M10.342 **Gout due to renal impairment,** left **hand**
     M10.349 **Gout due to renal impairment,** unspecified **hand**

✓6ᵗʰ **M10.35 Gout due to renal impairment,** hip
     M10.351 **Gout due to renal impairment,** right **hip**
     M10.352 **Gout due to renal impairment,** left **hip**
     M10.359 **Gout due to renal impairment,** unspecified **hip**

✓6ᵗʰ **M10.36 Gout due to renal impairment,** knee
     M10.361 **Gout due to renal impairment,** right **knee**
     M10.362 **Gout due to renal impairment,** left **knee**
     M10.369 **Gout due to renal impairment,** unspecified **knee**

✓6ᵗʰ **M10.37 Gout due to renal impairment,** ankle and foot
     M10.371 **Gout due to renal impairment,** right **ankle and foot**
     M10.372 **Gout due to renal impairment,** left **ankle and foot**
     M10.379 **Gout due to renal impairment,** unspecified **ankle and foot**

M10.38 Gout due to renal impairment, vertebrae
M10.39 Gout due to renal impairment, multiple sites

✓5ᵗʰ **M10.4 Other secondary gout**
     Code first associated condition

M10.40 Other secondary gout, unspecified site

✓6ᵗʰ **M10.41 Other secondary gout,** shoulder
     M10.411 **Other secondary gout,** right **shoulder**
     M10.412 **Other secondary gout,** left **shoulder**
     M10.419 **Other secondary gout,** unspecified **shoulder**

✓6ᵗʰ **M10.42 Other secondary gout,** elbow
     M10.421 **Other secondary gout,** right **elbow**
     M10.422 **Other secondary gout,** left **elbow**
     M10.429 **Other secondary gout,** unspecified **elbow**

✓6ᵗʰ **M10.43 Other secondary gout,** wrist
     M10.431 **Other secondary gout,** right **wrist**
     M10.432 **Other secondary gout,** left **wrist**
     M10.439 **Other secondary gout,** unspecified **wrist**

✓6ᵗʰ **M10.44 Other secondary gout,** hand
     M10.441 **Other secondary gout,** right **hand**
     M10.442 **Other secondary gout,** left **hand**
     M10.449 **Other secondary gout,** unspecified **hand**

✓6ᵗʰ **M10.45 Other secondary gout,** hip
     M10.451 **Other secondary gout,** right **hip**
     M10.452 **Other secondary gout,** left **hip**
     M10.459 **Other secondary gout,** unspecified **hip**

✓6ᵗʰ **M10.46 Other secondary gout,** knee
     M10.461 **Other secondary gout,** right **knee**
     M10.462 **Other secondary gout,** left **knee**
     M10.469 **Other secondary gout,** unspecified **knee**

✓6ᵗʰ **M10.47 Other secondary gout,** ankle and foot
     M10.471 **Other secondary gout,** right **ankle and foot**
     M10.472 **Other secondary gout,** left **ankle and foot**
     M10.479 **Other secondary gout,** unspecified **ankle and foot**

M10.48 Other secondary gout, vertebrae
M10.49 Other secondary gout, multiple sites

M10.9 Gout, unspecified
     Gout NOS

✓4ᵗʰ **M11 Other crystal arthropathies**

✓5ᵗʰ **M11.0 Hydroxyapatite deposition disease**
     DEF: Disease caused by deposits of calcium phosphate crystals in the soft tissues close to the joint (especially tendons) or in the joints. These calcifications can be mono or polyarticular and can cause destruction of the joint involved.

M11.00 Hydroxyapatite deposition disease, unspecified site

✓6ᵗʰ **M11.01 Hydroxyapatite deposition disease,** shoulder
     M11.011 **Hydroxyapatite deposition disease,** right **shoulder**
     M11.012 **Hydroxyapatite deposition disease,** left **shoulder**
     M11.019 **Hydroxyapatite deposition disease,** unspecified **shoulder**

✓6ᵗʰ **M11.02 Hydroxyapatite deposition disease,** elbow
     M11.021 **Hydroxyapatite deposition disease,** right **elbow**
     M11.022 **Hydroxyapatite deposition disease,** left **elbow**
     M11.029 **Hydroxyapatite deposition disease,** unspecified **elbow**

✓6ᵗʰ **M11.03 Hydroxyapatite deposition disease,** wrist
     M11.031 **Hydroxyapatite deposition disease,** right **wrist**
     M11.032 **Hydroxyapatite deposition disease,** left **wrist**
     M11.039 **Hydroxyapatite deposition disease,** unspecified **wrist**

✓6ᵗʰ **M11.04 Hydroxyapatite deposition disease,** hand
     M11.041 **Hydroxyapatite deposition disease,** right **hand**
     M11.042 **Hydroxyapatite deposition disease,** left **hand**
     M11.049 **Hydroxyapatite deposition disease,** unspecified **hand**

✓6ᵗʰ **M11.05 Hydroxyapatite deposition disease,** hip
     M11.051 **Hydroxyapatite deposition disease,** right **hip**
     M11.052 **Hydroxyapatite deposition disease,** left **hip**
     M11.059 **Hydroxyapatite deposition disease,** unspecified **hip**

✓6ᵗʰ **M11.06 Hydroxyapatite deposition disease,** knee
     M11.061 **Hydroxyapatite deposition disease,** right **knee**
     M11.062 **Hydroxyapatite deposition disease,** left **knee**
     M11.069 **Hydroxyapatite deposition disease,** unspecified **knee**

✓6ᵗʰ **M11.07 Hydroxyapatite deposition disease,** ankle and foot
     M11.071 **Hydroxyapatite deposition disease,** right **ankle and foot**

✓ Additional Character Required   ✓x7ᵗʰ Placeholder   Unacceptable PDx   Questionable PDx   Manifestation   **H1**-**H14** HAC   **HCC** CMS-HCC Dx   **HIV** HIV Dx

M11.072   Hydroxyapatite deposition disease, left ankle and foot

M11.079   Hydroxyapatite deposition disease, unspecified ankle and foot

M11.08   Hydroxyapatite deposition disease, vertebrae

M11.09   Hydroxyapatite deposition disease, multiple sites

✓5ᵗʰ **M11.1 Familial chondrocalcinosis**

M11.10   Familial chondrocalcinosis, unspecified site

✓6ᵗʰ M11.11   Familial chondrocalcinosis, shoulder

    M11.111   Familial chondrocalcinosis, right shoulder

    M11.112   Familial chondrocalcinosis, left shoulder

    M11.119   Familial chondrocalcinosis, unspecified shoulder

✓6ᵗʰ M11.12   Familial chondrocalcinosis, elbow

    M11.121   Familial chondrocalcinosis, right elbow

    M11.122   Familial chondrocalcinosis, left elbow

    M11.129   Familial chondrocalcinosis, unspecified elbow

✓6ᵗʰ M11.13   Familial chondrocalcinosis, wrist

    M11.131   Familial chondrocalcinosis, right wrist

    M11.132   Familial chondrocalcinosis, left wrist

    M11.139   Familial chondrocalcinosis, unspecified wrist

✓6ᵗʰ M11.14   Familial chondrocalcinosis, hand

    M11.141   Familial chondrocalcinosis, right hand

    M11.142   Familial chondrocalcinosis, left hand

    M11.149   Familial chondrocalcinosis, unspecified hand

✓6ᵗʰ M11.15   Familial chondrocalcinosis, hip

    M11.151   Familial chondrocalcinosis, right hip

    M11.152   Familial chondrocalcinosis, left hip

    M11.159   Familial chondrocalcinosis, unspecified hip

✓6ᵗʰ M11.16   Familial chondrocalcinosis, knee

    M11.161   Familial chondrocalcinosis, right knee

    M11.162   Familial chondrocalcinosis, left knee

    M11.169   Familial chondrocalcinosis, unspecified knee

✓6ᵗʰ M11.17   Familial chondrocalcinosis, ankle and foot

    M11.171   Familial chondrocalcinosis, right ankle and foot

    M11.172   Familial chondrocalcinosis, left ankle and foot

    M11.179   Familial chondrocalcinosis, unspecified ankle and foot

M11.18   Familial chondrocalcinosis, vertebrae

M11.19   Familial chondrocalcinosis, multiple sites

✓5ᵗʰ **M11.2 Other chondrocalcinosis**

Chondrocalcinosis NOS

M11.20   Other chondrocalcinosis, unspecified site

✓6ᵗʰ M11.21   Other chondrocalcinosis, shoulder

    M11.211   Other chondrocalcinosis, right shoulder

    M11.212   Other chondrocalcinosis, left shoulder

    M11.219   Other chondrocalcinosis, unspecified shoulder

✓6ᵗʰ M11.22   Other chondrocalcinosis, elbow

    M11.221   Other chondrocalcinosis, right elbow

    M11.222   Other chondrocalcinosis, left elbow

    M11.229   Other chondrocalcinosis, unspecified elbow

✓6ᵗʰ M11.23   Other chondrocalcinosis, wrist

    M11.231   Other chondrocalcinosis, right wrist

    M11.232   Other chondrocalcinosis, left wrist

    M11.239   Other chondrocalcinosis, unspecified wrist

✓6ᵗʰ M11.24   Other chondrocalcinosis, hand

    M11.241   Other chondrocalcinosis, right hand

    M11.242   Other chondrocalcinosis, left hand

    M11.249   Other chondrocalcinosis, unspecified hand

✓6ᵗʰ M11.25   Other chondrocalcinosis, hip

    M11.251   Other chondrocalcinosis, right hip

    M11.252   Other chondrocalcinosis, left hip

    M11.259   Other chondrocalcinosis, unspecified hip

✓6ᵗʰ M11.26   Other chondrocalcinosis, knee

    M11.261   Other chondrocalcinosis, right knee

    M11.262   Other chondrocalcinosis, left knee

    M11.269   Other chondrocalcinosis, unspecified knee

✓6ᵗʰ M11.27   Other chondrocalcinosis, ankle and foot

    M11.271   Other chondrocalcinosis, right ankle and foot

    M11.272   Other chondrocalcinosis, left ankle and foot

    M11.279   Other chondrocalcinosis, unspecified ankle and foot

M11.28   Other chondrocalcinosis, vertebrae

M11.29   Other chondrocalcinosis, multiple sites

✓5ᵗʰ **M11.8 Other specified crystal arthropathies**

M11.80   Other specified crystal arthropathies, unspecified site

✓6ᵗʰ M11.81   Other specified crystal arthropathies, shoulder

    M11.811   Other specified crystal arthropathies, right shoulder

    M11.812   Other specified crystal arthropathies, left shoulder

    M11.819   Other specified crystal arthropathies, unspecified shoulder

✓6ᵗʰ M11.82   Other specified crystal arthropathies, elbow

    M11.821   Other specified crystal arthropathies, right elbow

    M11.822   Other specified crystal arthropathies, left elbow

    M11.829   Other specified crystal arthropathies, unspecified elbow

✓6ᵗʰ M11.83   Other specified crystal arthropathies, wrist

    M11.831   Other specified crystal arthropathies, right wrist

    M11.832   Other specified crystal arthropathies, left wrist

    M11.839   Other specified crystal arthropathies, unspecified wrist

✓6ᵗʰ M11.84   Other specified crystal arthropathies, hand

    M11.841   Other specified crystal arthropathies, right hand

    M11.842   Other specified crystal arthropathies, left hand

    M11.849   Other specified crystal arthropathies, unspecified hand

✓6ᵗʰ M11.85   Other specified crystal arthropathies, hip

    M11.851   Other specified crystal arthropathies, right hip

    M11.852   Other specified crystal arthropathies, left hip

    M11.859   Other specified crystal arthropathies, unspecified hip

✓6ᵗʰ M11.86   Other specified crystal arthropathies, knee

    M11.861   Other specified crystal arthropathies, right knee

    M11.862   Other specified crystal arthropathies, left knee

    M11.869   Other specified crystal arthropathies, unspecified knee

✓6ᵗʰ M11.87   Other specified crystal arthropathies, ankle and foot

    M11.871   Other specified crystal arthropathies, right ankle and foot

    M11.872   Other specified crystal arthropathies, left ankle and foot

    M11.879   Other specified crystal arthropathies, unspecified ankle and foot

M11.88   Other specified crystal arthropathies, vertebrae

M11.89   Other specified crystal arthropathies, multiple sites

M11.9   Crystal arthropathy, unspecified

✓4ᵗʰ **M12 Other and unspecified arthropathy**

EXCLUDES 1   arthrosis (M15-M19)

    cricoarytenoid arthropathy (J38.7)

✓5ᵗʰ **M12.0 Chronic postrheumatic arthropathy [Jaccoud]**

M12.00   Chronic postrheumatic arthropathy [Jaccoud], HCC unspecified site

N Newborn: 0   P Pediatric: 0-17   M Maternity: 12-55   A Adult: 15-124   MCC Major Complication/Comorbidity   CC Complication/Comorbidity   SW Severe Wound Dx

758   ICD-10-CM 2019

✓6ᵗʰ **M12.01** **Chronic postrheumatic arthropathy [Jaccoud], shoulder**

     M12.011 **Chronic postrheumatic arthropathy [Jaccoud], right shoulder** `HCC`

     M12.012 **Chronic postrheumatic arthropathy [Jaccoud], left shoulder** `HCC`

     M12.019 **Chronic postrheumatic arthropathy [Jaccoud], unspecified shoulder** `HCC`

✓6ᵗʰ **M12.02** **Chronic postrheumatic arthropathy [Jaccoud], elbow**

     M12.021 **Chronic postrheumatic arthropathy [Jaccoud], right elbow** `HCC`

     M12.022 **Chronic postrheumatic arthropathy [Jaccoud], left elbow** `HCC`

     M12.029 **Chronic postrheumatic arthropathy [Jaccoud], unspecified elbow** `HCC`

✓6ᵗʰ **M12.03** **Chronic postrheumatic arthropathy [Jaccoud], wrist**

     M12.031 **Chronic postrheumatic arthropathy [Jaccoud], right wrist** `HCC`

     M12.032 **Chronic postrheumatic arthropathy [Jaccoud], left wrist** `HCC`

     M12.039 **Chronic postrheumatic arthropathy [Jaccoud], unspecified wrist** `HCC`

✓6ᵗʰ **M12.04** **Chronic postrheumatic arthropathy [Jaccoud], hand**

     M12.041 **Chronic postrheumatic arthropathy [Jaccoud], right hand** `HCC`

     M12.042 **Chronic postrheumatic arthropathy [Jaccoud], left hand** `HCC`

     M12.049 **Chronic postrheumatic arthropathy [Jaccoud], unspecified hand** `HCC`

✓6ᵗʰ **M12.05** **Chronic postrheumatic arthropathy [Jaccoud], hip**

     M12.051 **Chronic postrheumatic arthropathy [Jaccoud], right hip** `HCC`

     M12.052 **Chronic postrheumatic arthropathy [Jaccoud], left hip** `HCC`

     M12.059 **Chronic postrheumatic arthropathy [Jaccoud], unspecified hip** `HCC`

✓6ᵗʰ **M12.06** **Chronic postrheumatic arthropathy [Jaccoud], knee**

     M12.061 **Chronic postrheumatic arthropathy [Jaccoud], right knee** `HCC`

     M12.062 **Chronic postrheumatic arthropathy [Jaccoud], left knee** `HCC`

     M12.069 **Chronic postrheumatic arthropathy [Jaccoud], unspecified knee** `HCC`

✓6ᵗʰ **M12.07** **Chronic postrheumatic arthropathy [Jaccoud], ankle and foot**

     M12.071 **Chronic postrheumatic arthropathy [Jaccoud], right ankle and foot** `HCC`

     M12.072 **Chronic postrheumatic arthropathy [Jaccoud], left ankle and foot** `HCC`

     M12.079 **Chronic postrheumatic arthropathy [Jaccoud], unspecified ankle and foot** `HCC`

     M12.08 **Chronic postrheumatic arthropathy [Jaccoud], other specified site** `HCC`

         Chronic postrheumatic arthropathy [Jaccoud], vertebrae

     M12.09 **Chronic postrheumatic arthropathy [Jaccoud], multiple sites** `HCC`

✓6ᵗʰ **M12.1** **Kaschin-Beck disease**

     Osteochondroarthrosis deformans endemica

     M12.10 **Kaschin-Beck disease, unspecified site**

✓6ᵗʰ **M12.11** **Kaschin-Beck disease, shoulder**

     M12.111 **Kaschin-Beck disease, right shoulder**

     M12.112 **Kaschin-Beck disease, left shoulder**

     M12.119 **Kaschin-Beck disease, unspecified shoulder**

✓6ᵗʰ **M12.12** **Kaschin-Beck disease, elbow**

     M12.121 **Kaschin-Beck disease, right elbow**

     M12.122 **Kaschin-Beck disease, left elbow**

     M12.129 **Kaschin-Beck disease, unspecified elbow**

✓6ᵗʰ **M12.13** **Kaschin-Beck disease, wrist**

     M12.131 **Kaschin-Beck disease, right wrist**

     M12.132 **Kaschin-Beck disease, left wrist**

     M12.139 **Kaschin-Beck disease, unspecified wrist**

✓6ᵗʰ **M12.14** **Kaschin-Beck disease, hand**

     M12.141 **Kaschin-Beck disease, right hand**

     M12.142 **Kaschin-Beck disease, left hand**

     M12.149 **Kaschin-Beck disease, unspecified hand**

✓6ᵗʰ **M12.15** **Kaschin-Beck disease, hip**

     M12.151 **Kaschin-Beck disease, right hip**

     M12.152 **Kaschin-Beck disease, left hip**

     M12.159 **Kaschin-Beck disease, unspecified hip**

✓6ᵗʰ **M12.16** **Kaschin-Beck disease, knee**

     M12.161 **Kaschin-Beck disease, right knee**

     M12.162 **Kaschin-Beck disease, left knee**

     M12.169 **Kaschin-Beck disease, unspecified knee**

✓6ᵗʰ **M12.17** **Kaschin-Beck disease, ankle and foot**

     M12.171 **Kaschin-Beck disease, right ankle and foot**

     M12.172 **Kaschin-Beck disease, left ankle and foot**

     M12.179 **Kaschin-Beck disease, unspecified ankle and foot**

     M12.18 **Kaschin-Beck disease, vertebrae**

     M12.19 **Kaschin-Beck disease, multiple sites**

✓5ᵗʰ **M12.2** **Villonodular synovitis (pigmented)**

     M12.20 **Villonodular synovitis (pigmented), unspecified site**

✓6ᵗʰ **M12.21** **Villonodular synovitis (pigmented), shoulder**

     M12.211 **Villonodular synovitis (pigmented), right shoulder**

     M12.212 **Villonodular synovitis (pigmented), left shoulder**

     M12.219 **Villonodular synovitis (pigmented), unspecified shoulder**

✓6ᵗʰ **M12.22** **Villonodular synovitis (pigmented), elbow**

     M12.221 **Villonodular synovitis (pigmented), right elbow**

     M12.222 **Villonodular synovitis (pigmented), left elbow**

     M12.229 **Villonodular synovitis (pigmented), unspecified elbow**

✓6ᵗʰ **M12.23** **Villonodular synovitis (pigmented), wrist**

     M12.231 **Villonodular synovitis (pigmented), right wrist**

     M12.232 **Villonodular synovitis (pigmented), left wrist**

     M12.239 **Villonodular synovitis (pigmented), unspecified wrist**

✓6ᵗʰ **M12.24** **Villonodular synovitis (pigmented), hand**

     M12.241 **Villonodular synovitis (pigmented), right hand**

     M12.242 **Villonodular synovitis (pigmented), left hand**

     M12.249 **Villonodular synovitis (pigmented), unspecified hand**

✓6ᵗʰ **M12.25** **Villonodular synovitis (pigmented), hip**

     M12.251 **Villonodular synovitis (pigmented), right hip**

     M12.252 **Villonodular synovitis (pigmented), left hip**

     M12.259 **Villonodular synovitis (pigmented), unspecified hip**

✓6ᵗʰ **M12.26** **Villonodular synovitis (pigmented), knee**

     M12.261 **Villonodular synovitis (pigmented), right knee**

     M12.262 **Villonodular synovitis (pigmented), left knee**

     M12.269 **Villonodular synovitis (pigmented), unspecified knee**

✓6ᵗʰ **M12.27** **Villonodular synovitis (pigmented), ankle and foot**

     M12.271 **Villonodular synovitis (pigmented), right ankle and foot**

     M12.272 **Villonodular synovitis (pigmented), left ankle and foot**

     M12.279 **Villonodular synovitis (pigmented), unspecified ankle and foot**

     M12.28 **Villonodular synovitis (pigmented), other specified site**

         Villonodular synovitis (pigmented), vertebrae

     M12.29 **Villonodular synovitis (pigmented), multiple sites**

✓ Additional Character Required   ✓x7ᵗʰ Placeholder   Unacceptable PDx   Questionable PDx   Manifestation   H1–H14 HAC   HCC CMS-HCC Dx   HIV HIV Dx

ICD-10-CM 2019   759

√5ᵗʰ M12.3 Palindromic rheumatism
DEF: Sudden and recurring attacks of moderate to severe joint pain and swelling generally occurring in the hands or feet of unknown etiology. After the attack subsides, the joints appear normal again.

M12.30   Palindromic rheumatism, unspecified site

√6ᵗʰ M12.31   Palindromic rheumatism, shoulder
M12.311   Palindromic rheumatism, right shoulder
M12.312   Palindromic rheumatism, left shoulder
M12.319   Palindromic rheumatism, unspecified shoulder

√6ᵗʰ M12.32   Palindromic rheumatism, elbow
M12.321   Palindromic rheumatism, right elbow
M12.322   Palindromic rheumatism, left elbow
M12.329   Palindromic rheumatism, unspecified elbow

√6ᵗʰ M12.33   Palindromic rheumatism, wrist
M12.331   Palindromic rheumatism, right wrist
M12.332   Palindromic rheumatism, left wrist
M12.339   Palindromic rheumatism, unspecified wrist

√6ᵗʰ M12.34   Palindromic rheumatism, hand
M12.341   Palindromic rheumatism, right hand
M12.342   Palindromic rheumatism, left hand
M12.349   Palindromic rheumatism, unspecified hand

√6ᵗʰ M12.35   Palindromic rheumatism, hip
M12.351   Palindromic rheumatism, right hip
M12.352   Palindromic rheumatism, left hip
M12.359   Palindromic rheumatism, unspecified hip

√6ᵗʰ M12.36   Palindromic rheumatism, knee
M12.361   Palindromic rheumatism, right knee
M12.362   Palindromic rheumatism, left knee
M12.369   Palindromic rheumatism, unspecified knee

√6ᵗʰ M12.37   Palindromic rheumatism, ankle and foot
M12.371   Palindromic rheumatism, right ankle and foot
M12.372   Palindromic rheumatism, left ankle and foot
M12.379   Palindromic rheumatism, unspecified ankle and foot

M12.38   Palindromic rheumatism, other specified site
Palindromic rheumatism, vertebrae

M12.39   Palindromic rheumatism, multiple sites

√5ᵗʰ M12.4 Intermittent hydrarthrosis
M12.40   Intermittent hydrarthrosis, unspecified site

√6ᵗʰ M12.41   Intermittent hydrarthrosis, shoulder
M12.411   Intermittent hydrarthrosis, right shoulder
M12.412   Intermittent hydrarthrosis, left shoulder
M12.419   Intermittent hydrarthrosis, unspecified shoulder

√6ᵗʰ M12.42   Intermittent hydrarthrosis, elbow
M12.421   Intermittent hydrarthrosis, right elbow
M12.422   Intermittent hydrarthrosis, left elbow
M12.429   Intermittent hydrarthrosis, unspecified elbow

√6ᵗʰ M12.43   Intermittent hydrarthrosis, wrist
M12.431   Intermittent hydrarthrosis, right wrist
M12.432   Intermittent hydrarthrosis, left wrist
M12.439   Intermittent hydrarthrosis, unspecified wrist

√6ᵗʰ M12.44   Intermittent hydrarthrosis, hand
M12.441   Intermittent hydrarthrosis, right hand
M12.442   Intermittent hydrarthrosis, left hand
M12.449   Intermittent hydrarthrosis, unspecified hand

√6ᵗʰ M12.45   Intermittent hydrarthrosis, hip
M12.451   Intermittent hydrarthrosis, right hip
M12.452   Intermittent hydrarthrosis, left hip
M12.459   Intermittent hydrarthrosis, unspecified hip

√6ᵗʰ M12.46   Intermittent hydrarthrosis, knee
M12.461   Intermittent hydrarthrosis, right knee

M12.462   Intermittent hydrarthrosis, left knee
M12.469   Intermittent hydrarthrosis, unspecified knee

√6ᵗʰ M12.47   Intermittent hydrarthrosis, ankle and foot
M12.471   Intermittent hydrarthrosis, right ankle and foot
M12.472   Intermittent hydrarthrosis, left ankle and foot
M12.479   Intermittent hydrarthrosis, unspecified ankle and foot

M12.48   Intermittent hydrarthrosis, other site
M12.49   Intermittent hydrarthrosis, multiple sites

√5ᵗʰ M12.5 Traumatic arthropathy
EXCLUDES 1   current injury–see Alphabetic Index
post-traumatic osteoarthritis NOS (M19.1-)
post-traumatic osteoarthritis of first carpometacarpal joint (M18.2-M18.3)
post-traumatic osteoarthritis of hip (M16.4-M16.5)
post-traumatic osteoarthritis of knee (M17.2-M17.3)
post-traumatic osteoarthritis of other single joints (M19.1-)
AHA: 2015, 1Q, 17

M12.50   Traumatic arthropathy, unspecified site

√6ᵗʰ M12.51   Traumatic arthropathy, shoulder
M12.511   Traumatic arthropathy, right shoulder
M12.512   Traumatic arthropathy, left shoulder
M12.519   Traumatic arthropathy, unspecified shoulder

√6ᵗʰ M12.52   Traumatic arthropathy, elbow
M12.521   Traumatic arthropathy, right elbow
M12.522   Traumatic arthropathy, left elbow
M12.529   Traumatic arthropathy, unspecified elbow

√6ᵗʰ M12.53   Traumatic arthropathy, wrist
M12.531   Traumatic arthropathy, right wrist
M12.532   Traumatic arthropathy, left wrist
M12.539   Traumatic arthropathy, unspecified wrist

√6ᵗʰ M12.54   Traumatic arthropathy, hand
M12.541   Traumatic arthropathy, right hand
M12.542   Traumatic arthropathy, left hand
M12.549   Traumatic arthropathy, unspecified hand

√6ᵗʰ M12.55   Traumatic arthropathy, hip
M12.551   Traumatic arthropathy, right hip
M12.552   Traumatic arthropathy, left hip
M12.559   Traumatic arthropathy, unspecified hip

√6ᵗʰ M12.56   Traumatic arthropathy, knee
M12.561   Traumatic arthropathy, right knee
M12.562   Traumatic arthropathy, left knee
M12.569   Traumatic arthropathy, unspecified knee

√6ᵗʰ M12.57   Traumatic arthropathy, ankle and foot
M12.571   Traumatic arthropathy, right ankle and foot
M12.572   Traumatic arthropathy, left ankle and foot
M12.579   Traumatic arthropathy, unspecified ankle and foot

M12.58   Traumatic arthropathy, other specified site
Traumatic arthropathy, vertebrae

M12.59   Traumatic arthropathy, multiple sites

√5ᵗʰ M12.8 Other specific arthropathies, not elsewhere classified
Transient arthropathy

M12.80   Other specific arthropathies, not elsewhere classified, unspecified site

√6ᵗʰ M12.81   Other specific arthropathies, not elsewhere classified, shoulder
M12.811   Other specific arthropathies, not elsewhere classified, right shoulder
M12.812   Other specific arthropathies, not elsewhere classified, left shoulder
M12.819   Other specific arthropathies, not elsewhere classified, unspecified shoulder

√6ᵗʰ M12.82   Other specific arthropathies, not elsewhere classified, elbow
M12.821   Other specific arthropathies, not elsewhere classified, right elbow
M12.822   Other specific arthropathies, not elsewhere classified, left elbow

N Newborn: 0   **P** Pediatric: 0-17   **M** Maternity: 12-55   **A** Adult: 15-124   **MCC** Major Complication/Comorbidity   **CC** Complication/Comorbidity   **SW** Severe Wound Dx

760   ICD-10-CM 2019

M12.829   Other specific arthropathies, not elsewhere classified, unspecified elbow

✓6ᵗʰ **M12.83**   **Other specific arthropathies, not elsewhere classified,** wrist

M12.831   Other specific arthropathies, not elsewhere classified, right wrist

M12.832   Other specific arthropathies, not elsewhere classified, left wrist

M12.839   Other specific arthropathies, not elsewhere classified, unspecified wrist

✓6ᵗʰ **M12.84**   **Other specific arthropathies, not elsewhere classified,** hand

M12.841   Other specific arthropathies, not elsewhere classified, right hand

M12.842   Other specific arthropathies, not elsewhere classified, left hand

M12.849   Other specific arthropathies, not elsewhere classified, unspecified hand

✓6ᵗʰ **M12.85**   **Other specific arthropathies, not elsewhere classified,** hip

M12.851   Other specific arthropathies, not elsewhere classified, right hip

M12.852   Other specific arthropathies, not elsewhere classified, left hip

M12.859   Other specific arthropathies, not elsewhere classified, unspecified hip

✓6ᵗʰ **M12.86**   **Other specific arthropathies, not elsewhere classified,** knee

M12.861   Other specific arthropathies, not elsewhere classified, right knee

M12.862   Other specific arthropathies, not elsewhere classified, left knee

M12.869   Other specific arthropathies, not elsewhere classified, unspecified knee

✓6ᵗʰ **M12.87**   **Other specific arthropathies, not elsewhere classified,** ankle and foot

M12.871   Other specific arthropathies, not elsewhere classified, right ankle and foot

M12.872   Other specific arthropathies, not elsewhere classified, left ankle and foot

M12.879   Other specific arthropathies, not elsewhere classified, unspecified ankle and foot

M12.88   **Other specific arthropathies, not elsewhere classified,** other specified site

Other specific arthropathies, not elsewhere classified, vertebrae

M12.89   **Other specific arthropathies, not elsewhere classified,** multiple sites

M12.9   **Arthropathy,** unspecified

✓4ᵗʰ **M13**   **Other arthritis**

EXCLUDES 1   arthrosis (M15-M19)
osteoarthritis (M15-M19)

M13.0   **Polyarthritis, unspecified**

✓5ᵗʰ **M13.1**   **Monoarthritis, not elsewhere classified**

M13.10   Monoarthritis, not elsewhere classified, unspecified site

✓6ᵗʰ **M13.11**   **Monoarthritis, not elsewhere classified,** shoulder

M13.111   Monoarthritis, not elsewhere classified, right shoulder

M13.112   Monoarthritis, not elsewhere classified, left shoulder

M13.119   Monoarthritis, not elsewhere classified, unspecified shoulder

✓6ᵗʰ **M13.12**   **Monoarthritis, not elsewhere classified,** elbow

M13.121   Monoarthritis, not elsewhere classified, right elbow

M13.122   Monoarthritis, not elsewhere classified, left elbow

M13.129   Monoarthritis, not elsewhere classified, unspecified elbow

✓6ᵗʰ **M13.13**   **Monoarthritis, not elsewhere classified,** wrist

M13.131   Monoarthritis, not elsewhere classified, right wrist

M13.132   Monoarthritis, not elsewhere classified, left wrist

M13.139   Monoarthritis, not elsewhere classified, unspecified wrist

✓6ᵗʰ **M13.14**   **Monoarthritis, not elsewhere classified,** hand

M13.141   Monoarthritis, not elsewhere classified, right hand

M13.142   Monoarthritis, not elsewhere classified, left hand

M13.149   Monoarthritis, not elsewhere classified, unspecified hand

✓6ᵗʰ **M13.15**   **Monoarthritis, not elsewhere classified,** hip

M13.151   Monoarthritis, not elsewhere classified, right hip

M13.152   Monoarthritis, not elsewhere classified, left hip

M13.159   Monoarthritis, not elsewhere classified, unspecified hip

✓6ᵗʰ **M13.16**   **Monoarthritis, not elsewhere classified,** knee

M13.161   Monoarthritis, not elsewhere classified, right knee

M13.162   Monoarthritis, not elsewhere classified, left knee

M13.169   Monoarthritis, not elsewhere classified, unspecified knee

✓6ᵗʰ **M13.17**   **Monoarthritis, not elsewhere classified,** ankle and foot

M13.171   Monoarthritis, not elsewhere classified, right ankle and foot

M13.172   Monoarthritis, not elsewhere classified, left ankle and foot

M13.179   Monoarthritis, not elsewhere classified, unspecified ankle and foot

✓5ᵗʰ **M13.8**   **Other specified arthritis**

Allergic arthritis

EXCLUDES 1   osteoarthritis (M15-M19)

M13.80   **Other specified arthritis,** unspecified site

✓6ᵗʰ **M13.81**   **Other specified arthritis,** shoulder

M13.811   Other specified arthritis, right shoulder

M13.812   Other specified arthritis, left shoulder

M13.819   Other specified arthritis, unspecified shoulder

✓6ᵗʰ **M13.82**   **Other specified arthritis,** elbow

M13.821   Other specified arthritis, right elbow

M13.822   Other specified arthritis, left elbow

M13.829   Other specified arthritis, unspecified elbow

✓6ᵗʰ **M13.83**   **Other specified arthritis,** wrist

M13.831   Other specified arthritis, right wrist

M13.832   Other specified arthritis, left wrist

M13.839   Other specified arthritis, unspecified wrist

✓6ᵗʰ **M13.84**   **Other specified arthritis,** hand

M13.841   Other specified arthritis, right hand

M13.842   Other specified arthritis, left hand

M13.849   Other specified arthritis, unspecified hand

✓6ᵗʰ **M13.85**   **Other specified arthritis,** hip

M13.851   Other specified arthritis, right hip

M13.852   Other specified arthritis, left hip

M13.859   Other specified arthritis, unspecified hip

✓6ᵗʰ **M13.86**   **Other specified arthritis,** knee

M13.861   Other specified arthritis, right knee

M13.862   Other specified arthritis, left knee

M13.869   Other specified arthritis, unspecified knee

✓6ᵗʰ **M13.87**   **Other specified arthritis,** ankle and foot

M13.871   Other specified arthritis, right ankle and foot

M13.872   Other specified arthritis, left ankle and foot

M13.879   Other specified arthritis, unspecified ankle and foot

M13.88   **Other specified arthritis,** other site

M13.89   **Other specified arthritis,** multiple sites

✔ Additional Character Required   ✓x7ᵗʰ Placeholder   Unacceptable PDx   Questionable PDx   Manifestation   H1 - H14 HAC   HCC CMS-HCC Dx   HIV HIV Dx

ICD-10-CM 2019   761

Chapter 13. Diseases of the Musculoskeletal System and Connective Tissue *(left margin)*

✓4ᵗʰ **M14 Arthropathies in other diseases classified elsewhere**

> *EXCLUDES 1*   arthropathy in:
>> diabetes mellitus (E08-E13 with .61-)
>> hematological disorders (M36.2-M36.3)
>> hypersensitivity reactions (M36.4)
>> neoplastic disease (M36.1)
>> neurosyphillis (A52.16)
>> sarcoidosis (D86.86)
>> enteropathic arthropathies (M07.-)
>> juvenile psoriatic arthropathy (L40.54)
>> lipoid dermatoarthritis (E78.81)

✓5ᵗʰ **M14.6 Charcôt's joint**
> Neuropathic arthropathy
>> *EXCLUDES 1*   Charcôt's joint in diabetes mellitus (E08-E13 with .610-)
>> Charcôt's joint in tabes dorsalis (A52.16)
>
> **DEF:** Progressive neurologic arthropathy in which chronic degeneration of joints in the weight-bearing areas with peripheral hypertrophy occurs as a complication of a neuropathy disorder. Supporting structures relax from a loss of sensation resulting in chronic joint instability.

> **M14.60 Charcôt's joint,** unspecified site

✓6ᵗʰ **M14.61 Charcôt's joint,** shoulder
> **M14.611 Charcôt's joint,** right shoulder
> **M14.612 Charcôt's joint,** left shoulder
> **M14.619 Charcôt's joint,** unspecified shoulder

✓6ᵗʰ **M14.62 Charcôt's joint,** elbow
> **M14.621 Charcôt's joint,** right elbow
> **M14.622 Charcôt's joint,** left elbow
> **M14.629 Charcôt's joint,** unspecified elbow

✓6ᵗʰ **M14.63 Charcôt's joint,** wrist
> **M14.631 Charcôt's joint,** right wrist
> **M14.632 Charcôt's joint,** left wrist
> **M14.639 Charcôt's joint,** unspecified wrist

✓6ᵗʰ **M14.64 Charcôt's joint,** hand
> **M14.641 Charcôt's joint,** right hand
> **M14.642 Charcôt's joint,** left hand
> **M14.649 Charcôt's joint,** unspecified hand

✓6ᵗʰ **M14.65 Charcôt's joint,** hip
> **M14.651 Charcôt's joint,** right hip
> **M14.652 Charcôt's joint,** left hip
> **M14.659 Charcôt's joint,** unspecified hip

✓6ᵗʰ **M14.66 Charcôt's joint,** knee
> **M14.661 Charcôt's joint,** right knee
> **M14.662 Charcôt's joint,** left knee
> **M14.669 Charcôt's joint,** unspecified knee

✓6ᵗʰ **M14.67 Charcôt's joint,** ankle and foot
> **M14.671 Charcôt's joint,** right ankle and foot
> **M14.672 Charcôt's joint,** left ankle and foot
> **M14.679 Charcôt's joint,** unspecified ankle and foot

> **M14.68 Charcôt's joint,** vertebrae
> **M14.69 Charcôt's joint,** multiple sites

✓5ᵗʰ **M14.8 Arthropathies in other specified diseases classified elsewhere**
> Code first underlying disease, such as:
>> amyloidosis (E85.-)
>> erythema multiforme (L51.-)
>> erythema nodosum (L52)
>> hemochromatosis (E83.11-)
>> hyperparathyroidism (E21.-)
>> hypothyroidism (E00-E03)
>> sickle-cell disorders (D57.-)
>> thyrotoxicosis [hyperthyroidism] (E05.-)
>> Whipple's disease (K90.81)

> **M14.80 Arthropathies in other specified diseases classified elsewhere,** unspecified site

✓6ᵗʰ **M14.81 Arthropathies in other specified diseases classified elsewhere,** shoulder
> **M14.811 Arthropathies in other specified diseases classified elsewhere,** right shoulder
> **M14.812 Arthropathies in other specified diseases classified elsewhere,** left shoulder
> **M14.819 Arthropathies in other specified diseases classified elsewhere,** unspecified shoulder

✓6ᵗʰ **M14.82 Arthropathies in other specified diseases classified elsewhere,** elbow
> **M14.821 Arthropathies in other specified diseases classified elsewhere,** right elbow
> **M14.822 Arthropathies in other specified diseases classified elsewhere,** left elbow
> **M14.829 Arthropathies in other specified diseases classified elsewhere,** unspecified elbow

✓6ᵗʰ **M14.83 Arthropathies in other specified diseases classified elsewhere,** wrist
> **M14.831 Arthropathies in other specified diseases classified elsewhere,** right wrist
> **M14.832 Arthropathies in other specified diseases classified elsewhere,** left wrist
> **M14.839 Arthropathies in other specified diseases classified elsewhere,** unspecified wrist

✓6ᵗʰ **M14.84 Arthropathies in other specified diseases classified elsewhere,** hand
> **M14.841 Arthropathies in other specified diseases classified elsewhere,** right hand
> **M14.842 Arthropathies in other specified diseases classified elsewhere,** left hand
> **M14.849 Arthropathies in other specified diseases classified elsewhere,** unspecified hand

✓6ᵗʰ **M14.85 Arthropathies in other specified diseases classified elsewhere,** hip
> **M14.851 Arthropathies in other specified diseases classified elsewhere,** right hip
> **M14.852 Arthropathies in other specified diseases classified elsewhere,** left hip
> **M14.859 Arthropathies in other specified diseases classified elsewhere,** unspecified hip

✓6ᵗʰ **M14.86 Arthropathies in other specified diseases classified elsewhere,** knee
> **M14.861 Arthropathies in other specified diseases classified elsewhere,** right knee
> **M14.862 Arthropathies in other specified diseases classified elsewhere,** left knee
> **M14.869 Arthropathies in other specified diseases classified elsewhere,** unspecified knee

✓6ᵗʰ **M14.87 Arthropathies in other specified diseases classified elsewhere,** ankle and foot
> **M14.871 Arthropathies in other specified diseases classified elsewhere,** right ankle and foot
> **M14.872 Arthropathies in other specified diseases classified elsewhere,** left ankle and foot
> **M14.879 Arthropathies in other specified diseases classified elsewhere,** unspecified ankle and foot

> **M14.88 Arthropathies in other specified diseases classified elsewhere,** vertebrae
> **M14.89 Arthropathies in other specified diseases classified elsewhere,** multiple sites

Osteoarthritis (M15-M19)

> *EXCLUDES 2*   osteoarthritis of spine (M47.-)

TIP: Assign a primary osteoarthritis code when the type of osteoarthritis—primary, secondary, or generalized—is not specified in the documentation. Primary is considered the default.

✓4ᵗʰ **M15 Polyosteoarthritis**
> *INCLUDES*   arthritis of multiple sites
> *EXCLUDES 1*   bilateral involvement of single joint (M16-M19)

> **M15.0 Primary generalized (osteo)arthritis**

> **M15.1 Heberden's nodes (with arthropathy)**
>> Interphalangeal distal osteoarthritis

> **M15.2 Bouchard's nodes (with arthropathy)**
>> Juxtaphalangeal distal osteoarthritis

> **M15.3 Secondary multiple arthritis**
>> Post-traumatic polyosteoarthritis

> **M15.4 Erosive (osteo)arthritis**

> **M15.8 Other polyosteoarthritis**

> **M15.9 Polyosteoarthritis, unspecified**
>> Generalized osteoarthritis NOS

✓4ᵗʰ **M16 Osteoarthritis of** hip
> **AHA:** 2016, 4Q, 146

> **M16.0 Bilateral primary osteoarthritis of hip**
>> **AHA:** 2018, 2Q, 15

✓5ᵗʰ **M16.1 Unilateral primary osteoarthritis of hip**
>> Primary osteoarthritis of hip NOS
>> **AHA:** 2018, 2Q, 15

>> **M16.10 Unilateral primary osteoarthritis,** unspecified hip

---

N Newborn: 0   P Pediatric: 0-17   M Maternity: 12-55   A Adult: 15-124   MCC Major Complication/Comorbidity   CC Complication/Comorbidity   SW Severe Wound Dx

762   ICD-10-CM 2019

M16.11   **Unilateral primary osteoarthritis, right hip**

M16.12   **Unilateral primary osteoarthritis, left hip**

M16.2   **Bilateral osteoarthritis resulting from hip dysplasia**

✓5ᵗʰ   M16.3   Unilateral osteoarthritis resulting from hip dysplasia
Dysplastic osteoarthritis of hip NOS

     M16.30   **Unilateral osteoarthritis resulting from hip dysplasia, unspecified hip**

     M16.31   **Unilateral osteoarthritis resulting from hip dysplasia, right hip**

     M16.32   **Unilateral osteoarthritis resulting from hip dysplasia, left hip**

M16.4   **Bilateral post-traumatic osteoarthritis of hip**

✓5ᵗʰ   M16.5   Unilateral post-traumatic osteoarthritis of hip
Post-traumatic osteoarthritis of hip NOS

     M16.50   **Unilateral post-traumatic osteoarthritis, unspecified hip**

     M16.51   **Unilateral post-traumatic osteoarthritis, right hip**

     M16.52   **Unilateral post-traumatic osteoarthritis, left hip**

M16.6   Other bilateral secondary osteoarthritis of hip

M16.7   Other unilateral secondary osteoarthritis of hip
Secondary osteoarthritis of hip NOS

M16.9   **Osteoarthritis of hip, unspecified**

✓4ᵗʰ   **M17   Osteoarthritis of knee**
AHA: 2016, 4Q, 146-147

M17.0   Bilateral primary osteoarthritis of knee
AHA: 2018, 2Q, 15

✓5ᵗʰ   M17.1   Unilateral primary osteoarthritis of knee
Primary osteoarthritis of knee NOS
AHA: 2018, 2Q, 15

     M17.10   **Unilateral primary osteoarthritis, unspecified knee**

     M17.11   **Unilateral primary osteoarthritis, right knee**

     M17.12   **Unilateral primary osteoarthritis, left knee**

M17.2   Bilateral post-traumatic osteoarthritis of knee

✓5ᵗʰ   M17.3   Unilateral post-traumatic osteoarthritis of knee
Post-traumatic osteoarthritis of knee NOS

     M17.30   **Unilateral post-traumatic osteoarthritis, unspecified knee**

     M17.31   **Unilateral post-traumatic osteoarthritis, right knee**

     M17.32   **Unilateral post-traumatic osteoarthritis, left knee**

M17.4   Other bilateral secondary osteoarthritis of knee

M17.5   Other unilateral secondary osteoarthritis of knee
Secondary osteoarthritis of knee NOS

M17.9   **Osteoarthritis of knee, unspecified**

✓4ᵗʰ   **M18   Osteoarthritis of first carpometacarpal joint**

M18.0   Bilateral primary osteoarthritis of first carpometacarpal joints

✓5ᵗʰ   M18.1   Unilateral primary osteoarthritis of first carpometacarpal joint
Primary osteoarthritis of first carpometacarpal joint NOS

     M18.10   **Unilateral primary osteoarthritis of first carpometacarpal joint, unspecified hand**

     M18.11   **Unilateral primary osteoarthritis of first carpometacarpal joint, right hand**

     M18.12   **Unilateral primary osteoarthritis of first carpometacarpal joint, left hand**

M18.2   Bilateral post-traumatic osteoarthritis of first carpometacarpal joints

✓5ᵗʰ   M18.3   Unilateral post-traumatic osteoarthritis of first carpometacarpal joint
Post-traumatic osteoarthritis of first carpometacarpal joint NOS

     M18.30   **Unilateral post-traumatic osteoarthritis of first carpometacarpal joint, unspecified hand**

     M18.31   **Unilateral post-traumatic osteoarthritis of first carpometacarpal joint, right hand**

     M18.32   **Unilateral post-traumatic osteoarthritis of first carpometacarpal joint, left hand**

M18.4   Other bilateral secondary osteoarthritis of first carpometacarpal joints

✓5ᵗʰ   M18.5   Other unilateral secondary osteoarthritis of first carpometacarpal joint
Secondary osteoarthritis of first carpometacarpal joint NOS

     M18.50   **Other unilateral secondary osteoarthritis of first carpometacarpal joint, unspecified hand**

     M18.51   **Other unilateral secondary osteoarthritis of first carpometacarpal joint, right hand**

M18.52   **Other unilateral secondary osteoarthritis of first carpometacarpal joint, left hand**

M18.9   Osteoarthritis of first carpometacarpal joint, unspecified

✓4ᵗʰ   **M19   Other and unspecified osteoarthritis**
     EXCLUDES 1   polyarthritis (M15.-)
     EXCLUDES 2   arthrosis of spine (M47.-)
           hallux rigidus (M20.2)
           osteoarthritis of spine (M47.-)

✓5ᵗʰ   M19.0   Primary osteoarthritis of other joints
AHA: 2018, 2Q, 15; 2016, 4Q, 145

   ✓6ᵗʰ   M19.01   **Primary osteoarthritis, shoulder**

     M19.011   **Primary osteoarthritis, right shoulder**

     M19.012   **Primary osteoarthritis, left shoulder**

     M19.019   **Primary osteoarthritis, unspecified shoulder**

   ✓6ᵗʰ   M19.02   **Primary osteoarthritis, elbow**

     M19.021   **Primary osteoarthritis, right elbow**

     M19.022   **Primary osteoarthritis, left elbow**

     M19.029   **Primary osteoarthritis, unspecified elbow**

   ✓6ᵗʰ   M19.03   **Primary osteoarthritis, wrist**

     M19.031   **Primary osteoarthritis, right wrist**

     M19.032   **Primary osteoarthritis, left wrist**

     M19.039   **Primary osteoarthritis, unspecified wrist**

   ✓6ᵗʰ   M19.04   **Primary osteoarthritis, hand**
     EXCLUDES 2   primary osteoarthritis of first carpometacarpal joint (M18.0-, M18.1-)

     M19.041   **Primary osteoarthritis, right hand**

     M19.042   **Primary osteoarthritis, left hand**

     M19.049   **Primary osteoarthritis, unspecified hand**

   ✓6ᵗʰ   M19.07   **Primary osteoarthritis ankle and foot**

     M19.071   **Primary osteoarthritis, right ankle and foot**

     M19.072   **Primary osteoarthritis, left ankle and foot**

     M19.079   **Primary osteoarthritis, unspecified ankle and foot**

✓5ᵗʰ   M19.1   Post-traumatic osteoarthritis of other joints

   ✓6ᵗʰ   M19.11   **Post-traumatic osteoarthritis, shoulder**

     M19.111   **Post-traumatic osteoarthritis, right shoulder**

     M19.112   **Post-traumatic osteoarthritis, left shoulder**

     M19.119   **Post-traumatic osteoarthritis, unspecified shoulder**

   ✓6ᵗʰ   M19.12   **Post-traumatic osteoarthritis, elbow**

     M19.121   **Post-traumatic osteoarthritis, right elbow**

     M19.122   **Post-traumatic osteoarthritis, left elbow**

     M19.129   **Post-traumatic osteoarthritis, unspecified elbow**

   ✓6ᵗʰ   M19.13   **Post-traumatic osteoarthritis, wrist**

     M19.131   **Post-traumatic osteoarthritis, right wrist**

     M19.132   **Post-traumatic osteoarthritis, left wrist**

     M19.139   **Post-traumatic osteoarthritis, unspecified wrist**

   ✓6ᵗʰ   M19.14   **Post-traumatic osteoarthritis, hand**
     EXCLUDES 2   post-traumatic osteoarthritis of first carpometacarpal joint (M18.2-, M18.3-)

     M19.141   **Post-traumatic osteoarthritis, right hand**

     M19.142   **Post-traumatic osteoarthritis, left hand**

     M19.149   **Post-traumatic osteoarthritis, unspecified hand**

   ✓6ᵗʰ   M19.17   **Post-traumatic osteoarthritis, ankle and foot**

     M19.171   **Post-traumatic osteoarthritis, right ankle and foot**

     M19.172   **Post-traumatic osteoarthritis, left ankle and foot**

     M19.179   **Post-traumatic osteoarthritis, unspecified ankle and foot**

✓5ᵗʰ   M19.2   Secondary osteoarthritis of other joints

   ✓6ᵗʰ   M19.21   **Secondary osteoarthritis, shoulder**

     M19.211   **Secondary osteoarthritis, right shoulder**

     M19.212   **Secondary osteoarthritis, left shoulder**

     M19.219   **Secondary osteoarthritis, unspecified shoulder**

✓ Additional Character Required   ✓x7ᵗʰ Placeholder   Unacceptable PDx   Questionable PDx   Manifestation   H1 - H14 HAC   HCC CMS-HCC Dx   HIV HIV Dx

ICD-10-CM 2019   763

✓6th **M19.22 Secondary osteoarthritis, elbow**
    M19.221 Secondary osteoarthritis, right elbow
    M19.222 Secondary osteoarthritis, left elbow
    M19.229 Secondary osteoarthritis, unspecified elbow

✓6th **M19.23 Secondary osteoarthritis, wrist**
    M19.231 Secondary osteoarthritis, right wrist
    M19.232 Secondary osteoarthritis, left wrist
    M19.239 Secondary osteoarthritis, unspecified wrist

✓6th **M19.24 Secondary osteoarthritis, hand**
    M19.241 Secondary osteoarthritis, right hand
    M19.242 Secondary osteoarthritis, left hand
    M19.249 Secondary osteoarthritis, unspecified hand

✓6th **M19.27 Secondary osteoarthritis, ankle and foot**
    M19.271 Secondary osteoarthritis, right ankle and foot
    M19.272 Secondary osteoarthritis, left ankle and foot
    M19.279 Secondary osteoarthritis, unspecified ankle and foot

✓5th **M19.9 Osteoarthritis, unspecified site**
    M19.90 Unspecified osteoarthritis, unspecified site
      Arthrosis NOS
      Arthritis NOS
      Osteoarthritis NOS
      AHA: 2016, 4Q, 147
    M19.91 Primary osteoarthritis, unspecified site
      Primary osteoarthritis NOS
    M19.92 Post-traumatic osteoarthritis, unspecified site
      Post-traumatic osteoarthritis NOS
    M19.93 Secondary osteoarthritis, unspecified site
      Secondary osteoarthritis NOS

Other joint disorders (M20-M25)
EXCLUDES 2   joints of the spine (M40-M54)

✓4th **M20 Acquired deformities of fingers and toes**
    EXCLUDES 1   acquired absence of fingers and toes (Z89.-)
      congenital absence of fingers and toes (Q71.3-, Q72.3-)
      congenital deformities and malformations of fingers and toes (Q66-, Q68-Q70, Q74-)

✓5th **M20.0 Deformity of finger(s)**
    EXCLUDES 1   clubbing of fingers (R68.3)
      palmar fascial fibromatosis [Dupuytren] (M72.0)
      trigger finger (M65.3)

   ✓6th **M20.00 Unspecified deformity of finger(s)**
      M20.001 Unspecified deformity of right finger(s)
      M20.002 Unspecified deformity of left finger(s)
      M20.009 Unspecified deformity of unspecified finger(s)

   ✓6th **M20.01 Mallet finger**
      M20.011 Mallet finger of right finger(s)
      M20.012 Mallet finger of left finger(s)
      M20.019 Mallet finger of unspecified finger(s)

   ✓6th **M20.02 Boutonnière deformity**
      DEF: Deformity of the finger caused by flexion of the proximal interphalangeal joint and hyperextension of the distal joint. The deformity results from rheumatoid arthritis, osteoarthritis, or injury.
      M20.021 Boutonnière deformity of right finger(s)
      M20.022 Boutonnière deformity of left finger(s)
      M20.029 Boutonnière deformity of unspecified finger(s)

   ✓6th **M20.03 Swan-neck deformity**
      DEF: Flexed distal and hyperextended proximal interphalangeal joint most commonly caused by rheumatoid arthritis.
      M20.031 Swan-neck deformity of right finger(s)
      M20.032 Swan-neck deformity of left finger(s)
      M20.039 Swan-neck deformity of unspecified finger(s)

   ✓6th **M20.09 Other deformity of finger(s)**
      M20.091 Other deformity of right finger(s)
      M20.092 Other deformity of left finger(s)

      M20.099 Other deformity of finger(s), unspecified finger(s)

✓5th **M20.1 Hallux valgus (acquired)**
    EXCLUDES 2   bunion (M21.6-)
    AHA: 2016, 4Q, 38
    DEF: Deformity in which the great toe deviates toward the other toes and may even be positioned over or under the second toe.
    M20.10 Hallux valgus (acquired), unspecified foot
    M20.11 Hallux valgus (acquired), right foot
    M20.12 Hallux valgus (acquired), left foot

Hallux Valgus

Hallux valgus

Medial eminence of metatarsal bone

Right foot

✓5th **M20.2 Hallux rigidus**
    M20.20 Hallux rigidus, unspecified foot
    M20.21 Hallux rigidus, right foot
    M20.22 Hallux rigidus, left foot

✓5th **M20.3 Hallux varus (acquired)**
    DEF: Deformity in which the great toe deviates away from the other toes.
    M20.30 Hallux varus (acquired), unspecified foot
    M20.31 Hallux varus (acquired), right foot
    M20.32 Hallux varus (acquired), left foot

✓5th **M20.4 Other hammer toe(s) (acquired)**
    M20.40 Other hammer toe(s) (acquired), unspecified foot
    M20.41 Other hammer toe(s) (acquired), right foot
    M20.42 Other hammer toe(s) (acquired), left foot

✓5th **M20.5 Other deformities of toe(s) (acquired)**
   ✓6th **M20.5X Other deformities of toe(s) (acquired)**
      M20.5X1 Other deformities of toe(s) (acquired), right foot
      M20.5X2 Other deformities of toe(s) (acquired), left foot
      M20.5X9 Other deformities of toe(s) (acquired), unspecified foot

✓5th **M20.6 Acquired deformities of toe(s), unspecified**
    M20.60 Acquired deformities of toe(s), unspecified, unspecified foot
    M20.61 Acquired deformities of toe(s), unspecified, right foot
    M20.62 Acquired deformities of toe(s), unspecified, left foot

✓4th **M21 Other acquired deformities of limbs**
    EXCLUDES 1   acquired absence of limb (Z89.-)
      congenital absence of limbs (Q71-Q73)
      congenital deformities and malformations of limbs (Q65-Q66, Q68-Q74)
    EXCLUDES 2   acquired deformities of fingers or toes (M20.-)
      coxa plana (M91.2)

✓5th **M21.0 Valgus deformity, not elsewhere classified**
    EXCLUDES 1   metatarsus valgus (Q66.6)
      talipes calcaneovalgus (Q66.4)
    M21.00 Valgus deformity, not elsewhere classified, unspecified site

N Newborn: 0   **P** Pediatric: 0-17   **M** Maternity: 12-55   **A** Adult: 15-124   **MCC** Major Complication/Comorbidity   **CC** Complication/Comorbidity   **SW** Severe Wound Dx

764   ICD-10-CM 2019

✓6ᵗʰ **M21.02** Valgus deformity, not elsewhere classified, elbow
Cubitus valgus

     M21.021 Valgus deformity, not elsewhere classified, right elbow

     M21.022 Valgus deformity, not elsewhere classified, left elbow

     M21.029 Valgus deformity, not elsewhere classified, unspecified elbow

✓6ᵗʰ **M21.05** Valgus deformity, not elsewhere classified, hip

     M21.051 Valgus deformity, not elsewhere classified, right hip

     M21.052 Valgus deformity, not elsewhere classified, left hip

     M21.059 Valgus deformity, not elsewhere classified, unspecified hip

✓6ᵗʰ **M21.06** Valgus deformity, not elsewhere classified, knee
Genu valgum
Knock knee
DEF: Genu valga/valgum: Condition in which the thighs slant inward, causing the knees to be angled abnormally close together, leaving the space between the ankles wider than normal.

     M21.061 Valgus deformity, not elsewhere classified, right knee

     M21.062 Valgus deformity, not elsewhere classified, left knee

     M21.069 Valgus deformity, not elsewhere classified, unspecified knee

Genu Valga (knock-knee)

✓6ᵗʰ **M21.07** Valgus deformity, not elsewhere classified, ankle

     M21.071 Valgus deformity, not elsewhere classified, right ankle

     M21.072 Valgus deformity, not elsewhere classified, left ankle

     M21.079 Valgus deformity, not elsewhere classified, unspecified ankle

✓5ᵗʰ **M21.1** Varus deformity, not elsewhere classified
EXCLUDES 1   metatarsus varus (Q66.22)
            tibia vara (M92.5)

     M21.10 Varus deformity, not elsewhere classified, unspecified site

✓6ᵗʰ **M21.12** Varus deformity, not elsewhere classified, elbow
Cubitus varus, elbow

     M21.121 Varus deformity, not elsewhere classified, right elbow

     M21.122 Varus deformity, not elsewhere classified, left elbow

     M21.129 Varus deformity, not elsewhere classified, unspecified elbow

✓6ᵗʰ **M21.15** Varus deformity, not elsewhere classified, hip

     M21.151 Varus deformity, not elsewhere classified, right hip

     M21.152 Varus deformity, not elsewhere classified, left hip

     M21.159 Varus deformity, not elsewhere classified, unspecified

✓6ᵗʰ **M21.16** Varus deformity, not elsewhere classified, knee
Bow leg
Genu varum
DEF: Genu varus/varum: Condition in which the thighs and/or legs are bowed in an outward curve with an abnormally increased space between the knees.

     M21.161 Varus deformity, not elsewhere classified, right knee

     M21.162 Varus deformity, not elsewhere classified, left knee

     M21.169 Varus deformity, not elsewhere classified, unspecified knee

Genu Varus (bowleg)

✓6ᵗʰ **M21.17** Varus deformity, not elsewhere classified, ankle

     M21.171 Varus deformity, not elsewhere classified, right ankle

     M21.172 Varus deformity, not elsewhere classified, left ankle

     M21.179 Varus deformity, not elsewhere classified, unspecified ankle

✓5ᵗʰ **M21.2** Flexion deformity

     M21.20 Flexion deformity, unspecified site

✓6ᵗʰ **M21.21** Flexion deformity, shoulder

     M21.211 Flexion deformity, right shoulder

     M21.212 Flexion deformity, left shoulder

     M21.219 Flexion deformity, unspecified shoulder

✓6ᵗʰ **M21.22** Flexion deformity, elbow

     M21.221 Flexion deformity, right elbow

     M21.222 Flexion deformity, left elbow

     M21.229 Flexion deformity, unspecified elbow

✓6ᵗʰ **M21.23** Flexion deformity, wrist

     M21.231 Flexion deformity, right wrist

     M21.232 Flexion deformity, left wrist

     M21.239 Flexion deformity, unspecified wrist

✓6ᵗʰ **M21.24** Flexion deformity, finger joints

     M21.241 Flexion deformity, right finger joints

     M21.242 Flexion deformity, left finger joints

     M21.249 Flexion deformity, unspecified finger joints

✓6ᵗʰ **M21.25** Flexion deformity, hip

     M21.251 Flexion deformity, right hip

     M21.252 Flexion deformity, left hip

     M21.259 Flexion deformity, unspecified hip

✓6ᵗʰ **M21.26** Flexion deformity, knee

     M21.261 Flexion deformity, right knee

     M21.262 Flexion deformity, left knee

     M21.269 Flexion deformity, unspecified knee

✓6ᵗʰ **M21.27** Flexion deformity, ankle and toes

     M21.271 Flexion deformity, right ankle and toes

✔Additional Character Required   ✓x7ᵗʰ Placeholder   Unacceptable PDx   Questionable PDx   Manifestation   H1 - H14 HAC   HCC CMS-HCC Dx   HIV HIV Dx

ICD-10-CM 2019   **765**

            M21.272   Flexion deformity, left ankle and toes
            M21.279   Flexion deformity, unspecified ankle and toes

✓5th **M21.3 Wrist or foot drop (acquired)**

  ✓6th **M21.33 Wrist drop (acquired)**
        M21.331   Wrist drop, right wrist
        M21.332   Wrist drop, left wrist
        M21.339   Wrist drop, unspecified wrist

  ✓6th **M21.37 Foot drop (acquired)**
        M21.371   Foot drop, right foot
        M21.372   Foot drop, left foot
        M21.379   Foot drop, unspecified foot

✓5th **M21.4 Flat foot [pes planus] (acquired)**
    EXCLUDES 1   congenital pes planus (Q66.5-)
    M21.40   Flat foot [pes planus] (acquired), unspecified foot
    M21.41   Flat foot [pes planus] (acquired), right foot
    M21.42   Flat foot [pes planus] (acquired), left foot

✓5th **M21.5 Acquired clawhand, clubhand, clawfoot and clubfoot**
    EXCLUDES 1   clubfoot, not specified as acquired (Q66.89)

  ✓6th **M21.51 Acquired clawhand**
        M21.511   Acquired clawhand, right hand
        M21.512   Acquired clawhand, left hand
        M21.519   Acquired clawhand, unspecified hand

  ✓6th **M21.52 Acquired clubhand**
        M21.521   Acquired clubhand, right hand
        M21.522   Acquired clubhand, left hand
        M21.529   Acquired clubhand, unspecified hand

  ✓6th **M21.53 Acquired clawfoot**
        DEF: High foot arch with hyperextended toes at the metatarsophalangeal joint and flexed toes at the distal joints.
        M21.531   Acquired clawfoot, right foot
        M21.532   Acquired clawfoot, left foot
        M21.539   Acquired clawfoot, unspecified foot

  ✓6th **M21.54 Acquired clubfoot**
        DEF: Acquired anomaly of the foot with the heel elevated and rotated outward and the toes pointing inward.
        M21.541   Acquired clubfoot, right foot
        M21.542   Acquired clubfoot, left foot
        M21.549   Acquired clubfoot, unspecified foot

✓5th **M21.6 Other acquired deformities of foot**
    EXCLUDES 2   deformities of toe (acquired) (M20.1-M20.6-)
    AHA: 2016, 4Q, 38

  ✓6th **M21.61 Bunion**
        M21.611   Bunion of right foot
        M21.612   Bunion of left foot
        M21.619   Bunion of unspecified foot

  ✓6th **M21.62 Bunionette**
        M21.621   Bunionette of right foot
        M21.622   Bunionette of left foot
        M21.629   Bunionette of unspecified foot

  ✓6th **M21.6X Other acquired deformities of foot**
        M21.6X1   Other acquired deformities of right foot
        M21.6X2   Other acquired deformities of left foot
        M21.6X9   Other acquired deformities of unspecified foot

✓5th **M21.7 Unequal limb length (acquired)**
    NOTE   The site used should correspond to the shorter limb.
    M21.70   Unequal limb length (acquired), unspecified site

  ✓6th **M21.72 Unequal limb length (acquired), humerus**
        M21.721   Unequal limb length (acquired), right humerus
        M21.722   Unequal limb length (acquired), left humerus
        M21.729   Unequal limb length (acquired), unspecified humerus

  ✓6th **M21.73 Unequal limb length (acquired), ulna and radius**
        M21.731   Unequal limb length (acquired), right ulna
        M21.732   Unequal limb length (acquired), left ulna
        M21.733   Unequal limb length (acquired), right radius
        M21.734   Unequal limb length (acquired), left radius

        M21.739   Unequal limb length (acquired), unspecified ulna and radius

  ✓6th **M21.75 Unequal limb length (acquired), femur**
        M21.751   Unequal limb length (acquired), right femur
        M21.752   Unequal limb length (acquired), left femur
        M21.759   Unequal limb length (acquired), unspecified femur

  ✓6th **M21.76 Unequal limb length (acquired), tibia and fibula**
        M21.761   Unequal limb length (acquired), right tibia
        M21.762   Unequal limb length (acquired), left tibia
        M21.763   Unequal limb length (acquired), right fibula
        M21.764   Unequal limb length (acquired), left fibula
        M21.769   Unequal limb length (acquired), unspecified tibia and fibula

✓5th **M21.8 Other specified acquired deformities of limbs**
    EXCLUDES 2   coxa plana (M91.2)
    M21.80   Other specified acquired deformities of unspecified limb

  ✓6th **M21.82 Other specified acquired deformities of upper arm**
        M21.821   Other specified acquired deformities of right upper arm
        M21.822   Other specified acquired deformities of left upper arm
        M21.829   Other specified acquired deformities of unspecified upper arm

  ✓6th **M21.83 Other specified acquired deformities of forearm**
        M21.831   Other specified acquired deformities of right forearm
        M21.832   Other specified acquired deformities of left forearm
        M21.839   Other specified acquired deformities of unspecified forearm

  ✓6th **M21.85 Other specified acquired deformities of thigh**
        M21.851   Other specified acquired deformities of right thigh
        M21.852   Other specified acquired deformities of left thigh
        M21.859   Other specified acquired deformities of unspecified thigh

  ✓6th **M21.86 Other specified acquired deformities of lower leg**
        M21.861   Other specified acquired deformities of right lower leg
        M21.862   Other specified acquired deformities of left lower leg
        M21.869   Other specified acquired deformities of unspecified lower leg

✓5th **M21.9 Unspecified acquired deformity of limb and hand**
    M21.90   Unspecified acquired deformity of unspecified limb

  ✓6th **M21.92 Unspecified acquired deformity of upper arm**
        M21.921   Unspecified acquired deformity of right upper arm
        M21.922   Unspecified acquired deformity of left upper arm
        M21.929   Unspecified acquired deformity of unspecified upper arm

  ✓6th **M21.93 Unspecified acquired deformity of forearm**
        M21.931   Unspecified acquired deformity of right forearm
        M21.932   Unspecified acquired deformity of left forearm
        M21.939   Unspecified acquired deformity of unspecified forearm

  ✓6th **M21.94 Unspecified acquired deformity of hand**
        M21.941   Unspecified acquired deformity of hand, right hand
        M21.942   Unspecified acquired deformity of hand, left hand
        M21.949   Unspecified acquired deformity of hand, unspecified hand

  ✓6th **M21.95 Unspecified acquired deformity of thigh**
        M21.951   Unspecified acquired deformity of right thigh
        M21.952   Unspecified acquired deformity of left thigh

N Newborn: 0   **P** Pediatric: 0-17   **M** Maternity: 12-55   **A** Adult: 15-124   **MCC** Major Complication/Comorbidity   **CC** Complication/Comorbidity   **SW** Severe Wound Dx

766   ICD-10-CM 2019

M21.959   Unspecified acquired deformity of unspecified **thigh**

☑6ᵗʰ   **M21.96**   Unspecified acquired deformity of lower leg

    M21.961   Unspecified acquired deformity of right **lower leg**

    M21.962   Unspecified acquired deformity of left **lower leg**

    M21.969   Unspecified acquired deformity of unspecified **lower leg**

☑4ᵗʰ   **M22**   **Disorder of patella**

    EXCLUDES 1   *traumatic dislocation of patella (S83.0-)*

☑5ᵗʰ   **M22.0**   Recurrent dislocation of patella

    M22.00   Recurrent dislocation of patella, unspecified **knee**

    M22.01   Recurrent dislocation of patella, right **knee**

    M22.02   Recurrent dislocation of patella, left **knee**

☑5ᵗʰ   **M22.1**   Recurrent subluxation of patella
    Incomplete dislocation of patella

    M22.10   Recurrent subluxation of patella, unspecified **knee**

    M22.11   Recurrent subluxation of patella, right **knee**

    M22.12   Recurrent subluxation of patella, left **knee**

☑5ᵗʰ   **M22.2**   Patellofemoral disorders

    ☑6ᵗʰ   **M22.2X**   Patellofemoral disorders

      M22.2X1   Patellofemoral disorders, right **knee**

      M22.2X2   Patellofemoral disorders, left **knee**

      M22.2X9   Patellofemoral disorders, unspecified **knee**

☑5ᵗʰ   **M22.3**   Other derangements of patella

    ☑6ᵗʰ   **M22.3X**   Other derangements of patella

      M22.3X1   Other derangements of patella, right **knee**

      M22.3X2   Other derangements of patella, left **knee**

      M22.3X9   Other derangements of patella, unspecified **knee**

☑5ᵗʰ   **M22.4**   Chondromalacia patellae

    M22.40   Chondromalacia patellae, unspecified **knee**

    M22.41   Chondromalacia patellae, right **knee**

    M22.42   Chondromalacia patellae, left **knee**

☑5ᵗʰ   **M22.8**   Other disorders of patella

    ☑6ᵗʰ   **M22.8X**   Other disorders of patella

      M22.8X1   Other disorders of patella, right **knee**

      M22.8X2   Other disorders of patella, left **knee**

      M22.8X9   Other disorders of patella, unspecified **knee**

☑5ᵗʰ   **M22.9**   Unspecified disorder of patella

    M22.90   Unspecified disorder of patella, unspecified **knee**

    M22.91   Unspecified disorder of patella, right **knee**

    M22.92   Unspecified disorder of patella, left **knee**

☑4ᵗʰ   **M23**   **Internal derangement of knee**

    EXCLUDES 1   *ankylosis (M24.66)*
       current injury—see injury of knee and lower leg (S80-S89)
       deformity of knee (M21.-)
       osteochondritis dissecans (M93.2)
       recurrent dislocation or subluxation of joints (M24.4)
       recurrent dislocation or subluxation of patella (M22.0-M22.1)

☑5ᵗʰ   **M23.0**   Cystic meniscus

    ☑6ᵗʰ   **M23.00**   Cystic meniscus, unspecified **meniscus**
      Cystic meniscus, unspecified lateral meniscus
      Cystic meniscus, unspecified medial meniscus

      M23.000   Cystic meniscus, unspecified lateral meniscus, right **knee**

      M23.001   Cystic meniscus, unspecified lateral meniscus, left **knee**

      M23.002   Cystic meniscus, unspecified lateral meniscus, unspecified **knee**

      M23.003   Cystic meniscus, unspecified medial meniscus, right **knee**

      M23.004   Cystic meniscus, unspecified medial meniscus, left **knee**

      M23.005   Cystic meniscus, unspecified medial meniscus, unspecified **knee**

      M23.006   Cystic meniscus, unspecified meniscus, right **knee**

      M23.007   Cystic meniscus, unspecified meniscus, left **knee**

      M23.009   Cystic meniscus, unspecified meniscus, unspecified **knee**

☑6ᵗʰ   **M23.01**   Cystic meniscus, anterior horn of medial **meniscus**

    M23.011   Cystic meniscus, anterior horn of medial meniscus, right **knee**

    M23.012   Cystic meniscus, anterior horn of medial meniscus, left **knee**

    M23.019   Cystic meniscus, anterior horn of medial meniscus, unspecified **knee**

☑6ᵗʰ   **M23.02**   Cystic meniscus, posterior horn of medial **meniscus**

    M23.021   Cystic meniscus, posterior horn of medial meniscus, right **knee**

    M23.022   Cystic meniscus, posterior horn of medial meniscus, left **knee**

    M23.029   Cystic meniscus, posterior horn of medial meniscus, unspecified **knee**

☑6ᵗʰ   **M23.03**   Cystic meniscus, other medial meniscus

    M23.031   Cystic meniscus, other medial meniscus, right **knee**

    M23.032   Cystic meniscus, other medial meniscus, left **knee**

    M23.039   Cystic meniscus, other medial meniscus, unspecified **knee**

☑6ᵗʰ   **M23.04**   Cystic meniscus, anterior horn of lateral **meniscus**

    M23.041   Cystic meniscus, anterior horn of lateral meniscus, right **knee**

    M23.042   Cystic meniscus, anterior horn of lateral meniscus, left **knee**

    M23.049   Cystic meniscus, anterior horn of lateral meniscus, unspecified **knee**

☑6ᵗʰ   **M23.05**   Cystic meniscus, posterior horn of lateral **meniscus**

    M23.051   Cystic meniscus, posterior horn of lateral meniscus, right **knee**

    M23.052   Cystic meniscus, posterior horn of lateral meniscus, left **knee**

    M23.059   Cystic meniscus, posterior horn of lateral meniscus, unspecified **knee**

☑6ᵗʰ   **M23.06**   Cystic meniscus, other lateral **meniscus**

    M23.061   Cystic meniscus, other lateral meniscus, right **knee**

    M23.062   Cystic meniscus, other lateral meniscus, left **knee**

    M23.069   Cystic meniscus, other lateral meniscus, unspecified **knee**

☑5ᵗʰ   **M23.2**   **Derangement of meniscus due to old tear or injury**
    Old bucket-handle tear

    ☑6ᵗʰ   **M23.20**   Derangement of unspecified meniscus due to old tear or injury
      Derangement of unspecified lateral meniscus due to old tear or injury
      Derangement of unspecified medial meniscus due to old tear or injury

      M23.200   Derangement of unspecified lateral meniscus due to old tear or injury, right **knee**

      M23.201   Derangement of unspecified lateral meniscus due to old tear or injury, left **knee**

      M23.202   Derangement of unspecified lateral meniscus due to old tear or injury, unspecified **knee**

      M23.203   Derangement of unspecified medial meniscus due to old tear or injury, right **knee**

      M23.204   Derangement of unspecified medial meniscus due to old tear or injury, left **knee**

      M23.205   Derangement of unspecified medial meniscus due to old tear or injury, unspecified **knee**

      M23.206   Derangement of unspecified meniscus due to old tear or injury, right **knee**

      M23.207   Derangement of unspecified meniscus due to old tear or injury, left **knee**

      M23.209   Derangement of unspecified meniscus due to old tear or injury, unspecified **knee**

☑ Additional Character Required   ✓ˣ⁷ᵗʰ Placeholder   Unacceptable PDx   Questionable PDx   Manifestation   H1 – H14 HAC   HCC CMS-HCC Dx   HIV HIV Dx

ICD-10-CM 2019   767

Derangement of Meniscus

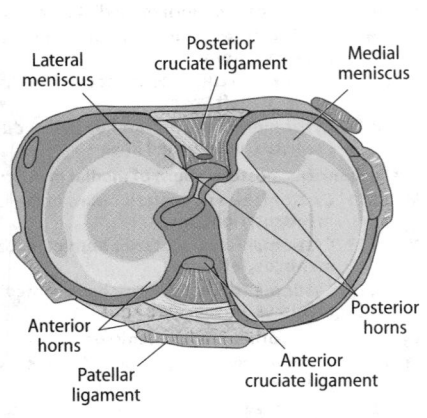

Overhead view of right knee

Bucket handle tear

Radial tear

Meniscus

✓6ᵗʰ **M23.21** **Derangement of** anterior horn of medial **meniscus due to old tear or injury**
     M23.211 Derangement of anterior horn of medial meniscus due to old tear or injury, right knee
     M23.212 Derangement of anterior horn of medial meniscus due to old tear or injury, left knee
     M23.219 Derangement of anterior horn of medial meniscus due to old tear or injury, unspecified knee

✓6ᵗʰ **M23.22** **Derangement of** posterior horn of medial **meniscus due to old tear or injury**
     M23.221 Derangement of posterior horn of medial meniscus due to old tear or injury, right knee
     M23.222 Derangement of posterior horn of medial meniscus due to old tear or injury, left knee
     M23.229 Derangement of posterior horn of medial meniscus due to old tear or injury, unspecified knee

✓6ᵗʰ **M23.23** **Derangement of** other medial **meniscus due to old tear or injury**
     M23.231 Derangement of other medial meniscus due to old tear or injury, right knee
     M23.232 Derangement of other medial meniscus due to old tear or injury, left knee
     M23.239 Derangement of other medial meniscus due to old tear or injury, unspecified knee

✓6ᵗʰ **M23.24** **Derangement of** anterior horn of lateral **meniscus due to old tear or injury**
     M23.241 Derangement of anterior horn of lateral meniscus due to old tear or injury, right knee
     M23.242 Derangement of anterior horn of lateral meniscus due to old tear or injury, left knee
     M23.249 Derangement of anterior horn of lateral meniscus due to old tear or injury, unspecified knee

✓6ᵗʰ **M23.25** **Derangement of** posterior horn of lateral **meniscus due to old tear or injury**
     M23.251 Derangement of posterior horn of lateral meniscus due to old tear or injury, right knee
     M23.252 Derangement of posterior horn of lateral meniscus due to old tear or injury, left knee
     M23.259 Derangement of posterior horn of lateral meniscus due to old tear or injury, unspecified knee

✓6ᵗʰ **M23.26** **Derangement of** other lateral **meniscus due to old tear or injury**
     M23.261 Derangement of other lateral meniscus due to old tear or injury, right knee
     M23.262 Derangement of other lateral meniscus due to old tear or injury, left knee
     M23.269 Derangement of other lateral meniscus due to old tear or injury, unspecified knee

✓5ᵗʰ **M23.3** **Other meniscus derangements**
     Degenerate meniscus
     Detached meniscus
     Retained meniscus

✓6ᵗʰ **M23.30** **Other meniscus derangements,** unspecified meniscus
     Other meniscus derangements, unspecified lateral meniscus
     Other meniscus derangements, unspecified medial meniscus
     M23.300 Other meniscus derangements, unspecified lateral meniscus, right knee
     M23.301 Other meniscus derangements, unspecified lateral meniscus, left knee
     M23.302 Other meniscus derangements, unspecified lateral meniscus, unspecified knee
     M23.303 Other meniscus derangements, unspecified medial meniscus, right knee
     M23.304 Other meniscus derangements, unspecified medial meniscus, left knee
     M23.305 Other meniscus derangements, unspecified medial meniscus, unspecified knee
     M23.306 Other meniscus derangements, unspecified meniscus, right knee
     M23.307 Other meniscus derangements, unspecified meniscus, left knee
     M23.309 Other meniscus derangements, unspecified meniscus, unspecified knee

✓6ᵗʰ **M23.31** **Other meniscus derangements,** anterior horn of medial **meniscus**
     M23.311 Other meniscus derangements, anterior horn of medial meniscus, right knee
     M23.312 Other meniscus derangements, anterior horn of medial meniscus, left knee
     M23.319 Other meniscus derangements, anterior horn of medial meniscus, unspecified knee

✓6ᵗʰ **M23.32** **Other meniscus derangements,** posterior horn of medial **meniscus**
     M23.321 Other meniscus derangements, posterior horn of medial meniscus, right knee
     M23.322 Other meniscus derangements, posterior horn of medial meniscus, left knee
     M23.329 Other meniscus derangements, posterior horn of medial meniscus, unspecified knee

✓6ᵗʰ **M23.33** **Other meniscus derangements,** other medial **meniscus**
     M23.331 Other meniscus derangements, other medial meniscus, right knee
     M23.332 Other meniscus derangements, other medial meniscus, left knee
     M23.339 Other meniscus derangements, other medial meniscus, unspecified knee

✓6ᵗʰ **M23.34** **Other meniscus derangements,** anterior horn of lateral **meniscus**
     M23.341 Other meniscus derangements, anterior horn of lateral meniscus, right knee
     M23.342 Other meniscus derangements, anterior horn of lateral meniscus, left knee
     M23.349 Other meniscus derangements, anterior horn of lateral meniscus, unspecified knee

✓6ᵗʰ **M23.35** **Other meniscus derangements,** posterior horn of lateral **meniscus**
     M23.351 Other meniscus derangements, posterior horn of lateral meniscus, right knee
     M23.352 Other meniscus derangements, posterior horn of lateral meniscus, left knee
     M23.359 Other meniscus derangements, posterior horn of lateral meniscus, unspecified knee

Ⓝ Newborn: 0   Ⓟ Pediatric: 0-17   Ⓜ Maternity: 12-55   Ⓐ Adult: 15-124   ᴹᶜᶜ Major Complication/Comorbidity   ᶜᶜ Complication/Comorbidity   ˢʷ Severe Wound Dx

768   ICD-10-CM 2019

✓6th **M23.36** **Other meniscus derangements,** other lateral meniscus

     M23.361 **Other meniscus derangements, other lateral meniscus,** right **knee**

     M23.362 **Other meniscus derangements, other lateral meniscus,** left **knee**

     M23.369 **Other meniscus derangements, other lateral meniscus,** unspecified **knee**

✓5th **M23.4** **Loose body in knee**

     M23.40 **Loose body in knee,** unspecified **knee**

     M23.41 **Loose body in knee,** right **knee**

     M23.42 **Loose body in knee,** left **knee**

✓5th **M23.5** **Chronic instability of knee**

     M23.50 **Chronic instability of knee,** unspecified **knee**

     M23.51 **Chronic instability of knee,** right **knee**

     M23.52 **Chronic instability of knee,** left **knee**

✓5th **M23.6** **Other spontaneous disruption of ligament(s) of knee**

  ✓6th **M23.60** **Other spontaneous disruption of** unspecified ligament **of knee**

     M23.601 **Other spontaneous disruption of unspecified ligament of** right **knee**

     M23.602 **Other spontaneous disruption of unspecified ligament of** left **knee**

     M23.609 **Other spontaneous disruption of unspecified ligament of** unspecified **knee**

  ✓6th **M23.61** **Other spontaneous disruption of** anterior cruciate **ligament of knee**

     M23.611 **Other spontaneous disruption of anterior cruciate ligament of** right **knee**

     M23.612 **Other spontaneous disruption of anterior cruciate ligament of** left **knee**

     M23.619 **Other spontaneous disruption of anterior cruciate ligament of** unspecified **knee**

  ✓6th **M23.62** **Other spontaneous disruption of** posterior cruciate **ligament of knee**

     M23.621 **Other spontaneous disruption of posterior cruciate ligament of** right **knee**

     M23.622 **Other spontaneous disruption of posterior cruciate ligament of** left **knee**

     M23.629 **Other spontaneous disruption of posterior cruciate ligament of** unspecified **knee**

  ✓6th **M23.63** **Other spontaneous disruption of** medial collateral **ligament of knee**

     M23.631 **Other spontaneous disruption of medial collateral ligament of** right **knee**

     M23.632 **Other spontaneous disruption of medial collateral ligament of** left **knee**

     M23.639 **Other spontaneous disruption of medial collateral ligament of** unspecified **knee**

  ✓6th **M23.64** **Other spontaneous disruption of** lateral collateral **ligament of knee**

     M23.641 **Other spontaneous disruption of lateral collateral ligament of** right **knee**

     M23.642 **Other spontaneous disruption of lateral collateral ligament of** left **knee**

     M23.649 **Other spontaneous disruption of lateral collateral ligament of** unspecified **knee**

  ✓6th **M23.67** **Other spontaneous disruption of** capsular **ligament of knee**

     M23.671 **Other spontaneous disruption of capsular ligament of** right **knee**

     M23.672 **Other spontaneous disruption of capsular ligament of** left **knee**

     M23.679 **Other spontaneous disruption of capsular ligament of** unspecified **knee**

✓5th **M23.8** **Other internal derangements of knee**

     Laxity of ligament of knee

     Snapping knee

  ✓6th **M23.8X** **Other internal derangements of knee**

     M23.8X1 **Other internal derangements of** right **knee**

     M23.8X2 **Other internal derangements of** left **knee**

     M23.8X9 **Other internal derangements of** unspecified **knee**

✓5th **M23.9** **Unspecified internal derangement of knee**

     M23.90 **Unspecified internal derangement of** unspecified **knee**

     M23.91 **Unspecified internal derangement of** right **knee**

     M23.92 **Unspecified internal derangement of** left **knee**

✓4th **M24** **Other specific joint derangements**

     EXCLUDES 1   current injury—see injury of joint by body region

     EXCLUDES 2   ganglion (M67.4)

               snapping knee (M23.8-)

               temporomandibular joint disorders (M26.6-)

✓5th **M24.0** **Loose body in joint**

     EXCLUDES 2   loose body in knee (M23.4)

     M24.00 **Loose body in** unspecified **joint**

  ✓6th **M24.01** **Loose body in** shoulder

     M24.011 **Loose body in** right **shoulder**

     M24.012 **Loose body in** left **shoulder**

     M24.019 **Loose body in** unspecified **shoulder**

  ✓6th **M24.02** **Loose body in** elbow

     M24.021 **Loose body in** right **elbow**

     M24.022 **Loose body in** left **elbow**

     M24.029 **Loose body in** unspecified **elbow**

  ✓6th **M24.03** **Loose body in** wrist

     M24.031 **Loose body in** right **wrist**

     M24.032 **Loose body in** left **wrist**

     M24.039 **Loose body in** unspecified **wrist**

  ✓6th **M24.04** **Loose body in** finger joints

     M24.041 **Loose body in** right **finger joint(s)**

     M24.042 **Loose body in** left **finger joint(s)**

     M24.049 **Loose body in** unspecified **finger joint(s)**

  ✓6th **M24.05** **Loose body in** hip

     M24.051 **Loose body in** right **hip**

     M24.052 **Loose body in** left **hip**

     M24.059 **Loose body in** unspecified **hip**

  ✓6th **M24.07** **Loose body in** ankle and toe joints

     M24.071 **Loose body in** right **ankle**

     M24.072 **Loose body in** left **ankle**

     M24.073 **Loose body in** unspecified **ankle**

     M24.074 **Loose body in** right **toe joint(s)**

     M24.075 **Loose body in** left **toe joint(s)**

     M24.076 **Loose body in** unspecified **toe joints**

     M24.08 **Loose body,** other site

✓5th **M24.1** **Other articular cartilage disorders**

     EXCLUDES 2   chondrocalcinosis (M11.1, M11.2-)

               internal derangement of knee (M23.-)

               metastatic calcification (E83.5)

               ochronosis (E70.2)

     M24.10 **Other articular cartilage disorders,** unspecified site

  ✓6th **M24.11** **Other articular cartilage disorders,** shoulder

     M24.111 **Other articular cartilage disorders,** right **shoulder**

     M24.112 **Other articular cartilage disorders,** left **shoulder**

     M24.119 **Other articular cartilage disorders,** unspecified **shoulder**

  ✓6th **M24.12** **Other articular cartilage disorders,** elbow

     M24.121 **Other articular cartilage disorders,** right **elbow**

     M24.122 **Other articular cartilage disorders,** left **elbow**

     M24.129 **Other articular cartilage disorders,** unspecified **elbow**

  ✓6th **M24.13** **Other articular cartilage disorders,** wrist

     M24.131 **Other articular cartilage disorders,** right **wrist**

     M24.132 **Other articular cartilage disorders,** left **wrist**

     M24.139 **Other articular cartilage disorders,** unspecified **wrist**

  ✓6th **M24.14** **Other articular cartilage disorders,** hand

     M24.141 **Other articular cartilage disorders,** right **hand**

     M24.142 **Other articular cartilage disorders,** left **hand**

✓ Additional Character Required   ✓x7th Placeholder   Unacceptable PDx   Questionable PDx   Manifestation   H1 -H14 HAC   HCC CMS-HCC Dx   HIV HIV Dx

ICD-10-CM 2019   769

Chapter 13. Diseases of the Musculoskeletal System and Connective Tissue

M24.149 **Other articular cartilage disorders, unspecified hand**

✓6th **M24.15 Other articular cartilage disorders, hip**
     M24.151 **Other articular cartilage disorders, right hip**
     M24.152 **Other articular cartilage disorders, left hip**
     M24.159 **Other articular cartilage disorders, unspecified hip**

✓6th **M24.17 Other articular cartilage disorders, ankle and foot**
     M24.171 **Other articular cartilage disorders, right ankle**
     M24.172 **Other articular cartilage disorders, left ankle**
     M24.173 **Other articular cartilage disorders, unspecified ankle**
     M24.174 **Other articular cartilage disorders, right foot**
     M24.175 **Other articular cartilage disorders, left foot**
     M24.176 **Other articular cartilage disorders, unspecified foot**

✓5th **M24.2 Disorder of ligament**
     Instability secondary to old ligament injury
     Ligamentous laxity NOS
     EXCLUDES 1   *familial ligamentous laxity (M35.7)*
     EXCLUDES 2   *internal derangement of knee (M23.5-M23.89)*

     M24.20 **Disorder of ligament, unspecified site**

✓6th **M24.21 Disorder of ligament, shoulder**
     M24.211 **Disorder of ligament, right shoulder**
     M24.212 **Disorder of ligament, left shoulder**
     M24.219 **Disorder of ligament, unspecified shoulder**

✓6th **M24.22 Disorder of ligament, elbow**
     M24.221 **Disorder of ligament, right elbow**
     M24.222 **Disorder of ligament, left elbow**
     M24.229 **Disorder of ligament, unspecified elbow**

✓6th **M24.23 Disorder of ligament, wrist**
     M24.231 **Disorder of ligament, right wrist**
     M24.232 **Disorder of ligament, left wrist**
     M24.239 **Disorder of ligament, unspecified wrist**

✓6th **M24.24 Disorder of ligament, hand**
     M24.241 **Disorder of ligament, right hand**
     M24.242 **Disorder of ligament, left hand**
     M24.249 **Disorder of ligament, unspecified hand**

✓6th **M24.25 Disorder of ligament, hip**
     M24.251 **Disorder of ligament, right hip**
     M24.252 **Disorder of ligament, left hip**
     M24.259 **Disorder of ligament, unspecified hip**

✓6th **M24.27 Disorder of ligament, ankle and foot**
     M24.271 **Disorder of ligament, right ankle**
     M24.272 **Disorder of ligament, left ankle**
     M24.273 **Disorder of ligament, unspecified ankle**
     M24.274 **Disorder of ligament, right foot**
     M24.275 **Disorder of ligament, left foot**
     M24.276 **Disorder of ligament, unspecified foot**

     M24.28 **Disorder of ligament, vertebrae**

✓5th **M24.3 Pathological dislocation of joint, not elsewhere classified**
     EXCLUDES 1   *congenital dislocation or displacement of joint—see congenital malformations and deformations of the musculoskeletal system (Q65-Q79)*
     current injury—see injury of joints and ligaments by body region
     recurrent dislocation of joint (M24.4-)

     M24.30 **Pathological dislocation of unspecified joint, not elsewhere classified**

✓6th **M24.31 Pathological dislocation of shoulder, not elsewhere classified**
     M24.311 **Pathological dislocation of right shoulder, not elsewhere classified**
     M24.312 **Pathological dislocation of left shoulder, not elsewhere classified**
     M24.319 **Pathological dislocation of unspecified shoulder, not elsewhere classified**

✓6th **M24.32 Pathological dislocation of elbow, not elsewhere classified**
     M24.321 **Pathological dislocation of right elbow, not elsewhere classified**
     M24.322 **Pathological dislocation of left elbow, not elsewhere classified**
     M24.329 **Pathological dislocation of unspecified elbow, not elsewhere classified**

✓6th **M24.33 Pathological dislocation of wrist, not elsewhere classified**
     M24.331 **Pathological dislocation of right wrist, not elsewhere classified**
     M24.332 **Pathological dislocation of left wrist, not elsewhere classified**
     M24.339 **Pathological dislocation of unspecified wrist, not elsewhere classified**

✓6th **M24.34 Pathological dislocation of hand, not elsewhere classified**
     M24.341 **Pathological dislocation of right hand, not elsewhere classified**
     M24.342 **Pathological dislocation of left hand, not elsewhere classified**
     M24.349 **Pathological dislocation of unspecified hand, not elsewhere classified**

✓6th **M24.35 Pathological dislocation of hip, not elsewhere classified**
     M24.351 **Pathological dislocation of right hip, not elsewhere classified**
     M24.352 **Pathological dislocation of left hip, not elsewhere classified**
     M24.359 **Pathological dislocation of unspecified hip, not elsewhere classified**

✓6th **M24.36 Pathological dislocation of knee, not elsewhere classified**
     M24.361 **Pathological dislocation of right knee, not elsewhere classified**
     M24.362 **Pathological dislocation of left knee, not elsewhere classified**
     M24.369 **Pathological dislocation of unspecified knee, not elsewhere classified**

✓6th **M24.37 Pathological dislocation of ankle and foot, not elsewhere classified**
     M24.371 **Pathological dislocation of right ankle, not elsewhere classified**
     M24.372 **Pathological dislocation of left ankle, not elsewhere classified**
     M24.373 **Pathological dislocation of unspecified ankle, not elsewhere classified**
     M24.374 **Pathological dislocation of right foot, not elsewhere classified**
     M24.375 **Pathological dislocation of left foot, not elsewhere classified**
     M24.376 **Pathological dislocation of unspecified foot, not elsewhere classified**

✓5th **M24.4 Recurrent dislocation of joint**
     Recurrent subluxation of joint
     EXCLUDES 2   *recurrent dislocation of patella (M22.0-M22.1)*
     recurrent vertebral dislocation (M43.3-, M43.4, M43.5-)

     M24.40 **Recurrent dislocation, unspecified joint**

✓6th **M24.41 Recurrent dislocation, shoulder**
     M24.411 **Recurrent dislocation, right shoulder**
     M24.412 **Recurrent dislocation, left shoulder**
     M24.419 **Recurrent dislocation, unspecified shoulder**

✓6th **M24.42 Recurrent dislocation, elbow**
     M24.421 **Recurrent dislocation, right elbow**
     M24.422 **Recurrent dislocation, left elbow**
     M24.429 **Recurrent dislocation, unspecified elbow**

✓6th **M24.43 Recurrent dislocation, wrist**
     M24.431 **Recurrent dislocation, right wrist**
     M24.432 **Recurrent dislocation, left wrist**
     M24.439 **Recurrent dislocation, unspecified wrist**

✓6th **M24.44 Recurrent dislocation, hand and finger(s)**
     M24.441 **Recurrent dislocation, right hand**
     M24.442 **Recurrent dislocation, left hand**
     M24.443 **Recurrent dislocation, unspecified hand**

N Newborn: 0   P Pediatric: 0-17   M Maternity: 12-55   A Adult: 15-124   MCC Major Complication/Comorbidity   CC Complication/Comorbidity   SW Severe Wound Dx

770   ICD-10-CM 2019

M24.444 Recurrent dislocation, right finger
M24.445 Recurrent dislocation, left finger
M24.446 Recurrent dislocation, unspecified finger

✓6ᵗʰ **M24.45 Recurrent dislocation, hip**
M24.451 Recurrent dislocation, right hip
M24.452 Recurrent dislocation, left hip
M24.459 Recurrent dislocation, unspecified hip

✓6ᵗʰ **M24.46 Recurrent dislocation, knee**
M24.461 Recurrent dislocation, right knee
M24.462 Recurrent dislocation, left knee
M24.469 Recurrent dislocation, unspecified knee

✓6ᵗʰ **M24.47 Recurrent dislocation, ankle, foot and toes**
M24.471 Recurrent dislocation, right ankle
M24.472 Recurrent dislocation, left ankle
M24.473 Recurrent dislocation, unspecified ankle
M24.474 Recurrent dislocation, right foot
M24.475 Recurrent dislocation, left foot
M24.476 Recurrent dislocation, unspecified foot
M24.477 Recurrent dislocation, right toe(s)
M24.478 Recurrent dislocation, left toe(s)
M24.479 Recurrent dislocation, unspecified toe(s)

✓5ᵗʰ **M24.5 Contracture of joint**
    EXCLUDES 1   contracture of muscle without contracture of joint (M62.4-)
              contracture of tendon (sheath) without contracture of joint (M62.4-)
              Dupuytren's contracture (M72.0)
    EXCLUDES 2   acquired deformities of limbs (M20-M21)
    AHA: 2016, 2Q, 6

M24.50 Contracture, unspecified joint

✓6ᵗʰ **M24.51 Contracture, shoulder**
M24.511 Contracture, right shoulder
M24.512 Contracture, left shoulder
M24.519 Contracture, unspecified shoulder

✓6ᵗʰ **M24.52 Contracture, elbow**
M24.521 Contracture, right elbow
M24.522 Contracture, left elbow
M24.529 Contracture, unspecified elbow

✓6ᵗʰ **M24.53 Contracture, wrist**
M24.531 Contracture, right wrist
M24.532 Contracture, left wrist
M24.539 Contracture, unspecified wrist

✓6ᵗʰ **M24.54 Contracture, hand**
M24.541 Contracture, right hand
M24.542 Contracture, left hand
M24.549 Contracture, unspecified hand

✓6ᵗʰ **M24.55 Contracture, hip**
M24.551 Contracture, right hip
M24.552 Contracture, left hip
M24.559 Contracture, unspecified hip

✓6ᵗʰ **M24.56 Contracture, knee**
M24.561 Contracture, right knee
M24.562 Contracture, left knee
M24.569 Contracture, unspecified knee

✓6ᵗʰ **M24.57 Contracture, ankle and foot**
M24.571 Contracture, right ankle
M24.572 Contracture, left ankle
M24.573 Contracture, unspecified ankle
M24.574 Contracture, right foot
M24.575 Contracture, left foot
M24.576 Contracture, unspecified foot

✓5ᵗʰ **M24.6 Ankylosis of joint**
    EXCLUDES 1   stiffness of joint without ankylosis (M25.6-)
    EXCLUDES 2   spine (M43.2-)
    DEF: Ankylosis: Abnormal union or fusion of bones in a joint, which is normally moveable.

M24.60 Ankylosis, unspecified joint

✓6ᵗʰ **M24.61 Ankylosis, shoulder**
M24.611 Ankylosis, right shoulder
M24.612 Ankylosis, left shoulder
M24.619 Ankylosis, unspecified shoulder

✓6ᵗʰ **M24.62 Ankylosis, elbow**
M24.621 Ankylosis, right elbow
M24.622 Ankylosis, left elbow
M24.629 Ankylosis, unspecified elbow

✓6ᵗʰ **M24.63 Ankylosis, wrist**
M24.631 Ankylosis, right wrist
M24.632 Ankylosis, left wrist
M24.639 Ankylosis, unspecified wrist

✓6ᵗʰ **M24.64 Ankylosis, hand**
M24.641 Ankylosis, right hand
M24.642 Ankylosis, left hand
M24.649 Ankylosis, unspecified hand

✓6ᵗʰ **M24.65 Ankylosis, hip**
M24.651 Ankylosis, right hip
M24.652 Ankylosis, left hip
M24.659 Ankylosis, unspecified hip

✓6ᵗʰ **M24.66 Ankylosis, knee**
M24.661 Ankylosis, right knee
M24.662 Ankylosis, left knee
M24.669 Ankylosis, unspecified knee

✓6ᵗʰ **M24.67 Ankylosis, ankle and foot**
M24.671 Ankylosis, right ankle
M24.672 Ankylosis, left ankle
M24.673 Ankylosis, unspecified ankle
M24.674 Ankylosis, right foot
M24.675 Ankylosis, left foot
M24.676 Ankylosis, unspecified foot

M24.7 Protrusio acetabuli
    DEF: Intrapelvic protrusion of the acetabulum characterized by the sinking of the floor of the acetabulum, causing the femoral head to protrude. It limits hip movement and is of unknown etiology. *Synonym(s): Otto's pelvis.*

✓5ᵗʰ **M24.8 Other specific joint derangements, not elsewhere classified**
    EXCLUDES 2   iliotibial band syndrome (M76.3)

M24.80 Other specific joint derangements of unspecified joint, not elsewhere classified

✓6ᵗʰ **M24.81 Other specific joint derangements of shoulder, not elsewhere classified**
M24.811 Other specific joint derangements of right shoulder, not elsewhere classified
M24.812 Other specific joint derangements of left shoulder, not elsewhere classified
M24.819 Other specific joint derangements of unspecified shoulder, not elsewhere classified

✓6ᵗʰ **M24.82 Other specific joint derangements of elbow, not elsewhere classified**
M24.821 Other specific joint derangements of right elbow, not elsewhere classified
M24.822 Other specific joint derangements of left elbow, not elsewhere classified
M24.829 Other specific joint derangements of unspecified elbow, not elsewhere classified

✓6ᵗʰ **M24.83 Other specific joint derangements of wrist, not elsewhere classified**
M24.831 Other specific joint derangements of right wrist, not elsewhere classified
M24.832 Other specific joint derangements of left wrist, not elsewhere classified
M24.839 Other specific joint derangements of unspecified wrist, not elsewhere classified

✓6ᵗʰ **M24.84 Other specific joint derangements of hand, not elsewhere classified**
M24.841 Other specific joint derangements of right hand, not elsewhere classified
M24.842 Other specific joint derangements of left hand, not elsewhere classified
M24.849 Other specific joint derangements of unspecified hand, not elsewhere classified

✓6ᵗʰ **M24.85 Other specific joint derangements of hip, not elsewhere classified**
Irritable hip
M24.851 Other specific joint derangements of right hip, not elsewhere classified

☑Additional Character Required   ✓7ᵗʰ Placeholder   Unacceptable PDx   Questionable PDx   Manifestation   **H1–H14** HAC   **HCC** CMS-HCC Dx   **HIV** HIV Dx

ICD-10-CM 2019   771

M24.444–M24.851

M24.852 **Other specific joint derangements of** left hip, not elsewhere classified

M24.859 **Other specific joint derangements of** unspecified **hip, not elsewhere classified**

√6ᵗʰ M24.87 **Other specific joint derangements of** ankle and foot, **not elsewhere classified**

M24.871 **Other specific joint derangements of** right ankle, **not elsewhere classified**

M24.872 **Other specific joint derangements of** left ankle, **not elsewhere classified**

M24.873 **Other specific joint derangements of** unspecified ankle, **not elsewhere classified**

M24.874 **Other specific joint derangements of** right foot, **not elsewhere classified**

M24.875 **Other specific joint derangements** left foot, **not elsewhere classified**

M24.876 **Other specific joint derangements of** unspecified foot, **not elsewhere classified**

M24.9 **Joint derangement,** unspecified

√4ᵗʰ **M25 Other joint disorder, not elsewhere classified**

EXCLUDES 2　*abnormality of gait and mobility (R26.-)*
acquired deformities of limb (M20-M21)
calcification of bursa (M71.4-)
calcification of shoulder (joint) (M75.3)
calcification of tendon (M65.2-)
difficulty in walking (R26.2)
temporomandibular joint disorder (M26.6-)

√5ᵗʰ **M25.0 Hemarthrosis**

EXCLUDES 1　*current injury—see injury of joint by body region*
hemophilic arthropathy (M36.2)

M25.00 **Hemarthrosis,** unspecified joint　　CC
　　CC Excl: PDX collection 868

√6ᵗʰ M25.01 **Hemarthrosis,** shoulder

　　CC Excl: For CC codes in subcategory M25.01:
　　PDX collection 869

M25.011 **Hemarthrosis,** right shoulder　CC
M25.012 **Hemarthrosis,** left shoulder　CC
M25.019 **Hemarthrosis,** unspecified shoulder　CC

√6ᵗʰ M25.02 **Hemarthrosis,** elbow

　　CC Excl: For CC codes in subcategory M25.02:
　　PDX collection 870

M25.021 **Hemarthrosis,** right elbow　CC
M25.022 **Hemarthrosis,** left elbow　CC
M25.029 **Hemarthrosis,** unspecified elbow　CC

√6ᵗʰ M25.03 **Hemarthrosis,** wrist

　　CC Excl: For CC codes in subcategory M25.03:
　　PDX collection 871

M25.031 **Hemarthrosis,** right wrist　CC
M25.032 **Hemarthrosis,** left wrist　CC
M25.039 **Hemarthrosis,** unspecified wrist　CC

√6ᵗʰ M25.04 **Hemarthrosis,** hand

　　CC Excl: For CC codes in subcategory M25.04:
　　PDX collection 872

M25.041 **Hemarthrosis,** right hand　CC
M25.042 **Hemarthrosis,** left hand　CC
M25.049 **Hemarthrosis,** unspecified hand　CC

√6ᵗʰ M25.05 **Hemarthrosis,** hip

　　CC Excl: For CC codes in subcategory M25.05:
　　PDX collection 868

M25.051 **Hemarthrosis,** right hip　CC
M25.052 **Hemarthrosis,** left hip　CC
M25.059 **Hemarthrosis,** unspecified hip　CC

√6ᵗʰ M25.06 **Hemarthrosis,** knee

　　CC Excl: For CC codes in subcategory M25.06:
　　PDX collection 873

M25.061 **Hemarthrosis,** right knee　CC
M25.062 **Hemarthrosis,** left knee　CC
M25.069 **Hemarthrosis,** unspecified knee　CC

√6ᵗʰ M25.07 **Hemarthrosis,** ankle and foot

　　CC Excl: For CC codes in subcategory M25.07:
　　PDX collection 873

M25.071 **Hemarthrosis,** right ankle　CC
M25.072 **Hemarthrosis,** left ankle　CC
M25.073 **Hemarthrosis,** unspecified ankle　CC
M25.074 **Hemarthrosis,** right foot　CC
M25.075 **Hemarthrosis,** left foot　CC
M25.076 **Hemarthrosis,** unspecified foot　CC

M25.08 **Hemarthrosis,** other specified site　CC
　　Hemarthrosis, vertebrae
　　CC Excl: PDX collection 868

√5ᵗʰ **M25.1 Fistula of joint**

M25.10 **Fistula,** unspecified joint　SW

√6ᵗʰ M25.11 **Fistula,** shoulder

M25.111 **Fistula,** right shoulder　SW
M25.112 **Fistula,** left shoulder　SW
M25.119 **Fistula,** unspecified shoulder　SW

√6ᵗʰ M25.12 **Fistula,** elbow

M25.121 **Fistula,** right elbow　SW
M25.122 **Fistula,** left elbow　SW
M25.129 **Fistula,** unspecified elbow　SW

√6ᵗʰ M25.13 **Fistula,** wrist

M25.131 **Fistula,** right wrist　SW
M25.132 **Fistula,** left wrist　SW
M25.139 **Fistula,** unspecified wrist　SW

√6ᵗʰ M25.14 **Fistula,** hand

M25.141 **Fistula,** right hand　SW
M25.142 **Fistula,** left hand　SW
M25.149 **Fistula,** unspecified hand　SW

√6ᵗʰ M25.15 **Fistula,** hip

M25.151 **Fistula,** right hip　SW
M25.152 **Fistula,** left hip　SW
M25.159 **Fistula,** unspecified hip　SW

√6ᵗʰ M25.16 **Fistula,** knee

M25.161 **Fistula,** right knee　SW
M25.162 **Fistula,** left knee　SW
M25.169 **Fistula,** unspecified knee　SW

√6ᵗʰ M25.17 **Fistula,** ankle and foot

M25.171 **Fistula,** right ankle　SW
M25.172 **Fistula,** left ankle　SW
M25.173 **Fistula,** unspecified ankle　SW
M25.174 **Fistula,** right foot　SW
M25.175 **Fistula,** left foot　SW
M25.176 **Fistula,** unspecified foot　SW

M25.18 **Fistula,** other specified site　SW
　　Fistula, vertebrae

√5ᵗʰ **M25.2 Flail joint**

DEF: Hinged joint that exhibits an abnormal or excessive degree of range and mobility.

M25.20 **Flail joint,** unspecified joint

√6ᵗʰ M25.21 **Flail joint,** shoulder

M25.211 **Flail joint,** right shoulder
M25.212 **Flail joint,** left shoulder
M25.219 **Flail joint,** unspecified shoulder

√6ᵗʰ M25.22 **Flail joint,** elbow

M25.221 **Flail joint,** right elbow
M25.222 **Flail joint,** left elbow
M25.229 **Flail joint,** unspecified elbow

√6ᵗʰ M25.23 **Flail joint,** wrist

M25.231 **Flail joint,** right wrist
M25.232 **Flail joint,** left wrist
M25.239 **Flail joint,** unspecified wrist

√6ᵗʰ M25.24 **Flail joint,** hand

M25.241 **Flail joint,** right hand
M25.242 **Flail joint,** left hand
M25.249 **Flail joint,** unspecified hand

√6ᵗʰ M25.25 **Flail joint,** hip

M25.251 **Flail joint,** right hip
M25.252 **Flail joint,** left hip
M25.259 **Flail joint,** unspecified hip

N Newborn: 0　　P Pediatric: 0-17　　M Maternity: 12-55　　A Adult: 15-124　　MCC Major Complication/Comorbidity　　CC Complication/Comorbidity　　SW Severe Wound Dx

772

ICD-10-CM 2019

√6ᵗʰ **M25.26 Flail joint,** knee
    M25.261 Flail joint, right **knee**
    M25.262 Flail joint, left **knee**
    M25.269 Flail joint, unspecified **knee**

√6ᵗʰ **M25.27 Flail joint,** ankle and foot
    M25.271 Flail joint, right **ankle and foot**
    M25.272 Flail joint, left **ankle and foot**
    M25.279 Flail joint, unspecified **ankle and foot**

M25.28 Flail joint, other site

√5ᵗʰ **M25.3 Other instability of joint**
    EXCLUDES 1   *instability of joint secondary to old ligament injury (M24.2-)*
            instability of joint secondary to removal of joint prosthesis (M96.8-)
    EXCLUDES 2   *spinal instabilities (M53.2-)*

M25.30 Other instability, unspecified **joint**

√6ᵗʰ **M25.31 Other instability,** shoulder
    M25.311 Other instability, right **shoulder**
    M25.312 Other instability, left **shoulder**
    M25.319 Other instability, unspecified **shoulder**

√6ᵗʰ **M25.32 Other instability,** elbow
    M25.321 Other instability, right **elbow**
    M25.322 Other instability, left **elbow**
    M25.329 Other instability, unspecified **elbow**

√6ᵗʰ **M25.33 Other instability,** wrist
    M25.331 Other instability, right **wrist**
    M25.332 Other instability, left **wrist**
    M25.339 Other instability, unspecified **wrist**

√6ᵗʰ **M25.34 Other instability,** hand
    M25.341 Other instability, right **hand**
    M25.342 Other instability, left **hand**
    M25.349 Other instability, unspecified **hand**

√6ᵗʰ **M25.35 Other instability,** hip
    M25.351 Other instability, right **hip**
    M25.352 Other instability, left **hip**
    M25.359 Other instability, unspecified **hip**

√6ᵗʰ **M25.36 Other instability,** knee
    M25.361 Other instability, right **knee**
    M25.362 Other instability, left **knee**
    M25.369 Other instability, unspecified **knee**

√6ᵗʰ **M25.37 Other instability,** ankle and foot
    M25.371 Other instability, right **ankle**
    M25.372 Other instability, left **ankle**
    M25.373 Other instability, unspecified **ankle**
    M25.374 Other instability, right **foot**
    M25.375 Other instability, left **foot**
    M25.376 Other instability, unspecified **foot**

√5ᵗʰ **M25.4 Effusion of joint**
    EXCLUDES 1   *hydrarthrosis in yaws (A66.6)*
            intermittent hydrarthrosis (M12.4-)
            other infective (teno)synovitis (M65.1-)

M25.40 Effusion, unspecified **joint**

√6ᵗʰ **M25.41 Effusion,** shoulder
    M25.411 Effusion, right **shoulder**
    M25.412 Effusion, left **shoulder**
    M25.419 Effusion, unspecified **shoulder**

√6ᵗʰ **M25.42 Effusion,** elbow
    M25.421 Effusion, right **elbow**
    M25.422 Effusion, left **elbow**
    M25.429 Effusion, unspecified **elbow**

√6ᵗʰ **M25.43 Effusion,** wrist
    M25.431 Effusion, right **wrist**
    M25.432 Effusion, left **wrist**
    M25.439 Effusion, unspecified **wrist**

√6ᵗʰ **M25.44 Effusion,** hand
    M25.441 Effusion, right **hand**
    M25.442 Effusion, left **hand**
    M25.449 Effusion, unspecified **hand**

√6ᵗʰ **M25.45 Effusion,** hip
    M25.451 Effusion, right **hip**
    M25.452 Effusion, left **hip**
    M25.459 Effusion, unspecified **hip**

√6ᵗʰ **M25.46 Effusion,** knee
    M25.461 Effusion, right **knee**
    M25.462 Effusion, left **knee**
    M25.469 Effusion, unspecified **knee**

√6ᵗʰ **M25.47 Effusion,** ankle and foot
    M25.471 Effusion, right **ankle**
    M25.472 Effusion, left **ankle**
    M25.473 Effusion, unspecified **ankle**
    M25.474 Effusion, right **foot**
    M25.475 Effusion, left **foot**
    M25.476 Effusion, unspecified **foot**

M25.48 Effusion, other site

√5ᵗʰ **M25.5 Pain in joint**
    EXCLUDES 2   *pain in hand (M79.64-)*
            pain in fingers (M79.64-)
            pain in foot (M79.67-)
            pain in limb (M79.6-)
            pain in toes (M79.67-)

M25.50 Pain in unspecified **joint**

√6ᵗʰ **M25.51 Pain in** shoulder
    M25.511 Pain in right **shoulder**
    M25.512 Pain in left **shoulder**
    M25.519 Pain in unspecified **shoulder**

√6ᵗʰ **M25.52 Pain in** elbow
    M25.521 Pain in right **elbow**
    M25.522 Pain in left **elbow**
    M25.529 Pain in unspecified **elbow**

√6ᵗʰ **M25.53 Pain in** wrist
    M25.531 Pain in right **wrist**
    M25.532 Pain in left **wrist**
    M25.539 Pain in unspecified **wrist**

√6ᵗʰ **M25.54 Pain in** joints of hand
    AHA: 2016, 4Q, 38
    M25.541 Pain in joints of right **hand**
    M25.542 Pain in joints of left **hand**
    M25.549 Pain in joints of unspecified **hand**
            Pain in joints of hand NOS

√6ᵗʰ **M25.55 Pain in** hip
    M25.551 Pain in right **hip**
    M25.552 Pain in left **hip**
    M25.559 Pain in unspecified **hip**

√6ᵗʰ **M25.56 Pain in** knee
    M25.561 Pain in right **knee**
    M25.562 Pain in left **knee**
    M25.569 Pain in unspecified **knee**

√6ᵗʰ **M25.57 Pain in** ankle and joints of foot
    M25.571 Pain in right **ankle and joints of right foot**
    M25.572 Pain in left **ankle and joints of left foot**
    M25.579 Pain in unspecified **ankle and joints of unspecified foot**

√5ᵗʰ **M25.6 Stiffness of joint, not elsewhere classified**
    EXCLUDES 1   *ankylosis of joint (M24.6-)*
            contracture of joint (M24.5-)

M25.60 Stiffness of unspecified **joint, not elsewhere classified**

√6ᵗʰ **M25.61 Stiffness of** shoulder, **not elsewhere classified**
    M25.611 Stiffness of right **shoulder, not elsewhere classified**
    M25.612 Stiffness of left **shoulder, not elsewhere classified**
    M25.619 Stiffness of unspecified **shoulder, not elsewhere classified**

√6ᵗʰ **M25.62 Stiffness of** elbow, **not elsewhere classified**
    M25.621 Stiffness of right **elbow, not elsewhere classified**
    M25.622 Stiffness of left **elbow, not elsewhere classified**
    M25.629 Stiffness of unspecified **elbow, not elsewhere classified**

√6ᵗʰ **M25.63 Stiffness of** wrist, **not elsewhere classified**
    M25.631 Stiffness of right **wrist, not elsewhere classified**
    M25.632 Stiffness of left **wrist, not elsewhere classified**

✓ Additional Character Required   √x7ᵗʰ Placeholder   Unacceptable PDx   Questionable PDx   Manifestation   H1 - H14 HAC   HCC CMS-HCC Dx   HIV HIV Dx

ICD-10-CM 2019   773

M25.639   Stiffness of unspecified wrist, not elsewhere classified

✓6th M25.64   Stiffness of hand, not elsewhere classified
- M25.641   Stiffness of right hand, not elsewhere classified
- M25.642   Stiffness of left hand, not elsewhere classified
- M25.649   Stiffness of unspecified hand, not elsewhere classified

✓6th M25.65   Stiffness of hip, not elsewhere classified
- M25.651   Stiffness of right hip, not elsewhere classified
- M25.652   Stiffness of left hip, not elsewhere classified
- M25.659   Stiffness of unspecified hip, not elsewhere classified

✓6th M25.66   Stiffness of knee, not elsewhere classified
- M25.661   Stiffness of right knee, not elsewhere classified
- M25.662   Stiffness of left knee, not elsewhere classified
- M25.669   Stiffness of unspecified knee, not elsewhere classified

✓6th M25.67   Stiffness of ankle and foot, not elsewhere classified
- M25.671   Stiffness of right ankle, not elsewhere classified
- M25.672   Stiffness of left ankle, not elsewhere classified
- M25.673   Stiffness of unspecified ankle, not elsewhere classified
- M25.674   Stiffness of right foot, not elsewhere classified
- M25.675   Stiffness of left foot, not elsewhere classified
- M25.676   Stiffness of unspecified foot, not elsewhere classified

✓5th M25.7   Osteophyte
- M25.70   Osteophyte, unspecified joint

✓6th M25.71   Osteophyte, shoulder
- M25.711   Osteophyte, right shoulder
- M25.712   Osteophyte, left shoulder
- M25.719   Osteophyte, unspecified shoulder

✓6th M25.72   Osteophyte, elbow
- M25.721   Osteophyte, right elbow
- M25.722   Osteophyte, left elbow
- M25.729   Osteophyte, unspecified elbow

✓6th M25.73   Osteophyte, wrist
- M25.731   Osteophyte, right wrist
- M25.732   Osteophyte, left wrist
- M25.739   Osteophyte, unspecified wrist

✓6th M25.74   Osteophyte, hand
- M25.741   Osteophyte, right hand
- M25.742   Osteophyte, left hand
- M25.749   Osteophyte, unspecified hand

✓6th M25.75   Osteophyte, hip
- M25.751   Osteophyte, right hip
- M25.752   Osteophyte, left hip
- M25.759   Osteophyte, unspecified hip

✓6th M25.76   Osteophyte, knee
- M25.761   Osteophyte, right knee
- M25.762   Osteophyte, left knee
- M25.769   Osteophyte, unspecified knee

✓6th M25.77   Osteophyte, ankle and foot
- M25.771   Osteophyte, right ankle
- M25.772   Osteophyte, left ankle
- M25.773   Osteophyte, unspecified ankle
- M25.774   Osteophyte, right foot
- M25.775   Osteophyte, left foot
- M25.776   Osteophyte, unspecified foot
- M25.78   Osteophyte, vertebrae

✓5th M25.8   Other specified joint disorders
- M25.80   Other specified joint disorders, unspecified joint

✓6th M25.81   Other specified joint disorders, shoulder
- M25.811   Other specified joint disorders, right shoulder
- M25.812   Other specified joint disorders, left shoulder
- M25.819   Other specified joint disorders, unspecified shoulder

✓6th M25.82   Other specified joint disorders, elbow
- M25.821   Other specified joint disorders, right elbow
- M25.822   Other specified joint disorders, left elbow
- M25.829   Other specified joint disorders, unspecified elbow

✓6th M25.83   Other specified joint disorders, wrist
- M25.831   Other specified joint disorders, right wrist
- M25.832   Other specified joint disorders, left wrist
- M25.839   Other specified joint disorders, unspecified wrist

✓6th M25.84   Other specified joint disorders, hand
- M25.841   Other specified joint disorders, right hand
- M25.842   Other specified joint disorders, left hand
- M25.849   Other specified joint disorders, unspecified hand

✓6th M25.85   Other specified joint disorders, hip
   AHA: 2014, 4Q, 25
- M25.851   Other specified joint disorders, right hip
- M25.852   Other specified joint disorders, left hip
- M25.859   Other specified joint disorders, unspecified hip

✓6th M25.86   Other specified joint disorders, knee
- M25.861   Other specified joint disorders, right knee
- M25.862   Other specified joint disorders, left knee
- M25.869   Other specified joint disorders, unspecified knee

✓6th M25.87   Other specified joint disorders, ankle and foot
- M25.871   Other specified joint disorders, right ankle and foot
- M25.872   Other specified joint disorders, left ankle and foot
- M25.879   Other specified joint disorders, unspecified ankle and foot

M25.9   Joint disorder, unspecified

Dentofacial anomalies [including malocclusion] and other disorders of jaw (M26-M27)

EXCLUDES 1   hemifacial atrophy or hypertrophy (Q67.4)
unilateral condylar hyperplasia or hypoplasia (M27.8)

✓4th M26   Dentofacial anomalies [including malocclusion]

✓5th M26.0   Major anomalies of jaw size
   EXCLUDES 1   acromegaly (E22.0)
   Robin's syndrome (Q87.0)
- M26.00   Unspecified anomaly of jaw size
- M26.01   Maxillary hyperplasia
- M26.02   Maxillary hypoplasia
   AHA: 2014, 3Q, 23
- M26.03   Mandibular hyperplasia
- M26.04   Mandibular hypoplasia
- M26.05   Macrogenia
- M26.06   Microgenia
- M26.07   Excessive tuberosity of jaw
   Entire maxillary tuberosity
- M26.09   Other specified anomalies of jaw size

✓5th M26.1   Anomalies of jaw-cranial base relationship
- M26.10   Unspecified anomaly of jaw-cranial base relationship
- M26.11   Maxillary asymmetry
- M26.12   Other jaw asymmetry
- M26.19   Other specified anomalies of jaw-cranial base relationship

✓5th M26.2   Anomalies of dental arch relationship
- M26.20   Unspecified anomaly of dental arch relationship

✓6th M26.21   Malocclusion, Angle's class
- M26.211   Malocclusion, Angle's class I
   Neutro-occlusion

N Newborn: 0   P Pediatric: 0-17   M Maternity: 12-55   A Adult: 15-124   MCC Major Complication/Comorbidity   CC Complication/Comorbidity   SW Severe Wound Dx

774   ICD-10-CM 2019

M26.212　**Malocclusion, Angle's class II**
Disto-occlusion Division I
Disto-occlusion Division II

M26.213　**Malocclusion, Angle's class III**
Mesio-occlusion

M26.219　**Malocclusion, Angle's class, unspecified**

✓6th M26.22　**Open occlusal relationship**

M26.220　**Open anterior occlusal relationship**
►Anterior open bite◄

M26.221　**Open posterior occlusal relationship**
►Posterior open bite◄

M26.23　**Excessive horizontal overlap**
Excessive horizontal overjet

M26.24　**Reverse articulation**
Crossbite (anterior) (posterior)

M26.25　**Anomalies of interarch distance**

M26.29　**Other anomalies of dental arch relationship**
Midline deviation of dental arch
Overbite (excessive) deep
Overbite (excessive) horizontal
Overbite (excessive) vertical
Posterior lingual occlusion of mandibular teeth

✓5th M26.3　**Anomalies of tooth position of fully erupted tooth or teeth**
EXCLUDES 2　embedded and impacted teeth (K01.-)

M26.30　**Unspecified anomaly of tooth position of fully erupted tooth or teeth**
Abnormal spacing of fully erupted tooth or teeth NOS
Displacement of fully erupted tooth or teeth NOS
Transposition of fully erupted tooth or teeth NOS

M26.31　**Crowding of fully erupted teeth**

M26.32　**Excessive spacing of fully erupted teeth**
Diastema of fully erupted tooth or teeth NOS

M26.33　**Horizontal displacement of fully erupted tooth or teeth**
Tipped tooth or teeth
Tipping of fully erupted tooth

M26.34　**Vertical displacement of fully erupted tooth or teeth**
Extruded tooth
Infraeruption of tooth or teeth
Supraeruption of tooth or teeth

M26.35　**Rotation of fully erupted tooth or teeth**

M26.36　**Insufficient interocclusal distance of fully erupted teeth (ridge)**
Lack of adequate intermaxillary vertical dimension of fully erupted teeth

M26.37　**Excessive interocclusal distance of fully erupted teeth**
Excessive intermaxillary vertical dimension of fully erupted teeth
Loss of occlusal vertical dimension of fully erupted teeth

M26.39　**Other anomalies of tooth position of fully erupted tooth or teeth**

M26.4　**Malocclusion, unspecified**

✓5th M26.5　**Dentofacial functional abnormalities**
EXCLUDES 1　bruxism (F45.8)
teeth-grinding NOS (F45.8)

M26.50　**Dentofacial functional abnormalities, unspecified**

M26.51　**Abnormal jaw closure**

M26.52　**Limited mandibular range of motion**

M26.53　**Deviation in opening and closing of the mandible**

M26.54　**Insufficient anterior guidance**
Insufficient anterior occlusal guidance

M26.55　**Centric occlusion maximum intercuspation discrepancy**
EXCLUDES 1　centric occlusion NOS (M26.59)

M26.56　**Non-working side interference**
Balancing side interference

M26.57　**Lack of posterior occlusal support**

M26.59　**Other dentofacial functional abnormalities**
Centric occlusion (of teeth) NOS
Malocclusion due to abnormal swallowing
Malocclusion due to mouth breathing
Malocclusion due to tongue, lip or finger habits

Temporomandibular Joint

Cutaway detail　　Upper joint space

Articular disc (meniscus)　　Lower joint space

Condyle

Mandible　　Cutaway view of temporomandibular joint (TMJ)

✓5th M26.6　**Temporomandibular joint disorders**
EXCLUDES 2　current temporomandibular joint dislocation (S03.0)
current temporomandibular joint sprain (S03.4)
AHA: 2016, 4Q, 38-39

✓6th M26.60　**Temporomandibular joint disorder, unspecified**

M26.601　**Right temporomandibular joint disorder, unspecified**

M26.602　**Left temporomandibular joint disorder, unspecified**

M26.603　**Bilateral temporomandibular joint disorder, unspecified**

M26.609　**Unspecified temporomandibular joint disorder, unspecified side**
Temporomandibular joint disorder NOS

✓6th M26.61　**Adhesions and ankylosis of temporomandibular joint**

M26.611　**Adhesions and ankylosis of right temporomandibular joint**

M26.612　**Adhesions and ankylosis of left temporomandibular joint**

M26.613　**Adhesions and ankylosis of bilateral temporomandibular joint**

M26.619　**Adhesions and ankylosis of temporomandibular joint, unspecified side**

✓6th M26.62　**Arthralgia of temporomandibular joint**

M26.621　**Arthralgia of right temporomandibular joint**

M26.622　**Arthralgia of left temporomandibular joint**

M26.623　**Arthralgia of bilateral temporomandibular joint**

M26.629　**Arthralgia of temporomandibular joint, unspecified side**

✓6th M26.63　**Articular disc disorder of temporomandibular joint**

M26.631　**Articular disc disorder of right temporomandibular joint**

M26.632　**Articular disc disorder of left temporomandibular joint**

M26.633　**Articular disc disorder of bilateral temporomandibular joint**

M26.639　**Articular disc disorder of temporomandibular joint, unspecified side**

M26.69　**Other specified disorders of temporomandibular joint**

✓5th M26.7　**Dental alveolar anomalies**

M26.70　**Unspecified alveolar anomaly**

M26.71　**Alveolar maxillary hyperplasia**

M26.72　**Alveolar mandibular hyperplasia**

M26.73　**Alveolar maxillary hypoplasia**

M26.74　**Alveolar mandibular hypoplasia**

M26.79　**Other specified alveolar anomalies**

✓5th M26.8　**Other dentofacial anomalies**

M26.81　**Anterior soft tissue impingement**
Anterior soft tissue impingement on teeth

M26.82　**Posterior soft tissue impingement**
Posterior soft tissue impingement on teeth

M26.89　**Other dentofacial anomalies**

M26.9　**Dentofacial anomaly, unspecified**

✓ Additional Character Required　　✓x7th Placeholder　　Unacceptable PDx　　Questionable PDx　　Manifestation　　**H1**-**H14** HAC　　**HCC** CMS-HCC Dx　　**HIV** HIV Dx

ICD-10-CM 2019　　　　**775**

✓4ᵗʰ **M27 Other diseases of jaws**

    M27.0 Developmental disorders of jaws
        Latent bone cyst of jaw
        Stafne's cyst
        Torus mandibularis
        Torus palatinus

    M27.1 Giant cell granuloma, central
        Giant cell granuloma NOS
        EXCLUDES 1   *peripheral giant cell granuloma (K06.8)*

    M27.2 Inflammatory conditions of jaws
        Osteitis of jaw(s)
        Osteomyelitis (neonatal) jaw(s)
        Osteoradionecrosis jaw(s)
        Periostitis jaw(s)
        Sequestrum of jaw bone
        Use additional code (W88-W90, X39.0) to identify radiation, if radiation-induced
        EXCLUDES 2   *osteonecrosis of jaw due to drug (M87.180)*

    M27.3 Alveolitis of jaws
        Alveolar osteitis
        Dry socket

✓5ᵗʰ   **M27.4 Other and unspecified cysts of jaw**
        EXCLUDES 1   *cysts of oral region (K09.-)*
                     latent bone cyst of jaw (M27.0)
                     Stafne's cyst (M27.0)

        M27.40 Unspecified cyst of jaw
            Cyst of jaw NOS

        M27.49 Other cysts of jaw
            Aneurysmal cyst of jaw
            Hemorrhagic cyst of jaw
            Traumatic cyst of jaw

✓5ᵗʰ   **M27.5 Periradicular pathology associated with previous endodontic treatment**
        M27.51 Perforation of root canal space due to endodontic treatment
        M27.52 Endodontic overfill
        M27.53 Endodontic underfill
        M27.59 Other periradicular pathology associated with previous endodontic treatment

✓5ᵗʰ   **M27.6 Endosseous dental implant failure**
        M27.61 Osseointegration failure of dental implant
            Hemorrhagic complications of dental implant placement
            Iatrogenic osseointegration failure of dental implant
            Osseointegration failure of dental implant due to complications of systemic disease
            Osseointegration failure of dental implant due to poor bone quality
            Pre-integration failure of dental implant NOS
            Pre-osseointegration failure of dental implant

        M27.62 Post-osseointegration biological failure of dental implant
            Failure of dental implant due to lack of attached gingiva
            Failure of dental implant due to occlusal trauma (caused by poor prosthetic design)
            Failure of dental implant due to parafunctional habits
            Failure of dental implant due to periodontal infection (peri-implantitis)
            Failure of dental implant due to poor oral hygiene
            Iatrogenic post-osseointegration failure of dental implant
            Post-osseointegration failure of dental implant due to complications of systemic disease

        M27.63 Post-osseointegration mechanical failure of dental implant
            Failure of dental prosthesis causing loss of dental implant
            Fracture of dental implant
            EXCLUDES 2   *cracked tooth (K03.81)*
                         fractured dental restorative material with loss of material (K08.531)
                         fractured dental restorative material without loss of material (K08.530)
                         fractured tooth (S02.5)

        M27.69 Other endosseous dental implant failure
            Dental implant failure NOS

    M27.8 Other specified diseases of jaws
        Cherubism
        Exostosis
        Fibrous dysplasia
        Unilateral condylar hyperplasia
        Unilateral condylar hypoplasia
        EXCLUDES 1   *jaw pain (R68.84)*

    M27.9 Disease of jaws, unspecified

Systemic connective tissue disorders (M30-M36)

INCLUDES   autoimmune disease NOS
             collagen (vascular) disease NOS
             systemic autoimmune disease
             systemic collagen (vascular) disease
EXCLUDES 1   *autoimmune disease, single organ or single cell-type—code to relevant condition category*

✓4ᵗʰ **M30 Polyarteritis nodosa and related conditions**
    EXCLUDES 1   *microscopic polyarteritis (M31.7)*

    CC Excl: For CC codes in category M30, unless otherwise noted: PDX collection 874

    M30.0 Polyarteritis nodosa   CC HCC

    M30.1 Polyarteritis with lung involvement [Churg-Strauss]   CC HCC
        Allergic granulomatous angiitis

    M30.2 Juvenile polyarteritis   CC HCC

    M30.3 Mucocutaneous lymph node syndrome [Kawasaki]   CC HCC
        CC Excl: PDX collection 875

    M30.8 Other conditions related to polyarteritis nodosa   CC HCC
        Polyangiitis overlap syndrome

✓4ᵗʰ **M31 Other necrotizing vasculopathies**

    CC Excl: For CC/MCC codes in category M31, unless otherwise noted: PDX collection 874

    M31.0 Hypersensitivity angiitis   CC HCC
        Goodpasture's syndrome

    M31.1 Thrombotic microangiopathy   MCC HCC
        Thrombotic thrombocytopenic purpura

    M31.2 Lethal midline granuloma   CC HCC

✓5ᵗʰ   **M31.3 Wegener's granulomatosis**
        Necrotizing respiratory granulomatosis

        M31.30 Wegener's granulomatosis without renal involvement   CC HCC
            Wegener's granulomatosis NOS

        M31.31 Wegener's granulomatosis with renal involvement   CC HCC

    M31.4 Aortic arch syndrome [Takayasu]   CC HCC

    M31.5 Giant cell arteritis with polymyalgia rheumatica   HCC

    M31.6 Other giant cell arteritis   HCC

    M31.7 Microscopic polyangiitis   CC HCC
        Microscopic polyarteritis
        EXCLUDES 1   *polyarteritis nodosa (M30.0)*

    M31.8 Other specified necrotizing vasculopathies   CC HCC
        Hypocomplementemic vasculitis
        Septic vasculitis
        CC Excl: PDX collection 712

    M31.9 Necrotizing vasculopathy, unspecified   CC HCC
        CC Excl: PDX collection 712

✓4ᵗʰ **M32 Systemic lupus erythematosus (SLE)**
    EXCLUDES 1   *lupus erythematosus (discoid) (NOS) (L93.0)*

    M32.0 Drug-induced systemic lupus erythematosus   HCC
        Use additional code for adverse effect, if applicable, to identify drug (T36-T50 with fifth or sixth character 5)

✓5ᵗʰ   **M32.1 Systemic lupus erythematosus with organ or system involvement**

        M32.10 Systemic lupus erythematosus, organ or system involvement unspecified   HCC

        M32.11 Endocarditis in systemic lupus erythematosus   CC HCC
            Libman-Sacks disease
            CC Excl: PDX collection 676

        M32.12 Pericarditis in systemic lupus erythematosus   CC HCC
            Lupus pericarditis
            CC Excl: PDX collection 673

        M32.13 Lung involvement in systemic lupus erythematosus   HCC
            Pleural effusion due to systemic lupus erythematosus

N Newborn: 0   P Pediatric: 0-17   M Maternity: 12-55   A Adult: 15-124   MCC Major Complication/Comorbidity   CC Complication/Comorbidity   SW Severe Wound Dx

776   ICD-10-CM 2019

M32.14 Glomerular disease in systemic lupus erythematosus   `HCC`
     Lupus renal disease NOS
     AHA: 2013, 4Q, 125

M32.15 Tubulo-interstitial nephropathy in systemic lupus erythematosus   `HCC`

M32.19 Other organ or system involvement in systemic lupus erythematosus   `HCC`

M32.8 Other forms of systemic lupus erythematosus   `HCC`

M32.9 Systemic lupus erythematosus, unspecified   `HCC`
     SLE NOS
     Systemic lupus erythematosus NOS
     Systemic lupus erythematosus without organ involvement

✓4th **M33 Dermatopolymyositis**
     AHA: 2017, 4Q, 18

> **CC Excl: For CC codes in category M33, unless otherwise noted:** PDX collection 876

✓5th **M33.0** Juvenile dermatomyositis

M33.00 Juvenile dermatomyositis, organ involvement unspecified   `CC` `HCC`

M33.01 Juvenile dermatomyositis with respiratory involvement   `CC` `HCC`

M33.02 Juvenile dermatomyositis with myopathy   `CC` `HCC`
     CC Excl: PDX collection 877

M33.03 Juvenile dermatomyositis without myopathy   `CC` `HCC`

M33.09 Juvenile dermatomyositis with other organ involvement   `CC` `HCC`

✓5th **M33.1** Other dermatomyositis
     Adult dermatomyositis

M33.10 Other dermatomyositis, organ involvement unspecified   `CC` `HCC`

M33.11 Other dermatomyositis with respiratory involvement   `CC` `HCC`

M33.12 Other dermatomyositis with myopathy   `CC` `HCC`
     CC Excl: PDX collection 877

M33.13 Other dermatomyositis without myopathy   `CC` `HCC`
     Dermatomyositis NOS

M33.19 Other dermatomyositis with other organ involvement   `CC` `HCC`

✓5th **M33.2** Polymyositis

> **CC Excl: For CC codes in subcategory M33.2, unless otherwise noted:** PDX collection 878

M33.20 Polymyositis, organ involvement unspecified   `CC` `HCC`

M33.21 Polymyositis with respiratory involvement   `CC` `HCC`

M33.22 Polymyositis with myopathy   `CC` `HCC`
     CC Excl: PDX collection 879

M33.29 Polymyositis with other organ involvement   `CC` `HCC`

✓5th **M33.9** Dermatopolymyositis, unspecified

M33.90 Dermatopolymyositis, unspecified, organ involvement unspecified   `CC` `HCC`

M33.91 Dermatopolymyositis, unspecified with respiratory involvement   `CC` `HCC`

M33.92 Dermatopolymyositis, unspecified with myopathy   `CC` `HCC`
     CC Excl: PDX collection 877

M33.93 Dermatopolymyositis, unspecified without myopathy   `CC` `HCC`

M33.99 Dermatopolymyositis, unspecified with other organ involvement   `CC` `HCC`

✓4th **M34 Systemic sclerosis [scleroderma]**
     EXCLUDES 1   circumscribed scleroderma (L94.0)
               neonatal scleroderma (P83.8)

M34.0 Progressive systemic sclerosis   `HCC`

M34.1 CR(E)ST syndrome   `HCC`
     Combination of calcinosis, Raynaud's phenomenon, esophageal dysfunction, sclerodactyly, telangiectasia

M34.2 Systemic sclerosis induced by drug and chemical   `HCC`
     Code first poisoning due to drug or toxin, if applicable (T36-T65 with fifth or sixth character 1-4 or 6)
     Use additional code for adverse effect, if applicable, to identify drug (T36-T50 with fifth or sixth character 5)

✓5th **M34.8** Other forms of systemic sclerosis

M34.81 Systemic sclerosis with lung involvement   `CC` `HCC`
     CC Excl: No excl

M34.82 Systemic sclerosis with myopathy   `CC` `HCC`
     CC Excl: PDX collection 867

M34.83 Systemic sclerosis with polyneuropathy   `HCC`

M34.89 Other systemic sclerosis   `HCC`

M34.9 Systemic sclerosis, unspecified   `HCC`

✓4th **M35 Other systemic involvement of connective tissue**
     EXCLUDES 1   reactive perforating collagenosis (L87.1)

✓5th **M35.0** Sicca syndrome [Sjögren]
     DEF: Autoimmune disease associated with keratoconjunctivitis, laryngopharyngitis, rhinitis, dry mouth, enlarged parotid gland, and chronic polyarthritis.

M35.00 Sicca syndrome, unspecified   `HCC`

M35.01 Sicca syndrome with keratoconjunctivitis   `HCC`

M35.02 Sicca syndrome with lung involvement   `HCC`

M35.03 Sicca syndrome with myopathy   `CC` `HCC`
     CC Excl: PDX collection 867

M35.04 Sicca syndrome with tubulo-interstitial nephropathy   `HCC`
     Renal tubular acidosis in sicca syndrome

M35.09 Sicca syndrome with other organ involvement   `CC` `HCC`

M35.1 Other overlap syndromes
     Mixed connective tissue disease
     EXCLUDES 1   polyangiitis overlap syndrome (M30.8)
     CC Excl: PDX collection 880

M35.2 Behçet's disease   `CC` `HCC`
     CC Excl: PDX collection 863

M35.3 Polymyalgia rheumatica   `HCC`
     EXCLUDES 1   polymyalgia rheumatica with giant cell arteritis (M31.5)

M35.4 Diffuse (eosinophilic) fasciitis

M35.5 Multifocal fibrosclerosis   `CC` `HCC`
     CC Excl: PDX collection 880

M35.6 Relapsing panniculitis [Weber-Christian]
     EXCLUDES 1   lupus panniculitis (L93.2)
               panniculitis NOS (M79.3-)

M35.7 Hypermobility syndrome
     Familial ligamentous laxity
     EXCLUDES 1   Ehlers-Danlos syndrome (Q79.6)
               ligamentous laxity, NOS (M24.2-)

M35.8 Other specified systemic involvement of connective tissue   `CC` `HCC`
     CC Excl: PDX collection 880

M35.9 Systemic involvement of connective tissue, unspecified   `HCC`
     Autoimmune disease (systemic) NOS
     Collagen (vascular) disease NOS

✓4th **M36 Systemic disorders of connective tissue in diseases classified elsewhere**
     EXCLUDES 2   arthropathies in diseases classified elsewhere (M14.-)

M36.0 *Dermato(poly)myositis in neoplastic disease*   `CC` `HCC`
     Code first underlying neoplasm (C00-D49)
     CC Excl: PDX collection 876

M36.1 *Arthropathy in neoplastic disease*
     Code first underlying neoplasm, such as:
         leukemia (C91-C95)
         malignant histiocytosis (C96.A)
         multiple myeloma (C90.0)

M36.2 *Hemophilic arthropathy*
     Hemarthrosis in hemophilic arthropathy
     Code first underlying disease, such as:
         factor VIII deficiency (D66)
             with vascular defect (D68.0)
         factor IX deficiency (D67)
         hemophilia (classical) (D66)
         hemophilia B (D67)
         hemophilia C (D68.1)

M36.3 *Arthropathy in other blood disorders*

M36.4 *Arthropathy in hypersensitivity reactions classified elsewhere*
     Code first underlying disease, such as:
         Henoch (-Schönlein) purpura (D69.0)
         serum sickness (T80.6-)

M36.8 *Systemic disorders of connective tissue in other diseases classified elsewhere*   `HCC`
     Code first underlying disease, such as:
         alkaptonuria (E70.2)
         hypogammaglobulinemia (D80.-)
         ochronosis (E70.2)

✓ Additional Character Required   ✓7th Placeholder   Unacceptable PDx   Questionable PDx   Manifestation   `H1`-`H14` HAC   `HCC` CMS-HCC Dx   `HIV` HIV Dx

ICD-10-CM 2019   **777**

DORSOPATHIES (M40-M54)

Deforming dorsopathies (M40-M43)

✓4th M40 Kyphosis and lordosis
> EXCLUDES 1   *congenital kyphosis and lordosis (Q76.4)*
> *kyphoscoliosis (M41.-)*
> *postprocedural kyphosis and lordosis (M96.-)*

✓5th M40.0 Postural kyphosis
> EXCLUDES 1   *osteochondrosis of spine (M42.-)*
- M40.00 Postural kyphosis, site unspecified
- M40.03 Postural kyphosis, cervicothoracic region
- M40.04 Postural kyphosis, thoracic region
- M40.05 Postural kyphosis, thoracolumbar region

✓5th M40.1 Other secondary kyphosis
- M40.10 Other secondary kyphosis, site unspecified
- M40.12 Other secondary kyphosis, cervical region
- M40.13 Other secondary kyphosis, cervicothoracic region
- M40.14 Other secondary kyphosis, thoracic region
- M40.15 Other secondary kyphosis, thoracolumbar region

✓5th M40.2 Other and unspecified kyphosis
- **✓6th M40.20 Unspecified kyphosis**
  - M40.202 Unspecified kyphosis, cervical region
  - M40.203 Unspecified kyphosis, cervicothoracic region
  - M40.204 Unspecified kyphosis, thoracic region
  - M40.205 Unspecified kyphosis, thoracolumbar region
  - M40.209 Unspecified kyphosis, site unspecified
- **✓6th M40.29 Other kyphosis**
  - M40.292 Other kyphosis, cervical region
  - M40.293 Other kyphosis, cervicothoracic region
  - M40.294 Other kyphosis, thoracic region
  - M40.295 Other kyphosis, thoracolumbar region
  - M40.299 Other kyphosis, site unspecified

✓5th M40.3 Flatback syndrome
- M40.30 Flatback syndrome, site unspecified
- M40.35 Flatback syndrome, thoracolumbar region
- M40.36 Flatback syndrome, lumbar region
- M40.37 Flatback syndrome, lumbosacral region

✓5th M40.4 Postural lordosis
> Acquired lordosis
- M40.40 Postural lordosis, site unspecified
- M40.45 Postural lordosis, thoracolumbar region
- M40.46 Postural lordosis, lumbar region
- M40.47 Postural lordosis, lumbosacral region

✓5th M40.5 Lordosis, unspecified
- M40.50 Lordosis, unspecified, site unspecified
- M40.55 Lordosis, unspecified, thoracolumbar region
- M40.56 Lordosis, unspecified, lumbar region
- M40.57 Lordosis, unspecified, lumbosacral region

✓4th M41 Scoliosis
> INCLUDES   kyphoscoliosis
> EXCLUDES 1   *congenital scoliosis due to bony malformation (Q76.3)*
> *congenital scoliosis NOS (Q67.5)*
> *kyphoscoliotic heart disease (I27.1)*
> *postprocedural scoliosis (M96.-)*
> *postural congenital scoliosis (Q67.5)*

✓5th M41.0 Infantile idiopathic scoliosis
> AHA: 2014, 4Q, 26
- M41.00 Infantile idiopathic scoliosis, site unspecified
- M41.02 Infantile idiopathic scoliosis, cervical region
- M41.03 Infantile idiopathic scoliosis, cervicothoracic region
- M41.04 Infantile idiopathic scoliosis, thoracic region
- M41.05 Infantile idiopathic scoliosis, thoracolumbar region
- M41.06 Infantile idiopathic scoliosis, lumbar region
- M41.07 Infantile idiopathic scoliosis, lumbosacral region
- M41.08 Infantile idiopathic scoliosis, sacral and sacrococcygeal region

✓5th M41.1 Juvenile and adolescent idiopathic scoliosis
- **✓6th M41.11 Juvenile idiopathic scoliosis**
  - AHA: 2014, 4Q, 28
  - M41.112 Juvenile idiopathic scoliosis, cervical region
  - M41.113 Juvenile idiopathic scoliosis, cervicothoracic region
  - M41.114 Juvenile idiopathic scoliosis, thoracic region
  - M41.115 Juvenile idiopathic scoliosis, thoracolumbar region
  - M41.116 Juvenile idiopathic scoliosis, lumbar region
  - M41.117 Juvenile idiopathic scoliosis, lumbosacral region
  - M41.119 Juvenile idiopathic scoliosis, site unspecified
- **✓6th M41.12 Adolescent scoliosis**
  - M41.122 Adolescent idiopathic scoliosis, cervical region
  - M41.123 Adolescent idiopathic scoliosis, cervicothoracic region
  - M41.124 Adolescent idiopathic scoliosis, thoracic region
  - M41.125 Adolescent idiopathic scoliosis, thoracolumbar region
  - M41.126 Adolescent idiopathic scoliosis, lumbar region
  - M41.127 Adolescent idiopathic scoliosis, lumbosacral region
  - M41.129 Adolescent idiopathic scoliosis, site unspecified

Scoliosis

Lateral curvature of spine

Kyphosis and Lordosis

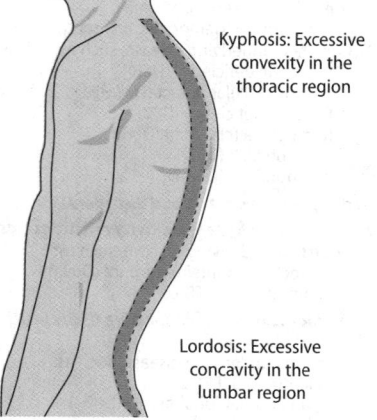

Kyphosis: Excessive convexity in the thoracic region

Lordosis: Excessive concavity in the lumbar region

N Newborn: 0   P Pediatric: 0-17   M Maternity: 12-55   A Adult: 15-124   MCC Major Complication/Comorbidity   CC Complication/Comorbidity   SW Severe Wound Dx

778   ICD-10-CM 2019

✓5ᵗʰ **M41.2** Other idiopathic **scoliosis**
- **M41.20** Other idiopathic scoliosis, site unspecified
- **M41.22** Other idiopathic scoliosis, cervical **region**
- **M41.23** Other idiopathic scoliosis, cervicothoracic **region**
- **M41.24** Other idiopathic scoliosis, thoracic **region**
- **M41.25** Other idiopathic scoliosis, thoracolumbar **region**
- **M41.26** Other idiopathic scoliosis, lumbar **region**
- **M41.27** Other idiopathic scoliosis, lumbosacral **region**

✓5ᵗʰ **M41.3** Thoracogenic **scoliosis**
- **M41.30** Thoracogenic scoliosis, site unspecified
- **M41.34** Thoracogenic scoliosis, thoracic **region**
- **M41.35** Thoracogenic scoliosis, thoracolumbar **region**

✓5ᵗʰ **M41.4** Neuromuscular **scoliosis**
Scoliosis secondary to cerebral palsy, Friedreich's ataxia, poliomyelitis and other neuromuscular disorders
Code also underlying condition
AHA: 2014, 4Q, 27
- **M41.40** Neuromuscular scoliosis, site unspecified
- **M41.41** Neuromuscular scoliosis, occipito-atlanto-axial **region**
- **M41.42** Neuromuscular scoliosis, cervical **region**
- **M41.43** Neuromuscular scoliosis, cervicothoracic **region**
- **M41.44** Neuromuscular scoliosis, thoracic **region**
- **M41.45** Neuromuscular scoliosis, thoracolumbar **region**
- **M41.46** Neuromuscular scoliosis, lumbar **region**
- **M41.47** Neuromuscular scoliosis, lumbosacral **region**

✓5ᵗʰ **M41.5** Other secondary **scoliosis**
- **M41.50** Other secondary scoliosis, site unspecified
- **M41.52** Other secondary scoliosis, cervical **region**
- **M41.53** Other secondary scoliosis, cervicothoracic **region**
- **M41.54** Other secondary scoliosis, thoracic **region**
- **M41.55** Other secondary scoliosis, thoracolumbar **region**
- **M41.56** Other secondary scoliosis, lumbar **region**
- **M41.57** Other secondary scoliosis, lumbosacral **region**

✓5ᵗʰ **M41.8** Other **forms of scoliosis**
- **M41.80** Other forms of scoliosis, site unspecified
- **M41.82** Other forms of scoliosis, cervical **region**
- **M41.83** Other forms of scoliosis, cervicothoracic **region**
- **M41.84** Other forms of scoliosis, thoracic **region**
- **M41.85** Other forms of scoliosis, thoracolumbar **region**
- **M41.86** Other forms of scoliosis, lumbar **region**
- **M41.87** Other forms of scoliosis, lumbosacral **region**

M41.9 Scoliosis, unspecified

✓4ᵗʰ **M42** Spinal osteochondrosis

✓5ᵗʰ **M42.0** Juvenile osteochondrosis of spine
Calvé's disease
Scheuermann's disease
EXCLUDES 1   postural kyphosis (M40.0)
- **M42.00** Juvenile osteochondrosis of spine, site unspecified
- **M42.01** Juvenile osteochondrosis of spine, occipito-atlanto-axial **region**
- **M42.02** Juvenile osteochondrosis of spine, cervical **region**
- **M42.03** Juvenile osteochondrosis of spine, cervicothoracic **region**
- **M42.04** Juvenile osteochondrosis of spine, thoracic **region**
- **M42.05** Juvenile osteochondrosis of spine, thoracolumbar **region**
- **M42.06** Juvenile osteochondrosis of spine, lumbar **region**
- **M42.07** Juvenile osteochondrosis of spine, lumbosacral **region**
- **M42.08** Juvenile osteochondrosis of spine, sacral and sacrococcygeal **region**
- **M42.09** Juvenile osteochondrosis of spine, multiple sites in spine

✓5ᵗʰ **M42.1** Adult osteochondrosis of spine
- **M42.10** Adult osteochondrosis of spine, site unspecified   Ⓐ
- **M42.11** Adult osteochondrosis of spine, occipito-atlanto-axial **region**   Ⓐ
- **M42.12** Adult osteochondrosis of spine, cervical **region**   Ⓐ
- **M42.13** Adult osteochondrosis of spine, cervicothoracic **region**   Ⓐ
- **M42.14** Adult osteochondrosis of spine, thoracic **region**   Ⓐ

- **M42.15** Adult osteochondrosis of spine, thoracolumbar **region**   Ⓐ
- **M42.16** Adult osteochondrosis of spine, lumbar **region**   Ⓐ
- **M42.17** Adult osteochondrosis of spine, lumbosacral **region**   Ⓐ
- **M42.18** Adult osteochondrosis of spine, sacral and sacrococcygeal **region**   Ⓐ
- **M42.19** Adult osteochondrosis of spine, multiple sites in spine   Ⓐ

M42.9 Spinal osteochondrosis, unspecified

✓4ᵗʰ **M43** Other deforming dorsopathies
EXCLUDES 1   congenital spondylolysis and spondylolisthesis (Q76.2)
hemivertebra (Q76.3-Q76.4)
Klippel-Feil syndrome (Q76.1)
lumbarization and sacralization (Q76.4)
platyspondylisis (Q76.4)
spina bifida occulta (Q76.0)
spinal curvature in osteoporosis (M80.-)
spinal curvature in Paget's disease of bone [osteitis deformans] (M88.-)

✓5ᵗʰ **M43.0** Spondylolysis
EXCLUDES 1   congenital spondylolysis (Q76.2)
spondylolisthesis (M43.1)
- **M43.00** Spondylolysis, site unspecified
- **M43.01** Spondylolysis, occipito-atlanto-axial **region**
- **M43.02** Spondylolysis, cervical **region**
- **M43.03** Spondylolysis, cervicothoracic **region**
- **M43.04** Spondylolysis, thoracic **region**
- **M43.05** Spondylolysis, thoracolumbar **region**
- **M43.06** Spondylolysis, lumbar **region**
- **M43.07** Spondylolysis, lumbosacral **region**
- **M43.08** Spondylolysis, sacral and sacrococcygeal **region**
- **M43.09** Spondylolysis, multiple sites in spine

✓5ᵗʰ **M43.1** Spondylolisthesis
EXCLUDES 1   acute traumatic of lumbosacral region (S33.1)
acute traumatic of sites other than lumbosacral— code to Fracture, vertebra, by region
congenital spondylolisthesis (Q76.2)
- **M43.10** Spondylolisthesis, site unspecified
- **M43.11** Spondylolisthesis, occipito-atlanto-axial **region**
- **M43.12** Spondylolisthesis, cervical **region**
- **M43.13** Spondylolisthesis, cervicothoracic **region**
- **M43.14** Spondylolisthesis, thoracic **region**
- **M43.15** Spondylolisthesis, thoracolumbar **region**
- **M43.16** Spondylolisthesis, lumbar **region**
- **M43.17** Spondylolisthesis, lumbosacral **region**
- **M43.18** Spondylolisthesis, sacral and sacrococcygeal **region**
- **M43.19** Spondylolisthesis, multiple sites in spine

✓5ᵗʰ **M43.2** Fusion of spine
Ankylosis of spinal joint
EXCLUDES 1   ankylosing spondylitis (M45.0-)
congenital fusion of spine (Q76.4)
EXCLUDES 2   arthrodesis status (Z98.1)
pseudoarthrosis after fusion or arthrodesis (M96.0)
- **M43.20** Fusion of spine, site unspecified
- **M43.21** Fusion of spine, occipito-atlanto-axial **region**
- **M43.22** Fusion of spine, cervical **region**
- **M43.23** Fusion of spine, cervicothoracic **region**
- **M43.24** Fusion of spine, thoracic **region**
- **M43.25** Fusion of spine, thoracolumbar **region**
- **M43.26** Fusion of spine, lumbar **region**
- **M43.27** Fusion of spine, lumbosacral **region**
- **M43.28** Fusion of spine, sacral and sacrococcygeal **region**

M43.3 Recurrent atlantoaxial dislocation with myelopathy

M43.4 Other recurrent atlantoaxial dislocation

✓5ᵗʰ **M43.5** Other recurrent vertebral dislocation
EXCLUDES 1   biomechanical lesions NEC (M99.-)
- ✓6ᵗʰ **M43.5X** Other recurrent vertebral dislocation
  - **M43.5X2** Other recurrent vertebral dislocation, cervical **region**
  - **M43.5X3** Other recurrent vertebral dislocation, cervicothoracic **region**
  - **M43.5X4** Other recurrent vertebral dislocation, thoracic **region**

M43.5X5 Other recurrent vertebral dislocation, **thoracolumbar region**

M43.5X6 Other recurrent vertebral dislocation, **lumbar region**

M43.5X7 Other recurrent vertebral dislocation, **lumbosacral region**

M43.5X8 Other recurrent vertebral dislocation, **sacral and sacrococcygeal region**

M43.5X9 Other recurrent vertebral dislocation, site unspecified

M43.6 Torticollis

EXCLUDES 1 congenital (sternomastoid) torticollis (Q68.0)
current injury—see Injury, of spine, by body region
ocular torticollis (R29.891)
psychogenic torticollis (F45.8)
spasmodic torticollis (G24.3)
torticollis due to birth injury (P15.2)

DEF: Twisted, unnatural position of the neck due to contracted cervical muscles that pull the head to one side.

✓5th M43.8 Other specified deforming dorsopathies

EXCLUDES 2 kyphosis and lordosis (M40.-)
scoliosis (M41.-)

✓6th M43.8X Other specified deforming dorsopathies

M43.8X1 Other specified deforming dorsopathies, **occipito-atlanto-axial region**

M43.8X2 Other specified deforming dorsopathies, **cervical region**

M43.8X3 Other specified deforming dorsopathies, **cervicothoracic region**

M43.8X4 Other specified deforming dorsopathies, **thoracic region**

M43.8X5 Other specified deforming dorsopathies, **thoracolumbar region**

M43.8X6 Other specified deforming dorsopathies, **lumbar region**

M43.8X7 Other specified deforming dorsopathies, **lumbosacral region**

M43.8X8 Other specified deforming dorsopathies, **sacral and sacrococcygeal region**

M43.8X9 Other specified deforming dorsopathies, site unspecified

M43.9 Deforming dorsopathy, unspecified
Curvature of spine NOS

Spondylopathies (M45-M49)

✓4th M45 Ankylosing spondylitis
Rheumatoid arthritis of spine

EXCLUDES 1 arthropathy in Reiter's disease (M02.3-)
juvenile (ankylosing) spondylitis (M08.1)

EXCLUDES 2 Behçet's disease (M35.2)

M45.0 Ankylosing spondylitis of multiple sites in spine `HCC`
M45.1 Ankylosing spondylitis of occipito-atlanto-axial region `HCC`
M45.2 Ankylosing spondylitis of cervical region `HCC`
M45.3 Ankylosing spondylitis of cervicothoracic region `HCC`
M45.4 Ankylosing spondylitis of thoracic region `HCC`
M45.5 Ankylosing spondylitis of thoracolumbar region `HCC`
M45.6 Ankylosing spondylitis lumbar region `HCC`
M45.7 Ankylosing spondylitis of lumbosacral region `HCC`
M45.8 Ankylosing spondylitis sacral and sacrococcygeal region `HCC`
M45.9 Ankylosing spondylitis of unspecified sites in spine `HCC`

✓4th M46 Other inflammatory spondylopathies

✓5th M46.0 Spinal enthesopathy
Disorder of ligamentous or muscular attachments of spine

M46.00 Spinal enthesopathy, site unspecified `HCC`
M46.01 Spinal enthesopathy, occipito-atlanto-axial region `HCC`
M46.02 Spinal enthesopathy, cervical region `HCC`
M46.03 Spinal enthesopathy, cervicothoracic region `HCC`
M46.04 Spinal enthesopathy, thoracic region `HCC`
M46.05 Spinal enthesopathy, thoracolumbar region `HCC`
M46.06 Spinal enthesopathy, lumbar region `HCC`
M46.07 Spinal enthesopathy, lumbosacral region `HCC`
M46.08 Spinal enthesopathy, sacral and sacrococcygeal region `HCC`
M46.09 Spinal enthesopathy, multiple sites in spine `HCC`

M46.1 Sacroiliitis, not elsewhere classified `HCC`
DEF: Inflammation of the sacroiliac joint (situated at the juncture of the sacrum and hip). Symptoms include pain in the buttocks or lower back that can extend down one or both legs.

✓5th M46.2 Osteomyelitis of vertebra

> **CC Excl: For CC codes in subcategory M46.2:**
> PDX collection 881

M46.20 Osteomyelitis of vertebra, site unspecified `CC` `HCC`
M46.21 Osteomyelitis of vertebra, occipito-atlanto-axial region `HCC`
M46.22 Osteomyelitis of vertebra, cervical region `CC` `HCC`
M46.23 Osteomyelitis of vertebra, cervicothoracic region `CC` `HCC`
M46.24 Osteomyelitis of vertebra, thoracic region `CC` `HCC`
M46.25 Osteomyelitis of vertebra, thoracolumbar region `CC` `HCC`
M46.26 Osteomyelitis of vertebra, lumbar region `CC` `HCC`
M46.27 Osteomyelitis of vertebra, lumbosacral region `CC` `HCC`
M46.28 Osteomyelitis of vertebra, sacral and sacrococcygeal region `CC` `HCC`

✓5th M46.3 Infection of intervertebral disc (pyogenic)
Use additional code (B95-B97) to identify infectious agent

> **CC Excl: For CC codes in subcategory M46.3:**
> PDX collection 882

M46.30 Infection of intervertebral disc (pyogenic), site unspecified `CC` `HCC`
M46.31 Infection of intervertebral disc (pyogenic), occipito-atlanto-axial region `CC` `HCC`
M46.32 Infection of intervertebral disc (pyogenic), cervical region `CC` `HCC`
M46.33 Infection of intervertebral disc (pyogenic), cervicothoracic region `CC` `HCC`
M46.34 Infection of intervertebral disc (pyogenic), thoracic region `CC` `HCC`
M46.35 Infection of intervertebral disc (pyogenic), thoracolumbar region `CC` `HCC`
M46.36 Infection of intervertebral disc (pyogenic), lumbar region `CC` `HCC`
M46.37 Infection of intervertebral disc (pyogenic), lumbosacral region `CC` `HCC`
M46.38 Infection of intervertebral disc (pyogenic), sacral and sacrococcygeal region `CC` `HCC`
M46.39 Infection of intervertebral disc (pyogenic), multiple sites in spine `CC` `HCC`

✓5th M46.4 Discitis, unspecified

M46.40 Discitis, unspecified, site unspecified
M46.41 Discitis, unspecified, occipito-atlanto-axial region
M46.42 Discitis, unspecified, cervical region
M46.43 Discitis, unspecified, cervicothoracic region
M46.44 Discitis, unspecified, thoracic region
M46.45 Discitis, unspecified, thoracolumbar region
M46.46 Discitis, unspecified, lumbar region
M46.47 Discitis, unspecified, lumbosacral region
M46.48 Discitis, unspecified, sacral and sacrococcygeal region
M46.49 Discitis, unspecified, multiple sites in spine

✓5th M46.5 Other infective spondylopathies

M46.50 Other infective spondylopathies, site unspecified `HCC`
M46.51 Other infective spondylopathies, occipito-atlanto-axial region `HCC`
M46.52 Other infective spondylopathies, cervical region `HCC`
M46.53 Other infective spondylopathies, cervicothoracic region `HCC`
M46.54 Other infective spondylopathies, thoracic region `HCC`
M46.55 Other infective spondylopathies, thoracolumbar region `HCC`
M46.56 Other infective spondylopathies, lumbar region `HCC`
M46.57 Other infective spondylopathies, lumbosacral region `HCC`

N Newborn: 0　　P Pediatric: 0-17　　M Maternity: 12-55　　A Adult: 15-124　　MCC Major Complication/Comorbidity　　CC Complication/Comorbidity　　SW Severe Wound Dx

780

ICD-10-CM 2019

M46.58   Other infective spondylopathies, sacral and sacrococcygeal region   `HCC`

M46.59   Other infective spondylopathies, multiple sites in spine   `HCC`

✓5th M46.8   Other specified inflammatory spondylopathies

M46.80   Other specified inflammatory spondylopathies, site unspecified   `HCC`

M46.81   Other specified inflammatory spondylopathies, occipito-atlanto-axial region   `HCC`

M46.82   Other specified inflammatory spondylopathies, cervical region   `HCC`

M46.83   Other specified inflammatory spondylopathies, cervicothoracic region   `HCC`

M46.84   Other specified inflammatory spondylopathies, thoracic region   `HCC`

M46.85   Other specified inflammatory spondylopathies, thoracolumbar region   `HCC`

M46.86   Other specified inflammatory spondylopathies, lumbar region   `HCC`

M46.87   Other specified inflammatory spondylopathies, lumbosacral region   `HCC`

M46.88   Other specified inflammatory spondylopathies, sacral and sacrococcygeal region   `HCC`

M46.89   Other specified inflammatory spondylopathies, multiple sites in spine   `HCC`

✓5th M46.9   Unspecified inflammatory spondylopathy

M46.90   Unspecified inflammatory spondylopathy, site unspecified   `HCC`

M46.91   Unspecified inflammatory spondylopathy, occipito-atlanto-axial region   `HCC`

M46.92   Unspecified inflammatory spondylopathy, cervical region   `HCC`

M46.93   Unspecified inflammatory spondylopathy, cervicothoracic region   `HCC`

M46.94   Unspecified inflammatory spondylopathy, thoracic region   `HCC`

M46.95   Unspecified inflammatory spondylopathy, thoracolumbar region   `HCC`

M46.96   Unspecified inflammatory spondylopathy, lumbar region   `HCC`

M46.97   Unspecified inflammatory spondylopathy, lumbosacral region   `HCC`

M46.98   Unspecified inflammatory spondylopathy, sacral and sacrococcygeal region   `HCC`

M46.99   Unspecified inflammatory spondylopathy, multiple sites in spine   `HCC`

✓4th M47   Spondylosis

INCLUDES   arthrosis or osteoarthritis of spine
degeneration of facet joints

✓5th M47.0   Anterior spinal and vertebral artery compression syndromes

> **CC Excl:** For CC codes in subcategory M47.0:
> PDX collection 883

✓6th M47.01   Anterior spinal artery compression syndromes

M47.011   Anterior spinal artery compression syndromes, occipito-atlanto-axial region   `CC`

M47.012   Anterior spinal artery compression syndromes, cervical region   `CC`

M47.013   Anterior spinal artery compression syndromes, cervicothoracic region   `CC`

M47.014   Anterior spinal artery compression syndromes, thoracic region   `CC`

M47.015   Anterior spinal artery compression syndromes, thoracolumbar region   `CC`

M47.016   Anterior spinal artery compression syndromes, lumbar region   `CC`

M47.019   Anterior spinal artery compression syndromes, site unspecified   `CC`

✓6th M47.02   Vertebral artery compression syndromes

M47.021   Vertebral artery compression syndromes, occipito-atlanto-axial region   `CC`

M47.022   Vertebral artery compression syndromes, cervical region   `CC`

M47.029   Vertebral artery compression syndromes, site unspecified   `CC`

✓5th M47.1   Other spondylosis with myelopathy
Spondylogenic compression of spinal cord
EXCLUDES 1   vertebral subluxation (M43.3-M43.5X9)

M47.10   Other spondylosis with myelopathy, site unspecified   `CC`
    CC Excl: PDX collection 884

M47.11   Other spondylosis with myelopathy, occipito-atlanto-axial region   `CC`
    CC Excl: PDX collection 883

M47.12   Other spondylosis with myelopathy, cervical region   `CC`
    CC Excl: PDX collection 883

M47.13   Other spondylosis with myelopathy, cervicothoracic region   `CC`
    CC Excl: PDX collection 883

M47.14   Other spondylosis with myelopathy, thoracic region   `CC`
    CC Excl: PDX collection 885

M47.15   Other spondylosis with myelopathy, thoracolumbar region   `CC`
    CC Excl: PDX collection 885

M47.16   Other spondylosis with myelopathy, lumbar region   `CC`
    CC Excl: PDX collection 886

✓5th M47.2   Other spondylosis with radiculopathy

M47.20   Other spondylosis with radiculopathy, site unspecified

M47.21   Other spondylosis with radiculopathy, occipito-atlanto-axial region

M47.22   Other spondylosis with radiculopathy, cervical region

M47.23   Other spondylosis with radiculopathy, cervicothoracic region

M47.24   Other spondylosis with radiculopathy, thoracic region

M47.25   Other spondylosis with radiculopathy, thoracolumbar region

M47.26   Other spondylosis with radiculopathy, lumbar region

M47.27   Other spondylosis with radiculopathy, lumbosacral region

M47.28   Other spondylosis with radiculopathy, sacral and sacrococcygeal region

✓5th M47.8   Other spondylosis

✓6th M47.81   Spondylosis without myelopathy or radiculopathy
AHA: 2018, 2Q, 14

M47.811   Spondylosis without myelopathy or radiculopathy, occipito-atlanto-axial region

M47.812   Spondylosis without myelopathy or radiculopathy, cervical region

M47.813   Spondylosis without myelopathy or radiculopathy, cervicothoracic region

M47.814   Spondylosis without myelopathy or radiculopathy, thoracic region

M47.815   Spondylosis without myelopathy or radiculopathy, thoracolumbar region

M47.816   Spondylosis without myelopathy or radiculopathy, lumbar region

M47.817   Spondylosis without myelopathy or radiculopathy, lumbosacral region

M47.818   Spondylosis without myelopathy or radiculopathy, sacral and sacrococcygeal region

M47.819   Spondylosis without myelopathy or radiculopathy, site unspecified

✓6th M47.89   Other spondylosis

M47.891   Other spondylosis, occipito-atlanto-axial region

M47.892   Other spondylosis, cervical region

M47.893   Other spondylosis, cervicothoracic region

M47.894   Other spondylosis, thoracic region

M47.895   Other spondylosis, thoracolumbar region

M47.896   Other spondylosis, lumbar region

M47.897   Other spondylosis, lumbosacral region

M47.898   Other spondylosis, sacral and sacrococcygeal region

✓ Additional Character Required   ✓7th Placeholder   Unacceptable PDx   Questionable PDx   Manifestation   H1-H14 HAC   HCC CMS-HCC Dx   HIV HIV Dx

ICD-10-CM 2019   781

M47.899   **Other spondylosis,** site unspecified

M47.9   **Spondylosis,** unspecified

✓4ᵗʰ **M48   Other spondylopathies**

✓5ᵗʰ   M48.0   **Spinal stenosis**
Caudal stenosis

    M48.00   **Spinal stenosis,** site unspecified

    M48.01   **Spinal stenosis,** occipito-atlanto-axial **region**

    M48.02   **Spinal stenosis,** cervical **region**

    M48.03   **Spinal stenosis,** cervicothoracic **region**

    M48.04   **Spinal stenosis,** thoracic **region**

    M48.05   **Spinal stenosis,** thoracolumbar **region**

✓6ᵗʰ   M48.06   **Spinal stenosis,** lumbar **region**
      AHA: 2017, 4Q, 18-19
      DEF: Spinal canal narrowing in the lumbar area with nerve root compression, causing muscle pain, fatigue, and weakness during extension of the lumbar spine. Pain is relieved by sitting or bending.

      M48.061   **Spinal stenosis, lumbar region** without **neurogenic claudication**
         Spinal stenosis, lumbar region NOS

      M48.062   **Spinal stenosis, lumbar region** with **neurogenic claudication**

    M48.07   **Spinal stenosis,** lumbosacral **region**

    M48.08   **Spinal stenosis,** sacral and sacrococcygeal **region**

✓5ᵗʰ   M48.1   **Ankylosing hyperostosis [Forestier]**
Diffuse idiopathic skeletal hyperostosis [DISH]

    M48.10   **Ankylosing hyperostosis [Forestier],** site unspecified

    M48.11   **Ankylosing hyperostosis [Forestier],** occipito-atlanto-axial **region**

    M48.12   **Ankylosing hyperostosis [Forestier],** cervical **region**

    M48.13   **Ankylosing hyperostosis [Forestier],** cervicothoracic **region**

    M48.14   **Ankylosing hyperostosis [Forestier],** thoracic **region**

    M48.15   **Ankylosing hyperostosis [Forestier],** thoracolumbar **region**

    M48.16   **Ankylosing hyperostosis [Forestier],** lumbar **region**

    M48.17   **Ankylosing hyperostosis [Forestier],** lumbosacral **region**

    M48.18   **Ankylosing hyperostosis [Forestier],** sacral and sacrococcygeal **region**

    M48.19   **Ankylosing hyperostosis [Forestier],** multiple sites in **spine**

✓5ᵗʰ   M48.2   **Kissing spine**

    M48.20   **Kissing spine,** site unspecified

    M48.21   **Kissing spine,** occipito-atlanto-axial **region**

    M48.22   **Kissing spine,** cervical **region**

    M48.23   **Kissing spine,** cervicothoracic **region**

    M48.24   **Kissing spine,** thoracic **region**

    M48.25   **Kissing spine,** thoracolumbar **region**

    M48.26   **Kissing spine,** lumbar **region**

    M48.27   **Kissing spine,** lumbosacral **region**

✓5ᵗʰ   M48.3   **Traumatic spondylopathy**

    CC Excl: For CC codes in subcategory M48.3:
    PDX collection 887

    M48.30   **Traumatic spondylopathy,** site unspecified   **CC**

    M48.31   **Traumatic spondylopathy,** occipito-atlanto-axial **region**   **CC**

    M48.32   **Traumatic spondylopathy,** cervical **region**   **CC**

    M48.33   **Traumatic spondylopathy,** cervicothoracic **region**   **CC**

    M48.34   **Traumatic spondylopathy,** thoracic **region**   **CC**

    M48.35   **Traumatic spondylopathy,** thoracolumbar **region**   **CC**

    M48.36   **Traumatic spondylopathy,** lumbar **region**   **CC**

    M48.37   **Traumatic spondylopathy,** lumbosacral **region**   **CC**

    M48.38   **Traumatic spondylopathy,** sacral and sacrococcygeal **region**   **CC**

✓5ᵗʰ   M48.4   **Fatigue fracture of vertebra**
Stress fracture of vertebra
EXCLUDES 1   *pathological fracture NOS (M84.-)*
      pathological fracture of vertebra due to neoplasm (M84.58)
      pathological fracture of vertebra due to other diagnosis (M84.68)
      pathological fracture of vertebra due to osteoporosis (M80.-)
      traumatic fracture of vertebrae (S12.0-S12.3-, S22.0-, S32.0-)

    The appropriate 7th character is to be added to each code from subcategory M48.4.
    A   initial encounter for fracture
    D   subsequent encounter for fracture with routine healing
    G   subsequent encounter for fracture with delayed healing
    S   sequela of fracture

    ✓x7ᵗʰ   M48.40   **Fatigue fracture of vertebra,** site unspecified

    ✓x7ᵗʰ   M48.41   **Fatigue fracture of vertebra,** occipito-atlanto-axial **region**

    ✓x7ᵗʰ   M48.42   **Fatigue fracture of vertebra,** cervical **region**

    ✓x7ᵗʰ   M48.43   **Fatigue fracture of vertebra,** cervicothoracic **region**

    ✓x7ᵗʰ   M48.44   **Fatigue fracture of vertebra,** thoracic **region**

    ✓x7ᵗʰ   M48.45   **Fatigue fracture of vertebra,** thoracolumbar **region**

    ✓x7ᵗʰ   M48.46   **Fatigue fracture of vertebra,** lumbar **region**

    ✓x7ᵗʰ   M48.47   **Fatigue fracture of vertebra,** lumbosacral **region**

    ✓x7ᵗʰ   M48.48   **Fatigue fracture of vertebra,** sacral and sacrococcygeal **region**

✓5ᵗʰ   M48.5   **Collapsed vertebra, not elsewhere classified**
Collapsed vertebra NOS
Compression fracture of vertebra NOS
Wedging of vertebra NOS
EXCLUDES 1   *current injury—see Injury of spine, by body region*
      fatigue fracture of vertebra (M48.4)
      pathological fracture of vertebra due to neoplasm (M84.58)
      pathological fracture of vertebra due to other diagnosis (M84.68)
      pathological fracture of vertebra due to osteoporosis (M80.-)
      pathological fracture NOS (M84.4-)
      stress fracture of vertebra (M48.4-)
      traumatic fracture of vertebra (S12-, S22-, S32-)

    The appropriate 7th character is to be added to each code from subcategory M48.5.
    A   initial encounter for fracture
    D   subsequent encounter for fracture with routine healing
    G   subsequent encounter for fracture with delayed healing
    S   sequela of fracture

    CC Excl: For CC codes in subcategory M48.5:
    PDX collection 888

    6   ✓x7ᵗʰ   M48.50   **Collapsed vertebra, not elsewhere classified,** site unspecified   **CC** **HCC**

    6   ✓x7ᵗʰ   M48.51   **Collapsed vertebra, not elsewhere classified,** occipito-atlanto-axial **region**   **CC** **HCC**

    6   ✓x7ᵗʰ   M48.52   **Collapsed vertebra, not elsewhere classified,** cervical **region**   **CC** **HCC**

    6   ✓x7ᵗʰ   M48.53   **Collapsed vertebra, not elsewhere classified,** cervicothoracic **region**   **CC** **HCC**

    6   ✓x7ᵗʰ   M48.54   **Collapsed vertebra, not elsewhere classified,** thoracic **region**   **CC** **HCC**

    6   ✓x7ᵗʰ   M48.55   **Collapsed vertebra, not elsewhere classified,** thoracolumbar **region**   **CC** **HCC**

    6   ✓x7ᵗʰ   M48.56   **Collapsed vertebra, not elsewhere classified,** lumbar **region**   **CC** **HCC**

    6   ✓x7ᵗʰ   M48.57   **Collapsed vertebra, not elsewhere classified,** lumbosacral **region**   **CC** **HCC**

    6   ✓x7ᵗʰ   M48.58   **Collapsed vertebra, not elsewhere classified,** sacral and sacrococcygeal **region**   **CC** **HCC**

N Newborn: 0   **P** Pediatric: 0-17   **M** Maternity: 12-55   **A** Adult: 15-124   **MCC** Major Complication/Comorbidity   **CC** Complication/Comorbidity   **SW** Severe Wound Dx

782   ICD-10-CM 2019

✓5ᵗʰ **M48.8 Other specified spondylopathies**
Ossification of posterior longitudinal ligament

   ✓6ᵗʰ **M48.8X Other specified spondylopathies**

      M48.8X1 Other specified spondylopathies, HCC
      occipito-atlanto-axial region

      M48.8X2 Other specified spondylopathies, HCC
      cervical region

      M48.8X3 Other specified spondylopathies, HCC
      cervicothoracic region

      M48.8X4 Other specified spondylopathies, HCC
      thoracic region

      M48.8X5 Other specified spondylopathies, HCC
      thoracolumbar region

      M48.8X6 Other specified spondylopathies, HCC
      lumbar region

      M48.8X7 Other specified spondylopathies, HCC
      lumbosacral region

      M48.8X8 Other specified spondylopathies, HCC
      sacral and sacrococcygeal region

      M48.8X9 Other specified spondylopathies, HCC
      site unspecified

   M48.9 Spondylopathy, unspecified

✓4ᵗʰ **M49 Spondylopathies in diseases classified elsewhere**

   INCLUDES   curvature of spine in diseases classified elsewhere
         deformity of spine in diseases classified elsewhere
         kyphosis in diseases classified elsewhere
         scoliosis in diseases classified elsewhere
         spondylopathy in diseases classified elsewhere

   Code first underlying disease, such as:
       brucellosis (A23.-)
       Charcôt-Marie-Tooth disease (G60.0)
       enterobacterial infections (A01-A04)
       osteitis fibrosa cystica (E21.0)

   EXCLUDES 1   *curvature of spine in tuberculosis [Pott's] (A18.01)*
         enteropathic arthropathies (M07.-)
         gonococcal spondylitis (A54.41)
         neuropathic [tabes dorsalis] spondylitis (A52.11)
         neuropathic spondylopathy in syringomyelia (G95.0)
         neuropathic spondylopathy in tabes dorsalis (A52.11)
         nonsyphilitic neuropathic spondylopathy NEC (G98.0)
         spondylitis in syphilis (acquired) (A52.77)
         tuberculous spondylitis (A18.01)
         typhoid fever spondylitis (A01.05)

  ✓5ᵗʰ **M49.8 Spondylopathy in diseases classified elsewhere**

     M49.80 Spondylopathy in diseases classified elsewhere, HCC
     site unspecified

     M49.81 Spondylopathy in diseases classified elsewhere, HCC
     occipito-atlanto-axial region

     M49.82 Spondylopathy in diseases classified elsewhere, HCC
     cervical region

     M49.83 Spondylopathy in diseases classified elsewhere, HCC
     cervicothoracic region

     M49.84 Spondylopathy in diseases classified elsewhere, HCC
     thoracic region

     M49.85 Spondylopathy in diseases classified elsewhere, HCC
     thoracolumbar region

     M49.86 Spondylopathy in diseases classified elsewhere, HCC
     lumbar region

     M49.87 Spondylopathy in diseases classified elsewhere, HCC
     lumbosacral region

     M49.88 Spondylopathy in diseases classified elsewhere, HCC
     sacral and sacrococcygeal region

     M49.89 Spondylopathy in diseases classified elsewhere, HCC
     multiple sites in spine

Other dorsopathies (M50-M54)

   EXCLUDES 1   current injury—see injury of spine by body region
         discitis NOS (M46.4-)

✓4ᵗʰ **M50 Cervical disc disorders**

   NOTE   Code to the most superior level of disorder.
   INCLUDES   cervicothoracic disc disorders with cervicalgia
         cervicothoracic disc disorders

   AHA: 2016, 4Q, 39-40; 2016, 1Q, 17

  ✓5ᵗʰ **M50.0 Cervical disc disorder with myelopathy**

     CC Excl: For CC codes in subcategory M50.0:
     PDX collection 889

     M50.00 Cervical disc disorder with myelopathy, CC
     unspecified cervical region

▲   **M50.01 Cervical disc disorder with myelopathy,** CC
     high cervical region
        C2-C3 disc disorder with myelopathy
        C3-C4 disc disorder with myelopathy

  ✓6ᵗʰ **M50.02 Cervical disc disorder with myelopathy,**
     mid-cervical region

     M50.020 Cervical disc disorder with CC
     myelopathy, mid-cervical region,
     unspecified level

     M50.021 Cervical disc disorder at C4-C5 level CC
     with myelopathy
        C4-C5 disc disorder with myelopathy

     M50.022 Cervical disc disorder at C5-C6 level CC
     with myelopathy
        C5-C6 disc disorder with myelopathy

     M50.023 Cervical disc disorder at C6-C7 level CC
     with myelopathy
        C6-C7 disc disorder with myelopathy

     M50.03 Cervical disc disorder with myelopathy, CC
     cervicothoracic region
        C7-T1 disc disorder with myelopathy

  ✓5ᵗʰ **M50.1 Cervical disc disorder with radiculopathy**

     EXCLUDES 2   *brachial radiculitis NOS (M54.13)*

     M50.10 Cervical disc disorder with radiculopathy,
     unspecified cervical region

▲   **M50.11 Cervical disc disorder with radiculopathy, high**
     cervical region
        C2-C3 disc disorder with radiculopathy
        C3 radiculopathy due to disc disorder
        C3-C4 disc disorder with radiculopathy
        C4 radiculopathy due to disc disorder

  ✓6ᵗʰ **M50.12 Cervical disc disorder with radiculopathy, mid-**
     cervical region

     M50.120 Mid-cervical disc disorder, unspecified

     M50.121 Cervical disc disorder at C4-C5 level with
     radiculopathy
        C4-C5 disc disorder with radiculopathy
        C5 radiculopathy due to disc disorder

     M50.122 Cervical disc disorder at C5-C6 level with
     radiculopathy
        C5-C6 disc disorder with radiculopathy
        C6 radiculopathy due to disc disorder

     M50.123 Cervical disc disorder at C6-C7 level with
     radiculopathy
        C6-C7 disc disorder with radiculopathy
        C7 radiculopathy due to disc disorder

     M50.13 Cervical disc disorder with radiculopathy,
     cervicothoracic region
        C7-T1 disc disorder with radiculopathy
        C8 radiculopathy due to disc disorder

  ✓5ᵗʰ **M50.2 Other cervical disc displacement**

     M50.20 Other cervical disc displacement, unspecified
     cervical region

▲   **M50.21 Other cervical disc displacement, high cervical**
     region
        Other C2-C3 cervical disc displacement
        Other C3-C4 cervical disc displacement

  ✓6ᵗʰ **M50.22 Other cervical disc displacement, mid-cervical region**

     M50.220 Other cervical disc displacement,
     mid-cervical region, unspecified level

     M50.221 Other cervical disc displacement at C4-C5
     level
        Other C4-C5 cervical disc displacement

     M50.222 Other cervical disc displacement at C5-C6
     level
        Other C5-C6 cervical disc displacement

     M50.223 Other cervical disc displacement at C6-C7
     level
        Other C6-C7 cervical disc displacement

     M50.23 Other cervical disc displacement, cervicothoracic
     region
        Other C7-T1 cervical disc displacement

  ✓5ᵗʰ **M50.3 Other cervical disc degeneration**

     M50.30 Other cervical disc degeneration, unspecified
     cervical region

▲   **M50.31 Other cervical disc degeneration, high cervical**
     region
        Other C2-C3 cervical disc degeneration
        Other C3-C4 cervical disc degeneration

✓ Additional Character Required   ✓x7ᵗʰ Placeholder   Unacceptable PDx   Questionable PDx   Manifestation   H1-H14 HAC   HCC CMS-HCC Dx   HIV HIV Dx

ICD-10-CM 2019   783

Chapter 13. Diseases of the Musculoskeletal System and Connective Tissue *(side margin)*

✓6ᵗʰ **M50.32 Other cervical disc degeneration,** mid-cervical region
- **M50.320 Other cervical disc degeneration, mid-cervical region,** unspecified level
- **M50.321 Other cervical disc degeneration at** C4-C5 level
  - Other C4-C5 cervical disc degeneration
- **M50.322 Other cervical disc degeneration at** C5-C6 level
  - Other C5-C6 cervical disc degeneration
- **M50.323 Other cervical disc degeneration at** C6-C7 level
  - Other C6-C7 cervical disc degeneration

M50.33 Other cervical disc degeneration, cervicothoracic region
- Other C7-T1 cervical disc degeneration

✓5ᵗʰ **M50.8 Other** cervical disc disorders
- **M50.80 Other cervical disc disorders,** unspecified cervical region
▲ **M50.81 Other cervical disc disorders,** high cervical region
  - Other C2-C3 cervical disc disorders
  - Other C3-C4 cervical disc disorders

✓6ᵗʰ **M50.82 Other cervical disc disorders,** mid-cervical region
- **M50.820 Other cervical disc disorders, mid-cervical region,** unspecified level
- **M50.821 Other cervical disc disorders at** C4-C5 level
  - Other C4-C5 cervical disc disorders
- **M50.822 Other cervical disc disorders at** C5-C6 level
  - Other C5-C6 cervical disc disorders
- **M50.823 Other cervical disc disorders at** C6-C7 level
  - Other C6-C7 cervical disc disorders

M50.83 Other cervical disc disorders, cervicothoracic region
- Other C7-T1 cervical disc disorders

✓5ᵗʰ **M50.9 Cervical disc disorder,** unspecified
- **M50.90 Cervical disc disorder, unspecified,** unspecified cervical region
▲ **M50.91 Cervical disc disorder, unspecified,** high cervical region
  - C2-C3 cervical disc disorder, unspecified
  - C3-C4 cervical disc disorder, unspecified

✓6ᵗʰ **M50.92 Cervical disc disorder, unspecified,** mid-cervical region
- **M50.920 Unspecified cervical disc disorder, mid-cervical region,** unspecified level
- **M50.921 Unspecified cervical disc disorder at** C4-C5 level
  - Unspecified C4-C5 cervical disc disorder
- **M50.922 Unspecified cervical disc disorder at** C5-C6 level
  - Unspecified C5-C6 cervical disc disorder
- **M50.923 Unspecified cervical disc disorder at** C6-C7 level
  - Unspecified C6-C7 cervical disc disorder

M50.93 Cervical disc disorder, unspecified, cervicothoracic region
- C7-T1 cervical disc disorder, unspecified

✓4ᵗʰ **M51 Thoracic, thoracolumbar, and lumbosacral intervertebral disc disorders**
> *EXCLUDES 2*   cervical and cervicothoracic disc disorders (M50.-)
> sacral and sacrococcygeal disorders (M53.3)

✓5ᵗʰ **M51.0 Thoracic, thoracolumbar and lumbosacral intervertebral disc disorders** with myelopathy
- **M51.04 Intervertebral disc disorders with myelopathy,** thoracic region   **CC**
  - **CC Excl:** PDX collection 890
- **M51.05 Intervertebral disc disorders with myelopathy,** thoracolumbar region   **CC**
  - **CC Excl:** PDX collection 890
- **M51.06 Intervertebral disc disorders with myelopathy,** lumbar region   **CC**
  - **CC Excl:** PDX collection 891

✓5ᵗʰ **M51.1 Thoracic, thoracolumbar and lumbosacral intervertebral disc disorders** with radiculopathy
- Sciatica due to intervertebral disc disorder
> *EXCLUDES 1*   lumbar radiculitis NOS (M54.16)
> sciatica NOS (M54.3)
- **M51.14 Intervertebral disc disorders with radiculopathy,** thoracic region

- **M51.15 Intervertebral disc disorders with radiculopathy,** thoracolumbar region
- **M51.16 Intervertebral disc disorders with radiculopathy,** lumbar region
- **M51.17 Intervertebral disc disorders with radiculopathy,** lumbosacral region

✓5ᵗʰ **M51.2 Other** thoracic, thoracolumbar and lumbosacral intervertebral disc displacement
- Lumbago due to displacement of intervertebral disc
- **M51.24 Other intervertebral disc displacement,** thoracic region
- **M51.25 Other intervertebral disc displacement,** thoracolumbar region
- **M51.26 Other intervertebral disc displacement,** lumbar region
- **M51.27 Other intervertebral disc displacement,** lumbosacral region

Displacement Intervertebral Disc

Normal Top View — Lamina, Ligamentum flavum, Disc annulus, Nucleus pulposus

Herniated Top View — Nucleus pulposus, Spinal cord, Herniates through annulus, Spinal nerve

✓5ᵗʰ **M51.3 Other** thoracic, thoracolumbar and lumbosacral intervertebral disc degeneration
- **AHA:** 2018, 2Q, 15; 2013, 3Q, 22
- **M51.34 Other intervertebral disc degeneration,** thoracic region
- **M51.35 Other intervertebral disc degeneration,** thoracolumbar region
- **M51.36 Other intervertebral disc degeneration,** lumbar region
- **M51.37 Other intervertebral disc degeneration,** lumbosacral region

✓5ᵗʰ **M51.4 Schmorl's nodes**
> **DEF:** Irregular bone defect in the margin of the vertebral body that causes herniation into the end plate of the vertebral body.
- **M51.44 Schmorl's nodes,** thoracic region
- **M51.45 Schmorl's nodes,** thoracolumbar region
- **M51.46 Schmorl's nodes,** lumbar region
- **M51.47 Schmorl's nodes,** lumbosacral region

✓5ᵗʰ **M51.8 Other** thoracic, thoracolumbar and lumbosacral intervertebral disc disorders
- **M51.84 Other intervertebral disc disorders,** thoracic region
- **M51.85 Other intervertebral disc disorders,** thoracolumbar region
- **M51.86 Other intervertebral disc disorders,** lumbar region
- **M51.87 Other intervertebral disc disorders,** lumbosacral region

M51.9 Unspecified thoracic, thoracolumbar and lumbosacral intervertebral disc disorder

✓4ᵗʰ **M53 Other and unspecified dorsopathies, not elsewhere classified**
- **M53.0 Cervicocranial syndrome**
  - Posterior cervical sympathetic syndrome
- **M53.1 Cervicobrachial syndrome**
> *EXCLUDES 2*   cervical disc disorder (M50.-)
> thoracic outlet syndrome (G54.0)

✓5ᵗʰ **M53.2 Spinal instabilities**
- ✓6ᵗʰ **M53.2X Spinal** instabilities
  - **M53.2X1 Spinal instabilities,** occipito-atlanto-axial region
  - **M53.2X2 Spinal instabilities,** cervical region
  - **M53.2X3 Spinal instabilities,** cervicothoracic region

*(side margin bottom)* M50.32–M53.2X3

                M53.2X4 **Spinal instabilities, thoracic region**

                M53.2X5 **Spinal instabilities, thoracolumbar region**

                M53.2X6 **Spinal instabilities, lumbar region**

                M53.2X7 **Spinal instabilities, lumbosacral region**

                M53.2X8 **Spinal instabilities, sacral and sacrococcygeal region**

                M53.2X9 **Spinal instabilities, site unspecified**

            M53.3 **Sacrococcygeal disorders, not elsewhere classified**
                Coccygodynia

    ✓5ᵗʰ **M53.8** Other specified dorsopathies

                M53.80 **Other specified dorsopathies, site unspecified**

                M53.81 **Other specified dorsopathies, occipito-atlanto-axial region**

                M53.82 **Other specified dorsopathies, cervical region**

                M53.83 **Other specified dorsopathies, cervicothoracic region**

                M53.84 **Other specified dorsopathies, thoracic region**

                M53.85 **Other specified dorsopathies, thoracolumbar region**

                M53.86 **Other specified dorsopathies, lumbar region**

                M53.87 **Other specified dorsopathies, lumbosacral region**

                M53.88 **Other specified dorsopathies, sacral and sacrococcygeal region**

            M53.9 **Dorsopathy, unspecified**

✓4ᵗʰ **M54 Dorsalgia**
          EXCLUDES 1   *psychogenic dorsalgia (F45.41)*

    ✓5ᵗʰ **M54.0** **Panniculitis affecting regions of neck and back**
              EXCLUDES 1   *lupus panniculitis (L93.2)*
                         panniculitis NOS (M79.3)
                         relapsing [Weber-Christian] panniculitis (M35.6)

                M54.00 **Panniculitis affecting regions of neck and back, site unspecified**

                M54.01 **Panniculitis affecting regions of neck and back, occipito-atlanto-axial region**

                M54.02 **Panniculitis affecting regions of neck and back, cervical region**

                M54.03 **Panniculitis affecting regions of neck and back, cervicothoracic region**

                M54.04 **Panniculitis affecting regions of neck and back, thoracic region**

                M54.05 **Panniculitis affecting regions of neck and back, thoracolumbar region**

                M54.06 **Panniculitis affecting regions of neck and back, lumbar region**

                M54.07 **Panniculitis affecting regions of neck and back, lumbosacral region**

                M54.08 **Panniculitis affecting regions of neck and back, sacral and sacrococcygeal region**

                M54.09 **Panniculitis affecting regions, neck and back, multiple sites in spine**

    ✓5ᵗʰ **M54.1** **Radiculopathy**
                Brachial neuritis or radiculitis NOS
                Lumbar neuritis or radiculitis NOS
                Lumbosacral neuritis or radiculitis NOS
                Thoracic neuritis or radiculitis NOS
                Radiculitis NOS
                EXCLUDES 1   *neuralgia and neuritis NOS (M79.2)*
                         radiculopathy with cervical disc disorder (M50.1)
                         radiculopathy with lumbar and other intervertebral disc disorder (M51.1-)
                         radiculopathy with spondylosis (M47.2-)

                M54.10 **Radiculopathy, site unspecified**

                M54.11 **Radiculopathy, occipito-atlanto-axial region**

                M54.12 **Radiculopathy, cervical region**

                M54.13 **Radiculopathy, cervicothoracic region**

                M54.14 **Radiculopathy, thoracic region**

                M54.15 **Radiculopathy, thoracolumbar region**

                M54.16 **Radiculopathy, lumbar region**

                M54.17 **Radiculopathy, lumbosacral region**

                M54.18 **Radiculopathy, sacral and sacrococcygeal region**

           M54.2 **Cervicalgia**
                EXCLUDES 1   *cervicalgia due to intervertebral cervical disc disorder (M50.-)*

    ✓5ᵗʰ **M54.3** **Sciatica**
                EXCLUDES 1   *lesion of sciatic nerve (G57.0)*
                         sciatica due to intervertebral disc disorder (M51.1-)
                         sciatica with lumbago (M54.4-)

                M54.30 **Sciatica, unspecified side**

                M54.31 **Sciatica, right side**

                M54.32 **Sciatica, left side**

    ✓5ᵗʰ **M54.4** **Lumbago with sciatica**
                EXCLUDES 1   *lumbago with sciatica due to intervertebral disc disorder (M51.1-)*
                AHA: 2016, 2Q, 7

                M54.40 **Lumbago with sciatica, unspecified side**

                M54.41 **Lumbago with sciatica, right side**

                M54.42 **Lumbago with sciatica, left side**

           M54.5 **Low back pain**
                Loin pain
                Lumbago NOS
                EXCLUDES 1   *low back strain (S39.012)*
                         lumbago due to intervertebral disc displacement (M51.2-)
                         lumbago with sciatica (M54.4-)

           M54.6 **Pain in thoracic spine**
                EXCLUDES 1   *pain in thoracic spine due to intervertebral disc disorder (M51.-)*

    ✓5ᵗʰ **M54.8** **Other dorsalgia**
                EXCLUDES 1   *dorsalgia in thoracic region (M54.6)*
                         low back pain (M54.5)

                M54.81 **Occipital neuralgia**

                M54.89 **Other dorsalgia**

           M54.9 **Dorsalgia, unspecified**
                Backache NOS
                Back pain NOS

SOFT TISSUE DISORDERS (M60-M79)

Disorders of muscles (M60-M63)

      EXCLUDES 1   *dermatopolymyositis (M33.-)*
                muscular dystrophies and myopathies (G71-G72)
                myopathy in amyloidosis (E85.-)
                myopathy in polyarteritis nodosa (M30.0)
                myopathy in rheumatoid arthritis (M05.32)
                myopathy in scleroderma (M34.-)
                myopathy in Sjögren's syndrome (M35.03)
                myopathy in systemic lupus erythematosus (M32.-)

✓4ᵗʰ **M60 Myositis**
          EXCLUDES 2   *inclusion body myositis [IBM] (G72.41)*

    ✓5ᵗʰ **M60.0** **Infective myositis**
                Tropical pyomyositis
                Use additional code (B95-B97) to identify infectious agent

              CC Excl: For CC codes in subcategory M60.0: PDX collection 806

      ✓6ᵗʰ **M60.00** **Infective myositis, unspecified site**

                M60.000 **Infective myositis, unspecified right arm**   CC
                         Infective myositis, right upper limb NOS

                M60.001 **Infective myositis, unspecified left arm**   CC
                         Infective myositis, left upper limb NOS

                M60.002 **Infective myositis, unspecified arm**   CC
                         Infective myositis, upper limb NOS

                M60.003 **Infective myositis, unspecified right leg**   CC
                         Infective myositis, right lower limb NOS

                M60.004 **Infective myositis, unspecified left leg**   CC
                         Infective myositis, left lower limb NOS

                M60.005 **Infective myositis, unspecified leg**   CC
                         Infective myositis, lower limb NOS

                M60.009 **Infective myositis, unspecified site**   CC

      ✓6ᵗʰ **M60.01** **Infective myositis, shoulder**

                M60.011 **Infective myositis, right shoulder**   CC
                M60.012 **Infective myositis, left shoulder**   CC
                M60.019 **Infective myositis, unspecified shoulder**   CC

      ✓6ᵗʰ **M60.02** **Infective myositis, upper arm**

                M60.021 **Infective myositis, right upper arm**   CC
                M60.022 **Infective myositis, left upper arm**   CC

✓ Additional Character Required   ✓x7ᵗʰ Placeholder   Unacceptable PDx   Questionable PDx   Manifestation   H1-H14 HAC   HCC CMS-HCC Dx   HIV HIV Dx

ICD-10-CM 2019   **785**

M60.029 Infective myositis, unspecified upper arm `CC`

✓6ᵗʰ M60.03 Infective myositis, forearm
     M60.031 Infective myositis, right forearm `CC`
     M60.032 Infective myositis, left forearm `CC`
     M60.039 Infective myositis, unspecified forearm `CC`

✓6ᵗʰ M60.04 Infective myositis, hand and fingers
     M60.041 Infective myositis, right hand `CC`
     M60.042 Infective myositis, left hand `CC`
     M60.043 Infective myositis, unspecified hand `CC`
     M60.044 Infective myositis, right finger(s) `CC`
     M60.045 Infective myositis, left finger(s) `CC`
     M60.046 Infective myositis, unspecified finger(s) `CC`

✓6ᵗʰ M60.05 Infective myositis, thigh
     M60.051 Infective myositis, right thigh `CC`
     M60.052 Infective myositis, left thigh `CC`
     M60.059 Infective myositis, unspecified thigh `CC`

✓6ᵗʰ M60.06 Infective myositis, lower leg
     M60.061 Infective myositis, right lower leg `CC`
     M60.062 Infective myositis, left lower leg `CC`
     M60.069 Infective myositis, unspecified lower leg `CC`

✓6ᵗʰ M60.07 Infective myositis, ankle, foot and toes
     M60.070 Infective myositis, right ankle `CC`
     M60.071 Infective myositis, left ankle `CC`
     M60.072 Infective myositis, unspecified ankle `CC`
     M60.073 Infective myositis, right foot `CC`
     M60.074 Infective myositis, left foot `CC`
     M60.075 Infective myositis, unspecified foot `CC`
     M60.076 Infective myositis, right toe(s) `CC`
     M60.077 Infective myositis, left toe(s) `CC`
     M60.078 Infective myositis, unspecified toe(s) `CC`

M60.08 Infective myositis, other site `CC`
M60.09 Infective myositis, multiple sites `CC`

M60.1 Interstitial myositis
M60.10 Interstitial myositis of unspecified site

✓6ᵗʰ M60.11 Interstitial myositis, shoulder
     M60.111 Interstitial myositis, right shoulder
     M60.112 Interstitial myositis, left shoulder
     M60.119 Interstitial myositis, unspecified shoulder

✓6ᵗʰ M60.12 Interstitial myositis, upper arm
     M60.121 Interstitial myositis, right upper arm
     M60.122 Interstitial myositis, left upper arm
     M60.129 Interstitial myositis, unspecified upper arm

✓6ᵗʰ M60.13 Interstitial myositis, forearm
     M60.131 Interstitial myositis, right forearm
     M60.132 Interstitial myositis, left forearm
     M60.139 Interstitial myositis, unspecified forearm

✓6ᵗʰ M60.14 Interstitial myositis, hand
     M60.141 Interstitial myositis, right hand
     M60.142 Interstitial myositis, left hand
     M60.149 Interstitial myositis, unspecified hand

✓6ᵗʰ M60.15 Interstitial myositis, thigh
     M60.151 Interstitial myositis, right thigh
     M60.152 Interstitial myositis, left thigh
     M60.159 Interstitial myositis, unspecified thigh

✓6ᵗʰ M60.16 Interstitial myositis, lower leg
     M60.161 Interstitial myositis, right lower leg
     M60.162 Interstitial myositis, left lower leg
     M60.169 Interstitial myositis, unspecified lower leg

✓6ᵗʰ M60.17 Interstitial myositis, ankle and foot
     M60.171 Interstitial myositis, right ankle and foot
     M60.172 Interstitial myositis, left ankle and foot
     M60.179 Interstitial myositis, unspecified ankle and foot

M60.18 Interstitial myositis, other site
M60.19 Interstitial myositis, multiple sites

✓5ᵗʰ M60.2 Foreign body granuloma of soft tissue, not elsewhere classified
     Use additional code to identify the type of retained foreign body (Z18.-)
     EXCLUDES 1   foreign body granuloma of skin and subcutaneous tissue (L92.3)

M60.20 Foreign body granuloma of soft tissue, not elsewhere classified, unspecified site

✓6ᵗʰ M60.21 Foreign body granuloma of soft tissue, not elsewhere classified, shoulder
     M60.211 Foreign body granuloma of soft tissue, not elsewhere classified, right shoulder
     M60.212 Foreign body granuloma of soft tissue, not elsewhere classified, left shoulder
     M60.219 Foreign body granuloma of soft tissue, not elsewhere classified, unspecified shoulder

✓6ᵗʰ M60.22 Foreign body granuloma of soft tissue, not elsewhere classified, upper arm
     M60.221 Foreign body granuloma of soft tissue, not elsewhere classified, right upper arm
     M60.222 Foreign body granuloma of soft tissue, not elsewhere classified, left upper arm
     M60.229 Foreign body granuloma of soft tissue, not elsewhere classified, unspecified upper arm

✓6ᵗʰ M60.23 Foreign body granuloma of soft tissue, not elsewhere classified, forearm
     M60.231 Foreign body granuloma of soft tissue, not elsewhere classified, right forearm
     M60.232 Foreign body granuloma of soft tissue, not elsewhere classified, left forearm
     M60.239 Foreign body granuloma of soft tissue, not elsewhere classified, unspecified forearm

✓6ᵗʰ M60.24 Foreign body granuloma of soft tissue, not elsewhere classified, hand
     M60.241 Foreign body granuloma of soft tissue, not elsewhere classified, right hand
     M60.242 Foreign body granuloma of soft tissue, not elsewhere classified, left hand
     M60.249 Foreign body granuloma of soft tissue, not elsewhere classified, unspecified hand

✓6ᵗʰ M60.25 Foreign body granuloma of soft tissue, not elsewhere classified, thigh
     M60.251 Foreign body granuloma of soft tissue, not elsewhere classified, right thigh
     M60.252 Foreign body granuloma of soft tissue, not elsewhere classified, left thigh
     M60.259 Foreign body granuloma of soft tissue, not elsewhere classified, unspecified thigh

✓6ᵗʰ M60.26 Foreign body granuloma of soft tissue, not elsewhere classified, lower leg
     M60.261 Foreign body granuloma of soft tissue, not elsewhere classified, right lower leg
     M60.262 Foreign body granuloma of soft tissue, not elsewhere classified, left lower leg
     M60.269 Foreign body granuloma of soft tissue, not elsewhere classified, unspecified lower leg

✓6ᵗʰ M60.27 Foreign body granuloma of soft tissue, not elsewhere classified, ankle and foot
     M60.271 Foreign body granuloma of soft tissue, not elsewhere classified, right ankle and foot
     M60.272 Foreign body granuloma of soft tissue, not elsewhere classified, left ankle and foot
     M60.279 Foreign body granuloma of soft tissue, not elsewhere classified, unspecified ankle and foot

M60.28 Foreign body granuloma of soft tissue, not elsewhere classified, other site

✓5ᵗʰ M60.8 Other myositis
M60.80 Other myositis, unspecified site

✓6ᵗʰ M60.81 Other myositis shoulder
     M60.811 Other myositis, right shoulder
     M60.812 Other myositis, left shoulder
     M60.819 Other myositis, unspecified shoulder

✓6ᵗʰ M60.82 Other myositis, upper arm
     M60.821 Other myositis, right upper arm
     M60.822 Other myositis, left upper arm

N Newborn: 0   P Pediatric: 0-17   M Maternity: 12-55   A Adult: 15-124   MCC Major Complication/Comorbidity   CC Complication/Comorbidity   SW Severe Wound Dx

786

ICD-10-CM 2019

M60.829   Other myositis, unspecified upper arm

✓6th **M60.83**   Other myositis, forearm
     M60.831   Other myositis, right forearm
     M60.832   Other myositis, left forearm
     M60.839   Other myositis, unspecified forearm

✓6th **M60.84**   Other myositis, hand
     M60.841   Other myositis, right hand
     M60.842   Other myositis, left hand
     M60.849   Other myositis, unspecified hand

✓6th **M60.85**   Other myositis, thigh
     M60.851   Other myositis, right thigh
     M60.852   Other myositis, left thigh
     M60.859   Other myositis, unspecified thigh

✓6th **M60.86**   Other myositis, lower leg
     M60.861   Other myositis, right lower leg
     M60.862   Other myositis, left lower leg
     M60.869   Other myositis, unspecified lower leg

✓6th **M60.87**   Other myositis, ankle and foot
     M60.871   Other myositis, right ankle and foot
     M60.872   Other myositis, left ankle and foot
     M60.879   Other myositis, unspecified ankle and foot

     M60.88   Other myositis, other site
     M60.89   Other myositis, multiple sites

M60.9   Myositis, unspecified

✓4th **M61**   **Calcification and ossification of muscle**

✓5th **M61.0**   **Myositis ossificans** traumatica
     M61.00   Myositis ossificans traumatica, unspecified site

✓6th **M61.01**   Myositis ossificans traumatica, shoulder
     M61.011   Myositis ossificans traumatica, right shoulder
     M61.012   Myositis ossificans traumatica, left shoulder
     M61.019   Myositis ossificans traumatica, unspecified shoulder

✓6th **M61.02**   Myositis ossificans traumatica, upper arm
     M61.021   Myositis ossificans traumatica, right upper arm
     M61.022   Myositis ossificans traumatica, left upper arm
     M61.029   Myositis ossificans traumatica, unspecified upper arm

✓6th **M61.03**   Myositis ossificans traumatica, forearm
     M61.031   Myositis ossificans traumatica, right forearm
     M61.032   Myositis ossificans traumatica, left forearm
     M61.039   Myositis ossificans traumatica, unspecified forearm

✓6th **M61.04**   Myositis ossificans traumatica, hand
     M61.041   Myositis ossificans traumatica, right hand
     M61.042   Myositis ossificans traumatica, left hand
     M61.049   Myositis ossificans traumatica, unspecified hand

✓6th **M61.05**   Myositis ossificans traumatica, thigh
     M61.051   Myositis ossificans traumatica, right thigh
     M61.052   Myositis ossificans traumatica, left thigh
     M61.059   Myositis ossificans traumatica, unspecified thigh

✓6th **M61.06**   Myositis ossificans traumatica, lower leg
     M61.061   Myositis ossificans traumatica, right lower leg
     M61.062   Myositis ossificans traumatica, left lower leg
     M61.069   Myositis ossificans traumatica, unspecified lower leg

✓6th **M61.07**   Myositis ossificans traumatica, ankle and foot
     M61.071   Myositis ossificans traumatica, right ankle and foot
     M61.072   Myositis ossificans traumatica, left ankle and foot
     M61.079   Myositis ossificans traumatica, unspecified ankle and foot

     M61.08   Myositis ossificans traumatica, other site

M61.09   Myositis ossificans traumatica, multiple sites

✓5th **M61.1**   **Myositis ossificans** progressiva
     Fibrodysplasia ossificans progressiva
     M61.10   Myositis ossificans progressiva, unspecified site

✓6th **M61.11**   Myositis ossificans progressiva, shoulder
     M61.111   Myositis ossificans progressiva, right shoulder
     M61.112   Myositis ossificans progressiva, left shoulder
     M61.119   Myositis ossificans progressiva, unspecified shoulder

✓6th **M61.12**   Myositis ossificans progressiva, upper arm
     M61.121   Myositis ossificans progressiva, right upper arm
     M61.122   Myositis ossificans progressiva, left upper arm
     M61.129   Myositis ossificans progressiva, unspecified arm

✓6th **M61.13**   Myositis ossificans progressiva, forearm
     M61.131   Myositis ossificans progressiva, right forearm
     M61.132   Myositis ossificans progressiva, left forearm
     M61.139   Myositis ossificans progressiva, unspecified forearm

✓6th **M61.14**   Myositis ossificans progressiva, hand and finger(s)
     M61.141   Myositis ossificans progressiva, right hand
     M61.142   Myositis ossificans progressiva, left hand
     M61.143   Myositis ossificans progressiva, unspecified hand
     M61.144   Myositis ossificans progressiva, right finger(s)
     M61.145   Myositis ossificans progressiva, left finger(s)
     M61.146   Myositis ossificans progressiva, unspecified finger(s)

✓6th **M61.15**   Myositis ossificans progressiva, thigh
     M61.151   Myositis ossificans progressiva, right thigh
     M61.152   Myositis ossificans progressiva, left thigh
     M61.159   Myositis ossificans progressiva, unspecified thigh

✓6th **M61.16**   Myositis ossificans progressiva, lower leg
     M61.161   Myositis ossificans progressiva, right lower leg
     M61.162   Myositis ossificans progressiva, left lower leg
     M61.169   Myositis ossificans progressiva, unspecified lower leg

✓6th **M61.17**   Myositis ossificans progressiva, ankle, foot and toe(s)
     M61.171   Myositis ossificans progressiva, right ankle
     M61.172   Myositis ossificans progressiva, left ankle
     M61.173   Myositis ossificans progressiva, unspecified ankle
     M61.174   Myositis ossificans progressiva, right foot
     M61.175   Myositis ossificans progressiva, left foot
     M61.176   Myositis ossificans progressiva, unspecified foot
     M61.177   Myositis ossificans progressiva, right toe(s)
     M61.178   Myositis ossificans progressiva, left toe(s)
     M61.179   Myositis ossificans progressiva, unspecified toe(s)

     M61.18   Myositis ossificans progressiva, other site
     M61.19   Myositis ossificans progressiva, multiple sites

✓5th **M61.2**   **Paralytic** calcification and ossification of muscle
     Myositis ossificans associated with quadriplegia or paraplegia
     M61.20   Paralytic calcification and ossification of muscle, unspecified site

✓6th **M61.21**   Paralytic calcification and ossification of muscle, shoulder
     M61.211   Paralytic calcification and ossification of muscle, right shoulder

✓ Additional Character Required   ✓x7th Placeholder   Unacceptable PDx   Questionable PDx   Manifestation   H1-H14 HAC   HCC CMS-HCC Dx   HIV HIV Dx

ICD-10-CM 2019

787

M61.212 Paralytic calcification and ossification of muscle, left shoulder

M61.219 Paralytic calcification and ossification of muscle, unspecified shoulder

✓6ᵗʰ M61.22 Paralytic calcification and ossification of muscle, upper arm

M61.221 Paralytic calcification and ossification of muscle, right upper arm

M61.222 Paralytic calcification and ossification of muscle, left upper arm

M61.229 Paralytic calcification and ossification of muscle, unspecified upper arm

✓6ᵗʰ M61.23 Paralytic calcification and ossification of muscle, forearm

M61.231 Paralytic calcification and ossification of muscle, right forearm

M61.232 Paralytic calcification and ossification of muscle, left forearm

M61.239 Paralytic calcification and ossification of muscle, unspecified forearm

✓6ᵗʰ M61.24 Paralytic calcification and ossification of muscle, hand

M61.241 Paralytic calcification and ossification of muscle, right hand

M61.242 Paralytic calcification and ossification of muscle, left hand

M61.249 Paralytic calcification and ossification of muscle, unspecified hand

✓6ᵗʰ M61.25 Paralytic calcification and ossification of muscle, thigh

M61.251 Paralytic calcification and ossification of muscle, right thigh

M61.252 Paralytic calcification and ossification of muscle, left thigh

M61.259 Paralytic calcification and ossification of muscle, unspecified thigh

✓6ᵗʰ M61.26 Paralytic calcification and ossification of muscle, lower leg

M61.261 Paralytic calcification and ossification of muscle, right lower leg

M61.262 Paralytic calcification and ossification of muscle, left lower leg

M61.269 Paralytic calcification and ossification of muscle, unspecified lower leg

✓6ᵗʰ M61.27 Paralytic calcification and ossification of muscle, ankle and foot

M61.271 Paralytic calcification and ossification of muscle, right ankle and foot

M61.272 Paralytic calcification and ossification of muscle, left ankle and foot

M61.279 Paralytic calcification and ossification of muscle, unspecified ankle and foot

M61.28 Paralytic calcification and ossification of muscle, other site

M61.29 Paralytic calcification and ossification of muscle, multiple sites

✓5ᵗʰ M61.3 Calcification and ossification of muscles associated with burns

Myositis ossificans associated with burns

M61.30 Calcification and ossification of muscles associated with burns, unspecified site

✓6ᵗʰ M61.31 Calcification and ossification of muscles associated with burns, shoulder

M61.311 Calcification and ossification of muscles associated with burns, right shoulder

M61.312 Calcification and ossification of muscles associated with burns, left shoulder

M61.319 Calcification and ossification of muscles associated with burns, unspecified shoulder

✓6ᵗʰ M61.32 Calcification and ossification of muscles associated with burns, upper arm

M61.321 Calcification and ossification of muscles associated with burns, right upper arm

M61.322 Calcification and ossification of muscles associated with burns, left upper arm

M61.329 Calcification and ossification of muscles associated with burns, unspecified upper arm

✓6ᵗʰ M61.33 Calcification and ossification of muscles associated with burns, forearm

M61.331 Calcification and ossification of muscles associated with burns, right forearm

M61.332 Calcification and ossification of muscles associated with burns, left forearm

M61.339 Calcification and ossification of muscles associated with burns, unspecified forearm

✓6ᵗʰ M61.34 Calcification and ossification of muscles associated with burns, hand

M61.341 Calcification and ossification of muscles associated with burns, right hand

M61.342 Calcification and ossification of muscles associated with burns, left hand

M61.349 Calcification and ossification of muscles associated with burns, unspecified hand

✓6ᵗʰ M61.35 Calcification and ossification of muscles associated with burns, thigh

M61.351 Calcification and ossification of muscles associated with burns, right thigh

M61.352 Calcification and ossification of muscles associated with burns, left thigh

M61.359 Calcification and ossification of muscles associated with burns, unspecified thigh

✓6ᵗʰ M61.36 Calcification and ossification of muscles associated with burns, lower leg

M61.361 Calcification and ossification of muscles associated with burns, right lower leg

M61.362 Calcification and ossification of muscles associated with burns, left lower leg

M61.369 Calcification and ossification of muscles associated with burns, unspecified lower leg

✓6ᵗʰ M61.37 Calcification and ossification of muscles associated with burns, ankle and foot

M61.371 Calcification and ossification of muscles associated with burns, right ankle and foot

M61.372 Calcification and ossification of muscles associated with burns, left ankle and foot

M61.379 Calcification and ossification of muscles associated with burns, unspecified ankle and foot

M61.38 Calcification and ossification of muscles associated with burns, other site

M61.39 Calcification and ossification of muscles associated with burns, multiple sites

✓5ᵗʰ M61.4 Other calcification of muscle

EXCLUDES 1   calcific tendinitis NOS (M65.2-)
calcific tendinitis of shoulder (M75.3)

M61.40 Other calcification of muscle, unspecified site

✓6ᵗʰ M61.41 Other calcification of muscle, shoulder

M61.411 Other calcification of muscle, right shoulder

M61.412 Other calcification of muscle, left shoulder

M61.419 Other calcification of muscle, unspecified shoulder

✓6ᵗʰ M61.42 Other calcification of muscle, upper arm

M61.421 Other calcification of muscle, right upper arm

M61.422 Other calcification of muscle, left upper arm

M61.429 Other calcification of muscle, unspecified upper arm

✓6ᵗʰ M61.43 Other calcification of muscle, forearm

M61.431 Other calcification of muscle, right forearm

M61.432 Other calcification of muscle, left forearm

M61.439 Other calcification of muscle, unspecified forearm

N Newborn: 0   P Pediatric: 0-17   M Maternity: 12-55   A Adult: 15-124   MCC Major Complication/Comorbidity   CC Complication/Comorbidity   SW Severe Wound Dx

788   ICD-10-CM 2019

✓6ᵗʰ **M61.44** Other calcification of muscle, hand
   M61.441 Other calcification of muscle, right hand
   M61.442 Other calcification of muscle, left hand
   M61.449 Other calcification of muscle, unspecified hand

✓6ᵗʰ **M61.45** Other calcification of muscle, thigh
   M61.451 Other calcification of muscle, right thigh
   M61.452 Other calcification of muscle, left thigh
   M61.459 Other calcification of muscle, unspecified thigh

✓6ᵗʰ **M61.46** Other calcification of muscle, lower leg
   M61.461 Other calcification of muscle, right lower leg
   M61.462 Other calcification of muscle, left lower leg
   M61.469 Other calcification of muscle, unspecified lower leg

✓6ᵗʰ **M61.47** Other calcification of muscle, ankle and foot
   M61.471 Other calcification of muscle, right ankle and foot
   M61.472 Other calcification of muscle, left ankle and foot
   M61.479 Other calcification of muscle, unspecified ankle and foot

   M61.48 Other calcification of muscle, other site
   M61.49 Other calcification of muscle, multiple sites

✓5ᵗʰ **M61.5** Other ossification of muscle
   M61.50 Other ossification of muscle, unspecified site

✓6ᵗʰ **M61.51** Other ossification of muscle, shoulder
   M61.511 Other ossification of muscle, right shoulder
   M61.512 Other ossification of muscle, left shoulder
   M61.519 Other ossification of muscle, unspecified shoulder

✓6ᵗʰ **M61.52** Other ossification of muscle, upper arm
   M61.521 Other ossification of muscle, right upper arm
   M61.522 Other ossification of muscle, left upper arm
   M61.529 Other ossification of muscle, unspecified upper arm

✓6ᵗʰ **M61.53** Other ossification of muscle, forearm
   M61.531 Other ossification of muscle, right forearm
   M61.532 Other ossification of muscle, left forearm
   M61.539 Other ossification of muscle, unspecified forearm

✓6ᵗʰ **M61.54** Other ossification of muscle, hand
   M61.541 Other ossification of muscle, right hand
   M61.542 Other ossification of muscle, left hand
   M61.549 Other ossification of muscle, unspecified hand

✓6ᵗʰ **M61.55** Other ossification of muscle, thigh
   M61.551 Other ossification of muscle, right thigh
   M61.552 Other ossification of muscle, left thigh
   M61.559 Other ossification of muscle, unspecified thigh

✓6ᵗʰ **M61.56** Other ossification of muscle, lower leg
   M61.561 Other ossification of muscle, right lower leg
   M61.562 Other ossification of muscle, left lower leg
   M61.569 Other ossification of muscle, unspecified lower leg

✓6ᵗʰ **M61.57** Other ossification of muscle, ankle and foot
   M61.571 Other ossification of muscle, right ankle and foot
   M61.572 Other ossification of muscle, left ankle and foot
   M61.579 Other ossification of muscle, unspecified ankle and foot

   M61.58 Other ossification of muscle, other site
   M61.59 Other ossification of muscle, multiple sites
M61.9 Calcification and ossification of muscle, unspecified

✓4ᵗʰ **M62** Other disorders of muscle
   EXCLUDES 1   alcoholic myopathy (G72.1)
     cramp and spasm (R25.2)
     drug-induced myopathy (G72.0)
     myalgia ►(M79.1-)◄
     stiff-man syndrome (G25.82)
   EXCLUDES 2   nontraumatic hematoma of muscle (M79.81)

✓5ᵗʰ **M62.0** Separation of muscle (nontraumatic)
   Diastasis of muscle
   EXCLUDES 1   diastasis recti complicating pregnancy, labor and delivery (O71.8)
     traumatic separation of muscle—see strain of muscle by body region
   M62.00 Separation of muscle (nontraumatic), unspecified site

✓6ᵗʰ **M62.01** Separation of muscle (nontraumatic), shoulder
   M62.011 Separation of muscle (nontraumatic), right shoulder
   M62.012 Separation of muscle (nontraumatic), left shoulder
   M62.019 Separation of muscle (nontraumatic), unspecified shoulder

✓6ᵗʰ **M62.02** Separation of muscle (nontraumatic), upper arm
   M62.021 Separation of muscle (nontraumatic), right upper arm
   M62.022 Separation of muscle (nontraumatic), left upper arm
   M62.029 Separation of muscle (nontraumatic), unspecified upper arm

✓6ᵗʰ **M62.03** Separation of muscle (nontraumatic), forearm
   M62.031 Separation of muscle (nontraumatic), right forearm
   M62.032 Separation of muscle (nontraumatic), left forearm
   M62.039 Separation of muscle (nontraumatic), unspecified forearm

✓6ᵗʰ **M62.04** Separation of muscle (nontraumatic), hand
   M62.041 Separation of muscle (nontraumatic), right hand
   M62.042 Separation of muscle (nontraumatic), left hand
   M62.049 Separation of muscle (nontraumatic), unspecified hand

✓6ᵗʰ **M62.05** Separation of muscle (nontraumatic), thigh
   M62.051 Separation of muscle (nontraumatic), right thigh
   M62.052 Separation of muscle (nontraumatic), left thigh
   M62.059 Separation of muscle (nontraumatic), unspecified thigh

✓6ᵗʰ **M62.06** Separation of muscle (nontraumatic), lower leg
   M62.061 Separation of muscle (nontraumatic), right lower leg
   M62.062 Separation of muscle (nontraumatic), left lower leg
   M62.069 Separation of muscle (nontraumatic), unspecified lower leg

✓6ᵗʰ **M62.07** Separation of muscle (nontraumatic), ankle and foot
   M62.071 Separation of muscle (nontraumatic), right ankle and foot
   M62.072 Separation of muscle (nontraumatic), left ankle and foot
   M62.079 Separation of muscle (nontraumatic), unspecified ankle and foot

   M62.08 Separation of muscle (nontraumatic), other site

✓5ᵗʰ **M62.1** Other rupture of muscle (nontraumatic)
   EXCLUDES 1   traumatic rupture of muscle—see strain of muscle by body region
   EXCLUDES 2   rupture of tendon (M66.-)
   M62.10 Other rupture of muscle (nontraumatic), unspecified site

✓6ᵗʰ **M62.11** Other rupture of muscle (nontraumatic), shoulder
   M62.111 Other rupture of muscle (nontraumatic), right shoulder
   M62.112 Other rupture of muscle (nontraumatic), left shoulder

✓Additional Character Required   ✓7ᵗʰ Placeholder   Unacceptable PDx   Questionable PDx   Manifestation   H1-H14 HAC   HCC CMS-HCC Dx   HIV HIV Dx

ICD-10-CM 2019   789

M62.119   Other rupture of muscle (nontraumatic), unspecified **shoulder**

✓6ᵗʰ   **M62.12**   **Other rupture of muscle (nontraumatic),** upper arm

M62.121   **Other rupture of muscle (nontraumatic),** right **upper arm**

M62.122   **Other rupture of muscle (nontraumatic),** left **upper arm**

M62.129   **Other rupture of muscle (nontraumatic),** unspecified **upper arm**

✓6ᵗʰ   **M62.13**   **Other rupture of muscle (nontraumatic),** forearm

M62.131   **Other rupture of muscle (nontraumatic),** right **forearm**

M62.132   **Other rupture of muscle (nontraumatic),** left **forearm**

M62.139   **Other rupture of muscle (nontraumatic),** unspecified **forearm**

✓6ᵗʰ   **M62.14**   **Other rupture of muscle (nontraumatic),** hand

M62.141   **Other rupture of muscle (nontraumatic),** right **hand**

M62.142   **Other rupture of muscle (nontraumatic),** left **hand**

M62.149   **Other rupture of muscle (nontraumatic),** unspecified **hand**

✓6ᵗʰ   **M62.15**   **Other rupture of muscle (nontraumatic),** thigh

M62.151   **Other rupture of muscle (nontraumatic),** right **thigh**

M62.152   **Other rupture of muscle (nontraumatic),** left **thigh**

M62.159   **Other rupture of muscle (nontraumatic),** unspecified **thigh**

✓6ᵗʰ   **M62.16**   **Other rupture of muscle (nontraumatic),** lower leg

M62.161   **Other rupture of muscle (nontraumatic),** right **lower leg**

M62.162   **Other rupture of muscle (nontraumatic),** left **lower leg**

M62.169   **Other rupture of muscle (nontraumatic),** unspecified **lower leg**

✓6ᵗʰ   **M62.17**   **Other rupture of muscle (nontraumatic),** ankle and foot

M62.171   **Other rupture of muscle (nontraumatic),** right **ankle and foot**

M62.172   **Other rupture of muscle (nontraumatic),** left **ankle and foot**

M62.179   **Other rupture of muscle (nontraumatic),** unspecified **ankle and foot**

M62.18   **Other rupture of muscle (nontraumatic),** other site

✓5ᵗʰ   **M62.2**   **Nontraumatic ischemic infarction of muscle**

> **EXCLUDES 1**   *compartment syndrome (traumatic) (T79.A-)*
> *nontraumatic compartment syndrome (M79.A-)*
> *rhabdomyolysis (M62.82)*
> *traumatic ischemia of muscle (T79.6)*
> *Volkmann's ischemic contracture (T79.6)*

M62.20   **Nontraumatic ischemic infarction of muscle, unspecified site**

✓6ᵗʰ   **M62.21**   **Nontraumatic ischemic infarction of muscle,** shoulder

M62.211   **Nontraumatic ischemic infarction of muscle,** right **shoulder**

M62.212   **Nontraumatic ischemic infarction of muscle,** left **shoulder**

M62.219   **Nontraumatic ischemic infarction of muscle,** unspecified **shoulder**

✓6ᵗʰ   **M62.22**   **Nontraumatic ischemic infarction of muscle,** upper arm

M62.221   **Nontraumatic ischemic infarction of muscle,** right **upper arm**

M62.222   **Nontraumatic ischemic infarction of muscle,** left **upper arm**

M62.229   **Nontraumatic ischemic infarction of muscle,** unspecified **upper arm**

✓6ᵗʰ   **M62.23**   **Nontraumatic ischemic infarction of muscle,** forearm

M62.231   **Nontraumatic ischemic infarction of muscle,** right **forearm**

M62.232   **Nontraumatic ischemic infarction of muscle,** left **forearm**

M62.239   **Nontraumatic ischemic infarction of muscle,** unspecified **forearm**

✓6ᵗʰ   **M62.24**   **Nontraumatic ischemic infarction of muscle,** hand

M62.241   **Nontraumatic ischemic infarction of muscle,** right **hand**

M62.242   **Nontraumatic ischemic infarction of muscle,** left **hand**

M62.249   **Nontraumatic ischemic infarction of muscle,** unspecified **hand**

✓6ᵗʰ   **M62.25**   **Nontraumatic ischemic infarction of muscle,** thigh

M62.251   **Nontraumatic ischemic infarction of muscle,** right **thigh**

M62.252   **Nontraumatic ischemic infarction of muscle,** left **thigh**

M62.259   **Nontraumatic ischemic infarction of muscle,** unspecified **thigh**

✓6ᵗʰ   **M62.26**   **Nontraumatic ischemic infarction of muscle,** lower leg

M62.261   **Nontraumatic ischemic infarction of muscle,** right **lower leg**

M62.262   **Nontraumatic ischemic infarction of muscle,** left **lower leg**

M62.269   **Nontraumatic ischemic infarction of muscle,** unspecified **lower leg**

✓6ᵗʰ   **M62.27**   **Nontraumatic ischemic infarction of muscle,** ankle and foot

M62.271   **Nontraumatic ischemic infarction of muscle,** right **ankle and foot**

M62.272   **Nontraumatic ischemic infarction of muscle,** left **ankle and foot**

M62.279   **Nontraumatic ischemic infarction of muscle,** unspecified **ankle and foot**

M62.28   **Nontraumatic ischemic infarction of muscle,** other site

M62.3   **Immobility syndrome (paraplegic)**

✓5ᵗʰ   **M62.4**   **Contracture of muscle**

> Contracture of tendon (sheath)
> **EXCLUDES 1**   *contracture of joint (M24.5-)*

M62.40   **Contracture of muscle,** unspecified site

✓6ᵗʰ   **M62.41**   **Contracture of muscle,** shoulder

M62.411   **Contracture of muscle,** right **shoulder**

M62.412   **Contracture of muscle,** left **shoulder**

M62.419   **Contracture of muscle,** unspecified **shoulder**

✓6ᵗʰ   **M62.42**   **Contracture of muscle,** upper arm

M62.421   **Contracture of muscle,** right **upper arm**

M62.422   **Contracture of muscle,** left **upper arm**

M62.429   **Contracture of muscle,** unspecified **upper arm**

✓6ᵗʰ   **M62.43**   **Contracture of muscle,** forearm

M62.431   **Contracture of muscle,** right **forearm**

M62.432   **Contracture of muscle,** left **forearm**

M62.439   **Contracture of muscle,** unspecified **forearm**

✓6ᵗʰ   **M62.44**   **Contracture of muscle,** hand

M62.441   **Contracture of muscle,** right **hand**

M62.442   **Contracture of muscle,** left **hand**

M62.449   **Contracture of muscle,** unspecified **hand**

✓6ᵗʰ   **M62.45**   **Contracture of muscle,** thigh

M62.451   **Contracture of muscle,** right **thigh**

M62.452   **Contracture of muscle,** left **thigh**

M62.459   **Contracture of muscle,** unspecified **thigh**

✓6ᵗʰ   **M62.46**   **Contracture of muscle,** lower leg

M62.461   **Contracture of muscle,** right **lower leg**

M62.462   **Contracture of muscle,** left **lower leg**

M62.469   **Contracture of muscle,** unspecified **lower leg**

✓6ᵗʰ   **M62.47**   **Contracture of muscle,** ankle and foot

M62.471   **Contracture of muscle,** right **ankle and foot**

M62.472   **Contracture of muscle,** left **ankle and foot**

M62.479   **Contracture of muscle,** unspecified **ankle and foot**

M62.48   **Contracture of muscle,** other site

M62.49   **Contracture of muscle,** multiple sites

N Newborn: 0   **P** Pediatric: 0-17   **M** Maternity: 12-55   **A** Adult: 15-124   **MCC** Major Complication/Comorbidity   **CC** Complication/Comorbidity   **SW** Severe Wound Dx

790   ICD-10-CM 2019

✓5th **M62.5 Muscle wasting and atrophy, not elsewhere classified**
Disuse atrophy NEC

EXCLUDES 1   *neuralgic amyotrophy (G54.5)*
progressive muscular atrophy (G12.21)
sarcopenia (M62.84)

EXCLUDES 2   *pelvic muscle wasting (N81.84)*

     M62.50 Muscle wasting and atrophy, not elsewhere classified, unspecified site

✓6th   **M62.51 Muscle wasting and atrophy, not elsewhere classified,** shoulder

     M62.511 Muscle wasting and atrophy, not elsewhere classified, right **shoulder**

     M62.512 Muscle wasting and atrophy, not elsewhere classified, left **shoulder**

     M62.519 Muscle wasting and atrophy, not elsewhere classified, unspecified **shoulder**

✓6th   **M62.52 Muscle wasting and atrophy, not elsewhere classified,** upper arm

     M62.521 Muscle wasting and atrophy, not elsewhere classified, right **upper arm**

     M62.522 Muscle wasting and atrophy, not elsewhere classified, left **upper arm**

     M62.529 Muscle wasting and atrophy, not elsewhere classified, unspecified **upper arm**

✓6th   **M62.53 Muscle wasting and atrophy, not elsewhere classified,** forearm

     M62.531 Muscle wasting and atrophy, not elsewhere classified, right **forearm**

     M62.532 Muscle wasting and atrophy, not elsewhere classified, left **forearm**

     M62.539 Muscle wasting and atrophy, not elsewhere classified, unspecified **forearm**

✓6th   **M62.54 Muscle wasting and atrophy, not elsewhere classified,** hand

     M62.541 Muscle wasting and atrophy, not elsewhere classified, right **hand**

     M62.542 Muscle wasting and atrophy, not elsewhere classified, left **hand**

     M62.549 Muscle wasting and atrophy, not elsewhere classified, unspecified **hand**

✓6th   **M62.55 Muscle wasting and atrophy, not elsewhere classified,** thigh

     M62.551 Muscle wasting and atrophy, not elsewhere classified, right **thigh**

     M62.552 Muscle wasting and atrophy, not elsewhere classified, left **thigh**

     M62.559 Muscle wasting and atrophy, not elsewhere classified, unspecified **thigh**

✓6th   **M62.56 Muscle wasting and atrophy, not elsewhere classified,** lower leg

     M62.561 Muscle wasting and atrophy, not elsewhere classified, right **lower leg**

     M62.562 Muscle wasting and atrophy, not elsewhere classified, left **lower leg**

     M62.569 Muscle wasting and atrophy, not elsewhere classified, unspecified **lower leg**

✓6th   **M62.57 Muscle wasting and atrophy, not elsewhere classified,** ankle and foot

     M62.571 Muscle wasting and atrophy, not elsewhere classified, right **ankle and foot**

     M62.572 Muscle wasting and atrophy, not elsewhere classified, left **ankle and foot**

     M62.579 Muscle wasting and atrophy, not elsewhere classified, unspecified **ankle and foot**

     M62.58 Muscle wasting and atrophy, not elsewhere classified, other site

     M62.59 Muscle wasting and atrophy, not elsewhere classified, multiple sites

✓5th **M62.8 Other specified disorders of muscle**

EXCLUDES 2   *nontraumatic hematoma of muscle (M79.81)*

     M62.81 Muscle weakness (generalized)

EXCLUDES 1   *muscle weakness in sarcopenia (M62.84)*

     M62.82 Rhabdomyolysis   CC

EXCLUDES 1   *traumatic rhabdomyolysis (T79.6)*

DEF: Rapid disintegration or destruction of skeletal muscle caused by direct or indirect injury, resulting in the excretion of muscle protein myoglobin into the urine.

CC Excl: PDX collection 892

✓6th   **M62.83 Muscle spasm**

     M62.830 Muscle spasm of back

     M62.831 Muscle spasm of calf
Charley-horse

     M62.838 Other **muscle spasm**

     M62.84 Sarcopenia
Age-related sarcopenia
Code first underlying disease, if applicable, such as:
     disorders of myoneural junction and muscle disease in diseases classified elsewhere (G73.-)
     other and unspecified myopathies (G72.-)
     primary disorders of muscles (G71.-)

AHA: 2016, 4Q, 41

     M62.89 Other specified disorders of muscle
Muscle (sheath) hernia

M62.9 Disorder of muscle, unspecified

✓4th **M63 Disorders of muscle in diseases classified elsewhere**
Code first underlying disease, such as:
leprosy (A30.-)
neoplasm (C49-, C79.89, D21-, D48.1)
schistosomiasis (B65.-)
trichinellosis (B75)

EXCLUDES 1   *myopathy in cysticercosis (B69.81)*
myopathy in endocrine diseases (G73.7)
myopathy in metabolic diseases (G73.7)
myopathy in sarcoidosis (D86.87)
myopathy in secondary syphilis (A51.49)
myopathy in syphilis (late) (A52.78)
myopathy in toxoplasmosis (B58.82)
myopathy in tuberculosis (A18.09)

✓5th **M63.8 Disorders of muscle in diseases classified elsewhere**

     M63.80 Disorders of muscle in diseases classified elsewhere, unspecified site

✓6th   **M63.81 Disorders of muscle in diseases classified elsewhere,** shoulder

     M63.811 Disorders of muscle in diseases classified elsewhere, right **shoulder**

     M63.812 Disorders of muscle in diseases classified elsewhere, left **shoulder**

     M63.819 Disorders of muscle in diseases classified elsewhere, unspecified **shoulder**

✓6th   **M63.82 Disorders of muscle in diseases classified elsewhere,** upper arm

     M63.821 Disorders of muscle in diseases classified elsewhere, right **upper arm**

     M63.822 Disorders of muscle in diseases classified elsewhere, left **upper arm**

     M63.829 Disorders of muscle in diseases classified elsewhere, unspecified **upper arm**

✓6th   **M63.83 Disorders of muscle in diseases classified elsewhere,** forearm

     M63.831 Disorders of muscle in diseases classified elsewhere, right **forearm**

     M63.832 Disorders of muscle in diseases classified elsewhere, left **forearm**

     M63.839 Disorders of muscle in diseases classified elsewhere, unspecified **forearm**

✓6th   **M63.84 Disorders of muscle in diseases classified elsewhere,** hand

     M63.841 Disorders of muscle in diseases classified elsewhere, right **hand**

     M63.842 Disorders of muscle in diseases classified elsewhere, left **hand**

     M63.849 Disorders of muscle in diseases classified elsewhere, unspecified **hand**

✓ Additional Character Required   ✓x7th Placeholder   Unacceptable PDx   Questionable PDx   Manifestation   H1 - H14 HAC   HCC CMS-HCC Dx   HIV HIV Dx

ICD-10-CM 2019   791

Chapter 13. Diseases of the Musculoskeletal System and Connective Tissue

✓6ᵗʰ **M63.85** **Disorders of muscle in diseases classified elsewhere, thigh**

    M63.851 *Disorders of muscle in diseases classified elsewhere, right thigh*

    M63.852 *Disorders of muscle in diseases classified elsewhere, left thigh*

    M63.859 *Disorders of muscle in diseases classified elsewhere, unspecified thigh*

✓6ᵗʰ **M63.86** **Disorders of muscle in diseases classified elsewhere, lower leg**

    M63.861 *Disorders of muscle in diseases classified elsewhere, right lower leg*

    M63.862 *Disorders of muscle in diseases classified elsewhere, left lower leg*

    M63.869 *Disorders of muscle in diseases classified elsewhere, unspecified lower leg*

✓6ᵗʰ **M63.87** **Disorders of muscle in diseases classified elsewhere, ankle and foot**

    M63.871 *Disorders of muscle in diseases classified elsewhere, right ankle and foot*

    M63.872 *Disorders of muscle in diseases classified elsewhere, left ankle and foot*

    M63.879 *Disorders of muscle in diseases classified elsewhere, unspecified ankle and foot*

  M63.88 *Disorders of muscle in diseases classified elsewhere, other site*

  M63.89 *Disorders of muscle in diseases classified elsewhere, multiple sites*

Disorders of synovium and tendon (M65-M67)

✓4ᵗʰ **M65** **Synovitis and tenosynovitis**

  EXCLUDES 1   chronic crepitant synovitis of hand and wrist (M70.0-)
               current injury—see injury of ligament or tendon by body region
               soft tissue disorders related to use, overuse and pressure (M70.-)

✓5ᵗʰ **M65.0** **Abscess of tendon sheath**

    Use additional code (B95-B96) to identify bacterial agent.

  M65.00 **Abscess of tendon sheath, unspecified site**

✓6ᵗʰ **M65.01** **Abscess of tendon sheath, shoulder**

    M65.011 **Abscess of tendon sheath, right shoulder**

    M65.012 **Abscess of tendon sheath, left shoulder**

    M65.019 **Abscess of tendon sheath, unspecified shoulder**

✓6ᵗʰ **M65.02** **Abscess of tendon sheath, upper arm**

    M65.021 **Abscess of tendon sheath, right upper arm**

    M65.022 **Abscess of tendon sheath, left upper arm**

    M65.029 **Abscess of tendon sheath, unspecified upper arm**

✓6ᵗʰ **M65.03** **Abscess of tendon sheath, forearm**

    M65.031 **Abscess of tendon sheath, right forearm**

    M65.032 **Abscess of tendon sheath, left forearm**

    M65.039 **Abscess of tendon sheath, unspecified forearm**

✓6ᵗʰ **M65.04** **Abscess of tendon sheath, hand**

    M65.041 **Abscess of tendon sheath, right hand**

    M65.042 **Abscess of tendon sheath, left hand**

    M65.049 **Abscess of tendon sheath, unspecified hand**

✓6ᵗʰ **M65.05** **Abscess of tendon sheath, thigh**

    M65.051 **Abscess of tendon sheath, right thigh**

    M65.052 **Abscess of tendon sheath, left thigh**

    M65.059 **Abscess of tendon sheath, unspecified thigh**

✓6ᵗʰ **M65.06** **Abscess of tendon sheath, lower leg**

    M65.061 **Abscess of tendon sheath, right lower leg**

    M65.062 **Abscess of tendon sheath, left lower leg**

    M65.069 **Abscess of tendon sheath, unspecified lower leg**

✓6ᵗʰ **M65.07** **Abscess of tendon sheath, ankle and foot**

    M65.071 **Abscess of tendon sheath, right ankle and foot**

    M65.072 **Abscess of tendon sheath, left ankle and foot**

    M65.079 **Abscess of tendon sheath, unspecified ankle and foot**

  M65.08 **Abscess of tendon sheath, other site**

✓5ᵗʰ **M65.1** **Other infective (teno)synovitis**

  M65.10 **Other infective (teno)synovitis, unspecified site**

✓6ᵗʰ **M65.11** **Other infective (teno)synovitis, shoulder**

    M65.111 **Other infective (teno)synovitis, right shoulder**

    M65.112 **Other infective (teno)synovitis, left shoulder**

    M65.119 **Other infective (teno)synovitis, unspecified shoulder**

✓6ᵗʰ **M65.12** **Other infective (teno)synovitis, elbow**

    M65.121 **Other infective (teno)synovitis, right elbow**

    M65.122 **Other infective (teno)synovitis, left elbow**

    M65.129 **Other infective (teno)synovitis, unspecified elbow**

✓6ᵗʰ **M65.13** **Other infective (teno)synovitis, wrist**

    M65.131 **Other infective (teno)synovitis, right wrist**

    M65.132 **Other infective (teno)synovitis, left wrist**

    M65.139 **Other infective (teno)synovitis, unspecified wrist**

✓6ᵗʰ **M65.14** **Other infective (teno)synovitis, hand**

    M65.141 **Other infective (teno)synovitis, right hand**

    M65.142 **Other infective (teno)synovitis, left hand**

    M65.149 **Other infective (teno)synovitis, unspecified hand**

✓6ᵗʰ **M65.15** **Other infective (teno)synovitis, hip**

    M65.151 **Other infective (teno)synovitis, right hip**

    M65.152 **Other infective (teno)synovitis, left hip**

    M65.159 **Other infective (teno)synovitis, unspecified hip**

✓6ᵗʰ **M65.16** **Other infective (teno)synovitis, knee**

    M65.161 **Other infective (teno)synovitis, right knee**

    M65.162 **Other infective (teno)synovitis, left knee**

    M65.169 **Other infective (teno)synovitis, unspecified knee**

✓6ᵗʰ **M65.17** **Other infective (teno)synovitis, ankle and foot**

    M65.171 **Other infective (teno)synovitis, right ankle and foot**

    M65.172 **Other infective (teno)synovitis, left ankle and foot**

    M65.179 **Other infective (teno)synovitis, unspecified ankle and foot**

  M65.18 **Other infective (teno)synovitis, other site**

  M65.19 **Other infective (teno)synovitis, multiple sites**

✓5ᵗʰ **M65.2** **Calcific tendinitis**

  EXCLUDES 1   tendinitis as classified in M75-M77
               calcified tendinitis of shoulder (M75.3)

  M65.20 **Calcific tendinitis, unspecified site**

✓6ᵗʰ **M65.22** **Calcific tendinitis, upper arm**

    M65.221 **Calcific tendinitis, right upper arm**

    M65.222 **Calcific tendinitis, left upper arm**

    M65.229 **Calcific tendinitis, unspecified upper arm**

✓6ᵗʰ **M65.23** **Calcific tendinitis, forearm**

    M65.231 **Calcific tendinitis, right forearm**

    M65.232 **Calcific tendinitis, left forearm**

    M65.239 **Calcific tendinitis, unspecified forearm**

✓6ᵗʰ **M65.24** **Calcific tendinitis, hand**

    M65.241 **Calcific tendinitis, right hand**

    M65.242 **Calcific tendinitis, left hand**

    M65.249 **Calcific tendinitis, unspecified hand**

✓6ᵗʰ **M65.25** **Calcific tendinitis, thigh**

    M65.251 **Calcific tendinitis, right thigh**

    M65.252 **Calcific tendinitis, left thigh**

    M65.259 **Calcific tendinitis, unspecified thigh**

✓6ᵗʰ **M65.26** **Calcific tendinitis, lower leg**

    M65.261 **Calcific tendinitis, right lower leg**

    M65.262 **Calcific tendinitis, left lower leg**

    M65.269 **Calcific tendinitis, unspecified lower leg**

✓6ᵗʰ **M65.27** **Calcific tendinitis, ankle and foot**

    M65.271 **Calcific tendinitis, right ankle and foot**

    M65.272 **Calcific tendinitis, left ankle and foot**

    M65.279 **Calcific tendinitis, unspecified ankle and foot**

N Newborn: 0   **P** Pediatric: 0-17   **M** Maternity: 12-55   **A** Adult: 15-124   **MCC** Major Complication/Comorbidity   **CC** Complication/Comorbidity   **SW** Severe Wound Dx

792

ICD-10-CM 2019

M65.28 Calcific tendinitis, other site
M65.29 Calcific tendinitis, multiple sites

✓5ᵗʰ **M65.3 Trigger finger**
Nodular tendinous disease
M65.30 Trigger finger, unspecified finger

✓6ᵗʰ **M65.31 Trigger** thumb
M65.311 Trigger thumb, right thumb
M65.312 Trigger thumb, left thumb
M65.319 Trigger thumb, unspecified thumb

✓6ᵗʰ **M65.32 Trigger finger,** index finger
M65.321 Trigger finger, right index finger
M65.322 Trigger finger, left index finger
M65.329 Trigger finger, unspecified index finger

✓6ᵗʰ **M65.33 Trigger finger,** middle finger
M65.331 Trigger finger, right middle finger
M65.332 Trigger finger, left middle finger
M65.339 Trigger finger, unspecified middle finger

✓6ᵗʰ **M65.34 Trigger finger,** ring finger
M65.341 Trigger finger, right ring finger
M65.342 Trigger finger, left ring finger
M65.349 Trigger finger, unspecified ring finger

✓6ᵗʰ **M65.35 Trigger finger,** little finger
M65.351 Trigger finger, right little finger
M65.352 Trigger finger, left little finger
M65.359 Trigger finger, unspecified little finger

M65.4 Radial styloid tenosynovitis [de Quervain]

✓5ᵗʰ **M65.8 Other synovitis and tenosynovitis**
M65.80 Other synovitis and tenosynovitis, unspecified site

✓6ᵗʰ **M65.81 Other synovitis and tenosynovitis,** shoulder
M65.811 Other synovitis and tenosynovitis, right shoulder
M65.812 Other synovitis and tenosynovitis, left shoulder
M65.819 Other synovitis and tenosynovitis, unspecified shoulder

✓6ᵗʰ **M65.82 Other synovitis and tenosynovitis,** upper arm
M65.821 Other synovitis and tenosynovitis, right upper arm
M65.822 Other synovitis and tenosynovitis, left upper arm
M65.829 Other synovitis and tenosynovitis, unspecified upper arm

✓6ᵗʰ **M65.83 Other synovitis and tenosynovitis,** forearm
M65.831 Other synovitis and tenosynovitis, right forearm
M65.832 Other synovitis and tenosynovitis, left forearm
M65.839 Other synovitis and tenosynovitis, unspecified forearm

✓6ᵗʰ **M65.84 Other synovitis and tenosynovitis,** hand
M65.841 Other synovitis and tenosynovitis, right hand
M65.842 Other synovitis and tenosynovitis, left hand
M65.849 Other synovitis and tenosynovitis, unspecified hand

✓6ᵗʰ **M65.85 Other synovitis and tenosynovitis,** thigh
M65.851 Other synovitis and tenosynovitis, right thigh
M65.852 Other synovitis and tenosynovitis, left thigh
M65.859 Other synovitis and tenosynovitis, unspecified thigh

✓6ᵗʰ **M65.86 Other synovitis and tenosynovitis,** lower leg
M65.861 Other synovitis and tenosynovitis, right lower leg
M65.862 Other synovitis and tenosynovitis, left lower leg
M65.869 Other synovitis and tenosynovitis, unspecified lower leg

✓6ᵗʰ **M65.87 Other synovitis and tenosynovitis,** ankle and foot
M65.871 Other synovitis and tenosynovitis, right ankle and foot

M65.872 Other synovitis and tenosynovitis, left ankle and foot
M65.879 Other synovitis and tenosynovitis, unspecified ankle and foot

M65.88 Other synovitis and tenosynovitis, other site
M65.89 Other synovitis and tenosynovitis, multiple sites
M65.9 Synovitis and tenosynovitis, unspecified

✓4ᵗʰ **M66 Spontaneous rupture of synovium and tendon**
[INCLUDES] rupture that occurs when a normal force is applied to tissues that are inferred to have less than normal strength
[EXCLUDES 2] rotator cuff syndrome (M75.1-)
rupture where an abnormal force is applied to normal tissue—see injury of tendon by body region

M66.0 Rupture of popliteal cyst

✓5ᵗʰ **M66.1 Rupture of** synovium
Rupture of synovial cyst
[EXCLUDES 2] rupture of popliteal cyst (M66.0)
M66.10 Rupture of synovium, unspecified joint

✓6ᵗʰ **M66.11 Rupture of synovium,** shoulder
M66.111 Rupture of synovium, right shoulder
M66.112 Rupture of synovium, left shoulder
M66.119 Rupture of synovium, unspecified shoulder

✓6ᵗʰ **M66.12 Rupture of synovium,** elbow
M66.121 Rupture of synovium, right elbow
M66.122 Rupture of synovium, left elbow
M66.129 Rupture of synovium, unspecified elbow

✓6ᵗʰ **M66.13 Rupture of synovium,** wrist
M66.131 Rupture of synovium, right wrist
M66.132 Rupture of synovium, left wrist
M66.139 Rupture of synovium, unspecified wrist

✓6ᵗʰ **M66.14 Rupture of synovium,** hand and fingers
M66.141 Rupture of synovium, right hand
M66.142 Rupture of synovium, left hand
M66.143 Rupture of synovium, unspecified hand
M66.144 Rupture of synovium, right finger(s)
M66.145 Rupture of synovium, left finger(s)
M66.146 Rupture of synovium, unspecified finger(s)

✓6ᵗʰ **M66.15 Rupture of synovium,** hip
M66.151 Rupture of synovium, right hip
M66.152 Rupture of synovium, left hip
M66.159 Rupture of synovium, unspecified hip

✓6ᵗʰ **M66.17 Rupture of synovium,** ankle, foot and toes
M66.171 Rupture of synovium, right ankle
M66.172 Rupture of synovium, left ankle
M66.173 Rupture of synovium, unspecified ankle
M66.174 Rupture of synovium, right foot
M66.175 Rupture of synovium, left foot
M66.176 Rupture of synovium, unspecified foot
M66.177 Rupture of synovium, right toe(s)
M66.178 Rupture of synovium, left toe(s)
M66.179 Rupture of synovium, unspecified toe(s)

M66.18 Rupture of synovium, other site

✓5ᵗʰ **M66.2 Spontaneous rupture of** extensor tendons
TIP: Refer to the Muscle/Tendon table at the beginning of this chapter.
M66.20 Spontaneous rupture of extensor tendons, unspecified site

✓6ᵗʰ **M66.21 Spontaneous rupture of extensor tendons,** shoulder
M66.211 Spontaneous rupture of extensor tendons, right shoulder
M66.212 Spontaneous rupture of extensor tendons, left shoulder
M66.219 Spontaneous rupture of extensor tendons, unspecified shoulder

✓6ᵗʰ **M66.22 Spontaneous rupture of extensor tendons,** upper arm
M66.221 Spontaneous rupture of extensor tendons, right upper arm
M66.222 Spontaneous rupture of extensor tendons, left upper arm
M66.229 Spontaneous rupture of extensor tendons, unspecified upper arm

✓6ᵗʰ **M66.23** Spontaneous rupture of extensor tendons, forearm

     M66.231 Spontaneous rupture of extensor tendons, right forearm

     M66.232 Spontaneous rupture of extensor tendons, left forearm

     M66.239 Spontaneous rupture of extensor tendons, unspecified forearm

✓6ᵗʰ **M66.24** Spontaneous rupture of extensor tendons, hand

     M66.241 Spontaneous rupture of extensor tendons, right hand

     M66.242 Spontaneous rupture of extensor tendons, left hand

     M66.249 Spontaneous rupture of extensor tendons, unspecified hand

✓6ᵗʰ **M66.25** Spontaneous rupture of extensor tendons, thigh

     M66.251 Spontaneous rupture of extensor tendons, right thigh

     M66.252 Spontaneous rupture of extensor tendons, left thigh

     M66.259 Spontaneous rupture of extensor tendons, unspecified thigh

✓6ᵗʰ **M66.26** Spontaneous rupture of extensor tendons, lower leg

     M66.261 Spontaneous rupture of extensor tendons, right lower leg

     M66.262 Spontaneous rupture of extensor tendons, left lower leg

     M66.269 Spontaneous rupture of extensor tendons, unspecified lower leg

✓6ᵗʰ **M66.27** Spontaneous rupture of extensor tendons, ankle and foot

     M66.271 Spontaneous rupture of extensor tendons, right ankle and foot

     M66.272 Spontaneous rupture of extensor tendons, left ankle and foot

     M66.279 Spontaneous rupture of extensor tendons, unspecified ankle and foot

M66.28 Spontaneous rupture of extensor tendons, other site

M66.29 Spontaneous rupture of extensor tendons, multiple sites

✓5ᵗʰ **M66.3** Spontaneous rupture of flexor tendons

     TIP: Refer to the Muscle/Tendon table at the beginning of this chapter.

     M66.30 Spontaneous rupture of flexor tendons, unspecified site

✓6ᵗʰ **M66.31** Spontaneous rupture of flexor tendons, shoulder

     M66.311 Spontaneous rupture of flexor tendons, right shoulder

     M66.312 Spontaneous rupture of flexor tendons, left shoulder

     M66.319 Spontaneous rupture of flexor tendons, unspecified shoulder

✓6ᵗʰ **M66.32** Spontaneous rupture of flexor tendons, upper arm

     M66.321 Spontaneous rupture of flexor tendons, right upper arm

     M66.322 Spontaneous rupture of flexor tendons, left upper arm

     M66.329 Spontaneous rupture of flexor tendons, unspecified upper arm

✓6ᵗʰ **M66.33** Spontaneous rupture of flexor tendons, forearm

     M66.331 Spontaneous rupture of flexor tendons, right forearm

     M66.332 Spontaneous rupture of flexor tendons, left forearm

     M66.339 Spontaneous rupture of flexor tendons, unspecified forearm

✓6ᵗʰ **M66.34** Spontaneous rupture of flexor tendons, hand

     M66.341 Spontaneous rupture of flexor tendons, right hand

     M66.342 Spontaneous rupture of flexor tendons, left hand

     M66.349 Spontaneous rupture of flexor tendons, unspecified hand

✓6ᵗʰ **M66.35** Spontaneous rupture of flexor tendons, thigh

     M66.351 Spontaneous rupture of flexor tendons, right thigh

     M66.352 Spontaneous rupture of flexor tendons, left thigh

     M66.359 Spontaneous rupture of flexor tendons, unspecified thigh

✓6ᵗʰ **M66.36** Spontaneous rupture of flexor tendons, lower leg

     M66.361 Spontaneous rupture of flexor tendons, right lower leg

     M66.362 Spontaneous rupture of flexor tendons, left lower leg

     M66.369 Spontaneous rupture of flexor tendons, unspecified lower leg

✓6ᵗʰ **M66.37** Spontaneous rupture of flexor tendons, ankle and foot

     M66.371 Spontaneous rupture of flexor tendons, right ankle and foot

     M66.372 Spontaneous rupture of flexor tendons, left ankle and foot

     M66.379 Spontaneous rupture of flexor tendons, unspecified ankle and foot

M66.38 Spontaneous rupture of flexor tendons, other site

M66.39 Spontaneous rupture of flexor tendons, multiple sites

✓5ᵗʰ **M66.8** Spontaneous rupture of other tendons

     TIP: Refer to the Muscle/Tendon table at the beginning of this chapter.

     M66.80 Spontaneous rupture of other tendons, unspecified site

✓6ᵗʰ **M66.81** Spontaneous rupture of other tendons, shoulder

     M66.811 Spontaneous rupture of other tendons, right shoulder

     M66.812 Spontaneous rupture of other tendons, left shoulder

     M66.819 Spontaneous rupture of other tendons, unspecified shoulder

✓6ᵗʰ **M66.82** Spontaneous rupture of other tendons, upper arm

     M66.821 Spontaneous rupture of other tendons, right upper arm

     M66.822 Spontaneous rupture of other tendons, left upper arm

     M66.829 Spontaneous rupture of other tendons, unspecified upper arm

✓6ᵗʰ **M66.83** Spontaneous rupture of other tendons, forearm

     M66.831 Spontaneous rupture of other tendons, right forearm

     M66.832 Spontaneous rupture of other tendons, left forearm

     M66.839 Spontaneous rupture of other tendons, unspecified forearm

✓6ᵗʰ **M66.84** Spontaneous rupture of other tendons, hand

     M66.841 Spontaneous rupture of other tendons, right hand

     M66.842 Spontaneous rupture of other tendons, left hand

     M66.849 Spontaneous rupture of other tendons, unspecified hand

✓6ᵗʰ **M66.85** Spontaneous rupture of other tendons, thigh

     M66.851 Spontaneous rupture of other tendons, right thigh

     M66.852 Spontaneous rupture of other tendons, left thigh

     M66.859 Spontaneous rupture of other tendons, unspecified thigh

✓6ᵗʰ **M66.86** Spontaneous rupture of other tendons, lower leg

     M66.861 Spontaneous rupture of other tendons, right lower leg

     M66.862 Spontaneous rupture of other tendons, left lower leg

     M66.869 Spontaneous rupture of other tendons, unspecified lower leg

✓6ᵗʰ **M66.87** Spontaneous rupture of other tendons, ankle and foot

     M66.871 Spontaneous rupture of other tendons, right ankle and foot

     M66.872 Spontaneous rupture of other tendons, left ankle and foot

     M66.879 Spontaneous rupture of other tendons, unspecified ankle and foot

M66.88 Spontaneous rupture of other tendons, other

Ⓝ Newborn: 0   Ⓟ Pediatric: 0-17   Ⓜ Maternity: 12-55   Ⓐ Adult: 15-124   ᴹᶜᶜ Major Complication/Comorbidity   ᶜᶜ Complication/Comorbidity   ˢᵂ Severe Wound Dx

794   ICD-10-CM 2019

M66.89   **Spontaneous rupture of other tendons,** multiple sites

M66.9   **Spontaneous rupture of** unspecified tendon
Rupture at musculotendinous junction, nontraumatic

✓4th **M67   Other disorders of synovium and tendon**
     EXCLUDES 1   *palmar fascial fibromatosis [Dupuytren] (M72.0)*
                 tendinitis NOS (M77.9-)
                 xanthomatosis localized to tendons (E78.2)

✓5th **M67.0   Short Achilles tendon (acquired)**

M67.00   **Short Achilles tendon (acquired),** unspecified ankle

M67.01   **Short Achilles tendon (acquired),** right ankle

M67.02   **Short Achilles tendon (acquired),** left ankle

✓5th **M67.2   Synovial hypertrophy, not elsewhere classified**
     EXCLUDES 1   *villonodular synovitis (pigmented) (M12.2-)*

M67.20   **Synovial hypertrophy, not elsewhere classified,** unspecified site

✓6th M67.21   **Synovial hypertrophy, not elsewhere classified,** shoulder

     M67.211   **Synovial hypertrophy, not elsewhere classified,** right shoulder

     M67.212   **Synovial hypertrophy, not elsewhere classified,** left shoulder

     M67.219   **Synovial hypertrophy, not elsewhere classified,** unspecified shoulder

✓6th M67.22   **Synovial hypertrophy, not elsewhere classified,** upper arm

     M67.221   **Synovial hypertrophy, not elsewhere classified,** right upper arm

     M67.222   **Synovial hypertrophy, not elsewhere classified,** left upper arm

     M67.229   **Synovial hypertrophy, not elsewhere classified,** unspecified upper arm

✓6th M67.23   **Synovial hypertrophy, not elsewhere classified,** forearm

     M67.231   **Synovial hypertrophy, not elsewhere classified,** right forearm

     M67.232   **Synovial hypertrophy, not elsewhere classified,** left forearm

     M67.239   **Synovial hypertrophy, not elsewhere classified,** unspecified forearm

✓6th M67.24   **Synovial hypertrophy, not elsewhere classified,** hand

     M67.241   **Synovial hypertrophy, not elsewhere classified,** right hand

     M67.242   **Synovial hypertrophy, not elsewhere classified,** left hand

     M67.249   **Synovial hypertrophy, not elsewhere classified,** unspecified hand

✓6th M67.25   **Synovial hypertrophy, not elsewhere classified,** thigh

     M67.251   **Synovial hypertrophy, not elsewhere classified,** right thigh

     M67.252   **Synovial hypertrophy, not elsewhere classified,** left thigh

     M67.259   **Synovial hypertrophy, not elsewhere classified,** unspecified thigh

✓6th M67.26   **Synovial hypertrophy, not elsewhere classified,** lower leg

     M67.261   **Synovial hypertrophy, not elsewhere classified,** right lower leg

     M67.262   **Synovial hypertrophy, not elsewhere classified,** left lower leg

     M67.269   **Synovial hypertrophy, not elsewhere classified,** unspecified lower leg

✓6th M67.27   **Synovial hypertrophy, not elsewhere classified,** ankle and foot

     M67.271   **Synovial hypertrophy, not elsewhere classified,** right ankle and foot

     M67.272   **Synovial hypertrophy, not elsewhere classified,** left ankle and foot

     M67.279   **Synovial hypertrophy, not elsewhere classified,** unspecified ankle and foot

M67.28   **Synovial hypertrophy, not elsewhere classified,** other site

M67.29   **Synovial hypertrophy, not elsewhere classified,** multiple sites

✓5th **M67.3   Transient synovitis**
Toxic synovitis
     EXCLUDES 1   *palindromic rheumatism (M12.3-)*

M67.30   **Transient synovitis,** unspecified site

✓6th M67.31   **Transient synovitis,** shoulder

     M67.311   **Transient synovitis,** right shoulder

     M67.312   **Transient synovitis,** left shoulder

     M67.319   **Transient synovitis,** unspecified shoulder

✓6th M67.32   **Transient synovitis,** elbow

     M67.321   **Transient synovitis,** right elbow

     M67.322   **Transient synovitis,** left elbow

     M67.329   **Transient synovitis,** unspecified elbow

✓6th M67.33   **Transient synovitis,** wrist

     M67.331   **Transient synovitis,** right wrist

     M67.332   **Transient synovitis,** left wrist

     M67.339   **Transient synovitis,** unspecified wrist

✓6th M67.34   **Transient synovitis,** hand

     M67.341   **Transient synovitis,** right hand

     M67.342   **Transient synovitis,** left hand

     M67.349   **Transient synovitis,** unspecified hand

✓6th M67.35   **Transient synovitis,** hip

     M67.351   **Transient synovitis,** right hip

     M67.352   **Transient synovitis,** left hip

     M67.359   **Transient synovitis,** unspecified hip

✓6th M67.36   **Transient synovitis,** knee

     M67.361   **Transient synovitis,** right knee

     M67.362   **Transient synovitis,** left knee

     M67.369   **Transient synovitis,** unspecified knee

✓6th M67.37   **Transient synovitis,** ankle and foot

     M67.371   **Transient synovitis,** right ankle and foot

     M67.372   **Transient synovitis,** left ankle and foot

     M67.379   **Transient synovitis,** unspecified ankle and foot

M67.38   **Transient synovitis,** other site

M67.39   **Transient synovitis,** multiple sites

✓5th **M67.4   Ganglion**
Ganglion of joint or tendon (sheath)
     EXCLUDES 1   *ganglion in yaws (A66.6)*
     EXCLUDES 2   *cyst of bursa (M71.2-M71.3)*
                 cyst of synovium (M71.2-M71.3)
     DEF: Fluid-filled, benign cyst appearing on a tendon sheath or aponeurosis, frequently connecting to an underlying joint.

M67.40   **Ganglion,** unspecified site

✓6th M67.41   **Ganglion,** shoulder

     M67.411   **Ganglion,** right shoulder

     M67.412   **Ganglion,** left shoulder

     M67.419   **Ganglion,** unspecified shoulder

✓6th M67.42   **Ganglion,** elbow

     M67.421   **Ganglion,** right elbow

     M67.422   **Ganglion,** left elbow

     M67.429   **Ganglion,** unspecified elbow

✓ Additional Character Required   ✓7th Placeholder   Unacceptable PDx   Questionable PDx   Manifestation   H1 - H14 HAC   HCC CMS-HCC Dx   HIV HIV Dx

ICD-10-CM 2019   795

Ganglion of Wrist

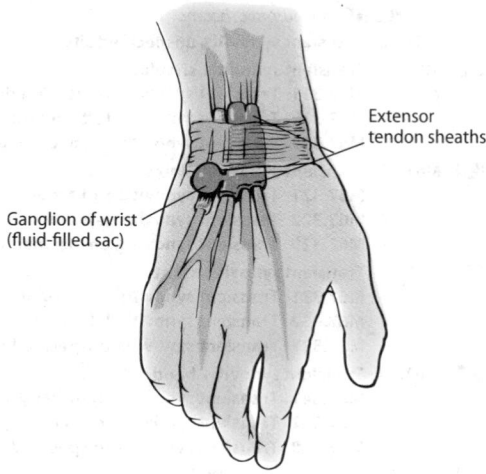

Extensor
tendon sheaths

Ganglion of wrist
(fluid-filled sac)

☑6ᵗʰ **M67.43 Ganglion,** wrist
    M67.431 Ganglion, right wrist
    M67.432 Ganglion, left wrist
    M67.439 Ganglion, unspecified wrist
☑6ᵗʰ **M67.44 Ganglion,** hand
    M67.441 Ganglion, right hand
    M67.442 Ganglion, left hand
    M67.449 Ganglion, unspecified hand
☑6ᵗʰ **M67.45 Ganglion,** hip
    M67.451 Ganglion, right hip
    M67.452 Ganglion, left hip
    M67.459 Ganglion, unspecified hip
☑6ᵗʰ **M67.46 Ganglion,** knee
    M67.461 Ganglion, right knee
    M67.462 Ganglion, left knee
    M67.469 Ganglion, unspecified knee
☑6ᵗʰ **M67.47 Ganglion,** ankle and foot
    M67.471 Ganglion, right ankle and foot
    M67.472 Ganglion, left ankle and foot
    M67.479 Ganglion, unspecified ankle and foot
  M67.48 Ganglion, other site
  M67.49 Ganglion, multiple sites
☑5ᵗʰ **M67.5 Plica syndrome**
    Plica knee
  M67.50 Plica syndrome, unspecified knee
  M67.51 Plica syndrome, right knee
  M67.52 Plica syndrome, left knee
☑5ᵗʰ **M67.8 Other specified disorders of synovium and tendon**
  M67.80 Other specified disorders of synovium and tendon, unspecified site
☑6ᵗʰ **M67.81 Other specified disorders of synovium and tendon,** shoulder
    M67.811 Other specified disorders of synovium, right shoulder
    M67.812 Other specified disorders of synovium, left shoulder
    M67.813 Other specified disorders of tendon, right shoulder
    M67.814 Other specified disorders of tendon, left shoulder
    M67.819 Other specified disorders of synovium and tendon, unspecified shoulder
☑6ᵗʰ **M67.82 Other specified disorders of synovium and tendon,** elbow
    M67.821 Other specified disorders of synovium, right elbow
    M67.822 Other specified disorders of synovium, left elbow
    M67.823 Other specified disorders of tendon, right elbow
    M67.824 Other specified disorders of tendon, left elbow

    M67.829 Other specified disorders of synovium and tendon, unspecified elbow
☑6ᵗʰ **M67.83 Other specified disorders of synovium and tendon,** wrist
    M67.831 Other specified disorders of synovium, right wrist
    M67.832 Other specified disorders of synovium, left wrist
    M67.833 Other specified disorders of tendon, right wrist
    M67.834 Other specified disorders of tendon, left wrist
    M67.839 Other specified disorders of synovium and tendon, unspecified forearm
☑6ᵗʰ **M67.84 Other specified disorders of synovium and tendon,** hand
    M67.841 Other specified disorders of synovium, right hand
    M67.842 Other specified disorders of synovium, left hand
    M67.843 Other specified disorders of tendon, right hand
    M67.844 Other specified disorders of tendon, left hand
    M67.849 Other specified disorders of synovium and tendon, unspecified hand
☑6ᵗʰ **M67.85 Other specified disorders of synovium and tendon,** hip
    M67.851 Other specified disorders of synovium, right hip
    M67.852 Other specified disorders of synovium, left hip
    M67.853 Other specified disorders of tendon, right hip
    M67.854 Other specified disorders of tendon, left hip
    M67.859 Other specified disorders of synovium and tendon, unspecified hip
☑6ᵗʰ **M67.86 Other specified disorders of synovium and tendon,** knee
    M67.861 Other specified disorders of synovium, right knee
    M67.862 Other specified disorders of synovium, left knee
    M67.863 Other specified disorders of tendon, right knee
    M67.864 Other specified disorders of tendon, left knee
    M67.869 Other specified disorders of synovium and tendon, unspecified knee
☑6ᵗʰ **M67.87 Other specified disorders of synovium and tendon,** ankle and foot
    M67.871 Other specified disorders of synovium, right ankle and foot
    M67.872 Other specified disorders of synovium, left ankle and foot
    M67.873 Other specified disorders of tendon, right ankle and foot
    M67.874 Other specified disorders of tendon, left ankle and foot
    M67.879 Other specified disorders of synovium and tendon, unspecified ankle and foot
  M67.88 Other specified disorders of synovium and tendon, other site
  M67.89 Other specified disorders of synovium and tendon, multiple sites
☑5ᵗʰ **M67.9 Unspecified disorder of synovium and tendon**
  M67.90 Unspecified disorder of synovium and tendon, unspecified site
☑6ᵗʰ **M67.91 Unspecified disorder of synovium and tendon,** shoulder
    M67.911 Unspecified disorder of synovium and tendon, right shoulder
    M67.912 Unspecified disorder of synovium and tendon, left shoulder
    M67.919 Unspecified disorder of synovium and tendon, unspecified shoulder

Ⓝ Newborn: 0   Ⓟ Pediatric: 0-17   Ⓜ Maternity: 12-55   Ⓐ Adult: 15-124   ᴹᶜᶜ Major Complication/Comorbidity   ᶜᶜ Complication/Comorbidity   ˢʷ Severe Wound Dx

796
ICD-10-CM 2019

✓6ᵗʰ M67.92 Unspecified disorder of synovium and tendon, upper arm

    M67.921 Unspecified disorder of synovium and tendon, right upper arm

    M67.922 Unspecified disorder of synovium and tendon, left upper arm

    M67.929 Unspecified disorder of synovium and tendon, unspecified upper arm

✓6ᵗʰ M67.93 Unspecified disorder of synovium and tendon, forearm

    M67.931 Unspecified disorder of synovium and tendon, right forearm

    M67.932 Unspecified disorder of synovium and tendon, left forearm

    M67.939 Unspecified disorder of synovium and tendon, unspecified forearm

✓6ᵗʰ M67.94 Unspecified disorder of synovium and tendon, hand

    M67.941 Unspecified disorder of synovium and tendon, right hand

    M67.942 Unspecified disorder of synovium and tendon, left hand

    M67.949 Unspecified disorder of synovium and tendon, unspecified hand

✓6ᵗʰ M67.95 Unspecified disorder of synovium and tendon, thigh

    M67.951 Unspecified disorder of synovium and tendon, right thigh

    M67.952 Unspecified disorder of synovium and tendon, left thigh

    M67.959 Unspecified disorder of synovium and tendon, unspecified thigh

✓6ᵗʰ M67.96 Unspecified disorder of synovium and tendon, lower leg

    M67.961 Unspecified disorder of synovium and tendon, right lower leg

    M67.962 Unspecified disorder of synovium and tendon, left lower leg

    M67.969 Unspecified disorder of synovium and tendon, unspecified lower leg

✓6ᵗʰ M67.97 Unspecified disorder of synovium and tendon, ankle and foot

    M67.971 Unspecified disorder of synovium and tendon, right ankle and foot

    M67.972 Unspecified disorder of synovium and tendon, left ankle and foot

    M67.979 Unspecified disorder of synovium and tendon, unspecified ankle and foot

    M67.98 Unspecified disorder of synovium and tendon, other site

    M67.99 Unspecified disorder of synovium and tendon, multiple sites

Other soft tissue disorders (M70-M79)

✓4ᵗʰ M70 Soft tissue disorders related to use, overuse and pressure

    INCLUDES soft tissue disorders of occupational origin

    Use additional external cause code to identify activity causing disorder (Y93.-)

    EXCLUDES 1 bursitis NOS (M71.9-)

    EXCLUDES 2 bursitis of shoulder (M75.5)
         enthesopathies (M76-M77)
         pressure ulcer (pressure area) (L89.-)

✓5ᵗʰ M70.0 Crepitant synovitis (acute) (chronic) of hand and wrist

  ✓6ᵗʰ M70.03 Crepitant synovitis (acute) (chronic), wrist

    M70.031 Crepitant synovitis (acute) (chronic), right wrist

    M70.032 Crepitant synovitis (acute) (chronic), left wrist

    M70.039 Crepitant synovitis (acute) (chronic), unspecified wrist

  ✓6ᵗʰ M70.04 Crepitant synovitis (acute) (chronic), hand

    M70.041 Crepitant synovitis (acute) (chronic), right hand

    M70.042 Crepitant synovitis (acute) (chronic), left hand

    M70.049 Crepitant synovitis (acute) (chronic), unspecified hand

✓5ᵗʰ M70.1 Bursitis of hand

    M70.10 Bursitis, unspecified hand

    M70.11 Bursitis, right hand

    M70.12 Bursitis, left hand

✓5ᵗʰ M70.2 Olecranon bursitis

    M70.20 Olecranon bursitis, unspecified elbow

    M70.21 Olecranon bursitis, right elbow

    M70.22 Olecranon bursitis, left elbow

✓5ᵗʰ M70.3 Other bursitis of elbow

    M70.30 Other bursitis of elbow, unspecified elbow

    M70.31 Other bursitis of elbow, right elbow

    M70.32 Other bursitis of elbow, left elbow

✓5ᵗʰ M70.4 Prepatellar bursitis

    M70.40 Prepatellar bursitis, unspecified knee

    M70.41 Prepatellar bursitis, right knee

    M70.42 Prepatellar bursitis, left knee

✓5ᵗʰ M70.5 Other bursitis of knee

    M70.50 Other bursitis of knee, unspecified knee

    M70.51 Other bursitis of knee, right knee

    M70.52 Other bursitis of knee, left knee

Knee Bursae

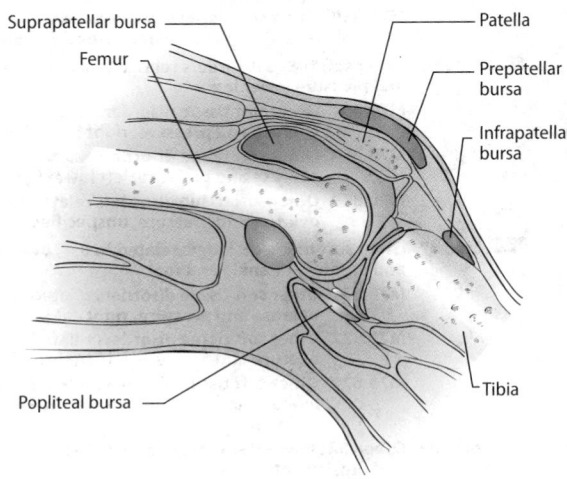

Suprapatellar bursa — Femur — Patella — Prepatellar bursa — Infrapatellar bursa — Popliteal bursa — Tibia

✓5ᵗʰ M70.6 Trochanteric bursitis
    Trochanteric tendinitis

    M70.60 Trochanteric bursitis, unspecified hip

    M70.61 Trochanteric bursitis, right hip

    M70.62 Trochanteric bursitis, left hip

✓5ᵗʰ M70.7 Other bursitis of hip
    Ischial bursitis

    M70.70 Other bursitis of hip, unspecified hip

    M70.71 Other bursitis of hip, right hip

    M70.72 Other bursitis of hip, left hip

✓5ᵗʰ M70.8 Other soft tissue disorders related to use, overuse and pressure

    M70.80 Other soft tissue disorders related to use, overuse and pressure of unspecified site

  ✓6ᵗʰ M70.81 Other soft tissue disorders related to use, overuse and pressure of shoulder

    M70.811 Other soft tissue disorders related to use, overuse and pressure, right shoulder

    M70.812 Other soft tissue disorders related to use, overuse and pressure, left shoulder

    M70.819 Other soft tissue disorders related to use, overuse and pressure, unspecified shoulder

  ✓6ᵗʰ M70.82 Other soft tissue disorders related to use, overuse and pressure of upper arm

    M70.821 Other soft tissue disorders related to use, overuse and pressure, right upper arm

    M70.822 Other soft tissue disorders related to use, overuse and pressure, left upper arm

    M70.829 Other soft tissue disorders related to use, overuse and pressure, unspecified upper arms

✓ Additional Character Required   ✓x7ᵗʰ Placeholder   Unacceptable PDx   Questionable PDx   Manifestation   H1-H14 HAC   HCC CMS-HCC Dx   HIV HIV Dx

ICD-10-CM 2019   797

✓6ᵗʰ **M70.83 Other soft tissue disorders related to use, overuse and pressure of** forearm

     M70.831 Other soft tissue disorders related to use, overuse and pressure, right forearm

     M70.832 Other soft tissue disorders related to use, overuse and pressure, left forearm

     M70.839 Other soft tissue disorders related to use, overuse and pressure, unspecified forearm

✓6ᵗʰ **M70.84 Other soft tissue disorders related to use, overuse and pressure of** hand

     M70.841 Other soft tissue disorders related to use, overuse and pressure, right hand

     M70.842 Other soft tissue disorders related to use, overuse and pressure, left hand

     M70.849 Other soft tissue disorders related to use, overuse and pressure, unspecified hand

✓6ᵗʰ **M70.85 Other soft tissue disorders related to use, overuse and pressure of** thigh

     M70.851 Other soft tissue disorders related to use, overuse and pressure, right thigh

     M70.852 Other soft tissue disorders related to use, overuse and pressure, left thigh

     M70.859 Other soft tissue disorders related to use, overuse and pressure, unspecified thigh

✓6ᵗʰ **M70.86 Other soft tissue disorders related to use, overuse and pressure** lower leg

     M70.861 Other soft tissue disorders related to use, overuse and pressure, right lower leg

     M70.862 Other soft tissue disorders related to use, overuse and pressure, left lower leg

     M70.869 Other soft tissue disorders related to use, overuse and pressure, unspecified leg

✓6ᵗʰ **M70.87 Other soft tissue disorders related to use, overuse and pressure of** ankle and foot

     M70.871 Other soft tissue disorders related to use, overuse and pressure, right ankle and foot

     M70.872 Other soft tissue disorders related to use, overuse and pressure, left ankle and foot

     M70.879 Other soft tissue disorders related to use, overuse and pressure, unspecified ankle and foot

M70.88 Other soft tissue disorders related to use, overuse and pressure other site

M70.89 Other soft tissue disorders related to use, overuse and pressure multiple sites

✓5ᵗʰ **M70.9 Unspecified soft tissue disorder related to use, overuse and pressure**

     M70.90 Unspecified soft tissue disorder related to use, overuse and pressure of unspecified site

✓6ᵗʰ   **M70.91 Unspecified soft tissue disorder related to use, overuse and pressure of** shoulder

     M70.911 Unspecified soft tissue disorder related to use, overuse and pressure, right shoulder

     M70.912 Unspecified soft tissue disorder related to use, overuse and pressure, left shoulder

     M70.919 Unspecified soft tissue disorder related to use, overuse and pressure, unspecified shoulder

✓6ᵗʰ   **M70.92 Unspecified soft tissue disorder related to use, overuse and pressure of** upper arm

     M70.921 Unspecified soft tissue disorder related to use, overuse and pressure, right upper arm

     M70.922 Unspecified soft tissue disorder related to use, overuse and pressure, left upper arm

     M70.929 Unspecified soft tissue disorder related to use, overuse and pressure, unspecified upper arm

✓6ᵗʰ   **M70.93 Unspecified soft tissue disorder related to use, overuse and pressure of** forearm

     M70.931 Unspecified soft tissue disorder related to use, overuse and pressure, right forearm

     M70.932 Unspecified soft tissue disorder related to use, overuse and pressure, left forearm

     M70.939 Unspecified soft tissue disorder related to use, overuse and pressure, unspecified forearm

✓6ᵗʰ **M70.94 Unspecified soft tissue disorder related to use, overuse and pressure of** hand

     M70.941 Unspecified soft tissue disorder related to use, overuse and pressure, right hand

     M70.942 Unspecified soft tissue disorder related to use, overuse and pressure, left hand

     M70.949 Unspecified soft tissue disorder related to use, overuse and pressure, unspecified hand

✓6ᵗʰ **M70.95 Unspecified soft tissue disorder related to use, overuse and pressure of** thigh

     M70.951 Unspecified soft tissue disorder related to use, overuse and pressure, right thigh

     M70.952 Unspecified soft tissue disorder related to use, overuse and pressure, left thigh

     M70.959 Unspecified soft tissue disorder related to use, overuse and pressure, unspecified thigh

✓6ᵗʰ **M70.96 Unspecified soft tissue disorder related to use, overuse and pressure** lower leg

     M70.961 Unspecified soft tissue disorder related to use, overuse and pressure, right lower leg

     M70.962 Unspecified soft tissue disorder related to use, overuse and pressure, left lower leg

     M70.969 Unspecified soft tissue disorder related to use, overuse and pressure, unspecified lower leg

✓6ᵗʰ **M70.97 Unspecified soft tissue disorder related to use, overuse and pressure of** ankle and foot

     M70.971 Unspecified soft tissue disorder related to use, overuse and pressure, right ankle and foot

     M70.972 Unspecified soft tissue disorder related to use, overuse and pressure, left ankle and foot

     M70.979 Unspecified soft tissue disorder related to use, overuse and pressure, unspecified ankle and foot

M70.98 Unspecified soft tissue disorder related to use, overuse and pressure other

M70.99 Unspecified soft tissue disorder related to use, overuse and pressure multiple sites

✓4ᵗʰ **M71 Other bursopathies**

     EXCLUDES 1   bunion (M20.1)

              bursitis related to use, overuse or pressure (M70.-)

              enthesopathies (M76-M77)

✓5ᵗʰ **M71.0 Abscess of bursa**

     Use additional code (B95.-, B96.-) to identify causative organism

     M71.00 Abscess of bursa, unspecified site

✓6ᵗʰ   **M71.01 Abscess of bursa,** shoulder

     M71.011 Abscess of bursa, right shoulder

     M71.012 Abscess of bursa, left shoulder

     M71.019 Abscess of bursa, unspecified shoulder

✓6ᵗʰ   **M71.02 Abscess of bursa,** elbow

     M71.021 Abscess of bursa, right elbow

     M71.022 Abscess of bursa, left elbow

     M71.029 Abscess of bursa, unspecified elbow

✓6ᵗʰ   **M71.03 Abscess of bursa,** wrist

     M71.031 Abscess of bursa, right wrist

     M71.032 Abscess of bursa, left wrist

     M71.039 Abscess of bursa, unspecified wrist

✓6ᵗʰ   **M71.04 Abscess of bursa,** hand

     M71.041 Abscess of bursa, right hand

     M71.042 Abscess of bursa, left hand

     M71.049 Abscess of bursa, unspecified hand

✓6ᵗʰ   **M71.05 Abscess of bursa,** hip

     M71.051 Abscess of bursa, right hip

     M71.052 Abscess of bursa, left hip

     M71.059 Abscess of bursa, unspecified hip

✓6ᵗʰ   **M71.06 Abscess of bursa,** knee

     M71.061 Abscess of bursa, right knee

     M71.062 Abscess of bursa, left knee

     M71.069 Abscess of bursa, unspecified knee

✓6ᵗʰ   **M71.07 Abscess of bursa,** ankle and foot

     M71.071 Abscess of bursa, right ankle and foot

N Newborn: 0   P Pediatric: 0-17   M Maternity: 12-55   A Adult: 15-124   MCC Major Complication/Comorbidity   CC Complication/Comorbidity   SW Severe Wound Dx

798   ICD-10-CM 2019

M71.072　Abscess of bursa, left ankle and foot
M71.079　Abscess of bursa, unspecified ankle and foot
M71.08　Abscess of bursa, other site
M71.09　Abscess of bursa, multiple sites

✓5ᵗʰ **M71.1　Other infective bursitis**
Use additional code (B95.-, B96.-) to identify causative organism
M71.10　Other infective bursitis, unspecified site

✓6ᵗʰ M71.11　Other infective bursitis, shoulder
M71.111　Other infective bursitis, right shoulder
M71.112　Other infective bursitis, left shoulder
M71.119　Other infective bursitis, unspecified shoulder

✓6ᵗʰ M71.12　Other infective bursitis, elbow
M71.121　Other infective bursitis, right elbow
M71.122　Other infective bursitis, left elbow
M71.129　Other infective bursitis, unspecified elbow

✓6ᵗʰ M71.13　Other infective bursitis, wrist
M71.131　Other infective bursitis, right wrist
M71.132　Other infective bursitis, left wrist
M71.139　Other infective bursitis, unspecified wrist

✓6ᵗʰ M71.14　Other infective bursitis, hand
M71.141　Other infective bursitis, right hand
M71.142　Other infective bursitis, left hand
M71.149　Other infective bursitis, unspecified hand

✓6ᵗʰ M71.15　Other infective bursitis, hip
M71.151　Other infective bursitis, right hip
M71.152　Other infective bursitis, left hip
M71.159　Other infective bursitis, unspecified hip

✓6ᵗʰ M71.16　Other infective bursitis, knee
M71.161　Other infective bursitis, right knee
M71.162　Other infective bursitis, left knee
M71.169　Other infective bursitis, unspecified knee

✓6ᵗʰ M71.17　Other infective bursitis, ankle and foot
M71.171　Other infective bursitis, right ankle and foot
M71.172　Other infective bursitis, left ankle and foot
M71.179　Other infective bursitis, unspecified ankle and foot
M71.18　Other infective bursitis, other site
M71.19　Other infective bursitis, multiple sites

✓5ᵗʰ **M71.2　Synovial cyst of popliteal space [Baker]**
EXCLUDES 1　synovial cyst of popliteal space with rupture (M66.0)
M71.20　Synovial cyst of popliteal space [Baker], unspecified knee
M71.21　Synovial cyst of popliteal space [Baker], right knee
M71.22　Synovial cyst of popliteal space [Baker], left knee

Baker's Cyst

Baker's cyst connected to knee joint synovial cavity

✓5ᵗʰ **M71.3　Other bursal cyst**
Synovial cyst NOS
EXCLUDES 1　synovial cyst with rupture (M66.1-)
M71.30　Other bursal cyst, unspecified site

✓6ᵗʰ M71.31　Other bursal cyst, shoulder
M71.311　Other bursal cyst, right shoulder
M71.312　Other bursal cyst, left shoulder
M71.319　Other bursal cyst, unspecified shoulder

✓6ᵗʰ M71.32　Other bursal cyst, elbow
M71.321　Other bursal cyst, right elbow
M71.322　Other bursal cyst, left elbow
M71.329　Other bursal cyst, unspecified elbow

✓6ᵗʰ M71.33　Other bursal cyst, wrist
M71.331　Other bursal cyst, right wrist
M71.332　Other bursal cyst, left wrist
M71.339　Other bursal cyst, unspecified wrist

✓6ᵗʰ M71.34　Other bursal cyst, hand
M71.341　Other bursal cyst, right hand
M71.342　Other bursal cyst, left hand
M71.349　Other bursal cyst, unspecified hand

✓6ᵗʰ M71.35　Other bursal cyst, hip
M71.351　Other bursal cyst, right hip
M71.352　Other bursal cyst, left hip
M71.359　Other bursal cyst, unspecified hip

✓6ᵗʰ M71.37　Other bursal cyst, ankle and foot
M71.371　Other bursal cyst, right ankle and foot
M71.372　Other bursal cyst, left ankle and foot
M71.379　Other bursal cyst, unspecified ankle and foot
M71.38　Other bursal cyst, other site
M71.39　Other bursal cyst, multiple sites

✓5ᵗʰ **M71.4　Calcium deposit in bursa**
EXCLUDES 2　calcium deposit in bursa of shoulder (M75.3)
M71.40　Calcium deposit in bursa, unspecified site

✓6ᵗʰ M71.42　Calcium deposit in bursa, elbow
M71.421　Calcium deposit in bursa, right elbow
M71.422　Calcium deposit in bursa, left elbow
M71.429　Calcium deposit in bursa, unspecified elbow

✓6ᵗʰ M71.43　Calcium deposit in bursa, wrist
M71.431　Calcium deposit in bursa, right wrist
M71.432　Calcium deposit in bursa, left wrist
M71.439　Calcium deposit in bursa, unspecified wrist

✓6ᵗʰ M71.44　Calcium deposit in bursa, hand
M71.441　Calcium deposit in bursa, right hand
M71.442　Calcium deposit in bursa, left hand
M71.449　Calcium deposit in bursa, unspecified hand

✓6ᵗʰ M71.45　Calcium deposit in bursa, hip
M71.451　Calcium deposit in bursa, right hip
M71.452　Calcium deposit in bursa, left hip
M71.459　Calcium deposit in bursa, unspecified hip

✓6ᵗʰ M71.46　Calcium deposit in bursa, knee
M71.461　Calcium deposit in bursa, right knee
M71.462　Calcium deposit in bursa, left knee
M71.469　Calcium deposit in bursa, unspecified knee

✓6ᵗʰ M71.47　Calcium deposit in bursa, ankle and foot
M71.471　Calcium deposit in bursa, right ankle and foot
M71.472　Calcium deposit in bursa, left ankle and foot
M71.479　Calcium deposit in bursa, unspecified ankle and foot
M71.48　Calcium deposit in bursa, other site
M71.49　Calcium deposit in bursa, multiple sites

☑5ᵗʰ **M71.5 Other bursitis, not elsewhere classified**
    EXCLUDES1 *bursitis NOS (M71.9-)*
    EXCLUDES2 *bursitis of shoulder (M75.5)*
           bursitis of tibial collateral [Pellegrini-Stieda] (M76.4-)

    M71.50 Other bursitis, not elsewhere classified, unspecified site

☑6ᵗʰ   **M71.52 Other bursitis, not elsewhere classified, elbow**
      M71.521 Other bursitis, not elsewhere classified, right elbow
      M71.522 Other bursitis, not elsewhere classified, left elbow
      M71.529 Other bursitis, not elsewhere classified, unspecified elbow

☑6ᵗʰ   **M71.53 Other bursitis, not elsewhere classified, wrist**
      M71.531 Other bursitis, not elsewhere classified, right wrist
      M71.532 Other bursitis, not elsewhere classified, left wrist
      M71.539 Other bursitis, not elsewhere classified, unspecified wrist

☑6ᵗʰ   **M71.54 Other bursitis, not elsewhere classified, hand**
      M71.541 Other bursitis, not elsewhere classified, right hand
      M71.542 Other bursitis, not elsewhere classified, left hand
      M71.549 Other bursitis, not elsewhere classified, unspecified hand

☑6ᵗʰ   **M71.55 Other bursitis, not elsewhere classified, hip**
      M71.551 Other bursitis, not elsewhere classified, right hip
      M71.552 Other bursitis, not elsewhere classified, left hip
      M71.559 Other bursitis, not elsewhere classified, unspecified hip

☑6ᵗʰ   **M71.56 Other bursitis, not elsewhere classified, knee**
      M71.561 Other bursitis, not elsewhere classified, right knee
      M71.562 Other bursitis, not elsewhere classified, left knee
      M71.569 Other bursitis, not elsewhere classified, unspecified knee

☑6ᵗʰ   **M71.57 Other bursitis, not elsewhere classified, ankle and foot**
      M71.571 Other bursitis, not elsewhere classified, right ankle and foot
      M71.572 Other bursitis, not elsewhere classified, left ankle and foot
      M71.579 Other bursitis, not elsewhere classified, unspecified ankle and foot

    M71.58 Other bursitis, not elsewhere classified, other site

☑5ᵗʰ **M71.8 Other specified bursopathies**
    M71.80 Other specified bursopathies, unspecified site

☑6ᵗʰ   **M71.81 Other specified bursopathies, shoulder**
      M71.811 Other specified bursopathies, right shoulder
      M71.812 Other specified bursopathies, left shoulder
      M71.819 Other specified bursopathies, unspecified shoulder

☑6ᵗʰ   **M71.82 Other specified bursopathies, elbow**
      M71.821 Other specified bursopathies, right elbow
      M71.822 Other specified bursopathies, left elbow
      M71.829 Other specified bursopathies, unspecified elbow

☑6ᵗʰ   **M71.83 Other specified bursopathies, wrist**
      M71.831 Other specified bursopathies, right wrist
      M71.832 Other specified bursopathies, left wrist
      M71.839 Other specified bursopathies, unspecified wrist

☑6ᵗʰ   **M71.84 Other specified bursopathies, hand**
      M71.841 Other specified bursopathies, right hand
      M71.842 Other specified bursopathies, left hand
      M71.849 Other specified bursopathies, unspecified hand

☑6ᵗʰ   **M71.85 Other specified bursopathies, hip**
      M71.851 Other specified bursopathies, right hip
      M71.852 Other specified bursopathies, left hip
      M71.859 Other specified bursopathies, unspecified hip

☑6ᵗʰ   **M71.86 Other specified bursopathies, knee**
      M71.861 Other specified bursopathies, right knee
      M71.862 Other specified bursopathies, left knee
      M71.869 Other specified bursopathies, unspecified knee

☑6ᵗʰ   **M71.87 Other specified bursopathies, ankle and foot**
      M71.871 Other specified bursopathies, right ankle and foot
      M71.872 Other specified bursopathies, left ankle and foot
      M71.879 Other specified bursopathies, unspecified ankle and foot

    M71.88 Other specified bursopathies, other site
    M71.89 Other specified bursopathies, multiple sites

M71.9 Bursopathy, unspecified
    Bursitis NOS

☑4ᵗʰ **M72 Fibroblastic disorders**
    EXCLUDES2 *retroperitoneal fibromatosis (D48.3)*

    M72.0 Palmar fascial fibromatosis [Dupuytren] 🅐
      DEF: Dupuytren's contracture: Flexion deformity of a finger, due to shortened, thickened fibrosing of palmar fascia. The cause is unknown, but it is associated with long-standing epilepsy.

    M72.1 Knuckle pads

    M72.2 Plantar fascial fibromatosis
      Plantar fasciitis
      DEF: Rapid-growing and multiplanar nodular swellings and pain in the foot that is not associated with contractures.

    M72.4 Pseudosarcomatous fibromatosis
      Nodular fasciitis

    M72.6 Necrotizing fasciitis MCC HCC
      Use additional code (B95.-, B96.-) to identify causative organism
      CC Excl: PDX collection 806

    M72.8 Other fibroblastic disorders
      Abscess of fascia
      Fasciitis NEC
      Other infective fasciitis
      Use additional code to (B95.-, B96.-) identify causative organism
      EXCLUDES1 *diffuse (eosinophilic) fasciitis (M35.4)*
           necrotizing fasciitis (M72.6)
           nodular fasciitis (M72.4)
           perirenal fasciitis NOS (N13.5)
           perirenal fasciitis with infection (N13.6)
           plantar fasciitis (M72.2)

    M72.9 Fibroblastic disorder, unspecified
      Fasciitis NOS
      Fibromatosis NOS

☑4ᵗʰ **M75 Shoulder lesions**
    EXCLUDES2 *shoulder-hand syndrome (M89.0-)*

☑5ᵗʰ   **M75.0 Adhesive capsulitis of shoulder**
      Frozen shoulder
      Periarthritis of shoulder
      AHA: 2015, 2Q, 23
      M75.00 Adhesive capsulitis of unspecified shoulder
      M75.01 Adhesive capsulitis of right shoulder
      M75.02 Adhesive capsulitis of left shoulder

☑5ᵗʰ   **M75.1 Rotator cuff tear or rupture, not specified as traumatic**
      Rotator cuff syndrome
      Supraspinatus syndrome
      Supraspinatus tear or rupture, not specified as traumatic
      EXCLUDES1 *tear of rotator cuff, traumatic (S46.01-)*

☑6ᵗʰ   **M75.10 Unspecified rotator cuff tear or rupture, not specified as traumatic**
      M75.100 Unspecified rotator cuff tear or rupture of unspecified shoulder, not specified as traumatic
      M75.101 Unspecified rotator cuff tear or rupture of right shoulder, not specified as traumatic
      M75.102 Unspecified rotator cuff tear or rupture of left shoulder, not specified as traumatic

✓6ᵗʰ **M75.11** Incomplete **rotator cuff tear or rupture not specified as traumatic**

     M75.110 Incomplete **rotator cuff tear or rupture of** unspecified **shoulder, not specified as traumatic**

     M75.111 Incomplete **rotator cuff tear or rupture of** right **shoulder, not specified as traumatic**

     M75.112 Incomplete **rotator cuff tear or rupture of** left **shoulder, not specified as traumatic**

✓6ᵗʰ **M75.12** Complete **rotator cuff tear or rupture not specified as traumatic**

     M75.120 Complete **rotator cuff tear or rupture of** unspecified **shoulder, not specified as traumatic**

     M75.121 Complete **rotator cuff tear or rupture of** right **shoulder, not specified as traumatic**

     M75.122 Complete **rotator cuff tear or rupture of** left **shoulder, not specified as traumatic**

✓5ᵗʰ **M75.2** Bicipital **tendinitis**

     M75.20 **Bicipital tendinitis,** unspecified **shoulder**

     M75.21 **Bicipital tendinitis,** right **shoulder**

     M75.22 **Bicipital tendinitis,** left **shoulder**

✓5ᵗʰ **M75.3** Calcific **tendinitis of shoulder**

     Calcified bursa of shoulder

     M75.30 **Calcific tendinitis of** unspecified **shoulder**

     M75.31 **Calcific tendinitis of** right **shoulder**

     M75.32 **Calcific tendinitis of** left **shoulder**

✓5ᵗʰ **M75.4** Impingement syndrome **of shoulder**

     M75.40 **Impingement syndrome of** unspecified **shoulder**

     M75.41 **Impingement syndrome of** right **shoulder**

     M75.42 **Impingement syndrome of** left **shoulder**

✓5ᵗʰ **M75.5** Bursitis **of shoulder**

     M75.50 **Bursitis of** unspecified **shoulder**

     M75.51 **Bursitis of** right **shoulder**

     M75.52 **Bursitis of** left **shoulder**

✓5ᵗʰ **M75.8** Other **shoulder lesions**

     M75.80 **Other shoulder lesions,** unspecified **shoulder**

     M75.81 **Other shoulder lesions,** right **shoulder**

     M75.82 **Other shoulder lesions,** left **shoulder**

✓5ᵗʰ **M75.9** Shoulder lesion, unspecified

     M75.90 **Shoulder lesion, unspecified,** unspecified **shoulder**

     M75.91 **Shoulder lesion, unspecified,** right **shoulder**

     M75.92 **Shoulder lesion, unspecified,** left **shoulder**

✓4ᵗʰ **M76 Enthesopathies, lower limb, excluding foot**

     EXCLUDES 2   *bursitis due to use, overuse and pressure (M70.-)*
                     enthesopathies of ankle and foot (M77.5-)

✓5ᵗʰ **M76.0** Gluteal **tendinitis**

     M76.00 **Gluteal tendinitis,** unspecified **hip**

     M76.01 **Gluteal tendinitis,** right **hip**

     M76.02 **Gluteal tendinitis,** left **hip**

✓5ᵗʰ **M76.1** Psoas **tendinitis**

     M76.10 **Psoas tendinitis,** unspecified **hip**

     M76.11 **Psoas tendinitis,** right **hip**

     M76.12 **Psoas tendinitis,** left **hip**

✓5ᵗʰ **M76.2** Iliac crest **spur**

     M76.20 **Iliac crest spur,** unspecified **hip**

     M76.21 **Iliac crest spur,** right **hip**

     M76.22 **Iliac crest spur,** left **hip**

✓5ᵗʰ **M76.3** Iliotibial band **syndrome**

     M76.30 **Iliotibial band syndrome,** unspecified **leg**

     M76.31 **Iliotibial band syndrome,** right **leg**

     M76.32 **Iliotibial band syndrome,** left **leg**

✓5ᵗʰ **M76.4** Tibial collateral **bursitis [Pellegrini-Stieda]**

     M76.40 **Tibial collateral bursitis [Pellegrini-Stieda],** unspecified **leg**

     M76.41 **Tibial collateral bursitis [Pellegrini-Stieda],** right **leg**

     M76.42 **Tibial collateral bursitis [Pellegrini-Stieda],** left **leg**

✓5ᵗʰ **M76.5** Patellar **tendinitis**

     M76.50 **Patellar tendinitis,** unspecified **knee**

     M76.51 **Patellar tendinitis,** right **knee**

     M76.52 **Patellar tendinitis,** left **knee**

✓5ᵗʰ **M76.6** Achilles **tendinitis**

     Achilles bursitis

     M76.60 **Achilles tendinitis,** unspecified **leg**

     M76.61 **Achilles tendinitis,** right **leg**

     M76.62 **Achilles tendinitis,** left **leg**

✓5ᵗʰ **M76.7** Peroneal **tendinitis**

     M76.70 **Peroneal tendinitis,** unspecified **leg**

     M76.71 **Peroneal tendinitis,** right **leg**

     M76.72 **Peroneal tendinitis,** left **leg**

✓5ᵗʰ **M76.8** Other **specified enthesopathies of lower limb, excluding foot**

     ✓6ᵗʰ **M76.81** Anterior tibial syndrome

         M76.811 **Anterior tibial syndrome,** right **leg**

         M76.812 **Anterior tibial syndrome,** left **leg**

         M76.819 **Anterior tibial syndrome,** unspecified **leg**

     ✓6ᵗʰ **M76.82** Posterior tibial tendinitis

         M76.821 **Posterior tibial tendinitis,** right **leg**

         M76.822 **Posterior tibial tendinitis,** left **leg**

         M76.829 **Posterior tibial tendinitis,** unspecified **leg**

     ✓6ᵗʰ **M76.89** Other **specified enthesopathies of** lower limb, excluding foot

         M76.891 **Other specified enthesopathies of** right **lower limb, excluding foot**

         M76.892 **Other specified enthesopathies of** left **lower limb, excluding foot**

         M76.899 **Other specified enthesopathies of** unspecified **lower limb, excluding foot**

     M76.9 Unspecified **enthesopathy, lower limb, excluding foot**

✓4ᵗʰ **M77 Other enthesopathies**

     EXCLUDES 1   *bursitis NOS (M71.9-)*

     EXCLUDES 2   *bursitis due to use, overuse and pressure (M70.-)*
                     osteophyte (M25.7)
                     spinal enthesopathy (M46.0-)

✓5ᵗʰ **M77.0** Medial **epicondylitis**

     M77.00 **Medial epicondylitis,** unspecified **elbow**

     M77.01 **Medial epicondylitis,** right **elbow**

     M77.02 **Medial epicondylitis,** left **elbow**

✓5ᵗʰ **M77.1** Lateral **epicondylitis**

     Tennis elbow

     M77.10 **Lateral epicondylitis,** unspecified **elbow**

     M77.11 **Lateral epicondylitis,** right **elbow**

     M77.12 **Lateral epicondylitis,** left **elbow**

✓5ᵗʰ **M77.2** Periarthritis **of wrist**

     M77.20 **Periarthritis,** unspecified **wrist**

     M77.21 **Periarthritis,** right **wrist**

     M77.22 **Periarthritis,** left **wrist**

✓5ᵗʰ **M77.3** Calcaneal **spur**

     DEF: Overgrowth of calcaneus bone on the underside of the heel that causes pain on walking. Calcaneal spur is due to a chronic avulsion injury of the plantar fascia from the calcaneus.

     M77.30 **Calcaneal spur,** unspecified **foot**

     M77.31 **Calcaneal spur,** right **foot**

     M77.32 **Calcaneal spur,** left **foot**

✓5ᵗʰ **M77.4** Metatarsalgia

     EXCLUDES 1   *Morton's metatarsalgia (G57.6)*

     M77.40 **Metatarsalgia,** unspecified **foot**

     M77.41 **Metatarsalgia,** right **foot**

     M77.42 **Metatarsalgia,** left **foot**

✓5ᵗʰ **M77.5** Other **enthesopathy of** foot

     M77.50 **Other enthesopathy of** unspecified **foot**

     M77.51 **Other enthesopathy of** right **foot**

     M77.52 **Other enthesopathy of** left **foot**

     M77.8 Other **enthesopathies, not elsewhere classified**

     M77.9 Enthesopathy, unspecified

     Bone spur NOS   Periarthritis NOS
     Capsulitis NOS   Tendinitis NOS

✓4ᵗʰ **M79 Other and unspecified soft tissue disorders, not elsewhere classified**

     EXCLUDES 1   *psychogenic rheumatism (F45.8)*
                     soft tissue pain, psychogenic (F45.41)

     M79.0 Rheumatism, unspecified

     EXCLUDES 1   *fibromyalgia (M79.7)*
                     palindromic rheumatism (M12.3-)

✔ Additional Character Required   ✓x7ᵗʰ Placeholder   Unacceptable PDx   Questionable PDx   Manifestation   H1 - H14 HAC   HCC CMS-HCC Dx   HIV HIV Dx

ICD-10-CM 2019   801

✓5th **M79.1 Myalgia**
     Myofascial pain syndrome
     EXCLUDES 1   *fibromyalgia (M79.7)*
                 myositis (M6Ø.-)

●   **M79.10 Myalgia, unspecified site**
●   **M79.11 Myalgia of mastication muscle**
●   **M79.12 Myalgia of auxiliary muscles, head and neck**
●   **M79.18 Myalgia, other site**

M79.2 Neuralgia and neuritis, unspecified
     EXCLUDES 1   *brachial radiculitis NOS (M54.1)*
                 lumbosacral radiculitis NOS (M54.1)
                 mononeuropathies (G56-G58)
                 radiculitis NOS (M54.1)
                 sciatica (M54.3-M54.4)

     TIP: Assign for documented neuropathic pain.

M79.3 Panniculitis, unspecified
     EXCLUDES 1   *lupus panniculitis (L93.2)*
                 neck and back panniculitis (M54.Ø-)
                 relapsing [Weber-Christian] panniculitis (M35.6)

M79.4 Hypertrophy of (infrapatellar) fat pad

M79.5 Residual foreign body in soft tissue
     EXCLUDES 1   *foreign body granuloma of skin and subcutaneous*
                     tissue (L92.3)
                 foreign body granuloma of soft tissue (M6Ø.2-)

✓5th **M79.6 Pain in limb, hand, foot, fingers and toes**
     EXCLUDES 2   *pain in joint (M25.5-)*

     ✓6th **M79.60 Pain in limb, unspecified**
         M79.601 Pain in right arm
              Pain in right upper limb NOS
         M79.602 Pain in left arm
              Pain in left upper limb NOS
         M79.603 Pain in arm, unspecified
              Pain in upper limb NOS
         M79.604 Pain in right leg
              Pain in right lower limb NOS
         M79.605 Pain in left leg
              Pain in left lower limb NOS
         M79.606 Pain in leg, unspecified
              Pain in lower limb NOS
         M79.609 Pain in unspecified limb
              Pain in limb NOS

     ✓6th **M79.62 Pain in upper arm**
         Pain in axillary region
         M79.621 Pain in right upper arm
         M79.622 Pain in left upper arm
         M79.629 Pain in unspecified upper arm

     ✓6th **M79.63 Pain in forearm**
         M79.631 Pain in right forearm
         M79.632 Pain in left forearm
         M79.639 Pain in unspecified forearm

     ✓6th **M79.64 Pain in hand and fingers**
         M79.641 Pain in right hand
         M79.642 Pain in left hand
         M79.643 Pain in unspecified hand
         M79.644 Pain in right finger(s)
         M79.645 Pain in left finger(s)
         M79.646 Pain in unspecified finger(s)

     ✓6th **M79.65 Pain in thigh**
         M79.651 Pain in right thigh
         M79.652 Pain in left thigh
         M79.659 Pain in unspecified thigh

     ✓6th **M79.66 Pain in lower leg**
         M79.661 Pain in right lower leg
         M79.662 Pain in left lower leg
         M79.669 Pain in unspecified lower leg

     ✓6th **M79.67 Pain in foot and toes**
         M79.671 Pain in right foot
         M79.672 Pain in left foot
         M79.673 Pain in unspecified foot
         M79.674 Pain in right toe(s)
         M79.675 Pain in left toe(s)
         M79.676 Pain in unspecified toe(s)

M79.7 Fibromyalgia
     Fibromyositis
     Fibrositis
     Myofibrositis

✓5th **M79.A Nontraumatic compartment syndrome**
     Code first, if applicable, associated postprocedural complication
     EXCLUDES 1   *compartment syndrome NOS (T79.A-)*
                 fibromyalgia (M79.7)
                 nontraumatic ischemic infarction of muscle (M62.2-)
                 traumatic compartment syndrome (T79.A-)

     ✓6th **M79.A1 Nontraumatic compartment syndrome of upper extremity**
         Nontraumatic compartment syndrome of shoulder, arm, forearm, wrist, hand, and fingers

         CC Excl: For CC codes in subcategory M79.A1: PDX collection 893

         M79.A11 Nontraumatic compartment syndrome CC **of right upper extremity**
         M79.A12 Nontraumatic compartment syndrome CC **of left upper extremity**
         M79.A19 Nontraumatic compartment syndrome CC **of unspecified upper extremity**

     ✓6th **M79.A2 Nontraumatic compartment syndrome of lower extremity**
         Nontraumatic compartment syndrome of hip, buttock, thigh, leg, foot, and toes

         CC Excl: For CC codes in subcategory M79.A2: PDX collection 894

         M79.A21 Nontraumatic compartment syndrome CC **of right lower extremity**
         M79.A22 Nontraumatic compartment syndrome CC **of left lower extremity**
         M79.A29 Nontraumatic compartment syndrome CC **of unspecified lower extremity**

     M79.A3 Nontraumatic compartment syndrome of abdomen CC
         CC Excl: PDX collection 895

     M79.A9 Nontraumatic compartment syndrome of other sites CC
         CC Excl: PDX collection 896

✓5th **M79.8 Other specified soft tissue disorders**
     M79.81 Nontraumatic hematoma of soft tissue
         Nontraumatic hematoma of muscle
         Nontraumatic seroma of muscle and soft tissue
     M79.89 Other specified soft tissue disorders
         Polyalgia

M79.9 Soft tissue disorder, unspecified

OSTEOPATHIES AND CHONDROPATHIES (M8Ø-M94)

Disorders of bone density and structure (M8Ø-M85)

✓4th **M8Ø Osteoporosis with current pathological fracture**
     INCLUDES   osteoporosis with current fragility fracture
     Use additional code to identify major osseous defect, if applicable (M89.7-)
     EXCLUDES 1   *collapsed vertebra NOS (M48.5)*
                 pathological fracture NOS (M84.4)
                 wedging of vertebra NOS (M48.5)
     EXCLUDES 2   *personal history of (healed) osteoporosis fracture (Z87.31Ø)*
     AHA: 2018, 2Q, 12
     TIP: The site codes in this category identify the site of the fracture, not the site of the osteoporosis.

     The appropriate 7th character is to be added to each code from category M8Ø.
     A   initial encounter for fracture
     D   subsequent encounter for fracture with routine healing
     G   subsequent encounter for fracture with delayed healing
     K   subsequent encounter for fracture with nonunion
     P   subsequent encounter for fracture with malunion
     S   sequela

     CC Excl: For CC codes in category M8Ø:
     CC with 7th character A: PDX collection 888
     CC with 7th character K or P: PDX collection 897

N Newborn: 0   P Pediatric: 0-17   M Maternity: 12-55   A Adult: 15-124   MCC Major Complication/Comorbidity   CC Complication/Comorbidity   SW Severe Wound Dx

802   ICD-10-CM 2019

☑5ᵗʰ **M80.0** Age-related **osteoporosis with current pathological fracture**
    Involutional osteoporosis with current pathological fracture
    Osteoporosis NOS with current pathological fracture
    Postmenopausal osteoporosis with current pathological fracture
    Senile osteoporosis with current pathological fracture

3 ☑x7ᵗʰ **M80.00** Age-related osteoporosis with current pathological fracture, unspecified site   cc A

☑6ᵗʰ **M80.01** Age-related osteoporosis with current pathological fracture, shoulder

  3 ☑7ᵗʰ **M80.011** Age-related osteoporosis with current pathological fracture, right shoulder   cc A

  3 ☑7ᵗʰ **M80.012** Age-related osteoporosis with current pathological fracture, left shoulder   cc A

  3 ☑7ᵗʰ **M80.019** Age-related osteoporosis with current pathological fracture, unspecified shoulder   cc A

☑6ᵗʰ **M80.02** Age-related osteoporosis with current pathological fracture, humerus

  3 ☑7ᵗʰ **M80.021** Age-related osteoporosis with current pathological fracture, right humerus   cc A

  3 ☑7ᵗʰ **M80.022** Age-related osteoporosis with current pathological fracture, left humerus   cc A

  3 ☑7ᵗʰ **M80.029** Age-related osteoporosis with current pathological fracture, unspecified humerus   cc A

☑6ᵗʰ **M80.03** Age-related osteoporosis with current pathological fracture, forearm
    Age-related osteoporosis with current pathological fracture of wrist

  3 ☑7ᵗʰ **M80.031** Age-related osteoporosis with current pathological fracture, right forearm   cc A

  3 ☑7ᵗʰ **M80.032** Age-related osteoporosis with current pathological fracture, left forearm   cc A

  3 ☑7ᵗʰ **M80.039** Age-related osteoporosis with current pathological fracture, unspecified forearm   cc A

☑6ᵗʰ **M80.04** Age-related osteoporosis with current pathological fracture, hand

  3 ☑7ᵗʰ **M80.041** Age-related osteoporosis with current pathological fracture, right hand   cc A

  3 ☑7ᵗʰ **M80.042** Age-related osteoporosis with current pathological fracture, left hand   cc A

  3 ☑7ᵗʰ **M80.049** Age-related osteoporosis with current pathological fracture, unspecified hand   cc A

☑6ᵗʰ **M80.05** Age-related osteoporosis with current pathological fracture, femur
    Age-related osteoporosis with current pathological fracture of hip

  3, 6 ☑7ᵗʰ **M80.051** Age-related osteoporosis with current pathological fracture, right femur   cc HCC A

  3, 6 ☑7ᵗʰ **M80.052** Age-related osteoporosis with current pathological fracture, left femur   cc HCC A

  3, 6 ☑7ᵗʰ **M80.059** Age-related osteoporosis with current pathological fracture, unspecified femur   cc HCC A

☑6ᵗʰ **M80.06** Age-related osteoporosis with current pathological fracture, lower leg

  3 ☑7ᵗʰ **M80.061** Age-related osteoporosis with current pathological fracture, right lower leg   cc A

  3 ☑7ᵗʰ **M80.062** Age-related osteoporosis with current pathological fracture, left lower leg   cc A

  3 ☑7ᵗʰ **M80.069** Age-related osteoporosis with current pathological fracture, unspecified lower leg   cc A

☑6ᵗʰ **M80.07** Age-related osteoporosis with current pathological fracture, ankle and foot

  3 ☑7ᵗʰ **M80.071** Age-related osteoporosis with current pathological fracture, right ankle and foot   cc A

  3 ☑7ᵗʰ **M80.072** Age-related osteoporosis with current pathological fracture, left ankle and foot   cc A

  3 ☑7ᵗʰ **M80.079** Age-related osteoporosis with current pathological fracture, unspecified ankle and foot   cc A

3, 6 ☑x7ᵗʰ **M80.08** Age-related osteoporosis with current pathological fracture, vertebra(e)   cc HCC

☑5ᵗʰ **M80.8** Other osteoporosis with current pathological fracture
    Drug-induced osteoporosis with current pathological fracture
    Idiopathic osteoporosis with current pathological fracture
    Osteoporosis of disuse with current pathological fracture
    Postoophorectomy osteoporosis with current pathological fracture
    Postsurgical malabsorption osteoporosis with current pathological fracture
    Post-traumatic osteoporosis with current pathological fracture
    Use additional code for adverse effect, if applicable, to identify drug (T36-T50 with fifth or sixth character 5)

3 ☑x7ᵗʰ **M80.80** Other osteoporosis with current pathological fracture, unspecified site   cc

☑6ᵗʰ **M80.81** Other osteoporosis with pathological fracture, shoulder

  3 ☑7ᵗʰ **M80.811** Other osteoporosis with current pathological fracture, right shoulder   cc

  3 ☑7ᵗʰ **M80.812** Other osteoporosis with current pathological fracture, left shoulder   cc

  3 ☑7ᵗʰ **M80.819** Other osteoporosis with current pathological fracture, unspecified shoulder   cc

☑6ᵗʰ **M80.82** Other osteoporosis with current pathological fracture, humerus

  3 ☑7ᵗʰ **M80.821** Other osteoporosis with current pathological fracture, right humerus   cc

  3 ☑7ᵗʰ **M80.822** Other osteoporosis with current pathological fracture, left humerus   cc

  3 ☑7ᵗʰ **M80.829** Other osteoporosis with current pathological fracture, unspecified humerus   cc

☑6ᵗʰ **M80.83** Other osteoporosis with pathological fracture, forearm
    Other osteoporosis with current pathological fracture of wrist

  3 ☑7ᵗʰ **M80.831** Other osteoporosis with current pathological fracture, right forearm   cc

  3 ☑7ᵗʰ **M80.832** Other osteoporosis with current pathological fracture, left forearm   cc

  3 ☑7ᵗʰ **M80.839** Other osteoporosis with current pathological fracture, unspecified forearm   cc

☑6ᵗʰ **M80.84** Other osteoporosis with current pathological fracture, hand

  3 ☑7ᵗʰ **M80.841** Other osteoporosis with current pathological fracture, right hand   cc

  3 ☑7ᵗʰ **M80.842** Other osteoporosis with current pathological fracture, left hand   cc

  3 ☑7ᵗʰ **M80.849** Other osteoporosis with current pathological fracture, unspecified hand   cc

☑6ᵗʰ **M80.85** Other osteoporosis with current pathological fracture, femur
    Other osteoporosis with current pathological fracture of hip

  3, 6 ☑7ᵗʰ **M80.851** Other osteoporosis with current pathological fracture, right femur   cc HCC

  3, 6 ☑7ᵗʰ **M80.852** Other osteoporosis with current pathological fracture, left femur   cc HCC

  3, 6 ☑7ᵗʰ **M80.859** Other osteoporosis with current pathological fracture, unspecified femur   cc HCC

☑ Additional Character Required   ☑x7ᵗʰ Placeholder   Unacceptable PDx   Questionable PDx   Manifestation   H1-H14 HAC   HCC CMS-HCC Dx   HIV HIV Dx

ICD-10-CM 2019   803

√6ᵗʰ **M80.86 Other osteoporosis with current pathological fracture, lower leg**

3 √7ᵗʰ **M80.861 Other osteoporosis with current pathological fracture, right lower leg** `CC`

3 √7ᵗʰ **M80.862 Other osteoporosis with current pathological fracture, left lower leg** `CC`

3 √7ᵗʰ **M80.869 Other osteoporosis with current pathological fracture, unspecified lower leg** `CC`

√6ᵗʰ **M80.87 Other osteoporosis with current pathological fracture, ankle and foot**

3 √7ᵗʰ **M80.871 Other osteoporosis with current pathological fracture, right ankle and foot** `CC`

3 √7ᵗʰ **M80.872 Other osteoporosis with current pathological fracture, left ankle and foot** `CC`

3 √7ᵗʰ **M80.879 Other osteoporosis with current pathological fracture, unspecified ankle and foot** `CC`

3, 6 √x7ᵗʰ **M80.88 Other osteoporosis with current pathological fracture, vertebra(e)** `CC` `HCC`

√4ᵗʰ **M81 Osteoporosis without current pathological fracture**
Use additional code to identify:
major osseous defect, if applicable (M89.7-)
personal history of (healed) osteoporosis fracture, if applicable (Z87.310)

EXCLUDES 1   *osteoporosis with current pathological fracture (M80.-)*
Sudeck's atrophy (M89.0)

M81.0 Age-related osteoporosis without current pathological fracture `A`
Involutional osteoporosis without current pathological fracture
Osteoporosis NOS
Postmenopausal osteoporosis without current pathological fracture
Senile osteoporosis without current pathological fracture

M81.6 Localized osteoporosis [Lequesne]
EXCLUDES 1   *Sudeck's atrophy (M89.0)*

M81.8 Other osteoporosis without current pathological fracture
Drug-induced osteoporosis without current pathological fracture
Idiopathic osteoporosis without current pathological fracture
Osteoporosis of disuse without current pathological fracture
Postoophorectomy osteoporosis without current pathological fracture
Postsurgical malabsorption osteoporosis without current pathological fracture
Post-traumatic osteoporosis without current pathological fracture
Use additional code for adverse effect, if applicable, to identify drug (T36-T50 with fifth or sixth character 5)

√4ᵗʰ **M83 Adult osteomalacia**
EXCLUDES 1   *infantile and juvenile osteomalacia (E55.0)*
renal osteodystrophy (N25.0)
rickets (active) (E55.0)
rickets (active) sequelae (E64.3)
vitamin D-resistant osteomalacia (E83.3)
vitamin D-resistant rickets (active) (E83.3)

M83.0 Puerperal osteomalacia `M`♀

M83.1 Senile osteomalacia `A`

M83.2 Adult osteomalacia due to malabsorption `A`
Postsurgical malabsorption osteomalacia in adults

M83.3 Adult osteomalacia due to malnutrition `A`

M83.4 Aluminum bone disease

M83.5 Other drug-induced osteomalacia in adults `A`
Use additional code for adverse effect, if applicable, to identify drug (T36-T50 with fifth or sixth character 5)

M83.8 Other adult osteomalacia `A`

M83.9 Adult osteomalacia, unspecified `A`

√4ᵗʰ **M84 Disorder of continuity of bone**
EXCLUDES 2   *traumatic fracture of bone-see fracture, by site*

√5ᵗʰ **M84.3 Stress fracture**
Fatigue fracture   Stress fracture NOS
March fracture   Stress reaction
Use additional external cause code(s) to identify the cause of the stress fracture
EXCLUDES 1   *pathological fracture NOS (M84.4-)*
pathological fracture due to osteoporosis (M80.-)
traumatic fracture (S12-, S22-, S32-, S42-, S52-, S62-, S72-, S82-, S92-)
EXCLUDES 2   *personal history of (healed) stress (fatigue) fracture (Z87.312)*
stress fracture of vertebra (M48.4-)

The appropriate 7th character is to be added to each code from subcategory M84.3.
A   initial encounter for fracture
D   subsequent encounter for fracture with routine healing
G   subsequent encounter for fracture with delayed healing
K   subsequent encounter for fracture with nonunion
P   subsequent encounter for fracture with malunion
S   sequela

CC Excl: For CC codes in subcategory M84.3:
CC with 7th character K or P: PDX collection 897

4 √x7ᵗʰ **M84.30 Stress fracture, unspecified site** `CC`

√6ᵗʰ **M84.31 Stress fracture, shoulder**
4 √7ᵗʰ **M84.311 Stress fracture, right shoulder** `CC`
4 √7ᵗʰ **M84.312 Stress fracture, left shoulder** `CC`
4 √7ᵗʰ **M84.319 Stress fracture, unspecified shoulder** `CC`

√6ᵗʰ **M84.32 Stress fracture, humerus**
4 √7ᵗʰ **M84.321 Stress fracture, right humerus** `CC`
4 √7ᵗʰ **M84.322 Stress fracture, left humerus** `CC`
4 √7ᵗʰ **M84.329 Stress fracture, unspecified humerus** `CC`

√6ᵗʰ **M84.33 Stress fracture, ulna and radius**
4 √7ᵗʰ **M84.331 Stress fracture, right ulna** `CC`
4 √7ᵗʰ **M84.332 Stress fracture, left ulna** `CC`
4 √7ᵗʰ **M84.333 Stress fracture, right radius** `CC`
4 √7ᵗʰ **M84.334 Stress fracture, left radius** `CC`
4 √7ᵗʰ **M84.339 Stress fracture, unspecified ulna and radius** `CC`

√6ᵗʰ **M84.34 Stress fracture, hand and fingers**
4 √7ᵗʰ **M84.341 Stress fracture, right hand** `CC`
4 √7ᵗʰ **M84.342 Stress fracture, left hand** `CC`
4 √7ᵗʰ **M84.343 Stress fracture, unspecified hand** `CC`
4 √7ᵗʰ **M84.344 Stress fracture, right finger(s)** `CC`
4 √7ᵗʰ **M84.345 Stress fracture, left finger(s)** `CC`
4 √7ᵗʰ **M84.346 Stress fracture, unspecified finger(s)** `CC`

√6ᵗʰ **M84.35 Stress fracture, pelvis and femur**
Stress fracture, hip
4 √7ᵗʰ **M84.350 Stress fracture, pelvis** `CC`
4 √7ᵗʰ **M84.351 Stress fracture, right femur** `CC`
4 √7ᵗʰ **M84.352 Stress fracture, left femur** `CC`
4 √7ᵗʰ **M84.353 Stress fracture, unspecified femur** `CC`
4 √7ᵗʰ **M84.359 Stress fracture, hip, unspecified** `CC`

√6ᵗʰ **M84.36 Stress fracture, tibia and fibula**
4 √7ᵗʰ **M84.361 Stress fracture, right tibia** `CC`
4 √7ᵗʰ **M84.362 Stress fracture, left tibia** `CC`
4 √7ᵗʰ **M84.363 Stress fracture, right fibula** `CC`
4 √7ᵗʰ **M84.364 Stress fracture, left fibula** `CC`
4 √7ᵗʰ **M84.369 Stress fracture, unspecified tibia and fibula** `CC`

√6ᵗʰ **M84.37 Stress fracture, ankle, foot and toes**
4 √7ᵗʰ **M84.371 Stress fracture, right ankle** `CC`
4 √7ᵗʰ **M84.372 Stress fracture, left ankle** `CC`
4 √7ᵗʰ **M84.373 Stress fracture, unspecified ankle** `CC`
4 √7ᵗʰ **M84.374 Stress fracture, right foot** `CC`
4 √7ᵗʰ **M84.375 Stress fracture, left foot** `CC`
4 √7ᵗʰ **M84.376 Stress fracture, unspecified foot** `CC`
4 √7ᵗʰ **M84.377 Stress fracture, right toe(s)** `CC`
4 √7ᵗʰ **M84.378 Stress fracture, left toe(s)** `CC`
4 √7ᵗʰ **M84.379 Stress fracture, unspecified toe(s)** `CC`

4 √x7ᵗʰ **M84.38 Stress fracture,** other site   `CC`

     EXCLUDES 2   *stress fracture of vertebra (M48.4-)*

√5ᵗʰ **M84.4 Pathological fracture,** not elsewhere classified
     Chronic fracture
     Pathological fracture NOS

     EXCLUDES 1   *collapsed vertebra NEC (M48.5)*
         pathological fracture in neoplastic disease (M84.5-)
         pathological fracture in osteoporosis (M80.-)
         pathological fracture in other disease (M84.6-)
         stress fracture (M84.3-)
         traumatic fracture (S12.-, S22.-, S32.-, S42.-, S52.-,
           S62.-, S72.-, S82.-, S92.-)

     EXCLUDES 2   *personal history of (healed) pathological fracture*
         (Z87.311)

     The appropriate 7th character is to be added to each code
     from subcategory M84.4.
     A   initial encounter for fracture
     D   subsequent encounter for fracture with routine healing
     G   subsequent encounter for fracture with delayed healing
     K   subsequent encounter for fracture with nonunion
     P   subsequent encounter for fracture with malunion
     S   sequela

     CC Excl: For CC codes in subcategory M84.4:
     CC with 7th character A: PDX collection 888
     CC with 7th character K or P: PDX collection 897

3 √x7ᵗʰ   **M84.40 Pathological fracture,** unspecified site   `CC`

√6ᵗʰ   **M84.41 Pathological fracture,** shoulder
   3   √7ᵗʰ   **M84.411 Pathological fracture,** right **shoulder**   `CC`
   3   √7ᵗʰ   **M84.412 Pathological fracture,** left **shoulder**   `CC`
   3   √7ᵗʰ   **M84.419 Pathological fracture,** unspecified **shoulder**   `CC`

√6ᵗʰ   **M84.42 Pathological fracture,** humerus
   3   √7ᵗʰ   **M84.421 Pathological fracture,** right **humerus**   `CC`
   3   √7ᵗʰ   **M84.422 Pathological fracture,** left **humerus**   `CC`
   3   √7ᵗʰ   **M84.429 Pathological fracture,** unspecified **humerus**   `CC`

√6ᵗʰ   **M84.43 Pathological fracture,** ulna and radius
   3   √7ᵗʰ   **M84.431 Pathological fracture,** right **ulna**   `CC`
   3   √7ᵗʰ   **M84.432 Pathological fracture,** left **ulna**   `CC`
   3   √7ᵗʰ   **M84.433 Pathological fracture,** right **radius**   `CC`
   3   √7ᵗʰ   **M84.434 Pathological fracture,** left **radius**   `CC`
   3   √7ᵗʰ   **M84.439 Pathological fracture,** unspecified **ulna and radius**   `CC`

√6ᵗʰ   **M84.44 Pathological fracture,** hand and fingers
   3   √7ᵗʰ   **M84.441 Pathological fracture,** right **hand**   `CC`
   3   √7ᵗʰ   **M84.442 Pathological fracture,** left **hand**   `CC`
   3   √7ᵗʰ   **M84.443 Pathological fracture,** unspecified **hand**   `CC`
   3   √7ᵗʰ   **M84.444 Pathological fracture,** right **finger(s)**   `CC`
   3   √7ᵗʰ   **M84.445 Pathological fracture,** left **finger(s)**   `CC`
   3   √7ᵗʰ   **M84.446 Pathological fracture,** unspecified **finger(s)**   `CC`

√6ᵗʰ   **M84.45 Pathological fracture,** femur and pelvis
     AHA: 2016, 4Q, 43
   3, 6   √7ᵗʰ   **M84.451 Pathological fracture,** right **femur**   `CC` `HCC`
   3, 6   √7ᵗʰ   **M84.452 Pathological fracture,** left **femur**   `CC` `HCC`
   3, 6   √7ᵗʰ   **M84.453 Pathological fracture,** unspecified **femur**   `CC` `HCC`
   3   √7ᵗʰ   **M84.454 Pathological fracture,** pelvis   `CC`
   3, 6   √7ᵗʰ   **M84.459 Pathological fracture,** hip, unspecified   `CC` `HCC`

√6ᵗʰ   **M84.46 Pathological fracture,** tibia and fibula
   3   √7ᵗʰ   **M84.461 Pathological fracture,** right **tibia**   `CC`
   3   √7ᵗʰ   **M84.462 Pathological fracture,** left **tibia**   `CC`
   3   √7ᵗʰ   **M84.463 Pathological fracture,** right **fibula**   `CC`
   3   √7ᵗʰ   **M84.464 Pathological fracture,** left **fibula**   `CC`
   3   √7ᵗʰ   **M84.469 Pathological fracture,** unspecified **tibia and fibula**   `CC`

√6ᵗʰ   **M84.47 Pathological fracture,** ankle, foot and toes
   3   √7ᵗʰ   **M84.471 Pathological fracture,** right **ankle**   `CC`
   3   √7ᵗʰ   **M84.472 Pathological fracture,** left **ankle**   `CC`
   3   √7ᵗʰ   **M84.473 Pathological fracture,** unspecified **ankle**   `CC`

---

   3   √7ᵗʰ   **M84.474 Pathological fracture,** right **foot**   `CC`
   3   √7ᵗʰ   **M84.475 Pathological fracture,** left **foot**   `CC`
   3   √7ᵗʰ   **M84.476 Pathological fracture,** unspecified **foot**   `CC`
   3   √7ᵗʰ   **M84.477 Pathological fracture,** right **toe(s)**   `CC`
   3   √7ᵗʰ   **M84.478 Pathological fracture,** left **toe(s)**   `CC`
   3   √7ᵗʰ   **M84.479 Pathological fracture,** unspecified **toe(s)**   `CC`

3 √x7ᵗʰ   **M84.48 Pathological fracture,** other site   `CC`

√5ᵗʰ **M84.5 Pathological fracture in** neoplastic disease
     Code also underlying neoplasm

     The appropriate 7th character is to be added to each code
     from subcategory M84.5.
     A   initial encounter for fracture
     D   subsequent encounter for fracture with routine healing
     G   subsequent encounter for fracture with delayed healing
     K   subsequent encounter for fracture with nonunion
     P   subsequent encounter for fracture with malunion
     S   sequela

     CC Excl: For CC codes in subcategory M84.5:
     CC with 7th character A: PDX collection 888
     CC with 7th character K or P: PDX collection 897

3 √x7ᵗʰ   **M84.50 Pathological fracture in neoplastic disease,** unspecified site   `CC`

√6ᵗʰ   **M84.51 Pathological fracture in neoplastic disease,** shoulder
   3   √7ᵗʰ   **M84.511 Pathological fracture in neoplastic disease,** right **shoulder**   `CC`
   3   √7ᵗʰ   **M84.512 Pathological fracture in neoplastic disease,** left **shoulder**   `CC`
   3   √7ᵗʰ   **M84.519 Pathological fracture in neoplastic disease,** unspecified **shoulder**

√6ᵗʰ   **M84.52 Pathological fracture in neoplastic disease,** humerus
   3   √7ᵗʰ   **M84.521 Pathological fracture in neoplastic disease,** right **humerus**   `CC`
   3   √7ᵗʰ   **M84.522 Pathological fracture in neoplastic disease,** left **humerus**   `CC`
   3   √7ᵗʰ   **M84.529 Pathological fracture in neoplastic disease,** unspecified **humerus**

√6ᵗʰ   **M84.53 Pathological fracture in neoplastic disease,** ulna and radius
   3   √7ᵗʰ   **M84.531 Pathological fracture in neoplastic disease,** right **ulna**   `CC`
   3   √7ᵗʰ   **M84.532 Pathological fracture in neoplastic disease,** left **ulna**   `CC`
   3   √7ᵗʰ   **M84.533 Pathological fracture in neoplastic disease,** right **radius**   `CC`
   3   √7ᵗʰ   **M84.534 Pathological fracture in neoplastic disease,** left **radius**   `CC`
   3   √7ᵗʰ   **M84.539 Pathological fracture in neoplastic disease,** unspecified **ulna and radius**

√6ᵗʰ   **M84.54 Pathological fracture in neoplastic disease,** hand
   3   √7ᵗʰ   **M84.541 Pathological fracture in neoplastic disease,** right **hand**   `CC`
   3   √7ᵗʰ   **M84.542 Pathological fracture in neoplastic disease,** left **hand**   `CC`
   3   √7ᵗʰ   **M84.549 Pathological fracture in neoplastic disease,** unspecified **hand**

√6ᵗʰ   **M84.55 Pathological fracture in neoplastic disease,** pelvis and femur
   3   √7ᵗʰ   **M84.550 Pathological fracture in neoplastic disease,** pelvis   `CC`
   3, 6   √7ᵗʰ   **M84.551 Pathological fracture in neoplastic disease,** right **femur**   `CC` `HCC`
   3, 6   √7ᵗʰ   **M84.552 Pathological fracture in neoplastic disease,** left **femur**   `CC` `HCC`
   3, 6   √7ᵗʰ   **M84.553 Pathological fracture in neoplastic disease,** unspecified **femur**   `CC` `HCC`
   3, 6   √7ᵗʰ   **M84.559 Pathological fracture in neoplastic disease,** hip, unspecified   `CC` `HCC`

√6ᵗʰ   **M84.56 Pathological fracture in neoplastic disease,** tibia and fibula
   3   √7ᵗʰ   **M84.561 Pathological fracture in neoplastic disease,** right **tibia**   `CC`
   3   √7ᵗʰ   **M84.562 Pathological fracture in neoplastic disease,** left **tibia**   `CC`

✓ Additional Character Required   √x7ᵗʰ Placeholder   Unacceptable PDx   Questionable PDx   Manifestation   H1 - H14 HAC   HCC CMS-HCC Dx   HIV HIV Dx

ICD-10-CM 2019   805

3   √7ᵗʰ   **M84.563**   **Pathological fracture in neoplastic disease,** right fibula   CC

3   √7ᵗʰ   **M84.564**   **Pathological fracture in neoplastic disease,** left fibula   CC

3   √7ᵗʰ   **M84.569**   **Pathological fracture in neoplastic disease,** unspecified tibia and fibula   CC

√6ᵗʰ   **M84.57**   **Pathological fracture in neoplastic disease,** ankle and foot

3   √7ᵗʰ   **M84.571**   **Pathological fracture in neoplastic disease,** right ankle   CC

3   √7ᵗʰ   **M84.572**   **Pathological fracture in neoplastic disease,** left ankle   CC

3   √7ᵗʰ   **M84.573**   **Pathological fracture in neoplastic disease,** unspecified ankle   CC

3   √7ᵗʰ   **M84.574**   **Pathological fracture in neoplastic disease,** right foot   CC

3   √7ᵗʰ   **M84.575**   **Pathological fracture in neoplastic disease,** left foot   CC

3   √7ᵗʰ   **M84.576**   **Pathological fracture in neoplastic disease,** unspecified foot   CC

3   √x7ᵗʰ   **M84.58**   **Pathological fracture in neoplastic disease, other specified site**   CC

      Pathological fracture in neoplastic disease, vertebrae

√5ᵗʰ   **M84.6**   **Pathological fracture** in other disease

    Code also underlying condition

    EXCLUDES 1   *pathological fracture in osteoporosis (M80.-)*

> The appropriate 7th character is to be added to each code from subcategory M84.6.
> A   initial encounter for fracture
> D   subsequent encounter for fracture with routine healing
> G   subsequent encounter for fracture with delayed healing
> K   subsequent encounter for fracture with nonunion
> P   subsequent encounter for fracture with malunion
> S   sequela

> CC Excl: For CC codes in subcategory M84.6:
> CC with 7th character A: PDX collection 888
> CC with 7th character K or P: PDX collection 897

3   √x7ᵗʰ   **M84.60**   **Pathological fracture in other disease, unspecified site**   CC

√6ᵗʰ   **M84.61**   **Pathological fracture in other disease,** shoulder

3   √7ᵗʰ   **M84.611**   **Pathological fracture in other disease,** right **shoulder**   CC

3   √7ᵗʰ   **M84.612**   **Pathological fracture in other disease,** left **shoulder**   CC

3   √7ᵗʰ   **M84.619**   **Pathological fracture in other disease,** unspecified **shoulder**   CC

√6ᵗʰ   **M84.62**   **Pathological fracture in other disease,** humerus

3   √7ᵗʰ   **M84.621**   **Pathological fracture in other disease,** right **humerus**   CC

3   √7ᵗʰ   **M84.622**   **Pathological fracture in other disease,** left **humerus**   CC

3   √7ᵗʰ   **M84.629**   **Pathological fracture in other disease,** unspecified **humerus**   CC

√6ᵗʰ   **M84.63**   **Pathological fracture in other disease,** ulna and radius

3   √7ᵗʰ   **M84.631**   **Pathological fracture in other disease,** right **ulna**   CC

3   √7ᵗʰ   **M84.632**   **Pathological fracture in other disease,** left **ulna**   CC

3   √7ᵗʰ   **M84.633**   **Pathological fracture in other disease,** right **radius**   CC

3   √7ᵗʰ   **M84.634**   **Pathological fracture in other disease,** left **radius**   CC

3   √7ᵗʰ   **M84.639**   **Pathological fracture in other disease,** unspecified **ulna and radius**   CC

√6ᵗʰ   **M84.64**   **Pathological fracture in other disease,** hand

3   √7ᵗʰ   **M84.641**   **Pathological fracture in other disease,** right **hand**   CC

3   √7ᵗʰ   **M84.642**   **Pathological fracture in other disease,** left **hand**   CC

3   √7ᵗʰ   **M84.649**   **Pathological fracture in other disease,** unspecified **hand**   CC

√6ᵗʰ   **M84.65**   **Pathological fracture in other disease,** pelvis and femur

3   √7ᵗʰ   **M84.650**   **Pathological fracture in other disease,** pelvis   CC

3, 6   √7ᵗʰ   **M84.651**   **Pathological fracture in other disease,** right femur   CC HCC

3, 6   √7ᵗʰ   **M84.652**   **Pathological fracture in other disease,** left femur   CC HCC

3, 6   √7ᵗʰ   **M84.653**   **Pathological fracture in other disease,** unspecified femur   CC HCC

3, 6   √7ᵗʰ   **M84.659**   **Pathological fracture in other disease,** hip, unspecified   CC HCC

√6ᵗʰ   **M84.66**   **Pathological fracture in other disease,** tibia and fibula

3   √7ᵗʰ   **M84.661**   **Pathological fracture in other disease,** right tibia   CC

3   √7ᵗʰ   **M84.662**   **Pathological fracture in other disease,** left tibia   CC

3   √7ᵗʰ   **M84.663**   **Pathological fracture in other disease,** right fibula   CC

3   √7ᵗʰ   **M84.664**   **Pathological fracture in other disease,** left fibula   CC

3   √7ᵗʰ   **M84.669**   **Pathological fracture in other disease,** unspecified **tibia and fibula**   CC

√6ᵗʰ   **M84.67**   **Pathological fracture in other disease,** ankle and foot

3   √7ᵗʰ   **M84.671**   **Pathological fracture in other disease,** right ankle   CC

3   √7ᵗʰ   **M84.672**   **Pathological fracture in other disease,** left ankle   CC

3   √7ᵗʰ   **M84.673**   **Pathological fracture in other disease,** unspecified ankle   CC

3   √7ᵗʰ   **M84.674**   **Pathological fracture in other disease,** right foot   CC

3   √7ᵗʰ   **M84.675**   **Pathological fracture in other disease,** left foot   CC

3   √7ᵗʰ   **M84.676**   **Pathological fracture in other disease,** unspecified foot   CC

3   √x7ᵗʰ   **M84.68**   **Pathological fracture in other disease,** other site   CC

√5ᵗʰ   **M84.7**   **Nontraumatic fracture, not elsewhere classified**

√6ᵗʰ   **M84.75**   **Atypical femoral fracture**

    AHA: 2016, 4Q, 41-42

> The appropriate 7th character is to be added to each code from subcategory M84.75.
> A   initial encounter for fracture
> D   subsequent encounter for fracture with routine healing
> G   subsequent encounter for fracture with delayed healing
> K   subsequent encounter for fracture with nonunion
> P   subsequent encounter for fracture with malunion
> S   sequela

> CC Excl: For CC codes in subcategory M84.75:
> CC with 7th character A: PDX collection 888
> CC with 7th character K or P: PDX collection 897

3   √7ᵗʰ   **M84.750**   **Atypical femoral fracture,** unspecified   CC

3   √7ᵗʰ   **M84.751**   **Incomplete atypical femoral fracture,** right **leg**   CC

3   √7ᵗʰ   **M84.752**   **Incomplete atypical femoral fracture,** left **leg**   CC

3   √7ᵗʰ   **M84.753**   **Incomplete atypical femoral fracture,** unspecified **leg**   CC

3, 6   √7ᵗʰ   **M84.754**   **Complete transverse atypical femoral fracture,** right **leg**   CC HCC

3, 6   √7ᵗʰ   **M84.755**   **Complete transverse atypical femoral fracture,** left **leg**   CC HCC

3, 6   √7ᵗʰ   **M84.756**   **Complete transverse atypical femoral fracture,** unspecified **leg**   CC HCC

3, 6   √7ᵗʰ   **M84.757**   **Complete oblique atypical femoral fracture,** right **leg**   CC HCC

3, 6   √7ᵗʰ   **M84.758**   **Complete oblique atypical femoral fracture,** left **leg**   CC HCC

3, 6   √7ᵗʰ   **M84.759**   **Complete oblique atypical femoral fracture,** unspecified **leg**   CC HCC

Ⓝ Newborn: 0   Ⓟ Pediatric: 0-17   Ⓜ Maternity: 12-55   Ⓐ Adult: 15-124   MCC Major Complication/Comorbidity   CC Complication/Comorbidity   SW Severe Wound Dx

806   ICD-10-CM 2019

✓5ᵗʰ **M84.8 Other disorders of continuity of bone**

    M84.80 Other disorders of continuity of bone, unspecified site

    ✓6ᵗʰ **M84.81 Other disorders of continuity of bone,** shoulder

        M84.811 Other disorders of continuity of bone, right **shoulder**

        M84.812 Other disorders of continuity of bone, left **shoulder**

        M84.819 Other disorders of continuity of bone, unspecified **shoulder**

    ✓6ᵗʰ **M84.82 Other disorders of continuity of bone,** humerus

        M84.821 Other disorders of continuity of bone, right **humerus**

        M84.822 Other disorders of continuity of bone, left **humerus**

        M84.829 Other disorders of continuity of bone, unspecified **humerus**

    ✓6ᵗʰ **M84.83 Other disorders of continuity of bone,** ulna and radius

        M84.831 Other disorders of continuity of bone, right **ulna**

        M84.832 Other disorders of continuity of bone, left **ulna**

        M84.833 Other disorders of continuity of bone, right **radius**

        M84.834 Other disorders of continuity of bone, left **radius**

        M84.839 Other disorders of continuity of bone, unspecified **ulna and radius**

    ✓6ᵗʰ **M84.84 Other disorders of continuity of bone,** hand

        M84.841 Other disorders of continuity of bone, right **hand**

        M84.842 Other disorders of continuity of bone, left **hand**

        M84.849 Other disorders of continuity of bone, unspecified **hand**

    ✓6ᵗʰ **M84.85 Other disorders of continuity of bone,** pelvic region and thigh

        M84.851 Other disorders of continuity of bone, right **pelvic region and thigh**

        M84.852 Other disorders of continuity of bone, left **pelvic region and thigh**

        M84.859 Other disorders of continuity of bone, unspecified **pelvic region and thigh**

    ✓6ᵗʰ **M84.86 Other disorders of continuity of bone,** tibia and fibula

        M84.861 Other disorders of continuity of bone, right **tibia**

        M84.862 Other disorders of continuity of bone, left **tibia**

        M84.863 Other disorders of continuity of bone, right **fibula**

        M84.864 Other disorders of continuity of bone, left **fibula**

        M84.869 Other disorders of continuity of bone, unspecified **tibia and fibula**

    ✓6ᵗʰ **M84.87 Other disorders of continuity of bone,** ankle and foot

        M84.871 Other disorders of continuity of bone, right **ankle and foot**

        M84.872 Other disorders of continuity of bone, left **ankle and foot**

        M84.879 Other disorders of continuity of bone, unspecified **ankle and foot**

    M84.88 Other disorders of continuity of bone, other site

  M84.9 Disorder of continuity of bone, unspecified

✓4ᵗʰ **M85 Other disorders of bone density and structure**

    EXCLUDES 1 osteogenesis imperfecta (Q78.0)
                 osteopetrosis (Q78.2)
                 osteopoikilosis (Q78.8)
                 polyostotic fibrous dysplasia (Q78.1)

  ✓5ᵗʰ **M85.0 Fibrous dysplasia (monostotic)**

    EXCLUDES 2 fibrous dysplasia of jaw (M27.8)

    M85.00 Fibrous dysplasia (monostotic), unspecified site

    ✓6ᵗʰ **M85.01 Fibrous dysplasia (monostotic),** shoulder

        M85.011 Fibrous dysplasia (monostotic), right **shoulder**

        M85.012 Fibrous dysplasia (monostotic), left **shoulder**

        M85.019 Fibrous dysplasia (monostotic), unspecified **shoulder**

    ✓6ᵗʰ **M85.02 Fibrous dysplasia (monostotic),** upper arm

        M85.021 Fibrous dysplasia (monostotic), right **upper arm**

        M85.022 Fibrous dysplasia (monostotic), left **upper arm**

        M85.029 Fibrous dysplasia (monostotic), unspecified **upper arm**

    ✓6ᵗʰ **M85.03 Fibrous dysplasia (monostotic),** forearm

        M85.031 Fibrous dysplasia (monostotic), right **forearm**

        M85.032 Fibrous dysplasia (monostotic), left **forearm**

        M85.039 Fibrous dysplasia (monostotic), unspecified **forearm**

    ✓6ᵗʰ **M85.04 Fibrous dysplasia (monostotic),** hand

        M85.041 Fibrous dysplasia (monostotic), right **hand**

        M85.042 Fibrous dysplasia (monostotic), left **hand**

        M85.049 Fibrous dysplasia (monostotic), unspecified **hand**

    ✓6ᵗʰ **M85.05 Fibrous dysplasia (monostotic),** thigh

        M85.051 Fibrous dysplasia (monostotic), right **thigh**

        M85.052 Fibrous dysplasia (monostotic), left **thigh**

        M85.059 Fibrous dysplasia (monostotic), unspecified **thigh**

    ✓6ᵗʰ **M85.06 Fibrous dysplasia (monostotic),** lower leg

        M85.061 Fibrous dysplasia (monostotic), right **lower leg**

        M85.062 Fibrous dysplasia (monostotic), left **lower leg**

        M85.069 Fibrous dysplasia (monostotic), unspecified **lower leg**

    ✓6ᵗʰ **M85.07 Fibrous dysplasia (monostotic),** ankle and foot

        M85.071 Fibrous dysplasia (monostotic), right **ankle and foot**

        M85.072 Fibrous dysplasia (monostotic), left **ankle and foot**

        M85.079 Fibrous dysplasia (monostotic), unspecified **ankle and foot**

    M85.08 Fibrous dysplasia (monostotic), other site

    M85.09 Fibrous dysplasia (monostotic), multiple sites

  ✓5ᵗʰ **M85.1 Skeletal fluorosis**

    M85.10 Skeletal fluorosis, unspecified site

    ✓6ᵗʰ **M85.11 Skeletal fluorosis,** shoulder

        M85.111 Skeletal fluorosis, right **shoulder**

        M85.112 Skeletal fluorosis, left **shoulder**

        M85.119 Skeletal fluorosis, unspecified **shoulder**

    ✓6ᵗʰ **M85.12 Skeletal fluorosis,** upper arm

        M85.121 Skeletal fluorosis, right **upper arm**

        M85.122 Skeletal fluorosis, left **upper arm**

        M85.129 Skeletal fluorosis, unspecified **upper arm**

    ✓6ᵗʰ **M85.13 Skeletal fluorosis,** forearm

        M85.131 Skeletal fluorosis, right **forearm**

        M85.132 Skeletal fluorosis, left **forearm**

        M85.139 Skeletal fluorosis, unspecified **forearm**

    ✓6ᵗʰ **M85.14 Skeletal fluorosis,** hand

        M85.141 Skeletal fluorosis, right **hand**

        M85.142 Skeletal fluorosis, left **hand**

        M85.149 Skeletal fluorosis, unspecified **hand**

    ✓6ᵗʰ **M85.15 Skeletal fluorosis,** thigh

        M85.151 Skeletal fluorosis, right **thigh**

        M85.152 Skeletal fluorosis, left **thigh**

        M85.159 Skeletal fluorosis, unspecified **thigh**

    ✓6ᵗʰ **M85.16 Skeletal fluorosis,** lower leg

        M85.161 Skeletal fluorosis, right **lower leg**

        M85.162 Skeletal fluorosis, left **lower leg**

        M85.169 Skeletal fluorosis, unspecified **lower leg**

    ✓6ᵗʰ **M85.17 Skeletal fluorosis,** ankle and foot

        M85.171 Skeletal fluorosis, right **ankle and foot**

        M85.172 Skeletal fluorosis, left **ankle and foot**

✔ Additional Character Required   ✓x7ᵗʰ Placeholder   Unacceptable PDx   Questionable PDx   Manifestation   H1–H14 HAC   HCC CMS-HCC Dx   HIV HIV Dx

ICD-10-CM 2019   807

Chapter 13. Diseases of the Musculoskeletal System and Connective Tissue

M84.8–M85.172

M85.179 Skeletal fluorosis, unspecified ankle and foot
M85.18 Skeletal fluorosis, other site
M85.19 Skeletal fluorosis, multiple sites
M85.2 Hyperostosis of skull
   DEF: Abnormal bone growth on the inner aspect of the cranial bones.
☑5th M85.3 Osteitis condensans
   M85.30 Osteitis condensans, unspecified site
   ☑6th M85.31 Osteitis condensans, shoulder
      M85.311 Osteitis condensans, right shoulder
      M85.312 Osteitis condensans, left shoulder
      M85.319 Osteitis condensans, unspecified shoulder
   ☑6th M85.32 Osteitis condensans, upper arm
      M85.321 Osteitis condensans, right upper arm
      M85.322 Osteitis condensans, left upper arm
      M85.329 Osteitis condensans, unspecified upper arm
   ☑6th M85.33 Osteitis condensans, forearm
      M85.331 Osteitis condensans, right forearm
      M85.332 Osteitis condensans, left forearm
      M85.339 Osteitis condensans, unspecified forearm
   ☑6th M85.34 Osteitis condensans, hand
      M85.341 Osteitis condensans, right hand
      M85.342 Osteitis condensans, left hand
      M85.349 Osteitis condensans, unspecified hand
   ☑6th M85.35 Osteitis condensans, thigh
      M85.351 Osteitis condensans, right thigh
      M85.352 Osteitis condensans, left thigh
      M85.359 Osteitis condensans, unspecified thigh
   ☑6th M85.36 Osteitis condensans, lower leg
      M85.361 Osteitis condensans, right lower leg
      M85.362 Osteitis condensans, left lower leg
      M85.369 Osteitis condensans, unspecified lower leg
   ☑6th M85.37 Osteitis condensans, ankle and foot
      M85.371 Osteitis condensans, right ankle and foot
      M85.372 Osteitis condensans, left ankle and foot
      M85.379 Osteitis condensans, unspecified ankle and foot
   M85.38 Osteitis condensans, other site
   M85.39 Osteitis condensans, multiple sites
☑5th M85.4 Solitary bone cyst
   EXCLUDES 2 solitary cyst of jaw (M27.4)
   M85.40 Solitary bone cyst, unspecified site
   ☑6th M85.41 Solitary bone cyst, shoulder
      M85.411 Solitary bone cyst, right shoulder
      M85.412 Solitary bone cyst, left shoulder
      M85.419 Solitary bone cyst, unspecified shoulder
   ☑6th M85.42 Solitary bone cyst, humerus
      M85.421 Solitary bone cyst, right humerus
      M85.422 Solitary bone cyst, left humerus
      M85.429 Solitary bone cyst, unspecified humerus
   ☑6th M85.43 Solitary bone cyst, ulna and radius
      M85.431 Solitary bone cyst, right ulna and radius
      M85.432 Solitary bone cyst, left ulna and radius
      M85.439 Solitary bone cyst, unspecified ulna and radius
   ☑6th M85.44 Solitary bone cyst, hand
      M85.441 Solitary bone cyst, right hand
      M85.442 Solitary bone cyst, left hand
      M85.449 Solitary bone cyst, unspecified hand
   ☑6th M85.45 Solitary bone cyst, pelvis
      M85.451 Solitary bone cyst, right pelvis
      M85.452 Solitary bone cyst, left pelvis
      M85.459 Solitary bone cyst, unspecified pelvis
   ☑6th M85.46 Solitary bone cyst, tibia and fibula
      M85.461 Solitary bone cyst, right tibia and fibula
      M85.462 Solitary bone cyst, left tibia and fibula
      M85.469 Solitary bone cyst, unspecified tibia and fibula
   ☑6th M85.47 Solitary bone cyst, ankle and foot
      M85.471 Solitary bone cyst, right ankle and foot

M85.472 Solitary bone cyst, left ankle and foot
M85.479 Solitary bone cyst, unspecified ankle and foot
M85.48 Solitary bone cyst, other site
☑5th M85.5 Aneurysmal bone cyst
   EXCLUDES 2 aneurysmal cyst of jaw (M27.4)
   DEF: Solitary bone lesion that bulges into the periosteum and is marked by a calcified rim.
   M85.50 Aneurysmal bone cyst, unspecified site
   ☑6th M85.51 Aneurysmal bone cyst, shoulder
      M85.511 Aneurysmal bone cyst, right shoulder
      M85.512 Aneurysmal bone cyst, left shoulder
      M85.519 Aneurysmal bone cyst, unspecified shoulder
   ☑6th M85.52 Aneurysmal bone cyst, upper arm
      M85.521 Aneurysmal bone cyst, right upper arm
      M85.522 Aneurysmal bone cyst, left upper arm
      M85.529 Aneurysmal bone cyst, unspecified upper arm
   ☑6th M85.53 Aneurysmal bone cyst, forearm
      M85.531 Aneurysmal bone cyst, right forearm
      M85.532 Aneurysmal bone cyst, left forearm
      M85.539 Aneurysmal bone cyst, unspecified forearm
   ☑6th M85.54 Aneurysmal bone cyst, hand
      M85.541 Aneurysmal bone cyst, right hand
      M85.542 Aneurysmal bone cyst, left hand
      M85.549 Aneurysmal bone cyst, unspecified hand
   ☑6th M85.55 Aneurysmal bone cyst, thigh
      M85.551 Aneurysmal bone cyst, right thigh
      M85.552 Aneurysmal bone cyst, left thigh
      M85.559 Aneurysmal bone cyst, unspecified thigh
   ☑6th M85.56 Aneurysmal bone cyst, lower leg
      M85.561 Aneurysmal bone cyst, right lower leg
      M85.562 Aneurysmal bone cyst, left lower leg
      M85.569 Aneurysmal bone cyst, unspecified lower leg
   ☑6th M85.57 Aneurysmal bone cyst, ankle and foot
      M85.571 Aneurysmal bone cyst, right ankle and foot
      M85.572 Aneurysmal bone cyst, left ankle and foot
      M85.579 Aneurysmal bone cyst, unspecified ankle and foot
   M85.58 Aneurysmal bone cyst, other site
   M85.59 Aneurysmal bone cyst, multiple sites
☑5th M85.6 Other cyst of bone
   EXCLUDES 1 cyst of jaw NEC (M27.4)
      osteitis fibrosa cystica generalisata [von Recklinghausen's disease of bone] (E21.0)
   M85.60 Other cyst of bone, unspecified site
   ☑6th M85.61 Other cyst of bone, shoulder
      M85.611 Other cyst of bone, right shoulder
      M85.612 Other cyst of bone, left shoulder
      M85.619 Other cyst of bone, unspecified shoulder
   ☑6th M85.62 Other cyst of bone, upper arm
      M85.621 Other cyst of bone, right upper arm
      M85.622 Other cyst of bone, left upper arm
      M85.629 Other cyst of bone, unspecified upper arm
   ☑6th M85.63 Other cyst of bone, forearm
      M85.631 Other cyst of bone, right forearm
      M85.632 Other cyst of bone, left forearm
      M85.639 Other cyst of bone, unspecified forearm
   ☑6th M85.64 Other cyst of bone, hand
      M85.641 Other cyst of bone, right hand
      M85.642 Other cyst of bone, left hand
      M85.649 Other cyst of bone, unspecified hand
   ☑6th M85.65 Other cyst of bone, thigh
      M85.651 Other cyst of bone, right thigh
      M85.652 Other cyst of bone, left thigh
      M85.659 Other cyst of bone, unspecified thigh
   ☑6th M85.66 Other cyst of bone, lower leg
      M85.661 Other cyst of bone, right lower leg
      M85.662 Other cyst of bone, left lower leg

M85.669   Other cyst of bone, unspecified lower leg

✓6ᵗʰ **M85.67**   Other cyst of bone, ankle and foot

     M85.671   Other cyst of bone, right ankle and foot

     M85.672   Other cyst of bone, left ankle and foot

     M85.679   Other cyst of bone, unspecified ankle and foot

M85.68   Other cyst of bone, other site

M85.69   Other cyst of bone, multiple sites

✓5ᵗʰ **M85.8**   **Other specified disorders of bone density and structure**

     Hyperostosis of bones, except skull

     Osteosclerosis, acquired

     EXCLUDES 1   diffuse idiopathic skeletal hyperostosis [DISH] (M48.1)

         osteosclerosis congenita (Q77.4)

         osteosclerosis fragilitas (generalista) (Q78.2)

         osteosclerosis myelofibrosis (D75.81)

     M85.80   Other specified disorders of bone density and structure, unspecified site

✓6ᵗʰ   **M85.81**   Other specified disorders of bone density and structure, shoulder

       M85.811   Other specified disorders of bone density and structure, right shoulder

       M85.812   Other specified disorders of bone density and structure, left shoulder

       M85.819   Other specified disorders of bone density and structure, unspecified shoulder

✓6ᵗʰ   **M85.82**   Other specified disorders of bone density and structure, upper arm

       M85.821   Other specified disorders of bone density and structure, right upper arm

       M85.822   Other specified disorders of bone density and structure, left upper arm

       M85.829   Other specified disorders of bone density and structure, unspecified upper arm

✓6ᵗʰ   **M85.83**   Other specified disorders of bone density and structure, forearm

       M85.831   Other specified disorders of bone density and structure, right forearm

       M85.832   Other specified disorders of bone density and structure, left forearm

       M85.839   Other specified disorders of bone density and structure, unspecified forearm

✓6ᵗʰ   **M85.84**   Other specified disorders of bone density and structure, hand

       M85.841   Other specified disorders of bone density and structure, right hand

       M85.842   Other specified disorders of bone density and structure, left hand

       M85.849   Other specified disorders of bone density and structure, unspecified hand

✓6ᵗʰ   **M85.85**   Other specified disorders of bone density and structure, thigh

       M85.851   Other specified disorders of bone density and structure, right thigh

       M85.852   Other specified disorders of bone density and structure, left thigh

       M85.859   Other specified disorders of bone density and structure, unspecified thigh

✓6ᵗʰ   **M85.86**   Other specified disorders of bone density and structure, lower leg

       M85.861   Other specified disorders of bone density and structure, right lower leg

       M85.862   Other specified disorders of bone density and structure, left lower leg

       M85.869   Other specified disorders of bone density and structure, unspecified lower leg

✓6ᵗʰ   **M85.87**   Other specified disorders of bone density and structure, ankle and foot

       M85.871   Other specified disorders of bone density and structure, right ankle and foot

       M85.872   Other specified disorders of bone density and structure, left ankle and foot

       M85.879   Other specified disorders of bone density and structure, unspecified ankle and foot

     M85.88   Other specified disorders of bone density and structure, other site

     M85.89   Other specified disorders of bone density and structure, multiple sites

M85.9   Disorder of bone density and structure, unspecified

Other osteopathies (M86-M90)

EXCLUDES 1   postprocedural osteopathies (M96.-)

✓4ᵗʰ **M86**   **Osteomyelitis**

     Use additional code (B95-B97) to identify infectious agent

     Use additional code to identify major osseous defect, if applicable (M89.7-)

     EXCLUDES 1   osteomyelitis due to:

         echinococcus (B67.2)

         gonococcus (A54.43)

         salmonella (A02.24)

     EXCLUDES 2   osteomyelitis of:

         orbit (H05.0-)

         petrous bone (H70.2-)

         vertebra (M46.2-)

✓5ᵗʰ **M86.0**   Acute hematogenous osteomyelitis

     M86.00   Acute hematogenous osteomyelitis, unspecified site   `CC` `HCC`

       CC Excl: PDX collection 898

✓6ᵗʰ   **M86.01**   Acute hematogenous osteomyelitis, shoulder

       CC Excl: For CC codes in subcategory M86.01: PDX collection 899

       M86.011   Acute hematogenous osteomyelitis, right shoulder   `CC` `HCC`

       M86.012   Acute hematogenous osteomyelitis, left shoulder   `CC` `HCC`

       M86.019   Acute hematogenous osteomyelitis, unspecified shoulder   `CC` `HCC`

✓6ᵗʰ   **M86.02**   Acute hematogenous osteomyelitis, humerus

       CC Excl: For CC codes in subcategory M86.02: PDX collection 900

       M86.021   Acute hematogenous osteomyelitis, right humerus   `CC` `HCC`

       M86.022   Acute hematogenous osteomyelitis, left humerus   `CC` `HCC`

       M86.029   Acute hematogenous osteomyelitis, unspecified humerus   `CC` `HCC`

✓6ᵗʰ   **M86.03**   Acute hematogenous osteomyelitis, radius and ulna

       CC Excl: For CC codes in subcategory M86.03: PDX collection 901

       M86.031   Acute hematogenous osteomyelitis, right radius and ulna   `CC` `HCC`

       M86.032   Acute hematogenous osteomyelitis, left radius and ulna   `CC` `HCC`

       M86.039   Acute hematogenous osteomyelitis, unspecified radius and ulna   `CC` `HCC`

✓6ᵗʰ   **M86.04**   Acute hematogenous osteomyelitis, hand

       CC Excl: For CC codes in subcategory M86.04: PDX collection 902

       M86.041   Acute hematogenous osteomyelitis, right hand   `CC` `HCC`

       M86.042   Acute hematogenous osteomyelitis, left hand   `CC` `HCC`

       M86.049   Acute hematogenous osteomyelitis, unspecified hand   `CC` `HCC`

✓6ᵗʰ   **M86.05**   Acute hematogenous osteomyelitis, femur

       CC Excl: For CC codes in subcategory M86.05: PDX collection 903

       M86.051   Acute hematogenous osteomyelitis, right femur   `CC` `HCC`

       M86.052   Acute hematogenous osteomyelitis, left femur   `CC` `HCC`

       M86.059   Acute hematogenous osteomyelitis, unspecified femur   `CC` `HCC`

✓6ᵗʰ   **M86.06**   Acute hematogenous osteomyelitis, tibia and fibula

       CC Excl: For CC codes in subcategory M86.06: PDX collection 904

       M86.061   Acute hematogenous osteomyelitis, right tibia and fibula   `CC` `HCC`

       M86.062   Acute hematogenous osteomyelitis, left tibia and fibula   `CC` `HCC`

✔ Additional Character Required   ✓x7ᵗʰ Placeholder   Unacceptable PDx   Questionable PDx   Manifestation   `H1`-`H14` HAC   `HCC` CMS-HCC Dx   `HIV` HIV Dx

ICD-10-CM 2019   **809**

M86.069 Acute hematogenous osteomyelitis, unspecified tibia and fibula `CC` `HCC`

✓6ᵗʰ **M86.07** Acute hematogenous osteomyelitis, ankle and foot

> **CC Excl:** For CC codes in subcategory M86.07: PDX collection 905

    M86.071 Acute hematogenous osteomyelitis, right ankle and foot `CC` `HCC`

    M86.072 Acute hematogenous osteomyelitis, left ankle and foot `CC` `HCC`

    M86.079 Acute hematogenous osteomyelitis, unspecified ankle and foot `CC` `HCC`

M86.08 Acute hematogenous osteomyelitis, other sites `CC` `HCC`
> **CC Excl:** PDX collection 882

M86.09 Acute hematogenous osteomyelitis, multiple sites `CC` `HCC`
> **CC Excl:** PDX collection 898

✓5ᵗʰ **M86.1** Other acute osteomyelitis

    M86.10 Other acute osteomyelitis, unspecified site `CC` `HCC`
> **CC Excl:** PDX collection 898

✓6ᵗʰ **M86.11** Other acute osteomyelitis, shoulder

> **CC Excl:** For CC codes in subcategory M86.11: PDX collection 899

    M86.111 Other acute osteomyelitis, right shoulder `CC` `HCC`

    M86.112 Other acute osteomyelitis, left shoulder `CC` `HCC`

    M86.119 Other acute osteomyelitis, unspecified shoulder `CC` `HCC`

✓6ᵗʰ **M86.12** Other acute osteomyelitis, humerus

> **CC Excl:** For CC codes in subcategory M86.12: PDX collection 900

    M86.121 Other acute osteomyelitis, right humerus `CC` `HCC`

    M86.122 Other acute osteomyelitis, left humerus `CC` `HCC`

    M86.129 Other acute osteomyelitis, unspecified humerus `CC` `HCC`

✓6ᵗʰ **M86.13** Other acute osteomyelitis, radius and ulna

> **CC Excl:** For CC codes in subcategory M86.13: PDX collection 901

    M86.131 Other acute osteomyelitis, right radius and ulna `CC` `HCC`

    M86.132 Other acute osteomyelitis, left radius and ulna `CC` `HCC`

    M86.139 Other acute osteomyelitis, unspecified radius and ulna `CC` `HCC`

✓6ᵗʰ **M86.14** Other acute osteomyelitis, hand

> **CC Excl:** For CC codes in subcategory M86.14: PDX collection 902

    M86.141 Other acute osteomyelitis, right hand `CC` `HCC`

    M86.142 Other acute osteomyelitis, left hand `CC` `HCC`

    M86.149 Other acute osteomyelitis, unspecified hand `CC` `HCC`

✓6ᵗʰ **M86.15** Other acute osteomyelitis, femur

> **CC Excl:** For CC codes in subcategory M86.15: PDX collection 903

    M86.151 Other acute osteomyelitis, right femur `CC` `HCC`

    M86.152 Other acute osteomyelitis, left femur `CC` `HCC`

    M86.159 Other acute osteomyelitis, unspecified femur `CC` `HCC`

✓6ᵗʰ **M86.16** Other acute osteomyelitis, tibia and fibula

> **CC Excl:** For CC codes in subcategory M86.16: PDX collection 904

    M86.161 Other acute osteomyelitis, right tibia and fibula `CC` `HCC`

    M86.162 Other acute osteomyelitis, left tibia and fibula `CC` `HCC`

M86.169 Other acute osteomyelitis, unspecified tibia and fibula `CC` `HCC`

✓6ᵗʰ **M86.17** Other acute osteomyelitis, ankle and foot

> **CC Excl:** For CC codes in subcategory M86.17: PDX collection 905

    M86.171 Other acute osteomyelitis, right ankle and foot `CC` `HCC`

    M86.172 Other acute osteomyelitis, left ankle and foot `CC` `HCC`

    M86.179 Other acute osteomyelitis, unspecified ankle and foot `CC` `HCC`

M86.18 Other acute osteomyelitis, other site `CC` `HCC`
> **CC Excl:** PDX collection 882

M86.19 Other acute osteomyelitis, multiple sites `CC` `HCC`
> **CC Excl:** PDX collection 898

✓5ᵗʰ **M86.2** Subacute osteomyelitis

    M86.20 Subacute osteomyelitis, unspecified site `CC` `HCC`
> **CC Excl:** PDX collection 898

✓6ᵗʰ **M86.21** Subacute osteomyelitis, shoulder

> **CC Excl:** For CC codes in subcategory M86.21: PDX collection 899

    M86.211 Subacute osteomyelitis, right shoulder `CC` `HCC`

    M86.212 Subacute osteomyelitis, left shoulder `CC` `HCC`

    M86.219 Subacute osteomyelitis, unspecified shoulder `CC` `HCC`

✓6ᵗʰ **M86.22** Subacute osteomyelitis, humerus

> **CC Excl:** For CC codes in subcategory M86.22: PDX collection 900

    M86.221 Subacute osteomyelitis, right humerus `CC` `HCC`

    M86.222 Subacute osteomyelitis, left humerus `CC` `HCC`

    M86.229 Subacute osteomyelitis, unspecified humerus `CC` `HCC`

✓6ᵗʰ **M86.23** Subacute osteomyelitis, radius and ulna

> **CC Excl:** For CC codes in subcategory M86.23: PDX collection 901

    M86.231 Subacute osteomyelitis, right radius and ulna `CC` `HCC`

    M86.232 Subacute osteomyelitis, left radius and ulna `CC` `HCC`

    M86.239 Subacute osteomyelitis, unspecified radius and ulna `CC` `HCC`

✓6ᵗʰ **M86.24** Subacute osteomyelitis, hand

> **CC Excl:** For CC codes in subcategory M86.24: PDX collection 902

    M86.241 Subacute osteomyelitis, right hand `CC` `HCC`

    M86.242 Subacute osteomyelitis, left hand `CC` `HCC`

    M86.249 Subacute osteomyelitis, unspecified hand `CC` `HCC`

✓6ᵗʰ **M86.25** Subacute osteomyelitis, femur

> **CC Excl:** For CC codes in subcategory M86.25: PDX collection 903

    M86.251 Subacute osteomyelitis, right femur `CC` `HCC`

    M86.252 Subacute osteomyelitis, left femur `CC` `HCC`

    M86.259 Subacute osteomyelitis, unspecified femur `CC` `HCC`

✓6ᵗʰ **M86.26** Subacute osteomyelitis, tibia and fibula

> **CC Excl:** For CC codes in subcategory M86.26: PDX collection 904

    M86.261 Subacute osteomyelitis, right tibia and fibula `CC` `HCC`

    M86.262 Subacute osteomyelitis, left tibia and fibula `CC` `HCC`

    M86.269 Subacute osteomyelitis, unspecified tibia and fibula `CC` `HCC`

Ⓝ Newborn: 0   Ⓟ Pediatric: 0-17   Ⓜ Maternity: 12-55   Ⓐ Adult: 15-124   `MCC` Major Complication/Comorbidity   `CC` Complication/Comorbidity   `SW` Severe Wound Dx

810   ICD-10-CM 2019

✓6ᵗʰ **M86.27** Subacute osteomyelitis, ankle and foot

> **CC Excl: For CC codes in subcategory M86.27:** PDX collection 905

     M86.271 Subacute osteomyelitis, right ankle and foot   `CC` `HCC`

     M86.272 Subacute osteomyelitis, left ankle and foot   `CC` `HCC`

     M86.279 Subacute osteomyelitis, unspecified ankle and foot   `CC` `HCC`

   M86.28 Subacute osteomyelitis, other site   `CC` `HCC`
> **CC Excl:** PDX collection 882

   M86.29 Subacute osteomyelitis, multiple sites   `CC` `HCC`
> **CC Excl:** PDX collection 898

✓5ᵗʰ **M86.3** Chronic multifocal osteomyelitis

> **CC Excl: For CC codes in subcategory M86.3, unless otherwise noted:** PDX collection 881

   M86.30 Chronic multifocal osteomyelitis, unspecified site   `CC` `HCC`
> **CC Excl:** PDX collection 906

✓6ᵗʰ **M86.31** Chronic multifocal osteomyelitis, shoulder

     M86.311 Chronic multifocal osteomyelitis, right shoulder   `CC` `HCC`

     M86.312 Chronic multifocal osteomyelitis, left shoulder   `CC` `HCC`

     M86.319 Chronic multifocal osteomyelitis, unspecified shoulder   `CC` `HCC`

✓6ᵗʰ **M86.32** Chronic multifocal osteomyelitis, humerus

     M86.321 Chronic multifocal osteomyelitis, right humerus   `CC` `HCC`

     M86.322 Chronic multifocal osteomyelitis, left humerus   `CC` `HCC`

     M86.329 Chronic multifocal osteomyelitis, unspecified humerus   `CC` `HCC`

✓6ᵗʰ **M86.33** Chronic multifocal osteomyelitis, radius and ulna

     M86.331 Chronic multifocal osteomyelitis, right radius and ulna   `CC` `HCC`

     M86.332 Chronic multifocal osteomyelitis, left radius and ulna   `CC` `HCC`

     M86.339 Chronic multifocal osteomyelitis, unspecified radius and ulna   `CC` `HCC`

✓6ᵗʰ **M86.34** Chronic multifocal osteomyelitis, hand

     M86.341 Chronic multifocal osteomyelitis, right hand   `CC` `HCC`

     M86.342 Chronic multifocal osteomyelitis, left hand   `CC` `HCC`

     M86.349 Chronic multifocal osteomyelitis, unspecified hand   `CC` `HCC`

✓6ᵗʰ **M86.35** Chronic multifocal osteomyelitis, femur

     M86.351 Chronic multifocal osteomyelitis, right femur   `CC` `HCC`

     M86.352 Chronic multifocal osteomyelitis, left femur   `CC` `HCC`

     M86.359 Chronic multifocal osteomyelitis, unspecified femur   `CC` `HCC`

✓6ᵗʰ **M86.36** Chronic multifocal osteomyelitis, tibia and fibula

     M86.361 Chronic multifocal osteomyelitis, right tibia and fibula   `CC` `HCC`

     M86.362 Chronic multifocal osteomyelitis, left tibia and fibula   `CC` `HCC`

     M86.369 Chronic multifocal osteomyelitis, unspecified tibia and fibula   `CC` `HCC`

✓6ᵗʰ **M86.37** Chronic multifocal osteomyelitis, ankle and foot

     M86.371 Chronic multifocal osteomyelitis, right ankle and foot   `CC` `HCC`

     M86.372 Chronic multifocal osteomyelitis, left ankle and foot   `CC` `HCC`

     M86.379 Chronic multifocal osteomyelitis, unspecified ankle and foot   `CC` `HCC`

   M86.38 Chronic multifocal osteomyelitis, other site   `CC` `HCC`

   M86.39 Chronic multifocal osteomyelitis, multiple sites   `CC` `HCC`

✓5ᵗʰ **M86.4** Chronic osteomyelitis with draining sinus

> **CC Excl: For CC codes in subcategory M86.4, unless otherwise noted:** PDX collection 881

   M86.40 Chronic osteomyelitis with draining sinus, unspecified site   `CC` `HCC`
> **CC Excl:** PDX collection 906

✓6ᵗʰ **M86.41** Chronic osteomyelitis with draining sinus, shoulder

     M86.411 Chronic osteomyelitis with draining sinus, right shoulder   `CC` `HCC`

     M86.412 Chronic osteomyelitis with draining sinus, left shoulder   `CC` `HCC`

     M86.419 Chronic osteomyelitis with draining sinus, unspecified shoulder   `CC` `HCC`

✓6ᵗʰ **M86.42** Chronic osteomyelitis with draining sinus, humerus

     M86.421 Chronic osteomyelitis with draining sinus, right humerus   `CC` `HCC`

     M86.422 Chronic osteomyelitis with draining sinus, left humerus   `CC` `HCC`

     M86.429 Chronic osteomyelitis with draining sinus, unspecified humerus   `CC` `HCC`

✓6ᵗʰ **M86.43** Chronic osteomyelitis with draining sinus, radius and ulna

     M86.431 Chronic osteomyelitis with draining sinus, right radius and ulna   `CC` `HCC`

     M86.432 Chronic osteomyelitis with draining sinus, left radius and ulna   `CC` `HCC`

     M86.439 Chronic osteomyelitis with draining sinus, unspecified radius and ulna   `CC` `HCC`

✓6ᵗʰ **M86.44** Chronic osteomyelitis with draining sinus, hand

     M86.441 Chronic osteomyelitis with draining sinus, right hand   `CC` `HCC`

     M86.442 Chronic osteomyelitis with draining sinus, left hand   `CC` `HCC`

     M86.449 Chronic osteomyelitis with draining sinus, unspecified hand   `CC` `HCC`

✓6ᵗʰ **M86.45** Chronic osteomyelitis with draining sinus, femur

     M86.451 Chronic osteomyelitis with draining sinus, right femur   `CC` `HCC`

     M86.452 Chronic osteomyelitis with draining sinus, left femur   `CC` `HCC`

     M86.459 Chronic osteomyelitis with draining sinus, unspecified femur   `CC` `HCC`

✓6ᵗʰ **M86.46** Chronic osteomyelitis with draining sinus, tibia and fibula

     M86.461 Chronic osteomyelitis with draining sinus, right tibia and fibula   `CC` `HCC`

     M86.462 Chronic osteomyelitis with draining sinus, left tibia and fibula   `CC` `HCC`

     M86.469 Chronic osteomyelitis with draining sinus, unspecified tibia and fibula   `CC` `HCC`

✓6ᵗʰ **M86.47** Chronic osteomyelitis with draining sinus, ankle and foot

     M86.471 Chronic osteomyelitis with draining sinus, right ankle and foot   `CC` `HCC`

     M86.472 Chronic osteomyelitis with draining sinus, left ankle and foot   `CC` `HCC`

     M86.479 Chronic osteomyelitis with draining sinus, unspecified ankle and foot   `CC` `HCC`

   M86.48 Chronic osteomyelitis with draining sinus, other site   `CC` `HCC`

   M86.49 Chronic osteomyelitis with draining sinus, multiple sites   `CC` `HCC`

✓5ᵗʰ **M86.5** Other chronic hematogenous osteomyelitis

> **CC Excl: For CC codes in subcategory M86.5, unless otherwise noted:** PDX collection 881

   M86.50 Other chronic hematogenous osteomyelitis, unspecified site   `CC` `HCC`
> **CC Excl:** PDX collection 906

✓6ᵗʰ **M86.51** Other chronic hematogenous osteomyelitis, shoulder

     M86.511 Other chronic hematogenous osteomyelitis, right shoulder   `CC` `HCC`

✓ Additional Character Required   ✓x7ᵗʰ Placeholder   Unacceptable PDx   Questionable PDx   Manifestation   **H1**-**H14** HAC   `HCC` CMS-HCC Dx   **HIV** HIV Dx

ICD-10-CM 2019   811

M86.512 Other chronic hematogenous osteomyelitis, left shoulder `CC` `HCC`

M86.519 Other chronic hematogenous osteomyelitis, unspecified shoulder `CC` `HCC`

✓6th **M86.52** Other chronic hematogenous osteomyelitis, humerus

M86.521 Other chronic hematogenous osteomyelitis, right humerus `CC` `HCC`

M86.522 Other chronic hematogenous osteomyelitis, left humerus `CC` `HCC`

M86.529 Other chronic hematogenous osteomyelitis, unspecified humerus `CC` `HCC`

✓6th **M86.53** Other chronic hematogenous osteomyelitis, radius and ulna

M86.531 Other chronic hematogenous osteomyelitis, right radius and ulna `CC` `HCC`

M86.532 Other chronic hematogenous osteomyelitis, left radius and ulna `CC` `HCC`

M86.539 Other chronic hematogenous osteomyelitis, unspecified radius and ulna `CC` `HCC`

✓6th **M86.54** Other chronic hematogenous osteomyelitis, hand

M86.541 Other chronic hematogenous osteomyelitis, right hand `CC` `HCC`

M86.542 Other chronic hematogenous osteomyelitis, left hand `CC` `HCC`

M86.549 Other chronic hematogenous osteomyelitis, unspecified hand `CC` `HCC`

✓6th **M86.55** Other chronic hematogenous osteomyelitis, femur

M86.551 Other chronic hematogenous osteomyelitis, right femur `CC` `HCC`

M86.552 Other chronic hematogenous osteomyelitis, left femur `CC` `HCC`

M86.559 Other chronic hematogenous osteomyelitis, unspecified femur `CC` `HCC`

✓6th **M86.56** Other chronic hematogenous osteomyelitis, tibia and fibula

M86.561 Other chronic hematogenous osteomyelitis, right tibia and fibula `CC` `HCC`

M86.562 Other chronic hematogenous osteomyelitis, left tibia and fibula `CC` `HCC`

M86.569 Other chronic hematogenous osteomyelitis, unspecified tibia and fibula `CC` `HCC`

✓6th **M86.57** Other chronic hematogenous osteomyelitis, ankle and foot

M86.571 Other chronic hematogenous osteomyelitis, right ankle and foot `CC` `HCC`

M86.572 Other chronic hematogenous osteomyelitis, left ankle and foot `CC` `HCC`

M86.579 Other chronic hematogenous osteomyelitis, unspecified ankle and foot `CC` `HCC`

M86.58 Other chronic hematogenous osteomyelitis, other site `CC` `HCC`

M86.59 Other chronic hematogenous osteomyelitis, multiple sites `CC` `HCC`

✓5th **M86.6** Other chronic osteomyelitis

> **CC Excl:** For CC codes in subcategory M86.6, unless otherwise noted: PDX collection 881

M86.60 Other chronic osteomyelitis, unspecified site `CC` `HCC`
    CC Excl: PDX collection 906

✓6th **M86.61** Other chronic osteomyelitis, shoulder

M86.611 Other chronic osteomyelitis, right shoulder `CC` `HCC`

M86.612 Other chronic osteomyelitis, left shoulder `CC` `HCC`

M86.619 Other chronic osteomyelitis, unspecified shoulder `CC` `HCC`

✓6th **M86.62** Other chronic osteomyelitis, humerus

▲ **M86.621** Other chronic osteomyelitis, right humerus `CC` `HCC`

▲ **M86.622** Other chronic osteomyelitis, left humerus `CC` `HCC`

▲ **M86.629** Other chronic osteomyelitis, unspecified humerus `CC` `HCC`

✓6th **M86.63** Other chronic osteomyelitis, radius and ulna

M86.631 Other chronic osteomyelitis, right radius and ulna `CC` `HCC`

M86.632 Other chronic osteomyelitis, left radius and ulna `CC` `HCC`

M86.639 Other chronic osteomyelitis, unspecified radius and ulna `CC` `HCC`

✓6th **M86.64** Other chronic osteomyelitis, hand

M86.641 Other chronic osteomyelitis, right hand `CC` `HCC`

M86.642 Other chronic osteomyelitis, left hand `CC` `HCC`

M86.649 Other chronic osteomyelitis, unspecified hand `CC` `HCC`

✓6th **M86.65** Other chronic osteomyelitis, thigh

M86.651 Other chronic osteomyelitis, right thigh `CC` `HCC`

M86.652 Other chronic osteomyelitis, left thigh `CC` `HCC`

M86.659 Other chronic osteomyelitis, unspecified thigh `CC` `HCC`

✓6th **M86.66** Other chronic osteomyelitis, tibia and fibula

M86.661 Other chronic osteomyelitis, right tibia and fibula `CC` `HCC`

M86.662 Other chronic osteomyelitis, left tibia and fibula `CC` `HCC`

M86.669 Other chronic osteomyelitis, unspecified tibia and fibula `CC` `HCC`

✓6th **M86.67** Other chronic osteomyelitis, ankle and foot

M86.671 Other chronic osteomyelitis, right ankle and foot `CC` `HCC`
    AHA: 2016, 1Q, 13

M86.672 Other chronic osteomyelitis, left ankle and foot `CC` `HCC`

M86.679 Other chronic osteomyelitis, unspecified ankle and foot `CC` `HCC`

M86.68 Other chronic osteomyelitis, other site `CC` `HCC`

M86.69 Other chronic osteomyelitis, multiple sites `CC` `HCC`

✓5th **M86.8** Other osteomyelitis
Brodie's abscess

> **CC Excl:** For CC codes in subcategory M86.8, unless otherwise noted: PDX collection 881

✓6th **M86.8X** Other osteomyelitis

M86.8X0 Other osteomyelitis, multiple sites `CC` `HCC`

M86.8X1 Other osteomyelitis, shoulder `CC` `HCC`

M86.8X2 Other osteomyelitis, upper arm `CC` `HCC`

M86.8X3 Other osteomyelitis, forearm `CC` `HCC`

M86.8X4 Other osteomyelitis, hand `CC` `HCC`

M86.8X5 Other osteomyelitis, thigh `CC` `HCC`

M86.8X6 Other osteomyelitis, lower leg `CC` `HCC`

M86.8X7 Other osteomyelitis, ankle and foot `CC` `HCC`

M86.8X8 Other osteomyelitis, other site `CC` `HCC`

M86.8X9 Other osteomyelitis, unspecified sites `CC` `HCC`
    CC Excl: PDX collection 906

M86.9 Osteomyelitis, unspecified `CC` `HCC`
Infection of bone NOS
Periostitis without osteomyelitis
CC Excl: PDX collection 906

✓4th **M87 Osteonecrosis**
`INCLUDES` avascular necrosis of bone
Use additional code to identify major osseous defect, if applicable (M89.7-)
`EXCLUDES 1` *juvenile osteonecrosis (M91-M92)*
osteochondropathies (M90-M93)

> **CC Excl:** For CC codes in category M87, unless otherwise noted: PDX collection 907

✓5th **M87.0** Idiopathic aseptic necrosis of bone

M87.00 Idiopathic aseptic necrosis of unspecified bone `CC` `HCC`

N Newborn: 0   **P** Pediatric: 0-17   **M** Maternity: 12-55   **A** Adult: 15-124   **MCC** Major Complication/Comorbidity   **CC** Complication/Comorbidity   **SW** Severe Wound Dx

812   ICD-10-CM 2019

☑6ᵗʰ **M87.01 Idiopathic aseptic necrosis of** shoulder
Idiopathic aseptic necrosis of clavicle and scapula

CC Excl: For CC codes in subcategory M87.01:
PDX collection 908

M87.011 Idiopathic aseptic necrosis of right `CC` `HCC`
shoulder

M87.012 Idiopathic aseptic necrosis of left `CC` `HCC`
shoulder

M87.019 Idiopathic aseptic necrosis of `CC` `HCC`
unspecified **shoulder**

☑6ᵗʰ **M87.02 Idiopathic aseptic necrosis of** humerus

CC Excl: For CC codes in subcategory M87.02:
PDX collection 908

M87.021 Idiopathic aseptic necrosis of right `CC` `HCC`
humerus

M87.022 Idiopathic aseptic necrosis of left `CC` `HCC`
humerus

M87.029 Idiopathic aseptic necrosis of `CC` `HCC`
unspecified **humerus**

☑6ᵗʰ **M87.03 Idiopathic aseptic necrosis of** radius, ulna and carpus

M87.031 Idiopathic aseptic necrosis of right `CC` `HCC`
radius

M87.032 Idiopathic aseptic necrosis of left `CC` `HCC`
radius

M87.033 Idiopathic aseptic necrosis of `CC` `HCC`
unspecified radius

M87.034 Idiopathic aseptic necrosis of `CC` `HCC`
right ulna

M87.035 Idiopathic aseptic necrosis of `CC` `HCC`
left ulna

M87.036 Idiopathic aseptic necrosis of `CC` `HCC`
unspecified ulna

M87.037 Idiopathic aseptic necrosis of right `CC` `HCC`
carpus

M87.038 Idiopathic aseptic necrosis of left `CC` `HCC`
carpus

M87.039 Idiopathic aseptic necrosis of `CC` `HCC`
unspecified carpus

☑6ᵗʰ **M87.04 Idiopathic aseptic necrosis of** hand and fingers
Idiopathic aseptic necrosis of metacarpals and
phalanges of hands

M87.041 Idiopathic aseptic necrosis of right `CC` `HCC`
hand

M87.042 Idiopathic aseptic necrosis of left `CC` `HCC`
hand

M87.043 Idiopathic aseptic necrosis of `CC` `HCC`
unspecified hand

M87.044 Idiopathic aseptic necrosis of right `CC` `HCC`
finger(s)

M87.045 Idiopathic aseptic necrosis of left `CC` `HCC`
finger(s)

M87.046 Idiopathic aseptic necrosis of `CC` `HCC`
unspecified finger(s)

☑6ᵗʰ **M87.05 Idiopathic aseptic necrosis of** pelvis and femur

M87.050 Idiopathic aseptic necrosis of `CC` `HCC`
pelvis

M87.051 Idiopathic aseptic necrosis of `CC` `HCC`
right femur
CC Excl: PDX collection 909

M87.052 Idiopathic aseptic necrosis of `CC` `HCC`
left femur
CC Excl: PDX collection 909

M87.059 Idiopathic aseptic necrosis of `CC` `HCC`
unspecified femur
Idiopathic aseptic necrosis of hip NOS
CC Excl: PDX collection 909

☑6ᵗʰ **M87.06 Idiopathic aseptic necrosis of** tibia and fibula

M87.061 Idiopathic aseptic necrosis of `CC` `HCC`
right tibia

M87.062 Idiopathic aseptic necrosis of `CC` `HCC`
left tibia

M87.063 Idiopathic aseptic necrosis of `CC` `HCC`
unspecified tibia

M87.064 Idiopathic aseptic necrosis of `CC` `HCC`
right fibula

M87.065 Idiopathic aseptic necrosis of `CC` `HCC`
left fibula

M87.066 Idiopathic aseptic necrosis of `CC` `HCC`
unspecified fibula

☑6ᵗʰ **M87.07 Idiopathic aseptic necrosis of** ankle, foot and toes
Idiopathic aseptic necrosis of metatarsus, tarsus, and
phalanges of toes

M87.071 Idiopathic aseptic necrosis of right `CC` `HCC`
ankle

M87.072 Idiopathic aseptic necrosis of left `CC` `HCC`
ankle

M87.073 Idiopathic aseptic necrosis of `CC` `HCC`
unspecified ankle

M87.074 Idiopathic aseptic necrosis of `CC` `HCC`
right foot
CC Excl: PDX collection 910

M87.075 Idiopathic aseptic necrosis of `CC` `HCC`
left foot
CC Excl: PDX collection 910

M87.076 Idiopathic aseptic necrosis of `CC` `HCC`
unspecified foot
CC Excl: PDX collection 910

M87.077 Idiopathic aseptic necrosis of `CC` `HCC`
right toe(s)

M87.078 Idiopathic aseptic necrosis of `CC` `HCC`
left toe(s)

M87.079 Idiopathic aseptic necrosis of `CC` `HCC`
unspecified toe(s)

M87.08 Idiopathic aseptic necrosis of bone, other `CC` `HCC`
site

M87.09 Idiopathic aseptic necrosis of bone, `CC` `HCC`
multiple sites

☑5ᵗʰ **M87.1 Osteonecrosis** due to drugs
Use additional code for adverse effect, if applicable, to identify
drug (T36-T50 with fifth or sixth character 5)

M87.10 Osteonecrosis due to drugs, unspecified `CC` `HCC`
bone

☑6ᵗʰ **M87.11 Osteonecrosis due to drugs,** shoulder

M87.111 Osteonecrosis due to drugs, right `CC` `HCC`
shoulder

M87.112 Osteonecrosis due to drugs, left `CC` `HCC`
shoulder

M87.119 Osteonecrosis due to drugs, `CC` `HCC`
unspecified **shoulder**

☑6ᵗʰ **M87.12 Osteonecrosis due to drugs,** humerus

CC Excl: For CC codes in subcategory M87.12:
PDX collection 908

M87.121 Osteonecrosis due to drugs, right `CC` `HCC`
humerus

M87.122 Osteonecrosis due to drugs, left `CC` `HCC`
humerus

M87.129 Osteonecrosis due to drugs, `CC` `HCC`
unspecified **humerus**

☑6ᵗʰ **M87.13 Osteonecrosis due to drugs of** radius, ulna and
carpus

M87.131 Osteonecrosis due to drugs of right `CC` `HCC`
radius

M87.132 Osteonecrosis due to drugs of left `CC` `HCC`
radius

M87.133 Osteonecrosis due to drugs of `CC` `HCC`
unspecified radius

M87.134 Osteonecrosis due to drugs of `CC` `HCC`
right ulna

M87.135 Osteonecrosis due to drugs of `CC` `HCC`
left ulna

M87.136 Osteonecrosis due to drugs of `CC` `HCC`
unspecified ulna

M87.137 Osteonecrosis due to drugs of right `CC` `HCC`
carpus

M87.138 Osteonecrosis due to drugs of left `CC` `HCC`
carpus

M87.139 Osteonecrosis due to drugs of `CC` `HCC`
unspecified carpus

☑6ᵗʰ **M87.14 Osteonecrosis due to drugs,** hand and fingers

M87.141 Osteonecrosis due to drugs, `CC` `HCC`
right hand

M87.142 Osteonecrosis due to drugs, left `CC` `HCC`
hand

M87.143 Osteonecrosis due to drugs, `CC` `HCC`
unspecified hand

☑ Additional Character Required   ✓x7ᵗʰ Placeholder   Unacceptable PDx   Questionable PDx   Manifestation   `H1`-`H14` HAC   `HCC` CMS-HCC Dx   `HIV` HIV Dx

ICD-10-CM 2019   **813**

M87.144 Osteonecrosis due to drugs, right finger(s) `CC` `HCC`

M87.145 Osteonecrosis due to drugs, left finger(s) `CC` `HCC`

M87.146 Osteonecrosis due to drugs, unspecified finger(s) `CC` `HCC`

✓6th M87.15 Osteonecrosis due to drugs, pelvis and femur

> **CC Excl: For CC codes in subcategory M87.15:** PDX collection 909

M87.150 Osteonecrosis due to drugs, pelvis `CC` `HCC`

M87.151 Osteonecrosis due to drugs, right femur `CC` `HCC`

M87.152 Osteonecrosis due to drugs, left femur `CC` `HCC`

M87.159 Osteonecrosis due to drugs, unspecified femur `CC` `HCC`

✓6th M87.16 Osteonecrosis due to drugs, tibia and fibula

M87.161 Osteonecrosis due to drugs, right tibia `CC` `HCC`

M87.162 Osteonecrosis due to drugs, left tibia `CC` `HCC`

M87.163 Osteonecrosis due to drugs, unspecified tibia `CC` `HCC`

M87.164 Osteonecrosis due to drugs, right fibula `CC` `HCC`

M87.165 Osteonecrosis due to drugs, left fibula `CC` `HCC`

M87.166 Osteonecrosis due to drugs, unspecified fibula `CC` `HCC`

✓6th M87.17 Osteonecrosis due to drugs, ankle, foot and toes

M87.171 Osteonecrosis due to drugs, right ankle `CC` `HCC`

M87.172 Osteonecrosis due to drugs, left ankle `CC` `HCC`

M87.173 Osteonecrosis due to drugs, unspecified ankle `CC` `HCC`

M87.174 Osteonecrosis due to drugs, right foot `CC` `HCC`
> **CC Excl:** PDX collection 910

M87.175 Osteonecrosis due to drugs, left foot `CC` `HCC`
> **CC Excl:** PDX collection 910

M87.176 Osteonecrosis due to drugs, unspecified foot `CC` `HCC`
> **CC Excl:** PDX collection 910

M87.177 Osteonecrosis due to drugs, right toe(s) `CC` `HCC`

M87.178 Osteonecrosis due to drugs, left toe(s) `CC` `HCC`

M87.179 Osteonecrosis due to drugs, unspecified toe(s) `CC` `HCC`

✓6th M87.18 Osteonecrosis due to drugs, other site

M87.180 Osteonecrosis due to drugs, jaw `CC` `HCC`

M87.188 Osteonecrosis due to drugs, other site `CC` `HCC`

M87.19 Osteonecrosis due to drugs, multiple sites `CC` `HCC`

✓5th **M87.2 Osteonecrosis due to previous trauma**

M87.20 Osteonecrosis due to previous trauma, unspecified bone `CC` `HCC`

✓6th M87.21 Osteonecrosis due to previous trauma, shoulder

M87.211 Osteonecrosis due to previous trauma, right shoulder `CC` `HCC`

M87.212 Osteonecrosis due to previous trauma, left shoulder `CC` `HCC`

M87.219 Osteonecrosis due to previous trauma, unspecified shoulder `CC` `HCC`

✓6th M87.22 Osteonecrosis due to previous trauma, humerus

> **CC Excl: For CC codes in subcategory M87.22:** PDX collection 908

M87.221 Osteonecrosis due to previous trauma, right humerus `CC` `HCC`

M87.222 Osteonecrosis due to previous trauma, left humerus `CC` `HCC`

M87.229 Osteonecrosis due to previous trauma, unspecified humerus `CC` `HCC`

✓6th M87.23 Osteonecrosis due to previous trauma of radius, ulna and carpus

M87.231 Osteonecrosis due to previous trauma of right radius `CC` `HCC`

M87.232 Osteonecrosis due to previous trauma of left radius `CC` `HCC`

M87.233 Osteonecrosis due to previous trauma of unspecified radius `CC` `HCC`

M87.234 Osteonecrosis due to previous trauma of right ulna `CC` `HCC`

M87.235 Osteonecrosis due to previous trauma of left ulna `CC` `HCC`

M87.236 Osteonecrosis due to previous trauma of unspecified ulna `CC` `HCC`

M87.237 Osteonecrosis due to previous trauma of right carpus `CC` `HCC`

M87.238 Osteonecrosis due to previous trauma of left carpus `CC` `HCC`

M87.239 Osteonecrosis due to previous trauma of unspecified carpus `CC` `HCC`

✓6th M87.24 Osteonecrosis due to previous trauma, hand and fingers

M87.241 Osteonecrosis due to previous trauma, right hand `CC` `HCC`

M87.242 Osteonecrosis due to previous trauma, left hand `CC` `HCC`

M87.243 Osteonecrosis due to previous trauma, unspecified hand `CC` `HCC`

M87.244 Osteonecrosis due to previous trauma, right finger(s) `CC` `HCC`

M87.245 Osteonecrosis due to previous trauma, left finger(s) `CC` `HCC`

M87.246 Osteonecrosis due to previous trauma, unspecified finger(s) `CC` `HCC`

✓6th M87.25 Osteonecrosis due to previous trauma, pelvis and femur

M87.250 Osteonecrosis due to previous trauma, pelvis `CC` `HCC`

M87.251 Osteonecrosis due to previous trauma, right femur `CC` `HCC`
> **CC Excl:** PDX collection 909

M87.252 Osteonecrosis due to previous trauma, left femur `CC` `HCC`
> **CC Excl:** PDX collection 909

M87.256 Osteonecrosis due to previous trauma, unspecified femur `CC` `HCC`
> **CC Excl:** PDX collection 909

✓6th M87.26 Osteonecrosis due to previous trauma, tibia and fibula

M87.261 Osteonecrosis due to previous trauma, right tibia `CC` `HCC`

M87.262 Osteonecrosis due to previous trauma, left tibia `CC` `HCC`

M87.263 Osteonecrosis due to previous trauma, unspecified tibia `CC` `HCC`

M87.264 Osteonecrosis due to previous trauma, right fibula `CC` `HCC`

M87.265 Osteonecrosis due to previous trauma, left fibula `CC` `HCC`

M87.266 Osteonecrosis due to previous trauma, unspecified fibula `CC` `HCC`

✓6th M87.27 Osteonecrosis due to previous trauma, ankle, foot and toes

M87.271 Osteonecrosis due to previous trauma, right ankle `CC` `HCC`

M87.272 Osteonecrosis due to previous trauma, left ankle `CC` `HCC`

M87.273 Osteonecrosis due to previous trauma, unspecified ankle `CC` `HCC`

M87.274 Osteonecrosis due to previous trauma, right foot `CC` `HCC`
> **CC Excl:** PDX collection 910

M87.275 Osteonecrosis due to previous trauma, left foot `CC` `HCC`
> **CC Excl:** PDX collection 910

M87.276 Osteonecrosis due to previous trauma, unspecified foot `CC` `HCC`
> **CC Excl:** PDX collection 910

N Newborn: 0   P Pediatric: 0-17   M Maternity: 12-55   A Adult: 15-124   MCC Major Complication/Comorbidity   CC Complication/Comorbidity   SW Severe Wound Dx

814   ICD-10-CM 2019

M87.277 **Osteonecrosis due to previous trauma,** right toe(s) `CC` `HCC`

M87.278 **Osteonecrosis due to previous trauma,** left toe(s) `CC` `HCC`

M87.279 **Osteonecrosis due to previous trauma,** unspecified toe(s) `CC` `HCC`

M87.28 **Osteonecrosis due to previous trauma, other site** `CC` `HCC`

M87.29 **Osteonecrosis due to previous trauma, multiple sites** `CC` `HCC`

✓5th **M87.3 Other secondary osteonecrosis**

M87.30 **Other secondary osteonecrosis, unspecified bone** `CC` `HCC`

✓6th **M87.31 Other secondary osteonecrosis,** shoulder

M87.311 **Other secondary osteonecrosis,** right shoulder `CC` `HCC`

M87.312 **Other secondary osteonecrosis,** left shoulder `CC` `HCC`

M87.319 **Other secondary osteonecrosis,** unspecified shoulder `CC` `HCC`

✓6th **M87.32 Other secondary osteonecrosis,** humerus

CC Excl: For CC codes in subcategory M87.32: PDX collection 908

M87.321 **Other secondary osteonecrosis,** right humerus `CC` `HCC`

M87.322 **Other secondary osteonecrosis,** left humerus `CC` `HCC`

M87.329 **Other secondary osteonecrosis,** unspecified humerus `CC` `HCC`

✓6th **M87.33 Other secondary osteonecrosis of** radius, ulna and carpus

M87.331 **Other secondary osteonecrosis of** right radius `CC` `HCC`

M87.332 **Other secondary osteonecrosis of** left radius `CC` `HCC`

M87.333 **Other secondary osteonecrosis of** unspecified radius `CC` `HCC`

M87.334 **Other secondary osteonecrosis of** right ulna `CC` `HCC`

M87.335 **Other secondary osteonecrosis of** left ulna `CC` `HCC`

M87.336 **Other secondary osteonecrosis of** unspecified ulna `CC` `HCC`

M87.337 **Other secondary osteonecrosis of** right carpus `CC` `HCC`

M87.338 **Other secondary osteonecrosis of** left carpus `CC` `HCC`

M87.339 **Other secondary osteonecrosis of** unspecified carpus `CC` `HCC`

✓6th **M87.34 Other secondary osteonecrosis,** hand and fingers

M87.341 **Other secondary osteonecrosis,** right hand `CC` `HCC`

M87.342 **Other secondary osteonecrosis,** left hand `CC` `HCC`

M87.343 **Other secondary osteonecrosis,** unspecified hand `CC` `HCC`

M87.344 **Other secondary osteonecrosis,** right finger(s) `CC` `HCC`

M87.345 **Other secondary osteonecrosis,** left finger(s) `CC` `HCC`

M87.346 **Other secondary osteonecrosis,** unspecified finger(s) `CC` `HCC`

✓6th **M87.35 Other secondary osteonecrosis,** pelvis and femur

CC Excl: For CC codes in subcategory M87.35: PDX collection 909

M87.350 **Other secondary osteonecrosis,** pelvis `CC` `HCC`

M87.351 **Other secondary osteonecrosis,** right femur `CC` `HCC`

M87.352 **Other secondary osteonecrosis,** left femur `CC` `HCC`

M87.353 **Other secondary osteonecrosis,** unspecified femur `CC` `HCC`

✓6th **M87.36 Other secondary osteonecrosis,** tibia and fibula

M87.361 **Other secondary osteonecrosis,** right tibia `CC` `HCC`

M87.362 **Other secondary osteonecrosis,** left tibia `CC` `HCC`

M87.363 **Other secondary osteonecrosis,** unspecified tibia `CC` `HCC`

M87.364 **Other secondary osteonecrosis,** right fibula `CC` `HCC`

M87.365 **Other secondary osteonecrosis,** left fibula `CC` `HCC`

M87.366 **Other secondary osteonecrosis,** unspecified fibula `CC` `HCC`

✓6th **M87.37 Other secondary osteonecrosis,** ankle and foot

M87.371 **Other secondary osteonecrosis,** right ankle `CC` `HCC`

M87.372 **Other secondary osteonecrosis,** left ankle `CC` `HCC`

M87.373 **Other secondary osteonecrosis,** unspecified ankle `CC` `HCC`

M87.374 **Other secondary osteonecrosis,** right foot `CC` `HCC`
CC Excl: PDX collection 910

M87.375 **Other secondary osteonecrosis,** left foot `CC` `HCC`
CC Excl: PDX collection 910

M87.376 **Other secondary osteonecrosis,** unspecified foot `CC` `HCC`
CC Excl: PDX collection 910

M87.377 **Other secondary osteonecrosis,** right toe(s) `CC` `HCC`

M87.378 **Other secondary osteonecrosis,** left toe(s) `CC` `HCC`

M87.379 **Other secondary osteonecrosis,** unspecified toe(s) `CC` `HCC`

M87.38 **Other secondary osteonecrosis,** other site `CC` `HCC`

M87.39 **Other secondary osteonecrosis,** multiple sites `CC` `HCC`

✓5th **M87.8 Other osteonecrosis**

M87.80 **Other osteonecrosis,** unspecified bone `CC` `HCC`

✓6th **M87.81 Other osteonecrosis,** shoulder

M87.811 **Other osteonecrosis,** right shoulder `CC` `HCC`

M87.812 **Other osteonecrosis,** left shoulder `CC` `HCC`

M87.819 **Other osteonecrosis,** unspecified shoulder `CC` `HCC`

✓6th **M87.82 Other osteonecrosis,** humerus

CC Excl: For CC codes in subcategory M87.82: PDX collection 908

M87.821 **Other osteonecrosis,** right humerus `CC` `HCC`

M87.822 **Other osteonecrosis,** left humerus `CC` `HCC`

M87.829 **Other osteonecrosis,** unspecified humerus `CC` `HCC`

✓6th **M87.83 Other osteonecrosis of** radius, ulna and carpus

M87.831 **Other osteonecrosis of** right radius `CC` `HCC`

M87.832 **Other osteonecrosis of** left radius `CC` `HCC`

M87.833 **Other osteonecrosis of** unspecified radius `CC` `HCC`

M87.834 **Other osteonecrosis of** right ulna `CC` `HCC`

M87.835 **Other osteonecrosis of** left ulna `CC` `HCC`

M87.836 **Other osteonecrosis of** unspecified ulna `CC` `HCC`

M87.837 **Other osteonecrosis of** right carpus `CC` `HCC`

M87.838 **Other osteonecrosis of** left carpus `CC` `HCC`

M87.839 **Other osteonecrosis of** unspecified carpus `CC` `HCC`

✓6th **M87.84 Other osteonecrosis,** hand and fingers

M87.841 **Other osteonecrosis,** right hand `CC` `HCC`

M87.842 **Other osteonecrosis,** left hand `CC` `HCC`

M87.843 **Other osteonecrosis,** unspecified hand `CC` `HCC`

M87.844 **Other osteonecrosis,** right finger(s) `CC` `HCC`

M87.845 **Other osteonecrosis,** left finger(s) `CC` `HCC`

M87.849 **Other osteonecrosis,** unspecified finger(s) `CC` `HCC`

✓ Additional Character Required   ✓x7th Placeholder   Unacceptable PDx   Questionable PDx   Manifestation   H1 - H14 HAC   HCC CMS-HCC Dx   HIV HIV Dx

ICD-10-CM 2019   815

√6ᵗʰ **M87.85 Other osteonecrosis, pelvis and femur**

> **CC Excl: For CC codes in subcategory M87.85:**
> PDX collection 909

     M87.850 Other osteonecrosis, pelvis CC HCC
     M87.851 Other osteonecrosis, right femur CC HCC
     M87.852 Other osteonecrosis, left femur CC HCC
     M87.859 Other osteonecrosis, unspecified femur CC HCC

√6ᵗʰ **M87.86 Other osteonecrosis, tibia and fibula**

     M87.861 Other osteonecrosis, right tibia CC HCC
     M87.862 Other osteonecrosis, left tibia CC HCC
     M87.863 Other osteonecrosis, unspecified tibia CC HCC
     M87.864 Other osteonecrosis, right fibula CC HCC
     M87.865 Other osteonecrosis, left fibula CC HCC
     M87.869 Other osteonecrosis, unspecified fibula CC HCC

√6ᵗʰ **M87.87 Other osteonecrosis, ankle, foot and toes**

     M87.871 Other osteonecrosis, right ankle CC HCC
     M87.872 Other osteonecrosis, left ankle CC HCC
     M87.873 Other osteonecrosis, unspecified ankle CC HCC
     M87.874 Other osteonecrosis, right foot CC HCC
> **CC Excl: PDX collection 910**
     M87.875 Other osteonecrosis, left foot CC HCC
> **CC Excl: PDX collection 910**
     M87.876 Other osteonecrosis, unspecified foot CC HCC
> **CC Excl: PDX collection 910**
     M87.877 Other osteonecrosis, right toe(s) CC HCC
     M87.878 Other osteonecrosis, left toe(s) CC HCC
     M87.879 Other osteonecrosis, unspecified toe(s) CC HCC

     M87.88 Other osteonecrosis, other site CC HCC
     M87.89 Other osteonecrosis, multiple sites CC HCC

M87.9 Osteonecrosis, unspecified CC HCC
     Necrosis of bone NOS

√4ᵗʰ **M88 Osteitis deformans [Paget's disease of bone]**

> EXCLUDES 1 osteitis deformans in neoplastic disease (M90.6)

DEF: Bone disease characterized by numerous cycles of bone resorption by the body. Resorption is followed by accelerated repair attempts, causing bone deformities and bowing, with associated fractures and pain.

M88.0 Osteitis deformans of skull

M88.1 Osteitis deformans of vertebrae

√5ᵗʰ **M88.8 Osteitis deformans of other bones**

√6ᵗʰ **M88.81 Osteitis deformans of shoulder**
     M88.811 Osteitis deformans of right shoulder
     M88.812 Osteitis deformans of left shoulder
     M88.819 Osteitis deformans of unspecified shoulder

√6ᵗʰ **M88.82 Osteitis deformans of upper arm**
     M88.821 Osteitis deformans of right upper arm
     M88.822 Osteitis deformans of left upper arm
     M88.829 Osteitis deformans of unspecified upper arm

√6ᵗʰ **M88.83 Osteitis deformans of forearm**
     M88.831 Osteitis deformans of right forearm
     M88.832 Osteitis deformans of left forearm
     M88.839 Osteitis deformans of unspecified forearm

√6ᵗʰ **M88.84 Osteitis deformans of hand**
     M88.841 Osteitis deformans of right hand
     M88.842 Osteitis deformans of left hand
     M88.849 Osteitis deformans of unspecified hand

√6ᵗʰ **M88.85 Osteitis deformans of thigh**
     M88.851 Osteitis deformans of right thigh
     M88.852 Osteitis deformans of left thigh
     M88.859 Osteitis deformans of unspecified thigh

√6ᵗʰ **M88.86 Osteitis deformans of lower leg**
     M88.861 Osteitis deformans of right lower leg
     M88.862 Osteitis deformans of left lower leg
     M88.869 Osteitis deformans of unspecified lower leg

√6ᵗʰ **M88.87 Osteitis deformans of ankle and foot**
     M88.871 Osteitis deformans of right ankle and foot
     M88.872 Osteitis deformans of left ankle and foot
     M88.879 Osteitis deformans of unspecified ankle and foot

     M88.88 Osteitis deformans of other bones
> EXCLUDES 2 osteitis deformans of skull (M88.0)
> osteitis deformans of vertebrae (M88.1)

     M88.89 Osteitis deformans of multiple sites

M88.9 Osteitis deformans of unspecified bone

√4ᵗʰ **M89 Other disorders of bone**

√5ᵗʰ **M89.0 Algoneurodystrophy**
     Shoulder-hand syndrome
     Sudeck's atrophy
> EXCLUDES 1 causalgia, lower limb (G57.7-)
> causalgia, upper limb (G56.4-)
> complex regional pain syndrome II, lower limb (G57.7-)
> complex regional pain syndrome II, upper limb (G56.4-)
> reflex sympathetic dystrophy (G90.5-)

     M89.00 Algoneurodystrophy, unspecified site

√6ᵗʰ **M89.01 Algoneurodystrophy, shoulder**
     M89.011 Algoneurodystrophy, right shoulder
     M89.012 Algoneurodystrophy, left shoulder
     M89.019 Algoneurodystrophy, unspecified shoulder

√6ᵗʰ **M89.02 Algoneurodystrophy, upper arm**
     M89.021 Algoneurodystrophy, right upper arm
     M89.022 Algoneurodystrophy, left upper arm
     M89.029 Algoneurodystrophy, unspecified upper arm

√6ᵗʰ **M89.03 Algoneurodystrophy, forearm**
     M89.031 Algoneurodystrophy, right forearm
     M89.032 Algoneurodystrophy, left forearm
     M89.039 Algoneurodystrophy, unspecified forearm

√6ᵗʰ **M89.04 Algoneurodystrophy, hand**
     M89.041 Algoneurodystrophy, right hand
     M89.042 Algoneurodystrophy, left hand
     M89.049 Algoneurodystrophy, unspecified hand

√6ᵗʰ **M89.05 Algoneurodystrophy, thigh**
     M89.051 Algoneurodystrophy, right thigh
     M89.052 Algoneurodystrophy, left thigh
     M89.059 Algoneurodystrophy, unspecified thigh

√6ᵗʰ **M89.06 Algoneurodystrophy, lower leg**
     M89.061 Algoneurodystrophy, right lower leg
     M89.062 Algoneurodystrophy, left lower leg
     M89.069 Algoneurodystrophy, unspecified lower leg

√6ᵗʰ **M89.07 Algoneurodystrophy, ankle and foot**
     M89.071 Algoneurodystrophy, right ankle and foot
     M89.072 Algoneurodystrophy, left ankle and foot
     M89.079 Algoneurodystrophy, unspecified ankle and foot

     M89.08 Algoneurodystrophy, other site
     M89.09 Algoneurodystrophy, multiple sites

√5ᵗʰ **M89.1 Physeal arrest**
     Arrest of growth plate
     Epiphyseal arrest
     Growth plate arrest

√6ᵗʰ **M89.12 Physeal arrest, humerus**
     M89.121 Complete physeal arrest, right proximal humerus
     M89.122 Complete physeal arrest, left proximal humerus
     M89.123 Partial physeal arrest, right proximal humerus
     M89.124 Partial physeal arrest, left proximal humerus
     M89.125 Complete physeal arrest, right distal humerus
     M89.126 Complete physeal arrest, left distal humerus
     M89.127 Partial physeal arrest, right distal humerus
     M89.128 Partial physeal arrest, left distal humerus
     M89.129 Physeal arrest, humerus, unspecified

N Newborn: 0   P Pediatric: 0-17   M Maternity: 12-55   A Adult: 15-124   MCC Major Complication/Comorbidity   CC Complication/Comorbidity   SW Severe Wound Dx

816   ICD-10-CM 2019

✓6ᵗʰ **M89.13** Physeal arrest, forearm
     M89.131 Complete physeal arrest, right distal radius
     M89.132 Complete physeal arrest, left distal radius
     M89.133 Partial physeal arrest, right distal radius
     M89.134 Partial physeal arrest, left distal radius
     M89.138 Other physeal arrest of forearm
     M89.139 Physeal arrest, forearm, unspecified

✓6ᵗʰ **M89.15** Physeal arrest, femur
     M89.151 Complete physeal arrest, right proximal femur
     M89.152 Complete physeal arrest, left proximal femur
     M89.153 Partial physeal arrest, right proximal femur
     M89.154 Partial physeal arrest, left proximal femur
     M89.155 Complete physeal arrest, right distal femur
     M89.156 Complete physeal arrest, left distal femur
     M89.157 Partial physeal arrest, right distal femur
     M89.158 Partial physeal arrest, left distal femur
     M89.159 Physeal arrest, femur, unspecified

✓6ᵗʰ **M89.16** Physeal arrest, lower leg
     M89.160 Complete physeal arrest, right proximal tibia
     M89.161 Complete physeal arrest, left proximal tibia
     M89.162 Partial physeal arrest, right proximal tibia
     M89.163 Partial physeal arrest, left proximal tibia
     M89.164 Complete physeal arrest, right distal tibia
     M89.165 Complete physeal arrest, left distal tibia
     M89.166 Partial physeal arrest, right distal tibia
     M89.167 Partial physeal arrest, left distal tibia
     M89.168 Other physeal arrest of lower leg
     M89.169 Physeal arrest, lower leg, unspecified

     M89.18 Physeal arrest, other site

✓5ᵗʰ **M89.2** Other disorders of bone development and growth
     M89.20 Other disorders of bone development and growth, unspecified site

✓6ᵗʰ **M89.21** Other disorders of bone development and growth, shoulder
     M89.211 Other disorders of bone development and growth, right shoulder
     M89.212 Other disorders of bone development and growth, left shoulder
     M89.219 Other disorders of bone development and growth, unspecified shoulder

✓6ᵗʰ **M89.22** Other disorders of bone development and growth, humerus
     M89.221 Other disorders of bone development and growth, right humerus
     M89.222 Other disorders of bone development and growth, left humerus
     M89.229 Other disorders of bone development and growth, unspecified humerus

✓6ᵗʰ **M89.23** Other disorders of bone development and growth, ulna and radius
     M89.231 Other disorders of bone development and growth, right ulna
     M89.232 Other disorders of bone development and growth, left ulna
     M89.233 Other disorders of bone development and growth, right radius
     M89.234 Other disorders of bone development and growth, left radius
     M89.239 Other disorders of bone development and growth, unspecified ulna and radius

✓6ᵗʰ **M89.24** Other disorders of bone development and growth, hand
     M89.241 Other disorders of bone development and growth, right hand
     M89.242 Other disorders of bone development and growth, left hand
     M89.249 Other disorders of bone development and growth, unspecified hand

✓6ᵗʰ **M89.25** Other disorders of bone development and growth, femur
     M89.251 Other disorders of bone development and growth, right femur
     M89.252 Other disorders of bone development and growth, left femur
     M89.259 Other disorders of bone development and growth, unspecified femur

✓6ᵗʰ **M89.26** Other disorders of bone development and growth, tibia and fibula
     M89.261 Other disorders of bone development and growth, right tibia
     M89.262 Other disorders of bone development and growth, left tibia
     M89.263 Other disorders of bone development and growth, right fibula
     M89.264 Other disorders of bone development and growth, left fibula
     M89.269 Other disorders of bone development and growth, unspecified lower leg

✓6ᵗʰ **M89.27** Other disorders of bone development and growth, ankle and foot
     M89.271 Other disorders of bone development and growth, right ankle and foot
     M89.272 Other disorders of bone development and growth, left ankle and foot
     M89.279 Other disorders of bone development and growth, unspecified ankle and foot

     M89.28 Other disorders of bone development and growth, other site

     M89.29 Other disorders of bone development and growth, multiple sites

✓5ᵗʰ **M89.3** Hypertrophy of bone
     M89.30 Hypertrophy of bone, unspecified site

✓6ᵗʰ **M89.31** Hypertrophy of bone, shoulder
     M89.311 Hypertrophy of bone, right shoulder
     M89.312 Hypertrophy of bone, left shoulder
     M89.319 Hypertrophy of bone, unspecified shoulder

✓6ᵗʰ **M89.32** Hypertrophy of bone, humerus
     M89.321 Hypertrophy of bone, right humerus
     M89.322 Hypertrophy of bone, left humerus
     M89.329 Hypertrophy of bone, unspecified humerus

✓6ᵗʰ **M89.33** Hypertrophy of bone, ulna and radius
     M89.331 Hypertrophy of bone, right ulna
     M89.332 Hypertrophy of bone, left ulna
     M89.333 Hypertrophy of bone, right radius
     M89.334 Hypertrophy of bone, left radius
     M89.339 Hypertrophy of bone, unspecified ulna and radius

✓6ᵗʰ **M89.34** Hypertrophy of bone, hand
     M89.341 Hypertrophy of bone, right hand
     M89.342 Hypertrophy of bone, left hand
     M89.349 Hypertrophy of bone, unspecified hand

✓6ᵗʰ **M89.35** Hypertrophy of bone, femur
     M89.351 Hypertrophy of bone, right femur
     M89.352 Hypertrophy of bone, left femur
     M89.359 Hypertrophy of bone, unspecified femur

✓6ᵗʰ **M89.36** Hypertrophy of bone, tibia and fibula
     M89.361 Hypertrophy of bone, right tibia
     M89.362 Hypertrophy of bone, left tibia
     M89.363 Hypertrophy of bone, right fibula
     M89.364 Hypertrophy of bone, left fibula
     M89.369 Hypertrophy of bone, unspecified tibia and fibula

✓6ᵗʰ **M89.37** Hypertrophy of bone, ankle and foot
     M89.371 Hypertrophy of bone, right ankle and foot
     M89.372 Hypertrophy of bone, left ankle and foot
     M89.379 Hypertrophy of bone, unspecified ankle and foot

     M89.38 Hypertrophy of bone, other site

     M89.39 Hypertrophy of bone, multiple sites

✓5th **M89.4 Other hypertrophic osteoarthropathy**
Marie-Bamberger disease
Pachydermoperiostosis

     M89.40 Other hypertrophic osteoarthropathy, unspecified site

     ✓6th **M89.41 Other hypertrophic osteoarthropathy, shoulder**
         M89.411 Other hypertrophic osteoarthropathy, right shoulder
         M89.412 Other hypertrophic osteoarthropathy, left shoulder
         M89.419 Other hypertrophic osteoarthropathy, unspecified shoulder

     ✓6th **M89.42 Other hypertrophic osteoarthropathy, upper arm**
         M89.421 Other hypertrophic osteoarthropathy, right upper arm
         M89.422 Other hypertrophic osteoarthropathy, left upper arm
         M89.429 Other hypertrophic osteoarthropathy, unspecified upper arm

     ✓6th **M89.43 Other hypertrophic osteoarthropathy, forearm**
         M89.431 Other hypertrophic osteoarthropathy, right forearm
         M89.432 Other hypertrophic osteoarthropathy, left forearm
         M89.439 Other hypertrophic osteoarthropathy, unspecified forearm

     ✓6th **M89.44 Other hypertrophic osteoarthropathy, hand**
         M89.441 Other hypertrophic osteoarthropathy, right hand
         M89.442 Other hypertrophic osteoarthropathy, left hand
         M89.449 Other hypertrophic osteoarthropathy, unspecified hand

     ✓6th **M89.45 Other hypertrophic osteoarthropathy, thigh**
         M89.451 Other hypertrophic osteoarthropathy, right thigh
         M89.452 Other hypertrophic osteoarthropathy, left thigh
         M89.459 Other hypertrophic osteoarthropathy, unspecified thigh

     ✓6th **M89.46 Other hypertrophic osteoarthropathy, lower leg**
         M89.461 Other hypertrophic osteoarthropathy, right lower leg
         M89.462 Other hypertrophic osteoarthropathy, left lower leg
         M89.469 Other hypertrophic osteoarthropathy, unspecified lower leg

     ✓6th **M89.47 Other hypertrophic osteoarthropathy, ankle and foot**
         M89.471 Other hypertrophic osteoarthropathy, right ankle and foot
         M89.472 Other hypertrophic osteoarthropathy, left ankle and foot
         M89.479 Other hypertrophic osteoarthropathy, unspecified ankle and foot

     M89.48 Other hypertrophic osteoarthropathy, other site
     M89.49 Other hypertrophic osteoarthropathy, multiple sites

✓5th **M89.5 Osteolysis**
Use additional code to identify major osseous defect, if applicable (M89.7-)
EXCLUDES 2   periprosthetic osteolysis of internal prosthetic joint (T84.05-)

     M89.50 Osteolysis, unspecified site

     ✓6th **M89.51 Osteolysis, shoulder**
         M89.511 Osteolysis, right shoulder
         M89.512 Osteolysis, left shoulder
         M89.519 Osteolysis, unspecified shoulder

     ✓6th **M89.52 Osteolysis, upper arm**
         M89.521 Osteolysis, right upper arm
         M89.522 Osteolysis, left upper arm
         M89.529 Osteolysis, unspecified upper arm

     ✓6th **M89.53 Osteolysis, forearm**
         M89.531 Osteolysis, right forearm
         M89.532 Osteolysis, left forearm
         M89.539 Osteolysis, unspecified forearm

     ✓6th **M89.54 Osteolysis, hand**
         M89.541 Osteolysis, right hand
         M89.542 Osteolysis, left hand
         M89.549 Osteolysis, unspecified hand

     ✓6th **M89.55 Osteolysis, thigh**
         M89.551 Osteolysis, right thigh
         M89.552 Osteolysis, left thigh
         M89.559 Osteolysis, unspecified thigh

     ✓6th **M89.56 Osteolysis, lower leg**
         M89.561 Osteolysis, right lower leg
         M89.562 Osteolysis, left lower leg
         M89.569 Osteolysis, unspecified lower leg

     ✓6th **M89.57 Osteolysis, ankle and foot**
         M89.571 Osteolysis, right ankle and foot
         M89.572 Osteolysis, left ankle and foot
         M89.579 Osteolysis, unspecified ankle and foot

     M89.58 Osteolysis, other site
     M89.59 Osteolysis, multiple sites

✓5th **M89.6 Osteopathy after poliomyelitis**
Use additional code (B91) to identify previous poliomyelitis
EXCLUDES 1   postpolio syndrome (G14)

     M89.60 Osteopathy after poliomyelitis, unspecified site `HCC`

     ✓6th **M89.61 Osteopathy after poliomyelitis, shoulder**
         M89.611 Osteopathy after poliomyelitis, right shoulder `HCC`
         M89.612 Osteopathy after poliomyelitis, left shoulder `HCC`
         M89.619 Osteopathy after poliomyelitis, unspecified shoulder `HCC`

     ✓6th **M89.62 Osteopathy after poliomyelitis, upper arm**
         M89.621 Osteopathy after poliomyelitis, right upper arm `HCC`
         M89.622 Osteopathy after poliomyelitis, left upper arm `HCC`
         M89.629 Osteopathy after poliomyelitis, unspecified upper arm `HCC`

     ✓6th **M89.63 Osteopathy after poliomyelitis, forearm**
         M89.631 Osteopathy after poliomyelitis, right forearm `HCC`
         M89.632 Osteopathy after poliomyelitis, left forearm `HCC`
         M89.639 Osteopathy after poliomyelitis, unspecified forearm `HCC`

     ✓6th **M89.64 Osteopathy after poliomyelitis, hand**
         M89.641 Osteopathy after poliomyelitis, right hand `HCC`
         M89.642 Osteopathy after poliomyelitis, left hand `HCC`
         M89.649 Osteopathy after poliomyelitis, unspecified hand `HCC`

     ✓6th **M89.65 Osteopathy after poliomyelitis, thigh**
         M89.651 Osteopathy after poliomyelitis, right thigh `HCC`
         M89.652 Osteopathy after poliomyelitis, left thigh `HCC`
         M89.659 Osteopathy after poliomyelitis, unspecified thigh `HCC`

     ✓6th **M89.66 Osteopathy after poliomyelitis, lower leg**
         M89.661 Osteopathy after poliomyelitis, right lower leg `HCC`
         M89.662 Osteopathy after poliomyelitis, left lower leg `HCC`
         M89.669 Osteopathy after poliomyelitis, unspecified lower leg `HCC`

     ✓6th **M89.67 Osteopathy after poliomyelitis, ankle and foot**
         M89.671 Osteopathy after poliomyelitis, right ankle and foot `HCC`
         M89.672 Osteopathy after poliomyelitis, left ankle and foot `HCC`
         M89.679 Osteopathy after poliomyelitis, unspecified ankle and foot `HCC`

     M89.68 Osteopathy after poliomyelitis, other site `HCC`
     M89.69 Osteopathy after poliomyelitis, multiple sites `HCC`

N Newborn: 0   P Pediatric: 0-17   M Maternity: 12-55   A Adult: 15-124   MCC Major Complication/Comorbidity   CC Complication/Comorbidity   SW Severe Wound Dx

818   ICD-10-CM 2019

✓5ᵗʰ M89.7 Major osseous defect
Code first underlying disease, if known, such as:
aseptic necrosis of bone (M87.-)
malignant neoplasm of bone (C40.-)
osteolysis (M89.5)
osteomyelitis (M86.-)
osteonecrosis (M87.-)
osteoporosis (M80.-, M81.-)
periprosthetic osteolysis (T84.05-)

M89.70   Major osseous defect, unspecified site

✓6ᵗʰ M89.71   Major osseous defect, shoulder region
Major osseous defect clavicle or scapula

M89.711   Major osseous defect, right shoulder region

M89.712   Major osseous defect, left shoulder region

M89.719   Major osseous defect, unspecified shoulder region

✓6ᵗʰ M89.72   Major osseous defect, humerus

M89.721   Major osseous defect, right humerus

M89.722   Major osseous defect, left humerus

M89.729   Major osseous defect, unspecified humerus

✓6ᵗʰ M89.73   Major osseous defect, forearm
Major osseous defect of radius and ulna

M89.731   Major osseous defect, right forearm

M89.732   Major osseous defect, left forearm

M89.739   Major osseous defect, unspecified forearm

✓6ᵗʰ M89.74   Major osseous defect, hand
Major osseous defect of carpus, fingers, metacarpus

M89.741   Major osseous defect, right hand

M89.742   Major osseous defect, left hand

M89.749   Major osseous defect, unspecified hand

✓6ᵗʰ M89.75   Major osseous defect, pelvic region and thigh
Major osseous defect of femur and pelvis

M89.751   Major osseous defect, right pelvic region and thigh

M89.752   Major osseous defect, left pelvic region and thigh

M89.759   Major osseous defect, unspecified pelvic region and thigh

✓6ᵗʰ M89.76   Major osseous defect, lower leg
Major osseous defect of fibula and tibia

M89.761   Major osseous defect, right lower leg

M89.762   Major osseous defect, left lower leg

M89.769   Major osseous defect, unspecified lower leg

✓6ᵗʰ M89.77   Major osseous defect, ankle and foot
Major osseous defect of metatarsus, tarsus, toes

M89.771   Major osseous defect, right ankle and foot

M89.772   Major osseous defect, left ankle and foot

M89.779   Major osseous defect, unspecified ankle and foot

M89.78   Major osseous defect, other site

M89.79   Major osseous defect, multiple sites

✓5ᵗʰ M89.8 Other specified disorders of bone
Infantile cortical hyperostoses
Post-traumatic subperiosteal ossification

✓6ᵗʰ M89.8X   Other specified disorders of bone

M89.8X0   Other specified disorders of bone, multiple sites

M89.8X1   Other specified disorders of bone, shoulder

M89.8X2   Other specified disorders of bone, upper arm

M89.8X3   Other specified disorders of bone, forearm

M89.8X4   Other specified disorders of bone, hand

M89.8X5   Other specified disorders of bone, thigh

M89.8X6   Other specified disorders of bone, lower leg

M89.8X7   Other specified disorders of bone, ankle and foot

M89.8X8   Other specified disorders of bone, other site

M89.8X9   Other specified disorders of bone, unspecified site

M89.9   Disorder of bone, unspecified

✓4ᵗʰ M90 Osteopathies in diseases classified elsewhere
EXCLUDES 1   osteochondritis, osteomyelitis, and osteopathy (in):
cryptococcosis (B45.3)
diabetes mellitus (E08-E13 with .69-)
gonococcal (A54.43)
neurogenic syphilis (A52.11)
renal osteodystrophy (N25.0)
salmonellosis (A02.24)
secondary syphilis (A51.46)
syphilis (late) (A52.77)

✓5ᵗʰ M90.5 Osteonecrosis in diseases classified elsewhere
Code first underlying disease, such as:
caisson disease (T70.3)
hemoglobinopathy (D50-D64)

CC Excl: For CC codes in subcategory M90.5, unless otherwise noted: PDX collection 907

M90.50   Osteonecrosis in diseases classified elsewhere, unspecified site   CC HCC

✓6ᵗʰ M90.51   Osteonecrosis in diseases classified elsewhere, shoulder

CC Excl: For CC codes in subcategory M90.51: PDX collection 908

M90.511   Osteonecrosis in diseases classified elsewhere, right shoulder   CC HCC

M90.512   Osteonecrosis in diseases classified elsewhere, left shoulder   CC HCC

M90.519   Osteonecrosis in diseases classified elsewhere, unspecified shoulder   CC HCC

✓6ᵗʰ M90.52   Osteonecrosis in diseases classified elsewhere, upper arm

M90.521   Osteonecrosis in diseases classified elsewhere, right upper arm   CC HCC

M90.522   Osteonecrosis in diseases classified elsewhere, left upper arm   CC HCC

M90.529   Osteonecrosis in diseases classified elsewhere, unspecified upper arm   CC HCC

✓6ᵗʰ M90.53   Osteonecrosis in diseases classified elsewhere, forearm

M90.531   Osteonecrosis in diseases classified elsewhere, right forearm   CC HCC

M90.532   Osteonecrosis in diseases classified elsewhere, left forearm   CC HCC

M90.539   Osteonecrosis in diseases classified elsewhere, unspecified forearm   CC HCC

✓6ᵗʰ M90.54   Osteonecrosis in diseases classified elsewhere, hand

M90.541   Osteonecrosis in diseases classified elsewhere, right hand   CC HCC

M90.542   Osteonecrosis in diseases classified elsewhere, left hand   CC HCC

M90.549   Osteonecrosis in diseases classified elsewhere, unspecified hand   CC HCC

✓6ᵗʰ M90.55   Osteonecrosis in diseases classified elsewhere, thigh

CC Excl: For CC codes in subcategory M90.55: PDX collection 909

M90.551   Osteonecrosis in diseases classified elsewhere, right thigh   CC HCC

M90.552   Osteonecrosis in diseases classified elsewhere, left thigh   CC HCC

M90.559   Osteonecrosis in diseases classified elsewhere, unspecified thigh   CC HCC

✓6ᵗʰ M90.56   Osteonecrosis in diseases classified elsewhere, lower leg

M90.561   Osteonecrosis in diseases classified elsewhere, right lower leg   CC HCC

M90.562   Osteonecrosis in diseases classified elsewhere, left lower leg   CC HCC

M90.569   Osteonecrosis in diseases classified elsewhere, unspecified lower leg   CC HCC

✓6ᵗʰ M90.57   Osteonecrosis in diseases classified elsewhere, ankle and foot

M90.571   Osteonecrosis in diseases classified elsewhere, right ankle and foot   CC HCC

M90.572   Osteonecrosis in diseases classified elsewhere, left ankle and foot   CC HCC

M90.579   Osteonecrosis in diseases classified elsewhere, unspecified ankle and foot   CC HCC

✓ Additional Character Required   ✓x7ᵗʰ Placeholder   Unacceptable PDx   Questionable PDx   Manifestation   H1-H14 HAC   HCC CMS-HCC Dx   HIV HIV Dx

ICD-10-CM 2019   819

Chapter 13. Diseases of the Musculoskeletal System and Connective Tissue

M89.7-M90.579

M90.58 **Osteonecrosis in diseases classified elsewhere,** *other site*   CC HCC

M90.59 **Osteonecrosis in diseases classified elsewhere,** *multiple sites*   CC HCC

✓6ᵗʰ **M90.6 Osteitis deformans in neoplastic diseases**
Osteitis deformans in malignant neoplasm of bone
Code first the neoplasm (C40-, C41-)
EXCLUDES 1 osteitis deformans [Paget's disease of bone] (M88.-)

M90.60 **Osteitis deformans in neoplastic diseases,** *unspecified site*

✓6ᵗʰ M90.61 **Osteitis deformans in neoplastic diseases,** shoulder
M90.611 *Osteitis deformans in neoplastic diseases, right shoulder*
M90.612 *Osteitis deformans in neoplastic diseases, left shoulder*
M90.619 *Osteitis deformans in neoplastic diseases, unspecified shoulder*

✓6ᵗʰ M90.62 **Osteitis deformans in neoplastic diseases,** upper arm
M90.621 *Osteitis deformans in neoplastic diseases, right upper arm*
M90.622 *Osteitis deformans in neoplastic diseases, left upper arm*
M90.629 *Osteitis deformans in neoplastic diseases, unspecified upper arm*

✓6ᵗʰ M90.63 **Osteitis deformans in neoplastic diseases,** forearm
M90.631 *Osteitis deformans in neoplastic diseases, right forearm*
M90.632 *Osteitis deformans in neoplastic diseases, left forearm*
M90.639 *Osteitis deformans in neoplastic diseases, unspecified forearm*

✓6ᵗʰ M90.64 **Osteitis deformans in neoplastic diseases,** hand
M90.641 *Osteitis deformans in neoplastic diseases, right hand*
M90.642 *Osteitis deformans in neoplastic diseases, left hand*
M90.649 *Osteitis deformans in neoplastic diseases, unspecified hand*

✓6ᵗʰ M90.65 **Osteitis deformans in neoplastic diseases,** thigh
M90.651 *Osteitis deformans in neoplastic diseases, right thigh*
M90.652 *Osteitis deformans in neoplastic diseases, left thigh*
M90.659 *Osteitis deformans in neoplastic diseases, unspecified thigh*

✓6ᵗʰ M90.66 **Osteitis deformans in neoplastic diseases,** lower leg
M90.661 *Osteitis deformans in neoplastic diseases, right lower leg*
M90.662 *Osteitis deformans in neoplastic diseases, left lower leg*
M90.669 *Osteitis deformans in neoplastic diseases, unspecified lower leg*

✓6ᵗʰ M90.67 **Osteitis deformans in neoplastic diseases,** ankle and foot
M90.671 *Osteitis deformans in neoplastic diseases, right ankle and foot*
M90.672 *Osteitis deformans in neoplastic diseases, left ankle and foot*
M90.679 *Osteitis deformans in neoplastic diseases, unspecified ankle and foot*

M90.68 **Osteitis deformans in neoplastic diseases,** *other site*

M90.69 **Osteitis deformans in neoplastic diseases,** *multiple sites*

✓5ᵗʰ **M90.8 Osteopathy in diseases classified elsewhere**
Code first underlying disease, such as:
rickets (E55.0)
vitamin-D-resistant rickets (E83.3)

M90.80 *Osteopathy in diseases classified elsewhere, unspecified site*

✓6ᵗʰ M90.81 **Osteopathy in diseases classified elsewhere,** shoulder
M90.811 *Osteopathy in diseases classified elsewhere, right shoulder*
M90.812 *Osteopathy in diseases classified elsewhere, left shoulder*
M90.819 *Osteopathy in diseases classified elsewhere, unspecified shoulder*

✓6ᵗʰ M90.82 **Osteopathy in diseases classified elsewhere,** upper arm
M90.821 *Osteopathy in diseases classified elsewhere, right upper arm*
M90.822 *Osteopathy in diseases classified elsewhere, left upper arm*
M90.829 *Osteopathy in diseases classified elsewhere, unspecified upper arm*

✓6ᵗʰ M90.83 **Osteopathy in diseases classified elsewhere,** forearm
M90.831 *Osteopathy in diseases classified elsewhere, right forearm*
M90.832 *Osteopathy in diseases classified elsewhere, left forearm*
M90.839 *Osteopathy in diseases classified elsewhere, unspecified forearm*

✓6ᵗʰ M90.84 **Osteopathy in diseases classified elsewhere,** hand
M90.841 *Osteopathy in diseases classified elsewhere, right hand*
M90.842 *Osteopathy in diseases classified elsewhere, left hand*
M90.849 *Osteopathy in diseases classified elsewhere, unspecified hand*

✓6ᵗʰ M90.85 **Osteopathy in diseases classified elsewhere,** thigh
M90.851 *Osteopathy in diseases classified elsewhere, right thigh*
M90.852 *Osteopathy in diseases classified elsewhere, left thigh*
M90.859 *Osteopathy in diseases classified elsewhere, unspecified thigh*

✓6ᵗʰ M90.86 **Osteopathy in diseases classified elsewhere,** lower leg
M90.861 *Osteopathy in diseases classified elsewhere, right lower leg*
M90.862 *Osteopathy in diseases classified elsewhere, left lower leg*
M90.869 *Osteopathy in diseases classified elsewhere, unspecified lower leg*

✓6ᵗʰ M90.87 **Osteopathy in diseases classified elsewhere,** ankle and foot
M90.871 *Osteopathy in diseases classified elsewhere, right ankle and foot*
M90.872 *Osteopathy in diseases classified elsewhere, left ankle and foot*
M90.879 *Osteopathy in diseases classified elsewhere, unspecified ankle and foot*

M90.88 **Osteopathy in diseases classified elsewhere,** *other site*

M90.89 **Osteopathy in diseases classified elsewhere,** *multiple sites*

Chondropathies (M91-M94)

EXCLUDES 1 postprocedural chondropathies (M96.-)

✓4ᵗʰ **M91 Juvenile osteochondrosis of** hip and pelvis
EXCLUDES 1 slipped upper femoral epiphysis (nontraumatic) (M93.0)

M91.0 Juvenile osteochondrosis of pelvis
Osteochondrosis (juvenile) of acetabulum
Osteochondrosis (juvenile) of iliac crest [Buchanan]
Osteochondrosis (juvenile) of ischiopubic synchondrosis [van Neck]
Osteochondrosis (juvenile) of symphysis pubis [Pierson]

✓5ᵗʰ **M91.1 Juvenile osteochondrosis of** head of femur [Legg-Calvé-Perthes]
M91.10 **Juvenile osteochondrosis of head of femur [Legg-Calvé-Perthes],** unspecified leg
M91.11 **Juvenile osteochondrosis of head of femur [Legg-Calvé-Perthes],** right leg
M91.12 **Juvenile osteochondrosis of head of femur [Legg-Calvé-Perthes],** left leg

✓5ᵗʰ **M91.2 Coxa plana**
Hip deformity due to previous juvenile osteochondrosis
M91.20 **Coxa plana,** unspecified hip
M91.21 **Coxa plana,** right hip
M91.22 **Coxa plana,** left hip

✓5ᵗʰ **M91.3 Pseudocoxalgia**
M91.30 **Pseudocoxalgia,** unspecified hip
M91.31 **Pseudocoxalgia,** right hip

M91.32 Pseudocoxalgia, left hip

✓5th **M91.4 Coxa magna**

    M91.40 Coxa magna, unspecified hip

    M91.41 Coxa magna, right hip

    M91.42 Coxa magna, left hip

✓5th **M91.8 Other juvenile osteochondrosis of hip and pelvis**

    Juvenile osteochondrosis after reduction of congenital dislocation of hip

    M91.80 Other juvenile osteochondrosis of hip and pelvis, unspecified leg

    M91.81 Other juvenile osteochondrosis of hip and pelvis, right leg

    M91.82 Other juvenile osteochondrosis of hip and pelvis, left leg

✓5th **M91.9 Juvenile osteochondrosis of hip and pelvis, unspecified**

    M91.90 Juvenile osteochondrosis of hip and pelvis, unspecified, unspecified leg

    M91.91 Juvenile osteochondrosis of hip and pelvis, unspecified, right leg

    M91.92 Juvenile osteochondrosis of hip and pelvis, unspecified, left leg

✓4th **M92 Other juvenile osteochondrosis**

✓5th **M92.0 Juvenile osteochondrosis of humerus**

    Osteochondrosis (juvenile) of capitulum of humerus [Panner]
    Osteochondrosis (juvenile) of head of humerus [Haas]

    M92.00 Juvenile osteochondrosis of humerus, unspecified arm

    M92.01 Juvenile osteochondrosis of humerus, right arm

    M92.02 Juvenile osteochondrosis of humerus, left arm

✓5th **M92.1 Juvenile osteochondrosis of radius and ulna**

    Osteochondrosis (juvenile) of lower ulna [Burns]
    Osteochondrosis (juvenile) of radial head [Brailsford]

    M92.10 Juvenile osteochondrosis of radius and ulna, unspecified arm

    M92.11 Juvenile osteochondrosis of radius and ulna, right arm

    M92.12 Juvenile osteochondrosis of radius and ulna, left arm

✓5th **M92.2 Juvenile osteochondrosis, hand**

    ✓6th **M92.20 Unspecified juvenile osteochondrosis, hand**

        M92.201 Unspecified juvenile osteochondrosis, right hand

        M92.202 Unspecified juvenile osteochondrosis, left hand

        M92.209 Unspecified juvenile osteochondrosis, unspecified hand

    ✓6th **M92.21 Osteochondrosis (juvenile) of carpal lunate [Kienböck]**

        M92.211 Osteochondrosis (juvenile) of carpal lunate [Kienböck], right hand

        M92.212 Osteochondrosis (juvenile) of carpal lunate [Kienböck], left hand

        M92.219 Osteochondrosis (juvenile) of carpal lunate [Kienböck], unspecified hand

    ✓6th **M92.22 Osteochondrosis (juvenile) of metacarpal heads [Mauclaire]**

        M92.221 Osteochondrosis (juvenile) of metacarpal heads [Mauclaire], right hand

        M92.222 Osteochondrosis (juvenile) of metacarpal heads [Mauclaire], left hand

        M92.229 Osteochondrosis (juvenile) of metacarpal heads [Mauclaire], unspecified hand

    ✓6th **M92.29 Other juvenile osteochondrosis, hand**

        M92.291 Other juvenile osteochondrosis, right hand

        M92.292 Other juvenile osteochondrosis, left hand

        M92.299 Other juvenile osteochondrosis, unspecified hand

✓5th **M92.3 Other juvenile osteochondrosis, upper limb**

    M92.30 Other juvenile osteochondrosis, unspecified upper limb

    M92.31 Other juvenile osteochondrosis, right upper limb

    M92.32 Other juvenile osteochondrosis, left upper limb

✓5th **M92.4 Juvenile osteochondrosis of patella**

    Osteochondrosis (juvenile) of primary patellar center [Köhler]
    Osteochondrosis (juvenile) of secondary patellar centre [Sinding Larsen]

    M92.40 Juvenile osteochondrosis of patella, unspecified knee

    M92.41 Juvenile osteochondrosis of patella, right knee

    M92.42 Juvenile osteochondrosis of patella, left knee

✓5th **M92.5 Juvenile osteochondrosis of tibia and fibula**

    Osteochondrosis (juvenile) of proximal tibia [Blount]
    Osteochondrosis (juvenile) of tibial tubercle [Osgood-Schlatter]
    Tibia vara

    M92.50 Juvenile osteochondrosis of tibia and fibula, unspecified leg

    M92.51 Juvenile osteochondrosis of tibia and fibula, right leg

    M92.52 Juvenile osteochondrosis of tibia and fibula, left leg

✓5th **M92.6 Juvenile osteochondrosis of tarsus**

    Osteochondrosis (juvenile) of calcaneum [Sever]
    Osteochondrosis (juvenile) of os tibiale externum [Haglund]
    Osteochondrosis (juvenile) of talus [Diaz]
    Osteochondrosis (juvenile) of tarsal navicular [Köhler]

    M92.60 Juvenile osteochondrosis of tarsus, unspecified ankle

    M92.61 Juvenile osteochondrosis of tarsus, right ankle

    M92.62 Juvenile osteochondrosis of tarsus, left ankle

✓5th **M92.7 Juvenile osteochondrosis of metatarsus**

    Osteochondrosis (juvenile) of fifth metatarsus [Iselin]
    Osteochondrosis (juvenile) of second metatarsus [Freiberg]

    M92.70 Juvenile osteochondrosis of metatarsus, unspecified foot

    M92.71 Juvenile osteochondrosis of metatarsus, right foot

    M92.72 Juvenile osteochondrosis of metatarsus, left foot

M92.8 Other specified juvenile osteochondrosis

    Calcaneal apophysitis

M92.9 Juvenile osteochondrosis, unspecified

    Juvenile apophysitis NOS
    Juvenile epiphysitis NOS
    Juvenile osteochondritis NOS
    Juvenile osteochondrosis NOS

✓4th **M93 Other osteochondropathies**

    EXCLUDES 2   osteochondrosis of spine (M42.-)

✓5th **M93.0 Slipped upper femoral epiphysis (nontraumatic)**

    Use additional code for associated chondrolysis (M94.3)

    ✓6th **M93.00 Unspecified slipped upper femoral epiphysis (nontraumatic)**

        M93.001 Unspecified slipped upper femoral epiphysis (nontraumatic), right hip

        M93.002 Unspecified slipped upper femoral epiphysis (nontraumatic), left hip

        M93.003 Unspecified slipped upper femoral epiphysis (nontraumatic), unspecified hip

    ✓6th **M93.01 Acute slipped upper femoral epiphysis (nontraumatic)**

        M93.011 Acute slipped upper femoral epiphysis (nontraumatic), right hip

        M93.012 Acute slipped upper femoral epiphysis (nontraumatic), left hip

        M93.013 Acute slipped upper femoral epiphysis (nontraumatic), unspecified hip

    ✓6th **M93.02 Chronic slipped upper femoral epiphysis (nontraumatic)**

        M93.021 Chronic slipped upper femoral epiphysis (nontraumatic), right hip

        M93.022 Chronic slipped upper femoral epiphysis (nontraumatic), left hip

        M93.023 Chronic slipped upper femoral epiphysis (nontraumatic), unspecified hip

    ✓6th **M93.03 Acute on chronic slipped upper femoral epiphysis (nontraumatic)**

        M93.031 Acute on chronic slipped upper femoral epiphysis (nontraumatic), right hip

        M93.032 Acute on chronic slipped upper femoral epiphysis (nontraumatic), left hip

        M93.033 Acute on chronic slipped upper femoral epiphysis (nontraumatic), unspecified hip

✓ Additional Character Required   ✓7th Placeholder   Unacceptable PDx   Questionable PDx   Manifestation   H1 - H14 HAC   HCC CMS-HCC Dx   HIV HIV Dx

ICD-10-CM 2019   821

M91.32–M93.033

M93.1 Kienböck's disease of adults   A
  Adult osteochondrosis of carpal lunates

✓5th **M93.2 Osteochondritis dissecans**
  DEF: Avascular necrosis caused by lack of blood flow to the bone and cartilage of a joint causing the bone to die. This can result in splinters or pieces of cartilage breaking off in the joint.

    M93.20 Osteochondritis dissecans of unspecified site

✓6th   **M93.21 Osteochondritis dissecans of** shoulder
    M93.211 Osteochondritis dissecans, right shoulder
    M93.212 Osteochondritis dissecans, left shoulder
    M93.219 Osteochondritis dissecans, unspecified **shoulder**

✓6th   **M93.22 Osteochondritis dissecans of** elbow
    M93.221 Osteochondritis dissecans, right elbow
    M93.222 Osteochondritis dissecans, left elbow
    M93.229 Osteochondritis dissecans, unspecified **elbow**

✓6th   **M93.23 Osteochondritis dissecans of** wrist
    M93.231 Osteochondritis dissecans, right wrist
    M93.232 Osteochondritis dissecans, left wrist
    M93.239 Osteochondritis dissecans, unspecified **wrist**

✓6th   **M93.24 Osteochondritis dissecans of joints of** hand
    M93.241 Osteochondritis dissecans, joints of right **hand**
    M93.242 Osteochondritis dissecans, joints of left **hand**
    M93.249 Osteochondritis dissecans, joints of unspecified **hand**

✓6th   **M93.25 Osteochondritis dissecans of** hip
    M93.251 Osteochondritis dissecans, right hip
    M93.252 Osteochondritis dissecans, left hip
    M93.259 Osteochondritis dissecans, unspecified **hip**

✓6th   **M93.26 Osteochondritis dissecans** knee
    M93.261 Osteochondritis dissecans, right knee
    M93.262 Osteochondritis dissecans, left knee
    M93.269 Osteochondritis dissecans, unspecified **knee**

✓6th   **M93.27 Osteochondritis dissecans of** ankle and joints of foot
    M93.271 Osteochondritis dissecans, right ankle and joints of **right** foot
    M93.272 Osteochondritis dissecans, left **ankle and joints of** left **foot**
    M93.279 Osteochondritis dissecans, unspecified **ankle and joints of foot**

    M93.28 Osteochondritis dissecans other site
    M93.29 Osteochondritis dissecans multiple sites

✓5th **M93.8 Other specified osteochondropathies**
    M93.80 Other specified osteochondropathies of unspecified site

✓6th   **M93.81 Other specified osteochondropathies of** shoulder
    M93.811 Other specified osteochondropathies, right shoulder
    M93.812 Other specified osteochondropathies, left **shoulder**
    M93.819 Other specified osteochondropathies, unspecified **shoulder**

✓6th   **M93.82 Other specified osteochondropathies of** upper arm
    M93.821 Other specified osteochondropathies, right upper arm
    M93.822 Other specified osteochondropathies, left upper arm
    M93.829 Other specified osteochondropathies, unspecified **upper arm**

✓6th   **M93.83 Other specified osteochondropathies of** forearm
    M93.831 Other specified osteochondropathies, right forearm
    M93.832 Other specified osteochondropathies, left forearm
    M93.839 Other specified osteochondropathies, unspecified **forearm**

✓6th   **M93.84 Other specified osteochondropathies of** hand
    M93.841 Other specified osteochondropathies, right hand

M93.842 Other specified osteochondropathies, left **hand**
M93.849 Other specified osteochondropathies, unspecified **hand**

✓6th **M93.85 Other specified osteochondropathies of** thigh
    M93.851 Other specified osteochondropathies, right thigh
    M93.852 Other specified osteochondropathies, left thigh
    M93.859 Other specified osteochondropathies, unspecified **thigh**

✓6th **M93.86 Other specified osteochondropathies** lower leg
    M93.861 Other specified osteochondropathies, right lower leg
    M93.862 Other specified osteochondropathies, left lower leg
    M93.869 Other specified osteochondropathies, unspecified **lower leg**

✓6th **M93.87 Other specified osteochondropathies of** ankle and foot
    M93.871 Other specified osteochondropathies, right ankle and foot
    M93.872 Other specified osteochondropathies, left ankle and foot
    M93.879 Other specified osteochondropathies, unspecified **ankle and foot**

  M93.88 Other specified osteochondropathies other site
  M93.89 Other specified osteochondropathies multiple sites

✓5th **M93.9 Osteochondropathy, unspecified**
  Apophysitis NOS   Osteochondritis NOS
  Epiphysitis NOS   Osteochondrosis NOS

    M93.90 Osteochondropathy, unspecified of unspecified site

✓6th   **M93.91 Osteochondropathy, unspecified of** shoulder
    M93.911 Osteochondropathy, unspecified, right shoulder
    M93.912 Osteochondropathy, unspecified, left shoulder
    M93.919 Osteochondropathy, unspecified, unspecified **shoulder**

✓6th   **M93.92 Osteochondropathy, unspecified of** upper arm
    M93.921 Osteochondropathy, unspecified, right upper arm
    M93.922 Osteochondropathy, unspecified, left upper arm
    M93.929 Osteochondropathy, unspecified, unspecified **upper arm**

✓6th   **M93.93 Osteochondropathy, unspecified of** forearm
    M93.931 Osteochondropathy, unspecified, right forearm
    M93.932 Osteochondropathy, unspecified, left forearm
    M93.939 Osteochondropathy, unspecified, unspecified **forearm**

✓6th   **M93.94 Osteochondropathy, unspecified of** hand
    M93.941 Osteochondropathy, unspecified, right hand
    M93.942 Osteochondropathy, unspecified, left hand
    M93.949 Osteochondropathy, unspecified, unspecified **hand**

✓6th   **M93.95 Osteochondropathy, unspecified of** thigh
    M93.951 Osteochondropathy, unspecified, right thigh
    M93.952 Osteochondropathy, unspecified, left thigh
    M93.959 Osteochondropathy, unspecified, unspecified **thigh**

✓6th   **M93.96 Osteochondropathy, unspecified** lower leg
    M93.961 Osteochondropathy, unspecified, right lower leg
    M93.962 Osteochondropathy, unspecified, left lower leg
    M93.969 Osteochondropathy, unspecified, unspecified **lower leg**

✓6th   **M93.97 Osteochondropathy, unspecified of** ankle and foot
    M93.971 Osteochondropathy, unspecified, right ankle and foot

N Newborn: 0   P Pediatric: 0-17   M Maternity: 12-55   A Adult: 15-124   MCC Major Complication/Comorbidity   CC Complication/Comorbidity   SW Severe Wound Dx

822   ICD-10-CM 2019

M93.972 Osteochondropathy, unspecified, left ankle and foot

M93.979 Osteochondropathy, unspecified, unspecified ankle and foot

M93.98 Osteochondropathy, unspecified other site

M93.99 Osteochondropathy, unspecified multiple sites

✅4th M94 Other disorders of cartilage

M94.0 Chondrocostal junction syndrome [Tietze]
Costochondritis

M94.1 Relapsing polychondritis

✅5th M94.2 Chondromalacia

EXCLUDES 1 chondromalacia patellae (M22.4)

M94.20 Chondromalacia, unspecified site

✅6th M94.21 Chondromalacia, shoulder
M94.211 Chondromalacia, right shoulder
M94.212 Chondromalacia, left shoulder
M94.219 Chondromalacia, unspecified shoulder

✅6th M94.22 Chondromalacia, elbow
M94.221 Chondromalacia, right elbow
M94.222 Chondromalacia, left elbow
M94.229 Chondromalacia, unspecified elbow

✅6th M94.23 Chondromalacia, wrist
M94.231 Chondromalacia, right wrist
M94.232 Chondromalacia, left wrist
M94.239 Chondromalacia, unspecified wrist

✅6th M94.24 Chondromalacia, joints of hand
M94.241 Chondromalacia, joints of right hand
M94.242 Chondromalacia, joints of left hand
M94.249 Chondromalacia, joints of unspecified hand

✅6th M94.25 Chondromalacia, hip
M94.251 Chondromalacia, right hip
M94.252 Chondromalacia, left hip
M94.259 Chondromalacia, unspecified hip

✅6th M94.26 Chondromalacia, knee
M94.261 Chondromalacia, right knee
M94.262 Chondromalacia, left knee
M94.269 Chondromalacia, unspecified knee

✅6th M94.27 Chondromalacia, ankle and joints of foot
M94.271 Chondromalacia, right ankle and joints of right foot
M94.272 Chondromalacia, left ankle and joints of left foot
M94.279 Chondromalacia, unspecified ankle and joints of foot

M94.28 Chondromalacia, other site

M94.29 Chondromalacia, multiple sites

✅5th M94.3 Chondrolysis
Code first any associated slipped upper femoral epiphysis (nontraumatic) (M93.0-)

✅6th M94.35 Chondrolysis, hip
M94.351 Chondrolysis, right hip
M94.352 Chondrolysis, left hip
M94.359 Chondrolysis, unspecified hip

✅5th M94.8 Other specified disorders of cartilage

✅6th M94.8X Other specified disorders of cartilage
M94.8X0 Other specified disorders of cartilage, multiple sites
M94.8X1 Other specified disorders of cartilage, shoulder
M94.8X2 Other specified disorders of cartilage, upper arm
M94.8X3 Other specified disorders of cartilage, forearm
M94.8X4 Other specified disorders of cartilage, hand
M94.8X5 Other specified disorders of cartilage, thigh
M94.8X6 Other specified disorders of cartilage, lower leg
M94.8X7 Other specified disorders of cartilage, ankle and foot
M94.8X8 Other specified disorders of cartilage, other site

M94.8X9 Other specified disorders of cartilage, unspecified sites

M94.9 Disorder of cartilage, unspecified

Other disorders of the musculoskeletal system and connective tissue (M95)

✅4th M95 Other acquired deformities of musculoskeletal system and connective tissue

EXCLUDES 2 acquired absence of limbs and organs (Z89-Z90)
acquired deformities of limbs (M20-M21)
congenital malformations and deformations of the musculoskeletal system (Q65-Q79)
deforming dorsopathies (M40-M43)
dentofacial anomalies [including malocclusion] (M26.-)
postprocedural musculoskeletal disorders (M96.-)

M95.0 Acquired deformity of nose
EXCLUDES 2 deviated nasal septum (J34.2)

✅5th M95.1 Cauliflower ear
EXCLUDES 2 other acquired deformities of ear (H61.1)
DEF: Acquired deformity of the external ear due to injury or subsequent perichondritis.
M95.10 Cauliflower ear, unspecified ear
M95.11 Cauliflower ear, right ear
M95.12 Cauliflower ear, left ear

M95.2 Other acquired deformity of head

M95.3 Acquired deformity of neck

M95.4 Acquired deformity of chest and rib
AHA: 2014, 4Q, 26-27

M95.5 Acquired deformity of pelvis
EXCLUDES 1 maternal care for known or suspected disproportion (O33.-)

M95.8 Other specified acquired deformities of musculoskeletal system

M95.9 Acquired deformity of musculoskeletal system, unspecified

Intraoperative and postprocedural complications and disorders of musculoskeletal system, not elsewhere classified (M96)

✅4th M96 Intraoperative and postprocedural complications and disorders of musculoskeletal system, not elsewhere classified

EXCLUDES 2 arthropathy following intestinal bypass (M02.0-)
complications of internal orthopedic prosthetic devices, implants and grafts (T84.-)
disorders associated with osteoporosis (M80)
periprosthetic fracture around internal prosthetic joint (M97.-)
presence of functional implants and other devices (Z96-Z97)

M96.0 Pseudarthrosis after fusion or arthrodesis   CC
CC Excl: No Excl

M96.1 Postlaminectomy syndrome, not elsewhere classified

M96.2 Postradiation kyphosis

M96.3 Postlaminectomy kyphosis

M96.4 Postsurgical lordosis

M96.5 Postradiation scoliosis

✅5th M96.6 Fracture of bone following insertion of orthopedic implant, joint prosthesis, or bone plate
Intraoperative fracture of bone during insertion of orthopedic implant, joint prosthesis, or bone plate
EXCLUDES 2 complication of internal orthopedic devices, implants or grafts (T84.-)

CC Excl: For CC codes in subcategory M96.6:
PDX collection 911

✅6th M96.62 Fracture of humerus following insertion of orthopedic implant, joint prosthesis, or bone plate
M96.621 Fracture of humerus following insertion of orthopedic implant, joint prosthesis, or bone plate, right arm   CC HCC
M96.622 Fracture of humerus following insertion of orthopedic implant, joint prosthesis, or bone plate, left arm   CC HCC
M96.629 Fracture of humerus following insertion of orthopedic implant, joint prosthesis, or bone plate, unspecified arm

✅6th M96.63 Fracture of radius or ulna following insertion of orthopedic implant, joint prosthesis, or bone plate
M96.631 Fracture of radius or ulna following insertion of orthopedic implant, joint prosthesis, or bone plate, right arm   CC HCC

✅ Additional Character Required   ✅x7th Placeholder   Unacceptable PDx   Questionable PDx   Manifestation   H1-H14 HAC   HCC CMS-HCC Dx   HIV HIV Dx

ICD-10-CM 2019   823

M96.632   **Fracture of radius or ulna** `CC` `HCC`
following insertion of orthopedic implant,
joint prosthesis, or bone plate, left arm

M96.639   **Fracture of radius or ulna** `CC` `HCC`
following insertion of orthopedic implant,
joint prosthesis, or bone plate,
unspecified arm

M96.65   **Fracture of pelvis following insertion of** `CC` `HCC`
orthopedic implant, joint prosthesis, or bone plate

✓6ᵗʰ **M96.66**   **Fracture of femur following insertion of orthopedic**
implant, joint prosthesis, or bone plate

M96.661   **Fracture of femur following** `CC` `HCC`
insertion of orthopedic implant, joint
prosthesis, or bone plate, right leg

M96.662   **Fracture of femur following** `CC` `HCC`
insertion of orthopedic implant, joint
prosthesis, or bone plate, left leg

M96.669   **Fracture of femur following** `CC` `HCC`
insertion of orthopedic implant, joint
prosthesis, or bone plate, unspecified leg

✓6ᵗʰ **M96.67**   **Fracture of tibia or fibula following insertion of**
orthopedic implant, joint prosthesis, or bone plate

M96.671   **Fracture of tibia or fibula** `CC` `HCC`
following insertion of orthopedic implant,
joint prosthesis, or bone plate, right leg

M96.672   **Fracture of tibia or fibula** `CC` `HCC`
following insertion of orthopedic implant,
joint prosthesis, or bone plate, left leg

M96.679   **Fracture of tibia or fibula** `CC` `HCC`
following insertion of orthopedic implant,
joint prosthesis, or bone plate,
unspecified leg

M96.69   **Fracture of other bone following insertion of** `CC` `HCC`
orthopedic implant, joint prosthesis, or bone plate

✓5ᵗʰ **M96.8**   **Other intraoperative and postprocedural complications and**
disorders of musculoskeletal system, not elsewhere classified
AHA: 2016, 4Q, 9-10

> **CC Excl: For CC codes in subcategory M96.8, unless**
> **otherwise noted:** PDX collection 912

✓6ᵗʰ **M96.81**   **Intraoperative hemorrhage and hematoma of a**
musculoskeletal structure complicating a procedure
> ***EXCLUDES 1***   *intraoperative hemorrhage and hematoma*
> *of a musculoskeletal structure due to*
> *accidental puncture and laceration*
> *during a procedure (M96.82-)*

M96.810   **Intraoperative hemorrhage and** `CC`
hematoma of a musculoskeletal structure
complicating a musculoskeletal system
procedure

M96.811   **Intraoperative hemorrhage and** `CC`
hematoma of a musculoskeletal structure
complicating other procedure

✓6ᵗʰ **M96.82**   **Accidental puncture and laceration of a**
musculoskeletal structure during a procedure

M96.820   **Accidental puncture and laceration of a** `CC`
musculoskeletal structure during a
musculoskeletal system procedure
    CC Excl: PDX collection 509

M96.821   **Accidental puncture and laceration of a** `CC`
musculoskeletal structure during other
procedure
    CC Excl: PDX collection 509

✓6ᵗʰ **M96.83**   **Postprocedural hemorrhage of a musculoskeletal**
structure following a procedure

M96.830   **Postprocedural hemorrhage of a** `CC`
musculoskeletal structure following a
musculoskeletal system procedure

M96.831   **Postprocedural hemorrhage of a** `CC`
musculoskeletal structure following
other procedure

✓6ᵗʰ **M96.84**   **Postprocedural hematoma and seroma of a**
musculoskeletal structure following a procedure

M96.840   **Postprocedural hematoma of a** `CC`
musculoskeletal structure following a
musculoskeletal system procedure

M96.841   **Postprocedural hematoma of a** `CC`
musculoskeletal structure following
other procedure
    AHA: 2016, 4Q, 10

M96.842   **Postprocedural seroma of a** `CC`
musculoskeletal structure following a
musculoskeletal system procedure

M96.843   **Postprocedural seroma of a** `CC`
musculoskeletal structure following
other procedure

M96.89   **Other intraoperative and postprocedural** `CC`
complications and disorders of the musculoskeletal
system
Instability of joint secondary to removal of joint
prosthesis
Use additional code, if applicable, to further specify
disorder
CC Excl: PDX collection 643

Periprosthetic fracture around internal prosthetic joint (M97)

✓4ᵗʰ **M97**   **Periprosthetic fracture around internal prosthetic joint**
> ***EXCLUDES 2***   *breakage (fracture) of prosthetic joint (T84.01-)*
> *fracture of bone following insertion of orthopedic implant, joint*
> *prosthesis or bone plate (M96.6-)*

AHA: 2016, 4Q, 42-43

> The appropriate 7th character is to be added to each code from
> category M97.
> A   initial encounter
> D   subsequent encounter
> S   sequela

> **CC Excl: For CC codes in category M97:** PDX collection 911

✓5ᵗʰ **M97.0**   **Periprosthetic fracture around internal prosthetic hip joint**
    AHA: 2018, 1Q, 21; 2016, 4Q, 42

✓x7ᵗʰ **M97.01**   **Periprosthetic fracture around internal** `CC` `HCC`
prosthetic right hip joint

✓x7ᵗʰ **M97.02**   **Periprosthetic fracture around internal** `CC` `HCC`
prosthetic left hip joint

✓5ᵗʰ **M97.1**   **Periprosthetic fracture around internal prosthetic knee joint**

✓x7ᵗʰ **M97.11**   **Periprosthetic fracture around internal** `CC`
prosthetic right knee joint

✓x7ᵗʰ **M97.12**   **Periprosthetic fracture around internal** `CC`
prosthetic left knee joint

✓5ᵗʰ **M97.2**   **Periprosthetic fracture around internal prosthetic ankle joint**

✓x7ᵗʰ **M97.21**   **Periprosthetic fracture around internal** `CC`
prosthetic right ankle joint

✓x7ᵗʰ **M97.22**   **Periprosthetic fracture around internal** `CC`
prosthetic left ankle joint

✓5ᵗʰ **M97.3**   **Periprosthetic fracture around internal prosthetic shoulder**
joint

✓x7ᵗʰ **M97.31**   **Periprosthetic fracture around internal** `CC`
prosthetic right shoulder joint

✓x7ᵗʰ **M97.32**   **Periprosthetic fracture around internal** `CC`
prosthetic left shoulder joint

✓5ᵗʰ **M97.4**   **Periprosthetic fracture around internal prosthetic elbow joint**

✓x7ᵗʰ **M97.41**   **Periprosthetic fracture around internal** `CC`
prosthetic right elbow joint

✓x7ᵗʰ **M97.42**   **Periprosthetic fracture around internal** `CC`
prosthetic left elbow joint

✓x7ᵗʰ **M97.8**   **Periprosthetic fracture around other internal prosthetic** `CC`
joint
Periprosthetic fracture around internal prosthetic finger joint
Periprosthetic fracture around internal prosthetic spinal joint
Periprosthetic fracture around internal prosthetic toe joint
Periprosthetic fracture around internal prosthetic wrist joint
Use additional code to identify the joint (Z96.6-)

✓x7ᵗʰ **M97.9**   **Periprosthetic fracture around unspecified internal** `CC`
prosthetic joint

Biomechanical lesions, not elsewhere classified (M99)

✓4ᵗʰ **M99**   **Biomechanical lesions, not elsewhere classified**
> **NOTE**   This category should not be used if the condition can be
> classified elsewhere.

DEF: Biomechanical lesion: Term used by osteopathic and chiropractic
physicians to describe musculoskeletal conditions treated that are not
more appropriately classified elsewhere.

✓5ᵗʰ **M99.0**   **Segmental and somatic dysfunction**

M99.00   **Segmental and somatic dysfunction of head region**

M99.01   **Segmental and somatic dysfunction of cervical**
region

N Newborn: 0   P Pediatric: 0-17   M Maternity: 12-55   A Adult: 15-124   **MCC** Major Complication/Comorbidity   **CC** Complication/Comorbidity   **SW** Severe Wound Dx

824   ICD-10-CM 2019

M99.02 Segmental and somatic dysfunction of thoracic region

M99.03 Segmental and somatic dysfunction of lumbar region

M99.04 Segmental and somatic dysfunction of sacral region

M99.05 Segmental and somatic dysfunction of pelvic region

M99.06 Segmental and somatic dysfunction of lower extremity

M99.07 Segmental and somatic dysfunction of upper extremity

M99.08 Segmental and somatic dysfunction of rib cage

M99.09 Segmental and somatic dysfunction of abdomen and other regions

✓5ᵗʰ **M99.1** Subluxation complex (vertebral)

> **CC Excl: For CC codes in subcategory M99.1, unless otherwise noted:** PDX collection 913

M99.10 Subluxation complex (vertebral) of head region   CC H5

M99.11 Subluxation complex (vertebral) of cervical region   CC H5

M99.12 Subluxation complex (vertebral) of thoracic region

M99.13 Subluxation complex (vertebral) of lumbar region

M99.14 Subluxation complex (vertebral) of sacral region

M99.15 Subluxation complex (vertebral) of pelvic region

M99.16 Subluxation complex (vertebral) of lower extremity

M99.17 Subluxation complex (vertebral) of upper extremity

M99.18 Subluxation complex (vertebral) of rib cage   CC H5

> **CC Excl:** PDX collection 914

M99.19 Subluxation complex (vertebral) of abdomen and other regions

✓5ᵗʰ **M99.2** Subluxation stenosis of neural canal

M99.20 Subluxation stenosis of neural canal of head region

M99.21 Subluxation stenosis of neural canal of cervical region

M99.22 Subluxation stenosis of neural canal of thoracic region

M99.23 Subluxation stenosis of neural canal of lumbar region

M99.24 Subluxation stenosis of neural canal of sacral region

M99.25 Subluxation stenosis of neural canal of pelvic region

M99.26 Subluxation stenosis of neural canal of lower extremity

M99.27 Subluxation stenosis of neural canal of upper extremity

M99.28 Subluxation stenosis of neural canal of rib cage

M99.29 Subluxation stenosis of neural canal of abdomen and other regions

✓5ᵗʰ **M99.3** Osseous stenosis of neural canal

M99.30 Osseous stenosis of neural canal of head region

M99.31 Osseous stenosis of neural canal of cervical region

M99.32 Osseous stenosis of neural canal of thoracic region

M99.33 Osseous stenosis of neural canal of lumbar region

M99.34 Osseous stenosis of neural canal of sacral region

M99.35 Osseous stenosis of neural canal of pelvic region

M99.36 Osseous stenosis of neural canal of lower extremity

M99.37 Osseous stenosis of neural canal of upper extremity

M99.38 Osseous stenosis of neural canal of rib cage

M99.39 Osseous stenosis of neural canal of abdomen and other regions

✓5ᵗʰ **M99.4** Connective tissue stenosis of neural canal

M99.40 Connective tissue stenosis of neural canal of head region

M99.41 Connective tissue stenosis of neural canal of cervical region

M99.42 Connective tissue stenosis of neural canal of thoracic region

M99.43 Connective tissue stenosis of neural canal of lumbar region

M99.44 Connective tissue stenosis of neural canal of sacral region

M99.45 Connective tissue stenosis of neural canal of pelvic region

M99.46 Connective tissue stenosis of neural canal of lower extremity

M99.47 Connective tissue stenosis of neural canal of upper extremity

M99.48 Connective tissue stenosis of neural canal of rib cage

M99.49 Connective tissue stenosis of neural canal of abdomen and other regions

✓5ᵗʰ **M99.5** Intervertebral disc stenosis of neural canal

M99.50 Intervertebral disc stenosis of neural canal of head region

M99.51 Intervertebral disc stenosis of neural canal of cervical region

M99.52 Intervertebral disc stenosis of neural canal of thoracic region

M99.53 Intervertebral disc stenosis of neural canal of lumbar region

M99.54 Intervertebral disc stenosis of neural canal of sacral region

M99.55 Intervertebral disc stenosis of neural canal of pelvic region

M99.56 Intervertebral disc stenosis of neural canal of lower extremity

M99.57 Intervertebral disc stenosis of neural canal of upper extremity

M99.58 Intervertebral disc stenosis of neural canal of rib cage

M99.59 Intervertebral disc stenosis of neural canal of abdomen and other regions

✓5ᵗʰ **M99.6** Osseous and subluxation stenosis of intervertebral foramina

M99.60 Osseous and subluxation stenosis of intervertebral foramina of head region

M99.61 Osseous and subluxation stenosis of intervertebral foramina of cervical region

M99.62 Osseous and subluxation stenosis of intervertebral foramina of thoracic region

M99.63 Osseous and subluxation stenosis of intervertebral foramina of lumbar region

M99.64 Osseous and subluxation stenosis of intervertebral foramina of sacral region

M99.65 Osseous and subluxation stenosis of intervertebral foramina of pelvic region

M99.66 Osseous and subluxation stenosis of intervertebral foramina of lower extremity

M99.67 Osseous and subluxation stenosis of intervertebral foramina of upper extremity

M99.68 Osseous and subluxation stenosis of intervertebral foramina of rib cage

M99.69 Osseous and subluxation stenosis of intervertebral foramina of abdomen and other regions

✓5ᵗʰ **M99.7** Connective tissue and disc stenosis of intervertebral foramina

M99.70 Connective tissue and disc stenosis of intervertebral foramina of head region

M99.71 Connective tissue and disc stenosis of intervertebral foramina of cervical region

M99.72 Connective tissue and disc stenosis of intervertebral foramina of thoracic region

M99.73 Connective tissue and disc stenosis of intervertebral foramina of lumbar region

M99.74 Connective tissue and disc stenosis of intervertebral foramina of sacral region

M99.75 Connective tissue and disc stenosis of intervertebral foramina of pelvic region

M99.76 Connective tissue and disc stenosis of intervertebral foramina of lower extremity

M99.77 Connective tissue and disc stenosis of intervertebral foramina of upper extremity

M99.78 Connective tissue and disc stenosis of intervertebral foramina of rib cage

M99.79 Connective tissue and disc stenosis of intervertebral foramina of abdomen and other regions

✓5ᵗʰ **M99.8** Other biomechanical lesions

M99.80 Other biomechanical lesions of head region

M99.81 Other biomechanical lesions of cervical region

M99.82 Other biomechanical lesions of thoracic region

M99.83 Other biomechanical lesions of lumbar region

M99.84 Other biomechanical lesions of sacral region

✔ Additional Character Required   ✓x7ᵗʰ Placeholder   Unacceptable PDx   Questionable PDx   Manifestation   H1-H14 HAC   HCC CMS-HCC Dx   HIV HIV Dx

ICD-10-CM 2019   **825**

M99.85   **Other biomechanical lesions of** pelvic region
M99.86   **Other biomechanical lesions of** lower extremity
M99.87   **Other biomechanical lesions of** upper extremity
M99.88   **Other biomechanical lesions of** rib cage
M99.89   **Other biomechanical lesions of** abdomen and other regions
M99.9   **Biomechanical lesion, unspecified**

N Newborn: 0   P Pediatric: 0-17   M Maternity: 12-55   A Adult: 15-124   MCC Major Complication/Comorbidity   CC Complication/Comorbidity   SW Severe Wound Dx

826   ICD-10-CM 2019

Chapter 14. Diseases of Genitourinary System (N00–N99)

Chapter Specific Guidelines with Coding Examples

The chapter specific guidelines from the ICD-10-CM Official Guidelines for Coding and Reporting have been provided below. Along with these guidelines are coding examples, contained in the shaded boxes, that have been developed to help illustrate the coding and/or sequencing guidance found in these guidelines.

a. Chronic kidney disease

1) Stages of chronic kidney disease (CKD)

The ICD-10-CM classifies CKD based on severity. The severity of CKD is designated by stages 1-5. Stage 2, code N18.2, equates to mild CKD; stage 3, code N18.3, equates to moderate CKD; and stage 4, code N18.4, equates to severe CKD. Code N18.6, End stage renal disease (ESRD), is assigned when the provider has documented end-stage-renal disease (ESRD).

If both a stage of CKD and ESRD are documented, assign code N18.6 only.

> Stage 5 chronic kidney disease with ESRD requiring chronic dialysis
>
> **N18.6**   **End stage renal disease**
>
> **Z99.2**   **Dependence on renal dialysis**
>
> *Explanation:* The diagnostic statement indicates the patient has chronic kidney disease, documented both as stage 5 and as ESRD requiring chronic dialysis. Code N18.6 End stage renal disease (ESRD), is assigned when the provider has documented end-stage-renal disease (ESRD). If both a stage of CKD and ESRD are documented, assign code N18.6 only.

2) Chronic kidney disease and kidney transplant status

Patients who have undergone kidney transplant may still have some form of chronic kidney disease (CKD) because the kidney transplant may not fully restore kidney function. Therefore, the presence of CKD alone does not constitute a transplant complication. Assign the appropriate N18 code for the patient's stage of CKD and code Z94.0, Kidney transplant status. If a transplant complication such as failure or rejection or other transplant complication is documented, see section I.C.19.g for information on coding complications of a kidney transplant. If the documentation is unclear as to whether the patient has a complication of the transplant, query the provider.

> Patient with residual chronic kidney disease stage 1 after kidney transplant
>
> **N18.1**   **Chronic kidney disease, stage 1**
>
> **Z94.0**   **Kidney transplant status**
>
> *Explanation:* Patients who have undergone kidney transplant may still have some form of chronic kidney disease (CKD) because the kidney transplant may not fully restore kidney function. The presence of CKD alone does not constitute a transplant complication. Assign the appropriate N18 code for the patient's stage of CKD and code Z94.0 Kidney transplant status.

3) Chronic kidney disease with other conditions

Patients with CKD may also suffer from other serious conditions, most commonly diabetes mellitus and hypertension. The sequencing of the CKD code in relationship to codes for other contributing conditions is based on the conventions in the Tabular List.

See I.C.9. Hypertensive chronic kidney disease.

See I.C.19. Chronic kidney disease and kidney transplant complications.

> Type 1 diabetic chronic kidney disease, stage 2
>
> **E10.22**   **Type 1 diabetes mellitus with diabetic chronic kidney disease**
>
> **N18.2**   **Chronic kidney disease, stage 2 (mild)**
>
> *Explanation:* Patients with CKD may also suffer from other serious conditions such as diabetes mellitus. The sequencing of the CKD code in relationship to codes for other contributing conditions is based on the conventions in the Tabular List. Diabetic CKD code E10.22 includes an instructional note to "Use additional code to identify stage of chronic kidney disease (N18.1–N18.6)," thus providing sequencing direction.

Chapter 14. Diseases of Genitourinary System *(left margin)*

Chapter 14. Diseases of the Genitourinary System (N00-N99)

EXCLUDES 2
certain conditions originating in the perinatal period (P04-P96)
certain infectious and parasitic diseases (A00-B99)
complications of pregnancy, childbirth and the puerperium (O00-O9A)
congenital malformations, deformations and chromosomal abnormalities (Q00-Q99)
endocrine, nutritional and metabolic diseases (E00-E88)
injury, poisoning and certain other consequences of external causes (S00-T88)
neoplasms (C00-D49)
symptoms, signs and abnormal clinical and laboratory findings, not elsewhere classified (R00-R94)

This chapter contains the following blocks:

N00-N08	Glomerular diseases
N10-N16	Renal tubulo-interstitial diseases
N17-N19	Acute kidney failure and chronic kidney disease
N20-N23	Urolithiasis
N25-N29	Other disorders of kidney and ureter
N30-N39	Other diseases of the urinary system
N40-N53	Diseases of male genital organs
N60-N65	Disorders of breast
N70-N77	Inflammatory diseases of female pelvic organs
N80-N98	Noninflammatory disorders of female genital tract
N99	Intraoperative and postprocedural complications and disorders of genitourinary system, not elsewhere classified

Glomerular diseases (N00-N08)

Code also any associated kidney failure (N17-N19).

EXCLUDES 1 hypertensive chronic kidney disease (I12.-)

DEF: Glomeruli: Clusters of microscopic blood vessels located within the kidneys containing small pores through which waste products are filtered from the blood and urine is formed.

DEF: Glomerulonephritis: Disease of the kidney with diffuse inflammation of the capillary loops of the glomeruli.

✓4ᵗʰ N00   Acute nephritic syndrome

INCLUDES
acute glomerular disease
acute glomerulonephritis
acute nephritis

EXCLUDES 1
acute tubulo-interstitial nephritis (N10)
nephritic syndrome NOS (N05.-)

CC Excl: For MCC codes in category N00, unless otherwise noted: PDX collection 915

N00.0 Acute nephritic syndrome with minor glomerular abnormality   `MCC`
Acute nephritic syndrome with minimal change lesion

N00.1 Acute nephritic syndrome with focal and segmental glomerular lesions   `MCC`
Acute nephritic syndrome with focal and segmental hyalinosis
Acute nephritic syndrome with focal and segmental sclerosis
Acute nephritic syndrome with focal glomerulonephritis

N00.2 Acute nephritic syndrome with diffuse membranous glomerulonephritis   `MCC`

N00.3 Acute nephritic syndrome with diffuse mesangial proliferative glomerulonephritis   `MCC`

N00.4 Acute nephritic syndrome with diffuse endocapillary proliferative glomerulonephritis   `MCC`

N00.5 Acute nephritic syndrome with diffuse mesangiocapillary glomerulonephritis   `MCC`
Acute nephritic syndrome with membranoproliferative glomerulonephritis, types 1 and 3, or NOS

N00.6 Acute nephritic syndrome with dense deposit disease   `MCC`
Acute nephritic syndrome with membranoproliferative glomerulonephritis, type 2

N00.7 Acute nephritic syndrome with diffuse crescentic glomerulonephritis   `MCC`
Acute nephritic syndrome with extracapillary glomerulonephritis

N00.8 Acute nephritic syndrome with other morphologic changes   `MCC`
Acute nephritic syndrome with proliferative glomerulonephritis NOS
CC Excl: PDX collection 916

N00.9 Acute nephritic syndrome with unspecified morphologic changes   `MCC`

✓4ᵗʰ N01   Rapidly progressive nephritic syndrome

INCLUDES
rapidly progressive glomerular disease
rapidly progressive glomerulonephritis
rapidly progressive nephritis

EXCLUDES 1 nephritic syndrome NOS (N05.-)

CC Excl: For MCC codes in category N01: PDX collection 915

N01.0 Rapidly progressive nephritic syndrome with minor glomerular abnormality   `MCC`
Rapidly progressive nephritic syndrome with minimal change lesion

N01.1 Rapidly progressive nephritic syndrome with focal and segmental glomerular lesions   `MCC`
Rapidly progressive nephritic syndrome with focal and segmental hyalinosis
Rapidly progressive nephritic syndrome with focal and segmental sclerosis
Rapidly progressive nephritic syndrome with focal glomerulonephritis

N01.2 Rapidly progressive nephritic syndrome with diffuse membranous glomerulonephritis   `MCC`

N01.3 Rapidly progressive nephritic syndrome with diffuse mesangial proliferative glomerulonephritis   `MCC`

N01.4 Rapidly progressive nephritic syndrome with diffuse endocapillary proliferative glomerulonephritis   `MCC`

N01.5 Rapidly progressive nephritic syndrome with diffuse mesangiocapillary glomerulonephritis   `MCC`
Rapidly progressive nephritic syndrome with membranoproliferative glomerulonephritis, types 1 and 3, or NOS

N01.6 Rapidly progressive nephritic syndrome with dense deposit disease   `MCC`
Rapidly progressive nephritic syndrome with membranoproliferative glomerulonephritis, type 2

N01.7 Rapidly progressive nephritic syndrome with diffuse crescentic glomerulonephritis   `MCC`
Rapidly progressive nephritic syndrome with extracapillary glomerulonephritis

N01.8 Rapidly progressive nephritic syndrome with other morphologic changes   `MCC`
Rapidly progressive nephritic syndrome with proliferative glomerulonephritis NOS

N01.9 Rapidly progressive nephritic syndrome with unspecified morphologic changes   `MCC`

✓4ᵗʰ N02   Recurrent and persistent hematuria

EXCLUDES 1
acute cystitis with hematuria (N30.01)
hematuria NOS (R31.9)
hematuria not associated with specified morphologic lesions (R31.-)

CC Excl: For CC codes in category N02, unless otherwise noted: PDX collection 917

N02.0 Recurrent and persistent hematuria with minor glomerular abnormality   `CC`
Recurrent and persistent hematuria with minimal change lesion

N02.1 Recurrent and persistent hematuria with focal and segmental glomerular lesions   `CC`
Recurrent and persistent hematuria with focal and segmental hyalinosis
Recurrent and persistent hematuria with focal and segmental sclerosis
Recurrent and persistent hematuria with focal glomerulonephritis

N02.2 Recurrent and persistent hematuria with diffuse membranous glomerulonephritis   `CC`

N02.3 Recurrent and persistent hematuria with diffuse mesangial proliferative glomerulonephritis   `CC`

N02.4 Recurrent and persistent hematuria with diffuse endocapillary proliferative glomerulonephritis   `CC`

N02.5 Recurrent and persistent hematuria with diffuse mesangiocapillary glomerulonephritis   `CC`
Recurrent and persistent hematuria with membranoproliferative glomerulonephritis, types 1 and 3, or NOS

N02.6 Recurrent and persistent hematuria with dense deposit disease   `CC`
Recurrent and persistent hematuria with membranoproliferative glomerulonephritis, type 2

N00-N02.6 *(left margin)*

N Newborn: 0   P Pediatric: 0-17   M Maternity: 12-55   A Adult: 15-124   MCC Major Complication/Comorbidity   CC Complication/Comorbidity   SW Severe Wound Dx

828   ICD-10-CM 2019

N02.7 **Recurrent and persistent hematuria with diffuse crescentic glomerulonephritis** `CC`
    Recurrent and persistent hematuria with extracapillary glomerulonephritis

N02.8 **Recurrent and persistent hematuria with other morphologic changes** `CC`
    Recurrent and persistent hematuria with proliferative glomerulonephritis NOS
    CC Excl: PDX collection 915

N02.9 **Recurrent and persistent hematuria with unspecified morphologic changes** `CC`
    AHA: 2017, 2Q, 5
    CC Excl: PDX collection 915

☑4ᵗʰ **N03** **Chronic nephritic syndrome**
    INCLUDES   chronic glomerular disease
                 chronic glomerulonephritis
                 chronic nephritis
    EXCLUDES 1   *chronic tubulo-interstitial nephritis (N11.-)*
                  diffuse sclerosing glomerulonephritis (N05.8-)
                  nephritic syndrome NOS (N05.-)
    DEF: Slow, progressive type of nephritis characterized by inflammation of the capillary loops in the glomeruli of the kidney, which leads to renal failure.

    CC Excl: For CC codes in catagory N03: PDX collection 918

N03.0 **Chronic nephritic syndrome with minor glomerular abnormality** `CC`
    Chronic nephritic syndrome with minimal change lesion

N03.1 **Chronic nephritic syndrome with focal and segmental glomerular lesions** `CC`
    Chronic nephritic syndrome with focal and segmental hyalinosis
    Chronic nephritic syndrome with focal and segmental sclerosis
    Chronic nephritic syndrome with focal glomerulonephritis

N03.2 **Chronic nephritic syndrome with diffuse membranous glomerulonephritis** `CC`

N03.3 **Chronic nephritic syndrome with diffuse mesangial proliferative glomerulonephritis** `CC`

N03.4 **Chronic nephritic syndrome with diffuse endocapillary proliferative glomerulonephritis** `CC`

N03.5 **Chronic nephritic syndrome with diffuse mesangiocapillary glomerulonephritis** `CC`
    Chronic nephritic syndrome with membranoproliferative glomerulonephritis, types 1 and 3, or NOS

N03.6 **Chronic nephritic syndrome with dense deposit disease** `CC`
    Chronic nephritic syndrome with membranoproliferative glomerulonephritis, type 2

N03.7 **Chronic nephritic syndrome with diffuse crescentic glomerulonephritis** `CC`
    Chronic nephritic syndrome with extracapillary glomerulonephritis

N03.8 **Chronic nephritic syndrome with other morphologic changes** `CC`
    Chronic nephritic syndrome with proliferative glomerulonephritis NOS

N03.9 **Chronic nephritic syndrome with unspecified morphologic changes** `CC`

☑4ᵗʰ **N04** **Nephrotic syndrome**
    INCLUDES   congenital nephrotic syndrome
                  lipoid nephrosis

    CC Excl: For CC codes in category N04, unless otherwise noted: PDX collection 917

N04.0 **Nephrotic syndrome with minor glomerular abnormality** `CC`
    Nephrotic syndrome with minimal change lesion

N04.1 **Nephrotic syndrome with focal and segmental glomerular lesions** `CC`
    Nephrotic syndrome with focal and segmental hyalinosis
    Nephrotic syndrome with focal and segmental sclerosis
    Nephrotic syndrome with focal glomerulonephritis

N04.2 **Nephrotic syndrome with diffuse membranous glomerulonephritis** `CC`

N04.3 **Nephrotic syndrome with diffuse mesangial proliferative glomerulonephritis** `CC`

N04.4 **Nephrotic syndrome with diffuse endocapillary proliferative glomerulonephritis** `CC`

N04.5 **Nephrotic syndrome with diffuse mesangiocapillary glomerulonephritis** `CC`
    Nephrotic syndrome with membranoproliferative glomerulonephritis, types 1 and 3, or NOS

N04.6 **Nephrotic syndrome with dense deposit disease** `CC`
    Nephrotic syndrome with membranoproliferative glomerulonephritis, type 2

N04.7 **Nephrotic syndrome with diffuse crescentic glomerulonephritis** `CC`
    Nephrotic syndrome with extracapillary glomerulonephritis
    CC Excl: PDX collection 915

N04.8 **Nephrotic syndrome with other morphologic changes** `CC`
    Nephrotic syndrome with proliferative glomerulonephritis NOS
    CC Excl: PDX collection 915

N04.9 **Nephrotic syndrome with unspecified morphologic changes** `CC`
    CC Excl: PDX collection 915

☑4ᵗʰ **N05** **Unspecified nephritic syndrome**
    INCLUDES   glomerular disease NOS
                  glomerulonephritis NOS
                  nephritis NOS
                  nephropathy NOS and renal disease NOS with morphological lesion specified in .0-.8
    EXCLUDES 1   *nephropathy NOS with no stated morphological lesion (N28.9)*
                  renal disease NOS with no stated morphological lesion (N28.9)
                  tubulo-interstitial nephritis NOS (N12)

    CC Excl: For CC codes in category N05: PDX collection 918

N05.0 **Unspecified nephritic syndrome with minor glomerular abnormality**
    Unspecified nephritic syndrome with minimal change lesion

N05.1 **Unspecified nephritic syndrome with focal and segmental glomerular lesions**
    Unspecified nephritic syndrome with focal and segmental hyalinosis
    Unspecified nephritic syndrome with focal and segmental sclerosis
    Unspecified nephritic syndrome with focal glomerulonephritis

N05.2 **Unspecified nephritic syndrome with diffuse membranous glomerulonephritis** `CC`

N05.3 **Unspecified nephritic syndrome with diffuse mesangial proliferative glomerulonephritis** `CC`

N05.4 **Unspecified nephritic syndrome with diffuse endocapillary proliferative glomerulonephritis** `CC`

N05.5 **Unspecified nephritic syndrome with diffuse mesangiocapillary glomerulonephritis** `CC`
    Unspecified nephritic syndrome with membranoproliferative glomerulonephritis, types 1 and 3, or NOS

N05.6 **Unspecified nephritic syndrome with dense deposit disease**
    Unspecified nephritic syndrome with membranoproliferative glomerulonephritis, type 2

N05.7 **Unspecified nephritic syndrome with diffuse crescentic glomerulonephritis**
    Unspecified nephritic syndrome with extracapillary glomerulonephritis

N05.8 **Unspecified nephritic syndrome with other morphologic changes**
    Unspecified nephritic syndrome with proliferative glomerulonephritis NOS

N05.9 **Unspecified nephritic syndrome with unspecified morphologic changes**

☑4ᵗʰ **N06** **Isolated proteinuria with specified morphological lesion**
    EXCLUDES 1   *proteinuria not associated with specific morphologic lesions (R80.0)*

    CC Excl: For CC codes in category N06: PDX collection 918

N06.0 **Isolated proteinuria with minor glomerular abnormality**
    Isolated proteinuria with minimal change lesion

N06.1 **Isolated proteinuria with focal and segmental glomerular lesions**
    Isolated proteinuria with focal and segmental hyalinosis
    Isolated proteinuria with focal and segmental sclerosis
    Isolated proteinuria with focal glomerulonephritis

N06.2 **Isolated proteinuria with diffuse membranous glomerulonephritis** `CC`

N06.3 **Isolated proteinuria with diffuse mesangial proliferative glomerulonephritis** `CC`

N06.4 **Isolated proteinuria with diffuse endocapillary proliferative glomerulonephritis** `CC`

N06.5 **Isolated proteinuria with diffuse mesangiocapillary glomerulonephritis** `CC`
    Isolated proteinuria with membranoproliferative glomerulonephritis, types 1 and 3, or NOS

N06.6 Isolated proteinuria with dense deposit disease
Isolated proteinuria with membranoproliferative glomerulonephritis, type 2

N06.7 Isolated proteinuria with diffuse crescentic glomerulonephritis
Isolated proteinuria with extracapillary glomerulonephritis

N06.8 Isolated proteinuria with other morphologic lesion
Isolated proteinuria with proliferative glomerulonephritis NOS

N06.9 Isolated proteinuria with unspecified morphologic lesion

✓4ᵗʰ **N07 Hereditary nephropathy, not elsewhere classified**
EXCLUDES 2   Alport's syndrome (Q87.81-)
hereditary amyloid nephropathy (E85.-)
nail patella syndrome (Q87.2)
non-neuropathic heredofamilial amyloidosis (E85.-)

CC Excl: For CC codes in category N07: PDX collection 918

N07.0 Hereditary nephropathy, not elsewhere classified with minor glomerular abnormality
Hereditary nephropathy, not elsewhere classified with minimal change lesion

N07.1 Hereditary nephropathy, not elsewhere classified with focal and segmental glomerular lesions
Hereditary nephropathy, not elsewhere classified with focal and segmental hyalinosis
Hereditary nephropathy, not elsewhere classified with focal and segmental sclerosis
Hereditary nephropathy, not elsewhere classified with focal glomerulonephritis

N07.2 Hereditary nephropathy, not elsewhere classified with diffuse membranous glomerulonephritis   CC

N07.3 Hereditary nephropathy, not elsewhere classified with diffuse mesangial proliferative glomerulonephritis   CC

N07.4 Hereditary nephropathy, not elsewhere classified with diffuse endocapillary proliferative glomerulonephritis   CC

N07.5 Hereditary nephropathy, not elsewhere classified with diffuse mesangiocapillary glomerulonephritis   CC
Hereditary nephropathy, not elsewhere classified with membranoproliferative glomerulonephritis, types 1 and 3, or NOS

N07.6 Hereditary nephropathy, not elsewhere classified with dense deposit disease
Hereditary nephropathy, not elsewhere classified with membranoproliferative glomerulonephritis, type 2

N07.7 Hereditary nephropathy, not elsewhere classified with diffuse crescentic glomerulonephritis
Hereditary nephropathy, not elsewhere classified with extracapillary glomerulonephritis

N07.8 Hereditary nephropathy, not elsewhere classified with other morphologic lesions
Hereditary nephropathy, not elsewhere classified with proliferative glomerulonephritis NOS

N07.9 Hereditary nephropathy, not elsewhere classified with unspecified morphologic lesions

N08 Glomerular disorders in diseases classified elsewhere
Glomerulonephritis
Nephritis
Nephropathy
Code first underlying disease, such as:
amyloidosis (E85.-)
congenital syphilis (A50.5)
cryoglobulinemia (D89.1)
disseminated intravascular coagulation (D65)
gout (M1A.-, M10.-)
microscopic polyangiitis (M31.7)
multiple myeloma (C90.0-)
sepsis (A40.0-A41.9)
sickle-cell disease (D57.0-D57.8)
EXCLUDES 1   glomerulonephritis, nephritis and nephropathy (in):
antiglomerular basement membrane disease (M31.0)
diabetes (E08-E13 with .21)
gonococcal (A54.21)
Goodpasture's syndrome (M31.0)
hemolytic-uremic syndrome (D59.3)
lupus (M32.14)
mumps (B26.83)
syphilis (A52.75)
systemic lupus erythematosus (M32.14)
Wegener's granulomatosis (M31.31)
pyelonephritis in diseases classified elsewhere (N16)
renal tubulo-interstitial disorders classified elsewhere (N16)

Renal tubulo-interstitial diseases (N10-N16)

INCLUDES   pyelonephritis
EXCLUDES 1   pyeloureteritis cystica (N28.85)

N10 Acute pyelonephritis   CC H6
Acute infectious interstitial nephritis
Acute pyelitis
Acute tubulo-interstitial nephritis
Hemoglobin nephrosis
Myoglobin nephrosis
Use additional code (B95-B97), to identify infectious agent
CC Excl: PDX collection 919

✓4ᵗʰ **N11 Chronic** tubulo-interstitial nephritis
INCLUDES   chronic infectious interstitial nephritis
chronic pyelitis
chronic pyelonephritis
Use additional code (B95-B97), to identify infectious agent

N11.0 Nonobstructive reflux-associated chronic pyelonephritis
Pyelonephritis (chronic) associated with (vesicoureteral) reflux
EXCLUDES 1   vesicoureteral reflux NOS (N13.70)

N11.1 Chronic obstructive **pyelonephritis**   CC
Pyelonephritis (chronic) associated with anomaly of pelviureteric junction
Pyelonephritis (chronic) associated with anomaly of pyeloureteric junction
Pyelonephritis (chronic) associated with crossing of vessel
Pyelonephritis (chronic) associated with kinking of ureter
Pyelonephritis (chronic) associated with obstruction of ureter
Pyelonephritis (chronic) associated with stricture of pelviureteric junction
Pyelonephritis (chronic) associated with stricture of ureter
EXCLUDES 1   calculous pyelonephritis (N20.9)
obstructive uropathy (N13.-)
CC Excl: PDX collection 920

N11.8 Other chronic tubulo-interstitial nephritis   CC
Nonobstructive chronic pyelonephritis NOS
CC Excl: PDX collection 921

N11.9 Chronic tubulo-interstitial nephritis, unspecified   CC H6
Chronic interstitial nephritis NOS
Chronic pyelitis NOS
Chronic pyelonephritis NOS
CC Excl: PDX collection 922

N12 Tubulo-interstitial nephritis, not specified as acute or chronic   CC H6
Interstitial nephritis NOS
Pyelitis NOS
Pyelonephritis NOS
EXCLUDES 1   calculous pyelonephritis (N20.9)
CC Excl: PDX collection 922

✓4ᵗʰ **N13 Obstructive and reflux uropathy**
EXCLUDES 2   calculus of kidney and ureter without hydronephrosis (N20.-)
congenital obstructive defects of renal pelvis and ureter (Q62.0-Q62.3)
hydronephrosis with ureteropelvic junction obstruction (Q62.11)
obstructive pyelonephritis (N11.1)
DEF: Hydronephrosis: Distension of the kidney caused by an accumulation of urine that cannot flow out due to an obstruction that may be caused by conditions such as kidney stones or vesicoureteral reflux.

CC Excl: For CC codes in category N13, unless otherwise noted: PDX collection 922

N13.0 Hydronephrosis with ureteropelvic junction obstruction   CC
Hydronephrosis due to acquired occlusion of ureteropelvic junction
EXCLUDES 2   hydronephrosis with ureteropelvic junction obstruction due to calculus (N13.2)
AHA: 2016, 4Q, 43

N13.1 Hydronephrosis with ureteral stricture, not elsewhere classified   CC
EXCLUDES 1   hydronephrosis with ureteral stricture with infection (N13.6)

N13.2 Hydronephrosis with renal and ureteral calculous obstruction   CC
EXCLUDES 1   hydronephrosis with renal and ureteral calculous obstruction with infection (N13.6)

✓5ᵗʰ **N13.3 Other and unspecified hydronephrosis**
EXCLUDES 1   hydronephrosis with infection (N13.6)

   N13.30 Unspecified hydronephrosis   CC
   N13.39 Other hydronephrosis   CC

N Newborn: 0   P Pediatric: 0-17   M Maternity: 12-55   A Adult: 15-124   MCC Major Complication/Comorbidity   CC Complication/Comorbidity   SW Severe Wound Dx

830   ICD-10-CM 2019

N06.6-N13.39

Hydronephrosis/UPJ Obstruction

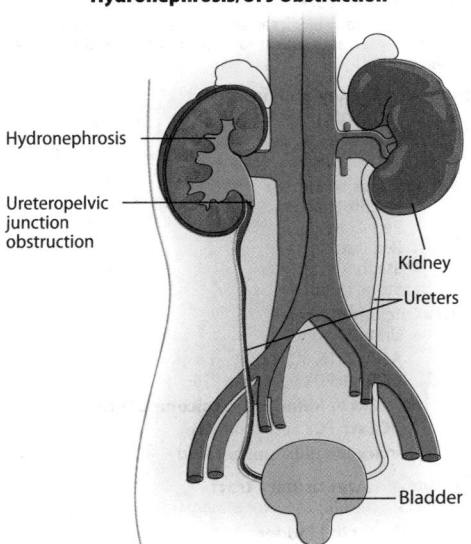

N13.4 **Hydroureter**   `CC`
     EXCLUDES 1   *congenital hydroureter (Q62.3-)*
                     hydroureter with infection (N13.6)
                     vesicoureteral-reflux with hydroureter (N13.73-)
     DEF: Abnormal enlargement or distension of the ureter with water or urine caused by an obstruction.
     CC Excl: PDX collection 923

N13.5 **Crossing vessel and stricture of ureter without hydronephrosis**
     Kinking and stricture of ureter without hydronephrosis
     EXCLUDES 1   *crossing vessel and stricture of ureter without hydronephrosis with infection (N13.6)*

N13.6 **Pyonephrosis**   `CC` `H6`
     Conditions in N13.0-N13.5 with infection
     Obstructive uropathy with infection
     Use additional code (B95-B97), to identify infectious agent
     AHA: 2018, 2Q, 21

✓5ᵗʰ N13.7 **Vesicoureteral-reflux**
     EXCLUDES 1   *reflux-associated pyelonephritis (N11.0)*
     DEF: Urine passage from the bladder flows backward up into the ureter and kidneys that can lead to bacterial infection and an increase in hydrostatic pressure, causing kidney damage.

     N13.70 **Vesicoureteral-reflux,** unspecified
           Vesicoureteral-reflux NOS

     N13.71 **Vesicoureteral-reflux** without reflux nephropathy

Vesicoureteral Reflux

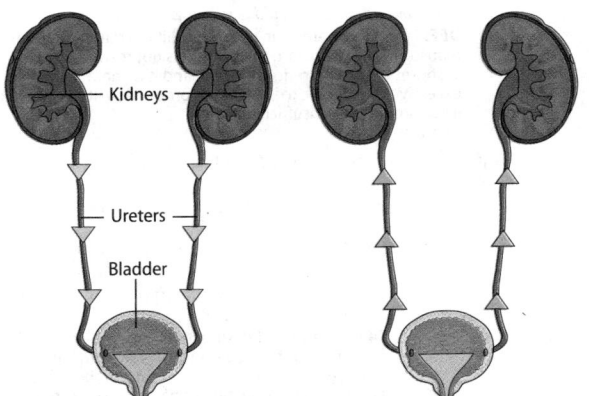

Normal flow of urine   Urine flowing the wrong way (VUR)

✓6ᵗʰ N13.72 **Vesicoureteral-reflux** with reflux nephropathy without hydroureter
     N13.721 **Vesicoureteral-reflux with reflux nephropathy without hydroureter,** unilateral
     N13.722 **Vesicoureteral-reflux with reflux nephropathy without hydroureter,** bilateral
     N13.729 **Vesicoureteral-reflux with reflux nephropathy without hydroureter,** unspecified

✓6ᵗʰ N13.73 **Vesicoureteral-reflux** with reflux nephropathy with hydroureter
     N13.731 **Vesicoureteral-reflux with reflux nephropathy with hydroureter,** unilateral
     N13.732 **Vesicoureteral-reflux with reflux nephropathy with hydroureter,** bilateral
     N13.739 **Vesicoureteral-reflux with reflux nephropathy with hydroureter,** unspecified

N13.8 **Other obstructive and reflux uropathy**   `CC`
     Urinary tract obstruction due to specified cause
     Code first, if applicable, any causal condition, such as:
           enlarged prostate (N40.1)
     CC Excl: PDX collection 920

N13.9 **Obstructive and reflux uropathy, unspecified**
     Urinary tract obstruction NOS

✓4ᵗʰ **N14** **Drug- and heavy-metal-induced tubulo-interstitial and tubular conditions**
     Code first poisoning due to drug or toxin, if applicable (T36-T65 with fifth or sixth character 1-4 or 6)
     Use additional code for adverse effect, if applicable, to identify drug (T36-T50 with fifth or sixth character 5)

     N14.0 **Analgesic nephropathy**

     N14.1 **Nephropathy induced by other drugs, medicaments and biological substances**

     N14.2 **Nephropathy induced by unspecified drug, medicament or biological substance**

     N14.3 **Nephropathy induced by heavy metals**

     N14.4 **Toxic nephropathy, not elsewhere classified**

✓4ᵗʰ **N15** **Other renal tubulo-interstitial diseases**

     N15.0 **Balkan nephropathy**
           Balkan endemic nephropathy

     N15.1 **Renal and perinephric abscess**   `MCC` `H6`
           CC Excl: PDX collection 919

     N15.8 **Other specified renal tubulo-interstitial diseases**

     N15.9 **Renal tubulo-interstitial disease, unspecified**
           Infection of kidney NOS
           EXCLUDES 1   *urinary tract infection NOS (N39.0)*

N16 ***Renal tubulo-interstitial disorders in diseases classified elsewhere***
     Pyelonephritis
     Tubulo-interstitial nephritis
     Code first underlying disease, such as:
           brucellosis (A23.0-A23.9)
           cryoglobulinemia (D89.1)
           glycogen storage disease (E74.0)
           leukemia (C91-C95)
           lymphoma (C81.0-C85.9, C96.0-C96.9)
           multiple myeloma (C90.0-)
           sepsis (A40.0-A41.9)
           Wilson's disease (E83.0)
     EXCLUDES 1   *diphtheritic pyelonephritis and tubulo-interstitial nephritis (A36.84)*
                     pyelonephritis and tubulo-interstitial nephritis in candidiasis (B37.49)
                     pyelonephritis and tubulo-interstitial nephritis in cystinosis (E72.04)
                     pyelonephritis and tubulo-interstitial nephritis in salmonella infection (A02.25)
                     pyelonephritis and tubulo-interstitial nephritis in sarcoidosis (D86.84)
                     pyelonephritis and tubulo-interstitial nephritis in sicca syndrome [Sjogren's] (M35.04)
                     pyelonephritis and tubulo-interstitial nephritis in systemic lupus erythematosus (M32.15)
                     pyelonephritis and tubulo-interstitial nephritis in toxoplasmosis (B58.83)
                     renal tubular degeneration in diabetes (E08-E13 with .29)
                     syphilitic pyelonephritis and tubulo-interstitial nephritis (A52.75)

✓ Additional Character Required   ✓ₓ7ᵗʰ Placeholder   Unacceptable PDx   Questionable PDx   Manifestation   **H1 - H14** HAC   **HCC** CMS-HCC Dx   **HIV** HIV Dx

ICD-10-CM 2019   **831**

Acute kidney failure and chronic kidney disease (N17-N19)

EXCLUDES 2   congenital renal failure (P96.0)
> drug- and heavy-metal-induced tubulo-interstitial and tubular conditions (N14.-)
> extrarenal uremia (R39.2)
> hemolytic-uremic syndrome (D59.3)
> hepatorenal syndrome (K76.7)
> postpartum hepatorenal syndrome (O90.4)
> posttraumatic renal failure (T79.5)
> prerenal uremia (R39.2)
> renal failure complicating abortion or ectopic or molar pregnancy (O00-O07, O08.4)
> renal failure following labor and delivery (O90.4)
> renal failure postprocedural (N99.0)

✓4th N17   Acute kidney failure

Code also associated underlying condition

EXCLUDES 1   posttraumatic renal failure (T79.5)

AHA: 2013, 4Q, 124

CC Excl: For CC/MCC codes in category N17, unless otherwise noted: PDX collection 924

N17.0   Acute kidney failure with tubular necrosis   MCC HCC
> Acute tubular necrosis
> Renal tubular necrosis
> Tubular necrosis NOS

N17.1   Acute kidney failure with acute cortical necrosis   MCC HCC
> Acute cortical necrosis
> Cortical necrosis NOS
> Renal cortical necrosis

N17.2   Acute kidney failure with medullary necrosis   MCC HCC
> Medullary [papillary] necrosis NOS
> Acute medullary [papillary] necrosis
> Renal medullary [papillary] necrosis

N17.8   Other acute kidney failure   CC HCC
> CC Excl: PDX collection 925

N17.9   Acute kidney failure, unspecified   CC HCC
> Acute kidney injury (nontraumatic)
> EXCLUDES 2   traumatic kidney injury (S37.0-)

✓4th N18   Chronic kidney disease (CKD)

Code first any associated:
> diabetic chronic kidney disease (E08.22, E09.22, E10.22, E11.22, E13.22)
> hypertensive chronic kidney disease (I12.-, I13-)

Use additional code to identify kidney transplant status, if applicable, (Z94.0)

AHA: 2013, 1Q, 24

N18.1   Chronic kidney disease, stage 1

N18.2   Chronic kidney disease, stage 2 (mild)

N18.3   Chronic kidney disease, stage 3 (moderate)

N18.4   Chronic kidney disease, stage 4 (severe)   CC HCC
> CC Excl: PDX collection 926

N18.5   Chronic kidney disease, stage 5   CC HCC
> EXCLUDES 1   chronic kidney disease, stage 5 requiring chronic dialysis (N18.6)
> DEF: End-stage renal disease (ESRD) with a GFR value of 15 ml/min or less not yet requiring chronic dialysis.
> TIP: When both ESRD and CKD 5 are documented, code only for ESRD.
> CC Excl: PDX collection 926

N18.6   End stage renal disease   MCC HCC
> Chronic kidney disease requiring chronic dialysis
> Use additional code to identify dialysis status (Z99.2)
> AHA: 2016, 3Q, 22; 2016, 1Q, 12; 2013, 4Q, 124-125
> TIP: When both ESRD and CKD 5 are documented, code only for ESRD.
> CC Excl: PDX collection 927

N18.9   Chronic kidney disease, unspecified
> Chronic renal disease
> Chronic renal failure NOS
> Chronic renal insufficiency
> Chronic uremia NOS
> Diffuse sclerosing glomerulonephritis NOS

N19   Unspecified kidney failure
> Uremia NOS
> EXCLUDES 1   acute kidney failure (N17.-)
> chronic kidney disease (N18.-)
> chronic uremia (N18.9)
> extrarenal uremia (R39.2)
> prerenal uremia (R39.2)
> renal insufficiency (acute) (N28.9)
> uremia of newborn (P96.0)

Urolithiasis (N20-N23)

AHA: 2017, 1Q, 5; 2015, 2Q, 8

TIP: Codes from this code block can be assigned based on the diagnosis listed in a radiology report when authenticated by a radiologist and available at the time of code assignment.

✓4th N20   Calculus of kidney and ureter
> Calculous pyelonephritis
> EXCLUDES 1   nephrocalcinosis (E83.5)
> that with hydronephrosis (N13.2)

N20.0   Calculus of kidney
> Nephrolithiasis NOS
> Renal calculus
> Renal stone
> Staghorn calculus
> Stone in kidney

N20.1   Calculus of ureter   CC
> Ureteric stone
> AHA: 2016, 3Q, 22
> CC Excl: PDX collection 928

N20.2   Calculus of kidney with calculus of ureter   CC
> CC Excl: PDX collection 928

N20.9   Urinary calculus, unspecified

✓4th N21   Calculus of lower urinary tract
> INCLUDES   calculus of lower urinary tract with cystitis and urethritis

N21.0   Calculus in bladder
> Calculus in diverticulum of bladder
> Urinary bladder stone
> EXCLUDES 2   staghorn calculus (N20.0)

N21.1   Calculus in urethra
> EXCLUDES 2   calculus of prostate (N42.0)

N21.8   Other lower urinary tract calculus

N21.9   Calculus of lower urinary tract, unspecified
> EXCLUDES 1   calculus of urinary tract NOS (N20.9)

N22   Calculus of urinary tract in diseases classified elsewhere
> Code first underlying disease, such as:
> gout (M1A.-, M10.-)
> schistosomiasis (B65.0-B65.9)

N23   Unspecified renal colic

Other disorders of kidney and ureter (N25-N29)

EXCLUDES 2   disorders of kidney and ureter with urolithiasis (N20-N23)

✓4th N25   Disorders resulting from impaired renal tubular function

N25.0   Renal osteodystrophy
> Azotemic osteodystrophy
> Phosphate-losing tubular disorders
> Renal rickets
> Renal short stature
> EXCLUDES 2   metabolic disorders classifiable to E70-E88
> DEF: Various bone diseases occurring when kidney function is impaired or fails. Abnormal levels of phosphorous and calcium can lead to osteomalacia, osteoporosis, or osteosclerosis.

N25.1   Nephrogenic diabetes insipidus   CC HCC
> EXCLUDES 1   diabetes insipidus NOS (E23.2)
> DEF: Type of diabetes due to the inability of renal tubules to reabsorb water back into the body. It is not responsive to vasopressin (antidiuretic hormone) and it is characterized by excessive thirst and excessive urine production. It may develop into chronic renal insufficiency.
> CC Excl: PDX collection 929

✓5th N25.8   Other disorders resulting from impaired renal tubular function

N25.81   Secondary hyperparathyroidism of renal origin   CC HCC
> EXCLUDES 1   secondary hyperparathyroidism, non-renal (E21.1)
> EXCLUDES 2   metabolic disorders classifiable to E70-E88
> DEF: Parathyroid dysfunction caused by chronic renal failure. Phosphate clearance and vitamin D production is impaired resulting in lowered calcium blood levels and an excessive production of parathyroid hormone.
> CC Excl: PDX collection 930

N25.89   Other disorders resulting from impaired renal tubular function
> Hypokalemic nephropathy
> Lightwood-Albright syndrome
> Renal tubular acidosis NOS

N Newborn: 0   P Pediatric: 0-17   M Maternity: 12-55   A Adult: 15-124   MCC Major Complication/Comorbidity   CC Complication/Comorbidity   SW Severe Wound Dx

832   ICD-10-CM 2019

N25.9   **Disorder resulting from impaired renal tubular function, unspecified**

☑4ᵗʰ **N26**   **Unspecified contracted kidney**
> EXCLUDES 1   contracted kidney due to hypertension (I12.-)
> diffuse sclerosing glomerulonephritis (N05.8-)
> hypertensive nephrosclerosis (arteriolar) (arteriosclerotic) (I12.-)
> small kidney of unknown cause (N27.-)

N26.1   **Atrophy of kidney (terminal)**

N26.2   **Page kidney**

N26.9   **Renal sclerosis, unspecified**

☑4ᵗʰ **N27**   **Small kidney of unknown cause**
> INCLUDES   oligonephronia

N27.0   **Small kidney, unilateral**

N27.1   **Small kidney, bilateral**

N27.9   **Small kidney, unspecified**

☑4ᵗʰ **N28**   **Other disorders of kidney and ureter, not elsewhere classified**

N28.0   **Ischemia and infarction of kidney**   `CC` `HCC`
> Renal artery embolism
> Renal artery obstruction
> Renal artery occlusion
> Renal artery thrombosis
> Renal infarct
> EXCLUDES 1   atherosclerosis of renal artery (extrarenal part) (I70.1)
> congenital stenosis of renal artery (Q27.1)
> Goldblatt's kidney (I70.1)
> **CC Excl:** PDX collection 931

N28.1   **Cyst of kidney, acquired**
> Cyst (multiple) (solitary) of kidney (acquired)
> EXCLUDES 1   cystic kidney disease (congenital) (Q61.-)

☑5ᵗʰ **N28.8**   **Other specified disorders of kidney and ureter**
> EXCLUDES 1   hydroureter (N13.4)
> ureteric stricture with hydronephrosis (N13.1)
> ureteric stricture without hydronephrosis (N13.5)

> **CC Excl: For CC codes in subcategory N28.8:**
> PDX collection 922

N28.81   **Hypertrophy of kidney**

N28.82   **Megaloureter**

N28.83   **Nephroptosis**

N28.84   **Pyelitis cystica**   `CC` `H6`

N28.85   **Pyeloureteritis cystica**   `CC` `H6`

N28.86   **Ureteritis cystica**   `CC` `H6`

N28.89   **Other specified disorders of kidney and ureter**

N28.9   **Disorder of kidney and ureter, unspecified**
> Nephropathy NOS
> Renal disease (acute) NOS
> Renal insufficiency (acute)
> EXCLUDES 1   chronic renal insufficiency (N18.9)
> unspecified nephritic syndrome (N05.-)
> **AHA:** 2016, 1Q, 13

N29   *Other disorders of kidney and ureter in diseases classified elsewhere*
> Code first underlying disease, such as:
> amyloidosis (E85.-)
> nephrocalcinosis (E83.5)
> schistosomiasis (B65.0-B65.9)
> EXCLUDES 1   disorders of kidney and ureter in:
> cystinosis (E72.0)
> gonorrhea (A54.21)
> syphilis (A52.75)
> tuberculosis (A18.11)

Other diseases of the urinary system (N30-N39)
> EXCLUDES 1   urinary infection (complicating):
> abortion or ectopic or molar pregnancy (O00-O07, O08.8)
> pregnancy, childbirth and the puerperium (O23-, O75.3, O86.2-)

☑4ᵗʰ **N30**   **Cystitis**
> Use additional code to identify infectious agent (B95-B97)
> EXCLUDES 1   prostatocystitis (N41.3)
> **AHA:** 2017, 1Q, 6
> **DEF:** Inflammation of the urinary bladder. Symptoms include dysuria, frequency of urination, urgency, and hematuria.

> **CC Excl: For CC codes in category N30:** PDX collection 932

☑5ᵗʰ **N30.0**   **Acute cystitis**
> EXCLUDES 1   irradiation cystitis (N30.4-)
> trigonitis (N30.3-)

N30.00   **Acute cystitis without hematuria**   `CC` `H6`

N30.01   **Acute cystitis with hematuria**   `CC` `H6`

☑5ᵗʰ **N30.1**   **Interstitial cystitis (chronic)**

N30.10   **Interstitial cystitis (chronic) without hematuria**

N30.11   **Interstitial cystitis (chronic) with hematuria**

☑5ᵗʰ **N30.2**   **Other chronic cystitis**

N30.20   **Other chronic cystitis without hematuria**

N30.21   **Other chronic cystitis with hematuria**

☑5ᵗʰ **N30.3**   **Trigonitis**
> Urethrotrigonitis

N30.30   **Trigonitis without hematuria**

N30.31   **Trigonitis with hematuria**

☑5ᵗʰ **N30.4**   **Irradiation cystitis**

N30.40   **Irradiation cystitis without hematuria**   `CC`

N30.41   **Irradiation cystitis with hematuria**   `CC`

☑5ᵗʰ **N30.8**   **Other cystitis**
> Abscess of bladder

N30.80   **Other cystitis without hematuria**

N30.81   **Other cystitis with hematuria**

☑5ᵗʰ **N30.9**   **Cystitis, unspecified**

N30.90   **Cystitis, unspecified without hematuria**

N30.91   **Cystitis, unspecified with hematuria**

☑4ᵗʰ **N31**   **Neuromuscular dysfunction of bladder, not elsewhere classified**
> Use additional code to identify any associated urinary incontinence (N39.3-N39.4-)
> EXCLUDES 1   cord bladder NOS (G95.89)
> neurogenic bladder due to cauda equina syndrome (G83.4)
> neuromuscular dysfunction due to spinal cord lesion (G95.89)

N31.0   **Uninhibited neuropathic bladder, not elsewhere classified**

N31.1   **Reflex neuropathic bladder, not elsewhere classified**

N31.2   **Flaccid neuropathic bladder, not elsewhere classified**
> Atonic (motor) (sensory) neuropathic bladder
> Autonomous neuropathic bladder
> Nonreflex neuropathic bladder

N31.8   **Other neuromuscular dysfunction of bladder**

N31.9   **Neuromuscular dysfunction of bladder, unspecified**
> Neurogenic bladder dysfunction NOS

☑4ᵗʰ **N32**   **Other disorders of bladder**
> EXCLUDES 2   calculus of bladder (N21.0)
> cystocele (N81.1-)
> hernia or prolapse of bladder, female (N81.1-)

N32.0   **Bladder-neck obstruction**
> Bladder-neck stenosis (acquired)
> EXCLUDES 1   congenital bladder-neck obstruction (Q64.3-)
> **DEF:** Bladder outlet and vesicourethral obstruction that occurs as a consequence of benign prostatic hypertrophy or prostatic cancer. It may also occur in either sex due to strictures, radiation, cystoscopy, catheterization, injury, infection, blood clots, bladder cancer, impaction, or other disease that compresses the bladder neck.

N32.1   **Vesicointestinal fistula**   `CC`
> Vesicorectal fistula
> **CC Excl:** PDX collection 933

N32.2   **Vesical fistula, not elsewhere classified**   `CC`
> EXCLUDES 1   fistula between bladder and female genital tract (N82.0-N82.1)
> **CC Excl:** PDX collection 933

N32.3   **Diverticulum of bladder**
> EXCLUDES 1   congenital diverticulum of bladder (Q64.6)
> diverticulitis of bladder (N30.8-)

☑5ᵗʰ **N32.8**   **Other specified disorders of bladder**

N32.81   **Overactive bladder**
> Detrusor muscle hyperactivity
> EXCLUDES 1   frequent urination due to specified bladder condition—code to condition
> **DEF:** Sudden involuntary contractions of the muscular wall of the bladder that results in a sudden, strong urge to urinate.

N32.89   **Other specified disorders of bladder**
> Bladder hemorrhage
> Bladder hypertrophy
> Calcified bladder
> Contracted bladder

N32.9   **Bladder disorder, unspecified**

☑ Additional Character Required   ✓x7ᵗʰ Placeholder   Unacceptable PDx   Questionable PDx   Manifestation   `H1`-`H14` HAC   `HCC` CMS-HCC Dx   `HIV` HIV Dx

ICD-10-CM 2019   **833**

Chapter 14. Diseases of Genitourinary System

N33 Bladder disorders in diseases classified elsewhere
Code first underlying disease, such as:
schistosomiasis (B65.0-B65.9)
EXCLUDES 1   bladder disorder in syphilis (A52.76)
bladder disorder in tuberculosis (A18.12)
candidal cystitis (B37.41)
chlamydial cystitis (A56.0)
cystitis in gonorrhea (A54.01)
cystitis in neurogenic bladder (N31.-)
diphtheritic cystitis (A36.85)
neurogenic bladder (N31.-)
syphilitic cystitis (A52.76)
trichomonal cystitis (A59.03)

N34 Urethritis and urethral syndrome
Use additional code (B95-B97), to identify infectious agent
EXCLUDES 2   Reiter's disease (M02.3-)
urethritis in diseases with a predominantly sexual mode of
transmission (A50-A64)
urethrotrigonitis (N30.3-)

AHA: 2017, 1Q, 6

N34.0 Urethral abscess   CC H6
Abscess (of) Cowper's gland
Abscess (of) Littrés gland
Abscess (of) urethral (gland)
Periurethral abscess
EXCLUDES 1   urethral caruncle (N36.2)
CC Excl: PDX collection 934

N34.1 Nonspecific urethritis
Nongonococcal urethritis
Nonvenereal urethritis

N34.2 Other urethritis
Meatitis, urethral
Postmenopausal urethritis
Ulcer of urethra (meatus)
Urethritis NOS

N34.3 Urethral syndrome, unspecified

N35 Urethral stricture
EXCLUDES 1   congenital urethral stricture (Q64.3-)
postprocedural urethral stricture (N99.1-)

N35.0 Post-traumatic urethral stricture
Urethral stricture due to injury
EXCLUDES 1   postprocedural urethral stricture (N99.1-)

N35.01 Post-traumatic urethral stricture, male
N35.010 Post-traumatic urethral stricture, male, meatal ♂
N35.011 Post-traumatic bulbous urethral stricture ♂
N35.012 Post-traumatic membranous urethral stricture ♂
N35.013 Post-traumatic anterior urethral stricture ♂
N35.014 Post-traumatic urethral stricture, male, unspecified ♂
N35.016 Post-traumatic urethral stricture, male, overlapping sites ♂

N35.02 Post-traumatic urethral stricture, female
N35.021 Urethral stricture due to childbirth ♀
N35.028 Other post-traumatic urethral stricture, female ♀

N35.1 Postinfective urethral stricture, not elsewhere classified
EXCLUDES 1   urethral stricture associated with schistosomiasis (B65-, N29)
gonococcal urethral stricture (A54.01)
syphilitic urethral stricture (A52.76)

N35.11 Postinfective urethral stricture, not elsewhere classified, male
N35.111 Postinfective urethral stricture, not elsewhere classified, male, meatal ♂
N35.112 Postinfective bulbous urethral stricture, not elsewhere classified, male ♂
N35.113 Postinfective membranous urethral stricture, not elsewhere classified, male ♂
N35.114 Postinfective anterior urethral stricture, not elsewhere classified, male ♂
N35.116 Postinfective urethral stricture, not elsewhere classified, male, overlapping sites ♂
N35.119 Postinfective urethral stricture, not elsewhere classified, male, unspecified ♂

N35.12 Postinfective urethral stricture, not elsewhere classified, female ♀

N35.8 Other urethral stricture
EXCLUDES 1   postprocedural urethral stricture (N99.1-)

N35.81 Other urethral stricture, male
N35.811 Other urethral stricture, male, meatal ♂
N35.812 Other urethral bulbous stricture, male ♂
N35.813 Other membranous urethral stricture, male ♂
N35.814 Other anterior urethral stricture, male, anterior ♂
N35.816 Other urethral stricture, male, overlapping sites ♂
N35.819 Other urethral stricture, male, unspecified site ♂

N35.82 Other urethral stricture, female ♀

N35.9 Urethral stricture, unspecified

N35.91 Urethral stricture, unspecified, male
N35.911 Unspecified urethral stricture, male, meatal ♂
N35.912 Unspecified bulbous urethral stricture, male ♂
N35.913 Unspecified membranous urethral stricture, male ♂
N35.914 Unspecified anterior urethral stricture, male ♂
N35.916 Unspecified urethral stricture, male, overlapping sites ♂
N35.919 Unspecified urethral stricture, male, unspecified site ♂
Pinhole meatus NOS
Urethral stricture NOS

N35.92 Unspecified urethral stricture, female ♀

N36 Other disorders of urethra
N36.0 Urethral fistula   CC
Urethroperineal fistula
Urethrorectal fistula
Urinary fistula NOS
EXCLUDES 1   urethroscrotal fistula (N50.89)
urethrovaginal fistula (N82.1)
urethrovesicovaginal fistula (N82.1)
CC Excl: PDX collection 935

N36.1 Urethral diverticulum

N36.2 Urethral caruncle

N36.4 Urethral functional and muscular disorders
Use additional code to identify associated urinary stress incontinence (N39.3)
N36.41 Hypermobility of urethra
N36.42 Intrinsic sphincter deficiency (ISD)
N36.43 Combined hypermobility of urethra and intrinsic sphincter deficiency
N36.44 Muscular disorders of urethra
Bladder sphincter dyssynergy

N36.5 Urethral false passage

N36.8 Other specified disorders of urethra
EXCLUDES 1   congenital urethrocele (Q64.7)
female urethrocele (N81.0)

N36.9 Urethral disorder, unspecified

N37 Urethral disorders in diseases classified elsewhere
Code first underlying disease
EXCLUDES 1   urethritis (in):
candidal infection (B37.41)
chlamydial (A56.01)
gonorrhea (A54.01)
syphilis (A52.76)
trichomonal infection (A59.03)
tuberculosis (A18.13)

✓4ᵗʰ **N39 Other disorders of urinary system**

    EXCLUDES 2 *hematuria NOS (R31.-)*
            recurrent or persistent hematuria (N02.-)
            recurrent or persistent hematuria with specified morphological
               lesion (N02.-)
            proteinuria NOS (R80.-)

N39.0 Urinary tract infection, site not specified   CC H6
    Use additional code (B95-B97), to identify infectious agent
    EXCLUDES 1 *candidiasis of urinary tract (B37.4-)*
            neonatal urinary tract infection (P39.3)
            urinary tract infection of specified site, such as:
              cystitis (N30.-)
              urethritis (N34.-)
    AHA: 2018, 2Q, 21, 22; 2018, 1Q, 16; 2017, 1Q, 6; 2012, 4Q, 94
    CC Excl: PDX collection 936

N39.3 Stress incontinence (female) (male)
    Code also any associated overactive bladder (N32.81)
    EXCLUDES 1 *mixed incontinence (N39.46)*

✓5ᵗʰ **N39.4 Other specified urinary incontinence**
    Code also any associated overactive bladder (N32.81)
    EXCLUDES 1 *enuresis NOS (R32)*
            functional urinary incontinence (R39.81)
            urinary incontinence associated with cognitive
              impairment (R39.81)
            urinary incontinence NOS (R32)
            urinary incontinence of nonorganic origin (F98.0)

    N39.41 Urge incontinence
        EXCLUDES 1 *mixed incontinence (N39.46)*

    N39.42 Incontinence without sensory awareness
        Insensible (urinary) incontinence

    N39.43 Post-void dribbling

    N39.44 Nocturnal enuresis

    N39.45 Continuous leakage

    N39.46 Mixed incontinence
        Urge and stress incontinence

  ✓6ᵗʰ **N39.49 Other specified urinary incontinence**
        AHA: 2016, 4Q, 44
        N39.490 Overflow incontinence
        N39.491 Coital incontinence
        N39.492 Postural (urinary) incontinence
        N39.498 Other specified urinary incontinence
            Reflex incontinence
            Total incontinence

N39.8 Other specified disorders of urinary system

N39.9 Disorder of urinary system, unspecified

Diseases of male genital organs (N40-N53)

✓4ᵗʰ **N40 Benign prostatic hyperplasia**
    INCLUDES adenofibromatous hypertrophy of prostate
            benign hypertrophy of the prostate
            benign prostatic hypertrophy
            BPH
            enlarged prostate
            nodular prostate
            polyp of prostate
    EXCLUDES 1 *benign neoplasms of prostate (adenoma, benign)*
            (fibroadenoma) (fibroma) (myoma) (D29.1)
    EXCLUDES 2 *malignant neoplasm of prostate (C61)*
    DEF: Enlargement of the prostate gland due to an abnormal proliferation
    of fibrostromal tissue in the paraurethral glands. This condition causes
    impingement of the urethra resulting in obstructed urinary flow.

    N40.0 Benign prostatic hyperplasia without lower   A ♂
        urinary tract symptoms
        Enlarged prostate NOS
        Enlarged prostate without LUTS

N40.1 Benign prostatic hyperplasia with lower urinary tract   A ♂
symptoms
    Enlarged prostate with LUTS
    Use additional code for associated symptoms, when specified:
        incomplete bladder emptying (R39.14)
        nocturia (R35.1)
        straining on urination (R39.16)
        urinary frequency (R35.0)
        urinary hesitancy (R39.11)
        urinary incontinence (N39.4-)
        urinary obstruction (N13.8)
        urinary retention (R33.8)
        urinary urgency (R39.15)
        weak urinary stream (R39.12)

N40.2 Nodular prostate without lower urinary tract symptoms   A ♂
    Nodular prostate without LUTS

N40.3 Nodular prostate with lower urinary tract symptoms   A ♂
    Use additional code for associated symptoms, when specified:
        incomplete bladder emptying (R39.14)
        nocturia (R35.1)
        straining on urination (R39.16)
        urinary frequency (R35.0)
        urinary hesitancy (R39.11)
        urinary incontinence (N39.4-)
        urinary obstruction (N13.8)
        urinary retention (R33.8)
        urinary urgency (R39.15)
        weak urinary stream (R39.12)

✓4ᵗʰ **N41 Inflammatory diseases of prostate**
    Use additional code (B95-B97), to identify infectious agent

    N41.0 Acute prostatitis   CC A ♂
        CC Excl: PDX collection 937

    N41.1 Chronic prostatitis   A ♂

    N41.2 Abscess of prostate   CC A ♂
        CC Excl: PDX collection 937

    N41.3 Prostatocystitis   A ♂

    N41.4 Granulomatous prostatitis   A ♂

    N41.8 Other inflammatory diseases of prostate   A ♂

    N41.9 Inflammatory disease of prostate, unspecified   A ♂
        Prostatitis NOS

✓4ᵗʰ **N42 Other and unspecified disorders of prostate**

    N42.0 Calculus of prostate   A ♂
        Prostatic stone
        DEF: Formation of a small, solid stone often composed of calcium
        carbonate or calcium phosphate in the prostate gland.

    N42.1 Congestion and hemorrhage of prostate   A ♂
        EXCLUDES 1 *enlarged prostate (N40.-)*
            hematuria (R31.-)
            hyperplasia of prostate (N40.-)
            inflammatory diseases of prostate (N41.-)

  ✓5ᵗʰ **N42.3 Dysplasia of prostate**
        AHA: 2016, 4Q, 44
        N42.30 Unspecified dysplasia of prostate   ♂
        N42.31 Prostatic intraepithelial neoplasia   ♂
            PIN
            Prostatic intraepithelial neoplasia I (PIN I)
            Prostatic intraepithelial neoplasia II (PIN II)
            EXCLUDES 1 *prostatic intraepithelial neoplasia III (PIN III)*
               (D07.5)
            DEF: Abnormality of shape and size of the intraepithelial
            tissues of the prostate. It is a premalignant condition
            characterized by stalks and absence of a basilar cell
            layer.
        N42.32 Atypical small acinar proliferation of prostate   ♂
        N42.39 Other dysplasia of prostate   ♂

  ✓5ᵗʰ **N42.8 Other specified disorders of prostate**
        N42.81 Prostatodynia syndrome   A ♂
            Painful prostate syndrome
        N42.82 Prostatosis syndrome   A ♂
        N42.83 Cyst of prostate   A ♂
        N42.89 Other specified disorders of prostate   A ♂
    N42.9 Disorder of prostate, unspecified   A ♂

✓4ᵗʰ **N43 Hydrocele and spermatocele**
    INCLUDES hydrocele of spermatic cord, testis or tunica vaginalis
    EXCLUDES 1 *congenital hydrocele (P83.5)*
    DEF: Hydrocele: Serous fluid that collects in the tunica vaginalis of the
    scrotum along the spermatic cord in males.
    N43.0 Encysted hydrocele   ♂

✔ Additional Character Required   ✓x7ᵗʰ Placeholder   Unacceptable PDx   Questionable PDx   Manifestation   H1-H14 HAC   HCC CMS-HCC Dx   HIV HIV Dx

ICD-10-CM 2019   **835**

Chapter 14. Diseases of Genitourinary System

N43.1   **Infected hydrocele**   CC ♂
Use additional code (B95-B97), to identify infectious agent
CC Excl: PDX collection 938

N43.2   **Other hydrocele**   ♂

N43.3   **Hydrocele, unspecified**   ♂

Hydrocele

Testicle
Scrotum

Normal   Noncommunicating hydrocele   Communicating hydrocele   Hydrocele of the cord

✓5th **N43.4**   **Spermatocele of epididymis**
Spermatic cyst
DEF: Spermatocele: Noncancerous accumulation of fluid and dead sperm cells normally located at the head of the epididymis that exhibits itself as a hard, smooth scrotal mass and do not normally require treatment unless they become enlarged or cause pain.

N43.40   **Spermatocele of epididymis, unspecified**   ♂

N43.41   **Spermatocele of epididymis, single**   ♂

N43.42   **Spermatocele of epididymis, multiple**   ♂

✓4th **N44**   **Noninflammatory disorders of testis**

CC Excl: For CC codes in category N44: PDX collection 939

✓5th **N44.0**   **Torsion of testis**

N44.00   **Torsion of testis, unspecified**   CC ♂

N44.01   **Extravaginal torsion of spermatic cord**   CC ♂
DEF: Torsion of the spermatic cord just below the tunica vaginalis attachments.

N44.02   **Intravaginal torsion of spermatic cord**   CC ♂
Torsion of spermatic cord NOS

N44.03   **Torsion of appendix testis**   CC ♂

N44.04   **Torsion of appendix epididymis**   CC ♂

N44.1   **Cyst of tunica albuginea testis**   ♂

N44.2   **Benign cyst of testis**   ♂

N44.8   **Other noninflammatory disorders of the testis**   ♂

✓4th **N45**   **Orchitis and epididymitis**
Use additional code (B95-B97), to identify infectious agent

N45.1   **Epididymitis**   ♂

N45.2   **Orchitis**   ♂

N45.3   **Epididymo-orchitis**   ♂

N45.4   **Abscess of epididymis or testis**   CC ♂
CC Excl: PDX collection 940

✓4th **N46**   **Male infertility**
EXCLUDES 1   vasectomy status (Z98.52)

✓5th **N46.0**   **Azoospermia**
Absolute male infertility
Male infertility due to germinal (cell) aplasia
Male infertility due to spermatogenic arrest (complete)

N46.01   **Organic azoospermia**   A ♂
Azoospermia NOS

✓6th **N46.02**   **Azoospermia due to extratesticular causes**
Code also associated cause

N46.021   **Azoospermia due to drug therapy**   A ♂

N46.022   **Azoospermia due to infection**   A ♂

N46.023   **Azoospermia due to obstruction of efferent ducts**   A ♂

N46.024   **Azoospermia due to radiation**   A ♂

N46.025   **Azoospermia due to systemic disease**   A ♂

N46.029   **Azoospermia due to other extratesticular causes**   A ♂

✓5th **N46.1**   **Oligospermia**
Male infertility due to germinal cell desquamation
Male infertility due to hypospermatogenesis
Male infertility due to incomplete spermatogenic arrest

N46.11   **Organic oligospermia**   A ♂
Oligospermia NOS

✓6th **N46.12**   **Oligospermia due to extratesticular causes**
Code also associated cause

N46.121   **Oligospermia due to drug therapy**   A ♂

N46.122   **Oligospermia due to infection**   A ♂

N46.123   **Oligospermia due to obstruction of efferent ducts**   A ♂

N46.124   **Oligospermia due to radiation**   A ♂

N46.125   **Oligospermia due to systemic disease**   A ♂

N46.129   **Oligospermia due to other extratesticular causes**   A ♂

N46.8   **Other male infertility**   A ♂

N46.9   **Male infertility, unspecified**   A ♂

✓4th **N47**   **Disorders of prepuce**

N47.0   **Adherent prepuce, newborn**   N ♂

N47.1   **Phimosis**   ♂
DEF: Condition in which the foreskin is contracted and cannot be drawn back behind the glans penis.

N47.2   **Paraphimosis**   ♂

N47.3   **Deficient foreskin**   ♂

N47.4   **Benign cyst of prepuce**   ♂

N47.5   **Adhesions of prepuce and glans penis**   ♂

N47.6   **Balanoposthitis**   ♂
Use additional code (B95-B97), to identify infectious agent
EXCLUDES 1   balanitis (N48.1)

N47.7   **Other inflammatory diseases of prepuce**   ♂
Use additional code (B95-B97), to identify infectious agent

N47.8   **Other disorders of prepuce**   ♂

✓4th **N48**   **Other disorders of penis**

N48.0   **Leukoplakia of penis**   ♂
Balanitis xerotica obliterans
Kraurosis of penis
Lichen sclerosus of external male genital organs
EXCLUDES 1   carcinoma in situ of penis (D07.4)

N48.1   **Balanitis**   ♂
Use additional code (B95-B97), to identify infectious agent
EXCLUDES 1   amebic balanitis (A06.8)
     balanitis xerotica obliterans (N48.0)
     candidal balanitis (B37.42)
     gonococcal balanitis (A54.23)
     herpesviral [herpes simplex] balanitis (A60.01)
DEF: Inflammation of the glans penis, most often affecting uncircumcised males.

✓5th **N48.2**   **Other inflammatory disorders of penis**
Use additional code (B95-B97), to identify infectious agent
EXCLUDES 1   balanitis (N48.1)
     balanitis xerotica obliterans (N48.0)
     balanoposthitis (N47.6)

N48.21   **Abscess of corpus cavernosum and penis**   ♂

N48.22   **Cellulitis of corpus cavernosum and penis**   ♂

N48.29   **Other inflammatory disorders of penis**   ♂

✓5th **N48.3**   **Priapism**
Painful erection
Code first underlying cause

CC Excl: For CC codes in subcategory N48.3: PDX collection 941

N48.30   **Priapism, unspecified**   CC ♂

N48.31   **Priapism due to trauma**   CC ♂

N48.32   *Priapism due to disease classified elsewhere*   CC ♂

N48.33   **Priapism, drug-induced**   CC ♂

N48.39   **Other priapism**   CC ♂

N48.5   **Ulcer of penis**   ♂

N48.6   **Induration penis plastica**   ♂
Peyronie's disease
Plastic induration of penis

✓5th **N48.8**   **Other specified disorders of penis**

N48.81   **Thrombosis of superficial vein of penis**   ♂

N Newborn: 0   P Pediatric: 0-17   M Maternity: 12-55   A Adult: 15-124   MCC Major Complication/Comorbidity   CC Complication/Comorbidity   SW Severe Wound Dx

836   ICD-10-CM 2019

N43.1–N48.81

N48.82   **Acquired torsion of penis**   ♂
Acquired torsion of penis NOS
EXCLUDES 1   *congenital torsion of penis (Q55.63)*

N48.83   **Acquired buried penis**   ♂
EXCLUDES 1   *congenital hidden penis (Q55.64)*

N48.89   **Other specified disorders of penis**   ♂

N48.9   **Disorder of penis, unspecified**   ♂

✓4ᵗʰ **N49**   **Inflammatory disorders of male genital organs, not elsewhere classified**
Use additional code (B95-B97), to identify infectious agent
EXCLUDES 1   *inflammation of penis (N48.1, N48.2-)*
orchitis and epididymitis (N45.-)

N49.0   **Inflammatory disorders of** seminal vesicle   ♂
Vesiculitis NOS

N49.1   **Inflammatory disorders of** spermatic cord, tunica vaginalis and vas deferens   ♂
Vasitis

N49.2   **Inflammatory disorders of** scrotum   ♂

N49.3   **Fournier gangrene**   ♂

N49.8   **Inflammatory disorders of** other specified male genital organs   ♂
Inflammation of multiple sites in male genital organs

N49.9   **Inflammatory disorder of** unspecified male genital organ   ♂
Abscess of unspecified male genital organ
Boil of unspecified male genital organ
Carbuncle of unspecified male genital organ
Cellulitis of unspecified male genital organ

✓4ᵗʰ **N50**   **Other and unspecified disorders of male genital organs**
EXCLUDES 2   *torsion of testis (N44.0-)*

N50.0   **Atrophy of testis**   ♂

N50.1   **Vascular disorders of male genital organs**   ♂
Hematocele, NOS, of male genital organs
Hemorrhage of male genital organs
Thrombosis of male genital organs

N50.3   **Cyst of epididymis**   ♂

✓5ᵗʰ **N50.8**   **Other specified disorders of male genital organs**
AHA: 2016, 4Q, 45

✓6ᵗʰ **N50.81**   Testicular pain
N50.811   Right testicular pain   ♂
N50.812   Left testicular pain   ♂
N50.819   Testicular pain, unspecified   ♂

N50.82   Scrotal pain   ♂

N50.89   Other specified disorders of the male genital organs   ♂
Atrophy of scrotum, seminal vesicle, spermatic cord, tunica vaginalis and vas deferens
Chylocele, tunica vaginalis (nonfilarial) NOS
Edema of scrotum, seminal vesicle, spermatic cord, tunica vaginalis and vas deferens
Hypertrophy of scrotum, seminal vesicle, spermatic cord, tunica vaginalis and vas deferens
Stricture of spermatic cord, tunica vaginalis, and vas deferens
Ulcer of scrotum, seminal vesicle, spermatic cord, testis, tunica vaginalis and vas deferens
Urethroscrotal fistula

N50.9   **Disorder of male genital organs, unspecified**   ♂

N51   *Disorders of male genital organs in diseases classified elsewhere*   ♂
Code first underlying disease, such as:
filariasis (B74.0-B74.9)
EXCLUDES 1   *amebic balanitis (A06.8)*
candidal balanitis (B37.42)
gonococcal balanitis (A54.23)
gonococcal prostatitis (A54.22)
herpesviral [herpes simplex] balanitis (A60.01)
trichomonal prostatitis (A59.02)
tuberculous prostatitis (A18.14)

✓4ᵗʰ **N52**   **Male erectile dysfunction**
EXCLUDES 1   *psychogenic impotence (F52.21)*

✓5ᵗʰ **N52.0**   **Vasculogenic erectile dysfunction**
N52.01   Erectile dysfunction due to arterial insufficiency   🅐 ♂
N52.02   Corporo-venous occlusive erectile dysfunction   🅐 ♂
N52.03   Combined arterial insufficiency and corporo-venous occlusive erectile dysfunction   🅐 ♂

N52.1   *Erectile dysfunction due to diseases classified elsewhere*   🅐 ♂
Code first underlying disease

N52.2   **Drug-induced erectile dysfunction**   🅐 ♂

✓5ᵗʰ **N52.3**   **Postprocedural erectile dysfunction**
AHA: 2016, 4Q, 45

N52.31   **Erectile dysfunction following** radical prostatectomy   🅐 ♂

N52.32   **Erectile dysfunction following** radical cystectomy   🅐 ♂

N52.33   **Erectile dysfunction following** urethral surgery   🅐 ♂

N52.34   **Erectile dysfunction following** simple prostatectomy   🅐 ♂

N52.35   **Erectile dysfunction following** radiation therapy   🅐 ♂

N52.36   **Erectile dysfunction following** interstitial seed therapy   🅐 ♂

N52.37   **Erectile dysfunction following** prostate ablative therapy   🅐 ♂
Erectile dysfunction following cryotherapy
Erectile dysfunction following other prostate ablative therapies
Erectile dysfunction following ultrasound ablative therapies

N52.39   Other and unspecified postprocedural erectile dysfunction   🅐 ♂

N52.8   Other male erectile dysfunction   🅐 ♂

N52.9   Male erectile dysfunction, unspecified   🅐 ♂
Impotence NOS

✓4ᵗʰ **N53**   **Other male sexual dysfunction**
EXCLUDES 1   *psychogenic sexual dysfunction (F52.-)*

✓5ᵗʰ **N53.1**   **Ejaculatory dysfunction**
EXCLUDES 1   *premature ejaculation (F52.4)*

N53.11   Retarded ejaculation   ♂
N53.12   Painful ejaculation   ♂
N53.13   Anejaculatory orgasm   ♂
N53.14   Retrograde ejaculation   ♂
DEF: Form of male sexual dysfunction in which the semen enters the bladder instead of going out through the urethra during ejaculation.

N53.19   Other ejaculatory dysfunction   ♂
Ejaculatory dysfunction NOS

N53.8   Other male sexual dysfunction   ♂

N53.9   Unspecified male sexual dysfunction   ♂

Disorders of breast (N60-N65)
EXCLUDES 1   *disorders of breast associated with childbirth (O91-O92)*

✓4ᵗʰ **N60**   **Benign mammary dysplasia**
INCLUDES   fibrocystic mastopathy

✓5ᵗʰ **N60.0**   **Solitary cyst of breast**
Cyst of breast
N60.01   Solitary cyst of right breast
N60.02   Solitary cyst of left breast
N60.09   Solitary cyst of unspecified breast

✓5ᵗʰ **N60.1**   **Diffuse cystic mastopathy**
Cystic breast
Fibrocystic disease of breast
EXCLUDES 1   *diffuse cystic mastopathy with epithelial proliferation (N60.3-)*

N60.11   Diffuse cystic mastopathy of right breast   🅐
N60.12   Diffuse cystic mastopathy of left breast   🅐
N60.19   Diffuse cystic mastopathy of unspecified breast   🅐

✓5ᵗʰ **N60.2**   **Fibroadenosis of breast**
Adenofibrosis of breast
EXCLUDES 2   *fibroadenoma of breast (D24.-)*

N60.21   Fibroadenosis of right breast
N60.22   Fibroadenosis of left breast
N60.29   Fibroadenosis of unspecified breast

✓5ᵗʰ **N60.3**   **Fibrosclerosis of breast**
Cystic mastopathy with epithelial proliferation
N60.31   Fibrosclerosis of right breast
N60.32   Fibrosclerosis of left breast
N60.39   Fibrosclerosis of unspecified breast

✓5ᵗʰ **N60.4**   **Mammary duct ectasia**
N60.41   Mammary duct ectasia of right breast

✓ Additional Character Required   ✓x7ᵗʰ Placeholder   Unacceptable PDx   Questionable PDx   Manifestation   H1 -H14 HAC   HCC CMS-HCC Dx   HIV HIV Dx

ICD-10-CM 2019   837

Chapter 14. Diseases of Genitourinary System

N60.42   Mammary duct ectasia of left breast

N60.49   Mammary duct ectasia of unspecified breast

☑5ᵗʰ **N60.8   Other benign mammary dysplasias**

N60.81   Other benign mammary dysplasias of right breast

N60.82   Other benign mammary dysplasias of left breast

N60.89   Other benign mammary dysplasias of unspecified breast

☑5ᵗʰ **N60.9   Unspecified benign mammary dysplasia**

N60.91   Unspecified benign mammary dysplasia of right breast

N60.92   Unspecified benign mammary dysplasia of left breast

N60.99   Unspecified benign mammary dysplasia of unspecified breast

☑4ᵗʰ **N61   Inflammatory disorders of breast**

EXCLUDES 1   inflammatory carcinoma of breast (C50.9)
inflammatory disorder of breast associated with childbirth (O91.-)
neonatal infective mastitis (P39.0)
thrombophlebitis of breast [Mondor's disease] (I80.8)

N61.0   Mastitis without abscess

Infective mastitis (acute) (nonpuerperal) (subacute)
Mastitis (acute) (nonpuerperal) (subacute) NOS
Cellulitis (acute) (nonpuerperal) (subacute) of breast NOS
Cellulitis (acute) (nonpuerperal) (subacute) of nipple NOS

N61.1   Abscess of the breast and nipple

Abscess (acute) (chronic) (nonpuerperal) of areola
Abscess (acute) (chronic) (nonpuerperal) of breast
Carbuncle of breast
Mastitis with abscess

N62   Hypertrophy of breast

Gynecomastia
Hypertrophy of breast NOS
Massive pubertal hypertrophy of breast

EXCLUDES 1   breast engorgement of newborn (P83.4)
disproportion of reconstructed breast (N65.1)

☑4ᵗʰ **N63   Unspecified lump in breast**

Nodule(s) NOS in breast

AHA: 2017, 4Q, 19

▲   **N63.0   Unspecified lump in unspecified breast**

☑5ᵗʰ **N63.1   Unspecified lump in the right breast**

N63.10   Unspecified lump in the right breast, unspecified quadrant

N63.11   Unspecified lump in the right breast, upper outer quadrant

N63.12   Unspecified lump in the right breast, upper inner quadrant

N63.13   Unspecified lump in the right breast, lower outer quadrant

N63.14   Unspecified lump in the right breast, lower inner quadrant

☑5ᵗʰ **N63.2   Unspecified lump in the left breast**

N63.20   Unspecified lump in the left breast, unspecified quadrant

N63.21   Unspecified lump in the left breast, upper outer quadrant

N63.22   Unspecified lump in the left breast, upper inner quadrant

N63.23   Unspecified lump in the left breast, lower outer quadrant

N63.24   Unspecified lump in the left breast, lower inner quadrant

☑5ᵗʰ **N63.3   Unspecified lump in axillary tail**

N63.31   Unspecified lump in axillary tail of the right breast

N63.32   Unspecified lump in axillary tail of the left breast

☑5ᵗʰ **N63.4   Unspecified lump in breast, subareolar**

N63.41   Unspecified lump in right breast, subareolar

N63.42   Unspecified lump in left breast, subareolar

☑4ᵗʰ **N64   Other disorders of breast**

EXCLUDES 2   mechanical complication of breast prosthesis and implant (T85.4-)

N64.0   Fissure and fistula of nipple

N64.1   Fat necrosis of breast

Fat necrosis (segmental) of breast
Code first breast necrosis due to breast graft (T85.898)

N64.2   Atrophy of breast

N64.3   Galactorrhea not associated with childbirth

N64.4   Mastodynia

☑5ᵗʰ **N64.5   Other signs and symptoms in breast**

EXCLUDES 2   abnormal findings on diagnostic imaging of breast (R92.-)

N64.51   Induration of breast

N64.52   Nipple discharge

EXCLUDES 1   abnormal findings in nipple discharge (R89.-)

N64.53   Retraction of nipple

N64.59   Other signs and symptoms in breast

☑5ᵗʰ **N64.8   Other specified disorders of breast**

N64.81   Ptosis of breast   **A**

EXCLUDES 1   ptosis of native breast in relation to reconstructed breast (N65.1)

N64.82   Hypoplasia of breast   **A**

Micromastia

EXCLUDES 1   congenital absence of breast (Q83.0)
hypoplasia of native breast in relation to reconstructed breast (N65.1)

N64.89   Other specified disorders of breast

Galactocele
Subinvolution of breast (postlactational)

AHA: 2018, 1Q, 3

N64.9   Disorder of breast, unspecified

☑4ᵗʰ **N65   Deformity and disproportion of reconstructed breast**

N65.0   Deformity of reconstructed breast   **A**

Contour irregularity in reconstructed breast
Excess tissue in reconstructed breast
Misshapen reconstructed breast

N65.1   Disproportion of reconstructed breast   **A**

Breast asymmetry between native breast and reconstructed breast
Disproportion between native breast and reconstructed breast

Inflammatory diseases of female pelvic organs (N70-N77)

EXCLUDES 1   inflammatory diseases of female pelvic organs complicating:
abortion or ectopic or molar pregnancy (O00-O07, O08.0)
pregnancy, childbirth and the puerperium (O23-, O75.3, O85, O86-)

☑4ᵗʰ **N70   Salpingitis and oophoritis**

INCLUDES   abscess (of) fallopian tube
abscess (of) ovary
pyosalpinx
salpingo-oophoritis
tubo-ovarian abscess
tubo-ovarian inflammatory disease

Use additional code (B95-B97), to identify infectious agent

EXCLUDES 1   gonococcal infection (A54.24)
tuberculous infection (A18.17)

CC Excl: For CC codes in category N70: PDX collection 942

☑5ᵗʰ **N70.0   Acute salpingitis and oophoritis**

N70.01   Acute salpingitis   **CC ♀**

N70.02   Acute oophoritis   **CC ♀**

N70.03   Acute salpingitis and oophoritis   **CC ♀**

☑5ᵗʰ **N70.1   Chronic salpingitis and oophoritis**

Hydrosalpinx

N70.11   Chronic salpingitis   **♀**

N70.12   Chronic oophoritis   **♀**

N70.13   Chronic salpingitis and oophoritis   **♀**

☑5ᵗʰ **N70.9   Salpingitis and oophoritis, unspecified**

N70.91   Salpingitis, unspecified   **♀**

N70.92   Oophoritis, unspecified   **♀**

N70.93   Salpingitis and oophoritis, unspecified   **♀**

☑4ᵗʰ **N71   Inflammatory disease of uterus, except cervix**

INCLUDES   endo (myo) metritis
metritis
myometritis
pyometra
uterine abscess

Use additional code (B95-B97), to identify infectious agent

EXCLUDES 1   hyperplastic endometritis (N85.0-)
infection of uterus following delivery (O85, O86.-)

N71.0   Acute inflammatory disease of uterus   **CC ♀**

CC Excl: PDX collection 943

N71.1   Chronic inflammatory disease of uterus   **♀**

N Newborn: 0   **P** Pediatric: 0-17   **M** Maternity: 12-55   **A** Adult: 15-124   **MCC** Major Complication/Comorbidity   **CC** Complication/Comorbidity   **SW** Severe Wound Dx

838   ICD-10-CM 2019

N71.9   Inflammatory disease of uterus, unspecified   ♀

N72   **Inflammatory disease of cervix uteri**   ♀
     INCLUDES   cervicitis (with or without erosion or ectropion)
             endocervicitis (with or without erosion or ectropion)
             exocervicitis (with or without erosion or ectropion)
     Use additional code (B95-B97), to identify infectious agent
     EXCLUDES 1   *erosion and ectropion of cervix without cervicitis (N86)*

✓4ᵗʰ **N73**   **Other female pelvic inflammatory diseases**
     Use additional code (B95-B97), to identify infectious agent

     CC Excl: For CC/MCC codes in category N73: PDX collection 942

     N73.0   Acute **parametritis and pelvic cellulitis**   CC
         Abscess of broad ligament
         Abscess of parametrium
         Pelvic cellulitis, female
         DEF: Parametritis: Inflammation of the parametrium.
     N73.1   Chronic **parametritis and pelvic cellulitis**   ♀
         Any condition in N73.0 specified as chronic
         EXCLUDES 1   *tuberculous parametritis and pelvic cellutis (A18.17)*
     N73.2   Unspecified **parametritis and pelvic cellulitis**   ♀
         Any condition in N73.0 unspecified whether acute or chronic
     N73.3   Female acute **pelvic peritonitis**   MCC ♀
     N73.4   Female chronic **pelvic peritonitis**   CC ♀
         EXCLUDES 1   *tuberculous pelvic (female) peritonitis (A18.17)*
     N73.5   Female pelvic peritonitis, unspecified   ♀
     N73.6   Female pelvic peritoneal adhesions (postinfective)   ♀
         EXCLUDES 2   *postprocedural pelvic peritoneal adhesions (N99.4)*
         AHA: 2014, 1Q, 6
     N73.8   Other specified female pelvic inflammatory diseases   ♀
     N73.9   Female pelvic inflammatory disease, unspecified   ♀
         Female pelvic infection or inflammation NOS

N74   *Female pelvic inflammatory disorders in diseases classified elsewhere*   ♀
     Code first underlying disease
     EXCLUDES 1   *chlamydial cervicitis (A56.02)*
               chlamydial pelvic inflammatory disease (A56.11)
               gonococcal cervicitis (A54.03)
               gonococcal pelvic inflammatory disease (A54.24)
               herpesviral [herpes simplex] cervicitis (A60.03)
               herpesviral [herpes simplex] pelvic inflammatory disease (A60.09)
               syphilitic cervicitis (A52.76)
               syphilitic pelvic inflammatory disease (A52.76)
               trichomonal cervicitis (A59.09)
               tuberculous cervicitis (A18.16)
               tuberculous pelvic inflammatory disease (A18.17)

✓4ᵗʰ **N75**   **Diseases of Bartholin's gland**
     DEF: Bartholin's gland: Mucous-producing gland found in the vestibular bulbs on either side of the vaginal orifice and connected to the mucosal membrane at the opening by a duct.
     N75.0   Cyst of Bartholin's gland   ♀
     N75.1   Abscess of Bartholin's gland   CC ♀
         CC Excl: PDX collection 944
     N75.8   Other diseases of Bartholin's gland   ♀
         Bartholinitis
     N75.9   Disease of Bartholin's gland, unspecified   ♀

✓4ᵗʰ **N76**   **Other inflammation of vagina and vulva**
     Use additional code (B95-B97), to identify infectious agent
     EXCLUDES 2   *senile (atrophic) vaginitis (N95.2)*
               vulvar vestibulitis (N94.810)
     N76.0   Acute vaginitis   ♀
         Acute vulvovaginitis   Vulvovaginitis NOS
         Vaginitis NOS
     N76.1   Subacute and chronic vaginitis   ♀
         Chronic vulvovaginitis
         Subacute vulvovaginitis
     N76.2   Acute vulvitis   ♀
         Vulvitis NOS
     N76.3   Subacute and chronic vulvitis   ♀
     N76.4   Abscess of vulva   CC ♀
         Furuncle of vulva
         CC Excl: PDX collection 944
     N76.5   Ulceration of vagina   ♀
     N76.6   Ulceration of vulva   ♀

✓5ᵗʰ **N76.8**   **Other specified inflammation of vagina and vulva**
     N76.81   Mucositis (ulcerative) of vagina and vulva   CC ♀
         Code also type of associated therapy, such as:
             antineoplastic and immunosuppressive drugs (T45.1X-)
             radiological procedure and radiotherapy (Y84.2)
         EXCLUDES 2   *gastrointestinal mucositis (ulcerative) (K92.81)*
                 nasal mucositis (ulcerative) (J34.81)
                 oral mucositis (ulcerative) (K12.3-)
         CC Excl: PDX collection 945
     N76.89   Other specified inflammation of vagina and vulva   ♀

✓4ᵗʰ **N77**   **Vulvovaginal ulceration and inflammation in diseases classified elsewhere**
     N77.0   *Ulceration of vulva in diseases classified elsewhere*   ♀
         Code first underlying disease, such as:
             Behçet's disease (M35.2)
         EXCLUDES 1   *ulceration of vulva in gonococcal infection (A54.02)*
                 ulceration of vulva in herpesviral [herpes simplex] infection (A60.04)
                 ulceration of vulva in syphilis (A51.0)
                 ulceration of vulva in tuberculosis (A18.18)
     N77.1   *Vaginitis, vulvitis and vulvovaginitis in diseases classified elsewhere*   ♀
         Code first underlying disease, such as:
             pinworm (B80)
         EXCLUDES 1   *candidal vulvovaginitis (B37.3)*
                 chlamydial vulvovaginitis (A56.02)
                 gonococcal vulvovaginitis (A54.02)
                 herpesviral [herpes simplex] vulvovaginitis (A60.04)
                 trichomonal vulvovaginitis (A59.01)
                 tuberculous vulvovaginitis (A18.18)
                 vulvovaginitis in early syphilis (A51.0)
                 vulvovaginitis in late syphilis (A52.76)

Noninflammatory disorders of female genital tract (N80-N98)

✓4ᵗʰ **N80**   **Endometriosis**
     DEF: Aberrant uterine mucosal tissue appearing in areas of the pelvic cavity outside of its normal location, lining the uterus, and inflaming surrounding tissues often resulting in infertility or spontaneous abortion.
     N80.0   Endometriosis of uterus   ♀
         Adenomyosis
         EXCLUDES 1   *stromal endometriosis (D39.0)*
     N80.1   Endometriosis of ovary   ♀
     N80.2   Endometriosis of fallopian tube   ♀
     N80.3   Endometriosis of pelvic peritoneum   ♀
     N80.4   Endometriosis of rectovaginal septum and vagina   ♀
     N80.5   Endometriosis of intestine   ♀
     N80.6   Endometriosis in cutaneous scar   ♀
     N80.8   Other endometriosis   ♀
         Endometriosis of thorax
     N80.9   Endometriosis, unspecified   ♀

✓4ᵗʰ **N81**   **Female genital prolapse**
     EXCLUDES 1   *genital prolapse complicating pregnancy, labor or delivery (O34.5-)*
               prolapse and hernia of ovary and fallopian tube (N83.4-)
               prolapse of vaginal vault after hysterectomy (N99.3)
     N81.0   Urethrocele   ♀
         EXCLUDES 1   *urethrocele with cystocele (N81.1-)*
                 urethrocele with prolapse of uterus (N81.2-N81.4)
     ✓5ᵗʰ **N81.1**   Cystocele
         Cystocele with urethrocele
         Cystourethrocele
         EXCLUDES 1   *cystocele with prolapse of uterus (N81.2-N81.4)*
         N81.10   Cystocele, unspecified   ♀
             Prolapse of (anterior) vaginal wall NOS
         N81.11   Cystocele, midline   ♀
         N81.12   Cystocele, lateral   ♀
             Paravaginal cystocele
             DEF: Detachment of the lateral support connections of the vagina at the arcus tendineus fasciae pelvis (ATFP) that results in bladder drop. The bladder herniates into the vagina laterally.
     N81.2   Incomplete uterovaginal prolapse   ♀
         First degree uterine prolapse
         Prolapse of cervix NOS
         Second degree uterine prolapse
         EXCLUDES 1   *cervical stump prolapse (N81.85)*

✔ Additional Character Required   ✓x7ᵗʰ Placeholder   Unacceptable PDx   Questionable PDx   Manifestation   H1-H14 HAC   HCC CMS-HCC Dx   HIV HIV Dx

ICD-10-CM 2019   839

N81.3 **Complete** uterovaginal prolapse ♀
Procidentia (uteri) NOS
Third degree uterine prolapse

N81.4 **Uterovaginal prolapse,** unspecified ♀
Prolapse of uterus NOS

N81.5 **Vaginal enterocele** ♀
EXCLUDES 1 *enterocele with prolapse of uterus (N81.2-N81.4)*

Types of Pelvic Organ Prolapse

N81.6 **Rectocele** ♀
Prolapse of posterior vaginal wall
Use additional code for any associated fecal incontinence, if applicable (R15.-)
EXCLUDES 2 *perineocele (N81.81)*
rectal prolapse (K62.3)
rectocele with prolapse of uterus (N81.2-N81.4)

✓5ᵗʰ **N81.8** **Other female genital prolapse**

N81.81 **Perineocele** ♀

N81.82 **Incompetence or weakening of** pubocervical tissue ♀

N81.83 **Incompetence or weakening of** rectovaginal tissue ♀

N81.84 **Pelvic muscle wasting** ♀
Disuse atrophy of pelvic muscles and anal sphincter

N81.85 **Cervical stump prolapse** ♀

N81.89 **Other female genital prolapse** ♀
Deficient perineum
Old laceration of muscles of pelvic floor

N81.9 **Female genital prolapse, unspecified** ♀

✓4ᵗʰ **N82** **Fistulae involving female genital tract**
EXCLUDES 1 *vesicointestinal fistulae (N32.1)*

CC Excl: For CC codes in category N82: PDX collection 946

N82.0 **Vesicovaginal** fistula CC SW ♀

N82.1 **Other female** urinary-genital tract **fistulae** CC ♀
Cervicovesical fistula   Uteroureteric fistula
Ureterovaginal fistula   Uterovesical fistula
Urethrovaginal fistula
AHA: 2017, 3Q, 3

N82.2 **Fistula of vagina to** small intestine CC SW ♀

N82.3 **Fistula of vagina to** large intestine CC SW ♀
Rectovaginal fistula

N82.4 **Other female** intestinal-genital tract **fistulae** CC SW ♀
Intestinouterine fistula

N82.5 **Female** genital tract-skin **fistulae** CC SW ♀
Uterus to abdominal wall fistula
Vaginoperineal fistula

N82.8 **Other** female genital tract **fistulae** CC ♀

N82.9 **Female genital tract fistula,** unspecified CC ♀

✓4ᵗʰ **N83** **Noninflammatory disorders of ovary, fallopian tube and broad ligament**
EXCLUDES 2 *hydrosalpinx (N70.1-)*
AHA: 2016, 4Q, 46

✓5ᵗʰ **N83.0** **Follicular cyst of ovary**
Cyst of graafian follicle
Hemorrhagic follicular cyst (of ovary)

N83.00 **Follicular cyst of ovary,** unspecified **side** ♀

N83.01 **Follicular cyst of** right **ovary** ♀

N83.02 **Follicular cyst of** left **ovary** ♀

✓5ᵗʰ **N83.1** **Corpus luteum cyst**
Hemorrhagic corpus luteum cyst

N83.10 **Corpus luteum cyst of ovary,** unspecified **side** ♀

N83.11 **Corpus luteum cyst of** right **ovary** ♀

N83.12 **Corpus luteum cyst of** left **ovary** ♀

✓5ᵗʰ **N83.2** **Other and unspecified ovarian cysts**
EXCLUDES 1 *developmental ovarian cyst (Q50.1)*
neoplastic ovarian cyst (D27.-)
polycystic ovarian syndrome (E28.2)
Stein-Leventhal syndrome (E28.2)

✓6ᵗʰ **N83.20** **Unspecified ovarian cysts**

N83.201 **Unspecified ovarian cyst,** right **side** ♀

N83.202 **Unspecified ovarian cyst,** left **side** ♀

N83.209 **Unspecified ovarian cyst,** unspecified **side** ♀
Ovarian cyst, NOS

✓6ᵗʰ **N83.29** **Other ovarian cysts**
Retention cyst of ovary
Simple cyst of ovary

N83.291 **Other ovarian cyst,** right **side** ♀

N83.292 **Other ovarian cyst,** left **side** ♀

N83.299 **Other ovarian cyst,** unspecified **side** ♀

✓5ᵗʰ **N83.3** **Acquired atrophy of ovary and fallopian tube**

✓6ᵗʰ **N83.31** **Acquired atrophy of** ovary

N83.311 **Acquired atrophy of** right **ovary** ♀

N83.312 **Acquired atrophy of** left **ovary** ♀

N83.319 **Acquired atrophy of ovary,** unspecified **side** ♀
Acquired atrophy of ovary, NOS

✓6ᵗʰ **N83.32** **Acquired atrophy of** fallopian tube

N83.321 **Acquired atrophy of** right **fallopian tube** ♀

N83.322 **Acquired atrophy of** left **fallopian tube** ♀

N83.329 **Acquired atrophy of fallopian tube,** unspecified **side** ♀
Acquired atrophy of fallopian tube, NOS

✓6ᵗʰ **N83.33** **Acquired atrophy of** ovary and fallopian tube

N83.331 **Acquired atrophy of** right **ovary and fallopian tube** ♀

N83.332 **Acquired atrophy of** left **ovary and fallopian tube** ♀

N83.339 **Acquired atrophy of ovary and fallopian tube,** unspecified **side** ♀
Acquired atrophy of ovary and fallopian tube, NOS

✓5ᵗʰ **N83.4** **Prolapse and hernia of ovary and fallopian tube**

N83.40 **Prolapse and hernia of ovary and fallopian tube,** unspecified **side** ♀
Prolapse and hernia of ovary and fallopian tube, NOS

N83.41 **Prolapse and hernia of** right **ovary and fallopian tube** ♀

N83.42 **Prolapse and hernia of** left **ovary and fallopian tube** ♀

✓5ᵗʰ **N83.5** **Torsion of ovary, ovarian pedicle and fallopian tube**
Torsion of accessory tube

CC Excl: For CC codes in subcategory N83.5: PDX collection 947

✓6ᵗʰ **N83.51** **Torsion of** ovary and ovarian pedicle

N83.511 **Torsion of** right **ovary and ovarian pedicle** CC ♀

N83.512 **Torsion of** left **ovary and ovarian pedicle** CC ♀

N83.519 **Torsion of ovary and ovarian pedicle,** unspecified **side** CC ♀
Torsion of ovary and ovarian pedicle, NOS

✓6ᵗʰ N83.52 Torsion of fallopian tube
Torsion of hydatid of Morgagni

     N83.521 Torsion of right fallopian tube `CC`♀

     N83.522 Torsion of left fallopian tube `CC`♀

     N83.529 Torsion of fallopian tube, unspecified side `CC`♀
        Torsion of fallopian tube, NOS

N83.53 Torsion of ovary, ovarian pedicle and fallopian tube `CC`♀

N83.6 Hematosalpinx ♀
   EXCLUDES 1   *hematosalpinx (with) (in):*
      hematocolpos (N89.7)
      hematometra (N85.7)
      tubal pregnancy (O00.1-)

N83.7 Hematoma of broad ligament ♀

N83.8 Other noninflammatory disorders of ovary, fallopian tube and broad ligament ♀
   Broad ligament laceration syndrome [Allen-Masters]

N83.9 Noninflammatory disorder of ovary, fallopian tube and broad ligament, unspecified ♀

✓4ᵗʰ N84 Polyp of female genital tract
   EXCLUDES 1   *adenomatous polyp (D28.-)*
      placental polyp (O90.89)

N84.0 Polyp of corpus uteri ♀
   Polyp of endometrium   Polyp of uterus NOS
   EXCLUDES 1   *polypoid endometrial hyperplasia (N85.0-)*

N84.1 Polyp of cervix uteri ♀
   Mucous polyp of cervix

N84.2 Polyp of vagina ♀

N84.3 Polyp of vulva ♀
   Polyp of labia

N84.8 Polyp of other parts of female genital tract ♀

N84.9 Polyp of female genital tract, unspecified ♀

✓4ᵗʰ N85 Other noninflammatory disorders of uterus, except cervix
   EXCLUDES 1   *endometriosis (N80.-)*
      inflammatory diseases of uterus (N71.-)
      noninflammatory disorders of cervix, except malposition (N86-N88)
      polyp of corpus uteri (N84.0)
      uterine prolapse (N81.-)

✓5ᵗʰ N85.0 Endometrial hyperplasia

     N85.00 Endometrial hyperplasia, unspecified ♀
       Hyperplasia (adenomatous) (cystic) (glandular) of endometrium
       Hyperplastic endometritis

     N85.01 Benign endometrial hyperplasia ♀
       Endometrial hyperplasia (complex) (simple) without atypia

     N85.02 Endometrial intraepithelial neoplasia [EIN] ♀
       Endometrial hyperplasia with atypia
       EXCLUDES 1   *malignant neoplasm of endometrium (with endometrial intraepithelial neoplasia [EIN]) (C54.1)*

N85.2 Hypertrophy of uterus ♀
   Bulky or enlarged uterus
   EXCLUDES 1   *puerperal hypertrophy of uterus (O90.89)*

N85.3 Subinvolution of uterus ♀
   EXCLUDES 1   *puerperal subinvolution of uterus (O90.89)*

N85.4 Malposition of uterus ♀
   Anteversion of uterus
   Retroflexion of uterus
   Retroversion of uterus
   EXCLUDES 1   *malposition of uterus complicating pregnancy, labor or delivery (O34.5-, O65.5)*

N85.5 Inversion of uterus ♀
   EXCLUDES 1   *current obstetric trauma (O71.2)*
      postpartum inversion of uterus (O71.2)
   DEF: Abnormality in which the uterus turns inside out.

Inversion of Uterus

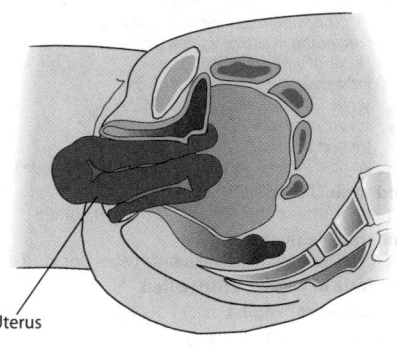

Uterus

N85.6 Intrauterine synechiae ♀

N85.7 Hematometra ♀
   Hematosalpinx with hematometra
   EXCLUDES 1   *hematometra with hematocolpos (N89.7)*
   DEF: Accumulation of blood within the uterus.

N85.8 Other specified noninflammatory disorders of uterus ♀
   Atrophy of uterus, acquired
   Fibrosis of uterus NOS

N85.9 Noninflammatory disorder of uterus, unspecified ♀
   Disorder of uterus NOS

N86 Erosion and ectropion of cervix uteri ♀
   Decubitus (trophic) ulcer of cervix
   Eversion of cervix
   EXCLUDES 1   *erosion and ectropion of cervix with cervicitis (N72)*

✓4ᵗʰ N87 Dysplasia of cervix uteri
   EXCLUDES 1   *abnormal results from cervical cytologic examination without histologic confirmation (R87.61-)*
      carcinoma in situ of cervix uteri (D06.-)
      cervical intraepithelial neoplasia III [CIN III] (D06.-)
      HGSIL of cervix (R87.613)
      severe dysplasia of cervix uteri (D06.-)

N87.0 Mild cervical dysplasia ♀
   Cervical intraepithelial neoplasia I [CIN I]

N87.1 Moderate cervical dysplasia ♀
   Cervical intraepithelial neoplasia II [CIN II]

N87.9 Dysplasia of cervix uteri, unspecified ♀
   Anaplasia of cervix
   Cervical atypism
   Cervical dysplasia NOS

✓4ᵗʰ N88 Other noninflammatory disorders of cervix uteri
   EXCLUDES 2   *inflammatory disease of cervix (N72)*
      polyp of cervix (N84.1)

N88.0 Leukoplakia of cervix uteri ♀

N88.1 Old laceration of cervix uteri ♀
   Adhesions of cervix
   EXCLUDES 1   *current obstetric trauma (O71.3)*

N88.2 Stricture and stenosis of cervix uteri ♀
   EXCLUDES 1   *stricture and stenosis of cervix uteri complicating labor (O65.5)*

N88.3 Incompetence of cervix uteri ♀
   Investigation and management of (suspected) cervical incompetence in a nonpregnant woman
   EXCLUDES 1   *cervical incompetence complicating pregnancy (O34.3-)*
   DEF: Inadequate functioning of the cervix marked by abnormal widening during pregnancy and causing premature birth or miscarriage.

N88.4 Hypertrophic elongation of cervix uteri ♀

N88.8 Other specified noninflammatory disorders of cervix uteri ♀
   EXCLUDES 1   *current obstetric trauma (O71.3)*

N88.9 Noninflammatory disorder of cervix uteri, unspecified ♀

✓ Additional Character Required   **✓x7ᵗʰ** Placeholder   Unacceptable PDx   Questionable PDx   Manifestation   **H1** - **H14** HAC   **HCC** CMS-HCC Dx   **HIV** HIV Dx

ICD-10-CM 2019   **841**

☑4th **N89** **Other noninflammatory disorders of vagina**

EXCLUDES 1   *abnormal results from vaginal cytologic examination without*
histologic confirmation (R87.62-)
carcinoma in situ of vagina (D07.2)
HGSIL of vagina (R87.623)
inflammation of vagina (N76.-)
senile (atrophic) vaginitis (N95.2)
severe dysplasia of vagina (D07.2)
trichomonal leukorrhea (A59.00)
vaginal intraepithelial neoplasia [VAIN], grade III (D07.2)

N89.0 **Mild** **vaginal dysplasia**   ♀
Vaginal intraepithelial neoplasia [VAIN], grade I

N89.1 **Moderate** **vaginal dysplasia**   ♀
Vaginal intraepithelial neoplasia [VAIN], grade II

N89.3 **Dysplasia of vagina, unspecified**   ♀

N89.4 **Leukoplakia of vagina**   ♀

N89.5 **Stricture and atresia of vagina**   ♀
Vaginal adhesions   Vaginal stenosis
EXCLUDES 1   *congenital atresia or stricture (Q52.4)*
postprocedural adhesions of vagina (N99.2)

N89.6 **Tight hymenal ring**   ♀
Rigid hymen
Tight introitus
EXCLUDES 1   *imperforate hymen (Q52.3)*

N89.7 **Hematocolpos**   ♀
Hematocolpos with hematometra or hematosalpinx
AHA: 2016, 4Q, 58

N89.8 **Other specified noninflammatory disorders of vagina**   ♀
Leukorrhea NOS
Old vaginal laceration
Pessary ulcer of vagina
EXCLUDES 1   *current obstetric trauma (O70-, O71.4, O71.7-O71.8)*
old laceration involving muscles of pelvic floor (N81.8)

N89.9 **Noninflammatory disorder of vagina, unspecified**

☑4th **N90** **Other noninflammatory disorders of vulva and perineum**

EXCLUDES 1   *anogenital (venereal) warts (A63.0)*
carcinoma in situ of vulva (D07.1)
condyloma acuminatum (A63.0)
current obstetric trauma (O70-, O71.7-O71.8)
inflammation of vulva (N76.-)
severe dysplasia of vulva (D07.1)
vulvar intraepithelial neoplasm III [VIN III] (D07.1)

N90.0 **Mild** **vulvar dysplasia**   ♀
Vulvar intraepithelial neoplasia [VIN], grade I

N90.1 **Moderate** **vulvar dysplasia**   ♀
Vulvar intraepithelial neoplasia [VIN], grade II

N90.3 **Dysplasia of vulva, unspecified**   ♀

N90.4 **Leukoplakia of vulva**   ♀
Dystrophy of vulva
Kraurosis of vulva
Lichen sclerosus of external female genital organs

N90.5 **Atrophy of vulva**   ♀
Stenosis of vulva

☑5th **N90.6** **Hypertrophy of vulva**
AHA: 2016, 4Q, 46

N90.60 **Unspecified hypertrophy of vulva**   ♀
Unspecified hypertrophy of labia

N90.61 **Childhood asymmetric labium majus enlargement** ♀
CALME

N90.69 **Other specified hypertrophy of vulva**   ♀
Other specified hypertrophy of labia

N90.7 **Vulvar cyst**   ♀

☑5th **N90.8** **Other specified noninflammatory disorders of vulva and perineum**

☑6th **N90.81** **Female genital mutilation status**
Female genital cutting status

N90.810 **Female genital mutilation status, unspecified**   ♀
Female genital cutting status, unspecified
Female genital mutilation status NOS

N90.811 **Female genital mutilation Type I status** ♀
Clitorectomy status
Female genital cutting Type I status

N90.812 **Female genital mutilation Type II status** ♀
Clitorectomy with excision of labia minora status
Female genital cutting Type II status

N90.813 **Female genital mutilation Type III status** ♀
Female genital cutting Type III status
Infibulation status

N90.818 **Other** **female genital mutilation status** ♀
Female genital cutting Type IV status
Female genital mutilation Type IV status
Other female genital cutting status

N90.89 **Other specified noninflammatory disorders of vulva and perineum**   ♀
Adhesions of vulva
Hypertrophy of clitoris

N90.9 **Noninflammatory disorder of vulva and perineum, unspecified**   ♀

☑4th **N91** **Absent, scanty and rare menstruation**
EXCLUDES 1   *ovarian dysfunction (E28.-)*

N91.0 **Primary amenorrhea**   ♀

N91.1 **Secondary amenorrhea**   ♀

N91.2 **Amenorrhea, unspecified**   ♀

N91.3 **Primary oligomenorrhea**   ♀

N91.4 **Secondary oligomenorrhea**   ♀

N91.5 **Oligomenorrhea, unspecified**   ♀
Hypomenorrhea NOS

☑4th **N92** **Excessive, frequent and irregular menstruation**
EXCLUDES 1   *postmenopausal bleeding (N95.0)*
precocious puberty (menstruation) (E30.1)

N92.0 **Excessive and frequent menstruation with regular cycle**   ♀
Heavy periods NOS
Menorrhagia NOS
Polymenorrhea

N92.1 **Excessive and frequent menstruation with irregular cycle**   ♀
Irregular intermenstrual bleeding
Irregular, shortened intervals between menstrual bleeding
Menometrorrhagia
Metrorrhagia

N92.2 **Excessive menstruation at puberty**   P♀
Excessive bleeding associated with onset of menstrual periods
Pubertal menorrhagia
Puberty bleeding

N92.3 **Ovulation bleeding**   ♀
Regular intermenstrual bleeding

N92.4 **Excessive bleeding in the premenopausal period**   ♀
Climacteric menorrhagia or metrorrhagia
Menopausal menorrhagia or metrorrhagia
Preclimacteric menorrhagia or metrorrhagia
Premenopausal menorrhagia or metrorrhagia

N92.5 **Other specified irregular menstruation**   ♀

N92.6 **Irregular menstruation, unspecified**   ♀
Irregular bleeding NOS
Irregular periods NOS
EXCLUDES 1   *irregular menstruation with:*
lengthened intervals or scanty bleeding (N91.3-N91.5)
shortened intervals or excessive bleeding (N92.1)

☑4th **N93** **Other abnormal uterine and vaginal bleeding**
EXCLUDES 1   *neonatal vaginal hemorrhage (P54.6)*
precocious puberty (menstruation) (E30.1)
pseudomenses (P54.6)

N93.0 **Postcoital and contact bleeding**   ♀

N93.1 **Pre-pubertal vaginal bleeding**
AHA: 2016, 4Q, 47

N93.8 **Other specified abnormal uterine and vaginal bleeding**   ♀
Dysfunctional or functional uterine or vaginal bleeding NOS

N93.9 **Abnormal uterine and vaginal bleeding, unspecified**   ♀

☑4th **N94** **Pain and other conditions associated with female genital organs and menstrual cycle**

N94.0 **Mittelschmerz**   ♀
DEF: One-sided, lower abdominal pain occurring between menstrual periods that is associated with ovulation.

☑5th **N94.1** **Dyspareunia**
EXCLUDES 1   *psychogenic dyspareunia (F52.6)*
AHA: 2016, 4Q, 47

N94.10 **Unspecified dyspareunia**   ♀

N94.11 **Superficial (introital) dyspareunia**   ♀

N94.12 **Deep dyspareunia**   ♀

N94.19 **Other specified dyspareunia**   ♀

N Newborn: 0   P Pediatric: 0-17   M Maternity: 12-55   A Adult: 15-124   MCC Major Complication/Comorbidity   CC Complication/Comorbidity   SW Severe Wound Dx

N94.2 Vaginismus ♀

     EXCLUDES1   psychogenic vaginismus (F52.5)

     DEF: Spontaneous contractions of the muscles surrounding the vagina, causing it to constrict or close.

N94.3 Premenstrual tension syndrome ♀

     Code also associated menstrual migraine (G43.82-, G43.83-)

     EXCLUDES1   premenstrual dysphoric disorder (F32.81)

N94.4 Primary dysmenorrhea ♀

N94.5 Secondary dysmenorrhea ♀

N94.6 Dysmenorrhea, unspecified ♀

     EXCLUDES1   psychogenic dysmenorrhea (F45.8)

✓5ᵗʰ **N94.8 Other specified conditions associated with female genital organs and menstrual cycle**

     ✓6ᵗʰ **N94.81 Vulvodynia**

         N94.810 Vulvar vestibulitis ♀

         N94.818 Other vulvodynia ♀

         N94.819 Vulvodynia, unspecified ♀

             Vulvodynia NOS

     N94.89 Other specified conditions associated with female ♀ **genital organs and menstrual cycle**

         DEF: Hydrocele: Serous fluid that collects in the canal of Nuck in females.

N94.9 Unspecified condition associated with female genital ♀ **organs and menstrual cycle**

✓4ᵗʰ **N95 Menopausal and other perimenopausal disorders**

     Menopausal and other perimenopausal disorders due to naturally occurring (age-related) menopause and perimenopause

     EXCLUDES1   excessive bleeding in the premenopausal period (N92.4)

                menopausal and perimenopausal disorders due to artificial or premature menopause (E89.4-, E28.31-)

                premature menopause (E28.31-)

     EXCLUDES2   postmenopausal osteoporosis (M81.0-)

                postmenopausal osteoporosis with current pathological fracture (M80.0-)

                postmenopausal urethritis (N34.2)

N95.0 Postmenopausal bleeding ♀

N95.1 Menopausal and female climacteric states ♀

     Symptoms such as flushing, sleeplessness, headache, lack of concentration, associated with natural (age-related) menopause

     Use additional code for associated symptoms

     EXCLUDES1   asymptomatic menopausal state (Z78.0)

                symptoms associated with artificial menopause (E89.41)

                symptoms associated with premature menopause (E28.310)

N95.2 Postmenopausal atrophic vaginitis ♀

     Senile (atrophic) vaginitis

N95.8 Other specified menopausal and perimenopausal ♀ **disorders**

N95.9 Unspecified menopausal and perimenopausal disorder ♀

N96 Recurrent pregnancy loss ♀

     Investigation or care in a nonpregnant woman with history of recurrent pregnancy loss

     EXCLUDES1   recurrent pregnancy loss with current pregnancy (O26.2-)

✓4ᵗʰ **N97 Female infertility**

     INCLUDES   inability to achieve a pregnancy

                sterility, female NOS

     EXCLUDES1   female infertility associated with:

                hypopituitarism (E23.0)

                Stein-Leventhal syndrome (E28.2)

     EXCLUDES2   incompetence of cervix uteri (N88.3)

     DEF: Infertility: Inability to conceive for at least one year with regular intercourse.

     DEF: Primary infertility: Infertility occurring in patients who have never conceived.

     DEF: Secondary infertility: Infertility occurring in patients who have previously conceived.

N97.0 Female infertility associated with anovulation ♀

N97.1 Female infertility of tubal origin ♀

     Female infertility associated with congenital anomaly of tube

     Female infertility due to tubal block

     Female infertility due to tubal occlusion

     Female infertility due to tubal stenosis

N97.2 Female infertility of uterine origin ♀

     Female infertility associated with congenital anomaly of uterus

     Female infertility due to nonimplantation of ovum

N97.8 Female infertility of other origin ♀

N97.9 Female infertility, unspecified ♀

✓4ᵗʰ **N98 Complications associated with artificial fertilization**

     CC Excl: For CC codes in category N98, unless otherwise noted: PDX collection 643

     N98.0 Infection associated with artificial insemination CC ♀

         CC Excl: PDX collection 948

     N98.1 Hyperstimulation of ovaries CC ♀

         Hyperstimulation of ovaries NOS

         Hyperstimulation of ovaries associated with induced ovulation

     N98.2 Complications of attempted introduction of fertilized CC ♀ **ovum following in vitro fertilization**

     N98.3 Complications of attempted introduction of embryo in CC ♀ **embryo transfer**

     N98.8 Other complications associated with artificial CC ♀ **fertilization**

     N98.9 Complication associated with artificial fertilization, CC ♀ **unspecified**

Intraoperative and postprocedural complications and disorders of genitourinary system, not elsewhere classified (N99)

✓4ᵗʰ **N99 Intraoperative and postprocedural complications and disorders of genitourinary system, not elsewhere classified**

     EXCLUDES2   irradiation cystitis (N30.4-)

                postoophorectomy osteoporosis with current pathological fracture (M80.8-)

                postoophorectomy osteoporosis without current pathological fracture (M81.8)

     N99.0 Postprocedural (acute) (chronic) kidney failure

         Use additional code for type of kidney disease

     ✓5ᵗʰ **N99.1 Postprocedural urethral stricture**

         Postcatheterization urethral stricture

         ✓6ᵗʰ **N99.11 Postprocedural urethral stricture, male**

             AHA: 2016, 4Q, 47-48

             N99.110 Postprocedural urethral stricture, male, ♂ **meatal**

             N99.111 Postprocedural bulbous urethral ♂ **stricture, male**

             N99.112 Postprocedural membranous urethral ♂ **stricture, male**

             N99.113 Postprocedural anterior bulbous ♂ **urethral stricture, male**

             N99.114 Postprocedural urethral stricture, ♂ **male, unspecified**

             N99.115 Postprocedural fossa navicularis ♂ **urethral stricture**

             N99.116 Postprocedural urethral stricture, ♂ **male, overlapping sites**

         N99.12 Postprocedural urethral stricture, female ♀

     N99.2 Postprocedural adhesions of vagina ♀

     N99.3 Prolapse of vaginal vault after hysterectomy ♀

     N99.4 Postprocedural pelvic peritoneal adhesions

         EXCLUDES2   pelvic peritoneal adhesions NOS (N73.6)

                postinfective pelvic peritoneal adhesions (N73.6)

     ✓5ᵗʰ **N99.5 Complications of stoma of urinary tract**

         EXCLUDES2   mechanical complication of urinary catheter (T83.0-)

         AHA: 2016, 4Q, 48

         ✓6ᵗʰ **N99.51 Complication of cystostomy**

             N99.510 Cystostomy hemorrhage CC HCC

                CC Excl: PDX collection 949

             N99.511 Cystostomy infection CC HCC

                CC Excl: PDX collection 950

             N99.512 Cystostomy malfunction CC HCC

                CC Excl: PDX collection 951

             N99.518 Other cystostomy complication CC HCC

                CC Excl: PDX collection 949

         ✓6ᵗʰ **N99.52 Complication of incontinent external stoma of urinary tract**

             N99.520 Hemorrhage of incontinent external HCC **stoma of urinary tract**

             N99.521 Infection of incontinent external HCC **stoma of urinary tract**

             N99.522 Malfunction of incontinent external HCC **stoma of urinary tract**

             N99.523 Herniation of incontinent stoma of HCC **urinary tract**

✓ Additional Character Required   ✓x7ᵗʰ Placeholder   Unacceptable PDx   Questionable PDx   Manifestation   H1-H14 HAC   HCC CMS-HCC Dx   HIV HIV Dx

ICD-10-CM 2019   843

Chapter 14. Diseases of Genitourinary System

N99.524   **Stenosis** of incontinent stoma of urinary tract   `HCC`

N99.528   **Other** complication of incontinent external stoma of urinary tract   `HCC`

✓6ᵗʰ **N99.53**   Complication of continent stoma of urinary tract

N99.530   **Hemorrhage** of continent stoma of urinary tract   `HCC`

N99.531   **Infection** of continent stoma of urinary tract   `HCC`

N99.532   **Malfunction** of continent stoma of urinary tract   `HCC`

N99.533   **Herniation** of continent stoma of urinary tract   `HCC`

N99.534   **Stenosis** of continent stoma of urinary tract   `HCC`

N99.538   **Other** complication of continent stoma of urinary tract   `HCC`

✓5ᵗʰ **N99.6**   Intraoperative hemorrhage and hematoma of a genitourinary system organ or structure complicating a procedure

> EXCLUDES 1   intraoperative hemorrhage and hematoma of a genitourinary system organ or structure due to accidental puncture or laceration during a procedure (N99.7-)

N99.61   **Intraoperative hemorrhage and hematoma of a genitourinary system organ or structure complicating a** genitourinary system procedure   `CC`
CC Excl: PDX collection 952

N99.62   **Intraoperative hemorrhage and hematoma of a genitourinary system organ or structure complicating** other procedure   `CC`
CC Excl: PDX collection 952

✓5ᵗʰ **N99.7**   Accidental puncture and laceration of a genitourinary system organ or structure during a procedure

N99.71   **Accidental puncture and laceration of a genitourinary system organ or structure during a** genitourinary system procedure   `CC`
CC Excl: PDX collection 509

N99.72   **Accidental puncture and laceration of a genitourinary system organ or structure during** other procedure   `CC`
CC Excl: PDX collection 509

✓5ᵗʰ **N99.8**   Other intraoperative and postprocedural complications and disorders of genitourinary system
AHA: 2016, 4Q, 9-10

> CC Excl: For CC codes in subcategory N99.8:
> PDX collection 952

N99.81   **Other intraoperative complications** of genitourinary system

✓6ᵗʰ **N99.82**   Postprocedural hemorrhage of a genitourinary system organ or structure following a procedure

N99.820   **Postprocedural hemorrhage of a genitourinary system organ or structure following a** genitourinary system procedure   `CC`

N99.821   **Postprocedural hemorrhage of a genitourinary system organ or structure following** other procedure   `CC`

N99.83   **Residual ovary syndrome**   ♀

✓6ᵗʰ **N99.84**   Postprocedural hematoma and seroma of a genitourinary system organ or structure following a procedure

N99.840   **Postprocedural** hematoma **of a genitourinary system organ or structure following a** genitourinary system procedure   `CC`

N99.841   **Postprocedural** hematoma **of a genitourinary system organ or structure following** other procedure   `CC`

N99.842   **Postprocedural** seroma **of a genitourinary system organ or structure following a** genitourinary system procedure   `CC`

N99.843   **Postprocedural** seroma **of a genitourinary system organ or structure following** other procedure   `CC`

N99.89   **Other postprocedural complications and disorders of genitourinary system**

N Newborn: 0   **P** Pediatric: 0-17   **M** Maternity: 12-55   **A** Adult: 15-124   `MCC` Major Complication/Comorbidity   `CC` Complication/Comorbidity   `SW` Severe Wound Dx

844   ICD-10-CM 2019

Chapter 15. Pregnancy, Childbirth and the Puerperium (O00–O9A)

Chapter Specific Guidelines with Coding Examples

The chapter specific guidelines from the ICD-10-CM Official Guidelines for Coding and Reporting have been provided below. Along with these guidelines are coding examples, contained in the shaded boxes, that have been developed to help illustrate the coding and/or sequencing guidance found in these guidelines.

a. General rules for obstetric cases

1) Codes from Chapter 15 and sequencing priority

Obstetric cases require codes from chapter 15, codes in the range O00–O9A, Pregnancy, Childbirth, and the Puerperium. Chapter 15 codes have sequencing priority over codes from other chapters. Additional codes from other chapters may be used in conjunction with chapter 15 codes to further specify conditions. Should the provider document that the pregnancy is incidental to the encounter, then code Z33.1, Pregnant state, incidental, should be used in place of any chapter 15 codes. It is the provider's responsibility to state that the condition being treated is not affecting the pregnancy.

> Pregnant patient at 25 weeks' gestation admitted for bladder abscess
>
> **O23.12**   **Infections of bladder in pregnancy, second trimester**
>
> **N30.80**   **Other cystitis without hematuria**
>
> **Z3A.25**   **25 weeks gestation of pregnancy**
>
> *Explanation:* The documentation does not indicate that the pregnancy is incidental or in any way unaffected by the bladder abscess; therefore, an obstetrics code should be sequenced first. An additional code was provided to identify the specific bladder condition as this information is not called out specifically in the obstetrics code.

2) Chapter 15 codes used only on the maternal record

Chapter 15 codes are to be used only on the maternal record, never on the record of the newborn.

3) Final character for trimester

The majority of codes in Chapter 15 have a final character indicating the trimester of pregnancy. The timeframes for the trimesters are indicated at the beginning of the chapter. If trimester is not a component of a code, it is because the condition always occurs in a specific trimester, or the concept of trimester of pregnancy is not applicable. Certain codes have characters for only certain trimesters because the condition does not occur in all trimesters, but it may occur in more than just one.

Assignment of the final character for trimester should be based on the provider's documentation of the trimester (or number of weeks) for the current admission/encounter. This applies to the assignment of trimester for pre-existing conditions as well as those that develop during or are due to the pregnancy. The provider's documentation of the number of weeks may be used to assign the appropriate code identifying the trimester.

Whenever delivery occurs during the current admission, and there is an "in childbirth" option for the obstetric complication being coded, the "in childbirth" code should be assigned.

> Pregnant patient at 21 weeks' gestation admitted with excessive vomiting
>
> **O21.2**   **Late vomiting of pregnancy**
>
> **Z3A.21**   **21 weeks gestation of pregnancy**
>
> *Explanation:* Category O21 classifies vomiting in pregnancy. Although code selection is based on whether the vomiting is before or after 20 completed weeks, these codes are not further classified by trimester. If vomiting only in the second trimester was documented, the provider should be queried for the specific week of gestation, as this will affect code selection.

4) Selection of trimester for inpatient admissions that encompass more than one trimester

In instances when a patient is admitted to a hospital for complications of pregnancy during one trimester and remains in the hospital into a subsequent trimester, the trimester character for the antepartum complication code should be assigned on the basis of the trimester when the complication developed, not the trimester of the discharge. If the condition developed prior to the current admission/encounter or represents a pre-existing condition, the trimester character for the trimester at the time of the admission/encounter should be assigned.

> Patient admitted at 27 6/7 weeks' gestation for hemorrhaging from partial placenta previa; three days after admission at 28 1/7 weeks' gestation, she developed gestational hypertension
>
> **O44.32**   **Partial placenta previa with hemorrhage, second trimester**
>
> **O13.3**   **Gestational [pregnancy-induced] hypertension without significant proteinuria, third trimester**
>
> **Z3A.27**   **27 weeks gestation of pregnancy**
>
> *Explanation:* The patient presented with hemorrhaging from partial placenta previa while still in her 27th week, which falls within the second trimester. The gestational hypertension did not occur until three days after admission, putting the patient in her 28th week of pregnancy or what is considered to be the third trimester. The weeks of gestation captured by a code from category Z3A should represent only the gestational weeks upon admission.

5) Unspecified trimester

Each category that includes codes for trimester has a code for "unspecified trimester." The "unspecified trimester" code should rarely be used, such as when the documentation in the record is insufficient to determine the trimester and it is not possible to obtain clarification.

6) 7th character for fetus identification

Where applicable, a 7th character is to be assigned for certain categories (O31, O32, O33.3 - O33.6, O35, O36, O40, O41, O60.1, O60.2, O64, and O69) to identify the fetus for which the complication code applies.

Assign 7th character "0":

- For single gestations
- When the documentation in the record is insufficient to determine the fetus affected and it is not possible to obtain clarification.
- When it is not possible to clinically determine which fetus is affected.

> Maternal patient with twin gestations is seen after ultrasound identifies fetus B to be in breech presentation
>
> **O32.1XX2**   **Maternal care for breech presentation, fetus 2**
>
> *Explanation:* The documentation indicates that although there are two fetuses, only one fetus is determined to be in breech presentation. Whether fetus 2 or fetus B is used, the coder can assign the seventh character of 2 to identify the second fetus as the one in breech.

b. Selection of OB principal or first-listed diagnosis

1) Routine outpatient prenatal visits

For routine outpatient prenatal visits when no complications are present, a code from category Z34, Encounter for supervision of normal pregnancy, should be used as the first-listed diagnosis. These codes should not be used in conjunction with chapter 15 codes.

2) Supervision of high-risk pregnancy

Codes from category O09, Supervision of high-risk pregnancy, are intended for use only during the prenatal period. For complications during the labor or delivery episode as a result of a high-risk pregnancy, assign the applicable complication codes from Chapter 15. If there are no complications during the labor or delivery episode, assign code O80, Encounter for full-term uncomplicated delivery.

For routine prenatal outpatient visits for patients with high-risk pregnancies, a code from category O09, Supervision of high-risk pregnancy, should be used as the first-listed diagnosis. Secondary chapter 15 codes may be used in conjunction with these codes if appropriate.

> 36-year-old admitted in labor with second child at 39 weeks' gestation, delivered a healthy baby, delivery complicated by tear of fourchette that was repaired
>
> **O70.0**   **First degree perineal laceration during delivery**
>
> **Z3A.39**   **39 weeks gestation of pregnancy**
>
> **Z37.0**   **Single live birth**
>
> Explanation: Although this patient is over 35 and having her second child (elderly multigravida), do not append a code from subcategory O09.52-. A code describing the tear of the fourchette, which complicated the delivery, should be used in addition to the applicable Z codes.

3) Episodes when no delivery occurs

In episodes when no delivery occurs, the principal diagnosis should correspond to the principal complication of the pregnancy which necessitated the encounter. Should more than one complication exist, all of which are treated or monitored, any of the complications codes may be sequenced first.

4) When a delivery occurs

When an obstetric patient is admitted and delivers during that admission, the condition that prompted the admission should be sequenced as the principal diagnosis. If multiple conditions prompted the admission, sequence the one most related to the delivery as the principal diagnosis. A code for any complication of the delivery should be assigned as an additional diagnosis. In cases of cesarean delivery, if the patient was admitted with a condition that resulted in the performance of a cesarean procedure, that condition should be selected as the principal diagnosis. If the reason for the admission was unrelated to the condition resulting in the cesarean delivery, the condition related to the reason for the admission should be selected as the principal diagnosis.

Maternal patient with diet-controlled gestational diabetes was admitted at 38 weeks' gestation in obstructed labor due to footling presentation; cesarean performed for the malpresentation

O64.8XX0	Obstructed labor due to other malposition and malpresentation, not applicable or unspecified
O24.420	Gestational diabetes mellitus in childbirth, diet controlled
Z3A.38	38 weeks gestation of pregnancy
Z37.0	Single live birth

Explanation: The obstructed labor necessitated the cesarean procedure.

At 39 weeks' gestation, a maternal patient presents with hemorrhage with coagulation defect; the next day the patient goes into labor and eventually delivers via cesarean section due to arrested active phase of labor

O46.003	Antepartum hemorrhage with coagulation defect, unspecified, third trimester
O62.1	Secondary uterine inertia
Z3A.39	39 weeks gestation of pregnancy
Z37.0	Single live birth

Explanation: The patient was admitted because of the antepartum hemorrhage with coagulation defect. The arrested active phase, although the reason for the cesarean delivery, did not develop until later into the stay.

5) Outcome of delivery

A code from category Z37, Outcome of delivery, should be included on every maternal record when a delivery has occurred. These codes are not to be used on subsequent records or on the newborn record.

c. Pre-existing conditions versus conditions due to the pregnancy

Certain categories in Chapter 15 distinguish between conditions of the mother that existed prior to pregnancy (pre-existing) and those that are a direct result of pregnancy. When assigning codes from Chapter 15, it is important to assess if a condition was pre-existing prior to pregnancy or developed during or due to the pregnancy in order to assign the correct code.

Categories that do not distinguish between pre-existing and pregnancy-related conditions may be used for either. It is acceptable to use codes specifically for the puerperium with codes complicating pregnancy and childbirth if a condition arises postpartum during the delivery encounter.

d. Pre-existing hypertension in pregnancy

Category O10, Pre-existing hypertension complicating pregnancy, childbirth and the puerperium, includes codes for hypertensive heart and hypertensive chronic kidney disease. When assigning one of the O10 codes that includes hypertensive heart disease or hypertensive chronic kidney disease, it is necessary to add a secondary code from the appropriate hypertension category to specify the type of heart failure or chronic kidney disease.

See Section I.C.9. Hypertension.

e. Fetal conditions affecting the management of the mother

1) Codes from categories O35 and O36

Codes from categories O35, Maternal care for known or suspected fetal abnormality and damage, and O36, Maternal care for other fetal problems, are assigned only when the fetal condition is actually responsible for modifying the management of the mother, i.e., by requiring diagnostic studies, additional observation, special care, or termination of pregnancy. The fact that the fetal condition exists does not justify assigning a code from this series to the mother's record.

A patient is seen in ED for spotting 15 weeks into her pregnancy; the doctors also suspect fetal hydrocephalus.

| O26.852 | Spotting complicating pregnancy, second trimester |
| Z3A.15 | 15 weeks gestation of pregnancy |

Explanation: Whether the fetal hydrocephalus was suspected or confirmed, an additional code is not warranted for this condition as the documentation does not indicate that this fetal condition is in any way altering the management of the mother or complicating her pregnancy.

2) In utero surgery

In cases when surgery is performed on the fetus, a diagnosis code from category O35, Maternal care for known or suspected fetal abnormality and damage, should be assigned identifying the fetal condition. Assign the appropriate procedure code for the procedure performed.

No code from Chapter 16, the perinatal codes, should be used on the mother's record to identify fetal conditions. Surgery performed in utero on a fetus is still to be coded as an obstetric encounter.

f. HIV infection in pregnancy, childbirth and the puerperium

During pregnancy, childbirth or the puerperium, a patient admitted because of an HIV-related illness should receive a principal diagnosis from subcategory O98.7-, Human immunodeficiency [HIV] disease complicating pregnancy, childbirth and the puerperium, followed by the code(s) for the HIV-related illness(es).

Patients with asymptomatic HIV infection status admitted during pregnancy, childbirth, or the puerperium should receive codes of O98.7- and Z21, Asymptomatic human immunodeficiency virus [HIV] infection status.

A previously asymptomatic HIV patient who is 13 weeks pregnant is admitted with oral thrush.

O98.711	Human immunodeficiency virus [HIV] disease complicating pregnancy, first trimester
B20	Human immunodeficiency virus [HIV] disease
B37.0	Candidal stomatitis
Z3A.13	13 weeks gestation of pregnancy

Explanation: Because oral thrush is an HIV-related condition, this patient is now considered to have HIV disease. An obstetrics code indicating that HIV is complicating the pregnancy is coded first, followed by B20 for HIV disease as well as a code for the oral thrush.

g. Diabetes mellitus in pregnancy

Diabetes mellitus is a significant complicating factor in pregnancy. Pregnant women who are diabetic should be assigned a code from category O24, Diabetes mellitus in pregnancy, childbirth, and the puerperium, first, followed by the appropriate diabetes code(s) (E08-E13) from Chapter 4.

h. Long term use of insulin and oral hypoglycemics

See section I.C.4.a.3 for information on the long term use of insulin and oral hypoglycemic.

i. Gestational (pregnancy induced) diabetes

Gestational (pregnancy induced) diabetes can occur during the second and third trimester of pregnancy in women who were not diabetic prior to pregnancy. Gestational diabetes can cause complications in the pregnancy similar to those of pre-existing diabetes mellitus. It also puts the woman at greater risk of developing diabetes after the pregnancy. Codes for gestational diabetes are in subcategory O24.4, Gestational diabetes mellitus. No other code from category O24, Diabetes mellitus in pregnancy, childbirth, and the puerperium, should be used with a code from O24.4.

The codes under subcategory O24.4 include diet controlled, insulin controlled, and controlled by oral hypoglycemic drugs. If a patient with gestational diabetes is treated with both diet and insulin, only the code for insulin-controlled is required. If a patient with gestational diabetes is treated with both diet and oral hypoglycemic medications, only the code for

"controlled by oral hypoglycemic drugs" is required. Code Z79.4, Long-term (current) use of insulin or code Z79.84, Long-term (current) use of oral hypoglycemic drugs, should not be assigned with codes from subcategory O24.4.

An abnormal glucose tolerance in pregnancy is assigned a code from subcategory O99.81, Abnormal glucose complicating pregnancy, childbirth, and the puerperium.

Patient at 39 weeks term pregnancy with gestational diabetes was admitted in labor and delivered a healthy newborn. Patient is on diabetes diet with daily metformin.

O24.425   **Gestational diabetes mellitus in childbirth, controlled by oral hypoglycemic drugs**

Z3A.39   **39 weeks gestation of pregnancy**

Z37.0   **Single live birth**

Explanation: When the patient is admitted for delivery and the patient's gestational diabetes is controlled by both diet and oral hypoglycemic medications, only the combination code in subcategory O24.4-Gestational diabetes mellitus, is reported. No code is added for diet controlled diabetes, and no Z code for long-term use of oral hypoglycemics is reported with the O24.4 combination codes.

---

j. Sepsis and septic shock complicating abortion, pregnancy, childbirth and the puerperium

When assigning a chapter 15 code for sepsis complicating abortion, pregnancy, childbirth, and the puerperium, a code for the specific type of infection should be assigned as an additional diagnosis. If severe sepsis is present, a code from subcategory R65.2, Severe sepsis, and code(s) for associated organ dysfunction(s) should also be assigned as additional diagnoses.

Patient is seen several days after a miscarriage with sepsis; cultures return MSSA

O03.87   **Sepsis following complete or unspecified spontaneous abortion**

B95.61   **Methicillin susceptible Staphylococcus aureus infection as the cause of diseases classified elsewhere**

Explanation: The type of infection that caused this patient to become septic was methicillin susceptible *Staphylococcus aureus* (MSSA), which as a secondary code helps capture all aspects related to this patient's septic condition.

---

k. Puerperal sepsis

Code O85, Puerperal sepsis, should be assigned with a secondary code to identify the causal organism (e.g., for a bacterial infection, assign a code from category B95-B96, Bacterial infections in conditions classified elsewhere). A code from category A40, Streptococcal sepsis, or A41, Other sepsis, should not be used for puerperal sepsis. If applicable, use additional codes to identify severe sepsis (R65.2-) and any associated acute organ dysfunction.

l. Alcohol, tobacco *and drug* use during pregnancy, childbirth and the puerperium

   1) Alcohol use during pregnancy, childbirth and the puerperium

Codes under subcategory O99.31, Alcohol use complicating pregnancy, childbirth, and the puerperium, should be assigned for any pregnancy case when a mother uses alcohol during the pregnancy or postpartum. A secondary code from category F10, Alcohol related disorders, should also be assigned to identify manifestations of the alcohol use.

   2) Tobacco use during pregnancy, childbirth and the puerperium

Codes under subcategory O99.33, Smoking (tobacco) complicating pregnancy, childbirth, and the puerperium, should be assigned for any pregnancy case when a mother uses any type of tobacco product during the pregnancy or postpartum. A secondary code from category F17, Nicotine dependence, should also be assigned to identify the type of nicotine dependence.

   3) Drug use during pregnancy, childbirth and the puerperium

Codes under subcategory O99.32, Drug use complicating pregnancy, childbirth, and the puerperium, should be assigned for any pregnancy case when a mother uses drugs during the pregnancy or postpartum. This can involve illegal drugs, or inappropriate use or abuse of prescription drugs. Secondary code(s) from categories F11-F16 and F18-F19 should also be assigned to identify manifestations of the drug use.

m. Poisoning, toxic effects, adverse effects and underdosing in a pregnant patient

A code from subcategory O9A.2, Injury, poisoning and certain other consequences of external causes complicating pregnancy, childbirth, and the puerperium, should be sequenced first, followed by the appropriate injury, poisoning, toxic effect, adverse effect or underdosing code, and then the additional code(s) that specifies the condition caused by the poisoning, toxic effect, adverse effect or underdosing.

See Section I.C.19. Adverse effects, poisoning, underdosing and toxic effects.

Patient admitted with accidental carbon monoxide poisoning from a gas heating implement; the patient is 18 weeks' pregnant

O9A.212   **Injury, poisoning and certain other consequences of external causes complicating pregnancy, second trimester**

T58.11XA   **Toxic effect of carbon monoxide from utility gas, accidental (unintentional), initial encounter**

Z3A.18   **18 weeks gestation of pregnancy**

Explanation: Although the carbon monoxide poisoning is the reason the patient was admitted, a code from the obstetrics chapter must be sequenced first. Chapter 15 codes have sequencing priority over codes from other chapters.

---

n. Normal delivery, code O80

   1) Encounter for full term uncomplicated delivery

Code O80 should be assigned when a woman is admitted for a full-term normal delivery and delivers a single, healthy infant without any complications antepartum, during the delivery, or postpartum during the delivery episode. Code O80 is always a principal diagnosis. It is not to be used if any other code from chapter 15 is needed to describe a current complication of the antenatal, delivery, or perinatal period. Additional codes from other chapters may be used with code O80 if they are not related to or are in any way complicating the pregnancy.

   2) Uncomplicated delivery with resolved antepartum complication

Code O80 may be used if the patient had a complication at some point during the pregnancy, but the complication is not present at the time of the admission for delivery.

Patient presents in labor at 39 weeks' gestation and delivers a healthy newborn; patient had abnormal glucose levels in her first trimester, which have since resolved

O80   **Encounter for full-term uncomplicated delivery**

Z37.0   **Single live birth**

Explanation: The abnormal glucose levels during the first trimester cannot be coded if they are not affecting the patient's current trimester. Without additional complications associated with the pregnancy, fetus, or mother, code O80 is appropriate.

---

   3) Outcome of delivery for O80

Z37.0, Single live birth, is the only outcome of delivery code appropriate for use with O80.

o. The peripartum and postpartum periods

   1) Peripartum and postpartum periods

The postpartum period begins immediately after delivery and continues for six weeks following delivery. The peripartum period is defined as the last month of pregnancy to five months postpartum.

   2) Peripartum and postpartum complication

A postpartum complication is any complication occurring within the six-week period.

   3) Pregnancy-related complications after 6 week period

Chapter 15 codes may also be used to describe pregnancy-related complications after the peripartum or postpartum period if the provider documents that a condition is pregnancy related.

Chapter 15. Pregnancy, Childbirth and the Puerperium

Patient admitted for varicose veins. She had a baby boy three months ago; the varicose veins started to appear one month ago. The doctor attributes the patient's pregnancy as the cause of the varicose veins, which continue to be painful and bother the patient. She is seeking surgical relief.

O87.4   Varicose veins of the lower extremity in the puerperium

Explanation: Although the varicose veins occurred several months after the delivery of the newborn, the doctor attributed the varicose veins to pregnancy and therefore a code from chapter 15 is appropriate.

4) Admission for routine postpartum care following delivery outside hospital

When the mother delivers outside the hospital prior to admission and is admitted for routine postpartum care and no complications are noted, code Z39.0, Encounter for care and examination of mother immediately after delivery, should be assigned as the principal diagnosis.

5) Pregnancy associated cardiomyopathy

Pregnancy associated cardiomyopathy, code O90.3, is unique in that it may be diagnosed in the third trimester of pregnancy but may continue to progress months after delivery. For this reason, it is referred to as peripartum cardiomyopathy. Code O90.3 is only for use when the cardiomyopathy develops as a result of pregnancy in a woman who did not have pre-existing heart disease.

p. Code O94, Sequelae of complication of pregnancy, childbirth, and the puerperium

1) Code O94

Code O94, Sequelae of complication of pregnancy, childbirth, and the puerperium, is for use in those cases when an initial complication of a pregnancy develops a sequelae requiring care or treatment at a future date.

2) After the initial postpartum period

This code may be used at any time after the initial postpartum period.

3) Sequencing of code O94

This code, like all sequela codes, is to be sequenced following the code describing the sequelae of the complication.

q. Termination of pregnancy and spontaneous abortions

1) Abortion with liveborn fetus

When an attempted termination of pregnancy results in a liveborn fetus, assign code Z33.2, Encounter for elective termination of pregnancy and a code from category Z37, Outcome of Delivery.

2) Retained products of conception following an abortion

Subsequent encounters for retained products of conception following a spontaneous abortion or elective termination of pregnancy, without complications are assigned O03.4, Incomplete spontaneous, abortion without complication, or code O07.4, Failed attempted termination of pregnancy without complication. This advice is appropriate even when the patient was discharged previously with a discharge diagnosis of complete abortion. If the patient has a specific complication associated with the spontaneous abortion or elective termination of pregnancy in addition to retained products of conception, assign the appropriate complication in category O03 or O07 instead of code O03.4 or O07.4

Patient was seen two days ago for complete spontaneous abortion but returns today for urinary tract infection (UTI) with ultrasound showing retained products of conception

O03.38   Urinary tract infection following incomplete spontaneous abortion

Explanation: Although the diagnosis from the patient's previous stay indicated that the patient had a complete abortion, it is now determined that there were actually retained products of conception (POC). An abortion with retained POC is considered incomplete and in this case resulted in the patient developing a UTI.

3) Complications leading to abortion

Codes from Chapter 15 may be used as additional codes to identify any documented complications of the pregnancy in conjunction with codes in categories in O04, O07 and O08.

r. Abuse in a pregnant patient

For suspected or confirmed cases of abuse of a pregnant patient, a code(s) from subcategories O9A.3, Physical abuse complicating pregnancy, childbirth, and the puerperium, O9A.4, Sexual abuse complicating pregnancy, childbirth, and the puerperium, and O9A.5, Psychological abuse complicating pregnancy, childbirth, and the puerperium, should be sequenced first, followed by the appropriate codes (if applicable) to identify any associated current injury due to physical abuse, sexual abuse, and the perpetrator of abuse.

See Section I.C.19. Adult and child abuse, neglect and other maltreatment.

Chapter 15. Pregnancy, Childbirth and the Puerperium (O00-O9A)

NOTE CODES FROM THIS CHAPTER ARE FOR USE ONLY ON MATERNAL RECORDS, NEVER ON NEWBORN RECORDS.

Codes from this chapter are for use for conditions related to or aggravated by the pregnancy, childbirth, or by the puerperium (maternal causes or obstetric causes).

NOTE Trimesters are counted from the first day of the last menstrual period. They are defined as follows:

1st trimester- less than 14 weeks Ø days
2nd trimester- 14 weeks Ø days to less than 28 weeks Ø days
3rd trimester- 28 weeks Ø days until delivery

Use additional code from category Z3A, Weeks of gestation, to identify the specific week of the pregnancy, if known

EXCLUDES 1 *supervision of normal pregnancy (Z34.-)*
EXCLUDES 2 *mental and behavioral disorders associated with the puerperium ▶(F53.-)◀*
obstetrical tetanus (A34)
postpartum necrosis of pituitary gland (E23.0)
puerperal osteomalacia (M83.0)

AHA: 2016, 1Q, 3-5; 2014, 3Q, 17

This chapter contains the following blocks:

O00-O08	Pregnancy with abortive outcome
O09	Supervision of high risk pregnancy
O10-O16	Edema, proteinuria and hypertensive disorders in pregnancy, childbirth and the puerperium
O20-O29	Other maternal disorders predominantly related to pregnancy
O30-O48	Maternal care related to the fetus and amniotic cavity and possible delivery problems
O60-O77	Complications of labor and delivery
O80, O82	Encounter for delivery
O85-O92	Complications predominantly related to the puerperium
O94-O9A	Other obstetric conditions, not elsewhere classified

Pregnancy with abortive outcome (O00-O08)

EXCLUDES 1 *continuing pregnancy in multiple gestation after abortion of one fetus or more (O31.1-, O31.3-)*

TIP: Do not assign a code from category Z3A with codes in this code block.

✓4ᵗʰ O00　Ectopic pregnancy
INCLUDES ruptured ectopic pregnancy
Use additional code from category O08 to identify any associated complication
AHA: 2016, 4Q, 48-50; 2014, 3Q, 17
DEF: Implantation of a fertilized egg outside the uterus, usually in the fallopian tube or abdomen that requires emergency treatment.

CC Excl: For CC codes in category O00: PDX collection 953

✓5ᵗʰ O00.0　Abdominal pregnancy
EXCLUDES 1 *maternal care for viable fetus in abdominal pregnancy (O36.7-)*

O00.00　Abdominal pregnancy without intrauterine pregnancy CC M♀
Abdominal pregnancy NOS

O00.01　Abdominal pregnancy with intrauterine pregnancy CC M♀

Ectopic Pregnancy

✓5ᵗʰ O00.1　Tubal pregnancy
Fallopian pregnancy
Rupture of (fallopian) tube due to pregnancy
Tubal abortion
AHA: 2017, 4Q, 20

✓6ᵗʰ O00.10　Tubal pregnancy without intrauterine pregnancy
Tubal pregnancy NOS

O00.101　Right tubal pregnancy without intrauterine pregnancy CC M♀

O00.102　Left tubal pregnancy without intrauterine pregnancy CC M♀

O00.109　Unspecified tubal pregnancy without intrauterine pregnancy CC M♀

✓6ᵗʰ O00.11　Tubal pregnancy with intrauterine pregnancy

O00.111　Right tubal pregnancy with intrauterine pregnancy CC M♀

O00.112　Left tubal pregnancy with intrauterine pregnancy CC M♀

O00.119　Unspecified tubal pregnancy with intrauterine pregnancy CC M♀

✓5ᵗʰ O00.2　Ovarian pregnancy
AHA: 2017, 4Q, 20

✓6ᵗʰ O00.20　Ovarian pregnancy without intrauterine pregnancy
Ovarian pregnancy NOS

O00.201　Right ovarian pregnancy without intrauterine pregnancy CC M♀

O00.202　Left ovarian pregnancy without intrauterine pregnancy CC M♀

O00.209　Unspecified ovarian pregnancy without intrauterine pregnancy CC M♀

✓6ᵗʰ O00.21　Ovarian pregnancy with intrauterine pregnancy

O00.211　Right ovarian pregnancy with intrauterine pregnancy CC M♀

O00.212　Left ovarian pregnancy with intrauterine pregnancy CC M♀

O00.219　Unspecified ovarian pregnancy with intrauterine pregnancy CC M♀

✓5ᵗʰ O00.8　Other ectopic pregnancy
Cervical pregnancy
Cornual pregnancy
Intraligamentous pregnancy
Mural pregnancy

O00.80　Other ectopic pregnancy without intrauterine pregnancy CC M♀
Other ectopic pregnancy NOS

O00.81　Other ectopic pregnancy with intrauterine pregnancy CC M♀

✓5ᵗʰ O00.9　Ectopic pregnancy, unspecified

O00.90　Unspecified ectopic pregnancy without intrauterine pregnancy CC M♀
Ectopic pregnancy NOS

O00.91　Unspecified ectopic pregnancy with intrauterine pregnancy CC M♀

✓4ᵗʰ O01　Hydatidiform mole
Use additional code from category O08 to identify any associated complication
EXCLUDES 1 *chorioadenoma (destruens) (D39.2)*
malignant hydatidiform mole (D39.2)
AHA: 2014, 3Q, 17
DEF: Abnormal product of pregnancy, marked by a mass of cysts resembling a bunch of grapes due to chorionic villi proliferation and dissolution. It must be surgically removed.

O01.0　Classical hydatidiform mole M♀
Complete hydatidiform mole

O01.1　Incomplete and partial hydatidiform mole M♀

O01.9　Hydatidiform mole, unspecified M♀
Trophoblastic disease NOS
Vesicular mole NOS

✓Additional Character Required　　✓x7ᵗʰ Placeholder　　Unacceptable PDx　　Questionable PDx　　Manifestation　　**H1**-**H14** HAC　　**HCC** CMS-HCC Dx　　**HIV** HIV Dx

ICD-10-CM 2019　　　　　　　　　　　　　　　　　　　　　　　　　　　**849**

Chapter 15. Pregnancy, Childbirth and the Puerperium *(side margin)*

✓4ᵗʰ **O02   Other abnormal products of conception**
Use additional code from category O08 to identify any associated complication
  EXCLUDES 1   papyraceous fetus (O31.0-)
  AHA: 2014, 3Q, 17

O02.0   Blighted ovum and nonhydatidiform mole   Ⓜ♀
Carneous mole
Fleshy mole
Intrauterine mole NOS
Molar pregnancy NEC
Pathological ovum

O02.1   Missed abortion   Ⓜ♀
Early fetal death, before completion of 20 weeks of gestation, with retention of dead fetus
  EXCLUDES 1   failed induced abortion (O07.-)
     fetal death (intrauterine) (late) (O36.4)
     missed abortion with blighted ovum (O02.0)
     missed abortion with hydatidiform mole (O01.-)
     missed abortion with nonhydatidiform (O02.0)
     missed abortion with other abnormal products of conception (O02.8-)
     missed delivery (O36.4)
     stillbirth (P95)

✓5ᵗʰ **O02.8   Other specified abnormal products of conception**
  EXCLUDES 1   abnormal products of conception with blighted ovum (O02.0)
     abnormal products of conception with hydatidiform mole (O01.-)
     abnormal products of conception with nonhydatidiform mole (O02.0)

O02.81   Inappropriate change in quantitative human chorionic gonadotropin (hCG) in early pregnancy   Ⓜ♀
Biochemical pregnancy
Chemical pregnancy
Inappropriate level of quantitative human chorionic gonadotropin (hCG) for gestational age in early pregnancy

O02.89   Other abnormal products of conception   Ⓜ♀

O02.9   Abnormal product of conception, unspecified   Ⓜ♀

✓4ᵗʰ **O03   Spontaneous abortion**
  NOTE   Incomplete abortion includes retained products of conception following spontaneous abortion
  INCLUDES   miscarriage

CC Excl: For CC/MCC codes in category O03: PDX collection 954

O03.0   Genital tract and pelvic infection following incomplete spontaneous abortion   ⒸⒸⓂ♀
Endometritis following incomplete spontaneous abortion
Oophoritis following incomplete spontaneous abortion
Parametritis following incomplete spontaneous abortion
Pelvic peritonitis following incomplete spontaneous abortion
Salpingitis following incomplete spontaneous abortion
Salpingo-oophoritis following incomplete spontaneous abortion
  EXCLUDES 1   sepsis following incomplete spontaneous abortion (O03.37)
     urinary tract infection following incomplete spontaneous abortion (O03.38)

O03.1   Delayed or excessive hemorrhage following incomplete spontaneous abortion   Ⓜ♀
Afibrinogenemia following incomplete spontaneous abortion
Defibrination syndrome following incomplete spontaneous abortion
Hemolysis following incomplete spontaneous abortion
Intravascular coagulation following incomplete spontaneous abortion

O03.2   Embolism following incomplete spontaneous abortion   ⓂⒸⒸⓂ♀
Air embolism following incomplete spontaneous abortion
Amniotic fluid embolism following incomplete spontaneous abortion
Blood-clot embolism following incomplete spontaneous abortion
Embolism NOS following incomplete spontaneous abortion
Fat embolism following incomplete spontaneous abortion
Pulmonary embolism following incomplete spontaneous abortion
Pyemic embolism following incomplete spontaneous abortion
Septic or septicopyemic embolism following incomplete spontaneous abortion
Soap embolism following incomplete spontaneous abortion

✓5ᵗʰ **O03.3   Other and unspecified complications following incomplete spontaneous abortion**

O03.30   Unspecified complication following incomplete spontaneous abortion   ⒸⒸⓂ♀

O03.31   Shock following incomplete spontaneous abortion   ⓂⒸⒸⓂ♀
Circulatory collapse following incomplete spontaneous abortion
Shock (postprocedural) following incomplete spontaneous abortion
  EXCLUDES 1   shock due to infection following incomplete spontaneous abortion (O03.37)

O03.32   Renal failure following incomplete spontaneous abortion   ⓂⒸⒸⓂ♀
Kidney failure (acute) following incomplete spontaneous abortion
Oliguria following incomplete spontaneous abortion
Renal shutdown following incomplete spontaneous abortion
Renal tubular necrosis following incomplete spontaneous abortion
Uremia following incomplete spontaneous abortion

O03.33   Metabolic disorder following incomplete spontaneous abortion   ⒸⒸⓂ♀

O03.34   Damage to pelvic organs following incomplete spontaneous abortion   ⒸⒸⓂ♀
Laceration, perforation, tear or chemical damage of bladder following incomplete spontaneous abortion
Laceration, perforation, tear or chemical damage of bowel following incomplete spontaneous abortion
Laceration, perforation, tear or chemical damage of broad ligament following incomplete spontaneous abortion
Laceration, perforation, tear or chemical damage of cervix following incomplete spontaneous abortion
Laceration, perforation, tear or chemical damage of periurethral tissue following incomplete spontaneous abortion
Laceration, perforation, tear or chemical damage of uterus following incomplete spontaneous abortion
Laceration, perforation, tear or chemical damage of vagina following incomplete spontaneous abortion

O03.35   Other venous complications following incomplete spontaneous abortion   ⒸⒸⓂ♀

O03.36   Cardiac arrest following incomplete spontaneous abortion   ⒸⒸⓂ♀

O03.37   Sepsis following incomplete spontaneous abortion   ⒸⒸⓂ♀
Use additional code to identify infectious agent (B95-B97)
Use additional code to identify severe sepsis, if applicable (R65.2-)
  EXCLUDES 1   septic or septicopyemic embolism following incomplete spontaneous abortion (O03.2)

O03.38   Urinary tract infection following incomplete spontaneous abortion   ⒸⒸⓂ♀
Cystitis following incomplete spontaneous abortion

O03.39   Incomplete spontaneous abortion with other complications   ⒸⒸⓂ♀

O03.4   Incomplete spontaneous abortion without complication   Ⓜ♀

Ⓝ Newborn: 0   Ⓟ Pediatric: 0-17   Ⓜ Maternity: 12-55   Ⓐ Adult: 15-124   ⓂⒸⒸ Major Complication/Comorbidity   ⒸⒸ Complication/Comorbidity   ⓈⓌ Severe Wound Dx

O03.5 **Genital tract and pelvic infection following complete** CC M♀
or unspecified spontaneous abortion
Endometritis following complete or unspecified spontaneous abortion
Oophoritis following complete or unspecified spontaneous abortion
Parametritis following complete or unspecified spontaneous abortion
Pelvic peritonitis following complete or unspecified spontaneous abortion
Salpingitis following complete or unspecified spontaneous abortion
Salpingo-oophoritis following complete or unspecified spontaneous abortion
> EXCLUDES 1   *sepsis following complete or unspecified spontaneous abortion (O03.87)*
> *urinary tract infection following complete or unspecified spontaneous abortion (O03.88)*

O03.6 **Delayed or excessive hemorrhage following complete or** M♀
unspecified spontaneous abortion
Afibrinogenemia following complete or unspecified spontaneous abortion
Defibrination syndrome following complete or unspecified spontaneous abortion
Hemolysis following complete or unspecified spontaneous abortion
Intravascular coagulation following complete or unspecified spontaneous abortion

O03.7 **Embolism following complete or unspecified** CC M♀
spontaneous abortion
Air embolism following complete or unspecified spontaneous abortion
Amniotic fluid embolism following complete or unspecified spontaneous abortion
Blood-clot embolism following complete or unspecified spontaneous abortion
Embolism NOS following complete or unspecified spontaneous abortion
Fat embolism following complete or unspecified spontaneous abortion
Pulmonary embolism following complete or unspecified spontaneous abortion
Pyemic embolism following complete or unspecified spontaneous abortion
Septic or septicopyemic embolism following complete or unspecified spontaneous abortion
Soap embolism following complete or unspecified spontaneous abortion

✓5ᵗʰ **O03.8** **Other and unspecified complications following complete or**
unspecified spontaneous abortion

O03.80 **Unspecified complication following complete** CC M♀
or unspecified spontaneous abortion

O03.81 **Shock following complete or unspecified** MCC M♀
spontaneous abortion
Circulatory collapse following complete or unspecified spontaneous abortion
Shock (postprocedural) following complete or unspecified spontaneous abortion
> EXCLUDES 1   *shock due to infection following complete or unspecified spontaneous abortion (O03.87)*

O03.82 **Renal failure following complete or** MCC M♀
unspecified spontaneous abortion
Kidney failure (acute) following complete or unspecified spontaneous abortion
Oliguria following complete or unspecified spontaneous abortion
Renal shutdown following complete or unspecified spontaneous abortion
Renal tubular necrosis following complete or unspecified spontaneous abortion
Uremia following complete or unspecified spontaneous abortion

O03.83 **Metabolic disorder following complete or** CC M♀
unspecified spontaneous abortion

O03.84 **Damage to pelvic organs following complete** CC M♀
or unspecified spontaneous abortion
Laceration, perforation, tear or chemical damage of bladder following complete or unspecified spontaneous abortion
Laceration, perforation, tear or chemical damage of bowel following complete or unspecified spontaneous abortion
Laceration, perforation, tear or chemical damage of broad ligament following complete or unspecified spontaneous abortion
Laceration, perforation, tear or chemical damage of cervix following complete or unspecified spontaneous abortion
Laceration, perforation, tear or chemical damage of periurethral tissue following complete or unspecified spontaneous abortion
Laceration, perforation, tear or chemical damage of uterus following complete or unspecified spontaneous abortion
Laceration, perforation, tear or chemical damage of vagina following complete or unspecified spontaneous abortion

O03.85 **Other venous complications following** CC M♀
complete or unspecified spontaneous abortion

O03.86 **Cardiac arrest following complete or** CC M♀
unspecified spontaneous abortion

O03.87 **Sepsis following complete or unspecified** CC M♀
spontaneous abortion
Use additional code to identify infectious agent (B95-B97)
Use additional code to identify severe sepsis, if applicable (R65.2-)
> EXCLUDES 1   *septic or septicopyemic embolism following complete or unspecified spontaneous abortion (O03.7)*

O03.88 **Urinary tract infection following complete or** CC M♀
unspecified spontaneous abortion
Cystitis following complete or unspecified spontaneous abortion

O03.89 **Complete or unspecified spontaneous** CC M♀
abortion with other complications

O03.9 **Complete or unspecified spontaneous abortion without** M♀
complication
Miscarriage NOS
Spontaneous abortion NOS

✓4ᵗʰ **O04** **Complications following (induced) termination of pregnancy**
> INCLUDES   complications following (induced) termination of pregnancy
> EXCLUDES 1   *encounter for elective termination of pregnancy, uncomplicated (Z33.2)*
> *failed attempted termination of pregnancy (O07.-)*

> **CC Excl: For CC/MCC codes in category O04, unless otherwise noted:** PDX collection 954

O04.5 **Genital tract and pelvic infection following (induced)** CC M♀
termination of pregnancy
Endometritis following (induced) termination of pregnancy
Oophoritis following (induced) termination of pregnancy
Parametritis following (induced) termination of pregnancy
Pelvic peritonitis following (induced) termination of pregnancy
Salpingitis following (induced) termination of pregnancy
Salpingo-oophoritis following (induced) termination of pregnancy
> EXCLUDES 1   *sepsis following (induced) termination of pregnancy (O04.87)*
> *urinary tract infection following (induced) termination of pregnancy (O04.88)*

O04.6 **Delayed or excessive hemorrhage following (induced)** M♀
termination of pregnancy
Afibrinogenemia following (induced) termination of pregnancy
Defibrination syndrome following (induced) termination of pregnancy
Hemolysis following (induced) termination of pregnancy
Intravascular coagulation following (induced) termination of pregnancy

✓ Additional Character Required   ✓x7ᵗʰ Placeholder   Unacceptable PDx   Questionable PDx   Manifestation   H1 - H14 HAC   HCC CMS-HCC Dx   HIV HIV Dx

ICD-10-CM 2019   851

O04.7 Embolism following (induced) termination of pregnancy MCC M♀
- Air embolism following (induced) termination of pregnancy
- Amniotic fluid embolism following (induced) termination of pregnancy
- Blood-clot embolism following (induced) termination of pregnancy
- Embolism NOS following (induced) termination of pregnancy
- Fat embolism following (induced) termination of pregnancy
- Pulmonary embolism following (induced) termination of pregnancy
- Pyemic embolism following (induced) termination of pregnancy
- Septic or septicopyemic embolism following (induced) termination of pregnancy
- Soap embolism following (induced) termination of pregnancy

✓5ᵗʰ **O04.8 (Induced) termination of pregnancy with other and unspecified complications**

O04.80 (Induced) termination of pregnancy with unspecified complications CC M♀

O04.81 Shock following (induced) termination of pregnancy MCC M♀
- Circulatory collapse following (induced) termination of pregnancy
- Shock (postprocedural) following (induced) termination of pregnancy
- EXCLUDES 1 *shock due to infection following (induced) termination of pregnancy (O04.87)*

O04.82 Renal failure following (induced) termination of pregnancy MCC M♀
- Kidney failure (acute) following (induced) termination of pregnancy
- Oliguria following (induced) termination of pregnancy
- Renal shutdown following (induced) termination of pregnancy
- Renal tubular necrosis following (induced) termination of pregnancy
- Uremia following (induced) termination of pregnancy

O04.83 Metabolic disorder following (induced) termination of pregnancy CC M♀

O04.84 Damage to pelvic organs following (induced) termination of pregnancy CC M♀
- Laceration, perforation, tear or chemical damage of bladder following (induced) termination of pregnancy
- Laceration, perforation, tear or chemical damage of bowel following (induced) termination of pregnancy
- Laceration, perforation, tear or chemical damage of broad ligament following (induced) termination of pregnancy
- Laceration, perforation, tear or chemical damage of cervix following (induced) termination of pregnancy
- Laceration, perforation, tear or chemical damage of periurethral tissue following (induced) termination of pregnancy
- Laceration, perforation, tear or chemical damage of uterus following (induced) termination of pregnancy
- Laceration, perforation, tear or chemical damage of vagina following (induced) termination of pregnancy

O04.85 Other venous complications following (induced) termination of pregnancy CC M♀

O04.86 Cardiac arrest following (induced) termination of pregnancy CC M♀

O04.87 Sepsis following (induced) termination of pregnancy CC M♀
- Use additional code to identify infectious agent (B95-B97)
- Use additional code to identify severe sepsis, if applicable (R65.2-)
- EXCLUDES 1 *septic or septicopyemic embolism following (induced) termination of pregnancy (O04.7)*
- CC Excl: PDX collection 955

O04.88 Urinary tract infection following (induced) termination of pregnancy CC M♀
- Cystitis following (induced) termination of pregnancy

O04.89 (Induced) termination of pregnancy with other complications CC M♀

✓4ᵗʰ **O07 Failed attempted termination of pregnancy**
- INCLUDES failure of attempted induction of termination of pregnancy
  - incomplete elective abortion
- EXCLUDES 1 *incomplete spontaneous abortion (O03.0-)*

O07.0 Genital tract and pelvic infection following failed attempted termination of pregnancy CC M♀
- Endometritis following failed attempted termination of pregnancy
- Oophoritis following failed attempted termination of pregnancy
- Parametritis following failed attempted termination of pregnancy
- Pelvic peritonitis following failed attempted termination of pregnancy
- Salpingitis following failed attempted termination of pregnancy
- Salpingo-oophoritis following failed attempted termination of pregnancy
- EXCLUDES 1 *sepsis following failed attempted termination of pregnancy (O07.37)*
  - *urinary tract infection following failed attempted termination of pregnancy (O07.38)*
- CC Excl: PDX collection 956

O07.1 Delayed or excessive hemorrhage following failed attempted termination of pregnancy CC M♀
- Afibrinogenemia following failed attempted termination of pregnancy
- Defibrination syndrome following failed attempted termination of pregnancy
- Hemolysis following failed attempted termination of pregnancy
- Intravascular coagulation following failed attempted termination of pregnancy
- CC Excl: PDX collection 957

O07.2 Embolism following failed attempted termination of pregnancy MCC M♀
- Air embolism following failed attempted termination of pregnancy
- Amniotic fluid embolism following failed attempted termination of pregnancy
- Blood-clot embolism following failed attempted termination of pregnancy
- Embolism NOS following failed attempted termination of pregnancy
- Fat embolism following failed attempted termination of pregnancy
- Pulmonary embolism following failed attempted termination of pregnancy
- Pyemic embolism following failed attempted termination of pregnancy
- Septic or septicopyemic embolism following failed attempted termination of pregnancy
- Soap embolism following failed attempted termination of pregnancy
- CC Excl: PDX collection 958

✓5ᵗʰ **O07.3 Failed attempted termination of pregnancy with other and unspecified complications**

CC Excl: For CC codes in subcategory O07.3, unless otherwise noted: PDX collection 954

O07.30 Failed attempted termination of pregnancy with unspecified complications CC M♀

O07.31 Shock following failed attempted termination of pregnancy MCC M♀
- Circulatory collapse following failed attempted termination of pregnancy
- Shock (postprocedural) following failed attempted termination of pregnancy
- EXCLUDES 1 *shock due to infection following failed attempted termination of pregnancy (O07.37)*
- CC Excl: PDX collection 959

O07.32 Renal failure following failed attempted termination of pregnancy MCC M♀
- Kidney failure (acute) following failed attempted termination of pregnancy
- Oliguria following failed attempted termination of pregnancy
- Renal shutdown following failed attempted termination of pregnancy
- Renal tubular necrosis following failed attempted termination of pregnancy
- Uremia following failed attempted termination of pregnancy
- CC Excl: PDX collection 960

O07.33 Metabolic disorder following failed attempted termination of pregnancy CC M♀

O07.34 Damage to pelvic organs following failed attempted termination of pregnancy CC M♀
Laceration, perforation, tear or chemical damage of bladder following failed attempted termination of pregnancy
Laceration, perforation, tear or chemical damage of bowel following failed attempted termination of pregnancy
Laceration, perforation, tear or chemical damage of broad ligament following failed attempted termination of pregnancy
Laceration, perforation, tear or chemical damage of cervix following failed attempted termination of pregnancy
Laceration, perforation, tear or chemical damage of periurethral tissue following failed attempted termination of pregnancy
Laceration, perforation, tear or chemical damage of uterus following failed attempted termination of pregnancy
Laceration, perforation, tear or chemical damage of vagina following failed attempted termination of pregnancy
CC Excl: PDX collection 961

O07.35 Other venous complications following failed attempted termination of pregnancy CC M♀

O07.36 Cardiac arrest following failed attempted termination of pregnancy CC M♀

O07.37 Sepsis following failed attempted termination of pregnancy CC M♀
Use additional code to identify infectious agent (B95-B97)
Use additional code to identify severe sepsis, if applicable (R65.2-)
EXCLUDES 1 *septic or septicopyemic embolism following failed attempted termination of pregnancy (O07.2)*
CC Excl: PDX collection 956

O07.38 Urinary tract infection following failed attempted termination of pregnancy CC M♀
Cystitis following failed attempted termination of pregnancy

O07.39 Failed attempted termination of pregnancy with other complications CC M♀

O07.4 Failed attempted termination of pregnancy without complication M♀

✓4th **O08 Complications following ectopic and molar pregnancy**
This category is for use with categories O00-O02 to identify any associated complications

CC Excl: For CC/MCC codes in category O08, unless otherwise noted: PDX collection 963

O08.0 Genital tract and pelvic infection following ectopic and molar pregnancy CC M♀
Endometritis following ectopic and molar pregnancy
Oophoritis following ectopic and molar pregnancy
Parametritis following ectopic and molar pregnancy
Pelvic peritonitis following ectopic and molar pregnancy
Salpingitis following ectopic and molar pregnancy
Salpingo-oophoritis following ectopic and molar pregnancy
EXCLUDES 1 *sepsis following ectopic and molar pregnancy (O08.82)*
urinary tract infection (O08.83)
CC Excl: PDX collection 85

O08.1 Delayed or excessive hemorrhage following ectopic and molar pregnancy CC M♀
Afibrinogenemia following ectopic and molar pregnancy
Defibrination syndrome following ectopic and molar pregnancy
Hemolysis following ectopic and molar pregnancy
Intravascular coagulation following ectopic and molar pregnancy
EXCLUDES 1 *delayed or excessive hemorrhage due to incomplete abortion (O03.1)*
CC Excl: PDX collection 962

O08.2 Embolism following ectopic and molar pregnancy MCC M♀
Air embolism following ectopic and molar pregnancy
Amniotic fluid embolism following ectopic and molar pregnancy
Blood-clot embolism following ectopic and molar pregnancy
Embolism NOS following ectopic and molar pregnancy
Fat embolism following ectopic and molar pregnancy
Pulmonary embolism following ectopic and molar pregnancy
Pyemic embolism following ectopic and molar pregnancy
Septic or septicopyemic embolism following ectopic and molar pregnancy
Soap embolism following ectopic and molar pregnancy

O08.3 Shock following ectopic and molar pregnancy MCC M♀
Circulatory collapse following ectopic and molar pregnancy
Shock (postprocedural) following ectopic and molar pregnancy
EXCLUDES 1 *shock due to infection following ectopic and molar pregnancy (O08.82)*

O08.4 Renal failure following ectopic and molar pregnancy MCC M♀
Kidney failure (acute) following ectopic and molar pregnancy
Oliguria following ectopic and molar pregnancy
Renal shutdown following ectopic and molar pregnancy
Renal tubular necrosis following ectopic and molar pregnancy
Uremia following ectopic and molar pregnancy

O08.5 Metabolic disorders following an ectopic and molar pregnancy CC M♀

O08.6 Damage to pelvic organs and tissues following an ectopic and molar pregnancy CC M♀
Laceration, perforation, tear or chemical damage of bladder following an ectopic and molar pregnancy
Laceration, perforation, tear or chemical damage of bowel following an ectopic and molar pregnancy
Laceration, perforation, tear or chemical damage of broad ligament following an ectopic and molar pregnancy
Laceration, perforation, tear or chemical damage of cervix following an ectopic and molar pregnancy
Laceration, perforation, tear or chemical damage of periurethral tissue following an ectopic and molar pregnancy
Laceration, perforation, tear or chemical damage of uterus following an ectopic and molar pregnancy
Laceration, perforation, tear or chemical damage of vagina following an ectopic and molar pregnancy

O08.7 Other venous complications following an ectopic and molar pregnancy CC M♀

✓5th **O08.8 Other complications following an ectopic and molar pregnancy**

O08.81 Cardiac arrest following an ectopic and molar pregnancy CC M♀

O08.82 Sepsis following ectopic and molar pregnancy CC M♀
Use additional code to identify infectious agent (B95-B97)
Use additional code to identify severe sepsis, if applicable (R65.2-)
EXCLUDES 1 *septic or septicopyemic embolism following ectopic and molar pregnancy (O08.2)*
CC Excl: PDX collection 85

O08.83 Urinary tract infection following an ectopic and molar pregnancy CC M♀
Cystitis following an ectopic and molar pregnancy

O08.89 Other complications following an ectopic and molar pregnancy CC M♀

O08.9 Unspecified complication following an ectopic and molar pregnancy CC M♀

Supervision of high risk pregnancy (O09)

✓4th **O09 Supervision of high risk pregnancy**
AHA: 2016, 4Q 48-50, 150

✓5th **O09.0 Supervision of pregnancy with history of infertility**
DEF: Infertility: Inability to conceive for at least one year with regular intercourse.

O09.00 Supervision of pregnancy with history of infertility, unspecified trimester M♀

O09.01 Supervision of pregnancy with history of infertility, first trimester M♀

O09.02 Supervision of pregnancy with history of infertility, second trimester M♀

O09.03 Supervision of pregnancy with history of infertility, third trimester M♀

Chapter 15. Pregnancy, Childbirth and the Puerperium

O09.1–O09.822

✓5ᵗʰ O09.1 Supervision of pregnancy with history of ectopic pregnancy

> **DEF:** Ectopic pregnancy: Implantation of a fertilized egg outside the uterus, usually in the fallopian tube or abdomen that requires emergency treatment.

- **O09.10 Supervision of pregnancy with history of ectopic pregnancy, unspecified trimester** Ⓜ♀
- **O09.11 Supervision of pregnancy with history of ectopic pregnancy, first trimester** Ⓜ♀
- **O09.12 Supervision of pregnancy with history of ectopic pregnancy, second trimester** Ⓜ♀
- **O09.13 Supervision of pregnancy with history of ectopic pregnancy, third trimester** Ⓜ♀

✓5ᵗʰ O09.A Supervision of pregnancy with history of molar pregnancy

> **DEF:** Molar pregnancy: Trophoblastic neoplasm that mimics pregnancy by proliferating from a pathologic ovum and resulting only in a mass of cysts resembling grapes, 80 percent of which are benign, but require surgical removal.

- **O09.A0 Supervision of pregnancy with history of molar pregnancy, unspecified trimester** Ⓜ♀
- **O09.A1 Supervision of pregnancy with history of molar pregnancy, first trimester** Ⓜ♀
- **O09.A2 Supervision of pregnancy with history of molar pregnancy, second trimester** Ⓜ♀
- **O09.A3 Supervision of pregnancy with history of molar pregnancy, third trimester** Ⓜ♀

✓5ᵗʰ O09.2 Supervision of pregnancy with other poor reproductive or obstetric history

> EXCLUDES 2 *pregnancy care for patient with history of recurrent pregnancy loss (O26.2-)*

✓6ᵗʰ O09.21 Supervision of pregnancy with history of pre-term labor

- **O09.211 Supervision of pregnancy with history of pre-term labor, first trimester** Ⓜ♀
- **O09.212 Supervision of pregnancy with history of pre-term labor, second trimester** Ⓜ♀
- **O09.213 Supervision of pregnancy with history of pre-term labor, third trimester** Ⓜ♀
- **O09.219 Supervision of pregnancy with history of pre-term labor, unspecified trimester** Ⓜ♀

✓6ᵗʰ O09.29 Supervision of pregnancy with other poor reproductive or obstetric history

> Supervision of pregnancy with history of neonatal death
> Supervision of pregnancy with history of stillbirth

- **O09.291 Supervision of pregnancy with other poor reproductive or obstetric history, first trimester** Ⓜ♀
- **O09.292 Supervision of pregnancy with other poor reproductive or obstetric history, second trimester** Ⓜ♀
- **O09.293 Supervision of pregnancy with other poor reproductive or obstetric history, third trimester** Ⓜ♀
- **O09.299 Supervision of pregnancy with other poor reproductive or obstetric history, unspecified trimester** Ⓜ♀

✓5ᵗʰ O09.3 Supervision of pregnancy with insufficient antenatal care

> Supervision of concealed pregnancy
> Supervision of hidden pregnancy

- **O09.30 Supervision of pregnancy with insufficient antenatal care, unspecified trimester** Ⓜ♀
- **O09.31 Supervision of pregnancy with insufficient antenatal care, first trimester** Ⓜ♀
- **O09.32 Supervision of pregnancy with insufficient antenatal care, second trimester** Ⓜ♀
- **O09.33 Supervision of pregnancy with insufficient antenatal care, third trimester** Ⓜ♀

✓5ᵗʰ O09.4 Supervision of pregnancy with grand multiparity

- **O09.40 Supervision of pregnancy with grand multiparity, unspecified trimester** Ⓜ♀
- **O09.41 Supervision of pregnancy with grand multiparity, first trimester** Ⓜ♀
- **O09.42 Supervision of pregnancy with grand multiparity, second trimester** Ⓜ♀
- **O09.43 Supervision of pregnancy with grand multiparity, third trimester** Ⓜ♀

✓5ᵗʰ O09.5 Supervision of elderly primigravida and multigravida

> Pregnancy for a female 35 years and older at expected date of delivery

✓6ᵗʰ O09.51 Supervision of elderly primigravida

- **O09.511 Supervision of elderly primigravida, first trimester** Ⓜ♀
- **O09.512 Supervision of elderly primigravida, second trimester** Ⓜ♀
- **O09.513 Supervision of elderly primigravida, third trimester** Ⓜ♀
- **O09.519 Supervision of elderly primigravida, unspecified trimester** Ⓜ♀

✓6ᵗʰ O09.52 Supervision of elderly multigravida

- **O09.521 Supervision of elderly multigravida, first trimester** Ⓜ♀
- **O09.522 Supervision of elderly multigravida, second trimester** Ⓜ♀
- **O09.523 Supervision of elderly multigravida, third trimester** Ⓜ♀
- **O09.529 Supervision of elderly multigravida, unspecified trimester** Ⓜ♀

✓5ᵗʰ O09.6 Supervision of young primigravida and multigravida

> Supervision of pregnancy for a female less than 16 years old at expected date of delivery

✓6ᵗʰ O09.61 Supervision of young primigravida

- **O09.611 Supervision of young primigravida, first trimester** Ⓜ♀
- **O09.612 Supervision of young primigravida, second trimester** Ⓜ♀
- **O09.613 Supervision of young primigravida, third trimester** Ⓜ♀
- **O09.619 Supervision of young primigravida, unspecified trimester** Ⓜ♀

✓6ᵗʰ O09.62 Supervision of young multigravida

- **O09.621 Supervision of young multigravida, first trimester** Ⓜ♀
- **O09.622 Supervision of young multigravida, second trimester** Ⓜ♀
- **O09.623 Supervision of young multigravida, third trimester** Ⓜ♀
- **O09.629 Supervision of young multigravida, unspecified trimester** Ⓜ♀

✓5ᵗʰ O09.7 Supervision of high risk pregnancy due to social problems

- **O09.70 Supervision of high risk pregnancy due to social problems, unspecified trimester** Ⓜ♀
- **O09.71 Supervision of high risk pregnancy due to social problems, first trimester** Ⓜ♀
- **O09.72 Supervision of high risk pregnancy due to social problems, second trimester** Ⓜ♀
- **O09.73 Supervision of high risk pregnancy due to social problems, third trimester** Ⓜ♀

✓5ᵗʰ O09.8 Supervision of other high risk pregnancies

✓6ᵗʰ O09.81 Supervision of pregnancy resulting from assisted reproductive technology

> Supervision of pregnancy resulting from in-vitro fertilization
>
> EXCLUDES 2 *gestational carrier status (Z33.3)*

- **O09.811 Supervision of pregnancy resulting from assisted reproductive technology, first trimester** Ⓜ♀
- **O09.812 Supervision of pregnancy resulting from assisted reproductive technology, second trimester** Ⓜ♀
- **O09.813 Supervision of pregnancy resulting from assisted reproductive technology, third trimester** Ⓜ♀
- **O09.819 Supervision of pregnancy resulting from assisted reproductive technology, unspecified trimester** Ⓜ♀

✓6ᵗʰ O09.82 Supervision of pregnancy with history of in utero procedure during previous pregnancy

- **O09.821 Supervision of pregnancy with history of in utero procedure during previous pregnancy, first trimester** Ⓜ♀
- **O09.822 Supervision of pregnancy with history of in utero procedure during previous pregnancy, second trimester** Ⓜ♀

Ⓝ Newborn: 0   Ⓟ Pediatric: 0-17   Ⓜ Maternity: 12-55   Ⓐ Adult: 15-124   **MCC** Major Complication/Comorbidity   **CC** Complication/Comorbidity   **SW** Severe Wound Dx

854   ICD-10-CM 2019

      O09.823 **Supervision of pregnancy with history** Ⓜ♀
of in utero procedure during previous
pregnancy, third trimester

      O09.829 **Supervision of pregnancy with history** Ⓜ♀
of in utero procedure during previous
pregnancy, unspecified trimester
       EXCLUDES 1   supervision of pregnancy affected
by in utero procedure during
current pregnancy (O35.7)

  ✓6ᵗʰ **O09.89** **Supervision of other high risk pregnancies**
      O09.891 **Supervision of other high risk** Ⓜ♀
pregnancies, first trimester
      O09.892 **Supervision of other high risk** Ⓜ♀
pregnancies, second trimester
      O09.893 **Supervision of other high risk** Ⓜ♀
pregnancies, third trimester
      O09.899 **Supervision of other high risk** Ⓜ♀
pregnancies, unspecified trimester

 ✓5ᵗʰ **O09.9** **Supervision of high risk pregnancy, unspecified**
      O09.90 **Supervision of high risk pregnancy,** Ⓜ♀
unspecified, unspecified trimester
      O09.91 **Supervision of high risk pregnancy,** Ⓜ♀
unspecified, first trimester
      O09.92 **Supervision of high risk pregnancy,** Ⓜ♀
unspecified, second trimester
      O09.93 **Supervision of high risk pregnancy,** Ⓜ♀
unspecified, third trimester

Edema, proteinuria and hypertensive disorders in pregnancy, childbirth and the puerperium (O10-O16)

AHA: 2016, 4Q, 50

✓4ᵗʰ **O10** **Pre-existing hypertension complicating pregnancy, childbirth and the puerperium**
     INCLUDES   pre-existing hypertension with pre-existing proteinuria
complicating pregnancy, childbirth and the puerperium
     EXCLUDES 2   pre-existing hypertension with superimposed pre-eclampsia
complicating pregnancy, childbirth and the puerperium
(O11.-)

     CC Excl: For CC/MCC codes in category O10: PDX collection 964

✓5ᵗʰ **O10.0** **Pre-existing essential hypertension complicating pregnancy, childbirth and the puerperium**
      Any condition in I10 specified as a reason for obstetric care
during pregnancy, childbirth or the puerperium

  ✓6ᵗʰ **O10.01** **Pre-existing essential hypertension complicating pregnancy**
      O10.011 **Pre-existing essential hypertension** ⒸⒸ Ⓜ♀
complicating pregnancy, first
trimester
      O10.012 **Pre-existing essential hypertension** ⒸⒸ Ⓜ♀
complicating pregnancy, second
trimester
      O10.013 **Pre-existing essential hypertension** ⒸⒸ Ⓜ♀
complicating pregnancy, third
trimester
      O10.019 **Pre-existing essential hypertension** Ⓜ♀
complicating pregnancy, unspecified
trimester
      O10.02 **Pre-existing essential hypertension** ⒸⒸ Ⓜ♀
complicating childbirth
      O10.03 **Pre-existing essential hypertension** Ⓜ♀
complicating the puerperium

 ✓5ᵗʰ **O10.1** **Pre-existing hypertensive heart disease complicating pregnancy, childbirth and the puerperium**
      Any condition in I11 specified as a reason for obstetric care
during pregnancy, childbirth or the puerperium
      Use additional code from I11 to identify the type of hypertensive
heart disease

  ✓6ᵗʰ **O10.11** **Pre-existing hypertensive heart disease complicating pregnancy**
      O10.111 **Pre-existing hypertensive heart** Ⓜ♀
disease complicating pregnancy,
first trimester
      O10.112 **Pre-existing hypertensive heart** Ⓜ♀
disease complicating pregnancy,
second trimester
      O10.113 **Pre-existing hypertensive heart** Ⓜ♀
disease complicating pregnancy,
third trimester

      O10.119 **Pre-existing hypertensive heart** Ⓜ♀
disease complicating pregnancy,
unspecified trimester
      O10.12 **Pre-existing hypertensive heart disease** Ⓜ♀
complicating childbirth
      O10.13 **Pre-existing hypertensive heart disease** Ⓜ♀
complicating the puerperium

✓5ᵗʰ **O10.2** **Pre-existing hypertensive chronic kidney disease complicating pregnancy, childbirth and the puerperium**
      Any condition in I12 specified as a reason for obstetric care
during pregnancy, childbirth or the puerperium
      Use additional code from I12 to identify the type of hypertensive
chronic kidney disease

  ✓6ᵗʰ **O10.21** **Pre-existing hypertensive chronic kidney disease complicating pregnancy**
      O10.211 **Pre-existing hypertensive chronic** Ⓜ♀
kidney disease complicating p
regnancy, first trimester
      O10.212 **Pre-existing hypertensive chronic** Ⓜ♀
kidney disease complicating
pregnancy, second trimester
      O10.213 **Pre-existing hypertensive chronic** Ⓜ♀
kidney disease complicating
pregnancy, third trimester
      O10.219 **Pre-existing hypertensive chronic** Ⓜ♀
kidney disease complicating pregnancy,
unspecified trimester
      O10.22 **Pre-existing hypertensive chronic kidney** Ⓜ♀
disease complicating childbirth
      O10.23 **Pre-existing hypertensive chronic kidney** Ⓜ♀
disease complicating the puerperium

✓5ᵗʰ **O10.3** **Pre-existing hypertensive heart and chronic kidney disease complicating pregnancy, childbirth and the puerperium**
      Any condition in I13 specified as a reason for obstetric care
during pregnancy, childbirth or the puerperium
      Use additional code from I13 to identify the type of hypertensive
heart and chronic kidney disease

  ✓6ᵗʰ **O10.31** **Pre-existing hypertensive heart and chronic kidney disease complicating pregnancy**
      O10.311 **Pre-existing hypertensive heart and** Ⓜ♀
chronic kidney disease complicating
pregnancy, first trimester
      O10.312 **Pre-existing hypertensive heart and** Ⓜ♀
chronic kidney disease complicating
pregnancy, second trimester
      O10.313 **Pre-existing hypertensive heart and** Ⓜ♀
chronic kidney disease complicating
pregnancy, third trimester
      O10.319 **Pre-existing hypertensive heart and** Ⓜ♀
chronic kidney disease complicating
pregnancy, unspecified trimester
      O10.32 **Pre-existing hypertensive heart and chronic** Ⓜ♀
kidney disease complicating childbirth
      O10.33 **Pre-existing hypertensive heart and chronic** Ⓜ♀
kidney disease complicating the puerperium

✓5ᵗʰ **O10.4** **Pre-existing secondary hypertension complicating pregnancy, childbirth and the puerperium**
      Any condition in I15 specified as a reason for obstetric care
during pregnancy, childbirth or the puerperium
      Use additional code from I15 to identify the type of secondary
hypertension

  ✓6ᵗʰ **O10.41** **Pre-existing secondary hypertension complicating pregnancy**
      O10.411 **Pre-existing secondary** ⒸⒸ Ⓜ♀
hypertension complicating
pregnancy, first trimester
      O10.412 **Pre-existing secondary** ⒸⒸ Ⓜ♀
hypertension complicating
pregnancy, second trimester
      O10.413 **Pre-existing secondary** ⒸⒸ Ⓜ♀
hypertension complicating
pregnancy, third trimester
      O10.419 **Pre-existing secondary hypertension** Ⓜ♀
complicating pregnancy, unspecified
trimester
      O10.42 **Pre-existing secondary hypertension** ⒹⒸⒸ Ⓜ♀
complicating childbirth
      O10.43 **Pre-existing secondary hypertension** ⒸⒸ Ⓜ♀
complicating the puerperium

✓5ᵗʰ **O10.9** Unspecified pre-existing hypertension complicating pregnancy, childbirth and the puerperium

    ✓6ᵗʰ **O10.91** Unspecified pre-existing hypertension complicating pregnancy

         O10.911 Unspecified pre-existing hypertension complicating pregnancy, **first trimester**   CC M ♀

         O10.912 Unspecified pre-existing hypertension complicating pregnancy, **second trimester**   CC M ♀

         O10.913 Unspecified pre-existing hypertension complicating pregnancy, **third trimester**   CC M ♀

         O10.919 Unspecified pre-existing hypertension complicating pregnancy, **unspecified trimester**   M ♀

    O10.92 Unspecified pre-existing hypertension complicating **childbirth**   CC M ♀

    O10.93 Unspecified pre-existing hypertension complicating the **puerperium**   M ♀

✓4ᵗʰ **O11** Pre-existing **hypertension** with pre-eclampsia

    INCLUDES   conditions in O10 complicated by pre-eclampsia
pre-eclampsia superimposed pre-existing hypertension

    Use additional code from O10 to identify the type of hypertension

    DEF: Complication of pregnancy manifesting in the development of borderline hypertension, protein in the urine, and unresponsive swelling between the 20th week of pregnancy and the end of the first week following birth in mild to moderate cases. Severe preeclampsia presents with hypertension, associated with marked swelling, proteinuria, abdominal pain, and/or visual changes.

    CC Excl: For MCC codes in category O11: PDX collection 964

    O11.1 Pre-existing hypertension with pre-eclampsia, **first trimester**   MCC M ♀

    O11.2 Pre-existing hypertension with pre-eclampsia, **second trimester**   MCC M ♀

    O11.3 Pre-existing hypertension with pre-eclampsia, **third trimester**   MCC M ♀

    O11.4 Pre-existing hypertension with pre-eclampsia, complicating **childbirth**   M ♀

    O11.5 Pre-existing hypertension with pre-eclampsia, complicating the **puerperium**   M ♀

    O11.9 Pre-existing hypertension with pre-eclampsia, **unspecified trimester**   M ♀

✓4ᵗʰ **O12** Gestational **[pregnancy-induced] edema and proteinuria** without hypertension

    CC Excl: For CC codes in category O12: PDX collection 965

    ✓5ᵗʰ **O12.0** Gestational **edema**

         O12.00 Gestational edema, **unspecified trimester**   M ♀

         O12.01 Gestational edema, **first trimester**   M ♀

         O12.02 Gestational edema, **second trimester**   M ♀

         O12.03 Gestational edema, **third trimester**   M ♀

         O12.04 Gestational edema, complicating **childbirth**   M ♀

         O12.05 Gestational edema, complicating the **puerperium**   M ♀

    ✓5ᵗʰ **O12.1** Gestational **proteinuria**

         O12.10 Gestational proteinuria, **unspecified trimester**   M ♀

         O12.11 Gestational proteinuria, **first trimester**   CC M ♀

         O12.12 Gestational proteinuria, **second trimester**   CC M ♀

         O12.13 Gestational proteinuria, **third trimester**   CC M ♀

         O12.14 Gestational proteinuria, complicating **childbirth**   M ♀

         O12.15 Gestational proteinuria, complicating the **puerperium**   M ♀

    ✓5ᵗʰ **O12.2** Gestational **edema with proteinuria**

         O12.20 Gestational edema with proteinuria, **unspecified trimester**   M ♀

         O12.21 Gestational edema with proteinuria, **first trimester**   CC M ♀

         O12.22 Gestational edema with proteinuria, **second trimester**   CC M ♀

         O12.23 Gestational edema with proteinuria, **third trimester**   CC M ♀

         O12.24 Gestational edema with proteinuria, complicating **childbirth**   M ♀

         O12.25 Gestational edema with proteinuria, complicating the **puerperium**   M ♀

✓4ᵗʰ **O13** Gestational **[pregnancy-induced] hypertension without significant proteinuria**

    INCLUDES   gestational hypertension NOS
transient hypertension of pregnancy

    AHA: 2016, 1Q, 5

    O13.1 Gestational [pregnancy-induced] hypertension without significant proteinuria, **first trimester**   M ♀

    O13.2 Gestational [pregnancy-induced] hypertension without significant proteinuria, **second trimester**   M ♀

    O13.3 Gestational [pregnancy-induced] hypertension without significant proteinuria, **third trimester**   M ♀

    O13.4 Gestational [pregnancy-induced] hypertension without significant proteinuria, complicating **childbirth**   M ♀

    O13.5 Gestational [pregnancy-induced] hypertension without significant proteinuria, complicating the **puerperium**   M ♀

    O13.9 Gestational [pregnancy-induced] hypertension without significant proteinuria, **unspecified trimester**   M ♀

✓4ᵗʰ **O14** Pre-eclampsia

    EXCLUDES 1   *pre-existing hypertension with pre-eclampsia (O11)*

    DEF: Complication of pregnancy manifesting in the development of borderline hypertension, protein in the urine, and unresponsive swelling between the 20th week of pregnancy and the end of the first week following birth in mild to moderate cases. Severe preeclampsia presents with hypertension, associated with marked swelling, proteinuria, abdominal pain, and/or visual changes.

    CC Excl: For CC/MCC codes in category O14: PDX collection 964

    ✓5ᵗʰ **O14.0** Mild to moderate **pre-eclampsia**

         O14.00 Mild to moderate pre-eclampsia, **unspecified trimester**   M ♀

         O14.02 Mild to moderate pre-eclampsia, **second trimester**   CC M ♀

         O14.03 Mild to moderate pre-eclampsia, **third trimester**   CC M ♀

         O14.04 Mild to moderate pre-eclampsia, complicating **childbirth**   M ♀

         O14.05 Mild to moderate pre-eclampsia, complicating the **puerperium**   M ♀

    ✓5ᵗʰ **O14.1** Severe **pre-eclampsia**

         EXCLUDES 1   *HELLP syndrome (O14.2-)*

         O14.10 Severe pre-eclampsia, **unspecified trimester**   M ♀

         O14.12 Severe pre-eclampsia, **second trimester**   MCC M ♀

         O14.13 Severe pre-eclampsia, **third trimester**   MCC M ♀

         O14.14 Severe pre-eclampsia complicating **childbirth**   M ♀

         O14.15 Severe pre-eclampsia, complicating the **puerperium**   M ♀

    ✓5ᵗʰ **O14.2** HELLP syndrome

         Severe pre-eclampsia with hemolysis, elevated liver enzymes and low platelet count (HELLP)

         O14.20 HELLP syndrome (HELLP), **unspecified trimester**   M ♀

         O14.22 HELLP syndrome (HELLP), **second trimester**   MCC M ♀

         O14.23 HELLP syndrome (HELLP), **third trimester**   MCC M ♀

         O14.24 HELLP syndrome, complicating **childbirth**   M ♀

         O14.25 HELLP syndrome, complicating the **puerperium**   M ♀

    ✓5ᵗʰ **O14.9** Unspecified **pre-eclampsia**

         O14.90 Unspecified pre-eclampsia, **unspecified trimester**   M ♀

         O14.92 Unspecified pre-eclampsia, **second trimester**   CC M ♀

         O14.93 Unspecified pre-eclampsia, **third trimester**   CC M ♀

         O14.94 Unspecified pre-eclampsia, complicating **childbirth**   M ♀

         O14.95 Unspecified pre-eclampsia, complicating the **puerperium**   M ♀

✓4ᵗʰ **O15** Eclampsia

    INCLUDES   convulsions following conditions in O10-O14 and O16

    DEF: Tetany and toxemia producing seizure activity or coma in a pregnant patient who most often has presented with prior preeclampsia (i.e., hypertension, albuminuria, and edema).

    CC Excl: For MCC codes in category O15: PDX collection 964

    ✓5ᵗʰ **O15.0** Eclampsia complicating **pregnancy**

         O15.00 Eclampsia complicating pregnancy, **unspecified trimester**   M ♀

N Newborn: 0   P Pediatric: 0-17   M Maternity: 12-55   A Adult: 15-124   MCC Major Complication/Comorbidity   CC Complication/Comorbidity   SW Severe Wound Dx

856   ICD-10-CM 2019

       O15.02   **Eclampsia complicating pregnancy, second trimester**   MCC M ♀

       O15.03   **Eclampsia complicating pregnancy, third trimester**   MCC M ♀

   O15.1   **Eclampsia complicating** labor   MCC M ♀

   O15.2   **Eclampsia complicating the** puerperium   MCC M ♀

   O15.9   **Eclampsia,** unspecified **as to time period**   M ♀
       Eclampsia NOS

✓4ᵗʰ **O16**   **Unspecified maternal hypertension**

> **CC Excl: For CC codes in category O16:** PDX collection 964

   O16.1   **Unspecified maternal hypertension,** first trimester   CC M ♀

   O16.2   **Unspecified maternal hypertension,** second trimester   CC M ♀

   O16.3   **Unspecified maternal hypertension,** third trimester   CC M ♀

   O16.4   **Unspecified maternal hypertension,** complicating childbirth   M ♀

   O16.5   **Unspecified maternal hypertension,** complicating the puerperium   M ♀

   O16.9   **Unspecified maternal hypertension,** unspecified trimester   M ♀

Other maternal disorders predominantly related to pregnancy (O20-O29)

> EXCLUDES 2   maternal care related to the fetus and amniotic cavity and possible delivery problems (O30-O48)
> maternal diseases classifiable elsewhere but complicating pregnancy, labor and delivery, and the puerperium (O98-O99)

✓4ᵗʰ **O20**   **Hemorrhage in early pregnancy**
       Hemorrhage before completion of 20 weeks gestation
> EXCLUDES 1   pregnancy with abortive outcome (O00-O08)

   O20.0   **Threatened abortion**   CC M ♀
       Hemorrhage specified as due to threatened abortion
       DEF: Bloody discharge during pregnancy. The cervix may be dilated and pregnancy threatened, but the pregnancy is not terminated.
       CC Excl: PDX collection 966

   O20.8   **Other hemorrhage in early pregnancy**   M ♀

   O20.9   **Hemorrhage in early pregnancy,** unspecified   CC M ♀
       CC Excl: PDX collection 966

✓4ᵗʰ **O21**   **Excessive vomiting in pregnancy**
   O21.0   Mild **hyperemesis gravidarum**   M ♀
       Hyperemesis gravidarum, mild or unspecified, starting before the end of the 20th week of gestation

   O21.1   **Hyperemesis gravidarum with** metabolic disturbance   M ♀
       Hyperemesis gravidarum, starting before the end of the 20th week of gestation, with metabolic disturbance such as carbohydrate depletion
       Hyperemesis gravidarum, starting before the end of the 20th week of gestation, with metabolic disturbance such as dehydration
       Hyperemesis gravidarum, starting before the end of the 20th week of gestation, with metabolic disturbance such as electrolyte imbalance

   O21.2   Late **vomiting of pregnancy**   M ♀
       Excessive vomiting starting after 20 completed weeks of gestation

   O21.8   Other **vomiting complicating pregnancy**   M ♀
       Vomiting due to diseases classified elsewhere, complicating pregnancy
       Use additional code to identify cause

   O21.9   **Vomiting of pregnancy,** unspecified   M ♀

✓4ᵗʰ **O22**   **Venous complications and hemorrhoids in pregnancy**
> EXCLUDES 1   venous complications of:
>   abortion NOS (O03.9)
>   ectopic or molar pregnancy (O08.7)
>   failed attempted abortion (O07.35)
>   induced abortion (O04.85)
>   spontaneous abortion (O03.89)
> EXCLUDES 2   obstetric pulmonary embolism (O88.-)
>   venous complications and hemorrhoids of childbirth and the puerperium (O87.-)

> **CC Excl: For CC/MCC codes in category O22:** PDX collection 967

✓5ᵗʰ **O22.0**   Varicose veins of lower extremity **in pregnancy**
       Varicose veins NOS in pregnancy
       DEF: Distended, tortuous veins of the lower extremities associated with pregnancy.

   O22.00   **Varicose veins of lower extremity in pregnancy,** unspecified trimester   M ♀

   O22.01   **Varicose veins of lower extremity in pregnancy,** first trimester   M ♀

   O22.02   **Varicose veins of lower extremity in pregnancy,** second trimester   M ♀

   O22.03   **Varicose veins of lower extremity in pregnancy,** third trimester   M ♀

✓5ᵗʰ **O22.1**   Genital varices **in pregnancy**
       Perineal varices in pregnancy
       Vaginal varices in pregnancy
       Vulval varices in pregnancy

   O22.10   **Genital varices in pregnancy,** unspecified trimester   M ♀

   O22.11   **Genital varices in pregnancy,** first trimester   M ♀

   O22.12   **Genital varices in pregnancy,** second trimester   M ♀

   O22.13   **Genital varices in pregnancy,** third trimester   M ♀

✓5ᵗʰ **O22.2**   Superficial thrombophlebitis **in pregnancy**
       Phlebitis in pregnancy NOS
       Thrombophlebitis of legs in pregnancy
       Thrombosis in pregnancy NOS
       Use additional code to identify the superficial thrombophlebitis (I80.0-)

   O22.20   **Superficial thrombophlebitis in pregnancy,** unspecified trimester   CC M ♀

   O22.21   **Superficial thrombophlebitis in pregnancy,** first trimester   CC M ♀

   O22.22   **Superficial thrombophlebitis in pregnancy,** second trimester   CC M ♀

   O22.23   **Superficial thrombophlebitis in pregnancy,** third trimester   CC M ♀

✓5ᵗʰ **O22.3**   Deep phlebothrombosis **in pregnancy**
       Deep vein thrombosis, antepartum
       Use additional code to identify the deep vein thrombosis (I82.4-, I82.5-, I82.62-, I82.72-)
       Use additional code, if applicable, for associated long-term (current) use of anticoagulants (Z79.01)

   O22.30   **Deep phlebothrombosis in pregnancy,** unspecified trimester   CC M ♀

   O22.31   **Deep phlebothrombosis in pregnancy,** first trimester   MCC M ♀

   O22.32   **Deep phlebothrombosis in pregnancy,** second trimester   MCC M ♀

   O22.33   **Deep phlebothrombosis in pregnancy,** third trimester   MCC M ♀

✓5ᵗʰ **O22.4**   Hemorrhoids **in pregnancy**
   O22.40   **Hemorrhoids in pregnancy,** unspecified trimester   CC M ♀

   O22.41   **Hemorrhoids in pregnancy,** first trimester   CC M ♀

   O22.42   **Hemorrhoids in pregnancy,** second trimester   CC M ♀

   O22.43   **Hemorrhoids in pregnancy,** third trimester   CC M ♀

✓5ᵗʰ **O22.5**   Cerebral venous thrombosis **in pregnancy**
       Cerebrovenous sinus thrombosis in pregnancy

   O22.50   **Cerebral venous thrombosis in pregnancy,** unspecified trimester   CC M ♀

   O22.51   **Cerebral venous thrombosis in pregnancy,** first trimester   CC M ♀

   O22.52   **Cerebral venous thrombosis in pregnancy,** second trimester   CC M ♀

   O22.53   **Cerebral venous thrombosis in pregnancy,** third trimester   CC M ♀

✓5ᵗʰ **O22.8**   Other venous complications **in pregnancy**
  ✓6ᵗʰ **O22.8X**   Other **venous complications in pregnancy**

      O22.8X1   **Other venous complications in pregnancy,** first trimester   CC M ♀

      O22.8X2   **Other venous complications in pregnancy,** second trimester   CC M ♀

      O22.8X3   **Other venous complications in pregnancy,** third trimester   CC M ♀

      O22.8X9   **Other venous complications in pregnancy,** unspecified trimester   CC M ♀

✓ Additional Character Required   ✓x7ᵗʰ Placeholder   Unacceptable PDx   Questionable PDx   Manifestation   H1 -H14 HAC   HCC CMS-HCC Dx   HIV HIV Dx

ICD-10-CM 2019   **857**

✓5ᵗʰ O22.9 Venous complication in pregnancy, unspecified
Gestational phlebitis NOS
Gestational phlebopathy NOS
Gestational thrombosis NOS

  O22.90 Venous complication in pregnancy, unspecified, unspecified trimester `CC` `M♀`

  O22.91 Venous complication in pregnancy, unspecified, first trimester `M♀`

  O22.92 Venous complication in pregnancy, unspecified, second trimester `M♀`

  O22.93 Venous complication in pregnancy, unspecified, third trimester `M♀`

✓4ᵗʰ O23 Infections of genitourinary tract in pregnancy
Use additional code to identify organism (B95.-, B96.-)

> EXCLUDES 2   gonococcal infections complicating pregnancy, childbirth and the puerperium (O98.2)
> infections with a predominantly sexual mode of transmission NOS complicating pregnancy, childbirth and the puerperium (O98.3)
> syphilis complicating pregnancy, childbirth and the puerperium (O98.1)
> tuberculosis of genitourinary system complicating pregnancy, childbirth and the puerperium (O98.0)
> venereal disease NOS complicating pregnancy, childbirth and the puerperium (O98.3)

AHA: 2018, 2Q, 20

CC Excl: For CC codes in category O23: PDX collection 968

✓5ᵗʰ O23.0 Infections of kidney in pregnancy
Pyelonephritis in pregnancy

  O23.00 Infections of kidney in pregnancy, unspecified trimester `M♀`

  O23.01 Infections of kidney in pregnancy, first trimester `CC` `M♀`

  O23.02 Infections of kidney in pregnancy, second trimester `CC` `M♀`

  O23.03 Infections of kidney in pregnancy, third trimester `CC` `M♀`

✓5ᵗʰ O23.1 Infections of bladder in pregnancy

  O23.10 Infections of bladder in pregnancy, unspecified trimester `M♀`

  O23.11 Infections of bladder in pregnancy, first trimester `CC` `M♀`

  O23.12 Infections of bladder in pregnancy, second trimester `CC` `M♀`

  O23.13 Infections of bladder in pregnancy, third trimester `CC` `M♀`

✓5ᵗʰ O23.2 Infections of urethra in pregnancy

  O23.20 Infections of urethra in pregnancy, unspecified trimester `M♀`

  O23.21 Infections of urethra in pregnancy, first trimester `CC` `M♀`

  O23.22 Infections of urethra in pregnancy, second trimester `CC` `M♀`

  O23.23 Infections of urethra in pregnancy, third trimester `CC` `M♀`

✓5ᵗʰ O23.3 Infections of other parts of urinary tract in pregnancy

  O23.30 Infections of other parts of urinary tract in pregnancy, unspecified trimester `M♀`

  O23.31 Infections of other parts of urinary tract in pregnancy, first trimester `CC` `M♀`

  O23.32 Infections of other parts of urinary tract in pregnancy, second trimester `CC` `M♀`

  O23.33 Infections of other parts of urinary tract in pregnancy, third trimester `CC` `M♀`

✓5ᵗʰ O23.4 Unspecified infection of urinary tract in pregnancy

  O23.40 Unspecified infection of urinary tract in pregnancy, unspecified trimester `M♀`

  O23.41 Unspecified infection of urinary tract in pregnancy, first trimester `CC` `M♀`

  O23.42 Unspecified infection of urinary tract in pregnancy, second trimester `CC` `M♀`

  O23.43 Unspecified infection of urinary tract in pregnancy, third trimester `CC` `M♀`

✓5ᵗʰ O23.5 Infections of the genital tract in pregnancy

  ✓6ᵗʰ O23.51 Infection of cervix in pregnancy

    O23.511 Infections of cervix in pregnancy, first trimester `CC` `M♀`

    O23.512 Infections of cervix in pregnancy, second trimester `CC` `M♀`

    O23.513 Infections of cervix in pregnancy, third trimester `CC` `M♀`

    O23.519 Infections of cervix in pregnancy, unspecified trimester `M♀`

  ✓6ᵗʰ O23.52 Salpingo-oophoritis in pregnancy
Oophoritis in pregnancy
Salpingitis in pregnancy

    O23.521 Salpingo-oophoritis in pregnancy, first trimester `CC` `M♀`

    O23.522 Salpingo-oophoritis in pregnancy, second trimester `CC` `M♀`

    O23.523 Salpingo-oophoritis in pregnancy, third trimester `CC` `M♀`

    O23.529 Salpingo-oophoritis in pregnancy, unspecified trimester `M♀`

  ✓6ᵗʰ O23.59 Infection of other part of genital tract in pregnancy

    O23.591 Infection of other part of genital tract in pregnancy, first trimester `CC` `M♀`

    O23.592 Infection of other part of genital tract in pregnancy, second trimester `CC` `M♀`

    O23.593 Infection of other part of genital tract in pregnancy, third trimester `CC` `M♀`

    O23.599 Infection of other part of genital tract in pregnancy, unspecified trimester `M♀`

✓5ᵗʰ O23.9 Unspecified genitourinary tract infection in pregnancy
Genitourinary tract infection in pregnancy NOS

  O23.90 Unspecified genitourinary tract infection in pregnancy, unspecified trimester `M♀`

  O23.91 Unspecified genitourinary tract infection in pregnancy, first trimester `CC` `M♀`

  O23.92 Unspecified genitourinary tract infection in pregnancy, second trimester `CC` `M♀`

  O23.93 Unspecified genitourinary tract infection in pregnancy, third trimester `CC` `M♀`

✓4ᵗʰ O24 Diabetes mellitus in pregnancy, childbirth, and the puerperium

CC Excl: For CC/MCC codes in category O24: PDX collection 969

✓5ᵗʰ O24.0 Pre-existing type 1 diabetes mellitus, in pregnancy, childbirth and the puerperium
Juvenile onset diabetes mellitus, in pregnancy, childbirth and the puerperium
Ketosis-prone diabetes mellitus in pregnancy, childbirth and the puerperium
Use additional code from category E10 to further identify any manifestations

  ✓6ᵗʰ O24.01 Pre-existing type 1 diabetes mellitus, in pregnancy

    O24.011 Pre-existing type 1 diabetes mellitus, in pregnancy, first trimester `CC` `M♀`

    O24.012 Pre-existing type 1 diabetes mellitus, in pregnancy, second trimester `CC` `M♀`

    O24.013 Pre-existing type 1 diabetes mellitus, in pregnancy, third trimester `CC` `M♀`

    O24.019 Pre-existing type 1 diabetes mellitus, in pregnancy, unspecified trimester `CC` `M♀`

  O24.02 Pre-existing type 1 diabetes mellitus, in childbirth `MCC` `M♀`

  O24.03 Pre-existing type 1 diabetes mellitus, in the puerperium `CC` `M♀`

✓5ᵗʰ O24.1 Pre-existing type 2 diabetes mellitus, in pregnancy, childbirth and the puerperium
Insulin-resistant diabetes mellitus in pregnancy, childbirth and the puerperium
Use additional code (for):
· from category E11 to further identify any manifestations
long-term (current) use of insulin (Z79.4)

  ✓6ᵗʰ O24.11 Pre-existing type 2 diabetes mellitus, in pregnancy

    O24.111 Pre-existing type 2 diabetes mellitus, in pregnancy, first trimester `CC` `M♀`

`N` Newborn: 0   `P` Pediatric: 0-17   `M` Maternity: 12-55   `A` Adult: 15-124   `MCC` Major Complication/Comorbidity   `CC` Complication/Comorbidity   `SW` Severe Wound Dx

858   ICD-10-CM 2019

O24.112   Pre-existing type 2 diabetes mellitus, in pregnancy, **second trimester**   `CC` `M` ♀

O24.113   Pre-existing type 2 diabetes mellitus, in pregnancy, **third trimester**   `CC` `M` ♀

O24.119   Pre-existing type 2 diabetes mellitus, in pregnancy, **unspecified trimester**   `CC` `M` ♀

O24.12   Pre-existing type 2 diabetes mellitus, in **childbirth**   `MCC` `M` ♀

O24.13   Pre-existing type 2 diabetes mellitus, in the **puerperium**   `CC` `M` ♀

✓5ᵗʰ **O24.3**   Unspecified pre-existing **diabetes mellitus in pregnancy, childbirth and the puerperium**

> Use additional code (for):
> from category E11 to further identify any manifestation
> long-term (current) use of insulin (Z79.4)

✓6ᵗʰ **O24.31**   Unspecified pre-existing diabetes mellitus in **pregnancy**

O24.311   Unspecified pre-existing diabetes mellitus in pregnancy, **first trimester**   `CC` `M` ♀

O24.312   Unspecified pre-existing diabetes mellitus in pregnancy, **second trimester**   `CC` `M` ♀

O24.313   Unspecified pre-existing diabetes mellitus in pregnancy, **third trimester**   `CC` `M` ♀

O24.319   Unspecified pre-existing diabetes mellitus in pregnancy, **unspecified trimester**   `CC` `M` ♀

O24.32   Unspecified pre-existing diabetes mellitus in **childbirth**   `MCC` `M` ♀

O24.33   Unspecified pre-existing diabetes mellitus in the **puerperium**   `CC` `M` ♀

✓5ᵗʰ **O24.4**   Gestational **diabetes mellitus**

> Diabetes mellitus arising in pregnancy
> Gestational diabetes mellitus NOS
> **AHA:** 2016, 4Q, 50

✓6ᵗʰ **O24.41**   Gestational diabetes mellitus in **pregnancy**

O24.410   Gestational diabetes mellitus in pregnancy, **diet controlled**   `M` ♀

O24.414   Gestational diabetes mellitus in pregnancy, **insulin controlled**   `M` ♀

O24.415   Gestational diabetes mellitus in pregnancy, **controlled by oral hypoglycemic drugs**   `M` ♀
> Gestational diabetes mellitus in pregnancy, controlled by oral antidiabetic drugs

O24.419   Gestational diabetes mellitus in pregnancy, **unspecified control**   `M` ♀
> **AHA:** 2015, 4Q, 34

✓6ᵗʰ **O24.42**   Gestational diabetes mellitus in **childbirth**
> **AHA:** 2016, 1Q, 5

O24.420   Gestational diabetes mellitus in childbirth, **diet controlled**   `M` ♀

O24.424   Gestational diabetes mellitus in childbirth, **insulin controlled**   `M` ♀

O24.425   Gestational diabetes mellitus in childbirth, **controlled by oral hypoglycemic drugs**   `M` ♀
> Gestational diabetes mellitus in childbirth, controlled by oral antidiabetic drugs

O24.429   Gestational diabetes mellitus in childbirth, **unspecified control**   `M` ♀
> **AHA:** 2015, 4Q, 34

✓6ᵗʰ **O24.43**   Gestational diabetes mellitus in the **puerperium**

O24.430   Gestational diabetes mellitus in the puerperium, **diet controlled**   `M` ♀

O24.434   Gestational diabetes mellitus in the puerperium, **insulin controlled**   `M` ♀

O24.435   Gestational diabetes mellitus in puerperium, **controlled by oral hypoglycemic drugs**   `M` ♀
> Gestational diabetes mellitus in puerperium, controlled by oral antidiabetic drugs

O24.439   Gestational diabetes mellitus in the puerperium, **unspecified control**   `M` ♀
> **AHA:** 2015, 4Q, 34

✓5ᵗʰ **O24.8**   Other pre-existing **diabetes mellitus in pregnancy, childbirth, and the puerperium**

> Use additional code (for):
> from categories E08, E09 and E13 to further identify any manifestation
> long-term (current) use of insulin (Z79.4)

✓6ᵗʰ **O24.81**   Other pre-existing diabetes mellitus in **pregnancy**

O24.811   Other pre-existing diabetes mellitus in pregnancy, **first trimester**   `CC` `M` ♀

O24.812   Other pre-existing diabetes mellitus in pregnancy, **second trimester**   `CC` `M` ♀

O24.813   Other pre-existing diabetes mellitus in pregnancy, **third trimester**   `CC` `M` ♀

O24.819   Other pre-existing diabetes mellitus in pregnancy, **unspecified trimester**   `CC` `M` ♀

O24.82   Other pre-existing diabetes mellitus in **childbirth**   `MCC` `M` ♀

O24.83   Other pre-existing diabetes mellitus in the **puerperium**   `CC` `M` ♀

✓5ᵗʰ **O24.9**   Unspecified **diabetes mellitus in pregnancy, childbirth and the puerperium**

> Use additional code for long-term (current) use of insulin (Z79.4)

✓6ᵗʰ **O24.91**   Unspecified diabetes mellitus in **pregnancy**

O24.911   Unspecified diabetes mellitus in pregnancy, **first trimester**   `CC` `M` ♀

O24.912   Unspecified diabetes mellitus in pregnancy, **second trimester**   `CC` `M` ♀

O24.913   Unspecified diabetes mellitus in pregnancy, **third trimester**   `CC` `M` ♀

O24.919   Unspecified diabetes mellitus in pregnancy, **unspecified trimester**   `CC` `M` ♀

O24.92   Unspecified diabetes mellitus in **childbirth**   `M` ♀

O24.93   Unspecified diabetes mellitus in the **puerperium**   `CC` `M` ♀

✓4ᵗʰ **O25**   **Malnutrition in pregnancy, childbirth and the puerperium**

✓5ᵗʰ **O25.1**   Malnutrition in **pregnancy**

O25.10   Malnutrition in pregnancy, **unspecified trimester** `M` ♀

O25.11   Malnutrition in pregnancy, **first trimester**   `M` ♀

O25.12   Malnutrition in pregnancy, **second trimester**   `M` ♀

O25.13   Malnutrition in pregnancy, **third trimester**   `M` ♀

O25.2   Malnutrition in **childbirth**   `M` ♀

O25.3   Malnutrition in the **puerperium**   `M` ♀

✓4ᵗʰ **O26**   **Maternal care for other conditions predominantly related to pregnancy**

✓5ᵗʰ **O26.0**   Excessive weight gain in pregnancy
> _EXCLUDES 2_   gestational edema (O12.0, O12.2)

O26.00   Excessive weight gain in pregnancy, **unspecified trimester**   `M` ♀

O26.01   Excessive weight gain in pregnancy, **first trimester**   `M` ♀

O26.02   Excessive weight gain in pregnancy, **second trimester**   `M` ♀

O26.03   Excessive weight gain in pregnancy, **third trimester**   `M` ♀

✓5ᵗʰ **O26.1**   Low weight gain in pregnancy

O26.10   Low weight gain in pregnancy, **unspecified trimester**   `M` ♀

O26.11   Low weight gain in pregnancy, **first trimester**   `M` ♀

O26.12   Low weight gain in pregnancy, **second trimester**   `M` ♀

O26.13   Low weight gain in pregnancy, **third trimester**   `M` ♀

✓5ᵗʰ **O26.2**   Pregnancy care for patient with recurrent pregnancy loss

O26.20   Pregnancy care for patient with recurrent pregnancy loss, **unspecified trimester**   `M` ♀

O26.21   Pregnancy care for patient with recurrent pregnancy loss, **first trimester**   `M` ♀

O26.22   Pregnancy care for patient with recurrent pregnancy loss, **second trimester**   `M` ♀

O26.23   Pregnancy care for patient with recurrent pregnancy loss, **third trimester**   `M` ♀

✓5ᵗʰ **O26.3**   Retained intrauterine contraceptive device in pregnancy

O26.30   Retained intrauterine contraceptive device in pregnancy, **unspecified trimester**   `M` ♀

O26.31   Retained intrauterine contraceptive device in pregnancy, **first trimester**   `M` ♀

✔ Additional Character Required   ✓x7ᵗʰ Placeholder   Unacceptable PDx   Questionable PDx   Manifestation   `H1`-`H14` HAC   `HCC` CMS-HCC Dx   `HIV` HIV Dx

ICD-10-CM 2019   859

Chapter 15. Pregnancy, Childbirth and the Puerperium

O26.32   **Retained intrauterine contraceptive device in pregnancy,** second trimester   M♀

O26.33   **Retained intrauterine contraceptive device in pregnancy,** third trimester   M♀

√5th **O26.4 Herpes gestationis**

    O26.40   **Herpes gestationis,** unspecified trimester   M♀

    O26.41   **Herpes gestationis,** first trimester   M♀

    O26.42   **Herpes gestationis,** second trimester   M♀

    O26.43   **Herpes gestationis,** third trimester   M♀

√5th **O26.5 Maternal hypotension syndrome**
     Supine hypotensive syndrome

    O26.50   **Maternal hypotension syndrome,** unspecified trimester   M♀

    O26.51   **Maternal hypotension syndrome,** first trimester   M♀

    O26.52   **Maternal hypotension syndrome,** second trimester   M♀

    O26.53   **Maternal hypotension syndrome,** third trimester   M♀

√5th **O26.6 Liver and biliary tract disorders in pregnancy, childbirth and the puerperium**
     Use additional code to identify the specific disorder
     EXCLUDES 2   hepatorenal syndrome following labor and delivery (O90.4)

    CC Excl: For CC codes in subcategory O26.6:
    PDX collection 972

    √6th O26.61   **Liver and biliary tract disorders in** pregnancy

       O26.611   **Liver and biliary tract disorders in pregnancy,** first trimester   CC M♀

       O26.612   **Liver and biliary tract disorders in pregnancy,** second trimester   CC M♀

       O26.613   **Liver and biliary tract disorders in pregnancy,** third trimester   CC M♀

       O26.619   **Liver and biliary tract disorders in pregnancy,** unspecified trimester   M♀

    O26.62   **Liver and biliary tract disorders in** childbirth   CC M♀

    O26.63   **Liver and biliary tract disorders in the** puerperium   M♀

√5th **O26.7 Subluxation of symphysis (pubis) in pregnancy, childbirth and the puerperium**
     EXCLUDES 1   traumatic separation of symphysis (pubis) during childbirth (O71.6)

    √6th O26.71   **Subluxation of symphysis (pubis) in pregnancy**

       O26.711   **Subluxation of symphysis (pubis) in pregnancy,** first trimester   M♀

       O26.712   **Subluxation of symphysis (pubis) in pregnancy,** second trimester   M♀

       O26.713   **Subluxation of symphysis (pubis) in pregnancy,** third trimester   M♀

       O26.719   **Subluxation of symphysis (pubis) in pregnancy,** unspecified trimester   M♀

    O26.72   **Subluxation of symphysis (pubis) in** childbirth   M♀

    O26.73   **Subluxation of symphysis (pubis) in the** puerperium   M♀

√5th **O26.8 Other specified pregnancy related conditions**

    √6th O26.81   **Pregnancy related exhaustion and fatigue**

       O26.811   **Pregnancy related exhaustion and fatigue,** first trimester   M♀

       O26.812   **Pregnancy related exhaustion and fatigue,** second trimester   M♀

       O26.813   **Pregnancy related exhaustion and fatigue,** third trimester   M♀

       O26.819   **Pregnancy related exhaustion and fatigue,** unspecified trimester   M♀

    √6th O26.82   **Pregnancy related peripheral neuritis**

       O26.821   **Pregnancy related peripheral neuritis,** first trimester   M♀

       O26.822   **Pregnancy related peripheral neuritis,** second trimester   M♀

       O26.823   **Pregnancy related peripheral neuritis,** third trimester   M♀

       O26.829   **Pregnancy related peripheral neuritis,** unspecified trimester   M♀

√6th O26.83   **Pregnancy related renal disease**
     Use additional code to identify the specific disorder

    CC Excl: For CC codes in subcategory O26.83:
    PDX collection 965

    O26.831   **Pregnancy related renal disease,** first trimester   CC M♀

    O26.832   **Pregnancy related renal disease,** second trimester   CC M♀

    O26.833   **Pregnancy related renal disease,** third trimester   CC M♀

    O26.839   **Pregnancy related renal disease,** unspecified trimester   M♀

√6th O26.84   **Uterine size-date discrepancy complicating pregnancy**
     EXCLUDES 1   encounter for suspected problem with fetal growth ruled out (Z03.74)

    O26.841   **Uterine size-date discrepancy,** first trimester   M♀

    O26.842   **Uterine size-date discrepancy,** second trimester   M♀

    O26.843   **Uterine size-date discrepancy,** third trimester   M♀

    O26.849   **Uterine size-date discrepancy,** unspecified trimester   M♀

√6th O26.85   **Spotting complicating pregnancy**

    O26.851   **Spotting complicating pregnancy,** first trimester   M♀

    O26.852   **Spotting complicating pregnancy,** second trimester   M♀

    O26.853   **Spotting complicating pregnancy,** third trimester   M♀

    O26.859   **Spotting complicating pregnancy,** unspecified trimester   M♀

    O26.86   **Pruritic urticarial papules and plaques of pregnancy (PUPPP)**   M♀
     Polymorphic eruption of pregnancy

√6th O26.87   **Cervical shortening**
     EXCLUDES 1   encounter for suspected cervical shortening ruled out (Z03.75)
     DEF: Cervix that has shortened to less than 25 mm before the 24th week of pregnancy. A shortened cervix is a warning sign for impending premature delivery and is treated by cervical cerclage placement or progesterone.

    CC Excl: For CC codes in subcategory O26.87:
    PDX collection 973

    O26.872   **Cervical shortening,** second trimester   CC M♀

    O26.873   **Cervical shortening,** third trimester   CC M♀

    O26.879   **Cervical shortening,** unspecified trimester   CC M♀

√6th O26.89   **Other specified pregnancy related conditions**
     AHA: 2015, 3Q, 40

    O26.891   **Other specified pregnancy related conditions,** first trimester   M♀

    O26.892   **Other specified pregnancy related conditions,** second trimester   M♀

    O26.893   **Other specified pregnancy related conditions,** third trimester   M♀

    O26.899   **Other specified pregnancy related conditions,** unspecified trimester   M♀

√5th **O26.9 Pregnancy related conditions, unspecified**

    O26.90   **Pregnancy related conditions, unspecified,** unspecified trimester   M♀

    O26.91   **Pregnancy related conditions, unspecified,** first trimester   M♀

    O26.92   **Pregnancy related conditions, unspecified,** second trimester   M♀

    O26.93   **Pregnancy related conditions, unspecified,** third trimester   M♀

√4th **O28 Abnormal findings on antenatal screening of mother**
     EXCLUDES 1   diagnostic findings classified elsewhere—see Alphabetical Index

    O28.0   **Abnormal** hematological **finding on antenatal screening of mother**   M♀

    O28.1   **Abnormal** biochemical **finding on antenatal screening of mother**   M♀

N Newborn: 0   P Pediatric: 0-17   M Maternity: 12-55   A Adult: 15-124   MCC Major Complication/Comorbidity   CC Complication/Comorbidity   SW Severe Wound Dx

860   ICD-10-CM 2019

O28.2 Abnormal cytological finding on antenatal screening of mother   M♀

O28.3 Abnormal ultrasonic finding on antenatal screening of mother   M♀

O28.4 Abnormal radiological finding on antenatal screening of mother   M♀

O28.5 Abnormal chromosomal and genetic finding on antenatal screening of mother   M♀

O28.8 Other abnormal findings on antenatal screening of mother   M♀

O28.9 Unspecified abnormal findings on antenatal screening of mother   M♀

✓4ᵗʰ **O29 Complications of anesthesia during pregnancy**

> INCLUDES   maternal complications arising from the administration of a general, regional or local anesthetic, analgesic or other sedation during pregnancy
>
> Use additional code, if necessary, to identify the complication
>
> EXCLUDES 2   complications of anesthesia during labor and delivery (O74.-)
> complications of anesthesia during the puerperium (O89.-)

✓5ᵗʰ **O29.0 Pulmonary complications of anesthesia during pregnancy**

  ✓6ᵗʰ **O29.01 Aspiration pneumonitis due to anesthesia during pregnancy**

    Inhalation of stomach contents or secretions NOS due to anesthesia during pregnancy
    Mendelson's syndrome due to anesthesia during pregnancy

    O29.011 Aspiration pneumonitis due to anesthesia during pregnancy, first trimester   M♀

    O29.012 Aspiration pneumonitis due to anesthesia during pregnancy, second trimester   M♀

    O29.013 Aspiration pneumonitis due to anesthesia during pregnancy, third trimester   M♀

    O29.019 Aspiration pneumonitis due to anesthesia during pregnancy, unspecified trimester   M♀

  ✓6ᵗʰ **O29.02 Pressure collapse of lung due to anesthesia during pregnancy**

    O29.021 Pressure collapse of lung due to anesthesia during pregnancy, first trimester   M♀

    O29.022 Pressure collapse of lung due to anesthesia during pregnancy, second trimester   M♀

    O29.023 Pressure collapse of lung due to anesthesia during pregnancy, third trimester   M♀

    O29.029 Pressure collapse of lung due to anesthesia during pregnancy, unspecified trimester   M♀

  ✓6ᵗʰ **O29.09 Other pulmonary complications of anesthesia during pregnancy**

    O29.091 Other pulmonary complications of anesthesia during pregnancy, first trimester   M♀

    O29.092 Other pulmonary complications of anesthesia during pregnancy, second trimester   M♀

    O29.093 Other pulmonary complications of anesthesia during pregnancy, third trimester   M♀

    O29.099 Other pulmonary complications of anesthesia during pregnancy, unspecified trimester   M♀

✓5ᵗʰ **O29.1 Cardiac complications of anesthesia during pregnancy**

  ✓6ᵗʰ **O29.11 Cardiac arrest due to anesthesia during pregnancy**

    O29.111 Cardiac arrest due to anesthesia during pregnancy, first trimester   M♀

    O29.112 Cardiac arrest due to anesthesia during pregnancy, second trimester   M♀

    O29.113 Cardiac arrest due to anesthesia during pregnancy, third trimester   M♀

    O29.119 Cardiac arrest due to anesthesia during pregnancy, unspecified trimester   M♀

  ✓6ᵗʰ **O29.12 Cardiac failure due to anesthesia during pregnancy**

    O29.121 Cardiac failure due to anesthesia during pregnancy, first trimester   M♀

    O29.122 Cardiac failure due to anesthesia during pregnancy, second trimester   M♀

    O29.123 Cardiac failure due to anesthesia during pregnancy, third trimester   M♀

    O29.129 Cardiac failure due to anesthesia during pregnancy, unspecified trimester   M♀

  ✓6ᵗʰ **O29.19 Other cardiac complications of anesthesia during pregnancy**

    O29.191 Other cardiac complications of anesthesia during pregnancy, first trimester   M♀

    O29.192 Other cardiac complications of anesthesia during pregnancy, second trimester   M♀

    O29.193 Other cardiac complications of anesthesia during pregnancy, third trimester   M♀

    O29.199 Other cardiac complications of anesthesia during pregnancy, unspecified trimester   M♀

✓5ᵗʰ **O29.2 Central nervous system complications of anesthesia during pregnancy**

  ✓6ᵗʰ **O29.21 Cerebral anoxia due to anesthesia during pregnancy**

    O29.211 Cerebral anoxia due to anesthesia during pregnancy, first trimester   M♀

    O29.212 Cerebral anoxia due to anesthesia during pregnancy, second trimester   M♀

    O29.213 Cerebral anoxia due to anesthesia during pregnancy, third trimester   M♀

    O29.219 Cerebral anoxia due to anesthesia during pregnancy, unspecified trimester   M♀

  ✓6ᵗʰ **O29.29 Other central nervous system complications of anesthesia during pregnancy**

    O29.291 Other central nervous system complications of anesthesia during pregnancy, first trimester   M♀

    O29.292 Other central nervous system complications of anesthesia during pregnancy, second trimester   M♀

    O29.293 Other central nervous system complications of anesthesia during pregnancy, third trimester   M♀

    O29.299 Other central nervous system complications of anesthesia during pregnancy, unspecified trimester   M♀

✓5ᵗʰ **O29.3 Toxic reaction to local anesthesia during pregnancy**

  ✓6ᵗʰ **O29.3X Toxic reaction to local anesthesia during pregnancy**

    O29.3X1 Toxic reaction to local anesthesia during pregnancy, first trimester   M♀

    O29.3X2 Toxic reaction to local anesthesia during pregnancy, second trimester   M♀

    O29.3X3 Toxic reaction to local anesthesia during pregnancy, third trimester   M♀

    O29.3X9 Toxic reaction to local anesthesia during pregnancy, unspecified trimester   M♀

✓5ᵗʰ **O29.4 Spinal and epidural anesthesia induced headache during pregnancy**

  O29.40 Spinal and epidural anesthesia induced headache during pregnancy, unspecified trimester   M♀

  O29.41 Spinal and epidural anesthesia induced headache during pregnancy, first trimester   M♀

  O29.42 Spinal and epidural anesthesia induced headache during pregnancy, second trimester   M♀

  O29.43 Spinal and epidural anesthesia induced headache during pregnancy, third trimester   M♀

✓5ᵗʰ **O29.5 Other complications of spinal and epidural anesthesia during pregnancy**

  ✓6ᵗʰ **O29.5X Other complications of spinal and epidural anesthesia during pregnancy**

    O29.5X1 Other complications of spinal and epidural anesthesia during pregnancy, first trimester   M♀

    O29.5X2 Other complications of spinal and epidural anesthesia during pregnancy, second trimester   M♀

    O29.5X3 Other complications of spinal and epidural anesthesia during pregnancy, third trimester   M♀

✓ Additional Character Required   ✓x7ᵗʰ Placeholder   Unacceptable PDx   Questionable PDx   Manifestation   H1 - H14 HAC   HCC CMS-HCC Dx   HIV HIV Dx

ICD-10-CM 2019   861

O29.5X9 Other complications of spinal and epidural anesthesia during pregnancy, unspecified trimester Ⓜ♀

✓5ᵗʰ **O29.6** Failed or difficult intubation for anesthesia during pregnancy

  O29.60 Failed or difficult intubation for anesthesia during pregnancy, unspecified trimester Ⓜ♀

  O29.61 Failed or difficult intubation for anesthesia during pregnancy, first trimester Ⓜ♀

  O29.62 Failed or difficult intubation for anesthesia during pregnancy, second trimester Ⓜ♀

  O29.63 Failed or difficult intubation for anesthesia during pregnancy, third trimester Ⓜ♀

✓5ᵗʰ **O29.8** Other complications of anesthesia during pregnancy

  ✓6ᵗʰ **O29.8X** Other complications of anesthesia during pregnancy

    O29.8X1 Other complications of anesthesia during pregnancy, first trimester Ⓜ♀

    O29.8X2 Other complications of anesthesia during pregnancy, second trimester Ⓜ♀

    O29.8X3 Other complications of anesthesia during pregnancy, third trimester Ⓜ♀

    O29.8X9 Other complications of anesthesia during pregnancy, unspecified trimester Ⓜ♀

✓5ᵗʰ **O29.9** Unspecified complication of anesthesia during pregnancy

  O29.90 Unspecified complication of anesthesia during pregnancy, unspecified trimester Ⓜ♀

  O29.91 Unspecified complication of anesthesia during pregnancy, first trimester Ⓜ♀

  O29.92 Unspecified complication of anesthesia during pregnancy, second trimester Ⓜ♀

  O29.93 Unspecified complication of anesthesia during pregnancy, third trimester Ⓜ♀

Maternal care related to the fetus and amniotic cavity and possible delivery problems (O30-O48)

✓4ᵗʰ **O30** Multiple gestation

Code also any complications specific to multiple gestation
AHA: 2016, 4Q, 51

> **CC Excl:** For CC codes in category O30: PDX collection 976

✓5ᵗʰ **O30.0** Twin pregnancy

  ✓6ᵗʰ **O30.00** Twin pregnancy, unspecified number of placenta and unspecified number of amniotic sacs

    O30.001 Twin pregnancy, unspecified number of placenta and unspecified number of amniotic sacs, first trimester Ⓜ♀

    O30.002 Twin pregnancy, unspecified number of placenta and unspecified number of amniotic sacs, second trimester Ⓜ♀

    O30.003 Twin pregnancy, unspecified number of placenta and unspecified number of amniotic sacs, third trimester Ⓜ♀

    O30.009 Twin pregnancy, unspecified number of placenta and unspecified number of amniotic sacs, unspecified trimester Ⓜ♀

Twin Gestation – Monochorionic/Monoamniotic

- 1 Chorionic sac
- 1 Amniotic sac
- 2 Fetuses
- 2 Umbilical cords
- 1 Placenta

✓6ᵗʰ **O30.01** Twin pregnancy, monochorionic/monoamniotic
Twin pregnancy, one placenta, one amniotic sac
> **EXCLUDES 1** conjoined twins (O30.02-)

  O30.011 Twin pregnancy, monochorionic/monoamniotic, first trimester Ⓜ♀

  O30.012 Twin pregnancy, monochorionic/monoamniotic, second trimester Ⓜ♀

  O30.013 Twin pregnancy, monochorionic/monoamniotic, third trimester Ⓜ♀

  O30.019 Twin pregnancy, monochorionic/monoamniotic, unspecified trimester Ⓜ♀

✓6ᵗʰ **O30.02** Conjoined twin pregnancy

  O30.021 Conjoined twin pregnancy, first trimester Ⓜ♀

  O30.022 Conjoined twin pregnancy, second trimester Ⓜ♀

  O30.023 Conjoined twin pregnancy, third trimester Ⓜ♀

  O30.029 Conjoined twin pregnancy, unspecified trimester Ⓜ♀

Twin Gestation – Monochorionic/Diamniotic

- 1 Chorionic sac
- 2 Amniotic sacs
- 2 Fetuses
- 2 Umbilical cords
- 1 Placenta

✓6ᵗʰ **O30.03** Twin pregnancy, monochorionic/diamniotic
Twin pregnancy, one placenta, two amniotic sacs

  O30.031 Twin pregnancy, monochorionic/diamniotic, first trimester Ⓜ♀

  O30.032 Twin pregnancy, monochorionic/diamniotic, second trimester Ⓜ♀

  O30.033 Twin pregnancy, monochorionic/diamniotic, third trimester Ⓜ♀

  O30.039 Twin pregnancy, monochorionic/diamniotic, unspecified trimester Ⓜ♀

Twin Gestation – Dichorionic/Diamniotic

- 2 Chorionic sacs
- 2 Amniotic sacs
- 2 Fetuses
- 2 Umbilical cords
- 2 Placentas

✓6ᵗʰ **O30.04** Twin pregnancy, dichorionic/diamniotic
Twin pregnancy, two placentae, two amniotic sacs

  O30.041 Twin pregnancy, dichorionic/diamniotic, first trimester Ⓜ♀

  O30.042 Twin pregnancy, dichorionic/diamniotic, second trimester Ⓜ♀

  O30.043 Twin pregnancy, dichorionic/diamniotic, third trimester Ⓜ♀

  O30.049 Twin pregnancy, dichorionic/diamniotic, unspecified trimester Ⓜ♀

Ⓝ Newborn: 0　　Ⓟ Pediatric: 0-17　　Ⓜ Maternity: 12-55　　Ⓐ Adult: 15-124　　ᴹᶜᶜ Major Complication/Comorbidity　　ᶜᶜ Complication/Comorbidity　　ˢᵂ Severe Wound Dx

862　　　　ICD-10-CM 2019

✓6ᵗʰ O30.09 Twin pregnancy, unable to determine number of placenta and number of amniotic sacs
- **O30.091** Twin pregnancy, unable to determine number of placenta and number of amniotic sacs, first trimester Ⓜ♀
- **O30.092** Twin pregnancy, unable to determine number of placenta and number of amniotic sacs, second trimester Ⓜ♀
- **O30.093** Twin pregnancy, unable to determine number of placenta and number of amniotic sacs, third trimester Ⓜ♀
- **O30.099** Twin pregnancy, unable to determine number of placenta and number of amniotic sacs, unspecified trimester Ⓜ♀

✓5ᵗʰ O30.1 Triplet pregnancy

✓6ᵗʰ O30.10 Triplet pregnancy, unspecified number of placenta and unspecified number of amniotic sacs
   AHA: 2016, 2Q, 8
- **O30.101** Triplet pregnancy, unspecified number of placenta and unspecified number of amniotic sacs, first trimester CC Ⓜ♀
- **O30.102** Triplet pregnancy, unspecified number of placenta and unspecified number of amniotic sacs, second trimester CC Ⓜ♀
- **O30.103** Triplet pregnancy, unspecified number of placenta and unspecified number of amniotic sacs, third trimester CC Ⓜ♀
- **O30.109** Triplet pregnancy, unspecified number of placenta and unspecified number of amniotic sacs, unspecified trimester Ⓜ♀

✓6ᵗʰ O30.11 Triplet pregnancy with two or more monochorionic fetuses
- **O30.111** Triplet pregnancy with two or more monochorionic fetuses, first trimester CC Ⓜ♀
- **O30.112** Triplet pregnancy with two or more monochorionic fetuses, second trimester CC Ⓜ♀
- **O30.113** Triplet pregnancy with two or more monochorionic fetuses, third trimester CC Ⓜ♀
- **O30.119** Triplet pregnancy with two or more monochorionic fetuses, unspecified trimester Ⓜ♀

✓6ᵗʰ O30.12 Triplet pregnancy with two or more monoamniotic fetuses
- **O30.121** Triplet pregnancy with two or more monoamniotic fetuses, first trimester CC Ⓜ♀
- **O30.122** Triplet pregnancy with two or more monoamniotic fetuses, second trimester CC Ⓜ♀
- **O30.123** Triplet pregnancy with two or more monoamniotic fetuses, third trimester CC Ⓜ♀
- **O30.129** Triplet pregnancy with two or more monoamniotic fetuses, unspecified trimester Ⓜ♀

✓6ᵗʰ O30.13 Triplet pregnancy, trichorionic/triamniotic
- **O30.131** Triplet pregnancy, trichorionic/triamniotic, first trimester CC Ⓜ♀
- **O30.132** Triplet pregnancy, trichorionic/triamniotic, second trimester CC Ⓜ♀
- **O30.133** Triplet pregnancy, trichorionic/triamniotic, third trimester CC Ⓜ♀
- **O30.139** Triplet pregnancy, trichorionic/triamniotic, unspecified trimester Ⓜ♀

✓6ᵗʰ O30.19 Triplet pregnancy, unable to determine number of placenta and number of amniotic sacs
- **O30.191** Triplet pregnancy, unable to determine number of placenta and number of amniotic sacs, first trimester CC Ⓜ♀
- **O30.192** Triplet pregnancy, unable to determine number of placenta and number of amniotic sacs, second trimester CC Ⓜ♀
- **O30.193** Triplet pregnancy, unable to determine number of placenta and number of amniotic sacs, third trimester CC Ⓜ♀
- **O30.199** Triplet pregnancy, unable to determine number of placenta and number of amniotic sacs, unspecified trimester Ⓜ♀

✓5ᵗʰ O30.2 Quadruplet pregnancy

✓6ᵗʰ O30.20 Quadruplet pregnancy, unspecified number of placenta and unspecified number of amniotic sacs
- **O30.201** Quadruplet pregnancy, unspecified number of placenta and unspecified number of amniotic sacs, first trimester CC Ⓜ♀
- **O30.202** Quadruplet pregnancy, unspecified number of placenta and unspecified number of amniotic sacs, second trimester CC Ⓜ♀
- **O30.203** Quadruplet pregnancy, unspecified number of placenta and unspecified number of amniotic sacs, third trimester CC Ⓜ♀
- **O30.209** Quadruplet pregnancy, unspecified number of placenta and unspecified number of amniotic sacs, unspecified trimester Ⓜ♀

✓6ᵗʰ O30.21 Quadruplet pregnancy with two or more monochorionic fetuses
- **O30.211** Quadruplet pregnancy with two or more monochorionic fetuses, first trimester CC Ⓜ♀
- **O30.212** Quadruplet pregnancy with two or more monochorionic fetuses, second trimester CC Ⓜ♀
- **O30.213** Quadruplet pregnancy with two or more monochorionic fetuses, third trimester CC Ⓜ♀
- **O30.219** Quadruplet pregnancy with two or more monochorionic fetuses, unspecified trimester Ⓜ♀

✓6ᵗʰ O30.22 Quadruplet pregnancy with two or more monoamniotic fetuses
- **O30.221** Quadruplet pregnancy with two or more monoamniotic fetuses, first trimester CC Ⓜ♀
- **O30.222** Quadruplet pregnancy with two or more monoamniotic fetuses, second trimester CC Ⓜ♀
- **O30.223** Quadruplet pregnancy with two or more monoamniotic fetuses, third trimester CC Ⓜ♀
- **O30.229** Quadruplet pregnancy with two or more monoamniotic fetuses, unspecified trimester Ⓜ♀

✓6ᵗʰ O30.23 Quadruplet pregnancy, quadrachorionic/quadra-amniotic
- **O30.231** Quadruplet pregnancy, quadrachorionic/quadra-amniotic, first trimester CC Ⓜ♀
- **O30.232** Quadruplet pregnancy, quadrachorionic/quadra-amniotic, second trimester CC Ⓜ♀
- **O30.233** Quadruplet pregnancy, quadrachorionic/quadra-amniotic, third trimester CC Ⓜ♀
- **O30.239** Quadruplet pregnancy, quadrachorionic/quadra-amniotic, unspecified trimester Ⓜ♀

✓ Additional Character Required   ✓x7ᵗʰ Placeholder   Unacceptable PDx   Questionable PDx   Manifestation   H1-H14 HAC   HCC CMS-HCC Dx   HIV HIV Dx

ICD-10-CM 2019   863

✓6ᵗʰ O30.29 Quadruplet pregnancy, unable to determine number of placenta and number of amniotic sacs

- **O30.291** Quadruplet pregnancy, unable to determine number of placenta and number of amniotic sacs, first trimester   cc M♀
- **O30.292** Quadruplet pregnancy, unable to determine number of placenta and number of amniotic sacs, second trimester   cc M♀
- **O30.293** Quadruplet pregnancy, unable to determine number of placenta and number of amniotic sacs, third trimester   cc M♀
- **O30.299** Quadruplet pregnancy, unable to determine number of placenta and number of amniotic sacs, unspecified trimester   M♀

✓5ᵗʰ O30.8 Other specified multiple gestation
Multiple gestation pregnancy greater than quadruplets

✓6ᵗʰ O30.80 Other specified multiple gestation, unspecified number of placenta and unspecified number of amniotic sacs

- **O30.801** Other specified multiple gestation, unspecified number of placenta and unspecified number of amniotic sacs, first trimester   cc M♀
- **O30.802** Other specified multiple gestation, unspecified number of placenta and unspecified number of amniotic sacs, second trimester   cc M♀
- **O30.803** Other specified multiple gestation, unspecified number of placenta and unspecified number of amniotic sacs, third trimester   cc M♀
- **O30.809** Other specified multiple gestation, unspecified number of placenta and unspecified number of amniotic sacs, unspecified trimester   M♀

✓6ᵗʰ O30.81 Other specified multiple gestation with two or more monochorionic fetuses

- **O30.811** Other specified multiple gestation with two or more monochorionic fetuses, first trimester   cc M♀
- **O30.812** Other specified multiple gestation with two or more monochorionic fetuses, second trimester   cc M♀
- **O30.813** Other specified multiple gestation with two or more monochorionic fetuses, third trimester   cc M♀
- **O30.819** Other specified multiple gestation with two or more monochorionic fetuses, unspecified trimester   M♀

✓6ᵗʰ O30.82 Other specified multiple gestation with two or more monoamniotic fetuses

- **O30.821** Other specified multiple gestation with two or more monoamniotic fetuses, first trimester   cc M♀
- **O30.822** Other specified multiple gestation with two or more monoamniotic fetuses, second trimester   cc M♀
- **O30.823** Other specified multiple gestation with two or more monoamniotic fetuses, third trimester   cc M♀
- **O30.829** Other specified multiple gestation with two or more monoamniotic fetuses, unspecified trimester   M♀

✓6ᵗʰ O30.83 Other specified multiple gestation, number of chorions and amnions are both equal to the number of fetuses
Pentachorionic, penta-amniotic pregnancy (quintuplets)
Hexachorionic, hexa-amniotic pregnancy (sextuplets)
Heptachorionic, hepta-amniotic pregnancy (septuplets)

- **O30.831** Other specified multiple gestation, number of chorions and amnions are both equal to the number of fetuses, first trimester   cc M♀
- **O30.832** Other specified multiple gestation, number of chorions and amnions are both equal to the number of fetuses, second trimester   cc M♀
- **O30.833** Other specified multiple gestation, number of chorions and amnions are both equal to the number of fetuses, third trimester   cc M♀
- **O30.839** Other specified multiple gestation, number of chorions and amnions are both equal to the number of fetuses, unspecified trimester   M♀

✓6ᵗʰ O30.89 Other specified multiple gestation, unable to determine number of placenta and number of amniotic sacs

- **O30.891** Other specified multiple gestation, unable to determine number of placenta and number of amniotic sacs, first trimester   cc M♀
- **O30.892** Other specified multiple gestation, unable to determine number of placenta and number of amniotic sacs, second trimester   cc M♀
- **O30.893** Other specified multiple gestation, unable to determine number of placenta and number of amniotic sacs, third trimester   cc M♀
- **O30.899** Other specified multiple gestation, unable to determine number of placenta and number of amniotic sacs, unspecified trimester   M♀

✓5ᵗʰ O30.9 Multiple gestation, unspecified
Multiple pregnancy NOS

- **O30.90** Multiple gestation, unspecified, unspecified trimester   M♀
- **O30.91** Multiple gestation, unspecified, first trimester   M♀
- **O30.92** Multiple gestation, unspecified, second trimester   M♀
- **O30.93** Multiple gestation, unspecified, third trimester   M♀

✓4ᵗʰ O31 Complications specific to multiple gestation

EXCLUDES 2   delayed delivery of second twin, triplet, etc. (O63.2)
malpresentation of one fetus or more (O32.9)
placental transfusion syndromes (O43.0-)

AHA: 2012, 4Q, 107

> One of the following 7th characters is to be assigned to each code under category O31. 7th character 0 is for single gestations and multiple gestations where the fetus is unspecified. 7th characters 1 through 9 are for cases of multiple gestations to identify the fetus for which the code applies. The appropriate code from category O30, Multiple gestation, must also be assigned when assigning a code from category O31 that has a 7th character of 1 through 9.
>
> | | | | |
> |---|---|---|---|
> | 0 | not applicable or unspecified | 3 | fetus 3 |
> | | | 4 | fetus 4 |
> | 1 | fetus 1 | 5 | fetus 5 |
> | 2 | fetus 2 | 9 | other fetus |

✓5ᵗʰ O31.0 Papyraceous fetus
Fetus compressus
DEF: Fetus that has died, but remains in utero for weeks before delivery, becoming compacted and mummified in appearance, with skin resembling parchment. Occurs most commonly in multigestational pregnancies. ***Synonym(s):*** *paper doll fetus.*

- **✓x7ᵗʰ O31.00** Papyraceous fetus, unspecified trimester   M♀
- **✓x7ᵗʰ O31.01** Papyraceous fetus, first trimester   M♀
- **✓x7ᵗʰ O31.02** Papyraceous fetus, second trimester   M♀
- **✓x7ᵗʰ O31.03** Papyraceous fetus, third trimester   M♀

✓5ᵗʰ O31.1 Continuing pregnancy after spontaneous abortion of one fetus or more

- **✓x7ᵗʰ O31.10** Continuing pregnancy after spontaneous abortion of one fetus or more, unspecified trimester   M♀
- **✓x7ᵗʰ O31.11** Continuing pregnancy after spontaneous abortion of one fetus or more, first trimester   M♀
- **✓x7ᵗʰ O31.12** Continuing pregnancy after spontaneous abortion of one fetus or more, second trimester   M♀
- **✓x7ᵗʰ O31.13** Continuing pregnancy after spontaneous abortion of one fetus or more, third trimester   M♀

N Newborn: 0   P Pediatric: 0-17   M Maternity: 12-55   A Adult: 15-124   MCC Major Complication/Comorbidity   CC Complication/Comorbidity   SW Severe Wound Dx

864   ICD-10-CM 2019

✓5ᵗʰ **O31.2 Continuing pregnancy** after intrauterine death of one fetus or more

    ✓x7ᵗʰ **O31.20 Continuing pregnancy after intrauterine death** Ⓜ♀
of one fetus or more, **unspecified trimester**

    ✓x7ᵗʰ **O31.21 Continuing pregnancy after intrauterine death** Ⓜ♀
of one fetus or more, **first trimester**

    ✓x7ᵗʰ **O31.22 Continuing pregnancy after intrauterine death** Ⓜ♀
of one fetus or more, **second trimester**

    ✓x7ᵗʰ **O31.23 Continuing pregnancy after intrauterine death** Ⓜ♀
of one fetus or more, **third trimester**

✓5ᵗʰ **O31.3 Continuing pregnancy after** elective fetal reduction **of one fetus or more**

    Continuing pregnancy after selective termination of one fetus or more

    ✓x7ᵗʰ **O31.30 Continuing pregnancy after elective fetal** Ⓜ♀
reduction of one fetus or more, unspecified trimester

    ✓x7ᵗʰ **O31.31 Continuing pregnancy after elective fetal** Ⓜ♀
reduction of one fetus or more, first trimester

    ✓x7ᵗʰ **O31.32 Continuing pregnancy after elective fetal** Ⓜ♀
reduction of one fetus or more, second trimester

    ✓x7ᵗʰ **O31.33 Continuing pregnancy after elective fetal** Ⓜ♀
reduction of one fetus or more, third trimester

✓5ᵗʰ **O31.8 Other complications specific to multiple gestation**

    ✓6ᵗʰ **O31.8X Other complications specific to multiple gestation**

      CC Excl: For CC codes in subcategory O31.8X: PDX collection 976

      ✓7ᵗʰ **O31.8X1 Other complications specific to** ⒸⒸ Ⓜ♀
multiple gestation, first trimester

      ✓7ᵗʰ **O31.8X2 Other complications specific to** ⒸⒸ Ⓜ♀
multiple gestation, second trimester

      ✓7ᵗʰ **O31.8X3 Other complications specific to** ⒸⒸ Ⓜ♀
multiple gestation, third trimester

      ✓7ᵗʰ **O31.8X9 Other complications specific to** Ⓜ♀
multiple gestation, unspecified trimester

Fetal Malpresentation

Breech

Shoulder
(arm prolapse)

Mother's pelvis

Compound
(extremity together with head)

Face
(mentum)

Oblique

✓4ᵗʰ **O32 Maternal care for malpresentation of fetus**

    INCLUDES the listed conditions as a reason for observation, hospitalization or other obstetric care of the mother, or for cesarean delivery before onset of labor

    EXCLUDES 1 *malpresentation of fetus with obstructed labor (O64.-)*

    AHA: 2012, 4Q, 107

    One of the following 7th characters is to be assigned to each code under category O32. 7th character Ø is for single gestations and multiple gestations where the fetus is unspecified. 7th characters 1 through 9 are for cases of multiple gestations to identify the fetus for which the code applies. The appropriate code from category O30, Multiple gestation, must also be assigned when assigning a code from category O32 that has a 7th character of 1 through 9.

    Ø   not applicable or   3   fetus 3
           unspecified   4   fetus 4
    1   fetus 1   5   fetus 5
    2   fetus 2   9   other fetus

    ✓x7ᵗʰ **O32.Ø Maternal care for** unstable lie   Ⓜ♀

    ✓x7ᵗʰ **O32.1 Maternal care for** breech presentation   Ⓜ♀
      Maternal care for buttocks presentation
      Maternal care for complete breech
      Maternal care for frank breech

      EXCLUDES 1 *footling presentation (O32.8)*
                        incomplete breech (O32.8)

      DEF: Fetus presentation in a longitudinal lie with the buttocks or feet closest to birth canal that may require external cephalic version or cesarean delivery.

    ✓x7ᵗʰ **O32.2 Maternal care for** transverse and oblique lie   Ⓜ♀
      Maternal care for oblique presentation
      Maternal care for transverse presentation

    ✓x7ᵗʰ **O32.3 Maternal care for** face, brow and chin presentation   Ⓜ♀

    ✓x7ᵗʰ **O32.4 Maternal care for** high head at term   Ⓜ♀
      Maternal care for failure of head to enter pelvic brim

    ✓x7ᵗʰ **O32.6 Maternal care for** compound presentation   Ⓜ♀

    ✓x7ᵗʰ **O32.8 Maternal care for** other malpresentation of fetus   Ⓜ♀
      Maternal care for footling presentation
      Maternal care for incomplete breech

    ✓x7ᵗʰ **O32.9 Maternal care for** malpresentation of fetus, unspecified   Ⓜ♀

✓4ᵗʰ **O33 Maternal care for disproportion**

    INCLUDES the listed conditions as a reason for observation, hospitalization or other obstetric care of the mother, or for cesarean delivery before onset of labor

    EXCLUDES 1 *disproportion with obstructed labor (O65-O66)*

    O33.Ø Maternal care for disproportion due to deformity of   ⒸⒸ Ⓜ♀
maternal pelvic bones
      Maternal care for disproportion due to pelvic deformity causing disproportion NOS

      CC Excl: PDX collection 977

    O33.1 Maternal care for disproportion due to generally   Ⓜ♀
contracted pelvis
      Maternal care for disproportion due to contracted pelvis NOS causing disproportion

    O33.2 Maternal care for disproportion due to inlet contraction   Ⓜ♀
of pelvis
      Maternal care for disproportion due to inlet contraction (pelvis) causing disproportion

    ✓x7ᵗʰ **O33.3 Maternal care for disproportion due to** outlet   Ⓜ♀
contraction of pelvis
      Maternal care for disproportion due to mid-cavity contraction (pelvis)
      Maternal care for disproportion due to outlet contraction (pelvis)

    One of the following 7th characters is to be assigned to code O33.3. 7th character Ø is for single gestations and multiple gestations where the fetus is unspecified. 7th characters 1 through 9 are for cases of multiple gestations to identify the fetus for which the code applies. The appropriate code from category O30, Multiple gestation, must also be assigned when assigning code O33.3 with a 7th character of 1 through 9.

    Ø   not applicable or   3   fetus 3
           unspecified   4   fetus 4
    1   fetus 1   5   fetus 5
    2   fetus 2   9   other fetus

    ✓x7ᵗʰ **O33.4 Maternal care for disproportion of mixed maternal and**   Ⓜ♀
fetal origin

    One of the following 7th characters is to be assigned to code O33.4. 7th character Ø is for single gestations and multiple gestations where the fetus is unspecified. 7th characters 1 through 9 are for cases of multiple gestations to identify the fetus for which the code applies. The appropriate code from category O30, Multiple gestation, must also be assigned when assigning code O33.4 with a 7th character of 1 through 9.

    Ø   not applicable or   3   fetus 3
           unspecified   4   fetus 4
    1   fetus 1   5   fetus 5
    2   fetus 2   9   other fetus

✔ Additional Character Required   ✓x7ᵗʰ Placeholder   Unacceptable PDx   Questionable PDx   Manifestation   H1-H14 HAC   HCC CMS-HCC Dx   HIV HIV Dx

ICD-10-CM 2019   865

√x7ᵗʰ O33.5 Maternal care for disproportion due to unusually large fetus Ⓜ♀

Maternal care for disproportion due to disproportion of fetal origin with normally formed fetus

Maternal care for disproportion due to fetal disproportion NOS

> One of the following 7th characters is to be assigned to code O33.5. 7th character Ø is for single gestations and multiple gestations where the fetus is unspecified. 7th characters 1 through 9 are for cases of multiple gestations to identify the fetus for which the code applies. The appropriate code from category O3Ø, Multiple gestation, must also be assigned when assigning code O33.5 with a 7th character of 1 through 9.
>
> | Ø | not applicable or unspecified | 3 | fetus 3 |
> | | | 4 | fetus 4 |
> | 1 | fetus 1 | 5 | fetus 5 |
> | 2 | fetus 2 | 9 | other fetus |

√x7ᵗʰ O33.6 Maternal care for disproportion due to hydrocephalic fetus Ⓜ♀

> One of the following 7th characters is to be assigned to code O33.6. 7th character Ø is for single gestations and multiple gestations where the fetus is unspecified. 7th characters 1 through 9 are for cases of multiple gestations to identify the fetus for which the code applies. The appropriate code from category O3Ø, Multiple gestation, must also be assigned when assigning code O33.6 with a 7th character of 1 through 9.
>
> | Ø | not applicable or unspecified | 3 | fetus 3 |
> | | | 4 | fetus 4 |
> | 1 | fetus 1 | 5 | fetus 5 |
> | 2 | fetus 2 | 9 | other fetus |

√x7ᵗʰ O33.7 Maternal care for disproportion due to other fetal deformities Ⓜ♀

Maternal care for disproportion due to fetal ascites

Maternal care for disproportion due to fetal hydrops

Maternal care for disproportion due to fetal meningomyelocele

Maternal care for disproportion due to fetal sacral teratoma

Maternal care for disproportion due to fetal tumor

EXCLUDES 1 obstructed labor due to other fetal deformities (O66.3)

AHA: 2016, 4Q, 51

> One of the following 7th characters is to be assigned to code O33.7. 7th character Ø is for single gestations and multiple gestations where the fetus is unspecified. 7th characters 1 through 9 are for cases of multiple gestations to identify the fetus for which the code applies. The appropriate code from category O3Ø, Multiple gestation, must also be assigned when assigning code O33.7 with a 7th character of 1 through 9.
>
> | Ø | not applicable or unspecified | 3 | fetus 3 |
> | | | 4 | fetus 4 |
> | 1 | fetus 1 | 5 | fetus 5 |
> | 2 | fetus 2 | 9 | other fetus |

O33.8 Maternal care for disproportion of other origin Ⓜ♀

O33.9 Maternal care for disproportion, unspecified Ⓜ♀

Maternal care for disproportion due to cephalopelvic disproportion NOS

Maternal care for disproportion due to fetopelvic disproportion NOS

√4ᵗʰ O34 Maternal care for abnormality of pelvic organs

INCLUDES the listed conditions as a reason for hospitalization or other obstetric care of the mother, or for cesarean delivery before onset of labor

Code first any associated obstructed labor (O65.5)

Use additional code for specific condition

√5ᵗʰ O34.Ø Maternal care for congenital malformation of uterus

Maternal care for double uterus

Maternal care for uterus bicornis

O34.ØØ Maternal care for unspecified congenital malformation of uterus, unspecified trimester Ⓜ♀

O34.Ø1 Maternal care for unspecified congenital malformation of uterus, first trimester Ⓜ♀

O34.Ø2 Maternal care for unspecified congenital malformation of uterus, second trimester Ⓜ♀

O34.Ø3 Maternal care for unspecified congenital malformation of uterus, third trimester Ⓜ♀

√5ᵗʰ O34.1 Maternal care for benign tumor of corpus uteri

EXCLUDES 2 maternal care for benign tumor of cervix (O34.4-)

maternal care for malignant neoplasm of uterus (O9A.1-)

O34.1Ø Maternal care for benign tumor of corpus uteri, unspecified trimester Ⓜ♀

O34.11 Maternal care for benign tumor of corpus uteri, first trimester Ⓜ♀

O34.12 Maternal care for benign tumor of corpus uteri, second trimester Ⓜ♀

O34.13 Maternal care for benign tumor of corpus uteri, third trimester Ⓜ♀

√5ᵗʰ O34.2 Maternal care due to uterine scar from previous surgery

AHA: 2016, 4Q, 76

√6ᵗʰ O34.21 Maternal care for scar from previous cesarean delivery

AHA: 2016, 4Q, 51-52

O34.211 Maternal care for low transverse scar from previous cesarean delivery Ⓜ♀

O34.212 Maternal care for vertical scar from previous cesarean delivery Ⓜ♀

Maternal care for classical scar from previous cesarean delivery

O34.219 Maternal care for unspecified type scar from previous cesarean delivery Ⓜ♀

O34.29 Maternal care due to uterine scar from other previous surgery Ⓜ♀

Maternal care due to uterine scar from other transmural uterine incision

√5ᵗʰ O34.3 Maternal care for cervical incompetence

Maternal care for cerclage with or without cervical incompetence

Maternal care for Shirodkar suture with or without cervical incompetence

DEF: Inadequate functioning of cervix marked by abnormal widening during pregnancy that may cause premature birth or miscarriage.

CC Excl: For MCC codes in subcategory O34.3:
PDX collection 973

O34.3Ø Maternal care for cervical incompetence, unspecified trimester Ⓜ♀

O34.31 Maternal care for cervical incompetence, first trimester ᴹᶜᶜ Ⓜ♀

O34.32 Maternal care for cervical incompetence, second trimester ᴹᶜᶜ Ⓜ♀

O34.33 Maternal care for cervical incompetence, third trimester ᴹᶜᶜ Ⓜ♀

√5ᵗʰ O34.4 Maternal care for other abnormalities of cervix

O34.4Ø Maternal care for other abnormalities of cervix, unspecified trimester Ⓜ♀

O34.41 Maternal care for other abnormalities of cervix, first trimester Ⓜ♀

O34.42 Maternal care for other abnormalities of cervix, second trimester Ⓜ♀

O34.43 Maternal care for other abnormalities of cervix, third trimester Ⓜ♀

√5ᵗʰ O34.5 Maternal care for other abnormalities of gravid uterus

√6ᵗʰ O34.51 Maternal care for incarceration of gravid uterus

O34.511 Maternal care for incarceration of gravid uterus, first trimester Ⓜ♀

O34.512 Maternal care for incarceration of gravid uterus, second trimester Ⓜ♀

O34.513 Maternal care for incarceration of gravid uterus, third trimester Ⓜ♀

O34.519 Maternal care for incarceration of gravid uterus, unspecified trimester Ⓜ♀

√6ᵗʰ O34.52 Maternal care for prolapse of gravid uterus

O34.521 Maternal care for prolapse of gravid uterus, first trimester Ⓜ♀

O34.522 Maternal care for prolapse of gravid uterus, second trimester Ⓜ♀

O34.523 Maternal care for prolapse of gravid uterus, third trimester Ⓜ♀

O34.529 Maternal care for prolapse of gravid uterus, unspecified trimester Ⓜ♀

√6ᵗʰ O34.53 Maternal care for retroversion of gravid uterus

O34.531 Maternal care for retroversion of gravid uterus, first trimester Ⓜ♀

O34.532 Maternal care for retroversion of gravid uterus, second trimester Ⓜ♀

O34.533 Maternal care for retroversion of gravid uterus, third trimester Ⓜ♀

Ⓝ Newborn: 0   Ⓟ Pediatric: 0-17   Ⓜ Maternity: 12-55   Ⓐ Adult: 15-124   ᴹᶜᶜ Major Complication/Comorbidity   ᶜᶜ Complication/Comorbidity   ˢᵂ Severe Wound Dx

866

ICD-10-CM 2019

O34.539   **Maternal care for retroversion of gravid uterus,** unspecified trimester   M♀

✓6ᵗʰ O34.59   **Maternal care for** other abnormalities of gravid uterus

O34.591   **Maternal care for other abnormalities of gravid uterus,** first trimester   M♀

O34.592   **Maternal care for other abnormalities of gravid uterus,** second trimester   M♀

O34.593   **Maternal care for other abnormalities of gravid uterus,** third trimester   M♀

O34.599   **Maternal care for other abnormalities of gravid uterus,** unspecified trimester   M♀

✓5ᵗʰ O34.6   **Maternal care for** abnormality of vagina

EXCLUDES 2   maternal care for vaginal varices in pregnancy (O22.1-)

O34.60   **Maternal care for abnormality of vagina,** unspecified trimester   M♀

O34.61   **Maternal care for abnormality of vagina,** first trimester   M♀

O34.62   **Maternal care for abnormality of vagina,** second trimester   M♀

O34.63   **Maternal care for abnormality of vagina,** third trimester   M♀

✓5ᵗʰ O34.7   **Maternal care for** abnormality of vulva and perineum

EXCLUDES 2   maternal care for perineal and vulval varices in pregnancy (O22.1-)

O34.70   **Maternal care for abnormality of vulva and perineum,** unspecified trimester   M♀

O34.71   **Maternal care for abnormality of vulva and perineum,** first trimester   M♀

O34.72   **Maternal care for abnormality of vulva and perineum,** second trimester   M♀

O34.73   **Maternal care for abnormality of vulva and perineum,** third trimester   M♀

✓5ᵗʰ O34.8   **Maternal care for** other abnormalities of pelvic organs

O34.80   **Maternal care for other abnormalities of pelvic organs,** unspecified trimester   M♀

O34.81   **Maternal care for other abnormalities of pelvic organs,** first trimester   M♀

O34.82   **Maternal care for other abnormalities of pelvic organs,** second trimester   M♀

O34.83   **Maternal care for other abnormalities of pelvic organs,** third trimester   M♀

✓5ᵗʰ O34.9   **Maternal care for abnormality of pelvic organ,** unspecified

O34.90   **Maternal care for abnormality of pelvic organ, unspecified,** unspecified trimester   M♀

O34.91   **Maternal care for abnormality of pelvic organ, unspecified,** first trimester   M♀

O34.92   **Maternal care for abnormality of pelvic organ, unspecified,** second trimester   M♀

O34.93   **Maternal care for abnormality of pelvic organ, unspecified,** third trimester   M♀

✓4ᵗʰ O35   **Maternal care for known or suspected fetal abnormality and damage**

INCLUDES   the listed conditions in the fetus as a reason for hospitalization or other obstetric care to the mother, or for termination of pregnancy

Code also any associated maternal condition

EXCLUDES 1   encounter for suspected maternal and fetal conditions ruled out (Z03.7-)

One of the following 7th characters is to be assigned to each code under category O35. 7th character Ø is for single gestations and multiple gestations where the fetus is unspecified. 7th characters 1 through 9 are for cases of multiple gestations to identify the fetus for which the code applies. The appropriate code from category O3Ø, Multiple gestation, must also be assigned when assigning a code from category O35 that has a 7th character of 1 through 9.

Ø	not applicable or unspecified	3	fetus 3
		4	fetus 4
1	fetus 1	5	fetus 5
2	fetus 2	9	other fetus

✓x7ᵗʰ O35.Ø   **Maternal care for (suspected)** central nervous system malformation in fetus   M♀

Maternal care for fetal anencephaly
Maternal care for fetal hydrocephalus
Maternal care for fetal spina bifida

EXCLUDES 2   chromosomal abnormality in fetus (O35.1)

✓x7ᵗʰ O35.1   **Maternal care for (suspected)** chromosomal abnormality in fetus   M♀

✓x7ᵗʰ O35.2   **Maternal care for (suspected)** hereditary disease in fetus   M♀

EXCLUDES 2   chromosomal abnormality in fetus (O35.1)

✓x7ᵗʰ O35.3   **Maternal care for (suspected)** damage to fetus from viral disease in mother   M♀

Maternal care for damage to fetus from maternal cytomegalovirus infection
Maternal care for damage to fetus from maternal rubella

✓x7ᵗʰ O35.4   **Maternal care for (suspected)** damage to fetus from alcohol   M♀

✓x7ᵗʰ O35.5   **Maternal care for (suspected)** damage to fetus by drugs   M♀

Maternal care for damage to fetus from drug addiction

✓x7ᵗʰ O35.6   **Maternal care for (suspected)** damage to fetus by radiation   M♀

✓x7ᵗʰ O35.7   **Maternal care for (suspected)** damage to fetus by other medical procedures   M♀

Maternal care for damage to fetus by amniocentesis
Maternal care for damage to fetus by biopsy procedures
Maternal care for damage to fetus by hematological investigation
Maternal care for damage to fetus by intrauterine contraceptive device
Maternal care for damage to fetus by intrauterine surgery

✓x7ᵗʰ O35.8   **Maternal care for other (suspected)** fetal abnormality and damage   M♀

Maternal care for damage to fetus from maternal listeriosis
Maternal care for damage to fetus from maternal toxoplasmosis

✓x7ᵗʰ O35.9   **Maternal care for (suspected)** fetal abnormality and damage, unspecified   M♀

✓4ᵗʰ O36   **Maternal care for other fetal problems**

INCLUDES   the listed conditions in the fetus as a reason for hospitalization or other obstetric care of the mother, or for termination of pregnancy

EXCLUDES 1   encounter for suspected maternal and fetal conditions ruled out (Z03.7-)
placental transfusion syndromes (O43.Ø-)

EXCLUDES 2   labor and delivery complicated by fetal stress (O77.-)

AHA: 2015, 3Q, 40

One of the following 7th characters is to be assigned to each code under category O36. 7th character Ø is for single gestations and multiple gestations where the fetus is unspecified. 7th characters 1 through 9 are for cases of multiple gestations to identify the fetus for which the code applies. The appropriate code from category O3Ø, Multiple gestation, must also be assigned when assigning a code from category O36 that has a 7th character of 1 through 9.

Ø	not applicable or unspecified	3	fetus 3
		4	fetus 4
1	fetus 1	5	fetus 5
2	fetus 2	9	other fetus

✓5ᵗʰ O36.Ø   **Maternal care for rhesus isoimmunization**

Maternal care for Rh incompatibility (with hydrops fetalis)

CC Excl: For CC codes in subcategory O36.Ø:
PDX collection 978

✓6ᵗʰ O36.Ø1   **Maternal care for** anti-D [Rh] antibodies

AHA: 2014, 4Q, 17

✓7ᵗʰ O36.Ø11   **Maternal care for anti-D [Rh] antibodies,** first trimester   CC M♀

✓7ᵗʰ O36.Ø12   **Maternal care for anti-D [Rh] antibodies,** second trimester   CC M♀

✓7ᵗʰ O36.Ø13   **Maternal care for anti-D [Rh] antibodies,** third trimester   CC M♀

✓7ᵗʰ O36.Ø19   **Maternal care for anti-D [Rh] antibodies,** unspecified **trimester**   M♀

✓6ᵗʰ O36.Ø9   **Maternal care for** other rhesus isoimmunization

✓7ᵗʰ O36.Ø91   **Maternal care for other rhesus isoimmunization,** first trimester   CC M♀

✓7ᵗʰ O36.Ø92   **Maternal care for other rhesus isoimmunization,** second trimester   CC M♀

✓7ᵗʰ O36.Ø93   **Maternal care for other rhesus isoimmunization,** third trimester   CC M♀

✓7ᵗʰ O36.Ø99   **Maternal care for other rhesus isoimmunization,** unspecified trimester   M♀

✔ Additional Character Required   ✓x7ᵗʰ Placeholder   Unacceptable PDx   Questionable PDx   Manifestation   H1 - H14 HAC   HCC CMS-HCC Dx   HIV HIV Dx

ICD-10-CM 2019   867

Chapter 15. Pregnancy, Childbirth and the Puerperium

√5ᵗʰ **O36.1 Maternal care for other isoimmunization**
Maternal care for ABO isoimmunization

√6ᵗʰ **O36.11 Maternal care for Anti-A sensitization**
Maternal care for isoimmunization NOS (with hydrops fetalis)

√7ᵗʰ **O36.111 Maternal care for Anti-A sensitization,** M♀
first trimester

√7ᵗʰ **O36.112 Maternal care for Anti-A sensitization,** M♀
second trimester

√7ᵗʰ **O36.113 Maternal care for Anti-A sensitization,** M♀
third trimester

√7ᵗʰ **O36.119 Maternal care for Anti-A sensitization,** M♀
unspecified trimester

√6ᵗʰ **O36.19 Maternal care for other isoimmunization**
Maternal care for Anti-B sensitization

√7ᵗʰ **O36.191 Maternal care for other** M♀
isoimmunization, first trimester

√7ᵗʰ **O36.192 Maternal care for other** M♀
isoimmunization, second trimester

√7ᵗʰ **O36.193 Maternal care for other** M♀
isoimmunization, third trimester

√7ᵗʰ **O36.199 Maternal care for other** M♀
isoimmunization, unspecified trimester

√5ᵗʰ **O36.2 Maternal care for hydrops fetalis**
Maternal care for hydrops fetalis NOS
Maternal care for hydrops fetalis not associated with isoimmunization

> **EXCLUDES 1** hydrops fetalis associated with ABO isoimmunization (O36.1-)
> hydrops fetalis associated with rhesus isoimmunization (O36.0-)

DEF: Hydrops fetalis: Abnormal fluid buildup in at least two of the following fetal organ spaces: the skin (edema), abdomen (ascites), around the heart (pericardia effusion), and around the lung (pleural effusion). Fluid accumulation may also occur in the mother as polyhydramnios and edema of the placenta.

√x7ᵗʰ **O36.20 Maternal care for hydrops fetalis, unspecified** M♀
trimester

√x7ᵗʰ **O36.21 Maternal care for hydrops fetalis, first trimester** M♀

√x7ᵗʰ **O36.22 Maternal care for hydrops fetalis, second** M♀
trimester

√x7ᵗʰ **O36.23 Maternal care for hydrops fetalis, third** M♀
trimester

√x7ᵗʰ **O36.4 Maternal care for intrauterine death** cc M♀
Maternal care for intrauterine fetal death NOS
Maternal care for intrauterine fetal death after completion of 20 weeks of gestation
Maternal care for late fetal death
Maternal care for missed delivery

> **EXCLUDES 1** missed abortion (O02.1)
> stillbirth (P95)

CC Excl: PDX collection 979

√5ᵗʰ **O36.5 Maternal care for known or suspected poor fetal growth**

√6ᵗʰ **O36.51 Maternal care for known or suspected placental insufficiency**

√7ᵗʰ **O36.511 Maternal care for known or** M♀
suspected placental insufficiency, first trimester

√7ᵗʰ **O36.512 Maternal care for known or** M♀
suspected placental insufficiency, second trimester

√7ᵗʰ **O36.513 Maternal care for known or** M♀
suspected placental insufficiency, third trimester

√7ᵗʰ **O36.519 Maternal care for known or suspected** M♀
placental insufficiency, unspecified trimester

√6ᵗʰ **O36.59 Maternal care for other known or suspected poor fetal growth**
Maternal care for known or suspected light-for-dates NOS
Maternal care for known or suspected small-for-dates NOS

√7ᵗʰ **O36.591 Maternal care for other known or** M♀
suspected poor fetal growth, first trimester

√7ᵗʰ **O36.592 Maternal care for other known or** M♀
suspected poor fetal growth, second trimester

√7ᵗʰ **O36.593 Maternal care for other known or** M♀
suspected poor fetal growth, third trimester

√7ᵗʰ **O36.599 Maternal care for other known or** M♀
suspected poor fetal growth, unspecified trimester

√5ᵗʰ **O36.6 Maternal care for excessive fetal growth**
Maternal care for known or suspected large-for-dates

√x7ᵗʰ **O36.60 Maternal care for excessive fetal growth,** M♀
unspecified trimester

√x7ᵗʰ **O36.61 Maternal care for excessive fetal growth,** M♀
first trimester

√x7ᵗʰ **O36.62 Maternal care for excessive fetal growth,** M♀
second trimester

√x7ᵗʰ **O36.63 Maternal care for excessive fetal growth,** M♀
third trimester

√5ᵗʰ **O36.7 Maternal care for viable fetus in abdominal pregnancy**

√x7ᵗʰ **O36.70 Maternal care for viable fetus in abdominal** M♀
pregnancy, unspecified trimester

√x7ᵗʰ **O36.71 Maternal care for viable fetus in abdominal** M♀
pregnancy, first trimester

√x7ᵗʰ **O36.72 Maternal care for viable fetus in abdominal** M♀
pregnancy, second trimester

√x7ᵗʰ **O36.73 Maternal care for viable fetus in abdominal** M♀
pregnancy, third trimester

√5ᵗʰ **O36.8 Maternal care for other specified fetal problems**

√x7ᵗʰ **O36.80 Pregnancy with inconclusive fetal viability** M♀
Encounter to determine fetal viability of pregnancy

√6ᵗʰ **O36.81 Decreased fetal movements**

√7ᵗʰ **O36.812 Decreased fetal movements, second** M♀
trimester

√7ᵗʰ **O36.813 Decreased fetal movements, third** M♀
trimester

√7ᵗʰ **O36.819 Decreased fetal movements,** M♀
unspecified trimester

√6ᵗʰ **O36.82 Fetal anemia and thrombocytopenia**

√7ᵗʰ **O36.821 Fetal anemia and thrombocytopenia,** M♀
first trimester

√7ᵗʰ **O36.822 Fetal anemia and thrombocytopenia,** M♀
second trimester

√7ᵗʰ **O36.823 Fetal anemia and thrombocytopenia,** M♀
third trimester

√7ᵗʰ **O36.829 Fetal anemia and thrombocytopenia,** M♀
unspecified trimester

√6ᵗʰ **O36.83 Maternal care for abnormalities of the fetal heart rate or rhythm**
AHA: 2017, 4Q, 20
TIP: Assign for documented fetal tachycardia, bradycardia, decelerations, or loss of variability detected during antenatal testing.

√7ᵗʰ **O36.831 Maternal care for abnormalities of the** M♀
fetal heart rate or rhythm, first trimester

√7ᵗʰ **O36.832 Maternal care for abnormalities of the** M♀
fetal heart rate or rhythm, second trimester

√7ᵗʰ **O36.833 Maternal care for abnormalities of the** M♀
fetal heart rate or rhythm, third trimester

√7ᵗʰ **O36.839 Maternal care for abnormalities of the** M♀
fetal heart rate or rhythm, unspecified trimester

√6ᵗʰ **O36.89 Maternal care for other specified fetal problems**

√7ᵗʰ **O36.891 Maternal care for other specified fetal** M♀
problems, first trimester

√7ᵗʰ **O36.892 Maternal care for other specified fetal** M♀
problems, second trimester

√7ᵗʰ **O36.893 Maternal care for other specified fetal** M♀
problems, third trimester

√7ᵗʰ **O36.899 Maternal care for other specified fetal** M♀
problems, unspecified trimester

√5ᵗʰ **O36.9 Maternal care for fetal problem, unspecified**

√x7ᵗʰ **O36.90 Maternal care for fetal problem, unspecified,** M♀
unspecified trimester

√x7ᵗʰ **O36.91 Maternal care for fetal problem, unspecified,** M♀
first trimester

N Newborn: 0   P Pediatric: 0-17   M Maternity: 12-55   A Adult: 15-124   MCC Major Complication/Comorbidity   CC Complication/Comorbidity   SW Severe Wound Dx

868   ICD-10-CM 2019

√x 7ᵗʰ **O36.92** **Maternal care for fetal problem, unspecified, second trimester** Ⓜ♀

√x 7ᵗʰ **O36.93** **Maternal care for fetal problem, unspecified, third trimester** Ⓜ♀

√4ᵗʰ **O40 Polyhydramnios**
     INCLUDES   hydramnios
     EXCLUDES 1   encounter for suspected maternal and fetal conditions ruled out (Z03.7-)
     AHA: 2016, 1Q, 4
     DEF: Excess amniotic fluid surrounding the fetus, typically defined as a total fluid volume of greater than 24.0 cc.

> One of the following 7th characters is to be assigned to each code under category O40. 7th character Ø is for single gestations and multiple gestations where the fetus is unspecified. 7th characters 1 through 9 are for cases of multiple gestations to identify the fetus for which the code applies. The appropriate code from category O3Ø, Multiple gestation, must also be assigned when assigning a code from category O40 that has a 7th character of 1 through 9.
> | Ø | not applicable or | 3 | fetus 3 |
> | | unspecified | 4 | fetus 4 |
> | 1 | fetus 1 | 5 | fetus 5 |
> | 2 | fetus 2 | 9 | other fetus |

√x 7ᵗʰ **O40.1** **Polyhydramnios,** first trimester Ⓜ♀

√x 7ᵗʰ **O40.2** **Polyhydramnios,** second trimester Ⓜ♀

√x 7ᵗʰ **O40.3** **Polyhydramnios,** third trimester Ⓜ♀

√x 7ᵗʰ **O40.9** **Polyhydramnios,** unspecified trimester Ⓜ♀

√4ᵗʰ **O41 Other disorders of amniotic fluid and membranes**
     EXCLUDES 1   encounter for suspected maternal and fetal conditions ruled out (Z03.7-)

> One of the following 7th characters is to be assigned to each code under category O41. 7th character Ø is for single gestations and multiple gestations where the fetus is unspecified. 7th characters 1 through 9 are for cases of multiple gestations to identify the fetus for which the code applies. The appropriate code from category O3Ø, Multiple gestation, must also be assigned when assigning a code from category O41 that has a 7th character of 1 through 9.
> | Ø | not applicable or | 3 | fetus 3 |
> | | unspecified | 4 | fetus 4 |
> | 1 | fetus 1 | 5 | fetus 5 |
> | 2 | fetus 2 | 9 | other fetus |

√5ᵗʰ **O41.0 Oligohydramnios**
     Oligohydramnios without rupture of membranes
     DEF: Low amniotic fluid, occurring most frequently in the last trimester.

> **CC Excl: For CC codes in subcategory O41.0:**
> PDX collection 982

√x 7ᵗʰ **O41.00** **Oligohydramnios,** unspecified trimester Ⓜ♀

√x 7ᵗʰ **O41.01** **Oligohydramnios,** first trimester CC Ⓜ♀

√x 7ᵗʰ **O41.02** **Oligohydramnios,** second trimester CC Ⓜ♀

√x 7ᵗʰ **O41.03** **Oligohydramnios,** third trimester CC Ⓜ♀

√5ᵗʰ **O41.1 Infection of amniotic sac and membranes**

> **CC Excl: For MCC codes in subcategory O41.1:**
> PDX collection 983

√6ᵗʰ **O41.10** **Infection of amniotic sac and membranes, unspecified**

     √7ᵗʰ **O41.101** **Infection of amniotic sac and membranes, unspecified,** first trimester MCC Ⓜ♀

     √7ᵗʰ **O41.102** **Infection of amniotic sac and membranes, unspecified,** second trimester MCC Ⓜ♀

     √7ᵗʰ **O41.103** **Infection of amniotic sac and membranes, unspecified,** third trimester MCC Ⓜ♀

     √7ᵗʰ **O41.109** **Infection of amniotic sac and membranes,** unspecified trimester Ⓜ♀

√6ᵗʰ **O41.12** **Chorioamnionitis**

     √7ᵗʰ **O41.121** **Chorioamnionitis,** first trimester MCC Ⓜ♀

     √7ᵗʰ **O41.122** **Chorioamnionitis,** second trimester MCC Ⓜ♀

     √7ᵗʰ **O41.123** **Chorioamnionitis,** third trimester MCC Ⓜ♀

     √7ᵗʰ **O41.129** **Chorioamnionitis,** unspecified trimester Ⓜ♀

√6ᵗʰ **O41.14** **Placentitis**

     √7ᵗʰ **O41.141** **Placentitis,** first trimester MCC Ⓜ♀

     √7ᵗʰ **O41.142** **Placentitis,** second trimester MCC Ⓜ♀

     √7ᵗʰ **O41.143** **Placentitis,** third trimester MCC Ⓜ♀

     √7ᵗʰ **O41.149** **Placentitis,** unspecified trimester Ⓜ♀

√5ᵗʰ **O41.8 Other specified disorders of amniotic fluid and membranes**

     √6ᵗʰ **O41.8X** **Other specified disorders of amniotic fluid and membranes**

         √7ᵗʰ **O41.8X1** **Other specified disorders of amniotic fluid and membranes,** first trimester Ⓜ♀

         √7ᵗʰ **O41.8X2** **Other specified disorders of amniotic fluid and membranes,** second trimester Ⓜ♀

         √7ᵗʰ **O41.8X3** **Other specified disorders of amniotic fluid and membranes,** third trimester Ⓜ♀

         √7ᵗʰ **O41.8X9** **Other specified disorders of amniotic fluid and membranes,** unspecified trimester Ⓜ♀

√5ᵗʰ **O41.9 Disorder of amniotic fluid and membranes, unspecified**

     √x 7ᵗʰ **O41.90** **Disorder of amniotic fluid and membranes, unspecified,** unspecified trimester Ⓜ♀

     √x 7ᵗʰ **O41.91** **Disorder of amniotic fluid and membranes, unspecified,** first trimester Ⓜ♀

     √x 7ᵗʰ **O41.92** **Disorder of amniotic fluid and membranes, unspecified,** second trimester Ⓜ♀

     √x 7ᵗʰ **O41.93** **Disorder of amniotic fluid and membranes, unspecified,** third trimester Ⓜ♀

√4ᵗʰ **O42 Premature rupture of membranes**
     AHA: 2016, 1Q, 3

√5ᵗʰ **O42.0 Premature rupture of membranes,** onset of labor within 24 hours of rupture

     O42.00 **Premature rupture of membranes, onset of labor within 24 hours of rupture,** unspecified weeks of gestation Ⓜ♀

     √6ᵗʰ **O42.01** **Preterm premature rupture of membranes, onset of labor within 24 hours of rupture**
         Premature rupture of membranes before 37 completed weeks of gestation

         O42.011 **Preterm premature rupture of membranes, onset of labor within 24 hours of rupture,** first trimester Ⓜ♀

         O42.012 **Preterm premature rupture of membranes, onset of labor within 24 hours of rupture,** second trimester Ⓜ♀

         O42.013 **Preterm premature rupture of membranes, onset of labor within 24 hours of rupture,** third trimester Ⓜ♀

         O42.019 **Preterm premature rupture of membranes, onset of labor within 24 hours of rupture,** unspecified trimester Ⓜ♀

     O42.02 **Full-term premature rupture of membranes,** onset of labor within 24 hours of rupture Ⓜ♀
         Premature rupture of membranes at or after 37 completed weeks of gestation, onset of labor within 24 hours of rupture

√5ᵗʰ **O42.1 Premature rupture of membranes,** onset of labor more than 24 hours following rupture
     AHA: 2016, 1Q, 5

     O42.10 **Premature rupture of membranes, onset of labor more than 24 hours following rupture,** unspecified weeks of gestation Ⓜ♀

     √6ᵗʰ **O42.11** **Preterm premature rupture of membranes, onset of labor more than 24 hours following rupture**
         Premature rupture of membranes before 37 completed weeks of gestation

         O42.111 **Preterm premature rupture of membranes, onset of labor more than 24 hours following rupture,** first trimester Ⓜ♀

         O42.112 **Preterm premature rupture of membranes, onset of labor more than 24 hours following rupture,** second trimester Ⓜ♀

         O42.113 **Preterm premature rupture of membranes, onset of labor more than 24 hours following rupture,** third trimester Ⓜ♀

✔ Additional Character Required   √x 7ᵗʰ Placeholder   Unacceptable PDx   Questionable PDx   Manifestation   H1 - H14 HAC   HCC CMS-HCC Dx   HIV HIV Dx

ICD-10-CM 2019   869

O42.119   **Preterm premature rupture of membranes, onset of labor more than 24 hours following rupture,** unspecified trimester   M♀

O42.12   Full-term **premature rupture of membranes, onset of labor more than 24 hours following rupture**   M♀
Premature rupture of membranes at or after 37 completed weeks of gestation, onset of labor more than 24 hours following rupture

✓5ᵗʰ **O42.9**   **Premature rupture of membranes,** unspecified as to length of time between rupture and onset of labor

     O42.90   **Premature rupture of membranes, unspecified as to length of time between rupture and onset of labor,** unspecified weeks of gestation   M♀

     ✓6ᵗʰ **O42.91**   Preterm **premature rupture of membranes, unspecified as to length of time between rupture and onset of labor**
Premature rupture of membranes before 37 completed weeks of gestation

       O42.911   **Preterm premature rupture of membranes, unspecified as to length of time between rupture and onset of labor,** first trimester   M♀

       O42.912   **Preterm premature rupture of membranes, unspecified as to length of time between rupture and onset of labor,** second trimester   M♀

       O42.913   **Preterm premature rupture of membranes, unspecified as to length of time between rupture and onset of labor,** third trimester   M♀

       O42.919   **Preterm premature rupture of membranes, unspecified as to length of time between rupture and onset of labor,** unspecified trimester   M♀

     O42.92   Full-term **premature rupture of membranes, unspecified as to length of time between rupture and onset of labor**   M♀
Premature rupture of membranes at or after 37 completed weeks of gestation, unspecified as to length of time between rupture and onset of labor

✓4ᵗʰ **O43**   **Placental disorders**
> EXCLUDES 2   *maternal care for poor fetal growth due to placental insufficiency (O36.5-)*
> *placenta previa (O44.-)*
> *placental polyp (O90.89)*
> *placentitis (O41.14-)*
> *premature separation of placenta [abruptio placentae] (O45.-)*

✓5ᵗʰ **O43.0**   **Placental transfusion syndromes**

     ✓6ᵗʰ **O43.01**   Fetomaternal **placental transfusion syndrome**
Maternofetal placental transfusion syndrome

       O43.011   **Fetomaternal placental transfusion syndrome,** first trimester   M♀

       O43.012   **Fetomaternal placental transfusion syndrome,** second trimester   M♀

       O43.013   **Fetomaternal placental transfusion syndrome,** third trimester   M♀

       O43.019   **Fetomaternal placental transfusion syndrome,** unspecified trimester   M♀

     ✓6ᵗʰ **O43.02**   Fetus-to-fetus **placental transfusion syndrome**
DEF: Condition in which an imbalance in amniotic fluid occurs due to uneven blood flow between twins sharing a placenta.

       O43.021   **Fetus-to-fetus placental transfusion syndrome,** first trimester   M♀

       O43.022   **Fetus-to-fetus placental transfusion syndrome,** second trimester   M♀

       O43.023   **Fetus-to-fetus placental transfusion syndrome,** third trimester   M♀

       O43.029   **Fetus-to-fetus placental transfusion syndrome,** unspecified trimester   M♀

Twin to Twin Transfusion Syndrome (TTTS)

Healthy twins   Twins with TTTS

✓5ᵗʰ **O43.1**   **Malformation of placenta**

     ✓6ᵗʰ **O43.10**   **Malformation of placenta,** unspecified
Abnormal placenta NOS

       O43.101   **Malformation of placenta, unspecified,** first trimester   M♀

       O43.102   **Malformation of placenta, unspecified,** second trimester   M♀

       O43.103   **Malformation of placenta, unspecified,** third trimester   M♀

       O43.109   **Malformation of placenta, unspecified,** unspecified trimester   M♀

     ✓6ᵗʰ **O43.11**   Circumvallate **placenta**

       O43.111   **Circumvallate placenta,** first trimester   M♀

       O43.112   **Circumvallate placenta,** second trimester   M♀

       O43.113   **Circumvallate placenta,** third trimester   M♀

       O43.119   **Circumvallate placenta,** unspecified trimester   M♀

     ✓6ᵗʰ **O43.12**   Velamentous insertion of umbilical cord

       O43.121   **Velamentous insertion of umbilical cord,** first trimester   M♀

       O43.122   **Velamentous insertion of umbilical cord,** second trimester   M♀

       O43.123   **Velamentous insertion of umbilical cord,** third trimester   M♀

       O43.129   **Velamentous insertion of umbilical cord,** unspecified trimester   M♀

     ✓6ᵗʰ **O43.19**   Other malformation of placenta

       O43.191   **Other malformation of placenta,** first trimester   M♀

       O43.192   **Other malformation of placenta,** second trimester   M♀

       O43.193   **Other malformation of placenta,** third trimester   M♀

       O43.199   **Other malformation of placenta,** unspecified trimester   M♀

✓5ᵗʰ **O43.2**   **Morbidly adherent placenta**
Code also associated third stage postpartum hemorrhage, if applicable (O72.0)
> EXCLUDES 1   *retained placenta (O73.-)*

     ✓6ᵗʰ **O43.21**   Placenta accreta
DEF: Condition where the placenta adheres too deeply to the uterine wall; often associated with placenta previa.

       O43.211   **Placenta accreta,** first trimester   M♀
       O43.212   **Placenta accreta,** second trimester   M♀
       O43.213   **Placenta accreta,** third trimester   M♀
       O43.219   **Placenta accreta,** unspecified trimester   M♀

     ✓6ᵗʰ **O43.22**   Placenta increta
DEF: Condition where the placenta adheres too deeply to the uterine wall and penetrates the muscle; often associated with placenta previa.

       O43.221   **Placenta increta,** first trimester   M♀
       O43.222   **Placenta increta,** second trimester   M♀
       O43.223   **Placenta increta,** third trimester   M♀

O43.229   **Placenta increta, unspecified**   M♀
trimester

☑6ᵗʰ   **O43.23**   **Placenta percreta**
DEF: Condition where the placenta attaches through the uterine muscle and may invade other organs, resulting in antenatal complications, premature delivery, retention of all or a portion of the placenta, or postpartum bleeding.

O43.231   **Placenta percreta, first trimester**   M♀
O43.232   **Placenta percreta, second trimester**   M♀
O43.233   **Placenta percreta, third trimester**   M♀
O43.239   **Placenta percreta, unspecified**   M♀
trimester

☑5ᵗʰ   **O43.8 Other placental disorders**
☑6ᵗʰ   **O43.81**   **Placental infarction**
O43.811   **Placental infarction, first trimester**   M♀
O43.812   **Placental infarction, second trimester**   M♀
O43.813   **Placental infarction, third trimester**   M♀
O43.819   **Placental infarction, unspecified**   M♀
trimester

☑6ᵗʰ   **O43.89**   **Other placental disorders**
Placental dysfunction
O43.891   **Other placental disorders, first**   M♀
trimester
O43.892   **Other placental disorders, second**   M♀
trimester
O43.893   **Other placental disorders, third**   M♀
trimester
O43.899   **Other placental disorders,**   M♀
unspecified trimester

☑5ᵗʰ   **O43.9 Unspecified placental disorder**
O43.90   **Unspecified placental disorder, unspecified**   M♀
trimester
O43.91   **Unspecified placental disorder, first trimester**   M♀
O43.92   **Unspecified placental disorder, second**   M♀
trimester
O43.93   **Unspecified placental disorder, third trimester**   M♀

☑4ᵗʰ   **O44**   **Placenta previa**
AHA: 2016, 4Q, 52-53
DEF: Placenta implanted in the lower segment of the uterus, which commonly causes hemorrhage in the last trimester of pregnancy.

CC Excl: For CC/MCC codes in category O44: PDX collection 966

☑5ᵗʰ   **O44.0 Complete placenta previa NOS or without hemorrhage**
Placenta previa NOS
O44.00   **Complete placenta previa NOS or without**   M♀
hemorrhage, unspecified trimester
O44.01   **Complete placenta previa NOS or without**   CC M♀
hemorrhage, first trimester
O44.02   **Complete placenta previa NOS or without**   CC M♀
hemorrhage, second trimester
O44.03   **Complete placenta previa NOS or without**   CC M♀
hemorrhage, third trimester

☑5ᵗʰ   **O44.1 Complete placenta previa with hemorrhage**
EXCLUDES 1   *labor and delivery complicated by hemorrhage from vasa previa (O69.4)*
O44.10   **Complete placenta previa with hemorrhage,**   M♀
unspecified trimester
O44.11   **Complete placenta previa with hemorrhage,**   MCC M♀
first trimester
O44.12   **Complete placenta previa with hemorrhage,**   MCC M♀
second trimester
O44.13   **Complete placenta previa with hemorrhage,**   MCC M♀
third trimester

☑5ᵗʰ   **O44.2 Partial placenta previa without hemorrhage**
Marginal placenta previa, NOS or without hemorrhage
O44.20   **Partial placenta previa NOS or without**   M♀
hemorrhage, unspecified trimester
O44.21   **Partial placenta previa NOS or without**   CC M♀
hemorrhage, first trimester
O44.22   **Partial placenta previa NOS or without**   CC M♀
hemorrhage, second trimester
O44.23   **Partial placenta previa NOS or without**   CC M♀
hemorrhage, third trimester

☑5ᵗʰ   **O44.3 Partial placenta previa with hemorrhage**
Marginal placenta previa with hemorrhage
O44.30   **Partial placenta previa with hemorrhage,**   M♀
unspecified trimester
O44.31   **Partial placenta previa with hemorrhage,**   MCC M♀
first trimester
O44.32   **Partial placenta previa with hemorrhage,**   MCC M♀
second trimester
O44.33   **Partial placenta previa with hemorrhage,**   MCC M♀
third trimester

☑5ᵗʰ   **O44.4 Low lying placenta NOS or without hemorrhage**
Low implantation of placenta NOS or without hemorrhage
O44.40   **Low lying placenta NOS or without**   M♀
hemorrhage, unspecified trimester
O44.41   **Low lying placenta NOS or without**   CC M♀
hemorrhage, first trimester
O44.42   **Low lying placenta NOS or without**   CC M♀
hemorrhage, second trimester
O44.43   **Low lying placenta NOS or without**   CC M♀
hemorrhage, third trimester

☑5ᵗʰ   **O44.5 Low lying placenta with hemorrhage**
Low implantation of placenta with hemorrhage
O44.50   **Low lying placenta with hemorrhage,**   M♀
unspecified trimester
O44.51   **Low lying placenta with hemorrhage, first**   MCC M♀
trimester
O44.52   **Low lying placenta with hemorrhage,**   MCC M♀
second trimester
O44.53   **Low lying placenta with hemorrhage, third**   MCC M♀
trimester

☑4ᵗʰ   **O45**   **Premature separation of placenta [abruptio placentae]**
☑5ᵗʰ   **O45.0 Premature separation of placenta with coagulation defect**

CC Excl: For MCC codes in subcategory O45.0: PDX collection 985

☑6ᵗʰ   **O45.00**   **Premature separation of placenta with coagulation defect, unspecified**
O45.001   **Premature separation of placenta**   MCC M♀
with coagulation defect, unspecified, first trimester
O45.002   **Premature separation of placenta**   MCC M♀
with coagulation defect, unspecified, second trimester
O45.003   **Premature separation of placenta**   MCC M♀
with coagulation defect, unspecified, third trimester
O45.009   **Premature separation of placenta**   M♀
with coagulation defect, unspecified, unspecified trimester

☑6ᵗʰ   **O45.01**   **Premature separation of placenta with afibrinogenemia**
Premature separation of placenta with hypofibrinogenemia
O45.011   **Premature separation of placenta**   MCC M♀
with afibrinogenemia, first trimester
O45.012   **Premature separation of placenta**   MCC M♀
with afibrinogenemia, second trimester
O45.013   **Premature separation of placenta**   MCC M♀
with afibrinogenemia, third trimester
O45.019   **Premature separation of placenta**   M♀
with afibrinogenemia, unspecified trimester

☑6ᵗʰ   **O45.02**   **Premature separation of placenta with disseminated intravascular coagulation**
O45.021   **Premature separation of placenta**   MCC M♀
with disseminated intravascular coagulation, first trimester
O45.022   **Premature separation of placenta**   MCC M♀
with disseminated intravascular coagulation, second trimester
O45.023   **Premature separation of placenta**   MCC M♀
with disseminated intravascular coagulation, third trimester
O45.029   **Premature separation of placenta**   M♀
with disseminated intravascular coagulation, unspecified trimester

☑ Additional Character Required   ✓ˣ7ᵗʰ Placeholder   Unacceptable PDx   Questionable PDx   Manifestation   H1 - H14 HAC   HCC CMS-HCC Dx   HIV HIV Dx

ICD-10-CM 2019   871

√6ᵗʰ **O45.09 Premature separation of placenta with** other **coagulation defect**

    O45.091 Premature separation of placenta MCC M♀ **with other coagulation defect, first trimester**

    O45.092 Premature separation of placenta MCC M♀ **with other coagulation defect, second trimester**

    O45.093 Premature separation of placenta MCC M♀ **with other coagulation defect, third trimester**

    O45.099 Premature separation of placenta M♀ **with other coagulation defect, unspecified trimester**

√5ᵗʰ **O45.8 Other premature separation** of placenta

> **CC Excl: For MCC codes in subcategory O45.8:** PDX collection 986

√6ᵗʰ **O45.8X Other premature separation of placenta**

    O45.8X1 Other premature separation of MCC M♀ **placenta, first trimester**

    O45.8X2 Other premature separation of MCC M♀ **placenta, second trimester**

    O45.8X3 Other premature separation of MCC M♀ **placenta, third trimester**

    O45.8X9 Other premature separation of M♀ **placenta, unspecified trimester**

√5ᵗʰ **O45.9 Premature separation of placenta,** unspecified
Abruptio placentae NOS

> **CC Excl: For MCC codes in subcategory O45.9:** PDX collection 986

    O45.90 Premature separation of placenta, unspecified, M♀ **unspecified trimester**

    O45.91 Premature separation of placenta, MCC M♀ **unspecified, first trimester**

    O45.92 Premature separation of placenta, MCC M♀ **unspecified, second trimester**

    O45.93 Premature separation of placenta, MCC M♀ **unspecified, third trimester**

√4ᵗʰ **O46 Antepartum hemorrhage, not elsewhere classified**

   EXCLUDES 1   *hemorrhage in early pregnancy (O20.-)*
          intrapartum hemorrhage NEC (O67.-)
          placenta previa (O44.-)
          premature separation of placenta [abruptio placentae] (O45.-)

   DEF: Uterine hemorrhage prior to delivery that is not related to placenta previa or abruptio placentae.

√5ᵗʰ **O46.0 Antepartum hemorrhage with** coagulation defect

> **CC Excl: For MCC codes in subcategory O46.0:** PDX collection 985

√6ᵗʰ **O46.00 Antepartum hemorrhage with coagulation defect, unspecified**

    O46.001 Antepartum hemorrhage with MCC M♀ **coagulation defect, unspecified, first trimester**

    O46.002 Antepartum hemorrhage with MCC M♀ **coagulation defect, unspecified, second trimester**

    O46.003 Antepartum hemorrhage with MCC M♀ **coagulation defect, unspecified, third trimester**

    O46.009 Antepartum hemorrhage with M♀ **coagulation defect, unspecified, unspecified trimester**

√6ᵗʰ **O46.01 Antepartum hemorrhage with** afibrinogenemia
Antepartum hemorrhage with hypofibrinogenemia

    O46.011 Antepartum hemorrhage with MCC M♀ **afibrinogenemia, first trimester**

    O46.012 Antepartum hemorrhage with MCC M♀ **afibrinogenemia, second trimester**

    O46.013 Antepartum hemorrhage with MCC M♀ **afibrinogenemia, third trimester**

    O46.019 Antepartum hemorrhage with M♀ **afibrinogenemia, unspecified trimester**

√6ᵗʰ **O46.02 Antepartum hemorrhage with** disseminated intravascular coagulation

    O46.021 Antepartum hemorrhage with MCC M♀ **disseminated intravascular coagulation, first trimester**

    O46.022 Antepartum hemorrhage with MCC M♀ **disseminated intravascular coagulation, second trimester**

    O46.023 Antepartum hemorrhage with MCC M♀ **disseminated intravascular coagulation, third trimester**

    O46.029 Antepartum hemorrhage with M♀ **disseminated intravascular coagulation, unspecified trimester**

√6ᵗʰ **O46.09 Antepartum hemorrhage with** other **coagulation defect**

    O46.091 Antepartum hemorrhage with MCC M♀ **other coagulation defect,** first **trimester**

    O46.092 Antepartum hemorrhage with MCC M♀ **other coagulation defect,** second **trimester**

    O46.093 Antepartum hemorrhage with MCC M♀ **other coagulation defect,** third **trimester**

    O46.099 Antepartum hemorrhage with other M♀ **coagulation defect,** unspecified **trimester**

√5ᵗʰ **O46.8 Other antepartum hemorrhage**

√6ᵗʰ **O46.8X** Other **antepartum hemorrhage**

    O46.8X1 Other antepartum hemorrhage, M♀ **first trimester**

    O46.8X2 Other antepartum hemorrhage, M♀ **second trimester**

    O46.8X3 Other antepartum hemorrhage, M♀ **third trimester**

    O46.8X9 Other antepartum hemorrhage, M♀ **unspecified trimester**

√5ᵗʰ **O46.9 Antepartum hemorrhage,** unspecified

    O46.90 Antepartum hemorrhage, unspecified, M♀ **unspecified trimester**

    O46.91 Antepartum hemorrhage, unspecified, M♀ **first trimester**

    O46.92 Antepartum hemorrhage, unspecified, M♀ **second trimester**

    O46.93 Antepartum hemorrhage, unspecified, M♀ **third trimester**

√4ᵗʰ **O47 False labor**

   INCLUDES   Braxton Hicks contractions
          threatened labor
   EXCLUDES 1   *preterm labor (O60.-)*

> **CC Excl: For CC codes in catagory O47:** PDX collection 987

√5ᵗʰ **O47.0 False labor** before 37 completed weeks of gestation

    O47.00 False labor before 37 completed weeks of M♀ **gestation,** unspecified trimester

    O47.02 False labor before 37 completed weeks of CC M♀ **gestation,** second trimester

    O47.03 False labor before 37 completed weeks of CC M♀ **gestation,** third trimester

   O47.1 False labor at or after 37 completed weeks of CC M♀ gestation

   O47.9 False labor, unspecified M♀

√4ᵗʰ **O48 Late pregnancy**

   O48.0 Post-term pregnancy M♀
Pregnancy over 40 completed weeks to 42 completed weeks gestation

   O48.1 Prolonged pregnancy M♀
Pregnancy which has advanced beyond 42 completed weeks gestation
AHA: 2016, 1Q, 5

N Newborn: 0   P Pediatric: 0-17   M Maternity: 12-55   A Adult: 15-124   MCC Major Complication/Comorbidity   CC Complication/Comorbidity   SW Severe Wound Dx

Complications of labor and delivery (O60-O77)

✓4ᵗʰ O60 Preterm labor

INCLUDES onset (spontaneous) of labor before 37 completed weeks of gestation

EXCLUDES 1 false labor (O47.0-)
           threatened labor NOS (O47.0-)

CC Excl: For CC/MCC codes in category O60: PDX collection 987

✓5ᵗʰ O60.0 Preterm labor without delivery

O60.00 Preterm labor without delivery, unspecified trimester   M♀

O60.02 Preterm labor without delivery, second trimester   MCC M♀

O60.03 Preterm labor without delivery, third trimester   MCC M♀

✓5ᵗʰ O60.1 Preterm labor with preterm delivery

AHA: 2016, 2Q, 10

> One of the following 7th characters is to be assigned to each code under subcategory O60.1. 7th character 0 is for single gestations and multiple gestations where the fetus is unspecified. 7th characters 1 through 9 are for cases of multiple gestations to identify the fetus for which the code applies. The appropriate code from category O30, Multiple gestation, must also be assigned when assigning a code from subcategory O60.1 that has a 7th character of 1 through 9.
>
> | 0 | not applicable or unspecified | 3 | fetus 3 |
> |---|---|---|---|
> | | | 4 | fetus 4 |
> | 1 | fetus 1 | 5 | fetus 5 |
> | 2 | fetus 2 | 9 | other fetus |

✓x7ᵗʰ O60.10 Preterm labor with preterm delivery, unspecified trimester   CC M♀
     Preterm labor with delivery NOS

✓x7ᵗʰ O60.12 Preterm labor second trimester with preterm delivery second trimester   MCC M♀

✓x7ᵗʰ O60.13 Preterm labor second trimester with preterm delivery third trimester   MCC M♀

✓x7ᵗʰ O60.14 Preterm labor third trimester with preterm delivery third trimester   MCC M♀

✓5ᵗʰ O60.2 Term delivery with preterm labor

> One of the following 7th characters is to be assigned to each code under subcategory O60.2. 7th character 0 is for single gestations and multiple gestations where the fetus is unspecified. 7th characters 1 through 9 are for cases of multiple gestations to identify the fetus for which the code applies. The appropriate code from category O30, Multiple gestation, must also be assigned when assigning a code from subcategory O60.2 that has a 7th character of 1 through 9.
>
> | 0 | not applicable or unspecified | 3 | fetus 3 |
> |---|---|---|---|
> | | | 4 | fetus 4 |
> | 1 | fetus 1 | 5 | fetus 5 |
> | 2 | fetus 2 | 9 | other fetus |

✓x7ᵗʰ O60.20 Term delivery with preterm labor, unspecified trimester   CC M♀

✓x7ᵗʰ O60.22 Term delivery with preterm labor, second trimester   MCC M♀

✓x7ᵗʰ O60.23 Term delivery with preterm labor, third trimester   MCC M♀

✓4ᵗʰ O61 Failed induction of labor

O61.0 Failed medical induction of labor   M♀
     Failed induction (of labor) by oxytocin
     Failed induction (of labor) by prostaglandins

O61.1 Failed instrumental induction of labor   M♀
     Failed mechanical induction (of labor)
     Failed surgical induction (of labor)

O61.8 Other failed induction of labor   M♀

O61.9 Failed induction of labor, unspecified   M♀

✓4ᵗʰ O62 Abnormalities of forces of labor

DEF: Uterine inertia: Weak or poorly coordinated contractions of the uterus during labor.

O62.0 Primary inadequate contractions   M♀
     Failure of cervical dilatation
     Primary hypotonic uterine dysfunction
     Uterine inertia during latent phase of labor

O62.1 Secondary uterine inertia   M♀
     Arrested active phase of labor
     Secondary hypotonic uterine dysfunction

O62.2 Other uterine inertia   M♀
     Atony of uterus without hemorrhage
     Atony of uterus NOS
     Desultory labor
     Hypotonic uterine dysfunction NOS
     Irregular labor
     Poor contractions
     Slow slope active phase of labor
     Uterine inertia NOS

     EXCLUDES 1 atony of uterus with hemorrhage (postpartum) (O72.1)
                postpartum atony of uterus without hemorrhage (O75.89)

     DEF: Uterine atony: Failure of the uterine muscles to contract after the fetus and placenta are delivered.

O62.3 Precipitate labor   M♀
     DEF: Rapid labor with delivery occurring in three hours or less from the onset of contractions.

O62.4 Hypertonic, incoordinate, and prolonged uterine contractions   M♀
     Cervical spasm
     Contraction ring dystocia
     Dyscoordinate labor
     Hour-glass contraction of uterus
     Hypertonic uterine dysfunction
     Incoordinate uterine action
     Tetanic contractions
     Uterine dystocia NOS
     Uterine spasm

     EXCLUDES 1 dystocia (fetal) (maternal) NOS (O66.9)

O62.8 Other abnormalities of forces of labor   M♀

O62.9 Abnormality of forces of labor, unspecified   M♀

✓4ᵗʰ O63 Long labor

O63.0 Prolonged first stage (of labor)   M♀

O63.1 Prolonged second stage (of labor)   M♀

O63.2 Delayed delivery of second twin, triplet, etc.   M♀

O63.9 Long labor, unspecified   CC M♀
     Prolonged labor NOS
     CC Excl: PDX collection 988

Fetal Malposition

Breech

Shoulder (arm prolapse)

Mother's pelvis

Compound (extremity together with head)

Face (mentum)

Oblique

✓4ᵗʰ O64 Obstructed labor due to malposition and malpresentation of fetus

> One of the following 7th characters is to be assigned to each code under category O64. 7th character 0 is for single gestations and multiple gestations where the fetus is unspecified. 7th characters 1 through 9 are for cases of multiple gestations to identify the fetus for which the code applies. The appropriate code from category O30, Multiple gestation, must also be assigned when assigning a code from category O64 that has a 7th character of 1 through 9.
>
> | 0 | not applicable or unspecified | 3 | fetus 3 |
> |---|---|---|---|
> | | | 4 | fetus 4 |
> | 1 | fetus 1 | 5 | fetus 5 |
> | 2 | fetus 2 | 9 | other fetus |

✓x7ᵗʰ O64.0 Obstructed labor due to incomplete rotation of fetal head   M♀
     Deep transverse arrest
     Obstructed labor due to persistent occipitoiliac (position)
     Obstructed labor due to persistent occipitoposterior (position)
     Obstructed labor due to persistent occipitosacral (position)
     Obstructed labor due to persistent occipitotransverse (position)

✓ Additional Character Required   ✓x7ᵗʰ Placeholder   Unacceptable PDx   Questionable PDx   Manifestation   H1 - H14 HAC   HCC CMS-HCC Dx   HIV HIV Dx

ICD-10-CM 2019   873

√x7ᵗʰ O64.1 Obstructed labor due to breech presentation M♀
Obstructed labor due to buttocks presentation
Obstructed labor due to complete breech presentation
Obstructed labor due to frank breech presentation

√x7ᵗʰ O64.2 Obstructed labor due to face presentation M♀
Obstructed labor due to chin presentation

√x7ᵗʰ O64.3 Obstructed labor due to brow presentation M♀

√x7ᵗʰ O64.4 Obstructed labor due to shoulder presentation M♀
Prolapsed arm
> EXCLUDES 1 *impacted shoulders (O66.Ø)*
> *shoulder dystocia (O66.Ø)*

√x7ᵗʰ O64.5 Obstructed labor due to compound presentation M♀

√x7ᵗʰ O64.8 Obstructed labor due to other malposition and malpresentation M♀
Obstructed labor due to footling presentation
Obstructed labor due to incomplete breech presentation

√x7ᵗʰ O64.9 Obstructed labor due to malposition and malpresentation, unspecified M♀

√4ᵗʰ O65 Obstructed labor due to maternal pelvic abnormality

O65.Ø Obstructed labor due to deformed pelvis M♀

O65.1 Obstructed labor due to generally contracted pelvis M♀

O65.2 Obstructed labor due to pelvic inlet contraction M♀

O65.3 Obstructed labor due to pelvic outlet and mid-cavity contraction M♀

O65.4 Obstructed labor due to fetopelvic disproportion, unspecified M♀
> EXCLUDES 1 *dystocia due to abnormality of fetus (O66.2-O66.3)*

O65.5 Obstructed labor due to abnormality of maternal pelvic organs M♀
Obstructed labor due to conditions listed in O34-
Use additional code to identify abnormality of pelvic organs (O34.-)

O65.8 Obstructed labor due to other maternal pelvic abnormalities M♀

O65.9 Obstructed labor due to maternal pelvic abnormality, unspecified M♀

√4ᵗʰ O66 Other obstructed labor

O66.Ø Obstructed labor due to shoulder dystocia M♀
Impacted shoulders
DEF: Obstructed labor due to impacted fetal shoulders. It is an emergency condition that may require cesarean section, forceps delivery, vacuum extraction, or symphysiotomy.

O66.1 Obstructed labor due to locked twins M♀

O66.2 Obstructed labor due to unusually large fetus M♀

O66.3 Obstructed labor due to other abnormalities of fetus M♀
Dystocia due to fetal ascites
Dystocia due to fetal hydrops
Dystocia due to fetal meningomyelocele
Dystocia due to fetal sacral teratoma
Dystocia due to fetal tumor
Dystocia due to hydrocephalic fetus
Use additional code to identify cause of obstruction

√5ᵗʰ O66.4 Failed trial of labor

O66.4Ø Failed trial of labor, unspecified M♀

O66.41 Failed attempted vaginal birth after previous cesarean delivery M♀
Code first rupture of uterus, if applicable (O71.Ø-, O71.1)

O66.5 Attempted application of vacuum extractor and forceps M♀
Attempted application of vacuum or forceps, with subsequent delivery by forceps or cesarean delivery

O66.6 Obstructed labor due to other multiple fetuses M♀

O66.8 Other specified obstructed labor M♀
Use additional code to identify cause of obstruction

O66.9 Obstructed labor, unspecified M♀
Dystocia NOS
Fetal dystocia NOS
Maternal dystocia NOS

√4ᵗʰ O67 Labor and delivery complicated by intrapartum hemorrhage, not elsewhere classified
> EXCLUDES 1 *antepartum hemorrhage NEC (O46.-)*
> *placenta previa (O44.-)*
> *premature separation of placenta [abruptio placentae] (O45.-)*
> EXCLUDES 2 *postpartum hemorrhage (O72.-)*

O67.Ø Intrapartum hemorrhage with coagulation defect MCC M♀
Intrapartum hemorrhage (excessive) associated with afibrinogenemia
Intrapartum hemorrhage (excessive) associated with disseminated intravascular coagulation
Intrapartum hemorrhage (excessive) associated with hyperfibrinolysis
Intrapartum hemorrhage (excessive) associated with hypofibrinogenemia
CC Excl: PDX collection 985

O67.8 Other intrapartum hemorrhage M♀
Excessive intrapartum hemorrhage

O67.9 Intrapartum hemorrhage, unspecified M♀

O68 Labor and delivery complicated by abnormality of fetal acid-base balance CC M♀
Fetal acidemia complicating labor and delivery
Fetal acidosis complicating labor and delivery
Fetal alkalosis complicating labor and delivery
Fetal metabolic acidemia complicating labor and delivery
> EXCLUDES 1 *fetal stress NOS (O77.9)*
> *labor and delivery complicated by electrocardiographic evidence of fetal stress (O77.8)*
> *labor and delivery complicated by ultrasonic evidence of fetal stress (O77.8)*
> EXCLUDES 2 *abnormality in fetal heart rate or rhythm (O76)*
> *labor and delivery complicated by meconium in amniotic fluid (O77.Ø)*
CC Excl: PDX collection 989

√4ᵗʰ O69 Labor and delivery complicated by umbilical cord complications
AHA: 2016, 1Q, 5

> One of the following 7th characters is to be assigned to each code under category O69. 7th character Ø is for single gestations and multiple gestations where the fetus is unspecified. 7th characters 1 through 9 are for cases of multiple gestations to identify the fetus for which the code applies. The appropriate code from category O3Ø, Multiple gestation, must also be assigned when assigning a code from category O69 that has a 7th character of 1 through 9.
> Ø   not applicable or   3   fetus 3
>   unspecified   4   fetus 4
> 1   fetus 1   5   fetus 5
> 2   fetus 2   9   other fetus

√x7ᵗʰ O69.Ø Labor and delivery complicated by prolapse of cord M♀
DEF: Abnormal presentation of the fetus marked by a protruding umbilical cord during labor. It can cause fetal death.

√x7ᵗʰ O69.1 Labor and delivery complicated by cord around neck, with compression M♀
> EXCLUDES 1 *labor and delivery complicated by cord around neck, without compression (O69.81)*

√x7ᵗʰ O69.2 Labor and delivery complicated by other cord entanglement, with compression M♀
Labor and delivery complicated by compression of cord NOS
Labor and delivery complicated by entanglement of cords of twins in monoamniotic sac
Labor and delivery complicated by knot in cord
> EXCLUDES 1 *labor and delivery complicated by other cord entanglement, without compression (O69.82)*

√x7ᵗʰ O69.3 Labor and delivery complicated by short cord M♀

√x7ᵗʰ O69.4 Labor and delivery complicated by vasa previa M♀
Labor and delivery complicated by hemorrhage from vasa previa

√x7ᵗʰ O69.5 Labor and delivery complicated by vascular lesion of cord M♀
Labor and delivery complicated by cord bruising
Labor and delivery complicated by cord hematoma
Labor and delivery complicated by thrombosis of umbilical vessels

√5ᵗʰ O69.8 Labor and delivery complicated by other cord complications

√x7ᵗʰ O69.81 Labor and delivery complicated by cord around neck, without compression M♀
AHA: 2016, 1Q, 5

√x7ᵗʰ O69.82 Labor and delivery complicated by other cord entanglement, without compression M♀

√x7ᵗʰ O69.89 Labor and delivery complicated by other cord complications M♀

✓x7ᵗʰ **O69.9 Labor and delivery complicated by cord complication,** Ⓜ♀
unspecified

✓4ᵗʰ **O70 Perineal laceration during delivery**
  INCLUDES episiotomy extended by laceration
  EXCLUDES 1 obstetric high vaginal laceration alone (O71.4)
  AHA: 2016, 2Q, 34; 2016, 1Q, 3-4, 5

O70.0 First degree perineal laceration during delivery   Ⓜ♀
  Perineal laceration, rupture or tear involving fourchette during delivery
  Perineal laceration, rupture or tear involving labia during delivery
  Perineal laceration, rupture or tear involving skin during delivery
  Perineal laceration, rupture or tear involving vagina during delivery
  Perineal laceration, rupture or tear involving vulva during delivery
  Slight perineal laceration, rupture or tear during delivery

O70.1 Second degree perineal laceration during delivery   Ⓜ♀
  Perineal laceration, rupture or tear during delivery as in O70.0, also involving pelvic floor
  Perineal laceration, rupture or tear during delivery as in O70.0, also involving perineal muscles
  Perineal laceration, rupture or tear during delivery as in O70.0, also involving vaginal muscles
  EXCLUDES 1 perineal laceration involving anal sphincter (O70.2)

✓5ᵗʰ **O70.2 Third degree perineal laceration during delivery**
  Perineal laceration, rupture or tear during delivery as in O70.1, also involving anal sphincter
  Perineal laceration, rupture or tear during delivery as in O70.1, also involving rectovaginal septum
  Perineal laceration, rupture or tear during delivery as in O70.1, also involving sphincter NOS
  EXCLUDES 1 anal sphincter tear during delivery without third degree perineal laceration (O70.4)
     perineal laceration involving anal or rectal mucosa (O70.3)

  AHA: 2016, 4Q, 53-54

  CC Excl: For CC codes in subcategory O70.2: PDX collection 990

  O70.20 Third degree perineal laceration during delivery, unspecified   cc Ⓜ♀

  O70.21 Third degree perineal laceration during delivery, IIIa   cc Ⓜ♀
     Third degree perineal laceration during delivery with less than 50% of external anal sphincter (EAS) thickness torn

  O70.22 Third degree perineal laceration during delivery, IIIb   cc Ⓜ♀
     Third degree perineal laceration during delivery with more than 50% external anal sphincter (EAS) thickness torn

  O70.23 Third degree perineal laceration during delivery, IIIc   cc Ⓜ♀
     Third degree perineal laceration during delivery with both external anal sphincter (EAS) and internal anal sphincter (IAS) torn

O70.3 Fourth degree perineal laceration during delivery   cc Ⓜ♀
  Perineal laceration, rupture or tear during delivery as in O70.2, also involving anal mucosa
  Perineal laceration, rupture or tear during delivery as in O70.2, also involving rectal mucosa
  CC Excl: PDX collection 991

O70.4 Anal sphincter tear complicating delivery, not associated with third degree laceration   cc Ⓜ♀
  EXCLUDES 1 anal sphincter tear with third degree perineal laceration (O70.2)
  CC Excl: PDX collection 992

O70.9 Perineal laceration during delivery, unspecified   Ⓜ♀

✓4ᵗʰ **O71 Other obstetric trauma**
  Obstetric damage from instruments

✓5ᵗʰ **O71.0 Rupture of uterus (spontaneous) before onset of labor**
  EXCLUDES 1 disruption of (current) cesarean delivery wound (O90.0)
     laceration of uterus, NEC (O71.81)

  O71.00 Rupture of uterus before onset of labor, unspecified trimester   Ⓜ♀

  O71.02 Rupture of uterus before onset of labor, second trimester   MCC Ⓜ♀
     CC Excl: PDX collection 993

  O71.03 Rupture of uterus before onset of labor, third trimester   MCC Ⓜ♀
     CC Excl: PDX collection 993

O71.1 Rupture of uterus during labor   MCC Ⓜ♀
  Rupture of uterus not stated as occurring before onset of labor
  EXCLUDES 1 disruption of cesarean delivery wound (O90.0)
     laceration of uterus, NEC (O71.81)
  CC Excl: PDX collection 993

O71.2 Postpartum inversion of uterus   cc Ⓜ♀
  CC Excl: PDX collection 994

O71.3 Obstetric laceration of cervix   cc Ⓜ♀
  Annular detachment of cervix
  CC Excl: PDX collection 995

O71.4 Obstetric high vaginal laceration alone   cc Ⓜ♀
  Laceration of vaginal wall without perineal laceration
  EXCLUDES 1 obstetric high vaginal laceration with perineal laceration (O70.-)
  AHA: 2016, 1Q, 5
  CC Excl: PDX collection 996

O71.5 Other obstetric injury to pelvic organs   cc Ⓜ♀
  Obstetric injury to bladder
  Obstetric injury to urethra
  EXCLUDES 2 obstetric periurethral trauma (O71.82)
  AHA: 2014, 4Q, 18
  CC Excl: PDX collection 993

O71.6 Obstetric damage to pelvic joints and ligaments   cc Ⓜ♀
  Obstetric avulsion of inner symphyseal cartilage
  Obstetric damage to coccyx
  Obstetric traumatic separation of symphysis (pubis)
  CC Excl: PDX collection 997

O71.7 Obstetric hematoma of pelvis   cc Ⓜ♀
  Obstetric hematoma of perineum
  Obstetric hematoma of vagina
  Obstetric hematoma of vulva
  CC Excl: PDX collection 998

✓5ᵗʰ **O71.8 Other specified obstetric trauma**

  O71.81 Laceration of uterus, not elsewhere classified   Ⓜ♀

  O71.82 Other specified trauma to perineum and vulva   Ⓜ♀
     Obstetric periurethral trauma
     AHA: 2016, 1Q, 4; 2014, 4Q, 18

  O71.89 Other specified obstetric trauma   Ⓜ♀

O71.9 Obstetric trauma, unspecified   Ⓜ♀

✓4ᵗʰ **O72 Postpartum hemorrhage**
  INCLUDES hemorrhage after delivery of fetus or infant

O72.0 Third-stage hemorrhage   cc Ⓜ♀
  Hemorrhage associated with retained, trapped or adherent placenta
  Retained placenta NOS
  Code also type of adherent placenta (O43.2-)
  CC Excl: PDX collection 999

O72.1 Other immediate postpartum hemorrhage   cc Ⓜ♀
  Hemorrhage following delivery of placenta
  Postpartum hemorrhage (atonic) NOS
  Uterine atony with hemorrhage
  EXCLUDES 1 uterine atony NOS (O62.2)
     uterine atony without hemorrhage (O62.2)
     postpartum atony of uterus without hemorrhage (O75.89)
  AHA: 2016, 1Q, 4
  DEF: Uterine atony: Failure of the uterine muscles to contract after the fetus and placenta are delivered.
  CC Excl: PDX collection 1000

O72.2 Delayed and secondary postpartum hemorrhage   cc Ⓜ♀
  Hemorrhage associated with retained portions of placenta or membranes after the first 24 hours following delivery of placenta
  Retained products of conception NOS, following delivery
  CC Excl: PDX collection 1001

O72.3 Postpartum coagulation defects   Ⓜ♀
  Postpartum afibrinogenemia
  Postpartum fibrinolysis

✓4ᵗʰ **O73 Retained placenta and membranes, without hemorrhage**

     EXCLUDES 1   *placenta accreta (O43.21-)*
                 placenta increta (O43.22-)
                 placenta percreta (O43.23-)

     DEF: Postpartum condition resulting from failure to expel placental membrane tissues due to failed contractions of the uterine wall.

     O73.0 Retained placenta without hemorrhage   M♀
         Adherent placenta, without hemorrhage
         Trapped placenta without hemorrhage

     O73.1 Retained portions of placenta and membranes, without hemorrhage   M♀
         Retained products of conception following delivery, without hemorrhage

✓4ᵗʰ **O74 Complications of anesthesia during labor and delivery**

     INCLUDES   maternal complications arising from the administration of a general, regional or local anesthetic, analgesic or other sedation during labor and delivery

     Use additional code, if applicable, to identify specific complication

     O74.0 Aspiration pneumonitis due to anesthesia during labor and delivery   M♀
         Inhalation of stomach contents or secretions NOS due to anesthesia during labor and delivery
         Mendelson's syndrome due to anesthesia during labor and delivery

     O74.1 Other pulmonary complications of anesthesia during labor and delivery   M♀

     O74.2 Cardiac complications of anesthesia during labor and delivery   M♀

     O74.3 Central nervous system complications of anesthesia during labor and delivery   M♀

     O74.4 Toxic reaction to local anesthesia during labor and delivery   M♀

     O74.5 Spinal and epidural anesthesia-induced headache during labor and delivery   M♀

     O74.6 Other complications of spinal and epidural anesthesia during labor and delivery   M♀

     O74.7 Failed or difficult intubation for anesthesia during labor and delivery   M♀

     O74.8 Other complications of anesthesia during labor and delivery   M♀

     O74.9 Complication of anesthesia during labor and delivery, unspecified   M♀

✓4ᵗʰ **O75 Other complications of labor and delivery, not elsewhere classified**

     EXCLUDES 2   *puerperal (postpartum) infection (O86.-)*
                 puerperal (postpartum) sepsis (O85)

     O75.0 Maternal distress during labor and delivery   M♀

     O75.1 Shock during or following labor and delivery   MCC M♀
         Obstetric shock following labor and delivery
         CC Excl: PDX collection 1002

     O75.2 Pyrexia during labor, not elsewhere classified   CC M♀
         CC Excl: PDX collection 1003

     O75.3 Other infection during labor   MCC M♀
         Sepsis during labor
         Use additional code (B95-B97), to identify infectious agent
         CC Excl: PDX collection 1004

     O75.4 Other complications of obstetric surgery and procedures   M♀
         Cardiac arrest following obstetric surgery or procedures
         Cardiac failure following obstetric surgery or procedures
         Cerebral anoxia following obstetric surgery or procedures
         Pulmonary edema following obstetric surgery or procedures
         Use additional code to identify specific complication
         EXCLUDES 2   *complications of anesthesia during labor and delivery (O74.-)*
                 disruption of obstetrical (surgical) wound (O90.0-O90.1)
                 hematoma of obstetrical (surgical) wound (O90.2)
                 infection of obstetrical (surgical) wound ▶(O86.0-)◀

     O75.5 Delayed delivery after artificial rupture of membranes   M♀

✓5ᵗʰ **O75.8 Other specified complications of labor and delivery**

         O75.81 Maternal exhaustion complicating labor and delivery   M♀

         O75.82 Onset (spontaneous) of labor after 37 completedweeks of gestation but before 39 completed weeks gestation, with delivery by (planned) cesarean section   M♀
             Delivery by (planned) cesarean section occurring after 37 completed weeks of gestation but before 39 completed weeks gestation due to (spontaneous) onset of labor
             Code first to specify reason for planned cesarean section such as:
                 cephalopelvic disproportion (normally formed fetus) (O33.9)
                 previous cesarean delivery (O34.21)

         O75.89 Other specified complications of labor and delivery   M♀

     O75.9 Complication of labor and delivery, unspecified   M♀

O76 Abnormality in fetal heart rate and rhythm complicating labor and delivery   M♀

     Depressed fetal heart rate tones complicating labor and delivery
     Fetal bradycardia complicating labor and delivery
     Fetal heart rate abnormal variability complicating labor and delivery
     Fetal heart rate decelerations complicating labor and delivery
     Fetal heart rate irregularity complicating labor and delivery
     Fetal tachycardia complicating labor and delivery
     Non-reassuring fetal heart rate or rhythm complicating labor and delivery

     EXCLUDES 1   *fetal stress NOS (O77.9)*
                 labor and delivery complicated by electrocardiographic evidence of fetal stress (O77.8)
                 labor and delivery complicated by ultrasonic evidence of fetal stress (O77.8)

     EXCLUDES 2   *fetal metabolic acidemia (O68)*
                 other fetal stress (O77.0-O77.1)

     AHA: 2013, 4Q, 118

✓4ᵗʰ **O77 Other fetal stress complicating labor and delivery**

     O77.0 Labor and delivery complicated by meconium in amniotic fluid   M♀
         AHA: 2013, 4Q, 117-118

     O77.1 Fetal stress in labor or delivery due to drug administration   M♀

     O77.8 Labor and delivery complicated by other evidence of fetal stress   M♀
         Labor and delivery complicated by electrocardiographic evidence of fetal stress
         Labor and delivery complicated by ultrasonic evidence of fetal stress
         EXCLUDES 1   *abnormality in fetal heart rate or rhythm (O76)*
                 abnormality of fetal acid-base balance (O68)
                 fetal metabolic acidemia (O68)

     O77.9 Labor and delivery complicated by fetal stress, unspecified   M♀
         EXCLUDES 1   *abnormality in fetal heart rate or rhythm (O76)*
                 abnormality of fetal acid-base balance (O68)
                 fetal metabolic acidemia (O68)

Encounter for delivery (O80-O82)

O80 Encounter for full-term uncomplicated delivery   M♀

     NOTE   Delivery requiring minimal or no assistance, with or without episiotomy, without fetal manipulation [e.g., rotation version] or instrumentation [forceps] of a spontaneous, cephalic, vaginal, full-term, single, live-born infant. This code is for use as a single diagnosis code and is not to be used with any other code from chapter 15.

     Use additional code to indicate outcome of delivery (Z37.0)
     AHA: 2016, 4Q, 150; 2014, 2Q, 9

O82 Encounter for cesarean delivery without indication   M♀

     Use additional code to indicate outcome of delivery (Z37.0)

N Newborn: 0   P Pediatric: 0-17   M Maternity: 12-55   A Adult: 15-124   MCC Major Complication/Comorbidity   CC Complication/Comorbidity   SW Severe Wound Dx

876   ICD-10-CM 2019

Complications predominantly related to the puerperium (O85-O92)

EXCLUDES 2   mental and behavioral disorders associated with the puerperium ▶(F53.-)◀
obstetrical tetanus (A34)
puerperal osteomalacia (M83.0)

O85   Puerperal sepsis   MCC M♀
Postpartum sepsis
Puerperal peritonitis
Puerperal pyemia
Use additional code (B95-B97), to identify infectious agent
Use additional code (R65.2-) to identify severe sepsis, if applicable
EXCLUDES 1   fever of unknown origin following delivery (O86.4)
genital tract infection following delivery (O86.1-)
obstetric pyemic and septic embolism (O88.3-)
puerperal septic thrombophlebitis (O86.81)
urinary tract infection following delivery (O86.2-)
EXCLUDES 2   sepsis during labor (O75.3)
CC Excl: PDX collection 1005

✓4th O86   Other puerperal infections
Use additional code (B95-B97), to identify infectious agent
EXCLUDES 2   infection during labor (O75.3)
obstetrical tetanus (A34)

CC Excl: For CC/MCC codes in category O86, unless otherwise noted: PDX collection 968

✓5th O86.0   Infection of obstetric surgical wound
Infected cesarean delivery wound following delivery
Infected perineal repair following delivery
EXCLUDES 1 ▶complications of procedures, not elsewhere classified (T81.4-)
postprocedural fever NOS (R50.82)
postprocedural retroperitoneal abscess (K68.11)◀

- O86.00   Infection of obstetric surgical wound, unspecified   M♀
- O86.01   Infection of obstetric surgical wound, superficial incisional site   M♀
  Subcutaneous abscess following an obstetrical procedure
  Stitch abscess following an obstetrical procedure
- O86.02   Infection of obstetric surgical wound, deep incisional site   M♀
  Intramuscular abscess following an obstetrical procedure
  Sub-fascial abscess following a procedure
- O86.03   Infection of obstetric surgical wound, organ and space site   M♀
  Intraabdominal abscess following an obstetrical procedure
  Subphrenic abscess following an obstetrical procedure
- O86.04   Sepsis following an obstetrical procedure   MCC M♀
  Use additional code to identify the sepsis
- O86.09   Infection of obstetric surgical wound, other surgical site   M♀

✓5th O86.1   Other infection of genital tract following delivery
- O86.11   Cervicitis following delivery   CC M♀
- O86.12   Endometritis following delivery   CC M♀
  CC Excl: PDX collection 1005
- O86.13   Vaginitis following delivery   CC M♀
- O86.19   Other infection of genital tract following delivery   CC M♀

✓5th O86.2   Urinary tract infection following delivery
- O86.20   Urinary tract infection following delivery, unspecified   CC M♀
  Puerperal urinary tract infection NOS
- O86.21   Infection of kidney following delivery   CC M♀
- O86.22   Infection of bladder following delivery   CC M♀
  Infection of urethra following delivery
- O86.29   Other urinary tract infection following delivery   CC M♀

O86.4   Pyrexia of unknown origin following delivery   CC M♀
Puerperal infection NOS following delivery
Puerperal pyrexia NOS following delivery
EXCLUDES 2   pyrexia during labor (O75.2)
DEF: Fever of unknown origin experienced by the mother after childbirth.
CC Excl: PDX collection 1006

✓5th O86.8   Other specified puerperal infections
- O86.81   Puerperal septic thrombophlebitis   MCC M♀
  CC Excl: PDX collection 1005
- O86.89   Other specified puerperal infections   MCC M♀
  CC Excl: PDX collection 1005

✓4th O87   Venous complications and hemorrhoids in the puerperium
INCLUDES   venous complications in labor, delivery and the puerperium
EXCLUDES 2   obstetric embolism (O88.-)
puerperal septic thrombophlebitis (O86.81)
venous complications in pregnancy (O22.-)

CC Excl: For CC/MCC codes in category O87: PDX collection 967

O87.0   Superficial thrombophlebitis in the puerperium   CC M♀
Puerperal phlebitis NOS
Puerperal thrombosis NOS

O87.1   Deep phlebothrombosis in the puerperium   MCC M♀
Deep vein thrombosis, postpartum
Pelvic thrombophlebitis, postpartum
Use additional code to identify the deep vein thrombosis (I82.4-, I82.5-, I82.62-. I82.72-)
Use additional code, if applicable, for associated long-term (current) use of anticoagulants (Z79.01)

O87.2   Hemorrhoids in the puerperium   CC M♀

O87.3   Cerebral venous thrombosis in the puerperium   CC M♀
Cerebrovenous sinus thrombosis in the puerperium

O87.4   Varicose veins of lower extremity in the puerperium   M♀

O87.8   Other venous complications in the puerperium   CC M♀
Genital varices in the puerperium

O87.9   Venous complication in the puerperium, unspecified   M♀
Puerperal phlebopathy NOS

✓4th O88   Obstetric embolism
EXCLUDES 1   embolism complicating abortion NOS (O03.2)
embolism complicating ectopic or molar pregnancy (O08.2)
embolism complicating failed attempted abortion (O07.2)
embolism complicating induced abortion (O04.7)
embolism complicating spontaneous abortion (O03.2, O03.7)

CC Excl: For CC/MCC codes in category O88: PDX collection 1007

✓5th O88.0   Obstetric air embolism
DEF: Sudden blocking of the pulmonary artery or right ventricle with air or nitrogen bubbles.

✓6th O88.01   Obstetric air embolism in pregnancy
- O88.011   Air embolism in pregnancy, first trimester   MCC M♀
- O88.012   Air embolism in pregnancy, second trimester   MCC M♀
- O88.013   Air embolism in pregnancy, third trimester   MCC M♀
- O88.019   Air embolism in pregnancy, unspecified trimester   M♀

O88.02   Air embolism in childbirth   MCC M♀
O88.03   Air embolism in the puerperium   MCC M♀

✓5th O88.1   Amniotic fluid embolism
Anaphylactoid syndrome in pregnancy

✓6th O88.11   Amniotic fluid embolism in pregnancy
- O88.111   Amniotic fluid embolism in pregnancy, first trimester   MCC M♀
- O88.112   Amniotic fluid embolism in pregnancy, second trimester   MCC M♀
- O88.113   Amniotic fluid embolism in pregnancy, third trimester   MCC M♀
- O88.119   Amniotic fluid embolism in pregnancy, unspecified trimester   M♀

O88.12   Amniotic fluid embolism in childbirth   MCC M♀
O88.13   Amniotic fluid embolism in the puerperium   MCC M♀

✓5th O88.2   Obstetric thromboembolism

✓6th O88.21   Thromboembolism in pregnancy
Obstetric (pulmonary) embolism NOS
- O88.211   Thromboembolism in pregnancy, first trimester   MCC M♀
- O88.212   Thromboembolism in pregnancy, second trimester   MCC M♀
- O88.213   Thromboembolism in pregnancy, third trimester   MCC M♀
- O88.219   Thromboembolism in pregnancy, unspecified trimester   M♀

O88.22   Thromboembolism in childbirth   MCC M♀

✓ Additional Character Required   √x7th Placeholder   Unacceptable PDx   Questionable PDx   Manifestation   H1 - H14 HAC   HCC CMS-HCC Dx   HIV HIV Dx

ICD-10-CM 2019   **877**

O88.23 **Thromboembolism in the** puerperium MCC M♀
　　Puerperal (pulmonary) embolism NOS

✓5ᵗʰ **O88.3** **Obstetric** pyemic and septic embolism

　✓6ᵗʰ **O88.31** **Pyemic and septic embolism in** pregnancy

　　　O88.311 **Pyemic and septic embolism in** MCC M♀
　　　　pregnancy, first trimester

　　　O88.312 **Pyemic and septic embolism in** MCC M♀
　　　　pregnancy, second trimester

　　　O88.313 **Pyemic and septic embolism in** MCC M♀
　　　　pregnancy, third trimester

　　　O88.319 **Pyemic and septic embolism in** CC M♀
　　　　pregnancy, unspecified trimester

　　O88.32 **Pyemic and septic embolism in** childbirth MCC M♀

　　O88.33 **Pyemic and septic embolism in the** MCC M♀
　　　puerperium

✓5ᵗʰ **O88.8** **Other** obstetric **embolism**
　　Obstetric fat embolism

　✓6ᵗʰ **O88.81** **Other embolism in** pregnancy

　　　O88.811 **Other embolism in pregnancy,** MCC M♀
　　　　first trimester

　　　O88.812 **Other embolism in pregnancy,** MCC M♀
　　　　second trimester

　　　O88.813 **Other embolism in pregnancy,** MCC M♀
　　　　third trimester

　　　O88.819 **Other embolism in pregnancy,** M♀
　　　　unspecified trimester

　　O88.82 **Other embolism in** childbirth MCC M♀

　　O88.83 **Other embolism in the** puerperium MCC M♀

✓4ᵗʰ **O89** **Complications of anesthesia during the puerperium**
　　INCLUDES　maternal complications arising from the administration of a
　　　general, regional or local anesthetic, analgesic or other
　　　sedation during the puerperium
　　Use additional code, if applicable, to identify specific complication

　✓5ᵗʰ **O89.0** **Pulmonary complications of anesthesia during the**
　　　puerperium

　　O89.01 **Aspiration pneumonitis** due to anesthesia M♀
　　　during the puerperium
　　　Inhalation of stomach contents or secretions NOS due
　　　to anesthesia during the puerperium
　　　Mendelson's syndrome due to anesthesia during the
　　　puerperium

　　O89.09 **Other pulmonary complications of anesthesia** M♀
　　　during the puerperium

　O89.1 **Cardiac complications of anesthesia during the** M♀
　　puerperium

　O89.2 **Central nervous system complications of anesthesia** M♀
　　during the puerperium

　O89.3 **Toxic reaction** to local anesthesia during the puerperium M♀

　O89.4 **Spinal and epidural anesthesia-induced headache** M♀
　　during the puerperium

　O89.5 **Other complications of** spinal and epidural anesthesia M♀
　　during the puerperium

　O89.6 **Failed or difficult intubation** for anesthesia during the M♀
　　puerperium

　O89.8 **Other complications of anesthesia during the puerperium** M♀

　O89.9 **Complication of anesthesia during the puerperium,** M♀
　　unspecified

✓4ᵗʰ **O90** **Complications of the puerperium, not elsewhere classified**

　O90.0 **Disruption of cesarean delivery wound** M♀
　　Dehiscence of cesarean delivery wound
　　EXCLUDES 1　rupture of uterus (spontaneous) before onset of labor
　　　　(O71.0-)
　　　　rupture of uterus during labor (O71.1)

　O90.1 **Disruption of perineal obstetric wound** M♀
　　Disruption of wound of episiotomy
　　Disruption of wound of perineal laceration
　　Secondary perineal tear

　O90.2 **Hematoma of obstetric wound** M♀

　O90.3 **Peripartum cardiomyopathy** MCC M♀
　　Conditions in I42- arising during pregnancy and the puerperium
　　EXCLUDES 1　pre-existing heart disease complicating pregnancy and
　　　　the puerperium (O99.4-)
　　DEF: Any structural or functional abnormality of the ventricular
　　myocardium. It is a noninflammatory disease of obscure or
　　unknown etiology with onset during the postpartum period.
　　CC Excl: PDX collection 1008

O90.4 **Postpartum acute kidney failure** MCC M♀
　　Hepatorenal syndrome following labor and delivery
　　CC Excl: PDX collection 1009

O90.5 **Postpartum thyroiditis** M♀

O90.6 **Postpartum mood disturbance** M♀
　　Postpartum blues
　　Postpartum dysphoria
　　Postpartum sadness
　　EXCLUDES 1　postpartum depression ▶(F53.0)◀
　　　　puerperal psychosis ▶(F53.1)◀

✓5ᵗʰ **O90.8** **Other complications of the puerperium, not elsewhere**
　　classified

　　O90.81 **Anemia of the puerperium** M♀
　　　Postpartum anemia NOS
　　　EXCLUDES 1　pre-existing anemia complicating the
　　　　　puerperium (O99.03)

　　O90.89 **Other complications of the puerperium, not** M♀
　　　elsewhere classified
　　　Placental polyp

O90.9 **Complication of the puerperium, unspecified** M♀

✓4ᵗʰ **O91** **Infections of breast associated with pregnancy, the puerperium**
　and lactation
　　Use additional code to identify infection

✓5ᵗʰ **O91.0** **Infection of nipple associated with pregnancy, the**
　　puerperium and lactation

　✓6ᵗʰ **O91.01** **Infection of nipple associated with** pregnancy
　　　Gestational abscess of nipple

　　　O91.011 **Infection of nipple associated with** M♀
　　　　pregnancy, first trimester

　　　O91.012 **Infection of nipple associated with** M♀
　　　　pregnancy, second trimester

　　　O91.013 **Infection of nipple associated with** M♀
　　　　pregnancy, third trimester

　　　O91.019 **Infection of nipple associated with** M♀
　　　　pregnancy, unspecified trimester

　　O91.02 **Infection of nipple associated with the** M♀
　　　puerperium
　　　Puerperal abscess of nipple

　　O91.03 **Infection of nipple associated with** lactation M♀
　　　Abscess of nipple associated with lactation

✓5ᵗʰ **O91.1** **Abscess of breast associated with pregnancy, the puerperium**
　　and lactation

　✓6ᵗʰ **O91.11** **Abscess of breast associated with** pregnancy
　　　Gestational mammary abscess
　　　Gestational purulent mastitis
　　　Gestational súbareolar abscess

　　　O91.111 **Abscess of breast associated with** M♀
　　　　pregnancy, first trimester

　　　O91.112 **Abscess of breast associated with** M♀
　　　　pregnancy, second trimester

　　　O91.113 **Abscess of breast associated with** M♀
　　　　pregnancy, third trimester

　　　O91.119 **Abscess of breast associated with** M♀
　　　　pregnancy, unspecified trimester

　　O91.12 **Abscess of breast associated with the** M♀
　　　puerperium
　　　Puerperal mammary abscess
　　　Puerperal purulent mastitis
　　　Puerperal subareolar abscess

　　O91.13 **Abscess of breast associated with** lactation M♀
　　　Mammary abscess associated with lactation
　　　Purulent mastitis associated with lactation
　　　Subareolar abscess associated with lactation

✓5ᵗʰ **O91.2** **Nonpurulent mastitis associated with pregnancy, the**
　　puerperium and lactation

　✓6ᵗʰ **O91.21** **Nonpurulent mastitis associated with** pregnancy
　　　Gestational interstitial mastitis
　　　Gestational lymphangitis of breast
　　　Gestational mastitis NOS
　　　Gestational parenchymatous mastitis

　　　O91.211 **Nonpurulent mastitis associated with** M♀
　　　　pregnancy, first trimester

　　　O91.212 **Nonpurulent mastitis associated with** M♀
　　　　pregnancy, second trimester

　　　O91.213 **Nonpurulent mastitis associated with** M♀
　　　　pregnancy, third trimester

　　　O91.219 **Nonpurulent mastitis associated with** M♀
　　　　pregnancy, unspecified trimester

N Newborn: 0　　P Pediatric: 0-17　　M Maternity: 12-55　　A Adult: 15-124　　MCC Major Complication/Comorbidity　　CC Complication/Comorbidity　　SW Severe Wound Dx

878　　ICD-10-CM 2019

O91.22   **Nonpurulent mastitis associated with the puerperium**   Ⓜ♀
  Puerperal interstitial mastitis
  Puerperal lymphangitis of breast
  Puerperal mastitis NOS
  Puerperal parenchymatous mastitis

O91.23   **Nonpurulent mastitis associated with lactation**   Ⓜ♀
  Interstitial mastitis associated with lactation
  Lymphangitis of breast associated with lactation
  Mastitis NOS associated with lactation
  Parenchymatous mastitis associated with lactation

✓4ᵗʰ **O92**   **Other disorders of breast and disorders of lactation associated with pregnancy and the puerperium**

✓5ᵗʰ **O92.0**   **Retracted nipple associated with pregnancy, the puerperium, and lactation**

✓6ᵗʰ **O92.01**   **Retracted nipple associated with pregnancy**

   O92.011   **Retracted nipple associated with pregnancy, first trimester**   Ⓜ♀

   O92.012   **Retracted nipple associated with pregnancy, second trimester**   Ⓜ♀

   O92.013   **Retracted nipple associated with pregnancy, third trimester**   Ⓜ♀

   O92.019   **Retracted nipple associated with pregnancy, unspecified trimester**   Ⓜ♀

O92.02   **Retracted nipple associated with the puerperium**   Ⓜ♀

O92.03   **Retracted nipple associated with lactation**   Ⓜ♀

✓5ᵗʰ **O92.1**   **Cracked nipple associated with pregnancy, the puerperium, and lactation**
  Fissure of nipple, gestational or puerperal

✓6ᵗʰ **O92.11**   **Cracked nipple associated with pregnancy**

   O92.111   **Cracked nipple associated with pregnancy, first trimester**   Ⓜ♀

   O92.112   **Cracked nipple associated with pregnancy, second trimester**   Ⓜ♀

   O92.113   **Cracked nipple associated with pregnancy, third trimester**   Ⓜ♀

   O92.119   **Cracked nipple associated with pregnancy, unspecified trimester**   Ⓜ♀

O92.12   **Cracked nipple associated with the puerperium**   Ⓜ♀

O92.13   **Cracked nipple associated with lactation**   Ⓜ♀

✓5ᵗʰ **O92.2**   **Other and unspecified disorders of breast associated with pregnancy and the puerperium**

O92.20   **Unspecified disorder of breast associated with pregnancy and the puerperium**   Ⓜ♀

O92.29   **Other disorders of breast associated with pregnancy and the puerperium**   Ⓜ♀

O92.3   **Agalactia**   Ⓜ♀
  Primary agalactia
  EXCLUDES 1   *elective agalactia (O92.5)*
       secondary agalactia (O92.5)
       therapeutic agalactia (O92.5)
  DEF: Absence of milk secretion in a female after delivery.

O92.4   **Hypogalactia**   Ⓜ♀

O92.5   **Suppressed lactation**   Ⓜ♀
  Elective agalactia
  Secondary agalactia
  Therapeutic agalactia
  EXCLUDES 1   *primary agalactia (O92.3)*

O92.6   **Galactorrhea**   Ⓜ♀
  DEF: Excessive or persistent milk secretion by the breast that may occur in the absence of nursing.

✓5ᵗʰ **O92.7**   **Other and unspecified disorders of lactation**

O92.70   **Unspecified disorders of lactation**   Ⓜ♀

O92.79   **Other disorders of lactation**   Ⓜ♀
  Puerperal galactocele

Other obstetric conditions, not elsewhere classified (O94-O9A)

O94   **Sequelae of complication of pregnancy, childbirth, and the puerperium**   Ⓜ♀
  NOTE   This category is to be used to indicate conditions in O00-O77.-, O85-O94 and O98-O9A.- as the cause of late effects. The sequelae include conditions specified as such, or as late effects, which may occur at any time after the puerperium.
  Code first condition resulting from (sequela) of complication of pregnancy, childbirth, and the puerperium

✓4ᵗʰ **O98**   **Maternal infectious and parasitic diseases classifiable elsewhere but complicating pregnancy, childbirth and the puerperium**
  INCLUDES   the listed conditions when complicating the pregnant state, when aggravated by the pregnancy, or as a reason for obstetric care
  Use additional code (Chapter 1), to identify specific infectious or parasitic disease
  EXCLUDES 2   *herpes gestationis (O26.4-)*
       infectious carrier state (O99.82-, O99.83-)
       obstetrical tetanus (A34)
       puerperal infection (O86.-)
       puerperal sepsis (O85)
       when the reason for maternal care is that the disease is known or suspected to have affected the fetus (O35-O36)

✓5ᵗʰ **O98.0**   **Tuberculosis complicating pregnancy, childbirth and the puerperium**
  Conditions in A15-A19

  CC Excl: For CC codes in subcategory O98.0:
  PDX collection 1011

✓6ᵗʰ **O98.01**   **Tuberculosis complicating pregnancy**

   O98.011   **Tuberculosis complicating pregnancy, first trimester**   CC Ⓜ♀

   O98.012   **Tuberculosis complicating pregnancy, second trimester**   CC Ⓜ♀

   O98.013   **Tuberculosis complicating pregnancy, third trimester**   CC Ⓜ♀

   O98.019   **Tuberculosis complicating pregnancy, unspecified trimester**   Ⓜ♀

O98.02   **Tuberculosis complicating childbirth**   CC Ⓜ♀

O98.03   **Tuberculosis complicating the puerperium**   CC Ⓜ♀

✓5ᵗʰ **O98.1**   **Syphilis complicating pregnancy, childbirth and the puerperium**
  Conditions in A50-A53

  CC Excl: For CC codes in subcategory O98.1:
  PDX collection 1012

✓6ᵗʰ **O98.11**   **Syphilis complicating pregnancy**

   O98.111   **Syphilis complicating pregnancy, first trimester**   CC Ⓜ♀

   O98.112   **Syphilis complicating pregnancy, second trimester**   CC Ⓜ♀

   O98.113   **Syphilis complicating pregnancy, third trimester**   CC Ⓜ♀

   O98.119   **Syphilis complicating pregnancy, unspecified trimester**   Ⓜ♀

O98.12   **Syphilis complicating childbirth**   CC Ⓜ♀

O98.13   **Syphilis complicating the puerperium**   CC Ⓜ♀

✓5ᵗʰ **O98.2**   **Gonorrhea complicating pregnancy, childbirth and the puerperium**
  Conditions in A54-

  CC Excl: For CC codes in subcategory O98.2:
  PDX collection 1012

✓6ᵗʰ **O98.21**   **Gonorrhea complicating pregnancy**

   O98.211   **Gonorrhea complicating pregnancy, first trimester**   CC Ⓜ♀

   O98.212   **Gonorrhea complicating pregnancy, second trimester**   CC Ⓜ♀

   O98.213   **Gonorrhea complicating pregnancy, third trimester**   CC Ⓜ♀

   O98.219   **Gonorrhea complicating pregnancy, unspecified trimester**   Ⓜ♀

O98.22   **Gonorrhea complicating childbirth**   CC Ⓜ♀

O98.23   **Gonorrhea complicating the puerperium**   CC Ⓜ♀

☑ Additional Character Required   ✓7ᵗʰ Placeholder   Unacceptable PDx   Questionable PDx   Manifestation   H1 - H14 HAC   HCC CMS-HCC Dx   HIV HIV Dx

ICD-10-CM 2019   879

Chapter 15. Pregnancy, Childbirth and the Puerperium

O98.3–O98.93

√5ᵗʰ **O98.3** Other infections with a predominantly sexual mode of transmission complicating pregnancy, childbirth and the puerperium
Conditions in A55-A64

> **CC Excl: For CC codes in subcategory O98.3:**
> PDX collection 1012

√6ᵗʰ **O98.31** Other infections with a predominantly sexual mode of transmission complicating pregnancy

O98.311 Other infections with a predominantly sexual mode of transmission complicating pregnancy, first trimester   CC M♀

O98.312 Other infections with a predominantly sexual mode of transmission complicating pregnancy, second trimester   CC M♀

O98.313 Other infections with a predominantly sexual mode of transmission complicating pregnancy, third trimester   CC M♀

O98.319 Other infections with a predominantly sexual mode of transmission complicating pregnancy, unspecified trimester   M♀

O98.32 Other infections with a predominantly sexual mode of transmission complicating childbirth   CC M♀

O98.33 Other infections with a predominantly sexual mode of transmission complicating the puerperium   CC M♀

√5ᵗʰ **O98.4** Viral hepatitis complicating pregnancy, childbirth and the puerperium
Conditions in B15-B19

> **CC Excl: For CC codes in subcategory O98.4:**
> PDX collection 1013

√6ᵗʰ **O98.41** Viral hepatitis complicating pregnancy

O98.411 Viral hepatitis complicating pregnancy, first trimester   CC M♀

O98.412 Viral hepatitis complicating pregnancy, second trimester   CC M♀

O98.413 Viral hepatitis complicating pregnancy, third trimester   CC M♀

O98.419 Viral hepatitis complicating pregnancy, unspecified trimester   M♀

O98.42 Viral hepatitis complicating childbirth   CC M♀

O98.43 Viral hepatitis complicating the puerperium   CC M♀

√5ᵗʰ **O98.5** Other viral diseases complicating pregnancy, childbirth and the puerperium
Conditions in A80-B09, B25-B34, R87.81-, R87.82-

> **EXCLUDES 1** human immunodeficiency virus [HIV] disease complicating pregnancy, childbirth and the puerperium (O98.7-)

> **CC Excl: For CC codes in subcategory O98.5:**
> PDX collection 1013

√6ᵗʰ **O98.51** Other viral diseases complicating pregnancy

O98.511 Other viral diseases complicating pregnancy, first trimester   CC M♀

O98.512 Other viral diseases complicating pregnancy, second trimester   CC M♀

O98.513 Other viral diseases complicating pregnancy, third trimester   CC M♀

O98.519 Other viral diseases complicating pregnancy, unspecified trimester   M♀

O98.52 Other viral diseases complicating childbirth   CC M♀

O98.53 Other viral diseases complicating the puerperium   CC M♀

√5ᵗʰ **O98.6** Protozoal diseases complicating pregnancy, childbirth and the puerperium
Conditions in B50-B64

> **CC Excl: For CC codes in subcategory O98.6, unless otherwise noted:** PDX collection 1014

√6ᵗʰ **O98.61** Protozoal diseases complicating pregnancy

O98.611 Protozoal diseases complicating pregnancy, first trimester   CC M♀

O98.612 Protozoal diseases complicating pregnancy, second trimester   CC M♀

O98.613 Protozoal diseases complicating pregnancy, third trimester   CC M♀

O98.619 Protozoal diseases complicating pregnancy, unspecified trimester   M♀

O98.62 Protozoal diseases complicating childbirth   CC M♀
     CC Excl: PDX collection 1015

O98.63 Protozoal diseases complicating the puerperium   CC M♀
     CC Excl: PDX collection 1015

√5ᵗʰ **O98.7** Human immunodeficiency virus [HIV] disease complicating pregnancy, childbirth and the puerperium
Use additional code to identify the type of HIV disease:
   acquired immune deficiency syndrome (AIDS) (B20)
   asymptomatic HIV status (Z21)
   HIV positive NOS (Z21)
   symptomatic HIV disease (B20)

> **CC Excl: For CC codes in subcategory O98.7:**
> PDX collection 1013

√6ᵗʰ **O98.71** Human immunodeficiency virus [HIV] disease complicating pregnancy

O98.711 Human immunodeficiency virus [HIV] disease complicating pregnancy, first trimester   CC M♀

O98.712 Human immunodeficiency virus [HIV] disease complicating pregnancy, second trimester   CC M♀

O98.713 Human immunodeficiency virus [HIV] disease complicating pregnancy, third trimester   CC M♀

O98.719 Human immunodeficiency virus [HIV] disease complicating pregnancy, unspecified trimester   M♀

O98.72 Human immunodeficiency virus [HIV] disease complicating childbirth   CC M♀

O98.73 Human immunodeficiency virus [HIV] disease complicating the puerperium   CC M♀

√5ᵗʰ **O98.8** Other maternal infectious and parasitic diseases complicating pregnancy, childbirth and the puerperium

> **CC Excl: For CC codes in subcategory O98.8:**
> PDX collection 1013

√6ᵗʰ **O98.81** Other maternal infectious and parasitic diseases complicating pregnancy

O98.811 Other maternal infectious and parasitic diseases complicating pregnancy, first trimester   CC M♀

O98.812 Other maternal infectious and parasitic diseases complicating pregnancy, second trimester   CC M♀

O98.813 Other maternal infectious and parasitic diseases complicating pregnancy, third trimester   CC M♀

O98.819 Other maternal infectious and parasitic diseases complicating pregnancy, unspecified trimester   M♀

O98.82 Other maternal infectious and parasitic diseases complicating childbirth   CC M♀

O98.83 Other maternal infectious and parasitic diseases complicating the puerperium   CC M♀

√5ᵗʰ **O98.9** Unspecified maternal infectious and parasitic disease complicating pregnancy, childbirth and the puerperium

> **CC Excl: For CC codes in subcategory O98.9:**
> PDX collection 1013

√6ᵗʰ **O98.91** Unspecified maternal infectious and parasitic disease complicating pregnancy

O98.911 Unspecified maternal infectious and parasitic disease complicating pregnancy, first trimester   CC M♀

O98.912 Unspecified maternal infectious and parasitic disease complicating pregnancy, second trimester   CC M♀

O98.913 Unspecified maternal infectious and parasitic disease complicating pregnancy, third trimester   CC M♀

O98.919 Unspecified maternal infectious and parasitic disease complicating pregnancy, unspecified trimester   M♀

O98.92 Unspecified maternal infectious and parasitic disease complicating childbirth   CC M♀

O98.93 Unspecified maternal infectious and parasitic disease complicating the puerperium   CC M♀

N Newborn: 0   P Pediatric: 0-17   M Maternity: 12-55   A Adult: 15-124   MCC Major Complication/Comorbidity   CC Complication/Comorbidity   SW Severe Wound Dx

880   ICD-10-CM 2019

☑️4ᵗʰ **O99 Other maternal diseases classifiable elsewhere but complicating pregnancy, childbirth and the puerperium**

INCLUDES   conditions which complicate the pregnant state, are aggravated by the pregnancy or are a main reason for obstetric care

Use additional code to identify specific condition

EXCLUDES 2   when the reason for maternal care is that the condition is known or suspected to have affected the fetus (O35-O36)

☑️5ᵗʰ **O99.0 Anemia complicating pregnancy, childbirth and the puerperium**

Conditions in D50-D64

EXCLUDES 1   anemia arising in the puerperium (O90.81)
postpartum anemia NOS (O90.81)

☑️6ᵗʰ **O99.01 Anemia complicating pregnancy**

AHA: 2016, 1Q, 4

     O99.011 Anemia complicating pregnancy, first trimester   M♀

     O99.012 Anemia complicating pregnancy, second trimester   M♀

     O99.013 Anemia complicating pregnancy, third trimester   M♀

     O99.019 Anemia complicating pregnancy, unspecified trimester   M♀

   O99.02 Anemia complicating childbirth   M♀

   O99.03 Anemia complicating the puerperium   M♀

EXCLUDES 1   postpartum anemia not pre-existing prior to delivery (O90.81)

☑️5ᵗʰ **O99.1 Other diseases of the blood and blood-forming organs and certain disorders involving the immune mechanism complicating pregnancy, childbirth and the puerperium**

Conditions in D65-D89

EXCLUDES 1   hemorrhage with coagulation defects (O45.-, O46.0-, O67.0, O72.3)

CC Excl: For CC codes in subcategory O99.1, unless otherwise noted: PDX collection 1016

☑️6ᵗʰ **O99.11 Other diseases of the blood and blood-forming organs and certain disorders involving the immune mechanism complicating pregnancy**

     O99.111 Other diseases of the blood and blood-forming organs and certain disorders involving the immune mechanism complicating pregnancy, first trimester   CC M♀

     O99.112 Other diseases of the blood and blood-forming organs and certain disorders involving the immune mechanism complicating pregnancy, second trimester   CC M♀

     O99.113 Other diseases of the blood and blood-forming organs and certain disorders involving the immune mechanism complicating pregnancy, third trimester   CC M♀

     O99.119 Other diseases of the blood and blood-forming organs and certain disorders involving the immune mechanism complicating pregnancy, unspecified trimester   CC M♀

CC Excl: PDX collection 1017

   O99.12 Other diseases of the blood and blood-forming organs and certain disorders involving the immune mechanism complicating childbirth   CC M♀

   O99.13 Other diseases of the blood and blood-forming organs and certain disorders involving the immune mechanism complicating the puerperium   CC M♀

☑️5ᵗʰ **O99.2 Endocrine, nutritional and metabolic diseases complicating pregnancy, childbirth and the puerperium**

Conditions in E00-E88

EXCLUDES 2   diabetes mellitus (O24.-)
malnutrition (O25.-)
postpartum thyroiditis (O90.5)

☑️6ᵗʰ **O99.21 Obesity complicating pregnancy, childbirth, and the puerperium**

Use additional code to identify the type of obesity (E66.-)

     O99.210 Obesity complicating pregnancy, unspecified trimester   M♀

     O99.211 Obesity complicating pregnancy, first trimester   M♀

     O99.212 Obesity complicating pregnancy, second trimester   M♀

     O99.213 Obesity complicating pregnancy, third trimester   M♀

     O99.214 Obesity complicating childbirth   M♀

     O99.215 Obesity complicating the puerperium   M♀

☑️6ᵗʰ **O99.28 Other endocrine, nutritional and metabolic diseases complicating pregnancy, childbirth and the puerperium**

     O99.280 Endocrine, nutritional and metabolic diseases complicating pregnancy, unspecified trimester   M♀

     O99.281 Endocrine, nutritional and metabolic diseases complicating pregnancy, first trimester   M♀

     O99.282 Endocrine, nutritional and metabolic diseases complicating pregnancy, second trimester   M♀

     O99.283 Endocrine, nutritional and metabolic diseases complicating pregnancy, third trimester   M♀

     O99.284 Endocrine, nutritional and metabolic diseases complicating childbirth   M♀

     O99.285 Endocrine, nutritional and metabolic diseases complicating the puerperium   M♀

☑️5ᵗʰ **O99.3 Mental disorders and diseases of the nervous system complicating pregnancy, childbirth and the puerperium**

CC Excl: For CC codes in subcategory O99.3, unless otherwise noted: PDX collection 1018

☑️6ᵗʰ **O99.31 Alcohol use complicating pregnancy, childbirth, and the puerperium**

Use additional code(s) from F10 to identify manifestations of the alcohol use

     O99.310 Alcohol use complicating pregnancy, unspecified trimester   M♀

     O99.311 Alcohol use complicating pregnancy, first trimester   M♀

     O99.312 Alcohol use complicating pregnancy, second trimester   M♀

     O99.313 Alcohol use complicating pregnancy, third trimester   M♀

     O99.314 Alcohol use complicating childbirth   M♀

     O99.315 Alcohol use complicating the puerperium   M♀

☑️6ᵗʰ **O99.32 Drug use complicating pregnancy, childbirth, and the puerperium**

Use additional code(s) from F11-F16 and F18-F19 to identify manifestations of the drug use

AHA: 2018, 2Q, 10

     O99.320 Drug use complicating pregnancy, unspecified trimester   M♀

     O99.321 Drug use complicating pregnancy, first trimester   CC M♀

     O99.322 Drug use complicating pregnancy, second trimester   CC M♀

     O99.323 Drug use complicating pregnancy, third trimester   CC M♀

     O99.324 Drug use complicating childbirth   CC M♀

     O99.325 Drug use complicating the puerperium   CC M♀

☑️6ᵗʰ **O99.33 Tobacco use disorder complicating pregnancy, childbirth, and the puerperium**

Smoking complicating pregnancy, childbirth, and the puerperium

Use additional code from category F17 to identify type of tobacco nicotine dependence

     O99.330 Smoking (tobacco) complicating pregnancy, unspecified trimester   M♀

     O99.331 Smoking (tobacco) complicating pregnancy, first trimester   M♀

     O99.332 Smoking (tobacco) complicating pregnancy, second trimester   M♀

     O99.333 Smoking (tobacco) complicating pregnancy, third trimester   M♀

     O99.334 Smoking (tobacco) complicating childbirth   M♀

     O99.335 Smoking (tobacco) complicating the puerperium   M♀

☑️ Additional Character Required   ☑️x7ᵗʰ Placeholder   Unacceptable PDx   Questionable PDx   Manifestation   H1-H14 HAC   HCC CMS-HCC Dx   HIV HIV Dx

Chapter 15. Pregnancy, Childbirth and the Puerperium (side tab)

O99.34–O99.810 (side tab)

✓6ᵗʰ **O99.34** Other mental disorders complicating pregnancy, childbirth, and the puerperium
Conditions in F01-F09 and F20-F99
EXCLUDES 2   *postpartum mood disturbance (O90.6)*
postnatal psychosis ▶(F53.1)◀
puerperal psychosis ▶(F53.1)◀

     O99.340 Other mental disorders complicating pregnancy, unspecified trimester   Ⓜ♀

     O99.341 Other mental disorders complicating pregnancy, first trimester   Ⓜ♀

     O99.342 Other mental disorders complicating pregnancy, second trimester   Ⓜ♀

     O99.343 Other mental disorders complicating pregnancy, third trimester   Ⓜ♀

     O99.344 Other mental disorders complicating childbirth   Ⓜ♀

     O99.345 Other mental disorders complicating the puerperium   Ⓜ♀

✓6ᵗʰ **O99.35** Diseases of the nervous system complicating pregnancy, childbirth, and the puerperium
Conditions in G00-G99
EXCLUDES 2   *pregnancy related peripheral neuritis (O26.8-)*

     O99.350 Diseases of the nervous system complicating pregnancy, unspecified trimester   Ⓜ♀

     O99.351 Diseases of the nervous system complicating pregnancy, first trimester   Ⓜ♀

     O99.352 Diseases of the nervous system complicating pregnancy, second trimester   Ⓜ♀

     O99.353 Diseases of the nervous system complicating pregnancy, third trimester   Ⓜ♀

     O99.354 Diseases of the nervous system complicating childbirth   CC Ⓜ♀
        CC Excl: PDX collection 1016

     O99.355 Diseases of the nervous system complicating the puerperium   CC Ⓜ♀
        CC Excl: PDX collection 1016

✓5ᵗʰ **O99.4** Diseases of the circulatory system complicating pregnancy, childbirth and the puerperium
Conditions in I00-I99
EXCLUDES 1   *peripartum cardiomyopathy (O90.3)*
EXCLUDES 2   *hypertensive disorders (O10-O16)*
obstetric embolism (O88.-)
venous complications and cerebrovenous sinus thrombosis in labor, childbirth and the puerperium (O87.-)
venous complications and cerebrovenous sinus thrombosis in pregnancy (O22.-)

AHA: 2016, 2Q, 8

CC Excl: For CC/MCC codes in subcategory O99.4, unless otherwise noted: PDX collection 1019

✓6ᵗʰ **O99.41** Diseases of the circulatory system complicating pregnancy

     O99.411 Diseases of the circulatory system complicating pregnancy, first trimester   CC Ⓜ♀

     O99.412 Diseases of the circulatory system complicating pregnancy, second trimester   CC Ⓜ♀

     O99.413 Diseases of the circulatory system complicating pregnancy, third trimester   CC Ⓜ♀

     O99.419 Diseases of the circulatory system complicating pregnancy, unspecified trimester   Ⓜ♀

     O99.42 Diseases of the circulatory system complicating childbirth   MCC Ⓜ♀
        CC Excl: PDX collection 1008

     O99.43 Diseases of the circulatory system complicating the puerperium   CC Ⓜ♀

✓5ᵗʰ **O99.5** Diseases of the respiratory system complicating pregnancy, childbirth and the puerperium
Conditions in J00-J99

✓6ᵗʰ **O99.51** Diseases of the respiratory system complicating pregnancy

     O99.511 Diseases of the respiratory system complicating pregnancy, first trimester   Ⓜ♀

     O99.512 Diseases of the respiratory system complicating pregnancy, second trimester   Ⓜ♀

     O99.513 Diseases of the respiratory system complicating pregnancy, third trimester   Ⓜ♀

     O99.519 Diseases of the respiratory system complicating pregnancy, unspecified trimester   Ⓜ♀

     O99.52 Diseases of the respiratory system complicating childbirth   Ⓜ♀

     O99.53 Diseases of the respiratory system complicating the puerperium   Ⓜ♀

✓6ᵗʰ **O99.6** Diseases of the digestive system complicating pregnancy, childbirth and the puerperium
Conditions in K00-K93
EXCLUDES 2   *hemorrhoids in pregnancy (O22.4-)*
liver and biliary tract disorders in pregnancy, childbirth and the puerperium (O26.6-)

✓6ᵗʰ **O99.61** Diseases of the digestive system complicating pregnancy
AHA: 2016, 1Q, 4

     O99.611 Diseases of the digestive system complicating pregnancy, first trimester   Ⓜ♀

     O99.612 Diseases of the digestive system complicating pregnancy, second trimester   Ⓜ♀

     O99.613 Diseases of the digestive system complicating pregnancy, third trimester   Ⓜ♀

     O99.619 Diseases of the digestive system complicating pregnancy, unspecified trimester   Ⓜ♀

     O99.62 Diseases of the digestive system complicating childbirth   Ⓜ♀

     O99.63 Diseases of the digestive system complicating the puerperium   Ⓜ♀

✓5ᵗʰ **O99.7** Diseases of the skin and subcutaneous tissue complicating pregnancy, childbirth and the puerperium
Conditions in L00-L99
EXCLUDES 2   *herpes gestationis (O26.4)*
pruritic urticarial papules and plaques of pregnancy (PUPPP) (O26.86)

✓6ᵗʰ **O99.71** Diseases of the skin and subcutaneous tissue complicating pregnancy

     O99.711 Diseases of the skin and subcutaneous tissue complicating pregnancy, first trimester   Ⓜ♀

     O99.712 Diseases of the skin and subcutaneous tissue complicating pregnancy, second trimester   Ⓜ♀

     O99.713 Diseases of the skin and subcutaneous tissue complicating pregnancy, third trimester   Ⓜ♀

     O99.719 Diseases of the skin and subcutaneous tissue complicating pregnancy, unspecified trimester   Ⓜ♀

     O99.72 Diseases of the skin and subcutaneous tissue complicating childbirth   Ⓜ♀

     O99.73 Diseases of the skin and subcutaneous tissue complicating the puerperium   Ⓜ♀

✓5ᵗʰ **O99.8** Other specified diseases and conditions complicating pregnancy, childbirth and the puerperium
Conditions in D00-D48, H00-H95, M00-N99, and Q00-Q99
Use additional code to identify condition
EXCLUDES 2   *genitourinary infections in pregnancy (O23.-)*
infection of genitourinary tract following delivery (O86.1-O86.3)
malignant neoplasm complicating pregnancy, childbirth and the puerperium (O9A.1-)
maternal care for known or suspected abnormality of maternal pelvic organs (O34.-)
postpartum acute kidney failure (O90.4)
traumatic injuries in pregnancy (O9A.2)

CC Excl: For CC codes in subcategory O99.8: PDX collection 1013

✓6ᵗʰ **O99.81** Abnormal glucose complicating pregnancy, childbirth and the puerperium
EXCLUDES 1   *gestational diabetes (O24.4-)*

     O99.810 Abnormal glucose complicating pregnancy   Ⓜ♀

Ⓝ Newborn: 0   Ⓟ Pediatric: 0-17   Ⓜ Maternity: 12-55   Ⓐ Adult: 15-124   MCC Major Complication/Comorbidity   CC Complication/Comorbidity   SW Severe Wound Dx

882   ICD-10-CM 2019

O99.814 Abnormal glucose complicating M♀
childbirth

O99.815 Abnormal glucose complicating the M♀
puerperium

✓6ᵗʰ **O99.82 Streptococcus B carrier state** complicating
pregnancy, childbirth and the puerperium
> EXCLUDES 1 carrier of streptococcus group B (GBS) in a
> nonpregnant woman (Z22.33Ø)

O99.82Ø Streptococcus B carrier state M♀
complicating pregnancy

O99.824 Streptococcus B carrier state M♀
complicating childbirth

O99.825 Streptococcus B carrier state M♀
complicating the puerperium

✓6ᵗʰ **O99.83 Other infection carrier state** complicating
pregnancy, childbirth and the puerperium
> Use additional code to identify the carrier state (Z22.-)

O99.83Ø Other infection carrier state CC M♀
complicating pregnancy

O99.834 Other infection carrier state CC M♀
complicating childbirth

O99.835 Other infection carrier state CC M♀
complicating the puerperium

✓6ᵗʰ **O99.84 Bariatric surgery status** complicating pregnancy,
childbirth and the puerperium
> Gastric banding status complicating pregnancy,
> childbirth and the puerperium
> Gastric bypass status for obesity complicating
> pregnancy, childbirth and the puerperium
> Obesity surgery status complicating pregnancy,
> childbirth and the puerperium

O99.84Ø Bariatric surgery status complicating M♀
pregnancy, unspecified trimester

O99.841 Bariatric surgery status complicating M♀
pregnancy, first trimester

O99.842 Bariatric surgery status complicating M♀
pregnancy, second trimester

O99.843 Bariatric surgery status complicating M♀
pregnancy, third trimester

O99.844 Bariatric surgery status complicating M♀
childbirth

O99.845 Bariatric surgery status complicating M♀
the puerperium

O99.89 Other specified diseases and conditions M♀
complicating pregnancy, childbirth and the
puerperium

✓4ᵗʰ **O9A Maternal malignant neoplasms, traumatic injuries and abuse
classifiable elsewhere but complicating pregnancy, childbirth
and the puerperium**

✓5ᵗʰ **O9A.1 Malignant neoplasm** complicating pregnancy, childbirth and
the puerperium
> Conditions in CØØ-C96
> Use additional code to identify neoplasm
> EXCLUDES 2 maternal care for benign tumor of corpus uteri (O34.1-)
> maternal care for benign tumor of cervix (O34.4-)

AHA: 2015, 3Q, 19

✓6ᵗʰ **O9A.11 Malignant neoplasm complicating** pregnancy

O9A.111 Malignant neoplasm complicating M♀
pregnancy, first trimester

O9A.112 Malignant neoplasm complicating M♀
pregnancy, second trimester

O9A.113 Malignant neoplasm complicating M♀
pregnancy, third trimester

O9A.119 Malignant neoplasm complicating M♀
pregnancy, unspecified trimester

O9A.12 Malignant neoplasm complicating childbirth M♀

O9A.13 Malignant neoplasm complicating the M♀
puerperium

✓5ᵗʰ **O9A.2 Injury, poisoning and** certain other consequences of external
causes complicating pregnancy, childbirth and the
puerperium
> Conditions in SØØ-T88, except T74 and T76
> Use additional code(s) to identify the injury or poisoning
> EXCLUDES 2 physical, sexual and psychological abuse complicating
> pregnancy, childbirth and the puerperium
> (O9A.3-, O9A.4-, O9A.5-)

✓6ᵗʰ **O9A.21 Injury, poisoning and certain other consequences of
external causes complicating** pregnancy

O9A.211 Injury, poisoning and certain other M♀
consequences of external causes
complicating pregnancy, first trimester

O9A.212 Injury, poisoning and certain other M♀
consequences of external causes
complicating pregnancy, second trimester

O9A.213 Injury, poisoning and certain other M♀
consequences of external causes
complicating pregnancy, third trimester

O9A.219 Injury, poisoning and certain other M♀
consequences of external causes
complicating pregnancy, unspecified
trimester

O9A.22 Injury, poisoning and certain other M♀
consequences of external causes complicating
childbirth

O9A.23 Injury, poisoning and certain other M♀
consequences of external causes complicating the
puerperium

✓5ᵗʰ **O9A.3 Physical abuse** complicating pregnancy, childbirth and the
puerperium
> Conditions in T74.11 or T76.11
> Use additional code (if applicable):
> to identify any associated current injury due to physical abuse
> to identify the perpetrator of abuse (YØ7.-)
> EXCLUDES 2 sexual abuse complicating pregnancy, childbirth and
> the puerperium (O9A.4)

✓6ᵗʰ **O9A.31 Physical abuse complicating** pregnancy

O9A.311 Physical abuse complicating M♀
pregnancy, first trimester

O9A.312 Physical abuse complicating M♀
pregnancy, second trimester

O9A.313 Physical abuse complicating M♀
pregnancy, third trimester

O9A.319 Physical abuse complicating M♀
pregnancy, unspecified trimester

O9A.32 Physical abuse complicating childbirth M♀

O9A.33 Physical abuse complicating the puerperium M♀

✓5ᵗʰ **O9A.4 Sexual abuse** complicating pregnancy, childbirth and the
puerperium
> Conditions in T74.21 or T76.21
> Use additional code (if applicable):
> to identify any associated current injury due to sexual abuse
> to identify the perpetrator of abuse (YØ7.-)

✓6ᵗʰ **O9A.41 Sexual abuse complicating** pregnancy

O9A.411 Sexual abuse complicating M♀
pregnancy, first trimester

O9A.412 Sexual abuse complicating M♀
pregnancy, second trimester

O9A.413 Sexual abuse complicating M♀
pregnancy, third trimester

O9A.419 Sexual abuse complicating M♀
pregnancy, unspecified trimester

O9A.42 Sexual abuse complicating childbirth M♀

O9A.43 Sexual abuse complicating the puerperium M♀

✓5ᵗʰ **O9A.5 Psychological abuse** complicating pregnancy, childbirth and
the puerperium
> Conditions in T74.31 or T76.31
> Use additional code to identify the perpetrator of abuse (YØ7.-)

✓6ᵗʰ **O9A.51 Psychological abuse complicating** pregnancy

O9A.511 Psychological abuse complicating M♀
pregnancy, first trimester

O9A.512 Psychological abuse complicating M♀
pregnancy, second trimester

O9A.513 Psychological abuse complicating M♀
pregnancy, third trimester

O9A.519 Psychological abuse complicating M♀
pregnancy, unspecified trimester

O9A.52 Psychological abuse complicating childbirth M♀

O9A.53 Psychological abuse complicating the M♀
puerperium

Chapter 16. Certain Conditions Originating in the Perinatal Period (P00–P96)

Chapter Specific Guidelines with Coding Examples

The chapter specific guidelines from the ICD-10-CM Official Guidelines for Coding and Reporting have been provided below. Along with these guidelines are coding examples, contained in the shaded boxes, that have been developed to help illustrate the coding and/or sequencing guidance found in these guidelines.

For coding and reporting purposes the perinatal period is defined as before birth through the 28th day following birth. The following guidelines are provided for reporting purposes

a. General perinatal rules

1) Use of Chapter 16 codes

Codes in this chapter are <u>never</u> for use on the maternal record. Codes from Chapter 15, the obstetric chapter, are never permitted on the newborn record. Chapter 16 codes may be used throughout the life of the patient if the condition is still present.

2) Principal diagnosis for birth record

When coding the birth episode in a newborn record, assign a code from category Z38, Liveborn infants according to place of birth and type of delivery, as the principal diagnosis. A code from category Z38 is assigned only once, to a newborn at the time of birth. If a newborn is transferred to another institution, a code from category Z38 should not be used at the receiving hospital.

A code from category Z38 is used only on the newborn record, not on the mother's record.

> Newborn delivered via vaginal delivery in Rural Hospital A, experienced meconium aspiration resulting in pneumonia. Rural Hospital A is not equipped to handle the extensive respiratory therapy this baby needs and transfers the patient to Metropolis Hospital B, where the pneumonia resolves and the newborn is eventually discharged.
>
> *Rural Hospital A*
>
> **Z38.00   Single liveborn infant, delivered vaginally**
>
> **P24.01   Meconium aspiration with respiratory symptoms**
>
> *Metropolis Hospital B*
>
> **P24.01   Meconium aspiration with respiratory symptoms**
>
> *Explanation:* A code from category Z38 is a one-time use only code. The hospital that actually delivered the newborn, in this case Rural Hospital A, can append a code from category Z38 but for the delivery admission only. Once the patient is transferred or discharged, the Z38 category no longer applies for that patient.
>
> The reason for the transfer to Metropolis Hospital B was for the respiratory symptoms (pneumonia) the newborn was exhibiting secondary to aspirating meconium.

3) Use of codes from other chapters with codes from Chapter 16

Codes from other chapters may be used with codes from chapter 16 if the codes from the other chapters provide more specific detail. Codes for signs and symptoms may be assigned when a definitive diagnosis has not been established. If the reason for the encounter is a perinatal condition, the code from chapter 16 should be sequenced first.

4) Use of Chapter 16 codes after the perinatal period

Should a condition originate in the perinatal period, and continue throughout the life of the patient, the perinatal code should continue to be used regardless of the patient's age.

> A 7-year-old patient with history of birth injury that resulted in Erb's palsy is seen for subscapularis release
>
> **P14.0   Erb's paralysis due to birth injury**
>
> *Explanation:* Although in this instance Erb's palsy is specifically related to a birth injury, it has not resolved and continues to be a health concern. A perinatal code is appropriate even though this patient is beyond the perinatal period.

5) Birth process or community acquired conditions

If a newborn has a condition that may be either due to the birth process or community acquired and the documentation does not indicate which it is, the default is due to the birth process and the code from Chapter 16 should be used. If the condition is community-acquired, a code from Chapter 16 should not be assigned.

6) Code all clinically significant conditions

All clinically significant conditions noted on routine newborn examination should be coded. A condition is clinically significant if it requires:

clinical evaluation; or

therapeutic treatment; or

diagnostic procedures; or

extended length of hospital stay; or

increased nursing care and/or monitoring; or

has implications for future health care needs

Note: The perinatal guidelines listed above are the same as the general coding guidelines for "additional diagnoses", except for the final point regarding implications for future health care needs. Codes should be assigned for conditions that have been specified by the provider as having implications for future health care needs.

b. Observation and evaluation of newborns for suspected conditions not found

1) Use of Z05 codes

Assign a code from category Z05, Observation and evaluation of newborns and infants for suspected conditions ruled out, to identify those instances when a healthy newborn is evaluated for a suspected condition that is determined after study not to be present. Do not use a code from category Z05 when the patient has identified signs or symptoms of a suspected problem; in such cases code the sign or symptom.

2) Z05 on Other than the birth record

A code from category Z05 may also be assigned as a principal or first-listed code for readmissions or encounters when the code from category Z38 code no longer applies. Codes from category Z05 are for use only for healthy newborns and infants for which no condition after study is found to be present.

3) Z05 on a birth record

A code from category Z05 is to be used as a secondary code after the code from category Z38, Liveborn infants according to place of birth and type of delivery.

> Newborn delivered via vaginal delivery; previous ultrasounds showed what appeared to be an abnormality of the right kidney. Kidney function tests were performed and ultrasounds taken and any genitourinary conditions ruled out.
>
> **Z38.00   Single liveborn infant, delivered vaginally**
>
> **Z05.6   Observation and evaluation of newborn for suspected genitourinary condition ruled out**
>
> Explanation: The newborn had no signs or symptoms of kidney or other genitourinary condition but was evaluated after delivery due to the abnormal prenatal ultrasound findings. A Z code describing the type and place of birth should be coded first, followed by a Z05 category code for the work performed to rule out a suspected genitourinary condition.

c. Coding additional perinatal diagnoses

1) Assigning codes for conditions that require treatment

Assign codes for conditions that require treatment or further investigation, prolong the length of stay, or require resource utilization.

Chapter 16. Certain Conditions Originating in the Perinatal Period

2) Codes for conditions specified as having implications for future health care needs

Assign codes for conditions that have been specified by the provider as having implications for future health care needs.

Note: This guideline should not be used for adult patients.

> An abnormal noise was heard in the left hip of a post-term newborn during a physical examination. The pediatrician would like to follow the patient after discharge as a hip click can be an early sign of hip dysplasia. The newborn was delivered via cesarean at 41 weeks.
>
> **Z38.01**   **Single liveborn infant, delivered by cesarean**
>
> **P08.21**   **Post-term newborn**
>
> **R29.4**   **Clicking hip**
>
> *Explanation:* The abnormal hip noise or click is appended as a secondary diagnosis not only because it is an abnormal finding upon examination, but also due to its potential to be part of a bigger health issue. The hip dysplasia has not yet been diagnosed and does not warrant a code at this time.

d. Prematurity and fetal growth retardation

Providers utilize different criteria in determining prematurity. A code for prematurity should not be assigned unless it is documented. Assignment of codes in categories P05, Disorders of newborn related to slow fetal growth and fetal malnutrition, and P07, Disorders of newborn related to short gestation and low birth weight, not elsewhere classified, should be based on the recorded birth weight and estimated gestational age.

When both birth weight and gestational age are available, two codes from category P07 should be assigned, with the code for birth weight sequenced before the code for gestational age.

e. Low birth weight and immaturity status

Codes from category P07, Disorders of newborn related to short gestation and low birth weight, not elsewhere classified, are for use for a child or adult who was premature or had a low birth weight as a newborn and this is affecting the patient's current health status.

See Section I.C.21. Factors influencing health status and contact with health services, Status.

> A 35-year-old patient, who weighed 659 grams at birth, is seen for heart disease documented as being a consequence of the low birth weight
>
> **I51.9**   **Heart disease, unspecified**
>
> **P07.02**   **Extremely low birth weight newborn, 500–749 grams**
>
> *Explanation:* A code from subcategories P07.0- and P07.1- is appropriate, regardless of the age of the patient, as long as the documentation provides a clear link between the patient's current illness and the low birth weight.

f. Bacterial sepsis of newborn

Category P36, Bacterial sepsis of newborn, includes congenital sepsis. If a perinate is documented as having sepsis without documentation of congenital or community acquired, the default is congenital and a code from category P36 should be assigned. If the P36 code includes the causal organism, an additional code from category B95, Streptococcus, Staphylococcus, and Enterococcus as the cause of diseases classified elsewhere, or B96, Other bacterial agents as the cause of diseases classified elsewhere, should not be assigned. If the P36 code does not include the causal organism, assign an additional code from category B96. If applicable, use additional codes to identify severe sepsis (R65.2-) and any associated acute organ dysfunction.

> A full-term infant develops severe sepsis 24 hours after discharge from the hospital and is readmitted; cultures identified *E. coli* as the infective agent
>
> **P36.4**   **Sepsis of newborn due to Escherichia coli**
>
> **R65.20**   **Severe sepsis without septic shock**
>
> *Explanation:* Even though this newborn was discharged and could have acquired *E. coli* from his/her external environment, due to the lack of documentation specifying specifically how this pathogen was acquired, the default is to code the *E. coli* sepsis as congenital. A code from chapter 1, "Certain Infectious and Parasitic Diseases," is not required because the perinatal sepsis code identifies both the sepsis and the bacteria causing the sepsis.

g. Stillbirth

Code P95, Stillbirth, is only for use in institutions that maintain separate records for stillbirths. No other code should be used with P95. Code P95 should not be used on the mother's record.

Chapter 16. Certain Conditions Originating in the Perinatal Period (P00-P96)

NOTE Codes from this chapter are for use on newborn records only, never on maternal records.

INCLUDES conditions that have their origin in the fetal or perinatal period (before birth through the first 28 days after birth) even if morbidity occurs later

EXCLUDES 2 *congenital malformations, deformations and chromosomal abnormalities (Q00-Q99)*
endocrine, nutritional and metabolic diseases (E00-E88)
injury, poisoning and certain other consequences of external causes (S00-T88)
neoplasms (C00-D49)
tetanus neonatorum (A33)

This chapter contains the following blocks:

P00-P04   Newborn affected by maternal factors and by complications of pregnancy, labor, and delivery
P05-P08   Disorders of newborn related to length of gestation and fetal growth
P09   Abnormal findings on neonatal screening
P10-P15   Birth trauma
P19-P29   Respiratory and cardiovascular disorders specific to the perinatal period
P35-P39   Infections specific to the perinatal period
P50-P61   Hemorrhagic and hematological disorders of newborn
P70-P74   Transitory endocrine and metabolic disorders specific to newborn
P76-P78   Digestive system disorders of newborn
P80-P83   Conditions involving the integument and temperature regulation of newborn
P84   Other problems with newborn
P90-P96   Other disorders originating in the perinatal period

Newborn affected by maternal factors and by complications of pregnancy, labor, and delivery (P00-P04)

NOTE These codes are for use when the listed maternal conditions are specified as the cause of confirmed morbidity or potential morbidity which have their origin in the perinatal period (before birth through the first 28 days after birth).

AHA: 2016, 4Q, 54-55

✓4ᵗʰ **P00 Newborn affected by maternal conditions that may be unrelated to present pregnancy**

Code first any current condition in newborn

EXCLUDES 2 *encounter for observation of newborn for suspected diseases and conditions ruled out (Z05.-)*
newborn affected by maternal complications of pregnancy (P01.-)
newborn affected by maternal endocrine and metabolic disorders (P70-P74)
newborn affected by noxious substances transmitted via placenta or breast milk (P04.-)

P00.0 Newborn affected by maternal hypertensive disorders
Newborn affected by maternal conditions classifiable to O10-O11, O13-O16

P00.1 Newborn affected by maternal renal and urinary tract diseases
Newborn affected by maternal conditions classifiable to N00-N39

P00.2 Newborn affected by maternal infectious and parasitic diseases
Newborn affected by maternal infectious disease classifiable to A00-B99, J09 and J10
EXCLUDES 1 *maternal genital tract or other localized infections (P00.8)*
EXCLUDES 2 *infections specific to the perinatal period (P35-P39)*
AHA: 2015, 3Q, 20

P00.3 Newborn affected by other maternal circulatory and respiratory diseases
Newborn affected by maternal conditions classifiable to I00-I99, J00-J99, Q20-Q34 and not included in P00.0, P00.2

P00.4 Newborn affected by maternal nutritional disorders
Newborn affected by maternal disorders classifiable to E40-E64
Maternal malnutrition NOS

P00.5 Newborn affected by maternal injury
Newborn affected by maternal conditions classifiable to O9A.2-

P00.6 Newborn affected by surgical procedure on mother
Newborn affected by amniocentesis
EXCLUDES 1 *Cesarean delivery for present delivery (P03.4)*
damage to placenta from amniocentesis, Cesarean delivery or surgical induction (P02.1)
previous surgery to uterus or pelvic organs (P03.89)
EXCLUDES 2 *newborn affected by complication of (fetal) intrauterine procedure (P96.5)*

P00.7 Newborn affected by other medical procedures on mother, not elsewhere classified
Newborn affected by radiation to mother
EXCLUDES 1 *damage to placenta from amniocentesis, cesarean delivery or surgical induction (P02.1)*
newborn affected by other complications of labor and delivery (P03.-)

✓5ᵗʰ **P00.8 Newborn affected by other maternal conditions**

P00.81 Newborn affected by periodontal disease in mother

P00.89 Newborn affected by other maternal conditions
Newborn affected by conditions classifiable to T80-T88
Newborn affected by maternal genital tract or other localized infections
Newborn affected by maternal systemic lupus erythematosus

P00.9 Newborn affected by unspecified maternal condition

✓4ᵗʰ **P01 Newborn affected by maternal complications of pregnancy**
Code first any current condition in newborn
EXCLUDES 2 *encounter for observation of newborn for suspected diseases and conditions ruled out (Z05.-)*

P01.0 Newborn affected by incompetent cervix

P01.1 Newborn affected by premature rupture of membranes

P01.2 Newborn affected by oligohydramnios
EXCLUDES 1 *oligohydramnios due to premature rupture of membranes (P01.1)*
DEF: Low amniotic fluid level, resulting in underdeveloped organs in the fetus.

P01.3 Newborn affected by polyhydramnios
Newborn affected by hydramnios
DEF: Polyhydramnios: Excess amniotic fluid surrounding the fetus, typically defined as a total fluid volume of greater than 24.0 cc.

P01.4 Newborn affected by ectopic pregnancy
Newborn affected by abdominal pregnancy

P01.5 Newborn affected by multiple pregnancy
Newborn affected by triplet (pregnancy)
Newborn affected by twin (pregnancy)

P01.6 Newborn affected by maternal death

P01.7 Newborn affected by malpresentation before labor
Newborn affected by breech presentation before labor
Newborn affected by external version before labor
Newborn affected by face presentation before labor
Newborn affected by transverse lie before labor
Newborn affected by unstable lie before labor

P01.8 Newborn affected by other maternal complications of pregnancy

P01.9 Newborn affected by maternal complication of pregnancy, unspecified

✓4ᵗʰ **P02 Newborn affected by complications of placenta, cord and membranes**
Code first any current condition in newborn
EXCLUDES 2 *encounter for observation of newborn for suspected diseases and conditions ruled out (Z05.-)*

P02.0 Newborn affected by placenta previa
DEF: Placenta developed in the lower segment of the uterus that can cause hemorrhaging leading to preterm delivery.

P02.1 Newborn affected by other forms of placental separation and hemorrhage
Newborn affected by abruptio placenta
Newborn affected by accidental hemorrhage
Newborn affected by antepartum hemorrhage
Newborn affected by damage to placenta from amniocentesis, cesarean delivery or surgical induction
Newborn affected by maternal blood loss
Newborn affected by premature separation of placenta

✓5ᵗʰ **P02.2 Newborn affected by other and unspecified morphological and functional abnormalities of placenta**

P02.20 Newborn affected by unspecified morphological and functional abnormalities of placenta

Chapter 16. Certain Conditions Originating in the Perinatal Period

P02.29   **Newborn affected by** other **morphological and functional** abnormalities **of placenta**
- Newborn affected by placental dysfunction
- Newborn affected by placental infarction
- Newborn affected by placental insufficiency

P02.3   **Newborn affected by** placental transfusion syndromes
- Newborn affected by placental and cord abnormalities resulting in twin-to-twin or other transplacental transfusion

P02.4   **Newborn affected by** prolapsed cord

P02.5   **Newborn affected by** other compression **of umbilical cord**
- Newborn affected by umbilical cord (tightly) around neck
- Newborn affected by entanglement of umbilical cord
- Newborn affected by knot in umbilical cord

✓5th **P02.6**   **Newborn affected by other and unspecified** conditions of **umbilical cord**

     P02.60   **Newborn affected by** unspecified **conditions of umbilical cord**

     P02.69   **Newborn affected by** other **conditions of umbilical cord**
- Newborn affected by short umbilical cord
- Newborn affected by vasa previa
- **EXCLUDES 1**   *newborn affected by single umbilical artery (Q27.0)*

✓5th **P02.7**   **Newborn affected by** chorioamnionitis
- ~~Newborn affected by amnionitis~~
- ~~Newborn affected by membranitis~~
- ~~Newborn affected by placentitis~~
- **DEF:** Inflammation of the fetal membranes due to maternal infection characterized by fetal tachycardia, respiratory distress, apnea, weak cries, and poor sucking.

     ● **P02.70**   **Newborn affected by** fetal inflammatory response syndrome
- Newborn affected by FIRS

     ● **P02.78**   **Newborn affected by** other **conditions from chorioamnionitis**
- Newborn affected by amnionitis
- Newborn affected by membranitis
- Newborn affected by placentitis

P02.8   **Newborn affected by** other abnormalities of membranes

P02.9   **Newborn affected by** abnormality of membranes, unspecified

✓4th **P03**   **Newborn affected by other complications of** labor and delivery
- Code first any current condition in newborn
- **EXCLUDES 2**   *encounter for observation of newborn for suspected diseases and conditions ruled out (Z05.-)*

P03.0   **Newborn affected by** breech delivery and extraction

P03.1   **Newborn affected by other** malpresentation, malposition **and disproportion during labor and delivery**
- Newborn affected by contracted pelvis
- Newborn affected by conditions classifiable to O64-O66
- Newborn affected by persistent occipitoposterior
- Newborn affected by transverse lie

P03.2   **Newborn affected by** forceps **delivery**

Forceps Assisted Birth

Forceps extractor

Vacuum Assisted Birth

Vacuum extractor

P03.3   **Newborn affected by delivery by** vacuum extractor **[ventouse]**

P03.4   **Newborn affected by** Cesarean **delivery**

P03.5   **Newborn affected by** precipitate **delivery**
- Newborn affected by rapid second stage

P03.6   **Newborn affected by** abnormal uterine contractions
- Newborn affected by conditions classifiable to O62.-, except O62.3
- Newborn affected by hypertonic labor
- Newborn affected by uterine inertia

✓5th **P03.8**   **Newborn affected by** other **specified complications of labor and delivery**

     ✓6th **P03.81**   **Newborn affected by** abnormality in fetal **(intrauterine) heart rate or rhythm**
- **EXCLUDES 1**   *neonatal cardiac dysrhythmia (P29.1-)*

         P03.810   **Newborn affected by abnormality in fetal (intrauterine) heart rate or rhythm** before **the onset of labor**

         P03.811   **Newborn affected by abnormality in fetal (intrauterine) heart rate or rhythm** during **labor**

         P03.819   **Newborn affected by abnormality in fetal (intrauterine) heart rate or rhythm, unspecified as to time of onset**

     P03.82   **Meconium passage during delivery**
- **EXCLUDES 1**   *meconium aspiration (P24.00, P24.01) meconium staining (P96.83)*
- **DEF:** Fetal intestinal activity that increases in response to a fetomaternal distressed state during delivery. The anal sphincter relaxes and meconium is passed into the amniotic fluid.

     P03.89   **Newborn affected by** other **specified complications of labor and delivery**
- Newborn affected by abnormality of maternal soft tissues
- Newborn affected by conditions classifiable to O60-O75 and by procedures used in labor and delivery not included in P02.- and P03.0-P03.6
- Newborn affected by induction of labor

P03.9   **Newborn affected by** complication of labor and delivery, unspecified

✓4th **P04**   **Newborn affected by** noxious substances transmitted via placenta or breast milk
- **INCLUDES**   nonteratogenic effects of substances transmitted via placenta
- **EXCLUDES 2**   *congenital malformations (Q00-Q99)*
  encounter for observation of newborn for suspected diseases and conditions ruled out (Z05.-)
  neonatal jaundice from excessive hemolysis due to drugs or toxins transmitted from mother (P58.4)
  newborn in contact with and (suspected) exposures hazardous to health not transmitted via placenta or breast milk (Z77.-)

P04.0   **Newborn affected by maternal** anesthesia and analgesia **in pregnancy, labor and delivery**
- ▶Newborn affected by reactions and intoxications from maternal opiates and tranquilizers administered for procedures during pregnancy or labor and delivery◀
- **EXCLUDES 2** ▶*newborn affected by other maternal medication (P04.1-)* ◀

N Newborn: 0   **P** Pediatric: 0-17   **M** Maternity: 12-55   **A** Adult: 15-124   **MCC** Major Complication/Comorbidity   **CC** Complication/Comorbidity   **SW** Severe Wound Dx

888   ICD-10-CM 2019

✓5ᵗʰ **P04.1 Newborn affected by** other maternal medication
Newborn affected by cancer chemotherapy
Newborn affected by cytotoxic drugs
▶Code first withdrawal symptoms from maternal use of drugs of addiction, if applicable (P96.1)◀

EXCLUDES 1　dysmorphism due to warfarin (Q86.2)
fetal hydantoin syndrome (Q86.1)
maternal use of drugs of addiction (P04.4-)

EXCLUDES 2　▶*maternal anesthesia and analgesia in pregnancy, labor and delivery (P04.0)*
maternal use of drugs of addiction (P04.4-)◀

● **P04.11 Newborn affected by maternal** antineoplastic chemotherapy

● **P04.12 Newborn affected by maternal** cytotoxic drugs

● **P04.13 Newborn affected by maternal use of** anticonvulsants

● **P04.14 Newborn affected by maternal use of** opiates

● **P04.15 Newborn affected by maternal use of** antidepressants

● **P04.16 Newborn affected by maternal use of** amphetamines

● **P04.17 Newborn affected by maternal use of** sedative-hypnotics

● **P04.1A Newborn affected by maternal use of** anxiolytics

● **P04.18 Newborn affected by** other maternal medication

● **P04.19 Newborn affected by maternal use of** unspecified medication

P04.2 Newborn affected by maternal use of tobacco
Newborn affected by exposure in utero to tobacco smoke
EXCLUDES 2　*newborn exposure to environmental tobacco smoke (P96.81)*

P04.3 Newborn affected by maternal use of alcohol
EXCLUDES 1　*fetal alcohol syndrome (Q86.0)*

✓5ᵗʰ **P04.4 Newborn affected by maternal use of** drugs of addiction

● **P04.40 Newborn affected by maternal use of** unspecified drugs of addiction

P04.41 Newborn affected by maternal use of cocaine
"Crack baby"

● **P04.42 Newborn affected by maternal use of** hallucinogens
EXCLUDES 2　*newborn affected by other maternal medication (P04.1-)*

P04.49 Newborn affected by maternal use of other drugs of addiction
EXCLUDES 2　*newborn affected by maternal anesthesia and analgesia (P04.0)*
withdrawal symptoms from maternal use of drugs of addiction (P96.1)

P04.5 Newborn affected by maternal use of nutritional chemical substances

P04.6 Newborn affected by maternal exposure to environmental chemical substances

✓5ᵗʰ **P04.8 Newborn affected by other maternal noxious substances**

● **P04.81 Newborn affected by maternal use of** cannabis

● **P04.89 Newborn affected by** other maternal noxious substances

P04.9 Newborn affected by maternal noxious substance, unspecified

Disorders of newborn related to length of gestation and fetal growth (P05-P08)

✓4ᵗʰ **P05 Disorders of newborn related to slow fetal growth and fetal malnutrition**
AHA: 2016, 4Q, 55-56

✓5ᵗʰ **P05.0 Newborn light for gestational age**
Newborn light-for-dates
Weight below but length above 10th percentile for gestational age

P05.00 Newborn light for gestational age, unspecified weight

P05.01 Newborn light for gestational age, less than 500 grams

P05.02 Newborn light for gestational age, 500-749 grams

P05.03 Newborn light for gestational age, 750-999 grams

P05.04 Newborn light for gestational age, 1000-1249 grams

P05.05 Newborn light for gestational age, 1250-1499 grams

P05.06 Newborn light for gestational age, 1500-1749 grams

P05.07 Newborn light for gestational age, 1750-1999 grams

P05.08 Newborn light for gestational age, 2000-2499 grams

P05.09 Newborn light for gestational age, 2500 grams and over
Newborn light for gestational age, other

✓5ᵗʰ **P05.1 Newborn small for gestational age**
Newborn small-and-light-for-dates
Newborn small-for-dates
Weight and length below 10th percentile for gestational age

P05.10 Newborn small for gestational age, unspecified weight

P05.11 Newborn small for gestational age, less than 500 grams

P05.12 Newborn small for gestational age, 500-749 grams

P05.13 Newborn small for gestational age, 750-999 grams

P05.14 Newborn small for gestational age, 1000-1249 grams

P05.15 Newborn small for gestational age, 1250-1499 grams

P05.16 Newborn small for gestational age, 1500-1749 grams

P05.17 Newborn small for gestational age, 1750-1999 grams

P05.18 Newborn small for gestational age, 2000-2499 grams

P05.19 Newborn small for gestational age, other
Newborn small for gestational age, 2500 grams and over

P05.2 Newborn affected by fetal (intrauterine) malnutrition **not light or small for gestational age**
Infant, not light or small for gestational age, showing signs of fetal malnutrition, such as dry, peeling skin and loss of subcutaneous tissue
EXCLUDES 1　*newborn affected by fetal malnutrition with light for gestational age (P05.0-)*
newborn affected by fetal malnutrition with small for gestational age (P05.1-)

P05.9 Newborn affected by slow intrauterine growth, **unspecified**
Newborn affected by fetal growth retardation NOS

✓4ᵗʰ **P07 Disorders of newborn related to short gestation and low birth weight, not elsewhere classified**
NOTE　When both birth weight and gestational age of the newborn are available, both should be coded with birth weight sequenced before gestational age
INCLUDES　the listed conditions, without further specification, as the cause of morbidity or additional care, in newborn

✓5ᵗʰ **P07.0 Extremely low birth weight newborn**
Newborn birth weight 999 g. or less
EXCLUDES 1　*low birth weight due to slow fetal growth and fetal malnutrition (P05.-)*

P07.00 Extremely low birth weight newborn, unspecified weight

P07.01 Extremely low birth weight newborn, less than 500 grams

P07.02 Extremely low birth weight newborn, 500-749 grams

P07.03 Extremely low birth weight newborn, 750-999 grams

✓5ᵗʰ **P07.1 Other low birth weight newborn**
Newborn birth weight 1000-2499 g.
EXCLUDES 1　*low birth weight due to slow fetal growth and fetal malnutrition (P05.-)*

P07.10 Other low birth weight newborn, unspecified weight

P07.14 Other low birth weight newborn, 1000-1249 grams

P07.15 Other low birth weight newborn, 1250-1499 grams

P07.16 Other low birth weight newborn, 1500-1749 grams

P07.17 Other low birth weight newborn, 1750-1999 grams

P07.18 Other low birth weight newborn, 2000-2499 grams

✓5ᵗʰ **P07.2 Extreme immaturity of newborn**
Less than 28 completed weeks (less than 196 completed days) of gestation.

P07.20 Extreme immaturity of newborn, unspecified weeks of gestation
Gestational age less than 28 completed weeks NOS

P07.21 Extreme immaturity of newborn, gestational age less than 23 completed weeks
Extreme immaturity of newborn, gestational age less than 23 weeks, 0 days

P07.22 **Extreme immaturity of newborn, gestational age 23 completed weeks**
Extreme immaturity of newborn, gestational age 23 weeks, 0 days through 23 weeks, 6 days

P07.23 **Extreme immaturity of newborn, gestational age 24 completed weeks**
Extreme immaturity of newborn, gestational age 24 weeks, 0 days through 24 weeks, 6 days

P07.24 **Extreme immaturity of newborn, gestational age 25 completed weeks**
Extreme immaturity of newborn, gestational age 25 weeks, 0 days through 25 weeks, 6 days

P07.25 **Extreme immaturity of newborn, gestational age 26 completed weeks**
Extreme immaturity of newborn, gestational age 26 weeks, 0 days through 26 weeks, 6 days

P07.26 **Extreme immaturity of newborn, gestational age 27 completed weeks**
Extreme immaturity of newborn, gestational age 27 weeks, 0 days through 27 weeks, 6 days

✓5ᵗʰ P07.3 **Preterm [premature] newborn [other]**
28 completed weeks or more but less than 37 completed weeks (196 completed days but less than 259 completed days) of gestation
Prematurity NOS
AHA: 2017, 3Q, 26

P07.30 **Preterm newborn, unspecified weeks of gestation**

P07.31 **Preterm newborn, gestational age 28 completed weeks**
Preterm newborn, gestational age 28 weeks, 0 days through 28 weeks, 6 days

P07.32 **Preterm newborn, gestational age 29 completed weeks**
Preterm newborn, gestational age 29 weeks, 0 days through 29 weeks, 6 days

P07.33 **Preterm newborn, gestational age 30 completed weeks**
Preterm newborn, gestational age 30 weeks, 0 days through 30 weeks, 6 days

P07.34 **Preterm newborn, gestational age 31 completed weeks**
Preterm newborn, gestational age 31 weeks, 0 days through 31 weeks, 6 days

P07.35 **Preterm newborn, gestational age 32 completed weeks**
Preterm newborn, gestational age 32 weeks, 0 days through 32 weeks, 6 days

P07.36 **Preterm newborn, gestational age 33 completed weeks**
Preterm newborn, gestational age 33 weeks, 0 days through 33 weeks, 6 days

P07.37 **Preterm newborn, gestational age 34 completed weeks**
Preterm newborn, gestational age 34 weeks, 0 days through 34 weeks, 6 days

P07.38 **Preterm newborn, gestational age 35 completed weeks**
Preterm newborn, gestational age 35 weeks, 0 days through 35 weeks, 6 days

P07.39 **Preterm newborn, gestational age 36 completed weeks**
Preterm newborn, gestational age 36 weeks, 0 days through 36 weeks, 6 days

✓4ᵗʰ P08 **Disorders of newborn related to long gestation and high birth weight**
NOTE When both birth weight and gestational age of the newborn are available, priority of assignment should be given to birth weight
INCLUDES the listed conditions, without further specification, as causes of morbidity or additional care, in newborn

P08.0 **Exceptionally large newborn baby**
Usually implies a birth weight of 4500 g. or more
EXCLUDES 1 syndrome of infant of diabetic mother (P70.1)
syndrome of infant of mother with gestational diabetes (P70.0)

P08.1 **Other heavy for gestational age newborn**
Other newborn heavy- or large-for-dates regardless of period of gestation
Usually implies a birth weight of 4000 g. to 4499 g.
EXCLUDES 1 newborn with a birth weight of 4500 or more (P08.0)
syndrome of infant of diabetic mother (P70.1)
syndrome of infant of mother with gestational diabetes (P70.0).

✓5ᵗʰ P08.2 **Late newborn, not heavy for gestational age**
AHA: 2014, 1Q, 14

P08.21 **Post-term newborn**
Newborn with gestation period over 40 completed weeks to 42 completed weeks

P08.22 **Prolonged gestation of newborn**
Newborn with gestation period over 42 completed weeks (294 days or more), not heavy- or large-for-dates.
Postmaturity NOS

Abnormal findings on neonatal screening (P09)

P09 **Abnormal findings on neonatal screening**
Use additional code to identify signs, symptoms and conditions associated with the screening
EXCLUDES 2 nonspecific serologic evidence of human immunodeficiency virus [HIV] (R75)

Birth trauma (P10-P15)

✓4ᵗʰ P10 **Intracranial laceration and hemorrhage due to birth injury**
EXCLUDES 1 intracranial hemorrhage of newborn NOS (P52.9)
intracranial hemorrhage of newborn due to anoxia or hypoxia (P52.-)
nontraumatic intracranial hemorrhage of newborn (P52.-)

CC Excl: For CC/MCC codes in category P10, unless otherwise noted: PDX collection 1020

P10.0 **Subdural hemorrhage due to birth injury**   MCC
Subdural hematoma (localized) due to birth injury
EXCLUDES 1 subdural hemorrhage accompanying tentorial tear (P10.4)

P10.1 **Cerebral hemorrhage due to birth injury**   MCC

P10.2 **Intraventricular hemorrhage due to birth injury**   CC
CC Excl: PDX collection 1021

P10.3 **Subarachnoid hemorrhage due to birth injury**   MCC
CC Excl: PDX collection 1022

P10.4 **Tentorial tear due to birth injury**   MCC

P10.8 **Other intracranial lacerations and hemorrhages due to birth injury**   MCC

P10.9 **Unspecified intracranial laceration and hemorrhage due to birth injury**   MCC

✓4ᵗʰ P11 **Other birth injuries to central nervous system**

CC Excl: For MCC codes in category P11: PDX collection 1020

P11.0 **Cerebral edema due to birth injury**   MCC

P11.1 **Other specified brain damage due to birth injury**

P11.2 **Unspecified brain damage due to birth injury**   MCC

P11.3 **Birth injury to facial nerve**
Facial palsy due to birth injury

P11.4 **Birth injury to other cranial nerves**

P11.5 **Birth injury to spine and spinal cord**
Fracture of spine due to birth injury

P11.9 **Birth injury to central nervous system, unspecified**   MCC

✓4ᵗʰ P12 **Birth injury to scalp**

P12.0 **Cephalhematoma due to birth injury**
DEF: Condition that occurs in a neonate when blood vessels between the skull and periosteum rupture and blood collects in the subperiosteal space (below the periosteum). It is typically caused by prolonged labor or trauma due to instrument-assisted delivery (e.g., forceps, vacuum extraction), although in rare circumstances, it may indicate a linear skull fracture with intracranial hemorrhage.

P12.1 **Chignon (from vacuum extraction) due to birth injury**
DEF: Artificial swelling of the scalp that occurs when a collection of interstitial fluid and blood forms in the area of the scalp where the suction cup was applied during a vacuum-assisted delivery.

P12.2 **Epicranial subaponeurotic hemorrhage due to birth injury**   CC
Subgaleal hemorrhage
CC Excl: PDX collection 1023

P12.3   Bruising of scalp due to birth injury

P12.4   Injury of scalp of newborn due to monitoring equipment
     Sampling incision of scalp of newborn
     Scalp clip (electrode) injury of newborn

√5ᵗʰ **P12.8**   Other birth injuries to scalp

     P12.81   Caput succedaneum
         DEF: Swelling of the scalp as a result of pressure being exerted on the head from the vaginal walls, uterus, or instrumentation used in assisting a delivery (e.g., vacuum).

     P12.89   Other birth injuries to scalp

P12.9   Birth injury to scalp, unspecified

Birth Injuries to Scalp

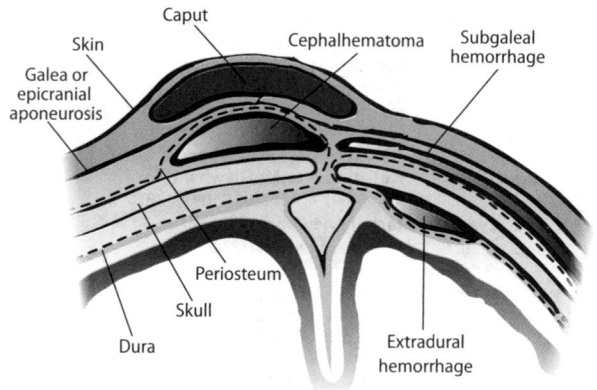

P13   **Birth injury to skeleton**
     EXCLUDES 2   birth injury to spine (P11.5)

P13.0   Fracture of skull due to birth injury

P13.1   Other birth injuries to skull
     EXCLUDES 1   cephalhematoma (P12.0)

P13.2   Birth injury to femur

P13.3   Birth injury to other long bones

P13.4   Fracture of clavicle due to birth injury

P13.8   Birth injuries to other parts of skeleton

P13.9   Birth injury to skeleton, unspecified

√4ᵗʰ **P14**   **Birth injury to peripheral nervous system**

P14.0   Erb's paralysis due to birth injury
     DEF: Erb's paralysis: Most common type of brachial plexus (peripheral nerve) injury in a neonate that involves nerve damage at the level of C5-C6. **Synonym(s):** Erb's palsy.

P14.1   Klumpke's paralysis due to birth injury

P14.2   Phrenic nerve paralysis due to birth injury

P14.3   Other brachial plexus birth injuries

P14.8   Birth injuries to other parts of peripheral nervous system

P14.9   Birth injury to peripheral nervous system, unspecified

√4ᵗʰ **P15**   **Other birth injuries**

P15.0   Birth injury to liver
     Rupture of liver due to birth injury

P15.1   Birth injury to spleen
     Rupture of spleen due to birth injury

P15.2   Sternomastoid injury due to birth injury

P15.3   Birth injury to eye
     Subconjunctival hemorrhage due to birth injury
     Traumatic glaucoma due to birth injury

P15.4   Birth injury to face
     Facial congestion due to birth injury

P15.5   Birth injury to external genitalia

P15.6   Subcutaneous fat necrosis due to birth injury

P15.8   Other specified birth injuries
     TIP: Use for any injury of newborn from scalpel.

P15.9   Birth injury, unspecified

Respiratory and cardiovascular disorders specific to the perinatal period (P19-P29)

√4ᵗʰ **P19**   **Metabolic acidemia in newborn**
     INCLUDES   metabolic acidemia in newborn

P19.0   Metabolic acidemia in newborn first noted before onset of labor

P19.1   Metabolic acidemia in newborn first noted during labor

P19.2   Metabolic acidemia noted at birth

P19.9   Metabolic acidemia, unspecified

√4ᵗʰ **P22**   **Respiratory distress of newborn**
     EXCLUDES 1   respiratory arrest of newborn (P28.81)
         respiratory failure of newborn NOS (P28.5)

P22.0   Respiratory distress syndrome of newborn   MCC
     Cardiorespiratory distress syndrome of newborn
     Hyaline membrane disease
     Idiopathic respiratory distress syndrome [IRDS or RDS] of newborn
     Pulmonary hypoperfusion syndrome
     Respiratory distress syndrome, type I
     DEF: Severe chest contractions upon air intake and expiratory grunting. The infant appears blue due to oxygen deficiency and has a rapid respiratory rate, formerly called hyaline membrane disease.
     CC Excl: PDX collection 748

P22.1   Transient tachypnea of newborn
     Idiopathic tachypnea of newborn
     Respiratory distress syndrome, type II
     Wet lung syndrome
     DEF: Rapid, labored breathing of a newborn. It is a short-term problem that begins after birth and lasts about three days.

P22.8   Other respiratory distress of newborn

P22.9   Respiratory distress of newborn, unspecified

√4ᵗʰ **P23**   **Congenital pneumonia**
     INCLUDES   infective pneumonia acquired in utero or during birth
     EXCLUDES 1   neonatal pneumonia resulting from aspiration (P24.-)

     CC Excl: For MCC codes in category P23: PDX collection 748

P23.0   Congenital pneumonia due to viral agent   MCC
     Use additional code (B97) to identify organism
     EXCLUDES 1   congenital rubella pneumonitis (P35.0)

P23.1   Congenital pneumonia due to Chlamydia   MCC

P23.2   Congenital pneumonia due to staphylococcus   MCC

P23.3   Congenital pneumonia due to streptococcus, group B   MCC

P23.4   Congenital pneumonia due to Escherichia coli   MCC

P23.5   Congenital pneumonia due to Pseudomonas   MCC

P23.6   Congenital pneumonia due to other bacterial agents   MCC
     Congenital pneumonia due to Hemophilus influenzae
     Congenital pneumonia due to Klebsiella pneumoniae
     Congenital pneumonia due to Mycoplasma
     Congenital pneumonia due to Streptococcus, except group B
     Use additional code (B95-B96) to identify organism

P23.8   Congenital pneumonia due to other organisms   MCC

P23.9   Congenital pneumonia, unspecified   MCC

√4ᵗʰ **P24**   **Neonatal aspiration**
     INCLUDES   aspiration in utero and during delivery

     CC Excl: For MCC codes in category P24: PDX collection 748

√5ᵗʰ **P24.0**   Meconium aspiration
     EXCLUDES 1   meconium passage (without aspiration) during delivery (P03.82)
         meconium staining (P96.83)

     P24.00   Meconium aspiration without respiratory symptoms
         Meconium aspiration NOS

     P24.01   Meconium aspiration with respiratory symptoms   MCC
         Meconium aspiration pneumonia
         Meconium aspiration pneumonitis
         Meconium aspiration syndrome NOS
         Use additional code to identify any secondary pulmonary hypertension, if applicable (I27.2-)
         DEF: Aspiration of fetal intestinal material during or prior to delivery. If is usually a complication of placental insufficiency, causing pneumonitis and bronchial obstruction (inflammatory reaction of lungs).

√5ᵗʰ **P24.1**   Neonatal aspiration of (clear) amniotic fluid and mucus
     Neonatal aspiration of liquor (amnii)

     P24.10   Neonatal aspiration of (clear) amniotic fluid and mucus without respiratory symptoms
         Neonatal aspiration of amniotic fluid and mucus NOS

✓ Additional Character Required   ✓x7ᵗʰ Placeholder   Unacceptable PDx   Questionable PDx   Manifestation   H1 - H14 HAC   HCC CMS-HCC Dx   HIV HIV Dx

ICD-10-CM 2019   891

Chapter 16. Certain Conditions Originating in the Perinatal Period

P24.11 **Neonatal aspiration of (clear) amniotic fluid and mucus** with respiratory symptoms `MCC`
Neonatal aspiration of amniotic fluid and mucus with pneumonia
Neonatal aspiration of amniotic fluid and mucus with pneumonitis
Use additional code to identify any secondary pulmonary hypertension, if applicable (I27.2-)

✓5th P24.2 **Neonatal aspiration of** blood

P24.20 **Neonatal aspiration of blood** without respiratory symptoms
Neonatal aspiration of blood NOS

P24.21 **Neonatal aspiration of blood** with respiratory symptoms `MCC`
Neonatal aspiration of blood with pneumonia
Neonatal aspiration of blood with pneumonitis
Use additional code to identify any secondary pulmonary hypertension, if applicable (I27.2-)

✓5th P24.3 **Neonatal aspiration of** milk **and regurgitated** food
Neonatal aspiration of stomach contents

P24.30 **Neonatal aspiration of milk and regurgitated food** without respiratory symptoms
Neonatal aspiration of milk and regurgitated food NOS

P24.31 **Neonatal aspiration of milk and regurgitated food** with respiratory symptoms `MCC`
Neonatal aspiration of milk and regurgitated food with pneumonia
Neonatal aspiration of milk and regurgitated food with pneumonitis
Use additional code to identify any secondary pulmonary hypertension, if applicable (I27.2-)

✓5th P24.8 **Other neonatal aspiration**

P24.80 **Other neonatal aspiration** without respiratory symptoms
Neonatal aspiration NEC

P24.81 **Other neonatal aspiration** with respiratory symptoms `MCC`
Neonatal aspiration pneumonia NEC
Neonatal aspiration with pneumonitis NEC
Neonatal aspiration with pneumonia NOS
Neonatal aspiration with pneumonitis NOS
Use additional code to identify any secondary pulmonary hypertension, if applicable (I27.2-)

P24.9 **Neonatal aspiration,** unspecified

✓4th P25 **Interstitial emphysema and related conditions originating in the perinatal period**

CC Excl: For MCC codes in category P25: PDX collection 748

P25.0 Interstitial emphysema **originating in the perinatal period** `MCC`

P25.1 Pneumothorax **originating in the perinatal period** `MCC`

P25.2 Pneumomediastinum **originating in the perinatal period** `MCC`

P25.3 Pneumopericardium **originating in the perinatal period** `MCC`

P25.8 Other **conditions related to interstitial emphysema originating in the perinatal period** `MCC`

✓4th P26 **Pulmonary hemorrhage originating in the perinatal period**
EXCLUDES 1 acute idiopathic hemorrhage in infants over 28 days old (R04.81)

CC Excl: For MCC codes in category P26: PDX collection 748

P26.0 Tracheobronchial **hemorrhage originating in the perinatal period** `MCC`

P26.1 Massive pulmonary **hemorrhage originating in the perinatal period** `MCC`

P26.8 Other pulmonary **hemorrhages originating in the perinatal period** `MCC`

P26.9 Unspecified **pulmonary hemorrhage originating in the perinatal period** `MCC`

✓4th P27 **Chronic respiratory disease originating in the perinatal period**
EXCLUDES 2 respiratory distress of newborn (P22.0-P22.9)

P27.0 **Wilson-Mikity syndrome** `MCC`
Pulmonary dysmaturity
DEF: Pulmonary insufficiency in newborn babies, especially those with low birth weight. Rapid onset of hypercapnia and cyanosis occur during the first month of life frequently resulting in death.

P27.1 **Bronchopulmonary dysplasia originating in the perinatal period** `MCC`

P27.8 **Other chronic respiratory diseases originating in the perinatal period** `MCC`
Congenital pulmonary fibrosis   Ventilator lung in newborn

P27.9 **Unspecified chronic respiratory disease originating in the perinatal period** `MCC`

✓4th P28 **Other respiratory conditions originating in the perinatal period**
EXCLUDES 1 congenital malformations of the respiratory system (Q30-Q34)

CC Excl: For CC/MCC codes in subcategory P28, unless otherwise noted: PDX collection 748

P28.0 **Primary atelectasis of newborn** `CC`
Primary failure to expand terminal respiratory units
Pulmonary hypoplasia associated with short gestation
Pulmonary immaturity NOS

✓5th P28.1 **Other and unspecified atelectasis of newborn**

P28.10 **Unspecified atelectasis of newborn** `CC`
Atelectasis of newborn NOS

P28.11 **Resorption atelectasis without respiratory distress syndrome** `CC`
EXCLUDES 1 resorption atelectasis with respiratory distress syndrome (P22.0)

P28.19 **Other atelectasis of newborn** `CC`
Partial atelectasis of newborn
Secondary atelectasis of newborn

P28.2 **Cyanotic attacks of newborn** `CC`
EXCLUDES 1 apnea of newborn (P28.3-P28.4)
CC Excl: PDX collection 1024

P28.3 **Primary sleep apnea of newborn** `CC`
Central sleep apnea of newborn
Obstructive sleep apnea of newborn
Sleep apnea of newborn NOS
DEF: Unexplained cessation of breathing when a neonate makes no respiratory effort for 20 seconds or longer or when a neonate's breathing cessation is accompanied by cyanosis, bradycardia, or hypotonia.
CC Excl: PDX collection 1025

P28.4 **Other apnea of newborn** `CC`
Apnea of prematurity
Obstructive apnea of newborn
EXCLUDES 1 obstructive sleep apnea of newborn (P28.3)
CC Excl: PDX collection 1026

P28.5 **Respiratory failure of newborn** `MCC`
EXCLUDES 1 respiratory arrest of newborn (P28.81)
respiratory distress of newborn (P22.0-)

✓5th P28.8 **Other specified respiratory conditions of newborn**

P28.81 **Respiratory arrest of newborn** `MCC`
CC Excl: PDX collection 1027

P28.89 **Other specified respiratory conditions of newborn**
Congenital laryngeal stridor
Sniffles in newborn
Snuffles in newborn
EXCLUDES 1 early congenital syphilitic rhinitis (A50.05)

P28.9 **Respiratory condition of newborn, unspecified**
Respiratory depression in newborn

✓4th P29 **Cardiovascular disorders originating in the perinatal period**
EXCLUDES 1 congenital malformations of the circulatory system (Q20-Q28)

P29.0 **Neonatal cardiac failure**

✓5th P29.1 **Neonatal cardiac dysrhythmia**

P29.11 **Neonatal** tachycardia

P29.12 **Neonatal** bradycardia

P29.2 **Neonatal hypertension**

✓5th P29.3 **Persistent fetal circulation**
AHA: 2017, 4Q, 20-21

P29.30 **Pulmonary hypertension of newborn** `MCC`
Persistent pulmonary hypertension of newborn
DEF: Condition that occurs when pressure within the pulmonary artery is elevated and vascular resistance is observed in the lungs.
CC Excl: PDX collection 1028

P29.38 **Other persistent fetal circulation** `MCC`
Delayed closure of ductus arteriosus
CC Excl: PDX collection 1028

P29.4 **Transient myocardial ischemia in newborn**

✓5th P29.8 **Other cardiovascular disorders originating in the perinatal period**

P29.81 **Cardiac arrest of newborn** `MCC`
CC Excl: PDX collection 1029

`N` Newborn: 0   `P` Pediatric: 0-17   `M` Maternity: 12-55   `A` Adult: 15-124   `MCC` Major Complication/Comorbidity   `CC` Complication/Comorbidity   `SW` Severe Wound Dx

P29.89   Other cardiovascular disorders originating in the perinatal period
AHA: 2014, 4Q, 23

P29.9   Cardiovascular disorder originating in the perinatal period, unspecified

Infections specific to the perinatal period (P35-P39)

Infections acquired in utero, during birth via the umbilicus, or during the first 28 days after birth

EXCLUDES 2   *asymptomatic human immunodeficiency virus [HIV] infection status (Z21)*
congenital gonococcal infection (A54.-)
congenital pneumonia (P23.-)
congenital syphilis (A50.-)
human immunodeficiency virus [HIV] disease (B20)
infant botulism (A48.51)
infectious diseases not specific to the perinatal period (A00-B99, J09, J10-)
intestinal infectious disease (A00-A09)
laboratory evidence of human immunodeficiency virus [HIV] (R75)
tetanus neonatorum (A33)

✓4ᵗʰ **P35   Congenital viral diseases**
INCLUDES   infections acquired in utero or during birth

CC Excl: For CC/MCC codes in category P35, unless otherwise noted: PDX collection 562

P35.0   Congenital rubella syndrome   CC
Congenital rubella pneumonitis
CC Excl: PDX collection 1030

P35.1   Congenital cytomegalovirus infection   MCC
CC Excl: PDX collection 1030

P35.2   Congenital herpesviral [herpes simplex] infection   MCC

P35.3   Congenital viral hepatitis   MCC

● **P35.4   Congenital Zika virus disease**   MCC
Use additional code to identify manifestations of congenital Zika virus disease

P35.8   Other congenital viral diseases   MCC
Congenital varicella [chickenpox]

P35.9   Congenital viral disease, unspecified   MCC

✓4ᵗʰ **P36   Bacterial sepsis of newborn**
INCLUDES   congenital sepsis
Use additional code(s), if applicable, to identify severe sepsis (R65.2-) and associated acute organ dysfunction(s)

CC Excl: For MCC codes in category P36: PDX collection 1031

P36.0   Sepsis of newborn due to streptococcus, group B   MCC HCC

✓5ᵗʰ **P36.1   Sepsis of newborn due to other and unspecified streptococci**

    P36.10   Sepsis of newborn due to unspecified streptococci   MCC HCC

    P36.19   Sepsis of newborn due to other streptococci   MCC HCC

P36.2   Sepsis of newborn due to Staphylococcus aureus   MCC HCC

✓5ᵗʰ **P36.3   Sepsis of newborn due to other and unspecified staphylococci**

    P36.30   Sepsis of newborn due to unspecified staphylococci   MCC HCC

    P36.39   Sepsis of newborn due to other staphylococci   MCC HCC

P36.4   Sepsis of newborn due to Escherichia coli   MCC HCC

P36.5   Sepsis of newborn due to anaerobes   MCC HCC

P36.8   Other bacterial sepsis of newborn   MCC HCC
Use additional code from category B96 to identify organism

P36.9   Bacterial sepsis of newborn, unspecified   MCC HCC

✓4ᵗʰ **P37   Other congenital infectious and parasitic diseases**
EXCLUDES 2   *congenital syphilis (A50.-)*
infectious neonatal diarrhea (A00-A09)
necrotizing enterocolitis in newborn (P77.-)
noninfectious neonatal diarrhea (P78.3)
ophthalmia neonatorum due to gonococcus (A54.31)
tetanus neonatorum (A33)

CC Excl: For MCC codes in category P37: PDX collection 562

P37.0   Congenital tuberculosis   MCC

P37.1   Congenital toxoplasmosis   MCC
Hydrocephalus due to congenital toxoplasmosis

P37.2   Neonatal (disseminated) listeriosis   MCC

P37.3   Congenital falciparum malaria   MCC

P37.4   Other congenital malaria   MCC

P37.5   Neonatal candidiasis

P37.8   Other specified congenital infectious and parasitic diseases   MCC

P37.9   Congenital infectious or parasitic disease, unspecified   MCC

✓4ᵗʰ **P38   Omphalitis of newborn**
EXCLUDES 1   *omphalitis not of newborn (L08.82)*
tetanus omphalitis (A33)
umbilical hemorrhage of newborn (P51.-)
DEF: Omphalitis: Infection and inflammation of the umbilical stump, often due to bacteria that can spread beyond the umbilical stump to the fascia, muscle, or even the umbilical vessels.

P38.1   Omphalitis with mild hemorrhage   CC
CC Excl: PDX collection 1032

P38.9   Omphalitis without hemorrhage   CC
Omphalitis of newborn NOS
CC Excl: PDX collection 1032

✓4ᵗʰ **P39   Other infections specific to the perinatal period**
Use additional code to identify organism or specific infection

CC Excl: For CC codes in category P39, unless otherwise noted: PDX collection 1033

P39.0   Neonatal infective mastitis   CC
EXCLUDES 1   *breast engorgement of newborn (P83.4)*
noninfective mastitis of newborn (P83.4)
CC Excl: PDX collection 1032

P39.1   Neonatal conjunctivitis and dacryocystitis
Neonatal chlamydial conjunctivitis
Ophthalmia neonatorum NOS
EXCLUDES 1   *gonococcal conjunctivitis (A54.31)*

P39.2   Intra-amniotic infection affecting newborn, not elsewhere classified   CC

P39.3   Neonatal urinary tract infection   CC
CC Excl: PDX collection 1034

P39.4   Neonatal skin infection   CC
Neonatal pyoderma
EXCLUDES 1   *pemphigus neonatorum (L00)*
staphylococcal scalded skin syndrome (L00)

P39.8   Other specified infections specific to the perinatal period   CC

P39.9   Infection specific to the perinatal period, unspecified   CC

Hemorrhagic and hematological disorders of newborn (P50-P61)

EXCLUDES 1   *congenital stenosis and stricture of bile ducts (Q44.3)*
Crigler-Najjar syndrome (E80.5)
Dubin-Johnson syndrome (E80.6)
Gilbert syndrome (E80.4)
hereditary hemolytic anemias (D55-D58)

✓4ᵗʰ **P50   Newborn affected by intrauterine (fetal) blood loss**
EXCLUDES 1   *congenital anemia from intrauterine (fetal) blood loss (P61.3)*

P50.0   Newborn affected by intrauterine (fetal) blood loss from vasa previa

P50.1   Newborn affected by intrauterine (fetal) blood loss from ruptured cord

P50.2   Newborn affected by intrauterine (fetal) blood loss from placenta

P50.3   Newborn affected by hemorrhage into co-twin

P50.4   Newborn affected by hemorrhage into maternal circulation

P50.5   Newborn affected by intrauterine (fetal) blood loss from cut end of co-twin's cord

P50.8   Newborn affected by other intrauterine (fetal) blood loss

P50.9   Newborn affected by intrauterine (fetal) blood loss, unspecified
Newborn affected by fetal hemorrhage NOS

✓4ᵗʰ **P51   Umbilical hemorrhage of newborn**
EXCLUDES 1   *omphalitis with mild hemorrhage (P38.1)*
umbilical hemorrhage from cut end of co-twins cord (P50.5)

P51.0   Massive umbilical hemorrhage of newborn

P51.8   Other umbilical hemorrhages of newborn
Slipped umbilical ligature NOS

P51.9   Umbilical hemorrhage of newborn, unspecified

✓4ᵗʰ **P52   Intracranial nontraumatic hemorrhage of newborn**
INCLUDES   intracranial hemorrhage due to anoxia or hypoxia
EXCLUDES 1   *intracranial hemorrhage due to birth injury (P10.-)*
intracranial hemorrhage due to other injury (S06.-)

✓ Additional Character Required   ✓x7ᵗʰ Placeholder   Unacceptable PDx   Questionable PDx   Manifestation   H1 - H14 HAC   HCC CMS-HCC Dx   HIV HIV Dx

ICD-10-CM 2019   **893**

P29.89–P52

Chapter 16. Certain Conditions Originating in the Perinatal Period

P52.0 **Intraventricular (nontraumatic) hemorrhage, grade 1, of newborn**   CC
Subependymal hemorrhage (without intraventricular extension)
Bleeding into germinal matrix
CC Excl: PDX collection 1021

P52.1 **Intraventricular (nontraumatic) hemorrhage, grade 2, of newborn**   CC
Subependymal hemorrhage with intraventricular extension
Bleeding into ventricle
CC Excl: PDX collection 1021

√5ᵗʰ **P52.2** **Intraventricular (nontraumatic) hemorrhage, grade 3 and grade 4, of newborn**

     P52.21 **Intraventricular (nontraumatic) hemorrhage, grade 3, of newborn**   MCC
       Subependymal hemorrhage with intraventricular extension with enlargement of ventricle
       CC Excl: PDX collection 1021

     P52.22 **Intraventricular (nontraumatic) hemorrhage, grade 4, of newborn**   MCC
       Bleeding into cerebral cortex
       Subependymal hemorrhage with intracerebral extension
       CC Excl: PDX collection 1021

P52.3 **Unspecified intraventricular (nontraumatic) hemorrhage of newborn**   CC
CC Excl: PDX collection 1021

P52.4 **Intracerebral (nontraumatic) hemorrhage of newborn**   MCC
CC Excl: PDX collection 1020

P52.5 **Subarachnoid (nontraumatic) hemorrhage of newborn**   MCC
CC Excl: PDX collection 1022

P52.6 **Cerebellar (nontraumatic) and posterior fossa hemorrhage of newborn**   MCC
CC Excl: PDX collection 1020

P52.8 **Other intracranial (nontraumatic) hemorrhages of newborn**   MCC
CC Excl: PDX collection 1020

P52.9 **Intracranial (nontraumatic) hemorrhage of newborn, unspecified**   MCC
CC Excl: PDX collection 1020

P53 **Hemorrhagic disease of newborn**   CC
Vitamin K deficiency of newborn
CC Excl: PDX collection 1035

√4ᵗʰ **P54** **Other neonatal hemorrhages**
   EXCLUDES 1   newborn affected by (intrauterine) blood loss (P50.-)
              pulmonary hemorrhage originating in the perinatal period (P26.-)

   CC Excl: For CC/MCC codes in category P54: PDX collection 1036

P54.0 **Neonatal hematemesis**
   EXCLUDES 1   neonatal hematemesis due to swallowed maternal blood (P78.2)

P54.1 **Neonatal melena**   MCC
   EXCLUDES 1   neonatal melena due to swallowed maternal blood (P78.2)

P54.2 **Neonatal rectal hemorrhage**   MCC

P54.3 **Other neonatal gastrointestinal hemorrhage**   MCC

P54.4 **Neonatal adrenal hemorrhage**   CC

P54.5 **Neonatal cutaneous hemorrhage**
Neonatal bruising
Neonatal ecchymoses
Neonatal petechiae
Neonatal superficial hematomata
   EXCLUDES 2   bruising of scalp due to birth injury (P12.3)
              cephalhematoma due to birth injury (P12.0)

P54.6 **Neonatal vaginal hemorrhage**   ♀
Neonatal pseudomenses

P54.8 **Other specified neonatal hemorrhages**

P54.9 **Neonatal hemorrhage, unspecified**

√4ᵗʰ **P55** **Hemolytic disease of newborn**

P55.0 **Rh isoimmunization of newborn**
DEF: Incompatible Rh fetal-maternal blood grouping that prematurely destroys red blood cells. Symptoms include jaundice, asphyxia, pulmonary hypertension, edema, respiratory distress, kernicterus, and coagulopathies. It is detected by a Coombs test.

P55.1 **ABO isoimmunization of newborn**
AHA: 2015, 3Q, 20

P55.8 **Other hemolytic diseases of newborn**

P55.9 **Hemolytic disease of newborn, unspecified**

√4ᵗʰ **P56** **Hydrops fetalis due to hemolytic disease**
   EXCLUDES 1   hydrops fetalis NOS (P83.2)

   CC Excl: For MCC codes in category P56: PDX collection 1037

P56.0 **Hydrops fetalis due to isoimmunization**   MCC

√5ᵗʰ **P56.9** **Hydrops fetalis due to other and unspecified hemolytic disease**

     P56.90 **Hydrops fetalis due to unspecified hemolytic disease**   MCC

     P56.99 **Hydrops fetalis due to other hemolytic disease**   MCC

√4ᵗʰ **P57** **Kernicterus**

P57.0 **Kernicterus due to isoimmunization**   MCC
DEF: Complication of erythroblastosis fetalis associated with severe neural symptoms, high blood bilirubin levels, and nerve cell destruction. It results in bilirubin-pigmented gray matter of the central nervous system.
CC Excl: PDX collection 1037

P57.8 **Other specified kernicterus**   MCC
   EXCLUDES 1   Crigler-Najjar syndrome (E80.5)
   CC Excl: PDX collection 1038

P57.9 **Kernicterus, unspecified**   MCC
CC Excl: PDX collection 1038

√4ᵗʰ **P58** **Neonatal jaundice due to other excessive hemolysis**
   EXCLUDES 1   jaundice due to isoimmunization (P55-P57)

P58.0 **Neonatal jaundice due to bruising**

P58.1 **Neonatal jaundice due to bleeding**

P58.2 **Neonatal jaundice due to infection**

P58.3 **Neonatal jaundice due to polycythemia**

√5ᵗʰ **P58.4** **Neonatal jaundice due to drugs or toxins transmitted from mother or given to newborn**
Code first poisoning due to drug or toxin, if applicable (T36-T65 with fifth or sixth character 1-4 or 6)
Use additional code for adverse effect, if applicable, to identify drug (T36-T50 with fifth or sixth character 5)

     P58.41 **Neonatal jaundice due to drugs or toxins transmitted from mother**

     P58.42 **Neonatal jaundice due to drugs or toxins given to newborn**

P58.5 **Neonatal jaundice due to swallowed maternal blood**

P58.8 **Neonatal jaundice due to other specified excessive hemolysis**

P58.9 **Neonatal jaundice due to excessive hemolysis, unspecified**

√4ᵗʰ **P59** **Neonatal jaundice from other and unspecified causes**
   EXCLUDES 1   jaundice due to inborn errors of metabolism (E70-E88)
              kernicterus (P57.-)

   CC Excl: For MCC codes in category P59: PDX collection 1038

P59.0 **Neonatal jaundice associated with preterm delivery**
Hyperbilirubinemia of prematurity
Jaundice due to delayed conjugation associated with preterm delivery

P59.1 **Inspissated bile syndrome**   MCC
DEF: Biliary obstruction in newborn resulting from obstruction of outflow tract.

√5ᵗʰ **P59.2** **Neonatal jaundice from other and unspecified hepatocellular damage**
   EXCLUDES 1   congenital viral hepatitis (P35.3)

     P59.20 **Neonatal jaundice from unspecified hepatocellular damage**   MCC

     P59.29 **Neonatal jaundice from other hepatocellular damage**   MCC
       Neonatal giant cell hepatitis
       Neonatal (idiopathic) hepatitis

P59.3 **Neonatal jaundice from breast milk inhibitor**

P59.8 **Neonatal jaundice from other specified causes**

P59.9 **Neonatal jaundice, unspecified**
Neonatal physiological jaundice (intense)(prolonged) NOS
AHA: 2015, 3Q, 20

P60 **Disseminated intravascular coagulation of newborn**   MCC
Defibrination syndrome of newborn
CC Excl: PDX collection 1035

Ⓝ Newborn: 0   Ⓟ Pediatric: 0-17   Ⓜ Maternity: 12-55   Ⓐ Adult: 15-124   MCC Major Complication/Comorbidity   CC Complication/Comorbidity   SW Severe Wound Dx

894   ICD-10-CM 2019

☑4ᵗʰ **P61 Other perinatal hematological disorders**
  EXCLUDES 1 transient hypogammaglobulinemia of infancy (D80.7)

  P61.0 Transient neonatal thrombocytopenia `MCC`
    Neonatal thrombocytopenia due to exchange transfusion
    Neonatal thrombocytopenia due to idiopathic maternal
      thrombocytopenia
    Neonatal thrombocytopenia due to isoimmunization
    DEF: Temporary decrease in blood platelets of a newborn that is
    secondary to placental insufficiency.
    CC Excl: PDX collection 1035

  P61.1 Polycythemia neonatorum
    DEF: Abnormal increase of total red blood cells of a newborn that
    results in hyperviscosity, which slows the flow of blood through
    small blood vessels.

  P61.2 Anemia of prematurity `CC`
    CC Excl: PDX collection 1039

  P61.3 Congenital anemia from fetal blood loss `CC`
    CC Excl: PDX collection 1039

  P61.4 Other congenital anemias, not elsewhere classified `CC`
    Congenital anemia NOS
    CC Excl: PDX collection 1039

  P61.5 Transient neonatal neutropenia `MCC`
    EXCLUDES 1 congenital neutropenia (nontransient) (D70.0)
    DEF: Low blood neutrophil counts of newborn that occurs due to
    maternal hypertension, sepsis, twin-twin transfusion,
    alloimmunization, and hemolytic disease.
    CC Excl: PDX collection 1040

  P61.6 Other transient neonatal disorders of coagulation `CC`
    CC Excl: PDX collection 1035

  P61.8 Other specified perinatal hematological disorders

  P61.9 Perinatal hematological disorder, unspecified

Transitory endocrine and metabolic disorders specific to newborn (P70-P74)

  INCLUDES transitory endocrine and metabolic disturbances caused by the
    infant's response to maternal endocrine and metabolic
    factors, or its adjustment to extrauterine environment
  AHA: 2018, 2Q, 6

☑4ᵗʰ **P70 Transitory disorders of carbohydrate metabolism specific to newborn**

  P70.0 Syndrome of infant of mother with gestational diabetes
    Newborn (with hypoglycemia) affected by maternal gestational
    diabetes
    EXCLUDES 1 newborn (with hypoglycemia) affected by maternal
        (pre-existing) diabetes mellitus (P70.1)
      syndrome of infant of a diabetic mother (P70.1)

  P70.1 Syndrome of infant of a diabetic mother
    Newborn (with hypoglycemia) affected by maternal (pre-
    existing) diabetes mellitus
    EXCLUDES 1 newborn (with hypoglycemia) affected by maternal
        gestational diabetes (P70.0)
      syndrome of infant of mother with gestational
        diabetes (P70.0)

  P70.2 Neonatal diabetes mellitus `CC`
    CC Excl: PDX collection 1041

  P70.3 Iatrogenic neonatal hypoglycemia

  P70.4 Other neonatal hypoglycemia
    Transitory neonatal hypoglycemia

  P70.8 Other transitory disorders of carbohydrate metabolism of newborn `CC`
    CC Excl: PDX collection 1042

  P70.9 Transitory disorder of carbohydrate metabolism of newborn, unspecified

☑4ᵗʰ **P71 Transitory neonatal disorders of calcium and magnesium metabolism**

  CC Excl: For CC codes in category P71: PDX collection 1041

  P71.0 Cow's milk hypocalcemia in newborn `CC`

  P71.1 Other neonatal hypocalcemia `CC`
    EXCLUDES 1 neonatal hypoparathyroidism (P71.4)

  P71.2 Neonatal hypomagnesemia `CC`

  P71.3 Neonatal tetany without calcium or magnesium deficiency `CC`
    Neonatal tetany NOS

  P71.4 Transitory neonatal hypoparathyroidism `CC`

  P71.8 Other transitory neonatal disorders of calcium and magnesium metabolism `CC`
    AHA: 2016, 4Q, 54

  P71.9 Transitory neonatal disorder of calcium and magnesium metabolism, unspecified `CC`

☑4ᵗʰ **P72 Other transitory neonatal endocrine disorders**
  EXCLUDES 1 congenital hypothyroidism with or without goiter (E03.0-E03.1)
    dyshormogenetic goiter (E07.1)
    Pendred's syndrome (E07.1)

  CC Excl: For CC codes in category P72, unless otherwise noted:
  PDX collection 1042

  P72.0 Neonatal goiter, not elsewhere classified `CC`
    Transitory congenital goiter with normal functioning

  P72.1 Transitory neonatal hyperthyroidism `CC`
    Neonatal thyrotoxicosis
    CC Excl: PDX collection 1041

  P72.2 Other transitory neonatal disorders of thyroid function, not elsewhere classified
    Transitory neonatal hypothyroidism

  P72.8 Other specified transitory neonatal endocrine disorders `CC`

  P72.9 Transitory neonatal endocrine disorder, unspecified

☑4ᵗʰ **P74 Other transitory neonatal electrolyte and metabolic disturbances**

  CC Excl: For CC codes in category P74: PDX collection 1042

  P74.0 Late metabolic acidosis of newborn `MCC`
    EXCLUDES 1 (fetal) metabolic acidosis of newborn (P19)
    CC Excl: PDX collection 1041

  P74.1 Dehydration of newborn

  ☑5ᵗʰ **P74.2 Disturbances of sodium balance of newborn**
    • **P74.21 Hypernatremia of newborn**
    • **P74.22 Hyponatremia of newborn**

  ☑5ᵗʰ **P74.3 Disturbances of potassium balance of newborn**
    • **P74.31 Hyperkalemia of newborn**
    • **P74.32 Hypokalemia of newborn**

  ☑5ᵗʰ **P74.4 Other transitory electrolyte disturbances of newborn**
    • **P74.41 Alkalosis of newborn** `CC`
        Hyperbicarbonatemia
    • ☑6ᵗʰ **P74.42 Disturbances of chlorine balance of newborn**
        • **P74.421 Hyperchloremia of newborn**
            Hyperchloremic metabolic acidosis
            EXCLUDES 2 late metabolic acidosis of the
                newborn (P77.0)
        • **P74.422 Hypochloremia of newborn**
    • **P74.49 Other transitory electrolyte disturbance of newborn**

  P74.5 Transitory tyrosinemia of newborn `CC`

  P74.6 Transitory hyperammonemia of newborn `CC`

  P74.8 Other transitory metabolic disturbances of newborn `CC`
    Amino-acid metabolic disorders described as transitory

  P74.9 Transitory metabolic disturbance of newborn, unspecified

Digestive system disorders of newborn (P76-P78)

☑4ᵗʰ **P76 Other intestinal obstruction of newborn**

  P76.0 Meconium plug syndrome
    Meconium ileus NOS
    EXCLUDES 1 meconium ileus in cystic fibrosis (E84.11)
    DEF: Meconium obstruction of a newborn's intestines, resulting
    from unusually thick or hard meconium.

  P76.1 Transitory ileus of newborn `CC`
    EXCLUDES 1 Hirschsprung's disease (Q43.1)
    CC Excl: PDX collection 1043

  P76.2 Intestinal obstruction due to inspissated milk

  P76.8 Other specified intestinal obstruction of newborn
    EXCLUDES 1 intestinal obstruction classifiable to K56-.

  P76.9 Intestinal obstruction of newborn, unspecified

☑4ᵗʰ **P77 Necrotizing enterocolitis of newborn**
    DEF: Serious intestinal infection and inflammation in preterm infants.
    Severity is measured by stages and may progress to life-threatening
    perforation or peritonitis. Resection surgical treatment may be necessary.

  CC Excl: For MCC codes in category P77: PDX collection 1044

  P77.1 Stage 1 necrotizing enterocolitis in newborn `MCC`
    Necrotizing enterocolitis without pneumatosis, without
    perforation
    DEF: Broad-spectrum symptoms with nonspecific signs, including
    feeding intolerance, abdominal distention, bradycardia, and
    metabolic abnormalities.

☑ Additional Character Required   √×7ᵗʰ Placeholder   Unacceptable PDx   Questionable PDx   Manifestation   H1-H14 HAC   HCC CMS-HCC Dx   HIV HIV Dx

P77.2 Stage 2 necrotizing enterocolitis in newborn `MCC`
Necrotizing enterocolitis with pneumatosis, without perforation
DEF: Radiographic confirmation of necrotizing enterocolitis showing intestinal dilatation, fixed loops of bowels, pneumatosis intestinalis, metabolic acidosis, and thrombocytopenia.

P77.3 Stage 3 necrotizing enterocolitis in newborn `MCC`
Necrotizing enterocolitis with perforation
Necrotizing enterocolitis with pneumatosis and perforation
DEF: Advanced stage in which an infant demonstrates signs of bowel perforation, septic shock, metabolic acidosis, ascites, disseminated intravascular coagulopathy, and neutropenia.

P77.9 Necrotizing enterocolitis in newborn, unspecified `MCC`
Necrotizing enterocolitis in newborn, NOS

✓4th P78 Other perinatal digestive system disorders
EXCLUDES 1 cystic fibrosis (E84.0-E84.9)
neonatal gastrointestinal hemorrhages (P54.0-P54.3)

P78.0 Perinatal intestinal perforation `MCC`
Meconium peritonitis
CC Excl: PDX collection 1044

P78.1 Other neonatal peritonitis
Neonatal peritonitis NOS

P78.2 Neonatal hematemesis and melena due to swallowed maternal blood

P78.3 Noninfective neonatal diarrhea
Neonatal diarrhea NOS

✓5th P78.8 Other specified perinatal digestive system disorders
P78.81 Congenital cirrhosis (of liver)
P78.82 Peptic ulcer of newborn
P78.83 Newborn esophageal reflux
Neonatal esophageal reflux
P78.84 Gestational alloimmune liver disease
GALD
Neonatal hemochromatosis
EXCLUDES 1 hemochromatosis (E83.11-)
AHA: 2017, 4Q, 21
DEF: Severe hepatic injury with onset during fetal development with manifestations beginning during fetal life. It is due to maternal antibodies to fetal hepatic cells (hepatocytes) that cross the placenta into the fetal circulation, causing hepatic cell necrosis.
P78.89 Other specified perinatal digestive system disorders
P78.9 Perinatal digestive system disorder, unspecified

Conditions involving the integument and temperature regulation of newborn (P80-P83)

✓4th P80 Hypothermia of newborn
DEF: Decrease in newborn body temperature due to their larger ratio of surface area to body weight, thin skin with blood vessels close to the surface, and a limited amount of subcutaneous fat.

P80.0 Cold injury syndrome
Severe and usually chronic hypothermia associated with a pink flushed appearance, edema and neurological and biochemical abnormalities.
EXCLUDES 1 mild hypothermia of newborn (P80.8)

P80.8 Other hypothermia of newborn
Mild hypothermia of newborn

P80.9 Hypothermia of newborn, unspecified

✓4th P81 Other disturbances of temperature regulation of newborn
P81.0 Environmental hyperthermia of newborn
P81.8 Other specified disturbances of temperature regulation of newborn
P81.9 Disturbance of temperature regulation of newborn, unspecified
Fever of newborn NOS

✓4th P83 Other conditions of integument specific to newborn
EXCLUDES 1 congenital malformations of skin and integument (Q80-Q84)
hydrops fetalis due to hemolytic disease (P56.-)
neonatal skin infection (P39.4)
staphylococcal scalded skin syndrome (L00)
EXCLUDES 2 cradle cap (L21.0)
diaper [napkin] dermatitis (L22)

P83.0 Sclerema neonatorum `CC`
DEF: Diffuse, rapidly progressing white, waxy, nonpitting hardening of tissue, usually of legs and feet that is life-threatening. It is found in preterm or debilitated infants. Etiology is unknown.
CC Excl: PDX collection 1045

P83.1 Neonatal erythema toxicum

P83.2 Hydrops fetalis not due to hemolytic disease `MCC`
Hydrops fetalis NOS
DEF: Severe, life-threatening problem of a newborn characterized by severe edema of the entire body. It is unrelated to immune response.
CC Excl: PDX collection 1046

✓5th P83.3 Other and unspecified edema specific to newborn
P83.30 Unspecified edema specific to newborn `CC`
CC Excl: PDX collection 1047
P83.39 Other edema specific to newborn `CC`
CC Excl: PDX collection 1047

P83.4 Breast engorgement of newborn
Noninfective mastitis of newborn

P83.5 Congenital hydrocele ♂
DEF: Hydrocele: Serous fluid that collects in the tunica vaginalis of the scrotum along the spermatic cord in males.

P83.6 Umbilical polyp of newborn

✓5th P83.8 Other specified conditions of integument specific to newborn
AHA: 2017, 4Q, 21-22
P83.81 Umbilical granuloma
EXCLUDES 2 granulomatous disorder of the skin and subcutaneous tissue, unspecified (L92.9)
P83.88 Other specified conditions of integument specific to newborn
Bronze baby syndrome
Neonatal scleroderma
Urticaria neonatorum

P83.9 Condition of the integument specific to newborn, unspecified

Other problems with newborn (P84)

P84 Other problems with newborn
Acidemia of newborn
Acidosis of newborn
Anoxia of newborn NOS
Asphyxia of newborn NOS
Hypercapnia of newborn
Hypoxemia of newborn
Hypoxia of newborn NOS
Mixed metabolic and respiratory acidosis of newborn
EXCLUDES 1 intracranial hemorrhage due to anoxia or hypoxia (P52.-)
hypoxic ischemic encephalopathy [HIE] (P91.6-)
late metabolic acidosis of newborn (P74.0)

Other disorders originating in the perinatal period (P90-P96)

P90 Convulsions of newborn `MCC`
EXCLUDES 1 benign myoclonic epilepsy in infancy (G40.3-)
benign neonatal convulsions (familial) (G40.3-)
CC Excl: PDX collection 1048

✓4th P91 Other disturbances of cerebral status of newborn

CC Excl: For CC/MCC codes in category P91, unless otherwise noted: PDX collection 1049

P91.0 Neonatal cerebral ischemia `MCC`
P91.1 Acquired periventricular cysts of newborn `MCC`
P91.2 Neonatal cerebral leukomalacia `MCC`
Periventricular leukomalacia
CC Excl: PDX collection 1022
P91.3 Neonatal cerebral irritability `MCC`
P91.4 Neonatal cerebral depression `MCC`
P91.5 Neonatal coma `MCC`

✓5th P91.6 Hypoxic ischemic encephalopathy [HIE]
EXCLUDES 1 neonatal cerebral depression (P91.4)
neonatal cerebral irritability (P91.3)
neonatal coma (P91.5)
AHA: 2017, 4Q, 22

CC Excl: For CC/MCC codes in subcategory P91.6: PDX collection 1050

P91.60 Hypoxic ischemic encephalopathy [HIE], unspecified `CC`
P91.61 Mild hypoxic ischemic encephalopathy [HIE] `CC`
P91.62 Moderate hypoxic ischemic encephalopathy [HIE] `CC`
P91.63 Severe hypoxic ischemic encephalopathy [HIE] `MCC`

N Newborn: 0   P Pediatric: 0-17   M Maternity: 12-55   A Adult: 15-124   MCC Major Complication/Comorbidity   CC Complication/Comorbidity   SW Severe Wound Dx

896   ICD-10-CM 2019

✓5ᵗʰ **P91.8** **Other specified disturbances of cerebral status of newborn**
        AHA: 2017, 4Q, 22

     ✓6ᵗʰ **P91.81** **Neonatal encephalopathy**

         P91.811 *Neonatal encephalopathy in diseases classified elsewhere*
            Code first underlying condition, if known, such as:
            congenital cirrhosis (of liver) ▶(P78.81)◀
            intracranial nontraumatic hemorrhage of newborn (P52.-)
            kernicterus (P57.-)

         P91.819 **Neonatal encephalopathy, unspecified**

        P91.88 **Other specified disturbances of cerebral status of newborn**

     P91.9 **Disturbance of cerebral status of newborn, unspecified**

✓4ᵗʰ **P92** **Feeding problems of newborn**
       EXCLUDES 1   *eating disorders (F50.-)*
            feeding problems in child over 28 days old (R63.3)
       AHA: 2016, 3Q, 19
       TIP: Continue to assign a code from this category for feeding problems in a patient greater than 28 days old when that feeding problem was initially diagnosed between day 0 and day 28. Do not assign code R63.3.

     ✓5ᵗʰ **P92.0** **Vomiting of newborn**
         EXCLUDES 1   *vomiting of child over 28 days old (R11.-)*

        P92.01 **Bilious vomiting of newborn**   `MCC`
           EXCLUDES 1   *bilious vomiting in child over 28 days old (R11.14)*
          CC Excl: PDX collection 1051

        P92.09 **Other vomiting of newborn**
           EXCLUDES 1   *regurgitation of food in newborn (P92.1)*

     P92.1 **Regurgitation and rumination of newborn**

     P92.2 **Slow feeding of newborn**

     P92.3 **Underfeeding of newborn**

     P92.4 **Overfeeding of newborn**

     P92.5 **Neonatal difficulty in feeding at breast**
         AHA: 2017, 1Q, 28

     P92.6 **Failure to thrive in newborn**
         EXCLUDES 1   *failure to thrive in child over 28 days old (R62.51)*

     P92.8 **Other feeding problems of newborn**

     P92.9 **Feeding problem of newborn, unspecified**

✓4ᵗʰ **P93** **Reactions and intoxications due to drugs administered to newborn**
       INCLUDES   reactions and intoxications due to drugs administered to fetus affecting newborn
       EXCLUDES 1   *jaundice due to drugs or toxins transmitted from mother or given to newborn (P58.4-)*
            reactions and intoxications from maternal opiates, tranquilizers and other medication ▶(P04.0-P04.1, P04.4-)◀
            withdrawal symptoms from maternal use of drugs of addiction (P96.1)
            withdrawal symptoms from therapeutic use of drugs in newborn (P96.2)

     P93.0 **Grey baby syndrome**   `CC`
         Grey syndrome from chloramphenicol administration in newborn
         CC Excl: PDX collection 1052

     P93.8 **Other reactions and intoxications due to drugs administered to newborn**   `CC`
         Use additional code for adverse effect, if applicable, to identify drug (T36-T50 with fifth or sixth character 5)
         CC Excl: PDX collection 1052

✓4ᵗʰ **P94** **Disorders of muscle tone of newborn**

     P94.0 **Transient neonatal myasthenia gravis**   `CC`
         EXCLUDES 1   *myasthenia gravis (G70.0)*
         CC Excl: PDX collection 1041

     P94.1 **Congenital hypertonia**

     P94.2 **Congenital hypotonia**
         Floppy baby syndrome, unspecified

     P94.8 **Other disorders of muscle tone of newborn**

     P94.9 **Disorder of muscle tone of newborn, unspecified**

P95 **Stillbirth**
       Deadborn fetus NOS
       Fetal death of unspecified cause
       Stillbirth NOS
       EXCLUDES 1   *maternal care for intrauterine death (O36.4)*
            missed abortion (O02.1)
            outcome of delivery, stillbirth (Z37.1, Z37.3, Z37.4, Z37.7)

✓4ᵗʰ **P96** **Other conditions originating in the perinatal period**

     P96.0 **Congenital renal failure**
         Uremia of newborn

     P96.1 **Neonatal withdrawal symptoms from maternal use of drugs of addiction**   `CC`
         Drug withdrawal syndrome in infant of dependent mother
         Neonatal abstinence syndrome
         EXCLUDES 1   *reactions and intoxications from maternal opiates and tranquilizers administered during labor and delivery (P04.0)*
         CC Excl: PDX collection 1052

     P96.2 **Withdrawal symptoms from therapeutic use of drugs in newborn**   `CC`
         CC Excl: PDX collection 1052

     P96.3 **Wide cranial sutures of newborn**
         Neonatal craniotabes

     P96.5 **Complication to newborn due to (fetal) intrauterine procedure**
         EXCLUDES 2   *newborn affected by amniocentesis (P00.6)*

     ✓5ᵗʰ **P96.8** **Other specified conditions originating in the perinatal period**

        P96.81 **Exposure to (parental) (environmental) tobacco smoke in the perinatal period**
           EXCLUDES 2   *newborn affected by in utero exposure to tobacco (P04.2)*
             exposure to environmental tobacco smoke after the perinatal period (Z77.22)

        P96.82 **Delayed separation of umbilical cord**

        P96.83 **Meconium staining**
           EXCLUDES 1   *meconium aspiration (P24.00, P24.01)*
             meconium passage during delivery (P03.82)
          DEF: Meconium passed in utero causing discoloration on the fetal skin and nails or on the umbilicus. This staining may be incidental or may be an indicator of significant fetal stress that could affect outcomes.

        P96.89 **Other specified conditions originating in the perinatal period**
          Use additional code to specify condition

     P96.9 **Condition originating in the perinatal period, unspecified**
         Congenital debility NOS

✅Additional Character Required   ✓x7ᵗʰ Placeholder   Unacceptable PDx   Questionable PDx   Manifestation   `H1`-`H14` HAC   `HCC` CMS-HCC Dx   `HIV` HIV Dx

Chapter 17. Congenital Malformations, Deformations and Chromosomal Abnormalities (Q00–Q99)

Chapter Specific Guidelines with Coding Examples

The chapter specific guidelines from the ICD-10-CM Official Guidelines for Coding and Reporting have been provided below. Along with these guidelines are coding examples, contained in the shaded boxes, that have been developed to help illustrate the coding and/or sequencing guidance found in these guidelines.

Assign an appropriate code(s) from categories Q00-Q99, Congenital malformations, deformations, and chromosomal abnormalities when a malformation/deformation or chromosomal abnormality is documented. A malformation/deformation or chromosomal abnormality may be the principal/first-listed diagnosis on a record or a secondary diagnosis.

When a malformation/deformation/or chromosomal abnormality does not have a unique code assignment, assign additional code(s) for any manifestations that may be present.

When the code assignment specifically identifies the malformation/deformation/or chromosomal abnormality, manifestations that are an inherent component of the anomaly should not be coded separately. Additional codes should be assigned for manifestations that are not an inherent component.

8-day-old infant with tetralogy of Fallot and pulmonary stenosis

Q21.3   **Tetralogy of Fallot**

Explanation: Pulmonary stenosis is inherent in the disease process of tetralogy of Fallot. When the code assignment specifically identifies the malformation/deformation/or chromosomal abnormality, manifestations that are inherent components of the anomaly should not be coded separately.

7-month-old infant with Down syndrome and common atrioventricular canal

Q90.9   **Down syndrome, unspecified**

Q21.2   **Atrioventricular septal defect**

Explanation: While a common atrioventricular canal is often associated with patients with Down syndrome, this manifestation is not an inherent component and may be reported separately. When the code assignment specifically identifies the anomaly, manifestations that are inherent components of the condition should not be coded separately. Additional codes should be assigned for manifestations that are not inherent components.

Codes from Chapter 17 may be used throughout the life of the patient. If a congenital malformation or deformity has been corrected, a personal history code should be used to identify the history of the malformation or deformity. Although present at birth, malformation/deformation/or chromosomal abnormality may not be identified until later in life. Whenever the condition is diagnosed by the physician, it is appropriate to assign a code from codes Q00-Q99. For the birth admission, the appropriate code from category Z38, Liveborn infants, according to place of birth and type of delivery, should be sequenced as the principal diagnosis, followed by any congenital anomaly codes, Q00- Q99.

Three-year-old with history of corrected ventricular septal defect

Z87.74   **Personal history of (corrected) congenital malformations of heart and circulatory system**

Explanation: If a congenital malformation or deformity has been corrected, a personal history code should be used to identify the history of the malformation or deformity.

Forty-year-old man with headaches diagnosed with congenital arteriovenous malformation by brain scan

Q28.2   **Arteriovenous malformation of cerebral vessels**

Explanation: Although present at birth, malformations may not be identified until later in life. Whenever the condition is diagnosed by the physician, it is appropriate to assign a code from the range Q00–Q99.

Newborn with anencephaly delivered vaginally in hospital

Z38.00   **Single liveborn infant, delivered vaginally**

Q00.0   **Anencephaly**

Explanation: For the birth admission, the appropriate code from category Z38 Liveborn infants, according to place of birth and type of delivery, should be sequenced as the principal diagnosis, followed by any congenital anomaly codes, Q00–Q99.

Chapter 17. Congenital Malformations, Deformations and Chromosomal Abnormalities(Q00-Q99)

NOTE ▶Codes from this chapter are not for use on maternal records◀

EXCLUDES 2 inborn errors of metabolism (E70-E88)

This chapter contains the following blocks:

Q00-Q07   Congenital malformations of the nervous system
Q10-Q18   Congenital malformations of eye, ear, face and neck
Q20-Q28   Congenital malformations of the circulatory system
Q30-Q34   Congenital malformations of the respiratory system
Q35-Q37   Cleft lip and cleft palate
Q38-Q45   Other congenital malformations of the digestive system
Q50-Q56   Congenital malformations of genital organs
Q60-Q64   Congenital malformations of the urinary system
Q65-Q79   Congenital malformations and deformations of the musculoskeletal system
Q80-Q89   Other congenital malformations
Q90-Q99   Chromosomal abnormalities, not elsewhere classified

Congenital malformations of the nervous system (Q00-Q07)

✓4ᵗʰ Q00 Anencephaly and similar malformations

> CC Excl: For MCC codes in category Q00: PDX collection 1053

Q00.0 Anencephaly `MCC` `HCC`
Acephaly
Acrania
Amyelencephaly
Hemianencephaly
Hemicephaly

Q00.1 Craniorachischisis `MCC` `HCC`

Q00.2 Iniencephaly `MCC` `HCC`

✓4ᵗʰ Q01 Encephalocele
INCLUDES Arnold-Chiari syndrome, type III
encephalocystocele
encephalomyelocele
hydroencephalocele
hydromeningocele, cranial
meningocele, cerebral
meningoencephalocele

EXCLUDES 1 Meckel-Gruber syndrome (Q61.9)

DEF: Congenital protrusion of brain tissue through a defect in the skull.

> CC Excl: For CC codes in category Q01: PDX collection 1054

Q01.0 Frontal encephalocele `CC` `HCC`

Q01.1 Nasofrontal encephalocele `CC` `HCC`

Q01.2 Occipital encephalocele `CC` `HCC`

Q01.8 Encephalocele of other sites `CC` `HCC`

Q01.9 Encephalocele, unspecified `CC` `HCC`

Q02 Microcephaly `HCC`
INCLUDES hydromicrocephaly
micrencephalon
▶Use additional code, if applicable, to identify congenital Zika virus disease◀
EXCLUDES 1 Meckel-Gruber syndrome (Q61.9)

DEF: Congenital disorder in which the head circumference is more than two standard deviations below the mean for age, sex, race, and gestation and associated with a decreased life expectancy.

✓4ᵗʰ Q03 Congenital hydrocephalus
INCLUDES hydrocephalus in newborn
EXCLUDES 1 Arnold-Chiari syndrome, type II (Q07.0-)
acquired hydrocephalus (G91.-)
hydrocephalus due to congenital toxoplasmosis (P37.1)
hydrocephalus with spina bifida (Q05.0-Q05.4)

Q03.0 Malformations of aqueduct of Sylvius `HCC`
Anomaly of aqueduct of Sylvius
Obstruction of aqueduct of Sylvius, congenital
Stenosis of aqueduct of Sylvius

Q03.1 Atresia of foramina of Magendie and Luschka `HCC`
Dandy-Walker syndrome

Q03.8 Other congenital hydrocephalus `HCC`

Q03.9 Congenital hydrocephalus, unspecified `HCC`

Congenital Hydrocephalus

Normal ventricles   Hydrocephalic ventricles

✓4ᵗʰ Q04 Other congenital malformations of brain
EXCLUDES 1 cyclopia (Q87.0)
macrocephaly (Q75.3)

> CC Excl: For MCC codes in category Q04: PDX collection 1054
> For CC codes in category Q04: PDX collection 1055

Q04.0 Congenital malformations of corpus callosum `MCC` `HCC`
Agenesis of corpus callosum

Q04.1 Arhinencephaly `MCC` `HCC`

Q04.2 Holoprosencephaly `MCC` `HCC`

Q04.3 Other reduction deformities of brain `MCC` `HCC`
Absence of part of brain
Agenesis of part of brain
Agyria
Aplasia of part of brain
Hydranencephaly
Hypoplasia of part of brain
Lissencephaly
Microgyria
Pachygyria
EXCLUDES 1 congenital malformations of corpus callosum (Q04.0)

Q04.4 Septo-optic dysplasia of brain `CC` `HCC`

Q04.5 Megalencephaly `CC` `HCC`

Q04.6 Congenital cerebral cysts `CC` `HCC`
Porencephaly
Schizencephaly
EXCLUDES 1 acquired porencephalic cyst (G93.0)

Q04.8 Other specified congenital malformations of brain `CC` `HCC`
Arnold-Chiari syndrome, type IV
Macrogyria

Q04.9 Congenital malformation of brain, unspecified `HCC`
Congenital anomaly NOS of brain
Congenital deformity NOS of brain
Congenital disease or lesion NOS of brain
Multiple anomalies NOS of brain, congenital

✓4ᵗʰ Q05 Spina bifida
Hydromeningocele (spinal)
Meningocele (spinal)
Meningomyelocele
Myelocele
Myelomeningocele
Rachischisis
Spina bifida (aperta)(cystica)
Syringomyelocele
Use additional code for any associated paraplegia (paraparesis) (G82.2-)
EXCLUDES 1 Arnold-Chiari syndrome, type II (Q07.0-)
spina bifida occulta (Q76.0)

DEF: Lack of closure in the vertebral column with protrusion of the spinal cord through the defect, often in the lumbosacral area. This condition can be recognized by the presence of alpha-fetoproteins in the amniotic fluid.

> CC Excl: For CC codes in category Q05: PDX collection 1056

Q05.0 Cervical spina bifida with hydrocephalus `CC` `HCC`

Q05.1 Thoracic spina bifida with hydrocephalus `CC` `HCC`
Dorsal spina bifida with hydrocephalus
Thoracolumbar spina bifida with hydrocephalus

Q05.2 Lumbar spina bifida with hydrocephalus `CC` `HCC`
Lumbosacral spina bifida with hydrocephalus

`N` Newborn: 0   `P` Pediatric: 0-17   `M` Maternity: 12-55   `A` Adult: 15-124   `MCC` Major Complication/Comorbidity   `CC` Complication/Comorbidity   `SW` Severe Wound Dx

900   ICD-10-CM 2019

Spina Bifida

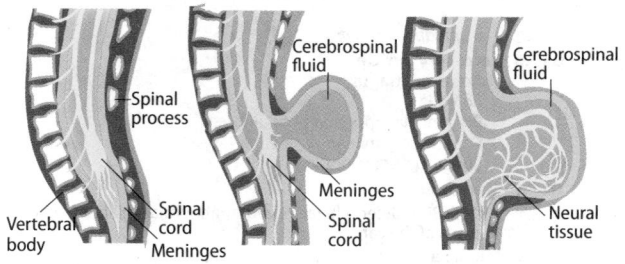

Spina bifida occulta   Meningocele   Myelomeningocele

Q05.3 Sacral **spina bifida** with hydrocephalus   `CC` `HCC`
Q05.4 Unspecified **spina bifida** with hydrocephalus   `CC` `HCC`
Q05.5 Cervical **spina bifida** without hydrocephalus   `HCC`
Q05.6 Thoracic **spina bifida** without hydrocephalus   `HCC`
  Dorsal spina bifida NOS
  Thoracolumbar spina bifida NOS
Q05.7 Lumbar **spina bifida** without hydrocephalus   `HCC`
  Lumbosacral spina bifida NOS
Q05.8 Sacral **spina bifida** without hydrocephalus   `HCC`
Q05.9 **Spina bifida,** unspecified   `HCC`

✓4ᵗʰ **Q06 Other congenital malformations of spinal cord**
Q06.0 Amyelia   `HCC`
Q06.1 Hypoplasia and dysplasia of spinal cord   `HCC`
  Atelomyelia
  Myelatelia
  Myelodysplasia of spinal cord
Q06.2 Diastematomyelia   `HCC`
  DEF: Rare congenital anomaly often associated with spina bifida. The spinal cord is separated into longitudinal halves by a bony, cartilaginous or fibrous septum, each half surrounded by a dural sac.
Q06.3 Other congenital cauda equina malformations   `HCC`
Q06.4 Hydromyelia   `HCC`
  Hydrorachis
Q06.8 Other specified congenital malformations of spinal cord   `HCC`
Q06.9 Congenital malformation of spinal cord, unspecified   `HCC`
  Congenital anomaly NOS of spinal cord
  Congenital deformity NOS of spinal cord
  Congenital disease or lesion NOS of spinal cord

✓4ᵗʰ **Q07 Other congenital malformations of nervous system**
  EXCLUDES 2 *congenital central alveolar hypoventilation syndrome (G47.35)*
    familial dysautonomia [Riley-Day] (G90.1)
    neurofibromatosis (nonmalignant) (Q85.0-)

  CC Excl: For CC codes in category Q07: PDX collection 1056

  ✓5ᵗʰ **Q07.0 Arnold-Chiari syndrome**
    Arnold-Chiari syndrome, type II
    EXCLUDES 1 *Arnold-Chiari syndrome, type III (Q01.-)*
      Arnold-Chiari syndrome, type IV (Q04.8)
    DEF: Congenital malformation of the brain in which the cerebellum protrudes through the foramen magnum into the spinal canal.
    Q07.00 **Arnold-Chiari syndrome** without spina bifida or hydrocephalus   `HCC`
    Q07.01 **Arnold-Chiari syndrome** with spina bifida   `HCC`
    Q07.02 **Arnold-Chiari syndrome** with hydrocephalus   `CC` `HCC`
    Q07.03 **Arnold-Chiari syndrome** with spina bifida and hydrocephalus   `CC` `HCC`
  Q07.8 Other specified congenital malformations of nervous system   `HCC`
    Agenesis of nerve
    Displacement of brachial plexus
    Jaw-winking syndrome
    Marcus Gunn's syndrome
  Q07.9 Congenital malformation of nervous system, unspecified   `HCC`
    Congenital anomaly NOS of nervous system
    Congenital deformity NOS of nervous system
    Congenital disease or lesion NOS of nervous system

Congenital malformations of eye, ear, face and neck (Q10-Q18)
  EXCLUDES 2 *cleft lip and cleft palate (Q35-Q37)*
    congenital malformation of cervical spine (Q05.0, Q05.5, Q67.5, Q76.0-Q76.4)
    congenital malformation of larynx (Q31.-)
    congenital malformation of lip NEC (Q38.0)
    congenital malformation of nose (Q30.-)
    congenital malformation of parathyroid gland (Q89.2)
    congenital malformation of thyroid gland (Q89.2)

✓4ᵗʰ **Q10 Congenital malformations of** eyelid, lacrimal apparatus and orbit
  EXCLUDES 1 *cryptophthalmos NOS (Q11.2)*
    cryptophthalmos syndrome (Q87.0)
  Q10.0 Congenital ptosis
    DEF: Congenital drooping of the eyelid. Ptosis is mostly idiopathic, but may occur genetically.
  Q10.1 Congenital ectropion
  Q10.2 Congenital entropion
  Q10.3 Other congenital malformations of eyelid
    Ablepharon
    Blepharophimosis, congenital
    Coloboma of eyelid
    Congenital absence or agenesis of cilia
    Congenital absence or agenesis of eyelid
    Congenital accessory eyelid
    Congenital accessory eye muscle
    Congenital malformation of eyelid NOS
  Q10.4 Absence and agenesis of lacrimal apparatus
    Congenital absence of punctum lacrimale
  Q10.5 Congenital stenosis and stricture of lacrimal duct
  Q10.6 Other congenital malformations of lacrimal apparatus
    Congenital malformation of lacrimal apparatus NOS
  Q10.7 Congenital malformation of orbit

✓4ᵗʰ **Q11 Anophthalmos, microphthalmos and macrophthalmos**
  Q11.0 Cystic eyeball
  Q11.1 Other anophthalmos
    Anophthalmos NOS
    Agenesis of eye
    Aplasia of eye
  Q11.2 Microphthalmos
    Cryptophthalmos NOS
    Dysplasia of eye
    Hypoplasia of eye
    Rudimentary eye
    EXCLUDES 1 *cryptophthalmos syndrome (Q87.0)*
  Q11.3 Macrophthalmos
    EXCLUDES 1 *macrophthalmos in congenital glaucoma (Q15.0)*

✓4ᵗʰ **Q12 Congenital lens malformations**
  Q12.0 Congenital cataract
  Q12.1 Congenital displaced lens
  Q12.2 Coloboma of lens

Coloboma of Lens

Coloboma

  Q12.3 Congenital aphakia
  Q12.4 Spherophakia
  Q12.8 Other congenital lens malformations
    Microphakia
  Q12.9 Congenital lens malformation, unspecified

Chapter 17. Congenital Malformations, Deformations and Chromosomal Abnormalities

Q13–Q20.3

✓4th Q13 Congenital malformations of anterior segment of eye

Q13.0 Coloboma of iris
Coloboma NOS
DEF: Defective or absent section of ocular tissue that may present as mild cupping or a small pit in the ocular disc due to extensive defects in the iris, ciliary body, choroids, and retina.

Q13.1 Absence of iris
Aniridia
Use additional code for associated glaucoma (H42)
DEF: Incompletely formed or absent iris. It affects both eyes and is a dominant trait.

Q13.2 Other congenital malformations of iris
Anisocoria, congenital
Atresia of pupil
Congenital malformation of iris NOS
Corectopia

Q13.3 Congenital corneal opacity

Q13.4 Other congenital corneal malformations
Congenital malformation of cornea NOS
Microcornea
Peter's anomaly

Q13.5 Blue sclera

✓5th Q13.8 Other congenital malformations of anterior segment of eye
  Q13.81 Rieger's anomaly
    Use additional code for associated glaucoma (H42)
  Q13.89 Other congenital malformations of anterior segment of eye

Q13.9 Congenital malformation of anterior segment of eye, unspecified

✓4th Q14 Congenital malformations of posterior segment of eye
EXCLUDES 2   optic nerve hypoplasia (H47.03-)

Q14.0 Congenital malformation of vitreous humor
Congenital vitreous opacity

Q14.1 Congenital malformation of retina
Congenital retinal aneurysm

Q14.2 Congenital malformation of optic disc
Coloboma of optic disc

Q14.3 Congenital malformation of choroid

Q14.8 Other congenital malformations of posterior segment of eye
Coloboma of the fundus

Q14.9 Congenital malformation of posterior segment of eye, unspecified

✓4th Q15 Other congenital malformations of eye
EXCLUDES 1   congenital nystagmus (H55.01)
      ocular albinism (E70.31-)
      optic nerve hypoplasia (H47.03-)
      retinitis pigmentosa (H35.52)

Q15.0 Congenital glaucoma
Axenfeld's anomaly
Buphthalmos
Glaucoma of childhood
Glaucoma of newborn
Hydrophthalmos
Keratoglobus, congenital, with glaucoma
Macrocornea with glaucoma
Macrophthalmos in congenital glaucoma
Megalocornea with glaucoma

Q15.8 Other specified congenital malformations of eye

Q15.9 Congenital malformation of eye, unspecified
Congenital anomaly of eye
Congenital deformity of eye

✓4th Q16 Congenital malformations of ear causing impairment of hearing
EXCLUDES 1   congenital deafness (H90.-)

Q16.0 Congenital absence of (ear) auricle

Q16.1 Congenital absence, atresia and stricture of auditory canal (external)
Congenital atresia or stricture of osseous meatus

Q16.2 Absence of eustachian tube

Q16.3 Congenital malformation of ear ossicles
Congenital fusion of ear ossicles

Q16.4 Other congenital malformations of middle ear
Congenital malformation of middle ear NOS

Q16.5 Congenital malformation of inner ear
Congenital anomaly of membranous labyrinth
Congenital anomaly of organ of Corti

Q16.9 Congenital malformation of ear causing impairment of hearing, unspecified
Congenital absence of ear NOS

✓4th Q17 Other congenital malformations of ear
EXCLUDES 1   congenital malformations of ear with impairment of hearing (Q16.0- Q16.9)
      preauricular sinus (Q18.1)

Q17.0 Accessory auricle
Accessory tragus
Polyotia
Preauricular appendage or tag
Supernumerary ear
Supernumerary lobule

Q17.1 Macrotia
DEF: Birth defect characterized by abnormal enlargement of the pinna of the ear.

Q17.2 Microtia

Q17.3 Other misshapen ear
Pointed ear

Q17.4 Misplaced ear
Low-set ears
EXCLUDES 1   cervical auricle (Q18.2)

Q17.5 Prominent ear
Bat ear

Q17.8 Other specified congenital malformations of ear
Congenital absence of lobe of ear

Q17.9 Congenital malformation of ear, unspecified
Congenital anomaly of ear NOS

✓4th Q18 Other congenital malformations of face and neck
EXCLUDES 1   cleft lip and cleft palate (Q35-Q37)
      conditions classified to Q67.0-Q67.4
      congenital malformations of skull and face bones (Q75.-)
      cyclopia (Q87.0)
      dentofacial anomalies [including malocclusion] (M26.-)
      malformation syndromes affecting facial appearance (Q87.0)
      persistent thyroglossal duct (Q89.2)

Q18.0 Sinus, fistula and cyst of branchial cleft
Branchial vestige

Q18.1 Preauricular sinus and cyst   **SW**
Fistula of auricle, congenital
Cervicoaural fistula

Q18.2 Other branchial cleft malformations
Branchial cleft malformation NOS
Cervical auricle
Otocephaly

Q18.3 Webbing of neck
Pterygium colli
DEF: Congenital malformation characterized by a thick, triangular skinfold that stretches from the lateral side of the neck across the shoulder. It is associated with genetic conditions such as Turner's and Noonan's syndromes.

Q18.4 Macrostomia
DEF: Rare congenital craniofacial bilateral or unilateral anomaly of the mouth due to malformed maxillary and mandibular processes. It results in an abnormally large mouth extending toward the ear.

Q18.5 Microstomia

Q18.6 Macrocheilia
Hypertrophy of lip, congenital

Q18.7 Microcheilia

Q18.8 Other specified congenital malformations of face and neck
Medial cyst of face and neck
Medial fistula of face and neck
Medial sinus of face and neck

Q18.9 Congenital malformation of face and neck, unspecified
Congenital anomaly NOS of face and neck

Congenital malformations of the circulatory system (Q20-Q28)

✓4th Q20 Congenital malformations of cardiac chambers and connections
EXCLUDES 1   dextrocardia with situs inversus (Q89.3)
      mirror-image atrial arrangement with situs inversus (Q89.3)

CC Excl: For CC/MCC codes in category Q20: PDX collection 1057

Q20.0 Common arterial trunk   **MCC**
Persistent truncus arteriosus
EXCLUDES 1   aortic septal defect (Q21.4)

Q20.1 Double outlet right ventricle   **MCC**
Taussig-Bing syndrome

Q20.2 Double outlet left ventricle   **MCC**

Q20.3 Discordant ventriculoarterial connection   **MCC**
Dextrotransposition of aorta
Transposition of great vessels (complete)

N Newborn: 0   **P** Pediatric: 0-17   **M** Maternity: 12-55   **A** Adult: 15-124   **MCC** Major Complication/Comorbidity   **CC** Complication/Comorbidity   **SW** Severe Wound Dx

902   ICD-10-CM 2019

Q20.4 Double inlet ventricle `MCC`
Common ventricle
Cor triloculare biatriatum
Single ventricle

Q20.5 Discordant atrioventricular connection `CC`
Corrected transposition
Levotransposition
Ventricular inversion

Q20.6 Isomerism of atrial appendages
Isomerism of atrial appendages with asplenia or polysplenia

Q20.8 Other congenital malformations of cardiac chambers and connections
Cor binoculare

Q20.9 Congenital malformation of cardiac chambers and connections, unspecified

✓4ᵗʰ **Q21 Congenital malformations of cardiac septa**
> *EXCLUDES 1*   acquired cardiac septal defect (I51.0)

> **CC Excl:** For CC/MCC codes in category Q21, unless otherwise noted: PDX collection 1057

Q21.0 Ventricular septal defect `CC`
Roger's disease

Q21.1 Atrial septal defect `CC`
Coronary sinus defect
Patent or persistent foramen ovale
Patent or persistent ostium secundum defect (type II)
Patent or persistent sinus venosus defect
CC Excl: PDX collection 1058

Q21.2 Atrioventricular septal defect `CC`
Common atrioventricular canal
Endocardial cushion defect
Ostium primum atrial septal defect (type I)

Ventricular Septal Defect

Atrial Septal Defect

Atrioventricular Septal Defect

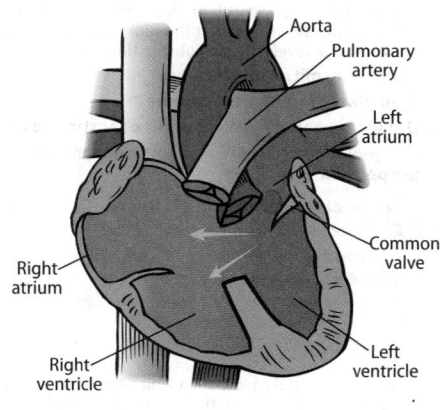

Q21.3 Tetralogy of Fallot `MCC`
Ventricular septal defect with pulmonary stenosis or atresia, dextroposition of aorta and hypertrophy of right ventricle.
AHA: 2014, 3Q, 16

Q21.4 Aortopulmonary septal defect
Aortic septal defect
Aortopulmonary window

Q21.8 Other congenital malformations of cardiac septa
Eisenmenger's defect
Pentalogy of Fallot
Code also if applicable:
Eisenmenger's complex (I27.83)
Eisenmenger's syndrome (I27.83)

Q21.9 Congenital malformation of cardiac septum, unspecified
Septal (heart) defect NOS

✓4ᵗʰ **Q22 Congenital malformations of pulmonary and tricuspid valves**

> **CC Excl:** For CC/MCC codes in category Q22, unless otherwise noted: PDX collection 1061

Q22.0 Pulmonary valve atresia `MCC`
CC Excl: PDX collection 1059

Q22.1 Congenital pulmonary valve stenosis `CC`
DEF: Stenosis of the opening between the pulmonary artery and right ventricle, causing obstructed blood outflow from the right ventricle.
CC Excl: PDX collection 1059

Q22.2 Congenital pulmonary valve insufficiency `CC`
Congenital pulmonary valve regurgitation
CC Excl: PDX collection 1060

Q22.3 Other congenital malformations of pulmonary valve `CC`
Congenital malformation of pulmonary valve NOS
Supernumerary cusps of pulmonary valve
CC Excl: PDX collection 1060

Q22.4 Congenital tricuspid stenosis `MCC`
Congenital tricuspid atresia

Q22.5 Ebstein's anomaly `MCC`
DEF: Malformation of the tricuspid valve characterized by septal and posterior leaflets attaching to the wall of the right ventricle. Ebstein's anomaly causes the right ventricle to fuse with the atrium into a large right atrium and a small ventricle and leads to heart failure and abnormal cardiac rhythm.

Q22.6 Hypoplastic right heart syndrome `MCC`

Q22.8 Other congenital malformations of tricuspid valve `MCC`

Q22.9 Congenital malformation of tricuspid valve, unspecified `MCC`

✓4ᵗʰ **Q23 Congenital malformations of aortic and mitral valves**

> **CC Excl:** For CC/MCC codes in category Q23: PDX collection 1061

Q23.0 Congenital stenosis of aortic valve `CC`
Congenital aortic atresia
Congenital aortic stenosis NOS
> *EXCLUDES 1*   congenital stenosis of aortic valve in hypoplastic left heart syndrome (Q23.4)
> congenital subaortic stenosis (Q24.4)
> supravalvular aortic stenosis (congenital) (Q25.3)

Q23.1 Congenital insufficiency of aortic valve `CC`
Bicuspid aortic valve
Congenital aortic insufficiency

☑ Additional Character Required   ✓x7ᵗʰ Placeholder   Unacceptable PDx   Questionable PDx   Manifestation   **H1**-**H14** HAC   **HCC** CMS-HCC Dx   **HIV** HIV Dx

ICD-10-CM 2019   **903**

Q23.2 Congenital mitral stenosis   `CC`
Congenital mitral atresia
DEF: Congenital stenosis of the mitral valve orifice between the left atrium and ventricle, at the supravalvular, valvular, or subvalvular levels, causing obstruction to left ventricular filling.

Q23.3 Congenital mitral insufficiency   `CC`
Q23.4 Hypoplastic left heart syndrome   `MCC`
Q23.8 Other congenital malformations of aortic and mitral **valves**
Q23.9 Congenital malformation of aortic and mitral **valves, unspecified**

✓4ᵗʰ **Q24 Other congenital malformations of** heart
EXCLUDES 1   endocardial fibroelastosis (I42.4)

Q24.0 Dextrocardia   `CC`
EXCLUDES 1   dextrocardia with situs inversus (Q89.3)
isomerism of atrial appendages (with asplenia or polysplenia) (Q20.6)
mirror-image atrial arrangement with situs inversus (Q89.3)
DEF: Congenital condition in which the heart is located on the right side of the chest rather than in its normal position on the left.
CC Excl: PDX collection 1062

Q24.1 Levocardia   `CC`
CC Excl: PDX collection 1062

Q24.2 Cor triatriatum   `MCC`
CC Excl: PDX collection 1063

Q24.3 Pulmonary infundibular stenosis   `CC`
Subvalvular pulmonic stenosis
CC Excl: PDX collection 1063

Q24.4 Congenital subaortic stenosis   `MCC`
DEF: Congenital heart defect characterized by stenosis of the left ventricular outflow tract due to a fibrous tissue ring or septal hypertrophy below the aortic valve.
CC Excl: PDX collection 1063

Q24.5 Malformation of coronary vessels   `CC`
Congenital coronary (artery) aneurysm
CC Excl: PDX collection 1064

Q24.6 Congenital heart block   `MCC`
CC Excl: PDX collection 1065

Q24.8 Other specified congenital malformations of heart
Congenital diverticulum of left ventricle
Congenital malformation of myocardium
Congenital malformation of pericardium
Malposition of heart
Uhl's disease

Q24.9 Congenital malformation of heart, unspecified
Congenital anomaly of heart
Congenital disease of heart

✓4ᵗʰ **Q25 Congenital malformations of** great arteries

Q25.0 Patent ductus arteriosus   `CC`
Patent ductus Botallo
Persistent ductus arteriosus
CC Excl: PDX collection 1066

Q25.1 Coarctation of aorta   `CC`
Coarctation of aorta (preductal) (postductal)
Stenosis of aorta
AHA: 2016, 4Q, 56-57
CC Excl: PDX collection 1067

Patent Ductus Arteriosus

Q25.2 Atresia of aorta   ✓5ᵗʰ
AHA: 2016, 4Q, 56-57

Q25.21 Interruption of aortic arch   `CC`
Atresia of aortic arch
CC Excl: PDX collection 1068

Q25.29 Other atresia of aorta   `CC`
Atresia of aorta
CC Excl: PDX collection 1068

Q25.3 Supravalvular aortic stenosis   `CC`
EXCLUDES 1   congenital aortic stenosis NOS (Q23.0)
congenital stenosis of aortic valve (Q23.0)
CC Excl: PDX collection 1068

Q25.4 Other congenital malformations of aorta   ✓5ᵗʰ
EXCLUDES 1   hypoplasia of aorta in hypoplastic left heart syndrome (Q23.4)
AHA: 2016, 4Q, 57

CC Excl: For CC codes in subcategory Q25.4:
PDX collection 1069

Q25.40 Congenital malformation of aorta unspecified   `CC`
Q25.41 Absence and aplasia of aorta   `CC`
Q25.42 Hypoplasia of aorta   `CC`
Q25.43 Congenital aneurysm of aorta   `CC`
Congenital aneurysm of aortic root
Congenital aneurysm of aortic sinus

Q25.44 Congenital dilation of aorta   `CC`
Q25.45 Double aortic arch   `CC`
Vascular ring of aorta

Aortic Arch Anomalies

Normal aortic arch

Double aortic arch   Right aortic arch

Q25.46 Tortuous aortic arch   `CC`
Persistent convolutions of aortic arch

Q25.47 Right aortic arch   `CC`
Persistent right aortic arch

Q25.48 Anomalous origin of subclavian artery   `CC`
Q25.49 Other congenital malformations of aorta   `CC`
Aortic arch
Bovine arch

Q25.5 Atresia of pulmonary artery   `MCC`
CC Excl: PDX collection 1070

Q25.6 Stenosis of pulmonary artery   `MCC`
Supravalvular pulmonary stenosis
CC Excl: PDX collection 1070

Q25.7 Other congenital malformations of pulmonary artery   ✓5ᵗʰ

CC Excl: For MCC codes in subcategory Q25.7:
PDX collection 1070

Q25.71 Coarctation of pulmonary artery   `MCC`
Q25.72 Congenital pulmonary arteriovenous malformation   `MCC`
Congenital pulmonary arteriovenous aneurysm

Q25.79 Other **congenital malformations of pulmonary** `MCC`
artery
Aberrant pulmonary artery
Agenesis of pulmonary artery
Congenital aneurysm of pulmonary artery
Congenital anomaly of pulmonary artery
Hypoplasia of pulmonary artery

Q25.8 **Other congenital malformations of** other great arteries `CC`
CC Excl: PDX collection 1069

Q25.9 **Congenital malformation of great arteries,** unspecified `CC`
CC Excl: PDX collection 1069

`✓4ᵗʰ` **Q26** **Congenital malformations of** great veins

Q26.0 **Congenital** stenosis of vena cava `CC`
Congenital stenosis of vena cava (inferior)(superior)
CC Excl: PDX collection 1071

Q26.1 **Persistent** left superior vena cava `CC`
CC Excl: PDX collection 1071

Q26.2 **Total** anomalous pulmonary venous connection `CC`
Total anomalous pulmonary venous return [TAPVR], subdiaphragmatic
Total anomalous pulmonary venous return [TAPVR], supradiaphragmatic
CC Excl: PDX collection 1072

Q26.3 **Partial** anomalous pulmonary venous connection `CC`
Partial anomalous pulmonary venous return
CC Excl: PDX collection 1073

Q26.4 **Anomalous** pulmonary venous connection, unspecified `CC`
CC Excl: PDX collection 1073

Q26.5 **Anomalous** portal venous connection

Q26.6 **Portal vein-hepatic** artery fistula

Q26.8 **Other congenital malformations of** great veins `CC`
Absence of vena cava (inferior) (superior)
Azygos continuation of inferior vena cava
Persistent left posterior cardinal vein
Scimitar syndrome
CC Excl: PDX collection 1071

Q26.9 **Congenital malformation of great vein,** unspecified `CC`
Congenital anomaly of vena cava (inferior) (superior) NOS
CC Excl: PDX collection 1074

`✓4ᵗʰ` **Q27** **Other congenital malformations of** peripheral vascular system
EXCLUDES 2 anomalies of cerebral and precerebral vessels (Q28.0–Q28.3)
anomalies of coronary vessels (Q24.5)
anomalies of pulmonary artery (Q25.5–Q25.7)
congenital retinal aneurysm (Q14.1)
hemangioma and lymphangioma (D18.-)

Q27.0 **Congenital** absence and hypoplasia of umbilical artery
Single umbilical artery

Q27.1 **Congenital** renal artery stenosis

Q27.2 **Other congenital malformations of** renal artery
Congenital malformation of renal artery NOS
Multiple renal arteries

`✓5ᵗʰ` **Q27.3** **Arteriovenous malformation (peripheral)**
Arteriovenous aneurysm
EXCLUDES 1 acquired arteriovenous aneurysm (I77.0)
EXCLUDES 2 arteriovenous malformation of cerebral vessels (Q28.2)
arteriovenous malformation of precerebral vessels (Q28.0)
DEF: Arteriovenous malformation: Connecting passage between an artery and a vein.

Q27.30 **Arteriovenous malformation,** site unspecified `CC`
CC Excl: PDX collection 1075

Q27.31 **Arteriovenous malformation of** vessel of upper limb

Q27.32 **Arteriovenous malformation of** vessel of lower limb

Q27.33 **Arteriovenous malformation of** digestive system vessel

Q27.34 **Arteriovenous malformation of** renal vessel

Q27.39 **Arteriovenous malformation,** other site

Q27.4 **Congenital** phlebectasia `CC`
CC Excl: PDX collection 1075

Q27.8 **Other specified congenital malformations of peripheral vascular system**
Absence of peripheral vascular system
Atresia of peripheral vascular system
Congenital aneurysm (peripheral)
Congenital stricture, artery
Congenital varix
EXCLUDES 1 arteriovenous malformation (Q27.3-)

Q27.9 **Congenital malformation of peripheral vascular system,** unspecified
Anomaly of artery or vein NOS

`✓4ᵗʰ` **Q28** **Other congenital malformations of** circulatory system
EXCLUDES 1 congenital aneurysm NOS (Q27.8)
congenital coronary aneurysm (Q24.5)
ruptured cerebral arteriovenous malformation (I60.8)
ruptured malformation of precerebral vessels (I72.0)
EXCLUDES 2 congenital peripheral aneurysm (Q27.8)
congenital pulmonary aneurysm (Q25.79)
congenital retinal aneurysm (Q14.1)

CC Excl: For CC/MCC codes in category Q28, unless otherwise noted: PDX collection 1075

Q28.0 **Arteriovenous malformation of** precerebral vessels `CC`
Congenital arteriovenous precerebral aneurysm (nonruptured)

Q28.1 **Other malformations of** precerebral vessels `CC`
Congenital malformation of precerebral vessels NOS
Congenital precerebral aneurysm (nonruptured)

Q28.2 **Arteriovenous malformation of** cerebral vessels `MCC`
Arteriovenous malformation of brain NOS
Congenital arteriovenous cerebral aneurysm (nonruptured)
CC Excl: PDX collection 1076

Q28.3 **Other malformations of** cerebral vessels `MCC`
Congenital cerebral aneurysm (nonruptured)
Congenital malformation of cerebral vessels NOS
Developmental venous anomaly
CC Excl: PDX collection 1076

Q28.8 **Other specified congenital malformations of circulatory** `CC`
system
Congenital aneurysm, specified site NEC
Spinal vessel anomaly

Q28.9 **Congenital malformation of circulatory system,** `CC`
unspecified
CC Excl: PDX collection 1077

Congenital malformations of the respiratory system (Q30–Q34)

`✓4ᵗʰ` **Q30** **Congenital malformations of** nose
EXCLUDES 1 congenital deviation of nasal septum (Q67.4)

Q30.0 **Choanal** atresia
Atresia of nares (anterior) (posterior)
Congenital stenosis of nares (anterior) (posterior)

Q30.1 **Agenesis and underdevelopment of nose**
Congenital absent of nose

Q30.2 **Fissured, notched and cleft nose**

Q30.3 **Congenital** perforated nasal septum

Q30.8 **Other congenital malformations of nose**
Accessory nose
Congenital anomaly of nasal sinus wall

Q30.9 **Congenital malformation of nose,** unspecified

`✓4ᵗʰ` **Q31** **Congenital malformations of** larynx
EXCLUDES 1 congenital laryngeal stridor NOS (P28.89)

CC Excl: For CC codes in category Q31: PDX collection 1078

Q31.0 **Web of larynx**
Glottic web of larynx
Subglottic web of larynx
Web of larynx NOS
DEF: Congenital malformation of the larynx marked by thin, translucent, or thick fibrotic membrane-like structure between the vocal folds. It is characterized by shortness of breath and stridor.

Q31.1 **Congenital** subglottic stenosis `CC`

Q31.2 **Laryngeal** hypoplasia `CC`

Q31.3 **Laryngocele** `CC`

Q31.5 **Congenital** laryngomalacia `CC`

Q31.8 **Other congenital malformations of larynx** `CC`
Absence of larynx
Agenesis of larynx
Atresia of larynx
Congenital cleft thyroid cartilage
Congenital fissure of epiglottis
Congenital stenosis of larynx NEC
Posterior cleft of cricoid cartilage

Q31.9 **Congenital malformation of larynx,** unspecified `CC`

✔ Additional Character Required   `✓x7ᵗʰ` Placeholder   Unacceptable PDx   Questionable PDx   Manifestation   `H1`-`H14` HAC   `HCC` CMS-HCC Dx   `HIV` HIV Dx

ICD-10-CM 2019   **905**

Chapter 17. Congenital Malformations, Deformations and Chromosomal Abnormalities

✓4ᵗʰ Q32 Congenital malformations of trachea and bronchus
   EXCLUDES 1   congenital bronchiectasis (Q33.4)

CC Excl: For CC codes in category Q32: PDX collection 1078

Q32.0 Congenital tracheomalacia   CC

Q32.1 Other congenital malformations of trachea   CC
   Atresia of trachea
   Congenital anomaly of tracheal cartilage
   Congenital dilatation of trachea
   Congenital malformation of trachea
   Congenital stenosis of trachea
   Congenital tracheocele

Q32.2 Congenital bronchomalacia   CC

Q32.3 Congenital stenosis of bronchus   CC

Q32.4 Other congenital malformations of bronchus   CC
   Absence of bronchus
   Agenesis of bronchus
   Atresia of bronchus
   Congenital diverticulum of bronchus
   Congenital malformation of bronchus NOS

✓4ᵗʰ Q33 Congenital malformations of lung

CC Excl: For CC/MCC codes in category Q33, unless otherwise noted: PDX collection 1079

Q33.0 Congenital cystic lung   CC
   Congenital cystic lung disease
   Congenital honeycomb lung
   Congenital polycystic lung disease
   EXCLUDES 1   cystic fibrosis (E84.0)
        cystic lung disease, acquired or unspecified (J98.4)

Q33.1 Accessory lobe of lung
   Azygos lobe (fissured), lung

Q33.2 Sequestration of lung   MCC

Q33.3 Agenesis of lung   MCC
   Congenital absence of lung (lobe)

Q33.4 Congenital bronchiectasis   CC
   CC Excl: PDX collection 1080

Q33.5 Ectopic tissue in lung

Q33.6 Congenital hypoplasia and dysplasia of lung   MCC
   EXCLUDES 1   pulmonary hypoplasia associated with short gestation (P28.0)

Q33.8 Other congenital malformations of lung

Q33.9 Congenital malformation of lung, unspecified

✓4ᵗʰ Q34 Other congenital malformations of respiratory system
   EXCLUDES 2   congenital central alveolar hypoventilation syndrome (G47.35)

Q34.0 Anomaly of pleura

Q34.1 Congenital cyst of mediastinum

Q34.8 Other specified congenital malformations of respiratory system
   Atresia of nasopharynx

Q34.9 Congenital malformation of respiratory system, unspecified
   Congenital absence of respiratory system
   Congenital anomaly of respiratory system NOS

Cleft lip and cleft palate (Q35-Q37)

Use additional code to identify associated malformation of the nose (Q30.2)
   EXCLUDES 1   Robin's syndrome (Q87.0)

✓4ᵗʰ Q35 Cleft palate
   INCLUDES   fissure of palate
        palatoschisis
   EXCLUDES 1   cleft palate with cleft lip (Q37.-)
   DEF: Congenital fissure or defect of the roof of the mouth opening to the nasal cavity due to failure of embryonic cells to fuse completely.

Q35.1 Cleft hard palate

Cleft Palate

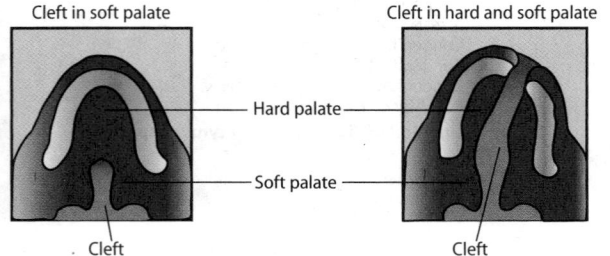

Cleft in soft palate   Cleft in hard and soft palate

Hard palate

Soft palate

Cleft   Cleft

Cleft Lip

Unilateral incomplete   Unilateral complete   Bilateral complete

Q35.3 Cleft soft palate

Q35.5 Cleft hard palate with cleft soft palate

Q35.7 Cleft uvula

Q35.9 Cleft palate, unspecified
   Cleft palate NOS

✓4ᵗʰ Q36 Cleft lip
   INCLUDES   cheiloschisis
        congenital fissure of lip
        harelip
        labium leporinum
   EXCLUDES 1   cleft lip with cleft palate (Q37.-)
   DEF: Congenital fissure or opening in the upper lip due to failure of embryonic cells to fuse completely.

Q36.0 Cleft lip, bilateral

Q36.1 Cleft lip, median

Q36.9 Cleft lip, unilateral
   Cleft lip NOS

✓4ᵗʰ Q37 Cleft palate with cleft lip
   INCLUDES   cheilopalatoschisis

Q37.0 Cleft hard palate with bilateral cleft lip

Q37.1 Cleft hard palate with unilateral cleft lip
   Cleft hard palate with cleft lip NOS

Q37.2 Cleft soft palate with bilateral cleft lip

Q37.3 Cleft soft palate with unilateral cleft lip
   Cleft soft palate with cleft lip NOS

Q37.4 Cleft hard and soft palate with bilateral cleft lip

Q37.5 Cleft hard and soft palate with unilateral cleft lip
   Cleft hard and soft palate with cleft lip NOS

Q37.8 Unspecified cleft palate with bilateral cleft lip

Q37.9 Unspecified cleft palate with unilateral cleft lip
   Cleft palate with cleft lip NOS

Other congenital malformations of the digestive system (Q38-Q45)

✓4ᵗʰ Q38 Other congenital malformations of tongue, mouth and pharynx
   EXCLUDES 1   dentofacial anomalies (M26.-)
        macrostomia (Q18.4)
        microstomia (Q18.5)

Q38.0 Congenital malformations of lips, not elsewhere classified
   Congenital fistula of lip
   Congenital malformation of lip NOS
   Van der Woude's syndrome
   EXCLUDES 1   cleft lip (Q36.-)
        cleft lip with cleft palate (Q37.-)
        macrocheilia (Q18.6)
        microcheilia (Q18.7)

Q38.1 Ankyloglossia
   Tongue tie

Q38.2 Macroglossia
   Congenital hypertrophy of tongue

Q38.3 Other congenital malformations of tongue
   Aglossia
   Bifid tongue
   Congenital adhesion of tongue
   Congenital fissure of tongue
   Congenital malformation of tongue NOS
   Double tongue
   Hypoglossia
   Hypoplasia of tongue
   Microglossia

Q38.4 Congenital malformations of salivary glands and ducts
   Atresia of salivary glands and ducts
   Congenital absence of salivary glands and ducts
   Congenital accessory salivary glands and ducts
   Congenital fistula of salivary gland

N Newborn: 0   P Pediatric: 0-17   M Maternity: 12-55   A Adult: 15-124   MCC Major Complication/Comorbidity   CC Complication/Comorbidity   SW Severe Wound Dx

906   ICD-10-CM 2019

Q38.5 Congenital malformations of palate, not elsewhere classified
Congenital absence of uvula
Congenital malformation of palate NOS
Congenital high arched palate
EXCLUDES1   cleft palate (Q35.-)
cleft palate with cleft lip (Q37.-)

Q38.6 Other congenital malformations of mouth
Congenital malformation of mouth NOS

Q38.7 Congenital pharyngeal pouch
Congenital diverticulum of pharynx
EXCLUDES1   pharyngeal pouch syndrome (D82.1)

Q38.8 Other congenital malformations of pharynx
Congenital malformation of pharynx NOS
Imperforate pharynx

✓4th Q39 Congenital malformations of esophagus

CC Excl: For MCC codes in category Q39: PDX collection 1081
For CC codes in category Q39: PDX collection 1082

Q39.0 Atresia of esophagus without fistula   MCC
Atresia of esophagus NOS

Q39.1 Atresia of esophagus with tracheo-esophageal fistula   MCC
Atresia of esophagus with broncho-esophageal fistula

Q39.2 Congenital tracheo-esophageal fistula without atresia   MCC
Congenital tracheo-esophageal fistula NOS

Q39.3 Congenital stenosis and stricture of esophagus   MCC

Q39.4 Esophageal web   MCC

Q39.5 Congenital dilatation of esophagus   CC
Congenital cardiospasm

Q39.6 Congenital diverticulum of esophagus   CC
Congenital esophageal pouch

Q39.8 Other congenital malformations of esophagus   CC
Congenital absence of esophagus
Congenital displacement of esophagus
Congenital duplication of esophagus

Q39.9 Congenital malformation of esophagus, unspecified   CC

✓4th Q40 Other congenital malformations of upper alimentary tract

Q40.0 Congenital hypertrophic pyloric stenosis
Congenital or infantile constriction
Congenital or infantile hypertrophy
Congenital or infantile spasm
Congenital or infantile stenosis
Congenital or infantile stricture

Q40.1 Congenital hiatus hernia
Congenital displacement of cardia through esophageal hiatus
EXCLUDES1   congenital diaphragmatic hernia (Q79.0)

Q40.2 Other specified congenital malformations of stomach
Congenital displacement of stomach
Congenital diverticulum of stomach
Congenital hourglass stomach
Congenital duplication of stomach
Megalogastria
Microgastria

Q40.3 Congenital malformation of stomach, unspecified

Q40.8 Other specified congenital malformations of upper alimentary tract

Q40.9 Congenital malformation of upper alimentary tract, unspecified
Congenital anomaly of upper alimentary tract
Congenital deformity of upper alimentary tract

✓4th Q41 Congenital absence, atresia and stenosis of small intestine
INCLUDES   congenital obstruction, occlusion or stricture of small intestine or intestine NOS
EXCLUDES1   cystic fibrosis with intestinal manifestation (E84.11)
meconium ileus NOS (without cystic fibrosis) (P76.0)

CC Excl: For CC codes in category Q41: PDX collection 1083

Q41.0 Congenital absence, atresia and stenosis of duodenum   CC

Q41.1 Congenital absence, atresia and stenosis of jejunum   CC
Apple peel syndrome
Imperforate jejunum

Q41.2 Congenital absence, atresia and stenosis of ileum   CC

Q41.8 Congenital absence, atresia and stenosis of other specified parts of small intestine   CC

Q41.9 Congenital absence, atresia and stenosis of small intestine, part unspecified   CC
Congenital absence, atresia and stenosis of intestine NOS

✓4th Q42 Congenital absence, atresia and stenosis of large intestine
INCLUDES   congenital obstruction, occlusion and stricture of large intestine

CC Excl: For CC codes in category Q42: PDX collection 1084

Q42.0 Congenital absence, atresia and stenosis of rectum with fistula   CC

Q42.1 Congenital absence, atresia and stenosis of rectum without fistula   CC
Imperforate rectum

Q42.2 Congenital absence, atresia and stenosis of anus with fistula   CC

Q42.3 Congenital absence, atresia and stenosis of anus without fistula   CC
Imperforate anus

Q42.8 Congenital absence, atresia and stenosis of other parts of large intestine   CC

Q42.9 Congenital absence, atresia and stenosis of large intestine, part unspecified   CC

✓4th Q43 Other congenital malformations of intestine

CC Excl: For CC codes in category Q43, unless otherwise noted:
PDX collection 1087

Q43.0 Meckel's diverticulum (displaced) (hypertrophic)
Persistent omphalomesenteric duct
Persistent vitelline duct
DEF: Congenital, abnormal remnant of embryonic digestive system development that leaves a sacculation or outpouching from the wall of the small intestine near the terminal part of the ileum made of acid-secreting tissue as in the stomach.

Q43.1 Hirschsprung's disease   CC
Aganglionosis
Congenital (aganglionic) megacolon
DEF: Congenital enlargement or dilation of the colon, with the absence of nerve cells in a segment of colon distally that causes the inability to defecate.
CC Excl: PDX collection 1085

Q43.2 Other congenital functional disorders of colon   CC
Congenital dilatation of colon
CC Excl: PDX collection 1085

Q43.3 Congenital malformations of intestinal fixation   CC
Congenital omental, anomalous adhesions [bands]
Congenital peritoneal adhesions [bands]
Incomplete rotation of cecum and colon
Insufficient rotation of cecum and colon
Jackson's membrane
Malrotation of colon
Rotation failure of cecum and colon
Universal mesentery
CC Excl: DX collection 1086

Q43.4 Duplication of intestine   CC

Q43.5 Ectopic anus   CC

Q43.6 Congenital fistula of rectum and anus   CC
EXCLUDES1   congenital fistula of anus with absence, atresia and stenosis (Q42.2)
congenital fistula of rectum with absence, atresia and stenosis (Q42.0)
congenital rectovaginal fistula (Q52.2)
congenital urethrorectal fistula (Q64.73)
pilonidal fistula or sinus (L05.-)

Q43.7 Persistent cloaca   CC
Cloaca NOS

Q43.8 Other specified congenital malformations of intestine   CC
Congenital blind loop syndrome
Congenital diverticulitis, colon
Congenital diverticulum, intestine
Dolichocolon
Megaloappendix
Megaloduodenum
Microcolon
Transposition of appendix
Transposition of colon
Transposition of intestine
AHA: 2013, 2Q, 31

Q43.9 Congenital malformation of intestine, unspecified   CC

✓4ᵗʰ Q44　Congenital malformations of gallbladder, bile ducts and liver

> CC Excl: For CC/MCC codes in category Q44, unless otherwise noted: PDX collection 1088

Q44.0　Agenesis, aplasia and hypoplasia of gallbladder　CC
Congenital absence of gallbladder

Q44.1　Other congenital malformations of gallbladder　CC
Congenital malformation of gallbladder NOS
Intrahepatic gallbladder

Q44.2　Atresia of bile ducts　MCC
CC Excl: PDX collection 1089

Q44.3　Congenital stenosis and stricture of bile ducts　MCC
CC Excl: PDX collection 1089

Q44.4　Choledochal cyst　CC

Q44.5　Other congenital malformations of bile ducts　CC
Accessory hepatic duct
Biliary duct duplication
Congenital malformation of bile duct NOS
Cystic duct duplication

Q44.6　Cystic disease of liver　CC
Fibrocystic disease of liver
CC Excl: PDX collection 1090

Q44.7　Other congenital malformations of liver　CC
Accessory liver
Alagille's syndrome
Congenital absence of liver
Congenital hepatomegaly
Congenital malformation of liver NOS

✓4ᵗʰ Q45　Other congenital malformations of digestive system

> EXCLUDES 2　congenital diaphragmatic hernia (Q79.0)
> congenital hiatus hernia (Q40.1)

> CC Excl: For CC codes in category Q45: PDX collection 1091

Q45.0　Agenesis, aplasia and hypoplasia of pancreas　CC
Congenital absence of pancreas

Q45.1　Annular pancreas　CC

Q45.2　Congenital pancreatic cyst　CC

Q45.3　Other congenital malformations of pancreas and pancreatic duct　CC
Accessory pancreas
Congenital malformation of pancreas or pancreatic duct NOS

> EXCLUDES 1　congenital diabetes mellitus (E10.-)
> cystic fibrosis (E84.0-E84.9)
> fibrocystic disease of pancreas (E84.-)
> neonatal diabetes mellitus (P70.2)

Q45.8　Other specified congenital malformations of digestive system
Absence (complete) (partial) of alimentary tract NOS
Duplication of digestive system
Malposition, congenital of digestive system

Q45.9　Congenital malformation of digestive system, unspecified
Congenital anomaly of digestive system
Congenital deformity of digestive system

Congenital malformations of genital organs (Q50-Q56)

> EXCLUDES 1　androgen insensitivity syndrome (E34.5-)
> syndromes associated with anomalies in the number and form of chromosomes (Q90-Q99)

✓4ᵗʰ Q50　Congenital malformations of ovaries, fallopian tubes and broad ligaments

✓5ᵗʰ Q50.0　Congenital absence of ovary
> EXCLUDES 1　Turner's syndrome (Q96.-)

　　Q50.01　Congenital absence of ovary, unilateral　♀
　　Q50.02　Congenital absence of ovary, bilateral　♀

Q50.1　Developmental ovarian cyst　♀

Q50.2　Congenital torsion of ovary　♀

✓5ᵗʰ Q50.3　Other congenital malformations of ovary
　　Q50.31　Accessory ovary　♀
　　Q50.32　Ovarian streak　♀
　　　　46, XX with streak gonads
　　Q50.39　Other congenital malformation of ovary　♀
　　　　Congenital malformation of ovary NOS

Q50.4　Embryonic cyst of fallopian tube　♀
Fimbrial cyst

Q50.5　Embryonic cyst of broad ligament　♀
Epoophoron cyst
Parovarian cyst

Q50.6　Other congenital malformations of fallopian tube and broad ligament　♀
Absence of fallopian tube and broad ligament
Accessory fallopian tube and broad ligament
Atresia of fallopian tube and broad ligament
Congenital malformation of fallopian tube or broad ligament NOS

✓4ᵗʰ Q51　Congenital malformations of uterus and cervix

Q51.0　Agenesis and aplasia of uterus　♀
Congenital absence of uterus

✓5ᵗʰ Q51.1　Doubling of uterus with doubling of cervix and vagina
　　Q51.10　Doubling of uterus with doubling of cervix and vagina without obstruction　♀
　　　　Doubling of uterus with doubling of cervix and vagina NOS
　　Q51.11　Doubling of uterus with doubling of cervix and vagina with obstruction　♀

✓5ᵗʰ Q51.2　Other doubling of uterus
Doubling of uterus NOS
▶Septate uterus◀
● 　**Q51.20　Other doubling of uterus, unspecified**　♀
　　　　Septate uterus, unspecified
● 　**Q51.21　Other complete doubling of uterus**　♀
　　　　Complete septate uterus
● 　**Q51.22　Other partial doubling of uterus**　♀
　　　　Partial septate uterus
● 　**Q51.28　Other doubling of uterus, other specified**　♀
　　　　Septate uterus, other specified

Q51.3　Bicornate uterus　♀
Bicornate uterus, complete or partial

Q51.4　Unicornate uterus　♀
Unicornate uterus with or without a separate uterine horn
Uterus with only one functioning horn

Q51.5　Agenesis and aplasia of cervix　♀
Congenital absence of cervix

Q51.6　Embryonic cyst of cervix　♀

Q51.7　Congenital fistulae between uterus and digestive and urinary tracts　♀

✓5ᵗʰ Q51.8　Other congenital malformations of uterus and cervix
　✓6ᵗʰ Q51.81　Other congenital malformations of uterus
　　　Q51.810　Arcuate uterus　♀
　　　　　Arcuatus uterus
　　　Q51.811　Hypoplasia of uterus　♀
　　　Q51.818　Other congenital malformations of uterus　♀
　　　　　Müllerian anomaly of uterus NEC
　✓6ᵗʰ Q51.82　Other congenital malformations of cervix
　　　Q51.820　Cervical duplication　♀
　　　Q51.821　Hypoplasia of cervix　♀
　　　Q51.828　Other congenital malformations of cervix　♀

Q51.9　Congenital malformation of uterus and cervix, unspecified　♀

✓4ᵗʰ Q52　Other congenital malformations of female genitalia

Q52.0　Congenital absence of vagina　♀
Vaginal agenesis, total or partial

✓5ᵗʰ Q52.1　Doubling of vagina
> EXCLUDES 1　doubling of vagina with doubling of uterus and cervix (Q51.1-)
　　Q52.10　Doubling of vagina, unspecified　♀
　　　　Septate vagina NOS
　　Q52.11　Transverse vaginal septum　♀
　✓6ᵗʰ Q52.12　Longitudinal vaginal septum
　　　AHA: 2016, 4Q, 58-59
　　　Q52.120　Longitudinal vaginal septum, nonobstructing　♀
　　　Q52.121　Longitudinal vaginal septum, obstructing, right side　♀
　　　Q52.122　Longitudinal vaginal septum, obstructing, left side　♀
　　　Q52.123　Longitudinal vaginal septum, microperforate, right side　♀
　　　Q52.124　Longitudinal vaginal septum, microperforate, left side　♀
　　　Q52.129　Other and unspecified longitudinal vaginal septum　♀

N Newborn: 0　P Pediatric: 0-17　M Maternity: 12-55　A Adult: 15-124　MCC Major Complication/Comorbidity　CC Complication/Comorbidity　SW Severe Wound Dx

908　　ICD-10-CM 2019

Q52.2 Congenital rectovaginal fistula   ♀
    EXCLUDES 1   cloaca (Q43.7)

Q52.3 Imperforate hymen   ♀
    DEF: Obstructive anomaly of vagina, characterized by complete closure of the membranous fold around the external opening of the vagina, obstructing the vaginal introitus.

Q52.4 Other congenital malformations of vagina   ♀
    Canal of Nuck cyst, congenital
    Congenital malformation of vagina NOS
    Embryonic vaginal cyst
    Gartner's duct cyst

Q52.5 Fusion of labia   ♀

Q52.6 Congenital malformation of clitoris   ♀

✓5ᵗʰ **Q52.7 Other and unspecified congenital malformations of** vulva   ♀
    Q52.70 Unspecified **congenital malformations of vulva**   ♀
       Congenital malformation of vulva NOS
    Q52.71 Congenital absence **of vulva**   ♀
    Q52.79 Other **congenital malformations of vulva**   ♀
       Congenital cyst of vulva

Q52.8 Other specified congenital malformations of female genitalia   ♀

Q52.9 Congenital malformation of female genitalia, unspecified   ♀

✓4ᵗʰ **Q53 Undescended and ectopic** testicle
    ✓5ᵗʰ **Q53.0 Ectopic** testis
       Q53.00 Ectopic testis, unspecified   ♂
       Q53.01 Ectopic testis, unilateral   ♂
       Q53.02 Ectopic testes, bilateral   ♂
    ✓5ᵗʰ **Q53.1 Undescended** testicle, unilateral
       AHA: 2017, 4Q, 22-23
       Q53.10 Unspecified **undescended testicle, unilateral**   ♂
       ✓6ᵗʰ **Q53.11** Abdominal **testis, unilateral**
          Q53.111 Unilateral intraabdominal **testis**   ♂
          Q53.112 Unilateral inguinal **testis**   ♂
       Q53.12 Ectopic perineal testis, unilateral   ♂
       Q53.13 Unilateral high scrotal testis   ♂
    ✓5ᵗʰ **Q53.2 Undescended** testicle, bilateral
       AHA: 2017, 4Q, 22-23
       Q53.20 Undescended testicle, unspecified, **bilateral**   ♂
       ✓6ᵗʰ **Q53.21** Abdominal **testis, bilateral**
          Q53.211 Bilateral intraabdominal **testes**   ♂
          Q53.212 Bilateral inguinal **testes**   ♂
       Q53.22 Ectopic perineal testis, bilateral   ♂
       Q53.23 Bilateral high scrotal testes   ♂
    Q53.9 Undescended testicle, unspecified   ♂
       Cryptorchism NOS

✓4ᵗʰ **Q54 Hypospadias**
    EXCLUDES 1   epispadias (Q64.0)
    DEF: Abnormal opening of the urethra on the ventral (underside) surface of the penis.

Q54.0 Hypospadias, balanic   ♂
    Hypospadias, coronal
    Hypospadias, glandular

Q54.1 Hypospadias, penile   ♂

Q54.2 Hypospadias, penoscrotal   ♂

Q54.3 Hypospadias, perineal   ♂

Hypospadias and Epispadias

Balanic (glanular, coronal) hypospadias
Subcoronal hypospadias
Penile hypospadias
Penile raphe
Penoscrotal hypospadius
Scrotal hypospadias
Scrotum
Scrotal raphe
Perineal hypospadias

Hypospadias (ventral view)

Normal external urethral orifice
Glans penis
Foreskin (retracted)
Epispadias

Epispadias (dorsal view)

Q54.4 Congenital chordee   ♂
    Chordee without hypospadias

Q54.8 Other hypospadias   ♂
    Hypospadias with intersex state

Q54.9 Hypospadias, unspecified   ♂

✓4ᵗʰ **Q55 Other congenital malformations of** male genital organs
    EXCLUDES 1   congenital hydrocele (P83.5)
               hypospadias (Q54.-)

Q55.0 Absence and aplasia of testis   ♂
    Monorchism

Q55.1 Hypoplasia of testis and scrotum   ♂
    Fusion of testes

✓5ᵗʰ **Q55.2 Other and unspecified congenital malformations of** testis and scrotum
    Q55.20 Unspecified **congenital malformations of testis and scrotum**   ♂
       Congenital malformation of testis or scrotum NOS
    Q55.21 Polyorchism   ♂
       DEF: Congenital anomaly in which there are more than two testes.
    Q55.22 Retractile **testis**   ♂
    Q55.23 Scrotal transposition   ♂
    Q55.29 Other **congenital malformations of testis and scrotum**   ♂

Q55.3 Atresia of vas deferens   ♂
    Code first any associated cystic fibrosis (E84.-)

Q55.4 Other congenital malformations of vas deferens, epididymis, seminal vesicles and prostate   ♂
    Absence or aplasia of prostate
    Absence or aplasia of spermatic cord
    Congenital malformation of vas deferens, epididymis, seminal vesicles or prostate NOS

Q55.5 Congenital absence and aplasia of penis   ♂

✓5ᵗʰ **Q55.6 Other congenital malformations of** penis
    Q55.61 Curvature of penis (lateral)   ♂
    Q55.62 Hypoplasia of penis   ♂
       Micropenis
    Q55.63 Congenital torsion of penis   ♂
       EXCLUDES 1   acquired torsion of penis (N48.82)
    Q55.64 Hidden **penis**   ♂
       Buried penis
       Concealed penis
       EXCLUDES 1   acquired buried penis (N48.83)
    Q55.69 Other **congenital malformation of penis**   ♂
       Congenital malformation of penis NOS

Q55.7 Congenital vasocutaneous fistula   ♂

Q55.8 Other specified congenital malformations of male genital organs   ♂

Q55.9 Congenital malformation of male genital organ, unspecified   ♂
    Congenital anomaly of male genital organ
    Congenital deformity of male genital organ

✓4ᵗʰ **Q56 Indeterminate sex and pseudohermaphroditism**
    EXCLUDES 1   46, XX true hermaphrodite (Q99.1)
               androgen insensitivity syndrome (E34.5-)
               chimera 46, XX/46, XY true hermaphrodite (Q99.0)
               female pseudohermaphroditism with adrenocortical disorder (E25.-)
               pseudohermaphroditism with specified chromosomal anomaly (Q96-Q99)
               pure gonadal dysgenesis (Q99.1)
    DEF: Indeterminate sex: External genitalia that is nondescript, lacking the physical appearance specific to either sex.
    DEF: Pseudohermaphroditism: Presence of gonads of one sex and external genitalia of another sex.

Q56.0 Hermaphroditism, not elsewhere classified
    Ovotestis

Q56.1 Male pseudohermaphroditism, not elsewhere classified   ♂
    46, XY with streak gonads
    Male pseudohermaphroditism NOS

Q56.2 Female pseudohermaphroditism, not elsewhere classified   ♀
    Female pseudohermaphroditism NOS

Q56.3 Pseudohermaphroditism, unspecified

Q56.4 Indeterminate sex, unspecified
    Ambiguous genitalia

✓ Additional Character Required   ✓x7ᵗʰ Placeholder   Unacceptable PDx   Questionable PDx   Manifestation   H1 - H14 HAC   HCC CMS-HCC Dx   HIV HIV Dx

ICD-10-CM 2019

909

Chapter 17. Congenital Malformations, Deformations and Chromosomal Abnormalities

Q52.2–Q56.4

Congenital malformations of the urinary system (Q60-Q64)

☑4ᵗʰ **Q60   Renal agenesis and other reduction defects of kidney**
  INCLUDES   congenital absence of kidney
            congenital atrophy of kidney
            infantile atrophy of kidney

  CC Excl: For CC codes in category Q60: PDX collection 1092

  Q60.0   Renal agenesis, unilateral   `CC`
  Q60.1   Renal agenesis, bilateral   `CC`
  Q60.2   Renal agenesis, unspecified   `CC`
  Q60.3   Renal hypoplasia, unilateral   `CC`
  Q60.4   Renal hypoplasia, bilateral   `CC`
  Q60.5   Renal hypoplasia, unspecified   `CC`
  Q60.6   Potter's syndrome   `CC`

☑4ᵗʰ **Q61   Cystic kidney disease**
  EXCLUDES 1   acquired cyst of kidney (N28.1)
              Potter's syndrome (Q60.6)

  ☑5ᵗʰ **Q61.0   Congenital renal cyst**
    Q61.00   Congenital renal cyst, unspecified   `CC`
              Cyst of kidney NOS (congenital)
              CC Excl: PDX collection 1093
    Q61.01   Congenital single renal cyst   `CC`
              CC Excl: PDX collection 1094
    Q61.02   Congenital multiple renal cysts   `CC`
              CC Excl: PDX collection 1095

  ☑5ᵗʰ **Q61.1   Polycystic kidney, infantile type**
              Polycystic kidney, autosomal recessive
    Q61.11   Cystic dilatation of collecting ducts   `CC`
              CC Excl: PDX collection 1096
    Q61.19   Other polycystic kidney, infantile type   `CC`
              CC Excl: PDX collection 1096

  Q61.2   Polycystic kidney, adult type   `CC`
            Polycystic kidney, autosomal dominant
            CC Excl: PDX collection 1096
  Q61.3   Polycystic kidney, unspecified   `CC`
            AHA: 2016, 3Q, 22
            CC Excl: PDX collection 1096
  Q61.4   Renal dysplasia   `CC`
            Multicystic dysplastic kidney
            Multicystic kidney (development)
            Multicystic kidney disease
            Multicystic renal dysplasia
            EXCLUDES 1   polycystic kidney disease (Q61.11-Q61.3)
            CC Excl: PDX collection 1097
  Q61.5   Medullary cystic kidney   `CC`
            Nephronopthisis
            Sponge kidney NOS
            DEF: Sponge kidney: Dilated collecting tubules that are usually
            asymptomatic. Calcinosis in tubules may cause renal insufficiency.
            CC Excl: PDX collection 1095
  Q61.8   Other cystic kidney diseases   `CC`
            Fibrocystic kidney
            Fibrocystic renal degeneration or disease
            CC Excl: PDX collection 1095
  Q61.9   Cystic kidney disease, unspecified   `CC`
            Meckel-Gruber syndrome
            CC Excl: PDX collection 1093

☑4ᵗʰ **Q62   Congenital obstructive defects of renal pelvis and congenital malformations of ureter**

  CC Excl: For CC codes in category Q62: PDX collection 1098

  Q62.0   Congenital hydronephrosis   `CC`
  ☑5ᵗʰ **Q62.1   Congenital occlusion of ureter**
              Atresia and stenosis of ureter
    Q62.10   Congenital occlusion of ureter, unspecified   `CC`
    Q62.11   Congenital occlusion of ureteropelvic junction   `CC`
    Q62.12   Congenital occlusion of ureterovesical orifice   `CC`
  Q62.2   Congenital megaureter   `CC`
            Congenital dilatation of ureter
  ☑5ᵗʰ **Q62.3   Other obstructive defects of renal pelvis and ureter**
    Q62.31   Congenital ureterocele, orthotopic   `CC`
    Q62.32   Cecoureterocele   `CC`
              Ectopic ureterocele
    Q62.39   Other obstructive defects of renal pelvis and ureter   `CC`
              Ureteropelvic junction obstruction NOS

  Q62.4   Agenesis of ureter
            Congenital absence ureter
  Q62.5   Duplication of ureter
            Accessory ureter
            Double ureter
  ☑5ᵗʰ **Q62.6   Malposition of ureter**
    Q62.60   Malposition of ureter, unspecified
    Q62.61   Deviation of ureter
    Q62.62   Displacement of ureter
    Q62.63   Anomalous implantation of ureter
              Ectopia of ureter
              Ectopic ureter
    Q62.69   Other malposition of ureter
  Q62.7   Congenital vesico-uretero-renal reflux
  Q62.8   Other congenital malformations of ureter
            Anomaly of ureter NOS

☑4ᵗʰ **Q63   Other congenital malformations of kidney**
  EXCLUDES 1   congenital nephrotic syndrome (N04.-)

  Q63.0   Accessory kidney
  Q63.1   Lobulated, fused and horseshoe kidney
  Q63.2   Ectopic kidney
            Congenital displaced kidney
            Malrotation of kidney
  Q63.3   Hyperplastic and giant kidney
            Compensatory hypertrophy of kidney
  Q63.8   Other specified congenital malformations of kidney
            Congenital renal calculi
  Q63.9   Congenital malformation of kidney, unspecified

☑4ᵗʰ **Q64   Other congenital malformations of urinary system**
  Q64.0   Epispadias
            EXCLUDES 1   hypospadias (Q54.-)
  ☑5ᵗʰ **Q64.1   Exstrophy of urinary bladder**

    CC Excl: For CC codes in subcategory Q64.1:
    PDX collection 1099

    Q64.10   Exstrophy of urinary bladder, unspecified   `CC`
              Ectopia vesicae
    Q64.11   Supravesical fissure of urinary bladder   `CC`
    Q64.12   Cloacal exstrophy of urinary bladder   `CC`
    Q64.19   Other exstrophy of urinary bladder   `CC`
              Extroversion of bladder
  Q64.2   Congenital posterior urethral valves   `CC`
            CC Excl: PDX collection 1100
  ☑5ᵗʰ **Q64.3   Other atresia and stenosis of urethra and bladder neck**

    CC Excl: For CC codes in subcategory Q64.3:
    PDX collection 1100

    Q64.31   Congenital bladder neck obstruction   `CC`
              Congenital obstruction of vesicourethral orifice
    Q64.32   Congenital stricture of urethra   `CC`
    Q64.33   Congenital stricture of urinary meatus   `CC`
    Q64.39   Other atresia and stenosis of urethra and bladder neck   `CC`
              Atresia and stenosis of urethra and bladder neck NOS
  Q64.4   Malformation of urachus
            Cyst of urachus
            Patent urachus
            Prolapse of urachus
  Q64.5   Congenital absence of bladder and urethra
  Q64.6   Congenital diverticulum of bladder
  ☑5ᵗʰ **Q64.7   Other and unspecified congenital malformations of bladder and urethra**
            EXCLUDES 1   congenital prolapse of bladder (mucosa) (Q79.4)
    Q64.70   Unspecified congenital malformation of bladder and urethra
              Malformation of bladder or urethra NOS
    Q64.71   Congenital prolapse of urethra
    Q64.72   Congenital prolapse of urinary meatus
    Q64.73   Congenital urethrorectal fistula
    Q64.74   Double urethra
    Q64.75   Double urinary meatus
    Q64.79   Other congenital malformations of bladder and urethra
  Q64.8   Other specified congenital malformations of urinary system

Q64.9 Congenital malformation of urinary system, unspecified
Congenital anomaly NOS of urinary system
Congenital deformity NOS of urinary system

Congenital malformations and deformations of the musculoskeletal system (Q65-Q79)

✓4ᵗʰ **Q65 Congenital deformities of** hip
    EXCLUDES 1 *clicking hip (R29.4)*

    ✓5ᵗʰ **Q65.0 Congenital** dislocation of hip, **unilateral**

       Q65.00 Congenital dislocation of unspecified **hip, unilateral**

       Q65.01 Congenital dislocation of right **hip, unilateral**

       Q65.02 Congenital dislocation of left **hip, unilateral**

    Q65.1 Congenital dislocation **of hip,** bilateral

    Q65.2 Congenital dislocation **of hip,** unspecified

    ✓5ᵗʰ **Q65.3 Congenital** partial dislocation **of hip,** unilateral

       Q65.30 Congenital partial dislocation of unspecified **hip, unilateral**

       Q65.31 Congenital partial dislocation of right **hip, unilateral**

       Q65.32 Congenital partial dislocation of left **hip, unilateral**

    Q65.4 Congenital partial dislocation **of hip,** bilateral

    Q65.5 Congenital partial dislocation **of hip,** unspecified

    Q65.6 Congenital unstable **hip**
       Congenital dislocatable hip

    ✓5ᵗʰ **Q65.8 Other** congenital deformities of hip

       Q65.81 Congenital coxa valga

       Q65.82 Congenital coxa vara

       Q65.89 Other specified congenital deformities of hip
          Anteversion of femoral neck
          Congenital acetabular dysplasia

    Q65.9 Congenital deformity of hip, unspecified

✓4ᵗʰ **Q66 Congenital deformities of** feet
    EXCLUDES 1 *reduction defects of feet (Q72.-)*
               valgus deformities (acquired) (M21.0-)
               varus deformities (acquired) (M21.1-)

    Q66.0 Congenital talipes equinovarus

    Q66.1 Congenital talipes calcaneovarus

    ✓5ᵗʰ **Q66.2 Congenital** metatarsus (primus) varus
       AHA: 2016, 4Q, 59

       Q66.21 Congenital metatarsus primus varus

       Q66.22 Congenital metatarsus adductus
          Congenital metatarsus varus

    Q66.3 Other congenital varus deformities of feet
       Hallux varus, congenital

    Q66.4 Congenital talipes calcaneovalgus

    ✓5ᵗʰ **Q66.5 Congenital** pes planus
       Congenital flat foot
       Congenital rigid flat foot
       Congenital spastic (everted) flat foot
       EXCLUDES 1 *pes planus, acquired (M21.4)*

       Q66.50 Congenital pes planus, unspecified **foot**

       Q66.51 Congenital pes planus, right **foot**

       Q66.52 Congenital pes planus, left **foot**

    Q66.6 Other congenital valgus deformities of feet
       Congenital metatarsus valgus

    Q66.7 Congenital pes cavus

    ✓5ᵗʰ **Q66.8 Other** congenital deformities of feet

       Q66.80 Congenital vertical talus deformity, unspecified **foot**

       Q66.81 Congenital vertical talus deformity, right **foot**

       Q66.82 Congenital vertical talus deformity, left **foot**

▲   **Q66.89 Other** specified congenital deformities of feet
          Congenital asymmetric talipes
          Congenital clubfoot NOS
          Congenital talipes NOS
          Congenital tarsal coalition
          Hammer toe, congenital
       DEF: Clubfoot: Congenital anomaly of the foot with the heel elevated and rotated outward and the toes pointing inward.

    Q66.9 Congenital deformity of feet, unspecified

✓4ᵗʰ **Q67 Congenital musculoskeletal deformities of** head, face, spine and chest
    EXCLUDES 1 *congenital malformation syndromes classified to Q87-*
               Potter's syndrome (Q60.6)

    Q67.0 Congenital facial asymmetry

    Q67.1 Congenital compression facies

    Q67.2 Dolichocephaly

    Q67.3 Plagiocephaly

    Q67.4 Other congenital deformities of skull, face and jaw
       Congenital depressions in skull
       Congenital hemifacial atrophy or hypertrophy
       Deviation of nasal septum, congenital
       Squashed or bent nose, congenital
       EXCLUDES 1 *dentofacial anomalies [including malocclusion]*
               (M26.-)
               syphilitic saddle nose (A50.5)
       DEF: Deviated septum: Condition in which the nasal septum, a thin wall composed of cartilage and bone that separates the two nostrils, is crooked or displaced from the midline.

    Q67.5 Congenital deformity of spine   `CC`
       Congenital postural scoliosis
       Congenital scoliosis NOS
       EXCLUDES 1 *infantile idiopathic scoliosis (M41.0)*
               scoliosis due to congenital bony malformation (Q76.3)
       AHA: 2014, 4Q, 26
       CC Excl: PDX collection 1101

    Q67.6 Pectus excavatum
       Congenital funnel chest

    Q67.7 Pectus carinatum
       Congenital pigeon chest

    Q67.8 Other congenital deformities of chest   `CC`
       Congenital deformity of chest wall NOS
       CC Excl: PDX collection 1102

✓4ᵗʰ **Q68 Other** congenital musculoskeletal deformities
    EXCLUDES 1 *reduction defects of limb(s) (Q71-Q73)*
    EXCLUDES 2 *congenital myotonic chondrodystrophy (G71.13)*

    Q68.0 Congenital deformity of sternocleidomastoid muscle
       Congenital contracture of sternocleidomastoid (muscle)
       Congenital (sternomastoid) torticollis
       Sternomastoid tumor (congenital)

    Q68.1 Congenital deformity of finger(s) and hand   `CC`
       Congenital clubfinger
       Spade-like hand (congenital)
       CC Excl: PDX collection 1102

    Q68.2 Congenital deformity of knee
       Congenital dislocation of knee
       Congenital genu recurvatum

    Q68.3 Congenital bowing of femur
       EXCLUDES 1 *anteversion of femur (neck) (Q65.89)*

    Q68.4 Congenital bowing of tibia and fibula

    Q68.5 Congenital bowing of long bones of leg, **unspecified**

    Q68.6 Discoid meniscus

    Q68.8 Other specified congenital musculoskeletal deformities
       Congenital deformity of clavicle
       Congenital deformity of elbow
       Congenital deformity of forearm
       Congenital deformity of scapula
       Congenital deformity of wrist
       Congenital dislocation of elbow
       Congenital dislocation of shoulder
       Congenital dislocation of wrist

✓4ᵗʰ **Q69** Polydactyly

    Q69.0 Accessory finger(s)

    Q69.1 Accessory thumb(s)

    Q69.2 Accessory toe(s)
       Accessory hallux

    Q69.9 Polydactyly, unspecified
       Supernumerary digit(s) NOS

✓4ᵗʰ **Q70** Syndactyly

    ✓5ᵗʰ **Q70.0** Fused fingers
       Complex syndactyly of fingers with synostosis

       Q70.00 Fused fingers, unspecified **hand**

       Q70.01 Fused fingers, right **hand**

       Q70.02 Fused fingers, left **hand**

       Q70.03 Fused fingers, bilateral

✓ Additional Character Required   ✓x7ᵗʰ Placeholder   Unacceptable PDx   Questionable PDx   Manifestation   **H1 - H14** HAC   **HCC** CMS-HCC Dx   **HIV** HIV Dx

ICD-10-CM 2019   911

√5ᵗʰ **Q70.1 Webbed fingers**
Simple syndactyly of fingers without synostosis
- **Q70.10 Webbed fingers, unspecified hand**
- **Q70.11 Webbed fingers, right hand**
- **Q70.12 Webbed fingers, left hand**
- **Q70.13 Webbed fingers, bilateral**

√5ᵗʰ **Q70.2 Fused toes**
Complex syndactyly of toes with synostosis
- **Q70.20 Fused toes, unspecified foot**
- **Q70.21 Fused toes, right foot**
- **Q70.22 Fused toes, left foot**
- **Q70.23 Fused toes, bilateral**

√5ᵗʰ **Q70.3 Webbed toes**
Simple syndactyly of toes without synostosis
- **Q70.30 Webbed toes, unspecified foot**
- **Q70.31 Webbed toes, right foot**
- **Q70.32 Webbed toes, left foot**
- **Q70.33 Webbed toes, bilateral**

Q70.4 Polysyndactyly, unspecified
> **EXCLUDES 1**   specified syndactyly of hand and feet—code to specified conditions (Q70.0-Q70.3-)

Q70.9 Syndactyly, unspecified
Symphalangy NOS

√4ᵗʰ **Q71 Reduction defects of upper limb**

√5ᵗʰ **Q71.0 Congenital complete absence of upper limb**
- **Q71.00 Congenital complete absence of unspecified upper limb**
- **Q71.01 Congenital complete absence of right upper limb**
- **Q71.02 Congenital complete absence of left upper limb**
- **Q71.03 Congenital complete absence of upper limb, bilateral**

√5ᵗʰ **Q71.1 Congenital absence of upper arm and forearm with hand present**
- **Q71.10 Congenital absence of unspecified upper arm and forearm with hand present**
- **Q71.11 Congenital absence of right upper arm and forearm with hand present**
- **Q71.12 Congenital absence of left upper arm and forearm with hand present**
- **Q71.13 Congenital absence of upper arm and forearm with hand present, bilateral**

√5ᵗʰ **Q71.2 Congenital absence of both forearm and hand**
- **Q71.20 Congenital absence of both forearm and hand, unspecified upper limb**
- **Q71.21 Congenital absence of both forearm and hand, right upper limb**
- **Q71.22 Congenital absence of both forearm and hand, left upper limb**
- **Q71.23 Congenital absence of both forearm and hand, bilateral**

√5ᵗʰ **Q71.3 Congenital absence of hand and finger**
- **Q71.30 Congenital absence of unspecified hand and finger**
- **Q71.31 Congenital absence of right hand and finger**
- **Q71.32 Congenital absence of left hand and finger**
- **Q71.33 Congenital absence of hand and finger, bilateral**

√5ᵗʰ **Q71.4 Longitudinal reduction defect of radius**
Clubhand (congenital)
Radial clubhand
- **Q71.40 Longitudinal reduction defect of unspecified radius**
- **Q71.41 Longitudinal reduction defect of right radius**
- **Q71.42 Longitudinal reduction defect of left radius**
- **Q71.43 Longitudinal reduction defect of radius, bilateral**

√5ᵗʰ **Q71.5 Longitudinal reduction defect of ulna**
- **Q71.50 Longitudinal reduction defect of unspecified ulna**
- **Q71.51 Longitudinal reduction defect of right ulna**
- **Q71.52 Longitudinal reduction defect of left ulna**
- **Q71.53 Longitudinal reduction defect of ulna, bilateral**

√5ᵗʰ **Q71.6 Lobster-claw hand**
- **Q71.60 Lobster-claw hand, unspecified hand**
- **Q71.61 Lobster-claw right hand**
- **Q71.62 Lobster-claw left hand**
- **Q71.63 Lobster-claw hand, bilateral**

√5ᵗʰ **Q71.8 Other reduction defects of upper limb**

√6ᵗʰ **Q71.81 Congenital shortening of upper limb**
- **Q71.811 Congenital shortening of right upper limb**
- **Q71.812 Congenital shortening of left upper limb**
- **Q71.813 Congenital shortening of upper limb, bilateral**
- **Q71.819 Congenital shortening of unspecified upper limb**

√6ᵗʰ **Q71.89 Other reduction defects of upper limb**
- **Q71.891 Other reduction defects of right upper limb**
- **Q71.892 Other reduction defects of left upper limb**
- **Q71.893 Other reduction defects of upper limb, bilateral**
- **Q71.899 Other reduction defects of unspecified upper limb**

√5ᵗʰ **Q71.9 Unspecified reduction defect of upper limb**
- **Q71.90 Unspecified reduction defect of unspecified upper limb**
- **Q71.91 Unspecified reduction defect of right upper limb**
- **Q71.92 Unspecified reduction defect of left upper limb**
- **Q71.93 Unspecified reduction defect of upper limb, bilateral**

√4ᵗʰ **Q72 Reduction defects of lower limb**

√5ᵗʰ **Q72.0 Congenital complete absence of lower limb**
- **Q72.00 Congenital complete absence of unspecified lower limb**
- **Q72.01 Congenital complete absence of right lower limb**
- **Q72.02 Congenital complete absence of left lower limb**
- **Q72.03 Congenital complete absence of lower limb, bilateral**

√5ᵗʰ **Q72.1 Congenital absence of thigh and lower leg with foot present**
- **Q72.10 Congenital absence of unspecified thigh and lower leg with foot present**
- **Q72.11 Congenital absence of right thigh and lower leg with foot present**
- **Q72.12 Congenital absence of left thigh and lower leg with foot present**
- **Q72.13 Congenital absence of thigh and lower leg with foot present, bilateral**

√5ᵗʰ **Q72.2 Congenital absence of both lower leg and foot**
- **Q72.20 Congenital absence of both lower leg and foot, unspecified lower limb**
- **Q72.21 Congenital absence of both lower leg and foot, right lower limb**
- **Q72.22 Congenital absence of both lower leg and foot, left lower limb**
- **Q72.23 Congenital absence of both lower leg and foot, bilateral**

√5ᵗʰ **Q72.3 Congenital absence of foot and toe(s)**
- **Q72.30 Congenital absence of unspecified foot and toe(s)**
- **Q72.31 Congenital absence of right foot and toe(s)**
- **Q72.32 Congenital absence of left foot and toe(s)**
- **Q72.33 Congenital absence of foot and toe(s), bilateral**

√5ᵗʰ **Q72.4 Longitudinal reduction defect of femur**
Proximal femoral focal deficiency
- **Q72.40 Longitudinal reduction defect of unspecified femur**
- **Q72.41 Longitudinal reduction defect of right femur**
- **Q72.42 Longitudinal reduction defect of left femur**
- **Q72.43 Longitudinal reduction defect of femur, bilateral**

√5ᵗʰ **Q72.5 Longitudinal reduction defect of tibia**
- **Q72.50 Longitudinal reduction defect of unspecified tibia**
- **Q72.51 Longitudinal reduction defect of right tibia**
- **Q72.52 Longitudinal reduction defect of left tibia**
- **Q72.53 Longitudinal reduction defect of tibia, bilateral**

√5ᵗʰ **Q72.6 Longitudinal reduction defect of fibula**
- **Q72.60 Longitudinal reduction defect of unspecified fibula**
- **Q72.61 Longitudinal reduction defect of right fibula**
- **Q72.62 Longitudinal reduction defect of left fibula**
- **Q72.63 Longitudinal reduction defect of fibula, bilateral**

√5ᵗʰ **Q72.7 Split foot**
- **Q72.70 Split foot, unspecified lower limb**
- **Q72.71 Split foot, right lower limb**
- **Q72.72 Split foot, left lower limb**

Ⓝ Newborn: 0   Ⓟ Pediatric: 0-17   Ⓜ Maternity: 12-55   Ⓐ Adult: 15-124   **MCC** Major Complication/Comorbidity   **CC** Complication/Comorbidity   **SW** Severe Wound Dx

912   ICD-10-CM 2019

Q72.73 **Split foot,** bilateral

✓5ᵗʰ Q72.8 Other **reduction defects of lower limb**

    ✓6ᵗʰ **Q72.81 Congenital** shortening **of lower limb**

        Q72.811 **Congenital shortening of** right **lower limb**

        Q72.812 **Congenital shortening of** left **lower limb**

        Q72.813 **Congenital shortening of lower limb,** bilateral

        Q72.819 **Congenital shortening of** unspecified **lower limb**

    ✓6ᵗʰ **Q72.89** Other **reduction defects of lower limb**

        Q72.891 **Other reduction defects of** right **lower limb**

        Q72.892 **Other reduction defects of** left **lower limb**

        Q72.893 **Other reduction defects of lower limb,** bilateral

        Q72.899 **Other reduction defects of** unspecified **lower limb**

✓5ᵗʰ Q72.9 Unspecified **reduction defect of lower limb**

    Q72.90 **Unspecified reduction defect of** unspecified **lower limb**

    Q72.91 **Unspecified reduction defect of** right **lower limb**

    Q72.92 **Unspecified reduction defect of** left **lower limb**

    Q72.93 **Unspecified reduction defect of lower limb,** bilateral

✓4ᵗʰ **Q73 Reduction defects of** unspecified **limb**

    Q73.0 Congenital absence **of unspecified limb(s)**
        Amelia NOS

    Q73.1 Phocomelia, **unspecified limb(s)**
        Phocomelia NOS

    Q73.8 Other **reduction defects of unspecified limb(s)**
        Longitudinal reduction deformity of unspecified limb(s)
        Ectromelia of limb NOS
        Hemimelia of limb NOS
        Reduction defect of limb NOS

✓4ᵗʰ **Q74** Other **congenital malformations of limb(s)**

    EXCLUDES 1 *polydactyly (Q69.-)*
                reduction defect of limb (Q71-Q73)
                syndactyly (Q70.-)

    Q74.0 Other congenital malformations of upper limb(s), **including shoulder girdle**
        Accessory carpal bones
        Cleidocranial dysostosis
        Congenital pseudarthrosis of clavicle
        Macrodactylia (fingers)
        Madelung's deformity
        Radioulnar synostosis
        Sprengel's deformity
        Triphalangeal thumb

    Q74.1 Congenital malformation of knee
        Congenital absence of patella
        Congenital dislocation of patella
        Congenital genu valgum
        Congenital genu varum
        Rudimentary patella
        EXCLUDES 1 *congenital dislocation of knee (Q68.2)*
                   congenital genu recurvatum (Q68.2)
                   nail patella syndrome (Q87.2)

    Q74.2 Other congenital malformations of lower limb(s), **including pelvic girdle**
        Congenital fusion of sacroiliac joint
        Congenital malformation of ankle joint
        Congenital malformation of sacroiliac joint
        EXCLUDES 1 *anteversion of femur (neck) (Q65.89)*

    Q74.3 Arthrogryposis multiplex congenita **cc**
        CC Excl: PDX collection 1102

    Q74.8 Other specified **congenital malformations of limb(s)**

    Q74.9 Unspecified **congenital malformation of limb(s)**
        Congenital anomaly of limb(s) NOS

✓4ᵗʰ **Q75 Other congenital malformations of** skull and face bones

    EXCLUDES 1 *congenital malformation of face NOS (Q18.-)*
                congenital malformation syndromes classified to Q87.-
                dentofacial anomalies [including malocclusion] (M26.-)
                musculoskeletal deformities of head and face (Q67.0-Q67.4)
                skull defects associated with congenital anomalies of brain
                    such as:
                    anencephaly (Q00.0)
                    encephalocele (Q01.-)
                    hydrocephalus (Q03.-)
                    microcephaly (Q02)

    Q75.0 Craniosynostosis
        Acrocephaly
        Imperfect fusion of skull
        Oxycephaly
        Trigonocephaly
        DEF: Congenital condition in which one or more of the cranial sutures fuse prematurely, creating a deformed or aberrant head shape.

    Q75.1 Craniofacial dysostosis
        Crouzon's disease

    Q75.2 Hypertelorism

    Q75.3 Macrocephaly

    Q75.4 Mandibulofacial dysostosis
        Franceschetti syndrome
        Treacher Collins syndrome

    Q75.5 Oculomandibular dysostosis

    Q75.8 Other specified congenital malformations of skull and face bones
        Absence of skull bone, congenital
        Congenital deformity of forehead
        Platybasia

    Q75.9 Congenital malformation of skull and face bones, unspecified
        Congenital anomaly of face bones NOS
        Congenital anomaly of skull NOS

✓4ᵗʰ **Q76 Congenital malformations of** spine and bony thorax

    EXCLUDES 1 *congenital musculoskeletal deformities of spine and chest (Q67.5-Q67.8)*

    Q76.0 Spina bifida occulta
        EXCLUDES 1 *meningocele (spinal) (Q05.-)*
                 spina bifida (aperta) (cystica) (Q05.-)

    Q76.1 Klippel-Feil syndrome
        Cervical fusion syndrome

    Q76.2 Congenital spondylolisthesis
        Congenital spondylolysis
        EXCLUDES 1 *spondylolisthesis (acquired) (M43.1-)*
                 spondylolysis (acquired) (M43.0-)

    Q76.3 Congenital scoliosis due to congenital bony malformation **cc**
        Hemivertebra fusion or failure of segmentation with scoliosis
        CC Excl: PDX collection 1101

✓5ᵗʰ **Q76.4 Other congenital malformations of spine, not associated with scoliosis**

        CC Excl: For CC codes in subcategory Q76.4:
        PDX collection 1101

    ✓6ᵗʰ **Q76.41 Congenital** kyphosis

        Q76.411 **Congenital kyphosis,** occipito-atlanto-axial **region**

        Q76.412 **Congenital kyphosis,** cervical **region**

        Q76.413 **Congenital kyphosis,** cervicothoracic **region**

        Q76.414 **Congenital kyphosis,** thoracic **region**

        Q76.415 **Congenital kyphosis,** thoracolumbar **region**

        Q76.419 **Congenital kyphosis,** unspecified **region**

    ✓6ᵗʰ **Q76.42 Congenital** lordosis

        Q76.425 **Congenital lordosis,** thoracolumbar **region** **cc**

        Q76.426 **Congenital lordosis,** lumbar **region** **cc**

        Q76.427 **Congenital lordosis,** lumbosacral **region** **cc**

        Q76.428 **Congenital lordosis,** sacral and sacrococcygeal **region** **cc**

        Q76.429 **Congenital lordosis,** unspecified **region** **cc**

✓ Additional Character Required   ✓x7ᵗʰ Placeholder   Unacceptable PDx   Questionable PDx   Manifestation   H1-H14 HAC   HCC CMS-HCC Dx   HIV HIV Dx

ICD-10-CM 2019   913

Q76.49 Other congenital malformations of spine, not associated with scoliosis
Congenital absence of vertebra NOS
Congenital fusion of spine NOS
Congenital malformation of lumbosacral (joint) (region) NOS
Congenital malformation of spine NOS
Hemivertebra NOS
Malformation of spine NOS
Platyspondylisis NOS
Supernumerary vertebra NOS

Q76.5 Cervical rib
Supernumerary rib in cervical region

Q76.6 Other congenital malformations of ribs   CC
Accessory rib
Congenital absence of rib
Congenital fusion of ribs
Congenital malformation of ribs NOS
EXCLUDES 1   *short rib syndrome (Q77.2)*
CC Excl: PDX collection 1103

Q76.7 Congenital malformation of sternum   CC
Congenital absence of sternum
Sternum bifidum
CC Excl: PDX collection 1103

Q76.8 Other congenital malformations of bony thorax   CC
CC Excl: PDX collection 1103

Q76.9 Congenital malformation of bony thorax, unspecified   CC
CC Excl: PDX collection 1103

✓4th **Q77 Osteochondrodysplasia with defects of growth of tubular bones and spine**
EXCLUDES 1   *mucopolysaccharidosis (E76.0-E76.3)*
EXCLUDES 2   *congenital myotonic chondrodystrophy (G71.13)*

Q77.0 Achondrogenesis
Hypochondrogenesis

Q77.1 Thanatophoric short stature

Q77.2 Short rib syndrome   CC
Asphyxiating thoracic dysplasia [Jeune]
CC Excl: PDX collection 1103

Q77.3 Chondrodysplasia punctata
EXCLUDES 1   *Rhizomelic chondrodysplasia punctata (E71.43)*

Q77.4 Achondroplasia
Hypochondroplasia
Osteosclerosis congenita

Q77.5 Diastrophic dysplasia

Q77.6 Chondroectodermal dysplasia
Ellis-van Creveld syndrome

Q77.7 Spondyloepiphyseal dysplasia

Q77.8 Other osteochondrodysplasia with defects of growth of tubular bones and spine

Q77.9 Osteochondrodysplasia with defects of growth of tubular bones and spine, unspecified

✓4th **Q78 Other osteochondrodysplasias**
EXCLUDES 2   *congenital myotonic chondrodystrophy (G71.13)*

Q78.0 Osteogenesis imperfecta   CC
Fragilitas ossium
Osteopsathyrosis
CC Excl: PDX collection 1104

Q78.1 Polyostotic fibrous dysplasia
Albright(-McCune)(-Sternberg) syndrome

Q78.2 Osteopetrosis   CC
Albers-Schönberg syndrome
Osteosclerosis NOS
DEF: Rare congenital condition in which the bones are excessively dense, resulting from a discrepancy in the formation and breakdown of bone.
CC Excl: PDX collection 1104

Q78.3 Progressive diaphyseal dysplasia
Camurati-Engelmann syndrome

Q78.4 Enchondromatosis
Maffucci's syndrome
Ollier's disease

Q78.5 Metaphyseal dysplasia
Pyle's syndrome

Q78.6 Multiple congenital exostoses
Diaphyseal aclasis

Q78.8 Other specified osteochondrodysplasias
Osteopoikilosis

Q78.9 Osteochondrodysplasia, unspecified
Chondrodystrophy NOS
Osteodystrophy NOS

✓4th **Q79 Congenital malformations of musculoskeletal system, not elsewhere classified**
EXCLUDES 2   *congenital (sternomastoid) torticollis (Q68.0)*

CC Excl: For CC/MCC codes in category Q79, unless otherwise noted: PDX collection 1106

Q79.0 Congenital diaphragmatic hernia   MCC
EXCLUDES 1   *congenital hiatus hernia (Q40.1)*
CC Excl: PDX collection 1105

Q79.1 Other congenital malformations of diaphragm   MCC
Absence of diaphragm
Congenital malformation of diaphragm NOS
Eventration of diaphragm
CC Excl: PDX collection 1105

Q79.2 Exomphalos   MCC
Omphalocele
EXCLUDES 1   *umbilical hernia (K42.-)*

Q79.3 Gastroschisis   MCC

Gastroschisis

Herniated small bowel (gastroschisis)
Rectus abdominus m.
Umbilicus
skin
distal
proximal
Defect

Q79.4 Prune belly syndrome   MCC
Congenital prolapse of bladder mucosa
Eagle-Barrett syndrome

✓5th **Q79.5 Other congenital malformations of abdominal wall**
EXCLUDES 1   *umbilical hernia (K42.-)*

Q79.51 Congenital hernia of bladder   MCC

Q79.59 Other congenital malformations of abdominal wall   MCC

Q79.6 Ehlers-Danlos syndrome   CC
DEF: Connective tissue disorder that causes hyperextended skin and joints and results in fragile blood vessels with bleeding, poor wound healing, and subcutaneous pseudotumors.
CC Excl: PDX collection 1107

Q79.8 Other congenital malformations of musculoskeletal system
Absence of muscle
Absence of tendon
Accessory muscle
Amyotrophia congenita
Congenital constricting bands
Congenital shortening of tendon
Poland syndrome

Q79.9 Congenital malformation of musculoskeletal system, unspecified
Congenital anomaly of musculoskeletal system NOS
Congenital deformity of musculoskeletal system NOS

Other congenital malformations (Q80-Q89)

✓4th **Q80 Congenital ichthyosis**
EXCLUDES 1   *Refsum's disease (G60.1)*
DEF: Excessive production of skin cells resulting in red, dry, scaly skin.

Q80.0 Ichthyosis vulgaris

Q80.1 X-linked ichthyosis

Q80.2 Lamellar ichthyosis
Collodion baby

Q80.3 Congenital bullous ichthyosiform erythroderma

Q80.4 Harlequin fetus

Q80.8 Other congenital ichthyosis

Q80.9 Congenital ichthyosis, unspecified

N Newborn: 0   P Pediatric: 0-17   M Maternity: 12-55   A Adult: 15-124   MCC Major Complication/Comorbidity   CC Complication/Comorbidity   SW Severe Wound Dx

914   ICD-10-CM 2019

✓4ᵗʰ Q81   Epidermolysis bullosa

Q81.0   Epidermolysis bullosa simplex
    EXCLUDES 1   *Cockayne's syndrome (Q87.1)*

Q81.1   Epidermolysis bullosa letalis
    Herlitz' syndrome

Q81.2   Epidermolysis bullosa dystrophica

Q81.8   Other epidermolysis bullosa

Q81.9   Epidermolysis bullosa, unspecified

✓4ᵗʰ Q82   Other congenital malformations of skin
    EXCLUDES 1   *acrodermatitis enteropathica (E83.2)*
        congenital erythropoietic porphyria (E80.0)
        pilonidal cyst or sinus (L05.-)
        Sturge-Weber (-Dimitri) syndrome (Q85.8)

Q82.0   Hereditary lymphedema

Q82.1   Xeroderma pigmentosum

Q82.2   Congenital cutaneous mastocytosis
    Congenital diffuse cutaneous mastocytosis
    Congenital maculopapular cutaneous mastocytosis
    Congenital urticaria pigmentosa
    EXCLUDES 1   *cutaneous mastocytosis NOS (D47.01)*
        diffuse cutaneous mastocytosis (with onset after
          newborn period) (D47.01)
        malignant mastocytosis (C96.2-)
        systemic mastocytosis (D47.02)
        urticaria pigmentosa (non-congenital) (with onset
          after newborn period) (D47.01)
    AHA: 2017, 4Q, 5

Q82.3   Incontinentia pigmenti

Q82.4   Ectodermal dysplasia (anhidrotic)
    EXCLUDES 1   *Ellis-van Creveld syndrome (Q77.6)*

Q82.5   Congenital non-neoplastic nevus
    Birthmark NOS
    Flammeus Nevus
    Portwine Nevus
    Sanguineous Nevus
    Strawberry Nevus
    Vascular Nevus NOS
    Verrucous Nevus
    EXCLUDES 2   *araneus nevus (I78.1)*
        café au lait spots (L81.3)
        lentigo (L81.4)
        melanocytic nevus (D22.-)
        nevus NOS (D22.-)
        pigmented nevus (D22.-)
        spider nevus (I78.1)
        stellar nevus (I78.1)

Q82.6   Congenital sacral dimple
    Parasacral dimple
    EXCLUDES 2   *pilonidal cyst with abscess (L05.01)*
        pilonidal cyst without abscess (L05.91)
    AHA: 2016, 4Q, 60

Q82.8   Other specified congenital malformations of skin
    Abnormal palmar creases
    Accessory skin tags
    Benign familial pemphigus [Hailey-Hailey]
    Congenital poikiloderma
    Cutis laxa (hyperelastica)
    Dermatoglyphic anomalies
    Inherited keratosis palmaris et plantaris
    Keratosis follicularis [Darier-White]
    EXCLUDES 1   *Ehlers-Danlos syndrome (Q79.6)*
    AHA: 2016, 1Q, 17

Q82.9   Congenital malformation of skin, unspecified

✓4ᵗʰ Q83   Congenital malformations of breast
    EXCLUDES 2   *absence of pectoral muscle (Q79.8)*
        hypoplasia of breast (N64.82)
        micromastia (N64.82)

Q83.0   Congenital absence of breast with absent nipple

Q83.1   Accessory breast
    Supernumerary breast

Q83.2   Absent nipple

Q83.3   Accessory nipple
    Supernumerary nipple

Q83.8   Other congenital malformations of breast

Q83.9   Congenital malformation of breast, unspecified

✓4ᵗʰ Q84   Other congenital malformations of integument

Q84.0   Congenital alopecia
    Congenital atrichosis

Q84.1   Congenital morphological disturbances of hair, not elsewhere classified
    Beaded hair
    Monilethrix
    Pili annulati
    EXCLUDES 1   *Menkes' kinky hair syndrome (E83.0)*

Q84.2   Other congenital malformations of hair
    Congenital hypertrichosis
    Congenital malformation of hair NOS
    Persistent lanugo

Q84.3   Anonychia
    EXCLUDES 1   *nail patella syndrome (Q87.2)*

Q84.4   Congenital leukonychia

Q84.5   Enlarged and hypertrophic nails
    Congenital onychauxis
    Pachyonychia

Q84.6   Other congenital malformations of nails
    Congenital clubnail
    Congenital koilonychia
    Congenital malformation of nail NOS

Q84.8   Other specified congenital malformations of integument
    Aplasia cutis congenita

Q84.9   Congenital malformation of integument, unspecified
    Congenital anomaly of integument NOS
    Congenital deformity of integument NOS

✓4ᵗʰ Q85   Phakomatoses, not elsewhere classified
    EXCLUDES 1   *ataxia telangiectasia [Louis-Bar] (G11.3)*
        familial dysautonomia [Riley-Day] (G90.1)

✓5ᵗʰ Q85.0   Neurofibromatosis (nonmalignant)

Q85.00   Neurofibromatosis, unspecified   `HCC`

Q85.01   Neurofibromatosis, type 1   `HCC`
    Von Recklinghausen disease

Q85.02   Neurofibromatosis, type 2   `HCC`
    Acoustic neurofibromatosis
    DEF: Inherited condition with cutaneous lesions, benign tumors of peripheral nerves, and bilateral 8th nerve masses.

Q85.03   Schwannomatosis   `HCC`
    DEF: Genetic mutation (SMARCB1/INI1) causing multiple benign tumors along the nerve pathways, except on the 8th cranial (vestibular) nerve.

Q85.09   Other neurofibromatosis   `HCC`

Q85.1   Tuberous sclerosis   `CC` `HCC`
    Bourneville's disease
    Epiloia
    CC Excl: PDX collection 1108

Q85.8   Other phakomatoses, not elsewhere classified   `CC` `HCC`
    Peutz-Jeghers Syndrome
    Sturge-Weber(-Dimitri) syndrome
    von Hippel-Lindau syndrome
    EXCLUDES 1   *Meckel-Gruber syndrome (Q61.9)*
    CC Excl: PDX collection 1109

Q85.9   Phakomatosis, unspecified   `CC` `HCC`
    Hamartosis NOS
    CC Excl: PDX collection 1109

✓4ᵗʰ Q86   Congenital malformation syndromes due to known exogenous causes, not elsewhere classified
    EXCLUDES 2   *iodine-deficiency-related hypothyroidism (E00-E02)*
        nonteratogenic effects of substances transmitted via placenta
        or breast milk (P04.-)

Q86.0   Fetal alcohol syndrome (dysmorphic)

Q86.1   Fetal hydantoin syndrome
    Meadow's syndrome

Q86.2   Dysmorphism due to warfarin

Q86.8   Other congenital malformation syndromes due to known exogenous causes

---

✓ Additional Character Required   ✓x7ᵗʰ Placeholder   Unacceptable PDx   Questionable PDx   Manifestation   H1 - H14 HAC   HCC CMS-HCC Dx   HIV HIV Dx

✓4ᵗʰ Q87 Other specified congenital malformation syndromes affecting multiple systems

Use additional code(s) to identify all associated manifestations

CC Excl: For CC codes in category Q87, unless otherwise noted: PDX collection 540

Q87.0 Congenital malformation syndromes predominantly affecting facial appearance
Acrocephalopolysyndactyly
Acrocephalosyndactyly [Apert]
Cryptophthalmos syndrome
Cyclopia
Goldenhar syndrome
Moebius syndrome
Oro-facial-digital syndrome
Robin syndrome
Whistling face

Q87.1 Congenital malformation syndromes predominantly associated with short stature CC
Aarskog syndrome
Cockayne syndrome
De Lange syndrome
Dubowitz syndrome
Noonan syndrome
Prader-Willi syndrome
Robinow-Silverman-Smith syndrome
Russell-Silver syndrome
Seckel syndrome
EXCLUDES 1 Ellis-van Creveld syndrome (Q77.6)
Smith-Lemli-Opitz syndrome (E78.72)
CC Excl: PDX collection 1110

Q87.2 Congenital malformation syndromes predominantly involving limbs CC
Holt-Oram syndrome
Klippel-Trenaunay-Weber syndrome
Nail patella syndrome
Rubinstein-Taybi syndrome
Sirenomelia syndrome
Thrombocytopenia with absent radius [TAR] syndrome
VATER syndrome

Q87.3 Congenital malformation syndromes involving early overgrowth CC
Beckwith-Wiedemann syndrome
Sotos syndrome
Weaver syndrome

✓5ᵗʰ Q87.4 Marfan's syndrome
DEF: Disorder that affects the connective tissue of multiple systems, including disproportionally long or abnormal bone structure and eye and cardiovascular complications.

CC Excl: For CC codes in subcategory Q87.4: PDX collection 1110

Q87.40 Marfan's syndrome, unspecified CC
✓6ᵗʰ Q87.41 Marfan's syndrome with cardiovascular manifestations
Q87.410 Marfan's syndrome with aortic dilation CC
Q87.418 Marfan's syndrome with other cardiovascular manifestations CC
Q87.42 Marfan's syndrome with ocular manifestations CC
Q87.43 Marfan's syndrome with skeletal manifestation CC
Q87.5 Other congenital malformation syndromes with other skeletal changes CC

✓5ᵗʰ Q87.8 Other specified congenital malformation syndromes, not elsewhere classified
EXCLUDES 1 Zellweger syndrome (E71.510)
Q87.81 Alport syndrome CC
Use additional code to identify stage of chronic kidney disease (N18.1-N18.6)
Q87.82 Arterial tortuosity syndrome CC
AHA: 2016, 4Q, 60-61
Q87.89 Other specified congenital malformation syndromes, not elsewhere classified CC
Laurence-Moon (-Bardet)-Biedl syndrome

✓4ᵗʰ Q89 Other congenital malformations, not elsewhere classified

✓5ᵗʰ Q89.0 Congenital absence and malformations of spleen
EXCLUDES 1 isomerism of atrial appendages (with asplenia or polysplenia) (Q20.6)
Q89.01 Asplenia (congenital) CC
CC Excl: PDX collection 1111

Q89.09 Congenital malformations of spleen CC
Congenital splenomegaly
CC Excl: PDX collection 1111

Q89.1 Congenital malformations of adrenal gland
EXCLUDES 1 adrenogenital disorders (E25.-)
congenital adrenal hyperplasia (E25.0)

Q89.2 Congenital malformations of other endocrine glands
Congenital malformation of parathyroid or thyroid gland
Persistent thyroglossal duct
Thyroglossal cyst
EXCLUDES 1 congenital goiter (E03.0)
congenital hypothyroidism (E03.1)

Q89.3 Situs inversus CC
Dextrocardia with situs inversus
Mirror-image atrial arrangement with situs inversus
Situs inversus or transversus abdominalis
Situs inversus or transversus thoracis
Transposition of abdominal viscera
Transposition of thoracic viscera
EXCLUDES 1 dextrocardia NOS (Q24.0)
DEF: Congenital anomaly in which the internal thoracic and abdominal organs are transposed laterally and found on the opposite side from the normal position.
CC Excl: PDX collection 1112

Q89.4 Conjoined twins MCC
Craniopagus
Dicephaly
Pygopagus
Thoracopagus
CC Excl: PDX collection 1113

Q89.7 Multiple congenital malformations, not elsewhere classified CC
Multiple congenital anomalies NOS
Multiple congenital deformities NOS
EXCLUDES 1 congenital malformation syndromes affecting multiple systems (Q87.-)
CC Excl: PDX collection 1112

Q89.8 Other specified congenital malformations CC
Use additional code(s) to identify all associated manifestations
CC Excl: PDX collection 540

Q89.9 Congenital malformation, unspecified
Congenital anomaly NOS
Congenital deformity NOS

Chromosomal abnormalities, not elsewhere classified (Q90-Q99)
EXCLUDES 2 mitochondrial metabolic disorders (E88.4-)

✓4ᵗʰ Q90 Down syndrome
Use additional code(s) to identify any associated physical conditions and degree of intellectual disabilities (F70-F79)
Q90.0 Trisomy 21, nonmosaicism (meiotic nondisjunction)
Q90.1 Trisomy 21, mosaicism (mitotic nondisjunction)
Q90.2 Trisomy 21, translocation
Q90.9 Down syndrome, unspecified
Trisomy 21 NOS

✓4ᵗʰ Q91 Trisomy 18 and Trisomy 13

CC Excl: For CC codes in category Q91: PDX collection 1114

Q91.0 Trisomy 18, nonmosaicism (meiotic nondisjunction) CC
Q91.1 Trisomy 18, mosaicism (mitotic nondisjunction) CC
Q91.2 Trisomy 18, translocation CC
Q91.3 Trisomy 18, unspecified CC
Q91.4 Trisomy 13, nonmosaicism (meiotic nondisjunction) CC
Q91.5 Trisomy 13, mosaicism (mitotic nondisjunction) CC
Q91.6 Trisomy 13, translocation CC
Q91.7 Trisomy 13, unspecified CC

✓4ᵗʰ Q92 Other trisomies and partial trisomies of the autosomes, not elsewhere classified
INCLUDES unbalanced translocations and insertions
EXCLUDES 1 trisomies of chromosomes 13, 18, 21 (Q90-Q91)
Q92.0 Whole chromosome trisomy, nonmosaicism (meiotic nondisjunction)
Q92.1 Whole chromosome trisomy, mosaicism (mitotic nondisjunction)
Q92.2 Partial trisomy
Less than whole arm duplicated
Whole arm or more duplicated
EXCLUDES 1 partial trisomy due to unbalanced translocation (Q92.5)

N Newborn: 0   **P** Pediatric: 0-17   **M** Maternity: 12-55   **A** Adult: 15-124   **MCC** Major Complication/Comorbidity   **CC** Complication/Comorbidity   **SW** Severe Wound Dx

916   ICD-10-CM 2019

Q92.5   **Duplications** with other complex rearrangements
      Partial trisomy due to unbalanced translocations
      Code also any associated deletions due to unbalanced
        translocations, inversions and insertions (Q93.7)

✓5ᵗʰ   Q92.6   **Marker chromosomes**
      Trisomies due to dicentrics
      Trisomies due to extra rings
      Trisomies due to isochromosomes
      Individual with marker heterochromatin

     Q92.61   **Marker chromosomes in normal individual**

     Q92.62   **Marker chromosomes in abnormal individual**

Q92.7   **Triploidy and polyploidy**

Q92.8   **Other specified trisomies and partial trisomies of autosomes**
      Duplications identified by fluorescence in situ hybridization
        (FISH)
      Duplications identified by in situ hybridization (ISH)
      Duplications seen only at prometaphase

Q92.9   **Trisomy and partial trisomy of autosomes, unspecified**

✓4ᵗʰ   **Q93**   **Monosomies and deletions from the autosomes, not elsewhere classified**

     CC Excl: For CC codes in category Q93, unless otherwise noted:
     PDX collection 1115

Q93.0   **Whole chromosome monosomy, nonmosaicism (meiotic nondisjunction)**

Q93.1   **Whole chromosome monosomy, mosaicism (mitotic nondisjunction)**

Q93.2   **Chromosome replaced with ring, dicentric or isochromosome**

Q93.3   **Deletion of short arm of chromosome 4**   `CC`
      Wolff-Hirschorn syndrome

Q93.4   **Deletion of short arm of chromosome 5**   `CC`
      Cri-du-chat syndrome
      CC Excl: PDX collection 1116

✓5ᵗʰ   Q93.5   **Other deletions of part of a chromosome**
      ~~Angelman syndrome~~

●   Q93.51   **Angelman syndrome**   `CC`

●   Q93.59   **Other deletions of part of a chromosome**   `CC`

Q93.7   **Deletions with other complex rearrangements**   `CC`
      Deletions due to unbalanced translocations, inversions and
        insertions
      Code also any associated duplications due to unbalanced
        translocations, inversions and insertions (Q92.5)

✓5ᵗʰ   Q93.8   **Other deletions from the autosomes**

     Q93.81   **Velo-cardio-facial syndrome**   `MCC`
        Deletion 22q11.2
        DEF: Microdeletion syndrome affecting multiple organs
        characterized by a cleft palate, heart defects, an
        elongated face with almond-shaped eyes, wide nose,
        small ears, weak immune system, weak musculature,
        hypothyroidism, short stature, and scoliosis. The
        deletion occurs at q11.2 on the long arm of the
        chromosome 22.
        CC Excl: PDX collection 1117

●   Q93.82   **Williams syndrome**   `CC`

     Q93.88   **Other microdeletions**   `CC`
        Miller-Dieker syndrome
        Smith-Magenis syndrome
        CC Excl: PDX collection 1118

     Q93.89   **Other deletions from the autosomes**   `CC`
        Deletions identified by fluorescence in situ
         hybridization (FISH)
        Deletions identified by in situ hybridization (ISH)
        Deletions seen only at prometaphase

Q93.9   **Deletion from autosomes, unspecified**   `CC`

✓4ᵗʰ   **Q95**   **Balanced rearrangements and structural markers, not elsewhere classified**
     `INCLUDES`   Robertsonian and balanced reciprocal translocations and
          insertions

Q95.0   **Balanced translocation and insertion in normal individual**

Q95.1   **Chromosome inversion in normal individual**

Q95.2   **Balanced autosomal rearrangement in abnormal individual**

Q95.3   **Balanced sex/autosomal rearrangement in abnormal individual**

Q95.5   **Individual with autosomal fragile site**

Q95.8   **Other balanced rearrangements and structural markers**

Q95.9   **Balanced rearrangement and structural marker, unspecified**

✓4ᵗʰ   **Q96**   **Turner's syndrome**
     `EXCLUDES 1`   *Noonan syndrome (Q87.1)*

Q96.0   **Karyotype 45, X**   ♀

Q96.1   **Karyotype 46, X iso (Xq)**   ♀
      Karyotype 46, isochromosome Xq

Q96.2   **Karyotype 46, X with abnormal sex chromosome, except iso (Xq)**   ♀
      Karyotype 46, X with abnormal sex chromosome, except
        isochromosome Xq

Q96.3   **Mosaicism, 45, X/46, XX or XY**   ♀

Q96.4   **Mosaicism, 45, X/other cell line(s) with abnormal sex chromosome**   ♀

Q96.8   **Other variants of Turner's syndrome**   ♀

Q96.9   **Turner's syndrome, unspecified**   ♀

✓4ᵗʰ   **Q97**   **Other sex chromosome abnormalities, female phenotype, not elsewhere classified**
     `EXCLUDES 1`   *Turner's syndrome (Q96.-)*

Q97.0   **Karyotype 47, XXX**   ♀

Q97.1   **Female with more than three X chromosomes**   ♀

Q97.2   **Mosaicism, lines with various numbers of X chromosomes**   ♀

Q97.3   **Female with 46, XY karyotype**   ♀

Q97.8   **Other specified sex chromosome abnormalities, female phenotype**   ♀

Q97.9   **Sex chromosome abnormality, female phenotype, unspecified**   ♀

✓4ᵗʰ   **Q98**   **Other sex chromosome abnormalities, male phenotype, not elsewhere classified**

Q98.0   **Klinefelter syndrome karyotype 47, XXY**   ♂

Q98.1   **Klinefelter syndrome, male with more than two X chromosomes**   ♂

Q98.3   **Other male with 46, XX karyotype**   ♂

Q98.4   **Klinefelter syndrome, unspecified**   ♂

Q98.5   **Karyotype 47, XYY**   ♂

Q98.6   **Male with structurally abnormal sex chromosome**   ♂

Q98.7   **Male with sex chromosome mosaicism**   ♂

Q98.8   **Other specified sex chromosome abnormalities, male phenotype**   ♂

Q98.9   **Sex chromosome abnormality, male phenotype, unspecified**   ♂

✓4ᵗʰ   **Q99**   **Other chromosome abnormalities, not elsewhere classified**

Q99.0   **Chimera 46, XX/46, XY**
      Chimera 46, XX/46, XY true hermaphrodite

Q99.1   **46, XX true hermaphrodite**
      46, XX with streak gonads
      46, XY with streak gonads
      Pure gonadal dysgenesis

Q99.2   **Fragile X chromosome**
      Fragile X syndrome

Q99.8   **Other specified chromosome abnormalities**

Q99.9   **Chromosomal abnormality, unspecified**

Chapter 17. Congenital Malformations, Deformations and Chromosomal Abnormalities

Q92.5–Q99.9

✓ Additional Character Required   ✓x7ᵗʰ Placeholder   Unacceptable PDx   Questionable PDx   Manifestation   `H1`-`H14` HAC   `HCC` CMS-HCC Dx   `HIV` HIV Dx

ICD-10-CM 2019   917

Chapter 18. Symptoms, Signs and Abnormal Clinical and Laboratory Findings, Not Elsewhere Classified (R00–R99)

Chapter Specific Guidelines with Coding Examples

The chapter specific guidelines from the ICD-10-CM Official Guidelines for Coding and Reporting have been provided below. Along with these guidelines are coding examples, contained in the shaded boxes, that have been developed to help illustrate the coding and/or sequencing guidance found in these guidelines.

Chapter 18 includes symptoms, signs, abnormal results of clinical or other investigative procedures, and ill-defined conditions regarding which no diagnosis classifiable elsewhere is recorded. Signs and symptoms that point to a specific diagnosis have been assigned to a category in other chapters of the classification.

a. Use of symptom codes

Codes that describe symptoms and signs are acceptable for reporting purposes when a related definitive diagnosis has not been established (confirmed) by the provider.

Chest pain of unknown origin

R07.9   Chest pain, unspecified

Explanation: Codes that describe symptoms such as chest pain are acceptable for reporting purposes when the provider has not established (confirmed) a related definitive diagnosis.

b. Use of a symptom code with a definitive diagnosis code

Codes for signs and symptoms may be reported in addition to a related definitive diagnosis when the sign or symptom is not routinely associated with that diagnosis, such as the various signs and symptoms associated with complex syndromes. The definitive diagnosis code should be sequenced before the symptom code.

Signs or symptoms that are associated routinely with a disease process should not be assigned as additional codes, unless otherwise instructed by the classification.

Pneumonia with hemoptysis

J18.9   Pneumonia, unspecified organism

R04.2   Hemoptysis

Explanation: Codes for signs and symptoms may be reported in addition to a related definitive diagnosis when the sign or symptom is not routinely associated with that diagnosis.

Abdominal pain due to acute appendicitis

K35.80   Unspecified acute appendicitis

Explanation: Codes for signs or symptoms routinely associated with a disease process should not be assigned unless the classification instructs otherwise.

c. Combination codes that include symptoms

ICD-10-CM contains a number of combination codes that identify both the definitive diagnosis and common symptoms of that diagnosis. When using one of these combination codes, an additional code should not be assigned for the symptom.

Acute gastritis with hemorrhage

K29.01   Acute gastritis with bleeding

Explanation: When a combination code identifies both the definitive diagnosis and the symptom, an additional code should not be assigned for the symptom.

d. Repeated falls

Code R29.6, Repeated falls, is for use for encounters when a patient has recently fallen and the reason for the fall is being investigated.

Code Z91.81, History of falling, is for use when a patient has fallen in the past and is at risk for future falls. When appropriate, both codes R29.6 and Z91.81 may be assigned together.

e. Coma scale

The coma scale codes (R40.2-) can be used in conjunction with traumatic brain injury codes, acute cerebrovascular disease or sequelae of cerebrovascular disease codes. These codes are primarily for use by trauma registries, but they may be used in any setting where this information is collected. The coma scale may also be used to assess the status of the central nervous system for other non-trauma conditions, such as monitoring patients in the intensive care unit regardless of medical condition. The coma scale codes should be sequenced after the diagnosis code(s).

These codes, one from each subcategory, are needed to complete the scale. The 7th character indicates when the scale was recorded. The 7th character should match for all three codes.

At a minimum, report the initial score documented on presentation at your facility. This may be a score from the emergency medicine technician (EMT) or in the emergency department. If desired, a facility may choose to capture multiple coma scale scores.

Assign code R40.24, Glasgow coma scale, total score, when only the total score is documented in the medical record and not the individual score(s).

Do not report codes for individual or total Glasgow coma scale scores for a patient with a medically induced coma or a sedated patient.

See Section I.B.14 for coma scale documentation by clinicians other than patient's provider

23-year-old man found down after unknown injury with skull fracture and with concussion and loss of consciousness of unknown duration. EMS evaluated the patient in the field and reported the individual Glasgow coma scores:

Eye opening response—3: eyes open to speech

Verbal response—4: confused but coherent speech

Motor response—6: obeys commands fully

S02.0XXA   Fracture of vault of skull, initial encounter for closed fracture

S06.0X9A   Concussion with loss of consciousness of unspecified duration, initial encounter

R40.2131   Coma scale, eyes open, to sound, in the field [EMT or ambulance]

R40.2241   Coma scale, best verbal response, confused conversation, in the field [EMT or ambulance]

R40.2361   Coma scale, best motor response, obeys commands, in the field [EMT or ambulance]

Explanation: When individual scores for the Glasgow coma scale are documented, one code from each category is needed to complete the scale. The seventh character indicates when the scale was recorded and should match for all three codes. Assign a code from subcategory R40.24- Glasgow coma scale, total score, when only the total and not the individual score(s) is documented.

Patient with intractable epilepsy with status epilepticus arrives to ED with alteration of consciousness. Coma scale performed en route by EMT documented total coma score as 11. Another coma score was performed upon hospital admission that was documented as 14.

G40.911   Epilepsy, unspecified, intractable, with status epilepticus

R40.2421   Glasgow coma scale score 9-12, in the field [EMT or ambulance]

R40.2413   Glasgow coma scale score 13-15, at hospital admission

Explanation: Coma scores may be used to assess mental status in non-trauma conditions. Use only code R40.24- Glasgow coma scale, total scores when individual scores are unavailable. Multiple scores may be reported with the seventh character representing where or when the assessment was made.

f. Functional quadriplegia

GUIDELINE HAS BEEN DELETED EFFECTIVE OCTOBER 1, 2017

g. SIRS due to non-infectious process

The systemic inflammatory response syndrome (SIRS) can develop as a result of certain non-infectious disease processes, such as trauma, malignant neoplasm, or pancreatitis. When SIRS is documented with a noninfectious condition, and no subsequent infection is documented, the code for the underlying condition, such as an injury, should be assigned, followed by code R65.1Ø, Systemic inflammatory response syndrome (SIRS) of non-infectious origin without acute organ dysfunction, or code R65.11, Systemic inflammatory response syndrome (SIRS) of non-infectious origin with acute organ dysfunction. If an associated acute organ dysfunction is documented, the appropriate code(s) for the specific type of organ dysfunction(s) should be assigned in addition to code R65.11. If acute organ dysfunction is documented, but it cannot be determined if the acute organ dysfunction is associated with SIRS or due to another condition (e.g., directly due to the trauma), the provider should be queried.

Systemic inflammatory response syndrome (SIRS) due to acute gallstone pancreatitis

| K85.1Ø | Biliary acute pancreatitis without necrosis or infection |
| R65.1Ø | Systemic inflammatory response syndrome (SIRS) of noninfectious origin without acute organ dysfunction |

Explanation: When SIRS is documented with a noninfectious condition without subsequent infection documented, the code for the underlying condition such as pancreatitis should be assigned followed by the appropriate code for SIRS of noninfectious origin, either with or without associated organ dysfunction.

h. Death NOS

Code R99, Ill-defined and unknown cause of mortality, is only for use in the very limited circumstance when a patient who has already died is brought into an emergency department or other healthcare facility and is pronounced dead upon arrival. It does not represent the discharge disposition of death.

i. NIHSS stroke scale

The NIH stroke scale (NIHSS) codes (R29.7- -) can be used in conjunction with acute stroke codes (I63) to identify the patient's neurological status and the severity of the stroke. The stroke scale codes should be sequenced after the acute stroke diagnosis code(s).

At a minimum, report the initial score documented. If desired, a facility may choose to capture multiple stroke scale scores.

See Section I.B.14 for NIHSS stroke scale documentation by clinicians other than patient's provider

Patient admitted with CVA seen by neurology consult who documents moderate to severe stroke, 17 on NIHSS stroke scale.

| I63.9 | Cerebral infarction, unspecified |
| R29.717 | NIHSS score 17 |

Explanation: Unspecified cerebral vascular accident (CVA) is sequenced before the NIHSS stroke scale score code. The stroke scale is an assessment tool to help measure stroke-related neurological deficits. Fifteen items are evaluated by trained observers and include such conditions as levels of consciousness, language, dysarthria, ataxia, and sensory loss. A facility may report multiple stroke scale scores if it wants to.

Chapter 18. Symptoms, Signs and Abnormal Clinical and Laboratory Findings, Not Elsewhere Classified (R00-R99)

NOTE This chapter includes symptoms, signs, abnormal results of clinical or other investigative procedures, and ill-defined conditions regarding which no diagnosis classifiable elsewhere is recorded.

Signs and symptoms that point rather definitely to a given diagnosis have been assigned to a category in other chapters of the classification. In general, categories in this chapter include the less well-defined conditions and symptoms that, without the necessary study of the case to establish a final diagnosis, point perhaps equally to two or more diseases or to two or more systems of the body. Practically all categories in the chapter could be designated "not otherwise specified", "unknown etiology" or "transient". The Alphabetical Index should be consulted to determine which symptoms and signs are to be allocated here and which to other chapters. The residual subcategories, numbered .8, are generally provided for other relevant symptoms that cannot be allocated elsewhere in the classification.

The conditions and signs or symptoms included in categories R00-R94 consist of:

(a) cases for which no more specific diagnosis can be made even after all the facts bearing on the case have been investigated;

(b) signs or symptoms existing at the time of initial encounter that proved to be transient and whose causes could not be determined;

(c) provisional diagnosis in a patient who failed to return for further investigation or care;

(d) cases referred elsewhere for investigation or treatment before the diagnosis was made;

(e) cases in which a more precise diagnosis was not available for any other reason;

(f) certain symptoms, for which supplementary information is provided, that represent important problems in medical care in their own right.

EXCLUDES 2 *abnormal findings on antenatal screening of mother (O28.-)*
certain conditions originating in the perinatal period (P04-P96)
signs and symptoms classified in the body system chapters
signs and symptoms of breast (N63, N64.5)

AHA: 2017, 1Q, 6, 7

This chapter contains the following blocks:

R00-R09	Symptoms and signs involving the circulatory and respiratory systems
R10-R19	Symptoms and signs involving the digestive system and abdomen
R20-R23	Symptoms and signs involving the skin and subcutaneous tissue
R25-R29	Symptoms and signs involving the nervous and musculoskeletal systems
R30-R39	Symptoms and signs involving the genitourinary system
R40-R46	Symptoms and signs involving cognition, perception, emotional state and behavior
R47-R49	Symptoms and signs involving speech and voice
R50-R69	General symptoms and signs
R70-R79	Abnormal findings on examination of blood, without diagnosis
R80-R82	Abnormal findings on examination of urine, without diagnosis
R83-R89	Abnormal findings on examination of other body fluids, substances and tissues, without diagnosis
R90-R94	Abnormal findings on diagnostic imaging and in function studies, without diagnosis
R97	Abnormal tumor markers
R99	Ill-defined and unknown cause of mortality

Symptoms and signs involving the circulatory and respiratory systems (R00-R09)

✓4th R00 Abnormalities of heart beat
     EXCLUDES 1 *abnormalities originating in the perinatal period (P29.1-)*
     EXCLUDES 2 *specified arrhythmias (I47-I49)*

     R00.0 Tachycardia, unspecified
         Rapid heart beat
         Sinoauricular tachycardia NOS
         Sinus [sinusal] tachycardia NOS
         EXCLUDES 1 *neonatal tachycardia (P29.11)*
                 paroxysmal tachycardia (I47.-)
         DEF: Excessively rapid heart rate of more than 100 beats per minute.

R00.1 Bradycardia, unspecified
     Sinoatrial bradycardia
     Sinus bradycardia
     Slow heart beat
     Vagal bradycardia
     Use additional code for adverse effect, if applicable, to identify drug (T36-T50 with fifth or sixth character 5)
     EXCLUDES 1 *neonatal bradycardia (P29.12)*

R00.2 Palpitations
     Awareness of heart beat

R00.8 Other abnormalities of heart beat

R00.9 Unspecified abnormalities of heart beat

✓4th R01 Cardiac murmurs and other cardiac sounds
     EXCLUDES 1 *cardiac murmurs and sounds originating in the perinatal period (P29.8)*

     R01.0 Benign and innocent cardiac murmurs
         Functional cardiac murmur

     R01.1 Cardiac murmur, unspecified
         Cardiac bruit NOS
         Heart murmur NOS
         Systolic murmur NOS

     R01.2 Other cardiac sounds
         Cardiac dullness, increased or decreased
         Precordial friction

✓4th R03 Abnormal blood-pressure reading, without diagnosis

     R03.0 Elevated blood-pressure reading, without diagnosis of hypertension
         NOTE This category is to be used to record an episode of elevated blood pressure in a patient in whom no formal diagnosis of hypertension has been made, or as an isolated incidental finding.

     R03.1 Nonspecific low blood-pressure reading
         EXCLUDES 1 *hypotension (I95.-)*
                 maternal hypotension syndrome (O26.5-)
                 neurogenic orthostatic hypotension (G90.3)

✓4th R04 Hemorrhage from respiratory passages

     CC Excl: For CC codes in category R04: PDX collection 1119

     R04.0 Epistaxis
         Hemorrhage from nose
         Nosebleed

     R04.1 Hemorrhage from throat
         EXCLUDES 2 *hemoptysis (R04.2)*

     R04.2 Hemoptysis   **CC**
         Blood-stained sputum
         Cough with hemorrhage
         AHA: 2013, 4Q, 118

     ✓5th R04.8 Hemorrhage from other sites in respiratory passages

         R04.81 Acute idiopathic pulmonary hemorrhage in infants   **CC P**
             AIPHI
             Acute idiopathic hemorrhage in infants over 28 days old
             EXCLUDES 1 *perinatal pulmonary hemorrhage (P26.-)*
                   von Willebrand's disease (D68.0)

         R04.89 Hemorrhage from other sites in respiratory passages   **CC**
             Pulmonary hemorrhage NOS

     R04.9 Hemorrhage from respiratory passages, unspecified   **CC**

R05 Cough
     EXCLUDES 1 *cough with hemorrhage (R04.2)*
                 smoker's cough (J41.0)
     AHA: 2016, 2Q, 33

✓4th R06 Abnormalities of breathing
     EXCLUDES 1 *acute respiratory distress syndrome (J80)*
                 respiratory arrest (R09.2)
                 respiratory arrest of newborn (P28.81)
                 respiratory distress syndrome of newborn (P22.-)
                 respiratory failure (J96.-)
                 respiratory failure of newborn (P28.5)

     ✓5th R06.0 Dyspnea
         EXCLUDES 1 *tachypnea NOS (R06.82)*
                 transient tachypnea of newborn (P22.1)

         R06.00 Dyspnea, unspecified
             AHA: 2017, 1Q, 26

         R06.01 Orthopnea

         R06.02 Shortness of breath

✓ Additional Character Required   ✓x7th Placeholder   Unacceptable PDx   Questionable PDx   Manifestation   **H1 -H14** HAC   **HCC** CMS-HCC Dx   **HIV** HIV Dx

ICD-10-CM 2019   921

R06.03   **Acute respiratory distress**
     AHA: 2017, 4Q, 23

R06.09   **Other** forms of dyspnea

R06.1   **Stridor**
    EXCLUDES 1   *congenital laryngeal stridor (P28.89)*
                laryngismus (stridulus) (J38.5)
    DEF: Certain type of wheezing described as a loud, constant, musical sound produced when breathing with an obstructed airway, like the inspiratory sound heard when laryngeal or esophageal obstruction is present.

R06.2   **Wheezing**
    EXCLUDES 1   *asthma (J45.-)*
    AHA: 2016, 2Q, 33
    DEF: High-pitched whistling sound during breathing due to stenosis of the respiratory passageway. Wheezing is associated with asthma, sleep apnea, bronchiectasis, bronchiolitis, COPD, and pleural effusion.

R06.3   **Periodic breathing**   CC
    Cheyne-Stokes breathing
    CC Excl: PDX collection 1120

R06.4   **Hyperventilation**
    EXCLUDES 1   *psychogenic hyperventilation (F45.8)*

R06.5   **Mouth breathing**
    EXCLUDES 2   *dry mouth NOS (R68.2)*

R06.6   **Hiccough**
    EXCLUDES 1   *psychogenic hiccough (F45.8)*

R06.7   **Sneezing**

✓5th   **R06.8**   **Other abnormalities of breathing**

    R06.81   **Apnea, not elsewhere classified**
        Apnea NOS
        EXCLUDES 1   *apnea (of) newborn (P28.4)*
                sleep apnea (G47.3-)
                sleep apnea of newborn (primary) (P28.3)

    R06.82   **Tachypnea, not elsewhere classified**
        Tachypnea NOS
        EXCLUDES 1   *transitory tachypnea of newborn (P22.1)*

    R06.83   **Snoring**

    R06.89   **Other abnormalities of breathing**
        Breath-holding (spells)
        Sighing

R06.9   **Unspecified** abnormalities of breathing

✓4th   **R07**   **Pain in throat and chest**
    EXCLUDES 1   *epidemic myalgia (B33.0)*
    EXCLUDES 2   *jaw pain (R68.84)*
                pain in breast (N64.4)

R07.0   **Pain in** throat
    EXCLUDES 1   *chronic sore throat (J31.2)*
                sore throat (acute) NOS (J02.9)
    EXCLUDES 2   *dysphagia (R13.1-)*
                pain in neck (M54.2)

R07.1   **Chest pain on breathing**
    Painful respiration

R07.2   **Precordial pain**
    DEF: Pain felt in the anterior (front) chest wall over the region of the heart. This type of pain is generally felt slightly to the left of the sternum, but may also extend into the surrounding chest wall region.

✓5th   **R07.8**   **Other chest pain**

    R07.81   **Pleurodynia**
        Pleurodynia NOS
        EXCLUDES 1   *epidemic pleurodynia (B33.0)*

    R07.82   **Intercostal pain**

    R07.89   **Other chest pain**
        Anterior chest-wall pain NOS

R07.9   **Chest pain, unspecified**

✓4th   **R09**   **Other symptoms and signs involving the circulatory and respiratory system**
    EXCLUDES 1   *acute respiratory distress syndrome (J80)*
                respiratory arrest of newborn (P28.81)
                respiratory distress syndrome of newborn (P22.0)
                respiratory failure (J96.-)
                respiratory failure of newborn (P28.5)

✓5th   **R09.0**   **Asphyxia and hypoxemia**
    EXCLUDES 1   *asphyxia due to carbon monoxide (T58.-)*
                asphyxia due to foreign body in respiratory tract (T17.-)
                birth (intrauterine) asphyxia (P84)
                hyperventilation (R06.4)
                traumatic asphyxia (T71.-)
    EXCLUDES 2   *hypercapnia (R06.89)*

    R09.01   **Asphyxia**   CC
        DEF: Interference of oxygen intake due to obstruction or injury of airways resulting in a lack of oxygen perfusion to the tissues or excessive carbon dioxide in the blood. Can cause unconsciousness or death.
        CC Excl: PDX collection 1121

    R09.02   **Hypoxemia**
        DEF: Insufficient oxygen in the arterial blood resulting in inadequate delivery of oxygen to the body tissues.

R09.1   **Pleurisy**
    EXCLUDES 1   *pleurisy with effusion (J90)*

[1]   **R09.2**   **Respiratory arrest**   MCC   HCC
    Cardiorespiratory failure
    EXCLUDES 1   *cardiac arrest (I46.-)*
                respiratory arrest of newborn (P28.81)
                respiratory distress of newborn (P22.0)
                respiratory failure (J96.-)
                respiratory failure of newborn (P28.5)
                respiratory insufficiency (R06.89)
                respiratory insufficiency of newborn (P28.5)
    CC Excl: PDX collection 1121

R09.3   **Abnormal sputum**
    Abnormal amount of sputum
    Abnormal color of sputum
    Abnormal odor of sputum
    Excessive sputum
    EXCLUDES 1   *blood-stained sputum (R04.2)*

✓5th   **R09.8**   **Other specified symptoms and signs involving the circulatory and respiratory systems**

    R09.81   **Nasal congestion**

    R09.82   **Postnasal drip**

    R09.89   **Other specified symptoms and signs involving the circulatory and respiratory systems**
        Abnormal chest percussion
        Bruit (arterial)
        Chest tympany
        Choking sensation
        Feeling of foreign body in throat
        Friction sounds in chest
        Rales
        Weak pulse
        EXCLUDES 2   *foreign body in throat (T17.2-)*
                wheezing (R06.2)

Symptoms and signs involving the digestive system and abdomen (R10-R19)

    EXCLUDES 2   *congenital or infantile pylorospasm (Q40.0)*
                gastrointestinal hemorrhage (K92.0-K92.2)
                intestinal obstruction (K56.-)
                newborn gastrointestinal hemorrhage (P54.0-P54.3)
                newborn intestinal obstruction (P76.-)
                pylorospasm (K31.3)
                signs and symptoms involving the urinary system (R30-R39)
                symptoms referable to female genital organs (N94.-)
                symptoms referable to male genital organs (N48-N50)

✓4th   **R10**   **Abdominal and pelvic pain**
    EXCLUDES 1   *renal colic (N23)*
    EXCLUDES 2   *dorsalgia (M54.-)*
                flatulence and related conditions (R14.-)

    R10.0   **Acute abdomen**
        Severe abdominal pain (generalized) (with abdominal rigidity)
        EXCLUDES 1   *abdominal rigidity NOS (R19.3)*
                generalized abdominal pain NOS (R10.84)
                localized abdominal pain (R10.1-R10.3-)

Abdominal Pain

Right upper
quadrant (RUQ)

Left upper
quadrant (LUQ)

Epigastric

Periumbilical

Right lower
quadrant (RLQ)

Left lower
quadrant (LLQ)

✓5ᵗʰ **R10.1** **Pain** localized to upper abdomen

R10.10 **Upper abdominal pain,** unspecified

R10.11 Right **upper quadrant pain**

R10.12 Left **upper quadrant pain**

R10.13 **Epigastric pain**
Dyspepsia
EXCLUDES 1 *functional dyspepsia (K30)*

R10.2 **Pelvic and perineal pain**
EXCLUDES 1 *vulvodynia (N94.81)*

✓5ᵗʰ **R10.3** **Pain** localized to other parts of lower abdomen

R10.30 **Lower abdominal pain,** unspecified

R10.31 Right **lower quadrant pain**

R10.32 Left **lower quadrant pain**

R10.33 **Periumbilical pain**

✓5ᵗʰ **R10.8** Other abdominal **pain**

✓6ᵗʰ **R10.81** **Abdominal** tenderness
Abdominal tenderness NOS

R10.811 Right upper **quadrant abdominal tenderness**

R10.812 Left upper **quadrant abdominal tenderness**

R10.813 Right lower **quadrant abdominal tenderness**

R10.814 Left lower **quadrant abdominal tenderness**

R10.815 Periumbilic **abdominal tenderness**

R10.816 Epigastric **abdominal tenderness**

R10.817 Generalized **abdominal tenderness**

R10.819 **Abdominal tenderness,** unspecified **site**

✓6ᵗʰ **R10.82** Rebound **abdominal tenderness**

R10.821 Right upper **quadrant rebound abdominal tenderness**

R10.822 Left upper **quadrant rebound abdominal tenderness**

R10.823 Right lower **quadrant rebound abdominal tenderness**

R10.824 Left lower **quadrant rebound abdominal tenderness**

R10.825 Periumbilic **rebound abdominal tenderness**

R10.826 Epigastric **rebound abdominal tenderness**

R10.827 Generalized **rebound abdominal tenderness**

R10.829 **Rebound abdominal tenderness,** unspecified **site**

R10.83 Colic P
Colic NOS
Infantile colic
EXCLUDES 1 *colic in adult and child over 12 months old (R10.84)*
DEF: Inconsolable crying in an otherwise well-fed and healthy infant for more than three hours a day, three days a week, for more than three weeks.

R10.84 Generalized **abdominal pain**
EXCLUDES 1 *generalized abdominal pain associated with acute abdomen (R10.0)*

R10.9 Unspecified **abdominal pain**

✓4ᵗʰ **R11** **Nausea and vomiting**
EXCLUDES 1 *cyclical vomiting associated with migraine (G43.A-)*
excessive vomiting in pregnancy (O21.-)
hematemesis (K92.0)
neonatal hematemesis (P54.0)
newborn vomiting (P92.0-)
psychogenic vomiting (F50.89)
vomiting associated with bulimia nervosa (F50.2)
vomiting following gastrointestinal surgery (K91.0)
AHA: 2017, 1Q, 28
TIP: Assign a code from this category along with K31.89 Other diseases of stomach and duodenum, to describe cyclical vomiting not due to migraine.

R11.0 **Nausea**
Nausea NOS
Nausea without vomiting

✓5ᵗʰ **R11.1** **Vomiting**

R11.10 **Vomiting,** unspecified
Vomiting NOS

R11.11 **Vomiting** without nausea

R11.12 Projectile **vomiting**

R11.13 **Vomiting** of fecal matter

R11.14 Bilious **vomiting**
Bilious emesis

R11.2 **Nausea with vomiting,** unspecified
Persistent nausea with vomiting NOS

R12 **Heartburn**
EXCLUDES 1 *dyspepsia NOS (R10.13)*
functional dyspepsia (K30)

✓4ᵗʰ **R13** **Aphagia and dysphagia**

R13.0 **Aphagia**
Inability to swallow
EXCLUDES 1 *psychogenic aphagia (F50.9)*

✓5ᵗʰ **R13.1** **Dysphagia**
Code first, if applicable, dysphagia following cerebrovascular disease (I69. with final characters -91)
EXCLUDES 1 *psychogenic dysphagia (F45.8)*

R13.10 **Dysphagia,** unspecified
Difficulty in swallowing NOS

R13.11 **Dysphagia,** oral **phase**

R13.12 **Dysphagia,** oropharyngeal **phase**

R13.13 **Dysphagia,** pharyngeal **phase**

R13.14 **Dysphagia,** pharyngoesophageal **phase**

R13.19 Other **dysphagia**
Cervical dysphagia
Neurogenic dysphagia

Swallowing Function

Bolus — Soft palate — Palatine tonsil

Oral phase

Epiglottis — Tongue — Bolus — Esophagus

Pharyngeal phase

Pharynx — Oral cavity — Bolus — Trachea

Oropharyngeal phase

Trachea — Bolus — Epiglottis

Pharyngoesophageal phase

✓ Additional Character Required ✓x7ᵗʰ Placeholder Unacceptable PDx Questionable PDx Manifestation **H1**-**H14** HAC **HCC** CMS-HCC Dx **HIV** HIV Dx

ICD-10-CM 2019 **923**

✓4ᵗʰ R14 Flatulence and related conditions
> EXCLUDES 1   *psychogenic aerophagy (F45.8)*

R14.0 Abdominal distension (gaseous)
> Bloating
> Tympanites (abdominal) (intestinal)

R14.1 Gas pain

R14.2 Eructation

R14.3 Flatulence

✓4ᵗʰ R15 Fecal incontinence
> INCLUDES   encopresis NOS
> EXCLUDES 1   *fecal incontinence of nonorganic origin (F98.1)*

R15.0 Incomplete defecation
> EXCLUDES 1   *constipation (K59.0-)*
> *fecal impaction (K56.41)*

R15.1 Fecal smearing
> Fecal soiling

R15.2 Fecal urgency

R15.9 Full incontinence of feces
> Fecal incontinence NOS

✓4ᵗʰ R16 Hepatomegaly and splenomegaly, not elsewhere classified

R16.0 Hepatomegaly, not elsewhere classified
> Hepatomegaly NOS

R16.1 Splenomegaly, not elsewhere classified
> Splenomegaly NOS

R16.2 Hepatomegaly with splenomegaly, not elsewhere classified
> Hepatosplenomegaly NOS

R17 Unspecified jaundice   CC
> EXCLUDES 1   *neonatal jaundice (P55, P57-P59)*
> **CC Excl:** PDX collection 1122

✓4ᵗʰ R18 Ascites
> INCLUDES   fluid in peritoneal cavity
> EXCLUDES 1   *ascites in alcoholic cirrhosis (K70.31)*
> *ascites in alcoholic hepatitis (K70.11)*
> *ascites in toxic liver disease with chronic active hepatitis (K71.51)*

R18.0 Malignant ascites   CC
> Code first malignancy, such as:
> malignant neoplasm of ovary (C56.-)
> secondary malignant neoplasm of retroperitoneum and peritoneum (C78.6)
> **CC Excl:** PDX collection 1123

R18.8 Other ascites   CC
> Ascites NOS
> Peritoneal effusion (chronic)
> **AHA:** 2018, 1Q, 4
> **CC Excl:** PDX collection 1123

✓4ᵗʰ R19 Other symptoms and signs involving the digestive system and abdomen
> EXCLUDES 1   *acute abdomen (R10.0)*

✓5ᵗʰ R19.0 Intra-abdominal and pelvic swelling, mass and lump
> EXCLUDES 1   *abdominal distension (gaseous) (R14.-)*
> *ascites (R18.-)*

R19.00 Intra-abdominal and pelvic swelling, mass and lump, unspecified site

R19.01 Right upper quadrant abdominal swelling, mass and lump

R19.02 Left upper quadrant abdominal swelling, mass and lump

R19.03 Right lower quadrant abdominal swelling, mass and lump

R19.04 Left lower quadrant abdominal swelling, mass and lump

R19.05 Periumbilic swelling, mass or lump
> Diffuse or generalized umbilical swelling or mass

R19.06 Epigastric swelling, mass or lump

R19.07 Generalized intra-abdominal and pelvic swelling, mass and lump
> Diffuse or generalized intra-abdominal swelling or mass NOS
> Diffuse or generalized pelvic swelling or mass NOS

R19.09 Other intra-abdominal and pelvic swelling, mass and lump

✓5ᵗʰ R19.1 Abnormal bowel sounds

R19.11 Absent bowel sounds

R19.12 Hyperactive bowel sounds

R19.15 Other abnormal bowel sounds
> Abnormal bowel sounds NOS

R19.2 Visible peristalsis
> Hyperperistalsis
> **DEF:** Visible movements of muscular attempts to move food through the digestive tract due to pyloric obstruction, stomach obstruction, or intestinal obstruction.

✓5ᵗʰ R19.3 Abdominal rigidity
> EXCLUDES 1   *abdominal rigidity with severe abdominal pain (R10.0)*

R19.30 Abdominal rigidity, unspecified site

R19.31 Right upper quadrant abdominal rigidity

R19.32 Left upper quadrant abdominal rigidity

R19.33 Right lower quadrant abdominal rigidity

R19.34 Left lower quadrant abdominal rigidity

R19.35 Periumbilic abdominal rigidity

R19.36 Epigastric abdominal rigidity

R19.37 Generalized abdominal rigidity

R19.4 Change in bowel habit
> EXCLUDES 1   *constipation (K59.0-)*
> *functional diarrhea (K59.1)*

R19.5 Other fecal abnormalities
> Abnormal stool color
> Bulky stools
> Mucus in stools
> Occult blood in feces
> Occult blood in stools
> EXCLUDES 1   *melena (K92.1)*
> *neonatal melena (P54.1)*

R19.6 Halitosis

R19.7 Diarrhea, unspecified
> Diarrhea NOS
> EXCLUDES 1   *functional diarrhea (K59.1)*
> *neonatal diarrhea (P78.3)*
> *psychogenic diarrhea (F45.8)*

R19.8 Other specified symptoms and signs involving the digestive system and abdomen

Symptoms and signs involving the skin and subcutaneous tissue (R20-R23)
> EXCLUDES 2   *symptoms relating to breast (N64.4-N64.5)*

✓4ᵗʰ R20 Disturbances of skin sensation
> EXCLUDES 1   *dissociative anesthesia and sensory loss (F44.6)*
> *psychogenic disturbances (F45.8)*

R20.0 Anesthesia of skin

R20.1 Hypoesthesia of skin

R20.2 Paresthesia of skin
> Formication
> Pins and needles
> Tingling skin
> EXCLUDES 1   *acroparesthesia (I73.8)*

R20.3 Hyperesthesia

R20.8 Other disturbances of skin sensation

R20.9 Unspecified disturbances of skin sensation

R21 Rash and other nonspecific skin eruption
> INCLUDES   rash NOS
> EXCLUDES 1   *specified type of rash—code to condition*
> *vesicular eruption (R23.8)*

✓4ᵗʰ R22 Localized swelling, mass and lump of skin and subcutaneous tissue
> INCLUDES   subcutaneous nodules (localized)(superficial)
> EXCLUDES 1   *abnormal findings on diagnostic imaging (R90-R93)*
> *edema (R60.-)*
> *enlarged lymph nodes (R59.-)*
> *localized adiposity (E65)*
> *swelling of joint (M25.4-)*

R22.0 Localized swelling, mass and lump, head

R22.1 Localized swelling, mass and lump, neck

R22.2 Localized swelling, mass and lump, trunk
> EXCLUDES 1   *intra-abdominal or pelvic mass and lump (R19.0-)*
> *intra-abdominal or pelvic swelling (R19.0-)*
> EXCLUDES 2   *breast mass and lump (N63)*

✓5ᵗʰ R22.3 Localized swelling, mass and lump, upper limb

R22.30 Localized swelling, mass and lump, unspecified upper limb

R22.31 Localized swelling, mass and lump, right upper limb

R22.32 Localized swelling, mass and lump, left upper limb

N Newborn: 0   P Pediatric: 0-17   M Maternity: 12-55   A Adult: 15-124   MCC Major Complication/Comorbidity   CC Complication/Comorbidity   SW Severe Wound Dx

R22.33 Localized swelling, mass and lump, upper limb, bilateral

✓5ᵗʰ **R22.4 Localized swelling, mass and lump, lower limb**

R22.40 Localized swelling, mass and lump, unspecified lower limb

R22.41 Localized swelling, mass and lump, right lower limb

R22.42 Localized swelling, mass and lump, left lower limb

R22.43 Localized swelling, mass and lump, lower limb, bilateral

R22.9 Localized swelling, mass and lump, unspecified

✓4ᵗʰ **R23 Other skin changes**

R23.0 **Cyanosis**
EXCLUDES 1 acrocyanosis (I73.8)
cyanotic attacks of newborn (P28.2)
DEF: Bluish or purplish discoloration of the skin due to an inadequate oxygen blood level.

R23.1 **Pallor**
Clammy skin

R23.2 **Flushing**
Excessive blushing
Code first, if applicable, menopausal and female climacteric states (N95.1)

R23.3 **Spontaneous ecchymoses**
Petechiae
EXCLUDES 1 ecchymoses of newborn (P54.5)
purpura (D69.-)

R23.4 **Changes in skin texture**
Desquamation of skin
Induration of skin
Scaling of skin
EXCLUDES 1 epidermal thickening NOS (L85.9)

R23.8 **Other skin changes**

R23.9 **Unspecified skin changes**

Symptoms and signs involving the nervous and musculoskeletal systems (R25-R29)

✓4ᵗʰ **R25 Abnormal involuntary movements**
EXCLUDES 1 specific movement disorders (G20-G26)
stereotyped movement disorders (F98.4)
tic disorders (F95.-)

R25.0 **Abnormal head movements**

R25.1 **Tremor, unspecified**
EXCLUDES 1 chorea NOS (G25.5)
essential tremor (G25.0)
hysterical tremor (F44.4)
intention tremor (G25.2)

R25.2 **Cramp and spasm**
EXCLUDES 2 carpopedal spasm (R29.0)
charley-horse (M62.831)
infantile spasms (G40.4-)
muscle spasm of back (M62.830)
muscle spasm of calf (M62.831)

R25.3 **Fasciculation**
Twitching NOS

R25.8 **Other abnormal involuntary movements**

R25.9 **Unspecified abnormal involuntary movements**

✓4ᵗʰ **R26 Abnormalities of gait and mobility**
EXCLUDES 1 ataxia NOS (R27.0)
hereditary ataxia (G11.-)
locomotor (syphilitic) ataxia (A52.11)
immobility syndrome (paraplegic) (M62.3)

R26.0 **Ataxic gait**
Staggering gait

R26.1 **Paralytic gait**
Spastic gait

R26.2 **Difficulty in walking, not elsewhere classified**
EXCLUDES 1 falling (R29.6)
unsteadiness on feet (R26.81)
AHA: 2016, 2Q, 7

✓5ᵗʰ R26.8 **Other abnormalities of gait and mobility**
R26.81 Unsteadiness on feet
R26.89 Other abnormalities of gait and mobility

R26.9 **Unspecified abnormalities of gait and mobility**

✓4ᵗʰ **R27 Other lack of coordination**
EXCLUDES 1 ataxic gait (R26.0)
hereditary ataxia (G11.-)
vertigo NOS (R42)

R27.0 **Ataxia, unspecified**
EXCLUDES 1 ataxia following cerebrovascular disease (I69. with final characters -93)

R27.8 **Other lack of coordination**

R27.9 **Unspecified lack of coordination**

✓4ᵗʰ **R29 Other symptoms and signs involving the nervous and musculoskeletal systems**

R29.0 **Tetany** CC
Carpopedal spasm
EXCLUDES 1 hysterical tetany (F44.5)
neonatal tetany (P71.3)
parathyroid tetany (E20.9)
post-thyroidectomy tetany (E89.2)
DEF: Calcium or other mineral imbalance causing voluntary muscles such as hands, feet, or larynx to spasm rhythmically.
CC Excl: PDX collection 1124

R29.1 **Meningismus** CC
CC Excl: PDX collection 1125

R29.2 **Abnormal reflex**
EXCLUDES 2 abnormal pupillary reflex (H57.0)
hyperactive gag reflex (J39.2)
vasovagal reaction or syncope (R55)

R29.3 **Abnormal posture**

R29.4 **Clicking hip**
EXCLUDES 1 congenital deformities of hip (Q65.-)

R29.5 **Transient paralysis** CC
Code first any associated spinal cord injury (S14.0, S14.1-, S24.0, S24.1-, S34.0-, S34.1-)
EXCLUDES 1 transient ischemic attack (G45.9)
CC Excl: PDX collection 1126

R29.6 **Repeated falls**
Falling
Tendency to fall
EXCLUDES 2 at risk for falling (Z91.81)
history of falling (Z91.81)
AHA: 2016, 2Q, 6
TIP: Code in addition to Parkinson's disease (G20), when documented.

✓5ᵗʰ R29.7 **National Institutes of Health Stroke Scale (NIHSS) score**
Code first the type of cerebral infarction (I63.-)
AHA: 2016, 4Q, 61-62

✓6ᵗʰ R29.70 NIHSS score 0-9
R29.700 NIHSS score 0
R29.701 NIHSS score 1
R29.702 NIHSS score 2
R29.703 NIHSS score 3
R29.704 NIHSS score 4
R29.705 NIHSS score 5
R29.706 NIHSS score 6
R29.707 NIHSS score 7
R29.708 NIHSS score 8
R29.709 NIHSS score 9

✓6ᵗʰ R29.71 NIHSS score 10-19
R29.710 NIHSS score 10
R29.711 NIHSS score 11
R29.712 NIHSS score 12
R29.713 NIHSS score 13
R29.714 NIHSS score 14
R29.715 NIHSS score 15
R29.716 NIHSS score 16
R29.717 NIHSS score 17
R29.718 NIHSS score 18
R29.719 NIHSS score 19

✓6ᵗʰ R29.72 NIHSS score 20-29
R29.720 NIHSS score 20
R29.721 NIHSS score 21
R29.722 NIHSS score 22
R29.723 NIHSS score 23
R29.724 NIHSS score 24
R29.725 NIHSS score 25
R29.726 NIHSS score 26

    R29.727   **NIHSS** score 27
    R29.728   **NIHSS** score 28
    R29.729   **NIHSS** score 29

✓6th   **R29.73**   **NIHSS** score 3Ø-39
    R29.73Ø   **NIHSS** score 3Ø
    R29.731   **NIHSS** score 31
    R29.732   **NIHSS** score 32
    R29.733   **NIHSS** score 33
    R29.734   **NIHSS** score 34
    R29.735   **NIHSS** score 35
    R29.736   **NIHSS** score 36
    R29.737   **NIHSS** score 37
    R29.738   **NIHSS** score 38
    R29.739   **NIHSS** score 39

✓6th   **R29.74**   **NIHSS** score 4Ø-42
    R29.74Ø   **NIHSS** score 4Ø
    R29.741   **NIHSS** score 41
    R29.742   **NIHSS** score 42

✓5th   **R29.8**   **Other symptoms and signs involving the nervous and musculoskeletal systems**

✓6th   **R29.81**   **Other symptoms and signs involving the nervous system**

    R29.81Ø   **Facial weakness**
      Facial droop
      EXCLUDES 1   *Bell's palsy (G51.Ø)*
      facial weakness following cerebrovascular disease (I69. with final characters -92)

    R29.818   **Other symptoms and signs involving the nervous system**

✓6th   **R29.89**   **Other symptoms and signs involving the musculoskeletal system**
      EXCLUDES 2   *pain in limb (M79.6-)*

    R29.89Ø   **Loss of height**
      EXCLUDES 1   *osteoporosis (M8Ø-M81)*

    R29.891   **Ocular torticollis**
      EXCLUDES 1   *congenital (sternomastoid) torticollis Q68.Ø*
      psychogenic torticollis (F45.8)
      spasmodic torticollis (G24.3)
      torticollis due to birth injury (P15.8)
      torticollis NOS M43.6

      DEF: Abnormal head posture as a result of a contracted state of cervical muscles to correct a visual disturbance, either double vision or a visual field defect.

    R29.898   **Other symptoms and signs involving the musculoskeletal system**

✓5th   **R29.9**   **Unspecified symptoms and signs involving the nervous and musculoskeletal systems**

    R29.9Ø   **Unspecified symptoms and signs involving the nervous system**

    R29.91   **Unspecified symptoms and signs involving the musculoskeletal system**

Symptoms and signs involving the genitourinary system (R3Ø-R39)

✓4th   **R3Ø**   **Pain associated with micturition**
    EXCLUDES 1   *psychogenic pain associated with micturition (F45.8)*

    R3Ø.Ø   **Dysuria**
      Strangury

    R3Ø.1   **Vesical tenesmus**
      DEF: Feeling of a full bladder even when there is little or no urine in the bladder.

    R3Ø.9   **Painful micturition, unspecified**
      Painful urination NOS

✓4th   **R31**   **Hematuria**
    EXCLUDES 1   *hematuria included with underlying conditions, such as:*
      acute cystitis with hematuria (N3Ø.Ø1)
      recurrent and persistent hematuria in glomerular diseases (NØ2.-)
    AHA: 2017, 1Q, 17

    R31.Ø   **Gross hematuria**

    R31.1   **Benign essential microscopic hematuria**

✓5th   **R31.2**   **Other microscopic hematuria**
      AHA: 2016, 4Q, 62

    R31.21   **Asymptomatic microscopic hematuria**
      AMH

    R31.29   **Other microscopic hematuria**

    R31.9   **Hematuria, unspecified**

R32   **Unspecified urinary incontinence**
    Enuresis NOS
    EXCLUDES 1   *functional urinary incontinence (R39.81)*
      nonorganic enuresis (F98.Ø)
      stress incontinence and other specified urinary incontinence (N39.3-N39.4-)
      urinary incontinence associated with cognitive impairment (R39.81)

✓4th   **R33**   **Retention of urine**
    EXCLUDES 1   *psychogenic retention of urine (F45.8)*

    R33.Ø   **Drug induced retention of urine**
      Use additional code for adverse effect, if applicable, to identify drug (T36-T5Ø with fifth or sixth character 5)

    R33.8   **Other retention of urine**
      Code first, if applicable, any causal condition, such as:
      enlarged prostate (N4Ø.1)

    R33.9   **Retention of urine, unspecified**

R34   **Anuria and oliguria**
    EXCLUDES 1   *anuria and oliguria complicating abortion or ectopic or molar pregnancy (OØØ-OØ7, OØ8.4)*
      anuria and oliguria complicating pregnancy (O26.83-)
      anuria and oliguria complicating the puerperium (O9Ø.4)

✓4th   **R35**   **Polyuria**
    Code first, if applicable, any causal condition, such as:
    enlarged prostate (N4Ø.1)
    EXCLUDES 1   *psychogenic polyuria (F45.8)*

    R35.Ø   **Frequency of micturition**

    R35.1   **Nocturia**

    R35.8   **Other polyuria**
      Polyuria NOS

✓4th   **R36**   **Urethral discharge**

    R36.Ø   **Urethral discharge without blood**

    R36.1   **Hematospermia** ♂

    R36.9   **Urethral discharge, unspecified**
      Penile discharge NOS
      Urethrorrhea

R37   **Sexual dysfunction, unspecified**

✓4th   **R39**   **Other and unspecified symptoms and signs involving the genitourinary system**

    R39.Ø   **Extravasation of urine**   CC
      CC Excl: PDX collection 1127

✓5th   **R39.1**   **Other difficulties with micturition**
      Code first, if applicable, any causal condition, such as:
      enlarged prostate (N4Ø.1)

    R39.11   **Hesitancy of micturition**

    R39.12   **Poor urinary stream**
      Weak urinary steam

    R39.13   **Splitting of urinary stream**

    R39.14   **Feeling of incomplete bladder emptying**

    R39.15   **Urgency of urination**
      EXCLUDES 1   *urge incontinence (N39.41, N39.46)*

    R39.16   **Straining to void**

✓6th   **R39.19**   **Other difficulties with micturition**
      AHA: 2016, 4Q, 63

    R39.191   **Need to immediately re-void**

    R39.192   **Position dependent micturition**

    R39.198   **Other difficulties with micturition**

    R39.2   **Extrarenal uremia**
      Prerenal uremia
      EXCLUDES 1   *uremia NOS (N19)*

Ⓝ Newborn: 0   Ⓟ Pediatric: 0-17   Ⓜ Maternity: 12-55   Ⓐ Adult: 15-124   MCC Major Complication/Comorbidity   CC Complication/Comorbidity   SW Severe Wound Dx

926   ICD-10-CM 2019

✓5ᵗʰ **R39.8** **Other symptoms and signs involving the genitourinary system**
    AHA: 2017, 4Q, 22-23

    R39.81 **Functional urinary incontinence**
        Urinary incontinence due to cognitive impairment, or severe physical disability or immobility
        EXCLUDES 1   *stress incontinence and other specified urinary incontinence (N39.3-N39.4-)*
                 urinary incontinence NOS (R32)

    R39.82 **Chronic bladder pain**
        AHA: 2016, 4Q, 64

    R39.83 **Unilateral non-palpable testicle**   ♂

    R39.84 **Bilateral non-palpable testicles**   ♂

    R39.89 **Other symptoms and signs involving the genitourinary system**

R39.9 **Unspecified symptoms and signs involving the genitourinary system**

Symptoms and signs involving cognition, perception, emotional state and behavior (R40-R46)

EXCLUDES 2   *symptoms and signs constituting part of a pattern of mental disorder (F01-F99)*

✓4ᵗʰ **R40** **Somnolence, stupor and coma**
    EXCLUDES 1   *neonatal coma (P91.5)*
            somnolence, stupor and coma in diabetes (E08-E13)
            somnolence, stupor and coma in hepatic failure (K72.-)
            somnolence, stupor and coma in hypoglycemia (nondiabetic) (E15)

    R40.0 **Somnolence**
        Drowsiness
        EXCLUDES 1   *coma (R40.2-)*

    R40.1 **Stupor**
        Catatonic stupor
        Semicoma
        EXCLUDES 1   *catatonic schizophrenia (F20.2)*
                 coma (R40.2-)
                 depressive stupor (F31-F33)
                 dissociative stupor (F44.2)
                 manic stupor (F30.2)

✓5ᵗʰ   **R40.2** **Coma**
        Code first any associated:
          fracture of skull (S02.-)
          intracranial injury (S06.-)
        NOTE   One code from each subcategory, R40.21-R40.23, is required to complete the coma scale
        AHA: 2017, 4Q, 23-25, 95; 2015, 2Q, 17; 2014, 1Q, 19

        CC Excl: For MCC codes in subcategory R40.2: PDX collection 515

      R40.20 **Unspecified coma**   MCC   HCC
          Coma NOS
          Unconsciousness NOS

✓6ᵗʰ   **R40.21** **Coma scale, eyes open**

        The following appropriate 7th character is to be added to subcategories R40.21-, R40.22-, R40.23-, and R40.24-.
        0   unspecified time
        1   in the field [EMT or ambulance]
        2   at arrival to emergency department
        3   at hospital admission
        4   24 hours or more after hospital admission

✓7ᵗʰ   **R40.211** **Coma scale, eyes open, never**   MCC   HCC
          ▶Coma scale eye opening score of 1◀

✓7ᵗʰ   **R40.212** **Coma scale, eyes open, to pain**   MCC   HCC
          ▶Coma scale eye opening score of 2◀

✓7ᵗʰ   **R40.213** **Coma scale, eyes open, to sound**
          ▶Coma scale eye opening score of 3◀

✓7ᵗʰ   **R40.214** **Coma scale, eyes open, spontaneous**
          ▶Coma scale eye opening score of 4◀

✓6ᵗʰ   **R40.22** **Coma scale, best verbal response**

✓7ᵗʰ   **R40.221** **Coma scale, best verbal response, none**   MCC   HCC
          ▶Coma scale verbal score of 1◀

✓7ᵗʰ   **R40.222** **Coma scale, best verbal response, incomprehensible words**   MCC   HCC
      ▶Coma scale verbal score of 2◀
      Incomprehensible sounds (2-5 years of age)
      Moans/grunts to pain; restless (< 2 years old)

✓7ᵗʰ   **R40.223** **Coma scale, best verbal response, inappropriate words**
      ▶Coma scale verbal score of 3◀
      Inappropriate crying or screaming (< 2 years of age)
      Screaming (2-5 years of age)

✓7ᵗʰ   **R40.224** **Coma scale, best verbal response, confused conversation**
      ▶Coma scale verbal score of 4◀
      Inappropriate words (2-5 years of age)
      Irritable cries (< 2 years of age)

✓7ᵗʰ   **R40.225** **Coma scale, best verbal response, oriented**
      ▶Coma scale verbal score of 5◀
      Cooing or babbling or crying appropriately (< 2 years of age)
      Uses appropriate words (2- 5 years of age)

✓6ᵗʰ **R40.23** **Coma scale, best motor response**

✓7ᵗʰ   **R40.231** **Coma scale, best motor response, none**   MCC   HCC
      ▶Coma scale motor score of 1◀

✓7ᵗʰ   **R40.232** **Coma scale, best motor response, extension**   MCC   HCC
      Abnormal extensor posturing to pain or noxious stimuli (< 2 years of age)
      ▶Coma scale motor score of 2◀
      Extensor posturing to pain or noxious stimuli (2-5 years of age)

✓7ᵗʰ   **R40.233** **Coma scale, best motor response, abnormal flexion**
      ▶Abnormal flexure posturing to pain or noxious stimuli (2-5 years of age)
      Coma scale motor score of 3◀
      Flexion/decorticate posturing (< 2 years of age)

✓7ᵗʰ   **R40.234** **Coma scale, best motor response, flexion withdrawal**   MCC   HCC
      ▶Coma scale motor score of 4
      Withdraws from pain or noxious stimuli (2-5 years of age)◀

✓7ᵗʰ   **R40.235** **Coma scale, best motor response, localizes pain**
      ▶Coma scale motor score of 5◀
      Localizes pain (2-5 years of age)
      Withdraws to touch (< 2 years of age)

✓7ᵗʰ   **R40.236** **Coma scale, best motor response, obeys commands**
      ▶Coma scale motor score of 6◀
      Normal or spontaneous movement (< 2 years of age)
      Obeys commands (2-5 years of age)

✓6ᵗʰ **R40.24** **Glasgow coma scale, total score**
      NOTE   Assign a code from subcategory R40.24, when only the total coma score is documented
      AHA: 2016, 4Q, 64-65

✓7ᵗʰ   **R40.241** **Glasgow coma scale score 13-15**

✓7ᵗʰ   **R40.242** **Glasgow coma scale score 9-12**

✓7ᵗʰ   **R40.243** **Glasgow coma scale score 3-8**   HCC

✓7ᵗʰ   **R40.244** **Other coma, without documented Glasgow coma scale score, or with partial score reported**   HCC

R40.3 **Persistent vegetative state**   CC   HCC
    DEF: Persistent wakefulness without consciousness due to a nonfunctioning cerebral cortex.
    CC Excl: PDX collection 515

R40.4 **Transient alteration of awareness**

✓ Additional Character Required   ✓x7ᵗʰ Placeholder   Unacceptable PDx   Questionable PDx   Manifestation   H1-H14 HAC   HCC CMS-HCC Dx   HIV HIV Dx

ICD-10-CM 2019   927

Chapter 18. Symptoms, Signs and Abnormal Clinical and Laboratory Findings, Not Elsewhere Classified (side margin)

R41–R46.89 (side margin)

✓4ᵗʰ R41 Other symptoms and signs involving cognitive functions and awareness

> EXCLUDES 1   *dissociative [conversion] disorders (F44.-)*
> *mild cognitive impairment, so stated (G31.84)*

R41.0 Disorientation, unspecified
Confusion NOS
Delirium NOS

R41.1 Anterograde amnesia

R41.2 Retrograde amnesia

R41.3 Other amnesia
Amnesia NOS
Memory loss NOS

> EXCLUDES 1   *amnestic disorder due to known physiologic condition (F04)*
> *amnestic syndrome due to psychoactive substance use (F10-F19 with 5th character .6)*
> *mild memory disturbance due to known physiological condition (F06.8)*
> *transient global amnesia (G45.4)*

R41.4 Neurologic neglect syndrome   CC
Asomatognosia
Hemi-akinesia
Hemi-inattention
Hemispatial neglect
Left-sided neglect
Sensory neglect
Visuospatial neglect

> EXCLUDES 1   *visuospatial deficit (R41.842)*

CC Excl: PDX collection 1128

✓5ᵗʰ R41.8 Other symptoms and signs involving cognitive functions and awareness

  R41.81 Age-related cognitive decline   A
    Senility NOS

  R41.82 Altered mental status, unspecified
    Change in mental status NOS
> EXCLUDES 1   *altered level of consciousness (R40.-)*
> *altered mental status due to known condition—code to condition delirium NOS (R41.0)*

    AHA: 2012, 4Q, 97

  R41.83 Borderline intellectual functioning
    IQ level 71 to 84
> EXCLUDES 1   *intellectual disabilities (F70-F79)*

  ✓6ᵗʰ R41.84 Other specified cognitive deficit
> EXCLUDES 1   *cognitive deficits as sequelae of cerebrovascular disease (I69.01-, I69.11-, I69.21-, I69.31-, I69.81-, I69.91-)*

    R41.840 Attention and concentration deficit
> EXCLUDES 1   *attention-deficit hyperactivity disorders (F90.-)*

    R41.841 Cognitive communication deficit

    R41.842 Visuospatial deficit

    R41.843 Psychomotor deficit

    R41.844 Frontal lobe and executive function deficit

  R41.89 Other symptoms and signs involving cognitive functions and awareness
    Anosognosia

R41.9 Unspecified symptoms and signs involving cognitive functions and awareness
Unspecified neurocognitive disorder

R42 Dizziness and giddiness
Light-headedness
Vertigo NOS

> EXCLUDES 1   *vertiginous syndromes (H81.-)*
> *vertigo from infrasound (T75.23)*

✓4ᵗʰ R43 Disturbances of smell and taste

R43.0 Anosmia
DEF: Permanent or transient absence of smell that may be congenital or acquired.

R43.1 Parosmia
DEF: Abnormal perception of smell usually triggered by environmental odors.

R43.2 Parageusia
DEF: Abnormal perception of taste.

R43.8 Other disturbances of smell and taste
Mixed disturbance of smell and taste

R43.9 Unspecified disturbances of smell and taste

✓4ᵗʰ R44 Other symptoms and signs involving general sensations and perceptions

> EXCLUDES 1   *alcoholic hallucinations (F1.5)*
> *hallucinations in drug psychosis (F11-F19 with .5)*
> *hallucinations in mood disorders with psychotic symptoms (F30.2, F31.5, F32.3, F33.3)*
> *hallucinations in schizophrenia, schizotypal and delusional disorders (F20-F29)*

> EXCLUDES 2   *disturbances of skin sensation (R20.-)*

CC Excl: For CC codes in category R44: PDX collection 1129

R44.0 Auditory hallucinations   CC

R44.1 Visual hallucinations

R44.2 Other hallucinations   CC

R44.3 Hallucinations, unspecified   CC

R44.8 Other symptoms and signs involving general sensations and perceptions

R44.9 Unspecified symptoms and signs involving general sensations and perceptions

✓4ᵗʰ R45 Symptoms and signs involving emotional state

R45.0 Nervousness
Nervous tension

R45.1 Restlessness and agitation

R45.2 Unhappiness

R45.3 Demoralization and apathy
> EXCLUDES 1   *anhedonia (R45.84)*

R45.4 Irritability and anger

R45.5 Hostility

R45.6 Violent behavior

R45.7 State of emotional shock and stress, unspecified

✓5ᵗʰ R45.8 Other symptoms and signs involving emotional state

  R45.81 Low self-esteem

  R45.82 Worries

  R45.83 Excessive crying of child, adolescent or adult
> EXCLUDES 1   *excessive crying of infant (baby) R68.11*

  R45.84 Anhedonia

  ✓6ᵗʰ R45.85 Homicidal and suicidal ideations
> EXCLUDES 1   *suicide attempt (T14.91)*

    R45.850 Homicidal ideations

    R45.851 Suicidal ideations   CC
      DEF: Thoughts of committing suicide but no actual attempt of suicide has been made.
      CC Excl: PDX collection 1130

  R45.86 Emotional lability

  R45.87 Impulsiveness

  R45.89 Other symptoms and signs involving emotional state

✓4ᵗʰ R46 Symptoms and signs involving appearance and behavior

> EXCLUDES 1   *appearance and behavior in schizophrenia, schizotypal and delusional disorders (F20-F29)*
> *mental and behavioral disorders (F01-F99)*

R46.0 Very low level of personal hygiene

R46.1 Bizarre personal appearance

R46.2 Strange and inexplicable behavior

R46.3 Overactivity

R46.4 Slowness and poor responsiveness
> EXCLUDES 1   *stupor (R40.1)*

R46.5 Suspiciousness and marked evasiveness

R46.6 Undue concern and preoccupation with stressful events

R46.7 Verbosity and circumstantial detail obscuring reason for contact

✓5ᵗʰ R46.8 Other symptoms and signs involving appearance and behavior

  R46.81 Obsessive-compulsive behavior
> EXCLUDES 1   *obsessive-compulsive disorder (F42-)*

  R46.89 Other symptoms and signs involving appearance and behavior

N Newborn: 0   P Pediatric: 0-17   M Maternity: 12-55   A Adult: 15-124   MCC Major Complication/Comorbidity   CC Complication/Comorbidity   SW Severe Wound Dx

928   ICD-10-CM 2019

Symptoms and signs involving speech and voice (R47-R49)

✓4ᵗʰ R47 Speech disturbances, not elsewhere classified
     EXCLUDES 1   *autism (F84.0)*
               cluttering (F80.81)
               specific developmental disorders of speech and language (F80.-)
               stuttering (F80.81)

✓5ᵗʰ R47.0 Dysphasia and aphasia

     R47.01 Aphasia   **cc**
         EXCLUDES 1   *aphasia following cerebrovascular disease*
                 (I69. with final characters -20)
                 progressive isolated aphasia (G31.01)
         CC Excl: PDX collection 1131

     R47.02 Dysphasia
         EXCLUDES 1   *dysphasia following cerebrovascular disease*
                 (I69. with final characters -21)

     R47.1 Dysarthria and anarthria
         EXCLUDES 1   *dysarthria following cerebrovascular disease (I69. with*
                 final characters -22)

✓5ᵗʰ R47.8 Other speech disturbances
     EXCLUDES 1   *dysarthria following cerebrovascular disease (I69. with*
                 final characters -28)

     R47.81 Slurred speech

     R47.82 *Fluency disorder in conditions classified elsewhere*
         Stuttering in conditions classified elsewhere
         Code first underlying disease or condition, such as:
         Parkinson's disease (G20)
         EXCLUDES 1   *adult onset fluency disorder (F98.5)*
                 childhood onset fluency disorder (F80.81)
                 fluency disorder (stuttering) following
                     cerebrovascular disease (I69. with final
                     characters-23)

     R47.89 Other speech disturbances

     R47.9 Unspecified speech disturbances

✓4ᵗʰ R48 Dyslexia and other symbolic dysfunctions, not elsewhere classified
     EXCLUDES 1   *specific developmental disorders of scholastic skills (F81.-)*

     R48.0 Dyslexia and alexia

     R48.1 Agnosia
         Astereognosia (astereognosis)
         Autotopagnosia
         EXCLUDES 1   *visual object agnosia (R48.3)*
         DEF: Inability to recognize common things such as faces, objects, smells, or voices.

     R48.2 Apraxia
         EXCLUDES 1   *apraxia following cerebrovascular disease (I69. with*
                 final characters -90)

     R48.3 Visual agnosia
         Prosopagnosia
         Simultanagnosia (asimultagnosia)

     R48.8 Other symbolic dysfunctions
         Acalculia
         Agraphia
         AHA: 2017, 1Q, 27

     R48.9 Unspecified symbolic dysfunctions

✓4ᵗʰ R49 Voice and resonance disorders
     EXCLUDES 1   *psychogenic voice and resonance disorders (F44.4)*

     R49.0 Dysphonia
         Hoarseness

     R49.1 Aphonia
         Loss of voice

✓5ᵗʰ R49.2 Hypernasality and hyponasality

     R49.21 Hypernasality

     R49.22 Hyponasality

     R49.8 Other voice and resonance disorders

     R49.9 Unspecified voice and resonance disorder
         Change in voice NOS
         Resonance disorder NOS

General symptoms and signs (R50-R69)

✓4ᵗʰ R50 Fever of other and unknown origin
     EXCLUDES 1   *chills without fever (R68.83)*
               febrile convulsions (R56.0-)
               fever of unknown origin during labor (O75.2)
               fever of unknown origin in newborn (P81.9)
               hypothermia due to illness (R68.0)
               malignant hyperthermia due to anesthesia (T88.3)
               puerperal pyrexia NOS (O86.4)

     R50.2 Drug induced fever
         Use additional code for adverse effect, if applicable, to identify drug (T36-T50 with fifth or sixth character 5)
         EXCLUDES 1   *postvaccination (postimmunization) fever (R50.83)*

✓5ᵗʰ R50.8 Other specified fever

     R50.81 *Fever presenting with conditions classified elsewhere*
         Code first underlying condition when associated fever is present, such as with:
         leukemia (C91-C95)
         neutropenia (D70.-)
         sickle-cell disease (D57.-)
         AHA: 2014, 4Q, 22

     R50.82 Postprocedural fever
         EXCLUDES 1   *postprocedural infection (T81.4-)*
                 posttransfusion fever (R50.84)
                 postvaccination (postimmunization) fever
                   (R50.83)

     R50.83 Postvaccination fever
         Postimmunization fever

     R50.84 Febrile nonhemolytic transfusion reaction
         FNHTR
         Posttransfusion fever

     R50.9 Fever, unspecified
         Fever NOS
         Fever of unknown origin [FUO]
         Fever with chills
         Fever with rigors
         Hyperpyrexia NOS
         Persistent fever
         Pyrexia NOS

R51 Headache
     Facial pain NOS
     EXCLUDES 1   *atypical face pain (G50.1)*
               migraine and other headache syndromes (G43-G44)
               trigeminal neuralgia (G50.0)

R52 Pain, unspecified
     Acute pain NOS
     Generalized pain NOS
     Pain NOS
     EXCLUDES 1   *acute and chronic pain, not elsewhere classified (G89.-)*
               localized pain, unspecified type—code to pain by site, such as:
                 abdomen pain (R10.-)
                 back pain (M54.9)
                 breast pain (N64.4)
                 chest pain (R07.1-R07.9)
                 ear pain (H92.0-)
                 eye pain (H57.1)
                 headache (R51)
                 joint pain (M25.5-)
                 limb pain (M79.6-)
                 lumbar region pain (M54.5)
                 pelvic and perineal pain (R10.2)
                 renal colic (N23)
                 shoulder pain (M25.51-)
                 spine pain (M54.-)
                 throat pain (R07.0)
                 tongue pain (K14.6)
                 tooth pain (K08.8)
               pain disorders exclusively related to psychological factors
                 (F45.41)

✓4ᵗʰ R53 Malaise and fatigue

     R53.0 Neoplastic (malignant) related fatigue
         Code first associated neoplasm

     R53.1 Weakness
         Asthenia NOS
         EXCLUDES 1   *age-related weakness (R54)*
                 muscle weakness (M62.8-)
                 sarcopenia (M62.84)
                 senile asthenia (R54)
         AHA: 2017, 1Q, 7; 2015, 1Q, 25

☑ Additional Character Required   ✓x7ᵗʰ Placeholder   Unacceptable PDx   Questionable PDx   Manifestation   **H1 - H14** HAC   **HCC** CMS-HCC Dx   **HIV** HIV Dx

ICD-10-CM 2019   929

Chapter 18. Symptoms, Signs and Abnormal Clinical and Laboratory Findings, Not Elsewhere Classified

R47–R53.1

R53.2 Functional quadriplegia `MCC` `HCC`
Complete immobility due to severe physical disability or frailty
> EXCLUDES 1   *frailty NOS (R54)*
> *hysterical paralysis (F44.4)*
> *immobility syndrome (M62.3)*
> *neurologic quadriplegia (G82.5-)*
> *quadriplegia (G82.50)*

AHA: 2016, 2Q, 6
DEF: Inability to move due to a nonphysiological condition, such as dementia. The patient has no mental ability to move independently.
CC Excl: PDX collection 595

R53.8 Other malaise and fatigue `✓5th`
> EXCLUDES 1   *combat exhaustion and fatigue (F43.0)*
> *congenital debility (P96.9)*
> *exhaustion and fatigue due to excessive exertion (T73.3)*
> *exhaustion and fatigue due to exposure (T73.2)*
> *exhaustion and fatigue due to heat (T67.-)*
> *exhaustion and fatigue due to pregnancy (O26.8-)*
> *exhaustion and fatigue due to recurrent depressive episode (F33)*
> *exhaustion and fatigue due to senile debility (R54)*

R53.81 Other malaise
Chronic debility
Debility NOS
General physical deterioration
Malaise NOS
Nervous debility
> EXCLUDES 1   *age-related physical debility (R54)*

R53.82 Chronic fatigue, unspecified
Chronic fatigue syndrome NOS
> EXCLUDES 1   *postviral fatigue syndrome (G93.3)*

R53.83 Other fatigue
Fatigue NOS
Lack of energy
Lethargy
Tiredness
> EXCLUDES 2   *exhaustion and fatigue due to depressive episode (F32.-)*

R54 Age-related physical debility `A`
Frailty   Senile asthenia
Old age   Senile debility
Senescence
> EXCLUDES 1   *age-related cognitive decline (R41.81)*
> *sarcopenia (M62.84)*
> *senile psychosis (F03)*
> *senility NOS (R41.81)*

R55 Syncope and collapse
Blackout
Fainting
Vasovagal attack
> EXCLUDES 1   *cardiogenic shock (R57.0)*
> *carotid sinus syncope (G90.01)*
> *heat syncope (T67.1)*
> *neurocirculatory asthenia (F45.8)*
> *neurogenic orthostatic hypotension (G90.3)*
> *orthostatic hypotension (I95.1)*
> *postprocedural shock (T81.1-)*
> *psychogenic syncope (F48.8)*
> *shock NOS (R57.9)*
> *shock complicating or following abortion or ectopic or molar pregnancy (O00-O07, O08.3)*
> *shock complicating or following labor and delivery (O75.1)*
> *Stokes-Adams attack (I45.9)*
> *unconsciousness NOS (R40.2-)*

R56 Convulsions, not elsewhere classified `✓4th`
> EXCLUDES 1   *dissociative convulsions and seizures (F44.5)*
> *epileptic convulsions and seizures (G40.-)*
> *newborn convulsions and seizures (P90)*

R56.0 Febrile convulsions `✓5th`

R56.00 Simple febrile convulsions `CC` `HCC`
Febrile convulsion NOS
Febrile seizure NOS
CC Excl: PDX collection 1132

R56.01 Complex febrile convulsions `CC` `HCC`
Atypical febrile seizure
Complex febrile seizure
Complicated febrile seizure
> EXCLUDES 1   *status epilepticus (G40.901)*

CC Excl: PDX collection 1132

R56.1 Post traumatic seizures `CC` `HCC`
> EXCLUDES 1   *post traumatic epilepsy (G40.-)*

CC Excl: PDX collection 582

R56.9 Unspecified convulsions `HCC`
Convulsion disorder
Fit NOS
Recurrent convulsions
Seizure(s) (convulsive) NOS

R57 Shock, not elsewhere classified `✓4th`
> EXCLUDES 1   *anaphylactic shock NOS (T78.2)*
> *anaphylactic reaction or shock due to adverse food reaction (T78.0-)*
> *anaphylactic shock due to adverse effect of correct drug or medicament properly administered (T88.6)*
> *anaphylactic shock due to serum (T80.5-)*
> *anesthetic shock (T88.3)*
> *electric shock (T75.4)*
> *obstetric shock (O75.1)*
> *postprocedural shock (T81.1-)*
> *psychic shock (F43.0)*
> *shock complicating or following ectopic or molar pregnancy (O00-O07, O08.3)*
> *shock due to lightning (T75.01)*
> *traumatic shock (T79.4)*
> *toxic shock syndrome (A48.3)*

> **CC Excl: For CC/MCC codes in category R57:** PDX collection 1133

[1] **R57.0 Cardiogenic shock** `MCC` `HCC`
> EXCLUDES 2   *septic shock (R65.21)*

DEF: Associated with myocardial infarction, cardiac tamponade, and massive pulmonary embolism. Symptoms include mental confusion, reduced blood pressure, tachycardia, pallor, and cold, clammy skin.

[1] **R57.1 Hypovolemic shock** `MCC` `HCC`

[1] **R57.8 Other shock** `MCC` `HCC`

R57.9 Shock, unspecified `CC` `HCC`
Failure of peripheral circulation NOS

R58 Hemorrhage, not elsewhere classified
Hemorrhage NOS
> EXCLUDES 1   *hemorrhage included with underlying conditions, such as:*
> *acute duodenal ulcer with hemorrhage (K26.0)*
> *acute gastritis with bleeding (K29.01)*
> *ulcerative enterocolitis with rectal bleeding (K51.01)*

R59 Enlarged lymph nodes `✓4th`
> INCLUDES   swollen glands
> EXCLUDES 1   *acute lymphadenitis (L04.-)*
> *chronic lymphadenitis (I88.1)*
> *lymphadenitis NOS (I88.9)*
> *mesenteric (acute) (chronic) lymphadenitis (I88.0)*

R59.0 Localized enlarged lymph nodes

R59.1 Generalized enlarged lymph nodes
Lymphadenopathy NOS

R59.9 Enlarged lymph nodes, unspecified

R60 Edema, not elsewhere classified `✓4th`
> EXCLUDES 1   *angioneurotic edema (T78.3)*
> *ascites (R18.-)*
> *cerebral edema (G93.6)*
> *cerebral edema due to birth injury (P11.0)*
> *edema of larynx (J38.4)*
> *edema of nasopharynx (J39.2)*
> *edema of pharynx (J39.2)*
> *gestational edema (O12.0-)*
> *hereditary edema (Q82.0)*
> *hydrops fetalis NOS (P83.2)*
> *hydrothorax (J94.8)*
> *hydrops fetalis NOS (P83.2)*
> *newborn edema (P83.3)*
> *pulmonary edema (J81.-)*

R60.0 Localized edema

R60.1 Generalized edema
> EXCLUDES 2   *nutritional edema (E40-E46)*

R60.9 Edema, unspecified
Fluid retention NOS

`N` Newborn: 0   `P` Pediatric: 0-17   `M` Maternity: 12-55   `A` Adult: 15-124   `MCC` Major Complication/Comorbidity   `CC` Complication/Comorbidity   `SW` Severe Wound Dx

930   ICD-10-CM 2019

R61 Generalized hyperhidrosis
Excessive sweating
Night sweats
Secondary hyperhidrosis
Code first, if applicable, menopausal and female climacteric states
(N95.1)
EXCLUDES 1   focal (primary) (secondary) hyperhidrosis (L74.5-)
Frey's syndrome (L74.52)
localized (primary) (secondary) hyperhidrosis (L74.5-)

√4ᵗʰ **R62 Lack of expected normal physiological development in childhood and adults**
EXCLUDES 1   delayed puberty (E30.0)
gonadal dysgenesis (Q99.1)
hypopituitarism (E23.0)

R62.0 Delayed milestone in childhood   P
Delayed attainment of expected physiological developmental
stage
Late talker
Late walker

√5ᵗʰ **R62.5 Other and unspecified lack of expected normal physiological development in childhood**
EXCLUDES 1   HIV disease resulting in failure to thrive (B20)
physical retardation due to malnutrition (E45)

R62.50 Unspecified lack of expected normal physiological development in childhood
Infantilism NOS

R62.51 Failure to thrive (child)   P
Failure to gain weight
EXCLUDES 1   failure to thrive in child under 28 days old
(P92.6)
DEF: Organic failure to thrive (FTT): Acute or chronic
illness that interferes with nutritional intake, absorption,
metabolism excretion, and energy requirements.
DEF: Nonorganic failure to thrive (FTT): Symptom of
neglect or abuse.

R62.52 Short stature (child)
Lack of growth
Physical retardation
Short stature NOS
EXCLUDES 1   short stature due to endocrine disorder
(E34.3)

R62.59 Other lack of expected normal physiological development in childhood

R62.7 Adult failure to thrive   A

√4ᵗʰ **R63 Symptoms and signs concerning food and fluid intake**
EXCLUDES 1   bulimia NOS (F50.2)
eating disorders of nonorganic origin (F50.-)
malnutrition (E40-E46)

R63.0 Anorexia
Loss of appetite
EXCLUDES 1   anorexia nervosa (F50.0-)
loss of appetite of nonorganic origin (F50.89)

R63.1 Polydipsia
Excessive thirst

R63.2 Polyphagia
Excessive eating
Hyperalimentation NOS

R63.3 Feeding difficulties
Feeding problem (elderly) (infant) NOS
Picky eater
EXCLUDES 1   eating disorders (F50.-)
feeding problems of newborn (P92.-)
infant feeding disorder of nonorganic origin (F98.2-)
AHA: 2017, 1Q, 28; 2016, 3Q, 19
TIP: Do not assign for feeding problems in a patient greater than
28 days old if the feeding problem was initially diagnosed
between day 0 and day 28. Use a code from category P92.

R63.4 Abnormal weight loss

R63.5 Abnormal weight gain
EXCLUDES 1   excessive weight gain in pregnancy (O26.0-)
obesity (E66.-)

R63.6 Underweight
Use additional code to identify body mass index (BMI), if known
(Z68.-)
EXCLUDES 1   abnormal weight loss (R63.4)
anorexia nervosa (F50.0-)
malnutrition (E40-E46)

R63.8 Other symptoms and signs concerning food and fluid intake

R64 Cachexia   CC HCC
Wasting syndrome
Code first underlying condition, if known
EXCLUDES 1   abnormal weight loss (R63.4)
nutritional marasmus (E41)
AHA: 2017, 3Q, 24
CC Excl: PDX collection 1134

√4ᵗʰ **R65 Symptoms and signs specifically associated with systemic inflammation and infection**
TIP: When documentation states SIRS with an infection, assign only a code
for the infection. ICD-10-CM does not offer a code for SIRS due to infectious
process. If sepsis is suspected, query the provider.

CC Excl: For CC/MCC codes in category R65, unless otherwise noted: PDX collection 71

√5ᵗʰ **R65.1 Systemic inflammatory response syndrome [SIRS] of non-infectious origin**
Code first underlying condition, such as:
heatstroke (T67.0)
injury and trauma (S00-T88)
EXCLUDES 1   sepsis—code to infection
severe sepsis (R65.2)

R65.10 Systemic inflammatory response syndrome [SIRS] of non-infectious origin without acute organ dysfunction   CC HCC
Systemic inflammatory response syndrome (SIRS) NOS

R65.11 Systemic inflammatory response syndrome [SIRS] of non-infectious origin with acute organ dysfunction   MCC HCC
Use additional code to identify specific acute organ
dysfunction, such as:
acute kidney failure (N17.-)
acute respiratory failure (J96.0-)
critical illness myopathy (G72.81)
critical illness polyneuropathy (G62.81)
disseminated intravascular coagulopathy [DIC]
(D65)
encephalopathy (metabolic) (septic) (G93.41)
hepatic failure (K72.0-)

√5ᵗʰ **R65.2 Severe sepsis**
Infection with associated acute organ dysfunction
Sepsis with acute organ dysfunction
Sepsis with multiple organ dysfunction
Systemic inflammatory response syndrome due to infectious
process with acute organ dysfunction
Code first underlying infection, such as:
infection following a procedure (T81.4-)
infections following infusion, transfusion and therapeutic
injection (T80.2-)
puerperal sepsis (O85)
sepsis following complete or unspecified spontaneous
abortion (O03.87)
sepsis following ectopic and molar pregnancy (O08.82)
sepsis following incomplete spontaneous abortion (O03.37)
sepsis following (induced) termination of pregnancy (O04.87)
sepsis NOS (A41.9)
Use additional code to identify specific acute organ dysfunction,
such as:
acute kidney failure (N17.-)
acute respiratory failure (J96.0-)
critical illness myopathy (G72.81)
critical illness polyneuropathy (G62.81)
disseminated intravascular coagulopathy [DIC] (D65)
encephalopathy (metabolic) (septic) (G93.41)
hepatic failure (K72.0-)
AHA: 2017, 4Q, 98-99; 2016, 3Q, 8

R65.20 Severe sepsis without septic shock   MCC HCC
Severe sepsis NOS
AHA: 2016, 3Q, 14; 2013, 4Q, 119

R65.21 Severe sepsis with septic shock   MCC HCC
CC Excl: PDX collection 1133

√4ᵗʰ **R68 Other general symptoms and signs**

R68.0 Hypothermia, not associated with low environmental temperature
EXCLUDES 1   hypothermia due to anesthesia (T88.51)
hypothermia due to low environmental temperature
(T68)
hypothermia NOS (accidental) (T68)
newborn hypothermia (P80.-)

✓5ᵗʰ R68.1 Nonspecific symptoms peculiar to infancy
> EXCLUDES 1   *colic, infantile (R10.83)*
> *neonatal cerebral irritability (P91.3)*
> *teething syndrome (K00.7)*

R68.11 Excessive crying of infant (baby)   P
> EXCLUDES 1   *excessive crying of child, adolescent, or adult (R45.83)*

R68.12 Fussy infant (baby)   P
> Irritable infant

R68.13 Apparent life threatening event in infant (ALTE)   P
> Apparent life threatening event in newborn
> Brief resolved unexplained event (BRUE)
> Code first confirmed diagnosis, if known
> Use additional code(s) for associated signs and symptoms if no confirmed diagnosis established, or if signs and symptoms are not associated routinely with confirmed diagnosis, or provide additional information for cause of ALTE

R68.19 Other nonspecific symptoms peculiar to infancy   P

R68.2 Dry mouth, unspecified
> EXCLUDES 1   *dry mouth due to dehydration (E86.0)*
> *dry mouth due to sicca syndrome [Sjögren] (M35.0-)*
> *salivary gland hyposecretion (K11.7)*

R68.3 Clubbing of fingers
> Clubbing of nails
> EXCLUDES 1   *congenital clubfinger (Q68.1)*
> **DEF:** Enlarged soft tissue of the distal fingers that usually occurs in heart and lung diseases.

✓5ᵗʰ R68.8 Other general symptoms and signs

R68.81 Early satiety
> **DEF:** Premature feeling of being full after eating only a small amount of food. The mechanism of satiety is multifactorial.

R68.82 Decreased libido   A
> Decreased sexual desire

R68.83 Chills (without fever)
> Chills NOS
> EXCLUDES 1   *chills with fever (R50.9)*

R68.84 Jaw pain
> Mandibular pain
> Maxilla pain
> EXCLUDES 1   *temporomandibular joint arthralgia (M26.62-)*

R68.89 Other general symptoms and signs

R69 Illness, unspecified
> Unknown and unspecified cases of morbidity

Abnormal findings on examination of blood, without diagnosis (R70-R79)

> EXCLUDES 2   *abnormal findings on antenatal screening of mother (O28.-)*
> *abnormalities of lipids (E78.-)*
> *abnormalities of platelets and thrombocytes (D69.-)*
> *abnormalities of white blood cells classified elsewhere (D70-D72)*
> *coagulation hemorrhagic disorders (D65-D68)*
> *diagnostic abnormal findings classified elsewhere—see Alphabetical Index*
> *hemorrhagic and hematological disorders of newborn (P50-P61)*

✓4ᵗʰ R70 Elevated erythrocyte sedimentation rate and abnormality of plasma viscosity

R70.0 Elevated erythrocyte sedimentation rate

R70.1 Abnormal plasma viscosity

✓4ᵗʰ R71 Abnormality of red blood cells
> EXCLUDES 1   *anemias (D50-D64)*
> *anemia of premature infant (P61.2)*
> *benign (familial) polycythemia (D75.0)*
> *congenital anemias (P61.2-P61.4)*
> *newborn anemia due to isoimmunization (P55.-)*
> *polycythemia neonatorum (P61.1)*
> *polycythemia NOS (D75.1)*
> *polycythemia vera (D45)*
> *secondary polycythemia (D75.1)*

R71.0 Precipitous drop in hematocrit   CC
> Drop (precipitous) in hemoglobin
> Drop in hematocrit
> **CC Excl:** PDX collection 1135

R71.8 Other abnormality of red blood cells
> Abnormal red-cell morphology NOS
> Abnormal red-cell volume NOS
> Anisocytosis
> Poikilocytosis

✓4ᵗʰ R73 Elevated blood glucose level
> EXCLUDES 1   *diabetes mellitus (E08-E13)*
> *diabetes mellitus in pregnancy, childbirth and the puerperium (O24.-)*
> *neonatal disorders (P70.0-P70.2)*
> *postsurgical hypoinsulinemia (E89.1)*

✓5ᵗʰ R73.0 Abnormal glucose
> EXCLUDES 1   *abnormal glucose in pregnancy (O99.81-)*
> *diabetes mellitus (E08-E13)*
> *dysmetabolic syndrome X (E88.81)*
> *gestational diabetes (O24.4-)*
> *glycosuria (R81)*
> *hypoglycemia (E16.2)*

R73.01 Impaired fasting glucose
> Elevated fasting glucose

R73.02 Impaired glucose tolerance (oral)
> Elevated glucose tolerance

R73.03 Prediabetes
> Latent diabetes
> **AHA:** 2016, 4Q, 65

R73.09 Other abnormal glucose
> Abnormal glucose NOS
> Abnormal non-fasting glucose tolerance

R73.9 Hyperglycemia, unspecified

✓4ᵗʰ R74 Abnormal serum enzyme levels

R74.0 Nonspecific elevation of levels of transaminase and lactic acid dehydrogenase [LDH]

R74.8 Abnormal levels of other serum enzymes
> Abnormal level of acid phosphatase
> Abnormal level of alkaline phosphatase
> Abnormal level of amylase
> Abnormal level of lipase [triacylglycerol lipase]
> **TIP:** Assign for documented abnormal or elevated troponin level when a definitive diagnosis has not been established.

R74.9 Abnormal serum enzyme level, unspecified

R75 Inconclusive laboratory evidence of human immunodeficiency virus [HIV]
> Nonconclusive HIV-test finding in infants
> EXCLUDES 1   *asymptomatic human immunodeficiency virus [HIV] infection status (Z21)*
> *human immunodeficiency virus [HIV] disease (B20)*
> **TIP:** Do not assign for patients previously diagnosed with an HIV-related illness. Assign code B20.

✓4ᵗʰ R76 Other abnormal immunological findings in serum

R76.0 Raised antibody titer
> EXCLUDES 1   *isoimmunization in pregnancy (O36.0-O36.1)*
> *isoimmunization affecting newborn (P55.-)*

✓5ᵗʰ R76.1 Nonspecific reaction to test for tuberculosis

R76.11 Nonspecific reaction to tuberculin skin test without active tuberculosis
> Abnormal result of Mantoux test
> PPD positive
> Tuberculin (skin test) positive
> Tuberculin (skin test) reactor
> EXCLUDES 1   *nonspecific reaction to cell mediated immunity measurement of gamma interferon antigen response without active tuberculosis (R76.12)*

R76.12 Nonspecific reaction to cell mediated immunity measurement of gamma interferon antigen response without active tuberculosis
> Nonspecific reaction to QuantiFERON-TB test (QFT) without active tuberculosis
> EXCLUDES 1   *nonspecific reaction to tuberculin skin test without active tuberculosis (R76.11)*
> *positive tuberculin skin test (R76.11)*

R76.8 Other specified abnormal immunological findings in serum
> Raised level of immunoglobulins NOS

R76.9 Abnormal immunological finding in serum, unspecified

✓4th **R77 Other abnormalities of plasma proteins**
> EXCLUDES 1   *disorders of plasma-protein metabolism ▶(E88.0-)◀*

R77.0 Abnormality of albumin

R77.1 Abnormality of globulin
> Hyperglobulinemia NOS

R77.2 Abnormality of alphafetoprotein

R77.8 Other **specified abnormalities of plasma proteins**

R77.9 Abnormality of plasma protein, unspecified

✓4th **R78 Findings of drugs and other substances, not normally found in blood**
> Use additional code to identify any retained foreign body, if applicable (Z18.-)
> EXCLUDES 1   *mental or behavioral disorders due to psychoactive substance use (F10-F19)*

R78.0 Finding of alcohol **in blood**
> Use additional external cause code (Y90.-), for detail regarding alcohol level

R78.1 Finding of opiate **drug in blood**

R78.2 Finding of cocaine **in blood**

R78.3 Finding of hallucinogen **in blood**

R78.4 Finding of other **drugs of** addictive potential **in blood**

R78.5 Finding of other psychotropic **drug in blood**

R78.6 Finding of steroid **agent in blood**

✓5th **R78.7 Finding of abnormal level of** heavy metals **in blood**

> **R78.71 Abnormal** lead **level in blood**
> > EXCLUDES 1   *lead poisoning (T56.0-)*

> **R78.79 Finding of abnormal level of** heavy metals **in blood**

✓5th **R78.8 Finding of other specified substances, not normally found in blood**

> **R78.81 Bacteremia**   `CC`
> > EXCLUDES 1   *sepsis—code to specified infection*
> > **DEF:** Laboratory finding of bacteria in the blood in the absence of two or more signs of sepsis. Transient in nature, it can progress to septicemia with a severe infectious process.
> > **CC Excl:** PDX collection 1136

> **R78.89 Finding of other specified substances, not normally found in blood**
> > Finding of abnormal level of lithium in blood

R78.9 Finding of unspecified **substance, not normally found in blood**

✓4th **R79 Other abnormal findings of blood chemistry**
> Use additional code to identify any retained foreign body, if applicable (Z18.-)
> EXCLUDES 1   *asymptomatic hyperuricemia (E79.0)*
> *hyperglycemia NOS (R73.9)*
> *hypoglycemia NOS (E16.2)*
> *neonatal hypoglycemia (P70.3-P70.4)*
> *specific findings indicating disorder of amino-acid metabolism (E70-E72)*
> *specific findings indicating disorder of carbohydrate metabolism (E73-E74)*
> *specific findings indicating disorder of lipid metabolism (E75.-)*

R79.0 Abnormal level of blood mineral
> Abnormal blood level of cobalt
> Abnormal blood level of copper
> Abnormal blood level of iron
> Abnormal blood level of magnesium
> Abnormal blood level of mineral NEC
> Abnormal blood level of zinc
> > EXCLUDES 1   *abnormal level of lithium (R78.89)*
> > *disorders of mineral metabolism (E83.-)*
> > *neonatal hypomagnesemia (P71.2)*
> > *nutritional mineral deficiency (E58-E61)*

R79.1 Abnormal coagulation profile
> Abnormal or prolonged bleeding time
> Abnormal or prolonged coagulation time
> Abnormal or prolonged partial thromboplastin time [PTT]
> Abnormal or prolonged prothrombin time [PT]
> > EXCLUDES 1   *coagulation defects (D68.-)*
> > EXCLUDES 2   *abnormality of fluid, electrolyte or acid-base balance (E86-E87)*

✓5th **R79.8 Other specified abnormal findings of blood chemistry**

> **R79.81 Abnormal** blood-gas **level**

> **R79.82** Elevated C-reactive protein [CRP]

R79.89 Other **specified abnormal findings of blood chemistry**
> **TIP:** Assign for positive Coombs test when not further clarified in the documentation.

R79.9 Abnormal finding of blood chemistry, unspecified

Abnormal findings on examination of urine, without diagnosis (R80-R82)

> EXCLUDES 1   *abnormal findings on antenatal screening of mother (O28.-)*
> *diagnostic abnormal findings classified elsewhere—see Alphabetical Index*
> *specific findings indicating disorder of amino-acid metabolism (E70-E72)*

✓4th **R80 Proteinuria**
> EXCLUDES 1   *gestational proteinuria (O12.1-)*

R80.0 Isolated **proteinuria**
> Idiopathic proteinuria
> > EXCLUDES 1   *isolated proteinuria with specific morphological lesion (N06.-)*

R80.1 Persistent **proteinuria, unspecified**

R80.2 Orthostatic **proteinuria, unspecified**
> Postural proteinuria

R80.3 Bence Jones **proteinuria**

R80.8 Other **proteinuria**

R80.9 Proteinuria, unspecified
> Albuminuria NOS

R81 Glycosuria
> EXCLUDES 1   *renal glycosuria (E74.8)*

✓4th **R82 Other and unspecified abnormal findings in urine**
> INCLUDES   chromoabnormalities in urine
> Use additional code to identify any retained foreign body, if applicable (Z18.-)
> EXCLUDES 2   *hematuria (R31.-)*

R82.0 Chyluria   `CC`
> > EXCLUDES 1   *filarial chyluria (B74.-)*
> **CC Excl:** PDX collection 1137

R82.1 Myoglobinuria   `CC`
> **CC Excl:** PDX collection 1138

R82.2 Biliuria

R82.3 Hemoglobinuria
> > EXCLUDES 1   *hemoglobinuria due to hemolysis from external causes NEC (D59.6)*
> > *hemoglobinuria due to paroxysmal nocturnal [Marchiafava-Micheli] (D59.5)*
> **DEF:** Free hemoglobin in blood due to rapid hemolysis of red blood cells. Causes include burns, crushed injury, sickle cell anemia, thalassemia, parasitic infections, or kidney infections.

R82.4 Acetonuria
> Ketonuria
> **DEF:** Excessive excretion of acetone in urine that commonly occurs in diabetic acidosis.

R82.5 Elevated urine levels of drugs, medicaments and biological substances
> Elevated urine levels of catecholamines
> Elevated urine levels of indoleacetic acid
> Elevated urine levels of 17-ketosteroids
> Elevated urine levels of steroids

R82.6 Abnormal urine levels of substances chiefly nonmedicinal as to source
> Abnormal urine level of heavy metals

✓5th **R82.7 Abnormal findings on microbiological examination of urine**
> EXCLUDES 1   *colonization status (Z22.-)*
> **AHA:** 2016, 4Q, 65

> **R82.71 Bacteriuria**

> **R82.79 Other abnormal findings on microbiological examination of urine**
> > Positive culture findings of urine

R82.8 Abnormal findings on cytological and histological examination of urine

✓5th **R82.9 Other and unspecified abnormal findings in urine**

> **R82.90 Unspecified abnormal findings in urine**

> **R82.91 Other chromoabnormalities of urine**
> > Chromoconversion (dipstick)
> > Idiopathic dipstick converts positive for blood with no cellular forms in sediment
> > > EXCLUDES 1   *hemoglobinuria (R82.3)*
> > > *myoglobinuria (R82.1)*

✔ Additional Character Required   ✓x7th Placeholder   Unacceptable PDx   Questionable PDx   Manifestation   H1 - H14 HAC   HCC CMS-HCC Dx   HIV HIV Dx

ICD-10-CM 2019   933

✓6ᵗʰ **R82.99**   **Other abnormal findings in urine**
~~Cells and casts in urine~~
~~Crystalluria~~
~~Melanuria~~

- **R82.991**   **Hypocitraturia**
- **R82.992**   **Hyperoxaluria**
  EXCLUDES 1   *primary hyperoxaluria (E72.53)*
- **R82.993**   **Hyperuricoscuria**
- **R82.994**   **Hypercalciuria**
  Idiopathic hypercalciuria
- **R82.998**   **Other abnormal findings in urine**
  Cells and casts in urine
  Crystalluria
  Melanuria

Abnormal findings on examination of other body fluids, substances and tissues, without diagnosis (R83-R89)

EXCLUDES 1   *abnormal findings on antenatal screening of mother (O28.-)*
diagnostic abnormal findings classified elsewhere—see Alphabetical Index
EXCLUDES 2   *abnormal findings on examination of blood, without diagnosis (R70-R79)*
abnormal findings on examination of urine, without diagnosis (R80-R82)
abnormal tumor markers (R97.-)

✓4ᵗʰ **R83   Abnormal findings in cerebrospinal fluid**

R83.0   **Abnormal level of enzymes in cerebrospinal fluid**

R83.1   **Abnormal level of hormones in cerebrospinal fluid**

R83.2   **Abnormal level of other drugs, medicaments and biological substances in cerebrospinal fluid**

R83.3   **Abnormal level of substances chiefly nonmedicinal as to source in cerebrospinal fluid**

R83.4   **Abnormal immunological findings in cerebrospinal fluid**

R83.5   **Abnormal microbiological findings in cerebrospinal fluid**
Positive culture findings in cerebrospinal fluid
EXCLUDES 1   *colonization status (Z22.-)*

R83.6   **Abnormal cytological findings in cerebrospinal fluid**

R83.8   **Other abnormal findings in cerebrospinal fluid**
Abnormal chromosomal findings in cerebrospinal fluid

R83.9   **Unspecified abnormal finding in cerebrospinal fluid**

Cerebrospinal Fluid

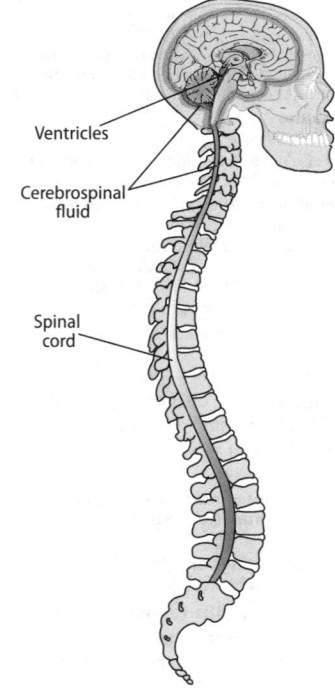

Ventricles

Cerebrospinal
fluid

Spinal
cord

✓4ᵗʰ **R84   Abnormal findings in specimens from respiratory organs and thorax**
INCLUDES   abnormal findings in bronchial washings
abnormal findings in nasal secretions
abnormal findings in pleural fluid
abnormal findings in sputum
abnormal findings in throat scrapings
EXCLUDES 1   *blood-stained sputum (R04.2)*

R84.0   **Abnormal level of enzymes in specimens from respiratory organs and thorax**

R84.1   **Abnormal level of hormones in specimens from respiratory organs and thorax**

R84.2   **Abnormal level of other drugs, medicaments and biological substances in specimens from respiratory organs and thorax**

R84.3   **Abnormal level of substances chiefly nonmedicinal as to source in specimens from respiratory organs and thorax**

R84.4   **Abnormal immunological findings in specimens from respiratory organs and thorax**

R84.5   **Abnormal microbiological findings in specimens from respiratory organs and thorax**
Positive culture findings in specimens from respiratory organs and thorax
EXCLUDES 1   *colonization status (Z22.-)*

R84.6   **Abnormal cytological findings in specimens from respiratory organs and thorax**

R84.7   **Abnormal histological findings in specimens from respiratory organs and thorax**

R84.8   **Other abnormal findings in specimens from respiratory organs and thorax**
Abnormal chromosomal findings in specimens from respiratory organs and thorax

R84.9   **Unspecified abnormal finding in specimens from respiratory organs and thorax**

✓4ᵗʰ **R85   Abnormal findings in specimens from digestive organs and abdominal cavity**
INCLUDES   abnormal findings in peritoneal fluid
abnormal findings in saliva
EXCLUDES 1   *cloudy peritoneal dialysis effluent (R88.0)*
fecal abnormalities (R19.5)

R85.0   **Abnormal level of enzymes in specimens from digestive organs and abdominal cavity**

R85.1   **Abnormal level of hormones in specimens from digestive organs and abdominal cavity**

R85.2   **Abnormal level of other drugs, medicaments and biological substances in specimens from digestive organs and abdominal cavity**

R85.3   **Abnormal level of substances chiefly nonmedicinal as to source in specimens from digestive organs and abdominal cavity**

R85.4   **Abnormal immunological findings in specimens from digestive organs and abdominal cavity**

R85.5   **Abnormal microbiological findings in specimens from digestive organs and abdominal cavity**
Positive culture findings in specimens from digestive organs and abdominal cavity
EXCLUDES 1   *colonization status (Z22.-)*

✓5ᵗʰ **R85.6**   **Abnormal cytological findings in specimens from digestive organs and abdominal cavity**

✓6ᵗʰ **R85.61**   **Abnormal cytologic smear of anus**
EXCLUDES 1   *abnormal cytological findings in specimens from other digestive organs and abdominal cavity (R85.69)*
anal intraepithelial neoplasia I [AIN I] (K62.82)
anal intraepithelial neoplasia II [AIN II] (K62.82)
anal intraepithelial neoplasia III [AIN III] (D01.3)
carcinoma in situ of anus (histologically confirmed) (D01.3)
dysplasia (mild) (moderate) of anus (histologically confirmed) (K62.82)
severe dysplasia of anus (histologically confirmed) (D01.3)
EXCLUDES 2   *anal high risk human papillomavirus (HPV) DNA test positive (R85.81)*
anal low risk human papillomavirus (HPV) DNA test positive (R85.82)

R85.610   **Atypical squamous cells of undetermined significance on cytologic smear of anus [ASC-US]**

R85.611 Atypical squamous cells cannot exclude high grade squamous intraepithelial lesion on cytologic smear of anus [ASC-H]

R85.612 Low grade squamous intraepithelial lesion on cytologic smear of anus [LGSIL]

R85.613 High grade squamous intraepithelial lesion on cytologic smear of anus [HGSIL]

R85.614 Cytologic evidence of malignancy on smear of anus

R85.615 Unsatisfactory cytologic smear of anus
Inadequate sample of cytologic smear of anus

R85.616 Satisfactory anal smear but lacking transformation zone

R85.618 Other abnormal cytological findings on specimens from anus

R85.619 Unspecified abnormal cytological findings in specimens from anus
Abnormal anal cytology NOS
Atypical glandular cells of anus NOS

R85.69 Abnormal cytological findings in specimens from other digestive organs and abdominal cavity

R85.7 Abnormal histological findings in specimens from digestive organs and abdominal cavity

✓5th R85.8 Other abnormal findings in specimens from digestive organs and abdominal cavity

R85.81 Anal high risk human papillomavirus [HPV] DNA test positive
EXCLUDES 1 anogenital warts due to human papillomavirus (HPV) (A63.0)
condyloma acuminatum (A63.0)

R85.82 Anal low risk human papillomavirus [HPV] DNA test positive
Use additional code for associated human papillomavirus (B97.7)

R85.89 Other abnormal findings in specimens from digestive organs and abdominal cavity
Abnormal chromosomal findings in specimens from digestive organs and abdominal cavity

R85.9 Unspecified abnormal finding in specimens from digestive organs and abdominal cavity

✓4th R86 Abnormal findings in specimens from male genital organs
INCLUDES abnormal findings in prostatic secretions
abnormal findings in semen, seminal fluid
abnormal spermatozoa
EXCLUDES 1 azoospermia (N46.0-)
oligospermia (N46.1-)

R86.0 Abnormal level of enzymes in specimens from male genital organs ♂

R86.1 Abnormal level of hormones in specimens from male genital organs ♂

R86.2 Abnormal level of other drugs, medicaments and biological substances in specimens from male genital organs ♂

R86.3 Abnormal level of substances chiefly nonmedicinal as to source in specimens from male genital organs ♂

R86.4 Abnormal immunological findings in specimens from male genital organs ♂

R86.5 Abnormal microbiological findings in specimens from male genital organs ♂
Positive culture findings in specimens from male genital organs
EXCLUDES 1 colonization status (Z22.-)

R86.6 Abnormal cytological findings in specimens from male genital organs ♂

R86.7 Abnormal histological findings in specimens from male genital organs ♂

R86.8 Other abnormal findings in specimens from male genital organs ♂
Abnormal chromosomal findings in specimens from male genital organs

R86.9 Unspecified abnormal finding in specimens from male genital organs ♂

✓4th R87 Abnormal findings in specimens from female genital organs
INCLUDES abnormal findings in secretion and smears from cervix uteri
abnormal findings in secretion and smears from vagina
abnormal findings in secretion and smears from vulva

R87.0 Abnormal level of enzymes in specimens from female genital organs ♀

R87.1 Abnormal level of hormones in specimens from female genital organs ♀

R87.2 Abnormal level of other drugs, medicaments and biological substances in specimens from female genital organs ♀

R87.3 Abnormal level of substances chiefly nonmedicinal as to source in specimens from female genital organs ♀

R87.4 Abnormal immunological findings in specimens from female genital organs ♀

R87.5 Abnormal microbiological findings in specimens from female genital organs ♀
Positive culture findings in specimens from female genital organs
EXCLUDES 1 colonization status (Z22.-)

✓5th R87.6 Abnormal cytological findings in specimens from female genital organs

✓6th R87.61 Abnormal cytological findings in specimens from cervix uteri
EXCLUDES 1 abnormal cytological findings in specimens from other female genital organs (R87.69)
abnormal cytological findings in specimens from vagina (R87.62-)
carcinoma in situ of cervix uteri (histologically confirmed) (D06.-)
cervical intraepithelial neoplasia I [CIN I] (N87.0)
cervical intraepithelial neoplasia II [CIN II] (N87.1)
cervical intraepithelial neoplasia III [CIN III] (D06.-)
dysplasia (mild) (moderate) of cervix uteri (histologically confirmed) (N87.-)
severe dysplasia of cervix uteri (histologically confirmed) (D06.-)
EXCLUDES 2 cervical high risk human papillomavirus (HPV) DNA test positive (R87.810)
cervical low risk human papillomavirus (HPV) DNA test positive (R87.820)

R87.610 Atypical squamous cells of undetermined significance on cytologic smear of cervix [ASC-US] ♀

R87.611 Atypical squamous cells cannot exclude high grade squamous intraepithelial lesion on cytologic smear of cervix [ASC-H] ♀

R87.612 Low grade squamous intraepithelial lesion on cytologic smear of cervix [LGSIL] ♀

R87.613 High grade squamous intraepithelial lesion on cytologic smear of cervix [HGSIL] ♀

R87.614 Cytologic evidence of malignancy on smear of cervix ♀

R87.615 Unsatisfactory cytologic smear of cervix ♀
Inadequate sample of cytologic smear of cervix

R87.616 Satisfactory cervical smear but lacking transformation zone ♀

R87.618 Other abnormal cytological findings on specimens from cervix uteri ♀

R87.619 Unspecified abnormal cytological findings in specimens from cervix uteri ♀
Abnormal cervical cytology NOS
Abnormal Papanicolaou smear of cervix NOS
Abnormal thin preparation smear of cervix NOS
Atypical endocervial cells of cervix NOS
Atypical endometrial cells of cervix NOS
Atypical glandular cells of cervix NOS

✓6ᵗʰ **R87.62 Abnormal cytological findings in specimens from vagina**
Use additional code to identify acquired absence of uterus and cervix, if applicable (Z90.71-)
> EXCLUDES 1   *abnormal cytological findings in specimens from cervix uteri (R87.61-)*
> *abnormal cytological findings in specimens from other female genital organs (R87.69)*
> *carcinoma in situ of vagina (histologically confirmed) (D07.2)*
> *dysplasia (mild) (moderate) of vagina (histologically confirmed) (N89.-)*
> *severe dysplasia of vagina (histologically confirmed) (D07.2)*
> *vaginal intraepithelial neoplasia I [VAIN I] (N89.0)*
> *vaginal intraepithelial neoplasia II [VAIN II] (N89.1)*
> *vaginal intraepithelial neoplasia III [VAIN III] (D07.2)*
>
> EXCLUDES 2   *vaginal high risk human papillomavirus (HPV) DNA test positive (R87.811)*
> *vaginal low risk human papillomavirus (HPV) DNA test positive (R87.821)*

   R87.620 Atypical squamous cells of undetermined significance on cytologic smear of vagina [ASC-US] ♀

   R87.621 Atypical squamous cells cannot exclude high grade squamous intraepithelial lesion on cytologic smear of vagina [ASC-H] ♀

   R87.622 Low grade squamous intraepithelial lesion on cytologic smear of vagina [LGSIL] ♀

   R87.623 High grade squamous intraepithelial lesion on cytologic smear of vagina [HGSIL] ♀

   R87.624 Cytologic evidence of malignancy on smear of vagina ♀

   R87.625 Unsatisfactory cytologic smear of vagina ♀
Inadequate sample of cytologic smear of vagina

   R87.628 Other abnormal cytological findings on specimens from vagina ♀

   R87.629 Unspecified abnormal cytological findings in specimens from vagina ♀
Abnormal Papanicolaou smear of vagina NOS
Abnormal thin preparation smear of vagina NOS
Abnormal vaginal cytology NOS
Atypical endocervical cells of vagina NOS
Atypical endometrial cells of vagina NOS
Atypical glandular cells of vagina NOS

R87.69 Abnormal cytological findings in specimens from other female genital organs ♀
Abnormal cytological findings in specimens from female genital organs NOS
> EXCLUDES 1   *dysplasia of vulva (histologically confirmed) (N90.0-N90.3)*

R87.7 Abnormal histological findings in specimens from female genital organs ♀
> EXCLUDES 1   *carcinoma in situ (histologically confirmed) of female genital organs (D06-D07.3)*
> *cervical intraepithelial neoplasia I [CIN I] (N87.0)*
> *cervical intraepithelial neoplasia II [CIN II] (N87.1)*
> *cervical intraepithelial neoplasia III [CIN III] (D06.-)*
> *dysplasia (mild) (moderate) of cervix uteri (histologically confirmed) (N87.-)*
> *dysplasia (mild) (moderate) of vagina (histologically confirmed) (N89.-)*
> *severe dysplasia of cervix uteri (histologically confirmed) (D06.-)*
> *severe dysplasia of vagina (histologically confirmed) (D07.2)*
> *vaginal intraepithelial neoplasia I [VAIN I] (N89.0)*
> *vaginal intraepithelial neoplasia II [VAIN II] (N89.1)*
> *vaginal intraepithelial neoplasia III [VAIN III] (D07.2)*

✓5ᵗʰ **R87.8 Other abnormal findings in specimens from female genital organs**

   ✓6ᵗʰ **R87.81 High risk human papillomavirus [HPV] DNA test positive from female genital organs**
> EXCLUDES 1   *anogenital warts due to human papillomavirus (HPV) (A63.0)*
> *condyloma acuminatum (A63.0)*

     R87.810 Cervical high risk human papillomavirus [HPV] DNA test positive ♀

     R87.811 Vaginal high risk human papillomavirus [HPV] DNA test positive ♀

   ✓6ᵗʰ **R87.82 Low risk human papillomavirus [HPV] DNA test positive from female genital organs**
Use additional code for associated human papillomavirus (B97.7)

     R87.820 Cervical low risk human papillomavirus [HPV] DNA test positive ♀

     R87.821 Vaginal low risk human papillomavirus [HPV] DNA test positive ♀

   R87.89 Other abnormal findings in specimens from female genital organs ♀
Abnormal chromosomal findings in specimens from female genital organs

R87.9 Unspecified abnormal finding in specimens from female genital organs ♀

✓4ᵗʰ **R88 Abnormal findings in other body fluids and substances**
R88.0 Cloudy (hemodialysis) (peritoneal) dialysis effluent
R88.8 Abnormal findings in other body fluids and substances

✓4ᵗʰ **R89 Abnormal findings in specimens from other organs, systems and tissues**
> INCLUDES   abnormal findings in nipple discharge
> abnormal findings in synovial fluid
> abnormal findings in wound secretions

R89.0 Abnormal level of enzymes in specimens from other organs, systems and tissues

R89.1 Abnormal level of hormones in specimens from other organs, systems and tissues

R89.2 Abnormal level of other drugs, medicaments and biological substances in specimens from other organs, systems and tissues

R89.3 Abnormal level of substances chiefly nonmedicinal as to source in specimens from other organs, systems and tissues

R89.4 Abnormal immunological findings in specimens from other organs, systems and tissues

R89.5 Abnormal microbiological findings in specimens from other organs, systems and tissues
Positive culture findings in specimens from other organs, systems and tissues
> EXCLUDES 1   *colonization status (Z22.-)*

R89.6 Abnormal cytological findings in specimens from other organs, systems and tissues

R89.7 Abnormal histological findings in specimens from other organs, systems and tissues

R89.8 Other abnormal findings in specimens from other organs, systems and tissues
Abnormal chromosomal findings in specimens from other organs, systems and tissues

R89.9 Unspecified abnormal finding in specimens from other organs, systems and tissues

N Newborn: 0   P Pediatric: 0-17   M Maternity: 12-55   A Adult: 15-124   MCC Major Complication/Comorbidity   CC Complication/Comorbidity   SW Severe Wound Dx
936   ICD-10-CM 2019
R87.62–R89.9

Abnormal findings on diagnostic imaging and in function studies, without diagnosis (R90-R94)

<u>INCLUDES</u> nonspecific abnormal findings on diagnostic imaging by computerized axial tomography [CAT scan]
nonspecific abnormal findings on diagnostic imaging by magnetic resonance imaging [MRI][NMR]
nonspecific abnormal findings on diagnostic imaging by positron emission tomography [PET scan]
nonspecific abnormal findings on diagnostic imaging by thermography
nonspecific abnormal findings on diagnostic imaging by ultrasound [echogram]
nonspecific abnormal findings on diagnostic imaging by X-ray examination

<u>EXCLUDES 1</u> *abnormal findings on antenatal screening of mother (O28.-)*
diagnostic abnormal findings classified elsewhere—see Alphabetical Index

✓4ᵗʰ **R90 Abnormal findings on diagnostic imaging of central nervous system**

R90.0 Intracranial space-occupying lesion found on diagnostic imaging of central nervous system

✓5ᵗʰ **R90.8 Other abnormal findings on diagnostic imaging of central nervous system**

R90.81 Abnormal echoencephalogram

R90.82 White matter disease, unspecified

R90.89 Other abnormal findings on diagnostic imaging of central nervous system
Other cerebrovascular abnormality found on diagnostic imaging of central nervous system

✓4ᵗʰ **R91 Abnormal findings on diagnostic imaging of lung**

R91.1 Solitary pulmonary nodule
Coin lesion lung
Solitary pulmonary nodule, subsegmental branch of the bronchial tree

R91.8 Other nonspecific abnormal finding of lung field
Lung mass NOS found on diagnostic imaging of lung
Pulmonary infiltrate NOS
Shadow, lung

✓4ᵗʰ **R92 Abnormal and inconclusive findings on diagnostic imaging of breast**

R92.0 Mammographic microcalcification found on diagnostic imaging of breast
<u>EXCLUDES 2</u> *mammographic calcification (calculus) found on diagnostic imaging of breast (R92.1)*
DEF: Calcium and cellular debris deposits in the breast that cannot be felt but can be detected on a mammogram. The deposits can be a sign of cancer, benign conditions, or changes in the breast tissue as a result of inflammation, injury, or an obstructed duct.

R92.1 Mammographic calcification found on diagnostic imaging of breast
Mammographic calculus found on diagnostic imaging of breast

R92.2 Inconclusive mammogram
Dense breasts NOS
Inconclusive mammogram NEC
Inconclusive mammography due to dense breasts
Inconclusive mammography NEC
AHA: 2015, 1Q, 24

R92.8 Other abnormal and inconclusive findings on diagnostic imaging of breast

✓4ᵗʰ **R93 Abnormal findings on diagnostic imaging of other body structures**

R93.0 Abnormal findings on diagnostic imaging of skull and head, not elsewhere classified
<u>EXCLUDES 1</u> *intracranial space-occupying lesion found on diagnostic imaging (R90.0)*

R93.1 Abnormal findings on diagnostic imaging of heart and coronary circulation
Abnormal echocardiogram NOS
Abnormal heart shadow

R93.2 Abnormal findings on diagnostic imaging of liver and biliary tract
Nonvisualization of gallbladder

R93.3 Abnormal findings on diagnostic imaging of other parts of digestive tract

✓5ᵗʰ **R93.4 Abnormal findings on diagnostic imaging of urinary organs**
<u>EXCLUDES 2</u> *hypertrophy of kidney (N28.81)*
AHA: 2016, 4Q, 66

R93.41 Abnormal radiologic findings on diagnostic imaging of renal pelvis, ureter, or bladder
Filling defect of bladder found on diagnostic imaging
Filling defect of renal pelvis found on diagnostic imaging
Filling defect of ureter found on diagnostic imaging

✓6ᵗʰ **R93.42 Abnormal radiologic findings on diagnostic imaging of kidney**

R93.421 Abnormal radiologic findings on diagnostic imaging of right kidney

R93.422 Abnormal radiologic findings on diagnostic imaging of left kidney

R93.429 Abnormal radiologic findings on diagnostic imaging of unspecified kidney

R93.49 Abnormal radiologic findings on diagnostic imaging of other urinary organs

R93.5 Abnormal findings on diagnostic imaging of other abdominal regions, including retroperitoneum

R93.6 Abnormal findings on diagnostic imaging of limbs
<u>EXCLUDES 2</u> *abnormal finding in skin and subcutaneous tissue* ▶*(R93.8-)*◀

R93.7 Abnormal findings on diagnostic imaging of other parts of musculoskeletal system
<u>EXCLUDES 2</u> *abnormal findings on diagnostic imaging of skull (R93.0)*

✓5ᵗʰ **R93.8 Abnormal findings on diagnostic imaging of other specified body structures**
~~Abnormal finding by radioisotope localization of placenta~~
~~Abnormal radiological finding in skin and subcutaneous tissue~~
~~Mediastinal shift~~

● ✓6ᵗʰ **R93.81 Abnormal radiologic findings on diagnostic imaging of testis**

● **R93.811 Abnormal radiologic findings on diagnostic imaging of right testicle** ♂

● **R93.812 Abnormal radiologic findings on diagnostic imaging of left testicle** ♂

● **R93.813 Abnormal radiologic findings on diagnostic imaging of testicles, bilateral** ♂

● **R93.819 Abnormal radiologic findings on diagnostic imaging of unspecified testicle** ♂

● **R93.89 Abnormal findings on diagnostic imaging of other specified body structures**
Abnormal finding by radioisotope localization of placenta
Abnormal radiological finding in skin and subcutaneous tissue
Mediastinal shift

R93.9 Diagnostic imaging inconclusive due to excess body fat of patient

✓4ᵗʰ **R94 Abnormal results of function studies**
<u>INCLUDES</u> abnormal results of radionuclide [radioisotope] uptake studies
abnormal results of scintigraphy

✓5ᵗʰ **R94.0 Abnormal results of function studies of central nervous system**

R94.01 Abnormal electroencephalogram [EEG]

R94.02 Abnormal brain scan

R94.09 Abnormal results of other function studies of central nervous system

✓5ᵗʰ **R94.1 Abnormal results of function studies of peripheral nervous system and special senses**

✓6ᵗʰ **R94.11 Abnormal results of function studies of eye**

R94.110 Abnormal electro-oculogram [EOG]

R94.111 Abnormal electroretinogram [ERG]
Abnormal retinal function study

R94.112 Abnormal visually evoked potential [VEP]

R94.113 Abnormal oculomotor study

R94.118 Abnormal results of other function studies of eye

☑ Additional Character Required   ✓x7ᵗʰ Placeholder   Unacceptable PDx   Questionable PDx   Manifestation   H1 - H14 HAC   HCC CMS-HCC Dx   HIV HIV Dx

ICD-10-CM 2019   937

✓6ᵗʰ **R94.12 Abnormal results of function studies of** ear and other special senses
AHA: 2016, 3Q, 17
R94.120 **Abnormal** auditory **function study**
R94.121 **Abnormal** vestibular **function study**
R94.128 **Abnormal results of** other **function studies of ear and other special senses**

✓6ᵗʰ **R94.13 Abnormal results of function studies of** peripheral nervous system
R94.130 **Abnormal response to** nerve stimulation, **unspecified**
R94.131 Abnormal electromyogram **[EMG]**
EXCLUDES 1 electromyogram of eye (R94.113)
R94.138 **Abnormal results of** other **function studies of peripheral nervous system**

R94.2 Abnormal results of pulmonary function **studies**
Reduced ventilatory capacity
Reduced vital capacity

✓5ᵗʰ **R94.3 Abnormal results of** cardiovascular function **studies**
R94.30 **Abnormal result of cardiovascular function study,** unspecified
R94.31 **Abnormal** electrocardiogram **[ECG] [EKG]**
EXCLUDES 1 long QT syndrome (I45.81)
R94.39 **Abnormal result of** other **cardiovascular function study**
Abnormal electrophysiological intracardiac studies
Abnormal phonocardiogram
Abnormal vectorcardiogram

R94.4 Abnormal results of kidney function **studies**
Abnormal renal function test

R94.5 Abnormal results of liver function **studies**

R94.6 Abnormal results of thyroid function **studies**

R94.7 Abnormal results of other endocrine function **studies**
EXCLUDES 2 abnormal glucose (R73.0-)

R94.8 Abnormal results of function studies of other organs and systems
Abnormal basal metabolic rate [BMR]
Abnormal bladder function test
Abnormal splenic function test

Abnormal tumor markers (R97)

✓4ᵗʰ **R97 Abnormal tumor markers**
Elevated tumor associated antigens [TAA]
Elevated tumor specific antigens [TSA]
R97.0 **Elevated carcinoembryonic antigen [CEA]**
R97.1 **Elevated cancer antigen 125 [CA 125]**
✓5ᵗʰ R97.2 **Elevated prostate specific antigen [PSA]**
AHA: 2016, 4Q, 66
R97.20 **Elevated prostate specific antigen [PSA]** A♂
R97.21 **Rising PSA following treatment for malignant neoplasm of prostate** A♂
R97.8 **Other abnormal tumor markers**

Ill-defined and unknown cause of mortality (R99)

R99 Ill-defined and unknown cause of mortality
Death (unexplained) NOS
Unspecified cause of mortality

Chapter 19. Injury, Poisoning and Certain Other Consequences of External Causes (S00–T88)

Chapter Specific Guidelines with Coding Examples

The chapter specific guidelines from the ICD-10-CM Official Guidelines for Coding and Reporting have been provided below. Along with these guidelines are coding examples, contained in the shaded boxes, that have been developed to help illustrate the coding and/or sequencing guidance found in these guidelines.

a. Application of 7th characters in Chapter 19

Most categories in chapter 19 have a 7th character requirement for each applicable code. Most categories in this chapter have three 7th character values (with the exception of fractures): A, initial encounter, D, subsequent encounter and S, sequela. Categories for traumatic fractures have additional 7th character values. While the patient may be seen by a new or different provider over the course of treatment for an injury, assignment of the 7th character is based on whether the patient is undergoing active treatment and not whether the provider is seeing the patient for the first time.

For complication codes, active treatment refers to treatment for the condition described by the code, even though it may be related to an earlier precipitating problem. For example, code T84.50XA, Infection and inflammatory reaction due to unspecified internal joint prosthesis, initial encounter, is used when active treatment is provided for the infection, even though the condition relates to the prosthetic device, implant or graft that was placed at a previous encounter.

7th character "A", initial encounter is used for each encounter where the patient is receiving active treatment for the condition.

> Patient admitted after fall from a skateboard onto the sidewalk, x-rays identify a nondisplaced fracture to the distal pole of the right scaphoid bone. The patient is placed in a cast.
>
> **S62.014A**   **Nondisplaced fracture of distal pole of navicular [scaphoid] bone of right wrist, initial encounter for closed fracture**
>
> **V00.131A**   **Fall from skateboard, initial encounter**
>
> **Y92.480**   **Sidewalk as the place of occurrence of the external cause**
>
> **Y93.51**   **Activity, roller skating (inline) and skateboarding**
>
> **Y99.8**   **Other external cause status**
>
> *Explanation:* This fracture would be coded with a seventh character A for initial encounter because the patient received x-rays to identify the site of the fracture and treatment was rendered; this would be considered active treatment.

7th character "D" subsequent encounter is used for encounters after the patient has completed active treatment of the condition and is receiving routine care for the condition during the healing or recovery phase.

> Patient admitted after fall from a skateboard onto the sidewalk resulted in casting of the right arm. X-rays are taken to evaluate how well the nondisplaced fracture to the distal pole of the right scaphoid bone is healing. The physician feels the fracture is healing appropriately; no adjustments to the cast are made.
>
> **S62.014D**   **Nondisplaced fracture of distal pole of navicular [scaphoid] bone of right wrist, subsequent encounter for fracture with routine healing**
>
> **V00.131D**   **Fall from skateboard, subsequent encounter**
>
> *Explanation:* This fracture would be coded with a seventh character D for subsequent encounter, whether the same physician who provided the initial cast application or a different physician is now seeing the patient. Although the patient received x-rays, the intent of the x-rays was to assess how the fracture was healing. There was no active treatment rendered and the visit is therefore considered a subsequent encounter.

The aftercare Z codes should not be used for aftercare for conditions such as injuries or poisonings, where 7th characters are provided to identify subsequent care. For example, for aftercare of an injury, assign the acute injury code with the 7th character "D" (subsequent encounter).

7th character "S", sequela, is for use for complications or conditions that arise as a direct result of a condition, such as scar formation after a burn. The scars are sequelae of the burn. When using 7th character "S", it is

necessary to use both the injury code that precipitated the sequela and the code for the sequela itself. The "S" is added only to the injury code, not the sequela code. The 7th character "S" identifies the injury responsible for the sequela. The specific type of sequela (e.g. scar) is sequenced first, followed by the injury code.

See Section I.B.10 Sequelae, (Late Effects)

> Patient with a history of a nondisplaced fracture to the distal pole of the right scaphoid bone due to a fall from a skateboard is admitted for evaluation of arthritis to the right wrist that has developed as a consequence of the traumatic fracture.
>
> **M12.531**   **Traumatic arthropathy, right wrist**
>
> **S62.014S**   **Nondisplaced fracture of distal pole of navicular [scaphoid] bone of right wrist, sequela**
>
> **V00.131S**   **Fall from skateboard, sequela**
>
> *Explanation:* The code identifying the specific sequela condition (traumatic arthritis) should be coded first followed by the injury that instigated the development of the sequela (fracture). The scaphoid fracture injury code is given a 7th character S for sequela to represent its role as the inciting injury. The fracture has healed and is not being managed or treated on this admit and therefore is not applicable as a first listed or principal diagnosis. However, it is directly related to the development of the arthritis and should be appended as a secondary code to signify this cause and effect relationship.

b. Coding of injuries

When coding injuries, assign separate codes for each injury unless a combination code is provided, in which case the combination code is assigned. Codes from category T07, Unspecified multiple injuries should not be assigned in the inpatient setting unless information for a more specific code is not available. Traumatic injury codes (S00-T14.9) are not to be used for normal, healing surgical wounds or to identify complications of surgical wounds.

The code for the most serious injury, as determined by the provider and the focus of treatment, is sequenced first.

1) Superficial injuries

Superficial injuries such as abrasions or contusions are not coded when associated with more severe injuries of the same site.

2) Primary injury with damage to nerves/blood vessels

When a primary injury results in minor damage to peripheral nerves or blood vessels, the primary injury is sequenced first with additional code(s) for injuries to nerves and spinal cord (such as category S04), and/or injury to blood vessels (such as category S15). When the primary injury is to the blood vessels or nerves, that injury should be sequenced first.

c. Coding of traumatic fractures

The principles of multiple coding of injuries should be followed in coding fractures. Fractures of specified sites are coded individually by site in accordance with both the provisions within categories S02, S12, S22, S32, S42, S49, S52, S59, S62, S72, S79, S82, S89, S92 and the level of detail furnished by medical record content.

A fracture not indicated as open or closed should be coded to closed. A fracture not indicated whether displaced or not displaced should be coded to displaced.

More specific guidelines are as follows:

1) Initial vs. subsequent encounter for fractures

Traumatic fractures are coded using the appropriate 7th character for initial encounter (A, B, C) for each encounter where the patient is receiving active treatment for the fracture. The appropriate 7th character for initial encounter should also be assigned for a patient who delayed seeking treatment for the fracture or nonunion.

Fractures are coded using the appropriate 7th character for subsequent care for encounters after the patient has completed active treatment of the fracture and is receiving routine care for the fracture during the healing or recovery phase.

Care for complications of surgical treatment for fracture repairs during the healing or recovery phase should be coded with the appropriate complication codes.

Care of complications of fractures, such as malunion and nonunion, should be reported with the appropriate 7th character for subsequent

care with nonunion (K, M, N,) or subsequent care with malunion (P, Q, R).

Malunion/nonunion: The appropriate 7th character for initial encounter should also be assigned for a patient who delayed seeking treatment for the fracture or nonunion.

> Female patient fell during a forest hiking excursion almost six months ago and until recently did not feel she needed to seek medical attention for her left ankle pain; x-rays show nonunion of lateral malleolus and surgery has been scheduled
>
> | Code | Description |
> |---|---|
> | S82.62XA | Displaced fracture of lateral malleolus of left fibula, initial encounter for closed fracture |
> | W01.0XXA | Fall on same level from slipping, tripping and stumbling without subsequent striking against object, initial encounter |
> | Y92.821 | Forest as place of occurrence of the external cause |
> | Y93.01 | Activity, walking, marching and hiking |
> | Y99.8 | Other external cause status |
>
> *Explanation:* A seventh character of A is used for the lateral malleolus nonunion fracture to signify that the fracture is receiving active treatment. The delayed care for the fracture has resulted in a nonunion, but capturing the nonunion in the seventh character is trumped by the provision of active care.

The open fracture designations in the assignment of the 7th character for fractures of the forearm, femur and lower leg, including ankle are based on the Gustilo open fracture classification. When the Gustilo classification type is not specified for an open fracture, the 7th character for open fracture type I or II should be assigned (B, E, H, M, Q).

> A 17-year-old arrives at the trauma center with open, displaced right forearm fracture with extensive soft tissue damage. He fell while being tackled playing football for his high school team. On-call orthopaedic specialist documents segmental type IIIA fracture of radial shaft with no need for plastic consult.
>
> | Code | Description |
> |---|---|
> | S52.361C | Displaced segmental fracture of shaft of radius, right arm, initial encounter for open fracture type IIIA, IIIB, or IIIC |
> | W03.XXXA | Other fall on same level due to collision with another person, initial encounter |
> | Y92.321 | Football field as the place of occurrence of the external cause |
> | Y93.61 | Activity, American tackle football |
>
> *Explanation:* The seventh character for forearm fractures capture the type of encounter and whether the fracture is open or closed; open fractures are broken down further by the type of fracture based on the Gustilo classification. The Gustilo classification describes the severity of open fracture and soft tissue injury. Type IIIA describes an open fracture with extensive soft tissue injury but adequate soft tissue remaining for wound coverage. A segmental fracture means that the bone is broken in two places, leaving at least one segment unattached to the bone. There is no need to report an additional code for the soft tissue injury as it is captured in the fracture code.

A code from category M80, not a traumatic fracture code, should be used for any patient with known osteoporosis who suffers a fracture, even if the patient had a minor fall or trauma, if that fall or trauma would not usually break a normal, healthy bone.

See Section I.C.13. Osteoporosis.

The aftercare Z codes should not be used for aftercare for traumatic fractures. For aftercare of a traumatic fracture, assign the acute fracture code with the appropriate 7th character.

2) Multiple fractures sequencing

Multiple fractures are sequenced in accordance with the severity of the fracture.

d. Coding of burns and corrosions

The ICD-10-CM makes a distinction between burns and corrosions. The burn codes are for thermal burns, except sunburns, that come from a heat source, such as a fire or hot appliance. The burn codes are also for burns resulting from electricity and radiation. Corrosions are burns due to chemicals. The guidelines are the same for burns and corrosions.

Current burns (T20-T25) are classified by depth, extent and by agent (X code). Burns are classified by depth as first degree (erythema), second degree (blistering), and third degree (full-thickness involvement). Burns of the eye and internal organs (T26-T28) are classified by site, but not by degree.

1) Sequencing of burn and related condition codes

Sequence first the code that reflects the highest degree of burn when more than one burn is present.

    a.   When the reason for the admission or encounter is for treatment of external multiple burns, sequence first the code that reflects the burn of the highest degree.

    b.   When a patient has both internal and external burns, the circumstances of admission govern the selection of the principal diagnosis or first-listed diagnosis.

    c.   When a patient is admitted for burn injuries and other related conditions such as smoke inhalation and/or respiratory failure, the circumstances of admission govern the selection of the principal or first-listed diagnosis.

> Patient admitted with minor first-degree burns to multiple sites of her right and left hands as well as severe smoke inhalation. While she was sleeping at home, a candle on her dresser lit the bedroom curtains on fire.
>
> | Code | Description |
> |---|---|
> | T59.811A | Toxic effect of smoke, accidental (unintentional), initial encounter |
> | J70.5 | Respiratory conditions due to smoke inhalation |
> | T23.191A | Burn of first degree of multiple sites of right wrist and hand, initial encounter |
> | T23.192A | Burn of first degree of multiple sites of left wrist and hand, initial encounter |
> | X08.8XXA | Exposure to other specified smoke, fire and flames, initial encounter |
> | Y92.003 | Bedroom of unspecified non-institutional (private) residence as the place of occurrence of the external cause |
> | Y93.84 | Activity, sleeping |
>
> *Explanation:* Based on the documentation, the inhalation injury is more severe than the first-degree burns and is sequenced first. The burns to the hands are appended as secondary diagnoses.

2) Burns of the same *anatomic* site

Classify burns of the same **anatomic** site **and on the same side** but of different degrees to the subcategory identifying the highest degree recorded in the diagnosis **(e.g., for second and third degree burns of right thigh, assign only code T24.311-).**

3) Non-healing burns

Non-healing burns are coded as acute burns.

Necrosis of burned skin should be coded as a non-healed burn.

4) Infected burn

For any documented infected burn site, use an additional code for the infection.

5) Assign separate codes for each burn site

When coding burns, assign separate codes for each burn site. Category T30, Burn and corrosion, body region unspecified is extremely vague and should rarely be used.

Codes for burns of "multiple sites" should only be assigned when the medical record documentation does not specify the individual sites.

> Patient is admitted with third-degree burns of the scalp as well as second-degree burns to the back of the right hand
>
> | Code | Description |
> |---|---|
> | T20.35XA | Burn of third degree of scalp [any part], initial encounter |
> | T23.261A | Burn of second degree of back of right hand, initial encounter |
>
> *Explanation:* Two codes may be reported as the hand and face represent distinct burn sites.

6) Burns and corrosions classified according to extent of body surface involved

Assign codes from category T31, Burns classified according to extent of body surface involved, or T32, Corrosions classified according to extent of body surface involved, when the site of the burn is not specified or when

there is a need for additional data. It is advisable to use category T31 as additional coding when needed to provide data for evaluating burn mortality, such as that needed by burn units. It is also advisable to use category T31 as an additional code for reporting purposes when there is mention of a third-degree burn involving 20 percent or more of the body surface.

Categories T31 and T32 are based on the classic "rule of nines" in estimating body surface involved: head and neck are assigned nine percent, each arm nine percent, each leg 18 percent, the anterior trunk 18 percent, posterior trunk 18 percent, and genitalia one percent. Providers may change these percentage assignments where necessary to accommodate infants and children who have proportionately larger heads than adults, and patients who have large buttocks, thighs, or abdomen that involve burns.

> Patient seen in burn unit for dressing change after he accidentally spilled acetic acid on himself two days ago. The second-degree burns to his right thigh, covering about 3 percent of his body surface, are healing appropriately.
>
> **T54.2X1D**   **Toxic effect of corrosive acids and acid-like substances, accidental (unintentional), subsequent encounter**
>
> **T24.611D**   **Corrosion of second degree of right thigh, subsequent encounter**
>
> **T32.0**   **Corrosions involving less than 10% of body surface**
>
> *Explanation:* Code T32.0 provides additional information as to how much of the patient's body was affected by the corrosive substance.

7) Encounters for treatment of sequela of burns

Encounters for the treatment of the late effects of burns or corrosions (i.e., scars or joint contractures) should be coded with a burn or corrosion code with the 7th character "S" for sequela.

8) Sequelae with a late effect code and current burn

When appropriate, both a code for a current burn or corrosion with 7th character "A" or "D" and a burn or corrosion code with 7th character "S" may be assigned on the same record (when both a current burn and sequelae of an old burn exist). Burns and corrosions do not heal at the same rate and a current healing wound may still exist with sequela of a healed burn or corrosion.

See Section I.B.10 Sequela (Late Effects)

> Female patient seen in ED for second-degree burn to the left ear; she also has significant scarring on her left elbow from a third-degree burn from childhood
>
> **T20.212A**   **Burn of second degree of left ear [any part, except ear drum], initial encounter**
>
> **L90.5**   **Scar conditions and fibrosis of skin**
>
> **T22.322S**   **Burn of third degree of left elbow, sequela**
>
> *Explanation:* The patient is being seen for management of a current second-degree burn, which is reflected in the code by appending the seventh character of A, indicating active treatment or management of this burn. The elbow scarring is a sequela of a previous third-degree burn. The sequela condition precedes the original burn injury, which is appended with a seventh character of S.

9) Use of an external cause code with burns and corrosions

An external cause code should be used with burns and corrosions to identify the source and intent of the burn, as well as the place where it occurred.

e. Adverse effects, poisoning, underdosing and toxic effects

Codes in categories T36-T65 are combination codes that include the substance that was taken as well as the intent. No additional external cause code is required for poisonings, toxic effects, adverse effects and underdosing codes.

1) Do not code directly from the Table of Drugs

Do not code directly from the Table of Drugs and Chemicals. Always refer back to the Tabular List.

2) Use as many codes as necessary to describe

Use as many codes as necessary to describe completely all drugs, medicinal or biological substances.

3) If the same code would describe the causative agent

If the same code would describe the causative agent for more than one adverse reaction, poisoning, toxic effect or underdosing, assign the code only once.

4) If two or more drugs, medicinal or biological substances

If two or more drugs, medicinal or biological substances are reported, code each individually unless a combination code is listed in the Table of Drugs and Chemicals.

5) The occurrence of drug toxicity is classified in ICD-10-CM as follows:

(a) Adverse effect

When coding an adverse effect of a drug that has been correctly prescribed and properly administered, assign the appropriate code for the nature of the adverse effect followed by the appropriate code for the adverse effect of the drug (T36-T50). The code for the drug should have a 5th or 6th character "5" (for example T36.0X5-) Examples of the nature of an adverse effect are tachycardia, delirium, gastrointestinal hemorrhaging, vomiting, hypokalemia, hepatitis, renal failure, or respiratory failure.

> Patient admitted for stomach pain and jaundice, indicated by physician as possible side-effects of Inderal, recently started for hypertension. Inderal was discontinued and the patient switched to Atenolol instead.
>
> **R10.9**   **Unspecified abdominal pain**
>
> **R17**   **Unspecified jaundice**
>
> **T44.7X5A**   **Adverse effect of beta-adrenoreceptor antagonists, initial encounter**
>
> **I10**   **Essential (primary) hypertension**
>
> *Explanation:* The side-effects caused by the drug are listed first, followed by the code for the adverse effect of the drug to capture the specific drug that was used.

(b) Poisoning

When coding a poisoning or reaction to the improper use of a medication (e.g., overdose, wrong substance given or taken in error, wrong route of administration), first assign the appropriate code from categories T36-T50. The poisoning codes have an associated intent as their 5th or 6th character (accidental, intentional self-harm, assault and undetermined. If the intent of the poisoning is unknown or unspecified, code the intent as accidental intent. The undetermined intent is only for use if the documentation in the record specifies that the intent cannot be determined. Use additional code(s) for all manifestations of poisonings.

> A 55-year-old female status post recent left knee replacement is admitted due to confusion, dizziness, and nausea. Her spouse brought in her prescribed Xanax, Ambien, and Percocet bottles but has no idea how many she took. It is suspected that her symptoms are due to an overdose of these medications.
>
> **T42.4X1A**   **Poisoning by benzodiazepines, accidental (unintentional), initial encounter**
>
> **T42.6X1A**   **Poisoning by other antiepileptic and sedative-hypnotic drugs, accidental (unintentional), initial encounter**
>
> **T40.2X1A**   **Poisoning by other opioids, accidental (unintentional), initial encounter**
>
> **R41.0**   **Disorientation, unspecified**
>
> **R42**   **Dizziness and giddiness**
>
> **R11.0**   **Nausea**
>
> *Explanation:* It was not documented whether the overdose of the drugs was accidental or intentional; therefore the correct reporting of the poisoning codes is accidental intent. The poisoning codes are sequenced first, followed by manifestations of the poisoning.

If there is also a diagnosis of abuse or dependence of the substance, the abuse or dependence is assigned as an additional code.

Examples of poisoning include:

(i)   Error was made in drug prescription

     Errors made in drug prescription or in the administration of the drug by provider, nurse, patient, or other person.

(ii)   Overdose of a drug intentionally taken

If an overdose of a drug was intentionally taken or administered and resulted in drug toxicity, it would be coded as a poisoning.

(iii) Nonprescribed drug taken with correctly prescribed and properly administered drug

If a nonprescribed drug or medicinal agent was taken in combination with a correctly prescribed and properly administered drug, any drug toxicity or other reaction resulting from the interaction of the two drugs would be classified as a poisoning.

(iv) Interaction of drug(s) and alcohol

When a reaction results from the interaction of a drug(s) and alcohol, this would be classified as poisoning.

See Section I.C.4. if poisoning is the result of insulin pump malfunctions.

(c) Underdosing

Underdosing refers to taking less of a medication than is prescribed by a provider or a manufacturer's instruction. **Discontinuing the use of a prescribed medication on the patient's own initiative (not directed by the patient's provider) is also classified as an underdosing.** For underdosing, assign the code from categories T36-T50 (fifth or sixth character "6").

Codes for underdosing should never be assigned as principal or first-listed codes. If a patient has a relapse or exacerbation of the medical condition for which the drug is prescribed because of the reduction in dose, then the medical condition itself should be coded.

Noncompliance (Z91.12-, Z91.13- **and Z91.14-**) or complication of care (Y63.6-Y63.9) codes are to be used with an underdosing code to indicate intent, if known.

> Patient admitted for atrial fibrillation with history of chronic atrial fibrillation for which she is prescribed amiodarone. Financial concerns have left the patient unable to pay for her prescriptions and she has been skipping her amiodarone dose every other day to offset the cost.
>
> | **I48.2** | **Chronic atrial fibrillation** |
> |---|---|
> | **T46.2X6A** | **Underdosing of other antidysrhythmic drugs, initial encounter** |
> | **Z91.120** | **Patient's intentional underdosing of medication regimen due to financial hardship** |
>
> *Explanation:* By skipping her amiodarone pill every other day, the patient's atrial fibrillation returned. The condition for which the drug was being taken is reported first, followed by an underdosing code to show that the patient was not adhering to her prescription regimen. The Z code helps elaborate on the patient's social and/or economic circumstances that led to the patient taking less then what she was prescribed.

(d) Toxic effects

When a harmful substance is ingested or comes in contact with a person, this is classified as a toxic effect. The toxic effect codes are in categories T51-T65.

Toxic effect codes have an associated intent: accidental, intentional self-harm, assault and undetermined.

f. Adult and child abuse, neglect and other maltreatment

Sequence first the appropriate code from categories T74.- (Adult and child abuse, neglect and other maltreatment, confirmed) or T76.- (Adult and child abuse, neglect and other maltreatment, suspected) for abuse, neglect and other maltreatment, followed by any accompanying mental health or injury code(s).

If the documentation in the medical record states abuse or neglect it is coded as confirmed (T74.-). It is coded as suspected if it is documented as suspected (T76.-).

For cases of confirmed abuse or neglect an external cause code from the assault section (X92-Y09) should be added to identify the cause of any physical injuries. A perpetrator code (Y07) should be added when the perpetrator of the abuse is known. For suspected cases of abuse or neglect, do not report external cause or perpetrator code.

If a suspected case of abuse, neglect or mistreatment is ruled out during an encounter code Z04.71, Encounter for examination and observation following alleged physical adult abuse, ruled out, or code Z04.72, Encounter for examination and observation following alleged child physical abuse, ruled out, should be used, not a code from T76.

If a suspected case of alleged rape or sexual abuse is ruled out during an encounter code Z04.41, Encounter for examination and observation following alleged adult rape or code Z04.42, Encounter for examination and observation following alleged child rape, should be used, not a code from T76.

If a suspected case of forced sexual exploitation or forced labor exploitation is ruled out during an encounter, code Z04.81, Encounter for examination and observation of victim following forced sexual exploitation, or code Z04.82, Encounter for examination and observation of victim following forced labor exploitation, should be used, not a code from T76.

See Section I.C.15. Abuse in a pregnant patient.

g. Complications of care

1) General guidelines for complications of care

(a) Documentation of complications of care

See Section I.B.16. for information on documentation of complications of care.

2) Pain due to medical devices

Pain associated with devices, implants or grafts left in a surgical site (for example painful hip prosthesis) is assigned to the appropriate code(s) found in Chapter 19, Injury, poisoning, and certain other consequences of external causes. Specific codes for pain due to medical devices are found in the T code section of the ICD-10-CM. Use additional code(s) from category G89 to identify acute or chronic pain due to presence of the device, implant or graft (G89.18 or G89.28).

> Chronic left breast pain secondary to breast implant
>
> | **T85.848A** | **Pain due to other internal prosthetic devices, implants and grafts, initial encounter** |
> |---|---|
> | **N64.4** | **Mastodynia** |
> | **G89.28** | **Other chronic postprocedural pain** |
>
> *Explanation:* As the pain is a complication related to the breast implant, the complication code is sequenced first. The T code does not describe the site or type of pain, so additional codes may be appended to indicate that the patient is experiencing chronic pain in the breast.

3) Transplant complications

(a) Transplant complications other than kidney

Codes under category T86, Complications of transplanted organs and tissues, are for use for both complications and rejection of transplanted organs. A transplant complication code is only assigned if the complication affects the function of the transplanted organ. Two codes are required to fully describe a transplant complication: the appropriate code from category T86 and a secondary code that identifies the complication.

Pre-existing conditions or conditions that develop after the transplant are not coded as complications unless they affect the function of the transplanted organs.

See I.C.21. for transplant organ removal status

See I.C.2. for malignant neoplasm associated with transplanted organ.

(b) Kidney transplant complications

Patients who have undergone kidney transplant may still have some form of chronic kidney disease (CKD) because the kidney transplant may not fully restore kidney function. Code T86.1- should be assigned for documented complications of a kidney transplant, such as transplant failure or rejection or other transplant complication. Code T86.1- should not be assigned for post kidney transplant patients who have chronic kidney (CKD) unless a transplant complication such as transplant failure or rejection is documented. If the documentation is unclear as to whether the patient has a complication of the transplant, query the provider.

Conditions that affect the function of the transplanted kidney, other than CKD, should be assigned a code from subcategory T86.1, Complications of transplanted organ, Kidney, and a secondary code that identifies the complication.

For patients with CKD following a kidney transplant, but who do not have a complication such as failure or rejection, *see section I.C.14. Chronic kidney disease and kidney transplant status.*

Patient with chronic kidney disease stage 2; history of successful kidney transplant with no complications identified

N18.2   **Chronic kidney disease, stage 2 (mild)**

Z94.Ø   **Kidney transplant status**

Explanation: This patient's stage 2 CKD is not indicated as being due to the transplanted kidney but instead is just the residual disease the patient had prior to the transplant.

4) Complication codes that include the external cause

As with certain other T codes, some of the complications of care codes have the external cause included in the code. The code includes the nature of the complication as well as the type of procedure that caused the complication. No external cause code indicating the type of procedure is necessary for these codes.

5) Complications of care codes within the body system chapters

Intraoperative and postprocedural complication codes are found within the body system chapters with codes specific to the organs and structures of that body system. These codes should be sequenced first, followed by a code(s) for the specific complication, if applicable.

During a spinal fusion procedure, the surgeon inadvertently punctured the dura. The midline durotomy was repaired, and the fusion procedure was completed.

G97.41   **Accidental puncture or laceration of dura during a procedure**

Explanation: The accidental durotomy is not coded to an injury code in chapter 19 but instead is categorized to the nervous system chapter.

Muscle/Tendon Table

ICD-10-CM categorizes certain muscles and tendons in the upper and lower extremities by their action (e.g., extension, flexion), their anatomical location (e.g., posterior, anterior), and/or whether they are intrinsic or extrinsic to a certain anatomical area. The Muscle/Tendon Table is provided at the beginning of chapters 13 and 19 as a resource to help users when code selection depends on one or more of these characteristics. Please note that this table is not all-inclusive, and proper code assignment should be based on the provider's documentation.

Body Region	Muscle	Extensor Tendon	Flexor Tendon	Other Tendon
Shoulder				
	Deltoid	Posterior deltoid	Anterior deltoid	
	Rotator cuff			
	Infraspinatus			Infraspinatus
	Subscapularis			Subscapularis
	Supraspinatus			Supraspinatus
	Teres minor			Teres minor
	Teres major	Teres major		
Upper arm				
	Anterior muscles			
	Biceps brachii — long head		Biceps brachii — long head	
	Biceps brachii — short head		Biceps brachii — short head	
	Brachialis		Brachialis	
	Coracobrachialis		Coracobrachialis	
	Posterior muscles			
	Triceps brachii	Triceps brachii		
Forearm				
	Anterior muscles			
	Flexors			
	Deep			
	Flexor digitorum profundus		Flexor digitorum profundus	
	Flexor pollicis longus		Flexor pollicis longus	
	Intermediate			
	Flexor digitorum superficialis		Flexor digitorum superficialis	
	Superficial			
	Flexor carpi radialis		Flexor carpi radialis	
	Flexor carpi ulnaris		Flexor carpi ulnaris	
	Palmaris longus		Palmaris longus	
	Pronators			
	Pronator quadratus			Pronator quadratus
	Pronator teres			Pronator teres
	Posterior muscles			
	Extensors			
	Deep			
	Abductor pollicis longus			Abductor pollicis longus
	Extensor indicis	Extensor indicis		
	Extensor pollicis brevis	Extensor pollicis brevis		
	Extensor pollicis longus	Extensor pollicis longus		
	Superficial			
	Brachioradialis			Brachioradialis
	Extensor carpi radialis brevis	Extensor carpi radialis brevis		
	Extensor carpi radialis longus	Extensor carpi radialis longus		
	Extensor carpi ulnaris	Extensor carpi ulnaris		
	Extensor digiti minimi	Extensor digiti minimi		
	Extensor digitorum	Extensor digitorum		
	Anconeus	Anconeus		
	Supinator			Supinator

Body Region	Muscle	Extensor Tendon	Flexor Tendon	Other Tendon
Hand				
Extrinsic — attach to a site in the forearm as well as a site in the hand with action related to hand movement at the wrist				
	Extensor carpi radialis brevis	Extensor carpi radialis brevis		
	Extensor carpi radialis longus	Extensor carpie radialis longus		
	Extensor carpi ulnaris	Extensor carpi ulnaris		
	Flexor carpi radialis		Flexor carpi radialis	
	Flexor carpi ulnaris		Flexor carpi ulnaris	
	Flexor digitorum superficialis		Flexor digitorum superficialis	
	Palmaris longus		Palmaris longus	
Extrinsic — attach to a site in the forearm as well as a site in the hand with action in the hand related to finger movement				
	Adductor pollicis longus			Adductor pollicis longus
	Extensor digiti minimi	Extensor digiti minimi		
	Extensor digitorum	Extensor digitorum		
	Extensor indicis	Extensor indicis		
	Flexor digitorum profundus		Flexor digitorum profundus	
	Flexor digitorum superficialis		Flexor digitorum superficialis	
Extrinsic — attach to a site in the forearm as well as a site in the hand with action in the hand related to thumb movement				
	Extensor pollicis brevis	Extensor pollicis brevis		
	Extensor pollicis longus	Extensor pollicis longus		
	Flexor pollicis longus		Flexor pollicis longus	
Intrinsic — found within the hand only				
	Adductor pollicis			Adductor pollicis
	Dorsal interossei	Dorsal interossei	Dorsal interossei	
	Lumbricals	Lumbricals	Lumbricals	
	Palmaris brevis			Palmaris brevis
	Palmar interossei	Palmar interossei	Palmar interossei	
	Hypothenar muscles			
	Abductor digiti minimi			Abductor digiti minimi
	Flexor digiti minimi brevis		Flexor digiti minimi brevis	
	Oppenens digiti minimi		Oppenens digiti minimi	
	Thenar muscles			
	Abductor pollicis brevis			Abductor pollicis brevis
	Flexor pollicis brevis		Flexor pollicis brevis	
	Oppenens pollicis		Oppenens pollicis	
Thigh				
	Anterior muscles			
	Iliopsoas		Iliopsoas	
	Pectineus		Pectineus	
	Quadriceps	Quadriceps		
	Rectus femoris	Rectus femoris — Extends knee	Rectus femoris — Flexes hip	
	Vastus intermedius	Vastus intermedius		
	Vastus lateralis	Vastus lateralis		
	Vastus medialis	Vastus medialis		
	Sartorius		Sartorius	
	Medial muscles			
	Adductor brevis			Adductor brevis
	Adductor longus			Adductor longus
	Adductor magnus			Adductor magnus
	Gracilis			Gracilis
	Obturator externus			Obturator externus
	Posterior muscles			
	Hamstring	Hamstring — Extends hip	Hamstring — Flexes knee	
	Biceps femoris	Biceps femoris	Biceps femoris	
	Semimembranosus	Semimembranosus	Semimembranosus	
	Semitendinosus	Semitendinosus	Semitendinosus	

Body Region	Muscle	Extensor Tendon	Flexor Tendon	Other Tendon
Lower leg				
	Anterior muscles			
	Extensor digitorum longus	Extensor digitorum longus		
	Extensor hallucis longus	Extensor hallucis longus		
	Fibularis (peroneus) tertius	Fibularis (peroneus) tertius		
	Tibialis anterior	Tibialis anterior		Tibialis anterior
	Lateral muscles			
	Fibularis (peroneus) brevis		Fibularis (peroneus) brevis	
	Fibularis (peroneus) longus		Fibularis (peroneus) longus	
	Posterior muscles			
	Deep			
	Flexor digitorum longus		Flexor digitorum longus	
	Flexor hallucis longus		Flexor hallucis longus	
	Popliteus		Popliteus	
	Tibialis posterior		Tibialis posterior	
	Superficial			
	Gastrocnemius		Gastrocnemius	
	Plantaris		Plantaris	
	Soleus		Soleus	
				Calcaneal (Achilles)
Ankle/Foot				
Extrinsic — attach to a site in the lower leg as well as a site in the foot with action related to foot movement at the ankle				
	Plantaris		Plantaris	
	Soleus		Soleus	
	Tibialis anterior	Tibialis anterior		
	Tibialis posterior		Tibialis posterior	
Extrinsic — attach to a site in the lower leg as well as a site in the foot with action in the foot related to toe movement				
	Extensor digitorum longus	Extensor digitorum longus		
	Extensor hallicus longus	Extensor hallicus longus		
	Flexor digitorum longus		Flexor digitorum longus	
	Flexor hallucis longus		Flexor hallucis longus	
Intrinsic — found within the ankle/foot only				
	Dorsal muscles			
	Extensor digitorum brevis	Extensor digitorum brevis		
	Extensor hallucis brevis	Extensor hallucis brevis		
	Plantar muscles			
	Abductor digiti minimi		Abductor digiti minimi	
	Abductor hallucis		Abductor hallucis	
	Dorsal interossei	Dorsal interossei	Dorsal interossei	
	Flexor digiti minimi brevis		Flexor digiti minimi brevis	
	Flexor digitorum brevis		Flexor digitorum brevis	
	Flexor hallucis brevis		Flexor hallucis brevis	
	Lumbricals	Lumbricals	Lumbricals	
	Quadratus plantae		Quadratus plantae	
	Plantar interossei	Plantar interossei	Plantar interossei	

Chapter 19. Injury, Poisoning and Certain Other Consequences of External Causes (S00-T88)

NOTE   Use secondary code(s) from Chapter 20, External causes of morbidity, to indicate cause of injury. Codes within the T section that include the external cause do not require an additional external cause code.

Use additional code to identify any retained foreign body, if applicable (Z18.-)

EXCLUDES 1   birth trauma (P10-P15)
obstetric trauma (O70-O71)

NOTE   The chapter uses the S-section for coding different types of injuries related to single body regions and the T-section to cover injuries to unspecified body regions as well as poisoning and certain other consequences of external causes.

AHA: 2016, 2Q, 3-7; 2015, 4Q, 35-38; 2015, 3Q, 37-39, 40; 2015, 2Q, 6; 2015, 1Q, 3-21

TIP: The specific site of an injury can be determined from the radiology report when authenticated by a radiologist and available at the time of code assignment.

This chapter contains the following blocks:

S00-S09	Injuries to the head
S10-S19	Injuries to the neck
S20-S29	Injuries to the thorax
S30-S39	Injuries to the abdomen, lower back, lumbar spine, pelvis and external genitals
S40-S49	Injuries to the shoulder and upper arm
S50-S59	Injuries to the elbow and forearm
S60-S69	Injuries to the wrist, hand and fingers
S70-S79	Injuries to the hip and thigh
S80-S89	Injuries to the knee and lower leg
S90-S99	Injuries to the ankle and foot
T07	Injuries involving multiple body regions
T14	Injury of unspecified body region
T15-T19	Effects of foreign body entering through natural orifice
T20-T25	Burns and corrosions of external body surface, specified by site
T26-T28	Burns and corrosions confined to eye and internal organs
T30-T32	Burns and corrosions of multiple and unspecified body regions
T33-T34	Frostbite
T36-T50	Poisoning by, adverse effect of and underdosing of drugs, medicaments and biological substances
T51-T65	Toxic effects of substances chiefly nonmedicinal as to source
T66-T78	Other and unspecified effects of external causes
T79	Certain early complications of trauma
T80-T88	Complications of surgical and medical care, not elsewhere classified

Injuries to the head (S00-S09)

INCLUDES   injuries of ear
injuries of eye
injuries of face [any part]
injuries of gum
injuries of jaw
injuries of oral cavity
injuries of palate
injuries of periocular area
injuries of scalp
injuries of temporomandibular joint area
injuries of tongue
injuries of tooth

Code also for any associated infection

EXCLUDES 2   burns and corrosions (T20-T32)
effects of foreign body in ear (T16)
effects of foreign body in larynx (T17.3)
effects of foreign body in mouth NOS (T18.0)
effects of foreign body in nose (T17.0-T17.1)
effects of foreign body in pharynx (T17.2)
effects of foreign body on external eye (T15.-)
frostbite (T33-T34)
insect bite or sting, venomous (T63.4)

√4ᵗʰ **S00**   **Superficial injury of head**
   EXCLUDES 1   diffuse cerebral contusion (S06.2-)
       focal cerebral contusion (S06.3-)
       injury of eye and orbit (S05.-)
       open wound of head (S01.-)

> The appropriate 7th character is to be added to each code from category S00.
> A   initial encounter
> D   subsequent encounter
> S   sequela

   √5ᵗʰ **S00.0**   **Superficial injury of** scalp
     √ₓ7ᵗʰ **S00.00**   Unspecified **superficial injury of scalp**
     √ₓ7ᵗʰ **S00.01**   Abrasion **of scalp**

√ₓ7ᵗʰ **S00.02**   Blister **(nonthermal) of scalp**
√ₓ7ᵗʰ **S00.03**   Contusion **of scalp**
     Bruise of scalp
     Hematoma of scalp
√ₓ7ᵗʰ **S00.04**   External constriction **of part of scalp**
√ₓ7ᵗʰ **S00.05**   Superficial foreign body **of scalp**
     Splinter in the scalp
√ₓ7ᵗʰ **S00.06**   Insect bite **(nonvenomous) of scalp**
√ₓ7ᵗʰ **S00.07**   Other **superficial** bite **of scalp**
     EXCLUDES 1   open bite of scalp (S01.05)

√5ᵗʰ **S00.1**   **Contusion of** eyelid and periocular area
     Black eye
     EXCLUDES 2   contusion of eyeball and orbital tissues (S05.1)
√ₓ7ᵗʰ **S00.10**   Contusion of unspecified **eyelid and periocular area**
√ₓ7ᵗʰ **S00.11**   Contusion of right **eyelid and periocular area**
√ₓ7ᵗʰ **S00.12**   Contusion of left **eyelid and periocular area**

√5ᵗʰ **S00.2**   **Other and unspecified superficial injuries of eyelid and periocular area**
     EXCLUDES 2   superficial injury of conjunctiva and cornea (S05.0-)
   √6ᵗʰ **S00.20**   Unspecified **superficial injury of eyelid and periocular area**
     √7ᵗʰ **S00.201**   **Unspecified superficial injury of** right **eyelid and periocular area**
     √7ᵗʰ **S00.202**   **Unspecified superficial injury of** left **eyelid and periocular area**
     √7ᵗʰ **S00.209**   **Unspecified superficial injury of** unspecified **eyelid and periocular area**
   √6ᵗʰ **S00.21**   Abrasion **of eyelid and periocular area**
     √7ᵗʰ **S00.211**   **Abrasion of** right **eyelid and periocular area**
     √7ᵗʰ **S00.212**   **Abrasion of** left **eyelid and periocular area**
     √7ᵗʰ **S00.219**   **Abrasion of** unspecified **eyelid and periocular area**
   √6ᵗʰ **S00.22**   Blister **(nonthermal) of eyelid and periocular area**
     √7ᵗʰ **S00.221**   **Blister (nonthermal) of** right **eyelid and periocular area**
     √7ᵗʰ **S00.222**   **Blister (nonthermal) of** left **eyelid and periocular area**
     √7ᵗʰ **S00.229**   **Blister (nonthermal) of** unspecified **eyelid and periocular area**
   √6ᵗʰ **S00.24**   External constriction **of eyelid and periocular area**
     √7ᵗʰ **S00.241**   **External constriction of** right **eyelid and periocular area**
     √7ᵗʰ **S00.242**   **External constriction of** left **eyelid and periocular area**
     √7ᵗʰ **S00.249**   **External constriction of** unspecified **eyelid and periocular area**
   √6ᵗʰ **S00.25**   **Superficial** foreign body **of eyelid and periocular area**
     Splinter of eyelid and periocular area
     EXCLUDES 2   retained foreign body in eyelid (H02.81-)
     √7ᵗʰ **S00.251**   **Superficial foreign body of** right **eyelid and periocular area**
     √7ᵗʰ **S00.252**   **Superficial foreign body of** left **eyelid and periocular area**
     √7ᵗʰ **S00.259**   **Superficial foreign body of** unspecified **eyelid and periocular area**
   √6ᵗʰ **S00.26**   Insect bite **(nonvenomous) of eyelid and periocular area**
     √7ᵗʰ **S00.261**   **Insect bite (nonvenomous) of** right **eyelid and periocular area**
     √7ᵗʰ **S00.262**   **Insect bite (nonvenomous) of** left **eyelid and periocular area**
     √7ᵗʰ **S00.269**   **Insect bite (nonvenomous) of** unspecified **eyelid and periocular area**
   √6ᵗʰ **S00.27**   Other **superficial** bite **of eyelid and periocular area**
     EXCLUDES 1   open bite of eyelid and periocular area (S01.15)
     √7ᵗʰ **S00.271**   **Other superficial bite of** right **eyelid and periocular area**
     √7ᵗʰ **S00.272**   **Other superficial bite of** left **eyelid and periocular area**
     √7ᵗʰ **S00.279**   **Other superficial bite of** unspecified **eyelid and periocular area**

√5ᵗʰ **S00.3** **Superficial injury of** nose

  √x7ᵗʰ **S00.30** **Unspecified superficial injury of** nose

  √x7ᵗʰ **S00.31** **Abrasion of** nose

  √x7ᵗʰ **S00.32** **Blister (nonthermal) of** nose

  √x7ᵗʰ **S00.33** **Contusion of** nose
       Bruise of nose
       Hematoma of nose

  √x7ᵗʰ **S00.34** **External constriction of** nose

  √x7ᵗʰ **S00.35** **Superficial** foreign body **of** nose
       Splinter in the nose

  √x7ᵗʰ **S00.36** **Insect bite (nonvenomous) of** nose

  √x7ᵗʰ **S00.37** **Other superficial** bite **of** nose
       EXCLUDES 1   *open bite of nose (S01.25)*

√5ᵗʰ **S00.4** **Superficial injury of** ear

  √6ᵗʰ **S00.40** **Unspecified superficial injury of** ear

    √7ᵗʰ **S00.401** **Unspecified superficial injury of** right **ear**

    √7ᵗʰ **S00.402** **Unspecified superficial injury of** left **ear**

    √7ᵗʰ **S00.409** **Unspecified superficial injury of** unspecified **ear**

  √6ᵗʰ **S00.41** **Abrasion of** ear

    √7ᵗʰ **S00.411** **Abrasion of** right **ear**

    √7ᵗʰ **S00.412** **Abrasion of** left **ear**

    √7ᵗʰ **S00.419** **Abrasion of** unspecified **ear**

  √6ᵗʰ **S00.42** **Blister (nonthermal) of** ear

    √7ᵗʰ **S00.421** **Blister (nonthermal) of** right **ear**

    √7ᵗʰ **S00.422** **Blister (nonthermal) of** left **ear**

    √7ᵗʰ **S00.429** **Blister (nonthermal) of** unspecified **ear**

  √6ᵗʰ **S00.43** **Contusion of** ear
       Bruise of ear
       Hematoma of ear

    √7ᵗʰ **S00.431** **Contusion of** right **ear**

    √7ᵗʰ **S00.432** **Contusion of** left **ear**

    √7ᵗʰ **S00.439** **Contusion of** unspecified **ear**

  √6ᵗʰ **S00.44** **External constriction of** ear

    √7ᵗʰ **S00.441** **External constriction of** right **ear**

    √7ᵗʰ **S00.442** **External constriction of** left **ear**

    √7ᵗʰ **S00.449** **External constriction of** unspecified **ear**

  √6ᵗʰ **S00.45** **Superficial** foreign body **of** ear
       Splinter in the ear

    √7ᵗʰ **S00.451** **Superficial foreign body of** right **ear**

    √7ᵗʰ **S00.452** **Superficial foreign body of** left **ear**

    √7ᵗʰ **S00.459** **Superficial foreign body of** unspecified **ear**

  √6ᵗʰ **S00.46** **Insect bite (nonvenomous) of** ear

    √7ᵗʰ **S00.461** **Insect bite (nonvenomous) of** right **ear**

    √7ᵗʰ **S00.462** **Insect bite (nonvenomous) of** left **ear**

    √7ᵗʰ **S00.469** **Insect bite (nonvenomous) of** unspecified **ear**

  √6ᵗʰ **S00.47** **Other superficial** bite **of ear**
       EXCLUDES 1   *open bite of ear (S01.35)*

    √7ᵗʰ **S00.471** **Other superficial bite of** right **ear**

    √7ᵗʰ **S00.472** **Other superficial bite of** left **ear**

    √7ᵗʰ **S00.479** **Other superficial bite of** unspecified **ear**

√5ᵗʰ **S00.5** **Superficial injury of** lip and oral cavity

  √6ᵗʰ **S00.50** **Unspecified superficial injury of** lip and oral cavity

    √7ᵗʰ **S00.501** **Unspecified superficial injury of** lip

    √7ᵗʰ **S00.502** **Unspecified superficial injury of** oral cavity

  √6ᵗʰ **S00.51** **Abrasion of** lip and oral cavity

    √7ᵗʰ **S00.511** **Abrasion of** lip

    √7ᵗʰ **S00.512** **Abrasion of** oral cavity

  √6ᵗʰ **S00.52** **Blister (nonthermal) of** lip and oral cavity

    √7ᵗʰ **S00.521** **Blister (nonthermal) of** lip

    √7ᵗʰ **S00.522** **Blister (nonthermal) of** oral cavity

  √6ᵗʰ **S00.53** **Contusion of** lip and oral cavity

    √7ᵗʰ **S00.531** **Contusion of** lip
         Bruise of lip
         Hematoma of lip

    √7ᵗʰ **S00.532** **Contusion of** oral cavity
         Bruise of oral cavity
         Hematoma of oral cavity

  √6ᵗʰ **S00.54** **External constriction of** lip and oral cavity

    √7ᵗʰ **S00.541** **External constriction of** lip

    √7ᵗʰ **S00.542** **External constriction of** oral cavity

  √6ᵗʰ **S00.55** **Superficial** foreign body **of** lip and oral cavity

    √7ᵗʰ **S00.551** **Superficial foreign body of** lip
         Splinter of lip and oral cavity

    √7ᵗʰ **S00.552** **Superficial foreign body of** oral cavity
         Splinter of lip and oral cavity

  √6ᵗʰ **S00.56** **Insect bite (nonvenomous) of** lip and oral cavity

    √7ᵗʰ **S00.561** **Insect bite (nonvenomous) of** lip

    √7ᵗʰ **S00.562** **Insect bite (nonvenomous) of** oral cavity

  √6ᵗʰ **S00.57** **Other superficial** bite **of** lip and oral cavity

    √7ᵗʰ **S00.571** **Other superficial bite of** lip
         EXCLUDES 1   *open bite of lip (S01.551)*

    √7ᵗʰ **S00.572** **Other superficial bite of** oral cavity
         EXCLUDES 1   *open bite of oral cavity (S01.552)*

√5ᵗʰ **S00.8** **Superficial injury of** other parts of head
     Superfical injuries of face [any part]

  √x7ᵗʰ **S00.80** **Unspecified superficial injury of other part of head**

  √x7ᵗʰ **S00.81** **Abrasion of other part of head**

  √x7ᵗʰ **S00.82** **Blister (nonthermal) of other part of head**

  √x7ᵗʰ **S00.83** **Contusion of other part of head**
       Bruise of other part of head
       Hematoma of other part of head

  √x7ᵗʰ **S00.84** **External constriction of other part of head**

  √x7ᵗʰ **S00.85** **Superficial** foreign body **of other part of head**
       Splinter in other part of head

  √x7ᵗʰ **S00.86** **Insect bite (nonvenomous) of other part of head**

  √x7ᵗʰ **S00.87** **Other superficial** bite **of other part of head**
       EXCLUDES 1   *open bite of other part of head (S01.85)*

√5ᵗʰ **S00.9** **Superficial injury of** unspecified part of head

  √x7ᵗʰ **S00.90** **Unspecified superficial injury of unspecified part of head**

  √x7ᵗʰ **S00.91** **Abrasion of unspecified part of head**

  √x7ᵗʰ **S00.92** **Blister (nonthermal) of unspecified part of head**

  √x7ᵗʰ **S00.93** **Contusion of unspecified part of head**
       Bruise of head
       Hematoma of head

  √x7ᵗʰ **S00.94** **External constriction of unspecified part of head**

  √x7ᵗʰ **S00.95** **Superficial** foreign body **of unspecified part of head**
       Splinter of head

  √x7ᵗʰ **S00.96** **Insect bite (nonvenomous) of unspecified part of head**

  √x7ᵗʰ **S00.97** **Other superficial** bite **of unspecified part of head**
       EXCLUDES 1   *open bite of head (S01.95)*

√4ᵗʰ **S01** **Open wound of head**
     Code also any associated:
       injury of cranial nerve (S04.-)
       injury of muscle and tendon of head (S09.1-)
       intracranial injury (S06.-)
       wound infection
     EXCLUDES 1   *open skull fracture (S02- with 7th B)*
     EXCLUDES 2   *injury of eye and orbit (S05.-)*
               traumatic amputation of part of head (S08.-)

> The appropriate 7th character is to be added to each code from category S01.
> A   initial encounter
> D   subsequent encounter
> S   sequela

√5ᵗʰ **S01.0** **Open wound of** scalp
     EXCLUDES 1   *avulsion of scalp (S08.0)*

  √x7ᵗʰ **S01.00** **Unspecified open wound of scalp**

  √x7ᵗʰ **S01.01** **Laceration without foreign body of scalp**

  √x7ᵗʰ **S01.02** **Laceration with foreign body of scalp**

  √x7ᵗʰ **S01.03** **Puncture wound without foreign body of scalp**

  √x7ᵗʰ **S01.04** **Puncture wound with foreign body of scalp**

  √x7ᵗʰ **S01.05** **Open bite of scalp**
       Bite of scalp NOS
       EXCLUDES 1   *superficial bite of scalp (S00.06, S00.07-)*

N Newborn: 0   **P** Pediatric: 0-17   **M** Maternity: 12-55   **A** Adult: 15-124   **MCC** Major Complication/Comorbidity   **CC** Complication/Comorbidity   **SW** Severe Wound Dx

948   ICD-10-CM 2019

√5ᵗʰ **S01.1** **Open wound of** eyelid and periocular area
Open wound of eyelid and periocular area with or without involvement of lacrimal passages

CC Excl: For CC codes in subcategory S01.1:
PDX collection 1139

√6ᵗʰ **S01.10** **Unspecified open wound of eyelid and periocular area**

√7ᵗʰ **S01.101** Unspecified open wound of right eyelid and periocular area   CC

√7ᵗʰ **S01.102** Unspecified open wound of left eyelid and periocular area   CC

√7ᵗʰ **S01.109** Unspecified open wound of unspecified eyelid and periocular area   CC

√6ᵗʰ **S01.11** **Laceration without foreign body of eyelid and periocular area**

√7ᵗʰ **S01.111** Laceration without foreign body of right eyelid and periocular area

√7ᵗʰ **S01.112** Laceration without foreign body of left eyelid and periocular area

√7ᵗʰ **S01.119** Laceration without foreign body of unspecified eyelid and periocular area

√6ᵗʰ **S01.12** **Laceration with foreign body of eyelid and periocular area**

√7ᵗʰ **S01.121** Laceration with foreign body of right eyelid and periocular area

√7ᵗʰ **S01.122** Laceration with foreign body of left eyelid and periocular area

√7ᵗʰ **S01.129** Laceration with foreign body of unspecified eyelid and periocular area

√6ᵗʰ **S01.13** **Puncture wound without foreign body of eyelid and periocular area**

√7ᵗʰ **S01.131** Puncture wound without foreign body of right eyelid and periocular area

√7ᵗʰ **S01.132** Puncture wound without foreign body of left eyelid and periocular area

√7ᵗʰ **S01.139** Puncture wound without foreign body of unspecified eyelid and periocular area

√6ᵗʰ **S01.14** **Puncture wound with foreign body of eyelid and periocular area**

√7ᵗʰ **S01.141** Puncture wound with foreign body of right eyelid and periocular area

√7ᵗʰ **S01.142** Puncture wound with foreign body of left eyelid and periocular area

√7ᵗʰ **S01.149** Puncture wound with foreign body of unspecified eyelid and periocular area

√6ᵗʰ **S01.15** **Open bite of eyelid and periocular area**
Bite of eyelid and periocular area NOS
EXCLUDES 1 *superficial bite of eyelid and periocular area (S00.26, S00.27)*

√7ᵗʰ **S01.151** Open bite of right eyelid and periocular area

√7ᵗʰ **S01.152** Open bite of left eyelid and periocular area

√7ᵗʰ **S01.159** Open bite of unspecified eyelid and periocular area

√5ᵗʰ **S01.2** **Open wound of** nose

√ₓ7ᵗʰ **S01.20** **Unspecified open wound of nose**

√ₓ7ᵗʰ **S01.21** **Laceration without foreign body of nose**

√ₓ7ᵗʰ **S01.22** **Laceration with foreign body of nose**

√ₓ7ᵗʰ **S01.23** **Puncture wound without foreign body of nose**

√ₓ7ᵗʰ **S01.24** **Puncture wound with foreign body of nose**

√ₓ7ᵗʰ **S01.25** **Open bite of nose**
Bite of nose NOS
EXCLUDES 1 *superficial bite of nose (S00.36, S00.37)*

√5ᵗʰ **S01.3** **Open wound of** ear

√6ᵗʰ **S01.30** **Unspecified open wound of ear**

√7ᵗʰ **S01.301** Unspecified open wound of right ear

√7ᵗʰ **S01.302** Unspecified open wound of left ear

√7ᵗʰ **S01.309** Unspecified open wound of unspecified ear

√6ᵗʰ **S01.31** **Laceration without foreign body of ear**

√7ᵗʰ **S01.311** Laceration without foreign body of right ear

√7ᵗʰ **S01.312** Laceration without foreign body of left ear

√7ᵗʰ **S01.319** Laceration without foreign body of unspecified ear

√6ᵗʰ **S01.32** **Laceration with foreign body of ear**

√7ᵗʰ **S01.321** Laceration with foreign body of right ear

√7ᵗʰ **S01.322** Laceration with foreign body of left ear

√7ᵗʰ **S01.329** Laceration with foreign body of unspecified ear

√6ᵗʰ **S01.33** **Puncture wound without foreign body of ear**

√7ᵗʰ **S01.331** Puncture wound without foreign body of right ear

√7ᵗʰ **S01.332** Puncture wound without foreign body of left ear

√7ᵗʰ **S01.339** Puncture wound without foreign body of unspecified ear

√6ᵗʰ **S01.34** **Puncture wound with foreign body of ear**

√7ᵗʰ **S01.341** Puncture wound with foreign body of right ear

√7ᵗʰ **S01.342** Puncture wound with foreign body of left ear

√7ᵗʰ **S01.349** Puncture wound with foreign body of unspecified ear

√6ᵗʰ **S01.35** **Open bite of ear**
Bite of ear NOS
EXCLUDES 1 *superficial bite of ear (S00.46, S00.47)*

√7ᵗʰ **S01.351** Open bite of right ear

√7ᵗʰ **S01.352** Open bite of left ear

√7ᵗʰ **S01.359** Open bite of unspecified ear

√5ᵗʰ **S01.4** **Open wound of** cheek and temporomandibular area

√6ᵗʰ **S01.40** **Unspecified open wound of cheek and temporomandibular area**

√7ᵗʰ **S01.401** Unspecified open wound of right cheek and temporomandibular area

√7ᵗʰ **S01.402** Unspecified open wound of left cheek and temporomandibular area

√7ᵗʰ **S01.409** Unspecified open wound of unspecified cheek and temporomandibular area

√6ᵗʰ **S01.41** **Laceration without foreign body of cheek and temporomandibular area**

√7ᵗʰ **S01.411** Laceration without foreign body of right cheek and temporomandibular area

√7ᵗʰ **S01.412** Laceration without foreign body of left cheek and temporomandibular area

√7ᵗʰ **S01.419** Laceration without foreign body of unspecified cheek and temporomandibular area

√6ᵗʰ **S01.42** **Laceration with foreign body of cheek and temporomandibular area**

√7ᵗʰ **S01.421** Laceration with foreign body of right cheek and temporomandibular area

√7ᵗʰ **S01.422** Laceration with foreign body of left cheek and temporomandibular area

√7ᵗʰ **S01.429** Laceration with foreign body of unspecified cheek and temporomandibular area

√6ᵗʰ **S01.43** **Puncture wound without foreign body of cheek and temporomandibular area**

√7ᵗʰ **S01.431** Puncture wound without foreign body of right cheek and temporomandibular area

√7ᵗʰ **S01.432** Puncture wound without foreign body of left cheek and temporomandibular area

√7ᵗʰ **S01.439** Puncture wound without foreign body of unspecified cheek and temporomandibular area

√6ᵗʰ **S01.44** **Puncture wound with foreign body of cheek and temporomandibular area**

√7ᵗʰ **S01.441** Puncture wound with foreign body of right cheek and temporomandibular area

√7ᵗʰ **S01.442** Puncture wound with foreign body of left cheek and temporomandibular area

√7ᵗʰ **S01.449** Puncture wound with foreign body of unspecified cheek and temporomandibular area

✓6ᵗʰ **S01.45** Open bite of cheek and temporomandibular area
Bite of cheek and temporomandibular area NOS
EXCLUDES 2 superficial bite of cheek and temporomandibular area (S00.86, S00.87)

    ✓7ᵗʰ **S01.451** Open bite of right cheek and temporomandibular area

    ✓7ᵗʰ **S01.452** Open bite of left cheek and temporomandibular area

    ✓7ᵗʰ **S01.459** Open bite of unspecified cheek and temporomandibular area

✓5ᵗʰ **S01.5** Open wound of lip and oral cavity
EXCLUDES 2 tooth dislocation (S03.2)
tooth fracture (S02.5)

    ✓6ᵗʰ **S01.50** Unspecified open wound of lip and oral cavity

      ✓7ᵗʰ **S01.501** Unspecified open wound of lip

      ✓7ᵗʰ **S01.502** Unspecified open wound of oral cavity

    ✓6ᵗʰ **S01.51** Laceration of lip and oral cavity without foreign body

      ✓7ᵗʰ **S01.511** Laceration without foreign body of lip

      ✓7ᵗʰ **S01.512** Laceration without foreign body of oral cavity

    ✓6ᵗʰ **S01.52** Laceration of lip and oral cavity with foreign body

      ✓7ᵗʰ **S01.521** Laceration with foreign body of lip

      ✓7ᵗʰ **S01.522** Laceration with foreign body of oral cavity

    ✓6ᵗʰ **S01.53** Puncture wound of lip and oral cavity without foreign body

      ✓7ᵗʰ **S01.531** Puncture wound without foreign body of lip

      ✓7ᵗʰ **S01.532** Puncture wound without foreign body of oral cavity

    ✓6ᵗʰ **S01.54** Puncture wound of lip and oral cavity with foreign body

      ✓7ᵗʰ **S01.541** Puncture wound with foreign body of lip

      ✓7ᵗʰ **S01.542** Puncture wound with foreign body of oral cavity

    ✓6ᵗʰ **S01.55** Open bite of lip and oral cavity

      ✓7ᵗʰ **S01.551** Open bite of lip
Bite of lip NOS
EXCLUDES 1 superficial bite of lip (S00.571)

      ✓7ᵗʰ **S01.552** Open bite of oral cavity
Bite of oral cavity NOS
EXCLUDES 1 superficial bite of oral cavity (S00.572)

✓5ᵗʰ **S01.8** Open wound of other parts of head

    ✓x7ᵗʰ **S01.80** Unspecified open wound of other part of head

    ✓x7ᵗʰ **S01.81** Laceration without foreign body of other part of head

    ✓x7ᵗʰ **S01.82** Laceration with foreign body of other part of head

    ✓x7ᵗʰ **S01.83** Puncture wound without foreign body of other part of head

    ✓x7ᵗʰ **S01.84** Puncture wound with foreign body of other part of head

    ✓x7ᵗʰ **S01.85** Open bite of other part of head
Bite of other part of head NOS
EXCLUDES 1 superficial bite of other part of head (S00.87)

✓5ᵗʰ **S01.9** Open wound of unspecified part of head

    ✓x7ᵗʰ **S01.90** Unspecified open wound of unspecified part of head

    ✓x7ᵗʰ **S01.91** Laceration without foreign body of unspecified part of head

    ✓x7ᵗʰ **S01.92** Laceration with foreign body of unspecified part of head

    ✓x7ᵗʰ **S01.93** Puncture wound without foreign body of unspecified part of head

    ✓x7ᵗʰ **S01.94** Puncture wound with foreign body of unspecified part of head

    ✓x7ᵗʰ **S01.95** Open bite of unspecified part of head
Bite of head NOS
EXCLUDES 1 superficial bite of head NOS (S00.97)

✓4ᵗʰ **S02** **Fracture of skull and facial bones**
NOTE A fracture not indicated as open or closed should be coded to closed.
Code also any associated intracranial injury (S06.-)
AHA: 2017, 1Q, 42; 2016, 4Q, 66-67

> The appropriate 7th character is to be added to each code from category S02.
> A   initial encounter for closed fracture
> B   initial encounter for open fracture
> D   subsequent encounter for fracture with routine healing
> G   subsequent encounter for fracture with delayed healing
> K   subsequent encounter for fracture with nonunion
> S   sequela

2,3,7 ✓x7ᵗʰ **S02.0** **Fracture of vault of skull**   MCC CC H5 HCC
Fracture of frontal bone
Fracture of parietal bone

> **CC Excl:** For codes in subcategory S02.0:
> **CC with 7th character A or MCC with 7th character B:** PDX collection 1140
> **CC with 7th character K:** PDX collection 897

✓5ᵗʰ **S02.1** **Fracture of base of skull**
EXCLUDES 1 orbit NOS (S02.8)
EXCLUDES 2 orbital floor (S02.3-)

> **CC Excl:** For codes in subcategory S02.1:
> **CC with 7th character A or MCC with 7th character B:** PDX collection 1140
> **CC with 7th character K:** PDX collection 897

    ✓6ᵗʰ **S02.10** Unspecified fracture of base of skull

      2,3,7 ✓7ᵗʰ **S02.101** Fracture of base of skull, right side   MCC CC H5 HCC

      2,3,7 ✓7ᵗʰ **S02.102** Fracture of base of skull, left side   MCC CC H5 HCC

      2,3,7 ✓7ᵗʰ **S02.109** Fracture of base of skull, unspecified side   MCC CC H5 HCC

    ✓6ᵗʰ **S02.11** Fracture of occiput

      2,3,7 ✓7ᵗʰ **S02.110** Type I occipital condyle fracture, unspecified side   MCC CC H5 HCC

      2,3,7 ✓7ᵗʰ **S02.111** Type II occipital condyle fracture, unspecified side   MCC CC H5 HCC

      2,3,7 ✓7ᵗʰ **S02.112** Type III occipital condyle fracture, unspecified side   MCC CC H5 HCC

      2,3,7 ✓7ᵗʰ **S02.113** Unspecified occipital condyle fracture   MCC CC H5 HCC

      2,3,7 ✓7ᵗʰ **S02.118** Other fracture of occiput, unspecified side   MCC CC H5 HCC

      2,3,7 ✓7ᵗʰ **S02.119** Unspecified fracture of occiput   MCC CC H5 HCC

      2,3,7 ✓7ᵗʰ **S02.11A** Type I occipital condyle fracture, right side   MCC CC H5 HCC

      2,3,7 ✓7ᵗʰ **S02.11B** Type I occipital condyle fracture, left side   MCC CC H5 HCC

      2,3,7 ✓7ᵗʰ **S02.11C** Type II occipital condyle fracture, right side   MCC CC H5 HCC

      2,3,7 ✓7ᵗʰ **S02.11D** Type II occipital condyle fracture, left side   MCC CC H5 HCC

      2,3,7 ✓7ᵗʰ **S02.11E** Type III occipital condyle fracture, right side   MCC CC H5 HCC

      2,3,7 ✓7ᵗʰ **S02.11F** Type III occipital condyle fracture, left side   MCC CC H5 HCC

      2,3,7 ✓7ᵗʰ **S02.11G** Other fracture of occiput, right side   MCC CC H5 HCC

      2,3,7 ✓7ᵗʰ **S02.11H** Other fracture of occiput, left side   MCC CC H5 HCC

    2,3,7 ✓x7ᵗʰ **S02.19** Other fracture of base of skull   MCC CC H5 HCC
Fracture of anterior fossa of base of skull
Fracture of ethmoid sinus
Fracture of frontal sinus
Fracture of middle fossa of base of skull
Fracture of orbital roof
Fracture of posterior fossa of base of skull
Fracture of sphenoid
Fracture of temporal bone

    3 ✓x7ᵗʰ **S02.2** **Fracture of nasal bones**   CC H5
CC Excl: CC with 7th character B: PDX collection 1141
CC Excl: CC with 7th character K: PDX collection 897

N Newborn: 0   P Pediatric: 0-17   M Maternity: 12-55   A Adult: 15-124   MCC Major Complication/Comorbidity   CC Complication/Comorbidity   SW Severe Wound Dx

950   ICD-10-CM 2019

✓5ᵗʰ **S02.3**   **Fracture of** orbital floor
    EXCLUDES 1   orbit NOS (S02.8)
    EXCLUDES 2   orbital roof (S02.1-)

> CC Excl: For codes in subcategory S02.3:
> CC with 7th character A or B: PDX collection 1142
> CC with 7th character K: PDX collection 897

3,7 ✓x7ᵗʰ **S02.30**   **Fracture of orbital floor, unspecified side** CC H5 HCC
3,7 ✓x7ᵗʰ **S02.31**   **Fracture of orbital floor, right side** CC H5 HCC
3,7 ✓x7ᵗʰ **S02.32**   **Fracture of orbital floor, left side** CC H5 HCC

✓5ᵗʰ **S02.4**   **Fracture of** malar, maxillary and zygoma bones
    Fracture of superior maxilla
    Fracture of upper jaw (bone)
    Fracture of zygomatic process of temporal bone

> CC Excl: For codes in subcategory S02.4, unless
> otherwise noted:
> CC with 7th character A or B: PDX collection 1143
> CC with 7th character K: PDX collection 897

✓6ᵗʰ **S02.40**   **Fracture of malar, maxillary and zygoma bones, unspecified**
3,7 ✓7ᵗʰ **S02.400**   **Malar fracture, unspecified side** CC H5 HCC
3,7 ✓7ᵗʰ **S02.401**   **Maxillary fracture, unspecified side** CC H5 HCC
3,7 ✓7ᵗʰ **S02.402**   **Zygomatic fracture, unspecified side** CC H5 HCC
3,7 ✓7ᵗʰ **S02.40A**   **Malar fracture, right side** CC H5 HCC
3,7 ✓7ᵗʰ **S02.40B**   **Malar fracture, left side** CC H5 HCC
3,7 ✓7ᵗʰ **S02.40C**   **Maxillary fracture, right side** CC H5 HCC
3,7 ✓7ᵗʰ **S02.40D**   **Maxillary fracture, left side** CC H5 HCC
3,7 ✓7ᵗʰ **S02.40E**   **Zygomatic fracture, right side** CC H5 HCC
3,7 ✓7ᵗʰ **S02.40F**   **Zygomatic fracture, left side** CC H5 HCC

✓6ᵗʰ **S02.41**   **LeFort fracture**
> **DEF:** Named for Rene Le Fort, these fractures describe
> different combinations of multiple fractures that occur
> from significant force to the midface. A common
> denominator in all three types of LeFort fractures is
> fracture of the pterygoid processes, which are two bony
> plates resembling wings that extend downward from
> the sphenoid bone.

3,7 ✓7ᵗʰ **S02.411**   **LeFort I fracture** CC H5 HCC
3,7 ✓7ᵗʰ **S02.412**   **LeFort II fracture** CC H5 HCC
3,7 ✓7ᵗʰ **S02.413**   **LeFort III fracture** CC H5 HCC

LeFort Fracture Types

Frontal bone   Nasal bone   Orbital floor
Type III
Type II
Type I
Maxilla
Zygomatic bone (malar) and arch

3,7 ✓x7ᵗʰ **S02.42**   **Fracture of alveolus of maxilla** CC H5 HCC
    CC Excl: CC with 7th character B: PDX collection 1141
    CC Excl: CC with 7th character K: PDX collection 897

4 ✓x7ᵗʰ **S02.5**   **Fracture of** tooth (traumatic) CC
    Broken tooth
    EXCLUDES 1   cracked tooth (nontraumatic) (K03.81)
    CC Excl: CC with 7th character K: PDX collection 897

✓5ᵗʰ **S02.6**   **Fracture of** mandible
    Fracture of lower jaw (bone)

> CC Excl: For codes in subcategory S02.6:
> CC with 7th character A or B: PDX collection 1143
> CC with 7th character K: PDX collection 897

✓6ᵗʰ **S02.60**   **Fracture of mandible, unspecified**
3,7 ✓7ᵗʰ **S02.600**   **Fracture of unspecified part of body of mandible, unspecified side** CC H5 HCC
3,7 ✓7ᵗʰ **S02.601**   **Fracture of unspecified part of body of right mandible** CC H5 HCC
3,7 ✓7ᵗʰ **S02.602**   **Fracture of unspecified part of body of left mandible** CC H5 HCC
3,7 ✓7ᵗʰ **S02.609**   **Fracture of mandible, unspecified** CC H5 HCC

✓6ᵗʰ **S02.61**   **Fracture of condylar process of mandible**
3,7 ✓7ᵗʰ **S02.610**   **Fracture of condylar process of mandible, unspecified side** CC H5 HCC
3,7 ✓7ᵗʰ **S02.611**   **Fracture of condylar process of right mandible** CC H5 HCC
3,7 ✓7ᵗʰ **S02.612**   **Fracture of condylar process of left mandible** CC H5 HCC

✓6ᵗʰ **S02.62**   **Fracture of subcondylar process of mandible**
3,7 ✓7ᵗʰ **S02.620**   **Fracture of subcondylar process of mandible, unspecified side** CC H5 HCC
3,7 ✓7ᵗʰ **S02.621**   **Fracture of subcondylar process of right mandible** CC H5 HCC
3,7 ✓7ᵗʰ **S02.622**   **Fracture of subcondylar process of left mandible** CC H5 HCC

✓6ᵗʰ **S02.63**   **Fracture of coronoid process of mandible**
3,7 ✓7ᵗʰ **S02.630**   **Fracture of coronoid process of mandible, unspecified side** CC H5 HCC
3,7 ✓7ᵗʰ **S02.631**   **Fracture of coronoid process of right mandible** CC H5 HCC
3,7 ✓7ᵗʰ **S02.632**   **Fracture of coronoid process of left mandible** CC H5 HCC

✓6ᵗʰ **S02.64**   **Fracture of ramus of mandible**
3,7 ✓7ᵗʰ **S02.640**   **Fracture of ramus of mandible, unspecified side** CC H5 HCC
3,7 ✓7ᵗʰ **S02.641**   **Fracture of ramus of right mandible** CC H5 HCC
3,7 ✓7ᵗʰ **S02.642**   **Fracture of ramus of left mandible** CC H5 HCC

✓6ᵗʰ **S02.65**   **Fracture of angle of mandible**
3,7 ✓7ᵗʰ **S02.650**   **Fracture of angle of mandible, unspecified side** CC H5 HCC
3,7 ✓7ᵗʰ **S02.651**   **Fracture of angle of right mandible** CC H5 HCC
3,7 ✓7ᵗʰ **S02.652**   **Fracture of angle of left mandible** CC H5 HCC

3,7 ✓x7ᵗʰ **S02.66**   **Fracture of symphysis of mandible** CC H5 HCC

✓6ᵗʰ **S02.67**   **Fracture of alveolus of mandible**
3,7 ✓7ᵗʰ **S02.670**   **Fracture of alveolus of mandible, unspecified side** CC H5 HCC
3,7 ✓7ᵗʰ **S02.671**   **Fracture of alveolus of right mandible** CC H5 HCC
3,7 ✓7ᵗʰ **S02.672**   **Fracture of alveolus of left mandible** CC H5 HCC

3,7 ✓x7ᵗʰ **S02.69**   **Fracture of mandible of other specified site** CC H5 HCC

✓5ᵗʰ **S02.8**   **Fractures of other specified skull and facial bones**
    Fracture of orbit NOS
    Fracture of palate
    EXCLUDES 1   fracture of orbital floor (S02.3-)
        fracture of orbital roof (S02.1-)

> CC Excl: For codes in subcategory S02.8:
> CC with 7th character A or B: PDX collection 1142
> CC with 7th character K: PDX collection 897

3,7 ✓x7ᵗʰ **S02.80**   **Fracture of other specified skull and facial bones, unspecified side** CC H5 HCC
3,7 ✓x7ᵗʰ **S02.81**   **Fracture of other specified skull and facial bones, right side** CC H5 HCC
3,7 ✓x7ᵗʰ **S02.82**   **Fracture of other specified skull and facial bones, left side** CC H5 HCC

✓ Additional Character Required   ✓x7ᵗʰ Placeholder   Unacceptable PDx   Questionable PDx   Manifestation   H1 - H14 HAC   HCC CMS-HCC Dx   HIV HIV Dx

ICD-10-CM 2019   **951**

Chapter 19. Injury, Poisoning and Certain Other Consequences of External Causes *(side margin)*

√5ᵗʰ S02.9 Fracture of unspecified skull and facial bones

2,3,7 **√7ᵗʰ S02.91 Unspecified fracture of skull** `MCC` `CC` `H5` `HCC`
     CC Excl: CC with 7th character A or MCC with 7th character B: PDX collection 1140
     CC with 7th character K: PDX collection 897

3,7 **√7ᵗʰ S02.92 Unspecified fracture of facial bones** `CC` `H5` `HCC`
     CC Excl: CC with 7th character A or B: PDX collection 1142
     CC with 7th character K: PDX collection 897

√4ᵗʰ S03 Dislocation and sprain of joints and ligaments of head
     INCLUDES   avulsion of joint (capsule) or ligament of head
         laceration of cartilage, joint (capsule) or ligament of head
         sprain of cartilage, joint (capsule) or ligament of head
         traumatic hemarthrosis of joint or ligament of head
         traumatic rupture of joint or ligament of head
         traumatic subluxation of joint or ligament of head
         traumatic tear of joint or ligament of head
     Code also any associated open wound
     EXCLUDES 2   *strain of muscle or tendon of head (S09.1)*

> The appropriate 7th character is to be added to each code from category S03.
> A   initial encounter
> D   subsequent encounter
> S   sequela

√5ᵗʰ S03.0 Dislocation of jaw
     Dislocation of jaw (cartilage) (meniscus)
     Dislocation of mandible
     Dislocation of temporomandibular (joint)
     AHA: 2016, 4Q, 67

   √x7ᵗʰ S03.00 Dislocation of jaw, unspecified side
   √x7ᵗʰ S03.01 Dislocation of jaw, right side
   √x7ᵗʰ S03.02 Dislocation of jaw, left side
   √x7ᵗʰ S03.03 Dislocation of jaw, bilateral

√x7ᵗʰ S03.1 Dislocation of septal cartilage of nose

√x7ᵗʰ S03.2 Dislocation of tooth

√5ᵗʰ S03.4 Sprain of jaw
     Sprain of temporomandibular (joint) (ligament)
     AHA: 2016, 4Q, 67

   √x7ᵗʰ S03.40 Sprain of jaw, unspecified side
   √x7ᵗʰ S03.41 Sprain of jaw, right side
   √x7ᵗʰ S03.42 Sprain of jaw, left side
   √x7ᵗʰ S03.43 Sprain of jaw, bilateral

√x7ᵗʰ S03.8 Sprain of joints and ligaments of other parts of head

√x7ᵗʰ S03.9 Sprain of joints and ligaments of unspecified parts of head

√4ᵗʰ S04 Injury of cranial nerve
     The selection of side should be based on the side of the body being affected
     Code first any associated intracranial injury (S06.-)
     Code also any associated:
         open wound of head (S01.-)
         skull fracture (S02.-)

> The appropriate 7th character is to be added to each code from category S04.
> A   initial encounter
> D   subsequent encounter
> S   sequela

√5ᵗʰ S04.0 Injury of optic nerve and pathways
     Use additional code to identify any visual field defect or blindness (H53.4-, H54.-)

     CC Excl: For CC codes in subcategory S04.0: PDX collection 1144

   √6ᵗʰ S04.01 Injury of optic nerve
     Injury of 2nd cranial nerve
     √7ᵗʰ S04.011 Injury of optic nerve, right eye `CC`
     √7ᵗʰ S04.012 Injury of optic nerve, left eye `CC`
     √7ᵗʰ S04.019 Injury of optic nerve, unspecified eye `CC`
         Injury of optic nerve NOS

   √x7ᵗʰ S04.02 Injury of optic chiasm `CC`

   √6ᵗʰ S04.03 Injury of optic tract and pathways
     Injury of optic radiation
     √7ᵗʰ S04.031 Injury of optic tract and pathways, right side `CC`

√7ᵗʰ S04.032 Injury of optic tract and pathways, left side `CC`

√7ᵗʰ S04.039 Injury of optic tract and pathways, unspecified side `CC`
     Injury of optic tract and pathways NOS

√6ᵗʰ S04.04 Injury of visual cortex
   √7ᵗʰ S04.041 Injury of visual cortex, right side `CC`
   √7ᵗʰ S04.042 Injury of visual cortex, left side `CC`
   √7ᵗʰ S04.049 Injury of visual cortex, unspecified side `CC`
     Injury of visual cortex NOS

√5ᵗʰ S04.1 Injury of oculomotor nerve
     Injury of 3rd cranial nerve

     CC Excl: For CC codes in subcategory S04.1: PDX collection 1145

   √x7ᵗʰ S04.10 Injury of oculomotor nerve, unspecified side `CC`
   √x7ᵗʰ S04.11 Injury of oculomotor nerve, right side `CC`
   √x7ᵗʰ S04.12 Injury of oculomotor nerve, left side `CC`

√5ᵗʰ S04.2 Injury of trochlear nerve
     Injury of 4th cranial nerve

     CC Excl: For CC codes in subcategory S04.2: PDX collection 1146

   √x7ᵗʰ S04.20 Injury of trochlear nerve, unspecified side `CC`
   √x7ᵗʰ S04.21 Injury of trochlear nerve, right side `CC`
   √x7ᵗʰ S04.22 Injury of trochlear nerve, left side `CC`

√5ᵗʰ S04.3 Injury of trigeminal nerve
     Injury of 5th cranial nerve

     CC Excl: For CC codes in subcategory S04.3: PDX collection 1147

   √x7ᵗʰ S04.30 Injury of trigeminal nerve, unspecified side `CC`
   √x7ᵗʰ S04.31 Injury of trigeminal nerve, right side `CC`
   √x7ᵗʰ S04.32 Injury of trigeminal nerve, left side `CC`

√5ᵗʰ S04.4 Injury of abducent nerve
     Injury of 6th cranial nerve

     CC Excl: For CC codes in subcategory S04.4: PDX collection 1148

   √x7ᵗʰ S04.40 Injury of abducent nerve, unspecified side `CC`
   √x7ᵗʰ S04.41 Injury of abducent nerve, right side `CC`
   √x7ᵗʰ S04.42 Injury of abducent nerve, left side `CC`

√5ᵗʰ S04.5 Injury of facial nerve
     Injury of 7th cranial nerve

     CC Excl: For CC codes in subcategory S04.5: PDX collection 1149

   √x7ᵗʰ S04.50 Injury of facial nerve, unspecified side `CC`
   √x7ᵗʰ S04.51 Injury of facial nerve, right side `CC`
   √x7ᵗʰ S04.52 Injury of facial nerve, left side `CC`

√5ᵗʰ S04.6 Injury of acoustic nerve
     Injury of auditory nerve
     Injury of 8th cranial nerve

     CC Excl: For CC codes in subcategory S04.6: PDX collection 1150

   √x7ᵗʰ S04.60 Injury of acoustic nerve, unspecified side `CC`
   √x7ᵗʰ S04.61 Injury of acoustic nerve, right side `CC`
   √x7ᵗʰ S04.62 Injury of acoustic nerve, left side `CC`

√5ᵗʰ S04.7 Injury of accessory nerve
     Injury of 11th cranial nerve

     CC Excl: For CC codes in subcategory S04.7: PDX collection 1151

   √x7ᵗʰ S04.70 Injury of accessory nerve, unspecified side `CC`
   √x7ᵗʰ S04.71 Injury of accessory nerve, right side `CC`
   √x7ᵗʰ S04.72 Injury of accessory nerve, left side `CC`

√5ᵗʰ S04.8 Injury of other cranial nerves

     CC Excl: For CC codes in subcategory S04.8: PDX collection 1152

   √6ᵗʰ S04.81 Injury of olfactory [1st] nerve
     √7ᵗʰ S04.811 Injury of olfactory [1st] nerve, right side `CC`

N Newborn: 0   **P** Pediatric: 0-17   **M** Maternity: 12-55   **A** Adult: 15-124   **MCC** Major Complication/Comorbidity   **CC** Complication/Comorbidity   **SW** Severe Wound Dx

952   ICD-10-CM 2019

√7ᵗʰ **S04.812** **Injury of olfactory [1st] nerve, left side** `CC`

√7ᵗʰ **S04.819** **Injury of olfactory [1st] nerve, unspecified side** `CC`

√6ᵗʰ **S04.89** **Injury of other cranial nerves**
Injury of vagus [10th] nerve

√7ᵗʰ **S04.891** **Injury of other cranial nerves, right side** `CC`

√7ᵗʰ **S04.892** **Injury of other cranial nerves, left side** `CC`

√7ᵗʰ **S04.899** **Injury of other cranial nerves, unspecified side** `CC`

√x7ᵗʰ **S04.9** **Injury of unspecified cranial nerve** `CC`
CC Excl: PDX collection 1152

√4ᵗʰ **S05** **Injury of eye and orbit**
INCLUDES open wound of eye and orbit
EXCLUDES 2 2nd cranial [optic] nerve injury (S04.0-)
3rd cranial [oculomotor] nerve injury (S04.1-)
open wound of eyelid and periocular area (S01.1-)
orbital bone fracture (S02.1-, S02.3-, S02.8-)
superficial injury of eyelid (S00.1-S00.2)

The appropriate 7th character is to be added to each code from category S05.
A   initial encounter
D   subsequent encounter
S   sequela

CC Excl: For CC codes in category S05, unless otherwise noted:
PDX collection 1139

√5ᵗʰ **S05.0** **Injury of conjunctiva and corneal abrasion without foreign body**
EXCLUDES 1 foreign body in conjunctival sac (T15.1)
foreign body in cornea (T15.0)

√x7ᵗʰ **S05.00** **Injury of conjunctiva and corneal abrasion without foreign body, unspecified eye**

√x7ᵗʰ **S05.01** **Injury of conjunctiva and corneal abrasion without foreign body, right eye**

√x7ᵗʰ **S05.02** **Injury of conjunctiva and corneal abrasion without foreign body, left eye**

√5ᵗʰ **S05.1** **Contusion of eyeball and orbital tissues**
Traumatic hyphema
EXCLUDES 2 black eye NOS (S00.1)
contusion of eyelid and periocular area (S00.1)

√x7ᵗʰ **S05.10** **Contusion of eyeball and orbital tissues, unspecified eye**

√x7ᵗʰ **S05.11** **Contusion of eyeball and orbital tissues, right eye**

√x7ᵗʰ **S05.12** **Contusion of eyeball and orbital tissues, left eye**

√5ᵗʰ **S05.2** **Ocular laceration and rupture with prolapse or loss of intraocular tissue**

√x7ᵗʰ **S05.20** **Ocular laceration and rupture with prolapse or loss of intraocular tissue, unspecified eye** `CC`

√x7ᵗʰ **S05.21** **Ocular laceration and rupture with prolapse or loss of intraocular tissue, right eye** `CC`

√x7ᵗʰ **S05.22** **Ocular laceration and rupture with prolapse or loss of intraocular tissue, left eye** `CC`

√5ᵗʰ **S05.3** **Ocular laceration without prolapse or loss of intraocular tissue**
Laceration of eye NOS
DEF: Tear in ocular tissue without displacing structures that is due to blunt trauma. It is characterized by pain, redness, and decreased vision.

√x7ᵗʰ **S05.30** **Ocular laceration without prolapse or loss of intraocular tissue, unspecified eye** `CC`

√x7ᵗʰ **S05.31** **Ocular laceration without prolapse or loss of intraocular tissue, right eye** `CC`

√x7ᵗʰ **S05.32** **Ocular laceration without prolapse or loss of intraocular tissue, left eye** `CC`

√5ᵗʰ **S05.4** **Penetrating wound of orbit with or without foreign body**
EXCLUDES 2 retained (old) foreign body following penetrating wound in orbit (H05.5-)

√x7ᵗʰ **S05.40** **Penetrating wound of orbit with or without foreign body, unspecified eye** `CC`

√x7ᵗʰ **S05.41** **Penetrating wound of orbit with or without foreign body, right eye** `CC`

√x7ᵗʰ **S05.42** **Penetrating wound of orbit with or without foreign body, left eye** `CC`

√5ᵗʰ **S05.5** **Penetrating wound with foreign body of eyeball**
EXCLUDES 2 retained (old) intraocular foreign body (H44.6-, H44.7)

CC Excl: For CC codes in subcategory S05.5:
PDX collection 1153

√x7ᵗʰ **S05.50** **Penetrating wound with foreign body of unspecified eyeball** `CC`

√x7ᵗʰ **S05.51** **Penetrating wound with foreign body of right eyeball** `CC`

√x7ᵗʰ **S05.52** **Penetrating wound with foreign body of left eyeball** `CC`

√5ᵗʰ **S05.6** **Penetrating wound without foreign body of eyeball**
Ocular penetration NOS

√x7ᵗʰ **S05.60** **Penetrating wound without foreign body of unspecified eyeball**

√x7ᵗʰ **S05.61** **Penetrating wound without foreign body of right eyeball**

√x7ᵗʰ **S05.62** **Penetrating wound without foreign body of left eyeball**

√5ᵗʰ **S05.7** **Avulsion of eye**
Traumatic enucleation

√x7ᵗʰ **S05.70** **Avulsion of unspecified eye** `CC`

√x7ᵗʰ **S05.71** **Avulsion of right eye** `CC`

√x7ᵗʰ **S05.72** **Avulsion of left eye** `CC`

√5ᵗʰ **S05.8** **Other injuries of eye and orbit**
Lacrimal duct injury

√6ᵗʰ **S05.8X** **Other injuries of eye and orbit**

√7ᵗʰ **S05.8X1** **Other injuries of right eye and orbit** `CC`

√7ᵗʰ **S05.8X2** **Other injuries of left eye and orbit** `CC`

√7ᵗʰ **S05.8X9** **Other injuries of unspecified eye and orbit** `CC`

√5ᵗʰ **S05.9** **Unspecified injury of eye and orbit**
Injury of eye NOS

√x7ᵗʰ **S05.90** **Unspecified injury of unspecified eye and orbit**

√x7ᵗʰ **S05.91** **Unspecified injury of right eye and orbit** `CC`

√x7ᵗʰ **S05.92** **Unspecified injury of left eye and orbit** `CC`

√4ᵗʰ **S06** **Intracranial injury**
NOTE 7th characters D and S do not apply to codes in category S06 with 6th character 7 – death due to brain injury prior to regaining consciousness, or 8 – death due to other cause prior to regaining consciousness
INCLUDES traumatic brain injury
Code also any associated:
open wound of head (S01.-)
skull fracture (S02.-)
EXCLUDES 1 head injury NOS (S09.90)
AHA: 2017, 4Q, 25; 2017, 1Q, 42; 2015, 3Q, 37
TIP: Do not assign Z87.820 Personal history of traumatic brain injury, when residual conditions persist after an intracranial injury. The codes for the residual conditions should be first listed, followed by a code from category S06 using seventh character S to identify sequelae.

The appropriate 7th character is to be added to each code from category S06.
A   initial encounter
D   subsequent encounter
S   sequela

CC Excl: For CC /MCC codes in category S06, unless otherwise noted: PDX collection 1154

√5ᵗʰ **S06.0** **Concussion**
Commotio cerebri
EXCLUDES 1 concussion with other intracranial injuries classified in subcategories S06.1- to S06.6-, S06.81 and S06.82- code to specified intracranial injury
AHA: 2016, 4Q, 67-68

√6ᵗʰ **S06.0X** **Concussion**

8 √7ᵗʰ **S06.0X0** **Concussion without loss of consciousness** `HCC`

8 √7ᵗʰ **S06.0X1** **Concussion with loss of consciousness of 30 minutes or less** `CC` `H5` `HCC`

8 √7ᵗʰ **S06.0X9** **Concussion with loss of consciousness of unspecified duration** `CC` `H5` `HCC`
Concussion NOS

✔ Additional Character Required   √x7ᵗʰ Placeholder   Unacceptable PDx   Questionable PDx   Manifestation   **H1**-**H14** HAC   **HCC** CMS-HCC Dx   **HIV** HIV Dx

ICD-10-CM 2019   953

Chapter 19. Injury, Poisoning and Certain Other Consequences of External Causes *(left margin)*

S06.1–S06.317 *(left margin, bottom)*

☑5th **S06.1** **Traumatic cerebral edema**
Diffuse traumatic cerebral edema
Focal traumatic cerebral edema

> **CC Excl:** For MCC codes in subcategory S06.1, unless otherwise noted: PDX collection 1155

☑6th **S06.1X** **Traumatic cerebral edema**

7 ☑7th **S06.1X0** **Traumatic cerebral edema** `MCC` `HCC`
without loss of consciousness
CC Excl: PDX collection 612

7 ☑7th **S06.1X1** **Traumatic cerebral edema** `MCC` `H5` `HCC`
with loss of consciousness
of 30 minutes or less

7 ☑7th **S06.1X2** **Traumatic cerebral edema** `MCC` `H5` `HCC`
with loss of consciousness
of 31 minutes to 59 minutes

7 ☑7th **S06.1X3** **Traumatic cerebral edema** `MCC` `H5` `HCC`
with loss of consciousness
of 1 hour to 5 hours 59 minutes

7 ☑7th **S06.1X4** **Traumatic cerebral edema** `MCC` `H5` `HCC`
with loss of consciousness
of 6 hours to 24 hours

7 ☑7th **S06.1X5** **Traumatic cerebral edema** `MCC` `H5` `HCC`
with loss of consciousness
greater than 24 hours with return
to pre-existing conscious level

7 ☑7th **S06.1X6** **Traumatic cerebral edema** `MCC` `H5` `HCC`
with loss of consciousness
greater than 24 hours without
return to pre-existing conscious
level with patient surviving
CC Excl: PDX collection 1154

☑7th **S06.1X7** **Traumatic cerebral edema with** `MCC` `H5`
loss of consciousness of
any duration with death due
to brain injury prior to regaining
consciousness
CC Excl: PDX collection 1154

☑7th **S06.1X8** **Traumatic cerebral edema with** `MCC` `H5`
loss of consciousness of
any duration with death due
to other cause prior to regaining
consciousness
CC Excl: PDX collection 1154

7 ☑7th **S06.1X9** **Traumatic cerebral edema** `MCC` `H5` `HCC`
with loss of consciousness
of unspecified duration
Traumatic cerebral edema NOS

☑5th **S06.2** **Diffuse traumatic brain injury**
Diffuse axonal brain injury
EXCLUDES 1 traumatic diffuse cerebral edema (S06.1X-)

☑6th **S06.2X** **Diffuse traumatic brain injury**

7 ☑7th **S06.2X0** **Diffuse traumatic brain injury** `HCC`
without loss of consciousness

7 ☑7th **S06.2X1** **Diffuse traumatic brain injury** `CC` `H5` `HCC`
with loss of consciousness of
30 minutes or less

7 ☑7th **S06.2X2** **Diffuse traumatic brain injury** `CC` `H5` `HCC`
with loss of consciousness of
31 minutes to 59 minutes

7 ☑7th **S06.2X3** **Diffuse traumatic brain injury** `CC` `H5` `HCC`
with loss of consciousness of
1 hour to 5 hours 59 minutes

7 ☑7th **S06.2X4** **Diffuse traumatic brain injury** `CC` `H5` `HCC`
with loss of consciousness of
6 hours to 24 hours

7 ☑7th **S06.2X5** **Diffuse traumatic brain injury** `CC` `H5` `HCC`
with loss of consciousness
greater than 24 hours with
return to pre-existing conscious levels

7 ☑7th **S06.2X6** **Diffuse traumatic brain injury** `MCC` `H5` `HCC`
with loss of consciousness
greater than 24 hours without
return to pre-existing conscious
level with patient surviving

☑7th **S06.2X7** **Diffuse traumatic brain injury** `MCC` `H5`
with loss of consciousness of any
duration with death due to brain
injury prior to regaining consciousness

☑7th **S06.2X8** **Diffuse traumatic brain injury** `MCC` `H5`
with loss of consciousness of any
duration with death due to other
cause prior to regaining consciousness

7 ☑7th **S06.2X9** **Diffuse traumatic brain injury** `CC` `H5` `HCC`
with loss of consciousness of
unspecified duration
Diffuse traumatic brain injury NOS

☑5th **S06.3** **Focal traumatic brain injury**
EXCLUDES 1 any condition classifiable to S06.4-S06.6
focal cerebral edema (S06.1)

☑6th **S06.30** **Unspecified focal traumatic brain injury**

7 ☑7th **S06.300** **Unspecified focal traumatic brain** `HCC`
injury without loss of consciousness

7 ☑7th **S06.301** **Unspecified focal traumatic** `CC` `H5` `HCC`
brain injury with loss of consciousness
of 30 minutes or less

7 ☑7th **S06.302** **Unspecified focal traumatic** `CC` `H5` `HCC`
brain injury with loss of consciousness
of 31 minutes to 59 minutes

7 ☑7th **S06.303** **Unspecified focal traumatic** `CC` `H5` `HCC`
brain injury with loss of consciousness
of 1 hour to 5 hours 59 minutes

7 ☑7th **S06.304** **Unspecified focal traumatic** `CC` `H5` `HCC`
brain injury with loss of consciousness
of 6 hours to 24 hours

7 ☑7th **S06.305** **Unspecified focal traumatic** `CC` `H5` `HCC`
brain injury with loss of consciousness
greater than 24 hours with return
to pre-existing conscious level

7 ☑7th **S06.306** **Unspecified focal traumatic** `MCC` `H5` `HCC`
brain injury with loss of consciousness
greater than 24 hours without return
to pre-existing conscious level with
patient surviving

☑7th **S06.307** **Unspecified focal traumatic** `MCC` `H5`
brain injury with loss of consciousness of
any duration with death due to brain
injury prior to regaining consciousness

☑7th **S06.308** **Unspecified focal traumatic brain** `MCC` `H5`
injury with loss of consciousness of
any duration with death due to other
cause prior to regaining consciousness

7 ☑7th **S06.309** **Unspecified focal traumatic** `CC` `H5` `HCC`
brain injury with loss of consciousness
of unspecified duration
Unspecified focal traumatic brain injury
NOS

☑6th **S06.31** **Contusion and laceration of right cerebrum**

7 ☑7th **S06.310** **Contusion and laceration of** `MCC` `H5` `HCC`
right cerebrum without loss of
consciousness

7 ☑7th **S06.311** **Contusion and laceration of** `MCC` `H5` `HCC`
right cerebrum with loss of
consciousness of 30 minutes or less

7 ☑7th **S06.312** **Contusion and laceration of** `MCC` `H5` `HCC`
right cerebrum with loss of
consciousness of 31 minutes
to 59 minutes

7 ☑7th **S06.313** **Contusion and laceration of** `MCC` `H5` `HCC`
right cerebrum with loss of
consciousness of 1 hour to
5 hours 59 minutes

7 ☑7th **S06.314** **Contusion and laceration of** `MCC` `H5` `HCC`
right cerebrum with loss of
consciousness of 6 hours to 24 hours

7 ☑7th **S06.315** **Contusion and laceration of** `MCC` `H5` `HCC`
right cerebrum with loss of consciousness
greater than 24 hours with return
to pre-existing conscious level

7 ☑7th **S06.316** **Contusion and laceration of** `MCC` `H5` `HCC`
right cerebrum with loss of
consciousness greater than 24 hours
without return to pre-existing
conscious level with patient surviving

☑7th **S06.317** **Contusion and laceration of right** `MCC` `H5`
cerebrum with loss of consciousness
of any duration with death due to
brain injury prior to regaining
consciousness

N Newborn: 0   P Pediatric: 0-17   M Maternity: 12-55   A Adult: 15-124   `MCC` Major Complication/Comorbidity   `CC` Complication/Comorbidity   `SW` Severe Wound Dx

954   ICD-10-CM 2019

✓7ᵗʰ **S06.318** **Contusion and laceration of right** MCC H5
cerebrum with loss of consciousness
of any duration with death due to other
cause prior to regaining consciousness

7 ✓7ᵗʰ **S06.319** **Contusion and laceration of** MCC H5 HCC
right cerebrum with loss of
consciousness of unspecified duration
Contusion and laceration of right cerebrum
NOS

✓6ᵗʰ **S06.32** **Contusion and laceration of** left cerebrum

7 ✓7ᵗʰ **S06.320** **Contusion and laceration of** MCC H5 HCC
left cerebrum without loss of
consciousness

7 ✓7ᵗʰ **S06.321** **Contusion and laceration of** MCC H5 HCC
left cerebrum with loss of
consciousness of 30 minutes or less

7 ✓7ᵗʰ **S06.322** **Contusion and laceration of** MCC H5 HCC
left cerebrum with loss of
consciousness of 31 minutes
to 59 minutes

7 ✓7ᵗʰ **S06.323** **Contusion and laceration of** MCC H5 HCC
left cerebrum with loss of
consciousness of 1 hour to
5 hours 59 minutes

7 ✓7ᵗʰ **S06.324** **Contusion and laceration of** MCC H5 HCC
left cerebrum with loss of
consciousness of 6 hours to 24 hours

7 ✓7ᵗʰ **S06.325** **Contusion and laceration of** MCC H5 HCC
left cerebrum with loss of consciousness
greater than 24 hours with return to
pre-existing conscious level

7 ✓7ᵗʰ **S06.326** **Contusion and laceration of** MCC H5 HCC
left cerebrum with loss of consciousness
greater than 24 hours without return
to pre-existing conscious level with
patient surviving

✓7ᵗʰ **S06.327** **Contusion and laceration of left** MCC H5
cerebrum with loss of consciousness
of any duration with death due to brain
injury prior to regaining consciousness

✓7ᵗʰ **S06.328** **Contusion and laceration of left** MCC H5
cerebrum with loss of consciousness
of any duration with death due to other
cause prior to regaining consciousness

7 ✓7ᵗʰ **S06.329** **Contusion and laceration of** MCC H5 HCC
left cerebrum with loss of
consciousness of unspecified duration
Contusion and laceration of left cerebrum
NOS

✓6ᵗʰ **S06.33** **Contusion and laceration of** cerebrum, unspecified

7 ✓7ᵗʰ **S06.330** **Contusion and laceration of** MCC H5 HCC
cerebrum, unspecified, without loss
of consciousness

7 ✓7ᵗʰ **S06.331** **Contusion and laceration of** MCC H5 HCC
cerebrum, unspecified, with loss of
consciousness of 30 minutes or less

7 ✓7ᵗʰ **S06.332** **Contusion and laceration of** MCC H5 HCC
cerebrum, unspecified, with loss of
consciousness of 31 minutes to 59 minutes

7 ✓7ᵗʰ **S06.333** **Contusion and laceration of** MCC H5 HCC
cerebrum, unspecified, with loss of
consciousness of 1 hour to 5 hours
59 minutes

7 ✓7ᵗʰ **S06.334** **Contusion and laceration of** MCC H5 HCC
cerebrum, unspecified, with loss of
consciousness of 6 hours to 24 hours

7 ✓7ᵗʰ **S06.335** **Contusion and laceration of** MCC H5 HCC
cerebrum, unspecified, with loss of
consciousness greater than 24 hours
with return to pre-existing conscious level

7 ✓7ᵗʰ **S06.336** **Contusion and laceration of** MCC H5 HCC
cerebrum, unspecified, with loss of
consciousness greater than 24 hours
without return to pre-existing
conscious level with patient surviving

✓7ᵗʰ **S06.337** **Contusion and laceration of** MCC H5
cerebrum, unspecified, with loss of
consciousness of any duration with
death due to brain injury prior to
regaining consciousness

✓7ᵗʰ **S06.338** **Contusion and laceration of** MCC H5
cerebrum, unspecified, with loss of
consciousness of any duration with
death due to other cause prior to
regaining consciousness

7 ✓7ᵗʰ **S06.339** **Contusion and laceration of** MCC H5 HCC
cerebrum, unspecified, with loss of
consciousness of unspecified duration
Contusion and laceration of cerebrum NOS

✓6ᵗʰ **S06.34** **Traumatic hemorrhage of** right cerebrum
Traumatic intracerebral hemorrhage and hematoma
of right cerebrum

7 ✓7ᵗʰ **S06.340** **Traumatic hemorrhage of** MCC H5 HCC
right cerebrum without loss of
consciousness

7 ✓7ᵗʰ **S06.341** **Traumatic hemorrhage of** MCC H5 HCC
right cerebrum with loss of
consciousness of 30 minutes or less

7 ✓7ᵗʰ **S06.342** **Traumatic hemorrhage of** MCC H5 HCC
right cerebrum with loss of
consciousness of 31 minutes
to 59 minutes

7 ✓7ᵗʰ **S06.343** **Traumatic hemorrhage of** MCC H5 HCC
right cerebrum with loss
of consciousness of 1 hours
to 5 hours 59 minutes

7 ✓7ᵗʰ **S06.344** **Traumatic hemorrhage of** MCC H5 HCC
right cerebrum with loss of
consciousness of 6 hours to 24 hours

7 ✓7ᵗʰ **S06.345** **Traumatic hemorrhage of** MCC H5 HCC
right cerebrum with loss of
consciousness greater than
24 hours with return
to pre-existing conscious level

7 ✓7ᵗʰ **S06.346** **Traumatic hemorrhage of right** MCC H5 HCC
cerebrum with loss of consciousness
greater than 24 hours without return
to pre-existing conscious level with
patient surviving

✓7ᵗʰ **S06.347** **Traumatic hemorrhage of right** MCC H5
cerebrum with loss of consciousness
of any duration with death due to
brain injury prior to regaining
consciousness

✓7ᵗʰ **S06.348** **Traumatic hemorrhage of right** MCC H5
cerebrum with loss of consciousness
of any duration with death due to
other cause prior to regaining
consciousness

7 ✓7ᵗʰ **S06.349** **Traumatic hemorrhage of right** MCC H5 HCC
cerebrum with loss of consciousness
of unspecified duration
Traumatic hemorrhage of right cerebrum
NOS

✓6ᵗʰ **S06.35** **Traumatic hemorrhage of** left cerebrum
Traumatic intracerebral hemorrhage and hematoma
of left cerebrum

7 ✓7ᵗʰ **S06.350** **Traumatic hemorrhage of left** MCC H5 HCC
cerebrum without loss of
consciousness

7 ✓7ᵗʰ **S06.351** **Traumatic hemorrhage of left** MCC H5 HCC
cerebrum with loss of consciousness
of 30 minutes or less

7 ✓7ᵗʰ **S06.352** **Traumatic hemorrhage of left** MCC H5 HCC
cerebrum with loss of consciousness
of 31 minutes to 59 minutes

7 ✓7ᵗʰ **S06.353** **Traumatic hemorrhage of left** MCC H5 HCC
cerebrum with loss of consciousness
of 1 hours to 5 hours 59 minutes

7 ✓7ᵗʰ **S06.354** **Traumatic hemorrhage of left** MCC H5 HCC
cerebrum with loss of consciousness
of 6 hours to 24 hours

7 ✓7ᵗʰ **S06.355** **Traumatic hemorrhage of left** MCC H5 HCC
cerebrum with loss of consciousness
greater than 24 hours with return
to pre-existing conscious level

7 ✓7ᵗʰ **S06.356** **Traumatic hemorrhage of left** MCC H5 HCC
cerebrum with loss of consciousness
greater than 24 hours without return
to pre-existing conscious level with
patient surviving

✔ Additional Character Required   ✓x7ᵗʰ Placeholder   Unacceptable PDx   Questionable PDx   Manifestation   H1 - H14 HAC   HCC CMS-HCC Dx   HIV HIV Dx

ICD-10-CM 2019   955

√7th **S06.357** Traumatic hemorrhage of left cerebrum with loss of consciousness of any duration with death due to brain injury prior to regaining consciousness `MCC` `H5`

√7th **S06.358** Traumatic hemorrhage of left cerebrum with loss of consciousness of any duration with death due to other cause prior to regaining consciousness `MCC` `H5`

7 √7th **S06.359** Traumatic hemorrhage of left cerebrum with loss of consciousness of unspecified duration `MCC` `H5` `HCC`
Traumatic hemorrhage of left cerebrum NOS

√6th **S06.36** Traumatic hemorrhage of cerebrum, unspecified
Traumatic intracerebral hemorrhage and hematoma, unspecified

7 √7th **S06.360** Traumatic hemorrhage of cerebrum, unspecified, without loss of consciousness `MCC` `H5` `HCC`

7 √7th **S06.361** Traumatic hemorrhage of cerebrum, unspecified, with loss of consciousness of 30 minutes or less `MCC` `H5` `HCC`

7 √7th **S06.362** Traumatic hemorrhage of cerebrum, unspecified, with loss of consciousness of 31 minutes to 59 minutes `MCC` `H5` `HCC`

7 √7th **S06.363** Traumatic hemorrhage of cerebrum, unspecified, with loss of consciousness of 1 hours to 5 hours 59 minutes `MCC` `H5` `HCC`

7 √7th **S06.364** Traumatic hemorrhage of cerebrum, unspecified, with loss of consciousness of 6 hours to 24 hours `MCC` `H5` `HCC`

7 √7th **S06.365** Traumatic hemorrhage of cerebrum, unspecified, with loss of consciousness greater than 24 hours with return to pre-existing conscious level `MCC` `H5` `HCC`

7 √7th **S06.366** Traumatic hemorrhage of cerebrum, unspecified, with loss of consciousness greater than 24 hours without return to pre-existing conscious level with patient surviving `MCC` `H5` `HCC`

√7th **S06.367** Traumatic hemorrhage of cerebrum, unspecified, with loss of consciousness of any duration with death due to brain injury prior to regaining consciousness `MCC` `H5`

√7th **S06.368** Traumatic hemorrhage of cerebrum, unspecified, with loss of consciousness of any duration with death due to other cause prior to regaining consciousness `MCC` `H5`

7 √7th **S06.369** Traumatic hemorrhage of cerebrum, unspecified, with loss of consciousness of unspecified duration `MCC` `H5` `HCC`
Traumatic hemorrhage of cerebrum NOS

√6th **S06.37** Contusion, laceration, and hemorrhage of cerebellum

7 √7th **S06.370** Contusion, laceration, and hemorrhage of cerebellum without loss of consciousness `MCC` `H5` `HCC`
CC Excl: No Excl

7 √7th **S06.371** Contusion, laceration, and hemorrhage of cerebellum with loss of consciousness of 30 minutes or less `CC` `H5` `HCC`

7 √7th **S06.372** Contusion, laceration, and hemorrhage of cerebellum with loss of consciousness of 31 minutes to 59 minutes `CC` `H5` `HCC`

7 √7th **S06.373** Contusion, laceration, and hemorrhage of cerebellum with loss of consciousness of 1 hour to 5 hours 59 minutes `CC` `H5` `HCC`

7 √7th **S06.374** Contusion, laceration, and hemorrhage of cerebellum with loss of consciousness of 6 hours to 24 hours `CC` `H5` `HCC`

7 √7th **S06.375** Contusion, laceration, and hemorrhage of cerebellum with loss of consciousness greater than 24 hours with return to pre-existing conscious level `CC` `H5` `HCC`

7 √7th **S06.376** Contusion, laceration, and hemorrhage of cerebellum with loss of consciousness greater than 24 hours without return to pre-existing conscious level with patient surviving `MCC` `H5` `HCC`

√7th **S06.377** Contusion, laceration, and hemorrhage of cerebellum with loss of consciousness of any duration with death due to brain injury prior to regaining consciousness `MCC` `H5`

√7th **S06.378** Contusion, laceration, and hemorrhage of cerebellum with loss of consciousness of any duration with death due to other cause prior to regaining consciousness `MCC` `H5`

7 √7th **S06.379** Contusion, laceration, and hemorrhage of cerebellum with loss of consciousness of unspecified duration `CC` `H5` `HCC`
Contusion, laceration, and hemorrhage of cerebellum NOS

√6th **S06.38** Contusion, laceration, and hemorrhage of brainstem

7 √7th **S06.380** Contusion, laceration, and hemorrhage of brainstem without loss of consciousness `MCC` `H5` `HCC`
CC Excl: No Excl

7 √7th **S06.381** Contusion, laceration, and hemorrhage of brainstem with loss of consciousness of 30 minutes or less `CC` `H5` `HCC`

7 √7th **S06.382** Contusion, laceration, and hemorrhage of brainstem with loss of consciousness of 31 minutes to 59 minutes `CC` `H5` `HCC`

7 √7th **S06.383** Contusion, laceration, and hemorrhage of brainstem with loss of consciousness of 1 hour to 5 hours 59 minutes `CC` `H5` `HCC`

7 √7th **S06.384** Contusion, laceration, and hemorrhage of brainstem with loss of consciousness of 6 hours to 24 hours `CC` `H5` `HCC`

7 √7th **S06.385** Contusion, laceration, and hemorrhage of brainstem with loss of consciousness greater than 24 hours with return to pre-existing conscious level `CC` `H5` `HCC`

7 √7th **S06.386** Contusion, laceration, and hemorrhage of brainstem with loss of consciousness greater than 24 hours without return to pre-existing conscious level with patient surviving `MCC` `H5` `HCC`

√7th **S06.387** Contusion, laceration, and hemorrhage of brainstem with loss of consciousness of any duration with death due to brain injury prior to regaining consciousness `MCC` `H5`

√7th **S06.388** Contusion, laceration, and hemorrhage of brainstem with loss of consciousness of any duration with death due to other cause prior to regaining consciousness `MCC` `H5`

7 √7th **S06.389** Contusion, laceration, and hemorrhage of brainstem with loss of consciousness of unspecified duration `CC` `H5` `HCC`
Contusion, laceration, and hemorrhage of brainstem NOS

√5th **S06.4** Epidural hemorrhage
Extradural hemorrhage NOS
Extradural hemorrhage (traumatic)
DEF: Epidural space: Space between the endosteum of the cranium (skull) and the dura mater, the outermost layer of a three-layer membrane that covers the brain.

√6th **S06.4X** Epidural hemorrhage

7 √7th **S06.4X0** Epidural hemorrhage without loss of consciousness `MCC` `H5` `HCC`

7 √7th **S06.4X1** Epidural hemorrhage with loss of consciousness of 30 minutes or less `MCC` `H5` `HCC`

7 √7th **S06.4X2** Epidural hemorrhage with loss of consciousness of 31 minutes to 59 minutes `MCC` `H5` `HCC`

7 ✓7th **S06.4X3 Epidural hemorrhage with loss of consciousness of 1 hour to 5 hours 59 minutes** `MCC` `H5` `HCC`

7 ✓7th **S06.4X4 Epidural hemorrhage with loss of consciousness of 6 hours to 24 hours** `MCC` `H5` `HCC`

7 ✓7th **S06.4X5 Epidural hemorrhage with loss of consciousness greater than 24 hours with return to pre-existing conscious level** `MCC` `H5` `HCC`

7 ✓7th **S06.4X6 Epidural hemorrhage with loss of consciousness greater than 24 hours without return to pre-existing conscious level with patient surviving** `MCC` `H5` `HCC`

✓7th **S06.4X7 Epidural hemorrhage with loss of consciousness of any duration with death due to brain injury prior to regaining consciousness** `MCC` `H5`

✓7th **S06.4X8 Epidural hemorrhage with loss of consciousness of any duration with death due to other causes prior to regaining consciousness** `MCC` `H5`

7 ✓7th **S06.4X9 Epidural hemorrhage with loss of consciousness of unspecified duration** `MCC` `H5` `HCC`
    Epidural hemorrhage NOS

✓5th **S06.5 Traumatic subdural hemorrhage**
    DEF: Subdural: Potential space between the dura mater and arachnoid membrane around the brain.

✓6th **S06.5X Traumatic subdural hemorrhage**

7 ✓7th **S06.5X0 Traumatic subdural hemorrhage without loss of consciousness** `MCC` `H5` `HCC`

7 ✓7th **S06.5X1 Traumatic subdural hemorrhage with loss of consciousness of 30 minutes or less** `MCC` `H5` `HCC`

7 ✓7th **S06.5X2 Traumatic subdural hemorrhage with loss of consciousness of 31 minutes to 59 minutes** `MCC` `H5` `HCC`

7 ✓7th **S06.5X3 Traumatic subdural hemorrhage with loss of consciousness of 1 hour to 5 hours 59 minutes** `MCC` `H5` `HCC`

7 ✓7th **S06.5X4 Traumatic subdural hemorrhage with loss of consciousness of 6 hours to 24 hours** `MCC` `H5` `HCC`

7 ✓7th **S06.5X5 Traumatic subdural hemorrhage with loss of consciousness greater than 24 hours with return to pre-existing conscious level** `MCC` `H5` `HCC`

7 ✓7th **S06.5X6 Traumatic subdural hemorrhage with loss of consciousness greater than 24 hours without return to pre-existing conscious level with patient surviving** `MCC` `H5` `HCC`

✓7th **S06.5X7 Traumatic subdural hemorrhage with loss of consciousness of any duration with death due to brain injury before regaining consciousness** `MCC` `H5`

✓7th **S06.5X8 Traumatic subdural hemorrhage with loss of consciousness of any duration with death due to other cause before regaining consciousness** `MCC` `H5`

7 ✓7th **S06.5X9 Traumatic subdural hemorrhage with loss of consciousness of unspecified duration** `MCC` `H5` `HCC`
    Traumatic subdural hemorrhage NOS

✓5th **S06.6 Traumatic subarachnoid hemorrhage**
    DEF: Subarachnoid: Space located between the arachnoid membrane and the pia mater that contains cerebrospinal fluid.

✓6th **S06.6X Traumatic subarachnoid hemorrhage**

7 ✓7th **S06.6X0 Traumatic subarachnoid hemorrhage without loss of consciousness** `MCC` `H5` `HCC`

7 ✓7th **S06.6X1 Traumatic subarachnoid hemorrhage with loss of consciousness of 30 minutes or less** `MCC` `H5` `HCC`

7 ✓7th **S06.6X2 Traumatic subarachnoid hemorrhage with loss of consciousness of 31 minutes to 59 minutes** `MCC` `H5` `HCC`

7 ✓7th **S06.6X3 Traumatic subarachnoid hemorrhage with loss of consciousness of 1 hour to 5 hours 59 minutes** `MCC` `H5` `HCC`

7 ✓7th **S06.6X4 Traumatic subarachnoid hemorrhage with loss of consciousness of 6 hours to 24 hours** `MCC` `H5` `HCC`

7 ✓7th **S06.6X5 Traumatic subarachnoid hemorrhage with loss of consciousness greater than 24 hours with return to pre-existing conscious level** `MCC` `H5` `HCC`

7 ✓7th **S06.6X6 Traumatic subarachnoid hemorrhage with loss of consciousness greater than 24 hours without return to pre-existing conscious level with patient surviving** `MCC` `H5` `HCC`

✓7th **S06.6X7 Traumatic subarachnoid hemorrhage with loss of consciousness of any duration with death due to brain injury prior to regaining consciousness** `MCC` `H5`

✓7th **S06.6X8 Traumatic subarachnoid hemorrhage with loss of consciousness of any duration with death due to other cause prior to regaining consciousness** `MCC` `H5`

7 ✓7th **S06.6X9 Traumatic subarachnoid hemorrhage with loss of consciousness of unspecified duration** `MCC` `H5` `HCC`
    Traumatic subarachnoid hemorrhage NOS

✓5th **S06.8 Other specified intracranial injuries**

✓6th **S06.81 Injury of right internal carotid artery, intracranial portion, not elsewhere classified**

7 ✓7th **S06.810 Injury of right internal carotid artery, intracranial portion, not elsewhere classified without loss of consciousness** `HCC`

7 ✓7th **S06.811 Injury of right internal carotid artery, intracranial portion, not elsewhere classified with loss of consciousness of 30 minutes or less** `CC` `H5` `HCC`

7 ✓7th **S06.812 Injury of right internal carotid artery, intracranial portion, not elsewhere classified with loss of consciousness of 31 minutes to 59 minutes** `CC` `H5` `HCC`

7 ✓7th **S06.813 Injury of right internal carotid artery, intracranial portion, not elsewhere classified with loss of consciousness of 1 hour to 5 hours 59 minutes** `CC` `H5` `HCC`

7 ✓7th **S06.814 Injury of right internal carotid artery, intracranial portion, not elsewhere classified with loss of consciousness of 6 hours to 24 hours** `CC` `H5` `HCC`

7 ✓7th **S06.815 Injury of right internal carotid artery, intracranial portion, not elsewhere classified with loss of consciousness greater than 24 hours with return to pre-existing conscious level** `CC` `H5` `HCC`

7 ✓7th **S06.816 Injury of right internal carotid artery, intracranial portion, not elsewhere classified with loss of consciousness greater than 24 hours without return to pre-existing conscious level with patient surviving** `MCC` `H5` `HCC`

✓7th **S06.817 Injury of right internal carotid artery, intracranial portion, not elsewhere classified with loss of consciousness of any duration with death due to brain injury prior to regaining consciousness** `MCC` `H5`

✓7th **S06.818 Injury of right internal carotid artery, intracranial portion, not elsewhere classified with loss of consciousness of any duration with death due to other cause prior to regaining consciousness** `MCC` `H5`

7 ✓7th **S06.819 Injury of right internal carotid artery, intracranial portion, not elsewhere classified with loss of consciousness of unspecified duration** `CC` `H5` `HCC`
    Injury of right internal carotid artery, intracranial portion, not elsewhere classified NOS

✓ Additional Character Required   ✓x7th Placeholder   Unacceptable PDx   Questionable PDx   Manifestation   `H1`-`H14` HAC   `HCC` CMS-HCC Dx   `HIV` HIV Dx

ICD-10-CM 2019   957

✓6ᵗʰ S06.82   **Injury of** left internal carotid artery, intracranial **portion, not elsewhere classified**

   7   ✓7ᵗʰ   **S06.820**   **Injury of left internal carotid artery, intracranial portion, not elsewhere classified** without loss of consciousness   HCC

   7   ✓7ᵗʰ   **S06.821**   **Injury of left internal carotid artery, intracranial portion, not elsewhere classified with loss of consciousness of** 30 minutes or less   CC H5 HCC

   7   ✓7ᵗʰ   **S06.822**   **Injury of left internal carotid artery, intracranial portion, not elsewhere classified with loss of consciousness of** 31 minutes to 59 minutes   CC H5 HCC

   7   ✓7ᵗʰ   **S06.823**   **Injury of left internal carotid artery, intracranial portion, not elsewhere classified with loss of consciousness of** 1 hour to 5 hours 59 minutes   CC H5 HCC

   7   ✓7ᵗʰ   **S06.824**   **Injury of left internal carotid artery, intracranial portion, not elsewhere classified with loss of consciousness of** 6 hours to 24 hours   CC H5 HCC

   7   ✓7ᵗʰ   **S06.825**   **Injury of left internal carotid artery, intracranial portion, not elsewhere classified with loss of consciousness** greater than 24 hours with return to pre-existing conscious level   CC H5 HCC

   7   ✓7ᵗʰ   **S06.826**   **Injury of left internal carotid artery, intracranial portion, not elsewhere classified with loss of consciousness** greater than 24 hours without return to pre-existing conscious level with patient surviving   MCC H5 HCC

   ✓7ᵗʰ   **S06.827**   **Injury of left internal carotid artery, intracranial portion, not elsewhere classified with loss of consciousness of** any duration with death due to brain injury prior to regaining consciousness   MCC H5

   ✓7ᵗʰ   **S06.828**   **Injury of left internal carotid artery, intracranial portion, not elsewhere classified with loss of consciousness of** any duration with death due to other cause prior to regaining consciousness   MCC H5

   7   ✓7ᵗʰ   **S06.829**   **Injury of left internal carotid artery, intracranial portion, not elsewhere classified with loss of consciousness of** unspecified duration   CC H5 HCC
       Injury of left internal carotid artery, intracranial portion, not elsewhere classified NOS

✓6ᵗʰ S06.89   **Other** specified intracranial injury
    EXCLUDES 1   concussion (S06.0X-)

   7   ✓7ᵗʰ   **S06.890**   **Other specified intracranial injury** without loss of consciousness   HCC

   7   ✓7ᵗʰ   **S06.891**   **Other specified intracranial injury with loss of consciousness of** 30 minutes or less   CC H5 HCC

   7   ✓7ᵗʰ   **S06.892**   **Other specified intracranial injury with loss of consciousness of** 31 minutes to 59 minutes   CC H5 HCC

   7   ✓7ᵗʰ   **S06.893**   **Other specified intracranial injury with loss of consciousness of** 1 hour to 5 hours 59 minutes   CC H5 HCC

   7   ✓7ᵗʰ   **S06.894**   **Other specified intracranial injury with loss of consciousness of** 6 hours to 24 hours   CC H5 HCC

   7   ✓7ᵗʰ   **S06.895**   **Other specified intracranial injury with loss of consciousness** greater than 24 hours with return to pre-existing conscious level   CC H5 HCC

   7   ✓7ᵗʰ   **S06.896**   **Other specified intracranial injury with loss of consciousness** greater than 24 hours without return to pre-existing conscious level with patient surviving   MCC H5 HCC

   ✓7ᵗʰ   **S06.897**   **Other specified intracranial injury with loss of consciousness of** any duration with death due to brain injury prior to regaining consciousness   MCC H5

   7   ✓7ᵗʰ   **S06.898**   **Other specified intracranial injury with loss of consciousness of** any duration with death due to other cause prior to regaining consciousness   MCC H5

   7   ✓7ᵗʰ   **S06.899**   **Other specified intracranial injury with loss of consciousness of** unspecified duration   CC H5 HCC

✓5ᵗʰ S06.9   **Unspecified intracranial injury**
    Brain injury NOS
    Head injury NOS with loss of consciousness
    Traumatic brain injury NOS
    EXCLUDES 1   conditions classifiable to S06.0- to S06.8- code to specified intracranial injury
       head injury NOS (S09.90)

   ✓6ᵗʰ   **S06.9X**   Unspecified **intracranial injury**

    7   ✓7ᵗʰ   **S06.9X0**   **Unspecified intracranial injury** without loss of consciousness   HCC

    7   ✓7ᵗʰ   **S06.9X1**   **Unspecified intracranial injury with loss of consciousness of** 30 minutes or less   CC H5 HCC

    7   ✓7ᵗʰ   **S06.9X2**   **Unspecified intracranial injury with loss of consciousness of** 31 minutes to 59 minutes   CC H5 HCC

    7   ✓7ᵗʰ   **S06.9X3**   **Unspecified intracranial injury with loss of consciousness of** 1 hour to 5 hours 59 minutes   CC H5 HCC

    7   ✓7ᵗʰ   **S06.9X4**   **Unspecified intracranial injury with loss of consciousness of** 6 hours to 24 hours   CC H5 HCC

    7   ✓7ᵗʰ   **S06.9X5**   **Unspecified intracranial injury with loss of consciousness** greater than 24 hours with return to pre-existing conscious level   CC H5 HCC

    7   ✓7ᵗʰ   **S06.9X6**   **Unspecified intracranial injury with loss of consciousness** greater than 24 hours without return to pre-existing conscious level with patient surviving   MCC H5 HCC

    ✓7ᵗʰ   **S06.9X7**   **Unspecified intracranial injury with loss of consciousness of** any duration with death due to brain injury prior to regaining consciousness   MCC H5

    ✓7ᵗʰ   **S06.9X8**   **Unspecified intracranial injury with loss of consciousness of** any duration with death due to other cause prior to regaining consciousness   MCC H5

    7   ✓7ᵗʰ   **S06.9X9**   **Unspecified intracranial injury with loss of consciousness of** unspecified duration   CC H5 HCC

✓4ᵗʰ S07   **Crushing injury of head**
    Use additional code for all associated injuries, such as:
      intracranial injuries (S06.-)
      skull fractures (S02.-)

    The appropriate 7th character is to be added to each code from category S07.
    A   initial encounter
    D   subsequent encounter
    S   sequela

    CC Excl: For CC codes in category S07: PDX collection 1156

   ✓x7ᵗʰ   **S07.0**   **Crushing injury of** face   CC H5

   ✓x7ᵗʰ   **S07.1**   **Crushing injury of** skull   CC H5

   ✓x7ᵗʰ   **S07.8**   **Crushing injury of** other **parts of head**   CC H5

   ✓x7ᵗʰ   **S07.9**   **Crushing injury of** head, part unspecified   CC H5

✓4ᵗʰ S08   **Avulsion and traumatic amputation of part of head**
    An amputation not identified as partial or complete should be coded to complete

    The appropriate 7th character is to be added to each code from category S08.
    A   initial encounter
    D   subsequent encounter
    S   sequela

   ✓x7ᵗʰ   **S08.0**   **Avulsion of** scalp

   ✓5ᵗʰ   **S08.1**   **Traumatic amputation of** ear

    ✓6ᵗʰ   **S08.11**   Complete **traumatic amputation of ear**

     ✓7ᵗʰ   **S08.111**   **Complete traumatic amputation of** right **ear**

N Newborn: 0   P Pediatric: 0-17   M Maternity: 12-55   A Adult: 15-124   MCC Major Complication/Comorbidity   CC Complication/Comorbidity   SW Severe Wound Dx

958   ICD-10-CM 2019

√7ᵗʰ   **S08.112**   **Complete** traumatic amputation of left **ear**

√7ᵗʰ   **S08.119**   **Complete** traumatic amputation of unspecified **ear**

√6ᵗʰ   **S08.12**   **Partial** traumatic amputation of ear

√7ᵗʰ   **S08.121**   **Partial** traumatic amputation of right **ear**

√7ᵗʰ   **S08.122**   **Partial** traumatic amputation of left **ear**

√7ᵗʰ   **S08.129**   **Partial** traumatic amputation of unspecified **ear**

√5ᵗʰ   **S08.8**   **Traumatic amputation of** other parts of head

√6ᵗʰ   **S08.81**   **Traumatic amputation of** nose

√7ᵗʰ   **S08.811**   **Complete** traumatic amputation of nose

√7ᵗʰ   **S08.812**   **Partial** traumatic amputation of nose

√x7ᵗʰ   **S08.89**   **Traumatic amputation of** other parts of head

√4ᵗʰ   **S09**   **Other and unspecified injuries of head**

> The appropriate 7th character is to be added to each code from category S09.
> A   initial encounter
> D   subsequent encounter
> S   sequela

> **CC Excl: For CC codes in category S09, unless otherwise noted:** PDX collection 1158

√x7ᵗʰ   **S09.0**   **Injury of** blood vessels **of head, not elsewhere classified**   CC

EXCLUDES 1   *injury of cerebral blood vessels (S06.-)*
           injury of precerebral blood vessels (S15.-)

CC Excl: PDX collection 1157

√5ᵗʰ   **S09.1**   **Injury of** muscle and tendon **of head**
Code also any associated open wound (S01.-)
EXCLUDES 2   *sprain to joints and ligament of head (S03.9)*

√x7ᵗʰ   **S09.10**   **Unspecified injury of muscle and tendon of head**
Injury of muscle and tendon of head NOS

√x7ᵗʰ   **S09.11**   **Strain of muscle and tendon of head**

√x7ᵗʰ   **S09.12**   **Laceration of muscle and tendon of head**

√x7ᵗʰ   **S09.19**   **Other specified injury of muscle and tendon of head**

√5ᵗʰ   **S09.2**   **Traumatic rupture of** ear drum
EXCLUDES 1   *traumatic rupture of ear drum due to blast injury (S09.31-)*

√x7ᵗʰ   **S09.20**   **Traumatic rupture of** unspecified **ear drum**   CC

√x7ᵗʰ   **S09.21**   **Traumatic rupture of** right **ear drum**   CC

√x7ᵗʰ   **S09.22**   **Traumatic rupture of** left **ear drum**   CC

√5ᵗʰ   **S09.3**   **Other specified and unspecified injury of middle and inner ear**
EXCLUDES 1   *injury to ear NOS (S09.91-)*
EXCLUDES 2   *injury to external ear (S00.4-, S01.3-, S08.1-)*

√6ᵗʰ   **S09.30**   **Unspecified injury of** middle and inner ear

√7ᵗʰ   **S09.301**   **Unspecified injury of** right **middle and inner ear**   CC

√7ᵗʰ   **S09.302**   **Unspecified injury of** left **middle and inner ear**   CC

√7ᵗʰ   **S09.309**   **Unspecified injury of** unspecified **middle and inner ear**   CC

√6ᵗʰ   **S09.31**   **Primary** blast injury **of ear**
Blast injury of ear NOS

√7ᵗʰ   **S09.311**   **Primary blast injury of** right **ear**   CC

√7ᵗʰ   **S09.312**   **Primary blast injury of** left **ear**   CC

√7ᵗʰ   **S09.313**   **Primary blast injury of ear,** bilateral   CC

√7ᵗʰ   **S09.319**   **Primary blast injury of** unspecified **ear**   CC

√6ᵗʰ   **S09.39**   **Other** specified injury of middle and inner ear
Secondary blast injury to ear

√7ᵗʰ   **S09.391**   **Other specified injury of** right **middle and inner ear**   CC

√7ᵗʰ   **S09.392**   **Other specified injury of** left **middle and inner ear**   CC

√7ᵗʰ   **S09.399**   **Other specified injury of** unspecified **middle and inner ear**   CC

√x7ᵗʰ   **S09.8**   **Other specified injuries of head**

√5ᵗʰ   **S09.9**   **Unspecified injury of face and head**

√x7ᵗʰ   **S09.90**   **Unspecified injury of** head
Head injury NOS
EXCLUDES 1   *brain injury NOS (S06.9-)*
         head injury NOS with loss of consciousness (S06.9-)
         intracranial injury NOS (S06.9-)

√x7ᵗʰ   **S09.91**   **Unspecified injury of** ear
Injury of ear NOS

√x7ᵗʰ   **S09.92**   **Unspecified injury of** nose
Injury of nose NOS

√x7ᵗʰ   **S09.93**   **Unspecified injury of** face
Injury of face NOS

Injuries to the neck (S10-S19)

INCLUDES   injuries of nape
         injuries of supraclavicular region
         injuries of throat
EXCLUDES 2   *burns and corrosions (T20-T32)*
         effects of foreign body in esophagus (T18.1)
         effects of foreign body in larynx (T17.3)
         effects of foreign body in pharynx (T17.2)
         effects of foreign body in trachea (T17.4)
         frostbite (T33-T34)
         insect bite or sting, venomous (T63.4)

√4ᵗʰ   **S10**   **Superficial injury of neck**

> The appropriate 7th character is to be added to each code from category S10.
> A   initial encounter
> D   subsequent encounter
> S   sequela

√x7ᵗʰ   **S10.0**   **Contusion of throat**
Contusion of cervical esophagus
Contusion of larynx
Contusion of pharynx
Contusion of trachea

√5ᵗʰ   **S10.1**   **Other and unspecified superficial injuries of throat**

√x7ᵗʰ   **S10.10**   **Unspecified superficial injuries of throat**

√x7ᵗʰ   **S10.11**   **Abrasion of throat**

√x7ᵗʰ   **S10.12**   **Blister (nonthermal) of throat**

√x7ᵗʰ   **S10.14**   **External constriction of part of throat**

√x7ᵗʰ   **S10.15**   **Superficial** foreign body **of throat**
Splinter in the throat

√x7ᵗʰ   **S10.16**   **Insect bite (nonvenomous) of throat**

√x7ᵗʰ   **S10.17**   **Other** superficial **bite of throat**
EXCLUDES 1   *open bite of throat (S11.85)*

√5ᵗʰ   **S10.8**   **Superficial injury of** other **specified parts of neck**

√x7ᵗʰ   **S10.80**   **Unspecified superficial injury of other specified part of neck**

√x7ᵗʰ   **S10.81**   **Abrasion of other specified part of neck**

√x7ᵗʰ   **S10.82**   **Blister (nonthermal) of other specified part of neck**

√x7ᵗʰ   **S10.83**   **Contusion of other specified part of neck**

√x7ᵗʰ   **S10.84**   **External constriction of other specified part of neck**

√x7ᵗʰ   **S10.85**   **Superficial** foreign body **of other specified part of neck**
Splinter in other specified part of neck

√x7ᵗʰ   **S10.86**   **Insect bite of other specified part of neck**

√x7ᵗʰ   **S10.87**   **Other** superficial **bite of other specified part of neck**
EXCLUDES 1   *open bite of other specified parts of neck (S11.85)*

√5ᵗʰ   **S10.9**   **Superficial injury of** unspecified **part of neck**

√x7ᵗʰ   **S10.90**   **Unspecified superficial injury of unspecified part of neck**

√x7ᵗʰ   **S10.91**   **Abrasion of unspecified part of neck**

√x7ᵗʰ   **S10.92**   **Blister (nonthermal) of unspecified part of neck**

√x7ᵗʰ   **S10.93**   **Contusion of unspecified part of neck**

√x7ᵗʰ   **S10.94**   **External constriction of unspecified part of neck**

√x7ᵗʰ   **S10.95**   **Superficial** foreign body **of unspecified part of neck**

√x7ᵗʰ   **S10.96**   **Insect bite of unspecified part of neck**

√x7ᵗʰ   **S10.97**   **Other** superficial **bite of unspecified part of neck**

✓4th **S11 Open wound of neck**
Code also any associated:
spinal cord injury (S14.Ø, S14.1-)
wound infection
EXCLUDES 2   *open fracture of vertebra (S12- with 7th B)*

> The appropriate 7th character is to be added to each code from
> category S11.
> A   initial encounter
> D   subsequent encounter
> S   sequela

✓5th **S11.Ø Open wound of larynx and trachea**

> CC Excl: For MCC codes in subcategory S11.Ø:
> PDX collection 1159

   ✓6th **S11.Ø1 Open wound of larynx**
     EXCLUDES 2   *open wound of vocal cord (S11.Ø3)*

     ✓7th **S11.Ø11 Laceration without foreign body of larynx** `MCC`

     ✓7th **S11.Ø12 Laceration with foreign body of larynx** `MCC`

     ✓7th **S11.Ø13 Puncture wound without foreign body of larynx** `MCC`

     ✓7th **S11.Ø14 Puncture wound with foreign body of larynx** `MCC`

     ✓7th **S11.Ø15 Open bite of larynx** `MCC`
       Bite of larynx NOS

     ✓7th **S11.Ø19 Unspecified open wound of larynx** `MCC`

   ✓6th **S11.Ø2 Open wound of trachea**
     Open wound of cervical trachea
     Open wound of trachea NOS
     EXCLUDES 2   *open wound of thoracic trachea (S27.5-)*

     ✓7th **S11.Ø21 Laceration without foreign body of trachea** `MCC`

     ✓7th **S11.Ø22 Laceration with foreign body of trachea** `MCC`

     ✓7th **S11.Ø23 Puncture wound without foreign body of trachea** `MCC`

     ✓7th **S11.Ø24 Puncture wound with foreign body of trachea** `MCC`

     ✓7th **S11.Ø25 Open bite of trachea** `MCC`
       Bite of trachea NOS

     ✓7th **S11.Ø29 Unspecified open wound of trachea** `MCC`

   ✓6th **S11.Ø3 Open wound of vocal cord**

     ✓7th **S11.Ø31 Laceration without foreign body of vocal cord** `MCC`

     ✓7th **S11.Ø32 Laceration with foreign body of vocal cord** `MCC`

     ✓7th **S11.Ø33 Puncture wound without foreign body of vocal cord** `MCC`

     ✓7th **S11.Ø34 Puncture wound with foreign body of vocal cord** `MCC`

     ✓7th **S11.Ø35 Open bite of vocal cord** `MCC`
       Bite of vocal cord NOS

     ✓7th **S11.Ø39 Unspecified open wound of vocal cord** `MCC`

✓5th **S11.1 Open wound of thyroid gland**

> CC Excl: For CC codes in subcategory S11.1, unless
> otherwise noted: PDX collection 116Ø

   ✓x7th **S11.1Ø Unspecified open wound of thyroid gland** `CC`

   ✓x7th **S11.11 Laceration without foreign body of thyroid gland** `CC`

   ✓x7th **S11.12 Laceration with foreign body of thyroid gland** `CC`
     CC Excl: PDX collection 1161

   ✓x7th **S11.13 Puncture wound without foreign body of thyroid gland** `CC`

   ✓x7th **S11.14 Puncture wound with foreign body of thyroid gland** `CC`
     CC Excl: PDX collection 1161

   ✓x7th **S11.15 Open bite of thyroid gland** `CC`
     Bite of thyroid gland NOS

✓5th **S11.2 Open wound of pharynx and cervical esophagus**
   EXCLUDES 1   *open wound of esophagus NOS (S27.8-)*

> CC Excl: For CC codes in subcategory S11.2, unless
> otherwise noted: PDX collection 1162

   ✓x7th **S11.2Ø Unspecified open wound of pharynx and cervical esophagus** `CC`

   ✓x7th **S11.21 Laceration without foreign body of pharynx and cervical esophagus** `CC`

   ✓x7th **S11.22 Laceration with foreign body of pharynx and cervical esophagus** `CC`
     CC Excl: PDX collection 1163

   ✓x7th **S11.23 Puncture wound without foreign body of pharynx and cervical esophagus** `CC`

   ✓x7th **S11.24 Puncture wound with foreign body of pharynx and cervical esophagus** `CC`
     CC Excl: PDX collection 1163

   ✓x7th **S11.25 Open bite of pharynx and cervical esophagus** `CC`
     Bite of pharynx and cervical esophagus NOS

✓5th **S11.8 Open wound of other specified parts of neck**

   ✓x7th **S11.8Ø Unspecified open wound of other specified part of neck**

   ✓x7th **S11.81 Laceration without foreign body of other specified part of neck**

   ✓x7th **S11.82 Laceration with foreign body of other specified part of neck**

   ✓x7th **S11.83 Puncture wound without foreign body of other specified part of neck**

   ✓x7th **S11.84 Puncture wound with foreign body of other specified part of neck**

   ✓x7th **S11.85 Open bite of other specified part of neck**
     Bite of other specified part of neck NOS
     EXCLUDES 1   *superficial bite of other specified part of neck (S1Ø.87)*

   ✓x7th **S11.89 Other open wound of other specified part of neck**

✓5th **S11.9 Open wound of unspecified part of neck**

   ✓x7th **S11.9Ø Unspecified open wound of unspecified part of neck**

   ✓x7th **S11.91 Laceration without foreign body of unspecified part of neck**

   ✓x7th **S11.92 Laceration with foreign body of unspecified part of neck**

   ✓x7th **S11.93 Puncture wound without foreign body of unspecified part of neck**

   ✓x7th **S11.94 Puncture wound with foreign body of unspecified part of neck**

   ✓x7th **S11.95 Open bite of unspecified part of neck**
     Bite of neck NOS
     EXCLUDES 1   *superficial bite of neck (S1Ø.97)*

✓4th **S12 Fracture of cervical vertebra and other parts of neck**
   NOTE   A fracture not indicated as nondisplaced or displaced
     should be classified to displaced.
     A fracture not indicated as open or closed should be coded
     to closed.
   INCLUDES   fracture of cervical neural arch
     fracture of cervical spine
     fracture of cervical spinous process
     fracture of cervical transverse process
     fracture of cervical vertebral arch
     fracture of neck
Code first any associated cervical spinal cord injury (S14.Ø, S14.1-)
AHA: 2018, 2Q, 12; 2015, 3Q, 37-39

> The appropriate 7th character is to be added to all codes from
> subcategories S12.Ø-S12.6.
> A   initial encounter for closed fracture
> B   initial encounter for open fracture
> D   subsequent encounter for fracture with routine healing
> G   subsequent encounter for fracture with delayed healing
> K   subsequent encounter for fracture with nonunion
> S   sequela

> CC Excl: For codes in category S12, unless otherwise noted:
> CC with 7th character A or MCC with 7th character B:
> PDX collection 1164
> CC with 7th character K: PDX collection 897

N Newborn: 0   P Pediatric: 0-17   M Maternity: 12-55   A Adult: 15-124   `MCC` Major Complication/Comorbidity   `CC` Complication/Comorbidity   `SW` Severe Wound Dx

960   ICD-10-CM 2019

✓5th **S12.0** **Fracture of first cervical vertebra**
Atlas

 ✓6th **S12.00** Unspecified **fracture of first cervical vertebra**

  2,3,6 ✓7th **S12.000** **Unspecified** displaced **fracture of first cervical vertebra** `MCC` `CC` `H5` `HCC`

  2,3,6 ✓7th **S12.001** **Unspecified** nondisplaced **fracture of first cervical vertebra** `MCC` `CC` `H5` `HCC`

 2,3,6 ✓x7th **S12.01** **Stable burst fracture of first cervical vertebra** `MCC` `CC` `H5` `HCC`

 2,3,6 ✓x7th **S12.02** **Unstable burst fracture of first cervical vertebra** `MCC` `CC` `H5` `HCC`

 ✓6th **S12.03** Posterior arch **fracture of first cervical vertebra**

  2,3,6 ✓7th **S12.030** Displaced posterior arch **fracture of first cervical vertebra** `MCC` `CC` `H5` `HCC`

  2,3,6 ✓7th **S12.031** Nondisplaced posterior arch **fracture of first cervical vertebra** `MCC` `CC` `H5` `HCC`

 ✓6th **S12.04** Lateral mass **fracture of first cervical vertebra**

  2,3,6 ✓7th **S12.040** Displaced lateral mass **fracture of first cervical vertebra** `MCC` `CC` `H5` `HCC`

  2,3,6 ✓7th **S12.041** Nondisplaced lateral mass **fracture of first cervical vertebra** `MCC` `CC` `H5` `HCC`

 ✓6th **S12.09** Other **fracture of first cervical vertebra**

  2,3,6 ✓7th **S12.090** Other displaced **fracture of first cervical vertebra** `MCC` `CC` `H5` `HCC`

  2,3,6 ✓7th **S12.091** Other nondisplaced **fracture of first cervical vertebra** `MCC` `CC` `H5` `HCC`

✓5th **S12.1** **Fracture of second cervical vertebra**
Axis

 ✓6th **S12.10** Unspecified **fracture of second cervical vertebra**

  2,3,6 ✓7th **S12.100** **Unspecified** displaced **fracture of second cervical vertebra** `MCC` `CC` `H5` `HCC`

  2,3,6 ✓7th **S12.101** **Unspecified** nondisplaced **fracture of second cervical vertebra** `MCC` `CC` `H5` `HCC`

 ✓6th **S12.11** Type II dens **fracture**

  2,3,6 ✓7th **S12.110** Anterior displaced Type II dens fracture `MCC` `CC` `H5` `HCC`

  2,3,6 ✓7th **S12.111** Posterior displaced Type II dens fracture `MCC` `CC` `H5` `HCC`

  2,3,6 ✓7th **S12.112** Nondisplaced Type II dens fracture `MCC` `CC` `H5` `HCC`

 ✓6th **S12.12** Other dens **fracture**

  2,3,6 ✓7th **S12.120** Other displaced dens fracture `MCC` `CC` `H5` `HCC`

  2,3,6 ✓7th **S12.121** Other nondisplaced dens fracture `MCC` `CC` `H5` `HCC`

 ✓6th **S12.13** Unspecified traumatic spondylolisthesis **of second cervical vertebra**

  2,3,6 ✓7th **S12.130** Unspecified traumatic displaced spondylolisthesis of second cervical vertebra `MCC` `CC` `H5` `HCC`

  2,3,6 ✓7th **S12.131** Unspecified traumatic nondisplaced spondylolisthesis of second cervical vertebra `MCC` `CC` `H5` `HCC`

 2,3,6 ✓x7th **S12.14** Type III traumatic spondylolisthesis **of second cervical vertebra** `MCC` `CC` `H5` `HCC`

 ✓6th **S12.15** Other traumatic spondylolisthesis **of second cervical vertebra**

  2,3,6 ✓7th **S12.150** Other traumatic displaced spondylolisthesis of second cervical vertebra `MCC` `CC` `H5` `HCC`

  2,3,6 ✓7th **S12.151** Other traumatic nondisplaced spondylolisthesis of second cervical vertebra `MCC` `CC` `H5` `HCC`

 ✓6th **S12.19** Other **fracture of second cervical vertebra**

  2,3,6 ✓7th **S12.190** Other displaced **fracture of second cervical vertebra** `MCC` `CC` `H5` `HCC`

  2,3,6 ✓7th **S12.191** Other nondisplaced fracture **of second cervical vertebra** `MCC` `CC` `H5` `HCC`

✓5th **S12.2** **Fracture of third cervical vertebra**

 ✓6th **S12.20** Unspecified **fracture of third cervical vertebra**

  2,3,6 ✓7th **S12.200** **Unspecified** displaced **fracture of third cervical vertebra** `MCC` `CC` `H5` `HCC`

  2,3,6 ✓7th **S12.201** **Unspecified** nondisplaced **fracture of third cervical vertebra** `MCC` `CC` `H5` `HCC`

 ✓6th **S12.23** Unspecified traumatic spondylolisthesis **of third cervical vertebra**

  2,3,6 ✓7th **S12.230** Unspecified traumatic displaced spondylolisthesis of third cervical vertebra `MCC` `CC` `H5` `HCC`

  2,3,6 ✓7th **S12.231** Unspecified traumatic nondisplaced spondylolisthesis of third cervical vertebra `MCC` `CC` `H5` `HCC`

 2,3,6 ✓x7th **S12.24** Type III traumatic spondylolisthesis **of third cervical vertebra** `MCC` `CC` `H5` `HCC`

 ✓6th **S12.25** Other traumatic spondylolisthesis **of third cervical vertebra**

  2,3,6 ✓7th **S12.250** Other traumatic displaced spondylolisthesis of third cervical vertebra `MCC` `CC` `H5` `HCC`

  2,3,6 ✓7th **S12.251** Other traumatic nondisplaced spondylolisthesis of third cervical vertebra `MCC` `CC` `H5` `HCC`

 ✓6th **S12.29** Other **fracture of third cervical vertebra**

  2,3,6 ✓7th **S12.290** Other displaced **fracture of third cervical vertebra** `MCC` `CC` `H5` `HCC`

  2,3,6 ✓7th **S12.291** Other nondisplaced fracture **of third cervical vertebra** `MCC` `CC` `H5` `HCC`

✓5th **S12.3** **Fracture of fourth cervical vertebra**

 ✓6th **S12.30** Unspecified **fracture of fourth cervical vertebra**

  2,3,6 ✓7th **S12.300** **Unspecified** displaced **fracture of fourth cervical vertebra** `MCC` `CC` `H5` `HCC`

  2,3,6 ✓7th **S12.301** **Unspecified** nondisplaced **fracture of fourth cervical vertebra** `MCC` `CC` `H5` `HCC`

 ✓6th **S12.33** Unspecified traumatic spondylolisthesis **of fourth cervical vertebra**

  2,3,6 ✓7th **S12.330** Unspecified traumatic displaced spondylolisthesis of fourth cervical vertebra `MCC` `CC` `H5` `HCC`

  2,3,6 ✓7th **S12.331** Unspecified traumatic nondisplaced spondylolisthesis of fourth cervical vertebra `MCC` `CC` `H5` `HCC`

 2,3,6 ✓x7th **S12.34** Type III traumatic spondylolisthesis **of fourth cervical vertebra** `MCC` `CC` `H5` `HCC`

 ✓6th **S12.35** Other traumatic spondylolisthesis **of fourth cervical vertebra**

  2,3,6 ✓7th **S12.350** Other traumatic displaced spondylolisthesis of fourth cervical vertebra `MCC` `CC` `H5` `HCC`

  2,3,6 ✓7th **S12.351** Other traumatic nondisplaced spondylolisthesis of fourth cervical vertebra `MCC` `CC` `H5` `HCC`

 ✓6th **S12.39** Other **fracture of fourth cervical vertebra**

  2,3,6 ✓7th **S12.390** Other displaced **fracture of fourth cervical vertebra** `MCC` `CC` `H5` `HCC`

  2,3,6 ✓7th **S12.391** Other nondisplaced fracture **of fourth cervical vertebra** `MCC` `CC` `H5` `HCC`

✓5th **S12.4** **Fracture of fifth cervical vertebra**

 ✓6th **S12.40** Unspecified **fracture of fifth cervical vertebra**

  2,3,6 ✓7th **S12.400** **Unspecified** displaced **fracture of fifth cervical vertebra** `MCC` `CC` `H5` `HCC`

  2,3,6 ✓7th **S12.401** **Unspecified** nondisplaced **fracture of fifth cervical vertebra** `MCC` `CC` `H5` `HCC`

 ✓6th **S12.43** Unspecified traumatic spondylolisthesis **of fifth cervical vertebra**

  2,3,6 ✓7th **S12.430** Unspecified traumatic displaced spondylolisthesis of fifth cervical vertebra `MCC` `CC` `H5` `HCC`

  2,3,6 ✓7th **S12.431** Unspecified traumatic nondisplaced spondylolisthesis of fifth cervical vertebra `MCC` `CC` `H5` `HCC`

 2,3,6 ✓x7th **S12.44** Type III traumatic spondylolisthesis **of fifth cervical vertebra** `MCC` `CC` `H5` `HCC`

 ✓6th **S12.45** Other traumatic spondylolisthesis **of fifth cervical vertebra**

  2,3,6 ✓7th **S12.450** Other traumatic displaced spondylolisthesis of fifth cervical vertebra `MCC` `CC` `H5` `HCC`

  2,3,6 ✓7th **S12.451** Other traumatic nondisplaced spondylolisthesis of fifth cervical vertebra `MCC` `CC` `H5` `HCC`

Chapter 19. Injury, Poisoning and Certain Other Consequences of External Causes

S12.0–S12.451

✓6ᵗʰ **S12.49** Other fracture of fifth cervical vertebra

  2,3,6 ✓7ᵗʰ **S12.490** Other displaced fracture of `MCC` `CC` `H5` `HCC`
fifth cervical vertebra

  2,3,6 ✓7ᵗʰ **S12.491** Other nondisplaced fracture `MCC` `CC` `H5` `HCC`
of fifth cervical vertebra

✓5ᵗʰ **S12.5** Fracture of sixth cervical vertebra

  ✓6ᵗʰ **S12.50** Unspecified fracture of sixth cervical vertebra

  2,3,6 ✓7ᵗʰ **S12.500** Unspecified displaced `MCC` `CC` `H5` `HCC`
fracture of sixth cervical vertebra

  2,3,6 ✓7ᵗʰ **S12.501** Unspecified nondisplaced `MCC` `CC` `H5` `HCC`
fracture of sixth cervical vertebra

  ✓6ᵗʰ **S12.53** Unspecified traumatic spondylolisthesis of sixth
cervical vertebra

  2,3,6 ✓7ᵗʰ **S12.530** Unspecified traumatic `MCC` `CC` `H5` `HCC`
displaced spondylolisthesis
of sixth cervical vertebra

  2,3,6 ✓7ᵗʰ **S12.531** Unspecified traumatic `MCC` `CC` `H5` `HCC`
nondisplaced spondylolisthesis
of sixth cervical vertebra

  2,3,6 ✓x7ᵗʰ **S12.54** Type III traumatic spondylolisthesis of `MCC` `CC` `H5` `HCC`
sixth cervical vertebra

  ✓6ᵗʰ **S12.55** Other traumatic spondylolisthesis of sixth cervical
vertebra

  2,3,6 ✓7ᵗʰ **S12.550** Other traumatic displaced `MCC` `CC` `H5` `HCC`
spondylolisthesis of sixth
cervical vertebra

  2,3,6 ✓7ᵗʰ **S12.551** Other traumatic `MCC` `CC` `H5` `HCC`
nondisplaced spondylolisthesis
of sixth cervicalvertebra

  ✓6ᵗʰ **S12.59** Other fracture of sixth cervical vertebra

  2,3,6 ✓7ᵗʰ **S12.590** Other displaced fracture of `MCC` `CC` `H5` `HCC`
sixth cervical vertebra

  2,3,6 ✓7ᵗʰ **S12.591** Other nondisplaced fracture `MCC` `CC` `H5` `HCC`
of sixth cervical vertebra

✓5ᵗʰ **S12.6** Fracture of seventh cervical vertebra

  ✓6ᵗʰ **S12.60** Unspecified fracture of seventh cervical vertebra

  2,3,6 ✓7ᵗʰ **S12.600** Unspecified displaced `MCC` `CC` `H5` `HCC`
fracture of seventh cervical vertebra

  2,3,6 ✓7ᵗʰ **S12.601** Unspecified nondisplaced `MCC` `CC` `H5` `HCC`
fracture of seventh cervical vertebra

  ✓6ᵗʰ **S12.63** Unspecified traumatic spondylolisthesis of seventh
cervical vertebra

  2,3,6 ✓7ᵗʰ **S12.630** Unspecified traumatic `MCC` `CC` `H5` `HCC`
displaced spondylolisthesis
of seventh cervical vertebra

  2,3,6 ✓7ᵗʰ **S12.631** Unspecified traumatic `MCC` `CC` `H5` `HCC`
nondisplaced spondylolisthesis
of seventh cervical vertebra

  2,3,6 ✓x7ᵗʰ **S12.64** Type III traumatic spondylolisthesis `MCC` `CC` `H5` `HCC`
of seventh cervical vertebra

  ✓6ᵗʰ **S12.65** Other traumatic spondylolisthesis of seventh
cervical vertebra

  2,3,6 ✓7ᵗʰ **S12.650** Other traumatic displaced `MCC` `CC` `H5` `HCC`
spondylolisthesis of seventh
cervical vertebra

  2,3,6 ✓7ᵗʰ **S12.651** Other traumatic `MCC` `CC` `H5` `HCC`
nondisplaced spondylolisthesis
of seventh cervical vertebra

  ✓6ᵗʰ **S12.69** Other fracture of seventh cervical vertebra

  2,3,6 ✓7ᵗʰ **S12.690** Other displaced fracture of `MCC` `CC` `H5` `HCC`
seventh cervical vertebra

  2,3,6 ✓7ᵗʰ **S12.691** Other nondisplaced `MCC` `CC` `H5` `HCC`
fracture of seventh cervical vertebra

6 ✓x7ᵗʰ **S12.8** Fracture of other parts of neck `MCC` `H5` `HCC`
Hyoid bone
Larynx
Thyroid cartilage
Trachea

> The appropriate 7th character is to be added to code S12.8.
> A   initial encounter
> D   subsequent encounter
> S   sequela

CC Excl: PDX collection 1165

6 ✓x7ᵗʰ **S12.9** Fracture of neck, unspecified `CC` `H5` `HCC`
Fracture of cervical spine NOS
Fracture of cervical vertebra NOS
Fracture of neck NOS

> The appropriate 7th character is to be added to code S12.9.
> A   initial encounter
> D   subsequent encounter
> S   sequela

CC Excl: PDX collection 1164

✓4ᵗʰ **S13** Dislocation and sprain of joints and ligaments at neck level

  `INCLUDES`   avulsion of joint or ligament at neck level
laceration of cartilage, joint or ligament at neck level
sprain of cartilage, joint or ligament at neck level
traumatic hemarthrosis of joint or ligament at neck level
traumatic rupture of joint or ligament at neck level
traumatic subluxation of joint or ligament at neck level
traumatic tear of joint or ligament at neck level

Code also any associated open wound

  EXCLUDES 2   *strain of muscle or tendon at neck level (S16.1)*

> The appropriate 7th character is to be added to each code from
> category S13.
> A   initial encounter
> D   subsequent encounter
> S   sequela

CC Excl: For CC codes in category S13: PDX collection 913

✓x7ᵗʰ **S13.0** Traumatic rupture of cervical intervertebral disc `CC` `H5`

  EXCLUDES 1   *rupture or displacement (nontraumatic) of cervical*
intervertebral disc NOS (M50.-)

✓5ᵗʰ **S13.1** Subluxation and dislocation of cervical vertebrae
Code also any associated:
  open wound of neck (S11.-)
  spinal cord injury (S14.1-)

  EXCLUDES 2   *fracture of cervical vertebrae (S12.0--S12.3-)*

  ✓6ᵗʰ **S13.10** Subluxation and dislocation of unspecified cervical
vertebrae

    ✓7ᵗʰ **S13.100** Subluxation of unspecified cervical `CC` `H5`
vertebrae

    ✓7ᵗʰ **S13.101** Dislocation of unspecified cervical `CC` `H5`
vertebrae

  ✓6ᵗʰ **S13.11** Subluxation and dislocation of C0/C1 cervical
vertebrae
Subluxation and dislocation of atlantooccipital joint
Subluxation and dislocation of atloidooccipital joint
Subluxation and dislocation of occipitoatloid joint

    ✓7ᵗʰ **S13.110** Subluxation of C0/C1 cervical `CC` `H5`
vertebrae

    ✓7ᵗʰ **S13.111** Dislocation of C0/C1 cervical `CC` `H5`
vertebrae

  ✓6ᵗʰ **S13.12** Subluxation and dislocation of C1/C2 cervical
vertebrae
Subluxation and dislocation of atlantoaxial joint

    ✓7ᵗʰ **S13.120** Subluxation of C1/C2 cervical `CC` `H5`
vertebrae

    ✓7ᵗʰ **S13.121** Dislocation of C1/C2 cervical `CC` `H5`
vertebrae

  ✓6ᵗʰ **S13.13** Subluxation and dislocation of C2/C3 cervical
vertebrae

    ✓7ᵗʰ **S13.130** Subluxation of C2/C3 cervical `CC` `H5`
vertebrae

    ✓7ᵗʰ **S13.131** Dislocation of C2/C3 cervical `CC` `H5`
vertebrae

  ✓6ᵗʰ **S13.14** Subluxation and dislocation of C3/C4 cervical
vertebrae

    ✓7ᵗʰ **S13.140** Subluxation of C3/C4 cervical `CC` `H5`
vertebrae

    ✓7ᵗʰ **S13.141** Dislocation of C3/C4 cervical `CC` `H5`
vertebrae

  ✓6ᵗʰ **S13.15** Subluxation and dislocation of C4/C5 cervical
vertebrae

    ✓7ᵗʰ **S13.150** Subluxation of C4/C5 cervical `CC` `H5`
vertebrae

    ✓7ᵗʰ **S13.151** Dislocation of C4/C5 cervical `CC` `H5`
vertebrae

N Newborn: 0   **P** Pediatric: 0-17   **M** Maternity: 12-55   **A** Adult: 15-124   **MCC** Major Complication/Comorbidity   **CC** Complication/Comorbidity   **SW** Severe Wound Dx

962   ICD-10-CM 2019

✓6ᵗʰ **S13.16 Subluxation and dislocation of C5/C6 cervical vertebrae**

    ✓7ᵗʰ **S13.160 Subluxation of C5/C6 cervical vertebrae** `CC` `H5`

    ✓7ᵗʰ **S13.161 Dislocation of C5/C6 cervical vertebrae** `CC` `H5`

✓6ᵗʰ **S13.17 Subluxation and dislocation of C6/C7 cervical vertebrae**

    ✓7ᵗʰ **S13.170 Subluxation of C6/C7 cervical vertebrae** `CC` `H5`

    ✓7ᵗʰ **S13.171 Dislocation of C6/C7 cervical vertebrae** `CC` `H5`

✓6ᵗʰ **S13.18 Subluxation and dislocation of C7/T1 cervical vertebrae**

    ✓7ᵗʰ **S13.180 Subluxation of C7/T1 cervical vertebrae** `CC` `H5`

    ✓7ᵗʰ **S13.181 Dislocation of C7/T1 cervical vertebrae** `CC` `H5`

✓5ᵗʰ **S13.2 Dislocation of other and unspecified parts of neck**

    S13.20 Dislocation of unspecified parts of neck `CC` `H5`

    S13.29 Dislocation of other parts of neck `CC` `H5`

✓x7ᵗʰ **S13.4 Sprain of ligaments of cervical spine**
Sprain of anterior longitudinal (ligament), cervical
Sprain of atlanto-axial (joints)
Sprain of atlanto-occipital (joints)
Whiplash injury of cervical spine

✓x7ᵗʰ **S13.5 Sprain of thyroid region**
Sprain of cricoarytenoid (joint) (ligament)
Sprain of cricothyroid (joint) (ligament)
Sprain of thyroid cartilage

✓x7ᵗʰ **S13.8 Sprain of joints and ligaments of other parts of neck**

✓x7ᵗʰ **S13.9 Sprain of joints and ligaments of unspecified parts of neck**

✓4ᵗʰ **S14 Injury of nerves and spinal cord at neck level**
    `NOTE`   Code to highest level of cervical cord injury.
Code also any associated:
    fracture of cervical vertebra (S12.0- – S12.6-)
    open wound of neck (S11.-)
    transient paralysis (R29.5)

> The appropriate 7th character is to be added to each code from category S14.
> A   initial encounter
> D   subsequent encounter
> S   sequela

> CC Excl: For MCC codes in category S14: PDX collection 1166

✓x7ᵗʰ **S14.0 Concussion and edema of cervical spinal cord** `MCC` `HCC`

✓5ᵗʰ **S14.1 Other and unspecified injuries of cervical spinal cord**

    ✓6ᵗʰ **S14.10 Unspecified injury of cervical spinal cord**

      ✓7ᵗʰ **S14.101 Unspecified injury at C1 level of cervical spinal cord** `MCC` `H5` `HCC`

      ✓7ᵗʰ **S14.102 Unspecified injury at C2 level of cervical spinal cord** `MCC` `H5` `HCC`

      ✓7ᵗʰ **S14.103 Unspecified injury at C3 level of cervical spinal cord** `MCC` `H5` `HCC`

      ✓7ᵗʰ **S14.104 Unspecified injury at C4 level of cervical spinal cord** `MCC` `H5` `HCC`

      ✓7ᵗʰ **S14.105 Unspecified injury at C5 level of cervical spinal cord** `MCC` `H5` `HCC`

      ✓7ᵗʰ **S14.106 Unspecified injury at C6 level of cervical spinal cord** `MCC` `H5` `HCC`

      ✓7ᵗʰ **S14.107 Unspecified injury at C7 level of cervical spinal cord** `MCC` `H5` `HCC`

      ✓7ᵗʰ **S14.108 Unspecified injury at C8 level of cervical spinal cord** `MCC` `HCC`

      ✓7ᵗʰ **S14.109 Unspecified injury at unspecified level of cervical spinal cord** `HCC`
        Injury of cervical spinal cord NOS

    ✓6ᵗʰ **S14.11 Complete lesion of cervical spinal cord**

      ✓7ᵗʰ **S14.111 Complete lesion at C1 level of cervical spinal cord** `MCC` `H5` `HCC`

      ✓7ᵗʰ **S14.112 Complete lesion at C2 level of cervical spinal cord** `MCC` `H5` `HCC`

      ✓7ᵗʰ **S14.113 Complete lesion at C3 level of cervical spinal cord** `MCC` `H5` `HCC`

      ✓7ᵗʰ **S14.114 Complete lesion at C4 level of cervical spinal cord** `MCC` `H5` `HCC`

      ✓7ᵗʰ **S14.115 Complete lesion at C5 level of cervical spinal cord** `MCC` `H5` `HCC`

      ✓7ᵗʰ **S14.116 Complete lesion at C6 level of cervical spinal cord** `MCC` `H5` `HCC`

      ✓7ᵗʰ **S14.117 Complete lesion at C7 level of cervical spinal cord** `MCC` `H5` `HCC`

      ✓7ᵗʰ **S14.118 Complete lesion at C8 level of cervical spinal cord** `MCC` `HCC`

      ✓7ᵗʰ **S14.119 Complete lesion at unspecified level of cervical spinal cord** `HCC`

    ✓6ᵗʰ **S14.12 Central cord syndrome of cervical spinal cord**

      ✓7ᵗʰ **S14.121 Central cord syndrome at C1 level of cervical spinal cord** `MCC` `H5` `HCC`

      ✓7ᵗʰ **S14.122 Central cord syndrome at C2 level of cervical spinal cord** `MCC` `H5` `HCC`

      ✓7ᵗʰ **S14.123 Central cord syndrome at C3 level of cervical spinal cord** `MCC` `H5` `HCC`

      ✓7ᵗʰ **S14.124 Central cord syndrome at C4 level of cervical spinal cord** `MCC` `H5` `HCC`

      ✓7ᵗʰ **S14.125 Central cord syndrome at C5 level of cervical spinal cord** `MCC` `H5` `HCC`

      ✓7ᵗʰ **S14.126 Central cord syndrome at C6 level of cervical spinal cord** `MCC` `H5` `HCC`

      ✓7ᵗʰ **S14.127 Central cord syndrome at C7 level of cervical spinal cord** `MCC` `H5` `HCC`

      ✓7ᵗʰ **S14.128 Central cord syndrome at C8 level of cervical spinal cord** `MCC` `HCC`

      ✓7ᵗʰ **S14.129 Central cord syndrome at unspecified level of cervical spinal cord** `HCC`

    ✓6ᵗʰ **S14.13 Anterior cord syndrome of cervical spinal cord**

      ✓7ᵗʰ **S14.131 Anterior cord syndrome at C1 level of cervical spinal cord** `MCC` `H5` `HCC`

      ✓7ᵗʰ **S14.132 Anterior cord syndrome at C2 level of cervical spinal cord** `MCC` `H5` `HCC`

      ✓7ᵗʰ **S14.133 Anterior cord syndrome at C3 level of cervical spinal cord** `MCC` `H5` `HCC`

      ✓7ᵗʰ **S14.134 Anterior cord syndrome at C4 level of cervical spinal cord** `MCC` `H5` `HCC`

      ✓7ᵗʰ **S14.135 Anterior cord syndrome at C5 level of cervical spinal cord** `MCC` `H5` `HCC`

      ✓7ᵗʰ **S14.136 Anterior cord syndrome at C6 level of cervical spinal cord** `MCC` `H5` `HCC`

      ✓7ᵗʰ **S14.137 Anterior cord syndrome at C7 level of cervical spinal cord** `MCC` `H5` `HCC`

      ✓7ᵗʰ **S14.138 Anterior cord syndrome at C8 level of cervical spinal cord** `MCC` `HCC`

      ✓7ᵗʰ **S14.139 Anterior cord syndrome at unspecified level of cervical spinal cord** `HCC`

    ✓6ᵗʰ **S14.14 Brown-Séquard syndrome of cervical spinal cord**

      ✓7ᵗʰ **S14.141 Brown-Séquard syndrome at C1 level of cervical spinal cord** `MCC` `HCC`

      ✓7ᵗʰ **S14.142 Brown-Séquard syndrome at C2 level of cervical spinal cord** `MCC` `HCC`

      ✓7ᵗʰ **S14.143 Brown-Séquard syndrome at C3 level of cervical spinal cord** `MCC` `HCC`

      ✓7ᵗʰ **S14.144 Brown-Séquard syndrome at C4 level of cervical spinal cord** `MCC` `HCC`

      ✓7ᵗʰ **S14.145 Brown-Séquard syndrome at C5 level of cervical spinal cord** `MCC` `HCC`

      ✓7ᵗʰ **S14.146 Brown-Séquard syndrome at C6 level of cervical spinal cord** `MCC` `HCC`

      ✓7ᵗʰ **S14.147 Brown-Séquard syndrome at C7 level of cervical spinal cord** `MCC` `HCC`

      ✓7ᵗʰ **S14.148 Brown-Séquard syndrome at C8 level of cervical spinal cord** `MCC` `HCC`

      ✓7ᵗʰ **S14.149 Brown-Séquard syndrome at unspecified level of cervical spinal cord** `HCC`

    ✓6ᵗʰ **S14.15 Other incomplete lesions of cervical spinal cord**
      Incomplete lesion of cervical spinal cord NOS
      Posterior cord syndrome of cervical spinal cord

      ✓7ᵗʰ **S14.151 Other incomplete lesion at C1 level of cervical spinal cord** `MCC` `H5` `HCC`

✓ Additional Character Required   ✓x7ᵗʰ Placeholder   Unacceptable PDx   Questionable PDx   Manifestation   `H1`-`H14` HAC   `HCC` CMS-HCC Dx   `HIV` HIV Dx

ICD-10-CM 2019   963

Chapter 19. Injury, Poisoning and Certain Other Consequences of External Causes

√7ᵗʰ **S14.152** Other incomplete lesion at **C2 level** of cervical spinal cord `MCC` `H5` `HCC`

√7ᵗʰ **S14.153** Other incomplete lesion at **C3 level** of cervical spinal cord `MCC` `H5` `HCC`

√7ᵗʰ **S14.154** Other incomplete lesion at **C4 level** of cervical spinal cord `MCC` `H5` `HCC`

√7ᵗʰ **S14.155** Other incomplete lesion at **C5 level** of cervical spinal cord `MCC` `H5` `HCC`

√7ᵗʰ **S14.156** Other incomplete lesion at **C6 level** of cervical spinal cord `MCC` `H5` `HCC`

√7ᵗʰ **S14.157** Other incomplete lesion at **C7 level** of cervical spinal cord `MCC` `H5` `HCC`

√7ᵗʰ **S14.158** Other incomplete lesion at **C8 level** of cervical spinal cord `MCC` `HCC`

√7ᵗʰ **S14.159** Other incomplete lesion at **unspecified level** of cervical spinal cord `HCC`

√x7ᵗʰ **S14.2 Injury of nerve root of cervical spine**

√x7ᵗʰ **S14.3 Injury of brachial plexus**

√x7ᵗʰ **S14.4 Injury of peripheral nerves of neck**

√x7ᵗʰ **S14.5 Injury of cervical sympathetic nerves**

√x7ᵗʰ **S14.8 Injury of other specified nerves of neck**

√x7ᵗʰ **S14.9 Injury of unspecified nerves of neck**

√4ᵗʰ **S15 Injury of blood vessels at neck level**
Code also any associated open wound (S11.-)

The appropriate 7th character is to be added to each code from category S15.
A   initial encounter
D   subsequent encounter
S   sequela

CC Excl: For CC codes in category S15, unless otherwise noted:
PDX collection 1157

√5ᵗʰ **S15.0 Injury of carotid artery of neck**
Injury of carotid artery (common) (external) (internal, extracranial portion)
Injury of carotid artery NOS
EXCLUDES 1 injury of internal carotid artery, intracranial portion (S06.8)

CC Excl: For CC codes in subcategory S15.0:
PDX collection 1167

√6ᵗʰ **S15.00 Unspecified injury of carotid artery**

√7ᵗʰ **S15.001** Unspecified injury of **right** carotid artery `CC`

√7ᵗʰ **S15.002** Unspecified injury of **left** carotid artery `CC`

√7ᵗʰ **S15.009** Unspecified injury of **unspecified** carotid artery `CC`

√6ᵗʰ **S15.01 Minor laceration of carotid artery**
Incomplete transection of carotid artery
Laceration of carotid artery NOS
Superficial laceration of carotid artery

√7ᵗʰ **S15.011** Minor laceration of **right** carotid artery `CC`

√7ᵗʰ **S15.012** Minor laceration of **left** carotid artery `CC`

√7ᵗʰ **S15.019** Minor laceration of **unspecified** carotid artery `CC`

√6ᵗʰ **S15.02 Major laceration of carotid artery**
Complete transection of carotid artery
Traumatic rupture of carotid artery

√7ᵗʰ **S15.021** Major laceration of **right** carotid artery `CC`

√7ᵗʰ **S15.022** Major laceration of **left** carotid artery `CC`

√7ᵗʰ **S15.029** Major laceration of **unspecified** carotid artery `CC`

√6ᵗʰ **S15.09 Other specified injury of carotid artery**

√7ᵗʰ **S15.091** Other specified injury of **right** carotid artery `CC`

√7ᵗʰ **S15.092** Other specified injury of **left** carotid artery `CC`

√7ᵗʰ **S15.099** Other specified injury of **unspecified** carotid artery `CC`

√5ᵗʰ **S15.1 Injury of vertebral artery**

√6ᵗʰ **S15.10 Unspecified injury of vertebral artery**

√7ᵗʰ **S15.101** Unspecified injury of **right** vertebral artery `CC`

√7ᵗʰ **S15.102** Unspecified injury of **left** vertebral artery `CC`

√7ᵗʰ **S15.109** Unspecified injury of **unspecified** vertebral artery `CC`

√6ᵗʰ **S15.11 Minor laceration of vertebral artery**
Incomplete transection of vertebral artery
Laceration of vertebral artery NOS
Superficial laceration of vertebral artery

√7ᵗʰ **S15.111** Minor laceration of **right** vertebral artery `CC`

√7ᵗʰ **S15.112** Minor laceration of **left** vertebral artery `CC`

√7ᵗʰ **S15.119** Minor laceration of **unspecified** vertebral artery `CC`

√6ᵗʰ **S15.12 Major laceration of vertebral artery**
Complete transection of vertebral artery
Traumatic rupture of vertebral artery

√7ᵗʰ **S15.121** Major laceration of **right** vertebral artery `CC`

√7ᵗʰ **S15.122** Major laceration of **left** vertebral artery `CC`

√7ᵗʰ **S15.129** Major laceration of **unspecified** vertebral artery `CC`

√6ᵗʰ **S15.19 Other specified injury of vertebral artery**

√7ᵗʰ **S15.191** Other specified injury of **right** vertebral artery `CC`

√7ᵗʰ **S15.192** Other specified injury of **left** vertebral artery `CC`

√7ᵗʰ **S15.199** Other specified injury of **unspecified** vertebral artery `CC`

√5ᵗʰ **S15.2 Injury of external jugular vein**

√6ᵗʰ **S15.20 Unspecified injury of external jugular vein**

√7ᵗʰ **S15.201** Unspecified injury of **right** external jugular vein `CC`

√7ᵗʰ **S15.202** Unspecified injury of **left** external jugular vein `CC`

√7ᵗʰ **S15.209** Unspecified injury of **unspecified** external jugular vein `CC`

√6ᵗʰ **S15.21 Minor laceration of external jugular vein**
Incomplete transection of external jugular vein
Laceration of external jugular vein NOS
Superficial laceration of external jugular vein

√7ᵗʰ **S15.211** Minor laceration of **right** external jugular vein `CC`

√7ᵗʰ **S15.212** Minor laceration of **left** external jugular vein `CC`

√7ᵗʰ **S15.219** Minor laceration of **unspecified** external jugular vein `CC`

√6ᵗʰ **S15.22 Major laceration of external jugular vein**
Complete transection of external jugular vein
Traumatic rupture of external jugular vein

√7ᵗʰ **S15.221** Major laceration of **right** external jugular vein `CC`

√7ᵗʰ **S15.222** Major laceration of **left** external jugular vein `CC`

√7ᵗʰ **S15.229** Major laceration of **unspecified** external jugular vein `CC`

√6ᵗʰ **S15.29 Other specified injury of external jugular vein**

√7ᵗʰ **S15.291** Other specified injury of **right** external jugular vein `CC`

√7ᵗʰ **S15.292** Other specified injury of **left** external jugular vein `CC`

√7ᵗʰ **S15.299** Other specified injury of **unspecified** external jugular vein `CC`

√5ᵗʰ **S15.3 Injury of internal jugular vein**

√6ᵗʰ **S15.30 Unspecified injury of internal jugular vein**

√7ᵗʰ **S15.301** Unspecified injury of **right** internal jugular vein `CC`

√7ᵗʰ **S15.302** Unspecified injury of **left** internal jugular vein `CC`

N Newborn: 0   P Pediatric: 0-17   M Maternity: 12-55   A Adult: 15-124   MCC Major Complication/Comorbidity   CC Complication/Comorbidity   SW Severe Wound Dx

964
ICD-10-CM 2019

☑7ᵗʰ **S15.3Ø9** **Unspecified injury of** unspecified internal jugular vein   `CC`

☑6ᵗʰ **S15.31** **Minor laceration of internal jugular vein**
Incomplete transection of internal jugular vein
Laceration of internal jugular vein NOS
Superficial laceration of internal jugular vein

  ☑7ᵗʰ **S15.311** **Minor laceration of** right **internal jugular vein**   `CC`

  ☑7ᵗʰ **S15.312** **Minor laceration of** left **internal jugular vein**   `CC`

  ☑7ᵗʰ **S15.319** **Minor laceration of** unspecified **internal jugular vein**   `CC`

☑6ᵗʰ **S15.32** **Major laceration of internal jugular vein**
Complete transection of internal jugular vein
Traumatic rupture of internal jugular vein

  ☑7ᵗʰ **S15.321** **Major laceration of** right **internal jugular vein**   `CC`

  ☑7ᵗʰ **S15.322** **Major laceration of** left **internal jugular vein**   `CC`

  ☑7ᵗʰ **S15.329** **Major laceration of** unspecified **internal jugular vein**   `CC`

☑6ᵗʰ **S15.39** **Other** specified injury of internal jugular vein

  ☑7ᵗʰ **S15.391** **Other specified injury of** right **internal jugular vein**   `CC`

  ☑7ᵗʰ **S15.392** **Other specified injury of** left **internal jugular vein**   `CC`

  ☑7ᵗʰ **S15.399** **Other specified injury of** unspecified **internal jugular vein**   `CC`

√x7ᵗʰ **S15.8** **Injury of other specified blood vessels at neck level**   `CC`

√x7ᵗʰ **S15.9** **Injury of unspecified blood vessel at neck level**   `CC`

☑4ᵗʰ **S16** **Injury of muscle, fascia and tendon at neck level**
Code also any associated open wound (S11.-)
EXCLUDES 2 *sprain of joint or ligament at neck level (S13.9)*

> The appropriate 7th character is to be added to each code from category S16.
> A   initial encounter
> D   subsequent encounter
> S   sequela

√x7ᵗʰ **S16.1** **Strain of muscle, fascia and tendon at neck level**

√x7ᵗʰ **S16.2** **Laceration of muscle, fascia and tendon at neck level**

√x7ᵗʰ **S16.8** **Other specified injury of muscle, fascia and tendon at neck level**

√x7ᵗʰ **S16.9** **Unspecified injury of muscle, fascia and tendon at neck level**

☑4ᵗʰ **S17** **Crushing injury of neck**
Use additional code for all associated injuries, such as:
injury of blood vessels (S15.-)
open wound of neck (S11.-)
spinal cord injury (S14.Ø, S14.1-)
vertebral fracture (S12.Ø- – S12.3-)

> The appropriate 7th character is to be added to each code from category S17.
> A   initial encounter
> D   subsequent encounter
> S   sequela

CC Excl: For CC codes in category S17: PDX collection 1156

√x7ᵗʰ **S17.Ø** **Crushing injury of larynx and trachea**   `CC` `H5`

√x7ᵗʰ **S17.8** **Crushing injury of other specified parts of neck**   `CC` `H5`

√x7ᵗʰ **S17.9** **Crushing injury of neck, part unspecified**   `CC` `H5`

☑4ᵗʰ **S19** **Other specified and unspecified injuries of neck**

> The appropriate 7th character is to be added to each code from category S19.
> A   initial encounter
> D   subsequent encounter
> S   sequela

√5ᵗʰ **S19.8** **Other specified injuries of neck**

 √x7ᵗʰ **S19.8Ø** **Other specified injuries of** unspecified **part of neck**

 √x7ᵗʰ **S19.81** **Other specified injuries of** larynx

 √x7ᵗʰ **S19.82** **Other specified injuries of** cervical trachea
   EXCLUDES 2 *other specified injury of thoracic trachea (S27.5-)*

 √x7ᵗʰ **S19.83** **Other specified injuries of** vocal cord

 √x7ᵗʰ **S19.84** **Other specified injuries of** thyroid gland

 √x7ᵗʰ **S19.85** **Other specified injuries of** pharynx and cervical esophagus

 √x7ᵗʰ **S19.89** **Other specified injuries of** other **specified part of neck**

√x7ᵗʰ **S19.9** **Unspecified injury of neck**

Injuries to the thorax (S2Ø-S29)

INCLUDES   injuries of breast
injuries of chest (wall)
injuries of interscapular area

EXCLUDES 2   *burns and corrosions (T2Ø-T32)*
effects of foreign body in bronchus (T17.5)
effects of foreign body in esophagus (T18.1)
effects of foreign body in lung (T17.8)
effects of foreign body in trachea (T17.4)
frostbite (T33-T34)
injuries of axilla
injuries of clavicle
injuries of scapular region
injuries of shoulder
insect bite or sting, venomous (T63.4)

☑4ᵗʰ **S2Ø** **Superficial injury of thorax**

> The appropriate 7th character is to be added to each code from category S2Ø.
> A   initial encounter
> D   subsequent encounter
> S   sequela

√5ᵗʰ **S2Ø.Ø** **Contusion of breast**

 √x7ᵗʰ **S2Ø.ØØ** **Contusion of breast,** unspecified **breast**

 √x7ᵗʰ **S2Ø.Ø1** **Contusion of** right **breast**

 √x7ᵗʰ **S2Ø.Ø2** **Contusion of** left **breast**

√5ᵗʰ **S2Ø.1** **Other and unspecified superficial injuries of breast**

 ☑6ᵗʰ **S2Ø.1Ø** **Unspecified superficial injuries of breast**

  ☑7ᵗʰ **S2Ø.1Ø1** **Unspecified superficial injuries of breast,** right **breast**

  ☑7ᵗʰ **S2Ø.1Ø2** **Unspecified superficial injuries of breast,** left **breast**

  ☑7ᵗʰ **S2Ø.1Ø9** **Unspecified superficial injuries of breast,** unspecified **breast**

 ☑6ᵗʰ **S2Ø.11** **Abrasion** of breast

  ☑7ᵗʰ **S2Ø.111** **Abrasion of breast,** right **breast**

  ☑7ᵗʰ **S2Ø.112** **Abrasion of breast,** left **breast**

  ☑7ᵗʰ **S2Ø.119** **Abrasion of breast,** unspecified **breast**

 ☑6ᵗʰ **S2Ø.12** **Blister** (nonthermal) of breast

  ☑7ᵗʰ **S2Ø.121** **Blister (nonthermal) of breast,** right **breast**

  ☑7ᵗʰ **S2Ø.122** **Blister (nonthermal) of breast,** left **breast**

  ☑7ᵗʰ **S2Ø.129** **Blister (nonthermal) of breast,** unspecified **breast**

 ☑6ᵗʰ **S2Ø.14** **External constriction** of part of breast

  ☑7ᵗʰ **S2Ø.141** **External constriction of part of breast,** right **breast**

  ☑7ᵗʰ **S2Ø.142** **External constriction of part of breast,** left **breast**

  ☑7ᵗʰ **S2Ø.149** **External constriction of part of breast,** unspecified **breast**

 ☑6ᵗʰ **S2Ø.15** **Superficial** foreign body **of breast**
   Splinter in the breast

  ☑7ᵗʰ **S2Ø.151** **Superficial foreign body of breast,** right **breast**

  ☑7ᵗʰ **S2Ø.152** **Superficial foreign body of breast,** left **breast**

  ☑7ᵗʰ **S2Ø.159** **Superficial foreign body of breast,** unspecified **breast**

 ☑6ᵗʰ **S2Ø.16** **Insect bite** (nonvenomous) of breast

  ☑7ᵗʰ **S2Ø.161** **Insect bite (nonvenomous) of breast,** right **breast**

  ☑7ᵗʰ **S2Ø.162** **Insect bite (nonvenomous) of breast,** left **breast**

  ☑7ᵗʰ **S2Ø.169** **Insect bite (nonvenomous) of breast,** unspecified **breast**

☑ Additional Character Required   √x7ᵗʰ Placeholder   Unacceptable PDx   Questionable PDx   Manifestation   `H1`-`H14` HAC   `HCC` CMS-HCC Dx   `HIV` HIV Dx

ICD-10-CM 2019   **965**

✓6ᵗʰ **S20.17** Other superficial **bite** of breast
     EXCLUDES 1   *open bite of breast (S21.05-)*

     ✓7ᵗʰ **S20.171** **Other superficial bite of breast, right breast**

     ✓7ᵗʰ **S20.172** **Other superficial bite of breast, left breast**

     ✓7ᵗʰ **S20.179** **Other superficial bite of breast, unspecified breast**

✓5ᵗʰ **S20.2** **Contusion of thorax**

   ✓x7ᵗʰ **S20.20** **Contusion of thorax, unspecified**

   ✓6ᵗʰ **S20.21** **Contusion of front wall of thorax**

     ✓7ᵗʰ **S20.211** **Contusion of right front wall of thorax**

     ✓7ᵗʰ **S20.212** **Contusion of left front wall of thorax**

     ✓7ᵗʰ **S20.219** **Contusion of unspecified front wall of thorax**

   ✓6ᵗʰ **S20.22** **Contusion of back wall of thorax**

     ✓7ᵗʰ **S20.221** **Contusion of right back wall of thorax**

     ✓7ᵗʰ **S20.222** **Contusion of left back wall of thorax**

     ✓7ᵗʰ **S20.229** **Contusion of unspecified back wall of thorax**

✓5ᵗʰ **S20.3** **Other and unspecified superficial injuries of front wall of thorax**

   ✓6ᵗʰ **S20.30** Unspecified superficial injuries of front wall of thorax

     ✓7ᵗʰ **S20.301** **Unspecified superficial injuries of right front wall of thorax**

     ✓7ᵗʰ **S20.302** **Unspecified superficial injuries of left front wall of thorax**

     ✓7ᵗʰ **S20.309** **Unspecified superficial injuries of unspecified front wall of thorax**

   ✓6ᵗʰ **S20.31** **Abrasion of front wall of thorax**

     ✓7ᵗʰ **S20.311** **Abrasion of right front wall of thorax**

     ✓7ᵗʰ **S20.312** **Abrasion of left front wall of thorax**

     ✓7ᵗʰ **S20.319** **Abrasion of unspecified front wall of thorax**

   ✓6ᵗʰ **S20.32** **Blister (nonthermal) of front wall of thorax**

     ✓7ᵗʰ **S20.321** **Blister (nonthermal) of right front wall of thorax**

     ✓7ᵗʰ **S20.322** **Blister (nonthermal) of left front wall of thorax**

     ✓7ᵗʰ **S20.329** **Blister (nonthermal) of unspecified front wall of thorax**

   ✓6ᵗʰ **S20.34** **External constriction of front wall of thorax**

     ✓7ᵗʰ **S20.341** **External constriction of right front wall of thorax**

     ✓7ᵗʰ **S20.342** **External constriction of left front wall of thorax**

     ✓7ᵗʰ **S20.349** **External constriction of unspecified front wall of thorax**

   ✓6ᵗʰ **S20.35** **Superficial foreign body of front wall of thorax**
     Splinter in front wall of thorax

     ✓7ᵗʰ **S20.351** **Superficial foreign body of right front wall of thorax**

     ✓7ᵗʰ **S20.352** **Superficial foreign body of left front wall of thorax**

     ✓7ᵗʰ **S20.359** **Superficial foreign body of unspecified front wall of thorax**

   ✓6ᵗʰ **S20.36** **Insect bite (nonvenomous) of front wall of thorax**

     ✓7ᵗʰ **S20.361** **Insect bite (nonvenomous) of right front wall of thorax**

     ✓7ᵗʰ **S20.362** **Insect bite (nonvenomous) of left front wall of thorax**

     ✓7ᵗʰ **S20.369** **Insect bite (nonvenomous) of unspecified front wall of thorax**

   ✓6ᵗʰ **S20.37** Other superficial **bite** of front wall of thorax
     EXCLUDES 1   *open bite of front wall of thorax (S21.14)*

     ✓7ᵗʰ **S20.371** **Other superficial bite of right front wall of thorax**

     ✓7ᵗʰ **S20.372** **Other superficial bite of left front wall of thorax**

     ✓7ᵗʰ **S20.379** **Other superficial bite of unspecified front wall of thorax**

✓5ᵗʰ **S20.4** **Other and unspecified superficial injuries of back wall of thorax**

   ✓6ᵗʰ **S20.40** Unspecified superficial injuries of back wall of thorax

     ✓7ᵗʰ **S20.401** **Unspecified superficial injuries of right back wall of thorax**

     ✓7ᵗʰ **S20.402** **Unspecified superficial injuries of left back wall of thorax**

     ✓7ᵗʰ **S20.409** **Unspecified superficial injuries of unspecified back wall of thorax**

   ✓6ᵗʰ **S20.41** **Abrasion of back wall of thorax**

     ✓7ᵗʰ **S20.411** **Abrasion of right back wall of thorax**

     ✓7ᵗʰ **S20.412** **Abrasion of left back wall of thorax**

     ✓7ᵗʰ **S20.419** **Abrasion of unspecified back wall of thorax**

   ✓6ᵗʰ **S20.42** **Blister (nonthermal) of back wall of thorax**

     ✓7ᵗʰ **S20.421** **Blister (nonthermal) of right back wall of thorax**

     ✓7ᵗʰ **S20.422** **Blister (nonthermal) of left back wall of thorax**

     ✓7ᵗʰ **S20.429** **Blister (nonthermal) of unspecified back wall of thorax**

   ✓6ᵗʰ **S20.44** **External constriction of back wall of thorax**

     ✓7ᵗʰ **S20.441** **External constriction of right back wall of thorax**

     ✓7ᵗʰ **S20.442** **External constriction of left back wall of thorax**

     ✓7ᵗʰ **S20.449** **External constriction of unspecified back wall of thorax**

   ✓6ᵗʰ **S20.45** **Superficial foreign body of back wall of thorax**
     Splinter of back wall of thorax

     ✓7ᵗʰ **S20.451** **Superficial foreign body of right back wall of thorax**

     ✓7ᵗʰ **S20.452** **Superficial foreign body of left back wall of thorax**

     ✓7ᵗʰ **S20.459** **Superficial foreign body of unspecified back wall of thorax**

   ✓6ᵗʰ **S20.46** **Insect bite (nonvenomous) of back wall of thorax**

     ✓7ᵗʰ **S20.461** **Insect bite (nonvenomous) of right back wall of thorax**

     ✓7ᵗʰ **S20.462** **Insect bite (nonvenomous) of left back wall of thorax**

     ✓7ᵗʰ **S20.469** **Insect bite (nonvenomous) of unspecified back wall of thorax**

   ✓6ᵗʰ **S20.47** Other superficial **bite** of back wall of thorax
     EXCLUDES 1   *open bite of back wall of thorax (S21.24)*

     ✓7ᵗʰ **S20.471** **Other superficial bite of right back wall of thorax**

     ✓7ᵗʰ **S20.472** **Other superficial bite of left back wall of thorax**

     ✓7ᵗʰ **S20.479** **Other superficial bite of unspecified back wall of thorax**

✓5ᵗʰ **S20.9** **Superficial injury of unspecified parts of thorax**
     EXCLUDES 1   *contusion of thorax NOS (S20.20)*

   ✓x7ᵗʰ **S20.90** **Unspecified superficial injury of unspecified parts of thorax**
     Superficial injury of thoracic wall NOS

   ✓x7ᵗʰ **S20.91** **Abrasion of unspecified parts of thorax**

   ✓x7ᵗʰ **S20.92** **Blister (nonthermal) of unspecified parts of thorax**

   ✓x7ᵗʰ **S20.94** **External constriction of unspecified parts of thorax**

   ✓x7ᵗʰ **S20.95** **Superficial foreign body of unspecified parts of thorax**
     Splinter in thorax NOS

   ✓x7ᵗʰ **S20.96** **Insect bite (nonvenomous) of unspecified parts of thorax**

   ✓x7ᵗʰ **S20.97** Other superficial **bite** of unspecified parts of thorax
     EXCLUDES 1   *open bite of thorax NOS (S21.95)*

N Newborn: 0   **P** Pediatric: 0-17   **M** Maternity: 12-55   **A** Adult: 15-124   **MCC** Major Complication/Comorbidity   **CC** Complication/Comorbidity   **SW** Severe Wound Dx

966   ICD-10-CM 2019

✓4ᵗʰ **S21**   **Open wound of thorax**

Code also any associated injury, such as:
injury of heart (S26.-)
injury of intrathoracic organs (S27.-)
rib fracture (S22.3-, S22.4-)
spinal cord injury (S24.0-, S24.1-)
traumatic hemopneumothorax (S27.3)
traumatic hemothorax (S27.1)
traumatic pneumothorax (S27.0)
wound infection

EXCLUDES 1   *traumatic amputation (partial) of thorax (S28.1)*

> The appropriate 7th character is to be added to each code from category S21.
> A   initial encounter
> D   subsequent encounter
> S   sequela

✓5ᵗʰ **S21.0**   **Open wound of breast**

   ✓6ᵗʰ **S21.00**   **Unspecified open wound of breast**

     ✓7ᵗʰ **S21.001**   **Unspecified open wound of right breast**

     ✓7ᵗʰ **S21.002**   **Unspecified open wound of left breast**

     ✓7ᵗʰ **S21.009**   **Unspecified open wound of unspecified breast**

   ✓6ᵗʰ **S21.01**   **Laceration without foreign body of breast**

     ✓7ᵗʰ **S21.011**   **Laceration without foreign body of right breast**

     ✓7ᵗʰ **S21.012**   **Laceration without foreign body of left breast**

     ✓7ᵗʰ **S21.019**   **Laceration without foreign body of unspecified breast**

   ✓6ᵗʰ **S21.02**   **Laceration with foreign body of breast**

     ✓7ᵗʰ **S21.021**   **Laceration with foreign body of right breast**

     ✓7ᵗʰ **S21.022**   **Laceration with foreign body of left breast**

     ✓7ᵗʰ **S21.029**   **Laceration with foreign body of unspecified breast**

   ✓6ᵗʰ **S21.03**   **Puncture wound without foreign body of breast**

     ✓7ᵗʰ **S21.031**   **Puncture wound without foreign body of right breast**

     ✓7ᵗʰ **S21.032**   **Puncture wound without foreign body of left breast**

     ✓7ᵗʰ **S21.039**   **Puncture wound without foreign body of unspecified breast**

   ✓6ᵗʰ **S21.04**   **Puncture wound with foreign body of breast**

     ✓7ᵗʰ **S21.041**   **Puncture wound with foreign body of right breast**

     ✓7ᵗʰ **S21.042**   **Puncture wound with foreign body of left breast**

     ✓7ᵗʰ **S21.049**   **Puncture wound with foreign body of unspecified breast**

   ✓6ᵗʰ **S21.05**   **Open bite of breast**
     Bite of breast NOS
     EXCLUDES 1   *superficial bite of breast (S20.17)*

     ✓7ᵗʰ **S21.051**   **Open bite of right breast**

     ✓7ᵗʰ **S21.052**   **Open bite of left breast**

     ✓7ᵗʰ **S21.059**   **Open bite of unspecified breast**

✓5ᵗʰ **S21.1**   **Open wound of front wall of thorax without penetration into thoracic cavity**
     Open wound of chest without penetration into thoracic cavity

> **CC Excl: For CC codes in subcategory S21.1:**
> PDX collection 1168

   ✓6ᵗʰ **S21.10**   **Unspecified open wound of front wall of thorax without penetration into thoracic cavity**

     ✓7ᵗʰ **S21.101**   **Unspecified open wound of right front wall of thorax without penetration into thoracic cavity** CC

     ✓7ᵗʰ **S21.102**   **Unspecified open wound of left front wall of thorax without penetration into thoracic cavity** CC

     ✓7ᵗʰ **S21.109**   **Unspecified open wound of unspecified front wall of thorax without penetration into thoracic cavity** CC

   ✓6ᵗʰ **S21.11**   **Laceration without foreign body of front wall of thorax without penetration into thoracic cavity**

     ✓7ᵗʰ **S21.111**   **Laceration without foreign body of right front wall of thorax without penetration into thoracic cavity** CC

     ✓7ᵗʰ **S21.112**   **Laceration without foreign body of left front wall of thorax without penetration into thoracic cavity** CC

     ✓7ᵗʰ **S21.119**   **Laceration without foreign body of unspecified front wall of thorax without penetration into thoracic cavity** CC

   ✓6ᵗʰ **S21.12**   **Laceration with foreign body of front wall of thorax without penetration into thoracic cavity**

     ✓7ᵗʰ **S21.121**   **Laceration with foreign body of right front wall of thorax without penetration into thoracic cavity** CC

     ✓7ᵗʰ **S21.122**   **Laceration with foreign body of left front wall of thorax without penetration into thoracic cavity** CC

     ✓7ᵗʰ **S21.129**   **Laceration with foreign body of unspecified front wall of thorax without penetration into thoracic cavity** CC

   ✓6ᵗʰ **S21.13**   **Puncture wound without foreign body of front wall of thorax without penetration into thoracic cavity**

     ✓7ᵗʰ **S21.131**   **Puncture wound without foreign body of right front wall of thorax without penetration into thoracic cavity** CC

     ✓7ᵗʰ **S21.132**   **Puncture wound without foreign body of left front wall of thorax without penetration into thoracic cavity** CC

     ✓7ᵗʰ **S21.139**   **Puncture wound without foreign body of unspecified front wall of thorax without penetration into thoracic cavity** CC

   ✓6ᵗʰ **S21.14**   **Puncture wound with foreign body of front wall of thorax without penetration into thoracic cavity**

     ✓7ᵗʰ **S21.141**   **Puncture wound with foreign body of right front wall of thorax without penetration into thoracic cavity** CC

     ✓7ᵗʰ **S21.142**   **Puncture wound with foreign body of left front wall of thorax without penetration into thoracic cavity** CC

     ✓7ᵗʰ **S21.149**   **Puncture wound with foreign body of unspecified front wall of thorax without penetration into thoracic cavity** CC

   ✓6ᵗʰ **S21.15**   **Open bite of front wall of thorax without penetration into thoracic cavity**
     Bite of front wall of thorax NOS
     EXCLUDES 1   *superficial bite of front wall of thorax (S20.37)*

     ✓7ᵗʰ **S21.151**   **Open bite of right front wall of thorax without penetration into thoracic cavity** CC

     ✓7ᵗʰ **S21.152**   **Open bite of left front wall of thorax without penetration into thoracic cavity** CC

     ✓7ᵗʰ **S21.159**   **Open bite of unspecified front wall of thorax without penetration into thoracic cavity** CC

✓5ᵗʰ **S21.2**   **Open wound of back wall of thorax without penetration into thoracic cavity**

   ✓6ᵗʰ **S21.20**   **Unspecified open wound of back wall of thorax without penetration into thoracic cavity**

     ✓7ᵗʰ **S21.201**   **Unspecified open wound of right back wall of thorax without penetration into thoracic cavity**

     ✓7ᵗʰ **S21.202**   **Unspecified open wound of left back wall of thorax without penetration into thoracic cavity**

     ✓7ᵗʰ **S21.209**   **Unspecified open wound of unspecified back wall of thorax without penetration into thoracic cavity**

   ✓6ᵗʰ **S21.21**   **Laceration without foreign body of back wall of thorax without penetration into thoracic cavity**

     ✓7ᵗʰ **S21.211**   **Laceration without foreign body of right back wall of thorax without penetration into thoracic cavity**

     ✓7ᵗʰ **S21.212**   **Laceration without foreign body of left back wall of thorax without penetration into thoracic cavity**

Chapter 19. Injury, Poisoning and Certain Other Consequences of External Causes

S21.219–S21.422

☑7ᵗʰ **S21.219** **Laceration without foreign body of** unspecified **back wall of thorax without penetration into thoracic cavity**

☑6ᵗʰ **S21.22** Laceration with foreign body **of back wall of thorax without penetration into thoracic cavity**

☑7ᵗʰ **S21.221** **Laceration with foreign body of** right **back wall of thorax without penetration into thoracic cavity**

☑7ᵗʰ **S21.222** **Laceration with foreign body of** left **back wall of thorax without penetration into thoracic cavity**

☑7ᵗʰ **S21.229** **Laceration with foreign body of** unspecified **back wall of thorax without penetration into thoracic cavity**

☑6ᵗʰ **S21.23** Puncture wound without foreign body **of back wall of thorax without penetration into thoracic cavity**

☑7ᵗʰ **S21.231** **Puncture wound without foreign body of** right **back wall of thorax without penetration into thoracic cavity**

☑7ᵗʰ **S21.232** **Puncture wound without foreign body of** left **back wall of thorax without penetration into thoracic cavity**

☑7ᵗʰ **S21.239** **Puncture wound without foreign body of** unspecified **back wall of thorax without penetration into thoracic cavity**

☑6ᵗʰ **S21.24** Puncture wound with foreign body **of back wall of thorax without penetration into thoracic cavity**

☑7ᵗʰ **S21.241** **Puncture wound with foreign body of** right **back wall of thorax without penetration into thoracic cavity**

☑7ᵗʰ **S21.242** **Puncture wound with foreign body of** left **back wall of thorax without penetration into thoracic cavity**

☑7ᵗʰ **S21.249** **Puncture wound with foreign body of** unspecified **back wall of thorax without penetration into thoracic cavity**

☑6ᵗʰ **S21.25** Open bite **of back wall of thorax without penetration into thoracic cavity**
Bite of back wall of thorax NOS
EXCLUDES 1 *superficial bite of back wall of thorax (S20.47)*

☑7ᵗʰ **S21.251** **Open bite of** right **back wall of thorax without penetration into thoracic cavity**

☑7ᵗʰ **S21.252** **Open bite of** left **back wall of thorax without penetration into thoracic cavity**

☑7ᵗʰ **S21.259** **Open bite of** unspecified **back wall of thorax without penetration into thoracic cavity**

☑5ᵗʰ **S21.3** **Open wound of** front wall of thorax with penetration **into thoracic cavity**
Open wound of chest with penetration into thoracic cavity

CC Excl: For MCC codes in subcategory S21.3, unless otherwise noted: PDX collection 1169

☑6ᵗʰ **S21.30** Unspecified **open wound of front wall of thorax with penetration into thoracic cavity**

☑7ᵗʰ **S21.301** **Unspecified open wound of** right **front wall of thorax with penetration into thoracic cavity** MCC

☑7ᵗʰ **S21.302** **Unspecified open wound of** left **front wall of thorax with penetration into thoracic cavity** MCC

☑7ᵗʰ **S21.309** **Unspecified open wound of** unspecified **front wall of thorax with penetration into thoracic cavity** MCC
CC Excl: PDX collection 1170

☑6ᵗʰ **S21.31** Laceration without foreign body **of front wall of thorax with penetration into thoracic cavity**

☑7ᵗʰ **S21.311** **Laceration without foreign body of** right **front wall of thorax with penetration into thoracic cavity** MCC

☑7ᵗʰ **S21.312** **Laceration without foreign body of** left **front wall of thorax with penetration into thoracic cavity** MCC

☑7ᵗʰ **S21.319** **Laceration without foreign body of** unspecified **front wall of thorax with penetration into thoracic cavity** MCC

☑6ᵗʰ **S21.32** Laceration with foreign body **of front wall of thorax with penetration into thoracic cavity**

☑7ᵗʰ **S21.321** **Laceration with foreign body of** right **front wall of thorax with penetration into thoracic cavity** MCC

☑7ᵗʰ **S21.322** **Laceration with foreign body of** left **front wall of thorax with penetration into thoracic cavity** MCC

☑7ᵗʰ **S21.329** **Laceration with foreign body of** unspecified **front wall of thorax with penetration into thoracic cavity** MCC

☑6ᵗʰ **S21.33** Puncture wound without foreign body **of front wall of thorax with penetration into thoracic cavity**

☑7ᵗʰ **S21.331** **Puncture wound without foreign body of** right **front wall of thorax with penetration into thoracic cavity** MCC

☑7ᵗʰ **S21.332** **Puncture wound without foreign body of** left **front wall of thorax with penetration into thoracic cavity** MCC

☑7ᵗʰ **S21.339** **Puncture wound without foreign body of** unspecified **front wall of thorax with penetration into thoracic cavity** MCC

☑6ᵗʰ **S21.34** Puncture wound with foreign body **of front wall of thorax with penetration into thoracic cavity**

☑7ᵗʰ **S21.341** **Puncture wound with foreign body of** right **front wall of thorax with penetration into thoracic cavity** MCC

☑7ᵗʰ **S21.342** **Puncture wound with foreign body of** left **front wall of thorax with penetration into thoracic cavity** MCC

☑7ᵗʰ **S21.349** **Puncture wound with foreign body of** unspecified **front wall of thorax with penetration into thoracic cavity** MCC

☑6ᵗʰ **S21.35** Open bite **of front wall of thorax with penetration into thoracic cavity**
EXCLUDES 1 *superficial bite of front wall of thorax (S20.37)*

☑7ᵗʰ **S21.351** **Open bite of** right **front wall of thorax with penetration into thoracic cavity** MCC

☑7ᵗʰ **S21.352** **Open bite of** left **front wall of thorax with penetration into thoracic cavity** MCC

☑7ᵗʰ **S21.359** **Open bite of** unspecified **front wall of thorax with penetration into thoracic cavity** MCC

☑5ᵗʰ **S21.4** **Open wound of** back wall of thorax with penetration **into thoracic cavity**

CC Excl: For MCC codes in subcategory S21.4: PDX collection 1169

☑6ᵗʰ **S21.40** Unspecified **open wound of back wall of thorax with penetration into thoracic cavity**

☑7ᵗʰ **S21.401** **Unspecified open wound of** right **back wall of thorax with penetration into thoracic cavity** MCC

☑7ᵗʰ **S21.402** **Unspecified open wound of** left **back wall of thorax with penetration into thoracic cavity** MCC

☑7ᵗʰ **S21.409** **Unspecified open wound of** unspecified **back wall of thorax with penetration into thoracic cavity** MCC

☑6ᵗʰ **S21.41** Laceration without foreign body **of back wall of thorax with penetration into thoracic cavity**

☑7ᵗʰ **S21.411** **Laceration without foreign body of** right **back wall of thorax with penetration into thoracic cavity** MCC

☑7ᵗʰ **S21.412** **Laceration without foreign body of** left **back wall of thorax with penetration into thoracic cavity** MCC

☑7ᵗʰ **S21.419** **Laceration without foreign body of** unspecified **back wall of thorax with penetration into thoracic cavity** MCC

☑6ᵗʰ **S21.42** Laceration with foreign body **of back wall of thorax with penetration into thoracic cavity**

☑7ᵗʰ **S21.421** **Laceration with foreign body of** right **back wall of thorax with penetration into thoracic cavity** MCC

☑7ᵗʰ **S21.422** **Laceration with foreign body of** left **back wall of thorax with penetration into thoracic cavity** MCC

√7ᵗʰ **S21.429** **Laceration with foreign body of** unspecified **back wall of thorax with penetration into thoracic cavity** `MCC`

√6ᵗʰ **S21.43** Puncture wound without foreign body **of back wall of thorax with penetration into thoracic cavity**

√7ᵗʰ **S21.431** **Puncture wound without foreign body of** right **back wall of thorax with penetration into thoracic cavity** `MCC`

√7ᵗʰ **S21.432** **Puncture wound without foreign body of** left **back wall of thorax with penetration into thoracic cavity** `MCC`

√7ᵗʰ **S21.439** **Puncture wound without foreign body of** unspecified **back wall of thorax with penetration into thoracic cavity** `MCC`

√6ᵗʰ **S21.44** Puncture wound with foreign body **of back wall of thorax with penetration into thoracic cavity**

√7ᵗʰ **S21.441** **Puncture wound with foreign body of** right **back wall of thorax with penetration into thoracic cavity** `MCC`

√7ᵗʰ **S21.442** **Puncture wound with foreign body of** left **back wall of thorax with penetration into thoracic cavity** `MCC`

√7ᵗʰ **S21.449** **Puncture wound with foreign body of** unspecified **back wall of thorax with penetration into thoracic cavity** `MCC`

√6ᵗʰ **S21.45** Open bite **of back wall of thorax with penetration into thoracic cavity**
Bite of back wall of thorax NOS
EXCLUDES 1 *superficial bite of back wall of thorax (S20.47)*

√7ᵗʰ **S21.451** **Open bite of** right **back wall of thorax with penetration into thoracic cavity** `MCC`

√7ᵗʰ **S21.452** **Open bite of** left **back wall of thorax with penetration into thoracic cavity** `MCC`

√7ᵗʰ **S21.459** **Open bite of** unspecified **back wall of thorax with penetration into thoracic cavity** `MCC`

√5ᵗʰ **S21.9** **Open wound of unspecified part of thorax**
Open wound of thoracic wall NOS

CC Excl: For CC codes in subcategory S21.9:
PDX collection 1168

√x 7ᵗʰ **S21.90** Unspecified **open wound of unspecified part of thorax** `CC`

√x 7ᵗʰ **S21.91** Laceration without foreign body **of unspecified part of thorax** `CC`

√x 7ᵗʰ **S21.92** Laceration with foreign body **of unspecified part of thorax** `CC`

√x 7ᵗʰ **S21.93** Puncture wound without foreign body **of unspecified part of thorax** `CC`

√x 7ᵗʰ **S21.94** Puncture wound with foreign body **of unspecified part of thorax** `CC`

√x 7ᵗʰ **S21.95** Open bite **of unspecified part of thorax** `CC`
EXCLUDES 1 *superficial bite of thorax (S20.97)*

√4ᵗʰ **S22** **Fracture of rib(s), sternum and thoracic spine**
NOTE A fracture not indicated as nondisplaced or displaced should be coded to displaced.
A fracture not indicated as open or closed should be coded to closed.
INCLUDES fracture of thoracic neural arch
fracture of thoracic spinous process
fracture of thoracic transverse process
fracture of thoracic vertebra
fracture of thoracic vertebral arch
Code first any associated:
injury of intrathoracic organ (S27.-)
spinal cord injury (S24.0-, S24.1-)
EXCLUDES 1 *transection of thorax (S28.1)*
EXCLUDES 2 *fracture of clavicle (S42.0-)*
fracture of scapula (S42.1-)
AHA: 2018, 2Q, 12; 2015, 3Q, 37-39

The appropriate 7th character is to be added to each code from category S22.
A   initial encounter for closed fracture
B   initial encounter for open fracture
D   subsequent encounter for fracture with routine healing
G   subsequent encounter for fracture with delayed healing
K   subsequent encounter for fracture with nonunion
S   sequela

√5ᵗʰ **S22.0** **Fracture of** thoracic vertebra

CC Excl: For codes in subcategory S22.0:
CC with 7th character A or MCC with 7th character B:
PDX collection 1171
CC with 7th character K: PDX collection 897

√6ᵗʰ **S22.00** **Fracture of** unspecified **thoracic vertebra**
2,3,6 √7ᵗʰ **S22.000** Wedge compression **fracture of unspecified thoracic vertebra** `MCC` `CC` `H5` `HCC`
2,3,6 √7ᵗʰ **S22.001** Stable burst **fracture of unspecified thoracic vertebra** `MCC` `CC` `H5` `HCC`
2,3,6 √7ᵗʰ **S22.002** Unstable burst **fracture of unspecified thoracic vertebra** `MCC` `CC` `H5` `HCC`
2,3,6 √7ᵗʰ **S22.008** Other **fracture of unspecified thoracic vertebra** `MCC` `CC` `H5` `HCC`
2,3,6 √7ᵗʰ **S22.009** Unspecified **fracture of unspecified thoracic vertebra** `MCC` `CC` `H5` `HCC`

√6ᵗʰ **S22.01** **Fracture of** first **thoracic vertebra**
2,3,6 √7ᵗʰ **S22.010** Wedge compression **fracture of first thoracic vertebra** `MCC` `CC` `H5` `HCC`
2,3,6 √7ᵗʰ **S22.011** Stable burst **fracture of first thoracic vertebra** `MCC` `CC` `H5` `HCC`
2,3,6 √7ᵗʰ **S22.012** Unstable burst **fracture of first thoracic vertebra** `MCC` `CC` `H5` `HCC`
2,3,6 √7ᵗʰ **S22.018** Other **fracture of first thoracic vertebra** `MCC` `CC` `H5` `HCC`
2,3,6 √7ᵗʰ **S22.019** Unspecified **fracture of first thoracic vertebra** `MCC` `CC` `H5` `HCC`

√6ᵗʰ **S22.02** **Fracture of** second **thoracic vertebra**
2,3,6 √7ᵗʰ **S22.020** Wedge compression **fracture of second thoracic vertebra** `MCC` `CC` `H5` `HCC`
2,3,6 √7ᵗʰ **S22.021** Stable burst **fracture of second thoracic vertebra** `MCC` `CC` `H5` `HCC`
2,3,6 √7ᵗʰ **S22.022** Unstable burst **fracture of second thoracic vertebra** `MCC` `CC` `H5` `HCC`
2,3,6 √7ᵗʰ **S22.028** Other **fracture of second thoracic vertebra** `MCC` `CC` `H5` `HCC`
2,3,6 √7ᵗʰ **S22.029** Unspecified **fracture of second thoracic vertebra** `MCC` `CC` `H5` `HCC`

√6ᵗʰ **S22.03** **Fracture of** third **thoracic vertebra**
2,3,6 √7ᵗʰ **S22.030** Wedge compression **fracture of third thoracic vertebra** `MCC` `CC` `H5` `HCC`
2,3,6 √7ᵗʰ **S22.031** Stable burst **fracture of third thoracic vertebra** `MCC` `CC` `H5` `HCC`
2,3,6 √7ᵗʰ **S22.032** Unstable burst **fracture of third thoracic vertebra** `MCC` `CC` `H5` `HCC`
2,3,6 √7ᵗʰ **S22.038** Other **fracture of third thoracic vertebra** `MCC` `CC` `H5` `HCC`
2,3,6 √7ᵗʰ **S22.039** Unspecified **fracture of third thoracic vertebra** `MCC` `CC` `H5` `HCC`

√6ᵗʰ **S22.04** **Fracture of** fourth **thoracic vertebra**
2,3,6 √7ᵗʰ **S22.040** Wedge compression **fracture of fourth thoracic vertebra** `MCC` `CC` `H5` `HCC`
2,3,6 √7ᵗʰ **S22.041** Stable burst **fracture of fourth thoracic vertebra** `MCC` `CC` `H5` `HCC`
2,3,6 √7ᵗʰ **S22.042** Unstable burst **fracture of fourth thoracic vertebra** `MCC` `CC` `H5` `HCC`
2,3,6 √7ᵗʰ **S22.048** Other **fracture of fourth thoracic vertebra** `MCC` `CC` `H5` `HCC`
2,3,6 √7ᵗʰ **S22.049** Unspecified **fracture of fourth thoracic vertebra** `MCC` `CC` `H5` `HCC`

√6ᵗʰ **S22.05** **Fracture of** T5-T6 **vertebra**
2,3,6 √7ᵗʰ **S22.050** Wedge compression **fracture of T5-T6 vertebra** `MCC` `CC` `H5` `HCC`
2,3,6 √7ᵗʰ **S22.051** Stable burst **fracture of T5-T6 vertebra** `MCC` `CC` `H5` `HCC`
2,3,6 √7ᵗʰ **S22.052** Unstable burst **fracture of T5-T6 vertebra** `MCC` `CC` `H5` `HCC`
2,3,6 √7ᵗʰ **S22.058** Other **fracture of T5-T6 vertebra** `MCC` `CC` `H5` `HCC`
2,3,6 √7ᵗʰ **S22.059** Unspecified **fracture of T5-T6 vertebra** `MCC` `CC` `H5` `HCC`

✓6ᵗʰ **S22.06** **Fracture of** T7-T8 **vertebra**

2,3,6 ✓7ᵗʰ **S22.060** **Wedge compression fracture of T7-T8 vertebra** `MCC` `CC` `H5` `HCC`

2,3,6 ✓7ᵗʰ **S22.061** **Stable burst fracture of T7-T8 vertebra** `MCC` `CC` `H5` `HCC`

2,3,6 ✓7ᵗʰ **S22.062** **Unstable burst fracture of T7-T8 vertebra** `MCC` `CC` `H5` `HCC`

2,3,6 ✓7ᵗʰ **S22.068** **Other fracture of T7-T8 thoracic vertebra** `MCC` `CC` `H5` `HCC`

2,3,6 ✓7ᵗʰ **S22.069** **Unspecified fracture of T7-T8 vertebra** `MCC` `CC` `H5` `HCC`

✓6ᵗʰ **S22.07** **Fracture of T9-T10 vertebra**

2,3,6 ✓7ᵗʰ **S22.070** **Wedge compression fracture of T9-T10 vertebra** `MCC` `CC` `H5` `HCC`

2,3,6 ✓7ᵗʰ **S22.071** **Stable burst fracture of T9-T10 vertebra** `MCC` `CC` `H5` `HCC`

2,3,6 ✓7ᵗʰ **S22.072** **Unstable burst fracture of T9-T10 vertebra** `MCC` `CC` `H5` `HCC`

2,3,6 ✓7ᵗʰ **S22.078** **Other fracture of T9-T10 vertebra** `MCC` `CC` `H5` `HCC`

2,3,6 ✓7ᵗʰ **S22.079** **Unspecified fracture of T9-T10 vertebra** `MCC` `CC` `H5` `HCC`

✓6ᵗʰ **S22.08** **Fracture of T11-T12 vertebra**

2,3,6 ✓7ᵗʰ **S22.080** **Wedge compression fracture of T11-T12 vertebra** `MCC` `CC` `H5` `HCC`

2,3,6 ✓7ᵗʰ **S22.081** **Stable burst fracture of T11-T12 vertebra** `MCC` `CC` `H5` `HCC`

2,3,6 ✓7ᵗʰ **S22.082** **Unstable burst fracture of T11-T12 vertebra** `MCC` `CC` `H5` `HCC`

2,3,6 ✓7ᵗʰ **S22.088** **Other fracture of T11-T12 vertebra** `MCC` `CC` `H5` `HCC`

2,3,6 ✓7ᵗʰ **S22.089** **Unspecified fracture of T11-T12 vertebra** `MCC` `CC` `H5` `HCC`

✓5ᵗʰ **S22.2** **Fracture of** sternum

DEF: Break in flat bone (breast bone) in the anterior thorax caused by blunt trauma to the anterior chest.

CC Excl: For codes in subcategory S22.2:
CC with 7th character A or MCC with 7th character B:
PDX collection 1172
CC with 7th character K: PDX collection 897

2,3 ✓7ᵗʰ **S22.20** **Unspecified fracture of sternum** `MCC` `CC` `H5`

2,3 ✓7ᵗʰ **S22.21** **Fracture of** manubrium `MCC` `CC` `H5`

2,3 ✓7ᵗʰ **S22.22** **Fracture of** body of sternum `MCC` `CC` `H5`

2,3 ✓7ᵗʰ **S22.23** **Sternal** manubrial dissociation `MCC` `CC` `H5`

2,3 ✓7ᵗʰ **S22.24** **Fracture of** xiphoid process `MCC` `CC` `H5`

✓5ᵗʰ **S22.3** **Fracture of** one rib

CC Excl: For codes in subcategory S22.3:
CC with 7th character A: PDX collection 1173
MCC with 7th character B: PDX collection 1174
CC with 7th character K: PDX collection 897

2,3 ✓7ᵗʰ **S22.31** **Fracture of one rib,** right **side** `MCC` `CC` `H5`

2,3 ✓7ᵗʰ **S22.32** **Fracture of one rib,** left **side** `MCC` `CC` `H5`

2,3 ✓7ᵗʰ **S22.39** **Fracture of one rib,** unspecified **side** `MCC` `CC` `H5`

✓5ᵗʰ **S22.4** **Multiple fractures of ribs**

Fractures of two or more ribs

EXCLUDES 1 flail chest (S22.5-)

CC Excl: For codes in subcategory S22.4, unless otherwise noted: CC with 7th character A or MCC with 7th character B: PDX collection 1174
CC with 7th character K: PDX collection 897

2,3 ✓7ᵗʰ **S22.41** **Multiple fractures of ribs,** right **side** `MCC` `CC` `H5`

2,3 ✓7ᵗʰ **S22.42** **Multiple fractures of ribs,** left **side** `MCC` `CC` `H5`

2,3 ✓7ᵗʰ **S22.43** **Multiple fractures of ribs,** bilateral `MCC` `CC` `H5`

2,3 ✓7ᵗʰ **S22.49** **Multiple fractures of ribs,** unspecified **side** `MCC` `CC` `H5`

CC Excl: CC with 7th character A: PDX collection 1174
MCC with 7th character B: No Excl
CC with 7th character K: PDX collection 897

4 ✓7ᵗʰ **S22.5** **Flail chest** `MCC` `CC` `H5`

CC Excl: MCC with 7th character A or B: PDX collection 1175
CC with 7th character K: PDX collection 897

2,3 ✓7ᵗʰ **S22.9** **Fracture of bony thorax, part unspecified** `MCC` `CC` `H5`

CC Excl: CC with 7th character A or
MCC with 7th character B: PDX collection 1176
CC with 7th character K: PDX collection 897

✓4ᵗʰ **S23** **Dislocation and sprain of joints and ligaments of thorax**

INCLUDES   avulsion of joint or ligament of thorax
laceration of cartilage, joint or ligament of thorax
sprain of cartilage, joint or ligament of thorax
traumatic hemarthrosis of joint or ligament of thorax
traumatic rupture of joint or ligament of thorax
traumatic subluxation of joint or ligament of thorax
traumatic tear of joint or ligament of thorax

Code also any associated open wound

EXCLUDES 2   dislocation, sprain of sternoclavicular joint (S43.2, S43.6)
strain of muscle or tendon of thorax (S29.01-)

The appropriate 7th character is to be added to each code from category S23.
A   initial encounter
D   subsequent encounter
S   sequela

✓x7ᵗʰ **S23.0** **Traumatic rupture of thoracic intervertebral disc**

EXCLUDES 1   rupture or displacement (nontraumatic) of thoracic intervertebral disc NOS (M51- with fifth character 4)

✓5ᵗʰ **S23.1** **Subluxation and dislocation of thoracic vertebra**

Code also any associated
open wound of thorax (S21.-)
spinal cord injury (S24.0-, S24.1-)

EXCLUDES 2   fracture of thoracic vertebrae (S22.0-)

✓6ᵗʰ **S23.10** **Subluxation and dislocation of** unspecified **thoracic vertebra**

✓7ᵗʰ **S23.100** **Subluxation** of unspecified thoracic vertebra

✓7ᵗʰ **S23.101** **Dislocation** of unspecified thoracic vertebra

✓6ᵗʰ **S23.11** **Subluxation and dislocation of** T1/T2 **thoracic vertebra**

✓7ᵗʰ **S23.110** **Subluxation** of T1/T2 thoracic vertebra

✓7ᵗʰ **S23.111** **Dislocation** of T1/T2 thoracic vertebra

✓6ᵗʰ **S23.12** **Subluxation and dislocation of** T2/T3-T3/T4 **thoracic vertebra**

✓7ᵗʰ **S23.120** **Subluxation** of T2/T3 thoracic vertebra

✓7ᵗʰ **S23.121** **Dislocation** of T2/T3 thoracic vertebra

✓7ᵗʰ **S23.122** **Subluxation** of T3/T4 thoracic vertebra

✓7ᵗʰ **S23.123** **Dislocation** of T3/T4 thoracic vertebra

✓6ᵗʰ **S23.13** **Subluxation and dislocation of** T4/T5-T5/T6 **thoracic vertebra**

✓7ᵗʰ **S23.130** **Subluxation** of T4/T5 thoracic vertebra

✓7ᵗʰ **S23.131** **Dislocation** of T4/T5 thoracic vertebra

✓7ᵗʰ **S23.132** **Subluxation** of T5/T6 thoracic vertebra

✓7ᵗʰ **S23.133** **Dislocation** of T5/T6 thoracic vertebra

✓6ᵗʰ **S23.14** **Subluxation and dislocation of** T6/T7-T7/T8 **thoracic vertebra**

✓7ᵗʰ **S23.140** **Subluxation** of T6/T7 thoracic vertebra

✓7ᵗʰ **S23.141** **Dislocation** of T6/T7 thoracic vertebra

✓7ᵗʰ **S23.142** **Subluxation** of T7/T8 thoracic vertebra

✓7ᵗʰ **S23.143** **Dislocation** of T7/T8 thoracic vertebra

✓6ᵗʰ **S23.15** **Subluxation and dislocation of** T8/T9-T9/T10 **thoracic vertebra**

✓7ᵗʰ **S23.150** **Subluxation** of T8/T9 thoracic vertebra

✓7ᵗʰ **S23.151** **Dislocation** of T8/T9 thoracic vertebra

✓7ᵗʰ **S23.152** **Subluxation** of T9/T10 thoracic vertebra

✓7ᵗʰ **S23.153** **Dislocation** of T9/T10 thoracic vertebra

✓6ᵗʰ **S23.16** **Subluxation and dislocation of** T10/T11-T11/T12 **thoracic vertebra**

✓7ᵗʰ **S23.160** **Subluxation** of T10/T11 thoracic vertebra

✓7ᵗʰ **S23.161** **Dislocation** of T10/T11 thoracic vertebra

✓7ᵗʰ **S23.162** **Subluxation** of T11/T12 thoracic vertebra

✓7ᵗʰ **S23.163** **Dislocation** of T11/T12 thoracic vertebra

✓6ᵗʰ **S23.17** **Subluxation and dislocation of** T12/L1 **thoracic vertebra**

✓7ᵗʰ **S23.170** **Subluxation** of T12/L1 thoracic vertebra

✓7ᵗʰ **S23.171** **Dislocation** of T12/L1 thoracic vertebra

✓5ᵗʰ **S23.2** **Dislocation of other and unspecified parts of thorax**

✓x7ᵗʰ **S23.20** **Dislocation of unspecified part of thorax**

✓x7ᵗʰ **S23.29** **Dislocation of other parts of thorax**

N Newborn: 0   P Pediatric: 0-17   M Maternity: 12-55   A Adult: 15-124   MCC Major Complication/Comorbidity   CC Complication/Comorbidity   SW Severe Wound Dx

970   ICD-10-CM 2019

√x7ᵗʰ **S23.3 Sprain of ligaments of thoracic spine**

√5ᵗʰ **S23.4 Sprain of ribs and sternum**

     √x7ᵗʰ **S23.41 Sprain of ribs**

     √6ᵗʰ **S23.42 Sprain of sternum**

         √7ᵗʰ **S23.420 Sprain of sternoclavicular (joint) (ligament)**

         √7ᵗʰ **S23.421 Sprain of chondrosternal joint**

         √7ᵗʰ **S23.428 Other sprain of sternum**

         √7ᵗʰ **S23.429 Unspecified sprain of sternum**

√x7ᵗʰ **S23.8 Sprain of other specified parts of thorax**

√x7ᵗʰ **S23.9 Sprain of unspecified parts of thorax**

√4ᵗʰ **S24 Injury of nerves and spinal cord at thorax level**

     NOTE   Code to highest level of thoracic spinal cord injury. Injuries to the spinal cord (S24.0 and S24.1) refer to the cord level and not bone level injury, and can affect nerve roots at and below the level given.

     Code also any associated:
       fracture of thoracic vertebra (S22.0-)
       open wound of thorax (S21.-)
       transient paralysis (R29.5)
     EXCLUDES 2   *injury of brachial plexus (S14.3)*

> The appropriate 7th character is to be added to each code from category S24.
> A   initial encounter
> D   subsequent encounter
> S   sequela

> **CC Excl: For MCC codes in category S24:** PDX collection 1177

√x7ᵗʰ **S24.0 Concussion and edema of thoracic spinal cord**   MCC HCC

√5ᵗʰ **S24.1 Other and unspecified injuries of thoracic spinal cord**

     √6ᵗʰ **S24.10 Unspecified injury of thoracic spinal cord**

         √7ᵗʰ **S24.101 Unspecified injury at T1 level of thoracic spinal cord**   MCC H5 HCC

         √7ᵗʰ **S24.102 Unspecified injury at T2-T6 level of thoracic spinal cord**   MCC H5 HCC

         √7ᵗʰ **S24.103 Unspecified injury at T7-T10 level of thoracic spinal cord**   MCC H5 HCC

         √7ᵗʰ **S24.104 Unspecified injury at T11-T12 level thoracic spinal cord**   MCC H5 HCC

         √7ᵗʰ **S24.109 Unspecified injury at unspecified level of thoracic spinal cord**   HCC
            Injury of thoracic spinal cord NOS

     √6ᵗʰ **S24.11 Complete lesion of thoracic spinal cord**

         √7ᵗʰ **S24.111 Complete lesion at T1 level of thoracic spinal cord**   MCC H5 HCC

         √7ᵗʰ **S24.112 Complete lesion at T2-T6 level of thoracic spinal cord**   MCC H5 HCC

         √7ᵗʰ **S24.113 Complete lesion at T7-T10 level of thoracic spinal cord**   MCC H5 HCC

         √7ᵗʰ **S24.114 Complete lesion at T11-T12 level of thoracic spinal cord**   MCC H5 HCC

         √7ᵗʰ **S24.119 Complete lesion at unspecified level of thoracic spinal cord**   HCC

     √6ᵗʰ **S24.13 Anterior cord syndrome of thoracic spinal cord**

         √7ᵗʰ **S24.131 Anterior cord syndrome at T1 level of thoracic spinal cord**   MCC H5 HCC

         √7ᵗʰ **S24.132 Anterior cord syndrome at T2-T6 level of thoracic spinal cord**   MCC H5 HCC

         √7ᵗʰ **S24.133 Anterior cord syndrome at T7-T10 level of thoracic spinal cord**   MCC H5 HCC

         √7ᵗʰ **S24.134 Anterior cord syndrome at T11-T12 level of thoracic spinal cord**   MCC H5 HCC

         √7ᵗʰ **S24.139 Anterior cord syndrome at unspecified level of thoracic spinal cord**   HCC

     √6ᵗʰ **S24.14 Brown-Séquard syndrome of thoracic spinal cord**

         √7ᵗʰ **S24.141 Brown-Séquard syndrome at T1 level of thoracic spinal cord**   MCC HCC

         √7ᵗʰ **S24.142 Brown-Séquard syndrome at T2-T6 level of thoracic spinal cord**   MCC HCC

         √7ᵗʰ **S24.143 Brown-Séquard syndrome at T7-T10 level of thoracic spinal cord**   MCC HCC

         √7ᵗʰ **S24.144 Brown-Séquard syndrome at T11-T12 level of thoracic spinal cord**   MCC HCC

         √7ᵗʰ **S24.149 Brown-Séquard syndrome at unspecified level of thoracic spinal cord**   HCC

     √6ᵗʰ **S24.15 Other incomplete lesions of thoracic spinal cord**
         Incomplete lesion of thoracic spinal cord NOS
         Posterior cord syndrome of thoracic spinal cord

         √7ᵗʰ **S24.151 Other incomplete lesion at T1 level of thoracic spinal cord**   MCC H5 HCC

         √7ᵗʰ **S24.152 Other incomplete lesion at T2-T6 level of thoracic spinal cord**   MCC H5 HCC

         √7ᵗʰ **S24.153 Other incomplete lesion at T7-T10 level of thoracic spinal cord**   MCC H5 HCC

         √7ᵗʰ **S24.154 Other incomplete lesion at T11-T12 level of thoracic spinal cord**   MCC H5 HCC

         √7ᵗʰ **S24.159 Other incomplete lesion at unspecified level of thoracic spinal cord**   HCC

√x7ᵗʰ **S24.2 Injury of nerve root of thoracic spine**

√x7ᵗʰ **S24.3 Injury of peripheral nerves of thorax**

√x7ᵗʰ **S24.4 Injury of thoracic sympathetic nervous system**
     Injury of cardiac plexus   Injury of stellate ganglion
     Injury of esophageal plexus   Injury of thoracic sympathetic
     Injury of pulmonary plexus   ganglion

√x7ᵗʰ **S24.8 Injury of other specified nerves of thorax**

√x7ᵗʰ **S24.9 Injury of unspecified nerve of thorax**

√4ᵗʰ **S25 Injury of blood vessels of thorax**
     Code also any associated open wound (S21.-)

> The appropriate 7th character is to be added to each code from category S25.
> A   initial encounter
> D   subsequent encounter
> S   sequela

√5ᵗʰ **S25.0 Injury of thoracic aorta**
     Injury of aorta NOS

> **CC Excl: For MCC codes in subcategory S25.0:**
> PDX collection 1178

     √x7ᵗʰ **S25.00 Unspecified injury of thoracic aorta**   MCC

     √x7ᵗʰ **S25.01 Minor laceration of thoracic aorta**   MCC
         Incomplete transection of thoracic aorta
         Laceration of thoracic aorta NOS
         Superficial laceration of thoracic aorta

     √x7ᵗʰ **S25.02 Major laceration of thoracic aorta**   MCC
         Complete transection of thoracic aorta
         Traumatic rupture of thoracic aorta

     √x7ᵗʰ **S25.09 Other specified injury of thoracic aorta**   MCC

√5ᵗʰ **S25.1 Injury of innominate or subclavian artery**

> **CC Excl: For MCC codes in subcategory S25.1:**
> PDX collection 1179

     √6ᵗʰ **S25.10 Unspecified injury of innominate or subclavian artery**

         √7ᵗʰ **S25.101 Unspecified injury of right innominate or subclavian artery**   MCC

         √7ᵗʰ **S25.102 Unspecified injury of left innominate or subclavian artery**   MCC

         √7ᵗʰ **S25.109 Unspecified injury of unspecified innominate or subclavian artery**   MCC

     √6ᵗʰ **S25.11 Minor laceration of innominate or subclavian artery**
         Incomplete transection of innominate or subclavian artery
         Laceration of innominate or subclavian artery NOS
         Superficial laceration of innominate or subclavian artery

         √7ᵗʰ **S25.111 Minor laceration of right innominate or subclavian artery**   MCC

         √7ᵗʰ **S25.112 Minor laceration of left innominate or subclavian artery**   MCC

         √7ᵗʰ **S25.119 Minor laceration of unspecified innominate or subclavian artery**   MCC

     √6ᵗʰ **S25.12 Major laceration of innominate or subclavian artery**
         Complete transection of innominate or subclavian artery
         Traumatic rupture of innominate or subclavian artery

         √7ᵗʰ **S25.121 Major laceration of right innominate or subclavian artery**   MCC

         √7ᵗʰ **S25.122 Major laceration of left innominate or subclavian artery**   MCC

✔ Additional Character Required   √x7ᵗʰ Placeholder   Unacceptable PDx   Questionable PDx   Manifestation   H1 - H14 HAC   HCC CMS-HCC Dx   HIV HIV Dx

ICD-10-CM 2019   971

Chapter 19. Injury, Poisoning and Certain Other Consequences of External Causes

√7ᵗʰ **S25.129**   **Major laceration of** unspecified **innominate or subclavian artery**   MCC

√6ᵗʰ **S25.19**   **Other** specified injury of innominate or subclavian **artery**

    √7ᵗʰ **S25.191**   **Other specified injury of** right **innominate or subclavian artery**   MCC

    √7ᵗʰ **S25.192**   **Other specified injury of** left **innominate or subclavian artery**   MCC

    √7ᵗʰ **S25.199**   **Other specified injury of** unspecified **innominate or subclavian artery**   MCC

√5ᵗʰ **S25.2**   **Injury of** superior vena cava
Injury of vena cava NOS

CC Excl: For MCC codes in subcategory S25.2:
PDX collection 1180

√x7ᵗʰ **S25.20**   **Unspecified injury of superior vena cava**   MCC

√x7ᵗʰ **S25.21**   **Minor laceration of superior vena cava**   MCC
Incomplete transection of superior vena cava
Laceration of superior vena cava NOS
Superficial laceration of superior vena cava

√x7ᵗʰ **S25.22**   **Major laceration of superior vena cava**   MCC
Complete transection of superior vena cava
Traumatic rupture of superior vena cava

√x7ᵗʰ **S25.29**   **Other** specified injury of superior vena cava   MCC

√5ᵗʰ **S25.3**   **Injury of** innominate or subclavian vein

CC Excl: For MCC codes in subcategory S25.3:
PDX collection 1181

√6ᵗʰ **S25.30**   **Unspecified injury of innominate or subclavian vein**

    √7ᵗʰ **S25.301**   **Unspecified injury of** right **innominate or subclavian vein**   MCC

    √7ᵗʰ **S25.302**   **Unspecified injury of** left **innominate or subclavian vein**   MCC

    √7ᵗʰ **S25.309**   **Unspecified injury of** unspecified **innominate or subclavian vein**   MCC

√6ᵗʰ **S25.31**   **Minor laceration of innominate or subclavian vein**
Incomplete transection of innominate or subclavian vein
Laceration of innominate or subclavian vein NOS
Superficial laceration of innominate or subclavian vein

    √7ᵗʰ **S25.311**   **Minor laceration of** right **innominate or subclavian vein**   MCC

    √7ᵗʰ **S25.312**   **Minor laceration of** left **innominate or subclavian vein**   MCC

    √7ᵗʰ **S25.319**   **Minor laceration of** unspecified **innominate or subclavian vein**   MCC

√6ᵗʰ **S25.32**   **Major laceration of innominate or subclavian vein**
Complete transection of innominate or subclavian vein
Traumatic rupture of innominate or subclavian vein

    √7ᵗʰ **S25.321**   **Major laceration of** right **innominate or subclavian vein**   MCC

    √7ᵗʰ **S25.322**   **Major laceration of** left **innominate or subclavian vein**   MCC

    √7ᵗʰ **S25.329**   **Major laceration of** unspecified **innominate or subclavian vein**   MCC

√6ᵗʰ **S25.39**   **Other** specified injury of innominate or subclavian **vein**

    √7ᵗʰ **S25.391**   **Other specified injury of** right **innominate or subclavian vein**   MCC

    √7ᵗʰ **S25.392**   **Other specified injury of** left **innominate or subclavian vein**   MCC

    √7ᵗʰ **S25.399**   **Other specified injury of** unspecified **innominate or subclavian vein**   MCC

√5ᵗʰ **S25.4**   **Injury of** pulmonary blood vessels

CC Excl: For MCC codes in subcategory S25.4, unless otherwise noted: PDX collection 1182

√6ᵗʰ **S25.40**   **Unspecified injury of pulmonary blood vessels**

    √7ᵗʰ **S25.401**   **Unspecified injury of** right **pulmonary blood vessels**   MCC

    √7ᵗʰ **S25.402**   **Unspecified injury of** left **pulmonary blood vessels**   MCC

    √7ᵗʰ **S25.409**   **Unspecified injury of** unspecified **pulmonary blood vessels**   MCC

√6ᵗʰ **S25.41**   **Minor laceration of pulmonary blood vessels**
Incomplete transection of pulmonary blood vessels
Laceration of pulmonary blood vessels NOS
Superficial laceration of pulmonary blood vessels

    √7ᵗʰ **S25.411**   **Minor laceration of** right **pulmonary blood vessels**   MCC

    √7ᵗʰ **S25.412**   **Minor laceration of** left **pulmonary blood vessels**   MCC

    √7ᵗʰ **S25.419**   **Minor laceration of** unspecified **pulmonary blood vessels**   MCC

√6ᵗʰ **S25.42**   **Major laceration of pulmonary blood vessels**
Complete transection of pulmonary blood vessels
Traumatic rupture of pulmonary blood vessels

    √7ᵗʰ **S25.421**   **Major laceration of** right **pulmonary blood vessels**   MCC
      CC Excl: PDX collection 1183

    √7ᵗʰ **S25.422**   **Major laceration of** left **pulmonary blood vessels**   MCC

    √7ᵗʰ **S25.429**   **Major laceration of** unspecified **pulmonary blood vessels**   MCC

√6ᵗʰ **S25.49**   **Other** specified injury of pulmonary blood vessels

    √7ᵗʰ **S25.491**   **Other specified injury of** right **pulmonary blood vessels**   MCC

    √7ᵗʰ **S25.492**   **Other specified injury of** left **pulmonary blood vessels**   MCC

    √7ᵗʰ **S25.499**   **Other specified injury of** unspecified **pulmonary blood vessels**   MCC

√5ᵗʰ **S25.5**   **Injury of** intercostal blood vessels

CC Excl: For CC codes in subcategory S25.5:
PDX collection 1184

√6ᵗʰ **S25.50**   **Unspecified injury of intercostal blood vessels**

    √7ᵗʰ **S25.501**   **Unspecified injury of intercostal blood vessels,** right **side**   CC

    √7ᵗʰ **S25.502**   **Unspecified injury of intercostal blood vessels,** left **side**   CC

    √7ᵗʰ **S25.509**   **Unspecified injury of intercostal blood vessels,** unspecified **side**   CC

√6ᵗʰ **S25.51**   **Laceration of intercostal blood vessels**

    √7ᵗʰ **S25.511**   **Laceration of intercostal blood vessels,** right **side**   CC

    √7ᵗʰ **S25.512**   **Laceration of intercostal blood vessels,** left **side**   CC

    √7ᵗʰ **S25.519**   **Laceration of intercostal blood vessels,** unspecified **side**   CC

√6ᵗʰ **S25.59**   **Other** specified injury of intercostal blood vessels

    √7ᵗʰ **S25.591**   **Other specified injury of intercostal blood vessels,** right **side**   CC

    √7ᵗʰ **S25.592**   **Other specified injury of intercostal blood vessels,** left **side**   CC

    √7ᵗʰ **S25.599**   **Other specified injury of intercostal blood vessels,** unspecified **side**   CC

√5ᵗʰ **S25.8**   **Injury of** other blood vessels of thorax
Injury of azygos vein
Injury of mammary artery or vein

CC Excl: For CC codes in subcategory S25.8:
PDX collection 1185

√6ᵗʰ **S25.80**   **Unspecified injury of other blood vessels of thorax**

    √7ᵗʰ **S25.801**   **Unspecified injury of other blood vessels of thorax,** right **side**   CC

    √7ᵗʰ **S25.802**   **Unspecified injury of other blood vessels of thorax,** left **side**   CC

    √7ᵗʰ **S25.809**   **Unspecified injury of other blood vessels of thorax,** unspecified **side**   CC

√6ᵗʰ **S25.81**   **Laceration of other blood vessels of thorax**

    √7ᵗʰ **S25.811**   **Laceration of other blood vessels of thorax,** right **side**   CC

    √7ᵗʰ **S25.812**   **Laceration of other blood vessels of thorax,** left **side**   CC

    √7ᵗʰ **S25.819**   **Laceration of other blood vessels of thorax,** unspecified **side**   CC

√6ᵗʰ **S25.89**   **Other** specified injury of other blood vessels of **thorax**

    √7ᵗʰ **S25.891**   **Other specified injury of other blood vessels of thorax,** right **side**   CC

N Newborn: 0   P Pediatric: 0-17   M Maternity: 12-55   A Adult: 15-124   MCC Major Complication/Comorbidity   CC Complication/Comorbidity   SW Severe Wound Dx

972   ICD-10-CM 2019

S25.129–S25.891

✓7ᵗʰ **S25.892** Other specified injury of other blood vessels of thorax, **left side**   CC

✓7ᵗʰ **S25.899** Other specified injury of other blood vessels of thorax, **unspecified side**   CC

✓5ᵗʰ **S25.9** Injury of **unspecified blood vessel of thorax**

CC Excl: For CC codes in subcategory S25.9:
PDX collection 1185

✓x7ᵗʰ **S25.90** **Unspecified** injury of unspecified blood vessel of thorax   CC

✓x7ᵗʰ **S25.91** **Laceration** of unspecified blood vessel of thorax   CC

✓x7ᵗʰ **S25.99** **Other** specified injury of unspecified blood vessel of thorax   CC

✓4ᵗʰ **S26** **Injury of heart**

Code also any associated:
     open wound of thorax (S21.-)
     traumatic hemopneumothorax (S27.2)
     traumatic hemothorax (S27.1)
     traumatic pneumothorax (S27.0)

The appropriate 7th character is to be added to each code from category S26.
A   initial encounter
D   subsequent encounter
S   sequela

CC Excl: For CC/MCC codes in category S26, unless otherwise noted: PDX collection 1187

✓5ᵗʰ **S26.0** **Injury of heart** with hemopericardium

✓x7ᵗʰ **S26.00** **Unspecified** injury of heart with hemopericardium   CC
     CC Excl: PDX collection 1186

✓x7ᵗʰ **S26.01** **Contusion** of heart with hemopericardium   CC

✓6ᵗʰ **S26.02** **Laceration** of heart with hemopericardium

✓7ᵗʰ **S26.020** **Mild laceration of heart with hemopericardium**   MCC
     Laceration of heart without penetration of heart chamber

✓7ᵗʰ **S26.021** **Moderate laceration of heart with hemopericardium**   MCC
     Laceration of heart with penetration of heart chamber

✓7ᵗʰ **S26.022** **Major laceration of heart with hemopericardium**   MCC
     Laceration of heart with penetration of multiple heart chambers

✓x7ᵗʰ **S26.09** **Other** injury of heart with hemopericardium   CC
     CC Excl: PDX collection 1186

✓5ᵗʰ **S26.1** **Injury of heart** without hemopericardium

✓x7ᵗʰ **S26.10** **Unspecified** injury of heart without hemopericardium   CC
     CC Excl: PDX collection 1186

✓x7ᵗʰ **S26.11** **Contusion** of heart without hemopericardium   CC

✓x7ᵗʰ **S26.12** **Laceration** of heart without hemopericardium   MCC

✓x7ᵗʰ **S26.19** **Other** injury of heart without hemopericardium   CC
     CC Excl: PDX collection 1186

✓5ᵗʰ **S26.9** **Injury of heart, unspecified** with or without hemopericardium

✓x7ᵗʰ **S26.90** **Unspecified** injury of heart, unspecified with or without hemopericardium   CC
     CC Excl: PDX collection 1186

✓x7ᵗʰ **S26.91** **Contusion** of heart, unspecified with or without hemopericardium   CC
     DEF: Bruising within the heart muscle, with no mention of an open wound, usually caused by blunt chest trauma in motor vehicle accidents, falling from great heights, or receiving CPR.

✓x7ᵗʰ **S26.92** **Laceration** of heart, unspecified with or without hemopericardium   MCC
     Laceration of heart NOS

✓x7ᵗʰ **S26.99** **Other** injury of heart, unspecified with or without hemopericardium   CC
     CC Excl: PDX collection 1186

✓4ᵗʰ **S27** **Injury of other and unspecified intrathoracic organs**

Code also any associated open wound of thorax (S21.-)

EXCLUDES 2   injury of cervical esophagus (S10-S19)
          injury of trachea (cervical) (S10-S19)

The appropriate 7th character is to be added to each code from category S27.
A   initial encounter
D   subsequent encounter
S   sequela

✓x7ᵗʰ **S27.0** **Traumatic pneumothorax**   CC
     EXCLUDES 1   spontaneous pneumothorax (J93.-)
     CC Excl: PDX collection 1188

✓x7ᵗʰ **S27.1** **Traumatic hemothorax**   MCC
     CC Excl: PDX collection 1188

✓x7ᵗʰ **S27.2** **Traumatic hemopneumothorax**   MCC
     CC Excl: PDX collection 1188

✓5ᵗʰ **S27.3** **Other and unspecified injuries of lung**

CC Excl: For CC/MCC codes in subcategory S27.3, unless otherwise noted: PDX collection 1189

✓6ᵗʰ **S27.30** **Unspecified** injury of lung

✓7ᵗʰ **S27.301** Unspecified injury of lung, **unilateral**   CC

✓7ᵗʰ **S27.302** Unspecified injury of lung, **bilateral**   CC

✓7ᵗʰ **S27.309** Unspecified injury of lung, **unspecified**   CC

✓6ᵗʰ **S27.31** **Primary blast injury of lung**
     Blast injury of lung NOS

✓7ᵗʰ **S27.311** Primary blast injury of lung, **unilateral**   CC

✓7ᵗʰ **S27.312** Primary blast injury of lung, **bilateral**   CC

✓7ᵗʰ **S27.319** Primary blast injury of lung, **unspecified**   CC

✓6ᵗʰ **S27.32** **Contusion of lung**
     DEF: Bruising of the lung without mention of an open wound.

✓7ᵗʰ **S27.321** Contusion of lung, **unilateral**   CC

✓7ᵗʰ **S27.322** Contusion of lung, **bilateral**   CC

✓7ᵗʰ **S27.329** Contusion of lung, **unspecified**   CC

✓6ᵗʰ **S27.33** **Laceration of lung**

CC Excl: For MCC codes in subcategory S27.33: PDX collection 1190

✓7ᵗʰ **S27.331** Laceration of lung, **unilateral**   MCC

✓7ᵗʰ **S27.332** Laceration of lung, **bilateral**   MCC

✓7ᵗʰ **S27.339** Laceration of lung, **unspecified**   MCC

✓6ᵗʰ **S27.39** **Other injuries of lung**
     Secondary blast injury of lung

✓7ᵗʰ **S27.391** Other injuries of lung, **unilateral**   CC

✓7ᵗʰ **S27.392** Other injuries of lung, **bilateral**   CC

✓7ᵗʰ **S27.399** Other injuries of lung, **unspecified**   CC

✓5ᵗʰ **S27.4** **Injury of bronchus**

CC Excl: For MCC codes in subcategory S27.4: PDX collection 1191

✓6ᵗʰ **S27.40** **Unspecified** injury of bronchus

✓7ᵗʰ **S27.401** Unspecified injury of bronchus, **unilateral**   MCC

✓7ᵗʰ **S27.402** Unspecified injury of bronchus, **bilateral**   MCC

✓7ᵗʰ **S27.409** Unspecified injury of bronchus, **unspecified**   MCC

✓6ᵗʰ **S27.41** **Primary blast injury of bronchus**
     Blast injury of bronchus NOS

✓7ᵗʰ **S27.411** Primary blast injury of bronchus, **unilateral**   MCC

✓7ᵗʰ **S27.412** Primary blast injury of bronchus, **bilateral**   MCC

✓7ᵗʰ **S27.419** Primary blast injury of bronchus, **unspecified**   MCC

✓6ᵗʰ **S27.42** **Contusion of bronchus**

✓7ᵗʰ **S27.421** Contusion of bronchus, **unilateral**   MCC

✓7ᵗʰ **S27.422** Contusion of bronchus, **bilateral**   MCC

✓7ᵗʰ **S27.429** Contusion of bronchus, **unspecified**   MCC

✓ Additional Character Required   ✓x7ᵗʰ Placeholder   Unacceptable PDx   Questionable PDx   Manifestation   H1-H14 HAC   HCC CMS-HCC Dx   HIV HIV Dx

ICD-10-CM 2019   973

Chapter 19. Injury, Poisoning and Certain Other Consequences of External Causes

✓6ᵗʰ **S27.43** **Laceration** of bronchus
- ✓7ᵗʰ **S27.431** **Laceration** of bronchus, unilateral   MCC
- ✓7ᵗʰ **S27.432** **Laceration** of bronchus, bilateral   MCC
- ✓7ᵗʰ **S27.439** **Laceration** of bronchus, unspecified   MCC

✓6ᵗʰ **S27.49** **Other** injury of bronchus
Secondary blast injury of bronchus
- ✓7ᵗʰ **S27.491** **Other** injury of bronchus, unilateral   MCC
- ✓7ᵗʰ **S27.492** **Other** injury of bronchus, bilateral   MCC
- ✓7ᵗʰ **S27.499** **Other** injury of bronchus, unspecified   MCC

✓5ᵗʰ **S27.5** **Injury** of thoracic trachea

CC Excl: For CC codes in subcategory S27.5:
PDX collection 1169

- ✓x7ᵗʰ **S27.50** **Unspecified** injury of thoracic trachea   CC
- ✓x7ᵗʰ **S27.51** **Primary blast** injury of thoracic trachea   CC
  Blast injury of thoracic trachea NOS
- ✓x7ᵗʰ **S27.52** **Contusion** of thoracic trachea   CC
- ✓x7ᵗʰ **S27.53** **Laceration** of thoracic trachea   CC
- ✓x7ᵗʰ **S27.59** **Other** injury of thoracic trachea   CC
  Secondary blast injury of thoracic trachea

✓5ᵗʰ **S27.6** **Injury** of pleura

CC Excl: For CC codes in subcategory S27.6:
PDX collection 1169

- ✓x7ᵗʰ **S27.60** **Unspecified** injury of pleura   CC
- ✓x7ᵗʰ **S27.63** **Laceration** of pleura   CC
- ✓x7ᵗʰ **S27.69** **Other** injury of pleura   CC

✓5ᵗʰ **S27.8** **Injury** of other specified intrathoracic organs
- ✓6ᵗʰ **S27.80** **Injury** of diaphragm

  CC Excl: For CC codes in subcategory S27.80:
  PDX collection 1192

  - ✓7ᵗʰ **S27.802** **Contusion** of diaphragm   CC
  - ✓7ᵗʰ **S27.803** **Laceration** of diaphragm   CC
  - ✓7ᵗʰ **S27.808** **Other** injury of diaphragm   CC
  - ✓7ᵗʰ **S27.809** **Unspecified** injury of diaphragm   CC

- ✓6ᵗʰ **S27.81** **Injury** of esophagus (thoracic part)

  CC Excl: For MCC codes in subcategory S27.81:
  PDX collection 1193

  - ✓7ᵗʰ **S27.812** **Contusion** of esophagus (thoracic part)   MCC
  - ✓7ᵗʰ **S27.813** **Laceration** of esophagus (thoracic part)   MCC
  - ✓7ᵗʰ **S27.818** **Other** injury of esophagus (thoracic part)   MCC
  - ✓7ᵗʰ **S27.819** **Unspecified** injury of esophagus (thoracic part)   MCC

- ✓6ᵗʰ **S27.89** **Injury** of other specified intrathoracic organs
  Injury of lymphatic thoracic duct
  Injury of thymus gland

  CC Excl: For CC codes in subcategory S27.89:
  PDX collection 1169

  - ✓7ᵗʰ **S27.892** **Contusion** of other specified intrathoracic organs   CC
  - ✓7ᵗʰ **S27.893** **Laceration** of other specified intrathoracic organs   CC
  - ✓7ᵗʰ **S27.898** **Other** injury of other specified intrathoracic organs   CC
  - ✓7ᵗʰ **S27.899** **Unspecified** injury of other specified intrathoracic organs   CC

✓x7ᵗʰ **S27.9** **Injury** of unspecified intrathoracic organ   CC
CC Excl: PDX collection 1194

✓4ᵗʰ **S28** **Crushing injury of thorax, and traumatic amputation of part of thorax**

The appropriate 7th character is to be added to each code from category S28.
A   initial encounter
D   subsequent encounter
S   sequela

✓x7ᵗʰ **S28.0** **Crushed chest**
Use additional code for all associated injuries
EXCLUDES 1   flail chest (S22.5)

✓x7ᵗʰ **S28.1** **Traumatic amputation (partial) of** part of thorax, except breast   CC
CC Excl: PDX collection 1168

✓5ᵗʰ **S28.2** **Traumatic amputation of** breast
- ✓6ᵗʰ **S28.21** **Complete** traumatic amputation of breast
  Traumatic amputation of breast NOS
  - ✓7ᵗʰ **S28.211** **Complete** traumatic amputation of right breast
  - ✓7ᵗʰ **S28.212** **Complete** traumatic amputation of left breast
  - ✓7ᵗʰ **S28.219** **Complete** traumatic amputation of unspecified breast

- ✓6ᵗʰ **S28.22** **Partial** traumatic amputation of breast
  - ✓7ᵗʰ **S28.221** **Partial** traumatic amputation of right breast
  - ✓7ᵗʰ **S28.222** **Partial** traumatic amputation of left breast
  - ✓7ᵗʰ **S28.229** **Partial** traumatic amputation of unspecified breast

✓4ᵗʰ **S29** **Other and unspecified injuries of thorax**
Code also any associated open wound (S21.-)

The appropriate 7th character is to be added to each code from category S29.
A   initial encounter
D   subsequent encounter
S   sequela

✓5ᵗʰ **S29.0** **Injury** of muscle and tendon at thorax level
- ✓6ᵗʰ **S29.00** **Unspecified** injury of muscle and tendon of thorax
  - ✓7ᵗʰ **S29.001** **Unspecified** injury of muscle and tendon of front wall of thorax
  - ✓7ᵗʰ **S29.002** **Unspecified** injury of muscle and tendon of back wall of thorax
  - ✓7ᵗʰ **S29.009** **Unspecified** injury of muscle and tendon of unspecified wall of thorax

- ✓6ᵗʰ **S29.01** **Strain** of muscle and tendon of thorax
  - ✓7ᵗʰ **S29.011** **Strain** of muscle and tendon of front wall of thorax
  - ✓7ᵗʰ **S29.012** **Strain** of muscle and tendon of back wall of thorax
  - ✓7ᵗʰ **S29.019** **Strain** of muscle and tendon of unspecified wall of thorax

- ✓6ᵗʰ **S29.02** **Laceration** of muscle and tendon of thorax
  - ✓7ᵗʰ **S29.021** **Laceration** of muscle and tendon of front wall of thorax   CC
    CC Excl: PDX collection 1168
  - ✓7ᵗʰ **S29.022** **Laceration** of muscle and tendon of back wall of thorax
  - ✓7ᵗʰ **S29.029** **Laceration** of muscle and tendon of unspecified wall of thorax   CC
    CC Excl: PDX collection 1168

- ✓6ᵗʰ **S29.09** **Other** injury of muscle and tendon of thorax
  - ✓7ᵗʰ **S29.091** **Other** injury of muscle and tendon of front wall of thorax
  - ✓7ᵗʰ **S29.092** **Other** injury of muscle and tendon of back wall of thorax
  - ✓7ᵗʰ **S29.099** **Other** injury of muscle and tendon of unspecified wall of thorax

✓x7ᵗʰ **S29.8** **Other specified injuries of thorax**

✓x7ᵗʰ **S29.9** **Unspecified injury of thorax**

Injuries to the abdomen, lower back, lumbar spine, pelvis and external genitals (S30-S39)

INCLUDES injuries to the abdominal wall
injuries to the anus
injuries to the buttock
injuries to the external genitalia
injuries to the flank
injuries to the groin

EXCLUDES 2 burns and corrosions (T20-T32)
effects of foreign body in anus and rectum (T18.5)
effects of foreign body in genitourinary tract (T19.-)
effects of foreign body in stomach, small intestine and colon (T18.2-T18.4)
frostbite (T33-T34)
insect bite or sting, venomous (T63.4)

✓4th S30 Superficial injury of abdomen, lower back, pelvis and external genitals

EXCLUDES 2 superficial injury of hip (S70.-)

The appropriate 7th character is to be added to each code from category S30.
A   initial encounter
D   subsequent encounter
S   sequela

✓x7th **S30.0 Contusion of lower back and pelvis**
Contusion of buttock

✓x7th **S30.1 Contusion of abdominal wall**
Contusion of flank
Contusion of groin

✓5th **S30.2 Contusion of external genital organs**

   ✓6th **S30.20 Contusion of unspecified external genital organ**

     ✓7th **S30.201 Contusion of unspecified external genital organ, male**   ♂

     ✓7th **S30.202 Contusion of unspecified external genital organ, female**   ♀

   ✓x7th **S30.21 Contusion of penis**   ♂

   ✓x7th **S30.22 Contusion of scrotum and testes**   ♂

   ✓x7th **S30.23 Contusion of vagina and vulva**   ♀

✓x7th **S30.3 Contusion of anus**

✓5th **S30.8 Other superficial injuries of abdomen, lower back, pelvis and external genitals**

   ✓6th **S30.81 Abrasion of abdomen, lower back, pelvis and external genitals**

     ✓7th **S30.810 Abrasion of lower back and pelvis**

     ✓7th **S30.811 Abrasion of abdominal wall**

     ✓7th **S30.812 Abrasion of penis**   ♂

     ✓7th **S30.813 Abrasion of scrotum and testes**   ♂

     ✓7th **S30.814 Abrasion of vagina and vulva**   ♀

     ✓7th **S30.815 Abrasion of unspecified external genital organs, male**   ♂

     ✓7th **S30.816 Abrasion of unspecified external genital organs, female**   ♀

     ✓7th **S30.817 Abrasion of anus**

   ✓6th **S30.82 Blister (nonthermal) of abdomen, lower back, pelvis and external genitals**

     ✓7th **S30.820 Blister (nonthermal) of lower back and pelvis**

     ✓7th **S30.821 Blister (nonthermal) of abdominal wall**

     ✓7th **S30.822 Blister (nonthermal) of penis**   ♂

     ✓7th **S30.823 Blister (nonthermal) of scrotum and testes**   ♂

     ✓7th **S30.824 Blister (nonthermal) of vagina and vulva**   ♀

     ✓7th **S30.825 Blister (nonthermal) of unspecified external genital organs, male**   ♂

     ✓7th **S30.826 Blister (nonthermal) of unspecified external genital organs, female**   ♀

     ✓7th **S30.827 Blister (nonthermal) of anus**

   ✓6th **S30.84 External constriction of abdomen, lower back, pelvis and external genitals**

     ✓7th **S30.840 External constriction of lower back and pelvis**

     ✓7th **S30.841 External constriction of abdominal wall**

     ✓7th **S30.842 External constriction of penis**   ♂
        Hair tourniquet syndrome of penis
        Use additional cause code to identify the constricting item (W49.0-)

     ✓7th **S30.843 External constriction of scrotum and testes**   ♂

     ✓7th **S30.844 External constriction of vagina and vulva**   ♀

     ✓7th **S30.845 External constriction of unspecified external genital organs, male**   ♂

     ✓7th **S30.846 External constriction of unspecified external genital organs, female**   ♀

   ✓6th **S30.85 Superficial foreign body of abdomen, lower back, pelvis and external genitals**
     Splinter in the abdomen, lower back, pelvis and external genitals

     ✓7th **S30.850 Superficial foreign body of lower back and pelvis**

     ✓7th **S30.851 Superficial foreign body of abdominal wall**

     ✓7th **S30.852 Superficial foreign body of penis**   ♂

     ✓7th **S30.853 Superficial foreign body of scrotum and testes**   ♂

     ✓7th **S30.854 Superficial foreign body of vagina and vulva**   ♀

     ✓7th **S30.855 Superficial foreign body of unspecified external genital organs, male**   ♂

     ✓7th **S30.856 Superficial foreign body of unspecified external genital organs, female**   ♀

     ✓7th **S30.857 Superficial foreign body of anus**

   ✓6th **S30.86 Insect bite (nonvenomous) of abdomen, lower back, pelvis and external genitals**

     ✓7th **S30.860 Insect bite (nonvenomous) of lower back and pelvis**

     ✓7th **S30.861 Insect bite (nonvenomous) of abdominal wall**

     ✓7th **S30.862 Insect bite (nonvenomous) of penis**   ♂

     ✓7th **S30.863 Insect bite (nonvenomous) of scrotum and testes**   ♂

     ✓7th **S30.864 Insect bite (nonvenomous) of vagina and vulva**   ♀

     ✓7th **S30.865 Insect bite (nonvenomous) of unspecified external genital organs, male**   ♂

     ✓7th **S30.866 Insect bite (nonvenomous) of unspecified external genital organs, female**   ♀

     ✓7th **S30.867 Insect bite (nonvenomous) of anus**

   ✓6th **S30.87 Other superficial bite of abdomen, lower back, pelvis and external genitals**

     EXCLUDES 1 open bite of abdomen, lower back, pelvis and external genitals (S31.05, S31.15, S31.25, S31.35, S31.45, S31.55)

     ✓7th **S30.870 Other superficial bite of lower back and pelvis**

     ✓7th **S30.871 Other superficial bite of abdominal wall**

     ✓7th **S30.872 Other superficial bite of penis**   ♂

     ✓7th **S30.873 Other superficial bite of scrotum and testes**   ♂

     ✓7th **S30.874 Other superficial bite of vagina and vulva**   ♀

     ✓7th **S30.875 Other superficial bite of unspecified external genital organs, male**   ♂

     ✓7th **S30.876 Other superficial bite of unspecified external genital organs, female**   ♀

     ✓7th **S30.877 Other superficial bite of anus**

✓5th **S30.9 Unspecified superficial injury of abdomen, lower back, pelvis and external genitals**

   ✓x7th **S30.91 Unspecified superficial injury of lower back and pelvis**

   ✓x7th **S30.92 Unspecified superficial injury of abdominal wall**

   ✓x7th **S30.93 Unspecified superficial injury of penis**   ♂

   ✓x7th **S30.94 Unspecified superficial injury of scrotum and testes**   ♂

✓ Additional Character Required   ✓x7th Placeholder   Unacceptable PDx   Questionable PDx   Manifestation   H1-H14 HAC   HCC CMS-HCC Dx   HIV HIV Dx

ICD-10-CM 2019   975

√x7th S30.95   **Unspecified superficial injury of** vagina and vulva   ♀

√x7th S30.96   **Unspecified superficial injury of** unspecified external genital organs, male   ♂

√x7th S30.97   **Unspecified superficial injury of** unspecified external genital organs, female   ♀

√x7th S30.98   **Unspecified superficial injury of** anus

√4th S31   **Open wound of abdomen, lower back, pelvis and external genitals**

Code also any associated:
    spinal cord injury (S24.0, S24.1-, S34.0-, S34.1-)
    wound infection

EXCLUDES 1   traumatic amputation of part of abdomen, lower back and pelvis (S38.2-, S38.3)

EXCLUDES 2   open wound of hip (S71.00-S71.02)
    open fracture of pelvis (S32.1- – S32.9 with 7th B)

The appropriate 7th character is to be added to each code from category S31.
A   initial encounter
D   subsequent encounter
S   sequela

CC Excl: For MCC codes in category S31: PDX collection 1195

√5th S31.0   **Open wound of** lower back and pelvis

  √6th S31.00   **Unspecified open wound** of lower back and pelvis

    √7th S31.000   **Unspecified open wound of lower back and pelvis** without penetration into retroperitoneum
      Unspecified open wound of lower back and pelvis NOS

    √7th S31.001   **Unspecified open wound of lower back and pelvis** with penetration into retroperitoneum   **MCC**

  √6th S31.01   **Laceration without foreign body** of lower back and pelvis

    √7th S31.010   **Laceration without foreign body of lower back and pelvis** without penetration into retroperitoneum
      Laceration without foreign body of lower back and pelvis NOS

    √7th S31.011   **Laceration without foreign body of lower back and pelvis** with penetration into retroperitoneum   **MCC**

  √6th S31.02   **Laceration with foreign body** of lower back and pelvis

    √7th S31.020   **Laceration with foreign body of lower back and pelvis** without penetration into retroperitoneum
      Laceration with foreign body of lower back and pelvis NOS

    √7th S31.021   **Laceration with foreign body of lower back and pelvis** with penetration into retroperitoneum   **MCC**

  √6th S31.03   **Puncture wound without foreign body** of lower back and pelvis

    √7th S31.030   **Puncture wound without foreign body of lower back and pelvis** without penetration into retroperitoneum
      Puncture wound without foreign body of lower back and pelvis NOS

    √7th S31.031   **Puncture wound without foreign body of lower back and pelvis** with penetration into retroperitoneum   **MCC**

  √6th S31.04   **Puncture wound with foreign body** of lower back and pelvis

    √7th S31.040   **Puncture wound with foreign body of lower back and pelvis** without penetration into retroperitoneum
      Puncture wound with foreign body of lower back and pelvis NOS

    √7th S31.041   **Puncture wound with foreign body of lower back and pelvis** with penetration into retroperitoneum   **MCC**

√6th S31.05   **Open bite of lower back and pelvis**
  Bite of lower back and pelvis NOS

  EXCLUDES 1   superficial bite of lower back and pelvis (S30.860, S30.870)

  √7th S31.050   **Open bite of lower back and pelvis** without penetration into retroperitoneum
    Open bite of lower back and pelvis NOS

  √7th S31.051   **Open bite of lower back and pelvis** with penetration into retroperitoneum   **MCC**

√5th S31.1   **Open wound of** abdominal wall without penetration into peritoneal cavity
  Open wound of abdominal wall NOS

  EXCLUDES 2   open wound of abdominal wall with penetration into peritoneal cavity (S31.6-)

  √6th S31.10   **Unspecified open wound of abdominal wall without penetration into peritoneal cavity**

    √7th S31.100   **Unspecified open wound of abdominal wall, right upper quadrant without penetration into peritoneal cavity**

    √7th S31.101   **Unspecified open wound of abdominal wall, left upper quadrant without penetration into peritoneal cavity**

    √7th S31.102   **Unspecified open wound of abdominal wall, epigastric region without penetration into peritoneal cavity**

    √7th S31.103   **Unspecified open wound of abdominal wall, right lower quadrant without penetration into peritoneal cavity**

    √7th S31.104   **Unspecified open wound of abdominal wall, left lower quadrant without penetration into peritoneal cavity**

    √7th S31.105   **Unspecified open wound of abdominal wall, periumbilic region without penetration into peritoneal cavity**

    √7th S31.109   **Unspecified open wound of abdominal wall, unspecified quadrant without penetration into peritoneal cavity**
      Unspecified open wound of abdominal wall NOS

  √6th S31.11   **Laceration without foreign body** of abdominal wall without penetration into peritoneal cavity

    √7th S31.110   **Laceration without foreign body of abdominal wall, right upper quadrant without penetration into peritoneal cavity**

    √7th S31.111   **Laceration without foreign body of abdominal wall, left upper quadrant without penetration into peritoneal cavity**

    √7th S31.112   **Laceration without foreign body of abdominal wall, epigastric region without penetration into peritoneal cavity**

    √7th S31.113   **Laceration without foreign body of abdominal wall, right lower quadrant without penetration into peritoneal cavity**

    √7th S31.114   **Laceration without foreign body of abdominal wall, left lower quadrant without penetration into peritoneal cavity**

    √7th S31.115   **Laceration without foreign body of abdominal wall, periumbilic region without penetration into peritoneal cavity**

    √7th S31.119   **Laceration without foreign body of abdominal wall, unspecified quadrant without penetration into peritoneal cavity**

  √6th S31.12   **Laceration with foreign body** of abdominal wall without penetration into peritoneal cavity

    √7th S31.120   **Laceration of abdominal wall with foreign body, right upper quadrant without penetration into peritoneal cavity**

    √7th S31.121   **Laceration of abdominal wall with foreign body, left upper quadrant without penetration into peritoneal cavity**

    √7th S31.122   **Laceration of abdominal wall with foreign body, epigastric region without penetration into peritoneal cavity**

    √7th S31.123   **Laceration of abdominal wall with foreign body, right lower quadrant without penetration into peritoneal cavity**

    √7th S31.124   **Laceration of abdominal wall with foreign body, left lower quadrant without penetration into peritoneal cavity**

N Newborn: 0   P Pediatric: 0-17   M Maternity: 12-55   A Adult: 15-124   MCC Major Complication/Comorbidity   CC Complication/Comorbidity   SW Severe Wound Dx

976   ICD-10-CM 2019

√7ᵗʰ **S31.125** Laceration of abdominal wall with foreign body, periumbilic region without penetration into peritoneal cavity

√7ᵗʰ **S31.129** Laceration of abdominal wall with foreign body, unspecified quadrant without penetration into peritoneal cavity

√6ᵗʰ **S31.13** Puncture wound of abdominal wall without foreign body without penetration into peritoneal cavity

√7ᵗʰ **S31.130** Puncture wound of abdominal wall without foreign body, right upper quadrant without penetration into peritoneal cavity

√7ᵗʰ **S31.131** Puncture wound of abdominal wall without foreign body, left upper quadrant without penetration into peritoneal cavity

√7ᵗʰ **S31.132** Puncture wound of abdominal wall without foreign body, epigastric region without penetration into peritoneal cavity

√7ᵗʰ **S31.133** Puncture wound of abdominal wall without foreign body, right lower quadrant without penetration into peritoneal cavity

√7ᵗʰ **S31.134** Puncture wound of abdominal wall without foreign body, left lower quadrant without penetration into peritoneal cavity

√7ᵗʰ **S31.135** Puncture wound of abdominal wall without foreign body, periumbilic region without penetration into peritoneal cavity

√7ᵗʰ **S31.139** Puncture wound of abdominal wall without foreign body, unspecified quadrant without penetration into peritoneal cavity

√6ᵗʰ **S31.14** Puncture wound of abdominal wall with foreign body without penetration into peritoneal cavity

√7ᵗʰ **S31.140** Puncture wound of abdominal wall with foreign body, right upper quadrant without penetration into peritoneal cavity

√7ᵗʰ **S31.141** Puncture wound of abdominal wall with foreign body, left upper quadrant without penetration into peritoneal cavity

√7ᵗʰ **S31.142** Puncture wound of abdominal wall with foreign body, epigastric region without penetration into peritoneal cavity

√7ᵗʰ **S31.143** Puncture wound of abdominal wall with foreign body, right lower quadrant without penetration into peritoneal cavity

√7ᵗʰ **S31.144** Puncture wound of abdominal wall with foreign body, left lower quadrant without penetration into peritoneal cavity

√7ᵗʰ **S31.145** Puncture wound of abdominal wall with foreign body, periumbilic region without penetration into peritoneal cavity

√7ᵗʰ **S31.149** Puncture wound of abdominal wall with foreign body, unspecified quadrant without penetration into peritoneal cavity

√6ᵗʰ **S31.15** Open bite of abdominal wall without penetration into peritoneal cavity
Bite of abdominal wall NOS
EXCLUDES 1   superficial bite of abdominal wall (S30.871)

√7ᵗʰ **S31.150** Open bite of abdominal wall, right upper quadrant without penetration into peritoneal cavity

√7ᵗʰ **S31.151** Open bite of abdominal wall, left upper quadrant without penetration into peritoneal cavity

√7ᵗʰ **S31.152** Open bite of abdominal wall, epigastric region without penetration into peritoneal cavity

√7ᵗʰ **S31.153** Open bite of abdominal wall, right lower quadrant without penetration into peritoneal cavity

√7ᵗʰ **S31.154** Open bite of abdominal wall, left lower quadrant without penetration into peritoneal cavity

√7ᵗʰ **S31.155** Open bite of abdominal wall, periumbilic region without penetration into peritoneal cavity

√7ᵗʰ **S31.159** Open bite of abdominal wall, unspecified quadrant without penetration into peritoneal cavity

√5ᵗʰ **S31.2** Open wound of penis

√x7ᵗʰ **S31.20** Unspecified open wound of penis   ♂

√x7ᵗʰ **S31.21** Laceration without foreign body of penis   ♂

√x7ᵗʰ **S31.22** Laceration with foreign body of penis   ♂

√x7ᵗʰ **S31.23** Puncture wound without foreign body of penis   ♂

√x7ᵗʰ **S31.24** Puncture wound with foreign body of penis   ♂

√x7ᵗʰ **S31.25** Open bite of penis   ♂
Bite of penis NOS
EXCLUDES 1   superficial bite of penis (S30.862, S30.872)

√5ᵗʰ **S31.3** Open wound of scrotum and testes

√x7ᵗʰ **S31.30** Unspecified open wound of scrotum and testes   ♂

√x7ᵗʰ **S31.31** Laceration without foreign body of scrotum and testes   ♂

√x7ᵗʰ **S31.32** Laceration with foreign body of scrotum and testes   ♂

√x7ᵗʰ **S31.33** Puncture wound without foreign body of scrotum and testes   ♂

√x7ᵗʰ **S31.34** Puncture wound with foreign body of scrotum and testes   ♂

√x7ᵗʰ **S31.35** Open bite of scrotum and testes   ♂
Bite of scrotum and testes NOS
EXCLUDES 1   superficial bite of scrotum and testes (S30.863, S30.873)

√5ᵗʰ **S31.4** Open wound of vagina and vulva
EXCLUDES 1   injury to vagina and vulva during delivery (O70-, O71.4)

√x7ᵗʰ **S31.40** Unspecified open wound of vagina and vulva   ♀

√x7ᵗʰ **S31.41** Laceration without foreign body of vagina and vulva   ♀

√x7ᵗʰ **S31.42** Laceration with foreign body of vagina and vulva   ♀

√x7ᵗʰ **S31.43** Puncture wound without foreign body of vagina and vulva   ♀

√x7ᵗʰ **S31.44** Puncture wound with foreign body of vagina and vulva   ♀

√x7ᵗʰ **S31.45** Open bite of vagina and vulva   ♀
Bite of vagina and vulva NOS
EXCLUDES 1   superficial bite of vagina and vulva (S30.864, S30.874)

√5ᵗʰ **S31.5** Open wound of unspecified external genital organs
EXCLUDES 1   traumatic amputation of external genital organs (S38.21, S38.22)

√6ᵗʰ **S31.50** Unspecified open wound of unspecified external genital organs

√7ᵗʰ **S31.501** Unspecified open wound of unspecified external genital organs, male   ♂

√7ᵗʰ **S31.502** Unspecified open wound of unspecified external genital organs, female   ♀

√6ᵗʰ **S31.51** Laceration without foreign body of unspecified external genital organs

√7ᵗʰ **S31.511** Laceration without foreign body of unspecified external genital organs, male   ♂

√7ᵗʰ **S31.512** Laceration without foreign body of unspecified external genital organs, female   ♀

√6ᵗʰ **S31.52** Laceration with foreign body of unspecified external genital organs

√7ᵗʰ **S31.521** Laceration with foreign body of unspecified external genital organs, male   ♂

√7ᵗʰ **S31.522** Laceration with foreign body of unspecified external genital organs, female   ♀

√6ᵗʰ **S31.53** Puncture wound without foreign body of unspecified external genital organs

√7ᵗʰ **S31.531** Puncture wound without foreign body of unspecified external genital organs, male   ♂

✔Additional Character Required   √x7ᵗʰ Placeholder   Unacceptable PDx   Questionable PDx   Manifestation   **H1**-**H14** HAC   **HCC** CMS-HCC Dx   **HIV** HIV Dx

ICD-10-CM 2019   **977**

√7ᵗʰ S31.532 Puncture wound without foreign body of unspecified external genital organs, female ♀

√6ᵗʰ S31.54 Puncture wound with foreign body of unspecified external genital organs

    √7ᵗʰ S31.541 Puncture wound with foreign body of unspecified external genital organs, male ♂

    √7ᵗʰ S31.542 Puncture wound with foreign body of unspecified external genital organs, female ♀

√6ᵗʰ S31.55 Open bite of unspecified external genital organs
    Bite of unspecified external genital organs NOS
    EXCLUDES 1   superficial bite of unspecified external genital organs (S30.865, S30.866, S30.875, S30.876)

    √7ᵗʰ S31.551 Open bite of unspecified external genital organs, male ♂

    √7ᵗʰ S31.552 Open bite of unspecified external genital organs, female ♀

√5ᵗʰ S31.6 Open wound of abdominal wall with penetration into peritoneal cavity

    √6ᵗʰ S31.60 Unspecified open wound of abdominal wall with penetration into peritoneal cavity

        √7ᵗʰ S31.600 Unspecified open wound of abdominal wall, right upper quadrant with penetration into peritoneal cavity   MCC

        √7ᵗʰ S31.601 Unspecified open wound of abdominal wall, left upper quadrant with penetration into peritoneal cavity   MCC

        √7ᵗʰ S31.602 Unspecified open wound of abdominal wall, epigastric region with penetration into peritoneal cavity   MCC

        √7ᵗʰ S31.603 Unspecified open wound of abdominal wall, right lower quadrant with penetration into peritoneal cavity   MCC

        √7ᵗʰ S31.604 Unspecified open wound of abdominal wall, left lower quadrant with penetration into peritoneal cavity   MCC

        √7ᵗʰ S31.605 Unspecified open wound of abdominal wall, periumbilic region with penetration into peritoneal cavity   MCC

        √7ᵗʰ S31.609 Unspecified open wound of abdominal wall, unspecified quadrant with penetration into peritoneal cavity   MCC

    √6ᵗʰ S31.61 Laceration without foreign body of abdominal wall with penetration into peritoneal cavity

        √7ᵗʰ S31.610 Laceration without foreign body of abdominal wall, right upper quadrant with penetration into peritoneal cavity   MCC

        √7ᵗʰ S31.611 Laceration without foreign body of abdominal wall, left upper quadrant with penetration into peritoneal cavity   MCC

        √7ᵗʰ S31.612 Laceration without foreign body of abdominal wall, epigastric region with penetration into peritoneal cavity   MCC

        √7ᵗʰ S31.613 Laceration without foreign body of abdominal wall, right lower quadrant with penetration into peritoneal cavity   MCC

        √7ᵗʰ S31.614 Laceration without foreign body of abdominal wall, left lower quadrant with penetration into peritoneal cavity   MCC

        √7ᵗʰ S31.615 Laceration without foreign body of abdominal wall, periumbilic region with penetration into peritoneal cavity   MCC

        √7ᵗʰ S31.619 Laceration without foreign body of abdominal wall, unspecified quadrant with penetration into peritoneal cavity   MCC

    √6ᵗʰ S31.62 Laceration with foreign body of abdominal wall with penetration into peritoneal cavity

        √7ᵗʰ S31.620 Laceration with foreign body of abdominal wall, right upper quadrant with penetration into peritoneal cavity   MCC

        √7ᵗʰ S31.621 Laceration with foreign body of abdominal wall, left upper quadrant with penetration into peritoneal cavity   MCC

        √7ᵗʰ S31.622 Laceration with foreign body of abdominal wall, epigastric region with penetration into peritoneal cavity   MCC

        √7ᵗʰ S31.623 Laceration with foreign body of abdominal wall, right lower quadrant with penetration into peritoneal cavity   MCC

        √7ᵗʰ S31.624 Laceration with foreign body of abdominal wall, left lower quadrant with penetration into peritoneal cavity   MCC

        √7ᵗʰ S31.625 Laceration with foreign body of abdominal wall, periumbilic region with penetration into peritoneal cavity   MCC

        √7ᵗʰ S31.629 Laceration with foreign body of abdominal wall, unspecified quadrant with penetration into peritoneal cavity   MCC

    √6ᵗʰ S31.63 Puncture wound without foreign body of abdominal wall with penetration into peritoneal cavity

        √7ᵗʰ S31.630 Puncture wound without foreign body of abdominal wall, right upper quadrant with penetration into peritoneal cavity   MCC

        √7ᵗʰ S31.631 Puncture wound without foreign body of abdominal wall, left upper quadrant with penetration into peritoneal cavity   MCC

        √7ᵗʰ S31.632 Puncture wound without foreign body of abdominal wall, epigastric region with penetration into peritoneal cavity   MCC

        √7ᵗʰ S31.633 Puncture wound without foreign body of abdominal wall, right lower quadrant with penetration into peritoneal cavity   MCC

        √7ᵗʰ S31.634 Puncture wound without foreign body of abdominal wall, left lower quadrant with penetration into peritoneal cavity   MCC

        √7ᵗʰ S31.635 Puncture wound without foreign body of abdominal wall, periumbilic region with penetration into peritoneal cavity   MCC

        √7ᵗʰ S31.639 Puncture wound without foreign body of abdominal wall, unspecified quadrant with penetration into peritoneal cavity   MCC

    √6ᵗʰ S31.64 Puncture wound with foreign body of abdominal wall with penetration into peritoneal cavity

        √7ᵗʰ S31.640 Puncture wound with foreign body of abdominal wall, right upper quadrant with penetration into peritoneal cavity   MCC

        √7ᵗʰ S31.641 Puncture wound with foreign body of abdominal wall, left upper quadrant with penetration into peritoneal cavity   MCC

        √7ᵗʰ S31.642 Puncture wound with foreign body of abdominal wall, epigastric region with penetration into peritoneal cavity   MCC

        √7ᵗʰ S31.643 Puncture wound with foreign body of abdominal wall, right lower quadrant with penetration into peritoneal cavity   MCC

        √7ᵗʰ S31.644 Puncture wound with foreign body of abdominal wall, left lower quadrant with penetration into peritoneal cavity   MCC

        √7ᵗʰ S31.645 Puncture wound with foreign body of abdominal wall, periumbilic region with penetration into peritoneal cavity   MCC

        √7ᵗʰ S31.649 Puncture wound with foreign body of abdominal wall, unspecified quadrant with penetration into peritoneal cavity   MCC

    √6ᵗʰ S31.65 Open bite of abdominal wall with penetration into peritoneal cavity
        EXCLUDES 1   superficial bite of abdominal wall (S30.861, S30.871)

        √7ᵗʰ S31.650 Open bite of abdominal wall, right upper quadrant with penetration into peritoneal cavity   MCC

        √7ᵗʰ S31.651 Open bite of abdominal wall, left upper quadrant with penetration into peritoneal cavity   MCC

N Newborn: 0   P Pediatric: 0-17   M Maternity: 12-55   A Adult: 15-124   MCC Major Complication/Comorbidity   CC Complication/Comorbidity   SW Severe Wound Dx

978   ICD-10-CM 2019

✓7ᵗʰ **S31.652 Open bite of abdominal wall, epigastric region with penetration into peritoneal cavity** MCC

✓7ᵗʰ **S31.653 Open bite of abdominal wall, right lower quadrant with penetration into peritoneal cavity** MCC

✓7ᵗʰ **S31.654 Open bite of abdominal wall, left lower quadrant with penetration into peritoneal cavity** MCC

✓7ᵗʰ **S31.655 Open bite of abdominal wall, periumbilic region with penetration into peritoneal cavity** MCC

✓7ᵗʰ **S31.659 Open bite of abdominal wall, unspecified quadrant with penetration into peritoneal cavity** MCC

✓5ᵗʰ **S31.8 Open wound of other parts of abdomen, lower back and pelvis**

✓6ᵗʰ **S31.80 Open wound of unspecified buttock**

✓7ᵗʰ **S31.801 Laceration without foreign body of unspecified buttock**

✓7ᵗʰ **S31.802 Laceration with foreign body of unspecified buttock**

✓7ᵗʰ **S31.803 Puncture wound without foreign body of unspecified buttock**

✓7ᵗʰ **S31.804 Puncture wound with foreign body of unspecified buttock**

✓7ᵗʰ **S31.805 Open bite of unspecified buttock**
Bite of buttock NOS
EXCLUDES 1   *superficial bite of buttock (S30.870)*

✓7ᵗʰ **S31.809 Unspecified open wound of unspecified buttock**

✓6ᵗʰ **S31.81 Open wound of right buttock**

✓7ᵗʰ **S31.811 Laceration without foreign body of right buttock**

✓7ᵗʰ **S31.812 Laceration with foreign body of right buttock**

✓7ᵗʰ **S31.813 Puncture wound without foreign body of right buttock**

✓7ᵗʰ **S31.814 Puncture wound with foreign body of right buttock**

✓7ᵗʰ **S31.815 Open bite of right buttock**
Bite of right buttock NOS
EXCLUDES 1   *superficial bite of buttock (S30.870)*

✓7ᵗʰ **S31.819 Unspecified open wound of right buttock**

✓6ᵗʰ **S31.82 Open wound of left buttock**

✓7ᵗʰ **S31.821 Laceration without foreign body of left buttock**

✓7ᵗʰ **S31.822 Laceration with foreign body of left buttock**

✓7ᵗʰ **S31.823 Puncture wound without foreign body of left buttock**

✓7ᵗʰ **S31.824 Puncture wound with foreign body of left buttock**

✓7ᵗʰ **S31.825 Open bite of left buttock**
Bite of left buttock NOS
EXCLUDES 1   *superficial bite of buttock (S30.870)*

✓7ᵗʰ **S31.829 Unspecified open wound of left buttock**

✓6ᵗʰ **S31.83 Open wound of anus**

✓7ᵗʰ **S31.831 Laceration without foreign body of anus**

✓7ᵗʰ **S31.832 Laceration with foreign body of anus**

✓7ᵗʰ **S31.833 Puncture wound without foreign body of anus**

✓7ᵗʰ **S31.834 Puncture wound with foreign body of anus**

✓7ᵗʰ **S31.835 Open bite of anus**
Bite of anus NOS
EXCLUDES 1   *superficial bite of anus (S30.877)*

✓7ᵗʰ **S31.839 Unspecified open wound of anus**

✓4ᵗʰ **S32 Fracture of lumbar spine and pelvis**

NOTE   A fracture not indicated as displaced or nondisplaced should be coded to displaced.
A fracture not indicated as opened or closed should be coded to closed.

INCLUDES   fracture of lumbosacral neural arch
fracture of lumbosacral spinous process
fracture of lumbosacral transverse process
fracture of lumbosacral vertebra
fracture of lumbosacral vertebral arch

Code first any associated spinal cord and spinal nerve injury (S34.-)

EXCLUDES 1   *transection of abdomen (S38.3)*

EXCLUDES 2   *fracture of hip NOS (S72.0-)*

AHA: 2018, 2Q, 12; 2015, 3Q, 37-39; 2012, 4Q, 93

The appropriate 7th character is to be added to each code from category S32.
A   initial encounter for closed fracture
B   initial encounter for open fracture
D   subsequent encounter for fracture with routine healing
G   subsequent encounter for fracture with delayed healing
K   subsequent encounter for fracture with nonunion
S   sequela

✓5ᵗʰ **S32.0 Fracture of lumbar vertebra**
Fracture of lumbar spine NOS

CC Excl: For codes in subcategory S32.0:
CC with 7th character A or MCC with 7th character B: PDX collection 1196
CC with 7th character K: PDX collection 897

✓6ᵗʰ **S32.00 Fracture of unspecified lumbar vertebra**

2,3,6 ✓7ᵗʰ **S32.000 Wedge compression fracture of unspecified lumbar vertebra** MCC CC H5 HCC

2,3,6 ✓7ᵗʰ **S32.001 Stable burst fracture of unspecified lumbar vertebra** MCC CC H5 HCC

2,3,6 ✓7ᵗʰ **S32.002 Unstable burst fracture of unspecified lumbar vertebra** MCC CC H5 HCC

2,3,6 ✓7ᵗʰ **S32.008 Other fracture of unspecified lumbar vertebra** MCC CC H5 HCC

2,3,6 ✓7ᵗʰ **S32.009 Unspecified fracture of unspecified lumbar vertebra** MCC CC H5 HCC

✓6ᵗʰ **S32.01 Fracture of first lumbar vertebra**

2,3,6 ✓7ᵗʰ **S32.010 Wedge compression fracture of first lumbar vertebra** MCC CC H5 HCC

2,3,6 ✓7ᵗʰ **S32.011 Stable burst fracture of first lumbar vertebra** MCC CC H5 HCC

2,3,6 ✓7ᵗʰ **S32.012 Unstable burst fracture of first lumbar vertebra** MCC CC H5 HCC

2,3,6 ✓7ᵗʰ **S32.018 Other fracture of first lumbar vertebra** MCC CC H5 HCC

2,3,6 ✓7ᵗʰ **S32.019 Unspecified fracture of first lumbar vertebra** MCC CC H5 HCC

✓6ᵗʰ **S32.02 Fracture of second lumbar vertebra**

2,3,6 ✓7ᵗʰ **S32.020 Wedge compression fracture of second lumbar vertebra** MCC CC H5 HCC

2,3,6 ✓7ᵗʰ **S32.021 Stable burst fracture of second lumbar vertebra** MCC CC H5 HCC

2,3,6 ✓7ᵗʰ **S32.022 Unstable burst fracture of second lumbar vertebra** MCC CC H5 HCC

2,3,6 ✓7ᵗʰ **S32.028 Other fracture of second lumbar vertebra** MCC CC H5 HCC

2,3,6 ✓7ᵗʰ **S32.029 Unspecified fracture of second lumbar vertebra** MCC CC H5 HCC

✓6ᵗʰ **S32.03 Fracture of third lumbar vertebra**

2,3,6 ✓7ᵗʰ **S32.030 Wedge compression fracture of third lumbar vertebra** MCC CC H5 HCC

2,3,6 ✓7ᵗʰ **S32.031 Stable burst fracture of third lumbar vertebra** MCC CC H5 HCC

2,3,6 ✓7ᵗʰ **S32.032 Unstable burst fracture of third lumbar vertebra** MCC CC H5 HCC

2,3,6 ✓7ᵗʰ **S32.038 Other fracture of third lumbar vertebra** MCC CC H5 HCC

2,3,6 ✓7ᵗʰ **S32.039 Unspecified fracture of third lumbar vertebra** MCC CC H5 HCC

✓6ᵗʰ **S32.04 Fracture of fourth lumbar vertebra**

2,3,6 ✓7ᵗʰ **S32.040 Wedge compression fracture of fourth lumbar vertebra** MCC CC H5 HCC

☑ Additional Character Required   ✓x7ᵗʰ Placeholder   Unacceptable PDx   Questionable PDx   Manifestation   H1 - H14 HAC   HCC CMS-HCC Dx   HIV HIV Dx

ICD-10-CM 2019   979

2,3,6 ✓7ᵗʰ **S32.041**   **Stable burst** fracture of fourth lumbar vertebra   MCC CC H5 HCC

2,3,6 ✓7ᵗʰ **S32.042**   **Unstable burst** fracture of fourth lumbar vertebra   MCC CC H5 HCC

2,3,6 ✓7ᵗʰ **S32.048**   **Other** fracture of fourth lumbar vertebra   MCC CC H5 HCC

2,3,6 ✓7ᵗʰ **S32.049**   **Unspecified** fracture of fourth lumbar vertebra   MCC CC H5 HCC

✓6ᵗʰ **S32.05**   Fracture of fifth lumbar vertebra

2,3,6 ✓7ᵗʰ **S32.050**   **Wedge compression** fracture of fifth lumbar vertebra   MCC CC H5 HCC

2,3,6 ✓7ᵗʰ **S32.051**   **Stable burst** fracture of fifth lumbar vertebra   MCC CC H5 HCC

2,3,6 ✓7ᵗʰ **S32.052**   **Unstable burst** fracture of fifth lumbar vertebra   MCC CC H5 HCC

2,3,6 ✓7ᵗʰ **S32.058**   **Other** fracture of fifth lumbar vertebra   MCC CC H5 HCC

2,3,6 ✓7ᵗʰ **S32.059**   **Unspecified** fracture of fifth lumbar vertebra   MCC CC H5 HCC

✓5ᵗʰ **S32.1**   **Fracture of** sacrum

> **NOTE**   For vertical fractures, code to most medial fracture extension.
> Use two codes if both a vertical and transverse fracture are present.
> Code also any associated fracture of pelvic ring (S32.8-)

> **CC Excl: For codes in subcategory S32.1:**
> **CC with 7th character A or MCC with 7th character B:** PDX collection 1197
> **CC with 7th character K:** PDX collection 897

2,3,6 ✓x7ᵗʰ **S32.10**   **Unspecified** fracture of sacrum   MCC CC H5 HCC

✓6ᵗʰ **S32.11**   **Zone I** fracture of sacrum
Vertical sacral ala fracture of sacrum

2,3,6 ✓7ᵗʰ **S32.110**   **Nondisplaced Zone I** fracture of sacrum   MCC CC H5 HCC

2,3,6 ✓7ᵗʰ **S32.111**   **Minimally displaced Zone I** fracture of sacrum   MCC CC H5 HCC

2,3,6 ✓7ᵗʰ **S32.112**   **Severely displaced Zone I** fracture of sacrum   MCC CC H5 HCC

2,3,6 ✓7ᵗʰ **S32.119**   **Unspecified Zone I** fracture of sacrum   MCC CC H5 HCC

Vertical Sacral Fracture Zones

Zones: ① ② ③

Transverse Sacral Fracture Types

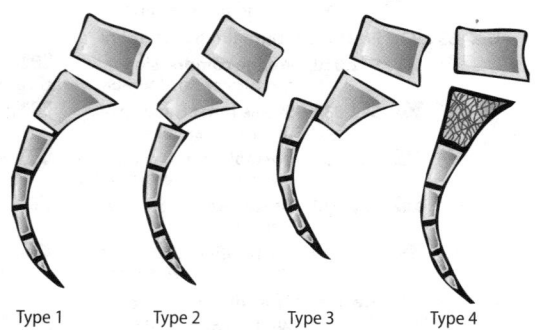

Type 1   Type 2   Type 3   Type 4

✓6ᵗʰ **S32.12**   **Zone II** fracture of sacrum
Vertical foraminal region fracture of sacrum

2,3,6 ✓7ᵗʰ **S32.120**   **Nondisplaced Zone II** fracture of sacrum   MCC CC H5 HCC

2,3,6 ✓7ᵗʰ **S32.121**   **Minimally displaced Zone II** fracture of sacrum   MCC CC H5 HCC

2,3,6 ✓7ᵗʰ **S32.122**   **Severely displaced Zone II** fracture of sacrum   MCC CC H5 HCC

2,3,6 ✓7ᵗʰ **S32.129**   **Unspecified Zone II** fracture of sacrum   MCC CC H5 HCC

✓6ᵗʰ **S32.13**   **Zone III** fracture of sacrum
Vertical fracture into spinal canal region of sacrum

2,3,6 ✓7ᵗʰ **S32.130**   **Nondisplaced Zone III** fracture of sacrum   MCC CC H5 HCC

2,3,6 ✓7ᵗʰ **S32.131**   **Minimally displaced Zone III** fracture of sacrum   MCC CC H5 HCC

2,3,6 ✓7ᵗʰ **S32.132**   **Severely displaced Zone III** fracture of sacrum   MCC CC H5 HCC

2,3,6 ✓7ᵗʰ **S32.139**   **Unspecified Zone III** fracture of sacrum   MCC CC H5 HCC

2,3,6 ✓x7ᵗʰ **S32.14**   **Type 1** fracture of sacrum   MCC CC H5 HCC
Transverse flexion fracture of sacrum without displacement

2,3,6 ✓x7ᵗʰ **S32.15**   **Type 2** fracture of sacrum   MCC CC H5 HCC
Transverse flexion fracture of sacrum with posterior displacement

2,3,6 ✓x7ᵗʰ **S32.16**   **Type 3** fracture of sacrum   MCC CC H5 HCC
Transverse extension fracture of sacrum with anterior displacement

2,3,6 ✓x7ᵗʰ **S32.17**   **Type 4** fracture of sacrum   MCC CC H5 HCC
Transverse segmental comminution of upper sacrum

2,3,6 ✓x7ᵗʰ **S32.19**   **Other** fracture of sacrum   MCC CC H5 HCC

2,3,6 ✓x7ᵗʰ **S32.2**   **Fracture of** coccyx   MCC CC H5 HCC
CC Excl: See code S32.1

✓5ᵗʰ **S32.3**   **Fracture of** ilium

> **EXCLUDES 1**   fracture of ilium with associated disruption of pelvic ring (S32.8-)

> **CC Excl: For codes in subcategory S32.3:**
> **CC with 7th character A:** PDX collection 1176
> **MCC with 7th character B:** PDX collection 1198
> **CC with 7th character K:** PDX collection 897

✓6ᵗʰ **S32.30**   **Unspecified** fracture of ilium

2,3,6 ✓7ᵗʰ **S32.301**   **Unspecified** fracture of **right** ilium   MCC CC H5 HCC

2,3,6 ✓7ᵗʰ **S32.302**   **Unspecified** fracture of **left** ilium   MCC CC H5 HCC

2,3,6 ✓7ᵗʰ **S32.309**   **Unspecified** fracture of **unspecified** ilium   MCC CC H5 HCC

✓6ᵗʰ **S32.31**   **Avulsion** fracture of ilium

2,3,6 ✓7ᵗʰ **S32.311**   **Displaced avulsion** fracture of **right** ilium   MCC CC H5 HCC

2,3,6 ✓7ᵗʰ **S32.312**   **Displaced avulsion** fracture of **left** ilium   MCC CC H5 HCC

2,3,6 ✓7ᵗʰ **S32.313**   **Displaced avulsion** fracture of **unspecified** ilium   MCC CC H5 HCC

2,3,6 ✓7ᵗʰ **S32.314**   **Nondisplaced avulsion** fracture of **right** ilium   MCC CC H5 HCC

2,3,6 ✓7ᵗʰ **S32.315**   **Nondisplaced avulsion** fracture of **left** ilium   MCC CC H5 HCC

2,3,6 ✓7ᵗʰ **S32.316**   **Nondisplaced avulsion** fracture of **unspecified** ilium   MCC CC H5 HCC

✓6ᵗʰ **S32.39**   **Other** fracture of ilium

2,3,6 ✓7ᵗʰ **S32.391**   **Other** fracture of **right** ilium   MCC CC H5 HCC

2,3,6 ✓7ᵗʰ **S32.392**   **Other** fracture of **left** ilium   MCC CC H5 HCC

2,3,6 ✓7ᵗʰ **S32.399**   **Other** fracture of **unspecified** ilium   MCC CC H5 HCC

N Newborn: 0   **P** Pediatric: 0-17   **M** Maternity: 12-55   **A** Adult: 15-124   **MCC** Major Complication/Comorbidity   **CC** Complication/Comorbidity   **SW** Severe Wound Dx

980   ICD-10-CM 2019

✓5th **S32.4**   **Fracture of** acetabulum

Code also any associated fracture of pelvic ring (S32.8-)

AHA: 2016, 3Q, 16

CC Excl: For codes in subcategory S32.4:
MCC with 7th character A: PDX collection 1199
MCC with 7th character B: PDX collection 1200
CC with 7th character K: PDX collection 897

✓6th **S32.40**   **Unspecified** fracture of acetabulum

4,6 ✓7th   **S32.401**   **Unspecified fracture of right** acetabulum   `MCC` `CC` `H5` `HCC`

4,6 ✓7th   **S32.402**   **Unspecified fracture of left** acetabulum   `MCC` `CC` `H5` `HCC`

4,6 ✓7th   **S32.409**   **Unspecified fracture of unspecified** acetabulum   `MCC` `CC` `H5` `HCC`

✓6th **S32.41**   **Fracture of** anterior wall **of acetabulum**

4,6 ✓7th   **S32.411**   **Displaced fracture of anterior wall of right acetabulum**   `MCC` `CC` `H5` `HCC`

4,6 ✓7th   **S32.412**   **Displaced fracture of anterior wall of left acetabulum**   `MCC` `CC` `H5` `HCC`

4,6 ✓7th   **S32.413**   **Displaced fracture of anterior wall of unspecified acetabulum**   `MCC` `CC` `H5` `HCC`

4,6 ✓7th   **S32.414**   **Nondisplaced fracture of anterior wall of right acetabulum**   `MCC` `CC` `H5` `HCC`

4,6 ✓7th   **S32.415**   **Nondisplaced fracture of anterior wall of left acetabulum**   `MCC` `CC` `H5` `HCC`

4,6 ✓7th   **S32.416**   **Nondisplaced fracture of anterior wall of unspecified acetabulum**   `MCC` `CC` `H5` `HCC`

✓6th **S32.42**   **Fracture of** posterior wall **of acetabulum**

4,6 ✓7th   **S32.421**   **Displaced fracture of posterior wall of right acetabulum**   `MCC` `CC` `H5` `HCC`

4,6 ✓7th   **S32.422**   **Displaced fracture of posteriorwall of left acetabulum**   `MCC` `CC` `H5` `HCC`

4,6 ✓7th   **S32.423**   **Displaced fracture of posterior wall of unspecified acetabulum**   `MCC` `CC` `H5` `HCC`

4,6 ✓7th   **S32.424**   **Nondisplaced fracture of posterior wall of right acetabulum**   `MCC` `CC` `H5` `HCC`

4,6 ✓7th   **S32.425**   **Nondisplaced fracture of posterior wall of left acetabulum**   `MCC` `CC` `H5` `HCC`

4,6 ✓7th   **S32.426**   **Nondisplaced fracture of posterior wall of unspecified acetabulum**   `MCC` `CC` `H5` `HCC`

✓6th **S32.43**   **Fracture of** anterior column [iliopubic] **of acetabulum**

4,6 ✓7th   **S32.431**   **Displaced fracture of anterior column [iliopubic] of right acetabulum**   `MCC` `CC` `H5` `HCC`

4,6 ✓7th   **S32.432**   **Displaced fracture of anterior column [iliopubic] of left acetabulum**   `MCC` `CC` `H5` `HCC`

4,6 ✓7th   **S32.433**   **Displaced fracture of anterior column [iliopubic] of unspecified acetabulum**   `MCC` `CC` `H5` `HCC`

4,6 ✓7th   **S32.434**   **Nondisplaced fracture of anterior column [iliopubic] of right acetabulum**   `MCC` `CC` `H5` `HCC`

4,6 ✓7th   **S32.435**   **Nondisplaced fracture of anterior column [iliopubic] of left acetabulum**   `MCC` `CC` `H5` `HCC`

4,6 ✓7th   **S32.436**   **Nondisplaced fracture of anterior column [iliopubic] of unspecified acetabulum**   `MCC` `CC` `H5` `HCC`

✓6th **S32.44**   **Fracture of** posterior column [ilioischial] **of acetabulum**

4,6 ✓7th   **S32.441**   **Displaced fracture of posterior column [ilioischial] of right acetabulum**   `MCC` `CC` `H5` `HCC`

4,6 ✓7th   **S32.442**   **Displaced fracture of posteriorcolumn [ilioischial] of left acetabulum**   `MCC` `CC` `H5` `HCC`

4,6 ✓7th   **S32.443**   **Displaced fracture of posterior column [ilioischial] of unspecified acetabulum**   `MCC` `CC` `H5` `HCC`

4,6 ✓7th   **S32.444**   **Nondisplaced fracture of posterior column [ilioischial] of right acetabulum**   `MCC` `CC` `H5` `HCC`

4,6 ✓7th   **S32.445**   **Nondisplaced fracture of posterior column [ilioischial] of left acetabulum**   `MCC` `CC` `H5` `HCC`

4,6 ✓7th   **S32.446**   **Nondisplaced fracture of posterior column [ilioischial] of unspecified acetabulum**   `MCC` `CC` `H5` `HCC`

✓6th **S32.45**   **Transverse** fracture of acetabulum

4,6 ✓7th   **S32.451**   **Displaced transverse fracture of right acetabulum**   `MCC` `CC` `H5` `HCC`

4,6 ✓7th   **S32.452**   **Displaced transverse fractureof left acetabulum**   `MCC` `CC` `H5` `HCC`

4,6 ✓7th   **S32.453**   **Displaced transverse fracture of unspecified acetabulum**   `MCC` `CC` `H5` `HCC`

4,6 ✓7th   **S32.454**   **Nondisplaced transverse fracture of right acetabulum**   `MCC` `CC` `H5` `HCC`

4,6 ✓7th   **S32.455**   **Nondisplaced transverse fracture of left acetabulum**   `MCC` `CC` `H5` `HCC`

4,6 ✓7th   **S32.456**   **Nondisplaced transverse fracture of unspecified acetabulum**   `MCC` `CC` `H5` `HCC`

✓6th **S32.46**   **Associated transverse-posterior** fracture of acetabulum

4,6 ✓7th   **S32.461**   **Displaced associated transverse-posterior fracture of right acetabulum**   `MCC` `CC` `H5` `HCC`

4,6 ✓7th   **S32.462**   **Displaced associated transverse-posterior fracture of left acetabulum**   `MCC` `CC` `H5` `HCC`

4,6 ✓7th   **S32.463**   **Displaced associated transverse-posterior fracture of unspecified acetabulum**   `MCC` `CC` `H5` `HCC`

4,6 ✓7th   **S32.464**   **Nondisplaced associated transverse-posterior fracture of right acetabulum**   `MCC` `CC` `H5` `HCC`

4,6 ✓7th   **S32.465**   **Nondisplaced associated transverse-posterior fracture of left acetabulum**   `MCC` `CC` `H5` `HCC`

4,6 ✓7th   **S32.466**   **Nondisplaced associated transverse-posterior fracture of unspecified acetabulum**   `MCC` `CC` `H5` `HCC`

✓6th **S32.47**   **Fracture of** medial wall **of acetabulum**

4,6 ✓7th   **S32.471**   **Displaced fracture of medial wall of right acetabulum**   `MCC` `CC` `H5` `HCC`

4,6 ✓7th   **S32.472**   **Displaced fracture of medial wall of left acetabulum**   `MCC` `CC` `H5` `HCC`

4,6 ✓7th   **S32.473**   **Displaced fracture of medial wall of unspecified acetabulum**   `MCC` `CC` `H5` `HCC`

4,6 ✓7th   **S32.474**   **Nondisplaced fracture of medial wall of right acetabulum**   `MCC` `CC` `H5` `HCC`

4,6 ✓7th   **S32.475**   **Nondisplaced fracture of medial wall of left acetabulum**   `MCC` `CC` `H5` `HCC`

4,6 ✓7th   **S32.476**   **Nondisplaced fracture of medial wall of unspecified acetabulum**   `MCC` `CC` `H5` `HCC`

✓6th **S32.48**   **Dome fracture of acetabulum**

4,6 ✓7th   **S32.481**   **Displaced dome fracture of right acetabulum**   `MCC` `CC` `H5` `HCC`

4,6 ✓7th   **S32.482**   **Displaced dome fracture of left acetabulum**   `MCC` `CC` `H5` `HCC`

4,6 ✓7th   **S32.483**   **Displaced dome fracture of unspecified acetabulum**   `MCC` `CC` `H5` `HCC`

4,6 ✓7th   **S32.484**   **Nondisplaced dome fracture of right acetabulum**   `MCC` `CC` `H5` `HCC`

4,6 ✓7th   **S32.485**   **Nondisplaced dome fracture of left acetabulum**   `MCC` `CC` `H5` `HCC`

4,6 ✓7th   **S32.486**   **Nondisplaced dome fracture of unspecified acetabulum**   `MCC` `CC` `H5` `HCC`

✓6th **S32.49**   **Other specified fracture of acetabulum**

4,6 ✓7th   **S32.491**   **Other specified fracture of right acetabulum**   `MCC` `CC` `H5` `HCC`

✓ Additional Character Required   ✓x7th Placeholder   Unacceptable PDx   Questionable PDx   Manifestation   `H1`-`H14` HAC   `HCC` CMS-HCC Dx   `HIV` HIV Dx

ICD-10-CM 2019   981

Chapter 19. Injury, Poisoning and Certain Other Consequences of External Causes

4,6 ✓7ᵗʰ **S32.492** Other specified fracture of left **acetabulum** `MCC` `CC` `H5` `HCC`

4,6 ✓7ᵗʰ **S32.499** Other specified fracture of unspecified **acetabulum** `MCC` `CC` `H5` `HCC`

✓5ᵗʰ **S32.5 Fracture of pubis**

> EXCLUDES 1   *fracture of pubis with associated disruption of pelvic ring (S32.8-)*

> **CC Excl: For codes in subcategory S32.5:**
> **CC with 7th character A or MCC with 7th character B:** PDX collection 1201
> **CC with 7th character K:** PDX collection 897

✓6ᵗʰ **S32.50** Unspecified fracture of pubis

2,3,6 ✓7ᵗʰ **S32.501** Unspecified fracture of right **pubis** `MCC` `CC` `H5` `HCC`

2,3,6 ✓7ᵗʰ **S32.502** Unspecified fracture of left **pubis** `MCC` `CC` `H5` `HCC`

2,3,6 ✓7ᵗʰ **S32.509** Unspecified fracture of unspecified **pubis** `MCC` `CC` `H5` `HCC`

✓6ᵗʰ **S32.51** Fracture of superior rim of pubis

2,3,6 ✓7ᵗʰ **S32.511** Fracture of superior rim of right **pubis** `MCC` `CC` `H5` `HCC`

2,3,6 ✓7ᵗʰ **S32.512** Fracture of superior rim of left **pubis** `MCC` `CC` `H5` `HCC`

2,3,6 ✓7ᵗʰ **S32.519** Fracture of superior rim of unspecified **pubis** `MCC` `CC` `H5` `HCC`

✓6ᵗʰ **S32.59** Other specified fracture of pubis

2,3,6 ✓7ᵗʰ **S32.591** Other specified fracture of right **pubis** `MCC` `CC` `H5` `HCC`

2,3,6 ✓7ᵗʰ **S32.592** Other specified fracture of left **pubis** `MCC` `CC` `H5` `HCC`

2,3,6 ✓7ᵗʰ **S32.599** Other specified fracture of unspecified **pubis** `MCC` `CC` `H5` `HCC`

✓5ᵗʰ **S32.6 Fracture of ischium**

> EXCLUDES 1   *fracture of ischium with associated disruption of pelvic ring (S32.8-)*

> **CC Excl: For codes in subcategory S32.6:**
> **CC with 7th character A:** PDX collection 1202
> **MCC with 7th character B:** PDX collection 1203
> **CC with 7th character K:** PDX collection 897

✓6ᵗʰ **S32.60** Unspecified fracture of ischium

2,3,6 ✓7ᵗʰ **S32.601** Unspecified fracture of right **ischium** `MCC` `CC` `H5` `HCC`

2,3,6 ✓7ᵗʰ **S32.602** Unspecified fracture of left **ischium** `MCC` `CC` `H5` `HCC`

2,3,6 ✓7ᵗʰ **S32.609** Unspecified fracture of unspecified **ischium** `MCC` `CC` `H5` `HCC`

✓6ᵗʰ **S32.61** Avulsion fracture of ischium

2,3,6 ✓7ᵗʰ **S32.611** Displaced avulsion fracture of right **ischium** `MCC` `CC` `H5` `HCC`

2,3,6 ✓7ᵗʰ **S32.612** Displaced avulsion fracture of left **ischium** `MCC` `CC` `H5` `HCC`

2,3,6 ✓7ᵗʰ **S32.613** Displaced avulsion fracture of unspecified **ischium** `MCC` `CC` `H5` `HCC`

2,3,6 ✓7ᵗʰ **S32.614** Nondisplaced avulsion fracture of right **ischium** `MCC` `CC` `H5` `HCC`

2,3,6 ✓7ᵗʰ **S32.615** Nondisplaced avulsion fracture of left **ischium** `MCC` `CC` `H5` `HCC`

2,3,6 ✓7ᵗʰ **S32.616** Nondisplaced avulsion fracture of unspecified **ischium** `MCC` `CC` `H5` `HCC`

✓6ᵗʰ **S32.69** Other specified fracture of ischium

2,3,6 ✓7ᵗʰ **S32.691** Other specified fracture of right **ischium** `MCC` `CC` `H5` `HCC`

2,3,6 ✓7ᵗʰ **S32.692** Other specified fracture of left **ischium** `MCC` `CC` `H5` `HCC`

2,3,6 ✓7ᵗʰ **S32.699** Other specified fracture of unspecified **ischium** `MCC` `CC` `H5` `HCC`

Fractures Disrupting Pelvic Circle

✓5ᵗʰ **S32.8 Fracture of other parts of pelvis**

> Code also any associated:
> fracture of acetabulum (S32.4-)
> sacral fracture (S32.1-)

✓6ᵗʰ **S32.81** Multiple fractures of pelvis with disruption of pelvic ring

> Multiple pelvic fractures with disruption of pelvic circle

> **CC Excl: For codes in subcategory S32.81:**
> **CC with 7th character A or MCC with 7th character B:** PDX collection 1204
> **CC with 7th character K:** PDX collection 897

2,3,6 ✓7ᵗʰ **S32.810** Multiple fractures of pelvis with stable disruption of pelvic ring `MCC` `CC` `H5` `HCC`

2,3,6 ✓7ᵗʰ **S32.811** Multiple fractures of pelvis with unstable disruption of pelvic ring `MCC` `CC` `H5` `HCC`

2,3,6 ✓x7ᵗʰ **S32.82** Multiple fractures of pelvis without disruption of pelvic ring `MCC` `CC` `H5` `HCC`

> Multiple pelvic fractures without disruption of pelvic circle

> **CC Excl: CC with 7th character A or MCC with 7th character B:** PDX collection 1205
> **CC with 7th character K:** PDX collection 897

2,3,6 ✓x7ᵗʰ **S32.89** Fracture of other parts of pelvis `MCC` `CC` `H5` `HCC`

> **CC Excl: CC with 7th character A or MCC with 7th character B:** PDX collection 1206
> **CC with 7th character K:** PDX collection 897

2,3,6 ✓x7ᵗʰ **S32.9 Fracture of unspecified parts of lumbosacral spine and pelvis** `MCC` `CC` `H5` `HCC`

> Fracture of lumbosacral spine NOS
> Fracture of pelvis NOS
> **AHA:** 2012, 4Q, 93
> **CC Excl: CC with 7th character A or MCC with 7th character B:** PDX collection 1204
> **CC with 7th character K:** PDX collection 897

✓4ᵗʰ **S33 Dislocation and sprain of joints and ligaments of lumbar spine and pelvis**

> INCLUDES   avulsion of joint or ligament of lumbar spine and pelvis
> laceration of cartilage, joint or ligament of lumbar spine and pelvis
> sprain of cartilage, joint or ligament of lumbar spine and pelvis
> traumatic hemarthrosis of joint or ligament of lumbar spine and pelvis
> traumatic rupture of joint or ligament of lumbar spine and pelvis
> traumatic subluxation of joint or ligament of lumbar spine and pelvis
> traumatic tear of joint or ligament of lumbar spine and pelvis

> Code also any associated open wound

> EXCLUDES 1   *nontraumatic rupture or displacement of lumbar intervertebral disc NOS (M51.-)*
> *obstetric damage to pelvic joints and ligaments (O71.6)*

> EXCLUDES 2   *dislocation and sprain of joints and ligaments of hip (S73.-)*
> *strain of muscle of lower back and pelvis (S39.01-)*

> The appropriate 7th character is to be added to each code from category S33.
> A   initial encounter
> D   subsequent encounter
> S   sequela

✓x7ᵗʰ **S33.0 Traumatic rupture of lumbar intervertebral disc**

> EXCLUDES 1   *rupture or displacement (nontraumatic) of lumbar intervertebral disc NOS (M51- with fifth character 6)*

N Newborn: 0   P Pediatric: 0-17   M Maternity: 12-55   A Adult: 15-124   MCC Major Complication/Comorbidity   CC Complication/Comorbidity   SW Severe Wound Dx

982   ICD-10-CM 2019

✓5ᵗʰ S33.1　Subluxation and dislocation of lumbar vertebra
　Code also any associated:
　　open wound of abdomen, lower back and pelvis (S31)
　　spinal cord injury (S24.0, S24.1-, S34.0-, S34.1-)
　　EXCLUDES 2　fracture of lumbar vertebrae (S32.0-)

　✓6ᵗʰ S33.10　Subluxation and dislocation of unspecified lumbar vertebra
　　✓7ᵗʰ S33.100　Subluxation of unspecified lumbar vertebra
　　✓7ᵗʰ S33.101　Dislocation of unspecified lumbar vertebra

　✓6ᵗʰ S33.11　Subluxation and dislocation of L1/L2 lumbar vertebra
　　✓7ᵗʰ S33.110　Subluxation of L1/L2 lumbar vertebra
　　✓7ᵗʰ S33.111　Dislocation of L1/L2 lumbar vertebra

　✓6ᵗʰ S33.12　Subluxation and dislocation of L2/L3 lumbar vertebra
　　✓7ᵗʰ S33.120　Subluxation of L2/L3 lumbar vertebra
　　✓7ᵗʰ S33.121　Dislocation of L2/L3 lumbar vertebra

　✓6ᵗʰ S33.13　Subluxation and dislocation of L3/L4 lumbar vertebra
　　✓7ᵗʰ S33.130　Subluxation of L3/L4 lumbar vertebra
　　✓7ᵗʰ S33.131　Dislocation of L3/L4 lumbar vertebra

　✓6ᵗʰ S33.14　Subluxation and dislocation of L4/L5 lumbar vertebra
　　✓7ᵗʰ S33.140　Subluxation of L4/L5 lumbar vertebra
　　✓7ᵗʰ S33.141　Dislocation of L4/L5 lumbar vertebra

✓x7ᵗʰ S33.2　Dislocation of sacroiliac and sacrococcygeal joint

✓5ᵗʰ S33.3　Dislocation of other and unspecified parts of lumbar spine and pelvis
　✓x7ᵗʰ S33.30　Dislocation of unspecified parts of lumbar spine and pelvis
　✓x7ᵗʰ S33.39　Dislocation of other parts of lumbar spine and pelvis

✓x7ᵗʰ S33.4　Traumatic rupture of symphysis pubis
✓x7ᵗʰ S33.5　Sprain of ligaments of lumbar spine
✓x7ᵗʰ S33.6　Sprain of sacroiliac joint
✓x7ᵗʰ S33.8　Sprain of other parts of lumbar spine and pelvis
✓x7ᵗʰ S33.9　Sprain of unspecified parts of lumbar spine and pelvis

✓4ᵗʰ S34　Injury of lumbar and sacral spinal cord and nerves at abdomen, lower back and pelvis level
　NOTE　Code to highest level of lumbar cord injury. Injuries to the spinal cord (S34.0 and S34.1) refer to the cord level and not bone level injury, and can affect nerve roots at and below the level given.
　Code also any associated:
　　fracture of vertebra (S22.0-, S32.0-)
　　open wound of abdomen, lower back and pelvis (S31.-)
　　transient paralysis (R29.5)

　The appropriate 7th character is to be added to each code from category S34.
　A　initial encounter
　D　subsequent encounter
　S　sequela

　CC Excl: For MCC codes in category S34, unless otherwise noted: PDX collection 1207

✓5ᵗʰ S34.0　Concussion and edema of lumbar and sacral spinal cord
　✓x7ᵗʰ S34.01　Concussion and edema of lumbar spinal cord MCC HCC
　✓x7ᵗʰ S34.02　Concussion and edema of sacral spinal cord MCC HCC
　　Concussion and edema of conus medullaris
　　CC Excl: PDX collection 1208

✓5ᵗʰ S34.1　Other and unspecified injury of lumbar and sacral spinal cord
　✓6ᵗʰ S34.10　Unspecified injury to lumbar spinal cord
　　✓7ᵗʰ S34.101　Unspecified injury to L1 level of lumbar spinal cord MCC H5 HCC
　　　Unspecified injury to lumbar spinal cord level 1
　　✓7ᵗʰ S34.102　Unspecified injury to L2 level of lumbar spinal cord MCC H5 HCC
　　　Unspecified injury to lumbar spinal cord level 2

　　✓7ᵗʰ S34.103　Unspecified injury to L3 level of lumbar spinal cord MCC H5 HCC
　　　Unspecified injury to lumbar spinal cord level 3
　　✓7ᵗʰ S34.104　Unspecified injury to L4 level of lumbar spinal cord MCC H5 HCC
　　　Unspecified injury to lumbar spinal cord level 4
　　✓7ᵗʰ S34.105　Unspecified injury to L5 level of lumbar spinal cord MCC H5 HCC
　　　Unspecified injury to lumbar spinal cord level 5
　　✓7ᵗʰ S34.109　Unspecified injury to unspecified level of lumbar spinal cord MCC H5 HCC

　✓6ᵗʰ S34.11　Complete lesion of lumbar spinal cord
　　✓7ᵗʰ S34.111　Complete lesion of L1 level of lumbar spinal cord MCC H5 HCC
　　　Complete lesion of lumbar spinal cord level 1
　　✓7ᵗʰ S34.112　Complete lesion of L2 level of lumbar spinal cord MCC H5 HCC
　　　Complete lesion of lumbar spinal cord level 2
　　✓7ᵗʰ S34.113　Complete lesion of L3 level of lumbar spinal cord MCC H5 HCC
　　　Complete lesion of lumbar spinal cord level 3
　　✓7ᵗʰ S34.114　Complete lesion of L4 level of lumbar spinal cord MCC H5 HCC
　　　Complete lesion of lumbar spinal cord level 4
　　✓7ᵗʰ S34.115　Complete lesion of L5 level of lumbar spinal cord MCC H5 HCC
　　　Complete lesion of lumbar spinal cord level 5
　　✓7ᵗʰ S34.119　Complete lesion of unspecified level of lumbar spinal cord MCC H5 HCC

　✓6ᵗʰ S34.12　Incomplete lesion of lumbar spinal cord
　　✓7ᵗʰ S34.121　Incomplete lesion of L1 level of lumbar spinal cord MCC H5 HCC
　　　Incomplete lesion of lumbar spinal cord level 1
　　✓7ᵗʰ S34.122　Incomplete lesion of L2 level of lumbar spinal cord MCC H5 HCC
　　　Incomplete lesion of lumbar spinal cord level 2
　　✓7ᵗʰ S34.123　Incomplete lesion of L3 level of lumbar spinal cord MCC H5 HCC
　　　Incomplete lesion of lumbar spinal cord level 3
　　✓7ᵗʰ S34.124　Incomplete lesion of L4 level of lumbar spinal cord MCC H5 HCC
　　　Incomplete lesion of lumbar spinal cord level 4
　　✓7ᵗʰ S34.125　Incomplete lesion of L5 level of lumbar spinal cord MCC H5 HCC
　　　Incomplete lesion of lumbar spinal cord level 5
　　✓7ᵗʰ S34.129　Incomplete lesion of unspecified level of lumbar spinal cord MCC H5 HCC

　✓6ᵗʰ S34.13　Other and unspecified injury to sacral spinal cord
　　Other injury to conus medullaris
　　CC Excl: For MCC codes in subcategory S34.13: PDX collection 1208
　　✓7ᵗʰ S34.131　Complete lesion of sacral spinal cord MCC H5 HCC
　　　Complete lesion of conus medullaris
　　✓7ᵗʰ S34.132　Incomplete lesion of sacral spinal cord MCC H5 HCC
　　　Incomplete lesion of conus medullaris
　　✓7ᵗʰ S34.139　Unspecified injury to sacral spinal cord MCC H5 HCC
　　　Unspecified injury of conus medullaris

✓5ᵗʰ S34.2　Injury of nerve root of lumbar and sacral spine
　✓x7ᵗʰ S34.21　Injury of nerve root of lumbar spine
　✓x7ᵗʰ S34.22　Injury of nerve root of sacral spine

6　✓x7ᵗʰ S34.3　Injury of cauda equina MCC H5 HCC
　CC Excl: PDX collection 1208

√x7ᵗʰ S34.4   **Injury of lumbosacral plexus**

√x7ᵗʰ S34.5   **Injury of lumbar, sacral and pelvic sympathetic nerves**
Injury of celiac ganglion or plexus
Injury of hypogastric plexus
Injury of mesenteric plexus (inferior) (superior)
Injury of splanchnic nerve

√x7ᵗʰ S34.6   **Injury of peripheral nerve(s) at abdomen, lower back and pelvis level**

√x7ᵗʰ S34.8   **Injury of other nerves at abdomen, lower back and pelvis level**

√x7ᵗʰ S34.9   **Injury of unspecified nerves at abdomen, lower back and pelvis level**

√4ᵗʰ S35   **Injury of blood vessels at abdomen, lower back and pelvis level**
Code also any associated open wound (S31.-)

> The appropriate 7th character is to be added to each code from category S35.
> A   initial encounter
> D   subsequent encounter
> S   sequela

√5ᵗʰ S35.0   **Injury of abdominal aorta**
> **EXCLUDES 1**   injury of aorta NOS (S25.0)

> **CC Excl: For MCC codes in subcategory S35.0:**
> PDX collection 1209

√x7ᵗʰ S35.00   **Unspecified injury of abdominal aorta**   MCC

√x7ᵗʰ S35.01   **Minor laceration of abdominal aorta**   MCC
Incomplete transection of abdominal aorta
Laceration of abdominal aorta NOS
Superficial laceration of abdominal aorta

√x7ᵗʰ S35.02   **Major laceration of abdominal aorta**   MCC
Complete transection of abdominal aorta
Traumatic rupture of abdominal aorta

√x7ᵗʰ S35.09   **Other injury of abdominal aorta**   MCC

√5ᵗʰ S35.1   **Injury of inferior vena cava**
Injury of hepatic vein
> **EXCLUDES 1**   injury of vena cava NOS (S25.2)

> **CC Excl: For MCC codes in subcategory S35.1:**
> PDX collection 1210

√x7ᵗʰ S35.10   **Unspecified injury of inferior vena cava**   MCC

√x7ᵗʰ S35.11   **Minor laceration of inferior vena cava**   MCC
Incomplete transection of inferior vena cava
Laceration of inferior vena cava NOS
Superficial laceration of inferior vena cava

√x7ᵗʰ S35.12   **Major laceration of inferior vena cava**   MCC
Complete transection of inferior vena cava
Traumatic rupture of inferior vena cava

√x7ᵗʰ S35.19   **Other injury of inferior vena cava**   MCC

√5ᵗʰ S35.2   **Injury of celiac or mesenteric artery and branches**

√6ᵗʰ S35.21   **Injury of celiac artery**

> **CC Excl: For MCC codes in subcategory S35.21:**
> PDX collection 1211

√7ᵗʰ S35.211   **Minor laceration of celiac artery**   MCC
Incomplete transection of celiac artery
Laceration of celiac artery NOS
Superficial laceration of celiac artery

√7ᵗʰ S35.212   **Major laceration of celiac artery**   MCC
Complete transection of celiac artery
Traumatic rupture of celiac artery

√7ᵗʰ S35.218   **Other injury of celiac artery**   MCC

√7ᵗʰ S35.219   **Unspecified injury of celiac artery**   MCC

√6ᵗʰ S35.22   **Injury of superior mesenteric artery**

> **CC Excl: For MCC codes in subcategory S35.22:**
> PDX collection 1212

√7ᵗʰ S35.221   **Minor laceration of superior mesenteric artery**   MCC
Incomplete transection of superior mesenteric artery
Laceration of superior mesenteric artery NOS
Superficial laceration of superior mesenteric artery

√7ᵗʰ S35.222   **Major laceration of superior mesenteric artery**   MCC
Complete transection of superior mesenteric artery
Traumatic rupture of superior mesenteric artery

√7ᵗʰ S35.228   **Other injury of superior mesenteric artery**   MCC

√7ᵗʰ S35.229   **Unspecified injury of superior mesenteric artery**   MCC

√6ᵗʰ S35.23   **Injury of inferior mesenteric artery**

> **CC Excl: For MCC codes in subcategory S35.23:**
> PDX collection 1213

√7ᵗʰ S35.231   **Minor laceration of inferior mesenteric artery**   MCC
Incomplete transection of inferior mesenteric artery
Laceration of inferior mesenteric artery NOS
Superficial laceration of inferior mesenteric artery

√7ᵗʰ S35.232   **Major laceration of inferior mesenteric artery**   MCC
Complete transection of inferior mesenteric artery
Traumatic rupture of inferior mesenteric artery

√7ᵗʰ S35.238   **Other injury of inferior mesenteric artery**   MCC

√7ᵗʰ S35.239   **Unspecified injury of inferior mesenteric artery**   MCC

√6ᵗʰ S35.29   **Injury of branches of celiac and mesenteric artery**
Injury of gastric artery
Injury of gastroduodenal artery
Injury of hepatic artery
Injury of splenic artery

√7ᵗʰ S35.291   **Minor laceration of branches of celiac and mesenteric artery**   MCC
Incomplete transection of branches of celiac and mesenteric artery
Laceration of branches of celiac and mesenteric artery NOS
Superficial laceration of branches of celiac and mesenteric artery
> **CC Excl:** PDX collection 1214

√7ᵗʰ S35.292   **Major laceration of branches of celiac and mesenteric artery**   MCC
Complete transection of branches of celiac and mesenteric artery
Traumatic rupture of branches of celiac and mesenteric artery
> **CC Excl:** PDX collection 1215

√7ᵗʰ S35.298   **Other injury of branches of celiac and mesenteric artery**   MCC
> **CC Excl:** PDX collection 1215

√7ᵗʰ S35.299   **Unspecified injury of branches of celiac and mesenteric artery**   MCC
> **CC Excl:** PDX collection 1216

√5ᵗʰ S35.3   **Injury of portal or splenic vein and branches**

√6ᵗʰ S35.31   **Injury of portal vein**

> **CC Excl: For MCC codes in subcategory S35.31:**
> PDX collection 1217

√7ᵗʰ S35.311   **Laceration of portal vein**   MCC
√7ᵗʰ S35.318   **Other specified injury of portal vein**   MCC
√7ᵗʰ S35.319   **Unspecified injury of portal vein**   MCC

√6ᵗʰ S35.32   **Injury of splenic vein**

> **CC Excl: For MCC codes in subcategory S35.32:**
> PDX collection 1218

√7ᵗʰ S35.321   **Laceration of splenic vein**   MCC
√7ᵗʰ S35.328   **Other specified injury of splenic vein**   MCC
√7ᵗʰ S35.329   **Unspecified injury of splenic vein**   MCC

√6ᵗʰ S35.33   **Injury of superior mesenteric vein**

> **CC Excl: For MCC codes in subcategory S35.33:**
> PDX collection 1219

√7ᵗʰ S35.331   **Laceration of superior mesenteric vein**   MCC

N Newborn: 0   P Pediatric: 0-17   M Maternity: 12-55   A Adult: 15-124   MCC Major Complication/Comorbidity   CC Complication/Comorbidity   SW Severe Wound Dx

984   ICD-10-CM 2019

✓7th **S35.338** Other specified injury of superior mesenteric vein `MCC`

✓7th **S35.339** Unspecified injury of superior mesenteric vein `MCC`

✓6th **S35.34** Injury of inferior mesenteric vein

CC Excl: For MCC codes in subcategory S35.34: PDX collection 1220

✓7th **S35.341** Laceration of inferior mesenteric vein `MCC`

✓7th **S35.348** Other specified injury of inferior mesenteric vein `MCC`

✓7th **S35.349** Unspecified injury of inferior mesenteric vein `MCC`

✓5th **S35.4** Injury of renal blood vessels

CC Excl: For MCC codes in subcategory S35.4, unless otherwise noted: PDX collection 1221

✓6th **S35.40** Unspecified injury of renal blood vessel

✓7th **S35.401** Unspecified injury of right renal artery `MCC`

✓7th **S35.402** Unspecified injury of left renal artery `MCC`

✓7th **S35.403** Unspecified injury of unspecified renal artery `MCC`

✓7th **S35.404** Unspecified injury of right renal vein `MCC`
CC Excl: PDX collection 1222

✓7th **S35.405** Unspecified injury of left renal vein `MCC`
CC Excl: PDX collection 1222

✓7th **S35.406** Unspecified injury of unspecified renal vein `MCC`
CC Excl: PDX collection 1222

✓6th **S35.41** Laceration of renal blood vessel

✓7th **S35.411** Laceration of right renal artery `MCC`

✓7th **S35.412** Laceration of left renal artery `MCC`

✓7th **S35.413** Laceration of unspecified renal artery `MCC`

✓7th **S35.414** Laceration of right renal vein `MCC`
CC Excl: PDX collection 1222

✓7th **S35.415** Laceration of left renal vein `MCC`
CC Excl: PDX collection 1222

✓7th **S35.416** Laceration of unspecified renal vein `MCC`
CC Excl: PDX collection 1222

✓6th **S35.49** Other specified injury of renal blood vessel

✓7th **S35.491** Other specified injury of right renal artery `MCC`

✓7th **S35.492** Other specified injury of left renal artery `MCC`

✓7th **S35.493** Other specified injury of unspecified renal artery `MCC`

✓7th **S35.494** Other specified injury of right renal vein `MCC`
CC Excl: PDX collection 1222

✓7th **S35.495** Other specified injury of left renal vein `MCC`
CC Excl: PDX collection 1222

✓7th **S35.496** Other specified injury of unspecified renal vein `MCC`
CC Excl: PDX collection 1222

✓5th **S35.5** Injury of iliac blood vessels

✓x7th **S35.50** Injury of unspecified iliac blood vessel(s) `MCC`
CC Excl: PDX collection 1223

✓6th **S35.51** Injury of iliac artery or vein
Injury of hypogastric artery or vein

✓7th **S35.511** Injury of right iliac artery `MCC`
CC Excl: PDX collection 1224

✓7th **S35.512** Injury of left iliac artery `MCC`
CC Excl: PDX collection 1224

✓7th **S35.513** Injury of unspecified iliac artery `MCC`
CC Excl: PDX collection 1224

✓7th **S35.514** Injury of right iliac vein `MCC`
CC Excl: PDX collection 1225

✓7th **S35.515** Injury of left iliac vein `MCC`
CC Excl: PDX collection 1225

✓7th **S35.516** Injury of unspecified iliac vein `MCC`
CC Excl: PDX collection 1225

✓6th **S35.53** Injury of uterine artery or vein

✓7th **S35.531** Injury of right uterine artery `CC` ♀
CC Excl: PDX collection 1226

✓7th **S35.532** Injury of left uterine artery `CC` ♀
CC Excl: PDX collection 1226

✓7th **S35.533** Injury of unspecified uterine artery `CC` ♀
CC Excl: PDX collection 1226

✓7th **S35.534** Injury of right uterine vein `CC` ♀
CC Excl: PDX collection 1227

✓7th **S35.535** Injury of left uterine vein `CC` ♀
CC Excl: PDX collection 1227

✓7th **S35.536** Injury of unspecified uterine vein `CC` ♀
CC Excl: PDX collection 1227

✓x7th **S35.59** Injury of other iliac blood vessels `MCC`
CC Excl: PDX collection 1223

✓5th **S35.8** Injury of other blood vessels at abdomen, lower back and pelvis level
Injury of ovarian artery or vein

✓6th **S35.8X** Injury of other blood vessels at abdomen, lower back and pelvis level

CC Excl: For CC codes in subcategory S35.8X: PDX collection 1228

✓7th **S35.8X1** Laceration of other blood vessels at abdomen, lower back and pelvis level `CC`

✓7th **S35.8X8** Other specified injury of other blood vessels at abdomen, lower back and pelvis level `CC`

✓7th **S35.8X9** Unspecified injury of other blood vessels at abdomen, lower back and pelvis level `CC`

✓5th **S35.9** Injury of unspecified blood vessel at abdomen, lower back and pelvis level

CC Excl: For CC codes in subcategory S35.9: PDX collection 1229

✓x7th **S35.90** Unspecified injury of unspecified blood vessel at abdomen, lower back and pelvis level `CC`

✓x7th **S35.91** Laceration of unspecified blood vessel at abdomen, lower back and pelvis level `CC`

✓x7th **S35.99** Other specified injury of unspecified blood vessel at abdomen, lower back and pelvis level `CC`

✓4th **S36** Injury of intra-abdominal organs
Code also any associated open wound (S31.-)

The appropriate 7th character is to be added to each code from category S36.
A   initial encounter
D   subsequent encounter
S   sequela

✓5th **S36.0** Injury of spleen
AHA: 2015, 2Q, 36; 2015, 1Q, 10

CC Excl: For CC/MCC codes in subcategory S36.0: PDX collection 1230

✓x7th **S36.00** Unspecified injury of spleen `CC`

✓6th **S36.02** Contusion of spleen

✓7th **S36.020** Minor contusion of spleen `CC`
Contusion of spleen less than 2 cm

✓7th **S36.021** Major contusion of spleen `CC`
Contusion of spleen greater than 2 cm

✓7th **S36.029** Unspecified contusion of spleen `CC`

✓6th **S36.03** Laceration of spleen

✓7th **S36.030** Superficial (capsular) laceration of spleen `CC`
Laceration of spleen less than 1cm
Minor laceration of spleen

✓7th **S36.031** Moderate laceration of spleen `MCC`
Laceration of spleen 1 to 3 cm

✓7th **S36.032** Major laceration of spleen `MCC`
Avulsion of spleen
Laceration of spleen greater than 3 cm
Massive laceration of spleen
Multiple moderate lacerations of spleen
Stellate laceration of spleen

✓7th **S36.039** Unspecified laceration of spleen `CC`

✓x7th **S36.09** Other injury of spleen `CC`

☑ Additional Character Required   ✓x7th Placeholder   Unacceptable PDx   Questionable PDx   Manifestation   H1-H14 HAC   HCC CMS-HCC Dx   HIV HIV Dx

ICD-10-CM 2019   985

Chapter 19. Injury, Poisoning and Certain Other Consequences of External Causes

√5ᵗʰ **S36.1** Injury of liver and gallbladder and bile duct

√6ᵗʰ   **S36.11** Injury of liver

> **CC Excl: For CC/MCC codes in subcategory S36.11:** PDX collection 1231

√7ᵗʰ   **S36.112** Contusion of liver   CC

√7ᵗʰ   **S36.113** Laceration of liver, unspecified degree   CC

√7ᵗʰ   **S36.114** Minor laceration of liver
Laceration involving capsule only, or, without significant involvement of hepatic parenchyma [i.e., less than 1cm deep]

√7ᵗʰ   **S36.115** Moderate laceration of liver   MCC
Laceration involving parenchyma but without major disruption of parenchyma [i.e., less than 10 cm long and less than 3 cm deep]

√7ᵗʰ   **S36.116** Major laceration of liver   MCC
Laceration with significant disruption of hepatic parenchyma [i.e., greater than 10 cm long and 3 cm deep]
Multiple moderate lacerations, with or without hematoma
Stellate laceration of liver

√7ᵗʰ   **S36.118** Other injury of liver   CC

√7ᵗʰ   **S36.119** Unspecified injury of liver   CC

√6ᵗʰ   **S36.12** Injury of gallbladder

> **CC Excl: For CC codes in subcategory S36.12:** PDX collection 1232

√7ᵗʰ   **S36.122** Contusion of gallbladder   CC

√7ᵗʰ   **S36.123** Laceration of gallbladder   CC

√7ᵗʰ   **S36.128** Other injury of gallbladder   CC

√7ᵗʰ   **S36.129** Unspecified injury of gallbladder   CC

√x7ᵗʰ   **S36.13** Injury of bile duct   CC
CC Excl: PDX collection 1232

√5ᵗʰ **S36.2** Injury of pancreas

> **CC Excl: For CC codes in subcategory S36.2:** PDX collection 1233

√6ᵗʰ   **S36.20** Unspecified injury of pancreas

√7ᵗʰ   **S36.200** Unspecified injury of head of pancreas   CC

√7ᵗʰ   **S36.201** Unspecified injury of body of pancreas   CC

√7ᵗʰ   **S36.202** Unspecified injury of tail of pancreas   CC

√7ᵗʰ   **S36.209** Unspecified injury of unspecified part of pancreas   CC

√6ᵗʰ   **S36.22** Contusion of pancreas

√7ᵗʰ   **S36.220** Contusion of head of pancreas   CC

√7ᵗʰ   **S36.221** Contusion of body of pancreas   CC

√7ᵗʰ   **S36.222** Contusion of tail of pancreas   CC

√7ᵗʰ   **S36.229** Contusion of unspecified part of pancreas   CC

√6ᵗʰ   **S36.23** Laceration of pancreas, unspecified degree

√7ᵗʰ   **S36.230** Laceration of head of pancreas, unspecified degree   CC

√7ᵗʰ   **S36.231** Laceration of body of pancreas, unspecified degree   CC

√7ᵗʰ   **S36.232** Laceration of tail of pancreas, unspecified degree   CC

√7ᵗʰ   **S36.239** Laceration of unspecified part of pancreas, unspecified degree   CC

√6ᵗʰ   **S36.24** Minor laceration of pancreas

√7ᵗʰ   **S36.240** Minor laceration of head of pancreas   CC

√7ᵗʰ   **S36.241** Minor laceration of body of pancreas   CC

√7ᵗʰ   **S36.242** Minor laceration of tail of pancreas   CC

√7ᵗʰ   **S36.249** Minor laceration of unspecified part of pancreas   CC

√6ᵗʰ   **S36.25** Moderate laceration of pancreas

√7ᵗʰ   **S36.250** Moderate laceration of head of pancreas   CC

√7ᵗʰ   **S36.251** Moderate laceration of body of pancreas

√7ᵗʰ   **S36.252** Moderate laceration of tail of pancreas   CC

√7ᵗʰ   **S36.259** Moderate laceration of unspecified part of pancreas   CC

√6ᵗʰ   **S36.26** Major laceration of pancreas

√7ᵗʰ   **S36.260** Major laceration of head of pancreas   CC

√7ᵗʰ   **S36.261** Major laceration of body of pancreas   CC

√7ᵗʰ   **S36.262** Major laceration of tail of pancreas   CC

√7ᵗʰ   **S36.269** Major laceration of unspecified part of pancreas   CC

√6ᵗʰ   **S36.29** Other injury of pancreas

√7ᵗʰ   **S36.290** Other injury of head of pancreas   CC

√7ᵗʰ   **S36.291** Other injury of body of pancreas   CC

√7ᵗʰ   **S36.292** Other injury of tail of pancreas   CC

√7ᵗʰ   **S36.299** Other injury of unspecified part of pancreas   CC

√5ᵗʰ **S36.3** Injury of stomach

> **CC Excl: For CC codes in subcategory S36.3:** PDX collection 1234

√x7ᵗʰ   **S36.30** Unspecified injury of stomach   CC

√x7ᵗʰ   **S36.32** Contusion of stomach   CC

√x7ᵗʰ   **S36.33** Laceration of stomach   CC

√x7ᵗʰ   **S36.39** Other injury of stomach   CC

√5ᵗʰ **S36.4** Injury of small intestine

> **CC Excl: For CC codes in subcategory S36.4:** PDX collection 1235

√6ᵗʰ   **S36.40** Unspecified injury of small intestine

√7ᵗʰ   **S36.400** Unspecified injury of duodenum   CC

√7ᵗʰ   **S36.408** Unspecified injury of other part of small intestine   CC

√7ᵗʰ   **S36.409** Unspecified injury of unspecified part of small intestine   CC

√6ᵗʰ   **S36.41** Primary blast injury of small intestine
Blast injury of small intestine NOS

√7ᵗʰ   **S36.410** Primary blast injury of duodenum   CC

√7ᵗʰ   **S36.418** Primary blast injury of other part of small intestine   CC

√7ᵗʰ   **S36.419** Primary blast injury of unspecified part of small intestine   CC

√6ᵗʰ   **S36.42** Contusion of small intestine

√7ᵗʰ   **S36.420** Contusion of duodenum   CC

√7ᵗʰ   **S36.428** Contusion of other part of small intestine   CC

√7ᵗʰ   **S36.429** Contusion of unspecified part of small intestine   CC

√6ᵗʰ   **S36.43** Laceration of small intestine

√7ᵗʰ   **S36.430** Laceration of duodenum   CC

√7ᵗʰ   **S36.438** Laceration of other part of small intestine   CC

√7ᵗʰ   **S36.439** Laceration of unspecified part of small intestine   CC

√6ᵗʰ   **S36.49** Other injury of small intestine

√7ᵗʰ   **S36.490** Other injury of duodenum   CC

√7ᵗʰ   **S36.498** Other injury of other part of small intestine   CC

√7ᵗʰ   **S36.499** Other injury of unspecified part of small intestine   CC

√5ᵗʰ **S36.5** Injury of colon
> EXCLUDES 2   injury of rectum (S36.6-)

> **CC Excl: For CC codes in subcategory S36.5:** PDX collection 1236

√6ᵗʰ   **S36.50** Unspecified injury of colon

√7ᵗʰ   **S36.500** Unspecified injury of ascending [right] colon   CC

√7ᵗʰ   **S36.501** Unspecified injury of transverse colon   CC

√7ᵗʰ   **S36.502** Unspecified injury of descending [left] colon   CC

√7ᵗʰ   **S36.503** Unspecified injury of sigmoid colon   CC

√7ᵗʰ   **S36.508** Unspecified injury of other part of colon   CC

√7ᵗʰ   **S36.509** Unspecified injury of unspecified part of colon   CC

N Newborn: 0   P Pediatric: 0-17   M Maternity: 12-55   A Adult: 15-124   MCC Major Complication/Comorbidity   CC Complication/Comorbidity   SW Severe Wound Dx

986   ICD-10-CM 2019

✓6ᵗʰ S36.51 Primary blast injury of colon
Blast injury of colon NOS

   ✓7ᵗʰ S36.510 Primary blast injury of ascending [right] colon CC

   ✓7ᵗʰ S36.511 Primary blast injury of transverse colon CC

   ✓7ᵗʰ S36.512 Primary blast injury of descending [left] colon CC

   ✓7ᵗʰ S36.513 Primary blast injury of sigmoid colon CC

   ✓7ᵗʰ S36.518 Primary blast injury of other part of colon CC

   ✓7ᵗʰ S36.519 Primary blast injury of unspecified part of colon CC

✓6ᵗʰ S36.52 Contusion of colon

   ✓7ᵗʰ S36.520 Contusion of ascending [right] colon CC
   ✓7ᵗʰ S36.521 Contusion of transverse colon CC
   ✓7ᵗʰ S36.522 Contusion of descending [left] colon CC
   ✓7ᵗʰ S36.523 Contusion of sigmoid colon CC
   ✓7ᵗʰ S36.528 Contusion of other part of colon CC
   ✓7ᵗʰ S36.529 Contusion of unspecified part of colon CC

✓6ᵗʰ S36.53 Laceration of colon

   ✓7ᵗʰ S36.530 Laceration of ascending [right] colon CC
   ✓7ᵗʰ S36.531 Laceration of transverse colon CC
   ✓7ᵗʰ S36.532 Laceration of descending [left] colon CC
   ✓7ᵗʰ S36.533 Laceration of sigmoid colon CC
   ✓7ᵗʰ S36.538 Laceration of other part of colon CC
   ✓7ᵗʰ S36.539 Laceration of unspecified part of colon CC

✓6ᵗʰ S36.59 Other injury of colon
Secondary blast injury of colon

   ✓7ᵗʰ S36.590 Other injury of ascending [right] colon CC
   ✓7ᵗʰ S36.591 Other injury of transverse colon CC
   ✓7ᵗʰ S36.592 Other injury of descending [left] colon CC
   ✓7ᵗʰ S36.593 Other injury of sigmoid colon CC
   ✓7ᵗʰ S36.598 Other injury of other part of colon CC
   ✓7ᵗʰ S36.599 Other injury of unspecified part of colon CC

✓5ᵗʰ S36.6 Injury of rectum

CC Excl: For CC codes in subcategory S36.6: PDX collection 1236

✓x7ᵗʰ S36.60 Unspecified injury of rectum CC
✓x7ᵗʰ S36.61 Primary blast injury of rectum CC
Blast injury of rectum NOS
✓x7ᵗʰ S36.62 Contusion of rectum CC
✓x7ᵗʰ S36.63 Laceration of rectum CC
✓x7ᵗʰ S36.69 Other injury of rectum CC
Secondary blast injury of rectum

✓5ᵗʰ S36.8 Injury of other intra-abdominal organs

CC Excl: For CC codes in subcategory S36.8: PDX collection 1195

✓x7ᵗʰ S36.81 Injury of peritoneum CC
✓6ᵗʰ S36.89 Injury of other intra-abdominal organs
Injury of retroperitoneum

   ✓7ᵗʰ S36.892 Contusion of other intra-abdominal organs CC
   ✓7ᵗʰ S36.893 Laceration of other intra-abdominal organs CC
   ✓7ᵗʰ S36.898 Other injury of other intra-abdominal organs CC
   ✓7ᵗʰ S36.899 Unspecified injury of other intra-abdominal organs CC

✓5ᵗʰ S36.9 Injury of unspecified intra-abdominal organ

CC Excl: For CC codes in subcategory S36.9: PDX collection 1195

✓x7ᵗʰ S36.90 Unspecified injury of unspecified intra-abdominal organ CC
✓x7ᵗʰ S36.92 Contusion of unspecified intra-abdominal organ CC
✓x7ᵗʰ S36.93 Laceration of unspecified intra-abdominal organ CC
✓x7ᵗʰ S36.99 Other injury of unspecified intra-abdominal organ

✓4ᵗʰ S37 Injury of urinary and pelvic organs
Code also any associated open wound (S31.-)
EXCLUDES 1 obstetric trauma to pelvic organs (O71.-)
EXCLUDES 2 injury of peritoneum (S36.81)
injury of retroperitoneum (S36.89-)

The appropriate 7th character is to be added to each code from category S37.
A initial encounter
D subsequent encounter
S sequela

✓5ᵗʰ S37.0 Injury of kidney
EXCLUDES 2 acute kidney injury (nontraumatic) (N17.9)

CC Excl: For CC/MCC codes in subcategory S37.0: PDX collection 1237

✓6ᵗʰ S37.00 Unspecified injury of kidney
   ✓7ᵗʰ S37.001 Unspecified injury of right kidney CC
   ✓7ᵗʰ S37.002 Unspecified injury of left kidney CC
   ✓7ᵗʰ S37.009 Unspecified injury of unspecified kidney CC

✓6ᵗʰ S37.01 Minor contusion of kidney
Contusion of kidney less than 2 cm
Contusion of kidney NOS
   ✓7ᵗʰ S37.011 Minor contusion of right kidney CC
   ✓7ᵗʰ S37.012 Minor contusion of left kidney CC
   ✓7ᵗʰ S37.019 Minor contusion of unspecified kidney CC

✓6ᵗʰ S37.02 Major contusion of kidney
Contusion of kidney greater than 2 cm
   ✓7ᵗʰ S37.021 Major contusion of right kidney CC
   ✓7ᵗʰ S37.022 Major contusion of left kidney CC
   ✓7ᵗʰ S37.029 Major contusion of unspecified kidney CC

✓6ᵗʰ S37.03 Laceration of kidney, unspecified degree
   ✓7ᵗʰ S37.031 Laceration of right kidney, unspecified degree CC
   ✓7ᵗʰ S37.032 Laceration of left kidney, unspecified degree CC
   ✓7ᵗʰ S37.039 Laceration of unspecified kidney, unspecified degree CC

✓6ᵗʰ S37.04 Minor laceration of kidney
Laceration of kidney less than 1 cm
   ✓7ᵗʰ S37.041 Minor laceration of right kidney CC
   ✓7ᵗʰ S37.042 Minor laceration of left kidney CC
   ✓7ᵗʰ S37.049 Minor laceration of unspecified kidney CC

✓6ᵗʰ S37.05 Moderate laceration of kidney
Laceration of kidney 1 to 3 cm
   ✓7ᵗʰ S37.051 Moderate laceration of right kidney CC
   ✓7ᵗʰ S37.052 Moderate laceration of left kidney CC
   ✓7ᵗʰ S37.059 Moderate laceration of unspecified kidney CC

✓6ᵗʰ S37.06 Major laceration of kidney
Avulsion of kidney
Laceration of kidney greater than 3 cm
Massive laceration of kidney
Multiple moderate lacerations of kidney
Stellate laceration of kidney
   ✓7ᵗʰ S37.061 Major laceration of right kidney MCC
   ✓7ᵗʰ S37.062 Major laceration of left kidney MCC
   ✓7ᵗʰ S37.069 Major laceration of unspecified kidney MCC

✓6ᵗʰ S37.09 Other injury of kidney
   ✓7ᵗʰ S37.091 Other injury of right kidney MCC
   ✓7ᵗʰ S37.092 Other injury of left kidney MCC
   ✓7ᵗʰ S37.099 Other injury of unspecified kidney MCC

✓5ᵗʰ S37.1 Injury of ureter

CC Excl: For CC codes in subcategory S37.1: PDX collection 1238

✓x7ᵗʰ S37.10 Unspecified injury of ureter CC
✓x7ᵗʰ S37.12 Contusion of ureter CC
✓x7ᵗʰ S37.13 Laceration of ureter CC
✓x7ᵗʰ S37.19 Other injury of ureter CC

√5ᵗʰ S37.2 Injury of bladder

> **CC Excl: For CC codes in subcategory S37.2:**
> PDX collection 1239

     √x7ᵗʰ **S37.20 Unspecified injury of bladder** `CC`

     √x7ᵗʰ **S37.22 Contusion of bladder** `CC`

     √x7ᵗʰ **S37.23 Laceration of bladder** `CC`

     √x7ᵗʰ **S37.29 Other injury of bladder** `CC`

√5ᵗʰ S37.3 Injury of urethra

> **CC Excl: For CC codes in subcategory S37.3:**
> PDX collection 1239

     √x7ᵗʰ **S37.30 Unspecified injury of urethra** `CC`

     √x7ᵗʰ **S37.32 Contusion of urethra** `CC`

     √x7ᵗʰ **S37.33 Laceration of urethra** `CC`

     √x7ᵗʰ **S37.39 Other injury of urethra** `CC`

√5ᵗʰ S37.4 Injury of ovary

     √6ᵗʰ **S37.40 Unspecified injury of ovary**

         √7ᵗʰ **S37.401 Unspecified injury of ovary, unilateral** ♀

         √7ᵗʰ **S37.402 Unspecified injury of ovary, bilateral** ♀

         √7ᵗʰ **S37.409 Unspecified injury of ovary, unspecified** ♀

     √6ᵗʰ **S37.42 Contusion of ovary**

         √7ᵗʰ **S37.421 Contusion of ovary, unilateral** ♀

         √7ᵗʰ **S37.422 Contusion of ovary, bilateral** ♀

         √7ᵗʰ **S37.429 Contusion of ovary, unspecified** ♀

     √6ᵗʰ **S37.43 Laceration of ovary**

         √7ᵗʰ **S37.431 Laceration of ovary, unilateral** ♀

         √7ᵗʰ **S37.432 Laceration of ovary, bilateral** ♀

         √7ᵗʰ **S37.439 Laceration of ovary, unspecified** ♀

     √6ᵗʰ **S37.49 Other injury of ovary**

         √7ᵗʰ **S37.491 Other injury of ovary, unilateral** ♀

         √7ᵗʰ **S37.492 Other injury of ovary, bilateral** ♀

         √7ᵗʰ **S37.499 Other injury of ovary, unspecified** ♀

√5ᵗʰ S37.5 Injury of fallopian tube

     √6ᵗʰ **S37.50 Unspecified injury of fallopian tube**

         √7ᵗʰ **S37.501 Unspecified injury of fallopian tube, unilateral** ♀

         √7ᵗʰ **S37.502 Unspecified injury of fallopian tube, bilateral** ♀

         √7ᵗʰ **S37.509 Unspecified injury of fallopian tube, unspecified** ♀

     √6ᵗʰ **S37.51 Primary blast injury of fallopian tube**
         Blast injury of fallopian tube NOS

         √7ᵗʰ **S37.511 Primary blast injury of fallopian tube, unilateral** ♀

         √7ᵗʰ **S37.512 Primary blast injury of fallopian tube, bilateral** ♀

         √7ᵗʰ **S37.519 Primary blast injury of fallopian tube, unspecified** ♀

     √6ᵗʰ **S37.52 Contusion of fallopian tube**

         √7ᵗʰ **S37.521 Contusion of fallopian tube, unilateral** ♀

         √7ᵗʰ **S37.522 Contusion of fallopian tube, bilateral** ♀

         √7ᵗʰ **S37.529 Contusion of fallopian tube, unspecified** ♀

     √6ᵗʰ **S37.53 Laceration of fallopian tube**

         √7ᵗʰ **S37.531 Laceration of fallopian tube, unilateral** ♀

         √7ᵗʰ **S37.532 Laceration of fallopian tube, bilateral** ♀

         √7ᵗʰ **S37.539 Laceration of fallopian tube, unspecified** ♀

     √6ᵗʰ **S37.59 Other injury of fallopian tube**
         Secondary blast injury of fallopian tube

         √7ᵗʰ **S37.591 Other injury of fallopian tube, unilateral** ♀

         √7ᵗʰ **S37.592 Other injury of fallopian tube, bilateral** ♀

         √7ᵗʰ **S37.599 Other injury of fallopian tube, unspecified** ♀

√5ᵗʰ S37.6 Injury of uterus

     EXCLUDES 1 *injury to gravid uterus (O9A.2-)*
                 injury to uterus during delivery (O71.-)

> **CC Excl: For CC codes in subcategory S37.6:**
> PDX collection 1240

     √x7ᵗʰ **S37.60 Unspecified injury of uterus** `CC` ♀

     √x7ᵗʰ **S37.62 Contusion of uterus** `CC` ♀

     √x7ᵗʰ **S37.63 Laceration of uterus** `CC` ♀

     √x7ᵗʰ **S37.69 Other injury of uterus** `CC` ♀

√5ᵗʰ S37.8 Injury of other urinary and pelvic organs

     √6ᵗʰ **S37.81 Injury of adrenal gland**

> **CC Excl: For CC codes in subcategory S37.81:**
> PDX collection 1241

         √7ᵗʰ **S37.812 Contusion of adrenal gland** `CC`

         √7ᵗʰ **S37.813 Laceration of adrenal gland** `CC`

         √7ᵗʰ **S37.818 Other injury of adrenal gland** `CC`

         √7ᵗʰ **S37.819 Unspecified injury of adrenal gland** `CC`

     √6ᵗʰ **S37.82 Injury of prostate**

         √7ᵗʰ **S37.822 Contusion of prostate** ♂

         √7ᵗʰ **S37.823 Laceration of prostate** ♂

         √7ᵗʰ **S37.828 Other injury of prostate** ♂

         √7ᵗʰ **S37.829 Unspecified injury of prostate** ♂

     √6ᵗʰ **S37.89 Injury of other urinary and pelvic organ**

> **CC Excl: For CC codes in subcategory S37.89:**
> PDX collection 1242

         √7ᵗʰ **S37.892 Contusion of other urinary and pelvic organ**

         √7ᵗʰ **S37.893 Laceration of other urinary and pelvic organ** `CC`

         √7ᵗʰ **S37.898 Other injury of other urinary and pelvic organ** `CC`

         √7ᵗʰ **S37.899 Unspecified injury of other urinary and pelvic organ** `CC`

√5ᵗʰ S37.9 Injury of unspecified urinary and pelvic organ

> **CC Excl: For CC codes in subcategory S37.9:**
> PDX collection 1242

     √x7ᵗʰ **S37.90 Unspecified injury of unspecified urinary and pelvic organ** `CC`

     √x7ᵗʰ **S37.92 Contusion of unspecified urinary and pelvic organ** `CC`

     √x7ᵗʰ **S37.93 Laceration of unspecified urinary and pelvic organ** `CC`

     √x7ᵗʰ **S37.99 Other injury of unspecified urinary and pelvic organ** `CC`

√4ᵗʰ S38 Crushing injury and traumatic amputation of abdomen, lower back, pelvis and external genitals

     An amputation not identified as partial or complete should be coded to complete.

> The appropriate 7th character is to be added to each code from category S38.
> A   initial encounter
> D   subsequent encounter
> S   sequela

√5ᵗʰ S38.0 Crushing injury of external genital organs
     Use additional code for any associated injuries

     √6ᵗʰ **S38.00 Crushing injury of unspecified external genital organs**

         √7ᵗʰ **S38.001 Crushing injury of unspecified external genital organs, male** ♂

         √7ᵗʰ **S38.002 Crushing injury of unspecified external genital organs, female** ♀

     √x7ᵗʰ **S38.01 Crushing injury of penis** ♂

     √x7ᵗʰ **S38.02 Crushing injury of scrotum and testis** ♂

     √x7ᵗʰ **S38.03 Crushing injury of vulva** ♀

√x7ᵗʰ S38.1 Crushing injury of abdomen, lower back, and pelvis

     Use additional code for all associated injuries, such as:
         fracture of thoracic or lumbar spine and pelvis (S22.0-, S32-)
         injury to intra-abdominal organs (S36.-)
         injury to urinary and pelvic organs (S37.-)
         open wound of abdominal wall (S31.-)
         spinal cord injury (S34.0, S34.1-)

     EXCLUDES 2 *crushing injury of external genital organs (S38.0-)*

Ⓝ Newborn: 0   Ⓟ Pediatric: 0-17   Ⓜ Maternity: 12-55   Ⓐ Adult: 15-124   `MCC` Major Complication/Comorbidity   `CC` Complication/Comorbidity   `SW` Severe Wound Dx

988   ICD-10-CM 2019

☑5ᵗʰ **S38.2** Traumatic amputation of external genital organs

  ☑6ᵗʰ **S38.21** **Traumatic amputation of** female **external genital organs**
    Traumatic amputation of clitoris
    Traumatic amputation of labium (majus) (minus)
    Traumatic amputation of vulva

    ☑7ᵗʰ **S38.211** Complete **traumatic amputation of female external genital organs** ♀

    ☑7ᵗʰ **S38.212** Partial **traumatic amputation of female external genital organs** ♀

  ☑6ᵗʰ **S38.22** **Traumatic amputation of** penis

    ☑7ᵗʰ **S38.221** Complete **traumatic amputation of penis** ♂

    ☑7ᵗʰ **S38.222** Partial **traumatic amputation of penis** ♂

  ☑6ᵗʰ **S38.23** **Traumatic amputation of** scrotum and testis

    ☑7ᵗʰ **S38.231** Complete **traumatic amputation of scrotum and testis** ♂

    ☑7ᵗʰ **S38.232** Partial **traumatic amputation of scrotum and testis** ♂

☑x7ᵗʰ **S38.3** **Transection (partial) of abdomen**

☑4ᵗʰ **S39** **Other and unspecified injuries of abdomen, lower back, pelvis and external genitals**
  Code also any associated open wound (S31.-)
  EXCLUDES 2 *sprain of joints and ligaments of lumbar spine and pelvis (S33.-)*

  The appropriate 7th character is to be added to each code from category S39.
  A   initial encounter
  D   subsequent encounter
  S   sequela

☑5ᵗʰ **S39.0** **Injury of muscle, fascia and tendon of abdomen, lower back and pelvis**

  ☑6ᵗʰ **S39.00** Unspecified **injury of muscle, fascia and tendon of abdomen, lower back and pelvis**

    ☑7ᵗʰ **S39.001** **Unspecified injury of muscle, fascia and tendon of** abdomen

    ☑7ᵗʰ **S39.002** **Unspecified injury of muscle, fascia and tendon of** lower back

    ☑7ᵗʰ **S39.003** **Unspecified injury of muscle, fascia and tendon of** pelvis

  ☑6ᵗʰ **S39.01** Strain **of muscle, fascia and tendon of abdomen, lower back and pelvis**

    ☑7ᵗʰ **S39.011** **Strain of muscle, fascia and tendon of** abdomen

    ☑7ᵗʰ **S39.012** **Strain of muscle, fascia and tendon of** lower back

    ☑7ᵗʰ **S39.013** **Strain of muscle, fascia and tendon of** pelvis

  ☑6ᵗʰ **S39.02** Laceration **of muscle, fascia and tendon of abdomen, lower back and pelvis**

    ☑7ᵗʰ **S39.021** **Laceration of muscle, fascia and tendon of** abdomen

    ☑7ᵗʰ **S39.022** **Laceration of muscle, fascia and tendon of** lower back

    ☑7ᵗʰ **S39.023** **Laceration of muscle, fascia and tendon of** pelvis

  ☑6ᵗʰ **S39.09** Other **injury of muscle, fascia and tendon of abdomen, lower back and pelvis**

    ☑7ᵗʰ **S39.091** **Other injury of muscle, fascia and tendon of** abdomen

    ☑7ᵗʰ **S39.092** **Other injury of muscle, fascia and tendon of** lower back

    ☑7ᵗʰ **S39.093** **Other injury of muscle, fascia and tendon of** pelvis

☑5ᵗʰ **S39.8** Other **specified injuries of abdomen, lower back, pelvis and external genitals**

  ☑x7ᵗʰ **S39.81** **Other specified injuries of** abdomen

  ☑x7ᵗʰ **S39.82** **Other specified injuries of** lower back

  ☑x7ᵗʰ **S39.83** **Other specified injuries of** pelvis

  ☑6ᵗʰ **S39.84** **Other specified injuries of** external genitals

    ☑7ᵗʰ **S39.840** **Fracture of** corpus cavernosum penis ♂

    ☑7ᵗʰ **S39.848** Other **specified injuries of external genitals**
      TIP: Assign for traumatic rupture of testis.

☑5ᵗʰ **S39.9** Unspecified **injury of abdomen, lower back, pelvis and external genitals**

  ☑x7ᵗʰ **S39.91** **Unspecified injury of** abdomen

  ☑x7ᵗʰ **S39.92** **Unspecified injury of** lower back

  ☑x7ᵗʰ **S39.93** **Unspecified injury of** pelvis

  ☑x7ᵗʰ **S39.94** **Unspecified injury of** external genitals

Injuries to the shoulder and upper arm (S40-S49)

INCLUDES   injuries of axilla
            injuries of scapular region
EXCLUDES 2   *burns and corrosions (T20-T32)*
            frostbite (T33-T34)
            injuries of elbow (S50-S59)
            insect bite or sting, venomous (T63.4)

☑4ᵗʰ **S40** **Superficial injury of shoulder and upper arm**

  The appropriate 7th character is to be added to each code from category S40.
  A   initial encounter
  D   subsequent encounter
  S   sequela

☑5ᵗʰ **S40.0** Contusion **of shoulder and upper arm**

  ☑6ᵗʰ **S40.01** **Contusion of** shoulder

    ☑7ᵗʰ **S40.011** **Contusion of** right **shoulder**

    ☑7ᵗʰ **S40.012** **Contusion of** left **shoulder**

    ☑7ᵗʰ **S40.019** **Contusion of** unspecified **shoulder**

  ☑6ᵗʰ **S40.02** **Contusion of** upper arm

    ☑7ᵗʰ **S40.021** **Contusion of** right **upper arm**

    ☑7ᵗʰ **S40.022** **Contusion of** left **upper arm**

    ☑7ᵗʰ **S40.029** **Contusion of** unspecified **upper arm**

☑5ᵗʰ **S40.2** Other **superficial injuries of shoulder**

  ☑6ᵗʰ **S40.21** Abrasion **of shoulder**

    ☑7ᵗʰ **S40.211** **Abrasion of** right **shoulder**

    ☑7ᵗʰ **S40.212** **Abrasion of** left **shoulder**

    ☑7ᵗʰ **S40.219** **Abrasion of** unspecified **shoulder**

  ☑6ᵗʰ **S40.22** Blister **(nonthermal) of shoulder**

    ☑7ᵗʰ **S40.221** **Blister (nonthermal) of** right **shoulder**

    ☑7ᵗʰ **S40.222** **Blister (nonthermal) of** left **shoulder**

    ☑7ᵗʰ **S40.229** **Blister (nonthermal) of** unspecified **shoulder**

  ☑6ᵗʰ **S40.24** External constriction **of shoulder**

    ☑7ᵗʰ **S40.241** **External constriction of** right **shoulder**

    ☑7ᵗʰ **S40.242** **External constriction of** left **shoulder**

    ☑7ᵗʰ **S40.249** **External constriction of** unspecified **shoulder**

  ☑6ᵗʰ **S40.25** Superficial foreign body **of shoulder**
    Splinter in the shoulder

    ☑7ᵗʰ **S40.251** **Superficial foreign body of** right **shoulder**

    ☑7ᵗʰ **S40.252** **Superficial foreign body of** left **shoulder**

    ☑7ᵗʰ **S40.259** **Superficial foreign body of** unspecified **shoulder**

  ☑6ᵗʰ **S40.26** Insect bite **(nonvenomous) of shoulder**

    ☑7ᵗʰ **S40.261** **Insect bite (nonvenomous) of** right **shoulder**

    ☑7ᵗʰ **S40.262** **Insect bite (nonvenomous) of** left **shoulder**

    ☑7ᵗʰ **S40.269** **Insect bite (nonvenomous) of** unspecified **shoulder**

  ☑6ᵗʰ **S40.27** Other superficial bite **of shoulder**
    EXCLUDES 1 *open bite of shoulder (S41.05)*

    ☑7ᵗʰ **S40.271** **Other superficial bite of** right **shoulder**

    ☑7ᵗʰ **S40.272** **Other superficial bite of** left **shoulder**

    ☑7ᵗʰ **S40.279** **Other superficial bite of** unspecified **shoulder**

☑5ᵗʰ **S40.8** Other **superficial injuries of upper arm**

  ☑6ᵗʰ **S40.81** Abrasion **of upper arm**

    ☑7ᵗʰ **S40.811** **Abrasion of** right **upper arm**

    ☑7ᵗʰ **S40.812** **Abrasion of** left **upper arm**

    ☑7ᵗʰ **S40.819** **Abrasion of** unspecified **upper arm**

  ☑6ᵗʰ **S40.82** Blister **(nonthermal) of upper arm**

    ☑7ᵗʰ **S40.821** **Blister (nonthermal) of** right **upper arm**

    ☑7ᵗʰ **S40.822** **Blister (nonthermal) of** left **upper arm**

☑ Additional Character Required   ☑x7ᵗʰ Placeholder   Unacceptable PDx   Questionable PDx   Manifestation   H1-H14 HAC   HCC CMS-HCC Dx   HIV HIV Dx

ICD-10-CM 2019   989

✓7th **S40.829** Blister (nonthermal) of unspecified upper arm

✓6th **S40.84** External constriction of upper arm

   ✓7th **S40.841** External constriction of right upper arm

   ✓7th **S40.842** External constriction of left upper arm

   ✓7th **S40.849** External constriction of unspecified upper arm

✓6th **S40.85** Superficial foreign body of upper arm
   Splinter in the upper arm

   ✓7th **S40.851** Superficial foreign body of right upper arm

   ✓7th **S40.852** Superficial foreign body of left upper arm

   ✓7th **S40.859** Superficial foreign body of unspecified upper arm

✓6th **S40.86** Insect bite (nonvenomous) of upper arm

   ✓7th **S40.861** Insect bite (nonvenomous) of right upper arm

   ✓7th **S40.862** Insect bite (nonvenomous) of left upper arm

   ✓7th **S40.869** Insect bite (nonvenomous) of unspecified upper arm

✓6th **S40.87** Other superficial bite of upper arm
   EXCLUDES 1 *open bite of upper arm (S41.14)*
   EXCLUDES 2 *other superficial bite of shoulder (S40.27-)*

   ✓7th **S40.871** Other superficial bite of right upper arm

   ✓7th **S40.872** Other superficial bite of left upper arm

   ✓7th **S40.879** Other superficial bite of unspecified upper arm

✓5th **S40.9** Unspecified superficial injury of shoulder and upper arm

✓6th **S40.91** Unspecified superficial injury of shoulder

   ✓7th **S40.911** Unspecified superficial injury of right shoulder

   ✓7th **S40.912** Unspecified superficial injury of left shoulder

   ✓7th **S40.919** Unspecified superficial injury of unspecified shoulder

✓6th **S40.92** Unspecified superficial injury of upper arm

   ✓7th **S40.921** Unspecified superficial injury of right upper arm

   ✓7th **S40.922** Unspecified superficial injury of left upper arm

   ✓7th **S40.929** Unspecified superficial injury of unspecified upper arm

✓4th **S41** **Open wound of shoulder and upper arm**
   Code also any associated wound infection
   EXCLUDES 1 *traumatic amputation of shoulder and upper arm (S48.-)*
   EXCLUDES 2 *open fracture of shoulder and upper arm (S42.- with 7th character B or C)*

> The appropriate 7th character is to be added to each code from category S41.
> A   initial encounter
> D   subsequent encounter
> S   sequela

✓5th **S41.0** Open wound of shoulder

✓6th **S41.00** Unspecified open wound of shoulder

   ✓7th **S41.001** Unspecified open wound of right shoulder

   ✓7th **S41.002** Unspecified open wound of left shoulder

   ✓7th **S41.009** Unspecified open wound of unspecified shoulder

✓6th **S41.01** Laceration without foreign body of shoulder

   ✓7th **S41.011** Laceration without foreign body of right shoulder

   ✓7th **S41.012** Laceration without foreign body of left shoulder

   ✓7th **S41.019** Laceration without foreign body of unspecified shoulder

✓6th **S41.02** Laceration with foreign body of shoulder

   ✓7th **S41.021** Laceration with foreign body of right shoulder

   ✓7th **S41.022** Laceration with foreign body of left shoulder

   ✓7th **S41.029** Laceration with foreign body of unspecified shoulder

✓6th **S41.03** Puncture wound without foreign body of shoulder

   ✓7th **S41.031** Puncture wound without foreign body of right shoulder

   ✓7th **S41.032** Puncture wound without foreign body of left shoulder

   ✓7th **S41.039** Puncture wound without foreign body of unspecified shoulder

✓6th **S41.04** Puncture wound with foreign body of shoulder

   ✓7th **S41.041** Puncture wound with foreign body of right shoulder

   ✓7th **S41.042** Puncture wound with foreign body of left shoulder

   ✓7th **S41.049** Puncture wound with foreign body of unspecified shoulder

✓6th **S41.05** Open bite of shoulder
   Bite of shoulder NOS
   EXCLUDES 1 *superficial bite of shoulder (S40.27)*

   ✓7th **S41.051** Open bite of right shoulder

   ✓7th **S41.052** Open bite of left shoulder

   ✓7th **S41.059** Open bite of unspecified shoulder

✓5th **S41.1** Open wound of upper arm

✓6th **S41.10** Unspecified open wound of upper arm
   AHA: 2016, 3Q, 24

   ✓7th **S41.101** Unspecified open wound of right upper arm

   ✓7th **S41.102** Unspecified open wound of left upper arm

   ✓7th **S41.109** Unspecified open wound of unspecified upper arm

✓6th **S41.11** Laceration without foreign body of upper arm

   ✓7th **S41.111** Laceration without foreign body of right upper arm

   ✓7th **S41.112** Laceration without foreign body of left upper arm

   ✓7th **S41.119** Laceration without foreign body of unspecified upper arm

✓6th **S41.12** Laceration with foreign body of upper arm

   ✓7th **S41.121** Laceration with foreign body of right upper arm

   ✓7th **S41.122** Laceration with foreign body of left upper arm

   ✓7th **S41.129** Laceration with foreign body of unspecified upper arm

✓6th **S41.13** Puncture wound without foreign body of upper arm
   AHA: 2016, 3Q, 24

   ✓7th **S41.131** Puncture wound without foreign body of right upper arm

   ✓7th **S41.132** Puncture wound without foreign body of left upper arm

   ✓7th **S41.139** Puncture wound without foreign body of unspecified upper arm

✓6th **S41.14** Puncture wound with foreign body of upper arm
   AHA: 2016, 3Q, 24

   ✓7th **S41.141** Puncture wound with foreign body of right upper arm

   ✓7th **S41.142** Puncture wound with foreign body of left upper arm

   ✓7th **S41.149** Puncture wound with foreign body of unspecified upper arm

✓6th **S41.15** Open bite of upper arm
   Bite of upper arm NOS
   EXCLUDES 1 *superficial bite of upper arm (S40.87)*

   ✓7th **S41.151** Open bite of right upper arm

   ✓7th **S41.152** Open bite of left upper arm

   ✓7th **S41.159** Open bite of unspecified upper arm

✓4th S42   Fracture of shoulder and upper arm

NOTE   A fracture not indicated as displaced or nondisplaced should be coded to displaced.
A fracture not indicated as open or closed should be coded to closed.

EXCLUDES 1   *traumatic amputation of shoulder and upper arm (S48.-)*

AHA: 2018, 2Q, 12; 2015, 3Q, 37-39

The appropriate 7th character is to be added to all codes from category S42 [unless otherwise indicated].
A   initial encounter for closed fracture
B   initial encounter for open fracture
D   subsequent encounter for fracture with routine healing
G   subsequent encounter for fracture with delayed healing
K   subsequent encounter for fracture with nonunion
P   subsequent encounter for fracture with malunion
S   sequela

✓5th S42.0   Fracture of clavicle

CC Excl: For codes in subcategory S42.0:
CC with 7th character B: PDX collection 1243
CC with 7th character K or P: PDX collection 897

✓6th S42.00   Fracture of unspecified part of clavicle

3 ✓7th **S42.001**   Fracture of unspecified part of right clavicle   **CC H5**

3 ✓7th **S42.002**   Fracture of unspecified part of left clavicle   **CC H5**

3 ✓7th **S42.009**   Fracture of unspecified part of unspecified clavicle   **CC H5**
    AHA: 2012, 4Q, 93

✓6th S42.01   Fracture of sternal end of clavicle

3 ✓7th **S42.011**   Anterior displaced fracture of sternal end of right clavicle   **CC H5**

3 ✓7th **S42.012**   Anterior displaced fracture of sternal end of left clavicle   **CC H5**

3 ✓7th **S42.013**   Anterior displaced fracture of sternal end of unspecified clavicle   **CC H5**
    Displaced fracture of sternal end of clavicle NOS

3 ✓7th **S42.014**   Posterior displaced fracture of sternal end of right clavicle   **CC H5**

3 ✓7th **S42.015**   Posterior displaced fracture of sternal end of left clavicle   **CC H5**

3 ✓7th **S42.016**   Posterior displaced fracture of sternal end of unspecified clavicle   **CC H5**

3 ✓7th **S42.013**   Nondisplaced fracture of sternal end of right clavicle   **CC H5**

3 ✓7th **S42.018**   Nondisplaced fracture of sternal end of left clavicle   **CC H5**

3 ✓7th **S42.019**   Nondisplaced fracture of sternal end of unspecified clavicle   **CC H5**

✓6th S42.02   Fracture of shaft of clavicle

3 ✓7th **S42.021**   Displaced fracture of shaft of right clavicle   **CC H5**

3 ✓7th **S42.022**   Displaced fracture of shaft of left clavicle   **CC H5**

3 ✓7th **S42.023**   Displaced fracture of shaft of unspecified clavicle   **CC H5**

3 ✓7th **S42.024**   Nondisplaced fracture of shaft of right clavicle   **CC H5**

3 ✓7th **S42.025**   Nondisplaced fracture of shaft of left clavicle   **CC H5**

3 ✓7th **S42.026**   Nondisplaced fracture of shaft of unspecified clavicle   **CC H5**

✓6th S42.03   Fracture of lateral end of clavicle
    Fracture of acromial end of clavicle

3 ✓7th **S42.031**   Displaced fracture of lateral end of right clavicle   **CC H5**

3 ✓7th **S42.032**   Displaced fracture of lateral end of left clavicle   **CC H5**

3 ✓7th **S42.033**   Displaced fracture of lateral end of unspecified clavicle   **CC H5**

3 ✓7th **S42.034**   Nondisplaced fracture of lateral end of right clavicle   **CC H5**

3 ✓7th **S42.035**   Nondisplaced fracture of lateral end of left clavicle   **CC H5**

3 ✓7th **S42.036**   Nondisplaced fracture of lateral end of unspecified clavicle   **CC H5**

✓5th S42.1   Fracture of scapula

CC Excl: For codes in subcategory S42.1:
CC with 7th character B: PDX collection 1244
CC with 7th character K or P: PDX collection 897

✓6th S42.10   Fracture of unspecified part of scapula

3 ✓7th **S42.101**   Fracture of unspecified part of scapula, right shoulder   **CC H5**

3 ✓7th **S42.102**   Fracture of unspecified part of scapula, left shoulder   **CC H5**

3 ✓7th **S42.109**   Fracture of unspecified part of scapula, unspecified shoulder   **CC H5**

✓6th S42.11   Fracture of body of scapula

3 ✓7th **S42.111**   Displaced fracture of body of scapula, right shoulder   **CC H5**

3 ✓7th **S42.112**   Displaced fracture of body of scapula, left shoulder   **CC H5**

3 ✓7th **S42.113**   Displaced fracture of body of scapula, unspecified shoulder   **CC H5**

3 ✓7th **S42.114**   Nondisplaced fracture of body of scapula, right shoulder   **CC H5**

3 ✓7th **S42.115**   Nondisplaced fracture of body of scapula, left shoulder   **CC H5**

3 ✓7th **S42.116**   Nondisplaced fracture of body of scapula, unspecified shoulder   **CC H5**

✓6th S42.12   Fracture of acromial process

3 ✓7th **S42.121**   Displaced fracture of acromial process, right shoulder   **CC H5**

3 ✓7th **S42.122**   Displaced fracture of acromial process, left shoulder   **CC H5**

3 ✓7th **S42.123**   Displaced fracture of acromial process, unspecified shoulder   **CC H5**

3 ✓7th **S42.124**   Nondisplaced fracture of acromial process, right shoulder   **CC H5**

3 ✓7th **S42.125**   Nondisplaced fracture of acromial process, left shoulder   **CC H5**

3 ✓7th **S42.126**   Nondisplaced fracture of acromial process, unspecified shoulder   **CC H5**

✓6th S42.13   Fracture of coracoid process

3 ✓7th **S42.131**   Displaced fracture of coracoid process, right shoulder   **CC H5**

3 ✓7th **S42.132**   Displaced fracture of coracoid process, left shoulder   **CC H5**

3 ✓7th **S42.133**   Displaced fracture of coracoid process, unspecified shoulder   **CC H5**

3 ✓7th **S42.134**   Nondisplaced fracture of coracoid process, right shoulder   **CC H5**

3 ✓7th **S42.135**   Nondisplaced fracture of coracoid process, left shoulder   **CC H5**

3 ✓7th **S42.136**   Nondisplaced fracture of coracoid process, unspecified shoulder   **CC H5**

✓6th S42.14   Fracture of glenoid cavity of scapula

3 ✓7th **S42.141**   Displaced fracture of glenoid cavity of scapula, right shoulder   **CC H5**

3 ✓7th **S42.142**   Displaced fracture of glenoid cavity of scapula, left shoulder   **CC H5**

3 ✓7th **S42.143**   Displaced fracture of glenoid cavity of scapula, unspecified shoulder   **CC H5**

3 ✓7th **S42.144**   Nondisplaced fracture of glenoid cavity of scapula, right shoulder   **CC H5**

3 ✓7th **S42.145**   Nondisplaced fracture of glenoid cavity of scapula, left shoulder   **CC H5**

3 ✓7th **S42.146**   Nondisplaced fracture of glenoid cavity of scapula, unspecified shoulder   **CC H5**

✓6th S42.15   Fracture of neck of scapula

3 ✓7th **S42.151**   Displaced fracture of neck of scapula, right shoulder   **CC H5**

3 ✓7th **S42.152**   Displaced fracture of neck of scapula, left shoulder   **CC H5**

3 ✓7th **S42.153**   Displaced fracture of neck of scapula, unspecified shoulder   **CC H5**

3 ✓7th **S42.154**   Nondisplaced fracture of neck of scapula, right shoulder   **CC H5**

3 ✓7th **S42.155**   Nondisplaced fracture of neck of scapula, left shoulder   **CC H5**

3 ✓7ᵗʰ **S42.156** Nondisplaced **fracture of neck of** scapula, unspecified **shoulder** `CC` `H5`

✓6ᵗʰ **S42.19** Fracture of other **part of scapula**

     3 ✓7ᵗʰ **S42.191** Fracture of other part of scapula, right **shoulder** `CC` `H5`

     3 ✓7ᵗʰ **S42.192** Fracture of other part of scapula, left **shoulder** `CC` `H5`

     3 ✓7ᵗʰ **S42.199** Fracture of other part of scapula, unspecified **shoulder** `CC` `H5`

✓5ᵗʰ **S42.2** Fracture of upper end **of humerus**
Fracture of proximal end of humerus

EXCLUDES 2   *fracture of shaft of humerus (S42.3-)*
           physeal fracture of upper end of humerus (S49.0-)

> **CC Excl: For CC/MCC codes in subcategory S42.2, unless otherwise noted:**
> **Right side:** See code S42.201
> **Left side:** See code S42.202
> **Unspecified side:** See code S42.209

✓6ᵗʰ **S42.20** Unspecified **fracture of upper end of humerus**

     2,3 ✓7ᵗʰ **S42.201** Unspecified fracture of upper end of right **humerus** `MCC` `CC` `H5`

> **CC Excl: CC with 7th character A:** PDX collection 1245
> **MCC with 7th character B:** PDX collection 1246
> **CC with 7th character K or P:** PDX collection 897

     2,3 ✓7ᵗʰ **S42.202** Unspecified fracture of upper end of left **humerus** `MCC` `CC` `H5`

> **CC Excl: CC with 7th character A:** PDX collection 1247
> **MCC with 7th character B:** PDX collection 1246
> **CC with 7th character K or P:** PDX collection 897

     2,3 ✓7ᵗʰ **S42.209** Unspecified fracture of upper end of unspecified **humerus** `MCC` `CC` `H5`

> **CC Excl: CC with 7th character A:** PDX collection 1248
> **MCC with 7th character B:** PDX collection 1246
> **CC with 7th character K or P:** PDX collection 897

✓6ᵗʰ **S42.21** Unspecified **fracture of surgical neck of humerus**
Fracture of neck of humerus NOS

     2,3 ✓7ᵗʰ **S42.211** Unspecified displaced **fracture of surgical neck of right humerus** `MCC` `CC` `H5`

     2,3 ✓7ᵗʰ **S42.212** Unspecified displaced **fracture of surgical neck of left humerus** `MCC` `CC` `H5`

     2,3 ✓7ᵗʰ **S42.213** Unspecified displaced **fracture of surgical neck of unspecified humerus** `MCC` `CC` `H5`

     2,3 ✓7ᵗʰ **S42.214** Unspecified nondisplaced **fracture of surgical neck of right humerus** `MCC` `CC` `H5`

     2,3 ✓7ᵗʰ **S42.215** Unspecified nondisplaced **fracture of surgical neck of left humerus** `MCC` `CC` `H5`

     2,3 ✓7ᵗʰ **S42.216** Unspecified nondisplaced **fracture of surgical neck of unspecified humerus** `MCC` `CC` `H5`

✓6ᵗʰ **S42.22** 2-part **fracture of surgical neck of humerus**

     2,3 ✓7ᵗʰ **S42.221** 2-part displaced **fracture of surgical neck of right humerus** `MCC` `CC` `H5`

     2,3 ✓7ᵗʰ **S42.222** 2-part displaced **fracture of surgical neck of left humerus** `MCC` `CC` `H5`

     2,3 ✓7ᵗʰ **S42.223** 2-part displaced **fracture of surgical neck of unspecified humerus** `MCC` `CC` `H5`

     2,3 ✓7ᵗʰ **S42.224** 2-part nondisplaced **fracture of surgical neck of right humerus** `MCC` `CC` `H5`

     2,3 ✓7ᵗʰ **S42.225** 2-part nondisplaced **fracture of surgical neck of left humerus** `MCC` `CC` `H5`

     2,3 ✓7ᵗʰ **S42.226** 2-part nondisplaced **fracture of surgical neck of unspecified humerus** `MCC` `CC` `H5`

✓6ᵗʰ **S42.23** 3-part **fracture of surgical neck of humerus**

     2,3 ✓7ᵗʰ **S42.231** 3-part fracture of surgical neck of right **humerus** `MCC` `CC` `H5`

     2,3 ✓7ᵗʰ **S42.232** 3-part fracture of surgical neck of left **humerus** `MCC` `CC` `H5`

     2,3 ✓7ᵗʰ **S42.239** 3-part fracture of surgical neck of unspecified **humerus** `MCC` `CC` `H5`

✓6ᵗʰ **S42.24** 4-part **fracture of surgical neck of humerus**

     2,3 ✓7ᵗʰ **S42.241** 4-part fracture of surgical neck of right **humerus** `MCC` `CC` `H5`

     2,3 ✓7ᵗʰ **S42.242** 4-part fracture of surgical neck of left **humerus** `MCC` `CC` `H5`

     2,3 ✓7ᵗʰ **S42.249** 4-part fracture of surgical neck of unspecified **humerus** `MCC` `CC` `H5`

✓6ᵗʰ **S42.25** Fracture of greater tuberosity **of humerus**

     2,3 ✓7ᵗʰ **S42.251** Displaced **fracture of greater tuberosity of right humerus** `MCC` `CC` `H5`

     2,3 ✓7ᵗʰ **S42.252** Displaced **fracture of greater tuberosity of left humerus** `MCC` `CC` `H5`

     2,3 ✓7ᵗʰ **S42.253** Displaced **fracture of greater tuberosity of unspecified humerus** `MCC` `CC` `H5`

     2,3 ✓7ᵗʰ **S42.254** Nondisplaced **fracture of greater tuberosity of right humerus** `MCC` `CC` `H5`

     2,3 ✓7ᵗʰ **S42.255** Nondisplaced **fracture of greater tuberosity of left humerus** `MCC` `CC` `H5`

     2,3 ✓7ᵗʰ **S42.256** Nondisplaced **fracture of greater tuberosity of unspecified humerus** `MCC` `CC` `H5`

✓6ᵗʰ **S42.26** Fracture of lesser tuberosity **of humerus**

     2,3 ✓7ᵗʰ **S42.261** Displaced **fracture of lesser tuberosity of right humerus** `MCC` `CC` `H5`

     2,3 ✓7ᵗʰ **S42.262** Displaced **fracture of lesser tuberosity of left humerus** `MCC` `CC` `H5`

     2,3 ✓7ᵗʰ **S42.263** Displaced **fracture of lesser tuberosity of unspecified humerus** `MCC` `CC` `H5`

     2,3 ✓7ᵗʰ **S42.264** Nondisplaced **fracture of lesser tuberosity of right humerus** `MCC` `CC` `H5`

     2,3 ✓7ᵗʰ **S42.265** Nondisplaced **fracture of lesser tuberosity of left humerus** `MCC` `CC` `H5`

     2,3 ✓7ᵗʰ **S42.266** Nondisplaced **fracture of lesser tuberosity of unspecified humerus** `MCC` `CC` `H5`

✓6ᵗʰ **S42.27** Torus **fracture of upper end of humerus**

> The appropriate 7th character is to be added to all codes in subcategory S42.27.
> A   initial encounter for closed fracture
> D   subsequent encounter for fracture with routine healing
> G   subsequent encounter for fracture with delayed healing
> K   subsequent encounter for fracture with nonunion
> P   subsequent encounter for fracture with malunion
> S   sequela

     3 ✓7ᵗʰ **S42.271** Torus fracture of upper end of right **humerus** `CC` `H5`

> **CC Excl: CC with 7th character A:** PDX collection 1245
> **CC with 7th character K or P:** PDX collection 897

     3 ✓7ᵗʰ **S42.272** Torus fracture of upper end of left **humerus** `CC` `H5`

> **CC Excl: CC with 7th character A:** PDX collection 1247
> **CC with 7th character K or P:** PDX collection 897

     3 ✓7ᵗʰ **S42.279** Torus fracture of upper end of unspecified **humerus** `CC` `H5`

> **CC Excl: CC with 7th character A:** PDX collection 1248
> **CC with 7th character K or P:** PDX collection 897

✓6ᵗʰ **S42.29** Other **fracture of upper end of humerus**
Fracture of anatomical neck of humerus
Fracture of articular head of humerus

     2,3 ✓7ᵗʰ **S42.291** Other displaced **fracture of upper end of right humerus** `MCC` `CC` `H5`

     2,3 ✓7ᵗʰ **S42.292** Other displaced **fracture of upper end of left humerus** `MCC` `CC` `H5`

     2,3 ✓7ᵗʰ **S42.293** Other displaced **fracture of upper end of unspecified humerus** `MCC` `CC` `H5`

     2,3 ✓7ᵗʰ **S42.294** Other nondisplaced **fracture of upper end of right humerus** `MCC` `CC` `H5`

N Newborn: 0   **P** Pediatric: 0-17   **M** Maternity: 12-55   **A** Adult: 15-124   `MCC` Major Complication/Comorbidity   `CC` Complication/Comorbidity   `SW` Severe Wound Dx

992   ICD-10-CM 2019

2,3 √7ᵗʰ **S42.295** Other nondisplaced fracture of `MCC` `CC` `H5`
upper end of left humerus

2,3 √7ᵗʰ **S42.296** Other nondisplaced fracture of `MCC` `CC` `H5`
upper end of unspecified humerus

√5ᵗʰ **S42.3** Fracture of shaft of humerus
Fracture of humerus NOS
Fracture of upper arm NOS
> *EXCLUDES 2*   physeal fractures of upper end of humerus (S49.0-)
> physeal fractures of lower end of humerus (S49.1-)

> **CC Excl: For CC/MCC codes in subcategory S42.3, unless otherwise noted:**
> **Right side:** See code S42.321
> **Left side:** See code S42.322
> **Unspecified side:** See code S42.323

√6ᵗʰ **S42.30** Unspecified fracture of shaft of humerus

2,3 √7ᵗʰ **S42.301** Unspecified fracture of shaft of `MCC` `CC` `H5`
humerus, right arm

2,3 √7ᵗʰ **S42.302** Unspecified fracture of shaft of `MCC` `CC` `H5`
humerus, left arm

2,3 √7ᵗʰ **S42.309** Unspecified fracture of shaft of `MCC` `CC` `H5`
humerus, unspecified arm

√6ᵗʰ **S42.31** Greenstick fracture of shaft of humerus

> The appropriate 7th character is to be added to all codes in subcategory S42.31.
> A   initial encounter for closed fracture
> D   subsequent encounter for fracture with routine healing
> G   subsequent encounter for fracture with delayed healing
> K   subsequent encounter for fracture with nonunion
> P   subsequent encounter for fracture with malunion
> S   sequela

3 √7ᵗʰ **S42.311** Greenstick fracture of shaft of `CC` `H5`
humerus, right arm
CC Excl: CC with 7th character A:
PDX collection 1249
CC with 7th character K or P:
PDX collection 897

3 √7ᵗʰ **S42.312** Greenstick fracture of shaft of `CC` `H5`
humerus, left arm
CC Excl: CC with 7th character A:
PDX collection 1250
CC with 7th character K or P:
PDX collection 897

3 √7ᵗʰ **S42.319** Greenstick fracture of shaft of `CC` `H5`
humerus, unspecified arm
CC Excl: CC with 7th character A:
PDX collection 1251
CC with 7th character K or P:
PDX collection 897

√6ᵗʰ **S42.32** Transverse fracture of shaft of humerus

2,3 √7ᵗʰ **S42.321** Displaced transverse fracture `MCC` `CC` `H5`
of shaft of humerus, right arm
CC Excl: CC with 7th character A:
PDX collection 1249
MCC with 7th character B:
PDX collection 1246
CC with 7th character K or P:
PDX collection 897

2,3 √7ᵗʰ **S42.322** Displaced transverse fracture `MCC` `CC` `H5`
of shaft of humerus, left arm
CC Excl: CC with 7th character A:
PDX collection 1250
MCC with 7th character B:
PDX collection 1246
CC with 7th character K or P:
PDX collection 897

2,3 √7ᵗʰ **S42.323** Displaced transverse fracture `MCC` `CC` `H5`
of shaft of humerus, unspecified arm
CC Excl: CC with 7th character A:
PDX collection 1251
MCC with 7th character B:
PDX collection 1246
CC with 7th character K or P:
PDX collection 897

2,3 √7ᵗʰ **S42.324** Nondisplaced transverse `MCC` `CC` `H5`
fracture of shaft of humerus, right arm

2,3 √7ᵗʰ **S42.325** Nondisplaced transverse `MCC` `CC` `H5`
fracture of shaft of humerus, left arm

2,3 √7ᵗʰ **S42.326** Nondisplaced transverse `MCC` `CC` `H5`
fracture of shaft of humerus, unspecified arm

√6ᵗʰ **S42.33** Oblique fracture of shaft of humerus

2,3 √7ᵗʰ **S42.331** Displaced oblique fracture of `MCC` `CC` `H5`
shaft of humerus, right arm

2,3 √7ᵗʰ **S42.332** Displaced oblique fracture of `MCC` `CC` `H5`
shaft of humerus, left arm

2,3 √7ᵗʰ **S42.333** Displaced oblique fracture of `MCC` `CC` `H5`
shaft of humerus, unspecified arm

2,3 √7ᵗʰ **S42.334** Nondisplaced oblique fracture `MCC` `CC` `H5`
of shaft of humerus, right arm

2,3 √7ᵗʰ **S42.335** Nondisplaced oblique fracture `MCC` `CC` `H5`
of shaft of humerus, left arm

2,3 √7ᵗʰ **S42.336** Nondisplaced oblique fracture `MCC` `CC` `H5`
of shaft of humerus, unspecified arm

√6ᵗʰ **S42.34** Spiral fracture of shaft of humerus

2,3 √7ᵗʰ **S42.341** Displaced spiral fracture of `MCC` `CC` `H5`
shaft of humerus, right arm

2,3 √7ᵗʰ **S42.342** Displaced spiral fracture of `MCC` `CC` `H5`
shaft of humerus, left arm

2,3 √7ᵗʰ **S42.343** Displaced spiral fracture of `MCC` `CC` `H5`
sharft of humerus, unspecified arm

2,3 √7ᵗʰ **S42.344** Nondisplaced spiral fracture `MCC` `CC` `H5`
of shaft of humerus, right arm

2,3 √7ᵗʰ **S42.345** Nondisplaced spiral fracture `MCC` `CC` `H5`
of shaft of humerus, left arm

2,3 √7ᵗʰ **S42.346** Nondisplaced spiral fracture `MCC` `CC` `H5`
of shaft of humerus, unspecified arm

√6ᵗʰ **S42.35** Comminuted fracture of shaft of humerus

2,3 √7ᵗʰ **S42.351** Displaced comminuted fracture `MCC` `CC` `H5`
of shaft of humerus, right arm

2,3 √7ᵗʰ **S42.352** Displaced comminuted fracture `MCC` `CC` `H5`
of shaft of humerus, left arm

2,3 √7ᵗʰ **S42.353** Displaced comminuted fracture `MCC` `CC` `H5`
of shaft of humerus, unspecified arm

2,3 √7ᵗʰ **S42.354** Nondisplaced comminuted `MCC` `CC` `H5`
fracture of shaft of humerus, right arm

2,3 √7ᵗʰ **S42.355** Nondisplaced comminuted `MCC` `CC` `H5`
fracture of shaft of humerus, left arm

2,3 √7ᵗʰ **S42.356** Nondisplaced comminuted `MCC` `CC` `H5`
fracture of shaft of humerus, unspecified arm

√6ᵗʰ **S42.36** Segmental fracture of shaft of humerus

2,3 √7ᵗʰ **S42.361** Displaced segmental fracture `MCC` `CC` `H5`
of shaft of humerus, right arm

2,3 √7ᵗʰ **S42.362** Displaced segmental fracture `MCC` `CC` `H5`
of shaft of humerus, left arm

2,3 √7ᵗʰ **S42.363** Displaced segmental fracture `MCC` `CC` `H5`
of shaft of humerus, unspecified arm

2,3 √7ᵗʰ **S42.364** Nondisplaced segmental `MCC` `CC` `H5`
fracture of shaft of humerus, right arm

2,3 √7ᵗʰ **S42.365** Nondisplaced segmental `MCC` `CC` `H5`
fracture of shaft of humerus, left arm

2,3 √7ᵗʰ **S42.366** Nondisplaced segmental `MCC` `CC` `H5`
fracture of shaft of humerus, unspecified arm

√6ᵗʰ **S42.39** Other fracture of shaft of humerus

2,3 √7ᵗʰ **S42.391** Other fracture of shaft of right `MCC` `CC` `H5`
humerus

2,3 √7ᵗʰ **S42.392** Other fracture of shaft of left `MCC` `CC` `H5`
humerus

2,3 √7ᵗʰ **S42.399** Other fracture of shaft of `MCC` `CC` `H5`
unspecified humerus

Chapter 19. Injury, Poisoning and Certain Other Consequences of External Causes

S42.295–S42.399

√5th S42.4 Fracture of lower end of humerus
Fracture of distal end of humerus
> EXCLUDES 2   fracture of shaft of humerus (S42.3-)
> physeal fracture of lower end of humerus (S49.1-)

CC Excl: For CC/MCC codes in subcategory S42.4, unless otherwise noted:
Right side: See code S42.201
Left side: See code S42.202
Unspecified side: See code S42.209

√6th S42.40 Unspecified fracture of lower end of humerus
Fracture of elbow NOS

2,3 √7th **S42.401** Unspecified fracture of lower end of right humerus   MCC CC H5

2,3 √7th **S42.402** Unspecified fracture of lower end of left humerus   MCC CC H5

2,3 √7th **S42.409** Unspecified fracture of lower end of unspecified humerus   MCC CC H5

√6th S42.41 Simple supracondylar fracture without intercondylar fracture of humerus

2,3 √7th **S42.411** Displaced simple supracondylar fracture without intercondylar fracture of right humerus   MCC CC H5

2,3 √7th **S42.412** Displaced simple supracondylar fracture without intercondylar fracture of left humerus   MCC CC H5

2,3 √7th **S42.413** Displaced simple supracondylar fracture without intercondylar fracture of unspecified humerus   MCC CC H5

2,3 √7th **S42.414** Nondisplaced simple supracondylar fracture without intercondylar fracture of right humerus   MCC CC H5

2,3 √7th **S42.415** Nondisplaced simple supracondylar fracture without intercondylar fracture of left humerus   MCC CC H5

2,3 √7th **S42.416** Nondisplaced simple supracondylar fracture without intercondylar fracture of unspecified humerus   MCC CC H5

√6th S42.42 Comminuted supracondylar fracture without intercondylar fracture of humerus

2,3 √7th **S42.421** Displaced comminuted supracondylar fracture without intercondylar fracture of right humerus   MCC CC H5

2,3 √7th **S42.422** Displaced comminuted supracondylar fracture without intercondylar fracture of left humerus   MCC CC H5

2,3 √7th **S42.423** Displaced comminuted supracondylar fracture without intercondylar fracture of unspecified humerus   MCC CC H5

2,3 √7th **S42.424** Nondisplaced comminuted supracondylar fracture without intercondylar fracture of right humerus   MCC CC H5

2,3 √7th **S42.425** Nondisplaced comminuted supracondylar fracture without intercondylar fracture of left humerus   MCC CC H5

2,3 √7th **S42.426** Nondisplaced comminuted supracondylar fracture without intercondylar fracture of unspecified humerus   MCC CC H5

√6th S42.43 Fracture (avulsion) of lateral epicondyle of humerus

2,3 √7th **S42.431** Displaced fracture (avulsion) of lateral epicondyle of right humerus   MCC CC H5

2,3 √7th **S42.432** Displaced fracture (avulsion) of lateral epicondyle of left humerus   MCC CC H5

2,3 √7th **S42.433** Displaced fracture (avulsion) of lateral epicondyle of unspecified humerus   MCC CC H5

2,3 √7th **S42.434** Nondisplaced fracture (avulsion) of lateral epicondyle of right humerus   MCC CC H5

2,3 √7th **S42.435** Nondisplaced fracture (avulsion) of lateral epicondyle of left humerus   MCC CC H5

2,3 √7th **S42.436** Nondisplaced fracture (avulsion) of lateral epicondyle of unspecified humerus   MCC CC H5

√6th S42.44 Fracture (avulsion) of medial epicondyle of humerus

2,3 √7th **S42.441** Displaced fracture (avulsion) of medial epicondyle of right humerus   MCC CC H5

2,3 √7th **S42.442** Displaced fracture (avulsion) of medial epicondyle of left humerus   MCC CC H5

2,3 √7th **S42.443** Displaced fracture (avulsion) of medial epicondyle of unspecified humerus   MCC CC H5

2,3 √7th **S42.444** Nondisplaced fracture (avulsion) of medial epicondyle of right humerus   MCC CC H5

2,3 √7th **S42.445** Nondisplaced fracture (avulsion) of medial epicondyle of left humerus   MCC CC H5

2,3 √7th **S42.446** Nondisplaced fracture (avulsion) medial epicondyle of unspecified of humerus   MCC CC H5

2,3 √7th **S42.447** Incarcerated fracture (avulsion) of medial epicondyle of right humerus   MCC CC H5

2,3 √7th **S42.448** Incarcerated fracture (avulsion) of medial epicondyle of left humerus   MCC CC H5

2,3 √7th **S42.449** Incarcerated fracture (avulsion) of medial epicondyle of unspecified humerus   MCC CC H5

√6th S42.45 Fracture of lateral condyle of humerus
Fracture of capitellum of humerus

2,3 √7th **S42.451** Displaced fracture of lateral condyle of right humerus   MCC CC H5

2,3 √7th **S42.452** Displaced fracture of lateral condyle of left humerus   MCC CC H5

2,3 √7th **S42.453** Displaced fracture of lateral condyle of unspecified humerus   MCC CC H5

2,3 √7th **S42.454** Nondisplaced fracture of lateral condyle of right humerus   MCC CC H5

2,3 √7th **S42.455** Nondisplaced fracture of lateral condyle of left humerus   MCC CC H5

2,3 √7th **S42.456** Nondisplaced fracture of lateral condyle of unspecified humerus   MCC CC H5

√6th S42.46 Fracture of medial condyle of humerus
Trochlea fracture of humerus

2,3 √7th **S42.461** Displaced fracture of medial condyle of right humerus   MCC CC H5

2,3 √7th **S42.462** Displaced fracture of medial condyle of left humerus   MCC CC H5

2,3 √7th **S42.463** Displaced fracture of medial condyle of unspecified humerus   MCC CC H5

2,3 √7th **S42.464** Nondisplaced fracture of medial condyle of right humerus   MCC CC H5

2,3 √7th **S42.465** Nondisplaced fracture of medial condyle of left humerus   MCC CC H5

2,3 √7th **S42.466** Nondisplaced fracture of medial condyle of unspecified humerus   MCC CC H5

√6th S42.47 Transcondylar fracture of humerus

2,3 √7th **S42.471** Displaced transcondylar fracture of right humerus   MCC CC H5

2,3 √7th **S42.472** Displaced transcondylar fracture of left humerus   MCC CC H5

2,3 √7th **S42.473** Displaced transcondylar fracture of unspecified humerus   MCC CC H5

2,3 √7th **S42.474** Nondisplaced transcondylar fracture of right humerus   MCC CC H5

2,3 √7th **S42.475** Nondisplaced transcondylar fracture of left humerus   MCC CC H5

2,3 √7th **S42.476** Nondisplaced transcondylar fracture of unspecified humerus   MCC CC H5

N Newborn: 0   P Pediatric: 0-17   M Maternity: 12-55   A Adult: 15-124   MCC Major Complication/Comorbidity   CC Complication/Comorbidity   SW Severe Wound Dx

994   ICD-10-CM 2019

S42.4–S42.476

✓6ᵗʰ S42.48 Torus fracture of lower end of humerus

> The appropriate 7th character is to be added to all codes in subcategory S42.48.
> A   initial encounter for closed fracture
> D   subsequent encounter for fracture with routine healing
> G   subsequent encounter for fracture with delayed healing
> K   subsequent encounter for fracture with nonunion
> P   subsequent encounter for fracture with malunion
> S   sequela

3 ✓7ᵗʰ **S42.481 Torus fracture of lower end of right humerus** `CC` `H5`

> **CC Excl: CC with 7th character A:**
> PDX collection 1245
> **CC with 7th character K or P:**
> PDX collection 897

3 ✓7ᵗʰ **S42.482 Torus fracture of lower end of left humerus** `CC` `H5`

> **CC Excl: CC with 7th character A:**
> PDX collection 1247
> **CC with 7th character K or P:**
> PDX collection 897

3 ✓7ᵗʰ **S42.489 Torus fracture of lower end of unspecified humerus** `CC` `H5`

> **CC Excl: CC with 7th character A:**
> PDX collection 1248
> **CC with 7th character K or P:**
> PDX collection 897

✓6ᵗʰ S42.49 Other fracture of lower end of humerus

2,3 ✓7ᵗʰ **S42.491 Other displaced fracture of lower end of right humerus** `MCC` `CC` `H5`

2,3 ✓7ᵗʰ **S42.492 Other displaced fracture of lower end of left humerus** `MCC` `CC` `H5`

2,3 ✓7ᵗʰ **S42.493 Other displaced fracture of lower end of unspecified humerus** `MCC` `CC` `H5`

2,3 ✓7ᵗʰ **S42.494 Other nondisplaced fracture of lower end of right humerus** `MCC` `CC` `H5`

2,3 ✓7ᵗʰ **S42.495 Other nondisplaced fracture of lower end of left humerus** `MCC` `CC` `H5`

2,3 ✓7ᵗʰ **S42.496 Other nondisplaced fracture of lower end of unspecified humerus** `MCC` `CC` `H5`

✓5ᵗʰ S42.9 Fracture of shoulder girdle, part unspecified
Fracture of shoulder NOS

> **CC Excl: For CC/MCC codes in subcategory S42.9:**
> See code S42.209

2,3 ✓x7ᵗʰ **S42.90 Fracture of unspecified shoulder girdle, part unspecified** `MCC` `CC` `H5`

2,3 ✓x7ᵗʰ **S42.91 Fracture of right shoulder girdle, part unspecified** `MCC` `CC` `H5`

2,3 ✓x7ᵗʰ **S42.92 Fracture of left shoulder girdle, part unspecified** `MCC` `CC` `H5`

✓4ᵗʰ S43 Dislocation and sprain of joints and ligaments of shoulder girdle

`INCLUDES` avulsion of joint or ligament of shoulder girdle
laceration of cartilage, joint or ligament of shoulder girdle
sprain of cartilage, joint or ligament of shoulder girdle
traumatic hemarthrosis of joint or ligament of shoulder girdle
traumatic rupture of joint or ligament of shoulder girdle
traumatic subluxation of joint or ligament of shoulder girdle
traumatic tear of joint or ligament of shoulder girdle

Code also any associated open wound

`EXCLUDES 2` *strain of muscle, fascia and tendon of shoulder and upper arm (S46.-)*

> The appropriate 7th character is to be added to each code from category S43.
> A   initial encounter
> D   subsequent encounter
> S   sequela

✓5ᵗʰ S43.0 Subluxation and dislocation of shoulder joint
Dislocation of glenohumeral joint
Subluxation of glenohumeral joint

✓6ᵗʰ S43.00 Unspecified subluxation and dislocation of shoulder joint
Dislocation of humerus NOS
Subluxation of humerus NOS

✓7ᵗʰ **S43.001 Unspecified subluxation of right shoulder joint**

✓7ᵗʰ **S43.002 Unspecified subluxation of left shoulder joint**

✓7ᵗʰ **S43.003 Unspecified subluxation of unspecified shoulder joint**

✓7ᵗʰ **S43.004 Unspecified dislocation of right shoulder joint**

✓7ᵗʰ **S43.005 Unspecified dislocation of left shoulder joint**

✓7ᵗʰ **S43.006 Unspecified dislocation of unspecified shoulder joint**

✓6ᵗʰ S43.01 Anterior subluxation and dislocation of humerus

✓7ᵗʰ **S43.011 Anterior subluxation of right humerus**

✓7ᵗʰ **S43.012 Anterior subluxation of left humerus**

✓7ᵗʰ **S43.013 Anterior subluxation of unspecified humerus**

✓7ᵗʰ **S43.014 Anterior dislocation of right humerus**

✓7ᵗʰ **S43.015 Anterior dislocation of left humerus**

✓7ᵗʰ **S43.016 Anterior dislocation of unspecified humerus**

✓6ᵗʰ S43.02 Posterior subluxation and dislocation of humerus

✓7ᵗʰ **S43.021 Posterior subluxation of right humerus**

✓7ᵗʰ **S43.022 Posterior subluxation of left humerus**

✓7ᵗʰ **S43.023 Posterior subluxation of unspecified humerus**

✓7ᵗʰ **S43.024 Posterior dislocation of right humerus**

✓7ᵗʰ **S43.025 Posterior dislocation of left humerus**

✓7ᵗʰ **S43.026 Posterior dislocation of unspecified humerus**

✓6ᵗʰ S43.03 Inferior subluxation and dislocation of humerus

✓7ᵗʰ **S43.031 Inferior subluxation of right humerus**

✓7ᵗʰ **S43.032 Inferior subluxation of left humerus**

✓7ᵗʰ **S43.033 Inferior subluxation of unspecified humerus**

✓7ᵗʰ **S43.034 Inferior dislocation of right humerus**

✓7ᵗʰ **S43.035 Inferior dislocation of left humerus**

✓7ᵗʰ **S43.036 Inferior dislocation of unspecified humerus**

✓6ᵗʰ S43.08 Other subluxation and dislocation of shoulder joint

✓7ᵗʰ **S43.081 Other subluxation of right shoulder joint**

✓7ᵗʰ **S43.082 Other subluxation of left shoulder joint**

✓7ᵗʰ **S43.083 Other subluxation of unspecified shoulder joint**

✓7ᵗʰ **S43.084 Other dislocation of right shoulder joint**

✓7ᵗʰ **S43.085 Other dislocation of left shoulder joint**

✓7ᵗʰ **S43.086 Other dislocation of unspecified shoulder joint**

✓5ᵗʰ S43.1 Subluxation and dislocation of acromioclavicular joint

✓6ᵗʰ S43.10 Unspecified dislocation of acromioclavicular joint

✓7ᵗʰ **S43.101 Unspecified dislocation of right acromioclavicular joint**

✓7ᵗʰ **S43.102 Unspecified dislocation of left acromioclavicular joint**

✓7ᵗʰ **S43.109 Unspecified dislocation of unspecified acromioclavicular joint**

✓6ᵗʰ S43.11 Subluxation of acromioclavicular joint

✓7ᵗʰ **S43.111 Subluxation of right acromioclavicular joint**

✓7ᵗʰ **S43.112 Subluxation of left acromioclavicular joint**

✓7ᵗʰ **S43.119 Subluxation of unspecified acromioclavicular joint**

✓6ᵗʰ S43.12 Dislocation of acromioclavicular joint, 100%-200% displacement

✓7ᵗʰ **S43.121 Dislocation of right acromioclavicular joint, 100%-200% displacement**

√7ᵗʰ S43.122 Dislocation of left acromioclavicular joint, 100%-200% displacement

√7ᵗʰ S43.129 Dislocation of unspecified acromioclavicular joint, 100%-200% displacement

√6ᵗʰ S43.13 Dislocation of acromioclavicular joint, greater than 200% displacement

  √7ᵗʰ S43.131 Dislocation of right acromioclavicular joint, greater than 200% displacement

  √7ᵗʰ S43.132 Dislocation of left acromioclavicular joint, greater than 200% displacement

  √7ᵗʰ S43.139 Dislocation of unspecified acromioclavicular joint, greater than 200% displacement

√6ᵗʰ S43.14 Inferior dislocation of acromioclavicular joint

  √7ᵗʰ S43.141 Inferior dislocation of right acromioclavicular joint

  √7ᵗʰ S43.142 Inferior dislocation of left acromioclavicular joint

  √7ᵗʰ S43.149 Inferior dislocation of unspecified acromioclavicular joint

√6ᵗʰ S43.15 Posterior dislocation of acromioclavicular joint

  √7ᵗʰ S43.151 Posterior dislocation of right acromioclavicular joint

  √7ᵗʰ S43.152 Posterior dislocation of left acromioclavicular joint

  √7ᵗʰ S43.159 Posterior dislocation of unspecified acromioclavicular joint

√5ᵗʰ S43.2 Subluxation and dislocation of sternoclavicular joint

> **CC Excl:** For CC codes in subcategory S43.2:
> **Right side:** PDX collection 1252
> **Left side:** PDX collection 1253
> **Unspecified side:** PDX collection 914

√6ᵗʰ S43.20 Unspecified subluxation and dislocation of sternoclavicular joint

  √7ᵗʰ S43.201 Unspecified subluxation of right sternoclavicular joint   CC H5

  √7ᵗʰ S43.202 Unspecified subluxation of left sternoclavicular joint   CC H5

  √7ᵗʰ S43.203 Unspecified subluxation of unspecified sternoclavicular joint   CC H5

  √7ᵗʰ S43.204 Unspecified dislocation of right sternoclavicular joint   CC H5

  √7ᵗʰ S43.205 Unspecified dislocation of left sternoclavicular joint   CC H5

  √7ᵗʰ S43.206 Unspecified dislocation of unspecified sternoclavicular joint   CC H5

√6ᵗʰ S43.21 Anterior subluxation and dislocation of sternoclavicular joint

  √7ᵗʰ S43.211 Anterior subluxation of right sternoclavicular joint   CC H5

  √7ᵗʰ S43.212 Anterior subluxation of left sternoclavicular joint   CC H5

  √7ᵗʰ S43.213 Anterior subluxation of unspecified sternoclavicular joint   CC H5

  √7ᵗʰ S43.214 Anterior dislocation of right sternoclavicular joint   CC H5

  √7ᵗʰ S43.215 Anterior dislocation of left sternoclavicular joint   CC H5

  √7ᵗʰ S43.216 Anterior dislocation of unspecified sternoclavicular joint   CC H5

√6ᵗʰ S43.22 Posterior subluxation and dislocation of sternoclavicular joint

  √7ᵗʰ S43.221 Posterior subluxation of right sternoclavicular joint   CC H5

  √7ᵗʰ S43.222 Posterior subluxation of left sternoclavicular joint   CC H5

  √7ᵗʰ S43.223 Posterior subluxation of unspecified sternoclavicular joint   CC H5

  √7ᵗʰ S43.224 Posterior dislocation of right sternoclavicular joint   CC H5

  √7ᵗʰ S43.225 Posterior dislocation of left sternoclavicular joint   CC H5

  √7ᵗʰ S43.226 Posterior dislocation of unspecified sternoclavicular joint   CC H5

√5ᵗʰ S43.3 Subluxation and dislocation of other and unspecified parts of shoulder girdle

√6ᵗʰ S43.30 Subluxation and dislocation of unspecified parts of shoulder girdle
> Dislocation of shoulder girdle NOS
> Subluxation of shoulder girdle NOS

  √7ᵗʰ S43.301 Subluxation of unspecified parts of right shoulder girdle

  √7ᵗʰ S43.302 Subluxation of unspecified parts of left shoulder girdle

  √7ᵗʰ S43.303 Subluxation of unspecified parts of unspecified shoulder girdle

  √7ᵗʰ S43.304 Dislocation of unspecified parts of right shoulder girdle

  √7ᵗʰ S43.305 Dislocation of unspecified parts of left shoulder girdle

  √7ᵗʰ S43.306 Dislocation of unspecified parts of unspecified shoulder girdle

√6ᵗʰ S43.31 Subluxation and dislocation of scapula

  √7ᵗʰ S43.311 Subluxation of right scapula

  √7ᵗʰ S43.312 Subluxation of left scapula

  √7ᵗʰ S43.313 Subluxation of unspecified scapula

  √7ᵗʰ S43.314 Dislocation of right scapula

  √7ᵗʰ S43.315 Dislocation of left scapula

  √7ᵗʰ S43.316 Dislocation of unspecified scapula

√6ᵗʰ S43.39 Subluxation and dislocation of other parts of shoulder girdle

  √7ᵗʰ S43.391 Subluxation of other parts of right shoulder girdle

  √7ᵗʰ S43.392 Subluxation of other parts of left shoulder girdle

  √7ᵗʰ S43.393 Subluxation of other parts of unspecified shoulder girdle

  √7ᵗʰ S43.394 Dislocation of other parts of right shoulder girdle

  √7ᵗʰ S43.395 Dislocation of other parts of left shoulder girdle

  √7ᵗʰ S43.396 Dislocation of other parts of unspecified shoulder girdle

√5ᵗʰ S43.4 Sprain of shoulder joint

√6ᵗʰ S43.40 Unspecified sprain of shoulder joint

  √7ᵗʰ S43.401 Unspecified sprain of right shoulder joint

  √7ᵗʰ S43.402 Unspecified sprain of left shoulder joint

  √7ᵗʰ S43.409 Unspecified sprain of unspecified shoulder joint

√6ᵗʰ S43.41 Sprain of coracohumeral (ligament)

  √7ᵗʰ S43.411 Sprain of right coracohumeral (ligament)

  √7ᵗʰ S43.412 Sprain of left coracohumeral (ligament)

  √7ᵗʰ S43.419 Sprain of unspecified coracohumeral (ligament)

√6ᵗʰ S43.42 Sprain of rotator cuff capsule
> **EXCLUDES 1** rotator cuff syndrome (complete) (incomplete), not specified as traumatic (M75.1-)
> **EXCLUDES 2** injury of tendon of rotator cuff (S46.0-)

  √7ᵗʰ S43.421 Sprain of right rotator cuff capsule

  √7ᵗʰ S43.422 Sprain of left rotator cuff capsule

  √7ᵗʰ S43.429 Sprain of unspecified rotator cuff capsule

√6ᵗʰ S43.43 Superior glenoid labrum lesion
> SLAP lesion
> **DEF:** Detachment injury of the superior aspect of the glenoid labrum, which is the ring of fibrocartilage attached to the rim of the glenoid cavity of the scapula.

  √7ᵗʰ S43.431 Superior glenoid labrum lesion of right shoulder

  √7ᵗʰ S43.432 Superior glenoid labrum lesion of left shoulder

  √7ᵗʰ S43.439 Superior glenoid labrum lesion of unspecified shoulder

√6ᵗʰ S43.49 Other sprain of shoulder joint

  √7ᵗʰ S43.491 Other sprain of right shoulder joint

  √7ᵗʰ S43.492 Other sprain of left shoulder joint

  √7ᵗʰ S43.499 Other sprain of unspecified shoulder joint

✓5ᵗʰ **S43.5** **Sprain of** acromioclavicular **joint**
Sprain of acromioclavicular ligament

 ✓x7ᵗʰ **S43.50** Sprain of unspecified acromioclavicular joint

 ✓x7ᵗʰ **S43.51** Sprain of right acromioclavicular joint

 ✓x7ᵗʰ **S43.52** Sprain of left acromioclavicular joint

✓5ᵗʰ **S43.6** **Sprain of** sternoclavicular **joint**

 ✓x7ᵗʰ **S43.60** Sprain of unspecified sternoclavicular joint

 ✓x7ᵗʰ **S43.61** Sprain of right sternoclavicular joint

 ✓x7ᵗʰ **S43.62** Sprain of left sternoclavicular joint

✓5ᵗʰ **S43.8** **Sprain of** other specified parts of shoulder girdle

 ✓x7ᵗʰ **S43.80** Sprain of other specified parts of unspecified shoulder girdle

 ✓x7ᵗʰ **S43.81** Sprain of other specified parts of right shoulder girdle

 ✓x7ᵗʰ **S43.82** Sprain of other specified parts of left shoulder girdle

✓5ᵗʰ **S43.9** **Sprain of** unspecified **parts of shoulder girdle**

 ✓x7ᵗʰ **S43.90** Sprain of unspecified parts of unspecified shoulder girdle
Sprain of shoulder girdle NOS

 ✓x7ᵗʰ **S43.91** Sprain of unspecified parts of right shoulder girdle

 ✓x7ᵗʰ **S43.92** Sprain of unspecified parts of left shoulder girdle

✓4ᵗʰ **S44** **Injury of nerves at shoulder and upper arm level**
Code also any associated open wound (S41.-)
EXCLUDES 2 injury of brachial plexus (S14.3-)

The appropriate 7th character is to be added to each code from category S44.
A   initial encounter
D   subsequent encounter
S   sequela

✓5ᵗʰ **S44.0** **Injury of** ulnar nerve **at upper arm level**
EXCLUDES 1 ulnar nerve NOS (S54.0)

 ✓x7ᵗʰ **S44.00** Injury of ulnar nerve at upper arm level, unspecified arm

 ✓x7ᵗʰ **S44.01** Injury of ulnar nerve at upper arm level, right arm

 ✓x7ᵗʰ **S44.02** Injury of ulnar nerve at upper arm level, left arm

✓5ᵗʰ **S44.1** **Injury of** median nerve **at upper arm level**
EXCLUDES 1 median nerve NOS (S54.1)

 ✓x7ᵗʰ **S44.10** Injury of median nerve at upper arm level, unspecified arm

 ✓x7ᵗʰ **S44.11** Injury of median nerve at upper arm level, right arm

 ✓x7ᵗʰ **S44.12** Injury of median nerve at upper arm level, left arm

✓5ᵗʰ **S44.2** **Injury of** radial nerve **at upper arm level**
EXCLUDES 1 radial nerve NOS (S54.2)

 ✓x7ᵗʰ **S44.20** Injury of radial nerve at upper arm level, unspecified arm

 ✓x7ᵗʰ **S44.21** Injury of radial nerve at upper arm level, right arm

 ✓x7ᵗʰ **S44.22** Injury of radial nerve at upper arm level, left arm

✓5ᵗʰ **S44.3** **Injury of** axillary nerve

 ✓x7ᵗʰ **S44.30** Injury of axillary nerve, unspecified arm

 ✓x7ᵗʰ **S44.31** Injury of axillary nerve, right arm

 ✓x7ᵗʰ **S44.32** Injury of axillary nerve, left arm

✓5ᵗʰ **S44.4** **Injury of** musculocutaneous nerve

 ✓x7ᵗʰ **S44.40** Injury of musculocutaneous nerve, unspecified arm

 ✓x7ᵗʰ **S44.41** Injury of musculocutaneous nerve, right arm

 ✓x7ᵗʰ **S44.42** Injury of musculocutaneous nerve, left arm

✓5ᵗʰ **S44.5** **Injury of** cutaneous sensory nerve **at shoulder and upper arm level**

 ✓x7ᵗʰ **S44.50** Injury of cutaneous sensory nerve at shoulder and upper arm level, unspecified arm

 ✓x7ᵗʰ **S44.51** Injury of cutaneous sensory nerve at shoulder and upper arm level, right arm

 ✓x7ᵗʰ **S44.52** Injury of cutaneous sensory nerve at shoulder and upper arm level, left arm

✓5ᵗʰ **S44.8** **Injury of other nerves at shoulder and upper arm level**

 ✓6ᵗʰ **S44.8X** Injury of other nerves at shoulder and upper arm level

  ✓7ᵗʰ **S44.8X1** Injury of other nerves at shoulder and upper arm level, right arm

  ✓7ᵗʰ **S44.8X2** Injury of other nerves at shoulder and upper arm level, left arm

  ✓7ᵗʰ **S44.8X9** Injury of other nerves at shoulder and upper arm level, unspecified arm

✓5ᵗʰ **S44.9** **Injury of** unspecified **nerve at shoulder and upper arm level**

 ✓x7ᵗʰ **S44.90** Injury of unspecified nerve at shoulder and upper arm level, unspecified arm

 ✓x7ᵗʰ **S44.91** Injury of unspecified nerve at shoulder and upper arm level, right arm

 ✓x7ᵗʰ **S44.92** Injury of unspecified nerve at shoulder and upper arm level, left arm

✓4ᵗʰ **S45** **Injury of blood vessels at shoulder and upper arm level**
Code also any associated open wound (S41.-)
EXCLUDES 2 injury of subclavian artery (S25.1)
injury of subclavian vein (S25.3)

The appropriate 7th character is to be added to each code from category S45.
A   initial encounter
D   subsequent encounter
S   sequela

✓5ᵗʰ **S45.0** **Injury of** axillary artery

CC Excl: For MCC codes in subcategory S45.0:
Right side: PDX collection 1254
Left side: PDX collection 1255
Unspecified side: PDX collection 1256

 ✓6ᵗʰ **S45.00** Unspecified injury of axillary artery

  ✓7ᵗʰ **S45.001** Unspecified injury of axillary artery, right side MCC

  ✓7ᵗʰ **S45.002** Unspecified injury of axillary artery, left side MCC

  ✓7ᵗʰ **S45.009** Unspecified injury of axillary artery, unspecified side MCC

 ✓6ᵗʰ **S45.01** Laceration of axillary artery

  ✓7ᵗʰ **S45.011** Laceration of axillary artery, right side MCC

  ✓7ᵗʰ **S45.012** Laceration of axillary artery, left side MCC

  ✓7ᵗʰ **S45.019** Laceration of axillary artery, unspecified side MCC

 ✓6ᵗʰ **S45.09** Other specified injury of axillary artery

  ✓7ᵗʰ **S45.091** Other specified injury of axillary artery, right side MCC

  ✓7ᵗʰ **S45.092** Other specified injury of axillary artery, left side MCC

  ✓7ᵗʰ **S45.099** Other specified injury of axillary artery, unspecified side MCC

✓5ᵗʰ **S45.1** **Injury of** brachial artery

CC Excl: For CC codes in subcategory S45.1:
Right side: PDX collection 1257
Left side: PDX collection 1258
Unspecified side: PDX collection 1259

 ✓6ᵗʰ **S45.10** Unspecified injury of brachial artery

  ✓7ᵗʰ **S45.101** Unspecified injury of brachial artery, right side CC

  ✓7ᵗʰ **S45.102** Unspecified injury of brachial artery, left side CC

  ✓7ᵗʰ **S45.109** Unspecified injury of brachial artery, unspecified side CC

 ✓6ᵗʰ **S45.11** Laceration of brachial artery

  ✓7ᵗʰ **S45.111** Laceration of brachial artery, right side CC

  ✓7ᵗʰ **S45.112** Laceration of brachial artery, left side CC

  ✓7ᵗʰ **S45.119** Laceration of brachial artery, unspecified side CC

 ✓6ᵗʰ **S45.19** Other specified injury of brachial artery

  ✓7ᵗʰ **S45.191** Other specified injury of brachial artery, right side CC

  ✓7ᵗʰ **S45.192** Other specified injury of brachial artery, left side CC

  ✓7ᵗʰ **S45.199** Other specified injury of brachial artery, unspecified side CC

✓5th **S45.2** **Injury of** axillary or brachial vein

> **CC Excl: For CC codes in subcategory S45.2:**
> **Right side:** PDX collection 1257
> **Left side:** PDX collection 1258
> **Unspecified side:** PDX collection 1259

✓6th **S45.20** Unspecified **injury of axillary or brachial vein**

✓7th **S45.201** Unspecified injury of axillary or brachial vein, right side `CC`

✓7th **S45.202** Unspecified injury of axillary or brachial vein, left side `CC`

✓7th **S45.209** Unspecified injury of axillary or brachial vein, unspecified side `CC`

✓6th **S45.21** Laceration **of axillary or brachial vein**

✓7th **S45.211** Laceration of axillary or brachial vein, right side `CC`

✓7th **S45.212** Laceration of axillary or brachial vein, left side `CC`

✓7th **S45.219** Laceration of axillary or brachial vein, unspecified side `CC`

✓6th **S45.29** Other **specified injury of axillary or brachial vein**

✓7th **S45.291** Other specified injury of axillary or brachial vein, right side `CC`

✓7th **S45.292** Other specified injury of axillary or brachial vein, left side `CC`

✓7th **S45.299** Other specified injury of axillary or brachial vein, unspecified side `CC`

✓5th **S45.3** **Injury of** superficial vein at shoulder and upper arm level

> **CC Excl: For CC codes in subcategory S45.3:**
> **Right side:** PDX collection 1260
> **Left side:** PDX collection 1261
> **Unspecified side:** PDX collection 1262

✓6th **S45.30** Unspecified **injury of superficial vein at shoulder and upper arm level**

✓7th **S45.301** Unspecified injury of superficial vein at shoulder and upper arm level, right arm `CC`

✓7th **S45.302** Unspecified injury of superficial vein at shoulder and upper arm level, left arm `CC`

✓7th **S45.309** Unspecified injury of superficial vein at shoulder and upper arm level, unspecified arm `CC`

✓6th **S45.31** Laceration **of superficial vein at shoulder and upper arm level**

✓7th **S45.311** Laceration of superficial vein at shoulder and upper arm level, right arm `CC`

✓7th **S45.312** Laceration of superficial vein at shoulder and upper arm level, left arm `CC`

✓7th **S45.319** Laceration of superficial vein at shoulder and upper arm level, unspecified arm `CC`

✓6th **S45.39** Other **specified injury of superficial vein at shoulder and upper arm level**

✓7th **S45.391** Other specified injury of superficial vein at shoulder and upper arm level, right arm `CC`

✓7th **S45.392** Other specified injury of superficial vein at shoulder and upper arm level, left arm `CC`

✓7th **S45.399** Other specified injury of superficial vein at shoulder and upper arm level, unspecified arm `CC`

✓5th **S45.8** **Injury of** other specified blood vessels **at shoulder and upper arm level**

> **CC Excl: For CC codes in subcategory S45.8:**
> **Right side:** PDX collection 1260
> **Left side:** PDX collection 1261
> **Unspecified side:** PDX collection 1262

✓6th **S45.80** Unspecified **injury of other specified blood vessels at shoulder and upper arm level**

✓7th **S45.801** Unspecified injury of other specified blood vessels at shoulder and upper arm level, right arm `CC`

✓7th **S45.802** Unspecified injury of other specified blood vessels at shoulder and upper arm level, left arm `CC`

✓7th **S45.809** Unspecified injury of other specified blood vessels at shoulder and upper arm level, unspecified arm `CC`

✓6th **S45.81** Laceration **of other specified blood vessels at shoulder and upper arm level**

✓7th **S45.811** Laceration of other specified blood vessels at shoulder and upper arm level, right arm `CC`

✓7th **S45.812** Laceration of other specified blood vessels at shoulder and upper arm level, left arm `CC`

✓7th **S45.819** Laceration of other specified blood vessels at shoulder and upper arm level, unspecified arm `CC`

✓6th **S45.89** Other **specified injury of other specified blood vessels at shoulder and upper arm level**

✓7th **S45.891** Other specified injury of other specified blood vessels at shoulder and upper arm level, right arm `CC`

✓7th **S45.892** Other specified injury of other specified blood vessels at shoulder and upper arm level, left arm `CC`

✓7th **S45.899** Other specified injury of other specified blood vessels at shoulder and upper arm level, unspecified arm `CC`

✓5th **S45.9** **Injury of** unspecified blood vessel **at shoulder and upper arm level**

> **CC Excl: For CC codes in subcategory S45.9:**
> **Right side:** PDX collection 1260
> **Left side:** PDX collection 1261
> **Unspecified side:** PDX collection 1262

✓6th **S45.90** Unspecified **injury of unspecified blood vessel at shoulder and upper arm level**

✓7th **S45.901** Unspecified injury of unspecified blood vessel at shoulder and upper arm level, right arm `CC`

✓7th **S45.902** Unspecified injury of unspecified blood vessel at shoulder and upper arm level, left arm `CC`

✓7th **S45.909** Unspecified injury of unspecified blood vessel at shoulder and upper arm level, unspecified arm `CC`

✓6th **S45.91** Laceration **of unspecified blood vessel at shoulder and upper arm level**

✓7th **S45.911** Laceration of unspecified blood vessel at shoulder and upper arm level, right arm `CC`

✓7th **S45.912** Laceration of unspecified blood vessel at shoulder and upper arm level, left arm `CC`

✓7th **S45.919** Laceration of unspecified blood vessel at shoulder and upper arm level, unspecified arm `CC`

✓6th **S45.99** Other **specified injury of unspecified blood vessel at shoulder and upper arm level**

✓7th **S45.991** Other specified injury of unspecified blood vessel at shoulder and upper arm level, right arm `CC`

✓7th **S45.992** Other specified injury of unspecified blood vessel at shoulder and upper arm level, left arm `CC`

✓7th **S45.999** Other specified injury of unspecified blood vessel at shoulder and upper arm level, unspecified arm `CC`

N Newborn: 0   P Pediatric: 0-17   M Maternity: 12-55   A Adult: 15-124   MCC Major Complication/Comorbidity   CC Complication/Comorbidity   SW Severe Wound Dx

998   ICD-10-CM 2019

☑4ᵗʰ **S46 Injury of muscle, fascia and tendon at shoulder and upper arm level**

Code also any associated open wound (S41.-)

EXCLUDES 2   *injury of muscle, fascia and tendon at elbow (S56.-)*
      sprain of joints and ligaments of shoulder girdle (S43.9)

TIP: Refer to the Muscle/Tendon table at the beginning of this chapter.

> The appropriate 7th character is to be added to each code from category S46.
> A   initial encounter
> D   subsequent encounter
> S   sequela

> **CC Excl: For CC codes in category S46:**
> **Right side:** PDX collection 1263
> **Left side:** PDX collection 1264
> **Unspecified side:** PDX collection 1265

☑5ᵗʰ **S46.0 Injury of muscle(s) and tendon(s) of the** rotator cuff **of shoulder**

     ☑6ᵗʰ **S46.00 Unspecified injury of muscle(s) and tendon(s) of the rotator cuff of shoulder**

         ☑7ᵗʰ **S46.001 Unspecified injury of muscle(s) and tendon(s) of the rotator cuff of** right **shoulder**

         ☑7ᵗʰ **S46.002 Unspecified injury of muscle(s) and tendon(s) of the rotator cuff of** left **shoulder**

         ☑7ᵗʰ **S46.009 Unspecified injury of muscle(s) and tendon(s) of the rotator cuff of** unspecified **shoulder**

     ☑6ᵗʰ **S46.01 Strain of muscle(s) and tendon(s) of the rotator cuff of shoulder**

         ☑7ᵗʰ **S46.011 Strain of muscle(s) and tendon(s) of the rotator cuff of** right **shoulder**

         ☑7ᵗʰ **S46.012 Strain of muscle(s) and tendon(s) of the rotator cuff of** left **shoulder**

         ☑7ᵗʰ **S46.019 Strain of muscle(s) and tendon(s) of the rotator cuff of** unspecified **shoulder**

     ☑6ᵗʰ **S46.02 Laceration of muscle(s) and tendon(s) of the rotator cuff of shoulder**

         ☑7ᵗʰ **S46.021 Laceration of muscle(s) and tendon(s)** CC **of the rotator cuff of** right **shoulder**

         ☑7ᵗʰ **S46.022 Laceration of muscle(s) and tendon(s)** CC **of the rotator cuff of** left **shoulder**

         ☑7ᵗʰ **S46.029 Laceration of muscle(s) and tendon(s)** CC **of the rotator cuff of** unspecified **shoulder**

     ☑6ᵗʰ **S46.09 Other injury of muscle(s) and tendon(s) of the rotator cuff of shoulder**

         ☑7ᵗʰ **S46.091 Other injury of muscle(s) and tendon(s) of the rotator cuff of** right **shoulder**

         ☑7ᵗʰ **S46.092 Other injury of muscle(s) and tendon(s) of the rotator cuff of** left **shoulder**

         ☑7ᵗʰ **S46.099 Other injury of muscle(s) and tendon(s) of the rotator cuff of** unspecified **shoulder**

☑5ᵗʰ **S46.1 Injury of muscle, fascia and tendon of** long head of biceps

     ☑6ᵗʰ **S46.10 Unspecified injury of muscle, fascia and tendon of long head of biceps**

         ☑7ᵗʰ **S46.101 Unspecified injury of muscle, fascia and tendon of long head of biceps,** right **arm**

         ☑7ᵗʰ **S46.102 Unspecified injury of muscle, fascia and tendon of long head of biceps,** left **arm**

         ☑7ᵗʰ **S46.109 Unspecified injury of muscle, fascia and tendon of long head of biceps,** unspecified **arm**

     ☑6ᵗʰ **S46.11 Strain of muscle, fascia and tendon of long head of biceps**

         ☑7ᵗʰ **S46.111 Strain of muscle, fascia and tendon of long head of biceps,** right **arm**

         ☑7ᵗʰ **S46.112 Strain of muscle, fascia and tendon of long head of biceps,** left **arm**

         ☑7ᵗʰ **S46.119 Strain of muscle, fascia and tendon of long head of biceps,** unspecified **arm**

     ☑6ᵗʰ **S46.12 Laceration of muscle, fascia and tendon of long head of biceps**

         ☑7ᵗʰ **S46.121 Laceration of muscle, fascia and** CC **tendon of long head of biceps,** right **arm**

         ☑7ᵗʰ **S46.122 Laceration of muscle, fascia and** CC **tendon of long head of biceps,** left **arm**

         ☑7ᵗʰ **S46.129 Laceration of muscle, fascia and** CC **tendon of long head of biceps,** unspecified **arm**

     ☑6ᵗʰ **S46.19 Other injury of muscle, fascia and tendon of long head of biceps**

         ☑7ᵗʰ **S46.191 Other injury of muscle, fascia and tendon of long head of biceps,** right **arm**

         ☑7ᵗʰ **S46.192 Other injury of muscle, fascia and tendon of long head of biceps,** left **arm**

         ☑7ᵗʰ **S46.199 Other injury of muscle, fascia and tendon of long head of biceps,** unspecified **arm**

☑5ᵗʰ **S46.2 Injury of muscle, fascia and tendon of** other parts **of** biceps

     ☑6ᵗʰ **S46.20 Unspecified injury of muscle, fascia and tendon of other parts of biceps**

         ☑7ᵗʰ **S46.201 Unspecified injury of muscle, fascia and tendon of other parts of biceps,** right **arm**

         ☑7ᵗʰ **S46.202 Unspecified injury of muscle, fascia and tendon of other parts of biceps,** left **arm**

         ☑7ᵗʰ **S46.209 Unspecified injury of muscle, fascia and tendon of other parts of biceps,** unspecified **arm**

     ☑6ᵗʰ **S46.21 Strain of muscle, fascia and tendon of other parts of biceps**

         ☑7ᵗʰ **S46.211 Strain of muscle, fascia and tendon of other parts of biceps,** right **arm**

         ☑7ᵗʰ **S46.212 Strain of muscle, fascia and tendon of other parts of biceps,** left **arm**

         ☑7ᵗʰ **S46.219 Strain of muscle, fascia and tendon of other parts of biceps,** unspecified **arm**

     ☑6ᵗʰ **S46.22 Laceration of muscle, fascia and tendon of other parts of biceps**

         ☑7ᵗʰ **S46.221 Laceration of muscle, fascia and** CC **tendon of other parts of biceps,** right **arm**

         ☑7ᵗʰ **S46.222 Laceration of muscle, fascia and** CC **tendon of other parts of biceps,** left **arm**

         ☑7ᵗʰ **S46.229 Laceration of muscle, fascia and** CC **tendon of other parts of biceps,** unspecified **arm**

     ☑6ᵗʰ **S46.29 Other injury of muscle, fascia and tendon of other parts of biceps**

         ☑7ᵗʰ **S46.291 Other injury of muscle, fascia and tendon of other parts of biceps,** right **arm**

         ☑7ᵗʰ **S46.292 Other injury of muscle, fascia and tendon of other parts of biceps,** left **arm**

         ☑7ᵗʰ **S46.299 Other injury of muscle, fascia and tendon of other parts of biceps,** unspecified **arm**

☑5ᵗʰ **S46.3 Injury of muscle, fascia and tendon of** triceps

     ☑6ᵗʰ **S46.30 Unspecified injury of muscle, fascia and tendon of triceps**

         ☑7ᵗʰ **S46.301 Unspecified injury of muscle, fascia and tendon of triceps,** right **arm**

         ☑7ᵗʰ **S46.302 Unspecified injury of muscle, fascia and tendon of triceps,** left **arm**

         ☑7ᵗʰ **S46.309 Unspecified injury of muscle, fascia and tendon of triceps,** unspecified **arm**

     ☑6ᵗʰ **S46.31 Strain of muscle, fascia and tendon of triceps**

         ☑7ᵗʰ **S46.311 Strain of muscle, fascia and tendon of triceps,** right **arm**

         ☑7ᵗʰ **S46.312 Strain of muscle, fascia and tendon of triceps,** left **arm**

         ☑7ᵗʰ **S46.319 Strain of muscle, fascia and tendon of triceps,** unspecified **arm**

     ☑6ᵗʰ **S46.32 Laceration of muscle, fascia and tendon of triceps**

         ☑7ᵗʰ **S46.321 Laceration of muscle, fascia and** CC **tendon of triceps,** right **arm**

         ☑7ᵗʰ **S46.322 Laceration of muscle, fascia and** CC **tendon of triceps,** left **arm**

         ☑7ᵗʰ **S46.329 Laceration of muscle, fascia and** CC **tendon of triceps,** unspecified **arm**

☑ Additional Character Required   ✗x7ᵗʰ Placeholder   Unacceptable PDx   Questionable PDx   Manifestation   H1-H14 HAC   HCC CMS-HCC Dx   HIV HIV Dx

ICD-10-CM 2019   999

✓6th S46.39 Other **injury of muscle, fascia and tendon of triceps**

    ✓7th S46.391 Other injury of muscle, fascia and tendon of triceps, right arm

    ✓7th S46.392 Other injury of muscle, fascia and tendon of triceps, left arm

    ✓7th S46.399 Other injury of muscle, fascia and tendon of triceps, unspecified arm

✓5th S46.8 **Injury of other muscles, fascia and tendons at shoulder and upper arm level**

  ✓6th S46.80 Unspecified **injury of other muscles, fascia and tendons at shoulder and upper arm level**

    ✓7th S46.801 Unspecified injury of other muscles, fascia and tendons at shoulder and upper arm level, right arm

    ✓7th S46.802 Unspecified injury of other muscles, fascia and tendons at shoulder and upper arm level, left arm

    ✓7th S46.809 Unspecified injury of other muscles, fascia and tendons at shoulder and upper arm level, unspecified arm

  ✓6th S46.81 Strain **of other muscles, fascia and tendons at shoulder and upper arm level**

    ✓7th S46.811 Strain of other muscles, fascia and tendons at shoulder and upper arm level, right arm

    ✓7th S46.812 Strain of other muscles, fascia and tendons at shoulder and upper arm level, left arm

    ✓7th S46.819 Strain of other muscles, fascia and tendons at shoulder and upper arm level, unspecified arm

  ✓6th S46.82 Laceration **of other muscles, fascia and tendons at shoulder and upper arm level**

    ✓7th S46.821 Laceration of other muscles, fascia and tendons at shoulder and upper arm level, right arm `CC`

    ✓7th S46.822 Laceration of other muscles, fascia and tendons at shoulder and upper arm level, left arm `CC`

    ✓7th S46.829 Laceration of other muscles, fascia and tendons at shoulder and upper arm level, unspecified arm `CC`

  ✓6th S46.89 Other **injury of other muscles, fascia and tendons at shoulder and upper arm level**

    ✓7th S46.891 Other injury of other muscles, fascia and tendons at shoulder and upper arm level, right arm

    ✓7th S46.892 Other injury of other muscles, fascia and tendons at shoulder and upper arm level, left arm

    ✓7th S46.899 Other injury of other muscles, fascia and tendons at shoulder and upper arm level, unspecified arm

✓5th S46.9 **Injury of** unspecified **muscle, fascia and tendon at shoulder and upper arm level**

  ✓6th S46.90 Unspecified **injury of unspecified muscle, fascia and tendon at shoulder and upper arm level**

    ✓7th S46.901 Unspecified injury of unspecified muscle, fascia and tendon at shoulder and upper arm level, right arm

    ✓7th S46.902 Unspecified injury of unspecified muscle, fascia and tendon at shoulder and upper arm level, left arm

    ✓7th S46.909 Unspecified injury of unspecified muscle, fascia and tendon at shoulder and upper arm level, unspecified arm

  ✓6th S46.91 Strain **of unspecified muscle, fascia and tendon at shoulder and upper arm level**

    ✓7th S46.911 Strain of unspecified muscle, fascia and tendon at shoulder and upper arm level, right arm

    ✓7th S46.912 Strain of unspecified muscle, fascia and tendon at shoulder and upper arm level, left arm

    ✓7th S46.919 Strain of unspecified muscle, fascia and tendon at shoulder and upper arm level, unspecified arm

✓6th S46.92 Laceration **of unspecified muscle, fascia and tendon at shoulder and upper arm level**

    ✓7th S46.921 Laceration of unspecified muscle, fascia and tendon at shoulder and upper arm level, right arm `CC`

    ✓7th S46.922 Laceration of unspecified muscle, fascia and tendon at shoulder and upper arm level, left arm `CC`

    ✓7th S46.929 Laceration of unspecified muscle, fascia and tendon at shoulder and upper arm level, unspecified arm `CC`

✓6th S46.99 Other **injury of unspecified muscle, fascia and tendon at shoulder and upper arm level**

    ✓7th S46.991 Other injury of unspecified muscle, fascia and tendon at shoulder and upper arm level, right arm

    ✓7th S46.992 Other injury of unspecified muscle, fascia and tendon at shoulder and upper arm level, left arm

    ✓7th S46.999 Other injury of unspecified muscle, fascia and tendon at shoulder and upper arm level, unspecified arm

✓4th S47 **Crushing injury of shoulder and upper arm**

Use additional code for all associated injuries

EXCLUDES 2 crushing injury of elbow (S57.0-)

> The appropriate 7th character is to be added to each code from category S47.
> A   initial encounter
> D   subsequent encounter
> S   sequela

✓x7th S47.1 **Crushing injury of** right **shoulder and upper arm**

✓x7th S47.2 **Crushing injury of** left **shoulder and upper arm**

✓x7th S47.9 **Crushing injury of shoulder and upper arm,** unspecified **arm**

✓4th S48 **Traumatic amputation of shoulder and upper arm**

An amputation not identified as partial or complete should be coded to complete.

EXCLUDES 1 traumatic amputation at elbow level (S58.0)

> The appropriate 7th character is to be added to each code from category S48.
> A   initial encounter
> D   subsequent encounter
> S   sequela

CC Excl: For CC codes in category S48:
Right side: PDX collection 1266
Left side: PDX collection 1267
Unspecified side: PDX collection 1268

✓5th S48.0 **Traumatic amputation at** shoulder joint

  ✓6th S48.01 Complete **traumatic amputation at shoulder joint**

    7 ✓7th S48.011 Complete traumatic amputation at right shoulder joint `CC` `HCC`

    7 ✓7th S48.012 Complete traumatic amputation at left shoulder joint `CC` `HCC`

    7 ✓7th S48.019 Complete traumatic amputation at unspecified shoulder joint `CC` `HCC`

  ✓6th S48.02 Partial **traumatic amputation at shoulder joint**

    7 ✓7th S48.021 Partial traumatic amputation at right shoulder joint `CC` `HCC`

    7 ✓7th S48.022 Partial traumatic amputation at left shoulder joint `CC` `HCC`

    7 ✓7th S48.029 Partial traumatic amputation at unspecified shoulder joint `CC` `HCC`

✓5th S48.1 **Traumatic amputation at** level between shoulder and elbow

  ✓6th S48.11 Complete **traumatic amputation at level between shoulder and elbow**

    7 ✓7th S48.111 Complete traumatic amputation at at level between right shoulder and elbow `CC` `HCC`

    7 ✓7th S48.112 Complete traumatic amputation at at level between left shoulder and elbow `CC` `HCC`

    7 ✓7th S48.119 Complete traumatic amputation at at level between unspecified shoulder and elbow `CC` `HCC`

N Newborn: 0   P Pediatric: 0-17   M Maternity: 12-55   A Adult: 15-124   MCC Major Complication/Comorbidity   CC Complication/Comorbidity   SW Severe Wound Dx

1000   ICD-10-CM 2019

√6ᵗʰ **S48.12** Partial traumatic amputation at level between shoulder and elbow

   7 √7ᵗʰ **S48.121** Partial traumatic amputation at level between right shoulder and elbow   CC HCC

   7 √7ᵗʰ **S48.122** Partial traumatic amputation at level between left shoulder and elbow   CC HCC

   7 √7ᵗʰ **S48.129** Partial traumatic amputation at level between unspecified shoulder and elbow   CC HCC

√5ᵗʰ **S48.9** Traumatic amputation of shoulder and upper arm, level unspecified

   √6ᵗʰ **S48.91** Complete traumatic amputation of shoulder and upper arm, level unspecified

    7 √7ᵗʰ **S48.911** Complete traumatic amputation of right shoulder and upper arm, level unspecified   CC HCC

    7 √7ᵗʰ **S48.912** Complete traumatic amputation of left shoulder and upper arm, level unspecified   CC HCC

    7 √7ᵗʰ **S48.919** Complete traumatic amputation of unspecified shoulder and upper arm, level unspecified   CC HCC

   √6ᵗʰ **S48.92** Partial traumatic amputation of shoulder and upper arm, level unspecified

    7 √7ᵗʰ **S48.921** Partial traumatic amputation of right shoulder and upper arm, level unspecified   CC HCC

    7 √7ᵗʰ **S48.922** Partial traumatic amputation of left shoulder and upper arm, level unspecified   CC HCC

    7 √7ᵗʰ **S48.929** Partial traumatic amputation of unspecified shoulder and upper arm, level unspecified   CC HCC

√4ᵗʰ **S49** **Other and unspecified injuries of shoulder and upper arm**
   AHA: 2018, 2Q, 12; 2018, 1Q, 3

> The appropriate 7th character is to be added to each code from subcategories S49.0 and S49.1.
> A   initial encounter for closed fracture
> D   subsequent encounter for fracture with routine healing
> G   subsequent encounter for fracture with delayed healing
> K   subsequent encounter for fracture with nonunion
> P   subsequent encounter for fracture with malunion
> S   sequela

> **CC Excl: For CC codes in category S49:**
> **Right side:** See code S49.001
> **Left side:** See code S49.002
> **Unspecified side:** See code S49.009

√5ᵗʰ **S49.0** Physeal fracture of upper end of humerus

   √6ᵗʰ **S49.00** Unspecified physeal fracture of upper end of humerus

    3 √7ᵗʰ **S49.001** Unspecified physeal fracture of upper end of humerus, right arm   CC H5
     CC Excl: CC with 7th character A: PDX collection 1245
     CC with 7th character K or P: PDX collection 897

    3 √7ᵗʰ **S49.002** Unspecified physeal fracture of upper end of humerus, left arm   CC H5
     CC Excl: CC with 7th character A: PDX collection 1247
     CC with 7th character K or P: PDX collection 897

    3 √7ᵗʰ **S49.009** Unspecified physeal fracture of upper end of humerus, unspecified arm   CC H5
     CC Excl: CC with 7th character A: PDX collection 1248
     CC with 7th character K or P: PDX collection 897

   √6ᵗʰ **S49.01** Salter-Harris Type I physeal fracture of upper end of humerus

    3 √7ᵗʰ **S49.011** Salter-Harris Type I physeal fracture of upper end of humerus, right arm   CC H5

    3 √7ᵗʰ **S49.012** Salter-Harris Type I physeal fracture of upper end of humerus, left arm   CC H5

    3 √7ᵗʰ **S49.019** Salter-Harris Type I physeal fracture of upper end of humerus, unspecified arm   CC H5

   √6ᵗʰ **S49.02** Salter-Harris Type II physeal fracture of upper end of humerus

    3 √7ᵗʰ **S49.021** Salter-Harris Type II physeal fracture of upper end of humerus, right arm   CC H5

    3 √7ᵗʰ **S49.022** Salter-Harris Type II physeal fracture of upper end of humerus, left arm   CC H5

    3 √7ᵗʰ **S49.029** Salter-Harris Type II physeal fracture of upper end of humerus, unspecified arm   CC H5

   √6ᵗʰ **S49.03** Salter-Harris Type III physeal fracture of upper end of humerus

    3 √7ᵗʰ **S49.031** Salter-Harris Type III physeal fracture of upper end of humerus, right arm   CC H5

    3 √7ᵗʰ **S49.032** Salter-Harris Type III physeal fracture of upper end of humerus, left arm   CC H5

    3 √7ᵗʰ **S49.039** Salter-Harris Type III physeal fracture of upper end of humerus, unspecified arm   CC H5

   √6ᵗʰ **S49.04** Salter-Harris Type IV physeal fracture of upper end of humerus

    3 √7ᵗʰ **S49.041** Salter-Harris Type IV physeal fracture of upper end of humerus, right arm   CC H5

    3 √7ᵗʰ **S49.042** Salter-Harris Type IV physeal fracture of upper end of humerus, left arm   CC H5

    3 √7ᵗʰ **S49.049** Salter-Harris Type IV physeal fracture of upper end of humerus, unspecified arm   CC H5

   √6ᵗʰ **S49.09** Other physeal fracture of upper end of humerus

    3 √7ᵗʰ **S49.091** Other physeal fracture of upper end of humerus, right arm   CC H5

    3 √7ᵗʰ **S49.092** Other physeal fracture of upper end of humerus, left arm   CC H5

    3 √7ᵗʰ **S49.099** Other physeal fracture of upper end of humerus, unspecified arm   CC H5

√5ᵗʰ **S49.1** Physeal fracture of lower end of humerus

   √6ᵗʰ **S49.10** Unspecified physeal fracture of lower end of humerus

    3 √7ᵗʰ **S49.101** Unspecified physeal fracture of lower end of humerus, right arm   CC H5

    3 √7ᵗʰ **S49.102** Unspecified physeal fracture of lower end of humerus, left arm   CC H5

    3 √7ᵗʰ **S49.109** Unspecified physeal fracture of lower end of humerus, unspecified arm   CC H5

   √6ᵗʰ **S49.11** Salter-Harris Type I physeal fracture of lower end of humerus

    3 √7ᵗʰ **S49.111** Salter-Harris Type I physeal fracture of lower end of humerus, right arm   CC H5

    3 √7ᵗʰ **S49.112** Salter-Harris Type I physeal fracture of lower end of humerus, left arm   CC H5

    3 √7ᵗʰ **S49.119** Salter-Harris Type I physeal fracture of lower end of humerus, unspecified arm   CC H5

   √6ᵗʰ **S49.12** Salter-Harris Type II physeal fracture of lower end of humerus

    3 √7ᵗʰ **S49.121** Salter-Harris Type II physeal fracture of lower end of humerus, right arm   CC H5

    3 √7ᵗʰ **S49.122** Salter-Harris Type II physeal fracture of lower end of humerus, left arm   CC H5

    3 √7ᵗʰ **S49.129** Salter-Harris Type II physeal fracture of lower end of humerus, unspecified arm   CC H5

   √6ᵗʰ **S49.13** Salter-Harris Type III physeal fracture of lower end of humerus

    3 √7ᵗʰ **S49.131** Salter-Harris Type III physeal fracture of lower end of humerus, right arm   CC H5

3 ✓7ᵗʰ **S49.132** **Salter-Harris Type III physeal fracture of lower end of humerus, left arm** `CC` `H5`

3 ✓7ᵗʰ **S49.139** **Salter-Harris Type III physeal fracture of lower end of humerus, unspecified arm** `CC` `H5`

✓6ᵗʰ **S49.14** Salter-Harris Type IV physeal fracture of lower end of humerus

3 ✓7ᵗʰ **S49.141** **Salter-Harris Type IV physeal fracture of lower end of humerus, right arm** `CC` `H5`

3 ✓7ᵗʰ **S49.142** **Salter-Harris Type IV physeal fracture of lower end of humerus, left arm** `CC` `H5`

3 ✓7ᵗʰ **S49.149** **Salter-Harris Type IV physeal fracture of lower end of humerus, unspecified arm** `CC` `H5`

✓6ᵗʰ **S49.19** Other physeal fracture of lower end of humerus

3 ✓7ᵗʰ **S49.191** **Other physeal fracture of lower end of humerus, right arm** `CC` `H5`

3 ✓7ᵗʰ **S49.192** **Other physeal fracture of lower end of humerus, left arm** `CC` `H5`

3 ✓7ᵗʰ **S49.199** **Other physeal fracture of lower end of humerus, unspecified arm** `CC` `H5`

✓5ᵗʰ **S49.8** **Other specified injuries of shoulder and upper arm**

> The appropriate 7th character is to be added to each code in subcategory S49.8.
> A   initial encounter
> D   subsequent encounter
> S   sequela

✓x7ᵗʰ **S49.80** **Other specified injuries of shoulder and upper arm, unspecified arm**

✓x7ᵗʰ **S49.81** **Other specified injuries of right shoulder and upper arm**

✓x7ᵗʰ **S49.82** **Other specified injuries of left shoulder and upper arm**

✓5ᵗʰ **S49.9** **Unspecified injury of shoulder and upper arm**

> The appropriate 7th character is to be added to each code in subcategory S49.9.
> A   initial encounter
> D   subsequent encounter
> S   sequela

✓x7ᵗʰ **S49.90** **Unspecified injury of shoulder and upper arm, unspecified arm**

✓x7ᵗʰ **S49.91** **Unspecified injury of right shoulder and upper arm**

✓x7ᵗʰ **S49.92** **Unspecified injury of left shoulder and upper arm**

Injuries to the elbow and forearm (S50-S59)

`EXCLUDES 2` *burns and corrosions (T20-T32)*
frostbite (T33-T34)
injuries of wrist and hand (S60-S69)
insect bite or sting, venomous (T63.4)

✓4ᵗʰ **S50** **Superficial injury of elbow and forearm**

`EXCLUDES 2` *superficial injury of wrist and hand (S60.-)*

> The appropriate 7th character is to be added to each code from category S50.
> A   initial encounter
> D   subsequent encounter
> S   sequela

✓5ᵗʰ **S50.0** **Contusion of elbow**

✓x7ᵗʰ **S50.00** **Contusion of unspecified elbow**

✓x7ᵗʰ **S50.01** **Contusion of right elbow**

✓x7ᵗʰ **S50.02** **Contusion of left elbow**

✓5ᵗʰ **S50.1** **Contusion of forearm**

✓x7ᵗʰ **S50.10** **Contusion of unspecified forearm**

✓x7ᵗʰ **S50.11** **Contusion of right forearm**

✓x7ᵗʰ **S50.12** **Contusion of left forearm**

✓5ᵗʰ **S50.3** **Other superficial injuries of elbow**

✓6ᵗʰ **S50.31** Abrasion of elbow

✓7ᵗʰ **S50.311** **Abrasion of right elbow**

✓7ᵗʰ **S50.312** **Abrasion of left elbow**

✓7ᵗʰ **S50.319** **Abrasion of unspecified elbow**

✓6ᵗʰ **S50.32** Blister (nonthermal) of elbow

✓7ᵗʰ **S50.321** **Blister (nonthermal) of right elbow**

✓7ᵗʰ **S50.322** **Blister (nonthermal) of left elbow**

✓7ᵗʰ **S50.329** **Blister (nonthermal) of unspecified elbow**

✓6ᵗʰ **S50.34** External constriction of elbow

✓7ᵗʰ **S50.341** **External constriction of right elbow**

✓7ᵗʰ **S50.342** **External constriction of left elbow**

✓7ᵗʰ **S50.349** **External constriction of unspecified elbow**

✓6ᵗʰ **S50.35** Superficial foreign body of elbow
Splinter in the elbow

✓7ᵗʰ **S50.351** **Superficial foreign body of right elbow**

✓7ᵗʰ **S50.352** **Superficial foreign body of left elbow**

✓7ᵗʰ **S50.359** **Superficial foreign body of unspecified elbow**

✓6ᵗʰ **S50.36** Insect bite (nonvenomous) of elbow

✓7ᵗʰ **S50.361** **Insect bite (nonvenomous) of right elbow**

✓7ᵗʰ **S50.362** **Insect bite (nonvenomous) of left elbow**

✓7ᵗʰ **S50.369** **Insect bite (nonvenomous) of unspecified elbow**

✓6ᵗʰ **S50.37** Other superficial bite of elbow
`EXCLUDES 1` *open bite of elbow (S51.04)*

✓7ᵗʰ **S50.371** **Other superficial bite of right elbow**

✓7ᵗʰ **S50.372** **Other superficial bite of left elbow**

✓7ᵗʰ **S50.379** **Other superficial bite of unspecified elbow**

✓5ᵗʰ **S50.8** **Other superficial injuries of forearm**

✓6ᵗʰ **S50.81** Abrasion of forearm

✓7ᵗʰ **S50.811** **Abrasion of right forearm**

✓7ᵗʰ **S50.812** **Abrasion of left forearm**

✓7ᵗʰ **S50.819** **Abrasion of unspecified forearm**

✓6ᵗʰ **S50.82** Blister (nonthermal) of forearm

✓7ᵗʰ **S50.821** **Blister (nonthermal) of right forearm**

✓7ᵗʰ **S50.822** **Blister (nonthermal) of left forearm**

✓7ᵗʰ **S50.829** **Blister (nonthermal) of unspecified forearm**

✓6ᵗʰ **S50.84** External constriction of forearm

✓7ᵗʰ **S50.841** **External constriction of right forearm**

✓7ᵗʰ **S50.842** **External constriction of left forearm**

✓7ᵗʰ **S50.849** **External constriction of unspecified forearm**

✓6ᵗʰ **S50.85** Superficial foreign body of forearm
Splinter in the forearm

✓7ᵗʰ **S50.851** **Superficial foreign body of right forearm**

✓7ᵗʰ **S50.852** **Superficial foreign body of left forearm**

✓7ᵗʰ **S50.859** **Superficial foreign body of unspecified forearm**

✓6ᵗʰ **S50.86** Insect bite (nonvenomous) of forearm

✓7ᵗʰ **S50.861** **Insect bite (nonvenomous) of right forearm**

✓7ᵗʰ **S50.862** **Insect bite (nonvenomous) of left forearm**

✓7ᵗʰ **S50.869** **Insect bite (nonvenomous) of unspecified forearm**

✓6ᵗʰ **S50.87** Other superficial bite of forearm
`EXCLUDES 1` *open bite of forearm (S51.84)*

✓7ᵗʰ **S50.871** **Other superficial bite of right forearm**

✓7ᵗʰ **S50.872** **Other superficial bite of left forearm**

✓7ᵗʰ **S50.879** **Other superficial bite of unspecified forearm**

✓5ᵗʰ **S50.9** **Unspecified superficial injury of elbow and forearm**

✓6ᵗʰ **S50.90** Unspecified superficial injury of elbow

✓7ᵗʰ **S50.901** **Unspecified superficial injury of right elbow**

✓7ᵗʰ **S50.902** **Unspecified superficial injury of left elbow**

✓7ᵗʰ **S50.909** **Unspecified superficial injury of unspecified elbow**

✓6ᵗʰ **S50.91** Unspecified superficial injury of forearm

✓7ᵗʰ **S50.911** **Unspecified superficial injury of right forearm**

✓7ᵗʰ **S50.912** **Unspecified superficial injury of left forearm**

✓7ᵗʰ **S50.919** **Unspecified superficial injury of unspecified forearm**

`N` Newborn: 0   `P` Pediatric: 0-17   `M` Maternity: 12-55   `A` Adult: 15-124   `MCC` Major Complication/Comorbidity   `CC` Complication/Comorbidity   `SW` Severe Wound Dx

1002   ICD-10-CM 2019

✓4ᵗʰ **S51**   **Open wound of elbow and forearm**
Code also any associated wound infection
EXCLUDES 1   open fracture of elbow and forearm (S52- with open fracture 7th character)
traumatic amputation of elbow and forearm (S58.-)
EXCLUDES 2   open wound of wrist and hand (S61.-)

> The appropriate 7th character is to be added to each code from category S51.
> A   initial encounter
> D   subsequent encounter
> S   sequela

✓5ᵗʰ **S51.0**   **Open wound of elbow**

   ✓6ᵗʰ **S51.00**   **Unspecified open wound of elbow**

     ✓7ᵗʰ **S51.001**   **Unspecified open wound of right elbow**
       AHA: 2012, 4Q, 108

     ✓7ᵗʰ **S51.002**   **Unspecified open wound of left elbow**

     ✓7ᵗʰ **S51.009**   **Unspecified open wound of unspecified elbow**
       Open wound of elbow NOS

   ✓6ᵗʰ **S51.01**   **Laceration without foreign body of elbow**

     ✓7ᵗʰ **S51.011**   **Laceration without foreign body of right elbow**

     ✓7ᵗʰ **S51.012**   **Laceration without foreign body of left elbow**

     ✓7ᵗʰ **S51.019**   **Laceration without foreign body of unspecified elbow**

   ✓6ᵗʰ **S51.02**   **Laceration with foreign body of elbow**

     ✓7ᵗʰ **S51.021**   **Laceration with foreign body of right elbow**

     ✓7ᵗʰ **S51.022**   **Laceration with foreign body of left elbow**

     ✓7ᵗʰ **S51.029**   **Laceration with foreign body of unspecified elbow**

   ✓6ᵗʰ **S51.03**   **Puncture wound without foreign body of elbow**

     ✓7ᵗʰ **S51.031**   **Puncture wound without foreign body of right elbow**

     ✓7ᵗʰ **S51.032**   **Puncture wound without foreign body of left elbow**

     ✓7ᵗʰ **S51.039**   **Puncture wound without foreign body of unspecified elbow**

   ✓6ᵗʰ **S51.04**   **Puncture wound with foreign body of elbow**

     ✓7ᵗʰ **S51.041**   **Puncture wound with foreign body of right elbow**

     ✓7ᵗʰ **S51.042**   **Puncture wound with foreign body of left elbow**

     ✓7ᵗʰ **S51.049**   **Puncture wound with foreign body of unspecified elbow**

   ✓6ᵗʰ **S51.05**   **Open bite of elbow**
     Bite of elbow NOS
     EXCLUDES 1   superficial bite of elbow (S50.36, S50.37)

     ✓7ᵗʰ **S51.051**   **Open bite, right elbow**

     ✓7ᵗʰ **S51.052**   **Open bite, left elbow**

     ✓7ᵗʰ **S51.059**   **Open bite, unspecified elbow**

✓5ᵗʰ **S51.8**   **Open wound of forearm**
   EXCLUDES 2   open wound of elbow (S51.0-)

   ✓6ᵗʰ **S51.80**   **Unspecified open wound of forearm**
     AHA: 2016, 3Q, 24

     ✓7ᵗʰ **S51.801**   **Unspecified open wound of right forearm**

     ✓7ᵗʰ **S51.802**   **Unspecified open wound of left forearm**

     ✓7ᵗʰ **S51.809**   **Unspecified open wound of unspecified forearm**
       Open wound of forearm NOS

   ✓6ᵗʰ **S51.81**   **Laceration without foreign body of forearm**

     ✓7ᵗʰ **S51.811**   **Laceration without foreign body of right forearm**

     ✓7ᵗʰ **S51.812**   **Laceration without foreign body of left forearm**

     ✓7ᵗʰ **S51.819**   **Laceration without foreign body of unspecified forearm**

   ✓6ᵗʰ **S51.82**   **Laceration with foreign body of forearm**

     ✓7ᵗʰ **S51.821**   **Laceration with foreign body of right forearm**

     ✓7ᵗʰ **S51.822**   **Laceration with foreign body of left forearm**

     ✓7ᵗʰ **S51.829**   **Laceration with foreign body of unspecified forearm**

   ✓6ᵗʰ **S51.83**   **Puncture wound without foreign body of forearm**
     AHA: 2016, 3Q, 24

     ✓7ᵗʰ **S51.831**   **Puncture wound without foreign body of right forearm**

     ✓7ᵗʰ **S51.832**   **Puncture wound without foreign body of left forearm**

     ✓7ᵗʰ **S51.839**   **Puncture wound without foreign body of unspecified forearm**

   ✓6ᵗʰ **S51.84**   **Puncture wound with foreign body of forearm**
     AHA: 2016, 3Q, 24

     ✓7ᵗʰ **S51.841**   **Puncture wound with foreign body of right forearm**

     ✓7ᵗʰ **S51.842**   **Puncture wound with foreign body of left forearm**

     ✓7ᵗʰ **S51.849**   **Puncture wound with foreign body of unspecified forearm**

   ✓6ᵗʰ **S51.85**   **Open bite of forearm**
     Bite of forearm NOS
     EXCLUDES 1   superficial bite of forearm (S50.86, S50.87)

     ✓7ᵗʰ **S51.851**   **Open bite of right forearm**

     ✓7ᵗʰ **S51.852**   **Open bite of left forearm**

     ✓7ᵗʰ **S51.859**   **Open bite of unspecified forearm**

✓4ᵗʰ **S52**   **Fracture of forearm**
   NOTE   A fracture not indicated as displaced or nondisplaced should be coded to displaced.
     A fracture not indicated as open or closed should be coded to closed.
     The open fracture designations are based on the Gustilo open fracture classification.
   EXCLUDES 1   traumatic amputation of forearm (S58.-)
   EXCLUDES 2   fracture at wrist and hand level (S62.-)
   AHA: 2018, 2Q, 12; 2016, 1Q, 33; 2015, 3Q, 37-39

> The appropriate 7th character is to be added to all codes from category S52 [unless otherwise indicated].
> A   initial encounter for closed fracture
> B   initial encounter for open fracture type I or II
>   initial encounter for open fracture NOS
> C   initial encounter for open fracture type IIIA, IIIB, or IIIC
> D   subsequent encounter for closed fracture with routine healing
> E   subsequent encounter for open fracture type I or II with routine healing
> F   subsequent encounter for open fracture type IIIA, IIIB, or IIIC with routine healing
> G   subsequent encounter for closed fracture with delayed healing
> H   subsequent encounter for open fracture type I or II with delayed healing
> J   subsequent encounter for open fracture type IIIA, IIIB, or IIIC with delayed healing
> K   subsequent encounter for closed fracture with nonunion
> M   subsequent encounter for open fracture type I or II with nonunion
> N   subsequent encounter for open fracture type IIIA, IIIB, or IIIC with nonunion
> P   subsequent encounter for closed fracture with malunion
> Q   subsequent encounter for open fracture type I or II with malunion
> R   subsequent encounter for open fracture type IIIA, IIIB, or IIIC with malunion
> S   sequela

✓5ᵗʰ **S52.0**   **Fracture of upper end of ulna**
   Fracture of proximal end of ulna
   EXCLUDES 2   fracture of elbow NOS (S42.40-)
     fractures of shaft of ulna (S52.2-)

   ✓6ᵗʰ **S52.00**   **Unspecified fracture of upper end of ulna**

> **CC Excl: For codes in subcatagory S52.00:**
> **MCC with 7th character B or C:**
> PDX collection 1269
> **CC with 7th character K, M, N, P, Q, or R:**
> PDX collection 897

     2,4 ✓7ᵗʰ **S52.001**   **Unspecified fracture of upper end of right ulna**   `MCC` `CC` `H5`

     2,4 ✓7ᵗʰ **S52.002**   **Unspecified fracture of upper end of left ulna**   `MCC` `CC` `H5`

2,4 √7ᵗʰ S52.009   Unspecified fracture of upper end of unspecified ulna   MCC CC H5

√6ᵗʰ S52.01   Torus fracture of upper end of ulna

> The appropriate 7th character is to be added to all codes in subcategory S52.01.
> A   initial encounter for closed fracture
> D   subsequent encounter for fracture with routine healing
> G   subsequent encounter for fracture with delayed healing
> K   subsequent encounter for fracture with nonunion
> P   subsequent encounter for fracture with malunion
> S   sequela

3 √7ᵗʰ S52.011   Torus fracture of upper end of right ulna   CC H5

> CC Excl: CC with 7th character A:
> PDX collection 1270
> CC with 7th character K or P:
> PDX collection 897

3 √7ᵗʰ S52.012   Torus fracture of upper end of left ulna   CC H5

> CC Excl: CC with 7th character A:
> PDX collection 1271
> CC with 7th character K or P:
> PDX collection 897

3 √7ᵗʰ S52.019   Torus fracture of upper end of unspecified ulna   CC H5

> CC Excl: CC with 7th character A:
> PDX collection 1272
> CC with 7th character K or P:
> PDX collection 897

√6ᵗʰ S52.02   Fracture of olecranon process without intraarticular extension of ulna

> CC Excl: For codes in subcatagory S52.02:
> MCC with 7th character B or C:
> PDX collection 1273
> CC with 7th character K, M, N, P, Q, or R:
> PDX collection 897

2,4 √7ᵗʰ S52.021   Displaced fracture of olecranon process without intraarticular extension of right ulna   MCC CC H5

2,4 √7ᵗʰ S52.022   Displaced fracture of olecranon process without intraarticular extension of left ulna   MCC CC H5

2,4 √7ᵗʰ S52.023   Displaced fracture of olecranon process without intraarticular extension of unspecified ulna   MCC CC H5

2,4 √7ᵗʰ S52.024   Nondisplaced fracture of olecranon process without intraarticular extension of right ulna   MCC CC H5

2,4 √7ᵗʰ S52.025   Nondisplaced fracture of olecranon process without intraarticular extension of left ulna   MCC CC H5

2,4 √7ᵗʰ S52.026   Nondisplaced fracture of olecranon process without intra-articular extension of unspecified ulna   MCC CC H5

√6ᵗʰ S52.03   Fracture of olecranon process with intraarticular extension of ulna

> CC Excl: For codes in subcatagory S52.03:
> MCC with 7th character B or C:
> PDX collection 1273
> CC with 7th character K, M, N, P, Q, or R:
> PDX collection 897

2,4 √7ᵗʰ S52.031   Displaced fracture of olecranon process with intraarticular extension of right ulna   MCC CC H5

2,4 √7ᵗʰ S52.032   Displaced fracture of olecranon process with intraarticular extension of left ulna   MCC CC H5

2,4 √7ᵗʰ S52.033   Displaced fracture of olecranon process with intraarticular extension of unspecified ulna   MCC CC H5

2,4 √7ᵗʰ S52.034   Nondisplaced fracture of olecranon process with intraarticular extension of right ulna   MCC CC H5

2,4 √7ᵗʰ S52.035   Nondisplaced fracture of olecranon process with intraarticular extension of left ulna   MCC CC H5

2,4 √7ᵗʰ S52.036   Nondisplaced fracture of olecranon process with intraarticular extension of unspecified ulna   MCC CC H5

√6ᵗʰ S52.04   Fracture of coronoid process of ulna

> CC Excl: For codes in subcatagory S52.04:
> MCC with 7th character B or C:
> PDX collection 1269
> CC with 7th character K, M, N, P, Q, or R:
> PDX collection 897

2,4 √7ᵗʰ S52.041   Displaced fracture of coronoid process of right ulna   MCC CC H5

2,4 √7ᵗʰ S52.042   Displaced fracture of coronoid process of left ulna   MCC CC H5

2,4 √7ᵗʰ S52.043   Displaced fracture of coronoid process of unspecified ulna   MCC CC H5

2,4 √7ᵗʰ S52.044   Nondisplaced fracture of coronoid process of right ulna   MCC CC H5

2,4 √7ᵗʰ S52.045   Nondisplaced fracture of coronoid process of left ulna   MCC CC H5

2,4 √7ᵗʰ S52.046   Nondisplaced fracture of coronoid process of unspecified ulna   MCC CC H5

√6ᵗʰ S52.09   Other fracture of upper end of ulna

> CC Excl: For codes in subcatagory S52.09:
> MCC with 7th character B or C:
> PDX collection 1269
> CC with 7th character K, M, N, P, Q, or R:
> PDX collection 897

2,4 √7ᵗʰ S52.091   Other fracture of upper end of right ulna   MCC CC H5

2,4 √7ᵗʰ S52.092   Other fracture of upper end of left ulna   MCC CC H5

2,4 √7ᵗʰ S52.099   Other fracture of upper end of unspecified ulna   MCC CC H5

√5ᵗʰ S52.1   Fracture of upper end of radius

Fracture of proximal end of radius

> EXCLUDES 2   physeal fractures of upper end of radius (S59.2-)
> fracture of shaft of radius (S52.3-)

> CC Excl: For codes in subcategory S52.1, unless otherwise noted:
> MCC with 7th character B or C: PDX collection 1269
> CC with 7th character K, M, N, P, Q, or R:
> PDX collection 897

√6ᵗʰ S52.10   Unspecified fracture of upper end of radius

2,4 √7ᵗʰ S52.101   Unspecified fracture of upper end of right radius   MCC CC H5

2,4 √7ᵗʰ S52.102   Unspecified fracture of upper end of left radius   MCC CC H5

2,4 √7ᵗʰ S52.109   Unspecified fracture of upper end of unspecified radius   MCC CC H5

√6ᵗʰ S52.11   Torus fracture of upper end of radius

> The appropriate 7th character is to be added to all codes in subcategory S52.11.
> A   initial encounter for closed fracture
> D   subsequent encounter for fracture with routine healing
> G   subsequent encounter for fracture with delayed healing
> K   subsequent encounter for fracture with nonunion
> P   subsequent encounter for fracture with malunion
> S   sequela

3 √7ᵗʰ S52.111   Torus fracture of upper end of right radius   CC H5

> CC Excl: CC with 7th character A:
> PDX collection 1270
> CC with 7th character K, P:
> PDX collection 897

N Newborn: 0   P Pediatric: 0-17   M Maternity: 12-55   A Adult: 15-124   MCC Major Complication/Comorbidity   CC Complication/Comorbidity   SW Severe Wound Dx

1004   ICD-10-CM 2019

³ ✓7ᵗʰ **S52.112** **Torus fracture of upper end of** left **radius**   `CC` `H5`

> CC Excl: CC with 7th character A:
> PDX collection 1271
> CC with 7th character K or P:
> PDX collection 897

³ ✓7ᵗʰ **S52.119** **Torus fracture of upper end of unspecified radius**   `CC` `H5`

> CC Excl: CC with 7th character A:
> PDX collection 1272
> CC Excl: CC with 7th character K or P:
> PDX collection 897

✓6ᵗʰ **S52.12** **Fracture of** head **of radius**

^{2,4} ✓7ᵗʰ **S52.121** **Displaced fracture of head of** right **radius**   `MCC` `CC` `H5`

^{2,4} ✓7ᵗʰ **S52.122** **Displaced fracture of head of** left **radius**   `MCC` `CC` `H5`

^{2,4} ✓7ᵗʰ **S52.123** **Displaced fracture of head of unspecified radius**   `MCC` `CC` `H5`

^{2,4} ✓7ᵗʰ **S52.124** **Nondisplaced fracture of head of** right **radius**   `MCC` `CC` `H5`

^{2,4} ✓7ᵗʰ **S52.125** **Nondisplaced fracture of head of** left **radius**   `MCC` `CC` `H5`

^{2,4} ✓7ᵗʰ **S52.126** **Nondisplaced fracture of head of unspecified radius**   `MCC` `CC` `H5`

✓6ᵗʰ **S52.13** **Fracture of** neck **of radius**

^{2,4} ✓7ᵗʰ **S52.131** **Displaced fracture of neck of** right **radius**   `MCC` `CC` `H5`

^{2,4} ✓7ᵗʰ **S52.132** **Displaced fracture of neck of** left **radius**   `MCC` `CC` `H5`

^{2,4} ✓7ᵗʰ **S52.133** **Displaced fracture of neck of unspecified radius**   `MCC` `CC` `H5`

^{2,4} ✓7ᵗʰ **S52.134** **Nondisplaced fracture of neck of** right **radius**   `MCC` `CC` `H5`

^{2,4} ✓7ᵗʰ **S52.135** **Nondisplaced fracture of neck of** left **radius**   `MCC` `CC` `H5`

^{2,4} ✓7ᵗʰ **S52.136** **Nondisplaced fracture of neck of unspecified radius**   `MCC` `CC` `H5`

✓6ᵗʰ **S52.18** Other **fracture of upper end of radius**

^{2,4} ✓7ᵗʰ **S52.181** **Other fracture of upper end of** right **radius**   `MCC` `CC` `H5`

^{2,4} ✓7ᵗʰ **S52.182** **Other fracture of upper end of** left **radius**   `MCC` `CC` `H5`

^{2,4} ✓7ᵗʰ **S52.189** **Other fracture of upper end of unspecified radius**   `MCC` `CC` `H5`

✓5ᵗʰ **S52.2** **Fracture of** shaft of ulna

> CC Excl: For CC/MCC codes in subcategory S52.2, unless otherwise noted:
> Right side: See code S52.201
> Left side: See code S52.202
> Unspecified side: See code S52.209

✓6ᵗʰ **S52.20** **Unspecified fracture of shaft of ulna**
Fracture of ulna NOS

^{2,3} ✓7ᵗʰ **S52.201** **Unspecified fracture of shaft of** right **ulna**   `MCC` `CC` `H5`

> CC Excl: CC with 7th character A:
> PDX collection 1270
> MCC with 7th character B or C:
> PDX collection 1269
> CC with 7th character K, M, N, P, Q or R:
> PDX collection 897

^{2,3} ✓7ᵗʰ **S52.202** **Unspecified fracture of shaft of** left **ulna**   `MCC` `CC` `H5`

> CC Excl: CC with 7th character A:
> PDX collection 1271
> MCC with 7th character B or C:
> PDX collection 1269
> CC with 7th character K, M, N, P, Q or R:
> PDX collection 897

^{2,3} ✓7ᵗʰ **S52.209** **Unspecified fracture of shaft of unspecified ulna**   `MCC` `CC` `H5`

> CC Excl: CC with 7th character A:
> PDX collection 1272
> MCC with 7th character B or C:
> PDX collection 1269
> CC with 7th character K, M, N, P, Q or R:
> PDX collection 897

✓6ᵗʰ **S52.21** Greenstick **fracture of shaft of ulna**

> The appropriate 7th character is to be added to all codes in subcategory S52.21.
> A   initial encounter for closed fracture
> D   subsequent encounter for fracture with routine healing
> G   subsequent encounter for fracture with delayed healing
> K   subsequent encounter for fracture with nonunion
> P   subsequent encounter for fracture with malunion
> S   sequela

³ ✓7ᵗʰ **S52.211** **Greenstick fracture of shaft of** right **ulna**   `CC` `H5`

> CC Excl: CC with 7th character A:
> PDX collection 1270
> CC with 7th character K or P:
> PDX collection 897

³ ✓7ᵗʰ **S52.212** **Greenstick fracture of shaft of** left **ulna**   `CC` `H5`

> CC Excl: CC with 7th character A:
> PDX collection 1271
> CC with 7th character K or P:
> PDX collection 897

³ ✓7ᵗʰ **S52.219** **Greenstick fracture of shaft of unspecified ulna**   `CC` `H5`

> CC Excl: CC with 7th character A:
> PDX collection 1272
> CC with 7th character K or P:
> PDX collection 897

✓6ᵗʰ **S52.22** Transverse **fracture of shaft of ulna**

^{2,3} ✓7ᵗʰ **S52.221** **Displaced transverse fracture of shaft of** right **ulna**   `MCC` `CC` `H5`

^{2,3} ✓7ᵗʰ **S52.222** **Displaced transverse fracture of shaft of** left **ulna**   `MCC` `CC` `H5`

^{2,3} ✓7ᵗʰ **S52.223** **Displaced transverse fracture of shaft of** unspecified **ulna**   `MCC` `CC` `H5`

^{2,3} ✓7ᵗʰ **S52.224** **Nondisplaced transverse fracture of shaft of** right **ulna**   `MCC` `CC` `H5`

^{2,3} ✓7ᵗʰ **S52.225** **Nondisplaced transverse fracture of shaft of** left **ulna**   `MCC` `CC` `H5`

^{2,3} ✓7ᵗʰ **S52.226** **Nondisplaced transverse fracture of shaft of** unspecified **ulna**   `MCC` `CC` `H5`

✓6ᵗʰ **S52.23** Oblique **fracture of shaft of ulna**

^{2,3} ✓7ᵗʰ **S52.231** **Displaced oblique fracture of shaft of** right **ulna**   `MCC` `CC` `H5`

^{2,3} ✓7ᵗʰ **S52.232** **Displaced oblique fracture of shaft of** left **ulna**   `MCC` `CC` `H5`

^{2,3} ✓7ᵗʰ **S52.233** **Displaced oblique fracture of shaft of** unspecified **ulna**   `MCC` `CC` `H5`

^{2,3} ✓7ᵗʰ **S52.234** **Nondisplaced oblique fracture of shaft of** right **ulna**   `MCC` `CC` `H5`

^{2,3} ✓7ᵗʰ **S52.235** **Nondisplaced oblique fracture of shaft of** left **ulna**   `MCC` `CC` `H5`

^{2,3} ✓7ᵗʰ **S52.236** **Nondisplaced oblique fracture of shaft of** unspecified **ulna**   `MCC` `CC` `H5`

✓6ᵗʰ **S52.24** Spiral **fracture of shaft of ulna**

^{2,3} ✓7ᵗʰ **S52.241** **Displaced spiral fracture of shaft of ulna,** right **arm**   `MCC` `CC` `H5`

^{2,3} ✓7ᵗʰ **S52.242** **Displaced spiral fracture of shaft of ulna,** left **arm**   `MCC` `CC` `H5`

^{2,3} ✓7ᵗʰ **S52.243** **Displaced spiral fracture of shaft of ulna,** unspecified **arm**   `MCC` `CC` `H5`

^{2,3} ✓7ᵗʰ **S52.244** **Nondisplaced spiral fracture of shaft of ulna,** right **arm**   `MCC` `CC` `H5`

^{2,3} ✓7ᵗʰ **S52.245** **Nondisplaced spiral fracture of shaft of ulna,** left **arm**   `MCC` `CC` `H5`

^{2,3} ✓7ᵗʰ **S52.246** **Nondisplaced spiral fracture of shaft of ulna,** unspecified **arm**   `MCC` `CC` `H5`

✓6ᵗʰ **S52.25** Comminuted **fracture of shaft of ulna**

^{2,3} ✓7ᵗʰ **S52.251** **Displaced comminuted fracture of shaft of ulna,** right **arm**   `MCC` `CC` `H5`

^{2,3} ✓7ᵗʰ **S52.252** **Displaced comminuted fracture of shaft of ulna,** left **arm**   `MCC` `CC` `H5`

^{2,3} ✓7ᵗʰ **S52.253** **Displaced comminuted fracture of shaft of ulna,** unspecified **arm**   `MCC` `CC` `H5`

✓ Additional Character Required   ✓x7ᵗʰ Placeholder   Unacceptable PDx   Questionable PDx   Manifestation   `H1`-`H14` HAC   `HCC` CMS-HCC Dx   `HIV` HIV Dx

ICD-10-CM 2019   **1005**

2,3 √7th S52.254 Nondisplaced comminuted fracture of shaft of ulna, right arm `MCC` `CC` `H5`

2,3 √7th S52.255 Nondisplaced comminuted fracture of shaft of ulna, left arm `MCC` `CC` `H5`

2,3 √7th S52.256 Nondisplaced comminuted fracture of shaft of ulna, unspecified arm `MCC` `CC` `H5`

√6th S52.26 Segmental fracture of shaft of ulna

2,3 √7th S52.261 Displaced segmental fracture of shaft of ulna, right arm `MCC` `CC` `H5`

2,3 √7th S52.262 Displaced segmental fracture of shaft of ulna, left arm `MCC` `CC` `H5`

2,3 √7th S52.263 Displaced segmental fracture of shaft of ulna, unspecified arm `MCC` `CC` `H5`

2,3 √7th S52.264 Nondisplaced segmental fracture of shaft of ulna, right arm `MCC` `CC` `H5`

2,3 √7th S52.265 Nondisplaced segmental fracture of shaft of ulna, left arm `MCC` `CC` `H5`

2,3 √7th S52.266 Nondisplaced segmental fracture of shaft of ulna, unspecified arm `MCC` `CC` `H5`

√6th S52.27 Monteggia's fracture of ulna
Fracture of upper shaft of ulna with dislocation of radial head

> CC Excl: For codes in subcategory S52.27:
> MCC with 7th character B or C:
> PDX collection 1269
> CC with 7th character K, M, N, P Q or R:
> PDX collection 897

2,4 √7th S52.271 Monteggia's fracture of right ulna `MCC` `CC` `H5`

2,4 √7th S52.272 Monteggia's fracture of left ulna `MCC` `CC` `H5`

2,4 √7th S52.279 Monteggia's fracture of unspecified ulna `MCC` `CC` `H5`

√6th S52.28 Bent bone of ulna

2,3 √7th S52.281 Bent bone of right ulna `MCC` `CC` `H5`

2,3 √7th S52.282 Bent bone of left ulna `MCC` `CC` `H5`

2,3 √7th S52.283 Bent bone of unspecified ulna `MCC` `CC` `H5`

√6th S52.29 Other fracture of shaft of ulna

2,3 √7th S52.291 Other fracture of shaft of right ulna `MCC` `CC` `H5`

2,3 √7th S52.292 Other fracture of shaft of left ulna `MCC` `CC` `H5`

2,3 √7th S52.299 Other fracture of shaft of unspecified ulna `MCC` `CC` `H5`

√5th S52.3 Fracture of shaft of radius

> CC Excl: For CC/MCC codes in subcategory S52.3, unless otherwise noted:
> Right side: See code S52.201
> Left side: See code S52.202
> Unspecified side: See code S52.209

√6th S52.30 Unspecified fracture of shaft of radius

2,3 √7th S52.301 Unspecified fracture of shaft of right radius `MCC` `CC` `H5`

2,3 √7th S52.302 Unspecified fracture of shaft of left radius `MCC` `CC` `H5`

2,3 √7th S52.309 Unspecified fracture of shaft of unspecified radius `MCC` `CC` `H5`

√6th S52.31 Greenstick fracture of shaft of radius

> The appropriate 7th character is to be added to all codes in subcategory S52.31.
> A   initial encounter for closed fracture
> D   subsequent encounter for fracture with routine healing
> G   subsequent encounter for fracture with delayed healing
> K   subsequent encounter for fracture with nonunion
> P   subsequent encounter for fracture with malunion
> S   sequela

3 √7th S52.311 Greenstick fracture of shaft of radius, right arm `CC` `H5`
CC Excl: See code: S52.211

3 √7th S52.312 Greenstick fracture of shaft of radius, left arm `CC` `H5`
CC Excl: See code: S52.212

3 √7th S52.319 Greenstick fracture of shaft of radius, unspecified arm `CC` `H5`
CC Excl: See code: S52.219

√6th S52.32 Transverse fracture of shaft of radius

2,3 √7th S52.321 Displaced transverse fracture of shaft of right radius `MCC` `CC` `H5`

2,3 √7th S52.322 Displaced transverse fracture of shaft of left radius `MCC` `CC` `H5`

2,3 √7th S52.323 Displaced transverse fracture of shaft of unspecified radius `MCC` `CC` `H5`

2,3 √7th S52.324 Nondisplaced transverse fracture of shaft of right radius `MCC` `CC` `H5`

2,3 √7th S52.325 Nondisplaced transverse fracture of shaft of left radius `MCC` `CC` `H5`

2,3 √7th S52.326 Nondisplaced transverse fracture of shaft of unspecified radius `MCC` `CC` `H5`

√6th S52.33 Oblique fracture of shaft of radius

2,3 √7th S52.331 Displaced oblique fracture of shaft of right radius `MCC` `CC` `H5`

2,3 √7th S52.332 Displaced oblique fracture of shaft of left radius `MCC` `CC` `H5`

2,3 √7th S52.333 Displaced oblique fracture of shaft of unspecified radius `MCC` `CC` `H5`

2,3 √7th S52.334 Nondisplaced oblique fracture of shaft of right radius `MCC` `CC` `H5`

2,3 √7th S52.335 Nondisplaced oblique fracture of shaft of left radius `MCC` `CC` `H5`

2,3 √7th S52.336 Nondisplaced oblique fracture of shaft of unspecified radius `MCC` `CC` `H5`

√6th S52.34 Spiral fracture of shaft of radius

2,3 √7th S52.341 Displaced spiral fracture of shaft of radius, right arm `MCC` `CC` `H5`

2,3 √7th S52.342 Displaced spiral fracture of shaft of radius, left arm `MCC` `CC` `H5`

2,3 √7th S52.343 Displaced spiral fracture of shaft of radius, unspecified arm `MCC` `CC` `H5`

2,3 √7th S52.344 Nondisplaced spiral fracture of shaft of radius, right arm `MCC` `CC` `H5`

2,3 √7th S52.345 Nondisplaced spiral fracture of shaft of radius, left arm `MCC` `CC` `H5`

2,3 √7th S52.346 Nondisplaced spiral fracture of shaft of radius, unspecified arm `MCC` `CC` `H5`

√6th S52.35 Comminuted fracture of shaft of radius

2,3 √7th S52.351 Displaced comminuted fracture of shaft of radius, right arm `MCC` `CC` `H5`

2,3 √7th S52.352 Displaced comminuted fracture of shaft of radius, left arm `MCC` `CC` `H5`

2,3 √7th S52.353 Displaced comminuted fracture of shaft of radius, unspecified arm `MCC` `CC` `H5`

2,3 √7th S52.354 Nondisplaced comminuted fracture of shaft of radius, right arm `MCC` `CC` `H5`

2,3 √7th S52.355 Nondisplaced comminuted fracture of shaft of radius, left arm `MCC` `CC` `H5`

2,3 √7th S52.356 Nondisplaced comminuted fracture of shaft of radius, unspecified arm `MCC` `CC` `H5`

√6th S52.36 Segmental fracture of shaft of radius

2,3 √7th S52.361 Displaced segmental fracture of shaft of radius, right arm `MCC` `CC` `H5`

2,3 √7th S52.362 Displaced segmental fracture of shaft of radius, left arm `MCC` `CC` `H5`

2,3 √7th S52.363 Displaced segmental fracture of shaft of radius, unspecified arm `MCC` `CC` `H5`

2,3 √7th S52.364 Nondisplaced segmental fracture of shaft of radius, right arm `MCC` `CC` `H5`

2,3 √7th S52.365 Nondisplaced segmental fracture of shaft of radius, left arm `MCC` `CC` `H5`

2,3 √7th S52.366 Nondisplaced segmental fracture of shaft of radius, unspecified arm `MCC` `CC` `H5`

✓6ᵗʰ **S52.37**   Galeazzi's **fracture**
     Fracture of lower shaft of radius with radioulnar joint dislocation

2,3 ✓7ᵗʰ **S52.371**   Galeazzi's fracture of right radius   `MCC` `CC` `H5`

2,3 ✓7ᵗʰ **S52.372**   Galeazzi's fracture of left radius   `MCC` `CC` `H5`

2,3 ✓7ᵗʰ **S52.379**   Galeazzi's fracture of unspecified radius   `MCC` `CC` `H5`

✓6ᵗʰ **S52.38**   Bent bone **of radius**

2,3 ✓7ᵗʰ **S52.381**   Bent bone of right radius   `MCC` `CC` `H5`

2,3 ✓7ᵗʰ **S52.382**   Bent bone of left radius   `MCC` `CC` `H5`

2,3 ✓7ᵗʰ **S52.389**   Bent bone of unspecified radius   `MCC` `CC` `H5`

✓6ᵗʰ **S52.39**   Other **fracture of shaft of radius**

2,3 ✓7ᵗʰ **S52.391**   Other fracture of shaft of radius, right arm   `MCC` `CC` `H5`

2,3 ✓7ᵗʰ **S52.392**   Other fracture of shaft of radius, left arm   `MCC` `CC` `H5`

2,3 ✓7ᵗʰ **S52.399**   Other fracture of shaft of radius, unspecified arm   `MCC` `CC` `H5`

✓5ᵗʰ **S52.5**   Fracture of lower end of radius
     Fracture of distal end of radius
     `EXCLUDES 2`   *physeal fractures of lower end of radius (S59.2-)*
     DEF: Fracture of the distal end of the radius above the wrist, most commonly caused by a fall onto an outstretched hand..

> **CC Excl: For CC/MCC codes in subcategory S52.5, unless otherwise noted:**
> **Right side:** See code S52.201
> **Left side:** See code S52.202
> **Unspecified side:** See code S52.209

✓6ᵗʰ **S52.50**   Unspecified **fracture of the lower end of radius**

2,3 ✓7ᵗʰ **S52.501**   Unspecified fracture of the lower end of right radius   `MCC` `CC` `H5`

2,3 ✓7ᵗʰ **S52.502**   Unspecified fracture of the lower end of left radius   `MCC` `CC` `H5`

2,3 ✓7ᵗʰ **S52.509**   Unspecified fracture of the lower nd of unspecified radius   `MCC` `CC` `H5`

✓6ᵗʰ **S52.51**   Fracture of radial styloid process

2,3 ✓7ᵗʰ **S52.511**   Displaced fracture of right radial styloid process   `MCC` `CC` `H5`

2,3 ✓7ᵗʰ **S52.512**   Displaced fracture of left radial styloid process   `MCC` `CC` `H5`

2,3 ✓7ᵗʰ **S52.513**   Displaced fracture of unspecified radial styloid process   `MCC` `CC` `H5`

2,3 ✓7ᵗʰ **S52.514**   Nondisplaced fracture of right radial styloid process   `MCC` `CC` `H5`

2,3 ✓7ᵗʰ **S52.515**   Nondisplaced fracture of left radial styloid process   `MCC` `CC` `H5`

2,3 ✓7ᵗʰ **S52.516**   Nondisplaced fracture of unspecified radial styloid process   `MCC` `CC` `H5`

✓6ᵗʰ **S52.52**   Torus **fracture of lower end of radius**

> The appropriate 7th character is to be added to all codes in subcategory S52.52.
> A   initial encounter for closed fracture
> D   subsequent encounter for fracture with routine healing
> G   subsequent encounter for fracture with delayed healing
> K   subsequent encounter for fracture with nonunion
> P   subsequent encounter for fracture with malunion
> S   sequela

3 ✓7ᵗʰ **S52.521**   Torus fracture of lower end of right radius   `CC` `H5`
     CC Excl: See code: S52.211

3 ✓7ᵗʰ **S52.522**   Torus fracture of lower end of left radius   `CC` `H5`
     CC Excl: See code: S52.212

3 ✓7ᵗʰ **S52.529**   Torus fracture of lower end of unspecified radius   `CC` `H5`
     CC Excl: See code: S52.219

✓6ᵗʰ **S52.53**   Colles' **fracture**
     DEF: Fracture of the radius at the wrist in which the distal fragment is pushed posteriorly. The dorsal angulation of the fragment results in the wrist cocking up.

2,3 ✓7ᵗʰ **S52.531**   Colles' fracture of right radius   `MCC` `CC` `H5`
     AHA: 2016, 2Q, 4

2,3 ✓7ᵗʰ **S52.532**   Colles' fracture of left radius   `MCC` `CC` `H5`

2,3 ✓7ᵗʰ **S52.539**   Colles' fracture of unspecified radius   `MCC` `CC` `H5`

✓6ᵗʰ **S52.54**   Smith's **fracture**

2,3 ✓7ᵗʰ **S52.541**   Smith's fracture of right radius   `MCC` `CC` `H5`

2,3 ✓7ᵗʰ **S52.542**   Smith's fracture of left radius   `MCC` `CC` `H5`

2,3 ✓7ᵗʰ **S52.549**   Smith's fracture of unspecified radius   `MCC` `CC` `H5`

✓6ᵗʰ **S52.55**   Other extraarticular **fracture of lower end of radius**

2,3 ✓7ᵗʰ **S52.551**   Other extraarticular fracture of lower end of right radius   `MCC` `CC` `H5`

2,3 ✓7ᵗʰ **S52.552**   Other extraarticular fracture of lower end of left radius   `MCC` `CC` `H5`

2,3 ✓7ᵗʰ **S52.559**   Other extraarticular fracture of lower end of unspecified radius   `MCC` `CC` `H5`

✓6ᵗʰ **S52.56**   Barton's **fracture**

2,3 ✓7ᵗʰ **S52.561**   Barton's fracture of right radius   `MCC` `CC` `H5`

2,3 ✓7ᵗʰ **S52.562**   Barton's fracture of left radius   `MCC` `CC` `H5`

2,3 ✓7ᵗʰ **S52.569**   Barton's fracture of unspecified radius   `MCC` `CC` `H5`

✓6ᵗʰ **S52.57**   Other intraarticular **fracture of lower end of radius**

2,3 ✓7ᵗʰ **S52.571**   Other intraarticular fracture of lower end of right radius   `MCC` `CC` `H5`

2,3 ✓7ᵗʰ **S52.572**   Other intraarticular fracture of lower end of left radius   `MCC` `CC` `H5`

2,3 ✓7ᵗʰ **S52.579**   Other intraarticular fracture of lower end of unspecified radius   `MCC` `CC` `H5`

✓6ᵗʰ **S52.59**   Other **fractures of lower end of radius**

2,3 ✓7ᵗʰ **S52.591**   Other fractures of lower end of right radius   `MCC` `CC` `H5`

2,3 ✓7ᵗʰ **S52.592**   Other fractures of lower end of left radius   `MCC` `CC` `H5`

2,3 ✓7ᵗʰ **S52.599**   Other fractures of lower end of unspecified radius   `MCC` `CC` `H5`

✓5ᵗʰ **S52.6**   Fracture of lower end of ulna

> **CC Excl: For CC/MCC codes in subcategory S52.6, unless otherwise noted:**
> **Right side:** See code S52.201
> **Left side:** See code S52.202
> **Unspecified side:** See code S52.209

✓6ᵗʰ **S52.60**   Unspecified **fracture of lower end of ulna**

2,3 ✓7ᵗʰ **S52.601**   Unspecified fracture of lower end of right ulna   `MCC` `CC` `H5`

2,3 ✓7ᵗʰ **S52.602**   Unspecified fracture of lower end of left ulna   `MCC` `CC` `H5`

2,3 ✓7ᵗʰ **S52.609**   Unspecified fracture of lower end of unspecified ulna   `MCC` `CC` `H5`

✓6ᵗʰ **S52.61**   Fracture of ulna styloid process

2,3 ✓7ᵗʰ **S52.611**   Displaced fracture of right ulna styloid process   `MCC` `CC` `H5`

2,3 ✓7ᵗʰ **S52.612**   Displaced fracture of left ulna styloid process   `MCC` `CC` `H5`

2,3 ✓7ᵗʰ **S52.613**   Displaced fracture of unspecified ulna styloid process   `MCC` `CC` `H5`

2,3 ✓7ᵗʰ **S52.614**   Nondisplaced fracture of right ulna styloid process   `MCC` `CC` `H5`

2,3 ✓7ᵗʰ **S52.615**   Nondisplaced fracture of left ulna styloid process   `MCC` `CC` `H5`

2,3 ✓7ᵗʰ **S52.616**   Nondisplaced fracture of unspecified ulna styloid process   `MCC` `CC` `H5`

✓ Additional Character Required   ✓xᵗʰ Placeholder   Unacceptable PDx   Questionable PDx   Manifestation   `H1`-`H14` HAC   `HCC` CMS-HCC Dx   `HIV` HIV Dx

ICD-10-CM 2019   **1007**

☑6th **S52.62** Torus fracture of lower end of ulna

> The appropriate 7th character is to be added to all codes in subcategory S52.62.
> A initial encounter for closed fracture
> D subsequent encounter for fracture with routine healing
> G subsequent encounter for fracture with delayed healing
> K subsequent encounter for fracture with nonunion
> P subsequent encounter for fracture with malunion
> S sequela

3 ☑7th **S52.621** Torus fracture of lower end of right ulna `CC` `H5`
   CC Excl: See code: S52.211

3 ☑7th **S52.622** Torus fracture of lower end of left ulna `CC` `H5`
   CC Excl: See code: S52.212

3 ☑7th **S52.629** Torus fracture of lower end of unspecified ulna `CC` `H5`
   CC Excl: See code: S52.219

☑6th **S52.69** Other fracture of lower end of ulna

2,3 ☑7th **S52.691** Other fracture of lower end of right ulna `MCC` `CC` `H5`

2,3 ☑7th **S52.692** Other fracture of lower end of left ulna `MCC` `CC` `H5`

2,3 ☑7th **S52.699** Other fracture of lower end of unspecified ulna `MCC` `CC` `H5`

☑5th **S52.9** Unspecified fracture of forearm

> CC Excl: For CC/MCC codes in subcategory S52.9: See code S52.209

2,3 ☑x7th **S52.90** Unspecified fracture of unspecified forearm `MCC` `CC` `H5`

2,3 ☑x7th **S52.91** Unspecified fracture of right forearm `MCC` `CC` `H5`

2,3 ☑x7th **S52.92** Unspecified fracture of left forearm `MCC` `CC` `H5`

☑4th **S53 Dislocation and sprain of joints and ligaments of elbow**

> `INCLUDES` avulsion of joint or ligament of elbow
> laceration of cartilage, joint or ligament of elbow
> sprain of cartilage, joint or ligament of elbow
> traumatic hemarthrosis of joint or ligament of elbow
> traumatic rupture of joint or ligament of elbow
> traumatic subluxation of joint or ligament of elbow
> traumatic tear of joint or ligament of elbow

Code also any associated open wound

> `EXCLUDES 2` strain of muscle, fascia and tendon at forearm level (S56.-)

> The appropriate 7th character is to be added to each code from category S53.
> A initial encounter
> D subsequent encounter
> S sequela

☑5th **S53.0** Subluxation and dislocation of radial head
   Dislocation of radiohumeral joint
   Subluxation of radiohumeral joint
   > `EXCLUDES 1` Monteggia's fracture-dislocation (S52.27-)

☑6th **S53.00** Unspecified subluxation and dislocation of radial head

☑7th **S53.001** Unspecified subluxation of right radial head

☑7th **S53.002** Unspecified subluxation of left radial head

☑7th **S53.003** Unspecified subluxation of unspecified radial head

☑7th **S53.004** Unspecified dislocation of right radial head

☑7th **S53.005** Unspecified dislocation of left radial head

☑7th **S53.006** Unspecified dislocation of unspecified radial head

☑6th **S53.01** Anterior subluxation and dislocation of radial head
   Anteriomedial subluxation and dislocation of radial head

☑7th **S53.011** Anterior subluxation of right radial head

☑7th **S53.012** Anterior subluxation of left radial head

☑7th **S53.013** Anterior subluxation of unspecified radial head

☑7th **S53.014** Anterior dislocation of right radial head

☑7th **S53.015** Anterior dislocation of left radial head

☑7th **S53.016** Anterior dislocation of unspecified radial head

☑6th **S53.02** Posterior subluxation and dislocation of radial head
   Posteriolateral subluxation and dislocation of radial head

☑7th **S53.021** Posterior subluxation of right radial head

☑7th **S53.022** Posterior subluxation of left radial head

☑7th **S53.023** Posterior subluxation of unspecified radial head

☑7th **S53.024** Posterior dislocation of right radial head

☑7th **S53.025** Posterior dislocation of left radial head

☑7th **S53.026** Posterior dislocation of unspecified radial head

☑6th **S53.03** Nursemaid's elbow

☑7th **S53.031** Nursemaid's elbow, right elbow

☑7th **S53.032** Nursemaid's elbow, left elbow

☑7th **S53.033** Nursemaid's elbow, unspecified elbow

☑6th **S53.09** Other subluxation and dislocation of radial head

☑7th **S53.091** Other subluxation of right radial head

☑7th **S53.092** Other subluxation of left radial head

☑7th **S53.093** Other subluxation of unspecified radial head

☑7th **S53.094** Other dislocation of right radial head

☑7th **S53.095** Other dislocation of left radial head

☑7th **S53.096** Other dislocation of unspecified radial head

☑5th **S53.1** Subluxation and dislocation of ulnohumeral joint
   Subluxation and dislocation of elbow NOS
   > `EXCLUDES 1` dislocation of radial head alone (S53.0-)

☑6th **S53.10** Unspecified subluxation and dislocation of ulnohumeral joint

☑7th **S53.101** Unspecified subluxation of right ulnohumeral joint

☑7th **S53.102** Unspecified subluxation of left ulnohumeral joint

☑7th **S53.103** Unspecified subluxation of unspecified ulnohumeral joint

☑7th **S53.104** Unspecified dislocation of right ulnohumeral joint

☑7th **S53.105** Unspecified dislocation of left ulnohumeral joint

☑7th **S53.106** Unspecified dislocation of unspecified ulnohumeral joint

☑6th **S53.11** Anterior subluxation and dislocation of ulnohumeral joint

☑7th **S53.111** Anterior subluxation of right ulnohumeral joint

☑7th **S53.112** Anterior subluxation of left ulnohumeral joint

☑7th **S53.113** Anterior subluxation of unspecified ulnohumeral joint

☑7th **S53.114** Anterior dislocation of right ulnohumeral joint
   AHA: 2012, 4Q, 108

☑7th **S53.115** Anterior dislocation of left ulnohumeral joint

☑7th **S53.116** Anterior dislocation of unspecified ulnohumeral joint

☑6th **S53.12** Posterior subluxation and dislocation of ulnohumeral joint

☑7th **S53.121** Posterior subluxation of right ulnohumeral joint

☑7th **S53.122** Posterior subluxation of left ulnohumeral joint

☑7th **S53.123** Posterior subluxation of unspecified ulnohumeral joint

☑7th **S53.124** Posterior dislocation of right ulnohumeral joint

☑7th **S53.125** Posterior dislocation of left ulnohumeral joint

☑7th **S53.126** Posterior dislocation of unspecified ulnohumeral joint

✓6ᵗʰ **S53.13** Medial **subluxation and dislocation of ulnohumeral joint**

    ✓7ᵗʰ **S53.131** **Medial** subluxation **of** right **ulnohumeral joint**

    ✓7ᵗʰ **S53.132** **Medial** subluxation **of** left **ulnohumeral joint**

    ✓7ᵗʰ **S53.133** **Medial** subluxation **of** unspecified **ulnohumeral joint**

    ✓7ᵗʰ **S53.134** **Medial** dislocation **of** right **ulnohumeral joint**

    ✓7ᵗʰ **S53.135** **Medial** dislocation **of** left **ulnohumeral joint**

    ✓7ᵗʰ **S53.136** **Medial** dislocation **of** unspecified **ulnohumeral joint**

✓6ᵗʰ **S53.14** Lateral **subluxation and dislocation of ulnohumeral joint**

    ✓7ᵗʰ **S53.141** **Lateral** subluxation **of** right **ulnohumeral joint**

    ✓7ᵗʰ **S53.142** **Lateral** subluxation **of** left **ulnohumeral joint**

    ✓7ᵗʰ **S53.143** **Lateral** subluxation **of** unspecified **ulnohumeral joint**

    ✓7ᵗʰ **S53.144** **Lateral** dislocation **of** right **ulnohumeral joint**

    ✓7ᵗʰ **S53.145** **Lateral** dislocation **of** left **ulnohumeral joint**

    ✓7ᵗʰ **S53.146** **Lateral** dislocation **of** unspecified **ulnohumeral joint**

✓6ᵗʰ **S53.19** Other **subluxation and dislocation of ulnohumeral joint**

    ✓7ᵗʰ **S53.191** **Other** subluxation **of** right **ulnohumeral joint**

    ✓7ᵗʰ **S53.192** **Other** subluxation **of** left **ulnohumeral joint**

    ✓7ᵗʰ **S53.193** **Other** subluxation **of** unspecified **ulnohumeral joint**

    ✓7ᵗʰ **S53.194** **Other** dislocation **of** right **ulnohumeral joint**

    ✓7ᵗʰ **S53.195** **Other** dislocation **of** left **ulnohumeral joint**

    ✓7ᵗʰ **S53.196** **Other** dislocation **of** unspecified **ulnohumeral joint**

✓5ᵗʰ **S53.2** **Traumatic rupture of** radial collateral ligament

    EXCLUDES 1   *sprain of radial collateral ligament NOS (S53.43-)*

    ✓x7ᵗʰ **S53.20** **Traumatic rupture of** unspecified **radial collateral ligament**

    ✓x7ᵗʰ **S53.21** **Traumatic rupture of** right **radial collateral ligament**

    ✓x7ᵗʰ **S53.22** **Traumatic rupture of** left **radial collateral ligament**

✓5ᵗʰ **S53.3** **Traumatic rupture of** ulnar collateral ligament

    EXCLUDES 1   *sprain of ulnar collateral ligament (S53.44-)*

    ✓x7ᵗʰ **S53.30** **Traumatic rupture of** unspecified **ulnar collateral ligament**

    ✓x7ᵗʰ **S53.31** **Traumatic rupture of** right **ulnar collateral ligament**

    ✓x7ᵗʰ **S53.32** **Traumatic rupture of** left **ulnar collateral ligament**

✓5ᵗʰ **S53.4** **Sprain of** elbow

    EXCLUDES 2   *traumatic rupture of radial collateral ligament (S53.2-)*
             traumatic rupture of ulnar collateral ligament (S53.3-)

    ✓6ᵗʰ **S53.40** Unspecified **sprain of elbow**

        ✓7ᵗʰ **S53.401** **Unspecified sprain of** right **elbow**

        ✓7ᵗʰ **S53.402** **Unspecified sprain of** left **elbow**

        ✓7ᵗʰ **S53.409** **Unspecified sprain of** unspecified **elbow**
                 Sprain of elbow NOS

    ✓6ᵗʰ **S53.41** Radiohumeral **(joint) sprain**

        ✓7ᵗʰ **S53.411** **Radiohumeral (joint) sprain of** right **elbow**

        ✓7ᵗʰ **S53.412** **Radiohumeral (joint) sprain of** left **elbow**

        ✓7ᵗʰ **S53.419** **Radiohumeral (joint) sprain of** unspecified **elbow**

    ✓6ᵗʰ **S53.42** Ulnohumeral **(joint) sprain**

        ✓7ᵗʰ **S53.421** **Ulnohumeral (joint) sprain of** right **elbow**

        ✓7ᵗʰ **S53.422** **Ulnohumeral (joint) sprain of** left **elbow**

        ✓7ᵗʰ **S53.429** **Ulnohumeral (joint) sprain of** unspecified **elbow**

✓6ᵗʰ **S53.43** Radial collateral ligament **sprain**

    ✓7ᵗʰ **S53.431** **Radial collateral ligament sprain of** right **elbow**

    ✓7ᵗʰ **S53.432** **Radial collateral ligament sprain of** left **elbow**

    ✓7ᵗʰ **S53.439** **Radial collateral ligament sprain of** unspecified **elbow**

✓6ᵗʰ **S53.44** Ulnar collateral ligament **sprain**

    ✓7ᵗʰ **S53.441** **Ulnar collateral ligament sprain of** right **elbow**

    ✓7ᵗʰ **S53.442** **Ulnar collateral ligament sprain of** left **elbow**

    ✓7ᵗʰ **S53.449** **Ulnar collateral ligament sprain of** unspecified **elbow**

✓6ᵗʰ **S53.49** Other **sprain of elbow**

    ✓7ᵗʰ **S53.491** **Other sprain of** right **elbow**

    ✓7ᵗʰ **S53.492** **Other sprain of** left **elbow**

    ✓7ᵗʰ **S53.499** **Other sprain of** unspecified **elbow**

✓4ᵗʰ **S54** **Injury of nerves at forearm level**

    Code also any associated open wound (S51.-)

    EXCLUDES 2   *injury of nerves at wrist and hand level (S64.-)*

> The appropriate 7th character is to be added to each code from category S54.
> A   initial encounter
> D   subsequent encounter
> S   sequela

✓5ᵗʰ **S54.0** **Injury of** ulnar **nerve at forearm level**
               Injury of ulnar nerve NOS

    ✓x7ᵗʰ **S54.00** **Injury of ulnar nerve at forearm level,** unspecified **arm**

    ✓x7ᵗʰ **S54.01** **Injury of ulnar nerve at forearm level,** right **arm**

    ✓x7ᵗʰ **S54.02** **Injury of ulnar nerve at forearm level,** left **arm**

✓5ᵗʰ **S54.1** **Injury of** median **nerve at forearm level**
               Injury of median nerve NOS

    ✓x7ᵗʰ **S54.10** **Injury of median nerve at forearm level,** unspecified **arm**

    ✓x7ᵗʰ **S54.11** **Injury of median nerve at forearm level,** right **arm**

    ✓x7ᵗʰ **S54.12** **Injury of median nerve at forearm level,** left **arm**

✓5ᵗʰ **S54.2** **Injury of** radial **nerve at forearm level**
               Injury of radial nerve NOS

    ✓x7ᵗʰ **S54.20** **Injury of radial nerve at forearm level,** unspecified **arm**

    ✓x7ᵗʰ **S54.21** **Injury of radial nerve at forearm level,** right **arm**

    ✓x7ᵗʰ **S54.22** **Injury of radial nerve at forearm level,** left **arm**

✓5ᵗʰ **S54.3** **Injury of** cutaneous sensory **nerve at forearm level**

    ✓x7ᵗʰ **S54.30** **Injury of cutaneous sensory nerve at forearm level,** unspecified **arm**

    ✓x7ᵗʰ **S54.31** **Injury of cutaneous sensory nerve at forearm level,** right **arm**

    ✓x7ᵗʰ **S54.32** **Injury of cutaneous sensory nerve at forearm level,** left **arm**

✓5ᵗʰ **S54.8** **Injury of** other **nerves at forearm level**

    ✓6ᵗʰ **S54.8X** **Injury of other nerves at forearm level**

        ✓7ᵗʰ **S54.8X1** **Injury of other nerves at forearm level,** right **arm**

        ✓7ᵗʰ **S54.8X2** **Injury of other nerves at forearm level,** left **arm**

        ✓7ᵗʰ **S54.8X9** **Injury of other nerves at forearm level,** unspecified **arm**

✓5ᵗʰ **S54.9** **Injury of** unspecified **nerve at forearm level**

    ✓x7ᵗʰ **S54.90** **Injury of unspecified nerve at forearm level,** unspecified **arm**

    ✓x7ᵗʰ **S54.91** **Injury of unspecified nerve at forearm level,** right **arm**

    ✓x7ᵗʰ **S54.92** **Injury of unspecified nerve at forearm level,** left **arm**

✓ Additional Character Required   ✓x7ᵗʰ Placeholder   Unacceptable PDx   Questionable PDx   Manifestation   **H1**-**H14** HAC   **HCC** CMS-HCC Dx   **HIV** HIV Dx

Chapter 19. Injury, Poisoning and Certain Other Consequences of External Causes

☑4ᵗʰ **S55   Injury of blood vessels at forearm level**

Code also any associated open wound (S51.-)

EXCLUDES 2   injury of blood vessels at wrist and hand level (S65.-)
            injury of brachial vessels (S45.1-S45.2)

> The appropriate 7th character is to be added to each code from category S55.
> A   initial encounter
> D   subsequent encounter
> S   sequela

☑5ᵗʰ **S55.0   Injury of ulnar artery at forearm level**

> **CC Excl: For CC codes in subcategory S55.0:**
> **Right side:** PDX collection 1274
> **Left side:** PDX collection 1275
> **Unspecified side:** PDX collection 1276

☑6ᵗʰ   **S55.00   Unspecified injury of ulnar artery at forearm level**

     ☑7ᵗʰ   **S55.001   Unspecified injury of ulnar artery at forearm level, right arm**   CC

     ☑7ᵗʰ   **S55.002   Unspecified injury of ulnar artery at forearm level, left arm**   CC

     ☑7ᵗʰ   **S55.009   Unspecified injury of ulnar artery at forearm level, unspecified arm**   CC

☑6ᵗʰ   **S55.01   Laceration of ulnar artery at forearm level**

     ☑7ᵗʰ   **S55.011   Laceration of ulnar artery at forearm level, right arm**   CC

     ☑7ᵗʰ   **S55.012   Laceration of ulnar artery at forearm level, left arm**   CC

     ☑7ᵗʰ   **S55.019   Laceration of ulnar artery at forearm level, unspecified arm**   CC

☑6ᵗʰ   **S55.09   Other specified injury of ulnar artery at forearm level**

     ☑7ᵗʰ   **S55.091   Other specified injury of ulnar artery at forearm level, right arm**   CC

     ☑7ᵗʰ   **S55.092   Other specified injury of ulnar artery at forearm level, left arm**   CC

     ☑7ᵗʰ   **S55.099   Other specified injury of ulnar artery at forearm level, unspecified arm**   CC

☑5ᵗʰ **S55.1   Injury of radial artery at forearm level**

> **CC Excl: For CC codes in subcategory S55.1:**
> **Right side:** PDX collection 1277
> **Left side:** PDX collection 1278
> **Unspecified side:** PDX collection 1279

☑6ᵗʰ   **S55.10   Unspecified injury of radial artery at forearm level**

     ☑7ᵗʰ   **S55.101   Unspecified injury of radial artery at forearm level, right arm**   CC

     ☑7ᵗʰ   **S55.102   Unspecified injury of radial artery at forearm level, left arm**   CC

     ☑7ᵗʰ   **S55.109   Unspecified injury of radial artery at forearm level, unspecified arm**   CC

☑6ᵗʰ   **S55.11   Laceration of radial artery at forearm level**

     ☑7ᵗʰ   **S55.111   Laceration of radial artery at forearm level, right arm**   CC

     ☑7ᵗʰ   **S55.112   Laceration of radial artery at forearm level, left arm**   CC

     ☑7ᵗʰ   **S55.119   Laceration of radial artery at forearm level, unspecified arm**   CC

☑6ᵗʰ   **S55.19   Other specified injury of radial artery at forearm level**

     ☑7ᵗʰ   **S55.191   Other specified injury of radial artery at forearm level, right arm**   CC

     ☑7ᵗʰ   **S55.192   Other specified injury of radial artery at forearm level, left arm**   CC

     ☑7ᵗʰ   **S55.199   Other specified injury of radial artery at forearm level, unspecified arm**   CC

☑5ᵗʰ **S55.2   Injury of vein at forearm level**

> **CC Excl: For CC codes in subcategory S55.2:**
> **Right side:** PDX collection 1260
> **Left side:** PDX collection 1261
> **Unspecified side:** PDX collection 1262

☑6ᵗʰ   **S55.20   Unspecified injury of vein at forearm level**

     ☑7ᵗʰ   **S55.201   Unspecified injury of vein at forearm level, right arm**   CC

     ☑7ᵗʰ   **S55.202   Unspecified injury of vein at forearm level, left arm**   CC

     ☑7ᵗʰ   **S55.209   Unspecified injury of vein at forearm level, unspecified arm**   CC

☑6ᵗʰ   **S55.21   Laceration of vein at forearm level**

     ☑7ᵗʰ   **S55.211   Laceration of vein at forearm level, right arm**   CC

     ☑7ᵗʰ   **S55.212   Laceration of vein at forearm level, left arm**   CC

     ☑7ᵗʰ   **S55.219   Laceration of vein at forearm level, unspecified arm**   CC

☑6ᵗʰ   **S55.29   Other specified injury of vein at forearm level**

     ☑7ᵗʰ   **S55.291   Other specified injury of vein at forearm level, right arm**   CC

     ☑7ᵗʰ   **S55.292   Other specified injury of vein at forearm level, left arm**   CC

     ☑7ᵗʰ   **S55.299   Other specified injury of vein at forearm level, unspecified arm**   CC

☑5ᵗʰ **S55.8   Injury of other blood vessels at forearm level**

> **CC Excl: For CC codes in subcategory S55.8:**
> **Right side:** PDX collection 1260
> **Left side:** PDX collection 1261
> **Unspecified side:** PDX collection 1262

☑6ᵗʰ   **S55.80   Unspecified injury of other blood vessels at forearm level**

     ☑7ᵗʰ   **S55.801   Unspecified injury of other blood vessels at forearm level, right arm**   CC

     ☑7ᵗʰ   **S55.802   Unspecified injury of other blood vessels at forearm level, left arm**   CC

     ☑7ᵗʰ   **S55.809   Unspecified injury of other blood vessels at forearm level, unspecified arm**   CC

☑6ᵗʰ   **S55.81   Laceration of other blood vessels at forearm level**

     ☑7ᵗʰ   **S55.811   Laceration of other blood vessels at forearm level, right arm**   CC

     ☑7ᵗʰ   **S55.812   Laceration of other blood vessels at forearm level, left arm**   CC

     ☑7ᵗʰ   **S55.819   Laceration of other blood vessels at forearm level, unspecified arm**   CC

☑6ᵗʰ   **S55.89   Other specified injury of other blood vessels at forearm level**

     ☑7ᵗʰ   **S55.891   Other specified injury of other blood vessels at forearm level, right arm**   CC

     ☑7ᵗʰ   **S55.892   Other specified injury of other blood vessels at forearm level, left arm**   CC

     ☑7ᵗʰ   **S55.899   Other specified injury of other blood vessels at forearm level, unspecified arm**   CC

☑5ᵗʰ **S55.9   Injury of unspecified blood vessel at forearm level**

> **CC Excl: For CC codes in subcategory S55.9:**
> **Right side:** PDX collection 1260
> **Left side:** PDX collection 1261
> **Unspecified side:** PDX collection 1262

☑6ᵗʰ   **S55.90   Unspecified injury of unspecified blood vessel at forearm level**

     ☑7ᵗʰ   **S55.901   Unspecified injury of unspecified blood vessel at forearm level, right arm**   CC

     ☑7ᵗʰ   **S55.902   Unspecified injury of unspecified blood vessel at forearm level, left arm**   CC

     ☑7ᵗʰ   **S55.909   Unspecified injury of unspecified blood vessel at forearm level, unspecified arm**   CC

☑6ᵗʰ   **S55.91   Laceration of unspecified blood vessel at forearm level**

     ☑7ᵗʰ   **S55.911   Laceration of unspecified blood vessel at forearm level, right arm**   CC

     ☑7ᵗʰ   **S55.912   Laceration of unspecified blood vessel at forearm level, left arm**   CC

     ☑7ᵗʰ   **S55.919   Laceration of unspecified blood vessel at forearm level, unspecified arm**   CC

☑6ᵗʰ   **S55.99   Other specified injury of unspecified blood vessel at forearm level**

     ☑7ᵗʰ   **S55.991   Other specified injury of unspecified blood vessel at forearm level, right arm**   CC

     ☑7ᵗʰ   **S55.992   Other specified injury of unspecified blood vessel at forearm level, left arm**   CC

N Newborn: 0   P Pediatric: 0-17   M Maternity: 12-55   A Adult: 15-124   MCC Major Complication/Comorbidity   CC Complication/Comorbidity   SW Severe Wound Dx

1010   ICD-10-CM 2019

√7ᵗʰ **S55.999** **Other specified injury of unspecified blood vessel at forearm level, unspecified arm** `CC`

√4ᵗʰ **S56** **Injury of muscle, fascia and tendon at forearm level**
Code also any associated open wound (S51.-)
EXCLUDES 2 *injury of muscle, fascia and tendon at or below wrist (S66.-)*
sprain of joints and ligaments of elbow (S53.4-)
TIP: Refer to the Muscle/Tendon table at the beginning of this chapter.

The appropriate 7th character is to be added to each code from category S56.
A   initial encounter
D   subsequent encounter
S   sequela

CC Excl: For CC codes in category S56:
Right side: PDX collection 1280
Left side: PDX collection 1281
Unspecified side: PDX collection 1282

√5ᵗʰ **S56.0** **Injury of flexor muscle, fascia and tendon of thumb at forearm level**

  √6ᵗʰ **S56.00** **Unspecified injury of flexor muscle, fascia and tendon of thumb at forearm level**

    √7ᵗʰ **S56.001** **Unspecified injury of flexor muscle, fascia and tendon of right thumb at forearm level**

    √7ᵗʰ **S56.002** **Unspecified injury of flexor muscle, fascia and tendon of left thumb at forearm level**

    √7ᵗʰ **S56.009** **Unspecified injury of flexor muscle, fascia and tendon of unspecified thumb at forearm level**

  √6ᵗʰ **S56.01** **Strain of flexor muscle, fascia and tendon of thumb at forearm level**

    √7ᵗʰ **S56.011** **Strain of flexor muscle, fascia and tendon of right thumb at forearm level**

    √7ᵗʰ **S56.012** **Strain of flexor muscle, fascia and tendon of left thumb at forearm level**

    √7ᵗʰ **S56.019** **Strain of flexor muscle, fascia and tendon of unspecified thumb at forearm level**

  √6ᵗʰ **S56.02** **Laceration of flexor muscle, fascia and tendon of thumb at forearm level**

    √7ᵗʰ **S56.021** **Laceration of flexor muscle, fascia and tendon of right thumb at forearm level** `CC`

    √7ᵗʰ **S56.022** **Laceration of flexor muscle, fascia and tendon of left thumb at forearm level** `CC`

    √7ᵗʰ **S56.029** **Laceration of flexor muscle, fascia and tendon of unspecified thumb at forearm level** `CC`

  √6ᵗʰ **S56.09** **Other injury of flexor muscle, fascia and tendon of thumb at forearm level**

    √7ᵗʰ **S56.091** **Other injury of flexor muscle, fascia and tendon of right thumb at forearm level**

    √7ᵗʰ **S56.092** **Other injury of flexor muscle, fascia and tendon of left thumb at forearm level**

    √7ᵗʰ **S56.099** **Other injury of flexor muscle, fascia and tendon of unspecified thumb at forearm level**

√5ᵗʰ **S56.1** **Injury of flexor muscle, fascia and tendon of other and unspecified finger at forearm level**

  √6ᵗʰ **S56.10** **Unspecified injury of flexor muscle, fascia and tendon of other and unspecified finger at forearm level**

    √7ᵗʰ **S56.101** **Unspecified injury of flexor muscle, fascia and tendon of right index finger at forearm level**

    √7ᵗʰ **S56.102** **Unspecified injury of flexor muscle, fascia and tendon of left index finger at forearm level**

    √7ᵗʰ **S56.103** **Unspecified injury of flexor muscle, fascia and tendon of right middle finger at forearm level**

    √7ᵗʰ **S56.104** **Unspecified injury of flexor muscle, fascia and tendon of left middle finger at forearm level**

    √7ᵗʰ **S56.105** **Unspecified injury of flexor muscle, fascia and tendon of right ring finger at forearm level**

    √7ᵗʰ **S56.106** **Unspecified injury of flexor muscle, fascia and tendon of left ring finger at forearm level**

    √7ᵗʰ **S56.107** **Unspecified injury of flexor muscle, fascia and tendon of right little finger at forearm level**

    √7ᵗʰ **S56.108** **Unspecified injury of flexor muscle, fascia and tendon of left little finger at forearm level**

    √7ᵗʰ **S56.109** **Unspecified injury of flexor muscle, fascia and tendon of unspecified finger at forearm level**

  √6ᵗʰ **S56.11** **Strain of flexor muscle, fascia and tendon of other and unspecified finger at forearm level**

    √7ᵗʰ **S56.111** **Strain of flexor muscle, fascia and tendon of right index finger at forearm level**

    √7ᵗʰ **S56.112** **Strain of flexor muscle, fascia and tendon of left index finger at forearm level**

    √7ᵗʰ **S56.113** **Strain of flexor muscle, fascia and tendon of right middle finger at forearm level**

    √7ᵗʰ **S56.114** **Strain of flexor muscle, fascia and tendon of left middle finger at forearm level**

    √7ᵗʰ **S56.115** **Strain of flexor muscle, fascia and tendon of right ring finger at forearm level**

    √7ᵗʰ **S56.116** **Strain of flexor muscle, fascia and tendon of left ring finger at forearm level**

    √7ᵗʰ **S56.117** **Strain of flexor muscle, fascia and tendon of right little finger at forearm level**

    √7ᵗʰ **S56.118** **Strain of flexor muscle, fascia and tendon of left little finger at forearm level**

    √7ᵗʰ **S56.119** **Strain of flexor muscle, fascia and tendon of finger of unspecified finger at forearm level**

  √6ᵗʰ **S56.12** **Laceration of flexor muscle, fascia and tendon of other and unspecified finger at forearm level**

    √7ᵗʰ **S56.121** **Laceration of flexor muscle, fascia and tendon of right index finger at forearm level** `CC`

    √7ᵗʰ **S56.122** **Laceration of flexor muscle, fascia and tendon of left index finger at forearm level** `CC`

    √7ᵗʰ **S56.123** **Laceration of flexor muscle, fascia and tendon of right middle finger at forearm level** `CC`

    √7ᵗʰ **S56.124** **Laceration of flexor muscle, fascia and tendon of left middle finger at forearm level** `CC`

    √7ᵗʰ **S56.125** **Laceration of flexor muscle, fascia and tendon of right ring finger at forearm level** `CC`

    √7ᵗʰ **S56.126** **Laceration of flexor muscle, fascia and tendon of left ring finger at forearm level** `CC`

    √7ᵗʰ **S56.127** **Laceration of flexor muscle, fascia and tendon of right little finger at forearm level** `CC`

    √7ᵗʰ **S56.128** **Laceration of flexor muscle, fascia and tendon of left little finger at forearm level** `CC`

    √7ᵗʰ **S56.129** **Laceration of flexor muscle, fascia and tendon of unspecified finger at forearm level** `CC`

  √6ᵗʰ **S56.19** **Other injury of flexor muscle, fascia and tendon of other and unspecified finger at forearm level**

    √7ᵗʰ **S56.191** **Other injury of flexor muscle, fascia and tendon of right index finger at forearm level**

    √7ᵗʰ **S56.192** **Other injury of flexor muscle, fascia and tendon of left index finger at forearm level**

    √7ᵗʰ **S56.193** **Other injury of flexor muscle, fascia and tendon of right middle finger at forearm level**

    √7ᵗʰ **S56.194** **Other injury of flexor muscle, fascia and tendon of left middle finger at forearm level**

    √7ᵗʰ **S56.195** **Other injury of flexor muscle, fascia and tendon of right ring finger at forearm level**

✔ Additional Character Required   √x7ᵗʰ Placeholder   Unacceptable PDx   Questionable PDx   Manifestation   H1 - H14 HAC   HCC CMS-HCC Dx   HIV HIV Dx

ICD-10-CM 2019   1011

✓7ᵗʰ **S56.196**   Other injury of flexor muscle, fascia and tendon of left ring finger at forearm level

✓7ᵗʰ **S56.197**   Other injury of flexor muscle, fascia and tendon of right little finger at forearm level

✓7ᵗʰ **S56.198**   Other injury of flexor muscle, fascia and tendon of left little finger at forearm level

✓7ᵗʰ **S56.199**   Other injury of flexor muscle, fascia and tendon of unspecified finger at forearm level

✓5ᵗʰ **S56.2**   Injury of other flexor muscle, fascia and tendon at forearm level

✓6ᵗʰ **S56.20**   Unspecified injury of other flexor muscle, fascia and tendon at forearm level

✓7ᵗʰ **S56.201**   Unspecified injury of other flexor muscle, fascia and tendon at forearm level, right arm

✓7ᵗʰ **S56.202**   Unspecified injury of other flexor muscle, fascia and tendon at forearm level, left arm

✓7ᵗʰ **S56.209**   Unspecified injury of other flexor muscle, fascia and tendon at forearm level, unspecified arm

✓6ᵗʰ **S56.21**   Strain of other flexor muscle, fascia and tendon at forearm level

✓7ᵗʰ **S56.211**   Strain of other flexor muscle, fascia and tendon at forearm level, right arm

✓7ᵗʰ **S56.212**   Strain of other flexor muscle, fascia and tendon at forearm level, left arm

✓7ᵗʰ **S56.219**   Strain of other flexor muscle, fascia and tendon at forearm level, unspecified arm

✓6ᵗʰ **S56.22**   Laceration of other flexor muscle, fascia and tendon at forearm level

✓7ᵗʰ **S56.221**   Laceration of other flexor muscle, fascia and tendon at forearm level, right arm   **CC**

✓7ᵗʰ **S56.222**   Laceration of other flexor muscle, fascia and tendon at forearm level, left arm   **CC**

✓7ᵗʰ **S56.229**   Laceration of other flexor muscle, fascia and tendon at forearm level, unspecified arm   **CC**

✓6ᵗʰ **S56.29**   Other injury of other flexor muscle, fascia and tendon at forearm level

✓7ᵗʰ **S56.291**   Other injury of other flexor muscle, fascia and tendon at forearm level, right arm

✓7ᵗʰ **S56.292**   Other injury of other flexor muscle, fascia and tendon at forearm level, left arm

✓7ᵗʰ **S56.299**   Other injury of other flexor muscle, fascia and tendon at forearm level, unspecified arm

✓5ᵗʰ **S56.3**   Injury of extensor or abductor muscles, fascia and tendons of thumb at forearm level

✓6ᵗʰ **S56.30**   Unspecified injury of extensor or abductor muscles, fascia and tendons of thumb at forearm level

✓7ᵗʰ **S56.301**   Unspecified injury of extensor or abductor muscles, fascia and tendons of right thumb at forearm level

✓7ᵗʰ **S56.302**   Unspecified injury of extensor or abductor muscles, fascia and tendons of left thumb at forearm level

✓7ᵗʰ **S56.309**   Unspecified injury of extensor or abductor muscles, fascia and tendons of unspecified thumb at forearm level

✓6ᵗʰ **S56.31**   Strain of extensor or abductor muscles, fascia and tendons of thumb at forearm level

✓7ᵗʰ **S56.311**   Strain of extensor or abductor muscles, fascia and tendons of right thumb at forearm level

✓7ᵗʰ **S56.312**   Strain of extensor or abductor muscles, fascia and tendons of left thumb at forearm level

✓7ᵗʰ **S56.319**   Strain of extensor or abductor muscles, fascia and tendons of unspecified thumb at forearm level

✓6ᵗʰ **S56.32**   Laceration of extensor or abductor muscles, fascia and tendons of thumb at forearm level

✓7ᵗʰ **S56.321**   Laceration of extensor or abductor muscles, fascia and tendons of right thumb at forearm level   **CC**

✓7ᵗʰ **S56.322**   Laceration of extensor or abductor muscles, fascia and tendons of left thumb at forearm level   **CC**

✓7ᵗʰ **S56.329**   Laceration of extensor or abductor muscles, fascia and tendons of unspecified thumb at forearm level   **CC**

✓6ᵗʰ **S56.39**   Other injury of extensor or abductor muscles, fascia and tendons of thumb at forearm level

✓7ᵗʰ **S56.391**   Other injury of extensor or abductor muscles, fascia and tendons of right thumb at forearm level

✓7ᵗʰ **S56.392**   Other injury of extensor or abductor muscles, fascia and tendons of left thumb at forearm level

✓7ᵗʰ **S56.399**   Other injury of extensor or abductor muscles, fascia and tendons of unspecified thumb at forearm level

✓5ᵗʰ **S56.4**   Injury of extensor muscle, fascia and tendon of other and unspecified finger at forearm level

✓6ᵗʰ **S56.40**   Unspecified injury of extensor muscle, fascia and tendon of other and unspecified finger at forearm level

✓7ᵗʰ **S56.401**   Unspecified injury of extensor muscle, fascia and tendon of right index finger at forearm level

✓7ᵗʰ **S56.402**   Unspecified injury of extensor muscle, fascia and tendon of left index finger at forearm level

✓7ᵗʰ **S56.403**   Unspecified injury of extensor muscle, fascia and tendon of right middle finger at forearm level

✓7ᵗʰ **S56.404**   Unspecified injury of extensor muscle, fascia and tendon of left middle finger at forearm level

✓7ᵗʰ **S56.405**   Unspecified injury of extensor muscle, fascia and tendon of right ring finger at forearm level

✓7ᵗʰ **S56.406**   Unspecified injury of extensor muscle, fascia and tendon of left ring finger at forearm level

✓7ᵗʰ **S56.407**   Unspecified injury of extensor muscle, fascia and tendon of right little finger at forearm level

✓7ᵗʰ **S56.408**   Unspecified injury of extensor muscle, fascia and tendon of left little finger at forearm level

✓7ᵗʰ **S56.409**   Unspecified injury of extensor muscle, fascia and tendon of unspecified finger at forearm level

✓6ᵗʰ **S56.41**   Strain of extensor muscle, fascia and tendon of other and unspecified finger at forearm level

✓7ᵗʰ **S56.411**   Strain of extensor muscle, fascia and tendon of right index finger at forearm level

✓7ᵗʰ **S56.412**   Strain of extensor muscle, fascia and tendon of left index finger at forearm level

✓7ᵗʰ **S56.413**   Strain of extensor muscle, fascia and tendon of right middle finger at forearm level

✓7ᵗʰ **S56.414**   Strain of extensor muscle, fascia and tendon of left middle finger at forearm level

✓7ᵗʰ **S56.415**   Strain of extensor muscle, fascia and tendon of right ring finger at forearm level

✓7ᵗʰ **S56.416**   Strain of extensor muscle, fascia and tendon of left ring finger at forearm level

✓7ᵗʰ **S56.417**   Strain of extensor muscle, fascia and tendon of right little finger at forearm level

✓7ᵗʰ **S56.418**   Strain of extensor muscle, fascia and tendon of left little finger at forearm level

N Newborn: 0   **P** Pediatric: 0-17   **M** Maternity: 12-55   **A** Adult: 15-124   **MCC** Major Complication/Comorbidity   **CC** Complication/Comorbidity   **SW** Severe Wound Dx

1012   ICD-10-CM 2019

✓7th **S56.419** **Strain of extensor muscle, fascia and tendon of finger,** unspecified finger **at forearm level**

✓6th **S56.42** Laceration **of extensor muscle, fascia and tendon of other and unspecified** finger **at forearm level**

    ✓7th **S56.421** **Laceration of extensor muscle, fascia and tendon of** right index finger **at forearm level** `CC`

    ✓7th **S56.422** **Laceration of extensor muscle, fascia and tendon of** left index finger **at forearm level** `CC`

    ✓7th **S56.423** **Laceration of extensor muscle, fascia and tendon of** right middle finger **at forearm level** `CC`

    ✓7th **S56.424** **Laceration of extensor muscle, fascia and tendon of** left middle finger **at forearm level** `CC`

    ✓7th **S56.425** **Laceration of extensor muscle, fascia and tendon of** right ring finger **at forearm level** `CC`

    ✓7th **S56.426** **Laceration of extensor muscle, fascia and tendon of** left ring finger **at forearm level** `CC`

    ✓7th **S56.427** **Laceration of extensor muscle, fascia and tendon of** right little finger **at forearm level** `CC`

    ✓7th **S56.428** **Laceration of extensor muscle, fascia and tendon of** left little finger **at forearm level** `CC`

    ✓7th **S56.429** **Laceration of extensor muscle, fascia and tendon of** unspecified finger **at forearm level** `CC`

✓6th **S56.49** Other **injury of extensor muscle, fascia and tendon of other and unspecified** finger **at forearm level**

    ✓7th **S56.491** **Other injury of extensor muscle, fascia and tendon of** right index finger **at forearm level**

    ✓7th **S56.492** **Other injury of extensor muscle, fascia and tendon of** left index finger **at forearm level**

    ✓7th **S56.493** **Other injury of extensor muscle, fascia and tendon of** right middle finger **at forearm level**

    ✓7th **S56.494** **Other injury of extensor muscle, fascia and tendon of** left middle finger **at forearm level**

    ✓7th **S56.495** **Other injury of extensor muscle, fascia and tendon of** right ring finger **at forearm level**

    ✓7th **S56.496** **Other injury of extensor muscle, fascia and tendon of** left ring finger **at forearm level**

    ✓7th **S56.497** **Other injury of extensor muscle, fascia and tendon of** right little finger **at forearm level**

    ✓7th **S56.498** **Other injury of extensor muscle, fascia and tendon of** left little finger **at forearm level**

    ✓7th **S56.499** **Other injury of extensor muscle, fascia and tendon of** unspecified finger **at forearm level**

✓5th **S56.5** **Injury of** other extensor **muscle, fascia and tendon at** forearm **level**

✓6th **S56.50** Unspecified **injury of other extensor muscle, fascia and tendon at forearm level**

    ✓7th **S56.501** **Unspecified injury of other extensor muscle, fascia and tendon at forearm level,** right arm

    ✓7th **S56.502** **Unspecified injury of other extensor muscle, fascia and tendon at forearm level,** left arm

    ✓7th **S56.509** **Unspecified injury of other extensor muscle, fascia and tendon at forearm level,** unspecified arm

✓6th **S56.51** Strain **of other extensor muscle, fascia and tendon at forearm level**

    ✓7th **S56.511** **Strain of other extensor muscle, fascia and tendon at forearm level,** right arm

    ✓7th **S56.512** **Strain of other extensor muscle, fascia and tendon at forearm level,** left arm

✓7th **S56.519** **Strain of other extensor muscle, fascia and tendon at forearm level,** unspecified arm

✓6th **S56.52** Laceration **of other extensor muscle, fascia and tendon at forearm level**

    ✓7th **S56.521** **Laceration of other extensor muscle, fascia and tendon at forearm level,** right arm `CC`

    ✓7th **S56.522** **Laceration of other extensor muscle, fascia and tendon at forearm level,** left arm `CC`

    ✓7th **S56.529** **Laceration of other extensor muscle, fascia and tendon at forearm level,** unspecified arm `CC`

✓6th **S56.59** Other **injury of other extensor muscle, fascia and tendon at forearm level**

    ✓7th **S56.591** **Other injury of other extensor muscle, fascia and tendon at forearm level,** right arm

    ✓7th **S56.592** **Other injury of other extensor muscle, fascia and tendon at forearm level,** left arm

    ✓7th **S56.599** **Other injury of other extensor muscle, fascia and tendon at forearm level,** unspecified arm

✓5th **S56.8** **Injury of** other muscles, fascia and tendons at forearm level

✓6th **S56.80** Unspecified **injury of other muscles, fascia and tendons at forearm level**

    ✓7th **S56.801** **Unspecified injury of other muscles, fascia and tendons at forearm level,** right arm

    ✓7th **S56.802** **Unspecified injury of other muscles, fascia and tendons at forearm level,** left arm

    ✓7th **S56.809** **Unspecified injury of other muscles, fascia and tendons at forearm level,** unspecified arm

✓6th **S56.81** Strain **of other muscles, fascia and tendons at forearm level**

    ✓7th **S56.811** **Strain of other muscles, fascia and tendons at forearm level,** right arm

    ✓7th **S56.812** **Strain of other muscles, fascia and tendons at forearm level,** left arm

    ✓7th **S56.819** **Strain of other muscles, fascia and tendons at forearm level,** unspecified arm

✓6th **S56.82** Laceration **of other muscles, fascia and tendons at forearm level**

    ✓7th **S56.821** **Laceration of other muscles, fascia and tendons at forearm level,** right arm `CC`

    ✓7th **S56.822** **Laceration of other muscles, fascia and tendons at forearm level,** left arm `CC`

    ✓7th **S56.829** **Laceration of other muscles, fascia and tendons at forearm level,** unspecified arm `CC`

✓6th **S56.89** Other **injury of other muscles, fascia and tendons at forearm level**

    ✓7th **S56.891** **Other injury of other muscles, fascia and tendons at forearm level,** right arm

    ✓7th **S56.892** **Other injury of other muscles, fascia and tendons at forearm level,** left arm

    ✓7th **S56.899** **Other injury of other muscles, fascia and tendons at forearm level,** unspecified arm

✓5th **S56.9** **Injury of** unspecified muscles, fascia and tendons at forearm **level**

✓6th **S56.90** Unspecified **injury of unspecified muscles, fascia and tendons at forearm level**

    ✓7th **S56.901** **Unspecified injury of unspecified muscles, fascia and tendons at forearm level,** right arm

    ✓7th **S56.902** **Unspecified injury of unspecified muscles, fascia and tendons at forearm level,** left arm

    ✓7th **S56.909** **Unspecified injury of unspecified muscles, fascia and tendons at forearm level,** unspecified arm

✓6th **S56.91** Strain **of unspecified muscles, fascia and tendons at forearm level**

    ✓7th **S56.911** **Strain of unspecified muscles, fascia and tendons at forearm level,** right arm

---

✓ Additional Character Required   ✓x7th Placeholder   Unacceptable PDx   Questionable PDx   Manifestation   `H1`-`H14` HAC   `HCC` CMS-HCC Dx   `HIV` HIV Dx

ICD-10-CM 2019   1013

√7ᵗʰ **S56.912** **Strain of unspecified muscles, fascia and tendons at forearm level,** left arm

√7ᵗʰ **S56.919** **Strain of unspecified muscles, fascia and tendons at forearm level,** unspecified arm

√6ᵗʰ **S56.92** **Laceration** of unspecified muscles, fascia and tendons at forearm level

√7ᵗʰ **S56.921** **Laceration of unspecified muscles, fascia and tendons at forearm level,** right arm   CC

√7ᵗʰ **S56.922** **Laceration of unspecified muscles, fascia and tendons at forearm level,** left arm   CC

√7ᵗʰ **S56.929** **Laceration of unspecified muscles, fascia and tendons at forearm level,** unspecified arm   CC

√6ᵗʰ **S56.99** **Other** injury of unspecified muscles, fascia and tendons at forearm level

√7ᵗʰ **S56.991** **Other injury of unspecified muscles, fascia and tendons at forearm level,** right arm

√7ᵗʰ **S56.992** **Other injury of unspecified muscles, fascia and tendons at forearm level,** left arm

√7ᵗʰ **S56.999** **Other injury of unspecified muscles, fascia and tendons at forearm level,** unspecified arm

√4ᵗʰ **S57** **Crushing injury of elbow and forearm**
Use additional code(s) for all associated injuries
EXCLUDES 2   *crushing injury of wrist and hand (S67.-)*

The appropriate 7th character is to be added to each code from category S57.
A   initial encounter
D   subsequent encounter
S   sequela

√5ᵗʰ **S57.Ø** **Crushing injury of** elbow

√x7ᵗʰ **S57.ØØ** **Crushing injury of** unspecified **elbow**

√x7ᵗʰ **S57.Ø1** **Crushing injury of** right **elbow**

√x7ᵗʰ **S57.Ø2** **Crushing injury of** left **elbow**

√5ᵗʰ **S57.8** **Crushing injury of** forearm

√x7ᵗʰ **S57.8Ø** **Crushing injury of** unspecified **forearm**

√x7ᵗʰ **S57.81** **Crushing injury of** right **forearm**

√x7ᵗʰ **S57.82** **Crushing injury of** left **forearm**

√4ᵗʰ **S58** **Traumatic amputation of elbow and forearm**
An amputation not identified as partial or complete should be coded to complete.
EXCLUDES 1   *traumatic amputation of wrist and hand (S68.-)*

The appropriate 7th character is to be added to each code from category S58.
A   initial encounter
D   subsequent encounter
S   sequela

CC Excl: For CC codes in category S58:
Right side: PDX collection 1266
Left side: PDX collection 1267
Unspecified side: PDX collection 1268

√5ᵗʰ **S58.Ø** **Traumatic amputation at** elbow **level**

√6ᵗʰ **S58.Ø1** **Complete** traumatic amputation at elbow level

7 √7ᵗʰ **S58.Ø11** **Complete traumatic amputation at elbow level,** right **arm**   CC HCC

7 √7ᵗʰ **S58.Ø12** **Complete traumatic amputation at elbow level,** left **arm**   CC HCC

7 √7ᵗʰ **S58.Ø19** **Complete traumatic amputation at elbow level,** unspecified **arm**   CC HCC

√6ᵗʰ **S58.Ø2** **Partial** traumatic amputation at elbow level

7 √7ᵗʰ **S58.Ø21** **Partial traumatic amputation at elbow level,** right **arm**   CC HCC

7 √7ᵗʰ **S58.Ø22** **Partial traumatic amputation at elbow level,** left **arm**   CC HCC

7 √7ᵗʰ **S58.Ø29** **Partial traumatic amputation at elbow level,** unspecified **arm**   CC HCC

√5ᵗʰ **S58.1** **Traumatic amputation at level** between elbow and wrist

√6ᵗʰ **S58.11** **Complete** traumatic amputation at level between elbow and wrist

7 √7ᵗʰ **S58.111** **Complete traumatic amputation at level between elbow and wrist,** right **arm**   CC HCC

7 √7ᵗʰ **S58.112** **Complete traumatic amputation at level between elbow and wrist,** left **arm**   CC HCC

7 √7ᵗʰ **S58.119** **Complete traumatic amputation at level between elbow and wrist,** unspecified **arm**   CC HCC

√6ᵗʰ **S58.12** **Partial** traumatic amputation at level between elbow and wrist

7 √7ᵗʰ **S58.121** **Partial traumatic amputation at level between elbow and wrist,** right **arm**   CC HCC

7 √7ᵗʰ **S58.122** **Partial traumatic amputation at level between elbow and wrist,** left **arm**   CC HCC

7 √7ᵗʰ **S58.129** **Partial traumatic amputation at level between elbow and wrist,** unspecified **arm**   CC HCC

√5ᵗʰ **S58.9** **Traumatic amputation of** forearm, level unspecified
EXCLUDES 1   *traumatic amputation of wrist (S68.-)*

√6ᵗʰ **S58.91** **Complete** traumatic amputation of forearm, level unspecified

7 √7ᵗʰ **S58.911** **Complete traumatic amputation of** right **forearm, level unspecified**   CC HCC

7 √7ᵗʰ **S58.912** **Complete traumatic amputation of** left **forearm, level unspecified**   CC HCC

7 √7ᵗʰ **S58.919** **Complete traumatic amputation of** unspecified **forearm, level unspecified**   CC HCC

√6ᵗʰ **S58.92** **Partial** traumatic amputation of forearm, level unspecified

7 √7ᵗʰ **S58.921** **Partial traumatic amputation of** right **forearm, level unspecified**   CC HCC

7 √7ᵗʰ **S58.922** **Partial traumatic amputation of** left **forearm, level unspecified**   CC HCC

7 √7ᵗʰ **S58.929** **Partial traumatic amputation of** unspecified **forearm, level unspecified**   CC HCC

√4ᵗʰ **S59** **Other and unspecified injuries of elbow and forearm**
EXCLUDES 2   *other and unspecified injuries of wrist and hand (S69.-)*
AHA: 2018, 2Q, 12; 2018, 1Q, 3; 2015, 3Q, 37-39

The appropriate 7th character is to be added to each code from subcategories S59.Ø, S59.1, and S59.2.
A   initial encounter for closed fracture
D   subsequent encounter for fracture with routine healing
G   subsequent encounter for fracture with delayed healing
K   subsequent encounter for fracture with nonunion
P   subsequent encounter for fracture with malunion
S   sequela

√5ᵗʰ **S59.Ø** **Physeal fracture of** lower end of ulna

CC Excl: For CC codes in subcategory S59.Ø:
Right side: See code S59.ØØ1
Left side: See code S59.ØØ2
Unspecified side: See code S59.ØØ9

√6ᵗʰ **S59.ØØ** **Unspecified** physeal fracture of lower end of ulna

3 √7ᵗʰ **S59.ØØ1** **Unspecified physeal fracture of lower end of ulna,** right **arm**   CC H5
CC Excl: CC with 7th character A: PDX collection 1270
CC with 7th character K or P: PDX collection 897

3 √7ᵗʰ **S59.ØØ2** **Unspecified physeal fracture of lower end of ulna,** left **arm**   CC H5
CC Excl: CC with 7th character A: PDX collection 1271
CC with 7th character K or P: PDX collection 897

3 √7ᵗʰ **S59.ØØ9** **Unspecified physeal fracture of lower end of ulna,** unspecified **arm**   CC H5
CC Excl: CC with 7th character A: PDX collection 1272
CC with 7th character K or P: PDX collection 897

√6ᵗʰ **S59.Ø1** **Salter-Harris Type I** physeal fracture of lower end of ulna

3 √7ᵗʰ **S59.Ø11** **Salter-Harris Type I physeal fracture of lower end of ulna,** right **arm**   CC H5

N Newborn: 0   P Pediatric: 0-17   M Maternity: 12-55   A Adult: 15-124   MCC Major Complication/Comorbidity   CC Complication/Comorbidity   SW Severe Wound Dx

1014   ICD-10-CM 2019

3 √7th **S59.012** Salter-Harris Type I physeal fracture `CC` `H5`
of lower end of ulna, left arm

3 √7th **S59.019** Salter-Harris Type I physeal fracture `CC` `H5`
of lower end of ulna, unspecified arm

√6th **S59.02** Salter-Harris Type II physeal fracture of lower end of
ulna

3 √7th **S59.021** Salter-Harris Type II physeal `CC` `H5`
fracture of lower end of ulna, right arm

3 √7th **S59.022** Salter-Harris Type II physeal `CC` `H5`
fracture of lower end of ulna, left arm

3 √7th **S59.029** Salter-Harris Type II physeal `CC` `H5`
fracture of lower end of ulna,
unspecified arm

√6th **S59.03** Salter-Harris Type III physeal fracture of lower end of
ulna

3 √7th **S59.031** Salter-Harris Type III physeal `CC` `H5`
fracture of lower end of ulna, right arm

3 √7th **S59.032** Salter-Harris Type III physeal `CC` `H5`
fracture of lower end of ulna, left arm

3 √7th **S59.039** Salter-Harris Type III physeal `CC` `H5`
fracture of lower end of ulna,
unspecified arm

√6th **S59.04** Salter-Harris Type IV physeal fracture of lower end of
ulna

3 √7th **S59.041** Salter-Harris Type IV physeal `CC` `H5`
fracture of lower end of ulna, right arm

3 √7th **S59.042** Salter-Harris Type IV physeal `CC` `H5`
fracture of lower end of ulna, left arm

3 √7th **S59.049** Salter-Harris Type IV physeal `CC` `H5`
fracture of lower end of ulna,
unspecified arm

√6th **S59.09** Other physeal fracture of lower end of ulna

3 √7th **S59.091** Other physeal fracture of lower end `CC` `H5`
of ulna, right arm

3 √7th **S59.092** Other physeal fracture of lower end `CC` `H5`
of ulna, left arm

3 √7th **S59.099** Other physeal fracture of lower end `CC` `H5`
of ulna, unspecified arm

√5th **S59.1** Physeal fracture of upper end of radius

> **CC Excl: For codes in subcategory S59.1:**
> **CC with 7th character K or P:** PDX collection 897

√6th **S59.10** Unspecified physeal fracture of upper end of radius

4 √7th **S59.101** Unspecified physeal fracture of upper `CC`
end of radius, right arm

4 √7th **S59.102** Unspecified physeal fracture of upper `CC`
end of radius, left arm

4 √7th **S59.109** Unspecified physeal fracture of upper `CC`
end of radius, unspecified arm

√6th **S59.11** Salter-Harris Type I physeal fracture of upper end of
radius

4 √7th **S59.111** Salter-Harris Type I physeal fracture `CC`
of upper end of radius, right arm

4 √7th **S59.112** Salter-Harris Type I physeal fracture `CC`
of upper end of radius, left arm

4 √7th **S59.119** Salter-Harris Type I physeal fracture `CC`
of upper end of radius, unspecified arm

√6th **S59.12** Salter-Harris Type II physeal fracture of upper end of
radius

4 √7th **S59.121** Salter-Harris Type II physeal fracture `CC`
of upper end of radius, right arm

4 √7th **S59.122** Salter-Harris Type II physeal fracture `CC`
of upper end of radius, left arm

4 √7th **S59.129** Salter-Harris Type II physeal fracture `CC`
of upper end of radius, unspecified arm

√6th **S59.13** Salter-Harris Type III physeal fracture of upper end
of radius

4 √7th **S59.131** Salter-Harris Type III physeal fracture `CC`
of upper end of radius, right arm

4 √7th **S59.132** Salter-Harris Type III physeal fracture `CC`
of upper end of radius, left arm

4 √7th **S59.139** Salter-Harris Type III physeal fracture `CC`
of upper end of radius, unspecified arm

√6th **S59.14** Salter-Harris Type IV physeal fracture of upper end
of radius

4 √7th **S59.141** Salter-Harris Type IV physeal fracture `CC`
of upper end of radius, right arm

4 √7th **S59.142** Salter-Harris Type IV physeal fracture `CC`
of upper end of radius, left arm

4 √7th **S59.149** Salter-Harris Type IV physeal fracture `CC`
of upper end of radius, unspecified arm

√6th **S59.19** Other physeal fracture of upper end of radius

4 √7th **S59.191** Other physeal fracture of upper end `CC`
of radius, right arm

4 √7th **S59.192** Other physeal fracture of upper end `CC`
of radius, left arm

4 √7th **S59.199** Other physeal fracture of upper end `CC`
of radius, unspecified arm

√5th **S59.2** Physeal fracture of lower end of radius

> **CC Excl: For CC codes in subcategory S59.2:**
> **Right side:** See code S59.201
> **Left side:** See code S59.202
> **Unspecified side:** See code S59.209

√6th **S59.20** Unspecified physeal fracture of lower end of radius

3 √7th **S59.201** Unspecified physeal fracture of `CC` `H5`
lower end of radius, right arm
> **CC Excl: CC with 7th character A:**
> PDX collection 1270
> **CC with 7th character K or P:**
> PDX collection 897

3 √7th **S59.202** Unspecified physeal fracture of `CC` `H5`
lower end of radius, left arm
> **CC Excl: CC with 7th character A:**
> PDX collection 1271
> **CC with 7th character K or P:**
> PDX collection 897

3 √7th **S59.209** Unspecified physeal fracture of `CC` `H5`
lower end of radius, unspecified arm
> **CC Excl: CC with 7th character A:**
> PDX collection 1272
> **CC with 7th character K or P:**
> PDX collection 897

√6th **S59.21** Salter-Harris Type I physeal fracture of lower end of
radius

3 √7th **S59.211** Salter-Harris Type I physeal `CC` `H5`
fracture of lower end of radius, right arm

3 √7th **S59.212** Salter-Harris Type I physeal `CC` `H5`
fracture of lower end of radius, left arm

3 √7th **S59.219** Salter-Harris Type I physeal `CC` `H5`
fracture of lower end of radius,
unspecified arm

√6th **S59.22** Salter-Harris Type II physeal fracture of lower end of
radius

3 √7th **S59.221** Salter-Harris Type II physeal `CC` `H5`
fracture of lower end of radius, right arm

3 √7th **S59.222** Salter-Harris Type II physeal `CC` `H5`
fracture of lower end of radius, left arm

3 √7th **S59.229** Salter-Harris Type II physeal `CC` `H5`
fracture of lower end of radius,
unspecified arm

√6th **S59.23** Salter-Harris Type III physeal fracture of lower end of
radius

3 √7th **S59.231** Salter-Harris Type III physeal `CC` `H5`
fracture of lower end of radius, right arm

3 √7th **S59.232** Salter-Harris Type III physeal `CC` `H5`
fracture of lower end of radius, left arm

3 √7th **S59.239** Salter-Harris Type III physeal `CC` `H5`
fracture of lower end of radius,
unspecified arm

√6th **S59.24** Salter-Harris Type IV physeal fracture of lower end of
radius

3 √7th **S59.241** Salter-Harris Type IV physeal `CC` `H5`
fracture of lower end of radius, right arm

3 √7th **S59.242** Salter-Harris Type IV physeal `CC` `H5`
fracture of lower end of radius, left arm

3 √7th **S59.249** Salter-Harris Type IV physeal `CC` `H5`
fracture of lower end of radius,
unspecified arm

✔ Additional Character Required   √x7th Placeholder   Unacceptable PDx   Questionable PDx   Manifestation   `H1`-`H14` HAC   `HCC` CMS-HCC Dx   `HIV` HIV Dx

☑6ᵗʰ **S59.29** Other physeal fracture of lower end of radius

   ³ ☑7ᵗʰ **S59.291** Other physeal fracture of lower end of radius, right arm   CC H5

   ³ ☑7ᵗʰ **S59.292** Other physeal fracture of lower end of radius, left arm   CC H5

   ³ ☑7ᵗʰ **S59.299** Other physeal fracture of lower end of radius, unspecified arm   CC H5

☑5ᵗʰ **S59.8** Other specified injuries of elbow and forearm

> The appropriate 7th character is to be added to each code in subcategory S59.8.
> A   initial encounter
> D   subsequent encounter
> S   sequela

☑6ᵗʰ **S59.80** Other specified injuries of elbow

   ☑7ᵗʰ **S59.801** Other specified injuries of right elbow

   ☑7ᵗʰ **S59.802** Other specified injuries of left elbow

   ☑7ᵗʰ **S59.809** Other specified injuries of unspecified elbow

☑6ᵗʰ **S59.81** Other specified injuries of forearm

   ☑7ᵗʰ **S59.811** Other specified injuries right forearm

   ☑7ᵗʰ **S59.812** Other specified injuries left forearm

   ☑7ᵗʰ **S59.819** Other specified injuries unspecified forearm

☑5ᵗʰ **S59.9** Unspecified injury of elbow and forearm

> The appropriate 7th character is to be added to each code in subcategory S59.9.
> A   initial encounter
> D   subsequent encounter
> S   sequela

☑6ᵗʰ **S59.90** Unspecified injury of elbow

   ☑7ᵗʰ **S59.901** Unspecified injury of right elbow

   ☑7ᵗʰ **S59.902** Unspecified injury of left elbow

   ☑7ᵗʰ **S59.909** Unspecified injury of unspecified elbow

☑6ᵗʰ **S59.91** Unspecified injury of forearm

   ☑7ᵗʰ **S59.911** Unspecified injury of right forearm

   ☑7ᵗʰ **S59.912** Unspecified injury of left forearm

   ☑7ᵗʰ **S59.919** Unspecified injury of unspecified forearm

Injuries to the wrist, hand and fingers (S60-S69)

EXCLUDES 2   burns and corrosions (T20-T32)
frostbite (T33-T34)
insect bite or sting, venomous (T63.4)

☑4ᵗʰ **S60** Superficial injury of wrist, hand and fingers

> The appropriate 7th character is to be added to each code from category S60.
> A   initial encounter
> D   subsequent encounter
> S   sequela

☑5ᵗʰ **S60.0** Contusion of finger without damage to nail

   EXCLUDES 1   contusion involving nail (matrix) (S60.1)

  ☑x7ᵗʰ **S60.00** Contusion of unspecified finger without damage to nail

     Contusion of finger(s) NOS

  ☑6ᵗʰ **S60.01** Contusion of thumb without damage to nail

   ☑7ᵗʰ **S60.011** Contusion of right thumb without damage to nail

   ☑7ᵗʰ **S60.012** Contusion of left thumb without damage to nail

   ☑7ᵗʰ **S60.019** Contusion of unspecified thumb without damage to nail

  ☑6ᵗʰ **S60.02** Contusion of index finger without damage to nail

   ☑7ᵗʰ **S60.021** Contusion of right index finger without damage to nail

   ☑7ᵗʰ **S60.022** Contusion of left index finger without damage to nail

   ☑7ᵗʰ **S60.029** Contusion of unspecified index finger without damage to nail

  ☑6ᵗʰ **S60.03** Contusion of middle finger without damage to nail

   ☑7ᵗʰ **S60.031** Contusion of right middle finger without damage to nail

   ☑7ᵗʰ **S60.032** Contusion of left middle finger without damage to nail

   ☑7ᵗʰ **S60.039** Contusion of unspecified middle finger without damage to nail

☑6ᵗʰ **S60.04** Contusion of ring finger without damage to nail

   ☑7ᵗʰ **S60.041** Contusion of right ring finger without damage to nail

   ☑7ᵗʰ **S60.042** Contusion of left ring finger without damage to nail

   ☑7ᵗʰ **S60.049** Contusion of unspecified ring finger without damage to nail

☑6ᵗʰ **S60.05** Contusion of little finger without damage to nail

   ☑7ᵗʰ **S60.051** Contusion of right little finger without damage to nail

   ☑7ᵗʰ **S60.052** Contusion of left little finger without damage to nail

   ☑7ᵗʰ **S60.059** Contusion of unspecified little finger without damage to nail

☑5ᵗʰ **S60.1** Contusion of finger with damage to nail

  ☑x7ᵗʰ **S60.10** Contusion of unspecified finger with damage to nail

  ☑6ᵗʰ **S60.11** Contusion of thumb with damage to nail

   ☑7ᵗʰ **S60.111** Contusion of right thumb with damage to nail

   ☑7ᵗʰ **S60.112** Contusion of left thumb with damage to nail

   ☑7ᵗʰ **S60.119** Contusion of unspecified thumb with damage to nail

  ☑6ᵗʰ **S60.12** Contusion of index finger with damage to nail

   ☑7ᵗʰ **S60.121** Contusion of right index finger with damage to nail

   ☑7ᵗʰ **S60.122** Contusion of left index finger with damage to nail

   ☑7ᵗʰ **S60.129** Contusion of unspecified index finger with damage to nail

  ☑6ᵗʰ **S60.13** Contusion of middle finger with damage to nail

   ☑7ᵗʰ **S60.131** Contusion of right middle finger with damage to nail

   ☑7ᵗʰ **S60.132** Contusion of left middle finger with damage to nail

   ☑7ᵗʰ **S60.139** Contusion of unspecified middle finger with damage to nail

  ☑6ᵗʰ **S60.14** Contusion of ring finger with damage to nail

   ☑7ᵗʰ **S60.141** Contusion of right ring finger with damage to nail

   ☑7ᵗʰ **S60.142** Contusion of left ring finger with damage to nail

   ☑7ᵗʰ **S60.149** Contusion of unspecified ring finger with damage to nail

  ☑6ᵗʰ **S60.15** Contusion of little finger with damage to nail

   ☑7ᵗʰ **S60.151** Contusion of right little finger with damage to nail

   ☑7ᵗʰ **S60.152** Contusion of left little finger with damage to nail

   ☑7ᵗʰ **S60.159** Contusion of unspecified little finger with damage to nail

☑5ᵗʰ **S60.2** Contusion of wrist and hand

   EXCLUDES 2   contusion of fingers (S60.0-, S60.1-)

  ☑6ᵗʰ **S60.21** Contusion of wrist

   ☑7ᵗʰ **S60.211** Contusion of right wrist

   ☑7ᵗʰ **S60.212** Contusion of left wrist

   ☑7ᵗʰ **S60.219** Contusion of unspecified wrist

  ☑6ᵗʰ **S60.22** Contusion of hand

   ☑7ᵗʰ **S60.221** Contusion of right hand

   ☑7ᵗʰ **S60.222** Contusion of left hand

   ☑7ᵗʰ **S60.229** Contusion of unspecified hand

☑5ᵗʰ **S60.3** Other superficial injuries of thumb

  ☑6ᵗʰ **S60.31** Abrasion of thumb

   ☑7ᵗʰ **S60.311** Abrasion of right thumb

   ☑7ᵗʰ **S60.312** Abrasion of left thumb

   ☑7ᵗʰ **S60.319** Abrasion of unspecified thumb

  ☑6ᵗʰ **S60.32** Blister (nonthermal) of thumb

   ☑7ᵗʰ **S60.321** Blister (nonthermal) of right thumb

   ☑7ᵗʰ **S60.322** Blister (nonthermal) of left thumb

   ☑7ᵗʰ **S60.329** Blister (nonthermal) of unspecified thumb

✓6ᵗʰ **S60.34** External constriction of thumb
    Hair tourniquet syndrome of thumb
    Use additional cause code to identify the constricting
    item (W49.0-)

    ✓7ᵗʰ **S60.341** External constriction of right thumb
    ✓7ᵗʰ **S60.342** External constriction of left thumb
    ✓7ᵗʰ **S60.349** External constriction of unspecified
        thumb

✓6ᵗʰ **S60.35** Superficial foreign body of thumb
    Splinter in the thumb

    ✓7ᵗʰ **S60.351** Superficial foreign body of right thumb
    ✓7ᵗʰ **S60.352** Superficial foreign body of left thumb
    ✓7ᵗʰ **S60.359** Superficial foreign body of unspecified
        thumb

✓6ᵗʰ **S60.36** Insect bite (nonvenomous) of thumb

    ✓7ᵗʰ **S60.361** Insect bite (nonvenomous) of right thumb
    ✓7ᵗʰ **S60.362** Insect bite (nonvenomous) of left thumb
    ✓7ᵗʰ **S60.369** Insect bite (nonvenomous) of unspecified
        thumb

✓6ᵗʰ **S60.37** Other superficial bite of thumb
    EXCLUDES 1   open bite of thumb (S61.05-, S61.15-)

    ✓7ᵗʰ **S60.371** Other superficial bite of right thumb
    ✓7ᵗʰ **S60.372** Other superficial bite of left thumb
    ✓7ᵗʰ **S60.379** Other superficial bite of unspecified
        thumb

✓6ᵗʰ **S60.39** Other superficial injuries of thumb

    ✓7ᵗʰ **S60.391** Other superficial injuries of right thumb
    ✓7ᵗʰ **S60.392** Other superficial injuries of left thumb
    ✓7ᵗʰ **S60.399** Other superficial injuries of unspecified
        thumb

✓5ᵗʰ **S60.4** Other superficial injuries of other fingers

  ✓6ᵗʰ **S60.41** Abrasion of fingers

    ✓7ᵗʰ **S60.410** Abrasion of right index finger
    ✓7ᵗʰ **S60.411** Abrasion of left index finger
    ✓7ᵗʰ **S60.412** Abrasion of right middle finger
    ✓7ᵗʰ **S60.413** Abrasion of left middle finger
    ✓7ᵗʰ **S60.414** Abrasion of right ring finger
    ✓7ᵗʰ **S60.415** Abrasion of left ring finger
    ✓7ᵗʰ **S60.416** Abrasion of right little finger
    ✓7ᵗʰ **S60.417** Abrasion of left little finger
    ✓7ᵗʰ **S60.418** Abrasion of other finger
        Abrasion of specified finger with
        unspecified laterality
    ✓7ᵗʰ **S60.419** Abrasion of unspecified finger

  ✓6ᵗʰ **S60.42** Blister (nonthermal) of fingers

    ✓7ᵗʰ **S60.420** Blister (nonthermal) of right index finger
    ✓7ᵗʰ **S60.421** Blister (nonthermal) of left index finger
    ✓7ᵗʰ **S60.422** Blister (nonthermal) of right middle finger
    ✓7ᵗʰ **S60.423** Blister (nonthermal) of left middle finger
    ✓7ᵗʰ **S60.424** Blister (nonthermal) of right ring finger
    ✓7ᵗʰ **S60.425** Blister (nonthermal) of left ring finger
    ✓7ᵗʰ **S60.426** Blister (nonthermal) of right little finger
    ✓7ᵗʰ **S60.427** Blister (nonthermal) of left little finger
    ✓7ᵗʰ **S60.428** Blister (nonthermal) of other finger
        Blister (nonthermal) of specified finger with
        unspecified laterality
    ✓7ᵗʰ **S60.429** Blister (nonthermal) of unspecified finger

  ✓6ᵗʰ **S60.44** External constriction of fingers
    Hair tourniquet syndrome of finger
    Use additional cause code to identify the constricting
    item (W49.0-)

    ✓7ᵗʰ **S60.440** External constriction of right index finger
    ✓7ᵗʰ **S60.441** External constriction of left index finger
    ✓7ᵗʰ **S60.442** External constriction of right middle
        finger
    ✓7ᵗʰ **S60.443** External constriction of left middle finger
    ✓7ᵗʰ **S60.444** External constriction of right ring finger
    ✓7ᵗʰ **S60.445** External constriction of left ring finger
    ✓7ᵗʰ **S60.446** External constriction of right little finger
    ✓7ᵗʰ **S60.447** External constriction of left little finger

    ✓7ᵗʰ **S60.448** External constriction of other finger
        External constriction of specified finger
        with unspecified laterality
    ✓7ᵗʰ **S60.449** External constriction of unspecified finger

✓6ᵗʰ **S60.45** Superficial foreign body of fingers
    Splinter in the finger(s)

    ✓7ᵗʰ **S60.450** Superficial foreign body of right index
        finger
    ✓7ᵗʰ **S60.451** Superficial foreign body of left index
        finger
    ✓7ᵗʰ **S60.452** Superficial foreign body of right middle
        finger
    ✓7ᵗʰ **S60.453** Superficial foreign body of left middle
        finger
    ✓7ᵗʰ **S60.454** Superficial foreign body of right ring
        finger
    ✓7ᵗʰ **S60.455** Superficial foreign body of left ring finger
    ✓7ᵗʰ **S60.456** Superficial foreign body of right little
        finger
    ✓7ᵗʰ **S60.457** Superficial foreign body of left little finger
    ✓7ᵗʰ **S60.458** Superficial foreign body of other finger
        Superficial foreign body of specified finger
        with unspecified laterality
    ✓7ᵗʰ **S60.459** Superficial foreign body of unspecified
        finger

✓6ᵗʰ **S60.46** Insect bite (nonvenomous) of fingers

    ✓7ᵗʰ **S60.460** Insect bite (nonvenomous) of right index
        finger
    ✓7ᵗʰ **S60.461** Insect bite (nonvenomous) of left index
        finger
    ✓7ᵗʰ **S60.462** Insect bite (nonvenomous) of right middle
        finger
    ✓7ᵗʰ **S60.463** Insect bite (nonvenomous) of left middle
        finger
    ✓7ᵗʰ **S60.464** Insect bite (nonvenomous) of right ring
        finger
    ✓7ᵗʰ **S60.465** Insect bite (nonvenomous) of left ring
        finger
    ✓7ᵗʰ **S60.466** Insect bite (nonvenomous) of right little
        finger
    ✓7ᵗʰ **S60.467** Insect bite (nonvenomous) of left little
        finger
    ✓7ᵗʰ **S60.468** Insect bite (nonvenomous) of other finger
        Insect bite (nonvenomous) of specified
        finger with unspecified laterality
    ✓7ᵗʰ **S60.469** Insect bite (nonvenomous) of unspecified
        finger

✓6ᵗʰ **S60.47** Other superficial bite of fingers
    EXCLUDES 1   open bite of fingers (S61.25-, S61.35-)

    ✓7ᵗʰ **S60.470** Other superficial bite of right index finger
    ✓7ᵗʰ **S60.471** Other superficial bite of left index finger
    ✓7ᵗʰ **S60.472** Other superficial bite of right middle
        finger
    ✓7ᵗʰ **S60.473** Other superficial bite of left middle finger
    ✓7ᵗʰ **S60.474** Other superficial bite of right ring finger
    ✓7ᵗʰ **S60.475** Other superficial bite of left ring finger
    ✓7ᵗʰ **S60.476** Other superficial bite of right little finger
    ✓7ᵗʰ **S60.477** Other superficial bite of left little finger
    ✓7ᵗʰ **S60.478** Other superficial bite of other finger
        Other superficial bite of specified finger
        with unspecified laterality
    ✓7ᵗʰ **S60.479** Other superficial bite of unspecified finger

✓5ᵗʰ **S60.5** Other superficial injuries of hand
    EXCLUDES 2   superficial injuries of fingers (S60.3-, S60.4-)

  ✓6ᵗʰ **S60.51** Abrasion of hand

    ✓7ᵗʰ **S60.511** Abrasion of right hand
    ✓7ᵗʰ **S60.512** Abrasion of left hand
    ✓7ᵗʰ **S60.519** Abrasion of unspecified hand

  ✓6ᵗʰ **S60.52** Blister (nonthermal) of hand

    ✓7ᵗʰ **S60.521** Blister (nonthermal) of right hand
    ✓7ᵗʰ **S60.522** Blister (nonthermal) of left hand
    ✓7ᵗʰ **S60.529** Blister (nonthermal) of unspecified hand

✓ Additional Character Required   ✓ₓ7ᵗʰ Placeholder   Unacceptable PDx   Questionable PDx   Manifestation   H1 - H14 HAC   HCC CMS-HCC Dx   HIV HIV Dx

ICD-10-CM 2019   **1017**

√6ᵗʰ **S60.54   External constriction** of hand
  √7ᵗʰ **S60.541   External constriction of right** hand
  √7ᵗʰ **S60.542   External constriction of left** hand
  √7ᵗʰ **S60.549   External constriction of unspecified** hand

√6ᵗʰ **S60.55   Superficial foreign body** of hand
      Splinter in the hand
  √7ᵗʰ **S60.551   Superficial foreign body of right** hand
  √7ᵗʰ **S60.552   Superficial foreign body of left** hand
  √7ᵗʰ **S60.559   Superficial foreign body of unspecified** hand

√6ᵗʰ **S60.56   Insect bite (nonvenomous)** of hand
  √7ᵗʰ **S60.561   Insect bite (nonvenomous) of right** hand
  √7ᵗʰ **S60.562   Insect bite (nonvenomous) of left** hand
  √7ᵗʰ **S60.569   Insect bite (nonvenomous) of unspecified** hand

√6ᵗʰ **S60.57   Other superficial bite** of hand
      EXCLUDES 1   *open bite of hand (S61.45-)*
  √7ᵗʰ **S60.571   Other superficial bite of hand of right** hand
  √7ᵗʰ **S60.572   Other superficial bite of hand of left** hand
  √7ᵗʰ **S60.579   Other superficial bite of hand of unspecified** hand

√5ᵗʰ **S60.8   Other superficial injuries of wrist**
  √6ᵗʰ **S60.81   Abrasion of wrist**
    √7ᵗʰ **S60.811   Abrasion of right** wrist
    √7ᵗʰ **S60.812   Abrasion of left** wrist
    √7ᵗʰ **S60.819   Abrasion of unspecified** wrist

  √6ᵗʰ **S60.82   Blister (nonthermal) of wrist**
    √7ᵗʰ **S60.821   Blister (nonthermal) of right** wrist
    √7ᵗʰ **S60.822   Blister (nonthermal) of left** wrist
    √7ᵗʰ **S60.829   Blister (nonthermal) of unspecified** wrist

  √6ᵗʰ **S60.84   External constriction of wrist**
    √7ᵗʰ **S60.841   External constriction of right** wrist
    √7ᵗʰ **S60.842   External constriction of left** wrist
    √7ᵗʰ **S60.849   External constriction of unspecified** wrist

  √6ᵗʰ **S60.85   Superficial foreign body of wrist**
      Splinter in the wrist
    √7ᵗʰ **S60.851   Superficial foreign body of right** wrist
    √7ᵗʰ **S60.852   Superficial foreign body of left** wrist
    √7ᵗʰ **S60.859   Superficial foreign body of unspecified** wrist

  √6ᵗʰ **S60.86   Insect bite (nonvenomous) of wrist**
    √7ᵗʰ **S60.861   Insect bite (nonvenomous) of right** wrist
    √7ᵗʰ **S60.862   Insect bite (nonvenomous) of left** wrist
    √7ᵗʰ **S60.869   Insect bite (nonvenomous) of unspecified** wrist

  √6ᵗʰ **S60.87   Other superficial bite of wrist**
      EXCLUDES 1   *open bite of wrist (S61.55)*
    √7ᵗʰ **S60.871   Other superficial bite of right** wrist
    √7ᵗʰ **S60.872   Other superficial bite of left** wrist
    √7ᵗʰ **S60.879   Other superficial bite of unspecified** wrist

√5ᵗʰ **S60.9   Unspecified superficial injury of wrist, hand and fingers**
  √6ᵗʰ **S60.91   Unspecified superficial injury of wrist**
    √7ᵗʰ **S60.911   Unspecified superficial injury of right** wrist
    √7ᵗʰ **S60.912   Unspecified superficial injury of left** wrist
    √7ᵗʰ **S60.919   Unspecified superficial injury of unspecified** wrist

  √6ᵗʰ **S60.92   Unspecified superficial injury of hand**
    √7ᵗʰ **S60.921   Unspecified superficial injury of right** hand
    √7ᵗʰ **S60.922   Unspecified superficial injury of left** hand
    √7ᵗʰ **S60.929   Unspecified superficial injury of unspecified** hand

  √6ᵗʰ **S60.93   Unspecified superficial injury of thumb**
    √7ᵗʰ **S60.931   Unspecified superficial injury of right** thumb
    √7ᵗʰ **S60.932   Unspecified superficial injury of left** thumb

  √7ᵗʰ **S60.939   Unspecified superficial injury of unspecified** thumb

  √6ᵗʰ **S60.94   Unspecified superficial injury of other fingers**
    √7ᵗʰ **S60.940   Unspecified superficial injury of right index** finger
    √7ᵗʰ **S60.941   Unspecified superficial injury of left index** finger
    √7ᵗʰ **S60.942   Unspecified superficial injury of right middle** finger
    √7ᵗʰ **S60.943   Unspecified superficial injury of left middle** finger
    √7ᵗʰ **S60.944   Unspecified superficial injury of right ring** finger
    √7ᵗʰ **S60.945   Unspecified superficial injury of left ring** finger
    √7ᵗʰ **S60.946   Unspecified superficial injury of right little** finger
    √7ᵗʰ **S60.947   Unspecified superficial injury of left little** finger
    √7ᵗʰ **S60.948   Unspecified superficial injury of other** finger
        Unspecified superficial injury of specified finger with unspecified laterality
    √7ᵗʰ **S60.949   Unspecified superficial injury of unspecified** finger

√4ᵗʰ **S61   Open wound of wrist, hand and fingers**
    Code also any associated wound infection
    EXCLUDES 1   *open fracture of wrist, hand and finger (S62- with 7th character B)*
                 traumatic amputation of wrist and hand (S68.-)

    The appropriate 7th character is to be added to each code from category S61.
    A   initial encounter
    D   subsequent encounter
    S   sequela

√5ᵗʰ **S61.0   Open wound of thumb without damage to nail**
      EXCLUDES 1   *open wound of thumb with damage to nail (S61.1-)*
  √6ᵗʰ **S61.00   Unspecified open wound of thumb without damage to nail**
    √7ᵗʰ **S61.001   Unspecified open wound of right** thumb without damage to nail
    √7ᵗʰ **S61.002   Unspecified open wound of left** thumb without damage to nail
    √7ᵗʰ **S61.009   Unspecified open wound of unspecified** thumb without damage to nail

  √6ᵗʰ **S61.01   Laceration without foreign body of thumb without damage to nail**
    √7ᵗʰ **S61.011   Laceration without foreign body of right** thumb without damage to nail
    √7ᵗʰ **S61.012   Laceration without foreign body of left** thumb without damage to nail
    √7ᵗʰ **S61.019   Laceration without foreign body of unspecified** thumb without damage to nail

  √6ᵗʰ **S61.02   Laceration with foreign body of thumb without damage to nail**
    √7ᵗʰ **S61.021   Laceration with foreign body of right** thumb without damage to nail
    √7ᵗʰ **S61.022   Laceration with foreign body of left** thumb without damage to nail
    √7ᵗʰ **S61.029   Laceration with foreign body of unspecified** thumb without damage to nail

  √6ᵗʰ **S61.03   Puncture wound without foreign body of thumb without damage to nail**
    √7ᵗʰ **S61.031   Puncture wound without foreign body of right** thumb without damage to nail
    √7ᵗʰ **S61.032   Puncture wound without foreign body of left** thumb without damage to nail
    √7ᵗʰ **S61.039   Puncture wound without foreign body of unspecified** thumb without damage to nail

  √6ᵗʰ **S61.04   Puncture wound with foreign body of thumb without damage to nail**
    √7ᵗʰ **S61.041   Puncture wound with foreign body of right** thumb without damage to nail

☑7ᵗʰ **S61.042** **Puncture wound with foreign body of** left **thumb without damage to nail**

☑7ᵗʰ **S61.049** **Puncture wound with foreign body of** unspecified **thumb without damage to nail**

☑6ᵗʰ **S61.05** Open bite **of thumb without damage to nail**
     Bite of thumb NOS
     EXCLUDES 1   *superficial bite of thumb (S60.36-, S60.37-)*

☑7ᵗʰ **S61.051** **Open bite of** right **thumb without damage to nail**

☑7ᵗʰ **S61.052** **Open bite of** left **thumb without damage to nail**

☑7ᵗʰ **S61.059** **Open bite of** unspecified **thumb without damage to nail**

☑5ᵗʰ **S61.1** **Open wound of** thumb with damage to nail

☑6ᵗʰ **S61.10** Unspecified **open wound of thumb with damage to nail**

☑7ᵗʰ **S61.101** **Unspecified open wound of** right **thumb with damage to nail**

☑7ᵗʰ **S61.102** **Unspecified open wound of** left **thumb with damage to nail**

☑7ᵗʰ **S61.109** **Unspecified open wound of** unspecified **thumb with damage to nail**

☑6ᵗʰ **S61.11** Laceration without foreign body **of thumb with damage to nail**

☑7ᵗʰ **S61.111** **Laceration without foreign body of** right **thumb with damage to nail**

☑7ᵗʰ **S61.112** **Laceration without foreign body of** left **thumb with damage to nail**

☑7ᵗʰ **S61.119** **Laceration without foreign body of** unspecified **thumb with damage to nail**

☑6ᵗʰ **S61.12** Laceration with foreign body **of thumb with damage to nail**

☑7ᵗʰ **S61.121** **Laceration with foreign body of** right **thumb with damage to nail**

☑7ᵗʰ **S61.122** **Laceration with foreign body of** left **thumb with damage to nail**

☑7ᵗʰ **S61.129** **Laceration with foreign body of** unspecified **thumb with damage to nail**

☑6ᵗʰ **S61.13** Puncture wound without foreign body **of thumb with damage to nail**

☑7ᵗʰ **S61.131** **Puncture wound without foreign body of** right **thumb with damage to nail**

☑7ᵗʰ **S61.132** **Puncture wound without foreign body of** left **thumb with damage to nail**

☑7ᵗʰ **S61.139** **Puncture wound without foreign body of** unspecified **thumb with damage to nail**

☑6ᵗʰ **S61.14** Puncture wound with foreign body **of thumb with damage to nail**

☑7ᵗʰ **S61.141** **Puncture wound with foreign body of** right **thumb with damage to nail**

☑7ᵗʰ **S61.142** **Puncture wound with foreign body of** left **thumb with damage to nail**

☑7ᵗʰ **S61.149** **Puncture wound with foreign body of** unspecified **thumb with damage to nail**

☑6ᵗʰ **S61.15** Open bite **of thumb** with damage to nail
     Bite of thumb with damage to nail NOS
     EXCLUDES 1   *superficial bite of thumb (S60.36-, S60.37-)*

☑7ᵗʰ **S61.151** **Open bite of** right **thumb with damage to nail**

☑7ᵗʰ **S61.152** **Open bite of** left **thumb with damage to nail**

☑7ᵗʰ **S61.159** **Open bite of** unspecified **thumb with damage to nail**

☑5ᵗʰ **S61.2** **Open wound of** other finger without damage to nail
     EXCLUDES 1   *open wound of finger involving nail (matrix) (S61.3-)*
     EXCLUDES 2   *open wound of thumb without damage to nail (S61.0-)*

☑6ᵗʰ **S61.20** Unspecified **open wound of other finger without damage to nail**

☑7ᵗʰ **S61.200** **Unspecified open wound of** right index **finger without damage to nail**

☑7ᵗʰ **S61.201** **Unspecified open wound of** left index **finger without damage to nail**

☑7ᵗʰ **S61.202** **Unspecified open wound of** right middle **finger without damage to nail**

☑7ᵗʰ **S61.203** **Unspecified open wound of** left middle **finger without damage to nail**

☑7ᵗʰ **S61.204** **Unspecified open wound of** right ring **finger without damage to nail**

☑7ᵗʰ **S61.205** **Unspecified open wound of** left ring **finger without damage to nail**

☑7ᵗʰ **S61.206** **Unspecified open wound of** right little **finger without damage to nail**

☑7ᵗʰ **S61.207** **Unspecified open wound of** left little **finger without damage to nail**

☑7ᵗʰ **S61.208** **Unspecified open wound of** other **finger without damage to nail**
     Unspecified open wound of specified finger with unspecified laterality without damage to nail

☑7ᵗʰ **S61.209** **Unspecified open wound of** unspecified **finger without damage to nail**

☑6ᵗʰ **S61.21** Laceration without foreign body **of finger without damage to nail**

☑7ᵗʰ **S61.210** **Laceration without foreign body of** right index **finger without damage to nail**

☑7ᵗʰ **S61.211** **Laceration without foreign body of** left index **finger without damage to nail**

☑7ᵗʰ **S61.212** **Laceration without foreign body of** right middle **finger without damage to nail**

☑7ᵗʰ **S61.213** **Laceration without foreign body of** left middle **finger without damage to nail**

☑7ᵗʰ **S61.214** **Laceration without foreign body of** right ring **finger without damage to nail**

☑7ᵗʰ **S61.215** **Laceration without foreign body of** left ring **finger without damage to nail**

☑7ᵗʰ **S61.216** **Laceration without foreign body of** right little **finger without damage to nail**

☑7ᵗʰ **S61.217** **Laceration without foreign body of** left little **finger without damage to nail**

☑7ᵗʰ **S61.218** **Laceration without foreign body of** other **finger without damage to nail**
     Laceration without foreign body of specified finger with unspecified laterality without damage to nail

☑7ᵗʰ **S61.219** **Laceration without foreign body of** unspecified **finger without damage to nail**

☑6ᵗʰ **S61.22** Laceration with foreign body **of finger without damage to nail**

☑7ᵗʰ **S61.220** **Laceration with foreign body of** right index **finger without damage to nail**

☑7ᵗʰ **S61.221** **Laceration with foreign body of** left index **finger without damage to nail**

☑7ᵗʰ **S61.222** **Laceration with foreign body of** right middle **finger without damage to nail**

☑7ᵗʰ **S61.223** **Laceration with foreign body of** left middle **finger without damage to nail**

☑7ᵗʰ **S61.224** **Laceration with foreign body of** right ring **finger without damage to nail**

☑7ᵗʰ **S61.225** **Laceration with foreign body of** left ring **finger without damage to nail**

☑7ᵗʰ **S61.226** **Laceration with foreign body of** right little **finger without damage to nail**

☑7ᵗʰ **S61.227** **Laceration with foreign body of** left little **finger without damage to nail**

☑7ᵗʰ **S61.228** **Laceration with foreign body of** other **finger without damage to nail**
     Laceration with foreign body of specified finger with unspecified laterality without damage to nail

☑7ᵗʰ **S61.229** **Laceration with foreign body of** unspecified **finger without damage to nail**

☑6ᵗʰ **S61.23** Puncture wound without foreign body **of finger without damage to nail**

☑7ᵗʰ **S61.230** **Puncture wound without foreign body of** right index **finger without damage to nail**

☑7ᵗʰ **S61.231** **Puncture wound without foreign body of** left index **finger without damage to nail**

☑7ᵗʰ **S61.232** **Puncture wound without foreign body of** right middle **finger without damage to nail**

☑Additional Character Required   ☑x7ᵗʰ Placeholder   Unacceptable PDx   Questionable PDx   Manifestation   **H1**-**H14** HAC   **HCC** CMS-HCC Dx   **HIV** HIV Dx

ICD-10-CM 2019   **1019**

Chapter 19. Injury, Poisoning and Certain Other Consequences of External Causes

S61.042–S61.232

√7ᵗʰ S61.233 Puncture wound without foreign body of left middle finger without damage to nail

√7ᵗʰ S61.234 Puncture wound without foreign body of right ring finger without damage to nail

√7ᵗʰ S61.235 Puncture wound without foreign body of left ring finger without damage to nail

√7ᵗʰ S61.236 Puncture wound without foreign body of right little finger without damage to nail

√7ᵗʰ S61.237 Puncture wound without foreign body of left little finger without damage to nail

√7ᵗʰ S61.238 Puncture wound without foreign body of other finger without damage to nail
Puncture wound without foreign body of specified finger with unspecified laterality without damage to nail

√7ᵗʰ S61.239 Puncture wound without foreign body of unspecified finger without damage to nail

√6ᵗʰ S61.24 Puncture wound with foreign body of finger without damage to nail

√7ᵗʰ S61.240 Puncture wound with foreign body of right index finger without damage to nail

√7ᵗʰ S61.241 Puncture wound with foreign body of left index finger without damage to nail

√7ᵗʰ S61.242 Puncture wound with foreign body of right middle finger without damage to nail

√7ᵗʰ S61.243 Puncture wound with foreign body of left middle finger without damage to nail

√7ᵗʰ S61.244 Puncture wound with foreign body of right ring finger without damage to nail

√7ᵗʰ S61.245 Puncture wound with foreign body of left ring finger without damage to nail

√7ᵗʰ S61.246 Puncture wound with foreign body of right little finger without damage to nail

√7ᵗʰ S61.247 Puncture wound with foreign body of left little finger without damage to nail

√7ᵗʰ S61.248 Puncture wound with foreign body of other finger without damage to nail
Puncture wound with foreign body of specified finger with unspecified laterality without damage to nail

√7ᵗʰ S61.249 Puncture wound with foreign body of unspecified finger without damage to nail

√6ᵗʰ S61.25 Open bite of finger without damage to nail
Bite of finger without damage to nail NOS
EXCLUDES 1 *superficial bite of finger (S60.46-, S60.47-)*

√7ᵗʰ S61.250 Open bite of right index finger without damage to nail

√7ᵗʰ S61.251 Open bite of left index finger without damage to nail

√7ᵗʰ S61.252 Open bite of right middle finger without damage to nail

√7ᵗʰ S61.253 Open bite of left middle finger without damage to nail

√7ᵗʰ S61.254 Open bite of right ring finger without damage to nail

√7ᵗʰ S61.255 Open bite of left ring finger without damage to nail

√7ᵗʰ S61.256 Open bite of right little finger without damage to nail

√7ᵗʰ S61.257 Open bite of left little finger without damage to nail

√7ᵗʰ S61.258 Open bite of other finger without damage to nail
Open bite of specified finger with unspecified laterality without damage to nail

√7ᵗʰ S61.259 Open bite of unspecified finger without damage to nail

√5ᵗʰ S61.3 Open wound of other finger with damage to nail

√6ᵗʰ S61.30 Unspecified open wound of finger with damage to nail

√7ᵗʰ S61.300 Unspecified open wound of right index finger with damage to nail

√7ᵗʰ S61.301 Unspecified open wound of left index finger with damage to nail

√7ᵗʰ S61.302 Unspecified open wound of right middle finger with damage to nail

√7ᵗʰ S61.303 Unspecified open wound of left middle finger with damage to nail

√7ᵗʰ S61.304 Unspecified open wound of right ring finger with damage to nail

√7ᵗʰ S61.305 Unspecified open wound of left ring finger with damage to nail

√7ᵗʰ S61.306 Unspecified open wound of right little finger with damage to nail

√7ᵗʰ S61.307 Unspecified open wound of left little finger with damage to nail

√7ᵗʰ S61.308 Unspecified open wound of other finger with damage to nail
Unspecified open wound of specified finger with unspecified laterality with damage to nail

√7ᵗʰ S61.309 Unspecified open wound of unspecified finger with damage to nail

√6ᵗʰ S61.31 Laceration without foreign body of finger with damage to nail

√7ᵗʰ S61.310 Laceration without foreign body of right index finger with damage to nail

√7ᵗʰ S61.311 Laceration without foreign body of left index finger with damage to nail

√7ᵗʰ S61.312 Laceration without foreign body of right middle finger with damage to nail

√7ᵗʰ S61.313 Laceration without foreign body of left middle finger with damage to nail

√7ᵗʰ S61.314 Laceration without foreign body of right ring finger with damage to nail

√7ᵗʰ S61.315 Laceration without foreign body of left ring finger with damage to nail

√7ᵗʰ S61.316 Laceration without foreign body of right little finger with damage to nail

√7ᵗʰ S61.317 Laceration without foreign body of left little finger with damage to nail

√7ᵗʰ S61.318 Laceration without foreign body of other finger with damage to nail
Laceration without foreign body of specified finger with unspecified laterality with damage to nail

√7ᵗʰ S61.319 Laceration without foreign body of unspecified finger with damage to nail

√6ᵗʰ S61.32 Laceration with foreign body of finger with damage to nail

√7ᵗʰ S61.320 Laceration with foreign body of right index finger with damage to nail

√7ᵗʰ S61.321 Laceration with foreign body of left index finger with damage to nail

√7ᵗʰ S61.322 Laceration with foreign body of right middle finger with damage to nail

√7ᵗʰ S61.323 Laceration with foreign body of left middle finger with damage to nail

√7ᵗʰ S61.324 Laceration with foreign body of right ring finger with damage to nail

√7ᵗʰ S61.325 Laceration with foreign body of left ring finger with damage to nail

√7ᵗʰ S61.326 Laceration with foreign body of right little finger with damage to nail

√7ᵗʰ S61.327 Laceration with foreign body of left little finger with damage to nail

√7ᵗʰ S61.328 Laceration with foreign body of other finger with damage to nail
Laceration with foreign body of specified finger with unspecified laterality with damage to nail

√7ᵗʰ S61.329 Laceration with foreign body of unspecified finger with damage to nail

√6ᵗʰ S61.33 Puncture wound without foreign body of finger with damage to nail

√7ᵗʰ S61.330 Puncture wound without foreign body of right index finger with damage to nail

√7ᵗʰ S61.331 Puncture wound without foreign body of left index finger with damage to nail

√7ᵗʰ S61.332 Puncture wound without foreign body of right middle finger with damage to nail

N Newborn: 0   **P** Pediatric: 0-17   **M** Maternity: 12-55   **A** Adult: 15-124   **MCC** Major Complication/Comorbidity   **CC** Complication/Comorbidity   **SW** Severe Wound Dx

1020   ICD-10-CM 2019

√7ᵗʰ **S61.333** **Puncture wound without foreign body of left middle finger with damage to nail**

√7ᵗʰ **S61.334** **Puncture wound without foreign body of right ring finger with damage to nail**

√7ᵗʰ **S61.335** **Puncture wound without foreign body of left ring finger with damage to nail**

√7ᵗʰ **S61.336** **Puncture wound without foreign body of right little finger with damage to nail**

√7ᵗʰ **S61.337** **Puncture wound without foreign body of left little finger with damage to nail**

√7ᵗʰ **S61.338** **Puncture wound without foreign body of other finger with damage to nail**
Puncture wound without foreign body of specified finger with unspecified laterality with damage to nail

√7ᵗʰ **S61.339** **Puncture wound without foreign body of unspecified finger with damage to nail**

√6ᵗʰ **S61.34** **Puncture wound with foreign body of finger with damage to nail**

√7ᵗʰ **S61.340** **Puncture wound with foreign body of right index finger with damage to nail**

√7ᵗʰ **S61.341** **Puncture wound with foreign body of left index finger with damage to nail**

√7ᵗʰ **S61.342** **Puncture wound with foreign body of right middle finger with damage to nail**

√7ᵗʰ **S61.343** **Puncture wound with foreign body of left middle finger with damage to nail**

√7ᵗʰ **S61.344** **Puncture wound with foreign body of right ring finger with damage to nail**

√7ᵗʰ **S61.345** **Puncture wound with foreign body of left ring finger with damage to nail**

√7ᵗʰ **S61.346** **Puncture wound with foreign body of right little finger with damage to nail**

√7ᵗʰ **S61.347** **Puncture wound with foreign body of left little finger with damage to nail**

√7ᵗʰ **S61.348** **Puncture wound with foreign body of other finger with damage to nail**
Puncture wound with foreign body of specified finger with unspecified laterality with damage to nail

√7ᵗʰ **S61.349** **Puncture wound with foreign body of unspecified finger with damage to nail**

√6ᵗʰ **S61.35** **Open bite of finger with damage to nail**
Bite of finger with damage to nail NOS
EXCLUDES 1 *superficial bite of finger (S60.46-, S60.47-)*

√7ᵗʰ **S61.350** **Open bite of right index finger with damage to nail**

√7ᵗʰ **S61.351** **Open bite of left index finger with damage to nail**

√7ᵗʰ **S61.352** **Open bite of right middle finger with damage to nail**

√7ᵗʰ **S61.353** **Open bite of left middle finger with damage to nail**

√7ᵗʰ **S61.354** **Open bite of right ring finger with damage to nail**

√7ᵗʰ **S61.355** **Open bite of left ring finger with damage to nail**

√7ᵗʰ **S61.356** **Open bite of right little finger with damage to nail**

√7ᵗʰ **S61.357** **Open bite of left little finger with damage to nail**

√7ᵗʰ **S61.358** **Open bite of other finger with damage to nail**
Open bite of specified finger with unspecified laterality with damage to nail

√7ᵗʰ **S61.359** **Open bite of unspecified finger with damage to nail**

√5ᵗʰ **S61.4** **Open wound of hand**

√6ᵗʰ **S61.40** **Unspecified open wound of hand**

√7ᵗʰ **S61.401** **Unspecified open wound of right hand**

√7ᵗʰ **S61.402** **Unspecified open wound of left hand**

√7ᵗʰ **S61.409** **Unspecified open wound of unspecified hand**

√6ᵗʰ **S61.41** **Laceration without foreign body of hand**

√7ᵗʰ **S61.411** **Laceration without foreign body of right hand**

√7ᵗʰ **S61.412** **Laceration without foreign body of left hand**

√7ᵗʰ **S61.419** **Laceration without foreign body of unspecified hand**

√6ᵗʰ **S61.42** **Laceration with foreign body of hand**

√7ᵗʰ **S61.421** **Laceration with foreign body of right hand**

√7ᵗʰ **S61.422** **Laceration with foreign body of left hand**

√7ᵗʰ **S61.429** **Laceration with foreign body of unspecified hand**

√6ᵗʰ **S61.43** **Puncture wound without foreign body of hand**

√7ᵗʰ **S61.431** **Puncture wound without foreign body of right hand**

√7ᵗʰ **S61.432** **Puncture wound without foreign body of left hand**

√7ᵗʰ **S61.439** **Puncture wound without foreign body of unspecified hand**

√6ᵗʰ **S61.44** **Puncture wound with foreign body of hand**

√7ᵗʰ **S61.441** **Puncture wound with foreign body of right hand**

√7ᵗʰ **S61.442** **Puncture wound with foreign body of left hand**

√7ᵗʰ **S61.449** **Puncture wound with foreign body of unspecified hand**

√6ᵗʰ **S61.45** **Open bite of hand**
Bite of hand NOS
EXCLUDES 1 *superficial bite of hand (S60.56-, S60.57-)*

√7ᵗʰ **S61.451** **Open bite of right hand**

√7ᵗʰ **S61.452** **Open bite of left hand**

√7ᵗʰ **S61.459** **Open bite of unspecified hand**

√5ᵗʰ **S61.5** **Open wound of wrist**

√6ᵗʰ **S61.50** **Unspecified open wound of wrist**

√7ᵗʰ **S61.501** **Unspecified open wound of right wrist**

√7ᵗʰ **S61.502** **Unspecified open wound of left wrist**

√7ᵗʰ **S61.509** **Unspecified open wound of unspecified wrist**

√6ᵗʰ **S61.51** **Laceration without foreign body of wrist**

√7ᵗʰ **S61.511** **Laceration without foreign body of right wrist**

√7ᵗʰ **S61.512** **Laceration without foreign body of left wrist**

√7ᵗʰ **S61.519** **Laceration without foreign body of unspecified wrist**

√6ᵗʰ **S61.52** **Laceration with foreign body of wrist**

√7ᵗʰ **S61.521** **Laceration with foreign body of right wrist**

√7ᵗʰ **S61.522** **Laceration with foreign body of left wrist**

√7ᵗʰ **S61.529** **Laceration with foreign body of unspecified wrist**

√6ᵗʰ **S61.53** **Puncture wound without foreign body of wrist**

√7ᵗʰ **S61.531** **Puncture wound without foreign body of right wrist**

√7ᵗʰ **S61.532** **Puncture wound without foreign body of left wrist**

√7ᵗʰ **S61.539** **Puncture wound without foreign body of unspecified wrist**

√6ᵗʰ **S61.54** **Puncture wound with foreign body of wrist**

√7ᵗʰ **S61.541** **Puncture wound with foreign body of right wrist**

√7ᵗʰ **S61.542** **Puncture wound with foreign body of left wrist**

√7ᵗʰ **S61.549** **Puncture wound with foreign body of unspecified wrist**

√6ᵗʰ **S61.55** **Open bite of wrist**
Bite of wrist NOS
EXCLUDES 1 *superficial bite of wrist (S60.86-, S60.87-)*

√7ᵗʰ **S61.551** **Open bite of right wrist**

√7ᵗʰ **S61.552** **Open bite of left wrist**

√7ᵗʰ **S61.559** **Open bite of unspecified wrist**

☑ Additional Character Required   √x7ᵗʰ Placeholder   Unacceptable PDx   Questionable PDx   Manifestation   **H1**-**H14** HAC   **HCC** CMS-HCC Dx   **HIV** HIV Dx

ICD-10-CM 2019   **1021**

✓4ᵗʰ S62 Fracture at wrist and hand level

NOTE A fracture not indicated as displaced or nondisplaced should be coded to displaced.
A fracture not indicated as open or closed should be coded to closed.

EXCLUDES 1 *traumatic amputation of wrist and hand (S68.-)*
EXCLUDES 2 *fracture of distal parts of ulna and radius (S52.-)*
AHA: 2018, 2Q, 12; 2015, 3Q, 37-39

The appropriate 7th character is to be added to each code from category S62.
A   initial encounter for closed fracture
B   initial encounter for open fracture
D   subsequent encounter for fracture with routine healing
G   subsequent encounter for fracture with delayed healing
K   subsequent encounter for fracture with nonunion
P   subsequent encounter for fracture with malunion
S   sequela

✓5ᵗʰ S62.0 Fracture of navicular [scaphoid] bone of wrist

CC Excl: For codes in subcategory S62.0:
CC with 7th character B: PDX collection 1283
CC with 7th character K or P: PDX collection 897

✓6ᵗʰ S62.00 Unspecified fracture of navicular [scaphoid] bone of wrist

3 ✓7ᵗʰ S62.001 Unspecified fracture of navicular [scaphoid] bone of right wrist   CC H5

3 ✓7ᵗʰ S62.002 Unspecified fracture of navicular [scaphoid] bone of left wrist   CC H5
AHA: 2012, 4Q, 106

3 ✓7ᵗʰ S62.009 Unspecified fracture of navicular [scaphoid] bone of unspecified wrist   CC H5

✓6ᵗʰ S62.01 Fracture of distal pole of navicular [scaphoid] bone of wrist
Fracture of volar tuberosity of navicular [scaphoid] bone of wrist

3 ✓7ᵗʰ S62.011 Displaced fracture of distal pole of navicular [scaphoid] bone of right wrist   CC H5

3 ✓7ᵗʰ S62.012 Displaced fracture of distal pole of navicular [scaphoid] bone of left wrist   CC H5

3 ✓7ᵗʰ S62.013 Displaced fracture of distal pole of navicular [scaphoid] bone of unspecified wrist   CC H5

3 ✓7ᵗʰ S62.014 Nondisplaced fracture of distal pole of navicular [scaphoid] bone of right wrist   CC H5

3 ✓7ᵗʰ S62.015 Nondisplaced fracture of distal pole of navicular [scaphoid] bone of left wrist   CC H5

3 ✓7ᵗʰ S62.016 Nondisplaced fracture of distal pole of navicular [scaphoid] bone of unspecified wrist   CC H5

✓6ᵗʰ S62.02 Fracture of middle third of navicular [scaphoid] bone of wrist

3 ✓7ᵗʰ S62.021 Displaced fracture of middle third of navicular [scaphoid] bone of right wrist   CC H5

3 ✓7ᵗʰ S62.022 Displaced fracture of middle third of navicular [scaphoid] bone of left wrist   CC H5

3 ✓7ᵗʰ S62.023 Displaced fracture of middle third of navicular [scaphoid] bone of unspecified wrist   CC H5

3 ✓7ᵗʰ S62.024 Nondisplaced fracture of middle third of navicular [scaphoid] bone of right wrist   CC H5

3 ✓7ᵗʰ S62.025 Nondisplaced fracture of middle third of navicular [scaphoid] bone of left wrist   CC H5

3 ✓7ᵗʰ S62.026 Nondisplaced fracture of middle third of navicular [scaphoid] bone of unspecified wrist   CC H5

✓6ᵗʰ S62.03 Fracture of proximal third of navicular [scaphoid] bone of wrist

3 ✓7ᵗʰ S62.031 Displaced fracture of proximal third of navicular [scaphoid] bone of right wrist   CC H5

3 ✓7ᵗʰ S62.032 Displaced fracture of proximal third of navicular [scaphoid] bone of left wrist   CC H5

3 ✓7ᵗʰ S62.033 Displaced fracture of proximal third of navicular [scaphoid] bone of unspecified wrist   CC H5

3 ✓7ᵗʰ S62.034 Nondisplaced fracture of proximal third of navicular [scaphoid] bone of right wrist   CC H5

3 ✓7ᵗʰ S62.035 Nondisplaced fracture of proximal third of navicular [scaphoid] bone of left wrist   CC H5

3 ✓7ᵗʰ S62.036 Nondisplaced fracture of proximal third of navicular [scaphoid] bone of unspecified wrist   CC H5

✓5ᵗʰ S62.1 Fracture of other and unspecified carpal bone(s)
EXCLUDES 2 *fracture of scaphoid of wrist (S62.0-)*

CC Excl: For codes in subcategory S62.1:
CC with 7th character B: PDX collection 1283
CC with 7th character K or P: PDX collection 897

✓6ᵗʰ S62.10 Fracture of unspecified carpal bone
Fracture of wrist NOS

3 ✓7ᵗʰ S62.101 Fracture of unspecified carpal bone, right wrist   CC H5

3 ✓7ᵗʰ S62.102 Fracture of unspecified carpal bone, left wrist   CC H5
AHA: 2012, 4Q, 95

3 ✓7ᵗʰ S62.109 Fracture of unspecified carpal bone, unspecified wrist   CC H5

✓6ᵗʰ S62.11 Fracture of triquetrum [cuneiform] bone of wrist

3 ✓7ᵗʰ S62.111 Displaced fracture of triquetrum [cuneiform] bone, right wrist   CC H5

3 ✓7ᵗʰ S62.112 Displaced fracture of triquetrum [cuneiform] bone, left wrist   CC H5

3 ✓7ᵗʰ S62.113 Displaced fracture of triquetrum [cuneiform] bone, unspecified wrist   CC H5

3 ✓7ᵗʰ S62.114 Nondisplaced fracture of triquetrum [cuneiform] bone, right wrist   CC H5

3 ✓7ᵗʰ S62.115 Nondisplaced fracture of triquetrum [cuneiform] bone, left wrist   CC H5

3 ✓7ᵗʰ S62.116 Nondisplaced fracture of triquetrum [cuneiform] bone, unspecified wrist   CC H5

✓6ᵗʰ S62.12 Fracture of lunate [semilunar]

3 ✓7ᵗʰ S62.121 Displaced fracture of lunate [semilunar], right wrist   CC H5

3 ✓7ᵗʰ S62.122 Displaced fracture of lunate [semilunar], left wrist   CC H5

3 ✓7ᵗʰ S62.123 Displaced fracture of lunate [semilunar], unspecified wrist   CC H5

3 ✓7ᵗʰ S62.124 Nondisplaced fracture of lunate [semilunar], right wrist   CC H5

3 ✓7ᵗʰ S62.125 Nondisplaced fracture of lunate [semilunar], left wrist   CC H5

3 ✓7ᵗʰ S62.126 Nondisplaced fracture of lunate [semilunar], unspecified wrist   CC H5

✓6ᵗʰ S62.13 Fracture of capitate [os magnum] bone

3 ✓7ᵗʰ S62.131 Displaced fracture of capitate [os magnum] bone, right wrist   CC H5

3 ✓7ᵗʰ S62.132 Displaced fracture of capitate [os magnum] bone, left wrist   CC H5

3 ✓7ᵗʰ S62.133 Displaced fracture of capitate [os magnum] bone, unspecified wrist   CC H5

3 ✓7ᵗʰ S62.134 Nondisplaced fracture of capitate [os magnum] bone, right wrist   CC H5

3 ✓7ᵗʰ S62.135 Nondisplaced fracture of capitate [os magnum] bone, left wrist   CC H5

3 ✓7ᵗʰ S62.136 Nondisplaced fracture of capitate [os magnum] bone, unspecified wrist   CC H5

✓6ᵗʰ S62.14 Fracture of body of hamate [unciform] bone
Fracture of hamate [unciform] bone NOS

3 ✓7ᵗʰ S62.141 Displaced fracture of body of hamate [unciform] bone, right wrist   CC H5

3 ✓7ᵗʰ S62.142 Displaced fracture of body of hamate [unciform] bone, left wrist   CC H5

3 ✓7ᵗʰ S62.143 Displaced fracture of body of hamate [unciform] bone, unspecified wrist   CC H5

3 ✓7ᵗʰ **S62.144** Nondisplaced **fracture of body of** **hamate [unciform] bone, right wrist** CC H5

3 ✓7ᵗʰ **S62.145** Nondisplaced **fracture of body of** **hamate [unciform] bone, left wrist** CC H5

3 ✓7ᵗʰ **S62.146** Nondisplaced **fracture of body of** **hamate [unciform] bone, unspecified wrist** CC H5

✓6ᵗʰ **S62.15** **Fracture of** hook process of hamate [unciform] **bone**
Fracture of unciform process of hamate [unciform] bone

3 ✓7ᵗʰ **S62.151** Displaced **fracture of hook process** CC H5 **of hamate [unciform] bone, right wrist**

3 ✓7ᵗʰ **S62.152** Displaced **fracture of hook process** CC H5 **of hamate [unciform] bone, left wrist**

3 ✓7ᵗʰ **S62.153** Displaced **fracture of hook process** CC H5 **of hamate [unciform] bone,** **unspecified wrist**

3 ✓7ᵗʰ **S62.154** Nondisplaced **fracture of hook** CC H5 **process of hamate [unciform] bone,** **right wrist**

3 ✓7ᵗʰ **S62.155** Nondisplaced **fracture of hook** CC H5 **process of hamate [unciform] bone,** **left wrist**

3 ✓7ᵗʰ **S62.156** Nondisplaced **fracture of hook** CC H5 **process of hamate [unciform] bone,** **unspecified wrist**

✓6ᵗʰ **S62.16** **Fracture of** pisiform

3 ✓7ᵗʰ **S62.161** Displaced **fracture of pisiform,** CC H5 **right wrist**

3 ✓7ᵗʰ **S62.162** Displaced **fracture of pisiform,** CC H5 **left wrist**

3 ✓7ᵗʰ **S62.163** Displaced **fracture of pisiform,** CC H5 **unspecified wrist**

3 ✓7ᵗʰ **S62.164** Nondisplaced **fracture of pisiform,** CC H5 **right wrist**

3 ✓7ᵗʰ **S62.165** Nondisplaced **fracture of pisiform,** CC H5 **left wrist**

3 ✓7ᵗʰ **S62.166** Nondisplaced **fracture of pisiform,** CC H5 **unspecified wrist**

✓6ᵗʰ **S62.17** **Fracture of** trapezium [larger multangular]

3 ✓7ᵗʰ **S62.171** Displaced **fracture of trapezium** CC H5 **[larger multangular], right wrist**

3 ✓7ᵗʰ **S62.172** Displaced **fracture of trapezium** CC H5 **[larger multangular], left wrist**

3 ✓7ᵗʰ **S62.173** Displaced **fracture of trapezium** CC H5 **[larger multangular], unspecified** **wrist**

3 ✓7ᵗʰ **S62.174** Nondisplaced **fracture of trapezium** CC H5 **[larger multangular], right wrist**

3 ✓7ᵗʰ **S62.175** Nondisplaced **fracture of trapezium** CC H5 **[larger multangular], left wrist**

3 ✓7ᵗʰ **S62.176** Nondisplaced **fracture of trapezium** CC H5 **[larger multangular], unspecified wrist**

✓6ᵗʰ **S62.18** **Fracture of** trapezoid [smaller multangular]

3 ✓7ᵗʰ **S62.181** Displaced **fracture of trapezoid** CC H5 **[smaller multangular], right wrist**

3 ✓7ᵗʰ **S62.182** Displaced **fracture of trapezoid** CC H5 **[smaller multangular], left wrist**

3 ✓7ᵗʰ **S62.183** Displaced **fracture of trapezoid** CC H5 **[smaller multangular], unspecified** **wrist**

3 ✓7ᵗʰ **S62.184** Nondisplaced **fracture of trapezoid** CC H5 **[smaller multangular], right wrist**

3 ✓7ᵗʰ **S62.185** Nondisplaced **fracture of trapezoid** CC H5 **[smaller multangular], left wrist**

3 ✓7ᵗʰ **S62.186** Nondisplaced **fracture of trapezoid** CC H5 **[smaller multangular], unspecified** **wrist**

✓5ᵗʰ **S62.2** **Fracture of** first metacarpal **bone**

> **CC Excl: For codes in subcategory S62.2:**
> **CC with 7th character B:** PDX collection 1284
> **CC with 7th character K or P:** PDX collection 897

✓6ᵗʰ **S62.20** Unspecified **fracture of first metacarpal bone**

3 ✓7ᵗʰ **S62.201** Unspecified **fracture of first** CC H5 **metacarpal bone, right hand**

3 ✓7ᵗʰ **S62.202** Unspecified **fracture of first** CC H5 **metacarpal bone, left hand**

3 ✓7ᵗʰ **S62.209** Unspecified **fracture of first** CC H5 **metacarpal bone, unspecified hand**

✓6ᵗʰ **S62.21** Bennett's **fracture**
> **DEF:** Intra-articular, two-part fracture at the base of the first metacarpal bone (thumb) on the ulnar side at the carpometacarpal (CMC) joint.

3 ✓7ᵗʰ **S62.211** **Bennett's fracture, right hand** CC H5

3 ✓7ᵗʰ **S62.212** **Bennett's fracture, left hand** CC H5

3 ✓7ᵗʰ **S62.213** **Bennett's fracture, unspecified** CC H5 **hand**

✓6ᵗʰ **S62.22** Rolando's **fracture**
> **DEF:** Comminuted, three part intra-articular fracture at the base of the thumb metacarpal.

3 ✓7ᵗʰ **S62.221** Displaced **Rolando's fracture,** CC H5 **right hand**

3 ✓7ᵗʰ **S62.222** Displaced **Rolando's fracture, left** CC H5 **hand**

3 ✓7ᵗʰ **S62.223** Displaced **Rolando's fracture,** CC H5 **unspecified hand**

3 ✓7ᵗʰ **S62.224** Nondisplaced **Rolando's fracture,** CC H5 **right hand**

3 ✓7ᵗʰ **S62.225** Nondisplaced **Rolando's fracture,** CC H5 **left hand**

3 ✓7ᵗʰ **S62.226** Nondisplaced **Rolando's fracture,** CC H5 **unspecified hand**

✓6ᵗʰ **S62.23** Other **fracture of** base of first metacarpal bone

3 ✓7ᵗʰ **S62.231** Other displaced **fracture of base of** CC H5 **first metacarpal bone, right hand**

3 ✓7ᵗʰ **S62.232** Other displaced **fracture of base of** CC H5 **first metacarpal bone, left hand**

3 ✓7ᵗʰ **S62.233** Other displaced **fracture of base of** CC H5 **first metacarpal bone, unspecified** **hand**

3 ✓7ᵗʰ **S62.234** Other nondisplaced **fracture of** CC H5 **base of first metacarpal bone, right hand**

3 ✓7ᵗʰ **S62.235** Other nondisplaced **fracture of** CC H5 **base of first metacarpal bone, left hand**

3 ✓7ᵗʰ **S62.236** Other nondisplaced **fracture of** CC H5 **base of first metacarpal bone,** **unspecified hand**

✓6ᵗʰ **S62.24** **Fracture of** shaft of first metacarpal bone

3 ✓7ᵗʰ **S62.241** Displaced **fracture of shaft of first** CC H5 **metacarpal bone, right hand**

3 ✓7ᵗʰ **S62.242** Displaced **fracture of shaft of first** CC H5 **metacarpal bone, left hand**

3 ✓7ᵗʰ **S62.243** Displaced **fracture of shaft of first** CC H5 **metacarpal bone, unspecified hand**

3 ✓7ᵗʰ **S62.244** Nondisplaced **fracture of shaft of** CC H5 **first metacarpal bone, right hand**

3 ✓7ᵗʰ **S62.245** Nondisplaced **fracture of shaft of** CC H5 **first metacarpal bone, left hand**

3 ✓7ᵗʰ **S62.246** Nondisplaced **fracture of shaft of** CC H5 **first metacarpal bone, unspecified** **hand**

✓6ᵗʰ **S62.25** **Fracture of** neck of first metacarpal bone

3 ✓7ᵗʰ **S62.251** Displaced **fracture of neck of first** CC H5 **metacarpal bone, right hand**

3 ✓7ᵗʰ **S62.252** Displaced **fracture of neck of first** CC H5 **metacarpal bone, left hand**

3 ✓7ᵗʰ **S62.253** Displaced **fracture of neck of first** CC H5 **metacarpal bone, unspecified hand**

3 ✓7ᵗʰ **S62.254** Nondisplaced **fracture of neck of** CC H5 **first metacarpal bone, right hand**

3 ✓7ᵗʰ **S62.255** Nondisplaced **fracture of neck of** CC H5 **first metacarpal bone, left hand**

3 ✓7ᵗʰ **S62.256** Nondisplaced **fracture of neck of** CC H5 **first metacarpal bone, unspecified** **hand**

✓6ᵗʰ **S62.29** Other **fracture of** first metacarpal bone

3 ✓7ᵗʰ **S62.291** Other **fracture of first metacarpal** CC H5 **bone, right hand**

3 ✓7ᵗʰ **S62.292** Other **fracture of first metacarpal** CC H5 **bone, left hand**

3 ✓7ᵗʰ **S62.299** Other **fracture of first metacarpal** CC H5 **bone, unspecified hand**

✔ Additional Character Required   ✓ₓ7ᵗʰ Placeholder   Unacceptable PDx   Questionable PDx   Manifestation   **H1**-**H14** HAC   **HCC** CMS-HCC Dx   **HIV** HIV Dx

ICD-10-CM 2019   **1023**

✓5ᵗʰ **S62.3** **Fracture of** other and unspecified metacarpal **bone**

> EXCLUDES 2   *fracture of first metacarpal bone (S62.2-)*

> **CC Excl: For codes in subcategory S62.3:**
> **CC with 7th character B:** PDX collection 1284
> **CC with 7th character K or P:** PDX collection 897

✓6ᵗʰ **S62.30** Unspecified **fracture of other metacarpal bone**

- 3 ✓7ᵗʰ **S62.300** **Unspecified fracture of** second **metacarpal bone, right hand**   CC H5
- 3 ✓7ᵗʰ **S62.301** **Unspecified fracture of** second **metacarpal bone, left hand**   CC H5
- 3 ✓7ᵗʰ **S62.302** **Unspecified fracture of** third **metacarpal bone, right hand**   CC H5
- 3 ✓7ᵗʰ **S62.303** **Unspecified fracture of** third **metacarpal bone, left hand**   CC H5
- 3 ✓7ᵗʰ **S62.304** **Unspecified fracture of** fourth **metacarpal bone, right hand**   CC H5
- 3 ✓7ᵗʰ **S62.305** **Unspecified fracture of** fourth **metacarpal bone, left hand**   CC H5
- 3 ✓7ᵗʰ **S62.306** **Unspecified fracture of** fifth **metacarpal bone, right hand**   CC H5
- 3 ✓7ᵗʰ **S62.307** **Unspecified fracture of** fifth **metacarpal bone, left hand**   CC H5
- 3 ✓7ᵗʰ **S62.308** **Unspecified fracture of** other **metacarpal bone**   CC H5
  > Unspecified fracture of specified metacarpal bone with unspecified laterality
- 3 ✓7ᵗʰ **S62.309** **Unspecified fracture of** unspecified **metacarpal bone**   CC H5

✓6ᵗʰ **S62.31** Displaced **fracture of** base **of other metacarpal bone**

- 3 ✓7ᵗʰ **S62.37** **Displaced fracture of base of** second **metacarpal bone, right hand**   CC H5
- 3 ✓7ᵗʰ **S62.311** **Displaced fracture of base of** second **metacarpal bone, left hand**   CC H5
- 3 ✓7ᵗʰ **S62.312** **Displaced fracture of base of** third **metacarpal bone, right hand**   CC H5
- 3 ✓7ᵗʰ **S62.313** **Displaced fracture of base of** third **metacarpal bone, left hand**   CC H5
- 3 ✓7ᵗʰ **S62.314** **Displaced fracture of base of** fourth **metacarpal bone, right hand**   CC H5
- 3 ✓7ᵗʰ **S62.315** **Displaced fracture of base of** fourth **metacarpal bone, left hand**   CC H5
- 3 ✓7ᵗʰ **S62.316** **Displaced fracture of base of** fifth **metacarpal bone, right hand**   CC H5
- 3 ✓7ᵗʰ **S62.317** **Displaced fracture of base of** fifth **metacarpal bone, left hand**   CC H5
- 3 ✓7ᵗʰ **S62.318** **Displaced fracture of base of** other **metacarpal bone**   CC H5
  > Displaced fracture of base of specified metacarpal bone with unspecified laterality
- 3 ✓7ᵗʰ **S62.319** **Displaced fracture of base of** unspecified **metacarpal bone**   CC H5

✓6ᵗʰ **S62.32** Displaced **fracture of** shaft **of other metacarpal bone**

- 3 ✓7ᵗʰ **S62.320** **Displaced fracture of shaft of** second **metacarpal bone, right hand**   CC H5
- 3 ✓7ᵗʰ **S62.321** **Displaced fracture of shaft of** second **metacarpal bone, left hand**   CC H5
- 3 ✓7ᵗʰ **S62.322** **Displaced fracture of shaft of** third **metacarpal bone, right hand**   CC H5
- 3 ✓7ᵗʰ **S62.323** **Displaced fracture of shaft of** third **metacarpal bone, left hand**   CC H5
- 3 ✓7ᵗʰ **S62.324** **Displaced fracture of shaft of** fourth **metacarpal bone, right hand**   CC H5
- 3 ✓7ᵗʰ **S62.325** **Displaced fracture of shaft of** fourth **metacarpal bone, left hand**   CC H5
- 3 ✓7ᵗʰ **S62.326** **Displaced fracture of shaft of** fifth **metacarpal bone, right hand**   CC H5
- 3 ✓7ᵗʰ **S62.327** **Displaced fracture of shaft of** fifth **metacarpal bone, left hand**   CC H5
- 3 ✓7ᵗʰ **S62.328** **Displaced fracture of shaft of** other **metacarpal bone**   CC H5
  > Displaced fracture of shaft of specified metacarpal bone with unspecified laterality

- 3 ✓7ᵗʰ **S62.329** **Displaced fracture of shaft of** unspecified **metacarpal bone**   CC H5

✓6ᵗʰ **S62.33** Displaced **fracture of neck of other metacarpal bone**

- 3 ✓7ᵗʰ **S62.330** **Displaced fracture of neck of** second **metacarpal bone, right hand**   CC H5
- 3 ✓7ᵗʰ **S62.331** **Displaced fracture of neck of** second **metacarpal bone, left hand**   CC H5
- 3 ✓7ᵗʰ **S62.332** **Displaced fracture of neck of** third **metacarpal bone, right hand**   CC H5
- 3 ✓7ᵗʰ **S62.333** **Displaced fracture of neck of** third **metacarpal bone, left hand**   CC H5
- 3 ✓7ᵗʰ **S62.334** **Displaced fracture of neck of** fourth **metacarpal bone, right hand**   CC H5
- 3 ✓7ᵗʰ **S62.335** **Displaced fracture of neck of** fourth **metacarpal bone, left hand**   CC H5
- 3 ✓7ᵗʰ **S62.336** **Displaced fracture of neck of** fifth **metacarpal bone, right hand**   CC H5
- 3 ✓7ᵗʰ **S62.337** **Displaced fracture of neck of** fifth **metacarpal bone, left hand**   CC H5
- 3 ✓7ᵗʰ **S62.338** **Displaced fracture of neck of** other **metacarpal bone**   CC H5
  > Displaced fracture of neck of specified metacarpal bone with unspecified laterality
- 3 ✓7ᵗʰ **S62.339** **Displaced fracture of neck of** unspecified **metacarpal bone**   CC H5

✓6ᵗʰ **S62.34** Nondisplaced **fracture of** base **of other metacarpal bone**

- 3 ✓7ᵗʰ **S62.340** **Nondisplaced fracture of base of** second **metacarpal bone, right hand**   CC H5
- 3 ✓7ᵗʰ **S62.341** **Nondisplaced fracture of base of** second **metacarpal bone, left hand**   CC H5
- 3 ✓7ᵗʰ **S62.342** **Nondisplaced fracture of base of** third **metacarpal bone, right hand**   CC H5
- 3 ✓7ᵗʰ **S62.343** **Nondisplaced fracture of base of** third **metacarpal bone, left hand**   CC H5
- 3 ✓7ᵗʰ **S62.344** **Nondisplaced fracture of base of** fourth **metacarpal bone, right hand**   CC H5
- 3 ✓7ᵗʰ **S62.345** **Nondisplaced fracture of base of** fourth **metacarpal bone, left hand**   CC H5
- 3 ✓7ᵗʰ **S62.346** **Nondisplaced fracture of base of** fifth **metacarpal bone, right hand**   CC H5
- 3 ✓7ᵗʰ **S62.347** **Nondisplaced fracture of base of** fifth **metacarpal bone, left hand**   CC H5
- 3 ✓7ᵗʰ **S62.348** **Nondisplaced fracture of base of** other **metacarpal bone**   CC H5
  > Nondisplaced fracture of base of specified metacarpal bone with unspecified laterality
- 3 ✓7ᵗʰ **S62.349** **Nondisplaced fracture of base of** unspecified **metacarpal bone**   CC H5

✓6ᵗʰ **S62.35** Nondisplaced **fracture of** shaft **of other metacarpal bone**

- 3 ✓7ᵗʰ **S62.350** **Nondisplaced fracture of shaft of** second **metacarpal bone, right hand**   CC H5
- 3 ✓7ᵗʰ **S62.351** **Nondisplaced fracture of shaft of** second **metacarpal bone, left hand**   CC H5
- 3 ✓7ᵗʰ **S62.352** **Nondisplaced fracture of shaft of** third **metacarpal bone, right hand**   CC H5
- 3 ✓7ᵗʰ **S62.353** **Nondisplaced fracture of shaft of** third **metacarpal bone, left hand**   CC H5
- 3 ✓7ᵗʰ **S62.354** **Nondisplaced fracture of shaft of** fourth **metacarpal bone, right hand**   CC H5
- 3 ✓7ᵗʰ **S62.355** **Nondisplaced fracture of shaft of** fourth **metacarpal bone, left hand**   CC H5
- 3 ✓7ᵗʰ **S62.356** **Nondisplaced fracture of shaft of** fifth **metacarpal bone, right hand**   CC H5
- 3 ✓7ᵗʰ **S62.357** **Nondisplaced fracture of shaft of** fifth **metacarpal bone, left hand**   CC H5
- 3 ✓7ᵗʰ **S62.358** **Nondisplaced fracture of shaft of** other **metacarpal bone**   CC H5
  > Nondisplaced fracture of shaft of specified metacarpal bone with unspecified laterality
- 3 ✓7ᵗʰ **S62.359** **Nondisplaced fracture of shaft of** unspecified **metacarpal bone**   CC H5

N Newborn: 0   P Pediatric: 0-17   M Maternity: 12-55   A Adult: 15-124   MCC Major Complication/Comorbidity   CC Complication/Comorbidity   SW Severe Wound Dx

1024   ICD-10-CM 2019

√6th **S62.36** Nondisplaced fracture of neck of other metacarpal bone

- 3   √7th   **S62.360**   **Nondisplaced fracture of neck of second metacarpal bone, right hand** `CC` `H5`
- 3   √7th   **S62.361**   **Nondisplaced fracture of neck of second metacarpal bone, left hand** `CC` `H5`
- 3   √7th   **S62.362**   **Nondisplaced fracture of neck of third metacarpal bone, right hand** `CC` `H5`
- 3   √7th   **S62.363**   **Nondisplaced fracture of neck of third metacarpal bone, left hand** `CC` `H5`
- 3   √7th   **S62.364**   **Nondisplaced fracture of neck of fourth metacarpal bone, right hand** `CC` `H5`
- 3   √7th   **S62.365**   **Nondisplaced fracture of neck of fourth metacarpal bone, left hand** `CC` `H5`
- 3   √7th   **S62.366**   **Nondisplaced fracture of neck of fifth metacarpal bone, right hand** `CC` `H5`
- 3   √7th   **S62.367**   **Nondisplaced fracture of neck of fifth metacarpal bone, left hand** `CC` `H5`
- 3   √7th   **S62.368**   **Nondisplaced fracture of neck of other metacarpal bone** `CC` `H5`
  Nondisplaced fracture of neck of specified metacarpal bone with unspecified laterality
- 3   √7th   **S62.369**   **Nondisplaced fracture of neck of unspecified metacarpal bone** `CC` `H5`

√6th **S62.39** Other fracture of other metacarpal bone

- 3   √7th   **S62.390**   **Other fracture of second metacarpal bone, right hand** `CC` `H5`
- 3   √7th   **S62.391**   **Other fracture of second metacarpal bone, left hand** `CC` `H5`
- 3   √7th   **S62.392**   **Other fracture of third metacarpal bone, right hand** `CC` `H5`
- 3   √7th   **S62.393**   **Other fracture of third metacarpal bone, left hand** `CC` `H5`
- 3   √7th   **S62.394**   **Other fracture of fourth metacarpal bone, right hand** `CC` `H5`
- 3   √7th   **S62.395**   **Other fracture of fourth metacarpal bone, left hand** `CC` `H5`
- 3   √7th   **S62.396**   **Other fracture of fifth metacarpal bone, right hand** `CC` `H5`
- 3   √7th   **S62.397**   **Other fracture of fifth metacarpal bone, left hand** `CC` `H5`
- 3   √7th   **S62.398**   **Other fracture of other metacarpal bone** `CC` `H5`
  Other fracture of specified metacarpal bone with unspecified laterality
- 3   √7th   **S62.399**   **Other fracture of unspecified metacarpal bone** `CC` `H5`

√5th **S62.5** Fracture of thumb

> **CC Excl: For codes in subcategory S62.5:**
> **CC with 7th character B:** PDX collection 1285
> **CC with 7th character K or P:** PDX collection 897

√6th **S62.50** Fracture of unspecified phalanx of thumb

- 3   √7th   **S62.501**   **Fracture of unspecified phalanx of right thumb** `CC` `H5`
- 3   √7th   **S62.502**   **Fracture of unspecified phalanx of left thumb** `CC` `H5`
- 3   √7th   **S62.509**   **Fracture of unspecified phalanx of unspecified thumb** `CC` `H5`

√6th **S62.51** Fracture of proximal phalanx of thumb

- 3   √7th   **S62.511**   **Displaced fracture of proximal phalanx of right thumb** `CC` `H5`
- 3   √7th   **S62.512**   **Displaced fracture of proximal phalanx of left thumb** `CC` `H5`
- 3   √7th   **S62.513**   **Displaced fracture of proximal phalanx of unspecified thumb** `CC` `H5`
- 3   √7th   **S62.514**   **Nondisplaced fracture of proximal phalanx of right thumb** `CC` `H5`
- 3   √7th   **S62.515**   **Nondisplaced fracture of proximal phalanx of left thumb** `CC` `H5`
- 3   √7th   **S62.516**   **Nondisplaced fracture of proximal phalanx of unspecified thumb** `CC` `H5`

√6th **S62.52** Fracture of distal phalanx of thumb

- 3   √7th   **S62.521**   **Displaced fracture of distal phalanx of right thumb** `CC` `H5`
- 3   √7th   **S62.522**   **Displaced fracture of distal phalanx of left thumb** `CC` `H5`
- 3   √7th   **S62.523**   **Displaced fracture of distal phalanx of unspecified thumb** `CC` `H5`
- 3   √7th   **S62.524**   **Nondisplaced fracture of distal phalanx of right thumb** `CC` `H5`
- 3   √7th   **S62.525**   **Nondisplaced fracture of distal phalanx of left thumb** `CC` `H5`
- 3   √7th   **S62.526**   **Nondisplaced fracture of distal phalanx of unspecified thumb** `CC` `H5`

√5th **S62.6** Fracture of other and unspecified finger(s)

    EXCLUDES 2   fracture of thumb (S62.5-)

> **CC Excl: For codes in subcategory S62.6:**
> **CC with 7th character B:** PDX collection 1285
> **CC with 7th character K or P:** PDX collection 897

√6th **S62.60** Fracture of unspecified phalanx of finger

- 3   √7th   **S62.600**   **Fracture of unspecified phalanx of right index finger** `CC` `H5`
- 3   √7th   **S62.601**   **Fracture of unspecified phalanx of left index finger** `CC` `H5`
- 3   √7th   **S62.602**   **Fracture of unspecified phalanx of right middle finger** `CC` `H5`
- 3   √7th   **S62.603**   **Fracture of unspecified phalanx of left middle finger** `CC` `H5`
- 3   √7th   **S62.604**   **Fracture of unspecified phalanx of right ring finger** `CC` `H5`
- 3   √7th   **S62.605**   **Fracture of unspecified phalanx of left ring finger** `CC` `H5`
- 3   √7th   **S62.606**   **Fracture of unspecified phalanx of right little finger** `CC` `H5`
- 3   √7th   **S62.607**   **Fracture of unspecified phalanx of left little finger** `CC` `H5`
- 3   √7th   **S62.608**   **Fracture of unspecified phalanx of other finger** `CC` `H5`
  Fracture of unspecified phalanx of specified finger with unspecified laterality
- 3   √7th   **S62.609**   **Fracture of unspecified phalanx of unspecified finger** `CC` `H5`

√6th **S62.61** Displaced fracture of proximal phalanx of finger

- 3   √7th   **S62.610**   **Displaced fracture of proximal phalanx of right index finger** `CC` `H5`
- 3   √7th   **S62.611**   **Displaced fracture of proximal phalanx of left index finger** `CC` `H5`
- 3   √7th   **S62.612**   **Displaced fracture of proximal phalanx of right middle finger** `CC` `H5`
- 3   √7th   **S62.613**   **Displaced fracture of proximal phalanx of left middle finger** `CC` `H5`
- 3   √7th   **S62.614**   **Displaced fracture of proximal phalanx of right ring finger** `CC` `H5`
- 3   √7th   **S62.615**   **Displaced fracture of proximal phalanx of left ring finger** `CC` `H5`
- 3   √7th   **S62.616**   **Displaced fracture of proximal phalanx of right little finger** `CC` `H5`
- 3   √7th   **S62.617**   **Displaced fracture of proximal phalanx of left little finger** `CC` `H5`
- 3   √7th   **S62.618**   **Displaced fracture of proximal phalanx of other finger** `CC` `H5`
  Displaced fracture of proximal phalanx of specified finger with unspecified laterality
- 3   √7th   **S62.619**   **Displaced fracture of proximal phalanx of unspecified finger** `CC` `H5`

√6th **S62.62** Displaced fracture of middle phalanx of finger

- 3   √7th   **S62.620**   **Displaced fracture of middle phalanx of right index finger** `CC` `H5`
- 3   √7th   **S62.621**   **Displaced fracture of middle phalanx of left index finger** `CC` `H5`
- 3   √7th   **S62.622**   **Displaced fracture of middle phalanx of right middle finger** `CC` `H5`
- 3   √7th   **S62.623**   **Displaced fracture of middle phalanx of left middle finger** `CC` `H5`
- 3   √7th   **S62.624**   **Displaced fracture of middle phalanx of right ring finger** `CC` `H5`
- 3   √7th   **S62.625**   **Displaced fracture of middle phalanx of left ring finger** `CC` `H5`

✓ Additional Character Required   √x7th Placeholder   Unacceptable PDx   Questionable PDx   Manifestation   `H1`-`H14` HAC   `HCC` CMS-HCC Dx   `HIV` HIV Dx

ICD-10-CM 2019   1025

▲   3   ✓7ᵗʰ   **S62.626**   **Displaced fracture of middle phalanx of right little finger**   `CC` `H5`

▲   3   ✓7ᵗʰ   **S62.627**   **Displaced fracture of middle phalanx of left little finger**   `CC` `H5`

▲   3   ✓7ᵗʰ   **S62.628**   **Displaced fracture of middle phalanx of other finger**   `CC` `H5`
    ▶Displaced fracture of middle phalanx of specified finger with unspecified laterality◀

▲   3   ✓7ᵗʰ   **S62.629**   **Displaced fracture of middle phalanx of unspecified finger**   `CC` `H5`

✓6ᵗʰ   **S62.63**   Displaced **fracture of distal phalanx** of finger

   3   ✓7ᵗʰ   **S62.630**   **Displaced fracture of distal phalanx of right index finger**   `CC` `H5`

   3   ✓7ᵗʰ   **S62.631**   **Displaced fracture of distal phalanx of left index finger**   `CC` `H5`

   3   ✓7ᵗʰ   **S62.632**   **Displaced fracture of distal phalanx of right middle finger**   `CC` `H5`

   3   ✓7ᵗʰ   **S62.633**   **Displaced fracture of distal phalanx of left middle finger**   `CC` `H5`

   3   ✓7ᵗʰ   **S62.634**   **Displaced fracture of distal phalanx of right ring finger**   `CC` `H5`

   3   ✓7ᵗʰ   **S62.635**   **Displaced fracture of distal phalanx of left ring finger**   `CC` `H5`

   3   ✓7ᵗʰ   **S62.636**   **Displaced fracture of distal phalanx of right little finger**   `CC` `H5`

   3   ✓7ᵗʰ   **S62.637**   **Displaced fracture of distal phalanx of left little finger**   `CC` `H5`

   3   ✓7ᵗʰ   **S62.638**   **Displaced fracture of distal phalanx of other finger**   `CC` `H5`
    Displaced fracture of distal phalanx of specified finger with unspecified laterality

   3   ✓7ᵗʰ   **S62.639**   **Displaced fracture of distal phalanx of unspecified finger**   `CC` `H5`

✓6ᵗʰ   **S62.64**   Nondisplaced **fracture of proximal phalanx** of finger

   3   ✓7ᵗʰ   **S62.640**   **Nondisplaced fracture of proximal phalanx of right index finger**   `CC` `H5`

   3   ✓7ᵗʰ   **S62.641**   **Nondisplaced fracture of proximal phalanx of left index finger**   `CC` `H5`

   3   ✓7ᵗʰ   **S62.642**   **Nondisplaced fracture of proximal phalanx of right middle finger**   `CC` `H5`

   3   ✓7ᵗʰ   **S62.643**   **Nondisplaced fracture of proximal phalanx of left middle finger**   `CC` `H5`

   3   ✓7ᵗʰ   **S62.644**   **Nondisplaced fracture of proximal phalanx of right ring finger**   `CC` `H5`

   3   ✓7ᵗʰ   **S62.645**   **Nondisplaced fracture of proximal phalanx of left ring finger**   `CC` `H5`

   3   ✓7ᵗʰ   **S62.646**   **Nondisplaced fracture of proximal phalanx of right little finger**   `CC` `H5`

   3   ✓7ᵗʰ   **S62.647**   **Nondisplaced fracture of proximal phalanx of left little finger**   `CC` `H5`

   3   ✓7ᵗʰ   **S62.648**   **Nondisplaced fracture of proximal phalanx of other finger**   `CC` `H5`
    Nondisplaced fracture of proximal phalanx of specified finger with unspecified laterality

   3   ✓7ᵗʰ   **S62.649**   **Nondisplaced fracture of proximal phalanx of unspecified finger**   `CC` `H5`

✓6ᵗʰ   **S62.65**   Nondisplaced **fracture of middle phalanx** of finger

   3   ✓7ᵗʰ   **S62.650**   **Nondisplaced fracture of middle phalanx of right index finger**   `CC` `H5`

   3   ✓7ᵗʰ   **S62.651**   **Nondisplaced fracture of middle phalanx of left index finger**   `CC` `H5`

   3   ✓7ᵗʰ   **S62.652**   **Nondisplaced fracture of middle phalanx of right middle finger**   `CC` `H5`

   3   ✓7ᵗʰ   **S62.653**   **Nondisplaced fracture of middle phalanx of left middle finger**   `CC` `H5`

▲   3   ✓7ᵗʰ   **S62.654**   **Nondisplaced fracture of middle phalanx of right ring finger**   `CC` `H5`

▲   3   ✓7ᵗʰ   **S62.655**   **Nondisplaced fracture of middle phalanx of left ring finger**   `CC` `H5`

▲   3   ✓7ᵗʰ   **S62.656**   **Nondisplaced fracture of middle phalanx of right little finger**   `CC` `H5`

▲   3   ✓7ᵗʰ   **S62.657**   **Nondisplaced fracture of middle phalanx of left little finger**   `CC` `H5`

▲   3   ✓7ᵗʰ   **S62.658**   **Nondisplaced fracture of middle phalanx of other finger**   `CC` `H5`
    ▶Nondisplaced fracture of middle phalanx of specified finger with unspecified laterality◀

▲   3   ✓7ᵗʰ   **S62.659**   **Nondisplaced fracture of middle phalanx of unspecified finger**   `CC` `H5`

✓6ᵗʰ   **S62.66**   Nondisplaced **fracture of distal phalanx** of finger

   3   ✓7ᵗʰ   **S62.660**   **Nondisplaced fracture of distal phalanx of right index finger**   `CC` `H5`

   3   ✓7ᵗʰ   **S62.661**   **Nondisplaced fracture of distal phalanx of left index finger**   `CC` `H5`

   3   ✓7ᵗʰ   **S62.662**   **Nondisplaced fracture of distal phalanx of right middle finger**   `CC` `H5`

   3   ✓7ᵗʰ   **S62.663**   **Nondisplaced fracture of distal phalanx of left middle finger**   `CC` `H5`

   3   ✓7ᵗʰ   **S62.664**   **Nondisplaced fracture of distal phalanx of right ring finger**   `CC` `H5`

   3   ✓7ᵗʰ   **S62.665**   **Nondisplaced fracture of distal phalanx of left ring finger**   `CC` `H5`

   3   ✓7ᵗʰ   **S62.666**   **Nondisplaced fracture of distal phalanx of right little finger**   `CC` `H5`

   3   ✓7ᵗʰ   **S62.667**   **Nondisplaced fracture of distal phalanx of left little finger**   `CC` `H5`

   3   ✓7ᵗʰ   **S62.668**   **Nondisplaced fracture of distal phalanx of other finger**   `CC` `H5`
    Nondisplaced fracture of distal phalanx of specified finger with unspecified laterality

   3   ✓7ᵗʰ   **S62.669**   **Nondisplaced fracture of distal phalanx of unspecified finger**   `CC` `H5`

✓5ᵗʰ   **S62.9**   **Unspecified fracture of wrist and hand**

   3   ✓x7ᵗʰ   **S62.90**   **Unspecified fracture of unspecified wrist and hand**   `CC` `H5`
    CC Excl: CC with 7th character B: PDX collection 1286
    CC with 7th character K or P: PDX collection 897

   3   ✓x7ᵗʰ   **S62.91**   **Unspecified fracture of right wrist and hand**   `CC` `H5`
    CC Excl: CC with 7th character B: PDX collection 1287
    CC with 7th character K or P: PDX collection 897

   3   ✓x7ᵗʰ   **S62.92**   **Unspecified fracture of left wrist and hand**   `CC` `H5`
    CC Excl: CC with 7th character B: PDX collection 1287
    CC with 7th character K or P: PDX collection 897

✓4ᵗʰ   **S63**   **Dislocation and sprain of joints and ligaments at wrist and hand level**

    `INCLUDES`   avulsion of joint or ligament at wrist and hand level
         laceration of cartilage, joint or ligament at wrist and hand level
         sprain of cartilage, joint or ligament at wrist and hand level
         traumatic hemarthrosis of joint or ligament at wrist and hand level
         traumatic rupture of joint or ligament at wrist and hand level
         traumatic subluxation of joint or ligament at wrist and hand level
         traumatic tear of joint or ligament at wrist and hand level

    Code also any associated open wound

    EXCLUDES 2   strain of muscle, fascia and tendon of wrist and hand (S66.-)

    The appropriate 7th character is to be added to each code from category S63.
    A   initial encounter
    D   subsequent encounter
    S   sequela

✓5ᵗʰ   **S63.0**   **Subluxation and dislocation of wrist and hand joints**

   ✓6ᵗʰ   **S63.00**   Unspecified **subluxation and dislocation of wrist and hand**
    Dislocation of carpal bone NOS
    Dislocation of distal end of radius NOS
    Subluxation of carpal bone NOS
    Subluxation of distal end of radius NOS

    ✓7ᵗʰ   **S63.001**   **Unspecified subluxation of right wrist and hand**

    ✓7ᵗʰ   **S63.002**   **Unspecified subluxation of left wrist and hand**

    ✓7ᵗʰ   **S63.003**   **Unspecified subluxation of unspecified wrist and hand**

    ✓7ᵗʰ   **S63.004**   **Unspecified dislocation of right wrist and hand**

    ✓7ᵗʰ   **S63.005**   **Unspecified dislocation of left wrist and hand**

N Newborn: 0   **P** Pediatric: 0-17   **M** Maternity: 12-55   **A** Adult: 15-124   **MCC** Major Complication/Comorbidity   **CC** Complication/Comorbidity   **SW** Severe Wound Dx

1026   ICD-10-CM 2019

☑6ᵗʰ **S63.006** **Unspecified** dislocation of unspecified **wrist and hand**

☑6ᵗʰ **S63.01** **Subluxation and dislocation of** distal radioulnar **joint**

☑7ᵗʰ **S63.011** Subluxation of distal radioulnar joint of right **wrist**

☑7ᵗʰ **S63.012** Subluxation of distal radioulnar joint of left **wrist**

☑7ᵗʰ **S63.013** Subluxation of distal radioulnar joint of unspecified **wrist**

☑7ᵗʰ **S63.014** Dislocation of distal radioulnar joint of right **wrist**

☑7ᵗʰ **S63.015** Dislocation of distal radioulnar joint of left **wrist**

☑7ᵗʰ **S63.016** Dislocation of distal radioulnar joint of unspecified **wrist**

☑6ᵗʰ **S63.02** **Subluxation and dislocation of** radiocarpal **joint**

☑7ᵗʰ **S63.021** Subluxation of radiocarpal joint of right **wrist**

☑7ᵗʰ **S63.022** Subluxation of radiocarpal joint of left **wrist**

☑7ᵗʰ **S63.023** Subluxation of radiocarpal joint of unspecified **wrist**

☑7ᵗʰ **S63.024** Dislocation of radiocarpal joint of right **wrist**

☑7ᵗʰ **S63.025** Dislocation of radiocarpal joint of left **wrist**

☑7ᵗʰ **S63.026** Dislocation of radiocarpal joint of unspecified **wrist**

☑6ᵗʰ **S63.03** **Subluxation and dislocation of** midcarpal **joint**

☑7ᵗʰ **S63.031** Subluxation of midcarpal joint of right **wrist**

☑7ᵗʰ **S63.032** Subluxation of midcarpal joint of left **wrist**

☑7ᵗʰ **S63.033** Subluxation of midcarpal joint of unspecified **wrist**

☑7ᵗʰ **S63.034** Dislocation of midcarpal joint of right **wrist**

☑7ᵗʰ **S63.035** Dislocation of midcarpal joint of left **wrist**

☑7ᵗʰ **S63.036** Dislocation of midcarpal joint of unspecified **wrist**

☑6ᵗʰ **S63.04** **Subluxation and dislocation of** carpometacarpal **joint of** thumb

    EXCLUDES 2   *interphalangeal subluxation and dislocation of thumb (S63.1-)*

☑7ᵗʰ **S63.041** Subluxation of carpometacarpal joint of right **thumb**

☑7ᵗʰ **S63.042** Subluxation of carpometacarpal joint of left **thumb**

☑7ᵗʰ **S63.043** Subluxation of carpometacarpal joint of unspecified **thumb**

☑7ᵗʰ **S63.044** Dislocation of carpometacarpal joint of right **thumb**

☑7ᵗʰ **S63.045** Dislocation of carpometacarpal joint of left **thumb**

☑7ᵗʰ **S63.046** Dislocation of carpometacarpal joint of unspecified **thumb**

☑6ᵗʰ **S63.05** **Subluxation and dislocation of** other carpometacarpal **joint**

    EXCLUDES 2   *subluxation and dislocation of carpometacarpal joint of thumb (S63.04-)*

☑7ᵗʰ **S63.051** Subluxation of other carpometacarpal joint of right **hand**

☑7ᵗʰ **S63.052** Subluxation of other carpometacarpal joint of left **hand**

☑7ᵗʰ **S63.053** Subluxation of other carpometacarpal joint of unspecified **hand**

☑7ᵗʰ **S63.054** Dislocation of other carpometacarpal joint of right **hand**

☑7ᵗʰ **S63.055** Dislocation of other carpometacarpal joint of left **hand**

☑7ᵗʰ **S63.056** Dislocation of other carpometacarpal joint of unspecified **hand**

☑6ᵗʰ **S63.06** **Subluxation and dislocation of** metacarpal (bone), proximal end

☑7ᵗʰ **S63.061** Subluxation of metacarpal (bone), proximal end of right **hand**

☑7ᵗʰ **S63.062** Subluxation of metacarpal (bone), proximal end of left **hand**

☑7ᵗʰ **S63.063** Subluxation of metacarpal (bone), proximal end of unspecified **hand**

☑7ᵗʰ **S63.064** Dislocation of metacarpal (bone), proximal end of right **hand**

☑7ᵗʰ **S63.065** Dislocation of metacarpal (bone), proximal end of left **hand**

☑7ᵗʰ **S63.066** Dislocation of metacarpal (bone), proximal end of unspecified **hand**

☑6ᵗʰ **S63.07** **Subluxation and dislocation of** distal end of ulna

☑7ᵗʰ **S63.071** Subluxation of distal end of right **ulna**

☑7ᵗʰ **S63.072** Subluxation of distal end of left **ulna**

☑7ᵗʰ **S63.073** Subluxation of distal end of unspecified **ulna**

☑7ᵗʰ **S63.074** Dislocation of distal end of right **ulna**

☑7ᵗʰ **S63.075** Dislocation of distal end of left **ulna**

☑7ᵗʰ **S63.076** Dislocation of distal end of unspecified **ulna**

☑6ᵗʰ **S63.09** **Other** subluxation and dislocation of wrist and hand

☑7ᵗʰ **S63.091** **Other** subluxation of right **wrist and hand**

☑7ᵗʰ **S63.092** **Other** subluxation of left **wrist and hand**

☑7ᵗʰ **S63.093** **Other** subluxation of unspecified **wrist and hand**

☑7ᵗʰ **S63.094** **Other** dislocation of right **wrist and hand**

☑7ᵗʰ **S63.095** **Other** dislocation of left **wrist and hand**

☑7ᵗʰ **S63.096** **Other** dislocation of unspecified **wrist and hand**

☑5ᵗʰ **S63.1** **Subluxation and dislocation of** thumb

☑6ᵗʰ **S63.10** **Unspecified** subluxation and dislocation of thumb

☑7ᵗʰ **S63.101** **Unspecified** subluxation of right **thumb**

☑7ᵗʰ **S63.102** **Unspecified** subluxation of left **thumb**

☑7ᵗʰ **S63.103** **Unspecified** subluxation of unspecified **thumb**

☑7ᵗʰ **S63.104** **Unspecified** dislocation of right **thumb**

☑7ᵗʰ **S63.105** **Unspecified** dislocation of left **thumb**

☑7ᵗʰ **S63.106** **Unspecified** dislocation of unspecified **thumb**

☑6ᵗʰ **S63.11** **Subluxation and dislocation of** metacarpophalangeal joint of thumb

☑7ᵗʰ **S63.111** Subluxation of metacarpophalangeal joint of right **thumb**

☑7ᵗʰ **S63.112** Subluxation of metacarpophalangeal joint of left **thumb**

☑7ᵗʰ **S63.113** Subluxation of metacarpophalangeal joint of unspecified **thumb**

☑7ᵗʰ **S63.114** Dislocation of metacarpophalangeal joint of right **thumb**

☑7ᵗʰ **S63.115** Dislocation of metacarpophalangeal joint of left **thumb**

☑7ᵗʰ **S63.116** Dislocation of metacarpophalangeal joint of unspecified **thumb**

☑6ᵗʰ **S63.12** **Subluxation and dislocation of** interphalangeal joint of thumb

☑7ᵗʰ **S63.121** Subluxation of interphalangeal joint of right **thumb**

☑7ᵗʰ **S63.122** Subluxation of interphalangeal joint of left **thumb**

☑7ᵗʰ **S63.123** Subluxation of interphalangeal joint of unspecified **thumb**

☑7ᵗʰ **S63.124** Dislocation of interphalangeal joint of right **thumb**

☑7ᵗʰ **S63.125** Dislocation of interphalangeal joint of left **thumb**

☑7ᵗʰ **S63.126** Dislocation of interphalangeal joint of unspecified **thumb**

☑ Additional Character Required   √ₓ7ᵗʰ Placeholder   Unacceptable PDx   Questionable PDx   Manifestation   **H1**-**H14** HAC   **HCC** CMS-HCC Dx   **HIV** HIV Dx

ICD-10-CM 2019   **1027**

S63.006–S63.126

√5ᵗʰ **S63.2**   **Subluxation and dislocation of** other finger(s)
- EXCLUDES 2   *subluxation and dislocation of thumb (S63.1-)*

√6ᵗʰ **S63.20**   **Unspecified subluxation of other finger**

√7ᵗʰ **S63.200**   **Unspecified subluxation of** right index finger

√7ᵗʰ **S63.201**   **Unspecified subluxation of** left index finger

√7ᵗʰ **S63.202**   **Unspecified subluxation of** right middle finger

√7ᵗʰ **S63.203**   **Unspecified subluxation of** left middle finger

√7ᵗʰ **S63.204**   **Unspecified subluxation of** right ring finger

√7ᵗʰ **S63.205**   **Unspecified subluxation of** left ring **finger**

√7ᵗʰ **S63.206**   **Unspecified subluxation of** right little finger

√7ᵗʰ **S63.207**   **Unspecified subluxation of** left little **finger**

√7ᵗʰ **S63.208**   **Unspecified subluxation of** other **finger**
    Unspecified subluxation of specified finger with unspecified laterality

√7ᵗʰ **S63.209**   **Unspecified subluxation of** unspecified finger

√6ᵗʰ **S63.21**   **Subluxation of** metacarpophalangeal joint **of finger**

√7ᵗʰ **S63.210**   **Subluxation of metacarpophalangeal joint of** right index **finger**

√7ᵗʰ **S63.211**   **Subluxation of metacarpophalangeal joint of** left index **finger**

√7ᵗʰ **S63.212**   **Subluxation of metacarpophalangeal joint of** right middle **finger**

√7ᵗʰ **S63.213**   **Subluxation of metacarpophalangeal joint of** left middle **finger**

√7ᵗʰ **S63.214**   **Subluxation of metacarpophalangeal joint of** right ring **finger**

√7ᵗʰ **S63.215**   **Subluxation of metacarpophalangeal joint of** left ring **finger**

√7ᵗʰ **S63.216**   **Subluxation of metacarpophalangeal joint of** right little **finger**

√7ᵗʰ **S63.217**   **Subluxation of metacarpophalangeal joint of** left little **finger**

√7ᵗʰ **S63.218**   **Subluxation of metacarpophalangeal joint of** other **finger**
    Subluxation of metacarpophalangeal joint of specified finger with unspecified laterality

√7ᵗʰ **S63.219**   **Subluxation of metacarpophalangeal joint of** unspecified **finger**

√6ᵗʰ **S63.22**   **Subluxation of unspecified** interphalangeal joint **of finger**

√7ᵗʰ **S63.220**   **Subluxation of unspecified interphalangeal joint of** right index **finger**

√7ᵗʰ **S63.221**   **Subluxation of unspecified interphalangeal joint of** left index **finger**

√7ᵗʰ **S63.222**   **Subluxation of unspecified interphalangeal joint of** right middle **finger**

√7ᵗʰ **S63.223**   **Subluxation of unspecified interphalangeal joint of** left middle **finger**

√7ᵗʰ **S63.224**   **Subluxation of unspecified interphalangeal joint of** right ring **finger**

√7ᵗʰ **S63.225**   **Subluxation of unspecified interphalangeal joint of** left ring **finger**

√7ᵗʰ **S63.226**   **Subluxation of unspecified interphalangeal joint of** right little **finger**

√7ᵗʰ **S63.227**   **Subluxation of unspecified interphalangeal joint of** left little **finger**

√7ᵗʰ **S63.228**   **Subluxation of unspecified interphalangeal joint of** other **finger**
    Subluxation of unspecified interphalangeal joint of specified finger with unspecified laterality

√7ᵗʰ **S63.229**   **Subluxation of unspecified inter-phalangeal joint of** unspecified **finger**

√6ᵗʰ **S63.23**   **Subluxation of** proximal interphalangeal **joint of finger**

√7ᵗʰ **S63.230**   **Subluxation of proximal interphalangeal joint of** right index **finger**

√7ᵗʰ **S63.231**   **Subluxation of proximal interphalangeal joint of** left index **finger**

√7ᵗʰ **S63.232**   **Subluxation of proximal interphalangeal joint of** right middle **finger**

√7ᵗʰ **S63.233**   **Subluxation of proximal interphalangeal joint of** left middle **finger**

√7ᵗʰ **S63.234**   **Subluxation of proximal interphalangeal joint of** right ring **finger**

√7ᵗʰ **S63.235**   **Subluxation of proximal interphalangeal joint of** left ring **finger**

√7ᵗʰ **S63.236**   **Subluxation of proximal interphalangeal joint of** right little **finger**

√7ᵗʰ **S63.237**   **Subluxation of proximal interphalangeal joint of** left little **finger**

√7ᵗʰ **S63.238**   **Subluxation of proximal interphalangeal joint of** other **finger**
    Subluxation of proximal interphalangeal joint of specified finger with unspecified laterality

√7ᵗʰ **S63.239**   **Subluxation of proximal interphalangeal joint of** unspecified **finger**

√6ᵗʰ **S63.24**   **Subluxation of** distal interphalangeal **joint of finger**

√7ᵗʰ **S63.240**   **Subluxation of distal interphalangeal joint of** right index **finger**

√7ᵗʰ **S63.241**   **Subluxation of distal interphalangeal joint of** left index **finger**

√7ᵗʰ **S63.242**   **Subluxation of distal interphalangeal joint of** right middle **finger**

√7ᵗʰ **S63.243**   **Subluxation of distal interphalangeal joint of** left middle **finger**

√7ᵗʰ **S63.244**   **Subluxation of distal interphalangeal joint of** right ring **finger**

√7ᵗʰ **S63.245**   **Subluxation of distal interphalangeal joint of** left ring **finger**

√7ᵗʰ **S63.246**   **Subluxation of distal interphalangeal joint of** right little **finger**

√7ᵗʰ **S63.247**   **Subluxation of distal interphalangeal joint of** left little **finger**

√7ᵗʰ **S63.248**   **Subluxation of distal interphalangeal joint of** other **finger**
    Subluxation of distal interphalangeal joint of specified finger with unspecified laterality

√7ᵗʰ **S63.249**   **Subluxation of distal interphalangeal joint of** unspecified **finger**

√6ᵗʰ **S63.25**   **Unspecified dislocation of** other finger

√7ᵗʰ **S63.250**   **Unspecified dislocation of** right index finger

√7ᵗʰ **S63.251**   **Unspecified dislocation of** left index finger

√7ᵗʰ **S63.252**   **Unspecified dislocation of** right middle finger

√7ᵗʰ **S63.253**   **Unspecified dislocation of** left middle finger

√7ᵗʰ **S63.254**   **Unspecified dislocation of** right ring finger

√7ᵗʰ **S63.255**   **Unspecified dislocation of** left ring finger

√7ᵗʰ **S63.256**   **Unspecified dislocation of** right little finger

√7ᵗʰ **S63.257**   **Unspecified dislocation of** left little finger

√7ᵗʰ **S63.258**   **Unspecified dislocation of** other finger
    Unspecified dislocation of specified finger with unspecified laterality

√7ᵗʰ **S63.259**   **Unspecified dislocation of** unspecified finger
    Unspecified dislocation of unspecified finger with unspecified laterality

√6ᵗʰ **S63.26**   **Dislocation of** metacarpophalangeal joint **of finger**

√7ᵗʰ **S63.260**   **Dislocation of metacarpophalangeal joint of** right index **finger**

√7ᵗʰ **S63.261**   **Dislocation of metacarpophalangeal joint of** left index **finger**

√7ᵗʰ **S63.262**   **Dislocation of metacarpophalangeal joint of** right middle **finger**

√7ᵗʰ **S63.263**   **Dislocation of metacarpophalangeal joint of** left middle **finger**

√7ᵗʰ **S63.264**   **Dislocation of metacarpophalangeal joint of** right ring **finger**

N Newborn: 0   P Pediatric: 0-17   M Maternity: 12-55   A Adult: 15-124   MCC Major Complication/Comorbidity   CC Complication/Comorbidity   SW Severe Wound Dx

1028

ICD-10-CM 2019

✓7ᵗʰ **S63.265** Dislocation of metacarpophalangeal joint of left ring finger

✓7ᵗʰ **S63.266** Dislocation of metacarpophalangeal joint of right little finger

✓7ᵗʰ **S63.267** Dislocation of metacarpophalangeal joint of left little finger

✓7ᵗʰ **S63.268** Dislocation of metacarpophalangeal joint of other finger
Dislocation of metacarpophalangeal joint of specified finger with unspecified laterality

✓7ᵗʰ **S63.269** Dislocation of metacarpophalangeal joint of unspecified finger

✓6ᵗʰ **S63.27** Dislocation of unspecified interphalangeal joint of finger

✓7ᵗʰ **S63.270** Dislocation of unspecified interphalangeal joint of right index finger

✓7ᵗʰ **S63.271** Dislocation of unspecified interphalangeal joint of left index finger

✓7ᵗʰ **S63.272** Dislocation of unspecified interphalangeal joint of right middle finger

✓7ᵗʰ **S63.273** Dislocation of unspecified interphalangeal joint of left middle finger

✓7ᵗʰ **S63.274** Dislocation of unspecified interphalangeal joint of right ring finger

✓7ᵗʰ **S63.275** Dislocation of unspecified interphalangeal joint of left ring finger

✓7ᵗʰ **S63.276** Dislocation of unspecified interphalangeal joint of right little finger

✓7ᵗʰ **S63.277** Dislocation of unspecified interphalangeal joint of left little finger

✓7ᵗʰ **S63.278** Dislocation of unspecified interphalangeal joint of other finger
Dislocation of unspecified interphalangeal joint of specified finger with unspecified laterality

✓7ᵗʰ **S63.279** Dislocation of unspecified interphalangeal joint of unspecified finger
Dislocation of unspecified interphalangeal joint of unspecified finger without specified laterality

✓6ᵗʰ **S63.28** Dislocation of proximal interphalangeal joint of finger

✓7ᵗʰ **S63.280** Dislocation of proximal interphalangeal joint of right index finger

✓7ᵗʰ **S63.281** Dislocation of proximal interphalangeal joint of left index finger

✓7ᵗʰ **S63.282** Dislocation of proximal interphalangeal joint of right middle finger

✓7ᵗʰ **S63.283** Dislocation of proximal interphalangeal joint of left middle finger

✓7ᵗʰ **S63.284** Dislocation of proximal interphalangeal joint of right ring finger

✓7ᵗʰ **S63.285** Dislocation of proximal interphalangeal joint of left ring finger

✓7ᵗʰ **S63.286** Dislocation of proximal interphalangeal joint of right little finger

✓7ᵗʰ **S63.287** Dislocation of proximal interphalangeal joint of left little finger

✓7ᵗʰ **S63.288** Dislocation of proximal interphalangeal joint of other finger
Dislocation of proximal interphalangeal joint of specified finger with unspecified laterality

✓7ᵗʰ **S63.289** Dislocation of proximal interphalangeal joint of unspecified finger

✓6ᵗʰ **S63.29** Dislocation of distal interphalangeal joint of finger

✓7ᵗʰ **S63.290** Dislocation of distal interphalangeal joint of right index finger

✓7ᵗʰ **S63.291** Dislocation of distal interphalangeal joint of left index finger

✓7ᵗʰ **S63.292** Dislocation of distal interphalangeal joint of right middle finger

✓7ᵗʰ **S63.293** Dislocation of distal interphalangeal joint of left middle finger

✓7ᵗʰ **S63.294** Dislocation of distal interphalangeal joint of right ring finger

✓7ᵗʰ **S63.295** Dislocation of distal interphalangeal joint of left ring finger

✓7ᵗʰ **S63.296** Dislocation of distal interphalangeal joint of right little finger

✓7ᵗʰ **S63.297** Dislocation of distal interphalangeal joint of left little finger

✓7ᵗʰ **S63.298** Dislocation of distal interphalangeal joint of other finger
Dislocation of distal interphalangeal joint of specified finger with unspecified laterality

✓7ᵗʰ **S63.299** Dislocation of distal interphalangeal joint of unspecified finger

✓5ᵗʰ **S63.3** Traumatic rupture of ligament of wrist

✓6ᵗʰ **S63.30** Traumatic rupture of unspecified ligament of wrist

✓7ᵗʰ **S63.301** Traumatic rupture of unspecified ligament of right wrist

✓7ᵗʰ **S63.302** Traumatic rupture of unspecified ligament of left wrist

✓7ᵗʰ **S63.309** Traumatic rupture of unspecified ligament of unspecified wrist

✓6ᵗʰ **S63.31** Traumatic rupture of collateral ligament of wrist

✓7ᵗʰ **S63.311** Traumatic rupture of collateral ligament of right wrist

✓7ᵗʰ **S63.312** Traumatic rupture of collateral ligament of left wrist

✓7ᵗʰ **S63.319** Traumatic rupture of collateral ligament of unspecified wrist

✓6ᵗʰ **S63.32** Traumatic rupture of radiocarpal ligament

✓7ᵗʰ **S63.321** Traumatic rupture of right radiocarpal ligament

✓7ᵗʰ **S63.322** Traumatic rupture of left radiocarpal ligament

✓7ᵗʰ **S63.329** Traumatic rupture of unspecified radiocarpal ligament

✓6ᵗʰ **S63.33** Traumatic rupture of ulnocarpal (palmar) ligament

✓7ᵗʰ **S63.331** Traumatic rupture of right ulnocarpal (palmar) ligament

✓7ᵗʰ **S63.332** Traumatic rupture of left ulnocarpal (palmar) ligament

✓7ᵗʰ **S63.339** Traumatic rupture of unspecified ulnocarpal (palmar) ligament

✓6ᵗʰ **S63.39** Traumatic rupture of other ligament of wrist

✓7ᵗʰ **S63.391** Traumatic rupture of other ligament of right wrist

✓7ᵗʰ **S63.392** Traumatic rupture of other ligament of left wrist

✓7ᵗʰ **S63.399** Traumatic rupture of other ligament of unspecified wrist

✓5ᵗʰ **S63.4** Traumatic rupture of ligament of finger at metacarpophalangeal and interphalangeal joint(s)

✓6ᵗʰ **S63.40** Traumatic rupture of unspecified ligament of finger at metacarpophalangeal and interphalangeal joint

✓7ᵗʰ **S63.400** Traumatic rupture of unspecified ligament of right index finger at metacarpophalangeal and interphalangeal joint

✓7ᵗʰ **S63.401** Traumatic rupture of unspecified ligament of left index finger at metacarpophalangeal and interphalangeal joint

✓7ᵗʰ **S63.402** Traumatic rupture of unspecified ligament of right middle finger at metacarpophalangeal and interphalangeal joint

✓7ᵗʰ **S63.403** Traumatic rupture of unspecified ligament of left middle finger at metacarpophalangeal and interphalangeal joint

✓7ᵗʰ **S63.404** Traumatic rupture of unspecified ligament of right ring finger at metacarpophalangeal and interphalangeal joint

✓ Additional Character Required   ✓x7ᵗʰ Placeholder   Unacceptable PDx   Questionable PDx   Manifestation   H1-H14 HAC   HCC CMS-HCC Dx   HIV HIV Dx

ICD-10-CM 2019   **1029**

✓7ᵗʰ **S63.405** **Traumatic rupture of unspecified ligament of left ring finger at metacarpophalangeal and interphalangeal joint**

✓7ᵗʰ **S63.406** **Traumatic rupture of unspecified ligament of right little finger at metacarpophalangeal and interphalangeal joint**

✓7ᵗʰ **S63.407** **Traumatic rupture of unspecified ligament of left little finger at metacarpophalangeal and interphalangeal joint**

✓7ᵗʰ **S63.408** **Traumatic rupture of unspecified ligament of other finger at metacarpophalangeal and interphalangeal joint**
Traumatic rupture of unspecified ligament of specified finger with unspecified laterality at metacarpophalangeal and interphalangeal joint

✓7ᵗʰ **S63.409** **Traumatic rupture of unspecified ligament of unspecified finger at metacarpophalangeal and interphalangeal joint**

✓6ᵗʰ **S63.41** **Traumatic rupture of collateral ligament of finger at metacarpophalangeal and interphalangeal joint**

✓7ᵗʰ **S63.410** **Traumatic rupture of collateral ligament of right index finger at metacarpophalangeal and interphalangeal joint**

✓7ᵗʰ **S63.411** **Traumatic rupture of collateral ligament of left index finger at metacarpophalangeal and interphalangeal joint**

✓7ᵗʰ **S63.412** **Traumatic rupture of collateral ligament of right middle finger at metacarpophalangeal and interphalangeal joint**

✓7ᵗʰ **S63.413** **Traumatic rupture of collateral ligament of left middle finger at metacarpophalangeal and interphalangeal joint**

✓7ᵗʰ **S63.414** **Traumatic rupture of collateral ligament of right ring finger at metacarpophalangeal and interphalangeal joint**

✓7ᵗʰ **S63.415** **Traumatic rupture of collateral ligament of left ring finger at metacarpophalangeal and interphalangeal joint**

✓7ᵗʰ **S63.416** **Traumatic rupture of collateral ligament of right little finger at metacarpophalangeal and interphalangeal joint**

✓7ᵗʰ **S63.417** **Traumatic rupture of collateral ligament of left little finger at metacarpophalangeal and interphalangeal joint**

✓7ᵗʰ **S63.418** **Traumatic rupture of collateral ligament of other finger at metacarpophalangeal and interphalangeal joint**
Traumatic rupture of collateral ligament of specified finger with unspecified laterality at metacarpophalangeal and interphalangeal joint

✓7ᵗʰ **S63.419** **Traumatic rupture of collateral ligament of unspecified finger at metacarpophalangeal and interphalangeal joint**

✓6ᵗʰ **S63.42** **Traumatic rupture of palmar ligament of finger at metacarpophalangeal and interphalangeal joint**

✓7ᵗʰ **S63.420** **Traumatic rupture of palmar ligament of right index finger at metacarpophalangeal and interphalangeal joint**

✓7ᵗʰ **S63.421** **Traumatic rupture of palmar ligament of left index finger at metacarpophalangeal and interphalangeal joint**

✓7ᵗʰ **S63.422** **Traumatic rupture of palmar ligament of right middle finger at metacarpophalangeal and interphalangeal joint**

✓7ᵗʰ **S63.423** **Traumatic rupture of palmar ligament of left middle finger at metacarpophalangeal and interphalangeal joint**

✓7ᵗʰ **S63.424** **Traumatic rupture of palmar ligament of right ring finger at metacarpophalangeal and interphalangeal joint**

✓7ᵗʰ **S63.425** **Traumatic rupture of palmar ligament of left ring finger at metacarpophalangeal and interphalangeal joint**

✓7ᵗʰ **S63.426** **Traumatic rupture of palmar ligament of right little finger at metacarpophalangeal and interphalangeal joint**

✓7ᵗʰ **S63.427** **Traumatic rupture of palmar ligament of left little finger at metacarpophalangeal and interphalangeal joint**

✓7ᵗʰ **S63.428** **Traumatic rupture of palmar ligament of other finger at metacarpophalangeal and interphalangeal joint**
Traumatic rupture of palmar ligament of specified finger with unspecified laterality at metacarpophalangeal and interphalangeal joint

✓7ᵗʰ **S63.429** **Traumatic rupture of palmar ligament of unspecified finger at metacarpophalangeal and interphalangeal joint**

✓6ᵗʰ **S63.43** **Traumatic rupture of volar plate of finger at metacarpophalangeal and interphalangeal joint**

✓7ᵗʰ **S63.430** **Traumatic rupture of volar plate of right index finger at metacarpophalangeal and interphalangeal joint**

✓7ᵗʰ **S63.431** **Traumatic rupture of volar plate of left index finger at metacarpophalangeal and interphalangeal joint**

✓7ᵗʰ **S63.432** **Traumatic rupture of volar plate of right middle finger at metacarpophalangeal and interphalangeal joint**

✓7ᵗʰ **S63.433** **Traumatic rupture of volar plate of left middle finger at metacarpophalangeal and interphalangeal joint**

✓7ᵗʰ **S63.434** **Traumatic rupture of volar plate of right ring finger at metacarpophalangeal and interphalangeal joint**

✓7ᵗʰ **S63.435** **Traumatic rupture of volar plate of left ring finger at metacarpophalangeal and interphalangeal joint**

✓7ᵗʰ **S63.436** **Traumatic rupture of volar plate of right little finger at metacarpophalangeal and interphalangeal joint**

✓7ᵗʰ **S63.437** **Traumatic rupture of volar plate of left little finger at metacarpophalangeal and interphalangeal joint**

✓7ᵗʰ **S63.438** **Traumatic rupture of volar plate of other finger at metacarpophalangeal and interphalangeal joint**
Traumatic rupture of volar plate of specified finger with unspecified laterality at metacarpophalangeal and interphalangeal joint

✓7ᵗʰ **S63.439** **Traumatic rupture of volar plate of unspecified finger at metacarpophalangeal and interphalangeal joint**

✓6ᵗʰ **S63.49** **Traumatic rupture of other ligament of finger at metacarpophalangeal and interphalangeal joint**

✓7ᵗʰ **S63.490** **Traumatic rupture of other ligament of right index finger at metacarpophalangeal and interphalangeal joint**

✓7ᵗʰ **S63.491** **Traumatic rupture of other ligament of left index finger at metacarpophalangeal and interphalangeal joint**

✓7ᵗʰ **S63.492** **Traumatic rupture of other ligament of right middle finger at metacarpophalangeal and interphalangeal joint**

Ⓝ Newborn: 0 　 Ⓟ Pediatric: 0-17 　 Ⓜ Maternity: 12-55 　 Ⓐ Adult: 15-124 　 ᴹᶜᶜ Major Complication/Comorbidity 　 ᶜᶜ Complication/Comorbidity 　 ˢʷ Severe Wound Dx

1030 ICD-10-CM 2019

✓7ᵗʰ **S63.493** **Traumatic rupture of other ligament of left middle finger at metacarpophalangeal and interphalangeal joint**

✓7ᵗʰ **S63.494** **Traumatic rupture of other ligament of right ring finger at metacarpophalangeal and interphalangeal joint**

✓7ᵗʰ **S63.495** **Traumatic rupture of other ligament of left ring finger at metacarpophalangeal and interphalangeal joint**

✓7ᵗʰ **S63.496** **Traumatic rupture of other ligament of right little finger at metacarpophalangeal and interphalangeal joint**

✓7ᵗʰ **S63.497** **Traumatic rupture of other ligament of left little finger at metacarpophalangeal and interphalangeal joint**

✓7ᵗʰ **S63.498** **Traumatic rupture of other ligament of other finger at metacarpophalangeal and interphalangeal joint**
Traumatic rupture of ligament of specified finger with unspecified laterality at metacarpophalangeal and interphalangeal joint

✓7ᵗʰ **S63.499** **Traumatic rupture of other ligament of unspecified finger at metacarpophalangeal and interphalangeal joint**

✓5ᵗʰ **S63.5** **Other and unspecified sprain of wrist**

  ✓6ᵗʰ **S63.50** **Unspecified sprain of wrist**

    ✓7ᵗʰ **S63.501** **Unspecified sprain of right wrist**

    ✓7ᵗʰ **S63.502** **Unspecified sprain of left wrist**

    ✓7ᵗʰ **S63.509** **Unspecified sprain of unspecified wrist**

  ✓6ᵗʰ **S63.51** **Sprain of carpal (joint)**

    ✓7ᵗʰ **S63.511** **Sprain of carpal joint of right wrist**

    ✓7ᵗʰ **S63.512** **Sprain of carpal joint of left wrist**

    ✓7ᵗʰ **S63.519** **Sprain of carpal joint of unspecified wrist**

  ✓6ᵗʰ **S63.52** **Sprain of radiocarpal joint**
    EXCLUDES 1   *traumatic rupture of radiocarpal ligament (S63.32-)*

    ✓7ᵗʰ **S63.521** **Sprain of radiocarpal joint of right wrist**

    ✓7ᵗʰ **S63.522** **Sprain of radiocarpal joint of left wrist**

    ✓7ᵗʰ **S63.529** **Sprain of radiocarpal joint of unspecified wrist**

  ✓6ᵗʰ **S63.59** **Other specified sprain of wrist**

    ✓7ᵗʰ **S63.591** **Other specified sprain of right wrist**

    ✓7ᵗʰ **S63.592** **Other specified sprain of left wrist**

    ✓7ᵗʰ **S63.599** **Other specified sprain of unspecified wrist**

✓5ᵗʰ **S63.6** **Other and unspecified sprain of finger(s)**
  EXCLUDES 1   *traumatic rupture of ligament of finger at metacarpophalangeal and interphalangeal joint(s) (S63.4-)*

  ✓6ᵗʰ **S63.60** **Unspecified sprain of thumb**

    ✓7ᵗʰ **S63.601** **Unspecified sprain of right thumb**

    ✓7ᵗʰ **S63.602** **Unspecified sprain of left thumb**

    ✓7ᵗʰ **S63.609** **Unspecified sprain of unspecified thumb**

  ✓6ᵗʰ **S63.61** **Unspecified sprain of other and unspecified finger(s)**

    ✓7ᵗʰ **S63.610** **Unspecified sprain of right index finger**

    ✓7ᵗʰ **S63.611** **Unspecified sprain of left index finger**

    ✓7ᵗʰ **S63.612** **Unspecified sprain of right middle finger**

    ✓7ᵗʰ **S63.613** **Unspecified sprain of left middle finger**

    ✓7ᵗʰ **S63.614** **Unspecified sprain of right ring finger**

    ✓7ᵗʰ **S63.615** **Unspecified sprain of left ring finger**

    ✓7ᵗʰ **S63.616** **Unspecified sprain of right little finger**

    ✓7ᵗʰ **S63.617** **Unspecified sprain of left little finger**

    ✓7ᵗʰ **S63.618** **Unspecified sprain of other finger**
Unspecified sprain of specified finger with unspecified laterality

    ✓7ᵗʰ **S63.619** **Unspecified sprain of unspecified finger**

  ✓6ᵗʰ **S63.62** **Sprain of interphalangeal joint of thumb**

    ✓7ᵗʰ **S63.621** **Sprain of interphalangeal joint of right thumb**

    ✓7ᵗʰ **S63.622** **Sprain of interphalangeal joint of left thumb**

    ✓7ᵗʰ **S63.629** **Sprain of interphalangeal joint of unspecified thumb**

  ✓6ᵗʰ **S63.63** **Sprain of interphalangeal joint of other and unspecified finger(s)**

    ✓7ᵗʰ **S63.630** **Sprain of interphalangeal joint of right index finger**

    ✓7ᵗʰ **S63.631** **Sprain of interphalangeal joint of left index finger**

    ✓7ᵗʰ **S63.632** **Sprain of interphalangeal joint of right middle finger**

    ✓7ᵗʰ **S63.633** **Sprain of interphalangeal joint of left middle finger**

    ✓7ᵗʰ **S63.634** **Sprain of interphalangeal joint of right ring finger**

    ✓7ᵗʰ **S63.635** **Sprain of interphalangeal joint of left ring finger**

    ✓7ᵗʰ **S63.636** **Sprain of interphalangeal joint of right little finger**

    ✓7ᵗʰ **S63.637** **Sprain of interphalangeal joint of left little finger**

    ✓7ᵗʰ **S63.638** **Sprain of interphalangeal joint of other finger**

    ✓7ᵗʰ **S63.639** **Sprain of interphalangeal joint of unspecified finger**

  ✓6ᵗʰ **S63.64** **Sprain of metacarpophalangeal joint of thumb**

    ✓7ᵗʰ **S63.641** **Sprain of metacarpophalangeal joint of right thumb**

    ✓7ᵗʰ **S63.642** **Sprain of metacarpophalangeal joint of left thumb**

    ✓7ᵗʰ **S63.649** **Sprain of metacarpophalangeal joint of unspecified thumb**

  ✓6ᵗʰ **S63.65** **Sprain of metacarpophalangeal joint of other and unspecified finger(s)**

    ✓7ᵗʰ **S63.650** **Sprain of metacarpophalangeal joint of right index finger**

    ✓7ᵗʰ **S63.651** **Sprain of metacarpophalangeal joint of left index finger**

    ✓7ᵗʰ **S63.652** **Sprain of metacarpophalangeal joint of right middle finger**

    ✓7ᵗʰ **S63.653** **Sprain of metacarpophalangeal joint of left middle finger**

    ✓7ᵗʰ **S63.654** **Sprain of metacarpophalangeal joint of right ring finger**

    ✓7ᵗʰ **S63.655** **Sprain of metacarpophalangeal joint of left ring finger**

    ✓7ᵗʰ **S63.656** **Sprain of metacarpophalangeal joint of right little finger**

    ✓7ᵗʰ **S63.657** **Sprain of metacarpophalangeal joint of left little finger**

    ✓7ᵗʰ **S63.658** **Sprain of metacarpophalangeal joint of other finger**
Sprain of metacarpophalangeal joint of specified finger with unspecified laterality

    ✓7ᵗʰ **S63.659** **Sprain of metacarpophalangeal joint of unspecified finger**

  ✓6ᵗʰ **S63.68** **Other sprain of thumb**

    ✓7ᵗʰ **S63.681** **Other sprain of right thumb**

    ✓7ᵗʰ **S63.682** **Other sprain of left thumb**

    ✓7ᵗʰ **S63.689** **Other sprain of unspecified thumb**

  ✓6ᵗʰ **S63.69** **Other sprain of other and unspecified finger(s)**

    ✓7ᵗʰ **S63.690** **Other sprain of right index finger**

    ✓7ᵗʰ **S63.691** **Other sprain of left index finger**

    ✓7ᵗʰ **S63.692** **Other sprain of right middle finger**

    ✓7ᵗʰ **S63.693** **Other sprain of left middle finger**

    ✓7ᵗʰ **S63.694** **Other sprain of right ring finger**

    ✓7ᵗʰ **S63.695** **Other sprain of left ring finger**

    ✓7ᵗʰ **S63.696** **Other sprain of right little finger**

    ✓7ᵗʰ **S63.697** **Other sprain of left little finger**

    ✓7ᵗʰ **S63.698** **Other sprain of other finger**
Other sprain of specified finger with unspecified laterality

    ✓7ᵗʰ **S63.699** **Other sprain of unspecified finger**

✓ Additional Character Required   ✓x7ᵗʰ Placeholder   Unacceptable PDx   Questionable PDx   Manifestation   H1-H14 HAC   HCC CMS-HCC Dx   HIV HIV Dx

ICD-10-CM 2019   1031

S63.493–S63.699

☑5ᵗʰ **S63.8 Sprain of other part of wrist and hand**

   ☑6ᵗʰ **S63.8X Sprain of other part of wrist and hand**

     ☑7ᵗʰ **S63.8X1 Sprain of other part of right wrist and hand**

     ☑7ᵗʰ **S63.8X2 Sprain of other part of left wrist and hand**

     ☑7ᵗʰ **S63.8X9 Sprain of other part of unspecified wrist and hand**

☑5ᵗʰ **S63.9 Sprain of unspecified part of wrist and hand**

   ☑7ᵗʰ **S63.90 Sprain of unspecified part of unspecified wrist and hand**

   ☑7ᵗʰ **S63.91 Sprain of unspecified part of right wrist and hand**

   ☑7ᵗʰ **S63.92 Sprain of unspecified part of left wrist and hand**

☑4ᵗʰ **S64 Injury of nerves at wrist and hand level**

Code also any associated open wound (S61.-)

> The appropriate 7th character is to be added to each code from category S64.
> A   initial encounter
> D   subsequent encounter
> S   sequela

☑5ᵗʰ **S64.0 Injury of ulnar nerve at wrist and hand level**

   ☑x7ᵗʰ **S64.00 Injury of ulnar nerve at wrist and hand level of unspecified arm**

   ☑x7ᵗʰ **S64.01 Injury of ulnar nerve at wrist and hand level of right arm**

   ☑x7ᵗʰ **S64.02 Injury of ulnar nerve at wrist and hand level of left arm**

☑5ᵗʰ **S64.1 Injury of median nerve at wrist and hand level**

   ☑x7ᵗʰ **S64.10 Injury of median nerve at wrist and hand level of unspecified arm**

   ☑x7ᵗʰ **S64.11 Injury of median nerve at wrist and hand level of right arm**

   ☑x7ᵗʰ **S64.12 Injury of median nerve at wrist and hand level of left arm**

☑5ᵗʰ **S64.2 Injury of radial nerve at wrist and hand level**

   ☑x7ᵗʰ **S64.20 Injury of radial nerve at wrist and hand level of unspecified arm**

   ☑x7ᵗʰ **S64.21 Injury of radial nerve at wrist and hand level of right arm**

   ☑x7ᵗʰ **S64.22 Injury of radial nerve at wrist and hand level of left arm**

☑5ᵗʰ **S64.3 Injury of digital nerve of thumb**

   ☑x7ᵗʰ **S64.30 Injury of digital nerve of unspecified thumb**

   ☑x7ᵗʰ **S64.31 Injury of digital nerve of right thumb**

   ☑x7ᵗʰ **S64.32 Injury of digital nerve of left thumb**

☑5ᵗʰ **S64.4 Injury of digital nerve of other and unspecified finger**

   ☑x7ᵗʰ **S64.40 Injury of digital nerve of unspecified finger**

   ☑6ᵗʰ **S64.49 Injury of digital nerve of other finger**

     ☑7ᵗʰ **S64.490 Injury of digital nerve of right index finger**

     ☑7ᵗʰ **S64.491 Injury of digital nerve of left index finger**

     ☑7ᵗʰ **S64.492 Injury of digital nerve of right middle finger**

     ☑7ᵗʰ **S64.493 Injury of digital nerve of left middle finger**

     ☑7ᵗʰ **S64.494 Injury of digital nerve of right ring finger**

     ☑7ᵗʰ **S64.495 Injury of digital nerve of left ring finger**

     ☑7ᵗʰ **S64.496 Injury of digital nerve of right little finger**

     ☑7ᵗʰ **S64.497 Injury of digital nerve of left little finger**

     ☑7ᵗʰ **S64.498 Injury of digital nerve of other finger**
Injury of digital nerve of specified finger with unspecified laterality

☑5ᵗʰ **S64.8 Injury of other nerves at wrist and hand level**

   ☑6ᵗʰ **S64.8X Injury of other nerves at wrist and hand level**

     ☑7ᵗʰ **S64.8X1 Injury of other nerves at wrist and hand level of right arm**

     ☑7ᵗʰ **S64.8X2 Injury of other nerves at wrist and hand level of left arm**

     ☑7ᵗʰ **S64.8X9 Injury of other nerves at wrist and hand level of unspecified arm**

☑5ᵗʰ **S64.9 Injury of unspecified nerve at wrist and hand level**

   ☑x7ᵗʰ **S64.90 Injury of unspecified nerve at wrist and hand level of unspecified arm**

   ☑x7ᵗʰ **S64.91 Injury of unspecified nerve at wrist and hand level of right arm**

   ☑x7ᵗʰ **S64.92 Injury of unspecified nerve at wrist and hand level of left arm**

☑4ᵗʰ **S65 Injury of blood vessels at wrist and hand level**

Code also any associated open wound (S61.-)

> The appropriate 7th character is to be added to each code from category S65.
> A   initial encounter
> D   subsequent encounter
> S   sequela

☑5ᵗʰ **S65.0 Injury of ulnar artery at wrist and hand level**

> **CC Excl: For CC codes in subcategory S65.0:**
> **Right side:** PDX collection 1274
> **Left side:** PDX collection 1275
> **Unspecified side:** PDX collection 1276

   ☑6ᵗʰ **S65.00 Unspecified injury of ulnar artery at wrist and hand level**

     ☑7ᵗʰ **S65.001 Unspecified injury of ulnar artery at wrist and hand level of right arm** CC

     ☑7ᵗʰ **S65.002 Unspecified injury of ulnar artery at wrist and hand level of left arm** CC

     ☑7ᵗʰ **S65.009 Unspecified injury of ulnar artery at wrist and hand level of unspecified arm** CC

   ☑6ᵗʰ **S65.01 Laceration of ulnar artery at wrist and hand level**

     ☑7ᵗʰ **S65.011 Laceration of ulnar artery at wrist and hand level of right arm** CC

     ☑7ᵗʰ **S65.012 Laceration of ulnar artery at wrist and hand level of left arm** CC

     ☑7ᵗʰ **S65.019 Laceration of ulnar artery at wrist and hand level of unspecified arm** CC

   ☑6ᵗʰ **S65.09 Other specified injury of ulnar artery at wrist and hand level**

     ☑7ᵗʰ **S65.091 Other specified injury of ulnar artery at wrist and hand level of right arm** CC

     ☑7ᵗʰ **S65.092 Other specified injury of ulnar artery at wrist and hand level of left arm** CC

     ☑7ᵗʰ **S65.099 Other specified injury of ulnar artery at wrist and hand level of unspecified arm** CC

☑5ᵗʰ **S65.1 Injury of radial artery at wrist and hand level**

> **CC Excl: For CC codes in subcategory S65.1:**
> **Right side:** PDX collection 1277
> **Left side:** PDX collection 1278
> **Unspecified side:** PDX collection 1279

   ☑6ᵗʰ **S65.10 Unspecified injury of radial artery at wrist and hand level**

     ☑7ᵗʰ **S65.101 Unspecified injury of radial artery at wrist and hand level of right arm** CC

     ☑7ᵗʰ **S65.102 Unspecified injury of radial artery at wrist and hand level of left arm** CC

     ☑7ᵗʰ **S65.109 Unspecified injury of radial artery at wrist and hand level of unspecified arm** CC

   ☑6ᵗʰ **S65.11 Laceration of radial artery at wrist and hand level**

     ☑7ᵗʰ **S65.111 Laceration of radial artery at wrist and hand level of right arm** CC

     ☑7ᵗʰ **S65.112 Laceration of radial artery at wrist and hand level of left arm** CC

     ☑7ᵗʰ **S65.119 Laceration of radial artery at wrist and hand level of unspecified arm** CC

   ☑6ᵗʰ **S65.19 Other specified injury of radial artery at wrist and hand level**

     ☑7ᵗʰ **S65.191 Other specified injury of radial artery at wrist and hand level of right arm** CC

     ☑7ᵗʰ **S65.192 Other specified injury of radial artery at wrist and hand level of left arm** CC

     ☑7ᵗʰ **S65.199 Other specified injury of radial artery at wrist and hand level of unspecified arm** CC

Ⓝ Newborn: 0   Ⓟ Pediatric: 0-17   Ⓜ Maternity: 12-55   Ⓐ Adult: 15-124   **MCC** Major Complication/Comorbidity   **CC** Complication/Comorbidity   **SW** Severe Wound Dx

1032   ICD-10-CM 2019

✓5th S65.2 Injury of superficial palmar arch

> **CC Excl: For CC codes in subcategory S65.2:**
> **Right side:** PDX collection 1288
> **Left side:** PDX collection 1289
> **Unspecified side:** PDX collection 1290

> **✓6th S65.20 Unspecified injury of superficial palmar arch**
> > ✓7th **S65.201 Unspecified injury of superficial palmar arch of right hand** CC
> > ✓7th **S65.202 Unspecified injury of superficial palmar arch of left hand** CC
> > ✓7th **S65.209 Unspecified injury of superficial palmar arch of unspecified hand** CC

> **✓6th S65.21 Laceration of superficial palmar arch**
> > ✓7th **S65.211 Laceration of superficial palmar arch of right hand** CC
> > ✓7th **S65.212 Laceration of superficial palmar arch of left hand** CC
> > ✓7th **S65.219 Laceration of superficial palmar arch of unspecified hand** CC

> **✓6th S65.29 Other specified injury of superficial palmar arch**
> > ✓7th **S65.291 Other specified injury of superficial palmar arch of right hand** CC
> > ✓7th **S65.292 Other specified injury of superficial palmar arch of left hand** CC
> > ✓7th **S65.299 Other specified injury of superficial palmar arch of unspecified hand** CC

✓5th S65.3 Injury of deep palmar arch

> **CC Excl: For CC codes in subcategory S65.3:**
> **Right side:** PDX collection 1288
> **Left side:** PDX collection 1289
> **Unspecified side:** PDX collection 1290

> **✓6th S65.30 Unspecified injury of deep palmar arch**
> > ✓7th **S65.301 Unspecified injury of deep palmar arch of right hand** CC
> > ✓7th **S65.302 Unspecified injury of deep palmar arch of left hand** CC
> > ✓7th **S65.309 Unspecified injury of deep palmar arch of unspecified hand** CC

> **✓6th S65.31 Laceration of deep palmar arch**
> > ✓7th **S65.311 Laceration of deep palmar arch of right hand** CC
> > ✓7th **S65.312 Laceration of deep palmar arch of left hand** CC
> > ✓7th **S65.319 Laceration of deep palmar arch of unspecified hand** CC

> **✓6th S65.39 Other specified injury of deep palmar arch**
> > ✓7th **S65.391 Other specified injury of deep palmar arch of right hand** CC
> > ✓7th **S65.392 Other specified injury of deep palmar arch of left hand** CC
> > ✓7th **S65.399 Other specified injury of deep palmar arch of unspecified hand** CC

✓5th S65.4 Injury of blood vessel of thumb

> **CC Excl: For CC codes in subcategory S65.4:**
> **Right side:** PDX collection 1291
> **Left side:** PDX collection 1292
> **Unspecified side:** PDX collection 1293

> **✓6th S65.40 Unspecified injury of blood vessel of thumb**
> > ✓7th **S65.401 Unspecified injury of blood vessel of right thumb** CC
> > ✓7th **S65.402 Unspecified injury of blood vessel of left thumb** CC
> > ✓7th **S65.409 Unspecified injury of blood vessel of unspecified thumb** CC

> **✓6th S65.41 Laceration of blood vessel of thumb**
> > ✓7th **S65.411 Laceration of blood vessel of right thumb** CC
> > ✓7th **S65.412 Laceration of blood vessel of left thumb** CC
> > ✓7th **S65.419 Laceration of blood vessel of unspecified thumb** CC

> > ✓6th **S65.49 Other specified injury of blood vessel of thumb**
> > ✓7th **S65.491 Other specified injury of blood vessel of right thumb** CC
> > ✓7th **S65.492 Other specified injury of blood vessel of left thumb** CC
> > ✓7th **S65.499 Other specified injury of blood vessel of unspecified thumb** CC

✓5th S65.5 Injury of blood vessel of other and unspecified finger

> **CC Excl: For CC codes in subcategory S65.5:**
> **Right side:** PDX collection 1291
> **Left side:** PDX collection 1292
> **Other or unspecified side:** PDX collection 1293

> **✓6th S65.50 Unspecified injury of blood vessel of other and unspecified finger**
> > ✓7th **S65.500 Unspecified injury of blood vessel of right index finger** CC
> > ✓7th **S65.501 Unspecified injury of blood vessel of left index finger** CC
> > ✓7th **S65.502 Unspecified injury of blood vessel of right middle finger** CC
> > ✓7th **S65.503 Unspecified injury of blood vessel of left middle finger** CC
> > ✓7th **S65.504 Unspecified injury of blood vessel of right ring finger** CC
> > ✓7th **S65.505 Unspecified injury of blood vessel of left ring finger** CC
> > ✓7th **S65.506 Unspecified injury of blood vessel of right little finger** CC
> > ✓7th **S65.507 Unspecified injury of blood vessel of left little finger** CC
> > ✓7th **S65.508 Unspecified injury of blood vessel of other finger** CC
> > > Unspecified injury of blood vessel of specified finger with unspecified laterality
> > ✓7th **S65.509 Unspecified injury of blood vessel of unspecified finger** CC

> **✓6th S65.51 Laceration of blood vessel of other and unspecified finger**
> > ✓7th **S65.510 Laceration of blood vessel of right index finger** CC
> > ✓7th **S65.511 Laceration of blood vessel of left index finger** CC
> > ✓7th **S65.512 Laceration of blood vessel of right middle finger** CC
> > ✓7th **S65.513 Laceration of blood vessel of left middle finger** CC
> > ✓7th **S65.514 Laceration of blood vessel of right ring finger** CC
> > ✓7th **S65.515 Laceration of blood vessel of left ring finger** CC
> > ✓7th **S65.516 Laceration of blood vessel of right little finger** CC
> > ✓7th **S65.517 Laceration of blood vessel of left little finger** CC
> > ✓7th **S65.518 Laceration of blood vessel of other finger** CC
> > > Laceration of blood vessel of specified finger with unspecified laterality
> > ✓7th **S65.519 Laceration of blood vessel of unspecified finger** CC

> **✓6th S65.59 Other specified injury of blood vessel of other and unspecified finger**
> > ✓7th **S65.590 Other specified injury of blood vessel of right index finger** CC
> > ✓7th **S65.591 Other specified injury of blood vessel of left index finger** CC
> > ✓7th **S65.592 Other specified injury of blood vessel of right middle finger** CC
> > ✓7th **S65.593 Other specified injury of blood vessel of left middle finger** CC
> > ✓7th **S65.594 Other specified injury of blood vessel of right ring finger** CC
> > ✓7th **S65.595 Other specified injury of blood vessel of left ring finger** CC

✓ Additional Character Required   ✓x7th Placeholder   Unacceptable PDx   Questionable PDx   Manifestation   H1-H14 HAC   HCC CMS-HCC Dx   HIV HIV Dx

ICD-10-CM 2019   1033

✓7ᵗʰ **S65.596** **Other specified injury of blood vessel of** right little **finger** CC

✓7ᵗʰ **S65.597** **Other specified injury of blood vessel of** left little **finger** CC

✓7ᵗʰ **S65.598** **Other specified injury of blood vessel of** other **finger** CC
Other specified injury of blood vessel of specified finger with unspecified laterality

✓7ᵗʰ **S65.599** **Other specified injury of blood vessel of** unspecified **finger** CC

✓5ᵗʰ **S65.8** **Injury of other blood vessels at** wrist and hand level

CC Excl: For CC codes in subcategory S65.8:
Right side: PDX collection 1260
Left side: PDX collection 1261
Unspecified side: PDX collection 1262

✓6ᵗʰ **S65.80** Unspecified **injury of other blood vessels at wrist and hand level**

✓7ᵗʰ **S65.801** **Unspecified injury of other blood vessels at wrist and hand level of** right **arm** CC

✓7ᵗʰ **S65.802** **Unspecified injury of other blood vessels at wrist and hand level of** left **arm** CC

✓7ᵗʰ **S65.809** **Unspecified injury of other blood vessels at wrist and hand level of** unspecified **arm** CC

✓6ᵗʰ **S65.81** Laceration **of other blood vessels at wrist and hand level**

✓7ᵗʰ **S65.811** **Laceration of other blood vessels at wrist and hand level of** right **arm** CC

✓7ᵗʰ **S65.812** **Laceration of other blood vessels at wrist and hand level of** left **arm** CC

✓7ᵗʰ **S65.819** **Laceration of other blood vessels at wrist and hand level of** unspecified **arm** CC

✓6ᵗʰ **S65.89** Other **specified injury of other blood vessels at wrist and hand level**

✓7ᵗʰ **S65.891** **Other specified injury of other blood vessels at wrist and hand level of** right **arm** CC

✓7ᵗʰ **S65.892** **Other specified injury of other blood vessels at wrist and hand level of** left **arm** CC

✓7ᵗʰ **S65.899** **Other specified injury of other blood vessels at wrist and hand level of** unspecified **arm** CC

✓5ᵗʰ **S65.9** **Injury of unspecified blood vessel at** wrist and hand level

CC Excl: For CC codes in subcategory S65.9:
Right side: PDX collection 1260
Left side: PDX collection 1261
Unspecified side: PDX collection 1262

✓6ᵗʰ **S65.90** Unspecified **injury of unspecified blood vessel at wrist and hand level**

✓7ᵗʰ **S65.901** **Unspecified injury of unspecified blood vessel at wrist and hand level of** right **arm** CC

✓7ᵗʰ **S65.902** **Unspecified injury of unspecified blood vessel at wrist and hand level of** left **arm** CC

✓7ᵗʰ **S65.909** **Unspecified injury of unspecified blood vessel at wrist and hand level of** unspecified **arm** CC

✓6ᵗʰ **S65.91** Laceration **of unspecified blood vessel at wrist and hand level**

✓7ᵗʰ **S65.911** **Laceration of unspecified blood vessel at wrist and hand level of** right **arm** CC

✓7ᵗʰ **S65.912** **Laceration of unspecified blood vessel at wrist and hand level of** left **arm** CC

✓7ᵗʰ **S65.919** **Laceration of unspecified blood vessel at wrist and hand level of** unspecified **arm** CC

✓6ᵗʰ **S65.99** Other **specified injury of unspecified blood vessel at wrist and hand level**

✓7ᵗʰ **S65.991** **Other specified injury of unspecified blood vessel at wrist and hand of** right **arm** CC

✓7ᵗʰ **S65.992** **Other specified injury of unspecified blood vessel at wrist and hand of** left **arm** CC

✓7ᵗʰ **S65.999** **Other specified injury of unspecified blood vessel at wrist and hand of** unspecified **arm** CC

✓4ᵗʰ **S66** **Injury of muscle, fascia and tendon at wrist and hand level**
Code also any associated open wound (S61.-)
EXCLUDES 2 *sprain of joints and ligaments of wrist and hand (S63.-)*
TIP: Refer to the Muscle/Tendon table at the beginning of this chapter.

The appropriate 7th character is to be added to each code from category S66.
A   initial encounter
D   subsequent encounter
S   sequela

CC Excl: For CC codes in category S66:
Right side: PDX collection 1294
Left side: PDX collection 1295
Other or unspecified side: PDX collection 1296

✓5ᵗʰ **S66.0** **Injury of** long flexor **muscle, fascia and tendon of** thumb **at wrist and hand level**

✓6ᵗʰ **S66.00** Unspecified **injury of long flexor muscle, fascia and tendon of thumb at wrist and hand level**

✓7ᵗʰ **S66.001** **Unspecified injury of long flexor muscle, fascia and tendon of** right **thumb at wrist and hand level**

✓7ᵗʰ **S66.002** **Unspecified injury of long flexor muscle, fascia and tendon of** left **thumb at wrist and hand level**

✓7ᵗʰ **S66.009** **Unspecified injury of long flexor muscle, fascia and tendon of** unspecified **thumb at wrist and hand level**

✓6ᵗʰ **S66.01** Strain **of long flexor muscle, fascia and tendon of thumb at wrist and hand level**

✓7ᵗʰ **S66.011** **Strain of long flexor muscle, fascia and tendon of** right **thumb at wrist and hand level**

✓7ᵗʰ **S66.012** **Strain of long flexor muscle, fascia and tendon of** left **thumb at wrist and hand level**

✓7ᵗʰ **S66.019** **Strain of long flexor muscle, fascia and tendon of** unspecified **thumb at wrist and hand level**

✓6ᵗʰ **S66.02** Laceration **of long flexor muscle, fascia and tendon of thumb at wrist and hand level**

✓7ᵗʰ **S66.021** **Laceration of long flexor muscle, fascia and tendon of** right **thumb at wrist and hand level** CC

✓7ᵗʰ **S66.022** **Laceration of long flexor muscle, fascia and tendon of** left **thumb at wrist and hand level** CC

✓7ᵗʰ **S66.029** **Laceration of long flexor muscle, fascia and tendon of** unspecified **thumb at wrist and hand level** CC

✓6ᵗʰ **S66.09** Other **specified injury of long flexor muscle, fascia and tendon of thumb at wrist and hand level**

✓7ᵗʰ **S66.091** **Other specified injury of long flexor muscle, fascia and tendon of** right **thumb at wrist and hand level**

✓7ᵗʰ **S66.092** **Other specified injury of long flexor muscle, fascia and tendon of** left **thumb at wrist and hand level**

✓7ᵗʰ **S66.099** **Other specified injury of long flexor muscle, fascia and tendon of** unspecified **thumb at wrist and hand level**

✓5ᵗʰ **S66.1** **Injury of** flexor muscle, **fascia and tendon of other and unspecified** finger **at wrist and hand level**

> EXCLUDES 2   *Injury of long flexor muscle, fascia and tendon of thumb at wrist and hand level (S66.0-)*

✓6ᵗʰ **S66.10** Unspecified **injury of flexor muscle, fascia and tendon of other and unspecified finger at wrist and hand level**

     ✓7ᵗʰ **S66.100** **Unspecified injury of flexor muscle, fascia and tendon of** right index **finger at wrist and hand level**

     ✓7ᵗʰ **S66.101** **Unspecified injury of flexor muscle, fascia and tendon of** left index **finger at wrist and hand level**

     ✓7ᵗʰ **S66.102** **Unspecified injury of flexor muscle, fascia and tendon of** right middle **finger at wrist and hand level**

     ✓7ᵗʰ **S66.103** **Unspecified injury of flexor muscle, fascia and tendon of** left middle **finger at wrist and hand level**

     ✓7ᵗʰ **S66.104** **Unspecified injury of flexor muscle, fascia and tendon of** right ring **finger at wrist and hand level**

     ✓7ᵗʰ **S66.105** **Unspecified injury of flexor muscle, fascia and tendon of** left ring **finger at wrist and hand level**

     ✓7ᵗʰ **S66.106** **Unspecified injury of flexor muscle, fascia and tendon of** right little **finger at wrist and hand level**

     ✓7ᵗʰ **S66.107** **Unspecified injury of flexor muscle, fascia and tendon of** left little **finger at wrist and hand level**

     ✓7ᵗʰ **S66.108** **Unspecified injury of flexor muscle, fascia and tendon of** other **finger at wrist and hand level**
> Unspecified injury of flexor muscle, fascia and tendon of specified finger with unspecified laterality at wrist and hand level

     ✓7ᵗʰ **S66.109** **Unspecified injury of flexor muscle, fascia and tendon of** unspecified **finger at wrist and hand level**

✓6ᵗʰ **S66.11** Strain **of flexor muscle, fascia and tendon of other and unspecified finger at wrist and hand level**

     ✓7ᵗʰ **S66.110** **Strain of flexor muscle, fascia and tendon of** right index **finger at wrist and hand level**

     ✓7ᵗʰ **S66.111** **Strain of flexor muscle, fascia and tendon of** left index **finger at wrist and hand level**

     ✓7ᵗʰ **S66.112** **Strain of flexor muscle, fascia and tendon of** right middle **finger at wrist and hand level**

     ✓7ᵗʰ **S66.113** **Strain of flexor muscle, fascia and tendon of** left middle **finger at wrist and hand level**

     ✓7ᵗʰ **S66.114** **Strain of flexor muscle, fascia and tendon of** right ring **finger at wrist and hand level**

     ✓7ᵗʰ **S66.115** **Strain of flexor muscle, fascia and tendon of** left ring **finger at wrist and hand level**

     ✓7ᵗʰ **S66.116** **Strain of flexor muscle, fascia and tendon of** right little **finger at wrist and hand level**

     ✓7ᵗʰ **S66.117** **Strain of flexor muscle, fascia and tendon of** left little **finger at wrist and hand level**

     ✓7ᵗʰ **S66.118** **Strain of flexor muscle, fascia and tendon of** other **finger at wrist and hand level**
> Strain of flexor muscle, fascia and tendon of specified finger with unspecified laterality at wrist and hand level

     ✓7ᵗʰ **S66.119** **Strain of flexor muscle, fascia and tendon of** unspecified **finger at wrist and hand level**

✓6ᵗʰ **S66.12** Laceration **of flexor muscle, fascia and tendon of other and unspecified finger at wrist and hand level**

     ✓7ᵗʰ **S66.120** **Laceration of flexor muscle, fascia and tendon of** right index **finger at wrist and hand level**   CC

     ✓7ᵗʰ **S66.121** **Laceration of flexor muscle, fascia and tendon of** left index **finger at wrist and hand level**   CC

     ✓7ᵗʰ **S66.122** **Laceration of flexor muscle, fascia and tendon of** right middle **finger at wrist and hand level**   CC

     ✓7ᵗʰ **S66.123** **Laceration of flexor muscle, fascia and tendon of** left middle **finger at wrist and hand level**   CC

     ✓7ᵗʰ **S66.124** **Laceration of flexor muscle, fascia and tendon of** right ring **finger at wrist and hand level**   CC

     ✓7ᵗʰ **S66.125** **Laceration of flexor muscle, fascia and tendon of** left ring **finger at wrist and hand level**   CC

     ✓7ᵗʰ **S66.126** **Laceration of flexor muscle, fascia and tendon of** right little **finger at wrist and hand level**   CC

     ✓7ᵗʰ **S66.127** **Laceration of flexor muscle, fascia and tendon of** left little **finger at wrist and hand level**   CC

     ✓7ᵗʰ **S66.128** **Laceration of flexor muscle, fascia and tendon of** other **finger at wrist and hand level**   CC
> Laceration of flexor muscle, fascia and tendon of specified finger with unspecified laterality at wrist and hand level

     ✓7ᵗʰ **S66.129** **Laceration of flexor muscle, fascia and tendon of** unspecified **finger at wrist and hand level**   CC

✓6ᵗʰ **S66.19** Other **injury of flexor muscle, fascia and tendon of other and unspecified finger at wrist and hand level**

     ✓7ᵗʰ **S66.190** **Other injury of flexor muscle, fascia and tendon of** right index **finger at wrist and hand level**

     ✓7ᵗʰ **S66.191** **Other injury of flexor muscle, fascia and tendon of** left index **finger at wrist and hand level**

     ✓7ᵗʰ **S66.192** **Other injury of flexor muscle, fascia and tendon of** right middle **finger at wrist and hand level**

     ✓7ᵗʰ **S66.193** **Other injury of flexor muscle, fascia and tendon of** left middle **finger at wrist and hand level**

     ✓7ᵗʰ **S66.194** **Other injury of flexor muscle, fascia and tendon of** right ring **finger at wrist and hand level**

     ✓7ᵗʰ **S66.195** **Other injury of flexor muscle, fascia and tendon of** left ring **finger at wrist and hand level**

     ✓7ᵗʰ **S66.196** **Other injury of flexor muscle, fascia and tendon of** right little **finger at wrist and hand level**

     ✓7ᵗʰ **S66.197** **Other injury of flexor muscle, fascia and tendon of** left little **finger at wrist and hand level**

     ✓7ᵗʰ **S66.198** **Other injury of flexor muscle, fascia and tendon of** other **finger at wrist and hand level**
> Other injury of flexor muscle, fascia and tendon of specified finger with unspecified laterality at wrist and hand level

     ✓7ᵗʰ **S66.199** **Other injury of flexor muscle, fascia and tendon of** unspecified **finger at wrist and hand level**

✓5ᵗʰ **S66.2** **Injury of** extensor muscle, **fascia and tendon of** thumb **at wrist and hand level**

✓6ᵗʰ **S66.20** Unspecified **injury of extensor muscle, fascia and tendon of thumb at wrist and hand level**

     ✓7ᵗʰ **S66.201** **Unspecified injury of extensor muscle, fascia and tendon of** right **thumb at wrist and hand level**

     ✓7ᵗʰ **S66.202** **Unspecified injury of extensor muscle, fascia and tendon of** left **thumb at wrist and hand level**

     ✓7ᵗʰ **S66.209** **Unspecified injury of extensor muscle, fascia and tendon of** unspecified **thumb at wrist and hand level**

✓ Additional Character Required   ✓x7ᵗʰ Placeholder   Unacceptable PDx   Questionable PDx   Manifestation   H1-H14 HAC   HCC CMS-HCC Dx   HIV HIV Dx

ICD-10-CM 2019   1035

√6ᵗʰ **S66.21** Strain of extensor muscle, fascia and tendon of thumb at wrist and hand level

    √7ᵗʰ **S66.211** Strain of extensor muscle, fascia and tendon of right thumb at wrist and hand level

    √7ᵗʰ **S66.212** Strain of extensor muscle, fascia and tendon of left thumb at wrist and hand level

    √7ᵗʰ **S66.219** Strain of extensor muscle, fascia and tendon of unspecified thumb at wrist and hand level

√6ᵗʰ **S66.22** Laceration of extensor muscle, fascia and tendon of thumb at wrist and hand level

    √7ᵗʰ **S66.221** Laceration of extensor muscle, fascia and tendon of right thumb at wrist and hand level   `CC`

    √7ᵗʰ **S66.222** Laceration of extensor muscle, fascia and tendon of left thumb at wrist and hand level   `CC`

    √7ᵗʰ **S66.229** Laceration of extensor muscle, fascia and tendon of unspecified thumb at wrist and hand level   `CC`

√6ᵗʰ **S66.29** Other specified injury of extensor muscle, fascia and tendon of thumb at wrist and hand level

    √7ᵗʰ **S66.291** Other specified injury of extensor muscle, fascia and tendon of right thumb at wrist and hand level

    √7ᵗʰ **S66.292** Other specified injury of extensor muscle, fascia and tendon of left thumb at wrist and hand level

    √7ᵗʰ **S66.299** Other specified injury of extensor muscle, fascia and tendon of unspecified thumb at wrist and hand level

√5ᵗʰ **S66.3** Injury of extensor muscle, fascia and tendon of other and unspecified finger at wrist and hand level

    EXCLUDES 2   injury of extensor muscle, fascia and tendon of thumb at wrist and hand level (S66.2-)

√6ᵗʰ **S66.30** Unspecified injury of extensor muscle, fascia and tendon of other and unspecified finger at wrist and hand level

    √7ᵗʰ **S66.300** Unspecified injury of extensor muscle, fascia and tendon of right index finger at wrist and hand level

    √7ᵗʰ **S66.301** Unspecified injury of extensor muscle, fascia and tendon of left index finger at wrist and hand level

    √7ᵗʰ **S66.302** Unspecified injury of extensor muscle, fascia and tendon of right middle finger at wrist and hand level

    √7ᵗʰ **S66.303** Unspecified injury of extensor muscle, fascia and tendon of left middle finger at wrist and hand level

    √7ᵗʰ **S66.304** Unspecified injury of extensor muscle, fascia and tendon of right ring finger at wrist and hand level

    √7ᵗʰ **S66.305** Unspecified injury of extensor muscle, fascia and tendon of left ring finger at wrist and hand level

    √7ᵗʰ **S66.306** Unspecified injury of extensor muscle, fascia and tendon of right little finger at wrist and hand level

    √7ᵗʰ **S66.307** Unspecified injury of extensor muscle, fascia and tendon of left little finger at wrist and hand level

    √7ᵗʰ **S66.308** Unspecified injury of extensor muscle, fascia and tendon of other finger at wrist and hand level
       Unspecified injury of extensor muscle, fascia and tendon of specified finger with unspecified laterality at wrist and hand level

    √7ᵗʰ **S66.309** Unspecified injury of extensor muscle, fascia and tendon of unspecified finger at wrist and hand level

√6ᵗʰ **S66.31** Strain of extensor muscle, fascia and tendon of other and unspecified finger at wrist and hand level

    √7ᵗʰ **S66.310** Strain of extensor muscle, fascia and tendon of right index finger at wrist and hand level

√7ᵗʰ **S66.311** Strain of extensor muscle, fascia and tendon of left index finger at wrist and hand level

√7ᵗʰ **S66.312** Strain of extensor muscle, fascia and tendon of right middle finger at wrist and hand level

√7ᵗʰ **S66.313** Strain of extensor muscle, fascia and tendon of left middle finger at wrist and hand level

√7ᵗʰ **S66.314** Strain of extensor muscle, fascia and tendon of right ring finger at wrist and hand level

√7ᵗʰ **S66.315** Strain of extensor muscle, fascia and tendon of left ring finger at wrist and hand level

√7ᵗʰ **S66.316** Strain of extensor muscle, fascia and tendon of right little finger at wrist and hand level

√7ᵗʰ **S66.317** Strain of extensor muscle, fascia and tendon of left little finger at wrist and hand level

√7ᵗʰ **S66.318** Strain of extensor muscle, fascia and tendon of other finger at wrist and hand level
       Strain of extensor muscle, fascia and tendon of specified finger with unspecified laterality at wrist and hand level

√7ᵗʰ **S66.319** Strain of extensor muscle, fascia and tendon of unspecified finger at wrist and hand level

√6ᵗʰ **S66.32** Laceration of extensor muscle, fascia and tendon of other and unspecified finger at wrist and hand level

    √7ᵗʰ **S66.320** Laceration of extensor muscle, fascia and tendon of right index finger at wrist and hand level   `CC`

    √7ᵗʰ **S66.321** Laceration of extensor muscle, fascia and tendon of left index finger at wrist and hand level   `CC`

    √7ᵗʰ **S66.322** Laceration of extensor muscle, fascia and tendon of right middle finger at wrist and hand level   `CC`

    √7ᵗʰ **S66.323** Laceration of extensor muscle, fascia and tendon of left middle finger at wrist and hand level   `CC`

    √7ᵗʰ **S66.324** Laceration of extensor muscle, fascia and tendon of right ring finger at wrist and hand level   `CC`

    √7ᵗʰ **S66.325** Laceration of extensor muscle, fascia and tendon of left ring finger at wrist and hand level   `CC`

    √7ᵗʰ **S66.326** Laceration of extensor muscle, fascia and tendon of right little finger at wrist and hand level   `CC`

    √7ᵗʰ **S66.327** Laceration of extensor muscle, fascia and tendon of left little finger at wrist and hand level   `CC`

    √7ᵗʰ **S66.328** Laceration of extensor muscle, fascia and tendon of other finger at wrist and hand level   `CC`
       Laceration of extensor muscle, fascia and tendon of specified finger with unspecified laterality at wrist and hand level

    √7ᵗʰ **S66.329** Laceration of extensor muscle, fascia and tendon of unspecified finger at wrist and hand level   `CC`

√6ᵗʰ **S66.39** Other injury of extensor muscle, fascia and tendon of other and unspecified finger at wrist and hand level

    √7ᵗʰ **S66.390** Other injury of extensor muscle, fascia and tendon of right index finger at wrist and hand level

    √7ᵗʰ **S66.391** Other injury of extensor muscle, fascia and tendon of left index finger at wrist and hand level

    √7ᵗʰ **S66.392** Other injury of extensor muscle, fascia and tendon of right middle finger at wrist and hand level

N Newborn: 0   **P** Pediatric: 0-17   **M** Maternity: 12-55   **A** Adult: 15-124   `MCC` Major Complication/Comorbidity   `CC` Complication/Comorbidity   `SW` Severe Wound Dx

1036   ICD-10-CM 2019

√7ᵗʰ **S66.393** Other injury of extensor muscle, fascia and tendon of left middle finger at wrist and hand level

√7ᵗʰ **S66.394** Other injury of extensor muscle, fascia and tendon of right ring finger at wrist and hand level

√7ᵗʰ **S66.395** Other injury of extensor muscle, fascia and tendon of left ring finger at wrist and hand level

√7ᵗʰ **S66.396** Other injury of extensor muscle, fascia and tendon of right little finger at wrist and hand level

√7ᵗʰ **S66.397** Other injury of extensor muscle, fascia and tendon of left little finger at wrist and hand level

√7ᵗʰ **S66.398** Other injury of extensor muscle, fascia and tendon of other finger at wrist and hand level
Other injury of extensor muscle, fascia and tendon of specified finger with unspecified laterality at wrist and hand level

√7ᵗʰ **S66.399** Other injury of extensor muscle, fascia and tendon of unspecified finger at wrist and hand level

√5ᵗʰ **S66.4 Injury of** intrinsic muscle, fascia and tendon of thumb at wrist and hand level

√6ᵗʰ **S66.40** Unspecified injury of intrinsic muscle, fascia and tendon of thumb at wrist and hand level

√7ᵗʰ **S66.401** Unspecified injury of intrinsic muscle, fascia and tendon of right thumb at wrist and hand level

√7ᵗʰ **S66.402** Unspecified injury of intrinsic muscle, fascia and tendon of left thumb at wrist and hand level

√7ᵗʰ **S66.409** Unspecified injury of intrinsic muscle, fascia and tendon of unspecified thumb at wrist and hand level

√6ᵗʰ **S66.41** Strain of intrinsic muscle, fascia and tendon of thumb at wrist and hand level

√7ᵗʰ **S66.411** Strain of intrinsic muscle, fascia and tendon of right thumb at wrist and hand level

√7ᵗʰ **S66.412** Strain of intrinsic muscle, fascia and tendon of left thumb at wrist and hand level

√7ᵗʰ **S66.419** Strain of intrinsic muscle, fascia and tendon of unspecified thumb at wrist and hand level

√6ᵗʰ **S66.42** Laceration of intrinsic muscle, fascia and tendon of thumb at wrist and hand level

√7ᵗʰ **S66.421** Laceration of intrinsic muscle, fascia and tendon of right thumb at wrist and hand level   CC

√7ᵗʰ **S66.422** Laceration of intrinsic muscle, fascia and tendon of left thumb at wrist and hand level   CC

√7ᵗʰ **S66.429** Laceration of intrinsic muscle, fascia and tendon of unspecified thumb at wrist and hand level   CC

√6ᵗʰ **S66.49** Other specified injury of intrinsic muscle, fascia and tendon of thumb at wrist and hand level

√7ᵗʰ **S66.491** Other specified injury of intrinsic muscle, fascia and tendon of right thumb at wrist and hand level

√7ᵗʰ **S66.492** Other specified injury of intrinsic muscle, fascia and tendon of left thumb at wrist and hand level

√7ᵗʰ **S66.499** Other specified injury of intrinsic muscle, fascia and tendon of unspecified thumb at wrist and hand level

√5ᵗʰ **S66.5 Injury of** intrinsic muscle, fascia and tendon of other and unspecified finger at wrist and hand level

EXCLUDES 2   injury of intrinsic muscle, fascia and tendon of thumb at wrist and hand level (S66.4-)

√6ᵗʰ **S66.50** Unspecified injury of intrinsic muscle, fascia and tendon of other and unspecified finger at wrist and hand level

√7ᵗʰ **S66.500** Unspecified injury of intrinsic muscle, fascia and tendon of right index finger at wrist and hand level

√7ᵗʰ **S66.501** Unspecified injury of intrinsic muscle, fascia and tendon of left index finger at wrist and hand level

√7ᵗʰ **S66.502** Unspecified injury of intrinsic muscle, fascia and tendon of right middle finger at wrist and hand level

√7ᵗʰ **S66.503** Unspecified injury of intrinsic muscle, fascia and tendon of left middle finger at wrist and hand level

√7ᵗʰ **S66.504** Unspecified injury of intrinsic muscle, fascia and tendon of right ring finger at wrist and hand level

√7ᵗʰ **S66.505** Unspecified injury of intrinsic muscle, fascia and tendon of left ring finger at wrist and hand level

√7ᵗʰ **S66.506** Unspecified injury of intrinsic muscle, fascia and tendon of right little finger at wrist and hand level

√7ᵗʰ **S66.507** Unspecified injury of intrinsic muscle, fascia and tendon of left little finger at wrist and hand level

√7ᵗʰ **S66.508** Unspecified injury of intrinsic muscle, fascia and tendon of other finger at wrist and hand level
Unspecified injury of intrinsic muscle, fascia and tendon of specified finger with unspecified laterality at wrist and hand level

√7ᵗʰ **S66.509** Unspecified injury of intrinsic muscle, fascia and tendon of unspecified finger at wrist and hand level

√6ᵗʰ **S66.51** Strain of intrinsic muscle, fascia and tendon of other and unspecified finger at wrist and hand level

√7ᵗʰ **S66.510** Strain of intrinsic muscle, fascia and tendon of right index finger at wrist and hand level

√7ᵗʰ **S66.511** Strain of intrinsic muscle, fascia and tendon of left index finger at wrist and hand level

√7ᵗʰ **S66.512** Strain of intrinsic muscle, fascia and tendon of right middle finger at wrist and hand level

√7ᵗʰ **S66.513** Strain of intrinsic muscle, fascia and tendon of left middle finger at wrist and hand level

√7ᵗʰ **S66.514** Strain of intrinsic muscle, fascia and tendon of right ring finger at wrist and hand level

√7ᵗʰ **S66.515** Strain of intrinsic muscle, fascia and tendon of left ring finger at wrist and hand level

√7ᵗʰ **S66.516** Strain of intrinsic muscle, fascia and tendon of right little finger at wrist and hand level

√7ᵗʰ **S66.517** Strain of intrinsic muscle, fascia and tendon of left little finger at wrist and hand level

√7ᵗʰ **S66.518** Strain of intrinsic muscle, fascia and tendon of other finger at wrist and hand level
Strain of intrinsic muscle, fascia and tendon of specified finger with unspecified laterality at wrist and hand level

√7ᵗʰ **S66.519** Strain of intrinsic muscle, fascia and tendon of unspecified finger at wrist and hand level

☑Additional Character Required   √x7ᵗʰ Placeholder   Unacceptable PDx   Questionable PDx   Manifestation   H1-H14 HAC   HCC CMS-HCC Dx   HIV HIV Dx

ICD-10-CM 2019   1037

☑6ᵗʰ **S66.52** Laceration of intrinsic muscle, fascia and tendon of other and unspecified finger at wrist and hand level

  ☑7ᵗʰ **S66.520** Laceration of intrinsic muscle, fascia and tendon of right index finger at wrist and hand level `CC`

  ☑7ᵗʰ **S66.521** Laceration of intrinsic muscle, fascia and tendon of left index finger at wrist and hand level `CC`

  ☑7ᵗʰ **S66.522** Laceration of intrinsic muscle, fascia and tendon of right middle finger at wrist and hand level `CC`

  ☑7ᵗʰ **S66.523** Laceration of intrinsic muscle, fascia and tendon of left middle finger at wrist and hand level `CC`

  ☑7ᵗʰ **S66.524** Laceration of intrinsic muscle, fascia and tendon of right ring finger at wrist and hand level `CC`

  ☑7ᵗʰ **S66.525** Laceration of intrinsic muscle, fascia and tendon of left ring finger at wrist and hand level `CC`

  ☑7ᵗʰ **S66.526** Laceration of intrinsic muscle, fascia and tendon of right little finger at wrist and hand level `CC`

  ☑7ᵗʰ **S66.527** Laceration of intrinsic muscle, fascia and tendon of left little finger at wrist and hand level `CC`

  ☑7ᵗʰ **S66.528** Laceration of intrinsic muscle, fascia and tendon of other finger at wrist and hand level `CC`

       Laceration of intrinsic muscle, fascia and tendon of specified finger with unspecified laterality at wrist and hand level

  ☑7ᵗʰ **S66.529** Laceration of intrinsic muscle, fascia and tendon of unspecified finger at wrist and hand level `CC`

☑6ᵗʰ **S66.59** Other injury of intrinsic muscle, fascia and tendon of other and unspecified finger at wrist and hand level

  ☑7ᵗʰ **S66.590** Other injury of intrinsic muscle, fascia and tendon of right index finger at wrist and hand level

  ☑7ᵗʰ **S66.591** Other injury of intrinsic muscle, fascia and tendon of left index finger at wrist and hand level

  ☑7ᵗʰ **S66.592** Other injury of intrinsic muscle, fascia and tendon of right middle finger at wrist and hand level

  ☑7ᵗʰ **S66.593** Other injury of intrinsic muscle, fascia and tendon of left middle finger at wrist and hand level

  ☑7ᵗʰ **S66.594** Other injury of intrinsic muscle, fascia and tendon of right ring finger at wrist and hand level

  ☑7ᵗʰ **S66.595** Other injury of intrinsic muscle, fascia and tendon of left ring finger at wrist and hand level

  ☑7ᵗʰ **S66.596** Other injury of intrinsic muscle, fascia and tendon of right little finger at wrist and hand level

  ☑7ᵗʰ **S66.597** Other injury of intrinsic muscle, fascia and tendon of left little finger at wrist and hand level

  ☑7ᵗʰ **S66.598** Other injury of intrinsic muscle, fascia and tendon of other finger at wrist and hand level

       Other injury of intrinsic muscle, fascia and tendon of specified finger with unspecified laterality at wrist and hand level

  ☑7ᵗʰ **S66.599** Other injury of intrinsic muscle, fascia and tendon of unspecified finger at wrist and hand level

☑5ᵗʰ **S66.8** Injury of other specified muscles, fascia and tendons at wrist and hand level

  ☑6ᵗʰ **S66.80** Unspecified injury of other specified muscles, fascia and tendons at wrist and hand level

    ☑7ᵗʰ **S66.801** Unspecified injury of other specified muscles, fascia and tendons at wrist and hand level, right hand

    ☑7ᵗʰ **S66.802** Unspecified injury of other specified muscles, fascia and tendons at wrist and hand level, left hand

    ☑7ᵗʰ **S66.809** Unspecified injury of other specified muscles, fascia and tendons at wrist and hand level, unspecified hand

  ☑6ᵗʰ **S66.81** Strain of other specified muscles, fascia and tendons at wrist and hand level

    ☑7ᵗʰ **S66.811** Strain of other specified muscles, fascia and tendons at wrist and hand level, right hand

    ☑7ᵗʰ **S66.812** Strain of other specified muscles, fascia and tendons at wrist and hand level, left hand

    ☑7ᵗʰ **S66.819** Strain of other specified muscles, fascia and tendons at wrist and hand level, unspecified hand

  ☑6ᵗʰ **S66.82** Laceration of other specified muscles, fascia and tendons at wrist and hand level

    ☑7ᵗʰ **S66.821** Laceration of other specified muscles, fascia and tendons at wrist and hand level, right hand `CC`

    ☑7ᵗʰ **S66.822** Laceration of other specified muscles, fascia and tendons at wrist and hand level, left hand `CC`

    ☑7ᵗʰ **S66.829** Laceration of other specified muscles, fascia and tendons at wrist and hand level, unspecified hand `CC`

  ☑6ᵗʰ **S66.89** Other injury of other specified muscles, fascia and tendons at wrist and hand level

    ☑7ᵗʰ **S66.891** Other injury of other specified muscles, fascia and tendons at wrist and hand level, right hand

    ☑7ᵗʰ **S66.892** Other injury of other specified muscles, fascia and tendons at wrist and hand level, left hand

    ☑7ᵗʰ **S66.899** Other injury of other specified muscles, fascia and tendons at wrist and hand level, unspecified hand

☑5ᵗʰ **S66.9** Injury of unspecified muscle, fascia and tendon at wrist and hand level

  ☑6ᵗʰ **S66.90** Unspecified injury of unspecified muscle, fascia and tendon at wrist and hand level

    ☑7ᵗʰ **S66.901** Unspecified injury of unspecified muscle, fascia and tendon at wrist and hand level, right hand

    ☑7ᵗʰ **S66.902** Unspecified injury of unspecified muscle, fascia and tendon at wrist and hand level, left hand

    ☑7ᵗʰ **S66.909** Unspecified injury of unspecified muscle, fascia and tendon at wrist and hand level, unspecified hand

  ☑6ᵗʰ **S66.91** Strain of unspecified muscle, fascia and tendon at wrist and hand level

    ☑7ᵗʰ **S66.911** Strain of unspecified muscle, fascia and tendon at wrist and hand level, right hand

    ☑7ᵗʰ **S66.912** Strain of unspecified muscle, fascia and tendon at wrist and hand level, left hand

    ☑7ᵗʰ **S66.919** Strain of unspecified muscle, fascia and tendon at wrist and hand level, unspecified hand

  ☑6ᵗʰ **S66.92** Laceration of unspecified muscle, fascia and tendon at wrist and hand level

    ☑7ᵗʰ **S66.921** Laceration of unspecified muscle, fascia and tendon at wrist and hand level, right hand `CC`

    ☑7ᵗʰ **S66.922** Laceration of unspecified muscle, fascia and tendon at wrist and hand level, left hand `CC`

    ☑7ᵗʰ **S66.929** Laceration of unspecified muscle, fascia and tendon at wrist and hand level, unspecified hand `CC`

  ☑6ᵗʰ **S66.99** Other injury of unspecified muscle, fascia and tendon at wrist and hand level

    ☑7ᵗʰ **S66.991** Other injury of unspecified muscle, fascia and tendon at wrist and hand level, right hand

---

Ⓝ Newborn: 0   Ⓟ Pediatric: 0-17   Ⓜ Maternity: 12-55   Ⓐ Adult: 15-124   `MCC` Major Complication/Comorbidity   `CC` Complication/Comorbidity   `SW` Severe Wound Dx

☑7ᵗʰ **S66.992**   **Other injury of unspecified muscle, fascia and tendon at wrist and hand level, left hand**

☑7ᵗʰ **S66.999**   **Other injury of unspecified muscle, fascia and tendon at wrist and hand level, unspecified hand**

✓4ᵗʰ **S67**   **Crushing injury of wrist, hand and fingers**

Use additional code for all associated injuries, such as:
fracture of wrist and hand (S62.-)
open wound of wrist and hand (S61.-)

The appropriate 7th character is to be added to each code from category S67.
A   initial encounter
D   subsequent encounter
S   sequela

✓5ᵗʰ **S67.0**   **Crushing injury of thumb**

✓x7ᵗʰ **S67.00**   **Crushing injury of unspecified thumb**

✓x7ᵗʰ **S67.01**   **Crushing injury of right thumb**

✓x7ᵗʰ **S67.02**   **Crushing injury of left thumb**

✓5ᵗʰ **S67.1**   **Crushing injury of other and unspecified finger(s)**
> EXCLUDES 2   *crushing injury of thumb (S67.0-)*

✓x7ᵗʰ **S67.10**   **Crushing injury of unspecified finger(s)**

✓6ᵗʰ **S67.19**   **Crushing injury of other finger(s)**

✓7ᵗʰ **S67.190**   **Crushing injury of right index finger**

✓7ᵗʰ **S67.191**   **Crushing injury of left index finger**

✓7ᵗʰ **S67.192**   **Crushing injury of right middle finger**

✓7ᵗʰ **S67.193**   **Crushing injury of left middle finger**

✓7ᵗʰ **S67.194**   **Crushing injury of right ring finger**

✓7ᵗʰ **S67.195**   **Crushing injury of left ring finger**

✓7ᵗʰ **S67.196**   **Crushing injury of right little finger**

✓7ᵗʰ **S67.197**   **Crushing injury of left little finger**

✓7ᵗʰ **S67.198**   **Crushing injury of other finger**
Crushing injury of specified finger with unspecified laterality

✓5ᵗʰ **S67.2**   **Crushing injury of hand**
> EXCLUDES 2   *crushing injury of fingers (S67.1-)*
> *crushing injury of thumb (S67.0-)*

✓x7ᵗʰ **S67.20**   **Crushing injury of unspecified hand**

✓x7ᵗʰ **S67.21**   **Crushing injury of right hand**

✓x7ᵗʰ **S67.22**   **Crushing injury of left hand**

✓5ᵗʰ **S67.3**   **Crushing injury of wrist**

✓x7ᵗʰ **S67.30**   **Crushing injury of unspecified wrist**

✓x7ᵗʰ **S67.31**   **Crushing injury of right wrist**

✓x7ᵗʰ **S67.32**   **Crushing injury of left wrist**

✓5ᵗʰ **S67.4**   **Crushing injury of wrist and hand**
> EXCLUDES 1   *crushing injury of hand alone (S67.2-)*
> *crushing injury of wrist alone (S67.3-)*
> EXCLUDES 2   *crushing injury of fingers (S67.1-)*
> *crushing injury of thumb (S67.0-)*

✓x7ᵗʰ **S67.40**   **Crushing injury of unspecified wrist and hand**

✓x7ᵗʰ **S67.41**   **Crushing injury of right wrist and hand**

✓x7ᵗʰ **S67.42**   **Crushing injury of left wrist and hand**

✓5ᵗʰ **S67.9**   **Crushing injury of unspecified part(s) of wrist, hand and fingers**

✓x7ᵗʰ **S67.90**   **Crushing injury of unspecified part(s) of unspecified wrist, hand and fingers**

✓x7ᵗʰ **S67.91**   **Crushing injury of unspecified part(s) of right wrist, hand and fingers**

✓x7ᵗʰ **S67.92**   **Crushing injury of unspecified part(s) of left wrist, hand and fingers**

✓4ᵗʰ **S68**   **Traumatic amputation of wrist, hand and fingers**

An amputation not identified as partial or complete should be coded to complete.

The appropriate 7th character is to be added to each code from category S68.
A   initial encounter
D   subsequent encounter
S   sequela

CC Excl: For CC codes in category S68:
Right side: PDX collection 1266
Left side: PDX collection 1267
Unspecified side: PDX collection 1268

✓5ᵗʰ **S68.0**   **Traumatic metacarpophalangeal amputation of thumb**
Traumatic amputation of thumb NOS

✓6ᵗʰ **S68.01**   **Complete traumatic metacarpophalangeal amputation of thumb**

8 ✓7ᵗʰ **S68.011**   **Complete traumatic metacarpophalangeal amputation of right thumb**   HCC

8 ✓7ᵗʰ **S68.012**   **Complete traumatic metacarpophalangeal amputation of left thumb**   HCC

8 ✓7ᵗʰ **S68.019**   **Complete traumatic metacarpophalangeal amputation of unspecified thumb**   HCC

✓6ᵗʰ **S68.02**   **Partial traumatic metacarpophalangeal amputation of thumb**

8 ✓7ᵗʰ **S68.021**   **Partial traumatic metacarpophalangeal amputation of right thumb**   HCC

8 ✓7ᵗʰ **S68.022**   **Partial traumatic metacarpophalangeal amputation of left thumb**   HCC

8 ✓7ᵗʰ **S68.029**   **Partial traumatic metacarpophalangeal amputation of unspecified thumb**   HCC

✓5ᵗʰ **S68.1**   **Traumatic metacarpophalangeal amputation of other and unspecified finger**
Traumatic amputation of finger NOS
> EXCLUDES 2   *traumatic metacarpophalangeal amputation of thumb (S68.0-)*

✓6ᵗʰ **S68.11**   **Complete traumatic metacarpophalangeal amputation of other and unspecified finger**

8 ✓7ᵗʰ **S68.110**   **Complete traumatic metacarpophalangeal amputation of right index finger**   HCC

8 ✓7ᵗʰ **S68.111**   **Complete traumatic metacarpophalangeal amputation of left index finger**   HCC

8 ✓7ᵗʰ **S68.112**   **Complete traumatic metacarpophalangeal amputation of right middle finger**   HCC

8 ✓7ᵗʰ **S68.113**   **Complete traumatic metacarpophalangeal amputation of left middle finger**   HCC

8 ✓7ᵗʰ **S68.114**   **Complete traumatic metacarpophalangeal amputation of right ring finger**   HCC

8 ✓7ᵗʰ **S68.115**   **Complete traumatic metacarpophalangeal amputation of left ring finger**   HCC

8 ✓7ᵗʰ **S68.116**   **Complete traumatic metacarpophalangeal amputation of right little finger**   HCC

8 ✓7ᵗʰ **S68.117**   **Complete traumatic metacarpophalangeal amputation of left little finger**   HCC

8 ✓7ᵗʰ **S68.118**   **Complete traumatic metacarpophalangeal amputation of other finger**   HCC
Complete traumatic metacarpophalangeal amputation of specified finger with unspecified laterality

8 ✓7ᵗʰ **S68.119**   **Complete traumatic metacarpophalangeal amputation of unspecified finger**   HCC

✓6ᵗʰ **S68.12**   **Partial traumatic metacarpophalangeal amputation of other and unspecified finger**

8 ✓7ᵗʰ **S68.120**   **Partial traumatic metacarpophalangeal amputation of right index finger**   HCC

☑ Additional Character Required   ✓x7ᵗʰ Placeholder   Unacceptable PDx   Questionable PDx   Manifestation   H1-H14 HAC   HCC CMS-HCC Dx   HIV HIV Dx

ICD-10-CM 2019   1039

8 √7ᵗʰ **S68.121** Partial traumatic metacarpo-phalangeal amputation of left index finger HCC

8 √7ᵗʰ **S68.122** Partial traumatic metacarpo-phalangeal amputation of right middle finger HCC

8 √7ᵗʰ **S68.123** Partial traumatic metacarpo-phalangeal amputation of left middle finger HCC

8 √7ᵗʰ **S68.124** Partial traumatic metacarpo-phalangeal amputation of right ring finger HCC

8 √7ᵗʰ **S68.125** Partial traumatic metacarpo-phalangeal amputation of left ring finger HCC

8 √7ᵗʰ **S68.126** Partial traumatic metacarpo-phalangeal amputation of right little finger HCC

8 √7ᵗʰ **S68.127** Partial traumatic metacarpo-phalangeal amputation of left little finger HCC

8 √7ᵗʰ **S68.128** Partial traumatic metacarpo-phalangeal amputation of other finger HCC
     Partial traumatic metacarpophalangeal amputation of specified finger with unspecified laterality

8 √7ᵗʰ **S68.129** Partial traumatic metacarpo-phalangeal amputation of unspecified finger HCC

√5ᵗʰ **S68.4** **Traumatic amputation of hand at wrist level**
     Traumatic amputation of hand NOS
     Traumatic amputation of wrist

     √6ᵗʰ **S68.41** **Complete traumatic amputation of hand at wrist level**

       7 √7ᵗʰ **S68.411** Complete traumatic amputation of right hand at wrist level CC HCC

       7 √7ᵗʰ **S68.412** Complete traumatic amputation of left hand at wrist level CC HCC

       7 √7ᵗʰ **S68.419** Complete traumatic amputation of unspecified hand at wrist level CC HCC

     √6ᵗʰ **S68.42** **Partial traumatic amputation of hand at wrist level**

       7 √7ᵗʰ **S68.421** Partial traumatic amputation of right hand at wrist level CC HCC

       7 √7ᵗʰ **S68.422** Partial traumatic amputation of left hand at wrist level CC HCC

       7 √7ᵗʰ **S68.429** Partial traumatic amputation of unspecified hand at wrist level CC HCC

√5ᵗʰ **S68.5** **Traumatic transphalangeal amputation of thumb**
     Traumatic interphalangeal joint amputation of thumb

     √6ᵗʰ **S68.51** **Complete traumatic transphalangeal amputation of thumb**

       8 √7ᵗʰ **S68.511** Complete traumatic transphalangeal amputation of right thumb HCC

       8 √7ᵗʰ **S68.512** Complete traumatic transphalangeal amputation of left thumb HCC

       8 √7ᵗʰ **S68.519** Complete traumatic transphalangeal amputation of unspecified thumb HCC

     √6ᵗʰ **S68.52** **Partial traumatic transphalangeal amputation of thumb**

       8 √7ᵗʰ **S68.521** Partial traumatic transphalangeal amputation of right thumb HCC

       8 √7ᵗʰ **S68.522** Partial traumatic transphalangeal amputation of left thumb HCC

       8 √7ᵗʰ **S68.529** Partial traumatic transphalangeal amputation of unspecified thumb HCC

√5ᵗʰ **S68.6** **Traumatic transphalangeal amputation of other and unspecified finger**

     √6ᵗʰ **S68.61** **Complete traumatic transphalangeal amputation of other and unspecified finger(s)**

       8 √7ᵗʰ **S68.610** Complete traumatic transphalangeal amputation of right index finger HCC

       8 √7ᵗʰ **S68.611** Complete traumatic transphalangeal amputation of left index finger HCC

       8 √7ᵗʰ **S68.612** Complete traumatic transphalangeal amputation of right middle finger HCC

8 √7ᵗʰ **S68.613** Complete traumatic transphalangeal amputation of left middle finger HCC

8 √7ᵗʰ **S68.614** Complete traumatic transphalangeal amputation of right ring finger HCC

8 √7ᵗʰ **S68.615** Complete traumatic transphalangeal amputation of left ring finger HCC

8 √7ᵗʰ **S68.616** Complete traumatic transphalangeal amputation of right little finger HCC

8 √7ᵗʰ **S68.617** Complete traumatic transphalangeal amputation of left little finger HCC

8 √7ᵗʰ **S68.618** Complete traumatic transphalangeal amputation of other finger HCC
     Complete traumatic transphalangeal amputation of specified finger with unspecified laterality

8 √7ᵗʰ **S68.619** Complete traumatic transphalangeal amputation of unspecified finger HCC

√6ᵗʰ **S68.62** **Partial traumatic transphalangeal amputation of other and unspecified finger**

     8 √7ᵗʰ **S68.620** Partial traumatic transphalangeal amputation of right index finger HCC

     8 √7ᵗʰ **S68.621** Partial traumatic transphalangeal amputation of left index finger HCC

     8 √7ᵗʰ **S68.622** Partial traumatic transphalangeal amputation of right middle finger HCC

     8 √7ᵗʰ **S68.623** Partial traumatic transphalangeal amputation of left middle finger HCC

     8 √7ᵗʰ **S68.624** Partial traumatic transphalangeal amputation of right ring finger HCC

     8 √7ᵗʰ **S68.625** Partial traumatic transphalangeal amputation of left ring finger HCC

     8 √7ᵗʰ **S68.626** Partial traumatic transphalangeal amputation of right little finger HCC

     8 √7ᵗʰ **S68.627** Partial traumatic transphalangeal amputation of left little finger HCC

     8 √7ᵗʰ **S68.628** Partial traumatic transphalangeal amputation of other finger HCC
       Partial traumatic transphalangeal amputation of specified finger with unspecified laterality

     8 √7ᵗʰ **S68.629** Partial traumatic transphalangeal amputation of unspecified finger HCC

√5ᵗʰ **S68.7** **Traumatic transmetacarpal amputation of hand**

     √6ᵗʰ **S68.71** **Complete traumatic transmetacarpal amputation of hand**

       7 √7ᵗʰ **S68.711** Complete traumatic transmetacarpal amputation of right hand CC HCC

       7 √7ᵗʰ **S68.712** Complete traumatic transmetacarpal amputation of left hand CC HCC

       7 √7ᵗʰ **S68.719** Complete traumatic transmetacarpal amputation of unspecified hand CC HCC

     √6ᵗʰ **S68.72** **Partial traumatic transmetacarpal amputation of hand**

       7 √7ᵗʰ **S68.721** Partial traumatic transmetacarpal amputation of right hand CC HCC

       7 √7ᵗʰ **S68.722** Partial traumatic transmetacarpal amputation of left hand CC HCC

       7 √7ᵗʰ **S68.729** Partial traumatic transmetacarpal amputation of unspecified hand CC HCC

√4ᵗʰ **S69** **Other and unspecified injuries of wrist, hand and finger(s)**

> The appropriate 7th character is to be added to each code from category S69.
> A   initial encounter
> D   subsequent encounter
> S   sequela

√5ᵗʰ **S69.8** **Other specified injuries of wrist, hand and finger(s)**

     √x7ᵗʰ **S69.80** Other specified injuries of unspecified wrist, hand and finger(s)

     √x7ᵗʰ **S69.81** Other specified injuries of right wrist, hand and finger(s)

     √x7ᵗʰ **S69.82** Other specified injuries of left wrist, hand and finger(s)

N Newborn: 0   P Pediatric: 0-17   M Maternity: 12-55   A Adult: 15-124   MCC Major Complication/Comorbidity   CC Complication/Comorbidity   SW Severe Wound Dx

1040   ICD-10-CM 2019

✓5th **S69.9** **Unspecified injury of wrist, hand and finger(s)**

     ✓x7th **S69.90** **Unspecified injury of** unspecified **wrist, hand and finger(s)**

     ✓x7th **S69.91** **Unspecified injury of** right **wrist, hand and finger(s)**

     ✓x7th **S69.92** **Unspecified injury of** left **wrist, hand and finger(s)**

Injuries to the hip and thigh (S70-S79)

EXCLUDES 2   burns and corrosions (T20-T32)
         frostbite (T33-T34)
         snake bite (T63.0-)
         venomous insect bite or sting (T63.4-)

✓4th **S70** **Superficial injury of hip and thigh**

> The appropriate 7th character is to be added to each code from category S70.
> A   initial encounter
> D   subsequent encounter
> S   sequela

   ✓5th **S70.0** **Contusion of** hip

     ✓x7th **S70.00** **Contusion of** unspecified **hip**

     ✓x7th **S70.01** **Contusion of** right **hip**

     ✓x7th **S70.02** **Contusion of** left **hip**

   ✓5th **S70.1** **Contusion of** thigh

     ✓x7th **S70.10** **Contusion of** unspecified **thigh**

     ✓x7th **S70.11** **Contusion of** right **thigh**

     ✓x7th **S70.12** **Contusion of** left **thigh**

   ✓5th **S70.2** **Other** superficial injuries of hip

     ✓6th **S70.21** **Abrasion** of hip

       ✓7th **S70.211** **Abrasion,** right **hip**

       ✓7th **S70.212** **Abrasion,** left **hip**

       ✓7th **S70.219** **Abrasion,** unspecified **hip**

     ✓6th **S70.22** **Blister** (nonthermal) of hip

       ✓7th **S70.221** **Blister (nonthermal),** right **hip**

       ✓7th **S70.222** **Blister (nonthermal),** left **hip**

       ✓7th **S70.229** **Blister (nonthermal),** unspecified **hip**

     ✓6th **S70.24** **External constriction** of hip

       ✓7th **S70.241** **External constriction,** right **hip**

       ✓7th **S70.242** **External constriction,** left **hip**

       ✓7th **S70.249** **External constriction,** unspecified **hip**

     ✓6th **S70.25** **Superficial** foreign body of hip
       Splinter in the hip

       ✓7th **S70.251** **Superficial foreign body,** right **hip**

       ✓7th **S70.252** **Superficial foreign body,** left **hip**

       ✓7th **S70.259** **Superficial foreign body,** unspecified **hip**

     ✓6th **S70.26** **Insect bite** (nonvenomous) of hip

       ✓7th **S70.261** **Insect bite (nonvenomous),** right **hip**

       ✓7th **S70.262** **Insect bite (nonvenomous),** left **hip**

       ✓7th **S70.269** **Insect bite (nonvenomous),** unspecified **hip**

     ✓6th **S70.27** **Other** superficial bite of hip
       EXCLUDES 1   open bite of hip (S71.05-)

       ✓7th **S70.271** **Other superficial bite of hip,** right **hip**

       ✓7th **S70.272** **Other superficial bite of hip,** left **hip**

       ✓7th **S70.279** **Other superficial bite of hip,** unspecified **hip**

   ✓5th **S70.3** **Other** superficial injuries of thigh

     ✓6th **S70.31** **Abrasion** of thigh

       ✓7th **S70.311** **Abrasion,** right **thigh**

       ✓7th **S70.312** **Abrasion,** left **thigh**

       ✓7th **S70.319** **Abrasion,** unspecified **thigh**

     ✓6th **S70.32** **Blister** (nonthermal) of thigh

       ✓7th **S70.321** **Blister (nonthermal),** right **thigh**

       ✓7th **S70.322** **Blister (nonthermal),** left **thigh**

       ✓7th **S70.329** **Blister (nonthermal),** unspecified **thigh**

     ✓6th **S70.34** **External constriction** of thigh

       ✓7th **S70.341** **External constriction,** right **thigh**

       ✓7th **S70.342** **External constriction,** left **thigh**

       ✓7th **S70.349** **External constriction,** unspecified **thigh**

     ✓6th **S70.35** **Superficial** foreign body of thigh
       Splinter in the thigh

       ✓7th **S70.351** **Superficial foreign body,** right **thigh**

       ✓7th **S70.352** **Superficial foreign body,** left **thigh**

       ✓7th **S70.359** **Superficial foreign body,** unspecified **thigh**

     ✓6th **S70.36** **Insect bite** (nonvenomous) of thigh

       ✓7th **S70.361** **Insect bite (nonvenomous),** right **thigh**

       ✓7th **S70.362** **Insect bite (nonvenomous),** left **thigh**

       ✓7th **S70.369** **Insect bite (nonvenomous),** unspecified **thigh**

     ✓6th **S70.37** **Other** superficial bite of thigh
       EXCLUDES 1   open bite of thigh (S71.15)

       ✓7th **S70.371** **Other superficial bite of** right **thigh**

       ✓7th **S70.372** **Other superficial bite of** left **thigh**

       ✓7th **S70.379** **Other superficial bite of** unspecified **thigh**

   ✓5th **S70.9** **Unspecified superficial injury of** hip and thigh

     ✓6th **S70.91** **Unspecified superficial injury of** hip

       ✓7th **S70.911** **Unspecified superficial injury of** right **hip**

       ✓7th **S70.912** **Unspecified superficial injury of** left **hip**

       ✓7th **S70.919** **Unspecified superficial injury of** unspecified **hip**

     ✓6th **S70.92** **Unspecified superficial injury of** thigh

       ✓7th **S70.921** **Unspecified superficial injury of** right **thigh**

       ✓7th **S70.922** **Unspecified superficial injury of** left **thigh**

       ✓7th **S70.929** **Unspecified superficial injury of** unspecified **thigh**

✓4th **S71** **Open wound of hip and thigh**
     Code also any associated wound infection
     EXCLUDES 1   open fracture of hip and thigh (S72.-)
            traumatic amputation of hip and thigh (S78.-)
     EXCLUDES 2   bite of venomous animal (T63.-)
            open wound of ankle, foot and toes (S91.-)
            open wound of knee and lower leg (S81.-)

> The appropriate 7th character is to be added to each code from category S71.
> A   initial encounter
> D   subsequent encounter
> S   sequela

   ✓5th **S71.0** **Open wound of** hip

     ✓6th **S71.00** **Unspecified** open wound of hip

       ✓7th **S71.001** **Unspecified open wound,** right **hip**

       ✓7th **S71.002** **Unspecified open wound,** left **hip**

       ✓7th **S71.009** **Unspecified open wound,** unspecified **hip**

     ✓6th **S71.01** **Laceration without foreign body** of hip

       ✓7th **S71.011** **Laceration without foreign body,** right **hip**

       ✓7th **S71.012** **Laceration without foreign body,** left **hip**

       ✓7th **S71.019** **Laceration without foreign body,** unspecified **hip**

     ✓6th **S71.02** **Laceration with foreign body** of hip

       ✓7th **S71.021** **Laceration with foreign body,** right **hip**

       ✓7th **S71.022** **Laceration with foreign body,** left **hip**

       ✓7th **S71.029** **Laceration with foreign body,** unspecified **hip**

     ✓6th **S71.03** **Puncture wound without foreign body** of hip

       ✓7th **S71.031** **Puncture wound without foreign body,** right **hip**

       ✓7th **S71.032** **Puncture wound without foreign body,** left **hip**

       ✓7th **S71.039** **Puncture wound without foreign body,** unspecified **hip**

     ✓6th **S71.04** **Puncture wound with foreign body** of hip

       ✓7th **S71.041** **Puncture wound with foreign body,** right **hip**

       ✓7th **S71.042** **Puncture wound with foreign body,** left **hip**

       ✓7th **S71.049** **Puncture wound with foreign body,** unspecified **hip**

✓Additional Character Required   ✓x7th Placeholder   Unacceptable PDx   Questionable PDx   Manifestation   H1 - H14 HAC   HCC CMS-HCC Dx   HIV HIV Dx

ICD-10-CM 2019   1041

√6ᵗʰ **S71.05 Open bite** of hip
Bite of hip NOS
EXCLUDES 1 superficial bite of hip (S70.26, S70.27)

√7ᵗʰ **S71.051 Open bite, right hip**
√7ᵗʰ **S71.052 Open bite, left hip**
√7ᵗʰ **S71.059 Open bite, unspecified hip**

√5ᵗʰ **S71.1 Open wound of thigh**

√6ᵗʰ **S71.10 Unspecified open wound of thigh**
AHA: 2016, 3Q, 24

√7ᵗʰ **S71.101 Unspecified open wound, right thigh**
√7ᵗʰ **S71.102 Unspecified open wound, left thigh**
√7ᵗʰ **S71.109 Unspecified open wound, unspecified thigh**

√6ᵗʰ **S71.11 Laceration without foreign body of thigh**

√7ᵗʰ **S71.111 Laceration without foreign body, right thigh**
√7ᵗʰ **S71.112 Laceration without foreign body, left thigh**
√7ᵗʰ **S71.119 Laceration without foreign body, unspecified thigh**

√6ᵗʰ **S71.12 Laceration with foreign body of thigh**

√7ᵗʰ **S71.121 Laceration with foreign body, right thigh**
√7ᵗʰ **S71.122 Laceration with foreign body, left thigh**
√7ᵗʰ **S71.129 Laceration with foreign body, unspecified thigh**

√6ᵗʰ **S71.13 Puncture wound without foreign body of thigh**
AHA: 2016, 3Q, 24

√7ᵗʰ **S71.131 Puncture wound without foreign body, right thigh**
√7ᵗʰ **S71.132 Puncture wound without foreign body, left thigh**
√7ᵗʰ **S71.139 Puncture wound without foreign body, unspecified thigh**

√6ᵗʰ **S71.14 Puncture wound with foreign body of thigh**
AHA: 2016, 3Q, 24

√7ᵗʰ **S71.141 Puncture wound with foreign body, right thigh**
√7ᵗʰ **S71.142 Puncture wound with foreign body, left thigh**
√7ᵗʰ **S71.149 Puncture wound with foreign body, unspecified thigh**

√6ᵗʰ **S71.15 Open bite of thigh**
Bite of thigh NOS
EXCLUDES 1 superficial bite of thigh (S70.37-)

√7ᵗʰ **S71.151 Open bite, right thigh**
√7ᵗʰ **S71.152 Open bite, left thigh**
√7ᵗʰ **S71.159 Open bite, unspecified thigh**

√4ᵗʰ **S72 Fracture of femur**
NOTE A fracture not indicated as displaced or nondisplaced should be coded to displaced.
The open fracture designations are based on the Gustilo open fracture classification A fracture not indicated as open or closed should be coded to closed.
EXCLUDES 1 traumatic amputation of hip and thigh (S78.-)
EXCLUDES 2 fracture of lower leg and ankle (S82.-)
fracture of foot (S92.-)
periprosthetic fracture of prosthetic implant of hip (M97.0-)

AHA: 2018, 2Q, 12; 2016, 1Q, 33; 2015, 3Q, 37-39; 2015, 1Q, 17; 2013, 4Q, 128

The appropriate 7th character is to be added to all codes from category S72 [unless otherwise indicated].
A   initial encounter for closed fracture
B   initial encounter for open fracture type I or II
     initial encounter for open fracture NOS
C   initial encounter for open fracture type IIIA, IIIB, or IIIC
D   subsequent encounter for closed fracture with routine healing
E   subsequent encounter for open fracture type I or II with routine healing
F   subsequent encounter for open fracture type IIIA, IIIB, or IIIC with routine healing
G   subsequent encounter for closed fracture with delayed healing
H   subsequent encounter for open fracture type I or II with delayed healing
J   subsequent encounter for open fracture type IIIA, IIIB, or IIIC with delayed healing
K   subsequent encounter for closed fracture with nonunion
M   subsequent encounter for open fracture type I or II with nonunion
N   subsequent encounter for open fracture type IIIA, IIIB, or IIIC with nonunion
P   subsequent encounter for closed fracture with malunion
Q   subsequent encounter for open fracture type I or II with malunion
R   subsequent encounter for open fracture type IIIA, IIIB, or IIIC with malunion
S   sequela

√5ᵗʰ **S72.0 Fracture of head and neck of femur**
EXCLUDES 2 physeal fracture of upper end of femur (S79.0-)
AHA: 2016, 3Q, 16

CC Excl: For CC/MCC codes in subcategory S72.0:
Right side: See code S72.001
Left side: See code S72.002
Unspecified side: See code S72.009

√6ᵗʰ **S72.00 Fracture of unspecified part of neck of femur**
Fracture of hip NOS
Fracture of neck of femur NOS

4,6 √7ᵗʰ **S72.001 Fracture of unspecified part** MCC CC H5 HCC **of neck of right femur**
CC Excl: MCC with 7th character A: PDX collection 1297
MCC with 7th character B or C: PDX collection 1298
CC with 7th character K, M, N, P, Q or R: PDX collection 897

4,6 √7ᵗʰ **S72.002 Fracture of unspecified part** MCC CC H5 HCC **of neck of left femur**
CC Excl: MCC with 7th character A: PDX collection 1299
MCC with 7th character B or C: PDX collection 1298
CC with 7th character K, M, N, P, Q or R: PDX collection 897

4,6 √7ᵗʰ **S72.009 Fracture of unspecified part** MCC CC H5 HCC **of neck of unspecified femur**
CC Excl: MCC with 7th character A, B or C: PDX collection 1298
CC with 7th character K, M, N, P, Q or R: PDX collection 897

√6ᵗʰ **S72.01 Unspecified intracapsular fracture of femur**
Subcapital fracture of femur

4,6 √7ᵗʰ **S72.011 Unspecified intracapsular fracture of right femur** MCC CC H5 HCC
4,6 √7ᵗʰ **S72.012 Unspecified intracapsular fracture of left femur** MCC CC H5 HCC
4,6 √7ᵗʰ **S72.019 Unspecified intracapsular fracture of unspecified femur** MCC CC H5 HCC

√6ᵗʰ **S72.02** **Fracture of** epiphysis (separation) (upper) **of femur**
Transepiphyseal fracture of femur
EXCLUDES 1 *capital femoral epiphyseal fracture (pediatric) of femur (S79.01-)*
Salter-Harris Type I physeal fracture of upper end of femur (S79.01-)

4,6 √7ᵗʰ **S72.021** **Displaced fracture of** epiphysis (separation) (upper) of right **femur** `MCC CC H5 HCC`

4,6 √7ᵗʰ **S72.022** **Displaced fracture of** epiphysis (separation) (upper) of left **femur** `MCC CC H5 HCC`

4,6 √7ᵗʰ **S72.023** **Displaced fracture of** epiphysis (separation) (upper) of unspecified **femur** `MCC CC H5 HCC`

4,6 √7ᵗʰ **S72.024** **Nondisplaced fracture of** epiphysis (separation) (upper) of right **femur** `MCC CC H5 HCC`

4,6 √7ᵗʰ **S72.025** **Nondisplaced fracture of** epiphysis (separation) (upper) of left **femur** `MCC CC H5 HCC`

4,6 √7ᵗʰ **S72.026** **Nondisplaced fracture of** epiphysis (separation) (upper) of unspecified **femur** `MCC CC H5 HCC`

√6ᵗʰ **S72.03** Midcervical **fracture of femur**
Transcervical fracture of femur NOS

4,6 √7ᵗʰ **S72.031** **Displaced** midcervical **fracture of** right **femur** `MCC CC H5 HCC`

4,6 √7ᵗʰ **S72.032** **Displaced** midcervical **fracture of** left **femur** `MCC CC H5 HCC`

4,6 √7ᵗʰ **S72.033** **Displaced** midcervical **fracture of** unspecified **femur** `MCC CC H5 HCC`

4,6 √7ᵗʰ **S72.034** **Nondisplaced** midcervical **fracture of** right **femur** `MCC CC H5 HCC`

4,6 √7ᵗʰ **S72.035** **Nondisplaced** midcervical **fracture of** left **femur** `MCC CC H5 HCC`

4,6 √7ᵗʰ **S72.036** **Nondisplaced** midcervical **fracture of** unspecified **femur** `MCC CC H5 HCC`

√6ᵗʰ **S72.04** **Fracture of** base of neck **of femur**
Cervicotrochanteric fracture of femur

4,6 √7ᵗʰ **S72.041** **Displaced fracture of base of neck of** right **femur** `MCC CC H5 HCC`

4,6 √7ᵗʰ **S72.042** **Displaced fracture of base of neck of** left **femur** `MCC CC H5 HCC`

4,6 √7ᵗʰ **S72.043** **Displaced fracture of base of neck of** unspecified **femur** `MCC CC H5 HCC`

4,6 √7ᵗʰ **S72.044** **Nondisplaced fracture of base of neck of** right **femur** `MCC CC H5 HCC`

4,6 √7ᵗʰ **S72.045** **Nondisplaced fracture of base of neck of** left **femur** `MCC CC H5 HCC`

4,6 √7ᵗʰ **S72.046** **Nondisplaced fracture of base of neck of** unspecified **femur** `MCC CC H5 HCC`

√6ᵗʰ **S72.05** Unspecified **fracture of** head **of femur**
Fracture of head of femur NOS

4,6 √7ᵗʰ **S72.051** **Unspecified fracture of head of** right **femur** `MCC CC H5 HCC`

4,6 √7ᵗʰ **S72.052** **Unspecified fracture of head of** left **femur** `MCC CC H5 HCC`

4,6 √7ᵗʰ **S72.059** **Unspecified fracture of head of** unspecified **femur** `MCC CC H5 HCC`

√6ᵗʰ **S72.06** Articular **fracture of head of femur**

4,6 √7ᵗʰ **S72.061** **Displaced articular fracture of head of** right **femur** `MCC CC H5 HCC`

4,6 √7ᵗʰ **S72.062** **Displaced articular fracture of head of** left **femur** `MCC CC H5 HCC`

4,6 √7ᵗʰ **S72.063** **Displaced articular fracture of head of** unspecified **femur** `MCC CC H5 HCC`

4,6 √7ᵗʰ **S72.064** **Nondisplaced articular fracture of head of** right **femur** `MCC CC H5 HCC`

4,6 √7ᵗʰ **S72.065** **Nondisplaced articular fracture of head of** left **femur** `MCC CC H5 HCC`

4,6 √7ᵗʰ **S72.066** **Nondisplaced articular fracture of head of** unspecified **femur** `MCC CC H5 HCC`

√6ᵗʰ **S72.09** **Other** fracture of head and neck **of femur**

4,6 √7ᵗʰ **S72.091** **Other fracture of head and neck of** right **femur** `MCC CC H5 HCC`

4,6 √7ᵗʰ **S72.092** **Other fracture of head and neck of** left **femur** `MCC CC H5 HCC`

4,6 √7ᵗʰ **S72.099** **Other fracture of head and neck of** unspecified **femur** `MCC CC H5 HCC`

√5ᵗʰ **S72.1** Pertrochanteric **fracture**
AHA: 2016, 3Q, 16

> **CC Excl:** For CC/MCC codes in subcategory S72.1:
> **Right side:** See code S72.001
> **Left side:** See code S72.002
> **Unspecified side:** See code S72.009

√6ᵗʰ **S72.10** Unspecified trochanteric **fracture of femur**
Fracture of trochanter NOS

4,6 √7ᵗʰ **S72.101** **Unspecified trochanteric fracture of** right **femur** `MCC CC H5 HCC`

4,6 √7ᵗʰ **S72.102** **Unspecified trochanteric fracture of** left **femur** `MCC CC H5 HCC`

4,6 √7ᵗʰ **S72.109** **Unspecified trochanteric fracture of** unspecified **femur** `MCC CC H5 HCC`

√6ᵗʰ **S72.11** **Fracture of** greater trochanter **of femur**

4,6 √7ᵗʰ **S72.111** **Displaced fracture of greater trochanter of** right **femur** `MCC CC H5 HCC`

4,6 √7ᵗʰ **S72.112** **Displaced fracture of greater trochanter of** left **femur** `MCC CC H5 HCC`

4,6 √7ᵗʰ **S72.113** **Displaced fracture of** greatertrochanter of unspecified **femur** `MCC CC H5 HCC`

4,6 √7ᵗʰ **S72.114** **Nondisplaced fracture of greater trochanter of** right **femur** `MCC CC H5 HCC`

4,6 √7ᵗʰ **S72.115** **Nondisplaced fracture of greater trochanter of** left **femur** `MCC CC H5 HCC`

4,6 √7ᵗʰ **S72.116** **Nondisplaced fracture of greater trochanter of** unspecified **femur** `MCC CC H5 HCC`

√6ᵗʰ **S72.12** **Fracture of** lesser trochanter **of femur**

4,6 √7ᵗʰ **S72.121** **Displaced fracture of lesser trochanter of** right **femur** `MCC CC H5 HCC`

4,6 √7ᵗʰ **S72.122** **Displaced fracture of lesser trochanter of** left **femur** `MCC CC H5 HCC`

4,6 √7ᵗʰ **S72.123** **Displaced fracture of lesser trochanter of** unspecified **femur** `MCC CC H5 HCC`

4,6 √7ᵗʰ **S72.124** **Nondisplaced fracture of lesser trochanter of** right **femur** `MCC CC H5 HCC`

4,6 √7ᵗʰ **S72.125** **Nondisplaced fracture of lesser trochanter of** left **femur** `MCC CC H5 HCC`

4,6 √7ᵗʰ **S72.126** **Nondisplaced fracture of lesser trochanter of** unspecified **femur** `MCC CC H5 HCC`

√6ᵗʰ **S72.13** Apophyseal **fracture of femur**
EXCLUDES 1 *chronic (nontraumatic) slipped upper femoral epiphysis (M93.0-)*

4,6 √7ᵗʰ **S72.131** **Displaced apophyseal fracture of** right **femur** `MCC CC H5 HCC`

4,6 √7ᵗʰ **S72.132** **Displaced apophyseal fracture of** left **femur** `MCC CC H5 HCC`

4,6 √7ᵗʰ **S72.133** **Displaced apophyseal fracture of** unspecified **femur** `MCC CC H5 HCC`

4,6 √7ᵗʰ **S72.134** **Nondisplaced apophyseal fracture of** right **femur** `MCC CC H5 HCC`

4,6 √7ᵗʰ **S72.135** **Nondisplaced apophyseal fractureof** left **femur** `MCC CC H5 HCC`

4,6 √7ᵗʰ **S72.136** **Nondisplaced apophyseal fracture of** unspecified **femur** `MCC CC H5 HCC`

√6ᵗʰ **S72.14** Intertrochanteric **fracture of femur**

4,6 √7ᵗʰ **S72.141** **Displaced intertrochanteric fracture of** right **femur** `MCC CC H5 HCC`

4,6 √7ᵗʰ **S72.142** **Displaced intertrochanteric fracture of** left **femur** `MCC CC H5 HCC`

4,6 √7ᵗʰ **S72.143** **Displaced intertrochanteric fracture of** unspecified **femur** `MCC CC H5 HCC`

4,6 √7ᵗʰ **S72.144** **Nondisplaced intertrochanteric fracture of** right **femur** `MCC CC H5 HCC`

☑ Additional Character Required   √x7ᵗʰ Placeholder   Unacceptable PDx   Questionable PDx   Manifestation   **H1**-**H14** HAC   **HCC** CMS-HCC Dx   **HIV** HIV Dx

4,6 ✓7th **S72.145** Nondisplaced intertrochanteric fracture of left femur   `MCC` `CC` `H5` `HCC`

4,6 ✓7th **S72.146** Nondisplaced intertrochanteric fracture of unspecified femur   `MCC` `CC` `H5` `HCC`

✓5th **S72.2** Subtrochanteric fracture of femur

> **CC Excl: For CC/MCC codes in subcategory S72.2:**
> **Right side:** See code S72.009
> **Left side:** See code S72.009
> **Unspecified side:** See code S72.009

4,6 ✓x7th **S72.21** Displaced subtrochanteric fracture of right femur   `MCC` `CC` `H5` `HCC`

4,6 ✓x7th **S72.22** Displaced subtrochanteric fracture of left femur   `MCC` `CC` `H5` `HCC`

4,6 ✓x7th **S72.23** Displaced subtrochanteric fracture of unspecified femur   `MCC` `CC` `H5` `HCC`

4,6 ✓x7th **S72.24** Nondisplaced subtrochanteric fracture of right femur   `MCC` `CC` `H5` `HCC`

4,6 ✓x7th **S72.25** Nondisplaced subtrochanteric fracture of left femur   `MCC` `CC` `H5` `HCC`

4,6 ✓x7th **S72.26** Nondisplaced subtrochanteric fracture of unspecified femur   `MCC` `CC` `H5` `HCC`

✓5th **S72.3** Fracture of shaft of femur

> **CC Excl: For CC/MCC codes in subcategory S72.3:**
> **Right side:** See code S72.001
> **Left side:** See code S72.002
> **Unspecified side:** See code S72.009

✓6th **S72.30** Unspecified fracture of shaft of femur

4,6 ✓7th **S72.301** Unspecified fracture of shaft of right femur   `MCC` `CC` `H5` `HCC`

4,6 ✓7th **S72.302** Unspecified fracture of shaft of left femur   `MCC` `CC` `H5` `HCC`

4,6 ✓7th **S72.309** Unspecified fracture of shaft of unspecified femur   `MCC` `CC` `H5` `HCC`

✓6th **S72.32** Transverse fracture of shaft of femur

4,6 ✓7th **S72.321** Displaced transverse fracture of shaft of right femur   `MCC` `CC` `H5` `HCC`

4,6 ✓7th **S72.322** Displaced transverse fracture of shaft of left femur   `MCC` `CC` `H5` `HCC`

4,6 ✓7th **S72.323** Displaced transverse fracture of shaft of unspecified femur   `MCC` `CC` `H5` `HCC`

4,6 ✓7th **S72.324** Nondisplaced transverse fracture of shaft of right femur   `MCC` `CC` `H5` `HCC`

4,6 ✓7th **S72.325** Nondisplaced transverse fracture of shaft of left femur   `MCC` `CC` `H5` `HCC`

4,6 ✓7th **S72.326** Nondisplaced transverse fracture of shaft of unspecified femur   `MCC` `CC` `H5` `HCC`

✓6th **S72.33** Oblique fracture of shaft of femur

4,6 ✓7th **S72.331** Displaced oblique fracture of shaft of right femur   `MCC` `CC` `H5` `HCC`

4,6 ✓7th **S72.332** Displaced oblique fracture of shaft of left femur   `MCC` `CC` `H5` `HCC`

4,6 ✓7th **S72.333** Displaced oblique fracture of shaft of unspecified femur   `MCC` `CC` `H5` `HCC`

4,6 ✓7th **S72.334** Nondisplaced oblique fracture of shaft of right femur   `MCC` `CC` `H5` `HCC`

4,6 ✓7th **S72.335** Nondisplaced oblique fracture of shaft of left femur   `MCC` `CC` `H5` `HCC`

4,6 ✓7th **S72.336** Nondisplaced oblique fracture of shaft of unspecified femur   `MCC` `CC` `H5` `HCC`

✓6th **S72.34** Spiral fracture of shaft of femur

4,6 ✓7th **S72.341** Displaced spiral fracture of shaft of right femur   `MCC` `CC` `H5` `HCC`

4,6 ✓7th **S72.342** Displaced spiral fracture of shaft of left femur   `MCC` `CC` `H5` `HCC`

4,6 ✓7th **S72.343** Displaced spiral fracture of shaft of unspecified femur   `MCC` `CC` `H5` `HCC`

4,6 ✓7th **S72.344** Nondisplaced spiral fracture of shaft of right femur   `MCC` `CC` `H5` `HCC`

4,6 ✓7th **S72.345** Nondisplaced spiral fracture of shaft of left femur   `MCC` `CC` `H5` `HCC`

4,6 ✓7th **S72.346** Nondisplaced spiral fracture of shaft of unspecified femur   `MCC` `CC` `H5` `HCC`

✓6th **S72.35** Comminuted fracture of shaft of femur

4,6 ✓7th **S72.351** Displaced comminuted fracture of shaft of right femur   `MCC` `CC` `H5` `HCC`

4,6 ✓7th **S72.352** Displaced comminuted fracture of shaft of left femur   `MCC` `CC` `H5` `HCC`

4,6 ✓7th **S72.353** Displaced comminuted fracture of shaft of unspecified femur   `MCC` `CC` `H5` `HCC`

4,6 ✓7th **S72.354** Nondisplaced comminuted fracture of shaft of right femur   `MCC` `CC` `H5` `HCC`

4,6 ✓7th **S72.355** Nondisplaced comminuted fracture of shaft of left femur   `MCC` `CC` `H5` `HCC`

4,6 ✓7th **S72.356** Nondisplaced comminuted fracture of shaft of unspecified femur   `MCC` `CC` `H5` `HCC`

✓6th **S72.36** Segmental fracture of shaft of femur

4,6 ✓7th **S72.361** Displaced segmental fracture of shaft of right femur   `MCC` `CC` `H5` `HCC`

4,6 ✓7th **S72.362** Displaced segmental fracture of shaft of left femur   `MCC` `CC` `H5` `HCC`

4,6 ✓7th **S72.363** Displaced segmental fracture of shaft of unspecified femur   `MCC` `CC` `H5` `HCC`

4,6 ✓7th **S72.364** Nondisplaced segmental fracture of shaft of right femur   `MCC` `CC` `H5` `HCC`

4,6 ✓7th **S72.365** Nondisplaced segmental fracture of shaft of left femur   `MCC` `CC` `H5` `HCC`

4,6 ✓7th **S72.366** Nondisplaced segmental fracture of shaft of unspecified femur   `MCC` `CC` `H5` `HCC`

✓6th **S72.39** Other fracture of shaft of femur

4,6 ✓7th **S72.391** Other fracture of shaft of right femur   `MCC` `CC` `H5` `HCC`

4,6 ✓7th **S72.392** Other fracture of shaft of left femur   `MCC` `CC` `H5` `HCC`

4,6 ✓7th **S72.399** Other fracture of shaft of unspecified femur   `MCC` `CC` `H5` `HCC`

✓5th **S72.4** Fracture of lower end of femur
Fracture of distal end of femur
EXCLUDES 2 fracture of shaft of femur (S72.3-)
physeal fracture of lower end of femur (S79.1-)
AHA: 2016, 4Q, 42

> **CC Excl: For CC/MCC codes in subcategory S72.4, unless otherwise noted:**
> **Right side:** See code S72.401
> **Left side:** See code S72.402
> **Unspecified side:** See code S72.409

✓6th **S72.40** Unspecified fracture of lower end of femur
AHA: 2018, 1Q, 21; 2016, 4Q, 42

2,3,6 ✓7th **S72.401** Unspecified fracture of lower end of right femur   `MCC` `CC` `H5` `HCC`
> **CC Excl: CC with 7th character A:**
> PDX collection 1300
> **MCC with 7th character B or C:**
> PDX collection 1301
> **CC with 7th character K, M, N, P, Q or R:**
> PDX collection 897

2,3,6 ✓7th **S72.402** Unspecified fracture of lower end of left femur   `MCC` `CC` `H5` `HCC`
> **CC Excl: CC with 7th character A:**
> PDX collection 1302
> **MCC with 7th character B or C:**
> PDX collection 1301
> **CC with 7th character K, M, N, P, Q or R:**
> PDX collection 897

2,3,6 ✓7th **S72.409** Unspecified fracture of lower end of unspecified femur   `MCC` `CC` `H5` `HCC`
> **CC Excl: CC with 7th character A or MCC with 7th character B or C:**
> PDX collection 1301
> **CC with 7th character K, M, N, P, Q or R:**
> PDX collection 897

✓6th **S72.41** Unspecified condyle fracture of lower end of femur
Condyle fracture of femur NOS

2,3,6 ✓7th **S72.411** Displaced unspecified condyle fracture of lower end of right femur   `MCC` `CC` `H5` `HCC`

2,3,6 ✓7th **S72.412** Displaced unspecified condyle fracture of lower end of left femur   `MCC` `CC` `H5` `HCC`

N Newborn: 0   **P** Pediatric: 0-17   **M** Maternity: 12-55   **A** Adult: 15-124   `MCC` Major Complication/Comorbidity   `CC` Complication/Comorbidity   `SW` Severe Wound Dx

1044   ICD-10-CM 2019

2,3,6 ✓7ᵗʰ **S72.413** Displaced unspecified condyle fracture of lower end of unspecified femur   `MCC` `CC` `H5` `HCC`

2,3,6 ✓7ᵗʰ **S72.414** Nondisplaced unspecified condyle fracture of lower end of right femur   `MCC` `CC` `H5` `HCC`

2,3,6 ✓7ᵗʰ **S72.415** Nondisplaced unspecified condyle fracture of lower end of left femur   `MCC` `CC` `H5` `HCC`

2,3,6 ✓7ᵗʰ **S72.416** Nondisplaced unspecified condyle fracture of lower end of unspecified femur   `MCC` `CC` `H5` `HCC`

✓6ᵗʰ **S72.42** Fracture of lateral condyle of femur

2,3,6 ✓7ᵗʰ **S72.421** Displaced fracture of lateral condyle of right femur   `MCC` `CC` `H5` `HCC`

2,3,6 ✓7ᵗʰ **S72.422** Displaced fracture of lateral condyle of left femur   `MCC` `CC` `H5` `HCC`

2,3,6 ✓7ᵗʰ **S72.423** Displaced fracture of lateral condyle of unspecified femur   `MCC` `CC` `H5` `HCC`

2,3,6 ✓7ᵗʰ **S72.424** Nondisplaced fracture of lateral condyle of right femur   `MCC` `CC` `H5` `HCC`

2,3,6 ✓7ᵗʰ **S72.425** Nondisplaced fracture of lateral condyle of left femur   `MCC` `CC` `H5` `HCC`

2,3,6 ✓7ᵗʰ **S72.426** Nondisplaced fracture of lateral condyle of unspecified femur   `MCC` `CC` `H5` `HCC`

✓6ᵗʰ **S72.43** Fracture of medial condyle of femur

2,3,6 ✓7ᵗʰ **S72.431** Displaced fracture of medial condyle of right femur   `MCC` `CC` `H5` `HCC`

2,3,6 ✓7ᵗʰ **S72.432** Displaced fracture of medial condyle of left femur   `MCC` `CC` `H5` `HCC`

2,3,6 ✓7ᵗʰ **S72.433** Displaced fracture of medial condyle of unspecified femur   `MCC` `CC` `H5` `HCC`

2,3,6 ✓7ᵗʰ **S72.434** Nondisplaced fracture of medial condyle of right femur   `MCC` `CC` `H5` `HCC`

2,3,6 ✓7ᵗʰ **S72.435** Nondisplaced fracture of medial condyle of left femur   `MCC` `CC` `H5` `HCC`

2,3,6 ✓7ᵗʰ **S72.436** Nondisplaced fracture of medial condyle of unspecified femur   `MCC` `CC` `H5` `HCC`

✓6ᵗʰ **S72.44** Fracture of lower epiphysis (separation) of femur

EXCLUDES 1 *Salter-Harris Type I physeal fracture of lower end of femur (S79.11-)*

2,3,6 ✓7ᵗʰ **S72.441** Displaced fracture of lower epiphysis (separation) of right femur   `MCC` `CC` `H5` `HCC`

2,3,6 ✓7ᵗʰ **S72.442** Displaced fracture of lower epiphysis (separation) of left femur   `MCC` `CC` `H5` `HCC`

2,3,6 ✓7ᵗʰ **S72.443** Displaced fracture of lower epiphysis (separation) of unspecified femur   `MCC` `CC` `H5` `HCC`

2,3,6 ✓7ᵗʰ **S72.444** Nondisplaced fracture of lowerepiphysis (separation) of right femur   `MCC` `CC` `H5` `HCC`

2,3,6 ✓7ᵗʰ **S72.445** Nondisplaced fracture of lower epiphysis (separation) of left femur   `MCC` `CC` `H5` `HCC`

2,3,6 ✓7ᵗʰ **S72.446** Nondisplaced fracture of lower epiphysis (separation) of unspecified femur   `MCC` `CC` `H5` `HCC`

✓6ᵗʰ **S72.45** Supracondylar fracture without intracondylar extension of lower end of femur

Supracondylar fracture of lower end of femur NOS

EXCLUDES 1 *supracondylar fracture with intracondylar extension of lower end of femur (S72.46-)*

2,3,6 ✓7ᵗʰ **S72.451** Displaced supracondylar fracture without intracondylar extension of lower end of right femur   `MCC` `CC` `H5` `HCC`

2,3,6 ✓7ᵗʰ **S72.452** Displaced supracondylar fracture without intracondylar extension of lower end of left femur   `MCC` `CC` `H5` `HCC`

2,3,6 ✓7ᵗʰ **S72.453** Displaced supracondylar fracture without intracondylar extension of lower end of unspecified femur   `MCC` `CC` `H5` `HCC`

2,3,6 ✓7ᵗʰ **S72.454** Nondisplaced supracondylar fracture without intracondylar extension of lower end of right femur   `MCC` `CC` `H5` `HCC`

2,3,6 ✓7ᵗʰ **S72.455** Nondisplaced supracondylar fracture without intracondylar extension of lower end of left femur   `MCC` `CC` `H5` `HCC`

2,3,6 ✓7ᵗʰ **S72.456** Nondisplaced supracondylar fracture without intracondylar extension of lower end of unspecified femur   `MCC` `CC` `H5` `HCC`

✓6ᵗʰ **S72.46** Supracondylar fracture with intracondylar extension of lower end of femur

EXCLUDES 1 *supracondylar fracture without intracondylar extension of lower end of femur (S72.45-)*

2,3,6 ✓7ᵗʰ **S72.461** Displaced supracondylar fracture with intracondylar extension of lower end of right femur   `MCC` `CC` `H5` `HCC`

2,3,6 ✓7ᵗʰ **S72.462** Displaced supracondylar fracture with intracondylar extension of lower end of left femur   `MCC` `CC` `H5` `HCC`

2,3,6 ✓7ᵗʰ **S72.463** Displaced supracondylar fracture with intracondylar extension of lower end of unspecified femur   `MCC` `CC` `H5` `HCC`

2,3,6 ✓7ᵗʰ **S72.464** Nondisplaced supracondylar fracture with intracondylar extension of lower end of right femur   `MCC` `CC` `H5` `HCC`

2,3,6 ✓7ᵗʰ **S72.465** Nondisplaced supracondylar fracture with intracondylar extension of lower end of left femur   `MCC` `CC` `H5` `HCC`

2,3,6 ✓7ᵗʰ **S72.466** Nondisplaced supracondylar fracture with intracondylar extension of lower end of unspecified femur   `MCC` `CC` `H5` `HCC`

✓6ᵗʰ **S72.47** Torus fracture of lower end of femur

> The appropriate 7th character is to be added to all codes in subcategory S72.47.
> A   initial encounter for closed fracture
> D   subsequent encounter for fracture with routine healing
> G   subsequent encounter for fracture with delayed healing
> K   subsequent encounter for fracture with nonunion
> P   subsequent encounter for fracture with malunion
> S   sequela

3,6 ✓7ᵗʰ **S72.471** Torus fracture of lower end of right femur   `CC` `H5` `HCC`

    CC Excl: CC with 7th character A: PDX collection 1300

    CC Excl: CC with 7th character K or P: PDX collection 897

3,6 ✓7ᵗʰ **S72.472** Torus fracture of lower end of left femur   `CC` `H5` `HCC`

    CC Excl: CC with 7th character A: PDX collection 1302

    CC Excl: CC with 7th character K or P: PDX collection 897

3,6 ✓7ᵗʰ **S72.479** Torus fracture of lower end of unspecified femur   `CC` `H5` `HCC`

    CC Excl: CC with 7th character A: PDX collection 1301

    CC Excl: CC with 7th character K or P: PDX collection 897

✓6ᵗʰ **S72.49** Other fracture of lower end of femur

2,3,6 ✓7ᵗʰ **S72.491** Other fracture of lower end of right femur   `MCC` `CC` `H5` `HCC`

    CC Excl: CC with 7th character A: PDX collection 1300

    MCC with 7th character B or C: PDX collection 1303

    CC with 7th character K, M, N, P, Q or R: PDX collection 897

✔ Additional Character Required   ✓x7ᵗʰ Placeholder   Unacceptable PDx   Questionable PDx   Manifestation   `H1`–`H14` HAC   `HCC` CMS-HCC Dx   `HIV` HIV Dx

ICD-10-CM 2019   1045

2,3,6 √7th **S72.492** **Other fracture of lower end** MCC CC H5 HCC
of left femur
CC Excl: CC with 7th character A:
PDX collection 1302
MCC with 7th character B or C:
PDX collection 1303
CC with 7th character K, M, N, P, Q or R:
PDX collection 897

2,3,6 √7th **S72.499** **Other fracture of lower end** MCC CC H5 HCC
of unspecified femur
CC Excl: CC with 7th character A:
PDX collection 1301
MCC with 7th character B or C:
PDX collection 1303
CC with 7th character K, M, N, P, Q or R:
PDX collection 897

√5th **S72.8** **Other fracture of femur**

√6th **S72.8X** **Other fracture of femur**

CC Excl: For codes in subcategory S72.8X:
MCC with 7th character A, B or C:
PDX collection 1298
CC with 7th character K, M, N, P, Q or R:
PDX collection 897

4,6 √7th **S72.8X1** **Other fracture of right** MCC CC H5 HCC
femur

4,6 √7th **S72.8X2** **Other fracture of left femur** MCC CC H5 HCC

4,6 √7th **S72.8X9** **Other fracture of** MCC CC H5 HCC
unspecified femur

√5th **S72.9** **Unspecified fracture of femur**
Fracture of thigh NOS
Fracture of upper leg NOS
EXCLUDES 1 *fracture of hip NOS (S72.00-, S72.01-)*

CC Excl: For codes in subcategory S72.9:
MCC with 7th character A, B or C:
PDX collection 1298
CC with 7th character K, M, N, P, Q or R:
PDX collection 897

4,6 √x7th **S72.90** **Unspecified fracture of unspecified** MCC CC H5 HCC
femur
AHA: 2012, 4Q, 93

4,6 √x7th **S72.91** **Unspecified fracture of right femur** MCC CC H5 HCC

4,6 √x7th **S72.92** **Unspecified fracture of left femur** MCC CC H5 HCC

√4th **S73** **Dislocation and sprain of joint and ligaments of hip**
INCLUDES avulsion of joint or ligament of hip
laceration of cartilage, joint or ligament of hip
sprain of cartilage, joint or ligament of hip
traumatic hemarthrosis of joint or ligament of hip
traumatic rupture of joint or ligament of hip
traumatic subluxation of joint or ligament of hip
traumatic tear of joint or ligament of hip

Code also any associated open wound
EXCLUDES 2 *strain of muscle, fascia and tendon of hip and thigh (S76.-)*

The appropriate 7th character is to be added to each code from
category S73.
A   initial encounter
D   subsequent encounter
S   sequela

√5th **S73.0** **Subluxation and dislocation of hip**
EXCLUDES 2 *dislocation and subluxation of hip prosthesis (T84.020,*
T84.021)

√6th **S73.00** **Unspecified subluxation and dislocation of hip**
Dislocation of hip NOS
Subluxation of hip NOS

CC Excl: For CC codes in subcategory S73.00:
Right side: PDX collection 1304
Left side: PDX collection 1305
Unspecified side: PDX collection 1306

6 √7th **S73.001** **Unspecified subluxation of** CC H5 HCC
right hip

6 √7th **S73.002** **Unspecified subluxation of** CC H5 HCC
left hip

6 √7th **S73.003** **Unspecified subluxation of** CC H5 HCC
unspecified hip

6 √7th **S73.004** **Unspecified dislocation of** CC H5 HCC
right hip

6 √7th **S73.005** **Unspecified dislocation of** CC H5 HCC
left hip

6 √7th **S73.006** **Unspecified dislocation of** CC H5 HCC
unspecified hip

√6th **S73.01** **Posterior subluxation and dislocation of hip**

CC Excl: For CC codes in subcategory S73.01:
Right side: PDX collection 1307
Left side: PDX collection 1308
Unspecified side: PDX collection 1309

6 √7th **S73.011** **Posterior subluxation of** CC H5 HCC
right hip

6 √7th **S73.012** **Posterior subluxation of left hip** CC H5 HCC

6 √7th **S73.013** **Posterior subluxation of** CC H5 HCC
unspecified hip

6 √7th **S73.014** **Posterior dislocation of right hip** CC H5 HCC

6 √7th **S73.015** **Posterior dislocation of left hip** CC H5 HCC

6 √7th **S73.016** **Posterior dislocation of** CC H5 HCC
unspecified hip

√6th **S73.02** **Obturator subluxation and dislocation of hip**

CC Excl: For CC codes in subcategory S73.02:
Right side: PDX collection 1310
Left side: PDX collection 1311
Unspecified side: PDX collection 1312

6 √7th **S73.021** **Obturator subluxation of** CC H5 HCC
right hip

6 √7th **S73.022** **Obturator subluxation of** CC H5 HCC
left hip

6 √7th **S73.023** **Obturator subluxation of** CC H5 HCC
unspecified hip

6 √7th **S73.024** **Obturator dislocation of** CC H5 HCC
right hip

6 √7th **S73.025** **Obturator dislocation of left hip** CC H5 HCC

6 √7th **S73.026** **Obturator dislocation of** CC H5 HCC
unspecified hip

√6th **S73.03** **Other anterior subluxation and dislocation of hip**

CC Excl: For CC codes in subcategory S73.03:
Right side: PDX collection 1313
Left side: PDX collection 1314
Unspecified side: PDX collection 1315

6 √7th **S73.031** **Other anterior subluxation** CC H5 HCC
of right hip

6 √7th **S73.032** **Other anterior subluxation** CC H5 HCC
of left hip

6 √7th **S73.033** **Other anterior subluxation** CC H5 HCC
of unspecified hip

6 √7th **S73.034** **Other anterior dislocation** CC H5 HCC
of right hip

6 √7th **S73.035** **Other anterior dislocation** CC H5 HCC
of left hip

6 √7th **S73.036** **Other anterior dislocation** CC H5 HCC
of unspecified hip

√6th **S73.04** **Central subluxation and dislocation of hip**

CC Excl: For CC codes in subcategory S73.04:
Right side: PDX collection 1304
Left side: PDX collection 1305
Unspecified side: PDX collection 1306

6 √7th **S73.041** **Central subluxation of right hip** CC H5 HCC

6 √7th **S73.042** **Central subluxation of left hip** CC H5 HCC

6 √7th **S73.043** **Central subluxation of** CC H5 HCC
unspecified hip

6 √7th **S73.044** **Central dislocation of right hip** CC H5 HCC

6 √7th **S73.045** **Central dislocation of left hip** CC H5 HCC

6 √7th **S73.046** **Central dislocation of** CC H5 HCC
unspecified hip

√5th **S73.1** **Sprain of hip**
AHA: 2014, 4Q, 25

√6th **S73.10** **Unspecified sprain of hip**

√7th **S73.101** **Unspecified sprain of right hip**

√7th **S73.102** **Unspecified sprain of left hip**

√7th **S73.109** **Unspecified sprain of unspecified hip**

√6th **S73.11** **Iliofemoral ligament sprain of hip**

√7th **S73.111** **Iliofemoral ligament sprain of right hip**

√7th **S73.112** **Iliofemoral ligament sprain of left hip**

N Newborn: 0   P Pediatric: 0-17   M Maternity: 12-55   A Adult: 15-124   MCC Major Complication/Comorbidity   CC Complication/Comorbidity   SW Severe Wound Dx

    ☑7th **S73.119**   **Iliofemoral ligament sprain of** unspecified
         hip

  ☑6th **S73.12**   **Ischiocapsular (ligament) sprain of hip**

    ☑7th **S73.121**   **Ischiocapsular ligament sprain of** right **hip**

    ☑7th **S73.122**   **Ischiocapsular ligament sprain of** left **hip**

    ☑7th **S73.129**   **Ischiocapsular ligament sprain of**
         unspecified **hip**

  ☑6th **S73.19**   **Other sprain of hip**

    ☑7th **S73.191**   **Other sprain of** right **hip**

    ☑7th **S73.192**   **Other sprain of** left **hip**

    ☑7th **S73.199**   **Other sprain of** unspecified **hip**

☑4th **S74**   **Injury of nerves at hip and thigh level**
     Code also any associated open wound (S71.-)
     EXCLUDES 2   injury of nerves at ankle and foot level (S94.-)
                injury of nerves at lower leg level (S84.-)

> The appropriate 7th character is to be added to each code from
> category S74.
> A   initial encounter
> D   subsequent encounter
> S   sequela

  ☑5th **S74.0**   **Injury of** sciatic nerve **at hip and thigh level**

    ☑x7th **S74.00**   **Injury of sciatic nerve at hip and thigh level,**
         unspecified **leg**

    ☑x7th **S74.01**   **Injury of sciatic nerve at hip and thigh level,** right **leg**

    ☑x7th **S74.02**   **Injury of sciatic nerve at hip and thigh level,** left **leg**

  ☑5th **S74.1**   **Injury of** femoral nerve **at hip and thigh level**

    ☑7th **S74.10**   **Injury of femoral nerve at hip and thigh level,**
         unspecified **leg**

    ☑x7th **S74.11**   **Injury of femoral nerve at hip and thigh level,** right
         leg

    ☑x7th **S74.12**   **Injury of femoral nerve at hip and thigh level,** left **leg**

  ☑5th **S74.2**   **Injury of** cutaneous sensory nerve **at hip and thigh level**

    ☑x7th **S74.20**   **Injury of cutaneous sensory nerve at hip and thigh
         level,** unspecified **leg**

    ☑x7th **S74.21**   **Injury of cutaneous sensory nerve at hip and high
         level,** right **leg**

    ☑x7th **S74.22**   **Injury of cutaneous sensory nerve at hip and thigh
         level,** left **leg**

  ☑5th **S74.8**   **Injury of** other nerves **at hip and thigh level**

    ☑6th **S74.8X**   **Injury of other nerves at hip and thigh level**

      ☑7th **S74.8X1**   **Injury of other nerves at hip and thigh
          level,** right **leg**

      ☑7th **S74.8X2**   **Injury of other nerves at hip and thigh
          level,** left **leg**

      ☑7th **S74.8X9**   **Injury of other nerves at hip and thigh
          level,** unspecified **leg**

  ☑5th **S74.9**   **Injury of** unspecified nerve **at hip and thigh level**

    ☑x7th **S74.90**   **Injury of unspecified nerve at hip and thigh level,**
         unspecified **leg**

    ☑x7th **S74.91**   **Injury of unspecified nerve at hip and thigh level,**
         right **leg**

    ☑x7th **S74.92**   **Injury of unspecified nerve at hip and thigh level,**
         left **leg**

☑4th **S75**   **Injury of blood vessels at hip and thigh level**
     Code also any associated open wound (S71.-)
     EXCLUDES 2   injury of blood vessels at lower leg level (S85.-)
                injury of popliteal artery (S85.0)

> The appropriate 7th character is to be added to each code from
> category S75.
> A   initial encounter
> D   subsequent encounter
> S   sequela

  ☑5th **S75.0**   **Injury of** femoral artery

> **CC Excl: For MCC codes in subcategory S75.0:**
> **Right side:** PDX collection 1316
> **Left side:** PDX collection 1317
> **Unspecified side:** PDX collection 1318

    ☑6th **S75.00**   **Unspecified injury of femoral artery**

      ☑7th **S75.001**   **Unspecified injury of femoral artery,** MCC
          right **leg**

      ☑7th **S75.002**   **Unspecified injury of femoral artery,** MCC
          left **leg**

      ☑7th **S75.009**   **Unspecified injury of femoral artery,** MCC
          unspecified **leg**

  ☑6th **S75.01**   **Minor laceration of femoral artery**
       Incomplete transection of femoral artery
       Laceration of femoral artery NOS
       Superficial laceration of femoral artery

    ☑7th **S75.011**   **Minor laceration of femoral artery,** MCC
         right **leg**

    ☑7th **S75.012**   **Minor laceration of femoral artery,** MCC
         left **leg**

    ☑7th **S75.019**   **Minor laceration of femoral artery,** MCC
         unspecified **leg**

  ☑6th **S75.02**   **Major laceration of femoral artery**
       Complete transection of femoral artery
       Traumatic rupture of femoral artery

    ☑7th **S75.021**   **Major laceration of femoral artery,** MCC
         right **leg**

    ☑7th **S75.022**   **Major laceration of femoral artery,** MCC
         left **leg**

    ☑7th **S75.029**   **Major laceration of femoral artery,** MCC
         unspecified **leg**

  ☑6th **S75.09**   **Other** specified injury of femoral artery

    ☑7th **S75.091**   **Other specified injury of femoral** MCC
         artery, right **leg**

    ☑7th **S75.092**   **Other specified injury of femoral** MCC
         artery, left **leg**

    ☑7th **S75.099**   **Other specified injury of femoral** MCC
         artery, unspecified **leg**

  ☑5th **S75.1**   **Injury of** femoral vein **at hip and thigh level**

> **CC Excl: For MCC codes in subcategory S75.1:**
> **Right side:** PDX collection 1319
> **Left side:** PDX collection 1320
> **Unspecified side:** PDX collection 1321

    ☑6th **S75.10**   **Unspecified injury of femoral vein at hip and thigh
         level**

    ☑7th **S75.101**   **Unspecified injury of femoral vein** MCC
         at hip and thigh level, right **leg**

    ☑7th **S75.102**   **Unspecified injury of femoral vein** MCC
         at hip and thigh level, left **leg**

    ☑7th **S75.109**   **Unspecified injury of femoral vein** MCC
         at hip and thigh level, unspecified **leg**

  ☑6th **S75.11**   **Minor laceration of femoral vein at hip and thigh
       level**
       Incomplete transection of femoral vein at hip and
         thigh level
       Laceration of femoral vein at hip and thigh level NOS
       Superficial laceration of femoral vein at hip and thigh
         level

    ☑7th **S75.111**   **Minor laceration of femoral vein at** MCC
         hip and thigh level, right **leg**

    ☑7th **S75.112**   **Minor laceration of femoral vein at** MCC
         hip and thigh level, left **leg**

    ☑7th **S75.119**   **Minor laceration of femoral vein at** MCC
         hip and thigh level, unspecified **leg**

  ☑6th **S75.12**   **Major laceration of femoral vein at hip and thigh
       level**
       Complete transection of femoral vein at hip and thigh
         level
       Traumatic rupture of femoral vein at hip and thigh
         level

    ☑7th **S75.121**   **Major laceration of femoral vein at** MCC
         hip and thigh level, right **leg**

    ☑7th **S75.122**   **Major laceration of femoral vein at** MCC
         hip and thigh level, left **leg**

    ☑7th **S75.129**   **Major laceration of femoral vein at** MCC
         hip and thigh level, unspecified **leg**

  ☑6th **S75.19**   **Other** specified injury of femoral vein at hip and
       thigh level

    ☑7th **S75.191**   **Other specified injury of femoral vein** MCC
         at hip and thigh level, right **leg**

    ☑7th **S75.192**   **Other specified injury of femoral vein** MCC
         at hip and thigh level, left **leg**

    ☑7th **S75.199**   **Other specified injury of femoral vein** MCC
         at hip and thigh level, unspecified **leg**

☑ Additional Character Required   ☑x7th Placeholder   Unacceptable PDx   Questionable PDx   Manifestation   H1 - H14 HAC   HCC CMS-HCC Dx   HIV HIV Dx

ICD-10-CM 2019   **1047**

✓5ᵗʰ **S75.2 Injury of** greater saphenous vein **at hip and thigh level**

EXCLUDES 1 *greater saphenous vein NOS (S85.3)*

CC Excl: For CC codes in subcategory S75.2:
Right side: PDX collection 1322
Left side: PDX collection 1323
Unspecified side: PDX collection 1324

✓6ᵗʰ **S75.20** Unspecified **injury of greater saphenous vein at hip and thigh level**

✓7ᵗʰ **S75.201 Unspecified injury of greater** CC **saphenous vein at hip and thigh level,** right **leg**

✓7ᵗʰ **S75.202 Unspecified injury of greater** CC **saphenous vein at hip and thigh level,** left **leg**

✓7ᵗʰ **S75.209 Unspecified injury of greater** CC **saphenous vein at hip and thigh level,** unspecified **leg**

✓6ᵗʰ **S75.21** Minor laceration **of greater saphenous vein at hip and thigh level**

Incomplete transection of greater saphenous vein at hip and thigh level
Laceration of greater saphenous vein at hip and thigh level NOS
Superficial laceration of greater saphenous vein at hip and thigh level

✓7ᵗʰ **S75.211 Minor laceration of greater saphenous** CC **vein at hip and thigh level,** right **leg**

✓7ᵗʰ **S75.212 Minor laceration of greater saphenous** CC **vein at hip and thigh level,** left **leg**

✓7ᵗʰ **S75.219 Minor laceration of greater saphenous** CC **vein at hip and thigh level,** unspecified **leg**

✓6ᵗʰ **S75.22** Major laceration **of greater saphenous vein at hip and thigh level**

Complete transection of greater saphenous vein at hip and thigh level
Traumatic rupture of greater saphenous vein at hip and thigh level

✓7ᵗʰ **S75.221 Major laceration of greater saphenous** CC **vein at hip and thigh level,** right **leg**

✓7ᵗʰ **S75.222 Major laceration of greater saphenous** CC **vein at hip and thigh level,** left **leg**

✓7ᵗʰ **S75.229 Major laceration of greater saphenous** CC **vein at hip and thigh level,** unspecified **leg**

✓6ᵗʰ **S75.29** Other specified injury of greater saphenous vein at hip and thigh level

✓7ᵗʰ **S75.291 Other specified injury of greater** CC **saphenous vein at hip and thigh level,** right **leg**

✓7ᵗʰ **S75.292 Other specified injury of greater** CC **saphenous vein at hip and thigh level,** left **leg**

✓7ᵗʰ **S75.299 Other specified injury of greater** CC **saphenous vein at hip and thigh level,** unspecified **leg**

✓5ᵗʰ **S75.8 Injury of** other blood vessels **at hip and thigh level**

CC Excl: For CC codes in subcategory S75.8:
Right side: PDX collection 1325
Left side: PDX collection 1326
Unspecified side: PDX collection 1327

✓6ᵗʰ **S75.80** Unspecified **injury of other blood vessels at hip and thigh level**

✓7ᵗʰ **S75.801 Unspecified injury of other blood** CC **vessels at hip and thigh level,** right **leg**

✓7ᵗʰ **S75.802 Unspecified injury of other blood** CC **vessels at hip and thigh level,** left **leg**

✓7ᵗʰ **S75.809 Unspecified injury of other blood** CC **vessels at hip and thigh level,** unspecified **leg**

✓6ᵗʰ **S75.81** Laceration **of other blood vessels at hip and thigh level**

✓7ᵗʰ **S75.811 Laceration of other blood vessels** CC **at hip and thigh level,** right **leg**

✓7ᵗʰ **S75.812 Laceration of other blood vessels at** CC **hip and thigh level,** left **leg**

✓7ᵗʰ **S75.819 Laceration of other blood vessels** CC **at hip and thigh level,** unspecified **leg**

✓6ᵗʰ **S75.89** Other **specified injury of other blood vessels at hip and thigh level**

✓7ᵗʰ **S75.891 Other specified injury of other blood** CC **vessels at hip and thigh level,** right **leg**

✓7ᵗʰ **S75.892 Other specified injury of other blood** CC **vessels at hip and thigh level,** left **leg**

✓7ᵗʰ **S75.899 Other specified injury of other blood** CC **vessels at hip and thigh level,** unspecified **leg**

✓5ᵗʰ **S75.9 Injury of unspecified blood vessel at hip and thigh level**

CC Excl: For CC codes in subcategory S75.9:
Right side: PDX collection 1325
Left side: PDX collection 1326
Unspecified side: PDX collection 1327

✓6ᵗʰ **S75.90** Unspecified **injury of unspecified blood vessel at hip and thigh level**

✓7ᵗʰ **S75.901 Unspecified injury of unspecified** CC **blood vessel at hip and thigh level,** right **leg**

✓7ᵗʰ **S75.902 Unspecified injury of unspecified** CC **blood vessel at hip and thigh level,** left **leg**

✓7ᵗʰ **S75.909 Unspecified injury of unspecified** CC **blood vessel at hip and thigh level,** unspecified **leg**

✓6ᵗʰ **S75.91** Laceration **of unspecified blood vessel at hip and thigh level**

✓7ᵗʰ **S75.911 Laceration of unspecified blood** CC **vessel at hip and thigh level,** right **leg**

✓7ᵗʰ **S75.912 Laceration of unspecified blood vessel** CC **at hip and thigh level,** left **leg**

✓7ᵗʰ **S75.919 Laceration of unspecified blood vessel** CC **at hip and thigh level,** unspecified **leg**

✓6ᵗʰ **S75.99** Other **specified injury of unspecified blood vessel at hip and thigh level**

✓7ᵗʰ **S75.991 Other specified injury of unspecified** CC **blood vessel at hip and thigh level,** right **leg**

✓7ᵗʰ **S75.992 Other specified injury of unspecified** CC **blood vessel at hip and thigh level,** left **leg**

✓7ᵗʰ **S75.999 Other specified injury of unspecified** CC **blood vessel at hip and thigh level,** unspecified **leg**

✓4ᵗʰ **S76 Injury of muscle, fascia and tendon at hip and thigh level**

Code also any associated open wound (S71.-)

EXCLUDES 2 *injury of muscle, fascia and tendon at lower leg level (S86)*
sprain of joint and ligament of hip (S73.1)

TIP: Refer to the Muscle/Tendon table at the beginning of this chapter.

The appropriate 7th character is to be added to each code from category S76.
A   initial encounter
D   subsequent encounter
S   sequela

CC Excl: For CC codes in category S76:
Right side: PDX collection 1328
Left side: PDX collection 1329
Unspecified side: PDX collection 1330

✓5ᵗʰ **S76.0 Injury of muscle, fascia and tendon of hip**

✓6ᵗʰ **S76.00** Unspecified **injury of muscle, fascia and tendon of hip**

✓7ᵗʰ **S76.001 Unspecified injury of muscle, fascia and tendon of** right **hip**

✓7ᵗʰ **S76.002 Unspecified injury of muscle, fascia and tendon of** left **hip**

✓7ᵗʰ **S76.009 Unspecified injury of muscle, fascia and tendon of** unspecified **hip**

✓6ᵗʰ **S76.01** Strain **of muscle, fascia and tendon of hip**

✓7ᵗʰ **S76.011 Strain of muscle, fascia and tendon of** right **hip**

✓7ᵗʰ **S76.012 Strain of muscle, fascia and tendon of** left **hip**

N Newborn: 0   P Pediatric: 0-17   M Maternity: 12-55   A Adult: 15-124   MCC Major Complication/Comorbidity   CC Complication/Comorbidity   SW Severe Wound Dx

1048   ICD-10-CM 2019

   ✓7ᵗʰ **S76.019**   **Strain of muscle, fascia and tendon of** unspecified **hip**

✓6ᵗʰ **S76.02**   Laceration **of muscle, fascia and tendon of hip**

   ✓7ᵗʰ **S76.021**   **Laceration of muscle, fascia and tendon of** right **hip**   `CC`

   ✓7ᵗʰ **S76.022**   **Laceration of muscle, fascia and tendon of** left **hip**   `CC`

   ✓7ᵗʰ **S76.029**   **Laceration of muscle, fascia and tendon of** unspecified **hip**   `CC`

✓6ᵗʰ **S76.09**   Other **specified injury of muscle, fascia and tendon of hip**

   ✓7ᵗʰ **S76.091**   **Other specified injury of muscle, fascia and tendon of** right **hip**

   ✓7ᵗʰ **S76.092**   **Other specified injury of muscle, fascia and tendon of** left **hip**

   ✓7ᵗʰ **S76.099**   **Other specified injury of muscle, fascia and tendon of** unspecified **hip**

✓5ᵗʰ **S76.1**   **Injury of** quadriceps **muscle, fascia and tendon**
Injury of patellar ligament (tendon)

✓6ᵗʰ **S76.10**   Unspecified **injury of quadriceps muscle, fascia and tendon**

   ✓7ᵗʰ **S76.101**   **Unspecified injury of** right **quadriceps muscle, fascia and tendon**

   ✓7ᵗʰ **S76.102**   **Unspecified injury of** left **quadriceps muscle, fascia and tendon**

   ✓7ᵗʰ **S76.109**   **Unspecified injury of** unspecified **quadriceps muscle, fascia and tendon**

✓6ᵗʰ **S76.11**   Strain **of quadriceps muscle, fascia and tendon**

   ✓7ᵗʰ **S76.111**   **Strain of** right **quadriceps muscle, fascia and tendon**

   ✓7ᵗʰ **S76.112**   **Strain of** left **quadriceps muscle, fascia and tendon**

   ✓7ᵗʰ **S76.119**   **Strain of** unspecified **quadriceps muscle, fascia and tendon**

✓6ᵗʰ **S76.12**   Laceration **of quadriceps muscle, fascia and tendon**

   ✓7ᵗʰ **S76.121**   **Laceration of** right **quadriceps muscle, fascia and tendon**   `CC`

   ✓7ᵗʰ **S76.122**   **Laceration of** left **quadriceps muscle, fascia and tendon**   `CC`

   ✓7ᵗʰ **S76.129**   **Laceration of** unspecified **quadriceps muscle, fascia and tendon**   `CC`

✓6ᵗʰ **S76.19**   Other **specified injury of quadriceps muscle, fascia and tendon**

   ✓7ᵗʰ **S76.191**   **Other specified injury of** right **quadriceps muscle, fascia and tendon**

   ✓7ᵗʰ **S76.192**   **Other specified injury of** left **quadriceps muscle, fascia and tendon**

   ✓7ᵗʰ **S76.199**   **Other specified injury of** unspecified **quadriceps muscle, fascia and tendon**

✓5ᵗʰ **S76.2**   **Injury of** adductor **muscle, fascia and tendon of** thigh

✓6ᵗʰ **S76.20**   Unspecified **injury of adductor muscle, fascia and tendon of thigh**

   ✓7ᵗʰ **S76.201**   **Unspecified injury of adductor muscle, fascia and tendon of** right **thigh**

   ✓7ᵗʰ **S76.202**   **Unspecified injury of adductor muscle, fascia and tendon of** left **thigh**

   ✓7ᵗʰ **S76.209**   **Unspecified injury of adductor muscle, fascia and tendon of** unspecified **thigh**

✓6ᵗʰ **S76.21**   Strain **of adductor muscle, fascia and tendon of thigh**

   ✓7ᵗʰ **S76.211**   **Strain of adductor muscle, fascia and tendon of** right **thigh**

   ✓7ᵗʰ **S76.212**   **Strain of adductor muscle, fascia and tendon of** left **thigh**

   ✓7ᵗʰ **S76.219**   **Strain of adductor muscle, fascia and tendon of** unspecified **thigh**

✓6ᵗʰ **S76.22**   Laceration **of adductor muscle, fascia and tendon of thigh**

   ✓7ᵗʰ **S76.221**   **Laceration of adductor muscle, fascia and tendon of** right **thigh**   `CC`

   ✓7ᵗʰ **S76.222**   **Laceration of adductor muscle, fascia and tendon of** left **thigh**   `CC`

   ✓7ᵗʰ **S76.229**   **Laceration of adductor muscle, fascia and tendon of** unspecified **thigh**   `CC`

✓6ᵗʰ **S76.29**   Other **injury of adductor muscle, fascia and tendon of thigh**

   ✓7ᵗʰ **S76.291**   **Other injury of adductor muscle, fascia and tendon of** right **thigh**

   ✓7ᵗʰ **S76.292**   **Other injury of adductor muscle, fascia and tendon of** left **thigh**

   ✓7ᵗʰ **S76.299**   **Other injury of adductor muscle, fascia and tendon of** unspecified **thigh**

✓5ᵗʰ **S76.3**   **Injury of muscle, fascia and tendon of the** posterior muscle group at thigh level

✓6ᵗʰ **S76.30**   Unspecified **injury of muscle, fascia and tendon of the posterior muscle group at thigh level**

   ✓7ᵗʰ **S76.301**   **Unspecified injury of muscle, fascia and tendon of the posterior muscle group at thigh level,** right **thigh**

   ✓7ᵗʰ **S76.302**   **Unspecified injury of muscle, fascia and tendon of the posterior muscle group at thigh level,** left **thigh**

   ✓7ᵗʰ **S76.309**   **Unspecified injury of muscle, fascia and tendon of the posterior muscle group at thigh level,** unspecified **thigh**

✓6ᵗʰ **S76.31**   Strain **of muscle, fascia and tendon of the posterior muscle group at thigh level**

   ✓7ᵗʰ **S76.311**   **Strain of muscle, fascia and tendon of the posterior muscle group at thigh level,** right **thigh**

   ✓7ᵗʰ **S76.312**   **Strain of muscle, fascia and tendon of the posterior muscle group at thigh level,** left **thigh**

   ✓7ᵗʰ **S76.319**   **Strain of muscle, fascia and tendon of the posterior muscle group at thigh level,** unspecified **thigh**

✓6ᵗʰ **S76.32**   Laceration **of muscle, fascia and tendon of the posterior muscle group at thigh level**

   ✓7ᵗʰ **S76.321**   **Laceration of muscle, fascia and tendon of the posterior muscle group at thigh level,** right **thigh**   `CC`

   ✓7ᵗʰ **S76.322**   **Laceration of muscle, fascia and tendon of the posterior muscle group at thigh level,** left **thigh**   `CC`

   ✓7ᵗʰ **S76.329**   **Laceration of muscle, fascia and tendon of the posterior muscle group at thigh level,** unspecified **thigh**   `CC`

✓6ᵗʰ **S76.39**   Other **specified injury of muscle, fascia and tendon of the posterior muscle group at thigh level**

   ✓7ᵗʰ **S76.391**   **Other specified injury of muscle, fascia and tendon of the posterior muscle group at thigh level,** right **thigh**

   ✓7ᵗʰ **S76.392**   **Other specified injury of muscle, fascia and tendon of the posterior muscle group at thigh level,** left **thigh**

   ✓7ᵗʰ **S76.399**   **Other specified injury of muscle, fascia and tendon of the posterior muscle group at thigh level,** unspecified **thigh**

✓5ᵗʰ **S76.8**   **Injury of** other specified **muscles, fascia and tendons at** thigh level

✓6ᵗʰ **S76.80**   Unspecified **injury of other specified muscles, fascia and tendons at thigh level**

   ✓7ᵗʰ **S76.801**   **Unspecified injury of other specified muscles, fascia and tendons at thigh level,** right **thigh**

   ✓7ᵗʰ **S76.802**   **Unspecified injury of other specified muscles, fascia and tendons at thigh level,** left **thigh**

   ✓7ᵗʰ **S76.809**   **Unspecified injury of other specified muscles, fascia and tendons at thigh level,** unspecified **thigh**

✓6ᵗʰ **S76.81**   Strain **of other specified muscles, fascia and tendons at thigh level**

   ✓7ᵗʰ **S76.811**   **Strain of other specified muscles, fascia and tendons at thigh level,** right **thigh**

   ✓7ᵗʰ **S76.812**   **Strain of other specified muscles, fascia and tendons at thigh level,** left **thigh**

   ✓7ᵗʰ **S76.819**   **Strain of other specified muscles, fascia and tendons at thigh level,** unspecified **thigh**

✔ Additional Character Required   ✓x7ᵗʰ Placeholder   Unacceptable PDx   Questionable PDx   Manifestation   **H1**-**H14** HAC   **HCC** CMS-HCC Dx   **HIV** HIV Dx

ICD-10-CM 2019   **1049**

✓6ᵗʰ **S76.82 Laceration** of other specified muscles, fascia and tendons at thigh level

✓7ᵗʰ **S76.821 Laceration** of other specified muscles, fascia and tendons at thigh level, right thigh `CC`

✓7ᵗʰ **S76.822 Laceration** of other specified muscles, fascia and tendons at thigh level, left thigh `CC`

✓7ᵗʰ **S76.829 Laceration** of other specified muscles, fascia and tendons at thigh level, unspecified thigh `CC`

✓6ᵗʰ **S76.89 Other** injury of other specified muscles, fascia and tendons at thigh level

✓7ᵗʰ **S76.891 Other** injury of other specified muscles, fascia and tendons at thigh level, right thigh

✓7ᵗʰ **S76.892 Other** injury of other specified muscles, fascia and tendons at thigh level, left thigh

✓7ᵗʰ **S76.899 Other** injury of other specified muscles, fascia and tendons at thigh level, unspecified thigh

✓5ᵗʰ **S76.9 Injury** of unspecified muscles, fascia and tendons at thigh level

✓6ᵗʰ **S76.90 Unspecified** injury of unspecified muscles, fascia and tendons at thigh level

✓7ᵗʰ **S76.901 Unspecified** injury of unspecified muscles, fascia and tendons at thigh level, right thigh

✓7ᵗʰ **S76.902 Unspecified** injury of unspecified muscles, fascia and tendons at thigh level, left thigh

✓7ᵗʰ **S76.909 Unspecified** injury of unspecified muscles, fascia and tendons at thigh level, unspecified thigh

✓6ᵗʰ **S76.91 Strain** of unspecified muscles, fascia and tendons at thigh level

✓7ᵗʰ **S76.911 Strain** of unspecified muscles, fascia and tendons at thigh level, right thigh

✓7ᵗʰ **S76.912 Strain** of unspecified muscles, fascia and tendons at thigh level, left thigh

✓7ᵗʰ **S76.919 Strain** of unspecified muscles, fascia and tendons at thigh level, unspecified thigh

✓6ᵗʰ **S76.92 Laceration** of unspecified muscles, fascia and tendons at thigh level

✓7ᵗʰ **S76.921 Laceration** of unspecified muscles, fascia and tendons at thigh level, right thigh `CC`

✓7ᵗʰ **S76.922 Laceration** of unspecified muscles, fascia and tendons at thigh level, left thigh `CC`

✓7ᵗʰ **S76.929 Laceration** of unspecified muscles, fascia and tendons at thigh level, unspecified thigh `CC`

✓6ᵗʰ **S76.99 Other** specified injury of unspecified muscles, fascia and tendons at thigh level

✓7ᵗʰ **S76.991 Other** specified injury of unspecified muscles, fascia and tendons at thigh level, right thigh

✓7ᵗʰ **S76.992 Other** specified injury of unspecified muscles, fascia and tendons at thigh level, left thigh

✓7ᵗʰ **S76.999 Other** specified injury of unspecified muscles, fascia and tendons at thigh level, unspecified thigh

✓4ᵗʰ **S77 Crushing injury** of hip and thigh

Use additional code(s) for all associated injuries

EXCLUDES 2   crushing injury of ankle and foot (S97.-)
               crushing injury of lower leg (S87.-)

The appropriate 7th character is to be added to each code from category S77.
A   initial encounter
D   subsequent encounter
S   sequela

✓5ᵗʰ **S77.0 Crushing injury** of hip

CC Excl: For CC codes in subcategory S77.0:
PDX collection 1331

✓x7ᵗʰ **S77.00 Crushing injury** of unspecified hip `CC` `H5`

✓x7ᵗʰ **S77.01 Crushing injury** of right hip `CC` `H5`

✓x7ᵗʰ **S77.02 Crushing injury** of left hip `CC` `H5`

✓5ᵗʰ **S77.1 Crushing injury** of thigh

CC Excl: For CC codes in subcategory S77.1:
PDX collection 1332

✓x7ᵗʰ **S77.10 Crushing injury** of unspecified thigh `CC` `H5`

✓x7ᵗʰ **S77.11 Crushing injury** of right thigh `CC` `H5`

✓x7ᵗʰ **S77.12 Crushing injury** of left thigh `CC` `H5`

✓5ᵗʰ **S77.2 Crushing injury** of hip with thigh

✓x7ᵗʰ **S77.20 Crushing injury** of unspecified hip with thigh

✓x7ᵗʰ **S77.21 Crushing injury** of right hip with thigh

✓x7ᵗʰ **S77.22 Crushing injury** of left hip with thigh

✓4ᵗʰ **S78 Traumatic amputation of hip and thigh**

An amputation not identified as partial or complete should be coded to complete.

EXCLUDES 1   traumatic amputation of knee (S88.0-)

The appropriate 7th character is to be added to each code from category S78.
A   initial encounter
D   subsequent encounter
S   sequela

CC Excl: For CC codes in category S78:
Right side: PDX collection 1333
Left side: PDX collection 1334
Unspecified side: PDX collection 1335

✓5ᵗʰ **S78.0 Traumatic amputation** at hip joint

✓6ᵗʰ **S78.01 Complete** traumatic amputation at hip joint

✓7ᵗʰ **S78.011 Complete** traumatic amputation at right hip joint `CC` `HCC`

✓7ᵗʰ **S78.012 Complete** traumatic amputation at left hip joint `CC` `HCC`

✓7ᵗʰ **S78.019 Complete** traumatic amputation at unspecified hip joint `CC` `HCC`

✓6ᵗʰ **S78.02 Partial** traumatic amputation at hip joint

✓7ᵗʰ **S78.021 Partial** traumatic amputation at right hip joint `CC` `HCC`

✓7ᵗʰ **S78.022 Partial** traumatic amputation at left hip joint `CC` `HCC`

✓7ᵗʰ **S78.029 Partial** traumatic amputation at unspecified hip joint `CC` `HCC`

✓5ᵗʰ **S78.1 Traumatic amputation** at level between hip and knee

EXCLUDES 1   traumatic amputation of knee (S88.0-)

✓6ᵗʰ **S78.11 Complete** traumatic amputation at level between hip and knee

✓7ᵗʰ **S78.111 Complete** traumatic amputation at level between right hip and knee `CC` `HCC`

✓7ᵗʰ **S78.112 Complete** traumatic amputation at level between left hip and knee `CC` `HCC`

✓7ᵗʰ **S78.119 Complete** traumatic amputation at level between unspecified hip and knee `CC` `HCC`

✓6ᵗʰ **S78.12 Partial** traumatic amputation at level between hip and knee

✓7ᵗʰ **S78.121 Partial** traumatic amputation at level between right hip and knee `CC` `HCC`

✓7ᵗʰ **S78.122 Partial** traumatic amputation at level between left hip and knee `CC` `HCC`

✓7ᵗʰ **S78.129 Partial** traumatic amputation at level between unspecified hip and knee `CC` `HCC`

✓5ᵗʰ **S78.9 Traumatic amputation** of hip and thigh, level unspecified

✓6ᵗʰ **S78.91 Complete** traumatic amputation of hip and thigh, level unspecified

✓7ᵗʰ **S78.911 Complete** traumatic amputation of right hip and thigh, level unspecified `CC` `HCC`

✓7ᵗʰ **S78.912 Complete** traumatic amputation of left hip and thigh, level unspecified `CC` `HCC`

Ⓝ Newborn: 0   Ⓟ Pediatric: 0-17   Ⓜ Maternity: 12-55   Ⓐ Adult: 15-124   `MCC` Major Complication/Comorbidity   `CC` Complication/Comorbidity   `SW` Severe Wound Dx

1050   ICD-10-CM 2019

√7th **S78.919 Complete traumatic amputation** `CC` `HCC`
of unspecified hip and thigh, level
unspecified

√6th **S78.92 Partial traumatic amputation of hip and thigh, level
unspecified**

√7th **S78.921 Partial traumatic amputation of** `CC` `HCC`
right hip and thigh, level unspecified

√7th **S78.922 Partial traumatic amputation of** `CC` `HCC`
left hip and thigh, level unspecified

√7th **S78.929 Partial traumatic amputation of** `CC` `HCC`
unspecified hip and thigh, level
unspecified

√4th **S79 Other and unspecified injuries of hip and thigh**
> **NOTE** A fracture not indicated as open or closed should
> be coded to closed.
AHA: 2018, 2Q, 12; 2018, 1Q, 3; 2015, 3Q, 37-39

The appropriate 7th character is to be added to each code from
subcategory S79.0 and S79.1
A   initial encounter for closed fracture
D   subsequent encounter for fracture with routine healing
G   subsequent encounter for fracture with delayed healing
K   subsequent encounter for fracture with nonunion
P   subsequent encounter for fracture with malunion
S   sequela

√5th **S79.0 Physeal fracture of upper end of femur**
> **EXCLUDES 1** apophyseal fracture of upper end of femur (S72.13-)
> nontraumatic slipped upper femoral epiphysis
> (M93.0-)

CC Excl: For CC/MCC codes in subcategory S79.0:
Right side: See code S79.001
Left side: See code S79.002
Unspecified side: See code S79.009

√6th **S79.00 Unspecified physeal fracture of upper end of femur**
4,6 √7th **S79.001 Unspecified physeal** `MCC` `CC` `H5` `HCC`
fracture of upper end
of right femur
> **CC Excl: MCC with 7th character A:**
> PDX collection 1297
> **CC with 7th character K or P:**
> PDX collection 897

4,6 √7th **S79.002 Unspecified physeal** `MCC` `CC` `H5` `HCC`
fracture of upper end
of left femur
> **CC Excl: MCC with 7th character A:**
> PDX collection 1299
> **CC with 7th character K or P:**
> PDX collection 897

4,6 √7th **S79.009 Unspecified physeal** `MCC` `CC` `H5` `HCC`
fracture of upper end of
unspecified femur
> **CC Excl: MCC with 7th character A:**
> PDX collection 1298
> **CC with 7th character K or P:**
> PDX collection 897

√6th **S79.01 Salter-Harris Type I physeal fracture of upper end of
femur**
Acute on chronic slipped capital femoral epiphysis
(traumatic)
Acute slipped capital femoral epiphysis (traumatic)
Capital femoral epiphyseal fracture
> **EXCLUDES 1** chronic slipped upper femoral epiphysis
> (nontraumatic) (M93.02-)

4,6 √7th **S79.011 Salter-Harris Type I physeal** `MCC` `CC` `H5` `HCC`
fracture of upper end of
right femur

4,6 √7th **S79.012 Salter-Harris Type I physeal** `MCC` `CC` `H5` `HCC`
fracture of upper end of
left femur

4,6 √7th **S79.019 Salter-Harris Type I physeal** `MCC` `CC` `H5` `HCC`
fracture of upper end of
unspecified femur

√6th **S79.09 Other physeal fracture of upper end of femur**
4,6 √7th **S79.091 Other physeal fracture of** `MCC` `CC` `H5` `HCC`
upper end of right femur

4,6 √7th **S79.092 Other physeal fracture of** `MCC` `CC` `H5` `HCC`
upper end of left femur

4,6 √7th **S79.099 Other physeal fracture of** `MCC` `CC` `H5` `HCC`
upper end of unspecified femur

√5th **S79.1 Physeal fracture of lower end of femur**

CC Excl: For CC codes in subcategory S79.1:
Right side: See code S79.101
Left side: See code S79.102
Unspecified side: See code S79.109

√6th **S79.10 Unspecified physeal fracture of lower end of femur**
3,6 √7th **S79.101 Unspecified physeal fracture of** `CC` `H5` `HCC`
lower end of right femur
> **CC Excl: CC with 7th character A:**
> PDX collection 1300
> **CC with 7th character K or P:**
> PDX collection 897

3,6 √7th **S79.102 Unspecified physeal fracture of** `CC` `H5` `HCC`
lower end of left femur
> **CC Excl: CC with 7th character A:**
> PDX collection 1302
> **CC with 7th character K or P:**
> PDX collection 897

3,6 √7th **S79.109 Unspecified physeal fracture of** `CC` `H5` `HCC`
lower end of unspecified femur
> **CC Excl: CC with 7th character A:**
> PDX collection 1301
> **CC with 7th character K or P:**
> PDX collection 897

√6th **S79.11 Salter-Harris Type I physeal fracture of lower end of
femur**
3,6 √7th **S79.111 Salter-Harris Type I physeal** `CC` `H5` `HCC`
fracture of lower end of right femur
3,6 √7th **S79.112 Salter-Harris Type I physeal** `CC` `H5` `HCC`
fracture of lower end of left femur
3,6 √7th **S79.119 Salter-Harris Type I physeal** `CC` `H5` `HCC`
fracture of lower end of unspecified femur

√6th **S79.12 Salter-Harris Type II physeal fracture of lower end of
femur**
3,6 √7th **S79.121 Salter-Harris Type II physeal** `CC` `H5` `HCC`
fracture of lower end of right femur
3,6 √7th **S79.122 Salter-Harris Type II physeal** `CC` `H5` `HCC`
fracture of lower end of left femur
3,6 √7th **S79.129 Salter-Harris Type II physeal** `CC` `H5` `HCC`
fracture of lower end of unspecified femur

√6th **S79.13 Salter-Harris Type III physeal fracture of lower end of
femur**
3,6 √7th **S79.131 Salter-Harris Type III physeal** `CC` `H5` `HCC`
fracture of lower end of right femur
3,6 √7th **S79.132 Salter-Harris Type III physeal** `CC` `H5` `HCC`
fracture of lower end of left femur
3,6 √7th **S79.139 Salter-Harris Type III physeal** `CC` `H5` `HCC`
fracture of lower end of unspecified femur

√6th **S79.14 Salter-Harris Type IV physeal fracture of lower end of
femur**
3,6 √7th **S79.141 Salter-Harris Type IV physeal** `CC` `H5` `HCC`
fracture of lower end of right femur
3,6 √7th **S79.142 Salter-Harris Type IV physeal** `CC` `H5` `HCC`
fracture of lower end of left femur
3,6 √7th **S79.149 Salter-Harris Type IV physeal** `CC` `H5` `HCC`
fracture of lower end of unspecified femur

√6th **S79.19 Other physeal fracture of lower end of femur**
3,6 √7th **S79.191 Other physeal fracture of lower** `CC` `H5` `HCC`
end of right femur
3,6 √7th **S79.192 Other physeal fracture of lower** `CC` `H5` `HCC`
end of left femur
3,6 √7th **S79.199 Other physeal fracture of lower** `CC` `H5` `HCC`
end of unspecified femur

√5th **S79.8 Other specified injuries of hip and thigh**

The appropriate 7th character is to be added to each code
in subcategory S79.8.
A   initial encounter
D   subsequent encounter
S   sequela

√6th **S79.81 Other specified injuries of hip**
√7th **S79.811 Other specified injuries of right hip**
√7th **S79.812 Other specified injuries of left hip**
√7th **S79.819 Other specified injuries of unspecified hip**

√6ᵗʰ **S79.82** Other specified injuries of thigh
- √7ᵗʰ **S79.821** Other specified injuries of right thigh
- √7ᵗʰ **S79.822** Other specified injuries of left thigh
- √7ᵗʰ **S79.829** Other specified injuries of unspecified thigh

√5ᵗʰ **S79.9** Unspecified injury of hip and thigh

> The appropriate 7th character is to be added to each code in subcategory S79.9.
> A   initial encounter
> D   subsequent encounter
> S   sequela

√6ᵗʰ **S79.91** Unspecified injury of hip
- √7ᵗʰ **S79.911** Unspecified injury of right hip
- √7ᵗʰ **S79.912** Unspecified injury of left hip
- √7ᵗʰ **S79.919** Unspecified injury of unspecified hip

√6ᵗʰ **S79.92** Unspecified injury of thigh
- √7ᵗʰ **S79.921** Unspecified injury of right thigh
- √7ᵗʰ **S79.922** Unspecified injury of left thigh
- √7ᵗʰ **S79.929** Unspecified injury of unspecified thigh

Injuries to the knee and lower leg (S8Ø-S89)

EXCLUDES 2   burns and corrosions (T2Ø-T32)
frostbite (T33-T34)
injuries of ankle and foot, except fracture of ankle and malleolus (S9Ø-S99)
insect bite or sting, venomous (T63.4)

√4ᵗʰ **S8Ø** **Superficial injury of knee and lower leg**
EXCLUDES 2   superficial injury of ankle and foot (S9Ø.-)

> The appropriate 7th character is to be added to each code from category S8Ø.
> A   initial encounter
> D   subsequent encounter
> S   sequela

√5ᵗʰ **S8Ø.Ø** Contusion of knee
- √x7ᵗʰ **S8Ø.ØØ** Contusion of unspecified knee
- √x7ᵗʰ **S8Ø.Ø1** Contusion of right knee
- √x7ᵗʰ **S8Ø.Ø2** Contusion of left knee

√5ᵗʰ **S8Ø.1** Contusion of lower leg
- √x7ᵗʰ **S8Ø.1Ø** Contusion of unspecified lower leg
- √x7ᵗʰ **S8Ø.11** Contusion of right lower leg
- √x7ᵗʰ **S8Ø.12** Contusion of left lower leg

√5ᵗʰ **S8Ø.2** Other superficial injuries of knee
- √6ᵗʰ **S8Ø.21** Abrasion of knee
  - √7ᵗʰ **S8Ø.211** Abrasion, right knee
  - √7ᵗʰ **S8Ø.212** Abrasion, left knee
  - √7ᵗʰ **S8Ø.219** Abrasion, unspecified knee
- √6ᵗʰ **S8Ø.22** Blister (nonthermal) of knee
  - √7ᵗʰ **S8Ø.221** Blister (nonthermal), right knee
  - √7ᵗʰ **S8Ø.222** Blister (nonthermal), left knee
  - √7ᵗʰ **S8Ø.229** Blister (nonthermal), unspecified knee
- √6ᵗʰ **S8Ø.24** External constriction of knee
  - √7ᵗʰ **S8Ø.241** External constriction, right knee
  - √7ᵗʰ **S8Ø.242** External constriction, left knee
  - √7ᵗʰ **S8Ø.249** External constriction, unspecified knee
- √6ᵗʰ **S8Ø.25** Superficial foreign body of knee
  Splinter in the knee
  - √7ᵗʰ **S8Ø.251** Superficial foreign body, right knee
  - √7ᵗʰ **S8Ø.252** Superficial foreign body, left knee
  - √7ᵗʰ **S8Ø.259** Superficial foreign body, unspecified knee
- √6ᵗʰ **S8Ø.26** Insect bite (nonvenomous) of knee
  - √7ᵗʰ **S8Ø.261** Insect bite (nonvenomous), right knee
  - √7ᵗʰ **S8Ø.262** Insect bite (nonvenomous), left knee
  - √7ᵗʰ **S8Ø.269** Insect bite (nonvenomous), unspecified knee
- √6ᵗʰ **S8Ø.27** Other superficial bite of knee
  EXCLUDES 1   open bite of knee (S81.Ø5-)
  - √7ᵗʰ **S8Ø.271** Other superficial bite of right knee
  - √7ᵗʰ **S8Ø.272** Other superficial bite of left knee
  - √7ᵗʰ **S8Ø.279** Other superficial bite of unspecified knee

√5ᵗʰ **S8Ø.8** Other superficial injuries of lower leg
- √6ᵗʰ **S8Ø.81** Abrasion of lower leg
  - √7ᵗʰ **S8Ø.811** Abrasion, right lower leg
  - √7ᵗʰ **S8Ø.812** Abrasion, left lower leg
  - √7ᵗʰ **S8Ø.819** Abrasion, unspecified lower leg
- √6ᵗʰ **S8Ø.82** Blister (nonthermal) of lower leg
  - √7ᵗʰ **S8Ø.821** Blister (nonthermal), right lower leg
  - √7ᵗʰ **S8Ø.822** Blister (nonthermal), left lower leg
  - √7ᵗʰ **S8Ø.829** Blister (nonthermal), unspecified lower leg
- √6ᵗʰ **S8Ø.84** External constriction of lower leg
  - √7ᵗʰ **S8Ø.841** External constriction, right lower leg
  - √7ᵗʰ **S8Ø.842** External constriction, left lower leg
  - √7ᵗʰ **S8Ø.849** External constriction, unspecified lower leg
- √6ᵗʰ **S8Ø.85** Superficial foreign body of lower leg
  Splinter in the lower leg
  - √7ᵗʰ **S8Ø.851** Superficial foreign body, right lower leg
  - √7ᵗʰ **S8Ø.852** Superficial foreign body, left lower leg
  - √7ᵗʰ **S8Ø.859** Superficial foreign body, unspecified lower leg
- √6ᵗʰ **S8Ø.86** Insect bite (nonvenomous) of lower leg
  - √7ᵗʰ **S8Ø.861** Insect bite (nonvenomous), right lower leg
  - √7ᵗʰ **S8Ø.862** Insect bite (nonvenomous), left lower leg
  - √7ᵗʰ **S8Ø.869** Insect bite (nonvenomous), unspecified lower leg
- √6ᵗʰ **S8Ø.87** Other superficial bite of lower leg
  EXCLUDES 1   open bite of lower leg (S81.85-)
  - √7ᵗʰ **S8Ø.871** Other superficial bite, right lower leg
  - √7ᵗʰ **S8Ø.872** Other superficial bite, left lower leg
  - √7ᵗʰ **S8Ø.879** Other superficial bite, unspecified lower leg

√5ᵗʰ **S8Ø.9** Unspecified superficial injury of knee and lower leg
- √6ᵗʰ **S8Ø.91** Unspecified superficial injury of knee
  - √7ᵗʰ **S8Ø.911** Unspecified superficial injury of right knee
  - √7ᵗʰ **S8Ø.912** Unspecified superficial injury of left knee
  - √7ᵗʰ **S8Ø.919** Unspecified superficial injury of unspecified knee
- √6ᵗʰ **S8Ø.92** Unspecified superficial injury of lower leg
  - √7ᵗʰ **S8Ø.921** Unspecified superficial injury of right lower leg
  - √7ᵗʰ **S8Ø.922** Unspecified superficial injury of left lower leg
  - √7ᵗʰ **S8Ø.929** Unspecified superficial injury of unspecified lower leg

√4ᵗʰ **S81** **Open wound of knee and lower leg**
Code also any associated wound infection
EXCLUDES 1   open fracture of knee and lower leg (S82.-)
traumatic amputation of lower leg (S88.-)
EXCLUDES 2   open wound of ankle and foot (S91.-)

> The appropriate 7th character is to be added to each code from category S81.
> A   initial encounter
> D   subsequent encounter
> S   sequela

√5ᵗʰ **S81.Ø** Open wound of knee
- √6ᵗʰ **S81.ØØ** Unspecified open wound of knee
  - √7ᵗʰ **S81.ØØ1** Unspecified open wound, right knee
  - √7ᵗʰ **S81.ØØ2** Unspecified open wound, left knee
  - √7ᵗʰ **S81.ØØ9** Unspecified open wound, unspecified knee
- √6ᵗʰ **S81.Ø1** Laceration without foreign body of knee
  - √7ᵗʰ **S81.Ø11** Laceration without foreign body, right knee
  - √7ᵗʰ **S81.Ø12** Laceration without foreign body, left knee
  - √7ᵗʰ **S81.Ø19** Laceration without foreign body, unspecified knee

N Newborn: 0   P Pediatric: 0-17   M Maternity: 12-55   A Adult: 15-124   MCC Major Complication/Comorbidity   CC Complication/Comorbidity   SW Severe Wound Dx

1052   ICD-10-CM 2019

☑6ᵗʰ **S81.02** Laceration with foreign body of knee
- ☑7ᵗʰ **S81.021** Laceration with foreign body, right knee
- ☑7ᵗʰ **S81.022** Laceration with foreign body, left knee
- ☑7ᵗʰ **S81.029** Laceration with foreign body, unspecified knee

☑6ᵗʰ **S81.03** Puncture wound without foreign body of knee
- ☑7ᵗʰ **S81.031** Puncture wound without foreign body, right knee
- ☑7ᵗʰ **S81.032** Puncture wound without foreign body, left knee
- ☑7ᵗʰ **S81.039** Puncture wound without foreign body, unspecified knee

☑6ᵗʰ **S81.04** Puncture wound with foreign body of knee
- ☑7ᵗʰ **S81.041** Puncture wound with foreign body, right knee
- ☑7ᵗʰ **S81.042** Puncture wound with foreign body, left knee
- ☑7ᵗʰ **S81.049** Puncture wound with foreign body, unspecified knee

☑6ᵗʰ **S81.05** Open bite of knee
  Bite of knee NOS
  EXCLUDES1 superficial bite of knee (S80.27-)
- ☑7ᵗʰ **S81.051** Open bite, right knee
- ☑7ᵗʰ **S81.052** Open bite, left knee
- ☑7ᵗʰ **S81.059** Open bite, unspecified knee

☑5ᵗʰ **S81.8** Open wound of lower leg

☑6ᵗʰ **S81.80** Unspecified open wound of lower leg
  AHA: 2016, 3Q, 24
- ☑7ᵗʰ **S81.801** Unspecified open wound, right lower leg
- ☑7ᵗʰ **S81.802** Unspecified open wound, left lower leg
- ☑7ᵗʰ **S81.809** Unspecified open wound, unspecified lower leg

☑6ᵗʰ **S81.81** Laceration without foreign body of lower leg
- ☑7ᵗʰ **S81.811** Laceration without foreign body, right lower leg
- ☑7ᵗʰ **S81.812** Laceration without foreign body, left lower leg
- ☑7ᵗʰ **S81.819** Laceration without foreign body, unspecified lower leg

☑6ᵗʰ **S81.82** Laceration with foreign body of lower leg
- ☑7ᵗʰ **S81.821** Laceration with foreign body, right lower leg
- ☑7ᵗʰ **S81.822** Laceration with foreign body, left lower leg
- ☑7ᵗʰ **S81.829** Laceration with foreign body, unspecified lower leg

☑6ᵗʰ **S81.83** Puncture wound without foreign body of lower leg
  AHA: 2016, 3Q, 24
- ☑7ᵗʰ **S81.831** Puncture wound without foreign body, right lower leg
- ☑7ᵗʰ **S81.832** Puncture wound without foreign body, left lower leg
- ☑7ᵗʰ **S81.839** Puncture wound without foreign body, unspecified lower leg

☑6ᵗʰ **S81.84** Puncture wound with foreign body of lower leg
  AHA: 2016, 3Q, 24
- ☑7ᵗʰ **S81.841** Puncture wound with foreign body, right lower leg
- ☑7ᵗʰ **S81.842** Puncture wound with foreign body, left lower leg
- ☑7ᵗʰ **S81.849** Puncture wound with foreign body, unspecified lower leg

☑6ᵗʰ **S81.85** Open bite of lower leg
  Bite of lower leg NOS
  EXCLUDES1 superficial bite of lower leg (S80.86-, S80.87-)
- ☑7ᵗʰ **S81.851** Open bite, right lower leg
- ☑7ᵗʰ **S81.852** Open bite, left lower leg
- ☑7ᵗʰ **S81.859** Open bite, unspecified lower leg

☑4ᵗʰ **S82** Fracture of lower leg, including ankle
  NOTE A fracture not indicated as displaced or nondisplaced should be coded to displaced.
  A fracture not designated as open or closed should be coded to closed.
  The open fracture designations are based on the Gustilo open fracture classification.
  INCLUDES fracture of malleolus
  EXCLUDES1 traumatic amputation of lower leg (S88.-)
  EXCLUDES2 fracture of foot, except ankle (S92.-)
  periprosthetic fracture of prosthetic implant of knee (M97.0-)
  AHA: 2018, 2Q, 12; 2016, 1Q, 33; 2015, 3Q, 37-39; 2015, 3Q, 37-39

The appropriate 7th character is to be added to all codes from category S82 [unless otherwise indicated].
A   initial encounter for closed fracture
B   initial encounter for open fracture type I or II
    initial encounter for open fracture NOS
C   initial encounter for open fracture type IIIA, IIIB, or IIIC
D   subsequent encounter for closed fracture with routine healing
E   subsequent encounter for open fracture type I or II with routine healing
F   subsequent encounter for open fracture type IIIA, IIIB, or IIIC with routine healing
G   subsequent encounter for closed fracture with delayed healing
H   subsequent encounter for open fracture type I or II with delayed healing
J   subsequent encounter for open fracture type IIIA, IIIB or IIIC with delayed healing
K   subsequent encounter for closed fracture with nonunion
M   subsequent encounter for open fracture type I or II with nonunion
N   subsequent encounter for open fracture type IIIA, IIIB or IIIC with nonunion
P   subsequent encounter for closed fracture with malunion
Q   subsequent encounter for open fracture type I or II with malunion
R   subsequent encounter for open fracture type IIIA, IIIB or IIIC with malunion
S   sequela

☑5ᵗʰ **S82.0** Fracture of patella
  Knee cap

  CC Excl: For CC codes in subcategory S82.0:
  Right side: See code S82.001
  Left side: See code S82.002
  Unspecified side: See code S82.009

☑6ᵗʰ **S82.00** Unspecified fracture of patella
- ³ ☑7ᵗʰ **S82.001** Unspecified fracture of right patella CC H5
  CC Excl: CC with 7th character A: PDX collection 1336
  CC with 7th character B or C: PDX collection 1337
  CC with 7th character K, M, N, P, Q or R: PDX collection 897
- ³ ☑7ᵗʰ **S82.002** Unspecified fracture of left patella CC H5
  CC Excl: CC with 7th character A: PDX collection 1338
  CC with 7th character B or C: PDX collection 1337
  CC with 7th character K, M, N, P, Q or R: PDX collection 897
- ³ ☑7ᵗʰ **S82.009** Unspecified fracture of unspecified patella CC H5
  CC Excl: CC with 7th character A: PDX collection 1339
  CC with 7th character B or C: PDX collection 1337
  CC with 7th character K, M, N, P, Q or R: PDX collection 897

☑6ᵗʰ **S82.01** Osteochondral fracture of patella
- ³ ☑7ᵗʰ **S82.011** Displaced osteochondral fracture of right patella CC H5
- ³ ☑7ᵗʰ **S82.012** Displaced osteochondral fracture of left patella CC H5
- ³ ☑7ᵗʰ **S82.013** Displaced osteochondral fracture of unspecified patella CC H5
- ³ ☑7ᵗʰ **S82.014** Nondisplaced osteochondral fracture of right patella CC H5
- ³ ☑7ᵗʰ **S82.015** Nondisplaced osteochondral fracture of left patella CC H5

3 ✓7th **S82.016** Nondisplaced **osteochondral fracture** of **unspecified patella** `CC` `H5`

✓6th **S82.02** Longitudinal **fracture of patella**

3 ✓7th **S82.021** Displaced **longitudinal fracture of** right **patella** `CC` `H5`

3 ✓7th **S82.022** Displaced **longitudinal fracture of** left **patella** `CC` `H5`

3 ✓7th **S82.023** Displaced **longitudinal fracture of unspecified patella** `CC` `H5`

3 ✓7th **S82.024** Nondisplaced **longitudinal fracture of** right **patella** `CC` `H5`

3 ✓7th **S82.025** Nondisplaced **longitudinal fracture of** left **patella** `CC` `H5`

3 ✓7th **S82.026** Nondisplaced **longitudinal fracture of unspecified patella** `CC` `H5`

✓6th **S82.03** Transverse **fracture of patella**

3 ✓7th **S82.031** Displaced **transverse fracture of** right **patella** `CC` `H5`

3 ✓7th **S82.032** Displaced **transverse fracture of** left **patella** `CC` `H5`

3 ✓7th **S82.033** Displaced **transverse fracture of unspecified patella** `CC` `H5`

3 ✓7th **S82.034** Nondisplaced **transverse fracture** of **right patella** `CC` `H5`

3 ✓7th **S82.035** Nondisplaced **transverse fracture** of **left patella** `CC` `H5`

3 ✓7th **S82.036** Nondisplaced **transverse fracture** of **unspecified patella** `CC` `H5`

✓6th **S82.04** Comminuted **fracture of patella**

3 ✓7th **S82.041** Displaced **comminuted fracture** of **right patella** `CC` `H5`

3 ✓7th **S82.042** Displaced **comminuted fracture of** left **patella** `CC` `H5`

3 ✓7th **S82.043** Displaced **comminuted fracture of unspecified patella** `CC` `H5`

3 ✓7th **S82.044** Nondisplaced **comminuted fracture** of **right patella** `CC` `H5`

3 ✓7th **S82.045** Nondisplaced **comminuted fracture** of **left patella** `CC` `H5`

3 ✓7th **S82.046** Nondisplaced **comminuted fracture** of **unspecified patella** `CC` `H5`

✓6th **S82.09** Other **fracture of patella**

3 ✓7th **S82.091** Other **fracture of** right **patella** `CC` `H5`

3 ✓7th **S82.092** Other **fracture of** left **patella** `CC` `H5`

3 ✓7th **S82.099** Other **fracture of unspecified patella** `CC` `H5`

✓5th **S82.1** Fracture of **upper end of tibia**
Fracture of proximal end of tibia

EXCLUDES 2   fracture of shaft of tibia (S82.2-)
physeal fracture of upper end of tibia (S89.0-)

CC Excl: For CC/MCC codes in subcategory S82.1, unless otherwise noted:
Right side: See code S82.101
Left side: See code S82.102
Unspecified side: See code S82.109

✓6th **S82.10** Unspecified **fracture of upper end of tibia**

2,3 ✓7th **S82.101** Unspecified **fracture of upper end of** right **tibia** `MCC` `CC` `H5`
CC Excl: CC with 7th character A:
PDX collection 1340
MCC with 7th character B or C:
PDX collection 1341
CC with 7th character K, M, N, P, Q or R:
PDX collection 897

2,3 ✓7th **S82.102** Unspecified **fracture of upper end of** left **tibia** `MCC` `CC` `H5`
CC Excl: CC with 7th character A:
PDX collection 1342
MCC with 7th character B or C:
PDX collection 1341
CC with 7th character K, M, N, P, Q or R:
PDX collection 897

2,3 ✓7th **S82.109** Unspecified **fracture of upper end of unspecified tibia** `MCC` `CC` `H5`
CC Excl:
CC or MCC with 7th character A, B or C:
PDX collection 1341
CC with 7th character K, M, N, P, Q or R:
PDX collection 897

✓6th **S82.11** Fracture of **tibial spine**

2,3 ✓7th **S82.111** Displaced **fracture of** right **tibial spine** `MCC` `CC` `H5`

2,3 ✓7th **S82.112** Displaced **fracture of** left **tibial spine** `MCC` `CC` `H5`

2,3 ✓7th **S82.113** Displaced **fracture of unspecified tibial spine** `MCC` `CC` `H5`

2,3 ✓7th **S82.114** Nondisplaced **fracture of** right **tibial spine** `MCC` `CC` `H5`

2,3 ✓7th **S82.115** Nondisplaced **fracture of** left **tibial spine** `MCC` `CC` `H5`

2,3 ✓7th **S82.116** Nondisplaced **fracture of unspecified tibial spine** `MCC` `CC` `H5`

✓6th **S82.12** Fracture of **lateral condyle** of tibia

2,3 ✓7th **S82.121** Displaced **fracture of lateral condyle of** right **tibia** `MCC` `CC` `H5`

2,3 ✓7th **S82.122** Displaced **fracture of lateral condyle of** left **tibia** `MCC` `CC` `H5`

2,3 ✓7th **S82.123** Displaced **fracture of lateral condyle of unspecified tibia** `MCC` `CC` `H5`

2,3 ✓7th **S82.124** Nondisplaced **fracture of lateral condyle of** right **tibia** `MCC` `CC` `H5`

2,3 ✓7th **S82.125** Nondisplaced **fracture of lateral condyle of** left **tibia** `MCC` `CC` `H5`

2,3 ✓7th **S82.126** Nondisplaced **fracture of lateral condyle of unspecified tibia** `MCC` `CC` `H5`

✓6th **S82.13** Fracture of **medial condyle** of tibia

2,3 ✓7th **S82.131** Displaced **fracture of medial condyle of** right **tibia** `MCC` `CC` `H5`

2,3 ✓7th **S82.132** Displaced **fracture of medial condyle of** left **tibia** `MCC` `CC` `H5`

2,3 ✓7th **S82.133** Displaced **fracture of medial condyle of unspecified tibia** `MCC` `CC` `H5`

2,3 ✓7th **S82.134** Nondisplaced **fracture of medial condyle of** right **tibia** `MCC` `CC` `H5`

2,3 ✓7th **S82.135** Nondisplaced **fracture of medial condyle of** left **tibia** `MCC` `CC` `H5`

2,3 ✓7th **S82.136** Nondisplaced **fracture of medial condyle of unspecified tibia** `MCC` `CC` `H5`

✓6th **S82.14** Bicondylar **fracture of tibia**
Fracture of tibial plateau NOS

2,3 ✓7th **S82.141** Displaced **bicondylar fracture of** right **tibia** `MCC` `CC` `H5`

2,3 ✓7th **S82.142** Displaced **bicondylar fracture of** left **tibia** `MCC` `CC` `H5`

2,3 ✓7th **S82.143** Displaced **bicondylar fracture of unspecified tibia** `MCC` `CC` `H5`

2,3 ✓7th **S82.144** Nondisplaced **bicondylar fracture of** right **tibia** `MCC` `CC` `H5`

2,3 ✓7th **S82.145** Nondisplaced **bicondylar fracture of** left **tibia** `MCC` `CC` `H5`

2,3 ✓7th **S82.146** Nondisplaced **bicondylar fracture of unspecified tibia** `MCC` `CC` `H5`

✓6th **S82.15** Fracture of **tibial tuberosity**

2,3 ✓7th **S82.151** Displaced **fracture of** right **tibial tuberosity** `MCC` `CC` `H5`

2,3 ✓7th **S82.152** Displaced **fracture of** left **tibial tuberosity** `MCC` `CC` `H5`

2,3 ✓7th **S82.153** Displaced **fracture of unspecified tibial tuberosity** `MCC` `CC` `H5`

2,3 ✓7th **S82.154** Nondisplaced **fracture of** right **tibial tuberosity** `MCC` `CC` `H5`

2,3 ✓7th **S82.155** Nondisplaced **fracture of** left **tibial tuberosity** `MCC` `CC` `H5`

2,3 ✓7th **S82.156** Nondisplaced **fracture of unspecified tibial tuberosity** `MCC` `CC` `H5`

`N` Newborn: 0   `P` Pediatric: 0-17   `M` Maternity: 12-55   `A` Adult: 15-124   `MCC` Major Complication/Comorbidity   `CC` Complication/Comorbidity   `SW` Severe Wound Dx

1054   ICD-10-CM 2019

√6th **S82.16** Torus **fracture of upper end of tibia**

> The appropriate 7th character is to be added to
> all codes in subcategory S82.16.
> A   initial encounter for closed fracture
> D   subsequent encounter for fracture with
>   routine healing
> G   subsequent encounter for fracture with
>   delayed healing
> K   subsequent encounter for fracture with
>   nonunion
> P   subsequent encounter for fracture with
>   malunion
> S   sequela

3 √7th **S82.161** **Torus fracture of upper end of** `CC` `H5`
                    right tibia
                    CC Excl: CC with 7th character A:
                    PDX collection 1343
                    CC with 7th character K or P:
                    PDX collection 897

3 √7th **S82.162** **Torus fracture of upper end of left** `CC` `H5`
                    tibia
                    CC Excl: CC with 7th character A:
                    PDX collection 1344
                    CC with 7th character K or P:
                    PDX collection 897

3 √7th **S82.169** **Torus fracture of upper end of** `CC` `H5`
                    unspecified tibia
                    CC Excl: CC with 7th character A:
                    PDX collection 1345
                    CC with 7th character K or P:
                    PDX collection 897

√6th **S82.19** Other **fracture of upper end of tibia**

2,3 √7th **S82.191** **Other fracture of upper end** `MCC` `CC` `H5`
                    of right tibia

2,3 √7th **S82.192** **Other fracture of upper end** `MCC` `CC` `H5`
                    of left tibia

2,3 √7th **S82.199** **Other fracture of upper end of** `MCC` `CC` `H5`
                    unspecified tibia

√5th **S82.2** **Fracture of shaft of tibia**

> **CC Excl: For CC/MCC codes in subcategory S82.2,
> unless otherwise noted:**
> **Right side:** See code S82.101
> **Left side:** See code S82.102
> **Unspecified side:** See code S82.109

√6th **S82.20** **Unspecified fracture of shaft of tibia**
                Fracture of tibia NOS

2,3 √7th **S82.201** **Unspecified fracture of shaft of** `MCC` `CC` `H5`
                    right tibia
                    CC Excl: CC with 7th character A:
                    PDX collection 1346
                    MCC with 7th character B or C:
                    PDX collection 1341
                    CC with 7th character K, M, N, P, Q or R:
                    PDX collection 897

2,3 √7th **S82.202** **Unspecified fracture of shaft** `MCC` `CC` `H5`
                    of left tibia
                    CC Excl: CC with 7th character A:
                    PDX collection 1342
                    MCC with 7th character B or C:
                    PDX collection 1341
                    CC with 7th character K, M, N, P, Q or R:
                    PDX collection 897

2,3 √7th **S82.209** **Unspecified fracture of shaft of** `MCC` `CC` `H5`
                    unspecified tibia
                    CC Excl:
                    CC or MCC with 7th character A, B or C:
                    PDX collection 1341
                    CC with 7th character K, M, N, P, Q or R:
                    PDX collection 897

√6th **S82.22** Transverse **fracture of shaft of tibia**

2,3 √7th **S82.221** **Displaced transverse fracture** `MCC` `CC` `H5`
                    of shaft of right tibia

2,3 √7th **S82.222** **Displaced transverse fracture** `MCC` `CC` `H5`
                    of shaft of left tibia

2,3 √7th **S82.223** **Displaced transverse fracture** `MCC` `CC` `H5`
                    of shaft of unspecified tibia

2,3 √7th **S82.224** **Nondisplaced transverse** `MCC` `CC` `H5`
                    fracture of shaft of right tibia

2,3 √7th **S82.225** **Nondisplaced transverse** `MCC` `CC` `H5`
                    fracture of shaft of left tibia

2,3 √7th **S82.226** **Nondisplaced transverse** `MCC` `CC` `H5`
                    fracture of shaft of unspecified tibia

√6th **S82.23** Oblique **fracture of shaft of tibia**

2,3 √7th **S82.231** **Displaced oblique fracture of** `MCC` `CC` `H5`
                    shaft of right tibia

2,3 √7th **S82.232** **Displaced oblique fracture of** `MCC` `CC` `H5`
                    shaft of left tibia

2,3 √7th **S82.233** **Displaced oblique fracture of** `MCC` `CC` `H5`
                    shaft of unspecified tibia

2,3 √7th **S82.234** **Nondisplaced oblique fracture** `MCC` `CC` `H5`
                    of shaft of right tibia

2,3 √7th **S82.235** **Nondisplaced oblique fracture** `MCC` `CC` `H5`
                    of shaft of left tibia

2,3 √7th **S82.236** **Nondisplaced oblique fracture** `MCC` `CC` `H5`
                    of shaft of unspecified tibia

√6th **S82.24** Spiral **fracture of shaft of tibia**
                Toddler fracture

2,3 √7th **S82.241** **Displaced spiral fracture of** `MCC` `CC` `H5`
                    shaft of right tibia

2,3 √7th **S82.242** **Displaced spiral fracture of** `MCC` `CC` `H5`
                    shaft of left tibia

2,3 √7th **S82.243** **Displaced spiral fracture of** `MCC` `CC` `H5`
                    shaft of unspecified tibia

2,3 √7th **S82.244** **Nondisplaced spiral fracture of** `MCC` `CC` `H5`
                    shaft of right tibia

2,3 √7th **S82.245** **Nondisplaced spiral fracture of** `MCC` `CC` `H5`
                    shaft of left tibia

2,3 √7th **S82.246** **Nondisplaced spiral fracture of** `MCC` `CC` `H5`
                    shaft of unspecified tibia

√6th **S82.25** Comminuted **fracture of shaft of tibia**

2,3 √7th **S82.251** **Displaced comminuted fracture** `MCC` `CC` `H5`
                    of shaft of right tibia

2,3 √7th **S82.252** **Displaced comminuted fracture** `MCC` `CC` `H5`
                    of shaft of left tibia

2,3 √7th **S82.253** **Displaced comminuted fracture** `MCC` `CC` `H5`
                    of shaft of unspecified tibia

2,3 √7th **S82.254** **Nondisplaced comminuted** `MCC` `CC` `H5`
                    fracture of shaft of right tibia

2,3 √7th **S82.255** **Nondisplaced comminuted** `MCC` `CC` `H5`
                    fracture of shaft of left tibia

2,3 √7th **S82.256** **Nondisplaced comminuted** `MCC` `CC` `H5`
                    **fracture of shaft of unspecified
                    tibia**

√6th **S82.26** Segmental **fracture of shaft of tibia**

2,3 √7th **S82.261** **Displaced segmental fracture** `MCC` `CC` `H5`
                    of shaft of right tibia

2,3 √7th **S82.262** **Displaced segmental fracture** `MCC` `CC` `H5`
                    of shaft of left tibia

2,3 √7th **S82.263** **Displaced segmental fracture** `MCC` `CC` `H5`
                    of shaft of unspecified tibia

2,3 √7th **S82.264** **Nondisplaced segmental** `MCC` `CC` `H5`
                    fracture of shaft of right tibia

2,3 √7th **S82.265** **Nondisplaced segmental** `MCC` `CC` `H5`
                    fracture of shaft of left tibia

2,3 √7th **S82.266** **Nondisplaced segmental** `MCC` `CC` `H5`
                    **fracture of shaft of unspecified
                    tibia**

√6th **S82.29** Other **fracture of shaft of tibia**

2,3 √7th **S82.291** **Other fracture of shaft of right** `MCC` `CC` `H5`
                    tibia

2,3 √7th **S82.292** **Other fracture of shaft of left** `MCC` `CC` `H5`
                    tibia

2,3 √7th **S82.299** **Other fracture of shaft of** `MCC` `CC` `H5`
                    unspecified tibia

✔Additional Character Required   √x7th Placeholder   Unacceptable PDx   Questionable PDx   Manifestation   `H1`-`H14` HAC   `HCC` CMS-HCC Dx   `HIV` HIV Dx

ICD-10-CM 2019   1055

Chapter 19. Injury, Poisoning and Certain Other Consequences of External Causes

✓5ᵗʰ **S82.3 Fracture of lower end of tibia**
> EXCLUDES 1   bimalleolar fracture of lower leg (S82.84-)
> fracture of medial malleolus alone (S82.5-)
> Maisonneuve's fracture (S82.86-)
> pilon fracture of distal tibia (S82.87-)
> trimalleolar fractures of lower leg (S82.85-)

✓6ᵗʰ **S82.30 Unspecified fracture of lower end of tibia**

> CC Excl: For codes in subcategory S82.30:
> CC with 7th character B or C: PDX collection 1347
> CC with 7th character K, M, N, P, Q or R:
> PDX collection 897

3 ✓7ᵗʰ **S82.301 Unspecified fracture of lower end of right tibia** `CC` `H5`

3 ✓7ᵗʰ **S82.302 Unspecified fracture of lower end of left tibia** `CC` `H5`

3 ✓7ᵗʰ **S82.309 Unspecified fracture of lower end of unspecified tibia** `CC` `H5`

✓6ᵗʰ **S82.31 Torus fracture of lower end of tibia**

> The appropriate 7th character is to be added to all codes in subcategory S82.31.
> A   initial encounter for closed fracture
> D   subsequent encounter for fracture with routine healing
> G   subsequent encounter for fracture with delayed healing
> K   subsequent encounter for fracture with nonunion
> P   subsequent encounter for fracture with malunion
> S   sequela

3 ✓7ᵗʰ **S82.311 Torus fracture of lower end of right tibia** `CC` `H5`
> CC Excl: CC with 7th character A:
> PDX collection 1343
> CC with 7th character K or P:
> PDX collection 897

3 ✓7ᵗʰ **S82.312 Torus fracture of lower end of left tibia** `CC` `H5`
> CC Excl: CC with 7th character A:
> PDX collection 1344
> CC with 7th character K or P:
> PDX collection 897

3 ✓7ᵗʰ **S82.319 Torus fracture of lower end of unspecified tibia** `CC` `H5`
> CC Excl: CC with 7th character A:
> PDX collection 1345
> CC with 7th character K or P:
> PDX collection 897

✓6ᵗʰ **S82.39 Other fracture of lower end of tibia**
> **AHA:** 2015, 1Q, 25

> CC Excl: For codes in subcategory S82.39:
> CC for codes with 7th character B or C:
> PDX collection 1347
> CC with 7th character K, M, N, P, Q or R:
> PDX collection 897

3 ✓7ᵗʰ **S82.391 Other fracture of lower end of right tibia** `CC` `H5`

3 ✓7ᵗʰ **S82.392 Other fracture of lower end of left tibia** `CC` `H5`

3 ✓7ᵗʰ **S82.399 Other fracture of lower end of unspecified tibia** `CC` `H5`

✓5ᵗʰ **S82.4 Fracture of shaft of fibula**
> EXCLUDES 2   fracture of lateral malleolus alone (S82.6-)

> CC Excl: For codes in subcategory S82.4:
> MCC for codes with 7th character B or C:
> PDX collection 1341
> CC with 7th character K, M, N, P, Q or R: PDX collection 897

✓6ᵗʰ **S82.40 Unspecified fracture of shaft of fibula**

2,4 ✓7ᵗʰ **S82.401 Unspecified fracture of shaft of right fibula** `MCC` `CC` `H5`

2,4 ✓7ᵗʰ **S82.402 Unspecified fracture of shaft of left fibula** `MCC` `CC` `H5`

2,4 ✓7ᵗʰ **S82.409 Unspecified fracture of shaft of unspecified fibula** `MCC` `CC` `H5`

✓6ᵗʰ **S82.42 Transverse fracture of shaft of fibula**

2,4 ✓7ᵗʰ **S82.421 Displaced transverse fracture of shaft of right fibula** `MCC` `CC` `H5`

2,4 ✓7ᵗʰ **S82.422 Displaced transverse fracture of shaft of left fibula** `MCC` `CC` `H5`

2,4 ✓7ᵗʰ **S82.423 Displaced transverse fracture of shaft of unspecified fibula** `MCC` `CC` `H5`

2,4 ✓7ᵗʰ **S82.424 Nondisplaced transverse fracture of shaft of right fibula** `MCC` `CC` `H5`

2,4 ✓7ᵗʰ **S82.425 Nondisplaced transverse fracture of shaft of left fibula** `MCC` `CC` `H5`

2,4 ✓7ᵗʰ **S82.426 Nondisplaced transverse fracture of shaft of unspecified fibula** `MCC` `CC` `H5`

✓6ᵗʰ **S82.43 Oblique fracture of shaft of fibula**

2,4 ✓7ᵗʰ **S82.431 Displaced oblique fracture of shaft of right fibula** `MCC` `CC` `H5`

2,4 ✓7ᵗʰ **S82.432 Displaced oblique fracture of shaft of left fibula** `MCC` `CC` `H5`

2,4 ✓7ᵗʰ **S82.433 Displaced oblique fracture of shaft of unspecified fibula** `MCC` `CC` `H5`

2,4 ✓7ᵗʰ **S82.434 Nondisplaced oblique fracture of shaft of right fibula** `MCC` `CC` `H5`

2,4 ✓7ᵗʰ **S82.435 Nondisplaced oblique fracture of shaft of left fibula** `MCC` `CC` `H5`

2,4 ✓7ᵗʰ **S82.436 Nondisplaced oblique fracture of shaft of unspecified fibula** `MCC` `CC` `H5`

✓6ᵗʰ **S82.44 Spiral fracture of shaft of fibula**

2,4 ✓7ᵗʰ **S82.441 Displaced spiral fracture of shaft of right fibula** `MCC` `CC` `H5`

2,4 ✓7ᵗʰ **S82.442 Displaced spiral fracture of shaft of left fibula** `MCC` `CC` `H5`

2,4 ✓7ᵗʰ **S82.443 Displaced spiral fracture of shaft of unspecified fibula** `MCC` `CC` `H5`

2,4 ✓7ᵗʰ **S82.444 Nondisplaced spiral fracture of shaft of right fibula** `MCC` `CC` `H5`

2,4 ✓7ᵗʰ **S82.445 Nondisplaced spiral fracture of shaft of left fibula** `MCC` `CC` `H5`

2,4 ✓7ᵗʰ **S82.446 Nondisplaced spiral fracture of shaft of unspecified fibula** `MCC` `CC` `H5`

✓6ᵗʰ **S82.45 Comminuted fracture of shaft of fibula**

2,4 ✓7ᵗʰ **S82.451 Displaced comminuted fracture of shaft of right fibula** `MCC` `CC` `H5`

2,4 ✓7ᵗʰ **S82.452 Displaced comminuted fracture of shaft of left fibula** `MCC` `CC` `H5`

2,4 ✓7ᵗʰ **S82.453 Displaced comminuted fracture of shaft of unspecified fibula** `MCC` `CC` `H5`

2,4 ✓7ᵗʰ **S82.454 Nondisplaced comminuted fracture of shaft of right fibula** `MCC` `CC` `H5`

2,4 ✓7ᵗʰ **S82.455 Nondisplaced comminuted fracture of shaft of left fibula** `MCC` `CC` `H5`

2,4 ✓7ᵗʰ **S82.456 Nondisplaced comminuted fracture of shaft of unspecified fibula** `MCC` `CC` `H5`

✓6ᵗʰ **S82.46 Segmental fracture of shaft of fibula**

2,4 ✓7ᵗʰ **S82.461 Displaced segmental fracture of shaft of right fibula** `MCC` `CC` `H5`

2,4 ✓7ᵗʰ **S82.462 Displaced segmental fracture of shaft of left fibula** `MCC` `CC` `H5`

2,4 ✓7ᵗʰ **S82.463 Displaced segmental fracture of shaft of unspecified fibula** `MCC` `CC` `H5`

2,4 ✓7ᵗʰ **S82.464 Nondisplaced segmental fracture of shaft of right fibula** `MCC` `CC` `H5`

2,4 ✓7ᵗʰ **S82.465 Nondisplaced segmental fracture of shaft of left fibula** `MCC` `CC` `H5`

2,4 ✓7ᵗʰ **S82.466 Nondisplaced segmental fracture of shaft of unspecified fibula** `MCC` `CC` `H5`

✓6ᵗʰ **S82.49 Other fracture of shaft of fibula**

2,4 ✓7ᵗʰ **S82.491 Other fracture of shaft of right fibula** `MCC` `CC` `H5`

2,4 ✓7ᵗʰ **S82.492 Other fracture of shaft of left fibula** `MCC` `CC` `H5`

2,4 ✓7ᵗʰ **S82.499 Other fracture of shaft of unspecified fibula** `MCC` `CC` `H5`

`N` Newborn: 0   `P` Pediatric: 0-17   `M` Maternity: 12-55   `A` Adult: 15-124   `MCC` Major Complication/Comorbidity   `CC` Complication/Comorbidity   `SW` Severe Wound Dx

1056   ICD-10-CM 2019

☑5ᵗʰ **S82.5** **Fracture of** medial malleolus

     EXCLUDES 1   *pilon fracture of distal tibia (S82.87-)*
                  Salter-Harris type III of lower end of tibia (S89.13-)
                  Salter-Harris type IV of lower end of tibia (S89.14-)

> **CC Excl: For codes in subcategory S82.5:**
> **CC with 7th character B or C:** PDX collection 1347
> **CC with 7th character K, M, N, P, Q or R:** PDX collection 897

3   ✓ₓ7ᵗʰ   **S82.51**   Displaced **fracture of medial malleolus of** right **tibia**   `CC` `H5`

3   ✓ₓ7ᵗʰ   **S82.52**   Displaced **fracture of medial malleolus of** left **tibia**   `CC` `H5`

3   ✓ₓ7ᵗʰ   **S82.53**   Displaced **fracture of medial malleolus of** unspecified **tibia**   `CC` `H5`

3   ✓ₓ7ᵗʰ   **S82.54**   Nondisplaced **fracture of medial malleolus of** right **tibia**   `CC` `H5`

3   ✓ₓ7ᵗʰ   **S82.55**   Nondisplaced **fracture of medial malleolus of** left **tibia**   `CC` `H5`

3   ✓ₓ7ᵗʰ   **S82.56**   Nondisplaced **fracture of medial malleolus of** unspecified **tibia**   `CC` `H5`

☑5ᵗʰ **S82.6** **Fracture of** lateral malleolus

     EXCLUDES 1   *pilon fracture of distal tibia (S82.87-)*

> **CC Excl: For codes in subcategory S82.6:**
> **CC with 7th character B or C:** PDX collection 1347
> **CC with 7th character K, M, N, P, Q or R:** PDX collection 897

3   ✓ₓ7ᵗʰ   **S82.61**   Displaced **fracture of lateral malleolus of** right **fibula**   `CC` `H5`

3   ✓ₓ7ᵗʰ   **S82.62**   Displaced **fracture of lateral malleolus of** left **fibula**   `CC` `H5`

3   ✓ₓ7ᵗʰ   **S82.63**   Displaced **fracture of lateral malleolus of** unspecified **fibula**   `CC` `H5`

3   ✓ₓ7ᵗʰ   **S82.64**   Nondisplaced **fracture of lateral malleolus of** right **fibula**   `CC` `H5`

3   ✓ₓ7ᵗʰ   **S82.65**   Nondisplaced **fracture of lateral malleolus of** left **fibula**   `CC` `H5`

3   ✓ₓ7ᵗʰ   **S82.66**   Nondisplaced **fracture of lateral malleolus of** unspecified **fibula**   `CC` `H5`

☑5ᵗʰ **S82.8** **Other fractures of** lower leg

   ☑6ᵗʰ **S82.81**   Torus **fracture of** upper end of fibula

> The appropriate 7th character is to be added to all codes in subcategory S82.81.
> A   initial encounter for closed fracture
> D   subsequent encounter for fracture with routine healing
> G   subsequent encounter for fracture with delayed healing
> K   subsequent encounter for fracture wit nonunion
> P   subsequent encounter for fracture with malunion
> S   sequela

> **CC Excl: For codes in subcategory S82.81:**
> **CC with 7th character K or P:** PDX collection 897

     4   ✓7ᵗʰ   **S82.811**   Torus **fracture of** upper end of right **fibula**   `CC`

     4   ✓7ᵗʰ   **S82.812**   Torus **fracture of** upper end of left **fibula**   `CC`

     4   ✓7ᵗʰ   **S82.819**   Torus **fracture of** upper end of unspecified **fibula**   `CC`

   ☑6ᵗʰ **S82.82**   Torus **fracture of** lower end of fibula

> The appropriate 7th character is to be added to all codes in subcategory S82.82.
> A   initial encounter for closed fracture
> D   subsequent encounter for fracture with routine healing
> G   subsequent encounter for fracture with delayed healing
> K   subsequent encounter for fracture with nonunion
> P   subsequent encounter for fracture with malunion
> S   sequela

> **CC Excl: For codes in subcatgory S82.82:**
> **CC with 7th character K or P:** PDX collection 897

---

4   ✓7ᵗʰ   **S82.821**   Torus fracture of lower end of right fibula   `CC`

4   ✓7ᵗʰ   **S82.822**   Torus fracture of lower end of left fibula   `CC`

4   ✓7ᵗʰ   **S82.829**   Torus fracture of lower end of unspecified fibula   `CC`

☑6ᵗʰ **S82.83**   Other **fracture of upper and lower end of fibula**
         AHA: 2015, 1Q, 25

> **CC Excl: For codes in subcatgory S82.83:**
> **MCC with 7th character B or C:**
> PDX collection 1341
> **CC with 7th character K, M, N, P, Q or R:**
> PDX collection 897

2,4   ✓7ᵗʰ   **S82.831**   Other fracture of upper and lower end of right fibula   `MCC` `CC` `H5`

2,4   ✓7ᵗʰ   **S82.832**   Other fracture of upper and lower end of left fibula   `MCC` `CC` `H5`

2,4   ✓7ᵗʰ   **S82.839**   Other fracture of upper and lower end of unspecified fibula   `MCC` `CC` `H5`

☑6ᵗʰ **S82.84**   Bimalleolar **fracture of lower leg**

> **CC Excl: For codes in subcategory S82.84:**
> **CC with 7th character B or C:** PDX collection 1347
> **CC with 7th character K, M, N, P, Q or R:**
> PDX collection 897

3   ✓7ᵗʰ   **S82.841**   Displaced **bimalleolar fracture of** right **lower leg**   `CC` `H5`

3   ✓7ᵗʰ   **S82.842**   Displaced **bimalleolar fracture of** left **lower leg**   `CC` `H5`

3   ✓7ᵗʰ   **S82.843**   Displaced **bimalleolar fracture of** unspecified **lower leg**   `H5`

3   ✓7ᵗʰ   **S82.844**   Nondisplaced **bimalleolar fracture of** right **lower leg**   `CC` `H5`

3   ✓7ᵗʰ   **S82.845**   Nondisplaced **bimalleolar fracture of** left **lower leg**   `CC` `H5`

3   ✓7ᵗʰ   **S82.846**   Nondisplaced **bimalleolar fracture of** unspecified **lower leg**   `CC` `H5`

Right Bimalleolar Fracture

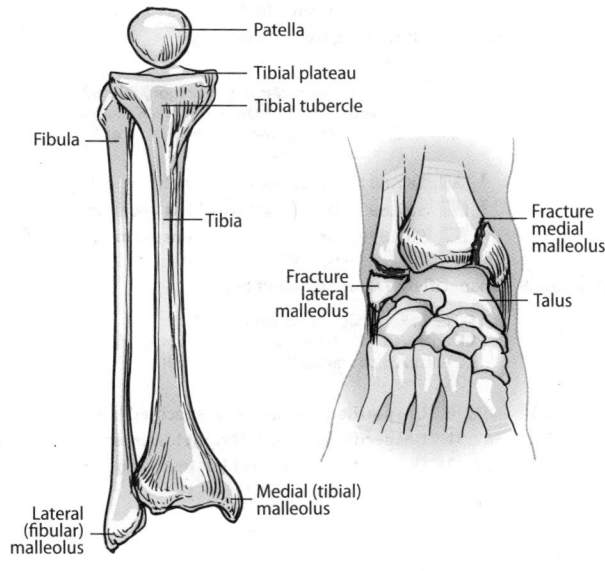

☑6ᵗʰ **S82.85**   Trimalleolar **fracture of lower leg**

> **CC Excl: For codes in subcatgory S82.85:**
> **CC with 7th character B or C:** PDX collection 1347
> **CC with 7th character K, M, N, P, Q or R:**
> PDX collection 897

3   ✓7ᵗʰ   **S82.851**   Displaced **trimalleolar fracture of** right **lower leg**   `CC` `H5`

3   ✓7ᵗʰ   **S82.852**   Displaced **trimalleolar fracture of** left **lower leg**   `CC` `H5`

3   ✓7ᵗʰ   **S82.853**   Displaced **trimalleolar fracture of** unspecified **lower leg**   `CC` `H5`

☑ Additional Character Required   ✓ₓ7ᵗʰ Placeholder   Unacceptable PDx   Questionable PDx   Manifestation   `H1`-`H14` HAC   `HCC` CMS-HCC Dx   `HIV` HIV Dx

ICD-10-CM 2019   1057

3 ✓7th **S82.854** Nondisplaced **trimalleolar** fracture of **right** lower leg   CC H5

3 ✓7th **S82.855** Nondisplaced **trimalleolar** fracture of **left** leg   CC H5

3 ✓7th **S82.856** Nondisplaced **trimalleolar** fracture of **unspecified** lower leg   CC H5

✓6th **S82.86** Maisonneuve's **fracture**

> **CC Excl:** For codes in subcatgory S82.86:
> **MCC with 7th character B or C:** PDX collection 1341
> **CC with 7th character K, M, N, P, Q or R:**
> PDX collection 897

2,4 ✓7th **S82.861** Displaced **Maisonneuve's** fracture of **right** leg   MCC CC H5

2,4 ✓7th **S82.862** Displaced **Maisonneuve's** fracture of **left** leg   MCC CC H5

2,4 ✓7th **S82.863** Displaced **Maisonneuve's** fracture of **unspecified** leg   MCC CC H5

2,4 ✓7th **S82.864** Nondisplaced **Maisonneuve's** fracture of **right** leg   MCC CC H5

2,4 ✓7th **S82.865** Nondisplaced **Maisonneuve's** fracture of **left** leg   MCC CC H5

2,4 ✓7th **S82.866** Nondisplaced **Maisonneuve's** fracture of **unspecified** leg   MCC CC H5

✓6th **S82.87** Pilon **fracture of tibia**

> **CC Excl:** For codes in subcatgory S82.87:
> **CC with 7th character B or C:** PDX collection 1347
> **CC with 7th character K, M, N, P, Q or R:**
> PDX collection 897

3 ✓7th **S82.871** Displaced **pilon fracture of right tibia**   CC H5

3 ✓7th **S82.872** Displaced **pilon fracture of left tibia**   CC H5

3 ✓7th **S82.873** Displaced **pilon fracture of unspecified tibia**   CC H5

3 ✓7th **S82.874** Nondisplaced **pilon fracture of right tibia**   CC H5

3 ✓7th **S82.875** Nondisplaced **pilon fracture of left tibia**   CC H5

3 ✓7th **S82.876** Nondisplaced **pilon fracture of unspecified tibia**   CC H5

✓6th **S82.89** Other **fractures of lower leg**
Fracture of ankle NOS

> **CC Excl:** For codes in subcatgory S82.89:
> **CC with 7th character B or C:** PDX collection 1347
> **CC with 7th character K, M, N, P, Q or R:**
> PDX collection 897

3 ✓7th **S82.891** Other fracture of **right** lower leg   CC H5

3 ✓7th **S82.892** Other fracture of **left** lower leg   CC H5

3 ✓7th **S82.899** Other fracture of **unspecified** lower leg   CC H5

✓5th **S82.9** Unspecified **fracture of lower leg**

> **CC Excl:** For codes in subcatgory S82.9:
> **CC with 7th character B or C:** PDX collection 1348
> **CC with 7th character K, M, N, P, Q or R:**
> PDX collection 897

3 ✓x7th **S82.90** Unspecified fracture of **unspecified** lower leg   CC H5

3 ✓x7th **S82.91** Unspecified fracture of **right** lower leg   CC H5

3 ✓x7th **S82.92** Unspecified fracture of **left** lower leg   CC H5

✓4th **S83** **Dislocation and sprain of joints and ligaments of knee**

> **INCLUDES** avulsion of joint or ligament of knee
> laceration of cartilage, joint or ligament of knee
> sprain of cartilage, joint or ligament of knee
> traumatic hemarthrosis of joint or ligament of knee
> traumatic rupture of joint or ligament of knee
> traumatic subluxation of joint or ligament of knee
> traumatic tear of joint or ligament of knee

Code also any associated open wound

> **EXCLUDES 1** derangement of patella (M22.0-M22.3)
> injury of patellar ligament (tendon) (S76.1-)
> internal derangement of knee (M23.-)
> old dislocation of knee (M24.36)
> pathological dislocation of knee (M24.36)
> recurrent dislocation of knee (M22.0)

> **EXCLUDES 2** strain of muscle, fascia and tendon of lower leg (S86.-)

> The appropriate 7th character is to be added to each code from category S83.
> A   initial encounter
> D   subsequent encounter
> S   sequela

✓5th **S83.0** **Subluxation and dislocation of patella**

✓6th **S83.00** Unspecified **subluxation and dislocation of patella**

✓7th **S83.001** Unspecified **subluxation** of **right** patella

✓7th **S83.002** Unspecified **subluxation** of **left** patella

✓7th **S83.003** Unspecified **subluxation** of **unspecified** patella

✓7th **S83.004** Unspecified **dislocation** of **right** patella

✓7th **S83.005** Unspecified **dislocation** of **left** patella

✓7th **S83.006** Unspecified **dislocation** of **unspecified** patella

✓6th **S83.01** Lateral **subluxation and dislocation of patella**

✓7th **S83.011** Lateral **subluxation** of **right** patella

✓7th **S83.012** Lateral **subluxation** of **left** patella

✓7th **S83.013** Lateral **subluxation** of **unspecified** patella

✓7th **S83.014** Lateral **dislocation** of **right** patella

✓7th **S83.015** Lateral **dislocation** of **left** patella

✓7th **S83.016** Lateral **dislocation** of **unspecified** patella

✓6th **S83.09** Other **subluxation and dislocation of patella**

✓7th **S83.091** Other **subluxation** of **right** patella

✓7th **S83.092** Other **subluxation** of **left** patella

✓7th **S83.093** Other **subluxation** of **unspecified** patella

✓7th **S83.094** Other **dislocation** of **right** patella

✓7th **S83.095** Other **dislocation** of **left** patella

✓7th **S83.096** Other **dislocation** of **unspecified** patella

✓5th **S83.1** **Subluxation and dislocation of knee**

> **EXCLUDES 2** instability of knee prosthesis (T84.022, T84.023)

✓6th **S83.10** Unspecified **subluxation and dislocation of knee**

✓7th **S83.101** Unspecified **subluxation** of **right** knee

✓7th **S83.102** Unspecified **subluxation** of **left** knee

✓7th **S83.103** Unspecified **subluxation** of **unspecified** knee

✓7th **S83.104** Unspecified **dislocation** of **right** knee

✓7th **S83.105** Unspecified **dislocation** of **left** knee

✓7th **S83.106** Unspecified **dislocation** of **unspecified** knee

✓6th **S83.11** Anterior **subluxation and dislocation of proximal end of tibia**
Posterior subluxation and dislocation of distal end of femur

✓7th **S83.111** Anterior **subluxation** of proximal end of tibia, **right** knee

✓7th **S83.112** Anterior **subluxation** of proximal end of tibia, **left** knee

✓7th **S83.113** Anterior **subluxation** of proximal end of tibia, **unspecified** knee

✓7th **S83.114** Anterior **dislocation** of proximal end of tibia, **right** knee

✓7th **S83.115** Anterior **dislocation** of proximal end of tibia, **left** knee

✓7th **S83.116** Anterior **dislocation** of proximal end of tibia, **unspecified** knee

N Newborn: 0   P Pediatric: 0-17   M Maternity: 12-55   A Adult: 15-124   MCC Major Complication/Comorbidity   CC Complication/Comorbidity   SW Severe Wound Dx

1058   ICD-10-CM 2019

✓6ᵗʰ **S83.12** Posterior **subluxation and dislocation of proximal end of tibia**
Anterior dislocation of distal end of femur

✓7ᵗʰ **S83.121** **Posterior** subluxation **of proximal end of tibia,** right **knee**

✓7ᵗʰ **S83.122** **Posterior** subluxation **of proximal end of tibia,** left **knee**

✓7ᵗʰ **S83.123** **Posterior** subluxation **of proximal end of tibia,** unspecified **knee**

✓7ᵗʰ **S83.124** **Posterior** dislocation **of proximal end of tibia,** right **knee**

✓7ᵗʰ **S83.125** **Posterior** dislocation **of proximal end of tibia,** left **knee**

✓7ᵗʰ **S83.126** **Posterior** dislocation **of proximal end of tibia,** unspecified **knee**

✓6ᵗʰ **S83.13** Medial **subluxation and dislocation of proximal end of tibia**

✓7ᵗʰ **S83.131** **Medial** subluxation **of proximal end of tibia,** right **knee**

✓7ᵗʰ **S83.132** **Medial** subluxation **of proximal end of tibia,** left **knee**

✓7ᵗʰ **S83.133** **Medial** subluxation **of proximal end of tibia,** unspecified **knee**

✓7ᵗʰ **S83.134** **Medial** dislocation **of proximal end of tibia,** right **knee**

✓7ᵗʰ **S83.135** **Medial** dislocation **of proximal end of tibia,** left **knee**

✓7ᵗʰ **S83.136** **Medial** dislocation **of proximal end of tibia,** unspecified **knee**

✓6ᵗʰ **S83.14** Lateral **subluxation and dislocation of proximal end of tibia**

✓7ᵗʰ **S83.141** **Lateral** subluxation **of proximal end of tibia,** right **knee**

✓7ᵗʰ **S83.142** **Lateral** subluxation **of proximal end of tibia,** left **knee**

✓7ᵗʰ **S83.143** **Lateral** subluxation **of proximal end of tibia,** unspecified **knee**

✓7ᵗʰ **S83.144** **Lateral** dislocation **of proximal end of tibia,** right **knee**

✓7ᵗʰ **S83.145** **Lateral** dislocation **of proximal end of tibia,** left **knee**

✓7ᵗʰ **S83.146** **Lateral** dislocation **of proximal end of tibia,** unspecified **knee**

✓6ᵗʰ **S83.19** Other **subluxation and dislocation of** knee

✓7ᵗʰ **S83.191** **Other** subluxation **of** right **knee**

✓7ᵗʰ **S83.192** **Other** subluxation **of** left **knee**

✓7ᵗʰ **S83.193** **Other** subluxation **of** unspecified **knee**

✓7ᵗʰ **S83.194** **Other** dislocation **of** right **knee**

✓7ᵗʰ **S83.195** **Other** dislocation **of** left **knee**

✓7ᵗʰ **S83.196** **Other** dislocation **of** unspecified **knee**

✓5ᵗʰ **S83.2** Tear of meniscus, **current injury**
EXCLUDES 1 old bucket-handle tear (M23.2)

✓6ᵗʰ **S83.20** **Tear of** unspecified **meniscus, current injury**
Tear of meniscus of knee NOS

✓7ᵗʰ **S83.200** Bucket-handle **tear of unspecified meniscus, current injury,** right **knee**

✓7ᵗʰ **S83.201** Bucket-handle **tear of unspecified meniscus, current injury,** left **knee**

✓7ᵗʰ **S83.202** Bucket-handle **tear of unspecified meniscus, current injury,** unspecified **knee**

✓7ᵗʰ **S83.203** Other **tear of unspecified meniscus, current injury,** right **knee**

✓7ᵗʰ **S83.204** Other **tear of unspecified meniscus, current injury,** left **knee**

✓7ᵗʰ **S83.205** Other **tear of unspecified meniscus, current injury,** unspecified **knee**

✓7ᵗʰ **S83.206** Unspecified **tear of unspecified meniscus, current injury,** right **knee**

✓7ᵗʰ **S83.207** Unspecified **tear of unspecified meniscus, current injury,** left **knee**

✓7ᵗʰ **S83.209** Unspecified **tear of unspecified meniscus, current injury,** unspecified **knee**

✓6ᵗʰ **S83.21** Bucket-handle **tear of** medial **meniscus, current injury**

✓7ᵗʰ **S83.211** **Bucket-handle tear of medial meniscus, current injury,** right **knee**

✓7ᵗʰ **S83.212** **Bucket-handle tear of medial meniscus, current injury,** left **knee**

✓7ᵗʰ **S83.219** **Bucket-handle tear of medial meniscus, current injury,** unspecified **knee**

✓6ᵗʰ **S83.22** Peripheral **tear of** medial **meniscus, current injury**

✓7ᵗʰ **S83.221** **Peripheral tear of medial meniscus, current injury,** right **knee**

✓7ᵗʰ **S83.222** **Peripheral tear of medial meniscus, current injury,** left **knee**

✓7ᵗʰ **S83.229** **Peripheral tear of medial meniscus, current injury,** unspecified **knee**

✓6ᵗʰ **S83.23** Complex **tear of** medial **meniscus, current injury**

✓7ᵗʰ **S83.231** **Complex tear of medial meniscus, current injury,** right **knee**

✓7ᵗʰ **S83.232** **Complex tear of medial meniscus, current injury,** left **knee**

✓7ᵗʰ **S83.239** **Complex tear of medial meniscus, current injury,** unspecified **knee**

✓6ᵗʰ **S83.24** Other **tear of** medial **meniscus, current injury**

✓7ᵗʰ **S83.241** **Other tear of medial meniscus, current injury,** right **knee**

✓7ᵗʰ **S83.242** **Other tear of medial meniscus, current injury,** left **knee**

✓7ᵗʰ **S83.249** **Other tear of medial meniscus, current injury,** unspecified **knee**

✓6ᵗʰ **S83.25** Bucket-handle **tear of** lateral **meniscus, current injury**

✓7ᵗʰ **S83.251** **Bucket-handle tear of lateral meniscus, current injury,** right **knee**

✓7ᵗʰ **S83.252** **Bucket-handle tear of lateral meniscus, current injury,** left **knee**

✓7ᵗʰ **S83.259** **Bucket-handle tear of lateral meniscus, current injury,** unspecified **knee**

✓6ᵗʰ **S83.26** Peripheral **tear of** lateral **meniscus, current injury**

✓7ᵗʰ **S83.261** **Peripheral tear of lateral meniscus, current injury,** right **knee**

✓7ᵗʰ **S83.262** **Peripheral tear of lateral meniscus, current injury,** left **knee**

✓7ᵗʰ **S83.269** **Peripheral tear of lateral meniscus, current injury,** unspecified **knee**

✓6ᵗʰ **S83.27** Complex **tear of** lateral **meniscus, current injury**

✓7ᵗʰ **S83.271** **Complex tear of lateral meniscus, current injury,** right **knee**

✓7ᵗʰ **S83.272** **Complex tear of lateral meniscus, current injury,** left **knee**

✓7ᵗʰ **S83.279** **Complex tear of lateral meniscus, current injury,** unspecified **knee**

✓6ᵗʰ **S83.28** Other **tear of** lateral **meniscus, current injury**

✓7ᵗʰ **S83.281** **Other tear of lateral meniscus, current injury,** right **knee**

✓7ᵗʰ **S83.282** **Other tear of lateral meniscus, current injury,** left **knee**

✓7ᵗʰ **S83.289** **Other tear of lateral meniscus, current injury,** unspecified **knee**

✓5ᵗʰ **S83.3** Tear of articular cartilage **of knee, current**

✓x7ᵗʰ **S83.30** **Tear of articular cartilage of** unspecified **knee, current**

✓x7ᵗʰ **S83.31** **Tear of articular cartilage of** right **knee, current**

✓x7ᵗʰ **S83.32** **Tear of articular cartilage of** left **knee, current**

✓5ᵗʰ **S83.4** Sprain of collateral ligament **of knee**

✓6ᵗʰ **S83.40** **Sprain of** unspecified **collateral ligament of knee**

✓7ᵗʰ **S83.401** **Sprain of unspecified collateral ligament of** right **knee**

✓7ᵗʰ **S83.402** **Sprain of unspecified collateral ligament of** left **knee**

✓7ᵗʰ **S83.409** **Sprain of unspecified collateral ligament of** unspecified **knee**

☑ Additional Character Required   ✓x7ᵗʰ Placeholder   Unacceptable PDx   Questionable PDx   Manifestation   **H1**-**H14** HAC   **HCC** CMS-HCC Dx   **HIV** HIV Dx

ICD-10-CM 2019   **1059**

✓6ᵗʰ S83.41 **Sprain of** medial **collateral ligament of knee**
Sprain of tibial collateral ligament

     ✓7ᵗʰ S83.411 **Sprain of medial collateral ligament of** right **knee**

     ✓7ᵗʰ S83.412 **Sprain of medial collateral ligament of** left **knee**

     ✓7ᵗʰ S83.419 **Sprain of medial collateral ligament of** unspecified **knee**

✓6ᵗʰ S83.42 **Sprain of** lateral **collateral ligament of knee**
Sprain of fibular collateral ligament

     ✓7ᵗʰ S83.421 **Sprain of lateral collateral ligament of** right **knee**

     ✓7ᵗʰ S83.422 **Sprain of lateral collateral ligament of** left **knee**

     ✓7ᵗʰ S83.429 **Sprain of lateral collateral ligament of** unspecified **knee**

✓5ᵗʰ S83.5 **Sprain of** cruciate ligament **of knee**
AHA: 2016, 2Q, 3

   ✓6ᵗʰ S83.50 **Sprain of** unspecified **cruciate ligament of knee**

     ✓7ᵗʰ S83.501 **Sprain of unspecified cruciate ligament of** right **knee**

     ✓7ᵗʰ S83.502 **Sprain of unspecified cruciate ligament of** left **knee**

     ✓7ᵗʰ S83.509 **Sprain of unspecified cruciate ligament of** unspecified **knee**

   ✓6ᵗʰ S83.51 **Sprain of** anterior **cruciate ligament of knee**

     ✓7ᵗʰ S83.511 **Sprain of anterior cruciate ligament of** right **knee**

     ✓7ᵗʰ S83.512 **Sprain of anterior cruciate ligament of** left **knee**

     ✓7ᵗʰ S83.519 **Sprain of anterior cruciate ligament of** unspecified **knee**

   ✓6ᵗʰ S83.52 **Sprain of** posterior **cruciate ligament of knee**

     ✓7ᵗʰ S83.521 **Sprain of posterior cruciate ligament of** right **knee**

     ✓7ᵗʰ S83.522 **Sprain of posterior cruciate ligament of** left **knee**

     ✓7ᵗʰ S83.529 **Sprain of posterior cruciate ligament of** unspecified **knee**

✓5ᵗʰ S83.6 **Sprain of the** superior tibiofibular **joint and ligament**

   ✓ₓ7ᵗʰ S83.60 **Sprain of the superior tibiofibular joint and ligament,** unspecified **knee**

   ✓ₓ7ᵗʰ S83.61 **Sprain of the superior tibiofibular joint and ligament,** right **knee**

   ✓ₓ7ᵗʰ S83.62 **Sprain of the superior tibiofibular joint and ligament,** left **knee**

✓5ᵗʰ S83.8 **Sprain of** other **specified parts of knee**

   ✓6ᵗʰ S83.8X **Sprain of other specified parts of knee**

     ✓7ᵗʰ S83.8X1 **Sprain of other specified parts of** right **knee**

     ✓7ᵗʰ S83.8X2 **Sprain of other specified parts of** left **knee**

     ✓7ᵗʰ S83.8X9 **Sprain of other specified parts of** unspecified **knee**

✓5ᵗʰ S83.9 **Sprain of** unspecified **site of knee**

   ✓ₓ7ᵗʰ S83.90 **Sprain of unspecified site of** unspecified **knee**

   ✓ₓ7ᵗʰ S83.91 **Sprain of unspecified site of** right **knee**

   ✓ₓ7ᵗʰ S83.92 **Sprain of unspecified site of** left **knee**

✓4ᵗʰ S84 **Injury of nerves at lower leg level**
Code also any associated open wound (S81.-)
EXCLUDES 2 *injury of nerves at ankle and foot level (S94.-)*

> The appropriate 7th character is to be added to each code from category S84.
> A   initial encounter
> D   subsequent encounter
> S   sequela

✓5ᵗʰ S84.0 **Injury of** tibial nerve **at lower leg level**

   ✓ₓ7ᵗʰ S84.00 **Injury of tibial nerve at lower leg level,** unspecified **leg**

   ✓ₓ7ᵗʰ S84.01 **Injury of tibial nerve at lower leg level,** right **leg**

   ✓ₓ7ᵗʰ S84.02 **Injury of tibial nerve at lower leg level,** left **leg**

✓5ᵗʰ S84.1 **Injury of** peroneal nerve **at lower leg level**

   ✓ₓ7ᵗʰ S84.10 **Injury of peroneal nerve at lower leg level,** unspecified **leg**

   ✓ₓ7ᵗʰ S84.11 **Injury of peroneal nerve at lower leg level,** right **leg**

   ✓ₓ7ᵗʰ S84.12 **Injury of peroneal nerve at lower leg level,** left **leg**

✓5ᵗʰ S84.2 **Injury of** cutaneous sensory nerve **at lower leg level**

   ✓ₓ7ᵗʰ S84.20 **Injury of cutaneous sensory nerve at lower leg level,** unspecified **leg**

   ✓ₓ7ᵗʰ S84.21 **Injury of cutaneous sensory nerve at lower leg level,** right **leg**

   ✓ₓ7ᵗʰ S84.22 **Injury of cutaneous sensory nerve at lower leg level,** left **leg**

✓5ᵗʰ S84.8 **Injury of** other nerves **at lower leg level**

   ✓6ᵗʰ S84.80 **Injury of other nerves at lower leg level**

     ✓7ᵗʰ S84.801 **Injury of other nerves at lower leg level,** right **leg**

     ✓7ᵗʰ S84.802 **Injury of other nerves at lower leg level,** left **leg**

     ✓7ᵗʰ S84.809 **Injury of other nerves at lower leg level,** unspecified **leg**

✓5ᵗʰ S84.9 **Injury of** unspecified nerve **at lower leg level**

   ✓ₓ7ᵗʰ S84.90 **Injury of unspecified nerve at lower leg level,** unspecified **leg**

   ✓ₓ7ᵗʰ S84.91 **Injury of unspecified nerve at lower leg level,** right **leg**

   ✓ₓ7ᵗʰ S84.92 **Injury of unspecified nerve at lower leg level,** left **leg**

✓4ᵗʰ S85 **Injury of blood vessels at lower leg level**
Code also any associated open wound (S81.-)
EXCLUDES 2 *injury of blood vessels at ankle and foot level (S95.-)*

> The appropriate 7th character is to be added to each code from category S85.
> A   initial encounter
> D   subsequent encounter
> S   sequela

✓5ᵗʰ S85.0 **Injury of** popliteal artery

> **CC Excl: For MCC codes in subcategory S85.0:**
> **Right side:** PDX collection 1349
> **Left side:** PDX collection 1350
> **Unspecified side:** PDX collection 1351

   ✓6ᵗʰ S85.00 Unspecified **injury of popliteal artery**

     ✓7ᵗʰ S85.001 **Unspecified injury of popliteal artery,** right **leg** `MCC`

     ✓7ᵗʰ S85.002 **Unspecified injury of popliteal artery,** left **leg** `MCC`

     ✓7ᵗʰ S85.009 **Unspecified injury of popliteal artery,** unspecified **leg** `MCC`

   ✓6ᵗʰ S85.01 Laceration **of popliteal artery**

     ✓7ᵗʰ S85.011 **Laceration of popliteal artery,** right **leg** `MCC`

     ✓7ᵗʰ S85.012 **Laceration of popliteal artery,** left **leg** `MCC`

     ✓7ᵗʰ S85.019 **Laceration of popliteal artery,** unspecified **leg** `MCC`

   ✓6ᵗʰ S85.09 Other **specified injury of popliteal artery**

     ✓7ᵗʰ S85.091 **Other specified injury of popliteal artery,** right **leg** `MCC`

     ✓7ᵗʰ S85.092 **Other specified injury of popliteal artery,** left **leg** `MCC`

     ✓7ᵗʰ S85.099 **Other specified injury of popliteal artery,** unspecified **leg** `MCC`

✓5ᵗʰ S85.1 **Injury of** tibial artery

   ✓6ᵗʰ S85.10 Unspecified **injury of** unspecified **tibial artery**
Injury of tibial artery NOS

     ✓7ᵗʰ S85.101 **Unspecified injury of unspecified tibial artery,** right **leg** `CC`
CC Excl: PDX collection 1352

     ✓7ᵗʰ S85.102 **Unspecified injury of unspecified tibial artery,** left **leg** `CC`
CC Excl: PDX collection 1353

     ✓7ᵗʰ S85.109 **Unspecified injury of unspecified tibial artery,** unspecified **leg** `CC`
CC Excl: PDX collection 1354

N Newborn: 0   **P** Pediatric: 0-17   **M** Maternity: 12-55   **A** Adult: 15-124   **MCC** Major Complication/Comorbidity   **CC** Complication/Comorbidity   **SW** Severe Wound Dx

1060   ICD-10-CM 2019

✓6ᵗʰ **S85.11** Laceration of unspecified tibial artery

  ✓7ᵗʰ **S85.111** Laceration of unspecified tibial artery, right leg `CC`
     CC Excl: PDX collection 1352

  ✓7ᵗʰ **S85.112** Laceration of unspecified tibial artery, left leg `CC`
     CC Excl: PDX collection 1353

  ✓7ᵗʰ **S85.119** Laceration of unspecified tibial artery, unspecified leg `CC`
     CC Excl: PDX collection 1354

✓6ᵗʰ **S85.12** Other specified injury of unspecified tibial artery

  ✓7ᵗʰ **S85.121** Other specified injury of unspecified tibial artery, right leg `CC`
     CC Excl: PDX collection 1352

  ✓7ᵗʰ **S85.122** Other specified injury of unspecified tibial artery, left leg `CC`
     CC Excl: PDX collection 1353

  ✓7ᵗʰ **S85.129** Other specified injury of unspecified tibial artery, unspecified leg `CC`
     CC Excl: PDX collection 1354

✓6ᵗʰ **S85.13** Unspecified injury of anterior tibial artery

  ✓7ᵗʰ **S85.131** Unspecified injury of anterior tibial artery, right leg `CC`
     CC Excl: PDX collection 1355

  ✓7ᵗʰ **S85.132** Unspecified injury of anterior tibial artery, left leg `CC`
     CC Excl: PDX collection 1356

  ✓7ᵗʰ **S85.139** Unspecified injury of anterior tibial artery, unspecified leg `CC`
     CC Excl: PDX collection 1357

✓6ᵗʰ **S85.14** Laceration of anterior tibial artery

  ✓7ᵗʰ **S85.141** Laceration of anterior tibial artery, right leg `CC`
     CC Excl: PDX collection 1355

  ✓7ᵗʰ **S85.142** Laceration of anterior tibial artery, left leg `CC`
     CC Excl: PDX collection 1356

  ✓7ᵗʰ **S85.149** Laceration of anterior tibial artery, unspecified leg `CC`
     CC Excl: PDX collection 1357

✓6ᵗʰ **S85.15** Other specified injury of anterior tibial artery

  ✓7ᵗʰ **S85.151** Other specified injury of anterior tibial artery, right leg `CC`
     CC Excl: PDX collection 1355

  ✓7ᵗʰ **S85.152** Other specified injury of anterior tibial artery, left leg `CC`
     CC Excl: PDX collection 1356

  ✓7ᵗʰ **S85.159** Other specified injury of anterior tibial artery, unspecified leg `CC`
     CC Excl: PDX collection 1357

✓6ᵗʰ **S85.16** Unspecified injury of posterior tibial artery

  ✓7ᵗʰ **S85.161** Unspecified injury of posterior tibial artery, right leg `CC`
     CC Excl: PDX collection 1358

  ✓7ᵗʰ **S85.162** Unspecified injury of posterior tibial artery, left leg `CC`
     CC Excl: PDX collection 1359

  ✓7ᵗʰ **S85.169** Unspecified injury of posterior tibial artery, unspecified leg `CC`
     CC Excl: PDX collection 1360

✓6ᵗʰ **S85.17** Laceration of posterior tibial artery

  ✓7ᵗʰ **S85.171** Laceration of posterior tibial artery, right leg `CC`
     CC Excl: PDX collection 1358

  ✓7ᵗʰ **S85.172** Laceration of posterior tibial artery, left leg `CC`
     CC Excl: PDX collection 1359

  ✓7ᵗʰ **S85.179** Laceration of posterior tibial artery, unspecified leg `CC`
     CC Excl: PDX collection 1360

✓6ᵗʰ **S85.18** Other specified injury of posterior tibial artery

  ✓7ᵗʰ **S85.181** Other specified injury of posterior tibial artery, right leg `CC`
     CC Excl: PDX collection 1358

  ✓7ᵗʰ **S85.182** Other specified injury of posterior tibial artery, left leg `CC`
     CC Excl: PDX collection 1359

  ✓7ᵗʰ **S85.189** Other specified injury of posterior tibial artery, unspecified leg `CC`
     CC Excl: PDX collection 1360

✓5ᵗʰ **S85.2** Injury of peroneal artery

> **CC Excl: For CC codes in subcategory S85.2:**
> **Right side:** PDX collection 1325
> **Left side:** PDX collection 1326
> **Unspecified side:** PDX collection 1327

✓6ᵗʰ **S85.20** Unspecified injury of peroneal artery

  ✓7ᵗʰ **S85.201** Unspecified injury of peroneal artery, right leg `CC`

  ✓7ᵗʰ **S85.202** Unspecified injury of peroneal artery, left leg `CC`

  ✓7ᵗʰ **S85.209** Unspecified injury of peroneal artery, unspecified leg `CC`

✓6ᵗʰ **S85.21** Laceration of peroneal artery

  ✓7ᵗʰ **S85.211** Laceration of peroneal artery, right leg `CC`

  ✓7ᵗʰ **S85.212** Laceration of peroneal artery, left leg `CC`

  ✓7ᵗʰ **S85.219** Laceration of peroneal artery, unspecified leg `CC`

✓6ᵗʰ **S85.29** Other specified injury of peroneal artery

  ✓7ᵗʰ **S85.291** Other specified injury of peroneal artery, right leg `CC`

  ✓7ᵗʰ **S85.292** Other specified injury of peroneal artery, left leg `CC`

  ✓7ᵗʰ **S85.299** Other specified injury of peroneal artery, unspecified leg `CC`

✓5ᵗʰ **S85.3** Injury of greater saphenous vein at lower leg level
Injury of greater saphenous vein NOS
Injury of saphenous vein NOS

> **CC Excl: For CC codes in subcategory S85.3:**
> **Right side:** PDX collection 1322
> **Left side:** PDX collection 1323
> **Unspecified side:** PDX collection 1324

✓6ᵗʰ **S85.30** Unspecified injury of greater saphenous vein at lower leg level

  ✓7ᵗʰ **S85.301** Unspecified injury of greater saphenous vein at lower leg level, right leg `CC`

  ✓7ᵗʰ **S85.302** Unspecified injury of greater saphenous vein at lower leg level, left leg `CC`

  ✓7ᵗʰ **S85.309** Unspecified injury of greater saphenous vein at lower leg level, unspecified leg `CC`

✓6ᵗʰ **S85.31** Laceration of greater saphenous vein at lower leg level

  ✓7ᵗʰ **S85.311** Laceration of greater saphenous vein at lower leg level, right leg `CC`

  ✓7ᵗʰ **S85.312** Laceration of greater saphenous vein at lower leg level, left leg `CC`

  ✓7ᵗʰ **S85.319** Laceration of greater saphenous vein at lower leg level, unspecified leg `CC`

✓6ᵗʰ **S85.39** Other specified injury of greater saphenous vein at lower leg level

  ✓7ᵗʰ **S85.391** Other specified injury of greater saphenous vein at lower leg level, right leg `CC`

  ✓7ᵗʰ **S85.392** Other specified injury of greater saphenous vein at lower leg level, left leg `CC`

  ✓7ᵗʰ **S85.399** Other specified injury of greater saphenous vein at lower leg level, unspecified leg `CC`

✓ Additional Character Required   ✓ˣ⁷ᵗʰ Placeholder   Unacceptable PDx   Questionable PDx   Manifestation   **H1**–**H14** HAC   **HCC** CMS-HCC Dx   **HIV** HIV Dx

ICD-10-CM 2019   **1061**

√5ᵗʰ S85.4   Injury of lesser saphenous vein **at lower leg level**

> **CC Excl: For CC codes in subcategory S85.4:**
> **Right side:** PDX collection 1322
> **Left side:** PDX collection 1323
> **Unspecified side:** PDX collection 1324

> **√6ᵗʰ S85.40   Unspecified injury of lesser saphenous vein at lower leg level**
>
> > **√7ᵗʰ S85.401   Unspecified injury of lesser saphenous vein at lower leg level, right leg**   CC
> >
> > **√7ᵗʰ S85.402   Unspecified injury of lesser saphenous vein at lower leg level, left leg**   CC
> >
> > **√7ᵗʰ S85.409   Unspecified injury of lesser saphenous vein at lower leg level, unspecified leg**   CC
>
> **√6ᵗʰ S85.41   Laceration of lesser saphenous vein at lower leg level**
>
> > **√7ᵗʰ S85.411   Laceration of lesser saphenous vein at lower leg level, right leg**   CC
> >
> > **√7ᵗʰ S85.412   Laceration of lesser saphenous vein at lower leg level, left leg**   CC
> >
> > **√7ᵗʰ S85.419   Laceration of lesser saphenous vein at lower leg level, unspecified leg**   CC
>
> **√6ᵗʰ S85.49   Other specified injury of lesser saphenous vein at lower leg level**
>
> > **√7ᵗʰ S85.491   Other specified injury of lesser saphenous vein at lower leg level, right leg**   CC
> >
> > **√7ᵗʰ S85.492   Other specified injury of lesser saphenous vein at lower leg level, left leg**   CC
> >
> > **√7ᵗʰ S85.499   Other specified injury of lesser saphenous vein at lower leg level, unspecified leg**   CC

√5ᵗʰ S85.5   Injury of popliteal vein

> **CC Excl: For MCC codes in subcategory S85.5:**
> **Right side:** PDX collection 1361
> **Left side:** PDX collection 1362
> **Unspecified side:** PDX collection 1363

> **√6ᵗʰ S85.50   Unspecified injury of popliteal vein**
>
> > **√7ᵗʰ S85.501   Unspecified injury of popliteal vein, right leg**   MCC
> >
> > **√7ᵗʰ S85.502   Unspecified injury of popliteal vein, left leg**   MCC
> >
> > **√7ᵗʰ S85.509   Unspecified injury of popliteal vein, unspecified leg**   MCC
>
> **√6ᵗʰ S85.51   Laceration of popliteal vein**
>
> > **√7ᵗʰ S85.511   Laceration of popliteal vein, right leg**   MCC
> >
> > **√7ᵗʰ S85.512   Laceration of popliteal vein, left leg**   MCC
> >
> > **√7ᵗʰ S85.519   Laceration of popliteal vein, unspecified leg**   MCC
>
> **√6ᵗʰ S85.59   Other specified injury of popliteal vein**
>
> > **√7ᵗʰ S85.591   Other specified injury of popliteal vein, right leg**   MCC
> >
> > **√7ᵗʰ S85.592   Other specified injury of popliteal vein, left leg**   MCC
> >
> > **√7ᵗʰ S85.599   Other specified injury of popliteal vein, unspecified leg**   MCC

√5ᵗʰ S85.8   Injury of other blood vessels **at lower leg level**

> **CC Excl: For CC codes in subcategory S85.8:**
> **Right side:** PDX collection 1325
> **Left side:** PDX collection 1326
> **Unspecified side:** PDX collection 1327

> **√6ᵗʰ S85.80   Unspecified injury of other blood vessels at lower leg level**
>
> > **√7ᵗʰ S85.801   Unspecified injury of other blood vessels at lower leg level, right leg**   CC
> >
> > **√7ᵗʰ S85.802   Unspecified injury of other blood vessels at lower leg level, left leg**   CC
> >
> > **√7ᵗʰ S85.809   Unspecified injury of other blood vessels at lower leg level, unspecified leg**   CC

> **√6ᵗʰ S85.81   Laceration of other blood vessels at lower leg level**
>
> > **√7ᵗʰ S85.811   Laceration of other blood vessels at lower leg level, right leg**   CC
> >
> > **√7ᵗʰ S85.812   Laceration of other blood vessels at lower leg level, left leg**   CC
> >
> > **√7ᵗʰ S85.819   Laceration of other blood vessels at lower leg level, unspecified leg**   CC
>
> **√6ᵗʰ S85.89   Other specified injury of other blood vessels at lower leg level**
>
> > **√7ᵗʰ S85.891   Other specified injury of other blood vessels at lower leg level, right leg**   CC
> >
> > **√7ᵗʰ S85.892   Other specified injury of other blood vessels at lower leg level, left leg**   CC
> >
> > **√7ᵗʰ S85.899   Other specified injury of other blood vessels at lower leg level, unspecified leg**   CC

√5ᵗʰ S85.9   Injury of unspecified blood vessel **at lower leg level**

> **CC Excl: For CC codes in subcategory S85.9:**
> **Right side:** PDX collection 1325
> **Left side:** PDX collection 1326
> **Unspecified side:** PDX collection 1327

> **√6ᵗʰ S85.90   Unspecified injury of unspecified blood vessel at lower leg level**
>
> > **√7ᵗʰ S85.901   Unspecified injury of unspecified blood vessel at lower leg level, right leg**   CC
> >
> > **√7ᵗʰ S85.902   Unspecified injury of unspecified blood vessel at lower leg level, left leg**   CC
> >
> > **√7ᵗʰ S85.909   Unspecified injury of unspecified blood vessel at lower leg level, unspecified leg**   CC
>
> **√6ᵗʰ S85.91   Laceration of unspecified blood vessel at lower leg level**
>
> > **√7ᵗʰ S85.911   Laceration of unspecified blood vessel at lower leg level, right leg**   CC
> >
> > **√7ᵗʰ S85.912   Laceration of unspecified blood vessel at lower leg level, left leg**   CC
> >
> > **√7ᵗʰ S85.919   Laceration of unspecified blood vessel at lower leg level, unspecified leg**   CC
>
> **√6ᵗʰ S85.99   Other specified injury of unspecified blood vessel at lower leg level**
>
> > **√7ᵗʰ S85.991   Other specified injury of unspecified blood vessel at lower leg level, right leg**   CC
> >
> > **√7ᵗʰ S85.992   Other specified injury of unspecified blood vessel at lower leg level, left leg**   CC
> >
> > **√7ᵗʰ S85.999   Other specified injury of unspecified blood vessel at lower leg level, unspecified leg**   CC

√4ᵗʰ S86   Injury of muscle, fascia and tendon at lower leg level

Code also any associated open wound (S81.-)

EXCLUDES 2   injury of muscle, fascia and tendon at ankle (S96.-)
injury of patellar ligament (tendon) (S76.1-)
sprain of joints and ligaments of knee (S83.-)

TIP: Refer to the Muscle/Tendon table at the beginning of this chapter

> The appropriate 7th character is to be added to each code from category S86.
> A   initial encounter
> D   subsequent encounter
> S   sequela

> **CC Excl: For CC codes in category S86:**
> **Right side:** PDX collection 1364
> **Left side:** PDX collection 1365
> **Unspecified side:** PDX collection 1366

√5ᵗʰ S86.0   Injury of Achilles tendon

> **√6ᵗʰ S86.00   Unspecified injury of Achilles tendon**
>
> > **√7ᵗʰ S86.001   Unspecified injury of right Achilles tendon**
> >
> > **√7ᵗʰ S86.002   Unspecified injury of left Achilles tendon**
> >
> > **√7ᵗʰ S86.009   Unspecified injury of unspecified Achilles tendon**

N Newborn: 0   **P** Pediatric: 0-17   **M** Maternity: 12-55   **A** Adult: 15-124   **MCC** Major Complication/Comorbidity   **CC** Complication/Comorbidity   **SW** Severe Wound Dx

1062

ICD-10-CM 2019

✓6ᵗʰ **S86.01 Strain of Achilles tendon**
 ✓7ᵗʰ **S86.011 Strain of right Achilles tendon**
 ✓7ᵗʰ **S86.012 Strain of left Achilles tendon**
 ✓7ᵗʰ **S86.019 Strain of unspecified Achilles tendon**

✓6ᵗʰ **S86.02 Laceration of Achilles tendon**
 ✓7ᵗʰ **S86.021 Laceration of right Achilles tendon** CC
 ✓7ᵗʰ **S86.022 Laceration of left Achilles tendon** CC
 ✓7ᵗʰ **S86.029 Laceration of unspecified Achilles tendon** CC

✓6ᵗʰ **S86.09 Other specified injury of Achilles tendon**
 ✓7ᵗʰ **S86.091 Other specified injury of right Achilles tendon**
 ✓7ᵗʰ **S86.092 Other specified injury of left Achilles tendon**
 ✓7ᵗʰ **S86.099 Other specified injury of unspecified Achilles tendon**

✓5ᵗʰ **S86.1 Injury of other muscle(s) and tendon(s) of posterior muscle group at lower leg level**

✓6ᵗʰ **S86.10 Unspecified injury of other muscle(s) and tendon(s) of posterior muscle group at lower leg level**
 ✓7ᵗʰ **S86.101 Unspecified injury of other muscle(s) and tendon(s) of posterior muscle group at lower leg level, right leg**
 ✓7ᵗʰ **S86.102 Unspecified injury of other muscle(s) and tendon(s) of posterior muscle group at lower leg level, left leg**
 ✓7ᵗʰ **S86.109 Unspecified injury of other muscle(s) and tendon(s) of posterior muscle group at lower leg level, unspecified leg**

✓6ᵗʰ **S86.11 Strain of other muscle(s) and tendon(s) of posterior muscle group at lower leg level**
 ✓7ᵗʰ **S86.111 Strain of other muscle(s) and tendon(s) of posterior muscle group at lower leg level, right leg**
 ✓7ᵗʰ **S86.112 Strain of other muscle(s) and tendon(s) of posterior muscle group at lower leg level, left leg**
 ✓7ᵗʰ **S86.119 Strain of other muscle(s) and tendon(s) of posterior muscle group at lower leg level, unspecified leg**

✓6ᵗʰ **S86.12 Laceration of other muscle(s) and tendon(s) of posterior muscle group at lower leg level**
 ✓7ᵗʰ **S86.121 Laceration of other muscle(s) and tendon(s) of posterior muscle group at lower leg level, right leg** CC
 ✓7ᵗʰ **S86.122 Laceration of other muscle(s) and tendon(s) of posterior muscle group at lower leg level, left leg** CC
 ✓7ᵗʰ **S86.129 Laceration of other muscle(s) and tendon(s) of posterior muscle group at lower leg level, unspecified leg** CC

✓6ᵗʰ **S86.19 Other injury of other muscle(s) and tendon(s) of posterior muscle group at lower leg level**
 ✓7ᵗʰ **S86.191 Other injury of other muscle(s) and tendon(s) of posterior muscle group at lower leg level, right leg**
 ✓7ᵗʰ **S86.192 Other injury of other muscle(s) and tendon(s) of posterior muscle group at lower leg level, left leg**
 ✓7ᵗʰ **S86.199 Other injury of other muscle(s) and tendon(s) of posterior muscle group at lower leg level, unspecified leg**

✓5ᵗʰ **S86.2 Injury of muscle(s) and tendon(s) of anterior muscle group at lower leg level**

✓6ᵗʰ **S86.20 Unspecified injury of muscle(s) and tendon(s) of anterior muscle group at lower leg level**
 ✓7ᵗʰ **S86.201 Unspecified injury of muscle(s) and tendon(s) of anterior muscle group at lower leg level, right leg**
 ✓7ᵗʰ **S86.202 Unspecified injury of muscle(s) and tendon(s) of anterior muscle group at lower leg level, left leg**
 ✓7ᵗʰ **S86.209 Unspecified injury of muscle(s) and tendon(s) of anterior muscle group at lower leg level, unspecified leg**

✓6ᵗʰ **S86.21 Strain of muscle(s) and tendon(s) of anterior muscle group at lower leg level**
 ✓7ᵗʰ **S86.211 Strain of muscle(s) and tendon(s) of anterior muscle group at lower leg level, right leg**
 ✓7ᵗʰ **S86.212 Strain of muscle(s) and tendon(s) of anterior muscle group at lower leg level, left leg**
 ✓7ᵗʰ **S86.219 Strain of muscle(s) and tendon(s) of anterior muscle group at lower leg level, unspecified leg**

✓6ᵗʰ **S86.22 Laceration of muscle(s) and tendon(s) of anterior muscle group at lower leg level**
 ✓7ᵗʰ **S86.221 Laceration of muscle(s) and tendon(s) of anterior muscle group at lower leg level, right leg** CC
 ✓7ᵗʰ **S86.222 Laceration of muscle(s) and tendon(s) of anterior muscle group at lower leg level, left leg** CC
 ✓7ᵗʰ **S86.229 Laceration of muscle(s) and tendon(s) of anterior muscle group at lower leg level, unspecified leg** CC

✓6ᵗʰ **S86.29 Other injury of muscle(s) and tendon(s) of anterior muscle group at lower leg level**
 ✓7ᵗʰ **S86.291 Other injury of muscle(s) and tendon(s) of anterior muscle group at lower leg level, right leg**
 ✓7ᵗʰ **S86.292 Other injury of muscle(s) and tendon(s) of anterior muscle group at lower leg level, left leg**
 ✓7ᵗʰ **S86.299 Other injury of muscle(s) and tendon(s) of anterior muscle group at lower leg level, unspecified leg**

✓5ᵗʰ **S86.3 Injury of muscle(s) and tendon(s) of peroneal muscle group at lower leg level**

✓6ᵗʰ **S86.30 Unspecified injury of muscle(s) and tendon(s) of peroneal muscle group at lower leg level**
 ✓7ᵗʰ **S86.301 Unspecified injury of muscle(s) and tendon(s) of peroneal muscle group at lower leg level, right leg**
 ✓7ᵗʰ **S86.302 Unspecified injury of muscle(s) and tendon(s) of peroneal muscle group at lower leg level, left leg**
 ✓7ᵗʰ **S86.309 Unspecified injury of muscle(s) and tendon(s) of peroneal muscle group at lower leg level, unspecified leg**

✓6ᵗʰ **S86.31 Strain of muscle(s) and tendon(s) of peroneal muscle group at lower leg level**
 ✓7ᵗʰ **S86.311 Strain of muscle(s) and tendon(s) of peroneal muscle group at lower leg level, right leg**
 ✓7ᵗʰ **S86.312 Strain of muscle(s) and tendon(s) of peroneal muscle group at lower leg level, left leg**
 ✓7ᵗʰ **S86.319 Strain of muscle(s) and tendon(s) of peroneal muscle group at lower leg level, unspecified leg**

✓6ᵗʰ **S86.32 Laceration of muscle(s) and tendon(s) of peroneal muscle group at lower leg level**
 ✓7ᵗʰ **S86.321 Laceration of muscle(s) and tendon(s) of peroneal muscle group at lower leg level, right leg** CC
 ✓7ᵗʰ **S86.322 Laceration of muscle(s) and tendon(s) of peroneal muscle group at lower leg level, left leg** CC
 ✓7ᵗʰ **S86.329 Laceration of muscle(s) and tendon(s) of peroneal muscle group at lower leg level, unspecified leg** CC

✓6ᵗʰ **S86.39 Other injury of muscle(s) and tendon(s) of peroneal muscle group at lower leg level**
 ✓7ᵗʰ **S86.391 Other injury of muscle(s) and tendon(s) of peroneal muscle group at lower leg level, right leg**
 ✓7ᵗʰ **S86.392 Other injury of muscle(s) and tendon(s) of peroneal muscle group at lower leg level, left leg**

✓Additional Character Required   ✓x7ᵗʰ Placeholder   Unacceptable PDx   Questionable PDx   Manifestation   H1–H14 HAC   HCC CMS-HCC Dx   HIV HIV Dx

ICD-10-CM 2019   1063

S86.01–S86.392

Chapter 19. Injury, Poisoning and Certain Other Consequences of External Causes

✓7th **S86.399** Other injury of muscle(s) and tendon(s) of peroneal muscle group at lower leg level, unspecified leg

✓5th **S86.8** Injury of other muscles and tendons at lower leg level

　✓6th **S86.80** Unspecified injury of other muscles and tendons at lower leg level

　　✓7th **S86.801** Unspecified injury of other muscle(s) and tendon(s) at lower leg level, right leg

　　✓7th **S86.802** Unspecified injury of other muscle(s) and tendon(s) at lower leg level, left leg

　　✓7th **S86.809** Unspecified injury of other muscle(s) and tendon(s) at lower leg level, unspecified leg

　✓6th **S86.81** Strain of other muscles and tendons at lower leg level

　　✓7th **S86.811** Strain of other muscle(s) and tendon(s) at lower leg level, right leg

　　✓7th **S86.812** Strain of other muscle(s) and tendon(s) at lower leg level, left leg

　　✓7th **S86.819** Strain of other muscle(s) and tendon(s) at lower leg level, unspecified leg

　✓6th **S86.82** Laceration of other muscles and tendons at lower leg level

　　✓7th **S86.821** Laceration of other muscle(s) and tendon(s) at lower leg level, right leg   CC

　　✓7th **S86.822** Laceration of other muscle(s) and tendon(s) at lower leg level, left leg   CC

　　✓7th **S86.829** Laceration of other muscle(s) and tendon(s) at lower leg level, unspecified leg   CC

　✓6th **S86.89** Other injury of other muscles and tendons at lower leg level

　　✓7th **S86.891** Other injury of other muscle(s) and tendon(s) at lower leg level, right leg

　　✓7th **S86.892** Other injury of other muscle(s) and tendon(s) at lower leg level, left leg

　　✓7th **S86.899** Other injury of other muscle(s) and tendon(s) at lower leg level, unspecified leg

✓5th **S86.9** Injury of unspecified muscle and tendon at lower leg level

　✓6th **S86.90** Unspecified injury of unspecified muscle and tendon at lower leg level

　　✓7th **S86.901** Unspecified injury of unspecified muscle(s) and tendon(s) at lower leg level, right leg

　　✓7th **S86.902** Unspecified injury of unspecified muscle(s) and tendon(s) at lower leg level, left leg

　　✓7th **S86.909** Unspecified injury of unspecified muscle(s) and tendon(s) at lower leg level, unspecified leg

　✓6th **S86.91** Strain of unspecified muscle and tendon at lower leg level

　　✓7th **S86.911** Strain of unspecified muscle(s) and tendon(s) at lower leg level, right leg

　　✓7th **S86.912** Strain of unspecified muscle(s) and tendon(s) at lower leg level, left leg

　　✓7th **S86.919** Strain of unspecified muscle(s) and tendon(s) at lower leg level, unspecified leg

　✓6th **S86.92** Laceration of unspecified muscle and tendon at lower leg level

　　✓7th **S86.921** Laceration of unspecified muscle(s) and tendon(s) at lower leg level, right leg   CC

　　✓7th **S86.922** Laceration of unspecified muscle(s) and tendon(s) at lower leg level, left leg   CC

　　✓7th **S86.929** Laceration of unspecified muscle(s) and tendon(s) at lower leg level, unspecified leg   CC

　✓6th **S86.99** Other injury of unspecified muscle and tendon at lower leg level

　　✓7th **S86.991** Other injury of unspecified muscle(s) and tendon(s) at lower leg level, right leg

✓7th **S86.992** Other injury of unspecified muscle(s) and tendon(s) at lower leg level, left leg

✓7th **S86.999** Other injury of unspecified muscle(s) and tendon(s) at lower leg level, unspecified leg

✓4th **S87** Crushing injury of lower leg

Use additional code(s) for all associated injuries

EXCLUDES 2　crushing injury of ankle and foot (S97.-)

The appropriate 7th character is to be added to each code from category S87.
A　initial encounter
D　subsequent encounter
S　sequela

✓5th **S87.0** Crushing injury of knee

　✓x7th **S87.00** Crushing injury of unspecified knee

　✓x7th **S87.01** Crushing injury of right knee

　✓x7th **S87.02** Crushing injury of left knee

✓5th **S87.8** Crushing injury of lower leg

　✓x7th **S87.80** Crushing injury of unspecified lower leg

　✓x7th **S87.81** Crushing injury of right lower leg

　✓x7th **S87.82** Crushing injury of left lower leg

✓4th **S88** Traumatic amputation of lower leg

An amputation not identified as partial or complete should be coded to complete.

EXCLUDES 1　traumatic amputation of ankle and foot (S98.-)

The appropriate 7th character is to be added to each code from category S88.
A　initial encounter
D　subsequent encounter
S　sequela

CC Excl: For CC codes in category S88:
Right side: PDX collection 1333
Left side: PDX collection 1334
Unspecified side: PDX collection 1335

✓5th **S88.0** Traumatic amputation at knee level

　✓6th **S88.01** Complete traumatic amputation at knee level

　　✓7th **S88.011** Complete traumatic amputation at knee level, right lower leg   CC HCC

　　✓7th **S88.012** Complete traumatic amputation at knee level, left lower leg   CC HCC

　　✓7th **S88.019** Complete traumatic amputation at knee level, unspecified lower leg   CC HCC

　✓6th **S88.02** Partial traumatic amputation at knee level

　　✓7th **S88.021** Partial traumatic amputation at knee level, right lower leg   CC HCC

　　✓7th **S88.022** Partial traumatic amputation at knee level, left lower leg   CC HCC

　　✓7th **S88.029** Partial traumatic amputation at knee level, unspecified lower leg   CC HCC

✓5th **S88.1** Traumatic amputation at level between knee and ankle

　✓6th **S88.11** Complete traumatic amputation at level between knee and ankle

　　✓7th **S88.111** Complete traumatic amputation at level between knee and ankle, right lower leg   CC HCC

　　✓7th **S88.112** Complete traumatic amputation at level between knee and ankle, left lower leg   CC HCC

　　✓7th **S88.119** Complete traumatic amputation at level between knee and ankle, unspecified lower leg   CC HCC

　✓6th **S88.12** Partial traumatic amputation at level between knee and ankle

　　✓7th **S88.121** Partial traumatic amputation at level between knee and ankle, right lower leg   CC HCC

　　✓7th **S88.122** Partial traumatic amputation at levelbetween knee and ankle, left lower leg   CC HCC

　　✓7th **S88.129** Partial traumatic amputation at level between knee and ankle, unspecified lower leg   CC HCC

✓5ᵗʰ **S88.9**   **Traumatic amputation of lower leg,** level unspecified

  ✓6ᵗʰ **S88.91**   Complete **traumatic amputation of lower leg, level unspecified**

    ✓7ᵗʰ **S88.911**   **Complete traumatic amputation of** right **lower leg, level unspecified**   `CC` `HCC`

    ✓7ᵗʰ **S88.912**   **Complete traumatic amputation of** left **lower leg, level unspecified**   `CC` `HCC`

    ✓7ᵗʰ **S88.919**   **Complete traumatic amputation of** unspecified **lower leg, level unspecified**   `CC` `HCC`

  ✓6ᵗʰ **S88.92**   Partial **traumatic amputation of lower leg, level unspecified**

    ✓7ᵗʰ **S88.921**   **Partial traumatic amputation of** right **lower leg, level unspecified**   `CC` `HCC`

    ✓7ᵗʰ **S88.922**   **Partial traumatic amputation of** left **lower leg, level unspecified**   `CC` `HCC`

    ✓7ᵗʰ **S88.929**   **Partial traumatic amputation of** unspecified **lower leg, level unspecified**   `CC` `HCC`

✓4ᵗʰ **S89**   **Other and unspecified injuries of lower leg**

  `NOTE`   A fracture not indicated as open or closed should be coded to closed.

  `EXCLUDES 2`   other and unspecified injuries of ankle and foot (S99.-)

  AHA: 2018, 2Q, 12; 2018, 1Q, 3; 2015, 3Q, 37-39

The appropriate 7th character is to be added to each code from subcategories S89.0, S89.1, S89.2, and S89.3.
A   initial encounter for closed fracture
D   subsequent encounter for fracture with routine healing
G   subsequent encounter for fracture with delayed healing
K   subsequent encounter for fracture with nonunion
P   subsequent encounter for fracture with malunion
S   sequela

✓5ᵗʰ **S89.0**   Physeal **fracture of** upper end of tibia

  CC Excl: For CC codes in subcategory S89.0:
  Right side: See code S89.001
  Left side: See code S89.002
  Unspecified side: See code S89.009

  ✓6ᵗʰ **S89.00**   Unspecified **physeal fracture of upper end of tibia**

    ³ ✓7ᵗʰ **S89.001**   **Unspecified physeal fracture of upper end of** right **tibia**   `CC` `H5`
      CC Excl: CC with 7th character A: PDX collection 1340
      CC with 7th character K or P: PDX collection 897

    ³ ✓7ᵗʰ **S89.002**   **Unspecified physeal fracture of upper end of** left **tibia**   `CC` `H5`
      CC Excl: CC with 7th character A: PDX collection 1342
      CC with 7th character K or P: PDX collection 897

    ³ ✓7ᵗʰ **S89.009**   **Unspecified physeal fracture of upper end of** unspecified **tibia**   `CC` `H5`
      CC Excl: CC with 7th character A: PDX collection 1341
      CC with 7th character K or P: PDX collection 897

  ✓6ᵗʰ **S89.01**   Salter-Harris Type I physeal fracture of upper end of tibia

    ³ ✓7ᵗʰ **S89.011**   **Salter-Harris Type I physeal fracture of upper end of** right **tibia**   `CC` `H5`

    ³ ✓7ᵗʰ **S89.012**   **Salter-Harris Type I physeal fracture of upper end of** left **tibia**   `CC` `H5`

    ³ ✓7ᵗʰ **S89.019**   **Salter-Harris Type I physeal fracture of upper end of** unspecified **tibia**   `CC` `H5`

  ✓6ᵗʰ **S89.02**   Salter-Harris Type II physeal fracture of upper end of tibia

    ³ ✓7ᵗʰ **S89.021**   **Salter-Harris Type II physeal fracture of upper end of** right **tibia**   `CC` `H5`

    ³ ✓7ᵗʰ **S89.022**   **Salter-Harris Type II physeal fracture of upper end of** left **tibia**   `CC` `H5`

    ³ ✓7ᵗʰ **S89.029**   **Salter-Harris Type II physeal fracture of upper end of** unspecified **tibia**   `CC` `H5`

  ✓6ᵗʰ **S89.03**   Salter-Harris Type III physeal fracture of upper end of tibia

    ³ ✓7ᵗʰ **S89.031**   **Salter-Harris Type III physeal fracture of upper end of** right **tibia**   `CC` `H5`

    ³ ✓7ᵗʰ **S89.032**   **Salter-Harris Type III physeal fracture of upper end of** left **tibia**   `CC` `H5`

    ³ ✓7ᵗʰ **S89.039**   **Salter-Harris Type III physeal fracture of upper end of** unspecified **tibia**   `CC` `H5`

  ✓6ᵗʰ **S89.04**   Salter-Harris Type IV physeal fracture of upper end of tibia

    ³ ✓7ᵗʰ **S89.041**   **Salter-Harris Type IV physeal fracture of upper end of** right **tibia**   `CC` `H5`

    ³ ✓7ᵗʰ **S89.042**   **Salter-Harris Type IV physeal fracture of upper end of** left **tibia**   `CC` `H5`

    ³ ✓7ᵗʰ **S89.049**   **Salter-Harris Type IV physeal fracture of upper end of** unspecified **tibia**   `CC` `H5`

  ✓6ᵗʰ **S89.09**   Other **physeal fracture of upper end of tibia**

    ³ ✓7ᵗʰ **S89.091**   **Other physeal fracture of upper end of** right **tibia**   `CC` `H5`

    ³ ✓7ᵗʰ **S89.092**   **Other physeal fracture of upper end of** left **tibia**   `CC` `H5`

    ³ ✓7ᵗʰ **S89.099**   **Other physeal fracture of upper end of** unspecified **tibia**   `CC` `H5`

✓5ᵗʰ **S89.1**   **Physeal fracture of** lower end of tibia

  CC Excl: For codes in subcategory S89.1:
  CC with 7th character K or P: PDX collection 897

  ✓6ᵗʰ **S89.10**   Unspecified **physeal fracture of lower end of tibia**

    ⁴ ✓7ᵗʰ **S89.101**   **Unspecified physeal fracture of lower end of** right **tibia**   `CC`

    ⁴ ✓7ᵗʰ **S89.102**   **Unspecified physeal fracture of lower end of** left **tibia**   `CC`

    ⁴ ✓7ᵗʰ **S89.109**   **Unspecified physeal fracture of lower end of** unspecified **tibia**   `CC`

  ✓6ᵗʰ **S89.11**   Salter-Harris Type I physeal fracture of ower end of tibia

    ⁴ ✓7ᵗʰ **S89.111**   **Salter-Harris Type I physeal fracture of lower end of** right **tibia**   `CC`

    ⁴ ✓7ᵗʰ **S89.112**   **Salter-Harris Type I physeal fracture oflower end of** left **tibia**   `CC`

    ⁴ ✓7ᵗʰ **S89.119**   **Salter-Harris Type I physeal fracture of lower end of** unspecified **tibia**   `CC`

  ✓6ᵗʰ **S89.12**   Salter-Harris Type II physeal fracture of lower end of tibia

    ⁴ ✓7ᵗʰ **S89.121**   **Salter-Harris Type II physeal fracture of lower end of** right **tibia**   `CC`

    ⁴ ✓7ᵗʰ **S89.122**   **Salter-Harris Type II physeal fracture of lower end of** left **tibia**   `CC`

    ⁴ ✓7ᵗʰ **S89.129**   **Salter-Harris Type II physeal fracture of lower end of** unspecified **tibia**   `CC`

  ✓6ᵗʰ **S89.13**   Salter-Harris Type III physeal fracture of lower end of tibia

    `EXCLUDES 1`   fracture of medial malleolus (adult) (S82.5-)

    ⁴ ✓7ᵗʰ **S89.131**   **Salter-Harris Type III physeal fracture of lower end of** right **tibia**   `CC`

    ⁴ ✓7ᵗʰ **S89.132**   **Salter-Harris Type III physeal fracture of lower end of** left **tibia**   `CC`

    ⁴ ✓7ᵗʰ **S89.139**   **Salter-Harris Type III physeal fracture of lower end of** unspecified **tibia**   `CC`

  ✓6ᵗʰ **S89.14**   Salter-Harris Type IV physeal fracture of lower end of tibia

    `EXCLUDES 1`   fracture of medial malleolus (adult) (S82.5-)

    ⁴ ✓7ᵗʰ **S89.141**   **Salter-Harris Type IV physeal fracture oflower end of** right **tibia**   `CC`

    ⁴ ✓7ᵗʰ **S89.142**   **Salter-Harris Type IV physeal fracture of lower end of** left **tibia**   `CC`

    ⁴ ✓7ᵗʰ **S89.149**   **Salter-Harris Type IV physeal fracture of lower end of** unspecified **tibia**   `CC`

  ✓6ᵗʰ **S89.19**   Other **physeal fracture of lower end of tibia**

    ⁴ ✓7ᵗʰ **S89.191**   **Other physeal fracture of lower end of** right **tibia**   `CC`

    ⁴ ✓7ᵗʰ **S89.192**   **Other physeal fracture of lower end of** left **tibia**   `CC`

    ⁴ ✓7ᵗʰ **S89.199**   **Other physeal fracture of lower end of** unspecified **tibia**   `CC`

✓ Additional Character Required   ✓x7ᵗʰ Placeholder   Unacceptable PDx   Questionable PDx   Manifestation   `H1`-`H14` HAC   `HCC` CMS-HCC Dx   `HIV` HIV Dx

ICD-10-CM 2019   **1065**

√5ᵗʰ S89.2 Physeal fracture of upper end of fibula

> **CC Excl:** For codes in subcategory S89.2:
> CC with 7th character K or P: PDX collection 897

    √6ᵗʰ S89.20 Unspecified physeal fracture of upper end of fibula

        4 √7ᵗʰ **S89.201** Unspecified physeal fracture of upper end of right fibula CC

        4 √7ᵗʰ **S89.202** Unspecified physeal fracture of upper end of left fibula CC

        4 √7ᵗʰ **S89.209** Unspecified physeal fracture of upper end of unspecified fibula CC

    √6ᵗʰ S89.21 Salter-Harris Type I physeal fracture of upper end of fibula

        4 √7ᵗʰ **S89.211** Salter-Harris Type I physeal fracture of upper end of right fibula CC

        4 √7ᵗʰ **S89.212** Salter-Harris Type I physeal fracture of upper end of left fibula CC

        4 √7ᵗʰ **S89.219** Salter-Harris Type I physeal fracture of upper end of unspecified fibula CC

    √6ᵗʰ S89.22 Salter-Harris Type II physeal fracture of upper end of fibula

        4 √7ᵗʰ **S89.221** Salter-Harris Type II physeal fracture of upper end of right fibula CC

        4 √7ᵗʰ **S89.222** Salter-Harris Type II physeal fracture of upper end of left fibula CC

        4 √7ᵗʰ **S89.229** Salter-Harris Type II physeal fracture of upper end of unspecified fibula CC

    √6ᵗʰ S89.29 Other physeal fracture of upper end of fibula

        4 √7ᵗʰ **S89.291** Other physeal fracture of upper end of right fibula CC

        4 √7ᵗʰ **S89.292** Other physeal fracture of upper end of left fibula CC

        4 √7ᵗʰ **S89.299** Other physeal fracture of upper end of unspecified fibula CC

√5ᵗʰ S89.3 Physeal fracture of lower end of fibula

> **CC Excl:** For codes in subcategory S89.3:
> CC with 7th character K or P: PDX collection 897

    √6ᵗʰ S89.30 Unspecified physeal fracture of lower end of fibula

        4 √7ᵗʰ **S89.301** Unspecified physeal fracture of lower end of right fibula CC

        4 √7ᵗʰ **S89.302** Unspecified physeal fracture of lower end of left fibula CC

        4 √7ᵗʰ **S89.309** Unspecified physeal fracture of lower end of unspecified fibula CC

    √6ᵗʰ S89.31 Salter-Harris Type I physeal fracture of lower end of fibula

        4 √7ᵗʰ **S89.311** Salter-Harris Type I physeal fracture of lower end of right fibula CC

        4 √7ᵗʰ **S89.312** Salter-Harris Type I physeal fracture of lower end of left fibula CC

        4 √7ᵗʰ **S89.319** Salter-Harris Type I physeal fracture of lower end of unspecified fibula CC

    √6ᵗʰ S89.32 Salter-Harris Type II physeal fracture of lower end of fibula

        4 √7ᵗʰ **S89.321** Salter-Harris Type II physeal fracture of lower end of right fibula CC

        4 √7ᵗʰ **S89.322** Salter-Harris Type II physeal fracture of lower end of left fibula CC

        4 √7ᵗʰ **S89.329** Salter-Harris Type II physeal fracture of lower end of unspecified fibula CC

    √6ᵗʰ S89.39 Other physeal fracture of lower end of fibula

        4 √7ᵗʰ **S89.391** Other physeal fracture of lower end of right fibula CC

        4 √7ᵗʰ **S89.392** Other physeal fracture of lower end of left fibula CC

        4 √7ᵗʰ **S89.399** Other physeal fracture of lower end of unspecified fibula CC

√5ᵗʰ S89.8 Other specified injuries of lower leg

> The appropriate 7th character is to be added to each code in subcategory S89.8.
> A   initial encounter
> D   subsequent encounter
> S   sequela

    √x7ᵗʰ **S89.80** Other specified injuries of unspecified lower leg

    √x7ᵗʰ **S89.81** Other specified injuries of right lower leg

    √x7ᵗʰ **S89.82** Other specified injuries of left lower leg

√5ᵗʰ S89.9 Unspecified injury of lower leg

> The appropriate 7th character is to be added to each code in subcategory S89.9.
> A   initial encounter
> D   subsequent encounter
> S   sequela

    √x7ᵗʰ **S89.90** Unspecified injury of unspecified lower leg

    √x7ᵗʰ **S89.91** Unspecified injury of right lower leg

    √x7ᵗʰ **S89.92** Unspecified injury of left lower leg

Injuries to the ankle and foot (S90-S99)

EXCLUDES 2   burns and corrosions (T20-T32)
                fracture of ankle and malleolus (S82.-)
                frostbite (T33-T34)
                insect bite or sting, venomous (T63.4)

√4ᵗʰ S90 Superficial injury of ankle, foot and toes

> The appropriate 7th character is to be added to each code from category S90.
> A   initial encounter
> D   subsequent encounter
> S   sequela

    √5ᵗʰ S90.0 Contusion of ankle

        √x7ᵗʰ **S90.00** Contusion of unspecified ankle

        √x7ᵗʰ **S90.01** Contusion of right ankle

        √x7ᵗʰ **S90.02** Contusion of left ankle

    √5ᵗʰ S90.1 Contusion of toe without damage to nail

        √6ᵗʰ S90.11 Contusion of great toe without damage to nail

            √7ᵗʰ **S90.111** Contusion of right great toe without damage to nail

            √7ᵗʰ **S90.112** Contusion of left great toe without damage to nail

            √7ᵗʰ **S90.119** Contusion of unspecified great toe without damage to nail

        √6ᵗʰ S90.12 Contusion of lesser toe without damage to nail

            √7ᵗʰ **S90.121** Contusion of right lesser toe(s) without damage to nail

            √7ᵗʰ **S90.122** Contusion of left lesser toe(s) without damage to nail

            √7ᵗʰ **S90.129** Contusion of unspecified lesser toe(s) without damage to nail
                Contusion of toe NOS

    √5ᵗʰ S90.2 Contusion of toe with damage to nail

        √6ᵗʰ S90.21 Contusion of great toe with damage to nail

            √7ᵗʰ **S90.211** Contusion of right great toe with damage to nail

            √7ᵗʰ **S90.212** Contusion of left great toe with damage to nail

            √7ᵗʰ **S90.219** Contusion of unspecified great toe with damage to nail

        √6ᵗʰ S90.22 Contusion of lesser toe with damage to nail

            √7ᵗʰ **S90.221** Contusion of right lesser toe(s) with damage to nail

            √7ᵗʰ **S90.222** Contusion of left lesser toe(s) with damage to nail

            √7ᵗʰ **S90.229** Contusion of unspecified lesser toe(s) with damage to nail

    √5ᵗʰ S90.3 Contusion of foot

        EXCLUDES 2   contusion of toes (S90.1-, S90.2-)

        √x7ᵗʰ **S90.30** Contusion of unspecified foot
                Contusion of foot NOS

        √x7ᵗʰ **S90.31** Contusion of right foot

        √x7ᵗʰ **S90.32** Contusion of left foot

N Newborn: 0   P Pediatric: 0-17   M Maternity: 12-55   A Adult: 15-124   MCC Major Complication/Comorbidity   CC Complication/Comorbidity   SW Severe Wound Dx

1066   ICD-10-CM 2019

✓5ᵗʰ **S90.4 Other superficial injuries of** toe
  ✓6ᵗʰ **S90.41 Abrasion** of toe
    ✓7ᵗʰ **S90.411 Abrasion,** right great **toe**
    ✓7ᵗʰ **S90.412 Abrasion,** left great **toe**
    ✓7ᵗʰ **S90.413 Abrasion,** unspecified great **toe**
    ✓7ᵗʰ **S90.414 Abrasion,** right lesser **toe(s)**
    ✓7ᵗʰ **S90.415 Abrasion,** left lesser **toe(s)**
    ✓7ᵗʰ **S90.416 Abrasion,** unspecified lesser **toe(s)**
  ✓6ᵗʰ **S90.42 Blister (nonthermal) of toe**
    ✓7ᵗʰ **S90.421 Blister (nonthermal),** right great **toe**
    ✓7ᵗʰ **S90.422 Blister (nonthermal),** left great **toe**
    ✓7ᵗʰ **S90.423 Blister (nonthermal),** unspecified great **toe**
    ✓7ᵗʰ **S90.424 Blister (nonthermal),** right lesser **toe(s)**
    ✓7ᵗʰ **S90.425 Blister (nonthermal),** left lesser **toe(s)**
    ✓7ᵗʰ **S90.426 Blister (nonthermal),** unspecified lesser **toe(s)**
  ✓6ᵗʰ **S90.44 External constriction of toe**
    Hair tourniquet syndrome of toe
    ✓7ᵗʰ **S90.441 External constriction,** right great **toe**
    ✓7ᵗʰ **S90.442 External constriction,** left great **toe**
    ✓7ᵗʰ **S90.443 External constriction,** unspecified great **toe**
    ✓7ᵗʰ **S90.444 External constriction,** right lesser **toe(s)**
    ✓7ᵗʰ **S90.445 External constriction,** left lesser **toe(s)**
    ✓7ᵗʰ **S90.446 External constriction,** unspecified lesser **toe(s)**
  ✓6ᵗʰ **S90.45 Superficial** foreign body **of toe**
    Splinter in the toe
    ✓7ᵗʰ **S90.451 Superficial foreign body,** right great **toe**
    ✓7ᵗʰ **S90.452 Superficial foreign body,** left great **toe**
    ✓7ᵗʰ **S90.453 Superficial foreign body,** unspecified great **toe**
    ✓7ᵗʰ **S90.454 Superficial foreign body,** right lesser **toe(s)**
    ✓7ᵗʰ **S90.455 Superficial foreign body,** left lesser **toe(s)**
    ✓7ᵗʰ **S90.456 Superficial foreign body,** unspecified lesser **toe(s)**
  ✓6ᵗʰ **S90.46 Insect bite (nonvenomous) of toe**
    ✓7ᵗʰ **S90.461 Insect bite (nonvenomous),** right great **toe**
    ✓7ᵗʰ **S90.462 Insect bite (nonvenomous),** left great **toe**
    ✓7ᵗʰ **S90.463 Insect bite (nonvenomous),** unspecified great **toe**
    ✓7ᵗʰ **S90.464 Insect bite (nonvenomous),** right lesser **toe(s)**
    ✓7ᵗʰ **S90.465 Insect bite (nonvenomous),** left lesser **toe(s)**
    ✓7ᵗʰ **S90.466 Insect bite (nonvenomous),** unspecified lesser **toe(s)**
  ✓6ᵗʰ **S90.47 Other** superficial bite **of toe**
    EXCLUDES 1 *open bite of toe (S91.15-, S91.25-)*
    ✓7ᵗʰ **S90.471 Other superficial bite of** right great **toe**
    ✓7ᵗʰ **S90.472 Other superficial bite of** left great **toe**
    ✓7ᵗʰ **S90.473 Other superficial bite of** unspecified great **toe**
    ✓7ᵗʰ **S90.474 Other superficial bite of** right lesser **toe(s)**
    ✓7ᵗʰ **S90.475 Other superficial bite of** left lesser **toe(s)**
    ✓7ᵗʰ **S90.476 Other superficial bite of** unspecified lesser **toe(s)**
✓5ᵗʰ **S90.5 Other superficial injuries of** ankle
  ✓6ᵗʰ **S90.51 Abrasion** of ankle
    ✓7ᵗʰ **S90.511 Abrasion,** right ankle
    ✓7ᵗʰ **S90.512 Abrasion,** left ankle
    ✓7ᵗʰ **S90.519 Abrasion,** unspecified ankle
  ✓6ᵗʰ **S90.52 Blister (nonthermal) of ankle**
    ✓7ᵗʰ **S90.521 Blister (nonthermal),** right ankle
    ✓7ᵗʰ **S90.522 Blister (nonthermal),** left ankle
    ✓7ᵗʰ **S90.529 Blister (nonthermal),** unspecified **ankle**
  ✓6ᵗʰ **S90.54 External constriction of ankle**
    ✓7ᵗʰ **S90.541 External constriction,** right ankle
    ✓7ᵗʰ **S90.542 External constriction,** left ankle

    ✓7ᵗʰ **S90.549 External constriction,** unspecified **ankle**
  ✓6ᵗʰ **S90.55 Superficial** foreign body **of ankle**
    Splinter in the ankle
    ✓7ᵗʰ **S90.551 Superficial foreign body,** right ankle
    ✓7ᵗʰ **S90.552 Superficial foreign body,** left ankle
    ✓7ᵗʰ **S90.559 Superficial foreign body,** unspecified **ankle**
  ✓6ᵗʰ **S90.56 Insect bite (nonvenomous) of ankle**
    ✓7ᵗʰ **S90.561 Insect bite (nonvenomous),** right ankle
    ✓7ᵗʰ **S90.562 Insect bite (nonvenomous),** left ankle
    ✓7ᵗʰ **S90.569 Insect bite (nonvenomous),** unspecified **ankle**
  ✓6ᵗʰ **S90.57 Other** superficial bite **of ankle**
    EXCLUDES 1 *open bite of ankle (S91.05-)*
    ✓7ᵗʰ **S90.571 Other superficial bite of ankle,** right ankle
    ✓7ᵗʰ **S90.572 Other superficial bite of ankle,** left ankle
    ✓7ᵗʰ **S90.579 Other superficial bite of ankle,** unspecified **ankle**
✓5ᵗʰ **S90.8 Other superficial injuries of** foot
  ✓6ᵗʰ **S90.81 Abrasion** of foot
    ✓7ᵗʰ **S90.811 Abrasion,** right **foot**
    ✓7ᵗʰ **S90.812 Abrasion,** left **foot**
    ✓7ᵗʰ **S90.819 Abrasion,** unspecified **foot**
  ✓6ᵗʰ **S90.82 Blister (nonthermal) of foot**
    ✓7ᵗʰ **S90.821 Blister (nonthermal),** right **foot**
    ✓7ᵗʰ **S90.822 Blister (nonthermal),** left **foot**
    ✓7ᵗʰ **S90.829 Blister (nonthermal),** unspecified **foot**
  ✓6ᵗʰ **S90.84 External constriction of foot**
    ✓7ᵗʰ **S90.841 External constriction,** right **foot**
    ✓7ᵗʰ **S90.842 External constriction,** left **foot**
    ✓7ᵗʰ **S90.849 External constriction,** unspecified **foot**
  ✓6ᵗʰ **S90.85 Superficial** foreign body **of foot**
    Splinter in the foot
    ✓7ᵗʰ **S90.851 Superficial foreign body,** right **foot**
    ✓7ᵗʰ **S90.852 Superficial foreign body,** left **foot**
    ✓7ᵗʰ **S90.859 Superficial foreign body,** unspecified **foot**
  ✓6ᵗʰ **S90.86 Insect bite (nonvenomous) of foot**
    ✓7ᵗʰ **S90.861 Insect bite (nonvenomous),** right **foot**
    ✓7ᵗʰ **S90.862 Insect bite (nonvenomous),** left **foot**
    ✓7ᵗʰ **S90.869 Insect bite (nonvenomous),** unspecified **foot**
  ✓6ᵗʰ **S90.87 Other** superficial bite **of foot**
    EXCLUDES 1 *open bite of foot (S91.35-)*
    ✓7ᵗʰ **S90.871 Other superficial bite of** right **foot**
    ✓7ᵗʰ **S90.872 Other superficial bite of** left **foot**
    ✓7ᵗʰ **S90.879 Other superficial bite of** unspecified **foot**
✓5ᵗʰ **S90.9 Unspecified superficial injury of** ankle, foot and toe
  ✓6ᵗʰ **S90.91 Unspecified superficial injury of** ankle
    ✓7ᵗʰ **S90.911 Unspecified superficial injury of** right **ankle**
    ✓7ᵗʰ **S90.912 Unspecified superficial injury of** left **ankle**
    ✓7ᵗʰ **S90.919 Unspecified superficial injury of** unspecified **ankle**
  ✓6ᵗʰ **S90.92 Unspecified superficial injury of** foot
    ✓7ᵗʰ **S90.921 Unspecified superficial injury of** right **foot**
    ✓7ᵗʰ **S90.922 Unspecified superficial injury of** left **foot**
    ✓7ᵗʰ **S90.929 Unspecified superficial injury of** unspecified **foot**
  ✓6ᵗʰ **S90.93 Unspecified superficial injury of** toes
    ✓7ᵗʰ **S90.931 Unspecified superficial injury of** right great **toe**
    ✓7ᵗʰ **S90.932 Unspecified superficial injury of** left great **toe**
    ✓7ᵗʰ **S90.933 Unspecified superficial injury of** unspecified great **toe**
    ✓7ᵗʰ **S90.934 Unspecified superficial injury of** right lesser **toe(s)**
    ✓7ᵗʰ **S90.935 Unspecified superficial injury of** left lesser **toe(s)**
    ✓7ᵗʰ **S90.936 Unspecified superficial injury of** unspecified lesser **toe(s)**

✓4ᵗʰ **S91** **Open wound of ankle, foot and toes**
Code also any associated wound infection
EXCLUDES 1   *open fracture of ankle, foot and toes (S92-with 7th B).*
traumatic amputation of ankle and foot (S98.-)

The appropriate 7th character is to be added to each code from category S91.
A   initial encounter
D   subsequent encounter
S   sequela

✓5ᵗʰ **S91.0**   **Open wound of** ankle
   ✓6ᵗʰ **S91.00**   **Unspecified open wound of ankle**
     ✓7ᵗʰ **S91.001**   **Unspecified open wound, right ankle**
     ✓7ᵗʰ **S91.002**   **Unspecified open wound, left ankle**
     ✓7ᵗʰ **S91.009**   **Unspecified open wound, unspecified ankle**
   ✓6ᵗʰ **S91.01**   **Laceration without foreign body of ankle**
     ✓7ᵗʰ **S91.011**   **Laceration without foreign body, right ankle**
     ✓7ᵗʰ **S91.012**   **Laceration without foreign body, left ankle**
     ✓7ᵗʰ **S91.019**   **Laceration without foreign body, unspecified ankle**
   ✓6ᵗʰ **S91.02**   **Laceration with foreign body of ankle**
     ✓7ᵗʰ **S91.021**   **Laceration with foreign body, right ankle**
     ✓7ᵗʰ **S91.022**   **Laceration with foreign body, left ankle**
     ✓7ᵗʰ **S91.029**   **Laceration with foreign body, unspecified ankle**
   ✓6ᵗʰ **S91.03**   **Puncture wound without foreign body of ankle**
     ✓7ᵗʰ **S91.031**   **Puncture wound without foreign body, right ankle**
     ✓7ᵗʰ **S91.032**   **Puncture wound without foreign body, left ankle**
     ✓7ᵗʰ **S91.039**   **Puncture wound without foreign body, unspecified ankle**
   ✓6ᵗʰ **S91.04**   **Puncture wound with foreign body of ankle**
     ✓7ᵗʰ **S91.041**   **Puncture wound with foreign body, right ankle**
     ✓7ᵗʰ **S91.042**   **Puncture wound with foreign body, left ankle**
     ✓7ᵗʰ **S91.049**   **Puncture wound with foreign body, unspecified ankle**
   ✓6ᵗʰ **S91.05**   **Open bite of ankle**
     EXCLUDES 1   *superficial bite of ankle (S90.56-, S90.57-)*
     ✓7ᵗʰ **S91.051**   **Open bite, right ankle**
     ✓7ᵗʰ **S91.052**   **Open bite, left ankle**
     ✓7ᵗʰ **S91.059**   **Open bite, unspecified ankle**
✓5ᵗʰ **S91.1**   **Open wound of** toe without damage to nail
   ✓6ᵗʰ **S91.10**   **Unspecified open wound of toe without damage to nail**
     ✓7ᵗʰ **S91.101**   **Unspecified open wound of right great toe without damage to nail**
     ✓7ᵗʰ **S91.102**   **Unspecified open wound of left great toe without damage to nail**
     ✓7ᵗʰ **S91.103**   **Unspecified open wound of unspecified great toe without damage to nail**
     ✓7ᵗʰ **S91.104**   **Unspecified open wound of right lesser toe(s) without damage to nail**
     ✓7ᵗʰ **S91.105**   **Unspecified open wound of left lesser toe(s) without damage to nail**
     ✓7ᵗʰ **S91.106**   **Unspecified open wound of unspecified lesser toe(s) without damage to nail**
     ✓7ᵗʰ **S91.109**   **Unspecified open wound of unspecified toe(s) without damage to nail**
   ✓6ᵗʰ **S91.11**   **Laceration without foreign body of toe without damage to nail**
     ✓7ᵗʰ **S91.111**   **Laceration without foreign body of right great toe without damage to nail**
     ✓7ᵗʰ **S91.112**   **Laceration without foreign body of left great toe without damage to nail**
     ✓7ᵗʰ **S91.113**   **Laceration without foreign body of unspecified great toe without damage to nail**

     ✓7ᵗʰ **S91.114**   **Laceration without foreign body of right lesser toe(s) without damage to nail**
     ✓7ᵗʰ **S91.115**   **Laceration without foreign body of left lesser toe(s) without damage to nail**
     ✓7ᵗʰ **S91.116**   **Laceration without foreign body of unspecified lesser toe(s) without damage to nail**
     ✓7ᵗʰ **S91.119**   **Laceration without foreign body of unspecified toe without damage to nail**
   ✓6ᵗʰ **S91.12**   **Laceration with foreign body of toe without damage to nail**
     ✓7ᵗʰ **S91.121**   **Laceration with foreign body of right great toe without damage to nail**
     ✓7ᵗʰ **S91.122**   **Laceration with foreign body of left great toe without damage to nail**
     ✓7ᵗʰ **S91.123**   **Laceration with foreign body of unspecified great toe without damage to nail**
     ✓7ᵗʰ **S91.124**   **Laceration with foreign body of right lesser toe(s) without damage to nail**
     ✓7ᵗʰ **S91.125**   **Laceration with foreign body of left lesser toe(s) without damage to nail**
     ✓7ᵗʰ **S91.126**   **Laceration with foreign body of unspecified lesser toe(s) without damage to nail**
     ✓7ᵗʰ **S91.129**   **Laceration with foreign body of unspecified toe(s) without damage to nail**
   ✓6ᵗʰ **S91.13**   **Puncture wound without foreign body of toe without damage to nail**
     ✓7ᵗʰ **S91.131**   **Puncture wound without foreign body of right great toe without damage to nail**
     ✓7ᵗʰ **S91.132**   **Puncture wound without foreign body of left great toe without damage to nail**
     ✓7ᵗʰ **S91.133**   **Puncture wound without foreign body of unspecified great toe without damage to nail**
     ✓7ᵗʰ **S91.134**   **Puncture wound without foreign body of right lesser toe(s) without damage to nail**
     ✓7ᵗʰ **S91.135**   **Puncture wound without foreign body of left lesser toe(s) without damage to nail**
     ✓7ᵗʰ **S91.136**   **Puncture wound without foreign body of unspecified lesser toe(s) without damage to nail**
     ✓7ᵗʰ **S91.139**   **Puncture wound without foreign body of unspecified toe(s) without damage to nail**
   ✓6ᵗʰ **S91.14**   **Puncture wound with foreign body of toe without damage to nail**
     ✓7ᵗʰ **S91.141**   **Puncture wound with foreign body of right great toe without damage to nail**
     ✓7ᵗʰ **S91.142**   **Puncture wound with foreign body of left great toe without damage to nail**
     ✓7ᵗʰ **S91.143**   **Puncture wound with foreign body of unspecified great toe without damage to nail**
     ✓7ᵗʰ **S91.144**   **Puncture wound with foreign body of right lesser toe(s) without damage to nail**
     ✓7ᵗʰ **S91.145**   **Puncture wound with foreign body of left lesser toe(s) without damage to nail**
     ✓7ᵗʰ **S91.146**   **Puncture wound with foreign body of unspecified lesser toe(s) without damage to nail**
     ✓7ᵗʰ **S91.149**   **Puncture wound with foreign body of unspecified toe(s) without damage to nail**
   ✓6ᵗʰ **S91.15**   **Open bite of toe without damage to nail**
     Bite of toe NOS
     EXCLUDES 1   *superficial bite of toe (S90.46-, S90.47-)*
     ✓7ᵗʰ **S91.151**   **Open bite of right great toe without damage to nail**
     ✓7ᵗʰ **S91.152**   **Open bite of left great toe without damage to nail**
     ✓7ᵗʰ **S91.153**   **Open bite of unspecified great toe without damage to nail**
     ✓7ᵗʰ **S91.154**   **Open bite of right lesser toe(s) without damage to nail**
     ✓7ᵗʰ **S91.155**   **Open bite of left lesser toe(s) without damage to nail**

N Newborn: 0   **P** Pediatric: 0-17   **M** Maternity: 12-55   **A** Adult: 15-124   **MCC** Major Complication/Comorbidity   **CC** Complication/Comorbidity   **SW** Severe Wound Dx

1068   ICD-10-CM 2019

S91–S91.155

☑7ᵗʰ **S91.156**   **Open bite of** unspecified lesser **toe(s) without damage to nail**

☑7ᵗʰ **S91.159**   **Open bite of** unspecified **toe(s) without damage to nail**

☑5ᵗʰ **S91.2**   Open wound of toe with damage to nail

  ☑6ᵗʰ **S91.20**   Unspecified open wound of toe with damage to nail

    ☑7ᵗʰ **S91.201**   **Unspecified open wound of** right great **toe with damage to nail**

    ☑7ᵗʰ **S91.202**   **Unspecified open wound of** left great **toe with damage to nail**

    ☑7ᵗʰ **S91.203**   **Unspecified open wound of** unspecified great **toe with damage to nail**

    ☑7ᵗʰ **S91.204**   **Unspecified open wound of** right lesser **toe(s) with damage to nail**

    ☑7ᵗʰ **S91.205**   **Unspecified open wound of** left lesser **toe(s) with damage to nail**

    ☑7ᵗʰ **S91.206**   **Unspecified open wound of** unspecified lesser **toe(s) with damage to nail**

    ☑7ᵗʰ **S91.209**   **Unspecified open wound of** unspecified **toe(s) with damage to nail**

  ☑6ᵗʰ **S91.21**   Laceration without foreign body of toe with damage to nail

    ☑7ᵗʰ **S91.211**   **Laceration without foreign body of** right great **toe with damage to nail**

    ☑7ᵗʰ **S91.212**   **Laceration without foreign body of** left great **toe with damage to nail**

    ☑7ᵗʰ **S91.213**   **Laceration without foreign body of** unspecified great **toe with damage to nail**

    ☑7ᵗʰ **S91.214**   **Laceration without foreign body of** right lesser **toe(s) with damage to nail**

    ☑7ᵗʰ **S91.215**   **Laceration without foreign body of** left lesser **toe(s) with damage to nail**

    ☑7ᵗʰ **S91.216**   **Laceration without foreign body of** unspecified lesser **toe(s) with damage to nail**

    ☑7ᵗʰ **S91.219**   **Laceration without foreign body of** unspecified **toe(s) with damage to nail**

  ☑6ᵗʰ **S91.22**   Laceration with foreign body of toe with damage to nail

    ☑7ᵗʰ **S91.221**   **Laceration with foreign body of** right great **toe with damage to nail**

    ☑7ᵗʰ **S91.222**   **Laceration with foreign body of** left great **toe with damage to nail**

    ☑7ᵗʰ **S91.223**   **Laceration with foreign body of** unspecified great **toe with damage to nail**

    ☑7ᵗʰ **S91.224**   **Laceration with foreign body of** right lesser **toe(s) with damage to nail**

    ☑7ᵗʰ **S91.225**   **Laceration with foreign body of** left lesser **toe(s) with damage to nail**

    ☑7ᵗʰ **S91.226**   **Laceration with foreign body of** unspecified lesser **toe(s) with damage to nail**

    ☑7ᵗʰ **S91.229**   **Laceration with foreign body of** unspecified **toe(s) with damage to nail**

  ☑6ᵗʰ **S91.23**   Puncture wound without foreign body of toe with damage to nail

    ☑7ᵗʰ **S91.231**   **Puncture wound without foreign body of** right great **toe with damage to nail**

    ☑7ᵗʰ **S91.232**   **Puncture wound without foreign body of** left great **toe with damage to nail**

    ☑7ᵗʰ **S91.233**   **Puncture wound without foreign body of** unspecified great **toe with damage to nail**

    ☑7ᵗʰ **S91.234**   **Puncture wound without foreign body of** right lesser **toe(s) with damage to nail**

    ☑7ᵗʰ **S91.235**   **Puncture wound without foreign body of** left lesser **toe(s) with damage to nail**

    ☑7ᵗʰ **S91.236**   **Puncture wound without foreign body of** unspecified lesser **toe(s) with damage to nail**

    ☑7ᵗʰ **S91.239**   **Puncture wound without foreign body of** unspecified **toe(s) with damage to nail**

  ☑6ᵗʰ **S91.24**   Puncture wound with foreign body of toe with damage to nail

    ☑7ᵗʰ **S91.241**   **Puncture wound with foreign body of** right great **toe with damage to nail**

    ☑7ᵗʰ **S91.242**   **Puncture wound with foreign body of** left great **toe with damage to nail**

    ☑7ᵗʰ **S91.243**   **Puncture wound with foreign body of** unspecified great **toe with damage to nail**

    ☑7ᵗʰ **S91.244**   **Puncture wound with foreign body of** right lesser **toe(s) with damage to nail**

    ☑7ᵗʰ **S91.245**   **Puncture wound with foreign body of** left lesser **toe(s) with damage to nail**

    ☑7ᵗʰ **S91.246**   **Puncture wound with foreign body of** unspecified lesser **toe(s) with damage to nail**

    ☑7ᵗʰ **S91.249**   **Puncture wound with foreign body of** unspecified **toe(s) with damage to nail**

  ☑6ᵗʰ **S91.25**   Open bite of toe with damage to nail
      Bite of toe with damage to nail NOS
      EXCLUDES 1   *superficial bite of toe (S90.46-, S90.47-)*

    ☑7ᵗʰ **S91.251**   **Open bite of** right great **toe with damage to nail**

    ☑7ᵗʰ **S91.252**   **Open bite of** left great **toe with damage to nail**

    ☑7ᵗʰ **S91.253**   **Open bite of** unspecified great **toe with damage to nail**

    ☑7ᵗʰ **S91.254**   **Open bite of** right lesser **toe(s) with damage to nail**

    ☑7ᵗʰ **S91.255**   **Open bite of** left lesser **toe(s) with damage to nail**

    ☑7ᵗʰ **S91.256**   **Open bite of** unspecified lesser **toe(s) with damage to nail**

    ☑7ᵗʰ **S91.259**   **Open bite of** unspecified **toe(s) with damage to nail**

☑5ᵗʰ **S91.3**   Open wound of foot

  ☑6ᵗʰ **S91.30**   Unspecified open wound of foot

    ☑7ᵗʰ **S91.301**   **Unspecified open wound,** right **foot**

    ☑7ᵗʰ **S91.302**   **Unspecified open wound,** left **foot**

    ☑7ᵗʰ **S91.309**   **Unspecified open wound,** unspecified **foot**

  ☑6ᵗʰ **S91.31**   Laceration without foreign body of foot

    ☑7ᵗʰ **S91.311**   **Laceration without foreign body,** right **foot**

    ☑7ᵗʰ **S91.312**   **Laceration without foreign body,** left **foot**

    ☑7ᵗʰ **S91.319**   **Laceration without foreign body,** unspecified **foot**

  ☑6ᵗʰ **S91.32**   Laceration with foreign body of foot

    ☑7ᵗʰ **S91.321**   **Laceration with foreign body,** right **foot**

    ☑7ᵗʰ **S91.322**   **Laceration with foreign body,** left **foot**

    ☑7ᵗʰ **S91.329**   **Laceration with foreign body,** unspecified **foot**

  ☑6ᵗʰ **S91.33**   Puncture wound without foreign body of foot

    ☑7ᵗʰ **S91.331**   **Puncture wound without foreign body,** right **foot**

    ☑7ᵗʰ **S91.332**   **Puncture wound without foreign body,** left **foot**

    ☑7ᵗʰ **S91.339**   **Puncture wound without foreign body,** unspecified **foot**

  ☑6ᵗʰ **S91.34**   Puncture wound with foreign body of foot

    ☑7ᵗʰ **S91.341**   **Puncture wound with foreign body,** right **foot**

    ☑7ᵗʰ **S91.342**   **Puncture wound with foreign body,** left **foot**

    ☑7ᵗʰ **S91.349**   **Puncture wound with foreign body,** unspecified **foot**

  ☑6ᵗʰ **S91.35**   Open bite of foot
      EXCLUDES 1   *superficial bite of foot (S90.86-, S90.87-)*

    ☑7ᵗʰ **S91.351**   **Open bite,** right **foot**

    ☑7ᵗʰ **S91.352**   **Open bite,** left **foot**

    ☑7ᵗʰ **S91.359**   **Open bite,** unspecified **foot**

☑ Additional Character Required   ☑x7ᵗʰ Placeholder   Unacceptable PDx   Questionable PDx   Manifestation   **H1**-**H14** HAC   **HCC** CMS-HCC Dx   **HIV** HIV Dx

ICD-10-CM 2019   1069

✓4ᵗʰ S92 Fracture of foot and toe, except ankle

> **NOTE** A fracture not indicated as displaced or nondisplaced should be coded to displaced.
> A fracture not indicated as open or closed should be coded to closed.

EXCLUDES 1 traumatic amputation of ankle and foot (S98.-)
EXCLUDES 2 fracture of ankle (S82.-)
fracture of malleolus (S82.-)

AHA: 2018, 2Q, 12; 2015, 3Q, 37-39

> The appropriate 7th character is to be added to each code from category S92.
> A   initial encounter for closed fracture
> B   initial encounter for open fracture
> D   subsequent encounter for fracture with routine healing
> G   subsequent encounter for fracture with delayed healing
> K   subsequent encounter for fracture with nonunion
> P   subsequent encounter for fracture with malunion
> S   sequela

✓5ᵗʰ S92.0 Fracture of calcaneus
Heel bone
Os calcis
EXCLUDES 2 physeal fracture of calcaneus (S99.0-)

> **CC Excl: For codes in subcategory S92.0:**
> **CC with 7th character B:** PDX collection 1367
> **CC with 7th character K or P:** PDX collection 897

✓6ᵗʰ S92.00 Unspecified fracture of calcaneus
- ³ ✓7ᵗʰ **S92.001** Unspecified fracture of right calcaneus `CC` `H5`
- ³ ✓7ᵗʰ **S92.002** Unspecified fracture of left calcaneus `CC` `H5`
- ³ ✓7ᵗʰ **S92.009** Unspecified fracture of unspecified calcaneus `CC` `H5`

✓6ᵗʰ S92.01 Fracture of body of calcaneus
- ³ ✓7ᵗʰ **S92.011** Displaced fracture of body of right calcaneus `CC` `H5`
- ³ ✓7ᵗʰ **S92.012** Displaced fracture of body of left calcaneus `CC` `H5`
- ³ ✓7ᵗʰ **S92.013** Displaced fracture of body of unspecified calcaneus `CC` `H5`
- ³ ✓7ᵗʰ **S92.014** Nondisplaced fracture of body of right calcaneus `CC` `H5`
- ³ ✓7ᵗʰ **S92.015** Nondisplaced fracture of body of left calcaneus `CC` `H5`
- ³ ✓7ᵗʰ **S92.016** Nondisplaced fracture of body of unspecified calcaneus `CC` `H5`

✓6ᵗʰ S92.02 Fracture of anterior process of calcaneus
- ³ ✓7ᵗʰ **S92.021** Displaced fracture of anterior process of right calcaneus `CC` `H5`
- ³ ✓7ᵗʰ **S92.022** Displaced fracture of anterior process of left calcaneus `CC` `H5`
- ³ ✓7ᵗʰ **S92.023** Displaced fracture of anterior process of unspecified calcaneus `CC` `H5`
- ³ ✓7ᵗʰ **S92.024** Nondisplaced fracture of anterior process of right calcaneus `CC` `H5`
- ³ ✓7ᵗʰ **S92.025** Nondisplaced fracture of anterior process of left calcaneus `CC` `H5`
- ³ ✓7ᵗʰ **S92.026** Nondisplaced fracture of anterior process of unspecified calcaneus `CC` `H5`

✓6ᵗʰ S92.03 Avulsion fracture of tuberosity of calcaneus
- ³ ✓7ᵗʰ **S92.031** Displaced avulsion fracture of tuberosity of right calcaneus `CC` `H5`
- ³ ✓7ᵗʰ **S92.032** Displaced avulsion fracture of tuberosity of left calcaneus `CC` `H5`
- ³ ✓7ᵗʰ **S92.033** Displaced avulsion fracture of tuberosity of unspecified calcaneus `CC` `H5`
- ³ ✓7ᵗʰ **S92.034** Nondisplaced avulsion fracture of tuberosity of right calcaneus `CC` `H5`
- ³ ✓7ᵗʰ **S92.035** Nondisplaced avulsion fracture of tuberosity of left calcaneus `CC` `H5`
- ³ ✓7ᵗʰ **S92.036** Nondisplaced avulsion fracture of tuberosity of unspecified calcaneus `CC` `H5`

✓6ᵗʰ S92.04 Other fracture of tuberosity of calcaneus
- ³ ✓7ᵗʰ **S92.041** Displaced other fracture of tuberosity of right calcaneus `CC` `H5`
- ³ ✓7ᵗʰ **S92.042** Displaced other fracture of tuberosity of left calcaneus `CC` `H5`

- ³ ✓7ᵗʰ **S92.043** Displaced other fracture of tuberosity of unspecified calcaneus `CC` `H5`
- ³ ✓7ᵗʰ **S92.044** Nondisplaced other fracture of tuberosity of right calcaneus `CC` `H5`
- ³ ✓7ᵗʰ **S92.045** Nondisplaced other fracture of tuberosity of left calcaneus `CC` `H5`
- ³ ✓7ᵗʰ **S92.046** Nondisplaced other fracture of tuberosity of unspecified calcaneus `CC` `H5`

✓6ᵗʰ S92.05 Other extraarticular fracture of calcaneus
- ³ ✓7ᵗʰ **S92.051** Displaced other extraarticular fracture of right calcaneus `CC` `H5`
- ³ ✓7ᵗʰ **S92.052** Displaced other extraarticular fracture of left calcaneus `CC` `H5`
- ³ ✓7ᵗʰ **S92.053** Displaced other extraarticular fracture of unspecified calcaneus `CC` `H5`
- ³ ✓7ᵗʰ **S92.054** Nondisplaced other extraarticular fracture of right calcaneus `CC` `H5`
- ³ ✓7ᵗʰ **S92.055** Nondisplaced other extraarticular fracture of left calcaneus `CC` `H5`
- ³ ✓7ᵗʰ **S92.056** Nondisplaced other extraarticular fracture of unspecified calcaneus `CC` `H5`

✓6ᵗʰ S92.06 Intraarticular fracture of calcaneus
- ³ ✓7ᵗʰ **S92.061** Displaced intraarticular fracture of right calcaneus `CC` `H5`
- ³ ✓7ᵗʰ **S92.062** Displaced intraarticular fracture of left calcaneus `CC` `H5`
- ³ ✓7ᵗʰ **S92.063** Displaced intraarticular fracture of unspecified calcaneus `CC` `H5`
- ³ ✓7ᵗʰ **S92.064** Nondisplaced intraarticular fracture of right calcaneus `CC` `H5`
- ³ ✓7ᵗʰ **S92.065** Nondisplaced intraarticular fracture of left calcaneus `CC` `H5`
- ³ ✓7ᵗʰ **S92.066** Nondisplaced intraarticular fracture of unspecified calcaneus `CC` `H5`

✓5ᵗʰ S92.1 Fracture of talus
Astragalus

> **CC Excl: For codes in subcategory S92.1:**
> **CC with 7th character B:** PDX collection 1368
> **CC with 7th character K or P:** PDX collection 897

✓6ᵗʰ S92.10 Unspecified fracture of talus
- ³ ✓7ᵗʰ **S92.101** Unspecified fracture of right talus `CC` `H5`
- ³ ✓7ᵗʰ **S92.102** Unspecified fracture of left talus `CC` `H5`
- ³ ✓7ᵗʰ **S92.109** Unspecified fracture of unspecified talus `CC` `H5`

✓6ᵗʰ S92.11 Fracture of neck of talus
- ³ ✓7ᵗʰ **S92.111** Displaced fracture of neck of right talus `CC` `H5`
- ³ ✓7ᵗʰ **S92.112** Displaced fracture of neck of left talus `CC` `H5`
- ³ ✓7ᵗʰ **S92.113** Displaced fracture of neck of unspecified talus `CC` `H5`
- ³ ✓7ᵗʰ **S92.114** Nondisplaced fracture of neck of right talus `CC` `H5`
- ³ ✓7ᵗʰ **S92.115** Nondisplaced fracture of neck of left talus `CC` `H5`
- ³ ✓7ᵗʰ **S92.116** Nondisplaced fracture of neck of unspecified talus `CC` `H5`

✓6ᵗʰ S92.12 Fracture of body of talus
- ³ ✓7ᵗʰ **S92.121** Displaced fracture of body of right talus `CC` `H5`
- ³ ✓7ᵗʰ **S92.122** Displaced fracture of body of left talus `CC` `H5`
- ³ ✓7ᵗʰ **S92.123** Displaced fracture of body of unspecified talus `CC` `H5`
- ³ ✓7ᵗʰ **S92.124** Nondisplaced fracture of body of right talus `CC` `H5`
- ³ ✓7ᵗʰ **S92.125** Nondisplaced fracture of body of left talus `CC` `H5`
- ³ ✓7ᵗʰ **S92.126** Nondisplaced fracture of body of unspecified talus `CC` `H5`

✓6ᵗʰ S92.13 Fracture of posterior process of talus
- ³ ✓7ᵗʰ **S92.131** Displaced fracture of posterior process of right talus `CC` `H5`
- ³ ✓7ᵗʰ **S92.132** Displaced fracture of posterior process of left talus `CC` `H5`

N Newborn: 0 **P** Pediatric: 0-17 **M** Maternity: 12-55 **A** Adult: 15-124 **MCC** Major Complication/Comorbidity **CC** Complication/Comorbidity **SW** Severe Wound Dx

1070 ICD-10-CM 2019

3 ☑7ᵗʰ **S92.133** Displaced fracture of posterior process of unspecified talus   CC H5

3 ☑7ᵗʰ **S92.134** Nondisplaced fracture of posterior process of right talus   CC H5

3 ☑7ᵗʰ **S92.135** Nondisplaced fracture of posterior process of left talus   CC H5

3 ☑7ᵗʰ **S92.136** Nondisplaced fracture of posterior process of unspecified talus   CC H5

☑6ᵗʰ **S92.14** Dome fracture of talus
> EXCLUDES 1   osteochondritis dissecans (M93.2)

3 ☑7ᵗʰ **S92.141** Displaced dome fracture of right talus   CC H5

3 ☑7ᵗʰ **S92.142** Displaced dome fracture of left talus   CC H5

3 ☑7ᵗʰ **S92.143** Displaced dome fracture of unspecified talus   CC H5

3 ☑7ᵗʰ **S92.144** Nondisplaced dome fracture of right talus   CC H5

3 ☑7ᵗʰ **S92.145** Nondisplaced dome fracture of left talus   CC H5

3 ☑7ᵗʰ **S92.146** Nondisplaced dome fracture of unspecified talus   CC H5

☑6ᵗʰ **S92.15** Avulsion fracture (chip fracture) of talus

3 ☑7ᵗʰ **S92.151** Displaced avulsion fracture (chip fracture) of right talus   CC H5

3 ☑7ᵗʰ **S92.152** Displaced avulsion fracture (chip fracture) of left talus   CC H5

3 ☑7ᵗʰ **S92.153** Displaced avulsion fracture (chip fracture) of unspecified talus   CC H5

3 ☑7ᵗʰ **S92.154** Nondisplaced avulsion fracture (chip fracture) of right talus   CC H5

3 ☑7ᵗʰ **S92.155** Nondisplaced avulsion fracture (chip fracture) of left talus   CC H5

3 ☑7ᵗʰ **S92.156** Nondisplaced avulsion fracture (chip fracture) of unspecified talus   CC H5

☑6ᵗʰ **S92.19** Other fracture of talus

3 ☑7ᵗʰ **S92.191** Other fracture of right talus   CC H5

3 ☑7ᵗʰ **S92.192** Other fracture of left talus   CC H5

3 ☑7ᵗʰ **S92.199** Other fracture of unspecified talus   CC H5

☑5ᵗʰ **S92.2** Fracture of other and unspecified tarsal bone(s)

> **CC Excl:** For codes in subcategory S92.2, unless otherwise noted:
> **CC with 7th character B:** PDX collection 1368
> **CC with 7th character K or P:** PDX collection 897

☑6ᵗʰ **S92.20** Fracture of unspecified tarsal bone(s)

> **CC Excl:** For codes in subcategory S92.20:
> **CC with 7th character B:** PDX collection 1369
> **CC with 7th character K or P:** PDX collection 897

3 ☑7ᵗʰ **S92.201** Fracture of unspecified tarsal bone(s) of right foot   CC H5

3 ☑7ᵗʰ **S92.202** Fracture of unspecified tarsal bone(s) of left foot   CC H5

3 ☑7ᵗʰ **S92.209** Fracture of unspecified tarsal bone(s) of unspecified foot   CC H5

☑6ᵗʰ **S92.21** Fracture of cuboid bone

3 ☑7ᵗʰ **S92.211** Displaced fracture of cuboid bone of right foot   CC H5

3 ☑7ᵗʰ **S92.212** Displaced fracture of cuboid bone of left foot   CC H5

3 ☑7ᵗʰ **S92.213** Displaced fracture of cuboid bone of unspecified foot   CC H5

3 ☑7ᵗʰ **S92.214** Nondisplaced fracture of cuboid bone of right foot   CC H5

3 ☑7ᵗʰ **S92.215** Nondisplaced fracture of cuboid bone of left foot   CC H5

3 ☑7ᵗʰ **S92.216** Nondisplaced fracture of cuboid bone of unspecified foot   CC H5

☑6ᵗʰ **S92.22** Fracture of lateral cuneiform

3 ☑7ᵗʰ **S92.221** Displaced fracture of lateral cuneiform of right foot   CC H5

3 ☑7ᵗʰ **S92.222** Displaced fracture of lateral cuneiform of left foot   CC H5

3 ☑7ᵗʰ **S92.223** Displaced fracture of lateral cuneiform of unspecified foot   CC H5

3 ☑7ᵗʰ **S92.224** Nondisplaced fracture of lateral cuneiform of right foot   CC H5

3 ☑7ᵗʰ **S92.225** Nondisplaced fracture of lateral cuneiform of left foot   CC H5

3 ☑7ᵗʰ **S92.226** Nondisplaced fracture of lateral cuneiform of unspecified foot   CC H5

☑6ᵗʰ **S92.23** Fracture of intermediate cuneiform

3 ☑7ᵗʰ **S92.231** Displaced fracture of intermediate cuneiform of right foot   CC H5

3 ☑7ᵗʰ **S92.232** Displaced fracture of intermediate cuneiform of left foot   CC H5

3 ☑7ᵗʰ **S92.233** Displaced fracture of intermediate cuneiform of unspecified foot   CC H5

3 ☑7ᵗʰ **S92.234** Nondisplaced fracture of intermediate cuneiform of right foot   CC H5

3 ☑7ᵗʰ **S92.235** Nondisplaced fracture of intermediate cuneiform of left foot   CC H5

3 ☑7ᵗʰ **S92.236** Nondisplaced fracture of intermediate cuneiform of unspecified foot   CC H5

☑6ᵗʰ **S92.24** Fracture of medial cuneiform

3 ☑7ᵗʰ **S92.241** Displaced fracture of medial cuneiform of right foot   CC H5

3 ☑7ᵗʰ **S92.242** Displaced fracture of medial cuneiform of left foot   CC H5

3 ☑7ᵗʰ **S92.243** Displaced fracture of medial cuneiform of unspecified foot   CC H5

3 ☑7ᵗʰ **S92.244** Nondisplaced fracture of medial cuneiform of right foot   CC H5

3 ☑7ᵗʰ **S92.245** Nondisplaced fracture of medial cuneiform of left foot   CC H5

3 ☑7ᵗʰ **S92.246** Nondisplaced fracture of medial cuneiform of unspecified foot   CC H5

☑6ᵗʰ **S92.25** Fracture of navicular [scaphoid] of foot

3 ☑7ᵗʰ **S92.251** Displaced fracture of navicular [scaphoid] of right foot   CC H5

3 ☑7ᵗʰ **S92.252** Displaced fracture of navicular [scaphoid] of left foot   CC H5

3 ☑7ᵗʰ **S92.253** Displaced fracture of navicular [scaphoid] of unspecified foot   CC H5

3 ☑7ᵗʰ **S92.254** Nondisplaced fracture of navicular [scaphoid] of right foot   CC H5

3 ☑7ᵗʰ **S92.255** Nondisplaced fracture of navicular [scaphoid] of left foot   CC H5

3 ☑7ᵗʰ **S92.256** Nondisplaced fracture of navicular [scaphoid] of unspecified foot   CC H5

☑5ᵗʰ **S92.3** Fracture of metatarsal bone(s)
> EXCLUDES 2   physeal fracture of metatarsal (S99.1-)
> **AHA:** 2018, 1Q, 3

> **CC Excl:** For codes in subcategory S92.3:
> **CC with 7th character B:** PDX collection 1368
> **CC with 7th character K or P:** PDX collection 897

☑6ᵗʰ **S92.30** Fracture of unspecified metatarsal bone(s)

3 ☑7ᵗʰ **S92.301** Fracture of unspecified metatarsal bone(s), right foot   CC H5

3 ☑7ᵗʰ **S92.302** Fracture of unspecified metatarsal bone(s), left foot   CC H5

3 ☑7ᵗʰ **S92.309** Fracture of unspecified metatarsal bone(s), unspecified foot   CC H5

☑6ᵗʰ **S92.31** Fracture of first metatarsal bone

3 ☑7ᵗʰ **S92.311** Displaced fracture of first metatarsal bone, right foot   CC H5

3 ☑7ᵗʰ **S92.312** Displaced fracture of first metatarsal bone, left foot   CC H5

3 ☑7ᵗʰ **S92.313** Displaced fracture of first metatarsal bone, unspecified foot   CC H5

3 ☑7ᵗʰ **S92.314** Nondisplaced fracture of first metatarsal bone, right foot   CC H5

3 ☑7ᵗʰ **S92.315** Nondisplaced fracture of first metatarsal bone, left foot   CC H5

3 ☑7ᵗʰ **S92.316** Nondisplaced fracture of first metatarsal bone, unspecified foot   CC H5

☑6ᵗʰ **S92.32** Fracture of second metatarsal bone

3 ☑7ᵗʰ **S92.321** Displaced fracture of second metatarsal bone, right foot   CC H5

☑ Additional Character Required   ☑7ᵗʰ Placeholder   Unacceptable PDx   Questionable PDx   Manifestation   H1-H14 HAC   HCC CMS-HCC Dx   HIV HIV Dx

ICD-10-CM 2019   1071

Chapter 19. Injury, Poisoning and Certain Other Consequences of External Causes

3 √7ᵗʰ **S92.322** Displaced **fracture of second metatarsal bone, left foot** `CC` `H5`

3 √7ᵗʰ **S92.323** Displaced **fracture of second metatarsal bone, unspecified foot** `CC` `H5`

3 √7ᵗʰ **S92.324** Nondisplaced **fracture of second metatarsal bone, right foot** `CC` `H5`

3 √7ᵗʰ **S92.325** Nondisplaced **fracture of second metatarsal bone, left foot** `CC` `H5`

3 √7ᵗʰ **S92.326** Nondisplaced **fracture of second metatarsal bone, unspecified foot** `CC` `H5`

√6ᵗʰ **S92.33** Fracture of **third metatarsal bone**

3 √7ᵗʰ **S92.331** Displaced **fracture of third metatarsal bone, right foot** `CC` `H5`

3 √7ᵗʰ **S92.332** Displaced **fracture of third metatarsal bone, left foot** `CC` `H5`

3 √7ᵗʰ **S92.333** Displaced **fracture of third metatarsal bone, unspecified foot** `CC` `H5`

3 √7ᵗʰ **S92.334** Nondisplaced **fracture of third metatarsal bone, right foot** `CC` `H5`

3 √7ᵗʰ **S92.335** Nondisplaced **fracture of third metatarsal bone, left foot** `CC` `H5`

3 √7ᵗʰ **S92.336** Nondisplaced **fracture of third metatarsal bone, unspecified foot** `CC` `H5`

√6ᵗʰ **S92.34** Fracture of **fourth metatarsal bone**

3 √7ᵗʰ **S92.341** Displaced **fracture of fourth metatarsal bone, right foot** `CC` `H5`

3 √7ᵗʰ **S92.342** Displaced **fracture of fourth metatarsal bone, left foot** `CC` `H5`

3 √7ᵗʰ **S92.343** Displaced **fracture of fourth metatarsal bone, unspecified foot** `CC` `H5`

3 √7ᵗʰ **S92.344** Nondisplaced **fracture of fourth metatarsal bone, right foot** `CC` `H5`

3 √7ᵗʰ **S92.345** Nondisplaced **fracture of fourth metatarsal bone, left foot** `CC` `H5`

3 √7ᵗʰ **S92.346** Nondisplaced **fracture of fourth metatarsal bone, unspecified foot** `CC` `H5`

√6ᵗʰ **S92.35** Fracture of **fifth metatarsal bone**

3 √7ᵗʰ **S92.351** Displaced **fracture of fifth metatarsal bone, right foot** `CC` `H5`

3 √7ᵗʰ **S92.352** Displaced **fracture of fifth metatarsal bone, left foot** `CC` `H5`

3 √7ᵗʰ **S92.353** Displaced **fracture of fifth metatarsal bone, unspecified foot** `CC` `H5`

3 √7ᵗʰ **S92.354** Nondisplaced **fracture of fifth metatarsal bone, right foot** `CC` `H5`

3 √7ᵗʰ **S92.355** Nondisplaced **fracture of fifth metatarsal bone, left foot** `CC` `H5`

3 √7ᵗʰ **S92.356** Nondisplaced **fracture of fifth metatarsal bone, unspecified foot** `CC` `H5`

√5ᵗʰ **S92.4** Fracture of **great toe**

EXCLUDES 2   *physeal fracture of phalanx of toe (S99.2-)*

CC Excl: For codes in subcategory S92.4:
CC with 7th character K or P: PDX collection 897

√6ᵗʰ **S92.40** Unspecified **fracture of great toe**

4 √7ᵗʰ **S92.401** Displaced **unspecified fracture of right great toe** `CC`

4 √7ᵗʰ **S92.402** Displaced **unspecified fracture of left great toe** `CC`

4 √7ᵗʰ **S92.403** Displaced **unspecified fracture of unspecified great toe** `CC`

4 √7ᵗʰ **S92.404** Nondisplaced **unspecified fracture of right great toe** `CC`

4 √7ᵗʰ **S92.405** Nondisplaced **unspecified fracture of left great toe** `CC`

4 √7ᵗʰ **S92.406** Nondisplaced **unspecified fracture of unspecified great toe** `CC`

√6ᵗʰ **S92.41** Fracture of **proximal phalanx of great toe**

4 √7ᵗʰ **S92.411** Displaced **fracture of proximal phalanx of right great toe** `CC`

4 √7ᵗʰ **S92.412** Displaced **fracture of proximal phalanx of left great toe** `CC`

4 √7ᵗʰ **S92.413** Displaced **fracture of proximal phalanx of unspecified great toe** `CC`

4 √7ᵗʰ **S92.414** Nondisplaced **fracture of proximal phalanx of right great toe** `CC`

4 √7ᵗʰ **S92.415** Nondisplaced **fracture of proximal phalanx of left great toe** `CC`

4 √7ᵗʰ **S92.416** Nondisplaced **fracture of proximal phalanx of unspecified great toe** `CC`

√6ᵗʰ **S92.42** Fracture of **distal phalanx of great toe**

4 √7ᵗʰ **S92.421** Displaced **fracture of distal phalanx of right great toe** `CC`

4 √7ᵗʰ **S92.422** Displaced **fracture of distal phalanx of left great toe** `CC`

4 √7ᵗʰ **S92.423** Displaced **fracture of distal phalanx of unspecified great toe** `CC`

4 √7ᵗʰ **S92.424** Nondisplaced **fracture of distal phalanx of right great toe** `CC`

4 √7ᵗʰ **S92.425** Nondisplaced **fracture of distal phalanx of left great toe** `CC`

4 √7ᵗʰ **S92.426** Nondisplaced **fracture of distal phalanx of unspecified great toe** `CC`

√6ᵗʰ **S92.49** Other **fracture of great toe**

4 √7ᵗʰ **S92.491** Other **fracture of right great toe** `CC`

4 √7ᵗʰ **S92.492** Other **fracture of left great toe** `CC`

4 √7ᵗʰ **S92.499** Other **fracture of unspecified great toe** `CC`

√5ᵗʰ **S92.5** Fracture of **lesser toe(s)**

EXCLUDES 2   *physeal fracture of phalanx of toe (S99.2-)*

CC Excl: For codes in subcategory S92.5:
CC with 7th character K or P: PDX collection 897

√6ᵗʰ **S92.50** Unspecified **fracture of lesser toe(s)**

4 √7ᵗʰ **S92.501** Displaced **unspecified fracture of right lesser toe(s)** `CC`

4 √7ᵗʰ **S92.502** Displaced **unspecified fracture of left lesser toe(s)** `CC`

4 √7ᵗʰ **S92.503** Displaced **unspecified fracture of unspecified lesser toe(s)** `CC`

4 √7ᵗʰ **S92.504** Nondisplaced **unspecified fracture of right lesser toe(s)** `CC`

4 √7ᵗʰ **S92.505** Nondisplaced **unspecified fracture of left lesser toe(s)** `CC`

4 √7ᵗʰ **S92.506** Nondisplaced **unspecified fracture of unspecified lesser toe(s)** `CC`

√6ᵗʰ **S92.51** Fracture of **proximal phalanx of lesser toe(s)**

4 √7ᵗʰ **S92.511** Displaced **fracture of proximal phalanx of right lesser toe(s)** `CC`

4 √7ᵗʰ **S92.512** Displaced **fracture of proximal phalanx of left lesser toe(s)** `CC`

4 √7ᵗʰ **S92.513** Displaced **fracture of proximal phalanx of unspecified lesser toe(s)** `CC`

4 √7ᵗʰ **S92.514** Nondisplaced **fracture of proximal phalanx of right lesser toe(s)** `CC`

4 √7ᵗʰ **S92.515** Nondisplaced **fracture of proximal phalanx of left lesser toe(s)** `CC`

4 √7ᵗʰ **S92.516** Nondisplaced **fracture of proximal phalanx of unspecified lesser toe(s)** `CC`

√6ᵗʰ **S92.52** Fracture of **middle phalanx of lesser toe(s)**

4 √7ᵗʰ **S92.521** Displaced **fracture of middle phalanx of right lesser toe(s)** `CC`

4 √7ᵗʰ **S92.522** Displaced **fracture of middle phalanx of left lesser toe(s)** `CC`

4 √7ᵗʰ **S92.523** Displaced **fracture of middle phalanx of unspecified lesser toe(s)** `CC`

4 √7ᵗʰ **S92.524** Nondisplaced **fracture of middle phalanx of right lesser toe(s)** `CC`

4 √7ᵗʰ **S92.525** Nondisplaced **fracture of middle phalanx of left lesser toe(s)** `CC`

4 √7ᵗʰ **S92.526** Nondisplaced **fracture of middle phalanx of unspecified lesser toe(s)** `CC`

√6ᵗʰ **S92.53** Fracture of **distal phalanx of lesser toe(s)**

4 √7ᵗʰ **S92.531** Displaced **fracture of distal phalanx of right lesser toe(s)** `CC`

4 √7ᵗʰ **S92.532** Displaced **fracture of distal phalanx of left lesser toe(s)** `CC`

4 √7ᵗʰ **S92.533** Displaced **fracture of distal phalanx of unspecified lesser toe(s)** `CC`

4 √7ᵗʰ **S92.534** Nondisplaced **fracture of distal phalanx of right lesser toe(s)** `CC`

Ⓝ Newborn: 0   Ⓟ Pediatric: 0-17   Ⓜ Maternity: 12-55   Ⓐ Adult: 15-124   `MCC` Major Complication/Comorbidity   `CC` Complication/Comorbidity   `SW` Severe Wound Dx

1072   ICD-10-CM 2019

4 ✓7ᵗʰ **S92.535** Nondisplaced **fracture of distal phalanx of** left lesser **toe(s)** `CC`

4 ✓7ᵗʰ **S92.536** Nondisplaced **fracture of distal phalanx of** unspecified lesser **toe(s)** `CC`

✓6ᵗʰ **S92.59** Other **fracture of lesser toe(s)**

4 ✓7ᵗʰ **S92.591** Other **fracture of** right lesser **toe(s)** `CC`

4 ✓7ᵗʰ **S92.592** Other **fracture of** left lesser **toe(s)** `CC`

4 ✓7ᵗʰ **S92.599** Other **fracture of** unspecified lesser **toe(s)** `CC`

✓5ᵗʰ **S92.8** Other **fracture of foot, except ankle**

✓6ᵗʰ **S92.81** Other **fracture of foot**
Sesamoid fracture of foot
AHA: 2016, 4Q, 68

> **CC Excl: For codes in subcategory S92.81:**
> **CC with 7th character B:** PDX collection 1369
> **CC with 7th character K or P:** PDX collection 897

3 ✓7ᵗʰ **S92.811** Other **fracture of** right **foot** `CC` `H5`

3 ✓7ᵗʰ **S92.812** Other **fracture of** left **foot** `CC` `H5`

3 ✓7ᵗʰ **S92.819** Other **fracture of** unspecified **foot** `CC` `H5`

✓5ᵗʰ **S92.9** Unspecified **fracture of foot and toe**

✓6ᵗʰ **S92.90** Unspecified **fracture of** foot

> **CC Excl: For codes in subcategory S92.90:**
> **CC with 7th character B:** PDX collection 1369
> **CC with 7th character K or P:** PDX collection 897

3 ✓7ᵗʰ **S92.901** Unspecified **fracture of** right **foot** `CC` `H5`

3 ✓7ᵗʰ **S92.902** Unspecified **fracture of** left **foot** `CC` `H5`

3 ✓7ᵗʰ **S92.909** Unspecified **fracture of** unspecified **foot** `CC` `H5`

✓6ᵗʰ **S92.91** Unspecified **fracture of** toe

> **CC Excl: For codes in subcategory S92.91:**
> **CC with 7th character K or P:** PDX collection 897

4 ✓7ᵗʰ **S92.911** Unspecified **fracture of** right **toe(s)** `CC`

4 ✓7ᵗʰ **S92.912** Unspecified **fracture of** left **toe(s)** `CC`

4 ✓7ᵗʰ **S92.919** Unspecified **fracture of** unspecified **toe(s)** `CC`

✓4ᵗʰ **S93** **Dislocation and sprain of joints and ligaments at ankle, foot and toe level**

INCLUDES   avulsion of joint or ligament of ankle, foot and toe
laceration of cartilage, joint or ligament of ankle, foot and toe
sprain of cartilage, joint or ligament of ankle, foot and toe
traumatic hemarthrosis of joint or ligament of ankle, foot and toe
traumatic rupture of joint or ligament of ankle, foot and toe
traumatic subluxation of joint or ligament of ankle, foot and toe
traumatic tear of joint or ligament of ankle, foot and toe

Code also any associated open wound

EXCLUDES 2   strain of muscle and tendon of ankle and foot (S96.-)

> The appropriate 7th character is to be added to each code from category S93.
> A   initial encounter
> D   subsequent encounter
> S   sequela

✓5ᵗʰ **S93.0** **Subluxation and dislocation of** ankle joint
Subluxation and dislocation of astragalus
Subluxation and dislocation of fibula, lower end
Subluxation and dislocation of talus
Subluxation and dislocation of tibia, lower end

✓×7ᵗʰ **S93.01** Subluxation **of** right **ankle joint**

✓×7ᵗʰ **S93.02** Subluxation **of** left **ankle joint**

✓×7ᵗʰ **S93.03** Subluxation **of** unspecified **ankle joint**

✓×7ᵗʰ **S93.04** Dislocation **of** right **ankle joint**

✓×7ᵗʰ **S93.05** Dislocation **of** left **ankle joint**

✓×7ᵗʰ **S93.06** Dislocation **of** unspecified **ankle joint**

✓5ᵗʰ **S93.1** **Subluxation and dislocation of** toe

✓6ᵗʰ **S93.10** Unspecified **subluxation and dislocation of toe**
Dislocation of toe NOS
Subluxation of toe NOS

✓7ᵗʰ **S93.101** Unspecified **subluxation of** right **toe(s)**

✓7ᵗʰ **S93.102** Unspecified **subluxation of** left **toe(s)**

✓7ᵗʰ **S93.103** Unspecified **subluxation of** unspecified **toe(s)**

✓7ᵗʰ **S93.104** Unspecified **dislocation of** right **toe(s)**

✓7ᵗʰ **S93.105** Unspecified **dislocation of** left **toe(s)**

✓7ᵗʰ **S93.106** Unspecified **dislocation of** unspecified **toe(s)**

✓6ᵗʰ **S93.11** Dislocation **of** interphalangeal joint

✓7ᵗʰ **S93.111** Dislocation of interphalangeal joint of right great **toe**

✓7ᵗʰ **S93.112** Dislocation of interphalangeal joint of left great **toe**

✓7ᵗʰ **S93.113** Dislocation of interphalangeal joint of unspecified great **toe**

✓7ᵗʰ **S93.114** Dislocation of interphalangeal joint of right lesser **toe(s)**

✓7ᵗʰ **S93.115** Dislocation of interphalangeal joint of left lesser **toe(s)**

✓7ᵗʰ **S93.116** Dislocation of interphalangeal joint of unspecified lesser **toe(s)**

✓7ᵗʰ **S93.119** Dislocation of interphalangeal joint of unspecified **toe(s)**

✓6ᵗʰ **S93.12** Dislocation **of** metatarsophalangeal joint

✓7ᵗʰ **S93.121** Dislocation of metatarsophalangeal joint of right great **toe**

✓7ᵗʰ **S93.122** Dislocation of metatarsophalangeal joint of left great **toe**

✓7ᵗʰ **S93.123** Dislocation of metatarsophalangeal joint of unspecified great **toe**

✓7ᵗʰ **S93.124** Dislocation of metatarsophalangeal joint of right lesser **toe(s)**

✓7ᵗʰ **S93.125** Dislocation of metatarsophalangeal joint of left lesser **toe(s)**

✓7ᵗʰ **S93.126** Dislocation of metatarsophalangeal joint of unspecified lesser **toe(s)**

✓7ᵗʰ **S93.129** Dislocation of metatarsophalangeal joint of unspecified **toe(s)**

✓6ᵗʰ **S93.13** Subluxation **of** interphalangeal joint

✓7ᵗʰ **S93.131** Subluxation of interphalangeal joint of right great **toe**

✓7ᵗʰ **S93.132** Subluxation of interphalangeal joint of left great **toe**

✓7ᵗʰ **S93.133** Subluxation of interphalangeal joint of unspecified great **toe**

✓7ᵗʰ **S93.134** Subluxation of interphalangeal joint of right lesser **toe(s)**

✓7ᵗʰ **S93.135** Subluxation of interphalangeal joint of left lesser **toe(s)**

✓7ᵗʰ **S93.136** Subluxation of interphalangeal joint of unspecified lesser **toe(s)**

✓7ᵗʰ **S93.139** Subluxation of interphalangeal joint of unspecified **toe(s)**

✓6ᵗʰ **S93.14** Subluxation **of** metatarsophalangeal joint

✓7ᵗʰ **S93.141** Subluxation of metatarsophalangeal joint of right great **toe**

✓7ᵗʰ **S93.142** Subluxation of metatarsophalangeal joint of left great **toe**

✓7ᵗʰ **S93.143** Subluxation of metatarsophalangeal joint of unspecified great **toe**

✓7ᵗʰ **S93.144** Subluxation of metatarsophalangeal joint of right lesser **toe(s)**

✓7ᵗʰ **S93.145** Subluxation of metatarsophalangeal joint of left lesser **toe(s)**

✓7ᵗʰ **S93.146** Subluxation of metatarsophalangeal joint of unspecified lesser **toe(s)**

✓7ᵗʰ **S93.149** Subluxation of metatarsophalangeal joint of unspecified **toe(s)**

✓5ᵗʰ **S93.3** **Subluxation and dislocation of foot**
EXCLUDES 2   dislocation of toe (S93.1-)

✓6ᵗʰ **S93.30** Unspecified **subluxation and dislocation of foot**
Dislocation of foot NOS
Subluxation of foot NOS

✓7ᵗʰ **S93.301** Unspecified **subluxation of** right **foot**

✓7ᵗʰ **S93.302** Unspecified **subluxation of** left **foot**

✓7ᵗʰ **S93.303** Unspecified **subluxation of** unspecified **foot**

✓7ᵗʰ **S93.304** Unspecified **dislocation of** right **foot**

☑Additional Character Required   ✓×7ᵗʰ Placeholder   Unacceptable PDx   Questionable PDx   Manifestation   `H1`-`H14` HAC   `HCC` CMS-HCC Dx   `HIV` HIV Dx

ICD-10-CM 2019   1073

√7th **S93.305** Unspecified dislocation of left foot

√7th **S93.306** Unspecified dislocation of unspecified foot

✓6th **S93.31** Subluxation and dislocation of tarsal joint

√7th **S93.311** Subluxation of tarsal joint of right foot

√7th **S93.312** Subluxation of tarsal joint of left foot

√7th **S93.313** Subluxation of tarsal joint of unspecified foot

√7th **S93.314** Dislocation of tarsal joint of right foot

√7th **S93.315** Dislocation of tarsal joint of left foot

√7th **S93.316** Dislocation of tarsal joint of unspecified foot

✓6th **S93.32** Subluxation and dislocation of tarsometatarsal joint

√7th **S93.321** Subluxation of tarsometatarsal joint of right foot

√7th **S93.322** Subluxation of tarsometatarsal joint of left foot

√7th **S93.323** Subluxation of tarsometatarsal joint of unspecified foot

√7th **S93.324** Dislocation of tarsometatarsal joint of right foot

√7th **S93.325** Dislocation of tarsometatarsal joint of left foot

√7th **S93.326** Dislocation of tarsometatarsal joint of unspecified foot

✓6th **S93.33** Other subluxation and dislocation of foot

√7th **S93.331** Other subluxation of right foot

√7th **S93.332** Other subluxation of left foot

√7th **S93.333** Other subluxation of unspecified foot

√7th **S93.334** Other dislocation of right foot

√7th **S93.335** Other dislocation of left foot

√7th **S93.336** Other dislocation of unspecified foot

✓5th **S93.4** Sprain of ankle

> EXCLUDES 2   injury of Achilles tendon (S86.0-)

✓6th **S93.40** Sprain of unspecified ligament of ankle
Sprain of ankle NOS
Sprained ankle NOS

√7th **S93.401** Sprain of unspecified ligament of right ankle

√7th **S93.402** Sprain of unspecified ligament of left ankle

√7th **S93.409** Sprain of unspecified ligament of unspecified ankle

✓6th **S93.41** Sprain of calcaneofibular ligament

√7th **S93.411** Sprain of calcaneofibular ligament of right ankle

√7th **S93.412** Sprain of calcaneofibular ligament of left ankle

√7th **S93.419** Sprain of calcaneofibular ligament of unspecified ankle

✓6th **S93.42** Sprain of deltoid ligament

√7th **S93.421** Sprain of deltoid ligament of right ankle

√7th **S93.422** Sprain of deltoid ligament of left ankle

√7th **S93.429** Sprain of deltoid ligament of unspecified ankle

✓6th **S93.43** Sprain of tibiofibular ligament

√7th **S93.431** Sprain of tibiofibular ligament of right ankle

√7th **S93.432** Sprain of tibiofibular ligament of left ankle

√7th **S93.439** Sprain of tibiofibular ligament of unspecified ankle

✓6th **S93.49** Sprain of other ligament of ankle
Sprain of internal collateral ligament
Sprain of talofibular ligament

√7th **S93.491** Sprain of other ligament of right ankle

√7th **S93.492** Sprain of other ligament of left ankle

√7th **S93.499** Sprain of other ligament of unspecified ankle

✓5th **S93.5** Sprain of toe

✓6th **S93.50** Unspecified sprain of toe

√7th **S93.501** Unspecified sprain of right great toe

√7th **S93.502** Unspecified sprain of left great toe

√7th **S93.503** Unspecified sprain of unspecified great toe

√7th **S93.504** Unspecified sprain of right lesser toe(s)

√7th **S93.505** Unspecified sprain of left lesser toe(s)

√7th **S93.506** Unspecified sprain of unspecified lesser toe(s)

√7th **S93.509** Unspecified sprain of unspecified toe(s)

✓6th **S93.51** Sprain of interphalangeal joint of toe

√7th **S93.511** Sprain of interphalangeal joint of right great toe

√7th **S93.512** Sprain of interphalangeal joint of left great toe

√7th **S93.513** Sprain of interphalangeal joint of unspecified great toe

√7th **S93.514** Sprain of interphalangeal joint of right lesser toe(s)

√7th **S93.515** Sprain of interphalangeal joint of left lesser toe(s)

√7th **S93.516** Sprain of interphalangeal joint of unspecified lesser toe(s)

√7th **S93.519** Sprain of interphalangeal joint of unspecified toe(s)

✓6th **S93.52** Sprain of metatarsophalangeal joint of toe

√7th **S93.521** Sprain of metatarsophalangeal joint of right great toe

√7th **S93.522** Sprain of metatarsophalangeal joint of left great toe

√7th **S93.523** Sprain of metatarsophalangeal joint of unspecified great toe

√7th **S93.524** Sprain of metatarsophalangeal joint of right lesser toe(s)

√7th **S93.525** Sprain of metatarsophalangeal joint of left lesser toe(s)

√7th **S93.526** Sprain of metatarsophalangeal joint of unspecified lesser toe(s)

√7th **S93.529** Sprain of metatarsophalangeal joint of unspecified toe(s)

✓5th **S93.6** Sprain of foot

> EXCLUDES 2   sprain of metatarsophalangeal joint of toe (S93.52-)
> sprain of toe (S93.5-)

✓6th **S93.60** Unspecified sprain of foot

√7th **S93.601** Unspecified sprain of right foot

√7th **S93.602** Unspecified sprain of left foot

√7th **S93.609** Unspecified sprain of unspecified foot

✓6th **S93.61** Sprain of tarsal ligament of foot

√7th **S93.611** Sprain of tarsal ligament of right foot

√7th **S93.612** Sprain of tarsal ligament of left foot

√7th **S93.619** Sprain of tarsal ligament of unspecified foot

✓6th **S93.62** Sprain of tarsometatarsal ligament of foot

√7th **S93.621** Sprain of tarsometatarsal ligament of right foot

√7th **S93.622** Sprain of tarsometatarsal ligament of left foot

√7th **S93.629** Sprain of tarsometatarsal ligament of unspecified foot

✓6th **S93.69** Other sprain of foot

√7th **S93.691** Other sprain of right foot

√7th **S93.692** Other sprain of left foot

√7th **S93.699** Other sprain of unspecified foot

✓4th **S94** Injury of nerves at ankle and foot level
Code also any associated open wound (S91.-)

> The appropriate 7th character is to be added to each code from category S94.
> A   initial encounter
> D   subsequent encounter
> S   sequela

✓5th **S94.0** Injury of lateral plantar nerve

√x7th **S94.00** Injury of lateral plantar nerve, unspecified leg

√x7th **S94.01** Injury of lateral plantar nerve, right leg

√x7th **S94.02** Injury of lateral plantar nerve, left leg

N Newborn: 0   **P** Pediatric: 0-17   **M** Maternity: 12-55   **A** Adult: 15-124   **MCC** Major Complication/Comorbidity   **CC** Complication/Comorbidity   **SW** Severe Wound Dx

1074   ICD-10-CM 2019

√5ᵗʰ **S94.1 Injury of medial plantar nerve**

√x7ᵗʰ **S94.10 Injury of medial plantar nerve, unspecified leg**

√x7ᵗʰ **S94.11 Injury of medial plantar nerve, right leg**

√x7ᵗʰ **S94.12 Injury of medial plantar nerve, left leg**

√5ᵗʰ **S94.2 Injury of deep peroneal nerve at ankle and foot level**
Injury of terminal, lateral branch of deep peroneal nerve

√x7ᵗʰ **S94.20 Injury of deep peroneal nerve at ankle and foot level, unspecified leg**

√x7ᵗʰ **S94.21 Injury of deep peroneal nerve at ankle and foot level, right leg**

√x7ᵗʰ **S94.22 Injury of deep peroneal nerve at ankle and foot level, left leg**

√5ᵗʰ **S94.3 Injury of cutaneous sensory nerve at ankle and foot level**

√x7ᵗʰ **S94.30 Injury of cutaneous sensory nerve at ankle and foot level, unspecified leg**

√x7ᵗʰ **S94.31 Injury of cutaneous sensory nerve at ankle and foot level, right leg**

√x7ᵗʰ **S94.32 Injury of cutaneous sensory nerve at ankle and foot level, left leg**

√5ᵗʰ **S94.8 Injury of other nerves at ankle and foot level**

√6ᵗʰ **S94.8X Injury of other nerves at ankle and foot level**

√7ᵗʰ **S94.8X1 Injury of other nerves at ankle and foot level, right leg**

√7ᵗʰ **S94.8X2 Injury of other nerves at ankle and foot level, left leg**

√7ᵗʰ **S94.8X9 Injury of other nerves at ankle and foot level, unspecified leg**

√5ᵗʰ **S94.9 Injury of unspecified nerve at ankle and foot level**

√x7ᵗʰ **S94.90 Injury of unspecified nerve at ankle and foot level, unspecified leg**

√x7ᵗʰ **S94.91 Injury of unspecified nerve at ankle and foot level, right leg**

√x7ᵗʰ **S94.92 Injury of unspecified nerve at ankle and foot level, left leg**

√4ᵗʰ **S95 Injury of blood vessels at ankle and foot level**
Code also any associated open wound (S91.-)
EXCLUDES 2 *injury of posterior tibial artery and vein (S85.1-, S85.8-)*

The appropriate 7th character is to be added to each code from category S95.
A   initial encounter
D   subsequent encounter
S   sequela

CC Excl: For CC codes in category S95, unless otherwise noted:
Right side: PDX collection 1325
Left side: PDX collection 1326
Unspecified side: PDX collection 1327

√5ᵗʰ **S95.0 Injury of dorsal artery of foot**

√6ᵗʰ **S95.00 Unspecified injury of dorsal artery of foot**

√7ᵗʰ **S95.001 Unspecified injury of dorsal artery of right foot** CC

√7ᵗʰ **S95.002 Unspecified injury of dorsal artery of left foot** CC

√7ᵗʰ **S95.009 Unspecified injury of dorsal artery of unspecified foot** CC

√6ᵗʰ **S95.01 Laceration of dorsal artery of foot**

√7ᵗʰ **S95.011 Laceration of dorsal artery of left foot** CC

√7ᵗʰ **S95.012 Laceration of dorsal artery of left foot** CC

√7ᵗʰ **S95.019 Laceration of dorsal artery of unspecified foot** CC

√6ᵗʰ **S95.09 Other specified injury of dorsal artery of foot**

√7ᵗʰ **S95.091 Other specified injury of dorsal artery of right foot** CC

√7ᵗʰ **S95.092 Other specified injury of dorsal artery of left foot** CC

√7ᵗʰ **S95.099 Other specified injury of dorsal artery of unspecified foot** CC

√5ᵗʰ **S95.1 Injury of plantar artery of foot**

CC Excl: For CC codes in subcategory S95.1:
Right side: PDX collection 1370
Left side: PDX collection 1371
Unspecified side: PDX collection 1372

√6ᵗʰ **S95.10 Unspecified injury of plantar artery of foot**

√7ᵗʰ **S95.101 Unspecified injury of plantar artery of right foot** CC

√7ᵗʰ **S95.102 Unspecified injury of plantar artery of left foot** CC

√7ᵗʰ **S95.109 Unspecified injury of plantar artery of unspecified foot** CC

√6ᵗʰ **S95.11 Laceration of plantar artery of foot**

√7ᵗʰ **S95.111 Laceration of plantar artery of right foot** CC

√7ᵗʰ **S95.112 Laceration of plantar artery of left foot** CC

√7ᵗʰ **S95.119 Laceration of plantar artery of unspecified foot** CC

√6ᵗʰ **S95.19 Other specified injury of plantar artery of foot**

√7ᵗʰ **S95.191 Other specified injury of plantar artery of right foot** CC

√7ᵗʰ **S95.192 Other specified injury of plantar artery of left foot** CC

√7ᵗʰ **S95.199 Other specified injury of plantar artery of unspecified foot** CC

√5ᵗʰ **S95.2 Injury of dorsal vein of foot**

√6ᵗʰ **S95.20 Unspecified injury of dorsal vein of foot**

√7ᵗʰ **S95.201 Unspecified injury of dorsal vein of right foot** CC

√7ᵗʰ **S95.202 Unspecified injury of dorsal vein of left foot** CC

√7ᵗʰ **S95.209 Unspecified injury of dorsal vein of unspecified foot** CC

√6ᵗʰ **S95.21 Laceration of dorsal vein of foot**

√7ᵗʰ **S95.211 Laceration of dorsal vein of right foot** CC

√7ᵗʰ **S95.212 Laceration of dorsal vein of left foot** CC

√7ᵗʰ **S95.219 Laceration of dorsal vein of unspecified foot** CC

√6ᵗʰ **S95.29 Other specified injury of dorsal vein of foot**

√7ᵗʰ **S95.291 Other specified injury of dorsal vein of right foot** CC

√7ᵗʰ **S95.292 Other specified injury of dorsal vein of left foot** CC

√7ᵗʰ **S95.299 Other specified injury of dorsal vein of unspecified foot** CC

√5ᵗʰ **S95.8 Injury of other blood vessels at ankle and foot level**

√6ᵗʰ **S95.80 Unspecified injury of other blood vessels at ankle and foot level**

√7ᵗʰ **S95.801 Unspecified injury of other blood vessels at ankle and foot level, right leg** CC

√7ᵗʰ **S95.802 Unspecified injury of other blood vessels at ankle and foot level, left leg** CC

√7ᵗʰ **S95.809 Unspecified injury of other blood vessels at ankle and foot level, unspecified leg** CC

√6ᵗʰ **S95.81 Laceration of other blood vessels at ankle and foot level**

√7ᵗʰ **S95.811 Laceration of other blood vessels at ankle and foot level, right leg** CC

√7ᵗʰ **S95.812 Laceration of other blood vessels at ankle and foot level, left leg** CC

√7ᵗʰ **S95.819 Laceration of other blood vessels at ankle and foot level, unspecified leg** CC

√6ᵗʰ **S95.89 Other specified injury of other blood vessels at ankle and foot level**

√7ᵗʰ **S95.891 Other specified injury of other blood vessels at ankle and foot level, right leg** CC

√7ᵗʰ **S95.892 Other specified injury of other blood vessels at ankle and foot level, left leg** CC

√7ᵗʰ **S95.899 Other specified injury of other blood vessels at ankle and foot level, unspecified leg** CC

✔ Additional Character Required   √x7ᵗʰ Placeholder   Unacceptable PDx   Questionable PDx   Manifestation   H1-H14 HAC   HCC CMS-HCC Dx   HIV HIV Dx

ICD-10-CM 2019   1075

✓5ᵗʰ **S95.9** **Injury of** unspecified blood vessel **at ankle and foot level**

     ✓6ᵗʰ **S95.90** Unspecified **injury of unspecified blood vessel at ankle and foot level**

         ✓7ᵗʰ **S95.901** **Unspecified injury of unspecified blood vessel at ankle and foot level,** right **leg** `CC`

         ✓7ᵗʰ **S95.902** **Unspecified injury of unspecified blood vessel at ankle and foot level,** left **leg** `CC`

         ✓7ᵗʰ **S95.909** **Unspecified injury of unspecified blood vessel at ankle and foot level,** unspecified **leg** `CC`

     ✓6ᵗʰ **S95.91** Laceration **of unspecified blood vessel at ankle and foot level**

         ✓7ᵗʰ **S95.911** **Laceration of unspecified blood vessel at ankle and foot level,** right **leg** `CC`

         ✓7ᵗʰ **S95.912** **Laceration of unspecified blood vessel at ankle and foot level,** left **leg** `CC`

         ✓7ᵗʰ **S95.919** **Laceration of unspecified blood vessel at ankle and foot level,** unspecified **leg** `CC`

     ✓6ᵗʰ **S95.99** Other **specified injury of unspecified blood vessel at ankle and foot level**

         ✓7ᵗʰ **S95.991** **Other specified injury of unspecified blood vessel at ankle and foot level,** right **leg** `CC`

         ✓7ᵗʰ **S95.992** **Other specified injury of unspecified blood vessel at ankle and foot level,** left **leg** `CC`

         ✓7ᵗʰ **S95.999** **Other specified injury of unspecified blood vessel at ankle and foot level,** unspecified **leg** `CC`

✓4ᵗʰ **S96** **Injury of muscle and tendon at ankle and foot level**

     Code also any associated open wound (S91.-)

     EXCLUDES 2   *injury of Achilles tendon (S86.0-)*
                    sprain of joints and ligaments of ankle and foot (S93.-)

     TIP: Refer to the Muscle/Tendon table at the beginning of this chapter

     The appropriate 7th character is to be added to each code from category S96.
     A   initial encounter
     D   subsequent encounter
     S   sequela

     CC Excl: For CC codes in category S96:
     Right side: PDX collection 1364
     Left side: PDX collection 1365
     Unspecified side: PDX collection 1366

     ✓5ᵗʰ **S96.0** **Injury of muscle and tendon of** long flexor muscle of toe **at ankle and foot level**

         ✓6ᵗʰ **S96.00** Unspecified **injury of muscle and tendon of long flexor muscle of toe at ankle and foot level**

             ✓7ᵗʰ **S96.001** **Unspecified injury of muscle and tendon of long flexor muscle of toe at ankle and foot level,** right **foot**

             ✓7ᵗʰ **S96.002** **Unspecified injury of muscle and tendon of long flexor muscle of toe at ankle and foot level,** left **foot**

             ✓7ᵗʰ **S96.009** **Unspecified injury of muscle and tendon of long flexor muscle of toe at ankle and foot level,** unspecified **foot**

         ✓6ᵗʰ **S96.01** Strain **of muscle and tendon of long flexor muscle of toe at ankle and foot level**

             ✓7ᵗʰ **S96.011** **Strain of muscle and tendon of long flexor muscle of toe at ankle and foot level,** right **foot**

             ✓7ᵗʰ **S96.012** **Strain of muscle and tendon of long flexor muscle of toe at ankle and foot level,** left **foot**

             ✓7ᵗʰ **S96.019** **Strain of muscle and tendon of long flexor muscle of toe at ankle and foot level,** unspecified **foot**

         ✓6ᵗʰ **S96.02** Laceration **of muscle and tendon of long flexor muscle of toe at ankle and foot level**

             ✓7ᵗʰ **S96.021** **Laceration of muscle and tendon of long flexor muscle of toe at ankle and foot level,** right **foot** `CC`

             ✓7ᵗʰ **S96.022** **Laceration of muscle and tendon of long flexor muscle of toe at ankle and foot level,** left **foot** `CC`

             ✓7ᵗʰ **S96.029** **Laceration of muscle and tendon of long flexor muscle of toe at ankle and foot level,** unspecified **foot** `CC`

         ✓6ᵗʰ **S96.09** Other **injury of muscle and tendon of long flexor muscle of toe at ankle and foot level**

             ✓7ᵗʰ **S96.091** **Other injury of muscle and tendon of long flexor muscle of toe at ankle and foot level,** right **foot**

             ✓7ᵗʰ **S96.092** **Other injury of muscle and tendon of long flexor muscle of toe at ankle and foot level,** left **foot**

             ✓7ᵗʰ **S96.099** **Other injury of muscle and tendon of long flexor muscle of toe at ankle and foot level,** unspecified **foot**

     ✓5ᵗʰ **S96.1** **Injury of muscle and tendon of** long extensor muscle of toe **at ankle and foot level**

         ✓6ᵗʰ **S96.10** Unspecified **injury of muscle and tendon of long extensor muscle of toe at ankle and foot level**

             ✓7ᵗʰ **S96.101** **Unspecified injury of muscle and tendon of long extensor muscle of toe at ankle and foot level,** right **foot**

             ✓7ᵗʰ **S96.102** **Unspecified injury of muscle and tendon of long extensor muscle of toe at ankle and foot level,** left **foot**

             ✓7ᵗʰ **S96.109** **Unspecified injury of muscle and tendon of long extensor muscle of toe at ankle and foot level,** unspecified **foot**

         ✓6ᵗʰ **S96.11** Strain **of muscle and tendon of long extensor muscle of toe at ankle and foot level**

             ✓7ᵗʰ **S96.111** **Strain of muscle and tendon of long extensor muscle of toe at ankle and foot level,** right **foot**

             ✓7ᵗʰ **S96.112** **Strain of muscle and tendon of long extensor muscle of toe at ankle and foot level,** left **foot**

             ✓7ᵗʰ **S96.119** **Strain of muscle and tendon of long extensor muscle of toe at ankle and foot level,** unspecified **foot**

         ✓6ᵗʰ **S96.12** Laceration **of muscle and tendon of long extensor muscle of toe at ankle and foot level**

             ✓7ᵗʰ **S96.121** **Laceration of muscle and tendon of long extensor muscle of toe at ankle and foot level,** right **foot** `CC`

             ✓7ᵗʰ **S96.122** **Laceration of muscle and tendon of long extensor muscle of toe at ankle and foot level,** left **foot** `CC`

             ✓7ᵗʰ **S96.129** **Laceration of muscle and tendon of long extensor muscle of toe at ankle and foot level,** unspecified **foot** `CC`

         ✓6ᵗʰ **S96.19** Other **specified injury of muscle and tendon of long extensor muscle of toe at ankle and foot level**

             ✓7ᵗʰ **S96.191** **Other specified injury of muscle and tendon of long extensor muscle of toe at ankle and foot level,** right **foot**

             ✓7ᵗʰ **S96.192** **Other specified injury of muscle and tendon of long extensor muscle of toe at ankle and foot level,** left **foot**

             ✓7ᵗʰ **S96.199** **Other specified injury of muscle and tendon of long extensor muscle of toe at ankle and foot level,** unspecified **foot**

     ✓5ᵗʰ **S96.2** **Injury of** intrinsic muscle and tendon **at ankle and foot level**

         ✓6ᵗʰ **S96.20** Unspecified **injury of intrinsic muscle and tendon at ankle and foot level**

             ✓7ᵗʰ **S96.201** **Unspecified injury of intrinsic muscle and tendon at ankle and foot level,** right **foot**

             ✓7ᵗʰ **S96.202** **Unspecified injury of intrinsic muscle and tendon at ankle and foot level,** left **foot**

             ✓7ᵗʰ **S96.209** **Unspecified injury of intrinsic muscle and tendon at ankle and foot level,** unspecified **foot**

✓6ᵗʰ **S96.21 Strain** of intrinsic muscle and tendon at ankle and foot level

   ✓7ᵗʰ **S96.211 Strain** of intrinsic muscle and tendon at ankle and foot level, **right** foot

   ✓7ᵗʰ **S96.212 Strain** of intrinsic muscle and tendon at ankle and foot level, **left** foot

   ✓7ᵗʰ **S96.219 Strain** of intrinsic muscle and tendon at ankle and foot level, **unspecified** foot

✓6ᵗʰ **S96.22 Laceration** of intrinsic muscle and tendon at ankle and foot level

   ✓7ᵗʰ **S96.221 Laceration** of intrinsic muscle and tendon at ankle and foot level, **right** foot CC

   ✓7ᵗʰ **S96.222 Laceration** of intrinsic muscle and tendon at ankle and foot level, **left** foot CC

   ✓7ᵗʰ **S96.229 Laceration** of intrinsic muscle and tendon at ankle and foot level, **unspecified** foot CC

✓6ᵗʰ **S96.29 Other** specified injury of intrinsic muscle and tendon at ankle and foot level

   ✓7ᵗʰ **S96.291 Other** specified injury of intrinsic muscle and tendon at ankle and foot level, **right** foot

   ✓7ᵗʰ **S96.292 Other** specified injury of intrinsic muscle and tendon at ankle and foot level, **left** foot

   ✓7ᵗʰ **S96.299 Other** specified injury of intrinsic muscle and tendon at ankle and foot level, **unspecified** foot

✓5ᵗʰ **S96.8 Injury** of other specified muscles and tendons at ankle and foot level

  ✓6ᵗʰ **S96.80 Unspecified** injury of other specified muscles and tendons at ankle and foot level

   ✓7ᵗʰ **S96.801 Unspecified** injury of other specified muscles and tendons at ankle and foot level, **right** foot

   ✓7ᵗʰ **S96.802 Unspecified** injury of other specified muscles and tendons at ankle and foot level, **left** foot

   ✓7ᵗʰ **S96.809 Unspecified** injury of other specified muscles and tendons at ankle and foot level, **unspecified** foot

  ✓6ᵗʰ **S96.81 Strain** of other specified muscles and tendons at ankle and foot level

   ✓7ᵗʰ **S96.811 Strain** of other specified muscles and tendons at ankle and foot level, **right** foot

   ✓7ᵗʰ **S96.812 Strain** of other specified muscles and tendons at ankle and foot level, **left** foot

   ✓7ᵗʰ **S96.819 Strain** of other specified muscles and tendons at ankle and foot level, **unspecified** foot

  ✓6ᵗʰ **S96.82 Laceration** of other specified muscles and tendons at ankle and foot level

   ✓7ᵗʰ **S96.821 Laceration** of other specified muscles and tendons at ankle and foot level, **right** foot CC

   ✓7ᵗʰ **S96.822 Laceration** of other specified muscles and tendons at ankle and foot level, **left** foot CC

   ✓7ᵗʰ **S96.829 Laceration** of other specified muscles and tendons at ankle and foot level, **unspecified** foot CC

  ✓6ᵗʰ **S96.89 Other** specified injury of other specified muscles and tendons at ankle and foot level

   ✓7ᵗʰ **S96.891 Other** specified injury of other specified muscles and tendons at ankle and foot level, **right** foot

   ✓7ᵗʰ **S96.892 Other** specified injury of other specified muscles and tendons at ankle and foot level, **left** foot

   ✓7ᵗʰ **S96.899 Other** specified injury of other specified muscles and tendons at ankle and foot level, **unspecified** foot

✓5ᵗʰ **S96.9 Injury** of unspecified muscle and tendon at ankle and foot level

  ✓6ᵗʰ **S96.90 Unspecified** injury of unspecified muscle and tendon at ankle and foot level

   ✓7ᵗʰ **S96.901 Unspecified** injury of unspecified muscle and tendon at ankle and foot level, **right** foot

   ✓7ᵗʰ **S96.902 Unspecified** injury of unspecified muscle and tendon at ankle and foot level, **left** foot

   ✓7ᵗʰ **S96.909 Unspecified** injury of unspecified muscle and tendon at ankle and foot level, **unspecified** foot

  ✓6ᵗʰ **S96.91 Strain** of unspecified muscle and tendon at ankle and foot level

   ✓7ᵗʰ **S96.911 Strain** of unspecified muscle and tendon at ankle and foot level, **right** foot

   ✓7ᵗʰ **S96.912 Strain** of unspecified muscle and tendon at ankle and foot level, **left** foot

   ✓7ᵗʰ **S96.919 Strain** of unspecified muscle and tendon at ankle and foot level, **unspecified** foot

  ✓6ᵗʰ **S96.92 Laceration** of unspecified muscle and tendon at ankle and foot level

   ✓7ᵗʰ **S96.921 Laceration** of unspecified muscle and tendon at ankle and foot level, **right** foot CC

   ✓7ᵗʰ **S96.922 Laceration** of unspecified muscle and tendon at ankle and foot level, **left** foot CC

   ✓7ᵗʰ **S96.929 Laceration** of unspecified muscle and tendon at ankle and foot level, **unspecified** foot CC

  ✓6ᵗʰ **S96.99 Other** specified injury of unspecified muscle and tendon at ankle and foot level

   ✓7ᵗʰ **S96.991 Other** specified injury of unspecified muscle and tendon at ankle and foot level, **right** foot

   ✓7ᵗʰ **S96.992 Other** specified injury of unspecified muscle and tendon at ankle and foot level, **left** foot

   ✓7ᵗʰ **S96.999 Other** specified injury of unspecified muscle and tendon at ankle and foot level, **unspecified** foot

✓4ᵗʰ **S97 Crushing injury of ankle and foot**
    Use additional code(s) for all associated injuries

> The appropriate 7th character is to be added to each code from category S97.
> A   initial encounter
> D   subsequent encounter
> S   sequela

✓5ᵗʰ **S97.0 Crushing injury** of ankle

  ✓x7ᵗʰ **S97.00 Crushing injury** of unspecified ankle

  ✓x7ᵗʰ **S97.01 Crushing injury** of right ankle

  ✓x7ᵗʰ **S97.02 Crushing injury** of left ankle

✓5ᵗʰ **S97.1 Crushing injury** of toe

  ✓6ᵗʰ **S97.10 Crushing injury** of unspecified toe(s)

   ✓7ᵗʰ **S97.101 Crushing injury** of unspecified right toe(s)

   ✓7ᵗʰ **S97.102 Crushing injury** of unspecified left toe(s)

   ✓7ᵗʰ **S97.109 Crushing injury** of unspecified toe(s)
      Crushing injury of toe NOS

  ✓6ᵗʰ **S97.11 Crushing injury** of great toe

   ✓7ᵗʰ **S97.111 Crushing injury** of right great toe

   ✓7ᵗʰ **S97.112 Crushing injury** of left great toe

   ✓7ᵗʰ **S97.119 Crushing injury** of unspecified great toe

  ✓6ᵗʰ **S97.12 Crushing injury** of lesser toe(s)

   ✓7ᵗʰ **S97.121 Crushing injury** of right lesser toe(s)

   ✓7ᵗʰ **S97.122 Crushing injury** of left lesser toe(s)

   ✓7ᵗʰ **S97.129 Crushing injury** of unspecified lesser toe(s)

✓5ᵗʰ **S97.8 Crushing injury** of foot

  ✓x7ᵗʰ **S97.80 Crushing injury** of unspecified foot
      Crushing injury of foot NOS

  ✓x7ᵗʰ **S97.81 Crushing injury** of right foot

  ✓x7ᵗʰ **S97.82 Crushing injury** of left foot

✓ Additional Character Required   ✓x7ᵗʰ Placeholder   Unacceptable PDx   Questionable PDx   Manifestation   H1-H14 HAC   HCC CMS-HCC Dx   HIV HIV Dx

ICD-10-CM 2019   **1077**

☑️4ᵗʰ **S98   Traumatic amputation of ankle and foot**

An amputation not identified as partial or complete should be coded to complete

> The appropriate 7th character is to be added to each code from category S98.
> A   initial encounter
> D   subsequent encounter
> S   sequela

> **CC Excl: For CC codes in category S98:**
> **Right side:** PDX collection 1333
> **Left side:** PDX collection 1334
> **Unspecified side:** PDX collection 1335

☑️5ᵗʰ **S98.Ø   Traumatic amputation of** foot at ankle level

   ☑️6ᵗʰ **S98.Ø1   Complete traumatic amputation of foot at ankle level**

     ☑️7ᵗʰ **S98.Ø11   Complete traumatic amputation of** right **foot at ankle level**   `CC` `HCC`

     ☑️7ᵗʰ **S98.Ø12   Complete traumatic amputation of** left **foot at ankle level**   `CC` `HCC`

     ☑️7ᵗʰ **S98.Ø19   Complete traumatic amputation of** unspecified **foot at ankle level**   `CC` `HCC`

   ☑️6ᵗʰ **S98.Ø2   Partial traumatic amputation of foot at ankle level**

     ☑️7ᵗʰ **S98.Ø21   Partial traumatic amputation of** right **foot at ankle level**   `CC` `HCC`

     ☑️7ᵗʰ **S98.Ø22   Partial traumatic amputation of** left **foot at ankle level**   `CC` `HCC`

     ☑️7ᵗʰ **S98.Ø29   Partial traumatic amputation of** unspecified **foot at ankle level**   `CC` `HCC`

☑️5ᵗʰ **S98.1   Traumatic amputation of** one toe

   ☑️6ᵗʰ **S98.11   Complete traumatic amputation of** great toe

     ☑️7ᵗʰ **S98.111   Complete traumatic amputation of** right **great toe**   `HCC`

     ☑️7ᵗʰ **S98.112   Complete traumatic amputation of** left **great toe**   `HCC`

     ☑️7ᵗʰ **S98.119   Complete traumatic amputation of** unspecified **great toe**   `HCC`

   ☑️6ᵗʰ **S98.12   Partial traumatic amputation of** great toe

     ☑️7ᵗʰ **S98.121   Partial traumatic amputation of** right **great toe**   `HCC`

     ☑️7ᵗʰ **S98.122   Partial traumatic amputation of** left **great toe**   `HCC`

     ☑️7ᵗʰ **S98.129   Partial traumatic amputation of** unspecified **great toe**   `HCC`

   ☑️6ᵗʰ **S98.13   Complete traumatic amputation of** one lesser toe
     Traumatic amputation of toe NOS

     ☑️7ᵗʰ **S98.131   Complete traumatic amputation of one** right **lesser toe**   `HCC`

     ☑️7ᵗʰ **S98.132   Complete traumatic amputation of one** left **lesser toe**   `HCC`

     ☑️7ᵗʰ **S98.139   Complete traumatic amputation of one** unspecified **lesser toe**   `HCC`

   ☑️6ᵗʰ **S98.14   Partial traumatic amputation of** one lesser toe

     ☑️7ᵗʰ **S98.141   Partial traumatic amputation of one** right **lesser toe**   `HCC`

     ☑️7ᵗʰ **S98.142   Partial traumatic amputation of one** left **lesser toe**   `HCC`

     ☑️7ᵗʰ **S98.149   Partial traumatic amputation of one** unspecified **lesser toe**   `HCC`

☑️5ᵗʰ **S98.2   Traumatic amputation of** two or more lesser toes

   ☑️6ᵗʰ **S98.21   Complete traumatic amputation of two or more lesser toes**

     ☑️7ᵗʰ **S98.211   Complete traumatic amputation of two or more** right **lesser toes**   `HCC`

     ☑️7ᵗʰ **S98.212   Complete traumatic amputation of two or more** left **lesser toes**   `HCC`

     ☑️7ᵗʰ **S98.219   Complete traumatic amputation of two or more** unspecified **lesser toes**   `HCC`

   ☑️6ᵗʰ **S98.22   Partial traumatic amputation of two or more lesser toes**

     ☑️7ᵗʰ **S98.221   Partial traumatic amputation of two or more** right **lesser toes**   `HCC`

     ☑️7ᵗʰ **S98.222   Partial traumatic amputation of two or more** left **lesser toes**   `HCC`

     ☑️7ᵗʰ **S98.229   Partial traumatic amputation of two or more** unspecified **lesser toes**   `HCC`

☑️5ᵗʰ **S98.3   Traumatic amputation of** midfoot

   ☑️6ᵗʰ **S98.31   Complete traumatic amputation of midfoot**

     ☑️7ᵗʰ **S98.311   Complete traumatic amputation of** right **midfoot**   `CC` `HCC`

     ☑️7ᵗʰ **S98.312   Complete traumatic amputation of** left **midfoot**   `CC` `HCC`

     ☑️7ᵗʰ **S98.319   Complete traumatic amputation of** unspecified **midfoot**   `CC` `HCC`

   ☑️6ᵗʰ **S98.32   Partial traumatic amputation of midfoot**

     ☑️7ᵗʰ **S98.321   Partial traumatic amputation of** right **midfoot**   `CC` `HCC`

     ☑️7ᵗʰ **S98.322   Partial traumatic amputation of** left **midfoot**   `CC` `HCC`

     ☑️7ᵗʰ **S98.329   Partial traumatic amputation of** unspecified **midfoot**   `CC` `HCC`

☑️5ᵗʰ **S98.9   Traumatic amputation of** foot, level unspecified

   ☑️6ᵗʰ **S98.91   Complete traumatic amputation of foot, level unspecified**

     ☑️7ᵗʰ **S98.911   Complete traumatic amputation of** right **foot, level unspecified**   `CC` `HCC`

     ☑️7ᵗʰ **S98.912   Complete traumatic amputation of** left **foot, level unspecified**   `CC` `HCC`

     ☑️7ᵗʰ **S98.919   Complete traumatic amputation of** unspecified **foot, level** unspecified   `CC` `HCC`

   ☑️6ᵗʰ **S98.92   Partial traumatic amputation of foot, level unspecified**

     ☑️7ᵗʰ **S98.921   Partial traumatic amputation of** right **foot, level unspecified**   `CC` `HCC`

     ☑️7ᵗʰ **S98.922   Partial traumatic amputation of** left **foot, level unspecified**   `CC` `HCC`

     ☑️7ᵗʰ **S98.929   Partial traumatic amputation of** unspecified **foot, level unspecified**   `CC` `HCC`

☑️4ᵗʰ **S99   Other and unspecified injuries of ankle and foot**

AHA: 2018, 2Q, 12; 2018, 1Q, 3; 2016, 4Q, 68-69

☑️5ᵗʰ **S99.Ø   Physeal fracture of** calcaneus

> The appropriate 7th character is to be added to each code from subcategories S99.Ø.
> A   initial encounter for closed fracture
> B   initial encounter for open fracture
> D   subsequent encounter for fracture with routine healing
> G   subsequent encounter for fracture with delayed healing
> K   subsequent encounter for fracture with nonunion
> P   subsequent encounter for fracture with malunion
> S   sequela

   ☑️6ᵗʰ **S99.ØØ   Unspecified physeal fracture of calcaneus**

     ☑️7ᵗʰ **S99.ØØ1   Unspecified physeal fracture of** right **calcaneus**

     ☑️7ᵗʰ **S99.ØØ2   Unspecified physeal fracture of** left **calcaneus**

     ☑️7ᵗʰ **S99.ØØ9   Unspecified physeal fracture of** unspecified **calcaneus**

   ☑️6ᵗʰ **S99.Ø1   Salter-Harris Type I physeal fracture of calcaneus**

     ☑️7ᵗʰ **S99.Ø11   Salter-Harris Type I physeal fracture of** right **calcaneus**

     ☑️7ᵗʰ **S99.Ø12   Salter-Harris Type I physeal fracture of** left **calcaneus**

     ☑️7ᵗʰ **S99.Ø19   Salter-Harris Type I physeal fracture of** unspecified **calcaneus**

   ☑️6ᵗʰ **S99.Ø2   Salter-Harris Type II physeal fracture of calcaneus**

     ☑️7ᵗʰ **S99.Ø21   Salter-Harris Type II physeal fracture of** right **calcaneus**

     ☑️7ᵗʰ **S99.Ø22   Salter-Harris Type II physeal fracture of** left **calcaneus**

     ☑️7ᵗʰ **S99.Ø29   Salter-Harris Type II physeal fracture of** unspecified **calcaneus**

   ☑️6ᵗʰ **S99.Ø3   Salter-Harris Type III physeal fracture of calcaneus**

     ☑️7ᵗʰ **S99.Ø31   Salter-Harris Type III physeal fracture of** right **calcaneus**

     ☑️7ᵗʰ **S99.Ø32   Salter-Harris Type III physeal fracture of** left **calcaneus**

     ☑️7ᵗʰ **S99.Ø39   Salter-Harris Type III physeal fracture of** unspecified **calcaneus**

◼ Newborn: 0   ◼ Pediatric: 0-17   ◼ Maternity: 12-55   ◼ Adult: 15-124   `MCC` Major Complication/Comorbidity   `CC` Complication/Comorbidity   `SW` Severe Wound Dx

1078   ICD-10-CM 2019

✓6ᵗʰ **S99.04** Salter-Harris Type IV physeal fracture of calcaneus

     ✓7ᵗʰ **S99.041** Salter-Harris Type IV physeal fracture of right calcaneus

     ✓7ᵗʰ **S99.042** Salter-Harris Type IV physeal fracture of left calcaneus

     ✓7ᵗʰ **S99.049** Salter-Harris Type IV physeal fracture of unspecified calcaneus

✓6ᵗʰ **S99.09** Other physeal fracture of calcaneus

     ✓7ᵗʰ **S99.091** Other physeal fracture of right calcaneus

     ✓7ᵗʰ **S99.092** Other physeal fracture of left calcaneus

     ✓7ᵗʰ **S99.099** Other physeal fracture of unspecified calcaneus

✓5ᵗʰ **S99.1** Physeal fracture of metatarsal

> The appropriate 7th character is to be added to each code from subcategories S99.1.
> A   initial encounter for closed fracture
> B   initial encounter for open fracture
> D   subsequent encounter for fracture with routine healing
> G   subsequent encounter for fracture with delayed healing
> K   subsequent encounter for fracture with nonunion
> P   subsequent encounter for fracture with malunion
> S   sequela

✓6ᵗʰ **S99.10** Unspecified physeal fracture of metatarsal

▲   ✓7ᵗʰ **S99.101** Unspecified physeal fracture of right metatarsal

     ✓7ᵗʰ **S99.102** Unspecified physeal fracture of left metatarsal

     ✓7ᵗʰ **S99.109** Unspecified physeal fracture of unspecified metatarsal

✓6ᵗʰ **S99.11** Salter-Harris Type I physeal fracture of metatarsal

     ✓7ᵗʰ **S99.111** Salter-Harris Type I physeal fracture of right metatarsal

     ✓7ᵗʰ **S99.112** Salter-Harris Type I physeal fracture of left metatarsal

     ✓7ᵗʰ **S99.119** Salter-Harris Type I physeal fracture of unspecified metatarsal

✓6ᵗʰ **S99.12** Salter-Harris Type II physeal fracture of metatarsal

     ✓7ᵗʰ **S99.121** Salter-Harris Type II physeal fracture of right metatarsal

     ✓7ᵗʰ **S99.122** Salter-Harris Type II physeal fracture of left metatarsal

     ✓7ᵗʰ **S99.129** Salter-Harris Type II physeal fracture of unspecified metatarsal

✓6ᵗʰ **S99.13** Salter-Harris Type III physeal fracture of metatarsal

     ✓7ᵗʰ **S99.131** Salter-Harris Type III physeal fracture of right metatarsal

     ✓7ᵗʰ **S99.132** Salter-Harris Type III physeal fracture of left metatarsal

     ✓7ᵗʰ **S99.139** Salter-Harris Type III physeal fracture of unspecified metatarsal

✓6ᵗʰ **S99.14** Salter-Harris Type IV physeal fracture of metatarsal

     ✓7ᵗʰ **S99.141** Salter-Harris Type IV physeal fracture of right metatarsal

     ✓7ᵗʰ **S99.142** Salter-Harris Type IV physeal fracture of left metatarsal

     ✓7ᵗʰ **S99.149** Salter-Harris Type IV physeal fracture of unspecified metatarsal

✓6ᵗʰ **S99.19** Other physeal fracture of metatarsal

     ✓7ᵗʰ **S99.191** Other physeal fracture of right metatarsal

     ✓7ᵗʰ **S99.192** Other physeal fracture of left metatarsal

     ✓7ᵗʰ **S99.199** Other physeal fracture of unspecified metatarsal

✓5ᵗʰ **S99.2** Physeal fracture of phalanx of toe

> The appropriate 7th character is to be added to each code from subcategories S99.2.
> A   initial encounter for closed fracture
> B   initial encounter for open fracture
> D   subsequent encounter for fracture with routine healing
> G   subsequent encounter for fracture with delayed healing
> K   subsequent encounter for fracture with nonunion
> P   subsequent encounter for fracture with malunion
> S   sequela

✓6ᵗʰ **S99.20** Unspecified physeal fracture of phalanx of toe

     ✓7ᵗʰ **S99.201** Unspecified physeal fracture of phalanx of right toe

     ✓7ᵗʰ **S99.202** Unspecified physeal fracture of phalanx of left toe

     ✓7ᵗʰ **S99.209** Unspecified physeal fracture of phalanx of unspecified toe

✓6ᵗʰ **S99.21** Salter-Harris Type I physeal fracture of phalanx of toe

     ✓7ᵗʰ **S99.211** Salter-Harris Type I physeal fracture of phalanx of right toe

     ✓7ᵗʰ **S99.212** Salter-Harris Type I physeal fracture of phalanx of left toe

     ✓7ᵗʰ **S99.219** Salter-Harris Type I physeal fracture of phalanx of unspecified toe

✓6ᵗʰ **S99.22** Salter-Harris Type II physeal fracture of phalanx of toe

     ✓7ᵗʰ **S99.221** Salter-Harris Type II physeal fracture of phalanx of right toe

     ✓7ᵗʰ **S99.222** Salter-Harris Type II physeal fracture of phalanx of left toe

     ✓7ᵗʰ **S99.229** Salter-Harris Type II physeal fracture of phalanx of unspecified toe

✓6ᵗʰ **S99.23** Salter-Harris Type III physeal fracture of phalanx of toe

     ✓7ᵗʰ **S99.231** Salter-Harris Type III physeal fracture of phalanx of right toe

     ✓7ᵗʰ **S99.232** Salter-Harris Type III physeal fracture of phalanx of left toe

     ✓7ᵗʰ **S99.239** Salter-Harris Type III physeal fracture of phalanx of unspecified toe

✓6ᵗʰ **S99.24** Salter-Harris Type IV physeal fracture of phalanx of toe

     ✓7ᵗʰ **S99.241** Salter-Harris Type IV physeal fracture of phalanx of right toe

     ✓7ᵗʰ **S99.242** Salter-Harris Type IV physeal fracture of phalanx of left toe

     ✓7ᵗʰ **S99.249** Salter-Harris Type IV physeal fracture of phalanx of unspecified toe

✓6ᵗʰ **S99.29** Other physeal fracture of phalanx of toe

     ✓7ᵗʰ **S99.291** Other physeal fracture of phalanx of right toe

     ✓7ᵗʰ **S99.292** Other physeal fracture of phalanx of left toe

     ✓7ᵗʰ **S99.299** Other physeal fracture of phalanx of unspecified toe

✓5ᵗʰ **S99.8** Other specified injuries of ankle and foot

> The appropriate 7th character is to be added to each code from subcategory S99.8.
> A   initial encounter
> D   subsequent encounter
> S   sequela

✓6ᵗʰ **S99.81** Other specified injuries of ankle

     ✓7ᵗʰ **S99.811** Other specified injuries of right ankle

     ✓7ᵗʰ **S99.812** Other specified injuries of left ankle

     ✓7ᵗʰ **S99.819** Other specified injuries of unspecified ankle

✓6ᵗʰ **S99.82** Other specified injuries of foot

     ✓7ᵗʰ **S99.821** Other specified injuries of right foot

     ✓7ᵗʰ **S99.822** Other specified injuries of left foot

     ✓7ᵗʰ **S99.829** Other specified injuries of unspecified foot

✓5ᵗʰ **S99.9** Unspecified injury of ankle and foot

> The appropriate 7th character is to be added to each code from subcategory S99.9.
> A   initial encounter
> D   subsequent encounter
> S   sequela

✓6ᵗʰ **S99.91** Unspecified injury of ankle

     ✓7ᵗʰ **S99.911** Unspecified injury of right ankle

     ✓7ᵗʰ **S99.912** Unspecified injury of left ankle

     ✓7ᵗʰ **S99.919** Unspecified injury of unspecified ankle

☑ Additional Character Required   ✓x7ᵗʰ Placeholder   Unacceptable PDx   Questionable PDx   Manifestation   H1-H14 HAC   HCC CMS-HCC Dx   HIV HIV Dx

ICD-10-CM 2019   1079

✓6ᵗʰ **S99.92**   **Unspecified injury of** foot
    ✓7ᵗʰ **S99.921**   **Unspecified injury of** right **foot**
    ✓7ᵗʰ **S99.922**   **Unspecified injury of** left **foot**
    ✓7ᵗʰ **S99.929**   **Unspecified injury of** unspecified **foot**

INJURY, POISONING AND CERTAIN OTHER CONSEQUENCES OF EXTERNAL CAUSES (TØ7-T88)

Injuries involving multiple body regions (TØ7)

EXCLUDES 1   burns and corrosions (T20-T32)
    frostbite (T33-T34)
    insect bite or sting, venomous (T63.4)
    sunburn (L55.-)

✓x7ᵗʰ **TØ7**   **Unspecified multiple injuries**
    EXCLUDES 1   injury NOS (T14.9Ø)
    AHA: 2017, 4Q, 26

> The appropriate 7th character is to be added to code TØ7.
> A   initial encounter
> D   subsequent encounter
> S   sequela

Injury of unspecified body region (T14)

✓4ᵗʰ **T14**   **Injury of unspecified body region**
    EXCLUDES 1   multiple unspecified injuries (TØ7)
    AHA: 2017, 4Q, 26

> The appropriate 7th character is to be added to each code from category T14.
> A   initial encounter
> D   subsequent encounter
> S   sequela

✓x7ᵗʰ **T14.8**   **Other injury of unspecified body region**
    Abrasion NOS   Skin injury NOS
    Contusion NOS   Vascular injury NOS
    Crush injury NOS   Wound NOS
    Fracture NOS

✓5ᵗʰ **T14.9**   **Unspecified injury**
    ✓x7ᵗʰ **T14.9Ø**   **Injury,** unspecified
       Injury NOS
    ✓x7ᵗʰ **T14.91**   **Suicide attempt**   HCC
       Attempted suicide NOS

Effects of foreign body entering through natural orifice (T15-T19)

EXCLUDES 2   foreign body accidentally left in operation wound (T81.5-)
    foreign body in penetrating wound—See open wound by body region
    residual foreign body in soft tissue (M79.5)
    splinter, without open wound—See superficial injury by body region

✓4ᵗʰ **T15**   **Foreign body on external eye**
    EXCLUDES 2   foreign body in penetrating wound of orbit and eye ball (SØ5.4-, SØ5.5-)
    open wound of eyelid and periocular area (SØ1.1-)
    retained foreign body in eyelid (HØ2.8-)
    retained (old) foreign body in penetrating wound of orbit and eye ball (HØ5.5-, H44.6-, H44.7-)
    superficial foreign body of eyelid and periocular area (SØØ.25-)

> The appropriate 7th character is to be added to each code from category T15.
> A   initial encounter
> D   subsequent encounter
> S   sequela

✓5ᵗʰ **T15.Ø**   **Foreign body in cornea**
    ✓x7ᵗʰ **T15.ØØ**   **Foreign body in cornea,** unspecified **eye**
    ✓x7ᵗʰ **T15.Ø1**   **Foreign body in cornea,** right **eye**
    ✓x7ᵗʰ **T15.Ø2**   **Foreign body in cornea,** left **eye**
✓5ᵗʰ **T15.1**   **Foreign body in conjunctival sac**
    ✓x7ᵗʰ **T15.1Ø**   **Foreign body in conjunctival sac,** unspecified **eye**
    ✓x7ᵗʰ **T15.11**   **Foreign body in conjunctival sac,** right **eye**
    ✓x7ᵗʰ **T15.12**   **Foreign body in conjunctival sac,** left **eye**
✓5ᵗʰ **T15.8**   **Foreign body in other and** multiple parts **of external eye**
    Foreign body in lacrimal punctum
    ✓x7ᵗʰ **T15.8Ø**   **Foreign body in other and multiple parts of external eye,** unspecified **eye**
    ✓x7ᵗʰ **T15.81**   **Foreign body in other and multiple parts of external eye,** right **eye**

    ✓x7ᵗʰ **T15.82**   **Foreign body in other and multiple parts of external eye,** left **eye**
✓5ᵗʰ **T15.9**   **Foreign body on external eye,** part unspecified
    ✓x7ᵗʰ **T15.9Ø**   **Foreign body on external eye, part unspecified,** unspecified **eye**
    ✓x7ᵗʰ **T15.91**   **Foreign body on external eye, part unspecified,** right **eye**
    ✓x7ᵗʰ **T15.92**   **Foreign body on external eye, part unspecified,** left **eye**

✓4ᵗʰ **T16**   **Foreign body in** ear
    INCLUDES   foreign body in auditory canal

> The appropriate 7th character is to be added to each code from category T16.
> A   initial encounter
> D   subsequent encounter
> S   sequela

✓x7ᵗʰ **T16.1**   **Foreign body in** right **ear**
✓x7ᵗʰ **T16.2**   **Foreign body in** left **ear**
✓x7ᵗʰ **T16.9**   **Foreign body in ear,** unspecified **ear**

✓4ᵗʰ **T17**   **Foreign body in respiratory tract**

> The appropriate 7th character is to be added to each code from category T17.
> A   initial encounter
> D   subsequent encounter
> S   sequela

✓x7ᵗʰ **T17.Ø**   **Foreign body in** nasal sinus
✓x7ᵗʰ **T17.1**   **Foreign body in** nostril
    Foreign body in nose NOS
✓5ᵗʰ **T17.2**   **Foreign body in** pharynx
    Foreign body in nasopharynx
    Foreign body in throat NOS
    ✓6ᵗʰ **T17.2Ø**   Unspecified **foreign body in pharynx**
       ✓7ᵗʰ **T17.2ØØ**   **Unspecified foreign body in pharynx causing asphyxiation**
       ✓7ᵗʰ **T17.2Ø8**   **Unspecified foreign body in pharynx causing other injury**
    ✓6ᵗʰ **T17.21**   **Gastric contents in pharynx**
       Aspiration of gastric contents into pharynx
       Vomitus in pharynx
       ✓7ᵗʰ **T17.21Ø**   **Gastric contents in pharynx** causing **asphyxiation**
       ✓7ᵗʰ **T17.218**   **Gastric contents in pharynx** causing **other injury**
    ✓6ᵗʰ **T17.22**   **Food in pharynx**
       Bones in pharynx
       Seeds in pharynx
       ✓7ᵗʰ **T17.22Ø**   **Food in pharynx** causing asphyxiation
       ✓7ᵗʰ **T17.228**   **Food in pharynx** causing other injury
    ✓6ᵗʰ **T17.29**   Other **foreign object in pharynx**
       ✓7ᵗʰ **T17.29Ø**   **Other foreign object in pharynx** causing **asphyxiation**
       ✓7ᵗʰ **T17.298**   **Other foreign object in pharynx** causing **other injury**
✓5ᵗʰ **T17.3**   **Foreign body in** larynx
    ✓6ᵗʰ **T17.3Ø**   Unspecified **foreign body in larynx**
       ✓7ᵗʰ **T17.3ØØ**   **Unspecified foreign body in larynx causing asphyxiation**
       ✓7ᵗʰ **T17.3Ø8**   **Unspecified foreign body in larynx causing other injury**
    ✓6ᵗʰ **T17.31**   **Gastric contents in larynx**
       Aspiration of gastric contents into larynx
       Vomitus in larynx
       ✓7ᵗʰ **T17.31Ø**   **Gastric contents in larynx** causing **asphyxiation**
       ✓7ᵗʰ **T17.318**   **Gastric contents in larynx** causing **other injury**
    ✓6ᵗʰ **T17.32**   **Food in larynx**
       Bones in larynx
       Seeds in larynx
       ✓7ᵗʰ **T17.32Ø**   **Food in larynx** causing asphyxiation
       ✓7ᵗʰ **T17.328**   **Food in larynx** causing other injury

☑6ᵗʰ **T17.39** Other **foreign object in larynx**

     ✓7ᵗʰ **T17.390** **Other foreign object in larynx** causing asphyxiation

     ✓7ᵗʰ **T17.398** **Other foreign object in larynx** causing other injury

☑5ᵗʰ **T17.4** **Foreign body in** trachea

> **CC Excl: For CC codes in subcategory T17.4:**
> PDX collection 1373

     ☑6ᵗʰ **T17.40** Unspecified **foreign body in trachea**

         ✓7ᵗʰ **T17.400** **Unspecified foreign body in trachea causing asphyxiation** `CC`

         ✓7ᵗʰ **T17.408** **Unspecified foreign body in trachea causing other injury** `CC`

     ☑6ᵗʰ **T17.41** **Gastric contents in trachea**
         Aspiration of gastric contents into trachea
         Vomitus in trachea

         ✓7ᵗʰ **T17.410** **Gastric contents in trachea** causing asphyxiation `CC`

         ✓7ᵗʰ **T17.418** **Gastric contents in trachea** causing other injury `CC`

     ☑6ᵗʰ **T17.42** **Food in trachea**
         Bones in trachea
         Seeds in trachea

         ✓7ᵗʰ **T17.420** **Food in trachea** causing asphyxiation `CC`

         ✓7ᵗʰ **T17.428** **Food in trachea** causing other injury `CC`

     ☑6ᵗʰ **T17.49** Other **foreign object in trachea**

         ✓7ᵗʰ **T17.490** **Other foreign object in trachea causing asphyxiation** `CC`

         ✓7ᵗʰ **T17.498** **Other foreign object in trachea causing other injury** `CC`

☑5ᵗʰ **T17.5** **Foreign body in** bronchus

> **CC Excl: For CC codes in subcategory T17.5:**
> PDX collection 1374

     ☑6ᵗʰ **T17.50** Unspecified **foreign body in bronchus**

         ✓7ᵗʰ **T17.500** **Unspecified foreign body in bronchus causing asphyxiation** `CC`

         ✓7ᵗʰ **T17.508** **Unspecified foreign body in bronchus causing other injury** `CC`

     ☑6ᵗʰ **T17.51** **Gastric contents in bronchus**
         Aspiration of gastric contents into bronchus
         Vomitus in bronchus

         ✓7ᵗʰ **T17.510** **Gastric contents in bronchus** causing asphyxiation `CC`

         ✓7ᵗʰ **T17.518** **Gastric contents in bronchus** causing other injury `CC`

     ☑6ᵗʰ **T17.52** **Food in bronchus**
         Bones in bronchus
         Seeds in bronchus

         ✓7ᵗʰ **T17.520** **Food in bronchus** causing asphyxiation `CC`

         ✓7ᵗʰ **T17.528** **Food in bronchus** causing other injury `CC`

     ☑6ᵗʰ **T17.59** Other **foreign object in bronchus**

         ✓7ᵗʰ **T17.590** **Other foreign object in bronchus causing asphyxiation** `CC`

         ✓7ᵗʰ **T17.598** **Other foreign object in bronchus causing other injury** `CC`

☑5ᵗʰ **T17.8** **Foreign body in** other parts **of respiratory tract**
     Foreign body in bronchioles
     Foreign body in lung

> **CC Excl: For CC codes in subcategory T17.8:**
> PDX collection 1374

     ☑6ᵗʰ **T17.80** Unspecified **foreign body in other parts of respiratory tract**

         ✓7ᵗʰ **T17.800** **Unspecified foreign body in other parts of respiratory tract** causing asphyxiation `CC`

         ✓7ᵗʰ **T17.808** **Unspecified foreign body in other parts of respiratory tract** causing other injury `CC`

☑6ᵗʰ **T17.81** **Gastric contents in other parts of respiratory tract**
     Aspiration of gastric contents into other parts of respiratory tract
     Vomitus in other parts of respiratory tract

     ✓7ᵗʰ **T17.810** **Gastric contents in other parts of respiratory tract** causing asphyxiation `CC`

     ✓7ᵗʰ **T17.818** **Gastric contents in other parts of respiratory tract** causing other injury `CC`

☑6ᵗʰ **T17.82** **Food in other parts of respiratory tract**
     Bones in other parts of respiratory tract
     Seeds in other parts of respiratory tract

     ✓7ᵗʰ **T17.820** **Food in other parts of respiratory tract** causing asphyxiation `CC`

     ✓7ᵗʰ **T17.828** **Food in other parts of respiratory tract** causing other injury `CC`

☑6ᵗʰ **T17.89** Other **foreign object in other parts of respiratory tract**

     ✓7ᵗʰ **T17.890** **Other foreign object in other parts of respiratory tract** causing asphyxiation `CC`

     ✓7ᵗʰ **T17.898** **Other foreign object in other parts of respiratory tract** causing other injury `CC`

☑5ᵗʰ **T17.9** **Foreign body in respiratory tract,** part unspecified

     ☑6ᵗʰ **T17.90** Unspecified **foreign body in respiratory tract, part unspecified**

         ✓7ᵗʰ **T17.900** **Unspecified foreign body in respiratory tract, part unspecified** causing asphyxiation

         ✓7ᵗʰ **T17.908** **Unspecified foreign body in respiratory tract, part unspecified** causing other injury

     ☑6ᵗʰ **T17.91** **Gastric contents in respiratory tract, part unspecified**
         Aspiration of gastric contents into respiratory tract, part unspecified
         Vomitus in trachea respiratory tract, part unspecified

         ✓7ᵗʰ **T17.910** **Gastric contents in respiratory tract, part unspecified** causing asphyxiation

         ✓7ᵗʰ **T17.918** **Gastric contents in respiratory tract, part unspecified** causing other injury

     ☑6ᵗʰ **T17.92** **Food in respiratory tract, part unspecified**
         Bones in respiratory tract, part unspecified
         Seeds in respiratory tract, part unspecified

         ✓7ᵗʰ **T17.920** **Food in respiratory tract, part unspecified** causing asphyxiation

         ✓7ᵗʰ **T17.928** **Food in respiratory tract, part unspecified** causing other injury

     ☑6ᵗʰ **T17.99** Other **foreign object in respiratory tract, part unspecified**

         ✓7ᵗʰ **T17.990** **Other foreign object in respiratory tract, part unspecified in** causing asphyxiation

         ✓7ᵗʰ **T17.998** **Other foreign object in respiratory tract, part unspecified** causing other injury

☑4ᵗʰ **T18** **Foreign body in alimentary tract**
     EXCLUDES 2   foreign body in pharynx (T17.2-)

> The appropriate 7th character is to be added to each code from category T18.
> A   initial encounter
> D   subsequent encounter
> S   sequela

✓x7ᵗʰ **T18.0** **Foreign body in** mouth

☑5ᵗʰ **T18.1** **Foreign body in** esophagus
     EXCLUDES 2   foreign body in respiratory tract (T17.-)

     ☑6ᵗʰ **T18.10** Unspecified **foreign body in esophagus**

         ✓7ᵗʰ **T18.100** **Unspecified foreign body in esophagus causing compression of trachea**
             Unspecified foreign body in esophagus causing obstruction of respiration

         ✓7ᵗʰ **T18.108** **Unspecified foreign body in esophagus causing other injury**

     ☑6ᵗʰ **T18.11** **Gastric contents in esophagus**
         Vomitus in esophagus

         ✓7ᵗʰ **T18.110** **Gastric contents in esophagus causing compression of trachea**
             Gastric contents in esophagus causing obstruction of respiration

         ✓7ᵗʰ **T18.118** **Gastric contents in esophagus causing other injury**

☑ Additional Character Required   ✓x7ᵗʰ Placeholder   Unacceptable PDx   Questionable PDx   Manifestation   H1-H14 HAC   HCC CMS-HCC Dx   HIV HIV Dx

ICD-10-CM 2019   **1081**

Chapter 19. Injury, Poisoning and Certain Other Consequences of External Causes

✓6th T18.12   **Food** in esophagus
Bones in esophagus   Seeds in esophagus

    ✓7th T18.120   **Food** in esophagus **causing compression**
of trachea
Food in esophagus causing obstruction of respiration

    ✓7th T18.128   **Food** in esophagus **causing other injury**

✓6th T18.19   **Other foreign object** in esophagus
AHA: 2015, 1Q, 23

    ✓7th T18.190   **Other foreign object** in esophagus
causing compression of trachea
Other foreign body in esophagus causing obstruction of respiration

    ✓7th T18.198   **Other foreign object** in esophagus
causing other injury

✓x7th T18.2   **Foreign body** in **stomach**

✓x7th T18.3   **Foreign body** in **small intestine**

✓x7th T18.4   **Foreign body** in **colon**

✓x7th T18.5   **Foreign body** in **anus and rectum**
Foreign body in rectosigmoid (junction)

✓x7th T18.8   **Foreign body** in **other parts** of alimentary tract

✓x7th T18.9   **Foreign body** of alimentary tract, **part unspecified**
Foreign body in digestive system NOS
Swallowed foreign body NOS

✓4th T19   **Foreign body in genitourinary tract**
EXCLUDES 2   *complications due to implanted mesh (T83.7-)*
mechanical complications of contraceptive device (intrauterine)
(vaginal) (T83.3-)
presence of contraceptive device (intrauterine) (vaginal) (Z97.5)

> The appropriate 7th character is to be added to each code from category T19.
> A   initial encounter
> D   subsequent encounter
> S   sequela

✓x7th T19.0   **Foreign body** in **urethra**

✓x7th T19.1   **Foreign body** in **bladder**

✓x7th T19.2   **Foreign body** in **vulva and vagina**   ♀

✓x7th T19.3   **Foreign body** in **uterus**   ♀

✓x7th T19.4   **Foreign body** in **penis**   ♂

✓x7th T19.8   **Foreign body** in **other parts** of genitourinary tract

✓x7th T19.9   **Foreign body** in genitourinary tract, **part unspecified**

Burns and corrosions (T20-T32)

INCLUDES   burns (thermal) from electrical heating appliances
burns (thermal) from electricity
burns (thermal) from flame
burns (thermal) from friction
burns (thermal) from hot air and hot gases
burns (thermal) from hot objects
burns (thermal) from lightning
burns (thermal) from radiation
chemical burn [corrosion] (external) (internal)
scalds

EXCLUDES 2   *erythema [dermatitis] ab igne (L59.0)*
radiation-related disorders of the skin and subcutaneous tissue (L55-L59)
sunburn (L55.-)

AHA: 2016, 2Q, 4

Burns and corrosions of external body surface, specified by site (T20-T25)

INCLUDES   burns and corrosions of first degree [erythema]
burns and corrosions of second degree [blisters] [epidermal loss]
burns and corrosions of third degree [deep necrosis of underlying tissue] [full-thickness skin loss]
Use additional code from category T31 or T32 to identify extent of body surface involved

✓4th T20   **Burn and corrosion of head, face, and neck**
EXCLUDES 2   *burn and corrosion of ear drum (T28.41, T28.91)*
burn and corrosion of eye and adnexa (T26.-)
burn and corrosion of mouth and pharynx (T28.0)

AHA: 2015, 1Q, 18-19

> The appropriate 7th character is to be added to each code from category T20.
> A   initial encounter
> D   subsequent encounter
> S   sequela

✓5th T20.0   **Burn of unspecified degree of head, face, and neck**
Use additional external cause code to identify the source, place and intent of the burn (X00-X19, X75-X77, X96-X98, Y92)

    ✓x7th T20.00   **Burn of unspecified degree of head, face, and neck, unspecified site**

    ✓6th T20.01   **Burn of unspecified degree of ear [any part, except ear drum]**
EXCLUDES 2   *burn of ear drum (T28.41-)*

      ✓7th T20.011   **Burn of unspecified degree of right ear [any part, except ear drum]**

      ✓7th T20.012   **Burn of unspecified degree of left ear [any part, except ear drum]**

      ✓7th T20.019   **Burn of unspecified degree of unspecified ear [any part, except ear drum]**

    ✓x7th T20.02   **Burn of unspecified degree of lip(s)**

    ✓x7th T20.03   **Burn of unspecified degree of chin**

    ✓x7th T20.04   **Burn of unspecified degree of nose (septum)**

    ✓x7th T20.05   **Burn of unspecified degree of scalp [any part]**

    ✓x7th T20.06   **Burn of unspecified degree of forehead and cheek**

    ✓x7th T20.07   **Burn of unspecified degree of neck**

    ✓x7th T20.09   **Burn of unspecified degree of multiple sites of head, face, and neck**

✓5th T20.1   **Burn of first degree of head, face, and neck**
Use additional external cause code to identify the source, place and intent of the burn (X00-X19, X75-X77, X96-X98, Y92)

    ✓x7th T20.10   **Burn of first degree of head, face, and neck, unspecified site**

Degree of Burns

Normal   First Degree Burn
Epidermis   Dermis   Subcutaneous
Second Degree Burn   Third Degree Burn
Epidermis   Dermis   Subcutaneous

    ✓6th T20.11   **Burn of first degree of ear [any part, except ear drum]**
EXCLUDES 2   *burn of ear drum (T28.41-)*

      ✓7th T20.111   **Burn of first degree of right ear [any part, except ear drum]**

      ✓7th T20.112   **Burn of first degree of left ear [any part, except ear drum]**

      ✓7th T20.119   **Burn of first degree of unspecified ear [any part, except ear drum]**

    ✓x7th T20.12   **Burn of first degree of lip(s)**

    ✓x7th T20.13   **Burn of first degree of chin**

    ✓x7th T20.14   **Burn of first degree of nose (septum)**

    ✓x7th T20.15   **Burn of first degree of scalp [any part]**

    ✓x7th T20.16   **Burn of first degree of forehead and cheek**

    ✓x7th T20.17   **Burn of first degree of neck**

    ✓x7th T20.19   **Burn of first degree of multiple sites of head, face, and neck**

N Newborn: 0   **P** Pediatric: 0-17   **M** Maternity: 12-55   **A** Adult: 15-124   **MCC** Major Complication/Comorbidity   **CC** Complication/Comorbidity   **SW** Severe Wound Dx

1082   ICD-10-CM 2019

✓5ᵗʰ **T20.2 Burn of second degree of head, face, and neck**
Use additional external cause code to identify the source, place and intent of the burn (X00-X19, X75-X77, X96-X98, Y92)

  ✓x7ᵗʰ **T20.20 Burn of second degree of head, face, and neck, unspecified site**

  ✓6ᵗʰ **T20.21 Burn of second degree of ear [any part, except ear drum]**
    EXCLUDES 2   burn of ear drum (T28.41-)

    ✓7ᵗʰ **T20.211 Burn of second degree of right ear [any part, except ear drum]**

    ✓7ᵗʰ **T20.212 Burn of second degree of left ear [any part, except ear drum]**

    ✓7ᵗʰ **T20.219 Burn of second degree of unspecified ear [any part, except ear drum]**

  ✓x7ᵗʰ **T20.22 Burn of second degree of lip(s)**

  ✓x7ᵗʰ **T20.23 Burn of second degree of chin**

  ✓x7ᵗʰ **T20.24 Burn of second degree of nose (septum)**

  ✓x7ᵗʰ **T20.25 Burn of second degree of scalp [any part]**

  ✓x7ᵗʰ **T20.26 Burn of second degree of forehead and cheek**

  ✓x7ᵗʰ **T20.27 Burn of second degree of neck**

  ✓x7ᵗʰ **T20.29 Burn of second degree of multiple sites of head, face, and neck**

✓5ᵗʰ **T20.3 Burn of third degree of head, face, and neck**
Use additional external cause code to identify the source, place and intent of the burn (X00-X19, X75-X77, X96-X98, Y92)

  ✓x7ᵗʰ **T20.30 Burn of third degree of head, face, and neck, unspecified site**   CC H5 SW
    CC Excl: PDX collection 1375

  ✓6ᵗʰ **T20.31 Burn of third degree of ear [any part, except ear drum]**
    EXCLUDES 2   burn of ear drum (T28.41-)
    AHA: 2015, 1Q, 18

    CC Excl: For CC codes in subcategory T20.31: PDX collection 1376

    ✓7ᵗʰ **T20.311 Burn of third degree of right ear [any part, except ear drum]**   CC H5 SW

    ✓7ᵗʰ **T20.312 Burn of third degree of left ear [any part, except ear drum]**   CC H5 SW

    ✓7ᵗʰ **T20.319 Burn of third degree of unspecified ear [any part, except ear drum]**   CC H5 SW

  ✓x7ᵗʰ **T20.32 Burn of third degree of lip(s)**   CC H5 SW
    CC Excl: PDX collection 1377

  ✓x7ᵗʰ **T20.33 Burn of third degree of chin**   CC H5 SW
    CC Excl: PDX collection 1378

  ✓x7ᵗʰ **T20.34 Burn of third degree of nose (septum)**   CC H5 SW
    CC Excl: PDX collection 1379

  ✓x7ᵗʰ **T20.35 Burn of third degree of scalp [any part]**   CC H5 SW
    CC Excl: PDX collection 1380

  ✓x7ᵗʰ **T20.36 Burn of third degree of forehead and cheek**   CC H5 SW
    CC Excl: PDX collection 1381

  ✓x7ᵗʰ **T20.37 Burn of third degree of neck**   CC H5 SW
    CC Excl: PDX collection 1382

  ✓x7ᵗʰ **T20.39 Burn of third degree of multiple sites of head, face, and neck**   CC H5 SW
    CC Excl: PDX collection 1383

✓5ᵗʰ **T20.4 Corrosion of unspecified degree of head, face, and neck**
Code first (T51-T65) to identify chemical and intent
Use additional external cause code to identify place (Y92)

  ✓x7ᵗʰ **T20.40 Corrosion of unspecified degree of head, face, and neck, unspecified site**

  ✓6ᵗʰ **T20.41 Corrosion of unspecified degree of ear [any part, except ear drum]**
    EXCLUDES 2   corrosion of ear drum (T28.91-)

    ✓7ᵗʰ **T20.411 Corrosion of unspecified degree of right ear [any part, except ear drum]**

    ✓7ᵗʰ **T20.412 Corrosion of unspecified degree of left ear [any part, except ear drum]**

    ✓7ᵗʰ **T20.419 Corrosion of unspecified degree of unspecified ear [any part, except ear drum]**

  ✓x7ᵗʰ **T20.42 Corrosion of unspecified degree of lip(s)**

  ✓x7ᵗʰ **T20.43 Corrosion of unspecified degree of chin**

  ✓x7ᵗʰ **T20.44 Corrosion of unspecified degree of nose (septum)**

  ✓x7ᵗʰ **T20.45 Corrosion of unspecified degree of scalp [any part]**

  ✓x7ᵗʰ **T20.46 Corrosion of unspecified degree of forehead and cheek**

  ✓x7ᵗʰ **T20.47 Corrosion of unspecified degree of neck**

  ✓x7ᵗʰ **T20.49 Corrosion of unspecified degree of multiple sites of head, face, and neck**

✓5ᵗʰ **T20.5 Corrosion of first degree of head, face, and neck**
Code first (T51-T65) to identify chemical and intent
Use additional external cause code to identify place (Y92)

  ✓x7ᵗʰ **T20.50 Corrosion of first degree of head, face, and neck, unspecified site**

  ✓6ᵗʰ **T20.51 Corrosion of first degree of ear [any part, except ear drum]**
    EXCLUDES 2   corrosion of ear drum (T28.91-)

    ✓7ᵗʰ **T20.511 Corrosion of first degree of right ear [any part, except ear drum]**

    ✓7ᵗʰ **T20.512 Corrosion of first degree of left ear [any part, except ear drum]**

    ✓7ᵗʰ **T20.519 Corrosion of first degree of unspecified ear [any part, except ear drum]**

  ✓x7ᵗʰ **T20.52 Corrosion of first degree of lip(s)**

  ✓x7ᵗʰ **T20.53 Corrosion of first degree of chin**

  ✓x7ᵗʰ **T20.54 Corrosion of first degree of nose (septum)**

  ✓x7ᵗʰ **T20.55 Corrosion of first degree of scalp [any part]**

  ✓x7ᵗʰ **T20.56 Corrosion of first degree of forehead and cheek**

  ✓x7ᵗʰ **T20.57 Corrosion of first degree of neck**

  ✓x7ᵗʰ **T20.59 Corrosion of first degree of multiple sites of head, face, and neck**

✓5ᵗʰ **T20.6 Corrosion of second degree of head, face, and neck**
Code first (T51-T65) to identify chemical and intent
Use additional external cause code to identify place (Y92)

  ✓x7ᵗʰ **T20.60 Corrosion of second degree of head, face, and neck, unspecified site**

  ✓6ᵗʰ **T20.61 Corrosion of second degree of ear [any part, except ear drum]**
    EXCLUDES 2   corrosion of ear drum (T28.91-)

    ✓7ᵗʰ **T20.611 Corrosion of second degree of right ear [any part, except ear drum]**

    ✓7ᵗʰ **T20.612 Corrosion of second degree of left ear [any part, except ear drum]**

    ✓7ᵗʰ **T20.619 Corrosion of second degree of unspecified ear [any part, except ear drum]**

  ✓x7ᵗʰ **T20.62 Corrosion of second degree of lip(s)**

  ✓x7ᵗʰ **T20.63 Corrosion of second degree of chin**

  ✓x7ᵗʰ **T20.64 Corrosion of second degree of nose (septum)**

  ✓x7ᵗʰ **T20.65 Corrosion of second degree of scalp [any part]**

  ✓x7ᵗʰ **T20.66 Corrosion of second degree of forehead and cheek**

  ✓x7ᵗʰ **T20.67 Corrosion of second degree of neck**

  ✓x7ᵗʰ **T20.69 Corrosion of second degree of multiple sites of head, face, and neck**

✓5ᵗʰ **T20.7 Corrosion of third degree of head, face, and neck**
Code first (T51-T65) to identify chemical and intent
Use additional external cause code to identify place (Y92)

  ✓x7ᵗʰ **T20.70 Corrosion of third degree of head, face, and neck, unspecified site**   CC H5 SW
    CC Excl: PDX collection 1375

  ✓6ᵗʰ **T20.71 Corrosion of third degree of ear [any part, except ear drum]**
    EXCLUDES 2   corrosion of ear drum (T28.91-)

    CC Excl: For CC codes in subcategory T20.71: PDX collection 1376

    ✓7ᵗʰ **T20.711 Corrosion of third degree of right ear [any part, except ear drum]**   CC H5 SW

    ✓7ᵗʰ **T20.712 Corrosion of third degree of left ear [any part, except ear drum]**   CC H5 SW

    ✓7ᵗʰ **T20.719 Corrosion of third degree of unspecified ear [any part, except ear drum]**   CC H5 SW

  ✓x7ᵗʰ **T20.72 Corrosion of third degree of lip(s)**   CC H5 SW
    CC Excl: PDX collection 1377

✓ Additional Character Required   ✓x7ᵗʰ Placeholder   Unacceptable PDx   Questionable PDx   Manifestation   H1-H14 HAC   HCC CMS-HCC Dx   HIV HIV Dx

ICD-10-CM 2019   1083

√x7ᵗʰ **T20.73** **Corrosion of third degree of chin** `CC` `H5` `SW`
CC Excl: PDX collection 1378

√x7ᵗʰ **T20.74** **Corrosion of third degree of nose (septum)** `CC` `H5` `SW`
CC Excl: PDX collection 1379

√x7ᵗʰ **T20.75** **Corrosion of third degree of scalp [any part]** `CC` `H5` `SW`
CC Excl: PDX collection 1380

√x7ᵗʰ **T20.76** **Corrosion of third degree of forehead and** `CC` `H5` `SW`
cheek
CC Excl: PDX collection 1381

√x7ᵗʰ **T20.77** **Corrosion of third degree of neck** `CC` `H5` `SW`
CC Excl: PDX collection 1382

√x7ᵗʰ **T20.79** **Corrosion of third degree of multiple sites** `CC` `H5` `SW`
of head, face, and neck
CC Excl: PDX collection 1383

√4ᵗʰ **T21** **Burn and corrosion of trunk**
INCLUDES   burns and corrosion of hip region
EXCLUDES 2   *burns and corrosion of axilla (T22.- with fifth character 4)*
burns and corrosion of scapular region (T22.- with fifth character 6)
burns and corrosion of shoulder (T22.- with fifth character 5)

The appropriate 7th character is to be added to each code from
category T21.
A   initial encounter
D   subsequent encounter
S   sequela

√5ᵗʰ **T21.0** **Burn of unspecified degree of trunk**
Use additional external cause code to identify the source, place
and intent of the burn (X00-X19, X75-X77, X96-X98, Y92)

√x7ᵗʰ **T21.00** **Burn of unspecified degree of trunk, unspecified site**

√x7ᵗʰ **T21.01** **Burn of unspecified degree of chest wall**
Burn of unspecified degree of breast

√x7ᵗʰ **T21.02** **Burn of unspecified degree of abdominal wall**
Burn of unspecified degree of flank
Burn of unspecified degree of groin

√x7ᵗʰ **T21.03** **Burn of unspecified degree of upper back**
Burn of unspecified degree of interscapular region

√x7ᵗʰ **T21.04** **Burn of unspecified degree of lower back**

√x7ᵗʰ **T21.05** **Burn of unspecified degree of buttock**
Burn of unspecified degree of anus

√x7ᵗʰ **T21.06** **Burn of unspecified degree of male genital region** ♂
Burn of unspecified degree of penis
Burn of unspecified degree of scrotum
Burn of unspecified degree of testis

√x7ᵗʰ **T21.07** **Burn of unspecified degree of female genital** ♀
region
Burn of unspecified degree of labium (majus) (minus)
Burn of unspecified degree of perineum
Burn of unspecified degree of vulva
EXCLUDES 2   *burn of vagina (T28.3)*

√x7ᵗʰ **T21.09** **Burn of unspecified degree of other site of trunk**

√5ᵗʰ **T21.1** **Burn of first degree of trunk**
Use additional external cause code to identify the source, place
and intent of the burn (X00-X19, X75-X77, X96-X98, Y92)

√x7ᵗʰ **T21.10** **Burn of first degree of trunk, unspecified site**

√x7ᵗʰ **T21.11** **Burn of first degree of chest wall**
Burn of first degree of breast

√x7ᵗʰ **T21.12** **Burn of first degree of abdominal wall**
Burn of first degree of flank
Burn of first degree of groin

√x7ᵗʰ **T21.13** **Burn of first degree of upper back**
Burn of first degree of interscapular region

√x7ᵗʰ **T21.14** **Burn of first degree of lower back**

√x7ᵗʰ **T21.15** **Burn of first degree of buttock**
Burn of first degree of anus

√x7ᵗʰ **T21.16** **Burn of first degree of male genital region** ♂
Burn of first degree of penis
Burn of first degree of scrotum
Burn of first degree of testis

√x7ᵗʰ **T21.17** **Burn of first degree of female genital region** ♀
Burn of first degree of labium (majus) (minus)
Burn of first degree of perineum
Burn of first degree of vulva
EXCLUDES 2   *burn of vagina (T28.3)*

√x7ᵗʰ **T21.19** **Burn of first degree of other site of trunk**

√5ᵗʰ **T21.2** **Burn of second degree of trunk**
Use additional external cause code to identify the source, place
and intent of the burn (X00-X19, X75-X77, X96-X98, Y92)

√x7ᵗʰ **T21.20** **Burn of second degree of trunk, unspecified site**

√x7ᵗʰ **T21.21** **Burn of second degree of chest wall**
Burn of second degree of breast

√x7ᵗʰ **T21.22** **Burn of second degree of abdominal wall**
Burn of second degree of flank
Burn of second degree of groin

√x7ᵗʰ **T21.23** **Burn of second degree of upper back**
Burn of second degree of interscapular region

√x7ᵗʰ **T21.24** **Burn of second degree of lower back**

√x7ᵗʰ **T21.25** **Burn of second degree of buttock**
Burn of second degree of anus

√x7ᵗʰ **T21.26** **Burn of second degree of male genital region** ♂
Burn of second degree of penis
Burn of second degree of scrotum
Burn of second degree of testis

√x7ᵗʰ **T21.27** **Burn of second degree of female genital region** ♀
Burn of second degree of labium (majus) (minus)
Burn of second degree of perineum
Burn of second degree of vulva
EXCLUDES 2   *burn of vagina (T28.3)*

√x7ᵗʰ **T21.29** **Burn of second degree of other site of trunk**

√5ᵗʰ **T21.3** **Burn of third degree of trunk**
Use additional external cause code to identify the source, place
and intent of the burn (X00-X19, X75-X77, X96-X98, Y92)

√x7ᵗʰ **T21.30** **Burn of third degree of trunk,** `CC` `H5` `SW`
unspecified site
CC Excl: PDX collection 1384

√x7ᵗʰ **T21.31** **Burn of third degree of chest wall** `CC` `H5` `SW`
Burn of third degree of breast
AHA: 2016, 2Q, 5
CC Excl: PDX collection 1385

√x7ᵗʰ **T21.32** **Burn of third degree of abdominal wall** `CC` `H5` `SW`
Burn of third degree of flank
Burn of third degree of groin
CC Excl: PDX collection 1386

√x7ᵗʰ **T21.33** **Burn of third degree of upper back** `CC` `H5` `SW`
Burn of third degree of interscapular region
CC Excl: PDX collection 1387

√x7ᵗʰ **T21.34** **Burn of third degree of lower back** `CC` `H5` `SW`
CC Excl: PDX collection 1387

√x7ᵗʰ **T21.35** **Burn of third degree of buttock** `CC` `H5` `SW`
Burn of third degree of anus
CC Excl: PDX collection 1387

√x7ᵗʰ **T21.36** **Burn of third degree of male genital** `CC` `H5` `SW` ♂
region
Burn of third degree of penis
Burn of third degree of scrotum
Burn of third degree of testis
CC Excl: PDX collection 1388

√x7ᵗʰ **T21.37** **Burn of third degree of female genital** `CC` `H5` `SW` ♀
region
Burn of third degree of labium (majus) (minus)
Burn of third degree of perineum
Burn of third degree of vulva
EXCLUDES 2   *burn of vagina (T28.3)*
CC Excl: PDX collection 1388

√x7ᵗʰ **T21.39** **Burn of third degree of other site of trunk** `CC` `H5` `SW`
CC Excl: PDX collection 1384

√5ᵗʰ **T21.4** **Corrosion of unspecified degree of trunk**
Code first (T51-T65) to identify chemical and intent
Use additional external cause code to identify place (Y92)

√x7ᵗʰ **T21.40** **Corrosion of unspecified degree of trunk,**
unspecified site

√x7ᵗʰ **T21.41** **Corrosion of unspecified degree of chest wall**
Corrosion of unspecified degree of breast

√x7ᵗʰ **T21.42** **Corrosion of unspecified degree of abdominal wall**
Corrosion of unspecified degree of flank
Corrosion of unspecified degree of groin

√x7ᵗʰ **T21.43** **Corrosion of unspecified degree of upper back**
Corrosion of unspecified degree of interscapular
region

√x7ᵗʰ **T21.44** **Corrosion of unspecified degree of lower back**

√x 7ᵗʰ **T21.45** **Corrosion of unspecified degree of** buttock
Corrosion of unspecified degree of anus

√x 7ᵗʰ **T21.46** **Corrosion of unspecified degree of** male genital ♂
region
Corrosion of unspecified degree of penis
Corrosion of unspecified degree of scrotum
Corrosion of unspecified degree of testis

√x 7ᵗʰ **T21.47** **Corrosion of unspecified degree of** female genital ♀
region
Corrosion of unspecified degree of labium (majus)
(minus)
Corrosion of unspecified degree of perineum
Corrosion of unspecified degree of vulva
EXCLUDES 2   corrosion of vagina (T28.8)

√x 7ᵗʰ **T21.49** **Corrosion of unspecified degree of** other site of
trunk

√5ᵗʰ **T21.5** **Corrosion of** first degree **of trunk**
Code first (T51-T65) to identify chemical and intent
Use additional external cause code to identify place (Y92)

√x 7ᵗʰ **T21.50** **Corrosion of first degree of trunk,** unspecified site

√x 7ᵗʰ **T21.51** **Corrosion of first degree of** chest wall
Corrosion of first degree of breast

√x 7ᵗʰ **T21.52** **Corrosion of first degree of** abdominal wall
Corrosion of first degree of flank
Corrosion of first degree of groin

√x 7ᵗʰ **T21.53** **Corrosion of first degree of** upper back
Corrosion of first degree of interscapular region

√x 7ᵗʰ **T21.54** **Corrosion of first degree of** lower back

√x 7ᵗʰ **T21.55** **Corrosion of first degree of** buttock
Corrosion of first degree of anus

√x 7ᵗʰ **T21.56** **Corrosion of first degree of** male genital region ♂
Corrosion of first degree of penis
Corrosion of first degree of scrotum
Corrosion of first degree of testis

√x 7ᵗʰ **T21.57** **Corrosion of first degree of** female genital region ♀
Corrosion of first degree of labium (majus) (minus)
Corrosion of first degree of perineum
Corrosion of first degree of vulva
EXCLUDES 2   corrosion of vagina (T28.8)

√x 7ᵗʰ **T21.59** **Corrosion of first degree of** other site **of trunk**

√5ᵗʰ **T21.6** **Corrosion of** second degree **of trunk**
Code first (T51-T65) to identify chemical and intent
Use additional external cause code to identify place (Y92)

√x 7ᵗʰ **T21.60** **Corrosion of second degree of trunk,**
unspecified site

√x 7ᵗʰ **T21.61** **Corrosion of second degree of** chest wall
Corrosion of second degree of breast

√x 7ᵗʰ **T21.62** **Corrosion of second degree of** abdominal wall
Corrosion of second degree of flank
Corrosion of second degree of groin

√x 7ᵗʰ **T21.63** **Corrosion of second degree of** upper back
Corrosion of second degree of interscapular region

√x 7ᵗʰ **T21.64** **Corrosion of second degree of** lower back

√x 7ᵗʰ **T21.65** **Corrosion of second degree of** buttock
Corrosion of second degree of anus

√x 7ᵗʰ **T21.66** **Corrosion of second degree of** male genital region ♂
Corrosion of second degree of penis
Corrosion of second degree of scrotum
Corrosion of second degree of testis

√x 7ᵗʰ **T21.67** **Corrosion of second degree of** female genital ♀
region
Corrosion of second degree of labium (majus) (minus)
Corrosion of second degree of perineum
Corrosion of second degree of vulva
EXCLUDES 2   corrosion of vagina (T28.8)

√x 7ᵗʰ **T21.69** **Corrosion of second degree of** other site **of trunk**

√5ᵗʰ **T21.7** **Corrosion of** third degree **of trunk**
Code first (T51-T65) to identify chemical and intent
Use additional external cause code to identify place (Y92)

√x 7ᵗʰ **T21.70** **Corrosion of third degree of trunk,**   CC H5 SW
unspecified site
CC Excl: PDX collection 1384

√x 7ᵗʰ **T21.71** **Corrosion of third degree of** chest wall   CC H5 SW
Corrosion of third degree of breast
CC Excl: PDX collection 1385

√x 7ᵗʰ **T21.72** **Corrosion of third degree of** abdominal   CC H5 SW
wall
Corrosion of third degree of flank
Corrosion of third degree of groin
CC Excl: PDX collection 1386

√x 7ᵗʰ **T21.73** **Corrosion of third degree of** upper back   CC H5 SW
Corrosion of third degree of interscapular region
CC Excl: PDX collection 1387

√x 7ᵗʰ **T21.74** **Corrosion of third degree of** lower back   CC H5 SW
CC Excl: PDX collection 1387

√x 7ᵗʰ **T21.75** **Corrosion of third degree of** buttock   CC H5 SW
Corrosion of third degree of anus
CC Excl: PDX collection 1387

√x 7ᵗʰ **T21.76** **Corrosion of third degree of** male genital   CC H5 SW ♂
region
Corrosion of third degree of penis
Corrosion of third degree of scrotum
Corrosion of third degree of testis
CC Excl: PDX collection 1388

√x 7ᵗʰ **T21.77** **Corrosion of third degree of** female   CC H5 SW ♀
genital region
Corrosion of third degree of labium (majus) (minus)
Corrosion of third degree of perineum
Corrosion of third degree of vulva
EXCLUDES 2   corrosion of vagina (T28.8)
CC Excl: PDX collection 1388

√x 7ᵗʰ **T21.79** **Corrosion of third degree of** other site of   CC H5 SW
trunk
CC Excl: PDX collection 1384

√4ᵗʰ **T22** **Burn and corrosion of shoulder and upper limb, except wrist and hand**
EXCLUDES 2   burn and corrosion of interscapular region (T21.-)
burn and corrosion of wrist and hand (T23.-)

The appropriate 7th character is to be added to each code from
category T22.
A   initial encounter
D   subsequent encounter
S   sequela

√5ᵗʰ **T22.0** **Burn of** unspecified degree **of shoulder and upper limb,**
except wrist and hand
Use additional external cause code to identify the source, place
and intent of the burn (X00-X19, X75-X77, X96-X98, Y92)

√x 7ᵗʰ **T22.00** **Burn of unspecified degree of shoulder and upper
limb, except wrist and hand,** unspecified site

√6ᵗʰ **T22.01** **Burn of unspecified degree of** forearm

√7ᵗʰ **T22.011** **Burn of unspecified degree of** right
forearm

√7ᵗʰ **T22.012** **Burn of unspecified degree of** left **forearm**

√7ᵗʰ **T22.019** **Burn of unspecified degree of**
unspecified **forearm**

√6ᵗʰ **T22.02** **Burn of unspecified degree of** elbow

√7ᵗʰ **T22.021** **Burn of unspecified degree of** right **elbow**

√7ᵗʰ **T22.022** **Burn of unspecified degree of** left **elbow**

√7ᵗʰ **T22.029** **Burn of unspecified degree of**
unspecified **elbow**

√6ᵗʰ **T22.03** **Burn of unspecified degree of** upper arm

√7ᵗʰ **T22.031** **Burn of unspecified degree of** right **upper
arm**

√7ᵗʰ **T22.032** **Burn of unspecified degree of** left **upper
arm**

√7ᵗʰ **T22.039** **Burn of unspecified degree of**
unspecified **upper arm**

√6ᵗʰ **T22.04** **Burn of unspecified degree of** axilla

√7ᵗʰ **T22.041** **Burn of unspecified degree of** right **axilla**

√7ᵗʰ **T22.042** **Burn of unspecified degree of** left **axilla**

√7ᵗʰ **T22.049** **Burn of unspecified degree of**
unspecified **axilla**

√6ᵗʰ **T22.05** **Burn of unspecified degree of** shoulder

√7ᵗʰ **T22.051** **Burn of unspecified degree of** right
shoulder

√7ᵗʰ **T22.052** **Burn of unspecified degree of** left
shoulder

√7ᵗʰ **T22.059** **Burn of unspecified degree of**
unspecified **shoulder**

✓6ᵗʰ T22.06 Burn of unspecified degree of scapular region

     ✓7ᵗʰ **T22.061** Burn of unspecified degree of right scapular region

     ✓7ᵗʰ **T22.062** Burn of unspecified degree of left scapular region

     ✓7ᵗʰ **T22.069** Burn of unspecified degree of unspecified scapular region

✓6ᵗʰ T22.09 Burn of unspecified degree of multiple sites of shoulder and upper limb, except wrist and hand

     ✓7ᵗʰ **T22.091** Burn of unspecified degree of multiple sites of right shoulder and upper limb, except wrist and hand

     ✓7ᵗʰ **T22.092** Burn of unspecified degree of multiple sites of left shoulder and upper limb, except wrist and hand

     ✓7ᵗʰ **T22.099** Burn of unspecified degree of multiple sites of unspecified shoulder and upper limb, except wrist and hand

✓5ᵗʰ T22.1 Burn of first degree of shoulder and upper limb, except wrist and hand

     Use additional external cause code to identify the source, place and intent of the burn (X00-X19, X75-X77, X96-X98, Y92)

✓x7ᵗʰ T22.10 Burn of first degree of shoulder and upper limb, except wrist and hand, unspecified site

✓6ᵗʰ T22.11 Burn of first degree of forearm

     ✓7ᵗʰ **T22.111** Burn of first degree of right forearm

     ✓7ᵗʰ **T22.112** Burn of first degree of left forearm

     ✓7ᵗʰ **T22.119** Burn of first degree of unspecified forearm

✓6ᵗʰ T22.12 Burn of first degree of elbow

     ✓7ᵗʰ **T22.121** Burn of first degree of right elbow

     ✓7ᵗʰ **T22.122** Burn of first degree of left elbow

     ✓7ᵗʰ **T22.129** Burn of first degree of unspecified elbow

✓6ᵗʰ T22.13 Burn of first degree of upper arm

     ✓7ᵗʰ **T22.131** Burn of first degree of right upper arm

     ✓7ᵗʰ **T22.132** Burn of first degree of left upper arm

     ✓7ᵗʰ **T22.139** Burn of first degree of unspecified upper arm

✓6ᵗʰ T22.14 Burn of first degree of axilla

     ✓7ᵗʰ **T22.141** Burn of first degree of right axilla

     ✓7ᵗʰ **T22.142** Burn of first degree of left axilla

     ✓7ᵗʰ **T22.149** Burn of first degree of unspecified axilla

✓6ᵗʰ T22.15 Burn of first degree of shoulder

     ✓7ᵗʰ **T22.151** Burn of first degree of right shoulder

     ✓7ᵗʰ **T22.152** Burn of first degree of left shoulder

     ✓7ᵗʰ **T22.159** Burn of first degree of unspecified shoulder

✓6ᵗʰ T22.16 Burn of first degree of scapular region

     ✓7ᵗʰ **T22.161** Burn of first degree of right scapular region

     ✓7ᵗʰ **T22.162** Burn of first degree of left scapular region

     ✓7ᵗʰ **T22.169** Burn of first degree of unspecified scapular region

✓6ᵗʰ T22.19 Burn of first degree of multiple sites of shoulder and upper limb, except wrist and hand

     ✓7ᵗʰ **T22.191** Burn of first degree of multiple sites of right shoulder and upper limb, except wrist and hand

     ✓7ᵗʰ **T22.192** Burn of first degree of multiple sites of left shoulder and upper limb, except wrist and hand

     ✓7ᵗʰ **T22.199** Burn of first degree of multiple sites of unspecified shoulder and upper limb, except wrist and hand

✓5ᵗʰ T22.2 Burn of second degree of shoulder and upper limb, except wrist and hand

     Use additional external cause code to identify the source, place and intent of the burn (X00-X19, X75-X77, X96-X98, Y92)

✓x7ᵗʰ T22.20 Burn of second degree of shoulder and upper limb, except wrist and hand, unspecified site

✓6ᵗʰ T22.21 Burn of second degree of forearm

     ✓7ᵗʰ **T22.211** Burn of second degree of right forearm

     ✓7ᵗʰ **T22.212** Burn of second degree of left forearm

     ✓7ᵗʰ **T22.219** Burn of second degree of unspecified forearm

✓6ᵗʰ T22.22 Burn of second degree of elbow

     ✓7ᵗʰ **T22.221** Burn of second degree of right elbow

     ✓7ᵗʰ **T22.222** Burn of second degree of left elbow

     ✓7ᵗʰ **T22.229** Burn of second degree of unspecified elbow

✓6ᵗʰ T22.23 Burn of second degree of upper arm

     ✓7ᵗʰ **T22.231** Burn of second degree of right upper arm

     ✓7ᵗʰ **T22.232** Burn of second degree of left upper arm

     ✓7ᵗʰ **T22.239** Burn of second degree of unspecified upper arm

✓6ᵗʰ T22.24 Burn of second degree of axilla

     ✓7ᵗʰ **T22.241** Burn of second degree of right axilla

     ✓7ᵗʰ **T22.242** Burn of second degree of left axilla

     ✓7ᵗʰ **T22.249** Burn of second degree of unspecified axilla

✓6ᵗʰ T22.25 Burn of second degree of shoulder

     ✓7ᵗʰ **T22.251** Burn of second degree of right shoulder

     ✓7ᵗʰ **T22.252** Burn of second degree of left shoulder

     ✓7ᵗʰ **T22.259** Burn of second degree of unspecified shoulder

✓6ᵗʰ T22.26 Burn of second degree of scapular region

     ✓7ᵗʰ **T22.261** Burn of second degree of right scapular region

     ✓7ᵗʰ **T22.262** Burn of second degree of left scapular region

     ✓7ᵗʰ **T22.269** Burn of second degree of unspecified scapular region

✓6ᵗʰ T22.29 Burn of second degree of multiple sites of shoulder and upper limb, except wrist and hand

     ✓7ᵗʰ **T22.291** Burn of second degree of multiple sites of right shoulder and upper limb, except wrist and hand

     ✓7ᵗʰ **T22.292** Burn of second degree of multiple sites of left shoulder and upper limb, except wrist and hand

     ✓7ᵗʰ **T22.299** Burn of second degree of multiple sites of unspecified shoulder and upper limb, except wrist and hand

✓5ᵗʰ T22.3 Burn of third degree of shoulder and upper limb, except wrist and hand

     Use additional external cause code to identify the source, place and intent of the burn (X00-X19, X75-X77, X96-X98, Y92)

✓x7ᵗʰ T22.30 Burn of third degree of shoulder and upper limb, except wrist and hand, unspecified site `CC` `H5` `SW`

     CC Excl: PDX collection 1389

✓6ᵗʰ T22.31 Burn of third degree of forearm

     CC Excl: For CC codes in subcategory T22.31: PDX collection 1390

     ✓7ᵗʰ **T22.311** Burn of third degree of right forearm `CC` `H5` `SW`

     ✓7ᵗʰ **T22.312** Burn of third degree of left forearm `CC` `H5` `SW`

     ✓7ᵗʰ **T22.319** Burn of third degree of unspecified forearm `CC` `H5` `SW`

✓6ᵗʰ T22.32 Burn of third degree of elbow

     CC Excl: For CC codes in subcategory T22.32: PDX collection 1391

     ✓7ᵗʰ **T22.321** Burn of third degree of right elbow `CC` `H5` `SW`

     ✓7ᵗʰ **T22.322** Burn of third degree of left elbow `CC` `H5` `SW`

     ✓7ᵗʰ **T22.329** Burn of third degree of unspecified elbow `CC` `H5` `SW`

✓6ᵗʰ T22.33 Burn of third degree of upper arm

     CC Excl: For CC codes in subcategory T22.33: PDX collection 1392

     ✓7ᵗʰ **T22.331** Burn of third degree of right upper arm `CC` `H5` `SW`

Ⓝ Newborn: 0   Ⓟ Pediatric: 0-17   Ⓜ Maternity: 12-55   Ⓐ Adult: 15-124   **MCC** Major Complication/Comorbidity   **CC** Complication/Comorbidity   **SW** Severe Wound Dx

1086   ICD-10-CM 2019

✓7ᵗʰ **T22.332** Burn of third degree of left upper arm `CC` `H5` `SW`

✓7ᵗʰ **T22.339** Burn of third degree of unspecified upper arm `CC` `H5` `SW`

✓6ᵗʰ **T22.34** Burn of third degree of axilla

> **CC Excl: For CC codes in subcategory T22.34:**
> PDX collection 1393

✓7ᵗʰ **T22.341** Burn of third degree of right axilla `CC` `H5` `SW`

✓7ᵗʰ **T22.342** Burn of third degree of left axilla `CC` `H5` `SW`

✓7ᵗʰ **T22.349** Burn of third degree of unspecified axilla `CC` `H5` `SW`

✓6ᵗʰ **T22.35** Burn of third degree of shoulder

> **CC Excl: For CC codes in subcategory T22.35:**
> PDX collection 1394

✓7ᵗʰ **T22.351** Burn of third degree of right shoulder `CC` `H5` `SW`

✓7ᵗʰ **T22.352** Burn of third degree of left shoulder `CC` `H5` `SW`

✓7ᵗʰ **T22.359** Burn of third degree of unspecified shoulder `CC` `H5` `SW`

✓6ᵗʰ **T22.36** Burn of third degree of scapular region

> **CC Excl: For CC codes in subcategory T22.36:**
> PDX collection 1395

✓7ᵗʰ **T22.361** Burn of third degree of right scapular region `CC` `H5` `SW`

✓7ᵗʰ **T22.362** Burn of third degree of left scapular region `CC` `H5` `SW`

✓7ᵗʰ **T22.369** Burn of third degree of unspecified scapular region `CC` `H5` `SW`

✓6ᵗʰ **T22.39** Burn of third degree of multiple sites of shoulder and upper limb, except wrist and hand

> **CC Excl: For CC codes in subcategory T22.39:**
> PDX collection 1389

✓7ᵗʰ **T22.391** Burn of third degree of multiple sites of right shoulder and upper limb, except wrist and hand `CC` `H5` `SW`

✓7ᵗʰ **T22.392** Burn of third degree of multiple sites of left shoulder and upper limb, except wrist and hand `CC` `H5` `SW`

✓7ᵗʰ **T22.399** Burn of third degree of multiple sites of unspecified shoulder and upper limb, except wrist and hand `CC` `H5` `SW`

✓5ᵗʰ **T22.4** Corrosion of unspecified degree of shoulder and upper limb, except wrist and hand

> Code first (T51-T65) to identify chemical and intent
> Use additional external cause code to identify place (Y92)

✓x7ᵗʰ **T22.40** Corrosion of unspecified degree of shoulder and upper limb, except wrist and hand, unspecified site

✓6ᵗʰ **T22.41** Corrosion of unspecified degree of forearm

✓7ᵗʰ **T22.411** Corrosion of unspecified degree of right forearm

✓7ᵗʰ **T22.412** Corrosion of unspecified degree of left forearm

✓7ᵗʰ **T22.419** Corrosion of unspecified degree of unspecified forearm

✓6ᵗʰ **T22.42** Corrosion of unspecified degree of elbow

✓7ᵗʰ **T22.421** Corrosion of unspecified degree of right elbow

✓7ᵗʰ **T22.422** Corrosion of unspecified degree of left elbow

✓7ᵗʰ **T22.429** Corrosion of unspecified degree of unspecified elbow

✓6ᵗʰ **T22.43** Corrosion of unspecified degree of upper arm

✓7ᵗʰ **T22.431** Corrosion of unspecified degree of right upper arm

✓7ᵗʰ **T22.432** Corrosion of unspecified degree of left upper arm

✓7ᵗʰ **T22.439** Corrosion of unspecified degree of unspecified upper arm

✓6ᵗʰ **T22.44** Corrosion of unspecified degree of axilla

✓7ᵗʰ **T22.441** Corrosion of unspecified degree of right axilla

✓7ᵗʰ **T22.442** Corrosion of unspecified degree of left axilla

✓7ᵗʰ **T22.449** Corrosion of unspecified degree of unspecified axilla

✓6ᵗʰ **T22.45** Corrosion of unspecified degree of shoulder

✓7ᵗʰ **T22.451** Corrosion of unspecified degree of right shoulder

✓7ᵗʰ **T22.452** Corrosion of unspecified degree of left shoulder

✓7ᵗʰ **T22.459** Corrosion of unspecified degree of unspecified shoulder

✓6ᵗʰ **T22.46** Corrosion of unspecified degree of scapular region

✓7ᵗʰ **T22.461** Corrosion of unspecified degree of right scapular region

✓7ᵗʰ **T22.462** Corrosion of unspecified degree of left scapular region

✓7ᵗʰ **T22.469** Corrosion of unspecified degree of unspecified scapular region

✓6ᵗʰ **T22.49** Corrosion of unspecified degree of multiple sites of shoulder and upper limb, except wrist and hand

✓7ᵗʰ **T22.491** Corrosion of unspecified degree of multiple sites of right shoulder and upper limb, except wrist and hand

✓7ᵗʰ **T22.492** Corrosion of unspecified degree of multiple sites of left shoulder and upper limb, except wrist and hand

✓7ᵗʰ **T22.499** Corrosion of unspecified degree of multiple sites of unspecified shoulder and upper limb, except wrist and hand

✓5ᵗʰ **T22.5** Corrosion of first degree of shoulder and upper limb, except wrist and hand

> Code first (T51-T65) to identify chemical and intent
> Use additional external cause code to identify place (Y92)

✓x7ᵗʰ **T22.50** Corrosion of first degree of shoulder and upper limb, except wrist and hand unspecified site

✓6ᵗʰ **T22.51** Corrosion of first degree of forearm

✓7ᵗʰ **T22.511** Corrosion of first degree of right forearm

✓7ᵗʰ **T22.512** Corrosion of first degree of left forearm

✓7ᵗʰ **T22.519** Corrosion of first degree of unspecified forearm

✓6ᵗʰ **T22.52** Corrosion of first degree of elbow

✓7ᵗʰ **T22.521** Corrosion of first degree of right elbow

✓7ᵗʰ **T22.522** Corrosion of first degree of left elbow

✓7ᵗʰ **T22.529** Corrosion of first degree of unspecified elbow

✓6ᵗʰ **T22.53** Corrosion of first degree of upper arm

✓7ᵗʰ **T22.531** Corrosion of first degree of right upper arm

✓7ᵗʰ **T22.532** Corrosion of first degree of left upper arm

✓7ᵗʰ **T22.539** Corrosion of first degree of unspecified upper arm

✓6ᵗʰ **T22.54** Corrosion of first degree of axilla

✓7ᵗʰ **T22.541** Corrosion of first degree of right axilla

✓7ᵗʰ **T22.542** Corrosion of first degree of left axilla

✓7ᵗʰ **T22.549** Corrosion of first degree of unspecified axilla

✓6ᵗʰ **T22.55** Corrosion of first degree of shoulder

✓7ᵗʰ **T22.551** Corrosion of first degree of right shoulder

✓7ᵗʰ **T22.552** Corrosion of first degree of left shoulder

✓7ᵗʰ **T22.559** Corrosion of first degree of unspecified shoulder

✓6ᵗʰ **T22.56** Corrosion of first degree of scapular region

✓7ᵗʰ **T22.561** Corrosion of first degree of right scapular region

✓7ᵗʰ **T22.562** Corrosion of first degree of left scapular region

✓7ᵗʰ **T22.569** Corrosion of first degree of unspecified scapular region

✓6ᵗʰ **T22.59** Corrosion of first degree of multiple sites of shoulder and upper limb, except wrist and hand

✓ Additional Character Required	✓x7ᵗʰ Placeholder	Unacceptable PDx	Questionable PDx	Manifestation	`H1` - `H14` HAC	`HCC` CMS-HCC Dx	`HIV` HIV Dx

ICD-10-CM 2019   **1087**

☑7ᵗʰ **T22.591** Corrosion of first degree of multiple sites of right shoulder and upper limb, except wrist and hand

☑7ᵗʰ **T22.592** Corrosion of first degree of multiple sites of left shoulder and upper limb, except wrist and hand

☑7ᵗʰ **T22.599** Corrosion of first degree of multiple sites of unspecified shoulder and upper limb, except wrist and hand

☑5ᵗʰ **T22.6** Corrosion of second degree of shoulder and upper limb, except wrist and hand

Code first (T51-T65) to identify chemical and intent
Use additional external cause code to identify place (Y92)

☑×7ᵗʰ **T22.60** Corrosion of second degree of shoulder and upper limb, except wrist and hand, unspecified site

☑6ᵗʰ **T22.61** Corrosion of second degree of forearm

☑7ᵗʰ **T22.611** Corrosion of second degree of right forearm

☑7ᵗʰ **T22.612** Corrosion of second degree of left forearm

☑7ᵗʰ **T22.619** Corrosion of second degree of unspecified forearm

☑6ᵗʰ **T22.62** Corrosion of second degree of elbow

☑7ᵗʰ **T22.621** Corrosion of second degree of right elbow

☑7ᵗʰ **T22.622** Corrosion of second degree of left elbow

☑7ᵗʰ **T22.629** Corrosion of second degree of unspecified elbow

☑6ᵗʰ **T22.63** Corrosion of second degree of upper arm

☑7ᵗʰ **T22.631** Corrosion of second degree of right upper arm

☑7ᵗʰ **T22.632** Corrosion of second degree of left upper arm

☑7ᵗʰ **T22.639** Corrosion of second degree of unspecified upper arm

☑6ᵗʰ **T22.64** Corrosion of second degree of axilla

☑7ᵗʰ **T22.641** Corrosion of second degree of right axilla

☑7ᵗʰ **T22.642** Corrosion of second degree of left axilla

☑7ᵗʰ **T22.649** Corrosion of second degree of unspecified axilla

☑6ᵗʰ **T22.65** Corrosion of second degree of shoulder

☑7ᵗʰ **T22.651** Corrosion of second degree of right shoulder

☑7ᵗʰ **T22.652** Corrosion of second degree of left shoulder

☑7ᵗʰ **T22.659** Corrosion of second degree of unspecified shoulder

☑6ᵗʰ **T22.66** Corrosion of second degree of scapular region

☑7ᵗʰ **T22.661** Corrosion of second degree of right scapular region

☑7ᵗʰ **T22.662** Corrosion of second degree of left scapular region

☑7ᵗʰ **T22.669** Corrosion of second degree of unspecified scapular region

☑6ᵗʰ **T22.69** Corrosion of second degree of multiple sites of shoulder and upper limb, except wrist and hand

☑7ᵗʰ **T22.691** Corrosion of second degree of multiple sites of right shoulder and upper limb, except wrist and hand

☑7ᵗʰ **T22.692** Corrosion of second degree of multiple sites of left shoulder and upper limb, except wrist and hand

☑7ᵗʰ **T22.699** Corrosion of second degree of multiple sites of unspecified shoulder and upper limb, except wrist and hand

☑5ᵗʰ **T22.7** Corrosion of third degree of shoulder and upper limb, except wrist and hand

Code first (T51-T65) to identify chemical and intent
Use additional external cause code to identify place (Y92)

☑×7ᵗʰ **T22.70** Corrosion of third degree of shoulder and upper limb, except wrist and hand, unspecified site `CC` `H5` `SW`
CC Excl: PDX collection 1389

☑6ᵗʰ **T22.71** Corrosion of third degree of forearm

CC Excl: **For CC codes in subcategory T22.71:**
PDX collection 1390

☑7ᵗʰ **T22.711** Corrosion of third degree of right forearm `CC` `H5` `SW`

☑7ᵗʰ **T22.712** Corrosion of third degree of left forearm `CC` `H5` `SW`

☑7ᵗʰ **T22.719** Corrosion of third degree of unspecified forearm `CC` `H5` `SW`

☑6ᵗʰ **T22.72** Corrosion of third degree of elbow

CC Excl: **For CC codes in subcategory T22.72:**
PDX collection 1391

☑7ᵗʰ **T22.721** Corrosion of third degree of right elbow `CC` `H5` `SW`

☑7ᵗʰ **T22.722** Corrosion of third degree of left elbow `CC` `H5` `SW`

☑7ᵗʰ **T22.729** Corrosion of third degree of unspecified elbow `CC` `H5` `SW`

☑6ᵗʰ **T22.73** Corrosion of third degree of upper arm

CC Excl: **For CC codes in subcategory T22.73:**
PDX collection 1392

☑7ᵗʰ **T22.731** Corrosion of third degree of right upper arm `CC` `H5` `SW`

☑7ᵗʰ **T22.732** Corrosion of third degree of left upper arm `CC` `H5` `SW`

☑7ᵗʰ **T22.739** Corrosion of third degree of unspecified upper arm `CC` `H5` `SW`

☑6ᵗʰ **T22.74** Corrosion of third degree of axilla

CC Excl: **For CC codes in subcategory T22.74:**
PDX collection 1393

☑7ᵗʰ **T22.741** Corrosion of third degree of right axilla `CC` `H5` `SW`

☑7ᵗʰ **T22.742** Corrosion of third degree of left axilla `CC` `H5` `SW`

☑7ᵗʰ **T22.749** Corrosion of third degree of unspecified axilla `CC` `H5` `SW`

☑6ᵗʰ **T22.75** Corrosion of third degree of shoulder

CC Excl: **For CC codes in subcategory T22.75:**
PDX collection 1394

☑7ᵗʰ **T22.751** Corrosion of third degree of right shoulder `CC` `H5` `SW`

☑7ᵗʰ **T22.752** Corrosion of third degree of left shoulder `CC` `H5` `SW`

☑7ᵗʰ **T22.759** Corrosion of third degree of unspecified shoulder `CC` `H5` `SW`

☑6ᵗʰ **T22.76** Corrosion of third degree of scapular region

CC Excl: **For CC codes in subcategory T22.76:**
PDX collection 1395

☑7ᵗʰ **T22.761** Corrosion of third degree of right scapular region `CC` `H5` `SW`

☑7ᵗʰ **T22.762** Corrosion of third degree of left scapular region `CC` `H5` `SW`

☑7ᵗʰ **T22.769** Corrosion of third degree of unspecified scapular region `CC` `H5` `SW`

☑6ᵗʰ **T22.79** Corrosion of third degree of multiple sites of shoulder and upper limb, except wrist and hand

CC Excl: **For CC codes in subcategory T22.79:**
PDX collection 1389

☑7ᵗʰ **T22.791** Corrosion of third degree of multiple sites of right shoulder and upper limb, except wrist and hand `CC` `H5` `SW`

☑7ᵗʰ **T22.792** Corrosion of third degree of multiple sites of left shoulder and upper limb, except wrist and hand `CC` `H5` `SW`

☑7ᵗʰ **T22.799** Corrosion of third degree of multiple sites of unspecified shoulder and upper limb, except wrist and hand `CC` `H5` `SW`

Ⓝ Newborn: 0   Ⓟ Pediatric: 0-17   Ⓜ Maternity: 12-55   Ⓐ Adult: 15-124   `MCC` Major Complication/Comorbidity   `CC` Complication/Comorbidity   `SW` Severe Wound Dx

1088   ICD-10-CM 2019

✓4ᵗʰ T23 Burn and corrosion of wrist and hand
AHA: 2015, 1Q, 19

The appropriate 7th character is to be added to each code from category T23.
A   initial encounter
D   subsequent encounter
S   sequela

✓5ᵗʰ T23.0 Burn of unspecified degree of wrist and hand
Use additional external cause code to identify the source, place and intent of the burn (X00-X19, X75-X77, X96-X98, Y92)

✓6ᵗʰ T23.00 Burn of unspecified degree of hand, unspecified site
- **✓7ᵗʰ T23.001** Burn of unspecified degree of right hand, unspecified site
- **✓7ᵗʰ T23.002** Burn of unspecified degree of left hand, unspecified site
- **✓7ᵗʰ T23.009** Burn of unspecified degree of unspecified hand, unspecified site

✓6ᵗʰ T23.01 Burn of unspecified degree of thumb (nail)
- **✓7ᵗʰ T23.011** Burn of unspecified degree of right thumb (nail)
- **✓7ᵗʰ T23.012** Burn of unspecified degree of left thumb (nail)
- **✓7ᵗʰ T23.019** Burn of unspecified degree of unspecified thumb (nail)

✓6ᵗʰ T23.02 Burn of unspecified degree of single finger (nail) except thumb
- **✓7ᵗʰ T23.021** Burn of unspecified degree of single right finger (nail) except thumb
- **✓7ᵗʰ T23.022** Burn of unspecified degree of single left finger (nail) except thumb
- **✓7ᵗʰ T23.029** Burn of unspecified degree of unspecified single finger (nail) except thumb

✓6ᵗʰ T23.03 Burn of unspecified degree of multiple fingers (nail), not including thumb
- **✓7ᵗʰ T23.031** Burn of unspecified degree of multiple right fingers (nail), not including thumb
- **✓7ᵗʰ T23.032** Burn of unspecified degree of multiple left fingers (nail), not including thumb
- **✓7ᵗʰ T23.039** Burn of unspecified degree of unspecified multiple fingers (nail), not including thumb

✓6ᵗʰ T23.04 Burn of unspecified degree of multiple fingers (nail), including thumb
- **✓7ᵗʰ T23.041** Burn of unspecified degree of multiple right fingers (nail), including thumb
- **✓7ᵗʰ T23.042** Burn of unspecified degree of multiple left fingers (nail), including thumb
- **✓7ᵗʰ T23.049** Burn of unspecified degree of unspecified multiple fingers (nail), including thumb

✓6ᵗʰ T23.05 Burn of unspecified degree of palm
- **✓7ᵗʰ T23.051** Burn of unspecified degree of right palm
- **✓7ᵗʰ T23.052** Burn of unspecified degree of left palm
- **✓7ᵗʰ T23.059** Burn of unspecified degree of unspecified palm

✓6ᵗʰ T23.06 Burn of unspecified degree of back of hand
- **✓7ᵗʰ T23.061** Burn of unspecified degree of back of right hand
- **✓7ᵗʰ T23.062** Burn of unspecified degree of back of left hand
- **✓7ᵗʰ T23.069** Burn of unspecified degree of back of unspecified hand

✓6ᵗʰ T23.07 Burn of unspecified degree of wrist
- **✓7ᵗʰ T23.071** Burn of unspecified degree of right wrist
- **✓7ᵗʰ T23.072** Burn of unspecified degree of left wrist
- **✓7ᵗʰ T23.079** Burn of unspecified degree of unspecified wrist

✓6ᵗʰ T23.09 Burn of unspecified degree of multiple sites of wrist and hand
- **✓7ᵗʰ T23.091** Burn of unspecified degree of multiple sites of right wrist and hand
- **✓7ᵗʰ T23.092** Burn of unspecified degree of multiple sites of left wrist and hand
- **✓7ᵗʰ T23.099** Burn of unspecified degree of multiple sites of unspecified wrist and hand

✓5ᵗʰ T23.1 Burn of first degree of wrist and hand
Use additional external cause code to identify the source, place and intent of the burn (X00-X19, X75-X77, X96-X98, Y92)

✓6ᵗʰ T23.10 Burn of first degree of hand, unspecified site
- **✓7ᵗʰ T23.101** Burn of first degree of right hand, unspecified site
- **✓7ᵗʰ T23.102** Burn of first degree of left hand, unspecified site
- **✓7ᵗʰ T23.109** Burn of first degree of unspecified hand, unspecified site

✓6ᵗʰ T23.11 Burn of first degree of thumb (nail)
- **✓7ᵗʰ T23.111** Burn of first degree of right thumb (nail)
- **✓7ᵗʰ T23.112** Burn of first degree of left thumb (nail)
- **✓7ᵗʰ T23.119** Burn of first degree of unspecified thumb (nail)

✓6ᵗʰ T23.12 Burn of first degree of single finger (nail) except thumb
- **✓7ᵗʰ T23.121** Burn of first degree of single right finger (nail) except thumb
- **✓7ᵗʰ T23.122** Burn of first degree of single left finger (nail) except thumb
- **✓7ᵗʰ T23.129** Burn of first degree of unspecified single finger (nail) except thumb

✓6ᵗʰ T23.13 Burn of first degree of multiple fingers (nail), not including thumb
- **✓7ᵗʰ T23.131** Burn of first degree of multiple right fingers (nail), not including thumb
- **✓7ᵗʰ T23.132** Burn of first degree of multiple left fingers (nail), not including thumb
- **✓7ᵗʰ T23.139** Burn of first degree of unspecified multiple fingers (nail), not including thumb

✓6ᵗʰ T23.14 Burn of first degree of multiple fingers (nail), including thumb
- **✓7ᵗʰ T23.141** Burn of first degree of multiple right fingers (nail), including thumb
- **✓7ᵗʰ T23.142** Burn of first degree of multiple left fingers (nail), including thumb
- **✓7ᵗʰ T23.149** Burn of first degree of unspecified multiple fingers (nail), including thumb

✓6ᵗʰ T23.15 Burn of first degree of palm
- **✓7ᵗʰ T23.151** Burn of first degree of right palm
- **✓7ᵗʰ T23.152** Burn of first degree of left palm
- **✓7ᵗʰ T23.159** Burn of first degree of unspecified palm

✓6ᵗʰ T23.16 Burn of first degree of back of hand
- **✓7ᵗʰ T23.161** Burn of first degree of back of right hand
- **✓7ᵗʰ T23.162** Burn of first degree of back of left hand
- **✓7ᵗʰ T23.169** Burn of first degree of back of unspecified hand

✓6ᵗʰ T23.17 Burn of first degree of wrist
- **✓7ᵗʰ T23.171** Burn of first degree of right wrist
- **✓7ᵗʰ T23.172** Burn of first degree of left wrist
- **✓7ᵗʰ T23.179** Burn of first degree of unspecified wrist

✓6ᵗʰ T23.19 Burn of first degree of multiple sites of wrist and hand
- **✓7ᵗʰ T23.191** Burn of first degree of multiple sites of right wrist and hand
- **✓7ᵗʰ T23.192** Burn of first degree of multiple sites of left wrist and hand
- **✓7ᵗʰ T23.199** Burn of first degree of multiple sites of unspecified wrist and hand

✓5ᵗʰ T23.2 Burn of second degree of wrist and hand
Use additional external cause code to identify the source, place and intent of the burn (X00-X19, X75-X77, X96-X98, Y92)

✓6ᵗʰ T23.20 Burn of second degree of hand, unspecified site
- **✓7ᵗʰ T23.201** Burn of second degree of right hand, unspecified site
- **✓7ᵗʰ T23.202** Burn of second degree of left hand, unspecified site
- **✓7ᵗʰ T23.209** Burn of second degree of unspecified hand, unspecified site

✓6ᵗʰ T23.21 Burn of second degree of thumb (nail)
- **✓7ᵗʰ T23.211** Burn of second degree of right thumb (nail)

✓ Additional Character Required   ✓7ᵗʰ Placeholder   Unacceptable PDx   Questionable PDx   Manifestation   H1 - H14 HAC   HCC CMS-HCC Dx   HIV HIV Dx

ICD-10-CM 2019   1089

√7ᵗʰ **T23.212** Burn of second degree of left thumb (nail)

√7ᵗʰ **T23.219** Burn of second degree of unspecified thumb (nail)

√6ᵗʰ **T23.22** Burn of second degree of single finger (nail) except thumb

√7ᵗʰ **T23.221** Burn of second degree of single right finger (nail) except thumb

√7ᵗʰ **T23.222** Burn of second degree of single left finger (nail) except thumb

√7ᵗʰ **T23.229** Burn of second degree of unspecified single finger (nail) except thumb

√6ᵗʰ **T23.23** Burn of second degree of multiple fingers (nail), not including thumb

√7ᵗʰ **T23.231** Burn of second degree of multiple right fingers (nail), not including thumb

√7ᵗʰ **T23.232** Burn of second degree of multiple left fingers (nail), not including thumb

√7ᵗʰ **T23.239** Burn of second degree of unspecified multiple fingers (nail), not including thumb

√6ᵗʰ **T23.24** Burn of second degree of multiple fingers (nail), including thumb

√7ᵗʰ **T23.241** Burn of second degree of multiple right fingers (nail), including thumb

√7ᵗʰ **T23.242** Burn of second degree of multiple left fingers (nail), including thumb

√7ᵗʰ **T23.249** Burn of second degree of unspecified multiple fingers (nail), including thumb

√6ᵗʰ **T23.25** Burn of second degree of palm

√7ᵗʰ **T23.251** Burn of second degree of right palm

√7ᵗʰ **T23.252** Burn of second degree of left palm

√7ᵗʰ **T23.259** Burn of second degree of unspecified palm

√6ᵗʰ **T23.26** Burn of second degree of back of hand

√7ᵗʰ **T23.261** Burn of second degree of back of right hand

√7ᵗʰ **T23.262** Burn of second degree of back of left hand

√7ᵗʰ **T23.269** Burn of second degree of back of unspecified hand

√6ᵗʰ **T23.27** Burn of second degree of wrist

√7ᵗʰ **T23.271** Burn of second degree of right wrist

√7ᵗʰ **T23.272** Burn of second degree of left wrist

√7ᵗʰ **T23.279** Burn of second degree of unspecified wrist

√6ᵗʰ **T23.29** Burn of second degree of multiple sites of wrist and hand

√7ᵗʰ **T23.291** Burn of second degree of multiple sites of right wrist and hand

√7ᵗʰ **T23.292** Burn of second degree of multiple sites of left wrist and hand

√7ᵗʰ **T23.299** Burn of second degree of multiple sites of unspecified wrist and hand

√5ᵗʰ **T23.3** Burn of third degree of wrist and hand

Use additional external cause code to identify the source, place and intent of the burn (X00-X19, X75-X77, X96-X98, Y92)

√6ᵗʰ **T23.30** Burn of third degree of hand, unspecified site
AHA: 2016, 2Q, 5

> **CC Excl: For CC codes in subcategory T23.30:**
> PDX collection 1396

√7ᵗʰ **T23.301** Burn of third degree of right hand, unspecified site   CC H5 SW

√7ᵗʰ **T23.302** Burn of third degree of left hand, unspecified site   CC H5 SW

√7ᵗʰ **T23.309** Burn of third degree of unspecified hand, unspecified site   CC H5 SW

√6ᵗʰ **T23.31** Burn of third degree of thumb (nail)

> **CC Excl: For CC codes in subcategory T23.31:**
> PDX collection 1397

√7ᵗʰ **T23.311** Burn of third degree of right thumb (nail)   CC H5 SW

√7ᵗʰ **T23.312** Burn of third degree of left thumb (nail)   CC H5 SW

√7ᵗʰ **T23.319** Burn of third degree of unspecified thumb (nail)   CC H5 SW

√6ᵗʰ **T23.32** Burn of third degree of single finger (nail) except thumb

> **CC Excl: For CC codes in subcategory T23.32:**
> PDX collection 1398

√7ᵗʰ **T23.321** Burn of third degree of single right finger (nail) except thumb   CC H5 SW

√7ᵗʰ **T23.322** Burn of third degree of single left finger (nail) except thumb   CC H5 SW

√7ᵗʰ **T23.329** Burn of third degree of unspecified single finger (nail) except thumb   CC H5 SW

√6ᵗʰ **T23.33** Burn of third degree of multiple fingers (nail), not including thumb

> **CC Excl: For CC codes in subcategory T23.33:**
> PDX collection 1399

√7ᵗʰ **T23.331** Burn of third degree of multiple right fingers (nail), not including thumb   CC H5 SW

√7ᵗʰ **T23.332** Burn of third degree of multiple left fingers (nail), not including thumb   CC H5 SW

√7ᵗʰ **T23.339** Burn of third degree of unspecified multiple fingers (nail), not including thumb   CC H5 SW

√6ᵗʰ **T23.34** Burn of third degree of multiple fingers (nail), including thumb

> **CC Excl: For CC codes in subcategory T23.34:**
> PDX collection 1400

√7ᵗʰ **T23.341** Burn of third degree of multiple right fingers (nail), including thumb   CC H5 SW

√7ᵗʰ **T23.342** Burn of third degree of multiple left fingers (nail), including thumb   CC H5 SW

√7ᵗʰ **T23.349** Burn of third degree of unspecified multiple fingers (nail), including thumb   CC H5 SW

√6ᵗʰ **T23.35** Burn of third degree of palm

> **CC Excl: For CC codes in subcategory T23.35:**
> PDX collection 1401

√7ᵗʰ **T23.351** Burn of third degree of right palm   CC H5 SW

√7ᵗʰ **T23.352** Burn of third degree of left palm   CC H5 SW

√7ᵗʰ **T23.359** Burn of third degree of unspecified palm   CC H5 SW

√6ᵗʰ **T23.36** Burn of third degree of back of hand

> **CC Excl: For CC codes in subcategory T23.36:**
> PDX collection 1402

√7ᵗʰ **T23.361** Burn of third degree of back of right hand   CC H5 SW

√7ᵗʰ **T23.362** Burn of third degree of back of left hand   CC H5 SW

√7ᵗʰ **T23.369** Burn of third degree of back of unspecified hand   CC H5 SW

√6ᵗʰ **T23.37** Burn of third degree of wrist

> **CC Excl: For CC codes in subcategory T23.37:**
> PDX collection 1403

√7ᵗʰ **T23.371** Burn of third degree of right wrist   CC H5 SW

√7ᵗʰ **T23.372** Burn of third degree of left wrist   CC H5 SW

√7ᵗʰ **T23.379** Burn of third degree of unspecified wrist   CC H5 SW

√6ᵗʰ **T23.39** Burn of third degree of multiple sites of wrist and hand

> **CC Excl: For CC codes in subcategory T23.39:**
> PDX collection 1396

√7ᵗʰ **T23.391** Burn of third degree of multiple sites of right wrist and hand   CC H5 SW

√7ᵗʰ **T23.392** Burn of third degree of multiple sites of left wrist and hand   CC H5 SW

√7ᵗʰ **T23.399** Burn of third degree of multiple sites of unspecified wrist and hand   CC H5 SW

N Newborn: 0   P Pediatric: 0-17   M Maternity: 12-55   A Adult: 15-124   MCC Major Complication/Comorbidity   CC Complication/Comorbidity   SW Severe Wound Dx

T23.212–T23.399

1090   ICD-10-CM 2019

✓5ᵗʰ **T23.4 Corrosion of** unspecified degree **of wrist and hand**
Code first (T51-T65) to identify chemical and intent
Use additional external cause code to identify place (Y92)

✓6ᵗʰ **T23.40 Corrosion of unspecified degree of hand,** unspecified site

✓7ᵗʰ **T23.401 Corrosion of unspecified degree of** right **hand, unspecified site**

✓7ᵗʰ **T23.402 Corrosion of unspecified degree of** left **hand, unspecified site**

✓7ᵗʰ **T23.409 Corrosion of unspecified degree of** unspecified **hand, unspecified site**

✓6ᵗʰ **T23.41 Corrosion of unspecified degree of** thumb **(nail)**

✓7ᵗʰ **T23.411 Corrosion of unspecified degree of** right **thumb (nail)**

✓7ᵗʰ **T23.412 Corrosion of unspecified degree of** left **thumb (nail)**

✓7ᵗʰ **T23.419 Corrosion of unspecified degree of** unspecified **thumb (nail)**

✓6ᵗʰ **T23.42 Corrosion of unspecified degree of** single finger **(nail) except thumb**

✓7ᵗʰ **T23.421 Corrosion of unspecified degree of single** right **finger (nail) except thumb**

✓7ᵗʰ **T23.422 Corrosion of unspecified degree of single** left **finger (nail) except thumb**

✓7ᵗʰ **T23.429 Corrosion of unspecified degree of** unspecified **single finger (nail) except thumb**

✓6ᵗʰ **T23.43 Corrosion of unspecified degree of** multiple fingers **(nail),** not including thumb

✓7ᵗʰ **T23.431 Corrosion of unspecified degree of multiple** right **fingers (nail), not including thumb**

✓7ᵗʰ **T23.432 Corrosion of unspecified degree of multiple** left **fingers (nail), not including thumb**

✓7ᵗʰ **T23.439 Corrosion of unspecified degree of** unspecified **multiple fingers (nail), not including thumb**

✓6ᵗʰ **T23.44 Corrosion of unspecified degree of** multiple fingers **(nail),** including thumb

✓7ᵗʰ **T23.441 Corrosion of unspecified degree of multiple** right **fingers (nail), including thumb**

✓7ᵗʰ **T23.442 Corrosion of unspecified degree of multiple** left **fingers (nail), including thumb**

✓7ᵗʰ **T23.449 Corrosion of unspecified degree of** unspecified **multiple fingers (nail), including thumb**

✓6ᵗʰ **T23.45 Corrosion of unspecified degree of** palm

✓7ᵗʰ **T23.451 Corrosion of unspecified degree of** right **palm**

✓7ᵗʰ **T23.452 Corrosion of unspecified degree of** left **palm**

✓7ᵗʰ **T23.459 Corrosion of unspecified degree of** unspecified **palm**

✓6ᵗʰ **T23.46 Corrosion of unspecified degree of** back of hand

✓7ᵗʰ **T23.461 Corrosion of unspecified degree of back of** right **hand**

✓7ᵗʰ **T23.462 Corrosion of unspecified degree of back of** left **hand**

✓7ᵗʰ **T23.469 Corrosion of unspecified degree of back of** unspecified **hand**

✓6ᵗʰ **T23.47 Corrosion of unspecified degree of** wrist

✓7ᵗʰ **T23.471 Corrosion of unspecified degree of** right **wrist**

✓7ᵗʰ **T23.472 Corrosion of unspecified degree of** left **wrist**

✓7ᵗʰ **T23.479 Corrosion of unspecified degree of** unspecified **wrist**

✓6ᵗʰ **T23.49 Corrosion of unspecified degree of** multiple sites **of wrist and hand**

✓7ᵗʰ **T23.491 Corrosion of unspecified degree of multiple sites of** right **wrist and hand**

✓7ᵗʰ **T23.492 Corrosion of unspecified degree of multiple sites of** left **wrist and hand**

✓7ᵗʰ **T23.499 Corrosion of unspecified degree of multiple sites of** unspecified **wrist and hand**

✓5ᵗʰ **T23.5 Corrosion of** first degree **of wrist and hand**
Code first (T51-T65) to identify chemical and intent
Use additional external cause code to identify place (Y92)

✓6ᵗʰ **T23.50 Corrosion of first degree of hand,** unspecified site

✓7ᵗʰ **T23.501 Corrosion of first degree of** right **hand, unspecified site**

✓7ᵗʰ **T23.502 Corrosion of first degree of** left **hand, unspecified site**

✓7ᵗʰ **T23.509 Corrosion of first degree of** unspecified **hand, unspecified site**

✓6ᵗʰ **T23.51 Corrosion of first degree of** thumb **(nail)**

✓7ᵗʰ **T23.511 Corrosion of first degree of** right **thumb (nail)**

✓7ᵗʰ **T23.512 Corrosion of first degree of** left **thumb (nail)**

✓7ᵗʰ **T23.519 Corrosion of first degree of** unspecified **thumb (nail)**

✓6ᵗʰ **T23.52 Corrosion of first degree of** single finger **(nail) except thumb**

✓7ᵗʰ **T23.521 Corrosion of first degree of single** right **finger (nail) except thumb**

✓7ᵗʰ **T23.522 Corrosion of first degree of single** left **finger (nail) except thumb**

✓7ᵗʰ **T23.529 Corrosion of first degree of** unspecified **single finger (nail) except thumb**

✓6ᵗʰ **T23.53 Corrosion of first degree of** multiple fingers **(nail),** not including thumb

✓7ᵗʰ **T23.531 Corrosion of first degree of multiple** right **fingers (nail), not including thumb**

✓7ᵗʰ **T23.532 Corrosion of first degree of multiple** left **fingers (nail), not including thumb**

✓7ᵗʰ **T23.539 Corrosion of first degree of** unspecified **multiple fingers (nail), not including thumb**

✓6ᵗʰ **T23.54 Corrosion of first degree of** multiple fingers **(nail),** including thumb

✓7ᵗʰ **T23.541 Corrosion of first degree of multiple** right **fingers (nail), including thumb**

✓7ᵗʰ **T23.542 Corrosion of first degree of multiple** left **fingers (nail), including thumb**

✓7ᵗʰ **T23.549 Corrosion of first degree of** unspecified **multiple fingers (nail), including thumb**

✓6ᵗʰ **T23.55 Corrosion of first degree of** palm

✓7ᵗʰ **T23.551 Corrosion of first degree of** right **palm**

✓7ᵗʰ **T23.552 Corrosion of first degree of** left **palm**

✓7ᵗʰ **T23.559 Corrosion of first degree of** unspecified **palm**

✓6ᵗʰ **T23.56 Corrosion of first degree of** back of hand

✓7ᵗʰ **T23.561 Corrosion of first degree of back of** right **hand**

✓7ᵗʰ **T23.562 Corrosion of first degree of back of** left **hand**

✓7ᵗʰ **T23.569 Corrosion of first degree of back of** unspecified **hand**

✓6ᵗʰ **T23.57 Corrosion of first degree of** wrist

✓7ᵗʰ **T23.571 Corrosion of first degree of** right **wrist**

✓7ᵗʰ **T23.572 Corrosion of first degree of** left **wrist**

✓7ᵗʰ **T23.579 Corrosion of first degree of** unspecified **wrist**

✓6ᵗʰ **T23.59 Corrosion of first degree of** multiple sites **of wrist and hand**

✓7ᵗʰ **T23.591 Corrosion of first degree of multiple sites of** right **wrist and hand**

✓7ᵗʰ **T23.592 Corrosion of first degree of multiple sites of** left **wrist and hand**

✓7ᵗʰ **T23.599 Corrosion of first degree of multiple sites of** unspecified **wrist and hand**

✔ Additional Character Required   ✔x7ᵗʰ Placeholder   Unacceptable PDx   Questionable PDx   Manifestation   H1-H14 HAC   HCC CMS-HCC Dx   HIV HIV Dx

ICD-10-CM 2019   1091

Chapter 19. Injury, Poisoning and Certain Other Consequences of External Causes

✓5ᵗʰ T23.6 Corrosion of second degree of wrist and hand
    Code first (T51-T65) to identify chemical and intent
    Use additional external cause code to identify place (Y92)

  ✓6ᵗʰ T23.60 Corrosion of second degree of hand, unspecified site
    ✓7ᵗʰ T23.601 Corrosion of second degree of right hand, unspecified site
    ✓7ᵗʰ T23.602 Corrosion of second degree of left hand, unspecified site
    ✓7ᵗʰ T23.609 Corrosion of second degree of unspecified hand, unspecified site

  ✓6ᵗʰ T23.61 Corrosion of second degree of thumb (nail)
    ✓7ᵗʰ T23.611 Corrosion of second degree of right thumb (nail)
    ✓7ᵗʰ T23.612 Corrosion of second degree of left thumb (nail)
    ✓7ᵗʰ T23.619 Corrosion of second degree of unspecified thumb (nail)

  ✓6ᵗʰ T23.62 Corrosion of second degree of single finger (nail) except thumb
    ✓7ᵗʰ T23.621 Corrosion of second degree of single right finger (nail) except thumb
    ✓7ᵗʰ T23.622 Corrosion of second degree of single left finger (nail) except thumb
    ✓7ᵗʰ T23.629 Corrosion of second degree of unspecified single finger (nail) except thumb

  ✓6ᵗʰ T23.63 Corrosion of second degree of multiple fingers (nail), not including thumb
    ✓7ᵗʰ T23.631 Corrosion of second degree of multiple right fingers (nail), not including thumb
    ✓7ᵗʰ T23.632 Corrosion of second degree of multiple left fingers (nail), not including thumb
    ✓7ᵗʰ T23.639 Corrosion of second degree of unspecified multiple fingers (nail), not including thumb

  ✓6ᵗʰ T23.64 Corrosion of second degree of multiple fingers (nail), including thumb
    ✓7ᵗʰ T23.641 Corrosion of second degree of multiple right fingers (nail), including thumb
    ✓7ᵗʰ T23.642 Corrosion of second degree of multiple left fingers (nail), including thumb
    ✓7ᵗʰ T23.649 Corrosion of second degree of unspecified multiple fingers (nail), including thumb

  ✓6ᵗʰ T23.65 Corrosion of second degree of palm
    ✓7ᵗʰ T23.651 Corrosion of second degree of right palm
    ✓7ᵗʰ T23.652 Corrosion of second degree of left palm
    ✓7ᵗʰ T23.659 Corrosion of second degree of unspecified palm

  ✓6ᵗʰ T23.66 Corrosion of second degree of back of hand
    ✓7ᵗʰ T23.661 Corrosion of second degree back of right hand
    ✓7ᵗʰ T23.662 Corrosion of second degree back of left hand
    ✓7ᵗʰ T23.669 Corrosion of second degree back of unspecified hand

  ✓6ᵗʰ T23.67 Corrosion of second degree of wrist
    ✓7ᵗʰ T23.671 Corrosion of second degree of right wrist
    ✓7ᵗʰ T23.672 Corrosion of second degree of left wrist
    ✓7ᵗʰ T23.679 Corrosion of second degree of unspecified wrist

  ✓6ᵗʰ T23.69 Corrosion of second degree of multiple sites of wrist and hand
    ✓7ᵗʰ T23.691 Corrosion of second degree of multiple sites of right wrist and hand
    ✓7ᵗʰ T23.692 Corrosion of second degree of multiple sites of left wrist and hand
    ✓7ᵗʰ T23.699 Corrosion of second degree of multiple sites of unspecified wrist and hand

✓5ᵗʰ T23.7 Corrosion of third degree of wrist and hand
    Code first (T51-T65) to identify chemical and intent
    Use additional external cause code to identify place (Y92)

  ✓6ᵗʰ T23.70 Corrosion of third degree of hand, unspecified site

    CC Excl: For CC codes in subcategory T23.70: PDX collection 1396

    ✓7ᵗʰ T23.701 Corrosion of third degree of right hand, unspecified site   CC H5 SW
    ✓7ᵗʰ T23.702 Corrosion of third degree of left hand, unspecified site   CC H5 SW
    ✓7ᵗʰ T23.709 Corrosion of third degree of unspecified hand, unspecified site   CC H5 SW

  ✓6ᵗʰ T23.71 Corrosion of third degree of thumb (nail)

    CC Excl: For CC codes in subcategory T23.71: PDX collection 1397

    ✓7ᵗʰ T23.711 Corrosion of third degree of right thumb (nail)   CC H5 SW
    ✓7ᵗʰ T23.712 Corrosion of third degree of left thumb (nail)   CC H5 SW
    ✓7ᵗʰ T23.719 Corrosion of third degree of unspecified thumb (nail)   CC H5 SW

  ✓6ᵗʰ T23.72 Corrosion of third degree of single finger (nail) except thumb

    CC Excl: For CC codes in subcategory T23.72: PDX collection 1398

    ✓7ᵗʰ T23.721 Corrosion of third degree of single right finger (nail) except thumb   CC H5 SW
    ✓7ᵗʰ T23.722 Corrosion of third degree of single left finger (nail) except thumb   CC H5 SW
    ✓7ᵗʰ T23.729 Corrosion of third degree of unspecified single finger (nail) except thumb   CC H5 SW

  ✓6ᵗʰ T23.73 Corrosion of third degree of multiple fingers (nail), not including thumb

    CC Excl: For CC codes in subcategory T23.73: PDX collection 1399

    ✓7ᵗʰ T23.731 Corrosion of third degree of multiple right fingers (nail), not including thumb   CC H5 SW
    ✓7ᵗʰ T23.732 Corrosion of third degree of multiple left fingers (nail), not including thumb   CC H5 SW
    ✓7ᵗʰ T23.739 Corrosion of third degree of unspecified multiple fingers (nail), not including thumb   CC H5 SW

  ✓6ᵗʰ T23.74 Corrosion of third degree of multiple fingers (nail), including thumb

    CC Excl: For CC codes in subcategory T23.74: PDX collection 1400

    ✓7ᵗʰ T23.741 Corrosion of third degree of multiple right fingers (nail), including thumb   CC H5 SW
    ✓7ᵗʰ T23.742 Corrosion of third degree of multiple left fingers (nail), including thumb   CC H5 SW
    ✓7ᵗʰ T23.749 Corrosion of third degree of unspecified multiple fingers (nail), including thumb   CC H5 SW

  ✓6ᵗʰ T23.75 Corrosion of third degree of palm

    CC Excl: For CC codes in subcategory T23.75: PDX collection 1401

    ✓7ᵗʰ T23.751 Corrosion of third degree of right palm   CC H5 SW
    ✓7ᵗʰ T23.752 Corrosion of third degree of left palm   CC H5 SW
    ✓7ᵗʰ T23.759 Corrosion of third degree of unspecified palm   CC H5 SW

N Newborn: 0   **P** Pediatric: 0-17   **M** Maternity: 12-55   **A** Adult: 15-124   **MCC** Major Complication/Comorbidity   **CC** Complication/Comorbidity   **SW** Severe Wound Dx

1092   ICD-10-CM 2019

√6ᵗʰ **T23.76** Corrosion of third degree of back of hand

> **CC Excl: For CC codes in subcategory T23.76:**
> PDX collection 1402

     √7ᵗʰ **T23.761** Corrosion of third degree of back of right hand   `CC` `H5` `SW`

     √7ᵗʰ **T23.762** Corrosion of third degree of back of left hand   `CC` `H5` `SW`

     √7ᵗʰ **T23.769** Corrosion of third degree back of unspecified hand   `CC` `H5` `SW`

√6ᵗʰ **T23.77** Corrosion of third degree of wrist

> **CC Excl: For CC codes in subcategory T23.77:**
> PDX collection 1403

     √7ᵗʰ **T23.771** Corrosion of third degree of right wrist   `CC` `H5` `SW`

     √7ᵗʰ **T23.772** Corrosion of third degree of left wrist   `CC` `H5` `SW`

     √7ᵗʰ **T23.779** Corrosion of third degree of unspecified wrist   `CC` `H5` `SW`

√6ᵗʰ **T23.79** Corrosion of third degree of multiple sites of wrist and hand

> **CC Excl: For CC codes in subcategory T23.79:**
> PDX collection 1396

     √7ᵗʰ **T23.791** Corrosion of third degree of multiple sites of right wrist and hand   `CC` `H5` `SW`

     √7ᵗʰ **T23.792** Corrosion of third degree of multiple sites of left wrist and hand   `CC` `H5` `SW`

     √7ᵗʰ **T23.799** Corrosion of third degree of multiple sites of unspecified wrist and hand   `CC` `H5` `SW`

√4ᵗʰ **T24** **Burn and corrosion of lower limb, except ankle and foot**

     EXCLUDES 2   burn and corrosion of ankle and foot (T25.-)
                 burn and corrosion of hip region (T21.-)

> The appropriate 7th character is to be added to each code from category T24.
> A   initial encounter
> D   subsequent encounter
> S   sequela

√5ᵗʰ **T24.0** **Burn of unspecified degree of lower limb, except ankle and foot**

> Use additional external cause code to identify the source, place and intent of the burn (X00-X19, X75-X77, X96-X98, Y92)

    √6ᵗʰ **T24.00** Burn of unspecified degree of unspecified site of lower limb, except ankle and foot

       √7ᵗʰ **T24.001** Burn of unspecified degree of unspecified site of right lower limb, except ankle and foot

       √7ᵗʰ **T24.002** Burn of unspecified degree of unspecified site of left lower limb, except ankle and foot

       √7ᵗʰ **T24.009** Burn of unspecified degree of unspecified site of unspecified lower limb, except ankle and foot

    √6ᵗʰ **T24.01** Burn of unspecified degree of thigh

       √7ᵗʰ **T24.011** Burn of unspecified degree of right thigh

       √7ᵗʰ **T24.012** Burn of unspecified degree of left thigh

       √7ᵗʰ **T24.019** Burn of unspecified degree of unspecified thigh

    √6ᵗʰ **T24.02** Burn of unspecified degree of knee

       √7ᵗʰ **T24.021** Burn of unspecified degree of right knee

       √7ᵗʰ **T24.022** Burn of unspecified degree of left knee

       √7ᵗʰ **T24.029** Burn of unspecified degree of unspecified knee

    √6ᵗʰ **T24.03** Burn of unspecified degree of lower leg

       √7ᵗʰ **T24.031** Burn of unspecified degree of right lower leg

       √7ᵗʰ **T24.032** Burn of unspecified degree of left lower leg

       √7ᵗʰ **T24.039** Burn of unspecified degree of unspecified lower leg

    √6ᵗʰ **T24.09** Burn of unspecified degree of multiple sites of lower limb, except ankle and foot

       √7ᵗʰ **T24.091** Burn of unspecified degree of multiple sites of right lower limb, except ankle and foot

       √7ᵗʰ **T24.092** Burn of unspecified degree of multiple sites of left lower limb, except ankle and foot

       √7ᵗʰ **T24.099** Burn of unspecified degree of multiple sites of unspecified lower limb, except ankle and foot

√5ᵗʰ **T24.1** **Burn of first degree of lower limb, except ankle and foot**

> Use additional external cause code to identify the source, place and intent of the burn (X00-X19, X75-X77, X96-X98, Y92)

    √6ᵗʰ **T24.10** Burn of first degree of unspecified site of lower limb, except ankle and foot

       √7ᵗʰ **T24.101** Burn of first degree of unspecified site of right lower limb, except ankle and foot

       √7ᵗʰ **T24.102** Burn of first degree of unspecified site of left lower limb, except ankle and foot

       √7ᵗʰ **T24.109** Burn of first degree of unspecified site of unspecified lower limb, except ankle and foot

    √6ᵗʰ **T24.11** Burn of first degree of thigh

       √7ᵗʰ **T24.111** Burn of first degree of right thigh

       √7ᵗʰ **T24.112** Burn of first degree of left thigh

       √7ᵗʰ **T24.119** Burn of first degree of unspecified thigh

    √6ᵗʰ **T24.12** Burn of first degree of knee

       √7ᵗʰ **T24.121** Burn of first degree of right knee

       √7ᵗʰ **T24.122** Burn of first degree of left knee

       √7ᵗʰ **T24.129** Burn of first degree of unspecified knee

    √6ᵗʰ **T24.13** Burn of first degree of lower leg

       √7ᵗʰ **T24.131** Burn of first degree of right lower leg

       √7ᵗʰ **T24.132** Burn of first degree of left lower leg

       √7ᵗʰ **T24.139** Burn of first degree of unspecified lower leg

    √6ᵗʰ **T24.19** Burn of first degree of multiple sites of lower limb, except ankle and foot

       √7ᵗʰ **T24.191** Burn of first degree of multiple sites of right lower limb, except ankle and foot

       √7ᵗʰ **T24.192** Burn of first degree of multiple sites of left lower limb, except ankle and foot

       √7ᵗʰ **T24.199** Burn of first degree of multiple sites of unspecified lower limb, except ankle and foot

√5ᵗʰ **T24.2** **Burn of second degree of lower limb, except ankle and foot**

> Use additional external cause code to identify the source, place and intent of the burn (X00-X19, X75-X77, X96-X98, Y92)

    √6ᵗʰ **T24.20** Burn of second degree of unspecified site of lower limb, except ankle and foot

       √7ᵗʰ **T24.201** Burn of second degree of unspecified site of right lower limb, except ankle and foot

       √7ᵗʰ **T24.202** Burn of second degree of unspecified site of left lower limb, except ankle and foot

       √7ᵗʰ **T24.209** Burn of second degree of unspecified site of unspecified lower limb, except ankle and foot

    √6ᵗʰ **T24.21** Burn of second degree of thigh

       √7ᵗʰ **T24.211** Burn of second degree of right thigh

       √7ᵗʰ **T24.212** Burn of second degree of left thigh

       √7ᵗʰ **T24.219** Burn of second degree of unspecified thigh

    √6ᵗʰ **T24.22** Burn of second degree of knee

       √7ᵗʰ **T24.221** Burn of second degree of right knee

       √7ᵗʰ **T24.222** Burn of second degree of left knee

       √7ᵗʰ **T24.229** Burn of second degree of unspecified knee

    √6ᵗʰ **T24.23** Burn of second degree of lower leg

       √7ᵗʰ **T24.231** Burn of second degree of right lower leg

       √7ᵗʰ **T24.232** Burn of second degree of left lower leg

       √7ᵗʰ **T24.239** Burn of second degree of unspecified lower leg

    √6ᵗʰ **T24.29** Burn of second degree of multiple sites of lower limb, except ankle and foot

       √7ᵗʰ **T24.291** Burn of second degree of multiple sites of right lower limb, except ankle and foot

       √7ᵗʰ **T24.292** Burn of second degree of multiple sites of left lower limb, except ankle and foot

☑ Additional Character Required   √x7ᵗʰ Placeholder   Unacceptable PDx   Questionable PDx   Manifestation   `H1`-`H14` HAC   `HCC` CMS-HCC Dx   `HIV` HIV Dx

ICD-10-CM 2019   **1093**

√7th **T24.299** Burn of second degree of multiple sites of unspecified lower limb, except ankle and foot

√5th **T24.3** Burn of third degree of lower limb, except ankle and foot

Use additional external cause code to identify the source, place and intent of the burn (X00-X19, X75-X77, X96-X98, Y92)

√6th **T24.30** Burn of third degree of unspecified site of lower limb, except ankle and foot

CC Excl: For CC codes in subcategory T24.30: PDX collection 1404

√7th **T24.301** Burn of third degree of unspecified site of right lower limb, except ankle and foot   CC H5 SW

√7th **T24.302** Burn of third degree of unspecified site of left lower limb, except ankle and foot   CC H5 SW

√7th **T24.309** Burn of third degree of unspecified site of unspecified lower limb, except ankle and foot   CC H5 SW

√6th **T24.31** Burn of third degree of thigh

CC Excl: For CC codes in subcategory T24.31: PDX collection 1405

√7th **T24.311** Burn of third degree of right thigh   CC H5 SW

√7th **T24.312** Burn of third degree of left thigh   CC H5 SW

√7th **T24.319** Burn of third degree of unspecified thigh   CC H5 SW

√6th **T24.32** Burn of third degree of knee

CC Excl: For CC codes in subcategory T24.32: PDX collection 1406

√7th **T24.321** Burn of third degree of right knee   CC H5 SW

√7th **T24.322** Burn of third degree of left knee   CC H5 SW

√7th **T24.329** Burn of third degree of unspecified knee   CC H5 SW

√6th **T24.33** Burn of third degree of lower leg

CC Excl: For CC codes in subcategory T24.33: PDX collection 1407

√7th **T24.331** Burn of third degree of right lower leg   CC H5 SW

√7th **T24.332** Burn of third degree of left lower leg   CC H5 SW

√7th **T24.339** Burn of third degree of unspecified lower leg   CC H5 SW

√6th **T24.39** Burn of third degree of multiple sites of lower limb, except ankle and foot

AHA: 2016, 2Q, 4

CC Excl: For CC codes in subcategory T24.39: PDX collection 1404

√7th **T24.391** Burn of third degree of multiple sites of right lower limb, except ankle and foot   CC H5 SW

√7th **T24.392** Burn of third degree of multiple sites of left lower limb, except ankle and foot   CC H5 SW

√7th **T24.399** Burn of third degree of multiple sites of unspecified lower limb, except ankle and foot   CC H5 SW

√5th **T24.4** Corrosion of unspecified degree of lower limb, except ankle and foot

Code first (T51-T65) to identify chemical and intent
Use additional external cause code to identify place (Y92)

√6th **T24.40** Corrosion of unspecified degree of unspecified site of lower limb, except ankle and foot

√7th **T24.401** Corrosion of unspecified degree of unspecified site of right lower limb, except ankle and foot

√7th **T24.402** Corrosion of unspecified degree of unspecified site of left lower limb, except ankle and foot

√7th **T24.409** Corrosion of unspecified degree of unspecified site of unspecified lower limb, except ankle and foot

√6th **T24.41** Corrosion of unspecified degree of thigh

√7th **T24.411** Corrosion of unspecified degree of right thigh

√7th **T24.412** Corrosion of unspecified degree of left thigh

√7th **T24.419** Corrosion of unspecified degree of unspecified thigh

√6th **T24.42** Corrosion of unspecified degree of knee

√7th **T24.421** Corrosion of unspecified degree of right knee

√7th **T24.422** Corrosion of unspecified degree of left knee

√7th **T24.429** Corrosion of unspecified degree of unspecified knee

√6th **T24.43** Corrosion of unspecified degree of lower leg

√7th **T24.431** Corrosion of unspecified degree of right lower leg

√7th **T24.432** Corrosion of unspecified degree of left lower leg

√7th **T24.439** Corrosion of unspecified degree of unspecified lower leg

√6th **T24.49** Corrosion of unspecified degree of multiple sites of lower limb, except ankle and foot

√7th **T24.491** Corrosion of unspecified degree of multiple sites of right lower limb, except ankle and foot

√7th **T24.492** Corrosion of unspecified degree of multiple sites of left lower limb, except ankle and foot

√7th **T24.499** Corrosion of unspecified degree of multiple sites of unspecified lower limb, except ankle and foot

√5th **T24.5** Corrosion of first degree of lower limb, except ankle and foot

Code first (T51-T65) to identify chemical and intent
Use additional external cause code to identify place (Y92)

√6th **T24.50** Corrosion of first degree of unspecified site of lower limb, except ankle and foot

√7th **T24.501** Corrosion of first degree of unspecified site of right lower limb, except ankle and foot

√7th **T24.502** Corrosion of first degree of unspecified site of left lower limb, except ankle and foot

√7th **T24.509** Corrosion of first degree of unspecified site of unspecified lower limb, except ankle and foot

√6th **T24.51** Corrosion of first degree of thigh

√7th **T24.511** Corrosion of first degree of right thigh

√7th **T24.512** Corrosion of first degree of left thigh

√7th **T24.519** Corrosion of first degree of unspecified thigh

√6th **T24.52** Corrosion of first degree of knee

√7th **T24.521** Corrosion of first degree of right knee

√7th **T24.522** Corrosion of first degree of left knee

√7th **T24.529** Corrosion of first degree of unspecified knee

√6th **T24.53** Corrosion of first degree of lower leg

√7th **T24.531** Corrosion of first degree of right lower leg

√7th **T24.532** Corrosion of first degree of left lower leg

√7th **T24.539** Corrosion of first degree of unspecified lower leg

√6th **T24.59** Corrosion of first degree of multiple sites of lower limb, except ankle and foot

√7th **T24.591** Corrosion of first degree of multiple sites of right lower limb, except ankle and foot

√7th **T24.592** Corrosion of first degree of multiple sites of left lower limb, except ankle and foot

√7th **T24.599** Corrosion of first degree of multiple sites of unspecified lower limb, except ankle and foot

N Newborn: 0   P Pediatric: 0-17   M Maternity: 12-55   A Adult: 15-124   MCC Major Complication/Comorbidity   CC Complication/Comorbidity   SW Severe Wound Dx

1094   ICD-10-CM 2019

✓5ᵗʰ **T24.6** **Corrosion of** second degree **of lower limb, except ankle and foot**
Code first (T51-T65) to identify chemical and intent
Use additional external cause code to identify place (Y92)

✓6ᵗʰ **T24.60** **Corrosion of second degree of** unspecified site **of lower limb, except ankle and foot**

✓7ᵗʰ **T24.601** **Corrosion of second degree of unspecified site of** right **lower limb, except ankle and foot**

✓7ᵗʰ **T24.602** **Corrosion of second degree of unspecified site of** left **lower limb, except ankle and foot**

✓7ᵗʰ **T24.609** **Corrosion of second degree of unspecified site of** unspecified **lower limb, except ankle and foot**

✓6ᵗʰ **T24.61** **Corrosion of second degree of** thigh

✓7ᵗʰ **T24.611** **Corrosion of second degree of** right **thigh**

✓7ᵗʰ **T24.612** **Corrosion of second degree of** left **thigh**

✓7ᵗʰ **T24.619** **Corrosion of second degree of** unspecified **thigh**

✓6ᵗʰ **T24.62** **Corrosion of second degree of** knee

✓7ᵗʰ **T24.621** **Corrosion of second degree of** right **knee**

✓7ᵗʰ **T24.622** **Corrosion of second degree of** left **knee**

✓7ᵗʰ **T24.629** **Corrosion of second degree of** unspecified **knee**

✓6ᵗʰ **T24.63** **Corrosion of second degree of** lower leg

✓7ᵗʰ **T24.631** **Corrosion of second degree of** right **lower leg**

✓7ᵗʰ **T24.632** **Corrosion of second degree of** left **lower leg**

✓7ᵗʰ **T24.639** **Corrosion of second degree of** unspecified **lower leg**

✓6ᵗʰ **T24.69** **Corrosion of second degree of** multiple sites **of lower limb, except ankle and foot**

✓7ᵗʰ **T24.691** **Corrosion of second degree of multiple sites of** right **lower limb, except ankle and foot**

✓7ᵗʰ **T24.692** **Corrosion of second degree of multiple sites of** left **lower limb, except ankle and foot**

✓7ᵗʰ **T24.699** **Corrosion of second degree of multiple sites of** unspecified **lower limb, except ankle and foot**

✓5ᵗʰ **T24.7** **Corrosion of** third degree **of lower limb, except ankle and foot**
Code first (T51-T65) to identify chemical and intent
Use additional external cause code to identify place (Y92)

✓6ᵗʰ **T24.70** **Corrosion of third degree of** unspecified site **of lower limb, except ankle and foot**

CC Excl: For CC codes in subcategory T24.70:
PDX collection 1404

✓7ᵗʰ **T24.701** **Corrosion of third degree of unspecified site of** right **lower limb, except ankle and foot** `CC` `H5` `SW`

✓7ᵗʰ **T24.702** **Corrosion of third degree of unspecified site of** left **lower limb, except ankle and foot** `CC` `H5` `SW`

✓7ᵗʰ **T24.709** **Corrosion of third degree of unspecified site of** unspecified **lower limb, except ankle and foot** `CC` `H5` `SW`

✓6ᵗʰ **T24.71** **Corrosion of third degree of** thigh

CC Excl: For CC codes in subcategory T24.71:
PDX collection 1405

✓7ᵗʰ **T24.711** **Corrosion of third degree of** right **thigh** `CC` `H5` `SW`

✓7ᵗʰ **T24.712** **Corrosion of third degree of** left **thigh** `CC` `H5` `SW`

✓7ᵗʰ **T24.719** **Corrosion of third degree of** unspecified **thigh** `CC` `H5` `SW`

✓6ᵗʰ **T24.72** **Corrosion of third degree of** knee

CC Excl: For CC codes in subcategory T24.72:
PDX collection 1406

✓7ᵗʰ **T24.721** **Corrosion of third degree of** right **knee** `CC` `H5` `SW`

✓7ᵗʰ **T24.722** **Corrosion of third degree of** left **knee** `CC` `H5` `SW`

✓7ᵗʰ **T24.729** **Corrosion of third degree of** unspecified **knee** `CC` `H5` `SW`

✓6ᵗʰ **T24.73** **Corrosion of third degree of** lower leg

CC Excl: For CC codes in subcategory T24.73:
PDX collection 1407

✓7ᵗʰ **T24.731** **Corrosion of third degree of** right **lower leg** `CC` `H5` `SW`

✓7ᵗʰ **T24.732** **Corrosion of third degree of** left **lower leg** `CC` `H5` `SW`

✓7ᵗʰ **T24.739** **Corrosion of third degree of** unspecified **lower leg** `CC` `H5` `SW`

✓6ᵗʰ **T24.79** **Corrosion of third degree of** multiple sites **of lower limb, except ankle and foot**

CC Excl: For CC codes in subcategory T24.79:
PDX collection 1404

✓7ᵗʰ **T24.791** **Corrosion of third degree of multiple sites of** right **lower limb, except ankle and foot** `CC` `H5` `SW`

✓7ᵗʰ **T24.792** **Corrosion of third degree of multiple sites of** left **lower limb, except ankle and foot** `CC` `H5` `SW`

✓7ᵗʰ **T24.799** **Corrosion of third degree of multiple sites of** unspecified **lower limb, except ankle and foot** `CC` `H5` `SW`

✓4ᵗʰ **T25** **Burn and corrosion of ankle and foot**

The appropriate 7th character is to be added to each code from category T25.
A   initial encounter
D   subsequent encounter
S   sequela

✓5ᵗʰ **T25.0** **Burn of** unspecified degree **of ankle and foot**
Use additional external cause code to identify the source, place and intent of the burn (X00-X19, X75-X77, X96-X98, Y92)

✓6ᵗʰ **T25.01** **Burn of unspecified degree of** ankle

✓7ᵗʰ **T25.011** **Burn of unspecified degree of** right **ankle**

✓7ᵗʰ **T25.012** **Burn of unspecified degree of** left **ankle**

✓7ᵗʰ **T25.019** **Burn of unspecified degree of** unspecified **ankle**

✓6ᵗʰ **T25.02** **Burn of unspecified degree of** foot
EXCLUDES 2   *burn of unspecified degree of toe(s) (nail) (T25.03-)*

✓7ᵗʰ **T25.021** **Burn of unspecified degree of** right **foot**

✓7ᵗʰ **T25.022** **Burn of unspecified degree of** left **foot**

✓7ᵗʰ **T25.029** **Burn of unspecified degree of** unspecified **foot**

✓6ᵗʰ **T25.03** **Burn of unspecified degree of** toe(s) (nail)

✓7ᵗʰ **T25.031** **Burn of unspecified degree of** right **toe(s) (nail)**

✓7ᵗʰ **T25.032** **Burn of unspecified degree of** left **toe(s) (nail)**

✓7ᵗʰ **T25.039** **Burn of unspecified degree of** unspecified **toe(s) (nail)**

✓6ᵗʰ **T25.09** **Burn of unspecified degree of** multiple sites **of ankle and foot**

✓7ᵗʰ **T25.091** **Burn of unspecified degree of multiple sites of** right **ankle and foot**

✓7ᵗʰ **T25.092** **Burn of unspecified degree of multiple sites of** left **ankle and foot**

✓7ᵗʰ **T25.099** **Burn of unspecified degree of multiple sites of** unspecified **ankle and foot**

✓5ᵗʰ **T25.1** **Burn of** first degree **of ankle and foot**
Use additional external cause code to identify the source, place and intent of the burn (X00-X19, X75-X77, X96-X98, Y92)

✓6ᵗʰ **T25.11** **Burn of first degree of** ankle

✓7ᵗʰ **T25.111** **Burn of first degree of** right **ankle**

✓7ᵗʰ **T25.112** **Burn of first degree of** left **ankle**

✓7ᵗʰ **T25.119** **Burn of first degree of** unspecified **ankle**

✓6ᵗʰ **T25.12** **Burn of first degree of** foot
EXCLUDES 2   *burn of first degree of toe(s) (nail) (T25.13-)*

✓7ᵗʰ **T25.121** **Burn of first degree of** right **foot**

✓ Additional Character Required   `✓x7ᵗʰ` Placeholder   Unacceptable PDx   Questionable PDx   Manifestation   `H1`-`H14` HAC   `HCC` CMS-HCC Dx   `HIV` HIV Dx

ICD-10-CM 2019   1095

Chapter 19. Injury, Poisoning and Certain Other Consequences of External Causes

✓7ᵗʰ T25.122   **Burn of first degree of** left **foot**

✓7ᵗʰ T25.129   **Burn of first degree of** unspecified **foot**

✓6ᵗʰ T25.13   **Burn of first degree of** toe(s) **(nail)**

     ✓7ᵗʰ T25.131   **Burn of first degree of** right **toe(s) (nail)**

     ✓7ᵗʰ T25.132   **Burn of first degree of** left **toe(s) (nail)**

     ✓7ᵗʰ T25.139   **Burn of first degree of** unspecified **toe(s) (nail)**

✓6ᵗʰ T25.19   **Burn of first degree of** multiple sites **of ankle and foot**

     ✓7ᵗʰ T25.191   **Burn of first degree of multiple sites of** right **ankle and foot**

     ✓7ᵗʰ T25.192   **Burn of first degree of multiple sites of** left **ankle and foot**

     ✓7ᵗʰ T25.199   **Burn of first degree of multiple sites of** unspecified **ankle and foot**

✓5ᵗʰ T25.2   **Burn of** second degree **of ankle and foot**

     Use additional external cause code to identify the source, place and intent of the burn (X00-X19, X75-X77, X96-X98, Y92)

✓6ᵗʰ T25.21   **Burn of second degree of** ankle

     ✓7ᵗʰ T25.211   **Burn of second degree of** right **ankle**

     ✓7ᵗʰ T25.212   **Burn of second degree of** left **ankle**

     ✓7ᵗʰ T25.219   **Burn of second degree of** unspecified **ankle**

✓6ᵗʰ T25.22   **Burn of second degree of** foot

     EXCLUDES 2   burn of second degree of toe(s) (nail) (T25.23-)

     ✓7ᵗʰ T25.221   **Burn of second degree of** right **foot**

     ✓7ᵗʰ T25.222   **Burn of second degree of** left **foot**

     ✓7ᵗʰ T25.229   **Burn of second degree of** unspecified **foot**

✓6ᵗʰ T25.23   **Burn of second degree of** toe(s) **(nail)**

     ✓7ᵗʰ T25.231   **Burn of second degree of** right **toe(s) (nail)**

     ✓7ᵗʰ T25.232   **Burn of second degree of** left **toe(s) (nail)**

     ✓7ᵗʰ T25.239   **Burn of second degree of** unspecified **toe(s) (nail)**

✓6ᵗʰ T25.29   **Burn of second degree of** multiple sites **of ankle and foot**

     ✓7ᵗʰ T25.291   **Burn of second degree of multiple sites of** right **ankle and foot**

     ✓7ᵗʰ T25.292   **Burn of second degree of multiple sites of** left **ankle and foot**

     ✓7ᵗʰ T25.299   **Burn of second degree of multiple sites of** unspecified **ankle and foot**

✓5ᵗʰ T25.3   **Burn of** third degree **of ankle and foot**

     Use additional external cause code to identify the source, place and intent of the burn (X00-X19, X75-X77, X96-X98, Y92)

✓6ᵗʰ T25.31   **Burn of third degree of** ankle

     CC Excl: For CC codes in subcategory T25.31:
     PDX collection 1408

     ✓7ᵗʰ T25.311   **Burn of third degree of** right **ankle** `CC` `H5` `SW`

     ✓7ᵗʰ T25.312   **Burn of third degree of** left **ankle** `CC` `H5` `SW`

     ✓7ᵗʰ T25.319   **Burn of third degree of** unspecified **ankle** `CC` `H5` `SW`

✓6ᵗʰ T25.32   **Burn of third degree of** foot

     EXCLUDES 2   burn of third degree of toe(s) (nail) (T25.33-)

     CC Excl: For CC codes in subcategory T25.32:
     PDX collection 1409

     ✓7ᵗʰ T25.321   **Burn of third degree of** right **foot** `CC` `H5` `SW`

     ✓7ᵗʰ T25.322   **Burn of third degree of** left **foot** `CC` `H5` `SW`

     ✓7ᵗʰ T25.329   **Burn of third degree of** unspecified **foot** `CC` `H5` `SW`

✓6ᵗʰ T25.33   **Burn of third degree of** toe(s) **(nail)**

     CC Excl: For CC codes in subcategory T25.33:
     PDX collection 1410

     ✓7ᵗʰ T25.331   **Burn of third degree of** right **toe(s) (nail)** `CC` `H5` `SW`

     ✓7ᵗʰ T25.332   **Burn of third degree of** left **toe(s) (nail)** `CC` `H5` `SW`

     ✓7ᵗʰ T25.339   **Burn of third degree of** unspecified **toe(s) (nail)** `CC` `H5` `SW`

✓6ᵗʰ T25.39   **Burn of third degree of** multiple sites **of ankle and foot**

     CC Excl: For CC codes in subcategory T25.39:
     PDX collection 1404

     ✓7ᵗʰ T25.391   **Burn of third degree of multiple sites of** right **ankle and foot** `CC` `H5` `SW`

     ✓7ᵗʰ T25.392   **Burn of third degree of multiple sites of** left **ankle and foot** `CC` `H5` `SW`

     ✓7ᵗʰ T25.399   **Burn of third degree of multiple sites of** unspecified **ankle and foot** `CC` `H5` `SW`

✓5ᵗʰ T25.4   **Corrosion of** unspecified degree **of ankle and foot**

     Code first (T51-T65) to identify chemical and intent
     Use additional external cause code to identify place (Y92)

✓6ᵗʰ T25.41   **Corrosion of unspecified degree of** ankle

     ✓7ᵗʰ T25.411   **Corrosion of unspecified degree of** right **ankle**

     ✓7ᵗʰ T25.412   **Corrosion of unspecified degree of** left **ankle**

     ✓7ᵗʰ T25.419   **Corrosion of unspecified degree of** unspecified **ankle**

✓6ᵗʰ T25.42   **Corrosion of unspecified degree of** foot

     EXCLUDES 2   corrosion of unspecified degree of toe(s) (nail) (T25.43-)

     ✓7ᵗʰ T25.421   **Corrosion of unspecified degree of** right **foot**

     ✓7ᵗʰ T25.422   **Corrosion of unspecified degree of** left **foot**

     ✓7ᵗʰ T25.429   **Corrosion of unspecified degree of** unspecified **foot**

✓6ᵗʰ T25.43   **Corrosion of unspecified degree of** toe(s) **(nail)**

     ✓7ᵗʰ T25.431   **Corrosion of unspecified degree of** right **toe(s) (nail)**

     ✓7ᵗʰ T25.432   **Corrosion of unspecified degree of** left **toe(s) (nail)**

     ✓7ᵗʰ T25.439   **Corrosion of unspecified degree of** unspecified **toe(s) (nail)**

✓6ᵗʰ T25.49   **Corrosion of unspecified degree of** multiple sites **of ankle and foot**

     ✓7ᵗʰ T25.491   **Corrosion of unspecified degree of multiple sites of** right **ankle and foot**

     ✓7ᵗʰ T25.492   **Corrosion of unspecified degree of multiple sites of** left **ankle and foot**

     ✓7ᵗʰ T25.499   **Corrosion of unspecified degree of multiple sites of** unspecified **ankle and foot**

✓5ᵗʰ T25.5   **Corrosion of** first degree **of ankle and foot**

     Code first (T51-T65) to identify chemical and intent
     Use additional external cause code to identify place (Y92)

✓6ᵗʰ T25.51   **Corrosion of first degree of** ankle

     ✓7ᵗʰ T25.511   **Corrosion of first degree of** right **ankle**

     ✓7ᵗʰ T25.512   **Corrosion of first degree of** left **ankle**

     ✓7ᵗʰ T25.519   **Corrosion of first degree of** unspecified **ankle**

✓6ᵗʰ T25.52   **Corrosion of first degree of** foot

     EXCLUDES 2   corrosion of first degree of toe(s) (nail) (T25.53-)

     ✓7ᵗʰ T25.521   **Corrosion of first degree of** right **foot**

     ✓7ᵗʰ T25.522   **Corrosion of first degree of** left **foot**

     ✓7ᵗʰ T25.529   **Corrosion of first degree of** unspecified **foot**

✓6ᵗʰ T25.53   **Corrosion of first degree of** toe(s) **(nail)**

     ✓7ᵗʰ T25.531   **Corrosion of first degree of** right **toe(s) (nail)**

     ✓7ᵗʰ T25.532   **Corrosion of first degree of** left **toe(s) (nail)**

     ✓7ᵗʰ T25.539   **Corrosion of first degree of** unspecified **toe(s) (nail)**

✓6ᵗʰ T25.59   **Corrosion of first degree of** multiple sites **of ankle and foot**

     ✓7ᵗʰ T25.591   **Corrosion of first degree of multiple sites of** right **ankle and foot**

     ✓7ᵗʰ T25.592   **Corrosion of first degree of multiple sites of** left **ankle and foot**

     ✓7ᵗʰ T25.599   **Corrosion of first degree of multiple sites of** unspecified **ankle and foot**

`N` Newborn: 0   `P` Pediatric: 0-17   `M` Maternity: 12-55   `A` Adult: 15-124   `MCC` Major Complication/Comorbidity   `CC` Complication/Comorbidity   `SW` Severe Wound Dx

✓5ᵗʰ **T25.6** **Corrosion of** second degree **of ankle and foot**
     Code first (T51-T65) to identify chemical and intent
     Use additional external cause code to identify place (Y92)

   ✓6ᵗʰ **T25.61** **Corrosion of second degree of** ankle

     ✓7ᵗʰ **T25.611** **Corrosion of second degree of** right **ankle**

     ✓7ᵗʰ **T25.612** **Corrosion of second degree of** left **ankle**

     ✓7ᵗʰ **T25.619** **Corrosion of second degree of** unspecified **ankle**

   ✓6ᵗʰ **T25.62** **Corrosion of second degree of** foot
     EXCLUDES 2 *corrosion of second degree of toe(s) (nail) (T25.63-)*

     ✓7ᵗʰ **T25.621** **Corrosion of second degree of** right **foot**

     ✓7ᵗʰ **T25.622** **Corrosion of second degree of** left **foot**

     ✓7ᵗʰ **T25.629** **Corrosion of second degree of** unspecified **foot**

   ✓6ᵗʰ **T25.63** **Corrosion of second degree of** toe(s) **(nail)**

     ✓7ᵗʰ **T25.631** **Corrosion of second degree of** right **toe(s) (nail)**

     ✓7ᵗʰ **T25.632** **Corrosion of second degree of** left **toe(s) (nail)**

     ✓7ᵗʰ **T25.639** **Corrosion of second degree of** unspecified **toe(s) (nail)**

   ✓6ᵗʰ **T25.69** **Corrosion of second degree of** multiple sites **of ankle and foot**

     ✓7ᵗʰ **T25.691** **Corrosion of second degree of** right **ankle and foot**

     ✓7ᵗʰ **T25.692** **Corrosion of second degree of** left **ankle and foot**

     ✓7ᵗʰ **T25.699** **Corrosion of second degree of** unspecified **ankle and foot**

✓5ᵗʰ **T25.7** **Corrosion of** third degree **of ankle and foot**
     Code first (T51-T65) to identify chemical and intent
     Use additional external cause code to identify place (Y92)

   ✓6ᵗʰ **T25.71** **Corrosion of third degree of** ankle

     CC Excl: For CC codes in subcategory T25.71:
     PDX collection 1408

     ✓7ᵗʰ **T25.711** **Corrosion of third degree of** right **ankle**   CC H5 SW

     ✓7ᵗʰ **T25.712** **Corrosion of third degree of** left **ankle**   CC H5 SW

     ✓7ᵗʰ **T25.719** **Corrosion of third degree of** unspecified **ankle**   CC H5 SW

   ✓6ᵗʰ **T25.72** **Corrosion of third degree of** foot
     EXCLUDES 2 *corrosion of third degree of toe(s) (nail) (T25.73-)*

     CC Excl: For CC codes in subcategory T25.72:
     PDX collection 1409

     ✓7ᵗʰ **T25.721** **Corrosion of third degree of** right **foot**   CC H5 SW

     ✓7ᵗʰ **T25.722** **Corrosion of third degree of** left **foot**   CC H5 SW

     ✓7ᵗʰ **T25.729** **Corrosion of third degree of** unspecified **foot**   CC H5 SW

   ✓6ᵗʰ **T25.73** **Corrosion of third degree of** toe(s) **(nail)**

     CC Excl: For CC codes in subcategory T25.73:
     PDX collection 1410

     ✓7ᵗʰ **T25.731** **Corrosion of third degree of** right **toe(s) (nail)**   CC H5 SW

     ✓7ᵗʰ **T25.732** **Corrosion of third degree of** left **toe(s) (nail)**   CC H5 SW

     ✓7ᵗʰ **T25.739** **Corrosion of third degree of** unspecified **toe(s) (nail)**   CC H5 SW

   ✓6ᵗʰ **T25.79** **Corrosion of third degree of** multiple sites **of ankle and foot**

     CC Excl: For CC codes in subcategory T25.79:
     PDX collection 1404

     ✓7ᵗʰ **T25.791** **Corrosion of third degree of multiple sites of** right **ankle and foot**   CC H5 SW

     ✓7ᵗʰ **T25.792** **Corrosion of third degree of multiple sites of** left **ankle and foot**   CC H5 SW

     ✓7ᵗʰ **T25.799** **Corrosion of third degree of multiple sites of** unspecified **ankle and foot**   CC H5 SW

Burns and corrosions confined to eye and internal organs (T26-T28)

✓4ᵗʰ **T26** **Burn and corrosion confined to eye and adnexa**

     The appropriate 7th character is to be added to each code from category T26.
     A   initial encounter
     D   subsequent encounter
     S   sequela

   ✓5ᵗʰ **T26.0** **Burn of** eyelid and periocular area
     Use additional external cause code to identify the source, place and intent of the burn (X00-X19, X75-X77, X96-X98, Y92)

     ✓x7ᵗʰ **T26.00** **Burn of** unspecified **eyelid and periocular area**

     ✓x7ᵗʰ **T26.01** **Burn of** right **eyelid and periocular area**

     ✓x7ᵗʰ **T26.02** **Burn of** left **eyelid and periocular area**

   ✓5ᵗʰ **T26.1** **Burn of** cornea and conjunctival sac
     Use additional external cause code to identify the source, place and intent of the burn (X00-X19, X75-X77, X96-X98, Y92)

     ✓x7ᵗʰ **T26.10** **Burn of cornea and conjunctival sac,** unspecified **eye**

     ✓x7ᵗʰ **T26.11** **Burn of cornea and conjunctival sac,** right **eye**

     ✓x7ᵗʰ **T26.12** **Burn of cornea and conjunctival sac,** left **eye**

   ✓5ᵗʰ **T26.2** **Burn with resulting** rupture and destruction of eyeball
     Use additional external cause code to identify the source, place and intent of the burn (X00-X19, X75-X77, X96-X98, Y92)

     ✓x7ᵗʰ **T26.20** **Burn with resulting rupture and destruction of** unspecified **eyeball**   CC H5
       CC Excl: No Excl

     ✓x7ᵗʰ **T26.21** **Burn with resulting rupture and destruction of** right **eyeball**   CC H5
       CC Excl: No Excl

     ✓x7ᵗʰ **T26.22** **Burn with resulting rupture and destruction of** left **eyeball**   CC H5
       CC Excl: No Excl

   ✓5ᵗʰ **T26.3** **Burns of** other specified parts **of eye and adnexa**
     Use additional external cause code to identify the source, place and intent of the burn (X00-X19, X75-X77, X96-X98, Y92)

     ✓x7ᵗʰ **T26.30** **Burns of other specified parts of** unspecified **eye and adnexa**

     ✓x7ᵗʰ **T26.31** **Burns of other specified parts of** right **eye and adnexa**

     ✓x7ᵗʰ **T26.32** **Burns of other specified parts of** left **eye and adnexa**

   ✓5ᵗʰ **T26.4** **Burn of eye and adnexa,** part unspecified
     Use additional external cause code to identify the source, place and intent of the burn (X00-X19, X75-X77, X96-X98, Y92)

     ✓x7ᵗʰ **T26.40** **Burn of** unspecified **eye and adnexa, part unspecified**

     ✓x7ᵗʰ **T26.41** **Burn of** right **eye and adnexa, part unspecified**

     ✓x7ᵗʰ **T26.42** **Burn of** left **eye and adnexa, part unspecified**

   ✓5ᵗʰ **T26.5** **Corrosion of** eyelid and periocular area
     Code first (T51-T65) to identify chemical and intent
     Use additional external cause code to identify place (Y92)

     ✓x7ᵗʰ **T26.50** **Corrosion of** unspecified **eyelid and periocular area**

     ✓x7ᵗʰ **T26.51** **Corrosion of** right **eyelid and periocular area**

     ✓x7ᵗʰ **T26.52** **Corrosion of** left **eyelid and periocular area**

   ✓5ᵗʰ **T26.6** **Corrosion of** cornea and conjunctival sac
     Code first (T51-T65) to identify chemical and intent
     Use additional external cause code to identify place (Y92)

     ✓x7ᵗʰ **T26.60** **Corrosion of cornea and conjunctival sac,** unspecified **eye**

     ✓x7ᵗʰ **T26.61** **Corrosion of cornea and conjunctival sac,** right **eye**

     ✓x7ᵗʰ **T26.62** **Corrosion of cornea and conjunctival sac,** left **eye**

   ✓5ᵗʰ **T26.7** **Corrosion with resulting** rupture and destruction of eyeball
     Code first (T51-T65) to identify chemical and intent
     Use additional external cause code to identify place (Y92)

     ✓x7ᵗʰ **T26.70** **Corrosion with resulting rupture and destruction of** unspecified **eyeball**   CC H5
       CC Excl: No Excl

     ✓x7ᵗʰ **T26.71** **Corrosion with resulting rupture and destruction of** right **eyeball**   CC H5
       CC Excl: No Excl

     ✓x7ᵗʰ **T26.72** **Corrosion with resulting rupture and destruction of** left **eyeball**   CC H5
       CC Excl: No Excl

✓ Additional Character Required   ✓x7ᵗʰ Placeholder   Unacceptable PDx   Questionable PDx   Manifestation   H1–H14 HAC   HCC CMS-HCC Dx   HIV HIV Dx

ICD-10-CM 2019   **1097**

Chapter 19. Injury, Poisoning and Certain Other Consequences of External Causes

T25.6–T26.72

✓5ᵗʰ **T26.8** **Corrosions of** other specified parts **of eye and adnexa**
    Code first (T51-T65) to identify chemical and intent
    Use additional external cause code to identify place (Y92)

    ✓x7ᵗʰ **T26.80** **Corrosions of other specified parts of** unspecified **eye and adnexa**

    ✓x7ᵗʰ **T26.81** **Corrosions of other specified parts of** right **eye and adnexa**

    ✓x7ᵗʰ **T26.82** **Corrosions of other specified parts of** left **eye and adnexa**

✓5ᵗʰ **T26.9** **Corrosion of eye and adnexa,** part unspecified
    Code first (T51-T65) to identify chemical and intent
    Use additional external cause code to identify place (Y92)

    ✓x7ᵗʰ **T26.90** **Corrosion of** unspecified **eye and adnexa, part unspecified**

    ✓x7ᵗʰ **T26.91** **Corrosion of** right **eye and adnexa, part unspecified**

    ✓x7ᵗʰ **T26.92** **Corrosion of** left **eye and adnexa, part unspecified**

✓4ᵗʰ **T27** **Burn and corrosion of respiratory tract**
    Use additional external cause code to identify the source and intent of the burn (X00-X19, X75-X77, X96-X98)
    Use additional external cause code to identify place (Y92)

> The appropriate 7th character is to be added to each code from category T27.
> A   initial encounter
> D   subsequent encounter
> S   sequela

> CC Excl: For CC codes in category T27: PDX collection 1411

    ✓x7ᵗʰ **T27.0** **Burn of larynx and trachea**   `CC` `H5`

    ✓x7ᵗʰ **T27.1** **Burn involving larynx and trachea with lung**   `CC` `H5`

    ✓x7ᵗʰ **T27.2** **Burn of other parts of respiratory tract**   `CC` `H5`
       Burn of thoracic cavity

    ✓x7ᵗʰ **T27.3** **Burn of respiratory tract,** part unspecified   `CC` `H5`

    ✓x7ᵗʰ **T27.4** **Corrosion of larynx and trachea**   `CC` `H5`
       Code first (T51-T65) to identify chemical and intent

    ✓x7ᵗʰ **T27.5** **Corrosion involving larynx and trachea with lung**   `CC` `H5`

    ✓x7ᵗʰ **T27.6** **Corrosion of other parts of respiratory tract**   `CC` `H5`
       Code first (T51-T65) to identify chemical and intent

    ✓x7ᵗʰ **T27.7** **Corrosion of respiratory tract,** part unspecified   `CC` `H5`
       Code first (T51-T65) to identify chemical and intent

✓4ᵗʰ **T28** **Burn and corrosion of other internal organs**
    Use additional external cause code to identify the source and intent of the burn (X00- X19, X75-X77, X96-X98)
    Use additional external cause code to identify place (Y92)

> The appropriate 7th character is to be added to each code from category T28.
> A   initial encounter
> D   subsequent encounter
> S   sequela

    ✓x7ᵗʰ **T28.0** **Burn of mouth and pharynx**

    ✓x7ᵗʰ **T28.1** **Burn of esophagus**   `CC` `H5`
       CC Excl: PDX collection 1412

    ✓x7ᵗʰ **T28.2** **Burn of other parts of alimentary tract**   `CC` `H5`
       CC Excl: PDX collection 1413

    ✓x7ᵗʰ **T28.3** **Burn of internal genitourinary organs**

    ✓5ᵗʰ **T28.4** **Burns of other and unspecified internal organs**
       Code first (T51-T65) to identify chemical and intent

       ✓x7ᵗʰ **T28.40** **Burn of** unspecified **internal organ**

       ✓6ᵗʰ **T28.41** **Burn of ear drum**

          ✓7ᵗʰ **T28.411** **Burn of** right **ear drum**

          ✓7ᵗʰ **T28.412** **Burn of** left **ear drum**

          ✓7ᵗʰ **T28.419** **Burn of** unspecified **ear drum**

       ✓x7ᵗʰ **T28.49** **Burn of** other **internal organ**

    ✓x7ᵗʰ **T28.5** **Corrosion of mouth and pharynx**
       Code first (T51-T65) to identify chemical and intent

    ✓x7ᵗʰ **T28.6** **Corrosion of esophagus**   `CC` `H5`
       Code first (T51-T65) to identify chemical and intent
       CC Excl: PDX collection 1412

    ✓x7ᵗʰ **T28.7** **Corrosion of other parts of alimentary tract**   `CC` `H5`
       Code first (T51-T65) to identify chemical and intent
       CC Excl: PDX collection 1413

✓x7ᵗʰ **T28.8** **Corrosion of internal** genitourinary organs
    Code first (T51-T65) to identify chemical and intent

✓5ᵗʰ **T28.9** **Corrosions of other and unspecified internal organs**
    Code first (T51-T65) to identify chemical and intent

    ✓x7ᵗʰ **T28.90** **Corrosions of** unspecified **internal organs**

    ✓6ᵗʰ **T28.91** **Corrosions of ear drum**

       ✓7ᵗʰ **T28.911** **Corrosions of** right **ear drum**

       ✓7ᵗʰ **T28.912** **Corrosions of** left **ear drum**

       ✓7ᵗʰ **T28.919** **Corrosions of** unspecified **ear drum**

    ✓x7ᵗʰ **T28.99** **Corrosions of** other **internal organs**

Burns and corrosions of multiple and unspecified body regions (T30-T32)

✓4ᵗʰ **T30** **Burn and corrosion, body region unspecified**

    T30.0 Burn **of unspecified body region, unspecified degree**
       This code is not for inpatient use. Code to specified site and degree of burns.
       Burn NOS
       Multiple burns NOS

    T30.4 Corrosion **of unspecified body region, unspecified degree**
       This code is not for inpatient use. Code to specified site and degree of corrosion.
       Corrosion NOS
       Multiple corrosion NOS

✓4ᵗʰ **T31** **Burns classified according to extent of body surface involved**
    NOTE   This category is to be used as the primary code only when the site of the burn is unspecified. It should be used as a supplementary code with categories T20-T25 when the site is specified.

> CC Excl: For CC/MCC codes in category T31: PDX collection 1414

    T31.0 **Burns involving** less than 10% **of body surface**

    ✓5ᵗʰ **T31.1** **Burns involving** 10-19% **of body surface**

       T31.10 **Burns involving 10-19% of body surface with** 0% to 9% third degree **burns**   `CC` `H5`
          Burns involving 10-19% of body surface NOS

       T31.11 **Burns involving 10-19% of body surface with** 10-19% third degree **burns**   `CC` `H5` `HCC`

    ✓5ᵗʰ **T31.2** **Burns involving** 20-29% **of body surface**

       T31.20 **Burns involving 20-29% of body surface with** 0% to 9% third degree **burns**   `CC` `H5`
          Burns involving 20-29% of body surface NOS

       T31.21 **Burns involving 20-29% of body surface with** 10-19% third degree **burns**   `MCC` `H5` `HCC`

       T31.22 **Burns involving 20-29% of body surface with** 20-29% third degree **burns**   `MCC` `H5` `HCC`

    ✓5ᵗʰ **T31.3** **Burns involving** 30-39% **of body surface**

       T31.30 **Burns involving 30-39% of body surface with** 0% to 9% third degree **burns**   `CC` `H5`
          Burns involving 30-39% of body surface NOS

       T31.31 **Burns involving 30-39% of body surface with** 10-19% third degree **burns**   `MCC` `H5` `HCC`

       T31.32 **Burns involving 30-39% of body surface with** 20-29% third degree **burns**   `MCC` `H5` `HCC`

       T31.33 **Burns involving 30-39% of body surface with** 30-39% third degree **burns**   `MCC` `H5` `HCC`

    ✓5ᵗʰ **T31.4** **Burns involving** 40-49% **of body surface**

       T31.40 **Burns involving 40-49% of body surface with** 0% to 9% third degree **burns**   `CC` `H5`
          Burns involving 40-49% of body surface NOS

       T31.41 **Burns involving 40-49% of body surface with** 10-19% third degree **burns**   `MCC` `H5` `HCC`

       T31.42 **Burns involving 40-49% of body surface with** 20-29% third degree **burns**   `MCC` `H5` `HCC`

       T31.43 **Burns involving 40-49% of body surface with** 30-39% third degree **burns**   `MCC` `H5` `HCC`

       T31.44 **Burns involving 40-49% of body surface with** 40-49% third degree **burns**   `MCC` `H5` `HCC`

    ✓5ᵗʰ **T31.5** **Burns involving** 50-59% **of body surface**

       T31.50 **Burns involving 50-59% of body surface with** 0% to 9% third degree **burns**   `CC` `H5`
          Burns involving 50-59% of body surface NOS

       T31.51 **Burns involving 50-59% of body surface with** 10-19% third degree **burns**   `MCC` `H5` `HCC`

T31.52 Burns involving 50-59% of body surface with 20-29% third degree burns `MCC` `H5` `HCC`

T31.53 Burns involving 50-59% of body surface with 30-39% third degree burns `MCC` `H5` `HCC`

T31.54 Burns involving 50-59% of body surface with 40-49% third degree burns `MCC` `H5` `HCC`

T31.55 Burns involving 50-59% of body surface with 50-59% third degree burns `MCC` `H5` `HCC`

✓5th **T31.6** Burns involving 60-69% of body surface

T31.60 Burns involving 60-69% of body surface with 0% to 9% third degree burns `CC` `H5`
Burns involving 60-69% of body surface NOS

T31.61 Burns involving 60-69% of body surface with 10-19% third degree burns `MCC` `H5` `HCC`

T31.62 Burns involving 60-69% of body surface with 20-29% third degree burns `MCC` `H5` `HCC`

T31.63 Burns involving 60-69% of body surface with 30-39% third degree burns `MCC` `H5` `HCC`

T31.64 Burns involving 60-69% of body surface with 40-49% third degree burns `MCC` `H5` `HCC`

T31.65 Burns involving 60-69% of body surface with 50-59% third degree burns `MCC` `H5` `HCC`

T31.66 Burns involving 60-69% of body surface with 60-69% third degree burns `MCC` `H5` `HCC`

✓5th **T31.7** Burns involving 70-79% of body surface

T31.70 Burns involving 70-79% of body surface with 0% to 9% third degree burns `CC` `H5`
Burns involving 70-79% of body surface NOS

T31.71 Burns involving 70-79% of body surface with 10-19% third degree burns `MCC` `H5` `HCC`

T31.72 Burns involving 70-79% of body surface with 20-29% third degree burns `MCC` `H5` `HCC`

T31.73 Burns involving 70-79% of body surface with 30-39% third degree burns `MCC` `H5` `HCC`

T31.74 Burns involving 70-79% of body surface with 40-49% third degree burns `MCC` `H5` `HCC`

T31.75 Burns involving 70-79% of body surface with 50-59% third degree burns `MCC` `H5` `HCC`

T31.76 Burns involving 70-79% of body surface with 60-69% third degree burns `MCC` `H5` `HCC`

T31.77 Burns involving 70-79% of body surface with 70-79% third degree burns `MCC` `H5` `HCC`

✓5th **T31.8** Burns involving 80-89% of body surface

T31.80 Burns involving 80-89% of body surface with 0% to 9% third degree burns `CC` `H5`
Burns involving 80-89% of body surface NOS

T31.81 Burns involving 80-89% of body surface with 10-19% third degree burns `MCC` `H5` `HCC`

T31.82 Burns involving 80-89% of body surface with 20-29% third degree burns `MCC` `H5` `HCC`

T31.83 Burns involving 80-89% of body surface with 30-39% third degree burns `MCC` `H5` `HCC`

T31.84 Burns involving 80-89% of body surface with 40-49% third degree burns `MCC` `H5` `HCC`

T31.85 Burns involving 80-89% of body surface with 50-59% third degree burns `MCC` `H5` `HCC`

T31.86 Burns involving 80-89% of body surface with 60-69% third degree burns `MCC` `H5` `HCC`

T31.87 Burns involving 80-89% of body surface with 70-79% third degree burns `MCC` `H5` `HCC`

T31.88 Burns involving 80-89% of body surface with 80-89% third degree burns `MCC` `H5` `HCC`

✓5th **T31.9** Burns involving 90% or more of body surface

T31.90 Burns involving 90% or more of body surface with 0% to 9% third degree burns `CC` `H5`
Burns involving 90% or more of body surface NOS

T31.91 Burns involving 90% or more of body surface with 10-19% third degree burns `MCC` `H5` `HCC`

T31.92 Burns involving 90% or more of body surface with 20-29% third degree burns `MCC` `H5` `HCC`

T31.93 Burns involving 90% or more of body surface with 30-39% third degree burns `MCC` `H5` `HCC`

T31.94 Burns involving 90% or more of body surface with 40-49% third degree burns `MCC` `H5` `HCC`

T31.95 Burns involving 90% or more of body surface with 50-59% third degree burns `MCC` `H5` `HCC`

T31.96 Burns involving 90% or more of body surface with 60-69% third degree burns `MCC` `H5` `HCC`

T31.97 Burns involving 90% or more of body surface with 70-79% third degree burns `MCC` `H5` `HCC`

T31.98 Burns involving 90% or more of body surface with 80-89% third degree burns `MCC` `H5` `HCC`

T31.99 Burns involving 90% or more of body surface with 90% or more third degree burns `MCC` `H5` `HCC`

Rule of Nines Estimation of Total Body Surface Burned

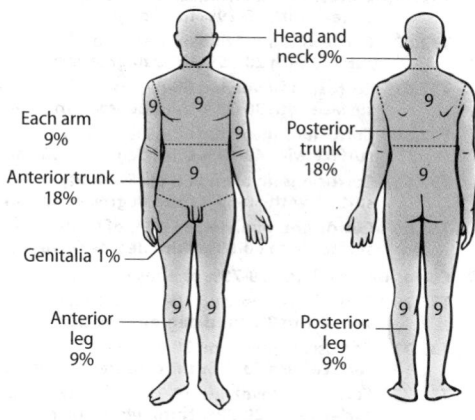

Head and neck 9%

Each arm 9%

Anterior trunk 18%

Posterior trunk 18%

Genitalia 1%

Anterior leg 9%

Posterior leg 9%

✓4th **T32** Corrosions classified according to extent of body surface involved

> **NOTE** This category is to be used as the primary code only when the site of the corrosion is unspecified. It may be used as a supplementary code with categories T20-T25 when the site is specified.

CC Excl: For CC/MCC codes in category T32: PDX collection 1414

T32.0 Corrosions involving less than 10% of body surface

✓5th **T32.1** Corrosions involving 10-19% of body surface

T32.10 Corrosions involving 10-19% of body surface with 0% to 9% third degree corrosion `CC` `H5`
Corrosions involving 10-19% of body surface NOS

T32.11 Corrosions involving 10-19% of body surface with 10-19% third degree corrosion `CC` `H5` `HCC`

✓5th **T32.2** Corrosions involving 20-29% of body surface

T32.20 Corrosions involving 20-29% of body surface with 0% to 9% third degree corrosion `CC` `H5`

T32.21 Corrosions involving 20-29% of body surface with 10-19% third degree corrosion `MCC` `H5` `HCC`

T32.22 Corrosions involving 20-29% of body surface with 20-29% third degree corrosion `MCC` `H5` `HCC`

✓5th **T32.3** Corrosions involving 30-39% of body surface

T32.30 Corrosions involving 30-39% of body surface with 0% to 9% third degree corrosion `CC` `H5`

T32.31 Corrosions involving 30-39% of body surface with 10-19% third degree corrosion `MCC` `H5` `HCC`

T32.32 Corrosions involving 30-39% of body surface with 20-29% third degree corrosion `MCC` `H5` `HCC`

T32.33 Corrosions involving 30-39% of body surface with 30-39% third degree corrosion `MCC` `H5` `HCC`

✓5th **T32.4** Corrosions involving 40-49% of body surface

T32.40 Corrosions involving 40-49% of body surface with 0% to 9% third degree corrosion `CC` `H5`

T32.41 Corrosions involving 40-49% of body surface with 10-19% third degree corrosion `MCC` `H5` `HCC`

T32.42 Corrosions involving 40-49% of body surface with 20-29% third degree corrosion `MCC` `H5` `HCC`

T32.43 Corrosions involving 40-49% of body surface with 30-39% third degree corrosion `MCC` `H5` `HCC`

T32.44 Corrosions involving 40-49% of body surface with 40-49% third degree corrosion `MCC` `H5` `HCC`

✓5th **T32.5** Corrosions involving 50-59% of body surface

T32.50 Corrosions involving 50-59% of body surface with 0% to 9% third degree corrosion `CC` `H5`

T32.51 Corrosions involving 50-59% of body surface with 10-19% third degree corrosion `MCC` `H5` `HCC`

T32.52 Corrosions involving 50-59% of body surface with 20-29% third degree corrosion `MCC` `H5` `HCC`

✔ Additional Character Required   ✓x7th Placeholder   Unacceptable PDx   Questionable PDx   Manifestation   `H1`-`H14` HAC   `HCC` CMS-HCC Dx   `HIV` HIV Dx

ICD-10-CM 2019   1099

T32.53 Corrosions involving 50-59% of body surface with 30-39% third degree corrosion `MCC` `H5` `HCC`

T32.54 Corrosions involving 50-59% of body surface with 40-49% third degree corrosion `MCC` `H5` `HCC`

T32.55 Corrosions involving 50-59% of body surface with 50-59% third degree corrosion `MCC` `H5` `HCC`

√5th T32.6 Corrosions involving 60-69% of body surface

T32.60 Corrosions involving 60-69% of body surface with 0% to 9% third degree corrosion `CC` `H5`

T32.61 Corrosions involving 60-69% of body surface with 10-19% third degree corrosion `MCC` `H5` `HCC`

T32.62 Corrosions involving 60-69% of body surface with 20-29% third degree corrosion `MCC` `H5` `HCC`

T32.63 Corrosions involving 60-69% of body surface with 30-39% third degree corrosion `MCC` `H5` `HCC`

T32.64 Corrosions involving 60-69% of body surface with 40-49% third degree corrosion `MCC` `H5` `HCC`

T32.65 Corrosions involving 60-69% of body surface with 50-59% third degree corrosion `MCC` `H5` `HCC`

T32.66 Corrosions involving 60-69% of body surface with 60-69% third degree corrosion `MCC` `H5` `HCC`

√5th T32.7 Corrosions involving 70-79% of body surface

T32.70 Corrosions involving 70-79% of body surface with 0% to 9% third degree corrosion `CC` `H5`

T32.71 Corrosions involving 70-79% of body surface with 10-19% third degree corrosion `MCC` `H5` `HCC`

T32.72 Corrosions involving 70-79% of body surface with 20-29% third degree corrosion `MCC` `H5` `HCC`

T32.73 Corrosions involving 70-79% of body surface with 30-39% third degree corrosion `MCC` `H5` `HCC`

T32.74 Corrosions involving 70-79% of body surface with 40-49% third degree corrosion `MCC` `H5` `HCC`

T32.75 Corrosions involving 70-79% of body surface with 50-59% third degree corrosion `MCC` `H5` `HCC`

T32.76 Corrosions involving 70-79% of body surface with 60-69% third degree corrosion `MCC` `H5` `HCC`

T32.77 Corrosions involving 70-79% of body surface with 70-79% third degree corrosion `MCC` `H5` `HCC`

√5th T32.8 Corrosions involving 80-89% of body surface

T32.80 Corrosions involving 80-89% of body surface with 0% to 9% third degree corrosion `CC` `H5`

T32.81 Corrosions involving 80-89% of body surface with 10-19% third degree corrosion `MCC` `H5` `HCC`

T32.82 Corrosions involving 80-89% of body surface with 20-29% third degree corrosion `MCC` `H5` `HCC`

T32.83 Corrosions involving 80-89% of body surface with 30-39% third degree corrosion `MCC` `H5` `HCC`

T32.84 Corrosions involving 80-89% of body surface with 40-49% third degree corrosion `MCC` `H5` `HCC`

T32.85 Corrosions involving 80-89% of body surface with 50-59% third degree corrosion `MCC` `H5` `HCC`

T32.86 Corrosions involving 80-89% of body surface with 60-69% third degree corrosion `MCC` `H5` `HCC`

T32.87 Corrosions involving 80-89% of body surface with 70-79% third degree corrosion `MCC` `H5` `HCC`

T32.88 Corrosions involving 80-89% of body surface with 80-89% third degree corrosion `MCC` `H5` `HCC`

√5th T32.9 Corrosions involving 90% or more of body surface

T32.90 Corrosions involving 90% or more of body surface with 0% to 9% third degree corrosion `CC` `H5`

T32.91 Corrosions involving 90% or more of body surface with 10-19% third degree corrosion `MCC` `H5` `HCC`

T32.92 Corrosions involving 90% or more of body surface with 20-29% third degree corrosion `MCC` `H5` `HCC`

T32.93 Corrosions involving 90% or more of body surface with 30-39% third degree corrosion `MCC` `H5` `HCC`

T32.94 Corrosions involving 90% or more of body surface with 40-49% third degree corrosion `MCC` `H5` `HCC`

T32.95 Corrosions involving 90% or more of body surface with 50-59% third degree corrosion `MCC` `H5` `HCC`

T32.96 Corrosions involving 90% or more of body surface with 60-69% third degree corrosion `MCC` `H5` `HCC`

T32.97 Corrosions involving 90% or more of body surface with 70-79% third degree corrosion `MCC` `H5` `HCC`

T32.98 Corrosions involving 90% or more of body surface with 80-89% third degree corrosion `MCC` `H5` `HCC`

T32.99 Corrosions involving 90% or more of body surface with 90% or more third degree corrosion `MCC` `H5` `HCC`

Frostbite (T33-T34)

EXCLUDES 2   *hypothermia and other effects of reduced temperature (T68, T69-)*

√4th **T33**   **Superficial** frostbite

INCLUDES   frostbite with partial thickness skin loss

The appropriate 7th character is to be added to each code from category T33.
A   initial encounter
D   subsequent encounter
S   sequela

CC Excl: For CC codes in category T33, unless otherwise noted: PDX collection 1416

√5th **T33.0**   Superficial frostbite of head

    CC Excl: For CC codes in subcategory T33.0: PDX collection 1415

    √6th T33.01   Superficial frostbite of ear
       √7th T33.011   Superficial frostbite of right ear `CC` `H5`
       √7th T33.012   Superficial frostbite of left ear `CC` `H5`
       √7th T33.019   Superficial frostbite of unspecified ear `CC` `H5`

    √x7th T33.02   Superficial frostbite of nose `CC` `H5`
    √x7th T33.09   Superficial frostbite of other part of head `CC` `H5`

√x7th **T33.1**   Superficial frostbite of neck `CC` `H5`
    CC Excl: PDX collection 1415

√x7th **T33.2**   Superficial frostbite of thorax `CC` `H5`

√x7th **T33.3**   Superficial frostbite of abdominal wall, lower back and pelvis `CC` `H5`

√5th **T33.4**   Superficial frostbite of arm
    EXCLUDES 2   *superficial frostbite of wrist and hand (T33.5-)*

    √x7th T33.40   Superficial frostbite of unspecified arm `CC` `H5`
    √x7th T33.41   Superficial frostbite of right arm `CC` `H5`
    √x7th T33.42   Superficial frostbite of left arm `CC` `H5`

√5th **T33.5**   Superficial frostbite of wrist, hand, and fingers

    CC Excl: For CC codes in subcategory T33.5: PDX collection 1417

    √6th T33.51   Superficial frostbite of wrist
       √7th T33.511   Superficial frostbite of right wrist `CC` `H5`
       √7th T33.512   Superficial frostbite of left wrist `CC` `H5`
       √7th T33.519   Superficial frostbite of unspecified wrist `CC` `H5`

    √6th T33.52   Superficial frostbite of hand
       EXCLUDES 2   *superficial frostbite of fingers (T33.53-)*
       √7th T33.521   Superficial frostbite of right hand `CC` `H5`
       √7th T33.522   Superficial frostbite of left hand `CC` `H5`
       √7th T33.529   Superficial frostbite of unspecified hand `CC` `H5`

    √6th T33.53   Superficial frostbite of finger(s)
       √7th T33.531   Superficial frostbite of right finger(s) `CC` `H5`
       √7th T33.532   Superficial frostbite of left finger(s) `CC` `H5`
       √7th T33.539   Superficial frostbite of unspecified finger(s) `CC` `H5`

√5th **T33.6**   Superficial frostbite of hip and thigh
    √x7th T33.60   Superficial frostbite of unspecified hip and thigh `CC` `H5`
    √x7th T33.61   Superficial frostbite of right hip and thigh `CC` `H5`
    √x7th T33.62   Superficial frostbite of left hip and thigh `CC` `H5`

√5th **T33.7**   Superficial frostbite of knee and lower leg
    EXCLUDES 2   *superficial frostbite of ankle and foot (T33.8-)*
    √x7th T33.70   Superficial frostbite of unspecified knee and lower leg `CC` `H5`
    √x7th T33.71   Superficial frostbite of right knee and lower leg `CC` `H5`
    √x7th T33.72   Superficial frostbite of left knee and lower leg `CC` `H5`

N Newborn: 0   P Pediatric: 0-17   M Maternity: 12-55   A Adult: 15-124   `MCC` Major Complication/Comorbidity   `CC` Complication/Comorbidity   `SW` Severe Wound Dx

1100   ICD-10-CM 2019

✓5ᵗʰ **T33.8** **Superficial frostbite of** ankle, foot, and toe(s)

> **CC Excl: For CC codes in subcategory T33.8:**
> PDX collection 1418

✓6ᵗʰ **T33.81** **Superficial frostbite of** ankle

✓7ᵗʰ **T33.811** **Superficial frostbite of** right **ankle** `CC` `H5`

✓7ᵗʰ **T33.812** **Superficial frostbite of** left **ankle** `CC` `H5`

✓7ᵗʰ **T33.819** **Superficial frostbite of** unspecified **ankle** `CC` `H5`

✓6ᵗʰ **T33.82** **Superficial frostbite of** foot

✓7ᵗʰ **T33.821** **Superficial frostbite of** right **foot** `CC` `H5`

✓7ᵗʰ **T33.822** **Superficial frostbite of** left **foot** `CC` `H5`

✓7ᵗʰ **T33.829** **Superficial frostbite of** unspecified **foot** `CC` `H5`

✓6ᵗʰ **T33.83** **Superficial frostbite of** toe(s)

✓7ᵗʰ **T33.831** **Superficial frostbite of** right **toe(s)** `CC` `H5`

✓7ᵗʰ **T33.832** **Superficial frostbite of** left **toe(s)** `CC` `H5`

✓7ᵗʰ **T33.839** **Superficial frostbite of** unspecified **toe(s)** `CC` `H5`

✓5ᵗʰ **T33.9** **Superficial frostbite of other and unspecified sites**

✓x7ᵗʰ **T33.90** **Superficial frostbite of** unspecified sites `CC` `H5`
Superficial frostbite NOS

✓x7ᵗʰ **T33.99** **Superficial frostbite of** other sites `CC` `H5`
Superficial frostbite of leg NOS
Superficial frostbite of trunk NOS

✓4ᵗʰ **T34** **Frostbite** with tissue necrosis

> The appropriate 7th character is to be added to each code from
> category T34.
> A   initial encounter
> D   subsequent encounter
> S   sequela

> **CC Excl: For CC codes in category T34, unless otherwise noted:**
> PDX collection 1416

✓5ᵗʰ **T34.0** **Frostbite with tissue necrosis of** head

> **CC Excl: For CC codes in subcategory T34.0:**
> PDX collection 1415

✓6ᵗʰ **T34.01** **Frostbite with tissue necrosis of** ear

✓7ᵗʰ **T34.011** **Frostbite with tissue necrosis of** right **ear** `CC` `H5`

✓7ᵗʰ **T34.012** **Frostbite with tissue necrosis of** left **ear** `CC` `H5`

✓7ᵗʰ **T34.019** **Frostbite with tissue necrosis of** unspecified **ear** `CC` `H5`

✓x7ᵗʰ **T34.02** **Frostbite with tissue necrosis of** nose `CC` `H5`

✓x7ᵗʰ **T34.09** **Frostbite with tissue necrosis of** other part of head `CC` `H5`

✓x7ᵗʰ **T34.1** **Frostbite with tissue necrosis of** neck `CC` `H5`
CC Excl: PDX collection 1415

✓x7ᵗʰ **T34.2** **Frostbite with tissue necrosis of** thorax `CC` `H5`

✓x7ᵗʰ **T34.3** **Frostbite with tissue necrosis of** abdominal wall, lower back and pelvis `CC` `H5`

✓5ᵗʰ **T34.4** **Frostbite with tissue necrosis of** arm
EXCLUDES 2   *frostbite with tissue necrosis of wrist and hand (T34.5-)*

✓x7ᵗʰ **T34.40** **Frostbite with tissue necrosis of** unspecified arm `CC` `H5`

✓x7ᵗʰ **T34.41** **Frostbite with tissue necrosis of** right arm `CC` `H5`

✓x7ᵗʰ **T34.42** **Frostbite with tissue necrosis of** left arm `CC` `H5`

✓5ᵗʰ **T34.5** **Frostbite with tissue necrosis of** wrist, hand, and finger(s)

> **CC Excl: For CC codes in subcategory T34.5:**
> PDX collection 1417

✓6ᵗʰ **T34.51** **Frostbite with tissue necrosis of** wrist

✓7ᵗʰ **T34.511** **Frostbite with tissue necrosis of** right **wrist** `CC` `H5`

✓7ᵗʰ **T34.512** **Frostbite with tissue necrosis of** left **wrist** `CC` `H5`

✓7ᵗʰ **T34.519** **Frostbite with tissue necrosis of** unspecified **wrist** `CC` `H5`

✓6ᵗʰ **T34.52** **Frostbite with tissue necrosis of** hand
EXCLUDES 2   *frostbite with tissue necrosis of finger(s) (T34.53-)*

✓7ᵗʰ **T34.521** **Frostbite with tissue necrosis of** right **hand** `CC` `H5`

✓7ᵗʰ **T34.522** **Frostbite with tissue necrosis of** left **hand** `CC` `H5`

✓7ᵗʰ **T34.529** **Frostbite with tissue necrosis of** unspecified **hand** `CC` `H5`

✓6ᵗʰ **T34.53** **Frostbite with tissue necrosis of** finger(s)

✓7ᵗʰ **T34.531** **Frostbite with tissue necrosis of** right **finger(s)** `CC` `H5`

✓7ᵗʰ **T34.532** **Frostbite with tissue necrosis of** left **finger(s)** `CC` `H5`

✓7ᵗʰ **T34.539** **Frostbite with tissue necrosis of** unspecified **finger(s)** `CC` `H5`

✓5ᵗʰ **T34.6** **Frostbite with tissue necrosis of** hip and thigh

✓x7ᵗʰ **T34.60** **Frostbite with tissue necrosis of** unspecified hip and thigh `CC` `H5`

✓x7ᵗʰ **T34.61** **Frostbite with tissue necrosis of** right hip and thigh `CC` `H5`

✓x7ᵗʰ **T34.62** **Frostbite with tissue necrosis of** left hip and thigh `CC` `H5`

✓5ᵗʰ **T34.7** **Frostbite with tissue necrosis of** knee and lower leg
EXCLUDES 2   *frostbite with tissue necrosis of ankle and foot (T34.8-)*

✓x7ᵗʰ **T34.70** **Frostbite with tissue necrosis of** unspecified knee and lower leg `CC` `H5`

✓x7ᵗʰ **T34.71** **Frostbite with tissue necrosis of** right knee and lower leg `CC` `H5`

✓x7ᵗʰ **T34.72** **Frostbite with tissue necrosis of** left knee and lower leg `CC` `H5`

✓5ᵗʰ **T34.8** **Frostbite with tissue necrosis of** ankle, foot, and toe(s)

> **CC Excl: For CC codes in subcategory T34.8:**
> PDX collection 1418

✓6ᵗʰ **T34.81** **Frostbite with tissue necrosis of** ankle

✓7ᵗʰ **T34.811** **Frostbite with tissue necrosis of** right **ankle** `CC` `H5`

✓7ᵗʰ **T34.812** **Frostbite with tissue necrosis of** left **ankle** `CC` `H5`

✓7ᵗʰ **T34.819** **Frostbite with tissue necrosis of** unspecified **ankle** `CC` `H5`

✓6ᵗʰ **T34.82** **Frostbite with tissue necrosis of** foot

✓7ᵗʰ **T34.821** **Frostbite with tissue necrosis of** right **foot** `CC` `H5`

✓7ᵗʰ **T34.822** **Frostbite with tissue necrosis of** left **foot** `CC` `H5`

✓7ᵗʰ **T34.829** **Frostbite with tissue necrosis of** unspecified **foot** `CC` `H5`

✓6ᵗʰ **T34.83** **Frostbite with tissue necrosis of** toe(s)

✓7ᵗʰ **T34.831** **Frostbite with tissue necrosis of** right **toe(s)** `CC` `H5`

✓7ᵗʰ **T34.832** **Frostbite with tissue necrosis of** left **toe(s)** `CC` `H5`

✓7ᵗʰ **T34.839** **Frostbite with tissue necrosis of** unspecified **toe(s)** `CC` `H5`

✓5ᵗʰ **T34.9** **Frostbite with tissue necrosis of other and unspecified sites**

✓x7ᵗʰ **T34.90** **Frostbite with tissue necrosis of** unspecified sites `CC` `H5`
Frostbite with tissue necrosis NOS

✓x7ᵗʰ **T34.99** **Frostbite with tissue necrosis of** other sites `CC` `H5`
Frostbite with tissue necrosis of leg NOS
Frostbite with tissue necrosis of trunk NOS

✓ Additional Character Required   ✓x7ᵗʰ Placeholder   Unacceptable PDx   Questionable PDx   Manifestation   **H1**-**H14** HAC   **HCC** CMS-HCC Dx   **HIV** HIV Dx

ICD-10-CM 2019   1101

Chapter 19. Injury, Poisoning and Certain Other Consequences of External Causes

Poisoning by, adverse effects of and underdosing of drugs, medicaments and biological substances (T36-T50)

INCLUDES   adverse effect of correct substance properly administered
poisoning by overdose of substance
poisoning by wrong substance given or taken in error
underdosing by (inadvertently) (deliberately) taking less substance than prescribed or instructed

Code first, for adverse effects, the nature of the adverse effect, such as:
adverse effect NOS (T88.7)
aspirin gastritis (K29.-)
blood disorders (D56-D76)
contact dermatitis (L23-L25)
dermatitis due to substances taken internally (L27.-)
nephropathy (N14.0-N14.2)

NOTE   The drug giving rise to the adverse effect should be identified by use of codes from categories T36-T50 with fifth or sixth character 5.

Use additional code(s) to specify:
manifestations of poisoning
underdosing or failure in dosage during medical and surgical care (Y63.6, Y63.8-Y63.9)
underdosing of medication regimen (Z91.12-, Z91.13-)

EXCLUDES 1   toxic reaction to local anesthesia in pregnancy (O29.3-)
EXCLUDES 2   abuse and dependence of psychoactive substances (F10-F19)
abuse of non-dependence-producing substances (F55.-)
drug reaction and poisoning affecting newborn (P00-P96)
pathological drug intoxication (inebriation) (F10-F19)

AHA: 2016, 2Q, 8; 2015, 3Q, 22

√4th **T36   Poisoning by, adverse effect of and underdosing of systemic antibiotics**

EXCLUDES 1   antineoplastic antibiotics (T45.1-)
locally applied antibiotic NEC (T49.0)
topically used antibiotic for ear, nose and throat (T49.6)
topically used antibiotic for eye (T49.5)

The appropriate 7th character is to be added to each code from category T36.
A   initial encounter
D   subsequent encounter
S   sequela

√5th **T36.0   Poisoning by, adverse effect of and underdosing of penicillins**

    √6th **T36.0X   Poisoning by, adverse effect of and underdosing of penicillins**

      √7th **T36.0X1   Poisoning by penicillins,** accidental (unintentional)
         Poisoning by penicillins NOS

      7 √7th **T36.0X2   Poisoning by penicillins,** intentional   HCC self-harm

      √7th **T36.0X3   Poisoning by penicillins,** assault

      √7th **T36.0X4   Poisoning by penicillins,** undetermined

      √7th **T36.0X5   Adverse effect** of penicillins

      √7th **T36.0X6   Underdosing** of penicillins

√5th **T36.1   Poisoning by, adverse effect of and underdosing of cephalosporins and other beta-lactam antibiotics**

    √6th **T36.1X   Poisoning by, adverse effect of and underdosing of cephalosporins and other beta-lactam antibiotics**

      √7th **T36.1X1   Poisoning by cephalosporins and other beta-lactam antibiotics,** accidental (unintentional)
         Poisoning by cephalosporins and other beta-lactam antibiotics NOS

      7 √7th **T36.1X2   Poisoning by cephalosporins and other beta-lactam antibiotics,** intentional self-harm   HCC

      √7th **T36.1X3   Poisoning by cephalosporins and other beta-lactam antibiotics,** assault

      √7th **T36.1X4   Poisoning by cephalosporins and other beta-lactam antibiotics,** undetermined

      √7th **T36.1X5   Adverse effect** of cephalosporins and other beta-lactam antibiotics

      √7th **T36.1X6   Underdosing** of cephalosporins and other beta-lactam antibiotics

√5th **T36.2   Poisoning by, adverse effect of and underdosing of chloramphenicol group**

    √6th **T36.2X   Poisoning by, adverse effect of and underdosing of chloramphenicol group**

      √7th **T36.2X1   Poisoning by chloramphenicol group,** accidental (unintentional)
         Poisoning by chloramphenicol group NOS

      7 √7th **T36.2X2   Poisoning by chloramphenicol group,**   HCC intentional self-harm

      √7th **T36.2X3   Poisoning by chloramphenicol group,** assault

      √7th **T36.2X4   Poisoning by chloramphenicol group,** undetermined

      √7th **T36.2X5   Adverse effect** of chloramphenicol group

      √7th **T36.2X6   Underdosing** of chloramphenicol group

√5th **T36.3   Poisoning by, adverse effect of and underdosing of macrolides**

    √6th **T36.3X   Poisoning by, adverse effect of and underdosing of macrolides**

      √7th **T36.3X1   Poisoning by macrolides,** accidental (unintentional)
         Poisoning by macrolides NOS

      7 √7th **T36.3X2   Poisoning by macrolides,** intentional   HCC self-harm

      √7th **T36.3X3   Poisoning by macrolides,** assault

      √7th **T36.3X4   Poisoning by macrolides,** undetermined

      √7th **T36.3X5   Adverse effect** of macrolides

      √7th **T36.3X6   Underdosing** of macrolides

√5th **T36.4   Poisoning by, adverse effect of and underdosing of tetracyclines**

    √6th **T36.4X   Poisoning by, adverse effect of and underdosing of tetracyclines**

      √7th **T36.4X1   Poisoning by tetracyclines,** accidental (unintentional)
         Poisoning by tetracyclines NOS

      7 √7th **T36.4X2   Poisoning by tetracyclines,** intentional self-harm   HCC

      √7th **T36.4X3   Poisoning by tetracyclines,** assault

      √7th **T36.4X4   Poisoning by tetracyclines,** undetermined

      √7th **T36.4X5   Adverse effect** of tetracyclines

      √7th **T36.4X6   Underdosing** of tetracyclines

√5th **T36.5   Poisoning by, adverse effect of and underdosing of aminoglycosides**
    Poisoning by, adverse effect of and underdosing of streptomycin

    √6th **T36.5X   Poisoning by, adverse effect of and underdosing of aminoglycosides**

      √7th **T36.5X1   Poisoning by aminoglycosides,** accidental (unintentional)
         Poisoning by aminoglycosides NOS

      7 √7th **T36.5X2   Poisoning by aminoglycosides,**   HCC intentional self-harm

      √7th **T36.5X3   Poisoning by aminoglycosides,** assault

      √7th **T36.5X4   Poisoning by aminoglycosides,** undetermined

      √7th **T36.5X5   Adverse effect** of aminoglycosides

      √7th **T36.5X6   Underdosing** of aminoglycosides

√5th **T36.6   Poisoning by, adverse effect of and underdosing of rifampicins**

    √6th **T36.6X   Poisoning by, adverse effect of and underdosing of rifampicins**

      √7th **T36.6X1   Poisoning by rifampicins,** accidental (unintentional)
         Poisoning by rifampicins NOS

      7 √7th **T36.6X2   Poisoning by rifampicins,** intentional   HCC self-harm

      √7th **T36.6X3   Poisoning by rifampicins,** assault

      √7th **T36.6X4   Poisoning by rifampicins,** undetermined

      √7th **T36.6X5   Adverse effect** of rifampicins

      √7th **T36.6X6   Underdosing** of rifampicins

√5th **T36.7   Poisoning by, adverse effect of and underdosing of antifungal antibiotics, systemically used**

    √6th **T36.7X   Poisoning by, adverse effect of and underdosing of antifungal antibiotics, systemically used**

      √7th **T36.7X1   Poisoning by antifungal antibiotics, systemically used,** accidental (unintentional)
         Poisoning by antifungal antibiotics, systemically used NOS

      7 √7th **T36.7X2   Poisoning by antifungal antibiotics,**   HCC **systemically used,** intentional self-harm

N Newborn: 0   P Pediatric: 0-17   M Maternity: 12-55   A Adult: 15-124   MCC Major Complication/Comorbidity   CC Complication/Comorbidity   SW Severe Wound Dx

ICD-10-CM 2019

1102

T36–T36.7X2

✓7th **T36.7X3** Poisoning by antifungal antibiotics, systemically used, assault

✓7th **T36.7X4** Poisoning by antifungal antibiotics, systemically used, undetermined

✓7th **T36.7X5** Adverse effect of antifungal antibiotics, systemically used

✓7th **T36.7X6** Underdosing of antifungal antibiotics, systemically used

✓5th **T36.8** Poisoning by, adverse effect of and underdosing of other systemic antibiotics

✓6th **T36.8X** Poisoning by, adverse effect of and underdosing of other systemic antibiotics

AHA: 2017, 1Q, 39

✓7th **T36.8X1** Poisoning by other systemic antibiotics, accidental (unintentional)

Poisoning by other systemic antibiotics NOS

7 ✓7th **T36.8X2** Poisoning by other systemic antibiotics, intentional self-harm   HCC

✓7th **T36.8X3** Poisoning by other systemic antibiotics, assault

✓7th **T36.8X4** Poisoning by other systemic antibiotics, undetermined

✓7th **T36.8X5** Adverse effect of other systemic antibiotics

✓7th **T36.8X6** Underdosing of other systemic antibiotics

✓5th **T36.9** Poisoning by, adverse effect of and underdosing of unspecified systemic antibiotic

✓x7th **T36.91** Poisoning by unspecified systemic antibiotic, accidental (unintentional)

Poisoning by systemic antibiotic NOS

7 ✓x7th **T36.92** Poisoning by unspecified systemic antibiotic, intentional self-harm   HCC

✓x7th **T36.93** Poisoning by unspecified systemic antibiotic, assault

✓x7th **T36.94** Poisoning by unspecified systemic antibiotic, undetermined

✓x7th **T36.95** Adverse effect of unspecified systemic antibiotic

✓x7th **T36.96** Underdosing of unspecified systemic antibiotic

▲✓4th **T37 Poisoning by, adverse effect of and underdosing of other systemic anti-infectives and antiparasitics**

EXCLUDES 1 anti-infectives topically used for ear, nose and throat (T49.6-)
anti-infectives topically used for eye (T49.5-)
locally applied anti-infectives NEC (T49.0-)

The appropriate 7th character is to be added to each code from category T37.
A   initial encounter
D   subsequent encounter
S   sequela

✓5th **T37.0** Poisoning by, adverse effect of and underdosing of sulfonamides

✓6th **T37.0X** Poisoning by, adverse effect of and underdosing of sulfonamides

✓7th **T37.0X1** Poisoning by sulfonamides, accidental (unintentional)

Poisoning by sulfonamides NOS

7 ✓7th **T37.0X2** Poisoning by sulfonamides, intentional self-harm   HCC

✓7th **T37.0X3** Poisoning by sulfonamides, assault

✓7th **T37.0X4** Poisoning by sulfonamides, undetermined

✓7th **T37.0X5** Adverse effect of sulfonamides

✓7th **T37.0X6** Underdosing of sulfonamides

✓5th **T37.1** Poisoning by, adverse effect of and underdosing of antimycobacterial drugs

EXCLUDES 1 rifampicins (T36.6-)
streptomycin (T36.5-)

✓6th **T37.1X** Poisoning by, adverse effect of and underdosing of antimycobacterial drugs

✓7th **T37.1X1** Poisoning by antimycobacterial drugs, accidental (unintentional)

Poisoning by antimycobacterial drugs NOS

7 ✓7th **T37.1X2** Poisoning by antimycobacterial drugs, intentional self-harm   HCC

✓7th **T37.1X3** Poisoning by antimycobacterial drugs, assault

✓7th **T37.1X4** Poisoning by antimycobacterial drugs, undetermined

✓7th **T37.1X5** Adverse effect of antimycobacterial drugs

✓7th **T37.1X6** Underdosing of antimycobacterial drugs

✓5th **T37.2** Poisoning by, adverse effect of and underdosing of antimalarials and drugs acting on other blood protozoa

EXCLUDES 1 hydroxyquinoline derivatives (T37.8-)

✓6th **T37.2X** Poisoning by, adverse effect of and underdosing of antimalarials and drugs acting on other blood protozoa

✓7th **T37.2X1** Poisoning by antimalarials and drugs acting on other blood protozoa, accidental (unintentional)

Poisoning by antimalarials and drugs acting on other blood protozoa NOS

7 ✓7th **T37.2X2** Poisoning by antimalarials and drugs   HCC acting on other blood protozoa, intentional self-harm

✓7th **T37.2X3** Poisoning by antimalarials and drugs acting on other blood protozoa, assault

✓7th **T37.2X4** Poisoning by antimalarials and drugs acting on other blood protozoa, undetermined

✓7th **T37.2X5** Adverse effect of antimalarials and drugs acting on other blood protozoa

✓7th **T37.2X6** Underdosing of antimalarials and drugs acting on other blood protozoa

✓5th **T37.3** Poisoning by, adverse effect of and underdosing of other antiprotozoal drugs

✓6th **T37.3X** Poisoning by, adverse effect of and underdosing of other antiprotozoal drugs

✓7th **T37.3X1** Poisoning by other antiprotozoal drugs, accidental (unintentional)

Poisoning by other antiprotozoal drugs NOS

7 ✓7th **T37.3X2** Poisoning by other antiprotozoal   HCC drugs, intentional self-harm

✓7th **T37.3X3** Poisoning by other antiprotozoal drugs, assault

✓7th **T37.3X4** Poisoning by other antiprotozoal drugs, undetermined

✓7th **T37.3X5** Adverse effect of other antiprotozoal drugs

✓7th **T37.3X6** Underdosing of other antiprotozoal drugs

✓5th **T37.4** Poisoning by, adverse effect of and underdosing of anthelminthics

✓6th **T37.4X** Poisoning by, adverse effect of and underdosing of anthelminthics

✓7th **T37.4X1** Poisoning by anthelminthics, accidental (unintentional)

Poisoning by anthelminthics NOS

7 ✓7th **T37.4X2** Poisoning by anthelminthics,   HCC intentional self-harm

✓7th **T37.4X3** Poisoning by anthelminthics, assault

✓7th **T37.4X4** Poisoning by anthelminthics, undetermined

✓7th **T37.4X5** Adverse effect of anthelminthics

✓7th **T37.4X6** Underdosing of anthelminthics

✓5th **T37.5** Poisoning by, adverse effect of and underdosing of antiviral drugs

EXCLUDES 1 amantadine (T42.8-)
cytarabine (T45.1-)

✓6th **T37.5X** Poisoning by, adverse effect of and underdosing of antiviral drugs

✓7th **T37.5X1** Poisoning by antiviral drugs, accidental (unintentional)

Poisoning by antiviral drugs NOS

7 ✓7th **T37.5X2** Poisoning by antiviral drugs,   HCC intentional self-harm

✓7th **T37.5X3** Poisoning by antiviral drugs, assault

✓7th **T37.5X4** Poisoning by antiviral drugs, undetermined

✓7th **T37.5X5** Adverse effect of antiviral drugs

✓7th **T37.5X6** Underdosing of antiviral drugs

✓ Additional Character Required   ✓x7th Placeholder   Unacceptable PDx   Questionable PDx   Manifestation   H1 - H14 HAC   HCC CMS-HCC Dx   HIV HIV Dx

ICD-10-CM 2019

1103

✓5ᵗʰ T37.8 **Poisoning by, adverse effect of and underdosing of other specified systemic anti-infectives and antiparasitics**
Poisoning by, adverse effect of and underdosing of hydroxyquinoline derivatives
> **EXCLUDES 1**   antimalarial drugs (T37.2-)

     ✓6ᵗʰ T37.8X **Poisoning by, adverse effect of and underdosing of other specified** systemic anti-infectives and antiparasitics

         ✓7ᵗʰ T37.8X1 **Poisoning by other specified systemic anti-infectives and antiparasitics, accidental (unintentional)**
Poisoning by other specified systemic anti-infectives and antiparasitics NOS

         7 **✓7ᵗʰ T37.8X2** **Poisoning by other specified systemic** HCC **anti-infectives and antiparasitics, intentional self-harm**

         ✓7ᵗʰ T37.8X3 **Poisoning by other specified systemic anti-infectives and antiparasitics, assault**

         ✓7ᵗʰ T37.8X4 **Poisoning by other specified systemic anti-infectives and antiparasitics, undetermined**

         ✓7ᵗʰ T37.8X5 **Adverse effect** of other specified systemic anti-infectives and antiparasitics

         ✓7ᵗʰ T37.8X6 **Underdosing** of other specified systemic anti-infectives and antiparasitics

✓5ᵗʰ T37.9 **Poisoning by, adverse effect of and underdosing of** unspecified systemic anti-infective and antiparasitics

     ✓x7ᵗʰ T37.91 **Poisoning by unspecified systemic anti-infective and antiparasitics, accidental (unintentional)**
Poisoning by, adverse effect of and underdosing of systemic anti-infective and antiparasitics NOS

     7 **✓x7ᵗʰ T37.92** **Poisoning by unspecified systemic** HCC **anti-infective and antiparasitics, intentional self-harm**

     ✓x7ᵗʰ T37.93 **Poisoning by unspecified systemic anti-infective and antiparasitics, assault**

     ✓x7ᵗʰ T37.94 **Poisoning by unspecified systemic anti-infective and antiparasitics, undetermined**

     ✓x7ᵗʰ T37.95 **Adverse effect** of unspecified systemic anti-infective and antiparasitic

     ✓x7ᵗʰ T37.96 **Underdosing** of unspecified systemic anti-infectives and antiparasitics

✓4ᵗʰ T38 **Poisoning by, adverse effect of and underdosing of hormones and their synthetic substitutes and antagonists, not elsewhere classified**
> **EXCLUDES 1**   mineralocorticoids and their antagonists (T50.0-)
> oxytocic hormones (T48.0-)
> parathyroid hormones and derivatives (T50.9-)

> The appropriate 7th character is to be added to each code from category T38.
> A   initial encounter
> D   subsequent encounter
> S   sequela

✓5ᵗʰ T38.0 **Poisoning by, adverse effect of and underdosing of glucocorticoids and synthetic analogues**
> **EXCLUDES 1**   glucocorticoids, topically used (T49.-)

     ✓6ᵗʰ T38.0X **Poisoning by, adverse effect of and underdosing of** glucocorticoids and synthetic analogues

         ✓7ᵗʰ T38.0X1 **Poisoning by glucocorticoids and synthetic analogues, accidental (unintentional)**
Poisoning by glucocorticoids and synthetic analogues NOS

         7 **✓7ᵗʰ T38.0X2** **Poisoning by glucocorticoids and** HCC **synthetic analogues, intentional self-harm**

         ✓7ᵗʰ T38.0X3 **Poisoning by glucocorticoids and synthetic analogues, assault**

         ✓7ᵗʰ T38.0X4 **Poisoning by glucocorticoids and synthetic analogues, undetermined**

         ✓7ᵗʰ T38.0X5 **Adverse effect** of glucocorticoids and synthetic analogues

         ✓7ᵗʰ T38.0X6 **Underdosing** of glucocorticoids and synthetic analogues

✓5ᵗʰ T38.1 **Poisoning by, adverse effect of and underdosing of thyroid hormones and substitutes**

     ✓6ᵗʰ T38.1X **Poisoning by, adverse effect of and underdosing of** thyroid hormones and substitutes

         ✓7ᵗʰ T38.1X1 **Poisoning by thyroid hormones and substitutes, accidental (unintentional)**
Poisoning by thyroid hormones and substitutes NOS

         7 **✓7ᵗʰ T38.1X2** **Poisoning by thyroid hormones and** HCC **substitutes, intentional self-harm**

         ✓7ᵗʰ T38.1X3 **Poisoning by thyroid hormones and substitutes, assault**

         ✓7ᵗʰ T38.1X4 **Poisoning by thyroid hormones and substitutes, undetermined**

         ✓7ᵗʰ T38.1X5 **Adverse effect** of thyroid hormones and substitutes

         ✓7ᵗʰ T38.1X6 **Underdosing** of thyroid hormones and substitutes

✓5ᵗʰ T38.2 **Poisoning by, adverse effect of and underdosing of antithyroid drugs**

     ✓6ᵗʰ T38.2X **Poisoning by, adverse effect of and underdosing of** antithyroid drugs

         ✓7ᵗʰ T38.2X1 **Poisoning by antithyroid drugs, accidental (unintentional)**
Poisoning by antithyroid drugs NOS

         7 **✓7ᵗʰ T38.2X2** **Poisoning by antithyroid drugs,** HCC **intentional self-harm**

         ✓7ᵗʰ T38.2X3 **Poisoning by antithyroid drugs, assault**

         ✓7ᵗʰ T38.2X4 **Poisoning by antithyroid drugs, undetermined**

         ✓7ᵗʰ T38.2X5 **Adverse effect** of antithyroid drugs

         ✓7ᵗʰ T38.2X6 **Underdosing** of antithyroid drugs

✓5ᵗʰ T38.3 **Poisoning by, adverse effect of and underdosing of insulin and oral hypoglycemic [antidiabetic] drugs**

     ✓6ᵗʰ T38.3X **Poisoning by, adverse effect of and underdosing of** insulin and oral hypoglycemic [antidiabetic] drugs

         ✓7ᵗʰ T38.3X1 **Poisoning by insulin and oral hypoglycemic [antidiabetic] drugs, accidental (unintentional)**
Poisoning by insulin and oral hypoglycemic [antidiabetic] drugs NOS

         7 **✓7ᵗʰ T38.3X2** **Poisoning by insulin and oral** HCC **hypoglycemic [antidiabetic] drugs, intentional self-harm**

         ✓7ᵗʰ T38.3X3 **Poisoning by insulin and oral hypoglycemic [antidiabetic] drugs, assault**

         ✓7ᵗʰ T38.3X4 **Poisoning by insulin and oral hypoglycemic [antidiabetic] drugs, undetermined**

         ✓7ᵗʰ T38.3X5 **Adverse effect** of insulin and oral hypoglycemic [antidiabetic] drugs

         ✓7ᵗʰ T38.3X6 **Underdosing** of insulin and oral hypoglycemic [antidiabetic] drugs

✓5ᵗʰ T38.4 **Poisoning by, adverse effect of and underdosing of oral contraceptives**
Poisoning by, adverse effect of and underdosing of multiple- and single-ingredient oral contraceptive preparations

     ✓6ᵗʰ T38.4X **Poisoning by, adverse effect of and underdosing of** oral contraceptives

         ✓7ᵗʰ T38.4X1 **Poisoning by oral contraceptives, accidental (unintentional)**
Poisoning by oral contraceptives NOS

         7 **✓7ᵗʰ T38.4X2** **Poisoning by oral contraceptives,** HCC **intentional self-harm**

         ✓7ᵗʰ T38.4X3 **Poisoning by oral contraceptives, assault**

         ✓7ᵗʰ T38.4X4 **Poisoning by oral contraceptives, undetermined**

         ✓7ᵗʰ T38.4X5 **Adverse effect** of oral contraceptives

         ✓7ᵗʰ T38.4X6 **Underdosing** of oral contraceptives

N Newborn: 0   **P** Pediatric: 0-17   **M** Maternity: 12-55   **A** Adult: 15-124   **MCC** Major Complication/Comorbidity   **CC** Complication/Comorbidity   **SW** Severe Wound Dx

1104   ICD-10-CM 2019

✓5th **T38.5 Poisoning by, adverse effect of and underdosing of other estrogens and progestogens**
Poisoning by, adverse effect of and underdosing of estrogens and progestogens mixtures and substitutes

✓6th **T38.5X Poisoning by, adverse effect of and underdosing of other estrogens and progestogens**

✓7th **T38.5X1 Poisoning by other estrogens and progestogens, accidental (unintentional)**
Poisoning by other estrogens and progestogens NOS

7 ✓7th **T38.5X2 Poisoning by other estrogens and progestogens, intentional self-harm** HCC

✓7th **T38.5X3 Poisoning by other estrogens and progestogens, assault**

✓7th **T38.5X4 Poisoning by other estrogens and progestogens, undetermined**

✓7th **T38.5X5 Adverse effect of other estrogens and progestogens**

✓7th **T38.5X6 Underdosing of other estrogens and progestogens**

✓5th **T38.6 Poisoning by, adverse effect of and underdosing of antigonadotrophins, antiestrogens, antiandrogens, not elsewhere classified**
Poisoning by, adverse effect of and underdosing of tamoxifen

✓6th **T38.6X Poisoning by, adverse effect of and underdosing of antigonadotrophins, antiestrogens, antiandrogens, not elsewhere classified**

✓7th **T38.6X1 Poisoning by antigonadotrophins, antiestrogens, antiandrogens, not elsewhere classified, accidental (unintentional)**
Poisoning by antigonadotrophins, antiestrogens, antiandrogens, not elsewhere classified NOS

7 ✓7th **T38.6X2 Poisoning by antigonadotrophins, antiestrogens, antiandrogens, not elsewhere classified, intentional self-harm** HCC

✓7th **T38.6X3 Poisoning by antigonadotrophins, antiestrogens, antiandrogens, not elsewhere classified, assault**

✓7th **T38.6X4 Poisoning by antigonadotrophins, antiestrogens, antiandrogens, not elsewhere classified, undetermined**

✓7th **T38.6X5 Adverse effect of antigonadotrophins, antiestrogens, antiandrogens, not elsewhere classified**

✓7th **T38.6X6 Underdosing of antigonadotrophins, antiestrogens, antiandrogens, not elsewhere classified**

✓5th **T38.7 Poisoning by, adverse effect of and underdosing of androgens and anabolic congeners**

✓6th **T38.7X Poisoning by, adverse effect of and underdosing of androgens and anabolic congeners**

✓7th **T38.7X1 Poisoning by androgens and anabolic congeners, accidental (unintentional)**
Poisoning by androgens and anabolic congeners NOS

7 ✓7th **T38.7X2 Poisoning by androgens and anabolic congeners, intentional self-harm** HCC

✓7th **T38.7X3 Poisoning by androgens and anabolic congeners, assault**

✓7th **T38.7X4 Poisoning by androgens and anabolic congeners, undetermined**

✓7th **T38.7X5 Adverse effect of androgens and anabolic congeners**

✓7th **T38.7X6 Underdosing of androgens and anabolic congeners**

✓5th **T38.8 Poisoning by, adverse effect of and underdosing of other and unspecified hormones and synthetic substitutes**

✓6th **T38.80 Poisoning by, adverse effect of and underdosing of unspecified hormones and synthetic substitutes**

✓7th **T38.801 Poisoning by unspecified hormones and synthetic substitutes, accidental (unintentional)**
Poisoning by unspecified hormones and synthetic substitutes NOS

7 ✓7th **T38.802 Poisoning by unspecified hormones and synthetic substitutes, intentional self-harm** HCC

✓7th **T38.803 Poisoning by unspecified hormones and synthetic substitutes, assault**

✓7th **T38.804 Poisoning by unspecified hormones and synthetic substitutes, undetermined**

✓7th **T38.805 Adverse effect of unspecified hormones and synthetic substitutes**

✓7th **T38.806 Underdosing of unspecified hormones and synthetic substitutes**

✓6th **T38.81 Poisoning by, adverse effect of and underdosing of anterior pituitary [adenohypophyseal] hormones**

✓7th **T38.811 Poisoning by anterior pituitary [adenohypophyseal] hormones, accidental (unintentional)**
Poisoning by anterior pituitary [adenohypophyseal] hormones NOS

7 ✓7th **T38.812 Poisoning by anterior pituitary [adenohypophyseal] hormones, intentional self-harm** HCC

✓7th **T38.813 Poisoning by anterior pituitary [adenohypophyseal] hormones, assault**

✓7th **T38.814 Poisoning by anterior pituitary [adenohypophyseal] hormones, undetermined**

✓7th **T38.815 Adverse effect of anterior pituitary [adenohypophyseal] hormones**

✓7th **T38.816 Underdosing of anterior pituitary [adenohypophyseal] hormones**

✓6th **T38.89 Poisoning by, adverse effect of and underdosing of other hormones and synthetic substitutes**

✓7th **T38.891 Poisoning by other hormones and synthetic substitutes, accidental (unintentional)**
Poisoning by other hormones and synthetic substitutes NOS

7 ✓7th **T38.892 Poisoning by other hormones and synthetic substitutes, intentional self-harm** HCC

✓7th **T38.893 Poisoning by other hormones and synthetic substitutes, assault**

✓7th **T38.894 Poisoning by other hormones and synthetic substitutes, undetermined**

✓7th **T38.895 Adverse effect of other hormones and synthetic substitutes**

✓7th **T38.896 Underdosing of other hormones and synthetic substitutes**

✓5th **T38.9 Poisoning by, adverse effect of and underdosing of other and unspecified hormone antagonists**

✓6th **T38.90 Poisoning by, adverse effect of and underdosing of unspecified hormone antagonists**

✓7th **T38.901 Poisoning by unspecified hormone antagonists, accidental (unintentional)**
Poisoning by unspecified hormone antagonists NOS

7 ✓7th **T38.902 Poisoning by unspecified hormone antagonists, intentional self-harm** HCC

✓7th **T38.903 Poisoning by unspecified hormone antagonists, assault**

✓7th **T38.904 Poisoning by unspecified hormone antagonists, undetermined**

✓7th **T38.905 Adverse effect of unspecified hormone antagonists**

✓7th **T38.906 Underdosing of unspecified hormone antagonists**

✓6th **T38.99 Poisoning by, adverse effect of and underdosing of other hormone antagonists**

✓7th **T38.991 Poisoning by other hormone antagonists, accidental (unintentional)**
Poisoning by other hormone antagonists NOS

7 ✓7th **T38.992 Poisoning by other hormone antagonists, intentional self-harm** HCC

✓7th **T38.993 Poisoning by other hormone antagonists, assault**

✓7th **T38.994 Poisoning by other hormone antagonists, undetermined**

✓ Additional Character Required   ✓x7th Placeholder   Unacceptable PDx   Questionable PDx   Manifestation   **H1 - H14** HAC   **HCC** CMS-HCC Dx   **HIV** HIV Dx

☑7ᵗʰ **T38.995** Adverse effect of other hormone antagonists

☑7ᵗʰ **T38.996** Underdosing of other hormone antagonists

☑4ᵗʰ **T39** **Poisoning by, adverse effect of and underdosing of nonopioid analgesics, antipyretics and antirheumatics**

> The appropriate 7th character is to be added to each code from category T39.
> A   initial encounter
> D   subsequent encounter
> S   sequela

☑5ᵗʰ **T39.0** Poisoning by, adverse effect of and underdosing of salicylates

☑6ᵗʰ **T39.01** Poisoning by, adverse effect of and underdosing of aspirin
> Poisoning by, adverse effect of and underdosing of acetylsalicylic acid

☑7ᵗʰ **T39.011** Poisoning by aspirin, accidental (unintentional)

7 ☑7ᵗʰ **T39.012** Poisoning by aspirin, intentional self-harm   **HCC**

☑7ᵗʰ **T39.013** Poisoning by aspirin, assault

☑7ᵗʰ **T39.014** Poisoning by aspirin, undetermined

☑7ᵗʰ **T39.015** Adverse effect of aspirin
> **AHA:** 2016, 1Q, 15

☑7ᵗʰ **T39.016** Underdosing of aspirin

☑6ᵗʰ **T39.09** Poisoning by, adverse effect of and underdosing of other salicylates

☑7ᵗʰ **T39.091** Poisoning by salicylates, accidental (unintentional)
> Poisoning by salicylates NOS

7 ☑7ᵗʰ **T39.092** Poisoning by salicylates, intentional self-harm   **HCC**

☑7ᵗʰ **T39.093** Poisoning by salicylates, assault

☑7ᵗʰ **T39.094** Poisoning by salicylates, undetermined

☑7ᵗʰ **T39.095** Adverse effect of salicylates

☑7ᵗʰ **T39.096** Underdosing of salicylates

☑5ᵗʰ **T39.1** Poisoning by, adverse effect of and underdosing of 4-Aminophenol derivatives

☑6ᵗʰ **T39.1X** Poisoning by, adverse effect of and underdosing of 4-Aminophenol derivatives

☑7ᵗʰ **T39.1X1** Poisoning by 4-Aminophenol derivatives, accidental (unintentional)
> Poisoning by 4-Aminophenol derivatives NOS

7 ☑7ᵗʰ **T39.1X2** Poisoning by 4-Aminophenol derivatives, intentional self-harm   **HCC**

☑7ᵗʰ **T39.1X3** Poisoning by 4-Aminophenol derivatives, assault

☑7ᵗʰ **T39.1X4** Poisoning by 4-Aminophenol derivatives, undetermined

☑7ᵗʰ **T39.1X5** Adverse effect of 4-Aminophenol derivatives

☑7ᵗʰ **T39.1X6** Underdosing of 4-Aminophenol derivatives

☑5ᵗʰ **T39.2** Poisoning by, adverse effect of and underdosing of pyrazolone derivatives

☑6ᵗʰ **T39.2X** Poisoning by, adverse effect of and underdosing of pyrazolone derivatives

☑7ᵗʰ **T39.2X1** Poisoning by pyrazolone derivatives, accidental (unintentional)
> Poisoning by pyrazolone derivatives NOS

7 ☑7ᵗʰ **T39.2X2** Poisoning by pyrazolone derivatives, intentional self-harm   **HCC**

☑7ᵗʰ **T39.2X3** Poisoning by pyrazolone derivatives, assault

☑7ᵗʰ **T39.2X4** Poisoning by pyrazolone derivatives, undetermined

☑7ᵗʰ **T39.2X5** Adverse effect of pyrazolone derivatives

☑7ᵗʰ **T39.2X6** Underdosing of pyrazolone derivatives

☑5ᵗʰ **T39.3** Poisoning by, adverse effect of and underdosing of other nonsteroidal anti-inflammatory drugs [NSAID]

☑6ᵗʰ **T39.31** Poisoning by, adverse effect of and underdosing of propionic acid derivatives
> Poisoning by, adverse effect of and underdosing of fenoprofen
> Poisoning by, adverse effect of and underdosing of flurbiprofen
> Poisoning by, adverse effect of and underdosing of ibuprofen
> Poisoning by, adverse effect of and underdosing of ketoprofen
> Poisoning by, adverse effect of and underdosing of naproxen
> Poisoning by, adverse effect of and underdosing of oxaprozin

☑7ᵗʰ **T39.311** Poisoning by propionic acid derivatives, accidental (unintentional)

7 ☑7ᵗʰ **T39.312** Poisoning by propionic acid derivatives, intentional self-harm   **HCC**

☑7ᵗʰ **T39.313** Poisoning by propionic acid derivatives, assault

☑7ᵗʰ **T39.314** Poisoning by propionic acid derivatives, undetermined

☑7ᵗʰ **T39.315** Adverse effect of propionic acid derivatives

☑7ᵗʰ **T39.316** Underdosing of propionic acid derivatives

☑6ᵗʰ **T39.39** Poisoning by, adverse effect of and underdosing of other nonsteroidal anti-inflammatory drugs [NSAID]

☑7ᵗʰ **T39.391** Poisoning by other nonsteroidal anti-inflammatory drugs [NSAID], accidental (unintentional)
> Poisoning by other nonsteroidal anti-inflammatory drugs NOS

7 ☑7ᵗʰ **T39.392** Poisoning by other nonsteroidal anti-inflammatory drugs [NSAID], intentional self-harm   **HCC**

☑7ᵗʰ **T39.393** Poisoning by other nonsteroidal anti-inflammatory drugs [NSAID], assault

☑7ᵗʰ **T39.394** Poisoning by other nonsteroidal anti-inflammatory drugs [NSAID], undetermined

☑7ᵗʰ **T39.395** Adverse effect of other nonsteroidal anti-inflammatory drugs [NSAID]

☑7ᵗʰ **T39.396** Underdosing of other nonsteroidal anti-inflammatory drugs [NSAID]

☑5ᵗʰ **T39.4** Poisoning by, adverse effect of and underdosing of antirheumatics, not elsewhere classified
> **EXCLUDES 1**   poisoning by, adverse effect of and underdosing of glucocorticoids (T38.0-)
> poisoning by, adverse effect of and underdosing of salicylates (T39.0-)

☑6ᵗʰ **T39.4X** Poisoning by, adverse effect of and underdosing of antirheumatics, not elsewhere classified

☑7ᵗʰ **T39.4X1** Poisoning by antirheumatics, not elsewhere classified, accidental (unintentional)
> Poisoning by antirheumatics, not elsewhere classified NOS

7 ☑7ᵗʰ **T39.4X2** Poisoning by antirheumatics, not elsewhere classified, intentional self-harm   **HCC**

☑7ᵗʰ **T39.4X3** Poisoning by antirheumatics, not elsewhere classified, assault

☑7ᵗʰ **T39.4X4** Poisoning by antirheumatics, not elsewhere classified, undetermined

☑7ᵗʰ **T39.4X5** Adverse effect of antirheumatics, not elsewhere classified

☑7ᵗʰ **T39.4X6** Underdosing of antirheumatics, not elsewhere classified

N Newborn: 0   P Pediatric: 0-17   M Maternity: 12-55   A Adult: 15-124   **MCC** Major Complication/Comorbidity   **CC** Complication/Comorbidity   **SW** Severe Wound Dx

1106   ICD-10-CM 2019

✓5ᵗʰ **T39.8** Poisoning by, adverse effect of and underdosing of other nonopioid analgesics and antipyretics, not elsewhere classified

✓6ᵗʰ **T39.8X** Poisoning by, adverse effect of and underdosing of other nonopioid analgesics and antipyretics, not elsewhere classified

✓7ᵗʰ **T39.8X1** Poisoning by other nonopioid analgesics and antipyretics, not elsewhere classified, accidental (unintentional)
Poisoning by other nonopioid analgesics and antipyretics, not elsewhere classified NOS

7 ✓7ᵗʰ **T39.8X2** Poisoning by other nonopioid   HCC analgesics and antipyretics, not elsewhere classified, intentional self-harm

✓7ᵗʰ **T39.8X3** Poisoning by other nonopioid analgesics and antipyretics, not elsewhere classified, assault

✓7ᵗʰ **T39.8X4** Poisoning by other nonopioid analgesics and antipyretics, not elsewhere classified, undetermined

✓7ᵗʰ **T39.8X5** Adverse effect of other nonopioid analgesics and antipyretics, not elsewhere classified

✓7ᵗʰ **T39.8X6** Underdosing of other nonopioid analgesics and antipyretics, not elsewhere classified

✓5ᵗʰ **T39.9** Poisoning by, adverse effect of and underdosing of unspecified nonopioid analgesic, antipyretic and antirheumatic

✓x7ᵗʰ **T39.91** Poisoning by unspecified nonopioid analgesic, antipyretic and antirheumatic, accidental (unintentional)
Poisoning by nonopioid analgesic, antipyretic and antirheumatic NOS

7 ✓x7ᵗʰ **T39.92** Poisoning by unspecified nonopioid   HCC analgesic, antipyretic and antirheumatic, intentional self-harm

✓x7ᵗʰ **T39.93** Poisoning by unspecified nonopioid analgesic, antipyretic and antirheumatic, assault

✓x7ᵗʰ **T39.94** Poisoning by unspecified nonopioid analgesic, antipyretic and antirheumatic, undetermined

✓x7ᵗʰ **T39.95** Adverse effect of unspecified nonopioid analgesic, antipyretic and antirheumatic

✓x7ᵗʰ **T39.96** Underdosing of unspecified nonopioid analgesic, antipyretic and antirheumatic

✓4ᵗʰ **T40** Poisoning by, adverse effect of and underdosing of narcotics and psychodysleptics [hallucinogens]

EXCLUDES 2 *drug dependence and related mental and behavioral disorders due to psychoactive substance use (F10-F19-)*

The appropriate 7th character is to be added to each code from category T40.
A   initial encounter
D   subsequent encounter
S   sequela

✓5ᵗʰ **T40.0** Poisoning by, adverse effect of and underdosing of opium

✓6ᵗʰ **T40.0X** Poisoning by, adverse effect of and underdosing of opium

✓7ᵗʰ **T40.0X1** Poisoning by opium, accidental (unintentional)
Poisoning by opium NOS

7 ✓7ᵗʰ **T40.0X2** Poisoning by opium, intentional   HCC self-harm

✓7ᵗʰ **T40.0X3** Poisoning by opium, assault

✓7ᵗʰ **T40.0X4** Poisoning by opium, undetermined

✓7ᵗʰ **T40.0X5** Adverse effect of opium

✓7ᵗʰ **T40.0X6** Underdosing of opium

✓5ᵗʰ **T40.1** Poisoning by and adverse effect of heroin

✓6ᵗʰ **T40.1X** Poisoning by and adverse effect of heroin

✓7ᵗʰ **T40.1X1** Poisoning by heroin, accidental (unintentional)
Poisoning by heroin NOS

7 ✓7ᵗʰ **T40.1X2** Poisoning by heroin, intentional   HCC self-harm

✓7ᵗʰ **T40.1X3** Poisoning by heroin, assault

✓7ᵗʰ **T40.1X4** Poisoning by heroin, undetermined

✓5ᵗʰ **T40.2** Poisoning by, adverse effect of and underdosing of other opioids

✓6ᵗʰ **T40.2X** Poisoning by, adverse effect of and underdosing of other opioids

✓7ᵗʰ **T40.2X1** Poisoning by other opioids, accidental (unintentional)
Poisoning by other opioids NOS

7 ✓7ᵗʰ **T40.2X2** Poisoning by other opioids,   HCC intentional self-harm

✓7ᵗʰ **T40.2X3** Poisoning by other opioids, assault

✓7ᵗʰ **T40.2X4** Poisoning by other opioids, undetermined

✓7ᵗʰ **T40.2X5** Adverse effect of other opioids

✓7ᵗʰ **T40.2X6** Underdosing of other opioids

✓5ᵗʰ **T40.3** Poisoning by, adverse effect of and underdosing of methadone

✓6ᵗʰ **T40.3X** Poisoning by, adverse effect of and underdosing of methadone

✓7ᵗʰ **T40.3X1** Poisoning by methadone, accidental (unintentional)
Poisoning by methadone NOS

7 ✓7ᵗʰ **T40.3X2** Poisoning by methadone, intentional   HCC self-harm

✓7ᵗʰ **T40.3X3** Poisoning by methadone, assault

✓7ᵗʰ **T40.3X4** Poisoning by methadone, undetermined

✓7ᵗʰ **T40.3X5** Adverse effect of methadone

✓7ᵗʰ **T40.3X6** Underdosing of methadone

✓5ᵗʰ **T40.4** Poisoning by, adverse effect of and underdosing of other synthetic narcotics

✓6ᵗʰ **T40.4X** Poisoning by, adverse effect of and underdosing of other synthetic narcotics

✓7ᵗʰ **T40.4X1** Poisoning by other synthetic narcotics, accidental (unintentional)
Poisoning by other synthetic narcotics NOS

7 ✓7ᵗʰ **T40.4X2** Poisoning by other synthetic   HCC narcotics, intentional self-harm

✓7ᵗʰ **T40.4X3** Poisoning by other synthetic narcotics, assault

✓7ᵗʰ **T40.4X4** Poisoning by other synthetic narcotics, undetermined

✓7ᵗʰ **T40.4X5** Adverse effect of other synthetic narcotics

✓7ᵗʰ **T40.4X6** Underdosing of other synthetic narcotics

✓5ᵗʰ **T40.5** Poisoning by, adverse effect of and underdosing of cocaine

✓6ᵗʰ **T40.5X** Poisoning by, adverse effect of and underdosing of cocaine

✓7ᵗʰ **T40.5X1** Poisoning by cocaine, accidental (unintentional)
Poisoning by cocaine NOS
AHA: 2016, 2Q, 8

7 ✓7ᵗʰ **T40.5X2** Poisoning by cocaine, intentional   HCC self-harm

✓7ᵗʰ **T40.5X3** Poisoning by cocaine, assault

✓7ᵗʰ **T40.5X4** Poisoning by cocaine, undetermined

✓7ᵗʰ **T40.5X5** Adverse effect of cocaine

✓7ᵗʰ **T40.5X6** Underdosing of cocaine

✓5ᵗʰ **T40.6** Poisoning by, adverse effect of and underdosing of other and unspecified narcotics

✓6ᵗʰ **T40.60** Poisoning by, adverse effect of and underdosing of unspecified narcotics

✓7ᵗʰ **T40.601** Poisoning by unspecified narcotics, accidental (unintentional)
Poisoning by narcotics NOS

7 ✓7ᵗʰ **T40.602** Poisoning by unspecified narcotics,   HCC intentional self-harm

✓7ᵗʰ **T40.603** Poisoning by unspecified narcotics, assault

✓7ᵗʰ **T40.604** Poisoning by unspecified narcotics, undetermined

✓7ᵗʰ **T40.605** Adverse effect of unspecified narcotics

✓7ᵗʰ **T40.606** Underdosing of unspecified narcotics

✓6ᵗʰ **T40.69** Poisoning by, adverse effect of and underdosing of other narcotics

✓7ᵗʰ **T40.691** Poisoning by other narcotics, accidental (unintentional)
Poisoning by other narcotics NOS

✓ Additional Character Required   ✓x7ᵗʰ Placeholder   Unacceptable PDx   Questionable PDx   Manifestation   H1-H14 HAC   HCC CMS-HCC Dx   HIV HIV Dx

ICD-10-CM 2019   **1107**

7 ✓7th **T40.692 Poisoning by other narcotics,** **HCC**
intentional self-harm

✓7th **T40.693 Poisoning by other narcotics,** assault

✓7th **T40.694 Poisoning by other narcotics,**
undetermined

✓7th **T40.695** Adverse effect **of other narcotics**

✓7th **T40.696** Underdosing **of other narcotics**

✓5th **T40.7 Poisoning by, adverse effect of and underdosing of cannabis
(derivatives)**

✓6th **T40.7X Poisoning by, adverse effect of and underdosing of
cannabis (derivatives)**

✓7th **T40.7X1 Poisoning by cannabis (derivatives),**
accidental **(unintentional)**
Poisoning by cannabis NOS

7 ✓7th **T40.7X2 Poisoning by cannabis (derivatives),** **HCC**
intentional self-harm

✓7th **T40.7X3 Poisoning by cannabis (derivatives),**
assault

✓7th **T40.7X4 Poisoning by cannabis (derivatives),**
undetermined

✓7th **T40.7X5** Adverse effect **of cannabis (derivatives)**

✓7th **T40.7X6** Underdosing **of cannabis (derivatives)**

✓5th **T40.8 Poisoning by and adverse effect of** lysergide [LSD]

✓6th **T40.8X Poisoning by and adverse effect of lysergide [LSD]**

✓7th **T40.8X1 Poisoning by lysergide [LSD],** accidental
(unintentional)
Poisoning by lysergide [LSD] NOS

7 ✓7th **T40.8X2 Poisoning by lysergide [LSD],** **HCC**
intentional self-harm

✓7th **T40.8X3 Poisoning by lysergide [LSD],** assault

✓7th **T40.8X4 Poisoning by lysergide [LSD],**
undetermined

✓5th **T40.9 Poisoning by, adverse effect of and underdosing of other and
unspecified psychodysleptics [hallucinogens]**

✓6th **T40.90 Poisoning by, adverse effect of and underdosing of
unspecified psychodysleptics [hallucinogens]**

✓7th **T40.901 Poisoning by unspecified
psychodysleptics [hallucinogens],
accidental (unintentional)**

7 ✓7th **T40.902 Poisoning by unspecified** **HCC**
**psychodysleptics [hallucinogens],
intentional self-harm**

✓7th **T40.903 Poisoning by unspecified
psychodysleptics [hallucinogens],** assault

✓7th **T40.904 Poisoning by unspecified
psychodysleptics [hallucinogens],**
undetermined

✓7th **T40.905** Adverse effect **of unspecified
psychodysleptics [hallucinogens]**

✓7th **T40.906** Underdosing **of unspecified
psychodysleptics**

✓6th **T40.99 Poisoning by, adverse effect of and underdosing of
other psychodysleptics [hallucinogens]**

✓7th **T40.991 Poisoning by other psychodysleptics
[hallucinogens],** accidental
(unintentional)
Poisoning by other psychodysleptics
[hallucinogens] NOS

7 ✓7th **T40.992 Poisoning by other psychodysleptics** **HCC**
[hallucinogens], intentional self-harm

✓7th **T40.993 Poisoning by other psychodysleptics
[hallucinogens],** assault

✓7th **T40.994 Poisoning by other psychodysleptics
[hallucinogens],** undetermined

✓7th **T40.995** Adverse effect **of other psychodysleptics
[hallucinogens]**

✓7th **T40.996** Underdosing **of other psychodysleptics**

✓4th **T41 Poisoning by, adverse effect of and underdosing of anesthetics
and therapeutic gases**

EXCLUDES 1 *benzodiazepines (T42.4-)*
cocaine (T40.5-)
complications of anesthesia during labor and delivery (O74.-)
complications of anesthesia during pregnancy (O29.-)
complications of anesthesia during the puerperium (O89.-)
opioids (T40.0-T40.2-)

The appropriate 7th character is to be added to each code from
category T41.
A   initial encounter
D   subsequent encounter
S   sequela

✓5th **T41.0 Poisoning by, adverse effect of and underdosing of inhaled
anesthetics**
EXCLUDES 1 *oxygen (T41.5-)*

✓6th **T41.0X Poisoning by, adverse effect of and underdosing of
inhaled anesthetics**

✓7th **T41.0X1 Poisoning by inhaled anesthetics,
accidental (unintentional)**
Poisoning by inhaled anesthetics NOS

7 ✓7th **T41.0X2 Poisoning by inhaled anesthetics,** **HCC**
intentional self-harm

✓7th **T41.0X3 Poisoning by inhaled anesthetics,** assault

✓7th **T41.0X4 Poisoning by inhaled anesthetics,**
undetermined

✓7th **T41.0X5** Adverse effect **of inhaled anesthetics**

✓7th **T41.0X6** Underdosing **of inhaled anesthetics**

✓5th **T41.1 Poisoning by, adverse effect of and underdosing of
intravenous anesthetics**
Poisoning by, adverse effect of and underdosing of
thiobarbiturates

✓6th **T41.1X Poisoning by, adverse effect of and underdosing of
intravenous anesthetics**

✓7th **T41.1X1 Poisoning by intravenous anesthetics,
accidental (unintentional)**
Poisoning by intravenous anesthetics NOS

7 ✓7th **T41.1X2 Poisoning by intravenous anesthetics,** **HCC**
intentional self-harm

✓7th **T41.1X3 Poisoning by intravenous anesthetics,**
assault

✓7th **T41.1X4 Poisoning by intravenous anesthetics,**
undetermined

✓7th **T41.1X5** Adverse effect **of intravenous anesthetics**

✓7th **T41.1X6** Underdosing **of intravenous anesthetics**

✓5th **T41.2 Poisoning by, adverse effect of and underdosing of other and
unspecified general anesthetics**

✓6th **T41.20 Poisoning by, adverse effect of and underdosing of
unspecified general anesthetics**

✓7th **T41.201 Poisoning by unspecified general
anesthetics,** accidental **(unintentional)**
Poisoning by general anesthetics NOS

7 ✓7th **T41.202 Poisoning by unspecified general** **HCC**
anesthetics, intentional self-harm

✓7th **T41.203 Poisoning by unspecified general
anesthetics,** assault

✓7th **T41.204 Poisoning by unspecified general
anesthetics,** undetermined

✓7th **T41.205** Adverse effect **of unspecified general
anesthetics**
AHA: 2016, 4Q, 73

✓7th **T41.206** Underdosing **of unspecified general
anesthetics**

✓6th **T41.29 Poisoning by, adverse effect of and underdosing of
other general anesthetics**

✓7th **T41.291 Poisoning by other general anesthetics,**
accidental **(unintentional)**
Poisoning by other general anesthetics NOS

7 ✓7th **T41.292 Poisoning by other general** **HCC**
anesthetics, intentional self-harm

✓7th **T41.293 Poisoning by other general anesthetics,**
assault

✓7th **T41.294 Poisoning by other general anesthetics,**
undetermined

✓7th **T41.295** Adverse effect **of other general
anesthetics**

N Newborn: 0   P Pediatric: 0-17   M Maternity: 12-55   A Adult: 15-124   MCC Major Complication/Comorbidity   CC Complication/Comorbidity   SW Severe Wound Dx

1108   ICD-10-CM 2019

✓7ᵗʰ **T41.296** Underdosing of other general anesthetics

✓5ᵗʰ **T41.3** Poisoning by, adverse effect of and underdosing of local anesthetics
  Cocaine (topical)
  EXCLUDES 2 poisoning by cocaine used as a central nervous system stimulant (T40.5X1-T40.5X4)

  ✓6ᵗʰ **T41.3X** Poisoning by, adverse effect of and underdosing of local anesthetics

    ✓7ᵗʰ **T41.3X1** Poisoning by local anesthetics, accidental (unintentional)
      Poisoning by local anesthetics NOS

    7 ✓7ᵗʰ **T41.3X2** Poisoning by local anesthetics, intentional self-harm   HCC

    ✓7ᵗʰ **T41.3X3** Poisoning by local anesthetics, assault

    ✓7ᵗʰ **T41.3X4** Poisoning by local anesthetics, undetermined

    ✓7ᵗʰ **T41.3X5** Adverse effect of local anesthetics

    ✓7ᵗʰ **T41.3X6** Underdosing of local anesthetics

✓5ᵗʰ **T41.4** Poisoning by, adverse effect of and underdosing of unspecified anesthetic

  ✓x7ᵗʰ **T41.41** Poisoning by unspecified anesthetic, accidental (unintentional)
    Poisoning by anesthetic NOS

  7 ✓x7ᵗʰ **T41.42** Poisoning by unspecified anesthetic, intentional self-harm   HCC

  ✓x7ᵗʰ **T41.43** Poisoning by unspecified anesthetic, assault

  ✓x7ᵗʰ **T41.44** Poisoning by unspecified anesthetic, undetermined

  ✓x7ᵗʰ **T41.45** Adverse effect of unspecified anesthetic

  ✓x7ᵗʰ **T41.46** Underdosing of unspecified anesthetics

✓5ᵗʰ **T41.5** Poisoning by, adverse effect of and underdosing of therapeutic gases

  ✓6ᵗʰ **T41.5X** Poisoning by, adverse effect of and underdosing of therapeutic gases

    ✓7ᵗʰ **T41.5X1** Poisoning by therapeutic gases, accidental (unintentional)
      Poisoning by therapeutic gases NOS

    7 ✓7ᵗʰ **T41.5X2** Poisoning by therapeutic gases, intentional self-harm   HCC

    ✓7ᵗʰ **T41.5X3** Poisoning by therapeutic gases, assault

    ✓7ᵗʰ **T41.5X4** Poisoning by therapeutic gases, undetermined

    ✓7ᵗʰ **T41.5X5** Adverse effect of therapeutic gases

    ✓7ᵗʰ **T41.5X6** Underdosing of therapeutic gases

✓4ᵗʰ **T42** Poisoning by, adverse effect of and underdosing of antiepileptic, sedative-hypnotic and antiparkinsonism drugs
  EXCLUDES 2 drug dependence and related mental and behavioral disorders due to psychoactive substance use (F10- – F19-)

  The appropriate 7th character is to be added to each code from category T42.
  A   initial encounter
  D   subsequent encounter
  S   sequela

✓5ᵗʰ **T42.0** Poisoning by, adverse effect of and underdosing of hydantoin derivatives

  ✓6ᵗʰ **T42.0X** Poisoning by, adverse effect of and underdosing of hydantoin derivatives

    ✓7ᵗʰ **T42.0X1** Poisoning by hydantoin derivatives, accidental (unintentional)
      Poisoning by hydantoin derivatives NOS

    7 ✓7ᵗʰ **T42.0X2** Poisoning by hydantoin derivatives, intentional self-harm   HCC

    ✓7ᵗʰ **T42.0X3** Poisoning by hydantoin derivatives, assault

    ✓7ᵗʰ **T42.0X4** Poisoning by hydantoin derivatives, undetermined

    ✓7ᵗʰ **T42.0X5** Adverse effect of hydantoin derivatives

    ✓7ᵗʰ **T42.0X6** Underdosing of hydantoin derivatives

✓5ᵗʰ **T42.1** Poisoning by, adverse effect of and underdosing of iminostilbenes
  Poisoning by, adverse effect of and underdosing of carbamazepine

  ✓6ᵗʰ **T42.1X** Poisoning by, adverse effect of and underdosing of iminostilbenes

    ✓7ᵗʰ **T42.1X1** Poisoning by iminostilbenes, accidental (unintentional)
      Poisoning by iminostilbenes NOS

    7 ✓7ᵗʰ **T42.1X2** Poisoning by iminostilbenes, intentional self-harm   HCC

    ✓7ᵗʰ **T42.1X3** Poisoning by iminostilbenes, assault

    ✓7ᵗʰ **T42.1X4** Poisoning by iminostilbenes, undetermined

    ✓7ᵗʰ **T42.1X5** Adverse effect of iminostilbenes

    ✓7ᵗʰ **T42.1X6** Underdosing of iminostilbenes

✓5ᵗʰ **T42.2** Poisoning by, adverse effect of and underdosing of succinimides and oxazolidinediones

  ✓6ᵗʰ **T42.2X** Poisoning by, adverse effect of and underdosing of succinimides and oxazolidinediones

    ✓7ᵗʰ **T42.2X1** Poisoning by succinimides and oxazolidinediones, accidental (unintentional)
      Poisoning by succinimides and oxazolidinediones NOS

    7 ✓7ᵗʰ **T42.2X2** Poisoning by succinimides and oxazolidinediones, intentional self-harm   HCC

    ✓7ᵗʰ **T42.2X3** Poisoning by succinimides and oxazolidinediones, assault

    ✓7ᵗʰ **T42.2X4** Poisoning by succinimides and oxazolidinediones, undetermined

    ✓7ᵗʰ **T42.2X5** Adverse effect of succinimides and oxazolidinediones

    ✓7ᵗʰ **T42.2X6** Underdosing of succinimides and oxazolidinediones

✓5ᵗʰ **T42.3** Poisoning by, adverse effect of and underdosing of barbiturates
  EXCLUDES 1 poisoning by, adverse effect of and underdosing of thiobarbiturates (T41.1-)

  ✓6ᵗʰ **T42.3X** Poisoning by, adverse effect of and underdosing of barbiturates

    ✓7ᵗʰ **T42.3X1** Poisoning by barbiturates, accidental (unintentional)
      Poisoning by barbiturates NOS

    7 ✓7ᵗʰ **T42.3X2** Poisoning by barbiturates, intentional self-harm   HCC

    ✓7ᵗʰ **T42.3X3** Poisoning by barbiturates, assault

    ✓7ᵗʰ **T42.3X4** Poisoning by barbiturates, undetermined

    ✓7ᵗʰ **T42.3X5** Adverse effect of barbiturates

    ✓7ᵗʰ **T42.3X6** Underdosing of barbiturates

✓5ᵗʰ **T42.4** Poisoning by, adverse effect of and underdosing of benzodiazepines

  ✓6ᵗʰ **T42.4X** Poisoning by, adverse effect of and underdosing of benzodiazepines

    ✓7ᵗʰ **T42.4X1** Poisoning by benzodiazepines, accidental (unintentional)
      Poisoning by benzodiazepines NOS

    7 ✓7ᵗʰ **T42.4X2** Poisoning by benzodiazepines, intentional self-harm   HCC

    ✓7ᵗʰ **T42.4X3** Poisoning by benzodiazepines, assault

    ✓7ᵗʰ **T42.4X4** Poisoning by benzodiazepines, undetermined

    ✓7ᵗʰ **T42.4X5** Adverse effect of benzodiazepines

    ✓7ᵗʰ **T42.4X6** Underdosing of benzodiazepines

✓5ᵗʰ **T42.5** Poisoning by, adverse effect of and underdosing of mixed antiepileptics

  ✓6ᵗʰ **T42.5X** Poisoning by, adverse effect of and underdosing of antiepileptics

    ✓7ᵗʰ **T42.5X1** Poisoning by mixed antiepileptics, accidental (unintentional)
      Poisoning by mixed antiepileptics NOS

    7 ✓7ᵗʰ **T42.5X2** Poisoning by mixed antiepileptics, intentional self-harm   HCC

    ✓7ᵗʰ **T42.5X3** Poisoning by mixed antiepileptics, assault

✓ Additional Character Required   ✓x7ᵗʰ Placeholder   Unacceptable PDx   Questionable PDx   Manifestation   H1-H14 HAC   HCC CMS-HCC Dx   HIV HIV Dx

ICD-10-CM 2019   **1109**

☑7ᵗʰ **T42.5X4 Poisoning by mixed antiepileptics,** undetermined

☑7ᵗʰ **T42.5X5** Adverse effect of mixed antiepileptics

☑7ᵗʰ **T42.5X6** Underdosing of mixed antiepileptics

☑5ᵗʰ **T42.6 Poisoning by, adverse effect of and underdosing of other antiepileptic and sedative-hypnotic drugs**
Poisoning by, adverse effect of and underdosing of methaqualone
Poisoning by, adverse effect of and underdosing of valproic acid
EXCLUDES 1 *poisoning by, adverse effect of and underdosing of carbamazepine (T42.1-)*

☑6ᵗʰ **T42.6X Poisoning by, adverse effect of and underdosing of** other antiepileptic and sedative-hypnotic **drugs**

☑7ᵗʰ **T42.6X1 Poisoning by other antiepileptic and sedative-hypnotic drugs,** accidental **(unintentional)**
Poisoning by other antiepileptic and sedative-hypnotic drugs NOS

7 ☑7ᵗʰ **T42.6X2 Poisoning by other antiepileptic and** [HCC] **sedative-hypnotic drugs,** intentional self-harm

☑7ᵗʰ **T42.6X3 Poisoning by other antiepileptic and sedative-hypnotic drugs,** assault

☑7ᵗʰ **T42.6X4 Poisoning by other antiepileptic and sedative-hypnotic drugs,** undetermined

☑7ᵗʰ **T42.6X5** Adverse effect of other antiepileptic and sedative-hypnotic drugs

☑7ᵗʰ **T42.6X6** Underdosing of other antiepileptic and sedative-hypnotic drugs

☑5ᵗʰ **T42.7 Poisoning by, adverse effect of and underdosing of** unspecified antiepileptic and sedative-hypnotic **drugs**

☑x7ᵗʰ **T42.71 Poisoning by unspecified antiepileptic and sedative-hypnotic drugs,** accidental **(unintentional)**
Poisoning by antiepileptic and sedative-hypnotic drugs NOS

7 ☑x7ᵗʰ **T42.72 Poisoning by unspecified antiepileptic and** [HCC] **sedative-hypnotic drugs,** intentional self-harm

☑x7ᵗʰ **T42.73 Poisoning by unspecified antiepileptic and sedative-hypnotic drugs,** assault

☑x7ᵗʰ **T42.74 Poisoning by unspecified antiepileptic and sedative-hypnotic drugs,** undetermined

☑x7ᵗʰ **T42.75** Adverse effect of unspecified antiepileptic and sedative-hypnotic drugs

☑x7ᵗʰ **T42.76** Underdosing of unspecified antiepileptic and sedative-hypnotic drugs

☑5ᵗʰ **T42.8 Poisoning by, adverse effect of and underdosing of antiparkinsonism drugs and other central muscle-tone depressants**
Poisoning by, adverse effect of and underdosing of amantadine

☑6ᵗʰ **T42.8X Poisoning by, adverse effect of and underdosing of** antiparkinsonism drugs and other central muscle-tone depressants

☑7ᵗʰ **T42.8X1 Poisoning by antiparkinsonism drugs and other central muscle-tone depressants,** accidental **(unintentional)**
Poisoning by antiparkinsonism drugs and other central muscle-tone depressants NOS

7 ☑7ᵗʰ **T42.8X2 Poisoning by antiparkinsonism drugs** [HCC] **and other central muscle-tone depressants,** intentional self-harm

☑7ᵗʰ **T42.8X3 Poisoning by antiparkinsonism drugs and other central muscle-tone depressants,** assault

☑7ᵗʰ **T42.8X4 Poisoning by antiparkinsonism drugs and other central muscle-tone depressants,** undetermined

☑7ᵗʰ **T42.8X5** Adverse effect of antiparkinsonism drugs and other central muscle-tone depressants

☑7ᵗʰ **T42.8X6** Underdosing of antiparkinsonism drugs and other central muscle-tone depressants

☑4ᵗʰ **T43 Poisoning by, adverse effect of and underdosing of psychotropic drugs, not elsewhere classified**
EXCLUDES 1 *appetite depressants (T50.5-)*
barbiturates (T42.3-)
benzodiazepines (T42.4-)
methaqualone (T42.6-)
psychodysleptics [hallucinogens] (T40.7-T40.9-)
EXCLUDES 2 *drug dependence and related mental and behavioral disorders due to psychoactive substance use (F10.- – F19.-)*

The appropriate 7th character is to be added to each code from category T43.
A   initial encounter
D   subsequent encounter
S   sequela

☑5ᵗʰ **T43.Ø Poisoning by, adverse effect of and underdosing of tricyclic and tetracyclic antidepressants**

☑6ᵗʰ **T43.Ø1 Poisoning by, adverse effect of and underdosing of** tricyclic antidepressants

☑7ᵗʰ **T43.Ø11 Poisoning by tricyclic antidepressants,** accidental **(unintentional)**
Poisoning by tricyclic antidepressants NOS

7 ☑7ᵗʰ **T43.Ø12 Poisoning by tricyclic** [HCC] **antidepressants,** intentional self-harm

☑7ᵗʰ **T43.Ø13 Poisoning by tricyclic antidepressants,** assault

☑7ᵗʰ **T43.Ø14 Poisoning by tricyclic antidepressants,** undetermined

☑7ᵗʰ **T43.Ø15** Adverse effect of tricyclic antidepressants

☑7ᵗʰ **T43.Ø16** Underdosing of tricyclic antidepressants

☑6ᵗʰ **T43.Ø2 Poisoning by, adverse effect of and underdosing of** tetracyclic antidepressants

☑7ᵗʰ **T43.Ø21 Poisoning by tetracyclic antidepressants,** accidental **(unintentional)**
Poisoning by tetracyclic antidepressants NOS

7 ☑7ᵗʰ **T43.Ø22 Poisoning by tetracyclic** [HCC] **antidepressants,** intentional self-harm

☑7ᵗʰ **T43.Ø23 Poisoning by tetracyclic antidepressants,** assault

☑7ᵗʰ **T43.Ø24 Poisoning by tetracyclic antidepressants,** undetermined

☑7ᵗʰ **T43.Ø25** Adverse effect of tetracyclic antidepressants

☑7ᵗʰ **T43.Ø26** Underdosing of tetracyclic antidepressants

☑5ᵗʰ **T43.1 Poisoning by, adverse effect of and underdosing of monoamine-oxidase-inhibitor antidepressants**

☑6ᵗʰ **T43.1X Poisoning by, adverse effect of and underdosing of** monoamine-oxidase-inhibitor antidepressants

☑7ᵗʰ **T43.1X1 Poisoning by monoamine-oxidase-inhibitor antidepressants,** accidental **(unintentional)**
Poisoning by monoamine-oxidase-inhibitor antidepressants NOS

7 ☑7ᵗʰ **T43.1X2 Poisoning by monoamine-oxidase-** [HCC] **inhibitor antidepressants,** intentional self-harm

☑7ᵗʰ **T43.1X3 Poisoning by monoamine-oxidase-inhibitor antidepressants,** assault

☑7ᵗʰ **T43.1X4 Poisoning by monoamine-oxidase-inhibitor antidepressants,** undetermined

☑7ᵗʰ **T43.1X5** Adverse effect of monoamine-oxidase-inhibitor antidepressants

☑7ᵗʰ **T43.1X6** Underdosing of monoamine-oxidase-inhibitor antidepressants

☑5ᵗʰ **T43.2 Poisoning by, adverse effect of and underdosing of other and unspecified antidepressants**

☑6ᵗʰ **T43.2Ø Poisoning by, adverse effect of and underdosing of** unspecified antidepressants

☑7ᵗʰ **T43.2Ø1 Poisoning by unspecified antidepressants,** accidental **(unintentional)**
Poisoning by antidepressants NOS

7 ☑7ᵗʰ **T43.2Ø2 Poisoning by unspecified** [HCC] **antidepressants,** intentional self-harm

☑7ᵗʰ **T43.2Ø3 Poisoning by unspecified antidepressants,** assault

✓7ᵗʰ **T43.204** Poisoning by unspecified antidepressants, undetermined

✓7ᵗʰ **T43.205** Adverse effect of unspecified antidepressants
     Antidepressant discontinuation syndrome

✓7ᵗʰ **T43.206** Underdosing of unspecified antidepressants

✓6ᵗʰ **T43.21** Poisoning by, adverse effect of and underdosing of selective serotonin and norepinephrine reuptake inhibitors
     Poisoning by, adverse effect of and underdosing of SSNRI antidepressants

     ✓7ᵗʰ **T43.211** Poisoning by selective serotonin and norepinephrine reuptake inhibitors, accidental (unintentional)

     7 ✓7ᵗʰ **T43.212** Poisoning by selective serotonin and norepinephrine reuptake inhibitors, intentional self-harm   HCC

     ✓7ᵗʰ **T43.213** Poisoning by selective serotonin and norepinephrine reuptake inhibitors, assault

     ✓7ᵗʰ **T43.214** Poisoning by selective serotonin and norepinephrine reuptake inhibitors, undetermined

     ✓7ᵗʰ **T43.215** Adverse effect of selective serotonin and norepinephrine reuptake inhibitors

     ✓7ᵗʰ **T43.216** Underdosing of selective serotonin and norepinephrine reuptake inhibitors

✓6ᵗʰ **T43.22** Poisoning by, adverse effect of and underdosing of selective serotonin reuptake inhibitors
     Poisoning by, adverse effect of and underdosing of SSRI antidepressants

     ✓7ᵗʰ **T43.221** Poisoning by selective serotonin reuptake inhibitors, accidental (unintentional)

     7 ✓7ᵗʰ **T43.222** Poisoning by selective serotonin reuptake inhibitors, intentional self-harm   HCC

     ✓7ᵗʰ **T43.223** Poisoning by selective serotonin reuptake inhibitors, assault

     ✓7ᵗʰ **T43.224** Poisoning by selective serotonin reuptake inhibitors, undetermined

     ✓7ᵗʰ **T43.225** Adverse effect of selective serotonin reuptake inhibitors

     ✓7ᵗʰ **T43.226** Underdosing of selective serotonin reuptake inhibitors

✓6ᵗʰ **T43.29** Poisoning by, adverse effect of and underdosing of other antidepressants

     ✓7ᵗʰ **T43.291** Poisoning by other antidepressants, accidental (unintentional)
         Poisoning by other antidepressants NOS

     7 ✓7ᵗʰ **T43.292** Poisoning by other antidepressants, intentional self-harm   HCC

     ✓7ᵗʰ **T43.293** Poisoning by other antidepressants, assault

     ✓7ᵗʰ **T43.294** Poisoning by other antidepressants, undetermined

     ✓7ᵗʰ **T43.295** Adverse effect of other antidepressants

     ✓7ᵗʰ **T43.296** Underdosing of other antidepressants

✓5ᵗʰ **T43.3** Poisoning by, adverse effect of and underdosing of phenothiazine antipsychotics and neuroleptics

   ✓6ᵗʰ **T43.3X** Poisoning by, adverse effect of and underdosing of phenothiazine antipsychotics and neuroleptics

     ✓7ᵗʰ **T43.3X1** Poisoning by phenothiazine antipsychotics and neuroleptics, accidental (unintentional)
         Poisoning by phenothiazine antipsychotics and neuroleptics NOS

     7 ✓7ᵗʰ **T43.3X2** Poisoning by phenothiazine antipsychotics and neuroleptics, intentional self-harm   HCC

     ✓7ᵗʰ **T43.3X3** Poisoning by phenothiazine antipsychotics and neuroleptics, assault

     ✓7ᵗʰ **T43.3X4** Poisoning by phenothiazine antipsychotics and neuroleptics, undetermined

     ✓7ᵗʰ **T43.3X5** Adverse effect of phenothiazine antipsychotics and neuroleptics

     ✓7ᵗʰ **T43.3X6** Underdosing of phenothiazine antipsychotics and neuroleptics

✓5ᵗʰ **T43.4** Poisoning by, adverse effect of and underdosing of butyrophenone and thiothixene neuroleptics

   ✓6ᵗʰ **T43.4X** Poisoning by, adverse effect of and underdosing of butyrophenone and thiothixene neuroleptics

     ✓7ᵗʰ **T43.4X1** Poisoning by butyrophenone and thiothixene neuroleptics, accidental (unintentional)
         Poisoning by butyrophenone and thiothixene neuroleptics NOS

     7 ✓7ᵗʰ **T43.4X2** Poisoning by butyrophenone and thiothixene neuroleptics, intentional self-harm   HCC

     ✓7ᵗʰ **T43.4X3** Poisoning by butyrophenone and thiothixene neuroleptics, assault

     ✓7ᵗʰ **T43.4X4** Poisoning by butyrophenone and thiothixene neuroleptics, undetermined

     ✓7ᵗʰ **T43.4X5** Adverse effect of butyrophenone and thiothixene neuroleptics

     ✓7ᵗʰ **T43.4X6** Underdosing of butyrophenone and thiothixene neuroleptics

✓5ᵗʰ **T43.5** Poisoning by, adverse effect of and underdosing of other and unspecified antipsychotics and neuroleptics
     EXCLUDES 1   *poisoning by, adverse effect of and underdosing of rauwolfia (T46.5-)*

   ✓6ᵗʰ **T43.50** Poisoning by, adverse effect of and underdosing of unspecified antipsychotics and neuroleptics

     ✓7ᵗʰ **T43.501** Poisoning by unspecified antipsychotics and neuroleptics, accidental (unintentional)
         Poisoning by antipsychotics and neuroleptics NOS

     7 ✓7ᵗʰ **T43.502** Poisoning by unspecified antipsychotics and neuroleptics, intentional self-harm   HCC

     ✓7ᵗʰ **T43.503** Poisoning by unspecified antipsychotics and neuroleptics, assault

     ✓7ᵗʰ **T43.504** Poisoning by unspecified antipsychotics and neuroleptics, undetermined

     ✓7ᵗʰ **T43.505** Adverse effect of unspecified antipsychotics and neuroleptics

     ✓7ᵗʰ **T43.506** Underdosing of unspecified antipsychotics and neuroleptics

   ✓6ᵗʰ **T43.59** Poisoning by, adverse effect of and underdosing of other antipsychotics and neuroleptics
     AHA: 2017, 1Q, 40

     ✓7ᵗʰ **T43.591** Poisoning by other antipsychotics and neuroleptics, accidental (unintentional)
         Poisoning by other antipsychotics and neuroleptics NOS

     7 ✓7ᵗʰ **T43.592** Poisoning by other antipsychotics and neuroleptics, intentional self-harm   HCC

     ✓7ᵗʰ **T43.593** Poisoning by other antipsychotics and neuroleptics, assault

     ✓7ᵗʰ **T43.594** Poisoning by other antipsychotics and neuroleptics, undetermined

     ✓7ᵗʰ **T43.595** Adverse effect of other antipsychotics and neuroleptics

     ✓7ᵗʰ **T43.596** Underdosing of other antipsychotics and neuroleptics

✓5ᵗʰ **T43.6** Poisoning by, adverse effect of and underdosing of psychostimulants
     EXCLUDES 1   *poisoning by, adverse effect of and underdosing of cocaine (T40.5-)*

   ✓6ᵗʰ **T43.60** Poisoning by, adverse effect of and underdosing of unspecified psychostimulant

     ✓7ᵗʰ **T43.601** Poisoning by unspecified psychostimulants, accidental (unintentional)
         Poisoning by psychostimulants NOS

     7 ✓7ᵗʰ **T43.602** Poisoning by unspecified psychostimulants, intentional self-harm   HCC

     ✓7ᵗʰ **T43.603** Poisoning by unspecified psychostimulants, assault

     ✓7ᵗʰ **T43.604** Poisoning by unspecified psychostimulants, undetermined

---

✓ Additional Character Required   ✓7ᵗʰ Placeholder   Unacceptable PDx   Questionable PDx   Manifestation   **H1**-**H14** HAC   **HCC** CMS-HCC Dx   **HIV** HIV Dx

√7ᵗʰ **T43.605** Adverse effect of unspecified psychostimulants

√7ᵗʰ **T43.606** Underdosing of unspecified psychostimulants

√6ᵗʰ **T43.61** Poisoning by, adverse effect of and underdosing of caffeine

√7ᵗʰ **T43.611** Poisoning by caffeine, accidental (unintentional)
Poisoning by caffeine NOS

7 √7ᵗʰ **T43.612** Poisoning by caffeine, intentional self-harm   **HCC**

√7ᵗʰ **T43.613** Poisoning by caffeine, assault

√7ᵗʰ **T43.614** Poisoning by caffeine, undetermined

√7ᵗʰ **T43.615** Adverse effect of caffeine

√7ᵗʰ **T43.616** Underdosing of caffeine

√6ᵗʰ **T43.62** Poisoning by, adverse effect of and underdosing of amphetamines
Poisoning by, adverse effect of and underdosing of methamphetamines

√7ᵗʰ **T43.621** Poisoning by amphetamines, accidental (unintentional)
Poisoning by amphetamines NOS

7 √7ᵗʰ **T43.622** Poisoning by amphetamines, intentional self-harm   **HCC**

√7ᵗʰ **T43.623** Poisoning by amphetamines, assault

√7ᵗʰ **T43.624** Poisoning by amphetamines, undetermined

√7ᵗʰ **T43.625** Adverse effect of amphetamines

√7ᵗʰ **T43.626** Underdosing of amphetamines

√6ᵗʰ **T43.63** Poisoning by, adverse effect of and underdosing of methylphenidate

√7ᵗʰ **T43.631** Poisoning by methylphenidate, accidental (unintentional)
Poisoning by methylphenidate NOS

7 √7ᵗʰ **T43.632** Poisoning by methylphenidate, intentional self-harm   **HCC**

√7ᵗʰ **T43.633** Poisoning by methylphenidate, assault

√7ᵗʰ **T43.634** Poisoning by methylphenidate, undetermined

√7ᵗʰ **T43.635** Adverse effect of methylphenidate

√7ᵗʰ **T43.636** Underdosing of methylphenidate

● √6ᵗʰ **T43.64** Poisoning by ecstasy
Poisoning by MDMA
Poisoning by 3,4-methylenedioxymethamphetamine

● √7ᵗʰ **T43.641** Poisoning by ecstasy, accidental (unintentional)
Poisoning by ecstasy NOS

● √7ᵗʰ **T43.642** Poisoning by ecstasy, intentional self-harm

● √7ᵗʰ **T43.643** Poisoning by ecstasy, assault

● √7ᵗʰ **T43.644** Poisoning by ecstasy, undetermined

√6ᵗʰ **T43.69** Poisoning by, adverse effect of and underdosing of other psychostimulants

√7ᵗʰ **T43.691** Poisoning by other psychostimulants, accidental (unintentional)
Poisoning by other psychostimulants NOS

7 √7ᵗʰ **T43.692** Poisoning by other psychostimulants, intentional self-harm   **HCC**

√7ᵗʰ **T43.693** Poisoning by other psychostimulants, assault

√7ᵗʰ **T43.694** Poisoning by other psychostimulants, undetermined

√7ᵗʰ **T43.695** Adverse effect of other psychostimulants

√7ᵗʰ **T43.696** Underdosing of other psychostimulants

√5ᵗʰ **T43.8** Poisoning by, adverse effect of and underdosing of other psychotropic drugs

√6ᵗʰ **T43.8X** Poisoning by, adverse effect of and underdosing of other psychotropic drugs

√7ᵗʰ **T43.8X1** Poisoning by other psychotropic drugs, accidental (unintentional)
Poisoning by other psychotropic drugs NOS

7 √7ᵗʰ **T43.8X2** Poisoning by other psychotropic drugs, intentional self-harm   **HCC**

√7ᵗʰ **T43.8X3** Poisoning by other psychotropic drugs, assault

√7ᵗʰ **T43.8X4** Poisoning by other psychotropic drugs, undetermined

√7ᵗʰ **T43.8X5** Adverse effect of other psychotropic drugs

√7ᵗʰ **T43.8X6** Underdosing of other psychotropic drugs

√5ᵗʰ **T43.9** Poisoning by, adverse effect of and underdosing of unspecified psychotropic drug

√x7ᵗʰ **T43.91** Poisoning by unspecified psychotropic drug, accidental (unintentional)
Poisoning by psychotropic drug NOS

7 √x7ᵗʰ **T43.92** Poisoning by unspecified psychotropic drug, intentional self-harm   **HCC**

√x7ᵗʰ **T43.93** Poisoning by unspecified psychotropic drug, assault

√x7ᵗʰ **T43.94** Poisoning by unspecified psychotropic drug, undetermined

√x7ᵗʰ **T43.95** Adverse effect of unspecified psychotropic drug

√x7ᵗʰ **T43.96** Underdosing of unspecified psychotropic drug

√4ᵗʰ **T44** Poisoning by, adverse effect of and underdosing of drugs primarily affecting the autonomic nervous system

> The appropriate 7th character is to be added to each code from category T44.
> A   initial encounter
> D   subsequent encounter
> S   sequela

√5ᵗʰ **T44.0** Poisoning by, adverse effect of and underdosing of anticholinesterase agents

√6ᵗʰ **T44.0X** Poisoning by, adverse effect of and underdosing of anticholinesterase agents

√7ᵗʰ **T44.0X1** Poisoning by anticholinesterase agents, accidental (unintentional)
Poisoning by anticholinesterase agents NOS

7 √7ᵗʰ **T44.0X2** Poisoning by anticholinesterase agents, intentional self-harm   **HCC**

√7ᵗʰ **T44.0X3** Poisoning by anticholinesterase agents, assault

√7ᵗʰ **T44.0X4** Poisoning by anticholinesterase agents, undetermined

√7ᵗʰ **T44.0X5** Adverse effect of anticholinesterase agents

√7ᵗʰ **T44.0X6** Underdosing of anticholinesterase agents

√5ᵗʰ **T44.1** Poisoning by, adverse effect of and underdosing of other parasympathomimetics [cholinergics]

√6ᵗʰ **T44.1X** Poisoning by, adverse effect of and underdosing of other parasympathomimetics [cholinergics]

√7ᵗʰ **T44.1X1** Poisoning by other parasympathomimetics [cholinergics], accidental (unintentional)
Poisoning by other parasympathomimetics [cholinergics] NOS

7 √7ᵗʰ **T44.1X2** Poisoning by other parasympathomimetics [cholinergics], intentional self-harm   **HCC**

√7ᵗʰ **T44.1X3** Poisoning by other parasympathomimetics [cholinergics], assault

√7ᵗʰ **T44.1X4** Poisoning by other parasympathomimetics [cholinergics], undetermined

√7ᵗʰ **T44.1X5** Adverse effect of other parasympathomimetics [cholinergics]

√7ᵗʰ **T44.1X6** Underdosing of other parasympathomimetics

√5ᵗʰ **T44.2** Poisoning by, adverse effect of and underdosing of ganglionic blocking drugs

√6ᵗʰ **T44.2X** Poisoning by, adverse effect of and underdosing of ganglionic blocking drugs

√7ᵗʰ **T44.2X1** Poisoning by ganglionic blocking drugs, accidental (unintentional)
Poisoning by ganglionic blocking drugs NOS

7 √7ᵗʰ **T44.2X2** Poisoning by ganglionic blocking drugs, intentional self-harm   **HCC**

√7ᵗʰ **T44.2X3** Poisoning by ganglionic blocking drugs, assault

N Newborn: 0   P Pediatric: 0-17   M Maternity: 12-55   A Adult: 15-124   **MCC** Major Complication/Comorbidity   **CC** Complication/Comorbidity   **SW** Severe Wound Dx

1112   ICD-10-CM 2019

√7th **T44.2X4** **Poisoning by ganglionic blocking drugs,** undetermined

√7th **T44.2X5** Adverse effect **of ganglionic blocking drugs**

√7th **T44.2X6** Underdosing **of ganglionic blocking drugs**

√5th **T44.3** **Poisoning by, adverse effect of and underdosing of other parasympatholytics [anticholinergics and antimuscarinics] and spasmolytics**
Poisoning by, adverse effect of and underdosing of papaverine

√6th **T44.3X** **Poisoning by, adverse effect of and underdosing of** other parasympatholytics [anticholinergics and antimuscarinics] and spasmolytics

√7th **T44.3X1** **Poisoning by other parasympatholytics [anticholinergics and antimuscarinics] and spasmolytics,** accidental (unintentional)
Poisoning by other parasympatholytics [anticholinergics and antimuscarinics] and spasmolytics NOS

7 √7th **T44.3X2** **Poisoning by other parasympatholytics [anticholinergics and antimuscarinics] and spasmolytics,** intentional self-harm   HCC

√7th **T44.3X3** **Poisoning by other parasympatholytics [anticholinergics and antimuscarinics] and spasmolytics,** assault

√7th **T44.3X4** **Poisoning by other parasympatholytics [anticholinergics and antimuscarinics] and spasmolytics,** undetermined

√7th **T44.3X5** Adverse effect **of other parasympatholytics [anticholinergics and antimuscarinics] and spasmolytics**

√7th **T44.3X6** Underdosing **of other parasympatholytics [anticholinergics and antimuscarinics] and spasmolytics**

√5th **T44.4** **Poisoning by, adverse effect of and underdosing of predominantly alpha-adrenoreceptor agonists**
Poisoning by, adverse effect of and underdosing of metaraminol

√6th **T44.4X** **Poisoning by, adverse effect of and underdosing of** predominantly alpha-adrenoreceptor agonists

√7th **T44.4X1** **Poisoning by predominantly alpha-adrenoreceptor agonists,** accidental (unintentional)
Poisoning by predominantly alpha-adrenoreceptor agonists NOS

7 √7th **T44.4X2** **Poisoning by predominantly alpha-adrenoreceptor agonists,** intentional self-harm   HCC

√7th **T44.4X3** **Poisoning by predominantly alpha-adrenoreceptor agonists,** assault

√7th **T44.4X4** **Poisoning by predominantly alpha-adrenoreceptor agonists,** undetermined

√7th **T44.4X5** Adverse effect **of predominantly alpha-adrenoreceptor agonists**

√7th **T44.4X6** Underdosing **of predominantly alpha-adrenoreceptor agonists**

√5th **T44.5** **Poisoning by, adverse effect of and underdosing of predominantly beta-adrenoreceptor agonists**
EXCLUDES 1   poisoning by, adverse effect of and underdosing of beta-adrenoreceptor agonists used in asthma therapy (T48.6-)

√6th **T44.5X** **Poisoning by, adverse effect of and underdosing of** predominantly beta-adrenoreceptor agonists

√7th **T44.5X1** **Poisoning by predominantly beta-adrenoreceptor agonists,** accidental (unintentional)
Poisoning by predominantly beta-adrenoreceptor agonists NOS

7 √7th **T44.5X2** **Poisoning by predominantly beta-adrenoreceptor agonists,** intentional self-harm   HCC

√7th **T44.5X3** **Poisoning by predominantly beta-adrenoreceptor agonists,** assault

√7th **T44.5X4** **Poisoning by predominantly beta-adrenoreceptor agonists,** undetermined

√7th **T44.5X5** Adverse effect **of predominantly beta-adrenoreceptor agonists**

√7th **T44.5X6** Underdosing **of predominantly beta-adrenoreceptor agonists**

√5th **T44.6** **Poisoning by, adverse effect of and underdosing of alpha-adrenoreceptor antagonists**
EXCLUDES 1   poisoning by, adverse effect of and underdosing of ergot alkaloids (T48.0)

√6th **T44.6X** **Poisoning by, adverse effect of and underdosing of** alpha-adrenoreceptor antagonists

√7th **T44.6X1** **Poisoning by alpha-adrenoreceptor antagonists,** accidental (unintentional)
Poisoning by alpha-adrenoreceptor antagonists NOS

7 √7th **T44.6X2** **Poisoning by alpha-adrenoreceptor antagonists,** intentional self-harm   HCC

√7th **T44.6X3** **Poisoning by alpha-adrenoreceptor antagonists,** assault

√7th **T44.6X4** **Poisoning by alpha-adrenoreceptor antagonists,** undetermined

√7th **T44.6X5** Adverse effect **of alpha-adrenoreceptor antagonists**

√7th **T44.6X6** Underdosing **of alpha-adrenoreceptor antagonists**

√5th **T44.7** **Poisoning by, adverse effect of and underdosing of beta-adrenoreceptor antagonists**

√6th **T44.7X** **Poisoning by, adverse effect of and underdosing of** beta-adrenoreceptor antagonists

√7th **T44.7X1** **Poisoning by beta-adrenoreceptor antagonists,** accidental (unintentional)
Poisoning by beta-adrenoreceptor antagonists NOS

7 √7th **T44.7X2** **Poisoning by beta-adrenoreceptor antagonists,** intentional self-harm   HCC

√7th **T44.7X3** **Poisoning by beta-adrenoreceptor antagonists,** assault

√7th **T44.7X4** **Poisoning by beta-adrenoreceptor antagonists,** undetermined

√7th **T44.7X5** Adverse effect **of beta-adrenoreceptor antagonists**

√7th **T44.7X6** Underdosing **of beta-adrenoreceptor antagonists**

√5th **T44.8** **Poisoning by, adverse effect of and underdosing of centrally-acting and adrenergic-neuron- blocking agents**
EXCLUDES 1   poisoning by, adverse effect of and underdosing of clonidine (T46.5)
poisoning by, adverse effect of and underdosing of guanethidine (T46.5)

√6th **T44.8X** **Poisoning by, adverse effect of and underdosing of** centrally-acting and adrenergic-neuron-blocking agents

√7th **T44.8X1** **Poisoning by centrally-acting and adrenergic-neuron-blocking agents,** accidental (unintentional)
Poisoning by centrally-acting and adrenergic-neuron-blocking agents NOS

7 √7th **T44.8X2** **Poisoning by centrally-acting and adrenergic-neuron-blocking agents,** intentional self-harm   HCC

√7th **T44.8X3** **Poisoning by centrally-acting and adrenergic-neuron-blocking agents,** assault

√7th **T44.8X4** **Poisoning by centrally-acting and adrenergic-neuron-blocking agents,** undetermined

√7th **T44.8X5** Adverse effect **of centrally-acting and adrenergic-neuron-blocking agents**

√7th **T44.8X6** Underdosing **of centrally-acting and adrenergic-neuron-blocking agents**

✓5ᵗʰ **T44.9** **Poisoning by, adverse effect of and underdosing of other and unspecified drugs** primarily affecting the autonomic nervous system

Poisoning by, adverse effect of and underdosing of drug stimulating both alpha and beta-adrenoreceptors

✓6ᵗʰ **T44.90** **Poisoning by, adverse effect of and underdosing of** unspecified **drugs primarily affecting the autonomic nervous system**

✓7ᵗʰ **T44.901** **Poisoning by unspecified drugs primarily affecting the autonomic nervous system,** accidental **(unintentional)**

Poisoning by unspecified drugs primarily affecting the autonomic nervous system NOS

7 ✓7ᵗʰ **T44.902** **Poisoning by unspecified drugs** HCC **primarily affecting the autonomic nervous system,** intentional self-harm

✓7ᵗʰ **T44.903** **Poisoning by unspecified drugs primarily affecting the autonomic nervous system,** assault

✓7ᵗʰ **T44.904** **Poisoning by unspecified drugs primarily affecting the autonomic nervous system,** undetermined

✓7ᵗʰ **T44.905** Adverse effect **of unspecified drugs primarily affecting the autonomic nervous system**

✓7ᵗʰ **T44.906** Underdosing **of unspecified drugs primarily affecting the autonomic nervous system**

✓6ᵗʰ **T44.99** **Poisoning by, adverse effect of and underdosing of** other **drugs primarily affecting the autonomic nervous system**

✓7ᵗʰ **T44.991** **Poisoning by other drug primarily affecting the autonomic nervous system,** accidental **(unintentional)**

Poisoning by other drugs primarily affecting the autonomic nervous system NOS

7 ✓7ᵗʰ **T44.992** **Poisoning by other drug primarily** HCC **affecting the autonomic nervous system,** intentional self-harm

✓7ᵗʰ **T44.993** **Poisoning by other drug primarily affecting the autonomic nervous system,** assault

✓7ᵗʰ **T44.994** **Poisoning by other drug primarily affecting the autonomic nervous system,** undetermined

✓7ᵗʰ **T44.995** Adverse effect **of other drug primarily affecting the autonomic nervous system**

✓7ᵗʰ **T44.996** Underdosing **of other drug primarily affecting the autonomic nervous system**

✓4ᵗʰ **T45** **Poisoning by, adverse effect of and underdosing of primarily systemic and hematological agents, not elsewhere classified**

The appropriate 7th character is to be added to each code from category T45.
A   initial encounter
D   subsequent encounter
S   sequela

✓5ᵗʰ **T45.0** **Poisoning by, adverse effect of and underdosing of antiallergic and antiemetic drugs**

EXCLUDES 1   poisoning by, adverse effect of and underdosing of phenothiazine-based neuroleptics (T43.3)

✓6ᵗʰ **T45.0X** **Poisoning by, adverse effect of and underdosing of** antiallergic and antiemetic **drugs**

✓7ᵗʰ **T45.0X1** **Poisoning by antiallergic and antiemetic drugs,** accidental **(unintentional)**

Poisoning by antiallergic and antiemetic drugs NOS

7 ✓7ᵗʰ **T45.0X2** **Poisoning by antiallergic and** HCC **antiemetic drugs,** intentional self-harm

✓7ᵗʰ **T45.0X3** **Poisoning by antiallergic and antiemetic drugs,** assault

✓7ᵗʰ **T45.0X4** **Poisoning by antiallergic and antiemetic drugs,** undetermined

✓7ᵗʰ **T45.0X5** Adverse effect **of antiallergic and antiemetic drugs**

✓7ᵗʰ **T45.0X6** Underdosing **of antiallergic and antiemetic drugs**

✓5ᵗʰ **T45.1** **Poisoning by, adverse effect of and underdosing of antineoplastic and immunosuppressive drugs**

EXCLUDES 1   poisoning by, adverse effect of and underdosing of tamoxifen (T38.6)

AHA: 2014, 4Q, 22

✓6ᵗʰ **T45.1X** **Poisoning by, adverse effect of and underdosing of** antineoplastic and immunosuppressive **drugs**

✓7ᵗʰ **T45.1X1** **Poisoning by antineoplastic and immunosuppressive drugs,** accidental **(unintentional)**

Poisoning by antineoplastic and immunosuppressive drugs NOS

7 ✓7ᵗʰ **T45.1X2** **Poisoning by antineoplastic and** HCC **immunosuppressive drugs,** intentional self-harm

✓7ᵗʰ **T45.1X3** **Poisoning by antineoplastic and immunosuppressive drugs,** assault

✓7ᵗʰ **T45.1X4** **Poisoning by antineoplastic and immunosuppressive drugs,** undetermined

✓7ᵗʰ **T45.1X5** Adverse effect **of antineoplastic and immunosuppressive drugs**

✓7ᵗʰ **T45.1X6** Underdosing **of antineoplastic and immunosuppressive drugs**

✓5ᵗʰ **T45.2** **Poisoning by, adverse effect of and underdosing of vitamins**

EXCLUDES 2   poisoning by, adverse effect of and underdosing of iron (T45.4)
poisoning by, adverse effect of and underdosing of nicotinic acid (derivatives) (T46.7)
poisoning by, adverse effect of and underdosing of vitamin K (T45.7)

✓6ᵗʰ **T45.2X** **Poisoning by, adverse effect of and underdosing of** vitamins

✓7ᵗʰ **T45.2X1** **Poisoning by vitamins,** accidental **(unintentional)**

Poisoning by vitamins NOS

7 ✓7ᵗʰ **T45.2X2** **Poisoning by vitamins,** intentional HCC self-harm

✓7ᵗʰ **T45.2X3** **Poisoning by vitamins,** assault

✓7ᵗʰ **T45.2X4** **Poisoning by vitamins,** undetermined

✓7ᵗʰ **T45.2X5** Adverse effect **of vitamins**

✓7ᵗʰ **T45.2X6** Underdosing **of vitamins**

EXCLUDES 1   vitamin deficiencies (E50-E56)

✓5ᵗʰ **T45.3** **Poisoning by, adverse effect of and underdosing of enzymes**

✓6ᵗʰ **T45.3X** **Poisoning by, adverse effect of and underdosing of** enzymes

✓7ᵗʰ **T45.3X1** **Poisoning by enzymes,** accidental **(unintentional)**

Poisoning by enzymes NOS

7 ✓7ᵗʰ **T45.3X2** **Poisoning by enzymes,** intentional HCC self-harm

✓7ᵗʰ **T45.3X3** **Poisoning by enzymes,** assault

✓7ᵗʰ **T45.3X4** **Poisoning by enzymes,** undetermined

✓7ᵗʰ **T45.3X5** Adverse effect **of enzymes**

✓7ᵗʰ **T45.3X6** Underdosing **of enzymes**

✓5ᵗʰ **T45.4** **Poisoning by, adverse effect of and underdosing of iron and its compounds**

✓6ᵗʰ **T45.4X** **Poisoning by, adverse effect of and underdosing of** iron and its compounds

✓7ᵗʰ **T45.4X1** **Poisoning by iron and its compounds,** accidental **(unintentional)**

Poisoning by iron and its compounds NOS

7 ✓7ᵗʰ **T45.4X2** **Poisoning by iron and its compounds,** HCC intentional self-harm

✓7ᵗʰ **T45.4X3** **Poisoning by iron and its compounds,** assault

✓7ᵗʰ **T45.4X4** **Poisoning by iron and its compounds,** undetermined

✓7ᵗʰ **T45.4X5** Adverse effect **of iron and its compounds**

✓7ᵗʰ **T45.4X6** Underdosing **of iron and its compounds**

EXCLUDES 1   iron deficiency (E61.1)

N Newborn: 0   P Pediatric: 0-17   M Maternity: 12-55   A Adult: 15-124   MCC Major Complication/Comorbidity   CC Complication/Comorbidity   SW Severe Wound Dx

1114   ICD-10-CM 2019

☑5ᵗʰ **T45.5** **Poisoning by, adverse effect of and underdosing of anticoagulants and antithrombotic drugs**

☑6ᵗʰ **T45.51** **Poisoning by, adverse effect of and underdosing of anticoagulants**

☑7ᵗʰ **T45.511** **Poisoning by anticoagulants, accidental (unintentional)**
Poisoning by anticoagulants NOS

7 ☑7ᵗʰ **T45.512** **Poisoning by anticoagulants, intentional self-harm** HCC

☑7ᵗʰ **T45.513** **Poisoning by anticoagulants, assault**

☑7ᵗʰ **T45.514** **Poisoning by anticoagulants, undetermined**

☑7ᵗʰ **T45.515** **Adverse effect of anticoagulants**
AHA: 2016, 1Q, 14; 2013, 2Q, 34

☑7ᵗʰ **T45.516** **Underdosing of anticoagulants**

☑6ᵗʰ **T45.52** **Poisoning by, adverse effect of and underdosing of antithrombotic drugs**
Poisoning by, adverse effect of and underdosing of antiplatelet drugs
EXCLUDES 2　*poisoning by, adverse effect of and underdosing of aspirin (T39.Ø1-)*
poisoning by, adverse effect of and underdosing of acetylsalicylic acid (T39.Ø1-)

☑7ᵗʰ **T45.521** **Poisoning by antithrombotic drugs, accidental (unintentional)**
Poisoning by antithrombotic drug NOS

7 ☑7ᵗʰ **T45.522** **Poisoning by antithrombotic drugs, intentional self-harm** HCC

☑7ᵗʰ **T45.523** **Poisoning by antithrombotic drugs, assault**

☑7ᵗʰ **T45.524** **Poisoning by antithrombotic drugs, undetermined**

☑7ᵗʰ **T45.525** **Adverse effect of antithrombotic drugs**
AHA: 2016, 1Q, 15

☑7ᵗʰ **T45.526** **Underdosing of antithrombotic drugs**

☑5ᵗʰ **T45.6** **Poisoning by, adverse effect of and underdosing of fibrinolysis-affecting drugs**

☑6ᵗʰ **T45.6Ø** **Poisoning by, adverse effect of and underdosing of unspecified fibrinolysis-affecting drugs**

☑7ᵗʰ **T45.6Ø1** **Poisoning by unspecified fibrinolysis-affecting drugs, accidental (unintentional)**
Poisoning by fibrinolysis-affecting drug NOS

7 ☑7ᵗʰ **T45.6Ø2** **Poisoning by unspecified fibrinolysis-affecting drugs, intentional self-harm** HCC

☑7ᵗʰ **T45.6Ø3** **Poisoning by unspecified fibrinolysis-affecting drugs, assault**

☑7ᵗʰ **T45.6Ø4** **Poisoning by unspecified fibrinolysis-affecting drugs, undetermined**

☑7ᵗʰ **T45.6Ø5** **Adverse effect of unspecified fibrinolysis-affecting drugs**

☑7ᵗʰ **T45.6Ø6** **Underdosing of unspecified fibrinolysis-affecting drugs**

☑6ᵗʰ **T45.61** **Poisoning by, adverse effect of and underdosing of thrombolytic drugs**

☑7ᵗʰ **T45.611** **Poisoning by thrombolytic drug, accidental (unintentional)**
Poisoning by thrombolytic drug NOS

7 ☑7ᵗʰ **T45.612** **Poisoning by thrombolytic drug, intentional self-harm** HCC

☑7ᵗʰ **T45.613** **Poisoning by thrombolytic drug, assault**

☑7ᵗʰ **T45.614** **Poisoning by thrombolytic drug, undetermined**

☑7ᵗʰ **T45.615** **Adverse effect of thrombolytic drugs**
AHA: 2017, 2Q, 9

☑7ᵗʰ **T45.616** **Underdosing of thrombolytic drugs**

☑6ᵗʰ **T45.62** **Poisoning by, adverse effect of and underdosing of hemostatic drugs**

☑7ᵗʰ **T45.621** **Poisoning by hemostatic drug, accidental (unintentional)**
Poisoning by hemostatic drug NOS

7 ☑7ᵗʰ **T45.622** **Poisoning by hemostatic drug, intentional self-harm** HCC

☑7ᵗʰ **T45.623** **Poisoning by hemostatic drug, assault**

☑7ᵗʰ **T45.624** **Poisoning by hemostatic drug, undetermined**

☑7ᵗʰ **T45.625** **Adverse effect of hemostatic drug**

☑7ᵗʰ **T45.626** **Underdosing of hemostatic drugs**

☑6ᵗʰ **T45.69** **Poisoning by, adverse effect of and underdosing of other fibrinolysis-affecting drugs**

☑7ᵗʰ **T45.691** **Poisoning by other fibrinolysis-affecting drugs, accidental (unintentional)**
Poisoning by other fibrinolysis-affecting drug NOS

7 ☑7ᵗʰ **T45.692** **Poisoning by other fibrinolysis-affecting drugs, intentional self-harm** HCC

☑7ᵗʰ **T45.693** **Poisoning by other fibrinolysis-affecting drugs, assault**

☑7ᵗʰ **T45.694** **Poisoning by other fibrinolysis-affecting drugs, undetermined**

☑7ᵗʰ **T45.695** **Adverse effect of other fibrinolysis-affecting drugs**

☑7ᵗʰ **T45.696** **Underdosing of other fibrinolysis-affecting drugs**

☑5ᵗʰ **T45.7** **Poisoning by, adverse effect of and underdosing of anticoagulant antagonists, vitamin K and other coagulants**

☑6ᵗʰ **T45.7X** **Poisoning by, adverse effect of and underdosing of anticoagulant antagonists, vitamin K and other coagulants**

☑7ᵗʰ **T45.7X1** **Poisoning by anticoagulant antagonists, vitamin K and other coagulants, accidental (unintentional)**
Poisoning by anticoagulant antagonists, vitamin K and other coagulants NOS

7 ☑7ᵗʰ **T45.7X2** **Poisoning by anticoagulant antagonists, vitamin K and other coagulants, intentional self-harm** HCC

☑7ᵗʰ **T45.7X3** **Poisoning by anticoagulant antagonists, vitamin K and other coagulants, assault**

☑7ᵗʰ **T45.7X4** **Poisoning by anticoagulant antagonists, vitamin K and other coagulants, undetermined**

☑7ᵗʰ **T45.7X5** **Adverse effect of anticoagulant antagonists, vitamin K and other coagulants**

☑7ᵗʰ **T45.7X6** **Underdosing of anticoagulant antagonist, vitamin K and other coagulants**
EXCLUDES 1　*vitamin K deficiency (E56.1)*

☑5ᵗʰ **T45.8** **Poisoning by, adverse effect of and underdosing of other primarily systemic and hematological agents**
Poisoning by, adverse effect of and underdosing of liver preparations and other antianemic agents
Poisoning by, adverse effect of and underdosing of natural blood and blood products
Poisoning by, adverse effect of and underdosing of plasma substitute
EXCLUDES 2　*poisoning by, adverse effect of and underdosing of immunoglobulin (T5Ø.Z1)*
poisoning by, adverse effect of and underdosing of iron (T45.4)
transfusion reactions (T8Ø.-)

☑6ᵗʰ **T45.8X** **Poisoning by, adverse effect of and underdosing of other primarily systemic and hematological agents**

☑7ᵗʰ **T45.8X1** **Poisoning by other primarily systemic and hematological agents, accidental (unintentional)**
Poisoning by other primarily systemic and hematological agents NOS

7 ☑7ᵗʰ **T45.8X2** **Poisoning by other primarily systemic and hematological agents, intentional self-harm** HCC

☑7ᵗʰ **T45.8X3** **Poisoning by other primarily systemic and hematological agents, assault**

☑7ᵗʰ **T45.8X4** **Poisoning by other primarily systemic and hematological agents, undetermined**

☑7ᵗʰ **T45.8X5** **Adverse effect of other primarily systemic and hematological agents**
AHA: 2016, 4Q, 42

☑7ᵗʰ **T45.8X6** **Underdosing of other primarily systemic and hematological agents**

✔ Additional Character Required　　✔x7ᵗʰ Placeholder　　Unacceptable PDx　　Questionable PDx　　Manifestation　　H1 - H14 HAC　　HCC CMS-HCC Dx　　HIV HIV Dx

ICD-10-CM 2019　　**1115**

✓5ᵗʰ **T45.9** **Poisoning by, adverse effect of and underdosing of** unspecified **primarily systemic and hematological agent**

     ✓x7ᵗʰ **T45.91** **Poisoning by unspecified primarily systemic and hematological agent,** accidental **(unintentional)**
         Poisoning by primarily systemic and hematological agent NOS

     7 ✓x7ᵗʰ **T45.92** **Poisoning by unspecified primarily systemic and hematological agent,** intentional self-harm   HCC

     ✓x7ᵗʰ **T45.93** **Poisoning by unspecified primarily systemic and hematological agent,** assault

     ✓x7ᵗʰ **T45.94** **Poisoning by unspecified primarily systemic and hematological agent,** undetermined

     ✓x7ᵗʰ **T45.95** Adverse effect **of unspecified primarily systemic and hematological agent**

     ✓x7ᵗʰ **T45.96** Underdosing **of unspecified primarily systemic and hematological agent**

✓4ᵗʰ **T46** **Poisoning by, adverse effect of and underdosing of agents primarily affecting the cardiovascular system**
     EXCLUDES 1   *poisoning by, adverse effect of and underdosing of metaraminol (T44.4)*

The appropriate 7th character is to be added to each code from category T46.
A   initial encounter
D   subsequent encounter
S   sequela

✓5ᵗʰ **T46.0** **Poisoning by, adverse effect of and underdosing of cardiac-stimulant glycosides and drugs of similar action**

     ✓6ᵗʰ **T46.0X** **Poisoning by, adverse effect of and underdosing of** cardiac-stimulant glycosides **and drugs of similar action**

         ✓7ᵗʰ **T46.0X1** **Poisoning by cardiac-stimulant glycosides and drugs of similar action,** accidental **(unintentional)**
             Poisoning by cardiac-stimulant glycosides and drugs of similar action NOS

         7 ✓7ᵗʰ **T46.0X2** **Poisoning by cardiac-stimulant glycosides and drugs of similar action,** intentional self-harm   HCC

         ✓7ᵗʰ **T46.0X3** **Poisoning by cardiac-stimulant glycosides and drugs of similar action,** assault

         ✓7ᵗʰ **T46.0X4** **Poisoning by cardiac-stimulant glycosides and drugs of similar action,** undetermined

         ✓7ᵗʰ **T46.0X5** Adverse effect **of cardiac-stimulant glycosides and drugs of similar action**

         ✓7ᵗʰ **T46.0X6** Underdosing **of cardiac-stimulant glycosides and drugs of similar action**

✓5ᵗʰ **T46.1** **Poisoning by, adverse effect of and underdosing of calcium-channel blockers**

     ✓6ᵗʰ **T46.1X** **Poisoning by, adverse effect of and underdosing of** calcium-channel blockers

         ✓7ᵗʰ **T46.1X1** **Poisoning by calcium-channel blockers,** accidental **(unintentional)**
             Poisoning by calcium-channel blockers NOS

         7 ✓7ᵗʰ **T46.1X2** **Poisoning by calcium-channel blockers,** intentional self-harm   HCC

         ✓7ᵗʰ **T46.1X3** **Poisoning by calcium-channel blockers,** assault

         ✓7ᵗʰ **T46.1X4** **Poisoning by calcium-channel blockers,** undetermined

         ✓7ᵗʰ **T46.1X5** Adverse effect **of calcium-channel blockers**

         ✓7ᵗʰ **T46.1X6** Underdosing **of calcium-channel blockers**

✓5ᵗʰ **T46.2** **Poisoning by, adverse effect of and underdosing of other antidysrhythmic drugs, not elsewhere classified**
     EXCLUDES 1   *poisoning by, adverse effect of and underdosing of beta-adrenoreceptor antagonists (T44.7-)*

     ✓6ᵗʰ **T46.2X** **Poisoning by, adverse effect of and underdosing of** other antidysrhythmic **drugs**

         ✓7ᵗʰ **T46.2X1** **Poisoning by other antidysrhythmic drugs,** accidental **(unintentional)**
             Poisoning by other antidysrhythmic drugs NOS

         7 ✓7ᵗʰ **T46.2X2** **Poisoning by other antidysrhythmic drugs,** intentional self-harm   HCC

         ✓7ᵗʰ **T46.2X3** **Poisoning by other antidysrhythmic drugs,** assault

         ✓7ᵗʰ **T46.2X4** **Poisoning by other antidysrhythmic drugs,** undetermined

         ✓7ᵗʰ **T46.2X5** Adverse effect **of other antidysrhythmic drugs**

         ✓7ᵗʰ **T46.2X6** Underdosing **of other antidysrhythmic drugs**

✓5ᵗʰ **T46.3** **Poisoning by, adverse effect of and underdosing of coronary vasodilators**
     Poisoning by, adverse effect of and underdosing of dipyridamole
     EXCLUDES 1   *poisoning by, adverse effect of and underdosing of calcium-channel blockers (T46.1)*

     ✓6ᵗʰ **T46.3X** **Poisoning by, adverse effect of and underdosing of** coronary vasodilators

         ✓7ᵗʰ **T46.3X1** **Poisoning by coronary vasodilators,** accidental **(unintentional)**
             Poisoning by coronary vasodilators NOS

         7 ✓7ᵗʰ **T46.3X2** **Poisoning by coronary vasodilators,** intentional self-harm   HCC

         ✓7ᵗʰ **T46.3X3** **Poisoning by coronary vasodilators,** assault

         ✓7ᵗʰ **T46.3X4** **Poisoning by coronary vasodilators,** undetermined

         ✓7ᵗʰ **T46.3X5** Adverse effect **of coronary vasodilators**

         ✓7ᵗʰ **T46.3X6** Underdosing **of coronary vasodilators**

✓5ᵗʰ **T46.4** **Poisoning by, adverse effect of and underdosing of angiotensin-converting-enzyme inhibitors**

     ✓6ᵗʰ **T46.4X** **Poisoning by, adverse effect of and underdosing of** angiotensin-converting-enzyme inhibitors

         ✓7ᵗʰ **T46.4X1** **Poisoning by angiotensin-converting-enzyme inhibitors,** accidental **(unintentional)**
             Poisoning by angiotensin-converting-enzyme inhibitors NOS

         7 ✓7ᵗʰ **T46.4X2** **Poisoning by angiotensin-converting-enzyme inhibitors,** intentional self-harm   HCC

         ✓7ᵗʰ **T46.4X3** **Poisoning by angiotensin-converting-enzyme inhibitors,** assault

         ✓7ᵗʰ **T46.4X4** **Poisoning by angiotensin-converting-enzyme inhibitors,** undetermined

         ✓7ᵗʰ **T46.4X5** Adverse effect **of angiotensin-converting-enzyme inhibitors**

         ✓7ᵗʰ **T46.4X6** Underdosing **of angiotensin-converting-enzyme inhibitors**

✓5ᵗʰ **T46.5** **Poisoning by, adverse effect of and underdosing of other antihypertensive drugs**
     EXCLUDES 2   *poisoning by, adverse effect of and underdosing of beta-adrenoreceptor antagonists (T44.7)*
                  poisoning by, adverse effect of and underdosing of calcium-channel blockers (T46.1)
                  poisoning by, adverse effect of and underdosing of diuretics (T50.0-T50.2)

     ✓6ᵗʰ **T46.5X** **Poisoning by, adverse effect of and underdosing of** other antihypertensive **drugs**

         ✓7ᵗʰ **T46.5X1** **Poisoning by other antihypertensive drugs,** accidental **(unintentional)**
             Poisoning by other antihypertensive drugs NOS

         7 ✓7ᵗʰ **T46.5X2** **Poisoning by other antihypertensive drugs,** intentional self-harm   HCC

         ✓7ᵗʰ **T46.5X3** **Poisoning by other antihypertensive drugs,** assault

         ✓7ᵗʰ **T46.5X4** **Poisoning by other antihypertensive drugs,** undetermined

         ✓7ᵗʰ **T46.5X5** Adverse effect **of other antihypertensive drugs**

         ✓7ᵗʰ **T46.5X6** Underdosing **of other antihypertensive drugs**

✓5ᵗʰ **T46.6** **Poisoning by, adverse effect of and underdosing of antihyperlipidemic and antiarteriosclerotic drugs**

  ✓6ᵗʰ **T46.6X** **Poisoning by, adverse effect of and underdosing of** antihyperlipidemic and antiarteriosclerotic **drugs**

    ✓7ᵗʰ **T46.6X1** **Poisoning by antihyperlipidemic and antiarteriosclerotic drugs,** accidental **(unintentional)**
      Poisoning by antihyperlipidemic and antiarteriosclerotic drugs NOS

    7 ✓7ᵗʰ **T46.6X2** **Poisoning by antihyperlipidemic and** HCC **antiarteriosclerotic drugs,** intentional self-harm

    ✓7ᵗʰ **T46.6X3** **Poisoning by antihyperlipidemic and antiarteriosclerotic drugs,** assault

    ✓7ᵗʰ **T46.6X4** **Poisoning by antihyperlipidemic and antiarteriosclerotic drugs,** undetermined

    ✓7ᵗʰ **T46.6X5** Adverse effect **of antihyperlipidemic and antiarteriosclerotic drugs**

    ✓7ᵗʰ **T46.6X6** Underdosing **of antihyperlipidemic and antiarteriosclerotic drugs**

✓5ᵗʰ **T46.7** **Poisoning by, adverse effect of and underdosing of peripheral vasodilators**
  Poisoning by, adverse effect of and underdosing of nicotinic acid (derivatives)
    EXCLUDES 1 *poisoning by, adverse effect of and underdosing of papaverine (T44.3)*

  ✓6ᵗʰ **T46.7X** **Poisoning by, adverse effect of and underdosing of** peripheral vasodilators

    ✓7ᵗʰ **T46.7X1** **Poisoning by peripheral vasodilators,** accidental **(unintentional)**
      Poisoning by peripheral vasodilators NOS

    7 ✓7ᵗʰ **T46.7X2** **Poisoning by peripheral vasodilators,** HCC intentional self-harm

    ✓7ᵗʰ **T46.7X3** **Poisoning by peripheral vasodilators,** assault

    ✓7ᵗʰ **T46.7X4** **Poisoning by peripheral vasodilators,** undetermined

    ✓7ᵗʰ **T46.7X5** Adverse effect **of peripheral vasodilators**

    ✓7ᵗʰ **T46.7X6** Underdosing **of peripheral vasodilators**

✓5ᵗʰ **T46.8** **Poisoning by, adverse effect of and underdosing of antivaricose drugs, including sclerosing agents**

  ✓6ᵗʰ **T46.8X** **Poisoning by, adverse effect of and underdosing of** antivaricose **drugs, including sclerosing agents**

    ✓7ᵗʰ **T46.8X1** **Poisoning by antivaricose drugs, including sclerosing agents,** accidental **(unintentional)**
      Poisoning by antivaricose drugs, including sclerosing agents NOS

    7 ✓7ᵗʰ **T46.8X2** **Poisoning by antivaricose drugs,** HCC **including sclerosing agents,** intentional self-harm

    ✓7ᵗʰ **T46.8X3** **Poisoning by antivaricose drugs, including sclerosing agents,** assault

    ✓7ᵗʰ **T46.8X4** **Poisoning by antivaricose drugs, including sclerosing agents,** undetermined

    ✓7ᵗʰ **T46.8X5** Adverse effect **of antivaricose drugs, including sclerosing agents**

    ✓7ᵗʰ **T46.8X6** Underdosing **of antivaricose drugs, including sclerosing agents**

✓5ᵗʰ **T46.9** **Poisoning by, adverse effect of and underdosing of other and unspecified** agents primarily affecting the cardiovascular system

  ✓6ᵗʰ **T46.90** **Poisoning by, adverse effect of and underdosing of** unspecified agents primarily affecting the cardiovascular system

    ✓7ᵗʰ **T46.901** **Poisoning by unspecified agents primarily affecting the cardiovascular system,** accidental **(unintentional)**

    7 ✓7ᵗʰ **T46.902** **Poisoning by unspecified agents** HCC **primarily affecting the cardiovascular system,** intentional self-harm

    ✓7ᵗʰ **T46.903** **Poisoning by unspecified agents primarily affecting the cardiovascular system,** assault

    ✓7ᵗʰ **T46.904** **Poisoning by unspecified agents primarily affecting the cardiovascular system,** undetermined

    ✓7ᵗʰ **T46.905** Adverse effect **of unspecified agents primarily affecting the cardiovascular system**

    ✓7ᵗʰ **T46.906** Underdosing **of unspecified agents primarily affecting the cardiovascular system**

  ✓6ᵗʰ **T46.99** **Poisoning by, adverse effect of and underdosing of** other agents primarily affecting the cardiovascular system

    ✓7ᵗʰ **T46.991** **Poisoning by other agents primarily affecting the cardiovascular system,** accidental **(unintentional)**

    7 ✓7ᵗʰ **T46.992** **Poisoning by other agents primarily** HCC **affecting the cardiovascular system,** intentional self-harm

    ✓7ᵗʰ **T46.993** **Poisoning by other agents primarily affecting the cardiovascular system,** assault

    ✓7ᵗʰ **T46.994** **Poisoning by other agents primarily affecting the cardiovascular system,** undetermined

    ✓7ᵗʰ **T46.995** Adverse effect **of other agents primarily affecting the cardiovascular system**

    ✓7ᵗʰ **T46.996** Underdosing **of other agents primarily affecting the cardiovascular system**

✓4ᵗʰ **T47** **Poisoning by, adverse effect of and underdosing of agents primarily affecting the gastrointestinal system**

> The appropriate 7th character is to be added to each code from category T47.
> A   initial encounter
> D   subsequent encounter
> S   sequela

✓5ᵗʰ **T47.0** **Poisoning by, adverse effect of and underdosing of histamine H2-receptor blockers**

  ✓6ᵗʰ **T47.0X** **Poisoning by, adverse effect of and underdosing of** histamine H2-receptor blockers

    ✓7ᵗʰ **T47.0X1** **Poisoning by histamine H2-receptor blockers,** accidental **(unintentional)**
      Poisoning by histamine H2-receptor blockers NOS

    7 ✓7ᵗʰ **T47.0X2** **Poisoning by histamine H2-receptor** HCC **blockers,** intentional self-harm

    ✓7ᵗʰ **T47.0X3** **Poisoning by histamine H2-receptor blockers,** assault

    ✓7ᵗʰ **T47.0X4** **Poisoning by histamine H2-receptor blockers,** undetermined

    ✓7ᵗʰ **T47.0X5** Adverse effect **of histamine H2-receptor blockers**

    ✓7ᵗʰ **T47.0X6** Underdosing **of histamine H2-receptor blockers**

✓5ᵗʰ **T47.1** **Poisoning by, adverse effect of and underdosing of other antacids and anti-gastric-secretion drugs**

  ✓6ᵗʰ **T47.1X** **Poisoning by, adverse effect of and underdosing of** other antacids and anti-gastric-secretion **drugs**

    ✓7ᵗʰ **T47.1X1** **Poisoning by other antacids and anti-gastric-secretion drugs,** accidental **(unintentional)**
      Poisoning by other antacids and anti-gastric-secretion drugs NOS

    7 ✓7ᵗʰ **T47.1X2** **Poisoning by other antacids and** HCC **anti-gastric-secretion drugs,** intentional self-harm

    ✓7ᵗʰ **T47.1X3** **Poisoning by other antacids and anti-gastric-secretion drugs,** assault

    ✓7ᵗʰ **T47.1X4** **Poisoning by other antacids and anti-gastric-secretion drugs,** undetermined

    ✓7ᵗʰ **T47.1X5** Adverse effect **of other antacids and anti-gastric-secretion drugs**

    ✓7ᵗʰ **T47.1X6** Underdosing **of other antacids and anti-gastric-secretion drugs**

✓5ᵗʰ **T47.2** **Poisoning by, adverse effect of and underdosing of stimulant laxatives**

  ✓6ᵗʰ **T47.2X** **Poisoning by, adverse effect of and underdosing of** stimulant laxatives

    ✓7ᵗʰ **T47.2X1** **Poisoning by stimulant laxatives,** accidental **(unintentional)**
      Poisoning by stimulant laxatives NOS

☑ Additional Character Required   ✓x7ᵗʰ Placeholder   Unacceptable PDx   Questionable PDx   Manifestation   H1-H14 HAC   HCC CMS-HCC Dx   HIV HIV Dx

ICD-10-CM 2019   **1117**

7 √7ᵗʰ **T47.2X2** **Poisoning by stimulant laxatives,** intentional self-harm　HCC

√7ᵗʰ **T47.2X3** **Poisoning by stimulant laxatives,** assault

√7ᵗʰ **T47.2X4** **Poisoning by stimulant laxatives,** undetermined

√7ᵗʰ **T47.2X5** Adverse effect **of stimulant laxatives**

√7ᵗʰ **T47.2X6** Underdosing **of stimulant laxatives**

√5ᵗʰ **T47.3** **Poisoning by, adverse effect of and underdosing of saline and osmotic laxatives**

√6ᵗʰ **T47.3X** **Poisoning by and adverse effect of** saline and osmotic laxatives

√7ᵗʰ **T47.3X1** **Poisoning by saline and osmotic laxatives,** accidental (unintentional)
Poisoning by saline and osmotic laxatives NOS

7 √7ᵗʰ **T47.3X2** **Poisoning by saline and osmotic laxatives,** intentional self-harm　HCC

√7ᵗʰ **T47.3X3** **Poisoning by saline and osmotic laxatives,** assault

√7ᵗʰ **T47.3X4** **Poisoning by saline and osmotic laxatives,** undetermined

√7ᵗʰ **T47.3X5** Adverse effect **of saline and osmotic laxatives**

√7ᵗʰ **T47.3X6** Underdosing **of saline and osmotic laxatives**

√5ᵗʰ **T47.4** **Poisoning by, adverse effect of and underdosing of other laxatives**

√6ᵗʰ **T47.4X** **Poisoning by, adverse effect of and underdosing of** other laxatives

√7ᵗʰ **T47.4X1** **Poisoning by other laxatives,** accidental (unintentional)
Poisoning by other laxatives NOS

7 √7ᵗʰ **T47.4X2** **Poisoning by other laxatives,** intentional self-harm　HCC

√7ᵗʰ **T47.4X3** **Poisoning by other laxatives,** assault

√7ᵗʰ **T47.4X4** **Poisoning by other laxatives,** undetermined

√7ᵗʰ **T47.4X5** Adverse effect **of other laxatives**

√7ᵗʰ **T47.4X6** Underdosing **of other laxatives**

√5ᵗʰ **T47.5** **Poisoning by, adverse effect of and underdosing of digestants**

√6ᵗʰ **T47.5X** **Poisoning by, adverse effect of and underdosing of** digestants

√7ᵗʰ **T47.5X1** **Poisoning by digestants,** accidental (unintentional)
Poisoning by digestants NOS

7 √7ᵗʰ **T47.5X2** **Poisoning by digestants,** intentional self-harm　HCC

√7ᵗʰ **T47.5X3** **Poisoning by digestants,** assault

√7ᵗʰ **T47.5X4** **Poisoning by digestants,** undetermined

√7ᵗʰ **T47.5X5** Adverse effect **of digestants**

√7ᵗʰ **T47.5X6** Underdosing **of digestants**

√5ᵗʰ **T47.6** **Poisoning by, adverse effect of and underdosing of antidiarrheal drugs**

EXCLUDES 2　poisoning by, adverse effect of and underdosing of systemic antibiotics and other anti-infectives (T36-T37)

√6ᵗʰ **T47.6X** **Poisoning by, adverse effect of and underdosing of** antidiarrheal drugs

√7ᵗʰ **T47.6X1** **Poisoning by antidiarrheal drugs,** accidental (unintentional)
Poisoning by antidiarrheal drugs NOS

7 √7ᵗʰ **T47.6X2** **Poisoning by antidiarrheal drugs,** intentional self-harm　HCC

√7ᵗʰ **T47.6X3** **Poisoning by antidiarrheal drugs,** assault

√7ᵗʰ **T47.6X4** **Poisoning by antidiarrheal drugs,** undetermined

√7ᵗʰ **T47.6X5** Adverse effect **of antidiarrheal drugs**

√7ᵗʰ **T47.6X6** Underdosing **of antidiarrheal drugs**

√5ᵗʰ **T47.7** **Poisoning by, adverse effect of and underdosing of emetics**

√6ᵗʰ **T47.7X** **Poisoning by, adverse effect of and underdosing of** emetics

√7ᵗʰ **T47.7X1** **Poisoning by emetics,** accidental (unintentional)
Poisoning by emetics NOS

7 √7ᵗʰ **T47.7X2** **Poisoning by emetics,** intentional self-harm　HCC

√7ᵗʰ **T47.7X3** **Poisoning by emetics,** assault

√7ᵗʰ **T47.7X4** **Poisoning by emetics,** undetermined

√7ᵗʰ **T47.7X5** Adverse effect **of emetics**

√7ᵗʰ **T47.7X6** Underdosing **of emetics**

√5ᵗʰ **T47.8** **Poisoning by, adverse effect of and underdosing of other agents primarily affecting gastrointestinal system**

√6ᵗʰ **T47.8X** **Poisoning by, adverse effect of and underdosing of** other agents primarily affecting gastrointestinal system

√7ᵗʰ **T47.8X1** **Poisoning by other agents primarily affecting gastrointestinal system,** accidental (unintentional)
Poisoning by other agents primarily affecting gastrointestinal system NOS

7 √7ᵗʰ **T47.8X2** **Poisoning by other agents primarily affecting gastrointestinal system,** intentional self-harm　HCC

√7ᵗʰ **T47.8X3** **Poisoning by other agents primarily affecting gastrointestinal system,** assault

√7ᵗʰ **T47.8X4** **Poisoning by other agents primarily affecting gastrointestinal system,** undetermined

√7ᵗʰ **T47.8X5** Adverse effect **of other agents primarily affecting gastrointestinal system**

√7ᵗʰ **T47.8X6** Underdosing **of other agents primarily affecting gastrointestinal system**

√5ᵗʰ **T47.9** **Poisoning by, adverse effect of and underdosing of** unspecified **agents primarily affecting the gastrointestinal system**

√x7ᵗʰ **T47.91** **Poisoning by unspecified agents primarily affecting the gastrointestinal system,** accidental (unintentional)
Poisoning by agents primarily affecting the gastrointestinal system NOS

7 √x7ᵗʰ **T47.92** **Poisoning by unspecified agents primarily affecting the gastrointestinal system,** intentional self-harm　HCC

√x7ᵗʰ **T47.93** **Poisoning by unspecified agents primarily affecting the gastrointestinal system,** assault

√x7ᵗʰ **T47.94** **Poisoning by unspecified agents primarily affecting the gastrointestinal system,** undetermined

√x7ᵗʰ **T47.95** Adverse effect **of unspecified agents primarily affecting the gastrointestinal system**

√x7ᵗʰ **T47.96** Underdosing **of unspecified agents primarily affecting the gastrointestinal system**

√4ᵗʰ **T48** **Poisoning by, adverse effect of and underdosing of agents primarily acting on smooth and skeletal muscles and the respiratory system**

The appropriate 7th character is to be added to each code from category T48.
A　initial encounter
D　subsequent encounter
S　sequela

√5ᵗʰ **T48.0** **Poisoning by, adverse effect of and underdosing of oxytocic drugs**

EXCLUDES 1　poisoning by, adverse effect of and underdosing of estrogens, progestogens and antagonists (T38.4-T38.6)

√6ᵗʰ **T48.0X** **Poisoning by, adverse effect of and underdosing of** oxytocic drugs

√7ᵗʰ **T48.0X1** **Poisoning by oxytocic drugs,** accidental (unintentional)
Poisoning by oxytocic drugs NOS

7 √7ᵗʰ **T48.0X2** **Poisoning by oxytocic drugs,** intentional self-harm　HCC

√7ᵗʰ **T48.0X3** **Poisoning by oxytocic drugs,** assault

√7ᵗʰ **T48.0X4** **Poisoning by oxytocic drugs,** undetermined

√7ᵗʰ **T48.0X5** Adverse effect **of oxytocic drugs**

√7ᵗʰ **T48.0X6** Underdosing **of oxytocic drugs**

N Newborn: 0　P Pediatric: 0-17　M Maternity: 12-55　A Adult: 15-124　MCC Major Complication/Comorbidity　CC Complication/Comorbidity　SW Severe Wound Dx

1118　　　ICD-10-CM 2019

✓5ᵗʰ **T48.1 Poisoning by, adverse effect of and underdosing of skeletal muscle relaxants [neuromuscular blocking agents]**

     ✓6ᵗʰ **T48.1X Poisoning by, adverse effect of and underdosing of skeletal muscle relaxants [neuromuscular blocking agents]**

         ✓7ᵗʰ **T48.1X1 Poisoning by skeletal muscle relaxants [neuromuscular blocking agents], accidental (unintentional)**
             Poisoning by skeletal muscle relaxants [neuromuscular blocking agents] NOS

         7 ✓7ᵗʰ **T48.1X2 Poisoning by skeletal muscle relaxants [neuromuscular blocking agents], intentional self-harm** HCC

         ✓7ᵗʰ **T48.1X3 Poisoning by skeletal muscle relaxants [neuromuscular blocking agents], assault**

         ✓7ᵗʰ **T48.1X4 Poisoning by skeletal muscle relaxants [neuromuscular blocking agents], undetermined**

         ✓7ᵗʰ **T48.1X5 Adverse effect of skeletal muscle relaxants [neuromuscular blocking agents]**

         ✓7ᵗʰ **T48.1X6 Underdosing of skeletal muscle relaxants [neuromuscular blocking agents]**

✓5ᵗʰ **T48.2 Poisoning by, adverse effect of and underdosing of other and unspecified drugs acting on muscles**

     ✓6ᵗʰ **T48.20 Poisoning by, adverse effect of and underdosing of unspecified drugs acting on muscles**

         ✓7ᵗʰ **T48.201 Poisoning by unspecified drugs acting on muscles, accidental (unintentional)**
             Poisoning by unspecified drugs acting on muscles NOS

         7 ✓7ᵗʰ **T48.202 Poisoning by unspecified drugs acting on muscles, intentional self-harm** HCC

         ✓7ᵗʰ **T48.203 Poisoning by unspecified drugs acting on muscles, assault**

         ✓7ᵗʰ **T48.204 Poisoning by unspecified drugs acting on muscles, undetermined**

         ✓7ᵗʰ **T48.205 Adverse effect of unspecified drugs acting on muscles**

         ✓7ᵗʰ **T48.206 Underdosing of unspecified drugs acting on muscles**

     ✓6ᵗʰ **T48.29 Poisoning by, adverse effect of and underdosing of other drugs acting on muscles**

         ✓7ᵗʰ **T48.291 Poisoning by other drugs acting on muscles, accidental (unintentional)**
             Poisoning by other drugs acting on muscles NOS

         7 ✓7ᵗʰ **T48.292 Poisoning by other drugs acting on muscles, intentional self-harm** HCC

         ✓7ᵗʰ **T48.293 Poisoning by other drugs acting on muscles, assault**

         ✓7ᵗʰ **T48.294 Poisoning by other drugs acting on muscles, undetermined**

         ✓7ᵗʰ **T48.295 Adverse effect of other drugs acting on muscles**

         ✓7ᵗʰ **T48.296 Underdosing of other drugs acting on muscles**

✓5ᵗʰ **T48.3 Poisoning by, adverse effect of and underdosing of antitussives**

     ✓6ᵗʰ **T48.3X Poisoning by, adverse effect of and underdosing of antitussives**

         ✓7ᵗʰ **T48.3X1 Poisoning by antitussives, accidental (unintentional)**
             Poisoning by antitussives NOS

         7 ✓7ᵗʰ **T48.3X2 Poisoning by antitussives, intentional self-harm** HCC

         ✓7ᵗʰ **T48.3X3 Poisoning by antitussives, assault**

         ✓7ᵗʰ **T48.3X4 Poisoning by antitussives, undetermined**

         ✓7ᵗʰ **T48.3X5 Adverse effect of antitussives**

         ✓7ᵗʰ **T48.3X6 Underdosing of antitussives**

✓5ᵗʰ **T48.4 Poisoning by, adverse effect of and underdosing of expectorants**

     ✓6ᵗʰ **T48.4X Poisoning by, adverse effect of and underdosing of expectorants**

         ✓7ᵗʰ **T48.4X1 Poisoning by expectorants, accidental (unintentional)**
             Poisoning by expectorants NOS

         7 ✓7ᵗʰ **T48.4X2 Poisoning by expectorants, intentional self-harm** HCC

         ✓7ᵗʰ **T48.4X3 Poisoning by expectorants, assault**

         ✓7ᵗʰ **T48.4X4 Poisoning by expectorants, undetermined**

         ✓7ᵗʰ **T48.4X5 Adverse effect of expectorants**

         ✓7ᵗʰ **T48.4X6 Underdosing of expectorants**

✓5ᵗʰ **T48.5 Poisoning by, adverse effect of and underdosing of other anti-common-cold drugs**
     Poisoning by, adverse effect of and underdosing of decongestants
     EXCLUDES 2   *poisoning by, adverse effect of and underdosing of antipyretics, NEC (T39.9-)*
             poisoning by, adverse effect of and underdosing of non-steroidal antiinflammatory drugs (T39.3-)
             poisoning by, adverse effect of and underdosing of salicylates (T39.0-)

     ✓6ᵗʰ **T48.5X Poisoning by, adverse effect of and underdosing of other anti-common-cold drugs**

         ✓7ᵗʰ **T48.5X1 Poisoning by other anti-common-cold drugs, accidental (unintentional)**
             Poisoning by other anti-common-cold drugs NOS

         7 ✓7ᵗʰ **T48.5X2 Poisoning by other anti-common-cold drugs, intentional self-harm** HCC

         ✓7ᵗʰ **T48.5X3 Poisoning by other anti-common-cold drugs, assault**

         ✓7ᵗʰ **T48.5X4 Poisoning by other anti-common-cold drugs, undetermined**

         ✓7ᵗʰ **T48.5X5 Adverse effect of other anti-common-cold drugs**

         ✓7ᵗʰ **T48.5X6 Underdosing of other anti-common-cold drugs**

✓5ᵗʰ **T48.6 Poisoning by, adverse effect of and underdosing of antiasthmatics, not elsewhere classified**
     Poisoning by, adverse effect of and underdosing of beta-adrenoreceptor agonists used in asthma therapy
     EXCLUDES 1   *poisoning by, adverse effect of and underdosing of anterior pituitary [adenohypophyseal] hormones (T38.8)*
             poisoning by, adverse effect of and underdosing of beta-adrenoreceptor agonists not used in asthma therapy (T44.5)

     ✓6ᵗʰ **T48.6X Poisoning by, adverse effect of and underdosing of antiasthmatics**

         ✓7ᵗʰ **T48.6X1 Poisoning by antiasthmatics, accidental (unintentional)**
             Poisoning by antiasthmatics NOS

         7 ✓7ᵗʰ **T48.6X2 Poisoning by antiasthmatics, intentional self-harm** HCC

         ✓7ᵗʰ **T48.6X3 Poisoning by antiasthmatics, assault**

         ✓7ᵗʰ **T48.6X4 Poisoning by antiasthmatics, undetermined**

         ✓7ᵗʰ **T48.6X5 Adverse effect of antiasthmatics**

         ✓7ᵗʰ **T48.6X6 Underdosing of antiasthmatics**

✓5ᵗʰ **T48.9 Poisoning by, adverse effect of and underdosing of other and unspecified agents primarily acting on the respiratory system**

     ✓6ᵗʰ **T48.90 Poisoning by, adverse effect of and underdosing of unspecified agents primarily acting on the respiratory system**

         ✓7ᵗʰ **T48.901 Poisoning by unspecified agents primarily acting on the respiratory system, accidental (unintentional)**

         7 ✓7ᵗʰ **T48.902 Poisoning by unspecified agents primarily acting on the respiratory system, intentional self-harm** HCC

         ✓7ᵗʰ **T48.903 Poisoning by unspecified agents primarily acting on the respiratory system, assault**

         ✓7ᵗʰ **T48.904 Poisoning by unspecified agents primarily acting on the respiratory system, undetermined**

         ✓7ᵗʰ **T48.905 Adverse effect of unspecified agents primarily acting on the respiratory system**

         ✓7ᵗʰ **T48.906 Underdosing of unspecified agents primarily acting on the respiratory system**

☑6ᵗʰ **T48.99** **Poisoning by, adverse effect of and underdosing of** other **agents primarily acting on the respiratory system**

    ☑7ᵗʰ **T48.991** **Poisoning by other agents primarily acting on the respiratory system,** accidental (unintentional)

    7 ☑7ᵗʰ **T48.992** **Poisoning by other agents primarily acting on the respiratory system,** intentional self-harm `HCC`

    ☑7ᵗʰ **T48.993** **Poisoning by other agents primarily acting on the respiratory system,** assault

    ☑7ᵗʰ **T48.994** **Poisoning by other agents primarily acting on the respiratory system,** undetermined

    ☑7ᵗʰ **T48.995** Adverse effect **of other agents primarily acting on the respiratory system**

    ☑7ᵗʰ **T48.996** Underdosing **of other agents primarily acting on the respiratory system**

☑4ᵗʰ **T49** **Poisoning by, adverse effect of and underdosing of topical agents primarily affecting skin and mucous membrane and by ophthalmological, otorhinolaryngological and dental drugs**

    INCLUDES   poisoning by, adverse effect of and underdosing of glucocorticoids, topically used

    The appropriate 7th character is to be added to each code from category T49.
    A   initial encounter
    D   subsequent encounter
    S   sequela

   ☑5ᵗʰ **T49.0** **Poisoning by, adverse effect of and underdosing of local antifungal, anti-infective and anti-inflammatory drugs**

    ☑6ᵗʰ **T49.0X** **Poisoning by, adverse effect of and underdosing of** local antifungal, anti-infective and anti-inflammatory **drugs**

      ☑7ᵗʰ **T49.0X1** **Poisoning by local antifungal, anti-infective and anti-inflammatory drugs,** accidental (unintentional)
       Poisoning by local antifungal, anti-infective and anti-inflammatory drugs NOS

      7 ☑7ᵗʰ **T49.0X2** **Poisoning by local antifungal, anti-infective and anti-inflammatory drugs,** intentional self-harm `HCC`

      ☑7ᵗʰ **T49.0X3** **Poisoning by local antifungal, anti-infective and anti-inflammatory drugs,** assault

      ☑7ᵗʰ **T49.0X4** **Poisoning by local antifungal, anti-infective and anti-inflammatory drugs,** undetermined

      ☑7ᵗʰ **T49.0X5** Adverse effect **of local antifungal, anti-infective and anti-inflammatory drugs**

      ☑7ᵗʰ **T49.0X6** Underdosing **of local antifungal, anti-infective and anti-inflammatory drugs**

   ☑5ᵗʰ **T49.1** **Poisoning by, adverse effect of and underdosing of antipruritics**

    ☑6ᵗʰ **T49.1X** **Poisoning by, adverse effect of and underdosing of** antipruritics

      ☑7ᵗʰ **T49.1X1** **Poisoning by antipruritics,** accidental (unintentional)
       Poisoning by antipruritics NOS

      7 ☑7ᵗʰ **T49.1X2** **Poisoning by antipruritics,** intentional self-harm `HCC`

      ☑7ᵗʰ **T49.1X3** **Poisoning by antipruritics,** assault

      ☑7ᵗʰ **T49.1X4** **Poisoning by antipruritics,** undetermined

      ☑7ᵗʰ **T49.1X5** Adverse effect **of antipruritics**

      ☑7ᵗʰ **T49.1X6** Underdosing **of antipruritics**

   ☑5ᵗʰ **T49.2** **Poisoning by, adverse effect of and underdosing of local astringents and local detergents**

    ☑6ᵗʰ **T49.2X** **Poisoning by, adverse effect of and underdosing of** local astringents and local detergents

      ☑7ᵗʰ **T49.2X1** **Poisoning by local astringents and local detergents,** accidental (unintentional)
       Poisoning by local astringents and local detergents NOS

      7 ☑7ᵗʰ **T49.2X2** **Poisoning by local astringents and local detergents,** intentional self-harm `HCC`

      ☑7ᵗʰ **T49.2X3** **Poisoning by local astringents and local detergents,** assault

      ☑7ᵗʰ **T49.2X4** **Poisoning by local astringents and local detergents,** undetermined

      ☑7ᵗʰ **T49.2X5** Adverse effect **of local astringents and local detergents**

      ☑7ᵗʰ **T49.2X6** Underdosing **of local astringents and local detergents**

   ☑5ᵗʰ **T49.3** **Poisoning by, adverse effect of and underdosing of emollients, demulcents and protectants**

    ☑6ᵗʰ **T49.3X** **Poisoning by, adverse effect of and underdosing of** emollients, demulcents and protectants

      ☑7ᵗʰ **T49.3X1** **Poisoning by emollients, demulcents and protectants,** accidental (unintentional)
       Poisoning by emollients, demulcents and protectants NOS

      7 ☑7ᵗʰ **T49.3X2** **Poisoning by emollients, demulcents and protectants,** intentional self-harm `HCC`

      ☑7ᵗʰ **T49.3X3** **Poisoning by emollients, demulcents and protectants,** assault

      ☑7ᵗʰ **T49.3X4** **Poisoning by emollients, demulcents and protectants,** undetermined

      ☑7ᵗʰ **T49.3X5** Adverse effect **of emollients, demulcents and protectants**

      ☑7ᵗʰ **T49.3X6** Underdosing **of emollients, demulcents and protectants**

   ☑5ᵗʰ **T49.4** **Poisoning by, adverse effect of and underdosing of keratolytics, keratoplastics, and other hair treatment drugs and preparations**

    ☑6ᵗʰ **T49.4X** **Poisoning by, adverse effect of and underdosing of** keratolytics, keratoplastics, and other hair treatment drugs and preparations

      ☑7ᵗʰ **T49.4X1** **Poisoning by keratolytics, keratoplastics, and other hair treatment drugs and preparations,** accidental (unintentional)
       Poisoning by keratolytics, keratoplastics, and other hair treatment drugs and preparations NOS

      7 ☑7ᵗʰ **T49.4X2** **Poisoning by keratolytics, keratoplastics, and other hair treatment drugs and preparations,** intentional self-harm `HCC`

      ☑7ᵗʰ **T49.4X3** **Poisoning by keratolytics, keratoplastics, and other hair treatment drugs and preparations,** assault

      ☑7ᵗʰ **T49.4X4** **Poisoning by keratolytics, keratoplastics, and other hair treatment drugs and preparations,** undetermined

      ☑7ᵗʰ **T49.4X5** Adverse effect **of keratolytics, keratoplastics, and other hair treatment drugs and preparations**

      ☑7ᵗʰ **T49.4X6** Underdosing **of keratolytics, keratoplastics, and other hair treatment drugs and preparations**

   ☑5ᵗʰ **T49.5** **Poisoning by, adverse effect of and underdosing of ophthalmological drugs and preparations**

    ☑6ᵗʰ **T49.5X** **Poisoning by, adverse effect of and underdosing of** ophthalmological **drugs and preparations**

      ☑7ᵗʰ **T49.5X1** **Poisoning by ophthalmological drugs and preparations,** accidental (unintentional)
       Poisoning by ophthalmological drugs and preparations NOS

      7 ☑7ᵗʰ **T49.5X2** **Poisoning by ophthalmological drugs and preparations,** intentional self-harm `HCC`

      ☑7ᵗʰ **T49.5X3** **Poisoning by ophthalmological drugs and preparations,** assault

      ☑7ᵗʰ **T49.5X4** **Poisoning by ophthalmological drugs and preparations,** undetermined

      ☑7ᵗʰ **T49.5X5** Adverse effect **of ophthalmological drugs and preparations**

      ☑7ᵗʰ **T49.5X6** Underdosing **of ophthalmological drugs and preparations**

N Newborn: 0   **P** Pediatric: 0-17   **M** Maternity: 12-55   **A** Adult: 15-124   **MCC** Major Complication/Comorbidity   **CC** Complication/Comorbidity   **SW** Severe Wound Dx

1120   ICD-10-CM 2019

√5th **T49.6** **Poisoning by, adverse effect of and underdosing of otorhinolaryngological drugs and preparations**

  √6th **T49.6X** **Poisoning by, adverse effect of and underdosing of otorhinolaryngological drugs and preparations**

    √7th **T49.6X1** **Poisoning by otorhinolaryngological drugs and preparations, accidental (unintentional)**
Poisoning by otorhinolaryngological drugs and preparations NOS

    7 √7th **T49.6X2** **Poisoning by otorhinolaryngological drugs and preparations, intentional self-harm** HCC

    √7th **T49.6X3** **Poisoning by otorhinolaryngological drugs and preparations, assault**

    √7th **T49.6X4** **Poisoning by otorhinolaryngological drugs and preparations, undetermined**

    √7th **T49.6X5** **Adverse effect of otorhinolaryngological drugs and preparations**

    √7th **T49.6X6** **Underdosing of otorhinolaryngological drugs and preparations**

√5th **T49.7** **Poisoning by, adverse effect of and underdosing of dental drugs, topically applied**

  √6th **T49.7X** **Poisoning by, adverse effect of and underdosing of dental drugs, topically applied**

    √7th **T49.7X1** **Poisoning by dental drugs, topically applied, accidental (unintentional)**
Poisoning by dental drugs, topically applied NOS

    7 √7th **T49.7X2** **Poisoning by dental drugs, topically applied, intentional self-harm** HCC

    √7th **T49.7X3** **Poisoning by dental drugs, topically applied, assault**

    √7th **T49.7X4** **Poisoning by dental drugs, topically applied, undetermined**

    √7th **T49.7X5** **Adverse effect of dental drugs, topically applied**

    √7th **T49.7X6** **Underdosing of dental drugs, topically applied**

√5th **T49.8** **Poisoning by, adverse effect of and underdosing of other topical agents**
Poisoning by, adverse effect of and underdosing of spermicides

  √6th **T49.8X** **Poisoning by, adverse effect of and underdosing of other topical agents**

    √7th **T49.8X1** **Poisoning by other topical agents, accidental (unintentional)**
Poisoning by other topical agents NOS

    7 √7th **T49.8X2** **Poisoning by other topical agents, intentional self-harm** HCC

    √7th **T49.8X3** **Poisoning by other topical agents, assault**

    √7th **T49.8X4** **Poisoning by other topical agents, undetermined**

    √7th **T49.8X5** **Adverse effect of other topical agents**

    √7th **T49.8X6** **Underdosing of other topical agents**

√5th **T49.9** **Poisoning by, adverse effect of and underdosing of unspecified topical agent**

  √x7th **T49.91** **Poisoning by unspecified topical agent, accidental (unintentional)**

  7 √x7th **T49.92** **Poisoning by unspecified topical agent, intentional self-harm** HCC

  √x7th **T49.93** **Poisoning by unspecified topical agent, assault**

  √x7th **T49.94** **Poisoning by unspecified topical agent, undetermined**

  √x7th **T49.95** **Adverse effect of unspecified topical agent**

  √x7th **T49.96** **Underdosing of unspecified topical agent**

√4th **T50** **Poisoning by, adverse effect of and underdosing of diuretics and other and unspecified drugs, medicaments and biological substances**

> The appropriate 7th character is to be added to each code from category T50.
> A   initial encounter
> D   subsequent encounter
> S   sequela

√5th **T50.0** **Poisoning by, adverse effect of and underdosing of mineralocorticoids and their antagonists**

  √6th **T50.0X** **Poisoning by, adverse effect of and underdosing of mineralocorticoids and their antagonists**

    √7th **T50.0X1** **Poisoning by mineralocorticoids and their antagonists, accidental (unintentional)**
Poisoning by mineralocorticoids and their antagonists NOS

    7 √7th **T50.0X2** **Poisoning by mineralocorticoids and their antagonists, intentional self-harm** HCC

    √7th **T50.0X3** **Poisoning by mineralocorticoids and their antagonists, assault**

    √7th **T50.0X4** **Poisoning by mineralocorticoids and their antagonists, undetermined**

    √7th **T50.0X5** **Adverse effect of mineralocorticoids and their antagonists**

    √7th **T50.0X6** **Underdosing of mineralocorticoids and their antagonists**

√5th **T50.1** **Poisoning by, adverse effect of and underdosing of loop [high-ceiling] diuretics**

  √6th **T50.1X** **Poisoning by, adverse effect of and underdosing of loop [high-ceiling] diuretics**

    √7th **T50.1X1** **Poisoning by loop [high-ceiling] diuretics, accidental (unintentional)**
Poisoning by loop [high-ceiling] diuretics NOS

    7 √7th **T50.1X2** **Poisoning by loop [high-ceiling] diuretics, intentional self-harm** HCC

    √7th **T50.1X3** **Poisoning by loop [high-ceiling] diuretics, assault**

    √7th **T50.1X4** **Poisoning by loop [high-ceiling] diuretics, undetermined**

    √7th **T50.1X5** **Adverse effect of loop [high-ceiling] diuretics**

    √7th **T50.1X6** **Underdosing of loop [high-ceiling] diuretics**

√5th **T50.2** **Poisoning by, adverse effect of and underdosing of carbonic-anhydrase inhibitors, benzothiadiazides and other diuretics**
Poisoning by, adverse effect of and underdosing of acetazolamide

  √6th **T50.2X** **Poisoning by, adverse effect of and underdosing of carbonic-anhydrase inhibitors, benzothiadiazides and other diuretics**

    √7th **T50.2X1** **Poisoning by carbonic-anhydrase inhibitors, benzothiadiazides and other diuretics, accidental (unintentional)**
Poisoning by carbonic-anhydrase inhibitors, benzothiadiazides and other diuretics NOS

    7 √7th **T50.2X2** **Poisoning by carbonic-anhydrase inhibitors, benzothiadiazides and other diuretics, intentional self-harm** HCC

    √7th **T50.2X3** **Poisoning by carbonic-anhydrase inhibitors, benzothiadiazides and other diuretics, assault**

    √7th **T50.2X4** **Poisoning by carbonic-anhydrase inhibitors, benzothiadiazides and other diuretics, undetermined**

    √7th **T50.2X5** **Adverse effect of carbonic-anhydrase inhibitors, benzothiadiazides and other diuretics**

    √7th **T50.2X6** **Underdosing of carbonic-anhydrase inhibitors, benzothiadiazides and other diuretics**

☑Additional Character Required   √x7th Placeholder   Unacceptable PDx   Questionable PDx   Manifestation   H1-H14 HAC   HCC CMS-HCC Dx   HIV HIV Dx

ICD-10-CM 2019   1121

✓5ᵗʰ T50.3 Poisoning by, adverse effect of and underdosing of electrolytic, caloric and water-balance agents
Poisoning by, adverse effect of and underdosing of oral rehydration salts

    ✓6ᵗʰ T50.3X Poisoning by, adverse effect of and underdosing of electrolytic, caloric and water-balance agents

        ✓7ᵗʰ T50.3X1 Poisoning by electrolytic, caloric and water-balance agents, accidental (unintentional)
Poisoning by electrolytic, caloric and water-balance agents NOS

        7 ✓7ᵗʰ T50.3X2 Poisoning by electrolytic, caloric and water-balance agents, intentional self-harm `HCC`

        ✓7ᵗʰ T50.3X3 Poisoning by electrolytic, caloric and water-balance agents, assault

        ✓7ᵗʰ T50.3X4 Poisoning by electrolytic, caloric and water-balance agents, undetermined

        ✓7ᵗʰ T50.3X5 Adverse effect of electrolytic, caloric and water-balance agents

        ✓7ᵗʰ T50.3X6 Underdosing of electrolytic, caloric and water-balance agents

✓5ᵗʰ T50.4 Poisoning by, adverse effect of and underdosing of drugs affecting uric acid metabolism

    ✓6ᵗʰ T50.4X Poisoning by, adverse effect of and underdosing of drugs affecting uric acid metabolism

        ✓7ᵗʰ T50.4X1 Poisoning by drugs affecting uric acid metabolism, accidental (unintentional)
Poisoning by drugs affecting uric acid metabolism NOS

        7 ✓7ᵗʰ T50.4X2 Poisoning by drugs affecting uric acid metabolism, intentional self-harm `HCC`

        ✓7ᵗʰ T50.4X3 Poisoning by drugs affecting uric acid metabolism, assault

        ✓7ᵗʰ T50.4X4 Poisoning by drugs affecting uric acid metabolism, undetermined

        ✓7ᵗʰ T50.4X5 Adverse effect of drugs affecting uric acid metabolism

        ✓7ᵗʰ T50.4X6 Underdosing of drugs affecting uric acid metabolism

✓5ᵗʰ T50.5 Poisoning by, adverse effect of and underdosing of appetite depressants

    ✓6ᵗʰ T50.5X Poisoning by, adverse effect of and underdosing of appetite depressants

        ✓7ᵗʰ T50.5X1 Poisoning by appetite depressants, accidental (unintentional)
Poisoning by appetite depressants NOS

        7 ✓7ᵗʰ T50.5X2 Poisoning by appetite depressants, intentional self-harm `HCC`

        ✓7ᵗʰ T50.5X3 Poisoning by appetite depressants, assault

        ✓7ᵗʰ T50.5X4 Poisoning by appetite depressants, undetermined

        ✓7ᵗʰ T50.5X5 Adverse effect of appetite depressants

        ✓7ᵗʰ T50.5X6 Underdosing of appetite depressants

✓5ᵗʰ T50.6 Poisoning by, adverse effect of and underdosing of antidotes and chelating agents
Poisoning by, adverse effect of and underdosing of alcohol deterrents

    ✓6ᵗʰ T50.6X Poisoning by, adverse effect of and underdosing of antidotes and chelating agents

        ✓7ᵗʰ T50.6X1 Poisoning by antidotes and chelating agents, accidental (unintentional)
Poisoning by antidotes and chelating agents NOS

        7 ✓7ᵗʰ T50.6X2 Poisoning by antidotes and chelating agents, intentional self-harm `HCC`

        ✓7ᵗʰ T50.6X3 Poisoning by antidotes and chelating agents, assault

        ✓7ᵗʰ T50.6X4 Poisoning by antidotes and chelating agents, undetermined

        ✓7ᵗʰ T50.6X5 Adverse effect of antidotes and chelating agents

        ✓7ᵗʰ T50.6X6 Underdosing of antidotes and chelating agents

✓5ᵗʰ T50.7 Poisoning by, adverse effect of and underdosing of analeptics and opioid receptor antagonists

    ✓6ᵗʰ T50.7X Poisoning by, adverse effect of and underdosing of analeptics and opioid receptor antagonists

        ✓7ᵗʰ T50.7X1 Poisoning by analeptics and opioid receptor antagonists, accidental (unintentional)
Poisoning by analeptics and opioid receptor antagonists NOS

        7 ✓7ᵗʰ T50.7X2 Poisoning by analeptics and opioid receptor antagonists, intentional self-harm `HCC`

        ✓7ᵗʰ T50.7X3 Poisoning by analeptics and opioid receptor antagonists, assault

        ✓7ᵗʰ T50.7X4 Poisoning by analeptics and opioid receptor antagonists, undetermined

        ✓7ᵗʰ T50.7X5 Adverse effect of analeptics and opioid receptor antagonists

        ✓7ᵗʰ T50.7X6 Underdosing of analeptics and opioid receptor antagonists

✓5ᵗʰ T50.8 Poisoning by, adverse effect of and underdosing of diagnostic agents

    ✓6ᵗʰ T50.8X Poisoning by, adverse effect of and underdosing of diagnostic agents

        ✓7ᵗʰ T50.8X1 Poisoning by diagnostic agents, accidental (unintentional)
Poisoning by diagnostic agents NOS

        7 ✓7ᵗʰ T50.8X2 Poisoning by diagnostic agents, intentional self-harm `HCC`

        ✓7ᵗʰ T50.8X3 Poisoning by diagnostic agents, assault

        ✓7ᵗʰ T50.8X4 Poisoning by diagnostic agents, undetermined

        ✓7ᵗʰ T50.8X5 Adverse effect of diagnostic agents

        ✓7ᵗʰ T50.8X6 Underdosing of diagnostic agents

✓5ᵗʰ T50.A Poisoning by, adverse effect of and underdosing of bacterial vaccines

    ✓6ᵗʰ T50.A1 Poisoning by, adverse effect of and underdosing of pertussis vaccine, including combinations with a pertussis component

        ✓7ᵗʰ T50.A11 Poisoning by pertussis vaccine, including combinations with a pertussis component, accidental (unintentional)

        7 ✓7ᵗʰ T50.A12 Poisoning by pertussis vaccine, including combinations with a pertussis component, intentional self-harm `HCC`

        ✓7ᵗʰ T50.A13 Poisoning by pertussis vaccine, including combinations with a pertussis component, assault

        ✓7ᵗʰ T50.A14 Poisoning by pertussis vaccine, including combinations with a pertussis component, undetermined

        ✓7ᵗʰ T50.A15 Adverse effect of pertussis vaccine, including combinations with a pertussis component

        ✓7ᵗʰ T50.A16 Underdosing of pertussis vaccine, including combinations with a pertussis component

    ✓6ᵗʰ T50.A2 Poisoning by, adverse effect of and underdosing of mixed bacterial vaccines without a pertussis component

        ✓7ᵗʰ T50.A21 Poisoning by mixed bacterial vaccines without a pertussis component, accidental (unintentional)

        7 ✓7ᵗʰ T50.A22 Poisoning by mixed bacterial vaccines without a pertussis component, intentional self-harm `HCC`

        ✓7ᵗʰ T50.A23 Poisoning by mixed bacterial vaccines without a pertussis component, assault

        ✓7ᵗʰ T50.A24 Poisoning by mixed bacterial vaccines without a pertussis component, undetermined

        ✓7ᵗʰ T50.A25 Adverse effect of mixed bacterial vaccines without a pertussis component

        ✓7ᵗʰ T50.A26 Underdosing of mixed bacterial vaccines without a pertussis component

N Newborn: 0   **P** Pediatric: 0-17   **M** Maternity: 12-55   **A** Adult: 15-124   **MCC** Major Complication/Comorbidity   **CC** Complication/Comorbidity   **SW** Severe Wound Dx

1122   ICD-10-CM 2019

√6th **T50.A9** Poisoning by, adverse effect of and underdosing of other bacterial vaccines

√7th **T50.A91** Poisoning by other bacterial vaccines, accidental (unintentional)

7 √7th **T50.A92** Poisoning by other bacterial vaccines, intentional self-harm   HCC

√7th **T50.A93** Poisoning by other bacterial vaccines, assault

√7th **T50.A94** Poisoning by other bacterial vaccines, undetermined

√7th **T50.A95** Adverse effect of other bacterial vaccines

√7th **T50.A96** Underdosing of other bacterial vaccines

√5th **T50.B** Poisoning by, adverse effect of and underdosing of viral vaccines

√6th **T50.B1** Poisoning by, adverse effect of and underdosing of smallpox vaccines

√7th **T50.B11** Poisoning by smallpox vaccines, accidental (unintentional)

7 √7th **T50.B12** Poisoning by smallpox vaccines, intentional self-harm   HCC

√7th **T50.B13** Poisoning by smallpox vaccines, assault

√7th **T50.B14** Poisoning by smallpox vaccines, undetermined

√7th **T50.B15** Adverse effect of smallpox vaccines

√7th **T50.B16** Underdosing of smallpox vaccines

√6th **T50.B9** Poisoning by, adverse effect of and underdosing of other viral vaccines

√7th **T50.B91** Poisoning by other viral vaccines, accidental (unintentional)

7 √7th **T50.B92** Poisoning by other viral vaccines, intentional self-harm   HCC

√7th **T50.B93** Poisoning by other viral vaccines, assault

√7th **T50.B94** Poisoning by other viral vaccines, undetermined

√7th **T50.B95** Adverse effect of other viral vaccines

√7th **T50.B96** Underdosing of other viral vaccines

√5th **T50.Z** Poisoning by, adverse effect of and underdosing of other vaccines and biological substances

√6th **T50.Z1** Poisoning by, adverse effect of and underdosing of immunoglobulin

√7th **T50.Z11** Poisoning by immunoglobulin, accidental (unintentional)

7 √7th **T50.Z12** Poisoning by immunoglobulin, intentional self-harm   HCC

√7th **T50.Z13** Poisoning by immunoglobulin, assault

√7th **T50.Z14** Poisoning by immunoglobulin, undetermined

√7th **T50.Z15** Adverse effect of immunoglobulin

√7th **T50.Z16** Underdosing of immunoglobulin

√6th **T50.Z9** Poisoning by, adverse effect of and underdosing of other vaccines and biological substances

√7th **T50.Z91** Poisoning by other vaccines and biological substances, accidental (unintentional)

7 √7th **T50.Z92** Poisoning by other vaccines and biological substances, intentional self-harm   HCC

√7th **T50.Z93** Poisoning by other vaccines and biological substances, assault

√7th **T50.Z94** Poisoning by other vaccines and biological substances, undetermined

√7th **T50.Z95** Adverse effect of other vaccines and biological substances

√7th **T50.Z96** Underdosing of other vaccines and biological substances

√5th **T50.9** Poisoning by, adverse effect of and underdosing of other and unspecified drugs, medicaments and biological substances
   AHA: 2016, 1Q, 38; 2015, 1Q, 21

√6th **T50.90** Poisoning by, adverse effect of and underdosing of unspecified drugs, medicaments and biological substances

√7th **T50.901** Poisoning by unspecified drugs, medicaments and biological substances, accidental (unintentional)

7 √7th **T50.902** Poisoning by unspecified drugs, medicaments and biological substances, intentional self-harm   HCC

√7th **T50.903** Poisoning by unspecified drugs, medicaments and biological substances, assault

√7th **T50.904** Poisoning by unspecified drugs, medicaments and biological substances, undetermined

√7th **T50.905** Adverse effect of unspecified drugs, medicaments and biological substances

√7th **T50.906** Underdosing of unspecified drugs, medicaments and biological substances

√6th **T50.99** Poisoning by, adverse effect of and underdosing of other drugs, medicaments and biological substances

√7th **T50.991** Poisoning by other drugs, medicaments and biological substances, accidental (unintentional)

7 √7th **T50.992** Poisoning by other drugs, medicaments and biological substances, intentional self-harm   HCC

√7th **T50.993** Poisoning by other drugs, medicaments and biological substances, assault

√7th **T50.994** Poisoning by other drugs, medicaments and biological substances, undetermined

√7th **T50.995** Adverse effect of other drugs, medicaments and biological substances

√7th **T50.996** Underdosing of other drugs, medicaments and biological substances

Toxic effects of substances chiefly nonmedicinal as to source (T51-T65)

NOTE   When no intent is indicated code to accidental. Undetermined intent is only for use when there is specific documentation in the record that the intent of the toxic effect cannot be determined.

Use additional code(s) for all associated manifestations of toxic effect, such as:
   personal history of foreign body fully removed (Z87.821)
   respiratory conditions due to external agents (J60-J70)
   to identify any retained foreign body, if applicable (Z18.-)
   EXCLUDES 1   contact with and (suspected) exposure to toxic substances (Z77.-)
AHA: 2017, 1Q, 39-40

√4th **T51** **Toxic effect of alcohol**

The appropriate 7th character is to be added to each code from category T51.
   A   initial encounter
   D   subsequent encounter
   S   sequela

√5th **T51.0** Toxic effect of ethanol
   Toxic effect of ethyl alcohol
   EXCLUDES 2   acute alcohol intoxication or 'hangover' effects (F10.129, F10.229, F10.929)
      drunkenness (F10.129, F10.229, F10.929)
      pathological alcohol intoxication (F10.129, F10.229, F10.929)

√6th **T51.0X** Toxic effect of ethanol

√7th **T51.0X1** Toxic effect of ethanol, accidental (unintentional)
   Toxic effect of ethanol NOS

7 √7th **T51.0X2** Toxic effect of ethanol, intentional self-harm   HCC

√7th **T51.0X3** Toxic effect of ethanol, assault

√7th **T51.0X4** Toxic effect of ethanol, undetermined

√5th **T51.1** Toxic effect of methanol
   Toxic effect of methyl alcohol

√6th **T51.1X** Toxic effect of methanol

√7th **T51.1X1** Toxic effect of methanol, accidental (unintentional)
   Toxic effect of methanol NOS

7 √7th **T51.1X2** Toxic effect of methanol, intentional self-harm   HCC

√7th **T51.1X3** Toxic effect of methanol, assault

√7th **T51.1X4** Toxic effect of methanol, undetermined

✔ Additional Character Required   √x7th Placeholder   Unacceptable PDx   Questionable PDx   Manifestation   H1 -H14 HAC   HCC CMS-HCC Dx   HIV HIV Dx

ICD-10-CM 2019   1123

Chapter 19. Injury, Poisoning and Certain Other Consequences of External Causes

T51.2–T53.0X4

✓5th **T51.2** **Toxic effect of 2-Propanol**
Toxic effect of isopropyl alcohol

    ✓6th **T51.2X** **Toxic effect of 2-Propanol**

      ✓7th **T51.2X1** **Toxic effect of 2-Propanol, accidental (unintentional)**
Toxic effect of 2-Propanol NOS

      7 ✓7th **T51.2X2** **Toxic effect of 2-Propanol, intentional self-harm**   HCC

      ✓7th **T51.2X3** **Toxic effect of 2-Propanol, assault**

      ✓7th **T51.2X4** **Toxic effect of 2-Propanol, undetermined**

✓5th **T51.3** **Toxic effect of fusel oil**
Toxic effect of amyl alcohol
Toxic effect of butyl [1-butanol] alcohol
Toxic effect of propyl [1-propanol] alcohol

    ✓6th **T51.3X** **Toxic effect of fusel oil**

      ✓7th **T51.3X1** **Toxic effect of fusel oil, accidental (unintentional)**
Toxic effect of fusel oil NOS

      7 ✓7th **T51.3X2** **Toxic effect of fusel oil, intentional self-harm**   HCC

      ✓7th **T51.3X3** **Toxic effect of fusel oil, assault**

      ✓7th **T51.3X4** **Toxic effect of fusel oil, undetermined**

✓5th **T51.8** **Toxic effect of other alcohols**

    ✓6th **T51.8X** **Toxic effect of other alcohols**

      ✓7th **T51.8X1** **Toxic effect of other alcohols, accidental (unintentional)**
Toxic effect of other alcohols NOS

      7 ✓7th **T51.8X2** **Toxic effect of other alcohols, intentional self-harm**   HCC

      ✓7th **T51.8X3** **Toxic effect of other alcohols, assault**

      ✓7th **T51.8X4** **Toxic effect of other alcohols, undetermined**

✓5th **T51.9** **Toxic effect of unspecified alcohol**

    ✓x7th **T51.91** **Toxic effect of unspecified alcohol, accidental (unintentional)**

    7 ✓x7th **T51.92** **Toxic effect of unspecified alcohol, intentional self-harm**   HCC

    ✓x7th **T51.93** **Toxic effect of unspecified alcohol, assault**

    ✓x7th **T51.94** **Toxic effect of unspecified alcohol, undetermined**

✓4th **T52** **Toxic effect of organic solvents**
EXCLUDES 1 *halogen derivatives of aliphatic and aromatic hydrocarbons (T53.-)*

The appropriate 7th character is to be added to each code from category T52.
A   initial encounter
D   subsequent encounter
S   sequela

✓5th **T52.0** **Toxic effects of petroleum products**
Toxic effects of ether petroleum
Toxic effects of gasoline [petrol]
Toxic effects of kerosene [paraffin oil]
Toxic effects of naphtha petroleum
Toxic effects of paraffin wax
Toxic effects of spirit petroleum

    ✓6th **T52.0X** **Toxic effects of petroleum products**

      ✓7th **T52.0X1** **Toxic effect of petroleum products, accidental (unintentional)**
Toxic effects of petroleum products NOS

      7 ✓7th **T52.0X2** **Toxic effect of petroleum products, intentional self-harm**   HCC

      ✓7th **T52.0X3** **Toxic effect of petroleum products, assault**

      ✓7th **T52.0X4** **Toxic effect of petroleum products, undetermined**

✓5th **T52.1** **Toxic effects of benzene**
EXCLUDES 1 *homologues of benzene (T52.2)*
nitroderivatives and aminoderivatives of benzene and its homologues (T65.3)

    ✓6th **T52.1X** **Toxic effects of benzene**

      ✓7th **T52.1X1** **Toxic effect of benzene, accidental (unintentional)**
Toxic effects of benzene NOS

      7 ✓7th **T52.1X2** **Toxic effect of benzene, intentional self-harm**   HCC

      ✓7th **T52.1X3** **Toxic effect of benzene, assault**

      ✓7th **T52.1X4** **Toxic effect of benzene, undetermined**

✓5th **T52.2** **Toxic effects of homologues of benzene**
Toxic effects of toluene [methylbenzene]
Toxic effects of xylene [dimethylbenzene]

    ✓6th **T52.2X** **Toxic effects of homologues of benzene**

      ✓7th **T52.2X1** **Toxic effect of homologues of benzene, accidental (unintentional)**
Toxic effects of homologues of benzene NOS

      7 ✓7th **T52.2X2** **Toxic effect of homologues of benzene, intentional self-harm**   HCC

      ✓7th **T52.2X3** **Toxic effect of homologues of benzene, assault**

      ✓7th **T52.2X4** **Toxic effect of homologues of benzene, undetermined**

✓5th **T52.3** **Toxic effects of glycols**

    ✓6th **T52.3X** **Toxic effects of glycols**

      ✓7th **T52.3X1** **Toxic effect of glycols, accidental (unintentional)**
Toxic effects of glycols NOS

      7 ✓7th **T52.3X2** **Toxic effect of glycols, intentional self-harm**   HCC

      ✓7th **T52.3X3** **Toxic effect of glycols, assault**

      ✓7th **T52.3X4** **Toxic effect of glycols, undetermined**

✓5th **T52.4** **Toxic effects of ketones**

    ✓6th **T52.4X** **Toxic effects of ketones**

      ✓7th **T52.4X1** **Toxic effect of ketones, accidental (unintentional)**
Toxic effects of ketones NOS

      7 ✓7th **T52.4X2** **Toxic effect of ketones, intentional self-harm**   HCC

      ✓7th **T52.4X3** **Toxic effect of ketones, assault**

      ✓7th **T52.4X4** **Toxic effect of ketones, undetermined**

✓5th **T52.8** **Toxic effects of other organic solvents**

    ✓6th **T52.8X** **Toxic effects of other organic solvents**

      ✓7th **T52.8X1** **Toxic effect of other organic solvents, accidental (unintentional)**
Toxic effects of other organic solvents NOS

      7 ✓7th **T52.8X2** **Toxic effect of other organic solvents, intentional self-harm**   HCC

      ✓7th **T52.8X3** **Toxic effect of other organic solvents, assault**

      ✓7th **T52.8X4** **Toxic effect of other organic solvents, undetermined**

✓5th **T52.9** **Toxic effects of unspecified organic solvent**

    ✓x7th **T52.91** **Toxic effect of unspecified organic solvent, accidental (unintentional)**

    7 ✓x7th **T52.92** **Toxic effect of unspecified organic solvent, intentional self-harm**   HCC

    ✓x7th **T52.93** **Toxic effect of unspecified organic solvent, assault**

    ✓x7th **T52.94** **Toxic effect of unspecified organic solvent, undetermined**

✓4th **T53** **Toxic effect of halogen derivatives of aliphatic and aromatic hydrocarbons**

The appropriate 7th character is to be added to each code from category T53.
A   initial encounter
D   subsequent encounter
S   sequela

✓5th **T53.0** **Toxic effects of carbon tetrachloride**
Toxic effects of tetrachloromethane

    ✓6th **T53.0X** **Toxic effects of carbon tetrachloride**

      ✓7th **T53.0X1** **Toxic effect of carbon tetrachloride, accidental (unintentional)**
Toxic effects of carbon tetrachloride NOS

      7 ✓7th **T53.0X2** **Toxic effect of carbon tetrachloride, intentional self-harm**   HCC

      ✓7th **T53.0X3** **Toxic effect of carbon tetrachloride, assault**

      ✓7th **T53.0X4** **Toxic effect of carbon tetrachloride, undetermined**

N Newborn: 0   **P** Pediatric: 0-17   **M** Maternity: 12-55   **A** Adult: 15-124   **MCC** Major Complication/Comorbidity   **CC** Complication/Comorbidity   **SW** Severe Wound Dx

1124   ICD-10-CM 2019

✓5th **T53.1 Toxic effects of chloroform**
Toxic effects of trichloromethane

    ✓6th **T53.1X Toxic effects of** chloroform

       ✓7th **T53.1X1 Toxic effect of chloroform,** accidental **(unintentional)**
Toxic effects of chloroform NOS

       7 ✓7th **T53.1X2 Toxic effect of chloroform,**   **HCC** intentional self-harm

       ✓7th **T53.1X3 Toxic effect of chloroform,** assault

       ✓7th **T53.1X4 Toxic effect of chloroform,** undetermined

✓5th **T53.2 Toxic effects of trichloroethylene**
Toxic effects of trichloroethene

    ✓6th **T53.2X Toxic effects of** trichloroethylene

       ✓7th **T53.2X1 Toxic effect of trichloroethylene,** accidental **(unintentional)**
Toxic effects of trichloroethylene NOS

       7 ✓7th **T53.2X2 Toxic effect of trichloroethylene,**   **HCC** intentional self-harm

       ✓7th **T53.2X3 Toxic effect of trichloroethylene,** assault

       ✓7th **T53.2X4 Toxic effect of trichloroethylene,** undetermined

✓5th **T53.3 Toxic effects of tetrachloroethylene**
Toxic effects of perchloroethylene
Toxic effect of tetrachloroethene

    ✓6th **T53.3X Toxic effects of** tetrachloroethylene

       ✓7th **T53.3X1 Toxic effect of tetrachloroethylene,** accidental **(unintentional)**
Toxic effects of tetrachloroethylene NOS

       7 ✓7th **T53.3X2 Toxic effect of tetrachloroethylene,**   **HCC** intentional self-harm

       ✓7th **T53.3X3 Toxic effect of tetrachloroethylene,** assault

       ✓7th **T53.3X4 Toxic effect of tetrachloroethylene,** undetermined

✓5th **T53.4 Toxic effects of dichloromethane**
Toxic effects of methylene chloride

    ✓6th **T53.4X Toxic effects of** dichloromethane

       ✓7th **T53.4X1 Toxic effect of dichloromethane,** accidental **(unintentional)**
Toxic effects of dichloromethane NOS

       7 ✓7th **T53.4X2 Toxic effect of dichloromethane,**   **HCC** intentional self-harm

       ✓7th **T53.4X3 Toxic effect of dichloromethane,** assault

       ✓7th **T53.4X4 Toxic effect of dichloromethane,** undetermined

✓5th **T53.5 Toxic effects of chlorofluorocarbons**

    ✓6th **T53.5X Toxic effects of** chlorofluorocarbons

       ✓7th **T53.5X1 Toxic effect of chlorofluorocarbons,** accidental **(unintentional)**
Toxic effects of chlorofluorocarbons NOS

       7 ✓7th **T53.5X2 Toxic effect of chlorofluorocarbons,**   **HCC** intentional self-harm

       ✓7th **T53.5X3 Toxic effect of chlorofluorocarbons,** assault

       ✓7th **T53.5X4 Toxic effect of chlorofluorocarbons,** undetermined

✓5th **T53.6 Toxic effects of other halogen derivatives of aliphatic hydrocarbons**

    ✓6th **T53.6X Toxic effects of other** halogen derivatives of aliphatic hydrocarbons

       ✓7th **T53.6X1 Toxic effect of other halogen derivatives of aliphatic hydrocarbons,** accidental **(unintentional)**
Toxic effects of other halogen derivatives of aliphatic hydrocarbons NOS

       7 ✓7th **T53.6X2 Toxic effect of other halogen derivatives of aliphatic hydrocarbons,**   **HCC** intentional self-harm

       ✓7th **T53.6X3 Toxic effect of other halogen derivatives of aliphatic hydrocarbons,** assault

       ✓7th **T53.6X4 Toxic effect of other halogen derivatives of aliphatic hydrocarbons,** undetermined

✓5th **T53.7 Toxic effects of other halogen derivatives of aromatic hydrocarbons**

    ✓6th **T53.7X Toxic effects of other** halogen derivatives of aromatic hydrocarbons

       ✓7th **T53.7X1 Toxic effect of other halogen derivatives of aromatic hydrocarbons,** accidental **(unintentional)**
Toxic effects of other halogen derivatives of aromatic hydrocarbons NOS

       7 ✓7th **T53.7X2 Toxic effect of other halogen**   **HCC** **derivatives of aromatic hydrocarbons,** intentional self-harm

       ✓7th **T53.7X3 Toxic effect of other halogen derivatives of aromatic hydrocarbons,** assault

       ✓7th **T53.7X4 Toxic effect of other halogen derivatives of aromatic hydrocarbons,** undetermined

✓5th **T53.9 Toxic effects of** unspecified halogen derivatives of aliphatic and aromatic hydrocarbons

    ✓x7th **T53.91 Toxic effect of unspecified halogen derivatives of aliphatic and aromatic hydrocarbons,** accidental **(unintentional)**

    7 ✓x7th **T53.92 Toxic effect of unspecified halogen derivatives**   **HCC** **of aliphatic and aromatic hydrocarbons,** intentional self-harm

    ✓x7th **T53.93 Toxic effect of unspecified halogen derivatives of aliphatic and aromatic hydrocarbons,** assault

    ✓x7th **T53.94 Toxic effect of unspecified halogen derivatives of aliphatic and aromatic hydrocarbons,** undetermined

✓4th **T54 Toxic effect of corrosive substances**

> The appropriate 7th character is to be added to each code from category T54.
> A   initial encounter
> D   subsequent encounter
> S   sequela

✓5th **T54.0 Toxic effects of phenol and phenol homologues**

    ✓6th **T54.0X Toxic effects of** phenol and phenol homologues

       ✓7th **T54.0X1 Toxic effect of phenol and phenol homologues,** accidental **(unintentional)**
Toxic effects of phenol and phenol homologues NOS

       7 ✓7th **T54.0X2 Toxic effect of phenol and phenol**   **HCC** **homologues,** intentional self-harm

       ✓7th **T54.0X3 Toxic effect of phenol and phenol homologues,** assault

       ✓7th **T54.0X4 Toxic effect of phenol and phenol homologues,** undetermined

✓5th **T54.1 Toxic effects of other corrosive organic compounds**

    ✓6th **T54.1X Toxic effects of** other corrosive organic compounds

       ✓7th **T54.1X1 Toxic effect of other corrosive organic compounds,** accidental **(unintentional)**
Toxic effects of other corrosive organic compounds NOS

       7 ✓7th **T54.1X2 Toxic effect of other corrosive organic** **HCC** **compounds,** intentional self-harm

       ✓7th **T54.1X3 Toxic effect of other corrosive organic compounds,** assault

       ✓7th **T54.1X4 Toxic effect of other corrosive organic compounds,** undetermined

✓5th **T54.2 Toxic effects of corrosive acids and acid-like substances**
Toxic effects of hydrochloric acid
Toxic effects of sulfuric acid

    ✓6th **T54.2X Toxic effects of corrosive** acids and acid-like substances

       ✓7th **T54.2X1 Toxic effect of corrosive acids and acid-like substances,** accidental **(unintentional)**
Toxic effects of corrosive acids and acid-like substances NOS

       7 ✓7th **T54.2X2 Toxic effect of corrosive acids and**   **HCC** **acid-like substances,** intentional self-harm

       ✓7th **T54.2X3 Toxic effect of corrosive acids and acid-like substances,** assault

       ✓7th **T54.2X4 Toxic effect of corrosive acids and acid-like substances,** undetermined

✓ Additional Character Required   ✓x7th Placeholder   Unacceptable PDx   Questionable PDx   Manifestation   H1 - H14 HAC   HCC CMS-HCC Dx   HIV HIV Dx

ICD-10-CM 2019   1125

√5ᵗʰ **T54.3 Toxic effects of corrosive alkalis and alkali-like substances**
Toxic effects of potassium hydroxide
Toxic effects of sodium hydroxide

√6ᵗʰ **T54.3X Toxic effects of corrosive** alkalis and alkali-like substances

√7ᵗʰ **T54.3X1 Toxic effect of corrosive alkalis and alkali-like substances,** accidental **(unintentional)**
Toxic effects of corrosive alkalis and alkali-like substances NOS

7 √7ᵗʰ **T54.3X2 Toxic effect of corrosive alkalis and alkali-like substances,** intentional self-harm   HCC

√7ᵗʰ **T54.3X3 Toxic effect of corrosive alkalis and alkali-like substances,** assault

√7ᵗʰ **T54.3X4 Toxic effect of corrosive alkalis and alkali-like substances,** undetermined

√5ᵗʰ **T54.9 Toxic effects of** unspecified **corrosive substance**

√x7ᵗʰ **T54.91 Toxic effect of unspecified corrosive substance,** accidental **(unintentional)**

7 √x7ᵗʰ **T54.92 Toxic effect of unspecified corrosive substance,** intentional self-harm   HCC

√x7ᵗʰ **T54.93 Toxic effect of unspecified corrosive substance,** assault

√x7ᵗʰ **T54.94 Toxic effect of unspecified corrosive substance,** undetermined

√4ᵗʰ **T55 Toxic effect of soaps and detergents**

The appropriate 7th character is to be added to each code from category T55.
A   initial encounter
D   subsequent encounter
S   sequela

√5ᵗʰ **T55.Ø Toxic effect of soaps**

√6ᵗʰ **T55.ØX Toxic effect of** soaps

√7ᵗʰ **T55.ØX1 Toxic effect of soaps,** accidental **(unintentional)**
Toxic effect of soaps NOS

7 √7ᵗʰ **T55.ØX2 Toxic effect of soaps,** intentional self-harm   HCC

√7ᵗʰ **T55.ØX3 Toxic effect of soaps,** assault

√7ᵗʰ **T55.ØX4 Toxic effect of soaps,** undetermined

√5ᵗʰ **T55.1 Toxic effect of detergents**

√6ᵗʰ **T55.1X Toxic effect of** detergents

√7ᵗʰ **T55.1X1 Toxic effect of detergents,** accidental **(unintentional)**
Toxic effect of detergents NOS

7 √7ᵗʰ **T55.1X2 Toxic effect of detergents,** intentional self-harm   HCC

√7ᵗʰ **T55.1X3 Toxic effect of detergents,** assault

√7ᵗʰ **T55.1X4 Toxic effect of detergents,** undetermined

√4ᵗʰ **T56 Toxic effect of metals**
INCLUDES   toxic effects of fumes and vapors of metals
toxic effects of metals from all sources, except medicinal substances
Use additional code to identify any retained metal foreign body, if applicable (Z18.Ø-, T18.1-)
EXCLUDES 1   arsenic and its compounds (T57.Ø)
manganese and its compounds (T57.2)

The appropriate 7th character is to be added to each code from category T56.
A   initial encounter
D   subsequent encounter
S   sequela

√5ᵗʰ **T56.Ø Toxic effects of lead and its compounds**

√6ᵗʰ **T56.ØX Toxic effects of** lead **and its compounds**

√7ᵗʰ **T56.ØX1 Toxic effect of lead and its compounds,** accidental **(unintentional)**
Toxic effects of lead and its compounds NOS

7 √7ᵗʰ **T56.ØX2 Toxic effect of lead and its compounds,** intentional self-harm   HCC

√7ᵗʰ **T56.ØX3 Toxic effect of lead and its compounds,** assault

√7ᵗʰ **T56.ØX4 Toxic effect of lead and its compounds,** undetermined

√5ᵗʰ **T56.1 Toxic effects of mercury and its compounds**

√6ᵗʰ **T56.1X Toxic effects of** mercury **and its compounds**

√7ᵗʰ **T56.1X1 Toxic effect of mercury and its compounds,** accidental **(unintentional)**
Toxic effects of mercury and its compounds NOS

7 √7ᵗʰ **T56.1X2 Toxic effect of mercury and its compounds,** intentional self-harm   HCC

√7ᵗʰ **T56.1X3 Toxic effect of mercury and its compounds,** assault

√7ᵗʰ **T56.1X4 Toxic effect of mercury and its compounds,** undetermined

√5ᵗʰ **T56.2 Toxic effects of chromium and its compounds**

√6ᵗʰ **T56.2X Toxic effects of** chromium **and its compounds**

√7ᵗʰ **T56.2X1 Toxic effect of chromium and its compounds,** accidental **(unintentional)**
Toxic effects of chromium and its compounds NOS

7 √7ᵗʰ **T56.2X2 Toxic effect of chromium and its compounds,** intentional self-harm   HCC

√7ᵗʰ **T56.2X3 Toxic effect of chromium and its compounds,** assault

√7ᵗʰ **T56.2X4 Toxic effect of chromium and its compounds,** undetermined

√5ᵗʰ **T56.3 Toxic effects of cadmium and its compounds**

√6ᵗʰ **T56.3X Toxic effects of cadmium and its compounds**

√7ᵗʰ **T56.3X1 Toxic effect of cadmium and its compounds,** accidental **(unintentional)**
Toxic effects of cadmium and its compounds NOS

7 √7ᵗʰ **T56.3X2 Toxic effect of cadmium and its compounds,** intentional self-harm   HCC

√7ᵗʰ **T56.3X3 Toxic effect of cadmium and its compounds,** assault

√7ᵗʰ **T56.3X4 Toxic effect of cadmium and its compounds,** undetermined

√5ᵗʰ **T56.4 Toxic effects of copper and its compounds**

√6ᵗʰ **T56.4X Toxic effects of** copper **and its compounds**

√7ᵗʰ **T56.4X1 Toxic effect of copper and its compounds,** accidental **(unintentional)**
Toxic effects of copper and its compounds NOS

7 √7ᵗʰ **T56.4X2 Toxic effect of copper and its compounds,** intentional self-harm   HCC

√7ᵗʰ **T56.4X3 Toxic effect of copper and its compounds,** assault

√7ᵗʰ **T56.4X4 Toxic effect of copper and its compounds,** undetermined

√5ᵗʰ **T56.5 Toxic effects of zinc and its compounds**

√6ᵗʰ **T56.5X Toxic effects of** zinc **and its compounds**

√7ᵗʰ **T56.5X1 Toxic effect of zinc and its compounds,** accidental **(unintentional)**
Toxic effects of zinc and its compounds NOS

7 √7ᵗʰ **T56.5X2 Toxic effect of zinc and its compounds,** intentional self-harm   HCC

√7ᵗʰ **T56.5X3 Toxic effect of zinc and its compounds,** assault

√7ᵗʰ **T56.5X4 Toxic effect of zinc and its compounds,** undetermined

√5ᵗʰ **T56.6 Toxic effects of tin and its compounds**

√6ᵗʰ **T56.6X Toxic effects of** tin **and its compounds**

√7ᵗʰ **T56.6X1 Toxic effect of tin and its compounds,** accidental **(unintentional)**
Toxic effects of tin and its compounds NOS

7 √7ᵗʰ **T56.6X2 Toxic effect of tin and its compounds,** intentional self-harm   HCC

√7ᵗʰ **T56.6X3 Toxic effect of tin and its compounds,** assault

√7ᵗʰ **T56.6X4 Toxic effect of tin and its compounds,** undetermined

N Newborn: 0   P Pediatric: 0-17   M Maternity: 12-55   A Adult: 15-124   MCC Major Complication/Comorbidity   CC Complication/Comorbidity   SW Severe Wound Dx

1126   ICD-10-CM 2019

√5th **T56.7 Toxic effects of beryllium and its compounds**

√6th **T56.7X Toxic effects of** beryllium **and its compounds**

√7th **T56.7X1 Toxic effect of beryllium and its compounds, accidental (unintentional)**
Toxic effects of beryllium and its compounds NOS

7 √7th **T56.7X2 Toxic effect of beryllium and its compounds, intentional self-harm** `HCC`

√7th **T56.7X3 Toxic effect of beryllium and its compounds, assault**

√7th **T56.7X4 Toxic effect of beryllium and its compounds, undetermined**

√5th **T56.8 Toxic effects of** other metals

√6th **T56.81 Toxic effect of** thallium

√7th **T56.811 Toxic effect of thallium, accidental (unintentional)**
Toxic effect of thallium NOS

7 √7th **T56.812 Toxic effect of thallium, intentional self-harm** `HCC`

√7th **T56.813 Toxic effect of thallium, assault**

√7th **T56.814 Toxic effect of thallium, undetermined**

√6th **T56.89 Toxic effects of** other metals

√7th **T56.891 Toxic effect of other metals, accidental (unintentional)**
Toxic effects of other metals NOS

7 √7th **T56.892 Toxic effect of other metals, intentional self-harm** `HCC`

√7th **T56.893 Toxic effect of other metals, assault**

√7th **T56.894 Toxic effect of other metals, undetermined**

√5th **T56.9 Toxic effects of** unspecified metal

√x7th **T56.91 Toxic effect of unspecified metal, accidental (unintentional)**

7 √x7th **T56.92 Toxic effect of unspecified metal, intentional self-harm** `HCC`

√x7th **T56.93 Toxic effect of unspecified metal, assault**

√x7th **T56.94 Toxic effect of unspecified metal, undetermined**

√4th **T57 Toxic effect of other inorganic substances**

> The appropriate 7th character is to be added to each code from category T57.
> A   initial encounter
> D   subsequent encounter
> S   sequela

√5th **T57.0 Toxic effect of arsenic and its compounds**

√6th **T57.0X Toxic effect of** arsenic **and its compounds**

√7th **T57.0X1 Toxic effect of arsenic and its compounds, accidental (unintentional)**
Toxic effect of arsenic and its compounds NOS

7 √7th **T57.0X2 Toxic effect of arsenic and its compounds, intentional self-harm** `HCC`

√7th **T57.0X3 Toxic effect of arsenic and its compounds, assault**

√7th **T57.0X4 Toxic effect of arsenic and its compounds, undetermined**

√5th **T57.1 Toxic effect of phosphorus and its compounds**
`EXCLUDES 1` organophosphate insecticides (T60.0)

√6th **T57.1X Toxic effect of** phosphorus **and its compounds**

√7th **T57.1X1 Toxic effect of phosphorus and its compounds, accidental (unintentional)**
Toxic effect of phosphorus and its compounds NOS

7 √7th **T57.1X2 Toxic effect of phosphorus and its compounds, intentional self-harm** `HCC`

√7th **T57.1X3 Toxic effect of phosphorus and its compounds, assault**

√7th **T57.1X4 Toxic effect of phosphorus and its compounds, undetermined**

√5th **T57.2 Toxic effect of manganese and its compounds**

√6th **T57.2X Toxic effect of** manganese **and its compounds**

√7th **T57.2X1 Toxic effect of** manganese **and its compounds, accidental (unintentional)**
Toxic effect of manganese and its compounds NOS

7 √7th **T57.2X2 Toxic effect of manganese and its compounds, intentional self-harm** `HCC`

√7th **T57.2X3 Toxic effect of manganese and its compounds, assault**

√7th **T57.2X4 Toxic effect of manganese and its compounds, undetermined**

√5th **T57.3 Toxic effect of hydrogen cyanide**

√6th **T57.3X Toxic effect of** hydrogen cyanide

√7th **T57.3X1 Toxic effect of hydrogen cyanide, accidental (unintentional)**
Toxic effect of hydrogen cyanide NOS

7 √7th **T57.3X2 Toxic effect of hydrogen cyanide, intentional self-harm** `HCC`

√7th **T57.3X3 Toxic effect of hydrogen cyanide, assault**

√7th **T57.3X4 Toxic effect of hydrogen cyanide, undetermined**

√5th **T57.8 Toxic effect of other specified inorganic substances**

√6th **T57.8X Toxic effect of** other **specified** inorganic substances

√7th **T57.8X1 Toxic effect of other specified inorganic substances, accidental (unintentional)**
Toxic effect of other specified inorganic substances NOS

7 √7th **T57.8X2 Toxic effect of other specified inorganic substances, intentional self-harm** `HCC`

√7th **T57.8X3 Toxic effect of other specified inorganic substances, assault**

√7th **T57.8X4 Toxic effect of other specified inorganic substances, undetermined**

√5th **T57.9 Toxic effect of** unspecified inorganic substance

√x7th **T57.91 Toxic effect of unspecified inorganic substance, accidental (unintentional)**

7 √x7th **T57.92 Toxic effect of unspecified inorganic substance, intentional self-harm** `HCC`

√x7th **T57.93 Toxic effect of unspecified inorganic substance, assault**

√x7th **T57.94 Toxic effect of unspecified inorganic substance, undetermined**

√4th **T58 Toxic effect of carbon monoxide**
`INCLUDES` asphyxiation from carbon monoxide
toxic effect of carbon monoxide from all sources

> The appropriate 7th character is to be added to each code from category T58.
> A   initial encounter
> D   subsequent encounter
> S   sequela

√5th **T58.0 Toxic effect of carbon monoxide** from motor vehicle exhaust
Toxic effect of exhaust gas from gas engine
Toxic effect of exhaust gas from motor pump

√x7th **T58.01 Toxic effect of carbon monoxide from motor vehicle exhaust, accidental (unintentional)**

7 √x7th **T58.02 Toxic effect of carbon monoxide from motor vehicle exhaust, intentional self-harm** `HCC`

√x7th **T58.03 Toxic effect of carbon monoxide from motor vehicle exhaust, assault**

√x7th **T58.04 Toxic effect of carbon monoxide from motor vehicle exhaust, undetermined**

√5th **T58.1 Toxic effect of carbon monoxide** from utility gas
Toxic effect of acetylene
Toxic effect of gas NOS used for lighting, heating, cooking
Toxic effect of water gas

√x7th **T58.11 Toxic effect of carbon monoxide from utility gas, accidental (unintentional)**

7 √x7th **T58.12 Toxic effect of carbon monoxide from utility gas, intentional self-harm** `HCC`

√x7th **T58.13 Toxic effect of carbon monoxide from utility gas, assault**

√x7th **T58.14 Toxic effect of carbon monoxide from utility gas, undetermined**

✓5th **T58.2** **Toxic effect of carbon monoxide** from incomplete combustion of other domestic fuels
> Toxic effect of carbon monoxide from incomplete combustion of coal, coke, kerosene, wood

    ✓6th **T58.2X** **Toxic effect of carbon monoxide from incomplete combustion of other domestic fuels**

        ✓7th **T58.2X1** **Toxic effect of carbon monoxide from incomplete combustion of other domestic fuels**, accidental (unintentional)

        7 ✓7th **T58.2X2** **Toxic effect of carbon monoxide from incomplete combustion of other domestic fuels**, intentional self-harm   HCC

        ✓7th **T58.2X3** **Toxic effect of carbon monoxide from incomplete combustion of other domestic fuels**, assault

        ✓7th **T58.2X4** **Toxic effect of carbon monoxide from incomplete combustion of other domestic fuels**, undetermined

✓5th **T58.8** **Toxic effect of carbon monoxide** from other source
> Toxic effect of carbon monoxide from blast furnace gas
> Toxic effect of carbon monoxide from fuels in industrial use
> Toxic effect of carbon monoxide from kiln vapor

    ✓6th **T58.8X** **Toxic effect of carbon monoxide from other source**

        ✓7th **T58.8X1** **Toxic effect of carbon monoxide from other source**, accidental (unintentional)

        7 ✓7th **T58.8X2** **Toxic effect of carbon monoxide from other source**, intentional self-harm   HCC

        ✓7th **T58.8X3** **Toxic effect of carbon monoxide from other source**, assault

        ✓7th **T58.8X4** **Toxic effect of carbon monoxide from other source**, undetermined

✓5th **T58.9** **Toxic effect of carbon monoxide** from unspecified source

    ✓x7th **T58.91** **Toxic effect of carbon monoxide from unspecified source**, accidental (unintentional)

    7 ✓x7th **T58.92** **Toxic effect of carbon monoxide from unspecified source**, intentional self-harm   HCC

    ✓x7th **T58.93** **Toxic effect of carbon monoxide from unspecified source**, assault

    ✓x7th **T58.94** **Toxic effect of carbon monoxide from unspecified source**, undetermined

✓4th **T59** **Toxic effect of other gases, fumes and vapors**
> INCLUDES   aerosol propellants
> EXCLUDES 1   *chlorofluorocarbons (T53.5)*

> The appropriate 7th character is to be added to each code from category T59.
> A   initial encounter
> D   subsequent encounter
> S   sequela

✓5th **T59.0** **Toxic effect of nitrogen oxides**

    ✓6th **T59.0X** **Toxic effect of nitrogen oxides**

        ✓7th **T59.0X1** **Toxic effect of nitrogen oxides**, accidental (unintentional)
> Toxic effect of nitrogen oxides NOS

        7 ✓7th **T59.0X2** **Toxic effect of nitrogen oxides**, intentional self-harm   HCC

        ✓7th **T59.0X3** **Toxic effect of nitrogen oxides**, assault

        ✓7th **T59.0X4** **Toxic effect of nitrogen oxides**, undetermined

✓5th **T59.1** **Toxic effect of sulfur dioxide**

    ✓6th **T59.1X** **Toxic effect of sulfur dioxide**

        ✓7th **T59.1X1** **Toxic effect of sulfur dioxide**, accidental (unintentional)
> Toxic effect of sulfur dioxide NOS

        7 ✓7th **T59.1X2** **Toxic effect of sulfur dioxide**, intentional self-harm   HCC

        ✓7th **T59.1X3** **Toxic effect of sulfur dioxide**, assault

        ✓7th **T59.1X4** **Toxic effect of sulfur dioxide**, undetermined

✓5th **T59.2** **Toxic effect of formaldehyde**

    ✓6th **T59.2X** **Toxic effect of** formaldehyde

        ✓7th **T59.2X1** **Toxic effect of formaldehyde**, accidental (unintentional)
> Toxic effect of formaldehyde NOS

        7 ✓7th **T59.2X2** **Toxic effect of formaldehyde**, intentional self-harm   HCC

        ✓7th **T59.2X3** **Toxic effect of formaldehyde**, assault

        ✓7th **T59.2X4** **Toxic effect of formaldehyde**, undetermined

✓5th **T59.3** **Toxic effect of lacrimogenic gas**
> Toxic effect of tear gas

    ✓6th **T59.3X** **Toxic effect of** lacrimogenic gas

        ✓7th **T59.3X1** **Toxic effect of lacrimogenic gas**, accidental (unintentional)
> Toxic effect of lacrimogenic gas NOS

        7 ✓7th **T59.3X2** **Toxic effect of lacrimogenic gas**, intentional self-harm   HCC

        ✓7th **T59.3X3** **Toxic effect of lacrimogenic gas**, assault

        ✓7th **T59.3X4** **Toxic effect of lacrimogenic gas**, undetermined

✓5th **T59.4** **Toxic effect of chlorine gas**

    ✓6th **T59.4X** **Toxic effect of** chlorine gas

        ✓7th **T59.4X1** **Toxic effect of chlorine gas**, accidental (unintentional)
> Toxic effect of chlorine gas NOS

        7 ✓7th **T59.4X2** **Toxic effect of chlorine gas**, intentional self-harm   HCC

        ✓7th **T59.4X3** **Toxic effect of chlorine gas**, assault

        ✓7th **T59.4X4** **Toxic effect of chlorine gas**, undetermined

✓5th **T59.5** **Toxic effect of fluorine gas and hydrogen fluoride**

    ✓6th **T59.5X** **Toxic effect of** fluorine gas and hydrogen fluoride

        ✓7th **T59.5X1** **Toxic effect of fluorine gas and hydrogen fluoride**, accidental (unintentional)
> Toxic effect of fluorine gas and hydrogen fluoride NOS

        7 ✓7th **T59.5X2** **Toxic effect of fluorine gas and hydrogen fluoride**, intentional self-harm   HCC

        ✓7th **T59.5X3** **Toxic effect of fluorine gas and hydrogen fluoride**, assault

        ✓7th **T59.5X4** **Toxic effect of fluorine gas and hydrogen fluoride**, undetermined

✓5th **T59.6** **Toxic effect of hydrogen sulfide**

    ✓6th **T59.6X** **Toxic effect of** hydrogen sulfide

        ✓7th **T59.6X1** **Toxic effect of hydrogen sulfide**, accidental (unintentional)
> Toxic effect of hydrogen sulfide NOS

        7 ✓7th **T59.6X2** **Toxic effect of hydrogen sulfide**, intentional self-harm   HCC

        ✓7th **T59.6X3** **Toxic effect of hydrogen sulfide**, assault

        ✓7th **T59.6X4** **Toxic effect of hydrogen sulfide**, undetermined

✓5th **T59.7** **Toxic effect of carbon dioxide**

    ✓6th **T59.7X** **Toxic effect of** carbon dioxide

        ✓7th **T59.7X1** **Toxic effect of carbon dioxide**, accidental (unintentional)
> Toxic effect of carbon dioxide NOS

        7 ✓7th **T59.7X2** **Toxic effect of carbon dioxide**, intentional self-harm   HCC

        ✓7th **T59.7X3** **Toxic effect of carbon dioxide**, assault

        ✓7th **T59.7X4** **Toxic effect of carbon dioxide**, undetermined

✓5th **T59.8** **Toxic effect of** other specified gases, fumes and vapors

    ✓6th **T59.81** **Toxic effect of** smoke
> Smoke inhalation
> EXCLUDES 2   *toxic effect of cigarette (tobacco) smoke (T65.22-)*

        ✓7th **T59.811** **Toxic effect of smoke**, accidental (unintentional)
> Toxic effect of smoke NOS
> **AHA:** 2013, 4Q, 121

        7 ✓7th **T59.812** **Toxic effect of smoke**, intentional self-harm   HCC

        ✓7th **T59.813** **Toxic effect of smoke**, assault

        ✓7th **T59.814** **Toxic effect of smoke**, undetermined

    ✓6th **T59.89** **Toxic effect of** other specified gases, fumes and vapors

        ✓7th **T59.891** **Toxic effect of other specified gases, fumes and vapors**, accidental (unintentional)

N Newborn: 0   P Pediatric: 0-17   M Maternity: 12-55   A Adult: 15-124   MCC Major Complication/Comorbidity   CC Complication/Comorbidity   SW Severe Wound Dx

1128   ICD-10-CM 2019

7 ✓7ᵗʰ **T59.892** **Toxic effect of other specified gases,** HCC
fumes and vapors, intentional self-harm

✓7ᵗʰ **T59.893** **Toxic effect of other specified gases,**
fumes and vapors, assault

✓7ᵗʰ **T59.894** **Toxic effect of other specified gases,**
fumes and vapors, undetermined

✓5ᵗʰ **T59.9** **Toxic effect of** unspecified **gases, fumes and vapors**

✓x7ᵗʰ **T59.91** **Toxic effect of unspecified gases, fumes and vapors,**
accidental **(unintentional)**

7 ✓x7ᵗʰ **T59.92** **Toxic effect of unspecified gases, fumes and** HCC
vapors, intentional self-harm

✓x7ᵗʰ **T59.93** **Toxic effect of unspecified gases, fumes and vapors,**
assault

✓x7ᵗʰ **T59.94** **Toxic effect of unspecified gases, fumes and vapors,**
undetermined

✓4ᵗʰ **T60** **Toxic effect of pesticides**
INCLUDES   toxic effect of wood preservatives

The appropriate 7th character is to be added to each code from
category T60.
A   initial encounter
D   subsequent encounter
S   sequela

✓5ᵗʰ **T60.0** **Toxic effect of organophosphate and carbamate insecticides**

✓6ᵗʰ **T60.0X** **Toxic effect of** organophosphate and carbamate
insecticides

✓7ᵗʰ **T60.0X1** **Toxic effect of organophosphate and**
carbamate insecticides, accidental
(unintentional)
Toxic effect of organophosphate and
carbamate insecticides NOS

7 ✓7ᵗʰ **T60.0X2** **Toxic effect of organophosphate and** HCC
carbamate insecticides, intentional self-
harm

✓7ᵗʰ **T60.0X3** **Toxic effect of organophosphate and**
carbamate insecticides, assault

✓7ᵗʰ **T60.0X4** **Toxic effect of organophosphate and**
carbamate insecticides, undetermined

✓5ᵗʰ **T60.1** **Toxic effect of halogenated insecticides**
EXCLUDES 1   chlorinated hydrocarbon (T53.-)

✓6ᵗʰ **T60.1X** **Toxic effect of** halogenated insecticides

✓7ᵗʰ **T60.1X1** **Toxic effect of halogenated insecticides,**
accidental **(unintentional)**
Toxic effect of halogenated insecticides
NOS

7 ✓7ᵗʰ **T60.1X2** **Toxic effect of halogenated** HCC
insecticides, intentional self-harm

✓7ᵗʰ **T60.1X3** **Toxic effect of halogenated insecticides,**
assault

✓7ᵗʰ **T60.1X4** **Toxic effect of halogenated insecticides,**
undetermined

✓5ᵗʰ **T60.2** **Toxic effect of other insecticides**

✓6ᵗʰ **T60.2X** **Toxic effect of** other insecticides

✓7ᵗʰ **T60.2X1** **Toxic effect of other insecticides,**
accidental **(unintentional)**
Toxic effect of other insecticides NOS

7 ✓7ᵗʰ **T60.2X2** **Toxic effect of other insecticides,** HCC
intentional self-harm

✓7ᵗʰ **T60.2X3** **Toxic effect of other insecticides,** assault

✓7ᵗʰ **T60.2X4** **Toxic effect of other insecticides,**
undetermined

✓5ᵗʰ **T60.3** **Toxic effect of herbicides and fungicides**

✓6ᵗʰ **T60.3X** **Toxic effect of** herbicides and fungicides

✓7ᵗʰ **T60.3X1** **Toxic effect of herbicides and fungicides,**
accidental **(unintentional)**
Toxic effect of herbicides and fungicides
NOS

7 ✓7ᵗʰ **T60.3X2** **Toxic effect of herbicides and** HCC
fungicides, intentional self-harm

✓7ᵗʰ **T60.3X3** **Toxic effect of herbicides and fungicides,**
assault

✓7ᵗʰ **T60.3X4** **Toxic effect of herbicides and fungicides,**
undetermined

✓5ᵗʰ **T60.4** **Toxic effect of rodenticides**
EXCLUDES 1   strychnine and its salts (T65.1)
thallium (T56.81-)

✓6ᵗʰ **T60.4X** **Toxic effect of** rodenticides

✓7ᵗʰ **T60.4X1** **Toxic effect of rodenticides,** accidental
(unintentional)
Toxic effect of rodenticides NOS

7 ✓7ᵗʰ **T60.4X2** **Toxic effect of rodenticides,** HCC
intentional self-harm

✓7ᵗʰ **T60.4X3** **Toxic effect of rodenticides,** assault

✓7ᵗʰ **T60.4X4** **Toxic effect of rodenticides,**
undetermined

✓5ᵗʰ **T60.8** **Toxic effect of other pesticides**

✓6ᵗʰ **T60.8X** **Toxic effect of** other pesticides

✓7ᵗʰ **T60.8X1** **Toxic effect of other pesticides,** accidental
(unintentional)
Toxic effect of other pesticides NOS

7 ✓7ᵗʰ **T60.8X2** **Toxic effect of other pesticides,** HCC
intentional self-harm

✓7ᵗʰ **T60.8X3** **Toxic effect of other pesticides,** assault

✓7ᵗʰ **T60.8X4** **Toxic effect of other pesticides,**
undetermined

✓5ᵗʰ **T60.9** **Toxic effect of** unspecified pesticide

✓x7ᵗʰ **T60.91** **Toxic effect of unspecified pesticide,** accidental
(unintentional)

7 ✓x7ᵗʰ **T60.92** **Toxic effect of unspecified pesticide,** HCC
intentional self-harm

✓x7ᵗʰ **T60.93** **Toxic effect of unspecified pesticide,** assault

✓x7ᵗʰ **T60.94** **Toxic effect of unspecified pesticide,** undetermined

✓4ᵗʰ **T61** **Toxic effect of noxious substances eaten as seafood**
EXCLUDES 1   allergic reaction to food, such as:
anaphylactic reaction or shock due to adverse food reaction
(T78.0-)
bacterial foodborne intoxications (A05.-)
dermatitis (L23.6, L25.4, L27.2)
food protein-induced enterocolitis syndrome (K52.21)
food protein-induced enteropathy (K52.22)
gastroenteritis (noninfective) (K52.29)
toxic effect of aflatoxin and other mycotoxins (T64)
toxic effect of cyanides (T65.0-)
toxic effect of harmful algae bloom (T65.82-)
toxic effect of hydrogen cyanide (T57.3-)
toxic effect of mercury (T56.1-)
toxic effect of red tide (T65.82-)

The appropriate 7th character is to be added to each code from
category T61.
A   initial encounter
D   subsequent encounter
S   sequela

✓5ᵗʰ **T61.0** Ciguatera fish **poisoning**

✓x7ᵗʰ **T61.01** **Ciguatera fish poisoning,** accidental **(unintentional)**

7 ✓x7ᵗʰ **T61.02** **Ciguatera fish poisoning,** intentional self-harm HCC

✓x7ᵗʰ **T61.03** **Ciguatera fish poisoning,** assault

✓x7ᵗʰ **T61.04** **Ciguatera fish poisoning,** undetermined

✓5ᵗʰ **T61.1** Scombroid fish **poisoning**
Histamine-like syndrome

✓x7ᵗʰ **T61.11** **Scombroid fish poisoning,** accidental **(unintentional)**

7 ✓x7ᵗʰ **T61.12** **Scombroid fish poisoning,** intentional self-harm HCC

✓x7ᵗʰ **T61.13** **Scombroid fish poisoning,** assault

✓x7ᵗʰ **T61.14** **Scombroid fish poisoning,** undetermined

✓5ᵗʰ **T61.7** Other **fish and shellfish poisoning**

✓6ᵗʰ **T61.77** **Other** fish **poisoning**

✓7ᵗʰ **T61.771** **Other fish poisoning,** accidental
(unintentional)

7 ✓7ᵗʰ **T61.772** **Other fish poisoning,** intentional HCC
self-harm

✓7ᵗʰ **T61.773** **Other fish poisoning,** assault

✓7ᵗʰ **T61.774** **Other fish poisoning,** undetermined

✓6ᵗʰ **T61.78** **Other** shellfish **poisoning**

✓7ᵗʰ **T61.781** **Other shellfish poisoning,** accidental
(unintentional)

7 ✓7ᵗʰ **T61.782** **Other shellfish poisoning,** intentional HCC
self-harm

Chapter 19. Injury, Poisoning and Certain Other Consequences of External Causes

✓7th **T61.783**   **Other shellfish poisoning,** assault
✓7th **T61.784**   **Other shellfish poisoning,** undetermined

✓5th **T61.8**   **Toxic effect of other seafood**
   ✓6th **T61.8X**   **Toxic effect of** other seafood
     ✓7th **T61.8X1**   **Toxic effect of other seafood,** accidental **(unintentional)**
     7 ✓7th **T61.8X2**   **Toxic effect of other seafood,** intentional self-harm   HCC
     ✓7th **T61.8X3**   **Toxic effect of other seafood,** assault
     ✓7th **T61.8X4**   **Toxic effect of other seafood,** undetermined

✓5th **T61.9**   **Toxic effect of** unspecified seafood
   ✓x7th **T61.91**   **Toxic effect of unspecified seafood,** accidental **(unintentional)**
   7 ✓x7th **T61.92**   **Toxic effect of unspecified seafood,** intentional self-harm   HCC
   ✓x7th **T61.93**   **Toxic effect of unspecified seafood,** assault
   ✓x7th **T61.94**   **Toxic effect of unspecified seafood,** undetermined

✓4th **T62**   **Toxic effect of other noxious substances eaten as food**
   EXCLUDES 1   allergic reaction to food, such as:
        anaphylactic shock (reaction) due to adverse food reaction (T78.0-)
        bacterial food borne intoxications (A05.-)
        dermatitis (L23.6, L25.4, L27.2)
        food protein-induced enterocolitis syndrome (K52.21)
        food protein-induced enteropathy (K52.22)
        gastroenteritis (noninfective) (K52.29)
     toxic effect of aflatoxin and other mycotoxins (T64)
     toxic effect of cyanides (T65.0-)
     toxic effect of hydrogen cyanide (T57.3-)
     toxic effect of mercury (T56.1-)

   The appropriate 7th character is to be added to each code from category T62.
     A   initial encounter
     D   subsequent encounter
     S   sequela

✓5th **T62.0**   **Toxic effect of ingested mushrooms**
   ✓6th **T62.0X**   **Toxic effect of** ingested mushrooms
     ✓7th **T62.0X1**   **Toxic effect of ingested mushrooms, accidental (unintentional)**
        Toxic effect of ingested mushrooms NOS
     7 ✓7th **T62.0X2**   **Toxic effect of ingested mushrooms,** intentional self-harm   HCC
     ✓7th **T62.0X3**   **Toxic effect of ingested mushrooms,** assault
     ✓7th **T62.0X4**   **Toxic effect of ingested mushrooms,** undetermined

✓5th **T62.1**   **Toxic effect of ingested berries**
   ✓6th **T62.1X**   **Toxic effect of** ingested berries
     ✓7th **T62.1X1**   **Toxic effect of ingested berries,** accidental **(unintentional)**
        Toxic effect of ingested berries NOS
     7 ✓7th **T62.1X2**   **Toxic effect of ingested berries,** intentional self-harm   HCC
     ✓7th **T62.1X3**   **Toxic effect of ingested berries,** assault
     ✓7th **T62.1X4**   **Toxic effect of ingested berries,** undetermined

✓5th **T62.2**   **Toxic effect of other ingested (parts of) plant(s)**
   ✓6th **T62.2X**   **Toxic effect of** other ingested **(parts of)** plant(s)
     ✓7th **T62.2X1**   **Toxic effect of other ingested (parts of) plant(s),** accidental **(unintentional)**
        Toxic effect of other ingested (parts of) plant(s) NOS
     7 ✓7th **T62.2X2**   **Toxic effect of other ingested (parts of) plant(s),** intentional self-harm   HCC
     ✓7th **T62.2X3**   **Toxic effect of other ingested (parts of) plant(s),** assault
     ✓7th **T62.2X4**   **Toxic effect of other ingested (parts of) plant(s),** undetermined

✓5th **T62.8**   **Toxic effect of other specified** noxious substances eaten as food
   ✓6th **T62.8X**   **Toxic effect of** other specified noxious substances eaten as food
     ✓7th **T62.8X1**   **Toxic effect of other specified noxious substances eaten as food,** accidental **(unintentional)**
        Toxic effect of other specified noxious substances eaten as food NOS
     7 ✓7th **T62.8X2**   **Toxic effect of other specified noxious substances eaten as food,** intentional self-harm   HCC
     ✓7th **T62.8X3**   **Toxic effect of other specified noxious substances eaten as food,** assault
     ✓7th **T62.8X4**   **Toxic effect of other specified noxious substances eaten as food,** undetermined

✓5th **T62.9**   **Toxic effect of** unspecified **noxious substance eaten as food**
   ✓x7th **T62.91**   **Toxic effect of unspecified noxious substance eaten as food,** accidental **(unintentional)**
        Toxic effect of unspecified noxious substance eaten as food NOS
   7 ✓x7th **T62.92**   **Toxic effect of unspecified noxious substance eaten as food,** intentional self-harm   HCC
   ✓x7th **T62.93**   **Toxic effect of unspecified noxious substance eaten as food,** assault
   ✓x7th **T62.94**   **Toxic effect of unspecified noxious substance eaten as food,** undetermined

✓4th **T63**   **Toxic effect of contact with venomous animals and plants**
   INCLUDES   bite or touch of venomous animal
         pricked or stuck by thorn or leaf
   EXCLUDES 2   ingestion of toxic animal or plant (T61.-, T62.-)

   The appropriate 7th character is to be added to each code from category T63.
     A   initial encounter
     D   subsequent encounter
     S   sequela

✓5th **T63.0**   **Toxic effect of** snake venom
   ✓6th **T63.00**   **Toxic effect of** unspecified snake venom
     ✓7th **T63.001**   **Toxic effect of unspecified snake venom,** accidental **(unintentional)**
        Toxic effect of unspecified snake venom NOS
     7 ✓7th **T63.002**   **Toxic effect of unspecified snake venom,** intentional self-harm   HCC
     ✓7th **T63.003**   **Toxic effect of unspecified snake venom,** assault
     ✓7th **T63.004**   **Toxic effect of unspecified snake venom,** undetermined
   ✓6th **T63.01**   **Toxic effect of** rattlesnake venom
     ✓7th **T63.011**   **Toxic effect of rattlesnake venom,** accidental **(unintentional)**
        Toxic effect of rattlesnake venom NOS
     7 ✓7th **T63.012**   **Toxic effect of rattlesnake venom,** intentional self-harm   HCC
     ✓7th **T63.013**   **Toxic effect of rattlesnake venom,** assault
     ✓7th **T63.014**   **Toxic effect of rattlesnake venom,** undetermined
   ✓6th **T63.02**   **Toxic effect of** coral snake venom
     ✓7th **T63.021**   **Toxic effect of coral snake venom,** accidental **(unintentional)**
        Toxic effect of coral snake venom NOS
     7 ✓7th **T63.022**   **Toxic effect of coral snake venom,** intentional self-harm   HCC
     ✓7th **T63.023**   **Toxic effect of coral snake venom,** assault
     ✓7th **T63.024**   **Toxic effect of coral snake venom,** undetermined
   ✓6th **T63.03**   **Toxic effect of** taipan venom
     ✓7th **T63.031**   **Toxic effect of taipan venom,** accidental **(unintentional)**
        Toxic effect of taipan venom NOS
     7 ✓7th **T63.032**   **Toxic effect of taipan venom,** intentional self-harm   HCC
     ✓7th **T63.033**   **Toxic effect of taipan venom,** assault
     ✓7th **T63.034**   **Toxic effect of taipan venom,** undetermined

N Newborn: 0   P Pediatric: 0-17   M Maternity: 12-55   A Adult: 15-124   MCC Major Complication/Comorbidity   CC Complication/Comorbidity   SW Severe Wound Dx

1130   ICD-10-CM 2019

Chapter 19. Injury, Poisoning and Certain Other Consequences of External Causes

✓6ᵗʰ **T63.04** **Toxic effect of** cobra **venom**

✓7ᵗʰ **T63.041** **Toxic effect of cobra venom, accidental (unintentional)**
Toxic effect of cobra venom NOS

⁷ ✓7ᵗʰ **T63.042** **Toxic effect of cobra venom, intentional self-harm**   HCC

✓7ᵗʰ **T63.043** **Toxic effect of cobra venom, assault**

✓7ᵗʰ **T63.044** **Toxic effect of cobra venom, undetermined**

✓6ᵗʰ **T63.06** **Toxic effect of venom of** other North and South American snake

✓7ᵗʰ **T63.061** **Toxic effect of venom of other North and South American snake, accidental (unintentional)**
Toxic effect of venom of other North and South American snake NOS

⁷ ✓7ᵗʰ **T63.062** **Toxic effect of venom of other North and South American snake, intentional self-harm**   HCC

✓7ᵗʰ **T63.063** **Toxic effect of venom of other North and South American snake, assault**

✓7ᵗʰ **T63.064** **Toxic effect of venom of other North and South American snake, undetermined**

✓6ᵗʰ **T63.07** **Toxic effect of venom of** other Australian snake

✓7ᵗʰ **T63.071** **Toxic effect of venom of other Australian snake, accidental (unintentional)**
Toxic effect of venom of other Australian snake NOS

⁷ ✓7ᵗʰ **T63.072** **Toxic effect of venom of other Australian snake, intentional self-harm**   HCC

✓7ᵗʰ **T63.073** **Toxic effect of venom of other Australian snake, assault**

✓7ᵗʰ **T63.074** **Toxic effect of venom of other Australian snake, undetermined**

✓6ᵗʰ **T63.08** **Toxic effect of venom of** other African and Asian snake

✓7ᵗʰ **T63.081** **Toxic effect of venom of other African and Asian snake, accidental (unintentional)**
Toxic effect of venom of other African and Asian snake NOS

⁷ ✓7ᵗʰ **T63.082** **Toxic effect of venom of other African and Asian snake, intentional self-harm**   HCC

✓7ᵗʰ **T63.083** **Toxic effect of venom of other African and Asian snake, assault**

✓7ᵗʰ **T63.084** **Toxic effect of venom of other African and Asian snake, undetermined**

✓6ᵗʰ **T63.09** **Toxic effect of venom of** other snake

✓7ᵗʰ **T63.091** **Toxic effect of venom of other snake, accidental (unintentional)**
Toxic effect of venom of other snake NOS

⁷ ✓7ᵗʰ **T63.092** **Toxic effect of venom of other snake, intentional self-harm**   HCC

✓7ᵗʰ **T63.093** **Toxic effect of venom of other snake, assault**

✓7ᵗʰ **T63.094** **Toxic effect of venom of other snake, undetermined**

✓5ᵗʰ **T63.1** **Toxic effect of venom of** other reptiles

✓6ᵗʰ **T63.11** **Toxic effect of venom of** gila monster

✓7ᵗʰ **T63.111** **Toxic effect of venom of gila monster, accidental (unintentional)**
Toxic effect of venom of gila monster NOS

⁷ ✓7ᵗʰ **T63.112** **Toxic effect of venom of gila monster, intentional self-harm**   HCC

✓7ᵗʰ **T63.113** **Toxic effect of venom of gila monster, assault**

✓7ᵗʰ **T63.114** **Toxic effect of venom of gila monster, undetermined**

✓6ᵗʰ **T63.12** **Toxic effect of venom of** other venomous lizard

✓7ᵗʰ **T63.121** **Toxic effect of venom of other venomous lizard, accidental (unintentional)**
Toxic effect of venom of other venomous lizard NOS

⁷ ✓7ᵗʰ **T63.122** **Toxic effect of venom of other venomous lizard, intentional self-harm**   HCC

✓7ᵗʰ **T63.123** **Toxic effect of venom of other venomous lizard, assault**

✓7ᵗʰ **T63.124** **Toxic effect of venom of other venomous lizard, undetermined**

✓6ᵗʰ **T63.19** **Toxic effect of venom of** other reptiles

✓7ᵗʰ **T63.191** **Toxic effect of venom of other reptiles, accidental (unintentional)**
Toxic effect of venom of other reptiles NOS

⁷ ✓7ᵗʰ **T63.192** **Toxic effect of venom of other reptiles, intentional self-harm**   HCC

✓7ᵗʰ **T63.193** **Toxic effect of venom of other reptiles, assault**

✓7ᵗʰ **T63.194** **Toxic effect of venom of other reptiles, undetermined**

✓5ᵗʰ **T63.2** **Toxic effect of venom of** scorpion

✓6ᵗʰ **T63.2X** **Toxic effect of venom of scorpion**

✓7ᵗʰ **T63.2X1** **Toxic effect of venom of scorpion, accidental (unintentional)**
Toxic effect of venom of scorpion NOS

⁷ ✓7ᵗʰ **T63.2X2** **Toxic effect of venom of scorpion, intentional self-harm**   HCC

✓7ᵗʰ **T63.2X3** **Toxic effect of venom of scorpion, assault**

✓7ᵗʰ **T63.2X4** **Toxic effect of venom of scorpion, undetermined**

✓5ᵗʰ **T63.3** **Toxic effect of venom of** spider

✓6ᵗʰ **T63.30** **Toxic effect of** unspecified **spider venom**

✓7ᵗʰ **T63.301** **Toxic effect of unspecified spider venom, accidental (unintentional)**

⁷ ✓7ᵗʰ **T63.302** **Toxic effect of unspecified spider venom, intentional self-harm**   HCC

✓7ᵗʰ **T63.303** **Toxic effect of unspecified spider venom, assault**

✓7ᵗʰ **T63.304** **Toxic effect of unspecified spider venom, undetermined**

✓6ᵗʰ **T63.31** **Toxic effect of venom of** black widow **spider**

✓7ᵗʰ **T63.311** **Toxic effect of venom of black widow spider, accidental (unintentional)**

⁷ ✓7ᵗʰ **T63.312** **Toxic effect of venom of black widow spider, intentional self-harm**   HCC

✓7ᵗʰ **T63.313** **Toxic effect of venom of black widow spider, assault**

✓7ᵗʰ **T63.314** **Toxic effect of venom of black widow spider, undetermined**

✓6ᵗʰ **T63.32** **Toxic effect of venom of** tarantula

✓7ᵗʰ **T63.321** **Toxic effect of venom of tarantula, accidental (unintentional)**

⁷ ✓7ᵗʰ **T63.322** **Toxic effect of venom of tarantula, intentional self-harm**   HCC

✓7ᵗʰ **T63.323** **Toxic effect of venom of tarantula, assault**

✓7ᵗʰ **T63.324** **Toxic effect of venom of tarantula, undetermined**

✓6ᵗʰ **T63.33** **Toxic effect of venom of** brown recluse **spider**

✓7ᵗʰ **T63.331** **Toxic effect of venom of brown recluse spider, accidental (unintentional)**

⁷ ✓7ᵗʰ **T63.332** **Toxic effect of venom of brown recluse spider, intentional self-harm**   HCC

✓7ᵗʰ **T63.333** **Toxic effect of venom of brown recluse spider, assault**

✓7ᵗʰ **T63.334** **Toxic effect of venom of brown recluse spider, undetermined**

✓6ᵗʰ **T63.39** **Toxic effect of venom of** other spider

✓7ᵗʰ **T63.391** **Toxic effect of venom of other spider, accidental (unintentional)**

⁷ ✓7ᵗʰ **T63.392** **Toxic effect of venom of other spider, intentional self-harm**   HCC

✓7ᵗʰ **T63.393** **Toxic effect of venom of other spider, assault**

✓7ᵗʰ **T63.394** **Toxic effect of venom of other spider, undetermined**

✓5ᵗʰ **T63.4** **Toxic effect of venom of** other arthropods

✓6ᵗʰ **T63.41** **Toxic effect of venom of** centipedes and venomous millipedes

✓7ᵗʰ **T63.411** **Toxic effect of venom of centipedes and venomous millipedes, accidental (unintentional)**

✔ Additional Character Required   ✓ₓ7ᵗʰ Placeholder   Unacceptable PDx   Questionable PDx   Manifestation   **H1**-**H14** HAC   HCC CMS-HCC Dx   HIV HIV Dx

7 ☑7ᵗʰ **T63.412 Toxic effect of venom of centipedes and venomous millipedes,** *intentional self-harm* HCC

☑7ᵗʰ **T63.413 Toxic effect of venom of centipedes and venomous millipedes,** *assault*

☑7ᵗʰ **T63.414 Toxic effect of venom of centipedes and venomous millipedes,** *undetermined*

☑6ᵗʰ **T63.42 Toxic effect of venom of** ants

    ☑7ᵗʰ **T63.421 Toxic effect of venom of ants,** *accidental* **(unintentional)**

    7 ☑7ᵗʰ **T63.422 Toxic effect of venom of ants,** *intentional self-harm* HCC

    ☑7ᵗʰ **T63.423 Toxic effect of venom of ants,** *assault*

    ☑7ᵗʰ **T63.424 Toxic effect of venom of ants,** *undetermined*

☑6ᵗʰ **T63.43 Toxic effect of venom of** caterpillars

    ☑7ᵗʰ **T63.431 Toxic effect of venom of caterpillars,** *accidental* **(unintentional)**

    7 ☑7ᵗʰ **T63.432 Toxic effect of venom of caterpillars,** *intentional self-harm* HCC

    ☑7ᵗʰ **T63.433 Toxic effect of venom of caterpillars,** *assault*

    ☑7ᵗʰ **T63.434 Toxic effect of venom of caterpillars,** *undetermined*

☑6ᵗʰ **T63.44 Toxic effect of venom of** bees

    ☑7ᵗʰ **T63.441 Toxic effect of venom of bees,** *accidental* **(unintentional)**

    7 ☑7ᵗʰ **T63.442 Toxic effect of venom of bees,** *intentional self-harm* HCC

    ☑7ᵗʰ **T63.443 Toxic effect of venom of bees,** *assault*

    ☑7ᵗʰ **T63.444 Toxic effect of venom of bees,** *undetermined*

☑6ᵗʰ **T63.45 Toxic effect of venom of** hornets

    ☑7ᵗʰ **T63.451 Toxic effect of venom of hornets,** *accidental* **(unintentional)**

    7 ☑7ᵗʰ **T63.452 Toxic effect of venom of hornets,** *intentional self-harm* HCC

    ☑7ᵗʰ **T63.453 Toxic effect of venom of hornets,** *assault*

    ☑7ᵗʰ **T63.454 Toxic effect of venom of hornets,** *undetermined*

☑6ᵗʰ **T63.46 Toxic effect of venom of** wasps
    Toxic effect of yellow jacket

    ☑7ᵗʰ **T63.461 Toxic effect of venom of wasps,** *accidental* **(unintentional)**

    7 ☑7ᵗʰ **T63.462 Toxic effect of venom of wasps,** *intentional self-harm* HCC

    ☑7ᵗʰ **T63.463 Toxic effect of venom of wasps,** *assault*

    ☑7ᵗʰ **T63.464 Toxic effect of venom of wasps,** *undetermined*

☑6ᵗʰ **T63.48 Toxic effect of venom of** other arthropod

    ☑7ᵗʰ **T63.481 Toxic effect of venom of other arthropod,** *accidental* **(unintentional)**

    7 ☑7ᵗʰ **T63.482 Toxic effect of venom of other arthropod,** *intentional self-harm* HCC

    ☑7ᵗʰ **T63.483 Toxic effect of venom of other arthropod,** *assault*

    ☑7ᵗʰ **T63.484 Toxic effect of venom of other arthropod,** *undetermined*

☑5ᵗʰ **T63.5 Toxic effect of contact with** venomous fish
    EXCLUDES 2   poisoning by ingestion of fish (T61.-)

☑6ᵗʰ **T63.51 Toxic effect of contact with** stingray

    ☑7ᵗʰ **T63.511 Toxic effect of contact with stingray,** *accidental* **(unintentional)**

    7 ☑7ᵗʰ **T63.512 Toxic effect of contact with stingray,** *intentional self-harm* HCC

    ☑7ᵗʰ **T63.513 Toxic effect of contact with stingray,** *assault*

    ☑7ᵗʰ **T63.514 Toxic effect of contact with stingray,** *undetermined*

☑6ᵗʰ **T63.59 Toxic effect of contact with** other venomous fish

    ☑7ᵗʰ **T63.591 Toxic effect of contact with other venomous fish,** *accidental* **(unintentional)**

    7 ☑7ᵗʰ **T63.592 Toxic effect of contact with other venomous fish,** *intentional self-harm* HCC

☑7ᵗʰ **T63.593 Toxic effect of contact with other venomous fish,** *assault*

☑7ᵗʰ **T63.594 Toxic effect of contact with other venomous fish,** *undetermined*

☑5ᵗʰ **T63.6 Toxic effect of contact with** other venomous marine animals
    EXCLUDES 1   sea-snake venom (T63.09)
    EXCLUDES 2   poisoning by ingestion of shellfish (T61.78-)

☑6ᵗʰ **T63.61 Toxic effect of contact with** Portugese Man-o-war
    Toxic effect of contact with bluebottle

    ☑7ᵗʰ **T63.611 Toxic effect of contact with Portugese Man-o-war,** *accidental* **(unintentional)**

    7 ☑7ᵗʰ **T63.612 Toxic effect of contact with Portugese Man-o-war,** *intentional self-harm* HCC

    ☑7ᵗʰ **T63.613 Toxic effect of contact with Portugese Man-o-war,** *assault*

    ☑7ᵗʰ **T63.614 Toxic effect of contact with Portugese Man-o-war,** *undetermined*

☑6ᵗʰ **T63.62 Toxic effect of contact with** other jellyfish

    ☑7ᵗʰ **T63.621 Toxic effect of contact with other jellyfish,** *accidental* **(unintentional)**

    7 ☑7ᵗʰ **T63.622 Toxic effect of contact with other jellyfish,** *intentional self-harm* HCC

    ☑7ᵗʰ **T63.623 Toxic effect of contact with other jellyfish,** *assault*

    ☑7ᵗʰ **T63.624 Toxic effect of contact with other jellyfish,** *undetermined*

☑6ᵗʰ **T63.63 Toxic effect of contact with** sea anemone

    ☑7ᵗʰ **T63.631 Toxic effect of contact with sea anemone,** *accidental* **(unintentional)**

    7 ☑7ᵗʰ **T63.632 Toxic effect of contact with sea anemone,** *intentional self-harm* HCC

    ☑7ᵗʰ **T63.633 Toxic effect of contact with sea anemone,** *assault*

    ☑7ᵗʰ **T63.634 Toxic effect of contact with sea anemone,** *undetermined*

☑6ᵗʰ **T63.69 Toxic effect of contact with** other venomous marine animals

    ☑7ᵗʰ **T63.691 Toxic effect of contact with other venomous marine animals,** *accidental* **(unintentional)**

    7 ☑7ᵗʰ **T63.692 Toxic effect of contact with other venomous marine animals,** *intentional self-harm* HCC

    ☑7ᵗʰ **T63.693 Toxic effect of contact with other venomous marine animals,** *assault*

    ☑7ᵗʰ **T63.694 Toxic effect of contact with other venomous marine animals,** *undetermined*

☑5ᵗʰ **T63.7 Toxic effect of contact with** venomous plant

☑6ᵗʰ **T63.71 Toxic effect of contact with venomous** marine plant

    ☑7ᵗʰ **T63.711 Toxic effect of contact with venomous marine plant,** *accidental* **(unintentional)**

    7 ☑7ᵗʰ **T63.712 Toxic effect of contact with venomous marine plant,** *intentional self-harm* HCC

    ☑7ᵗʰ **T63.713 Toxic effect of contact with venomous marine plant,** *assault*

    ☑7ᵗʰ **T63.714 Toxic effect of contact with venomous marine plant,** *undetermined*

☑6ᵗʰ **T63.79 Toxic effect of contact with** other venomous plant

    ☑7ᵗʰ **T63.791 Toxic effect of contact with other venomous plant,** *accidental* **(unintentional)**

    7 ☑7ᵗʰ **T63.792 Toxic effect of contact with other venomous plant,** *intentional self-harm* HCC

    ☑7ᵗʰ **T63.793 Toxic effect of contact with other venomous plant,** *assault*

    ☑7ᵗʰ **T63.794 Toxic effect of contact with other venomous plant,** *undetermined*

☑5ᵗʰ **T63.8 Toxic effect of contact with** other venomous animals

☑6ᵗʰ **T63.81 Toxic effect of contact with** venomous frog
    EXCLUDES 1   contact with nonvenomous frog (W62.0)

    ☑7ᵗʰ **T63.811 Toxic effect of contact with venomous frog,** *accidental* **(unintentional)**

    7 ☑7ᵗʰ **T63.812 Toxic effect of contact with venomous frog,** *intentional self-harm* HCC

N Newborn: 0   P Pediatric: 0-17   M Maternity: 12-55   A Adult: 15-124   MCC Major Complication/Comorbidity   CC Complication/Comorbidity   SW Severe Wound Dx

1132   ICD-10-CM 2019

√7ᵗʰ **T63.813** **Toxic effect of contact with venomous frog,** assault

√7ᵗʰ **T63.814** **Toxic effect of contact with venomous frog,** undetermined

√6ᵗʰ **T63.82** **Toxic effect of contact with venomous** toad
    EXCLUDES 1   contact with nonvenomous toad (W62.1)

√7ᵗʰ **T63.821** **Toxic effect of contact with venomous toad,** accidental **(unintentional)**

7 √7ᵗʰ **T63.822** **Toxic effect of contact with venomous** HCC **toad,** intentional self-harm

√7ᵗʰ **T63.823** **Toxic effect of contact with venomous toad,** assault

√7ᵗʰ **T63.824** **Toxic effect of contact with venomous toad,** undetermined

√6ᵗʰ **T63.83** **Toxic effect of contact with** other **venomous** amphibian
    EXCLUDES 1   contact with nonvenomous amphibian (W62.9)

√7ᵗʰ **T63.831** **Toxic effect of contact with other venomous amphibian,** accidental **(unintentional)**

7 √7ᵗʰ **T63.832** **Toxic effect of contact with other** HCC **venomous amphibian,** intentional self-harm

√7ᵗʰ **T63.833** **Toxic effect of contact with other venomous amphibian,** assault

√7ᵗʰ **T63.834** **Toxic effect of contact with other venomous amphibian,** undetermined

√6ᵗʰ **T63.89** **Toxic effect of contact with** other **venomous** animals

√7ᵗʰ **T63.891** **Toxic effect of contact with other venomous animals,** accidental **(unintentional)**

7 √7ᵗʰ **T63.892** **Toxic effect of contact with other** HCC **venomous animals,** intentional self-harm

√7ᵗʰ **T63.893** **Toxic effect of contact with other venomous animals,** assault

√7ᵗʰ **T63.894** **Toxic effect of contact with other venomous animals,** undetermined

√5ᵗʰ **T63.9** **Toxic effect of contact with** unspecified **venomous** animal

√x7ᵗʰ **T63.91** **Toxic effect of contact with unspecified venomous animal,** accidental **(unintentional)**

7 √x7ᵗʰ **T63.92** **Toxic effect of contact with unspecified** HCC **venomous animal,** intentional self-harm

√x7ᵗʰ **T63.93** **Toxic effect of contact with unspecified venomous animal,** assault

√x7ᵗʰ **T63.94** **Toxic effect of contact with unspecified venomous animal,** undetermined

√4ᵗʰ **T64** **Toxic effect of aflatoxin and other mycotoxin food contaminants**

> The appropriate 7th character is to be added to each code from category T64.
> A   initial encounter
> D   subsequent encounter
> S   sequela

√5ᵗʰ **T64.0** **Toxic effect of** aflatoxin

√x7ᵗʰ **T64.01** **Toxic effect of aflatoxin,** accidental **(unintentional)**

7 √x7ᵗʰ **T64.02** **Toxic effect of aflatoxin,** intentional self-harm HCC

√x7ᵗʰ **T64.03** **Toxic effect of aflatoxin,** assault

√x7ᵗʰ **T64.04** **Toxic effect of aflatoxin,** undetermined

√5ᵗʰ **T64.8** **Toxic effect of** other mycotoxin **food contaminants**

√x7ᵗʰ **T64.81** **Toxic effect of other mycotoxin food contaminants,** accidental **(unintentional)**

7 √x7ᵗʰ **T64.82** **Toxic effect of other mycotoxin food** HCC **contaminants,** intentional self-harm

√x7ᵗʰ **T64.83** **Toxic effect of other mycotoxin food contaminants,** assault

√x7ᵗʰ **T64.84** **Toxic effect of other mycotoxin food contaminants,** undetermined

√4ᵗʰ **T65** **Toxic effect of other and unspecified substances**

> The appropriate 7th character is to be added to each code from category T65.
> A   initial encounter
> D   subsequent encounter
> S   sequela

√5ᵗʰ **T65.0** **Toxic effect of** cyanides
    EXCLUDES 1   hydrogen cyanide (T57.3-)

√6ᵗʰ **T65.0X** **Toxic effect of cyanides**

√7ᵗʰ **T65.0X1** **Toxic effect of cyanides,** accidental **(unintentional)**
      Toxic effect of cyanides NOS

7 √7ᵗʰ **T65.0X2** **Toxic effect of cyanides,** intentional HCC **self-harm**

√7ᵗʰ **T65.0X3** **Toxic effect of cyanides,** assault

√7ᵗʰ **T65.0X4** **Toxic effect of cyanides,** undetermined

√5ᵗʰ **T65.1** **Toxic effect of** strychnine **and its salts**

√6ᵗʰ **T65.1X** **Toxic effect of strychnine and its salts**

√7ᵗʰ **T65.1X1** **Toxic effect of strychnine and its salts,** accidental **(unintentional)**
      Toxic effect of strychnine and its salts NOS

7 √7ᵗʰ **T65.1X2** **Toxic effect of strychnine and its salts,** HCC **intentional self-harm**

√7ᵗʰ **T65.1X3** **Toxic effect of strychnine and its salts,** assault

√7ᵗʰ **T65.1X4** **Toxic effect of strychnine and its salts,** undetermined

√5ᵗʰ **T65.2** **Toxic effect of** tobacco and nicotine
    EXCLUDES 2   nicotine dependence (F17.-)

√6ᵗʰ **T65.21** **Toxic effect of** chewing tobacco

√7ᵗʰ **T65.211** **Toxic effect of chewing tobacco,** accidental **(unintentional)**
      Toxic effect of chewing tobacco NOS

7 √7ᵗʰ **T65.212** **Toxic effect of chewing tobacco,** HCC **intentional self-harm**

√7ᵗʰ **T65.213** **Toxic effect of chewing tobacco,** assault

√7ᵗʰ **T65.214** **Toxic effect of chewing tobacco,** undetermined

√6ᵗʰ **T65.22** **Toxic effect of** tobacco cigarettes
    Toxic effect of tobacco smoke
    Use additional code for exposure to second hand tobacco smoke (Z57.31, Z77.22)

√7ᵗʰ **T65.221** **Toxic effect of tobacco cigarettes,** accidental **(unintentional)**
      Toxic effect of tobacco cigarettes NOS

7 √7ᵗʰ **T65.222** **Toxic effect of tobacco cigarettes,** HCC **intentional self-harm**

√7ᵗʰ **T65.223** **Toxic effect of tobacco cigarettes,** assault

√7ᵗʰ **T65.224** **Toxic effect of tobacco cigarettes,** undetermined

√6ᵗʰ **T65.29** **Toxic effect of** other tobacco and nicotine

√7ᵗʰ **T65.291** **Toxic effect of other tobacco and nicotine,** accidental **(unintentional)**
      Toxic effect of other tobacco and nicotine NOS

7 √7ᵗʰ **T65.292** **Toxic effect of other tobacco and** HCC **nicotine,** intentional self-harm

√7ᵗʰ **T65.293** **Toxic effect of other tobacco and nicotine,** assault

√7ᵗʰ **T65.294** **Toxic effect of other tobacco and nicotine,** undetermined

√5ᵗʰ **T65.3** **Toxic effect of** nitroderivatives and aminoderivatives of benzene and its homologues
    Toxic effect of anilin [benzenamine]
    Toxic effect of nitrobenzene
    Toxic effect of trinitrotoluene

√6ᵗʰ **T65.3X** **Toxic effect of nitroderivatives and aminoderivatives of benzene and its homologues**

√7ᵗʰ **T65.3X1** **Toxic effect of nitroderivatives and aminoderivatives of benzene and its homologues,** accidental **(unintentional)**
      Toxic effect of nitroderivatives and aminoderivatives of benzene and its homologues NOS

✔Additional Character Required   √x7ᵗʰ Placeholder   Unacceptable PDx   Questionable PDx   Manifestation   H1 - H14 HAC   HCC CMS-HCC Dx   HIV HIV Dx

ICD-10-CM 2019   1133

7 ✓7ᵗʰ **T65.3X2** **Toxic effect of nitroderivatives and aminoderivatives of benzene and its homologues,** intentional self-harm   HCC

✓7ᵗʰ **T65.3X3** **Toxic effect of nitroderivatives and aminoderivatives of benzene and its homologues,** assault

✓7ᵗʰ **T65.3X4** **Toxic effect of nitroderivatives and aminoderivatives of benzene and its homologues,** undetermined

✓5ᵗʰ **T65.4** **Toxic effect of** carbon disulfide

  ✓6ᵗʰ **T65.4X** **Toxic effect of carbon disulfide**

    ✓7ᵗʰ **T65.4X1** **Toxic effect of carbon disulfide,** accidental (unintentional)
        Toxic effect of carbon disulfide NOS

    7 ✓7ᵗʰ **T65.4X2** **Toxic effect of carbon disulfide,** intentional self-harm   HCC

    ✓7ᵗʰ **T65.4X3** **Toxic effect of carbon disulfide,** assault

    ✓7ᵗʰ **T65.4X4** **Toxic effect of carbon disulfide,** undetermined

✓5ᵗʰ **T65.5** **Toxic effect of** nitroglycerin and other nitric acids and esters
  Toxic effect of 1,2,3-Propanetriol trinitrate

  ✓6ᵗʰ **T65.5X** **Toxic effect of nitroglycerin and other nitric acids and esters**

    ✓7ᵗʰ **T65.5X1** **Toxic effect of nitroglycerin and other nitric acids and esters,** accidental (unintentional)
        Toxic effect of nitroglycerin and other nitric acids and esters NOS

    7 ✓7ᵗʰ **T65.5X2** **Toxic effect of nitroglycerin and other nitric acids and esters,** intentional self-harm   HCC

    ✓7ᵗʰ **T65.5X3** **Toxic effect of nitroglycerin and other nitric acids and esters,** assault

    ✓7ᵗʰ **T65.5X4** **Toxic effect of nitroglycerin and other nitric acids and esters,** undetermined

✓5ᵗʰ **T65.6** **Toxic effect of** paints and dyes, not elsewhere classified

  ✓6ᵗʰ **T65.6X** **Toxic effect of paints and dyes, not elsewhere classified**

    ✓7ᵗʰ **T65.6X1** **Toxic effect of paints and dyes, not elsewhere classified,** accidental (unintentional)
        Toxic effect of paints and dyes NOS

    7 ✓7ᵗʰ **T65.6X2** **Toxic effect of paints and dyes, not elsewhere classified,** intentional self-harm   HCC

    ✓7ᵗʰ **T65.6X3** **Toxic effect of paints and dyes, not elsewhere classified,** assault

    ✓7ᵗʰ **T65.6X4** **Toxic effect of paints and dyes, not elsewhere classified,** undetermined

✓5ᵗʰ **T65.8** **Toxic effect of** other specified substances

  ✓6ᵗʰ **T65.81** **Toxic effect of** latex

    ✓7ᵗʰ **T65.811** **Toxic effect of latex,** accidental (unintentional)
        Toxic effect of latex NOS

    7 ✓7ᵗʰ **T65.812** **Toxic effect of latex,** intentional self-harm   HCC

    ✓7ᵗʰ **T65.813** **Toxic effect of latex,** assault

    ✓7ᵗʰ **T65.814** **Toxic effect of latex,** undetermined

  ✓6ᵗʰ **T65.82** **Toxic effect of** harmful algae and algae toxins
    Toxic effect of (harmful) algae bloom NOS
    Toxic effect of blue-green algae bloom
    Toxic effect of brown tide
    Toxic effect of cyanobacteria bloom
    Toxic effect of Florida red tide
    Toxic effect of pfiesteria piscicida
    Toxic effect of red tide

    ✓7ᵗʰ **T65.821** **Toxic effect of harmful algae and algae toxins,** accidental (unintentional)
        Toxic effect of harmful algae and algae toxins NOS

    7 ✓7ᵗʰ **T65.822** **Toxic effect of harmful algae and algae toxins,** intentional self-harm   HCC

    ✓7ᵗʰ **T65.823** **Toxic effect of harmful algae and algae toxins,** assault

    ✓7ᵗʰ **T65.824** **Toxic effect of harmful algae and algae toxins,** undetermined

✓6ᵗʰ **T65.83** **Toxic effect of** fiberglass

    ✓7ᵗʰ **T65.831** **Toxic effect of fiberglass,** accidental (unintentional)
        Toxic effect of fiberglass NOS

    7 ✓7ᵗʰ **T65.832** **Toxic effect of fiberglass,** intentional self-harm   HCC

    ✓7ᵗʰ **T65.833** **Toxic effect of fiberglass,** assault

    ✓7ᵗʰ **T65.834** **Toxic effect of fiberglass,** undetermined

✓6ᵗʰ **T65.89** **Toxic effect of** other specified substances

    ✓7ᵗʰ **T65.891** **Toxic effect of other specified substances,** accidental (unintentional)
        Toxic effect of other specified substances NOS
        AHA: 2018, 1Q, 5

    7 ✓7ᵗʰ **T65.892** **Toxic effect of other specified substances,** intentional self-harm   HCC

    ✓7ᵗʰ **T65.893** **Toxic effect of other specified substances,** assault

    ✓7ᵗʰ **T65.894** **Toxic effect of other specified substances,** undetermined

✓5ᵗʰ **T65.9** **Toxic effect of** unspecified substance

  ✓×7ᵗʰ **T65.91** **Toxic effect of unspecified substance,** accidental (unintentional)
    Poisoning NOS

  7 ✓×7ᵗʰ **T65.92** **Toxic effect of unspecified substance,** intentional self-harm   HCC

  ✓×7ᵗʰ **T65.93** **Toxic effect of unspecified substance,** assault

  ✓×7ᵗʰ **T65.94** **Toxic effect of unspecified substance,** undetermined

Other and unspecified effects of external causes (T66-T78)

✓×7ᵗʰ **T66** **Radiation sickness, unspecified**
  EXCLUDES 1   specified adverse effects of radiation, such as:
    burns (T20-T31)
    leukemia (C91-C95)
    radiation gastroenteritis and colitis (K52.0)
    radiation pneumonitis (J70.0)
    radiation related disorders of the skin and subcutaneous tissue (L55-L59)
    radiation sunburn (L55.-)

> The appropriate 7th character is to be added to code T66.
> A   initial encounter
> D   subsequent encounter
> S   sequela

✓4ᵗʰ **T67** **Effects of heat and light**
  EXCLUDES 1   erythema [dermatitis] ab igne (L59.0)
    malignant hyperpyrexia due to anesthesia (T88.3)
    radiation-related disorders of the skin and subcutaneous tissue (L55-L59)
  EXCLUDES 2   burns (T20-T31)
    sunburn (L55.-)
    sweat disorder due to heat (L74-L75)

> The appropriate 7th character is to be added to each code from category T67.
> A   initial encounter
> D   subsequent encounter
> S   sequela

✓×7ᵗʰ **T67.0** **Heatstroke and sunstroke**   CC H5
  Heat apoplexy   Siriasis
  Heat pyrexia   Thermoplegia
  Use additional code(s) to identify any associated complications of heatstroke, such as:
    coma and stupor (R40.-)
    systemic inflammatory response syndrome (R65.1-)
  DEF: Headache, vertigo, cramps, and elevated body temperature due to prolonged exposure to high environmental temperatures that requires emergency intervention.
  CC Excl: PDX collection 1419

✓×7ᵗʰ **T67.1** **Heat** syncope
  Heat collapse

✓×7ᵗʰ **T67.2** **Heat** cramp

✓×7ᵗʰ **T67.3** **Heat exhaustion,** anhydrotic
  Heat prostration due to water depletion
  EXCLUDES 1   heat exhaustion due to salt depletion (T67.4)

✓×7ᵗʰ **T67.4** **Heat exhaustion** due to salt depletion
  Heat prostration due to salt (and water) depletion

N Newborn: 0   **P** Pediatric: 0-17   **M** Maternity: 12-55   **A** Adult: 15-124   **MCC** Major Complication/Comorbidity   **CC** Complication/Comorbidity   **SW** Severe Wound Dx

1134   ICD-10-CM 2019

√x7ᵗʰ **T67.5** **Heat exhaustion,** unspecified
    Heat prostration NOS

√x7ᵗʰ **T67.6** **Heat** fatigue, **transient**

√x7ᵗʰ **T67.7** **Heat** edema

√x7ᵗʰ **T67.8** **Other effects of heat and light**

√x7ᵗʰ **T67.9** **Effect of heat and light, unspecified**

√x7ᵗʰ **T68** **Hypothermia**
    Accidental hypothermia
    Hypothermia NOS
    Use additional code to identify source of exposure:
       exposure to excessive cold of man-made origin (W93)
       exposure to excessive cold of natural origin (X31)
       EXCLUDES 1   *hypothermia following anesthesia (T88.51)*
                hypothermia not associated with low environmental
                    temperature (R68.0)
                hypothermia of newborn (P80.-)
       EXCLUDES 2   *frostbite (T33-T34)*

> The appropriate 7th character is to be added to code T68.
> A   initial encounter
> D   subsequent encounter
> S   sequela

√4ᵗʰ **T69** **Other effects of reduced temperature**
    Use additional code to identify source of exposure:
       exposure to excessive cold of man-made origin (W93)
       exposure to excessive cold of natural origin (X31)
       EXCLUDES 2   *frostbite (T33-T34)*

> The appropriate 7th character is to be added to each code from
> category T69.
> A   initial encounter
> D   subsequent encounter
> S   sequela

√5ᵗʰ **T69.0** **Immersion hand and foot**

√6ᵗʰ **T69.01** **Immersion** hand

√7ᵗʰ **T69.011** **Immersion hand,** right **hand**

√7ᵗʰ **T69.012** **Immersion hand,** left **hand**

√7ᵗʰ **T69.019** **Immersion hand,** unspecified **hand**

√6ᵗʰ **T69.02** **Immersion** foot
    Trench foot

> **CC Excl: For CC codes in subcategory T69.02:**
> PDX collection 1420

√7ᵗʰ **T69.021** **Immersion foot,** right **foot**   CC H5

√7ᵗʰ **T69.022** **Immersion foot,** left **foot**   CC H5

√7ᵗʰ **T69.029** **Immersion foot,** unspecified **foot**   CC H5

√x7ᵗʰ **T69.1** **Chilblains**
    DEF: Red, swollen, itchy skin primarily affecting the fingers and
    toes, nose and ears, and legs. Chilblains follows damp-cold
    exposure, and can also be associated with pruritus and a burning
    feeling.

√x7ᵗʰ **T69.8** **Other specified effects of reduced temperature**

√x7ᵗʰ **T69.9** **Effect of reduced temperature, unspecified**

√4ᵗʰ **T70** **Effects of air pressure and water pressure**

> The appropriate 7th character is to be added to each code from
> category T70.
> A   initial encounter
> D   subsequent encounter
> S   sequela

√x7ᵗʰ **T70.0** **Otitic barotrauma**
    Aero-otitis media
    Effects of change in ambient atmospheric pressure or water
       pressure on ears

√x7ᵗʰ **T70.1** **Sinus barotrauma**
    Aerosinusitis
    Effects of change in ambient atmospheric pressure on sinuses

√5ᵗʰ **T70.2** **Other and unspecified effects of high altitude**
       EXCLUDES 2   *polycythemia due to high altitude (D75.1)*

√x7ᵗʰ **T70.20** **Unspecified effects of high altitude**

√x7ᵗʰ **T70.29** **Other effects of high altitude**
    Alpine sickness   Hypobaropathy
    Anoxia due to high altitude   Mountain sickness
    Barotrauma NOS

√x7ᵗʰ **T70.3** **Caisson disease [decompression sickness]**   CC H5
    Compressed-air disease
    Diver's palsy or paralysis
    DEF: Rapid reduction in air pressure while breathing compressed
    air. Symptoms include skin lesions, joint pains, and respiratory and
    neurological problems.
    CC Excl: PDX collection 1421

√x7ᵗʰ **T70.4** **Effects of high-pressure fluids**
    Hydraulic jet injection (industrial)
    Pneumatic jet injection (industrial)
    Traumatic jet injection (industrial)

√x7ᵗʰ **T70.8** **Other effects of air pressure and water pressure**

√x7ᵗʰ **T70.9** **Effect of air pressure and water pressure, unspecified**

√4ᵗʰ **T71** **Asphyxiation**
    Mechanical suffocation
    Traumatic suffocation
       EXCLUDES 1   *acute respiratory distress (syndrome) (J80)*
                anoxia due to high altitude (T70.2)
                asphyxia NOS (R09.01)
                asphyxia from carbon monoxide (T58.-)
                asphyxia from inhalation of food or foreign body (T17.-)
                asphyxia from other gases, fumes and vapors (T59.-)
                respiratory distress (syndrome) in newborn (P22.-)

> The appropriate 7th character is to be added to each code from
> category T71.
> A   initial encounter
> D   subsequent encounter
> S   sequela

> **CC Excl: For CC codes in category T71:** PDX collection 1422

√5ᵗʰ **T71.1** **Asphyxiation due to** mechanical threat to breathing
    Suffocation due to mechanical threat to breathing

√6ᵗʰ **T71.11** **Asphyxiation due to** smothering under pillow

√7ᵗʰ **T71.111** **Asphyxiation due to smothering**   CC H5
    under pillow, accidental
       Asphyxiation due to smothering under
          pillow NOS

7 √7ᵗʰ **T71.112** **Asphyxiation due to**   CC H5 HCC
    smothering under pillow,
    intentional self-harm

√7ᵗʰ **T71.113** **Asphyxiation due to smothering**   CC H5
    under pillow, assault

√7ᵗʰ **T71.114** **Asphyxiation due to smothering**   CC H5
    under pillow, undetermined

√6ᵗʰ **T71.12** **Asphyxiation due to** plastic bag

√7ᵗʰ **T71.121** **Asphyxiation due to plastic bag,**   CC H5
    accidental
       Asphyxiation due to plastic bag NOS

7 √7ᵗʰ **T71.122** **Asphyxiation due to plastic**   CC H5 HCC
    bag, intentional self-harm

√7ᵗʰ **T71.123** **Asphyxiation due to plastic bag,**   CC H5
    assault

√7ᵗʰ **T71.124** **Asphyxiation due to plastic bag,**   CC H5
    undetermined

√6ᵗʰ **T71.13** **Asphyxiation due to being** trapped in bed linens

√7ᵗʰ **T71.131** **Asphyxiation due to being trapped**   CC H5
    in bed linens, accidental
       Asphyxiation due to being trapped in bed
          linens NOS

7 √7ᵗʰ **T71.132** **Asphyxiation due to being**   CC H5 HCC
    trapped in bed linens, intentional
    self-harm

√7ᵗʰ **T71.133** **Asphyxiation due to being trapped**   CC H5
    in bed linens, assault

√7ᵗʰ **T71.134** **Asphyxiation due to being trapped**   CC H5
    in bed linens, undetermined

√6ᵗʰ **T71.14** **Asphyxiation due to** smothering under another
    person's body (in bed)

√7ᵗʰ **T71.141** **Asphyxiation due to smothering**   CC H5
    under another person's body (in bed),
    accidental
       Asphyxiation due to smothering under
          another person's body (in bed) NOS

√7ᵗʰ **T71.143** **Asphyxiation due to smothering**   CC H5
    under another person's body (in bed),
    assault

✔ Additional Character Required   √x7ᵗʰ Placeholder   Unacceptable PDx   Questionable PDx   Manifestation   H1 - H14 HAC   HCC CMS-HCC Dx   HIV HIV Dx

ICD-10-CM 2019   **1135**

✓7th **T71.144** **Asphyxiation due to smothering** `CC` `H5` **under another person's body (in bed), undetermined**

✓6th **T71.15** **Asphyxiation due to** smothering in furniture

✓7th **T71.151** **Asphyxiation due to smothering in** `CC` `H5` **furniture,** accidental
Asphyxiation due to smothering in furniture NOS

7 ✓7th **T71.152** **Asphyxiation due to** `CC` `H5` `HCC` **smothering in furniture,** intentional self-harm

✓7th **T71.153** **Asphyxiation due to smothering in** `CC` `H5` **furniture,** assault

✓7th **T71.154** **Asphyxiation due to smothering in** `CC` `H5` **furniture,** undetermined

✓6th **T71.16** **Asphyxiation due to** hanging
Hanging by window shade cord
Use additional code for any associated injuries, such as:
  crushing injury of neck (S17.-)
  fracture of cervical vertebrae (S12.0-S12.2-)
  open wound of neck (S11.-)

✓7th **T71.161** **Asphyxiation due to hanging,** `CC` `H5` accidental
Asphyxiation due to hanging NOS
Hanging NOS

7 ✓7th **T71.162** **Asphyxiation due to hanging,** `CC` `H5` `HCC` intentional self-harm

✓7th **T71.163** **Asphyxiation due to hanging,** `CC` `H5` assault

✓7th **T71.164** **Asphyxiation due to hanging,** `CC` `H5` undetermined

✓6th **T71.19** **Asphyxiation due to mechanical threat to breathing** due to other causes

✓7th **T71.191** **Asphyxiation due to mechanical** `CC` `H5` **threat to breathing due to other causes,** accidental
Asphyxiation due to other causes NOS

7 ✓7th **T71.192** **Asphyxiation due to mechanical** `CC` `H5` `HCC` **threat to breathing due to other causes,** intentional self-harm

✓7th **T71.193** **Asphyxiation due to mechanical** `CC` `H5` **threat to breathing due to other causes,** assault

✓7th **T71.194** **Asphyxiation due to mechanical** `CC` `H5` **threat to breathing due to other causes,** undetermined

✓5th **T71.2** **Asphyxiation due to** systemic oxygen deficiency due to low oxygen content in ambient air
Suffocation due to systemic oxygen deficiency due to low oxygen content in ambient air

✓x7th **T71.20** **Asphyxiation due to systemic oxygen** `CC` `H5` **deficiency due to low oxygen content in ambient air due to** unspecified cause

✓x7th **T71.21** **Asphyxiation due to** cave-in or falling earth `CC` `H5`
Use additional code for any associated cataclysm (X34-X38)

✓6th **T71.22** **Asphyxiation due to** being trapped in a car trunk

✓7th **T71.221** **Asphyxiation due to being trapped in** `CC` **a car trunk,** accidental

7 ✓7th **T71.222** **Asphyxiation due to being trapped** `CC` `HCC` **in a car trunk,** intentional self-harm

✓7th **T71.223** **Asphyxiation due to being trapped in** `CC` **a car trunk,** assault

✓7th **T71.224** **Asphyxiation due to being trapped in** `CC` **a car trunk,** undetermined

✓6th **T71.23** **Asphyxiation due to being** trapped in a (discarded) refrigerator

✓7th **T71.231** **Asphyxiation due to being trapped in** `CC` **a (discarded) refrigerator,** accidental

7 ✓7th **T71.232** **Asphyxiation due to being trapped** `CC` `HCC` **in a (discarded) refrigerator,** intentional self-harm

✓7th **T71.233** **Asphyxiation due to being trapped** `CC` **in a (discarded) refrigerator,** assault

✓7th **T71.234** **Asphyxiation due to being trapped** `CC` **in a (discarded) refrigerator,** undetermined

✓x7th **T71.29** **Asphyxiation due to being trapped in** other `CC` `H5` **low oxygen environment**

✓x7th **T71.9** **Asphyxiation due to** unspecified cause `CC` `H5`
Suffocation (by strangulation) due to unspecified cause
Suffocation NOS
Systemic oxygen deficiency due to low oxygen content in ambient air due to unspecified cause
Systemic oxygen deficiency due to mechanical threat to breathing due to unspecified cause
Traumatic asphyxia NOS

✓4th **T73** **Effects of other deprivation**

> The appropriate 7th character is to be added to each code from category T73.
> A   initial encounter
> D   subsequent encounter
> S   sequela

✓x7th **T73.0** **Starvation**
Deprivation of food

✓x7th **T73.1** **Deprivation of water**

✓x7th **T73.2** **Exhaustion due to exposure**

✓x7th **T73.3** **Exhaustion due to excessive exertion**
Exhaustion due to overexertion

✓x7th **T73.8** **Other effects of deprivation**

✓x7th **T73.9** **Effect of deprivation, unspecified**

✓4th **T74** **Adult and child abuse, neglect and other maltreatment, confirmed**
Use additional code, if applicable, to identify any associated current injury
Use additional external cause code to identify perpetrator, if known (Y07.-)
EXCLUDES 1   *abuse and maltreatment in pregnancy (O9A.3-, O9A.4-, O9A.5-)*
         adult and child maltreatment, suspected (T76.-)

> The appropriate 7th character is to be added to each code from category T74.
> A   initial encounter
> D   subsequent encounter
> S   sequela

> **CC Excl: For CC codes in category T74, unless otherwise noted:**
> PDX collection 1423

✓5th **T74.0** **Neglect or abandonment, confirmed**

✓x7th **T74.01** **Adult** neglect or abandonment, confirmed `CC` `A`

✓x7th **T74.02** **Child** neglect or abandonment, confirmed `CC` `P`

✓5th **T74.1** **Physical abuse, confirmed**
EXCLUDES 2   *sexual abuse (T74.2-)*

✓x7th **T74.11** **Adult** physical abuse, confirmed `CC` `A`

✓x7th **T74.12** **Child** physical abuse, confirmed `CC` `P`
EXCLUDES 2   *shaken infant syndrome (T74.4)*

✓5th **T74.2** **Sexual abuse, confirmed**
Rape, confirmed
Sexual assault, confirmed

✓x7th **T74.21** **Adult** sexual abuse, confirmed `CC` `A`

✓x7th **T74.22** **Child** sexual abuse, confirmed `CC` `P`

✓5th **T74.3** **Psychological abuse, confirmed**
▶Bullying and intimidation, confirmed
Intimidation through social media, confirmed◀

✓x7th **T74.31** **Adult** psychological abuse, confirmed `A`

✓x7th **T74.32** **Child** psychological abuse, confirmed `CC` `P`

✓x7th **T74.4** **Shaken infant syndrome** `CC` `P`

● ✓5th **T74.5** **Forced sexual exploitation, confirmed**

● ✓x7th **T74.51** **Adult** forced sexual exploitation, confirmed

● ✓x7th **T74.52** **Child** sexual exploitation, confirmed

● ✓5th **T74.6** **Forced labor exploitation, confirmed**

● ✓x7th **T74.61** **Adult** forced labor exploitation, confirmed

● ✓x7th **T74.62** **Child** forced labor exploitation, confirmed

✓5th **T74.9** **Unspecified maltreatment, confirmed**

✓x7th **T74.91** **Unspecified** adult **maltreatment, confirmed** `CC` `A`
CC Excl: PDX collection 1424

✓x7th **T74.92** **Unspecified** child **maltreatment, confirmed** `CC` `P`

`N` Newborn: 0   `P` Pediatric: 0-17   `M` Maternity: 12-55   `A` Adult: 15-124   `MCC` Major Complication/Comorbidity   `CC` Complication/Comorbidity   `SW` Severe Wound Dx

1136   ICD-10-CM 2019

√4th **T75   Other and unspecified effects of other external causes**
  EXCLUDES1 adverse effects NEC (T78.-)
  EXCLUDES2 burns (electric) (T20-T31)

  The appropriate 7th character is to be added to each code from category T75.
  A   initial encounter
  D   subsequent encounter
  S   sequela

√5th **T75.0   Effects of lightning**
        Struck by lightning
    √x7th **T75.00   Unspecified effects of lightning**
            Struck by lightning NOS
    √x7th **T75.01   Shock due to being struck by lightning**
    √x7th **T75.09   Other effects of lightning**
            Use additional code for other effects of lightning

√x7th **T75.1   Unspecified effects of drowning and nonfatal** CC H5
        submersion
        Immersion
        EXCLUDES1 specified effects of drowning—code to effects
        CC Excl: PDX collection 1425

√5th **T75.2   Effects of vibration**
    √x7th **T75.20   Unspecified effects of vibration**
    √x7th **T75.21   Pneumatic hammer syndrome**
    √x7th **T75.22   Traumatic vasospastic syndrome**
    √x7th **T75.23   Vertigo from infrasound**
            EXCLUDES1 vertigo NOS (R42)
    √x7th **T75.29   Other effects of vibration**

√x7th **T75.3   Motion sickness**
        Airsickness
        Seasickness
        Travel sickness
        Use additional external cause code to identify vehicle or type of motion (Y92.81-, Y93.5-)

√x7th **T75.4   Electrocution**
        Shock from electric current
        Shock from electroshock gun (taser)

√5th **T75.8   Other specified effects of external causes**
    √x7th **T75.81   Effects of abnormal gravitation [G] forces**
    √x7th **T75.82   Effects of weightlessness**
    √x7th **T75.89   Other specified effects of external causes**

√4th **T76   Adult and child abuse, neglect and other maltreatment, suspected**
        Use additional code, if applicable, to identify any associated current injury
        EXCLUDES1 adult and child maltreatment, confirmed (T74.-)
                suspected abuse and maltreatment in pregnancy (O9A.3-, O9A.4-, O9A.5-)
                suspected adult physical and sexual abuse, ruled out (Z04.71)
                suspected adult sexual abused, ruled out (Z04.41)
                suspected child physical abuse, ruled out (Z04.72)
                suspected child sexual abuse, ruled out (Z04.42)

  The appropriate 7th character is to be added to each code from category T76.
  A   initial encounter
  D   subsequent encounter
  S   sequela

  CC Excl: For CC codes in category T76, unless otherwise noted: PDX collection 1423

√5th **T76.0   Neglect or abandonment, suspected**
    √x7th **T76.01   Adult neglect or abandonment, suspected** CC A
    √x7th **T76.02   Child neglect or abandonment, suspected** CC P
√5th **T76.1   Physical abuse, suspected**
    √x7th **T76.11   Adult physical abuse, suspected** CC A
    √x7th **T76.12   Child physical abuse, suspected** CC P
√5th **T76.2   Sexual abuse, suspected**
        Rape, suspected
        EXCLUDES1 alleged abuse, ruled out (Z04.7)
    √x7th **T76.21   Adult sexual abuse, suspected** CC A
    √x7th **T76.22   Child sexual abuse, suspected** CC P

√5th **T76.3   Psychological abuse, suspected**
        ▶Bullying and intimidation, suspected
        Intimidation through social media, suspected◀
    √x7th **T76.31   Adult psychological abuse, suspected** A
    √x7th **T76.32   Child psychological abuse, suspected** CC P
● √5th **T76.5   Forced sexual exploitation, suspected**
●   √x7th **T76.51   Adult forced sexual exploitation, suspected**
●   √x7th **T76.52   Child sexual exploitation, suspected**
● √5th **T76.6   Forced labor exploitation, suspected**
●   √x7th **T76.61   Adult forced labor exploitation, suspected**
●   √x7th **T76.62   Child forced labor exploitation, suspected**
√5th **T76.9   Unspecified maltreatment, suspected**
    √x7th **T76.91   Unspecified adult maltreatment, suspected** CC A
            CC Excl: PDX collection 1424
    √x7th **T76.92   Unspecified child maltreatment, suspected** CC P

√4th **T78   Adverse effects, not elsewhere classified**
        EXCLUDES2 complications of surgical and medical care NEC (T80-T88)

  The appropriate 7th character is to be added to each code from category T78.
  A   initial encounter
  D   subsequent encounter
  S   sequela

  CC Excl: For CC codes in category T78: PDX collection 1426

√5th **T78.0   Anaphylactic reaction due to food**
        Anaphylactic reaction due to adverse food reaction
        Anaphylactic shock or reaction due to nonpoisonous foods
        Anaphylactoid reaction due to food
    √x7th **T78.00   Anaphylactic reaction due to unspecified food** CC
    √x7th **T78.01   Anaphylactic reaction due to peanuts** CC
    √x7th **T78.02   Anaphylactic reaction due to shellfish (crustaceans)** CC
    √x7th **T78.03   Anaphylactic reaction due to other fish** CC
    √x7th **T78.04   Anaphylactic reaction due to fruits and vegetables** CC
    √x7th **T78.05   Anaphylactic reaction due to tree nuts and seeds** CC
            EXCLUDES2 anaphylactic reaction due to peanuts (T78.01)
    √x7th **T78.06   Anaphylactic reaction due to food additives** CC
    √x7th **T78.07   Anaphylactic reaction due to milk and dairy products** CC
    √x7th **T78.08   Anaphylactic reaction due to eggs** CC
    √x7th **T78.09   Anaphylactic reaction due to other food products** CC

√x7th **T78.1   Other adverse food reactions, not elsewhere classified**
        Use additional code to identify the type of reaction, if applicable
        EXCLUDES1 anaphylactic reaction or shock due to adverse food reaction (T78.0-)
                anaphylactic reaction due to food (T78.0-)
                bacterial food borne intoxications (A05.-)
        EXCLUDES2 allergic and dietetic gastroenteritis and colitis (K52.29)
                allergic rhinitis due to food (J30.5)
                dermatitis due to food in contact with skin (L23.6, L24.6, L25.4)
                dermatitis due to ingested food (L27.2)
                food protein-induced enterocolitis syndrome (K52.21)
                food protein-induced enteropathy (K52.22)

√x7th **T78.2   Anaphylactic shock, unspecified** CC
        Allergic shock
        Anaphylactic reaction
        Anaphylaxis
        EXCLUDES1 anaphylactic reaction or shock due to adverse effect of correct medicinal substance properly administered (T88.6)
                anaphylactic reaction or shock due to adverse food reaction (T78.0-)
                anaphylactic reaction or shock due to serum (T80.5-)

√x7th **T78.3   Angioneurotic edema**
        Allergic angioedema
        Giant urticaria
        Quincke's edema
        EXCLUDES1 serum urticaria (T80.6-)
                urticaria (L50.-)

✔Additional Character Required   •√x7th Placeholder   Unacceptable PDx   Questionable PDx   Manifestation   H1 - H14 HAC   HCC CMS-HCC Dx   HIV HIV Dx

ICD-10-CM 2019   1137

√5ᵗʰ T78.4 Other and unspecified allergy

> EXCLUDES 1   specified types of allergic reaction such as:
> allergic diarrhea (K52.29)
> allergic gastroenteritis and colitis (K52.29)
> dermatitis (L23-L25, L27-)
> food protein-induced enterocolitis syndrome (K52.21)
> food protein-induced enteropathy (K52.22)
> hay fever (J30.1)

√x7ᵗʰ T78.40 Allergy, unspecified
Allergic reaction NOS
Hypersensitivity NOS

√x7ᵗʰ T78.41 Arthus phenomenon
Arthus reaction

√x7ᵗʰ T78.49 Other allergy

√x7ᵗʰ T78.8 Other adverse effects, not elsewhere classified

Certain early complications of trauma (T79)

√4ᵗʰ T79 Certain early complications of trauma, not elsewhere classified

> EXCLUDES 2   acute respiratory distress syndrome (J80)
> complications occurring during or following medical procedures (T80-T88)
> complications of surgical and medical care NEC (T80-T88)
> newborn respiratory distress syndrome (P22.0)

> The appropriate 7th character is to be added to each code from category T79.
> A   initial encounter
> D   subsequent encounter
> S   sequela

6 √x7ᵗʰ T79.0 Air embolism (traumatic)   MCC HCC

> EXCLUDES 1   air embolism complicating abortion or ectopic or molar pregnancy (O00-O07, O08.2)
> air embolism complicating pregnancy, childbirth and the puerperium (O88.0)
> air embolism following infusion, transfusion, and therapeutic injection (T80.0)
> air embolism following procedure NEC (T81.7-)

> **DEF:** Arterial or venous obstruction due to the introduction of air bubbles into the blood vessels following surgery or trauma.
> **CC Excl:** PDX collection 1427

6 √x7ᵗʰ T79.1 Fat embolism (traumatic)   MCC HCC

> EXCLUDES 1   fat embolism complicating:
> abortion or ectopic or molar pregnancy (O00-O07, O08.2)
> pregnancy, childbirth and the puerperium (O88.8)

> **DEF:** Arterial blockage due to the entrance of fat into the circulatory system after a fracture of the large bones or administration of corticosteroids.
> **CC Excl:** PDX collection 1428

6 √x7ᵗʰ T79.2 Traumatic secondary and recurrent hemorrhage and seroma   CC HCC
> **CC Excl:** PDX collection 1429

6 √x7ᵗʰ T79.4 Traumatic shock   MCC HCC
Shock (immediate) (delayed) following injury

> EXCLUDES 1   anaphylactic shock due to adverse food reaction (T78.0-)
> anaphylactic shock due to correct medicinal substance properly administered (T88.6)
> anaphylactic shock due to serum (T80.5-)
> anaphylactic shock NOS (T78.2)
> anesthetic shock (T88.2)
> electric shock (T75.4)
> nontraumatic shock NEC (R57.-)
> obstetric shock (O75.1)
> postprocedural shock (T81.1-)
> septic shock (R65.21)
> shock complicating abortion or ectopic or molar pregnancy (O00-O07, O08.3)
> shock due to lightning (T75.01)
> shock NOS (R57.9)

> **CC Excl:** PDX collection 1430

6 √x7ᵗʰ T79.5 Traumatic anuria   MCC HCC
Crush syndrome
Renal failure following crushing
> **CC Excl:** PDX collection 1431

6 √x7ᵗʰ T79.6 Traumatic ischemia of muscle   HCC
Traumatic rhabdomyolysis
Volkmann's ischemic contracture

> EXCLUDES 2   anterior tibial syndrome (M76.8)
> compartment syndrome (traumatic) (T79.A-)
> nontraumatic ischemia of muscle (M62.2-)

6 √x7ᵗʰ T79.7 Traumatic subcutaneous emphysema   CC HCC

> EXCLUDES 1   emphysema NOS (J43)
> emphysema (subcutaneous) resulting from a procedure (T81.82)

> **CC Excl:** PDX collection 1432

√5ᵗʰ T79.A Traumatic compartment syndrome

> EXCLUDES 1   fibromyalgia (M79.7)
> nontraumatic compartment syndrome (M79.A-)
> traumatic ischemic infarction of muscle (T79.6)

> **DEF:** Compression of nerves and blood vessels within an enclosed muscle space due to previous trauma, which leads to impaired blood flow and muscle and nerve damage.

6 √x7ᵗʰ T79.A0 Compartment syndrome, unspecified   CC HCC
Compartment syndrome NOS
> **CC Excl:** PDX collection 896

√6ᵗʰ T79.A1 Traumatic compartment syndrome of upper extremity
Traumatic compartment syndrome of shoulder, arm, forearm, wrist, hand, and fingers

> **CC Excl:** For CC codes in category T79.A1: PDX collection 1433

6 √7ᵗʰ T79.A11 Traumatic compartment syndrome of right upper extremity   CC HCC

6 √7ᵗʰ T79.A12 Traumatic compartment syndrome of left upper extremity   CC HCC

6 √7ᵗʰ T79.A19 Traumatic compartment syndrome of unspecified upper extremity   CC HCC

√6ᵗʰ T79.A2 Traumatic compartment syndrome of lower extremity
Traumatic compartment syndrome of hip, buttock, thigh, leg, foot, and toes

> **CC Excl:** For CC codes in category T79.A2: PDX collection 1433

6 √7ᵗʰ T79.A21 Traumatic compartment syndrome of right lower extremity   CC HCC

6 √7ᵗʰ T79.A22 Traumatic compartment syndrome of left lower extremity   CC HCC

6 √7ᵗʰ T79.A29 Traumatic compartment syndrome of unspecified lower extremity   CC HCC

6 √x7ᵗʰ T79.A3 Traumatic compartment syndrome of abdomen   CC HCC
> **CC Excl:** PDX collection 1434

6 √x7ᵗʰ T79.A9 Traumatic compartment syndrome of other sites   CC HCC
> **CC Excl:** PDX collection 896

6 √x7ᵗʰ T79.8 Other early complications of trauma   HCC

6 √x7ᵗʰ T79.9 Unspecified early complication of trauma   HCC

N Newborn: 0   P Pediatric: 0-17   M Maternity: 12-55   A Adult: 15-124   MCC Major Complication/Comorbidity   CC Complication/Comorbidity   SW Severe Wound Dx

1138   ICD-10-CM 2019

Complications of surgical and medical care, not elsewhere classified (T80-T88)

Use additional code for adverse effect, if applicable, to identify drug (T36-T50 with fifth or sixth character 5)

Use additional code(s) to identify the specified condition resulting from the complication

Use additional code to identify devices involved and details of circumstances (Y62-Y82)

EXCLUDES 2   *any encounters with medical care for postprocedural conditions in which no complications are present, such as:*
     artificial opening status (Z93.-)
     closure of external stoma (Z43.-)
     fitting and adjustment of external prosthetic device (Z44.-)
   burns and corrosions from local applications and irradiation (T20-T32)
   complications of surgical procedures during pregnancy, childbirth and the puerperium (O00-O9A)
   mechanical complication of respirator [ventilator] (J95.850)
   poisoning and toxic effects of drugs and chemicals (T36-T65 with fifth or sixth character 1-4 or 6)
   postprocedural fever (R50.82)
   specified complications classified elsewhere, such as:
     cerebrospinal fluid leak from spinal puncture (G97.0)
     colostomy malfunction (K94.0-)
     disorders of fluid and electrolyte imbalance (E86-E87)
     functional disturbances following cardiac surgery (I97.0-I97.1)
     intraoperative and postprocedural complications of specified body systems (D78.-, E36.-, E89.-, G97.3-, G97.4, H59.3-, H59.-, H95.2-, H95.3, I97.4-, I97.5, J95.6-, J95.7, K91.6-, L76.-, M96.-, N99.-)
     ostomy complications (J95.0-, K94-, N99.5-)
     postgastric surgery syndromes (K91.1)
     postlaminectomy syndrome NEC (M96.1)
     postmastectomy lymphedema syndrome (I97.2)
     postsurgical blind-loop syndrome (K91.2)
     ventilator associated pneumonia (J95.851)

AHA: 2015, 1Q, 15

✓4th **T80 Complications following infusion, transfusion and therapeutic injection**

INCLUDES   complications following perfusion

EXCLUDES 2   *bone marrow transplant rejection (T86.01)*
   febrile nonhemolytic transfusion reaction (R50.84)
   fluid overload due to transfusion (E87.71)
   posttransfusion purpura (D69.51)
   transfusion associated circulatory overload (TACO) (E87.71)
   transfusion (red blood cell) associated hemochromatosis (E83.111)
   transfusion related acute lung injury (TRALI) (J95.84)

> The appropriate 7th character is to be added to each code from category T80.
> A   initial encounter
> D   subsequent encounter
> S   sequela

✓x7th **T80.0 Air embolism following infusion, transfusion and therapeutic injection**   MCC H2

     CC Excl: PDX collection 1435

✓x7th **T80.1 Vascular complications following infusion, transfusion and therapeutic injection**   CC

     Use additional code to identify the vascular complication

     EXCLUDES 2   *extravasation of vesicant agent (T80.81-)*
       infiltration of vesicant agent (T80.81-)
       postprocedural vascular complications (T81.7-)
       vascular complications specified as due to prosthetic devices, implants and grafts (T82.8-, T83.8-, T84.8-, T85.8-)

     CC Excl: PDX collection 1436

✓5th **T80.2 Infections following infusion, transfusion and therapeutic injection**

     Use additional code to identify the specific infection, such as: sepsis (A41.9)

     Use additional code (R65.2-) to identify severe sepsis, if applicable

     EXCLUDES 2   *infections specified as due to prosthetic devices, implants and grafts (T82.6-T82.7, T83.5-T83.6, T84.5-T84.7, T85.7)*
       postprocedural infections (T81.4-)

     CC Excl: For CC codes in subcategory T80.2:
     PDX collection 948

✓6th **T80.21 Infection due to central venous catheter**

     Infection due to pulmonary artery catheter (Swan-Ganz catheter)

✓7th **T80.211 Bloodstream infection due to central venous catheter**   CC H7

     Catheter-related bloodstream infection (CRBSI) NOS
     Central line-associated bloodstream infection (CLABSI)
     Bloodstream infection due to Hickman catheter
     Bloodstream infection due to peripherally inserted central catheter (PICC)
     Bloodstream infection due to portacath (port-a-cath)
     Bloodstream infection due to pulmonary artery catheter
     Bloodstream infection due to triple lumen catheter
     Bloodstream infection due to umbilical venous catheter

✓7th **T80.212 Local infection due to central venous catheter**   CC H7

     Exit or insertion site infection
     Local infection due to Hickman catheter
     Local infection due to peripherally inserted central catheter (PICC)
     Local infection due to portacath (port-a-cath)
     Local infection due to pulmonary artery catheter
     Local infection due to triple lumen catheter
     Local infection due to umbilical venous catheter
     Port or reservoir infection
     Tunnel infection

✓7th **T80.218 Other infection due to central venous catheter**   CC H7

     Other central line-associated infection
     Other infection due to Hickman catheter
     Other infection due to peripherally inserted central catheter (PICC)
     Other infection due to portacath (port-a-cath)
     Other infection due to pulmonary artery catheter
     Other infection due to triple lumen catheter
     Other infection due to umbilical venous catheter

✓7th **T80.219 Unspecified infection due to central venous catheter**   CC H7

     Central line-associated infection NOS
     Unspecified infection due to Hickman catheter
     Unspecified infection due to peripherally inserted central catheter (PICC)
     Unspecified infection due to portacath (port-a-cath)
     Unspecified infection due to pulmonary artery catheter
     Unspecified infection due to triple lumen catheter
     Unspecified infection due to umbilical venous catheter

✓x7th **T80.22 Acute infection following transfusion, infusion, or injection of blood and blood products**   CC

✓x7th **T80.29 Infection following other infusion, transfusion and therapeutic injection**   CC

✓5th **T80.3 ABO incompatibility reaction due to transfusion of blood or blood products**

     EXCLUDES 1 ▶ *minor blood group antigens reactions (Duffy) (E) (K) (Kell) (Kidd) (Lewis) (M) (N) (P) (S) (T80.A-)* ◀

     CC Excl: For CC codes in subcategory T80.3:
     PDX collection 1437

✓x7th **T80.30 ABO incompatibility reaction due to transfusion of blood or blood products, unspecified**   CC H3

     ABO incompatibility blood transfusion NOS
     Reaction to ABO incompatibility from transfusion NOS

☑ Additional Character Required   ✓x7th Placeholder   Unacceptable PDx   Questionable PDx   Manifestation   H1-H14 HAC   HCC CMS-HCC Dx   HIV HIV Dx

ICD-10-CM 2019   1139

T80–T80.30

✓6ᵗʰ T80.31 ABO incompatibility with hemolytic transfusion reaction

    ✓7ᵗʰ T80.310 ABO incompatibility with acute **hemolytic transfusion reaction**   `CC` `H3`
        ABO incompatibility with hemolytic transfusion reaction less than 24 hours after transfusion
        Acute hemolytic transfusion reaction (AHTR) due to ABO incompatibility

    ✓7ᵗʰ T80.311 ABO incompatibility with delayed **hemolytic transfusion reaction**   `CC` `H3`
        ABO incompatibility with hemolytic transfusion reaction 24 hours or more after transfusion
        Delayed hemolytic transfusion reaction (DHTR) due to ABO incompatibility

    ✓7ᵗʰ T80.319 ABO incompatibility with hemolytic transfusion reaction, unspecified   `CC` `H3`
        ABO incompatibility with hemolytic transfusion reaction at unspecified time after transfusion
        Hemolytic transfusion reaction (HTR) due to ABO incompatibility NOS

✓x7ᵗʰ T80.39 Other ABO incompatibility reaction due to transfusion of blood or blood products   `CC` `H3`
    Delayed serologic transfusion reaction (DSTR) from ABO incompatibility
    Other ABO incompatible blood transfusion
    Other reaction to ABO incompatible blood transfusion

✓5ᵗʰ T80.4 Rh incompatibility reaction due to transfusion of blood or blood products
    Reaction due to incompatibility of Rh antigens (C) (c) (D) (E) (e)

> **CC Excl: For CC codes in subcategory T80.4, unless otherwise noted:** PDX collection 1437

✓x7ᵗʰ T80.40 Rh incompatibility reaction due to transfusion of blood or blood products, unspecified   `CC`
    Reaction due to Rh factor in transfusion NOS
    Rh incompatible blood transfusion NOS

✓6ᵗʰ T80.41 Rh incompatibility with hemolytic transfusion reaction

    ✓7ᵗʰ T80.410 Rh incompatibility with acute **hemolytic transfusion reaction**   `CC`
        Acute hemolytic transfusion reaction (AHTR) due to Rh incompatibility
        Rh incompatibility with hemolytic transfusion reaction less than 24 hours after transfusion

    ✓7ᵗʰ T80.411 Rh incompatibility with delayed **hemolytic transfusion reaction**   `CC`
        Delayed hemolytic transfusion reaction (DHTR) due to Rh incompatibility
        Rh incompatibility with hemolytic transfusion reaction 24 hours or more after transfusion

    ✓7ᵗʰ T80.419 Rh incompatibility with hemolytic transfusion reaction, unspecified   `CC`
        Hemolytic transfusion reaction (HTR) due to Rh incompatibility NOS
        Rh incompatibility with hemolytic transfusion reaction at unspecified time after transfusion

✓x7ᵗʰ T80.49 Other Rh incompatibility reaction due to transfusion of blood or blood products   `CC`
    Delayed serologic transfusion reaction (DSTR) from Rh incompatibility
    Other reaction to Rh incompatible blood transfusion
    CC Excl: PDX collection 1438

✓5ᵗʰ T80.A Non-ABO incompatibility reaction due to transfusion of blood or blood products
    Reaction due to incompatibility of minor antigens (Duffy) (Kell) (Kidd) (Lewis) (M) (N) (P) (S)

> **CC Excl: For CC codes in subcategory T80.A, unless otherwise noted:** PDX collection 1438

✓x7ᵗʰ T80.A0 Non-ABO incompatibility reaction due to transfusion of blood or blood products, unspecified   `CC`
    Non-ABO antigen incompatibility reaction from transfusion NOS

✓6ᵗʰ T80.A1 Non-ABO incompatibility with hemolytic transfusion reaction

    ✓7ᵗʰ T80.A10 Non-ABO incompatibility with acute **hemolytic transfusion reaction**   `CC`
        Acute hemolytic transfusion reaction (AHTR) due to non-ABO incompatibility
        Non-ABO incompatibility with hemolytic transfusion reaction less than 24 hours after transfusion

    ✓7ᵗʰ T80.A11 Non-ABO incompatibility with delayed **hemolytic transfusion reaction**   `CC`
        Delayed hemolytic transfusion reaction (DHTR) due to non-ABO incompatibility
        Non-ABO incompatibility with hemolytic transfusion reaction 24 or more hours after transfusion

    ✓7ᵗʰ T80.A19 Non-ABO incompatibility with hemolytic transfusion reaction, unspecified   `CC`
        Hemolytic transfusion reaction (HTR) due to non-ABO incompatibility NOS
        Non-ABO incompatibility with hemolytic transfusion reaction at unspecified time after transfusion

✓x7ᵗʰ T80.A9 Other non-ABO incompatibility reaction due to transfusion of blood or blood products   `CC`
    Delayed serologic transfusion reaction (DSTR) from non-ABO incompatibility
    Other reaction to non-ABO incompatible blood transfusion
    CC Excl: PDX collection 1437

✓5ᵗʰ T80.5 Anaphylactic reaction due to serum
    Allergic shock due to serum
    Anaphylactic shock due to serum
    Anaphylactoid reaction due to serum
    Anaphylaxis due to serum

    EXCLUDES 1   *ABO incompatibility reaction due to transfusion of blood or blood products (T80.3-)*
        allergic reaction or shock NOS (T78.2)
        anaphylactic reaction or shock NOS (T78.2)
        anaphylactic reaction or shock due to adverse effect of correct medicinal substance properly administered (T88.6)
        other serum reaction (T80.6-)

    DEF: Life-threatening hypersensitivity to a foreign serum causing respiratory distress, vascular collapse, and shock.

> **CC Excl: For CC codes in subcategory T80.5:** PDX collection 1439

✓x7ᵗʰ T80.51 Anaphylactic reaction due to administration of blood and blood products   `CC`

✓x7ᵗʰ T80.52 Anaphylactic reaction due to vaccination   `CC`

✓x7ᵗʰ T80.59 Anaphylactic reaction due to other serum   `CC`

✓5ᵗʰ T80.6 Other serum reactions

Intoxication by serum	Serum sickness
Protein sickness	Serum urticaria
Serum rash	

    EXCLUDES 2   *serum hepatitis (B16-B19)*

    DEF: Serum sickness: Hypersensitivity to a foreign serum that causes fever, hives, swelling, and lymphadenopathy.

> **CC Excl: For CC codes in subcategory T80.6, unless otherwise noted:** PDX collection 1439

✓x7ᵗʰ T80.61 Other serum reaction due to administration of blood and blood products   `CC`

✓x7ᵗʰ T80.62 Other serum reaction due to vaccination   `CC`

✓x7ᵗʰ T80.69 Other serum reaction due to other serum   `CC`
    Code also, if applicable, arthropathy in hypersensitivity reactions classified elsewhere (M36.4)
    CC Excl: PDX collection 1440

✓5ᵗʰ T80.8 Other complications following infusion, transfusion and therapeutic injection

    ✓6ᵗʰ T80.81 Extravasation of vesicant agent
        Infiltration of vesicant agent

        ✓7ᵗʰ T80.810 Extravasation of vesicant antineoplastic chemotherapy   `CC`
            Infiltration of vesicant antineoplastic chemotherapy
            CC Excl: PDX collection 1436

N Newborn: 0   **P** Pediatric: 0-17   **M** Maternity: 12-55   **A** Adult: 15-124   **MCC** Major Complication/Comorbidity   **CC** Complication/Comorbidity   **SW** Severe Wound Dx

1140   ICD-10-CM 2019

√7ᵗʰ T80.818 Extravasation of other vesicant agent `CC`
Infiltration of other vesicant agent
CC Excl: PDX collection 1436

√x7ᵗʰ T80.89 Other complications following infusion, transfusion and therapeutic injection
Delayed serologic transfusion reaction (DSTR), unspecified incompatibility
Use additional code to identify graft-versus-host reaction, if applicable, (D89.81-)

√5ᵗʰ T80.9 Unspecified complication following infusion, transfusion and therapeutic injection

√x7ᵗʰ T80.90 Unspecified complication following infusion and therapeutic injection

√6ᵗʰ T80.91 Hemolytic transfusion reaction, unspecified incompatibility
> *EXCLUDES 1*   *ABO incompatibility with hemolytic transfusion reaction (T80.31-)*
> *Non-ABO incompatibility with hemolytic transfusion reaction (T80.A1-)*
> *Rh incompatibility with hemolytic transfusion reaction (T80.41-)*

> **CC Excl: For CC codes in subcategory T80.91:** PDX collection 1437

√7ᵗʰ T80.910 Acute hemolytic transfusion reaction, unspecified incompatibility `CC`

√7ᵗʰ T80.911 Delayed hemolytic transfusion reaction, unspecified incompatibility `CC`

√7ᵗʰ T80.919 Hemolytic transfusion reaction, unspecified incompatibility, unspecified as acute or delayed `CC`
Hemolytic transfusion reaction NOS

√x7ᵗʰ T80.92 Unspecified transfusion reaction
Transfusion reaction NOS

√4ᵗʰ T81 Complications of procedures, not elsewhere classified
Use additional code for adverse effect, if applicable, to identify drug (T36-T50 with fifth or sixth character 5)
> *EXCLUDES 2*   *complications following immunization (T88.0-T88.1)*
> *complications following infusion, transfusion and therapeutic injection (T80.-)*
> *complications of transplanted organs and tissue (T86.-)*
> *specified complications classified elsewhere, such as:*
> *complication of prosthetic devices, implants and grafts (T82-T85)*
> *dermatitis due to drugs and medicaments (L23.3, L24.4, L25.1, L27.0-L27.1)*
> *endosseous dental implant failure (M27.6-)*
> *floppy iris syndrome (IFIS) (intraoperative) (H21.81)*
> *intraoperative and postprocedural complications of specific body system (D78.-, E36.-, E89.-, G97.3-, G97.4, H59.3-, H59.-, H95.2-, H95.3, I97.4-, I97.5, J95.-, K91.-, L76.-, M96.-, N99.-)*
> *ostomy complications (J95.0-, K94.-, N99.5-)*
> *plateau iris syndrome (post-iridectomy) (postprocedural) (H21.82)*
> *poisoning and toxic effects of drugs and chemicals (T36-T65 with fifth or sixth character 1-4 or 6)*

> The appropriate 7th character is to be added to each code from category T81.
> A   initial encounter
> D   subsequent encounter
> S   sequela

√5ᵗʰ T81.1 Postprocedural shock
Shock during or resulting from a procedure, not elsewhere classified
> *EXCLUDES 1*   *anaphylactic shock due to correct substance properly administered (T88.6)*
> *anaphylactic shock due to serum (T80.5-)*
> *anaphylactic shock NOS (T78.2)*
> *anesthetic shock (T88.2)*
> *electric shock (T75.4)*
> *obstetric shock (O75.1)*
> *septic shock (R65.21)*
> *shock following abortion or ectopic or molar pregnancy (O00-O07, O08.3)*
> *traumatic shock (T79.4)*

> **CC Excl: For CC/MCC codes in subcategory T81.1:** PDX collection 1441

√x7ᵗʰ T81.10 Postprocedural shock unspecified `CC`
Collapse NOS during or resulting from a procedure, not elsewhere classified
Postprocedural failure of peripheral circulation
Postprocedural shock NOS

▲   6 **√x7ᵗʰ T81.11 Postprocedural cardiogenic shock** `MCC` `HCC`

6 **√x7ᵗʰ T81.12 Postprocedural septic shock** `MCC` `HCC`
Postprocedural endotoxic shock resulting from a procedure, not elsewhere classified
Postprocedural gram-negative shock resulting from a procedure, not elsewhere classified
Code first underlying infection
Use additional code, to identify any associated acute organ dysfunction, if applicable

√x7ᵗʰ T81.19 Other postprocedural shock `MCC`
Postprocedural hypovolemic shock

√5ᵗʰ T81.3 Disruption of wound, not elsewhere classified
Disruption of any suture materials or other closure methods
> *EXCLUDES 1*   *breakdown (mechanical) of permanent sutures (T85.612)*
> *displacement of permanent sutures (T85.622)*
> *disruption of cesarean delivery wound (O90.0)*
> *disruption of perineal obstetric wound (O90.1)*
> *mechanical complication of permanent sutures NEC (T85.692)*

AHA: 2014, 1Q, 23

> **CC Excl: For CC codes in subcategory T81.3:** PDX collection 1442

√x7ᵗʰ T81.30 Disruption of wound, unspecified `CC` `SW`
Disruption of wound NOS

√x7ᵗʰ T81.31 Disruption of external operation (surgical) wound, not elsewhere classified `CC` `SW`
Dehiscence of operation wound NOS
Disruption of operation wound NOS
Disruption or dehiscence of closure of cornea
Disruption or dehiscence of closure of mucosa
Disruption or dehiscence of closure of skin and subcutaneous tissue
Full-thickness skin disruption or dehiscence
Superficial disruption or dehiscence of operation wound
> *EXCLUDES 1*   *dehiscence of amputation stump (T87.81)*

√x7ᵗʰ T81.32 Disruption of internal operation (surgical) wound, not elsewhere classified `CC` `SW`
Deep disruption or dehiscence of operation wound NOS
Disruption or dehiscence of closure of internal organ or other internal tissue
Disruption or dehiscence of closure of muscle or muscle flap
Disruption or dehiscence of closure of ribs or rib cage
Disruption or dehiscence of closure of skull or craniotomy
Disruption or dehiscence of closure of sternum or sternotomy
Disruption or dehiscence of closure of tendon or ligament
Disruption or dehiscence of closure of superficial or muscular fascia
AHA: 2017, 3Q, 4

√x7ᵗʰ T81.33 Disruption of traumatic injury wound repair `CC`
Disruption or dehiscence of closure of traumatic laceration (external) (internal)

✓5ᵗʰ **T81.4 Infection following a procedure**
~~Intra-abdominal abscess following a procedure~~
~~Postprocedural infection, not elsewhere classified~~
~~Sepsis following a procedure~~
~~Stitch abscess following a procedure~~
~~Subphrenic abscess following a procedure~~
Wound abscess following a procedure
Use additional code to identify infection
Use additional code (R65.2-) to identify severe sepsis, if applicable

EXCLUDES 1 ~~obstetric surgical wound infection (O86.0)~~
~~postprocedural fever NOS (R50.82)~~
~~postprocedural retroperitoneal abscess (K68.11)~~

EXCLUDES 2 bleb associated endophthalmitis (H59.4-)
infection due to infusion, transfusion and therapeutic injection (T80.2-)
infection due to prosthetic devices, implants and grafts (T82.6-T82.7, T83.5-T83.6, T84.5-T84.7, T85.7)
▶obstetric surgical wound infection (O86.0-)
postprocedural fever NOS (R50.82)
postprocedural retroperitoneal abscess (K68.11)◀

AHA: 2014, 1Q, 23

- ✓✗7ᵗʰ **T81.40 Infection following a procedure, unspecified** `CC`
- ✓✗7ᵗʰ **T81.41 Infection following a procedure, superficial incisional surgical site** `CC`
Subcutaneous abscess following a procedure
Stitch abscess following a procedure
- ✓✗7ᵗʰ **T81.42 Infection following a procedure, deep incisional surgical site** `CC`
Intra-muscular abscess following a procedure
- ✓✗7ᵗʰ **T81.43 Infection following a procedure, organ and space surgical site** `CC`
Intra-abdominal abscess following a procedure
Subphrenic abscess following a procedure
- ✓✗7ᵗʰ **T81.44 Sepsis following a procedure** `CC`
Use additional code to identify the sepsis
- ✓✗7ᵗʰ **T81.49 Infection following a procedure, other surgical site** `CC`

✓5ᵗʰ **T81.5 Complications of foreign body accidentally left in body following procedure**
AHA: 2014, 4Q, 24

CC Excl: For CC codes in subcategory T81.5:
PDX collection 1443

✓6ᵗʰ **T81.50 Unspecified complication of foreign body accidentally left in body following procedure**
- ✓7ᵗʰ **T81.500 Unspecified complication of foreign body accidentally left in body following surgical operation** `CC` `H1`
- ✓7ᵗʰ **T81.501 Unspecified complication of foreign body accidentally left in body following infusion or transfusion** `CC` `H1`
- ✓7ᵗʰ **T81.502 Unspecified complication of foreign body accidentally left in body following kidney dialysis** `CC` `H1` `HCC`
- ✓7ᵗʰ **T81.503 Unspecified complication of foreign body accidentally left in body following injection or immunization** `CC` `H1`
- ✓7ᵗʰ **T81.504 Unspecified complication of foreign body accidentally left in body following endoscopic examination** `CC` `H1`
- ✓7ᵗʰ **T81.505 Unspecified complication of foreign body accidentally left in body following heart catheterization** `CC` `H1`
- ✓7ᵗʰ **T81.506 Unspecified complication of foreign body accidentally left in body following aspiration, puncture or other catheterization** `CC` `H1`
- ✓7ᵗʰ **T81.507 Unspecified complication of foreign body accidentally left in body following removal of catheter or packing** `CC` `H1`
- ✓7ᵗʰ **T81.508 Unspecified complication of foreign body accidentally left in body following other procedure** `CC` `H1`
- ✓7ᵗʰ **T81.509 Unspecified complication of foreign body accidentally left in body following unspecified procedure** `CC` `H1`

✓6ᵗʰ **T81.51 Adhesions due to foreign body accidentally left in body following procedure**
- ✓7ᵗʰ **T81.510 Adhesions due to foreign body accidentally left in body following surgical operation** `CC` `H1`
- ✓7ᵗʰ **T81.511 Adhesions due to foreign body accidentally left in body following infusion or transfusion** `CC` `H1`
- ✓7ᵗʰ **T81.512 Adhesions due to foreign body accidentally left in body following kidney dialysis** `CC` `H1` `HCC`
- ✓7ᵗʰ **T81.513 Adhesions due to foreign body accidentally left in body following injection or immunization** `CC` `H1`
- ✓7ᵗʰ **T81.514 Adhesions due to foreign body accidentally left in body following endoscopic examination** `CC` `H1`
- ✓7ᵗʰ **T81.515 Adhesions due to foreign body accidentally left in body following heart catheterization** `CC` `H1`
- ✓7ᵗʰ **T81.516 Adhesions due to foreign body accidentally left in body following aspiration, puncture or other catheterization** `CC` `H1`
- ✓7ᵗʰ **T81.517 Adhesions due to foreign body accidentally left in body following removal of catheter or packing** `CC` `H1`
- ✓7ᵗʰ **T81.518 Adhesions due to foreign body accidentally left in body following other procedure** `CC` `H1`
- ✓7ᵗʰ **T81.519 Adhesions due to foreign body accidentally left in body following unspecified procedure** `CC` `H1`

✓6ᵗʰ **T81.52 Obstruction due to foreign body accidentally left in body following procedure**
- ✓7ᵗʰ **T81.520 Obstruction due to foreign body accidentally left in body following surgical operation** `CC` `H1`
- ✓7ᵗʰ **T81.521 Obstruction due to foreign body accidentally left in body following infusion or transfusion** `CC` `H1`
- ✓7ᵗʰ **T81.522 Obstruction due to foreign body accidentally left in body following kidney dialysis** `CC` `H1` `HCC`
- ✓7ᵗʰ **T81.523 Obstruction due to foreign body accidentally left in body following injection or immunization** `CC` `H1`
- ✓7ᵗʰ **T81.524 Obstruction due to foreign body accidentally left in body following endoscopic examination** `CC` `H1`
- ✓7ᵗʰ **T81.525 Obstruction due to foreign body accidentally left in body following heart catheterization** `CC` `H1`
- ✓7ᵗʰ **T81.526 Obstruction due to foreign body accidentally left in body following aspiration, puncture or other catheterization** `CC` `H1`
- ✓7ᵗʰ **T81.527 Obstruction due to foreign body accidentally left in body following removal of catheter or packing** `CC` `H1`
- ✓7ᵗʰ **T81.528 Obstruction due to foreign body accidentally left in body following other procedure** `CC` `H1`
- ✓7ᵗʰ **T81.529 Obstruction due to foreign body accidentally left in body following unspecified procedure** `CC` `H1`

✓6ᵗʰ **T81.53 Perforation due to foreign body accidentally left in body following procedure**
- ✓7ᵗʰ **T81.530 Perforation due to foreign body accidentally left in body following surgical operation** `CC` `H1`
- ✓7ᵗʰ **T81.531 Perforation due to foreign body accidentally left in body following infusion or transfusion** `CC` `H1`
- ✓7ᵗʰ **T81.532 Perforation due to foreign body accidentally left in body following kidney dialysis** `CC` `H1` `HCC`

√7ᵗʰ **T81.533** **Perforation due to foreign body accidentally left in body following injection or immunization** `CC` `H1`

√7ᵗʰ **T81.534** **Perforation due to foreign body accidentally left in body following endoscopic examination** `CC` `H1`

√7ᵗʰ **T81.535** **Perforation due to foreign body accidentally left in body following heart catheterization** `CC` `H1`

√7ᵗʰ **T81.536** **Perforation due to foreign body accidentally left in body following aspiration, puncture or other catheterization** `CC` `H1`

√7ᵗʰ **T81.537** **Perforation due to foreign body accidentally left in body following removal of catheter or packing** `CC` `H1`

√7ᵗʰ **T81.538** **Perforation due to foreign body accidentally left in body following other procedure** `CC` `H1`

√7ᵗʰ **T81.539** **Perforation due to foreign body accidentally left in body following unspecified procedure** `CC` `H1`

√6ᵗʰ **T81.59** **Other complications of foreign body accidentally left in body following procedure**
    EXCLUDES 2   *obstruction or perforation due to prosthetic devices and implants intentionally left in body (T82.0-T82.5, T83.0-T83.4, T83.7, T84.0-T84.4, T85.0-T85.6)*

√7ᵗʰ **T81.590** **Other complications of foreign body accidentally left in body following surgical operation** `CC` `H1`

√7ᵗʰ **T81.591** **Other complications of foreign body accidentally left in body following infusion or transfusion** `CC` `H1`

√7ᵗʰ **T81.592** **Other complications of foreign body accidentally left in body following kidney dialysis** `CC` `H1` `HCC`

√7ᵗʰ **T81.593** **Other complications of foreign body accidentally left in body following injection or immunization** `CC` `H1`

√7ᵗʰ **T81.594** **Other complications of foreign body accidentally left in body following endoscopic examination** `CC` `H1`

√7ᵗʰ **T81.595** **Other complications of foreign body accidentally left in body following heart catheterization** `CC` `H1`

√7ᵗʰ **T81.596** **Other complications of foreign body accidentally left in body following aspiration, puncture or other catheterization** `CC` `H1`

√7ᵗʰ **T81.597** **Other complications of foreign body accidentally left in body following removal of catheter or packing** `CC` `H1`

√7ᵗʰ **T81.598** **Other complications of foreign body accidentally left in body following other procedure** `CC` `H1`

√7ᵗʰ **T81.599** **Other complications of foreign body accidentally left in body following unspecified procedure** `CC` `H1`

√5ᵗʰ **T81.6** **Acute reaction to foreign substance accidentally left during a procedure**
    EXCLUDES 2   *complications of foreign body accidentally left in body cavity or operation wound following procedure (T81.5-)*

    CC Excl: For CC codes in subcategory T81.6:
    PDX collection 1444

√x7ᵗʰ **T81.60** **Unspecified acute reaction to foreign substance accidentally left during a procedure** `CC` `H1`

√x7ᵗʰ **T81.61** **Aseptic peritonitis due to foreign substance accidentally left during a procedure** `CC` `H1`
    Chemical peritonitis

√x7ᵗʰ **T81.69** **Other acute reaction to foreign substance accidentally left during a procedure** `CC` `H1`

√5ᵗʰ **T81.7** **Vascular complications following a procedure, not elsewhere classified**
    Air embolism following procedure NEC
    Phlebitis or thrombophlebitis resulting from a procedure
    EXCLUDES 1   *embolism complicating abortion or ectopic or molar pregnancy (O00-O07, O08.2)*
          embolism complicating pregnancy, childbirth and the puerperium (O88.-)
          traumatic embolism (T79.0)
    EXCLUDES 2   *embolism due to prosthetic devices, implants and grafts (T82.8-, T83.81, T84.8-, T85.81-)*
          embolism following infusion, transfusion and therapeutic injection (T80.0)

√6ᵗʰ **T81.71** **Complication of artery following a procedure, not elsewhere classified**

√7ᵗʰ **T81.710** **Complication of mesenteric artery following a procedure, not elsewhere classified** `CC`
         CC Excl: PDX collection 1445

√7ᵗʰ **T81.711** **Complication of renal artery following a procedure, not elsewhere classified** `CC`
         CC Excl: PDX collection 1445

√7ᵗʰ **T81.718** **Complication of other artery following a procedure, not elsewhere classified** `CC`
         CC Excl: PDX collection 1446

√7ᵗʰ **T81.719** **Complication of unspecified artery following a procedure, not elsewhere classified** `CC`
         CC Excl: PDX collection 1446

√x7ᵗʰ **T81.72** **Complication of vein following a procedure, not elsewhere classified** `CC`
         CC Excl: PDX collection 1446

√5ᵗʰ **T81.8** **Other complications of procedures, not elsewhere classified**
    EXCLUDES 2   *hypothermia following anesthesia (T88.51)*
          malignant hyperpyrexia due to anesthesia (T88.3)

√x7ᵗʰ **T81.81** **Complication of inhalation therapy**

√x7ᵗʰ **T81.82** **Emphysema (subcutaneous) resulting from a procedure**

√x7ᵗʰ **T81.83** **Persistent postprocedural fistula** `CC` `SW`
    AHA: 2017, 3Q, 3-4
    CC Excl: PDX collection 1447

√x7ᵗʰ **T81.89** **Other complications of procedures, not elsewhere classified** `SW`
    Use additional code to specify complication, such as:
        postprocedural delirium (F05)
    AHA: 2014, 1Q, 23

√x7ᵗʰ **T81.9** **Unspecified complication of procedure**

√4ᵗʰ **T82** **Complications of cardiac and vascular prosthetic devices, implants and grafts**
    EXCLUDES 2   *failure and rejection of transplanted organs and tissue (T86.-)*

    The appropriate 7th character is to be added to each code from category T82.
    A   initial encounter
    D   subsequent encounter
    S   sequela

√5ᵗʰ **T82.0** **Mechanical complication of heart valve prosthesis**
    Mechanical complication of artificial heart valve
    EXCLUDES 1   *mechanical complication of biological heart valve graft (T82.22-)*

    CC Excl: For CC codes in subcategory T82.0:
    PDX collection 1448

√x7ᵗʰ **T82.01** **Breakdown (mechanical) of heart valve prosthesis** `CC`

√x7ᵗʰ **T82.02** **Displacement of heart valve prosthesis** `CC`
    Malposition of heart valve prosthesis

√x7ᵗʰ **T82.03** **Leakage of heart valve prosthesis** `CC`

√x7ᵗʰ **T82.09** **Other mechanical complication of heart valve prosthesis** `CC`
    Obstruction (mechanical) of heart valve prosthesis
    Perforation of heart valve prosthesis
    Protrusion of heart valve prosthesis

✔Additional Character Required   √x7ᵗʰ Placeholder   Unacceptable PDx   Questionable PDx   Manifestation   `H1`-`H14` HAC   `HCC`CMS-HCC Dx   `HIV` HIV Dx

ICD-10-CM 2019   1143

Chapter 19. Injury, Poisoning and Certain Other Consequences of External Causes

T82.1–T82.49

√5th **T82.1** Mechanical complication of cardiac electronic device

> CC Excl: For CC codes in subcategory T82.1, unless otherwise noted: PDX collection 1449

√6th **T82.11** Breakdown (mechanical) of cardiac electronic device

√7th **T82.110** Breakdown (mechanical) of cardiac electrode   CC

√7th **T82.111** Breakdown (mechanical) of cardiac pulse generator (battery)   CC

√7th **T82.118** Breakdown (mechanical) of other cardiac electronic device   CC
> CC Excl: PDX collection 1450

√7th **T82.119** Breakdown (mechanical) of unspecified cardiac electronic device   CC
> CC Excl: No Excl

√6th **T82.12** Displacement of cardiac electronic device
> Malposition of cardiac electronic device

√7th **T82.120** Displacement of cardiac electrode   CC

√7th **T82.121** Displacement of cardiac pulse generator (battery)   CC

√7th **T82.128** Displacement of other cardiac electronic device   CC
> CC Excl: PDX collection 1450

√7th **T82.129** Displacement of unspecified cardiac electronic device   CC
> CC Excl: No Excl

√6th **T82.19** Other mechanical complication of cardiac electronic device
> Leakage of cardiac electronic device
> Obstruction of cardiac electronic device
> Perforation of cardiac electronic device
> Protrusion of cardiac electronic device

√7th **T82.190** Other mechanical complication of cardiac electrode   CC

√7th **T82.191** Other mechanical complication of cardiac pulse generator (battery)   CC

√7th **T82.198** Other mechanical complication of other cardiac electronic device   CC
> CC Excl: PDX collection 1450

√7th **T82.199** Other mechanical complication of unspecified cardiac device   CC
> CC Excl: No Excl

√5th **T82.2** Mechanical complication of coronary artery bypass graft and biological heart valve graft
> EXCLUDES 1   mechanical complication of artificial heart valve prosthesis (T82.0-)

√6th **T82.21** Mechanical complication of coronary artery bypass graft

> CC Excl: For CC codes in subcategory T82.21: PDX collection 1451

√7th **T82.211** Breakdown (mechanical) of coronary artery bypass graft   CC

√7th **T82.212** Displacement of coronary artery bypass graft   CC
> Malposition of coronary artery bypass graft

√7th **T82.213** Leakage of coronary artery bypass graft   CC

√7th **T82.218** Other mechanical complication of coronary artery bypass graft
> Obstruction, mechanical of coronary artery bypass graft
> Perforation of coronary artery bypass graft
> Protrusion of coronary artery bypass graft

√6th **T82.22** Mechanical complication of biological heart valve graft

> CC Excl: For CC codes in subcategory T82.22: PDX collection 1450

√7th **T82.221** Breakdown (mechanical) of biological heart valve graft   CC

√7th **T82.222** Displacement of biological heart valve graft   CC
> Malposition of biological heart valve graft

√7th **T82.223** Leakage of biological heart valve graft   CC

√7th **T82.228** Other mechanical complication of biological heart valve graft   CC
> Obstruction of biological heart valve graft
> Perforation of biological heart valve graft
> Protrusion of biological heart valve graft

√5th **T82.3** Mechanical complication of other vascular grafts

> CC Excl: For CC codes in subcategory T82.3: PDX collection 1452

√6th **T82.31** Breakdown (mechanical) of other vascular grafts

6 √7th **T82.310** Breakdown (mechanical) of aortic (bifurcation) graft (replacement)   CC HCC

6 √7th **T82.311** Breakdown (mechanical) of carotid arterial graft (bypass)   CC HCC

6 √7th **T82.312** Breakdown (mechanical) of femoral arterial graft (bypass)   CC HCC

6 √7th **T82.318** Breakdown (mechanical) of other vascular grafts   CC HCC

6 √7th **T82.319** Breakdown (mechanical) of unspecified vascular grafts   CC HCC

√6th **T82.32** Displacement of other vascular grafts
> Malposition of other vascular grafts

6 √7th **T82.320** Displacement of aortic (bifurcation) graft (replacement)   CC HCC

6 √7th **T82.321** Displacement of carotid arterial graft (bypass)   CC HCC

6 √7th **T82.322** Displacement of femoral arterial graft (bypass)   CC HCC

6 √7th **T82.328** Displacement of other vascular grafts   CC HCC

6 √7th **T82.329** Displacement of unspecified vascular grafts   CC HCC

√6th **T82.33** Leakage of other vascular grafts

6 √7th **T82.330** Leakage of aortic (bifurcation) graft (replacement)   CC HCC

6 √7th **T82.331** Leakage of carotid arterial graft (bypass)   CC HCC

6 √7th **T82.332** Leakage of femoral arterial graft (bypass)   CC HCC

6 √7th **T82.338** Leakage of other vascular grafts   CC HCC

6 √7th **T82.339** Leakage of unspecified vascular graft   CC HCC

√6th **T82.39** Other mechanical complication of other vascular grafts
> Obstruction (mechanical) of other vascular grafts
> Perforation of other vascular grafts
> Protrusion of other vascular grafts

6 √7th **T82.390** Other mechanical complication of aortic (bifurcation) graft (replacement)   CC HCC

6 √7th **T82.391** Other mechanical complication of carotid arterial graft (bypass)   CC HCC

6 √7th **T82.392** Other mechanical complication of femoral arterial graft (bypass)   CC HCC

6 √7th **T82.398** Other mechanical complication of other vascular grafts   CC HCC

6 √7th **T82.399** Other mechanical complication of unspecified vascular grafts   CC HCC

√5th **T82.4** Mechanical complication of vascular dialysis catheter
> Mechanical complication of hemodialysis catheter
> EXCLUDES 1   mechanical complication of intraperitoneal dialysis catheter (T85.62)

> CC Excl: For CC codes in subcategory T82.4: PDX collection 1452

√x7th **T82.41** Breakdown (mechanical) of vascular dialysis catheter   CC HCC

√x7th **T82.42** Displacement of vascular dialysis catheter   CC HCC
> Malposition of vascular dialysis catheter

√x7th **T82.43** Leakage of vascular dialysis catheter   CC HCC

√x7th **T82.49** Other complication of vascular dialysis catheter   CC HCC
> Obstruction (mechanical) of vascular dialysis catheter
> Perforation of vascular dialysis catheter
> Protrusion of vascular dialysis catheter

N Newborn: 0   P Pediatric: 0-17   M Maternity: 12-55   A Adult: 15-124   MCC Major Complication/Comorbidity   CC Complication/Comorbidity   SW Severe Wound Dx

1144   ICD-10-CM 2019

✓5ᵗʰ T82.5 **Mechanical complication of** other cardiac and vascular devices and implants

> EXCLUDES 2   mechanical complication of epidural and subdural infusion catheter (T85.61)

> **CC Excl: For CC codes in subcategory T82.5, unless otherwise noted:** PDX collection 1452

✓6ᵗʰ T82.51 Breakdown (mechanical) of other cardiac and vascular devices and implants

6   **✓7ᵗʰ T82.510** **Breakdown (mechanical) of** surgically created arteriovenous fistula   `CC` `HCC`

6   **✓7ᵗʰ T82.511** **Breakdown (mechanical) of** surgically created arteriovenous shunt   `CC` `HCC`

✓7ᵗʰ T82.512 **Breakdown (mechanical) of** artificial heart   `CC`
> **CC Excl:** PDX collection 1450

6   **✓7ᵗʰ T82.513** **Breakdown (mechanical) of** balloon (counterpulsation) device   `CC` `HCC`

6   **✓7ᵗʰ T82.514** **Breakdown (mechanical) of** infusion catheter   `CC` `HCC`

6   **✓7ᵗʰ T82.515** **Breakdown (mechanical) of** umbrella device   `CC` `HCC`

6   **✓7ᵗʰ T82.518** **Breakdown (mechanical) of** other cardiac and vascular devices and implants   `CC` `HCC`

✓7ᵗʰ T82.519 **Breakdown (mechanical) of** unspecified cardiac and vascular devices and implants   `CC`
> **CC Excl:** PDX collection 1453

✓6ᵗʰ T82.52 Displacement of other cardiac and vascular devices and implants
> Malposition of other cardiac and vascular devices and implants

6   **✓7ᵗʰ T82.520** **Displacement of** surgically created arteriovenous fistula   `CC` `HCC`

6   **✓7ᵗʰ T82.521** **Displacement of** surgically created arteriovenous shunt   `CC` `HCC`

✓7ᵗʰ T82.522 **Displacement of** artificial heart   `CC`
> **CC Excl:** PDX collection 1450

6   **✓7ᵗʰ T82.523** **Displacement of** balloon (counterpulsation) device   `CC` `HCC`

6   **✓7ᵗʰ T82.524** **Displacement of** infusion catheter   `CC` `HCC`

6   **✓7ᵗʰ T82.525** **Displacement of** umbrella device   `CC` `HCC`

6   **✓7ᵗʰ T82.528** **Displacement of** other cardiac and vascular devices and implants   `CC` `HCC`

✓7ᵗʰ T82.529 **Displacement of** unspecified cardiac and vascular devices and implants   `CC`

✓6ᵗʰ T82.53 Leakage of other cardiac and vascular devices and implants

6   **✓7ᵗʰ T82.530** **Leakage of** surgically created arteriovenous fistula   `CC` `HCC`

6   **✓7ᵗʰ T82.531** **Leakage of** surgically created arteriovenous shunt   `CC` `HCC`

✓7ᵗʰ T82.532 **Leakage of** artificial heart   `CC`
> **CC Excl:** PDX collection 1450

6   **✓7ᵗʰ T82.533** **Leakage of** balloon (counterpulsation) device   `CC` `HCC`

6   **✓7ᵗʰ T82.534** **Leakage of** infusion catheter   `CC` `HCC`

6   **✓7ᵗʰ T82.535** **Leakage of** umbrella device   `CC` `HCC`

6   **✓7ᵗʰ T82.538** **Leakage of** other cardiac and vascular devices and implants   `CC` `HCC`

✓7ᵗʰ T82.539 **Leakage of** unspecified cardiac and vascular devices and implants   `CC`
> **CC Excl:** PDX collection 1453

✓6ᵗʰ T82.59 Other mechanical complication of other cardiac and vascular devices and implants
> Obstruction (mechanical) of other cardiac and vascular devices and implants
> Perforation of other cardiac and vascular devices and implants
> Protrusion of other cardiac and vascular devices and implants

6   **✓7ᵗʰ T82.590** **Other mechanical complication of** surgically created arteriovenous fistula   `CC` `HCC`

6   **✓7ᵗʰ T82.591** **Other mechanical complication of** surgically created arteriovenous shunt   `CC` `HCC`

6   **✓7ᵗʰ T82.592** **Other mechanical complication of** artificial heart   `CC`
> **CC Excl:** PDX collection 1450

6   **✓7ᵗʰ T82.593** **Other mechanical complication of** balloon (counterpulsation) device   `CC` `HCC`

6   **✓7ᵗʰ T82.594** **Other mechanical complication of** infusion catheter   `CC` `HCC`
> **CC Excl:** PDX collection 1450

6   **✓7ᵗʰ T82.595** **Other mechanical complication of** umbrella device   `CC` `HCC`

6   **✓7ᵗʰ T82.598** **Other mechanical complication of** other cardiac and vascular devices and implants   `CC` `HCC`
> **CC Excl:** PDX collection 1450

✓7ᵗʰ T82.599 **Other mechanical complication of** unspecified cardiac and vascular devices and implants   `CC`
> **CC Excl:** PDX collection 1453

6   **✓x7ᵗʰ T82.6** Infection and inflammatory reaction due to cardiac valveprosthesis   `CC` `H13` `HCC`
> Use additional code to identify infection
> **CC Excl:** PDX collection 1454

6   **✓x7ᵗʰ T82.7** Infection and inflammatory reaction due to other cardiac and vascular devices, implants and grafts   `CC` `H13` `HCC`
> Use additional code to identify infection
> **CC Excl:** PDX collection 1454

✓5ᵗʰ T82.8 Other specified complications of cardiac and vascular prosthetic devices, implants and grafts
> **AHA:** 2016, 4Q, 70

✓6ᵗʰ T82.81 Embolism due to cardiac and vascular prosthetic devices, implants and grafts

✓7ᵗʰ T82.817 **Embolism due to** cardiac prosthetic devices, implants and grafts   `CC`
> **CC Excl:** PDX collection 1455

6   **✓7ᵗʰ T82.818** **Embolism due to** vascular prosthetic devices, implants and grafts   `CC` `HCC`
> **CC Excl:** PDX collection 1454

✓6ᵗʰ T82.82 Fibrosis due to cardiac and vascular prosthetic devices, implants and grafts

✓7ᵗʰ T82.827 **Fibrosis due to** cardiac prosthetic devices, implants and grafts   `CC`
> **CC Excl:** PDX collection 1455

6   **✓7ᵗʰ T82.828** **Fibrosis due to** vascular prosthetic devices, implants and grafts   `CC` `HCC`
> **CC Excl:** PDX collection 1454

✓6ᵗʰ T82.83 Hemorrhage due to cardiac and vascular prosthetic devices, implants and grafts

✓7ᵗʰ T82.837 **Hemorrhage due to** cardiac prosthetic devices, implants and grafts   `CC`
> **CC Excl:** PDX collection 1455

✓7ᵗʰ T82.838 **Hemorrhage due to** vascular prosthetic devices, implants and grafts   `CC` `HCC`
> **CC Excl:** PDX collection 1454

✓6ᵗʰ T82.84 Pain due to cardiac and vascular prosthetic devices, implants and grafts

✓7ᵗʰ T82.847 **Pain due to** cardiac prosthetic devices, implants and grafts   `CC`
> **CC Excl:** PDX collection 1455

6   **✓7ᵗʰ T82.848** **Pain due to** vascular prosthetic devices, implants and grafts   `CC` `HCC`
> **CC Excl:** PDX collection 1454

✓6ᵗʰ T82.85 Stenosis due to cardiac and vascular prosthetic devices, implants and grafts

✓7ᵗʰ T82.855 **Stenosis of** coronary artery stent   `CC`
> In-stent stenosis (restenosis) of coronary artery stent
> Restenosis of coronary artery stent
> **CC Excl:** PDX collection 1455

6   **✓7ᵗʰ T82.856** **Stenosis of** peripheral vascular stent   `CC` `HCC`
> In-stent stenosis (restenosis) of peripheral vascular stent
> Restenosis of peripheral vascular stent
> **CC Excl:** PDX collection 1454

✓7ᵗʰ T82.857 **Stenosis of** other cardiac prosthetic devices, implants and grafts   `CC`
> **CC Excl:** PDX collection 1455

✓ Additional Character Required   ✓x7ᵗʰ Placeholder   Unacceptable PDx   Questionable PDx   Manifestation   `H1`-`H14` HAC   `HCC` CMS-HCC Dx   `HIV` HIV Dx

ICD-10-CM 2019   1145

6 ✓7ᵗʰ **T82.858** Stenosis of other vascular `CC` `HCC`
prostheticdevices, implants and grafts
CC Excl: PDX collection 1454

✓6ᵗʰ **T82.86** **Thrombosis of cardiac and vascular prosthetic devices, implants and grafts**

    ✓7ᵗʰ **T82.867** Thrombosis due to cardiac prosthetic `CC`
devices, implants and grafts
CC Excl: PDX collection 1455

    6 ✓7ᵗʰ **T82.868** Thrombosis due to vascular `CC` `HCC`
prosthetic devices, implants and grafts
CC Excl: PDX collection 1454

✓6ᵗʰ **T82.89** **Other specified complication of cardiac and vascular prosthetic devices, implants and grafts**

    ✓7ᵗʰ **T82.897** Other specified complication of `CC`
cardiac prosthetic devices, implants and grafts
CC Excl: PDX collection 1455

    6 ✓7ᵗʰ **T82.898** Other specified complication of `CC` `HCC`
vascular prosthetic devices, implants and grafts
CC Excl: PDX collection 1454

✓×7ᵗʰ **T82.9** **Unspecified complication of cardiac and vascular** `CC`
prosthetic device, implant and graft
CC Excl: PDX collection 1455

✓4ᵗʰ **T83** **Complications of genitourinary prosthetic devices, implants and grafts**
    `EXCLUDES 2` *failure and rejection of transplanted organs and tissue (T86.-)*
    AHA: 2016, 4Q, 70-71

> The appropriate 7th character is to be added to each code from category T83.
> A   initial encounter
> D   subsequent encounter
> S   sequela

> **CC Excl:** For CC codes in category T83, unless otherwise noted:
> PDX collection 1456

✓5ᵗʰ **T83.0** **Mechanical complication of urinary catheter**
    `EXCLUDES 2` *complications of stoma of urinary tract (N99.5-)*

✓6ᵗʰ **T83.01** **Breakdown (mechanical) of urinary catheter**

    6 ✓7ᵗʰ **T83.010** Breakdown (mechanical) of `CC` `HCC`
cystostomy catheter

    6 ✓7ᵗʰ **T83.011** Breakdown (mechanical) of `HCC`
indwelling urethral catheter

    6 ✓7ᵗʰ **T83.012** Breakdown (mechanical) of `HCC`
nephrostomy catheter

    6 ✓7ᵗʰ **T83.018** Breakdown (mechanical) of other `HCC`
urinary catheter
Breakdown (mechanical) of Hopkins catheter
Breakdown (mechanical) of ileostomy catheter
Breakdown (mechanical) urostomy catheter

✓6ᵗʰ **T83.02** **Displacement of urinary catheter**
Malposition of urinary catheter

    6 ✓7ᵗʰ **T83.020** Displacement of cystostomy `CC` `HCC`
catheter

    6 ✓7ᵗʰ **T83.021** Displacement of indwelling urethral `HCC`
catheter

    6 ✓7ᵗʰ **T83.022** Displacement of nephrostomy `HCC`
catheter

    6 ✓7ᵗʰ **T83.028** Displacement of other urinary `HCC`
catheter
Displacement of Hopkins catheter
Displacement of ileostomy catheter
Displacement of urostomy catheter

✓6ᵗʰ **T83.03** **Leakage of urinary catheter**

    6 ✓7ᵗʰ **T83.030** Leakage of cystostomy catheter `CC` `HCC`

    6 ✓7ᵗʰ **T83.031** Leakage of indwelling urethral `HCC`
catheter

    6 ✓7ᵗʰ **T83.032** Leakage of nephrostomy catheter `HCC`

    6 ✓7ᵗʰ **T83.038** Leakage of other urinary catheter `HCC`
Leakage of Hopkins catheter
Leakage of ileostomy catheter
Leakage of urostomy catheter

✓6ᵗʰ **T83.09** **Other mechanical complication of urinary catheter**
Obstruction (mechanical) of urinary catheter
Perforation of urinary catheter
Protrusion of urinary catheter

6 ✓7ᵗʰ **T83.090** Other mechanical complication of `CC` `HCC`
cystostomy catheter

6 ✓7ᵗʰ **T83.091** Other mechanical complication of `HCC`
indwelling urethral catheter

6 ✓7ᵗʰ **T83.092** Other mechanical complication of `HCC`
nephrostomy catheter

6 ✓7ᵗʰ **T83.098** Other mechanical complication of `HCC`
other urinary catheter
Other mechanical complication of Hopkins catheter
Other mechanical complication of ileostomy catheter
Other mechanical complication of urostomy catheter

✓5ᵗʰ **T83.1** **Mechanical complication of other urinary devices and implants**

✓6ᵗʰ **T83.11** **Breakdown (mechanical) of other urinary devices and implants**

    6 ✓7ᵗʰ **T83.110** Breakdown (mechanical) of urinary `CC` `HCC`
electronic stimulator device
    `EXCLUDES 2` *breakdown (mechanical) of electrode (lead) for sacral nerve neurostimulator (T85.111)*
breakdown (mechanical) of implanted electronic sacral neurostimulator, pulse generator or receiver (T85.113)

    6 ✓7ᵗʰ **T83.111** Breakdown (mechanical) of `CC` `HCC`
implanted urinary sphincter

    6 ✓7ᵗʰ **T83.112** Breakdown (mechanical) of `CC` `HCC`
indwelling ureteral stent

    6 ✓7ᵗʰ **T83.113** Breakdown (mechanical) of other `CC` `HCC`
urinary stents
Breakdown (mechanical) of ileal conduit stent
Breakdown (mechanical) of nephroureteral stent

    6 ✓7ᵗʰ **T83.118** Breakdown (mechanical) of other `CC` `HCC`
urinary devices and implants

✓6ᵗʰ **T83.12** **Displacement of other urinary devices and implants**
Malposition of other urinary devices and implants

    6 ✓7ᵗʰ **T83.120** Displacement of urinary electronic `CC` `HCC`
stimulator device
    `EXCLUDES 2` *displacement of electrode (lead) for sacral nerve neurostimulator (T85.121)*
displacement of implanted electronic sacral neurostimulator, pulse generator or receiver (T85.123)

    6 ✓7ᵗʰ **T83.121** Displacement of implanted `CC` `HCC`
urinary sphincter

    6 ✓7ᵗʰ **T83.122** Displacement of indwelling `CC` `HCC`
ureteral stent

    6 ✓7ᵗʰ **T83.123** Displacement of other urinary `CC` `HCC`
stents
Displacement of ileal conduit stent
Displacement of nephroureteral stent

    6 ✓7ᵗʰ **T83.128** Displacement of other urinary `CC` `HCC`
devices and implants

✓6ᵗʰ **T83.19** **Other mechanical complication of other urinary devices and implants**
Leakage of other urinary devices and implants
Obstruction (mechanical) of other urinary devices and implants
Perforation of other urinary devices and implants
Protrusion of other urinary devices and implants

    6 ✓7ᵗʰ **T83.190** Other mechanical complication of `CC` `HCC`
urinary electronic stimulator device
    `EXCLUDES 2` *other mechanical complication of electrode (lead) for sacral nerve neurostimulator (T85.191)*
other mechanical complication of implanted electronic sacral neurostimulator, pulse generator or receiver (T85.193)

---

6 ✓7ᵗʰ **T83.191** **Other mechanical complication of** CC HCC
implanted urinary sphincter

6 ✓7ᵗʰ **T83.192** **Other mechanical complication of** CC HCC
indwelling ureteral stent

6 ✓7ᵗʰ **T83.193** **Other mechanical complication of** CC HCC
other urinary stent
   Other mechanical complication of ileal
     conduit stent
   Other mechanical complication of
     nephroureteral stent

6 ✓7ᵗʰ **T83.198** **Other mechanical complication of** CC HCC
other urinary devices and implants

✓5ᵗʰ **T83.2** **Mechanical complication of** graft of urinary organ

6 ✓x7ᵗʰ **T83.21** **Breakdown (mechanical) of graft of urinary** CC HCC
organ

6 ✓x7ᵗʰ **T83.22** **Displacement of graft of urinary organ** CC HCC
   Malposition of graft of urinary organ

6 ✓x7ᵗʰ **T83.23** **Leakage of graft of urinary organ** CC HCC

6 ✓x7ᵗʰ **T83.24** **Erosion of graft of urinary organ** CC HCC

6 ✓x7ᵗʰ **T83.25** **Exposure of graft of urinary organ** CC HCC

6 ✓x7ᵗʰ **T83.29** **Other mechanical complication of graft of** CC HCC
urinary organ
   Obstruction (mechanical) of graft of urinary organ
   Perforation of graft of urinary organ
   Protrusion of graft of urinary organ

✓5ᵗʰ **T83.3** **Mechanical complication of** intrauterine contraceptive device

✓x7ᵗʰ **T83.31** **Breakdown (mechanical) of intrauterine** ♀
contraceptive device

✓x7ᵗʰ **T83.32** **Displacement of intrauterine contraceptive** ♀
device
   Malposition of intrauterine contraceptive device
   Missing string of intrauterine contraceptive device
   AHA: 2018, 1Q, 5

✓x7ᵗʰ **T83.39** **Other mechanical complication of intrauterine** ♀
contraceptive device
   Leakage of intrauterine contraceptive device
   Obstruction (mechanical) of intrauterine contraceptive
     device
   Perforation of intrauterine contraceptive device
   Protrusion of intrauterine contraceptive device

✓5ᵗʰ **T83.4** **Mechanical complication of** other prosthetic devices,
implants and grafts of genital tract

✓6ᵗʰ **T83.41** **Breakdown (mechanical) of other prosthetic**
devices, implants and grafts of genital tract

6 ✓7ᵗʰ **T83.410** **Breakdown (mechanical) of** CC HCC ♂
implanted penile prosthesis
   Breakdown (mechanical) of penile
     prosthesis cylinder
   Breakdown (mechanical) of penile
     prosthesis pump
   Breakdown (mechanical) of penile
     prosthesis reservoir

6 ✓7ᵗʰ **T83.411** **Breakdown (mechanical) of** CC HCC
implanted testicular prosthesis

6 ✓7ᵗʰ **T83.418** **Breakdown (mechanical) of** other CC HCC
prosthetic devices, implants and grafts
of genital tract

✓6ᵗʰ **T83.42** **Displacement of other prosthetic devices, implants**
and grafts of genital tract
   Malposition of other prosthetic devices, implants and
     grafts of genital tract

6 ✓7ᵗʰ **T83.420** **Displacement of** implanted CC HCC ♂
penile prosthesis
   Displacement of penile prosthesis cylinder
   Displacement of penile prosthesis pump
   Displacement of penile prosthesis reservoir

6 ✓7ᵗʰ **T83.421** **Displacement of** implanted CC HCC
testicular prosthesis

6 ✓7ᵗʰ **T83.428** **Displacement of** other **prosthetic** CC HCC
devices, implants and grafts of genital
tract
   AHA: 2018, 1Q, 5

✓6ᵗʰ **T83.49** **Other** mechanical complication of other prosthetic
devices, implants and grafts of genital tract
   Leakage of other prosthetic devices, implants and
     grafts of genital tract
   Obstruction, mechanical of other prosthetic devices,
     implants and grafts of genital tract
   Perforation of other prosthetic devices, implants and
     grafts of genital tract
   Protrusion of other prosthetic devices, implants and
     grafts of genital tract

6 ✓7ᵗʰ **T83.490** **Other mechanical complication** CC HCC ♂
of implanted penile prosthesis
   Other mechanical complication of penile
     prosthesis cylinder
   Other mechanical complication of penile
     prosthesis pump
   Other mechanical complication of penile
     prosthesis reservoir

6 ✓7ᵗʰ **T83.491** **Other mechanical complication of** CC HCC
implanted testicular prosthesis

6 ✓7ᵗʰ **T83.498** **Other mechanical complication of** CC HCC
other **prosthetic devices, implants and**
grafts of genital tract

✓5ᵗʰ **T83.5** **Infection and inflammatory reaction due to prosthetic device,**
implant and graft in urinary system
   Use additional code to identify infection

> **CC Excl: For CC codes in subcategory T83.5, unless**
> **otherwise noted:** PDX collection 1458

✓6ᵗʰ **T83.51** **Infection and inflammatory reaction due to** urinary
catheter
   EXCLUDES 2 *complications of stoma of urinary tract*
     (N99.5-)

6 ✓7ᵗʰ **T83.510** **Infection and inflammatory** CC HCC
reaction due to cystostomy **catheter**

6 ✓7ᵗʰ **T83.511** **Infection and inflammatory** CC H5 HCC
reaction due to indwelling urethral
catheter
   CC Excl: PDX collection 1457

6 ✓7ᵗʰ **T83.512** **Infection and inflammatory** CC HCC
reaction due to nephrostomy **catheter**

6 ✓7ᵗʰ **T83.518** **Infection and inflammatory** CC H5 HCC
reaction due to other **urinary catheter**
   Infection and inflammatory reaction due to
     Hopkins catheter
   Infection and inflammatory reaction due to
     ileostomy catheter
   Infection and inflammatory reaction due to
     urostomy catheter

✓6ᵗʰ **T83.59** **Infection and inflammatory reaction due to**
prosthetic device, implant and graft in urinary
system

6 ✓7ᵗʰ **T83.590** **Infection and inflammatory** CC HCC
reaction due to implanted urinary
neurostimulation device
   EXCLUDES 2 *infection and inflammatory*
     reaction due to electrode
     lead of sacral nerve
     neurostimulator (T85.732)
     infection and inflammatory
     reaction due to pulse
     generator or receiver of
     sacral nerve neurostimulator
     (T85.734)

6 ✓7ᵗʰ **T83.591** **Infection and inflammatory** CC HCC
reaction due to implanted urinary
sphincter

6 ✓7ᵗʰ **T83.592** **Infection and inflammatory** CC HCC
reaction due to indwelling ureteral stent

6 ✓7ᵗʰ **T83.593** **Infection and inflammatory** CC HCC
reaction due to other urinary stents
   Infection and inflammatory reaction due to
     ileal conduit stents
   Infection and inflammatory reaction due to
     nephroureteral stent

6 ✓7ᵗʰ **T83.598** **Infection and inflammatory** CC HCC
reaction due to other **prosthetic device,**
implant and graft in urinary system

✓ Additional Character Required   ✓x7ᵗʰ Placeholder   Unacceptable PDx   Questionable PDx   Manifestation   H1 - H14 HAC   HCC CMS-HCC Dx   HIV HIV Dx

ICD-10-CM 2019   **1147**

T83.191–T83.598

√5th **T83.6** **Infection and inflammatory reaction due to prosthetic device, implant and graft in** genital tract
> Use additional code to identify infection

> **CC Excl:** For CC codes in subcategory T83.6:
> PDX collection 1458

6 √x7th **T83.61** **Infection and inflammatory reaction due to implanted** penile prosthesis   CC HCC
> Infection and inflammatory reaction due to penile prosthesis cylinder
> Infection and inflammatory reaction due to penile prosthesis pump
> Infection and inflammatory reaction due to penile prosthesis reservoir

6 √x7th **T83.62** **Infection and inflammatory reaction due to implanted** testicular prosthesis   CC HCC

6 √x7th **T83.69** **Infection and inflammatory reaction due to other** prosthetic device, implant and graft in genital tract   CC HCC

√5th **T83.7** **Complications due to** implanted mesh and other prosthetic materials

√6th **T83.71** **Erosion of implanted mesh and other prosthetic materials to surrounding organ or tissue**

6 √7th **T83.711** **Erosion of implanted** vaginal **mesh to surrounding organ or tissue**   HCC ♀
> Erosion of implanted vaginal mesh into pelvic floor muscles

6 √7th **T83.712** **Erosion of implanted** urethral **mesh to surrounding organ or tissue**   CC HCC
> Erosion of implanted female urethral sling
> Erosion of implanted male urethral sling
> Erosion of implanted urethral mesh into pelvic floor muscles

6 √7th **T83.713** **Erosion of implanted** urethral bulking agent **to surrounding organ or tissue**   CC HCC

6 √7th **T83.714** **Erosion of implanted** ureteral bulking agent **to surrounding organ or tissue**   CC HCC

6 √7th **T83.718** **Erosion of** other implanted mesh **to organ or tissue**   CC HCC

6 √7th **T83.719** **Erosion of** other prosthetic materials **to surrounding organ or tissue**   CC HCC

√6th **T83.72** **Exposure** of implanted mesh and other prosthetic materials into surrounding organ or tissue
> Extrusion of implanted mesh

6 √7th **T83.721** **Exposure of implanted** vaginal mesh **into** vagina   HCC ♀
> Exposure of implanted vaginal mesh through vaginal wall

6 √7th **T83.722** **Exposure of implanted** urethral mesh **into** urethra   CC HCC
> Exposure of implanted female urethral sling
> Exposure of implanted male urethral sling
> Exposure of implanted urethral mesh through urethral wall

6 √7th **T83.723** **Exposure of implanted** urethral bulking agent **into** urethra   CC HCC

6 √7th **T83.724** **Exposure of implanted** ureteral bulking agent **into** ureter   CC HCC

6 √7th **T83.728** **Exposure of** other implanted mesh **into organ or tissue**   CC HCC

6 √7th **T83.729** **Exposure of** other prosthetic materials **into organ or tissue**   CC HCC

6 √x7th **T83.79** **Other specified complications due to other genitourinary prosthetic materials**   CC HCC
> **CC Excl:** PDX collection 1458

√5th **T83.8** **Other specified complications of** genitourinary prosthetic devices, implants and grafts

> **CC Excl:** For CC codes in subcategory T83.8:
> PDX collection 1458

6 √x7th **T83.81** **Embolism due to genitourinary prosthetic devices, implants and grafts**   CC HCC

6 √x7th **T83.82** **Fibrosis due to genitourinary prosthetic devices, implants and grafts**   CC HCC

6 √x7th **T83.83** **Hemorrhage due to genitourinary prosthetic devices, implants and grafts**   CC HCC

6 √x7th **T83.84** **Pain due to genitourinary prosthetic devices,** CC HCC **implants and grafts**

6 √x7th **T83.85** **Stenosis due to genitourinary prosthetic devices, implants and grafts**   CC HCC

6 √x7th **T83.86** **Thrombosis due to genitourinary prosthetic devices, implants and grafts**   CC HCC

6 √x7th **T83.89** **Other** specified complication of genitourinary prosthetic devices, implants and grafts   CC HCC

6 √x7th **T83.9** **Unspecified complication of genitourinary prosthetic device, implant and graft**   CC HCC
> **CC Excl:** PDX collection 1458

√4th **T84** **Complications of internal orthopedic prosthetic devices, implants and grafts**
> EXCLUDES 2   failure and rejection of transplanted organs and tissues (T86.-)
> fracture of bone following insertion of orthopedic implant, joint prosthesis or bone plate (M96.6)

> The appropriate 7th character is to be added to each code from category T84.
> A   initial encounter
> D   subsequent encounter
> S   sequela

> **CC Excl:** For CC codes in category T84, unless otherwise noted:
> PDX collection 911

√5th **T84.0** **Mechanical complication of** internal joint prosthesis

√6th **T84.01** **Broken** internal joint prosthesis
> Breakage (fracture) of prosthetic joint
> Broken prosthetic joint implant
> EXCLUDES 1   periprosthetic joint implant fracture (M97-)
> **AHA:** 2016, 4Q, 42

6 √7th **T84.010** **Broken internal** right hip **prosthesis** CC HCC

6 √7th **T84.011** **Broken internal** left hip **prosthesis** CC HCC

6 √7th **T84.012** **Broken internal** right knee **prosthesis** CC HCC

6 √7th **T84.013** **Broken internal** left knee **prosthesis** CC HCC

6 √7th **T84.018** **Broken internal joint prosthesis, other** site   CC HCC
> Use additional code to identify the joint (Z96.6-)

6 √7th **T84.019** **Broken internal joint prosthesis, unspecified** site   CC HCC

√6th **T84.02** **Dislocation** of internal joint prosthesis
> Instability of internal joint prosthesis
> Subluxation of internal joint prosthesis

6 √7th **T84.020** **Dislocation of internal** right hip **prosthesis** CC HCC

6 √7th **T84.021** **Dislocation of internal** left hip **prosthesis** CC HCC

6 √7th **T84.022** **Instability of internal** right knee **prosthesis** CC HCC

6 √7th **T84.023** **Instability of internal** left knee **prosthesis** CC HCC

6 √7th **T84.028** **Dislocation of** other internal joint **prosthesis** CC HCC
> Use additional code to identify the joint (Z96.6-)

6 √7th **T84.029** **Dislocation of** unspecified internal joint prosthesis   CC HCC

√6th **T84.03** **Mechanical loosening** of internal prosthetic joint
> Aseptic loosening of prosthetic joint

6 √7th **T84.030** **Mechanical loosening of internal** right hip **prosthetic joint** CC HCC

6 √7th **T84.031** **Mechanical loosening of internal** left hip **prosthetic joint** CC HCC

6 √7th **T84.032** **Mechanical loosening of internal** right knee **prosthetic joint** CC HCC

6 √7th **T84.033** **Mechanical loosening of internal** left knee **prosthetic joint** CC HCC

6 √7th **T84.038** **Mechanical loosening of** other internal prosthetic joint   CC HCC
> Use additional code to identify the joint (Z96.6-)

6 √7th **T84.039** **Mechanical loosening of** unspecified internal prosthetic joint   CC HCC

N Newborn: 0   P Pediatric: 0-17   M Maternity: 12-55   A Adult: 15-124   MCC Major Complication/Comorbidity   CC Complication/Comorbidity   SW Severe Wound Dx

1148   ICD-10-CM 2019

✓6ᵗʰ **T84.05** Periprosthetic osteolysis of internal prosthetic joint
  Use additional code to identify major osseous defect, if applicable (M89.7-)

    6 ✓7ᵗʰ **T84.050** Periprosthetic osteolysis of internal prosthetic right hip joint   CC HCC

    6 ✓7ᵗʰ **T84.051** Periprosthetic osteolysis of internal prosthetic left hip joint   CC HCC

    6 ✓7ᵗʰ **T84.052** Periprosthetic osteolysis of internal prosthetic right knee joint   CC HCC

    6 ✓7ᵗʰ **T84.053** Periprosthetic osteolysis of internal prosthetic left knee joint   CC HCC

    6 ✓7ᵗʰ **T84.058** Periprosthetic osteolysis of other internal prosthetic joint   CC HCC
  Use additional code to identify the joint (Z96. 6-)

    6 ✓7ᵗʰ **T84.059** Periprosthetic osteolysis of unspecified internal prosthetic joint   CC HCC

✓6ᵗʰ **T84.06** Wear of articular bearing surface of internal prosthetic joint

    6 ✓7ᵗʰ **T84.060** Wear of articular bearing surface of internal prosthetic right hip joint   CC HCC

    6 ✓7ᵗʰ **T84.061** Wear of articular bearing surface of internal prosthetic left hip joint   CC HCC

    6 ✓7ᵗʰ **T84.062** Wear of articular bearing surface of internal prosthetic right knee joint   CC HCC

    6 ✓7ᵗʰ **T84.063** Wear of articular bearing surface of internal prosthetic left knee joint   CC HCC

    6 ✓7ᵗʰ **T84.068** Wear of articular bearing surface of other internal prosthetic joint   CC HCC
  Use additional code to identify the joint (Z96.6-)

    6 ✓7ᵗʰ **T84.069** Wear of articular bearing surface of unspecified internal prosthetic joint   CC HCC

✓6ᵗʰ **T84.09** Other mechanical complication of internal joint prosthesis
  Prosthetic joint implant failure NOS

    6 ✓7ᵗʰ **T84.090** Other mechanical complication of internal right hip prosthesis   CC HCC

    6 ✓7ᵗʰ **T84.091** Other mechanical complication of internal left hip prosthesis   CC HCC

    6 ✓7ᵗʰ **T84.092** Other mechanical complication of internal right knee prosthesis   CC HCC

    6 ✓7ᵗʰ **T84.093** Other mechanical complication of internal left knee prosthesis   CC HCC

    6 ✓7ᵗʰ **T84.098** Other mechanical complication of other internal joint prosthesis   CC HCC
  Use additional code to identify the joint (Z96.6-)

    6 ✓7ᵗʰ **T84.099** Other mechanical complication of unspecified internal joint prosthesis   CC HCC

✓5ᵗʰ **T84.1** Mechanical complication of internal fixation device of bones of limb

    EXCLUDES 2   *mechanical complication of internal fixation device of bones of feet (T84.2-)*
  mechanical complication of internal fixation device of bones of fingers (T84.2-)
  mechanical complication of internal fixation device of bones of hands (T84.2-)
  mechanical complication of internal fixation device of bones of toes (T84.2-)

✓6ᵗʰ **T84.11** Breakdown (mechanical) of internal fixation device of bones of limb

    6 ✓7ᵗʰ **T84.110** Breakdown (mechanical) of internal fixation device of right humerus   CC HCC

    6 ✓7ᵗʰ **T84.111** Breakdown (mechanical) of internal fixation device of left humerus   CC HCC

    6 ✓7ᵗʰ **T84.112** Breakdown (mechanical) of internal fixation device of bone of right forearm   CC HCC

    6 ✓7ᵗʰ **T84.113** Breakdown (mechanical) of internal fixation device of bone of left forearm   CC HCC

    6 ✓7ᵗʰ **T84.114** Breakdown (mechanical) of internal fixation device of right femur   CC HCC

    6 ✓7ᵗʰ **T84.115** Breakdown (mechanical) of internal fixation device of left femur   CC HCC

    6 ✓7ᵗʰ **T84.116** Breakdown (mechanical) of internal fixation device of bone of right lower leg   CC HCC

    6 ✓7ᵗʰ **T84.117** Breakdown (mechanical) of internal fixation device of bone of left lower leg   CC HCC

    6 ✓7ᵗʰ **T84.119** Breakdown (mechanical) of internal fixation device of unspecified bone of limb   CC HCC

✓6ᵗʰ **T84.12** Displacement of internal fixation device of bones of limb
  Malposition of internal fixation device of bones of limb

    6 ✓7ᵗʰ **T84.120** Displacement of internal fixation device of right humerus   CC HCC

    6 ✓7ᵗʰ **T84.121** Displacement of internal fixation device of left humerus   CC HCC

    6 ✓7ᵗʰ **T84.122** Displacement of internal fixation device of bone of right forearm   CC HCC

    6 ✓7ᵗʰ **T84.123** Displacement of internal fixation device of bone of left forearm   CC HCC

    6 ✓7ᵗʰ **T84.124** Displacement of internal fixation device of right femur   CC HCC

    6 ✓7ᵗʰ **T84.125** Displacement of internal fixation device of left femur   CC HCC

    6 ✓7ᵗʰ **T84.126** Displacement of internal fixation device of bone of right lower leg   CC HCC

    6 ✓7ᵗʰ **T84.127** Displacement of internal fixation device of bone of left lower leg   CC HCC

    6 ✓7ᵗʰ **T84.129** Displacement of internal fixation device of unspecified bone of limb   CC HCC

✓6ᵗʰ **T84.19** Other mechanical complication of internal fixation device of bones of limb
  Obstruction (mechanical) of internal fixation device of bones of limb
  Perforation of internal fixation device of bones of limb
  Protrusion of internal fixation device of bones of limb

    6 ✓7ᵗʰ **T84.190** Other mechanical complication of internal fixation device of right humerus   CC HCC

    6 ✓7ᵗʰ **T84.191** Other mechanical complication of internal fixation device of left humerus   CC HCC

    6 ✓7ᵗʰ **T84.192** Other mechanical complication of internal fixation device of bone of right forearm   CC HCC

    6 ✓7ᵗʰ **T84.193** Other mechanical complication of internal fixation device of bone of left forearm   CC HCC

    6 ✓7ᵗʰ **T84.194** Other mechanical complication of internal fixation device of right femur   CC HCC

    6 ✓7ᵗʰ **T84.195** Other mechanical complication of internal fixation device of left femur   CC HCC

    6 ✓7ᵗʰ **T84.196** Other mechanical complication of internal fixation device of bone of right lower leg   CC HCC

    6 ✓7ᵗʰ **T84.197** Other mechanical complication of internal fixation device of bone of left lower leg   CC HCC

    6 ✓7ᵗʰ **T84.199** Other mechanical complication of internal fixation device of unspecified bone of limb   CC HCC

✓5ᵗʰ **T84.2** Mechanical complication of internal fixation device of other bones

✓6ᵗʰ **T84.21** Breakdown (mechanical) of internal fixation device of other bones

    6 ✓7ᵗʰ **T84.210** Breakdown (mechanical) of internal fixation device of bones of hand and fingers   CC HCC

    6 ✓7ᵗʰ **T84.213** Breakdown (mechanical) of internal fixation device of bones of foot and toes   CC HCC

    6 ✓7ᵗʰ **T84.216** Breakdown (mechanical) of internal fixation device of vertebrae   CC HCC

    6 ✓7ᵗʰ **T84.218** Breakdown (mechanical) of internal fixation device of other bones   CC HCC

✓ Additional Character Required   ✓7ᵗʰ Placeholder   Unacceptable PDx   Questionable PDx   Manifestation   H1-H14 HAC   HCC CMS-HCC Dx   HIV HIV Dx

ICD-10-CM 2019   1149

√6ᵗʰ **T84.22** Displacement of internal fixation device of other bones
　Malposition of internal fixation device of other bones

　6 √7ᵗʰ **T84.220** Displacement of internal fixation device of bones of hand and fingers `CC` `HCC`

　6 √7ᵗʰ **T84.223** Displacement of internal fixation device of bones of foot and toes `CC` `HCC`

　6 √7ᵗʰ **T84.226** Displacement of internal fixation device of vertebrae `CC` `HCC`

　6 √7ᵗʰ **T84.228** Displacement of internal fixation device of other bones `CC` `HCC`

√6ᵗʰ **T84.29** Other mechanical complication of internal fixation device of other bones
　Obstruction (mechanical) of internal fixation device of other bones
　Perforation of internal fixation device of other bones
　Protrusion of internal fixation device of other bones

　6 √7ᵗʰ **T84.290** Other mechanical complication of internal fixation device of bones of hand and fingers `CC` `HCC`

　6 √7ᵗʰ **T84.293** Other mechanical complication of internal fixation device of bones of foot and toes `CC` `HCC`

　6 √7ᵗʰ **T84.296** Other mechanical complication of internal fixation device of vertebrae `CC` `HCC`

　6 √7ᵗʰ **T84.298** Other mechanical complication of internal fixation device of other bones `CC` `HCC`

√5ᵗʰ **T84.3** Mechanical complication of other bone devices, implants and grafts
　EXCLUDES 2　other complications of bone graft (T86.83-)

　√6ᵗʰ **T84.31** Breakdown (mechanical) of other bone devices, implants and grafts

　　6 √7ᵗʰ **T84.310** Breakdown (mechanical) of electronic bone stimulator `CC` `HCC`

　　6 √7ᵗʰ **T84.318** Breakdown (mechanical) of other bone devices, implants and grafts `CC` `HCC`

　√6ᵗʰ **T84.32** Displacement of other bone devices, implants and grafts
　　Malposition of other bone devices, implants and grafts

　　6 √7ᵗʰ **T84.320** Displacement of electronic bone stimulator `CC` `HCC`

　　6 √7ᵗʰ **T84.328** Displacement of other bone devices, implants and grafts `CC` `HCC`
　　　AHA: 2014, 4Q, 28

　√6ᵗʰ **T84.39** Other mechanical complication of other bone devices, implants and grafts
　　Obstruction (mechanical) of other bone devices, implants and grafts
　　Perforation of other bone devices, implants and grafts
　　Protrusion of other bone devices, implants and grafts

　　6 √7ᵗʰ **T84.390** Other mechanical complication of electronic bone stimulator `CC` `HCC`

　　6 √7ᵗʰ **T84.398** Other mechanical complication of other bone devices, implants and grafts `CC` `HCC`

√5ᵗʰ **T84.4** Mechanical complication of other internal orthopedic devices, implants and grafts

　√6ᵗʰ **T84.41** Breakdown (mechanical) of other internal orthopedic devices, implants and grafts

　　6 √7ᵗʰ **T84.410** Breakdown (mechanical) of muscle and tendon graft `CC` `HCC`

　　6 √7ᵗʰ **T84.418** Breakdown (mechanical) of other internal orthopedic devices, implants and grafts `CC` `HCC`

　√6ᵗʰ **T84.42** Displacement of other internal orthopedic devices, implants and grafts
　　Malposition of other internal orthopedic devices, implants and grafts

　　6 √7ᵗʰ **T84.420** Displacement of muscle and tendon graft `CC` `HCC`

　　6 √7ᵗʰ **T84.428** Displacement of other internal orthopedic devices, implants and grafts `CC` `HCC`

√6ᵗʰ **T84.49** Other mechanical complication of other internal orthopedic devices, implants and grafts
　Mechanical complication of other internal orthopedic devices, implants and grafts NOS
　Obstruction (mechanical) of other internal orthopedic devices, implants and grafts
　Perforation of other internal orthopedic devices, implants and grafts
　Protrusion of other internal orthopedic devices, implants and grafts

　6 √7ᵗʰ **T84.490** Other mechanical complication of muscle and tendon graft `CC` `HCC`

　6 √7ᵗʰ **T84.498** Other mechanical complication of other internal orthopedic devices, implants and grafts `CC` `HCC`

√5ᵗʰ **T84.5** Infection and inflammatory reaction due to internal joint prosthesis
　Use additional code to identify infection
　AHA: 2015, 1Q, 16

　CC Excl: For CC codes in subcategory T84.5:
　PDX collection 1459

　6 √x7ᵗʰ **T84.50** Infection and inflammatory reaction due to unspecified internal joint prosthesis `CC` `HCC`

　6 √x7ᵗʰ **T84.51** Infection and inflammatory reaction due to internal right hip prosthesis `CC` `HCC`

　6 √x7ᵗʰ **T84.52** Infection and inflammatory reaction due to internal left hip prosthesis `CC` `HCC`

　6 √x7ᵗʰ **T84.53** Infection and inflammatory reaction due to internal right knee prosthesis `CC` `HCC`

　6 √x7ᵗʰ **T84.54** Infection and inflammatory reaction due to internal left knee prosthesis `CC` `HCC`

　6 √x7ᵗʰ **T84.59** Infection and inflammatory reaction due to other internal joint prosthesis `CC` `HCC`

√5ᵗʰ **T84.6** Infection and inflammatory reaction due to internal fixation device
　Use additional code to identify infection

　CC Excl: For CC codes in subcategory T84.6:
　PDX collection 1459

　6 √x7ᵗʰ **T84.60** Infection and inflammatory reaction due to internal fixation device of unspecified site `CC` `H12` `HCC`

　√6ᵗʰ **T84.61** Infection and inflammatory reaction due to internal fixation device of arm

　　6 √7ᵗʰ **T84.610** Infection and inflammatory reaction due to internal fixation device of right humerus `CC` `H12` `HCC`

　　6 √7ᵗʰ **T84.611** Infection and inflammatory reaction due to internal fixation device of left humerus `CC` `H12` `HCC`

　　6 √7ᵗʰ **T84.612** Infection and inflammatory reaction due to internal fixation device of right radius `CC` `H12` `HCC`

　　6 √7ᵗʰ **T84.613** Infection and inflammatory reaction due to internal fixation device of left radius `CC` `H12` `HCC`

　　6 √7ᵗʰ **T84.614** Infection and inflammatory reaction due to internal fixation device of right ulna `CC` `H12` `HCC`

　　6 √7ᵗʰ **T84.615** Infection and inflammatory reaction due to internal fixation device of left ulna `CC` `H12` `HCC`

　　6 √7ᵗʰ **T84.619** Infection and inflammatory reaction due to internal fixation device of unspecified bone of arm `CC` `H12` `HCC`

　√6ᵗʰ **T84.62** Infection and inflammatory reaction due to internal fixation device of leg

　　6 √7ᵗʰ **T84.620** Infection and inflammatory reaction due to internal fixation device of right femur `CC` `HCC`

　　6 √7ᵗʰ **T84.621** Infection and inflammatory reaction due to internal fixation device of left femur `CC` `HCC`

　　6 √7ᵗʰ **T84.622** Infection and inflammatory reaction due to internal fixation device of right tibia `CC` `HCC`

　　6 √7ᵗʰ **T84.623** Infection and inflammatory reaction due to internal fixation device of left tibia `CC` `HCC`

Ⓝ Newborn: 0　　Ⓟ Pediatric: 0-17　　Ⓜ Maternity: 12-55　　Ⓐ Adult: 15-124　　`MCC` Major Complication/Comorbidity　　`CC` Complication/Comorbidity　　`SW` Severe Wound Dx

1150　　ICD-10-CM 2019

6 ✓7ᵗʰ **T84.624** **Infection and inflammatory** `CC` `HCC`
reaction due to internal fixation
device of **right fibula**

6 ✓7ᵗʰ **T84.625** **Infection and inflammatory** `CC` `HCC`
reaction due to internal fixation
device of **left fibula**

6 ✓7ᵗʰ **T84.629** **Infection and inflammatory** `CC` `HCC`
reaction due to internal fixation
device of **unspecified bone** of leg

6 ✓x7ᵗʰ **T84.63** **Infection and inflammatory reaction due** `CC` `H12` `HCC`
to internal fixation device of **spine**

6 ✓x7ᵗʰ **T84.69** **Infection and inflammatory reaction due** `CC` `H12` `HCC`
to internal fixation device of **other site**

6 ✓x7ᵗʰ **T84.7** **Infection and inflammatory reaction due to** other `CC` `H12` `HCC`
internal orthopedic prosthetic devices, implants
and grafts

> Use additional code to identify infection
> **CC Excl:** PDX collection 1459

✓5ᵗʰ **T84.8** **Other specified complications of internal orthopedic**
prosthetic devices, implants and grafts

> **CC Excl: For CC codes in subcategory T84.8:**
> PDX collection 1459

6 ✓x7ᵗʰ **T84.81** **Embolism** due to internal orthopedic `CC` `HCC`
prosthetic devices, implants and grafts

6 ✓x7ᵗʰ **T84.82** **Fibrosis** due to internal orthopedic `CC` `HCC`
prosthetic devices, implants and grafts

6 ✓x7ᵗʰ **T84.83** **Hemorrhage** due to internal orthopedic `CC` `HCC`
prosthetic devices, implants and grafts

6 ✓x7ᵗʰ **T84.84** **Pain** due to internal orthopedic prosthetic `CC` `HCC`
devices, implants and grafts

6 ✓x7ᵗʰ **T84.85** **Stenosis** due to internal orthopedic `CC` `HCC`
prosthetic devices, implants and grafts

6 ✓x7ᵗʰ **T84.86** **Thrombosis** due to internal orthopedic `CC` `HCC`
prosthetic devices, implants and grafts

6 ✓x7ᵗʰ **T84.89** **Other** specified complication of internal `CC` `HCC`
orthopedic prosthetic devices, implants
and grafts

6 ✓x7ᵗʰ **T84.9** **Unspecified complication of internal orthopedic** `CC` `HCC`
prosthetic device, implant and graft

> **CC Excl:** PDX collection 1459

✓4ᵗʰ **T85** **Complications of other internal prosthetic devices, implants and**
grafts

> **EXCLUDES 2** *failure and rejection of transplanted organs and tissue (T86.-)*
> **AHA:** 2016, 4Q, 71-72

> The appropriate 7th character is to be added to each code from
> category T85.
> A   initial encounter
> D   subsequent encounter
> S   sequela

✓5ᵗʰ **T85.0** **Mechanical complication of** ventricular intracranial
(communicating) shunt

> **CC Excl: For CC codes in subcategory T85.0:**
> PDX collection 1460

6 ✓x7ᵗʰ **T85.01** **Breakdown (mechanical) of ventricular** `CC` `HCC`
intracranial (communicating) shunt

6 ✓x7ᵗʰ **T85.02** **Displacement** of ventricular intracranial `CC` `HCC`
(communicating) shunt
> Malposition of ventricular intracranial
> (communicating) shunt

6 ✓x7ᵗʰ **T85.03** **Leakage** of ventricular intracranial `CC` `HCC`
(communicating) shunt

6 ✓x7ᵗʰ **T85.09** **Other** mechanical complication of ventricular `CC` `HCC`
intracranial (communicating) shunt
> Obstruction (mechanical) of ventricular intracranial
> (communicating) shunt
> Perforation of ventricular intracranial
> (communicating) shunt
> Protrusion of ventricular intracranial (communicating)
> shunt

✓5ᵗʰ **T85.1** **Mechanical complication of** implanted electronic stimulator
of nervous system

> **CC Excl: For CC codes in subcategory T85.1:**
> PDX collection 1460

✓6ᵗʰ **T85.11** **Breakdown (mechanical) of implanted electronic**
stimulator of nervous system

6 ✓7ᵗʰ **T85.110** **Breakdown (mechanical) of** `CC` `HCC`
implanted electronic neurostimulator
of brain electrode (lead)

6 ✓7ᵗʰ **T85.111** **Breakdown (mechanical) of** `CC` `HCC`
implanted electronic neurostimulator
of peripheral nerve electrode (lead)
> Breakdown of electrode (lead) for cranial
> nerve neurostimulators
> Breakdown of electrode (lead) for gastric
> neurostimulator
> Breakdown of electrode (lead) for sacral
> nerve neurostimulator
> Breakdown of electrode (lead) for vagal
> nerve neurostimulators

6 ✓7ᵗʰ **T85.112** **Breakdown (mechanical) of** `CC` `HCC`
implanted electronic neurostimulator
of spinal cord electrode (lead)

6 ✓7ᵗʰ **T85.113** **Breakdown (mechanical) of** `CC` `HCC`
implanted electronic neurostimulator,
generator
> ▶Breakdown (mechanical) of implanted
> electronic neurostimulator generator,
> brain, peripheral, gastric, spinal◀
> Breakdown (mechanical) of implanted
> electronic sacral neurostimulator,
> pulse generator or receiver

6 ✓7ᵗʰ **T85.118** **Breakdown (mechanical) of other** `CC` `HCC`
implanted electronic stimulator
of nervous system

✓6ᵗʰ **T85.12** **Displacement of implanted electronic stimulator of**
nervous system
> Malposition of implanted electronic stimulator of
> nervous system

6 ✓7ᵗʰ **T85.120** **Displacement of implanted** `CC` `HCC`
electronic neurostimulator
of brain electrode (lead)

6 ✓7ᵗʰ **T85.121** **Displacement of implanted** `CC` `HCC`
electronic neurostimulator of
peripheral nerve electrode (lead)
> Displacement of electrode (lead) for cranial
> nerve neurostimulators
> Displacement of electrode (lead) for gastric
> neurostimulator
> Displacement of electrode (lead) for sacral
> nerve neurostimulator
> Displacement of electrode (lead) for vagal
> nerve neurostimulators

6 ✓7ᵗʰ **T85.122** **Displacement of implanted** `CC` `HCC`
electronic neurostimulator of
spinal cord electrode (lead)

6 ✓7ᵗʰ **T85.123** **Displacement of implanted** `CC` `HCC`
electronic neurostimulator, generator
> Displacement of implanted electronic
> neurostimulator generator, brain,
> peripheral, gastric, spinal
> Displacement of implanted electronic
> sacral neurostimulator, pulse
> generator or receiver

6 ✓7ᵗʰ **T85.128** **Displacement of other implanted** `CC` `HCC`
electronic stimulator of nervous system

✓6ᵗʰ **T85.19** **Other** mechanical complication of implanted
electronic stimulator of nervous system
> Leakage of implanted electronic stimulator of nervous
> system
> Obstruction (mechanical) of implanted electronic
> stimulator of nervous system
> Perforation of implanted electronic stimulator of
> nervous system
> Protrusion of implanted electronic stimulator of
> nervous system

6 ✓7ᵗʰ **T85.190** **Other mechanical complication of** `CC` `HCC`
implanted electronic neurostimulator
of brain electrode (lead)

6 ☑7ᵗʰ **T85.191** **Other mechanical complication of** CC HCC
implanted electronic neurostimulator
of peripheral nerve electrode (lead)
Other mechanical complication of
electrode (lead) for cranial nerve
neurostimulators
Other mechanical complication of
electrode (lead) for gastric
neurostimulator
Other mechanical complication of
electrode (lead) for sacral nerve
neurostimulator
Other mechanical complication of
electrode (lead) for vagal nerve
neurostimulators

6 ☑7ᵗʰ **T85.192** **Other mechanical complication of** CC HCC
implanted electronic neurostimulator
of spinal cord electrode (lead)

6 ☑7ᵗʰ **T85.193** **Other mechanical complication of** CC HCC
implanted electronic neurostimulator,
generator
Other mechanical complication of
implanted electronic neurostimulator
generator, brain, peripheral, gastric,
spinal
Other mechanical complication of
implanted electronic sacral
neurostimulator, pulse generator or
receiver

6 ☑7ᵗʰ **T85.199** **Other mechanical complication of** CC HCC
other implanted electronic stimulator
of nervous system

☑5ᵗʰ **T85.2** **Mechanical complication of intraocular lens**

> **CC Excl: For CC codes in subcategory T85.2:**
> PDX collection 1461

☑x7ᵗʰ **T85.21** **Breakdown (mechanical) of intraocular lens** CC

☑x7ᵗʰ **T85.22** **Displacement of intraocular lens** CC
Malposition of intraocular lens

☑x7ᵗʰ **T85.29** **Other mechanical complication of intraocular** CC
lens
Obstruction (mechanical) of intraocular lens
Perforation of intraocular lens
Protrusion of intraocular lens

☑5ᵗʰ **T85.3** **Mechanical complication of other ocular prosthetic devices,**
implants and grafts
> EXCLUDES 2   other complications of corneal graft (T86.84-)

> **CC Excl: For CC codes in subcategory T85.3:**
> PDX collection 1462

☑6ᵗʰ **T85.31** **Breakdown (mechanical) of other ocular prosthetic**
devices, implants and grafts

☑7ᵗʰ **T85.310** **Breakdown (mechanical) of prosthetic** CC
orbit of right eye

☑7ᵗʰ **T85.311** **Breakdown (mechanical) of prosthetic** CC
orbit of left eye

☑7ᵗʰ **T85.318** **Breakdown (mechanical) of other ocular**
prosthetic devices, implants and grafts

☑6ᵗʰ **T85.32** **Displacement of other ocular prosthetic devices,**
implants and grafts
Malposition of other ocular prosthetic devices,
implants and grafts

☑7ᵗʰ **T85.320** **Displacement of prosthetic orbit of** CC
right eye

☑7ᵗʰ **T85.321** **Displacement of prosthetic orbit of** CC
left eye

☑7ᵗʰ **T85.328** **Displacement of other ocular prosthetic**
devices, implants and grafts

☑6ᵗʰ **T85.39** **Other mechanical complication of other ocular**
prosthetic devices, implants and grafts
Obstruction (mechanical) of other ocular prosthetic
devices, implants and grafts
Perforation of other ocular prosthetic devices,
implants and grafts
Protrusion of other ocular prosthetic devices, implants
and grafts

☑7ᵗʰ **T85.390** **Other mechanical complication of** CC
prosthetic orbit of right eye

☑7ᵗʰ **T85.391** **Other mechanical complication of** CC
prosthetic orbit of left eye

☑7ᵗʰ **T85.398** **Other mechanical complication of other**
ocular prosthetic devices, implants and
grafts

☑5ᵗʰ **T85.4** **Mechanical complication of breast prosthesis and implant**

> **CC Excl: For CC codes in subcategory T85.4:**
> PDX collection 1463

☑x7ᵗʰ **T85.41** **Breakdown (mechanical) of breast prosthesis** CC
and implant

☑x7ᵗʰ **T85.42** **Displacement of breast prosthesis and implant** CC
Malposition of breast prosthesis and implant

☑x7ᵗʰ **T85.43** **Leakage of breast prosthesis and implant** CC

☑x7ᵗʰ **T85.44** **Capsular contracture of breast implant** CC

☑x7ᵗʰ **T85.49** **Other mechanical complication of breast** CC
prosthesis and implant
Obstruction (mechanical) of breast prosthesis and
implant
Perforation of breast prosthesis and implant
Protrusion of breast prosthesis and implant

☑5ᵗʰ **T85.5** **Mechanical complication of gastrointestinal prosthetic**
devices, implants and grafts

> **CC Excl: For CC codes in subcategory T85.5:**
> PDX collection 1464

☑6ᵗʰ **T85.51** **Breakdown (mechanical) of gastrointestinal**
prosthetic devices, implants and grafts

☑7ᵗʰ **T85.510** **Breakdown (mechanical) of bile duct** CC
prosthesis

☑7ᵗʰ **T85.511** **Breakdown (mechanical) of** CC
esophageal anti-reflux device

☑7ᵗʰ **T85.518** **Breakdown (mechanical) of other** CC
gastrointestinal prosthetic devices,
implants and grafts

☑6ᵗʰ **T85.52** **Displacement of gastrointestinal prosthetic devices,**
implants and grafts
Malposition of gastrointestinal prosthetic devices,
implants and grafts

☑7ᵗʰ **T85.520** **Displacement of bile duct prosthesis** CC

☑7ᵗʰ **T85.521** **Displacement of esophageal** CC
anti-reflux device

☑7ᵗʰ **T85.528** **Displacement of other gastrointestinal** CC
prosthetic devices, implants and grafts

☑6ᵗʰ **T85.59** **Other mechanical complication of gastrointestinal**
prosthetic devices, implants and grafts
Obstruction, mechanical of gastrointestinal prosthetic
devices, implants and grafts
Perforation of gastrointestinal prosthetic devices,
implants and grafts
Protrusion of gastrointestinal prosthetic devices,
implants and grafts

☑7ᵗʰ **T85.590** **Other mechanical complication of bile** CC
duct prosthesis

☑7ᵗʰ **T85.591** **Other mechanical complication of** CC
esophageal anti-reflux device

☑7ᵗʰ **T85.598** **Other mechanical complication of**
other gastrointestinal prosthetic
devices, implants and grafts

☑5ᵗʰ **T85.6** **Mechanical complication of other specified internal and**
external prosthetic devices, implants and grafts

☑6ᵗʰ **T85.61** **Breakdown (mechanical) of other specified internal**
prosthetic devices, implants and grafts

☑7ᵗʰ **T85.610** **Breakdown (mechanical) of cranial** CC
or spinal infusion catheter
Breakdown (mechanical) of epidural
infusion catheter
Breakdown (mechanical) of intrathecal
infusion catheter
Breakdown (mechanical) of subarachnoid
infusion catheter
Breakdown (mechanical) of subdural
infusion catheter
CC Excl: PDX collection 1465

☑7ᵗʰ **T85.611** **Breakdown (mechanical) of** CC HCC
intraperitoneal dialysis catheter
> EXCLUDES 1   mechanical complication of
> vascular dialysis catheter
> (T82.4-)
CC Excl: PDX collection 1466

N Newborn: 0   P Pediatric: 0-17   M Maternity: 12-55   A Adult: 15-124   MCC Major Complication/Comorbidity   CC Complication/Comorbidity   SW Severe Wound Dx

1152   ICD-10-CM 2019

Twin Gestation–Monochorionic–Diamniotic (MO-DI)

1 Chorionic sac

2 Amniotic sacs

2 Fetuses

2 Umbilical cords

1 Placenta

Twin Gestation–Monochorionic–Monoamniotic (MO-MO)

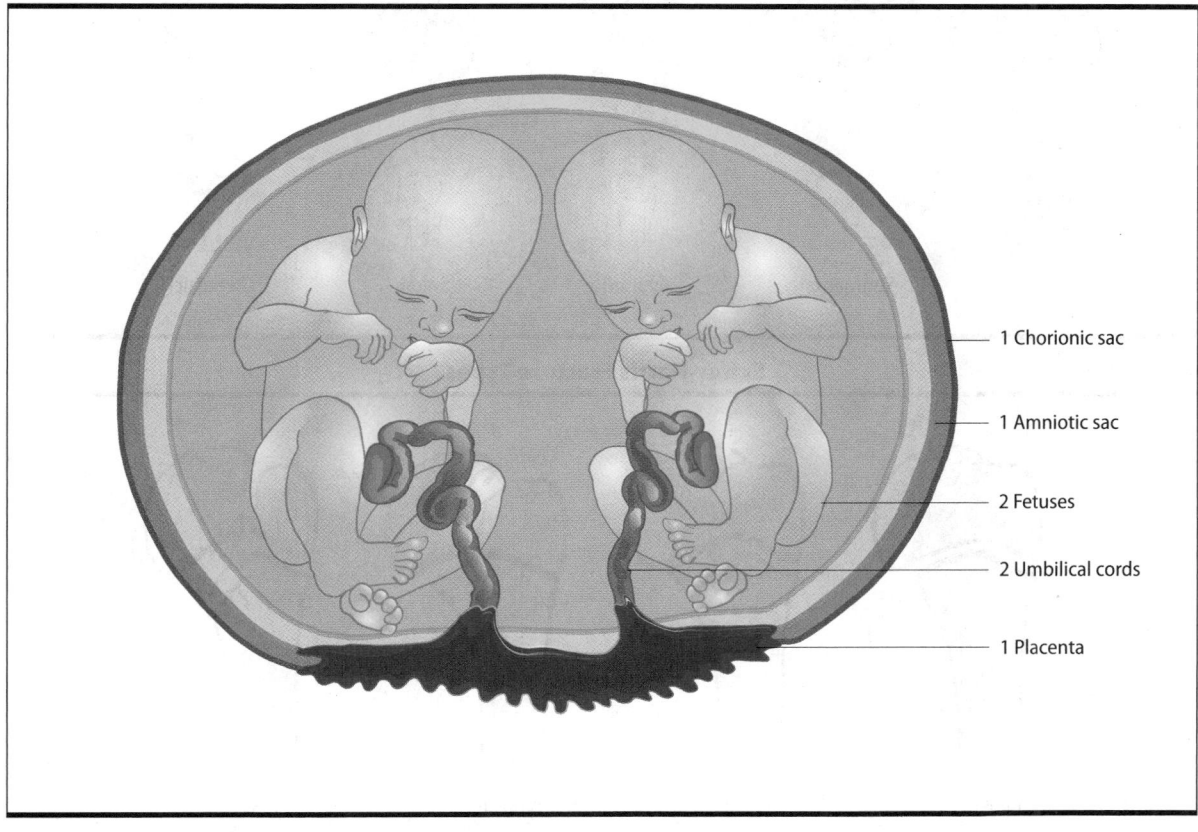

1 Chorionic sac

1 Amniotic sac

2 Fetuses

2 Umbilical cords

1 Placenta

Types of Fractures

Normal   Transverse   Open/Compound   Oblique   Oblique displaced

Comminuted   Segmental   Avulsed   Spiral   Greenstick

Salter-Harris Fracture Types

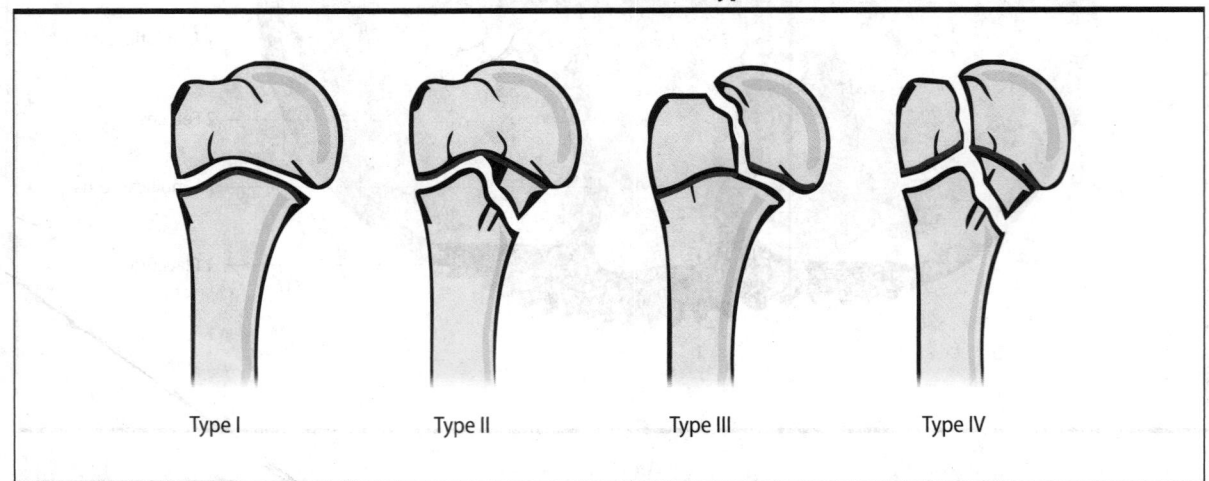

Type I   Type II   Type III   Type IV

Twin Gestation–Monochorionic–Diamniotic (MO-DI)

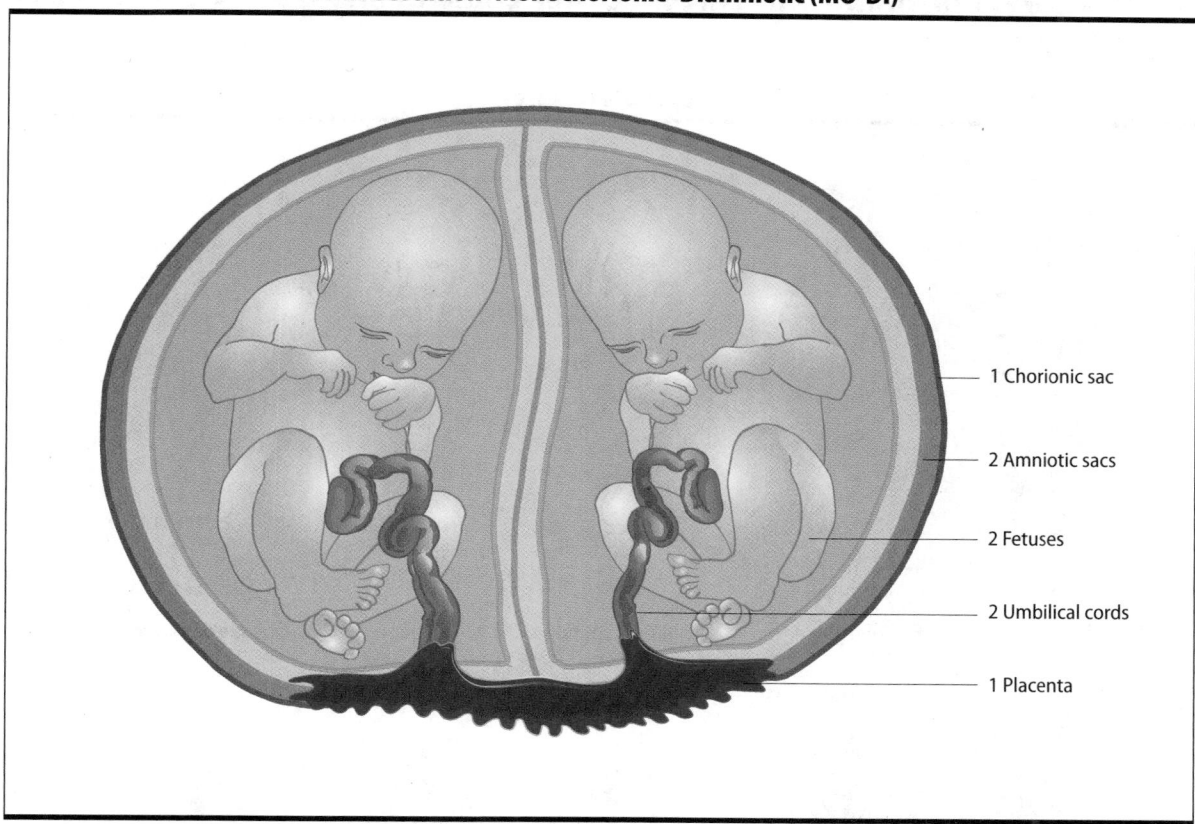

1 Chorionic sac

2 Amniotic sacs

2 Fetuses

2 Umbilical cords

1 Placenta

Twin Gestation–Monochorionic–Monoamniotic (MO-MO)

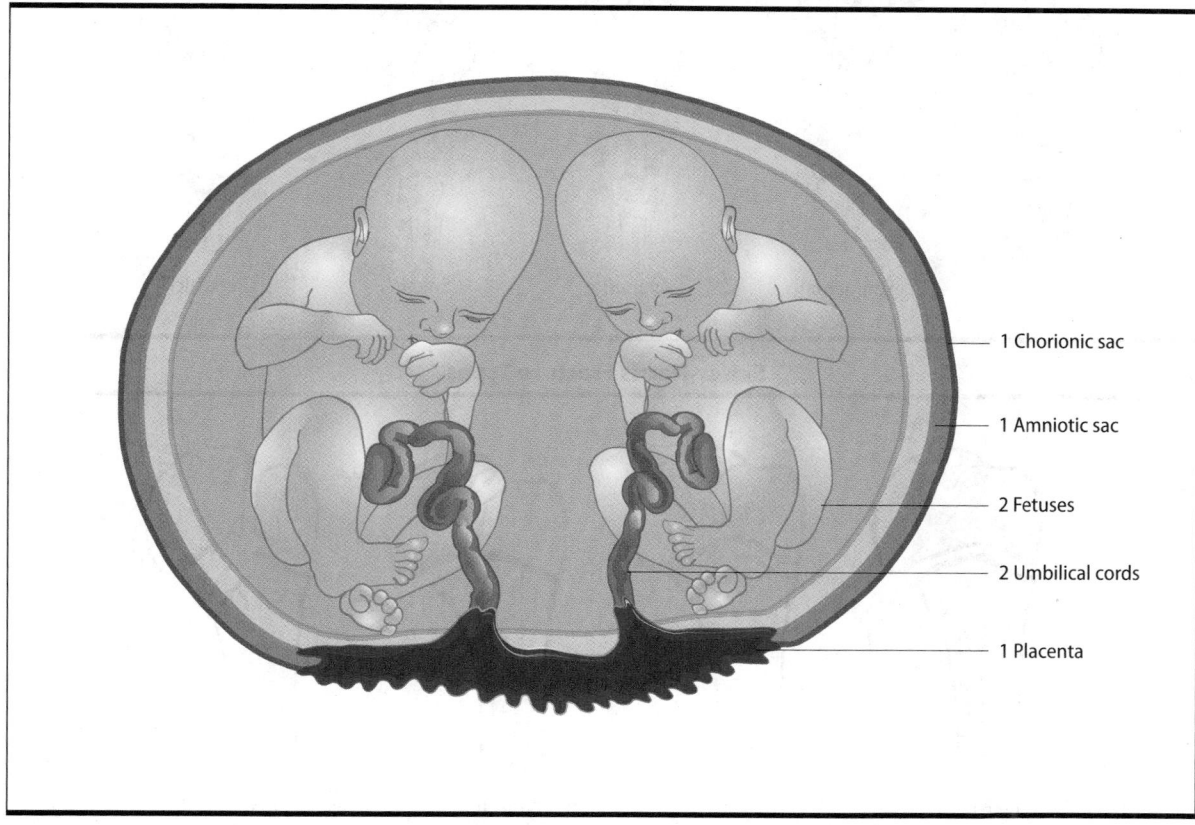

1 Chorionic sac

1 Amniotic sac

2 Fetuses

2 Umbilical cords

1 Placenta

Chapter 19. Injury, Poisoning and Certain Other Consequences of External Causes (S00–T88)

Types of Fractures

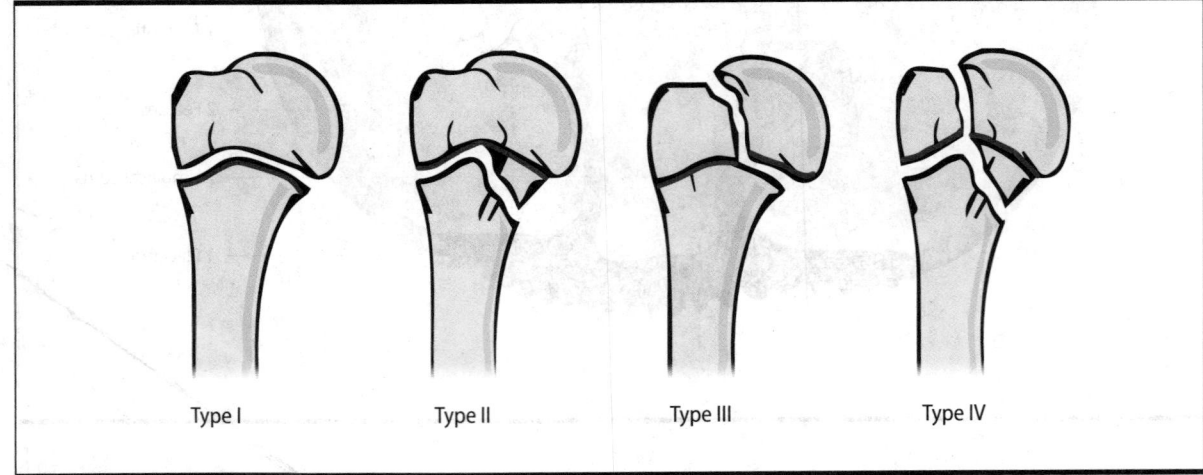

Salter-Harris Fracture Types

√7ᵗʰ **T85.612** **Breakdown (mechanical) of**   CC
permanent sutures
> EXCLUDES 1   *mechanical complication of permanent (wire) suture used in bone repair (T84.1-T84.2)*

CC Excl: PDX collection 1467

√7ᵗʰ **T85.613** **Breakdown (mechanical) of artificial**   CC
skin graft and decellularized allodermis
Failure of artificial skin graft and decellularized allodermis
Non-adherence of artificial skin graft and decellularized allodermis
Poor incorporation of artificial skin graft and decellularized allodermis
Shearing of artificial skin graft and decellularized allodermis

CC Excl: PDX collection 1468

√7ᵗʰ **T85.614** **Breakdown (mechanical) of insulin**   CC
pump

CC Excl: PDX collection 1469

6 √7ᵗʰ **T85.615** **Breakdown (mechanical) of other**   CC HCC
nervous system device, implant or graft
Breakdown (mechanical) of intrathecal infusion pump

CC Excl: PDX collection 1467

√7ᵗʰ **T85.618** **Breakdown (mechanical) of other**   CC
specified internal prosthetic devices, implants and grafts

CC Excl: PDX collection 1467

√6ᵗʰ **T85.62** **Displacement of other specified internal prosthetic devices, implants and grafts**
Malposition of other specified internal prosthetic devices, implants and grafts

√7ᵗʰ **T85.620** **Displacement of cranial or spinal**   CC
infusion catheter
Displacement of epidural infusion catheter
Displacement of intrathecal infusion catheter
Displacement of subarachnoid infusion catheter
Displacement of subdural infusion catheter

CC Excl: PDX collection 1465

√7ᵗʰ **T85.621** **Displacement of intraperitoneal**   CC HCC
dialysis catheter
> EXCLUDES 1   *mechanical complication of vascular dialysis catheter (T82.4-)*

CC Excl: PDX collection 1466

√7ᵗʰ **T85.622** **Displacement of permanent sutures**   CC
> EXCLUDES 1   *mechanical complication of permanent (wire) suture used in bone repair (T84.1-T84.2)*

CC Excl: PDX collection 1467

√7ᵗʰ **T85.623** **Displacement of artificial skin graft**   CC
and decellularized allodermis
Dislodgement of artificial skin graft and decellularized allodermis

CC Excl: PDX collection 1468

√7ᵗʰ **T85.624** **Displacement of insulin pump**   CC

CC Excl: PDX collection 1469

6 √7ᵗʰ **T85.625** **Displacement of other nervous**   CC HCC
system device, implant or graft
Displacement of intrathecal infusion pump

CC Excl: PDX collection 1467

√7ᵗʰ **T85.628** **Displacement of other specified**   CC
internal prosthetic devices, implants and grafts

CC Excl: PDX collection 1467

√6ᵗʰ **T85.63** **Leakage of other specified internal prosthetic devices, implants and grafts**

√7ᵗʰ **T85.630** **Leakage of cranial or spinal infusion**   CC
catheter
Leakage of epidural infusion catheter
Leakage of intrathecal infusion catheter infusion catheter
Leakage of subdural infusion catheter
Leakage of subarachnoid infusion catheter

CC Excl: PDX collection 1465

√7ᵗʰ **T85.631** **Leakage of intraperitoneal dialysis**   CC HCC
catheter
> EXCLUDES 1   *mechanical complication of vascular dialysis catheter (T82.4)*

CC Excl: PDX collection 1466

√7ᵗʰ **T85.633** **Leakage of insulin pump**   CC

CC Excl: PDX collection 1469

6 √7ᵗʰ **T85.635** **Leakage of other nervous system**   CC HCC
device, implant or graft
Leakage of intrathecal infusion pump

CC Excl: PDX collection 1467

√7ᵗʰ **T85.638** **Leakage of other specified internal**   CC
prosthetic devices, implants and grafts

CC Excl: PDX collection 1467

√6ᵗʰ **T85.69** **Other mechanical complication of other specified internal prosthetic devices, implants and grafts**
Obstruction, mechanical of other specified internal prosthetic devices, implants and grafts
Perforation of other specified internal prosthetic devices, implants and grafts
Protrusion of other specified internal prosthetic devices, implants and grafts

√7ᵗʰ **T85.690** **Other mechanical complication of**   CC
cranial or spinal infusion catheter
Other mechanical complication of epidural infusion catheter
Other mechanical complication of intrathecal infusion catheter
Other mechanical complication of subarachnoid infusion catheter
Other mechanical complication of subdural infusion catheter

CC Excl: PDX collection 1465

√7ᵗʰ **T85.691** **Other mechanical complication of**   CC HCC
intraperitoneal dialysis catheter
> EXCLUDES 1   *mechanical complication of vascular dialysis catheter (T82.4)*

CC Excl: PDX collection 1466

√7ᵗʰ **T85.692** **Other mechanical complication of**   CC
permanent sutures
> EXCLUDES 1   *mechanical complication of permanent (wire) suture used in bone repair (T84.1-T84.2)*

CC Excl: PDX collection 1467

√7ᵗʰ **T85.693** **Other mechanical complication of**   CC
artificial skin graft and decellularized allodermis

CC Excl: PDX collection 1468

√7ᵗʰ **T85.694** **Other mechanical complication of**   CC
insulin pump

CC Excl: PDX collection 1469

6 √7ᵗʰ **T85.695** **Other mechanical complication of**   CC HCC
other nervous system device, implant or graft
Other mechanical complication of intrathecal infusion pump

CC Excl: PDX collection 1467

√7ᵗʰ **T85.698** **Other mechanical complication of**   CC
other specified internal prosthetic devices, implants and grafts
Mechanical complication of nonabsorbable surgical material NOS

CC Excl: PDX collection 1467

√5ᵗʰ **T85.7** **Infection and inflammatory reaction due to other internal prosthetic devices, implants and grafts**
Use additional code to identify infection

> **CC Excl: For CC codes in subcategory T85.7, unless otherwise noted:** PDX collection 1470

√x7ᵗʰ **T85.71** **Infection and inflammatory reaction due to**   CC HCC
peritoneal dialysis catheter

CC Excl: PDX collection 1467

6 √x7ᵗʰ **T85.72** **Infection and inflammatory reaction due to**   CC HCC
insulin pump

✔ Additional Character Required   √x7ᵗʰ Placeholder   Unacceptable PDx   Questionable PDx   Manifestation   H1–H14 HAC   HCC CMS-HCC Dx   HIV HIV Dx

ICD-10-CM 2019   1153

✓6ᵗʰ **T85.73 Infection and inflammatory reaction due to** nervous system **devices, implants and graft**

6 ✓7ᵗʰ **T85.730 Infection and inflammatory reaction due to** ventricular intracranial (communicating) shunt   `CC` `HCC`

6 ✓7ᵗʰ **T85.731 Infection and inflammatory reaction due to implanted electronic neurostimulator of** brain, electrode (lead)   `CC` `HCC`

6 ✓7ᵗʰ **T85.732 Infection and inflammatory reaction due to implanted electronic neurostimulator of** peripheral nerve, electrode (lead)   `CC` `HCC`
> Infection and inflammatory reaction due to electrode (lead) for cranial nerve neurostimulators
> Infection and inflammatory reaction due to electrode (lead) for gastric neurostimulator
> Infection and inflammatory reaction due to electrode (lead) for sacral nerve neurostimulator
> Infection and inflammatory reaction due to electrode (lead) for vagal nerve neurostimulators

6 ✓7ᵗʰ **T85.733 Infection and inflammatory reaction due to implanted electronic neurostimulator of** spinal cord, electrode (lead)   `CC` `HCC`

6 ✓7ᵗʰ **T85.734 Infection and inflammatory reaction due to implanted electronic neurostimulator,** generator   `CC` `HCC`
> Generator pocket infection

6 ✓7ᵗʰ **T85.735 Infection and inflammatory reaction due to** cranial or spinal infusion catheter   `CC` `HCC`
> Infection and inflammatory reaction due to epidural catheter
> Infection and inflammatory reaction due to intrathecal infusion catheter
> Infection and inflammatory reaction due to subarachnoid catheter
> Infection and inflammatory reaction due to subdural catheter

6 ✓7ᵗʰ **T85.738 Infection and inflammatory reaction due to** other nervous system **device, implant or graft**   `CC` `HCC`
> Infection and inflammatory reaction due to intrathecal infusion pump

6 ✓x7ᵗʰ **T85.79 Infection and inflammatory reaction due to** other internal prosthetic devices, implants and grafts   `CC` `HCC`

✓5ᵗʰ **T85.8 Other specified complications of internal prosthetic devices, implants and grafts, not elsewhere classified**

> **CC Excl: For CC codes in subcategory T85.8:**
> **CC with 7th character A or D:** PDX collection 1470

✓6ᵗʰ **T85.81 Embolism due to internal prosthetic devices, implants and grafts, not elsewhere classified**

5,6 ✓7ᵗʰ **T85.810 Embolism due to** nervous system **prosthetic devices, implants and grafts**   `CC` `HCC`

✓7ᵗʰ **T85.818 Embolism due to** other **internal prosthetic devices, implants and grafts**

✓6ᵗʰ **T85.82 Fibrosis due to internal prosthetic devices, implants and grafts, not elsewhere classified**

5,6 ✓7ᵗʰ **T85.820 Fibrosis due to** nervous system **prosthetic devices, implants and grafts**   `CC` `HCC`

✓7ᵗʰ **T85.828 Fibrosis due to** other **internal prosthetic devices, implants and grafts**

✓6ᵗʰ **T85.83 Hemorrhage due to internal prosthetic devices, implants and grafts, not elsewhere classified**

5,6 ✓7ᵗʰ **T85.830 Hemorrhage due to** nervous system **prosthetic devices, implants and grafts**   `CC` `HCC`

✓7ᵗʰ **T85.838 Hemorrhage due to** other **internal prosthetic devices, implants and grafts**

✓6ᵗʰ **T85.84 Pain due to internal prosthetic devices, implants and grafts, not elsewhere classified**

5,6 ✓7ᵗʰ **T85.840 Pain due to** nervous system **prosthetic devices, implants and grafts**   `CC` `HCC`

✓7ᵗʰ **T85.848 Pain due to** other **internal prosthetic devices, implants and grafts**

✓6ᵗʰ **T85.85 Stenosis due to internal prosthetic devices, implants and grafts, not elsewhere classified**

5,6 ✓7ᵗʰ **T85.850 Stenosis due to** nervous system **prosthetic devices, implants and grafts**   `CC` `HCC`

✓7ᵗʰ **T85.858 Stenosis due to** other **internal prosthetic devices, implants and grafts**

✓6ᵗʰ **T85.86 Thrombosis due to internal prosthetic devices, implants and grafts, not elsewhere classified**

5,6 ✓7ᵗʰ **T85.860 Thrombosis due to** nervous system **prosthetic devices, implants and grafts**   `CC` `HCC`

✓7ᵗʰ **T85.868 Thrombosis due to** other **internal prosthetic devices, implants and grafts**

✓6ᵗʰ **T85.89 Other specified complication of internal prosthetic devices, implants and grafts, not elsewhere classified**
> Erosion or breakdown of subcutaneous device pocket

5,6 ✓7ᵗʰ **T85.890 Other specified complication of** nervous system **prosthetic devices, implants and grafts**   `CC` `HCC`

✓7ᵗʰ **T85.898 Other specified complication of** other **internal prosthetic devices, implants and grafts**

✓x7ᵗʰ **T85.9 Unspecified complication of internal prosthetic device, implant and graft**
> Complication of internal prosthetic device, implant and graft NOS

✓4ᵗʰ **T86 Complications of transplanted organs and tissue**
> Use additional code to identify other transplant complications, such as:
> graft-versus-host disease (D89.81-)
> malignancy associated with organ transplant (C80.2)
> post-transplant lymphoproliferative disorders (PTLD) (D47.Z1)

✓5ᵗʰ **T86.0 Complications of** bone marrow **transplant**

> **CC Excl: For CC codes in subcategory T86.0:**
> PDX collection 514

T86.00 Unspecified complication of bone marrow transplant   `CC` `HCC`

T86.01 Bone marrow transplant rejection   `CC` `HCC`

T86.02 Bone marrow transplant failure   `CC` `HCC`

T86.03 Bone marrow transplant infection   `CC` `HCC`

T86.09 Other complications of bone marrow transplant   `CC` `HCC`

✓5ᵗʰ **T86.1 Complications of** kidney **transplant**

> **CC Excl: For CC codes in subcategory T86.1:**
> PDX collection 1471

T86.10 Unspecified complication of kidney transplant   `CC`

T86.11 Kidney transplant rejection   `CC`

T86.12 Kidney transplant failure   `CC`
> **AHA:** 2013, 1Q, 24

T86.13 Kidney transplant infection   `CC`
> Use additional code to specify infection

T86.19 Other complication of kidney transplant   `CC`

✓5ᵗʰ **T86.2 Complications of** heart **transplant**
> *EXCLUDES 1*   complication of:
> artificial heart device (T82.5)
> heart-lung transplant (T86.3)

> **CC Excl: For CC codes in subcategory T86.2:**
> PDX collection 1472

T86.20 Unspecified complication of heart transplant   `CC` `HCC`

T86.21 Heart transplant rejection   `CC` `HCC`

T86.22 Heart transplant failure   `CC` `HCC`

T86.23 Heart transplant infection   `CC` `HCC`
> Use additional code to specify infection

✓6ᵗʰ **T86.29 Other complications of heart transplant**

T86.290 Cardiac allograft vasculopathy   `CC` `HCC`
> *EXCLUDES 1*   atherosclerosis of coronary arteries (I25.75-, I25.76-, I25.81-)

T86.298 Other complications of heart transplant   `CC` `HCC`

N Newborn: 0   **P** Pediatric: 0-17   **M** Maternity: 12-55   **A** Adult: 15-124   `MCC` Major Complication/Comorbidity   `CC` Complication/Comorbidity   `SW` Severe Wound Dx

✓5th **T86.3** **Complications of** heart-lung **transplant**

CC Excl: For CC codes in subcategory T86.3:
PDX collection 1472

T86.30 Unspecified **complication of heart-lung transplant** `CC` `HCC`

T86.31 **Heart-lung transplant** rejection `CC` `HCC`

T86.32 **Heart-lung transplant** failure `CC` `HCC`

T86.33 **Heart-lung transplant** infection `CC` `HCC`
Use additional code to specify infection

T86.39 Other **complications of heart-lung transplant** `CC` `HCC`

✓5th **T86.4** **Complications of** liver **transplant**

CC Excl: For CC codes in subcategory T86.4:
PDX collection 1473

T86.40 Unspecified **complication of liver transplant** `CC` `HCC`

T86.41 **Liver transplant** rejection `CC` `HCC`

T86.42 **Liver transplant** failure `CC` `HCC`

T86.43 **Liver transplant** infection `CC` `HCC`
Use additional code to identify infection, such as:
cytomegalovirus (CMV) infection (B25.-)

T86.49 Other **complications of liver transplant** `CC` `HCC`

T86.5 **Complications of** stem cell **transplant** `CC` `HCC`
Complications from stem cells from peripheral blood
Complications from stem cells from umbilical cord
CC Excl: PDX collection 1474

✓5th **T86.8** **Complications of** other **transplanted organs and tissues**

✓6th **T86.81** **Complications of** lung **transplant**
`EXCLUDES 1` *complication of heart-lung transplant (T86.3-)*

CC Excl: For CC codes in subcategory T86.81:
PDX collection 1475

T86.810 **Lung transplant** rejection `CC` `HCC`

T86.811 **Lung transplant** failure `CC` `HCC`

T86.812 **Lung transplant** infection `CC` `HCC`
Use additional code to specify infection

T86.818 Other **complications of lung transplant** `CC` `HCC`

T86.819 Unspecified **complication of lung transplant** `CC` `HCC`

✓6th **T86.82** **Complications of** skin graft (allograft) (autograft)
`EXCLUDES 2` *complication of artificial skin graft (T85.693)*

CC Excl: For CC codes in subcategory T86.82:
PDX collection 1476

T86.820 **Skin graft (allograft)** rejection `CC`

T86.821 **Skin graft (allograft) (autograft)** failure `CC`

T86.822 **Skin graft (allograft) (autograft)** infection `CC`
Use additional code to specify infection

T86.828 Other **complications of skin graft (allograft) (autograft)** `CC`

T86.829 Unspecified **complication of skin graft (allograft) (autograft)** `CC`

✓6th **T86.83** **Complications of** bone graft
`EXCLUDES 2` *mechanical complications of bone graft (T84.3-)*

CC Excl: For CC codes in subcategory T86.83:
PDX collection 1477

T86.830 **Bone graft** rejection `CC`

T86.831 **Bone graft** failure `CC`

T86.832 **Bone graft** infection `CC`
Use additional code to specify infection

T86.838 Other **complications of bone graft** `CC`

T86.839 Unspecified **complication of bone graft** `CC`

✓6th **T86.84** **Complications of** corneal **transplant**
`EXCLUDES 2` *mechanical complications of corneal graft (T85.3-)*

T86.840 **Corneal transplant** rejection `CC`
CC Excl: PDX collection 1478

T86.841 **Corneal transplant** failure `CC`
CC Excl: PDX collection 1478

T86.842 **Corneal transplant** infection `CC` `HCC`
Use additional code to specify infection
CC Excl: PDX collection 1479

T86.848 Other **complications of corneal transplant** `CC`
CC Excl: PDX collection 1479

T86.849 Unspecified **complication of corneal transplant** `CC`
CC Excl: PDX collection 1479

✓6th **T86.85** **Complication of** intestine **transplant**

CC Excl: For CC codes in subcategory T86.85:
PDX collection 495

T86.850 **Intestine transplant** rejection `CC` `HCC`

T86.851 **Intestine transplant** failure `CC` `HCC`

T86.852 **Intestine transplant** infection `CC` `HCC`
Use additional code to specify infection

T86.858 Other **complications of intestine transplant** `CC` `HCC`

T86.859 Unspecified **complication of intestine transplant** `CC` `HCC`

✓6th **T86.89** **Complications of** other **transplanted** tissue
Transplant failure or rejection of pancreas

CC Excl: For CC codes in subcategory T86.89:
PDX collection 1480

T86.890 **Other transplanted tissue** rejection `CC`

T86.891 **Other transplanted tissue** failure `CC`

T86.892 **Other transplanted tissue** infection `CC`
Use additional code to specify infection

T86.898 Other **complications of other transplanted tissue** `CC`

T86.899 Unspecified **complication of other transplanted tissue** `CC`

✓5th **T86.9** **Complication of** unspecified **transplanted** organ and tissue

CC Excl: For CC codes in subcategory T86.9:
PDX collection 495

T86.90 Unspecified **complication of** unspecified **transplanted organ and tissue** `CC`

T86.91 Unspecified **transplanted organ and tissue** rejection `CC`

T86.92 Unspecified **transplanted organ and tissue** failure `CC`

T86.93 Unspecified **transplanted organ and tissue** infection `CC`
Use additional code to specify infection

T86.99 Other **complications of unspecified transplanted organ and tissue** `CC`

✓4th **T87** **Complications peculiar to reattachment and amputation**

✓5th **T87.0** **Complications of reattached (part of)** upper extremity

✓6th **T87.0X** **Complications of reattached (part of) upper extremity**

CC Excl: For CC codes in subcategory T87.0X:
PDX collection 1481

T87.0X1 **Complications of reattached (part of)** right **upper extremity** `CC` `HCC`

T87.0X2 **Complications of reattached (part of)** left **upper extremity** `CC` `HCC`

T87.0X9 **Complications of reattached (part of)** unspecified **upper extremity** `CC` `HCC`

✓5th **T87.1** **Complications of reattached (part of)** lower extremity

✓6th **T87.1X** **Complications of reattached (part of) lower extremity**

CC Excl: For CC codes in subcategory T87.1X:
PDX collection 1482

T87.1X1 **Complications of reattached (part of)** right **lower extremity** `CC` `HCC`

T87.1X2 **Complications of reattached (part of)** left **lower extremity** `CC` `HCC`

T87.1X9 **Complications of reattached (part of)** unspecified **lower extremity** `CC` `HCC`

T87.2 **Complications of** other **reattached** body part `CC` `HCC`
CC Excl: PDX collection 1483

✓ Additional Character Required   ✓x7th Placeholder   Unacceptable PDx   Questionable PDx   Manifestation   `H1`-`H14` HAC   `HCC` CMS-HCC Dx   `HIV` HIV Dx

✓5th **T87.3 Neuroma of amputation stump**
DEF: Non-neoplastic tumor generated at the proximal end of severed, partially transected, or injured nerve following amputation.

T87.30 **Neuroma of amputation stump,** unspecified extremity   HCC

T87.31 **Neuroma of amputation stump,** right upper extremity   HCC

T87.32 **Neuroma of amputation stump,** left upper extremity   HCC

T87.33 **Neuroma of amputation stump,** right lower extremity   HCC

T87.34 **Neuroma of amputation stump,** left lower extremity   HCC

✓5th **T87.4 Infection of amputation stump**

CC Excl: For CC codes in subcategory T87.4: PDX collection 1484

T87.40 **Infection of amputation stump,** unspecified extremity   CC HCC

T87.41 **Infection of amputation stump,** right upper extremity   CC HCC

T87.42 **Infection of amputation stump,** left upper extremity   CC HCC

T87.43 **Infection of amputation stump,** right lower extremity   CC HCC

T87.44 **Infection of amputation stump,** left lower extremity   CC HCC

✓5th **T87.5 Necrosis of amputation stump**

T87.50 **Necrosis of amputation stump,** unspecified extremity   HCC

T87.51 **Necrosis of amputation stump,** right upper extremity   HCC

T87.52 **Necrosis of amputation stump,** left upper extremity   HCC

T87.53 **Necrosis of amputation stump,** right lower extremity   HCC

T87.54 **Necrosis of amputation stump,** left lower extremity   HCC

✓5th **T87.8 Other complications of amputation stump**

T87.81 **Dehiscence of amputation stump**   HCC

T87.89 **Other complications of amputation stump**   HCC
Amputation stump contracture
Amputation stump contracture of next proximal joint
Amputation stump flexion
Amputation stump edema
Amputation stump hematoma
EXCLUDES 2   *phantom limb syndrome (G54.6-G54.7)*

T87.9 Unspecified complications of amputation stump   HCC

✓4th **T88 Other complications of surgical and medical care, not elsewhere classified**
EXCLUDES 2   *complication following infusion, transfusion and therapeutic injection (T80.-)*
complication following procedure NEC (T81.-)
complications of anesthesia in labor and delivery (O74.-)
complications of anesthesia in pregnancy (O29.-)
complications of anesthesia in puerperium (O89.-)
complications of devices, implants and grafts (T82-T85)
complications of obstetric surgery and procedure (O75.4)
dermatitis due to drugs and medicaments (L23.3, L24.4, L25.1, L27.0-L27.1)
poisoning and toxic effects of drugs and chemicals (T36-T65 with fifth or sixth character 1-4 or 6)
specified complications classified elsewhere

The appropriate 7th character is to be added to each code from category T88.
A   initial encounter
D   subsequent encounter
S   sequela

✓x7th **T88.0 Infection following immunization**   CC
Sepsis following immunization
CC Excl: PDX collection 948

✓x7th **T88.1 Other complications following immunization, not elsewhere classified**   CC
Generalized vaccinia
Rash following immunization
EXCLUDES 1   *vaccinia not from vaccine (B08.011)*
EXCLUDES 2   *anaphylactic shock due to serum (T80.5-)*
other serum reactions (T80.6-)
postimmunization arthropathy (M02.2)
postimmunization encephalitis (G04.02)
postimmunization fever (R50.83)
CC Excl: PDX collection 1485

✓x7th **T88.2 Shock due to anesthesia**   CC
Use additional code for adverse effect, if applicable, to identify drug (T41.- with fifth or sixth character 5)
EXCLUDES 1   *complications of anesthesia (in):*
labor and delivery (O74.-)
postprocedural shock NOS (T81.1-)
pregnancy (O29.-)
puerperium (O89.-)
CC Excl: PDX collection 1441

✓x7th **T88.3 Malignant hyperthermia due to anesthesia**   CC
Use additional code for adverse effect, if applicable, to identify drug (T41.- with fifth or sixth character 5)
CC Excl: PDX collection 1486

✓x7th **T88.4 Failed or difficult intubation**

✓5th **T88.5 Other complications of anesthesia**
Use additional code for adverse effect, if applicable, to identify drug (T41.- with fifth or sixth character 5)

✓x7th **T88.51 Hypothermia following anesthesia**

✓x7th **T88.52 Failed moderate sedation during procedure**
Failed conscious sedation during procedure
EXCLUDES 2   *personal history of failed moderate sedation (Z92.83)*

✓x7th **T88.53 Unintended awareness under general anesthesia during procedure**
EXCLUDES 2   *personal history of unintended awareness under general anesthesia (Z92.84)*
AHA: 2016, 4Q, 72-73

✓x7th **T88.59 Other complications of anesthesia**

✓x7th **T88.6 Anaphylactic reaction due to adverse effect of correct drug or medicament properly administered**   CC
Anaphylactic shock due to adverse effect of correct drug or medicament properly administered
Anaphylactoid reaction NOS
Use additional code for adverse effect, if applicable, to identify drug (T41.- with fifth or sixth character 5)
EXCLUDES 1   *anaphylactic reaction due to serum (T80.5-)*
anaphylactic shock or reaction due to adverse food reaction (T78.0-)
CC Excl: PDX collection 1426

✓x7th **T88.7 Unspecified adverse effect of drug or medicament**
Drug hypersensitivity NOS
Drug reaction NOS
Use additional code for adverse effect, if applicable, to identify drug (T41.- with fifth or sixth character 5)
EXCLUDES 1   *specified adverse effects of drugs and medicaments (A00-R94 and T80-T88.6, T88.8)*

✓x7th **T88.8 Other specified complications of surgical and medical care, not elsewhere classified**
Use additional code to identify the complication

✓x7th **T88.9 Complication of surgical and medical care, unspecified**

Chapter 20. External Causes of Morbidity (V00–Y99)

Chapter Specific Guidelines with Coding Examples

The chapter specific guidelines from the ICD-10-CM Official Guidelines for Coding and Reporting have been provided below. Along with these guidelines are coding examples, contained in the shaded boxes, that have been developed to help illustrate the coding and/or sequencing guidance found in these guidelines.

The external causes of morbidity codes should never be sequenced as the first-listed or principal diagnosis.

External cause codes are intended to provide data for injury research and evaluation of injury prevention strategies. These codes capture how the injury or health condition happened (cause), the intent (unintentional or accidental; or intentional, such as suicide or assault), the place where the event occurred the activity of the patient at the time of the event, and the person's status (e.g., civilian, military).

There is no national requirement for mandatory ICD-10-CM external cause code reporting. Unless a provider is subject to a state-based external cause code reporting mandate or these codes are required by a particular payer, reporting of ICD-10-CM codes in Chapter 20, External Causes of Morbidity, is not required. In the absence of a mandatory reporting requirement, providers are encouraged to voluntarily report external cause codes, as they provide valuable data for injury research and evaluation of injury prevention strategies.

a. General external cause coding guidelines

1) Used with any code in the range of A00.0–T88.9, Z00–Z99

An external cause code may be used with any code in the range of A00.0–T88.9, Z00-Z99, classification that represents a health condition due to an external cause. Though they are most applicable to injuries, they are also valid for use with such things as infections or diseases due to an external source, and other health conditions, such as a heart attack that occurs during strenuous physical activity.

> Actinic reticuloid due to tanning bed use
>
> **L57.1**   **Actinic reticuloid**
>
> **W89.1XXA**   **Exposure to tanning bed, initial encounter**
>
> *Explanation:* An external cause code may be used with any code in the range of A00.0–T88.9, Z00–Z99, classifications that describe health conditions due to an external cause. Code W89.1 Exposure to tanning bed requires a seventh character of A to report this initial encounter, with a placeholder X for the fifth and sixth characters.

2) External cause code used for length of treatment

Assign the external cause code, with the appropriate 7th character (initial encounter, subsequent encounter or sequela) for each encounter for which the injury or condition is being treated.

Most categories in chapter 20 have a 7th character requirement for each applicable code. Most categories in this chapter have three 7th character values: A, initial encounter, D, subsequent encounter and S, sequela. While the patient may be seen by a new or different provider over the course of treatment for an injury or condition, assignment of the 7th character for external cause should match the 7th character of the code assigned for the associated injury or condition for the encounter.

3) Use the full range of external cause codes

Use the full range of external cause codes to completely describe the cause, the intent, the place of occurrence, and if applicable, the activity of the patient at the time of the event, and the patient's status, for all injuries, and other health conditions due to an external cause.

4) Assign as many external cause codes as necessary

Assign as many external cause codes as necessary to fully explain each cause. If only one external code can be recorded, assign the code most related to the principal diagnosis.

5) The selection of the appropriate external cause code

The selection of the appropriate external cause code is guided by the Alphabetic Index of External Causes and by Inclusion and Exclusion notes in the Tabular List.

6) External cause code can never be a principal diagnosis

An external cause code can never be a principal (first-listed) diagnosis.

7) Combination external cause codes

Certain of the external cause codes are combination codes that identify sequential events that result in an injury, such as a fall which results in striking against an object. The injury may be due to either event or both.

The combination external cause code used should correspond to the sequence of events regardless of which caused the most serious injury.

> Toddler tripped and fell while walking and struck his head on an end table, sustaining a scalp contusion
>
> **S00.03XA**   **Contusion of scalp, initial encounter**
>
> **W01.190A**   **Fall on same level from slipping, tripping and stumbling with subsequent striking against furniture, initial encounter**
>
> *Explanation:* Combination external cause codes identify sequential events that result in an injury, such as a fall resulting in striking against an object. The injury may be due to either or both events.

8) No external cause code needed in certain circumstances

No external cause code from Chapter 20 is needed if the external cause and intent are included in a code from another chapter (e.g. T36.0X1-Poisoning by penicillins, accidental (unintentional)).

b. Place of occurrence guideline

Codes from category Y92, Place of occurrence of the external cause, are secondary codes for use after other external cause codes to identify the location of the patient at the time of injury or other condition.

Generally, a place of occurrence code is assigned only once, at the initial encounter for treatment. However, in the rare instance that a new injury occurs during hospitalization, an additional place of occurrence code may be assigned. No 7th characters are used for Y92.

Do not use place of occurrence code Y92.9 if the place is not stated or is not applicable.

> A farmer was working in his barn and sustained a foot contusion when the horse stepped on his left foot
>
> **S90.32XA**   **Contusion of left foot, initial encounter**
>
> **W55.19XA**   **Other contact with horse, initial encounter**
>
> **Y92.71**   **Barn as the place of occurrence of the external cause**
>
> *Explanation:* A place-of-occurrence code from category Y92 is assigned at the initial encounter to identify the location of the patient at the time the injury occurred.

c. Activity code

Assign a code from category Y93, Activity code, to describe the activity of the patient at the time the injury or other health condition occurred.

An activity code is used only once, at the initial encounter for treatment. Only one code from Y93 should be recorded on a medical record.

The activity codes are not applicable to poisonings, adverse effects, misadventures or sequela.

Do not assign Y93.9, Unspecified activity, if the activity is not stated.

A code from category Y93 is appropriate for use with external cause and intent codes if identifying the activity provides additional information about the event.

> Ranch hand who was grooming a horse sustained a foot contusion when the horse stepped on his left foot
>
> **S90.32XA**   **Contusion of left foot, initial encounter**
>
> **W55.19XA**   **Other contact with horse, initial encounter**
>
> **Y93.K3**   **Activity, grooming and shearing an animal**
>
> *Explanation:* One activity code from category Y93 is assigned at the initial encounter only to describe the activity of the patient at the time the injury occurred.

d. Place of occurrence, activity, and status codes used with other external cause code

When applicable, place of occurrence, activity, and external cause status codes are sequenced after the main external cause code(s). Regardless of the number of external cause codes assigned, generally there should be only one place of occurrence code, one activity code, and one external cause status code assigned to an encounter. However, in the rare instance that a new injury occurs during hospitalization, an additional place of occurrence code may be assigned.

e. If the reporting format limits the number of external cause codes

If the reporting format limits the number of external cause codes that can be used in reporting clinical data, report the code for the cause/intent most related to the principal diagnosis. If the format permits capture of additional external cause codes, the cause/intent, including medical misadventures, of the additional events should be reported rather than the codes for place, activity, or external status.

f. Multiple external cause coding guidelines

More than one external cause code is required to fully describe the external cause of an illness or injury. The assignment of external cause codes should be sequenced in the following priority:

If two or more events cause separate injuries, an external cause code should be assigned for each cause. The first-listed external cause code will be selected in the following order:

External codes for child and adult abuse take priority over all other external cause codes.

See Section I.C.19., Child and Adult abuse guidelines.

External cause codes for terrorism events take priority over all other external cause codes except child and adult abuse.

External cause codes for cataclysmic events take priority over all other external cause codes except child and adult abuse and terrorism.

External cause codes for transport accidents take priority over all other external cause codes except cataclysmic events, child and adult abuse and terrorism.

Activity and external cause status codes are assigned following all causal (intent) external cause codes.

The first-listed external cause code should correspond to the cause of the most serious diagnosis due to an assault, accident, or self-harm, following the order of hierarchy listed above..

30-year-old man accidentally discharged his hunting rifle, sustaining an open gunshot wound to the right thigh, which caused him to fall down the stairs, resulting in closed displaced comminuted fracture of his left radial shaft	
S71.101A	**Unspecified open wound, right thigh, initial encounter**
W33.02XA	**Accidental discharge of hunting rifle, initial encounter**
S52.352A	**Displaced comminuted fracture of shaft of radius, left arm, initial encounter for closed fracture**
W10.9XXA	**Fall (on) (from) unspecified stairs and steps, initial encounter**

Explanation: If two or more events cause separate injuries, an external cause code should be assigned for each cause.

g. Child and adult abuse guideline

Adult and child abuse, neglect and maltreatment are classified as assault. Any of the assault codes may be used to indicate the external cause of any injury resulting from the confirmed abuse.

For confirmed cases of abuse, neglect and maltreatment, when the perpetrator is known, a code from Y07, Perpetrator of maltreatment and neglect, should accompany any other assault codes.

See Section I.C.19. Adult and child abuse, neglect and other maltreatment

h. Unknown or undetermined intent guideline

If the intent (accident, self-harm, assault) of the cause of an injury or other condition is unknown or unspecified, code the intent as accidental intent. All transport accident categories assume accidental intent.

1) Use of undetermined intent

External cause codes for events of undetermined intent are only for use if the documentation in the record specifies that the intent cannot be determined.

i. Sequelae (late effects) of external cause guidelines

1) Sequelae external cause codes

Sequelae are reported using the external cause code with the 7th character "S" for sequela. These codes should be used with any report of a late effect or sequela resulting from a previous injury.

See Section I.B.10 Sequela (Late Effects)

2) Sequela external cause code with a related current injury

A sequela external cause code should never be used with a related current nature of injury code.

3) Use of sequela external cause codes for subsequent visits

Use a late effect external cause code for subsequent visits when a late effect of the initial injury is being treated. Do not use a late effect external cause code for subsequent visits for follow-up care (e.g., to assess healing, to receive rehabilitative therapy) of the injury when no late effect of the injury has been documented.

j. Terrorism guidelines

1) Cause of injury identified by the Federal Government (FBI) as terrorism

When the cause of an injury is identified by the Federal Government (FBI) as terrorism, the first-listed external cause code should be a code from category Y38, Terrorism. The definition of terrorism employed by the FBI is found at the inclusion note at the beginning of category Y38. Use additional code for place of occurrence (Y92.-). More than one Y38 code may be assigned if the injury is the result of more than one mechanism of terrorism.

2) Cause of an injury is suspected to be the result of terrorism

When the cause of an injury is suspected to be the result of terrorism a code from category Y38 should not be assigned. Suspected cases should be classified as assault.

3) Code Y38.9, Terrorism, secondary effects

Assign code Y38.9, Terrorism, secondary effects, for conditions occurring subsequent to the terrorist event. This code should not be assigned for conditions that are due to the initial terrorist act.

It is acceptable to assign code Y38.9 with another code from Y38 if there is an injury due to the initial terrorist event and an injury that is a subsequent result of the terrorist event.

k. External cause status

A code from category Y99, External cause status, should be assigned whenever any other external cause code is assigned for an encounter, including an Activity code, except for the events noted below. Assign a code from category Y99, External cause status, to indicate the work status of the person at the time the event occurred. The status code indicates whether the event occurred during military activity, whether a non-military person was at work, whether an individual including a student or volunteer was involved in a non-work activity at the time of the causal event.

A code from Y99, External cause status, should be assigned, when applicable, with other external cause codes, such as transport accidents and falls. The external cause status codes are not applicable to poisonings, adverse effects, misadventures or late effects.

Do not assign a code from category Y99 if no other external cause codes (cause, activity) are applicable for the encounter.

An external cause status code is used only once, at the initial encounter for treatment. Only one code from Y99 should be recorded on a medical record.

Do not assign code Y99.9, Unspecified external cause status, if the status is not stated.

Chapter 20. External Causes of Morbidity (V00-Y99)

NOTE This chapter permits the classification of environmental events and circumstances as the cause of injury, and other adverse effects. Where a code from this section is applicable, it is intended that it shall be used secondary to a code from another chapter of the Classification indicating the nature of the condition. Most often, the condition will be classifiable to Chapter 19, Injury, poisoning and certain other consequences of external causes (S00-T88). Other conditions that may be stated to be due to external causes are classified in Chapters I to XVIII. For these conditions, codes from Chapter 20 should be used to provide additional information as to the cause of the condition.

This chapter contains the following blocks:

V00-X58	Accidents
V00-V99	Transport accidents
V00-V09	Pedestrian injured in transport accident
V10-V19	Pedal cycle rider injured in transport accident
V20-V29	Motorcycle rider injured in transport accident
V30-V39	Occupant of three-wheeled motor vehicle injured in transport accident
V40-V49	Car occupant injured in transport accident
V50-V59	Occupant of pick-up truck or van injured in transport accident
V60-V69	Occupant of heavy transport vehicle injured in transport accident
V70-V79	Bus occupant injured in transport accident
V80-V89	Other land transport accidents
V90-V94	Water transport accidents
V95-V97	Air and space transport accidents
V98-V99	Other and unspecified transport accidents
W00-X58	Other external causes of accidental injury
W00-W19	Slipping, tripping, stumbling and falls
W20-W49	Exposure to inanimate mechanical forces
W50-W64	Exposure to animate mechanical forces
W65-W74	Accidental non-transport drowning and submersion
W85-W99	Exposure to electric current, radiation and extreme ambient air temperature and pressure
X00-X08	Exposure to smoke, fire and flames
X10-X19	Contact with heat and hot substances
X30-X39	Exposure to forces of nature
▶X50	Overexertion and strenuous or repetitive movements◀
X52-X58	Accidental exposure to other specified factors
X71-X83	Intentional self-harm
X92-Y09	Assault
Y21-Y33	Event of undetermined intent
Y35-Y38	Legal intervention, operations of war, military operations, and terrorism
Y62-Y84	Complications of medical and surgical care
Y62-Y69	Misadventures to patients during surgical and medical care
Y70-Y82	Medical devices associated with adverse incidents in diagnostic and therapeutic use
Y83-Y84	Surgical and other medical procedures as the cause of abnormal reaction of the patient, or of later complication, without mention of misadventure at the time of the procedure
Y90-Y99	Supplementary factors related to causes of morbidity classified elsewhere

ACCIDENTS (V00-X58)

AHA: 2018, 2Q, 7-8

Transport accidents (V00-V99)

NOTE This section is structured in 12 groups. Those relating to land transport accidents (V00-V89) reflect the victim's mode of transport and are subdivided to identify the victim's 'counterpart' or the type of event. The vehicle of which the injured person is an occupant is identified in the first two characters since it is seen as the most important factor to identify for prevention purposes. A transport accident is one in which the vehicle involved must be moving or running or in use for transport purposes at the time of the accident.

Use additional code to identify:
airbag injury (W22.1)
type of street or road (Y92.4-)
use of cellular telephone and other electronic equipment at the time of the transport accident (Y93.C-)

EXCLUDES 1 *agricultural vehicles in stationary use or maintenance (W31.-)*
assault by crashing of motor vehicle (Y03.-)
automobile or motor cycle in stationary use or maintenance—code to type of accident
crashing of motor vehicle, undetermined intent (Y32)
intentional self-harm by crashing of motor vehicle (X82)
EXCLUDES 2 *transport accidents due to cataclysm (X34-X38)*

NOTE Definitions related to transport accidents:

(a) A transport accident (V00-V99) is any accident involving a device designed primarily for, or used at the time primarily for, conveying persons or good from one place to another.

(b) A public highway [trafficway] or street is the entire width between property lines (or other boundary lines) of land open to the public as a matter of right or custom for purposes of moving persons or property from one place to another. A roadway is that part of the public highway designed, improved and customarily used for vehicular traffic.

(c) A traffic accident is any vehicle accident occurring on the public highway [i.e. originating on, terminating on, or involving a vehicle partially on the highway]. A vehicle accident is assumed to have occurred on the public highway unless another place is specified, except in the case of accidents involving only off-road motor vehicles, which are classified as nontraffic accidents unless the contrary is stated.

(d) A nontraffic accident is any vehicle accident that occurs entirely in any place other than a public highway.

▶(e) A pedestrian is any person involved in an accident who was not at the time of the accident riding in or on a motor vehicle, railway train, streetcar or animal-drawn or other vehicle, or on a pedal cycle or animal. This includes, a person changing a tire, working on a parked car, or a person on foot. It also includes the user of a pedestrian conveyance such as a baby stroller, ice-skates, skis, sled, roller skates, a skateboard, nonmotorized or motorized wheelchair, motorized mobility scooter, or nonmotorized scooter.◀

(f) A driver is an occupant of a transport vehicle who is operating or intending to operate it.

(g) A passenger is any occupant of a transport vehicle other than the driver, except a person traveling on the outside of the vehicle.

(h) A person on the outside of a vehicle is any person being transported by a vehicle but not occupying the space normally reserved for the driver or passengers, or the space intended for the transport of property. This includes a person travelling on the bodywork, bumper, fender, roof, running board or step of a vehicle, as well as, hanging on the outside of the vehicle.

(i) A pedal cycle is any land transport vehicle operated solely by nonmotorized pedals including a bicycle or tricycle.

(j) A pedal cyclist is any person riding a pedal cycle or in a sidecar or trailer attached to a pedal cycle.

(k) A motorcycle is a two-wheeled motor vehicle with one or two riding saddles and sometimes with a third wheel for the support of a sidecar. The sidecar is considered part of the motorcycle. This includes a moped, motor scooter, or motorized bicycle.

(l) A motorcycle rider is any person riding a motorcycle or in a sidecar or trailer attached to the motorcycle.

(m) A three-wheeled motor vehicle is a motorized tricycle designed primarily for on-road use. This includes a motor-driven tricycle, a motorized rickshaw, or a three-wheeled motor car.

(n) A car [automobile] is a four-wheeled motor vehicle designed primarily for carrying up to 7 persons. A trailer being towed by the car is considered part of the car. It does not include a van or minivan - see definition (o).

(o) A pick-up truck or van is a four or six-wheeled motor vehicle designed for carrying passengers as well as property or cargo weighing less than the local limit for classification as a heavy goods vehicle, and not requiring a special driver's license. This includes a minivan and a sport-utility vehicle (SUV).

(p) A heavy transport vehicle is a motor vehicle designed primarily for carrying property, meeting local criteria for classification as a heavy goods vehicle in terms of weight and requiring a special driver's license.

(q) A bus (coach) is a motor vehicle designed or adapted primarily for carrying more than 10 passengers, and requiring a special driver's license.

(r) A railway train or railway vehicle is any device, with or without freight or passenger cars couple to it, designed for traffic on a railway track. This includes subterranean (subways) or elevated trains.

(s) A streetcar, is a device designed and used primarily for transporting passengers within a municipality, running on rails, usually subject to normal traffic control signals, and operated principally on a right-of-way that forms part of the roadway. This includes a tram or trolley that runs on rails. A trailer being towed by a streetcar is considered part of the streetcar.

(t) A special vehicle mainly used on industrial premises is a motor vehicle designed primarily for use within the buildings and premises of industrial or commercial establishments. This includes battery-powered airport passenger vehicles or baggage/mail trucks, forklifts, coal-cars in a coal mine, logging cars and trucks used in mines or quarries.

✓Additional Character Required   √x7ᵗʰ Placeholder   Unacceptable PDx   Questionable PDx   Wrong Procedure   Manifestation   **H1**-**H14** HAC   **HCC** CMS-HCC Dx   **HIV** HIV Dx

ICD-10-CM 2019   **1159**

(u) A special vehicle mainly used in agriculture is a motor vehicle designed specifically for use in farming and agriculture (horticulture), to work the land, tend and harvest crops and transport materials on the farm. This includes harvesters, farm machinery and tractor and trailers.

(v) A special construction vehicle is a motor vehicle designed specifically for use on construction and demolition sites. This includes bulldozers, diggers, earth levellers, dump trucks. backhoes, front-end loaders, pavers, and mechanical shovels.

(w) A special all-terrain vehicle is a motor vehicle of special design to enable it to negotiate over rough or soft terrain, snow or sand. Examples of special design are high construction, special wheels and tires, tracks, and support on a cushion of air. This includes snow mobiles, All-terrain vehicles (ATV), and dune buggies. It does not include passenger vehicle designated as Sport Utility Vehicles. (SUV)

(x) A watercraft is any device designed for transporting passengers or goods on water. This includes motor or sailboats, ships, and hovercraft.

(y) An aircraft is any device for transporting passengers or goods in the air. This includes hot-air balloons, gliders, helicopters and airplanes.

(z) A military vehicle is any motorized vehicle operating on a public roadway owned by the military and being operated by a member of the military

AHA: 2018, 2Q, 7-8

Pedestrian injured in transport accident (V00-V09)

INCLUDES   person changing tire on transport vehicle
person examining engine of vehicle broken down in (on side of) road

EXCLUDES 1   *fall due to non-transport collision with other person (W03)*
pedestrian on foot falling (slipping) on ice and snow (W00.-)
struck or bumped by another person (W51)

> The appropriate 7th character is to be added to each code from categories V00-V09.
> A   initial encounter
> D   subsequent encounter
> S   sequela

✓4th **V00 Pedestrian conveyance accident**

Use additional place of occurrence and activity external cause codes, if known (Y92-, Y93-)

EXCLUDES 1   *collision with another person without fall (W51)*
fall due to person on foot colliding with another person on foot (W03)
fall from non-moving wheelchair, nonmotorized scooter and motorized mobility scooter without collision (W05.-)
pedestrian (conveyance) collision with other land transport vehicle (V01-V09)
pedestrian on foot falling (slipping) on ice and snow (W00.-)

✓5th **V00.0 Pedestrian on foot injured in collision with pedestrian conveyance**

✓x7th **V00.01 Pedestrian on foot injured in collision with** roller-skater

✓x7th **V00.02 Pedestrian on foot injured in collision with** skateboarder

✓x7th **V00.09 Pedestrian on foot injured in collision with** other pedestrian conveyance

✓5th **V00.1 Rolling-type pedestrian conveyance accident**

EXCLUDES 1 ▶ *accident with baby stroller◀ (V00.82-)*
accident with motorized mobility scooter (V00.83-)
accident with wheelchair (powered) (V00.81-)

✓6th **V00.11 In-line roller-skate accident**

✓7th **V00.111 Fall from in-line roller-skates**

✓7th **V00.112 In-line roller-skater** colliding with stationary object

✓7th **V00.118 Other in-line roller-skate accident**
EXCLUDES 1 *roller-skater collision with other land transport vehicle (V01-V09 with 5th character 1)*

✓6th **V00.12 Non-in- line roller-skate accident**

✓7th **V00.121 Fall from non-in-line roller-skates**

✓7th **V00.122 Non-in-line roller-skater** colliding with stationary object

✓7th **V00.128 Other non-in-line roller-skating accident**
EXCLUDES 1 *roller-skater collision with other land transport vehicle (V01-V09 with 5th character 1)*

✓6th **V00.13 Skateboard accident**

✓7th **V00.131 Fall from skateboard**

✓7th **V00.132 Skateboarder** colliding with stationary object

✓7th **V00.138 Other skateboard accident**
EXCLUDES 1 *skateboarder collision with other land transport vehicle (V01-V09 with 5th character 2)*

✓6th **V00.14 Scooter (nonmotorized) accident**
EXCLUDES 1 ▶ *motor scooter accident◀ (V20-V29)*

✓7th **V00.141 Fall from scooter (nonmotorized)**

✓7th **V00.142 Scooter (nonmotorized)** colliding with stationary object

✓7th **V00.148 Other scooter (nonmotorized) accident**
EXCLUDES 1 *scooter (nonmotorized) collision with other land transport vehicle (V01-V09 with fifth character 9)*

✓6th **V00.15 Heelies accident**
Rolling shoe
Wheeled shoe
Wheelies accident

✓7th **V00.151 Fall from heelies**

✓7th **V00.152 Heelies** colliding with stationary object

✓7th **V00.158 Other heelies accident**

✓6th **V00.18 Accident on other rolling-type pedestrian conveyance**

✓7th **V00.181 Fall from other rolling-type pedestrian conveyance**

✓7th **V00.182 Pedestrian on other rolling-type pedestrian conveyance** colliding with stationary object

✓7th **V00.188 Other accident on other rolling-type pedestrian conveyance**

✓5th **V00.2 Gliding-type pedestrian conveyance accident**

✓6th **V00.21 Ice-skates accident**

✓7th **V00.211 Fall from ice-skates**

✓7th **V00.212 Ice-skater** colliding with stationary object

✓7th **V00.218 Other ice-skates accident**
EXCLUDES 1 *ice-skater collision with other land transport vehicle ▶(V01-V09 with 5th character 9)◀*

✓6th **V00.22 Sled accident**

✓7th **V00.221 Fall from sled**

✓7th **V00.222 Sledder** colliding with stationary object

✓7th **V00.228 Other sled accident**
EXCLUDES 1 *sled collision with other land transport vehicle ▶(V01-V09 with 5th character 9)◀*

✓6th **V00.28 Other gliding-type pedestrian conveyance accident**

✓7th **V00.281 Fall from other gliding-type pedestrian conveyance**

✓7th **V00.282 Pedestrian on other gliding-type pedestrian conveyance** colliding with stationary object

✓7th **V00.288 Other accident on other gliding-type pedestrian conveyance**
EXCLUDES 1 *gliding-type pedestrian conveyance collision with other land transport vehicle ▶(V01-V09 with 5th character 9)◀*

✓5th **V00.3 Flat-bottomed pedestrian conveyance accident**

✓6th **V00.31 Snowboard accident**

✓7th **V00.311 Fall from snowboard**

✓7th **V00.312 Snowboarder** colliding with stationary object

✓7th **V00.318 Other snowboard accident**
EXCLUDES 1 *snowboarder collision with other land transport vehicle ▶(V01-V09 with 5th character 9)◀*

✓6th **V00.32 Snow-ski accident**

✓7th **V00.321 Fall from snow-skis**

✓7th **V00.322 Snow-skier** colliding with stationary object

N Newborn: 0   P Pediatric: 0-17   M Maternity: 12-55   A Adult: 15-124   MCC Major Complication/Comorbidity   CC Complication/Comorbidity   SW Severe Wound Dx

1160

ICD-10-CM 2019

✓7ᵗʰ **V00.328** Other snow-ski accident
  EXCLUDES 1 *snow-skier collision with other land transport vehicle ▶(V01-V09 with 5th character 9)◀*

✓6ᵗʰ **V00.38** Other flat-bottomed pedestrian conveyance accident

  ✓7ᵗʰ **V00.381** Fall from other flat-bottomed pedestrian conveyance

  ✓7ᵗʰ **V00.382** Pedestrian on other flat-bottomed pedestrian conveyance colliding with stationary object

  ✓7ᵗʰ **V00.388** Other accident on other flat-bottomed pedestrian conveyance

✓5ᵗʰ **V00.8** Accident on other pedestrian conveyance

  ✓6ᵗʰ **V00.81** Accident with wheelchair (powered)

    ✓7ᵗʰ **V00.811** Fall from moving wheelchair (powered)
      EXCLUDES 1 *fall from non-moving wheelchair (W05.0)*

    ✓7ᵗʰ **V00.812** Wheelchair (powered) colliding with stationary object

    ✓7ᵗʰ **V00.818** Other accident with wheelchair (powered)

  ▲ ✓6ᵗʰ **V00.82** Accident with baby stroller

    ▲ ✓7ᵗʰ **V00.821** Fall from baby stroller

    ▲ ✓7ᵗʰ **V00.822** Baby stroller colliding with stationary object

    ▲ ✓7ᵗʰ **V00.828** Other accident with baby stroller

  ✓6ᵗʰ **V00.83** Accident with motorized mobility scooter

    ✓7ᵗʰ **V00.831** Fall from motorized mobility scooter
      EXCLUDES 1 *fall from non-moving motorized mobility scooter (W05.2)*

    ✓7ᵗʰ **V00.832** Motorized mobility scooter colliding with stationary object

    ✓7ᵗʰ **V00.838** Other accident with motorized mobility scooter

  ✓6ᵗʰ **V00.89** Accident on other pedestrian conveyance

    ✓7ᵗʰ **V00.891** Fall from other pedestrian conveyance

    ✓7ᵗʰ **V00.892** Pedestrian on other pedestrian conveyance colliding with stationary object

    ✓7ᵗʰ **V00.898** Other accident on other pedestrian conveyance
      EXCLUDES 1 *other pedestrian (conveyance) collision with other land transport vehicle ▶(V01-V09 with 5th character 9)◀*

✓4ᵗʰ **V01** Pedestrian injured in collision with pedal cycle

  ✓5ᵗʰ **V01.0** Pedestrian injured in collision with pedal cycle in nontraffic accident

    ✓x7ᵗʰ **V01.00** Pedestrian on foot injured in collision with pedal cycle in nontraffic accident
      Pedestrian NOS injured in collision with pedal cycle in nontraffic accident

    ✓x7ᵗʰ **V01.01** Pedestrian on roller-skates injured in collision with pedal cycle in nontraffic accident

    ✓x7ᵗʰ **V01.02** Pedestrian on skateboard injured in collision with pedal cycle in nontraffic accident

    ✓x7ᵗʰ **V01.09** Pedestrian with other conveyance injured in collision with pedal cycle in nontraffic accident
      ▶Pedestrian with baby stroller injured in collision with pedal cycle in nontraffic accident◀
      Pedestrian on ice-skates injured in collision with pedal cycle in nontraffic accident
      Pedestrian on nonmotorized scooter injured in collision with pedal cycle in nontraffic accident
      Pedestrian on sled injured in collision with pedal cycle in nontraffic accident
      Pedestrian on snowboard injured in collision with pedal cycle in nontraffic accident
      Pedestrian on snow-skis injured in collision with pedal cycle in nontraffic accident
      Pedestrian in wheelchair (powered) injured in collision with pedal cycle in nontraffic accident
      Pedestrian in motorized mobility scooter injured in collision with pedal cycle in nontraffic accident

  ✓5ᵗʰ **V01.1** Pedestrian injured in collision with pedal cycle in traffic accident

    ✓x7ᵗʰ **V01.10** Pedestrian on foot injured in collision with pedal cycle in traffic accident
      Pedestrian NOS injured in collision with pedal cycle in traffic accident

    ✓x7ᵗʰ **V01.11** Pedestrian on roller-skates injured in collision with pedal cycle in traffic accident

    ✓x7ᵗʰ **V01.12** Pedestrian on skateboard injured in collision with pedal cycle in traffic accident

    ✓x7ᵗʰ **V01.19** Pedestrian with other conveyance injured in collision with pedal cycle in traffic accident
      ▶Pedestrian with baby stroller injured in collision with pedal cycle in traffic accident◀
      Pedestrian on ice-skates injured in collision with pedal cycle in traffic accident
      Pedestrian on nonmotorized scooter injured in collision with pedal cycle in traffic accident
      Pedestrian on sled injured in collision with pedal cycle in traffic accident
      Pedestrian on snowboard injured in collision with pedal cycle in traffic accident
      Pedestrian on snow-skis injured in collision with pedal cycle in traffic accident
      Pedestrian in wheelchair (powered) injured in collision with pedal cycle in traffic accident
      Pedestrian in motorized mobility scooter injured in collision with pedal cycle in traffic accident

  ✓5ᵗʰ **V01.9** Pedestrian injured in collision with pedal cycle, unspecified whether traffic or nontraffic accident

    ✓x7ᵗʰ **V01.90** Pedestrian on foot injured in collision with pedal cycle, unspecified whether traffic or nontraffic accident
      Pedestrian NOS injured in collision with pedal cycle, unspecified whether traffic or nontraffic accident

    ✓x7ᵗʰ **V01.91** Pedestrian on roller-skates injured in collision with pedal cycle, unspecified whether traffic or nontraffic accident

    ✓x7ᵗʰ **V01.92** Pedestrian on skateboard injured in collision with pedal cycle, unspecified whether traffic or nontraffic accident

    ✓x7ᵗʰ **V01.99** Pedestrian with other conveyance injured in collision with pedal cycle, unspecified whether traffic or nontraffic accident
      ▶Pedestrian with baby stroller injured in collision with pedal cycle, unspecified whether traffic or nontraffic accident◀
      Pedestrian on ice-skates injured in collision with pedal cycle unspecified, whether traffic or nontraffic accident
      Pedestrian on nonmotorized scooter injured in collision with pedal cycle, unspecified whether traffic or nontraffic accident
      Pedestrian on sled injured in collision with pedal cycle unspecified, whether traffic or nontraffic accident
      Pedestrian on snowboard injured in collision with pedal cycle, unspecified whether traffic or nontraffic accident
      Pedestrian on snow-skis injured in collision with pedal cycle, unspecified whether traffic or nontraffic accident
      Pedestrian in wheelchair (powered) injured in collision with pedal cycle, unspecified whether traffic or nontraffic accident
      Pedestrian in motorized mobility scooter injured in collision with pedal cycle, unspecified whether traffic or nontraffic accident

✓4ᵗʰ **V02** Pedestrian injured in collision with two- or three-wheeled motor vehicle

  ✓5ᵗʰ **V02.0** Pedestrian injured in collision with two- or three-wheeled motor vehicle in nontraffic accident

    ✓x7ᵗʰ **V02.00** Pedestrian on foot injured in collision with two- or three-wheeled motor vehicle in nontraffic accident
      Pedestrian NOS injured in collision with two- or three-wheeled motor vehicle in nontraffic accident

    ✓x7ᵗʰ **V02.01** Pedestrian on roller-skates injured in collision with two- or three-wheeled motor vehicle in nontraffic accident

    ✓x7ᵗʰ **V02.02** Pedestrian on skateboard injured in collision with two- or three-wheeled motor vehicle in nontraffic accident

√x7ᵗʰ **V02.09** **Pedestrian with other conveyance injured in collision with two- or three-wheeled motor vehicle in nontraffic accident**
▶Pedestrian with baby stroller injured in collision with two- or three-wheeled motor vehicle in nontraffic accident◀
Pedestrian on ice-skates injured in collision with two- or three-wheeled motor vehicle in nontraffic accident
Pedestrian on nonmotorized scooter injured in collision with two- or three-wheeled motor vehicle in nontraffic accident
Pedestrian on sled injured in collision with two- or three-wheeled motor vehicle in nontraffic accident
Pedestrian on snowboard injured in collision with two- or three-wheeled motor vehicle in nontraffic accident
Pedestrian on snow-skis injured in collision with two- or three-wheeled motor vehicle in nontraffic accident
Pedestrian in wheelchair (powered) injured in collision with two- or three-wheeled motor vehicle in nontraffic accident
Pedestrian in motorized mobility scooter injured in collision with two- or three-wheeled motor vehicle in nontraffic accident

√5ᵗʰ **V02.1** **Pedestrian injured in collision with two- or three-wheeled motor vehicle in traffic accident**

√x7ᵗʰ **V02.10** **Pedestrian on foot injured in collision with two- or three-wheeled motor vehicle in traffic accident**
Pedestrian NOS injured in collision with two- or three-wheeled motor vehicle in traffic accident

√x7ᵗʰ **V02.11** **Pedestrian on roller-skates injured in collision with two- or three-wheeled motor vehicle in traffic accident**

√x7ᵗʰ **V02.12** **Pedestrian on skateboard injured in collision with two- or three-wheeled motor vehicle in traffic accident**

√x7ᵗʰ **V02.19** **Pedestrian with other conveyance injured in collision with two- or three-wheeled motor vehicle in traffic accident**
▶Pedestrian with baby stroller injured in collision with two- or three-wheeled motor vehicle in traffic accident◀
Pedestrian on ice-skates injured in collision with two- or three-wheeled motor vehicle in traffic accident
Pedestrian on nonmotorized scooter injured in collision with two- or three-wheeled motor vehicle in traffic accident
Pedestrian on sled injured in collision with two- or three-wheeled motor vehicle in traffic accident
Pedestrian on snowboard injured in collision with two- or three-wheeled motor vehicle in traffic accident
Pedestrian on snow-skis injured in collision with two- or three-wheeled motor vehicle in traffic accident
Pedestrian in wheelchair (powered) injured in collision with two- or three-wheeled motor vehicle in traffic accident
Pedestrian in motorized mobility scooter injured in collision with two- or three-wheeled motor vehicle in traffic accident

√5ᵗʰ **V02.9** **Pedestrian injured in collision with two- or three-wheeled motor vehicle, unspecified whether traffic or nontraffic accident**

√x7ᵗʰ **V02.90** **Pedestrian on foot injured in collision with two- or three-wheeled motor vehicle, unspecified whether traffic or nontraffic accident**
Pedestrian NOS injured in collision with two- or three-wheeled motor vehicle, unspecified whether traffic or nontraffic accident

√x7ᵗʰ **V02.91** **Pedestrian on roller-skates injured in collision with two- or three-wheeled motor vehicle, unspecified whether traffic or nontraffic accident**

√x7ᵗʰ **V02.92** **Pedestrian on skateboard injured in collision with two- or three-wheeled motor vehicle, unspecified whether traffic or nontraffic accident**

√x7ᵗʰ **V02.99** **Pedestrian with other conveyance injured in collision with two- or three-wheeled motor vehicle, unspecified whether traffic or nontraffic accident**
▶Pedestrian with baby stroller injured in collision with two- or three-wheeled motor vehicle, unspecified whether traffic or nontraffic accident◀
Pedestrian on ice-skates injured in collision with two- or three-wheeled motor vehicle, unspecified whether traffic or nontraffic accident
Pedestrian on nonmotorized scooter injured in collision with two- or three-wheeled motor vehicle, unspecified whether traffic or nontraffic accident
Pedestrian on sled injured in collision with two- or three-wheeled motor vehicle, unspecified whether traffic or nontraffic accident
Pedestrian on snowboard injured in collision with two- or three-wheeled motor vehicle, unspecified whether traffic or nontraffic accident
Pedestrian on snow-skis injured in collision with two- or three-wheeled motor vehicle, unspecified whether traffic or nontraffic accident
Pedestrian in wheelchair (powered) injured in collision with two- or three-wheeled motor vehicle, unspecified whether traffic or nontraffic accident
Pedestrian in motorized mobility scooter injured in collision with two- or three-wheeled motor vehicle, unspecified whether traffic or nontraffic accident

√4ᵗʰ **V03** **Pedestrian injured in collision with car, pick-up truck or van**

√5ᵗʰ **V03.0** **Pedestrian injured in collision with car, pick-up truck or van in nontraffic accident**

√x7ᵗʰ **V03.00** **Pedestrian on foot injured in collision with car, pick-up truck or van in nontraffic accident**
Pedestrian NOS injured in collision with car, pick-up truck or van in nontraffic accident

√x7ᵗʰ **V03.01** **Pedestrian on roller-skates injured in collision with car, pick-up truck or van in nontraffic accident**

√x7ᵗʰ **V03.02** **Pedestrian on skateboard injured in collision with car, pick-up truck or van in nontraffic accident**

√x7ᵗʰ **V03.09** **Pedestrian with other conveyance injured in collision with car, pick-up truck or van in nontraffic accident**
▶Pedestrian with baby stroller injured in collision with car, pick-up truck or van in nontraffic accident◀
Pedestrian on ice-skates injured in collision with car, pick-up truck or van in nontraffic accident
Pedestrian on nonmotorized scooter injured in collision with car, pick-up truck or van in nontraffic accident
Pedestrian on sled injured in collision with car, pick-up truck or van in nontraffic accident
Pedestrian on snowboard injured in collision with car, pick-up truck or van in nontraffic accident
Pedestrian on snow-skis injured in collision with car, pick-up truck or van in nontraffic accident
Pedestrian in wheelchair (powered) injured in collision with car, pick-up truck or van in nontraffic accident
Pedestrian in motorized mobility scooter injured in collision with car, pick-up truck or van in nontraffic accident

√5ᵗʰ **V03.1** **Pedestrian injured in collision with car, pick-up truck or van in traffic accident**

√x7ᵗʰ **V03.10** **Pedestrian on foot injured in collision with car, pick-up truck or van in traffic accident**
Pedestrian NOS injured in collision with car, pick-up truck or van in traffic accident

√x7ᵗʰ **V03.11** **Pedestrian on roller-skates injured in collision with car, pick-up truck or van in traffic accident**

√x7ᵗʰ **V03.12** **Pedestrian on skateboard injured in collision with car, pick-up truck or van in traffic accident**

✓x7ᵗʰ **V03.19 Pedestrian with other conveyance injured in collision with car, pick-up truck or van in traffic accident**
▸Pedestrian with baby stroller injured in collision with car, pick-up truck or van in traffic accident◂
Pedestrian on ice-skates injured in collision with car, pick-up truck or van in traffic accident
Pedestrian on nonmotorized scooter injured in collision with car, pick-up truck or van in traffic accident
Pedestrian on sled injured in collision with car, pick-up truck or van in traffic accident
Pedestrian on snowboard injured in collision with car, pick-up truck or van in traffic accident
Pedestrian on snow-skis injured in collision with car, pick-up truck or van in traffic accident
Pedestrian in wheelchair (powered) injured in collision with car, pick-up truck or van in traffic accident
Pedestrian in motorized mobility scooter injured in collision with car, pick-up truck or van in traffic accident

✓5ᵗʰ **V03.9 Pedestrian injured in collision with car, pick-up truck or van, unspecified whether traffic or nontraffic accident**

✓x7ᵗʰ **V03.90 Pedestrian on foot injured in collision with car, pick-up truck or van, unspecified whether traffic or nontraffic accident**
Pedestrian NOS injured in collision with car, pick-up truck or van, unspecified whether traffic or nontraffic accident

✓x7ᵗʰ **V03.91 Pedestrian on roller-skates injured in collision with car, pick-up truck or van, unspecified whether traffic or nontraffic accident**

✓x7ᵗʰ **V03.92 Pedestrian on skateboard injured in collision with car, pick-up truck or van, unspecified whether traffic or nontraffic accident**

✓x7ᵗʰ **V03.99 Pedestrian with other conveyance injured in collision with car, pick-up truck or van, unspecified whether traffic or nontraffic accident**
▸Pedestrian with baby stroller injured in collision with car, pick-up truck or van, unspecified whether traffic or nontraffic accident◂
Pedestrian on ice-skates injured in collision with car, pick-up truck or van, unspecified whether traffic or nontraffic accident
Pedestrian on nonmotorized scooter injured in collision with car, pick-up truck or van, unspecified whether traffic or nontraffic accident
Pedestrian on sled injured in collision with car, pick-up truck or van in nontraffic accident
Pedestrian on snowboard injured in collision with car, pick-up truck or van, unspecified whether traffic or nontraffic accident
Pedestrian on snow-skis injured in collision with car, pick-up truck or van, unspecified whether traffic or nontraffic accident
Pedestrian in wheelchair (powered) injured in collision with car, pick-up truck or van, unspecified whether traffic or nontraffic accident
Pedestrian in motorized mobility scooter injured in collision with car, pick-up truck or van, unspecified whether traffic or nontraffic accident

✓4ᵗʰ **V04 Pedestrian injured in collision with heavy transport vehicle or bus**
EXCLUDES 1 *pedestrian injured in collision with military vehicle (V09.01, V09.21)*

✓5ᵗʰ **V04.0 Pedestrian injured in collision with heavy transport vehicle or bus in nontraffic accident**

✓x7ᵗʰ **V04.00 Pedestrian on foot injured in collision with heavy transport vehicle or bus in nontraffic accident**
Pedestrian NOS injured in collision with heavy transport vehicle or bus in nontraffic accident

✓x7ᵗʰ **V04.01 Pedestrian on roller-skates injured in collision with heavy transport vehicle or bus in nontraffic accident**

✓x7ᵗʰ **V04.02 Pedestrian on skateboard injured in collision with heavy transport vehicle or bus in nontraffic accident**

✓x7ᵗʰ **V04.09 Pedestrian with other conveyance injured in collision with heavy transport vehicle or bus in nontraffic accident**
▸Pedestrian with baby stroller injured in collision with heavy transport vehicle or bus in nontraffic accident◂
Pedestrian on ice-skates injured in collision with heavy transport vehicle or bus in nontraffic accident
Pedestrian on nonmotorized scooter injured in collision with heavy transport vehicle or bus in nontraffic accident
Pedestrian on sled injured in collision with heavy transport vehicle or bus in nontraffic accident
Pedestrian on snowboard injured in collision with heavy transport vehicle or bus in nontraffic accident
Pedestrian on snow-skis injured in collision with heavy transport vehicle or bus in nontraffic accident
Pedestrian in wheelchair (powered) injured in collision with heavy transport vehicle or bus in nontraffic accident
Pedestrian in motorized mobility scooter injured in collision with heavy transport vehicle or bus in nontraffic accident

✓5ᵗʰ **V04.1 Pedestrian injured in collision with heavy transport vehicle or bus in traffic accident**

✓x7ᵗʰ **V04.10 Pedestrian on foot injured in collision with heavy transport vehicle or bus in traffic accident**
Pedestrian NOS injured in collision with heavy transport vehicle or bus in traffic accident

✓x7ᵗʰ **V04.11 Pedestrian on roller-skates injured in collision with heavy transport vehicle or bus in traffic accident**

✓x7ᵗʰ **V04.12 Pedestrian on skateboard injured in collision with heavy transport vehicle or bus in traffic accident**

✓x7ᵗʰ **V04.19 Pedestrian with other conveyance injured in collision with heavy transport vehicle or bus in traffic accident**
▸Pedestrian with baby stroller injured in collision with heavy transport vehicle or bus in traffic accident◂
Pedestrian on ice-skates injured in collision with heavy transport vehicle or bus in traffic accident
Pedestrian on nonmotorized scooter injured in collision with heavy transport vehicle or bus in traffic accident
Pedestrian on sled injured in collision with heavy transport vehicle or bus in traffic accident
Pedestrian on snowboard injured in collision with heavy transport vehicle or bus in traffic accident
Pedestrian on snow-skis injured in collision with heavy transport vehicle or bus in traffic accident
Pedestrian in wheelchair (powered) injured in collision with heavy transport vehicle or bus in traffic accident
Pedestrian in motorized mobility scooter injured in collision with heavy transport vehicle or bus in traffic accident

✓5ᵗʰ **V04.9 Pedestrian injured in collision with heavy transport vehicle or bus, unspecified whether traffic or nontraffic accident**

✓x7ᵗʰ **V04.90 Pedestrian on foot injured in collision with heavy transport vehicle or bus, unspecified whether traffic or nontraffic accident**
Pedestrian NOS injured in collision with heavy transport vehicle or bus, unspecified whether traffic or nontraffic accident

✓x7ᵗʰ **V04.91 Pedestrian on roller-skates injured in collision with heavy transport vehicle or bus, unspecified whether traffic or nontraffic accident**

✓x7ᵗʰ **V04.92 Pedestrian on skateboard injured in collision with heavy transport vehicle or bus, unspecified whether traffic or nontraffic accident**

✓x7ᵗʰ **V04.99 Pedestrian** with other conveyance **injured in collision with heavy transport vehicle or bus, unspecified whether traffic or nontraffic accident**
▶Pedestrian with baby stroller injured in collision with heavy transport vehicle or bus, unspecified whether traffic or nontraffic accident◀
Pedestrian on ice-skates injured in collision with heavy transport vehicle or bus, unspecified whether traffic or nontraffic accident
Pedestrian on nonmotorized scooter injured in collision with heavy transport vehicle or bus, unspecified whether traffic or nontraffic accident
Pedestrian on sled injured in collision with heavy transport vehicle or bus, unspecified whether traffic or nontraffic accident
Pedestrian on snowboard injured in collision with heavy transport vehicle or bus, unspecified whether traffic or nontraffic accident
Pedestrian on snow-skis injured in collision with heavy transport vehicle or bus, unspecified whether traffic or nontraffic accident
Pedestrian in wheelchair (powered) injured in collision with heavy transport vehicle or bus, unspecified whether traffic or nontraffic accident
Pedestrian in motorized mobility scooter injured in collision with heavy transport vehicle or bus, unspecified whether traffic or nontraffic accident

✓4ᵗʰ **V05 Pedestrian injured in collision with railway train or railway vehicle**

✓5ᵗʰ **V05.0 Pedestrian injured in collision with railway train or railway vehicle** in nontraffic accident

  ✓x7ᵗʰ **V05.00 Pedestrian** on foot **injured in collision with railway train or railway vehicle in nontraffic accident**
Pedestrian NOS injured in collision with railway train or railway vehicle in nontraffic accident

  ✓x7ᵗʰ **V05.01 Pedestrian** on roller-skates **injured in collision with railway train or railway vehicle in nontraffic accident**

  ✓x7ᵗʰ **V05.02 Pedestrian** on skateboard **injured in collision with railway train or railway vehicle in nontraffic accident**

  ✓x7ᵗʰ **V05.09 Pedestrian** with other conveyance **injured in collision with railway train or railway vehicle in nontraffic accident**
▶Pedestrian with baby stroller injured in collision with railway train or railway vehicle in nontraffic accident◀
Pedestrian on ice-skates injured in collision with railway train or railway vehicle in nontraffic accident
Pedestrian on nonmotorized scooter injured in collision with railway train or railway vehicle in nontraffic accident
Pedestrian on sled injured in collision with railway train or railway vehicle in nontraffic accident
Pedestrian on snowboard injured in collision with railway train or railway vehicle in nontraffic accident
Pedestrian on snow-skis injured in collision with railway train or railway vehicle in nontraffic accident
Pedestrian in wheelchair (powered) injured in collision with railway train or railway vehicle in nontraffic accident
Pedestrian in motorized mobility scooter injured in collision with railway train or railway vehicle in nontraffic accident

✓5ᵗʰ **V05.1 Pedestrian injured in collision with railway train or railway vehicle** in traffic accident

  ✓x7ᵗʰ **V05.10 Pedestrian** on foot **injured in collision with railway train or railway vehicle in traffic accident**
Pedestrian NOS injured in collision with railway train or railway vehicle in traffic accident

  ✓x7ᵗʰ **V05.11 Pedestrian** on roller-skates **injured in collision with railway train or railway vehicle in traffic accident**

  ✓x7ᵗʰ **V05.12 Pedestrian** on skateboard **injured in collision with railway train or railway vehicle in traffic accident**

✓x7ᵗʰ **V05.19 Pedestrian** with other conveyance **injured in collision with railway train or railway vehicle in traffic accident**
▶Pedestrian with baby stroller injured in collision with railway train or railway vehicle in traffic accident◀
Pedestrian on ice-skates injured in collision with railway train or railway vehicle in traffic accident
Pedestrian on nonmotorized scooter injured in collision with railway train or railway vehicle in traffic accident
Pedestrian on sled injured in collision with railway train or railway vehicle in traffic accident
Pedestrian on snowboard injured in collision with railway train or railway vehicle in traffic accident
Pedestrian on snow-skis injured in collision with railway train or railway vehicle in traffic accident
Pedestrian in wheelchair (powered) injured in collision with railway train or railway vehicle in traffic accident
Pedestrian in motorized mobility scooter injured in collision with railway train or railway vehicle in traffic accident

✓5ᵗʰ **V05.9 Pedestrian injured in collision with railway train or railway vehicle,** unspecified whether traffic or nontraffic accident

  ✓x7ᵗʰ **V05.90 Pedestrian** on foot **injured in collision with railway train or railway vehicle, unspecified whether traffic or nontraffic accident**
Pedestrian NOS injured in collision with railway train or railway vehicle, unspecified whether traffic or nontraffic accident

  ✓x7ᵗʰ **V05.91 Pedestrian** on roller-skates **injured in collision with railway train or railway vehicle, unspecified whether traffic or nontraffic accident**

  ✓x7ᵗʰ **V05.92 Pedestrian** on skateboard **injured in collision with railway train or railway vehicle, unspecified whether traffic or nontraffic accident**

  ✓x7ᵗʰ **V05.99 Pedestrian** with other conveyance **injured in collision with railway train or railway vehicle, unspecified whether traffic or nontraffic accident**
▶Pedestrian with baby stroller injured in collision with railway train or railway vehicle, unspecified whether traffic or nontraffic◀
Pedestrian on ice-skates injured in collision with railway train or railway vehicle, unspecified whether traffic or nontraffic
Pedestrian on nonmotorized scooter injured in collision with railway train or railway vehicle, unspecified whether traffic or nontraffic
Pedestrian on sled injured in collision with railway train or railway vehicle, unspecified whether traffic or nontraffic
Pedestrian on snowboard injured in collision with railway train or railway vehicle, unspecified whether traffic or nontraffic
Pedestrian on snow-skis injured in collision with railway train or railway vehicle, unspecified whether traffic or nontraffic
Pedestrian in wheelchair (powered) injured in collision with railway train or railway vehicle, unspecified whether traffic or nontraffic
Pedestrian in motorized mobility scooter injured in collision with railway train or railway vehicle, unspecified whether traffic or nontraffic

✓4ᵗʰ **V06 Pedestrian injured in collision with other nonmotor vehicle**
INCLUDES collision with animal-drawn vehicle, animal being ridden, nonpowered streetcar
EXCLUDES 1 pedestrian injured in collision with pedestrian conveyance (V00.0-)

✓5ᵗʰ **V06.0 Pedestrian injured in collision with other nonmotor vehicle** in nontraffic accident

  ✓x7ᵗʰ **V06.00 Pedestrian** on foot **injured in collision with other nonmotor vehicle in nontraffic accident**
Pedestrian NOS injured in collision with other nonmotor vehicle in nontraffic accident

  ✓x7ᵗʰ **V06.01 Pedestrian** on roller-skates **injured in collision with other nonmotor vehicle in nontraffic accident**

  ✓x7ᵗʰ **V06.02 Pedestrian** on skateboard **injured in collision with other nonmotor vehicle in nontraffic accident**

√x 7ᵗʰ **V06.09 Pedestrian with other conveyance injured in collision with other nonmotor vehicle in nontraffic accident**
▶Pedestrian with baby stroller injured in collision with other nonmotor vehicle in nontraffic accident◀
Pedestrian on ice-skates injured in collision with other nonmotor vehicle in nontraffic accident
Pedestrian on nonmotorized scooter injured in collision with other nonmotor vehicle in nontraffic accident
Pedestrian on sled injured in collision with other nonmotor vehicle in nontraffic accident
Pedestrian on snowboard injured in collision with other nonmotor vehicle in nontraffic accident
Pedestrian on snow-skis injured in collision with other nonmotor vehicle in nontraffic accident
Pedestrian in wheelchair (powered) injured in collision with other nonmotor vehicle in nontraffic accident
Pedestrian in motorized mobility scooter injured in collision with other nonmotor vehicle in nontraffic accident

√5ᵗʰ **V06.1 Pedestrian injured in collision with other nonmotor vehicle in traffic accident**

√x 7ᵗʰ **V06.10 Pedestrian on foot injured in collision with other nonmotor vehicle in traffic accident**
Pedestrian NOS injured in collision with other nonmotor vehicle in traffic accident

√x 7ᵗʰ **V06.11 Pedestrian on roller-skates injured in collision with other nonmotor vehicle in traffic accident**

√x 7ᵗʰ **V06.12 Pedestrian on skateboard injured in collision with other nonmotor vehicle in traffic accident**

√x 7ᵗʰ **V06.19 Pedestrian with other conveyance injured in collision with other nonmotor vehicle in traffic accident**
▶Pedestrian with baby stroller injured in collision with other nonmotor vehicle in nontraffic accident◀
Pedestrian on ice-skates injured in collision with other nonmotor vehicle in traffic accident
Pedestrian on nonmotorized scooter injured in collision with other nonmotor vehicle in traffic accident
Pedestrian on sled injured in collision with other nonmotor vehicle in traffic accident
Pedestrian on snowboard injured in collision with other nonmotor vehicle in traffic accident
Pedestrian on snow-skis injured in collision with other nonmotor vehicle in traffic accident
Pedestrian in wheelchair (powered) injured in collision with other nonmotor vehicle in traffic accident
Pedestrian in motorized mobility scooter injured in collision with other nonmotor vehicle in traffic accident

√5ᵗʰ **V06.9 Pedestrian injured in collision with other nonmotor vehicle, unspecified whether traffic or nontraffic accident**

√x 7ᵗʰ **V06.90 Pedestrian on foot injured in collision with other nonmotor vehicle, unspecified whether traffic or nontraffic accident**
Pedestrian NOS injured in collision with other nonmotor vehicle, unspecified whether traffic or nontraffic accident

√x 7ᵗʰ **V06.91 Pedestrian on roller-skates injured in collision with other nonmotor vehicle, unspecified whether traffic or nontraffic accident**

√x 7ᵗʰ **V06.92 Pedestrian on skateboard injured in collision with other nonmotor vehicle, unspecified whether traffic or nontraffic accident**

√x 7ᵗʰ **V06.99 Pedestrian with other conveyance injured in collision with other nonmotor vehicle, unspecified whether traffic or nontraffic accident**
▶Pedestrian with baby stroller injured in collision with other nonmotor vehicle, unspecified whether traffic or nontraffic accident◀
Pedestrian on ice-skates injured in collision with other nonmotor vehicle, unspecified whether traffic or nontraffic accident
Pedestrian on nonmotorized scooter injured in collision with other nonmotor vehicle, unspecified whether traffic or nontraffic accident
Pedestrian on sled injured in collision with other nonmotor vehicle, unspecified whether traffic or nontraffic accident
Pedestrian on snowboard injured in collision with other nonmotor vehicle, unspecified whether traffic or nontraffic accident
Pedestrian on snow-skis injured in collision with other nonmotor vehicle, unspecified whether traffic or nontraffic accident
Pedestrian in wheelchair (powered) injured in collision with other nonmotor vehicle, unspecified whether traffic or nontraffic accident
Pedestrian in motorized mobility scooter injured in collision with other nonmotor vehicle, unspecified whether traffic or nontraffic accident

√4ᵗʰ **V09 Pedestrian injured in other and unspecified transport accidents**

√5ᵗʰ **V09.0 Pedestrian injured in nontraffic accident involving other and unspecified motor vehicles**

√x 7ᵗʰ **V09.00 Pedestrian injured in nontraffic accident involving unspecified motor vehicles**

√x 7ᵗʰ **V09.01 Pedestrian injured in nontraffic accident involving military vehicle**

√x 7ᵗʰ **V09.09 Pedestrian injured in nontraffic accident involving other motor vehicles**
Pedestrian injured in nontraffic accident by special vehicle

√x 7ᵗʰ **V09.1 Pedestrian injured in unspecified nontraffic accident**

√5ᵗʰ **V09.2 Pedestrian injured in traffic accident involving other and unspecified motor vehicles**

√x 7ᵗʰ **V09.20 Pedestrian injured in traffic accident involving unspecified motor vehicles**

√x 7ᵗʰ **V09.21 Pedestrian injured in traffic accident involving military vehicle**

√x 7ᵗʰ **V09.29 Pedestrian injured in traffic accident involving other motor vehicles**

√x 7ᵗʰ **V09.3 Pedestrian injured in unspecified traffic accident**

√x 7ᵗʰ **V09.9 Pedestrian injured in unspecified transport accident**

Pedal cycle rider injured in transport accident (V10-V19)

INCLUDES any non-motorized vehicle, excluding an animal-drawn vehicle, or a sidecar or trailer attached to the pedal cycle
EXCLUDES 2 rupture of pedal cycle tire (W37.0)

The appropriate 7th character is to be added to each code from categories V10-V19.
A   initial encounter
D   subsequent encounter
S   sequela

√4ᵗʰ **V10 Pedal cycle rider injured in collision with pedestrian or animal**
EXCLUDES 1 pedal cycle rider collision with animal-drawn vehicle or animal being ridden (V16.-)

√x 7ᵗʰ **V10.0 Pedal cycle driver injured in collision with pedestrian or animal in nontraffic accident**

√x 7ᵗʰ **V10.1 Pedal cycle passenger injured in collision with pedestrian or animal in nontraffic accident**

√x 7ᵗʰ **V10.2 Unspecified pedal cyclist injured in collision with pedestrian or animal in nontraffic accident**

√x 7ᵗʰ **V10.3 Person boarding or alighting a pedal cycle injured in collision with pedestrian or animal**

√x 7ᵗʰ **V10.4 Pedal cycle driver injured in collision with pedestrian or animal in traffic accident**

√x 7ᵗʰ **V10.5 Pedal cycle passenger injured in collision with pedestrian or animal in traffic accident**

√x 7ᵗʰ **V10.9 Unspecified pedal cyclist injured in collision with pedestrian or animal in traffic accident**

✔ Additional Character Required   √x 7ᵗʰ Placeholder   Unacceptable PDx   Questionable PDx   Wrong Procedure   Manifestation   H1-H14 HAC   HCC CMS-HCC Dx   HIV HIV Dx

ICD-10-CM 2019   1165

Chapter 20. External Causes of Morbidity

☑4ᵗʰ **V11 Pedal cycle rider injured in collision with other pedal cycle**

☑x7ᵗʰ **V11.0** Pedal cycle driver injured in collision with other pedal cycle in nontraffic accident

☑x7ᵗʰ **V11.1** Pedal cycle passenger injured in collision with other pedal cycle in nontraffic accident

☑x7ᵗʰ **V11.2** Unspecified pedal cyclist injured in collision with other pedal cycle in nontraffic accident

☑x7ᵗʰ **V11.3** Person boarding or alighting a pedal cycle injured in collision with other pedal cycle

☑x7ᵗʰ **V11.4** Pedal cycle driver injured in collision with other pedal cycle in traffic accident

☑x7ᵗʰ **V11.5** Pedal cycle passenger injured in collision with other pedal cycle in traffic accident

☑x7ᵗʰ **V11.9** Unspecified pedal cyclist injured in collision with other pedal cycle in traffic accident

☑4ᵗʰ **V12 Pedal cycle rider injured in collision with two- or three-wheeled motor vehicle**

☑x7ᵗʰ **V12.0** Pedal cycle driver injured in collision with two- or three-wheeled motor vehicle in nontraffic accident

☑x7ᵗʰ **V12.1** Pedal cycle passenger injured in collision with two- or three-wheeled motor vehicle in nontraffic accident

☑x7ᵗʰ **V12.2** Unspecified pedal cyclist injured in collision with two- or three-wheeled motor vehicle in nontraffic accident

☑x7ᵗʰ **V12.3** Person boarding or alighting a pedal cycle injured in collision with two- or three-wheeled motor vehicle

☑x7ᵗʰ **V12.4** Pedal cycle driver injured in collision with two- or three-wheeled motor vehicle in traffic accident

☑x7ᵗʰ **V12.5** Pedal cycle passenger injured in collision with two- or three-wheeled motor vehicle in traffic accident

☑x7ᵗʰ **V12.9** Unspecified pedal cyclist injured in collision with two- or three-wheeled motor vehicle in traffic accident

☑4ᵗʰ **V13 Pedal cycle rider injured in collision with car, pick-up truck or van**

☑x7ᵗʰ **V13.0** Pedal cycle driver injured in collision with car, pick-up truck or van in nontraffic accident

☑x7ᵗʰ **V13.1** Pedal cycle passenger injured in collision with car, pick-up truck or van in nontraffic accident

☑x7ᵗʰ **V13.2** Unspecified pedal cyclist injured in collision with car, pick-up truck or van in nontraffic accident

☑x7ᵗʰ **V13.3** Person boarding or alighting a pedal cycle injured in collision with car, pick-up truck or van

☑x7ᵗʰ **V13.4** Pedal cycle driver injured in collision with car, pick-up truck or van in traffic accident

☑x7ᵗʰ **V13.5** Pedal cycle passenger injured in collision with car, pick-up truck or van in traffic accident

☑x7ᵗʰ **V13.9** Unspecified pedal cyclist injured in collision with car, pick-up truck or van in traffic accident

☑4ᵗʰ **V14 Pedal cycle rider injured in collision with heavy transport vehicle or bus**

EXCLUDES 1 *pedal cycle rider injured in collision with military vehicle (V19.81)*

☑x7ᵗʰ **V14.0** Pedal cycle driver injured in collision with heavy transport vehicle or bus in nontraffic accident

☑x7ᵗʰ **V14.1** Pedal cycle passenger injured in collision with heavy transport vehicle or bus in nontraffic accident

☑x7ᵗʰ **V14.2** Unspecified pedal cyclist injured in collision with heavy transport vehicle or bus in nontraffic accident

☑x7ᵗʰ **V14.3** Person boarding or alighting a pedal cycle injured in collision with heavy transport vehicle or bus

☑x7ᵗʰ **V14.4** Pedal cycle driver injured in collision with heavy transport vehicle or bus in traffic accident

☑x7ᵗʰ **V14.5** Pedal cycle passenger injured in collision with heavy transport vehicle or bus in traffic accident

☑x7ᵗʰ **V14.9** Unspecified pedal cyclist injured in collision with heavy transport vehicle or bus in traffic accident

☑4ᵗʰ **V15 Pedal cycle rider injured in collision with railway train or railway vehicle**

☑x7ᵗʰ **V15.0** Pedal cycle driver injured in collision with railway train or railway vehicle in nontraffic accident

☑x7ᵗʰ **V15.1** Pedal cycle passenger injured in collision with railway train or railway vehicle in nontraffic accident

☑x7ᵗʰ **V15.2** Unspecified pedal cyclist injured in collision with railway train or railway vehicle in nontraffic accident

☑x7ᵗʰ **V15.3** Person boarding or alighting a pedal cycle injured in collision with railway train or railway vehicle

☑x7ᵗʰ **V15.4** Pedal cycle driver injured in collision with railway train or railway vehicle in traffic accident

☑x7ᵗʰ **V15.5** Pedal cycle passenger injured in collision with railway train or railway vehicle in traffic accident

☑x7ᵗʰ **V15.9** Unspecified pedal cyclist injured in collision with railway train or railway vehicle in traffic accident

☑4ᵗʰ **V16 Pedal cycle rider injured in collision with other nonmotor vehicle**

INCLUDES collision with animal-drawn vehicle, animal being ridden, streetcar

☑x7ᵗʰ **V16.0** Pedal cycle driver injured in collision with other nonmotor vehicle in nontraffic accident

☑x7ᵗʰ **V16.1** Pedal cycle passenger injured in collision with other nonmotor vehicle in nontraffic accident

☑x7ᵗʰ **V16.2** Unspecified pedal cyclist injured in collision with other nonmotor vehicle in nontraffic accident

☑x7ᵗʰ **V16.3** Person boarding or alighting a pedal cycle injured in collision with other nonmotor vehicle in nontraffic accident

☑x7ᵗʰ **V16.4** Pedal cycle driver injured in collision with other nonmotor vehicle in traffic accident

☑x7ᵗʰ **V16.5** Pedal cycle passenger injured in collision with other nonmotor vehicle in traffic accident

☑x7ᵗʰ **V16.9** Unspecified pedal cyclist injured in collision with other nonmotor vehicle in traffic accident

☑4ᵗʰ **V17 Pedal cycle rider injured in collision with fixed or stationary object**

☑x7ᵗʰ **V17.0** Pedal cycle driver injured in collision with fixed or stationary object in nontraffic accident

☑x7ᵗʰ **V17.1** Pedal cycle passenger injured in collision with fixed or stationary object in nontraffic accident

☑x7ᵗʰ **V17.2** Unspecified pedal cyclist injured in collision with fixed or stationary object in nontraffic accident

☑x7ᵗʰ **V17.3** Person boarding or alighting a pedal cycle injured in collision with fixed or stationary object

☑x7ᵗʰ **V17.4** Pedal cycle driver injured in collision with fixed or stationary object in traffic accident

☑x7ᵗʰ **V17.5** Pedal cycle passenger injured in collision with fixed or stationary object in traffic accident

☑x7ᵗʰ **V17.9** Unspecified pedal cyclist injured in collision with fixed or stationary object in traffic accident

☑4ᵗʰ **V18 Pedal cycle rider injured in noncollision transport accident**

INCLUDES fall or thrown from pedal cycle (without antecedent collision)
overturning pedal cycle NOS
overturning pedal cycle without collision

☑x7ᵗʰ **V18.0** Pedal cycle driver injured in noncollision transport accident in nontraffic accident

☑x7ᵗʰ **V18.1** Pedal cycle passenger injured in noncollision transport accident in nontraffic accident

☑x7ᵗʰ **V18.2** Unspecified pedal cyclist injured in noncollision transport accident in nontraffic accident

☑x7ᵗʰ **V18.3** Person boarding or alighting a pedal cycle injured in noncollision transport accident

☑x7ᵗʰ **V18.4** Pedal cycle driver injured in noncollision transport accident in traffic accident

☑x7ᵗʰ **V18.5** Pedal cycle passenger injured in noncollision transport accident in traffic accident

☑x7ᵗʰ **V18.9** Unspecified pedal cyclist injured in noncollision transport accident in traffic accident

☑4ᵗʰ **V19 Pedal cycle rider injured in other and unspecified transport accidents**

☑5ᵗʰ **V19.0** Pedal cycle driver injured in collision with other and unspecified motor vehicles in nontraffic accident

☑x7ᵗʰ **V19.00** Pedal cycle driver injured in collision with unspecified motor vehicles in nontraffic accident

☑x7ᵗʰ **V19.09** Pedal cycle driver injured in collision with other motor vehicles in nontraffic accident

☑5ᵗʰ **V19.1** Pedal cycle passenger injured in collision with other and unspecified motor vehicles in nontraffic accident

☑x7ᵗʰ **V19.10** Pedal cycle passenger injured in collision with unspecified motor vehicles in nontraffic accident

☑x7ᵗʰ **V19.19** Pedal cycle passenger injured in collision with other motor vehicles in nontraffic accident

Ⓝ Newborn: 0   Ⓟ Pediatric: 0-17   Ⓜ Maternity: 12-55   Ⓐ Adult: 15-124   **MCC** Major Complication/Comorbidity   **CC** Complication/Comorbidity   **SW** Severe Wound Dx

1166   ICD-10-CM 2019

✓5ᵗʰ **V19.2 Unspecified pedal cyclist injured in collision with** other and unspecified motor vehicles in nontraffic accident

    ✓x7ᵗʰ **V19.20 Unspecified pedal cyclist injured in collision with** unspecified **motor vehicles in nontraffic accident**
           Pedal cycle collision NOS, nontraffic

    ✓x7ᵗʰ **V19.29 Unspecified pedal cyclist injured in collision with** other **motor vehicles in nontraffic accident**

✓x7ᵗʰ **V19.3 Pedal cyclist (driver) (passenger) injured in unspecified nontraffic accident**
     Pedal cycle accident NOS, nontraffic
     Pedal cyclist injured in nontraffic accident NOS

✓5ᵗʰ **V19.4 Pedal cycle** driver **injured in collision with other and unspecified motor vehicles in traffic accident**

    ✓x7ᵗʰ **V19.40 Pedal cycle driver injured in collision with** unspecified **motor vehicles in traffic accident**

    ✓x7ᵗʰ **V19.49 Pedal cycle driver injured in collision with** other **motor vehicles in traffic accident**

✓5ᵗʰ **V19.5 Pedal cycle** passenger **injured in collision with other and unspecified motor vehicles in traffic accident**

    ✓x7ᵗʰ **V19.50 Pedal cycle passenger injured in collision with** unspecified **motor vehicles in traffic accident**

    ✓x7ᵗʰ **V19.59 Pedal cycle passenger injured in collision with** other **motor vehicles in traffic accident**

✓5ᵗʰ **V19.6 Unspecified pedal cyclist injured in collision with** other and unspecified **motor vehicles in traffic accident**

    ✓x7ᵗʰ **V19.60 Unspecified pedal cyclist injured in collision with** unspecified **motor vehicles in traffic accident**
           Pedal cycle collision NOS (traffic)

    ✓x7ᵗʰ **V19.69 Unspecified pedal cyclist injured in collision with** other **motor vehicles in traffic accident**

✓5ᵗʰ **V19.8 Pedal cyclist (driver) (passenger) injured in** other specified transport accidents

    ✓x7ᵗʰ **V19.81 Pedal cyclist (driver) (passenger) injured in transport accident with** military vehicle

    ✓x7ᵗʰ **V19.88 Pedal cyclist (driver) (passenger) injured in** other **specified transport accidents**

✓x7ᵗʰ **V19.9 Pedal cyclist (driver) (passenger) injured in unspecified traffic accident**
     Pedal cycle accident NOS

Motorcycle rider injured in transport accident (V20-V29)

INCLUDES   moped
           motorcycle with sidecar
           motorized bicycle
           motor scooter

EXCLUDES 1   *three-wheeled motor vehicle (V30-V39)*

> The appropriate 7th character is to be added to each code from categories V20-V29.
> A   initial encounter
> D   subsequent encounter
> S   sequela

✓4ᵗʰ **V20 Motorcycle rider injured in collision with pedestrian or animal**

    EXCLUDES 1   *motorcycle rider collision with animal-drawn vehicle or animal being ridden (V26.-)*

✓x7ᵗʰ **V20.0 Motorcycle** driver **injured in collision with pedestrian or animal** in nontraffic accident

✓x7ᵗʰ **V20.1 Motorcycle** passenger **injured in collision with pedestrian or animal** in nontraffic accident

✓x7ᵗʰ **V20.2 Unspecified motorcycle rider injured in collision with pedestrian or animal** in nontraffic accident

✓x7ᵗʰ **V20.3 Person boarding or alighting a motorcycle injured in collision with pedestrian or animal**

✓x7ᵗʰ **V20.4 Motorcycle** driver **injured in collision with pedestrian or animal** in traffic accident

✓x7ᵗʰ **V20.5 Motorcycle** passenger **injured in collision with pedestrian or animal** in traffic accident

✓x7ᵗʰ **V20.9 Unspecified motorcycle rider injured in collision with pedestrian or animal** in traffic accident

✓4ᵗʰ **V21 Motorcycle rider injured in collision with pedal cycle**

✓x7ᵗʰ **V21.0 Motorcycle** driver **injured in collision with pedal cycle** in nontraffic accident

✓x7ᵗʰ **V21.1 Motorcycle** passenger **injured in collision with pedal cycle** in nontraffic accident

✓x7ᵗʰ **V21.2 Unspecified motorcycle rider injured in collision with pedal cycle** in nontraffic accident

✓x7ᵗʰ **V21.3 Person boarding or alighting a motorcycle injured in collision with pedal cycle**

✓x7ᵗʰ **V21.4 Motorcycle** driver **injured in collision with pedal cycle in traffic accident**

✓x7ᵗʰ **V21.5 Motorcycle** passenger **injured in collision with pedal cycle in traffic accident**

✓x7ᵗʰ **V21.9 Unspecified motorcycle rider injured in collision with pedal cycle in traffic accident**

✓4ᵗʰ **V22 Motorcycle rider injured in collision with two- or three-wheeled motor vehicle**

✓x7ᵗʰ **V22.0 Motorcycle** driver **injured in collision with two- or three-wheeled motor vehicle** in nontraffic accident

✓x7ᵗʰ **V22.1 Motorcycle** passenger **injured in collision with two- or three-wheeled motor vehicle** in nontraffic accident

✓x7ᵗʰ **V22.2 Unspecified motorcycle rider injured in collision with two- or three-wheeled motor vehicle** in nontraffic accident

✓x7ᵗʰ **V22.3 Person boarding or alighting a motorcycle injured in collision with two- or three-wheeled motor vehicle**

✓x7ᵗʰ **V22.4 Motorcycle** driver **injured in collision with two- or three-wheeled motor vehicle** in traffic accident

✓x7ᵗʰ **V22.5 Motorcycle** passenger **injured in collision with two- or three-wheeled motor vehicle** in traffic accident

✓x7ᵗʰ **V22.9 Unspecified motorcycle rider injured in collision with two- or three-wheeled motor vehicle** in traffic accident

✓4ᵗʰ **V23 Motorcycle rider injured in collision with car, pick-up truck or van**

✓x7ᵗʰ **V23.0 Motorcycle** driver **injured in collision with car, pick-up truck or van** in nontraffic accident

✓x7ᵗʰ **V23.1 Motorcycle** passenger **injured in collision with car, pick-up truck or van** in nontraffic accident

✓x7ᵗʰ **V23.2 Unspecified motorcycle rider injured in collision with car, pick-up truck or van** in nontraffic accident

✓x7ᵗʰ **V23.3 Person boarding or alighting a motorcycle injured in collision with car, pick-up truck or van**

✓x7ᵗʰ **V23.4 Motorcycle** driver **injured in collision with car, pick-up truck or van** in traffic accident

✓x7ᵗʰ **V23.5 Motorcycle** passenger **injured in collision with car, pick-up truck or van** in traffic accident

✓x7ᵗʰ **V23.9 Unspecified motorcycle rider injured in collision with car, pick-up truck or van** in traffic accident

✓4ᵗʰ **V24 Motorcycle rider injured in collision with heavy transport vehicle or bus**

    EXCLUDES 1   *motorcycle rider injured in collision with military vehicle (V29.81)*

✓x7ᵗʰ **V24.0 Motorcycle** driver **injured in collision with heavy transport vehicle or bus** in nontraffic accident

✓x7ᵗʰ **V24.1 Motorcycle** passenger **injured in collision with heavy transport vehicle or bus** in nontraffic accident

✓x7ᵗʰ **V24.2 Unspecified motorcycle rider injured in collision with heavy transport vehicle or bus** in nontraffic accident

✓x7ᵗʰ **V24.3 Person boarding or alighting a motorcycle injured in collision with heavy transport vehicle or bus**

✓x7ᵗʰ **V24.4 Motorcycle** driver **injured in collision with heavy transport vehicle or bus** in traffic accident

✓x7ᵗʰ **V24.5 Motorcycle** passenger **injured in collision with heavy transport vehicle or bus** in traffic accident

✓x7ᵗʰ **V24.9 Unspecified motorcycle rider injured in collision with heavy transport vehicle or bus** in traffic accident

✓4ᵗʰ **V25 Motorcycle rider injured in collision with railway train or railway vehicle**

✓x7ᵗʰ **V25.0 Motorcycle** driver **injured in collision with railway train or railway vehicle** in nontraffic accident

✓x7ᵗʰ **V25.1 Motorcycle** passenger **injured in collision with railway train or railway vehicle** in nontraffic accident

✓x7ᵗʰ **V25.2 Unspecified motorcycle rider injured in collision with railway train or railway vehicle** in nontraffic accident

✓x7ᵗʰ **V25.3 Person boarding or alighting a motorcycle injured in collision with railway train or railway vehicle**

✓x7ᵗʰ **V25.4 Motorcycle** driver **injured in collision with railway train or railway vehicle** in traffic accident

✓x7ᵗʰ **V25.5 Motorcycle** passenger **injured in collision with railway train or railway vehicle** in traffic accident

✔ Additional Character Required   ✓x7ᵗʰ Placeholder   Unacceptable PDx   Questionable PDx   Wrong Procedure   Manifestation   H1-H14 HAC   HCC CMS-HCC Dx   HIV HIV Dx

ICD-10-CM 2019   1167

√x7ᵗʰ **V25.9** Unspecified motorcycle rider injured in collision with railway train or railway vehicle in traffic accident

√4ᵗʰ **V26** **Motorcycle rider injured in collision with other nonmotor vehicle**
INCLUDES collision with animal-drawn vehicle, animal being ridden, streetcar

√x7ᵗʰ **V26.0** Motorcycle driver injured in collision with other nonmotor vehicle in nontraffic accident

√x7ᵗʰ **V26.1** Motorcycle passenger injured in collision with other nonmotor vehicle in nontraffic accident

√x7ᵗʰ **V26.2** Unspecified motorcycle rider injured in collision with other nonmotor vehicle in nontraffic accident

√x7ᵗʰ **V26.3** Person boarding or alighting a motorcycle injured in collision with other nonmotor vehicle

√x7ᵗʰ **V26.4** Motorcycle driver injured in collision with other nonmotor vehicle in traffic accident

√x7ᵗʰ **V26.5** Motorcycle passenger injured in collision with other nonmotor vehicle in traffic accident

√x7ᵗʰ **V26.9** Unspecified motorcycle rider injured in collision with other nonmotor vehicle in traffic accident

√4ᵗʰ **V27** **Motorcycle rider injured in collision with fixed or stationary object**

√x7ᵗʰ **V27.0** Motorcycle driver injured in collision with fixed or stationary object in nontraffic accident

√x7ᵗʰ **V27.1** Motorcycle passenger injured in collision with fixed or stationary object in nontraffic accident

√x7ᵗʰ **V27.2** Unspecified motorcycle rider injured in collision with fixed or stationary object in nontraffic accident

√x7ᵗʰ **V27.3** Person boarding or alighting a motorcycle injured in collision with fixed or stationary object

√x7ᵗʰ **V27.4** Motorcycle driver injured in collision with fixed or stationary object in traffic accident

√x7ᵗʰ **V27.5** Motorcycle passenger injured in collision with fixed or stationary object in traffic accident

√x7ᵗʰ **V27.9** Unspecified motorcycle rider injured in collision with fixed or stationary object in traffic accident

√4ᵗʰ **V28** **Motorcycle rider injured in noncollision transport accident**
INCLUDES fall or thrown from motorcycle (without antecedent collision)
overturning motorcycle NOS
overturning motorcycle without collision

√x7ᵗʰ **V28.0** Motorcycle driver injured in noncollision transport accident in nontraffic accident

√x7ᵗʰ **V28.1** Motorcycle passenger injured in noncollision transport accident in nontraffic accident

√x7ᵗʰ **V28.2** Unspecified motorcycle rider injured in noncollision transport accident in nontraffic accident

√x7ᵗʰ **V28.3** Person boarding or alighting a motorcycle injured in noncollision transport accident

√x7ᵗʰ **V28.4** Motorcycle driver injured in noncollision transport accident in traffic accident

√x7ᵗʰ **V28.5** Motorcycle passenger injured in noncollision transport accident in traffic accident

√x7ᵗʰ **V28.9** Unspecified motorcycle rider injured in noncollision transport accident in traffic accident

√4ᵗʰ **V29** **Motorcycle rider injured in other and unspecified transport accidents**

√5ᵗʰ **V29.0** Motorcycle driver injured in collision with other and unspecified motor vehicles in nontraffic accident

√x7ᵗʰ **V29.00** Motorcycle driver injured in collision with unspecified motor vehicles in nontraffic accident

√x7ᵗʰ **V29.09** Motorcycle driver injured in collision with other motor vehicles in nontraffic accident

√5ᵗʰ **V29.1** Motorcycle passenger injured in collision with other and unspecified motor vehicles in nontraffic accident

√x7ᵗʰ **V29.10** Motorcycle passenger injured in collision with unspecified motor vehicles in nontraffic accident

√x7ᵗʰ **V29.19** Motorcycle passenger injured in collision with other motor vehicles in nontraffic accident

√5ᵗʰ **V29.2** Unspecified motorcycle rider injured in collision with other and unspecified motor vehicles in nontraffic accident

√x7ᵗʰ **V29.20** Unspecified motorcycle rider injured in collision with unspecified motor vehicles in nontraffic accident
Motorcycle collision NOS, nontraffic

√x7ᵗʰ **V29.29** Unspecified motorcycle rider injured in collision with other motor vehicles in nontraffic accident

√x7ᵗʰ **V29.3** Motorcycle rider (driver) (passenger) injured in unspecified nontraffic accident
Motorcycle accident NOS, nontraffic
Motorcycle rider injured in nontraffic accident NOS

√5ᵗʰ **V29.4** Motorcycle driver injured in collision with other and unspecified motor vehicles in traffic accident

√x7ᵗʰ **V29.40** Motorcycle driver injured in collision with unspecified motor vehicles in traffic accident

√x7ᵗʰ **V29.49** Motorcycle driver injured in collision with other motor vehicles in traffic accident

√5ᵗʰ **V29.5** Motorcycle passenger injured in collision with other and unspecified motor vehicles in traffic accident

√x7ᵗʰ **V29.50** Motorcycle passenger injured in collision with unspecified motor vehicles in traffic accident

√x7ᵗʰ **V29.59** Motorcycle passenger injured in collision with other motor vehicles in traffic accident

√5ᵗʰ **V29.6** Unspecified motorcycle rider injured in collision with other and unspecified motor vehicles in traffic accident

√x7ᵗʰ **V29.60** Unspecified motorcycle rider injured in collision with unspecified motor vehicles in traffic accident
Motorcycle collision NOS (traffic)

√x7ᵗʰ **V29.69** Unspecified motorcycle rider injured in collision with other motor vehicles in traffic accident

√5ᵗʰ **V29.8** Motorcycle rider (driver) (passenger) injured in other specified transport accidents

√x7ᵗʰ **V29.81** Motorcycle rider (driver) (passenger) injured in transport accident with military vehicle

√x7ᵗʰ **V29.88** Motorcycle rider (driver) (passenger) injured in other specified transport accidents

√x7ᵗʰ **V29.9** Motorcycle rider (driver) (passenger) injured in unspecified traffic accident
Motorcycle accident NOS

Occupant of three-wheeled motor vehicle injured in transport accident (V30-V39)

INCLUDES motorized tricycle
motorized rickshaw
three-wheeled motor car
EXCLUDES 1 all-terrain vehicles (V86.-)
motorcycle with sidecar (V20-V29)
vehicle designed primarily for off-road use (V86.-)

The appropriate 7th character is to be added to each code from categories V30-V39.
A initial encounter
D subsequent encounter
S sequela

√4ᵗʰ **V30** **Occupant of three-wheeled motor vehicle injured in collision with pedestrian or animal**
EXCLUDES 1 three-wheeled motor vehicle collision with animal-drawn vehicle or animal being ridden (V36.-)

√x7ᵗʰ **V30.0** Driver of three-wheeled motor vehicle injured in collision with pedestrian or animal in nontraffic accident

√x7ᵗʰ **V30.1** Passenger in three-wheeled motor vehicle injured in collision with pedestrian or animal in nontraffic accident

√x7ᵗʰ **V30.2** Person on outside of three-wheeled motor vehicle injured in collision with pedestrian or animal in nontraffic accident

√x7ᵗʰ **V30.3** Unspecified occupant of three-wheeled motor vehicle injured in collision with pedestrian or animal in nontraffic accident

√x7ᵗʰ **V30.4** Person boarding or alighting a three-wheeled motor vehicle injured in collision with pedestrian or animal

√x7ᵗʰ **V30.5** Driver of three-wheeled motor vehicle injured in collision with pedestrian or animal in traffic accident

√x7ᵗʰ **V30.6** Passenger in three-wheeled motor vehicle injured in collision with pedestrian or animal in traffic accident

√x7ᵗʰ **V30.7** Person on outside of three-wheeled motor vehicle injured in collision with pedestrian or animal in traffic accident

√x7ᵗʰ **V30.9** Unspecified occupant of three-wheeled motor vehicle injured in collision with pedestrian or animal in traffic accident

√4ᵗʰ **V31** **Occupant of three-wheeled motor vehicle injured in collision with pedal cycle**

√x7ᵗʰ **V31.0** Driver of three-wheeled motor vehicle injured in collision with pedal cycle in nontraffic accident

Ⓝ Newborn: 0 Ⓟ Pediatric: 0-17 Ⓜ Maternity: 12-55 Ⓐ Adult: 15-124 MCC Major Complication/Comorbidity CC Complication/Comorbidity SW Severe Wound Dx

1168 | ICD-10-CM 2019

☑x7ᵗʰ **V31.1** Passenger in three-wheeled motor vehicle injured in collision with pedal cycle in nontraffic accident

☑x7ᵗʰ **V31.2** Person on outside of three-wheeled motor vehicle injured in collision with pedal cycle in nontraffic accident

☑x7ᵗʰ **V31.3** Unspecified occupant of three-wheeled motor vehicle injured in collision with pedal cycle in nontraffic accident

☑x7ᵗʰ **V31.4** Person boarding or alighting a three-wheeled motor vehicle injured in collision with pedal cycle

☑x7ᵗʰ **V31.5** Driver of three-wheeled motor vehicle injured in collision with pedal cycle in traffic accident

☑x7ᵗʰ **V31.6** Passenger in three-wheeled motor vehicle injured in collision with pedal cycle in traffic accident

☑x7ᵗʰ **V31.7** Person on outside of three-wheeled motor vehicle injured in collision with pedal cycle in traffic accident

☑x7ᵗʰ **V31.9** Unspecified occupant of three-wheeled motor vehicle injured in collision with pedal cycle in traffic accident

☑4ᵗʰ **V32 Occupant of three-wheeled motor vehicle injured in collision with two- or three-wheeled motor vehicle**

☑x7ᵗʰ **V32.0** Driver of three-wheeled motor vehicle injured in collision with two- or three-wheeled motor vehicle in nontraffic accident

☑x7ᵗʰ **V32.1** Passenger in three-wheeled motor vehicle injured in collision with two- or three-wheeled motor vehicle in nontraffic accident

☑x7ᵗʰ **V32.2** Person on outside of three-wheeled motor vehicle injured in collision with two- or three-wheeled motor vehicle in nontraffic accident

☑x7ᵗʰ **V32.3** Unspecified occupant of three-wheeled motor vehicle injured in collision with two- or three-wheeled motor vehicle in nontraffic accident

☑x7ᵗʰ **V32.4** Person boarding or alighting a three-wheeled motor vehicle injured in collision with two- or three-wheeled motor vehicle

☑x7ᵗʰ **V32.5** Driver of three-wheeled motor vehicle injured in collision with two- or three-wheeled motor vehicle in traffic accident

☑x7ᵗʰ **V32.6** Passenger in three-wheeled motor vehicle injured in collision with two- or three-wheeled motor vehicle in traffic accident

☑x7ᵗʰ **V32.7** Person on outside of three-wheeled motor vehicle injured in collision with two- or three-wheeled motor vehicle in traffic accident

☑x7ᵗʰ **V32.9** Unspecified occupant of three-wheeled motor vehicle injured in collision with two- or three-wheeled motor vehicle in traffic accident

☑4ᵗʰ **V33 Occupant of three-wheeled motor vehicle injured in collision with car, pick-up truck or van**

☑x7ᵗʰ **V33.0** Driver of three-wheeled motor vehicle injured in collision with car, pick-up truck or van in nontraffic accident

☑x7ᵗʰ **V33.1** Passenger in three-wheeled motor vehicle injured in collision with car, pick-up truck or van in nontraffic accident

☑x7ᵗʰ **V33.2** Person on outside of three-wheeled motor vehicle injured in collision with car, pick-up truck or van in nontraffic accident

☑x7ᵗʰ **V33.3** Unspecified occupant of three-wheeled motor vehicle injured in collision with car, pick-up truck or van in nontraffic accident

☑x7ᵗʰ **V33.4** Person boarding or alighting a three-wheeled motor vehicle injured in collision with car, pick-up truck or van

☑x7ᵗʰ **V33.5** Driver of three-wheeled motor vehicle injured in collision with car, pick-up truck or van in traffic accident

☑x7ᵗʰ **V33.6** Passenger in three-wheeled motor vehicle injured in collision with car, pick-up truck or van in traffic accident

☑x7ᵗʰ **V33.7** Person on outside of three-wheeled motor vehicle injured in collision with car, pick-up truck or van in traffic accident

☑x7ᵗʰ **V33.9** Unspecified occupant of three-wheeled motor vehicle injured in collision with car, pick-up truck or van in traffic accident

☑4ᵗʰ **V34 Occupant of three-wheeled motor vehicle injured in collision with heavy transport vehicle or bus**

EXCLUDES 1 *occupant of three-wheeled motor vehicle injured in collision with military vehicle (V39.81)*

☑x7ᵗʰ **V34.0** Driver of three-wheeled motor vehicle injured in collision with heavy transport vehicle or bus in nontraffic accident

☑x7ᵗʰ **V34.1** Passenger in three-wheeled motor vehicle injured in collision with heavy transport vehicle or bus in nontraffic accident

☑x7ᵗʰ **V34.2** Person on outside of three-wheeled motor vehicle injured in collision with heavy transport vehicle or bus in nontraffic accident

☑x7ᵗʰ **V34.3** Unspecified occupant of three-wheeled motor vehicle injured in collision with heavy transport vehicle or bus in nontraffic accident

☑x7ᵗʰ **V34.4** Person boarding or alighting a three-wheeled motor vehicle injured in collision with heavy transport vehicle or bus

☑x7ᵗʰ **V34.5** Driver of three-wheeled motor vehicle injured in collision with heavy transport vehicle or bus in traffic accident

☑x7ᵗʰ **V34.6** Passenger in three-wheeled motor vehicle injured in collision with heavy transport vehicle or bus in traffic accident

☑x7ᵗʰ **V34.7** Person on outside of three-wheeled motor vehicle injured in collision with heavy transport vehicle or bus in traffic accident

☑x7ᵗʰ **V34.9** Unspecified occupant of three-wheeled motor vehicle injured in collision with heavy transport vehicle or bus in traffic accident

☑4ᵗʰ **V35 Occupant of three-wheeled motor vehicle injured in collision with railway train or railway vehicle**

☑x7ᵗʰ **V35.0** Driver of three-wheeled motor vehicle injured in collision with railway train or railway vehicle in nontraffic accident

☑x7ᵗʰ **V35.1** Passenger in three-wheeled motor vehicle injured in collision with railway train or railway vehicle in nontraffic accident

☑x7ᵗʰ **V35.2** Person on outside of three-wheeled motor vehicle injured in collision with railway train or railway vehicle in nontraffic accident

☑x7ᵗʰ **V35.3** Unspecified occupant of three-wheeled motor vehicle injured in collision with railway train or railway vehicle in nontraffic accident

☑x7ᵗʰ **V35.4** Person boarding or alighting a three-wheeled motor vehicle injured in collision with railway train or railway vehicle

☑x7ᵗʰ **V35.5** Driver of three-wheeled motor vehicle injured in collision with railway train or railway vehicle in traffic accident

☑x7ᵗʰ **V35.6** Passenger in three-wheeled motor vehicle injured in collision with railway train or railway vehicle in traffic accident

☑x7ᵗʰ **V35.7** Person on outside of three-wheeled motor vehicle injured in collision with railway train or railway vehicle in traffic accident

☑x7ᵗʰ **V35.9** Unspecified occupant of three-wheeled motor vehicle injured in collision with railway train or railway vehicle in traffic accident

☑4ᵗʰ **V36 Occupant of three-wheeled motor vehicle injured in collision with other nonmotor vehicle**

INCLUDES collision with animal-drawn vehicle, animal being ridden, streetcar

☑x7ᵗʰ **V36.0** Driver of three-wheeled motor vehicle injured in collision with other nonmotor vehicle in nontraffic accident

☑x7ᵗʰ **V36.1** Passenger in three-wheeled motor vehicle injured in collision with other nonmotor vehicle in nontraffic accident

☑x7ᵗʰ **V36.2** Person on outside of three-wheeled motor vehicle injured in collision with other nonmotor vehicle in nontraffic accident

☑x7ᵗʰ **V36.3** Unspecified occupant of three-wheeled motor vehicle injured in collision with other nonmotor vehicle in nontraffic accident

☑x7ᵗʰ **V36.4** Person boarding or alighting a three-wheeled motor vehicle injured in collision with other nonmotor vehicle

☑x7ᵗʰ **V36.5** Driver of three-wheeled motor vehicle injured in collision with other nonmotor vehicle in traffic accident

☑x7ᵗʰ **V36.6** Passenger in three-wheeled motor vehicle injured in collision with other nonmotor vehicle in traffic accident

☑x7ᵗʰ **V36.7** Person on outside of three-wheeled motor vehicle injured in collision with other nonmotor vehicle in traffic accident

☑x7ᵗʰ **V36.9** Unspecified occupant of three-wheeled motor vehicle injured in collision with other nonmotor vehicle in traffic accident

☑4ᵗʰ **V37 Occupant of three-wheeled motor vehicle injured in collision with fixed or stationary object**

☑x7ᵗʰ **V37.0** Driver of three-wheeled motor vehicle injured in collision with fixed or stationary object in nontraffic accident

☑x7ᵗʰ **V37.1** Passenger in three-wheeled motor vehicle injured in collision with fixed or stationary object in nontraffic accident

☑x7ᵗʰ **V37.2** Person on outside of three-wheeled motor vehicle injured in collision with fixed or stationary object in nontraffic accident

☑x7ᵗʰ **V37.3** Unspecified occupant of three-wheeled motor vehicle injured in collision with fixed or stationary object in nontraffic accident

☑x7ᵗʰ **V37.4** Person boarding or alighting a three-wheeled motor vehicle injured in collision with fixed or stationary object

☑Additional Character Required   ☑x7ᵗʰ Placeholder   Unacceptable PDx   Questionable PDx   Wrong Procedure   Manifestation   H1 - H14 HAC   HCC CMS-HCC Dx   HIV HIV Dx

ICD-10-CM 2019   1169

√x7ᵗʰ **V37.5** **Driver** of three-wheeled motor vehicle injured in collision with fixed or stationary object **in traffic accident**

√x7ᵗʰ **V37.6** **Passenger** in three-wheeled motor vehicle injured in collision with fixed or stationary object **in traffic accident**

√x7ᵗʰ **V37.7** **Person on outside** of three-wheeled motor vehicle injured in collision with fixed or stationary object **in traffic accident**

√x7ᵗʰ **V37.9** **Unspecified** occupant of three-wheeled motor vehicle injured in collision with fixed or stationary object **in traffic accident**

√4ᵗʰ **V38** **Occupant of three-wheeled motor vehicle injured in noncollision transport accident**

     INCLUDES   fall or thrown from three-wheeled motor vehicle
                   overturning of three-wheeled motor vehicle NOS
                   overturning of three-wheeled motor vehicle without collision

√x7ᵗʰ **V38.0** **Driver** of three-wheeled motor vehicle injured in noncollision transport accident **in nontraffic accident**

√x7ᵗʰ **V38.1** **Passenger** in three-wheeled motor vehicle injured in noncollision transport accident **in nontraffic accident**

√x7ᵗʰ **V38.2** **Person on outside** of three-wheeled motor vehicle injured in noncollision transport accident **in nontraffic accident**

√x7ᵗʰ **V38.3** **Unspecified** occupant of three-wheeled motor vehicle injured in noncollision transport accident **in nontraffic accident**

√x7ᵗʰ **V38.4** **Person boarding or alighting** a three-wheeled motor vehicle injured in noncollision transport accident

√x7ᵗʰ **V38.5** **Driver** of three-wheeled motor vehicle injured in noncollision transport accident **in traffic accident**

√x7ᵗʰ **V38.6** **Passenger** in three-wheeled motor vehicle injured in noncollision transport accident **in traffic accident**

√x7ᵗʰ **V38.7** **Person on outside** of three-wheeled motor vehicle injured in noncollision transport accident **in traffic accident**

√x7ᵗʰ **V38.9** **Unspecified** occupant of three-wheeled motor vehicle injured in noncollision transport accident **in traffic accident**

√4ᵗʰ **V39** **Occupant of three-wheeled motor vehicle injured in other and unspecified transport accidents**

√5ᵗʰ **V39.0** **Driver** of three-wheeled motor vehicle injured in collision with other and unspecified motor vehicles **in nontraffic accident**

     √x7ᵗʰ **V39.00** **Driver** of three-wheeled motor vehicle injured in collision with **unspecified** motor vehicles in **nontraffic accident**

     √x7ᵗʰ **V39.09** **Driver** of three-wheeled motor vehicle injured in collision with **other** motor vehicles in **nontraffic accident**

√5ᵗʰ **V39.1** **Passenger** in three-wheeled motor vehicle injured in collision with other and unspecified motor vehicles **in nontraffic accident**

     √x7ᵗʰ **V39.10** **Passenger** in three-wheeled motor vehicle injured in collision with **unspecified** motor vehicles in **nontraffic accident**

     √x7ᵗʰ **V39.19** **Passenger** in three-wheeled motor vehicle injured in collision with **other** motor vehicles in **nontraffic accident**

√5ᵗʰ **V39.2** **Unspecified** occupant of three-wheeled motor vehicle injured in collision with other and unspecified motor vehicles **in nontraffic accident**

     √x7ᵗʰ **V39.20** **Unspecified** occupant of three-wheeled motor vehicle injured in collision with **unspecified** motor vehicles in **nontraffic accident**
             Collision NOS involving three-wheeled motor vehicle, nontraffic

     √x7ᵗʰ **V39.29** **Unspecified** occupant of three-wheeled motor vehicle injured in collision with **other** motor vehicles in **nontraffic accident**

√x7ᵗʰ **V39.3** **Occupant (driver) (passenger)** of three-wheeled motor vehicle injured in unspecified **nontraffic accident**
         Accident NOS involving three-wheeled motor vehicle, nontraffic
         Occupant of three-wheeled motor vehicle injured in nontraffic accident NOS

√5ᵗʰ **V39.4** **Driver** of three-wheeled motor vehicle injured in collision with other and unspecified motor vehicles **in traffic accident**

     √x7ᵗʰ **V39.40** **Driver** of three-wheeled motor vehicle injured in collision with **unspecified** motor vehicles in traffic accident

     √x7ᵗʰ **V39.49** **Driver** of three-wheeled motor vehicle injured in collision with **other** motor vehicles in traffic accident

√5ᵗʰ **V39.5** **Passenger** in three-wheeled motor vehicle injured in collision with other and unspecified motor vehicles **in traffic accident**

     √x7ᵗʰ **V39.50** **Passenger** in three-wheeled motor vehicle injured in collision with **unspecified** motor vehicles in traffic accident

     √x7ᵗʰ **V39.59** **Passenger** in three-wheeled motor vehicle injured in collision with **other** motor vehicles in traffic accident

√5ᵗʰ **V39.6** **Unspecified** occupant of three-wheeled motor vehicle injured in collision with other and unspecified motor vehicles in **traffic accident**

     √x7ᵗʰ **V39.60** **Unspecified** occupant of three-wheeled motor vehicle injured in collision with **unspecified** motor vehicles in traffic accident
             Collision NOS involving three-wheeled motor vehicle (traffic)

     √x7ᵗʰ **V39.69** **Unspecified** occupant of three-wheeled motor vehicle injured in collision with **other** motor vehicles in traffic accident

√5ᵗʰ **V39.8** **Occupant (driver) (passenger)** of three-wheeled motor vehicle injured in **other specified transport accidents**

     √x7ᵗʰ **V39.81** **Occupant (driver) (passenger)** of three-wheeled motor vehicle injured in transport accident with **military vehicle**

     √x7ᵗʰ **V39.89** **Occupant (driver) (passenger)** of three-wheeled motor vehicle injured in **other specified** transport accidents

√x7ᵗʰ **V39.9** **Occupant (driver) (passenger)** of three-wheeled motor vehicle injured in **unspecified traffic accident**
         Accident NOS involving three-wheeled motor vehicle

Car occupant injured in transport accident (V40-V49)

     INCLUDES   a four-wheeled motor vehicle designed primarily for carrying passengers
                 automobile (pulling a trailer or camper)

     EXCLUDES 1   *bus (V50-V59)*
                 minibus (V50-V59)
                 minivan (V50-V59)
                 motorcoach (V70-V79)
                 pick-up truck (V50-V59)
                 sport utility vehicle (SUV) (V50-V59)

> The appropriate 7th character is to be added to each code from categories V40-V49.
> A   initial encounter
> D   subsequent encounter
> S   sequela

√4ᵗʰ **V40** **Car occupant injured in collision with pedestrian or animal**
     EXCLUDES 1   *car collision with animal-drawn vehicle or animal being ridden (V46.-)*

√x7ᵗʰ **V40.0** **Car driver** injured in collision with pedestrian or animal **in nontraffic accident**

√x7ᵗʰ **V40.1** **Car passenger** injured in collision with pedestrian or animal **in nontraffic accident**

√x7ᵗʰ **V40.2** **Person on outside** of car injured in collision with pedestrian or animal **in nontraffic accident**

√x7ᵗʰ **V40.3** **Unspecified** car occupant injured in collision with pedestrian or animal **in nontraffic accident**

√x7ᵗʰ **V40.4** **Person boarding or alighting** a car injured in collision with pedestrian or animal

√x7ᵗʰ **V40.5** **Car driver** injured in collision with pedestrian or animal **in traffic accident**

√x7ᵗʰ **V40.6** **Car passenger** injured in collision with pedestrian or animal **in traffic accident**

√x7ᵗʰ **V40.7** **Person on outside** of car injured in collision with pedestrian or animal **in traffic accident**

√x7ᵗʰ **V40.9** **Unspecified** car occupant injured in collision with pedestrian or animal **in traffic accident**

√4ᵗʰ **V41** **Car occupant injured in collision with pedal cycle**

√x7ᵗʰ **V41.0** **Car driver** injured in collision with pedal cycle **in nontraffic accident**

√x7ᵗʰ **V41.1** **Car passenger** injured in collision with pedal cycle **in nontraffic accident**

√x7ᵗʰ **V41.2** **Person on outside** of car injured in collision with pedal cycle **in nontraffic accident**

√x7ᵗʰ **V41.3** **Unspecified** car occupant injured in collision with pedal cycle **in nontraffic accident**

N Newborn: 0   P Pediatric: 0-17   M Maternity: 12-55   A Adult: 15-124   MCC Major Complication/Comorbidity   CC Complication/Comorbidity   SW Severe Wound Dx

1170   ICD-10-CM 2019

☑x7ᵗʰ **V41.4** Person boarding or alighting a car injured in collision with pedal cycle

☑x7ᵗʰ **V41.5** Car driver injured in collision with pedal cycle in traffic accident

☑x7ᵗʰ **V41.6** Car passenger injured in collision with pedal cycle in traffic accident

☑x7ᵗʰ **V41.7** Person on outside of car injured in collision with pedal cycle in traffic accident

☑x7ᵗʰ **V41.9** Unspecified car occupant injured in collision with pedal cycle in traffic accident

☑4ᵗʰ **V42** Car occupant injured in collision with two- or three-wheeled motor vehicle

☑x7ᵗʰ **V42.0** Car driver injured in collision with two- or three-wheeled motor vehicle in nontraffic accident

☑x7ᵗʰ **V42.1** Car passenger injured in collision with two- or three-wheeled motor vehicle in nontraffic accident

☑x7ᵗʰ **V42.2** Person on outside of car injured in collision with two- or three-wheeled motor vehicle in nontraffic accident

☑x7ᵗʰ **V42.3** Unspecified car occupant injured in collision with two- or three-wheeled motor vehicle in nontraffic accident

☑x7ᵗʰ **V42.4** Person boarding or alighting a car injured in collision with two- or three-wheeled motor vehicle

☑x7ᵗʰ **V42.5** Car driver injured in collision with two- or three-wheeled motor vehicle in traffic accident

☑x7ᵗʰ **V42.6** Car passenger injured in collision with two- or three-wheeled motor vehicle in traffic accident

☑x7ᵗʰ **V42.7** Person on outside of car injured in collision with two- or three-wheeled motor vehicle in traffic accident

☑x7ᵗʰ **V42.9** Unspecified car occupant injured in collision with two- or three-wheeled motor vehicle in traffic accident

☑4ᵗʰ **V43** Car occupant injured in collision with car, pick-up truck or van

☑5ᵗʰ **V43.0** Car driver injured in collision with car, pick-up truck or van in nontraffic accident

☑x7ᵗʰ **V43.01** Car driver injured in collision with sport utility vehicle in nontraffic accident

☑x7ᵗʰ **V43.02** Car driver injured in collision with other type car in nontraffic accident

☑x7ᵗʰ **V43.03** Car driver injured in collision with pick-up truck in nontraffic accident

☑x7ᵗʰ **V43.04** Car driver injured in collision with van in nontraffic accident

☑5ᵗʰ **V43.1** Car passenger injured in collision with car, pick-up truck or van in nontraffic accident

☑x7ᵗʰ **V43.11** Car passenger injured in collision with sport utility vehicle in nontraffic accident

☑x7ᵗʰ **V43.12** Car passenger injured in collision with other type car in nontraffic accident

☑x7ᵗʰ **V43.13** Car passenger injured in collision with pick-up in nontraffic accident

☑x7ᵗʰ **V43.14** Car passenger injured in collision with van in nontraffic accident

☑5ᵗʰ **V43.2** Person on outside of car injured in collision with car, pick-up truck or van in nontraffic accident

☑x7ᵗʰ **V43.21** Person on outside of car injured in collision with sport utility vehicle in nontraffic accident

☑x7ᵗʰ **V43.22** Person on outside of car injured in collision with other type car in nontraffic accident

☑x7ᵗʰ **V43.23** Person on outside of car injured in collision with pick-up truck in nontraffic accident

☑x7ᵗʰ **V43.24** Person on outside of car injured in collision with van in nontraffic accident

☑5ᵗʰ **V43.3** Unspecified car occupant injured in collision with car, pick-up truck or van in nontraffic accident

☑x7ᵗʰ **V43.31** Unspecified car occupant injured in collision with sport utility vehicle in nontraffic accident

☑x7ᵗʰ **V43.32** Unspecified car occupant injured in collision with other type car in nontraffic accident

☑x7ᵗʰ **V43.33** Unspecified car occupant injured in collision with pick-up truck in nontraffic accident

☑x7ᵗʰ **V43.34** Unspecified car occupant injured in collision with van in nontraffic accident

☑5ᵗʰ **V43.4** Person boarding or alighting a car injured in collision with car, pick-up truck or van

☑x7ᵗʰ **V43.41** Person boarding or alighting a car injured in collision with sport utility vehicle

☑x7ᵗʰ **V43.42** Person boarding or alighting a car injured in collision with other type car

☑x7ᵗʰ **V43.43** Person boarding or alighting a car injured in collision with pick-up truck

☑x7ᵗʰ **V43.44** Person boarding or alighting a car injured in collision with van

☑5ᵗʰ **V43.5** Car driver injured in collision with car, pick-up truck or van in traffic accident

☑x7ᵗʰ **V43.51** Car driver injured in collision with sport utility vehicle in traffic accident

☑x7ᵗʰ **V43.52** Car driver injured in collision with other type car in traffic accident

☑x7ᵗʰ **V43.53** Car driver injured in collision with pick-up truck in traffic accident

☑x7ᵗʰ **V43.54** Car driver injured in collision with van in traffic accident

☑5ᵗʰ **V43.6** Car passenger injured in collision with car, pick-up truck or van in traffic accident

☑x7ᵗʰ **V43.61** Car passenger injured in collision with sport utility vehicle in traffic accident

☑x7ᵗʰ **V43.62** Car passenger injured in collision with other type car in traffic accident

☑x7ᵗʰ **V43.63** Car passenger injured in collision with pick-up truck in traffic accident

☑x7ᵗʰ **V43.64** Car passenger injured in collision with van in traffic accident

☑5ᵗʰ **V43.7** Person on outside of car injured in collision with car, pick-up truck or van in traffic accident

☑x7ᵗʰ **V43.71** Person on outside of car injured in collision with sport utility vehicle in traffic accident

☑x7ᵗʰ **V43.72** Person on outside of car injured in collision with other type car in traffic accident

☑x7ᵗʰ **V43.73** Person on outside of car injured in collision with pick-up truck in traffic accident

☑x7ᵗʰ **V43.74** Person on outside of car injured in collision with van in traffic accident

☑5ᵗʰ **V43.9** Unspecified car occupant injured in collision with car, pick-up truck or van in traffic accident

☑x7ᵗʰ **V43.91** Unspecified car occupant injured in collision with sport utility vehicle in traffic accident

☑x7ᵗʰ **V43.92** Unspecified car occupant injured in collision with other type car in traffic accident

☑x7ᵗʰ **V43.93** Unspecified car occupant injured in collision with pick-up truck in traffic accident

☑x7ᵗʰ **V43.94** Unspecified car occupant injured in collision with van in traffic accident

☑4ᵗʰ **V44** Car occupant injured in collision with heavy transport vehicle or bus

> **EXCLUDES 1** car occupant injured in collision with military vehicle (V49.81)

☑x7ᵗʰ **V44.0** Car driver injured in collision with heavy transport vehicle or bus in nontraffic accident

☑x7ᵗʰ **V44.1** Car passenger injured in collision with heavy transport vehicle or bus in nontraffic accident

☑x7ᵗʰ **V44.2** Person on outside of car injured in collision with heavy transport vehicle or bus in nontraffic accident

☑x7ᵗʰ **V44.3** Unspecified car occupant injured in collision with heavy transport vehicle or bus in nontraffic accident

☑x7ᵗʰ **V44.4** Person boarding or alighting a car injured in collision with heavy transport vehicle or bus

☑x7ᵗʰ **V44.5** Car driver injured in collision with heavy transport vehicle or bus in traffic accident

☑x7ᵗʰ **V44.6** Car passenger injured in collision with heavy transport vehicle or bus in traffic accident

☑x7ᵗʰ **V44.7** Person on outside of car injured in collision with heavy transport vehicle or bus in traffic accident

☑x7ᵗʰ **V44.9** Unspecified car occupant injured in collision with heavy transport vehicle or bus in traffic accident

☑ Additional Character Required   ☑x7ᵗʰ Placeholder   Unacceptable PDx   Questionable PDx   Wrong Procedure   Manifestation   H1 - H14 HAC   HCC CMS-HCC Dx   HIV HIV Dx

ICD-10-CM 2019   1171

Chapter 20. External Causes of Morbidity *(side tab)*

✓4ᵗʰ **V45** **Car occupant injured in collision with railway train or railway vehicle**

  ✓x7ᵗʰ **V45.0** Car **driver** injured in collision with railway train or railway vehicle in nontraffic accident

  ✓x7ᵗʰ **V45.1** Car **passenger** injured in collision with railway train or railway vehicle in nontraffic accident

  ✓x7ᵗʰ **V45.2** Person on outside of car injured in collision with railway train or railway vehicle in nontraffic accident

  ✓x7ᵗʰ **V45.3** Unspecified car occupant injured in collision with railway train or railway vehicle in nontraffic accident

  ✓x7ᵗʰ **V45.4** Person boarding or alighting a car injured in collision with railway train or railway vehicle

  ✓x7ᵗʰ **V45.5** Car **driver** injured in collision with railway train or railway vehicle in traffic accident

  ✓x7ᵗʰ **V45.6** Car **passenger** injured in collision with railway train or railway vehicle in traffic accident

  ✓x7ᵗʰ **V45.7** Person on outside of car injured in collision with railway train or railway vehicle in traffic accident

  ✓x7ᵗʰ **V45.9** Unspecified car occupant injured in collision with railway train or railway vehicle in traffic accident

✓4ᵗʰ **V46** **Car occupant injured in collision with other nonmotor vehicle**
   INCLUDES collision with animal-drawn vehicle, animal being ridden, streetcar

  ✓x7ᵗʰ **V46.0** Car **driver** injured in collision with other nonmotor vehicle in nontraffic accident

  ✓x7ᵗʰ **V46.1** Car **passenger** injured in collision with other nonmotor vehicle in nontraffic accident

  ✓x7ᵗʰ **V46.2** Person on outside of car injured in collision with other nonmotor vehicle in nontraffic accident

  ✓x7ᵗʰ **V46.3** Unspecified car occupant injured in collision with other nonmotor vehicle in nontraffic accident

  ✓x7ᵗʰ **V46.4** Person boarding or alighting a car injured in collision with other nonmotor vehicle

  ✓x7ᵗʰ **V46.5** Car **driver** injured in collision with other nonmotor vehicle in traffic accident

  ✓x7ᵗʰ **V46.6** Car **passenger** injured in collision with other nonmotor vehicle in traffic accident

  ✓x7ᵗʰ **V46.7** Person on outside of car injured in collision with other nonmotor vehicle in traffic accident

  ✓x7ᵗʰ **V46.9** Unspecified car occupant injured in collision with other nonmotor vehicle in traffic accident

✓4ᵗʰ **V47** **Car occupant injured in collision with fixed or stationary object**
   AHA: 2016, 4Q, 73

  ✓x7ᵗʰ **V47.0** Car driver injured in collision with fixed or stationary object in nontraffic accident

  ✓x7ᵗʰ **V47.1** Car **passenger** injured in collision with fixed or stationary object in nontraffic accident

  ✓x7ᵗʰ **V47.2** Person on outside of car injured in collision with fixed or stationary object in nontraffic accident

  ✓x7ᵗʰ **V47.3** Unspecified car occupant injured in collision with fixed or stationary object in nontraffic accident

  ✓x7ᵗʰ **V47.4** Person boarding or alighting a car injured in collision with fixed or stationary object

  ✓x7ᵗʰ **V47.5** Car **driver** injured in collision with fixed or stationary object in traffic accident

  ✓x7ᵗʰ **V47.6** Car **passenger** injured in collision with fixed or stationary object in traffic accident

  ✓x7ᵗʰ **V47.7** Person on outside of car injured in collision with fixed or stationary object in traffic accident

  ✓x7ᵗʰ **V47.9** Unspecified car occupant injured in collision with fixed or stationary object in traffic accident

✓4ᵗʰ **V48** **Car occupant injured in noncollision transport accident**
   INCLUDES overturning car NOS
               overturning car without collision

  ✓x7ᵗʰ **V48.0** Car **driver** injured in noncollision transport accident in nontraffic accident

  ✓x7ᵗʰ **V48.1** Car **passenger** injured in noncollision transport accident in nontraffic accident

  ✓x7ᵗʰ **V48.2** Person on outside of car injured in noncollision transport accident in nontraffic accident

  ✓x7ᵗʰ **V48.3** Unspecified car occupant injured in noncollision transport accident in nontraffic accident

  ✓x7ᵗʰ **V48.4** Person boarding or alighting a car injured in noncollision transport accident

  ✓x7ᵗʰ **V48.5** Car **driver** injured in noncollision transport accident in traffic accident

  ✓x7ᵗʰ **V48.6** Car **passenger** injured in noncollision transport accident in traffic accident

  ✓x7ᵗʰ **V48.7** Person on outside of car injured in noncollision transport accident in traffic accident

  ✓x7ᵗʰ **V48.9** Unspecified car occupant injured in noncollision transport accident in traffic accident

✓4ᵗʰ **V49** **Car occupant injured in other and unspecified transport accidents**

  ✓5ᵗʰ **V49.0** Driver injured in collision with other and unspecified motor vehicles in nontraffic accident

    ✓x7ᵗʰ **V49.00** Driver injured in collision with unspecified motor vehicles in nontraffic accident

    ✓x7ᵗʰ **V49.09** Driver injured in collision with other motor vehicles in nontraffic accident

  ✓5ᵗʰ **V49.1** Passenger injured in collision with other and unspecified motor vehicles in nontraffic accident

    ✓x7ᵗʰ **V49.10** Passenger injured in collision with unspecified motor vehicles in nontraffic accident

    ✓x7ᵗʰ **V49.19** Passenger injured in collision with other motor vehicles in nontraffic accident

  ✓5ᵗʰ **V49.2** Unspecified car occupant injured in collision with other and unspecified motor vehicles in nontraffic accident

    ✓x7ᵗʰ **V49.20** Unspecified car occupant injured in collision with unspecified motor vehicles in nontraffic accident
         Car collision NOS, nontraffic

    ✓x7ᵗʰ **V49.29** Unspecified car occupant injured in collision with other motor vehicles in nontraffic accident

  ✓x7ᵗʰ **V49.3** Car occupant (driver) (passenger) injured in unspecified nontraffic accident
       Car accident NOS, nontraffic
       Car occupant injured in nontraffic accident NOS

  ✓5ᵗʰ **V49.4** Driver injured in collision with other and unspecified motor vehicles in traffic accident

    ✓x7ᵗʰ **V49.40** Driver injured in collision with unspecified motor vehicles in traffic accident

    ✓x7ᵗʰ **V49.49** Driver injured in collision with other motor vehicles in traffic accident

  ✓5ᵗʰ **V49.5** Passenger injured in collision with other and unspecified motor vehicles in traffic accident

    ✓x7ᵗʰ **V49.50** Passenger injured in collision with unspecified motor vehicles in traffic accident

    ✓x7ᵗʰ **V49.59** Passenger injured in collision with other motor vehicles in traffic accident

  ✓5ᵗʰ **V49.6** Unspecified car occupant injured in collision with other and unspecified motor vehicles in traffic accident

    ✓x7ᵗʰ **V49.60** Unspecified car occupant injured in collision with unspecified motor vehicles in traffic accident
         Car collision NOS (traffic)

    ✓x7ᵗʰ **V49.69** Unspecified car occupant injured in collision with other motor vehicles in traffic accident

  ✓5ᵗʰ **V49.8** Car occupant (driver) (passenger) injured in other specified transport accidents

    ✓x7ᵗʰ **V49.81** Car occupant (driver) (passenger) injured in transport accident with military vehicle

    ✓x7ᵗʰ **V49.88** Car occupant (driver) (passenger) injured in other specified transport accidents

  ✓x7ᵗʰ **V49.9** Car occupant (driver) (passenger) injured in unspecified traffic accident
       Car accident NOS

Ⓝ Newborn: 0   Ⓟ Pediatric: 0-17   Ⓜ Maternity: 12-55   Ⓐ Adult: 15-124   **MCC** Major Complication/Comorbidity   **CC** Complication/Comorbidity   **SW** Severe Wound Dx

1172   ICD-10-CM 2019

V45–V49.9 *(side tab)*

Occupant of pick-up truck or van injured in transport accident (V50-V59)

INCLUDES a four or six wheel motor vehicle designed primarily for carrying passengers and property but weighing less than the local limit for classification as a heavy goods vehicle

minibus
minivan
sport utility vehicle (SUV)
truck
van

EXCLUDES 1 *heavy transport vehicle (V60-V69)*

The appropriate 7th character is to be added to each code from categories V50-V59.
A   initial encounter
D   subsequent encounter
S   sequela

☑4ᵗʰ **V50 Occupant of pick-up truck or van injured in collision with pedestrian or animal**
EXCLUDES 1 *pick-up truck or van collision with animal-drawn vehicle or animal being ridden (V56.-)*

☑x7ᵗʰ **V50.0 Driver** of pick-up truck or van injured in collision with pedestrian or animal **in nontraffic accident**

☑x7ᵗʰ **V50.1 Passenger** in pick-up truck or van injured in collision with pedestrian or animal **in nontraffic accident**

☑x7ᵗʰ **V50.2 Person on outside** of pick-up truck or van injured in collision with pedestrian or animal **in nontraffic accident**

☑x7ᵗʰ **V50.3 Unspecified occupant** of pick-up truck or van injured in collision with pedestrian or animal **in nontraffic accident**

☑x7ᵗʰ **V50.4 Person boarding or alighting** a pick-up truck or van injured in collision with pedestrian or animal

☑x7ᵗʰ **V50.5 Driver** of pick-up truck or van injured in collision with pedestrian or animal **in traffic accident**

☑x7ᵗʰ **V50.6 Passenger** in pick-up truck or van injured in collision with pedestrian or animal **in traffic accident**

☑x7ᵗʰ **V50.7 Person on outside** of pick-up truck or van injured in collision with pedestrian or animal **in traffic accident**

☑x7ᵗʰ **V50.9 Unspecified occupant** of pick-up truck or van injured in collision with pedestrian or animal **in traffic accident**

☑4ᵗʰ **V51 Occupant of pick-up truck or van injured in collision with pedal cycle**

☑x7ᵗʰ **V51.0 Driver** of pick-up truck or van injured in collision with pedal cycle **in nontraffic accident**

☑x7ᵗʰ **V51.1 Passenger** in pick-up truck or van injured in collision with pedal cycle **in nontraffic accident**

☑x7ᵗʰ **V51.2 Person on outside** of pick-up truck or van injured in collision with pedal cycle **in nontraffic accident**

☑x7ᵗʰ **V51.3 Unspecified occupant** of pick-up truck or van injured in collision with pedal cycle **in nontraffic accident**

☑x7ᵗʰ **V51.4 Person boarding or alighting** a pick-up truck or van injured in collision with pedal cycle

☑x7ᵗʰ **V51.5 Driver** of pick-up truck or van injured in collision with pedal cycle **in traffic accident**

☑x7ᵗʰ **V51.6 Passenger** in pick-up truck or van injured in collision with pedal cycle **in traffic accident**

☑x7ᵗʰ **V51.7 Person on outside** of pick-up truck or van injured in collision with pedal cycle **in traffic accident**

☑x7ᵗʰ **V51.9 Unspecified occupant** of pick-up truck or van injured in collision with pedal cycle **in traffic accident**

☑4ᵗʰ **V52 Occupant of pick-up truck or van injured in collision with two- or three-wheeled motor vehicle**

☑x7ᵗʰ **V52.0 Driver** of pick-up truck or van injured in collision with two- or three-wheeled motor vehicle **in nontraffic accident**

☑x7ᵗʰ **V52.1 Passenger** in pick-up truck or van injured in collision with two- or three-wheeled motor vehicle **in nontraffic accident**

☑x7ᵗʰ **V52.2 Person on outside** of pick-up truck or van injured in collision with two- or three-wheeled motor vehicle **in nontraffic accident**

☑x7ᵗʰ **V52.3 Unspecified occupant** of pick-up truck or van injured in collision with two- or three-wheeled motor vehicle **in nontraffic accident**

☑x7ᵗʰ **V52.4 Person boarding or alighting** a pick-up truck or van injured in collision with two- or three-wheeled motor vehicle

☑x7ᵗʰ **V52.5 Driver** of pick-up truck or van injured in collision with two- or three-wheeled motor vehicle **in traffic accident**

☑x7ᵗʰ **V52.6 Passenger** in pick-up truck or van injured in collision with two- or three-wheeled motor vehicle **in traffic accident**

☑x7ᵗʰ **V52.7 Person on outside** of pick-up truck or van injured in collision with two- or three-wheeled motor vehicle **in traffic accident**

☑x7ᵗʰ **V52.9 Unspecified occupant** of pick-up truck or van injured in collision with two- or three-wheeled motor vehicle **in traffic accident**

☑4ᵗʰ **V53 Occupant of pick-up truck or van injured in collision with car, pick-up truck or van**

☑x7ᵗʰ **V53.0 Driver** of pick-up truck or van injured in collision with car, pick-up truck or van **in nontraffic accident**

☑x7ᵗʰ **V53.1 Passenger** in pick-up truck or van injured in collision with car, pick-up truck or van **in nontraffic accident**

☑x7ᵗʰ **V53.2 Person on outside** of pick-up truck or van injured in collision with car, pick-up truck or van **in nontraffic accident**

☑x7ᵗʰ **V53.3 Unspecified occupant** of pick-up truck or van injured in collision with car, pick-up truck or van **in nontraffic accident**

☑x7ᵗʰ **V53.4 Person boarding or alighting** a pick-up truck or van injured in collision with car, pick-up truck or van

☑x7ᵗʰ **V53.5 Driver** of pick-up truck or van injured in collision with car, pick-up truck or van **in traffic accident**

☑x7ᵗʰ **V53.6 Passenger** in pick-up truck or van injured in collision with car, pick-up truck or van **in traffic accident**

☑x7ᵗʰ **V53.7 Person on outside** of pick-up truck or van injured in collision with car, pick-up truck or van **in traffic accident**

☑x7ᵗʰ **V53.9 Unspecified occupant** of pick-up truck or van injured in collision with car, pick-up truck or van **in traffic accident**

☑4ᵗʰ **V54 Occupant of pick-up truck or van injured in collision with heavy transport vehicle or bus**
EXCLUDES 1 *occupant of pick-up truck or van injured in collision with military vehicle (V59.81)*

☑x7ᵗʰ **V54.0 Driver** of pick-up truck or van injured in collision with heavy transport vehicle or bus **in nontraffic accident**

☑x7ᵗʰ **V54.1 Passenger** in pick-up truck or van injured in collision with heavy transport vehicle or bus **in nontraffic accident**

☑x7ᵗʰ **V54.2 Person on outside** of pick-up truck or van injured in collision with heavy transport vehicle or bus **in nontraffic accident**

☑x7ᵗʰ **V54.3 Unspecified occupant** of pick-up truck or van injured in collision with heavy transport vehicle or bus **in nontraffic accident**

☑x7ᵗʰ **V54.4 Person boarding or alighting** a pick-up truck or van injured in collision with heavy transport vehicle or bus

☑x7ᵗʰ **V54.5 Driver** of pick-up truck or van injured in collision with heavy transport vehicle or bus **in traffic accident**

☑x7ᵗʰ **V54.6 Passenger** in pick-up truck or van injured in collision with heavy transport vehicle or bus **in traffic accident**

☑x7ᵗʰ **V54.7 Person on outside** of pick-up truck or van injured in collision with heavy transport vehicle or bus **in traffic accident**

☑x7ᵗʰ **V54.9 Unspecified occupant** of pick-up truck or van injured in collision with heavy transport vehicle or bus **in traffic accident**

☑4ᵗʰ **V55 Occupant of pick-up truck or van injured in collision with railway train or railway vehicle**

☑x7ᵗʰ **V55.0 Driver** of pick-up truck or van injured in collision with railway train or railway vehicle **in nontraffic accident**

☑x7ᵗʰ **V55.1 Passenger** in pick-up truck or van injured in collision with railway train or railway vehicle **in nontraffic accident**

☑x7ᵗʰ **V55.2 Person on outside** of pick-up truck or van injured in collision with railway train or railway vehicle **in nontraffic accident**

☑x7ᵗʰ **V55.3 Unspecified occupant** of pick-up truck or van injured in collision with railway train or railway vehicle **in nontraffic accident**

☑x7ᵗʰ **V55.4 Person boarding or alighting** a pick-up truck or van injured in collision with railway train or railway vehicle

☑x7ᵗʰ **V55.5 Driver** of pick-up truck or van injured in collision with railway train or railway vehicle **in traffic accident**

☑x7ᵗʰ **V55.6 Passenger** in pick-up truck or van injured in collision with railway train or railway vehicle **in traffic accident**

☑x7ᵗʰ **V55.7 Person on outside** of pick-up truck or van injured in collision with railway train or railway vehicle **in traffic accident**

☑x7ᵗʰ **V55.9 Unspecified occupant** of pick-up truck or van injured in collision with railway train or railway vehicle **in traffic accident**

☑ Additional Character Required   ☑x7ᵗʰ Placeholder   Unacceptable PDx   Questionable PDx   Wrong Procedure   Manifestation   H1-H14 HAC   HCC CMS-HCC Dx   HIV HIV Dx

ICD-10-CM 2019   1173

✓4th V56 Occupant of pick-up truck or van injured in collision with other nonmotor vehicle

INCLUDES   collision with animal-drawn vehicle, animal being ridden, streetcar

✓x7th **V56.0** Driver of pick-up truck or van injured in collision with other nonmotor vehicle in nontraffic accident

✓x7th **V56.1** Passenger in pick-up truck or van injured in collision with other nonmotor vehicle in nontraffic accident

✓x7th **V56.2** Person on outside of pick-up truck or van injured in collision with other nonmotor vehicle in nontraffic accident

✓x7th **V56.3** Unspecified occupant of pick-up truck or van injured in collision with other nonmotor vehicle in nontraffic accident

✓x7th **V56.4** Person boarding or alighting a pick-up truck or van injured in collision with other nonmotor vehicle

✓x7th **V56.5** Driver of pick-up truck or van injured in collision with other nonmotor vehicle in traffic accident

✓x7th **V56.6** Passenger in pick-up truck or van injured in collision with other nonmotor vehicle in traffic accident

✓x7th **V56.7** Person on outside of pick-up truck or van injured in collision with other nonmotor vehicle in traffic accident

✓x7th **V56.9** Unspecified occupant of pick-up truck or van injured in collision with other nonmotor vehicle in traffic accident

✓4th V57 Occupant of pick-up truck or van injured in collision with fixed or stationary object

✓x7th **V57.0** Driver of pick-up truck or van injured in collision with fixed or stationary object in nontraffic accident

✓x7th **V57.1** Passenger in pick-up truck or van injured in collision with fixed or stationary object in nontraffic accident

✓x7th **V57.2** Person on outside of pick-up truck or van injured in collision with fixed or stationary object in nontraffic accident

✓x7th **V57.3** Unspecified occupant of pick-up truck or van injured in collision with fixed or stationary object in nontraffic accident

✓x7th **V57.4** Person boarding or alighting a pick-up truck or van injured in collision with fixed or stationary object

✓x7th **V57.5** Driver of pick-up truck or van injured in collision with fixed or stationary object in traffic accident

✓x7th **V57.6** Passenger in pick-up truck or van injured in collision with fixed or stationary object in traffic accident

✓x7th **V57.7** Person on outside of pick-up truck or van injured in collision with fixed or stationary object in traffic accident

✓x7th **V57.9** Unspecified occupant of pick-up truck or van injured in collision with fixed or stationary object in traffic accident

✓4th V58 Occupant of pick-up truck or van injured in noncollision transport accident

INCLUDES   overturning pick-up truck or van NOS
overturning pick-up truck or van without collision

✓x7th **V58.0** Driver of pick-up truck or van injured in noncollision transport accident in nontraffic accident

✓x7th **V58.1** Passenger in pick-up truck or van injured in noncollision transport accident in nontraffic accident

✓x7th **V58.2** Person on outside of pick-up truck or van injured in noncollision transport accident in nontraffic accident

✓x7th **V58.3** Unspecified occupant of pick-up truck or van injured in noncollision transport accident in nontraffic accident

✓x7th **V58.4** Person boarding or alighting a pick-up truck or van injured in noncollision transport accident

✓x7th **V58.5** Driver of pick-up truck or van injured in noncollision transport accident in traffic accident

✓x7th **V58.6** Passenger in pick-up truck or van injured in noncollision transport accident in traffic accident

✓x7th **V58.7** Person on outside of pick-up truck or van injured in noncollision transport accident in traffic accident

✓x7th **V58.9** Unspecified occupant of pick-up truck or van injured in noncollision transport accident in traffic accident

✓4th V59 Occupant of pick-up truck or van injured in other and unspecified transport accidents

✓5th **V59.0** Driver of pick-up truck or van injured in collision with other and unspecified motor vehicles in nontraffic accident

✓x7th **V59.00** Driver of pick-up truck or van injured in collision with unspecified motor vehicles in nontraffic accident

✓x7th **V59.09** Driver of pick-up truck or van injured in collision with other motor vehicles in nontraffic accident

✓5th **V59.1** Passenger in pick-up truck or van injured in collision with other and unspecified motor vehicles in nontraffic accident

✓x7th **V59.10** Passenger in pick-up truck or van injured in collision with unspecified motor vehicles in nontraffic accident

✓x7th **V59.19** Passenger in pick-up truck or van injured in collision with other motor vehicles in nontraffic accident

✓5th **V59.2** Unspecified occupant of pick-up truck or van injured in collision with other and unspecified motor vehicles in nontraffic accident

✓x7th **V59.20** Unspecified occupant of pick-up truck or van injured in collision with unspecified motor vehicles in nontraffic accident
Collision NOS involving pick-up truck or van, nontraffic

✓x7th **V59.29** Unspecified occupant of pick-up truck or van injured in collision with other motor vehicles in nontraffic accident

✓x7th **V59.3** Occupant (driver) (passenger) of pick-up truck or van injured in unspecified nontraffic accident
Accident NOS involving pick-up truck or van, nontraffic
Occupant of pick-up truck or van injured in nontraffic accident NOS

✓5th **V59.4** Driver of pick-up truck or van injured in collision with other and unspecified motor vehicles in traffic accident

✓x7th **V59.40** Driver of pick-up truck or van injured in collision with unspecified motor vehicles in traffic accident

✓x7th **V59.49** Driver of pick-up truck or van injured in collision with other motor vehicles in traffic accident

✓5th **V59.5** Passenger in pick-up truck or van injured in collision with other and unspecified motor vehicles in traffic accident

✓x7th **V59.50** Passenger in pick-up truck or van injured in collision with unspecified motor vehicles in traffic accident

✓x7th **V59.59** Passenger in pick-up truck or van injured in collision with other motor vehicles in traffic accident

✓5th **V59.6** Unspecified occupant of pick-up truck or van injured in collision with other and unspecified motor vehicles in traffic accident

✓x7th **V59.60** Unspecified occupant of pick-up truck or van injured in collision with unspecified motor vehicles in traffic accident
Collision NOS involving pick-up truck or van (traffic)

✓x7th **V59.69** Unspecified occupant of pick-up truck or van injured in collision with other motor vehicles in traffic accident

✓5th **V59.8** Occupant (driver) (passenger) of pick-up truck or van injured in other specified transport accidents

✓x7th **V59.81** Occupant (driver) (passenger) of pick-up truck or van injured in transport accident with military vehicle

✓x7th **V59.88** Occupant (driver) (passenger) of pick-up truck or van injured in other specified transport accidents

✓x7th **V59.9** Occupant (driver) (passenger) of pick-up truck or van injured in unspecified traffic accident
Accident NOS involving pick-up truck or van

Occupant of heavy transport vehicle injured in transport accident (V60-V69)

INCLUDES   18 wheeler
armored car
panel truck

EXCLUDES 1   bus
motorcoach

The appropriate 7th character is to be added to each code from categories V60-V69.
A   initial encounter
D   subsequent encounter
S   sequela

✓4th V60 Occupant of heavy transport vehicle injured in collision with pedestrian or animal

EXCLUDES 1   heavy transport vehicle collision with animal-drawn vehicle or animal being ridden (V66.-)

✓x7th **V60.0** Driver of heavy transport vehicle injured in collision with pedestrian or animal in nontraffic accident

✓x7th **V60.1** Passenger in heavy transport vehicle injured in collision with pedestrian or animal in nontraffic accident

✓x7th **V60.2** Person on outside of heavy transport vehicle injured in collision with pedestrian or animal in nontraffic accident

---

N Newborn: 0   P Pediatric: 0-17   M Maternity: 12-55   A Adult: 15-124   MCC Major Complication/Comorbidity   CC Complication/Comorbidity   SW Severe Wound Dx

1174   ICD-10-CM 2019

✓x7ᵗʰ **V60.3** Unspecified occupant of heavy transport vehicle injured in collision with pedestrian or animal in nontraffic accident

✓x7ᵗʰ **V60.4** Person boarding or alighting a heavy transport vehicle injured in collision with pedestrian or animal

✓x7ᵗʰ **V60.5** Driver of heavy transport vehicle injured in collision with pedestrian or animal in traffic accident

✓x7ᵗʰ **V60.6** Passenger in heavy transport vehicle injured in collision with pedestrian or animal in traffic accident

✓x7ᵗʰ **V60.7** Person on outside of heavy transport vehicle injured in collision with pedestrian or animal in traffic accident

✓x7ᵗʰ **V60.9** Unspecified occupant of heavy transport vehicle injured in collision with pedestrian or animal in traffic accident

✓4ᵗʰ **V61** Occupant of heavy transport vehicle injured in collision with pedal cycle

✓x7ᵗʰ **V61.0** Driver of heavy transport vehicle injured in collision with pedal cycle in nontraffic accident

✓x7ᵗʰ **V61.1** Passenger in heavy transport vehicle injured in collision with pedal cycle in nontraffic accident

✓x7ᵗʰ **V61.2** Person on outside of heavy transport vehicle injured in collision with pedal cycle in nontraffic accident

✓x7ᵗʰ **V61.3** Unspecified occupant of heavy transport vehicle injured in collision with pedal cycle in nontraffic accident

✓x7ᵗʰ **V61.4** Person boarding or alighting a heavy transport vehicle injured in collision with pedal cycle while boarding or alighting

✓x7ᵗʰ **V61.5** Driver of heavy transport vehicle injured in collision with pedal cycle in traffic accident

✓x7ᵗʰ **V61.6** Passenger in heavy transport vehicle injured in collision with pedal cycle in traffic accident

✓x7ᵗʰ **V61.7** Person on outside of heavy transport vehicle injured in collision with pedal cycle in traffic accident

✓x7ᵗʰ **V61.9** Unspecified occupant of heavy transport vehicle injured in collision with pedal cycle in traffic accident

✓4ᵗʰ **V62** Occupant of heavy transport vehicle injured in collision with two- or three-wheeled motor vehicle

✓x7ᵗʰ **V62.0** Driver of heavy transport vehicle injured in collision with two- or three-wheeled motor vehicle in nontraffic accident

✓x7ᵗʰ **V62.1** Passenger in heavy transport vehicle injured in collision with two- or three-wheeled motor vehicle in nontraffic accident

✓x7ᵗʰ **V62.2** Person on outside of heavy transport vehicle injured in collision with two- or three-wheeled motor vehicle in nontraffic accident

✓x7ᵗʰ **V62.3** Unspecified occupant of heavy transport vehicle injured in collision with two- or three-wheeled motor vehicle in nontraffic accident

✓x7ᵗʰ **V62.4** Person boarding or alighting a heavy transport vehicle injured in collision with two- or three-wheeled motor vehicle

✓x7ᵗʰ **V62.5** Driver of heavy transport vehicle injured in collision with two- or three-wheeled motor vehicle in traffic accident

✓x7ᵗʰ **V62.6** Passenger in heavy transport vehicle injured in collision with two- or three-wheeled motor vehicle in traffic accident

✓x7ᵗʰ **V62.7** Person on outside of heavy transport vehicle injured in collision with two- or three-wheeled motor vehicle in traffic accident

✓x7ᵗʰ **V62.9** Unspecified occupant of heavy transport vehicle injured in collision with two- or three-wheeled motor vehicle in traffic accident

✓4ᵗʰ **V63** Occupant of heavy transport vehicle injured in collision with car, pick-up truck or van

✓x7ᵗʰ **V63.0** Driver of heavy transport vehicle injured in collision with car, pick-up truck or van in nontraffic accident

✓x7ᵗʰ **V63.1** Passenger in heavy transport vehicle injured in collision with car, pick-up truck or van in nontraffic accident

✓x7ᵗʰ **V63.2** Person on outside of heavy transport vehicle injured in collision with car, pick-up truck or van in nontraffic accident

✓x7ᵗʰ **V63.3** Unspecified occupant of heavy transport vehicle injured in collision with car, pick-up truck or van in nontraffic accident

✓x7ᵗʰ **V63.4** Person boarding or alighting a heavy transport vehicle injured in collision with car, pick-up truck or van

✓x7ᵗʰ **V63.5** Driver of heavy transport vehicle injured in collision with car, pick-up truck or van in traffic accident

✓x7ᵗʰ **V63.6** Passenger in heavy transport vehicle injured in collision with car, pick-up truck or van in traffic accident

✓x7ᵗʰ **V63.7** Person on outside of heavy transport vehicle injured in collision with car, pick-up truck or van in traffic accident

✓x7ᵗʰ **V63.9** Unspecified occupant of heavy transport vehicle injured in collision with car, pick-up truck or van in traffic accident

✓4ᵗʰ **V64** Occupant of heavy transport vehicle injured in collision with heavy transport vehicle or bus
　　　EXCLUDES 1 occupant of heavy transport vehicle injured in collision with military vehicle (V69.81)

✓x7ᵗʰ **V64.0** Driver of heavy transport vehicle injured in collision with heavy transport vehicle or bus in nontraffic accident

✓x7ᵗʰ **V64.1** Passenger in heavy transport vehicle injured in collision with heavy transport vehicle or bus in nontraffic accident

✓x7ᵗʰ **V64.2** Person on outside of heavy transport vehicle injured in collision with heavy transport vehicle or bus in nontraffic accident

✓x7ᵗʰ **V64.3** Unspecified occupant of heavy transport vehicle injured in collision with heavy transport vehicle or bus in nontraffic accident

✓x7ᵗʰ **V64.4** Person boarding or alighting a heavy transport vehicle injured in collision with heavy transport vehicle or bus while boarding or alighting

✓x7ᵗʰ **V64.5** Driver of heavy transport vehicle injured in collision with heavy transport vehicle or bus in traffic accident

✓x7ᵗʰ **V64.6** Passenger in heavy transport vehicle injured in collision with heavy transport vehicle or bus in traffic accident

✓x7ᵗʰ **V64.7** Person on outside of heavy transport vehicle injured in collision with heavy transport vehicle or bus in traffic accident

✓x7ᵗʰ **V64.9** Unspecified occupant of heavy transport vehicle injured in collision with heavy transport vehicle or bus in traffic accident

✓4ᵗʰ **V65** Occupant of heavy transport vehicle injured in collision with railway train or railway vehicle

✓x7ᵗʰ **V65.0** Driver of heavy transport vehicle injured in collision with railway train or railway vehicle in nontraffic accident

✓x7ᵗʰ **V65.1** Passenger in heavy transport vehicle injured in collision with railway train or railway vehicle in nontraffic accident

✓x7ᵗʰ **V65.2** Person on outside of heavy transport vehicle injured in collision with railway train or railway vehicle in nontraffic accident

✓x7ᵗʰ **V65.3** Unspecified occupant of heavy transport vehicle injured in collision with railway train or railway vehicle in nontraffic accident

✓x7ᵗʰ **V65.4** Person boarding or alighting a heavy transport vehicle injured in collision with railway train or railway vehicle

✓x7ᵗʰ **V65.5** Driver of heavy transport vehicle injured in collision with railway train or railway vehicle in traffic accident

✓x7ᵗʰ **V65.6** Passenger in heavy transport vehicle injured in collision with railway train or railway vehicle in traffic accident

✓x7ᵗʰ **V65.7** Person on outside of heavy transport vehicle injured in collision with railway train or railway vehicle in traffic accident

✓x7ᵗʰ **V65.9** Unspecified occupant of heavy transport vehicle injured in collision with railway train or railway vehicle in traffic accident

✓4ᵗʰ **V66** Occupant of heavy transport vehicle injured in collision with other nonmotor vehicle
　　　INCLUDES collision with animal-drawn vehicle, animal being ridden, streetcar

✓x7ᵗʰ **V66.0** Driver of heavy transport vehicle injured in collision with other nonmotor vehicle in nontraffic accident

✓x7ᵗʰ **V66.1** Passenger in heavy transport vehicle injured in collision with other nonmotor vehicle in nontraffic accident

✓x7ᵗʰ **V66.2** Person on outside of heavy transport vehicle injured in collision with other nonmotor vehicle in nontraffic accident

✓x7ᵗʰ **V66.3** Unspecified occupant of heavy transport vehicle injured in collision with other nonmotor vehicle in nontraffic accident

✓x7ᵗʰ **V66.4** Person boarding or alighting a heavy transport vehicle injured in collision with other nonmotor vehicle

✓x7ᵗʰ **V66.5** Driver of heavy transport vehicle injured in collision with other nonmotor vehicle in traffic accident

✓x7ᵗʰ **V66.6** Passenger in heavy transport vehicle injured in collision with other nonmotor vehicle in traffic accident

✓x7ᵗʰ **V66.7** Person on outside of heavy transport vehicle injured in collision with other nonmotor vehicle in traffic accident

✓ Additional Character Required　　✓x7ᵗʰ Placeholder　　Unacceptable PDx　　Questionable PDx　　Wrong Procedure　　Manifestation　　H1-H14 HAC　　HCC CMS-HCC Dx　　HIV HIV Dx

ICD-10-CM 2019　　　　　　　　　　　　　　　　　　　　　　　　　　　　　　　　　1175

Chapter 20. External Causes of Morbidity

V60.3–V66.7

√x7ᵗʰ **V66.9** Unspecified **occupant of heavy transport vehicle injured in collision with other nonmotor vehicle** in traffic accident

√4ᵗʰ **V67** **Occupant of heavy transport vehicle injured in collision with fixed or stationary object**

√x7ᵗʰ **V67.0** Driver **of heavy transport vehicle injured in collision with fixed or stationary object** in nontraffic accident

√x7ᵗʰ **V67.1** Passenger **in heavy transport vehicle injured in collision with fixed or stationary object** in nontraffic accident

√x7ᵗʰ **V67.2** Person on outside **of heavy transport vehicle injured in collision with fixed or stationary object** in nontraffic accident

√x7ᵗʰ **V67.3** Unspecified **occupant of heavy transport vehicle injured in collision with fixed or stationary object** in nontraffic accident

√x7ᵗʰ **V67.4** Person boarding or alighting **a heavy transport vehicle injured in collision with fixed or stationary object**

√x7ᵗʰ **V67.5** Driver **of heavy transport vehicle injured in collision with fixed or stationary object** in traffic accident

√x7ᵗʰ **V67.6** Passenger **in heavy transport vehicle injured in collision with fixed or stationary object** in traffic accident

√x7ᵗʰ **V67.7** Person on outside **of heavy transport vehicle injured in collision with fixed or stationary object** in traffic accident

√x7ᵗʰ **V67.9** Unspecified **occupant of heavy transport vehicle injured in collision with fixed or stationary object** in traffic accident

√4ᵗʰ **V68** **Occupant of heavy transport vehicle injured in noncollision transport accident**
INCLUDES overturning heavy transport vehicle NOS
overturning heavy transport vehicle without collision

√x7ᵗʰ **V68.0** Driver **of heavy transport vehicle injured in noncollision transport accident** in nontraffic accident

√x7ᵗʰ **V68.1** Passenger **in heavy transport vehicle injured in noncollision transport accident** in nontraffic accident

√x7ᵗʰ **V68.2** Person on outside **of heavy transport vehicle injured in noncollision transport accident** in nontraffic accident

√x7ᵗʰ **V68.3** Unspecified **occupant of heavy transport vehicle injured in noncollision transport accident** in nontraffic accident

√x7ᵗʰ **V68.4** Person boarding or alighting **a heavy transport vehicle injured in noncollision transport accident**

√x7ᵗʰ **V68.5** Driver **of heavy transport vehicle injured in noncollision transport accident** in traffic accident

√x7ᵗʰ **V68.6** Passenger **in heavy transport vehicle injured in noncollision transport accident** in traffic accident

√x7ᵗʰ **V68.7** Person on outside **of heavy transport vehicle injured in noncollision transport accident** in traffic accident

√x7ᵗʰ **V68.9** Unspecified **occupant of heavy transport vehicle injured in noncollision transport accident** in traffic accident

√4ᵗʰ **V69** **Occupant of heavy transport vehicle injured in other and unspecified transport accidents**

√5ᵗʰ **V69.0** Driver **of heavy transport vehicle injured in collision with other and unspecified motor vehicles** in nontraffic accident

√x7ᵗʰ **V69.00** Driver of heavy transport vehicle injured in collision with unspecified motor vehicles in nontraffic accident

√x7ᵗʰ **V69.09** Driver of heavy transport vehicle injured in collision with other motor vehicles in nontraffic accident

√5ᵗʰ **V69.1** Passenger **in heavy transport vehicle injured in collision with other and unspecified motor vehicles** in nontraffic accident

√x7ᵗʰ **V69.10** Passenger in heavy transport vehicle injured in collision with unspecified motor vehicles in nontraffic accident

√x7ᵗʰ **V69.19** Passenger in heavy transport vehicle injured in collision with other motor vehicles in nontraffic accident

√5ᵗʰ **V69.2** Unspecified **occupant of heavy transport vehicle injured in collision with other and unspecified motor vehicles** in nontraffic accident

√x7ᵗʰ **V69.20** Unspecified occupant of heavy transport vehicle injured in collision with unspecified motor vehicles in nontraffic accident
Collision NOS involving heavy transport vehicle, nontraffic

√x7ᵗʰ **V69.29** Unspecified occupant of heavy transport vehicle injured in collision with other motor vehicles in nontraffic accident

√x7ᵗʰ **V69.3** Occupant (driver) (passenger) **of heavy transport vehicle injured in** unspecified nontraffic accident
Accident NOS involving heavy transport vehicle, nontraffic
Occupant of heavy transport vehicle injured in nontraffic accident NOS

√5ᵗʰ **V69.4** Driver **of heavy transport vehicle injured in collision with other and unspecified motor vehicles** in traffic accident

√x7ᵗʰ **V69.40** Driver of heavy transport vehicle injured in collision with unspecified motor vehicles in traffic accident

√x7ᵗʰ **V69.49** Driver of heavy transport vehicle injured in collision with other motor vehicles in traffic accident

√5ᵗʰ **V69.5** Passenger **in heavy transport vehicle injured in collision with other and unspecified motor vehicles** in traffic accident

√x7ᵗʰ **V69.50** Passenger in heavy transport vehicle injured in collision with unspecified motor vehicles in traffic accident

√x7ᵗʰ **V69.59** Passenger in heavy transport vehicle injured in collision with other motor vehicles in traffic accident

√5ᵗʰ **V69.6** Unspecified **occupant of heavy transport vehicle injured in collision with other and unspecified motor vehicles** in traffic accident

√x7ᵗʰ **V69.60** Unspecified occupant of heavy transport vehicle injured in collision with unspecified motor vehicles in traffic accident
Collision NOS involving heavy transport vehicle (traffic)

√x7ᵗʰ **V69.69** Unspecified occupant of heavy transport vehicle injured in collision with other motor vehicles in traffic accident

√5ᵗʰ **V69.8** Occupant (driver) (passenger) **of heavy transport vehicle injured in other specified transport accidents**

√x7ᵗʰ **V69.81** Occupant (driver) (passenger) of heavy transport vehicle injured in transport accidents with military vehicle

√x7ᵗʰ **V69.88** Occupant (driver) (passenger) of heavy transport vehicle injured in other specified transport accidents

√x7ᵗʰ **V69.9** Occupant (driver) (passenger) **of heavy transport vehicle injured in** unspecified traffic accident
Accident NOS involving heavy transport vehicle

Bus occupant injured in transport accident (V70-V79)
INCLUDES motorcoach
EXCLUDES 1 minibus (V50-V59)

The appropriate 7th character is to be added to each code from categories V70-V79.
A   initial encounter
D   subsequent encounter
S   sequela

√4ᵗʰ **V70** **Bus occupant injured in collision with pedestrian or animal**
EXCLUDES 1 bus collision with animal-drawn vehicle or animal being ridden (V76.-)

√x7ᵗʰ **V70.0** Driver **of bus injured in collision with pedestrian or animal** in nontraffic accident

√x7ᵗʰ **V70.1** Passenger **on bus injured in collision with pedestrian or animal** in nontraffic accident

√x7ᵗʰ **V70.2** Person on outside **of bus injured in collision with pedestrian or animal** in nontraffic accident

√x7ᵗʰ **V70.3** Unspecified **occupant of bus injured in collision with pedestrian or animal** in nontraffic accident

√x7ᵗʰ **V70.4** Person boarding or alighting **from bus injured in collision with pedestrian or animal**

√x7ᵗʰ **V70.5** Driver **of bus injured in collision with pedestrian or animal** in traffic accident

√x7ᵗʰ **V70.6** Passenger **on bus injured in collision with pedestrian or animal** in traffic accident

√x7ᵗʰ **V70.7** Person on outside **of bus injured in collision with pedestrian or animal** in traffic accident

√x7ᵗʰ **V70.9** Unspecified **occupant of bus injured in collision with pedestrian or animal** in traffic accident

√4ᵗʰ **V71** **Bus occupant injured in collision with pedal cycle**

√x7ᵗʰ **V71.0** Driver **of bus injured in collision with pedal cycle** in nontraffic accident

√x7ᵗʰ **V71.1** Passenger **on bus injured in collision with pedal cycle** in nontraffic accident

√x7ᵗʰ **V71.2** Person on outside of bus injured in collision with pedal cycle in nontraffic accident

√x7ᵗʰ **V71.3** Unspecified occupant of bus injured in collision with pedal cycle in nontraffic accident

√x7ᵗʰ **V71.4** Person boarding or alighting from bus injured in collision with pedal cycle

√x7ᵗʰ **V71.5** Driver of bus injured in collision with pedal cycle in traffic accident

√x7ᵗʰ **V71.6** Passenger on bus injured in collision with pedal cycle in traffic accident

√x7ᵗʰ **V71.7** Person on outside of bus injured in collision with pedal cycle in traffic accident

√x7ᵗʰ **V71.9** Unspecified occupant of bus injured in collision with pedal cycle in traffic accident

✓4ᵗʰ **V72 Bus occupant injured in collision with two- or three-wheeled motor vehicle**

√x7ᵗʰ **V72.0** Driver of bus injured in collision with two- or three-wheeled motor vehicle in nontraffic accident

√x7ᵗʰ **V72.1** Passenger on bus injured in collision with two- or three-wheeled motor vehicle in nontraffic accident

√x7ᵗʰ **V72.2** Person on outside of bus injured in collision with two- or three-wheeled motor vehicle in nontraffic accident

√x7ᵗʰ **V72.3** Unspecified occupant of bus injured in collision with two- or three-wheeled motor vehicle in nontraffic accident

√x7ᵗʰ **V72.4** Person boarding or alighting from bus injured in collision with two- or three-wheeled motor vehicle

√x7ᵗʰ **V72.5** Driver of bus injured in collision with two- or three-wheeled motor vehicle in traffic accident

√x7ᵗʰ **V72.6** Passenger on bus injured in collision with two- or three-wheeled motor vehicle in traffic accident

√x7ᵗʰ **V72.7** Person on outside of bus injured in collision with two- or three-wheeled motor vehicle in traffic accident

√x7ᵗʰ **V72.9** Unspecified occupant of bus injured in collision with two- or three-wheeled motor vehicle in traffic accident

✓4ᵗʰ **V73 Bus occupant injured in collision with car, pick-up truck or van**

√x7ᵗʰ **V73.0** Driver of bus injured in collision with car, pick-up truck or van in nontraffic accident

√x7ᵗʰ **V73.1** Passenger on bus injured in collision with car, pick-up truck or van in nontraffic accident

√x7ᵗʰ **V73.2** Person on outside of bus injured in collision with car, pick-up truck or van in nontraffic accident

√x7ᵗʰ **V73.3** Unspecified occupant of bus injured in collision with car, pick-up truck or van in nontraffic accident

√x7ᵗʰ **V73.4** Person boarding or alighting from bus injured in collision with car, pick-up truck or van

√x7ᵗʰ **V73.5** Driver of bus injured in collision with car, pick-up truck or van in traffic accident

√x7ᵗʰ **V73.6** Passenger on bus injured in collision with car, pick-up truck or van in traffic accident

√x7ᵗʰ **V73.7** Person on outside of bus injured in collision with car, pick-up truck or van in traffic accident

√x7ᵗʰ **V73.9** Unspecified occupant of bus injured in collision with car, pick-up truck or van in traffic accident

✓4ᵗʰ **V74 Bus occupant injured in collision with heavy transport vehicle or bus**

     EXCLUDES1   bus occupant injured in collision with military vehicle (V79.81)

√x7ᵗʰ **V74.0** Driver of bus injured in collision with heavy transport vehicle or bus in nontraffic accident

√x7ᵗʰ **V74.1** Passenger on bus injured in collision with heavy transport vehicle or bus in nontraffic accident

√x7ᵗʰ **V74.2** Person on outside of bus injured in collision with heavy transport vehicle or bus in nontraffic accident

√x7ᵗʰ **V74.3** Unspecified occupant of bus injured in collision with heavy transport vehicle or bus in nontraffic accident

√x7ᵗʰ **V74.4** Person boarding or alighting from bus injured in collision with heavy transport vehicle or bus

√x7ᵗʰ **V74.5** Driver of bus injured in collision with heavy transport vehicle or bus in traffic accident

√x7ᵗʰ **V74.6** Passenger on bus injured in collision with heavy transport vehicle or bus in traffic accident

√x7ᵗʰ **V74.7** Person on outside of bus injured in collision with heavy transport vehicle or bus in traffic accident

√x7ᵗʰ **V74.9** Unspecified occupant of bus injured in collision with heavy transport vehicle or bus in traffic accident

✓4ᵗʰ **V75 Bus occupant injured in collision with railway train or railway vehicle**

√x7ᵗʰ **V75.0** Driver of bus injured in collision with railway train or railway vehicle in nontraffic accident

√x7ᵗʰ **V75.1** Passenger on bus injured in collision with railway train or railway vehicle in nontraffic accident

√x7ᵗʰ **V75.2** Person on outside of bus injured in collision with railway train or railway vehicle in nontraffic accident

√x7ᵗʰ **V75.3** Unspecified occupant of bus injured in collision with railway train or railway vehicle in nontraffic accident

√x7ᵗʰ **V75.4** Person boarding or alighting from bus injured in collision with railway train or railway vehicle

√x7ᵗʰ **V75.5** Driver of bus injured in collision with railway train or railway vehicle in traffic accident

√x7ᵗʰ **V75.6** Passenger on bus injured in collision with railway train or railway vehicle in traffic accident

√x7ᵗʰ **V75.7** Person on outside of bus injured in collision with railway train or railway vehicle in traffic accident

√x7ᵗʰ **V75.9** Unspecified occupant of bus injured in collision with railway train or railway vehicle in traffic accident

✓4ᵗʰ **V76 Bus occupant injured in collision with other nonmotor vehicle**

     INCLUDES   collision with animal-drawn vehicle, animal being ridden, streetcar

√x7ᵗʰ **V76.0** Driver of bus injured in collision with other nonmotor vehicle in nontraffic accident

√x7ᵗʰ **V76.1** Passenger on bus injured in collision with other nonmotor vehicle in nontraffic accident

√x7ᵗʰ **V76.2** Person on outside of bus injured in collision with other nonmotor vehicle in nontraffic accident

√x7ᵗʰ **V76.3** Unspecified occupant of bus injured in collision with other nonmotor vehicle in nontraffic accident

√x7ᵗʰ **V76.4** Person boarding or alighting from bus injured in collision with other nonmotor vehicle

√x7ᵗʰ **V76.5** Driver of bus injured in collision with other nonmotor vehicle in traffic accident

√x7ᵗʰ **V76.6** Passenger on bus injured in collision with other nonmotor vehicle in traffic accident

√x7ᵗʰ **V76.7** Person on outside of bus injured in collision with other nonmotor vehicle in traffic accident

√x7ᵗʰ **V76.9** Unspecified occupant of bus injured in collision with other nonmotor vehicle in traffic accident

✓4ᵗʰ **V77 Bus occupant injured in collision with fixed or stationary object**

√x7ᵗʰ **V77.0** Driver of bus injured in collision with fixed or stationary object in nontraffic accident

√x7ᵗʰ **V77.1** Passenger on bus injured in collision with fixed or stationary object in nontraffic accident

√x7ᵗʰ **V77.2** Person on outside of bus injured in collision with fixed or stationary object in nontraffic accident

√x7ᵗʰ **V77.3** Unspecified occupant of bus injured in collision with fixed or stationary object in nontraffic accident

√x7ᵗʰ **V77.4** Person boarding or alighting from bus injured in collision with fixed or stationary object

√x7ᵗʰ **V77.5** Driver of bus injured in collision with fixed or stationary object in traffic accident

√x7ᵗʰ **V77.6** Passenger on bus injured in collision with fixed or stationary object in traffic accident

√x7ᵗʰ **V77.7** Person on outside of bus injured in collision with fixed or stationary object in traffic accident

√x7ᵗʰ **V77.9** Unspecified occupant of bus injured in collision with fixed or stationary object in traffic accident

✓4ᵗʰ **V78 Bus occupant injured in noncollision transport accident**

     INCLUDES   overturning bus NOS
                     overturning bus without collision

√x7ᵗʰ **V78.0** Driver of bus injured in noncollision transport accident in nontraffic accident

√x7ᵗʰ **V78.1** Passenger on bus injured in noncollision transport accident in nontraffic accident

√x7ᵗʰ **V78.2** Person on outside of bus injured in noncollision transport accident in nontraffic accident

√x7ᵗʰ **V78.3** Unspecified occupant of bus injured in noncollision transport accident in nontraffic accident

☑ Additional Character Required   √x7ᵗʰ Placeholder   Unacceptable PDx   Questionable PDx   Wrong Procedure   Manifestation   H1 - H14 HAC   HCC CMS-HCC Dx   HIV HIV Dx

ICD-10-CM 2019   1177

✓x7ᵗʰ **V78.4** Person boarding or alighting from bus injured in noncollision transport accident

✓x7ᵗʰ **V78.5** Driver of bus injured in noncollision transport accident in traffic accident

✓x7ᵗʰ **V78.6** Passenger on bus injured in noncollision transport accident in traffic accident

✓x7ᵗʰ **V78.7** Person on outside of bus injured in noncollision transport accident in traffic accident

✓x7ᵗʰ **V78.9** Unspecified occupant of bus injured in noncollision transport accident in traffic accident

✓4ᵗʰ **V79** **Bus occupant injured in other and unspecified transport accidents**

✓5ᵗʰ **V79.0** Driver of bus injured in collision with other and unspecified motor vehicles in nontraffic accident

　✓x7ᵗʰ **V79.00** Driver of bus injured in collision with unspecified motor vehicles in nontraffic accident

　✓x7ᵗʰ **V79.09** Driver of bus injured in collision with other motor vehicles in nontraffic accident

✓5ᵗʰ **V79.1** Passenger on bus injured in collision with other and unspecified motor vehicles in nontraffic accident

　✓x7ᵗʰ **V79.10** Passenger on bus injured in collision with unspecified motor vehicles in nontraffic accident

　✓x7ᵗʰ **V79.19** Passenger on bus injured in collision with other motor vehicles in nontraffic accident

✓5ᵗʰ **V79.2** Unspecified bus occupant injured in collision with other and unspecified motor vehicles in nontraffic accident

　✓x7ᵗʰ **V79.20** Unspecified bus occupant injured in collision with unspecified motor vehicles in nontraffic accident
　　Bus collision NOS, nontraffic

　✓x7ᵗʰ **V79.29** Unspecified bus occupant injured in collision with other motor vehicles in nontraffic accident

✓x7ᵗʰ **V79.3** Bus occupant (driver) (passenger) injured in unspecified nontraffic accident
　Bus accident NOS, nontraffic
　Bus occupant injured in nontraffic accident NOS

✓5ᵗʰ **V79.4** Driver of bus injured in collision with other and unspecified motor vehicles in traffic accident

　✓x7ᵗʰ **V79.40** Driver of bus injured in collision with unspecified motor vehicles in traffic accident

　✓x7ᵗʰ **V79.49** Driver of bus injured in collision with other motor vehicles in traffic accident

✓5ᵗʰ **V79.5** Passenger on bus injured in collision with other and unspecified motor vehicles in traffic accident

　✓x7ᵗʰ **V79.50** Passenger on bus injured in collision with unspecified motor vehicles in traffic accident

　✓x7ᵗʰ **V79.59** Passenger on bus injured in collision with other motor vehicles in traffic accident

✓5ᵗʰ **V79.6** Unspecified bus occupant injured in collision with other and unspecified motor vehicles in traffic accident

　✓x7ᵗʰ **V79.60** Unspecified bus occupant injured in collision with unspecified motor vehicles in traffic accident
　　Bus collision NOS (traffic)

　✓x7ᵗʰ **V79.69** Unspecified bus occupant injured in collision with other motor vehicles in traffic accident

✓5ᵗʰ **V79.8** Bus occupant (driver) (passenger) injured in other specified transport accidents

　✓x7ᵗʰ **V79.81** Bus occupant (driver) (passenger) injured in transport accidents with military vehicle

　✓x7ᵗʰ **V79.88** Bus occupant (driver) (passenger) injured in other specified transport accidents

✓x7ᵗʰ **V79.9** Bus occupant (driver) (passenger) injured in unspecified traffic accident
　Bus accident NOS

Other land transport accidents (V80–V89)

The appropriate 7th character is to be added to each code from categories V80-V89.
A　initial encounter
D　subsequent encounter
S　sequela

✓4ᵗʰ **V80** **Animal-rider or occupant of animal-drawn vehicle injured in transport accident**

✓5ᵗʰ **V80.0** Animal-rider or occupant of animal drawn vehicle injured by fall from or being thrown from animal or animal-drawn vehicle in noncollision accident

　✓6ᵗʰ **V80.01** Animal-rider injured by fall from or being thrown from animal in noncollision accident

　　✓7ᵗʰ **V80.010** Animal-rider injured by fall from or being thrown from horse in noncollision accident

　　✓7ᵗʰ **V80.018** Animal-rider injured by fall from or being thrown from other animal in noncollision accident

　✓x7ᵗʰ **V80.02** Occupant of animal-drawn vehicle injured by fall from or being thrown from animal-drawn vehicle in noncollision accident
　　Overturning animal-drawn vehicle NOS
　　Overturning animal-drawn vehicle without collision

✓5ᵗʰ **V80.1** Animal-rider or occupant of animal-drawn vehicle injured in collision with pedestrian or animal
　　EXCLUDES 1 animal-rider or animal-drawn vehicle collision with animal-drawn vehicle or animal being ridden (V80.7)

　✓x7ᵗʰ **V80.11** Animal-rider injured in collision with pedestrian or animal

　✓x7ᵗʰ **V80.12** Occupant of animal-drawn vehicle injured in collision with pedestrian or animal

✓5ᵗʰ **V80.2** Animal-rider or occupant of animal-drawn vehicle injured in collision with pedal cycle

　✓x7ᵗʰ **V80.21** Animal-rider injured in collision with pedal cycle

　✓x7ᵗʰ **V80.22** Occupant of animal-drawn vehicle injured in collision with pedal cycle

✓5ᵗʰ **V80.3** Animal-rider or occupant of animal-drawn vehicle injured in collision with two- or three-wheeled motor vehicle

　✓x7ᵗʰ **V80.31** Animal-rider injured in collision with two- or three-wheeled motor vehicle

　✓x7ᵗʰ **V80.32** Occupant of animal-drawn vehicle injured in collision with two- or three-wheeled motor vehicle

✓5ᵗʰ **V80.4** Animal-rider or occupant of animal-drawn vehicle injured in collision with car, pick-up truck, van, heavy transport vehicle or bus
　　EXCLUDES 1 animal-rider injured in collision with military vehicle (V80.910)
　　occupant of animal-drawn vehicle injured in collision with military vehicle (V80.920)

　✓x7ᵗʰ **V80.41** Animal-rider injured in collision with car, pick-up truck, van, heavy transport vehicle or bus

　✓x7ᵗʰ **V80.42** Occupant of animal-drawn vehicle injured in collision with car, pick-up truck, van, heavy transport vehicle or bus

✓5ᵗʰ **V80.5** Animal-rider or occupant of animal-drawn vehicle injured in collision with other specified motor vehicle

　✓x7ᵗʰ **V80.51** Animal-rider injured in collision with other specified motor vehicle

　✓x7ᵗʰ **V80.52** Occupant of animal-drawn vehicle injured in collision with other specified motor vehicle

✓5ᵗʰ **V80.6** Animal-rider or occupant of animal-drawn vehicle injured in collision with railway train or railway vehicle

　✓x7ᵗʰ **V80.61** Animal-rider injured in collision with railway train or railway vehicle

　✓x7ᵗʰ **V80.62** Occupant of animal-drawn vehicle injured in collision with railway train or railway vehicle

✓5ᵗʰ **V80.7** Animal-rider or occupant of animal-drawn vehicle injured in collision with other nonmotor vehicles

　✓6ᵗʰ **V80.71** Animal-rider or occupant of animal-drawn vehicle injured in collision with animal being ridden

　　✓7ᵗʰ **V80.710** Animal-rider injured in collision with other animal being ridden

N Newborn: 0　P Pediatric: 0-17　M Maternity: 12-55　A Adult: 15-124　MCC Major Complication/Comorbidity　CC Complication/Comorbidity　SW Severe Wound Dx

1178

ICD-10-CM 2019

☑7ᵗʰ **V80.711** Occupant of animal-drawn vehicle injured in collision with animal being ridden

☑6ᵗʰ **V80.72** Animal-rider or occupant of animal-drawn vehicle injured in collision with other animal-drawn vehicle

☑7ᵗʰ **V80.720** Animal-rider injured in collision with animal-drawn vehicle

☑7ᵗʰ **V80.721** Occupant of animal-drawn vehicle injured in collision with other animal-drawn vehicle

☑6ᵗʰ **V80.73** Animal-rider or occupant of animal-drawn vehicle injured in collision with streetcar

☑7ᵗʰ **V80.730** Animal-rider injured in collision with streetcar

☑7ᵗʰ **V80.731** Occupant of animal-drawn vehicle injured in collision with streetcar

☑6ᵗʰ **V80.79** Animal-rider or occupant of animal-drawn vehicle injured in collision with other nonmotor vehicles

☑7ᵗʰ **V80.790** Animal-rider injured in collision with other nonmotor vehicles

☑7ᵗʰ **V80.791** Occupant of animal-drawn vehicle injured in collision with other nonmotor vehicles

☑5ᵗʰ **V80.8** Animal-rider or occupant of animal-drawn vehicle injured in collision with fixed or stationary object

☑x7ᵗʰ **V80.81** Animal-rider injured in collision with fixed or stationary object

☑x7ᵗʰ **V80.82** Occupant of animal-drawn vehicle injured in collision with fixed or stationary object

☑5ᵗʰ **V80.9** Animal-rider or occupant of animal-drawn vehicle injured in other and unspecified transport accidents

☑6ᵗʰ **V80.91** Animal-rider injured in other and unspecified transport accidents

☑7ᵗʰ **V80.910** Animal-rider injured in transport accident with military vehicle

☑7ᵗʰ **V80.918** Animal-rider injured in other transport accident

☑7ᵗʰ **V80.919** Animal-rider injured in unspecified transport accident
Animal rider accident NOS

☑6ᵗʰ **V80.92** Occupant of animal-drawn vehicle injured in other and unspecified transport accidents

☑7ᵗʰ **V80.920** Occupant of animal-drawn vehicle injured in transport accident with military vehicle

☑7ᵗʰ **V80.928** Occupant of animal-drawn vehicle injured in other transport accident

☑7ᵗʰ **V80.929** Occupant of animal-drawn vehicle injured in unspecified transport accident
Animal-drawn vehicle accident NOS

☑4ᵗʰ **V81** Occupant of railway train or railway vehicle injured in transport accident
INCLUDES   derailment of railway train or railway vehicle
person on outside of train
EXCLUDES 1   streetcar (V82.-)

☑x7ᵗʰ **V81.0** Occupant of railway train or railway vehicle injured in collision with motor vehicle in nontraffic accident
EXCLUDES 1   occupant of railway train or railway vehicle injured due to collision with military vehicle (V81.83)

☑x7ᵗʰ **V81.1** Occupant of railway train or railway vehicle injured in collision with motor vehicle in traffic accident
EXCLUDES 1   occupant of railway train or railway vehicle injured due to collision with military vehicle (V81.83)

☑x7ᵗʰ **V81.2** Occupant of railway train or railway vehicle injured in collision with or hit by rolling stock

☑x7ᵗʰ **V81.3** Occupant of railway train or railway vehicle injured in collision with other object
Railway collision NOS

☑x7ᵗʰ **V81.4** Person injured while boarding or alighting from railway train or railway vehicle

☑x7ᵗʰ **V81.5** Occupant of railway train or railway vehicle injured by fall in railway train or railway vehicle

☑x7ᵗʰ **V81.6** Occupant of railway train or railway vehicle injured by fall from railway train or railway vehicle

☑x7ᵗʰ **V81.7** Occupant of railway train or railway vehicle injured in derailment without antecedent collision

☑5ᵗʰ **V81.8** Occupant of railway train or railway vehicle injured in other specified railway accidents

☑x7ᵗʰ **V81.81** Occupant of railway train or railway vehicle injured due to explosion or fire on train

☑x7ᵗʰ **V81.82** Occupant of railway train or railway vehicle injured due to object falling onto train
Occupant of railway train or railway vehicle injured due to falling earth onto train
Occupant of railway train or railway vehicle injured due to falling rocks onto train
Occupant of railway train or railway vehicle injured due to falling snow onto train
Occupant of railway train or railway vehicle injured due to falling trees onto train

☑x7ᵗʰ **V81.83** Occupant of railway train or railway vehicle injured due to collision with military vehicle

☑x7ᵗʰ **V81.89** Occupant of railway train or railway vehicle injured due to other specified railway accident

☑x7ᵗʰ **V81.9** Occupant of railway train or railway vehicle injured in unspecified railway accident
Railway accident NOS

☑4ᵗʰ **V82** Occupant of powered streetcar injured in transport accident
INCLUDES   interurban electric car
person on outside of streetcar
tram (car)
trolley (car)
EXCLUDES 1   bus (V70-V79)
motorcoach (V70-V79)
nonpowered streetcar (V76.-)
train (V81.-)

☑x7ᵗʰ **V82.0** Occupant of streetcar injured in collision with motor vehicle in nontraffic accident

☑x7ᵗʰ **V82.1** Occupant of streetcar injured in collision with motor vehicle in traffic accident

☑x7ᵗʰ **V82.2** Occupant of streetcar injured in collision with or hit by rolling stock

☑x7ᵗʰ **V82.3** Occupant of streetcar injured in collision with other object
EXCLUDES 1   collision with animal-drawn vehicle or animal being ridden (V82.8)

☑x7ᵗʰ **V82.4** Person injured while boarding or alighting from streetcar

☑x7ᵗʰ **V82.5** Occupant of streetcar injured by fall in streetcar
EXCLUDES 1   fall in streetcar:
while boarding or alighting (V82.4)
with antecedent collision (V82.0-V82.3)

☑x7ᵗʰ **V82.6** Occupant of streetcar injured by fall from streetcar
EXCLUDES 1   fall from streetcar:
while boarding or alighting (V82.4)
with antecedent collision (V82.0-V82.3)

☑x7ᵗʰ **V82.7** Occupant of streetcar injured in derailment without antecedent collision
EXCLUDES 1   occupant of streetcar injured in derailment with antecedent collision (V82.0-V82.3)

☑x7ᵗʰ **V82.8** Occupant of streetcar injured in other specified transport accidents
Streetcar collision with military vehicle
Streetcar collision with train or nonmotor vehicles

☑x7ᵗʰ **V82.9** Occupant of streetcar injured in unspecified traffic accident
Streetcar accident NOS

☑4ᵗʰ **V83** Occupant of special vehicle mainly used on industrial premises injured in transport accident
INCLUDES   battery-powered airport passenger vehicle
battery-powered truck (baggage) (mail)
coal-car in mine
forklift (truck)
logging car
self-propelled industrial truck
station baggage truck (powered)
tram, truck, or tub (powered) in mine or quarry
EXCLUDES 1   special construction vehicles (V85.-)
special industrial vehicle in stationary use or maintenance (W31.-)

☑x7ᵗʰ **V83.0** Driver of special industrial vehicle injured in traffic accident

☑x7ᵗʰ **V83.1** Passenger of special industrial vehicle injured in traffic accident

☑x7ᵗʰ **V83.2** Person on outside of special industrial vehicle injured in traffic accident

☑x7ᵗʰ **V83.3** Unspecified occupant of special industrial vehicle injured in traffic accident

✔Additional Character Required   ☑x7ᵗʰ Placeholder   Unacceptable PDx   Questionable PDx   **Wrong Procedure**   Manifestation   **H1-H14** HAC   **HCC** CMS-HCC Dx   **HIV** HIV Dx

ICD-10-CM 2019   1179

Chapter 20. External Causes of Morbidity

V80.711–V83.3

√x7ᵗʰ **V83.4** **Person injured while** boarding or alighting **from special industrial vehicle**

√x7ᵗʰ **V83.5** **Driver** of special industrial vehicle injured in nontraffic accident

√x7ᵗʰ **V83.6** **Passenger** of special industrial vehicle injured in nontraffic accident

√x7ᵗʰ **V83.7** **Person on outside** of special industrial vehicle injured in nontraffic accident

√x7ᵗʰ **V83.9** **Unspecified occupant** of special industrial vehicle injured in nontraffic accident
Special-industrial-vehicle accident NOS

√4ᵗʰ **V84** **Occupant of special vehicle mainly used in agriculture injured in transport accident**
INCLUDES   self-propelled farm machinery
tractor (and trailer)
EXCLUDES 1   animal-powered farm machinery accident (W30.8-)
contact with combine harvester (W30.0)
special agricultural vehicle in stationary use or maintenance (W30.-)

√x7ᵗʰ **V84.0** **Driver** of special agricultural vehicle injured in traffic accident

√x7ᵗʰ **V84.1** **Passenger** of special agricultural vehicle injured in traffic accident

√x7ᵗʰ **V84.2** **Person on outside** of special agricultural vehicle injured in traffic accident

√x7ᵗʰ **V84.3** **Unspecified** occupant of special agricultural vehicle injured in traffic accident

√x7ᵗʰ **V84.4** **Person injured while** boarding or alighting **from special agricultural vehicle**

√x7ᵗʰ **V84.5** **Driver** of special agricultural vehicle injured in nontraffic accident

√x7ᵗʰ **V84.6** **Passenger** of special agricultural vehicle injured in nontraffic accident

√x7ᵗʰ **V84.7** **Person on outside** of special agricultural vehicle injured in nontraffic accident

√x7ᵗʰ **V84.9** **Unspecified** occupant of special agricultural vehicle injured in nontraffic accident
Special-agricultural vehicle accident NOS

√4ᵗʰ **V85** **Occupant of special construction vehicle injured in transport accident**
INCLUDES   bulldozer
digger
dump truck
earth-leveller
mechanical shovel
road-roller
EXCLUDES 1   special industrial vehicle (V83.-)
special construction vehicle in stationary use or maintenance (W31.-)

√x7ᵗʰ **V85.0** **Driver** of special construction vehicle injured in traffic accident

√x7ᵗʰ **V85.1** **Passenger** of special construction vehicle injured in traffic accident

√x7ᵗʰ **V85.2** **Person on outside** of special construction vehicle injured in traffic accident

√x7ᵗʰ **V85.3** **Unspecified** occupant of special construction vehicle injured in traffic accident

√x7ᵗʰ **V85.4** **Person injured while** boarding or alighting **from special construction vehicle**

√x7ᵗʰ **V85.5** **Driver** of special construction vehicle injured in nontraffic accident

√x7ᵗʰ **V85.6** **Passenger** of special construction vehicle injured in nontraffic accident

√x7ᵗʰ **V85.7** **Person on outside** of special construction vehicle injured in nontraffic accident

√x7ᵗʰ **V85.9** **Unspecified** occupant of special construction vehicle injured in nontraffic accident
Special-construction-vehicle accident NOS

√4ᵗʰ **V86** **Occupant of special all-terrain or other off-road motor vehicle, injured in transport accident**
EXCLUDES 1   special all-terrain vehicle in stationary use or maintenance (W31.-)
sport-utility vehicle (V50-V59)
three-wheeled motor vehicle designed for on-road use (V30-V39)
AHA: 2017, 4Q, 26

√5ᵗʰ **V86.0** **Driver** of special all-terrain or other off-road motor vehicle injured in traffic accident

√x7ᵗʰ **V86.01** **Driver of** ambulance **or** fire engine **injured in traffic accident**

√x7ᵗʰ **V86.02** **Driver of** snowmobile **injured in traffic accident**

√x7ᵗʰ **V86.03** **Driver of** dune buggy **injured in traffic accident**

√x7ᵗʰ **V86.04** **Driver of** military vehicle **injured in traffic accident**

√x7ᵗʰ **V86.05** **Driver of** 3- or 4- wheeled all-terrain vehicle (ATV) **injured in traffic accident**

√x7ᵗʰ **V86.06** **Driver of** dirt bike or motor/cross bike **injured in traffic accident**

√x7ᵗʰ **V86.09** **Driver of** other special all-terrain or other off-road motor vehicle injured in traffic accident
Driver of dirt bike injured in traffic accident
Driver of go cart injured in traffic accident
Driver of golf cart injured in traffic accident

√5ᵗʰ **V86.1** **Passenger** of special all-terrain or other off-road motor vehicle injured in traffic accident

√x7ᵗʰ **V86.11** **Passenger of** ambulance **or** fire engine **injured in traffic accident**

√x7ᵗʰ **V86.12** **Passenger of** snowmobile **injured in traffic accident**

√x7ᵗʰ **V86.13** **Passenger of** dune buggy **injured in traffic accident**

√x7ᵗʰ **V86.14** **Passenger of** military vehicle **injured in traffic accident**

√x7ᵗʰ **V86.15** **Passenger of** 3- or 4- wheeled all-terrain vehicle (ATV) **injured in traffic accident**

√x7ᵗʰ **V86.16** **Passenger of** dirt bike or motor/cross bike **injured in traffic accident**

√x7ᵗʰ **V86.19** **Passenger of** other special all-terrain or other off-road motor vehicle injured in traffic accident
Passenger of dirt bike injured in traffic accident
Passenger of go cart injured in traffic accident
Passenger of golf cart injured in traffic accident

√5ᵗʰ **V86.2** **Person on outside** of special all-terrain or other off-road motor vehicle injured in traffic accident

√x7ᵗʰ **V86.21** **Person on outside of** ambulance **or** fire engine **injured in traffic accident**

√x7ᵗʰ **V86.22** **Person on outside of** snowmobile **injured in traffic accident**

√x7ᵗʰ **V86.23** **Person on outside of** dune buggy **injured in traffic accident**

√x7ᵗʰ **V86.24** **Person on outside of** military vehicle **injured in traffic accident**

√x7ᵗʰ **V86.25** **Person on outside of** 3- or 4- wheeled all-terrain vehicle (ATV) **injured in traffic accident**

√x7ᵗʰ **V86.26** **Person on outside of** dirt bike or motor/cross bike **injured in traffic accident**

√x7ᵗʰ **V86.29** **Person on outside of** other special all-terrain or other off-road motor vehicle injured in traffic accident
Person on outside of dirt bike injured in traffic accident
Person on outside of go cart injured in traffic accident
Person on outside of golf cart injured in traffic accident

√5ᵗʰ **V86.3** **Unspecified occupant** of special all-terrain or other off-road motor vehicle injured in traffic accident

√x7ᵗʰ **V86.31** **Unspecified occupant of** ambulance **or** fire engine **injured in traffic accident**

√x7ᵗʰ **V86.32** **Unspecified occupant of** snowmobile **injured in traffic accident**

√x7ᵗʰ **V86.33** **Unspecified occupant of** dune buggy **injured in traffic accident**

√x7ᵗʰ **V86.34** **Unspecified occupant of** military vehicle **injured in traffic accident**

√x7ᵗʰ **V86.35** **Unspecified occupant of** 3- or 4- wheeled all-terrain vehicle (ATV) **injured in traffic accident**

√x7ᵗʰ **V86.36** **Unspecified occupant of** dirt bike or motor/cross bike **injured in traffic accident**

√x7ᵗʰ **V86.39** Unspecified occupant of other special all-terrain or other off-road motor vehicle injured in traffic accident
> Unspecified occupant of dirt bike injured in traffic accident
> Unspecified occupant of go cart injured in traffic accident
> Unspecified occupant of golf cart injured in traffic accident

√5ᵗʰ **V86.4** Person injured while boarding or alighting from special all-terrain or other off-road motor vehicle

√x7ᵗʰ **V86.41** Person injured while boarding or alighting from ambulance or fire engine

√x7ᵗʰ **V86.42** Person injured while boarding or alighting from snowmobile

√x7ᵗʰ **V86.43** Person injured while boarding or alighting from dune buggy

√x7ᵗʰ **V86.44** Person injured while boarding or alighting from military vehicle

√x7ᵗʰ **V86.45** Person injured while boarding or alighting from a 3- or 4- wheeled all-terrain vehicle (ATV)

√x7ᵗʰ **V86.46** Person injured while boarding or alighting from a dirt bike or motor/cross bike

√x7ᵗʰ **V86.49** Person injured while boarding or alighting from other special all-terrain or other off-road motor vehicle
> Person injured while boarding or alighting from dirt bike
> Person injured while boarding or alighting from go cart
> Person injured while boarding or alighting from golf cart

√5ᵗʰ **V86.5** Driver of special all-terrain or other off-road motor vehicle injured in nontraffic accident

√x7ᵗʰ **V86.51** Driver of ambulance or fire engine injured in nontraffic accident

√x7ᵗʰ **V86.52** Driver of snowmobile injured in nontraffic accident

√x7ᵗʰ **V86.53** Driver of dune buggy injured in nontraffic accident

√x7ᵗʰ **V86.54** Driver of military vehicle injured in nontraffic accident

√x7ᵗʰ **V86.55** Driver of 3- or 4- wheeled all-terrain vehicle (ATV) injured in nontraffic accident

√x7ᵗʰ **V86.56** Driver of dirt bike or motor/cross bike injured in nontraffic accident

√x7ᵗʰ **V86.59** Driver of other special all-terrain or other off-road motor vehicle injured in nontraffic accident
> Driver of dirt bike injured in nontraffic accident
> Driver of go cart injured in nontraffic accident
> Driver of golf cart injured in nontraffic accident

√5ᵗʰ **V86.6** Passenger of special all-terrain or other off-road motor vehicle injured in nontraffic accident

√x7ᵗʰ **V86.61** Passenger of ambulance or fire engine injured in nontraffic accident

√x7ᵗʰ **V86.62** Passenger of snowmobile injured in nontraffic accident

√x7ᵗʰ **V86.63** Passenger of dune buggy injured in nontraffic accident

√x7ᵗʰ **V86.64** Passenger of military vehicle injured in nontraffic accident

√x7ᵗʰ **V86.65** Passenger of 3- or 4- wheeled all-terrain vehicle (ATV) injured in nontraffic accident

√x7ᵗʰ **V86.66** Passenger of dirt bike or motor/cross bike injured in nontraffic accident

√x7ᵗʰ **V86.69** Passenger of other special all-terrain or other off-road motor vehicle injured in nontraffic accident
> Passenger of dirt bike injured in nontraffic accident
> Passenger of go cart injured in nontraffic accident
> Passenger of golf cart injured in nontraffic accident

√5ᵗʰ **V86.7** Person on outside of special all-terrain or other off-road motor vehicle injured in nontraffic accident

√x7ᵗʰ **V86.71** Person on outside of ambulance or fire engine injured in nontraffic accident

√x7ᵗʰ **V86.72** Person on outside of snowmobile injured in nontraffic accident

√x7ᵗʰ **V86.73** Person on outside of dune buggy injured in nontraffic accident

√x7ᵗʰ **V86.74** Person on outside of military vehicle injured in nontraffic accident

√x7ᵗʰ **V86.75** Person on outside of 3- or 4- wheeled all-terrain vehicle (ATV) injured in nontraffic accident

√x7ᵗʰ **V86.76** Person on outside of dirt bike or motor/cross bike injured in nontraffic accident

√x7ᵗʰ **V86.79** Person on outside of other special all-terrain or other off-road motor vehicles injured in nontraffic accident
> Person on outside of dirt bike injured in nontraffic accident
> Person on outside of go cart injured in nontraffic accident
> Person on outside of golf cart injured in nontraffic accident

√5ᵗʰ **V86.9** Unspecified occupant of special all-terrain or other off-road motor vehicle injured in nontraffic accident

√x7ᵗʰ **V86.91** Unspecified occupant of ambulance or fire engine injured in nontraffic accident

√x7ᵗʰ **V86.92** Unspecified occupant of snowmobile injured in nontraffic accident

√x7ᵗʰ **V86.93** Unspecified occupant of dune buggy injured in nontraffic accident

√x7ᵗʰ **V86.94** Unspecified occupant of military vehicle injured in nontraffic accident

√x7ᵗʰ **V86.95** Unspecified occupant of 3- or 4- wheeled all-terrain vehicle (ATV) injured in nontraffic accident

√x7ᵗʰ **V86.96** Unspecified occupant of dirt bike or motor/cross bike injured in nontraffic accident

√x7ᵗʰ **V86.99** Unspecified occupant of other special all-terrain or other off-road motor vehicle injured in nontraffic accident
> Off-road motor-vehicle accident NOS
> Other motor-vehicle accident NOS
> Unspecified occupant of go cart injured in nontraffic accident
> Unspecified occupant of golf cart injured in nontraffic accident

√4ᵗʰ **V87** Traffic accident of specified type but victim's mode of transport unknown
> **EXCLUDES 1** collision involving:
> pedal cycle (V10-V19)
> pedestrian (V01-V09)

√x7ᵗʰ **V87.0** Person injured in collision between car and two- or three-wheeled powered vehicle (traffic)

√x7ᵗʰ **V87.1** Person injured in collision between other motor vehicle and two- or three-wheeled motor vehicle (traffic)

√x7ᵗʰ **V87.2** Person injured in collision between car and pick-up truck or van (traffic)

√x7ᵗʰ **V87.3** Person injured in collision between car and bus (traffic)

√x7ᵗʰ **V87.4** Person injured in collision between car and heavy transport vehicle (traffic)

√x7ᵗʰ **V87.5** Person injured in collision between heavy transport vehicle and bus (traffic)

√x7ᵗʰ **V87.6** Person injured in collision between railway train or railway vehicle and car (traffic)

√x7ᵗʰ **V87.7** Person injured in collision between other specified motor vehicles (traffic)

√x7ᵗʰ **V87.8** Person injured in other specified noncollision transport accidents involving motor vehicle (traffic)

√x7ᵗʰ **V87.9** Person injured in other specified (collision)(noncollision) transport accidents involving nonmotor vehicle (traffic)

√4ᵗʰ **V88** Nontraffic accident of specified type but victim's mode of transport unknown
> **EXCLUDES 1** collision involving:
> pedal cycle (V10-V19)
> pedestrian (V01-V09)

√x7ᵗʰ **V88.0** Person injured in collision between car and two- or three-wheeled motor vehicle, nontraffic

√x7ᵗʰ **V88.1** Person injured in collision between other motor vehicle and two- or three-wheeled motor vehicle, nontraffic

√x7ᵗʰ **V88.2** Person injured in collision between car and pick-up truck or van, nontraffic

√x7ᵗʰ **V88.3** Person injured in collision between car and bus, nontraffic

√x7ᵗʰ **V88.4** Person injured in collision between car and heavy transport vehicle, nontraffic

☑ Additional Character Required √x7ᵗʰ Placeholder Unacceptable PDx Questionable PDx Wrong Procedure Manifestation H1-H14 HAC HCC CMS-HCC Dx HIV HIV Dx

ICD-10-CM 2019 1181

√x7ᵗʰ **V88.5** **Person injured in collision between** heavy transport vehicle and bus, **nontraffic**

√x7ᵗʰ **V88.6** **Person injured in collision between** railway train or railway vehicle and car, **nontraffic**

√x7ᵗʰ **V88.7** **Person injured in collision between** other specified motor vehicle, **nontraffic**

√x7ᵗʰ **V88.8** **Person injured in** other specified noncollision transport accidents **involving motor vehicle, nontraffic**

√x7ᵗʰ **V88.9** **Person injured in** other specified (collision)(noncollision) transport accidents **involving** nonmotor vehicle, **nontraffic**

√4ᵗʰ **V89** **Motor- or nonmotor-vehicle accident, type of vehicle unspecified**

√x7ᵗʰ **V89.0** **Person injured in unspecified** motor-vehicle **accident,** nontraffic
Motor-vehicle accident NOS, nontraffic

√x7ᵗʰ **V89.1** **Person injured in unspecified** nonmotor-vehicle **accident,** nontraffic
Nonmotor-vehicle accident NOS (nontraffic)

√x7ᵗʰ **V89.2** **Person injured in** unspecified motor-vehicle **accident,** traffic
Motor-vehicle accident [MVA] NOS
Road (traffic) accident [RTA] NOS

√x7ᵗʰ **V89.3** **Person injured in** unspecified nonmotor-vehicle **accident,** traffic
Nonmotor-vehicle traffic accident NOS

√x7ᵗʰ **V89.9** **Person injured in** unspecified vehicle accident
Collision NOS

Water transport accidents (V90-V94)

The appropriate 7th character is to be added to each code from categories V90-V94.
A   initial encounter
D   subsequent encounter
S   sequela

√4ᵗʰ **V90** **Drowning and submersion due to accident to watercraft**
EXCLUDES 1 civilian water transport accident involving military watercraft (V94.81-)
fall into water not from watercraft (W16.-)
military watercraft accident in military or war operations (Y36.0-, Y37.0-)
water-transport-related drowning or submersion without accident to watercraft (V92.-)

√5ᵗʰ **V90.0** **Drowning and submersion due to** watercraft overturning

√x7ᵗʰ **V90.00** **Drowning and submersion due to** merchant ship **overturning**

√x7ᵗʰ **V90.01** **Drowning and submersion due to** passenger ship **overturning**
Drowning and submersion due to Ferry-boat overturning
Drowning and submersion due to Liner overturning

√x7ᵗʰ **V90.02** **Drowning and submersion due to** fishing boat **overturning**

√x7ᵗʰ **V90.03** **Drowning and submersion due to** other powered watercraft **overturning**
Drowning and submersion due to Hovercraft (on open water) overturning
Drowning and submersion due to Jet ski overturning

√x7ᵗʰ **V90.04** **Drowning and submersion due to** sailboat **overturning**

√x7ᵗʰ **V90.05** **Drowning and submersion due to** canoe or kayak **overturning**

√x7ᵗʰ **V90.06** **Drowning and submersion due to** (nonpowered) inflatable craft **overturning**

√x7ᵗʰ **V90.08** **Drowning and submersion due to** other unpowered watercraft **overturning**
Drowning and submersion due to windsurfer overturning

√x7ᵗʰ **V90.09** **Drowning and submersion due to** unspecified watercraft **overturning**
Drowning and submersion due to boat NOS overturning
Drowning and submersion due to ship NOS overturning
Drowning and submersion due to watercraft NOS overturning

√5ᵗʰ **V90.1** **Drowning and submersion due to** watercraft sinking

√x7ᵗʰ **V90.10** **Drowning and submersion due to** merchant ship **sinking**

√x7ᵗʰ **V90.11** **Drowning and submersion due to** passenger ship **sinking**
Drowning and submersion due to Ferry-boat sinking
Drowning and submersion due to Liner sinking

√x7ᵗʰ **V90.12** **Drowning and submersion due to** fishing boat **sinking**

√x7ᵗʰ **V90.13** **Drowning and submersion due to** other powered watercraft **sinking**
Drowning and submersion due to Hovercraft (on open water) sinking
Drowning and submersion due to Jet ski sinking

√x7ᵗʰ **V90.14** **Drowning and submersion due to** sailboat **sinking**

√x7ᵗʰ **V90.15** **Drowning and submersion due to** canoe or kayak **sinking**

√x7ᵗʰ **V90.16** **Drowning and submersion due to** (nonpowered) inflatable craft **sinking**

√x7ᵗʰ **V90.18** **Drowning and submersion due to** other unpowered watercraft **sinking**

√x7ᵗʰ **V90.19** **Drowning and submersion due to** unspecified watercraft **sinking**
Drowning and submersion due to boat NOS sinking
Drowning and submersion due to ship NOS sinking
Drowning and submersion due to watercraft NOS sinking

√5ᵗʰ **V90.2** **Drowning and submersion due to** falling or jumping from burning **watercraft**

√x7ᵗʰ **V90.20** **Drowning and submersion due to falling or jumping from burning** merchant ship

√x7ᵗʰ **V90.21** **Drowning and submersion due to falling or jumping from burning** passenger ship
Drowning and submersion due to falling or jumping from burning Ferry-boat
Drowning and submersion due to falling or jumping from burning Liner

√x7ᵗʰ **V90.22** **Drowning and submersion due to falling or jumping from burning** fishing boat

√x7ᵗʰ **V90.23** **Drowning and submersion due to falling or jumping from** other burning powered watercraft
Drowning and submersion due to falling and jumping from burning Hovercraft (on open water)
Drowning and submersion due to falling and jumping from burning Jet ski

√x7ᵗʰ **V90.24** **Drowning and submersion due to falling or jumping from burning** sailboat

√x7ᵗʰ **V90.25** **Drowning and submersion due to falling or jumping from burning** canoe or kayak

√x7ᵗʰ **V90.26** **Drowning and submersion due to falling or jumping from burning** (nonpowered) inflatable craft

√x7ᵗʰ **V90.27** **Drowning and submersion due to falling or jumping from burning** water-skis

√x7ᵗʰ **V90.28** **Drowning and submersion due to falling or jumping from** other burning unpowered watercraft
Drowning and submersion due to falling and jumping from burning surf-board
Drowning and submersion due to falling and jumping from burning windsurfer

√x7ᵗʰ **V90.29** **Drowning and submersion due to falling or jumping from** unspecified burning watercraft
Drowning and submersion due to falling or jumping from burning boat NOS
Drowning and submersion due to falling or jumping from burning ship NOS
Drowning and submersion due to falling or jumping from burning watercraft NOS

√5ᵗʰ **V90.3** **Drowning and submersion due to** falling or jumping from crushed watercraft

√x7ᵗʰ **V90.30** **Drowning and submersion due to falling or jumping from crushed** merchant ship

√x7ᵗʰ **V90.31** **Drowning and submersion due to falling or jumping from crushed** passenger ship
Drowning and submersion due to falling and jumping from crushed Ferry boat
Drowning and submersion due to falling and jumping from crushed Liner

√x7ᵗʰ **V90.32** **Drowning and submersion due to falling or jumping from crushed** fishing boat

Ⓝ Newborn: 0   Ⓟ Pediatric: 0-17   Ⓜ Maternity: 12-55   Ⓐ Adult: 15-124   **MCC** Major Complication/Comorbidity   **CC** Complication/Comorbidity   **SW** Severe Wound Dx

1182
ICD-10-CM 2019

√x7ᵗʰ **V90.33** **Drowning and submersion due to falling or jumping from** other crushed powered **watercraft**
Drowning and submersion due to falling and jumping from crushed Hovercraft
Drowning and submersion due to falling and jumping from crushed Jet ski

√x7ᵗʰ **V90.34** **Drowning and submersion due to falling or jumping from crushed** sailboat

√x7ᵗʰ **V90.35** **Drowning and submersion due to falling or jumping from crushed** canoe or kayak

√x7ᵗʰ **V90.36** **Drowning and submersion due to falling or jumping from crushed (nonpowered)** inflatable craft

√x7ᵗʰ **V90.37** **Drowning and submersion due to falling or jumping from crushed** water-skis

√x7ᵗʰ **V90.38** **Drowning and submersion due to falling or jumping from** other crushed unpowered **watercraft**
Drowning and submersion due to falling and jumping from crushed surf-board
Drowning and submersion due to falling and jumping from crushed windsurfer

√x7ᵗʰ **V90.39** **Drowning and submersion due to falling or jumping from crushed** unspecified **watercraft**
Drowning and submersion due to falling and jumping from crushed boat NOS
Drowning and submersion due to falling and jumping from crushed ship NOS
Drowning and submersion due to falling and jumping from crushed watercraft NOS

√5ᵗʰ **V90.8** **Drowning and submersion due to** other accident to watercraft

√x7ᵗʰ **V90.80** **Drowning and submersion due to other accident to** merchant ship

√x7ᵗʰ **V90.81** **Drowning and submersion due to other accident to** passenger ship
Drowning and submersion due to other accident to Ferry-boat
Drowning and submersion due to other accident to Liner

√x7ᵗʰ **V90.82** **Drowning and submersion due to other accident to** fishing boat

√x7ᵗʰ **V90.83** **Drowning and submersion due to other accident to** other powered **watercraft**
Drowning and submersion due to other accident to Hovercraft (on open water)
Drowning and submersion due to other accident to Jet ski

√x7ᵗʰ **V90.84** **Drowning and submersion due to other accident to** sailboat

√x7ᵗʰ **V90.85** **Drowning and submersion due to other accident to** canoe or kayak

√x7ᵗʰ **V90.86** **Drowning and submersion due to other accident to (nonpowered)** inflatable craft

√x7ᵗʰ **V90.87** **Drowning and submersion due to other accident to** water-skis

√x7ᵗʰ **V90.88** **Drowning and submersion due to other accident to** other unpowered **watercraft**
Drowning and submersion due to other accident to surf-board
Drowning and submersion due to other accident to windsurfer

√x7ᵗʰ **V90.89** **Drowning and submersion due to other accident to** unspecified **watercraft**
Drowning and submersion due to other accident to boat NOS
Drowning and submersion due to other accident to ship NOS
Drowning and submersion due to other accident to watercraft NOS

√4ᵗʰ **V91** **Other injury due to accident to watercraft**
INCLUDES   any injury except drowning and submersion as a result of an accident to watercraft
EXCLUDES 1   civilian water transport accident involving military watercraft (V94.81-)
military watercraft accident in military or war operations (Y36, Y37.-)
EXCLUDES 2   drowning and submersion due to accident to watercraft (V90.-)

√5ᵗʰ **V91.0** **Burn due to watercraft on fire**
EXCLUDES 1   burn from localized fire or explosion on board ship without accident to watercraft (V93.-)

√x7ᵗʰ **V91.00** **Burn due to** merchant ship **on fire**

√x7ᵗʰ **V91.01** **Burn due to** passenger ship **on fire**
Burn due to Ferry-boat on fire
Burn due to Liner on fire

√x7ᵗʰ **V91.02** **Burn due to** fishing boat **on fire**

√x7ᵗʰ **V91.03** **Burn due to** other powered **watercraft on fire**
Burn due to Hovercraft (on open water) on fire
Burn due to Jet ski on fire

√x7ᵗʰ **V91.04** **Burn due to** sailboat **on fire**

√x7ᵗʰ **V91.05** **Burn due to** canoe or kayak **on fire**

√x7ᵗʰ **V91.06** **Burn due to (nonpowered)** inflatable craft **on fire**

√x7ᵗʰ **V91.07** **Burn due to** water-skis **on fire**

√x7ᵗʰ **V91.08** **Burn due to** other unpowered **watercraft on fire**

√x7ᵗʰ **V91.09** **Burn due to** unspecified **watercraft on fire**
Burn due to boat NOS on fire
Burn due to ship NOS on fire
Burn due to watercraft NOS on fire

√5ᵗʰ **V91.1** **Crushed between watercraft and other watercraft or other object due to collision**
Crushed by lifeboat after abandoning ship in a collision
NOTE   Select the specified type of watercraft that the victim was on at the time of the collision

√x7ᵗʰ **V91.10** **Crushed between** merchant ship **and other watercraft or other object due to collision**

√x7ᵗʰ **V91.11** **Crushed between** passenger ship **and other watercraft or other object due to collision**
Crushed between Ferry-boat and other watercraft or other object due to collision
Crushed between Liner and other watercraft or other object due to collision

√x7ᵗʰ **V91.12** **Crushed between** fishing boat **and other watercraft or other object due to collision**

√x7ᵗʰ **V91.13** **Crushed between** other powered **watercraft and other watercraft or other object due to collision**
Crushed between Hovercraft (on open water) and other watercraft or other object due to collision
Crushed between Jet ski and other watercraft or other object due to collision

√x7ᵗʰ **V91.14** **Crushed between** sailboat **and other watercraft or other object due to collision**

√x7ᵗʰ **V91.15** **Crushed between** canoe or kayak **and other watercraft or other object due to collision**

√x7ᵗʰ **V91.16** **Crushed between (nonpowered)** inflatable craft **and other watercraft or other object due to collision**

√x7ᵗʰ **V91.18** **Crushed between other** unpowered **watercraft and other watercraft or other object due to collision**
Crushed between surfboard and other watercraft or other object due to collision
Crushed between windsurfer and other watercraft or other object due to collision

√x7ᵗʰ **V91.19** **Crushed between** unspecified **watercraft and other watercraft or other object due to collision**
Crushed between boat NOS and other watercraft or other object due to collision
Crushed between ship NOS and other watercraft or other object due to collision
Crushed between watercraft NOS and other watercraft or other object due to collision

√5ᵗʰ **V91.2** **Fall due to collision between watercraft and other watercraft or other object**
Fall while remaining on watercraft after collision
NOTE   Select the specified type of watercraft that the victim was on at the time of the collision.
EXCLUDES 1   crushed between watercraft and other watercraft and other object due to collision (V91.1-)
drowning and submersion due to falling from crushed watercraft (V90.3-)

√x7ᵗʰ **V91.20** **Fall due to collision between** merchant ship **and other watercraft or other object**

√x7ᵗʰ **V91.21** **Fall due to collision between** passenger ship **and other watercraft or other object**
Fall due to collision between Ferry-boat and other watercraft or other object
Fall due to collision between Liner and other watercraft or other object

√x7ᵗʰ **V91.22** **Fall due to collision between** fishing boat **and other watercraft or other object**

☑ Additional Character Required   √x7ᵗʰ Placeholder   Unacceptable PDx   Questionable PDx   Wrong Procedure   Manifestation   H1 -H14 HAC   HCC CMS-HCC Dx   HIV HIV Dx

Chapter 20. External Causes of Morbidity *(side margin)*

V91.23–V92.09 *(side margin)*

√x7ᵗʰ **V91.23** **Fall due to collision between** other powered watercraft **and other watercraft or other object**
     Fall due to collision between Hovercraft (on open water) and other watercraft or other object
     Fall due to collision between Jet ski and other watercraft or other object

√x7ᵗʰ **V91.24** **Fall due to collision between** sailboat **and other watercraft or other object**

√x7ᵗʰ **V91.25** **Fall due to collision between** canoe or kayak **and other watercraft or other object**

√x7ᵗʰ **V91.26** **Fall due to collision between (nonpowered)** inflatable craft **and other watercraft or other object**

√x7ᵗʰ **V91.29** **Fall due to collision between** unspecified **watercraft and other watercraft or other object**
     Fall due to collision between boat NOS and other watercraft or other object
     Fall due to collision between ship NOS and other watercraft or other object
     Fall due to collision between watercraft NOS and other watercraft or other object

√5ᵗʰ **V91.3** **Hit or struck by falling object due to accident to watercraft**
     Hit or struck by falling object (part of damaged watercraft or other object) after falling or jumping from damaged watercraft
     EXCLUDES 2   *drowning or submersion due to fall or jumping from damaged watercraft (V90.2-, V90.3-)*

√x7ᵗʰ **V91.30** **Hit or struck by falling object due to accident to** merchant ship

√x7ᵗʰ **V91.31** **Hit or struck by falling object due to accident to** passenger ship
     Hit or struck by falling object due to accident to Ferry-boat
     Hit or struck by falling object due to accident to Liner

√x7ᵗʰ **V91.32** **Hit or struck by falling object due to accident to** fishing boat

√x7ᵗʰ **V91.33** **Hit or struck by falling object due to accident to** other powered **watercraft**
     Hit or struck by falling object due to accident to Hovercraft (on open water)
     Hit or struck by falling object due to accident to Jet ski

√x7ᵗʰ **V91.34** **Hit or struck by falling object due to accident to** sailboat

√x7ᵗʰ **V91.35** **Hit or struck by falling object due to accident to** canoe or kayak

√x7ᵗʰ **V91.36** **Hit or struck by falling object due to accident to (nonpowered)** inflatable craft

√x7ᵗʰ **V91.37** **Hit or struck by falling object due to accident to** water-skis
     Hit by water-skis after jumping off of waterskis

√x7ᵗʰ **V91.38** **Hit or struck by falling object due to accident to** other unpowered **watercraft**
     Hit or struck by surf-board after falling off damaged surf-board
     Hit or struck by object after falling off damaged windsurfer

√x7ᵗʰ **V91.39** **Hit or struck by falling object due to accident to** unspecified **watercraft**
     Hit or struck by falling object due to accident to boat NOS
     Hit or struck by falling object due to accident to ship NOS
     Hit or struck by falling object due to accident to watercraft NOS

√5ᵗʰ **V91.8** **Other injury due to other accident to watercraft**

√x7ᵗʰ **V91.80** **Other injury due to other accident to** merchant ship

√x7ᵗʰ **V91.81** **Other injury due to other accident to** passenger ship
     Other injury due to other accident to Ferry-boat
     Other injury due to other accident to Liner

√x7ᵗʰ **V91.82** **Other injury due to other accident to** fishing boat

√x7ᵗʰ **V91.83** **Other injury due to other accident to** other powered **watercraft**
     Other injury due to other accident to Hovercraft (on open water)
     Other injury due to other accident to Jet ski

√x7ᵗʰ **V91.84** **Other injury due to other accident to** sailboat

√x7ᵗʰ **V91.85** **Other injury due to other accident to** canoe or kayak

√x7ᵗʰ **V91.86** **Other injury due to other accident to (nonpowered)** inflatable craft

√x7ᵗʰ **V91.87** **Other injury due to other accident to** water-skis

√x7ᵗʰ **V91.88** **Other injury due to other accident to** other unpowered **watercraft**
     Other injury due to other accident to surf-board
     Other injury due to other accident to windsurfer

√x7ᵗʰ **V91.89** **Other injury due to other accident to** unspecified **watercraft**
     Other injury due to other accident to boat NOS
     Other injury due to other accident to ship NOS
     Other injury due to other accident to watercraft NOS

√4ᵗʰ **V92** **Drowning and submersion due to accident on board watercraft, without accident to watercraft**
     EXCLUDES 1   *civilian water transport accident involving military watercraft (V94.81-)*
     drowning or submersion due to accident to watercraft (V90-V91)
     drowning or submersion of diver who voluntarily jumps from boat not involved in an accident (W16.711, W16.721)
     fall into water without watercraft (W16.-)
     military watercraft accident in military or war operations (Y36, Y37)

√5ᵗʰ **V92.0** **Drowning and submersion due to** fall off **watercraft**
     Drowning and submersion due to fall from gangplank of watercraft
     Drowning and submersion due to fall overboard watercraft
     EXCLUDES 2   *hitting head on object or bottom of body of water due to fall from watercraft (V94.0-)*

√x7ᵗʰ **V92.00** **Drowning and submersion due to fall off** merchant ship

√x7ᵗʰ **V92.01** **Drowning and submersion due to fall off** passenger ship
     Drowning and submersion due to fall off Ferry-boat
     Drowning and submersion due to fall off Liner

√x7ᵗʰ **V92.02** **Drowning and submersion due to fall off** fishing boat

√x7ᵗʰ **V92.03** **Drowning and submersion due to fall off** other powered **watercraft**
     Drowning and submersion due to fall off Hovercraft (on open water)
     Drowning and submersion due to fall off Jet ski

√x7ᵗʰ **V92.04** **Drowning and submersion due to fall off** sailboat

√x7ᵗʰ **V92.05** **Drowning and submersion due to fall off** canoe or kayak

√x7ᵗʰ **V92.06** **Drowning and submersion due to fall off (nonpowered)** inflatable craft

√x7ᵗʰ **V92.07** **Drowning and submersion due to fall off** water-skis
     EXCLUDES 1   *drowning and submersion due to falling off burning water-skis (V90.27)*
     drowning and submersion due to falling off crushed water-skis (V90.37)
     hit by boat while water-skiing NOS (V94.X)

√x7ᵗʰ **V92.08** **Drowning and submersion due to fall off** other unpowered **watercraft**
     Drowning and submersion due to fall off surf-board
     Drowning and submersion due to fall off windsurfer
     EXCLUDES 1   *drowning and submersion due to fall off burning unpowered watercraft (V90.28)*
     drowning and submersion due to fall off crushed unpowered watercraft (V90.38)
     drowning and submersion due to fall off damaged unpowered watercraft (V90.88)
     drowning and submersion due to rider of nonpowered watercraft being hit by other watercraft (V94.-)
     other injury due to rider of nonpowered watercraft being hit by other watercraft (V94.-)

√x7ᵗʰ **V92.09** **Drowning and submersion due to fall off** unspecified **watercraft**
     Drowning and submersion due to fall off boat NOS
     Drowning and submersion due to fall off ship
     Drowning and submersion due to fall off watercraft NOS

Ⓝ Newborn: 0   Ⓟ Pediatric: 0-17   Ⓜ Maternity: 12-55   Ⓐ Adult: 15-124   MCC Major Complication/Comorbidity   CC Complication/Comorbidity   SW Severe Wound Dx

1184   ICD-10-CM 2019

☑5ᵗʰ V92.1 Drowning and submersion due to being thrown overboard by motion of watercraft

> EXCLUDES 1   *drowning and submersion due to fall off surf-board (V92.08)*
> *drowning and submersion due to fall off water-skis (V92.07)*
> *drowning and submersion due to fall off windsurfer (V92.08)*

☑x7ᵗʰ **V92.10 Drowning and submersion due to being thrown overboard by motion of merchant ship**

☑x7ᵗʰ **V92.11 Drowning and submersion due to being thrown overboard by motion of passenger ship**
> Drowning and submersion due to being thrown overboard by motion of Ferry-boat
> Drowning and submersion due to being thrown overboard by motion of Liner

☑x7ᵗʰ **V92.12 Drowning and submersion due to being thrown overboard by motion of fishing boat**

☑x7ᵗʰ **V92.13 Drowning and submersion due to being thrown overboard by motion of other powered watercraft**
> Drowning and submersion due to being thrown overboard by motion of Hovercraft

☑x7ᵗʰ **V92.14 Drowning and submersion due to being thrown overboard by motion of sailboat**

☑x7ᵗʰ **V92.15 Drowning and submersion due to being thrown overboard by motion of canoe or kayak**

☑x7ᵗʰ **V92.16 Drowning and submersion due to being thrown overboard by motion of (nonpowered) inflatable craft**

☑x7ᵗʰ **V92.19 Drowning and submersion due to being thrown overboard by motion of unspecified watercraft**
> Drowning and submersion due to being thrown overboard by motion of boat NOS
> Drowning and submersion due to being thrown overboard by motion of ship NOS
> Drowning and submersion due to being thrown overboard by motion of watercraft NOS

☑5ᵗʰ V92.2 Drowning and submersion due to being washed overboard from watercraft

> Code first any associated cataclysm (X37.0-)

☑x7ᵗʰ **V92.20 Drowning and submersion due to being washed overboard from merchant ship**

☑x7ᵗʰ **V92.21 Drowning and submersion due to being washed overboard from passenger ship**
> Drowning and submersion due to being washed overboard from Ferry-boat
> Drowning and submersion due to being washed overboard from Liner

☑x7ᵗʰ **V92.22 Drowning and submersion due to being washed overboard from fishing boat**

☑x7ᵗʰ **V92.23 Drowning and submersion due to being washed overboard from other powered watercraft**
> Drowning and submersion due to being washed overboard from Hovercraft (on open water)
> Drowning and submersion due to being washed overboard from Jet ski

☑x7ᵗʰ **V92.24 Drowning and submersion due to being washed overboard from sailboat**

☑x7ᵗʰ **V92.25 Drowning and submersion due to being washed overboard from canoe or kayak**

☑x7ᵗʰ **V92.26 Drowning and submersion due to being washed overboard from (nonpowered) inflatable craft**

☑x7ᵗʰ **V92.27 Drowning and submersion due to being washed overboard from water-skis**
> EXCLUDES 1   *drowning and submersion due to fall off water-skis (V92.07)*

☑x7ᵗʰ **V92.28 Drowning and submersion due to being washed overboard from other unpowered watercraft**
> Drowning and submersion due to being washed overboard from surf-board
> Drowning and submersion due to being washed overboard from windsurfer

☑x7ᵗʰ **V92.29 Drowning and submersion due to being washed overboard from unspecified watercraft**
> Drowning and submersion due to being washed overboard from boat NOS
> Drowning and submersion due to being washed overboard from ship NOS
> Drowning and submersion due to being washed overboard from watercraft NOS

☑4ᵗʰ V93 Other injury due to accident on board watercraft, without accident to watercraft

> EXCLUDES 1   *civilian water transport accident involving military watercraft (V94.81-)*
> *other injury due to accident to watercraft (V91.-)*
> *military watercraft accident in military or war operations (Y36, Y37.-)*
> EXCLUDES 2   *drowning and submersion due to accident on board watercraft, without accident to watercraft (V92.-)*

☑5ᵗʰ V93.0 Burn due to localized fire on board watercraft
> EXCLUDES 1   *burn due to watercraft on fire (V91.0-)*

☑x7ᵗʰ **V93.00 Burn due to localized fire on board merchant vessel**

☑x7ᵗʰ **V93.01 Burn due to localized fire on board passenger vessel**
> Burn due to localized fire on board Ferry-boat
> Burn due to localized fire on board Liner

☑x7ᵗʰ **V93.02 Burn due to localized fire on board fishing boat**

☑x7ᵗʰ **V93.03 Burn due to localized fire on board other powered watercraft**
> Burn due to localized fire on board Hovercraft
> Burn due to localized fire on board Jet ski

☑x7ᵗʰ **V93.04 Burn due to localized fire on board sailboat**

☑x7ᵗʰ **V93.09 Burn due to localized fire on board unspecified watercraft**
> Burn due to localized fire on board boat NOS
> Burn due to localized fire on board ship NOS
> Burn due to localized fire on board watercraft NOS

☑5ᵗʰ V93.1 Other burn on board watercraft
> Burn due to source other than fire on board watercraft
> EXCLUDES 1   *burn due to watercraft on fire (V91.0-)*

☑x7ᵗʰ **V93.10 Other burn on board merchant vessel**

☑x7ᵗʰ **V93.11 Other burn on board passenger vessel**
> Other burn on board Ferry-boat
> Other burn on board Liner

☑x7ᵗʰ **V93.12 Other burn on board fishing boat**

☑x7ᵗʰ **V93.13 Other burn on board other powered watercraft**
> Other burn on board Hovercraft
> Other burn on board Jet ski

☑x7ᵗʰ **V93.14 Other burn on board sailboat**

☑x7ᵗʰ **V93.19 Other burn on board unspecified watercraft**
> Other burn on board boat NOS
> Other burn on board ship NOS
> Other burn on board watercraft NOS

☑5ᵗʰ V93.2 Heat exposure on board watercraft
> EXCLUDES 1   *exposure to man-made heat not aboard watercraft (W92)*
> *exposure to natural heat while on board watercraft (X30)*
> *exposure to sunlight while on board watercraft (X32)*
> EXCLUDES 2   *burn due to fire on board watercraft (V93.0-)*

☑x7ᵗʰ **V93.20 Heat exposure on board merchant ship**

☑x7ᵗʰ **V93.21 Heat exposure on board passenger ship**
> Heat exposure on board Ferry-boat
> Heat exposure on board Liner

☑x7ᵗʰ **V93.22 Heat exposure on board fishing boat**

☑x7ᵗʰ **V93.23 Heat exposure on board other powered watercraft**
> Heat exposure on board hovercraft

☑x7ᵗʰ **V93.24 Heat exposure on board sailboat**

☑x7ᵗʰ **V93.29 Heat exposure on board unspecified watercraft**
> Heat exposure on board boat NOS
> Heat exposure on board ship NOS
> Heat exposure on board watercraft NOS

☑5ᵗʰ V93.3 Fall on board watercraft
> EXCLUDES 1   *fall due to collision of watercraft (V91.2-)*

☑x7ᵗʰ **V93.30 Fall on board merchant ship**

☑x7ᵗʰ **V93.31 Fall on board passenger ship**
> Fall on board Ferry-boat
> Fall on board Liner

☑x7ᵗʰ **V93.32 Fall on board fishing boat**

☑x7ᵗʰ **V93.33 Fall on board other powered watercraft**
> Fall on board Hovercraft (on open water)
> Fall on board Jet ski

☑x7ᵗʰ **V93.34 Fall on board sailboat**

☑x7ᵗʰ **V93.35 Fall on board canoe or kayak**

☑x7ᵗʰ **V93.36 Fall on board (nonpowered) inflatable craft**

☑x7ᵗʰ **V93.38 Fall on board other unpowered watercraft**

✔Additional Character Required   ☑x7ᵗʰ Placeholder   Unacceptable PDx   Questionable PDx   Wrong Procedure   Manifestation   H1 - H14 HAC   HCC CMS-HCC Dx   HIV HIV Dx

√x7ᵗʰ **V93.39 Fall on board unspecified watercraft**
Fall on board boat NOS
Fall on board ship NOS
Fall on board watercraft NOS

√5ᵗʰ **V93.4 Struck by falling object on board watercraft**
Hit by falling object on board watercraft
EXCLUDES 1 *struck by falling object due to accident to watercraft (V91.3)*

√x7ᵗʰ **V93.40 Struck by falling object on merchant ship**

√x7ᵗʰ **V93.41 Struck by falling object on passenger ship**
Struck by falling object on Ferry-boat
Struck by falling object on Liner

√x7ᵗʰ **V93.42 Struck by falling object on fishing boat**

√x7ᵗʰ **V93.43 Struck by falling object on other powered watercraft**
Struck by falling object on Hovercraft

√x7ᵗʰ **V93.44 Struck by falling object on sailboat**

√x7ᵗʰ **V93.48 Struck by falling object on other unpowered watercraft**

√x7ᵗʰ **V93.49 Struck by falling object on unspecified watercraft**

√5ᵗʰ **V93.5 Explosion on board watercraft**
Boiler explosion on steamship
EXCLUDES 2 *fire on board watercraft (V93.0-)*

√x7ᵗʰ **V93.50 Explosion on board merchant ship**

√x7ᵗʰ **V93.51 Explosion on board passenger ship**
Explosion on board Ferry-boat
Explosion on board Liner

√x7ᵗʰ **V93.52 Explosion on board fishing boat**

√x7ᵗʰ **V93.53 Explosion on board other powered watercraft**
Explosion on board Hovercraft
Explosion on board Jet ski

√x7ᵗʰ **V93.54 Explosion on board sailboat**

√x7ᵗʰ **V93.59 Explosion on board unspecified watercraft**
Explosion on board boat NOS
Explosion on board ship NOS
Explosion on board watercraft NOS

√5ᵗʰ **V93.6 Machinery accident on board watercraft**
EXCLUDES 1 *machinery explosion on board watercraft (V93.4-)*
machinery fire on board watercraft (V93.0-)

√x7ᵗʰ **V93.60 Machinery accident on board merchant ship**

√x7ᵗʰ **V93.61 Machinery accident on board passenger ship**
Machinery accident on board Ferry-boat
Machinery accident on board Liner

√x7ᵗʰ **V93.62 Machinery accident on board fishing boat**

√x7ᵗʰ **V93.63 Machinery accident on board other powered watercraft**
Machinery accident on board Hovercraft

√x7ᵗʰ **V93.64 Machinery accident on board sailboat**

√x7ᵗʰ **V93.69 Machinery accident on board unspecified watercraft**
Machinery accident on board boat NOS
Machinery accident on board ship NOS
Machinery accident on board watercraft NOS

√5ᵗʰ **V93.8 Other injury due to other accident on board watercraft**
Accidental poisoning by gases or fumes on watercraft

√x7ᵗʰ **V93.80 Other injury due to other accident on board merchant ship**

√x7ᵗʰ **V93.81 Other injury due to other accident on board passenger ship**
Other injury due to other accident on board Ferry-boat
Other injury due to other accident on board Liner

√x7ᵗʰ **V93.82 Other injury due to other accident on board fishing boat**

√x7ᵗʰ **V93.83 Other injury due to other accident on board other powered watercraft**
Other injury due to other accident on board Hovercraft
Other injury due to other accident on board Jet ski

√x7ᵗʰ **V93.84 Other injury due to other accident on board sailboat**

√x7ᵗʰ **V93.85 Other injury due to other accident on board canoe or kayak**

√x7ᵗʰ **V93.86 Other injury due to other accident on board (nonpowered) inflatable craft**

√x7ᵗʰ **V93.87 Other injury due to other accident on board water-skis**
Hit or struck by object while waterskiing

√x7ᵗʰ **V93.88 Other injury due to other accident on board other unpowered watercraft**
Hit or struck by object while surfing
Hit or struck by object while on board windsurfer

√x7ᵗʰ **V93.89 Other injury due to other accident on board unspecified watercraft**
Other injury due to other accident on board boat NOS
Other injury due to other accident on board ship NOS
Other injury due to other accident on board watercraft NOS

√4ᵗʰ **V94 Other and unspecified water transport accidents**
EXCLUDES 1 *military watercraft accidents in military or war operations (Y36, Y37)*

√x7ᵗʰ **V94.0 Hitting object or bottom of body of water due to fall from watercraft**
EXCLUDES 2 *drowning and submersion due to fall from watercraft (V92.0-)*

√5ᵗʰ **V94.1 Bather struck by watercraft**
Swimmer hit by watercraft

√x7ᵗʰ **V94.11 Bather struck by powered watercraft**

√x7ᵗʰ **V94.12 Bather struck by nonpowered watercraft**

√5ᵗʰ **V94.2 Rider of nonpowered watercraft struck by other watercraft**

√x7ᵗʰ **V94.21 Rider of nonpowered watercraft struck by other nonpowered watercraft**
Canoer hit by other nonpowered watercraft
Surfer hit by other nonpowered watercraft
Windsurfer hit by other nonpowered watercraft

√x7ᵗʰ **V94.22 Rider of nonpowered watercraft struck by powered watercraft**
Canoer hit by motorboat
Surfer hit by motorboat
Windsurfer hit by motorboat

√5ᵗʰ **V94.3 Injury to rider of (inflatable) watercraft being pulled behind other watercraft**

√x7ᵗʰ **V94.31 Injury to rider of (inflatable) recreational watercraft being pulled behind other watercraft**
Injury to rider of inner-tube pulled behind motor boat

√x7ᵗʰ **V94.32 Injury to rider of non-recreational watercraft being pulled behind other watercraft**
Injury to occupant of dingy being pulled behind boat or ship
Injury to occupant of life-raft being pulled behind boat or ship

√x7ᵗʰ **V94.4 Injury to barefoot water-skier**
Injury to person being pulled behind boat or ship

√5ᵗʰ **V94.8 Other water transport accident**

√6ᵗʰ **V94.81 Water transport accident involving military watercraft**

√7ᵗʰ **V94.810 Civilian watercraft involved in water transport accident with military watercraft**
Passenger on civilian watercraft injured due to accident with military watercraft

√7ᵗʰ **V94.811 Civilian in water injured by military watercraft**

√7ᵗʰ **V94.818 Other water transport accident involving military watercraft**

√x7ᵗʰ **V94.89 Other water transport accident**

√x7ᵗʰ **V94.9 Unspecified water transport accident**
Water transport accident NOS

Air and space transport accidents (V95-V97)

EXCLUDES 1 *military aircraft accidents in military or war operations (Y36, Y37)*

The appropriate 7th character is to be added to each code from categories V95-V97.
A   initial encounter
D   subsequent encounter
S   sequela

√4ᵗʰ **V95 Accident to powered aircraft causing injury to occupant**

√5ᵗʰ **V95.0 Helicopter accident injuring occupant**

√x7ᵗʰ **V95.00 Unspecified helicopter accident injuring occupant**

√x7ᵗʰ **V95.01 Helicopter crash injuring occupant**

√x7ᵗʰ **V95.02 Forced landing of helicopter injuring occupant**

√x7ᵗʰ **V95.03** Helicopter collision injuring occupant
Helicopter collision with any object, fixed, movable or moving

√x7ᵗʰ **V95.04** Helicopter fire injuring occupant

√x7ᵗʰ **V95.05** Helicopter explosion injuring occupant

√x7ᵗʰ **V95.09** Other helicopter accident injuring occupant

√5ᵗʰ **V95.1** Ultralight, microlight or powered-glider accident injuring occupant

√x7ᵗʰ **V95.10** Unspecified ultralight, microlight or powered-glider accident injuring occupant

√x7ᵗʰ **V95.11** Ultralight, microlight or powered-glider crash injuring occupant

√x7ᵗʰ **V95.12** Forced landing of ultralight, microlight or powered-glider injuring occupant

√x7ᵗʰ **V95.13** Ultralight, microlight or powered-glider collision injuring occupant
Ultralight, microlight or powered-glider collision with any object, fixed, movable or moving

√x7ᵗʰ **V95.14** Ultralight, microlight or powered-glider fire injuring occupant

√x7ᵗʰ **V95.15** Ultralight, microlight or powered-glider explosion injuring occupant

√x7ᵗʰ **V95.19** Other ultralight, microlight or powered-glider accident injuring occupant

√5ᵗʰ **V95.2** Other private fixed-wing aircraft accident injuring occupant

√x7ᵗʰ **V95.20** Unspecified accident to other private fixed-wing aircraft, injuring occupant

√x7ᵗʰ **V95.21** Other private fixed-wing aircraft crash injuring occupant

√x7ᵗʰ **V95.22** Forced landing of other private fixed-wing aircraft injuring occupant

√x7ᵗʰ **V95.23** Other private fixed-wing aircraft collision injuring occupant
Other private fixed-wing aircraft collision with any object, fixed, movable or moving

√x7ᵗʰ **V95.24** Other private fixed-wing aircraft fire injuring occupant

√x7ᵗʰ **V95.25** Other private fixed-wing aircraft explosion injuring occupant

√x7ᵗʰ **V95.29** Other accident to other private fixed-wing aircraft injuring occupant

√5ᵗʰ **V95.3** Commercial fixed-wing aircraft accident injuring occupant

√x7ᵗʰ **V95.30** Unspecified accident to commercial fixed-wing aircraft injuring occupant

√x7ᵗʰ **V95.31** Commercial fixed-wing aircraft crash injuring occupant

√x7ᵗʰ **V95.32** Forced landing of commercial fixed-wing aircraft injuring occupant

√x7ᵗʰ **V95.33** Commercial fixed-wing aircraft collision injuring occupant
Commercial fixed-wing aircraft collision with any object, fixed, movable or moving

√x7ᵗʰ **V95.34** Commercial fixed-wing aircraft fire injuring occupant

√x7ᵗʰ **V95.35** Commercial fixed-wing aircraft explosion injuring occupant

√x7ᵗʰ **V95.39** Other accident to commercial fixed-wing aircraft injuring occupant

√5ᵗʰ **V95.4** Spacecraft accident injuring occupant

√x7ᵗʰ **V95.40** Unspecified spacecraft accident injuring occupant

√x7ᵗʰ **V95.41** Spacecraft crash injuring occupant

√x7ᵗʰ **V95.42** Forced landing of spacecraft injuring occupant

√x7ᵗʰ **V95.43** Spacecraft collision injuring occupant
Spacecraft collision with any object, fixed, moveable or moving

√x7ᵗʰ **V95.44** Spacecraft fire injuring occupant

√x7ᵗʰ **V95.45** Spacecraft explosion injuring occupant

√x7ᵗʰ **V95.49** Other spacecraft accident injuring occupant

√x7ᵗʰ **V95.8** Other powered aircraft accidents injuring occupant

√x7ᵗʰ **V95.9** Unspecified aircraft accident injuring occupant
Aircraft accident NOS
Air transport accident NOS

√4ᵗʰ **V96** Accident to nonpowered aircraft causing injury to occupant

√5ᵗʰ **V96.0** Balloon accident injuring occupant

√x7ᵗʰ **V96.00** Unspecified balloon accident injuring occupant

√x7ᵗʰ **V96.01** Balloon crash injuring occupant

√x7ᵗʰ **V96.02** Forced landing of balloon injuring occupant

√x7ᵗʰ **V96.03** Balloon collision injuring occupant
Balloon collision with any object, fixed, moveable or moving

√x7ᵗʰ **V96.04** Balloon fire injuring occupant

√x7ᵗʰ **V96.05** Balloon explosion injuring occupant

√x7ᵗʰ **V96.09** Other balloon accident injuring occupant

√5ᵗʰ **V96.1** Hang-glider accident injuring occupant

√x7ᵗʰ **V96.10** Unspecified hang-glider accident injuring occupant

√x7ᵗʰ **V96.11** Hang-glider crash injuring occupant

√x7ᵗʰ **V96.12** Forced landing of hang-glider injuring occupant

√x7ᵗʰ **V96.13** Hang-glider collision injuring occupant
Hang-glider collision with any object, fixed, moveable or moving

√x7ᵗʰ **V96.14** Hang-glider fire injuring occupant

√x7ᵗʰ **V96.15** Hang-glider explosion injuring occupant

√x7ᵗʰ **V96.19** Other hang-glider accident injuring occupant

√5ᵗʰ **V96.2** Glider (nonpowered) accident injuring occupant

√x7ᵗʰ **V96.20** Unspecified glider (nonpowered) accident injuring occupant

√x7ᵗʰ **V96.21** Glider (nonpowered) crash injuring occupant

√x7ᵗʰ **V96.22** Forced landing of glider (nonpowered) injuring occupant

√x7ᵗʰ **V96.23** Glider (nonpowered) collision injuring occupant
Glider (nonpowered) collision with any object, fixed, moveable or moving

√x7ᵗʰ **V96.24** Glider (nonpowered) fire injuring occupant

√x7ᵗʰ **V96.25** Glider (nonpowered) explosion injuring occupant

√x7ᵗʰ **V96.29** Other glider (nonpowered) accident injuring occupant

√x7ᵗʰ **V96.8** Other nonpowered-aircraft accidents injuring occupant
Kite carrying a person accident injuring occupant

√x7ᵗʰ **V96.9** Unspecified nonpowered-aircraft accident injuring occupant
Nonpowered-aircraft accident NOS

√4ᵗʰ **V97** Other specified air transport accidents

√x7ᵗʰ **V97.0** Occupant of aircraft injured in other specified air transport accidents
Fall in, on or from aircraft in air transport accident
EXCLUDES 1 *accident while boarding or alighting aircraft (V97.1)*

√x7ᵗʰ **V97.1** Person injured while boarding or alighting from aircraft

√5ᵗʰ **V97.2** Parachutist accident

√x7ᵗʰ **V97.21** Parachutist entangled in object
Parachutist landing in tree

√x7ᵗʰ **V97.22** Parachutist injured on landing

√x7ᵗʰ **V97.29** Other parachutist accident

√5ᵗʰ **V97.3** Person on ground injured in air transport accident

√x7ᵗʰ **V97.31** Hit by object falling from aircraft
Hit by crashing aircraft
Injured by aircraft hitting house
Injured by aircraft hitting car

√x7ᵗʰ **V97.32** Injured by rotating propeller

√x7ᵗʰ **V97.33** Sucked into jet engine

√x7ᵗʰ **V97.39** Other injury to person on ground due to air transport accident

√5ᵗʰ **V97.8** Other air transport accidents, not elsewhere classified
EXCLUDES 1 *aircraft accident NOS (V95.9)*
exposure to changes in air pressure during ascent or descent (W94.-)

√6ᵗʰ **V97.81** Air transport accident involving military aircraft

√7ᵗʰ **V97.810** Civilian aircraft involved in air transport accident with military aircraft
Passenger in civilian aircraft injured due to accident with military aircraft

√7ᵗʰ **V97.811** Civilian injured by military aircraft

√7ᵗʰ **V97.818** Other air transport accident involving military aircraft

---

☑Additional Character Required   √x7ᵗʰ Placeholder   Unacceptable PDx   Questionable PDx   Wrong Procedure   Manifestation   **H1**-**H14** HAC   **HCC** CMS-HCC Dx   **HIV** HIV Dx

√x7ᵗʰ **V97.89 Other air transport accidents, not elsewhere classified**
Injury from machinery on aircraft

Other and unspecified transport accidents (V98-V99)

EXCLUDES 1   *vehicle accident, type of vehicle unspecified (V89.-)*

The appropriate 7th character is to be added to each code from categories V98-V99.
A   initial encounter
D   subsequent encounter
S   sequela

√4ᵗʰ **V98 Other specified transport accidents**

√x7ᵗʰ **V98.0 Accident to, on or involving cable-car, not on rails**
Caught or dragged by cable-car, not on rails
Fall or jump from cable-car, not on rails
Object thrown from or in cable-car, not on rails

√x7ᵗʰ **V98.1 Accident to, on or involving land-yacht**

√x7ᵗʰ **V98.2 Accident to, on or involving ice yacht**

√x7ᵗʰ **V98.3 Accident to, on or involving ski lift**
Accident to, on or involving ski chair-lift
Accident to, on or involving ski-lift with gondola

√x7ᵗʰ **V98.8 Other specified transport accidents**

√x7ᵗʰ **V99 Unspecified transport accident**

OTHER EXTERNAL CAUSES OF ACCIDENTAL INJURY (W00-X58)

Slipping, tripping, stumbling and falls (W00-W19)

EXCLUDES 1   *assault involving a fall (Y01-Y02)*
fall from animal (V80.-)
fall (in) (from) machinery (in operation) (W28-W31)
fall (in) (from) transport vehicle (V01-V99)
intentional self-harm involving a fall (X80-X81)
EXCLUDES 2   *at risk for fall (history of fall) (Z91.81)*
fall (in) (from) burning building (X00.-)
fall into fire (X00-X04, X08)

The appropriate 7th character is to be added to each code from category W00-W19.
A   initial encounter
D   subsequent encounter
S   sequela

√4ᵗʰ **W00 Fall due to ice and snow**
INCLUDES   pedestrian on foot falling (slipping) on ice and snow
EXCLUDES 1   *fall on (from) ice and snow involving pedestrian conveyance (V00.-)*
fall from stairs and steps not due to ice and snow (W10.-)
AHA: 2016, 2Q, 4

√x7ᵗʰ **W00.0 Fall on same level due to ice and snow**

√x7ᵗʰ **W00.1 Fall from stairs and steps due to ice and snow**

√x7ᵗʰ **W00.2 Other fall from one level to another due to ice and snow**

√x7ᵗʰ **W00.9 Unspecified fall due to ice and snow**

√4ᵗʰ **W01 Fall on same level from slipping, tripping and stumbling**
INCLUDES   fall on moving sidewalk
EXCLUDES 1   *fall due to bumping (striking) against object (W18.0-)*
fall in shower or bathtub (W18.2-)
fall on same level NOS (W18.30)
fall on same level from slipping, tripping and stumbling due to ice or snow (W00.0)
fall off or from toilet (W18.1-)
slipping, tripping and stumbling NOS (W18.40)
slipping, tripping and stumbling without falling (W18.4-)

√x7ᵗʰ **W01.0 Fall on same level from slipping, tripping and stumbling without subsequent striking against object**
Falling over animal

√5ᵗʰ **W01.1 Fall on same level from slipping, tripping and stumbling with subsequent striking against object**

√x7ᵗʰ **W01.10 Fall on same level from slipping, tripping and stumbling with subsequent striking against unspecified object**

√6ᵗʰ **W01.11 Fall on same level from slipping, tripping and stumbling with subsequent striking against sharp object**

√7ᵗʰ **W01.110 Fall on same level from slipping, tripping and stumbling with subsequent striking against sharp glass**

√7ᵗʰ **W01.111 Fall on same level from slipping, tripping and stumbling with subsequent striking against power tool or machine**

√7ᵗʰ **W01.118 Fall on same level from slipping, tripping and stumbling with subsequent striking against other sharp object**

√7ᵗʰ **W01.119 Fall on same level from slipping, tripping and stumbling with subsequent striking against unspecified sharp object**

√6ᵗʰ **W01.19 Fall on same level from slipping, tripping and stumbling with subsequent striking against other object**

√7ᵗʰ **W01.190 Fall on same level from slipping, tripping and stumbling with subsequent striking against furniture**

√7ᵗʰ **W01.198 Fall on same level from slipping, tripping and stumbling with subsequent striking against other object**

√x7ᵗʰ **W03 Other fall on same level due to collision with another person**
Fall due to non-transport collision with other person
EXCLUDES 1   *collision with another person without fall (W51)*
crushed or pushed by a crowd or human stampede (W52)
fall involving pedestrian conveyance (V00-V09)
fall due to ice or snow (W00)
fall on same level NOS (W18.30)
AHA: 2012, 4Q, 108

√x7ᵗʰ **W04 Fall while being carried or supported by other persons**
Accidentally dropped while being carried

√4ᵗʰ **W05 Fall from non-moving wheelchair, nonmotorized scooter and motorized mobility scooter**
EXCLUDES 1   *fall from moving motorized mobility scooter (V00.831)*
fall from moving wheelchair (powered) (V00.811)
fall from nonmotorized scooter (V00.141)

√x7ᵗʰ **W05.0 Fall from non-moving wheelchair**

√x7ᵗʰ **W05.1 Fall from non-moving nonmotorized scooter**

√x7ᵗʰ **W05.2 Fall from non-moving motorized mobility scooter**

√x7ᵗʰ **W06 Fall from bed**

√x7ᵗʰ **W07 Fall from chair**

√x7ᵗʰ **W08 Fall from other furniture**

√4ᵗʰ **W09 Fall on and from playground equipment**
EXCLUDES 1   *fall involving recreational machinery (W31)*

√x7ᵗʰ **W09.0 Fall on or from playground slide**

√x7ᵗʰ **W09.1 Fall from playground swing**

√x7ᵗʰ **W09.2 Fall on or from jungle gym**

√x7ᵗʰ **W09.8 Fall on or from other playground equipment**

√4ᵗʰ **W10 Fall on and from stairs and steps**
EXCLUDES 1   *Fall from stairs and steps due to ice and snow (W00.1)*

√x7ᵗʰ **W10.0 Fall (on)(from) escalator**

√x7ᵗʰ **W10.1 Fall (on)(from) sidewalk curb**

√x7ᵗʰ **W10.2 Fall (on)(from) incline**
Fall (on) (from) ramp

√x7ᵗʰ **W10.8 Fall (on) (from) other stairs and steps**

√x7ᵗʰ **W10.9 Fall (on) (from) unspecified stairs and steps**

√x7ᵗʰ **W11 Fall on and from ladder**

√x7ᵗʰ **W12 Fall on and from scaffolding**

√4ᵗʰ **W13 Fall from, out of or through building or structure**

√x7ᵗʰ **W13.0 Fall from, out of or through balcony**
Fall from, out of or through railing

√x7ᵗʰ **W13.1 Fall from, out of or through bridge**

√x7ᵗʰ **W13.2 Fall from, out of or through roof**

√x7ᵗʰ **W13.3 Fall through floor**

√x7ᵗʰ **W13.4 Fall from, out of or through window**
EXCLUDES 2   *fall with subsequent striking against sharp glass (W01.110)*

√x7ᵗʰ **W13.8 Fall from, out of or through other building or structure**
Fall from, out of or through viaduct
Fall from, out of or through wall
Fall from, out of or through flag-pole

√x7ᵗʰ **W13.9 Fall from, out of or through building, not otherwise specified**
EXCLUDES 1   *collapse of a building or structure (W20.-)*
fall or jump from burning building or structure (X00.-)

N Newborn: 0   **P** Pediatric: 0-17   **M** Maternity: 12-55   **A** Adult: 15-124   **MCC** Major Complication/Comorbidity   **CC** Complication/Comorbidity   **SW** Severe Wound Dx

1188   ICD-10-CM 2019

√x7th **W14 Fall from tree**

√x7th **W15 Fall from cliff**

√4th **W16 Fall, jump or diving into water**

> EXCLUDES 1   accidental non-watercraft drowning and submersion not involving fall (W65-W74)
> effects of air pressure from diving (W94.-)
> fall into water from watercraft (V90-V94)
> hitting an object or against bottom when falling from watercraft (V94.0)
>
> EXCLUDES 2   striking or hitting diving board (W21.4)

√5th **W16.0 Fall into swimming pool**
> Fall into swimming pool NOS
> EXCLUDES 1   fall into empty swimming pool (W17.3)

√6th **W16.01 Fall into swimming pool striking water surface**

√7th **W16.011 Fall into swimming pool striking water surface causing drowning and submersion**
> EXCLUDES 1   drowning and submersion while in swimming pool without fall (W67)

√7th **W16.012 Fall into swimming pool striking water surface causing other injury**

√6th **W16.02 Fall into swimming pool striking bottom**

√7th **W16.021 Fall into swimming pool striking bottom causing drowning and submersion**
> EXCLUDES 1   drowning and submersion while in swimming pool without fall (W67)

√7th **W16.022 Fall into swimming pool striking bottom causing other injury**

√6th **W16.03 Fall into swimming pool striking wall**

√7th **W16.031 Fall into swimming pool striking wall causing drowning and submersion**
> EXCLUDES 1   drowning and submersion while in swimming pool without fall (W67)

√7th **W16.032 Fall into swimming pool striking wall causing other injury**

√5th **W16.1 Fall into natural body of water**
> Fall into laker
> Fall into open sea
> Fall into river
> Fall into stream

√6th **W16.11 Fall into natural body of water striking water surface**

√7th **W16.111 Fall into natural body of water striking water surface causing drowning and submersion**
> EXCLUDES 1   drowning and submersion while in natural body of water without fall (W69)

√7th **W16.112 Fall into natural body of water striking water surface causing other injury**

√6th **W16.12 Fall into natural body of water striking bottom**

√7th **W16.121 Fall into natural body of water striking bottom causing drowning and submersion**
> EXCLUDES 1   drowning and submersion while in natural body of water without fall (W69)

√7th **W16.122 Fall into natural body of water striking bottom causing other injury**

√6th **W16.13 Fall into natural body of water striking side**

√7th **W16.131 Fall into natural body of water striking side causing drowning and submersion**
> EXCLUDES 1   drowning and submersion while in natural body of water without fall (W69)

√7th **W16.132 Fall into natural body of water striking side causing other injury**

√5th **W16.2 Fall in (into) filled bathtub or bucket of water**

√6th **W16.21 Fall in (into) filled bathtub**
> EXCLUDES 1   fall into empty bathtub (W18.2)

√7th **W16.211 Fall in (into) filled bathtub causing drowning and submersion**
> EXCLUDES 1   drowning and submersion while in filled bathtub without fall (W65)

√7th **W16.212 Fall in (into) filled bathtub causing other injury**

√6th **W16.22 Fall in (into) bucket of water**

√7th **W16.221 Fall in (into) bucket of water causing drowning and submersion**

√7th **W16.222 Fall in (into) bucket of water causing other injury**

√5th **W16.3 Fall into other water**
> Fall into fountain
> Fall into reservoir

√6th **W16.31 Fall into other water striking water surface**

√7th **W16.311 Fall into other water striking water surface causing drowning and submersion**
> EXCLUDES 1   drowning and submersion while in other water without fall (W73)

√7th **W16.312 Fall into other water striking water surface causing other injury**

√6th **W16.32 Fall into other water striking bottom**

√7th **W16.321 Fall into other water striking bottom causing drowning and submersion**
> EXCLUDES 1   drowning and submersion while in other water without fall (W73)

√7th **W16.322 Fall into other water striking bottom causing other injury**

√6th **W16.33 Fall into other water striking wall**

√7th **W16.331 Fall into other water striking wall causing drowning and submersion**
> EXCLUDES 1   drowning and submersion while in other water without fall (W73)

√7th **W16.332 Fall into other water striking wall causing other injury**

√5th **W16.4 Fall into unspecified water**

√x7th **W16.41 Fall into unspecified water causing drowning and submersion**

√x7th **W16.42 Fall into unspecified water causing other injury**

√5th **W16.5 Jumping or diving into swimming pool**

√6th **W16.51 Jumping or diving into swimming pool striking water surface**

√7th **W16.511 Jumping or diving into swimming pool striking water surface causing drowning and submersion**
> EXCLUDES 1   drowning and submersion while in swimming pool without jumping or diving (W67)

√7th **W16.512 Jumping or diving into swimming pool striking water surface causing other injury**

√6th **W16.52 Jumping or diving into swimming pool striking bottom**

√7th **W16.521 Jumping or diving into swimming pool striking bottom causing drowning and submersion**
> EXCLUDES 1   drowning and submersion while in swimming pool without jumping or diving (W67)

√7th **W16.522 Jumping or diving into swimming pool striking bottom causing other injury**

√6th **W16.53 Jumping or diving into swimming pool striking wall**

√7th **W16.531 Jumping or diving into swimming pool striking wall causing drowning and submersion**
> EXCLUDES 1   drowning and submersion while in swimming pool without jumping or diving (W67)

√7th **W16.532 Jumping or diving into swimming pool striking wall causing other injury**

✓Additional Character Required   √x7th Placeholder   Unacceptable PDx   Questionable PDx   Wrong Procedure   Manifestation   H1-H14 HAC   HCC CMS-HCC Dx   HIV HIV Dx

Chapter 20. External Causes of Morbidity

W16.6–W19

✓5th **W16.6 Jumping or diving into** natural body of water
Jumping or diving into lake
Jumping or diving into open sea
Jumping or diving into river
Jumping or diving into stream

  ✓6th **W16.61 Jumping or diving into natural body of water striking water surface**

    ✓7th **W16.611 Jumping or diving into natural body of water striking water surface causing** drowning **and submersion**
EXCLUDES 1 *drowning and submersion while in natural body of water without jumping or diving (W69)*

    ✓7th **W16.612 Jumping or diving into natural body of water striking water surface causing** other injury

  ✓6th **W16.62 Jumping or diving into natural body of water striking bottom**

    ✓7th **W16.621 Jumping or diving into natural body of water striking bottom causing** drowning **and submersion**
EXCLUDES 1 *drowning and submersion while in natural body of water without jumping or diving (W69)*

    ✓7th **W16.622 Jumping or diving into natural body of water striking bottom causing** other injury

✓5th **W16.7 Jumping or diving** from boat
EXCLUDES 1 *fall from boat into water—see watercraft accident (V90-V94)*

  ✓6th **W16.71 Jumping or diving from boat** striking water surface

    ✓7th **W16.711 Jumping or diving from boat striking water surface causing** drowning **and submersion**

    ✓7th **W16.712 Jumping or diving from boat striking water surface causing** other injury

  ✓6th **W16.72 Jumping or diving from boat** striking bottom

    ✓7th **W16.721 Jumping or diving from boat striking bottom causing** drowning **and submersion**

    ✓7th **W16.722 Jumping or diving from boat striking bottom causing** other injury

✓5th **W16.8 Jumping or diving** into other water
Jumping or diving into fountain
Jumping or diving into reservoir

  ✓6th **W16.81 Jumping or diving into other water** striking water surface

    ✓7th **W16.811 Jumping or diving into other water striking water surface causing** drowning **and submersion**
EXCLUDES 1 *drowning and submersion while in other water without jumping or diving (W73)*

    ✓7th **W16.812 Jumping or diving into other water striking water surface causing** other injury

  ✓6th **W16.82 Jumping or diving into other water** striking bottom

    ✓7th **W16.821 Jumping or diving into other water striking bottom causing** drowning **and submersion**
EXCLUDES 1 *drowning and submersion while in other water without jumping or diving (W73)*

    ✓7th **W16.822 Jumping or diving into other water striking bottom causing** other injury

  ✓6th **W16.83 Jumping or diving into other water** striking wall

    ✓7th **W16.831 Jumping or diving into other water striking wall causing** drowning **and submersion**
EXCLUDES 1 *drowning and submersion while in other water without jumping or diving (W73)*

    ✓7th **W16.832 Jumping or diving into other water striking wall causing** other injury

✓5th **W16.9 Jumping or diving into** unspecified water

  ✓x7th **W16.91 Jumping or diving into unspecified water causing** drowning **and submersion**

  ✓x7th **W16.92 Jumping or diving into unspecified water causing** other injury

✓4th **W17 Other fall from one level to another**

  ✓x7th **W17.0 Fall into well**

  ✓x7th **W17.1 Fall into storm drain or manhole**

  ✓x7th **W17.2 Fall into hole**
Fall into pit

  ✓x7th **W17.3 Fall into empty swimming pool**
EXCLUDES 1 *fall into filled swimming pool (W16.0-)*

  ✓x7th **W17.4 Fall from dock**

  ✓5th **W17.8 Other fall from one level to another**

    ✓x7th **W17.81 Fall down embankment (hill)**

    ✓x7th **W17.82 Fall from (out of) grocery cart**
Fall due to grocery cart tipping over

    ✓x7th **W17.89 Other fall from one level to another**
Fall from cherry picker
Fall from lifting device
Fall from mobile elevated work platform [MEWP]
Fall from sky lift
AHA: 2015, 2Q, 6

✓4th **W18 Other slipping, tripping and stumbling and falls**

  ✓5th **W18.0 Fall due to bumping against object**
Striking against object with subsequent fall
EXCLUDES 1 *fall on same level due to slipping, tripping, or stumbling with subsequent striking against object (W01.1-)*

    ✓x7th **W18.00 Striking against** unspecified **object with subsequent fall**

    ✓x7th **W18.01 Striking against** sports equipment **with subsequent fall**

    ✓x7th **W18.02 Striking against** glass **with subsequent fall**

    ✓x7th **W18.09 Striking against** other **object with subsequent fall**

  ✓5th **W18.1 Fall from or off toilet**

    ✓x7th **W18.11 Fall from or off toilet** without subsequent striking against object
Fall from (off) toilet NOS

    ✓x7th **W18.12 Fall from or off toilet** with subsequent striking against object

  ✓x7th **W18.2 Fall in (into) shower or empty bathtub**
EXCLUDES 1 *fall in full bathtub causing drowning or submersion (W16.21-)*

  ✓5th **W18.3 Other and unspecified fall on same level**

    ✓x7th **W18.30 Fall on same level, unspecified**

    ✓x7th **W18.31 Fall on same level due to stepping on an object**
Fall on same level due to stepping on an animal
EXCLUDES 1 *slipping, tripping and stumbling without fall due to stepping on animal (W18.41)*

    ✓x7th **W18.39 Other fall on same level**

  ✓5th **W18.4 Slipping, tripping and stumbling without falling**
EXCLUDES 1 *collision with another person without fall (W51)*

    ✓x7th **W18.40 Slipping, tripping and stumbling without falling, unspecified**

    ✓x7th **W18.41 Slipping, tripping and stumbling without falling due to** stepping on object
Slipping, tripping and stumbling without falling due to stepping on animal
EXCLUDES 1 *slipping, tripping and stumbling with fall due to stepping on animal (W18.31)*

    ✓x7th **W18.42 Slipping, tripping and stumbling without falling due to** stepping into hole or opening

    ✓x7th **W18.43 Slipping, tripping and stumbling without falling due to** stepping from one level to another

    ✓x7th **W18.49 Other** slipping, tripping and stumbling without falling

✓x7th **W19 Unspecified fall**
Accidental fall NOS
AHA: 2012, 4Q, 95

N Newborn: 0   P Pediatric: 0-17   M Maternity: 12-55   A Adult: 15-124   MCC Major Complication/Comorbidity   CC Complication/Comorbidity   SW Severe Wound Dx

1190   ICD-10-CM 2019

Exposure to inanimate mechanical forces (W20-W49)

EXCLUDES 1   assault (X92-Y09)
     contact or collision with animals or persons (W50-W64)
     exposure to inanimate mechanical forces involving military or war
        operations (Y36.-, Y37.-)
     intentional self-harm (X71-X83)

The appropriate 7th character is to be added to each code from categories
W20-W49.
A   initial encounter
D   subsequent encounter
S   sequela

✓4th W20 Struck by thrown, projected or falling object

Code first any associated:
     cataclysm (X34-X39)
     lightning strike (T75.00)

EXCLUDES 1   falling object in machinery accident (W24, W28-W31)
     falling object in transport accident (V01-V99)
     object set in motion by explosion (W35-W40)
     object set in motion by firearm (W32-W34)
     struck by thrown sports equipment (W21.-)

✓x7th **W20.0 Struck by falling object in cave-in**
     EXCLUDES 2   asphyxiation due to cave-in (T71.21)

✓x7th **W20.1 Struck by object due to collapse of building**
     EXCLUDES 1   struck by object due to collapse of burning building
         (X00.2, X02.2)

✓x7th **W20.8 Other cause of strike by thrown, projected or falling object**
     EXCLUDES 1   struck by thrown sports equipment (W21.-)

✓4th W21 Striking against or struck by sports equipment

EXCLUDES 1   assault with sports equipment (Y08.0-)
     striking against or struck by sports equipment with subsequent
        fall (W18.01)

✓5th **W21.0 Struck by hit or thrown ball**

   ✓x7th **W21.00 Struck by hit or thrown ball, unspecified type**

   ✓x7th **W21.01 Struck by football**

   ✓x7th **W21.02 Struck by soccer ball**

   ✓x7th **W21.03 Struck by baseball**

   ✓x7th **W21.04 Struck by golf ball**

   ✓x7th **W21.05 Struck by basketball**

   ✓x7th **W21.06 Struck by volleyball**

   ✓x7th **W21.07 Struck by softball**

   ✓x7th **W21.09 Struck by other hit or thrown ball**

✓5th **W21.1 Struck by bat, racquet or club**

   ✓x7th **W21.11 Struck by baseball bat**

   ✓x7th **W21.12 Struck by tennis racquet**

   ✓x7th **W21.13 Struck by golf club**

   ✓x7th **W21.19 Struck by other bat, racquet or club**

✓5th **W21.2 Struck by hockey stick or puck**

   ✓6th **W21.21 Struck by hockey stick**

     ✓7th **W21.210 Struck by ice hockey stick**

     ✓7th **W21.211 Struck by field hockey stick**

   ✓6th **W21.22 Struck by hockey puck**

     ✓7th **W21.220 Struck by ice hockey puck**

     ✓7th **W21.221 Struck by field hockey puck**

✓5th **W21.3 Struck by sports foot wear**

   ✓x7th **W21.31 Struck by shoe cleats**
       Stepped on by shoe cleats

   ✓x7th **W21.32 Struck by skate blades**
       Skated over by skate blades

   ✓x7th **W21.39 Struck by other sports foot wear**

✓x7th **W21.4 Striking against diving board**
     Use additional code for subsequent falling into water, if
       applicable (W16.-)

✓5th **W21.8 Striking against or struck by other sports equipment**

   ✓x7th **W21.81 Striking against or struck by football helmet**

   ✓x7th **W21.89 Striking against or struck by other sports equipment**

✓x7th **W21.9 Striking against or struck by unspecified sports equipment**

✓4th W22 Striking against or struck by other objects

EXCLUDES 1   striking against or struck by object with subsequent fall
     (W18.09)

✓5th **W22.0 Striking against stationary object**
     EXCLUDES 1   striking against stationary sports equipment (W21.8)

   ✓x7th **W22.01 Walked into wall**

   ✓x7th **W22.02 Walked into lamppost**

   ✓x7th **W22.03 Walked into furniture**

   ✓6th **W22.04 Striking against wall of swimming pool**

     ✓7th **W22.041 Striking against wall of swimming pool
         causing drowning and submersion**
         EXCLUDES 1   drowning and submersion while
             swimming without striking
             against wall (W67)

     ✓7th **W22.042 Striking against wall of swimming pool
         causing other injury**

   ✓x7th **W22.09 Striking against other stationary object**

✓5th **W22.1 Striking against or struck by automobile airbag**

   ✓x7th **W22.10 Striking against or struck by unspecified automobile
       airbag**

   ✓x7th **W22.11 Striking against or struck by driver side automobile
       airbag**

   ✓x7th **W22.12 Striking against or struck by front passenger side
       automobile airbag**

   ✓x7th **W22.19 Striking against or struck by other automobile
       airbag**

✓x7th **W22.8 Striking against or struck by other objects**
     Striking against or struck by object NOS
     EXCLUDES 1   struck by thrown, projected or falling object (W20.-)

✓4th W23 Caught, crushed, jammed or pinched in or between objects

EXCLUDES 1   injury caused by cutting or piercing instruments (W25-W27)
     injury caused by firearms malfunction (W32.1, W33.1-, W34.1-)
     injury caused by lifting and transmission devices (W24.-)
     injury caused by machinery (W28-W31)
     injury caused by nonpowered hand tools (W27.-)
     injury caused by transport vehicle being used as a means of
        transportation (V01-V99)
     injury caused by struck by thrown, projected or falling object
        (W20.-)

✓x7th **W23.0 Caught, crushed, jammed, or pinched between moving
     objects**

✓x7th **W23.1 Caught, crushed, jammed, or pinched between stationary
     objects**

✓4th W24 Contact with lifting and transmission devices, not elsewhere classified

EXCLUDES 1   transport accidents (V01-V99)

✓x7th **W24.0 Contact with lifting devices, not elsewhere classified**
     Contact with chain hoist
     Contact with drive belt
     Contact with pulley (block)

✓x7th **W24.1 Contact with transmission devices, not elsewhere classified**
     Contact with transmission belt or cable

✓x7th W25 Contact with sharp glass

Code first any associated:
     injury due to flying glass from explosion or firearm discharge (W32-
       W40)
     transport accident (V00-V99)

EXCLUDES 1   fall on same level due to slipping, tripping and stumbling with
        subsequent striking against sharp glass (W01.10)
     striking against sharp glass with subsequent fall (W18.02)

EXCLUDES 2   glass embedded in skin (W45)

✓4th W26 Contact with other sharp objects

EXCLUDES 2   sharp object(s) embedded in skin (W45)

AHA: 2016, 4Q, 73

✓x7th **W26.0 Contact with knife**
     EXCLUDES 1   contact with electric knife (W29.1)

✓x7th **W26.1 Contact with sword or dagger**

✓x7th **W26.2 Contact with edge of stiff paper**
     Paper cut

✓x7th **W26.8 Contact with other sharp object(s), not elsewhere classified**
     Contact with tin can lid

✓x7th **W26.9 Contact with unspecified sharp object(s)**

✓Additional Character Required   ✓x7th Placeholder   Unacceptable PDx   Questionable PDx   Wrong Procedure   Manifestation   H1 -H14 HAC   HCC CMS-HCC Dx   HIV HIV Dx

ICD-10-CM 2019   1191

☑4ᵗʰ **W27 Contact with nonpowered hand tool**

  √x7ᵗʰ **W27.0 Contact with workbench tool**
Contact with auger   Contact with handsaw
Contact with axe   Contact with screwdriver
Contact with chisel

  √x7ᵗʰ **W27.1 Contact with garden tool**
Contact with hoe
Contact with nonpowered lawn mower
Contact with pitchfork
Contact with rake

  √x7ᵗʰ **W27.2 Contact with scissors**

  √x7ᵗʰ **W27.3 Contact with needle (sewing)**
    EXCLUDES 1   *contact with hypodermic needle (W46.-)*

  √x7ᵗʰ **W27.4 Contact with kitchen utensil**
Contact with fork
Contact with ice-pick
Contact with can-opener NOS

  √x7ᵗʰ **W27.5 Contact with paper-cutter**

  √x7ᵗʰ **W27.8 Contact with other nonpowered hand tool**
Contact with nonpowered sewing machine
Contact with shovel

√x7ᵗʰ **W28 Contact with powered lawn mower**
Powered lawn mower (commercial) (residential)
  EXCLUDES 1   *contact with nonpowered lawn mower (W27.1)*
  EXCLUDES 2   *exposure to electric current (W86.-)*

☑4ᵗʰ **W29 Contact with other powered hand tools and household machinery**
  EXCLUDES 1   *contact with commercial machinery (W31.82)*
        contact with hot household appliance (X15)
        contact with nonpowered hand tool (W27.-)
        exposure to electric current (W86)

  √x7ᵗʰ **W29.0 Contact with powered kitchen appliance**
Contact with blender   Contact with garbage disposal
Contact with can-opener   Contact with mixer

  √x7ᵗʰ **W29.1 Contact with electric knife**

  √x7ᵗʰ **W29.2 Contact with other powered household machinery**
Contact with electric fan
Contact with powered dryer (clothes) (powered)
Contact with washing-machine
Contact with sewing machine

  √x7ᵗʰ **W29.3 Contact with powered garden and outdoor hand tools and machinery**
Contact with chainsaw
Contact with edger
Contact with garden cultivator (tiller)
Contact with hedge trimmer
Contact with other powered garden tool
    EXCLUDES 1   *contact with powered lawn mower (W28)*

  √x7ᵗʰ **W29.4 Contact with nail gun**

  √x7ᵗʰ **W29.8 Contact with other powered hand tools and household machinery**
Contact with do-it-yourself tool NOS

☑4ᵗʰ **W30 Contact with agricultural machinery**
  INCLUDES   animal-powered farm machine
  EXCLUDES 1   *agricultural transport vehicle accident (V01-V99)*
        explosion of grain store (W40.8)
        exposure to electric current (W86.-)

  √x7ᵗʰ **W30.0 Contact with combine harvester**
Contact with reaper   Contact with thresher

  √x7ᵗʰ **W30.1 Contact with power take-off devices (PTO)**

  √x7ᵗʰ **W30.2 Contact with hay derrick**

  √x7ᵗʰ **W30.3 Contact with grain storage elevator**
    EXCLUDES 1   *explosion of grain store (W40.8)*

  √5ᵗʰ **W30.8 Contact with other specified agricultural machinery**

    √x7ᵗʰ **W30.81 Contact with agricultural transport vehicle in stationary use**
Contact with agricultural transport vehicle under repair, not on public roadway
      EXCLUDES 1   *agricultural transport vehicle accident (V01-V99)*

    √x7ᵗʰ **W30.89 Contact with other specified agricultural machinery**

  √x7ᵗʰ **W30.9 Contact with unspecified agricultural machinery**
Contact with farm machinery NOS

☑4ᵗʰ **W31 Contact with other and unspecified machinery**
  EXCLUDES 1   *contact with agricultural machinery (W30.-)*
        contact with machinery in transport under own power or being towed by a vehicle (V01-V99)
        exposure to electric current (W86)

  √x7ᵗʰ **W31.0 Contact with mining and earth-drilling machinery**
Contact with bore or drill (land) (seabed)
Contact with shaft hoist
Contact with shaft lift
Contact with undercutter

  √x7ᵗʰ **W31.1 Contact with metalworking machines**
Contact with abrasive wheel
Contact with forging machine
Contact with lathe
Contact with mechanical shears
Contact with metal drilling machine
Contact with milling machine
Contact with power press
Contact with rolling-mill
Contact with metal sawing machine

  √x7ᵗʰ **W31.2 Contact with powered woodworking and forming machines**
Contact with band saw   Contact with overhead plane
Contact with bench saw   Contact with powered saw
Contact with circular saw   Contact with radial saw
Contact with molding machine   Contact with sander
    EXCLUDES 1   *nonpowered woodworking tools (W27.0)*

  √x7ᵗʰ **W31.3 Contact with prime movers**
Contact with gas turbine
Contact with internal combustion engine
Contact with steam engine
Contact with water driven turbine

  √5ᵗʰ **W31.8 Contact with other specified machinery**

    √x7ᵗʰ **W31.81 Contact with recreational machinery**
Contact with roller coaster

    √x7ᵗʰ **W31.82 Contact with other commercial machinery**
Contact with commercial electric fan
Contact with commercial kitchen appliances
Contact with commercial powered dryer (clothes) (powered) (spin)
Contact with commercial washing-machine
Contact with commercial sewing machine
      EXCLUDES 1   *contact with household machinery (W29.-)*
          contact with powered lawn mower (W28)

    √x7ᵗʰ **W31.83 Contact with special construction vehicle in stationary use**
Contact with special construction vehicle under repair, not on public roadway
      EXCLUDES 1   *special construction vehicle accident (V01-V99)*

    √x7ᵗʰ **W31.89 Contact with other specified machinery**

  √x7ᵗʰ **W31.9 Contact with unspecified machinery**
Contact with machinery NOS

☑4ᵗʰ **W32 Accidental handgun discharge and malfunction**
  INCLUDES   accidental discharge and malfunction of gun for single hand use
        accidental discharge and malfunction of pistol
        accidental discharge and malfunction of revolver
        handgun discharge and malfunction NOS
  EXCLUDES 1   *accidental airgun discharge and malfunction (W34.010, W34.110)*
        accidental BB gun discharge and malfunction (W34.010, W34.110)
        accidental pellet gun discharge and malfunction (W34.010, W34.110)
        accidental shotgun discharge and malfunction (W33.01, W33.11)
        assault by handgun discharge (X93)
        handgun discharge involving legal intervention (Y35.0-)
        handgun discharge involving military or war operations (Y36.4-)
        intentional self-harm by handgun discharge (X72)
        Very pistol discharge and malfunction (W34.09, W34.19)

  √x7ᵗʰ **W32.0 Accidental handgun discharge**

  √x7ᵗʰ **W32.1 Accidental handgun malfunction**
Injury due to explosion of handgun (parts)
Injury due to malfunction of mechanism or component of handgun
Injury due to recoil of handgun
Powder burn from handgun

N Newborn: 0   **P** Pediatric: 0-17   **M** Maternity: 12-55   **A** Adult: 15-124   **MCC** Major Complication/Comorbidity   **CC** Complication/Comorbidity   **SW** Severe Wound Dx

1192   ICD-10-CM 2019

✅4ᵗʰ **W33 Accidental** rifle, shotgun and larger firearm **discharge and malfunction**

> INCLUDES   rifle, shotgun and larger firearm discharge and malfunction NOS
>
> EXCLUDES 1   *accidental airgun discharge and malfunction (W34.010, W34.110)*
> *accidental BB gun discharge and malfunction (W34.010, W34.110)*
> *accidental handgun discharge and malfunction (W32.-)*
> *accidental pellet gun discharge and malfunction (W34.010, W34.110)*
> *assault by rifle, shotgun and larger firearm discharge (X94)*
> *firearm discharge involving legal intervention (Y35.0-)*
> *firearm discharge involving military or war operations (Y36.4-)*
> *intentional self-harm by rifle, shotgun and larger firearm discharge (X73)*

✅5ᵗʰ **W33.0 Accidental rifle, shotgun and larger firearm** discharge

   ✓x7ᵗʰ **W33.00 Accidental discharge of** unspecified **larger firearm**
     Discharge of unspecified larger firearm NOS

   ✓x7ᵗʰ **W33.01 Accidental discharge of** shotgun
     Discharge of shotgun NOS

   ✓x7ᵗʰ **W33.02 Accidental discharge of** hunting rifle
     Discharge of hunting rifle NOS

   ✓x7ᵗʰ **W33.03 Accidental discharge of** machine gun
     Discharge of machine gun NOS

   ✓x7ᵗʰ **W33.09 Accidental discharge of** other **larger firearm**
     Discharge of other larger firearm NOS

✅5ᵗʰ **W33.1 Accidental rifle, shotgun and larger firearm** malfunction

     Injury due to explosion of rifle, shotgun and larger firearm (parts)
     Injury due to malfunction of mechanism or component of rifle, shotgun and larger firearm
     Injury due to piercing, cutting, crushing or pinching due to (by) slide trigger mechanism, scope or other gun part
     Injury due to recoil of rifle, shotgun and larger firearm
     Powder burn from rifle, shotgun and larger firearm

   ✓x7ᵗʰ **W33.10 Accidental malfunction of** unspecified **larger firearm**
     Malfunction of unspecified larger firearm NOS

   ✓x7ᵗʰ **W33.11 Accidental malfunction of** shotgun
     Malfunction of shotgun NOS

   ✓x7ᵗʰ **W33.12 Accidental malfunction of** hunting rifle
     Malfunction of hunting rifle NOS

   ✓x7ᵗʰ **W33.13 Accidental malfunction of** machine gun
     Malfunction of machine gun NOS

   ✓x7ᵗʰ **W33.19 Accidental malfunction of** other **larger firearm**
     Malfunction of other larger firearm NOS

✅4ᵗʰ **W34 Accidental discharge and malfunction from other and unspecified firearms and guns**

✅5ᵗʰ **W34.0 Accidental** discharge **from other and unspecified firearms and guns**

   ✓x7ᵗʰ **W34.00 Accidental discharge from** unspecified **firearms or gun**
     Discharge from firearm NOS
     Gunshot wound NOS
     Shot NOS

   ✓6ᵗʰ **W34.01 Accidental discharge of** gas, air or spring-operated **guns**

     ✓7ᵗʰ **W34.010 Accidental discharge of** airgun
       Accidental discharge of BB gun
       Accidental discharge of pellet gun

     ✓7ᵗʰ **W34.011 Accidental discharge of** paintball gun
       Accidental injury due to paintball discharge

     ✓7ᵗʰ **W34.018 Accidental discharge of** other **gas, air or spring-operated gun**

   ✓x7ᵗʰ **W34.09 Accidental discharge from** other **specified firearms**
     Accidental discharge from Very pistol [flare]

✅5ᵗʰ **W34.1 Accidental** malfunction **from other and unspecified firearms and guns**

   ✓x7ᵗʰ **W34.10 Accidental malfunction from** unspecified **firearms or gun**
     Firearm malfunction NOS

   ✓6ᵗʰ **W34.11 Accidental malfunction of** gas, air or spring-**operated guns**

     ✓7ᵗʰ **W34.110 Accidental malfunction of** airgun
       Accidental malfunction of BB gun
       Accidental malfunction of pellet gun

     ✓7ᵗʰ **W34.111 Accidental malfunction of** paintball gun
       Accidental injury due to paintball gun malfunction

     ✓7ᵗʰ **W34.118 Accidental malfunction of** other **gas, air or spring-operated gun**

   ✓x7ᵗʰ **W34.19 Accidental malfunction from** other **specified firearms**
     Accidental malfunction from Very pistol [flare]

✓x7ᵗʰ **W35 Explosion and rupture of boiler**

> EXCLUDES 1   *explosion and rupture of boiler on watercraft (V93.4)*

✅4ᵗʰ **W36 Explosion and rupture of** gas cylinder

   ✓x7ᵗʰ **W36.1 Explosion and rupture of** aerosol can

   ✓x7ᵗʰ **W36.2 Explosion and rupture of** air tank

   ✓x7ᵗʰ **W36.3 Explosion and rupture of** pressurized-gas tank

   ✓x7ᵗʰ **W36.8 Explosion and rupture of** other **gas cylinder**

   ✓x7ᵗʰ **W36.9 Explosion and rupture of** unspecified **gas cylinder**

✅4ᵗʰ **W37 Explosion and rupture of** pressurized tire, pipe or hose

   ✓x7ᵗʰ **W37.0 Explosion of** bicycle tire

   ✓x7ᵗʰ **W37.8 Explosion and rupture of** other pressurized tire, pipe or hose

✓x7ᵗʰ **W38 Explosion and rupture of** other **specified** pressurized devices

✓x7ᵗʰ **W39 Discharge of** firework

✅4ᵗʰ **W40 Explosion of** other **materials**

> EXCLUDES 1   *assault by explosive material (X96)*
> *explosion involving legal intervention (Y35.1-)*
> *explosion involving military or war operations (Y36.0-, Y36.2-)*
> *intentional self-harm by explosive material (X75)*

   ✓x7ᵗʰ **W40.0 Explosion of** blasting material
     Explosion of blasting cap
     Explosion of detonator
     Explosion of dynamite
     Explosion of explosive (any) used in blasting operations

   ✓x7ᵗʰ **W40.1 Explosion of** explosive gases

Explosion of acetylene	Explosion of fire damp
Explosion of butane	Explosion of gasoline fumes
Explosion of coal gas	Explosion of methane
Explosion in mine NOS	Explosion of propane
Explosion of explosive gas	

   ✓x7ᵗʰ **W40.8 Explosion of** other **specified explosive materials**

Explosion in dump NOS	Explosion in grain store
Explosion in factory NOS	Explosion in munitions

> EXCLUDES 1   *explosion involving legal intervention (Y35.1-)*
> *explosion involving military or war operations (Y36.0-, Y36.2-)*

   ✓x7ᵗʰ **W40.9 Explosion of** unspecified **explosive materials**
     Explosion NOS

✅4ᵗʰ **W42 Exposure to noise**

   ✓x7ᵗʰ **W42.0 Exposure to supersonic waves**

   ✓x7ᵗʰ **W42.9 Exposure to other noise**
     Exposure to sound waves NOS

✅4ᵗʰ **W45 Foreign body or object entering through skin**

> INCLUDES   foreign body or object embedded in skin
> nail embedded in skin
>
> EXCLUDES 2   *contact with hand tools (nonpowered) (powered) (W27-W29)*
> *contact with other sharp object(s) (W26.-)*
> *contact with sharp glass (W25.-)*
> *struck by objects (W20-W22)*

   ✓x7ᵗʰ **W45.0 Nail entering through skin**

   ✓x7ᵗʰ **W45.8 Other foreign body or object entering through skin**
     Splinter in skin NOS

✅4ᵗʰ **W46 Contact with hypodermic needle**

   ✓x7ᵗʰ **W46.0 Contact with hypodermic needle**
     Hypodermic needle stick NOS

   ✓x7ᵗʰ **W46.1 Contact with** contaminated **hypodermic needle**

✅4ᵗʰ **W49 Exposure to other inanimate mechanical forces**

> INCLUDES   exposure to abnormal gravitational [G] forces
> exposure to inanimate mechanical forces NEC
>
> EXCLUDES 1   *exposure to inanimate mechanical forces involving military or war operations (Y36.-, Y37.-)*

   ✅5ᵗʰ **W49.0 Item causing** external constriction

     ✓x7ᵗʰ **W49.01 Hair causing external constriction**

     ✓x7ᵗʰ **W49.02 String or thread causing external constriction**

     ✓x7ᵗʰ **W49.03 Rubber band causing external constriction**

✔ Additional Character Required   ✓x7ᵗʰ Placeholder   Unacceptable PDx   Questionable PDx   Wrong Procedure   Manifestation   H1-H14 HAC   HCC CMS-HCC Dx   HIV HIV Dx

ICD-10-CM 2019   1193

✓x7th **W49.04** Ring or other jewelry **causing external constriction**

✓x7th **W49.09** Other **specified item causing external constriction**

✓x7th **W49.9 Exposure to other inanimate mechanical forces**

Exposure to animate mechanical forces (W50-W64)

EXCLUDES 1 *Toxic effect of contact with venomous animals and plants (T63.-)*

The appropriate 7th character is to be added to each code from categories W50-W64.
A   initial encounter
D   subsequent encounter
S   sequela

✓4th **W50 Accidental hit, strike, kick, twist, bite or scratch by another person**
INCLUDES hit, strike, kick, twist, bite, or scratch by another person NOS
EXCLUDES 1 *assault by bodily force (Y04)*
struck by objects (W20-W22)

✓x7th **W50.0 Accidental hit or strike by another person**
Hit or strike by another person NOS

✓x7th **W50.1 Accidental kick by another person**
Kick by another person NOS

✓x7th **W50.2 Accidental twist by another person**
Twist by another person NOS

✓x7th **W50.3 Accidental bite by another person**
Human bite   Bite by another person NOS

✓x7th **W50.4 Accidental scratch by another person**
Scratch by another person NOS

✓x7th **W51 Accidental striking against or bumped into by another person**
EXCLUDES 1 *assault by striking against or bumping into by another person (Y04.2)*
fall due to collision with another person (W03)

✓x7th **W52 Crushed, pushed or stepped on by crowd or human stampede**
Crushed, pushed or stepped on by crowd or human stampede with or without fall

✓4th **W53 Contact with rodent**
INCLUDES contact with saliva, feces or urine of rodent

✓5th **W53.0 Contact with mouse**

✓x7th **W53.01 Bitten by mouse**

✓x7th **W53.09 Other contact with mouse**

✓5th **W53.1 Contact with rat**

✓x7th **W53.11 Bitten by rat**

✓x7th **W53.19 Other contact with rat**

✓5th **W53.2 Contact with squirrel**

✓x7th **W53.21 Bitten by squirrel**

✓x7th **W53.29 Other contact with squirrel**

✓5th **W53.8 Contact with other rodent**

✓x7th **W53.81 Bitten by other rodent**

✓x7th **W53.89 Other contact with other rodent**

✓4th **W54 Contact with dog**
INCLUDES contact with saliva, feces or urine of dog

✓x7th **W54.0 Bitten by dog**

✓x7th **W54.1 Struck by dog**
Knocked over by dog

✓x7th **W54.8 Other contact with dog**

✓4th **W55 Contact with other mammals**
INCLUDES contact with saliva, feces or urine of mammal
EXCLUDES 1 *animal being ridden—see transport accidents*
bitten or struck by dog (W54)
bitten or struck by rodent (W53.-)
contact with marine mammals (W56.-)

✓5th **W55.0 Contact with cat**

✓x7th **W55.01 Bitten by cat**

✓x7th **W55.03 Scratched by cat**

✓x7th **W55.09 Other contact with cat**

✓5th **W55.1 Contact with horse**

✓x7th **W55.11 Bitten by horse**

✓x7th **W55.12 Struck by horse**

✓x7th **W55.19 Other contact with horse**

✓5th **W55.2 Contact with cow**
Contact with bull

✓x7th **W55.21 Bitten by cow**

✓x7th **W55.22 Struck by cow**
Gored by bull

✓x7th **W55.29 Other contact with cow**

✓5th **W55.3 Contact with other hoof stock**
Contact with goats
Contact with sheep

✓x7th **W55.31 Bitten by other hoof stock**

✓x7th **W55.32 Struck by other hoof stock**
Gored by goat
Gored by ram

✓x7th **W55.39 Other contact with other hoof stock**

✓5th **W55.4 Contact with pig**

✓x7th **W55.41 Bitten by pig**

✓x7th **W55.42 Struck by pig**

✓x7th **W55.49 Other contact with pig**

✓5th **W55.5 Contact with raccoon**

✓x7th **W55.51 Bitten by raccoon**

✓x7th **W55.52 Struck by raccoon**

✓x7th **W55.59 Other contact with raccoon**

✓5th **W55.8 Contact with other mammals**

✓x7th **W55.81 Bitten by other mammals**

✓x7th **W55.82 Struck by other mammals**

✓x7th **W55.89 Other contact with other mammals**

✓4th **W56 Contact with nonvenomous marine animal**
EXCLUDES 1 *contact with venomous marine animal (T63.-)*

✓5th **W56.0 Contact with dolphin**

✓x7th **W56.01 Bitten by dolphin**

✓x7th **W56.02 Struck by dolphin**

✓x7th **W56.09 Other contact with dolphin**

✓5th **W56.1 Contact with sea lion**

✓x7th **W56.11 Bitten by sea lion**

✓x7th **W56.12 Struck by sea lion**

✓x7th **W56.19 Other contact with sea lion**

✓5th **W56.2 Contact with orca**
Contact with killer whale

✓x7th **W56.21 Bitten by orca**

✓x7th **W56.22 Struck by orca**

✓x7th **W56.29 Other contact with orca**

✓5th **W56.3 Contact with other marine mammals**

✓x7th **W56.31 Bitten by other marine mammals**

✓x7th **W56.32 Struck by other marine mammals**

✓x7th **W56.39 Other contact with other marine mammals**

✓5th **W56.4 Contact with shark**

✓x7th **W56.41 Bitten by shark**

✓x7th **W56.42 Struck by shark**

✓x7th **W56.49 Other contact with shark**

✓5th **W56.5 Contact with other fish**

✓x7th **W56.51 Bitten by other fish**

✓x7th **W56.52 Struck by other fish**

✓x7th **W56.59 Other contact with other fish**

✓5th **W56.8 Contact with other nonvenomous marine animals**

✓x7th **W56.81 Bitten by other nonvenomous marine animals**

✓x7th **W56.82 Struck by other nonvenomous marine animals**

✓x7th **W56.89 Other contact with other nonvenomous marine animals**

✓x7th **W57 Bitten or stung by nonvenomous insect and other nonvenomous arthropods**
EXCLUDES 1 *contact with venomous insects and arthropods (T63.2-, T63.3-, T63.4-)*

✓4th **W58 Contact with crocodile or alligator**

✓5th **W58.0 Contact with alligator**

✓x7th **W58.01 Bitten by alligator**

✓x7th **W58.02 Struck by alligator**

✓x7th **W58.03 Crushed by alligator**

✓x7th **W58.09 Other contact with alligator**

N Newborn: 0   P Pediatric: 0-17   M Maternity: 12-55   A Adult: 15-124   MCC Major Complication/Comorbidity   CC Complication/Comorbidity   SW Severe Wound Dx

1194   ICD-10-CM 2019

✓5ᵗʰ **W58.1 Contact with** crocodile

    ✓x7ᵗʰ **W58.11 Bitten by crocodile**

    ✓x7ᵗʰ **W58.12 Struck by crocodile**

    ✓x7ᵗʰ **W58.13 Crushed by crocodile**

    ✓x7ᵗʰ **W58.19 Other contact with crocodile**

✓4ᵗʰ **W59 Contact with other nonvenomous reptiles**

    EXCLUDES 1   contact with venomous reptile (T63.0-, T63.1-)

  ✓5ᵗʰ **W59.0 Contact with nonvenomous** lizards

    ✓x7ᵗʰ **W59.01 Bitten by nonvenomous lizards**

    ✓x7ᵗʰ **W59.02 Struck by nonvenomous lizards**

    ✓x7ᵗʰ **W59.09 Other contact with nonvenomous lizards**
         Exposure to nonvenomous lizards

  ✓5ᵗʰ **W59.1 Contact with nonvenomous** snakes

    ✓x7ᵗʰ **W59.11 Bitten by nonvenomous snake**

    ✓x7ᵗʰ **W59.12 Struck by nonvenomous snake**

    ✓x7ᵗʰ **W59.13 Crushed by nonvenomous snake**

    ✓x7ᵗʰ **W59.19 Other contact with nonvenomous snake**

  ✓5ᵗʰ **W59.2 Contact with** turtles

    EXCLUDES 1   contact with tortoises (W59.8-)

    ✓x7ᵗʰ **W59.21 Bitten by turtle**

    ✓x7ᵗʰ **W59.22 Struck by turtle**

    ✓x7ᵗʰ **W59.29 Other contact with turtle**
         Exposure to turtles

  ✓5ᵗʰ **W59.8 Contact with other nonvenomous reptiles**

    ✓x7ᵗʰ **W59.81 Bitten by other nonvenomous reptiles**

    ✓x7ᵗʰ **W59.82 Struck by other nonvenomous reptiles**

    ✓x7ᵗʰ **W59.83 Crushed by other nonvenomous reptiles**

    ✓x7ᵗʰ **W59.89 Other contact with other nonvenomous reptiles**

✓x7ᵗʰ **W60 Contact with nonvenomous plant thorns and spines and sharp leaves**

    EXCLUDES 1   contact with venomous plants (T63.7-)

✓4ᵗʰ **W61 Contact with birds (domestic) (wild)**

    INCLUDES   contact with excreta of birds

  ✓5ᵗʰ **W61.0 Contact with** parrot

    ✓x7ᵗʰ **W61.01 Bitten by parrot**

    ✓x7ᵗʰ **W61.02 Struck by parrot**

    ✓x7ᵗʰ **W61.09 Other contact with parrot**
         Exposure to parrots

  ✓5ᵗʰ **W61.1 Contact with** macaw

    ✓x7ᵗʰ **W61.11 Bitten by macaw**

    ✓x7ᵗʰ **W61.12 Struck by macaw**

    ✓x7ᵗʰ **W61.19 Other contact with macaw**
         Exposure to macaws

  ✓5ᵗʰ **W61.2 Contact with other** psittacines

    ✓x7ᵗʰ **W61.21 Bitten by other psittacines**

    ✓x7ᵗʰ **W61.22 Struck by other psittacines**

    ✓x7ᵗʰ **W61.29 Other contact with other psittacines**
         Exposure to other psittacines

  ✓5ᵗʰ **W61.3 Contact with** chicken

    ✓x7ᵗʰ **W61.32 Struck by chicken**

    ✓x7ᵗʰ **W61.33 Pecked by chicken**

    ✓x7ᵗʰ **W61.39 Other contact with chicken**
         Exposure to chickens

  ✓5ᵗʰ **W61.4 Contact with** turkey

    ✓x7ᵗʰ **W61.42 Struck by turkey**

    ✓x7ᵗʰ **W61.43 Pecked by turkey**

    ✓x7ᵗʰ **W61.49 Other contact with turkey**

  ✓5ᵗʰ **W61.5 Contact with** goose

    ✓x7ᵗʰ **W61.51 Bitten by goose**

    ✓x7ᵗʰ **W61.52 Struck by goose**

    ✓x7ᵗʰ **W61.59 Other contact with goose**

  ✓5ᵗʰ **W61.6 Contact with** duck

    ✓x7ᵗʰ **W61.61 Bitten by duck**

    ✓x7ᵗʰ **W61.62 Struck by duck**

    ✓x7ᵗʰ **W61.69 Other contact with duck**

  ✓5ᵗʰ **W61.9 Contact with** other birds

    ✓x7ᵗʰ **W61.91 Bitten by other birds**

    ✓x7ᵗʰ **W61.92 Struck by other birds**

    ✓x7ᵗʰ **W61.99 Other contact with other birds**
         Contact with bird NOS

✓4ᵗʰ **W62 Contact with nonvenomous amphibians**

    EXCLUDES 1   contact with venomous amphibians (T63.81-R63.83)

  ✓x7ᵗʰ **W62.0 Contact with nonvenomous** frogs

  ✓x7ᵗʰ **W62.1 Contact with nonvenomous** toads

  ✓x7ᵗʰ **W62.9 Contact with other nonvenomous** amphibians

✓x7ᵗʰ **W64 Exposure to other animate mechanical forces**

    INCLUDES   exposure to nonvenomous animal NOS

    EXCLUDES 1   contact with venomous animal (T63.-)

Accidental non-transport drowning and submersion (W65-W74)

    EXCLUDES 1   accidental drowning and submersion due to fall into water (W16.-)
         accidental drowning and submersion due to water transport accident (V90.-, V92.-)

    EXCLUDES 2   accidental drowning and submersion due to cataclysm (X34-X39)

> The appropriate 7th character is to be added to each code from categories W65-W74.
> A   initial encounter
> D   subsequent encounter
> S   sequela

✓x7ᵗʰ **W65 Accidental drowning and submersion while in** bath-tub

    EXCLUDES 1   accidental drowning and submersion due to fall in (into) bathtub (W16.211)

✓x7ᵗʰ **W67 Accidental drowning and submersion while in** swimming-pool

    EXCLUDES 1   accidental drowning and submersion due to fall into swimming pool (W16.011, W16.021, W16.031)
         accidental drowning and submersion due to striking into wall of swimming pool (W22.041)

✓x7ᵗʰ **W69 Accidental drowning and submersion while in** natural water

     Accidental drowning and submersion while in lake
     Accidental drowning and submersion while in open sea
     Accidental drowning and submersion while in river
     Accidental drowning and submersion while in stream

    EXCLUDES 1   accidental drowning and submersion due to fall into natural body of water (W16.111, W16.121, W16.131)

✓x7ᵗʰ **W73 Other specified cause of accidental non-transport drowning and submersion**

     Accidental drowning and submersion while in quenching tank
     Accidental drowning and submersion while in reservoir

    EXCLUDES 1   accidental drowning and submersion due to fall into other water (W16.311, W16.321, W16.331)

✓x7ᵗʰ **W74 Unspecified cause of accidental drowning and submersion**

     Drowning NOS

Exposure to electric current, radiation and extreme ambient air temperature and pressure (W85-W99)

    EXCLUDES 1   exposure to:
         failure in dosage of radiation or temperature during surgical and medical care (Y63.2-Y63.5)
         lightning (T75.0-)
         natural cold (X31)
         natural heat (X30)
         natural radiation NOS (X39)
         radiological procedure and radiotherapy (Y84.2)
         sunlight (X32)

AHA: 2018, 2Q, 7-8

> The appropriate 7th character is to be added to each code from categories W85-W99.
> A   initial encounter
> D   subsequent encounter
> S   sequela

✓x7ᵗʰ **W85 Exposure to electric transmission lines**

     Broken power line

✓4ᵗʰ **W86 Exposure to other specified electric current**

  ✓x7ᵗʰ **W86.0 Exposure to domestic wiring and appliances**

  ✓x7ᵗʰ **W86.1 Exposure to industrial wiring, appliances and electrical machinery**

     Exposure to conductors
     Exposure to control apparatus
     Exposure to electrical equipment and machinery
     Exposure to transformers

✓ Additional Character Required   ✓x7ᵗʰ Placeholder   Unacceptable PDx   Questionable PDx   Wrong Procedure   Manifestation   H1-H14 HAC   HCC CMS-HCC Dx   HIV HIV Dx

ICD-10-CM 2019   1195

Chapter 20. External Causes of Morbidity

✓x7ᵗʰ **W86.8 Exposure to other electric current**
Exposure to wiring and appliances in or on farm (not farmhouse)
Exposure to wiring and appliances outdoors
Exposure to wiring and appliances in or on public building
Exposure to wiring and appliances in or on residential institutions
Exposure to wiring and appliances in or on schools

✓4ᵗʰ **W88 Exposure to ionizing radiation**
    EXCLUDES 1   *exposure to sunlight (X32)*

✓x7ᵗʰ **W88.0 Exposure to X-rays**

✓x7ᵗʰ **W88.1 Exposure to radioactive isotopes**

✓x7ᵗʰ **W88.8 Exposure to other ionizing radiation**

✓4ᵗʰ **W89 Exposure to man-made visible and ultraviolet light**
    INCLUDES   exposure to welding light (arc)
    EXCLUDES 1   *exposure to sunlight (X32)*

✓x7ᵗʰ **W89.0 Exposure to welding light (arc)**

✓x7ᵗʰ **W89.1 Exposure to tanning bed**

✓x7ᵗʰ **W89.8 Exposure to other man-made visible and ultraviolet light**

✓x7ᵗʰ **W89.9 Exposure to unspecified man-made visible and ultraviolet light**

✓4ᵗʰ **W90 Exposure to other nonionizing radiation**
    EXCLUDES 1   *exposure to sunlight (X32)*

✓x7ᵗʰ **W90.0 Exposure to radiofrequency**

✓x7ᵗʰ **W90.1 Exposure to infrared radiation**

✓x7ᵗʰ **W90.2 Exposure to laser radiation**

✓x7ᵗʰ **W90.8 Exposure to other nonionizing radiation**

✓x7ᵗʰ **W92 Exposure to excessive heat of man-made origin**

✓4ᵗʰ **W93 Exposure to excessive cold of man-made origin**

  ✓5ᵗʰ **W93.0 Contact with or inhalation of dry ice**

    ✓x7ᵗʰ **W93.01 Contact with dry ice**

    ✓x7ᵗʰ **W93.02 Inhalation of dry ice**

  ✓5ᵗʰ **W93.1 Contact with or inhalation of liquid air**

    ✓x7ᵗʰ **W93.11 Contact with liquid air**
        Contact with liquid hydrogen
        Contact with liquid nitrogen

    ✓x7ᵗʰ **W93.12 Inhalation of liquid air**
        Inhalation of liquid hydrogen
        Inhalation of liquid nitrogen

  ✓x7ᵗʰ **W93.2 Prolonged exposure in deep freeze unit or refrigerator**

  ✓x7ᵗʰ **W93.8 Exposure to other excessive cold of man-made origin**

✓4ᵗʰ **W94 Exposure to high and low air pressure and changes in air pressure**

  ✓x7ᵗʰ **W94.0 Exposure to prolonged high air pressure**

  ✓5ᵗʰ **W94.1 Exposure to prolonged low air pressure**

    ✓x7ᵗʰ **W94.11 Exposure to residence or prolonged visit at high altitude**

    ✓x7ᵗʰ **W94.12 Exposure to other prolonged low air pressure**

  ✓5ᵗʰ **W94.2 Exposure to rapid changes in air pressure during ascent**

    ✓x7ᵗʰ **W94.21 Exposure to reduction in atmospheric pressure while surfacing from deep-water diving**

    ✓x7ᵗʰ **W94.22 Exposure to reduction in atmospheric pressure while surfacing from underground**

    ✓x7ᵗʰ **W94.23 Exposure to sudden change in air pressure in aircraft during ascent**

    ✓x7ᵗʰ **W94.29 Exposure to other rapid changes in air pressure during ascent**

  ✓5ᵗʰ **W94.3 Exposure to rapid changes in air pressure during descent**

    ✓x7ᵗʰ **W94.31 Exposure to sudden change in air pressure in aircraft during descent**

    ✓x7ᵗʰ **W94.32 Exposure to high air pressure from rapid descent in water**

    ✓x7ᵗʰ **W94.39 Exposure to other rapid changes in air pressure during descent**

✓x7ᵗʰ **W99 Exposure to other man-made environmental factors**

Exposure to smoke, fire and flames (X00-X08)

  EXCLUDES 1   *arson (X97)*
  EXCLUDES 2   *explosions (W35-W40)*
      lightning (T75.0-)
      transport accident (V01-V99)
  AHA: 2018, 2Q, 7-8

> The appropriate 7th character is to be added to each code from categories X00-X08.
> A   initial encounter
> D   subsequent encounter
> S   sequela

✓4ᵗʰ **X00 Exposure to uncontrolled fire in building or structure**
    INCLUDES   conflagration in building or structure
    Code first any associated cataclysm
    EXCLUDES 2   *exposure to ignition or melting of nightwear (X05)*
        exposure to ignition or melting of other clothing and apparel (X06.-)
        exposure to other specified smoke, fire and flames (X08.-)
    AHA: 2016, 2Q, 5

  ✓x7ᵗʰ **X00.0 Exposure to flames in uncontrolled fire in building or structure**

  ✓x7ᵗʰ **X00.1 Exposure to smoke in uncontrolled fire in building or structure**

  ✓x7ᵗʰ **X00.2 Injury due to collapse of burning building or structure in uncontrolled fire**
      EXCLUDES 1   *injury due to collapse of building not on fire (W20.1)*

  ✓x7ᵗʰ **X00.3 Fall from burning building or structure in uncontrolled fire**

  ✓x7ᵗʰ **X00.4 Hit by object from burning building or structure in uncontrolled fire**
      AHA: 2016, 2Q, 4

  ✓x7ᵗʰ **X00.5 Jump from burning building or structure in uncontrolled fire**

  ✓x7ᵗʰ **X00.8 Other exposure to uncontrolled fire in building or structure**

✓4ᵗʰ **X01 Exposure to uncontrolled fire, not in building or structure**
    INCLUDES   exposure to forest fire

  ✓x7ᵗʰ **X01.0 Exposure to flames in uncontrolled fire, not in building or structure**

  ✓x7ᵗʰ **X01.1 Exposure to smoke in uncontrolled fire, not in building or structure**

  ✓x7ᵗʰ **X01.3 Fall due to uncontrolled fire, not in building or structure**

  ✓x7ᵗʰ **X01.4 Hit by object due to uncontrolled fire, not in building or structure**

  ✓x7ᵗʰ **X01.8 Other exposure to uncontrolled fire, not in building or structure**

✓4ᵗʰ **X02 Exposure to controlled fire in building or structure**
    INCLUDES   exposure to fire in fireplace
        exposure to fire in stove

  ✓x7ᵗʰ **X02.0 Exposure to flames in controlled fire in building or structure**

  ✓x7ᵗʰ **X02.1 Exposure to smoke in controlled fire in building or structure**

  ✓x7ᵗʰ **X02.2 Injury due to collapse of burning building or structure in controlled fire**
      EXCLUDES 1   *injury due to collapse of building not on fire (W20.1)*

  ✓x7ᵗʰ **X02.3 Fall from burning building or structure in controlled fire**

  ✓x7ᵗʰ **X02.4 Hit by object from burning building or structure in controlled fire**

  ✓x7ᵗʰ **X02.5 Jump from burning building or structure in controlled fire**

  ✓x7ᵗʰ **X02.8 Other exposure to controlled fire in building or structure**

✓4ᵗʰ **X03 Exposure to controlled fire, not in building or structure**
    INCLUDES   exposure to bon fire
        exposure to camp-fire
        exposure to trash fire

  ✓x7ᵗʰ **X03.0 Exposure to flames in controlled fire, not in building or structure**

  ✓x7ᵗʰ **X03.1 Exposure to smoke in controlled fire, not in building or structure**

  ✓x7ᵗʰ **X03.3 Fall due to controlled fire, not in building or structure**

  ✓x7ᵗʰ **X03.4 Hit by object due to controlled fire, not in building or structure**

  ✓x7ᵗʰ **X03.8 Other exposure to controlled fire, not in building or structure**

Ⓝ Newborn: 0   Ⓟ Pediatric: 0-17   Ⓜ Maternity: 12-55   Ⓐ Adult: 15-124   **MCC** Major Complication/Comorbidity   **CC** Complication/Comorbidity   **SW** Severe Wound Dx

1196   ICD-10-CM 2019

√x7th X04 Exposure to ignition of highly flammable material
Exposure to ignition of gasoline
Exposure to ignition of kerosene
Exposure to ignition of petrol
> EXCLUDES 2   exposure to ignition or melting of nightwear (X05)
> exposure to ignition or melting of other clothing and apparel (X06)

AHA: 2016, 2Q, 4

√x7th X05 Exposure to ignition or melting of nightwear
> EXCLUDES 2   exposure to uncontrolled fire in building or structure (X00.-)
> exposure to uncontrolled fire, not in building or structure (X01.-)
> exposure to controlled fire in building or structure (X02.-)
> exposure to controlled fire, not in building or structure (X03.-)
> exposure to ignition of highly flammable materials (X04.-)

√4th X06 Exposure to ignition or melting of other clothing and apparel
> EXCLUDES 2   exposure to uncontrolled fire in building or structure (X00.-)
> exposure to uncontrolled fire, not in building or structure (X01.-)
> exposure to controlled fire in building or structure (X02.-)
> exposure to controlled fire, not in building or structure (X03.-)
> exposure to ignition of highly flammable materials (X04.-)

√x7th **X06.0** Exposure to ignition of plastic jewelry
√x7th **X06.1** Exposure to melting of plastic jewelry
√x7th **X06.2** Exposure to ignition of other clothing and apparel
√x7th **X06.3** Exposure to melting of other clothing and apparel

√4th X08 Exposure to other specified smoke, fire and flames
√5th **X08.0** Exposure to bed fire
Exposure to mattress fire
√x7th **X08.00** Exposure to bed fire due to unspecified burning material
√x7th **X08.01** Exposure to bed fire due to burning cigarette
√x7th **X08.09** Exposure to bed fire due to other burning material

√5th **X08.1** Exposure to sofa fire
√x7th **X08.10** Exposure to sofa fire due to unspecified burning material
√x7th **X08.11** Exposure to sofa fire due to burning cigarette
√x7th **X08.19** Exposure to sofa fire due to other burning material

√5th **X08.2** Exposure to other furniture fire
√x7th **X08.20** Exposure to other furniture fire due to unspecified burning material
√x7th **X08.21** Exposure to other furniture fire due to burning cigarette
√x7th **X08.29** Exposure to other furniture fire due to other burning material

√x7th **X08.8** Exposure to other specified smoke, fire and flames

Contact with heat and hot substances (X10-X19)
> EXCLUDES 1   exposure to excessive natural heat (X30)
> exposure to fire and flames (X00-X08)

AHA: 2018, 2Q, 7-8

The appropriate 7th character is to be added to each code from categories X10-X19.
A   initial encounter
D   subsequent encounter
S   sequela

√4th X10 Contact with hot drinks, food, fats and cooking oils
√x7th **X10.0** Contact with hot drinks
√x7th **X10.1** Contact with hot food
√x7th **X10.2** Contact with fats and cooking oils

√4th X11 Contact with hot tap-water
> INCLUDES   contact with boiling tap-water
> contact with boiling water NOS
> EXCLUDES 1   contact with water heated on stove (X12)

√x7th **X11.0** Contact with hot water in bath or tub
> EXCLUDES 1   contact with running hot water in bath or tub (X11.1)

√x7th **X11.1** Contact with running hot water
Contact with hot water running out of hose
Contact with hot water running out of tap

√x7th **X11.8** Contact with other hot tap-water
Contact with hot water in bucket
Contact with hot tap-water NOS

√x7th X12 Contact with other hot fluids
Contact with water heated on stove
> EXCLUDES 1   hot (liquid) metals (X18)

√4th X13 Contact with steam and other hot vapors
√x7th **X13.0** Inhalation of steam and other hot vapors
√x7th **X13.1** Other contact with steam and other hot vapors

√4th X14 Contact with hot air and other hot gases
√x7th **X14.0** Inhalation of hot air and gases
√x7th **X14.1** Other contact with hot air and other hot gases

√4th X15 Contact with hot household appliances
> EXCLUDES 1   contact with heating appliances (X16)
> contact with powered household appliances (W29.-)
> exposure to controlled fire in building or structure due to household appliance (X02.8)
> exposure to household appliances electrical current (W86.0)

√x7th **X15.0** Contact with hot stove (kitchen)
√x7th **X15.1** Contact with hot toaster
√x7th **X15.2** Contact with hotplate
√x7th **X15.3** Contact with hot saucepan or skillet
√x7th **X15.8** Contact with other hot household appliances
Contact with cooker
Contact with kettle
Contact with light bulbs

√x7th X16 Contact with hot heating appliances, radiators and pipes
> EXCLUDES 1   contact with powered appliances (W29.-)
> exposure to controlled fire in building or structure due to appliance (X02.8)
> exposure to industrial appliances electrical current (W86.1)

√x7th X17 Contact with hot engines, machinery and tools
> EXCLUDES 1   contact with hot heating appliances, radiators and pipes (X16)
> contact with hot household appliances (X15)

√x7th X18 Contact with other hot metals
Contact with liquid metal

√x7th X19 Contact with other heat and hot substances
> EXCLUDES 1   objects that are not normally hot, e.g., an object made hot by a house fire (X00-X08)

Exposure to forces of nature (X30-X39)
AHA: 2018, 2Q, 7-8

The appropriate 7th character is to be added to each code from categories X30-X39.
A   initial encounter
D   subsequent encounter
S   sequela

√x7th X30 Exposure to excessive natural heat
Exposure to excessive heat as the cause of sunstroke
Exposure to heat NOS
> EXCLUDES 1   excessive heat of man-made origin (W92)
> exposure to man-made radiation (W89)
> exposure to sunlight (X32)
> exposure to tanning bed (W89)

√x7th X31 Exposure to excessive natural cold
Excessive cold as the cause of chilblains NOS
Excessive cold as the cause of immersion foot or hand
Exposure to cold NOS
Exposure to weather conditions
> EXCLUDES 1   cold of man-made origin (W93.-)
> contact with or inhalation of dry ice (W93.-)
> contact with or inhalation of liquefied gas (W93.-)

√x7th X32 Exposure to sunlight
> EXCLUDES 1   man-made radiation (tanning bed) (W89)
> EXCLUDES 2   radiation-related disorders of the skin and subcutaneous tissue (L55-L59)

√x7th X34 Earthquake
> EXCLUDES 2   tidal wave (tsunami) due to earthquake (X37.41)

√x7th X35 Volcanic eruption
> EXCLUDES 2   tidal wave (tsunami) due to volcanic eruption (X37.41)

✔ Additional Character Required   √x7th Placeholder   Unacceptable PDx   Questionable PDx   Wrong Procedure   Manifestation   H1 - H14 HAC   HCC CMS-HCC Dx   HIV HIV Dx

ICD-10-CM 2019   1197

Chapter 20. External Causes of Morbidity

✓4ᵗʰ **X36 Avalanche, landslide and other earth movements**
     INCLUDES victim of mudslide of cataclysmic nature
     EXCLUDES 1 *earthquake (X34)*
     EXCLUDES 2 *transport accident involving collision with avalanche or landslide not in motion (V01-V99)*

   ✓x7ᵗʰ **X36.0 Collapse of dam or man-made structure causing earth movement**

   ✓x7ᵗʰ **X36.1 Avalanche, landslide, or mudslide**

✓4ᵗʰ **X37 Cataclysmic storm**

   ✓x7ᵗʰ **X37.0 Hurricane**
     Storm surge
     Typhoon

   ✓x7ᵗʰ **X37.1 Tornado**
     Cyclone
     Twister

   ✓x7ᵗʰ **X37.2 Blizzard (snow)(ice)**

   ✓x7ᵗʰ **X37.3 Dust storm**

   ✓5ᵗʰ **X37.4 Tidalwave**

     ✓x7ᵗʰ **X37.41 Tidal wave due to earthquake or volcanic eruption**
       Tidal wave NOS
       Tsunami

     ✓x7ᵗʰ **X37.42 Tidal wave due to storm**

     ✓x7ᵗʰ **X37.43 Tidal wave due to landslide**

   ✓x7ᵗʰ **X37.8 Other cataclysmic storms**
     Cloudburst
     Torrential rain
     EXCLUDES 2 *flood (X38)*

   ✓x7ᵗʰ **X37.9 Unspecified cataclysmic storm**
     Storm NOS
     EXCLUDES 1 *collapse of dam or man-made structure causing earth movement ▶(X36.0)◀*

✓x7ᵗʰ **X38 Flood**
     Flood arising from remote storm
     Flood of cataclysmic nature arising from melting snow
     Flood resulting directly from storm
     EXCLUDES 1 *collapse of dam or man-made structure causing earth movement ▶(X36.0)◀*
       tidal wave NOS (X37.41)
       tidal wave caused by storm ▶(X37.42)◀

✓4ᵗʰ **X39 Exposure to other forces of nature**

   ✓5ᵗʰ **X39.0 Exposure to natural radiation**
     EXCLUDES 1 *▶contact with and (suspected) exposure to radon and other naturally occurring radiation◀ (Z77.123)*
       exposure to man-made radiation (W88-W90)
       exposure to sunlight (X32)

     ✓x7ᵗʰ **X39.01 Exposure to radon**

     ✓x7ᵗʰ **X39.08 Exposure to other natural radiation**

   ✓x7ᵗʰ **X39.8 Other exposure to forces of nature**

Overexertion and strenuous or repetitive movements (X50)

✓4ᵗʰ **X50 Overexertion and strenuous or repetitive movements**
     AHA: 2018, 2Q, 7-8; 2016, 4Q, 73-74

     The appropriate 7th character is to be added to each code from category X50.
     A   initial encounter
     D   subsequent encounter
     S   sequela

   ✓x7ᵗʰ **X50.0 Overexertion from strenuous movement or load**
     Lifting heavy objects
     Lifting weights

   ✓x7ᵗʰ **X50.1 Overexertion from prolonged static or awkward postures**
     Prolonged bending
     Prolonged kneeling
     Prolonged reaching
     Prolonged sitting
     Prolonged standing
     Prolonged twisting
     Static bending
     Static kneeling
     Static reaching
     Static sitting
     Static standing
     Static twisting

   ✓x7ᵗʰ **X50.3 Overexertion from repetitive movements**
     Use of hand as hammer
     EXCLUDES 2 *overuse from prolonged static or awkward postures (X50.1)*

   ✓x7ᵗʰ **X50.9 Other and unspecified overexertion or strenuous movements or postures**
     Contact pressure
     Contact stress

Accidental exposure to other specified factors (X52-X58)

AHA: 2018, 2Q, 7-8

The appropriate 7th character is to be added to each code from categories X52 and X58.
A   initial encounter
D   subsequent encounter
S   sequela

✓x7ᵗʰ **X52 Prolonged stay in weightless environment**
     Weightlessness in spacecraft (simulator)

✓x7ᵗʰ **X58 Exposure to other specified factors**
     Accident NOS
     Exposure NOS

Intentional self-harm (X71-X83)

Purposely self-inflicted injury
Suicide (attempted)

The appropriate 7th character is to be added to each code from categories X71-X83.
A   initial encounter
D   subsequent encounter
S   sequela

✓4ᵗʰ **X71 Intentional self-harm by drowning and submersion**

   ✓x7ᵗʰ **X71.0 Intentional self-harm by drowning and submersion while in bathtub**   HCC

   ✓x7ᵗʰ **X71.1 Intentional self-harm by drowning and submersion while in swimming pool**   HCC

   ✓x7ᵗʰ **X71.2 Intentional self-harm by drowning and submersion after jump into swimming pool**   HCC

   ✓x7ᵗʰ **X71.3 Intentional self-harm by drowning and submersion in natural water**   HCC

   ✓x7ᵗʰ **X71.8 Other intentional self-harm by drowning and submersion**   HCC

   ✓x7ᵗʰ **X71.9 Intentional self-harm by drowning and submersion, unspecified**   HCC

✓x7ᵗʰ **X72 Intentional self-harm by handgun discharge**   HCC
     Intentional self-harm by gun for single hand use
     Intentional self-harm by pistol
     Intentional self-harm by revolver
     EXCLUDES 1 *Very pistol (X74.8)*

✓4ᵗʰ **X73 Intentional self-harm by rifle, shotgun and larger firearm discharge**
     EXCLUDES 1 *airgun (X74.01)*

   ✓x7ᵗʰ **X73.0 Intentional self-harm by shotgun discharge**   HCC

   ✓x7ᵗʰ **X73.1 Intentional self-harm by hunting rifle discharge**   HCC

   ✓x7ᵗʰ **X73.2 Intentional self-harm by machine gun discharge**   HCC

   ✓x7ᵗʰ **X73.8 Intentional self-harm by other larger firearm discharge**   HCC

   ✓x7ᵗʰ **X73.9 Intentional self-harm by unspecified larger firearm discharge**   HCC

✓4ᵗʰ **X74 Intentional self-harm by other and unspecified firearm and gun discharge**

   ✓5ᵗʰ **X74.0 Intentional self-harm by gas, air or spring-operated guns**

     ✓x7ᵗʰ **X74.01 Intentional self-harm by airgun**   HCC
       Intentional self-harm by BB gun discharge
       Intentional self-harm by pellet gun discharge

     ✓x7ᵗʰ **X74.02 Intentional self-harm by paintball gun**   HCC

     ✓x7ᵗʰ **X74.09 Intentional self-harm by other gas, air or spring-operated gun**   HCC

   ✓x7ᵗʰ **X74.8 Intentional self-harm by other firearm discharge**   HCC
     Intentional self-harm by Very pistol [flare] discharge

   ✓x7ᵗʰ **X74.9 Intentional self-harm by unspecified firearm discharge**   HCC

✓x7ᵗʰ **X75 Intentional self-harm by explosive material**   HCC

✓x7ᵗʰ **X76 Intentional self-harm by smoke, fire and flames**   HCC

N Newborn: 0   P Pediatric: 0-17   M Maternity: 12-55   A Adult: 15-124   MCC Major Complication/Comorbidity   CC Complication/Comorbidity   SW Severe Wound Dx

1198   ICD-10-CM 2019

✓4ᵗʰ X77 Intentional self-harm by steam, hot vapors and hot objects
- ✓x7ᵗʰ X77.0 Intentional self-harm by steam or hot vapors   HCC
- ✓x7ᵗʰ X77.1 Intentional self-harm by hot tap water   HCC
- ✓x7ᵗʰ X77.2 Intentional self-harm by other hot fluids   HCC
- ✓x7ᵗʰ X77.3 Intentional self-harm by hot household appliances   HCC
- ✓x7ᵗʰ X77.8 Intentional self-harm by other hot objects   HCC
- ✓x7ᵗʰ X77.9 Intentional self-harm by unspecified hot objects   HCC

✓4ᵗʰ X78 Intentional self-harm by sharp object
- ✓x7ᵗʰ X78.0 Intentional self-harm by sharp glass   HCC
- ✓x7ᵗʰ X78.1 Intentional self-harm by knife   HCC
- ✓x7ᵗʰ X78.2 Intentional self-harm by sword or dagger   HCC
- ✓x7ᵗʰ X78.8 Intentional self-harm by other sharp object   HCC
- ✓x7ᵗʰ X78.9 Intentional self-harm by unspecified sharp object   HCC

✓x7ᵗʰ X79 Intentional self-harm by blunt object   HCC

✓x7ᵗʰ X80 Intentional self-harm by jumping from a high place   HCC
Intentional fall from one level to another

✓4ᵗʰ X81 Intentional self-harm by jumping or lying in front of moving object
- ✓x7ᵗʰ X81.0 Intentional self-harm by jumping or lying in front of motor vehicle   HCC
- ✓x7ᵗʰ X81.1 Intentional self-harm by jumping or lying in front of (subway) train   HCC
- ✓x7ᵗʰ X81.8 Intentional self-harm by jumping or lying in front of other moving object   HCC

✓4ᵗʰ X82 Intentional self-harm by crashing of motor vehicle
- ✓x7ᵗʰ X82.0 Intentional collision of motor vehicle with other motor vehicle   HCC
- ✓x7ᵗʰ X82.1 Intentional collision of motor vehicle with train   HCC
- ✓x7ᵗʰ X82.2 Intentional collision of motor vehicle with tree   HCC
- ✓x7ᵗʰ X82.8 Other intentional self-harm by crashing of motor vehicle   HCC

✓4ᵗʰ X83 Intentional self-harm by other specified means
EXCLUDES 1 intentional self-harm by poisoning or contact with toxic substance—see Table of Drugs and Chemicals
- ✓x7ᵗʰ X83.0 Intentional self-harm by crashing of aircraft   HCC
- ✓x7ᵗʰ X83.1 Intentional self-harm by electrocution   HCC
- ✓x7ᵗʰ X83.2 Intentional self-harm by exposure to extremes of cold   HCC
- ✓x7ᵗʰ X83.8 Intentional self-harm by other specified means   HCC

Assault (X92-Y09)

INCLUDES   homicide
injuries inflicted by another person with intent to injure or kill, by any means
EXCLUDES 1 injuries due to legal intervention (Y35.-)
injuries due to operations of war (Y36.-)
injuries due to terrorism (Y38.-)

The appropriate 7th character is to be added to each code from categories X92-Y04 and Y08.
A   initial encounter
D   subsequent encounter
S   sequela

✓4ᵗʰ X92 Assault by drowning and submersion
- ✓x7ᵗʰ X92.0 Assault by drowning and submersion while in bathtub
- ✓x7ᵗʰ X92.1 Assault by drowning and submersion while in swimming pool
- ✓x7ᵗʰ X92.2 Assault by drowning and submersion after push into swimming pool
- ✓x7ᵗʰ X92.3 Assault by drowning and submersion in natural water
- ✓x7ᵗʰ X92.8 Other assault by drowning and submersion
- ✓x7ᵗʰ X92.9 Assault by drowning and submersion, unspecified

✓x7ᵗʰ X93 Assault by handgun discharge
Assault by discharge of gun for single hand use
Assault by discharge of pistol
Assault by discharge of revolver
EXCLUDES 1 Very pistol (X95.8)

✓4ᵗʰ X94 Assault by rifle, shotgun and larger firearm discharge
EXCLUDES 1 airgun (X95.01)
- ✓x7ᵗʰ X94.0 Assault by shotgun
- ✓x7ᵗʰ X94.1 Assault by hunting rifle
- ✓x7ᵗʰ X94.2 Assault by machine gun

- ✓x7ᵗʰ X94.8 Assault by other larger firearm discharge
- ✓x7ᵗʰ X94.9 Assault by unspecified larger firearm discharge

✓4ᵗʰ X95 Assault by other and unspecified firearm and gun discharge
- ✓5ᵗʰ X95.0 Assault by gas, air or spring-operated guns
  - ✓x7ᵗʰ X95.01 Assault by airgun discharge
    Assault by BB gun discharge
    Assault by pellet gun discharge
  - ✓x7ᵗʰ X95.02 Assault by paintball gun discharge
  - ✓x7ᵗʰ X95.09 Assault by other gas, air or spring-operated gun
- ✓x7ᵗʰ X95.8 Assault by other firearm discharge
  Assault by Very pistol [flare] discharge
- ✓x7ᵗʰ X95.9 Assault by unspecified firearm discharge

✓4ᵗʰ X96 Assault by explosive material
EXCLUDES 1 incendiary device (X97)
terrorism involving explosive material (Y38.2-)
- ✓x7ᵗʰ X96.0 Assault by antipersonnel bomb
  EXCLUDES 1 antipersonnel bomb use in military or war (Y36.2-)
- ✓x7ᵗʰ X96.1 Assault by gasoline bomb
- ✓x7ᵗʰ X96.2 Assault by letter bomb
- ✓x7ᵗʰ X96.3 Assault by fertilizer bomb
- ✓x7ᵗʰ X96.4 Assault by pipe bomb
- ✓x7ᵗʰ X96.8 Assault by other specified explosive
- ✓x7ᵗʰ X96.9 Assault by unspecified explosive

✓x7ᵗʰ X97 Assault by smoke, fire and flames
Assault by arson
Assault by cigarettes
Assault by incendiary device

✓4ᵗʰ X98 Assault by steam, hot vapors and hot objects
- ✓x7ᵗʰ X98.0 Assault by steam or hot vapors
- ✓x7ᵗʰ X98.1 Assault by hot tap water
- ✓x7ᵗʰ X98.2 Assault by hot fluids
- ✓x7ᵗʰ X98.3 Assault by hot household appliances
- ✓x7ᵗʰ X98.8 Assault by other hot objects
- ✓x7ᵗʰ X98.9 Assault by unspecified hot objects

✓4ᵗʰ X99 Assault by sharp object
EXCLUDES 1 assault by strike by sports equipment (Y08.0-)
- ✓x7ᵗʰ X99.0 Assault by sharp glass
- ✓x7ᵗʰ X99.1 Assault by knife
- ✓x7ᵗʰ X99.2 Assault by sword or dagger
- ✓x7ᵗʰ X99.8 Assault by other sharp object
- ✓x7ᵗʰ X99.9 Assault by unspecified sharp object
  Assault by stabbing NOS

✓x7ᵗʰ Y00 Assault by blunt object
EXCLUDES 1 assault by strike by sports equipment (Y08.0-)

✓x7ᵗʰ Y01 Assault by pushing from high place

✓4ᵗʰ Y02 Assault by pushing or placing victim in front of moving object
- ✓x7ᵗʰ Y02.0 Assault by pushing or placing victim in front of motor vehicle
- ✓x7ᵗʰ Y02.1 Assault by pushing or placing victim in front of (subway) train
- ✓x7ᵗʰ Y02.8 Assault by pushing or placing victim in front of other moving object

✓4ᵗʰ Y03 Assault by crashing of motor vehicle
- ✓x7ᵗʰ Y03.0 Assault by being hit or run over by motor vehicle
- ✓x7ᵗʰ Y03.8 Other assault by crashing of motor vehicle

✓4ᵗʰ Y04 Assault by bodily force
EXCLUDES 1 assault by:
submersion (X92.-)
use of weapon (X93-X95, X99, Y00)
- ✓x7ᵗʰ Y04.0 Assault by unarmed brawl or fight
- ✓x7ᵗʰ Y04.1 Assault by human bite
- ✓x7ᵗʰ Y04.2 Assault by strike against or bumped into by another person
- ✓x7ᵗʰ Y04.8 Assault by other bodily force
  Assault by bodily force NOS

Chapter 20. External Causes of Morbidity

✓4ᵗʰ Y07 Perpetrator of assault, maltreatment and neglect

> **NOTE** Codes from this category are for use only in cases of confirmed abuse (T74.-)
> Selection of the correct perpetrator code is based on the relationship between the perpetrator and the victim
>
> **INCLUDES** perpetrator of abandonment
> perpetrator of emotional neglect
> perpetrator of mental cruelty
> perpetrator of physical abuse
> perpetrator of physical neglect
> perpetrator of sexual abuse
> perpetrator of torture

✓5ᵗʰ Y07.0 Spouse or partner, perpetrator of maltreatment and neglect
> Spouse or partner, perpetrator of maltreatment and neglect against spouse or partner

    Y07.01 Husband, perpetrator of maltreatment and neglect

    Y07.02 Wife, perpetrator of maltreatment and neglect

    Y07.03 Male partner, perpetrator of maltreatment and neglect

    Y07.04 Female partner, perpetrator of maltreatment and neglect

✓5ᵗʰ Y07.1 Parent (adoptive) (biological), perpetrator of maltreatment and neglect

    Y07.11 Biological father, perpetrator of maltreatment and neglect

    Y07.12 Biological mother, perpetrator of maltreatment and neglect

    Y07.13 Adoptive father, perpetrator of maltreatment and neglect

    Y07.14 Adoptive mother, perpetrator of maltreatment and neglect

✓5ᵗʰ Y07.4 Other family member, perpetrator of maltreatment and neglect

    ✓6ᵗʰ Y07.41 Sibling, perpetrator of maltreatment and neglect
> **EXCLUDES 1** *stepsibling, perpetrator of maltreatment and neglect (Y07.435, Y07.436)*

        Y07.410 Brother, perpetrator of maltreatment and neglect

        Y07.411 Sister, perpetrator of maltreatment and neglect

    ✓6ᵗʰ Y07.42 Foster parent, perpetrator of maltreatment and neglect

        Y07.420 Foster father, perpetrator of maltreatment and neglect

        Y07.421 Foster mother, perpetrator of maltreatment and neglect

    ✓6ᵗʰ Y07.43 Stepparent or stepsibling, perpetrator of maltreatment and neglect

        Y07.430 Stepfather, perpetrator of maltreatment and neglect

        Y07.432 Male friend of parent (co-residing in household), perpetrator of maltreatment and neglect

        Y07.433 Stepmother, perpetrator of maltreatment and neglect

        Y07.434 Female friend of parent (co-residing in household), perpetrator of maltreatment and neglect

        Y07.435 Stepbrother, perpetrator or maltreatment and neglect

        Y07.436 Stepsister, perpetrator of maltreatment and neglect

    ✓6ᵗʰ Y07.49 Other family member, perpetrator of maltreatment and neglect

        Y07.490 Male cousin, perpetrator of maltreatment and neglect

        Y07.491 Female cousin, perpetrator of maltreatment and neglect

        Y07.499 Other family member, perpetrator of maltreatment and neglect

✓5ᵗʰ Y07.5 Non-family member, perpetrator of maltreatment and neglect

    Y07.50 Unspecified non-family member, perpetrator of maltreatment and neglect

    ✓6ᵗʰ Y07.51 Daycare provider, perpetrator of maltreatment and neglect

        Y07.510 At-home childcare provider, perpetrator of maltreatment and neglect

        Y07.511 Daycare center childcare provider, perpetrator of maltreatment and neglect

        Y07.512 At-home adultcare provider, perpetrator of maltreatment and neglect

        Y07.513 Adultcare center provider, perpetrator of maltreatment and neglect

        Y07.519 Unspecified daycare provider, perpetrator of maltreatment and neglect

    ✓6ᵗʰ Y07.52 Healthcare provider, perpetrator of maltreatment and neglect

        Y07.521 Mental health provider, perpetrator of maltreatment and neglect

        Y07.528 Other therapist or healthcare provider, perpetrator of maltreatment and neglect
> Nurse, perpetrator of maltreatment and neglect
> Occupational therapist, perpetrator of maltreatment and neglect
> Physical therapist, perpetrator of maltreatment and neglect
> Speech therapist, perpetrator of maltreatment and neglect

        Y07.529 Unspecified healthcare provider, perpetrator of maltreatment and neglect

    Y07.53 Teacher or instructor, perpetrator of maltreatment and neglect
> Coach, perpetrator of maltreatment and neglect

    Y07.59 Other non-family member, perpetrator of maltreatment and neglect

● **Y07.6 Multiple perpetrators of maltreatment and neglect**

    Y07.9 Unspecified perpetrator of maltreatment and neglect

✓4ᵗʰ Y08 Assault by other specified means

✓5ᵗʰ Y08.0 Assault by strike by sport equipment

    ✓x7ᵗʰ Y08.01 Assault by strike by hockey stick

    ✓x7ᵗʰ Y08.02 Assault by strike by baseball bat

    ✓x7ᵗʰ Y08.09 Assault by strike by other specified type of sport equipment

✓5ᵗʰ Y08.8 Assault by other specified means

    ✓x7ᵗʰ Y08.81 Assault by crashing of aircraft

    ✓x7ᵗʰ Y08.89 Assault by other specified means

Y09 Assault by unspecified means
> Assassination (attempted) NOS
> Homicide (attempted) NOS
> Manslaughter (attempted) NOS
> Murder (attempted) NOS

Event of undetermined intent (Y21-Y33)

Undetermined intent is only for use when there is specific documentation in the record that the intent of the injury cannot be determined. If no such documentation is present, code to accidental (unintentional)

> The appropriate 7th character is to be added to each code from categories Y21-Y33.
> A   initial encounter
> D   subsequent encounter
> S   sequela

✓4ᵗʰ Y21 Drowning and submersion, undetermined intent

    ✓x7ᵗʰ Y21.0 Drowning and submersion while in bathtub, undetermined intent

    ✓x7ᵗʰ Y21.1 Drowning and submersion after fall into bathtub, undetermined intent

    ✓x7ᵗʰ Y21.2 Drowning and submersion while in swimming pool, undetermined intent

    ✓x7ᵗʰ Y21.3 Drowning and submersion after fall into swimming pool, undetermined intent

    ✓x7ᵗʰ Y21.4 Drowning and submersion in natural water, undetermined intent

    ✓x7ᵗʰ Y21.8 Other drowning and submersion, undetermined intent

    ✓x7ᵗʰ Y21.9 Unspecified drowning and submersion, undetermined intent

Ⓝ Newborn: 0   Ⓟ Pediatric: 0-17   Ⓜ Maternity: 12-55   Ⓐ Adult: 15-124   **MCC** Major Complication/Comorbidity   **CC** Complication/Comorbidity   **SW** Severe Wound Dx

1200   ICD-10-CM 2019

√x7ᵗʰ **Y22 Handgun discharge, undetermined intent**
     Discharge of gun for single hand use, undetermined intent
     Discharge of pistol, undetermined intent
     Discharge of revolver, undetermined intent
     EXCLUDES 2   Very pistol (Y24.8)

√4ᵗʰ **Y23 Rifle, shotgun and larger firearm discharge, undetermined intent**
     EXCLUDES 2   airgun (Y24.0)

   √x7ᵗʰ **Y23.0 Shotgun discharge, undetermined intent**

   √x7ᵗʰ **Y23.1 Hunting rifle discharge, undetermined intent**

   √x7ᵗʰ **Y23.2 Military firearm discharge, undetermined intent**

   √x7ᵗʰ **Y23.3 Machine gun discharge, undetermined intent**

   √x7ᵗʰ **Y23.8 Other larger firearm discharge, undetermined intent**

   √x7ᵗʰ **Y23.9 Unspecified larger firearm discharge, undetermined intent**

√4ᵗʰ **Y24 Other and unspecified firearm discharge, undetermined intent**

   √x7ᵗʰ **Y24.0 Airgun discharge, undetermined intent**
       BB gun discharge, undetermined intent
       Pellet gun discharge, undetermined intent

   √x7ᵗʰ **Y24.8 Other firearm discharge, undetermined intent**
       Paintball gun discharge, undetermined intent
       Very pistol [flare] discharge, undetermined intent

   √x7ᵗʰ **Y24.9 Unspecified firearm discharge, undetermined intent**

√x7ᵗʰ **Y25 Contact with explosive material, undetermined intent**

√x7ᵗʰ **Y26 Exposure to smoke, fire and flames, undetermined intent**

√4ᵗʰ **Y27 Contact with steam, hot vapors and hot objects, undetermined intent**

   √x7ᵗʰ **Y27.0 Contact with steam and hot vapors, undetermined intent**

   √x7ᵗʰ **Y27.1 Contact with hot tap water, undetermined intent**

   √x7ᵗʰ **Y27.2 Contact with hot fluids, undetermined intent**

   √x7ᵗʰ **Y27.3 Contact with hot household appliance, undetermined intent**

   √x7ᵗʰ **Y27.8 Contact with other hot objects, undetermined intent**

   √x7ᵗʰ **Y27.9 Contact with unspecified hot objects, undetermined intent**

√4ᵗʰ **Y28 Contact with sharp object, undetermined intent**

   √x7ᵗʰ **Y28.0 Contact with sharp glass, undetermined intent**

   √x7ᵗʰ **Y28.1 Contact with knife, undetermined intent**

   √x7ᵗʰ **Y28.2 Contact with sword or dagger, undetermined intent**

   √x7ᵗʰ **Y28.8 Contact with other sharp object, undetermined intent**

   √x7ᵗʰ **Y28.9 Contact with unspecified sharp object, undetermined intent**

√x7ᵗʰ **Y29 Contact with blunt object, undetermined intent**

√x7ᵗʰ **Y30 Falling, jumping or pushed from a high place, undetermined intent**
     Victim falling from one level to another, undetermined intent

√x7ᵗʰ **Y31 Falling, lying or running before or into moving object, undetermined intent**

√x7ᵗʰ **Y32 Crashing of motor vehicle, undetermined intent**

√x7ᵗʰ **Y33 Other specified events, undetermined intent**

Legal intervention, operations of war, military operations, and terrorism (Y35-Y38)

> The appropriate 7th character is to be added to each code from categories Y35-Y38.
> A   initial encounter
> D   subsequent encounter
> S   sequela

√4ᵗʰ **Y35 Legal intervention**
   INCLUDES   any injury sustained as a result of an encounter with any law enforcement official, serving in any capacity at the time of the encounter, whether on-duty or off-duty. Includes: injury to law enforcement official, suspect and bystander

   √5ᵗʰ **Y35.0 Legal intervention involving firearm discharge**

     √6ᵗʰ **Y35.00 Legal intervention involving unspecified firearm discharge**
        Legal intervention involving gunshot wound
        Legal intervention involving shot NOS

       √7ᵗʰ **Y35.001 Legal intervention involving unspecified firearm discharge, law enforcement official injured**

       √7ᵗʰ **Y35.002 Legal intervention involving unspecified firearm discharge, bystander injured**

       √7ᵗʰ **Y35.003 Legal intervention involving unspecified firearm discharge, suspect injured**

     √6ᵗʰ **Y35.01 Legal intervention involving injury by machine gun**

       √7ᵗʰ **Y35.011 Legal intervention involving injury by machine gun, law enforcement official injured**

       √7ᵗʰ **Y35.012 Legal intervention involving injury by machine gun, bystander injured**

       √7ᵗʰ **Y35.013 Legal intervention involving injury by machine gun, suspect injured**

     √6ᵗʰ **Y35.02 Legal intervention involving injury by handgun**

       √7ᵗʰ **Y35.021 Legal intervention involving injury by handgun, law enforcement official injured**

       √7ᵗʰ **Y35.022 Legal intervention involving injury by handgun, bystander injured**

       √7ᵗʰ **Y35.023 Legal intervention involving injury by handgun, suspect injured**

     √6ᵗʰ **Y35.03 Legal intervention involving injury by rifle pellet**

       √7ᵗʰ **Y35.031 Legal intervention involving injury by rifle pellet, law enforcement official injured**

       √7ᵗʰ **Y35.032 Legal intervention involving injury by rifle pellet, bystander injured**

       √7ᵗʰ **Y35.033 Legal intervention involving injury by rifle pellet, suspect injured**

     √6ᵗʰ **Y35.04 Legal intervention involving injury by rubber bullet**

       √7ᵗʰ **Y35.041 Legal intervention involving injury by rubber bullet, law enforcement official injured**

       √7ᵗʰ **Y35.042 Legal intervention involving injury by rubber bullet, bystander injured**

       √7ᵗʰ **Y35.043 Legal intervention involving injury by rubber bullet, suspect injured**

     √6ᵗʰ **Y35.09 Legal intervention involving other firearm discharge**

       √7ᵗʰ **Y35.091 Legal intervention involving other firearm discharge, law enforcement official injured**

       √7ᵗʰ **Y35.092 Legal intervention involving other firearm discharge, bystander injured**

       √7ᵗʰ **Y35.093 Legal intervention involving other firearm discharge, suspect injured**

   √5ᵗʰ **Y35.1 Legal intervention involving explosives**

     √6ᵗʰ **Y35.10 Legal intervention involving unspecified explosives**

       √7ᵗʰ **Y35.101 Legal intervention involving unspecified explosives, law enforcement official injured**

       √7ᵗʰ **Y35.102 Legal intervention involving unspecified explosives, bystander injured**

       √7ᵗʰ **Y35.103 Legal intervention involving unspecified explosives, suspect injured**

     √6ᵗʰ **Y35.11 Legal intervention involving injury by dynamite**

       √7ᵗʰ **Y35.111 Legal intervention involving injury by dynamite, law enforcement official injured**

       √7ᵗʰ **Y35.112 Legal intervention involving injury by dynamite, bystander injured**

       √7ᵗʰ **Y35.113 Legal intervention involving injury by dynamite, suspect injured**

     √6ᵗʰ **Y35.12 Legal intervention involving injury by explosive shell**

       √7ᵗʰ **Y35.121 Legal intervention involving injury by explosive shell, law enforcement official injured**

       √7ᵗʰ **Y35.122 Legal intervention involving injury by explosive shell, bystander injured**

       √7ᵗʰ **Y35.123 Legal intervention involving injury by explosive shell, suspect injured**

     √6ᵗʰ **Y35.19 Legal intervention involving other explosives**
        Legal intervention involving injury by grenade
        Legal intervention involving injury by mortar bomb

       √7ᵗʰ **Y35.191 Legal intervention involving other explosives, law enforcement official injured**

       √7ᵗʰ **Y35.192 Legal intervention involving other explosives, bystander injured**

       √7ᵗʰ **Y35.193 Legal intervention involving other explosives, suspect injured**

✓5th **Y35.2** **Legal intervention involving** gas
Legal intervention involving asphyxiation by gas
Legal intervention involving poisoning by gas

  ✓6th **Y35.20** **Legal intervention involving** unspecified gas

    ✓7th **Y35.201** **Legal intervention involving unspecified gas,** law enforcement **official injured**

    ✓7th **Y35.202** **Legal intervention involving unspecified gas,** bystander **injured**

    ✓7th **Y35.203** **Legal intervention involving unspecified gas,** suspect **injured**

  ✓6th **Y35.21** **Legal intervention involving injury by** tear gas

    ✓7th **Y35.211** **Legal intervention involving injury by tear gas,** law enforcement **official injured**

    ✓7th **Y35.212** **Legal intervention involving injury by tear gas,** bystander **injured**

    ✓7th **Y35.213** **Legal intervention involving injury by tear gas,** suspect **injured**

  ✓6th **Y35.29** **Legal intervention involving** other gas

    ✓7th **Y35.291** **Legal intervention involving other gas,** law enforcement **official injured**

    ✓7th **Y35.292** **Legal intervention involving other gas,** bystander **injured**

    ✓7th **Y35.293** **Legal intervention involving other gas,** suspect **injured**

✓5th **Y35.3** **Legal intervention involving** blunt objects
Legal intervention involving being hit or struck by blunt object

  ✓6th **Y35.30** **Legal intervention involving** unspecified blunt objects

    ✓7th **Y35.301** **Legal intervention involving unspecified blunt objects,** law enforcement **official injured**

    ✓7th **Y35.302** **Legal intervention involving unspecified blunt objects,** bystander **injured**

    ✓7th **Y35.303** **Legal intervention involving unspecified blunt objects,** suspect **injured**

  ✓6th **Y35.31** **Legal intervention involving** baton

    ✓7th **Y35.311** **Legal intervention involving baton,** law enforcement **official injured**

    ✓7th **Y35.312** **Legal intervention involving baton,** bystander **injured**

    ✓7th **Y35.313** **Legal intervention involving baton,** suspect **injured**

  ✓6th **Y35.39** **Legal intervention involving** other blunt objects

    ✓7th **Y35.391** **Legal intervention involving other blunt objects,** law enforcement **official injured**

    ✓7th **Y35.392** **Legal intervention involving other blunt objects,** bystander **injured**

    ✓7th **Y35.393** **Legal intervention involving other blunt objects,** suspect **injured**

✓5th **Y35.4** **Legal intervention involving** sharp objects
Legal intervention involving being cut by sharp objects
Legal intervention involving being stabbed by sharp objects

  ✓6th **Y35.40** **Legal intervention involving** unspecified sharp objects

    ✓7th **Y35.401** **Legal intervention involving unspecified sharp objects,** law enforcement **official injured**

    ✓7th **Y35.402** **Legal intervention involving unspecified sharp objects,** bystander **injured**

    ✓7th **Y35.403** **Legal intervention involving unspecified sharp objects,** suspect **injured**

  ✓6th **Y35.41** **Legal intervention involving** bayonet

    ✓7th **Y35.411** **Legal intervention involving bayonet,** law enforcement **official injured**

    ✓7th **Y35.412** **Legal intervention involving bayonet,** bystander **injured**

    ✓7th **Y35.413** **Legal intervention involving bayonet,** suspect **injured**

  ✓6th **Y35.49** **Legal intervention involving** other sharp objects

    ✓7th **Y35.491** **Legal intervention involving other sharp objects,** law enforcement **official injured**

    ✓7th **Y35.492** **Legal intervention involving other sharp objects,** bystander **injured**

    ✓7th **Y35.493** **Legal intervention involving other sharp objects,** suspect **injured**

✓5th **Y35.8** **Legal intervention involving** other specified means

  ✓6th **Y35.81** **Legal intervention involving** manhandling

    ✓7th **Y35.811** **Legal intervention involving manhandling,** law enforcement **official injured**

    ✓7th **Y35.812** **Legal intervention involving manhandling,** bystander **injured**

    ✓7th **Y35.813** **Legal intervention involving manhandling,** suspect **injured**

  ✓6th **Y35.89** **Legal intervention involving** other specified means

    ✓7th **Y35.891** **Legal intervention involving other specified means,** law enforcement **official injured**

    ✓7th **Y35.892** **Legal intervention involving other specified means,** bystander **injured**

    ✓7th **Y35.893** **Legal intervention involving other specified means,** suspect **injured**
        AHA: 2018, 1Q, 5

✓5th **Y35.9** **Legal intervention, means** unspecified

  ✓x7th **Y35.91** **Legal intervention, means unspecified,** law enforcement **official injured**

  ✓x7th **Y35.92** **Legal intervention, means unspecified,** bystander **injured**

  ✓x7th **Y35.93** **Legal intervention, means unspecified,** suspect **injured**

✓4th **Y36** **Operations of war**
  INCLUDES injuries to military personnel and civilians caused by war, civil insurrection, and peacekeeping missions
  EXCLUDES 1 *injury to military personnel occurring during peacetime military operations (Y37.-)*
        military vehicles involved in transport accidents with non-military vehicle during peacetime (V09.01, V09.21, V19.81, V29.81, V39.81, V49.81, V59.81, V69.81, V79.81)
  AHA: 2014, 3Q, 4

✓5th **Y36.0** **War operations involving** explosion of marine weapons

  ✓6th **Y36.00** **War operations involving explosion of** unspecified marine weapon
      War operations involving underwater blast NOS

    ✓7th **Y36.000** **War operations involving explosion of unspecified marine weapon,** military personnel

    ✓7th **Y36.001** **War operations involving explosion of unspecified marine weapon,** civilian

  ✓6th **Y36.01** **War operations involving explosion of** depth-charge

    ✓7th **Y36.010** **War operations involving explosion of depth-charge,** military personnel

    ✓7th **Y36.011** **War operations involving explosion of depth-charge,** civilian

  ✓6th **Y36.02** **War operations involving explosion of** marine mine
      War operations involving explosion of marine mine, at sea or in harbor

    ✓7th **Y36.020** **War operations involving explosion of marine mine,** military personnel

    ✓7th **Y36.021** **War operations involving explosion of marine mine,** civilian

  ✓6th **Y36.03** **War operations involving explosion of** sea-based artillery shell

    ✓7th **Y36.030** **War operations involving explosion of sea-based artillery shell,** military personnel

    ✓7th **Y36.031** **War operations involving explosion of sea-based artillery shell,** civilian

  ✓6th **Y36.04** **War operations involving explosion of** torpedo

    ✓7th **Y36.040** **War operations involving explosion of torpedo,** military personnel

    ✓7th **Y36.041** **War operations involving explosion of torpedo,** civilian

  ✓6th **Y36.05** **War operations involving** accidental detonation of onboard marine weapons

    ✓7th **Y36.050** **War operations involving accidental detonation of onboard marine weapons,** military personnel

    ✓7th **Y36.051** **War operations involving accidental detonation of onboard marine weapons,** civilian

✓6ᵗʰ **Y36.09** **War operations involving explosion of** other marine weapons

     ✓7ᵗʰ **Y36.090** **War operations involving explosion of other marine weapons,** military personnel

     ✓7ᵗʰ **Y36.091** **War operations involving explosion of other marine weapons,** civilian

✓5ᵗʰ **Y36.1** **War operations involving** destruction of aircraft

   ✓6ᵗʰ **Y36.10** **War operations involving** unspecified **destruction of aircraft**

     ✓7ᵗʰ **Y36.100** **War operations involving unspecified destruction of aircraft,** military personnel

     ✓7ᵗʰ **Y36.101** **War operations involving unspecified destruction of aircraft,** civilian

   ✓6ᵗʰ **Y36.11** **War operations involving destruction of aircraft due to** enemy fire or explosives

     War operations involving destruction of aircraft due to air to air missile
     War operations involving destruction of aircraft due to explosive placed on aircraft
     War operations involving destruction of aircraft due to rocket propelled grenade [RPG]
     War operations involving destruction of aircraft due to small arms fire
     War operations involving destruction of aircraft due to surface to air missile

     ✓7ᵗʰ **Y36.110** **War operations involving destruction of aircraft due to enemy fire or explosives, military personnel**

     ✓7ᵗʰ **Y36.111** **War operations involving destruction of aircraft due to enemy fire or explosives,** civilian

   ✓6ᵗʰ **Y36.12** **War operations involving destruction of aircraft due to** collision with other aircraft

     ✓7ᵗʰ **Y36.120** **War operations involving destruction of aircraft due to collision with other aircraft,** military personnel

     ✓7ᵗʰ **Y36.121** **War operations involving destruction of aircraft due to collision with other aircraft,** civilian

   ✓6ᵗʰ **Y36.13** **War operations involving destruction of aircraft due to** onboard fire

     ✓7ᵗʰ **Y36.130** **War operations involving destruction of aircraft due to onboard fire,** military personnel

     ✓7ᵗʰ **Y36.131** **War operations involving destruction of aircraft due to onboard fire,** civilian

   ✓6ᵗʰ **Y36.14** **War operations involving destruction of aircraft due to** accidental detonation of onboard munitions and explosives

     ✓7ᵗʰ **Y36.140** **War operations involving destruction of aircraft due to accidental detonation of onboard munitions and explosives,** military personnel

     ✓7ᵗʰ **Y36.141** **War operations involving destruction of aircraft due to accidental detonation of onboard munitions and explosives,** civilian

   ✓6ᵗʰ **Y36.19** **War operations involving** other **destruction of aircraft**

     ✓7ᵗʰ **Y36.190** **War operations involving other destruction of aircraft,** military personnel

     ✓7ᵗʰ **Y36.191** **War operations involving other destruction of aircraft,** civilian

✓5ᵗʰ **Y36.2** **War operations involving** other **explosions and fragments**

     EXCLUDES 1   *war operations involving explosion of aircraft (Y36.1-)*
        war operations involving explosion of marine weapons (Y36.0-)
        war operations involving explosion of nuclear weapons (Y36.5-)
        war operations involving explosion occurring after cessation of hostilities (Y36.8-)

✓6ᵗʰ **Y36.20** **War operations involving** unspecified **explosion and fragments**

     War operations involving air blast NOS
     War operations involving blast NOS
     War operations involving blast fragments NOS
     War operations involving blast wave NOS
     War operations involving blast wind NOS
     War operations involving explosion NOS
     War operations involving explosion of bomb NOS

     ✓7ᵗʰ **Y36.200** **War operations involving unspecified explosion and fragments,** military personnel

     ✓7ᵗʰ **Y36.201** **War operations involving unspecified explosion and fragments,** civilian

✓6ᵗʰ **Y36.21** **War operations involving explosion of** aerial bomb

     ✓7ᵗʰ **Y36.210** **War operations involving explosion of aerial bomb,** military personnel

     ✓7ᵗʰ **Y36.211** **War operations involving explosion of aerial bomb,** civilian

✓6ᵗʰ **Y36.22** **War operations involving explosion of** guided missile

     ✓7ᵗʰ **Y36.220** **War operations involving explosion of guided missile,** military personnel

     ✓7ᵗʰ **Y36.221** **War operations involving explosion of guided missile,** civilian

✓6ᵗʰ **Y36.23** **War operations involving explosion of** improvised explosive device [IED]

     War operations involving explosion of person-borne improvised explosive device [IED]
     War operations involving explosion of vehicle-borne improvised explosive device [IED]
     War operations involving explosion of roadside improvised explosive device [IED]

     ✓7ᵗʰ **Y36.230** **War operations involving explosion of improvised explosive device [IED],** military personnel

     ✓7ᵗʰ **Y36.231** **War operations involving explosion of improvised explosive device [IED],** civilian

✓6ᵗʰ **Y36.24** **War operations involving explosion due to** accidental detonation and discharge of own munitions or munitions launch device

     ✓7ᵗʰ **Y36.240** **War operations involving explosion due to accidental detonation and discharge of own munitions or munitions launch device,** military personnel

     ✓7ᵗʰ **Y36.241** **War operations involving explosion due to accidental detonation and discharge of own munitions or munitions launch device,** civilian

✓6ᵗʰ **Y36.25** **War operations involving** fragments from munitions

     ✓7ᵗʰ **Y36.250** **War operations involving fragments from munitions,** military personnel

     ✓7ᵗʰ **Y36.251** **War operations involving fragments from munitions,** civilian

✓6ᵗʰ **Y36.26** **War operations involving fragments of** improvised explosive device [IED]

     War operations involving fragments of person-borne improvised explosive device [IED]
     War operations involving fragments of vehicle-borne improvised explosive device [IED]
     War operations involving fragments of roadside improvised explosive device [IED]

     ✓7ᵗʰ **Y36.260** **War operations involving fragments of improvised explosive device [IED],** military personnel

     ✓7ᵗʰ **Y36.261** **War operations involving fragments of improvised explosive device [IED],** civilian

✓6ᵗʰ **Y36.27** **War operations involving** fragments from weapons

     ✓7ᵗʰ **Y36.270** **War operations involving fragments from weapons,** military personnel

     ✓7ᵗʰ **Y36.271** **War operations involving fragments from weapons,** civilian

✓6ᵗʰ **Y36.29** **War operations involving** other **explosions and fragments**

     War operations involving explosion of grenade
     War operations involving explosions of land mine
     War operations involving shrapnel NOS

     ✓7ᵗʰ **Y36.290** **War operations involving other explosions and fragments,** military personnel

✅ Additional Character Required   ✓×7ᵗʰ Placeholder   Unacceptable PDx   Questionable PDx   Wrong Procedure   Manifestation   **H1**-**H14** HAC   **HCC** CMS-HCC Dx   **HIV** HIV Dx

ICD-10-CM 2019   **1203**

√7ᵗʰ **Y36.291** **War operations involving other explosions and fragments,** civilian

√5ᵗʰ **Y36.3** **War operations involving** fires, conflagrations and hot substance
     War operations involving smoke, fumes, and heat from fires, conflagrations and hot substances
     EXCLUDES 1   *war operations involving fires and conflagrations aboard military aircraft (Y36.1-)*
         war operations involving fires and conflagrations aboard military watercraft (Y36.0-)
         war operations involving fires and conflagrations caused indirectly by conventional weapons (Y36.2-)
         war operations involving fires and thermal effects of nuclear weapons (Y36.53-)

√6ᵗʰ **Y36.30** **War operations involving** unspecified **fire, conflagration and hot substance**

√7ᵗʰ **Y36.300** **War operations involving unspecified fire, conflagration and hot substance,** military personnel

√7ᵗʰ **Y36.301** **War operations involving unspecified fire, conflagration and hot substance,** civilian

√6ᵗʰ **Y36.31** **War operations involving** gasoline bomb
     War operations involving incendiary bomb
     War operations involving petrol bomb

√7ᵗʰ **Y36.310** **War operations involving gasoline bomb,** military personnel

√7ᵗʰ **Y36.311** **War operations involving gasoline bomb,** civilian

√6ᵗʰ **Y36.32** **War operations involving** incendiary bullet

√7ᵗʰ **Y36.320** **War operations involving incendiary bullet,** military personnel

√7ᵗʰ **Y36.321** **War operations involving incendiary bullet,** civilian

√6ᵗʰ **Y36.33** **War operations involving** flamethrower

√7ᵗʰ **Y36.330** **War operations involving flamethrower,** military personnel

√7ᵗʰ **Y36.331** **War operations involving flamethrower,** civilian

√6ᵗʰ **Y36.39** **War operations involving other fires,** conflagrations and hot substances

√7ᵗʰ **Y36.390** **War operations involving other fires, conflagrations and hot substances,** military personnel

√7ᵗʰ **Y36.391** **War operations involving other fires, conflagrations and hot substances,** civilian

√5ᵗʰ **Y36.4** **War operations involving firearm discharge and other forms of conventional warfare**

√6ᵗʰ **Y36.41** **War operations involving** rubber bullets

√7ᵗʰ **Y36.410** **War operations involving rubber bullets,** military personnel

√7ᵗʰ **Y36.411** **War operations involving rubber bullets,** civilian

√6ᵗʰ **Y36.42** **War operations involving** firearms pellets

√7ᵗʰ **Y36.420** **War operations involving firearms pellets,** military personnel

√7ᵗʰ **Y36.421** **War operations involving firearms pellets,** civilian

√6ᵗʰ **Y36.43** **War operations involving** other **firearms discharge**
     War operations involving bullets NOS
     EXCLUDES 1   *war operations involving munitions fragments (Y36.25-)*
         war operations involving incendiary bullets (Y36.32-)

√7ᵗʰ **Y36.430** **War operations involving other firearms discharge,** military personnel

√7ᵗʰ **Y36.431** **War operations involving other firearms discharge,** civilian

√6ᵗʰ **Y36.44** **War operations involving** unarmed hand to hand combat
     EXCLUDES 1   *war operations involving combat using blunt or piercing object (Y36.45-)*
         war operations involving intentional restriction of air and airway (Y36.46-)
         war operations involving unintentional restriction of air and airway (Y36.47-)

√7ᵗʰ **Y36.440** **War operations involving unarmed hand to hand combat,** military personnel

√7ᵗʰ **Y36.441** **War operations involving unarmed hand to hand combat,** civilian

√6ᵗʰ **Y36.45** **War operations involving combat using blunt or piercing object**

√7ᵗʰ **Y36.450** **War operations involving combat using blunt or piercing object,** military personnel

√7ᵗʰ **Y36.451** **War operations involving combat using blunt or piercing object,** civilian

√6ᵗʰ **Y36.46** **War operations involving** intentional restriction of air and airway

√7ᵗʰ **Y36.460** **War operations involving intentional restriction of air and airway,** military personnel

√7ᵗʰ **Y36.461** **War operations involving intentional restriction of air and airway,** civilian

√6ᵗʰ **Y36.47** **War operations involving** unintentional restriction of air and airway

√7ᵗʰ **Y36.470** **War operations involving unintentional restriction of air and airway,** military personnel

√7ᵗʰ **Y36.471** **War operations involving unintentional restriction of air and airway,** civilian

√6ᵗʰ **Y36.49** **War operations involving** other forms of conventional warfare

√7ᵗʰ **Y36.490** **War operations involving other forms of conventional warfare,** military personnel

√7ᵗʰ **Y36.491** **War operations involving other forms of conventional warfare,** civilian

√5ᵗʰ **Y36.5** **War operations involving** nuclear weapons
     War operations involving dirty bomb NOS

√6ᵗʰ **Y36.50** **War operations involving** unspecified **effect of nuclear weapon**

√7ᵗʰ **Y36.500** **War operations involving unspecified effect of nuclear weapon,** military personnel

√7ᵗʰ **Y36.501** **War operations involving unspecified effect of nuclear weapon,** civilian

√6ᵗʰ **Y36.51** **War operations involving** direct blast **effect of nuclear weapon**
     War operations involving blast pressure of nuclear weapon

√7ᵗʰ **Y36.510** **War operations involving direct blast effect of nuclear weapon,** military personnel

√7ᵗʰ **Y36.511** **War operations involving direct blast effect of nuclear weapon,** civilian

√6ᵗʰ **Y36.52** **War operations involving** indirect blast **effect of nuclear weapon**
     War operations involving being thrown by blast of nuclear weapon
     War operations involving being struck or crushed by blast debris of nuclear weapon

√7ᵗʰ **Y36.520** **War operations involving indirect blast effect of nuclear weapon,** military personnel

√7ᵗʰ **Y36.521** **War operations involving indirect blast effect of nuclear weapon,** civilian

√6ᵗʰ **Y36.53** **War operations involving** thermal radiation **effect of nuclear weapon**
     War operations involving direct heat from nuclear weapon
     War operation involving fireball effects from nuclear weapon

√7ᵗʰ **Y36.530** **War operations involving thermal radiation effect of nuclear weapon,** military personnel

---

☑7ᵗʰ **Y36.531** **War operations involving thermal radiation effect of nuclear weapon,** civilian

☑6ᵗʰ **Y36.54** **War operation involving** nuclear radiation **effects of nuclear weapon**
War operation involving acute radiation exposure from nuclear weapon
War operation involving exposure to immediate ionizing radiation from nuclear weapon
War operation involving fallout exposure from nuclear weapon
War operation involving secondary effects of nuclear weapons

☑7ᵗʰ **Y36.540** **War operation involving nuclear radiation effects of nuclear weapon,** military personnel

☑7ᵗʰ **Y36.541** **War operation involving nuclear radiation effects of nuclear weapon,** civilian

☑6ᵗʰ **Y36.59** **War operation involving** other **effects of nuclear weapons**

☑7ᵗʰ **Y36.590** **War operation involving other effects of nuclear weapons,** military personnel

☑7ᵗʰ **Y36.591** **War operation involving other effects of nuclear weapons,** civilian

☑5ᵗʰ **Y36.6** **War operations involving biological weapons**

☑6ᵗʰ **Y36.6X** **War operations involving** biological weapons

☑7ᵗʰ **Y36.6X0** **War operations involving biological weapons,** military personnel

☑7ᵗʰ **Y36.6X1** **War operations involving biological weapons,** civilian

☑5ᵗʰ **Y36.7** **War operations involving chemical weapons and other forms of unconventional warfare**
    EXCLUDES 1   war operations involving incendiary devices (Y36.3-, Y36.5-)

☑6ᵗʰ **Y36.7X** **War operations involving** chemical weapons **and** other **forms of** unconventional warfare

☑7ᵗʰ **Y36.7X0** **War operations involving chemical weapons and other forms of unconventional warfare,** military personnel

☑7ᵗʰ **Y36.7X1** **War operations involving chemical weapons and other forms of unconventional warfare,** civilian

☑5ᵗʰ **Y36.8** **War operations occurring** after cessation of hostilities
War operations classifiable to categories Y36.0-Y36.8 but occurring after cessation of hostilities

☑6ᵗʰ **Y36.81** **Explosion of** mine **placed during war operations but exploding after cessation of hostilities**

☑7ᵗʰ **Y36.810** **Explosion of mine placed during war operations but exploding after cessation of hostilities,** military personnel

☑7ᵗʰ **Y36.811** **Explosion of mine placed during war operations but exploding after cessation of hostilities,** civilian

☑6ᵗʰ **Y36.82** **Explosion of** bomb **placed during war operations but exploding after cessation of hostilities**

☑7ᵗʰ **Y36.820** **Explosion of bomb placed during war operations but exploding after cessation of hostilities,** military personnel

☑7ᵗʰ **Y36.821** **Explosion of bomb placed during war operations but exploding after cessation of hostilities,** civilian

☑6ᵗʰ **Y36.88** Other **war operations occurring after cessation of hostilities**

☑7ᵗʰ **Y36.880** **Other war operations occurring after cessation of hostilities,** military personnel

☑7ᵗʰ **Y36.881** **Other war operations occurring after cessation of hostilities,** civilian

☑6ᵗʰ **Y36.89** Unspecified **war operations occurring after cessation of hostilities**

☑7ᵗʰ **Y36.890** **Unspecified war operations occurring after cessation of hostilities,** military personnel

☑7ᵗʰ **Y36.891** **Unspecified war operations occurring after cessation of hostilities,** civilian

☑5ᵗʰ **Y36.9** **Other and unspecified war operations**

☑x7ᵗʰ **Y36.90** **War operations,** unspecified

☑x7ᵗʰ **Y36.91** **War operations** involving unspecified weapon of mass destruction [WMD]

☑x7ᵗʰ **Y36.92** **War operations** involving friendly fire

☑4ᵗʰ **Y37** **Military operations**
  INCLUDES   injuries to military personnel and civilians occurring during peacetime on military property and during routine military exercises and operations
  EXCLUDES 1   *military aircraft involved in aircraft accident with civilian aircraft (V97.81-)*
military vehicles involved in transport accident with civilian vehicle (V09.01, V09.21, V19.81, V29.81, V39.81, V49.81, V59.81, V69.81, V79.81)
military watercraft involved in water transport accident with civilian watercraft (V94.81-)
war operations (Y36.-)

☑5ᵗʰ **Y37.0** **Military operations involving** explosion of marine weapons

☑6ᵗʰ **Y37.00** **Military operations involving explosion of** unspecified **marine weapon**
Military operations involving underwater blast NOS

☑7ᵗʰ **Y37.000** **Military operations involving explosion of unspecified marine weapon,** military personnel

☑7ᵗʰ **Y37.001** **Military operations involving explosion of unspecified marine weapon,** civilian

☑6ᵗʰ **Y37.01** **Military operations involving explosion of** depth-charge

☑7ᵗʰ **Y37.010** **Military operations involving explosion of depth-charge,** military personnel

☑7ᵗʰ **Y37.011** **Military operations involving explosion of depth-charge,** civilian

☑6ᵗʰ **Y37.02** **Military operations involving explosion of** marine mine
Military operations involving explosion of marine mine, at sea or in harbor

☑7ᵗʰ **Y37.020** **Military operations involving explosion of marine mine,** military personnel

☑7ᵗʰ **Y37.021** **Military operations involving explosion of marine mine,** civilian

☑6ᵗʰ **Y37.03** **Military operations involving explosion of** sea-based artillery shell

☑7ᵗʰ **Y37.030** **Military operations involving explosion of sea-based artillery shell,** military personnel

☑7ᵗʰ **Y37.031** **Military operations involving explosion of sea-based artillery shell,** civilian

☑6ᵗʰ **Y37.04** **Military operations involving explosion of** torpedo

☑7ᵗʰ **Y37.040** **Military operations involving explosion of torpedo,** military personnel

☑7ᵗʰ **Y37.041** **Military operations involving explosion of torpedo,** civilian

☑6ᵗʰ **Y37.05** **Military operations involving accidental detonation of** onboard marine weapons

☑7ᵗʰ **Y37.050** **Military operations involving accidental detonation of onboard marine weapons,** military personnel

☑7ᵗʰ **Y37.051** **Military operations involving accidental detonation of onboard marine weapons,** civilian

☑6ᵗʰ **Y37.09** **Military operations involving explosion of** other marine weapons

☑7ᵗʰ **Y37.090** **Military operations involving explosion of other marine weapons,** military personnel

☑7ᵗʰ **Y37.091** **Military operations involving explosion of other marine weapons,** civilian

☑5ᵗʰ **Y37.1** **Military operations involving** destruction of aircraft

☑6ᵗʰ **Y37.10** **Military operations involving** unspecified **destruction of aircraft**

☑7ᵗʰ **Y37.100** **Military operations involving unspecified destruction of aircraft,** military personnel

☑7ᵗʰ **Y37.101** **Military operations involving unspecified destruction of aircraft,** civilian

☑ Additional Character Required   ☑x7ᵗʰ Placeholder   Unacceptable PDx   Questionable PDx   Wrong Procedure   Manifestation   H1-H14 HAC   HCC CMS-HCC Dx   HIV HIV Dx

ICD-10-CM 2019   1205

✓6ᵗʰ Y37.11 Military operations involving destruction of aircraft due to enemy fire or explosives

Military operations involving destruction of aircraft due to air to air missile

Military operations involving destruction of aircraft due to explosive placed on aircraft

Military operations involving destruction of aircraft due to rocket propelled grenade [RPG]

Military operations involving destruction of aircraft due to small arms fire

Military operations involving destruction of aircraft due to surface to air missile

✓7ᵗʰ Y37.110 Military operations involving destruction of aircraft due to enemy fire or explosives, military personnel

✓7ᵗʰ Y37.111 Military operations involving destruction of aircraft due to enemy fire or explosives, civilian

✓6ᵗʰ Y37.12 Military operations involving destruction of aircraft due to collision with other aircraft

✓7ᵗʰ Y37.120 Military operations involving destruction of aircraft due to collision with other aircraft, military personnel

✓7ᵗʰ Y37.121 Military operations involving destruction of aircraft due to collision with other aircraft, civilian

✓6ᵗʰ Y37.13 Military operations involving destruction of aircraft due to onboard fire

✓7ᵗʰ Y37.130 Military operations involving destruction of aircraft due to onboard fire, military personnel

✓7ᵗʰ Y37.131 Military operations involving destruction of aircraft due to onboard fire, civilian

✓6ᵗʰ Y37.14 Military operations involving destruction of aircraft due to accidental detonation of onboard munitions and explosives

✓7ᵗʰ Y37.140 Military operations involving destruction of aircraft due to accidental detonation of onboard munitions and explosives, military personnel

✓7ᵗʰ Y37.141 Military operations involving destruction of aircraft due to accidental detonation of onboard munitions and explosives, civilian

✓6ᵗʰ Y37.19 Military operations involving other destruction of aircraft

✓7ᵗʰ Y37.190 Military operations involving other destruction of aircraft, military personnel

✓7ᵗʰ Y37.191 Military operations involving other destruction of aircraft, civilian

✓5ᵗʰ Y37.2 Military operations involving other explosions and fragments

EXCLUDES 1   military operations involving explosion of aircraft (Y37.1-)

military operations involving explosion of marine weapons (Y37.0-)

military operations involving explosion of nuclear weapons (Y37.5-)

✓6ᵗʰ Y37.20 Military operations involving unspecified **explosion and fragments**

Military operations involving air blast NOS

Military operations involving blast NOS

Military operations involving blast fragments NOS

Military operations involving blast wave NOS

Military operations involving blast wind NOS

Military operations involving explosion NOS

Military operations involving explosion of bomb NOS

✓7ᵗʰ Y37.200 Military operations involving unspecified explosion and fragments, military personnel

✓7ᵗʰ Y37.201 Military operations involving unspecified explosion and fragments, civilian

✓6ᵗʰ Y37.21 Military operations involving explosion of aerial bomb

✓7ᵗʰ Y37.210 Military operations involving explosion of aerial bomb, military personnel

✓7ᵗʰ Y37.211 Military operations involving explosion of aerial bomb, civilian

✓6ᵗʰ Y37.22 Military operations involving explosion of guided missile

✓7ᵗʰ Y37.220 Military operations involving explosion of guided missile, military personnel

✓7ᵗʰ Y37.221 Military operations involving explosion of guided missile, civilian

✓6ᵗʰ Y37.23 Military operations involving explosion of improvised explosive device **[IED]**

Military operations involving explosion of person-borne improvised explosive device [IED]

Military operations involving explosion of vehicle-borne improvised explosive device [IED]

Military operations involving explosion of roadside improvised explosive device [IED]

✓7ᵗʰ Y37.230 Military operations involving explosion of improvised explosive device [IED], military personnel

✓7ᵗʰ Y37.231 Military operations involving explosion of improvised explosive device [IED], civilian

✓6ᵗʰ Y37.24 Military operations involving explosion due to accidental detonation and discharge of own munitions or munitions launch device

✓7ᵗʰ Y37.240 Military operations involving explosion due to accidental detonation and discharge of own munitions or munitions launch device, military personnel

✓7ᵗʰ Y37.241 Military operations involving explosion due to accidental detonation and discharge of own munitions or munitions launch device, civilian

✓6ᵗʰ Y37.25 Military operations involving fragments from munitions

✓7ᵗʰ Y37.250 Military operations involving fragments from munitions, military personnel

✓7ᵗʰ Y37.251 Military operations involving fragments from munitions, civilian

✓6ᵗʰ Y37.26 Military operations involving fragments of improvised explosive device **[IED]**

Military operations involving fragments of person-borne improvised explosive device [IED]

Military operations involving fragments of vehicle-borne improvised explosive device [IED]

Military operations involving fragments of roadside improvised explosive device [IED]

✓7ᵗʰ Y37.260 Military operations involving fragments of improvised explosive device [IED], military personnel

✓7ᵗʰ Y37.261 Military operations involving fragments of improvised explosive device [IED], civilian

✓6ᵗʰ Y37.27 Military operations involving fragments from weapons

✓7ᵗʰ Y37.270 Military operations involving fragments from weapons, military personnel

✓7ᵗʰ Y37.271 Military operations involving fragments from weapons, civilian

✓6ᵗʰ Y37.29 Military operations involving other **explosions and fragments**

Military operations involving explosion of grenade

Military operations involving explosions of land mine

Military operations involving shrapnel NOS

✓7ᵗʰ Y37.290 Military operations involving other explosions and fragments, military personnel

✓7ᵗʰ Y37.291 Military operations involving other explosions and fragments, civilian

N Newborn: 0   **P** Pediatric: 0-17   **M** Maternity: 12-55   **A** Adult: 15-124   **MCC** Major Complication/Comorbidity   **CC** Complication/Comorbidity   **SW** Severe Wound Dx

1206

ICD-10-CM 2019

☑5ᵗʰ Y37.3 Military operations involving fires, conflagrations and hot substances

Military operations involving smoke, fumes, and heat from fires, conflagrations and hot substances

> **EXCLUDES 1**   *military operations involving fires and conflagrations aboard military aircraft (Y37.1-)*
> *military operations involving fires and conflagrations aboard military watercraft (Y37.0-)*
> *military operations involving fires and conflagrations caused indirectly by conventional weapons (Y37.2-)*
> *military operations involving fires and thermal effects of nuclear weapons (Y36.53-)*

☑6ᵗʰ Y37.30 Military operations involving unspecified **fire, conflagration and hot substance**

> **☑7ᵗʰ Y37.300 Military operations involving unspecified fire, conflagration and hot substance,** military personnel

> **☑7ᵗʰ Y37.301 Military operations involving unspecified fire, conflagration and hot substance,** civilian

☑6ᵗʰ Y37.31 Military operations involving gasoline bomb

Military operations involving incendiary bomb
Military operations involving petrol bomb

> **☑7ᵗʰ Y37.310 Military operations involving gasoline bomb,** military personnel

> **☑7ᵗʰ Y37.311 Military operations involving gasoline bomb,** civilian

☑6ᵗʰ Y37.32 Military operations involving incendiary bullet

> **☑7ᵗʰ Y37.320 Military operations involving incendiary bullet,** military personnel

> **☑7ᵗʰ Y37.321 Military operations involving incendiary bullet,** civilian

☑6ᵗʰ Y37.33 Military operations involving flamethrower

> **☑7ᵗʰ Y37.330 Military operations involving flamethrower,** military personnel

> **☑7ᵗʰ Y37.331 Military operations involving flamethrower,** civilian

☑6ᵗʰ Y37.39 Military operations involving other **fires, conflagrations and hot substances**

> **☑7ᵗʰ Y37.390 Military operations involving other fires, conflagrations and hot substances,** military personnel

> **☑7ᵗʰ Y37.391 Military operations involving other fires, conflagrations and hot substances,** civilian

☑5ᵗʰ Y37.4 Military operations involving firearm discharge and other forms of conventional warfare

☑6ᵗʰ Y37.41 Military operations involving rubber bullets

> **☑7ᵗʰ Y37.410 Military operations involving rubber bullets,** military personnel

> **☑7ᵗʰ Y37.411 Military operations involving rubber bullets,** civilian

☑6ᵗʰ Y37.42 Military operations involving firearms pellets

> **☑7ᵗʰ Y37.420 Military operations involving firearms pellets,** military personnel

> **☑7ᵗʰ Y37.421 Military operations involving firearms pellets,** civilian

☑6ᵗʰ Y37.43 Military operations involving other firearms discharge

Military operations involving bullets NOS

> **EXCLUDES 1**   *military operations involving munitions fragments (Y37.25-)*
> *military operations involving incendiary bullets (Y37.32-)*

> **☑7ᵗʰ Y37.430 Military operations involving other firearms discharge,** military personnel

> **☑7ᵗʰ Y37.431 Military operations involving other firearms discharge,** civilian

☑6ᵗʰ Y37.44 Military operations involving unarmed hand to hand combat

> **EXCLUDES 1**   *military operations involving combat using blunt or piercing object (Y37.45-)*
> *military operations involving intentional restriction of air and airway (Y37.46-)*
> *military operations involving unintentional restriction of air and airway (Y37.47-)*

> **☑7ᵗʰ Y37.440 Military operations involving unarmed hand to hand combat,** military personnel

> **☑7ᵗʰ Y37.441 Military operations involving unarmed hand to hand combat,** civilian

☑6ᵗʰ Y37.45 Military operations involving combat using blunt or piercing object

> **☑7ᵗʰ Y37.450 Military operations involving combat using blunt or piercing object,** military personnel

> **☑7ᵗʰ Y37.451 Military operations involving combat using blunt or piercing object,** civilian

☑6ᵗʰ Y37.46 Military operations involving intentional restriction of air and airway

> **☑7ᵗʰ Y37.460 Military operations involving intentional restriction of air and airway,** military personnel

> **☑7ᵗʰ Y37.461 Military operations involving intentional restriction of air and airway,** civilian

☑6ᵗʰ Y37.47 Military operations involving unintentional restriction of air and airway

> **☑7ᵗʰ Y37.470 Military operations involving unintentional restriction of air and airway,** military personnel

> **☑7ᵗʰ Y37.471 Military operations involving unintentional restriction of air and airway,** civilian

☑6ᵗʰ Y37.49 Military operations involving other forms of conventional warfare

> **☑7ᵗʰ Y37.490 Military operations involving other forms of conventional warfare,** military personnel

> **☑7ᵗʰ Y37.491 Military operations involving other forms of conventional warfare,** civilian

☑5ᵗʰ Y37.5 Military operations involving nuclear weapons

Military operation involving dirty bomb NOS

☑6ᵗʰ Y37.50 Military operations involving unspecified effect of nuclear weapon

> **☑7ᵗʰ Y37.500 Military operations involving unspecified effect of nuclear weapon,** military personnel

> **☑7ᵗʰ Y37.501 Military operations involving unspecified effect of nuclear weapon,** civilian

☑6ᵗʰ Y37.51 Military operations involving direct blast effect of nuclear weapon

Military operations involving blast pressure of nuclear weapon

> **☑7ᵗʰ Y37.510 Military operations involving direct blast effect of nuclear weapon,** military personnel

> **☑7ᵗʰ Y37.511 Military operations involving direct blast effect of nuclear weapon,** civilian

☑6ᵗʰ Y37.52 Military operations involving indirect blast effect of nuclear weapon

Military operations involving being thrown by blast of nuclear weapon
Military operations involving being struck or crushed by blast debris of nuclear weapon

> **☑7ᵗʰ Y37.520 Military operations involving indirect blast effect of nuclear weapon,** military personnel

> **☑7ᵗʰ Y37.521 Military operations involving indirect blast effect of nuclear weapon,** civilian

☑6ᵗʰ Y37.53 Military operations involving thermal radiation effect of nuclear weapon

Military operations involving direct heat from nuclear weapon
Military operation involving fireball effects from nuclear weapon

> **☑7ᵗʰ Y37.530 Military operations involving thermal radiation effect of nuclear weapon,** military personnel

---

☑ Additional Character Required   ☑×7ᵗʰ Placeholder   Unacceptable PDx   Questionable PDx   Wrong Procedure   Manifestation   **H1**-**H14** HAC   **HCC** CMS-HCC Dx   **HIV** HIV Dx

ICD-10-CM 2019   **1207**

Chapter 20. External Causes of Morbidity

✓7ᵗʰ **Y37.531 Military operations involving thermal radiation effect of nuclear weapon, civilian**

✓6ᵗʰ **Y37.54 Military operation involving nuclear radiation effects of nuclear weapon**
Military operation involving acute radiation exposure from nuclear weapon
Military operation involving exposure to immediate ionizing radiation from nuclear weapon
Military operation involving fallout exposure from nuclear weapon
Military operation involving secondary effects of nuclear weapons

✓7ᵗʰ **Y37.540 Military operation involving nuclear radiation effects of nuclear weapon, military personnel**

✓7ᵗʰ **Y37.541 Military operation involving nuclear radiation effects of nuclear weapon, civilian**

✓6ᵗʰ **Y37.59 Military operation involving other effects of nuclear weapons**

✓7ᵗʰ **Y37.590 Military operation involving other effects of nuclear weapons, military personnel**

✓7ᵗʰ **Y37.591 Military operation involving other effects of nuclear weapons, civilian**

✓5ᵗʰ **Y37.6 Military operations involving biological weapons**

✓6ᵗʰ **Y37.6X Military operations involving biological weapons**

✓7ᵗʰ **Y37.6X0 Military operations involving biological weapons, military personnel**

✓7ᵗʰ **Y37.6X1 Military operations involving biological weapons, civilian**

✓5ᵗʰ **Y37.7 Military operations involving chemical weapons and other forms of unconventional warfare**
EXCLUDES 1 *military operations involving incendiary devices (Y36.3-, Y36.5-)*

✓6ᵗʰ **Y37.7X Military operations involving chemical weapons and other forms of unconventional warfare**

✓7ᵗʰ **Y37.7X0 Military operations involving chemical weapons and other forms of unconventional warfare, military personnel**

✓7ᵗʰ **Y37.7X1 Military operations involving chemical weapons and other forms of unconventional warfare, civilian**

✓5ᵗʰ **Y37.9 Other and unspecified military operations**

✓x7ᵗʰ **Y37.90 Military operations, unspecified**

✓x7ᵗʰ **Y37.91 Military operations involving unspecified weapon of mass destruction [WMD]**

✓x7ᵗʰ **Y37.92 Military operations involving friendly fire**

✓4ᵗʰ **Y38 Terrorism**
NOTE These codes are for use to identify injuries resulting from the unlawful use of force or violence against persons or property to intimidate or coerce a Government, the civilian population, or any segment thereof, in furtherance of political or social objective.
Use additional code for place of occurrence (Y92.-)

✓5ᵗʰ **Y38.0 Terrorism involving explosion of marine weapons**
Terrorism involving depth-charge
Terrorism involving marine mine
Terrorism involving mine NOS, at sea or in harbor
Terrorism involving sea-based artillery shell
Terrorism involving torpedo
Terrorism involving underwater blast

✓6ᵗʰ **Y38.0X Terrorism involving explosion of marine weapons**

✓7ᵗʰ **Y38.0X1 Terrorism involving explosion of marine weapons, public safety official injured**

✓7ᵗʰ **Y38.0X2 Terrorism involving explosion of marine weapons, civilian injured**

✓7ᵗʰ **Y38.0X3 Terrorism involving explosion of marine weapons, terrorist injured**

✓5ᵗʰ **Y38.1 Terrorism involving destruction of aircraft**
Terrorism involving aircraft burned
Terrorism involving aircraft exploded
Terrorism involving aircraft being shot down
Terrorism involving aircraft used as a weapon

✓6ᵗʰ **Y38.1X Terrorism involving destruction of aircraft**

✓7ᵗʰ **Y38.1X1 Terrorism involving destruction of aircraft, public safety official injured**

✓7ᵗʰ **Y38.1X2 Terrorism involving destruction of aircraft, civilian injured**

✓7ᵗʰ **Y38.1X3 Terrorism involving destruction of aircraft, terrorist injured**

✓5ᵗʰ **Y38.2 Terrorism involving other explosions and fragments**
Terrorism involving antipersonnel (fragments) bomb
Terrorism involving blast NOS
Terrorism involving explosion NOS
Terrorism involving explosion of breech block
Terrorism involving explosion of cannon block
Terrorism involving explosion (fragments) of artillery shell
Terrorism involving explosion (fragments) of bomb
Terrorism involving explosion (fragments) of grenade
Terrorism involving explosion (fragments) of guided missile
Terrorism involving explosion (fragments) of land mine
Terrorism involving explosion of mortar bomb
Terrorism involving explosion of munitions
Terrorism involving explosion (fragments) of rocket
Terrorism involving explosion (fragments) of shell
Terrorism involving shrapnel
Terrorism involving mine NOS, on land
EXCLUDES 1 *terrorism involving explosion of nuclear weapon (Y38.5)*
terrorism involving suicide bomber (Y38.81)

✓6ᵗʰ **Y38.2X Terrorism involving other explosions and fragments**

✓7ᵗʰ **Y38.2X1 Terrorism involving other explosions and fragments, public safety official injured**

✓7ᵗʰ **Y38.2X2 Terrorism involving other explosions and fragments, civilian injured**

✓7ᵗʰ **Y38.2X3 Terrorism involving other explosions and fragments, terrorist injured**

✓5ᵗʰ **Y38.3 Terrorism involving fires, conflagration and hot substances**
Terrorism involving conflagration NOS
Terrorism involving fire NOS
Terrorism involving petrol bomb
EXCLUDES 1 *terrorism involving fire or heat of nuclear weapon (Y38.5)*

✓6ᵗʰ **Y38.3X Terrorism involving fires, conflagration and hot substances**

✓7ᵗʰ **Y38.3X1 Terrorism involving fires, conflagration and hot substances, public safety official injured**

✓7ᵗʰ **Y38.3X2 Terrorism involving fires, conflagration and hot substances, civilian injured**

✓7ᵗʰ **Y38.3X3 Terrorism involving fires, conflagration and hot substances, terrorist injured**

✓5ᵗʰ **Y38.4 Terrorism involving firearms**
Terrorism involving carbine bullet
Terrorism involving machine gun bullet
Terrorism involving pellets (shotgun)
Terrorism involving pistol bullet
Terrorism involving rifle bullet
Terrorism involving rubber (rifle) bullet

✓6ᵗʰ **Y38.4X Terrorism involving firearms**

✓7ᵗʰ **Y38.4X1 Terrorism involving firearms, public safety official injured**

✓7ᵗʰ **Y38.4X2 Terrorism involving firearms, civilian injured**

✓7ᵗʰ **Y38.4X3 Terrorism involving firearms, terrorist injured**

✓5ᵗʰ **Y38.5 Terrorism involving nuclear weapons**
Terrorism involving blast effects of nuclear weapon
Terrorism involving exposure to ionizing radiation from nuclear weapon
Terrorism involving fireball effect of nuclear weapon
Terrorism involving heat from nuclear weapon

✓6ᵗʰ **Y38.5X Terrorism involving nuclear weapons**

✓7ᵗʰ **Y38.5X1 Terrorism involving nuclear weapons, public safety official injured**

☑7ᵗʰ **Y38.5X2** Terrorism involving nuclear weapons, civilian injured

☑7ᵗʰ **Y38.5X3** Terrorism involving nuclear weapons, terrorist injured

☑5ᵗʰ **Y38.6** Terrorism involving biological weapons
Terrorism involving anthrax
Terrorism involving cholera
Terrorism involving smallpox

☑6ᵗʰ **Y38.6X** Terrorism involving biological weapons

☑7ᵗʰ **Y38.6X1** Terrorism involving biological weapons, public safety official injured

☑7ᵗʰ **Y38.6X2** Terrorism involving biological weapons, civilian injured

☑7ᵗʰ **Y38.6X3** Terrorism involving biological weapons, terrorist injured

☑5ᵗʰ **Y38.7** Terrorism involving chemical weapons
Terrorism involving gases, fumes, chemicals
Terrorism involving hydrogen cyanide
Terrorism involving phosgene
Terrorism involving sarin

☑6ᵗʰ **Y38.7X** Terrorism involving chemical weapons

☑7ᵗʰ **Y38.7X1** Terrorism involving chemical weapons, public safety official injured

☑7ᵗʰ **Y38.7X2** Terrorism involving chemical weapons, civilian injured

☑7ᵗʰ **Y38.7X3** Terrorism involving chemical weapons, terrorist injured

☑5ᵗʰ **Y38.8** Terrorism involving other and unspecified means

☑x7ᵗʰ **Y38.80** Terrorism involving unspecified means
Terrorism NOS

☑6ᵗʰ **Y38.81** Terrorism involving suicide bomber

☑7ᵗʰ **Y38.811** Terrorism involving suicide bomber, public safety official injured

☑7ᵗʰ **Y38.812** Terrorism involving suicide bomber, civilian injured

☑6ᵗʰ **Y38.89** Terrorism involving other means
Terrorism involving drowning and submersion
Terrorism involving lasers
Terrorism involving piercing or stabbing instruments

☑7ᵗʰ **Y38.891** Terrorism involving other means, public safety official injured

☑7ᵗʰ **Y38.892** Terrorism involving other means, civilian injured

☑7ᵗʰ **Y38.893** Terrorism involving other means, terrorist injured

☑5ᵗʰ **Y38.9** Terrorism, secondary effects
NOTE This code is for use to identify injuries occurring subsequent to a terrorist attack, not those that are due to the initial terrorist attack.

☑6ᵗʰ **Y38.9X** Terrorism, secondary effects

☑7ᵗʰ **Y38.9X1** Terrorism, secondary effects, public safety official injured

☑7ᵗʰ **Y38.9X2** Terrorism, secondary effects, civilian injured

COMPLICATIONS OF MEDICAL AND SURGICAL CARE (Y62-Y84)

INCLUDES complications of medical devices
surgical and medical procedures as the cause of abnormal reaction of the patient, or of later complication, without mention of misadventure at the time of the procedure

Misadventures to patients during surgical and medical care (Y62-Y69)

EXCLUDES 1 surgical and medical procedures as the cause of abnormal reaction of the patient, without mention of misadventure at the time of the procedure (Y83-Y84)

EXCLUDES 2 breakdown or malfunctioning of medical device (during procedure) (after implantation) (ongoing use) (Y70-Y82)

☑4ᵗʰ **Y62** Failure of sterile precautions during surgical and medical care

Y62.0 Failure of sterile precautions during surgical operation

Y62.1 Failure of sterile precautions during infusion or transfusion

Y62.2 Failure of sterile precautions during kidney dialysis and other perfusion ᴴᶜᶜ

Y62.3 Failure of sterile precautions during injection or immunization

Y62.4 Failure of sterile precautions during endoscopic examination

Y62.5 Failure of sterile precautions during heart catheterization

Y62.6 Failure of sterile precautions during aspiration, puncture and other catheterization

Y62.8 Failure of sterile precautions during other surgical and medical care

Y62.9 Failure of sterile precautions during unspecified surgical and medical care

☑4ᵗʰ **Y63** Failure in dosage during surgical and medical care
EXCLUDES 2 accidental overdose of drug or wrong drug given in error (T36-T50)

Y63.0 Excessive amount of blood or other fluid given during transfusion or infusion

Y63.1 Incorrect dilution of fluid used during infusion

Y63.2 Overdose of radiation given during therapy

Y63.3 Inadvertent exposure of patient to radiation during medical care

Y63.4 Failure in dosage in electroshock or insulin-shock therapy

Y63.5 Inappropriate temperature in local application and packing

Y63.6 Underdosing and nonadministration of necessary drug, medicament or biological substance

Y63.8 Failure in dosage during other surgical and medical care

Y63.9 Failure in dosage during unspecified surgical and medical care

☑4ᵗʰ **Y64** Contaminated medical or biological substances

Y64.0 Contaminated medical or biological substance, transfused or infused

Y64.1 Contaminated medical or biological substance, injected or used for immunization

Y64.8 Contaminated medical or biological substance administered by other means

Y64.9 Contaminated medical or biological substance administered by unspecified means
Administered contaminated medical or biological substance NOS

☑4ᵗʰ **Y65** Other misadventures during surgical and medical care

Y65.0 Mismatched blood in transfusion

Y65.1 Wrong fluid used in infusion

Y65.2 Failure in suture or ligature during surgical operation

Y65.3 Endotracheal tube wrongly placed during anesthetic procedure

Y65.4 Failure to introduce or to remove other tube or instrument

☑5ᵗʰ **Y65.5** Performance of wrong procedure (operation)

Y65.51 Performance of wrong procedure (operation) on correct patient
Wrong device implanted into correct surgical site
EXCLUDES 1 performance of correct procedure (operation) on wrong side or body part (Y65.53)

Y65.52 Performance of procedure (operation) on patient not scheduled for surgery
Performance of procedure (operation) intended for another patient
Performance of procedure (operation) on wrong patient

Y65.53 Performance of correct procedure (operation) on wrong side or body part
Performance of correct procedure (operation) on wrong side
Performance of correct procedure (operation) on wrong site

Y65.8 Other specified misadventures during surgical and medical care

Y66 Nonadministration of surgical and medical care
Premature cessation of surgical and medical care
EXCLUDES 1 DNR status (Z66)
palliative care (Z51.5)

Y69 Unspecified misadventure during surgical and medical care

---

☑ Additional Character Required ☑7ᵗʰ Placeholder Unacceptable PDx Questionable PDx Wrong Procedure Manifestation **H1 - H14** HAC **HCC** CMS-HCC Dx **HIV** HIV Dx

Chapter 20. External Causes of Morbidity

Y70–Y81.Ø

Medical devices associated with adverse incidents in diagnostic and therapeutic use (Y70–Y82)

INCLUDES   breakdown or malfunction of medical devices (during use) (after implantation) (ongoing use)

EXCLUDES 2   ~~breakdown or malfunctioning of medical device (after implantation) (during procedure) (ongoing use) (Y70-Y82)~~

later complications following use of medical devices without breakdown or malfunctioning of device (Y83-Y84)

misadventure to patients during surgical and medical care, classifiable to (Y62-Y69)

surgical and other medical procedures as the cause of abnormal reaction of the patient, or of later complication, without mention of misadventure at the time of the procedure (Y83-Y84)

✓4ᵗʰ **Y70 Anesthesiology devices associated with adverse incidents**

     Y70.Ø Diagnostic and monitoring **anesthesiology devices associated with adverse incidents**

     Y70.1 Therapeutic **(nonsurgical)** and rehabilitative **anesthesiology devices associated with adverse incidents**

     Y70.2 Prosthetic and other implants, **materials and accessory anesthesiology devices associated with adverse incidents**

     Y70.3 Surgical instruments, materials **and anesthesiology devices (including sutures) associated with adverse incidents**

     Y70.8 Miscellaneous **anesthesiology devices associated with adverse incidents, not elsewhere classified**

✓4ᵗʰ **Y71 Cardiovascular devices associated with adverse incidents**

     Y71.Ø Diagnostic and monitoring **cardiovascular devices associated with adverse incidents**

     Y71.1 Therapeutic **(nonsurgical)** and rehabilitative **cardiovascular devices associated with adverse incidents**

     Y71.2 Prosthetic and other implants, **materials and accessory cardiovascular devices associated with adverse incidents**

     Y71.3 Surgical instruments, materials **and cardiovascular devices (including sutures) associated with adverse incidents**

     Y71.8 Miscellaneous **cardiovascular devices associated with adverse incidents, not elsewhere classified**

✓4ᵗʰ **Y72 Otorhinolaryngological devices associated with adverse incidents**

     Y72.Ø Diagnostic and monitoring **otorhinolaryngological devices associated with adverse incidents**

     Y72.1 Therapeutic **(nonsurgical)** and rehabilitative **otorhinolaryngological devices associated with adverse incidents**

     Y72.2 Prosthetic and other implants, **materials and accessory otorhinolaryngological devices associated with adverse incidents**

     Y72.3 Surgical instruments, materials **and otorhinolaryngological devices (including sutures) associated with adverse incidents**

     Y72.8 Miscellaneous **otorhinolaryngological devices associated with adverse incidents, not elsewhere classified**

✓4ᵗʰ **Y73 Gastroenterology and urology devices associated with adverse incidents**

     Y73.Ø Diagnostic and monitoring **gastroenterology and urology devices associated with adverse incidents**

     Y73.1 Therapeutic **(nonsurgical)** and rehabilitative **gastroenterology and urology devices associated with adverse incidents**

     Y73.2 Prosthetic and other implants, **materials and accessory gastroenterology and urology devices associated with adverse incidents**

     Y73.3 Surgical instruments, materials **and gastroenterology and urology devices (including sutures) associated with adverse incidents**

     Y73.8 Miscellaneous **gastroenterology and urology devices associated with adverse incidents, not elsewhere classified**

✓4ᵗʰ **Y74 General hospital and personal-use devices associated with adverse incidents**

     Y74.Ø Diagnostic and monitoring **general hospital and personal-use devices associated with adverse incidents**

     Y74.1 Therapeutic **(nonsurgical)** and rehabilitative **general hospital and personal-use devices associated with adverse incidents**

     Y74.2 Prosthetic and other implants, **materials and accessory general hospital and personal-use devices associated with adverse incidents**

     Y74.3 Surgical instruments, materials **and general hospital and personal-use devices (including sutures) associated with adverse incidents**

     Y74.8 Miscellaneous **general hospital and personal-use devices associated with adverse incidents, not elsewhere classified**

✓4ᵗʰ **Y75 Neurological devices associated with adverse incidents**

     Y75.Ø Diagnostic and monitoring **neurological devices associated with adverse incidents**

     Y75.1 Therapeutic **(nonsurgical)** and rehabilitative **neurological devices associated with adverse incidents**

     Y75.2 Prosthetic and other implants, **materials and neurological devices associated with adverse incidents**

     Y75.3 Surgical instruments, materials **and neurological devices (including sutures) associated with adverse incidents**

     Y75.8 Miscellaneous **neurological devices associated with adverse incidents, not elsewhere classified**

✓4ᵗʰ **Y76 Obstetric and gynecological devices associated with adverse incidents**

     Y76.Ø Diagnostic and monitoring **obstetric and gynecological devices associated with adverse incidents** ♀

     Y76.1 Therapeutic **(nonsurgical)** and rehabilitative **obstetric and gynecological devices associated with adverse incidents** ♀

     Y76.2 Prosthetic and other implants, **materials and accessory obstetric and gynecological devices associated with adverse incidents** ♀

     Y76.3 Surgical instruments, materials **and obstetric and gynecological devices (including sutures) associated with adverse incidents** ♀

     Y76.8 Miscellaneous **obstetric and gynecological devices associated with adverse incidents, not elsewhere classified** ♀

✓4ᵗʰ **Y77 Ophthalmic devices associated with adverse incidents**

     Y77.Ø Diagnostic and monitoring **ophthalmic devices associated with adverse incidents**

     Y77.1 Therapeutic **(nonsurgical)** and rehabilitative **ophthalmic devices associated with adverse incidents**

     Y77.2 Prosthetic and other implants, **materials and accessory ophthalmic devices associated with adverse incidents**

     Y77.3 Surgical instruments, materials **and ophthalmic devices (including sutures) associated with adverse incidents**

     Y77.8 Miscellaneous **ophthalmic devices associated with adverse incidents, not elsewhere classified**

✓4ᵗʰ **Y78 Radiological devices associated with adverse incidents**

     Y78.Ø Diagnostic and monitoring **radiological devices associated with adverse incidents**

     Y78.1 Therapeutic **(nonsurgical)** and rehabilitative **radiological devices associated with adverse incidents**

     Y78.2 Prosthetic and other implants, **materials and accessory radiological devices associated with adverse incidents**

     Y78.3 Surgical instruments, materials **and radiological devices (including sutures) associated with adverse incidents**

     Y78.8 Miscellaneous **radiological devices associated with adverse incidents, not elsewhere classified**

✓4ᵗʰ **Y79 Orthopedic devices associated with adverse incidents**

     Y79.Ø Diagnostic and monitoring **orthopedic devices associated with adverse incidents**

     Y79.1 Therapeutic **(nonsurgical)** and rehabilitative **orthopedic devices associated with adverse incidents**

     Y79.2 Prosthetic and other implants, **materials and accessory orthopedic devices associated with adverse incidents**

     Y79.3 Surgical instruments, materials **and orthopedic devices (including sutures) associated with adverse incidents**

     Y79.8 Miscellaneous **orthopedic devices associated with adverse incidents, not elsewhere classified**

✓4ᵗʰ **Y80 Physical medicine devices associated with adverse incidents**

     Y80.Ø Diagnostic and monitoring **physical medicine devices associated with adverse incidents**

     Y80.1 Therapeutic **(nonsurgical)** and rehabilitative **physical medicine devices associated with adverse incidents**

     Y80.2 Prosthetic and other implants, **materials and accessory physical medicine devices associated with adverse incidents**

     Y80.3 Surgical instruments, materials **and physical medicine devices (including sutures) associated with adverse incidents**

     Y80.8 Miscellaneous **physical medicine devices associated with adverse incidents, not elsewhere classified**

✓4ᵗʰ **Y81 General- and plastic-surgery devices associated with adverse incidents**

     Y81.Ø Diagnostic and monitoring **general- and plastic-surgery devices associated with adverse incidents**

N Newborn: 0   **P** Pediatric: 0-17   **M** Maternity: 12-55   **A** Adult: 15-124   **MCC** Major Complication/Comorbidity   **CC** Complication/Comorbidity   **SW** Severe Wound Dx

1210   ICD-10-CM 2019

Y81.1 Therapeutic (nonsurgical) and rehabilitative general- and plastic-surgery devices associated with adverse incidents

Y81.2 Prosthetic and other implants, materials and accessory general- and plastic-surgery devices associated with adverse incidents

Y81.3 Surgical instruments, materials and general- and plastic-surgery devices (including sutures) associated with adverse incidents

Y81.8 Miscellaneous general- and plastic-surgery devices associated with adverse incidents, not elsewhere classified

✓4ᵗʰ **Y82** **Other and unspecified medical devices associated with adverse incidents**

Y82.8 Other medical devices associated with adverse incidents

Y82.9 Unspecified medical devices associated with adverse incidents

Surgical and other medical procedures as the cause of abnormal reaction of the patient, or of later complication, without mention of misadventure at the time of the procedure (Y83-Y84)

> EXCLUDES 1   misadventures to patients during surgical and medical care, classifiable to (Y62-Y69)
>
> EXCLUDES 2   breakdown or malfunctioning of medical device (after implantation) (during procedure) (ongoing use) (Y70-Y82)

✓4ᵗʰ **Y83** **Surgical operation and other surgical procedures as the cause of abnormal reaction of the patient, or of later complication, without mention of misadventure at the time of the procedure**

Y83.0 Surgical operation with transplant of whole organ as the cause of abnormal reaction of the patient, or of later complication, without mention of misadventure at the time of the procedure

Y83.1 Surgical operation with implant of artificial internal device as the cause of abnormal reaction of the patient, or of later complication, without mention of misadventure at the time of the procedure

Y83.2 Surgical operation with anastomosis, bypass or graft as the cause of abnormal reaction of the patient, or of later complication, without mention of misadventure at the time of the procedure

Y83.3 Surgical operation with formation of external stoma as the cause of abnormal reaction of the patient, or of later complication, without mention of misadventure at the time of the procedure

Y83.4 Other reconstructive surgery as the cause of abnormal reaction of the patient, or of later complication, without mention of misadventure at the time of the procedure

Y83.5 Amputation of limb(s) as the cause of abnormal reaction of the patient, or of later complication, without mention of misadventure at the time of the procedure

Y83.6 Removal of other organ (partial) (total) as the cause of abnormal reaction of the patient, or of later complication, without mention of misadventure at the time of the procedure

Y83.8 Other surgical procedures as the cause of abnormal reaction of the patient, or of later complication, without mention of misadventure at the time of the procedure

Y83.9 Surgical procedure, unspecified as the cause of abnormal reaction of the patient, or of later complication, without mention of misadventure at the time of the procedure

✓4ᵗʰ **Y84** **Other medical procedures as the cause of abnormal reaction of the patient, or of later complication, without mention of misadventure at the time of the procedure**

Y84.0 Cardiac catheterization as the cause of abnormal reaction of the patient, or of later complication, without mention of misadventure at the time of the procedure

Y84.1 Kidney dialysis as the cause of abnormal reaction of the patient, or of later complication, without mention of misadventure at the time of the procedure

Y84.2 Radiological procedure and radiotherapy as the cause of abnormal reaction of the patient, or of later complication, without mention of misadventure at the time of the procedure
> AHA: 2017, 1Q, 33

Y84.3 Shock therapy as the cause of abnormal reaction of the patient, or of later complication, without mention of misadventure at the time of the procedure

Y84.4 Aspiration of fluid as the cause of abnormal reaction of the patient, or of later complication, without mention of misadventure at the time of the procedure

Y84.5 Insertion of gastric or duodenal sound as the cause of abnormal reaction of the patient, or of later complication, without mention of misadventure at the time of the procedure

Y84.6 Urinary catheterization as the cause of abnormal reaction of the patient, or of later complication, without mention of misadventure at the time of the procedure

Y84.7 Blood-sampling as the cause of abnormal reaction of the patient, or of later complication, without mention of misadventure at the time of the procedure

Y84.8 Other medical procedures as the cause of abnormal reaction of the patient, or of later complication, without mention of misadventure at the time of the procedure
> AHA: 2014, 4Q, 24

Y84.9 Medical procedure, unspecified as the cause of abnormal reaction of the patient, or of later complication, without mention of misadventure at the time of the procedure

Supplementary factors related to causes of morbidity classified elsewhere (Y90-Y99)

> NOTE   These categories may be used to provide supplementary information concerning causes of morbidity. They are not to be used for single-condition coding.

✓4ᵗʰ **Y90** **Evidence of alcohol involvement determined by blood alcohol level**
> Code first any associated alcohol related disorders (F10)

Y90.0 Blood alcohol level of less than 20 mg/100 ml

Y90.1 Blood alcohol level of 20-39 mg/100 ml

Y90.2 Blood alcohol level of 40-59 mg/100 ml

Y90.3 Blood alcohol level of 60-79 mg/100 ml

Y90.4 Blood alcohol level of 80-99 mg/100 ml

Y90.5 Blood alcohol level of 100-119 mg/100 ml

Y90.6 Blood alcohol level of 120-199 mg/100 ml

Y90.7 Blood alcohol level of 200-239 mg/100 ml

Y90.8 Blood alcohol level of 240 mg/100 ml or more

Y90.9 Presence of alcohol in blood, level not specified

✓4ᵗʰ **Y92** **Place of occurrence of the external cause**
> The following category is for use, when relevant, to identify the place of occurrence of the external cause. Use in conjunction with an activity code.
>
> Place of occurrence should be recorded only at the initial encounter for treatment

✓5ᵗʰ **Y92.0** **Non-institutional (private) residence as the place of occurrence of the external cause**
> EXCLUDES 1   abandoned or derelict house (Y92.89)
> home under construction but not yet occupied (Y92.6-)
> institutional place of residence (Y92.1-)

✓6ᵗʰ **Y92.00** **Unspecified non-institutional (private) residence as the place of occurrence of the external cause**

Y92.000 Kitchen of unspecified non-institutional (private) residence as the place of occurrence of the external cause

Y92.001 Dining room of unspecified non-institutional (private) residence as the place of occurrence of the external cause

Y92.002 Bathroom of unspecified non-institutional (private) residence single-family (private) house as the place of occurrence of the external cause

Y92.003 Bedroom of unspecified non-institutional (private) residence as the place of occurrence of the external cause

Y92.007 Garden or yard of unspecified non-institutional (private) residence as the place of occurrence of the external cause

Y92.008 Other place in unspecified non-institutional (private) residence as the place of occurrence of the external cause

Y92.009 Unspecified place in unspecified non-institutional (private) residence as the place of occurrence of the external cause
> Home (NOS) as the place of occurrence of the external cause

✓ Additional Character Required   ✓x7ᵗʰ Placeholder   Unacceptable PDx   Questionable PDx   **Wrong Procedure**   Manifestation   **H1**-**H14** HAC   **HCC** CMS-HCC Dx   **HIV** HIV Dx

ICD-10-CM 2019   **1211**

Y81.1–Y92.009

Chapter 20. External Causes of Morbidity

☑6ᵗʰ **Y92.01** Single-family non-institutional (private) house as the place of occurrence of the external cause

Farmhouse as the place of occurrence of the external cause

EXCLUDES 1 barn (Y92.71)
chicken coop or hen house (Y92.72)
farm field (Y92.73)
orchard (Y92.74)
single family mobile home or trailer (Y92.02-)
slaughter house (Y92.86)

Y92.010 Kitchen of single-family (private) house as the place of occurrence of the external cause

Y92.011 Dining room of single-family (private) house as the place of occurrence of the external cause

Y92.012 Bathroom of single-family (private) house as the place of occurrence of the external cause

Y92.013 Bedroom of single-family (private) house as the place of occurrence of the external cause

Y92.014 Private driveway to single-family (private) house as the place of occurrence of the external cause

Y92.015 Private garage of single-family (private) house as the place of occurrence of the external cause

Y92.016 Swimming-pool in single-family (private) house or garden as the place of occurrence of the external cause

Y92.017 Garden or yard in single-family (private) house as the place of occurrence of the external cause

Y92.018 Other place in single-family (private) house as the place of occurrence of the external cause

Y92.019 Unspecified place in single-family (private) house as the place of occurrence of the external cause

☑6ᵗʰ **Y92.02** Mobile home as the place of occurrence of the external cause

Y92.020 Kitchen in mobile home as the place of occurrence of the external cause

Y92.021 Dining room in mobile home as the place of occurrence of the external cause

Y92.022 Bathroom in mobile home as the place of occurrence of the external cause

Y92.023 Bedroom in mobile home as the place of occurrence of the external cause

Y92.024 Driveway of mobile home as the place of occurrence of the external cause

Y92.025 Garage of mobile home as the place of occurrence of the external cause

Y92.026 Swimming-pool of mobile home as the place of occurrence of the external cause

Y92.027 Garden or yard of mobile home as the place of occurrence of the external cause

Y92.028 Other place in mobile home as the place of occurrence of the external cause

Y92.029 Unspecified place in mobile home as the place of occurrence of the external cause

☑6ᵗʰ **Y92.03** Apartment as the place of occurrence of the external cause

Condominium as the place of occurrence of the external cause

Co-op apartment as the place of occurrence of the external cause

Y92.030 Kitchen in apartment as the place of occurrence of the external cause

Y92.031 Bathroom in apartment as the place of occurrence of the external cause

Y92.032 Bedroom in apartment as the place of occurrence of the external cause

Y92.038 Other place in apartment as the place of occurrence of the external cause

Y92.039 Unspecified place in apartment as the place of occurrence of the external cause

☑6ᵗʰ **Y92.04** Boarding-house as the place of occurrence of the external cause

Y92.040 Kitchen in boarding-house as the place of occurrence of the external cause

Y92.041 Bathroom in boarding-house as the place of occurrence of the external cause

Y92.042 Bedroom in boarding-house as the place of occurrence of the external cause

Y92.043 Driveway of boarding-house as the place of occurrence of the external cause

Y92.044 Garage of boarding-house as the place of occurrence of the external cause

Y92.045 Swimming-pool of boarding-house as the place of occurrence of the external cause

Y92.046 Garden or yard of boarding-house as the place of occurrence of the external cause

Y92.048 Other place in boarding-house as the place of occurrence of the external cause

Y92.049 Unspecified place in boarding-house as the place of occurrence of the external cause

☑6ᵗʰ **Y92.09** Other non-institutional residence as the place of occurrence of the external cause

AHA: 2017, 2Q, 10

Y92.090 Kitchen in other non-institutional residence as the place of occurrence of the external cause

Y92.091 Bathroom in other non-institutional residence as the place of occurrence of the external cause

Y92.092 Bedroom in other non-institutional residence as the place of occurrence of the external cause

Y92.093 Driveway of other non-institutional residence as the place of occurrence of the external cause

Y92.094 Garage of other non-institutional residence as the place of occurrence of the external cause

Y92.095 Swimming-pool of other non-institutional residence as the place of occurrence of the external cause

Y92.096 Garden or yard of other non-institutional residence as the place of occurrence of the external cause

Y92.098 Other place in other non-institutional residence as the place of occurrence of the external cause

Y92.099 Unspecified place in other non-institutional residence as the place of occurrence of the external cause

☑5ᵗʰ **Y92.1** Institutional (nonprivate) residence as the place of occurrence of the external cause

Y92.10 Unspecified residential institution as the place of occurrence of the external cause

☑6ᵗʰ **Y92.11** Children's home and orphanage as the place of occurrence of the external cause

Y92.110 Kitchen in children's home and orphanage as the place of occurrence of the external cause

Y92.111 Bathroom in children's home and orphanage as the place of occurrence of the external cause

Y92.112 Bedroom in children's home and orphanage as the place of occurrence of the external cause

Y92.113 Driveway of children's home and orphanage as the place of occurrence of the external cause

Y92.114 Garage of children's home and orphanage as the place of occurrence of the external cause

Y92.115 Swimming-pool of children's home and orphanage as the place of occurrence of the external cause

Y92.116 Garden or yard of children's home and orphanage as the place of occurrence of the external cause

Y92.118 Other place in children's home and orphanage as the place of occurrence of the external cause

Ⓝ Newborn: 0   Ⓟ Pediatric: 0-17   Ⓜ Maternity: 12-55   Ⓐ Adult: 15-124   **MCC** Major Complication/Comorbidity   **CC** Complication/Comorbidity   **SW** Severe Wound Dx

1212   ICD-10-CM 2019

Y92.119 Unspecified place in children's home and orphanage as the place of occurrence of the external cause

☑6ᵗʰ **Y92.12** Nursing home as the place of occurrence of the external cause
Home for the sick as the place of occurrence of the external cause
Hospice as the place of occurrence of the external cause
AHA: 2017, 2Q, 10

Y92.120 Kitchen in nursing home as the place of occurrence of the external cause

Y92.121 Bathroom in nursing home as the place of occurrence of the external cause

Y92.122 Bedroom in nursing home as the place of occurrence of the external cause

Y92.123 Driveway of nursing home as the place of occurrence of the external cause

Y92.124 Garage of nursing home as the place of occurrence of the external cause

Y92.125 Swimming-pool of nursing home as the place of occurrence of the external cause

Y92.126 Garden or yard of nursing home as the place of occurrence of the external cause

Y92.128 Other place in nursing home as the place of occurrence of the external cause

Y92.129 Unspecified place in nursing home as the place of occurrence of the external cause

☑6ᵗʰ **Y92.13** Military base as the place of occurrence of the external cause
EXCLUDES 1 *military training grounds (Y92.83)*

Y92.130 Kitchen on military base as the place of occurrence of the external cause

Y92.131 Mess hall on military base as the place of occurrence of the external cause

Y92.133 Barracks on military base as the place of occurrence of the external cause

Y92.135 Garage on military base as the place of occurrence of the external cause

Y92.136 Swimming-pool on military base as the place of occurrence of the external cause

Y92.137 Garden or yard on military base as the place of occurrence of the external cause

Y92.138 Other place on military base as the place of occurrence of the external cause

Y92.139 Unspecified place military base as the place of occurrence of the external cause

☑6ᵗʰ **Y92.14** Prison as the place of occurrence of the external cause

Y92.140 Kitchen in prison as the place of occurrence of the external cause

Y92.141 Dining room in prison as the place of occurrence of the external cause

Y92.142 Bathroom in prison as the place of occurrence of the external cause

Y92.143 Cell of prison as the place of occurrence of the external cause

Y92.146 Swimming-pool of prison as the place of occurrence of the external cause

Y92.147 Courtyard of prison as the place of occurrence of the external cause

Y92.148 Other place in prison as the place of occurrence of the external cause

Y92.149 Unspecified place in prison as the place of occurrence of the external cause

☑6ᵗʰ **Y92.15** Reform school as the place of occurrence of the external cause

Y92.150 Kitchen in reform school as the place of occurrence of the external cause

Y92.151 Dining room in reform school as the place of occurrence of the external cause

Y92.152 Bathroom in reform school as the place of occurrence of the external cause

Y92.153 Bedroom in reform school as the place of occurrence of the external cause

Y92.154 Driveway of reform school as the place of occurrence of the external cause

Y92.155 Garage of reform school as the place of occurrence of the external cause

Y92.156 Swimming-pool of reform school as the place of occurrence of the external cause

Y92.157 Garden or yard of reform school as the place of occurrence of the external cause

Y92.158 Other place in reform school as the place of occurrence of the external cause

Y92.159 Unspecified place in reform school as the place of occurrence of the external cause

☑6ᵗʰ **Y92.16** School dormitory as the place of occurrence of the external cause
EXCLUDES 1 *reform school as the place of occurrence of the external cause (Y92.15-)*
school buildings and grounds as the place of occurrence of the external cause (Y92.2-)
school sports and athletic areas as the place of occurrence of the external cause (Y92.3-)

Y92.160 Kitchen in school dormitory as the place of occurrence of the external cause

Y92.161 Dining room in school dormitory as the place of occurrence of the external cause

Y92.162 Bathroom in school dormitory as the place of occurrence of the external cause

Y92.163 Bedroom in school dormitory as the place of occurrence of the external cause

Y92.168 Other place in school dormitory as the place of occurrence of the external cause

Y92.169 Unspecified place in school dormitory as the place of occurrence of the external cause

☑6ᵗʰ **Y92.19** Other specified residential institution as the place of occurrence of the external cause
AHA: 2017, 2Q, 10

Y92.190 Kitchen in other specified residential institution as the place of occurrence of the external cause

Y92.191 Dining room in other specified residential institution as the place of occurrence of the external cause

Y92.192 Bathroom in other specified residential institution as the place of occurrence of the external cause

Y92.193 Bedroom in other specified residential institution as the place of occurrence of the external cause

Y92.194 Driveway of other specified residential institution as the place of occurrence of the external cause

Y92.195 Garage of other specified residential institution as the place of occurrence of the external cause

Y92.196 Pool of other specified residential institution as the place of occurrence of the external cause

Y92.197 Garden or yard of other specified residential institution as the place of occurrence of the external cause

Y92.198 Other place in other specified residential institution as the place of occurrence of the external cause

Y92.199 Unspecified place in other specified residential institution as the place of occurrence of the external cause

☑5ᵗʰ **Y92.2** School, other institution and public administrative area as the place of occurrence of the external cause
Building and adjacent grounds used by the general public or by a particular group of the public
EXCLUDES 1 *building under construction as the place of occurrence of the external cause (Y92.6)*
residential institution as the place of occurrence of the external cause (Y92.1)
school dormitory as the place of occurrence of the external cause (Y92.16-)
sports and athletics area of schools as the place of occurrence of the external cause (Y92.3-)

☑6ᵗʰ **Y92.21** School (private) (public) (state) as the place of occurrence of the external cause

Y92.210 Daycare center as the place of occurrence of the external cause

☑ Additional Character Required   ☑x7ᵗʰ Placeholder   Unacceptable PDx   Questionable PDx   **Wrong Procedure**   Manifestation   **H1**-**H14** HAC   **HCC** CMS-HCC Dx   **HIV** HIV Dx

ICD-10-CM 2019   1213

Chapter 20. External Causes of Morbidity

Y92.211   **Elementary school** as the place of occurrence of the external cause
Kindergarten as the place of occurrence of the external cause

Y92.212   **Middle school** as the place of occurrence of the external cause

Y92.213   **High school** as the place of occurrence of the external cause
AHA: 2012, 4Q, 108

Y92.214   **College** as the place of occurrence of the external cause
University as the place of occurrence of the external cause

Y92.215   **Trade school** as the place of occurrence of the external cause

Y92.218   **Other** school as the place of occurrence of the external cause

Y92.219   **Unspecified** school as the place of occurrence of the external cause

Y92.22   **Religious institution** as the place of occurrence of the external cause
Church as the place of occurrence of the external cause
Mosque as the place of occurrence of the external cause
Synagogue as the place of occurrence of the external cause

✓6ᵗʰ Y92.23   **Hospital** as the place of occurrence of the external cause
EXCLUDES 1 *ambulatory (outpatient) health services establishments (Y92.53-)*
home for the sick as the place of occurrence of the external cause (Y92.12-)
hospice as the place of occurrence of the external cause (Y92.12-)
nursing home as the place of occurrence of the external cause (Y92.12-)

Y92.230   **Patient room** in hospital as the place of occurrence of the external cause

Y92.231   **Patient bathroom** in hospital as the place of occurrence of the external cause

Y92.232   **Corridor** of hospital as the place of occurrence of the external cause

Y92.233   **Cafeteria** of hospital as the place of occurrence of the external cause

Y92.234   **Operating room** of hospital as the place of occurrence of the external cause

Y92.238   **Other** place in hospital as the place of occurrence of the external cause

Y92.239   **Unspecified** place in hospital as the place of occurrence of the external cause

✓6ᵗʰ Y92.24   **Public administrative building** as the place of occurrence of the external cause

Y92.240   **Courthouse** as the place of occurrence of the external cause

Y92.241   **Library** as the place of occurrence of the external cause

Y92.242   **Post office** as the place of occurrence of the external cause

Y92.243   **City hall** as the place of occurrence of the external cause

Y92.248   **Other** public administrative building as the place of occurrence of the external cause

✓6ᵗʰ Y92.25   **Cultural building** as the place of occurrence of the external cause

Y92.250   **Art Gallery** as the place of occurrence of the external cause

Y92.251   **Museum** as the place of occurrence of the external cause

Y92.252   **Music hall** as the place of occurrence of the external cause

Y92.253   **Opera house** as the place of occurrence of the external cause

Y92.254   **Theater** (live) as the place of occurrence of the external cause

Y92.258   **Other** cultural public building as the place of occurrence of the external cause

Y92.26   **Movie house or cinema** as the place of occurrence of the external cause

Y92.29   **Other** specified public building as the place of occurrence of the external cause
Assembly hall as the place of occurrence of the external cause
Clubhouse as the place of occurrence of the external cause

✓5ᵗʰ Y92.3   **Sports and athletics area** as the place of occurrence of the external cause

✓6ᵗʰ Y92.31   **Athletic court** as the place of occurrence of the external cause
EXCLUDES 1 *tennis court in private home or garden (Y92.09)*

Y92.310   **Basketball** court as the place of occurrence of the external cause

Y92.311   **Squash** court as the place of occurrence of the external cause

Y92.312   **Tennis** court as the place of occurrence of the external cause

Y92.318   **Other** athletic court as the place of occurrence of the external cause

✓6ᵗʰ Y92.32   **Athletic field** as the place of occurrence of the external cause

Y92.320   **Baseball** field as the place of occurrence of the external cause

Y92.321   **Football** field as the place of occurrence of the external cause

Y92.322   **Soccer** field as the place of occurrence of the external cause

Y92.328   **Other** athletic field as the place of occurrence of the external cause
Cricket field as the place of occurrence of the external cause
Hockey field as the place of occurrence of the external cause

✓6ᵗʰ Y92.33   **Skating rink** as the place of occurrence of the external cause

Y92.330   **Ice skating rink** (indoor) (outdoor) as the place of occurrence of the external cause

Y92.331   **Roller skating rink** as the place of occurrence of the external cause

Y92.34   **Swimming pool** (public) as the place of occurrence of the external cause
EXCLUDES 1 *swimming pool in private home or garden (Y92.016)*

Y92.39   **Other** specified sports and athletic area as the place of occurrence of the external cause
Golf-course as the place of occurrence of the external cause
Gymnasium as the place of occurrence of the external cause
Riding-school as the place of occurrence of the external cause
Stadium as the place of occurrence of the external cause

✓5ᵗʰ Y92.4   **Street, highway and other paved roadways** as the place of occurrence of the external cause
EXCLUDES 1 *private driveway of residence (Y92.014, Y92.024, Y92.043, Y92.093, Y92.113, Y92.123, Y92.154, Y92.194)*

✓6ᵗʰ Y92.41   **Street and highway** as the place of occurrence of the external cause

Y92.410   **Unspecified** street and highway as the place of occurrence of the external cause
Road NOS as the place of occurrence of the external cause

Y92.411   **Interstate** highway as the place of occurrence of the external cause
Freeway as the place of occurrence of the external cause
Motorway as the place of occurrence of the external cause

Y92.412   **Parkway** as the place of occurrence of the external cause

Y92.413   **State road** as the place of occurrence of the external cause

Y92.414   **Local residential or business street** as the place of occurrence of the external cause

Y92.415   **Exit ramp or entrance ramp** of street or highway as the place of occurrence of the external cause

N Newborn: 0   P Pediatric: 0-17   M Maternity: 12-55   A Adult: 15-124   MCC Major Complication/Comorbidity   CC Complication/Comorbidity   SW Severe Wound Dx

1214   ICD-10-CM 2019

✓6ᵗʰ **Y92.48** **Other paved roadways** as the place of occurrence of the external cause

    Y92.480 **Sidewalk** as the place of occurrence of the external cause

    Y92.481 **Parking lot** as the place of occurrence of the external cause

    Y92.482 **Bike path** as the place of occurrence of the external cause

    Y92.488 **Other** paved roadways as the place of occurrence of the external cause

✓5ᵗʰ **Y92.5** **Trade and service area** as the place of occurrence of the external cause

    EXCLUDES 1   *garage in private home (Y92.015)*
        schools and other public administration buildings (Y92.2-)

✓6ᵗʰ **Y92.51** **Private commercial establishments** as the place of occurrence of the external cause

    Y92.510 **Bank** as the place of occurrence of the external cause

    Y92.511 **Restaurant** or **café** as the place of occurrence of the external cause

    Y92.512 **Supermarket, store** or **market** as the place of occurrence of the external cause

    Y92.513 **Shop (commercial)** as the place of occurrence of the external cause

✓6ᵗʰ **Y92.52** **Service areas** as the place of occurrence of the external cause

    Y92.520 **Airport** as the place of occurrence of the external cause

    Y92.521 **Bus station** as the place of occurrence of the external cause

    Y92.522 **Railway station** as the place of occurrence of the external cause

    Y92.523 **Highway rest stop** as the place of occurrence of the external cause

    Y92.524 **Gas station** as the place of occurrence of the external cause

        Petroleum station as the place of occurrence of the external cause

        Service station as the place of occurrence of the external cause

✓6ᵗʰ **Y92.53** **Ambulatory health services establishments** as the place of occurrence of the external cause

    Y92.530 **Ambulatory surgery center** as the place of occurrence of the external cause

        Outpatient surgery center, including that connected with a hospital as the place of occurrence of the external cause

        Same day surgery center, including that connected with a hospital as the place of occurrence of the external cause

    Y92.531 **Health care provider office** as the place of occurrence of the external cause

        Physician office as the place of occurrence of the external cause

    Y92.532 **Urgent care center** as the place of occurrence of the external cause

    Y92.538 **Other ambulatory** health services establishments as the place of occurrence of the external cause

    Y92.59 **Other trade areas** as the place of occurrence of the external cause

        Office building as the place of occurrence of the external cause

        Casino as the place of occurrence of the external cause

        Garage (commercial) as the place of occurrence of the external cause

        Hotel as the place of occurrence of the external cause

        Radio or television station as the place of occurrence of the external cause

        Shopping mall as the place of occurrence of the external cause

        Warehouse as the place of occurrence of the external cause

✓5ᵗʰ **Y92.6** **Industrial and construction area** as the place of occurrence of the external cause

    Y92.61 **Building [any] under construction** as the place of occurrence of the external cause

    Y92.62 **Dock or shipyard** as the place of occurrence of the external cause

        Dockyard as the place of occurrence of the external cause

        Dry dock as the place of occurrence of the external cause

        Shipyard as the place of occurrence of the external cause

    Y92.63 **Factory** as the place of occurrence of the external cause

        Factory building as the place of occurrence of the external cause

        Factory premises as the place of occurrence of the external cause

        Industrial yard as the place of occurrence of the external cause

    Y92.64 **Mine or pit** as the place of occurrence of the external cause

        Mine as the place of occurrence of the external cause

    Y92.65 **Oil rig** as the place of occurrence of the external cause

        Pit (coal) (gravel) (sand) as the place of occurrence of the external cause

    Y92.69 **Other** specified industrial and construction area as the place of occurrence of the external cause

        Gasworks as the place of occurrence of the external cause

        Power-station (coal) (nuclear) (oil) as the place of occurrence of the external cause

        Tunnel under construction as the place of occurrence of the external cause

        Workshop as the place of occurrence of the external cause

✓5ᵗʰ **Y92.7** **Farm** as the place of occurrence of the external cause

    Ranch as the place of occurrence of the external cause

    EXCLUDES 1   *farmhouse and home premises of farm (Y92.01-)*

    Y92.71 **Barn** as the place of occurrence of the external cause

    Y92.72 **Chicken coop** as the place of occurrence of the external cause

        Hen house as the place of occurrence of the external cause

    Y92.73 **Farm field** as the place of occurrence of the external cause

    Y92.74 **Orchard** as the place of occurrence of the external cause

    Y92.79 **Other** farm location as the place of occurrence of the external cause

✓5ᵗʰ **Y92.8** **Other places** as the place of occurrence of the external cause

✓6ᵗʰ **Y92.81** **Transport vehicle** as the place of occurrence of the external cause

    EXCLUDES 1   *transport accidents (V00-V99)*

    Y92.810 **Car** as the place of occurrence of the external cause

    Y92.811 **Bus** as the place of occurrence of the external cause

    Y92.812 **Truck** as the place of occurrence of the external cause

    Y92.813 **Airplane** as the place of occurrence of the external cause

    Y92.814 **Boat** as the place of occurrence of the external cause

    Y92.815 **Train** as the place of occurrence of the external cause

    Y92.816 **Subway car** as the place of occurrence of the external cause

    Y92.818 **Other** transport vehicle as the place of occurrence of the external cause

✓6ᵗʰ **Y92.82** **Wilderness area**

    Y92.820 **Desert** as the place of occurrence of the external cause

    Y92.821 **Forest** as the place of occurrence of the external cause

✔ Additional Character Required   ✓7ᵗʰ Placeholder   Unacceptable PDx   Questionable PDx   Wrong Procedure   Manifestation   H1–H14 HAC   HCC CMS-HCC Dx   HIV HIV Dx

ICD-10-CM 2019   1215

Y92.828   **Other wilderness area as the place of occurrence of the external cause**
     Swamp as the place of occurrence of the external cause
     Mountain as the place of occurrence of the external cause
     Marsh as the place of occurrence of the external cause
     Prairie as the place of occurrence of the external cause

✓6ᵗʰ **Y92.83**   **Recreation area as the place of occurrence of the external cause**

Y92.830   **Public park as the place of occurrence of the external cause**

Y92.831   **Amusement park as the place of occurrence of the external cause**

Y92.832   **Beach as the place of occurrence of the external cause**
     Seashore as the place of occurrence of the external cause

Y92.833   **Campsite as the place of occurrence of the external cause**

Y92.834   **Zoological garden (Zoo) as the place of occurrence of the external cause**

Y92.838   **Other recreation area as the place of occurrence of the external cause**

Y92.84   **Military training ground as the place of occurrence of the external cause**

Y92.85   **Railroad track as the place of occurrence of the external cause**

Y92.86   **Slaughter house as the place of occurrence of the external cause**

Y92.89   **Other specified places as the place of occurrence of the external cause**
     Derelict house as the place of occurrence of the external cause

Y92.9   **Unspecified place or not applicable**

✓4ᵗʰ **Y93**   **Activity codes**

> **NOTE**   Category Y93 is provided for use to indicate the activity of the person seeking healthcare for an injury or health condition, such as a heart attack while shoveling snow, which resulted from, or was contributed to, by the activity. These codes are appropriate for use for both acute injuries, such as those from chapter 19, and conditions that are due to the long-term, cumulative effects of an activity, such as those from chapter 13. They are also appropriate for use with external cause codes for cause and intent if identifying the activity provides additional information on the event. These codes should be used in conjunction with codes for external cause status (Y99) and place of occurrence (Y92).

This section contains the following broad activity categories:

Y93.Ø	Activities involving walking and running
Y93.1	Activities involving water and water craft
Y93.2	Activities involving ice and snow
Y93.3	Activities involving climbing, rappelling, and jumping off
Y93.4	Activities involving dancing and other rhythmic movement
Y93.5	Activities involving other sports and athletics played individually
Y93.6	Activities involving other sports and athletics played as a team or group
Y93.7	Activities involving other specified sports and athletics
Y93.A	Activities involving other cardiorespiratory exercise
Y93.B	Activities involving other muscle strengthening exercises
Y93.C	Activities involving computer technology and electronic devices
Y93.D	Activities involving arts and handcrafts
Y93.E	Activities involving personal hygiene and interior property and clothing maintenance
Y93.F	Activities involving caregiving
Y93.G	Activities involving food preparation, cooking and grilling
Y93.H	Activities involving exterior property and land maintenance, building and construction
Y93.I	Activities involving roller coasters and other types of external motion
Y93.J	Activities involving playing musical instrument
Y93.K	Activities involving animal care
Y93.8	Activities, other specified
Y93.9	Activity, unspecified

✓5ᵗʰ **Y93.Ø**   **Activities involving walking and running**
> **EXCLUDES 1**   activity, walking an animal (Y93.K1)
>   activity, walking or running on a treadmill (Y93.A1)

Y93.Ø1   **Activity, walking, marching and hiking**
     Activity, walking, marching and hiking on level or elevated terrain
> **EXCLUDES 1**   activity, mountain climbing (Y93.31)

Y93.Ø2   **Activity, running**

✓5ᵗʰ **Y93.1**   **Activities involving water and water craft**
> **EXCLUDES 1**   activities involving ice (Y93.2-)

Y93.11   **Activity, swimming**

Y93.12   **Activity, springboard and platform diving**

Y93.13   **Activity, water polo**

Y93.14   **Activity, water aerobics and water exercise**

Y93.15   **Activity, underwater diving and snorkeling**
     Activity, SCUBA diving

Y93.16   **Activity, rowing, canoeing, kayaking, rafting and tubing**
     Activity, canoeing, kayaking, rafting and tubing in calm and turbulent water

Y93.17   **Activity, water skiing and wake boarding**

Y93.18   **Activity, surfing, windsurfing and boogie boarding**
     Activity, water sliding

Y93.19   **Activity, other involving water and watercraft**
     Activity involving water NOS
     Activity, parasailing
     Activity, water survival training and testing

✓5ᵗʰ **Y93.2**   **Activities involving ice and snow**
> **EXCLUDES 1**   activity, shoveling ice and snow (Y93.H1)

Y93.21   **Activity, ice skating**
     Activity, figure skating (singles) (pairs)
     Activity, ice dancing
> **EXCLUDES 1**   activity, ice hockey (Y93.22)

Y93.22   **Activity, ice hockey**

Y93.23   **Activity, snow (alpine) (downhill) skiing, snowboarding, sledding, tobogganing and snow tubing**
> **EXCLUDES 1**   activity, cross country skiing (Y93.24)

Y93.24   **Activity, cross country skiing**
     Activity, nordic skiing

Y93.29   **Activity, other involving ice and snow**
     Activity involving ice and snow NOS

✓5ᵗʰ **Y93.3**   **Activities involving climbing, rappelling and jumping off**
> **EXCLUDES 1**   activity, hiking on level or elevated terrain (Y93.Ø1)
>   activity, jumping rope (Y93.56)
>   activity, trampoline jumping (Y93.44)

Y93.31   **Activity, mountain climbing, rock climbing and wall climbing**

Y93.32   **Activity, rappelling**

Y93.33   **Activity, BASE jumping**
     Activity, Building, Antenna, Span, Earth jumping

Y93.34   **Activity, bungee jumping**

Y93.35   **Activity, hang gliding**

Y93.39   **Activity, other involving climbing, rappelling and jumping off**

✓5ᵗʰ **Y93.4**   **Activities involving dancing and other rhythmic movement**
> **EXCLUDES 1**   activity, martial arts (Y93.75)

Y93.41   **Activity, dancing**
     AHA: 2012, 4Q, 108

Y93.42   **Activity, yoga**

Y93.43   **Activity, gymnastics**
     Activity, rhythmic gymnastics
> **EXCLUDES 1**   activity, trampolining (Y93.44)

Y93.44   **Activity, trampolining**

Y93.45   **Activity, cheerleading**

Y93.49   **Activity, other involving dancing and other rhythmic movements**

✓5ᵗʰ **Y93.5**   **Activities involving other sports and athletics played individually**
> **EXCLUDES 1**   activity, dancing (Y93.41)
>   activity, gymnastic (Y93.43)
>   activity, trampolining (Y93.44)
>   activity, yoga (Y93.42)

Y93.51   **Activity, roller skating (inline) and skateboarding**

Y93.52   **Activity, horseback riding**

Y93.53   **Activity, golf**

N Newborn: 0   P Pediatric: 0-17   M Maternity: 12-55   A Adult: 15-124   MCC Major Complication/Comorbidity   CC Complication/Comorbidity   SW Severe Wound Dx

1216   ICD-10-CM 2019

Y93.54 **Activity,** bowling

Y93.55 **Activity,** bike riding

Y93.56 **Activity,** jumping rope

Y93.57 **Activity,** non-running track and field events
    EXCLUDES 1   *activity, running (any form) (Y93.02)*

Y93.59 **Activity,** other involving other sports and athletics played individually
    EXCLUDES 1   *activities involving climbing, rappelling, and jumping (Y93.3-)*
        activities involving ice and snow (Y93.2-)
        activities involving walking and running (Y93.0-)
        activities involving water and watercraft (Y93.1-)

✓5th **Y93.6** **Activities involving other sports and athletics played as a team or group**
    EXCLUDES 1   *activity, ice hockey (Y93.22)*
        activity, water polo (Y93.13)

Y93.61 **Activity,** American tackle football
    Activity, football NOS

Y93.62 **Activity,** American flag or touch football

Y93.63 **Activity,** rugby

Y93.64 **Activity,** baseball
    Activity, softball

Y93.65 **Activity,** lacrosse and field hockey

Y93.66 **Activity,** soccer

Y93.67 **Activity,** basketball

Y93.68 **Activity,** volleyball (beach) (court)

Y93.6A **Activity,** physical games generally associated with school recess, summer camp and children
    Activity, capture the flag   Activity, four square
    Activity, dodge ball   Activity, kickball

Y93.69 **Activity,** other involving other sports and athletics played as a team or group
    Activity, cricket

✓5th **Y93.7** **Activities involving other specified sports and athletics**

Y93.71 **Activity,** boxing

Y93.72 **Activity,** wrestling

Y93.73 **Activity,** racquet and hand sports
    Activity, handball   Activity, squash
    Activity, racquetball   Activity, tennis

Y93.74 **Activity,** frisbee
    Activity, ultimate frisbee

Y93.75 **Activity,** martial arts
    Activity, combatives

Y93.79 **Activity,** other specified sports and athletics
    EXCLUDES 1   *sports and athletics activities specified in categories Y93.0-Y93.6*

✓5th **Y93.A** **Activities involving other cardiorespiratory exercise**
    Activities involving physical training

Y93.A1 **Activity,** exercise machines primarily for cardiorespiratory conditioning
    Activity, elliptical and stepper machines
    Activity, stationary bike
    Activity, treadmill

Y93.A2 **Activity,** calisthenics
    Activity, jumping jacks
    Activity, warm up and cool down

Y93.A3 **Activity,** aerobic and step exercise

Y93.A4 **Activity,** circuit training

Y93.A5 **Activity,** obstacle course
    Activity, challenge course
    Activity, confidence course

Y93.A6 **Activity,** grass drills
    Activity, guerilla drills

Y93.A9 **Activity,** other involving cardiorespiratory exercise
    EXCLUDES 1   *activities involving cardiorespiratory exercise specified in categories Y93.0-Y93.7*

✓5th **Y93.B** **Activities involving other muscle strengthening exercises**

Y93.B1 **Activity,** exercise machines primarily for muscle strengthening

Y93.B2 **Activity,** push-ups, pull-ups, sit-ups

Y93.B3 **Activity,** free weights
    Activity, barbells
    Activity, dumbbells

Y93.B4 **Activity,** pilates

Y93.B9 **Activity,** other involving muscle strengthening exercises
    EXCLUDES 1   *activities involving muscle strengthening specified in categories Y93.0-Y93.A*

✓5th **Y93.C** **Activities involving computer technology and electronic devices**
    EXCLUDES 1   *activity, electronic musical keyboard or instruments (Y93.J-)*

Y93.C1 **Activity,** computer keyboarding
    Activity, electronic game playing using keyboard or other stationary device

Y93.C2 **Activity,** hand held interactive electronic device
    Activity, cellular telephone and communication device
    Activity, electronic game playing using interactive device
    EXCLUDES 1   *activity, electronic game playing using keyboard or other stationary device (Y93.C1)*

Y93.C9 **Activity,** other involving computer technology and electronic devices

✓5th **Y93.D** **Activities involving arts and handcrafts**
    EXCLUDES 1   *activities involving playing musical instrument (Y93.J-)*

Y93.D1 **Activity,** knitting and crocheting

Y93.D2 **Activity,** sewing

Y93.D3 **Activity,** furniture building and finishing
    Activity, furniture repair

Y93.D9 **Activity,** other involving arts and handcrafts

✓5th **Y93.E** **Activities involving personal hygiene and interior property and clothing maintenance**
    EXCLUDES 1   *activities involving cooking and grilling (Y93.G-)*
        activities involving exterior property and land maintenance, building and construction (Y93.H-)
        activities involving caregiving (Y93.F-)
        activity, dishwashing (Y93.G1)
        activity, food preparation (Y93.G1)
        activity, gardening (Y93.H2)

Y93.E1 **Activity,** personal bathing and showering

Y93.E2 **Activity,** laundry

Y93.E3 **Activity,** vacuuming

Y93.E4 **Activity,** ironing

Y93.E5 **Activity,** floor mopping and cleaning

Y93.E6 **Activity,** residential relocation
    Activity, packing up and unpacking involved in moving to a new residence

Y93.E8 **Activity,** other personal hygiene

Y93.E9 **Activity,** other interior property and clothing maintenance

✓5th **Y93.F** **Activities involving caregiving**
    Activity involving the provider of caregiving

Y93.F1 **Activity,** caregiving, bathing

Y93.F2 **Activity,** caregiving, lifting

Y93.F9 **Activity,** other caregiving

✓5th **Y93.G** **Activities involving food preparation, cooking and grilling**

Y93.G1 **Activity,** food preparation and clean up
    Activity, dishwashing

Y93.G2 **Activity,** grilling and smoking food

Y93.G3 **Activity,** cooking and baking
    Activity, use of stove, oven and microwave oven

Y93.G9 **Activity,** other involving cooking and grilling

✓5th **Y93.H** **Activities involving exterior property and land maintenance, building and construction**

Y93.H1 **Activity,** digging, shoveling and raking
    Activity, dirt digging
    Activity, raking leaves
    Activity, snow shoveling

Y93.H2 **Activity,** gardening and landscaping
    Activity, pruning, trimming shrubs, weeding

Y93.H3 **Activity,** building and construction

Y93.H9 **Activity,** other involving exterior property and land maintenance, building and construction

✓5th **Y93.I** **Activities involving roller coasters and other types of external motion**

Y93.I1 **Activity,** rollercoaster riding

Y93.I9 **Activity,** other involving external motion

✔ Additional Character Required   ✓x7th Placeholder   Unacceptable PDx   Questionable PDx   Wrong Procedure   Manifestation   H1-H14 HAC   HCC CMS-HCC Dx   HIV HIV Dx

ICD-10-CM 2019   1217

✓5ᵗʰ Y93.J   Activities involving playing musical instrument
       Activity involving playing electric musical instrument

     Y93.J1   Activity, piano playing
           Activity, musical keyboard (electronic) playing

     Y93.J2   Activity, drum and other percussion instrument playing

     Y93.J3   Activity, string instrument playing

     Y93.J4   Activity, winds and brass instrument playing

✓5ᵗʰ Y93.K   Activities involving animal care
       EXCLUDES 1   activity, horseback riding (Y93.52)

     Y93.K1   Activity, walking an animal

     Y93.K2   Activity, milking an animal

     Y93.K3   Activity, grooming and shearing an animal

     Y93.K9   Activity, other involving animal care

✓5ᵗʰ Y93.8   Activities, other specified

     Y93.81   Activity, refereeing a sports activity

     Y93.82   Activity, spectator at an event

     Y93.83   Activity, rough housing and horseplay

     Y93.84   Activity, sleeping

     Y93.85   Activity, choking game
           Activity, blackout game
           Activity, fainting game
           Activity, pass out game
           AHA: 2016, 4Q, 74-76

     Y93.89   Activity, other specified

   Y93.9   Activity, unspecified

Y95   Nosocomial condition
     AHA: 2013, 4Q, 119

✓4ᵗʰ Y99   External cause status
     NOTE   A single code from category Y99 should be used in conjunction with the external cause code(s) assigned to a record to indicate the status of the person at the time the event occurred.

   Y99.0   Civilian activity done for income or pay
       Civilian activity done for financial or other compensation
       EXCLUDES 1   military activity (Y99.1)
                 volunteer activity (Y99.2)

   Y99.1   Military activity
       EXCLUDES 1   activity of off duty military personnel (Y99.8)

   Y99.2   Volunteer activity
       EXCLUDES 1   activity of child or other family member assisting in compensated work of other family member (Y99.8)

   Y99.8   Other external cause status
       Activity NEC
       Activity of child or other family member assisting in compensated work of other family member
       Hobby not done for income
       Leisure activity
       Off-duty activity of military personnel
       Recreation or sport not for income or while a student
       Student activity
       EXCLUDES 1   civilian activity done for income or compensation (Y99.0)
                 military activity (Y99.1)
       AHA: 2012, 4Q, 108

   Y99.9   Unspecified external cause status

N Newborn: 0   P Pediatric: 0-17   M Maternity: 12-55   A Adult: 15-124   MCC Major Complication/Comorbidity   CC Complication/Comorbidity   SW Severe Wound Dx

1218   ICD-10-CM 2019

Chapter 21. Factors Influencing Health Status and Contact with Health Services (Z00–Z99)

Chapter Specific Guidelines with Coding Examples

The chapter specific guidelines from the ICD-10-CM Official Guidelines for Coding and Reporting have been provided below. Along with these guidelines are coding examples, contained in the shaded boxes, that have been developed to help illustrate the coding and/or sequencing guidance found in these guidelines.

Note: The chapter specific guidelines provide additional information about the use of Z codes for specified encounters.

a. Use of Z codes in any healthcare setting

Z codes are for use in any healthcare setting. Z codes may be used as either a first-listed (principal diagnosis code in the inpatient setting) or secondary code, depending on the circumstances of the encounter. Certain Z codes may only be used as first-listed or principal diagnosis.

> Patient with middle lobe lung cancer admitted for initiation of chemotherapy
>
> **Z51.11**   **Encounter for antineoplastic chemotherapy**
>
> **C34.2**   **Malignant neoplasm of middle lobe, bronchus or lung**
>
> *Explanation:* A Z code can be used as first-listed in this situation based on guidelines in this chapter as well as chapter 2, "Neoplasms."

b. Z codes indicate a reason for an encounter

Z codes are not procedure codes. A corresponding procedure code must accompany a Z code to describe any procedure performed.

c. Categories of Z codes

1) Contact/exposure

Category Z20 indicates contact with, and suspected exposure to, communicable diseases. These codes are for patients who do not show any sign or symptom of a disease but are suspected to have been exposed to it by close personal contact with an infected individual or are in an area where a disease is epidemic.

Category Z77, Other contact with and (suspected) exposures hazardous to health, indicates contact with and suspected exposures hazardous to health.

Contact/exposure codes may be used as a first-listed code to explain an encounter for testing, or, more commonly, as a secondary code to identify a potential risk.

2) Inoculations and vaccinations

Code Z23 is for encounters for inoculations and vaccinations. It indicates that a patient is being seen to receive a prophylactic inoculation against a disease. Procedure codes are required to identify the actual administration of the injection and the type(s) of immunizations given. Code Z23 may be used as a secondary code if the inoculation is given as a routine part of preventive health care, such as a well-baby visit.

3) Status

Status codes indicate that a patient is either a carrier of a disease or has the sequelae or residual of a past disease or condition. This includes such things as the presence of prosthetic or mechanical devices resulting from past treatment. A status code is informative, because the status may affect the course of treatment and its outcome. A status code is distinct from a history code. The history code indicates that the patient no longer has the condition.

A status code should not be used with a diagnosis code from one of the body system chapters, if the diagnosis code includes the information provided by the status code. For example, code Z94.1, Heart transplant status, should not be used with a code from subcategory T86.2, Complications of heart transplant. The status code does not provide additional information. The complication code indicates that the patient is a heart transplant patient.

For encounters for weaning from a mechanical ventilator, assign a code from subcategory J96.1, Chronic respiratory failure, followed by code Z99.11, Dependence on respirator [ventilator] status.

The status Z codes/categories are:

     Z14   Genetic carrier

             Genetic carrier status indicates that a person carries a gene, associated with a particular disease, which may be passed to offspring who may develop that disease. The person does not have the disease and is not at risk of developing the disease.

     Z15   Genetic susceptibility to disease

             Genetic susceptibility indicates that a person has a gene that increases the risk of that person developing the disease.

             Codes from category Z15 should not be used as principal or first-listed codes. If the patient has the condition to which he/she is susceptible, and that condition is the reason for the encounter, the code for the current condition should be sequenced first. If the patient is being seen for follow-up after completed treatment for this condition, and the condition no longer exists, a follow-up code should be sequenced first, followed by the appropriate personal history and genetic susceptibility codes. If the purpose of the encounter is genetic counseling associated with procreative management, code Z31.5, Encounter for genetic counseling, should be assigned as the first-listed code, followed by a code from category Z15. Additional codes should be assigned for any applicable family or personal history.

     Z16   Resistance to antimicrobial drugs

             This code indicates that a patient has a condition that is resistant to antimicrobial drug treatment. Sequence the infection code first.

> Penicillin resistant streptococcus pneumoniae meningitis
>
> **G00.1**   **Pneumococcal meningitis**
>
> **Z16.11**   **Resistance to penicillins**
>
> *Explanation:* The status Z code is used to describe the presence of a drug-resistant organism that most likely altered how the meningitis was treated.

     Z17   Estrogen receptor status

     Z18   Retained foreign body fragments

     Z19   Hormone sensitivity malignancy status

     Z21   Asymptomatic HIV infection status

             This code indicates that a patient has tested positive for HIV but has manifested no signs or symptoms of the disease.

     Z22   Carrier of infectious disease

             Carrier status indicates that a person harbors the specific organisms of a disease without manifest symptoms and is capable of transmitting the infection.

     Z28.3   Underimmunization status

     Z33.1   Pregnant state, incidental

             This code is a secondary code only for use when the pregnancy is in no way complicating the reason for visit. Otherwise, a code from the obstetric chapter is required.

     Z66   Do not resuscitate

             This code may be used when it is documented by the provider that a patient is on do not resuscitate status at any time during the stay.

     Z67   Blood type

     Z68   Body mass index (BMI)

             BMI codes should only be assigned when the associated diagnosis (such as overweight or obesity) meets the definition of a reportable diagnosis (see Section III, Reporting Additional Diagnoses). **Do not assign BMI codes during pregnancy. *See Section I.B.14 for BMI documentation by clinicians other than the patient's provider.***

     Z74.01   Bed confinement status

     Z76.82   Awaiting organ transplant status

     Z78   Other specified health status

             Code Z78.1, Physical restraint status, may be used when it is documented by the provider that a patient has been put in restraints during the current encounter. Please note that this code should not be reported when it is documented by the provider that a patient is temporarily restrained during a procedure.

Z79   Long-term (current) drug therapy

Codes from this category indicate a patient's continuous use of a prescribed drug (including such things as aspirin therapy) for the long-term treatment of a condition or for prophylactic use. It is not for use for patients who have addictions to drugs. This subcategory is not for use of medications for detoxification or maintenance programs to prevent withdrawal symptoms in patients with drug dependence (e.g., methadone maintenance for opiate dependence). Assign the appropriate code for the drug dependence instead.

Assign a code from Z79 if the patient is receiving a medication for an extended period as a prophylactic measure (such as for the prevention of deep vein thrombosis) or as treatment of a chronic condition (such as arthritis) or a disease requiring a lengthy course of treatment (such as cancer). Do not assign a code from category Z79 for medication being administered for a brief period of time to treat an acute illness or injury (such as a course of antibiotics to treat acute bronchitis).

Z88   Allergy status to drugs, medicaments and biological substances

Except: Z88.9, Allergy status to unspecified drugs, medicaments and biological substances status

Z89   Acquired absence of limb

Z90   Acquired absence of organs, not elsewhere classified

Z91.0-   Allergy status, other than to drugs and biological substances

Z92.82   Status post administration of tPA (rtPA) in a different facility within the last 24 hours prior to admission to a current facility

Assign code Z92.82, Status post administration of tPA (rtPA) in a different facility within the last 24 hours prior to admission to current facility, as a secondary diagnosis when a patient is received by transfer into a facility and documentation indicates they were administered tissue plasminogen activator (tPA) within the last 24 hours prior to admission to the current facility.

This guideline applies even if the patient is still receiving the tPA at the time they are received into the current facility.

The appropriate code for the condition for which the tPA was administered (such as cerebrovascular disease or myocardial infarction) should be assigned first.

Code Z92.82 is only applicable to the receiving facility record and not to the transferring facility record.

Z93   Artificial opening status

Z94   Transplanted organ and tissue status

Z95   Presence of cardiac and vascular implants and grafts

Z96   Presence of other functional implants

Z97   Presence of other devices

Z98   Other postprocedural states

Assign code Z98.85, Transplanted organ removal status, to indicate that a transplanted organ has been previously removed. This code should not be assigned for the encounter in which the transplanted organ is removed. The complication necessitating removal of the transplant organ should be assigned for that encounter.

See section I.C19. for information on the coding of organ transplant complications.

Z99   Dependence on enabling machines and devices, not elsewhere classified

Note: Categories Z89-Z90 and Z93-Z99 are for use only if there are no complications or malfunctions of the organ or tissue replaced, the amputation site or the equipment on which the patient is dependent.

4) History (of)

There are two types of history Z codes, personal and family. Personal history codes explain a patient's past medical condition that no longer exists and is not receiving any treatment, but that has the potential for recurrence, and therefore may require continued monitoring.

Family history codes are for use when a patient has a family member(s) who has had a particular disease that causes the patient to be at higher risk of also contracting the disease.

Personal history codes may be used in conjunction with follow-up codes and family history codes may be used in conjunction with screening codes to explain the need for a test or procedure. History codes are also acceptable on any medical record regardless of the reason for visit. A history of an illness, even if no longer present, is important information that may alter the type of treatment ordered.

The history Z code categories are:

Z80   Family history of primary malignant neoplasm

Z81   Family history of mental and behavioral disorders

Z82   Family history of certain disabilities and chronic diseases (leading to disablement)

Z83   Family history of other specific disorders

Z84   Family history of other conditions

Z85   Personal history of malignant neoplasm

Z86   Personal history of certain other diseases

Z87   Personal history of other diseases and conditions

Z91.4-   Personal history of psychological trauma, not elsewhere classified

Z91.5   Personal history of self-harm

Z91.81   History of falling

Z91.82   Personal history of military deployment

Z92   Personal history of medical treatment

Except: Z92.0, Personal history of contraception

Except: Z92.82, Status post administration of tPA (rtPA) in a different facility within the last 24 hours prior to admission to a current facility

Patient has chronic lymphocytic leukemia for which the patient had previous chemotherapy and is now in remission

C91.11   Chronic lymphocytic leukemia of B-cell type in remission

Z92.21   Personal history of antineoplastic chemotherapy

Explanation: The personal history Z code is used to describe a secondary (supplementary) diagnosis to identify that this patient has had chemotherapy in the past.

5) Screening

Screening is the testing for disease or disease precursors in seemingly well individuals so that early detection and treatment can be provided for those who test positive for the disease (e.g., screening mammogram).

The testing of a person to rule out or confirm a suspected diagnosis because the patient has some sign or symptom is a diagnostic examination, not a screening. In these cases, the sign or symptom is used to explain the reason for the test.

A screening code may be a first-listed code if the reason for the visit is specifically the screening exam. It may also be used as an additional code if the screening is done during an office visit for other health problems. A screening code is not necessary if the screening is inherent to a routine examination, such as a pap smear done during a routine pelvic examination.

Should a condition be discovered during the screening then the code for the condition may be assigned as an additional diagnosis.

The Z code indicates that a screening exam is planned. A procedure code is required to confirm that the screening was performed.

The screening Z codes/categories:

Z11   Encounter for screening for infectious and parasitic diseases

Z12   Encounter for screening for malignant neoplasms

Z13   Encounter for screening for other diseases and disorders

Except: Z13.9, Encounter for screening, unspecified

Z36   Encounter for antenatal screening for mother

6) Observation

There are three observation Z code categories. They are for use in very limited circumstances when a person is being observed for a suspected condition that is ruled out. The observation codes are not for use if an injury or illness or any signs or symptoms related to the suspected condition are present. In such cases the diagnosis/symptom code is used with the corresponding external cause code.

The observation codes are to be used as principal diagnosis only. The only exception to this is when the principal diagnosis is required to be a code from category Z38, Liveborn infants according to place of birth and type of delivery. Then a code from category Z05, Encounter for observation and evaluation of newborn for suspected diseases and conditions ruled out, is sequenced after the Z38 code. Additional codes may be used in addition to the observation code but only if they are unrelated to the suspected condition being observed.

Codes from subcategory Z03.7, Encounter for suspected maternal and fetal conditions ruled out, may either be used as a first-listed or as an additional code assignment depending on the case. They are for use in very limited circumstances on a maternal record when an encounter is for a suspected maternal or fetal condition that is ruled out during that encounter (for example, a maternal or fetal condition may be suspected

due to an abnormal test result). These codes should not be used when the condition is confirmed. In those cases, the confirmed condition should be coded. In addition, these codes are not for use if an illness or any signs or symptoms related to the suspected condition or problem are present. In such cases the diagnosis/symptom code is used.

Additional codes may be used in addition to the code from subcategory Z03.7, but only if they are unrelated to the suspected condition being evaluated.

Codes from subcategory Z03.7 may not be used for encounters for antenatal screening of mother. *See Section I.C.21. Screening.*

For encounters for suspected fetal condition that are inconclusive following testing and evaluation, assign the appropriate code from category O35, O36, O40 or O41.

The observation Z code categories:

Z03	Encounter for medical observation for suspected diseases and conditions ruled out
Z04	Encounter for examination and observation for other reasons
	Except: Z04.9, Encounter for examination and observation for unspecified reason
Z05	Encounter for observation and evaluation of newborn for suspected diseases and conditions ruled out

> Upon initial examination, a heart murmur was heard in a newborn infant delivered vaginally in the hospital; however, after further observation, any serious cardiac conditions were ruled out.
>
> **Z38.00   Single liveborn infant, delivered vaginally**
>
> **Z05.0   Observation and evaluation of newborn for suspected cardiac condition ruled out**
>
> *Explanation:* Normally an observation code is used as the principal diagnosis except when the patient is a newborn. A code from category Z38 Liveborn infants according to place of birth and type of delivery code would be sequenced first, followed by the encounter for observation and evaluation of newborn for suspected diseases and conditions ruled out.

7) Aftercare

Aftercare visit codes cover situations when the initial treatment of a disease has been performed and the patient requires continued care during the healing or recovery phase, or for the long-term consequences of the disease. The aftercare Z code should not be used if treatment is directed at a current, acute disease. The diagnosis code is to be used in these cases. Exceptions to this rule are codes Z51.0, Encounter for antineoplastic radiation therapy, and codes from subcategory Z51.1, Encounter for antineoplastic chemotherapy and immunotherapy. These codes are to be first-listed, followed by the diagnosis code when a patient's encounter is solely to receive radiation therapy, chemotherapy, or immunotherapy for the treatment of a neoplasm. If the reason for the encounter is more than one type of antineoplastic therapy, code Z51.0 and a code from subcategory Z51.1 may be assigned together, in which case one of these codes would be reported as a secondary diagnosis.

The aftercare Z codes should also not be used for aftercare for injuries. For aftercare of an injury, assign the acute injury code with the appropriate 7th character (for subsequent encounter).

The aftercare codes are generally first-listed to explain the specific reason for the encounter. An aftercare code may be used as an additional code when some type of aftercare is provided in addition to the reason for admission and no diagnosis code is applicable. An example of this would be the closure of a colostomy during an encounter for treatment of another condition.

Aftercare codes should be used in conjunction with other aftercare codes or diagnosis codes to provide better detail on the specifics of an aftercare encounter visit, unless otherwise directed by the classification. Should a patient receive multiple types of antineoplastic therapy during the same encounter, code Z51.0, Encounter for antineoplastic radiation therapy, and codes from subcategory Z51.1, Encounter for antineoplastic chemotherapy and immunotherapy, may be used together on a record. The sequencing of multiple aftercare codes depends on the circumstances of the encounter.

Certain aftercare Z code categories need a secondary diagnosis code to describe the resolving condition or sequelae. For others, the condition is included in the code title.

Additional Z code aftercare category terms include fitting and adjustment, and attention to artificial openings.

Status Z codes may be used with aftercare Z codes to indicate the nature of the aftercare. For example code Z95.1, Presence of aortocoronary bypass graft, may be used with code Z48.812, Encounter for surgical aftercare following surgery on the circulatory system, to indicate the

surgery for which the aftercare is being performed. A status code should not be used when the aftercare code indicates the type of status, such as using Z43.0, Encounter for attention to tracheostomy, with Z93.0, Tracheostomy status.

The aftercare Z category/codes:

Z42	Encounter for plastic and reconstructive surgery following medical procedure or healed injury
Z43	Encounter for attention to artificial openings
Z44	Encounter for fitting and adjustment of external prosthetic device
Z45	Encounter for adjustment and management of implanted device
Z46	Encounter for fitting and adjustment of other devices
Z47	Orthopedic aftercare
Z48	Encounter for other postprocedural aftercare
Z49	Encounter for care involving renal dialysis
Z51	Encounter for other aftercare and medical care

8) Follow-up

The follow-up codes are used to explain continuing surveillance following completed treatment of a disease, condition, or injury. They imply that the condition has been fully treated and no longer exists. They should not be confused with aftercare codes, or injury codes with a 7th character for subsequent encounter, that explain ongoing care of a healing condition or its sequelae. Follow-up codes may be used in conjunction with history codes to provide the full picture of the healed condition and its treatment. The follow-up code is sequenced first, followed by the history code.

A follow-up code may be used to explain multiple visits. Should a condition be found to have recurred on the follow-up visit, then the diagnosis code for the condition should be assigned in place of the follow-up code.

The follow-up Z code categories:

Z08	Encounter for follow-up examination after completed treatment for malignant neoplasm
Z09	Encounter for follow-up examination after completed treatment for conditions other than malignant neoplasm
Z39	Encounter for maternal postpartum care and examination

9) Donor

Codes in category Z52, Donors of organs and tissues, are used for living individuals who are donating blood or other body tissue. These codes are only for individuals donating for others, not for self-donations. They are not used to identify cadaveric donations.

10) Counseling

Counseling Z codes are used when a patient or family member receives assistance in the aftermath of an illness or injury, or when support is required in coping with family or social problems.

The counseling Z codes/categories:

Z30.0-	Encounter for general counseling and advice on contraception
Z31.5	Encounter for procreative genetic counseling
Z31.6-	Encounter for general counseling and advice on procreation
Z32.2	Encounter for childbirth instruction
Z32.3	Encounter for childcare instruction
Z69	Encounter for mental health services for victim and perpetrator of abuse
Z70	Counseling related to sexual attitude, behavior and orientation
Z71	Persons encountering health services for other counseling and medical advice, not elsewhere classified
Z76.81	Expectant mother prebirth pediatrician visit

11) Encounters for obstetrical and reproductive services

See Section I.C.15. Pregnancy, Childbirth, and the Puerperium, for further instruction on the use of these codes.

Z codes for pregnancy are for use in those circumstances when none of the problems or complications included in the codes from the Obstetrics chapter exist (a routine prenatal visit or postpartum care). Codes in category Z34, Encounter for supervision of normal pregnancy, are always first-listed and are not to be used with any other code from the OB chapter.

Codes in category Z3A, Weeks of gestation, may be assigned to provide additional information about the pregnancy. Category Z3A codes should not be assigned for pregnancies with abortive outcomes (categories O00-O08), elective termination of pregnancy (code Z33.2), nor for postpartum conditions, as category Z3A is not applicable to these conditions. The date of the admission should be used to determine weeks of gestation for inpatient admissions that encompass more than one gestational week.

The outcome of delivery, category Z37, should be included on all maternal delivery records. It is always a secondary code. Codes in category Z37 should not be used on the newborn record.

Z codes for family planning (contraceptive) or procreative management and counseling should be included on an obstetric record either during the pregnancy or the postpartum stage, if applicable.

Z codes/categories for obstetrical and reproductive services:

Z30	Encounter for contraceptive management
Z31	Encounter for procreative management
Z32.2	Encounter for childbirth instruction
Z32.3	Encounter for childcare instruction
Z33	Pregnant state
Z34	Encounter for supervision of normal pregnancy
Z36	Encounter for antenatal screening of mother
Z3A	Weeks of gestation
Z37	Outcome of delivery
Z39	Encounter for maternal postpartum care and examination
Z76.81	Expectant mother prebirth pediatrician visit

12) Newborns and infants

See Section I.C.16. Newborn (Perinatal) Guidelines, for further instruction on the use of these codes.

Newborn Z codes/categories:

Z76.1	Encounter for health supervision and care of foundling
Z00.1-	Encounter for routine child health examination
Z38	Liveborn infants according to place of birth and type of delivery

13) Routine and administrative examinations

The Z codes allow for the description of encounters for routine examinations, such as, a general check-up, or, examinations for administrative purposes, such as, a pre-employment physical. The codes are not to be used if the examination is for diagnosis of a suspected condition or for treatment purposes. In such cases the diagnosis code is used. During a routine exam, should a diagnosis or condition be discovered, it should be coded as an additional code. Pre-existing and chronic conditions and history codes may also be included as additional codes as long as the examination is for administrative purposes and not focused on any particular condition.

Some of the codes for routine health examinations distinguish between "with" and "without" abnormal findings. Code assignment depends on the information that is known at the time the encounter is being coded. For example, if no abnormal findings were found during the examination, but the encounter is being coded before test results are back, it is acceptable to assign the code for "without abnormal findings." When assigning a code for "with abnormal findings," additional code(s) should be assigned to identify the specific abnormal finding(s).

Pre-operative examination and pre-procedural laboratory examination Z codes are for use only in those situations when a patient is being cleared for a procedure or surgery and no treatment is given.

The Z codes/categories for routine and administrative examinations:

Z00	Encounter for general examination without complaint, suspected or reported diagnosis
Z01	Encounter for other special examination without complaint, suspected or reported diagnosis
Z02	Encounter for administrative examination
	Except: Z02.9, Encounter for administrative examinations, unspecified
Z32.0-	Encounter for pregnancy test

14) Miscellaneous Z codes

The miscellaneous Z codes capture a number of other health care encounters that do not fall into one of the other categories. Certain of these codes identify the reason for the encounter; others are for use as additional codes that provide useful information on circumstances that may affect a patient's care and treatment.

Prophylactic organ removal

For encounters specifically for prophylactic removal of an organ (such as prophylactic removal of breasts due to a genetic susceptibility to cancer or a family history of cancer), the principal or first-listed code should be a code from category Z40, Encounter for prophylactic surgery, followed by the appropriate codes to identify the associated risk factor (such as genetic susceptibility or family history).

If the patient has a malignancy of one site and is having prophylactic removal at another site to prevent either a new primary malignancy or metastatic disease, a code for the malignancy should also be assigned in addition to a code from subcategory Z40.0, Encounter for prophylactic surgery for risk factors related to malignant neoplasms. A Z40.0 code should not be assigned if the patient is having organ removal for treatment of a malignancy, such as the removal of the testes for the treatment of prostate cancer.

Female patient with cancer in lower inner quadrant of right breast and positive BRCA 1 noted on testing is admitted for mastectomy of right breast and prophylactic removal of left breast

C50.311	**Malignant neoplasm of lower-inner quadrant of right female breast**
Z40.01	**Encounter for prophylactic removal of breast**
Z15.01	**Genetic susceptibility to malignant neoplasm of breast**

Explanation: Removal of the current neoplastic disease in the right breast was the focus of treatment for this admission and is sequenced first. The removal of the left breast was not required to treat a current disease process but as a means of prevention. The two Z codes are informational; they capture the reason behind the removal of what is currently a healthy left breast.

Miscellaneous Z codes/categories:

Z28	Immunization not carried out
	Except: Z28.3, Underimmunization status
Z29	Encounter for other prophylactic measures
Z40	Encounter for prophylactic surgery
Z41	Encounter for procedures for purposes other than remedying health state
	Except: Z41.9, Encounter for procedure for purposes other than remedying health state, unspecified
Z53	Persons encountering health services for specific procedures and treatment, not carried out
Z55	Problems related to education and literacy
Z56	Problems related to employment and unemployment
Z57	Occupational exposure to risk factors
Z58	Problems related to physical environment
Z59	Problems related to housing and economic circumstances
Z60	Problems related to social environment
Z62	Problems related to upbringing
Z63	Other problems related to primary support group, including family circumstances
Z64	Problems related to certain psychosocial circumstances
Z65	Problems related to other psychosocial circumstances
Z72	Problems related to lifestyle
	Note: These codes should be assigned only when the documentation specifies that the patient has an associated problem
Z73	Problems related to life management difficulty
Z74	Problems related to care provider dependency
	Except: Z74.01, Bed confinement status
Z75	Problems related to medical facilities and other health care
Z76.0	Encounter for issue of repeat prescription
Z76.3	Healthy person accompanying sick person
Z76.4	Other boarder to healthcare facility
Z76.5	Malingerer [conscious simulation]
Z91.1-	Patient's noncompliance with medical treatment and regimen
Z91.83	Wandering in diseases classified elsewhere
Z91.84-	Oral health risk factors
Z91.89	Other specified personal risk factors, not elsewhere classified

See Section I.B.14 for Z55-Z65 Persons with potential health hazards related to socioeconomic and psychosocial circumstances, documentation by clinicians other than the patient's provider

15) Nonspecific Z codes

Certain Z codes are so non-specific, or potentially redundant with other codes in the classification, that there can be little justification for their use in the inpatient setting. Their use in the outpatient setting should be limited to those instances when there is no further documentation to permit more precise coding. Otherwise, any sign or symptom or any other reason for visit that is captured in another code should be used.

Nonspecific Z codes/categories:

Z02.9	Encounter for administrative examinations, unspecified
Z04.9	Encounter for examination and observation for unspecified reason
Z13.9	Encounter for screening, unspecified
Z41.9	Encounter for procedure for purposes other than remedying health state, unspecified
Z52.9	Donor of unspecified organ or tissue
Z86.59	Personal history of other mental and behavioral disorders
Z88.9	Allergy status to unspecified drugs, medicaments and biological substances status
Z92.0	Personal history of contraception

16) Z codes that may only be principal/first-listed diagnosis

The following Z codes/categories may only be reported as the principal/first-listed diagnosis, except when there are multiple encounters on the same day and the medical records for the encounters are combined:

Z00	Encounter for general examination without complaint, suspected or reported diagnosis
	Except: Z00.6
Z01	Encounter for other special examination without complaint, suspected or reported diagnosis
Z02	Encounter for administrative examination
Z03	Encounter for medical observation for suspected diseases and conditions ruled out

Z04	Encounter for examination and observation for other reasons
Z33.2	Encounter for elective termination of pregnancy
Z31.81	Encounter for male factor infertility in female patient
Z31.83	Encounter for assisted reproductive fertility procedure cycle
Z31.84	Encounter for fertility preservation procedure
Z34	Encounter for supervision of normal pregnancy
Z39	Encounter for maternal postpartum care and examination
Z38	Liveborn infants according to place of birth and type of delivery
Z40	Encounter for prophylactic surgery
Z42	Encounter for plastic and reconstructive surgery following medical procedure or healed injury
Z51.0	Encounter for antineoplastic radiation therapy
Z51.1-	Encounter for antineoplastic chemotherapy and immunotherapy
Z52	Donors of organs and tissues
	Except: Z52.9, Donor of unspecified organ or tissue
Z76.1	Encounter for health supervision and care of foundling
Z76.2	Encounter for health supervision and care of other healthy infant and child
Z99.12	Encounter for respirator [ventilator] dependence during power failure

Chapter 21. Factors Influencing Health Status and Contact With Health Services (Z00-Z99)

NOTE Z codes represent reasons for encounters. A corresponding procedure code must accompany a Z code if a procedure is performed. Categories Z00-Z99 are provided for occasions when circumstances other than a disease, injury or external cause classifiable to categories A00-Y89 are recorded as "diagnoses" or "problems". This can arise in two main ways:

(a) When a person who may or may not be sick encounters the health services for some specific purpose, such as to receive limited care or service for a current condition, to donate an organ or tissue, to receive prophylactic vaccination (immunization), or to discuss a problem which is in itself not a disease or injury.

(b) When some circumstance or problem is present which influences the person's health status but is not in itself a current illness or injury.

This chapter contains the following blocks:

Z00-Z13	Persons encountering health services for examinations
Z14-Z15	Genetic carrier and genetic susceptibility to disease
Z16	Resistance to antimicrobial drugs
Z17	Estrogen receptor status
Z18	Retained foreign body fragments
▶Z19	Hormone sensitivity malignancy status◀
Z20-Z29	Persons with potential health hazards related to communicable diseases
Z30-Z39	Persons encountering health services in circumstances related to reproduction
Z40-Z53	Encounters for other specific health care
Z55-Z65	Persons with potential health hazards related to socioeconomic and psychosocial circumstances
Z66	Do not resuscitate status
Z67	Blood type
Z68	Body mass index (BMI)
Z69-Z76	Persons encountering health services in other circumstances
Z77-Z99	Persons with potential health hazards related to family and personal history and certain conditions influencing health status

Persons encountering health services for examinations (Z00-Z13)

NOTE Nonspecific abnormal findings disclosed at the time of these examinations are classified to categories R70-R94.

EXCLUDES 1 examinations related to pregnancy and reproduction (Z30-Z36, Z39-)

√4ᵗʰ **Z00** **Encounter for general examination without complaint, suspected or reported diagnosis**

    EXCLUDES 1 encounter for examination for administrative purposes (Z02.-)

    EXCLUDES 2 encounter for pre-procedural examinations (Z01.81-)
        special screening examinations (Z11-Z13)

    AHA: 2017, 4Q, 95

  √5ᵗʰ **Z00.0** **Encounter for general adult medical examination**

    Encounter for adult periodic examination (annual) (physical) and any associated laboratory and radiologic examinations

    EXCLUDES 1 encounter for examination of sign or symptom—code to sign or symptom
        general health check-up of infant or child (Z00.12-)

    Z00.00 **Encounter for general adult medical examination without abnormal findings** Ⓐ
        Encounter for adult health check-up NOS
        AHA: 2016, 1Q, 36

    Z00.01 **Encounter for general adult medical examination with abnormal findings** Ⓐ
        Use additional code to identify abnormal findings
        AHA: 2016, 1Q, 35-36

  √5ᵗʰ **Z00.1** **Encounter for newborn, infant and child health examinations**

    √6ᵗʰ **Z00.11** **Newborn health examination**
        Health check for child under 29 days old
        Use additional code to identify any abnormal findings
        EXCLUDES 1 health check for child over 28 days old (Z00.12-)

      Z00.110 **Health examination for newborn under 8 days old** Ⓝ
          Health check for newborn under 8 days old

      Z00.111 **Health examination for newborn 8 to 28 days old** Ⓝ
          Health check for newborn 8 to 28 days old
          Newborn weight check

    √6ᵗʰ **Z00.12** **Encounter for routine child health examination**
        Encounter for development testing of infant or child
        Health check (routine) for child over 28 days old
        ▶Immunizations appropriate for age
        Routine developmental screening of infant or child
        Routine vision and hearing testing◀
        EXCLUDES 1 health check for child under 29 days old (Z00.11-)
            health supervision of foundling or other healthy infant or child (Z76.1-Z76.2)
            newborn health examination (Z00.11-)

      Z00.121 **Encounter for routine child health examination with abnormal findings** Ⓟ
          Use additional code to identify abnormal findings
          AHA: 2016, 1Q, 34-35

      Z00.129 **Encounter for routine child health examination without abnormal findings** Ⓟ
          Encounter for routine child health examination NOS
          AHA: 2016, 1Q, 34

  Z00.2 **Encounter for examination for period of rapid growth in childhood** Ⓟ

  Z00.3 **Encounter for examination for adolescent development state** Ⓟ
    Encounter for puberty development state

  Z00.5 **Encounter for examination of potential donor of organ and tissue**

  Z00.6 **Encounter for examination for normal comparison and control in clinical research program**
    Examination of participant or control in clinical research program

  √5ᵗʰ **Z00.7** **Encounter for examination for period of delayed growth in childhood**

    Z00.70 **Encounter for examination for period of delayed growth in childhood without abnormal findings** Ⓟ

    Z00.71 **Encounter for examination for period of delayed growth in childhood with abnormal findings** Ⓟ
        Use additional code to identify abnormal findings

  Z00.8 **Encounter for other general examination**
    Encounter for health examination in population surveys

√4ᵗʰ **Z01** **Encounter for other special examination without complaint, suspected or reported diagnosis**

    INCLUDES routine examination of specific system

    NOTE Codes from category Z01 represent the reason for the encounter. A separate procedure code is required to identify any examinations or procedures performed.

    EXCLUDES 1 encounter for examination for administrative purposes (Z02.-)
        encounter for examination for suspected conditions, proven not to exist (Z03.-)
        encounter for laboratory and radiologic examinations as a component of general medical examinations (Z00.0-)
        encounter for laboratory, radiologic and imaging examinations for sign(s) and symptom(s)—code to the sign(s) or symptom(s)

    EXCLUDES 2 screening examinations (Z11-Z13)

  √5ᵗʰ **Z01.0** **Encounter for examination of eyes and vision**
    EXCLUDES 1 examination for driving license (Z02.4)

    Z01.00 **Encounter for examination of eyes and vision without abnormal findings**
        Encounter for examination of eyes and vision NOS

    Z01.01 **Encounter for examination of eyes and vision with abnormal findings**
        Use additional code to identify abnormal findings
        AHA: 2016, 4Q, 21

  √5ᵗʰ **Z01.1** **Encounter for examination of ears and hearing**
    Z01.10 **Encounter for examination of ears and hearing without abnormal findings**
        Encounter for examination of ears and hearing NOS
        AHA: 2016, 4Q, 24

    √6ᵗʰ **Z01.11** **Encounter for examination of ears and hearing with abnormal findings**
        AHA: 2016, 3Q, 17-18

      Z01.110 **Encounter for hearing examination following failed hearing screening**

      Z01.118 **Encounter for examination of ears and hearing with other abnormal findings**
          Use additional code to identify abnormal findings

    Z01.12 **Encounter for hearing conservation and treatmen**

Ⓝ Newborn: 0   Ⓟ Pediatric: 0-17   Ⓜ Maternity: 12-55   Ⓐ Adult: 15-124   **MCC** Major Complication/Comorbidity   **CC** Complication/Comorbidity   **SW** Severe Wound Dx

1224   ICD-10-CM 2019

✓5ᵗʰ Z01.2 Encounter for dental examination and cleaning

> **Z01.20 Encounter for dental examination and cleaning** without abnormal findings
>> Encounter for dental examination and cleaning NOS

> **Z01.21 Encounter for dental examination and cleaning** with abnormal findings
>> Use additional code to identify abnormal findings

✓5ᵗʰ Z01.3 Encounter for examination of blood pressure

> **Z01.30 Encounter for examination of blood pressure** without abnormal findings
>> Encounter for examination of blood pressure NOS

> **Z01.31 Encounter for examination of blood pressure** with abnormal findings
>> Use additional code to identify abnormal findings

✓5ᵗʰ Z01.4 Encounter for gynecological **examination**

> *EXCLUDES 2*   pregnancy examination or test (Z32.0-)
>   routine examination for contraceptive maintenance (Z30.4-)

> **✓6ᵗʰ Z01.41 Encounter for** routine **gynecological examination**
>> Encounter for general gynecological examination with or without cervical smear
>> Encounter for gynecological examination (general) (routine) NOS
>> Encounter for pelvic examination (annual) (periodic)
>> Use additional code:
>>> for screening for human papillomavirus, if applicable, (Z11.51)
>>> for screening vaginal pap smear, if applicable (Z12.72)
>>> to identify acquired absence of uterus, if applicable (Z90.71-)
>> *EXCLUDES 1*   gynecologic examination status-post hysterectomy for malignant condition (Z08)
>>   screening cervical pap smear not a part of a routine gynecological examination (Z12.4)

>> **Z01.411 Encounter for gynecological examination (general) (routine)** with abnormal findings ♀
>>> Use additional code to identify abnormal findings

>> **Z01.419 Encounter for gynecological examination (general) (routine)** without abnormal findings ♀

> **Z01.42 Encounter for** cervical smear to confirm findings **of recent normal smear following initial abnormal smear** ♀

✓5ᵗʰ Z01.8 Encounter for other specified special **examinations**

> **✓6ᵗʰ Z01.81 Encounter for** preprocedural **examinations**
>> Encounter for preoperative examinations
>> Encounter for radiological and imaging examinations as part of preprocedural examination

>> **Z01.810 Encounter for preprocedural** cardiovascular **examination**

>> **Z01.811 Encounter for preprocedural** respiratory **examination**

>> **Z01.812 Encounter for preprocedural** laboratory **examination**
>>> Blood and urine tests prior to treatment or procedure

>> **Z01.818 Encounter for** other preprocedural **examination**
>>> Encounter for preprocedural examination NOS
>>> Encounter for examinations prior to antineoplastic chemotherapy

> **Z01.82 Encounter for** allergy testing
>> *EXCLUDES 1*   encounter for antibody response examination (Z01.84)

> **Z01.83 Encounter for** blood typing
>> Encounter for Rh typing

> **Z01.84 Encounter for** antibody response examination
>> Encounter for immunity status testing
>> *EXCLUDES 1*   encounter for allergy testing (Z01.82)

> **Z01.89 Encounter for** other **specified special examinations**

✓4ᵗʰ Z02 Encounter for administrative **examination**

> **Z02.0 Encounter for examination for** admission to educational institution
>> Encounter for examination for admission to preschool (education)
>> Encounter for examination for re-admission to school following illness or medical treatment

> **Z02.1 Encounter for** pre-employment **examination**

> **Z02.2 Encounter for examination for** admission to residential institution
>> *EXCLUDES 1*   examination for admission to prison (Z02.89)

> **Z02.3 Encounter for examination for** recruitment to armed forces

> **Z02.4 Encounter for examination for** driving license

> **Z02.5 Encounter for examination for** participation in sport
>> *EXCLUDES 1*   blood-alcohol and blood-drug test (Z02.83)

> **Z02.6 Encounter for examination for** insurance purposes

> **✓5ᵗʰ Z02.7 Encounter for** issue of medical certificate
>> *EXCLUDES 1*   encounter for general medical examination (Z00–Z01, Z02.0–Z02.6, Z02.8–Z02.9)

>> **Z02.71 Encounter for** disability determination
>>> Encounter for issue of medical certificate of incapacity
>>> Encounter for issue of medical certificate of invalidity

>> **Z02.79 Encounter for issue of** other **medical certificate**

> **✓5ᵗʰ Z02.8 Encounter for** other administrative examinations

>> **Z02.81 Encounter for** paternity testing

>> **Z02.82 Encounter for** adoption services

>> **Z02.83 Encounter for** blood-alcohol and blood-drug test
>>> Use additional code for findings of alcohol or drugs in blood (R78.-)

>> **Z02.89 Encounter for** other administrative examinations
>>> Encounter for examination for admission to prison
>>> Encounter for examination for admission to summer camp
>>> Encounter for immigration examination
>>> Encounter for naturalization examination
>>> Encounter for premarital examination
>>> *EXCLUDES 1*   health supervision of foundling or other healthy infant or child (Z76.1–Z76.2)

> **Z02.9 Encounter for administrative examinations,** unspecified

✓4ᵗʰ Z03 Encounter for medical observation **for suspected diseases and conditions ruled out**

> *NOTE*   This category is to be used when a person without a diagnosis is suspected of having an abnormal condition, without signs or symptoms, which requires study, but after examination and observation, is ruled out. This category is also for use for administrative and legal observation status.
> *EXCLUDES 1*   contact with and (suspected) exposures hazardous to health (Z77.-)
>   encounter for observation and evaluation of newborn for suspected diseases and conditions ruled out ▶(Z05.-)◀
>   person with feared complaint in whom no diagnosis is made (Z71.1)
>   signs or symptoms under study—code to signs or symptoms
> **AHA:** 2018, 2Q, 7-8; 2017, 4Q, 27

> **Z03.6 Encounter for observation for suspected** toxic effect from ingested substance **ruled out**
>> Encounter for observation for suspected adverse effect from drug
>> Encounter for observation for suspected poisoning

> **✓5ᵗʰ Z03.7 Encounter for suspected** maternal and fetal conditions **ruled out**
>> Encounter for suspected maternal and fetal conditions not found
>> *EXCLUDES 1*   known or suspected fetal anomalies affecting management of mother, not ruled out (O26-, O35-, O36-, O40-, O41-)

>> **Z03.71 Encounter for suspected problem with** amniotic cavity and membrane **ruled out** M♀
>>> Encounter for suspected oligohydramnios ruled out
>>> Encounter for suspected polyhydramnios ruled out

>> **Z03.72 Encounter for suspected** placental problem **ruled out** M♀

>> **Z03.73 Encounter for suspected** fetal anomaly **ruled out** M♀

>> **Z03.74 Encounter for suspected** problem with fetal growth **ruled out** M♀

>> **Z03.75 Encounter for suspected** cervical shortening **ruled out** M♀

☑ Additional Character Required   ✓ˣ⁷ᵗʰ Placeholder   Unacceptable PDx   Questionable PDx   Manifestation   **H1 - H14** HAC   **HCC** CMS-HCC Dx   **HIV** HIV Dx

ICD-10-CM 2019   **1225**

Chapter 21. Factors Influencing Health Status and Contact with Health Services

Z01.2–Z03.75

Z03.79 Encounter for other suspected maternal and fetal conditions ruled out   Ⓜ♀

✓5ᵗʰ **Z03.8** Encounter for observation for other suspected diseases and conditions ruled out

   ✓6ᵗʰ **Z03.81** Encounter for observation for suspected exposure to biological agents ruled out

       Z03.810 Encounter for observation for suspected exposure to anthrax ruled out

       Z03.818 Encounter for observation for suspected exposure to other biological agents ruled out

     Z03.89 Encounter for observation for other suspected diseases and conditions ruled out

✓4ᵗʰ **Z04** Encounter for examination and observation for other reasons

    INCLUDES encounter for examination for medicolegal reasons

    This category is to be used when a person without a diagnosis is suspected of having an abnormal condition, without signs or symptoms, which requires study, but after examination and observation, is ruled-out. This category is also for use for administrative and legal observation status.

    AHA: 2018, 2Q, 7-8

   Z04.1 Encounter for examination and observation following transport accident

     EXCLUDES 1   encounter for examination and observation following work accident (Z04.2)

     AHA: 2018, 2Q, 8

   Z04.2 Encounter for examination and observation following work accident

   Z04.3 Encounter for examination and observation following other accident

✓5ᵗʰ **Z04.4** Encounter for examination and observation following alleged rape

    Encounter for examination and observation of victim following alleged rape

    Encounter for examination and observation of victim following alleged sexual abuse

     Z04.41 Encounter for examination and observation following alleged adult rape   Ⓐ

       Suspected adult rape, ruled out

       Suspected adult sexual abuse, ruled out

     Z04.42 Encounter for examination and observation following alleged child rape   Ⓟ

       Suspected child rape, ruled out

       Suspected child sexual abuse, ruled out

   Z04.6 Encounter for general psychiatric examination, requested by authority

✓5ᵗʰ **Z04.7** Encounter for examination and observation following alleged physical abuse

     Z04.71 Encounter for examination and observation following alleged adult physical abuse   Ⓐ

       Suspected adult physical abuse, ruled out

       EXCLUDES 1   confirmed case of adult physical abuse (T74.-)

            encounter for examination and observation following alleged adult sexual abuse (Z04.41)

            suspected case of adult physical abuse, not ruled out (T76.-)

     Z04.72 Encounter for examination and observation following alleged child physical abuse   Ⓟ

       Suspected child physical abuse, ruled out

       EXCLUDES 1   confirmed case of child physical abuse (T74.-)

            encounter for examination and observation following alleged child sexual abuse (Z04.42)

            suspected case of child physical abuse, not ruled out (T76.-)

✓5ᵗʰ **Z04.8** Encounter for examination and observation for other specified reasons

    Encounter for examination and observation for request for expert evidence

●   **Z04.81** Encounter for examination and observation of victim following forced sexual exploitation

●   **Z04.82** Encounter for examination and observation of victim following forced labor exploitation

●   **Z04.89** Encounter for examination and observation for other specified reasons

   Z04.9 Encounter for examination and observation for unspecified reason

    Encounter for observation NOS

✓4ᵗʰ **Z05** Encounter for observation of newborn for suspected diseases and conditions ruled out

    This category is to be used for newborns, within the neonatal period (the first 28 days of life), who are suspected of having an abnormal condition, but without signs or symptoms, and which, after examination and observation, is ruled out.

    AHA: 2017, 4Q, 27; 2016, 4Q, 77

   Z05.0 Observation and evaluation of newborn for suspected cardiac condition ruled out   Ⓝ

   Z05.1 Observation and evaluation of newborn for suspected infectious condition ruled out   Ⓝ

   Z05.2 Observation and evaluation of newborn for suspected neurological condition ruled out   Ⓝ

   Z05.3 Observation and evaluation of newborn for suspected respiratory condition ruled out   Ⓝ

✓5ᵗʰ **Z05.4** Observation and evaluation of newborn for suspected genetic, metabolic or immunologic condition ruled out

     Z05.41 Observation and evaluation of newborn for suspected genetic condition ruled out   Ⓝ

       AHA: 2016, 4Q, 55

     Z05.42 Observation and evaluation of newborn for suspected metabolic condition ruled out   Ⓝ

     Z05.43 Observation and evaluation of newborn for suspected immunologic condition ruled out   Ⓝ

   Z05.5 Observation and evaluation of newborn for suspected gastrointestinal condition ruled out   Ⓝ

   Z05.6 Observation and evaluation of newborn for suspected genitourinary condition ruled out   Ⓝ

✓5ᵗʰ **Z05.7** Observation and evaluation of newborn for suspected skin, subcutaneous, musculoskeletal and connective tissue condition ruled out

     Z05.71 Observation and evaluation of newborn for suspected skin and subcutaneous tissue condition ruled out   Ⓝ

     Z05.72 Observation and evaluation of newborn for suspected musculoskeletal condition ruled out   Ⓝ

     Z05.73 Observation and evaluation of newborn for suspected connective tissue condition ruled out   Ⓝ

   Z05.8 Observation and evaluation of newborn for other specified suspected condition ruled out   Ⓝ

   Z05.9 Observation and evaluation of newborn for unspecified suspected condition ruled out   Ⓝ

Z08 Encounter for follow-up examination after completed treatment for malignant neoplasm

    Medical surveillance following completed treatment

    Use additional code to identify any acquired absence of organs (Z90.-)

    Use additional code to identify the personal history of malignant neoplasm (Z85.-)

    EXCLUDES 1   aftercare following medical care (Z43-Z49, Z51)

Z09 Encounter for follow-up examination after completed treatment for conditions other than malignant neoplasm

    Medical surveillance following completed treatment

    Use additional code to identify any applicable history of disease code (Z86-. Z87-)

    EXCLUDES 1   aftercare following medical care (Z43-Z49, Z51)

            surveillance of contraception (Z30.4-)

            surveillance of prosthetic and other medical devices (Z44-Z46)

    AHA: 2017, 1Q, 9; 2015, 1Q, 8

✓4ᵗʰ **Z11** Encounter for screening for infectious and parasitic diseases

    Screening is the testing for disease or disease precursors in asymptomatic individuals so that early detection and treatment can be provided for those who test positive for the disease.

    EXCLUDES 1   encounter for diagnostic examination—code to sign or symptom

   Z11.0 Encounter for screening for intestinal infectious diseases

   Z11.1 Encounter for screening for respiratory tuberculosis

   Z11.2 Encounter for screening for other bacterial diseases

   Z11.3 Encounter for screening for infections with a predominantly sexual mode of transmission

     EXCLUDES 2   encounter for screening for human immunodeficiency virus [HIV] (Z11.4)

            encounter for screening for human papillomavirus (Z11.51)

   Z11.4 Encounter for screening for human immunodeficiency virus [HIV]

Ⓝ Newborn: 0   Ⓟ Pediatric: 0-17   Ⓜ Maternity: 12-55   Ⓐ Adult: 15-124   MCC Major Complication/Comorbidity   CC Complication/Comorbidity   SW Severe Wound Dx

1226   ICD-10-CM 2019

Z11.5 ☑5ᵗʰ **Encounter for screening for** other viral **diseases**

> *EXCLUDES 2* *encounter for screening for viral intestinal disease (Z11.0)*

Z11.51 **Encounter for screening for** human papillomavirus (HPV)

Z11.59 **Encounter for screening for** other viral **diseases**

Z11.6 **Encounter for screening for** other protozoal diseases and helminthiases

> *EXCLUDES 2* *encounter for screening for protozoal intestinal disease (Z11.0)*

Z11.8 **Encounter for screening for** other infectious and parasitic **diseases**

> Encounter for screening for chlamydia
> Encounter for screening for rickettsial
> Encounter for screening for spirochetal
> Encounter for screening for mycoses

Z11.9 **Encounter for screening for infectious and parasitic diseases,** unspecified

Z12 ☑4ᵗʰ **Encounter for** screening **for** malignant neoplasms

> Screening is the testing for disease or disease precursors in asymptomatic individuals so that early detection and treatment can be provided for those who test positive for the disease.
> Use additional code to identify any family history of malignant neoplasm (Z80.-)
> *EXCLUDES 1* *encounter for diagnostic examination—code to sign or symptom*

Z12.0 **Encounter for screening for malignant neoplasm of** stomach

Z12.1 ☑5ᵗʰ **Encounter for screening for malignant neoplasm of** intestinal tract

> **AHA:** 2017, 1Q, 8, 9

Z12.10 **Encounter for screening for malignant neoplasm of intestinal tract,** unspecified

Z12.11 **Encounter for screening for malignant neoplasm of** colon

> Encounter for screening colonoscopy NOS
> **AHA:** 2018, 1Q, 6

Z12.12 **Encounter for screening for malignant neoplasm of** rectum

> **AHA:** 2018, 1Q, 6

Z12.13 **Encounter for screening for malignant neoplasm of** small intestine

Z12.2 **Encounter for screening for malignant neoplasm of** respiratory organs

Z12.3 ☑5ᵗʰ **Encounter for screening for malignant neoplasm of** breast

Z12.31 **Encounter for screening** mammogram **for malignant neoplasm of breast**

> *EXCLUDES 1* *inconclusive mammogram (R92.2)*
> **AHA:** 2015, 1Q, 24

Z12.39 **Encounter for** other **screening for malignant neoplasm of breast**

Z12.4 **Encounter for screening for malignant neoplasm of** cervix ♀

> Encounter for screening pap smear for malignant neoplasm of cervix
> *EXCLUDES 1* *when screening is part of general gynecological examination (Z01.4-)*
> *EXCLUDES 2* *encounter for screening for human papillomavirus (Z11.51)*

Z12.5 **Encounter for screening for malignant neoplasm of** prostate ♂

Z12.6 **Encounter for screening for malignant neoplasm of** bladder

Z12.7 ☑5ᵗʰ **Encounter for screening for malignant neoplasm of** other genitourinary organs

Z12.71 **Encounter for screening for malignant neoplasm of** testis ♂

Z12.72 **Encounter for screening for malignant neoplasm of** vagina ♀

> Vaginal pap smear status-post hysterectomy for non-malignant condition
> Use additional code to identify acquired absence of uterus (Z90.71-)
> *EXCLUDES 1* *vaginal pap smear status-post hysterectomy for malignant conditions (Z08)*

Z12.73 **Encounter for screening for malignant neoplasm of** ovary ♀

Z12.79 **Encounter for screening for malignant neoplasm of** other genitourinary organs

Z12.8 ☑5ᵗʰ **Encounter for screening for malignant neoplasm of** other sites

Z12.81 **Encounter for screening for malignant neoplasm of** oral cavity

Z12.82 **Encounter for screening for malignant neoplasm of** nervous system

Z12.83 **Encounter for screening for malignant neoplasm of** skin

Z12.89 **Encounter for screening for malignant neoplasm of** other sites

Z12.9 **Encounter for screening for malignant neoplasm, site** unspecified

Z13 ☑4ᵗʰ **Encounter for screening for** other diseases and disorders

> Screening is the testing for disease or disease precursors in asymptomatic individuals so that early detection and treatment can be provided for those who test positive for the disease.
> *EXCLUDES 1* *encounter for diagnostic examination—code to sign or symptom*

Z13.0 **Encounter for screening for diseases of the** blood and blood-forming organs **and certain disorders involving the** immune mechanism

Z13.1 **Encounter for screening for** diabetes mellitus

Z13.2 ☑5ᵗʰ **Encounter for screening for nutritional, metabolic and other endocrine disorders**

Z13.21 **Encounter for screening for** nutritional **disorder**

Z13.22 ☑6ᵗʰ **Encounter for screening for** metabolic **disorder**

Z13.220 **Encounter for screening for** lipoid **disorders**

> Encounter for screening for cholesterol level
> Encounter for screening for hypercholesterolemia
> Encounter for screening for hyperlipidemia

Z13.228 **Encounter for screening for other metabolic disorders**

Z13.29 **Encounter for screening for** other suspected **endocrine disorder**

> *EXCLUDES 1* *encounter for screening for diabetes mellitus (Z13.1)*

Z13.3 ☑5ᵗʰ **Encounter for screening examination for** mental health and behavioral **disorders**

Z13.30 **Encounter for screening examination for mental health and behavioral disorders,** unspecified

Z13.31 **Encounter for screening for** depression

> Encounter for screening for depression, adult
> Encounter for screening for depression for child or adolescent

Z13.32 **Encounter for screening for** maternal depression ♀

> Encounter for screening for perinatal depression

Z13.39 **Encounter for screening examination for** other **mental health and behavioral disorders**

> Encounter for screening for alcoholism
> Encounter for screening for intellectual disabilities

Z13.4 ☑5ᵗʰ **Encounter for screening for certain** developmental **disorders in** childhood

> ►Encounter for development testing of infant or child◄
> Encounter for screening for developmental handicaps in early childhood
> *EXCLUDES 1* ~~*routine development testing of infant or child (Z00.1-)*~~
> *EXCLUDES 2* ►*encounter for routine child health examination (Z00.12-)*◄

Z13.40 **Encounter for screening for** unspecified **developmental delays**

Z13.41 **Encounter for** autism **screening**

Z13.42 **Encounter for screening for** global developmental delays **(milestones)**

> Encounter for screening for developmental handicaps in early childhood

Z13.49 **Encounter for screening for** other **developmental delays**

Z13.5 **Encounter for screening for** eye and ear **disorders**

> *EXCLUDES 2* *encounter for general hearing examination (Z01.1-)*
> *encounter for general vision examination (Z01.0-)*
> **AHA:** 2016, 3Q, 17

Z13.6 **Encounter for screening for** cardiovascular **disorders**

☑ Additional Character Required   ☑7ᵗʰ Placeholder   Unacceptable PDx   Questionable PDx   Manifestation   H1 - H14 HAC   HCC CMS-HCC Dx   HIV HIV Dx

ICD-10-CM 2019   1227

✓5ᵗʰ **Z13.7** **Encounter for screening for genetic and chromosomal anomalies**
    EXCLUDES 1   *genetic testing for procreative management (Z31.4-)*

  Z13.71 **Encounter for nonprocreative screening for genetic disease carrier status**

  Z13.79 **Encounter for other screening for genetic and chromosomal anomalies**

✓5ᵗʰ **Z13.8** **Encounter for screening for other specified diseases and disorders**
    EXCLUDES 2   *screening for malignant neoplasms (Z12.-)*

  ✓6ᵗʰ **Z13.81** **Encounter for screening for digestive system disorders**

    Z13.810 **Encounter for screening for upper gastrointestinal disorder**

    Z13.811 **Encounter for screening for lower gastrointestinal disorder**
      EXCLUDES 1   *encounter for screening for intestinal infectious disease (Z11.0)*

    Z13.818 **Encounter for screening for other digestive system disorders**

  ✓6ᵗʰ **Z13.82** **Encounter for screening for musculoskeletal disorder**

    Z13.820 **Encounter for screening for osteoporosis**

    Z13.828 **Encounter for screening for other musculoskeletal disorder**

  Z13.83 **Encounter for screening for respiratory disorder NEC**
    EXCLUDES 1   *encounter for screening for respiratory tuberculosis (Z11.1)*

  Z13.84 **Encounter for screening for dental disorders**

  ✓6ᵗʰ **Z13.85** **Encounter for screening for nervous system disorders**

    Z13.850 **Encounter for screening for traumatic brain injury**

    Z13.858 **Encounter for screening for other nervous system disorders**

  Z13.88 **Encounter for screening for disorder due to exposure to contaminants**
    EXCLUDES 1   *those exposed to contaminants without suspected disorders (Z57-Z77-)*

  Z13.89 **Encounter for screening for other disorder**
    Encounter for screening for genitourinary disorders

Z13.9 **Encounter for screening, unspecified**

Genetic carrier and genetic susceptibility to disease (Z14-Z15)

✓4ᵗʰ **Z14** **Genetic carrier**
  DEF: Individuals carrying a gene mutation associated with a certain disease that typically do not develop the disease but are able to pass the mutated genes to offspring.

  ✓5ᵗʰ **Z14.0** **Hemophilia A carrier**

    Z14.01 **Asymptomatic hemophilia A carrier**

    Z14.02 **Symptomatic hemophilia A carrier**

  Z14.1 **Cystic fibrosis carrier**

  Z14.8 **Genetic carrier of other disease**

✓4ᵗʰ **Z15** **Genetic susceptibility to disease**
  INCLUDES   confirmed abnormal gene
  Use additional code, if applicable, for any associated family history of the disease (Z80-Z84)
    EXCLUDES 1   *chromosomal anomalies (Q90-Q99)*

  ✓5ᵗʰ **Z15.0** **Genetic susceptibility to malignant neoplasm**
    Code first, if applicable, any current malignant neoplasm (C00-C75, C81-C96)
    Use additional code, if applicable, for any personal history of malignant neoplasm (Z85.-)

    Z15.01 **Genetic susceptibility to malignant neoplasm of breast**

    Z15.02 **Genetic susceptibility to malignant neoplasm of ovary** ♀

    Z15.03 **Genetic susceptibility to malignant neoplasm of prostate** ♂

    Z15.04 **Genetic susceptibility to malignant neoplasm of endometrium** ♀

    Z15.09 **Genetic susceptibility to other malignant neoplasm**

✓5ᵗʰ **Z15.8** **Genetic susceptibility to other disease**

  Z15.81 **Genetic susceptibility to multiple endocrine neoplasia [MEN]**
    EXCLUDES 1   *multiple endocrine neoplasia [MEN] syndromes (E31.2-)*

  Z15.89 **Genetic susceptibility to other disease**

Resistance to antimicrobial drugs (Z16)

✓4ᵗʰ **Z16** **Resistance to antimicrobial drugs**
  NOTE   The codes in this category are provided for use as additional codes to identify the resistance and non-responsiveness of a condition to antimicrobial drugs.
  Code first the infection
    EXCLUDES 1   *Methicillin resistant Staphylococcus aureus infection (A49.02)*
      Methicillin resistant Staphylococcus aureus pneumonia (J15.212)
      sepsis due to Methicillin resistant Staphylococcus aureus (A41.02)

  ✓5ᵗʰ **Z16.1** **Resistance to beta lactam antibiotics**

    Z16.10 **Resistance to unspecified beta lactam antibiotics**

    Z16.11 **Resistance to penicillins**
      Resistance to amoxicillin
      Resistance to ampicillin

    Z16.12 **Extended spectrum beta lactamase (ESBL) resistance**
      EXCLUDES 2   *Methicillin resistant Staphylococcus aureus infection in diseases classified elsewhere (B95.62)*

    Z16.19 **Resistance to other specified beta lactam antibiotics**
      Resistance to cephalosporins

  ✓5ᵗʰ **Z16.2** **Resistance to other antibiotics**

    Z16.20 **Resistance to unspecified antibiotic**
      Resistance to antibiotics NOS

    Z16.21 **Resistance to vancomycin**

    Z16.22 **Resistance to vancomycin related antibiotics**

    Z16.23 **Resistance to quinolones and fluoroquinolones**

    Z16.24 **Resistance to multiple antibiotics**

    Z16.29 **Resistance to other single specified antibiotic**
      Resistance to aminoglycosides
      Resistance to macrolides
      Resistance to sulfonamides
      Resistance to tetracyclines

  ✓5ᵗʰ **Z16.3** **Resistance to other antimicrobial drugs**
    EXCLUDES 1   *resistance to antibiotics (Z16.1-, Z16.2-)*

    Z16.30 **Resistance to unspecified antimicrobial drugs**
      Drug resistance NOS

    Z16.31 **Resistance to antiparasitic drug(s)**
      Resistance to quinine and related compounds

    Z16.32 **Resistance to antifungal drug(s)**

    Z16.33 **Resistance to antiviral drug(s)**

    ✓6ᵗʰ **Z16.34** **Resistance to antimycobacterial drug(s)**
      Resistance to tuberculostatics

      Z16.341 **Resistance to single antimycobacterial drug**
        Resistance to antimycobacterial drug NOS

      Z16.342 **Resistance to multiple antimycobacterial drugs**

    Z16.35 **Resistance to multiple antimicrobial drugs**
      EXCLUDES 1   *Resistance to multiple antibiotics only (Z16.24)*

    Z16.39 **Resistance to other specified antimicrobial drug**

Estrogen receptor status (Z17)

✓4ᵗʰ **Z17** **Estrogen receptor status**
  Code first malignant neoplasm of breast (C50.-)
  DEF: Receptor status of breast cancer cells for the hormone estrogen that is used to help determine treatment and evaluate prognosis. ER+ breast cancer responds to hormone therapies while ER- breast cancer does not.

  Z17.0 **Estrogen receptor positive status [ER+]**

  Z17.1 **Estrogen receptor negative status [ER-]**

N Newborn: 0   P Pediatric: 0-17   M Maternity: 12-55   A Adult: 15-124   MCC Major Complication/Comorbidity   CC Complication/Comorbidity   SW Severe Wound Dx

1228   ICD-10-CM 2019

Retained foreign body fragment (Z18)

✓4th Z18 Retained foreign body fragments

> INCLUDES embedded fragment (status)
> embedded splinter (status)
> retained foreign body status
>
> EXCLUDES 1 *artificial joint prosthesis status (Z96.6-)*
> *foreign body accidentally left during a procedure (T81.5-)*
> *foreign body entering through orifice (T15-T19)*
> *in situ cardiac device (Z95.-)*
> *organ or tissue replaced by means other than transplant (Z96.-, Z97.-)*
> *organ or tissue replaced by transplant (Z94.-)*
> *personal history of retained foreign body fully removed (Z87.821)*
> *superficial foreign body (non-embedded splinter)—code to superficial foreign body, by site*
>
> **DEF:** Embedded or retained fragment, splinter, or foreign body, natural or synthetic that can cause infection.

✓5th Z18.0 Retained radioactive fragments
- **Z18.01 Retained depleted uranium fragments**
- **Z18.09 Other retained radioactive fragments**
  - Other retained depleted isotope fragments
  - Retained nontherapeutic radioactive fragments

✓5th Z18.1 Retained metal fragments
> EXCLUDES 1 *retained radioactive metal fragments (Z18.01-Z18.09)*
- **Z18.10 Retained metal fragments, unspecified**
  - Retained metal fragment NOS
- **Z18.11 Retained magnetic metal fragments**
- **Z18.12 Retained nonmagnetic metal fragments**

Z18.2 Retained plastic fragments
- Acrylics fragments
- ▶Diethylhexyl phthalates fragments◀
- Isocyanate fragments

✓5th Z18.3 Retained organic fragments
- **Z18.31 Retained animal quills or spines**
- **Z18.32 Retained tooth**
- **Z18.33 Retained wood fragments**
- **Z18.39 Other retained organic fragments**

✓5th Z18.8 Other specified retained foreign body
- **Z18.81 Retained glass fragments**
- **Z18.83 Retained stone or crystalline fragments**
  - Retained concrete or cement fragments
- **Z18.89 Other specified retained foreign body fragments**

Z18.9 Retained foreign body fragments, unspecified material

Hormone sensitivity malignancy status (Z19)

✓4th Z19 Hormone sensitivity malignancy status

> Code first malignant neoplasm — see Table of Neoplasms, by site, malignant
>
> **AHA:** 2016, 4Q, 76

- **Z19.1 Hormone sensitive malignancy status**
- **Z19.2 Hormone resistant malignancy status**
  - Castrate resistant prostate malignancy status

Persons with potential health hazards related to communicable diseases (Z20-Z29)

✓4th Z20 Contact with and (suspected) exposure to communicable diseases

> EXCLUDES 1 *carrier of infectious disease (Z22.-)*
> *diagnosed current infectious or parasitic disease—see Alphabetic Index*
>
> EXCLUDES 2 *personal history of infectious and parasitic diseases (Z86.1-)*

✓5th Z20.0 Contact with and (suspected) exposure to intestinal infectious diseases
- **Z20.01 Contact with and (suspected) exposure to intestinal infectious diseases due to Escherichia coli (E. coli)**
- **Z20.09 Contact with and (suspected) exposure to other intestinal infectious diseases**

Z20.1 Contact with and (suspected) exposure to tuberculosis

Z20.2 Contact with and (suspected) exposure to infections with a predominantly sexual mode of transmission

Z20.3 Contact with and (suspected) exposure to rabies

Z20.4 Contact with and (suspected) exposure to rubella

Z20.5 Contact with and (suspected) exposure to viral hepatitis

Z20.6 Contact with and (suspected) exposure to human immunodeficiency virus [HIV]
> EXCLUDES 1 *asymptomatic human immunodeficiency virus [HIV] HIV infection status (Z21)*

Z20.7 Contact with and (suspected) exposure to pediculosis, acariasis and other infestations

✓5th Z20.8 Contact with and (suspected) exposure to other communicable diseases

✓6th Z20.81 Contact with and (suspected) exposure to other bacterial communicable diseases
- **Z20.810 Contact with and (suspected) exposure to anthrax**
- **Z20.811 Contact with and (suspected) exposure to meningococcus**
- **Z20.818 Contact with and (suspected) exposure to other bacterial communicable diseases**

✓6th Z20.82 Contact with and (suspected) exposure to other viral communicable diseases
- **Z20.820 Contact with and (suspected) exposure to varicella**
- **Z20.821 Contact with and (suspected) exposure to Zika virus**
- **Z20.828 Contact with and (suspected) exposure to other viral communicable diseases**

Z20.89 Contact with and (suspected) exposure to other communicable diseases

Z20.9 Contact with and (suspected) exposure to unspecified communicable disease

Z21 Asymptomatic human immunodeficiency virus [HIV] infection status HCC

> HIV positive NOS
> Code first human immunodeficiency virus [HIV] disease complicating pregnancy, childbirth and the puerperium, if applicable (O98.7-)
>
> EXCLUDES 1 *acquired immunodeficiency syndrome (B20)*
> *contact with human immunodeficiency virus [HIV] (Z20.6)*
> *exposure to human immunodeficiency virus [HIV] (Z20.6)*
> *human immunodeficiency virus [HIV] disease (B20)*
> *inconclusive laboratory evidence of human immunodeficiency virus [HIV] (R75)*
>
> **DEF:** Phase of human immunodeficiency virus (HIV) infection with no clinical symptoms. This phase may last for 10 years or more.

✓4th Z22 Carrier of infectious disease

> INCLUDES colonization status
> suspected carrier
>
> EXCLUDES 2 *carrier of viral hepatitis (B18.-)*

Z22.0 Carrier of typhoid

Z22.1 Carrier of other intestinal infectious diseases

Z22.2 Carrier of diphtheria

✓5th Z22.3 Carrier of other specified bacterial diseases
- **Z22.31 Carrier of bacterial disease due to meningococci**

✓6th Z22.32 Carrier of bacterial disease due to staphylococci
- **Z22.321 Carrier or suspected carrier of Methicillin susceptible Staphylococcus aureus**
  - MSSA colonization
- **Z22.322 Carrier or suspected carrier of Methicillin resistant Staphylococcus aureus**
  - MRSA colonization
  - **DEF:** Carriers (colonization) of methicillin resistant *Staphylococcus aureus* (MRSA) have MRSA on their skin or in their body but do not exhibit signs of infection. These individuals are able to pass MRSA on to others who may develop an infection.

✓6th Z22.33 Carrier of bacterial disease due to streptococci
- **Z22.330 Carrier of Group B streptococcus**
  - EXCLUDES 1 *carrier of streptococcus group B (GBS) complicating pregnancy, childbirth and the puerperium (O99.82-)*
- **Z22.338 Carrier of other streptococcus**
- **Z22.39 Carrier of other specified bacterial diseases**

Z22.4 Carrier of infections with a predominantly sexual mode of transmission

Z22.6 Carrier of human T-lymphotropic virus type-1 [HTLV-1] infection

Z22.8 Carrier of other infectious diseases

Z22.9 Carrier of infectious disease, unspecified

✓ Additional Character Required   ✓7th Placeholder   Unacceptable PDx   Questionable PDx   Manifestation   H1-H14 HAC   HCC CMS-HCC Dx   HIV HIV Dx

ICD-10-CM 2019   1229

Z23   **Encounter for immunization**
      Code first any routine childhood examination
      NOTE   Procedure codes are required to identify the types of immunizations given

✓4ᵗʰ **Z28**   **Immunization not carried out and underimmunization status**
      INCLUDES   vaccination not carried out

   ✓5ᵗʰ **Z28.0**   **Immunization not carried out because of** contraindication
      DEF: Contraindication: Situation where a drug, surgery, or other procedure may negatively affect or cause harm to a patient.

      Z28.01   **Immunization not carried out because of** acute illness **of patient**

      Z28.02   **Immunization not carried out because of** chronic illness **or condition of patient**

      Z28.03   **Immunization not carried out because of** immune compromised state **of patient**

      Z28.04   **Immunization not carried out because of patient** allergy to vaccine or component

      Z28.09   **Immunization not carried out because of** other contraindication

   Z28.1   **Immunization not carried out because of patient decision for** reasons of belief or group pressure
      Immunization not carried out because of religious belief

   ✓5ᵗʰ **Z28.2**   **Immunization not carried out because of patient decision for** other and unspecified **reason**

      Z28.20   **Immunization not carried out because of patient decision for** unspecified **reason**

      Z28.21   **Immunization not carried out because of patient refusal**

      Z28.29   **Immunization not carried out because of patient decision for** other reason

   Z28.3   **Underimmunization status**
      Delinquent immunization status
      Lapsed immunization schedule status

   ✓5ᵗʰ **Z28.8**   **Immunization not carried out for other reason**

      Z28.81   **Immunization not carried out due to** patient having had the disease

      Z28.82   **Immunization not carried out because of** caregiver refusal
        Immunization not carried out because of guardian refusal
        Immunization not carried out because of parent refusal
        EXCLUDES 1   *immunization not carried out because of caregiver refusal because of religious belief (Z28.1)*

  ●   **Z28.83**   **Immunization not carried out due to** unavailability of vaccine
        Delay in delivery of vaccine
        Lack of availability of vaccine
        Manufacturer delay of vaccine

      Z28.89   **Immunization not carried out for** other **reason**

   Z28.9   **Immunization not carried out for** unspecified **reason**

✓4ᵗʰ **Z29**   **Encounter for other prophylactic measures**
      EXCLUDES 1   *desensitization to allergens (Z51.6)*
                 prophylactic surgery (Z40.-)
      AHA: 2016, 4Q, 78-79

   ✓5ᵗʰ **Z29.1**   **Encounter for prophylactic immunotherapy**
      Encounter for administration of immunoglobulin

      Z29.11   **Encounter for prophylactic immunotherapy for** respiratory syncytial virus (RSV)

      Z29.12   **Encounter for prophylactic** antivenin

      Z29.13   **Encounter for prophylactic** Rho(D) immune globulin

      Z29.14   **Encounter for prophylactic** rabies immune globin

   Z29.3   **Encounter for prophylactic** fluoride **administration**

   Z29.8   **Encounter for** other **specified prophylactic measures**

   Z29.9   **Encounter for prophylactic measures,** unspecified

Persons encountering health services in circumstances related to reproduction (Z30-Z39)

✓4ᵗʰ **Z30**   **Encounter for contraceptive management**
      AHA: 2016, 4Q, 78
      DEF: Contraceptive management to prevent pregnancy. Methods include oral medications, intrauterine devices, and surgical procedures for males and females (sterilization).

   ✓5ᵗʰ **Z30.0**   **Encounter for general counseling and advice on** contraception

      ✓6ᵗʰ **Z30.01**   **Encounter for** initial prescription **of contraceptives**
        EXCLUDES 1   *encounter for surveillance of contraceptives (Z30.4-)*

        Z30.011   **Encounter for** initial prescription **of contraceptive pills** ♀

        Z30.012   **Encounter for prescription of** emergency **contraception** ♀
          Encounter for postcoital contraception

        Z30.013   **Encounter for initial prescription of** injectable **contraceptive** ♀

        Z30.014   **Encounter for initial prescription of** intrauterine **contraceptive device** ♀
          EXCLUDES 1   *encounter for insertion of intrauterine contraceptive device (Z30.430, Z30.432)*

        Z30.015   **Encounter for initial prescription of** vaginal ring hormonal **contraceptive** ♀

        Z30.016   **Encounter for initial prescription of** transdermal patch hormonal **contraceptive device** ♀

        Z30.017   **Encounter for initial prescription of** implantable subdermal **contraceptive** ♀

        Z30.018   **Encounter for initial prescription of** other **contraceptives** ♀
          Encounter for initial prescription of barrier contraception
          Encounter for initial prescription of diaphragm

        Z30.019   **Encounter for initial prescription of contraceptives,** unspecified ♀

      Z30.02   **Counseling and instruction in** natural family planning **to avoid pregnancy**

      Z30.09   **Encounter for** other general **counseling and advice on contraception**
        Encounter for family planning advice NOS

   Z30.2   **Encounter for** sterilization

   ✓5ᵗʰ **Z30.4**   **Encounter for** surveillance **of contraceptives**

      Z30.40   **Encounter for surveillance of contraceptives,** unspecified

      Z30.41   **Encounter for surveillance of contraceptive** pills ♀
        Encounter for repeat prescription for contraceptive pill

      Z30.42   **Encounter for surveillance of** injectable **contraceptive** ♀

      ✓6ᵗʰ **Z30.43**   **Encounter for surveillance of** intrauterine **contraceptive device**

        Z30.430   **Encounter for** insertion **of intrauterine contraceptive device** ♀

        Z30.431   **Encounter for** routine checking **of intrauterine contraceptive device** ♀

        Z30.432   **Encounter for** removal **of intrauterine contraceptive device** ♀

        Z30.433   **Encounter for** removal and reinsertion **of intrauterine contraceptive device** ♀
          Encounter for replacement of intrauterine contraceptive device

      Z30.44   **Encounter for surveillance of** vaginal ring hormonal **contraceptive device** ♀

      Z30.45   **Encounter for surveillance of** transdermal patch hormonal **contraceptive device** ♀

      Z30.46   **Encounter for surveillance of** implantable subdermal **contraceptive** ♀
        Encounter for checking, reinsertion or removal of implantable subdermal contraceptive

      Z30.49   **Encounter for** surveillance **of other contraceptives** ♀
        Encounter for surveillance of barrier contraception
        Encounter for surveillance of diaphragm

Ⓝ Newborn: 0   Ⓟ Pediatric: 0-17   Ⓜ Maternity: 12-55   Ⓐ Adult: 15-124   **MCC** Major Complication/Comorbidity   **CC** Complication/Comorbidity   **SW** Severe Wound Dx

1230   ICD-10-CM 2019

Z30.8 **Encounter for other contraceptive management**
Encounter for postvasectomy sperm count
Encounter for routine examination for contraceptive maintenance
> *EXCLUDES 1*   *sperm count following sterilization reversal (Z31.42)*
> *sperm count for fertility testing (Z31.41)*

Z30.9 **Encounter for contraceptive management, unspecified**

✓4th **Z31** **Encounter for procreative management**
> *EXCLUDES 1*   *complications associated with artificial fertilization (N98.-)*
> *female infertility (N97.-)*
> *male infertility (N46.-)*

Z31.0 **Encounter for reversal of previous sterilization**

✓5th **Z31.4** **Encounter for procreative investigation and testing**
> *EXCLUDES 1*   *postvasectomy sperm count (Z30.8)*

     Z31.41 **Encounter for fertility testing**
Encounter for fallopian tube patency testing
Encounter for sperm count for fertility testing

     Z31.42 **Aftercare following sterilization reversal**
Sperm count following sterilization reversal

     ✓6th **Z31.43** **Encounter for genetic testing of female for procreative management**
Use additional code for recurrent pregnancy loss, if applicable (N96, O26.2-)
> *EXCLUDES 1*   *nonprocreative genetic testing (Z13.7-)*

       Z31.430 **Encounter of female for testing for genetic disease carrier status for procreative management** ♀

       Z31.438 **Encounter for other genetic testing of female for procreative management** ♀

     ✓6th **Z31.44** **Encounter for genetic testing of male for procreative management**
> *EXCLUDES 1*   *nonprocreative genetic testing (Z13.7-)*

       Z31.440 **Encounter of male for testing for genetic disease carrier status for procreative management** ♂

       Z31.441 **Encounter for testing of male partner of patient with recurrent pregnancy loss** A♂

       Z31.448 **Encounter for other genetic testing of male for procreative management** A♂

     Z31.49 **Encounter for other procreative investigation and testing**

Z31.5 **Encounter for procreative genetic counseling**
AHA: 2017, 4Q, 27

✓5th **Z31.6** **Encounter for general counseling and advice on procreation**
     Z31.61 **Procreative counseling and advice using natural family planning**

     Z31.62 **Encounter for fertility preservation counseling**
Encounter for fertility preservation counseling prior to cancer therapy
Encounter for fertility preservation counseling prior to surgical removal of gonads

     Z31.69 **Encounter for other general counseling and advice on procreation**

Z31.7 **Encounter for procreative management and counseling for gestational carrier** ♀
> *EXCLUDES 1*   *pregnant state, gestational carrier (Z33.3)*
AHA: 2016, 4Q, 78

✓5th **Z31.8** **Encounter for other procreative management**
     Z31.81 **Encounter for male factor infertility in female patient** ♀

     Z31.82 **Encounter for Rh incompatibility status** ♀
AHA: 2015, 3Q, 40; 2014, 4Q, 17

     Z31.83 **Encounter for assisted reproductive fertility procedure cycle** ♀
Patient undergoing in vitro fertilization cycle
Use additional code to identify the type of infertility
> *EXCLUDES 1*   *pre-cycle diagnosis and testing—code to reason for encounter*

     Z31.84 **Encounter for fertility preservation procedure**
Encounter for fertility preservation procedure prior to cancer therapy
Encounter for fertility preservation procedure prior to surgical removal of gonads

     Z31.89 **Encounter for other procreative management**

Z31.9 **Encounter for procreative management, unspecified**

✓4th **Z32** **Encounter for pregnancy test and childbirth and childcare instruction**
✓5th **Z32.0** **Encounter for pregnancy test**
     Z32.00 **Encounter for pregnancy test, result unknown** ♀
Encounter for pregnancy test NOS

     Z32.01 **Encounter for pregnancy test, result positive** M♀

     Z32.02 **Encounter for pregnancy test, result negative** ♀

Z32.2 **Encounter for childbirth instruction**

Z32.3 **Encounter for childcare instruction**
Encounter for prenatal or postpartum childcare instruction

✓4th **Z33** **Pregnant state**
Z33.1 **Pregnant state, incidental** M♀
Pregnant state NOS
> *EXCLUDES 1*   *complications of pregnancy (O00-O9A)*
> *pregnant state, gestational carrier (Z33.3)*

Z33.2 **Encounter for elective termination of pregnancy** M♀
> *EXCLUDES 1*   *early fetal death with retention of dead fetus (O02.1)*
> *late fetal death (O36.4)*
> *spontaneous abortion (O03)*
> **TIP:** Do not assign a code from category Z3A with this code.

Z33.3 **Pregnant state, gestational carrier** M♀
> *EXCLUDES 1*   *encounter for procreative management and counseling for gestational carrier (Z31.7)*
AHA: 2016, 4Q, 78

✓4th **Z34** **Encounter for supervision of normal pregnancy**
> *EXCLUDES 1*   *any complication of pregnancy (O00-O9A)*
> *encounter for pregnancy test (Z32.0-)*
> *encounter for supervision of high risk pregnancy (O09.-)*
AHA: 2014, 4Q, 17

✓5th **Z34.0** **Encounter for supervision of normal first pregnancy**
     Z34.00 **Encounter for supervision of normal first pregnancy, unspecified trimester** M♀

     Z34.01 **Encounter for supervision of normal first pregnancy, first trimester** M♀

     Z34.02 **Encounter for supervision of normal first pregnancy, second trimester** M♀

     Z34.03 **Encounter for supervision of normal first pregnancy, third trimester** M♀

✓5th **Z34.8** **Encounter for supervision of other normal pregnancy**
     Z34.80 **Encounter for supervision of other normal pregnancy, unspecified trimester** M♀

     Z34.81 **Encounter for supervision of other normal pregnancy, first trimester** M♀

     Z34.82 **Encounter for supervision of other normal pregnancy, second trimester** M♀

     Z34.83 **Encounter for supervision of other normal pregnancy, third trimester** M♀

✓5th **Z34.9** **Encounter for supervision of normal pregnancy, unspecified**
     Z34.90 **Encounter for supervision of normal pregnancy, unspecified, unspecified trimester** M♀

     Z34.91 **Encounter for supervision of normal pregnancy, unspecified, first trimester** M♀

     Z34.92 **Encounter for supervision of normal pregnancy, unspecified, second trimester** M♀

     Z34.93 **Encounter for supervision of normal pregnancy, unspecified, third trimester** M♀

✓4th **Z36** **Encounter for antenatal screening of mother**
> *INCLUDES*   encounter for placental sample (taken vaginally)
> screening is the testing for disease or disease precursors in asymptomatic individuals so that early detection and treatment can be provided for those who test positive for the disease
> *EXCLUDES 1*   *diagnostic examination—code to sign or symptom*
> *encounter for suspected maternal and fetal conditions ruled out (Z03.7-)*
> *suspected fetal condition affecting management of pregnancy—code to condition in Chapter 15*
> *EXCLUDES 2*   *abnormal findings on antenatal screening of mother (O28.-)*
> *genetic counseling and testing (Z31.43-, Z31.5)*
> *routine prenatal care (Z34)*
AHA: 2017, 4Q, 28

Z36.0 **Encounter for antenatal screening for chromosomal anomalies** M♀

Z36.1 Encounter for antenatal screening for raised alphafetoprotein level   M♀

     Encounter for antenatal screening for elevated maternal serum alphafetoprotein level

     DEF: High levels of alpha-fetoprotein (AFP) that may indicate a possibility of spina bifida and other neural tube defects, anencephaly, or omphalocele in the fetus.

Z36.2 Encounter for other antenatal screening follow-up   M♀

     Non-visualized anatomy on a previous scan

Z36.3 Encounter for antenatal screening for malformations   M♀

     Screening for a suspected anomaly

Z36.4 Encounter for antenatal screening for fetal growth retardation   M♀

     Intrauterine growth restriction (IUGR)/small-for-dates

Z36.5 Encounter for antenatal screening for isoimmunization   M♀

✓5ᵗʰ **Z36.8 Encounter for other antenatal screening**

     Z36.81 Encounter for antenatal screening for hydrops fetalis   M♀

         DEF: Hydrops fetalis: Abnormal accumulation of fluid in two or more parts of the fetus, such as ascites, effusion of the pleural or pericardial tissues, or edema.

     Z36.82 Encounter for antenatal screening for nuchal translucency   M♀

     Z36.83 Encounter for fetal screening for congenital cardiac abnormalities   M♀

     Z36.84 Encounter for antenatal screening for fetal lung maturity   M♀

     Z36.85 Encounter for antenatal screening for Streptococcus B   M♀

     Z36.86 Encounter for antenatal screening for cervical length   M♀

         Screening for risk of pre-term labor

     Z36.87 Encounter for antenatal screening for uncertain dates   M♀

     Z36.88 Encounter for antenatal screening for fetal macrosomia   M♀

         Screening for large-for-dates

     Z36.89 Encounter for other specified antenatal screening   M♀

     Z36.8A Encounter for antenatal screening for other genetic defects   M♀

Z36.9 Encounter for antenatal screening, unspecified   M♀

✓4ᵗʰ **Z3A Weeks of gestation**

     NOTE   Codes from category Z3A are for use, only on the maternal record, to indicate the weeks of gestation of the pregnancy, if known.

     Code first complications of pregnancy, childbirth and the puerperium (O09-O9A)

     AHA: 2016, 2Q, 34; 2014, 3Q, 17; 2014, 2Q, 9; 2013, 2Q, 33

     TIP: Do not assign a code from this category with codes from categories O00-O08 or code Z33.2.

✓5ᵗʰ **Z3A.0 Weeks of gestation of pregnancy,** unspecified or less than 10 weeks

     Z3A.00 Weeks of gestation of pregnancy not specified   M♀

     Z3A.01 Less than 8 weeks **gestation of pregnancy**   M♀

     Z3A.08 8 weeks **gestation of pregnancy**   M♀

     Z3A.09 9 weeks **gestation of pregnancy**   M♀

✓5ᵗʰ **Z3A.1 Weeks of gestation of pregnancy, weeks** 10-19

     Z3A.10 10 weeks **gestation of pregnancy**   M♀

     Z3A.11 11 weeks **gestation of pregnancy**   M♀

     Z3A.12 12 weeks **gestation of pregnancy**   M♀

     Z3A.13 13 weeks **gestation of pregnancy**   M♀

     Z3A.14 14 weeks **gestation of pregnancy**   M♀

     Z3A.15 15 weeks **gestation of pregnancy**   M♀

     Z3A.16 16 weeks **gestation of pregnancy**   M♀

     Z3A.17 17 weeks **gestation of pregnancy**   M♀

     Z3A.18 18 weeks **gestation of pregnancy**   M♀

     Z3A.19 19 weeks **gestation of pregnancy**   M♀

✓5ᵗʰ **Z3A.2 Weeks of gestation of pregnancy, weeks** 20-29

     Z3A.20 20 weeks **gestation of pregnancy**   M♀

     Z3A.21 21 weeks **gestation of pregnancy**   M♀

     Z3A.22 22 weeks **gestation of pregnancy**   M♀

     Z3A.23 23 weeks **gestation of pregnancy**   M♀

     Z3A.24 24 weeks **gestation of pregnancy**   M♀

     Z3A.25 25 weeks **gestation of pregnancy**   M♀

     Z3A.26 26 weeks **gestation of pregnancy**   M♀

     Z3A.27 27 weeks **gestation of pregnancy**   M♀

     Z3A.28 28 weeks **gestation of pregnancy**   M♀

     Z3A.29 29 weeks **gestation of pregnancy**   M♀

✓5ᵗʰ **Z3A.3 Weeks of gestation of pregnancy, weeks** 30-39

     Z3A.30 30 weeks **gestation of pregnancy**   M♀

     Z3A.31 31 weeks **gestation of pregnancy**   M♀

     Z3A.32 32 weeks **gestation of pregnancy**   M♀

     Z3A.33 33 weeks **gestation of pregnancy**   M♀

     Z3A.34 34 weeks **gestation of pregnancy**   M♀

     Z3A.35 35 weeks **gestation of pregnancy**   M♀

     Z3A.36 36 weeks **gestation of pregnancy**   M♀

     Z3A.37 37 weeks **gestation of pregnancy**   M♀

     Z3A.38 38 weeks **gestation of pregnancy**   M♀

     Z3A.39 39 weeks **gestation of pregnancy**   M♀

✓5ᵗʰ **Z3A.4 Weeks of gestation of pregnancy, weeks** 40 or greater

     AHA: 2014, 4Q, 23

     Z3A.40 40 weeks **gestation of pregnancy**   M♀

     Z3A.41 41 weeks **gestation of pregnancy**   M♀

     Z3A.42 42 weeks **gestation of pregnancy**   M♀

     Z3A.49 Greater than 42 weeks **gestation of pregnancy**   M♀

✓4ᵗʰ **Z37 Outcome of delivery**

     This category is intended for use as an additional code to identify the outcome of delivery on the mother's record. It is not for use on the newborn record.

     EXCLUDES 1   stillbirth (P95)

Z37.0 Single live birth   M♀

     AHA: 2016, 2Q, 34; 2014, 2Q, 9

Z37.1 Single stillbirth   M♀

Z37.2 Twins, both liveborn   M♀

Z37.3 Twins, one liveborn and one stillborn   M♀

Z37.4 Twins, both stillborn   M♀

✓5ᵗʰ **Z37.5 Other multiple births, all liveborn**

     Z37.50 Multiple births, unspecified, all liveborn   M♀

     Z37.51 Triplets, all liveborn   M♀

     Z37.52 Quadruplets, all liveborn   M♀

     Z37.53 Quintuplets, all liveborn   M♀

     Z37.54 Sextuplets, all liveborn   M♀

     Z37.59 Other multiple births, all liveborn   M♀

✓5ᵗʰ **Z37.6 Other multiple births, some liveborn**

     Z37.60 Multiple births, unspecified, some liveborn   M♀

     Z37.61 Triplets, some liveborn   M♀

     Z37.62 Quadruplets, some liveborn   M♀

     Z37.63 Quintuplets, some liveborn   M♀

     Z37.64 Sextuplets, some liveborn   M♀

     Z37.69 Other multiple births, some liveborn   M♀

Z37.7 Other multiple births, all stillborn   M♀

Z37.9 Outcome of delivery, unspecified   M♀

     Multiple birth NOS

     Single birth NOS

✓4ᵗʰ **Z38 Liveborn infants according to place of birth and type of delivery**

     This category is for use as the principal code on the initial record of a newborn baby. It is to be used for the initial birth record only. It is not to be used on the mother's record.

     AHA: 2017, 2Q, 5-7; 2016, 3Q, 18; 2015, 2Q, 15

✓5ᵗʰ **Z38.0 Single liveborn infant,** born in hospital

     Single liveborn infant, born in birthing center or other health care facility

     Z38.00 Single liveborn infant, delivered vaginally   N

     Z38.01 Single liveborn infant, delivered by cesarean   N

Z38.1 Single liveborn infant, born outside hospital   N

Z38.2 Single liveborn infant, unspecified as to place of birth   N

     Single liveborn infant NOS

✓5ᵗʰ **Z38.3 Twin liveborn infant,** born in hospital

     Z38.30 Twin liveborn infant, delivered vaginally   N

     Z38.31 Twin liveborn infant, delivered by cesarean   N

Z38.4 Twin liveborn infant, born outside hospital   N

Z38.5 Twin liveborn infant, unspecified as to place of birth   N

✓5ᵗʰ **Z38.6 Other multiple liveborn infant, born in hospital**

     Z38.61 Triplet liveborn infant, delivered vaginally   N

     Z38.62 Triplet liveborn infant, delivered by cesarean   N

     Z38.63 Quadruplet liveborn infant, delivered vaginally   N

N Newborn: 0   P Pediatric: 0-17   M Maternity: 12-55   A Adult: 15-124   MCC Major Complication/Comorbidity   CC Complication/Comorbidity   SW Severe Wound Dx

1232   ICD-10-CM 2019

Z38.64   Quadruplet **liveborn infant, delivered by cesarean**   N

Z38.65   Quintuplet **liveborn infant, delivered** vaginally   N

Z38.66   Quintuplet **liveborn infant, delivered by** cesarean   N

Z38.68   Other **multiple liveborn infant, delivered** vaginally   N

Z38.69   Other **multiple liveborn infant, delivered by cesarean**   N

Z38.7   Other multiple liveborn infant, born outside hospital   N

Z38.8   Other multiple liveborn infant, unspecified as to place of birth   N

✓4ᵗʰ **Z39   Encounter for maternal postpartum care and examination**

   Z39.0   Encounter for care and examination of mother immediately after delivery   M♀

     Care and observation in uncomplicated cases when the delivery occurs outside a healthcare facility

     EXCLUDES 1   *care for postpartum complication—see Alphabetic index*

   Z39.1   Encounter for care and examination of lactating mother   M♀

     Encounter for supervision of lactation

     EXCLUDES 1   *disorders of lactation (O92.-)*

   Z39.2   Encounter for routine postpartum **follow-up**   M♀

Encounters for other specific health care (Z40-Z53)

Categories Z40-Z53 are intended for use to indicate a reason for care. They may be used for patients who have already been treated for a disease or injury, but who are receiving aftercare or prophylactic care, or care to consolidate the treatment, or to deal with a residual state.

   EXCLUDES 2   *follow-up examination for medical surveillance after treatment (Z08-Z09)*

✓4ᵗʰ **Z40   Encounter for prophylactic surgery**

     EXCLUDES 1   *organ donations (Z52.-)*

       therapeutic organ removal—code to condition

   ✓5ᵗʰ **Z40.0   Encounter for prophylactic surgery for** risk factors related to malignant neoplasms

     Admission for prophylactic organ removal

     Use additional code to identify risk factor

     AHA: 2017, 4Q, 28-29

     Z40.00   Encounter for prophylactic removal of unspecified organ

     Z40.01   Encounter for prophylactic removal of breast

     Z40.02   Encounter for prophylactic removal of ovary(s)   ♀

       Encounter for prophylactic removal of ovary(s) and fallopian tube(s)

▲   **Z40.03   Encounter for prophylactic removal of** fallopian tube(s)   ♀

     Z40.09   Encounter for prophylactic removal of other organ

   Z40.8   Encounter for other prophylactic surgery

   Z40.9   Encounter for prophylactic surgery, unspecified

✓4ᵗʰ **Z41   Encounter for procedures for purposes other than remedying health state**

   Z41.1   Encounter for cosmetic surgery

     Encounter for cosmetic breast implant

     Encounter for cosmetic procedure

     EXCLUDES 1   *encounter for plastic and reconstructive surgery following medical procedure or healed injury (Z42.-)*

       encounter for post-mastectomy breast implantation (Z42.1)

   Z41.2   Encounter for routine and ritual male circumcision   ♂

   Z41.3   Encounter for ear piercing

   Z41.8   Encounter for other procedures for purposes other than remedying health state

   Z41.9   Encounter for procedure for purposes other than remedying health state, unspecified

✓4ᵗʰ **Z42   Encounter for plastic and reconstructive surgery following medical procedure or healed injury**

     EXCLUDES 1   *encounter for cosmetic plastic surgery (Z41.1)*

       encounter for plastic surgery for treatment of current injury—code to relevant injury

   Z42.1   Encounter for breast reconstruction following mastectomy   A

     EXCLUDES 1   *deformity and disproportion of reconstructed breast (N65.1-)*

   Z42.8   Encounter for other plastic and reconstructive surgery **following medical procedure or healed injury**

     AHA: 2017, 1Q, 42

✓4ᵗʰ **Z43   Encounter for attention to artificial openings**

     INCLUDES   closure of artificial openings

       passage of sounds or bougies through artificial openings

       reforming artificial openings

       removal of catheter from artificial openings

       toilet or cleansing of artificial openings

     EXCLUDES 1   *complications of external stoma (J95.0-, K94.-, N99.5-)*

     EXCLUDES 2   *fitting and adjustment of prosthetic and other devices (Z44-Z46)*

   Z43.0   Encounter for attention to tracheostomy   HCC

   Z43.1   Encounter for attention to gastrostomy   CC HCC

     EXCLUDES 2   *artificial opening status only, without need for care (Z93.-)*

     CC Excl: PDX collection 1487

   Z43.2   Encounter for attention to ileostomy   HCC

   Z43.3   Encounter for attention to colostomy   HCC

   Z43.4   Encounter for attention to other artificial openings of digestive tract   HCC

   Z43.5   Encounter for attention to cystostomy   HCC

   Z43.6   Encounter for attention to other artificial openings of urinary tract   HCC

     Encounter for attention to nephrostomy

     Encounter for attention to ureterostomy

     Encounter for attention to urethrostomy

   Z43.7   Encounter for attention to artificial vagina

   Z43.8   Encounter for attention to other artificial openings   HCC

   Z43.9   Encounter for attention to unspecified artificial opening   HCC

✓4ᵗʰ **Z44   Encounter for fitting and adjustment of external prosthetic device**

     INCLUDES   removal or replacement of external prosthetic device

     EXCLUDES 1   *malfunction or other complications of device—see Alphabetical Index*

       presence of prosthetic device (Z97.-)

   ✓5ᵗʰ **Z44.0   Encounter for fitting and adjustment of** artificial arm

     ✓6ᵗʰ **Z44.00   Encounter for fitting and adjustment of** unspecified artificial arm

       Z44.001   Encounter for fitting and adjustment of unspecified right artificial arm

       Z44.002   Encounter for fitting and adjustment of unspecified left artificial arm

       Z44.009   Encounter for fitting and adjustment of unspecified artificial arm, unspecified arm

     ✓6ᵗʰ **Z44.01   Encounter for fitting and adjustment of** complete artificial arm

       Z44.011   Encounter for fitting and adjustment of complete right artificial arm

       Z44.012   Encounter for fitting and adjustment of complete left artificial arm

       Z44.019   Encounter for fitting and adjustment of complete artificial arm, unspecified arm

     ✓6ᵗʰ **Z44.02   Encounter for fitting and adjustment of** partial artificial arm

       Z44.021   Encounter for fitting and adjustment of partial artificial right arm

       Z44.022   Encounter for fitting and adjustment of partial artificial left arm

       Z44.029   Encounter for fitting and adjustment of partial artificial arm, unspecified arm

   ✓5ᵗʰ **Z44.1   Encounter for fitting and adjustment of** artificial leg

     ✓6ᵗʰ **Z44.10   Encounter for fitting and adjustment of** unspecified artificial leg

       Z44.101   Encounter for fitting and adjustment of unspecified right artificial leg   HCC

       Z44.102   Encounter for fitting and adjustment of unspecified left artificial leg   HCC

       Z44.109   Encounter for fitting and adjustment of unspecified artificial leg, unspecified leg   HCC

     ✓6ᵗʰ **Z44.11   Encounter for fitting and adjustment of** complete artificial leg

       Z44.111   Encounter for fitting and adjustment of complete right artificial leg   HCC

       Z44.112   Encounter for fitting and adjustment of complete left artificial leg   HCC

✓ Additional Character Required   ✓x7ᵗʰ Placeholder   Unacceptable PDx   Questionable PDx   Manifestation   H1-H14 HAC   HCC CMS-HCC Dx   HIV HIV Dx

ICD-10-CM 2019   1233

Z44.119   **Encounter for fitting and adjustment** `HCC`
     of complete artificial leg, unspecified leg

✓6ᵗʰ   **Z44.12**   **Encounter for fitting and adjustment of partial
artificial leg**

Z44.121   **Encounter for fitting and adjustment** `HCC`
     of partial artificial right leg

Z44.122   **Encounter for fitting and adjustment** `HCC`
     of partial artificial left leg

Z44.129   **Encounter for fitting and adjustment** `HCC`
     of partial artificial leg, unspecified leg

✓5ᵗʰ   **Z44.2**   **Encounter for fitting and adjustment of artificial eye**
     EXCLUDES 1   mechanical complication of ocular prosthesis (T85.3)

Z44.20   **Encounter for fitting and adjustment of artificial
eye, unspecified**

Z44.21   **Encounter for fitting and adjustment of artificial
right eye**

Z44.22   **Encounter for fitting and adjustment of artificial left
eye**

✓5ᵗʰ   **Z44.3**   **Encounter for fitting and adjustment of external breast
prosthesis**
     EXCLUDES 1   complications of breast implant (T85.4-)
          encounter for adjustment or removal of breast implant
            (Z45.81-)
          encounter for initial breast implant insertion for
            cosmetic breast augmentation (Z41.1)
          encounter for breast reconstruction following
            mastectomy (Z42.1)

Z44.30   **Encounter for fitting and adjustment of external
breast prosthesis, unspecified breast**

Z44.31   **Encounter for fitting and adjustment of external
right breast prosthesis**

Z44.32   **Encounter for fitting and adjustment of external
left breast prosthesis**

Z44.8   **Encounter for fitting and adjustment of other external
prosthetic devices**

Z44.9   **Encounter for fitting and adjustment of unspecified external
prosthetic device**

✓4ᵗʰ   **Z45**   **Encounter for adjustment and management of implanted device**
     `INCLUDES`   removal or replacement of implanted device
     EXCLUDES 1   malfunction or other complications of device – see Alphabetical
          Index
     EXCLUDES 2   encounter for fitting and adjustment of non-implanted device
          (Z46.-)

✓5ᵗʰ   **Z45.0**   **Encounter for adjustment and management of cardiac device**

✓6ᵗʰ   **Z45.01**   **Encounter for adjustment and management of
cardiac pacemaker**
     Encounter for adjustment and management of cardiac
     resynchronization therapy pacemaker (CRT-P)
     EXCLUDES 1   encounter for adjustment and management
          of automatic implantable cardiac
          defibrillator with synchronous cardiac
          pacemaker (Z45.02)

Z45.010   **Encounter for checking and testing of
cardiac pacemaker pulse generator
[battery]**
     Encounter for replacing cardiac pacemaker
     pulse generator [battery]

Z45.018   **Encounter for adjustment and
management of other part of cardiac
pacemaker**
     EXCLUDES 2   presence of prosthetic and other
          devices (Z95-Z97)

Z45.02   **Encounter for adjustment and management of
automatic implantable cardiac defibrillator**
     Encounter for adjustment and management of
     automatic implantable cardiac defibrillator with
     synchronous cardiac pacemaker
     Encounter for adjustment and management of cardiac
     resynchronization therapy defibrillator (CRT-D)

Z45.09   **Encounter for adjustment and management of other
cardiac device**

Z45.1   **Encounter for adjustment and management of infusion pump**

Z45.2   **Encounter for adjustment and management of vascular
access device**
     Encounter for adjustment and management of vascular
     catheters
     EXCLUDES 1   encounter for adjustment and management of renal
          dialysis catheter (Z49.01)

✓5ᵗʰ   **Z45.3**   **Encounter for adjustment and management of implanted
devices of the special senses**

Z45.31   **Encounter for adjustment and management of
implanted visual substitution device**

✓6ᵗʰ   **Z45.32**   **Encounter for adjustment and management of
implanted hearing device**
     EXCLUDES 1   encounter for fitting and adjustment of
          hearing aide (Z46.1)

Z45.320   **Encounter for adjustment and
management of bone conduction device**

Z45.321   **Encounter for adjustment and
management of cochlear device**

Z45.328   **Encounter for adjustment and
management of other implanted hearing
device**

✓5ᵗʰ   **Z45.4**   **Encounter for adjustment and management of implanted
nervous system device**

Z45.41   **Encounter for adjustment and management of
cerebrospinal fluid drainage device**
     Encounter for adjustment and management of
     cerebral ventricular (communicating) shunt

Z45.42   **Encounter for adjustment and management of
neuropacemaker (brain) (peripheral nerve) (spinal
cord)**

Z45.49   **Encounter for adjustment and management of other
implanted nervous system device**
     AHA: 2014, 3Q, 19

✓5ᵗʰ   **Z45.8**   **Encounter for adjustment and management of other
implanted devices**

✓6ᵗʰ   **Z45.81**   **Encounter for adjustment or removal of breast
implant**
     Encounter for elective implant exchange (different
     material) (different size)
     Encounter removal of tissue expander without
     synchronous insertion of permanent implant
     EXCLUDES 1   complications of breast implant (T85.4-)
          encounter for initial breast implant insertion
            for cosmetic breast augmentation
            (Z41.1)
          encounter for breast reconstruction following
            mastectomy (Z42.1)

Z45.811   **Encounter for adjustment or removal
of right breast implant**

Z45.812   **Encounter for adjustment or removal
of left breast implant**

Z45.819   **Encounter for adjustment or removal
of unspecified breast implant**

Z45.82   **Encounter for adjustment or removal of
myringotomy device (stent) (tube)**

Z45.89   **Encounter for adjustment and management of
other implanted devices**
     AHA: 2014, 4Q, 26-28

Z45.9   **Encounter for adjustment and management of unspecified
implanted device**

✓4ᵗʰ   **Z46**   **Encounter for fitting and adjustment of other devices**
     `INCLUDES`   removal or replacement of other device
     EXCLUDES 1   malfunction or other complications of device—see Alphabetical
          Index
     EXCLUDES 2   encounter for fitting and management of implanted devices
          (Z45.-)
          issue of repeat prescription only (Z76.0)
          presence of prosthetic and other devices (Z95-Z97)

Z46.0   **Encounter for fitting and adjustment of spectacles and
contact lenses**

Z46.1   **Encounter for fitting and adjustment of hearing aid**
     EXCLUDES 1   encounter for adjustment and management of
          implanted hearing device (Z45.32-)

Z46.2   **Encounter for fitting and adjustment of other devices related
to nervous system and special senses**
     EXCLUDES 2   encounter for adjustment and management of
          implanted nervous system device (Z45.4-)
          encounter for adjustment and management of
          implanted visual substitution device (Z45.31)

Z46.3   **Encounter for fitting and adjustment of dental prosthetic
device**
     Encounter for fitting and adjustment of dentures

Z46.4   **Encounter for fitting and adjustment of orthodontic device**

N Newborn: 0   P Pediatric: 0-17   M Maternity: 12-55   A Adult: 15-124   MCC Major Complication/Comorbidity   CC Complication/Comorbidity   SW Severe Wound Dx

1234   ICD-10-CM 2019

✓5ᵗʰ Z46.5   **Encounter for fitting and adjustment of other gastrointestinal appliance and device**
> **EXCLUDES 1**   *encounter for attention to artificial openings of digestive tract (Z43.1-Z43.4)*

     Z46.51   **Encounter for fitting and adjustment of gastric lap band**

     Z46.59   **Encounter for fitting and adjustment of other gastrointestinal appliance and device**

Z46.6   **Encounter for fitting and adjustment of urinary device**
> **EXCLUDES 2**   *attention to artificial openings of urinary tract (Z43.5, Z43.6)*

✓5ᵗʰ Z46.8   **Encounter for fitting and adjustment of other specified devices**

     Z46.81   **Encounter for fitting and adjustment of insulin pump**
         Encounter for insulin pump instruction and training
         Encounter for insulin pump titration

     Z46.82   **Encounter for fitting and adjustment of non-vascular catheter**

     Z46.89   **Encounter for fitting and adjustment of other specified devices**
         Encounter for fitting and adjustment of wheelchair
         AHA: 2014, 4Q, 26-28

Z46.9   **Encounter for fitting and adjustment of unspecified device**

✓4ᵗʰ Z47   **Orthopedic aftercare**
> **EXCLUDES 1**   *aftercare for healing fracture—code to fracture with 7th character D*

Z47.1   **Aftercare following joint replacement surgery**
     Use additional code to identify the joint (Z96.6-)

Z47.2   **Encounter for removal of internal fixation device**
> **EXCLUDES 1**   *encounter for adjustment of internal fixation device for fracture treatment—code to fracture with appropriate 7th character*
> *encounter for removal of external fixation device—code to fracture with 7th character D*
> *infection or inflammatory reaction to internal fixation device (T84.6-)*
> *mechanical complication of internal fixation device (T84.1-)*

✓5ᵗʰ Z47.3   **Aftercare following explantation of joint prosthesis**
     Aftercare following explantation of joint prosthesis, staged procedure
     Encounter for joint prosthesis insertion following prior explantation of joint prosthesis
     AHA: 2015, 1Q, 16

     Z47.31   **Aftercare following explantation of shoulder joint prosthesis**
>   **EXCLUDES 1**   *acquired absence of shoulder joint following prior explantation of shoulder joint prosthesis (Z89.23-)*
>   *shoulder joint prosthesis explantation status (Z89.23-)*

     Z47.32   **Aftercare following explantation of hip joint prosthesis**
>   **EXCLUDES 1**   *acquired absence of hip joint following prior explantation of hip joint prosthesis (Z89.62-)*
>   *hip joint prosthesis explantation status (Z89.62-)*

     Z47.33   **Aftercare following explantation of knee joint prosthesis**
>   **EXCLUDES 1**   *acquired absence of knee joint following prior explantation of knee prosthesis (Z89.52-)*
>   *knee joint prosthesis explantation status (Z89.52-)*

✓5ᵗʰ Z47.8   **Encounter for other orthopedic aftercare**

     Z47.81   **Encounter for orthopedic aftercare following surgical amputation**
         Use additional code to identify the limb amputated (Z89.-)

     Z47.82   **Encounter for orthopedic aftercare following scoliosis surgery**

     Z47.89   **Encounter for other orthopedic aftercare**
         AHA: 2015, 1Q, 8

✓4ᵗʰ Z48   **Encounter for other postprocedural aftercare**
> **EXCLUDES 1**   *encounter for aftercare following injury – code to Injury, by site, with appropriate 7th character for subsequent encounter*
> *encounter for follow-up examination after completed treatment (Z08-Z09)*
> **EXCLUDES 2**   *encounter for attention to artificial openings (Z43.-)*
> *encounter for fitting and adjustment of prosthetic and other devices (Z44-Z46)*
> **AHA:** 2015, 4Q, 38; 2015, 1Q, 6-7

✓5ᵗʰ Z48.0   **Encounter for attention to dressings, sutures and drains**
> **EXCLUDES 1**   *encounter for planned postprocedural wound closure (Z48.1)*

     Z48.00   **Encounter for change or removal of nonsurgical wound dressing**
         Encounter for change or removal of wound dressing NOS

     Z48.01   **Encounter for change or removal of surgical wound dressing**

     Z48.02   **Encounter for removal of sutures**
         Encounter for removal of staples

     Z48.03   **Encounter for change or removal of drains**

Z48.1   **Encounter for planned postprocedural wound closure**
> **EXCLUDES 1**   *encounter for attention to dressings and sutures (Z48.0-)*

✓5ᵗʰ Z48.2   **Encounter for aftercare following organ transplant**

     Z48.21   **Encounter for aftercare following heart transplant**   `CC` `HCC`
         CC Excl: PDX collection 1488

     Z48.22   **Encounter for aftercare following kidney transplant**   `CC`
         CC Excl: PDX collection 1489

     Z48.23   **Encounter for aftercare following liver transplant**   `CC` `HCC`
         CC Excl: PDX collection 1490

     Z48.24   **Encounter for aftercare following lung transplant**   `CC` `HCC`
         CC Excl: PDX collection 1491

     ✓6ᵗʰ Z48.28   **Encounter for aftercare following multiple organ transplant**

         Z48.280   **Encounter for aftercare following heart-lung transplant**   `CC` `HCC`
             CC Excl: PDX collection 1488

         Z48.288   **Encounter for aftercare following multiple organ transplant**

     ✓6ᵗʰ Z48.29   **Encounter for aftercare following other organ transplant**

         Z48.290   **Encounter for aftercare following bone marrow transplant**   `CC` `HCC`
             CC Excl: PDX collection 1492

         Z48.298   **Encounter for aftercare following other organ transplant**

Z48.3   **Aftercare following surgery for neoplasm**
     Use additional code to identify the neoplasm

✓5ᵗʰ Z48.8   **Encounter for other specified postprocedural aftercare**

     ✓6ᵗʰ Z48.81   **Encounter for surgical aftercare following surgery on specified body systems**
>   **NOTE**   These codes identify the body system requiring aftercare. They are for use in conjunction with other aftercare codes to fully explain the aftercare encounter. The condition treated should also be coded if still present.
>   **EXCLUDES 1**   *aftercare for injury—code the injury with 7th character D*
>   *aftercare following surgery for neoplasm (Z48.3)*
>   **EXCLUDES 2**   *aftercare following organ transplant (Z48.2-)*
>   *orthopedic aftercare (Z47.-)*
>   **AHA:** 2015, 4Q, 38

         Z48.810   **Encounter for surgical aftercare following surgery on the sense organs**

         Z48.811   **Encounter for surgical aftercare following surgery on the nervous system**
>   **EXCLUDES 2**   *encounter for surgical aftercare following surgery on the sense organs (Z48.810)*

         Z48.812   **Encounter for surgical aftercare following surgery on the circulatory system**
             AHA: 2012, 4Q, 96

✓ Additional Character Required   ✓x7ᵗʰ Placeholder   Unacceptable PDx   Questionable PDx   Manifestation   **H1**-**H14** HAC   **HCC** CMS-HCC Dx   **HIV** HIV Dx

Z48.813 Encounter for surgical aftercare following surgery on the respiratory system

Z48.814 Encounter for surgical aftercare following surgery on the teeth or oral cavity

Z48.815 Encounter for surgical aftercare following surgery on the digestive system

Z48.816 Encounter for surgical aftercare following surgery on the genitourinary system
> **EXCLUDES 1** encounter for aftercare following sterilization reversal (Z31.42)

Z48.817 Encounter for surgical aftercare following surgery on the skin and subcutaneous tissue

Z48.89 Encounter for other specified surgical aftercare

✓4ᵗʰ Z49 Encounter for care involving renal dialysis
Code also associated end stage renal disease (N18.6)

✓5ᵗʰ Z49.0 Preparatory care for renal dialysis
Encounter for dialysis instruction and training

Z49.01 Encounter for fitting and adjustment of extracorporeal dialysis catheter   HCC
Removal or replacement of renal dialysis catheter
Toilet or cleansing of renal dialysis catheter

Z49.02 Encounter for fitting and adjustment of peritoneal dialysis catheter   HCC

✓5ᵗʰ Z49.3 Encounter for adequacy testing for dialysis

Z49.31 Encounter for adequacy testing for hemodialysis   HCC

Z49.32 Encounter for adequacy testing for peritoneal dialysis   HCC
Encounter for peritoneal equilibration test

✓4ᵗʰ Z51 Encounter for other aftercare and medical care
Code also condition requiring care
> **EXCLUDES 1** follow-up examination after treatment (Z08-Z09)

Z51.0 Encounter for antineoplastic radiation therapy
AHA: 2017, 4Q, 103
TIP: Do not assign when admission is for insertion/implantation of radioactive elements. Assign a code for the malignancy instead. Any complications related to the radioactive elements should be assigned as secondary diagnoses.

✓5ᵗʰ Z51.1 Encounter for antineoplastic chemotherapy and immunotherapy
> **EXCLUDES 2** encounter for chemotherapy and immunotherapy for nonneoplastic condition—code to condition

Z51.11 Encounter for antineoplastic chemotherapy
AHA: 2015, 3Q, 19

Z51.12 Encounter for antineoplastic immunotherapy

Z51.5 Encounter for palliative care
AHA: 2017, 1Q, 48

Z51.6 Encounter for desensitization to allergens
AHA: 2016, 4Q, 77

✓5ᵗʰ Z51.8 Encounter for other specified aftercare
> **EXCLUDES 1** holiday relief care (Z75.5)

Z51.81 Encounter for therapeutic drug level monitoring
Code also any long-term (current) drug therapy (Z79.-)
> **EXCLUDES 1** encounter for blood-drug test for administrative or medicolegal reasons (Z02.83)

DEF: Drug monitoring: Measurement of the level of a specific drug in the body or measurement of a specific function to assess effectiveness of a drug.

Z51.89 Encounter for other specified aftercare
AHA: 2012, 4Q, 95-97
TIP: Unacceptable principal diagnosis edit applies if a secondary diagnosis is not present.

✓4ᵗʰ Z52 Donors of organs and tissues
> **INCLUDES** autologous and other living donors
> **EXCLUDES 1** cadaveric donor—omit code examination of potential donor (Z00.5)
AHA: 2012, 4Q, 99

✓5ᵗʰ Z52.0 Blood donor

✓6ᵗʰ Z52.00 Unspecified blood donor
Z52.000 Unspecified donor, whole blood
Z52.001 Unspecified donor, stem cells
Z52.008 Unspecified donor, other blood

✓6ᵗʰ Z52.01 Autologous blood donor
Z52.010 Autologous donor, whole blood
Z52.011 Autologous donor, stem cells
Z52.018 Autologous donor, other blood

✓6ᵗʰ Z52.09 Other blood donor
Volunteer donor
Z52.090 Other blood donor, whole blood
Z52.091 Other blood donor, stem cells
Z52.098 Other blood donor, other blood

✓5ᵗʰ Z52.1 Skin donor
Z52.10 Skin donor, unspecified
Z52.11 Skin donor, autologous
Z52.19 Skin donor, other

✓5ᵗʰ Z52.2 Bone donor
Z52.20 Bone donor, unspecified
Z52.21 Bone donor, autologous
Z52.29 Bone donor, other

Z52.3 Bone marrow donor

Z52.4 Kidney donor

Z52.5 Cornea donor

Z52.6 Liver donor

✓5ᵗʰ Z52.8 Donor of other specified organs or tissues

✓6ᵗʰ Z52.81 Egg (Oocyte) donor
Z52.810 Egg (Oocyte) donor under age 35, anonymous recipient   ♀
Egg donor under age 35 NOS
Z52.811 Egg (Oocyte) donor under age 35, designated recipient   ♀
Z52.812 Egg (Oocyte) donor age 35 and over, anonymous recipient   ♀
Egg donor age 35 and over NOS
Z52.813 Egg (Oocyte) donor age 35 and over, designated recipient   ♀
Z52.819 Egg (Oocyte) donor, unspecified   ♀

Z52.89 Donor of other specified organs or tissues

Z52.9 Donor of unspecified organ or tissue
Donor NOS

✓4ᵗʰ Z53 Persons encountering health services for specific procedures and treatment, not carried out

✓5ᵗʰ Z53.0 Procedure and treatment not carried out because of contraindication

Z53.01 Procedure and treatment not carried out due to patient smoking

Z53.09 Procedure and treatment not carried out because of other contraindication

Z53.1 Procedure and treatment not carried out because of patient's decision for reasons of belief and group pressure

✓5ᵗʰ Z53.2 Procedure and treatment not carried out because of patient's decision for other and unspecified reasons

Z53.20 Procedure and treatment not carried out because of patient's decision for unspecified reasons

Z53.21 Procedure and treatment not carried out due to patient leaving prior to being seen by health care provider

Z53.29 Procedure and treatment not carried out because of patient's decision for other reasons

✓5ᵗʰ Z53.3 Procedure converted to open procedure
AHA: 2016, 4Q, 79

Z53.31 Laparoscopic surgical procedure converted to open procedure

Z53.32 Thoracoscopic surgical procedure converted to open procedure

Z53.33 Arthroscopic surgical procedure converted to open procedure

Z53.39 Other specified procedure converted to open procedure

Z53.8 Procedure and treatment not carried out for other reasons

Z53.9 Procedure and treatment not carried out, unspecified reason

---

Ⓝ Newborn: 0   Ⓟ Pediatric: 0-17   Ⓜ Maternity: 12-55   Ⓐ Adult: 15-124   MCC Major Complication/Comorbidity   CC Complication/Comorbidity   SW Severe Wound Dx

1236   ICD-10-CM 2019

Persons with potential health hazards related to socioeconomic and psychosocial circumstances (Z55-Z65)

AHA: 2018, 1Q, 18
TIP: Codes from this code block can be assigned based on documentation from clinicians other than the diagnosing provider.

☑4ᵗʰ **Z55 Problems related to education and literacy**
> EXCLUDES 1 *disorders of psychological development (F80-F89)*

Z55.0 Illiteracy and low-level literacy

Z55.1 Schooling unavailable and unattainable

Z55.2 Failed school examinations

Z55.3 Underachievement in school

Z55.4 Educational maladjustment and discord with teachers and classmates

Z55.8 Other problems related to education and literacy
> Problems related to inadequate teaching

Z55.9 Problems related to education and literacy, unspecified
> Academic problems NOS

☑4ᵗʰ **Z56 Problems related to employment and unemployment**
> EXCLUDES 2 *occupational exposure to risk factors (Z57.-)*
> *problems related to housing and economic circumstances (Z59.-)*

Z56.0 Unemployment, unspecified

Z56.1 Change of job Ⓐ

Z56.2 Threat of job loss

Z56.3 Stressful work schedule

Z56.4 Discord with boss and workmates

Z56.5 Uncongenial work environment
> Difficult conditions at work

Z56.6 Other physical and mental strain related to work

☑5ᵗʰ **Z56.8 Other problems related to employment**

    Z56.81 Sexual harassment on the job

    Z56.82 Military deployment status
> Individual (civilian or military) currently deployed in theater or in support of military war, peacekeeping and humanitarian operations

    Z56.89 Other problems related to employment

Z56.9 Unspecified problems related to employment
> Occupational problems NOS

☑4ᵗʰ **Z57 Occupational exposure to risk factors**

Z57.0 Occupational exposure to noise

Z57.1 Occupational exposure to radiation

Z57.2 Occupational exposure to dust

☑5ᵗʰ **Z57.3 Occupational exposure to other air contaminants**

    Z57.31 Occupational exposure to environmental tobacco smoke
> EXCLUDES 2 *exposure to environmental tobacco smoke (Z77.22)*

    Z57.39 Occupational exposure to other air contaminants

Z57.4 Occupational exposure to toxic agents in agriculture
> Occupational exposure to solids, liquids, gases or vapors in agriculture

Z57.5 Occupational exposure to toxic agents in other industries
> Occupational exposure to solids, liquids, gases or vapors in other industries

Z57.6 Occupational exposure to extreme temperature

Z57.7 Occupational exposure to vibration

Z57.8 Occupational exposure to other risk factors

Z57.9 Occupational exposure to unspecified risk factor

☑4ᵗʰ **Z59 Problems related to housing and economic circumstances**
> EXCLUDES 2 *problems related to upbringing (Z62.-)*

Z59.0 Homelessness

Z59.1 Inadequate housing
> Lack of heating
> Restriction of space
> Technical defects in home preventing adequate care
> Unsatisfactory surroundings
> EXCLUDES 1 *problems related to the natural and physical environment (Z77.1-)*

Z59.2 Discord with neighbors, lodgers and landlord

Z59.3 Problems related to living in residential institution
> Boarding-school resident
> EXCLUDES 1 *institutional upbringing (Z62.2)*

Z59.4 Lack of adequate food and safe drinking water
> Inadequate drinking water supply
> EXCLUDES 1 *effects of hunger (T73.0)*
> *inappropriate diet or eating habits (Z72.4)*
> *malnutrition (E40-E46)*

Z59.5 Extreme poverty

Z59.6 Low income

Z59.7 Insufficient social insurance and welfare support

Z59.8 Other problems related to housing and economic circumstances
> Foreclosure on loan   Problems with creditors
> Isolated dwelling

Z59.9 Problem related to housing and economic circumstances, unspecified

☑4ᵗʰ **Z60 Problems related to social environment**

Z60.0 Problems of adjustment to life-cycle transitions
> Empty nest syndrome
> Phase of life problem
> Problem with adjustment to retirement [pension]

Z60.2 Problems related to living alone

Z60.3 Acculturation difficulty
> Problem with migration
> Problem with social transplantation
> **DEF:** Problem adapting to a different culture or environment not based on any coexisting mental disorder.

Z60.4 Social exclusion and rejection
> Exclusion and rejection on the basis of personal characteristics, such as unusual physical appearance, illness or behavior.
> EXCLUDES 1 *target of adverse discrimination such as for racial or religious reasons (Z60.5)*

Z60.5 Target of (perceived) adverse discrimination and persecution
> EXCLUDES 1 *social exclusion and rejection (Z60.4)*

Z60.8 Other problems related to social environment

Z60.9 Problem related to social environment, unspecified

☑4ᵗʰ **Z62 Problems related to upbringing**
> INCLUDES current and past negative life events in childhood
> current and past problems of a child related to upbringing
> EXCLUDES 2 *maltreatment syndrome (T74.-)*
> *problems related to housing and economic circumstances (Z59.-)*

Z62.0 Inadequate parental supervision and control

Z62.1 Parental overprotection

☑5ᵗʰ **Z62.2 Upbringing away from parents**
> EXCLUDES 1 *problems with boarding school (Z59.3)*

    Z62.21 Child in welfare custody Ⓟ
> Child in care of non-parental family member
> Child in foster care
> EXCLUDES 2 *problem for parent due to child in welfare custody (Z63.5)*

    Z62.22 Institutional upbringing
> Child living in orphanage or group home

    Z62.29 Other upbringing away from parents

Z62.3 Hostility towards and scapegoating of child Ⓟ

Z62.6 Inappropriate (excessive) parental pressure

☑5ᵗʰ **Z62.8 Other specified problems related to upbringing**

  ☑6ᵗʰ **Z62.81 Personal history of abuse in childhood**

      Z62.810 Personal history of physical and sexual abuse in childhood
> EXCLUDES 1 *current child physical abuse (T74.12, T76.12)*
> *current child sexual abuse (T74.22, T76.22)*

      Z62.811 Personal history of psychological abuse in childhood
> EXCLUDES 1 *current child psychological abuse (T74.32, T76.32)*

      Z62.812 Personal history of neglect in childhood
> EXCLUDES 1 *current child neglect (T74.02, T76.02)*

      Z62.813 Personal history of forced labor or sexual exploitation in childhood

      Z62.819 Personal history of unspecified abuse in childhood
> EXCLUDES 1 *current child abuse NOS (T74.92, T76.92)*

☑ Additional Character Required   ✓x7ᵗʰ Placeholder   Unacceptable PDx   Questionable PDx   Manifestation   H1 - H14 HAC   HCC CMS-HCC Dx   HIV HIV Dx

ICD-10-CM 2019   1237

Chapter 21. Factors Influencing Health Status and Contact with Health Services

√6th **Z62.82 Parent-child conflict**
    Z62.820 Parent-biological child conflict
        Parent-child problem NOS
    Z62.821 Parent-adopted child conflict
    Z62.822 Parent-foster child conflict
√6th **Z62.89 Other specified problems related to upbringing**
    Z62.890 Parent-child estrangement NEC
    Z62.891 Sibling rivalry
    Z62.898 Other specified problems related to upbringing
  Z62.9 Problem related to upbringing, unspecified

√4th **Z63 Other problems related to primary support group, including family circumstances**
    EXCLUDES 2   maltreatment syndrome (T74-, T76)
        parent-child problems (Z62.-)
        problems related to negative life events in childhood (Z62.-)
        problems related to upbringing (Z62.-)
  Z63.0 Problems in relationship with spouse or partner
    Relationship distress with spouse or intimate partner
    EXCLUDES 1   counseling for spousal or partner abuse problems (Z69.1)
        counseling related to sexual attitude, behavior, and orientation (Z70.-)
  Z63.1 Problems in relationship with in-laws
√5th **Z63.3 Absence of family member**
    EXCLUDES 1   absence of family member due to disappearance and death (Z63.4)
        absence of family member due to separation and divorce (Z63.5)
    Z63.31 Absence of family member due to military deployment
        Individual or family affected by other family member being on military deployment
        EXCLUDES 1   family disruption due to return of family member from military deployment (Z63.71)
    Z63.32 Other absence of family member
  Z63.4 Disappearance and death of family member
    Assumed death of family member
    Bereavement
    AHA: 2014, 1Q, 25
  Z63.5 Disruption of family by separation and divorce
    Marital estrangement
  Z63.6 Dependent relative needing care at home
√5th **Z63.7 Other stressful life events affecting family and household**
    Z63.71 Stress on family due to return of family member from military deployment
        Individual or family affected by family member having returned from military deployment (current or past conflict)
    Z63.72 Alcoholism and drug addiction in family
    Z63.79 Other stressful life events affecting family and household
        Anxiety (normal) about sick person in family
        Health problems within family
        Ill or disturbed family member
        Isolated family
  Z63.8 Other specified problems related to primary support group
    Family discord NOS
    Family estrangement NOS
    High expressed emotional level within family
    Inadequate family support NOS
    Inadequate or distorted communication within family
  Z63.9 Problem related to primary support group, unspecified
    Relationship disorder NOS

√4th **Z64 Problems related to certain psychosocial circumstances**
  Z64.0 Problems related to unwanted pregnancy ♀
  Z64.1 Problems related to multiparity ♀
  Z64.4 Discord with counselors
    Discord with probation officer
    Discord with social worker

√4th **Z65 Problems related to other psychosocial circumstances**
  Z65.0 Conviction in civil and criminal proceedings without imprisonment
  Z65.1 Imprisonment and other incarceration
  Z65.2 Problems related to release from prison
  Z65.3 Problems related to other legal circumstances
    Arrest
    Child custody or support proceedings
    Litigation
    Prosecution
  Z65.4 Victim of crime and terrorism
    Victim of torture
  Z65.5 Exposure to disaster, war and other hostilities
    EXCLUDES 1   target of perceived discrimination or persecution (Z60.5)
  Z65.8 Other specified problems related to psychosocial circumstances
    Religious or spiritual problem
  Z65.9 Problem related to unspecified psychosocial circumstances

Do not resuscitate status (Z66)

Z66 Do not resuscitate
  DNR status
  DEF: Medical order written by a physician that instructs others not to perform cardiopulmonary resuscitation (CPR), intubation, or advanced life support (ACLS). It prevents unnecessary invasive treatment to prolong life should breathing stop or cardiac arrest occur.

Blood type (Z67)

√4th **Z67 Blood type**
  AHA: 2015, 3Q, 40
√5th **Z67.1 Type A blood**
    Z67.10 Type A blood, Rh positive
    Z67.11 Type A blood, Rh negative
√5th **Z67.2 Type B blood**
    Z67.20 Type B blood, Rh positive
    Z67.21 Type B blood, Rh negative
√5th **Z67.3 Type AB blood**
    Z67.30 Type AB blood, Rh positive
    Z67.31 Type AB blood, Rh negative
√5th **Z67.4 Type O blood**
    Z67.40 Type O blood, Rh positive
    Z67.41 Type O blood, Rh negative
√5th **Z67.9 Unspecified blood type**
    Z67.90 Unspecified blood type, Rh positive
    Z67.91 Unspecified blood type, Rh negative

Blood Types

Antigen A   Antigen B
Blood Type A   Blood Type B
Anti-B antibody   Anti-A antibody
Blood Type AB   NO ANTIBODIES   NO ANTIGENS
Antigen A   Antigen B   Blood Type O

N Newborn: 0   P Pediatric: 0-17   M Maternity: 12-55   A Adult: 15-124   MCC Major Complication/Comorbidity   CC Complication/Comorbidity   SW Severe Wound Dx

1238   ICD-10-CM 2019

Body mass index [BMI] (Z68)

✓4ᵗʰ Z68 Body mass index [BMI]

Kilograms per meters squared

NOTE   BMI adult codes are for use for persons 21 years of age or older.
BMI pediatric codes are for use for persons 2-20 years of age. These percentiles are based on the growth charts published by the Centers for Disease Control and Prevention (CDC)

AHA: 2017, 1Q, 39

DEF: Index used to help determine whether an individual is underweight, a healthy weight, overweight, or obese.

TIP: BMI may be assigned to support an associated condition based on medical record documentation from clinicians who are not the patient's provider.

TIP: Do not assign when used in association with fluctuations in body fluid during an encounter, such as fluid overload or fluid retention.

Z68.1 Body mass index [BMI] 19.9 or less, adult   CC A
     CC Excl: PDX collection 1493

✓5ᵗʰ Z68.2 Body mass index [BMI] 20-29, adult

Z68.20	Body mass index [BMI] 20.0-20.9, adult	A
Z68.21	Body mass index [BMI] 21.0-21.9, adult	A
Z68.22	Body mass index [BMI] 22.0-22.9, adult	A
Z68.23	Body mass index [BMI] 23.0-23.9, adult	A
Z68.24	Body mass index [BMI] 24.0-24.9, adult	A
Z68.25	Body mass index [BMI] 25.0-25.9, adult	A
Z68.26	Body mass index [BMI] 26.0-26.9, adult	A
Z68.27	Body mass index [BMI] 27.0-27.9, adult	A
Z68.28	Body mass index [BMI] 28.0-28.9, adult	A
Z68.29	Body mass index [BMI] 29.0-29.9, adult	A

✓5ᵗʰ Z68.3 Body mass index [BMI] 30-39, adult

Z68.30	Body mass index [BMI] 30.0-30.9, adult	A
Z68.31	Body mass index [BMI] 31.0-31.9, adult	A
Z68.32	Body mass index [BMI] 32.0-32.9, adult	A
Z68.33	Body mass index [BMI] 33.0-33.9, adult	A
Z68.34	Body mass index [BMI] 34.0-34.9, adult	A
Z68.35	Body mass index [BMI] 35.0-35.9, adult	A
Z68.36	Body mass index [BMI] 36.0-36.9, adult	A
Z68.37	Body mass index [BMI] 37.0-37.9, adult	A
Z68.38	Body mass index [BMI] 38.0-38.9, adult	A
Z68.39	Body mass index [BMI] 39.0-39.9, adult	A

✓5ᵗʰ Z68.4 Body mass index [BMI] 40 or greater, adult

     CC Excl: For CC codes in subcategory Z68.4: PDX collection 1494

Z68.41	Body mass index [BMI] 40.0-44.9, adult	CC HCC A
Z68.42	Body mass index [BMI] 45.0-49.9, adult	CC HCC A
Z68.43	Body mass index [BMI] 50-59.9, adult	CC HCC A
Z68.44	Body mass index [BMI] 60.0-69.9, adult	CC HCC A
Z68.45	Body mass index [BMI] 70 or greater, adult	CC HCC A

✓5ᵗʰ Z68.5 Body mass index [BMI] pediatric

Z68.51	Body mass index [BMI] pediatric, less than 5th percentile for age
Z68.52	Body mass index [BMI] pediatric, 5th percentile to less than 85th percentile for age
Z68.53	Body mass index [BMI] pediatric, 85th percentile to less than 95th percentile for age
Z68.54	Body mass index [BMI] pediatric, greater than or equal to 95th percentile for age

Persons encountering health services in other circumstances (Z69-Z76)

✓4ᵗʰ Z69 Encounter for mental health services for victim and perpetrator of abuse

INCLUDES counseling for victims and perpetrators of abuse

✓5ᵗʰ Z69.0 Encounter for mental health services for child abuse problems

✓6ᵗʰ Z69.01 Encounter for mental health services for parental child abuse

Z69.010 Encounter for mental health services for victim of parental child abuse   P
Encounter for mental health services for victim of child abuse by parent
Encounter for mental health services for victim of child neglect by parent
Encounter for mental health services for victim of child psychological abuse by parent
Encounter for mental health services for victim of child sexual abuse by parent

Z69.011 Encounter for mental health services for perpetrator of parental child abuse
Encounter for mental health services for perpetrator of parental child neglect
Encounter for mental health services for perpetrator of parental child psychological abuse
Encounter for mental health services for perpetrator of parental child sexual abuse
EXCLUDES 1 encounter for mental health services for non-parental child abuse (Z69.02-)

✓6ᵗʰ Z69.02 Encounter for mental health services for non-parental child abuse

Z69.020 Encounter for mental health services for victim of non-parental child abuse   P
Encounter for mental health services for victim of non-parental child neglect
Encounter for mental health services for victim of non-parental child psychological abuse
Encounter for mental health services for victim of non-parental child sexual abuse

Z69.021 Encounter for mental health services for perpetrator of non-parental child abuse
Encounter for mental health services for perpetrator of non-parental child neglect
Encounter for mental health services for perpetrator of non-parental child psychological abuse
Encounter for mental health services for perpetrator of non-parental child sexual abuse

✓5ᵗʰ Z69.1 Encounter for mental health services for spousal or partner abuse problems

Z69.11 Encounter for mental health services for victim of spousal or partner abuse
Encounter for mental health services for victim of spouse or partner neglect
Encounter for mental health services for victim of spouse or partner psychological abuse
Encounter for mental health services for victim of spouse or partner violence, physical

Z69.12 Encounter for mental health services for perpetrator of spousal or partner abuse
Encounter for mental health services for perpetrator of spouse or partner neglect
Encounter for mental health services for perpetrator of spouse or partner psychological abuse
Encounter for mental health services for perpetrator of spouse or partner violence, physical
Encounter for mental health services for perpetrator of spouse or partner violence, sexual

✓ Additional Character Required   ✓x7ᵗʰ Placeholder   Unacceptable PDx   Questionable PDx   Manifestation   H1-H14 HAC   HCC CMS-HCC Dx   HIV HIV Dx

ICD-10-CM 2019   **1239**

✓5ᵗʰ **Z69.8** **Encounter for mental health services for victim or perpetrator of other abuse**

Z69.81 **Encounter for mental health services for victim of other abuse**
Encounter for mental health services for perpetrator of non-spousal adult abuse
Encounter for mental health services for victim of non-spousal adult abuse
Encounter for mental health services for victim of spouse or partner violence, sexual
Encounter for rape victim counseling

Z69.82 **Encounter for mental health services for perpetrator of other abuse**

✓4ᵗʰ **Z70** **Counseling related to sexual attitude, behavior and orientation**
INCLUDES   encounter for mental health services for sexual attitude, behavior and orientation
EXCLUDES 2   *contraceptive or procreative counseling (Z30-Z31)*

Z70.0 **Counseling related to sexual attitude**

Z70.1 **Counseling related to patient's sexual behavior and orientation**
Patient concerned regarding impotence
Patient concerned regarding non-responsiveness
Patient concerned regarding promiscuity
Patient concerned regarding sexual orientation

Z70.2 **Counseling related to sexual behavior and orientation of third party**
Advice sought regarding sexual behavior and orientation of child
Advice sought regarding sexual behavior and orientation of partner
Advice sought regarding sexual behavior and orientation of spouse

Z70.3 **Counseling related to combined concerns regarding sexual attitude, behavior and orientation**

Z70.8 **Other sex counseling**
Encounter for sex education

Z70.9 **Sex counseling, unspecified**

✓4ᵗʰ **Z71** **Persons encountering health services for other counseling and medical advice, not elsewhere classified**
EXCLUDES 2   *contraceptive or procreation counseling (Z30-Z31)*
    sex counseling (Z70.-)

Z71.0 **Person encountering health services to consult on behalf of another person**
Person encountering health services to seek advice or treatment for non-attending third party
EXCLUDES 2   *anxiety (normal) about sick person in family (Z63.7)*
    expectant (adoptive) parent(s) pre-birth pediatrician visit (Z76.81)

Z71.1 **Person with feared health complaint in whom no diagnosis is made**
Person encountering health services with feared condition which was not demonstrated
Person encountering health services in which problem was normal state
"Worried well"
EXCLUDES 1   *medical observation for suspected diseases and conditions proven not to exist (Z03.-)*

Z71.2 **Person consulting for explanation of examination or test findings**

Z71.3 **Dietary counseling and surveillance**
Use additional code for any associated underlying medical condition
Use additional code to identify body mass index (BMI), if known (Z68.-)

✓5ᵗʰ **Z71.4** **Alcohol abuse counseling and surveillance**
Use additional code for alcohol abuse or dependence (F10.-)

Z71.41 **Alcohol abuse counseling and surveillance of alcoholic**

Z71.42 **Counseling for family member of alcoholic**
Counseling for significant other, partner, or friend of alcoholic

✓5ᵗʰ **Z71.5** **Drug abuse counseling and surveillance**
Use additional code for drug abuse or dependence (F11-F16, F18-F19)

Z71.51 **Drug abuse counseling and surveillance of drug abuser**

Z71.52 **Counseling for family member of drug abuser**
Counseling for significant other, partner, or friend of drug abuser

Z71.6 **Tobacco abuse counseling**
Use additional code for nicotine dependence (F17.-)

Z71.7 **Human immunodeficiency virus [HIV] counseling**

✓5ᵗʰ **Z71.8** **Other specified counseling**
EXCLUDES 2   *counseling for contraception (Z30.0-)*
AHA: 2017, 4Q, 27

Z71.81 **Spiritual or religious counseling**

Z71.82 **Exercise counseling**

Z71.83 **Encounter for nonprocreative genetic counseling**
EXCLUDES 1   *counseling for procreative genetics (Z31.5)*
    counseling for procreative management (Z31.6)

Z71.89 **Other specified counseling**

Z71.9 **Counseling, unspecified**
Encounter for medical advice NOS

✓4ᵗʰ **Z72** **Problems related to lifestyle**
EXCLUDES 2   *problems related to life-management difficulty (Z73.-)*
    problems related to socioeconomic and psychosocial circumstances (Z55-Z65)

Z72.0 **Tobacco use**
Tobacco use NOS
EXCLUDES 1   *history of tobacco dependence (Z87.891)*
    nicotine dependence (F17.2-)
    tobacco dependence (F17.2-)
    tobacco use during pregnancy (O99.33-)

Z72.3 **Lack of physical exercise**

Z72.4 **Inappropriate diet and eating habits**
EXCLUDES 1   *behavioral eating disorders of infancy or childhood (F98.2- F98.3)*
    eating disorders (F50.-)
    lack of adequate food (Z59.4)
    malnutrition and other nutritional deficiencies (E40-E64)

✓5ᵗʰ **Z72.5** **High risk sexual behavior**
Promiscuity
EXCLUDES 1   *paraphilias (F65)*

Z72.51 **High risk heterosexual behavior**

Z72.52 **High risk homosexual behavior**

Z72.53 **High risk bisexual behavior**

Z72.6 **Gambling and betting**
EXCLUDES 1   *compulsive or pathological gambling (F63.0)*

Z72.8 **Other problems related to lifestyle**

✓6ᵗʰ **Z72.81** **Antisocial behavior**
EXCLUDES 1   *conduct disorders (F91.-)*

Z72.810 **Child and adolescent antisocial behavior**   P
Antisocial behavior (child) (adolescent) without manifest psychiatric disorder
Delinquency NOS
Group delinquency
Offenses in the context of gang membership
Stealing in company with others
Truancy from school

Z72.811 **Adult antisocial behavior**   A
Adult antisocial behavior without manifest psychiatric disorder

✓6ᵗʰ **Z72.82** **Problems related to sleep**

Z72.820 **Sleep deprivation**
Lack of adequate sleep
EXCLUDES 1   *insomnia (G47.0-)*

Z72.821 **Inadequate sleep hygiene**
Bad sleep habits
Irregular sleep habits
Unhealthy sleep wake schedule
EXCLUDES 1   *insomnia (F51.0-, G47.0-)*

Z72.89 **Other problems related to lifestyle**
Self-damaging behavior

Z72.9 **Problem related to lifestyle, unspecified**

✓4ᵗʰ **Z73** **Problems related to life management difficulty**
EXCLUDES 2   *problems related to socioeconomic and psychosocial circumstances (Z55-Z65)*
DEF: State of emotional, mental, and physical exhaustion causing difficulties in managing personal, school, or work circumstances. It is usually due to prolonged stress or poor interpersonal relationship skills or parenting skills.

Z73.0 **Burn-out**

Z73.1 **Type A behavior pattern**

Z73.2 **Lack of relaxation and leisure**

Z73.3 **Stress, not elsewhere classified**
Physical and mental strain NOS
EXCLUDES 1   *stress related to employment or unemployment (Z56.-)*

Z73.4 **Inadequate social skills, not elsewhere classified**

Z73.5 **Social role conflict, not elsewhere classified**

Z73.6 **Limitation of activities due to disability**
EXCLUDES 1   *care-provider dependency (Z74.-)*

✓5th **Z73.8** **Other problems related to life management difficulty**

✓6th **Z73.81** **Behavioral insomnia of childhood**
DEF: Behaviors on the part of the child or caregivers that cause negative compliance with a child's sleep schedule resulting in lack of adequate sleep.

Z73.810 **Behavioral insomnia of childhood, sleep-onset association type**   P

Z73.811 **Behavioral insomnia of childhood, limit setting type**   P

Z73.812 **Behavioral insomnia of childhood, combined type**   P

Z73.819 **Behavioral insomnia of childhood, unspecified type**   P

Z73.82 **Dual sensory impairment**

Z73.89 **Other problems related to life management difficulty**

Z73.9 **Problem related to life management difficulty, unspecified**

✓4th **Z74** **Problems related to care provider dependency**
EXCLUDES 2   *dependence on enabling machines or devices NEC (Z99.-)*

✓5th **Z74.0** **Reduced mobility**

Z74.01 **Bed confinement status**
Bedridden

Z74.09 **Other reduced mobility**
Chair ridden
Reduced mobility NOS
EXCLUDES 2   *wheelchair dependence (Z99.3)*

Z74.1 **Need for assistance with personal care**

Z74.2 **Need for assistance at home and no other household member able to render care**

Z74.3 **Need for continuous supervision**

Z74.8 **Other problems related to care provider dependency**

Z74.9 **Problem related to care provider dependency, unspecified**

✓4th **Z75** **Problems related to medical facilities and other health care**

Z75.0 **Medical services not available in home**
EXCLUDES 1   *no other household member able to render care (Z74.2)*

Z75.1 **Person awaiting admission to adequate facility elsewhere**

Z75.2 **Other waiting period for investigation and treatment**

Z75.3 **Unavailability and inaccessibility of health-care facilities**
EXCLUDES 1   *bed unavailable (Z75.1)*

Z75.4 **Unavailability and inaccessibility of other helping agencies**

Z75.5 **Holiday relief care**

Z75.8 **Other problems related to medical facilities and other health care**

Z75.9 **Unspecified problem related to medical facilities and other health care**

✓4th **Z76** **Persons encountering health services in other circumstances**

Z76.0 **Encounter for issue of repeat prescription**
Encounter for issue of repeat prescription for appliance
Encounter for issue of repeat prescription for medicaments
Encounter for issue of repeat prescription for spectacles
EXCLUDES 2   *issue of medical certificate (Z02.7)*
repeat prescription for contraceptive (Z30.4-)

Z76.1 **Encounter for health supervision and care of foundling**

Z76.2 **Encounter for health supervision and care of other healthy infant and child**   P
Encounter for medical or nursing care or supervision of healthy infant under circumstances such as adverse socioeconomic conditions at home
Encounter for medical or nursing care or supervision of healthy infant under circumstances such as awaiting foster or adoptive placement
Encounter for medical or nursing care or supervision of healthy infant under circumstances such as maternal illness
Encounter for medical or nursing care or supervision of healthy infant under circumstances such as number of children at home preventing or interfering with normal care

Z76.3 **Healthy person accompanying sick person**

Z76.4 **Other boarder to healthcare facility**
EXCLUDES 1   *homelessness (Z59.0)*

Z76.5 **Malingerer [conscious simulation]**
Person feigning illness (with obvious motivation)
EXCLUDES 1   *factitious disorder ▶(F68.1-, F68.A)◄*
peregrinating patient (F68.1-)
DEF: Act of intentionally exaggerating an illness or disability in order to receive personal gain or to avoid punishment or responsibility.

✓5th **Z76.8** **Persons encountering health services in other specified circumstances**

Z76.81 **Expectant parent(s) prebirth pediatrician visit**
Pre-adoption pediatrician visit for adoptive parent(s)

Z76.82 **Awaiting organ transplant status**
Patient waiting for organ availability

Z76.89 **Persons encountering health services in other specified circumstances**
Persons encountering health services NOS
AHA: 2014, 2Q, 10

Persons with potential health hazards related to family and personal history and certain conditions influencing health status (Z77-Z99)

Code also any follow-up examination (Z08-Z09)

✓4th **Z77** **Other contact with and (suspected) exposures hazardous to health**
INCLUDES   contact with and (suspected) exposures to potential hazards to health
EXCLUDES 2   *contact with and (suspected) exposure to communicable diseases (Z20.-)*
exposure to (parental) (environmental) tobacco smoke in the perinatal period (P96.81)
newborn affected by noxious substances transmitted via placenta or breast milk (P04.-)
occupational exposure to risk factors (Z57.-)
retained foreign body (Z18.-)
retained foreign body fully removed (Z87.821)
toxic effects of substances chiefly nonmedicinal as to source (T51-T65)

✓5th **Z77.0** **Contact with and (suspected) exposure to hazardous, chiefly nonmedicinal, chemicals**

✓6th **Z77.01** **Contact with and (suspected) exposure to hazardous metals**

Z77.010 **Contact with and (suspected) exposure to arsenic**

Z77.011 **Contact with and (suspected) exposure to lead**

Z77.012 **Contact with and (suspected) exposure to uranium**
EXCLUDES 1   *retained depleted uranium fragments (Z18.01)*

Z77.018 **Contact with and (suspected) exposure to other hazardous metals**
Contact with and (suspected) exposure to chromium compounds
Contact with and (suspected) exposure to nickel dust

✓6th **Z77.02** **Contact with and (suspected) exposure to hazardous aromatic compounds**

Z77.020 **Contact with and (suspected) exposure to aromatic amines**

Z77.021 **Contact with and (suspected) exposure to benzene**

Z77.028 **Contact with and (suspected) exposure to other hazardous aromatic compounds**
Aromatic dyes NOS
Polycyclic aromatic hydrocarbons

✓6th **Z77.09** **Contact with and (suspected) exposure to other hazardous, chiefly nonmedicinal, chemicals**

Z77.090 **Contact with and (suspected) exposure to asbestos**

Z77.098 **Contact with and (suspected) exposure to other hazardous, chiefly nonmedicinal, chemicals**
Dyes NOS

✔ Additional Character Required   ✓x7th Placeholder   Unacceptable PDx   Questionable PDx   Manifestation   H1-H14 HAC   HCC CMS-HCC Dx   HIV HIV Dx

ICD-10-CM 2019   **1241**

☑5ᵗʰ Z77.1 Contact with and (suspected) exposure to environmental pollution and hazards in the physical environment

   ☑6ᵗʰ Z77.11 Contact with and (suspected) exposure to environmental pollution

      Z77.110 Contact with and (suspected) exposure to air **pollution**

      Z77.111 Contact with and (suspected) exposure to water **pollution**

      Z77.112 Contact with and (suspected) exposure to soil **pollution**

      Z77.118 Contact with and (suspected) exposure to other **environmental pollution**

   ☑6ᵗʰ Z77.12 Contact with and (suspected) exposure to hazards in the physical environment

      Z77.120 Contact with and (suspected) exposure to mold (toxic)

      Z77.121 Contact with and (suspected) exposure to harmful algae and algae toxins

        Contact with and (suspected) exposure to (harmful) algae bloom NOS

        Contact with and (suspected) exposure to blue-green algae bloom

        Contact with and (suspected) exposure to brown tide

        Contact with and (suspected) exposure to cyanobacteria bloom

        Contact with and (suspected) exposure to Florida red tide

        Contact with and (suspected) exposure to pfiesteria piscicida

        Contact with and (suspected) exposure to red tide

      Z77.122 Contact with and (suspected) exposure to noise

      ▲ **Z77.123 Contact with and (suspected) exposure to** radon and other naturally occurring radiation

        EXCLUDES 2   *radiation exposure as the cause of a confirmed condition (W88-W90, X39.0-)*

            radiation sickness NOS (T66)

      Z77.128 Contact with and (suspected) exposure to other **hazards in the physical environment**

▲ **☑5ᵗʰ Z77.2 Contact with and (suspected) exposure to** other **hazardous substances**

   Z77.21 Contact with and (suspected) exposure to potentially hazardous body fluids

   Z77.22 Contact with and (suspected) exposure to environmental tobacco smoke **(acute) (chronic)**

      Exposure to second hand tobacco smoke (acute) (chronic)

      Passive smoking (acute) (chronic)

      EXCLUDES 1   *nicotine dependence (F17.-)*

           tobacco use (Z72.0)

      EXCLUDES 2   *occupational exposure to environmental tobacco smoke (Z57.31)*

   ▲ **Z77.29 Contact with and (suspected) exposure to** other **hazardous substances**

      AHA: 2016, 2Q, 33

   Z77.9 Other **contact with and (suspected) exposures hazardous to health**

☑4ᵗʰ Z78 Other specified health status

   EXCLUDES 2   *asymptomatic human immunodeficiency virus [HIV] infection status (Z21)*

         postprocedural status (Z93- Z99)

         sex reassignment status (Z87.890)

   Z78.0 Asymptomatic menopausal state   ▲♀

      Menopausal state NOS

      Postmenopausal status NOS

      EXCLUDES 2   *symptomatic menopausal state (N95.1)*

   Z78.1 Physical restraint status

      EXCLUDES 1   *physical restraint due to a procedure - omit code*

      DEF: Application of mechanical restraining devices or manual restraints to limit physical mobility of a patient.

   Z78.9 Other specified health status

☑4ᵗʰ Z79 Long term (current) drug therapy

   INCLUDES long term (current) drug use for prophylactic purposes

   Code also any therapeutic drug level monitoring (Z51.81)

   EXCLUDES 2   *drug abuse and dependence (F11-F19)*

         drug use complicating pregnancy, childbirth, and the puerperium (O99.32-)

         long term (current) use of oral antidiabetic drugs (Z79.84)

         long term (current) use of oral hypoglycemic drugs (Z79.84)

   ☑5ᵗʰ Z79.0 Long term (current) use of anticoagulants and antithrombotics/antiplatelets

      EXCLUDES 2   *long term (current) use of aspirin (Z79.82)*

      Z79.01 Long term (current) use of anticoagulants

      Z79.02 Long term (current) use of antithrombotics/antiplatelets

   Z79.1 Long term (current) use of non-steroidal anti-inflammatories **(NSAID)**

      EXCLUDES 2   *long term (current) use of aspirin (Z79.82)*

   Z79.2 Long term (current) use of antibiotics

   Z79.3 Long term (current) use of hormonal contraceptives

      Long term (current) use of birth control pill or patch

   Z79.4 Long term (current) use of insulin   HCC

      TIP: When both long-term (current) insulin and long-term (current) oral hypoglycemic use is documented, assign a code only for the long-term insulin use.

   ☑5ᵗʰ Z79.5 Long term (current) use of steroids

      Z79.51 Long term (current) use of inhaled steroids

      Z79.52 Long term (current) use of systemic steroids

   ☑5ᵗʰ Z79.8 Other long term (current) drug therapy

   ☑6ᵗʰ Z79.81 Long term (current) use of agents affecting estrogen receptors and estrogen levels

      Code first, if applicable:

        malignant neoplasm of breast (C50.-)

        malignant neoplasm of prostate (C61)

      Use additional code, if applicable, to identify:

        estrogen receptor positive status (Z17.0)

        family history of breast cancer (Z80.3)

        genetic susceptibility to malignant neoplasm (cancer) (Z15.0-)

        personal history of breast cancer (Z85.3)

        personal history of prostate cancer (Z85.46)

        postmenopausal status (Z78.0)

      EXCLUDES 1   *hormone replacement therapy (Z79.890)*

      Z79.810 Long term (current) use of selective estrogen receptor modulators (SERMs)

        Long term (current) use of raloxifene (Evista)

        Long term (current) use of tamoxifen (Nolvadex)

        Long term (current) use of toremifene (Fareston)

      Z79.811 Long term (current) use of aromatase inhibitors

        Long term (current) use of anastrozole (Arimidex)

        Long term (current) use of exemestane (Aromasin)

        Long term (current) use of letrozole (Femara)

      Z79.818 Long term (current) use of other **agents affecting estrogen receptors and estrogen levels**

        Long term (current) use of estrogen receptor downregulators

        Long term (current) use of fulvestrant (Faslodex)

        Long term (current) use of gonadotropin-releasing hormone (GnRH) agonist

        Long term (current) use of goserelin acetate (Zoladex)

        Long term (current) use of leuprolide acetate (leuprorelin) (Lupron)

        Long term (current) use of megestrol acetate (Megace)

   Z79.82 Long term (current) use of aspirin

   Z79.83 Long term (current) use of bisphosphonates

      AHA: 2016, 4Q, 42

N Newborn: 0   P Pediatric: 0-17   M Maternity: 12-55   A Adult: 15-124   MCC Major Complication/Comorbidity   CC Complication/Comorbidity   SW Severe Wound Dx

1242   ICD-10-CM 2019

Z79.84 **Long term (current) use of** oral hypoglycemic drugs
Long term (current) use of oral antidiabetic drugs
EXCLUDES 2 *long term (current) use of insulin (Z79.4)*
AHA: 2016, 4Q, 76
TIP: When both long-term (current) insulin and long term (current) oral hypoglycemic use is documented, assign only code Z79.4 for the long-term (current) insulin use.

✓6th **Z79.89** **Other long term (current) drug therapy**
Z79.890 Hormone replacement therapy
Z79.891 **Long term (current) use of** opiate analgesic
Long term (current) use of methadone for pain management
EXCLUDES 1 *methodone use NOS (F11.9-)*
use of methodone for treatment of heroin addiction (F11.2-)
Z79.899 Other long term (current) drug therapy
AHA: 2015, 4Q, 34; 2015, 3Q, 21

✓4th **Z80** **Family history of primary malignant neoplasm**
Z80.0 **Family history of malignant neoplasm of** digestive organs
Conditions classifiable to C15-C26
AHA: 2018, 1Q, 6

Z80.1 **Family history of malignant neoplasm of** trachea, bronchus and lung
Conditions classifiable to C33-C34

Z80.2 **Family history of malignant neoplasm of** other respiratory and intrathoracic organs
Conditions classifiable to C30-C32, C37-C39

Z80.3 **Family history of malignant neoplasm of** breast
Conditions classifiable to C50-

✓5th **Z80.4** **Family history of malignant neoplasm of genital organs**
Conditions classifiable to C51-C63
Z80.41 **Family history of malignant neoplasm of** ovary
Z80.42 **Family history of malignant neoplasm of** prostate
Z80.43 **Family history of malignant neoplasm of** testis
Z80.49 **Family history of malignant neoplasm of** other genital organs

✓5th **Z80.5** **Family history of malignant neoplasm of urinary tract**
Conditions classifiable to C64-C68
Z80.51 **Family history of malignant neoplasm of** kidney
Z80.52 **Family history of malignant neoplasm of** bladder
Z80.59 **Family history of malignant neoplasm of** other urinary tract organ

Z80.6 **Family history of** leukemia
Conditions classifiable to C91-C95

Z80.7 **Family history of** other **malignant neoplasms of** lymphoid, hematopoietic and related tissues
Conditions classifiable to C81-C90, C96-

Z80.8 **Family history of malignant neoplasm of** other organs or systems
Conditions classifiable to C00-C14, C40-C49, C69-C79

Z80.9 **Family history of malignant neoplasm,** unspecified
Conditions classifiable to C80.1

✓4th **Z81** **Family history of mental and behavioral disorders**
Z81.0 **Family history of** intellectual disabilities
Conditions classifiable to F70-F79

Z81.1 **Family history of** alcohol abuse and dependence
Conditions classifiable to F10-

Z81.2 **Family history of** tobacco abuse and dependence
Conditions classifiable to F17-

Z81.3 **Family history of** other psychoactive substance abuse and dependence
Conditions classifiable to F11-F16, F18-F19

Z81.4 **Family history of other** substance abuse and dependence
Conditions classifiable to F55

Z81.8 **Family history of other** mental and behavioral **disorders**
Conditions classifiable elsewhere in F01-F99

✓4th **Z82** **Family history of certain disabilities and chronic diseases (leading to disablement)**
Z82.0 **Family history of** epilepsy **and other diseases of the nervous system**
Conditions classifiable to G00-G99

Z82.1 **Family history of** blindness and visual loss
Conditions classifiable to H54-

Z82.2 **Family history of** deafness and hearing loss
Conditions classifiable to H90-H91

Z82.3 **Family history of** stroke
Conditions classifiable to I60-I64

✓5th **Z82.4** **Family history of ischemic heart disease and other diseases of the circulatory system**
Conditions classifiable to I00-I52, I65-I99
Z82.41 **Family history of** sudden cardiac death
Z82.49 **Family history of** ischemic heart disease **and other diseases of the circulatory system**

Z82.5 **Family history of** asthma **and other chronic lower respiratory diseases**
Conditions classifiable to J40-J47
EXCLUDES 2 *family history of other diseases of the respiratory system (Z83.6)*

✓5th **Z82.6** **Family history of arthritis and other diseases of the musculoskeletal system and connective tissue**
Conditions classifiable to M00-M99
Z82.61 **Family history of** arthritis
Z82.62 **Family history of** osteoporosis
Z82.69 **Family history of** other **diseases of the musculoskeletal system and connective tissue**

✓5th **Z82.7** **Family history of congenital malformations, deformations and chromosomal abnormalities**
Conditions classifiable to Q00-Q99
Z82.71 **Family history of** polycystic kidney
Z82.79 **Family history of** other **congenital malformations, deformations and chromosomal abnormalities**

Z82.8 **Family history of** other disabilities and chronic diseases leading to disablement, **not elsewhere classified**

✓4th **Z83** **Family history of other specific disorders**
EXCLUDES 2 *contact with and (suspected) exposure to communicable disease in the family (Z20.-)*
Z83.0 **Family history of** human immunodeficiency virus [HIV] **disease**
Conditions classifiable to B20

Z83.1 **Family history of other** infectious and parasitic diseases
Conditions classifiable to A00-B19, B25-B94, B99

Z83.2 **Family history of diseases of the** blood and blood-forming organs **and certain disorders involving the immune mechanism**
Conditions classifiable to D50-D89

Z83.3 **Family history of** diabetes mellitus
Conditions classifiable to E08-E13

✓5th **Z83.4** **Family history of other endocrine, nutritional and metabolic diseases**
Conditions classifiable to E00-E07, E15-E88
Z83.41 **Family history of** multiple endocrine neoplasia [MEN] syndrome
Z83.42 **Family history of** familial hypercholesterolemia
AHA: 2016, 4Q, 77

● ✓6th **Z83.43** **Family history of other disorder of lipoprotein metabolism and other lipidemias**
● **Z83.430** **Family history of** elevated lipoprotein(a)
Family history of elevated Lp(a)
● **Z83.438** **Family history of other disorder of lipoprotein metabolism and other lipidemia**
Family history of familial combined hyperlipidemia

Z83.49 **Family history of** other **endocrine, nutritional and metabolic diseases**

✓5th **Z83.5** **Family history of eye and ear disorders**
✓6th **Z83.51** **Family history of** eye **disorders**
Conditions classifiable to H00-H53, H55-H59
EXCLUDES 2 *family history of blindness and visual loss (Z82.1)*
Z83.511 **Family history of** glaucoma
Z83.518 **Family history of** other **specified eye disorder**
Z83.52 **Family history of** ear **disorders**
Conditions classifiable to H60-H83, H92-H95
EXCLUDES 2 *family history of deafness and hearing loss (Z82.2)*

Z83.6 **Family history of other diseases of the** respiratory system
Conditions classifiable to J00-J39, J60-J99
EXCLUDES 2 *family history of asthma and other chronic lower respiratory diseases (Z82.5)*

✔ Additional Character Required   ✓x7th Placeholder   Unacceptable PDx   Questionable PDx   Manifestation   **H1**-**H14** HAC   **HCC** CMS-HCC Dx   **HIV** HIV Dx

ICD-10-CM 2019   1243

✓5ᵗʰ Z83.7 Family history of diseases of the digestive system
Conditions classifiable to K00-K93

Z83.71 Family history of colonic polyps
EXCLUDES 2 *family history of malignant neoplasm of digestive organs (Z80.0)*

Z83.79 Family history of other diseases of the digestive system

✓4ᵗʰ Z84 Family history of other conditions

Z84.0 Family history of diseases of the skin and subcutaneous tissue
Conditions classifiable to L00-L99

Z84.1 Family history of disorders of kidney and ureter
Conditions classifiable to N00-N29

Z84.2 Family history of other diseases of the genitourinary system
Conditions classifiable to N30-N99

Z84.3 Family history of consanguinity

✓5ᵗʰ Z84.8 Family history of other specified conditions

Z84.81 Family history of carrier of genetic disease

Z84.82 Family history of sudden infant death syndrome
Family history of SIDS
AHA: 2016, 4Q, 77

Z84.89 Family history of other specified conditions

✓4ᵗʰ Z85 Personal history of malignant neoplasm
Code first any follow-up examination after treatment of malignant neoplasm (Z08)
Use additional code to identify:
  alcohol use and dependence (F10.-)
  exposure to environmental tobacco smoke (Z77.22)
  history of tobacco dependence (Z87.891)
  occupational exposure to environmental tobacco smoke (Z57.31)
  tobacco dependence (F17.-)
  tobacco use (Z72.0)
EXCLUDES 2 *personal history of benign neoplasm (Z86.01-)*
personal history of carcinoma-in-situ (Z86.00-)

✓5ᵗʰ Z85.0 Personal history of malignant neoplasm of digestive organs
AHA: 2017, 1Q, 9

Z85.00 Personal history of malignant neoplasm of unspecified digestive organ

Z85.01 Personal history of malignant neoplasm of esophagus
Conditions classifiable to C15

✓6ᵗʰ Z85.02 Personal history of malignant neoplasm of stomach

Z85.020 Personal history of malignant carcinoid tumor of stomach
Conditions classifiable to C7A.092

Z85.028 Personal history of other malignant neoplasm of stomach
Conditions classifiable to C16

✓6ᵗʰ Z85.03 Personal history of malignant neoplasm of large intestine

Z85.030 Personal history of malignant carcinoid tumor of large intestine
Conditions classifiable to C7A.022-C7A.025, C7A.029

Z85.038 Personal history of other malignant neoplasm of large intestine
Conditions classifiable to C18

✓6ᵗʰ Z85.04 Personal history of malignant neoplasm of rectum, rectosigmoid junction, and anus

Z85.040 Personal history of malignant carcinoid tumor of rectum
Conditions classifiable to C7A.026

Z85.048 Personal history of other malignant neoplasm of rectum, rectosigmoid junction, and anus
Conditions classifiable to C19-C21

Z85.05 Personal history of malignant neoplasm of liver
Conditions classifiable to C22

✓6ᵗʰ Z85.06 Personal history of malignant neoplasm of small intestine

Z85.060 Personal history of malignant carcinoid tumor of small intestine
Conditions classifiable to C7A.01-

Z85.068 Personal history of other malignant neoplasm of small intestine
Conditions classifiable to C17

Z85.07 Personal history of malignant neoplasm of pancreas
Conditions classifiable to C25

Z85.09 Personal history of malignant neoplasm of other digestive organs

✓5ᵗʰ Z85.1 Personal history of malignant neoplasm of trachea, bronchus and lung

✓6ᵗʰ Z85.11 Personal history of malignant neoplasm of bronchus and lung

Z85.110 Personal history of malignant carcinoid tumor of bronchus and lung
Conditions classifiable to C7A.090

Z85.118 Personal history of other malignant neoplasm of bronchus and lung
Conditions classifiable to C34

Z85.12 Personal history of malignant neoplasm of trachea
Conditions classifiable to C33

✓5ᵗʰ Z85.2 Personal history of malignant neoplasm of other respiratory and intrathoracic organs

Z85.20 Personal history of malignant neoplasm of unspecified respiratory organ

Z85.21 Personal history of malignant neoplasm of larynx
Conditions classifiable to C32

Z85.22 Personal history of malignant neoplasm of nasal cavities, middle ear, and accessory sinuses
Conditions classifiable to C30-C31

✓6ᵗʰ Z85.23 Personal history of malignant neoplasm of thymus

Z85.230 Personal history of malignant carcinoid tumor of thymus
Conditions classifiable to C7A.091

Z85.238 Personal history of other malignant neoplasm of thymus
Conditions classifiable to C37

Z85.29 Personal history of malignant neoplasm of other respiratory and intrathoracic organs

Z85.3 Personal history of malignant neoplasm of breast
Conditions classifiable to C50.-

✓5ᵗʰ Z85.4 Personal history of malignant neoplasm of genital organs
Conditions classifiable to C51-C63

Z85.40 Personal history of malignant neoplasm of unspecified female genital organ ♀

Z85.41 Personal history of malignant neoplasm of cervix uteri ♀

Z85.42 Personal history of malignant neoplasm of other parts of uterus ♀

Z85.43 Personal history of malignant neoplasm of ovary ♀

Z85.44 Personal history of malignant neoplasm of other female genital organs ♀

Z85.45 Personal history of malignant neoplasm of unspecified male genital organ ♂

Z85.46 Personal history of malignant neoplasm of prostate ♂

Z85.47 Personal history of malignant neoplasm of testis ♂

Z85.48 Personal history of malignant neoplasm of epididymis ♂

Z85.49 Personal history of malignant neoplasm of other male genital organs ♂

✓5ᵗʰ Z85.5 Personal history of malignant neoplasm of urinary tract
Conditions classifiable to C64-C68

Z85.50 Personal history of malignant neoplasm of unspecified urinary tract organ

Z85.51 Personal history of malignant neoplasm of bladder

✓6ᵗʰ Z85.52 Personal history of malignant neoplasm of kidney
EXCLUDES 1 *personal history of malignant neoplasm of renal pelvis (Z85.53)*

Z85.520 Personal history of malignant carcinoid tumor of kidney
Conditions classifiable to C7A.093

Z85.528 Personal history of other malignant neoplasm of kidney
Conditions classifiable to C64

Z85.53 Personal history of malignant neoplasm of renal pelvis

Z85.54 Personal history of malignant neoplasm of ureter

Z85.59 Personal history of malignant neoplasm of other urinary tract organ

Z85.6 Personal history of leukemia
Conditions classifiable to C91-C95
EXCLUDES 1 *leukemia in remission C91.0-C95.9 with 5th character 1*

Ⓝ Newborn: 0   Ⓟ Pediatric: 0-17   Ⓜ Maternity: 12-55   Ⓐ Adult: 15-124   MCC Major Complication/Comorbidity   CC Complication/Comorbidity   SW Severe Wound Dx

1244   ICD-10-CM 2019

☑5ᵗʰ **Z85.7** **Personal history of other malignant neoplasms of lymphoid, hematopoietic and related tissues**

   Z85.71 **Personal history of** Hodgkin lymphoma
     Conditions classifiable to C81

   Z85.72 **Personal history of** non-Hodgkin lymphomas
     Conditions classifiable to C82-C85

   Z85.79 **Personal history of** other **malignant neoplasms of lymphoid, hematopoietic and related tissues**
     Conditions classifiable to C88-C90, C96
     EXCLUDES 1 *multiple myeloma in remission (C90.01)*
        plasma cell leukemia in remission (C90.11)
        plasmacytoma in remission (C90.21)

☑5ᵗʰ **Z85.8** **Personal history of malignant neoplasms of other organs and systems**
     Conditions classifiable to C00-C14, C40-C49, C69-C75, C7A.098, C76-C79

  ☑6ᵗʰ **Z85.81** **Personal history of malignant neoplasm of** lip, oral cavity, and pharynx

    Z85.810 **Personal history of malignant neoplasm of** tongue

    Z85.818 **Personal history of malignant neoplasm of** other **sites of** lip, oral cavity, and pharynx

    Z85.819 **Personal history of malignant neoplasm of** unspecified **site of** lip, oral cavity, and pharynx

  ☑6ᵗʰ **Z85.82** **Personal history of malignant neoplasm of** skin

    Z85.820 **Personal history of malignant** melanoma **of skin**
      Conditions classifiable to C43

    Z85.821 **Personal history of** Merkel cell carcinoma
      Conditions classifiable to C4A

    Z85.828 **Personal history of** other **malignant neoplasm of skin**
      Conditions classifiable to C44

  ☑6ᵗʰ **Z85.83** **Personal history of malignant neoplasm of** bone and soft tissue

    Z85.830 **Personal history of malignant neoplasm of** bone

    Z85.831 **Personal history of malignant neoplasm of** soft tissue
      EXCLUDES 2 *personal history of malignant neoplasm of skin (Z85.82-)*

  ☑6ᵗʰ **Z85.84** **Personal history of malignant neoplasm of** eye and nervous tissue

    Z85.840 **Personal history of malignant neoplasm of** eye

    Z85.841 **Personal history of malignant neoplasm of** brain

    Z85.848 **Personal history of malignant neoplasm of** other **parts of nervous tissue**

  ☑6ᵗʰ **Z85.85** **Personal history of malignant neoplasm of** endocrine glands

    Z85.850 **Personal history of malignant neoplasm of** thyroid

    Z85.858 **Personal history of malignant neoplasm of** other **endocrine glands**

   Z85.89 **Personal history of malignant neoplasm of** other **organs and systems**

 Z85.9 **Personal history of malignant neoplasm,** unspecified
     Conditions classifiable to C7A.00, C80.1

☑4ᵗʰ **Z86** **Personal history of certain other diseases**
    Code first any follow-up examination after treatment (Z09)

☑5ᵗʰ **Z86.0** **Personal history of in-situ and benign neoplasms and neoplasms of uncertain behavior**
    EXCLUDES 2 *personal history of malignant neoplasms (Z85.-)*
    AHA: 2017, 1Q, 9

  ☑6ᵗʰ **Z86.00** **Personal history of** in-situ neoplasm
      Conditions classifiable to D00-D09

    Z86.000 **Personal history of in-situ neoplasm of** breast

    Z86.001 **Personal history of in-situ neoplasm of** ♀ cervix uteri
      Personal history of cervical intraepithelial neoplasia III [CIN III]

    Z86.008 **Personal history of in-situ neoplasm of** other **site**
      Personal history of vaginal intraepithelial neoplasia III [VAIN III]
      Personal history of vulvar intraepithelial neoplasia III [VIN III]

  ☑6ᵗʰ **Z86.01** **Personal history of** benign neoplasm

    Z86.010 **Personal history of** colonic polyps
      AHA: 2017, 1Q, 14

    Z86.011 **Personal history of benign neoplasm of the** brain

    Z86.012 **Personal history of benign** carcinoid tumor

    Z86.018 **Personal history of** other **benign neoplasm**
      AHA: 2017, 1Q, 14

  Z86.03 **Personal history of** neoplasm of uncertain behavior

☑5ᵗʰ **Z86.1** **Personal history of** infectious and parasitic diseases
    Conditions classifiable to A00-B89, B99
    EXCLUDES 1 *personal history of infectious diseases specific to a body system*
        sequelae of infectious and parasitic diseases (B90-B94)

  Z86.11 **Personal history of** tuberculosis

  Z86.12 **Personal history of** poliomyelitis

  Z86.13 **Personal history of** malaria

  Z86.14 **Personal history of** Methicillin resistant Staphylococcus aureus **infection**
     Personal history of MRSA infection

  Z86.19 **Personal history of** other **infectious and parasitic diseases**

Z86.2 **Personal history of diseases of the** blood and blood-forming organs **and certain disorders involving the** immune mechanism
    Conditions classifiable to D50-D89

☑5ᵗʰ **Z86.3** **Personal history of** endocrine, nutritional and metabolic diseases
    Conditions classifiable to E00-E88

  Z86.31 **Personal history of** diabetic foot ulcer
     EXCLUDES 2 *current diabetic foot ulcer (E08.621, E09.621, E10.621, E11.621, E13.621)*

  Z86.32 **Personal history of** gestational diabetes   ♀
     Personal history of conditions classifiable to O24.4-
     EXCLUDES 1 *gestational diabetes mellitus in current pregnancy (O24.4-)*

  Z86.39 **Personal history of** other **endocrine, nutritional and metabolic disease**

☑5ᵗʰ **Z86.5** **Personal history of** mental and behavioral disorders
    Conditions classifiable to F40-F59

  Z86.51 **Personal history of** combat and operational stress reaction   Ⓐ

  Z86.59 **Personal history of** other **mental and behavioral disorders**

☑5ᵗʰ **Z86.6** **Personal history of diseases of the** nervous system and sense organs
    Conditions classifiable to G00-G99, H00-H95
    EXCLUDES 2 *personal history of anaphylactic shock (Z87.892)*

  Z86.61 **Personal history of** infections of the central nervous system
     Personal history of encephalitis
     Personal history of meningitis

  Z86.69 **Personal history of** other **diseases of the nervous system and sense organs**
     AHA: 2016, 4Q, 24

☑5ᵗʰ **Z86.7** **Personal history of diseases of the** circulatory system
    Conditions classifiable to I00-I99
    EXCLUDES 2 *old myocardial infarction (I25.2)*
        personal history of anaphylactic shock (Z87.892)
        postmyocardial infarction syndrome (I24.1)

  ☑6ᵗʰ **Z86.71** **Personal history of** venous thrombosis and embolism

    Z86.711 **Personal history of** pulmonary **embolism**

    Z86.718 **Personal history of** other **venous thrombosis and embolism**

  Z86.72 **Personal history of** thrombophlebitis

☑ Additional Character Required   ✓x7ᵗʰ Placeholder   Unacceptable PDx   Questionable PDx   Manifestation   H1 - H14 HAC   HCC CMS-HCC Dx   HIV HIV Dx

ICD-10-CM 2019   **1245**

Z86.73 **Personal history of** transient ischemic attack **(TIA), and cerebral infarction without residual deficits**
Personal history of prolonged reversible ischemic neurological deficit (PRIND)
Personal history of stroke NOS without residual deficits
EXCLUDES 1 *personal history of traumatic brain injury (Z87.820)*
sequelae of cerebrovascular disease (I69.-)
AHA: 2012, 4Q, 92

Z86.74 **Personal history of** sudden cardiac arrest
Personal history of sudden cardiac death successfully resuscitated

Z86.79 **Personal history of** other **diseases of the circulatory system**

✓4ᵗʰ **Z87** **Personal history of other diseases and conditions**
Code first any follow-up examination after treatment (Z09)

✓5ᵗʰ **Z87.0** **Personal history of diseases of the** respiratory system
Conditions classifiable to J00-J99

Z87.01 **Personal history of** pneumonia (recurrent)

Z87.09 **Personal history of** other **diseases of the respiratory system**

✓5ᵗʰ **Z87.1** **Personal history of diseases of the** digestive system
Conditions classifiable to K00-K93

Z87.11 **Personal history of** peptic ulcer **disease**

Z87.19 **Personal history of** other **diseases of the digestive system**
AHA: 2017, 1Q, 14

Z87.2 **Personal history of diseases of the** skin and subcutaneous tissue
Conditions classifiable to L00-L99
EXCLUDES 2 *personal history of diabetic foot ulcer (Z86.31)*

✓5ᵗʰ **Z87.3** **Personal history of diseases of the** musculoskeletal system and connective tissue
Conditions classifiable to M00-M99
EXCLUDES 2 *personal history of (healed) traumatic fracture (Z87.81)*

✓6ᵗʰ **Z87.31** **Personal history of (healed)** nontraumatic fracture

Z87.310 **Personal history of (healed)** osteoporosis fracture
Personal history of (healed) fragility fracture
Personal history of (healed) collapsed vertebra due to osteoporosis
TIP: Assign for history of osteoporosis fractures that have resolved, even when a code from category M80 indicating current osteoporosis fracture is also listed.

Z87.311 **Personal history of (healed)** other **pathological fracture**
Personal history of (healed) collapsed vertebra NOS
EXCLUDES 2 *personal history of osteoporosis fracture (Z87.310)*

Z87.312 **Personal history of (healed)** stress **fracture**
Personal history of (healed) fatigue fracture

Z87.39 **Personal history of** other **diseases of the musculoskeletal system and connective tissue**

✓5ᵗʰ **Z87.4** **Personal history of diseases of** genitourinary system
Conditions classifiable to N00-N99

✓6ᵗʰ **Z87.41** **Personal history of** dysplasia of the female genital tract
EXCLUDES 1 *personal history of intraepithelial neoplasia III of female genital tract (Z86.001, Z86.008)*
personal history of malignant neoplasm of female genital tract (Z85.40-Z85.44)

Z87.410 **Personal history of** cervical **dysplasia** ♀
Z87.411 **Personal history of** vaginal **dysplasia** ♀
Z87.412 **Personal history of** vulvar **dysplasia** ♀

Z87.42 **Personal history of** other **diseases of the** female **genital tract** ♀

✓6ᵗʰ **Z87.43** **Personal history of diseases of the** male genital organs

Z87.430 **Personal history of** prostatic **dysplasia** ♂
EXCLUDES 1 *personal history of malignant neoplasm of prostate (Z85.46)*

Z87.438 **Personal history of** other **diseases of** male **genital organs** ♂

✓6ᵗʰ **Z87.44** **Personal history of diseases of the** urinary system
EXCLUDES 1 *personal history of malignant neoplasm of cervix uteri (Z85.41)*

Z87.440 **Personal history of urinary (tract) infections**

Z87.441 **Personal history of** nephrotic syndrome

Z87.442 **Personal history of** urinary calculi
Personal history of kidney stones

Z87.448 **Personal history of** other **diseases of urinary system**

✓5ᵗʰ **Z87.5** **Personal history of complications of** pregnancy, childbirth and the puerperium
Conditions classifiable to O00-O9A
EXCLUDES 2 *recurrent pregnancy loss (N96)*

Z87.51 **Personal history of** pre-term labor ♀
EXCLUDES 1 *current pregnancy with history of pre-term labor (O09.21-)*

Z87.59 **Personal history of** other **complications of pregnancy, childbirth and the puerperium** ♀
Personal history of trophoblastic disease

✓5ᵗʰ **Z87.7** **Personal history of (corrected)** congenital malformations
Conditions classifiable to Q00-Q89 that have been repaired or corrected
EXCLUDES 1 *congenital malformations that have been partially corrected or repaired but which still require medical treatment—code to condition*
EXCLUDES 2 *other postprocedural states (Z98.-)*
personal history of medical treatment (Z92.-)
presence of cardiac and vascular implants and grafts (Z95.-)
presence of other devices (Z97.-)
presence of other functional implants (Z96.-)
transplanted organ and tissue status (Z94.-)

✓6ᵗʰ **Z87.71** **Personal history of (corrected) congenital malformations of** genitourinary system

Z87.710 **Personal history of (corrected) hypospadias** ♂

Z87.718 **Personal history of** other **specified (corrected) congenital malformations of genitourinary system**

✓6ᵗʰ **Z87.72** **Personal history of (corrected) congenital malformations of** nervous system and sense organs

Z87.720 **Personal history of (corrected) congenital malformations of** eye

Z87.721 **Personal history of (corrected) congenital malformations of** ear

Z87.728 **Personal history of** other **specified (corrected) congenital malformations of nervous system and sense organs**

✓6ᵗʰ **Z87.73** **Personal history of (corrected) congenital malformations of** digestive system

Z87.730 **Personal history of (corrected)** cleft lip and palate

Z87.738 **Personal history of** other **specified (corrected) congenital malformations of digestive system**

Z87.74 **Personal history of (corrected) congenital malformations of** heart and circulatory system

Z87.75 **Personal history of (corrected) congenital malformations of** respiratory system

Z87.76 **Personal history of (corrected) congenital malformations of** integument, limbs and musculoskeletal system

✓6ᵗʰ **Z87.79** **Personal history of** other **(corrected) congenital malformations**

Z87.790 **Personal history of (corrected) congenital malformations of** face and neck

Z87.798 **Personal history of** other **(corrected) congenital malformations**

✓5ᵗʰ **Z87.8** **Personal history of other specified conditions**
EXCLUDES 2 *personal history of self harm (Z91.5)*

Z87.81 **Personal history of (healed)** traumatic fracture
EXCLUDES 2 *personal history of (healed) nontraumatic fracture (Z87.31-)*

| N Newborn: 0 | P Pediatric: 0-17 | M Maternity: 12-55 | A Adult: 15-124 | MCC Major Complication/Comorbidity | CC Complication/Comorbidity | SW Severe Wound Dx |

1246　　　ICD-10-CM 2019

✓6ᵗʰ Z87.82 **Personal history of other (healed)** physical injury and trauma
    Conditions classifiable to S00-T88, except traumatic fractures

Z87.820 **Personal history of traumatic** brain injury
    EXCLUDES 1 *personal history of transient ischemic attack (TIA), and cerebral infarction without residual deficits (Z86.73)*

Z87.821 **Personal history of** retained foreign body fully removed

Z87.828 **Personal history of** other (healed) physical injury and trauma

✓6ᵗʰ Z87.89 **Personal history of** other specified conditions

Z87.890 **Personal history of** sex reassignment

Z87.891 **Personal history of** nicotine dependence
    EXCLUDES 1 *current nicotine dependence (F17.2-)*
    AHA: 2017, 2Q, 27

Z87.892 **Personal history of** anaphylaxis
    Code also allergy status such as:
        allergy status to drugs, medicaments and biological substances (Z88.-)
        allergy status, other than to drugs and biological substances (Z91.0-)

Z87.898 **Personal history of** other specified conditions
    AHA: 2013, 1Q, 21

✓4ᵗʰ Z88 **Allergy status to drugs, medicaments and biological substances**
    EXCLUDES 2 *allergy status, other than to drugs and biological substances (Z91.0-)*
    AHA: 2015, 3Q, 23

Z88.0 **Allergy status to** penicillin

Z88.1 **Allergy status to** other antibiotic agents status

Z88.2 **Allergy status to** sulfonamides status

Z88.3 **Allergy status to** other anti-infective agents status

Z88.4 **Allergy status to** anesthetic agent status

Z88.5 **Allergy status to** narcotic agent status

Z88.6 **Allergy status to** analgesic agent status

Z88.7 **Allergy status to** serum and vaccine status

Z88.8 **Allergy status to** other drugs, medicaments and biological substances status

Z88.9 **Allergy status to** unspecified drugs, medicaments and biological substances status

✓4ᵗʰ Z89 **Acquired absence of limb**
    INCLUDES amputation status
        postprocedural loss of limb
        post-traumatic loss of limb
    EXCLUDES 1 *acquired deformities of limbs (M20-M21)*
        congenital absence of limbs (Q71-Q73)

✓5ᵗʰ Z89.0 **Acquired absence of** thumb and other finger(s)

✓6ᵗʰ Z89.01 **Acquired absence of** thumb

Z89.011 **Acquired absence of** right thumb

Z89.012 **Acquired absence of** left thumb

Z89.019 **Acquired absence of** unspecified thumb

✓6ᵗʰ Z89.02 **Acquired absence of** other finger(s)
    EXCLUDES 2 *acquired absence of thumb (Z89.01-)*

Z89.021 **Acquired absence of** right finger(s)

Z89.022 **Acquired absence of** left finger(s)

Z89.029 **Acquired absence of** unspecified finger(s)

✓5ᵗʰ Z89.1 **Acquired absence of** hand and wrist

✓6ᵗʰ Z89.11 **Acquired absence of** hand

Z89.111 **Acquired absence of** right hand

Z89.112 **Acquired absence of** left hand

Z89.119 **Acquired absence of** unspecified hand

✓6ᵗʰ Z89.12 **Acquired absence of** wrist
    Disarticulation at wrist

Z89.121 **Acquired absence of** right wrist

Z89.122 **Acquired absence of** left wrist

Z89.129 **Acquired absence of** unspecified wrist

✓5ᵗʰ Z89.2 **Acquired absence of** upper limb above wrist

✓6ᵗʰ Z89.20 **Acquired absence of** upper limb, unspecified level

Z89.201 **Acquired absence of** right upper limb, unspecified level

Z89.202 **Acquired absence of** left upper limb, unspecified level

Z89.209 **Acquired absence of** unspecified upper limb, unspecified level
    Acquired absence of arm NOS

✓6ᵗʰ Z89.21 **Acquired absence of** upper limb below elbow

Z89.211 **Acquired absence of** right upper limb below elbow

Z89.212 **Acquired absence of** left upper limb below elbow

Z89.219 **Acquired absence of** unspecified upper limb below elbow

✓6ᵗʰ Z89.22 **Acquired absence of** upper limb above elbow
    Disarticulation at elbow

Z89.221 **Acquired absence of** right upper limb above elbow

Z89.222 **Acquired absence of** left upper limb above elbow

Z89.229 **Acquired absence of** unspecified upper limb above elbow

✓6ᵗʰ Z89.23 **Acquired absence of** shoulder
    Acquired absence of shoulder joint following explantation of shoulder joint prosthesis, with or without presence of antibiotic-impregnated cement spacer

Z89.231 **Acquired absence of** right shoulder

Z89.232 **Acquired absence of** left shoulder

Z89.239 **Acquired absence of** unspecified shoulder

✓5ᵗʰ Z89.4 **Acquired absence of** toe(s), foot, and ankle

✓6ᵗʰ Z89.41 **Acquired absence of** great toe

Z89.411 **Acquired absence of** right great toe   **HCC**

Z89.412 **Acquired absence of** left great toe   **HCC**

Z89.419 **Acquired absence of** unspecified great toe   **HCC**

✓6ᵗʰ Z89.42 **Acquired absence of** other toe(s)
    EXCLUDES 2 *acquired absence of great toe (Z89.41-)*

Z89.421 **Acquired absence of** other right toe(s)   **HCC**

Z89.422 **Acquired absence of** other left toe(s)   **HCC**

Z89.429 **Acquired absence of** other toe(s), unspecified side   **HCC**

✓6ᵗʰ Z89.43 **Acquired absence of** foot

Z89.431 **Acquired absence of** right foot   **HCC**

Z89.432 **Acquired absence of** left foot   **HCC**

Z89.439 **Acquired absence of** unspecified foot   **HCC**

✓6ᵗʰ Z89.44 **Acquired absence of** ankle
    Disarticulation of ankle

Z89.441 **Acquired absence of** right ankle   **HCC**

Z89.442 **Acquired absence of** left ankle   **HCC**

Z89.449 **Acquired absence of** unspecified ankle   **HCC**

✓5ᵗʰ Z89.5 **Acquired absence of** leg below knee

✓6ᵗʰ Z89.51 **Acquired absence of** leg below knee

Z89.511 **Acquired absence of** right leg below knee   **HCC**

Z89.512 **Acquired absence of** left leg below knee   **HCC**

Z89.519 **Acquired absence of** unspecified leg below knee   **HCC**

✓6ᵗʰ Z89.52 **Acquired absence of** knee
    Acquired absence of knee joint following explantation of knee joint prosthesis, with or without presence of antibiotic-impregnated cement spacer

Z89.521 **Acquired absence of** right knee

Z89.522 **Acquired absence of** left knee

Z89.529 **Acquired absence of** unspecified knee

✓5ᵗʰ Z89.6 **Acquired absence of** leg above knee

✓6ᵗʰ Z89.61 **Acquired absence of** leg above knee
    Acquired absence of leg NOS
    Disarticulation at knee

Z89.611 **Acquired absence of** right leg above knee   **HCC**

Z89.612 **Acquired absence of** left leg above knee   **HCC**

Z89.619 **Acquired absence of** unspecified leg above knee   **HCC**

✓ Additional Character Required   **✓x7ᵗʰ** Placeholder   Unacceptable PDx   Questionable PDx   Manifestation   **H1 - H14** HAC   **HCC** CMS-HCC Dx   **HIV** HIV Dx

ICD-10-CM 2019   **1247**

✓6ᵗʰ **Z89.62** **Acquired absence of** hip
Acquired absence of hip joint following explantation of hip joint prosthesis, with or without presence of antibiotic-impregnated cement spacer
Disarticulation at hip

     Z89.621 **Acquired absence of** right **hip joint**

     Z89.622 **Acquired absence of** left **hip joint**

     Z89.629 **Acquired absence of** unspecified **hip joint**

Z89.9 **Acquired absence of limb,** unspecified

✓4ᵗʰ **Z90** **Acquired absence of organs, not elsewhere classified**
   INCLUDES   postprocedural or post-traumatic loss of body part NEC
   EXCLUDES 1   congenital absence—see Alphabetical Index
   EXCLUDES 2   postprocedural absence of endocrine glands (E89.-)

✓5ᵗʰ **Z90.0** **Acquired absence of part of** head and neck

     Z90.01 **Acquired absence of** eye

     Z90.02 **Acquired absence of** larynx

     Z90.09 **Acquired absence of** other **part of head and neck**
       Acquired absence of nose
       EXCLUDES 2   teeth (K08.1)

✓5ᵗʰ **Z90.1** **Acquired absence of** breast and nipple

     Z90.10 **Acquired absence of** unspecified **breast and nipple**

     Z90.11 **Acquired absence of** right **breast and nipple**

     Z90.12 **Acquired absence of** left **breast and nipple**

     Z90.13 **Acquired absence of** bilateral **breasts and nipples**

Z90.2 **Acquired absence of** lung [part of]

Z90.3 **Acquired absence of** stomach [part of]

✓5ᵗʰ **Z90.4** **Acquired absence of** other **specified parts of digestive tract**

   ✓6ᵗʰ **Z90.41** **Acquired absence of** pancreas
       Code also exocrine pancreatic insufficiency (K86.81)
       Use additional code to identify any associated:
         insulin use (Z79.4)
         diabetes mellitus, postpancreatectomy (E13.-)

     Z90.410 **Acquired** total absence **of pancreas**
       Acquired absence of pancreas NOS

     Z90.411 **Acquired** partial absence **of pancreas**

     Z90.49 **Acquired absence of** other **specified parts of digestive tract**

Z90.5 **Acquired absence of** kidney

Z90.6 **Acquired absence of** other parts of urinary tract
   Acquired absence of bladder

✓5ᵗʰ **Z90.7** **Acquired absence of** genital organ(s)
   EXCLUDES 1   personal history of sex reassignment (Z87.890)
   EXCLUDES 2   female genital mutilation status (N90.81-)

   ✓6ᵗʰ **Z90.71** **Acquired absence of** cervix and uterus

     Z90.710 **Acquired absence of** both cervix and uterus   ♀
       Acquired absence of uterus NOS
       Status post total hysterectomy

     Z90.711 **Acquired absence of uterus** with remaining cervical stump   ♀
       Status post partial hysterectomy with remaining cervical stump

     Z90.712 **Acquired absence of cervix with** remaining uterus   ♀

   ✓6ᵗʰ **Z90.72** **Acquired absence of** ovaries

     Z90.721 **Acquired absence of ovaries,** unilateral   ♀

     Z90.722 **Acquired absence of ovaries,** bilateral   ♀

     Z90.79 **Acquired absence of** other **genital organ(s)**

✓5ᵗʰ **Z90.8** **Acquired absence of** other **organs**

     Z90.81 **Acquired absence of** spleen

     Z90.89 **Acquired absence of** other **organs**

✓4ᵗʰ **Z91** **Personal risk factors, not elsewhere classified**
   EXCLUDES 2   contact with and (suspected) exposures hazardous to health (Z77.-)
       exposure to pollution and other problems related to physical environment (Z77.1-)
       female genital mutilation status (N90.81-)
       personal history of physical injury and trauma (Z87.81, Z87.82-)
       occupational exposure to risk factors (Z57.-)

✓5ᵗʰ **Z91.0** **Allergy status, other than to drugs and biological substances**
   EXCLUDES 2   allergy status to drugs, medicaments, and biological substances (Z88.-)

   ✓6ᵗʰ **Z91.01** **Food allergy status**
     EXCLUDES 2   food additives allergy status (Z91.02)

     Z91.010 **Allergy to** peanuts

     Z91.011 **Allergy to** milk products
       EXCLUDES 1   lactose intolerance (E73.-)

     Z91.012 **Allergy to** eggs

     Z91.013 **Allergy to** seafood
       Allergy to shellfish
       Allergy to octopus or squid ink

     Z91.018 **Allergy to** other **foods**
       Allergy to nuts other than peanuts

   Z91.02 **Food additives allergy status**

   ✓6ᵗʰ **Z91.03** **Insect allergy status**

     Z91.030 **Bee allergy status**

     Z91.038 **Other insect allergy status**

   ✓6ᵗʰ **Z91.04** **Nonmedicinal substance allergy status**

     Z91.040 **Latex allergy status**
       Latex sensitivity status

     Z91.041 **Radiographic dye allergy status**
       Allergy status to contrast media used for diagnostic X-ray procedure

     Z91.048 **Other nonmedicinal substance allergy status**

   Z91.09 **Other allergy status, other than to drugs and biological substances**

✓5ᵗʰ **Z91.1** **Patient's noncompliance with medical treatment and regimen**

   Z91.11 **Patient's noncompliance with** dietary regimen

   ✓6ᵗʰ **Z91.12** **Patient's** intentional underdosing of medication regimen
     Code first underdosing of medication (T36-T50) with fifth or sixth character 6
     EXCLUDES 1   adverse effect of prescribed drug taken as directed—code to adverse effect
       poisoning (overdose)—code to poisoning

     Z91.120 **Patient's intentional underdosing of medication regimen due to** financial hardship

     Z91.128 **Patient's intentional underdosing of medication regimen for** other reason

   ✓6ᵗʰ **Z91.13** **Patient's** unintentional underdosing of medication regimen
     Code first underdosing of medication (T36-T50) with fifth or sixth character 6
     EXCLUDES 1   adverse effect of prescribed drug taken as directed—code to adverse effect
       poisoning (overdose)—code to poisoning

     Z91.130 **Patient's unintentional underdosing of medication regimen due to** age-related debility

     Z91.138 **Patient's unintentional underdosing of medication regimen for** other reason

   Z91.14 **Patient's** other **noncompliance with medication regimen**
     Patient's underdosing of medication NOS

   Z91.15 **Patient's noncompliance with** renal dialysis   HCC

   Z91.19 **Patient's noncompliance with** other **medical treatment and regimen**
     Nonadherence to medical treatment

✓5ᵗʰ **Z91.4** **Personal history of psychological trauma, not elsewhere classified**

   ✓6ᵗʰ **Z91.41** **Personal history of** adult abuse
     EXCLUDES 2   personal history of abuse in childhood (Z62.81-)

     Z91.410 **Personal history of adult** physical and sexual **abuse**   A
       EXCLUDES 1   current adult physical abuse (T74.11, T76.11)
         current adult sexual abuse (T74.21, T76.11)

     Z91.411 **Personal history of adult** psychological **abuse**   A

     Z91.412 **Personal history of** adult neglect   A
       EXCLUDES 1   current adult neglect (T74.01, T76.01)

     Z91.419 **Personal history of** unspecified **adult abuse**   A

●   **Z91.42** **Personal history of** forced labor **or** sexual exploitation

   Z91.49 **Other personal history of psychological trauma, not elsewhere classified**

N Newborn: 0   P Pediatric: 0-17   M Maternity: 12-55   A Adult: 15-124   MCC Major Complication/Comorbidity   CC Complication/Comorbidity   SW Severe Wound Dx

1248   ICD-10-CM 2019

Z91.5   **Personal history of self-harm**
Personal history of parasuicide
Personal history of self-poisoning
Personal history of suicide attempt

✓5ᵗʰ **Z91.8**   **Other specified personal risk factors, not elsewhere classified**

     Z91.81   **History of falling**
       At risk for falling

     Z91.82   **Personal history of military deployment**   Ⓐ
       Individual (civilian or military) with past history of military war, peacekeeping and humanitarian deployment (current or past conflict)
       Returned from military deployment

     Z91.83   *Wandering in diseases classified elsewhere*
       Code first underlying disorder such as:
       Alzheimer's disease (G3Ø.-)
       autism or pervasive developmental disorder (F84.-)
       intellectual disabilities (F7Ø-F79)
       unspecified dementia with behavioral disturbance (FØ3.9-)

   ✓6ᵗʰ **Z91.84**   **Oral health risk factors**
       AHA: 2017, 4Q, 29

       Z91.841   **Risk for dental caries, low**
       Z91.842   **Risk for dental caries, moderate**
       Z91.843   **Risk for dental caries, high**
       Z91.849   **Unspecified risk for dental caries**

     Z91.89   **Other specified personal risk factors, not elsewhere classified**
       AHA: 2017, 1Q, 45

✓4ᵗʰ **Z92**   **Personal history of medical treatment**
     EXCLUDES 2   *postprocedural states (Z98.-)*

     Z92.Ø   **Personal history of contraception**
       EXCLUDES 1   *counseling or management of current contraceptive practices (Z3Ø.-)*
              long term (current) use of contraception (Z79.3)
              presence of (intrauterine) contraceptive device (Z97.5)

   ✓5ᵗʰ **Z92.2**   **Personal history of drug therapy**
       EXCLUDES 2   *long term (current) drug therapy (Z79.-)*

     Z92.21   **Personal history of antineoplastic chemotherapy**
     Z92.22   **Personal history of monoclonal drug therapy**
     Z92.23   **Personal history of estrogen therapy**
   ✓6ᵗʰ **Z92.24**   **Personal history of steroid therapy**

       Z92.24Ø   **Personal history of inhaled steroid therapy**
       Z92.241   **Personal history of systemic steroid therapy**
              Personal history of steroid therapy NOS

     Z92.25   **Personal history of immunosupression therapy**
       EXCLUDES 2   *personal history of steroid therapy (Z92.24)*

     Z92.29   **Personal history of other drug therapy**

     Z92.3   **Personal history of irradiation**
       Personal history of exposure to therapeutic radiation
       EXCLUDES 1   *exposure to radiation in the physical environment (Z77.12)*
              occupational exposure to radiation (Z57.1)

   ✓5ᵗʰ **Z92.8**   **Personal history of other medical treatment**

     Z92.81   **Personal history of extracorporeal membrane oxygenation (ECMO)**

     Z92.82   **Status post administration of tPA (rtPA) in a different facility within the last 24 hours prior to admission to current facility**
       Code first condition requiring tPA administration, such as:
       acute cerebral infarction (I63.-)
       acute myocardial infarction (I21.-, I22.-)
       AHA: 2013, 4Q, 124

     Z92.83   **Personal history of failed moderate sedation**
       Personal history of failed conscious sedation
       EXCLUDES 2   *failed moderate sedation during procedure (T88.52)*

     Z92.84   **Personal history of unintended awareness under general anesthesia**
       EXCLUDES 2   *unintended awareness under general anesthesia during procedure (T88.53)*
       AHA: 2016, 4Q, 72-73, 77

     Z92.89   **Personal history of other medical treatment**

✓4ᵗʰ **Z93**   **Artificial opening status**
     EXCLUDES 1   *artificial openings requiring attention or management (Z43.-)*
              complications of external stoma (J95.Ø-, K94.-, N99.5-)

     Z93.Ø   **Tracheostomy status**   HCC
       AHA: 2013, 4Q, 129

     Z93.1   **Gastrostomy status**   HCC
     Z93.2   **Ileostomy status**   HCC
     Z93.3   **Colostomy status**   HCC
     Z93.4   **Other artificial openings of gastrointestinal tract status**   HCC

   ✓5ᵗʰ **Z93.5**   **Cystostomy status**

     Z93.50   **Unspecified cystostomy status**   HCC
     Z93.51   **Cutaneous-vesicostomy status**   HCC
     Z93.52   **Appendico-vesicostomy status**   HCC
     Z93.59   **Other cystostomy status**   HCC

     Z93.6   **Other artificial openings of urinary tract status**   HCC
       Nephrostomy status
       Ureterostomy status
       Urethrostomy status

     Z93.8   **Other artificial opening status**   HCC
     Z93.9   **Artificial opening status, unspecified**   HCC

✓4ᵗʰ **Z94**   **Transplanted organ and tissue status**
     INCLUDES   organ or tissue replaced by heterogenous or homogenous transplant
     EXCLUDES 1   *complications of transplanted organ or tissue—see Alphabetical Index*
     EXCLUDES 2   *presence of vascular grafts (Z95.-)*

     Z94.Ø   **Kidney transplant status**   CC
       CC Excl: PDX collection 1489

     Z94.1   **Heart transplant status**   CC HCC
       EXCLUDES 1   *artificial heart status (Z95.812)*
              heart-valve replacement status (Z95.2-Z95.4)
       CC Excl: PDX collection 1488

     Z94.2   **Lung transplant status**   CC HCC
       CC Excl: PDX collection 1491

     Z94.3   **Heart and lungs transplant status**   CC HCC
       CC Excl: PDX collection 1488

     Z94.4   **Liver transplant status**   CC HCC
       CC Excl: PDX collection 149Ø

     Z94.5   **Skin transplant status**
       Autogenous skin transplant status

     Z94.6   **Bone transplant status**
     Z94.7   **Corneal transplant status**

   ✓5ᵗʰ **Z94.8**   **Other transplanted organ and tissue status**

     Z94.81   **Bone marrow transplant status**   CC HCC
       CC Excl: PDX collection 1492

     Z94.82   **Intestine transplant status**   CC HCC
       CC Excl: PDX collection 1495

     Z94.83   **Pancreas transplant status**   CC HCC
       CC Excl: PDX collection 1496

     Z94.84   **Stem cells transplant status**   CC HCC
       CC Excl: PDX collection 1497

     Z94.89   **Other transplanted organ and tissue status**
     Z94.9   **Transplanted organ and tissue status, unspecified**

✓4ᵗʰ **Z95**   **Presence of cardiac and vascular implants and grafts**
     EXCLUDES 2   *complications of cardiac and vascular devices, implants and grafts (T82.-)*

     Z95.Ø   **Presence of cardiac pacemaker**
       Presence of cardiac resynchronization therapy (CRT-P) pacemaker
       EXCLUDES 1   *adjustment or management of cardiac device (Z45.Ø-)*
              adjustment or management of cardiac pacemaker (Z45.Ø)
              presence of automatic (implantable) cardiac defibrillator with synchronous cardiac pacemaker (Z95.81Ø)

     Z95.1   **Presence of aortocoronary bypass graft**
       Presence of coronary artery bypass graft

     Z95.2   **Presence of prosthetic heart valve**
       Presence of heart valve NOS

     Z95.3   **Presence of xenogenic heart valve**
     Z95.4   **Presence of other heart-valve replacement**
     Z95.5   **Presence of coronary angioplasty implant and graft**
       EXCLUDES 1   *coronary angioplasty status without implant and graft (Z98.61)*

☑ Additional Character Required   ✓x7ᵗʰ Placeholder   Unacceptable PDx   Questionable PDx   Manifestation   H1-H14 HAC   HCC CMS-HCC Dx   HIV HIV Dx

ICD-10-CM 2019   **1249**

☑5th **Z95.8 Presence of other cardiac and vascular implants and grafts**

     ☑6th **Z95.81 Presence of** other **cardiac implants and grafts**

         Z95.810 Presence of automatic (implantable) cardiac defibrillator

             Presence of automatic (implantable) cardiac defibrillator with synchronous cardiac pacemaker

             Presence of cardiac resynchronization therapy defibrillator (CRT-D)

             ►Presence of cardioverter-defibrillator (ICD)◄

         Z95.811 Presence of heart assist device **CC HCC**

             CC Excl: PDX collection 1498

         Z95.812 Presence of fully implantable artificial heart **CC HCC**

             CC Excl: PDX collection 1498

         Z95.818 Presence of other **cardiac implants and grafts**

     ☑6th **Z95.82 Presence of other vascular implants and grafts**

         Z95.820 Peripheral vascular angioplasty status **with implants and grafts**

             EXCLUDES 1 *peripheral vascular angioplasty without implant and graft (Z98.62)*

         Z95.828 Presence of other **vascular implants and grafts**

             Presence of intravascular prosthesis NEC

     Z95.9 Presence of cardiac and vascular implant and graft, unspecified

☑4th **Z96 Presence of other functional implants**

     EXCLUDES 2 *complications of internal prosthetic devices, implants and grafts (T82-T85)*

         fitting and adjustment of prosthetic and other devices (Z44-Z46)

     Z96.0 Presence of urogenital **implants**

     Z96.1 Presence of intraocular lens

         Presence of pseudophakia

     ☑5th **Z96.2 Presence of** otological and audiological **implants**

         Z96.20 Presence of otological and audiological implant, unspecified

         Z96.21 Cochlear implant status

         Z96.22 Myringotomy tube(s) status

         Z96.29 Presence of other **otological and audiological implants**

             Presence of bone-conduction hearing device

             Presence of eustachian tube stent

             Stapes replacement

     Z96.3 Presence of artificial larynx

     ☑5th **Z96.4 Presence of** endocrine **implants**

         Z96.41 Presence of insulin pump **(external) (internal)**

         Z96.49 Presence of other **endocrine implants**

     Z96.5 Presence of tooth-root and mandibular **implants**

     ☑5th **Z96.6 Presence of** orthopedic joint **implants**

         Z96.60 Presence of unspecified **orthopedic joint implant**

     ☑6th **Z96.61 Presence of** artificial shoulder joint

         Z96.611 Presence of right **artificial shoulder joint**

         Z96.612 Presence of left **artificial shoulder joint**

         Z96.619 Presence of unspecified **artificial shoulder joint**

     ☑6th **Z96.62 Presence of** artificial elbow joint

         Z96.621 Presence of right **artificial elbow joint**

         Z96.622 Presence of left **artificial elbow joint**

         Z96.629 Presence of unspecified **artificial elbow joint**

     ☑6th **Z96.63 Presence of** artificial wrist joint

         Z96.631 Presence of right **artificial wrist joint**

         Z96.632 Presence of left **artificial wrist joint**

         Z96.639 Presence of unspecified **artificial wrist joint**

     ☑6th **Z96.64 Presence of** artificial hip joint

         Hip-joint replacement (partial) (total)

         Z96.641 Presence of right **artificial hip joint**

         Z96.642 Presence of left **artificial hip joint**

         Z96.643 Presence of artificial hip joint, bilateral

         Z96.649 Presence of unspecified **artificial hip joint**

     ☑6th **Z96.65 Presence of** artificial knee joint

         Z96.651 Presence of right **artificial knee joint**

         Z96.652 Presence of left **artificial knee joint**

         Z96.653 Presence of artificial knee joint, bilateral

         Z96.659 Presence of unspecified **artificial knee joint**

     ☑6th **Z96.66 Presence of** artificial ankle joint

         Z96.661 Presence of right **artificial ankle joint**

         Z96.662 Presence of left **artificial ankle joint**

         Z96.669 Presence of unspecified **artificial ankle joint**

     ☑6th **Z96.69 Presence of** other orthopedic joint **implants**

         Z96.691 Finger-joint replacement of right **hand**

         Z96.692 Finger-joint replacement of left **hand**

         Z96.693 Finger-joint replacement, bilateral

         Z96.698 Presence of other **orthopedic joint implants**

     Z96.7 Presence of other bone and tendon implants

         Presence of skull plate

     ☑5th **Z96.8 Presence of other specified functional implants**

         Z96.81 Presence of artificial skin

         Z96.89 Presence of other specified functional implants

     Z96.9 Presence of functional implant, unspecified

☑4th **Z97 Presence of other devices**

     EXCLUDES 1 *complications of internal prosthetic devices, implants and grafts (T82-T85)*

         fitting and adjustment of prosthetic and other devices (Z44-Z46)

     EXCLUDES 2 *presence of cerebrospinal fluid drainage device (Z98.2)*

     Z97.0 Presence of artificial eye

     ☑5th **Z97.1 Presence of** artificial limb (complete) (partial)

         Z97.10 Presence of artificial limb (complete) (partial), unspecified

         Z97.11 Presence of artificial right arm **(complete) (partial)**

         Z97.12 Presence of artificial left arm **(complete) (partial)**

         Z97.13 Presence of artificial right leg **(complete) (partial)**

         Z97.14 Presence of artificial left leg **(complete) (partial)**

         Z97.15 Presence of artificial arms, bilateral **(complete) (partial)**

         Z97.16 Presence of artificial legs, bilateral **(complete) (partial)**

     Z97.2 Presence of dental prosthetic device **(complete) (partial)**

         Presence of dentures (complete) (partial)

     Z97.3 Presence of spectacles and contact lenses

     Z97.4 Presence of external hearing-aid

     Z97.5 Presence of (intrauterine) contraceptive device   ♀

         EXCLUDES 1 *checking, reinsertion or removal of implantable subdermal contraceptive (Z30.46)*

             checking, reinsertion or removal of intrauterine contraceptive device (Z30.43-)

     Z97.8 Presence of other specified devices

☑4th **Z98 Other postprocedural states**

     EXCLUDES 2 *aftercare (Z43-Z49, Z51)*

         follow-up medical care (Z08- Z09)

         postprocedural complication—see Alphabetical Index

     Z98.0 Intestinal bypass and anastomosis status

         EXCLUDES 2 *bariatric surgery status (Z98.84)*

             gastric bypass status (Z98.84)

             obesity surgery status (Z98.84)

     Z98.1 Arthrodesis status

     Z98.2 Presence of cerebrospinal fluid drainage device

         Presence of CSF shunt

     Z98.3 Post therapeutic collapse of lung status

         Code first underlying disease

     ☑5th **Z98.4 Cataract extraction status**

         Use additional code to identify intraocular lens implant status (Z96.1)

         EXCLUDES 1 *aphakia (H27.0)*

         Z98.41 Cataract extraction status, right **eye**

         Z98.42 Cataract extraction status, left **eye**

         Z98.49 Cataract extraction status, unspecified **eye**

     ☑5th **Z98.5 Sterilization status**

         EXCLUDES 1 *female infertility (N97.-)*

             male infertility (N46.-)

         Z98.51 Tubal ligation status   ♀

         Z98.52 Vasectomy status   A ♂

N Newborn: 0   P Pediatric: 0-17   M Maternity: 12-55   A Adult: 15-124   MCC Major Complication/Comorbidity   CC Complication/Comorbidity   SW Severe Wound Dx

1250   ICD-10-CM 2019

✅5ᵗʰ **Z98.6** **Angioplasty status**

  Z98.61 **Coronary angioplasty status**
    EXCLUDES 1   *coronary angioplasty status with implant and graft (Z95.5)*

  Z98.62 **Peripheral vascular angioplasty status**
    EXCLUDES 1   *peripheral vascular angioplasty status with implant and graft (Z95.820)*

✅5ᵗʰ **Z98.8** **Other specified postprocedural states**

  ✅6ᵗʰ **Z98.81** **Dental procedure status**
    Z98.810 **Dental sealant status**
    Z98.811 **Dental restoration status**
      Dental crown status
      Dental fillings status
    Z98.818 **Other dental procedure status**

  Z98.82 **Breast implant status**
    EXCLUDES 1   *breast implant removal status (Z98.86)*

  Z98.83 **Filtering (vitreous) bleb after glaucoma surgery status**
    EXCLUDES 1   *inflammation (infection) of postprocedural bleb (H59.4-)*

  Z98.84 **Bariatric surgery status**
    Gastric banding status
    Gastric bypass status for obesity
    Obesity surgery status
    EXCLUDES 1   *bariatric surgery status complicating pregnancy, childbirth, or the puerperium (O99.84)*
    EXCLUDES 2   *intestinal bypass and anastomosis status (Z98.0)*

  Z98.85 **Transplanted organ removal status**
    Transplanted organ previously removed due to complication, failure, rejection or infection
    EXCLUDES 1   *encounter for removal of transplanted organ—code to complication of transplanted organ (T86.-)*

  Z98.86 **Personal history of breast implant removal**

  ✅6ᵗʰ **Z98.87** **Personal history of in utero procedure**
    Z98.870 **Personal history of in utero procedure during pregnancy** ♀
      EXCLUDES 2   *complications from in utero procedure for current pregnancy (O35.7)*
        supervision of current pregnancy with history of in utero procedure during previous pregnancy (O09.82-)
    Z98.871 **Personal history of in utero procedure while a fetus**

  ✅6ᵗʰ **Z98.89** **Other specified postprocedural states**
    Z98.890 **Other specified postprocedural states**
      Personal history of surgery, not elsewhere classified
    Z98.891 **History of uterine scar from previous surgery** ♀
      EXCLUDES 1   *maternal care due to uterine scar from previous surgery (O34.2-)*
      AHA: 2016, 4Q, 51-52, 76

✅4ᵗʰ **Z99** **Dependence on enabling machines and devices, not elsewhere classified**
  EXCLUDES 1   *cardiac pacemaker status (Z95.0)*

  Z99.0 **Dependence on aspirator**

  ✅5ᵗʰ **Z99.1** **Dependence on respirator**
    Dependence on ventilator
    Z99.11 **Dependence on respirator [ventilator] status** CC HCC
      AHA: 2015, 1Q, 21
      CC Excl: PDX collection 759
    Z99.12 **Encounter for respirator [ventilator] dependence during power failure** CC HCC
      EXCLUDES 1   *mechanical complication of respirator [ventilator] (J95.850)*
      CC Excl: PDX collection 759

  Z99.2 **Dependence on renal dialysis** HCC
    Hemodialysis status
    Peritoneal dialysis status
    Presence of arteriovenous shunt for dialysis
    Renal dialysis status NOS
    EXCLUDES 1   *encounter for fitting and adjustment of dialysis catheter (Z49.0-)*
    EXCLUDES 2   *noncompliance with renal dialysis (Z91.15)*
    AHA: 2016, 1Q, 12; 2013, 4Q, 125

  Z99.3 **Dependence on wheelchair**
    Wheelchair confinement status
    Code first cause of dependence, such as:
      muscular dystrophy ▶(G71.0-)◀
      obesity (E66.-)

  ✅5ᵗʰ **Z99.8** **Dependence on other enabling machines and devices**
    Z99.81 **Dependence on supplemental oxygen**
      Dependence on long-term oxygen
      AHA: 2013, 4Q, 129
    Z99.89 **Dependence on other enabling machines and devices**
      Dependence on machine or device NOS

✅ Additional Character Required   ✓x7ᵗʰ Placeholder   Unacceptable PDx   Questionable PDx   Manifestation   H1 - H14 HAC   HCC CMS-HCC Dx   HIV HIV Dx

Illustrations

Chapter 3. Diseases of the Blood and Blood-forming Organs and Certain Disorders Involving the Immune Mechanism (D5Ø–D89)

Red Blood Cells

White Blood Cell

Platelet

Coagulation

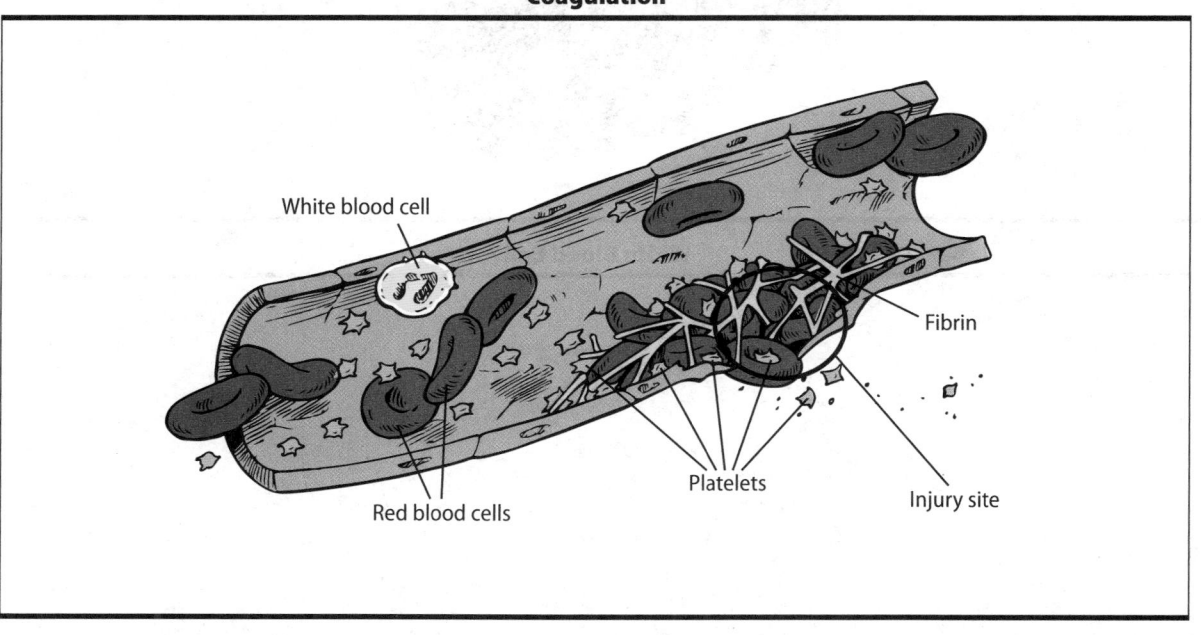

Spleen Anatomical Location and External Structures

Spleen Interior Structures

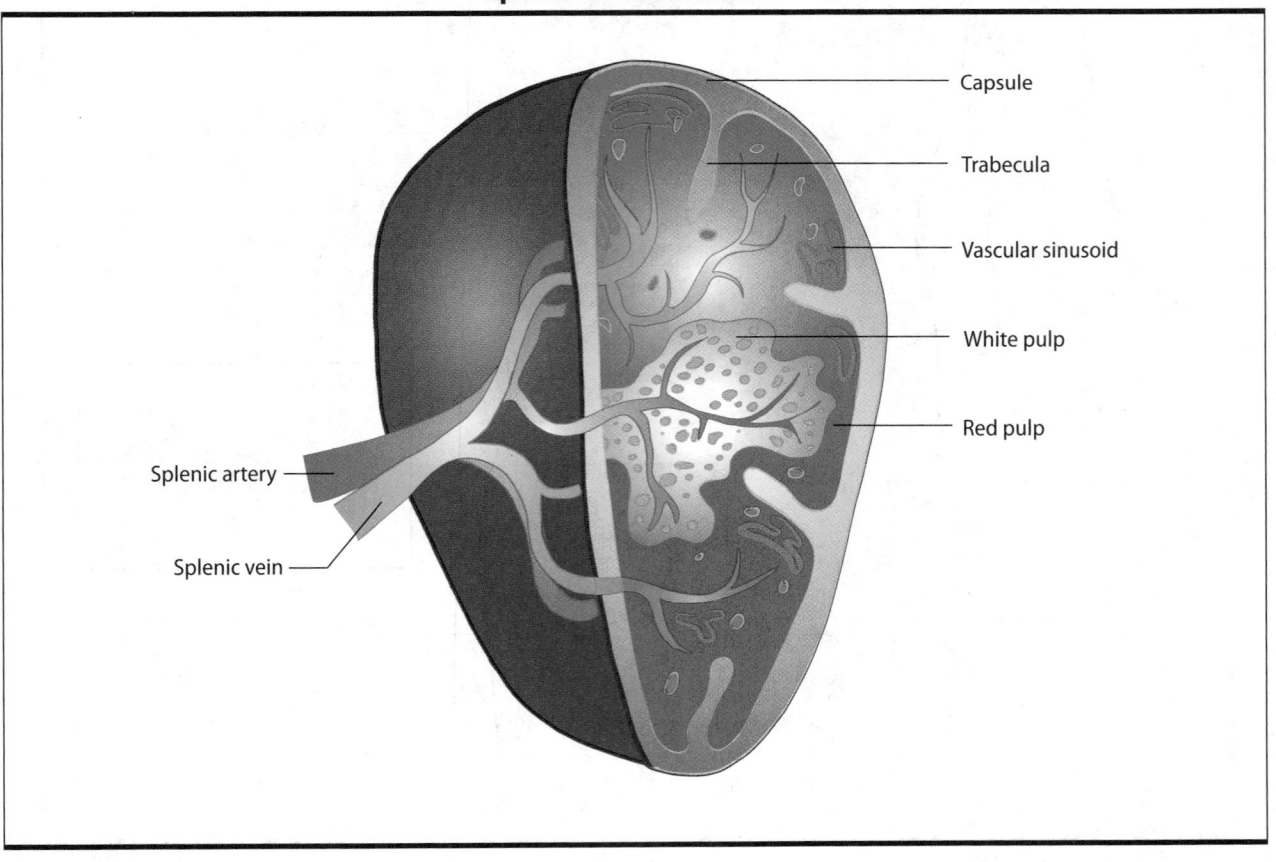

Chapter 4. Endocrine, Nutritional and Metabolic Diseases (E00–E89)

Endocrine System

Thyroid

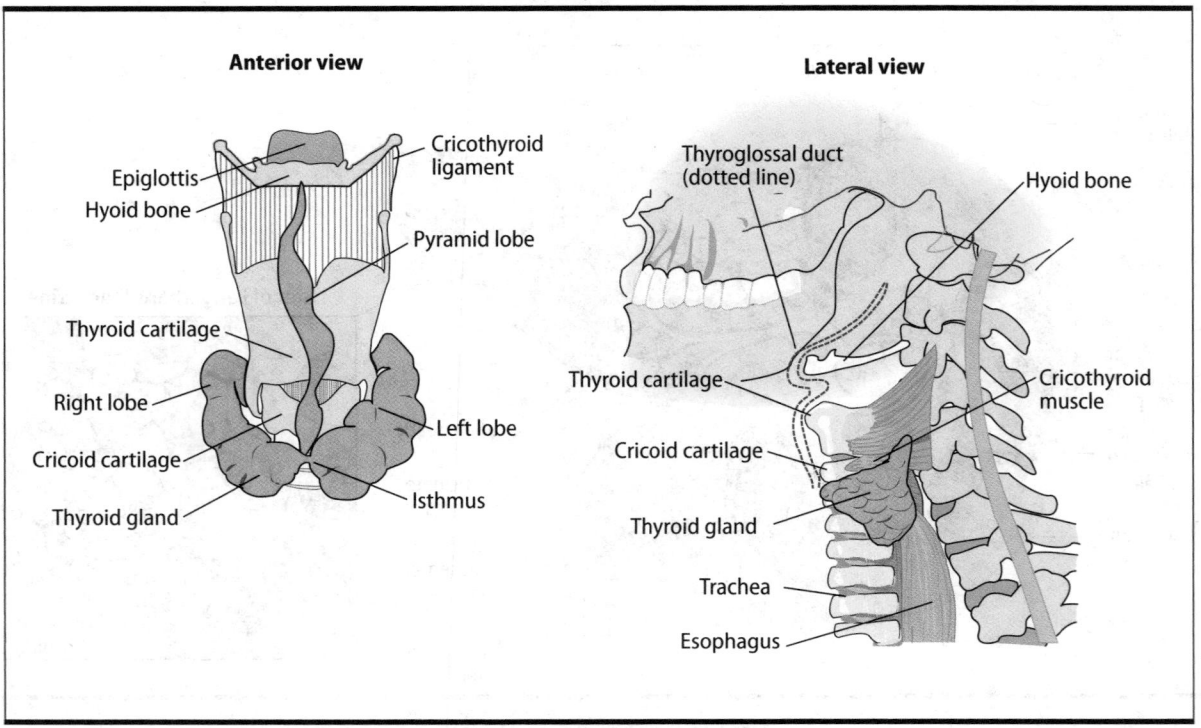

Anterior view

- Epiglottis
- Hyoid bone
- Cricothyroid ligament
- Pyramid lobe
- Thyroid cartilage
- Right lobe
- Left lobe
- Cricoid cartilage
- Isthmus
- Thyroid gland

Lateral view

- Thyroglossal duct (dotted line)
- Hyoid bone
- Thyroid cartilage
- Cricothyroid muscle
- Cricoid cartilage
- Thyroid gland
- Trachea
- Esophagus

Thyroid and Parathyroid Glands

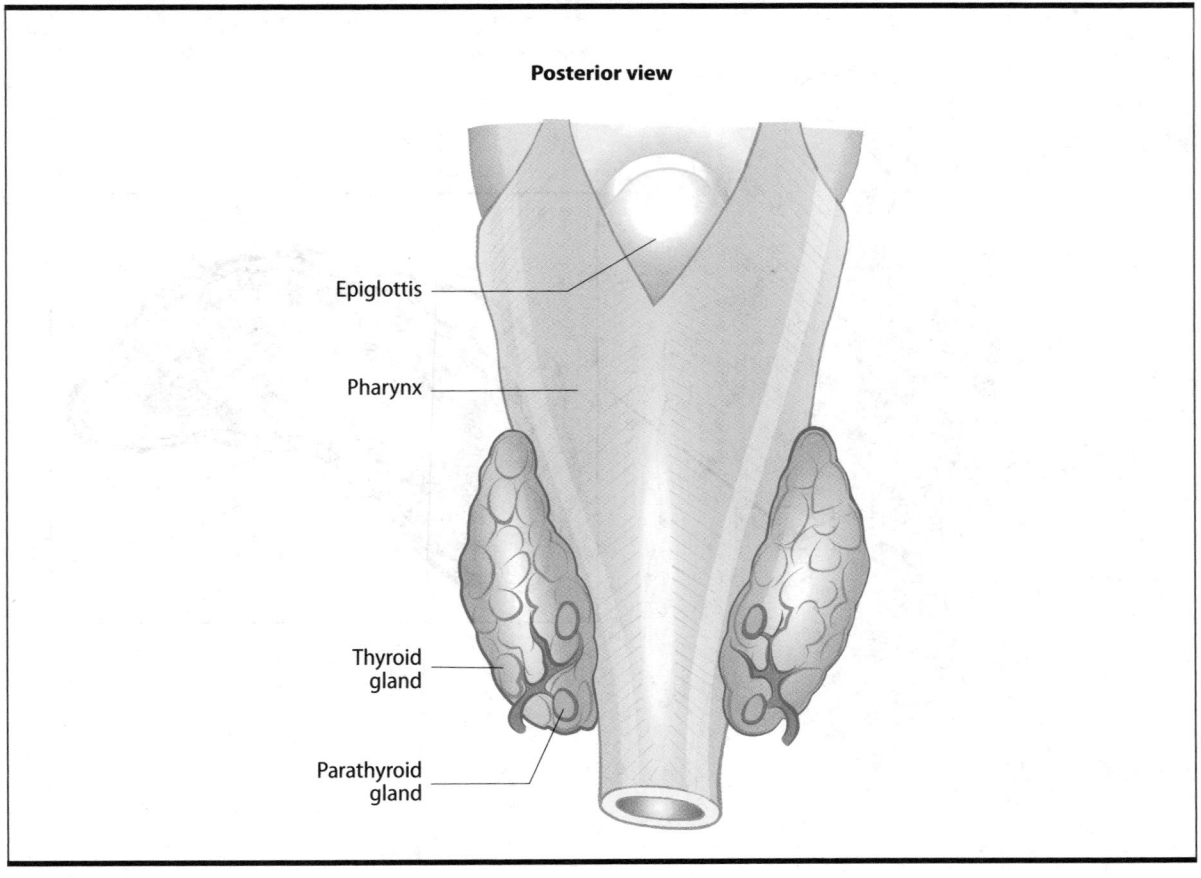

Posterior view

- Epiglottis
- Pharynx
- Thyroid gland
- Parathyroid gland

Pancreas

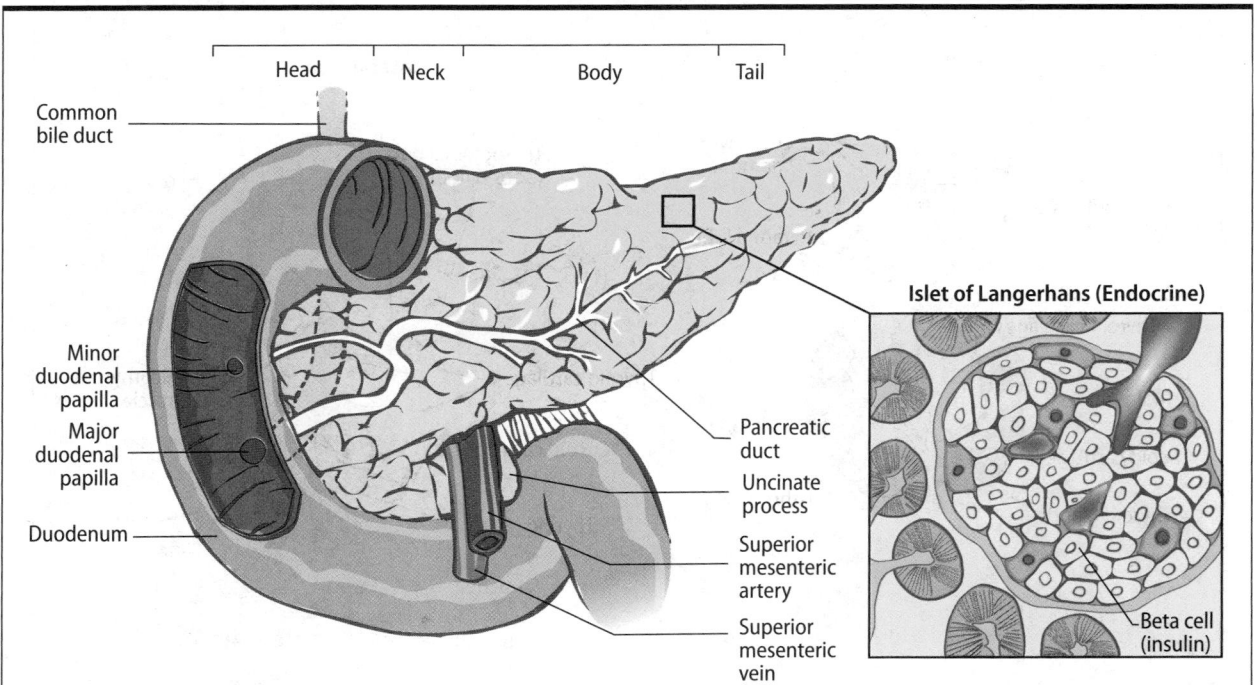

Anatomy of the Adrenal Gland

Structure of an Ovary

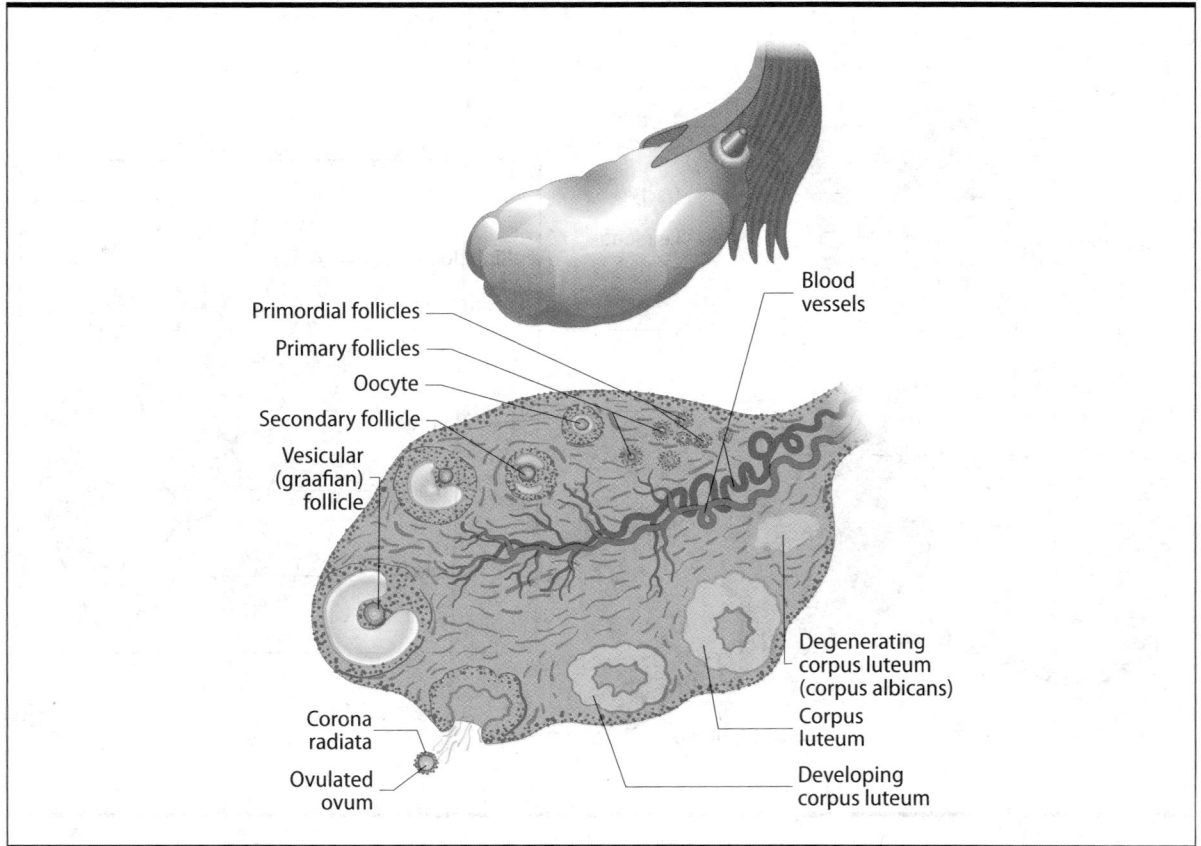

Testis and Associated Structures

Thymus

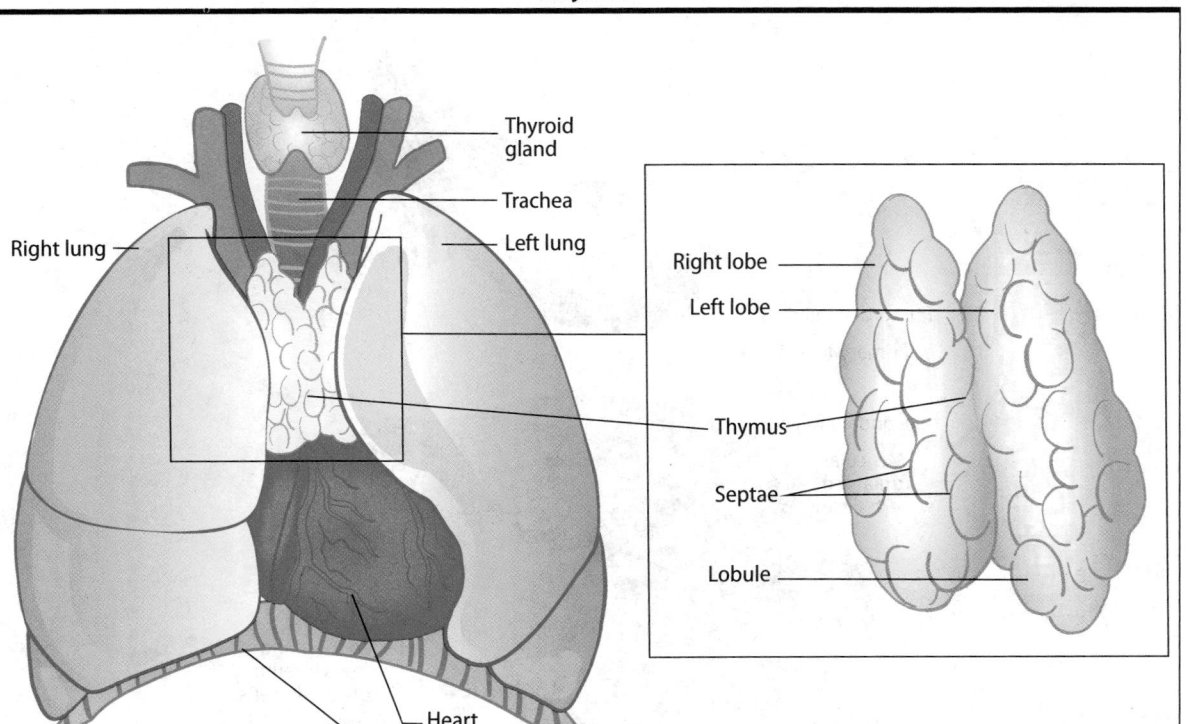

Chapter 6. Diseases of the Nervous System (G00–G99)

Brain

Cranial Nerves

Peripheral Nervous System

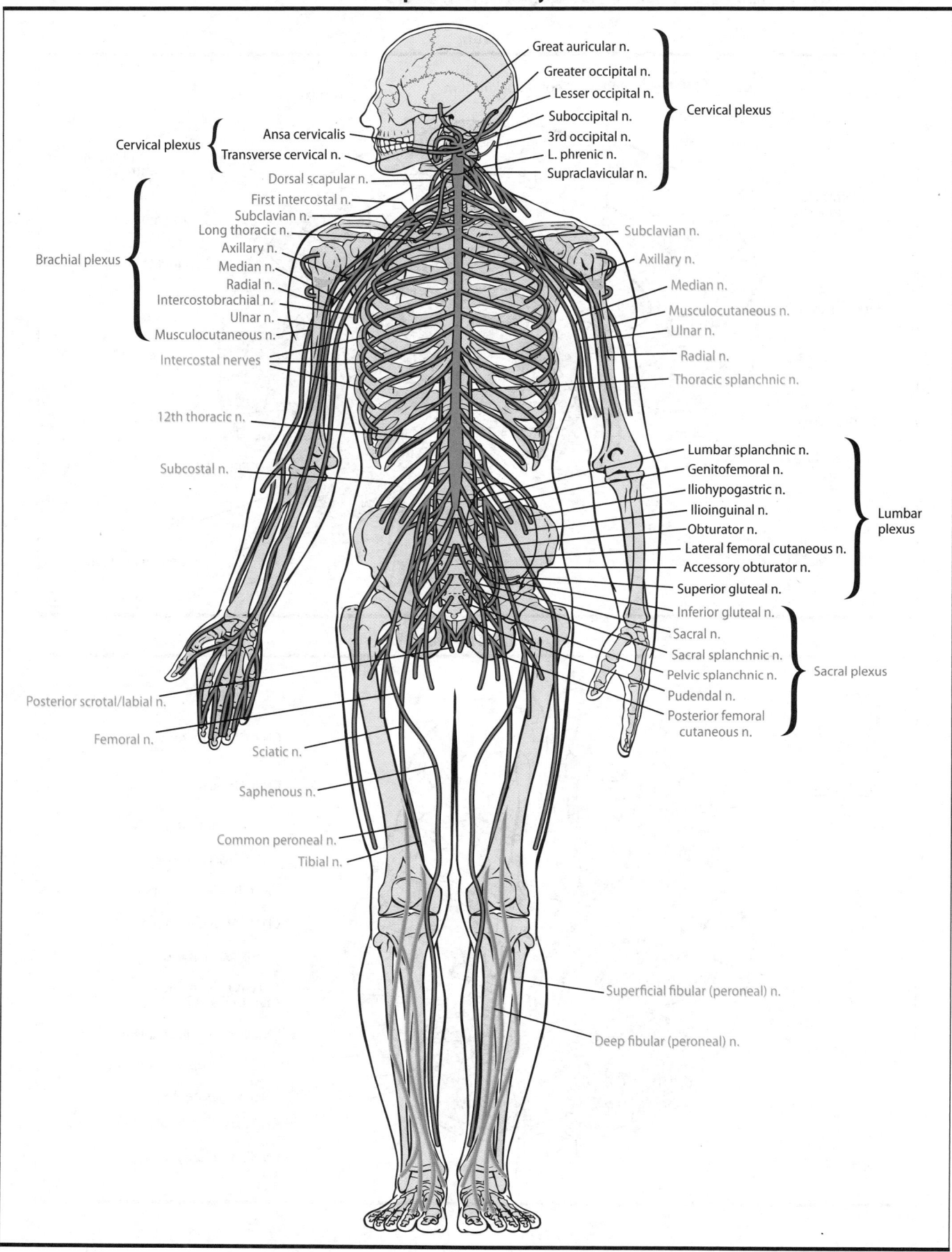

Cervical plexus

Ansa cervicalis
Transverse cervical n.
Dorsal scapular n.
First intercostal n.
Subclavian n.
Long thoracic n.
Axillary n.
Median n.
Radial n.
Intercostobrachial n.
Ulnar n.
Musculocutaneous n.
Intercostal nerves

Brachial plexus

12th thoracic n.
Subcostal n.

Posterior scrotal/labial n.
Femoral n.
Sciatic n.
Saphenous n.
Common peroneal n.
Tibial n.

Great auricular n.
Greater occipital n.
Lesser occipital n.
Suboccipital n.
3rd occipital n.
L. phrenic n.
Supraclavicular n.

Cervical plexus

Subclavian n.
Axillary n.
Median n.
Musculocutaneous n.
Ulnar n.
Radial n.
Thoracic splanchnic n.

Lumbar splanchnic n.
Genitofemoral n.
Iliohypogastric n.
Ilioinguinal n.
Obturator n.
Lateral femoral cutaneous n.
Accessory obturator n.
Superior gluteal n.

Lumbar plexus

Inferior gluteal n.
Sacral n.
Sacral splanchnic n.
Pelvic splanchnic n.
Pudendal n.
Posterior femoral cutaneous n.

Sacral plexus

Superficial fibular (peroneal) n.
Deep fibular (peroneal) n.

Spinal Cord and Spinal Nerves

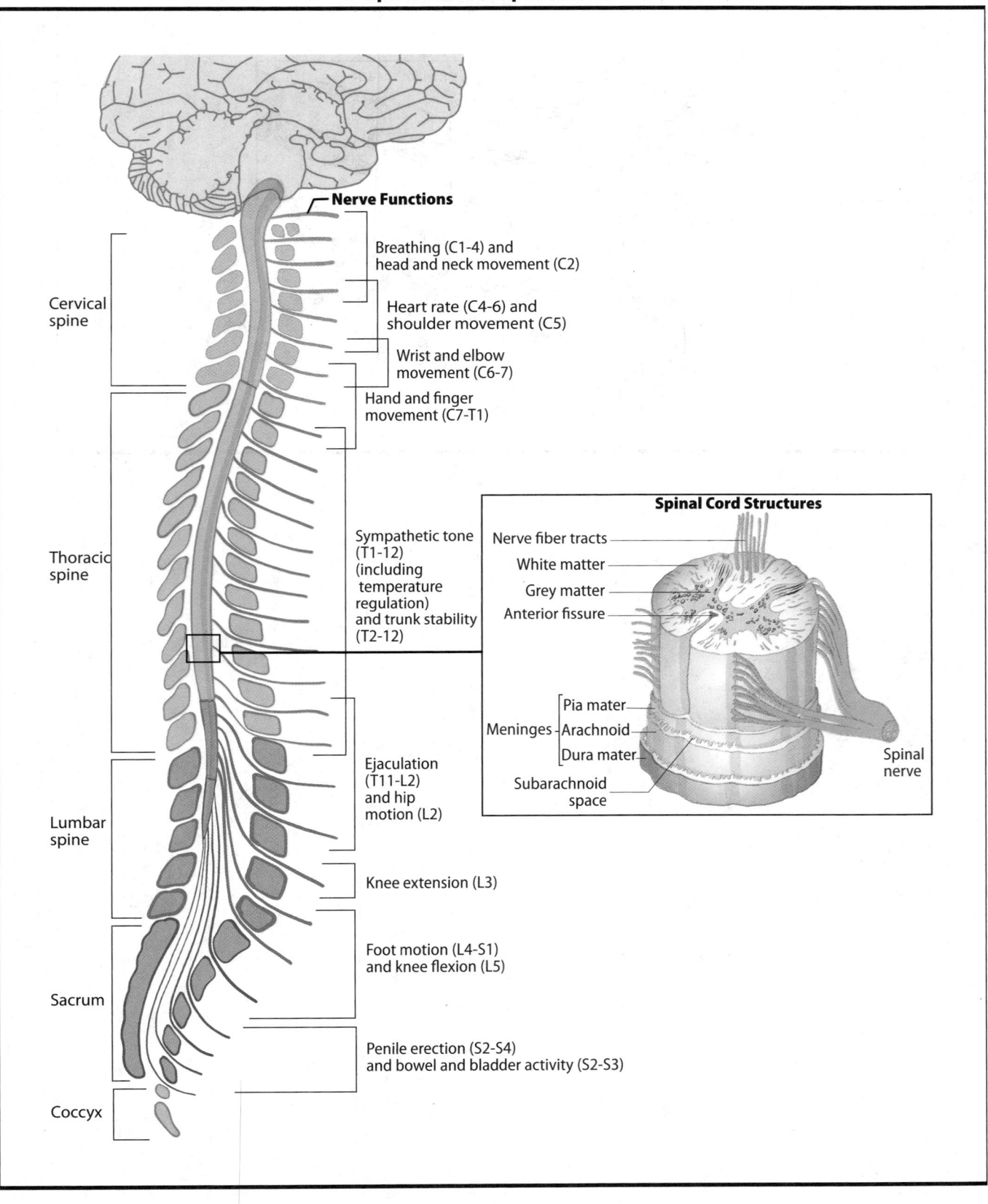

Nerve Functions

Breathing (C1-4) and
head and neck movement (C2)

Heart rate (C4-6) and
shoulder movement (C5)

Wrist and elbow
movement (C6-7)

Hand and finger
movement (C7-T1)

Cervical
spine

Thoracic
spine

Sympathetic tone
(T1-12)
(including
temperature
regulation)
and trunk stability
(T2-12)

Ejaculation
(T11-L2)
and hip
motion (L2)

Lumbar
spine

Knee extension (L3)

Foot motion (L4-S1)
and knee flexion (L5)

Sacrum

Penile erection (S2-S4)
and bowel and bladder activity (S2-S3)

Coccyx

Spinal Cord Structures

Nerve fiber tracts

White matter

Grey matter

Anterior fissure

Pia mater
Meninges — Arachnoid
Dura mater

Subarachnoid
space

Spinal
nerve

Nerve Cell

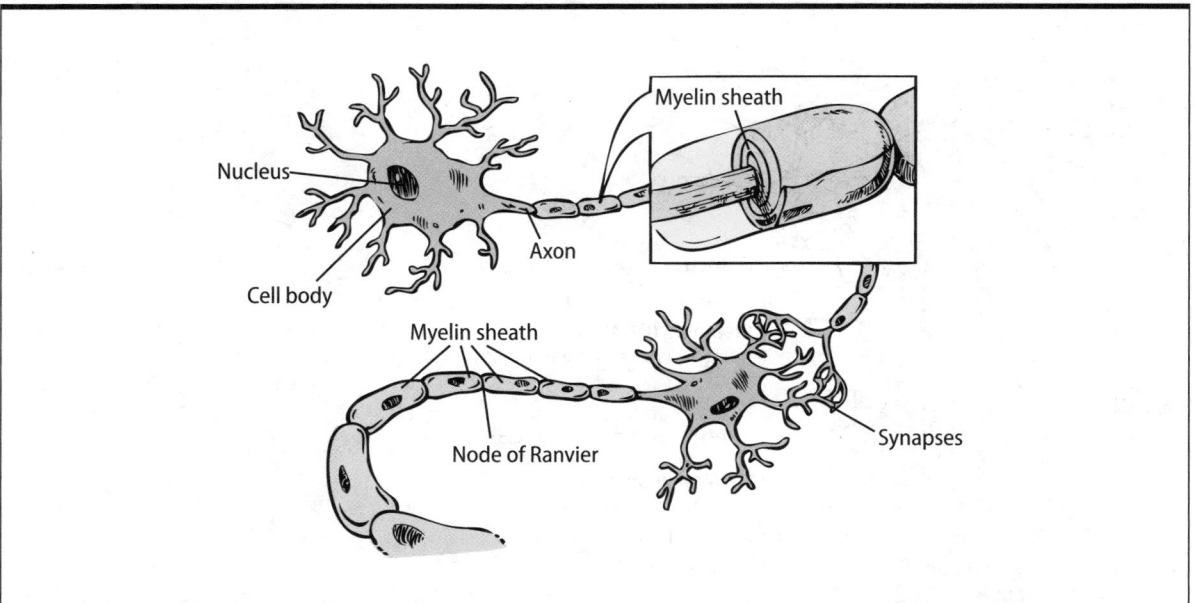

Chapter 7. Diseases of the Eye and Adnexa (H00–H59)

Eye

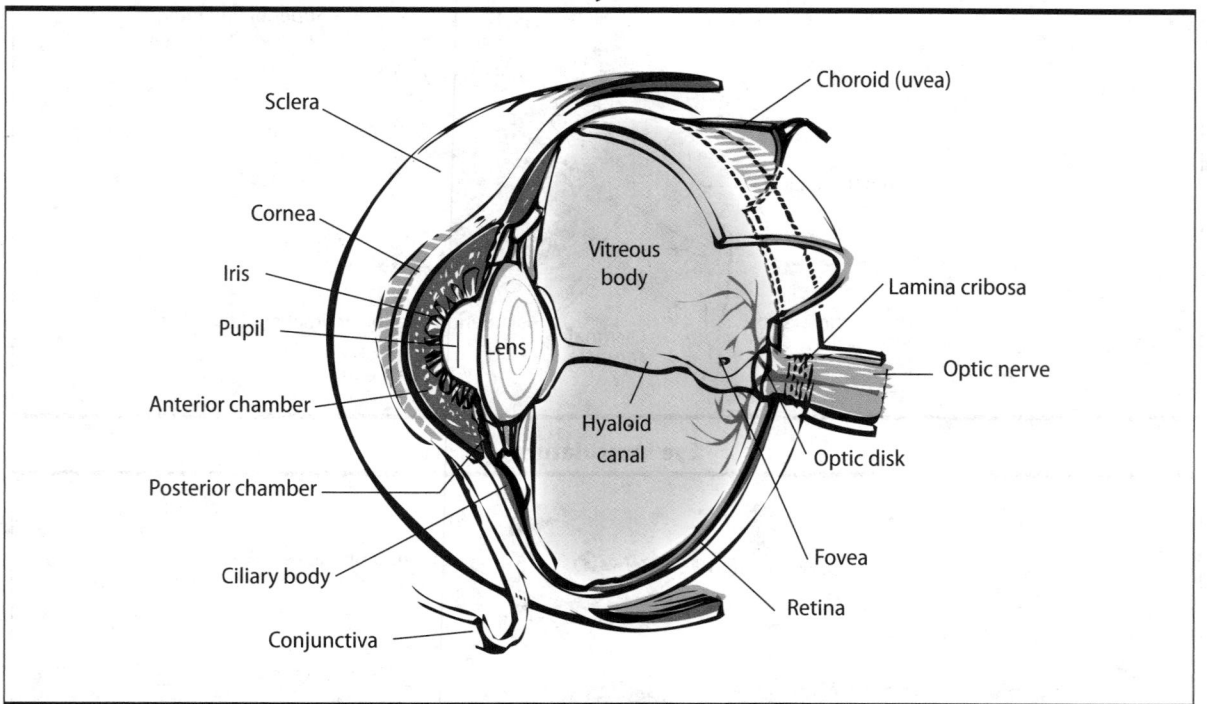

Posterior Pole of Globe/Flow of Aqueous Humor

Lacrimal System

Eye Musculature

Eyelid Structures

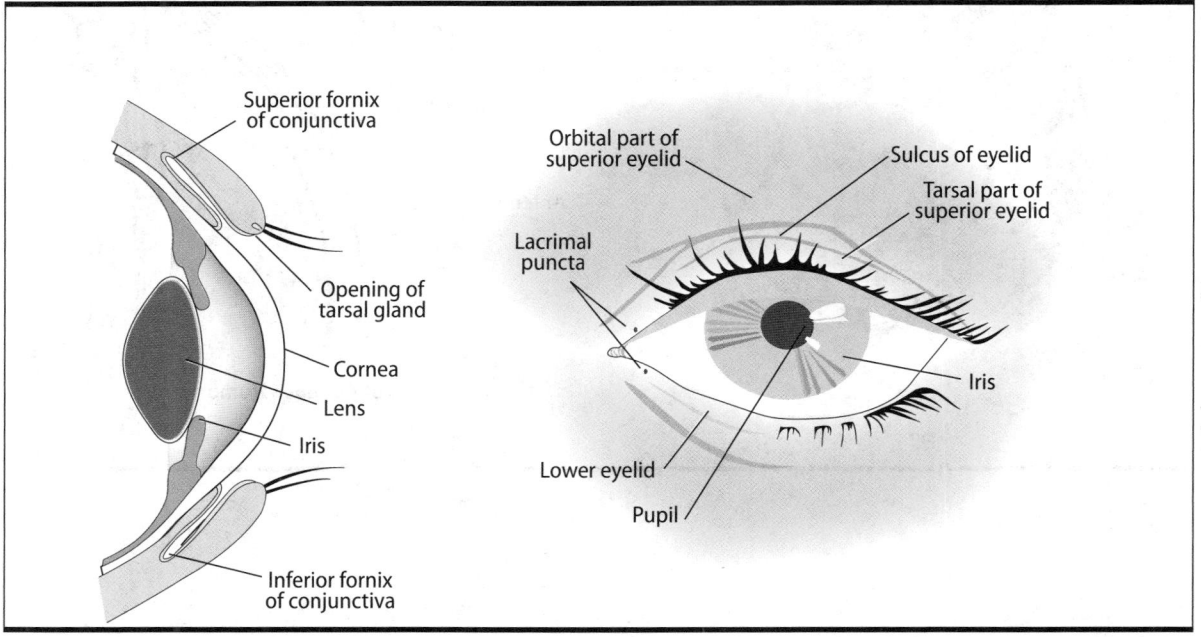

Chapter 8. Diseases of the Ear and Mastoid Process (H60–H95)

Ear Anatomy

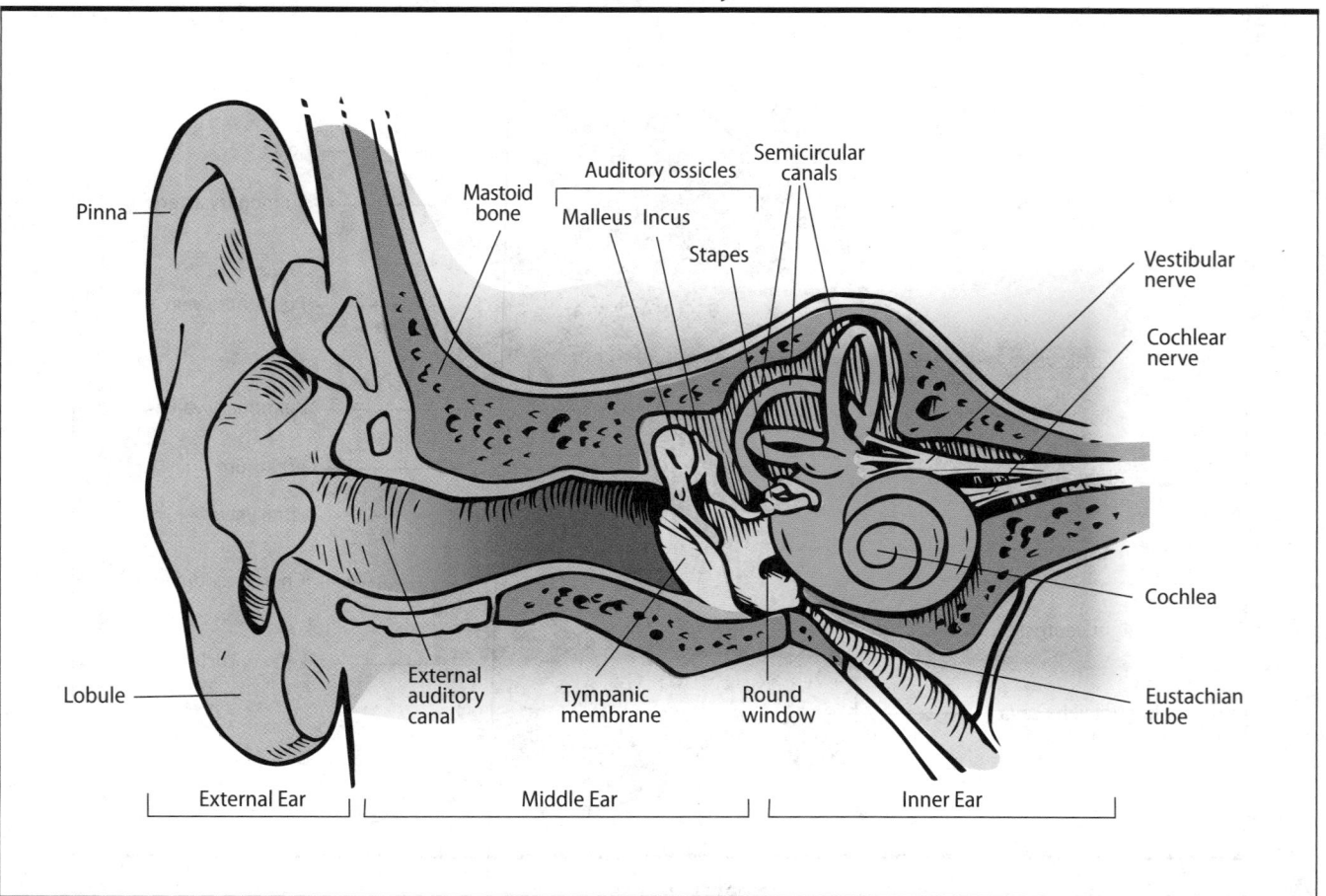

Chapter 9. Diseases of the Circulatory System (I00–I99)

Anatomy of the Heart

Heart Cross Section

Heart Valves

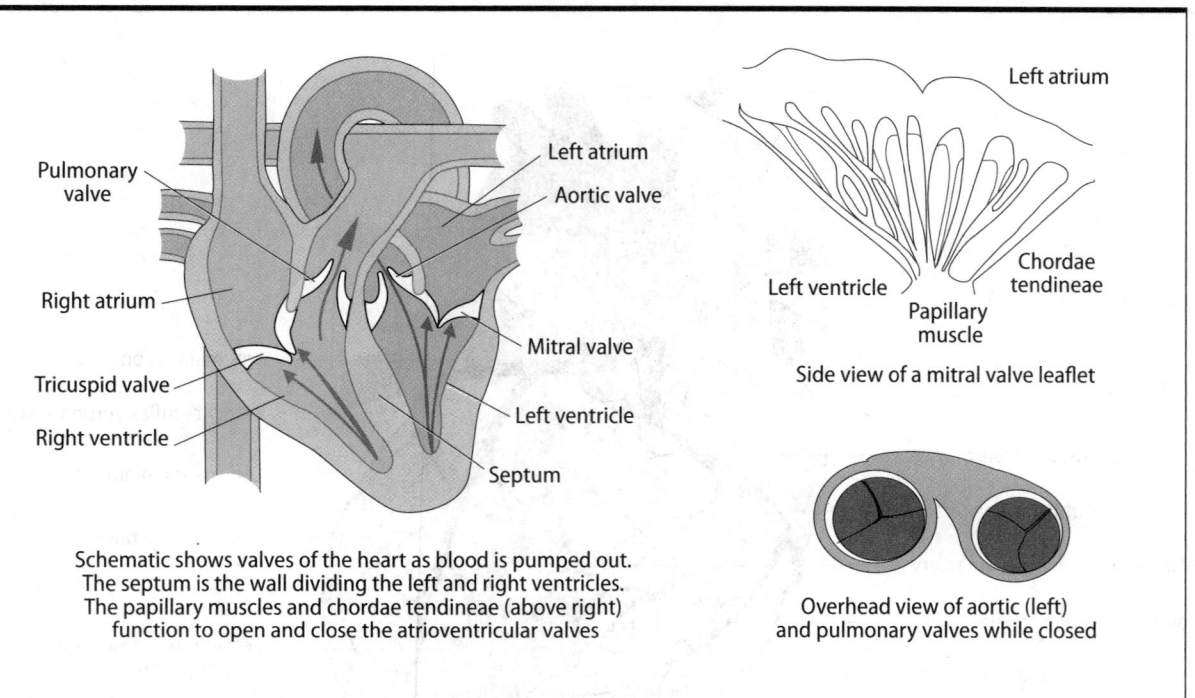

Schematic shows valves of the heart as blood is pumped out.
The septum is the wall dividing the left and right ventricles.
The papillary muscles and chordae tendineae (above right)
function to open and close the atrioventricular valves

Side view of a mitral valve leaflet

Overhead view of aortic (left)
and pulmonary valves while closed

Heart Conduction System

Coronary Arteries

Arteries

Veins

Superficial temporal v.

Vertebral v.

Internal jugular v.

External jugular v.

Subclavian v.

Innominate v.

Azygos v.

Axillary v.

Hemiazygos v.

Brachial v.

Cephalic v.

Inferior vena cava

Basilic v.

Common hepatic v.

Esophageal v.

Portal v.

L. gastric v.

R. gastric v.

Splenic v.

Renal v.

R. colic v.

Inferior mesenteric v.

Superior mesenteric v.

Radial v.

L. colic v.

Ulnar v.

Common iliac v.

Internal iliac v. (Hypogastric v.)

External iliac v.

Internal pudendal v.

Rectal venous plexus

Femoral v.

Greater saphenous v.

Popliteal v.

Lesser saphenous v.

Anterior tibial v.

Lesser saphenous v.

Posterior tibial v.

Greater saphenous v.

Internal Carotid and Vertebral Arteries and Branches

Side View

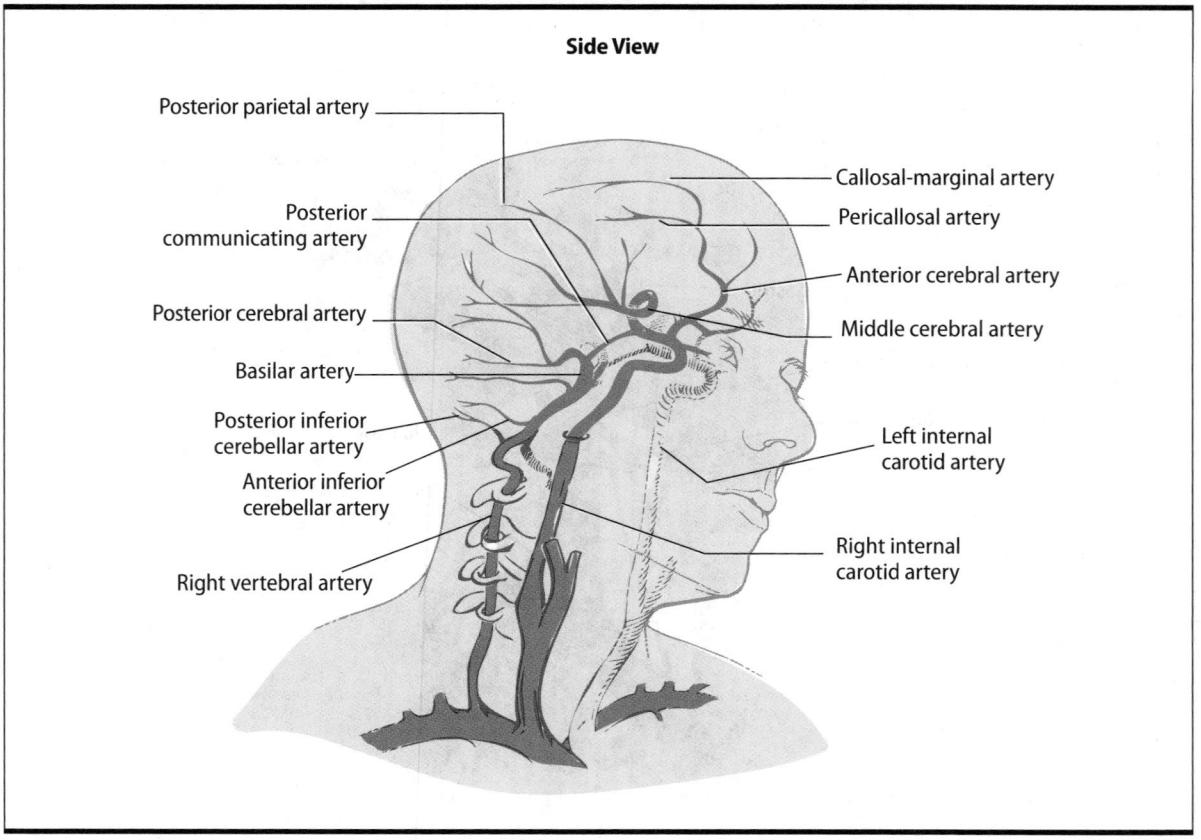

External Carotid Artery and Branches

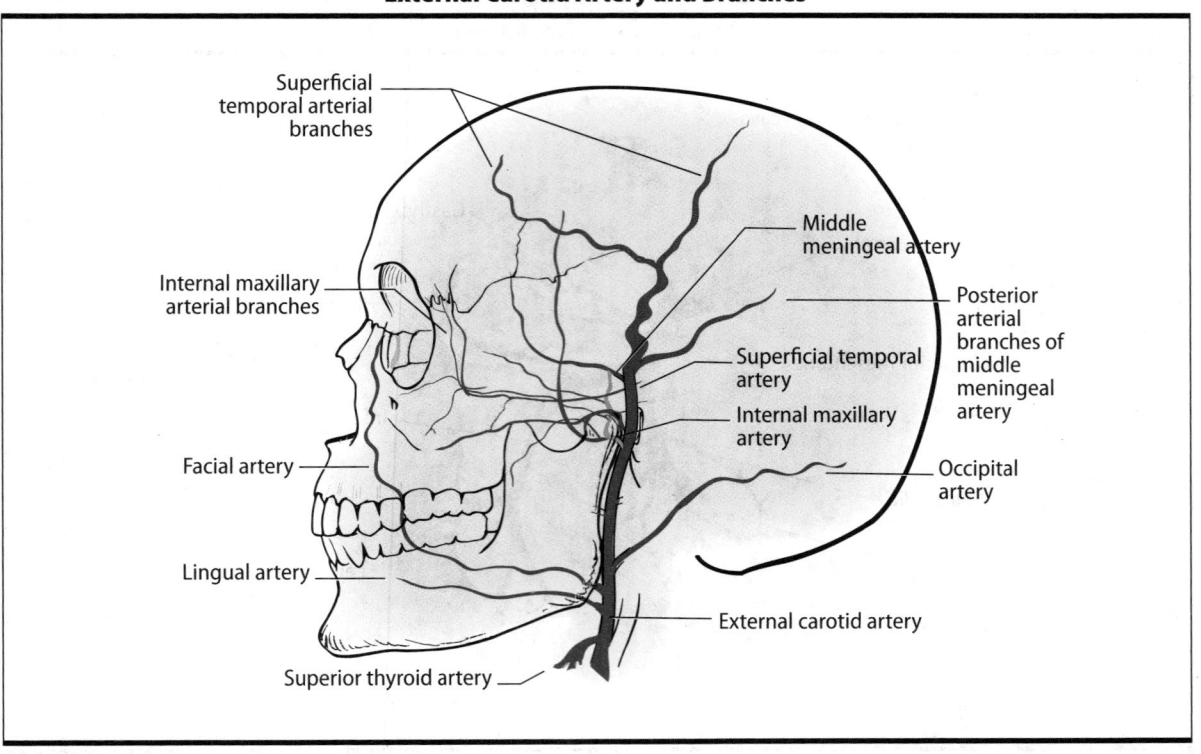

Branches of Abdominal Aorta

Portal Venous Circulation

Lymphatic System

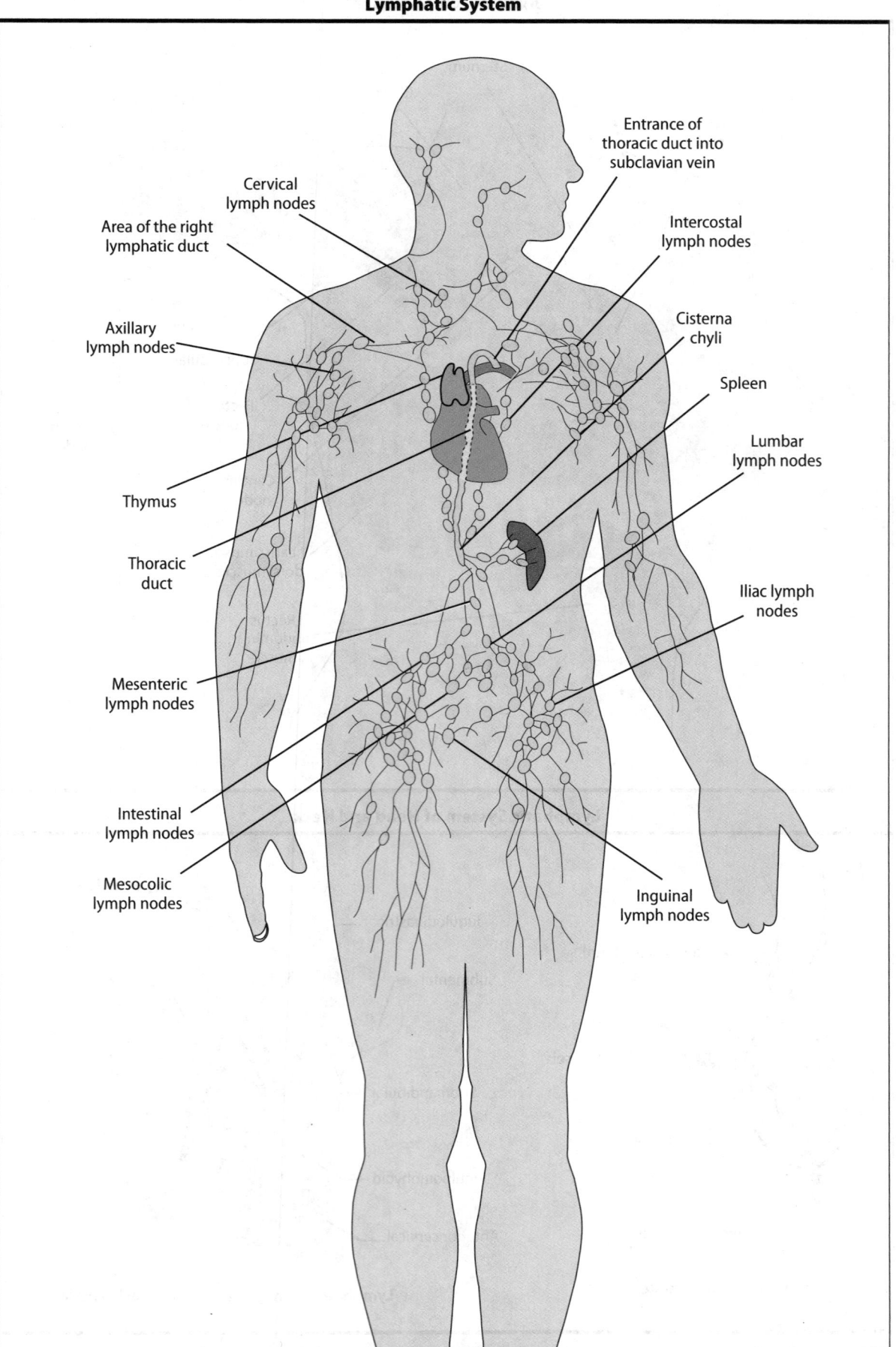

Cervical
lymph nodes

Area of the right
lymphatic duct

Axillary
lymph nodes

Thymus

Thoracic
duct

Mesenteric
lymph nodes

Intestinal
lymph nodes

Mesocolic
lymph nodes

Entrance of
thoracic duct into
subclavian vein

Intercostal
lymph nodes

Cisterna
chyli

Spleen

Lumbar
lymph nodes

Iliac lymph
nodes

Inguinal
lymph nodes

Axillary Lymph Nodes

Parasternal nodes

Sternum

Clavicle

Deltoid muscle

Brachialis muscle

Lateral nodes

Subscapular nodes

Pectoral nodes

Axillary lymph nodes

Central nodes

Latissimus dorsi muscle

Rectus abdominis muscle

Lymphatic System of Head and Neck

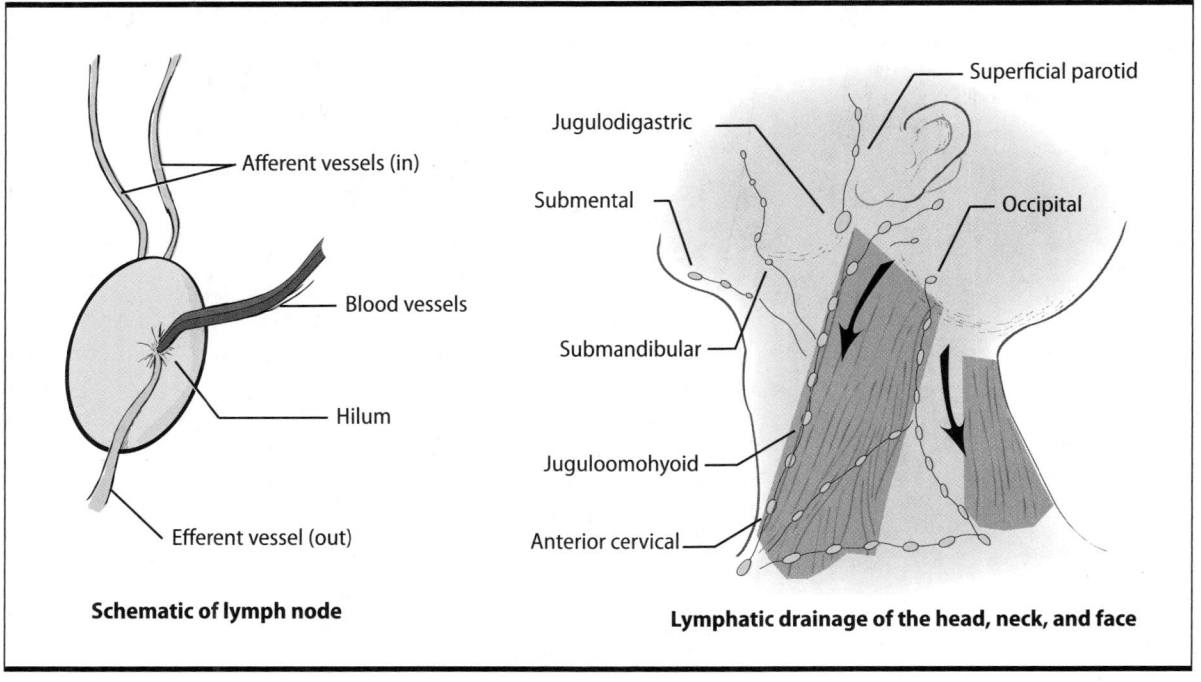

Afferent vessels (in)

Blood vessels

Hilum

Efferent vessel (out)

Jugulodigastric

Superficial parotid

Submental

Occipital

Submandibular

Juguloomohyoid

Anterior cervical

Schematic of lymph node

Lymphatic drainage of the head, neck, and face

Lymphatic Capillaries

Schematic of lymphatic capillaries

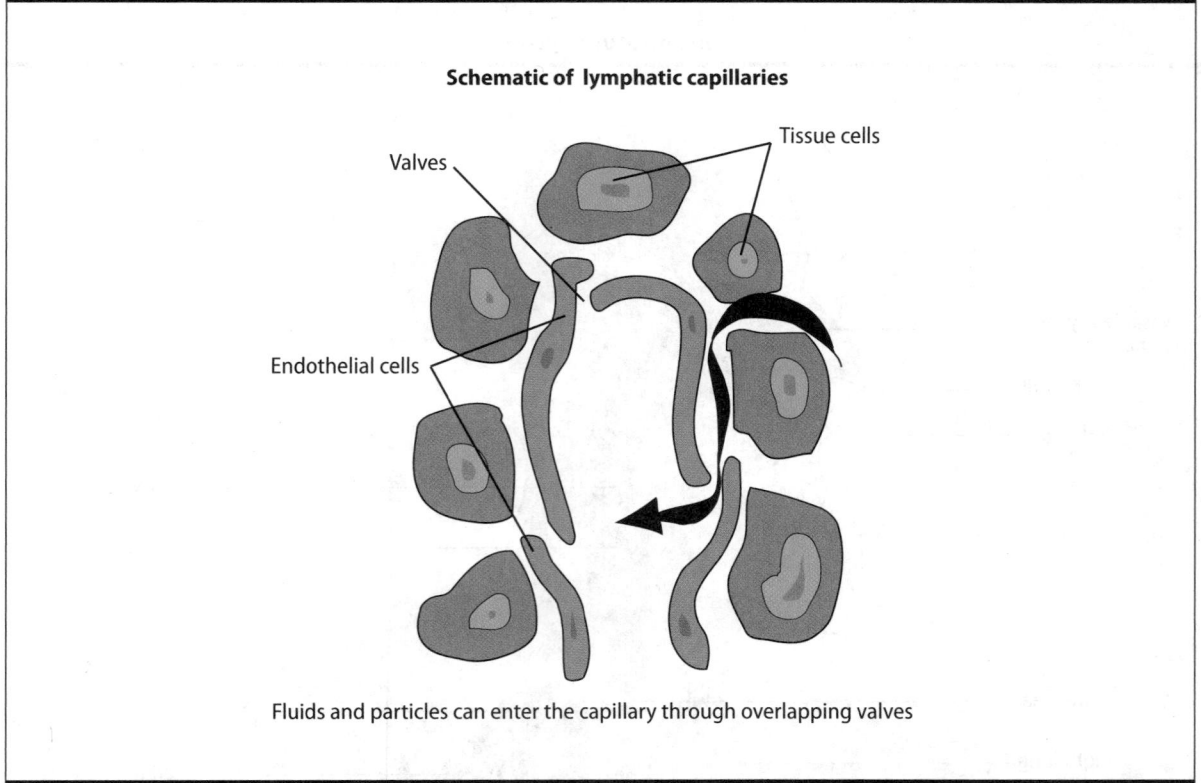

Tissue cells

Valves

Endothelial cells

Fluids and particles can enter the capillary through overlapping valves

Lymphatic Drainage

Lymphatic drainage of the colon follows blood supply

Middle colic nodes

Paracolic nodes

Left colic nodes

Ascending colon

Cecum

Rectum

Chapter 10. Diseases of the Respiratory System (JØØ–J99)

Respiratory System

Upper Respiratory System

Lower Respiratory System

Paranasal Sinuses

Lung Segments

Alveoli

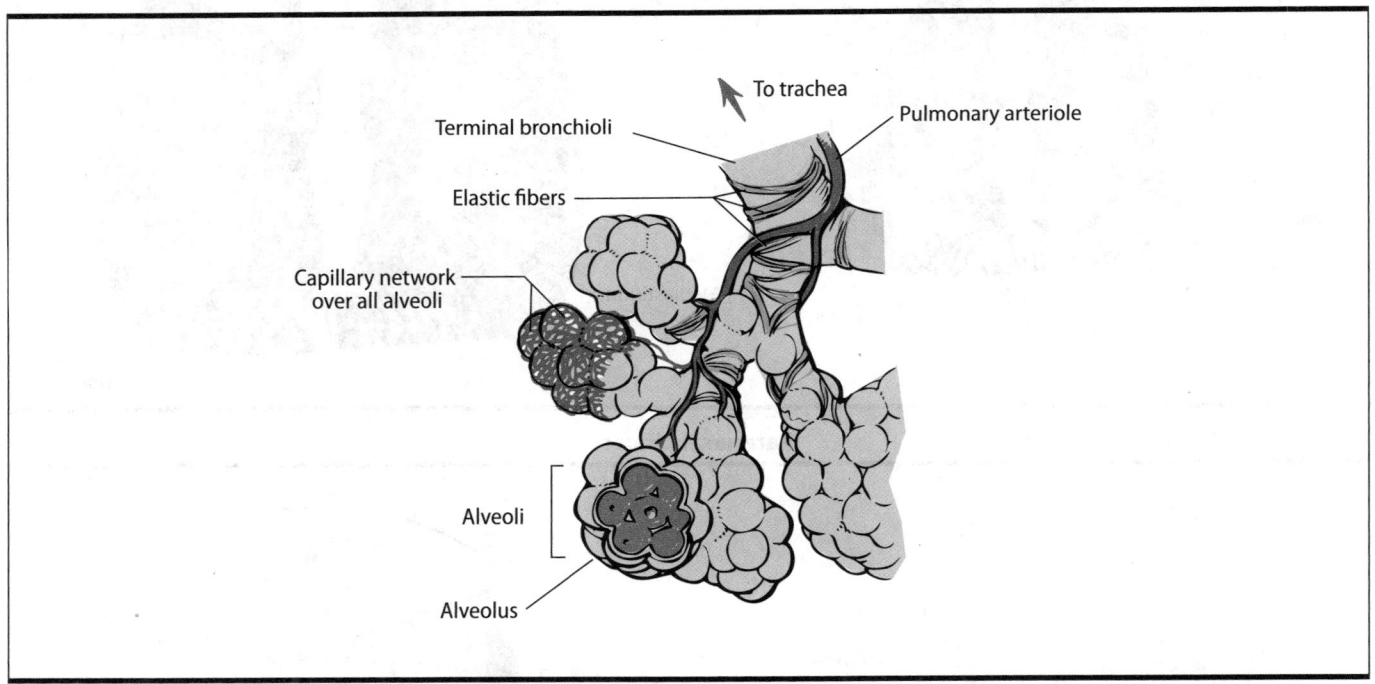

Chapter 11. Diseases of the Digestive System (K00–K95)

Digestive System

Omentum and Mesentery

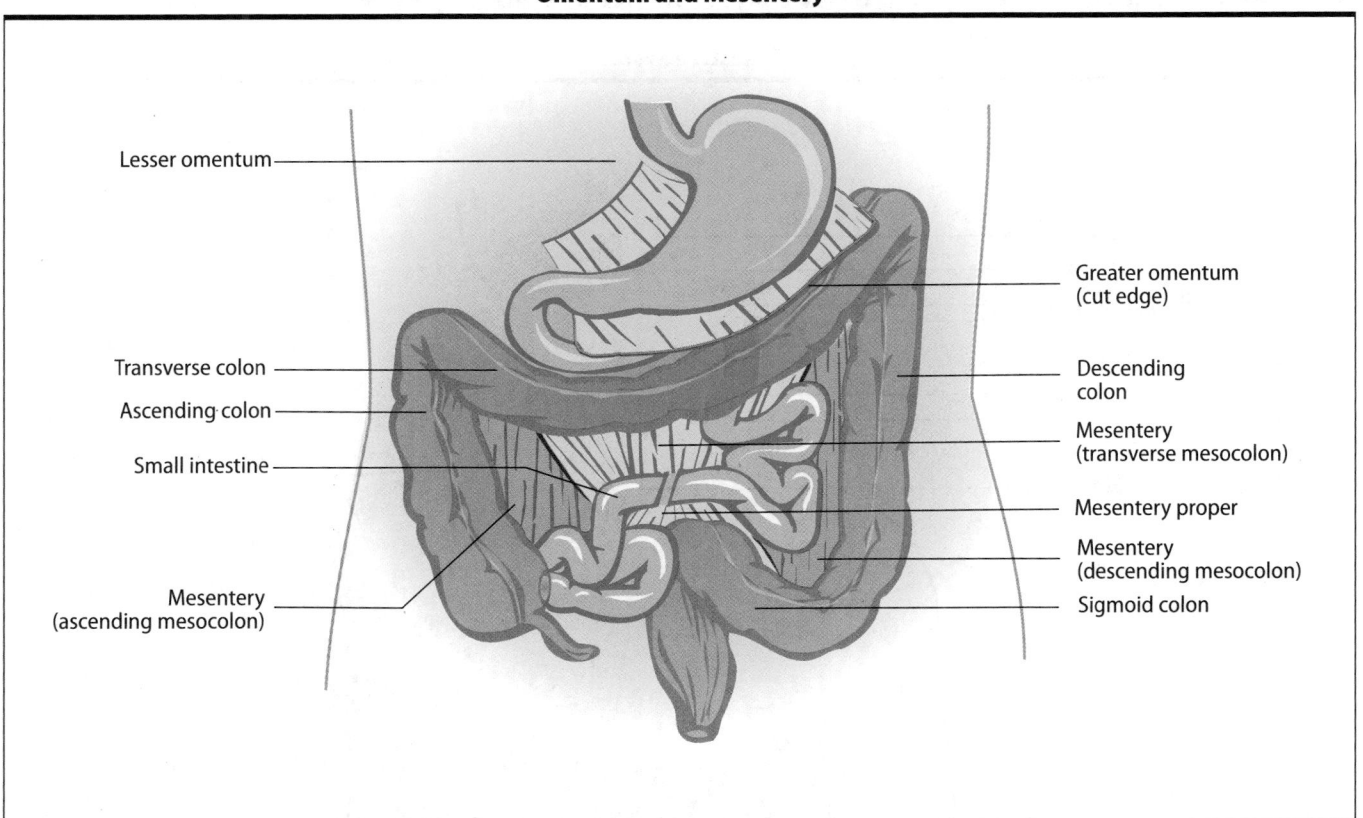

Lesser omentum

Greater omentum (cut edge)

Transverse colon

Descending colon

Ascending colon

Mesentery (transverse mesocolon)

Small intestine

Mesentery proper

Mesentery (descending mesocolon)

Mesentery (ascending mesocolon)

Sigmoid colon

Peritoneum and Retroperitoneum

Diaphragm

Liver

Pancreas

Lesser omentum

Duodenum

Stomach

Kidney

Transverse colon

Parietal peritoneum (lines abdomen and pelvis)

Ureter

Peritoneal cavity

Retroperitoneal space

Visceral peritoneum (covers organs)

Mesentery

Greater omentum

Small intestine

Sigmoid colon

Bladder

Rectum

Chapter 12. Diseases of the Skin and Subcutaneous Tissue (LØØ–L99)

Nail Anatomy

Skin and Subcutaneous Tissue

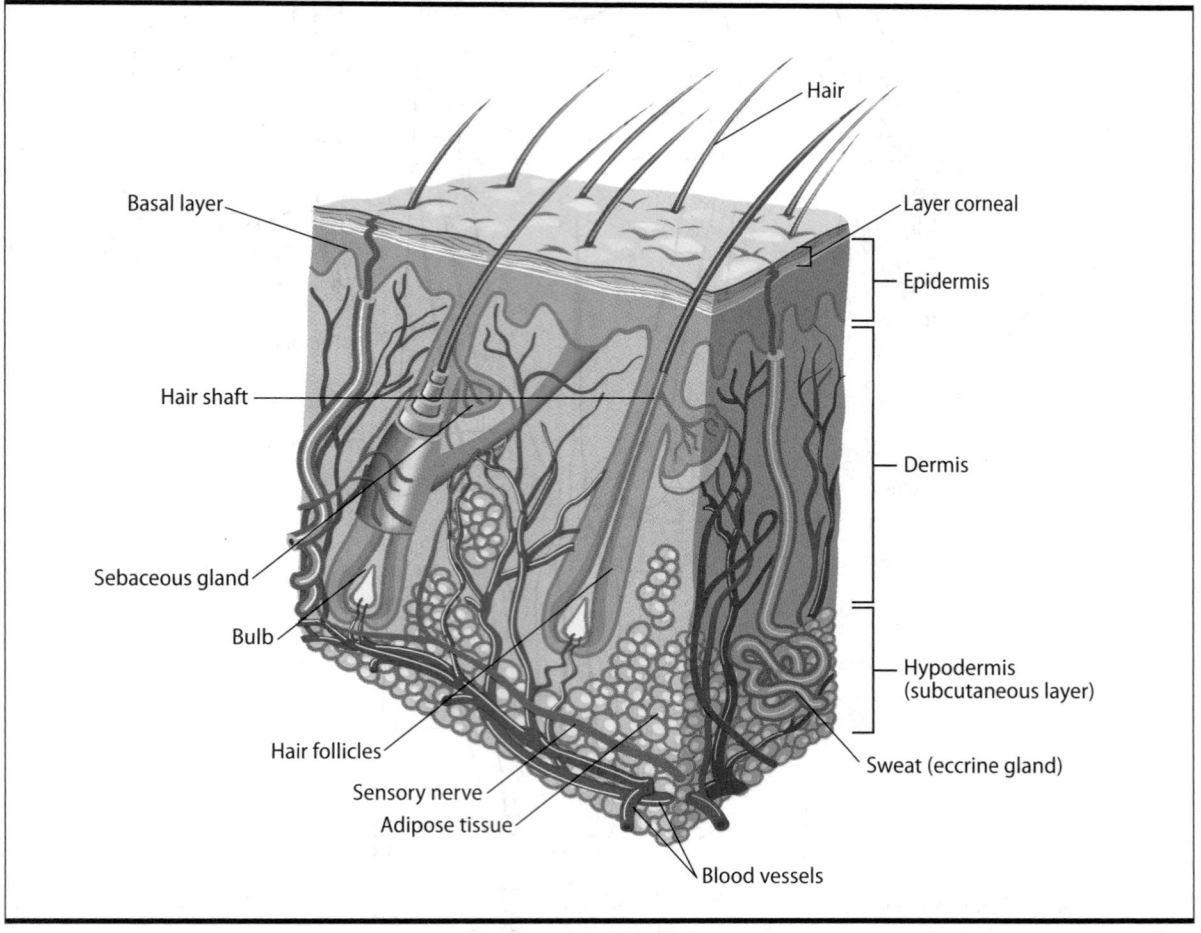

Chapter 13. Diseases of the Musculoskeletal System and Connective Tissue (MØØ–M99)

Bones and Joints

Shoulder Anterior View

Shoulder Posterior View

Elbow Anterior View

Shoulder Posterior View

Hand

Hip Anterior View

Hip Posterior View

Knee Anterior View

Knee Posterior View

Foot

Muscles

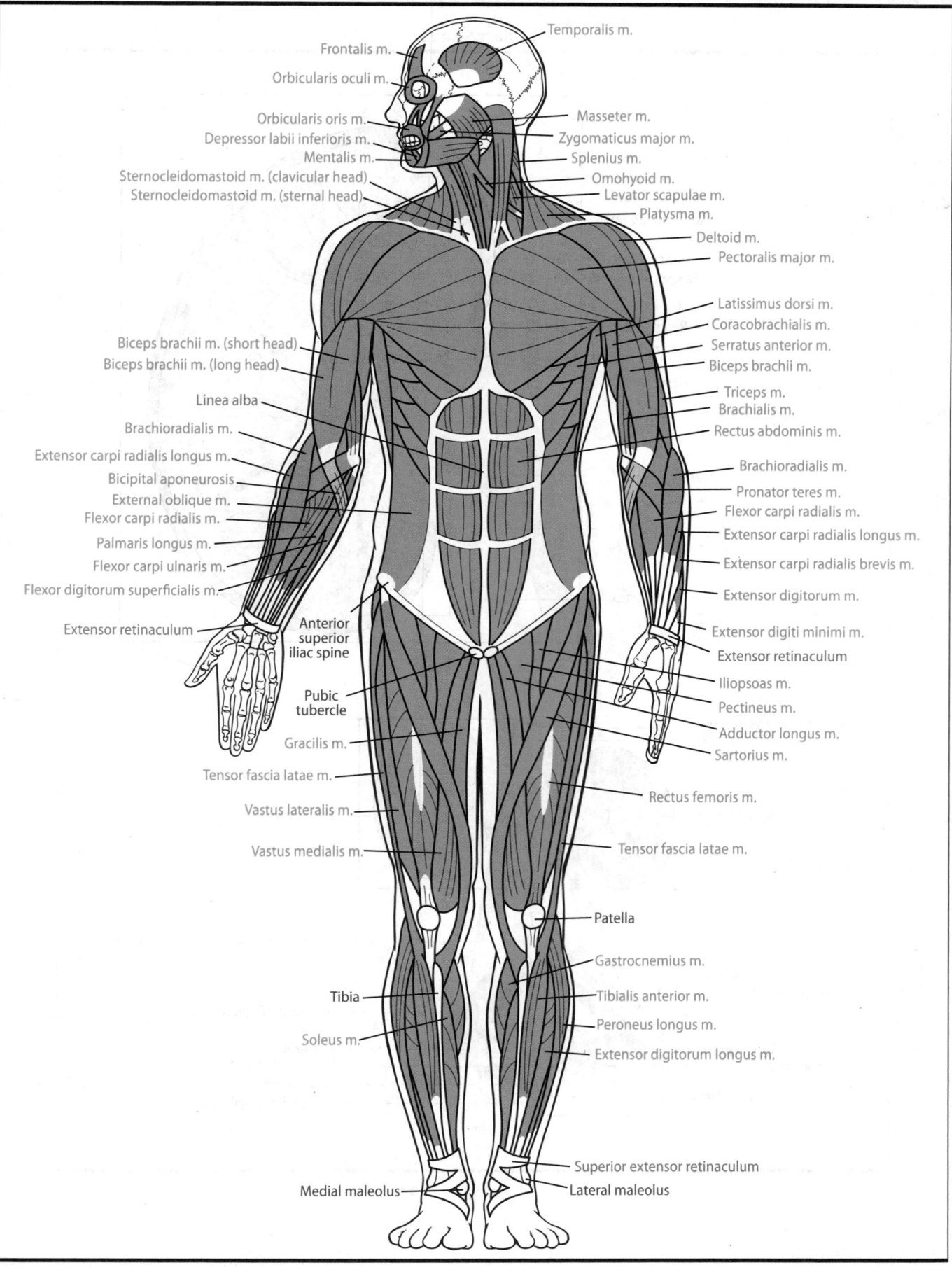

Chapter 14. Diseases of the Genitourinary System (N00–N99)

Urinary System

Male Genitourinary System

Female Internal Genitalia

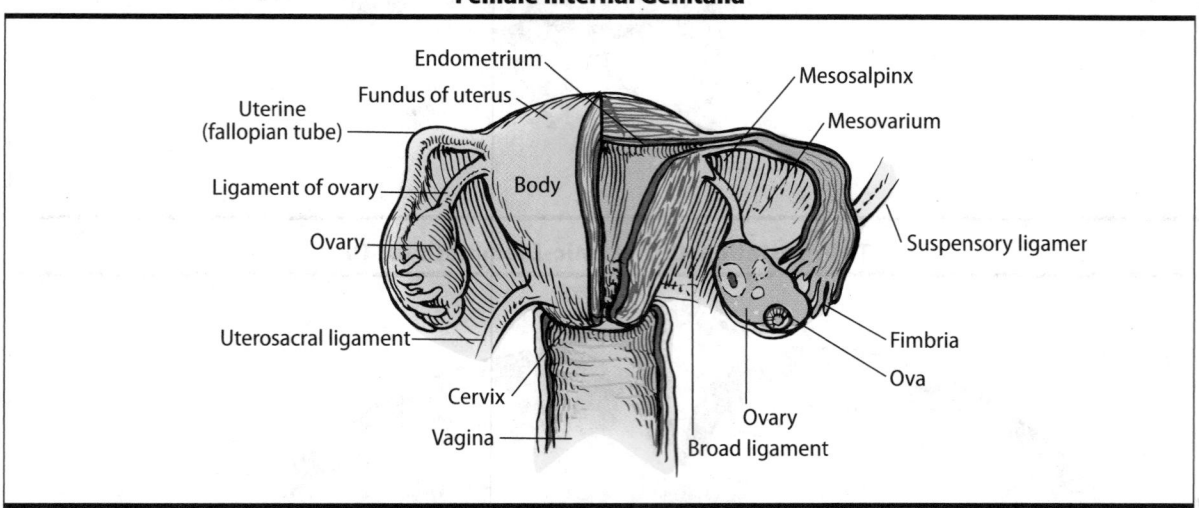

Female Genitourinary Tract Lateral View

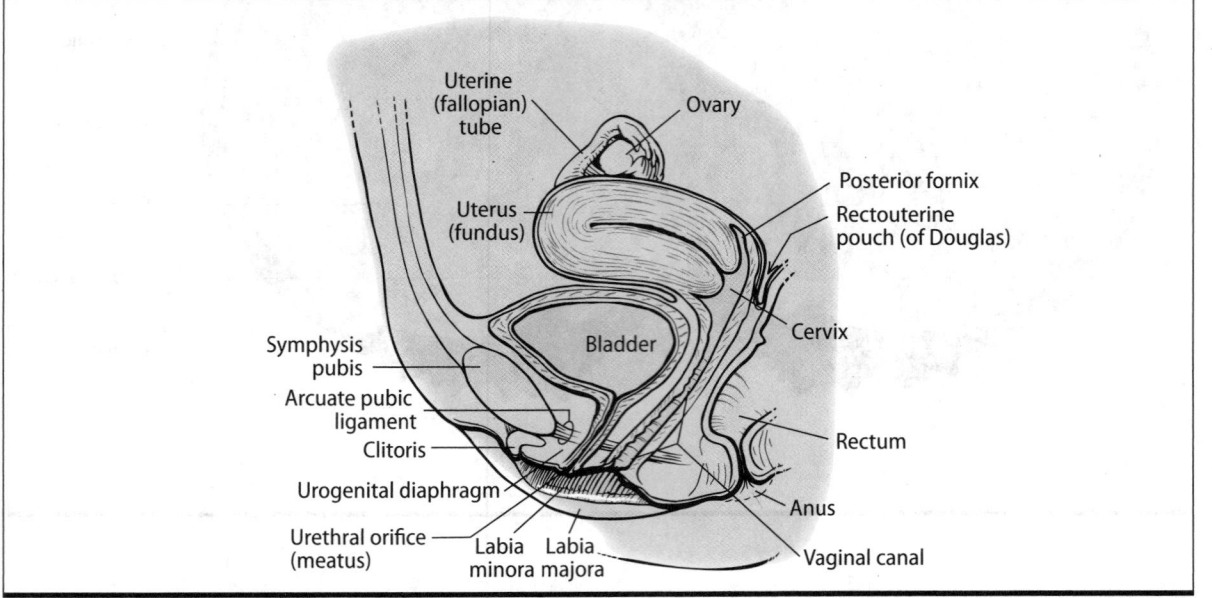

Chapter 15. Pregnancy, Childbirth and the Puerperium (O00–O9A)

Term Pregnancy – Single Gestation

- Placenta
- Umbilical cord
- Amniotic fluid
- Amniotic sac
- Uterus
- Cervix
- Mucous plug
- Vagina
- Pubic bone

Twin Gestation–Dichorionic–Diamniotic (DI DI)

- 2 Chorionic sacs
- 2 Amniotic sacs
- 2 Fetuses
- 2 Umbilical cords
- 2 Placentas